27th Edition

DORLAND'S ILLUSTRATED

Medical Dictionary

W.B. SAUNDERS COMPANY
Harcourt Brace Jovanovich, Inc.

Philadelphia London Toronto
Montreal Sydney Tokyo

Dorland's illustrated medical dictionary.
Philadelphia: W.B. Saunders Co.,

v.: ill.; 27 cm.

Irregular.
Began publication with 23rd ed.
Description based on: 26th ed.
Continues: American illustrated medical dictionary.

1. Medicine—Dictionaries.   I. Dorland, W.A. Newman
(William Alexander Newman), 1864–1956.
[DNLM: 1. Dictionaries, Medical.   2. Reference Books,
Medical]

R121.D73   610'.3'21—dc19   0-6383
                                   AACR 2   MARC-S

Library of Congress   [8607r85]rev6

W.B. SAUNDERS COMPANY
Harcourt Brace Jovanovich, Inc.

The Curtis Center
Independence Square West
Philadelphia, PA 19106

Listed here are the latest translated editions of this book together with the languages for the translations and the publishers.

Italian *(26th Edition, revised)*—Edizioni Scientifiche Internazionali (ESI), Milan, Italy

Japanese *(26th Edition)*—Hirokawa Publishing Company, Tokyo, Japan

Spanish *(26th Edition)* (Adaption)—Nueva Editorial Interamericana, Mexico City, Mexico

Managing Editor, Dictionaries: Elizabeth J. Taylor
Editors: Douglas M. Anderson, Joseph M. Patwell, Katharine Plaut, Kathleen McCullough
Production Manager: Carolyn Naylor
Illustrator: Sharon Iwanczuk
Illustration Coordinator: Walt Verbitski
Mechanical Artist: Melissa Walter

Dorland's Illustrated Medical Dictionary   ISBN 0–7216–3154–1

Preface

In the eighty-eight years of its existence, *Dorland's Illustrated Medical Dictionary* has served the needs of countless students and practitioners of medicine and related fields as an up-to-date source, in readily accessible form, of definitions of the terms they use every day. We have borne in mind in the preparation of this 27th Edition the basis on which any dictionary stands—that is, the need for a repository of agreed-upon vocabulary for the interchange of ideas. The challenge has been to maintain the standards of currency and usefulness set by our predecessors in the face of today's enormous increase of knowledge in medicine and science, the ever deepening complexity of the concepts, the rapidity with which the knowledge becomes available, and the greater number of forums for the presentation of newly discovered facts.

For the 27th Edition we eliminated hundreds of obsolete terms to make room for many more new terms and for more expansive definitions of existing terms warranted by advances in knowledge and understanding. These additions and changes have been made throughout the work. Furthermore, exhaustive review produced major changes in such particular categories of information as immunology, bacteriology, infectious diseases, enzymology, endocrinology, dermatology, tropical medicine, psychiatry, and psychology. Surgery, genetics, genetic diseases, dentistry, mathematics, and statistics also were given detailed attention. The plates, illustrations, and tables were carefully evaluated, and much of the artwork was redrawn in a more modern style. Several tables of useful information, including "Laboratory Values of Clinical Importance," were added as appendices to the work. And, finally, with this edition there is a change in policy with regard to the placement of certain entries: acids can be found at the names of the individual acids, enzymes should be sought at individual names rather than class names, and enzyme deficiencies are found following the specific enzyme involved (see "Main Entries and Subentries" in the "Notes on the Use of this Dictionary").

Every lexicographer finds himself occasionally embroiled in the debate whether a dictionary should simply reflect usage or offer itself as a set of standards. Our resolution of this quandary has been that *Dorland's* must reflect terms encountered in everyday use, but there is often an opportunity to show preference for properly constructed and unambiguous terms by placing the definitions with them and showing cross references to them at the entries for less etymologically acceptable synonyms. We believe that a dictionary has some role in upholding the principle that accurate and efficient expression of ideas requires integrity of language. We have in some cases yielded entirely to usage, however, when to ignore a term that has become entrenched among a community of users would leave our collection of entries suspect as to currency and completeness.

We have not set ourselves as arbiters of stylistic questions that arise in writing and editing, such as the use of diphthongs or the hyphenation of compound words, and we have made no attempt to present every stylistic variation that might be acceptable.

We hope you will find that the 27th Edition of this Dictionary meets your need for a current and useful source of medical and scientific information.

ACKNOWLEDGMENTS

To our consultants, whose names are listed on the following page, we acknowledge a huge debt; their help made wisdom of selection, contemporaneity of definition, and accuracy of infor-

iii

mation possible. We mention particularly our gratitude to Rex Conn for permission to include "Laboratory Values of Clinical Importance" in the Appendices. We are grateful, too, to the many others who have made valuable suggestions for improvement of the Dictionary. We hope all those who have provided help will find that we have repaid our debt to them by integrating the separate elements of information they have supplied into a useful, authoritative body of data.

As in the preceding edition, the definitions of the various anatomical structures are placed on the NA terms, that is, on the terms as they appear in the *Nomina Anatomica* as approved by the Eleventh International Congress of Anatomists at Mexico City, 1980.

In enzyme nomenclature, we have relied heavily on the Recommendations of the Nomenclature Committee of the International Union of Biochemistry on the Nomenclature and Classification of Enzyme-Catalysed Reactions.

In bacteriology, we have used as a guide *Bergey's Manual of Systematic Bacteriology*, Volume 1 (1984) and *Bergey's Manual of Determinative Bacteriology,* 8th Edition (1974).

We have referred to the *Journal of Protozoology* for information about the classification of Protozoa.

For psychiatric terms, we have been guided in many instances by *Diagnostic and Statistical Manual of Mental Disorders*, 3rd Edition-Revised (1987), published by the American Psychiatric Association.

In pharmacology, as noted on the copyright page, we have made use of portions of the text of the *United States Pharmacopeia*, the *National Formulary*, and *USAN and the USP Dictionary of Drug Names*, all publications of the United States Pharmacopeial Convention, Inc.

In acknowledging our indebtedness to the compilers, editors, and publishers of the aforementioned publications, we emphasize that any inaccuracies that may have arisen from our transcription or interpretation of this material are our sole responsibility.

ELIZABETH J. TAYLOR

Editor

Consultants

DANIEL M. ALBERT, M.D.
David C. Cogan Professor of Ophthalmology, Harvard Medical School; Director, Howe Laboratory of Ophthalmology, Massachusetts Eye and Ear Infirmary, Boston, Massachusetts

NICHOLAS P. CHRISTY, M.D.
Chief of Staff, Veterans Administration Medical Center, Brooklyn, New York; Professor of Medicine, Health Science Center at Brooklyn, State University of New York

REX B. CONN, M.D.
Professor and Vice Chairman, Department of Pathology, Jefferson Medical College of Thomas Jefferson University, Philadelphia, Pennsylvania

JULIUS M. CRUSE, D. MICROBIOL., M.D., PH.D., F.A.A.M., F.R.S.H.
Professor of Pathology, Director of Immunopathology and Transplantation Immunology, Director of Graduate Studies in Pathology, Associate Professor of Microbiology, The University of Mississippi Medical Center, Jackson, Mississippi

G.E. ERIKSON, PH.D.
Professor of Medical Science and Founding Chairman, Section of Morphology, Brown University, Providence, Rhode Island

JOAN JOHNSON, R.N.
Nurse Practitioner, Department of Dermatology, Hospital of the University of Pennsylvania, Philadelphia, Pennsylvania

ROBERT E. LEWIS, JR., B.A., M.S., PH.D., F.R.S.H.
Associate Professor of Pathology, Co-Director of the Clinical Immunopathology Laboratory, Co-Director of the Tissue Typing Laboratory, Director of the HLA Paternity Testing Laboratory, The University of Mississippi Medical Center, Jackson, Mississippi

JAMES J. LEYDEN, M.D.
Professor of Dermatology, University of Pennsylvania Medical School; Staff Physician, Department of Dermatology, Hospital of the University of Pennsylvania, Philadelphia, Pennsylvania

CHARLES McCABE, M.D.
Assistant Professor of Surgery, Harvard Medical School; Associate Visiting Surgeon and Associate Director of Emergency Medical Services, Massachusetts General Hospital, Boston, Massachusetts

ROBERT W. McGILVERY, PH.D.
Professor Emeritus of Biochemistry, University of Virginia School of Medicine, Charlottesville, Virginia

KARIN L. McGOWAN, PH.D.
Microbiology Laboratory, Children's Hospital of Philadelphia; Assistant Professor of Pediatrics, University of Pennsylvania Medical School, Philadelphia, Pennsylvania

THEODORE MILLON, PH.D.
Professor of Psychology and Psychiatry and Director, Clinical Training, University of Miami; Consultant, Veterans Administration Medical Center and Jackson Memorial Hospital, Miami, Florida

RALPH W. PHILLIPS, M.S., D.SC.
Associate Dean for Research and Research Professor of Dental Materials, Indiana University School of Dentistry, Indianapolis, Indiana

STANLEY SCHOR, PH.D.
Executive Director, Biostatistics and Research Data Systems, Merck Sharp & Dohme Research Laboratories, West Point, Pennsylvania

G. THOMAS STRICKLAND, M.D., PH.D.
Director, International Health Program and Professor of Microbiology, University of Maryland School of Medicine, Baltimore, Maryland

MARGARET W. THOMPSON, PH.D., F.C.C.M.G.
Professor of Medical Genetics, University of Toronto; Senior Staff Geneticist, The Hospital for Sick Children, Toronto, Ontario

DOROTHY WHITCOMB, B.A., M. LIB. SCI.
Historical Librarian, University of Wisconsin Health Science Center Libraries and William S. Middleton Library, University of Wisconsin, Madison, Wisconsin

Contents

Index to Tables

Index to Plates

Notes on the Use of This Dictionary

MAIN ENTRIES AND SUBENTRIES

Main entries appear in boldface type, without distortion by accents or other indications of syllabication. Terms consisting of two or more words are ordinarily given as subentries under the *noun*, as is traditional in medical dictionaries. According to this scheme, *Heinz-Ehrlich bodies*, *Howell-Jolly bodies*, and *Leishman-Donovan bodies* are all defined under the main entry *body*, and *carotid pulse*, *dicrotic pulse*, and *paradoxical pulse* are to be found under the main entry *pulse*. Subentries are set in the same boldface type as the main entry and are run on in the same paragraph.

In a subentry, the main entry word is represented only by the initial letter (e.g., *blast c.* under *cell*), unless it occurs in the plural form. Regular English plurals are represented by adding *'s* to the initial letter (e.g., *b's* for *bones* under *bone*). Irregular plurals and Latin plurals are spelled out (e.g., *teeth* under *tooth*, and *ossa* under *os²*).

Although this arrangement may be confusing at first to the user accustomed to general dictionaries, it has the advantage of allowing related terms to be grouped together (for example, all the lymphocyte entries will be found under *lymphocyte*). Because of the present multiplicity of terminology, it is important that the user keep in mind that a phrase that does not appear under one main entry should be sought under a synonymous main entry. For example, the same entity may be referred to as a disease or a syndrome (as *Fabry's disease—Fabry's syndrome*), or as a sign or a phenomenon (as *Gowers' sign—Gowers' phenomenon*).

Exceptions to the use of subentries are made for specific acids and for enzymes and enzyme deficiencies. Names of specific acids will be found under the first word of the name, e.g., *sulfuric acid* under *S*, as will enzyme names, e.g., *alkaline phosphatase* under *A*. Entries for enzyme deficiencies will be found immediately following the entry for the enzyme in question, e.g., *carbamoyl-phosphate synthetase deficiency* after *carbamoyl-phosphate synthetase*.

SEQUENCE OF ENTRIES

Main entries will be found alphabetized on the sequence of letters, regardless of spaces or hyphens that may occur between them. (Special rules govern eponymic terms; see below.) Thus the following sequences will be found:

formboard	heart
form-class	heart block
forme	heartburn
form-family	heart failure

Subentries, like the main entries, are alphabetized letter by letter. However, the main entry word, whether it is an abbreviation or a spelled-out plural, is ignored in alphabetizing subentries, as are prepositions, conjunctions, and articles. (For eponymic terms, see below.) Thus the subentries under *ganglion* (column 1), and *prolapse* (column 2) have the following order:

ganglia trunci sympathici	anal p.
tympanic g.	p. of anus
tympanic g. of Valentin	p. of cord
g. tympanicum	frank p.
upper g.	p. of iris

Eponymic terms constitute an exception to this scheme of alphabetization. For eponyms, the following rules apply, both in main entries and in subentries:

1. The *'s*, if one occurs, is not counted for alphabetization, nor are any words that follow the *'s*, unless the first word is the same. Thus, *Addison's planes* precedes *addisonian.*

2. The second name in a compound eponymic term does not count for alphabetization unless the terms are the same in all other respects. Thus, these terms appear in the following order: *Babinski's law, Babinski-Froelich syndrome, Babinski-Nageotte syndrome, Babinski-Vaquez syndrome.*

3. Umlauts (*ö, ü*) are ignored in alphabetization, as in the following sequence: *Löwe's ring, Lowe's syndrome, Löwenberg's canal, Löwenthal's tract, Lower's rings.*

4. Proper names beginning *Mc* or *Mac* are alphabetized as though spelled *Mac* in every instance, the sequence being determined by the letters immediately following the *c.*

Proper nouns (or capitalized entries) commonly appear before common nouns (or lower case entries). Thus *Diplococcus* precedes *diplococcus* and *Micrococcus* precedes *micrococcus.*

In the alphabetization of chemical terms, italic prefixes (e.g., *o-, p-, m-, trans-, cis-*) are ignored, as are numbers, Greek letters, and the prefixes L-, D-, *l-, d-,* (+)-, and (−)-. In the case of pharmaceutical names in which the prefix is spelled out, the term will be found under the fully spelled out form; for example, *levodopa* will be found under *L.*

INDICATION OF PRONUNCIATION

A phonetic spelling of a term appears in parentheses after the bold face entry. The pronunciation is provided for all main entries; it is generally not given for subentries but does appear in some subentries that are foreign words. As a rule only the most common pronunciation is given, with no effort to list variants. The phonetic spelling is presented in the simplest possible form, in a very broad transcription with few diacritical marks.

There are four basic rules:

1. An unmarked vowel ending a syllable (an "open" syllable) is long; thus *ma* represents the pronunciation of *may;* *ne,* that of *knee;* ri, of *rye* or *wry;* so, of *sew* or *so;* too, of *two, too,* or *to;* and *vu,* of *view.*

2. An unmarked vowel in a syllable ending with a consonant (a "closed" syllable) is short; thus kat represents *cat;* bed, *bed;* hit, *hit;* not, *not* or *knot;* foot, *foot;* and kusp, *cusp.*

3. A long vowel in a closed syllable is indicated by a macron; thus māt stands for *mate,* sēd for *seed,* bīl for *bile,* mōl for *mole,* fūm for *fume,* and fool for *fool.*

4. A short vowel that ends or itself constitutes a syllable is indicated by a breve; thus ĕ-fekt′ for *effect,* ĭ-mūn′ for *immune,* and ŏ-klood′ for *occlude.*

The digraph *ah* has two uses: (1) It represents the long open vowel of father; so bahm for *balm.* (2) It represents *schwa,* the indefinite vowel of sofa; thus ah-bāt′ for *abate.* Both values of the digraph appear in fahr′mah-se, *pharmacy.* The three digraphs oi (as in *oil*), ou (as in *out*), and aw (as in *paw*) complete the vocalic system.

Primary (′) and secondary (″) accents are shown in polysyllabic words, with unstressed syllables followed by hyphens, as in pol″e-sĭ-lab′ik. Monosyllables, even when part of a compound term, have no stress mark. Primary accents are also given as part of the bold face subentry for Latin phrases.

It is impossible with Dorland's simplified phonetics to represent the native pronunciations of many foreign words and proper names. These are shown as closely as possible in English phonetics.

PRESENTATION OF PLURALS AND OTHER INFLECTIONS

For main entries, the plural of an irregular noun and the original and anglicized plurals of a foreign noun or adjective are given after the phonetic spelling, for example,

stoma (sto′mah), pl. *sto′mas* or *sto′mata* . . . .

The original foreign plural is often given a separate bold face listing in proper alphabetical order, for example,

stomata (sto′mah-tah) [Gr.] plural of *stoma*.

Latin is used, especially in anatomy, to form phrases of the type "the X of Y," for example, *arcus aortae*, "the arch of the aorta." The prepositional phrase introduced by "of" corresponds to the Latin genitive case (abbreviated *gen.*); therefore Latin genitive case-forms are also frequently listed, for example:

papilla . . . gen. and pl. *papil′lae*

os[1] . . . gen. *o′ris*, pl. *o′ra*

os[2] . . . gen. *os′sis*, pl. *os′sa*

Other Latin inflected forms are found in subentries; these forms will be the objects in a prepositional phrase. For example, under the main entry **fissura** there is the subentry **f. in ano:** *ano* is the object of the preposition *in* and is one of the half dozen or so different inflected forms of *anus*, which is a main entry in the Dictionary and has listed with it the genitive and plural form *ani*. As in all subentries, differences in singular and plural forms do not count for alphabetizing, nor do prepositions and conjunctions (i.e., *et* "and"); thus under the main entry **fissura,** the subentry **f. in ano** precedes **f. antitrogohelicina.**

ETYMOLOGY

Information on the origin of a word appears in brackets after the phonetic spelling or a plural form of the entry when that is given. The information is necessarily brief, and the reader must often reason from the etymon, the original word from which other words are derived, to the meaning. For example, for the main entry **dualism,** the etymological section reads [L. *duo* two]. L. stands for Latin (languages may be either abbreviated or spelled out; see Abbreviations Used in This Dictionary on page xvi). The word *duo* is the etymon, and "two" is the English translation of the etymon, not of the entry. The reader proceeds from *duo* to *dual* to *dualism*, or vice versa. Furthermore, space limitations preclude the listing of all the stages in the passage from the etymon to the modern derivative (i.e., the entry). For example, the etymological part of the entry for **vein** is simply [L. *vena*]; in full, it would be [Middle English *veine*, from Old Fr., from L. *vena*].

For those foreign words or phrases taken into English entire, only the language is given, with the translation within quotation marks, for example: **déjà vu,** [Fr. "already seen"].

There are four further additions: (1) As a guide to related vocabulary, especially for anatomical terms, the main entry may be followed in brackets by its Greek and/or Latin equivalent, such as **kidney** . . . [L. *ren;* Gr. *nephros*]. (2) Many technical terms of Greek or Latin derivation are listed twice as main entries (and both times with etymology, meaning, and cross references), first as an independent word, and then as a combining form, for example, *metra* and *metra*-. (3) There is an essay *Fundamentals of Medical Etymology* (page xvii), which explains the basic rules for the derivation and composition of Greek, Latin, or Greco-Latin terms in medicine. At the end of the essay there is an analytical word list of Greek and Latin roots, prefixes, and combining forms; the list is an aid for the analysis of existing medical terms and the creation of new ones. (4) The prefixes (e.g., *hyper*-, *hypo*-), suffixes (e.g., *-ia, -oid*), and combining forms (e.g., *actino*-, *-emia*) from the analytical word list are also listed as main entries in the vocabulary.

OFFICIAL PUBLICATIONS

Certain terms listed in official publications are identified by an abbreviation in brackets. These abbreviations usually appear after the etymology (or after the phonetic spelling if no etymology is given) in main entries or after the bold face subentry. When a term has more than one meaning, the abbreviation will be placed at the beginning of the definition to which it applies. The following abbreviations are used:

[DSM-III-R]	*Diagnostic and Statistical Manual of Mental Disorders* of the American Psychiatric Association, 3rd edition-Revised (1987)
[EC]	Enzyme Commission number (e.g., **aspartate aminotransferase** . . . [EC 2.6.1.1]), from the Recommendations of the Nomenclature Committee of the International Union of Biochemistry on the Nomenclature and Classification of Enzyme-Catalyzed Reactions published in *Enzyme Nomenclature* (1984)
[NA]	*Nomina Anatomica*, 5th edition (1980)
[NF]	*The National Formulary*, 16th edition (1985)
[USP]	*The United States Pharmacopeia*, 21st revision (1985)

PLACEMENT OF DEFINITIONS AND CROSS REFERENCES

With few exceptions, a definition is given in only one place for two or more synonymous terms. Entries for the other terms provide cross references to the term where the definition is to be found. Such cross references are in place of a definition and are set in roman type:

mastoplasty (mas′to-plas″te) mammaplasty.

The definition will be found at *mammaplasty*. In many cases, synonyms for defined terms are listed at the end of the entry with the phrase "called also."

Cross references are also given to related entries or to entries where additional information may be found and are identified by the use of "see also," "cf.," and "q.v." All cross references with introductory phrases (including synonyms listed with "called also") are set in italic type.

Cross references from one subentry to another subentry under the same main heading use the abbreviated form of the main entry, for example:

syndrome

hypersomnia-bulima s., Klein-Levin s.

For certain classes of words, the definition will occur in a predictable place (synonyms will, of course, have cross references). Names of anatomical terms for which an official name is given in the fifth edition of the *Nomina Anatomica* [NA] (1980) are defined on the NA term. Drug names included in the twenty-first revision of *The United States Pharmacopeia* and the sixteenth edition of *The National Formulary* are defined on the official terms. Enzymes are defined at the name adopted in the fifth edition of *Enzyme Nomenclature* (1984). Definitions for bacteria, parasitic organisms, and most plants are found under the genus and species; for bacteria, the name follows the classification given in the eighth edition of *Bergey's Manual of Determinative Bacteriology* (1974) and *Bergey's Manual of Systemic Bacteriology*, vol. 1 (1984). For all genera and species, official spellings (e.g., *Haemophilus*, not *Hemophilus*) are used. Mental disorders are defined on the term given in *DSM-III-R*.

Chemical compounds embodying the name of an element will be found as subentries under the element: *aluminum acetate, aluminum hydroxide,* and *aluminum sulfate* are defined under *aluminum; calcium carbonate, calcium oxide,* and *calcium sulfate* are defined under *calcium*.

Also, names of salts and esters will be found as subentries under the first word of the compound name; if that word is not a main entry, then the entire compound will be a main entry alphabetized by the first word of the compound. For example, *prednisolone acetate, prednisolone sodium phosphate,* and *prednisolone succinate* appear under *prednisolone; diatrizoate sodium* appears under *diatrizoate;* and *mercaptomerin sodium* appears as a main entry under *M.*

Eponymic terms are generally entered twice. Biographical information is given at the personal name (or the initial name, if the eponym is compound) and the definition is given at the operative noun. This necessitates the use of cross references at eponymic entries, such as *"Apgar score . . . see under score."* If biographical information for an individual is not given (as *Mozer's disease),* there will be only one entry, under the operative noun, in this case *disease.*

The practice of cross referencing is also followed for earlier terms that have been supplanted and for variant spellings of a term. In most such instances, the term on which the definition appears is the currently preferred term or spelling. However, in some instances, the shade of preference may be very slight or nonexistent, while in others, some authorities may even prefer a term that has only a cross-reference to the defined term. In such cases, the practice of defining words only at one place has been adhered to as a means of keeping down the size of the Dictionary by avoiding duplication of definitions, and the user should remember that the appearance of a cross reference or a definition does not always indicate preference for one form or synonym over another.

FORM OF EPONYMS

The use of the possessive form ending in *'s* for eponyms is becoming progressively less common, and the entries for eponymic terms in this Dictionary reflect this ongoing change in usage. New terms and terms revised since the appearance of the previous edition generally omit the *'s.* But because the amount of time that would be needed to check and change every occurrence of *'s* would far exceed the amount of time available, it was decided that only new entries or entries that were to be changed in some additional way would appear without the *'s.* (Of course compound eponyms and some terms like *Apgar score* had no *'s* to begin with.) The Dictionary therefore presents an inconsistent mixture of forms, even in the cross references. Users should be aware that although the use of the nonpossessive form for eponyms is increasingly common, it is by no means universal, and should also remember that the variation in forms seen in the Dictionary is only a reflection of change and *not* a prescription for the use of possessive and nonpossessive forms.

SYMBOLS AND ABBREVIATIONS

Symbols and abbreviations are included as main entries; definitions consist of the term for which the symbol or the abbreviation (in most cases without the phrase "abbreviation for") stands, with a translation if the term is a foreign language. These terms will usually be found at the appropriate places in the vocabulary (with the abbreviation given at the end of the definition). Some terms, however, are self-explanatory and have no entry, such as the names of organizations and phrases like the following:

q.h. abbreviation for L. qua′que ho′ra, every hour.

Abbreviations appear both with and without periods. This should not be taken to denote proper usage, since abbreviations may appear either way; the trend at the moment is away from the use of the period for most abbreviations.

ABBREVIATIONS USED IN THIS DICTIONARY

a.	artery (L. *arteria*); agar		l.	ligament (L. *ligamentum*)
aa.	arteries (L. *arteriae*)		lat.	lateral
ant.	anterior		m.	muscle (L. *musculus*)
Ar.	Arabic		med.	medial, median
A.S.	Anglo-Saxon		n.	nerve (L. *nervus*)
c.	about (L. *circa*)		NA	Nomina Anatomica
cf.	compare (L. *confer*)		neg.	negative
def.	definition		NF	National Formulary
dim.	diminutive		obs.	obsolete
EC	Enzyme Commission		pl.	plural
e.g.	for example (L. *exampli gratia*)		Port.	Portuguese
Fr.	French		post.	posterior
gen.	genitive		q.v.	which see (L. *quod vide*)
Ger.	German		sing.	singular
Gr.	Greek		Sp.	Spanish
i.e.	that is (L. *id est*)		sup.	superior
inf.	inferior		USP	United States Pharmacopeia
It.	Italian		v.	vein (L. *vena*)
L.	Latin			

Fundamentals of Medical Etymology

By JOSEPH M. PATWELL, PH.D.

Twenty-six hundred years ago the Asiatic Greeks of Ionia and the Italian Greeks in Magna Graecia began the speculative and investigational sciences, pushing the then Greek to its limits, pushing beyond those limits, riveting new meanings onto old words, smithing new words for new ideas and discoveries—*philosophia*, "the love of wisdom," was supposedly first used by Pythagoras.

The sciences still go their robust way, iconoclastic but also indebted to and respectful of their ancient tradition. In anatomy, surgery, clinical medicine, and laboratory medicine, Greek, Latin, and Greco-Latin have always formed well over ninety per cent of the technical terms. Knowing the fundamentals of Greek and Latin word formation is immensely helpful in learning the vocabulary of modern medicine or of any modern science and is absolutely necessary for anyone coining a word for a new hypothesis, theory, process, or entity. The purpose of this introduction is to present those fundamentals in as practical and concise a form as possible; any statements contrary to historical and comparative linguistic fact that are made in the following pages are deliberate in keeping with this purpose.

ALPHABET AND PRONUNCIATION

The Latin alphabet is a modification of one of the many Greek alphabets. The order and shape of the Latin letters is the same as ours except that the Classical Latin alphabet has no *j*, *u*, or *w*, which are improvements dating from the Middle Ages.

The consonants of the Latin alphabet have about the same values as the English except that *c*, *ch*, *g*, *s*, *t*, and *v* are pronounced as in cold, *ch*rome, *g*et, *s*o, *t*in, and *w*ine, and not as in cent, *ch*ill, *g*em, rose, men*t*ion, and *v*ine. *Ph* and *th* may be pronounced as in *ph*ilosophy and *th*eology.

Latin vowels may be long or short. The short vowels are pronounced very much like the American w*a*nder, b*e*d, *i*t, h*o*pe, and p*u*t; short *y* sounds like the *ü* in German d*ü*nn. The long vowels are pronounced as in f*a*ther, h*e*y, mar*i*ne, st*o*ve, and r*u*de; long *y* is pronounced like the *ü* in the German *ü*ber.

Words are stressed on the next-to-last syllable, called the penult, if that syllable contains a long vowel or diphthong or is followed by two or more consonants, otherwise on the syllable before the penult.

The Greek alphabet used today is based on that used in Athens by the end of the fifth century B.C. The accompanying table shows one modern English pronunciation of each ancient Greek character in terms of English.

CAPITAL	SMALL LETTER	SOUND	NAME	TRANSCRIPTION
A	α	*a*rchaic	alpha	a
B	β	*b*arbarism	beta	b
Γ	γ	*g*rammar	gamma	g
Δ	δ	*d*ogma	delta	d
E	ε	*e*lephant	epsilon	e
Z	ζ	*z*oology	zeta	z
H	η	*a*ir	eta	ē
Θ	θ, ϑ	*th*eist	theta	th
I	ι	ma*ch*ine	iota	i
K	κ	s*k*eleton	kappa	c (Latin), k (Dorland's)
Λ	λ	*l*ithograph	lambda	l
M	μ	*m*usic	mu	m
N	ν	*n*eolithic	nu	n
Ξ	ξ	e*x*egesis	xi	x
O	ο	*o*belisk	omicron	o
Π	π	s*p*asm	pi	p
P	ρ	a*r*achnid	rho	r
Σ	σ, ς	*s*ymbol	sigma	s
T	τ	s*t*adium	tau	t
Υ	υ	*ü* über (German)	upsilon	y
Φ	φ	*ph*oto	phi	ph
X	χ	Ba*ch* (German)	chi	ch
Ψ	ψ	di*ps*omania	psi	ps
Ω	ω	*o*cher, Sh*aw*	omega	ō

The vowels are α, ε, η, ι, ο, υ, ω, most of which may be followed by ι, or υ to form diphthongs, the most common of which are shown below.

DIPHTHONG	SOUND	TRANSCRIPTION
αι	*ai*sle	ae, e, or ai
αυ	*ou*t	au
ει	*ei*ght	i, or ei
ευ	*eu*phony	eu
οι	*oi*	oe, e, or oi
ου	gh*ou*l	ou or u
υι	s*ui*te	ui, l*ui* (French)

TRANSLITERATION

The Romans transliterated kappa with *c*, not *k*, and chi with *ch*, not *kh;* thus *ch*aracter, not *kh*arakter. This Dictionary transliterates kappa with *k* in its etymologies in order to make immediately clear the nature of the underlying Greek sound: Spelling *cystis* for *kystis*, cyst, could cause doubt whether the sound was "kystis" or "systis." Similar difficulties with chi are less likely, and therefore Dorland's retains the traditional *ch;* hence our etymological spelling is *charakter.*

Classical Greek ει was pronounced as in *skein*, but by the end of the fourth century B.C. it was pronounced as in *seize;* thus the city that Alexander the Greek founded in Egypt, *Alexandreia*, became Alexandria in Latin. English generally prefers the Latin transliteration, but the use of *ei* for ει is growing. This Dictionary transliterates ει with *ei* in its etymologies.

The Romans transliterated Greek αι and οι with their own *ae* and *oe*, which had nearly the same pronunciation. By late antiquity the Greek and Latin diphthongs had become simple vowels, having gone through the regular progression *ai*sle to *ai*r to *ai*m, and the spelling wavered between the old diphthongs and the new pronunciation. This vacillation persists in English: the British prefer the diphthongs (*oe*dema, *ha*emorrhage); the Americans, the simple vowel (*e*dema, hemorrhage). In official nomenclature, e.g., the *Nomina Anatomica*, the *Index nominum genericorum (plantarum)*, and the *International Code of Nomenclature of Bacteria*, the official orthography fluctuates from edition to edition, swinging from *oesophagus* to *esophagus* and

Haemophilus to *Hemophilus* and back again. In the etymologies of this Dictionary Greek αι and οι are transliterated by *ai* and *oi*, and Latin *ae* and *oe* retained, for clarity's sake.

The Greeks especially but also the Romans had the same troubles with aitch (*h*) that Cockneys do, dropping it where it belonged and adding it where it did not. In Greek, initial *h-* ordinarily remained in simple words (*haima*, blood) but would either assimilate with or disappear before a prefix. For assimilation, *hypo* and *haima* make *hyphaimos*, suffused with blood (first appearing in Hippocrates); for disappearance, *a-, an-* and *haima* make *anaimia*, anemia (first appearing in Aristotle), not *ahaimia* and *ahemia*.

Latin usually preserved initial *h-* even after prefixes (*homo habilis, habilitas, inhabilitas; honor, honestus, inhonestus*), but very much of our Latin has come through French with inconsistent (to say the least) spellings and pronunciations: *able, ability,* and *inability,* not *hable, hability,* and *inhability; honor* and *honest,* not *onor* and *onest.*

Speakers of American English generally have no difficulty with *h-* and treat it as a full consonant when adding prefixes; thus we have *inharmonious,* not *anarmonious; ahaptoglobinemia,* not *anaptoglobinemia;* and *anhydride,* not *anydride* or *ahydride.*

Greek words are written with several accents that now indicate the stressed syllable. Words beginning with a vowel, diphthong, or *rho* (ρ) are written with a so-called breathing mark over the initial vowel or *rho* or over the second element of the diphthong (ἑτεροδοξία, heterodoxia; αἰσθητικός, aisthētikos; ῥυθμός, rhythmos). The *rough* breathing mark (ʽ) indicates that the syllable begins with an aspiration (aitch) as in *heterodoxia,* above, and words beginning with the rough breathing are usually transcribed into English with an initial *h.* Words beginning with a rho or an upsilon always have a rough breathing (ὑπέρ, hyper; ῥεῦμα, rheuma). The smooth breathing (ʼ) shows the absence of aspiration and so has no effect on pronunciation (ἀρωματικός, arōmatikos; αὐτογράφος, autographos).

The other conventions for transliterations from Greek are gamma (γ), which before gamma (γ), kappa (κ), chi (χ), or xi (ξ) has the sound of *n* as in *finger,* is transcribed as *n.** Initial *rho* and its rough breathing (ῥ) are transcribed as *rh* not *hr,* as *rheuma,* above; double *rho* (ρρ) is transcribed as *rrh* (διάρροια, diarrhoea, diarrhea). *Upsilon* (υ) is transcribed as *y* (ῥυθμός, rhythmos) except in diphthongs, where it is reproduced by *u* (ῥεῦμα, rheuma).

A few Greek words have come into English unchanged (σκελετόν, skeleton; αὐτόματον, automaton); most Greek words have passed into English through Latin, undergoing slight change (Greek στέρνον, sternon; Latin sternum); and some Greek words have passed through a secondary intermediary language, such as French, with still further change (Greek χειρουργία, cheirourgia; Latin chirurgia; French cirurgerie; English surgery). Other changes are accounted for by our tendency to drop Greek and Latin inflectional endings (ἀξίωμα, axioma, becomes axiom; *dorsalis* becomes dorsal) or replace them with a final mute *e* as if the words had come into English through French (γονοφόρος, gonophoros, becomes gonophore; *spina* becomes spine).

WORD FORMATION

The most frequent, the most important, and the seemingly most capricious changes in Greek or Latin words (or in English words, for that matter) arise not when the words pass from Greek or Latin into English, but when these words are first formed in the original language.

Many words in English and nearly all words in the Classical languages are combinations of roots and affixes. The root of a word contains the basic, lexical meaning, and the affixes give the root its shape as a word. (Affixes for the most part are prefixes and suffixes, including the inflections, added before or after the root, respectively.)

For example, in the English *love, loves, lover, lovers, loving, loved, lovingly, unloved,* and

---

*During World War II, *Ancistrodon* (from ἄγκιστρον, fishhook and ὀδοντ-. tooth) was reformed to *Agkistrodon,* which is the official spelling. *Ancistrodon* and *Ankistrodon* are both correct, but not *Agkistrodon:* Greek ἄγγελος (messenger) becomes *angelus* in Latin and *angel* in English, not *aggelus* and *aggel.*

unlovable, the root is *love*, and the various prefixes (*un-*) and suffixes (*-s, -r, -r-s, -ing, -ing, -ing-ly*, etc.) form the root into a word and modify that word for use in an utterance.

In English a root may very often function as an independent word, as *love, hate, smile, frown, milk;* these "root words" are extremely rare in the Classical languages. Nearly always in Latin and Greek, and usually in English, a word is a complex consisting of a form of a root and one or more affixes, which are not independent words themselves but may be used only to modify the root in some way (as *un-, -er, -ed*); such words are called "derived words."

When the root remains unchanged from derived word to derived word (a "regular" or "weak" root) and the affixes remain unaffected in their surroundings, the entire system of derived words has a transparent, instantly comprehended simplicity, as in *love* and its forms. So in Latin and Greek: there is a systematic clarity to the derivations of the Latin root *laud-* (praise)—the nouns *laudis* and *laudator* (praise, praiser); the principal parts of the regular verb, *laudo* (I praise), *laudare* (to praise); and the adjectives *laudabilis* and *laudatorius* (laudable, laudatory). There is also a regular system in the Greek root *pau-* (stop): the nouns *pausis* (pause) and *paustēr* (reliever, calmer); the regular principal parts of the verb *pauō* (I stop), *pausō* (I shall stop); and the adjectives *pausteon* (to be ended) and *paustērios* (relieving, calming).

Difficulties arise in English, Latin, and Greek with roots that change from word to word ("irregular" or "strong" roots) as in the English *sing, sang, sung, song;* and one says *singer*, not *songer; unsung*, not *unsing;* and *unsingable*, not *unsungable*. One example will suffice. The root *ten-* (stretch) appears in Latin and Greek (and also in English as *thin*). In Latin the root is as regular as the English *talk*, and the derivations are obvious: *ten*do (tendon), *ten*sio (tension), *ten*ius (tenuous, thin), ex*ten*uatus (stretched out, thinned out, weakened). In Greek, however, the same root appears as *ten-, tein-, ton-, ta-, tan-*, and *tain-*. Indeed, the rules for ancient Greek word formation would make a heavy book, and therefore, for efficiency's sake, the analytical word list, which follows this essay, gives examples of which affixes are attached to which forms of the root, for both the methodical Latin and the exuberant Greek.

In the Latin system there is an inconsistency affecting many common Latin and therefore English words: Latin roots with short vowels will have the normal, strong vowel in simple, unprefixed, words but a reduced, weakened vowel in prefixed words.

Consider the Latin root *făc-* (do, make). The normal *ă* remains in unprefixed words; hence the principal parts of the verb are:

făcio	I make
făcere	to make
făctus	made

Other unprefixed derivatives are:

facies	thing made or formed, face, "facies"
factor	factor
factura	as in manu*facture*
faction-	faction
factiosus	factious
facil-	doable, feasible, easy

From *facil-* are derived in turn:

facultat-	faculty
facilitat-	facility

Now let us add the prefix *ex* to the root *fac-*. *Ex* assimilates to *ef-* before *f* and changes the meaning of *fac-* to "complete." This or any prefix will cause a short *ă* to become a short *ĭ* before one consonant and a short *ĕ* before two consonants. Note the changes in the principal parts of the prefixed verb:

efficio	from	*exfacio*
efficere	from	*exfacere*
effectus	from	*exfactus*

It is from words like *efficio* that one can most clearly understand the derivations of Latin words. One forms the present participle by dropping the final *-re* from the present active infinitive, which is the form used in the etymologies of Dorland's, and adding *-nt* (verbs like *efficio* drop the final *-ere* and add *-ient*). The present participle of *efficio, efficere* is *efficient-* (efficient). And from the present participle is derived the noun *efficientia* (efficiency).

From the last principal part, *effectus*, one forms derivatives by dropping the *-us* and adding other suffixes. Thus from *effect-* one derives

effectum	effect
effector	effector
effectivus	effective

Occasionally the Romans would recompose a prefixed form according to the unprefixed norm. The most common example, and perfect for medical use, is *calefacio*, I warm, not *caleficio*, and therefore *calefacient-* not *caleficient-*.

Alas, there are exceptions. *Tenant* comes to English not directly from the Latin *tenēre*, to hold, which would give us *tenent*, but through the French *tenir*, and in French all verbs form their present participles in *-ant*, therefore *tenant;* a *locum tenens* is a *lieu tenant*.

Assimilation may affect the consonants between roots and affixes. In English the *v* in drive and thrive becomes voiceless and changes to *f* before the voiceless suffix *-t* that forms the nouns *drift* and *thrift*. In Latin, assimilation is usually minimal and obvious: *scribo* ("I write") and *scriba* ("writer, scribe") alternate with *scripsi* ("I wrote") and *scriptura* ("writing, scripture"). Occasionally the assimilation between Latin roots, prefixes, and suffixes may cause enough distortion to result in confusion. Below are listed some common Latin prefixes (most of them are also used as prepositions) showing the assimilation of the prefix to the following element. Note that the prefix *in-* has two sources and hence two uses: as a spatial prefix meaning *in, on,* or *into* (*in*scribe, *im*bibe, *il*luminate, *ir*radiate) and the antonymous prefix (*in*sensitive, *im*mature, *il*legible, *ir*reverent).

	Consonant Changes	English
ad-	before *c* becomes *ac-*	*ac*celerate
ad-	before *f* becomes *af-*	*af*finity
ad-	before *g* becomes *ag-*	*ag*glutinant
ad-	before *p* becomes *ap-*	*ap*pendix
ad-	before *s* becomes *as-*	*as*similate
ad-	before *t* becomes *at-*	*at*trition
ex-	before *f* becomes *ef-*	*ef*fusion
in-	before *l* becomes *il-*	*il*linition
in-	before *m* becomes *im-*	*im*mersion
in-	before *r* becomes *ir-*	*ir*radiation
ob-	before *c* becomes *oc-*	*oc*clusion
sub-	before *f* becomes *suf-*	*suf*focate
sub-	before *p* becomes *sup-*	*sup*pository
trans-	before *s* becomes *trans-*	*trans*piration

In Greek, assimilation may cause drastic changes to a word, and the phonetic laws governing these assimilations are far beyond the limits of this Dictionary. Fortunately, however, Greek prefixes are fairly regular. Like Latin prefixes, they may also function as prepositions of motion or location. Most Greek prefixes end in a vowel, which is maintained when the following element begins with a consonant and is lost (elided) when that element begins with a vowel: for example, the iota in *epi* ("on, upon") is unchanged in "epidemic" and is elided before *o* in "eponychium" ("cuticle"). When a Greek prefix ends in a consonant and the following element begins with a consonant, assimilation takes place with results as in Latin: the nu (*n*) of *syn* ("with") changes in *symphatheia* and *syllogismos* (sympathy and syllogism). Note that the prevocalic prefix *an-* has two sources and therefore two uses: it is the spatial preposition *ana* ("up, back"), as in *an*abolism and *an*ode; and it is the antonymous prefix *a-, an-,* as in *a*theist and *an*odyne, coming from the same source as Latin and English antonymous prefixes *in-* and *un-*.

Below are listed some common Greek prefixes with examples of elision and assimilation.

PREPOSITION	COMBINING FORMS	ENGLISH
amphi	amphi-	*amphi*crania
	amph-	*amph*eclexis
ana	ana-	*ana*bolism
	an-	*an*ode
anti	anti-	*anti*gen
	ant-	*ant*helminthic
apo	apo-	*apo*physis
	ap-	*ap*andria
dia	dia-	*dia*thermy
	di-	*di*uretic
ek	ek-	*ec*topia
ex	ex-	*ex*osmosis
en	en-	*en*ostosis
	em-	*em*bolus
epi	epi-	*epi*nephrine
	ep-	*ep*arterial
hyper	hyper-	*hyper*trophy
hypo	hypo-	*hypo*dermic
	hyp-	*hyp*axial
kata	kata-	*cata*lepsy
	kat-	*cat*ion
meta	meta-	*meta*morphosis
	met-	*met*encephalon
para	para-	*para*mastoid
	par-	*par*otid
peri	peri-	*peri*toneum
pro	pro-	*pro*gnosis
syn	syn-	*syn*thesis
	sym-	*sym*physis
	syl-	*syl*lepsis
	sy-	*sy*stole

Many Latin suffixes have been naturalized in English for centuries, and little comment is needed on their morphology and use. Some common suffixes of particular use in medicine are listed below with their English derivatives. Note that the suffixes *-abilis* and *-alis/-aris* are attached to verb stems of the first conjugation (the infinitives end in *-āre*, as in *laudāre* to praise); and *-ibilis* and *-ilis* are used with the other conjugations (*vidēre, visibilis; legĕre, legibilis; audīre, audibilis*).

LATIN COMPONENTS	ENGLISH
avis + -arium	avi*ary*
dormio (dormitus) + -orium	dormit*ory*
nutrio (nutritus) + -io	nutri*tion*
moveo (motus) + -or	mot*or*
porosus + -tas	porosi*ty*
frio + -abilis	fri*able*
edo + -ibilis	ed*ible*
corpus (corporis) + -alis	corpor*al*
febris + -ilis	febr*ile*
oculus + -aris	ocul*ar*
cilium + -arius	cili*ary*
sensus + -orius	sens*ory*
reticulum + -atus	reticul*ate*
morbus + -idus	morb*id*
aborior (abortus) + -ivus	abort*ive*
squama + -osus	squam*ous*
adeps (adipis) + -osus	adip*ose*
prae + caveo (cautus) + -io + -arius	precauti*onary*

Greek suffixes in general have not been naturalized in English as the Latin have, with the spectacular exception of the family of suffixes represented by verbs in *-izō* (-ize), agent nouns in *-istēs* (-ist), and verbal nouns in *-ismos* (-ism).

So far we have examined the various forms of roots, root words, and derived words; only compound words remain. A compound word is one formed from two (or more) independent words, the first word modifying, dependent upon, or being object of the next. In English, *housewife, kidney transplant, salesman, schoolboy, store-bought, backbreaking,* and *anteater* are compound words. In English the individual elements undergo little if any change from their basic, lexical forms but remain isolated, as it were, and receive their new meaning solely from juxtaposition (an example is the difference between *house guest* and *guest house*).

The conditions are vastly different in Latin and Greek; in the Classical languages one must use so-called combining forms of substantives (i.e., nouns and adjectives including past participles) that are often considerably different from the lexical forms.

In Latin all native compound words ordinarily will consist of the stem of the first word; then the connecting vowel, usually -i-, sometimes -u-; then the stem of the second word; then the inflection: magn-i-ficient-ia, *magnificientia*, magnificence. In science there are many compounds like *dorsoradial* and *frenosecretory* with Latin words and Greek connecting vowels; the true Latin forms for such compounds would be *dorsiradialis* and *frenisecretorius*.

In Greek the rules for forming compound words are much more complicated. If the first substantive of a Greek compound ends in *-a* (but not *-ma*) or *-ē*, one nearly always changes that vowel to *-o-*:

  glōssa, tongue + *ptōsis* fall = glossoptosis
  phōnē, voice, sound, + *logos*, word, reason, study = *phōnologia*, phonology

Substantives ending in *-on, -os,* or *-ys* usually drop the final consonant and leave the vowel unchanged:

  osteon, bone + *arthritis*, gout (first appears in Hippocrates) = osteoarthritis
  myelos marrow + *poiēsis* production = myelopoiesis
  pachys, thick + *derma* skin = pachydermia (first appears in Hippocrates)

If the second element begins with a vowel, one merely drops the final *-a* or *-ē* from the first element without adding *-o-*:

  archē, beginning, chief, rule + *enteron* intestine = archenteron
  bradys, slow, dull + *akusis*, hearing = bradyacousia

There are exceptions:

  idea, idea + *logos* = ideology is regular,

but

  genea, family, lineage + *logos* = *genealogia*, genealogy is irregular, as are
  architektōn not *archotektōn*, architect
  archetypos not *archotypos*, archetype

Indeed the regular *archo-* is extremely rare compared with *arche-* and *archi-* and is therefore "irregular."

Forming compounds from other substantives is complicated by the fact that one cannot generally predict the combining form of a substantive from the lexical entry, and in fact one usually predicts the lexical entry from the combining form, not vice versa.

In Greek, substantives ending in *-ma* have a stem or combining form in *-mat-;* so *haima* (blood), *haimat-* and *poiēsis* (making, "poesy") make *haimatopoiēsis*, hematopoiesis. But Hippocrates himself uses *haimorrhagia*, hemorrhage, not *haimatorrhagia*. And no one could predict from the nominative *gynē* (woman), which looks like a regular noun, a combining form *gynaik-*, whence gynecology; or from *gala* (milk), *galakt-*, whence galactophorous.

Latin is not so irregular, but even so *lac* (milk) has a combining stem *lact-* (lactacidemia); *cor* (heart), one in *cord-* (cordial); *miles* (soldier), *milit-* (military); *rex* (king), *reg-* (regicide); *nomen* (name), *nomin-* (nominate). The combining form of *homo* (human being, man) is *homin-* (hominoid ape), but Cicero himself uses *homicida* (murderer, homicide), not *hominicida*.

ANALYTICAL WORD LIST

The following list includes those Greek and Latin words occurring most frequently in this Dictionary, arranged alphabetically under their English combining forms as rubrics. The dash appended to a combining form indicates that it is not a complete word and, if the dash precedes the combining form, that it commonly appears as the terminal element of a compound. Infrequently a combining form is both preceded and followed by a dash, showing that it usually appears between two other elements. Closely related forms are shown in one entry by the use of parentheses: thus carbo(n)-, showing it may be either carbo-, as in *carbo*hydrate, or carbon-, as in *carbon*uria.

Following each combining form the first item of information is the Greek or Latin word, identified by [Gr.] and [L.], from which it is derived. Occasionally both a Greek and a Latin word are given. Presence of a dash before or after such an element indicates that it does not occur as an independent word in the original language. Information necessary to the understanding of the form appears next in parentheses. Then the meaning or meanings of the word are given, followed where appropriate by reference to a synonymous combining form in the other language, that is, on a combining form of Latin derivation, to the synonymous form of Greek derivation, and vice versa. Finally, an example is given to illustrate use of the combining form in a compound English derivative.

If this list is used in close conjunction with the etymological information given in the body of the Dictionary, no confusion should be caused by the similarity of elements in such words as *mel*algia, *mel*ancholia, and *mel*icera, where the similarity is only apparent and the derivation of each word is different.

a-   a- [L.] (*n* is added before words beginning with a vowel) negative prefix. Cf. in-³. a*metria*

ab-   ab [L.] away from. Cf. apo-. *ab*ducent

abdomin-   abdomen, abdominis [L.] abdomen. *abdomino*scopy

ac-   See ad-. *ac*cretion

acet-   acetum [L.] vinegar. *acet*ometer

acid-   acidus [L.] sour. *acid*uric

acou-   akouō [Gr.] hear. *acou*ethesia. (Also spelled acu-)

acr-   akron [Gr.] extremity, peak, *acro*megaly

act-   ago, actus [L.] do, drive. *act*. re*action*

actin-   aktis, aktinos [Gr.] ray, radius. Cf. radi-. *actin*ogenesis

acu-   See acou-. osteo*acusis*

ad-   ad [L.] (*d* changes to *c, f, g, p, s,* or *t* before words beginning with those consonants) to. *ad*renal

aden-   adēn [Gr.] gland. Cf. gland-. *aden*oma

adip-   adeps, adipis [L.] fat. Cf. lip- and stear-. *adip*ocellular

aer-   aēr [Gr.] air. an*aer*obiosis

aesthe-   See esthe-. *aesthe*sioneurosis

af-   See ad-. *af*ferent

ag-   See ad-. *ag*glutinant

-agogue   agōgos [Gr.] leading, inducing. ga*lactagogue*

-agra   agra [Gr.] catching, seizure. po*dagra*

alb-   albus [L.] white. Cf. leuk-. *alb*ocinereous

alg-   algos [Gr.] pain. neur*algia*

all-   allos [Gr.] other, different, *all*ergy

alve-   alveus [L.] trough, channel, cavity. *alve*olar

amph-   See amphi-. *amph*eclexis

amphi-   amphi [Gr.] (*i* is dropped before words beginning with a vowel) both, doubly. *amphi*celous

amyl-   amylon [Gr.] starch. *amyl*osynthesis

an-¹   See ana-. *an*agogic

an-²   See a-. *an*omalous

ana-   ana [Gr.] (final *a* is dropped before words beginning with a vowel) up, positive. *ana*phoresis

ancyl-   See ankyl-. *ancylo*stomiasis

andr-   anēr, andros [Gr.] man. gyn*andr*oid

angi-   angeion [Gr.] vessel. Cf. vas-. *angi*emphraxis

ankyl-   ankylos [Gr.] crooked, looped. *ankylo*dactylia. (Also spelled ancyl-)

ant-   See anti-. *ant*ophthalmic

ante-   ante [L.] before. *ante*flexion

anti-   anti [Gr.] (*i* is dropped before words beginning with a vowel) against, counter. Cf. contra*anti*pyogenic

antr-   antron [Gr.] cavern. *antr*odynia

ap-¹   See apo-. *ap*heter

ap-²   See ad-. *ap*pend

-aph   haptō, haph- [Gr.] touch. dys*aph*ia. (See also hapt-)

apo-   apo [Gr.] (*o* is dropped before words beginning with a vowel) away from, detached. Cf. ab-. *apo*physis

arachn-   arachnē [Gr.] spider. *arachn*odactyly

arch-   archē [Gr.] beginning, origin. *ar*chenteron

arter(i)-   *arteria* [Gr.] windpipe, artery. *ar-teri*osclerosis, peri*arteri*tis

arthr-   *arthron* [Gr.] joint. Cf. articul-. syn-*arthr*osis

articul-   *articulus* [L.] joint. Cf. arthr-. dis-*articul*ation

as-   See ad-. *as*similation

at-   See ad-. *at*trition

aur-   *auris* [L.] ear. Cf. ot-. *aur*inasal

aux-   *auxō* [Gr.] increase. enter*aux*e

ax-   *axōn* [Gr.] or *axis* [L.] axis. *axo*-fugal

axon-   *axōn* [Gr.] axis. *axon*ometer

ba-   *bainō, ba-* [Gr.] go, walk, stand. hypno*ba*tia

bacill-   *bacillus* [L.] small staff, rod. Cf. bacter-. actino*bacill*osis

bacter-   *bactērion* [Gr.] small staff, rod. Cf. bacill-. *bacter*iophage

ball-   *ballō, bol-* [Gr.] throw. *ball*istics. (See also bol-)

bar-   *baros* [Gr.] weight. pedo*bar*ometer

bi-¹   *bios* [Gr.] life. Cf. vit-. aero*bi*c

bi-²   *bi-* [L.] two (see also di-¹). *bi*lobate

bil-   *bilis* [L.] bile. Cf. chol-. *bil*iary

blast-   *blastos* [Gr.] bud, child, a growing thing in its early stages. Cf. germ-. *blast*oma, zygoto*blast*

blep-   *blepō* [Gr.] look, see. hemia*blep*sia

blephar-   *blepharon* [Gr.] (from *blepō;* see blep-) eyelid. Cf. cili-. *blephar*-oncus

bol-   See ball-. em*bol*ism

brachi-   *brachiōn* [Gr.] arm. *brachi*ocephalic

brachy-   *brachys* [Gr.] short. *brachy*cephalic

brady-   *bradys* [Gr.] slow. *brady*cardia

brom-   *brōmos* [Gr.] stench. podo*brom*idrosis

bronch-   *bronchos* [Gr.] windpipe. *bronch*oscopy

bry-   *bryō* [Gr.] be full of life. em*bry*onic

bucc-   *bucca* [L.] cheek. disto*bucc*al

cac-   *kakos* [Gr.] bad, abnormal. Cf. mal-. *cac*odontia, arthro*cac*e. (See also dys-)

calc-¹   *calx, calcis* [L.] stone (cf. lith-), limestone, lime. *calc*ipexy

calc-²   *calx, calcis* [L.] heel. *calc*aneotibial

calor-   *calor* [L.] heat. Cf. therm-. *calor*imeter

cancr-   *cancer, cancri* [L.] crab, cancer. Cf. carcin-. *cancr*ology. (Also spelled chancr-)

capit-   *caput, capitis* [L.] head. Cf. cephal-. de*capit*ator

caps-   *capsa* [L.] (from *capio;* see cept-) container. en*caps*ulation

carbo(n)-   *carbo, carbonis* [L.] coal, charcoal. *carbo*hydrate, *carbon*uria

carcin-   *karkinos* [Gr.] crab, cancer. Cf. cancr-. *carcin*oma

cardi-   *kardia* [Gr.] heart. lipo*cardi*ac

cary-   See kary-. *cary*okinesis

cat-   See cata-. *cat*hode

cata-   *kata* [Gr.] (final *a* is dropped before words beginning with a vowel) down, negative. *cata*batic

caud-   *cauda* [L.] tail. *caud*ad

cav-   *cavus* [L.] hollow. Cf. coel-. con*cav*e

cec-   *caecus* [L.] blind. Cf. typhl-. *cec*opexy

cel-¹   See coel-. amphi*cel*ous

cel-²   See -cele. *cel*ectome

-cele   *kēlē* [Gr.] tumor, hernia. gastro*cele*

cell-   *cella* [L.] room, cell. Cf. cyt-. *cell*iferous

cen-   *koinos* [Gr.] common. *cen*esthesia

cent-   *centum* [L.] hundred. Cf. hect-. Indicates fraction in metric system. [This exemplifies the custom in the metric system of identifying fractions of units by stems from the Latin, as centimeter, decimeter, millimeter, and multiples of units by the similar stems from the Greek, as hectometer, decameter, and kilometer.] *cent*imeter, *cent*ipede

cente-   *kenteō* [Gr.] to puncture. Cf. punct-. entero*cente*sis

centr-   *kentron* [Gr.] or *centrum* [L.] point, center. neuro*centr*al

cephal-   *kephalē* [Gr.] head. Cf. capit-. en*cephal*itis

cept-   *capio, -cipientis, -ceptus* [L.] take, receive, re*cept*or

cer-   *kēros* [Gr.] or *cera* [L.] wax. *cer*oplasty, *cer*omel

cerat-   See kerat-. a*cerat*osis

cerebr-   *cerebrum* [L.] brain. *cerebr*ospinal

cervic-   *cervix, cervicis* [L.] neck. Cf. trachel-. *cervic*itis

chancr-   See cancr-. *chancr*iform

cheil-   *cheilos* [Gr.] lip. Cf. labi-. *cheil*oschisis

cheir-   *cheir* [Gr.] hand. Cf. man-. macro*cheir*ia. (Also spelled chir-)

chir-   See cheir-. *chir*omegaly

chlor-   *chlōros* [Gr.] green. a*chlor*opsia

chol-   *cholē* [Gr.] bile. Cf. bil-. hepato*chol*angeitis

chondr-   *chondros* [Gr.] cartilage. *chondr*omalacia

chord-   *chordē* [Gr.] string, cord. peri*chord*al

chori-   *chorion* [Gr.] protective fetal membrane. endo*chori*on

chro-   *chrōs* [Gr.] color. poly*chro*matic

chron-   *chronos* [Gr.] time. syn*chron*ous

chy-   *cheō, chy-* [Gr.] pour. ec*chy*mosis

-cid(e)   *caedo, -cisus* [L.] cut, kill. infanti*cide*, germi*cid*al

cili-   *cilium* [L.] eyelid. Cf. blephar-. super*cili*ary

cine-   See kine-. auto*cine*sis

-cipient   See cept-. in*cipient*

circum-   *circum* [L.] around. Cf. peri-. *circum*ferential

-cis-   *caedo. -cisus* [L.] cut, kill. ex*cis*ion

clas-   *klaō* [Gr.] break, cranio*clas*t

clin-   *klinō* [Gr.] bend, incline, make lie down. *clin*ometer

clus-   *claudo, -clusus* [L.] shut. Maloc-*clus*ion

co-   See con-. *co*hesion

cocc-   *kokkos* [Gr.] seed, pill. gonococcus

coel-   *koilos* [Gr.] hollow. Cf. cav-. *coel*enteron. (Also spelled cel-)

col-¹   See colon-. *col*ic

col-²   See con-. *col*lapse

colon-   *kolon* [Gr.] lower intestine, *colon*ic

colp-   *kolpos* [Gr.] hollow, vagina. Cf. sin-. endo*colp*itis

com-   See con-. *com*masculation

con-   *con-* [L.] (becomes co- before vowels or *h;* col- before *l;* com- before *b, m,* or *p;* cor- before *r*) with, together. Cf. syn-. *con*traction

contra-   *contra* [L.] against, counter. Cf. anti-. *contra*indication

copr-   *kopros* [Gr.] dung. Cf. sterco-. *copr*oma

cor-¹   *korē* [Gr.] doll, little image, pupil. iso*cor*ia

cor-²   See con-. *cor*rugator

corpor-   *corpus, corporis* [L.] body. Cf. somat-. intra*corpor*al

cortic-   *cortex, corticis* [L.] bark, rind. *cortic*osterone

cost-   *costa* [L.] rib. Cf. pleur-. inter*cost*al

crani-   *kranion* [Gr.] or *cranium* [L.] skull. peri*crani*um

creat-   *kreas, kreato-* [Gr.] meat, flesh. *creat*orrhea

-crescent   *cresco, crescentis, cretus* [L.] grow. ex*crescent*

cret-¹   *cerno, cretus* [L.] distinguish, separate off. Cf. crin-. dis*cret*e

cret-²   See -crescent. ac*cret*ion

crin-   *krinō* [Gr.] distinguish, separate off. Cf. cret-¹. endo*crin*ology

crur-   *crus, cruris* [L.] shin, leg. brachio*crur*al

cry-   *kryos* [Gr.] cold. *cry*esthesia

crypt-   *kryptō* [Gr.] hide, conceal. *crypt*orchism

cult-   *colo, cultus* [L.] tend, cultivate. *cult*ure

cune-   *cuneus* [L.] wedge. Cf. sphen-. *cune*iform

cut-   *cutis* [L.] skin. Cf. derm(at)-. sub*cut*aneous

cyan-   *kyanos* [Gr.] blue, antho*cyan*in

cycl-   *kyklos* [Gr.] circle, cycle, *cyclo*phoria

cyst-   *kystis* [Gr.] bladder. Cf. vesic-. nephro*cyst*itis

cyt-   *kytos* [Gr.] cell. Cf. cell-. plasmo*cyt*oma

dacry-   *dakry* [Gr.] tear. *dacry*ocyst

dactyl-   *daktylos* [Gr.] finger, toe. Cf. digit-. hexa*dactyl*ism

de-   *de* [L.] down from. *de*composition

dec-¹   *deka* [Gr.] ten. Indicates multiple in metric system. Cf. dec-². *dec*agram

dec-²   *decem* [L.] ten. Indicates fraction in metric system. Cf. dec-¹. *deci*para, *deci*meter

dendr-   *dendron* [Gr.] tree. neuro*dendr*ite

dent-   *dens, dentis* [L.] tooth. Cf. odont-. inter*dent*al

derm(at)-   *derma, dermatos* [Gr.] skin. Cf. cut-. endo*derm*, *dermat*itis

desm-   *desmos* [Gr.] band, ligament. syn*desm*opexy

dextr-   *dexter, dextr-* [L.] right-hand. ambi*dextr*ous

di-¹   *di-* [Gr.] two. *di*morphic. (See also bi-²)

di-²   See dia-. *di*uresis

di-³   See dis-. *di*vergent

dia-   *dia* [Gr.] (*a* is dropped before words beginning with a vowel) through, apart. Cf. per-. *dia*gnosis

didym-   *didymos* [Gr.] twin. Cf. gemin-. epi*didym*al

digit-   *digitus* [L.] finger, toe. Cf. dactyl-. *digit*igrade

diplo-   *diploos* [Gr.] double. *diplo*myelia

dis-   *dis-* [L.] (*s* may be dropped before a word beginning with a consonant) apart, away from. *dis*location

disc-   *diskos* [Gr.] or *discus* [L.] disk. *disc*oplacenta

dors-   *dorsum* [L.] back. ventro*dors*al

drom-   *dromos* [Gr.] course, hemo*drom*ometer

-ducent   See duct-. ad*ducent*

-duct   *duco, ducentis, ductus* [L.] lead, conduct. ovi*duct*

dur-   *durus* [L.] hard. Cf. scler-. in*dur*ation

dynam(i)-   *dynamis* [Gr.] power. *dynam*oneure, neuro*dynam*ic

dys-   *dys-* [Gr.] bad, improper. Cf. mal-. *dys*trophic. (See also cac-)

e-   *e* [L.] out from. Cf. ec- and ex-. *e*mission

ec-   *ek* [Gr.] out of. Cf. e-. *ec*centric

-ech-   *echō* [Gr.] have, hold, be. syn*ech*otomy

ect-   *ektos* [Gr.] outside. Cf. extra-. *ect*oplasm

ede-   *oideō* [Gr.] swell. *ede*matous

ef-   See ex-. *ef*florescent

-elc-   *helkos* [Gr.] sore, ulcer. enter*elc*osis. (See also helc-)

electr-   *ēlectron* [Gr.] amber. *electr*otherapy

em-   See en-. *em*bolism, *em*pathy, *em*phlysis

-em-   *haima* [Gr.] blood. an*em*ia. (See also hem(at)-)

en-   *en* [Gr.] (*n* changes to *m* before *b, p* or *ph*) in, on. Cf. in-². *en*celitis

end-   *endon* [Gr.] inside. Cf. intra-. *end*angium

enter-   *enteron* [Gr.] intestine. dys*enter*y

ep-   See epi-. *ep*axial

epi-   *epi* [Gr.] (*i* is dropped before words beginning with a vowel) upon, after, in addition. *epi*glottis

erg-   *ergon* [Gr.] work, deed. en*erg*y

erythr-   *erythros* [Gr.] red. Cf. rub(r)-. *erythr*ochromia

eso-   *esō* [Gr.] inside. Cf. intra-. *eso*phylactic

esthe-   *aisthanomai, aisthē-* [Gr.] perceive, feel. Cf. sens-. an*esthe*sia

eu-   *eu* [Gr.] good, normal, *eu*pepsia

ex-   *ex* [Gr.] or *ex* [L.] out of. Cf. e-. *ex*cretion

exo-   *exō* [Gr.] outside. Cf. extra-. *exo*pathic

extra-	*extra* [L.] outside of, beyond. Cf. ect- and exo-. *extra*cellular
faci-	*facies* [L.] face. Cf. prosop-. brachio*faci*olingual
-facient	*facio, facientis, factus, -fectus* [L.] make. Cf. poie-. cale*facient*
-fact-	See facient-. arte*fact*
fasci-	*fascia* [L.] band. *fasci*orrhaphy
febr-	*febris* [L.] fever. Cf. pyr-. *febr*icide
-fect-	See -facient. de*fect*ive
-ferent	*fero, ferentis, latus* [L.] bear, carry. Cf. phor-. ef*ferent*
ferr-	*ferrum* [L.] iron. *ferr*oprotein
fibr-	*fibra* [L.] fiber. Cf. in-¹. chondro*fi-broma*
fil-	*filum* [L.] thread, *fil*iform
fiss-	*findo, fissus* [L.] split. Cf. schis-. *fiss*ion
flagell-	*flagellum* [L.] whip. *flagell*ation
flav-	*flavus* [L.] yellow. Cf. xanth-. ribo*flav*in
-flect-	*flecto, flexus* [L.] bend, divert. de*flect*ion
-flex-	See -flect-. re*flex*ometer
flu-	*fluo, fluxus* [L.] flow. Cf. rhe-. *flu*id
flux-	See flu-. af*flux*ion
for-	*foris* [L.] door, opening, per*for*ated
-form	*forma* [L.] shape. Cf. -oid. ossi*form*
fract-	*frango, fractus* [L.] break. re*fract*ive
front-	*frons, frontis* [L.] forehead, front. naso*front*al
-fug(e)	*fugio* [L.] flee, avoid. vermi*fuge*, centri*fug*al
funct-	*fungor, functus* [L.] perform, serve, function. mal*funct*ion
fund-	*fundo, fusus* [L.] pour. in*fund*ibulum
fus-	See fund-. dif*fus*ible
galact-	*gala, galactos* [Gr.] milk. Cf. lact-. dys*galact*ia
gam-	*gamos* [Gr.] marriage, reproductive union. a*gam*ont
gangli-	*ganglion* [Gr.] swelling, plexus. neuro*gangli*itis
gastr-	*gastēr, gastros* [Gr.] stomach. cholangio*gastr*ostomy
gelat-	*gelo, gelatus* [L.] freeze, congeal. *gelat*in
gemin-	*geminus* [L.] twin, double. Cf. didym-. quadri*gemin*al
gen-	*gignomai, gen-, gon-* [Gr.] become, be produced, originate, or *gennaō* [Gr.] produce, originate. cyto*gen*ic
germ-	*germen, germinis* [L.] bud, a growing thing in its early stages. Cf. blast-. *germ*inal, ovi*germ*
gest-	*gero, gerentis, gestus* [L.] bear, carry. con*gest*ion
gland-	*glans, glandis* [L.] acorn. Cf. aden-. intra*gland*ular
-glia	*glia* [Gr.] glue. neuro*glia*
gloss-	*glōssa* [Gr.] tongue. Cf. lingu-. tricho*gloss*ia
glott-	*glōtta* [Gr.] tongue, language. *glott*ic
gluc-	See glyc(y)-. *gluc*ophenetidin
glutin-	*gluten, glutinis* [L.] glue. ag*glutin*ation
glyc(y)-	*glykys* [Gr.] sweet. *glyc*emia, *glyc*yrrhizin. (Also spelled gluc-)
gnath-	*gnathos* [Gr.] jaw. ortho*gnath*ous
gno-	*gignōsiō, gnō-* [Gr.] know, discern. dia*gno*sis
gon-	See gen-. anphi*gon*y
grad-	*gradior* [L.] walk, take steps. retro*grad*e
-gram	*gramma* [Gr.] letter, drawing. cardio*gram*
gran-	*granum* [L.] grain, particle. lipo*gran*uloma
graph-	*graphō* [Gr.] scratch, write, record. histo*graph*y
grav-	*gravis* [L.] heavy. multi*grav*ida
gyn(ec)-	*gynē, gynaikos* [Gr.] woman, wife, andro*gyn*y, *gynec*ologic
gyr-	*gyros* [Gr.] ring, circle, *gyr*ospasm
haem(at)-	See hem(at)-. *haem*orrhagia, *haem*atoxylon
hapt-	*haptō* [Gr.] touch. *hapt*ometer
hect-	*hekt-* [Gr.] hundred. Cf. cent-. Indicates multiple in metric system. *hect*ometer
helc-	*helkos* [Gr.] sore, ulcer, *helc*osis
hem(at)-	*haima, haimatos* [Gr.] blood. Cf. sanguin-. *hem*angioma, *hemat*ocyturia. (See also -em-)
hemi-	*hēmi-* [Gr.] half. Cf. semi-. *hemi*ageusia
hen-	*heis, henos* [Gr.] one. Cf. un-. *hen*ogenesis
hepat-	*hēpar, hēpatos* [Gr.] liver. gastro*hepat*ic
hept(a)-	*hepta* [Gr.] seven. Cf. sept-². *hept*atomic, *hept*avalent
hered-	*heres, heredis* [L.] heir, *hered*oimmunity
hex-¹	*hex* [Gr.] six. Cf. sex-. *hex*yl-. An *a* is added in some combinations
hex-²	*echō, hex-* [Gr.] (added to *s* becomes hex-) have, hold, be. cache*x*ia
hexa-	See hex-¹. *hexa*chromic
hidr-	*hidros* [Gr.] sweat. hyper*hidr*osis
hist-	*histos* [Gr.] web, tissue. *hist*odialysis
hod-	*hodos* [Gr.] road, path. *hod*oneuromere. (See also od- and -ode¹)
hom-	*homos* [Gr.] common, same. *hom*omorphic
horm-	*ormē* [Gr.] impetus, impulse. *horm*one
hydat-	*hydōr, hydatos* [Gr.] water. *hydat*ism
hydr-	*hydōr, hydr-* [Gr.] water. Cf. lymph-. anchlor*hydr*ia
hyp-	See hypo-. *hyp*axial
hyper-	*hyper* [Gr.] above, beyond, extreme. Cf. super-. *hyper*trophy
hypn-	*hypnos* [Gr.] sleep. *hypn*otic
hypo-	*hypo* [Gr.] (*o* is dropped before words beginning with a vowel) under, below. Cf. sub-. *hypo*metabolism
hyster-	*hystera* [Gr.] womb. colpo*hyster*opexy
iatr-	*iatros* [Gr.] physician, ped*iatr*ics

idi-   *idios* [Gr.] peculiar, separate, distinct. *idi*osyncrasy

il-   See in-[2,3]. *il*linition (in, on), *il*legible (negative prefix)

ile-   See ili- [ile- is commonly used to refer to the portion of the intestines known as the ileum]. *ile*ostomy

ili-   *ilium (ileum)* [L.] lower abdomen, intestines [ili- is commonly used to refer to the flaring part of the hip bone known as the ilium]. *ili*osacral

im-   See in-[2,3]. *im*mersion (in, on), *im*perforation (negative prefix)

in-[1]   *is, inos* [Gr.] fiber. Cf. fibr-. *ino*steatoma

in-[2]   *in* [L.] (*n* changes to *l, m,* or *r* before words beginning with those consonants) in, on. Cf. en-. *in*sertion

in-[3]   *in-* [L.] (*n* changes to *l, m,* or *r* before words beginning with those consonants) negative prefix. Cf. a-. *in*valid

infra-   *infra* [L.] beneath. *infra*orbital

insul-   *insula* [L.] island. *insul*in

inter-   *inter* [L.] among, between. *inter*carpal

intra-   *intra* [L.] inside. Cf. end- and eso-. *intra*venous

ir-   See in-[2,3]. *ir*radiation (in, on), *ir*reducible (negative prefix)

irid-   *iris, iridos* [Gr.] rainbow, colored circle. kerato*irid*ocyclitis

is-   *isos* [Gr.] equal. *is*otope

ischi-   *ischion* [Gr.] hip, haunch, *ischio*pubic

jact-   *iacio, iactus* [L.] throw. *jact*itation

-ject   *iacio, -iectus* [L.] throw. in*ject*ion

jejun-   *ieiunus* [L.] hungry, not partaking of food. gastro*jejun*ostomy

jug-   *iugum* [L.] yoke. con*jug*ation

junct-   *iungo, iunctus* [L.] yoke, join. con*junct*iva

kary-   *karyon* [Gr.] nut, kernel, nucleus. Cf. nucle-. mega*kary*ocyte. (Also spelled cary-)

kerat-   *keras, keratos* [Gr.] horn. *kerat*olysis. (Also spelled cerat-)

kil-   *chilioi* [Gr.] one thousand. Cf. mill-. Indicates multiple in metric system. *kil*ogram

kine-   *kineō* [Gr.] move. *kine*matograph. (Also spelled cine-)

labi-   *labrium* [L.] lip. Cf. cheil-. gingivo*labi*al

lact-   *lac, lactis* [L.] milk. Cf. galact-. gluco*lact*one

lal-   *laleō* [Gr.] talk, babble. glosso*lal*ia

lapar-   *lapara* [Gr.] flank. *lapar*otomy

laryng-   *larynx, laryngos* [Gr.] windpipe. *laryng*endoscope

lat-   *fero, latus* [L.] bear, carry. See -ferent. trans*lat*ion

later-   *latus, lateris* [L.] side. ventro*later*al

lent-   *lens, lentis* [L.] lentil. Cf. phac-. *lent*iconus

lep-   *lambanō, lēp* [Gr.] take, seize. cat*alep*tic

leuc-   See leuk-. *leuc*inuria

leuk-   *leukos* [Gr.] white. Cf. alb-. *leuk*orrhea. (Also spelled leuc-)

lien-   *lien* [L.] spleen. Cf. splen-. *lien*ocele

lig-   *ligo* [L.] tie, bind. *lig*ate

lingu-   *lingua* [L.] tongue. Cf. gloss-. sub*lingu*al

lip-   *lipos* [Gr.] fat. Cf. adip-. glyco*lip*in

lith-   *lithos* [Gr.] stone. Cf. calc-[1]. neph*ro*lith*otomy

loc-   *locus* [L.] place. Cf. top-. *loc*omotion

log-   *legō, log-* [Gr.] speak, given an account. *log*orrhea, embryo*log*y

lumb-   *lumbus* [L.] loin. dorso*lumb*ar

lute-   *luteus* [L.] yellow. Cf. xanth-. *lute*oma

ly-   *lyō* [Gr.] loose, dissolve. Cf. solut-. kerato*ly*sis

lymph-   *lympha* [Gr.] water. Cf. hydr-. *lymph*adenosis

macr-   *makros* [Gr.] long, large, *macr*omyeloblast

mal-   *malus* [L.] bad, abnormal. Cf. cacand dys-. *mal*function

malac-   *malakos* [Gr.] soft. osteo*malac*ia

mamm-   *mamma* [L.] breast. Cf. mast-. sub*mamm*ary

man-   *manus* [L.] hand. Cf. cheir-. *man*iphalanx

mani-   *mania* [Gr.] mental aberration. *mani*graphy, klepto*mani*a

mast-   *mastos* [Gr.] breast. Cf. mamm-. hyper*mast*ia

medi-   *medius* [L.] middle. Cf. mes-. *med*ifrontal

mega-   *megas* [Gr.] great, large. Also indicates multiple (1,000,000) in metric system. *mega*colon, *mega*dyne. (See also megal-)

megal-   *megas, megalou* [Gr.] great, large. acro*megal*y

mel-   *melos* [Gr.] limb, member. sym*mel*ia

melan-   *melas, melanos* [Gr.] black. hippo*melan*in

men-   *mēn* [Gr.] month. dys*men*orrhea

mening-   *mēninx, mēningos* [Gr.] membrane. encephalo*mening*itis

ment-   *mens, mentis* [L.] mind. Cf. phren-, psych- and thym-. de*ment*ia

mer-   *meros* [Gr.] part. poly*mer*ic

mes-   *mesos* [Gr.] middle. Cf. medi-. *mes*oderm

met-   See meta-. *met*allergy

meta-   *meta* [Gr.] (*a* is dropped before words beginning with a vowel) after, beyond, accompanying. *meta*carpal

metr-[1]   *metron* [Gr.] measure. stereo*metr*y

metr-[2]   *metra* [Gr.] womb. endo*metr*itis

micr-   *mikros* [Gr.] small. photo*micr*ograph

mill-   *mille* [L.] one thousand. Cf. kil-. Indicates fraction in metric system. *mill*igram, *mill*ipede

miss-	See -mittent. intro*miss*ion
-mittent	*mitto, mittentis, missus* [L.] send. inter*mittent*
mne-	*mimnērcō, mnē-* [Gr.] remember. pseudo*mne*sia
mon-	*monos* [Gr.] only, sole. *mon*oplegia
morph-	*morphē* [Gr.] form, shape. poly*morph*onuclear
mot-	*moveo, motus* [L.] move. vaso*mot*or
my-	*mys, myos* [Gr.] muscle. inoleio*my*oma
-myces	*mykēs, mykētos* [Gr.] fungus. myelo*myces*
myc(et)-	See -myces. asco*myce*tes, strepto*myc*in
myel-	*myelos* [Gr.] marrow. polio*myel*itis
myx-	*myxa* [Gr.] mucus. *myx*edema
narc-	*narkē* [Gr.] numbness. topo*narc*osis
nas-	*nasus* [L.] nose. Cf. rhin-. palato*nas*al
ne-	*neos* [Gr.] new, young. *ne*ocyte
necr-	*nekros* [Gr.] corpse. *necr*ocytosis
nephr-	*nephros* [Gr.] kidney. Cf. ren-. par*anephr*ic
neur-	*neuron* [Gr.] nerve. esthesio*neur*e
nod-	*nodus* [L.] knot. *nod*osity
nom-	*nomos* [Gr.] (from *nemō* deal out, distribute) law, custom. taxo*nom*y
non-	*nona* [L.] nine. *non*acosane
nos-	*nosos* [Gr.] disease. *nos*ology
nucle-	*nucleus* [L.] (from *nux, nucis* nut) kernel. Cf. kary-. *nucle*ide
nutri-	*nutrio* [L.] nourish. mal*nutri*tion
ob-	*ob* [L.] (*b* changes to *c* before words beginning with that consonant) against, toward, etc. *ob*tuse
oc-	See ob-. *oc*clude
ocul-	*oculus* [L.] eye. Cf. ophthalm-. *ocul*omotor
-od¹	See -ode¹. peri*od*ic
-ode¹	*hodos* [Gr.] road, path. cath*ode*. (See also hod-)
-ode²	See -oid. nemat*ode*
odont-	*odous, odontos* [Gr.] tooth. Cf. dent-. orth*odont*ia
-odyn-	*odynē* [Gr.] pain, distress. gastro*dyn*ia
-oid	*eidos* [Gr.] form. Cf. -form. hy*oid*
-ol	See ole-. cholester*ol*
ole-	*oleum* [L.] oil. *ole*oresin
olig-	*oligos* [Gr.] few, small. *olig*ospermia
omphal-	*omphalos* [Gr.] navel. peri*omphal*ic
onc-	*onkos* [Gr.] bulk, mass. hemat*onc*ometry
onych-	*onyx, onychos* [Gr.] claw, nail. an*onych*ia
oo-	*ōon* [Gr.] egg. Cf. ov-. peri*oo*thecitis
op-	*horaō, op-* [Gr.] see. erythr*op*sia
ophthalm-	*ophthalmos* [Gr.] eye. Cf. ocul-. ex*ophthalm*ic
or-	*os, oris* [L.] mouth. Cf. stom(at)-. intra*or*al
orb-	*orbis* [L.] circle. sub*orb*ital
orchi-	*orchis* [Gr.] testicle. Cf. test-. *orchi*opathy
organ-	*organon* [Gr.] implement, instrument. *organ*oleptic
orth-	*orthos* [Gr.] straight, right, normal. *orth*opedics
oss-	*os, ossis* [L.] bone. Cf. ost(e)-. *oss*iphone
ost(e)-	*osteon* [Gr.] bone. Cf. oss-. en*osto*sis, *oste*anaphysis
ot-	*ous, ōtos* [Gr.] ear. Cf. aur-. par*ot*id
ov-	*ovum* [L.] egg. Cf. oo-. syn*ov*ia
oxy-	*oxys* [Gr.] sharp. *oxy*cephalic
pachy(n)-	*pachynō* [Gr.] thicken. *pachy*derma, myo*pachyn*sis
pag-	*pēgnymi, pag-* [Gr.] fix, make fast. thoraco*pag*us
par-¹	*pario* [L.] bear, give birth to. primi*par*ous
par-²	See para-. *par*epigastric
para-	*para* [Gr.] (final *a* is dropped before words beginning with a vowel) beside, beyond. *para*mastoid
part-	*pario, partus* [L.] bear, give birth to. *part*urition
path-	*pathos* [Gr.] that which one undergoes, sickness. psycho*path*ic
pec-	*pēgnymi, pēg-* [Gr.] (*pēk-* before *t*) fix, make fast. sym*pec*tothiene. (See also pex-)
ped-	*pais, paidos* [Gr.] child. ortho*ped*ic
pell-	*pellis* [L.] skin, hide. *pell*agra
-pellent	*pello, pellentis, pulsus* [L.] drive. re*pellent*
pen-	*penomai* [Gr.] need, lack. erythrocyto*pen*ia
pend-	*pendeo* [L.] hang down. ap*pend*ix
pent(a)-	*pente* [Gr.] five. Cf. quinque-. *pent*ose, *penta*ploid
peps-	*peptō, peps-* [Gr.] digest. brady*peps*ia
pept-	*peptō* [Gr.] digest. dys*pept*ic
per-	*per* [L.] through. Cf. dia-. *per*nasal
peri-	*peri* [Gr.] around. Cf. circum-. *peri*phery
pet-	*peto* [L.] seek, tend toward. centri*pet*al
pex-	*pēgnumi, pēg-* [Gr.] (added to *s* becomes *pēx*) fix, make fast. hepato*pex*y
pha-	*phēmi, pha-* [Gr.] say, speak. dys*pha*sia
phac-	*phakos* [Gr.] lentil, lens. Cf. lent-. *phac*osclerosis. (Also spelled phak-)
phag-	*phagein* [Gr.] eat. lipo*phag*ic
phak-	See phac-. *phak*itis
phan-	See phen-. dia*phan*oscopy
pharmac-	*pharmakon* [Gr.] drug. *pharmac*ognosy
pharyng-	*pharynx, pharyng-* [Gr.] throat. glosso*pharyng*eal
phen-	*phainō, phan-* [Gr.] show, be seen. phos*phen*e
pher-	*pherō, phor-* [Gr.] bear, support. peri*pher*y
phil-	*phileō* [Gr.] like, have affinity for. eosino*phil*ia
phleb-	*phleps, phlebos* [Gr.] vein. peri*phleb*itis
phleg-	*phlogō, phlog-* [Gr.] burn, inflame. adeno*phleg*mon
phlog-	See phleg-. anti*phlog*istic

phob-　　　　*phobos* [Gr.] fear, dread. claustro*phob*ia

phon-　　　*phōne* [Gr.] sound. echo*phon*y

phor-　　　See pher-. Cf. -ferent. exo*phor*ia

phos-　　　See phot-. *phos*phorus

phot-　　　*phōs, phōtos* [Gr.] light. *phot*erythrous

phrag-　　*phrassō, phrag-* [Gr.] fence, wall off, stop up. Cf. sept-[1]. dia*phrag*m

phrax-　　*phrassō, phrag-* [Gr.] (added to *s* becomes *phrax-*) fence, wall off, stop up. em*phrax*is

phren-　　*phrēn* [Gr.] mind, midriff. Cf. ment-. meta*phren*ia, meta*phren*on

phthi-　　*phthinō* [Gr.] decay, waste away. *phthi*sis

phy-　　　　*phyō* [Gr.] beget, bring forth, produce, be by nature. noso*phy*te

phyl-　　　*phylon* [Gr.] tribe, kind. *phyl*ogeny

-phyll　　*phyllon* [Gr.] leaf. xantho*phyll*

phylac-　*phylax* [Gr.] guard. pro*phylac*tic

phys(a)-　*physaō* [Gr.] blow, inflate. *phys*ocele, *phys*alis

physe-　　*physaō, physē-* [Gr.] blow, inflate. em*physe*ma

pil-　　　　*pilus* [L.] hair. e*pil*ation

pituit-　　*pituita* [L.] phlegm, rheum. *pituit*ous

placent-　*placenta* [L.] (from *plakous* [Gr.]) cake. extra*placent*al

plas-　　　*plassō* [Gr.] mold, shape. cine*plas*ty

platy-　　*platys* [Gr.] broad, flat. *platy*rrhine

pleg-　　　*plēssō* [Gr.] strike. di*pleg*ia

plet-　　　*pleo, -pletus* [L.] fill. de*plet*ion

pleur-　　*pleura* [Gr.] rib, side. Cf. cost-. peri*pleur*al

plex-　　　*plēssō, plēg-* (added to *s* becomes *plēx-*) strike. apo*plex*y

plic-　　　*plico* [L.] fold. compli*plic*ation

pne-　　　*pneuma, pneumatos* [Gr.] breathing. traumato*pne*a

pneum(at)-　*pneuma, pneumatos* [Gr.] breath, air. *pneum*odynamics, *pneuma*tothorax

pneumo(n)-　*pneumōn* [Gr.] lung. Cf. pulmo(n)-. *pneumo*centesis, *pneumo*notomy

pod-　　　*pous, podos* [Gr.] foot. *pod*iatry

poie-　　　*poieō* [Gr.] make, produce. Cf. -facient. sarco*poie*tic

pol-　　　　*polos* [Gr.] axis of a sphere. peri*pol*ar

poly-　　　*polys* [Gr.] much, many. *poly*spermia

pont-　　　*pons, pontis* [L.] bridge. *pont*ocerebellar

por-[1]　　*poros* [Gr.] passage. myelo*por*e

por-[2]　　*pōros* [Gr.] callus. *por*ocele

posit-　　*pono, positus* [L.] put, place. re*posit*or

post-　　　*post* [L.] after, behind in time or place. *post*natal, *post*oral

pre-　　　*prae* [L.] before in time or place. *pre*natal, *pre*vesical

press-　　*premo, pressus* [L.] press. *press*oreceptive

pro-　　　*pro* [Gr.] or *pro* [L.] before in time or place. *pro*gamous, *pro*cheilon, *pro*lapse

proct-　　*prōktos* [Gr.] anus. entero*proct*ia

prosop-　*prosōpon* [Gr.] face. Cf. faci-. di*pro*sopus

pseud-　　*pseudēs* [Gr.] false. *pseud*oparaplegia

psych-　　*psychē* [Gr.] soul, mind. Cf. ment-. *psych*osomatic

pto-　　　　*piptō, ptō* [Gr.] fall. nephro*pto*sis

pub-　　　*pubes* and *puber, puberis* [L.] adult. ischio*pub*ic. (See also puber-)

puber-　　*puber* [L.] adult. *puber*ty

pulmo(n)-　*pulmo, pulmonis* [L.] lung. Cf. pneumo(n)-. *pulmo*lith, cardio*pulmon*ary

puls-　　　*pello, pellentis, pulsus* [L.] drive, pro*puls*ion

punct-　　*pungo, punctus* [L.] prick, pierce. Cf. cente-. *punct*iform

pur-　　　　*pus, puris* [L.] pus. Cf. py-. sup*pur*ation

py-　　　　*pyon* [Gr.] pus. Cf. pur-. nephro*py*osis

pyel-　　　*pyelos* [Gr.] trough, basin, pelvis. nephro*pyel*itis

pyl-　　　　*pylē* [Gr.] door, orifice. *pyl*ephlebitis

pyr-　　　　*pyr* [Gr.] fire. Cf. febr-. galacto*pyr*a

quadr-　　*quadr-* [L.] four. Cf. tetra-. *quadr*igeminal

quinque-　*quinque* [L.] five. Cf. pent(a)-. *quinque*cuspid

rachi-　　*rachis* [Gr.] spine. Cf. spin-. encephalo*rachi*dian

radi-　　　*radius* [L.] ray. Cf. actin-. ir*radi*ation

re-　　　　*re-* [L.] back, again. *re*traction

ren-　　　*renes* [L.] kidneys. Cf. nephr-. ad*ren*al

ret-　　　*rete* [L.] net. *ret*othelium

retro-　　*retro* [L.] backwards. *retro*deviation

rhag-　　*rhēgnymi, rhag-* [Gr.] break, burst. hemor*rhag*ic

rhaph-　*rhaphē* [Gr.] suture. gastror*rhaph*y

rhe-　　　*rhaphē* [Gr.] flow. Cf. flu-. diar*rhe*al

rhex-　　*rhēgnymi, rhēg-* [Gr.] (added to *s* becomes *rhēx*) break, -burst. metror*rhex*is

rhin-　　*rhis, rhinos* [Gr.] nose. Cf. nas-. basi*rhin*al

rot-　　　*rota* [L.] wheel. *rot*ator

rub(r)-　*ruber, rubri* [L.] red. Cf. erythr-. bili*rub*in, *rub*rospinal

salping-　*salpinx, salpingos* [Gr.] tube, trumpet. *salping*itis

sanguin-　*sanguis, sanguinis* [L.] blood. Cf. hem(at)-. *sanguin*eous

sarc-　　*sarx, sarkos* [Gr.] flesh. *sarc*oma

schis-　*schizō, schid-* [Gr.] (before *t* or added to *s* becomes *schis-*) split. Cf. fiss-. *schis*torachis, rachi*schis*is

scler-　*sklēros* [Gr.] hard. Cf. dur-. *scler*osis

scop-　　*skopeō* [Gr.] look at, observe. endo*scop*e

sect-　　*seco, sectus* [L.] cut. Cf. tom-. *sect*ile

semi-　　*semi* [L.] half. Cf. hemi-. *semi*flexion

sens-   *sentio, sensus* [L.] perceive, feel. Cf. esthe-. *sens*ory

sep-   *sepō* [Gr.] rot, decay. *seps*is

sept-[1]   *saepio, saeptus* [L.] fence, wall off, stop up. Cf. phrag-. naso*sept*al

sept-[2]   *septem* [L.] seven. Cf. hept(a)-. *sept*an

ser-   *serum* [L.] whey, watery substance, *ser*osynovitis

sex-   *sex* [L.] six. Cf. hex-[1]. *sex*digitate

sial-   *sialon* [Gr.] saliva. poly*sial*ia

sin-   *sinus* [L.] hallow, fold. Cf. colp-. *sin*obronchitis

sit-   *sitos* [Gr.] food. para*sit*ic

solut-   *solvo, solventis, solutus* [L.] loose, dissolve, set free. Cf. ly-. dis*solut*ion

-solvent   See solut-. dis*solvent*

somat-   *sōma, somatos* [Gr.] body. Cf. corpor-. psycho*somat*ic

-some   See somat-. dictyo*some*

spas-   *spaō, spas-* [Gr.] draw, pull. *spas*m, *spas*tic

spectr-   *spectrum* [L.] -appearance, what is seen. micro*spectr*oscope

sperm(at)-   *sperma, spermatos* [Gr.] seed. *sperm*acrasia, *spermat*ozoon

spers-   *spargo, -spersus* [L.] scatter. dis*pers*ion

sphen-   *sphēn* [Gr.] wedge. Cf. cune-. *sphen*oid

spher-   *sphaira* [Gr.] ball. hemi*spher*e

sphygm-   *sphygmos* [Gr.] pulsation. *sphygm*omanometer

spin-   *spina* [L.] spine. Cf. rachi-. cerebro*spin*al

spirat-   *spiro, spiratus* [L.] breathe. in*spirat*ory

splanchn-   *splanchna* [Gr.] entrails, viscera. neuro*splanchn*ic

splen-   *splēn* [Gr.] spleen. Cf. lien-. *splen*omegaly

spor-   *sporos* [Gr.] seed. *spor*ophyte, zygo*spor*e

squam-   *squama* [L.] scale. de*squam*ation

sta-   *histēmi, sta-* [Gr.] make stand, stop. genesi*stas*is

stal-   *stellō, stal-* [Gr.] send. peri*stal*sis. (See also stol-)

staphyl-   *staphylē* [Gr.] bunch of grapes, uvula. *staphyl*ococcus, *staphyl*ectomy

stear-   *stear, steatos* [Gr.] fat. Cf. adip-. *stear*odermia

steat-   See stear-. *steat*opygous

sten-   *stenos* [Gr.] narrow, compressed. *sten*ocardia

ster-   *stereos* [Gr.] solid. chole*ster*ol

sterc-   *stercus* [L.] dung. Cf. copr-. *ster*coporphyrin

sthen-   *sthenos* [Gr.] strength. a*sthen*ia

stol-   *stellō, stol-* [Gr.] send. dia*stol*e

stom(at)-   *stoma, stomatos* [Gr.] mouth, orifice. Cf. or-. ana*stom*osis, *stomat*ogastric

strep(h)-   *strephō, strep-* (before *t*) [Gr.] twist. Cf. tors-. *strep*hosymbolia, *strep*tomycin. (See also stroph-)

strict-   *stringo, stringentis, strictus* [L.] draw tight, compress, cause pain. con*strict*ion

-stringent   See strict-. a*stringent*

stroph-   *strephō, stroph-* [Gr.] twist. ana*stroph*ic. (See also strep(h)-)

struct-   *struo, structus* [L.] pile up (against). ob*struct*ion

sub-   *sub* [L.] (*b* changes to *f* or *p* before words beginning with those consonants) under, below. Cf. hypo-. *sub*lumbar

suf-   See sub-. *suf*fusion

sup-   See sub-. *sup*pository

super-   *super* [L.] above, beyond, extreme. Cf. hyper-. *super*motility

sy-   See syn-. *sy*stole

syl-   See syn-. *syl*lepsiology

sym-   See syn-. *sym*biosis, *sym*metry, *sym*pathetic, *sym*physis

syn-   *syn* [Gr.] (*n* disappears before *s*, changes to *l* before *l*, and changes to *m* before *b, m, p,* and *ph*) with, together. Cf. con-. myo*syn*izesis

ta-   See ton-. *ta*ectasis

tac-   *tassō, tag-* [Gr.] (*tak-* before *t*) order, arrange. a*tac*tic

tact-   *tango, tactus* [L.] touch. con*tact*

tax-   *tassō, tag-* [Gr.] (added to *s* becomes *tax-*) order, arrange. a*tax*ia

tect-   See teg-. *tect*protective

teg-   *tego, tectus* [L.] cover. in*teg*ument

tel-   *telos* [Gr.] end. *tel*osynapsis

tele-   *tēle* [Gr.] at a distance. *tele*ceptor

tempor-   *tempus, temporis* [L.] time, timely or fatal spot, temple. *tempor*omalar

ten(ont)-   *tenōn, tenontos* [Gr.] (from *teinō* stretch) tight stretched band. *ten*odynia, *ten*onitis, *tenont*agra

tens-   *tendo, tensus* [L.] stretch. Cf. ton-. ex*tens*or

test-   *testis* [L.] testicle. Cf. orchi-. *test*itis

tetra-   *tetra-* [Gr.] four. Cf. quadr-. *tetra*genous

the-   *tithēmi, thē-* [Gr.] put, place. syn*the*sis

thec-   *thēkē* [Gr.] repository, case. *thec*ostegnosis

thel-   *thēlē* [Gr.] teat, nipple. *thel*erethism

therap-   *therapeia* [Gr.] treatment. hydro*therap*y

therm-   *thermē* [Gr.] heat. Cf. calor-. dia*therm*y

thi-   *theion* [Gr.] sulfur. *thi*ogenic

thorac-   *thōrax, thōrakos* [Gr.] chest. *thorac*oplasty

thromb-   *thrombos* [Gr.] lump, clot. *thromb*openia

thym-   *thymos* [Gr.] spirit. Cf. ment-. dys*thym*ia

thyr-   *thyreos* [Gr.] shield (shaped like a door *thyra*). *thyr*oid

tme-   *temnō, tmē-* [Gr.] cut. axono*tme*sis

toc-   *tokos* [Gr.] childbirth, dys*toc*ia

tom-   *temnō, tom-* [Gr.] cut. Cf. sect-. ap*pendec*tomy

ton-   *teino, ton-* [Gr.] stretch, put under tension. Cf. *tens-*. peri*ton*eum

top-   *topos* [Gr.] place. Cf. *loc-*. *topes*thesia

tors-   *torqueo, torsus* [L.] twist. Cf. *strep-*. ec*tors*ion

tox-   *toxicon* [Gr.] (from *toxon* bow) arrow poison, poison. *tox*emia

trache-   *tracheia* [Gr.] windpipe. *tracheot*omy

trachel-   *trachēlos* [Gr.] neck. Cf. *cervic-*. *trachel*opexy

tract-   *traho, tractus* [L.] draw, drag. pro*tract*ion

traumat-   *trauma, traumatos* [Gr.] wound. *traumat*ic

tri-   *treis, tria* [Gr.] or *tri-* [L.] three. *tri*gonid

trich-   *thrix, trichos* [Gr.] hair. *trich*oid

trip-   *tribō* [Gr.] rub. en*trip*sis

trop-   *trepō, trop-* [Gr.] turn, react. sito*trop*ism

troph-   *trepō, troph-* [Gr.] nurture. a*troph*y

tuber-   *tuber* [L.] swelling, node. *tuber*cle

typ-   *typos* [Gr.] (from *typto* strike) type. a*typ*ical

typh-   *typhos* [Gr.] fog, stupor. adeno*typh*us

typhl-   *typhlos* [Gr.] blind. Cf. *cec-*. *typhl*ectasis

un-   *unus* [L.] one. Cf. *hen-*. *uni*oval

ur-   *ouron* [Gr.] urine. poly*ur*ia

vacc-   *vacca* [L.] cow. *vacc*ine

vagin-   *vagina* [L.] sheath. in*vagin*ated

vas-   *vas* [L.] vessel. Cf. *angi-*. *vas*cular

vers-   See *vert-*. in*vers*ion

vert-   *verto, versus* [L.] turn. di*vert*iculum

vesic-   *vesica* [L.] bladder. Cf. *cyst-*. *vesic*ovaginal

vit-   *vita* [L.] life. Cf. *bi-*[1]. de*vit*alize

vuls-   *vello, vulsus* [L.] pull, twitch. con*vuls*ion

xanth-   *xanthos* [Gr.] yellow, blond. Cf. *flav-* and *lute-*. *xanth*ophyll

-yl-   *hyte* [Gr.] substance. cacod*yl*

zo-   *zoē* [Gr.] life, *zōon* [Gr.] animal. mi*cro*zoaria

zyg-   *zygon* [Gr.] yoke, union. *zyg*odactyly

zym-   *zymē* [Gr.] ferment, enzyme

DORLAND'S ILLUSTRATED

MEDICAL DICTIONARY

Å symbol for *Angström unit* or *angstrom*.

A symbol for *adenine* or *adenosine* (in nucleotides and nucleic acids), *ampere*, or *amplitude of accommodation*, as a subscript, symbol for *alveolar gas*.

A symbol for *absorbance, activity* (radioactivity), *area,* or *mass number*.

A₂ aortic second sound.

a symbol for *atto-;* as a subscript, symbol for *arterial blood.*

a. Abbreviation for L. aqua and arteria.

a symbol for *specific absorptivity, acceleration,* or *activity* (thermodynamic activity of a chemical species).

a- 1. [Gr.] an inseparable prefix denoting want or absence; appears as *an-*before stems beginning with a vowel or with *h.* 2. [L.] a prefix denoting separation, or away from.

α a prefix designating (1) an anomer of a carbohydrate, e.g., α-D-glucose; (2) a plasma protein migrating with the α band (subdivided into the α, and α 2 bands) in protein electrophoresis, e.g., α-fetoprotein; (3) a substituent group of a steroid that projects below the plane of the ring, e.g., 3 α-hydroxy-5α-androstan-17-one (androsterone); (4) the carbon atom next to the principal functional group, e.g., α-amino acid, succeeding letters, β, γ, δ, etc., being used to designate succeeding carbon atoms in the chain; and (5) one of a group of related compounds having the same trivial name, e.g., -tocopherol.

A.A. achievement age; Alcoholics Anonymous.

AA amino acid; aminoacyl.

aa. abbreviation for L. *arteriae,* arteries.

ĀĀ, āā [Gr. *ana* of each] an abbreviation used in prescription writing, following the names of two or more ingredients and signifying "of each"; also written *ana.*

A.A.A. American Association of Anatomists.

A.A.A.S. American Association for the Advancement of Science.

A.A.B.B. American Association of Blood Banks.

A.A.C.P. American Academy of Child Psychiatry.

A.A.D. American Academy of Dermatology.

A.A.D.P. American Academy of Denture Prosthetics.

A.A.D.R. American Academy of Dental Radiology.

A.A.D.S. American Association of Dental Schools.

A.A.E. American Association of Endodontists.

A.A.F.P. American Academy of Family Physicians.

A.A.I. American Association of Immunologists.

A.A.I.D. American Academy of Implant Dentistry.

A.A.I.N. American Association of Industrial Nurses.

A.A.M.A. American Association of Medical Assistants.

A.A.M.C. American Association of Medical Colleges.

A.A.M.D. American Association on Mental Deficiency.

A.A.N. American Academy of Neurology.

A.A.O. American Association of Orthodontists; American Academy of Ophthalmology; American Academy of Otolaryngology.

A.A.O.P. American Academy of Oral Pathology.

A.A.O.S. American Academy of Orthopaedic Surgeons.

A.A.P. American Academy of Pediatrics; American Academy of Pedodontics; American Academy of Periodontology; American Association of Pathologists.

A.A.P.A. American Academy of Physician Assistants.

A.A.P.B. American Association of Pathologists and Bacteriologists.

A.A.P.M.R. American Academy of Physical Medicine and Rehabilitation.

Aarane (ār'ān) trademark for a preparation of cromolyn sodium.

Aaron's sign (ār'onz) [Charles Dettie *Aaron,* American physician, 1866–1951] see under *sign.*

Aarskog syndrome (ars'kog) [D. *Aarskog*] see under *syndrome.*

Aarskog-Scott syndrome (ars'kog-skot) [D. *Aarskog;* C. I. *Scott,* Jr.] Aarskog syndrome.

Aase syndrome (ahz) [J. M. *Aase*] see under *syndrome.*

aasmus (a-as'mus) [Gr. *aasmos* breathing] (*obs.*) asthma.

AAV adeno-associated virus.

A.B. abbreviation for L. *Artium Baccalaureus,* Bachelor of Arts.

Ab abbreviation for antibody.

ab Latin preposition meaning from.

ab- [L. *ab* from] prefix meaning *away from, from*

abacterial (a″bak-te′re-al) free from bacteria.

Abadie's sign (ah-bah-dēz′) [1. Charles *Abadie,* ophthalmologist in Paris, 1842–1932. 2. Jean *Abadie,* Bordeaux neurologist, 1873–1946] see under *sign.*

abaissement (ah-bās-mawn′) [Fr.] 1. a lowering or a depressing. 2. couching.

abaptiston (ah″bap-tis′ton), pl. *abaptis′ta* [a neg. + Gr. *baptein* to dip] a trephine so shaped that it will not penetrate the brain.

abarognosis (a″bar-og-no′sis) [a neg. + Gr. *baros* weight + *gnōsis* knowledge] loss of weight sense; baragnosis.

abarthrosis (ab″ar-thro′sis) [*ab-* + L. *arthrosis*] diarthrosis.

abarticular (ab″ar-tik′u-lar) 1. not affecting a joint. 2. remote from a joint.

abarticulation (ab″ar-tik″u-la′shun) [*ab-* + L. *articulatio* joint] 1. a dislocation of a joint. 2. junctura synovialis.

abasia (ah-ba′zhe-ah) [a neg. + Gr. *basis* step + *-ia*] inability to walk. **a. asta′sia,** astasia-abasia. **a. atac′tica,** abasia characterized by uncertainty of movement, due to a defect of coordination. **choreic a.,** a form due to chorea of the legs. **paralytic a.,** a form due to paralysis of the leg muscles. **paroxysmal trepidant a.,** astasia-abasia caused by spastic stiffening of the legs on attempting to stand; called also *spastic a.* **spastic a.,** paroxysmal trepidant a. **trembling a., a. trep′idans,** abasia due to trembling of the legs.

abasic (ah-ba′sik) pertaining to abasia.

abate (ah-bāt′) to lessen or decrease.

abatement (ah-bāt′ment) a decrease in the severity of a pain or a symptom.

abatic (ah-bat′ik) abasic.

abbau (ahp′bow) [Ger. "decomposition," "breakdown"] 1. exergonic breakdown of chemical substances. 2. decomposition of chemical substances. 3. catabolic products.

Abbé's condenser (ah-bāz′) [Ernst Karl *Abbé,* German physicist, 1840–1905] see under *condenser.*

Abbé's flap, operation (ab′ēz) [Robert *Abbe,* New York surgeon, 1851–1928] see under *flap* and *operation.*

Abbé-Zeiss counting cell, counting chamber [E. K.

Abbé; Carl *Zeiss,* German optician, 1816–1888] see *Thom-a-Zeiss counting chamber,* under *chamber.*

Abbocillin-DC (ab″bo-sil′lin) trademark for preparations of penicillin G procaine.

Abbott's method (ab′ots) [Edville Gerhardt *Abbott,* surgeon in Portland, Maine, 1870–1938] see under *method.*

Abbott-Miller tube (ab′ot-mil′er) [William Osler *Abbott,* American physician, 1902–1943; T. Grier *Miller,* Philadelphia physician, 1886–1981] see *Miller-Abbott tube,* under *tube.*

Abbott-Rawson tube (ab′ot-raw′son) [William Osler *Abbott;* Arthur J. *Rawson,* American medical physicist] see under *tube.*

ABC aspiration biopsy cytology.

ABCD a regimen of Adriamycin (doxorubicin), bleomycin, CCNU (lomustine), and dacarbazine, used in cancer chemotherapy.

abdomen (ab-do′men) [L., possibly from *abdere* to hide] that portion of the body which lies between the thorax and the pelvis; called also *belly* and *venter.* It contains a cavity (*abdominal cavity*) separated by the diaphragm from the thoracic cavity, above and by the plane of the pelvic inlet from the pelvic cavity below, and lined with a serous membrane, the peritoneum. This cavity contains the abdominal viscera (see Plate accompanying *viscera*) and is enclosed by a wall (*abdominal wall* or *parietes*) formed by the abdominal muscles, vertebral column, and the ilia. It is divided into nine regions by four imaginary lines projected onto the anterior wall, of which two pass horizontally around the body (the upper at the level of the cartilages of the ninth ribs, the lower at the tops of the crests of the ilia), and two extend vertically on each side of the body from the cartilage of the eighth rib to the center of the inguinal ligament, as in A below. The regions are: three upper—right hypochondriac, epigastric, left hypochondriac; three middle—right lateral, umbilical, left lateral; and three lower—right inguinal, pubic, left inguinal. **acute a.,** an abdominal condition of

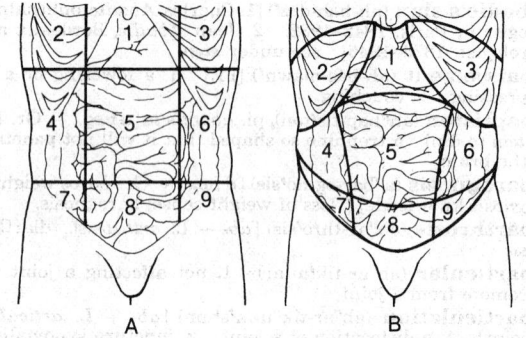

Regions of abdomen bounded according to (A) the standard and (B) a variant system: 1, epigastric; 2, right hypochondriac; 3, left hypochondriac; 4, right lateral (or lumbar); 5, umbilical; 6, left lateral (or lumbar); 7, right inguinal (or iliac); 8, pubic (hypogastric); 9, left inguinal (or iliac).

abrupt onset usually associated with abdominal pain due to inflammation, perforation, obstruction, infarction, or rupture of intra-abdominal organs. Emergency surgical intervention is usually required. Examples are acute cholecystitis or appendicitis, perforated peptic ulcer, strangulated hernia, superior mesenteric artery thrombosis, and splenic rupture. Called also *surgical a.* **boat-shaped a.,** scaphoid a. **carinate a.,** scaphoid a. **navicular a.,** scaphoid a. **a. obsti′pum,** congenital shortness of the rectus abdominis muscle. **pendulous a.,** a relaxed condition of the abdominal wall, so that the anterior abdominal wall hangs over the pubis; called also *venter propendens.* **scaphoid a.,** an abdomen whose anterior wall is hollowed out; seen in children with cerebral disease. Called also *boat-shaped a., carinate a.,* and *navicular a.* **surgical a.,** acute a.

abdominal (ab-dom′ĭ-nal) [L. *abdominalis*] pertaining to the abdomen.

abdomin(o)- [L. *abdomen,* q.v.] a combining form denoting relationship to the abdomen.

abdominoanterior (ab-dom″ĭ-no-an-te′re-or) (*obs.*) with the abdomen forward (denoting a position of the fetus in utero).

abdominocentesis (ab-dom″ĭ-no-sen-te′sis) [*abdomino-* + Gr. *kentēsis* puncture] paracentesis.

abdominocystic (ab-dom″ĭ-no-sis′tik) pertaining to the abdomen and gallbladder.

abdominogenital (ab-dom″ĭ-no-jen′ĭ-tal) pertaining to the abdomen and the reproductive organs.

abdominohysterectomy (ab-dom″ĭ-no-his″ter-ek′to-me) hysterectomy performed through an abdominal incision.

abdominohysterotomy (ab-dom″ĭ-no-his″ter-ot′o-me) hysterotomy performed through an abdominal incision; called also *abdominouterotomy.*

abdominoposterior (ab-dom″ĭ-no-pos-te′re-or) (*obs.*) having the abdomen turned backward (denoting a position of the fetus in utero).

abdominoscopy (ab-dom″ĭ-nos′ko-pe) [*abdomino-* + Gr. *skopein* to inspect] inspection or examination of the abdominal cavity, particularly direct examination of the abdominal organs by endoscopy; peritoneoscopy; laparoscopy.

abdominoscrotal (ab-dom″ĭ-no-skro′tal) pertaining to the abdomen and scrotum.

abdominothoracic (ab-dom″ĭ-no-tho-ras′ik) pertaining to the abdomen and thorax.

abdominouterotomy (ab-dom″ĭ-no-u″ter-ot′o-me) abdominohysterotomy.

abdominovaginal (ab-dom″ĭ-no-vaj′ĭ-nal) pertaining to the abdomen and the vagina.

abdominovesical (ab-dom″ĭ-no-ves′ĭ-k'l) pertaining to the abdomen and urinary bladder.

abducens (ab-du′senz) [L. "drawing away"] Latin adjective used in names of structures (e.g., nervus abducens) which serve to abduct a part.

abducent (ab-du′sent) [L. *abducens*] abducting, or effecting a separation, as an abducent nerve.

abduct (ab-dukt′) [*ab-* + L. *ducere* to draw] to draw away from the median plane or (in the digits) from the axial line of a limb.

abduction (ab-duk′shun) the act of abducting or state of being abducted.

abductor (ab-duk′tor) [L.] that which abducts; see *Table of Musculi.*

Abegg's rule (ab′egz) [Richard *Abegg,* Polish chemist, 1869–1910] see under *rule.*

abembryonic (ab″em-bre-on′ik) [*ab-* + Gr. *embryon* embryo] away from the embryo.

abepithymia (ab″ep-ĭ-thi′me-ah) [*ab-* + Gr. *epithymia* desire] paralysis of the solar plexus.

abequose (ab′ĕ-kwōs) an unusual sugar found to be a polysaccharide somatic antigen of *Salmonella* species.

Abercrombie's degeneration (syndrome) (ab′er-krom″bēz) [John *Abercrombie,* Scottish physician, 1780–1844] see *amyloid degeneration,* under *degeneration.*

Abernethy's fascia, sarcoma (ab′er-ne″thēz) [John *Abernethy,* British surgeon and anatomist, 1764–1831] see *fascia iliaca,* under *fascia,* and see under *sarcoma.*

aberrant (ab-er′ant) [L. *aberrans, ab* from + *errare* to wander] wandering or deviating from the usual or normal course.

aberratio (ab″er-a′she-o) [L., from *aberrare* to wander away from] aberration. **a. tes′tis,** situation of the testis in a part distant from the path which it takes in normal descent.

aberration (ab″er-a′shun) [*ab-* + L. *errare* to wander] 1. deviation from the usual course or condition. 2. unequal refraction or focalization of light rays by a lens, resulting in degradation of the image they produce. **chromatic a.,** unequal deviation of light rays of different wavelengths passing through a refractive medium, resulting in fringes of color around the image produced; called also *newtonian a.* **chromatic a., lateral,** difference in magnification due to differences in position of the principal points for light of different wavelengths; also a difference of focal length. **chromatic a., longitudinal,** difference in position along the axis for the focal points of light, produced by unequal deviation of light rays of different wavelengths by a lens. **chromosome a.,** an irregularity in the number or structure of chromosomes that may alter the course of development of the embryo, usually in the form of a gain (duplication), loss (deletion), exchange (translocation), or alteration in sequence (inversion) of genetic material. See also *genetic disease,* under *disease.* **dioptric a.,** spherical a. **distantial a.,** a blurring of vision for distant objects. **lateral a.,** deviation of a ray from the focal point, measured on a line perpendicular to the axis at the focal point. **longitudinal a.,** deviation of a ray from the focal point, measured along the optic axis. **mental a.,** any pathological deviation from normal mental activity, usually limited to a circumscribed deviation in an otherwise adapted individual. **meridional a.,** unequal refraction of light rays as a result of variation of refractive power in different portions of the same meridian of a lens. **newtonian a.,** chromatic a. **penta-X chromosomal a.,** one in which there are five X chromosomes in a female. **spherical a.,** zonal aberration in relation to an axial point; see *spherical a., negative,* and *spherical a., positive.* Called also *dioptric a.* **spherical a., negative,** unequal refraction of light rays by a lens, the peripheral rays being focused farther from the lens than the paraxial rays. **spherical a., positive,** unequal refraction of light rays by a lens, the peripheral rays being focused closer to the lens than the paraxial rays. **tetra-X chromosomal a.,** one in which there are four X chromosomes in a female or tetra-X Y in the male. **triple-X chromosomal a.,** one in which there are three X chromosomes in a female or triple-X Y in the male. **zonal a.,** unequal refraction of light rays by a lens, the rays passing through different zones being focused at different distances from the lens.

aberrometer (ab″er-om′ĕ-ter) [*aberration* + Gr. *metron* measure] an instrument for measuring errors in delicate experiments or observations.

abetalipoproteinemia (a-ba″tah-lip″o-pro-te″in-e′me-ah) see *familial lipoprotein deficiency,* under *deficiency.*

abeyance (ah-ba′ans) a suspension of function or of action; a state of suspended activity.

ABG arterial blood gases.

abiatrophy (ah″bi-at′ro-fe) premature and endogenous loss of vitality or tissue substance. See also *abiotrophy.*

abient (ab′e-ent) avoiding the source of stimulation; said of a response to a stimulus. Cf. *adient.*

abiogenesis (ab″e-o-jen′ĕ-sis) [*a* neg. + Gr. *bios* life + Gr. *genesis* generation] the spontaneous generation of life; the origin of living things from things inanimate. Cf. *biogenesis.*

abiogenetic (ab″e-o-jĕ-net′ik) pertaining to or marked by spontaneous generation.

abiogenous (ab″e-oj′ĕ-nus) abiogenetic.

abiologic, abiological (ab″bi-o-loj′ik, a″bi-o-loj′e-k'l) (*obs.*) pertaining to abiology.

abiology (a″bi-ol′o-je) [*a* neg. + Gr. *bios* life + *-logy*] (*obs.*) the study of nonliving things; anorganology.

abionergy (ab″e-on′er-je) [*a* neg. + Gr. *bios* life + *ergon* work] abiotrophy.

abiophysiology (ab″e-o-fiz″e-ol′o-je) [*a* neg. + Gr. *bios* life + *physiology*] the study of inorganic processes in living organisms.

abiosis (ab″e-o′sis) [*a* neg. + Gr. *bios* life + *-osis*] 1. absence or deficiency of life. 2. abiotrophy.

abiotic (ab″e-ot′ik) pertaining to or characterized by absence of life; incapable of living; antagonistic to life.

abiotrophia (ab″e-o-tro′fe-ah) abiotrophy.

abiotrophic (ab″e-o-trof′ik) pertaining to or characterized by abiotrophy.

abiotrophy (ab″e-ot′ro-fe) [*a* neg. + Gr. *bios* life + *trophē* nutrition] progressive loss of vitality of certain tissues or organs leading to disorders or loss of function; applied especially to degenerative hereditary diseases of late onset, e.g., Huntington's chorea. **retinal a.,** a general term for a group of degenerative diseases of the retina, such as retinitis pigmentosa and amaurotic familial idiocy.

abirritant (ab-ir′rĭ-tant) [*ab-* + L. *irritans* irritating] 1. diminishing or relieving irritation; soothing. 2. an agent that relieves irritation.

abirritation (ab″ir-rĭ-ta′shun) 1. diminished responsiveness to stimulation. 2. atony.

abirritative (ab-ir′rĭ-ta″tiv) reducing irritability; soothing.

abiuret (ah-bi′u-ret) [*a* neg. + *biuret*] not giving a positive reaction to the biuret test.

abiuretic (ah-bi″u-ret′ik) not responsive to the biuret test.

ablactation (ab″lak-ta′shun) [L. *ablactatio,* from *ab* from + *lactare* to give milk] the weaning of a child or the cessation of milk secretion.

ablastemic (a-blas-tem′ik) [*a* neg. + Gr. *blastēma* a shoot] not concerned with germination.

ablastin (ah-blas′tin) an antibody, produced by rats infected with trypanosomes, that inhibits reproduction of trypanosomes; it has no other known function and is neither a lysin nor an opsonin.

ablate (ab-lāt′) [L. *ablatus* removed] to remove, especially by cutting; to extirpate.

ablatio (ab-la′she-o) [L.] ablation. **a. placen′tae,** premature detachment of a placenta. **a. re′tinae** detachment of the retina.

ablation (ab-la′shun) [L. *ablatio*] 1. separation or detachment; extirpation; eradication. 2. removal of a part, especially by cutting.

ablepharia (ah″blef-a′re-ah) cryptophthalmos.

ablepharon (ah-blef′ah-ron) ablepharia.

ablepharous (ah-blef′ah-rus) pertaining to ablepharia.

ablephary (ah-blef′ah-re) ablepharia.

ablepsia (ah-blep′se-ah) [*a* neg. + Gr. *blepsis* sight + *-ia*] lack or loss of sight; blindness.

ablepsy (ah-blep′se) ablepsia.

abluent (ab′lu-ent) [*ab-* + L. *luens* washing] 1. detergent. 2. a cleansing agent.

abluminal (ab-loo′mĭ-nal) directed away from the lumen of a tubular structure.

ablution (ab-lu′shun) [L. *ablutio* a washing] the act of washing or cleansing; the application of water by the hand, which may be covered with a bath mitt or towel.

ablutomania (ab-lu″to-ma′ne-ah) [L. *ablutio* a washing + *mania*] obsessional preoccupation with cleanliness, washing, or bathing, often accompanied by compulsive rituals, a common symptom in obsessive-compulsive disorder.

abmortal (ab-mor′tal) situated or directed away from a dead or injured part; applied especially to electric currents set up in injured tissue.

abnormal (ab-nor′mal) [*ab-* + L. *norma* rule] not normal; contrary to the usual structure, position, condition, behavior, or rule.

abnormality (ab″nor-mal′ĭ-te) 1. the quality or fact of being abnormal. 2. a malformation or deformity; see also *abnormity* and *anomaly.* **potential a. of glucose tolerance (pot AGT),** a statistical classification containing individuals who have a statistical risk of developing diabetes mellitus, e.g., identical twins of non-insulin-dependent diabetics. **previous a. of glucose tolerance (prev AGT),** a statistical classification containing individuals once diagnosed as having diabetes mellitus (DM), gestational diabetes (GDM), or impaired glucose tolerance (IGT), who now have normal glucose tolerance.

abnormity (ab-nor′mĭ-te) 1. abnormality; deformity. 2. monstrosity.

abomasitis (ab″o-mah-si′tis) inflammation of the abomasum.

abomasum (ab″o-ma′sum) [*ab-* + L. *omasum* paunch] the fourth stomach of a ruminant animal.

aborad (ab-o′rad) directed away from the mouth.

aboral (ab-o′ral) opposite to, away from, or remote from the mouth.

aboriginal (ab-ŏ-rij′ĭ-nal) native to the place inhabited.

abort (ah-bort′) [L. *aboriri* to miscarry] 1. to check the usual course of a disease. 2. to miscarry before the fetus is viable. 3. an abortion. 4. to become checked in development.

aborticide (ah-bor′tĭ-sīd) [L. *aboriri* to miscarry + *caedere* to kill] abortifacient.

abortient (ah-bor′shent) abortifacient.

abortifacient (ah-bor″tĭ-fa′shent) [L. *abortio* abortion + *facere* to make] 1. causing abortion. 2. an agent which causes abortion; called also *abortient* and *aborticide.*

abortin (ah-bor′tin) a preparation of *Brucella abortus* antigens formerly used in skin testing for brucellosis.

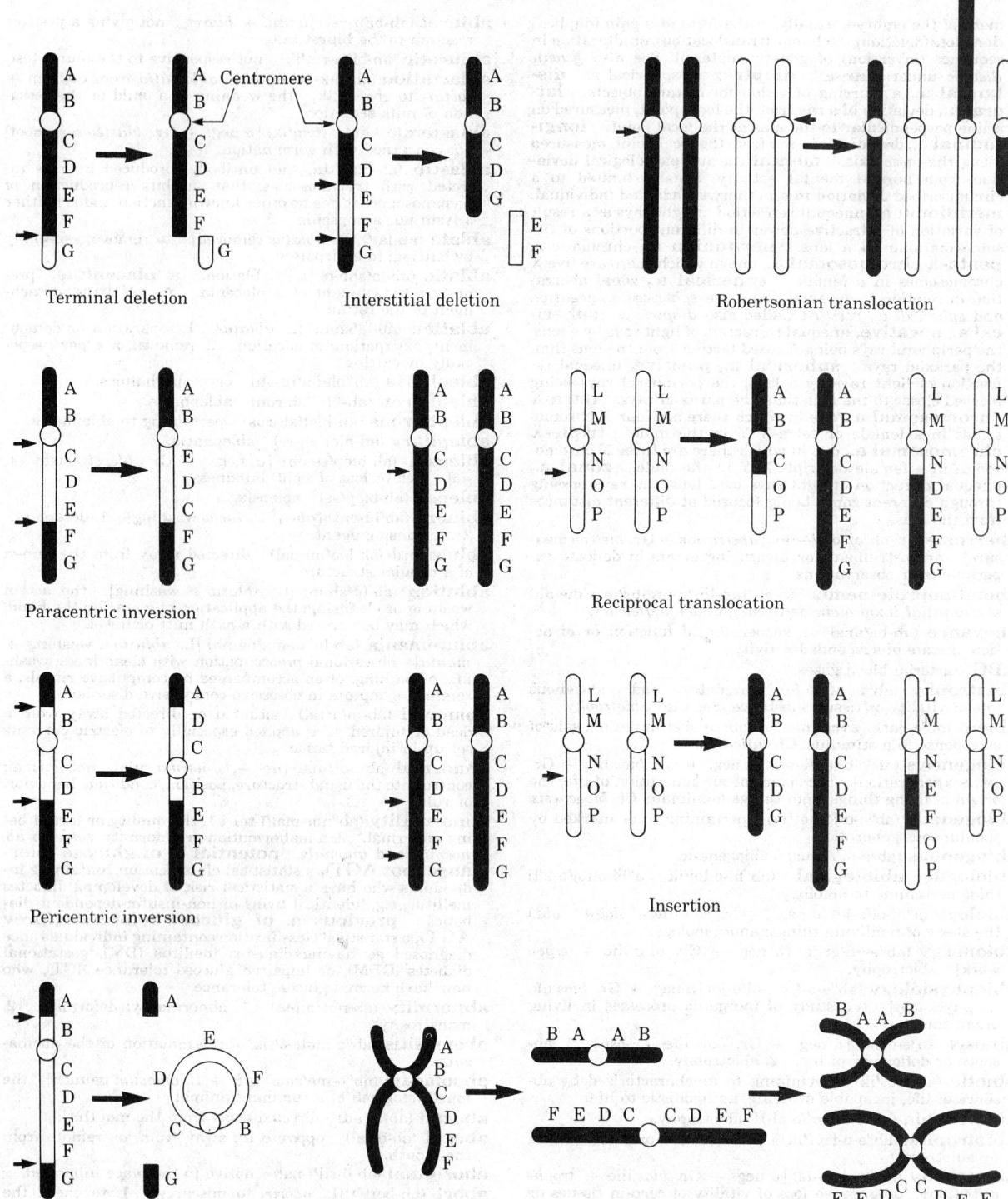

PLATE 1 —CHROMOSOME ABERRATIONS.

Genes are indicated by letters; breaks are indicated by small arrows.

4

abortion (ah-bor′shun) [L. *abortio*] 1. the premature expulsion from the uterus of the products of conception—of the embryo, or of a nonviable fetus. The four classic symptoms, usually present in each type of abortion, are uterine contractions, uterine hemorrhage, softening and dilatation of the cervix, and presentation or expulsion of all or part of the products of conception. 2. premature stoppage of a natural or a pathological process. **accidental a.,** an abortion which is due to an accident. **ampullar a.,** a variety of tubal abortion occurring from the ampulla of the oviduct. **artificial a.,** induced abortion; an abortion which is brought on intentionally. **complete a.,** abortion in which all of the products of conception have been expelled from the uterus and identified. **contagious a.,** in cattle, infectious a., def. 1. **contagious equine a.,** infectious a., def. 2. **enzootic of cattle,** an infectious abortion caused by organisms of the genus *Chlamydia;* also known as *foothill abortion* in western United States. **enzootic a. of ewes,** abortion in ewes, usually late in the gestation period, caused by *Chlamydia psittaci.* **equine epizootic a.,** an infectious abortion of horses, caused by the virus of equine rhinopneumonitis. **equine virus a.,** see under *rhinopneumonitis.* **foothill a.,** enzootic a. of cattle. **habitual a.,** the spontaneous expulsion of a dead or nonviable fetus in three or more consecutive pregnancies, at about the same period of development. **idiopathic a.,** abortion for which no recognized organic cause can be found. **imminent a.,** impending abortion in which the bleeding is profuse, the cervix softened and dilated, and the uterine contractions approach the character of labor pains. **incomplete a.,** abortion in which the uterus is not entirely emptied of its contents. **induced a.,** abortion brought on intentionally; called also *artificial* or *therapeutic a.* **inevitable a.,** a condition in which vaginal bleeding has been profuse or prolonged and the cervix has become effaced or dilated, and abortion will proceed naturally. **infected a.,** abortion associated with infection of the genital tract. **infectious a.,** 1. an infectious disease of cattle caused by *Brucella abortus,* marked by inflammatory changes in the uterine mucosa and fetal membranes, resulting in premature expulsion of the fetus. 2. an infectious disease of horses due to *Salmonella abortusequi* and of sheep due to *S. abortusovis.* Called also (in horses) *contagious equine a.* **justifiable a.,** therapeutic a. **missed a.,** retention in the uterus of an abortus that has been dead for at least eight weeks, indicated either by cessation of growth and hardening of the uterus or by actual diminution of its size; absence of fetal heart tones after they have been heard is also definitive; more accurate information of fetal death is obtainable by fetal electrocardiography and ultrasonography. **a. in progress,** a condition marked by profuse hemorrhage from the uterus and pains resembling those of labor, with softening and dilatation of the cervix, going on to expulsion of the products of conception. **recurrent a.,** habitual a. **septic a.,** abortion associated with serious infection of the uterus, leading to generalized infection; more common after criminal abortion. **spontaneous a.,** abortion occurring naturally. **therapeutic a.,** abortion induced to save the life or health (physical or mental) of a pregnant woman; sometimes performed after rape or incest. Called also *justifiable a.* **threatened a.,** a condition in which there is bloody discharge from the uterus but the loss of blood is less than in inevitable abortion and there is no dilatation of the cervix; it may proceed to actual abortion or the symptoms may subside and the pregnancy go to full term. **tubal a.,** extrusion of the conceptus through the open end of the uterine tube into the abdominal cavity, occurring in tubal (ectopic) pregnancy. **vibrio a.,** an infectious abortion of cattle, sheep, and goats, caused by *Campylobacter* (*Vibrio*) *fetus.*

abortionist (ah-bor′shun-ist) one who makes a business of inducing illegal abortions.

abortive (ah-bor′tiv) [L. *abortivus*] 1. incompletely developed. 2. effecting an abortion; abortifacient. 3. cutting short the course of a disease.

abortus (ah-bor′tus) [L.] a fetus weighing less than 500 gm. (17 oz.) or being of less than 20 weeks' gestational age at the time of expulsion from the uterus, having no chance of survival.

abouchement (ah-bōōsh-maw′) [Fr.] the termination of a vessel in a larger one.

aboulia (ah-boo′le-ah) abulia.

ABP   arterial blood pressure.

abrachia (ah-bra′ke-ah) [*a* neg. + Gr. *brachiōn* arm + *-ia*] congenital absence of the arms.

abrachiatism (ah-bra′ke-ah-tizm″)   abrachia.

abrachiocephalia (ah-bra″ke-o-sĕ-fa′le-ah) [*a* neg. + Gr. *brachiōn* arm + *kephalē* head + *-ia*] congenital absence of the arms and head.

abrachiocephalus (ah-bra″ke-o-sef′ah-lus) a monster exhibiting abrachiocephalia.

abrachius (ah-bra′ke-us) an individual exhibiting abrachia.

abradant (ah-bra′dant) abrasive.

abrade (ah-brād′) to rub away the external covering or layer of a part; see also *planing.*

Abrahams' sign (a′brah-hamz) [Robert *Abrahams,* New York physician, 1861–1935] see under *sign.*

Abrami's disease (ah-brahm′ēz) [Pierre *Abrami,* French physician, 1879–1943] hemolytic anemia.

Abrams' (heart) reflex (a′bramz) [Albert *Abrams,* physician in San Francisco, 1863–1924] see under *reflex.*

abrasio (ah-bra′se-o) [L.] abrasion. **a. cor′neae,** a rubbing off of the superficial layers of the cornea.

abrasion (ah-bra′zhun) [L. *abrasio*] 1. the wearing away of a substance or structure (such as the skin or the teeth) through some unusual or abnormal mechanical process; see also *planing.* 2. an area of body surface denuded of skin or mucous membrane by some unusual or abnormal mechanical process.

abrasive (ah-bra′siv) 1. causing abrasion. 2. a substance used for abrading, grinding, or polishing.

abrasor (ah-bra′zor) an instrument used for abrasion.

abreaction (ab″re-ak′shun) [*ab-* + *reaction*] the reliving of an experience in such a way that previously repressed emotions associated with it are released. **motor a.,** an abreaction achieved through motor or muscular expression.

abreuography (ab″roo-og′rah-fe) [Manoel de *Abreu,* Brazilian physician, 1892–1962] (*obs.*) photofluorography.

Abrikosov's (Abrikossoff's) tumor (ab″rĭ-kos′ofs) [Aleksei Ivanovich *Abrikosov,* Moscow pathologist, 1875–1955] granular cell tumor.

abrin (a′brin) a powerful phytotoxin or toxalbumin present in the seeds of *Abrus precatorius* L., Leguminosae; once used topically in certain chronic eye disorders. The plant is also known as jequirity or precatory bean, and rosary pea.

abrism (a′brizm) poisoning by jequirity; see *abrin.*

abrosia (ah-bro′ze-ah) [Gr. *abrōsia* fasting] lack of food.

abruptio (ab-rup′she-o) [L., from *abrumpere* to break off from] a rending asunder. **a. placen′tae,** premature detachment of a placenta, often attended by maternal systemic reactions in the form of shock, oliguria, and fibrinogenopenia.

Abrus precatorius L. (Leguminosae) (a′brus pre-kah-to′re-us) a species of tree native to tropical Asia, also found in Central America and Florida. Its seeds, called rosary beads, crab eyes, or jequirity beans, contain a toxalbumin (abrin) that is extremely irritant to mucous membranes. Used for jewelry and rosary beads.

abs- [L. *abs,* variant of *ab*] a prefix meaning away, from.

abscess (ab′ses) [L. *abscessus,* from *ab* away + *cedere* to go] a localized collection of pus caused by suppuration buried in tissues, organs, or confined spaces. **acute a.,** one which

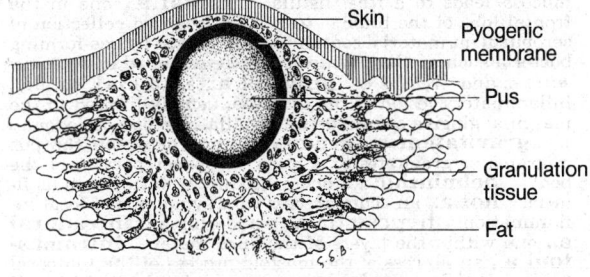

Cross section of abscess.

runs a relatively short course, producing some fever and a painful local inflammation. **acute dentoalveolar a.,** alveolar a. **alveolar a.,** apical a., def. 2. **amebic a.,** an abscess cavity of the liver resulting from liquefaction necrosis due to entrance of *Entamoeba histolytica* into the portal circulation in amebiasis; amebic abscesses may also involve lungs, spleen, and brain. **apical a.,** 1. one situated at the apex of an organ. 2. acute or chronic inflammation of tissues surrounding the apical portion of a tooth, associated with the collection of pus, resulting from infection following pulp infection through a carious lesion or as a result of an injury causing pulp necrosis. Called also *alveolar a., dentoalveolar a.,* and *periapical a.* **apical a., acute,** an acute inflammatory reaction involving the tissues surrounding the apical portion of a tooth, characterized by rapid onset, acute pain, tenderness of the tooth to touch and pressure, pus formation, and swelling of tissues in a later stage. Pulpal necrosis may be a cause. Called also *acute alveolar a., acute dentoalveolar a.,* and *acute periapical a.* **apical a., chronic,** a chronic inflammatory reaction of the tissues surrounding the apical portion of a tooth, characterized by an intermittent discharge of pus through a sinus tract, with gradual onset, little or no swelling of the affected tissue, and slight discomfort, if any. Pulpal necrosis may be a cause. Called also *chronic alveolar a., chronic dentoalveolar a., chronic periapical a.,* and *suppurative apical periodontitis.* **appendiceal a., appendicular a.,** abscess resulting from perforation of an acutely inflamed appendix. **arthrifluent a.,** a wandering abscess which has its point of origin in a diseased joint. **bartholinian a.,** abscess of the excretory duct of Bartholin's gland. **Bezold's a.,** an abscess deep in the neck resulting from a complication of acute mastoiditis in which pus tracts deep to the superior portion of the sternocleidomastoid muscle. **bicameral a.,** one which has two chambers or pockets; see *shirt-stud a.* **bile duct a.,** cholangitic a. **biliary a.,** abscess of the gallbladder or some part of the biliary tract. **bone a.,** osteomyelitis; suppurative periostitis. **brain a.,** one affecting the brain as a result of extension of an infection (e.g., otitis media) from an adjacent area or through bloodborne infection. **broad ligament a.,** an abscess between the folds of the broad ligament of the uterus; called also *parametric* or *parametrial a.* **Brodie's a.,** a roughly spherical region of bone destruction, filled with pus or connective tissue, usually found in the metaphyseal region of long bones and caused by *Staphylococcus aureus* or *albus.* **canalicular a.,** a mammary abscess communicating with a milk duct. **caseous a.,** one containing a cottage cheese–like material. Called also *cheesy a.* **cheesy a.,** caseous a. **cholangitic a.,** intrahepatic abscess complicating bacterial cholangitis; called also *bile duct a.* **chronic a.,** cold a., def. 1. **circumtonsillar a.,** peritonsillar a. **cold a.,** 1. an abscess of comparatively slow development with little evidence of inflammation. Called also *chronic a.* 2. tuberculous a. **collar-button a.,** shirt-stud a. **dental a.,** an abscess in or about a tooth. **dentoalveolar a.,** apical a., def. 2. **diffuse a.,** an uncircumscribed abscess, the pus of which is diffused in the surrounding tissues. **Douglas' a.,** an abscess in the rectouterine pouch. **dry a.,** one that disappears without pointing or breaking. **Dubois' a.,** abscess(es) of the thymus in congenital syphilis; called also *Dubois' disease* and *thymic a.* **epidural a.,** extradural a. **epiploic a.,** an abscess in the omentum. **extradural a.,** an abscess of the brain situated between the dura and the cranial bone; called also *epidural a.* **fecal a.,** an abscess, usually pericolic or perirectal, resulting from lower bowel perforation and containing pus and fecal matter; extension to the skin or mucosa leads to a fecal fistula. **frontal a.,** one in the frontal lobe of the brain. **gas a.,** a localized collection of seropurulent material containing gas, caused by gas-forming bacteria such as *Clostridium perfringens.* Called also *tympanitic a.* and *Welch's a.* **gingival a.,** a localized, painful, inflammatory lesion of the gingivae, usually limited to the marginal gingiva or interdental papilla. See also *periodontal a.* **gravitation a., gravity a.,** one in which the pus migrates or gravitates to a lower or deeper portion of the body. **helminthic a.,** one caused by a worm, such as filaria. **hot a.,** an acute abscess with symptoms of local inflammation. **hypostatic a.,** wandering a. **intradural a.,** one within the layers of the dura mater. **intramastoid a.,** an abscess of the mastoid process of the temporal bone. **ischiorectal a.,** one located in the ischiorectal fossa. **kidney a.,** renal a. **lacrimal a.,** one in or around the lacrimal sac. **lacunar a.,** one in the lacunae of the urethra. **lateral a., lateral alveolar a.,** peri-

odontal a. **mammary a.,** see accompanying illustration. **mastoid a.,** suppuration within the cells of the mastoid

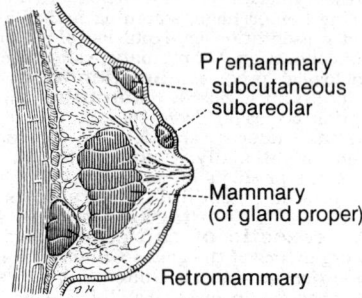

Premammary
subcutaneous
subareolar

Mammary
(of gland proper)

Retromammary

Abscesses of breast.

portion of the temporal bone. **metastatic a.,** a secondary abscess, usually of embolic origin, in which organisms are carried by the circulation to a point distant from the primary lesion. **metastatic tuberculous a.,** tuberculous gumma. **migrating a.,** wandering a. **miliary a.,** one of a set of small multiple abscesses. **Munro a.,** see under *microabscess.* **orbital a.,** suppuration in the orbit. **palatal a.,** an apical abscess of a maxillary tooth which erupts or extends toward the palate. **pancreatic a.,** an abscess formed following secondary bacterial contamination of necrotic pancreatic debris and hemorrhagic exudate; it is a serious complication of severe acute pancreatitis and of postoperative pancreatitis. **parafrenal a.,** abscess of the preputial gland. **parametrial a., parametric a.,** broad ligament a. **paranephric a.,** one in the tissues around the kidney. **parietal a.,** periodontal a. **Pautrier's a.,** see under *microabscess.* **pelvic a.,** abscess of the pelvic peritoneum, usually of the rectouterine pouch. **pelvirectal a.,** one lying immediately above the levator ani muscle, in close relation to the wall of the rectum. **periapical a.,** apical a., def. 2. **pericoronal a.,** an abscess around the crown of a partially erupted tooth. **peridental a.,** periodontal a. **perinephric a.,** one in the tissues immediately around the kidney. **periodontal a.,** an acute or chronic localized collection of purulent material in the periodontal tissue; it may involve the supporting periodontal tissue or the soft tissue wall of a periodontal pocket. Called also *lateral a., lateral alveolar a., parietal a.,* and *peridental a.* See also *gingival a.* **peripleuritic a.,** abscess between the parietal pleura and the chest wall. **peritoneal a.,** a confined collection of inflammatory exudate in peritonitis. **peritonsillar a.,** an abscess in the peritonsillar tissue extending into the tonsil capsule, resulting from suppuration of the tonsil; called also *quinsy.* **periureteral a.,** one around the ureter. **phlegmonous a.,** one associated with acute inflammation of the subcutaneous connective tissues. **phoenix a.,** an abscess with symptoms identical to those of an acute apical abscess, developing from a chronic apical granuloma and suddenly becoming symptomatic. **Pott's a.,** one associated with tuberculosis of the spine. **premammary a.,** see accompanying illustration. **psoas a.,** one which arises from disease of the lumbar or lower dorsal vertebrae, the pus descending in the sheath of the psoas muscle. **pulp a., pulpal a.,** 1. an acute or chronic inflammation of the dental pulp, associated with a circumscribed collection of necrotic tissue and pus arising from breakdown of leukocytes and bacteria, sometimes walled off with connective tissue. 2. an abscess of the tissues of the pulp of a finger; see also *felon.* **pyemic a.,** one due to pyemia. Called also *septicemic a.* **renal a.,** a localized renal parenchymal suppuration consequent to bacterial infection. **residual a.,** one recurring at the site where an incompletely resolved abscess occurred previously. **retromammary a.,** see accompanying illustration. **retroperitoneal a.,** subperitoneal a. **retropharyngeal a.,** a suppurative inflammation of the lymph nodes in the posterior and lateral walls of the pharynx; called also *hippocratic angina.* **retrotonsillar a.,** an abscess behind a tonsil caused by any of the common pyogenic bacteria, usually occurring with or closely following acute tonsillitis or pharyngitis. **ring a.,** a ring-shaped purulent infiltration at the periphery of the cornea. **root a.,** a chronic or acute pustular condition affecting the supporting structures of the root of a tooth; when it is of endodontic origin, called *apical abscess;* when periodontal in origin, called *periodontal abscess.* **satellite a.,** a secondary abscess arising from a primary one and situated near the latter. **septicemic a.,** pyemic a. **serous a.,** periostitis albuminosa. **shirt-stud a.,** a superficial abscess connected with a deeper one by a passage; called also *collar-button a.* **spermatic a.,** one in the seminiferous tubules. **splenic a.,** an abscess of the spleen. **stercoraceous a., stercoral a.,** fecal a. **sterile a.,** one not due to pathogenic microorganisms. **stitch a.,** one that develops adjacent to a stitch or suture. **strumous a.,** tuberculous a. **subaponeurotic a.,** one beneath an aponeurosis or fascia. **subareolar a.,** a subcutaneous abscess of the areola of the nipple. **subdiaphragmatic a.,** one beneath the diaphragm. **subdural a.,** a brain abscess situated just under the dura mater. **subfascial a.,** one beneath a fascia. **subgaleal a.,** one under the galea aponeurotica. **submammary a.,** one beneath the mammary gland. **subpectoral a.,** one beneath the pectoral muscles. **subperiosteal a.,** a bone abscess situated just below the periosteum. **subperitoneal a.,** one between the parietal peritoneum and the abdominal wall. **subphrenic a.,** one beneath the diaphragm. **subscapular a.,** one between the serratus anterior and the posterior thoracic wall. **sudoriparous a.,** an abscess arising in a sweat gland. **superficial a.,** one occurring near the surface. **suprahepatic a.,** one situated in the suspensory ligament between the liver and the diaphragm. **sympathetic a.,** one arising some distance from the exciting cause. **syphilitic a.,** one occurring in the bones during tertiary syphilis. **thecal a.,** one arising in an enveloping sheath, such as a tendon sheath. **thymic a.,** Dubois' a. **Tornwaldt (Thornwaldt) a.,** an abscess of the adenoids, usually associated with adenoid hyperplasia. **tuberculous a.,** one due to infection with tubercle bacilli (*Mycobacterium tuberculosis*); called also *cold a., scrofulous a.,* and *strumous a.* **tuboovarian a.,** abscess of the uterine tube and ovary resulting from extension of infection along the tube. **tympanitic a.,** gas a. **tympanocervical a.,** one arising in the tympanum and extending to the neck. **tympanomastoid a.,** a combined abscess of the tympanum and the mastoid. **urethral a.,** an abscess of the urethra. **urinary a.,** one caused by extravasation of infected urine. **verminous a.,** one which contains insect larvae or other animal parasites. **vitreous a.,** abscess of the vitreous humor of the eye due to infection, trauma, or foreign body. **von Bezold's a.,** Bezold's a. **wandering a.,** one that burrows in the tissues and finally points at a distance from the site of origin; called also *hypostatic a.* and *migrating a.* **Welch's a.,** gas a. **worm a.,** one caused by or containing worms.

abscessus (ab-ses'us) [L.] abscess.

abscise (ab-sīz') to cut off or remove.

abscissa (ab-sis'ah) [L. (*linea*) *abscissa* cut-off line, from *abscindere* to cut off] the horizontal coordinate in a two-dimensional coordinate system; the horizontal distance of a point from *y-* (or vertical) axis. Denoted by *x.* Cf. *ordinate.*

abscission (ab-sish'un) [L. *ab* from + *scindere* to cut] removal by cutting. **corneal a.,** excision of the prominence of the cornea in staphyloma.

absconsio (ab-skon'se-o), pl. *absconsio'nes* [L.] the cavity of a bone receiving and concealing the head of another bone.

abscopal (ab-sko'p'l) pertaining to the effect on nonirradiated tissue resulting from irradiation of other tissue of the organism.

absence (ab'sens) see *petit mal epilepsy,* under *epilepsy.*

abs. feb. abbreviation for L. *absen'te feb're,* while fever is absent. Cf. *adst. feb.*

Absidia (ab-sid'e-ah) a genus of fungi of the family Mucoraceae, order Mucorales. *A. corymbifera* (*Mucor rhizopodiformis*) and several other species are pathogenic for laboratory animals and may cause localized or generalized mycosis in man. *A. ramosa* (*Mucor ramosus*) is a pathogenic species that grows on bread and decaying vegetation, and causes otomycosis and sometimes mucormycosis. Formerly called *Leptomitus* and *Lichtheimia.* See also *mucormycosis.*

absinthe (ab'sinth) an extract of absinthium and other bitter herbs, containing 60 per cent alcohol; prolonged ingestion causes nervousness, convulsions, trismus, amblyopia, optic neuritis, and mental deterioration.

absinthin (ab-sin'thin) a crystalline compound, $C_{30}H_{40}O_6$, the chief bitter principle of wormwood (*Artemisia absinthium* L.), used as a flavoring in alcoholic beverages; formerly used as an anthelmintic and bitter tonic.

absinthium (ab-sinth'e-um) wormwood; the dead leaves and flowering tops of *Artemisia absinthium* L. (Compositae).

absolute (ab'so-lūt) [L. *absolutus,* from *absolvere* to set loose] free from limitations; unlimited; uncombined.

absorb (ab-sorb') [L. *absorbēre*] to take in or assimilate, as to take up substances into or across tissues, e.g., the skin, intestine, or kidney tubules, or to react with radiation energy so as to attenuate it.

absorbance (ab-sor'bans) 1. the analytical chemistry, the negative logarithm of the transmittance, $-\log_{10} (I/I_0)$, where I is the light intensity transmitted by the solution under analysis and I_0 is the intensity transmitted by the pure solvent or other reference solution. Symbol *A.* Formerly referred to as *absorbancy* or *optical density.* 2. in radiation physics, the negative logarithm of the transmittance, defined in this case as the ratio of the radiant energy transmitted by an object (I) to the incident radiant energy (I_0).

absorbefacient (ab-sor"be-fa'shent) [L. *absorbere* to absorb + *facere* to make] 1. causing or promoting absorption. 2. a medicine or an agent that promotes absorption.

absorbency (ab-sor'ben-se) absorbance.

absorbent (ab-sor'bent) [L. *absorbens,* from *ab* away + *sorbere* to suck] 1. able to take in, or suck up and incorporate. 2. a tissue structure involved in absorption. 3. a substance that absorbs or acts as an absorbefacient.

absorptiometer (ab-sorp"she-om'ĕ-ter) [*absorption* + Gr. *metron* measure] 1. an instrument for measuring the solubility of gas in a liquid. 2. a device for measuring the layer of liquid absorbed between two glass plates; used as a hematoscope.

absorption (ab-sorp'shun) [L. *absorptio*] 1. the uptake of substances into or across tissues, e.g., skin, intestine, and kidney tubules. 2. in psychology, devotion of thought to one object or activity, with inattention to others. 3. in radiology, the taking up of energy by matter with which the radiation interacts. Cf. *attenuation,* def. 3. **agglutinin a.,** the removal of antibody from an immune serum by treatment with particulate antigen (usually bacteria) homologous to that antibody, followed by centrifugation and separation of the antigen-antibody complex. **enteral a.,** internal a. **excrementitial a.,** pathologic a. **external a.,** the absorption of foods, poisons, or other agents through the skin or mucous membrane. **internal a.,** the normal absorption of foods, water, etc., in digestion. **interstitial a.,** removal of waste matter by the absorbent system. **intestinal a.,** the uptake from the intestinal lumen of fluids, solutes, proteins, fats, and other nutrients into the intestinal epithelial cells, blood, lymph, or interstitial fluids of the intestine. **net a.,** the difference between uptake and efflux from a tissue or cell. **parenteral a.,** absorption otherwise than through the digestive tract. **pathologic a., pathological a.,** the absorption into the blood of any bodily excretion or morbid product, such as bile or pus.

absorptive (ab-sorp'tiv) capable of absorbing; absorbent; pertaining to absorption.

absorptivity (ab"sorp-tiv'ĭ-te) a measure of the amount of light absorbed by a solution, defined as the absorbance per unit concentration per unit length of light path. By Beer's law (q.v.) absorptivity is proportional to the concentration of the absorbing solute. Formerly called *absorbancy index, absorption constant, absorption coefficient,* and *extinction coefficient.* **molar a.,** absorptivity defined in terms of concentrations expressed in moles per liter. Symbol E. **specific a.,** absorptivity defined in terms of concentrations expressed in grams per liter. Symbol *a.*

abst., abstr. abstract.

abstergent (ab-ster'jent) [L. *abstergere* to cleanse] 1. cleansing or purifying. 2. a cleansing application or medicine.

abstinence (ab'stĭ-nens) a refraining from the use of or indulgence in food, stimulants, or sexual intercourse. **alimentary a.,** fasting, hunger, or starvation.

abstr. abstract.

abstract (ab'strakt) [L. *abstractum,* from *abstrahere* to draw off] a summary or epitome of a book, paper, or case history.

abstraction (ab-strak'shun) [L. *abstractus*, past participle of *abstrahere* to draw away] 1. the withdrawal of any ingredient from a compound. 2. a condition in which the teeth or other maxillary and mandibular structures are lower than the normal position, away from the occlusal plane, thereby lengthening the face. Cf. *attraction*, def. 2.

abterminal (ab-ter'mĭ-nal) [*ab-* + L. *terminus* end] moving from the terminus toward the center; said of electric currents in muscular substance.

abtorsion (ab-tor'shun) extorsion.

Abulcasis (ah″bool-kas'is) Albucasis.

abulia (ah-bu'le-ah) [*a* neg. + Gr. *boulē* will + *-ia*] lack of will or willpower; inability to make decisions.

abulic (ah-bu'lik) affected with or pertaining to abulia.

Abulkasim (ah″bool-kas'im) Albucasis.

abuse (ah-būs′) misuse or wrong use, particularly excessive use of anything. **child a.**, physical, emotional, or sexual abuse of children, usually by parents, relatives, or caretakers. See also *battered child syndrome*, under *syndrome*. **drug a.**, see *dependence*. **psychoactive substance a.** [DSM III-R], use of a substance that modifies mood or behavior in a manner characterized by a maladaptive pattern of use (e.g., continued use despite knowledge of having a social, occupational, psychological, or physical problem caused or exacerbated by use of the substance, or use in situations when use is physically hazardous, as driving while intoxicated). Psychoactive substance abuse in conjunction with tolerance or withdrawal constitutes psychoactive substance dependence. DSM III-R includes specific abuse disorders for alcohol, amphetamines or similarly acting sympathomimetics, cannabis, cocaine, hallucinogens, inhalants, opioids, phencyclidine (PCP) or similarly acting arylcyclohexylamines, sedatives, hypnotics, and anxiolytics. **substance a.**, see *psychoactive substance a.*

abut (ah-but′) to touch, adjoin, or border upon.

abutment (ah-but′ment) 1. that on which or the point at which abutting occurs. 2. a part of a structure that sustains thrust or pressure. 3. a tooth or root used as an anchorage for either a fixed or a removable dental prosthesis, or any other device serving the same purpose. See also under *tooth*. **auxiliary a.**, secondary a. **implant a.** that part of a subperiosteal, intraperiosteal, or intraosseous implant that protrudes into the oral cavity and serves as an abutment for retaining and stabilizing a denture. Called also *abutment post*. **intermediate a.**, a natural tooth or root, without other natural teeth in proximal contact, that is used as an abutment, in addition to two terminal abutments. Called also *pier*. **isolated a.**, an intermediate abutment, particularly one used to support a removable partial denture. **multiple a.**, one resulting from the fixed splinting of two or more adjacent natural teeth to serve as a unit in the support and retention of a fixed or removable partial denture. **primary a.**, a tooth used for direct support of a denture. **secondary a.**, a natural tooth used in addition to the primary abutments to provide support or indirect retention for a removable partial denture; called also *auxiliary a.* **terminal a.**, a natural tooth located at an extremity of a fixed partial denture and used for the support and retention of the prosthesis.

ABVD a regimen consisting of Adriamycin (doxorubicin), bleomycin, vinblastine, and dacarbazine, used in cancer chemotherapy.

A.C. air conduction; alternating current; aortic closure; anodal closure; axiocervical; acromioclavicular.

AC a regimen of Adriamycin (doxorubicin) and CCNU (lomustine), used in a cancer chemotherapy.

Ac chemical symbol for *actinium*.

a.c. abbreviation for L. *an′te ci′bum*, before meals.

A.C.A. American College of Angiology; American College of Apothecaries.

Acacia (ah-ka′she-ah) [L.; Gr. *akakia*] a genus of leguminous shrubs or trees containing several economically and medically important species; e.g., *A. senegal* yields acacia (gum arabic). **A. cat′echu** Willd. (Leguminosae), a small tree native to India and Burma, which is a source of catechu. **A. georgi′nae** F. M. Bail. (Leguminosae), a tree in northern Australia; the fluoroacetate content of its leaves is fatal to sheep and cattle.

acacia (ah-ka′shah) [NF] the dried, gummy exudate from the stems and branches of *Acacia senegal* and other African species of *Acacia*, prepared as a mucilage or syrup; formerly used intravenously in the treatment of shock and now employed as a suspending agent, emollient, and demulcent for pharmaceutical preparations. Called also *gum arabic* and *gum senegal*.

acalcerosis (ah-kal″ser-o′sis) a deficiency of calcium in the system.

acalcicosis (ah-kal″sĭ-ko′sis) a condition caused by a deficiency of calcium in the diet.

acalculia (ah″kal-ku′le-ah) [*a* neg. + L. *calculare* to reckon + *-ia*] inability to do simple arithmetical calculations.

acampsia (ah-kamp′se-ah) [*a* neg. + Gr. *kamptein* to bend + *-ia*] rigidity or inflexibility of a part or of a joint.

acantha (ah-kan′thah) [Gr. *akantha* thorn] 1. the spine. 2. the spinous process of a vertebra.

acanthaceous (ak″an-tha′shus) bearing prickles or spines.

acanthamebiasis (ah-kan″thah-me-bi′ah-sis) infection with *Acanthamoeba castellani*.

Acanthamoeba (ah-kan″thah-me′bah) [*acanth-* + Gr. *amoibē* change] a genus of free-living ameboid protozoa (suborder Acanthopodina, order Amoebida) found usually in fresh water or moist soil. Certain species, such as *A. castellani*, *A. polyphaga*, *A. astronyxis*, and *A. culbertsoni*, may occur as opportunistic human pathogens, causing an acute fatal or chronic infection of the eye, brain, liver, kidney, lung, pancreas, and skin in patients with underlying disease or in immunocompromised patients. One of the most frequent forms of acanthamebiasis is granulomatous amebic encephalitis. The organisms may also be associated with nonfatal infections of the ear and respiratory tract in nonimmunocompromised hosts.

Acantharea (ah″kan-thār′re-ah) [Gr. *akantha* thorn, prickle] a class of marine, usually planktonic protozoa (superclass Actinopoda, subphylum Sarcodina), characterized by the presence of skeleton composed of strontium sulfate and usually consisting of 20 radial or 10 diametral spines that are more or less joined in the cell center; an extracellular cortex (*calymma*) and an inner envelope (*capsular membrane*) often closely lining the central cell mass are usually present. It includes five orders: Holacanthida, Symphyacanthida, Chaunacanthida, Arthracanthida, and Actineliida.

acantharian (ah-kan-thār′e-an) any protozoan of the class Acantharea. Cf. *radiolarian*.

acanthesthesia (ah-kan″thes-the′ze-ah) [*acantho-* + Gr. *aisthēsis* sensation + *-ia*] perverted sensibility with a feeling as of pressure of a sharp point.

Acanthia lectularia (ah-kan′the-ah lek″tu-la′re-ah) *Cimex lectularius*.

acanthion (ah-kan′the-on) [Gr. *akanthion* little thorn] a point at the base of the anterior nasal spine.

acanth(o)- [Gr. *akantha*, q.v.] a combining form meaning thorny or spiny, or denoting a relationship to a sharp spine or thorn.

Acanthobdellidea (ah-kan″tho-del-lid′e-ah) an order of leeches of the class Hirudinea, characterized by the presence of spines on the surface of the body.

Acanthocephala (ah-kan″tho-sef′ah-lah) [*acantho-* + Gr. *kephalē* head] a phylum of animal parasites, the thorny-headed or spiny-head worms, so called because of the proboscis which projects anteriorly, and is covered with thornlike recurved spines for attachment to the digestive tract of the host. In some systems of classification, they are considered to be a class of the phylum Nemathelminthes.

acanthocephalan (ah-kan″tho-sef′ah-lan) any individual of the phylum Acanthocephala.

acanthocephaliasis (ah-kan″tho-sef″ah-li′ah-sis) infestation with any species of the phylum Acanthocephala.

acanthocephalous (ah-kan″tho-sef′ah-lus) pertaining to or caused by worms of the phylum Acanthocephala.

Acanthocephalus (ah-kan″tho-sef′ah-lus) a genus of parasitic worms of the phylum Acanthocephala.

Acanthocheilonema (ah-kan″tho-ki″lo-ne′mah) a genus of filarial nematodes. **A. per′stans**, *Mansonella perstans*. **A. streptocer′ca**, *Mansonella streptocerca*.

acanthocheilonemiasis (ah-kan″tho-ki″lo-ne-mi′ah-sis) mansonellosis.

acanthocyte (ah-kan′tho-sīt) [*acantho-* + Gr. *kytos* cell] a distorted erythrocyte characterized by protoplasmic projections of varying sizes and shapes, irregularly spaced, which give the cell a "thorny" appearance; seen in abetalipoproteinemia.

acanthocytosis (ah-kan″tho-si-to′sis) [*acanthocyte* + *-osis*] the presence in the blood of acanthocytes; see familial *lipoprotein deficiency,* under *deficiency.*

acanthoid (ah-kan′thoid) [*acantho-* + Gr. *eidos* form] resembling a spine; spinous.

acantholysis (ak″an-thol′ĭ-sis) [*acantho-* + Gr. *lysis* a loosening] disruption of the intercellular connections between keratinocytes of the epidermis, caused by lysis of intercellular cement substance, resulting in secondary disruption of desmosomes and often in a defined sequence of cellular degenerative events; it is associated with the formation of epidermal vesicles in such conditions as pemphigus vulgaris, pemphigus foliaceus, and other skin disorders.

acantholytic (ah-kan″tho-lit′ik) pertaining or relating to acantholysis.

acanthoma (ak″an-tho′mah, a″kan-tho′mah), pl. *acantho′mas* or *acantho′mata* [*acantho-* + *-oma*] a tumor composed of epidermal or squamous cells. **a. adenoi′des cys′ticum,** trichoepithelioma papillosum cysticum.

acanthopelvis (ah-kan″tho-pel′vis) [*acantho-* + Gr. *pelyx* bowl] a pelvis with a very sharp and prominent pubic crest; called also *acanthopelyx.*

acanthopelyx (ah-kan″tho-pel′iks) acanthopelvis.

Acanthophacetus (ah-kan″tho-fah-se′tus) a genus of small fish. **A. reticula′tus,** *Lebistes reticulatus.*

Acanthophis (ah-kan′tho-fis) a genus of elapid snakes; see table accompanying *snake.* **A. antarc′tica,** a widespread, live-bearing elapid snake of Australia and New Guinea, remarkable for its viper-like form; next to the tiger snake it is the most feared snake in Australia. Called also *death adder.*

Acanthopodina (ah-kan″tho-po-di′nah) [*acantho-* + Gr. *pous* foot] a suborder of ameboid protozoa (order Amoebida, subclass Gymnamoebia), characterized by the presence of more or less finely tipped, sometimes filiform, often furcate hyaline subpseudopodia produced from a broad hyaline lobe. *Acanthamoeba* is a representative genus.

Acanthopterygii (ah-kan″tho-tĕ-rij′e-i) a superorder of spiny-finned teleosts.

acanthosis (ak″an-tho′sis) [*acanth-* + *-osis*] diffuse hyperplasia of the spinous layer of the skin. Called also *hyperacanthosis.* **a. ni′gricans,** diffuse velvety acanthosis with gray, brown, or black pigmentation, chiefly in axillae and other body folds, occurring in an adult form, often associated with an internal carcinoma (called *malignant acanthosis nigricans*), and in a benign, nevoid form, more or less generalized. A benign juvenile form associated with obesity, which is sometimes due to endocrine disturbance, is called *pseudoacanthosis nigricans.*

acanthotic (ak″an-thot′ik) marked by acanthosis.

acanthrocyte (ah-kan′thro-sīt) acanthocyte.

acanthrocytosis (ah-kan″thro-si-to′sis) acanthocytosis.

a cap′ite ad cal′cem (ah kap′ĭ-te ad kal′sĕm) [L.] from head to heel, the classic order for describing symptoms.

acapnia (ah-kap′ne-ah) [*a* neg. + Gr. *kapnos* smoke + *-ia*] a condition of diminished carbon dioxide in blood; hypocapnia.

acapnial (ah-kap′ne-al) acapnic.

acapnic (ah-kap′nik) pertaining to or characterized by acapnia.

Acarapis (a-kar′ah-pis) a genus of mites, including *A. woodi,* the tracheal mite of the honeybee, which causes Isle of Wight disease.

acarbia (ah-kar′be-ah) a condition in which the blood bicarbonate is lowered.

acardia (a-kar′de-ah) [*a* neg. + Gr. *kardia* heart] congenital absence of the heart.

acardiac (a-kar′de-ak) having no heart.

acardiacus (ah″kar-di′ah-kus) acardius.

acardius (ah-kar′de-us) [*a* neg. + Gr. *kardia* heart] an imperfectly formed free twin fetus, lacking a heart and invariably lacking other body parts as well; called also *fetus acardiacus.* **a. aceph′alus,** holoacardius acephalus.

a. acor′mus, holoacardius acormus. **a. amor′phus,** holoacardius amorphus. **a. an′ceps,** hemiacardius.

acari (ak′ah-ri) [L.] plural of *acarus,* a mite.

acarian (ah-ka′re-an) pertaining to the acarids or mites.

acariasis (ak″ah-ri′ah-sis) [Gr. *akari* mite + *-iasis*] an infestation with acarids, or mites; types of acariasis are known as chorioptic, demodectic, psoroptic, sarcoptic, and so on, depending on the mite causing the disease. Called also *acarinosis.* See also *itch, mange,* and *scabies.*

acaricide (ah-kar′ĭ-sīd) [L. *acarus* mite + *caedere* to slay] 1. destructive to mites. 2. an agent that destroys mites.

acarid (ak′ah-rid) a mite or tick of the order Acarina, or a mite of the family Acaridae.

Acaridae (ah-kar′ĭ-de) a family of small mites of the order Acarina; several species cause skin rashes, such as grocers' itch, copra itch, and vanillism.

acaridan (ah-kar′ĭ-dan) acarid.

acaridiasis (ah-kar″ĭ-di′ah-sis) acariasis.

Acarina (ak″ah-ri′nah) an order of the class Arachnida, including the ticks and mites.

acarine (ak′ah-rīn) any member of the order Acarina.

acarinosis (ah-kar″ĭ-no′sis) any disease caused by mites; acariasis.

acariosis (ah-kar″e-o′sis) acariasis.

acar(o)- [Gr. *akari;* L. *acarus,* a mite] a combining form denoting relationship to mites.

acarodermatitis (ak″ah-ro-der″mah-ti′tis) any skin inflammation caused by mites. **a. urticarioi′des,** grain itch.

acaroid (ak′ah-roid) [Gr. *akari* a mite + *eidos* form] resembling a mite.

acarologist (ak″ah-rol′o-jist) a specialist in acarology.

acarology (ak″ah-rol′o-je) [*acaro-* + *-logy*] the scientific study of mites and ticks.

acarophobia (ak″ah-ro-fo′be-ah) [*acaro-* + *phobia*] irrational fear of mites or of other minute animate (insects, worms) or inanimate (pins, needles) objects, sometimes accompanied by fear of parasites crawling beneath the skin.

acarotoxic (ak″ah-ro-tok′sik) destructive to mites.

Acarpomyxea (ah-kar″po-mik′se-ah) [*a* neg. + Gr. *karpos* fruit + *myxa* mucus] a class of ameboid protozoa (superclass Rhizopoda, subphylum Sarcodina) comprising small plasmodia or much expanded similar uninucleate forms, usually branching, sometimes forming a reticulum of coarse branches; no spores or fruiting bodies are known. It includes two orders: Leptomyxida and Stereomyxida.

Acartomyia (ah-kar″to-mi′yah) a genus of culicine mosquitoes.

Acarus (ak′ah-rus) [L.; Gr. *akari* a mite] a genus of small mites, often ectoparasitic; they cause itch, mange, and other skin diseases. **A. folliculo′rum,** *Demodex folliculorum.* **A. galli′nae,** *Dermanyssus gallinae.* **A. hor′dei,** the barley bug, a mite which burrows under the skin of man. **A. rhyzoglyp′ticus hyacin′thi,** the onion mite which occurs on decaying onions and produces a dermatitis (onion-mite dermatitis) on persons who handle them. **A. scabie′i,** *Sarcoptes scabiei.* **A. si′ro,** a mite that causes vanillism in vanilla pod handlers; called also *Tyrophagus siro* and *Tyroglyphus siro.* **A. trit′ici,** former name for *Pyemotes ventricosus.*

acarus (ak′ah-rus), pl. *ac′ari* [L.] a mite.

acaryote (ah-kār′e-ōt) akaryocyte.

acatalasemia (a″kat-ah-la-se′me-ah) [*a* neg. + *catalase* + Gr. *haima* blood] deficiency of catalase in the blood; now called *acatalasia* (q.v.).

acatalasia (a″kat-ah-la′ze-ah) a rare autosomal recessive disease caused by congenital absence of the catalase and observed mainly in Japan and Switzerland. It is usually characterized by gingivitis and infections of associated oral structures. Called also *acatalasemia* and *Takahara's disease.*

acatalepsia (ah-kat″ah-lep′se-ah) [*a* neg. + Gr. *katalēpsis* comprehension] (*obs.*) 1. impairment of reasoning or comprehension; dementia. 2. uncertainty of diagnosis or prognosis.

acatalepsy (ah-kat′ah-lep′se) acatalepsia.

acataleptic (ah-kat″ah-lep′tik) characterized by acatalepsy.

acatamathesia (a-kat″ah-mah-the′ze-ah) [*a* neg. + Gr. *katamathēsis* understanding + *-ia*] 1. loss or impairment of the power to understand speech. 2. impairment of any one of the perceptive faculties, due to a central lesion.

acataphasia (a-kat″ah-fa′ze-ah) [*a* neg. + Gr. *kataphasis* orderly utterance + *-ia*] inability to express one's thoughts in a connected manner, due to a central lesion.

acataposis (a-kat″ah-po′sis) [*a* neg. + Gr. *kata* down + *posis* drinking] (*obs.*) dysphagia.

acatastasia (ak″ah-tas-ta′ze-ah) [*a* neg. + Gr. *katastasis* stability + *-ia*] irregularity; variation from the normal.

acatastatic (ak″ah-tas-tat′ik) irregular; varying from the normal.

acathectic (ak″ah-thek′tik) [*a* neg. + Gr. *kathexis* a retention] pertaining to or characterized by acathexia.

acathexia (ak″ah-thek′se-ah) inability to retain bodily secretions.

acathexis (ah″kah-thek′sis) a lack of the emotional charge (cathexis) with which an object or idea would normally be invested; detachment of feelings from thoughts and ideas.

acathisia (ak″ah-thiz′e-ah) akathisia.

acaudal (a-kaw′dal) acaudate.

acaudate (a-kaw′dāt) [*a* neg. + L. *cauda* tail] lacking a tail.

acauline (a-kaw′lin) [*a* neg. + L. *caulis* stem] (*obs.*) having no stem, as certain fungi.

acaulinosis (a-kaw″lĭ-no′sis) infection with a fungus of the genus *Acaulium* (*Scopulariopsis*); scopulariopsosis.

Acaulium (ah-kaw′le-um) former name for *Scopulariopsis*.

A.C.C. American College of Cardiology.

ACC anodal closure contraction.

Acc. accommodation.

accelerans (ak-sel′er-anz) [L. "hastening"] (*obs.*) an autonomic nerve, stimulation of which hastens the heart's action.

accelerant (ak-sel′er-ant) a catalyst.

acceleration (ak-sel″er-a′shun) [L. *acceleratio*, from *ad* intensification + *celerare* to quicken] 1. a quickening, as of the pulse rate or respiration. 2. in physics, the time rate of change of velocity. **negative a.,** a slowing.

accelerator (ak-sel′er-a″tor) [L. "hastener"] 1. an agent or apparatus that is used to increase the rate at which an object proceeds or a substance acts, or at which some reaction occurs. 2. any nerve or muscle which hastens the performance of a function. 3. any of a group of chemicals used in the vulcanization of rubber or other polymerizations; they frequently cause dermatitis in workers. **C3b inactivator a.,** factor H. **linear a.,** an apparatus for the acceleration of subatomic particles, using alternating hollow electrodes in a straight vacuum tube, so arranged that when their high frequency potentials are properly varied the particles traveling through them receive successive increases in energy. **serum prothrombin conversion a. (SPCA),** Factor VII; see *coagulation factors*, under *factor*. **serum thrombotic a.,** a factor in serum which possesses procoagulant properties and the ability, when infused experimentally into locally arrested flow systems, to induce blood coagulation; its precise nature and role in normal blood coagulation has not been delineated and hence it has not been assigned a number in the conventional scheme of blood coagulation factors. **a. uri′nae,** musculus bulbospongiosus; see *Table of Musculi*.

accelerin (ak-sel′er-in) Factor VI; see *coagulation factors*, under *factor*.

accelerometer (ak-sel′er-om′ĕ-ter) an instrument for measuring the acceleration (rate of change of velocity) of an object.

accentuation (ak-sen″chu-a′shun) [L. *accentus* accent] increased loudness or distinctness; intensification.

acceptor (ak-sep′tor) a substance which unites with another substance; specifically a substance which unites with hydrogen or oxygen in an oxidoreduction reaction and so enables the reaction to proceed. Cf. *donor*. **hydrogen a.,** the substance that is reduced in the oxidation and reduction occurring anaerobically in the body tissues. **oxygen a.,** a substance that is oxidized.

accès pernicieux (ak-sa′ păr-nis-yuh′) [Fr. "pernicious attack"] a sudden and severe paroxysm in falciparum malaria.

accessiflexor (ak-ses′ĕ-flek″sor) any accessory flexor muscle.

accessorius (ak″ses-o′re-us) [L. "supplementary"] accessory; used in naming certain structures thought to serve a supplementary function.

accessory (ak-ses′o-re) [L. *accessorius*] supplementary or affording aid to another similar and generally more important thing; complementary; concomitant.

accident (ak′sĭ-dent) an unforeseen occurrence, especially one of an injurious character; an unexpected complicating occurrence in the regular course of a disease. **cerebrovascular a.,** stroke syndrome.

accidentalism (ak″sĭ-den′tal-izm) the medical theory that disease is only an accidental change from normal health and can be avoided or cured by changing external conditions; thus one treats only symptoms and ignores etiology and pathology.

accident prone (ak′sĭ-dent prōn) specially susceptible to accidents owing to psychological factors.

ACCl anodal closure clonus.

acclimatation (ah-kli″mah-ta′shun) acclimation.

acclimation (ak″li-ma′shun) physiological or psychological adjustment to a new environment.

acclimatization (ah-kli″mah-ti-za′shun) acclimation.

accolé see *appliqué form*, under *form*.

accommodation (ah-kom″o-da′shun) [L. *accommodare* to fit to] adjustment, especially that of the eye for various distances (see illustration). **absolute a.,** the accommoda-

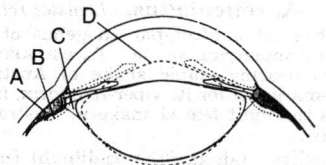

Changes during accomodation: A, contraction of ciliary muscles; B, approximation of ciliary muscles to lens; C, relaxation of suspensory ligament; D, increased curvature of anterior surface of lens.

tion of either eye separately. **binocular a.,** accommodation in both eyes in coordination with convergence. **excessive a.,** accommodation of the eye which is persistently above the normal. **histologic a.,** a group of changes in the morphology and function of cells following changed conditions. **negative a.,** adjustment of the eye for long distances by relaxation of the ciliary muscle. **nerve a.,** the rise in the threshold during the passage of a constant, direct electric current because of which only the make and break of the current stimulates the nerve. **positive a.,** adjustment of the eye for short distances by contraction of the ciliary muscle. **relative a.,** the change in accommodation that is possible with a fixed amount of convergence. **subnormal a.,** insufficient power of accommodation of the eye.

accommodative (ah-kom′o-da″tiv) pertaining to, of the nature of, or affecting accommodation.

accommodometer (ah-kom″o-dom′ĕ-ter) [*accommod*ation + *-meter*] a device for measuring the accommodative capacity of the eye.

accomplice (ak-om-plēs′) [Fr.] a bacterium which accompanies the chief infecting agent in a mixed infection and which influences the virulence of the chief organism.

accouchement (ah-kōōsh-maw′) [Fr.] delivery. **a. forcé** (ah-koosh-maw′ for-sa′), rapid forcible delivery from below by any one of several methods; originally applied to rapid dilatation of the cervix with the hands, followed immediately by version and extraction of the fetus.

accoucheur (ah-koosh-er′) [Fr.] one skilled in obstetrics; an obstetrician.

accoucheuse (ah-koosh-ez′) [Fr.] a midwife.

A.C.C.P. American College of Chest Physicians.

accrementition (ak″re-men-tish′un) [L. *ad* to + *crementum* increase] growth or increase by the addition of similar tissue.

accretio (ah-kre′she-o) [L.] abnormal adhesion of parts normally separate. **a. cor′dis, a. pericar′dii,** a form of adhesive pericarditis in which adhesions extend from the pericardium to the pleurae, diaphragm, and chest wall.

accretion (ah-kre′shun) [L. *ad* to + *crescere* to grow] 1. growth by addition of material. 2. accumulation. 3. adherence of parts normally separated.

accuracy (ak′u-rah-se) the closeness of the expected value to the true value of the measured quantity; a measure of bias. Sometimes called *validity*. Cf. *precision*, def. 1.

ACD acid citrate dextrose.

ACE 1. angiotensin converting enzyme. See *dipeptidyl carboxypeptidase I.* 2. adrenocortical extract.

acebutolol (ah″se-bu′to-lōl) a cardioselective β_1-adrenergic blocking agent with uses similar to those of propranolol.

acecainide hydrochloride (as″ē-ka′nīd) chemical name: 4-(acetylamino)-*N*-[2-(diethylamino)ethyl]benzamide monohydrochloride; an antiarrhythmic cardiac depressant, $C_{15}H_{23}N_3O_2 \cdot HCl$.

aceclidine (as-sek′lĭ-dēn) a synthetic cholinergic agonist similar to the natural alkaloids arecoline and pilocarpine; used to reduce intraocular pressure in glaucoma.

acedapsone (as-ĕ-dap′sōn) chemical name: 4′,4‴-sulfonylbis[acetanilide]. The diacetyl derivative of dapsone, $C_{16}H_{16}N_2O_4S$, having actions similar to those of the parent compound; used as a leprostatic and antimalarial. Called also *diacetyl diaminodiphenylsulfone (DADDS).*

acedia (ah-se′de-ah) [*a* neg. + Gr. *kēdos* care + *-ia*] (*obs.*) a state of apathy and depression.

acellular (a-sel′u-lar) not made up of or containing cells.

acelomate (a-se′lo-māt) not having a coelom or body cavity.

acelous (a-se′lus) [*a* neg. + Gr. *koilos* hollow] not concave on either surface; said of the vertebrae of certain animals.

acenesthesia (ah-sen″es-the′ze-ah) [*a* neg. + *cenesthesia*] absence of the normal sense of physical existence and well-being and of the regular functioning of the bodily organs.

acenocoumarin (ah-se″no-koo′mah-rin) acenoumarol.

acenocoumarol (ah-se″no-koo′mah-rol) chemical name: 2*H*-1-benzopyran-2-one-4-hydroxy-3-[1-4(4-nitrophenyl)-3-oxobutyl]-3-α-(acetonyl-*p*-nitrobenzyl)-4-hydroxycoumarin. One of the synthetic coumarin anticoagulants, $C_{19}H_{15}NO_6$, occurring as an off-white to light tan powder, having a rapid onset, intermediate duration of action, and little cumulative effect; administered orally.

acentric (ah-sen′trik) [Gr. *akentrikos* not centric] 1. not central; not located in the center. 2. a chromosome lacking a centromere, so that the chromosome will not survive subsequent cell divisions.

ACEP American College of Emergency Physicians.

acephalia (ah″sĕ-fa′le-ah) [*a* neg. + Gr. *kephalē* head] congenital absence of the head.

Acephalina (ah-sef″ah-li′nah) [*a* neg. + Gr. *kephalē* head] in former systems of classification, a suborder of protozoa (order Eugregarinida) comprising aseptate gregarines, i.e., those in which the body is not compartmentalized. These organisms have been assigned to the suborders Blastogregarinina and Aseptatina.

acephalism (ah-sef′ah-lizm) acephalia.

acephalobrachia (ah-sef″ah-lo-bra′ke-ah) [*a* neg. + Gr. *kephalē* head + *brachiōn* arm + *-ia*] congenital absence of the head and arms.

acephalobrachius (ah-sef″ah-lo-bra′ke-us) a monster exhibiting acephalobrachia.

acephalocardia (ah-sef″ah-lo-kar′de-ah) [*a* neg. + Gr. *kephalē* head + *kardia* heart + *-ia*] congenital absence of the head and heart.

acephalocardius (ah-sef″ah-lo-kar′de-us) a monster exhibiting acephalocardia.

acephalochiria (ah-sef″ah-lo-ki′re-ah) [*a* neg. + Gr. *kephalē* head + *cheir* hand + *-ia*] congenital absence of the head and hands.

acephalochirus (ah-sef″ah-lo-ki′rus) a monster exhibiting acephalochiria.

acephalocyst (ah-sef″ah-lo′sist) [*a* neg. + Gr. *kephalē* head + *kystis* bladder] sterile cyst.

acephalogaster (ah-sef″ah-lo-gas′ter) [*a* neg. + Gr. *kephalē*

head + *gastēr* belly] a monster exhibiting acephalogastria.

acephalogastria (ah-sef″ah-lo-gas′tre-ah) congenital absence of the head, chest, and upper part of the abdomen.

acephalopodia (ah-sef″ah-lo-po′de-ah) [*a* neg. + Gr. *kephalē* head + *pous* foot + *-ia*] congenital absence of the head and feet.

acephalopodius (ah-sef″ah-lo-po′de-us) a monster exhibiting acephalopodia.

acephalorhachia (ah-sef″ah-lo-ra′ke-ah) [*a* neg. + Gr. *kephalē* head + *rhachis* spine + *-ia*] congenital absence of the head and vertebral column.

acephalostomia (ah-sef″ah-lo-sto′me-ah) [*a* neg. + Gr. *kephalē* head + *stoma* mouth + *-ia*] congenital absence of the head, yet with a kind of mouth on the superior aspect.

acephalostomus (ah-sef″ah-los′to-mus) a monster exhibiting acephalostomia.

acephalothoracia (ah-sef″ah-lo-tho-ra′se-ah) [*a* neg. + Gr. *kephalē* head + *thōrax* chest + *-ia*] congenital absence of the head and chest.

acephalothorus (ah-sef″ah-lo-tho′rus) a monster exhibiting acephalothoracia.

acephalous (ah-sef′ah-lus) headless.

acephalus (ah-sef′ah-lus), pl. *aceph′ali* [*a* neg. + Gr. *kephalē* head] a headless monster. **a. dibra′chius,** an acephalus with both upper limbs more or less undeveloped. **a. di′pus,** an acephalus with both lower limbs more or less undeveloped. **a. monobra′chius,** an acephalus with only one upper limb. **a. mon′opus,** an acephalus with only one foot or lower limb. **a. paraceph′alus,** a monster with a partially formed skull but no brain. **a. sym′pus,** an acephalus with the two lower limbs fused into one.

acephaly (ah-sef′ah-le) acephalia.

acepromazine maleate (ah″se-pro′mah-zēn) 1-[10-[3-(dimethylamino)propyl]-10*H*-phenothiazin-2-yl]ethanone (*Z*)-2-butenedioate(1:1). A tranquilizer, $C_{19}H_{22}N_2OS \cdot C_4H_4O_4$, used in veterinary medicine to immobilize large animals.

Aceraria (as″ĕ-ra′re-ah) a genus of nematode parasites. **A. spira′lis,** a nematode parasite occurring in growths in the esophagus of fowls.

acerin (ah′ser-in) an extract from the dried fruit of the Norway maple, *Acer plantanoides* L. (Aceraceae); effective against *Escherichia coli* and the vaccinia virus.

acerola (ah-sĕ-ro′lah) the West Indian cherry fruit (*Malpighia punicifolia* L., Malpighiaceae), thought to be the richest natural source of vitamin C (about 1690 mg. per 100 grams of pitted fruit). It is given in the diet of individuals allergic to citrus fruits.

acervuli (ah-ser′vu-li) [L.] plural of *acervulus.*

acervuline (ah-ser′vu-līn) [L. *acervulus* little heap] aggregated; said of certain glands.

acervulus (ah-ser′vu-lus), pl. *acer′vuli* [L., dim. of *acervus* a heap] the mass of gritty matter which lies in or near the pineal body, the choroid plexus, and other parts of the brain; called also *acervulus cerebri, brain sand,* and *sand bodies.*

acescence (ah-ses′ens) [L. *acescere* to become sour] 1. sourness. 2. the process of becoming sour.

acescent (ah-ses′ent) somewhat or slightly acid.

acesodyne (ah-ses′o-dīn) [Gr. *akesis* cure + *odynē* pain] anodyne; allaying pain.

acestoma (ah″ses-to′mah) [Gr. *akesis* cure + *-oma*] (*obs.*) a mass of granulations.

acetabula (as″ĕ-tab′u-lah) plural of *acetabulum.*

acetabular (as″ĕ-tab′u-lar) pertaining to the acetabulum.

Acetabularia (as″ĕ-tab″u-la′re-ah) a genus of large single-celled green algae having a foot, a stalk, and a cap. *A. mediterra′nea* and *A. crenula′ta* have been used in genetic experiments.

acetabulectomy (as″ĕ-tab″u-lek′to-me) [*acetabulum* + Gr. *ektomē* excision] excision of the acetabulum.

acetabuloplasty (as″ĕ-tab′u-lo-plas″te) [*acetabulum* + Gr. *plassein* to form] plastic reconstruction of the acetabulum.

acetabulum (as″ĕ-tab′u-lum), pl. *acetab′ula* [L. "vinegar-cruet," from *acetum* vinegar] [NA] the large cup-shaped cavity on the lateral surface of the os coxae in which the head of the femur articulates; called also *acetabular bone, cotyloid cavity,* and *os acetabuli.* **sunken a.,** Otto pelvis.

acetal (as′ĕ-tal) an organic compound formed by a combination of an aldehyde with an alcohol.

acetaldehyde (as″et-al′dĕ-hīd″) a colorless flammable liquid, CH_3CHO, with a pungent odor, used in the manufacture of acetic acid, perfumes, and flavors. It is also an intermediate in the metabolism of alcohol. Acetaldehyde may cause irritation of mucous membranes, lacrimation, photophobia, conjunctivitis, corneal injury, rhinitis, anosmia, bronchitis, pneumonia, pleurisy, headache, and unconsciousness. Called also *acetic aldehyde, ethanal,* and *ethylaldehyde.*

acetaldehyde dehydrogenase (as″ĕ-tal′dĕ-hīd de-hi′-dro-jen-ās) aldehyde dehydrogenase (NAD^+).

acetaldehyde reductase (as″ĕ-tal′dĕ-hīd re-duk′tās) alcohol dehydrogenase (NAD^+).

acetamide (ah-set′ah-mīd) a white crystalline substance, CH_3CONH_2, used in organic synthesis and as a general solvent when melted.

acetamidine (as″et-am′ĭ-dīn) chemical name: α-amino-α-iminoethane. The imine, $CH_3CH(NH)NH_2$, of acetamide, used in the synthesis of imidazoles and pyrimidines.

p-acetamidobenzene sulfonamide (as″et-am″ĭ-do-ben′zēn sul-fon′ah-mīd) one of the conjugated forms in which benzene sulfonamide is excreted in the urine.

acetaminophen (ah-set″ah-me′no-fen) [USP] chemical name: *N*-(4-hydroxyphenyl) acetamide. The amide of acetic acid and *p*-aminophenol, a nonprescription drug having analgesic and antipyretic effects similar to aspirin but only weak anti-inflammatory effects. Called also *paractamol* [INN, BAN].

acetanilid (as″et-an′il-id) [*acetic* + *aniline*] chemical name: *N*-phenylacetamide; it is a white, crystalline, sublimable solid, $C_6H_5NH \cdot OC \cdot CH_3$, produced by combining glacial acetic acid with aniline. It is the parent drug of the para-aminophenol derivatives (phenacetin, acetaminophen); it has analgesic and antipyretic actions but is excessively toxic. Called also *acetylaminobenzene, acetaniline,* and *antifebrin.*

acetaniline (as″et-an′il-ēn) acetanilid.

acetannin (as″ĕ-tan′in) acetyltannic acid.

acetarsol (as″et-ar′sol) acetarsone.

acetarsone (as″et-ar′sōn) chemical name: 3-acetamido-hydroxyphenyl arsonic acid. A pentavalent arsenical, $C_8H_{10}As-NO_5$, occurring as a white, crystalline powder. It is used orally in the treatment of intestinal amebiasis, orally and topically in necrotizing ulcerative gingivitis, and topically in trichomonas vaginitis. Called also *acetphenarsine.*

acetas (ah-se′tas) [L.] acetate.

acetate (as′ĕ-tāt) a salt or ester or the conjugate base of acetic acid.

acetazolamide (as″et-ah-zol′ah-mīd) [USP] chemical name: *N*-[5-(aminosulfonyl)-1,3,4-thiadiazol-2-yl]acetamide. A white to faintly yellowish white crystalline powder, $C_4H_6-N_4O_3S_2$, it is a diuretic of the carbonic anhydrase inhibitor type, useful in treatment of carbon dioxide retention in chronic lung disease, to reduce intraocular pressure in glaucoma, and formerly in management of edema associated with heart disease. **sodium a., sterile** [USP], a preparation suitable for parenteral use, prepared from acetazolamide with the aid of sodium hydroxide, $C_4H_5N_4NaO_3S_2$, and containing between 95 and 110 per cent of the labeled amount of acetazolamide.

acetenyl (ah-se′tĕ-nil) ethynyl.

Acetest (ah′sĕ-test) trademark for reagent tablets containing sodium nitroprusside, aminoacetic acid, disodium phosphate, and lactose. A drop of urine is placed on a tablet on a sheet of white paper; if significant quantities of acetone are present the tablet changes from a purple tint (1+), to lavender (2+), to moderate purple (3+), or deep purple (4+).

aceteugenol (as″et-u′jĕ-nol) an essential oil from oil of cloves: 1-ethyl, 3-methoxy, 4-acetoxy benzene.

acetic (ah-se′tik, ah-set′ik) pertaining to vinegar or its acid; sour. **a. aldehyde,** acetaldehyde.

acetic acid (ah-se′tik) the two-carbon carboxylic acid, CH_3COOH, which is the characteristic component of vinegar; and, mostly in the form of acetylcoenzyme A, an important biochemical intermediate. Systematic name: *ethanoic acid.* **glacial a.a.,** 99.8 per cent pure acetic acid.

aceticoceptor (ah-se″te-ko-sep′tor) a ceptor or side chain having specific affinity for the acetic acid radical.

acetify (ah-set′ĭ-fi) to turn into acetic acid or vinegar.

acetimeter (as″ĕ-tim′ĕ-ter) [L. *acetum* vinegar + Gr. *metron* measure] an apparatus for determining the amount of acetic acid present in a solution.

acetin (as′ĕ-tin) a glyceryl acetate; it may contain one, two, or three acetyl groups.

Acetivibrio (ah-se″tĭ-vib′re-o) [*aceto-* + *vibrio*] a genus of anaerobic, gram-negative, straight or slightly curved rod-shaped bacteria of the family Bacteroidaceae, made up of cells that are motile with flagella and produce acetic acid as the principal acid from carbohydrates. The organisms are found in the intestines of pigs. The type species is *A. cellulolyticus.*

acetoacetic acid (ah-se″to-ah-se′tik; as″ĕ-to-ah-se′tik) 3-oxobutanoic acid, CH_3COCH_2COOH, one of the ketone bodies (q.v.) produced in diabetic ketoacidosis; called also *diacetic acid* and *β-ketobutyric acid.*

acetoacetyl-CoA (as″ĕ-to-as′ĕ-til, ah-se′to-as-ĕ-tēl″) acetoacetyl coenzyme A.

acetoacetyl-CoA reductase (as″ĕ-to-as′ĕ-til ko′a re-duk′tās) [EC 1.1.1.36] an enzyme of the oxidoreductase class that catalyzes the reaction 3-oxoacyl-CoA + NADPH = D-3-hydroxyacyl-CoA + $NADP^+$. It is a part of the fatty acid synthase complex.

acetoacetyl-CoA thiolase (as″ĕ-to-as′ĕ-til, ah-se′to-as-ĕ-tēl″ ko″a′ thi′o-lās) acetyl-CoA acetyltransferase.

acetoacetyl coenzyme A (ah-se″to-as′ĕ-til, ah-se′to-as-ĕ-tēl″ ko-en′zīm) a thioester of acetoacetic acid and coenzyme A. It is an important metabolic intermediate in the oxidation of fatty acids, as a fuel for the citric acid cycle in brain and nervous tissue, and as a precursor of cholesterol. Abbreviated acetoacetyl-CoA.

acetoacetyl thiolase (as″ĕ-to-as′ĕ-til, ah-se′to-as-ĕ-tēl thi′ol-ās) acetyl-CoA acetyltransferase.

Acetobacter (ah-se″to-bak′ter) [L. *acetum* vinegar + Gr. *baktron* a rod] a genus of gram-negative, aerobic, rod-shaped bacteria of the family Acetobacteraceae made up of nonsporogenous organisms that produce acetic acid from ethanol. They are found in fruits, vegetables, souring juices, and alcoholic beverages. The type species is *A. aceti.*

Acetobacteraceae (ah-se″to-bak-tĕ-ra′se-e) a family of gram-negative, aerobic, ellipsoidal to rod-shaped bacteria that form acetic acid. It includes the genera *Acetobacter* and *Gluconobacter.*

acetoform (ah-se′to-form) methenamine.

acetohexamide (as″ĕ-to-heks′ah-mīd) [USP] a first-generation sulphonylurea, an oral hypoglycemic agent with uses and actions similar to those of chlorpropamide.

acetohydroxamic acid (as″ĕ-to-hi″droks-am′ik as′id) a bacterial enzyme blocker used in the treatment of struvite renal calculi.

acetoin (ah-set′o-in) acetylmethylcarbinol: a ketone product formed in the fermentation of glucose by certain bacteria, especially species of Enterobacteriaceae, and detected by the Voges-Proskauer reaction.

acetokinase (as″ĕ-to-ki′nās) acetate kinase.

acetolysis (as″ĕ-tol′ĭ-sis) combined hydrolysis and acetylation.

acetomeroctol (as″ĕ-to-mer-ok′tol) chemical name: 2-acetoxymercuri-4(1,1,3,3-tetramethylbutyl) phenol; a crystalline substance, $C_{16}H_{24}HgO_3$, formerly used as a topical antiseptic.

acetometer (as″ĕ-tom′ĕ-ter) acetimeter.

acetomorphine (as″ĕ-to-mor′fēn) diacetylmorphine.

acetonaphthone (as″e-to-naf′thōn) an acetyl derivative of naphthalene, $C_{10}H_7COCH_3$, occurring in two isomeric forms. The 2-acetonaphthone isomer is a mosquito repellent; derivatives are used as bactericides and as an antitubercular agent.

acetonasthma (as″ĕ-tōn-az′mah) (*obs.*) air hunger due to acidosis.

acetonation (as″ĕ-to-na′shun) combination with acetone.

acetone (as′ĕ-tōn) dimethyl ketone, CH_3COCH_3, a flammable colorless, volatile liquid with a pleasant ethereal odor, which is a commonly used solvent and one of the ketone bodies (q.v.) produced in diabetic ketoacidosis. **a. diethyl-sulfone,** sulfonmethane.

acetonemia (as″ĕ-to-ne′me-ah) [*acetone* + Gr. *haima* blood

+ -ia] an excess of acetone bodies in the blood; now called *ketonemia.*

acetonemic (as″ĕ-to-ne′mik) pertaining to or marked by acetonemia.

acetonglycosuria (as″ĕ-tōn″gli-ko-su′re-ah) glycosuria due to acetone poisoning.

acetonitrile (as″ĕ-to-ni′tril) a poisonous colorless liquid, CH_3CN, with an ether-like odor; see also *Hunt's reaction,* under *reaction.*

acetonum (as″ĕ-to′num) [L.] acetone.

acetonumerator (as″ĕ-to-nu″mer-a″tor) an instrument for estimating the amount of acetone in the urine.

acetonuria (as″ĕ-to-nu′re-ah) an excess of acetone bodies in the urine; it occurs in diabetes, fever, starvation, carcinoma, and digestive disorders. Now called *ketonuria.*

aceto-orcein (as′ĕ-to-or′se-in) orcein dissolved in acetic acid, used in making squash preparations of polytene chromosomes.

acetophenazine maleate (as″ĕ-to-fen′ah-zēn) [USP] chemical name: 10-[3-[4-(2-hydroxyethyl)-1-piperazinyl]propyl]phenothiazin-2-yl methyl ketone maleate. A fine, yellow powder, $C_{23}H_{29}N_3O_2S \cdot 2C_4H_4O_4$, used as a major tranquilizer.

acetophenetidin (as″ĕ-to-fĕ-net′ĭ-din) phenacetin.

acetosal (ah-se′to-sal) aspirin.

acetosoluble (as″ĕ-to-sol′u-b'l) soluble in acetic acid.

acetosulfone sodium (as″ĕ-to-sul′fōn) chemical name: N-[[5-amino-2-[(4-aminophenyl)sulfonyl]phenyl]sulfonyl]acetamide monosodium salt. An antibacterial derivative of dapsone, $C_{14}N_{14}N_3NaO_5S_2$, having actions similar to those of the parent compound, occurring as a white to pinkish-white crystalline powder; used as leprostatic in lepromatous and tuberculoid leprosy and as a dermatitis herpetiformis suppressant, administered orally.

acetous (as′ĕ-tus) [L. *acetosus*] pertaining to, producing, or resembling acetic acid.

acetphenarsine (as″et-fen-ar′sēn) acetarsone.

acetphenetidin (as″et-fĕ-net′ĭ-din) phenacetin.

acetpyrogall (as″et-pi′ro-gal) chemical name: pyrogallol triacetate. A white crystalline compound, $C_6H_3(CH_3CO_2)_3$, used as a topical caustic and keratolytic.

acetract (as′ĕ-trakt) (*obs.*) an extract of a drug made with a menstruum containing acetic acid.

acetrizoate (as″ĕ-tri-zo′āt) a water-soluble, iodinated radiographic contrast medium, used as *sodium acetrizoate* in hysterosalpingography.

acetrizoic acid (as″ĕ-tri-zo′ik) the free acid of acetrizoate.

acetum (ah-se′tum), pl. *ace′ta* [L.] 1. vinegar. 2. a medicinal solution of a drug in dilute acetic acid. **a. plum′bi, a. satur′ni,** lead subacetate solution.

aceturate (ah-set′u-rāt) USAN contraction for N-acetylglycinate.

acetyl (as′ĕ-til) [L. *acetum* vinegar + Gr. *hylē* matter] the monovalent radical, CH_3CO. **a. chloride,** a colorless liquid, $CH_3 \cdot CO \cdot Cl$, used as a reagent for forming acetate esters of alcohols. **a. peroxide,** diacetyl peroxide. **a. sulfisoxazole,** chemical name: N^1-acetyl-N^1-(3,4-dimethyl-5-isoxazolyl)sulfanilamide. Tasteless crystals, $C_{13}H_{15}N_3O_4S$, used as an antimicrobial.

acetylaminobenzene (as″ĕ-til-am″ĭ-no-ben′zēn) acetanilid.

acetylaminobenzene sulfonate (as″ĕ-til-am″ĭ-no-ben′zēn) a compound, $CH_3 \cdot CO \cdot NH \cdot C_6H_4 \cdot SO_2 \cdot NH_2$, the form in which sulfanilamide is excreted.

acetylaminofluorene (as″ĕ-til-am″ĭ-no-floo′o-rēn) a compound, $C_6H_4CH_2C_6H_3NH \cdot CO \cdot CH_3$, which is carcinogenic when ingested.

acetylase (ah-set′ĭ-las) *acetyltransferase.*

acetylation (ah-set″ĭ-la′shun) the introduction of an acetyl group into the molecule of an organic compound.

acetylator (ah-set″ĭ-la′tor) an organism capable of metabolic acetylation; in man, acetylator status (fast or slow) is determined by the rate of acetylation of sulfamethazine.

acetylcholine (as″ĕ-til-ko′lēn) a reversible acetic acid ester of choline, $CH_3 \cdot CO \cdot O \cdot CH_2 \cdot CH_2 \cdot N(CH_3)_3 \cdot OH$, and a cholinergic agonist serving as a neurotransmitter at the myoneural junctions of striated muscles, at autonomic effector cells innervated by parasympathetic nerves, at the preganglionic synapses of the sympathetic and parasympathetic nervous systems, and at various sites in the central nervous system. ACh has few therapeutic applications owing to its diffuse action and rapid hydrolysis by acetylcholinesterase (AChE); synthetic derivatives are used for more specific, prolonged action. **a. chloride,** a miotic administered by instillation into the anterior chamber of the eye.

acetylcholinesterase (as″ĕ-til-ko″lin-es′ter-ās, as-ĕ-tēl′ko-lin-es″ter-ās) [EC 3.1.1.7] an enzyme of the hydrolase class that catalyzes the reaction acetylcholine $+ H_2O =$ choline $+$ acetate. It is found in the gray matter of nerve tissue, in red blood cells, and in the motor endplates of skeletal muscle. The reaction destroys acetylcholine released at neurohumoral junctions, thus permitting recovery for transmission of further impulses. Called also *choline esterase I* and *true cholineaterase.* Abbreviated AChE. Cf. *cholineaterase.*

acetyl-CoA acetylcoenzyme A.

acetyl-CoA acetyltransferase (as′ĕ-til, as-ĕ-tēl′, ko″a′ as″ĕ-til, as-ĕ-tēl′, trans′fer-ās) [EC 2.3.1.9] an enzyme of the transferase class that catalyzes the reaction acetoacetyl-coenzyme A $+$ CoA $=$ acetyl-CoA $+$ acetyl-CoA. The reaction generates two-carbon units from the four-carbon product of fatty acid oxidation. The reverse reaction occurs in the synthesis of acetoacetate or cholesterol. Called also *acetoacetyl-CoA thiolase* and *acetoacetyl thiolase.*

acetyl-CoA acyltransferase (as′ĕ-til, as-ĕ-tēl′, ko″a′ a″sil-trans′fer-ās) [EC 2.3.1.16] an enzyme of the transferase class that catalyzes the reaction 3-oxoacyl coenzyme A $+$ CoA $=$ acyl-CoA $+$ acetyl-CoA. It catalyzes the conversion of fatty acid chains to two-carbon units during fatty acid oxidation.

acetyl-CoA carboxylase (as′ĕ-til, as-ĕ-tēl, ko″a′ karbok′sĭ-lās) [EC 6.4.1.2] an enzyme of the ligase class that catalyzes the reaction ATP $+$ acetyl-CoA $+$ CO_2 $+$ H_2O = ADP $+$ orthophosphate $+$ malonyl-CoA. It is a biotin-protein. The reaction is the key rate-controlling step in the synthesis of fatty acids from acetyl groups.

acetyl-CoA: α-glucosaminide-N-acetyltransferase (as′ĕ-til, as-ĕ-tēl, ko″a′ gloo″kōs-am″ĭ-nīd as′ĕ-til, as-ĕ-tēl″trans′fer-ās) heparan-α-glucosaminide acetyltransferase.

acetyl-CoA: heparan-α-D-glucosaminide N-acetyltransferase (as′ĕ-til, as-ĕ-tēl″, ko″a′ hep′ah-ran gloo″kōs-am″ĭ-nīd as′ĕ-til, as-ĕtēl″, trans″fer-ās) heparan-α-glucosaminide acetyltransferase.

acetyl coenzyme A (as″ĕ-til, as-ĕ-tēl″, ko-en′zīm) acetyl-CoA, a thiol ester of coenzyme A and acetic acid. Acetyl groups derived from carbohydrates, fatty acids, and amino acids appear as acetyl coenzyme A, then enter the citric (tricarboxylic) acid cycle where they are oxidized to CO_2 and H_2O. Excess acetyl coenzyme A may be converted to fats for storage.

acetylcysteine (as″ĕ-til-sis′te-in) [USP] chemical name: N-acetyl-L-cysteine. A white, crystalline powder, $C_5H_9NO_3S$, used as a mucolytic agent for adjunct therapy in bronchopulmonary disorders to reduce the viscosity of mucus and facilitate its removal. Administered by instillation or nebulization.

acetyldigitoxin (as″ĕ-til-dij″ĭ-tok′sin) chemical name: $(3,\beta,5,\beta)$-3-[(O-2,6-dideoxy-β-D-*ribo*-hexopyranosyl-(1 → 4)-O-2,6-dideoxy-β-D-*ribo*-hexopyranosyl)-1(1 → 4)-2,6-dideoxy-β-D-ribo-hexopyranosyl)oxy]-14-hydroxy-card-20(22)-enolide monoacetate. A derivative of digitalis, $C_{43}H_{66}O_{14}$, obtained from lantoside A, composed of the aglycone digitoxigenin and three molecules of digitoxose, to one of which an acetyl group is attached; used as a cardiotonic.

acetylene (ah-set′ĭ-lēn) a colorless, volatile, explosive gas, C_2H_4; it is the simplest of a class of unsaturated (triple-bonded) hydrocarbons, the alkynes.

N-acetylgalactosamine-4-sulfatase (as″ĕ-til, as-ĕ-tēl″, gah-lak-to′sah-mēn sul′fah′tās) [EC 3.1.6.12] an enzyme that catalyzes the reaction N-acetylgalactosamine-4-sulfate $+$ H_2O = N-acetylgalactosamine $+$ sulfate. A genetic deficiency of the enzyme, transmitted as an autosomal recessive trait, results in mucopolysaccharidosis type VI (see *Maroteaux-Lamy syndrome,* under *syndrome*).

N-acetylgalactosamine-4-sulfatase deficiency Maroteaux-Lamy syndrome.

N-acetylgalactosamine-6-sulfatase (as″ĕ-til, as-ĕ-tēl″,

gah-lak-tōs'ah-mēn sul'fah-tās) [EC 3.1.6.4]   an enzyme of the hydrolase class that catalyzes the hydrolysis of 6-sulfate groups of the *N*-acetyl-D-galactosamine 6-sulfate units of chondroitin sulfate and of the D-galactose 6-sulfate units of keratan sulfate. Deficiency of the enzyme, transmitted as an autosomal recessive trait, results in Morquio's syndrome type A (mucopolysaccharidosis IV A). Called also *chondroitinsulfatase*.

α-N-acetylgalactosaminidase (as''ĕ-til, as-ĕ-tēl'', gah-lak''tōs-ah-min'ĭ-dās) [EC 3.2.1.49]   an enzyme of the hydrolase class that catalyzes the hydrolysis of terminal nonreducing *N*-acetyl-D-galactosamine residues in *N*-acetyl-α-D-galactosaminides. Called also *α-D-galactosidase B*.

β-N-acetylgalactosaminidase (as'e-til, as-e-tēl'', galak''tōs-ah-min'i-dās) [EC 3.2.1.53]   an enzyme of the hydrolase class that catalyzes the reaction R-2-acetamido-2-deoxy-β-D-galactoside H_2O = ROH + 2-acetamido-2-deoxy-D-galactose. The reaction breaks down the GM_2 gangliosides of sphingolipids. The enzyme occurs as two isozymes, A (α$β_2$) and B B$_4$ (hexosaminidases A and B). An autosomal recessive genetic defect in isozyme A (α-chain) results in Tay-Sachs disease. A genetic defect in isozymes A and B (β-chains), also an autosomal recessive trait, results in Sandhoff's disease. Called also *N-acetyl-β-hexosaminidase A*.

N-acetylglucosamine-6-sulfatase (as''ĕ-til, as-ĕ-tēl'', gloo-kōs'ah-mēn sul'fah-tās) [EC 3.1.6.14]   an enzyme of the hydrolase class that catalyzes the hydrolysis of the *N*-acetyl-D-glucosamine-6-sulfate groups of heparan sulfate and keratan sulfate. The reaction is a step in the degradation of heparan sulfate. A defect in the enzyme, an autosomal recessive trait, results in the Sanfilippo syndrome, type D. Called also *N-acetyl-α-D-glucosaminide-6-sulfatase*.

α-N-acetylglucosaminidase (as'e-til, as-ĕ-tēl'', gloo-kōs''ah-min'i-dās) [EC 3.2.1.50]   an enzyme of the hydrolase class that catalyzes the reaction R-2-acetamido-2-deoxy-α-D-glucoside + H_2O = ROH + 2-acetamido-2-deoxy-D-glucose. The reaction is necessary for the breakdown of heparan sulfate. A genetic defect in the enzyme, transmitted as an autosomal recessive trait, results in Sanfilippo syndrome, type B.

N-acetyl-α-D-glucosaminide-6-sulfatase (as''ĕ-til, as-ĕ-tēl'', gloo-kōs'ah-min-īd'')   *N*-acetylglucosamine-6-sulfatase.

N-acetylglucosaminylphosphotransferase (as''ĕ-til, as-ĕ-tēl'', gloo-kōs-am''ĭ-nil-fos''fo-trans'fer-ās)   UDP-*N*-acetylglucosamine-lysosomal-enzyme *N*-acetylglucosaminephosphotransferase.

N-acetyl-β-hexosaminidase A (as''ĕ-til, as-ĕ-tēl'', hek''sōs-am-in'ĭ-dās)   β-*N*-acetyl-D-galactosaminidase, isoenzyme A.

acetylization (ah-set''il-i-za'shun)   acetylation.

acetylmethadol (as''ĕ-til-meth'ah-dol)   methadyl acetate.

N-acetylneuraminate lyase (as''ĕ-til, as-ĕ-tēl'', nūr'-am''ĭ-nāt li'ās) [EC 4.1.3.3]   an enzyme of the lyase class that catalyzes the reaction *N*-acetylneuraminate-2-acetamido-2-deoxy-D-mannose + pyruvate. The substrate is a sialic acid anion.

N-acetylneuraminic acid (as''ĕ-til-nu''rah-min'ĭk)   a complex amino sugar occurring in many glycoproteins and polysaccharrides; it is formed by condensation of *N*-acetyl-D-mannosamine and pyruvate.

acetylphenylhydrazine (as''ĕ-til-fen''il-hi-dra'zēn)   chemical name: β-acetylphenylhydrazine. A compound, $C_8H_{10}N_2O$, that has been used as an oral erythrocyte depressant in the treatment of polycythemia vera and was once used as an antipyretic. Called also *hydracetin*.

acetylsalicylic acid (ah-se'til-sal''ah-sil''ik)   chemical name for aspirin. Abbreviated ASA.

acetylstrophanthidin (as''ĕ-til-stro-fan'thĭ-din)   a synthetic fast-acting digitalis-like preparation.

acetylsulfadiazine (as''ĕ-til-sul''fah-di'ah-zēn)   the form in which sulfadiazine is excreted in the urine, often occurring in dark green crystalline spheres.

acetylsulfaguanidine (as''ĕ-til-sul''fah-gwan'ĭ-dēn)   the form in which sulfaguanidine is excreted in the urine, often occurring in thin oblong crystalline plates.

acetylsulfanilamide (as''ĕ-til-sul''fah-nil'ah-mīd)   1. N^1-acetylsulfanilamide (see *sulfacetamide*). 2. N^4-acetyl-

sulfanilamide, $C_8H_{10}O_3S$, the acetylated (unconjugated) sulfanilamide as it appears in the body after administration.

acetylsulfathiazole (as''ĕ-til-sul''fah-thi'ah-zōl)   the form in which sulfathiazole is excreted in the urine, often occurring in the form of sheaves-of-wheat crystals.

acetyltannic acid (as''e-tēl-tan'ik)   the diacetyl ester of tannic acid; formerly used as an antiperistaltic in the treatment of diarrhea.

acetyltannin (as''ĕ-til-tan'in)   acetyltannic acid.

acetyltransferase (as''ĕ-til-trans'fer-ās) [EC 2.3.1]   one of a sub-subclass of enzymes of the transferase class that catalyze the transfer of an acetyl group, often acetyl-CoA, to another compound. Those forming esters or amides are also called *acetylases*.

A.C.G.   American College of Gastroenterology; angiocardiography.

AcG   accelerator globulin (coagulation Factor V; see under *factor*).

ACh   acetylcholine.

A.C.H.A.   American College of Hospital Administrators.

achalasia (ak''ah-la'ze-ah) [*a* neg + Gr. *chalasis* relaxation + -*ia*]   failure to relax of the smooth muscle fibers of the gastrointestinal tract at any point of junction of one part with another. Especially the failure of the esophagogastric sphincter to relax with swallowing, due to degeneration of ganglion cells in the wall of the organ. The thoracic esophagus also loses its normal peristaltic activity and becomes dilated (megaesophagus). Called also *cardiospasm*. **pelvirectal a.,** congenital megacolon. **sphincteral a.,** failure of any sphincter of a tubular organ to relax in response to a normal physiological stimulus.

Achard's syndrome (ash-arz')   [Émile Charles *Achard*, French physician, 1860–1941]   see under *syndrome*.

Achard-Thiers syndrome (ash-ar' tērz')   [Émile Charles *Achard*; Joseph *Thiers*, French physician, born 1885]   see under *syndrome*.

Achatina (ak''ah-ti'nah)   a genus of very large land snails. **A. fuli'ca,** a giant land snail that serves as an intermediate host of the rat lungworm, *Angiostrongylus cantonensis*, the causative agent of eosinophilic meningitis.

AChE   acetylcholinesterase.

ache (āk)   1. to suffer a continuous pain. 2. a continuous, fixed pain, as distinguished from twinges.

acheilia (ah-ki''le-ah) [*a* neg. + Gr. *cheilos* lip + -*ia*]   congenital absence of one or both lips.

acheilous (ah-ki'lus)   lacking lips; exhibiting acheilia.

acheiria (ah-ki''re-ah) [*a* neg. + Gr. *cheir* hand + -*ia*]   congenital absence of one or both hands.

acheiropodia (ah-ki''ro-po'de-ah) [*a* neg. + Gr. *cheir* hand + *pous* foot + -*ia*]   congenital absence of hands and feet.

acheirus (ah-ki'rus) [L.]   an individual exhibiting acheiria.

Achillea (ak''ĭ-le'ah) [L.; Gr. *achilleia*]   a genus of composite-flowered plants. *A. millefolium*, milfoil, has been used as a bitter and stimulant tonic; it contains an essential oil and a bitter alkaloid, achilleine.

Achilles bursa, jerk (reflex), tendon (ah-kil'ēz) [Gr. *Achilleus* Greek hero, whose mother held him by the ankle to dip him in the Styx]   see *bursa tendinis calcanei* [*Achillis*], *triceps surae* jerk, under *jerk*, and *tendo calcaneus*.

Achillini (ak''ĭ-le'ne)   Alessandro (1463–1512)   a celebrated Bolognese physician and philosopher who left several works on anatomy.

achillobursitis (ah-kil''o-bur-si'tis) [*Achilles* + Gr. *byrsa* bursa + -*itis*]   inflammation and thickening of the bursae about the Achilles tendon, especially of the bursa in front of it; called also *achillodynia*.

achillodynia (ak''ĭ-lo-din'e-ah) [*Achilles* (tendon) + Gr. *odynē* pain + -*ia*]   pain in the Achilles tendon or in its bursa; achilloburitis.

achillorrhaphy (ak''ĭ-lor'ah-fe) [*Achilles* (tendon) + Gr. *rhaphē* suture]   suture of the Achilles tendon.

achillotenotomy (ah-kil''o-ten-ot'o-me) [*Achilles* + Gr. *tenōn* tendon + *tomē* cut]   surgical division of the Achilles tendon. **plastic a.,** elongation of the Achilles tendon by plastic operation.

achillotomy (ak''ĭ-lot'o-me)   achillotenotomy.

achiria (ah-ki're-ah)   acheiria.

achirus (ah-ki′rus) acheirus.

achlorhydria (ah″klor-hi′dre-ah) [*a* neg. + *chlorhydria*] absence of hydrochloric acid from maximally stimulated gastric secretions; a result of gastric mucosal atrophy. Called also *gastric anacidity*. **a. apep′sia** (*obs.*), absence of pepsinogens in secretions of the stomach.

achlorhydric (ah″klor-hi′drik) characterized by achlorhydria.

Achlya (ak′le-ah) a genus of phycomycetous fungi of the order Saprolegniales, subclass Oomycetes, which form molds on certain fish and insects.

Acholeplasma (a″ko-le-plaz′mah)[*a*-neg. + Gr. *cholē*bile + *plasma*] a genus of bacteria of the family Acholeplasmataceae, order Mycoplasmatales, class Mollicutes, made up of spherical cells bounded by a triple-layered membrane but lacking a cell wall, and not requiring serum or cholesterol for growth. **A. granula′rum**, a species found in the nasal cavities of swine and reported to have been isolated from the synovial fluid of arthritic pigs. Called also *Mycoplasma granularum*. **A. laidlaw′ii**, a species isolated from various human clinical specimens, from the body cavities of cattle, swine, and birds, and from soils. Called also *M. laidlawii*.

Acholeplasmataceae (a-ko″le-plaz″mah-ta′se-e) a family of bacteria of the order Mycoplasmatales, class Mollicutes, made up of organisms that do not require sterol for growth. It contains the genus *Acholeplasma*.

acholia (ah-ko′le-ah) [*a* neg. + Gr. *cholē* bile + *-ia*] absence or failure of secretion of bile.

acholic (ah-kol′ik) free from bile.

acholuria (ah-ko-lu′re-ah)[*a* neg. + Gr. *cholē* bile + *ouron* urine + *-ia*] lack of bile pigment in the urine.

acholuric (ah-ko-lu′rik) pertaining to or characterized by acholuria, as acholuric jaundice.

achondrogenesis (ah-kon″dro-jen′ĕ-sis) a hereditary disorder characterized by hypoplasia of bone, resulting in markedly shortened limbs; the head and trunk are normal.

achondroplasia (ah-kon″dro-pla′ze-ah) [*a* neg. + Gr. *chondros* cartilage + *plassein* to form + *-ia*] a hereditary, congenital disturbance of epiphyseal chondroblastic growth and maturation, causing inadequate enchondral bone formation and resulting in a peculiar form of dwarfism with short limbs, normal trunk, small face, normal vault, lordosis, and trident hand. It may be accompanied by other anomalies. See also *achondroplastic dwarf*, under *dwarf*.

achondroplastic (ah-kon″dro-plas′tik) pertaining to, or affected with, achondroplasia.

achondroplasty (ah-kon′dro-plas″te) achondroplasia.

achordal (a-kor′dal) achordate.

achordate (a-kor′dāt) without a notochord; used with reference to animals which are not chordates.

achoresis (ak″o-re′sis) [*a* neg. + Gr. *chōrein* to hold] (*obs.*) diminution of the capacity of a hollow organ.

Achorion (ah-ko′re-on) *Trichophyton*.

achrestic (ah-kres′tik) [Gr. *achrēstia* the nonusance of a thing] pertaining to the lack of use of a principle which is present in the body, as in achrestic anemia, a condition in which the body is unable to use the antianemic principle.

achroacytosis (ak″ro″ah-si-to′sis)[*a* neg. + Gr. *chroa* color + *kytos* hollow vessel + *-osis*] a term once used to designate pathologically excessive numbers of lymphocytes in organs, as in Mikulicz's disease.

achromasia (ak″ro-ma′se-ah)[*a* neg. + Gr. *chrōma* color + *-ia*] 1. lack of normal pigmentation of the skin. 2. absence of the usual staining reaction in a tissue or cell.

achromat (ak′ro-mat) [*a* neg. + *chromatic*] 1. an achromatic objective. 2. monochromat.

achromate (ah-kro′māt) monochromat.

Achromatiaceae (ak″ro-ma″she-a′se-e) a family of gliding bacteria of uncertain affiliation, made up of cells that are spherical to ovoid, or short cylinders with hemispherical ends, not possessing photosynthetic pigments. It includes a single genus, *Achromatium*.

achromatic (ak″ro-mat′ik) [*a* neg. + Gr. *chrōmatikos* pertaining to color] 1. producing no discoloration. 2. staining with difficulty. 3. containing achromatin. 4. refracting light without decomposing it into its component colors. 5. monochromatic, def. 2.

achromatin (ah-kro′mah-tin) [*a* neg. + Gr. *chrōma* color] the faintly staining substance forming the karyolymph, linin, and nuclear membrane of the nucleus of a cell.

achromatinic (ah-kro″mah-tin′ik) pertaining to or containing achromatin.

achromatism (ah-kro″mah-tizm″) 1. the quality or condition of being achromatic. 2. monochromatism.

Achromatium (ak″ro-ma′she-um) [*a* neg. + Gr. *chrōma* color] a genus of gliding bacteria of the provisional family Achromatiaceae, found in fresh water and marine mud, made up of spherical to ovoid or cylindrical cells, sometimes containing sulfur and calcium carbonate inclusions. The type species is *A. oxalif′erum*.

achromatize (ah-kro′mah-tīz) to render achromatic.

achromatolysis (ah-kro″mah-tol′ĭ-sis) [*achromatin* + Gr. *lysis* dissolution] disorganization of the achromatin of a cell.

achromatophil (ah″kro-mat′o-fil) [*a* neg. + Gr. *chrōma* color + *philein* to love] 1. having no affinity for stains. 2. an organism or tissue element that does not stain easily.

achromatophilia (ah-kro″mah-to-fil′e-ah) the property of resisting the coloring action of stains.

achromatopsia (ah-kro″mah-top′se-ah) monochromatism.

achromatosis (ah-kro″mah-to′sis) [*a* neg. + Gr. *chrōma* color + *-osis*] 1. deficiency of pigmentation in the tissues, as in the skin and the iris. 2. lack of staining power in a cell or tissue.

achromatous (ah-kro′mah-tus) having no color; colorless.

achromaturia (ah-kro″mah-tu′re-ah)[*a* neg. + Gr. *chrōma* color + *ouron* urine + *-ia*] the excretion of colorless urine.

achromia (ah-kro′me-ah)[*a* neg. + Gr. *chrōma* color + *-ia*] the lack or absence of normal color or pigmentation, as of the skin. **cortical a.**, a condition in which an area of the cerebral cortex shows disappearance of ganglion cells. **a. parasit′ica**, a variant of tinea versicolor occurring in dark-skinned infants, particularly in the tropics, which begins in the diaper region and spreads rapidly, causing marked depigmentation of the skin.

achromic (ah-kro′mik) pertaining to or characterized by achromia.

achromin (ah-kro′min) achromatin.

Achromobacter (ah-kro′mo-bak′ter) [*a* neg. + Gr. *chrōma* color + *baktron* a rod] a genus of gram-negative, nonfermentative, peritrichously flagellated, rod-shaped bacteria of uncertain affiliation, found in water and the human intestinal tract. They have been isolated from various clinical sources, sometimes associated with significant infections. Organisms of this genus are sometimes classified in the genus *Alcaligenes*.

achromocyte (ah-kro′mo-sīt) a red cell artifact in the shape of a quarter moon which stains more faintly than intact red cells; called also *selenoid* or *crescent body*.

achromophil (ah-kro′mo-fil) [*a* neg. + Gr. *chrōma* color + *philein* to love] achromatophil.

achromophilous (ah″kro-mof′ĭ-lus) having no affinity for stains.

Achromycin (ak′ro-mi″sin) trademark for preparations of tetracycline.

achrooamyloid (a-kro″o-am′ĭ-loid) [Gr. *achroos* uncolored + *amyloid*] amyloid in its early nonstainable stage.

achrocytosis (ah-kro″o-si-to′sis) achroacytosis.

achroodextrin (ah-kro″o-dek′strin) [Gr. *achroos* uncolored + *dextrin*] a kind of lower-molecular-weight dextrin not colored by iodine.

Achroonema (ah″kro-o-ne′mah)[*a*-neg. + Gr. *chroa* color + *nēma* thread] a genus of gliding bacteria of the provisional family Pelonemataceae, found in water, made up of cylindrical cells in colorless unbranched filaments. The type species is *A. spiroideum*.

Achucárro's stain (ach″oo-kah′rōz) [Nicolás *Achucárro*, Spanish histologist, 1881–1918] see *Table of Stains*.

achylia (ah-ki′le-ah) [Gr. *achylos* juiceless + *-ia*] absence of hydrochloric acid and pepsinogens (pepsin) in the gastric juice (*a. gas′trica*). **a. gas′trica hemorrha′gica** (*obs.*), absence of hydrochloric acid from, and presence of occult blood in, the stomach. **a. pancreat′ica** (*obs.*), absence of exocrine pancreatic secretion, occurring in pancreatic ductal obstruction, pancreatic atrophy, or chronic pancreatitis with pancreatic insufficiency.

achylous (ah-ki'lus) [Gr. *achylos* juiceless] (*obs.*) deficient in chyle.

achymia (ah-ki'me-ah) imperfect, insufficient, or absence of formation of chyme.

achymosis (ak"i-mo'sis) achymia.

acicular (ah-sik'u-lar) [L. *acicularis*] shaped like a needle or needle point.

aciculum (ah-sik'u-lum) a bent, finger-like spine or bristle found in certain flagellates.

acid (as'id) [L. *acidum* from *acidus* sharp, sour] any of a large class of chemical substances defined by three chemical concepts of increasing generality. An *Arrhenius acid* is a substance that lowers the pH (increases the hydrogen ion concentration) when added to an aqueous solution; such substances have a sour taste, turn litmus red, and react with alkalis to form salts. A *Bronsted-Lowry acid* is a species that acts as a proton donor in solution; e.g., the ammonium ion (NH_4^+) can donate a proton leaving ammonia (NH_3); such species are termed conjugate acid-base pairs. A *Lewis acid* is a species that can accept a pair of electrons to form a covalent bond; e.g., BF_3 in the reaction $BF_3 + NH_3 \rightarrow BF_3 \cdot NH_3$. Aqueous solutions of certain compounds that dissociate in solution, e.g., hydrogen chloride, are designated as acids by names beginning with *hydro-*, e.g., hydrochloric a. Most other common inorganic acids are *oxo acids* (q.v.); common organic acids include carboxylic acids, sulfonic acids, and phenols. The name of the anion formed by the removal of hydrogen from an acid (its conjugate base) and the names of salts and esters of acids are formed by removing the suffix *-ic* and the word *acid* and adding the suffix *-ate*, except for oxo acids ending in *-ous*, when the suffix is *-ite*. For particular acids, see the specific name. **amino a.,** any organic compound containing an amino and a carboxyl group. See *amino acid*. **bile a's,** steroid acids derived from cholesterol. The primary bile acids, cholic and chenodeoxycholic acids, are formed in the liver and conjugated to glycine or taurine forming bile salts (e.g., cholylglycine), which are secreted in the bile and aid in the digestion of fats. Secondarily bile acids, deoxycholic, lithocholic, and ursodeoxycholic acids, are formed from the primary bile acids by the action of intestinal bacteria, either as bile salts or as deconjugated bile acids. Most of the bile acids are reabsorbed and returned to the liver via enterohepatic circulation, where, after free acids are reconjugated, they are again excreted. Because the lithocholyl conjugates are relatively insoluble they are excreted mostly in the form of sulfate esters (e.g., sulfolithocholylglycine) produced by the liver. **binary a.,** an acid which contains only two elements, e.g., HCl; called also *hydracid*. **carboxylic a.,** any organic acid containing the carboxy (—COOH) group, including amino acids and fatty acids. **choleic a's,** complexes of fatty acids with deoxycholeic acid. **a. citrate dextrose (ACD),** an anticoagulant solution containing citric acid, sodium citrate, and dextrose formerly used for the preservation of stored whole blood but now primarily for plateletpheresis. Called also *anticoagulant citrate dextrose solution* [USP]. **conjugate a.,** a chemical species that is formed from its conjugate base by addition of a proton, e.g., ammonium (NH_4^+) is the conjugate acid of ammonia (NH_3). **fatty a.,** see under *F*. **haloid a.,** an acid which contains no oxygen in the molecule, but is composed of hydrogen and a halogen element; called also *hydracid* and *hydrohalogen a.* **inorganic a.,** one containing no carbon atoms. **monobasic a.,** an acid having but one replaceable hydrogen atom and therefore yielding only one series of salts, e.g., HCl. **muconic a.,** a dibasic acid, COOH·(CH)₄·COOH, found in the urine of dogs that have been given benzene. **noncarbonic a's,** all acids other than carbonic acid; called also *fixed (nonvolatile) acids*. **nucleic a.,** see under *N*. **organic a.,** any acid the radical of which is a carbon derivative; a compound in which a hydrocarbon radical is united to COOH (a carboxylic acid) or to SO₃H (a sulfonic acid). **oxo a.,** 1. an inorganic acid in which a central atom is bonded to one or more oxygen atoms some of which are also bonded to a hydrogen atom. When there are two common oxo acids having the same central atom the one in which the central atom has the higher oxidation number is designated by the suffix *-ic* and the other by *-ous*. When there are more oxidation states, the prefix *hypo-* may be used to indicate a lower state and *per-* to indicate a higher state; e.g., hypochlorous acid (HClO), chlorous acid ($HClO_2$), chloric acid ($HClO_3$), and perchloric acid ($HClO_4$). Called also *oxacid* and *oxyacid*. 2. keto acid. **oxygen a.,** an acid that contains oxygen; an oxyacid. **polybasic a.,** an acid which contains two or more hydrogen atoms which may be neutralized by alkalies and replaced by organic radicals. **sulfo-a.,** an acid in which oxygen or carbon is replaced by sulfur. **ternary a.,** an acid which contains three distinct radicals; called also *oxacid*. **thio a.,** one formed by replacement of an oxygen atom in an oxo acid or carboxylic acid by a sulfur atom, e.g., thiophosphoric acid (H_3PSO_3) or thioacetic acid (CH_3COSH). **tribasic a.,** an acid that has three replaceable hydrogen atoms.

acidalbumin (as"id-al'bu-min) a protein that dissolves in acids and shows an acid reaction.

Acidaminococcus (as"id-ah-me"no-kok'us) [*acid* + *amino* + *coccus*] a genus of bacteria of the family Veillonellaceae, found in the intestinal tract of normal humans and pigs, made up of gram-negative anaerobic cocci. The type species is *A. fermentans.*

acidaminuria (as"id-am"i-nu're-ah) aminoaciduria.

acidemia (as"i-de'me-ah) [*acid* + Gr. *haima* blood + *-ia*] a decreased pH (increased hydrogen ion concentration) of the blood. **argininosuccinic a.,** argininosuccinicaciduria. **glutaric a.,** glutaric aciduria I. **isovaleric a.,** a genetic aminoacidopathy due to an enzyme deficiency in isovaleryl CoA dehydrogenase in the third step of the catabolism of the branched-chain amino acids (BCAAs). Isovaleric acid accumulates in the blood and urine and causes a smell like sweaty feet; isovalerylglycine is excreted in the urine. Two clinical, possibly allelic, forms are known: the *acute neonatal form* accounts for one half the cases, has neonatal onset, and causes acidosis, pernicious vomiting, tremors, lethargy, cyanosis, coma, and death within a few weeks; the *chronic intermittent form* shows episodes of ketoacidosis with intervening asymptomatic periods and can be treated with glucose infusions; 70 per cent of the children have normal psychomotor development. Called also *isovaleric acid CoA dehydrogenase deficiency*. **methylmalonic a.,** an inborn error of metabolism characterized by excretion of excessive amounts of methylmalonic acid in the urine, recurrent vomiting, failure to thrive, developmental retardation, hepatomegaly, intermittent neutropenia, and thrombocytopenia, and often by severe metabolic acidosis. It is due to defective methylmalonyl-CoA mutase or cob(1)alamin adenosyltransferase. **propionic a.,** an excess of propionic acid in the blood, due to defective methylmalonyl-CoA decarboxylase and characterized by ketosis, acidosis, and hyperglycinemia and, in the absence of dietary controls, by developmental retardation, electrocardiogram abnormalities, and osteoporosis.

acid-fast (as'id-fast) not readily decolorized by acid after staining, a characteristic of certain bacteria, particularly *Mycobacterium tuberculosis, Mycobacterium leprae,* and some species of *Nocardia.* See *Table of Stains and Staining Methods.*

acidic (ah-sid'ik) of or pertaining to an acid; acid-forming.

acidifiable (ah-sid'i-fi"ah-b'l) susceptible of being made acid.

acidifier (ah-sid"i-fi'er) an agent that causes acidity; a substance used to increase gastric acidity.

acidify (ah-sid'i-fi) 1. to render acid, as by addition of a strong acid. 2. to become acid.

acidimeter (as"i-dim'ĕ-ter) [L. *acidum* acid + Gr. *metron* measure] an instrument used in performing acidimetry.

acidimetry (as-i-dim'ĕ-tre) the determination of the amount of free acid in a solution.

acidism (as'i-dizm) a condition due to introduction into the body of acids from outside; called also *acidismus.*

acidismus (as"i-diz'mus) acidism.

acidity (ah-sid'i-te) [L. *aciditas*] the quality of being acid or sour; containing acid (hydrogen ions).

acid-maltase deficiency (as'id mawl'tās) glycogen storage disease, type II.

acidocyte (as'i-do-sīt") (*obs.*) 1. acidophil (def. 1). 2. eosinophil.

acidogenic (as"i-do-jen'ik) producing acid or acidity, especially acidity of the urine.

Acidol (a′sĭ-dol) trademark for a preparation of betaine hydrochloride.

acidophil (as′id-o-fil″) [L. *acidum* acid + Gr. *philein* to love] 1. a structure, cell, or other histologic element staining readily with acid dyes. 2. an alpha cell of the adenohypophysis; see also *carminophil* and *orangeophil*. 3. an organism that grows well in highly acid media. 4. acidophilic. **alpha a.,** orangeophil, def. 3. **epsilon a.,** carminophil, def. 3.

acidophile (as′id-o-fīl″) acidophil.

acidophilic (as″ĭ-do-fil′ik) 1. readily stained with acid dyes. 2. growing in highly acid media; said of microorganisms.

acidophilism (as″ĭ-dof′ĭ-lizm) the condition produced by acidophilic adenoma of the pituitary, resulting in acromegaly.

acidosic (as″ĭ-do′sik) acidotic.

acidosis (as″ĭ-do′sis) a pathologic condition resulting from accumulation of acid or depletion of the alkaline reserve (bicarbonate content) in the blood and body tissues, and characterized by an increase in hydrogen ion concentration (decrease in pH). Cf. *alkalosis*. **compensated a.,** a condition in which the compensatory mechanisms have returned the pH toward normal; see *metabolic a., compensated,* and *respiratory a., compensated.* **diabetic a.,** a variety of metabolic acidosis produced by accumulation of ketone bodies resulting from uncontrolled diabetes mellitus. **hypercapnic a.,** respiratory a. **hyperchloremic a.,** metabolic acidosis accompanied by elevated plasma chloride. **metabolic a.,** a disturbance in which the acid-base status of the body shifts toward the acid side because of loss of base or retention of noncarbonic, or fixed (nonvolatile), acids; called also *nonrespiratory a.* **metabolic a., compensated,** a state of metabolic acidosis in which the pH of the blood has been returned toward normal by respiratory compensatory mechanisms. **nonrespiratory a.,** metabolic a. **renal hyperchloremia a.,** renal tubular a. **renal tubular a.,** a variety of metabolic acidosis resulting from impairment of renal function. **respiratory a.,** a state due to excess retention of carbon dioxide in the body; called also *hypercapnic a.* **respiratory a., compensated,** respiratory acidosis in which the pH of the blood has been returned toward normal by renal compensatory mechanisms. **starvation a.,** a variety of metabolic acidosis produced by accumulation of ketone bodies which may accompany a caloric deficit. **uremic a.,** the condition in chronic renal disease in which the ability to excrete acid is decreased, causing acidosis.

acidosteophyte (as″ĭ-dos′te-o-fīt″) [Gr. *akis* point + *osteon* bone + *phyton* plant] a sharp-pointed osteophyte.

acidotic (as″ĭ-dot′ik) pertaining to or characterized by acidosis.

acid phosphatase (fos′fah-tās) [EC 3.1.3.2] an enzyme of the hydrolase class that catalyzes the reaction orthophosphoric monoester + H₂O = alcohol + orthophosphate, with optimal activity at a pH below 7.0. The enzyme is found in mammalian liver, spleen, and bone marrow, in plasma and formed blood elements, and especially in the prostate gland. The determination of serum acid phosphatase is an important diagnostic test. The enzyme is markedly elevated in metastasized prostatic cancer. Moderate elevation occurs in Paget's disease, hyperparathyroidism, bone cancer, and other pathological conditions. Called also *acid phosphomonoesterase*. Abbreviated ACP.

acidulated (ah-sid′u-lāt″ed) rendered acid in reaction.

Acidulin (ah-sid′u-lin) trademark for a preparation of glutamic acid hydrochloride.

acidulous (ah-sid′u-lus) somewhat acid.

acidum (as′ĭ-dum), gen. *ac′idi,* pl. *ac′ida* [L., from *acidus* sour] acid (def. 2).

aciduria (as″ĭ-du′re-ah) the presence of acid in the urine. **acetoacetic a.,** diaceturia. **argininosuccinic a.,** argininosuccinate lyase deficiency. **beta-aminoisobutyric a.,** excessive excretion of β-aminoisobutyric acid in the urine; it occurs as a benign genetic metabolic variant and in certain illnesses. **ethylmalonic-adipic a.,** glutaric aciduria IIB. **glutaric a. (GA),** a rare genetic aminoacidopathy due to enzyme deficiencies in the third step of branched-chain amino acid (BCAA) catabolism. There are three known types: *GA I* has onset in infancy and causes

glutaric aciduria, acidemia, and progressive choreoathetosis. Called also *glutaric acidemia I. GA II* causes glutaric, lactic, ethylmalonic, butyric, isobutyric, 2-methybutyric, and isovaleric aciduria; it occurs in two forms: the *neonatal form* (*GA IIA*) is X-linked and causes quick death; *GA IIB* causes glutaric and ethylmalonic aciduria and recurrent hypoglycemia without ketosis and shows a less severe course than GA IIA; patients survive to their late teens. Called also *ethylmalonic-adipic aciduria* (*EMA*). **methylmalonic a.,** excretion of excessive amounts of methylmalonic acid in the urine; a characteristic symptom of methylmalonic acidemia. **orotic a.,** an inborn error of pyrimidine metabolism of autosomal recessive inheritance due to defective orotate phosphoribosyltransferase (OPRT) or orotidine 5′-phosphate dicarboxylase (ODC). Manifestations include crystalluria and excessive excretion of orotic acid in the urine, megaloblastic anemia with hypochromic, microcytic circulating erythrocytes, and physical and mental growth retardation. There are two biochemical types: type 1, due to deficient OPRT and ODC; and type 2, due to deficient ODC only. **pyroglutamic a.,** 5-oxoprolinuria.

aciduric (as″ĭ-du′rik) [L. *acidum* acid + *durare* to endure] acid-tolerant; said of bacteria which are able to withstand a degree of acidity usually fatal to nonsporulating bacteria.

acidyl (as′ĭ-dil) any acid radical.

acidylation (ah-sid″ĭ-la′shun) acylation.

acies (a′se-ēz) [L.] edge, margin, or border. **a. thal′ami op′tici** (*obs.*), stria medullaris thalami.

acinar (as′ĭ-nar) pertaining to or affecting an acinus or acini.

acinesia (as″ĭ-ne′ze-ah) akinesia.

acinetic (as″ĭ-net′ik) akinetic (def. 1).

Acinetobacter (as″ĭ-net″o-bak′ter) [*a-* neg. + *cineto-* + Gr. *baktron* a rod] a genus of bacteria of the family Neisseriaceae, consisting of gram-negative, paired coccobacilli that are aerobic, catalase-positive, and oxidase-negative. The organisms are widely distributed in nature and are part of the normal mammalian flora, but can cause severe primary infections in compromised hosts. The single species is *A. calcoaceticus.* **A. anitra′tus,** *A. calcoaceticus.* **A. calcoace′ticus,** the type species of the genus *Acinetobacter.* Called also *A. anitratus, A. lwoffi, Herellea vaginicola, Mima polymorpha,* and *Moraxella lwoffi.* **A. lwof′fi,** *A. calcoaceticus.*

acini (as′ĭ-ni) [L.] genitive and plural of *acinus.*

acinic (ah-sin′ik) pertaining to an acinus.

aciniform (ah-sin′ĭ-form) [L. *acinus* grape + *forma* form] shaped like an acinus, or grape.

acinitis (as″ĭ-ni′tis) inflammation of the acini of a gland.

acinitrazole (as″ĭ-ni′tro-zōl) aminitrazole.

acinose (as′ĭ-nōs) [L. *acinosus* grape-like] 1. made up of acini. 2. acinar.

acinotubular (as″ĭ-no-tu′bu-lar) composed of tubular acini or of tubules ending in acini.

acinous (as′ĭ-nus) 1. resembling a grape. 2. acinar.

acinus (as′ĭ-nus), gen. and pl. *ac′ini* [L. "grape"] a general term used in anatomical nomenclature to designate a small saclike dilatation, particularly one found in various glands; see also *alveolus.* **liver a.,** a functional unit of the liver, smaller than a portal lobule, being a diamond-shaped mass of liver parenchyma that is supplied by a terminal branch of the portal vein and of the hepatic artery and drained by a terminal branch of the bile duct. **a. rena′lis [malpig′hii],** corpuscula renis. **a. re′nis [malpig′hii],** corpuscula renis.

acipenserin (as″ĭ-pen′ser-in) a toxic substance from the gonads of the sturgeon, *Acipenser.*

ackee (ah′ke) akee.

acladiosis (ah-klad″e-o′sis) an ulcerative dermatomycosis caused by *Acladium castellani,* occurring in Sri Lanka, the Malay States, and Macedonia, and marked by the formation of roundish or oval ulcers with sharply defined edges and a granulating fundus.

Acladium (ah-kla′de-um) a genus of imperfect fungi of the family Moniliaceae, order Moniliales, sometimes found in human infection; possibly identical with *Olpitrichum* or *Oidium.*

aclasia (ah-kla′ze-ah) aclasis.

aclasis (ah′klah-sis) [*a* neg. + Gr. *klasis* a breaking] pathologic continuity of structure, as in enchondromatosis. **diaphyseal a.**, multiple exostoses. **tarsoepiphyseal a.**, dysplasia epiphysealis hemimelica.

aclastic (a-klas′tik) [*a* neg. + Gr. *klan* to break] 1. pertaining to or characterized by aclasis. 2. not refracting.

acleistocardia (ah-klīs″to-kar′de-ah) [*a* neg. + Gr. *kleistos* closed + *kardia* heart] an open condition of the foramen ovale cordis.

aclusion (ah-kloo′zhun) [*a*-neg. + *occlusion*] absence of occlusion of the opposing tooth surfaces.

acmastic (ak-mas′tik) (*obs.*) pertaining to acme; having a period of increase (*epacmastic*) followed by a period of decline (*paracmastic*).

acme (ak′me) [Gr. *akmē* point] the crisis or critical stage of a disease.

acmesthesia (ak″mes-the′ze-ah) [Gr. *akmē* + *aisthēsis* perception + *-ia*] a sensation of a sharp point touching the skin.

acne (ak′ne) [possibly a corruption of Greek *akmē* a point or of *achnē* chaff] an inflammatory disease of the pilosebaceous unit, the specific type usually being indicated by a modifying term; frequently used alone to designate common acne, or *acne vulgaris*. **a. atroph′ica,** acne in which, after the disappearance of small papular lesions, there is left a stippling of tiny atrophic pits and scars. **bromide a.**, an acneiform eruption without comedones, one of the most constant symptoms of brominism. **chlorine a.**, chloracne. **common a.**, a. vulgaris. **a. congloba′ta, conglobate a.**, a severe, chronic form of acne seen almost exclusively in males, beginning during late puberty and often continuing in later life, and characterized by the presence of numerous comedones (often double or triple), large abscesses with interconnecting sinuses, and cysts containing clear or seropurulent material; pronounced and disfiguring scarring remains after healing. **contact a.**, a. venenata. **contagious a. of horses,** a contagious disease of the skin in horses caused by infection with *Corynebacterium pseudotuberculosis*, and characterized by the development of groups of pustules, especially in areas coming in contact with the harness which when ruptured release a greenish pus that dries with crust formation. Called also *contagious pustular acne*. **a. cosmet′ica,** a persistent, low-grade type of acne usually involving the chin and cheeks of women who use cosmetics, the lesions of which present as closed comedones and papulopustules, which are thought to be caused by comedogenic substances in the cosmetics. **cystic a.**, acne with the formation of cysts enclosing a mixture of keratin and sebum in varying proportions. **a. deter′gicans,** aggravation of the existing lesions of acne by too frequent washing with comedogenic soaps and rough cloths and abrasive pads. **epidemic a.**, keratosis follicularis contagiosa. **a. estiva′lis,** a form of acne characterized by the presence of keratotic papules that occurs in the summer or following a vacation in the sun. Called also *Mallorca a.* **excoriated a., a. excoriée des filles, a. excoriée des jeunes filles,** a superficial type of acne usually seen in girls and young women caused by the compulsive neurotic habit of picking and squeezing minute, trivial, or nonexistent facial lesions, producing secondary lesions that may leave scars. Called also *picker's a.* **a. fronta′lis,** a. varioliformis. **a. ful′minans,** a rare form of extremely severe cystic acne occurring primarily in teenage boys, characterized by the presence of highly inflammatory nodules and plaques that undergo suppurative degeneration leaving ulcerations, fever, weight loss, anemia, leukocytosis, elevated erythrocyte sedimentation rate, and polyarthritis. **halogen a.**, an acneiform eruption due to ingestion of the simple salts of bromine and iodine, usually as halogen-containing cold remedies, expectorants, sedatives, analgesics, and vitamins. **a. indura′ta,** a progression of papular acne, with deep-seated and destructive lesions that may produce severe scarring. **infantile a.**, a. neonatorum. **iodide a.**, an eruption caused by the use of iodide compounds. **a. keloid,** dermatitis papillaris capillitii. **Mallorca a.**, a. estivalis. **a. mechan′ica, mechanical a.**, aggravation of the existing lesions of acne by mechanical factors that deform the skin, including friction, rubbing, stretching, pressure, pinching, and pulling, which may be provoked by such factors as chin straps, articles of clothing, orthopedic casts, backpacks, and chair and car or bus seats. **a. necrot′ica milia′ris,**

a rare and chronic form of folliculitis of the scalp, occurring principally in adults, with formation of tiny superficial pustules which are destroyed by scratching. See also *a. varioliformis*. **neonatal a., a. neonata′rum,** acne vulgaris occurring in infants, usually in males before 3 months of age, chiefly characterized by the presence of papules, pustules, and open and closed comedones on the face; the affected child may be predisposed to more severe acne in adolescence. Called also *infantile a.* **occupational a.**, see *contact a.* **a. papulo′sa,** a type of acne vulgaris in which the lesions are typically numerous inflammatory papules; this type often progresses into acne indurata. **picker's a.**, excoriated a. **pomade a.**, acne vulgaris occurring almost exclusively in blacks who groom their scalp and facial hair with greasy lubricants, and characterized by the presence of closed comedones and occasional papulopustules on the forehead, temples, cheeks, and chin. **premenstrual a.**, acne of a cyclic nature, appearing shortly before (rarely after) the onset of menses. **a. pustulo′sa,** acne in which the lesions show central suppuration. **a. rosa′cea,** rosacea. **a. scorbu′tica** (*obs.*), a papular eruption in scurvy. **a. scrofuloso′rum,** papulonecrotic tuberculid. **tropical a., a. tropica′lis,** severe acne vulgaris occurring in the tropics when the weather is hot and humid, and characterized by the presence of large and painful cysts, nodules, and pustules that lead to the formation of conglobate abscesses and frequent scarring and tend to localize on the back, nape of the neck, buttocks, thighs, and upper arms and usually sparing the face. It tends to affect those who have had acne vulgaris at an earlier age. **a. urtica′ta,** an acneiform eruption characterized by edematous papular wheals, resembling acne papules. **a. variolifor′mis,** a rare condition, with persistent brown papulopustules, usually localized to the brow and scalp; probably a deep variant of acne necrotica miliaris. Called also *a. frontalis* and *folliculitis varioliformis*. **a. venena′ta,** acne produced by contact with a great variety of acnegenic chemicals, including those used in cosmetic and grooming agents and industry (*occupational a.*), including many oils and tars, waxes, and chlorinated hydrocarbons (*chloracne*). Called also *contact a.* **a. vulga′ris,** a chronic inflammatory disease of the pilosebaceous apparatus, the lesions occurring most frequently on the face, chest, and back. The inflamed glands may form small pink papules, which sometimes surround comedones so that they have black centers, or form pustules or cysts; the cause is unknown, but it has been suggested that many factors, including stress, hereditary factors, hormones, drugs, and bacteria, especially *Propionibacterium acnes, Staphylococcus albus,* and *Pityrosporon ovale,* play an etiologic role. Called also *common a.*

acneform (ak′ne-form) acneiform.

acnegen (ak′ne-jen) a substance that causes acne.

acnegenic (ak″ne-jen′ĭk) [*acne* + Gr. *gennan* to produce] causing or capable of producing acne.

acneiform (ak-ne′ĭ-form″) resembling acne.

acnemia (ak-ne′me-ah) [*a* neg. + Gr. *knēmē* leg] atrophy of the calves of the legs.

acnitis (ak-ni′tis) [*acne* + *-itis*] a term applied to a variant of papulonecrotic tuberculid occurring on the face.

A.C.N.M. American College of Nurse-Midwives; see *nurse-midwife* and *nurse-midwifery*.

acoasma (a″ko-as′mah) acousma.

Acocanthera (ak″o-kan-the′rah) [Gr. *akōkē* a point, edge + *anthēros* blooming] a genus of apocynaceous plants of African origin whose members yield a juice from stems and leaves which is used by natives to prepare arrow poison. *A. schimperi* (A.D.C.) Schwf. and other species yield the toxic glycoside ouabain (acocantherin).

acocantherin (ak″o-kan′ther-in) ouabain.

Acoela (ah-se′lah) an order of the class Turbellaria, made up of minute marine flatworms with no intestines that receive food into a porous mass of endodermal tissue.

acoelomate (ah-sēl′o-māt) 1. lacking a body cavity. 2. an animal lacking a body cavity, as the platyhelminths.

acoenesthesia (ah-sen″es-the′ze-ah) acenesthesia.

A.C.O.G. American College of Obstetricians and Gynecologists.

acognosia (ak″og-no′se-ah) [Gr. *akos* cure + *gnōsis* knowledge] knowledge of or study of remedies.

acognosy (ah-kog′no-se) acognosia.

Acokanthera (ak″o-kan-the′rah) *Acocanthera*.

acology (ah-kol′o-je) [Gr. *akos* cure + *-logy*] the science of remedies; therapeutics, def. 1.

Acon (a′kon) trademark for a preparation of vitamin A.

aconative (ah-kon′ah-tiv) without conation; lacking any desire or impulse to act.

Aconchulinida (ah-kon″chu-lin′ĭ-dah) an order of ameboid protozoa (class Filosea, superclass Rhizopoda), the organisms of which have no external skeletal material and produce filopodia from the main cell mass, not from a hyaline lobe. They are ectoparasites of various algae.

aconine (ak′o-nin) an alkaloid, $C_{25}H_{41}NO_9$, from aconitine, much less toxic than aconitine.

aconitase (ah-kon′ĭ-tās) aconitate hydratase.

aconitate hydratase (ah-kon′ĭ-tāt hi′drah-tās) [EC 4.2.1.3] an enzyme of the lyase class that catalyzes the reaction citrate = *cis*-aconitate + H_2O. It also interconverts isocitrate and *cis*-aconitate. It is an iron-containing (Fe^{2+}) hydro-lyase that is a part of the citric (tricarboxylic) acid cycle. Called also *aconitase*.

aconite (ak′o-nīt) [L *aconitum;* Gr. *akoniton*] a poisonous drug, from the dried tuberous root of *Aconitum napellus,* which contains several closely related alkaloids, the major one being aconitine. It was once given internally as a febrifuge and gastric anesthetic. Called also *monkshood* and *wolfsbane*.

aconitine (ah-kon′ĭ-tin) [L. *aconitina, aconitia*] a poisonous white crystalline alkaloid, $C_{34}H_{47}O_{11}N$, the active principle of aconite.

Aconitum (ak-o-ni′tum), gen. *aconi′ti* [L.] a genus of poisonous ranunculaceous herbs; *A. napellus* is the source of aconite.

aconuresis (ak″on-u-re′sis) [Gr. *akōn* unwilling + *ourēsis* urination] the involuntary passage of urine.

acoprosis (ak″o-pro′sis) [*a* neg. + Gr. *kopros* excrement] absence of fecal matter from the intestine.

acoprous (ah-kop′rus) having no fecal matter in the intestine.

acor (a′kor) [L.] 1. acidity. 2. acrimony or bitterness.

acorea (ah″ko-re′ah) [*a* neg. + Gr. *korē* pupil] absence of the pupil of the eye.

acoria (ah-ko′re-ah) [*a* neg. + Gr. *koros* satiety + *-ia*] a form of polyphagia due to loss of the sensation of satiety, a condition in which the patient never feels that he has enough, although the appetite may not be large.

acorin (ak′o-rin) a bitter glycoside, $C_{36}H_{60}O_6$, from calamus; it splits into oil of calamus and sugar.

acortan (a-kor′tan) corticotropin.

Acorus (ak′o-rus) [L.; Gr. *akoros*] a genus of araceous plants; see *calamus*, def. 2.

A.C.O.S. American College of Osteopathic Surgeons.

acosmia (a-koz′me-ah) [*a* neg. + Gr. *kosmos* order + *-ia*] (*obs.*) ill health.

Acosta's disease (ah-kos′tas) [José *d'Acosta*, 1539–1600, a Jesuit priest who first described it after his travels in Peru in 1590] acute mountain sickness.

acou- [Gr. *akouein* to hear] a combining form denoting relationship to hearing.

acouasm (ah-koo′azm) acousma.

acousma (ah-kōōs′mah), pl. *acous′mata* [Gr. *akousma* a thing heard] a simple auditory hallucination, e.g., buzzing or ringing sounds.

acousmatamnesia (ah-kōōs″mat-am-ne′ze-ah) [Gr. *akousma* hearing + *amnēsia* forgetfulness] failure of the memory to call up the images of sounds.

acoustic (ah-kōōs′tik) [Gr. *akoustikos*] pertaining to sound.

acousticophobia (ah-koos″tĕ-ko-fo′be-ah) [Gr. *akoustos* heard + *phobia*] irrational fear of sounds.

acoustics (ah-kōōs′tiks) the science of sounds.

acoustigram (ah-koos′tĭ-gram) acoustogram.

acoustogram (ah-koos′to-gram) the graphic tracing of the curves, delineated in frequencies per second and decibel levels, of sounds produced by motion of a joint. Applied to the knee joint, an acoustogram will show the sound of the moving semilunar cartilages, the moving contact between the articu-

lar surfaces of the femur and tibia, and the circulation of the synovia.

A.C.P. American College of Physicians.

acquired (ah-kwīrd′) [L. *acquirere* to obtain] not genetic, but produced by influences originating outside the organism.

acquisition (ah″kwĭ-zĭ′shun) in psychology, the period in learning during which progressive increments in response strength can be measured. Also the process involved in such learning.

acquisitus (ah-kwis′ĕ-tus) [L.] acquired.

A.C.R. American College of Radiology.

acragnosis (ak″rag-no′sis) acroagnosis.

acral (ak′ral) [Gr. *akron* extremity] pertaining to an extremity or apex; affecting the extremities.

acrania (ah-kra′ne-ah) [*a* neg. + Gr. *kranion* skull + *-ia*] a developmental anomaly characterized by partial or complete absence of the cranium, or skull.

acranial (ah-kra′ne-al) having no cranium.

Acraniata (ah-kra″ne-a′tah) a subphylum of Chordata comprising species without a true skull.

acranius (ah-kra′ne-us) a monster exhibiting acrania.

Acrasia (ah-kra′se-ah) [Gr. *akrasia* bad mixture] a class of protozoa (superclass Rhizopoda, subphylum Sarcodina) found free-living in soil, dung, and vegetative matter, characterized by a life cycle that includes during the growth state amebae with eruptive lobose pseudopodia (myxamebae) produced from spores, and a reproductive stage in which the myxamebae become aggregated to form a pseudoplasmodium that gives rise to a fruiting body lacking a stalk tube. It includes one order: Acrasida. See also *Mycetozoida*.

acrasia (ah-kra′ze-ah) (*obs.*) lack of self-control; intemperance.

Acrasida (ah-kra′sĭ-dah) an order of ameboid protozoa (class Acrasia, superclass Rhizopoda) having characters of the class. *Acrasis* is a representative genus.

Acrasis (ah-kra′sis) a genus of ameboid protozoa (order Acrasida, class Acrasia).

acratia (ah-kra′she-ah) [*a* neg. + Gr. *kratos* power + *-ia*] (*obs.*) loss of power or strength.

acraturesis (ah-krat″u-re′sis) [Gr. *akratēs* feeble + *ourēsis* urination] difficult urination due to atony of the bladder or to obstruction of the urethra, as in prostatism.

Acrel's ganglion (ak′relz) [Olof (or Olaf) *Acrel*, Swedish surgeon, 1717–1806] see under *ganglion*.

Acremoniella (ak″rĕ-mo-ne-el′ah) a genus of dematiacious imperfect fungi of the order Moniliales, resembling *Acremonium;* reportedly isolated from lesions of the lung.

acremoniosis (ak″rĕ-mo-ne-o′sis) infection with the fungus *Acremonium*, producing a state marked by fever and the formation of gumma-like swellings.

Acremonium (ak″rĕ-mo′ne-um) a genus of imperfect fungi of the family Moniliaceae, order Moniliales, rarely isolated from human infection. **A. kilien′se,** an etiologic agent of eumycotic mycetoma; called also *Cephalosporium falciforme*.

acribometer (ak″rĭ-bom′ĕ-ter) [Gr. *akribēs* exact + *metron* measure] an instrument for measuring minute objects.

acrid (ak′rid) [L. *acer, acris* sharp] pungent; producing an irritation.

acridine (ak′rĭ-din) a dibenzopyridine, $CH:(C_6H_4)_2:N$, used in the synthesis of dyes and drugs; its derivatives are mostly fluorescent yellow dyes (acridine dyes), and those used in medicine (as antiseptic agents) are acriflavine hydrochloride, acriflavine base, and proflavine. **a. orange,** tetramethyl acridine, $CH[N(CH_3)_2C_6H_3]_2N$, a fluorescent basic dye; sometimes used for vital staining.

acriflavine (ak″rĭ-fla′vin) a mixture of 3,6-diamino-10-methylacridinium chloride and 3,6-diaminoacridine, occurring as a deep orange granular powder; used in solution as a topical antiseptic for the skin and mucous membranes, and has been used orally as a urinary antiseptic. Called also *chromoflavine, euflavine, neutral acriflavine,* and *neutroflavine*. **a. hydrochloride,** a mixture of the hydrochloride salts of 3,6-diamino-10-methylacridinium chloride and 3,6-diaminoacridine, occurring as a brownish red, crystalline powder; used like the base. This substance was originally prepared by Benda in 1911 for use in trypanosomiasis, and was by him given the name of *trypaflavine*. It has also been called *flavine*. Its use is rapidly diminishing in modern medicine. **neutral a.,** acriflavine.

acrimony (ak′rĭ-mo″ne) [L. *acrimonia*] an acrid quality, property, or condition; called also *acor*.

acrinyl sulfocyanate (ak-ri′nil sul″fo-si′ah-nāt) an acrid vesicating principle found in white mustard.

acrisorcin (ak-rĭ-sor′sin) [USP] an acridine derivative applied topically to treat tinea versicolor.

acritical (ah-krit′ĭ-kal) [*a* neg. + Gr. *krisis* a crisis] having no crisis, said especially of febrile diseases ending by lysis.

acritochromacy (ah-krit″o-kro′mah-se) monochromatism.

A.C.R.M. American Congress of Rehabilitation Medicine.

acr(o)- [Gr. *akron* extremity, from *akros* extreme] a combining form denoting relation to an extremity, top, or summit, or to an extreme.

acroagnosis (ak″ro-ag-no′sis) [acro- + *a* neg. + Gr. *gnōsis* knowledge] lack of sensory recognition of a limb; lack of acrognosis. Called also *acragnosis*.

acroanesthesia (ak′ro-an″es-the′ze-ah) [acro- + *anesthesia*] loss of sensation in the extremities.

acroarthritis (ak″ro-ar-thri′tis) [acro- + *arthritis*] arthritis affecting the extremities.

acroasphyxia (ak″ro-as-fik′se-ah) [acro- + *asphyxia*] (*obs.*) acrocyanosis.

acroblast (ak′ro-blast) [acro- + Gr. *blastos* germ] Golgi material in the spermatid from which arises the acrosome.

acrobrachycephaly (ak″ro-brak″ĕ-sef′ah-le) [acro- + Gr. *brachys* short + *kephalē* head] a condition resulting from fusion of the coronal suture, causing abnormal shortening of the anteroposterior diameter of the skull.

acrobystiolith (ak″ro-bis′te-o-lith) [Gr. *akrobystia* prepuce + *lithos* stone] postholith.

acrobystitis (ak″ro-bis-ti′tis) [Gr. *akrobystia* prepuce + *-itis*] inflammation of the prepuce.

acrocentric (ak″ro-sen′trik) [acro- + Gr. *kentron,* L. *centrum* center] a type of chromosome having the centromere near one end of the replicating chromosome, so that one arm is much longer than the other. Cf. *metacentric* and *submetacentric*.

acrocephalia (ak″ro-sĕ-fa′le-ah) [Gr. *akra* point + *kephalē* head + *-ia*] oxycephaly.

acrocephalic (ak″ro-sĕ-fal′ik) oxycephalic.

acrocephalopolysyndactyly (ACPS) (ak″ro-sef″ah-lo-pol″e-sin-dak′tĭ-le) [*acrocephaly* + *polysyndactyly*] acrocephalosyndactyly with polydactyly as an additional feature. Four types are known: *type I* (*ACPS I; Noack syndrome*), autosomal dominant, is the same as acrocephalosyndactyly type V (Pfeiffer type); *type II* (*ACPS II; Carpenter syndrome*), with mental retardation and brachydactyly is autosomal recessive; *type III* (*ACPS with leg hypoplasia; Sakati-Nyhan syndrome*), with hypoplastic tibias and deformed, displaced fibulas, is autosomal dominant; *type IV* (*ACPS IV; Goodman syndrome*), with congenital heart defects, clinodactyly, camptodactyly, and ulnar deviation, but with unimpaired intelligence, is autosomal recessive.

acrocephalosyndactylia (ak″ro-sef″ah-lo-sin″dak-til′e-ah) acrocephalosyndactyly.

acrocephalosyndactylism (ak″ro-sef″ah-lo-sin-dak′tĭ-lizm) acrocephalosyndactyly.

acrocephalosyndactyly (ak″ro-sef″ah-lo-sin-dak′tĭ-le) [*acrocephaly* + *syndactyly*] craniostenosis characterized by acrocephaly and syndactyly, probably occurring as an autosomal dominant trait and usually as a new mutation; called also *a. type I, Apert syndrome, Apert-Crouzon disease,* and *Vogt's cephalodactyly*. It also occurs with other anomalies, which have been designated *Chotzen syndrome* (type III) and *Pfeiffer type acrocephalosyndactyly* (type V), which is the same as acrocephalopolysyndactyly type I.

acrocephalous (ak″ro-sef′ah-lus) oxycephalic.

acrocephaly (ak″ro-sef′ah-le) oxycephaly. **a.-syndactyly,** the characteristic shape of the head seen in acrocephalosyndactyly.

acrochordon (ak″ro-kor′don) [acro- + Gr. *chordē* string] a skin-colored to light brown papillomatous cutaneous lesion usually occurring on the neck, upper chest, and axillae of middle-aged women, characterized histologically by a hyperplastic epidermis enclosing a dermal connective tissue stalk composed of loose, edematous collagen fibers; larger lesions may be pedunculated (*soft fibromas*). Called also *cutaneous papilloma* or *tag* and *skin tag*.

acrocinesis (ak″ro-si-ne′sis) [acro- + Gr. *kinēsis* motion] excessive motility; abnormal freedom of movement. Called also *acrokinesia*.

acrocinetic (ak″ro-si-net′ik) affected with acrocinesis.

acrocontracture (ak″ro-kon-trak′chūr) [acro- + *contracture*] contracture of an extremity; contracture of muscles of the hand or foot.

acrocyanosis (ak″ro-si″ah-no′sis) [acro- + *cyanosis*] a condition marked by symmetrical cyanosis of the extremities, with persistent, uneven, mottled blue or red discoloration of the skin of the digits, wrists, and ankles and with profuse sweating and coldness of the digits. Called also *Raynaud's sign*.

acrodermatitis (ak″ro-der″mah-ti′tis) [acro- + *dermatitis*] inflammation involving the skin of the extremities, especially the hands and feet. **a. chron′ica atroph′icans,** a diffuse chronic idiopathic skin disease usually confined to the extremities, occurring almost exclusively in Northern, Central, and Eastern Europe, most often in women, and characterized initially by an erythematous, edematous, pruritic phase followed by sclerosis and atrophy. **a. contin′ua,** a variant of pustular psoriasis characterized by a chronic distinctive inflammatory eruption of the digits, palms, and soles, sometimes becoming more generalized, with a thin annular vesiculopustular border that gradually extends and recurs, leaving inflamed mildly exfoliating skin. Called also *a. perstans, Hallopeau's a.,* and *dermatitis repens.* **a. enteropath′ica,** a severe gastrointestinal and cutaneous disease of early childhood, due to an autosomal recessive disorder of zinc uptake and characterized by a vesiculopustulous dermatitis, preferentially located around the body orifices and on the head, hands, and feet, with diarrhea, true steatorrhea, and loss of hair. **Hallopeau's a.,** a. continua. **infantile a.,** Gianotti-Crosti syndrome. **papular a. of childhood, a. papulo′sa infan′tum,** Gianotti-Crosti syndrome. **a. per′stans,** a. continua.

acrodermatoses (ak″ro-der″mah-to′sēz) plural of *acrodermatosis*.

acrodermatosis (ak″ro-der″mah-to′sis), pl. *acrodermato′ses* [acro- + *dermatosis*] any disease involving the skin of the extremities.

acrodolichomelia (ak″ro-dol″ĕ-ko-me′le-ah) [acro- + Gr. *dolichos* long + *melos* limb + *-ia*] abnormal or disproportionate length of hands and feet.

acrodont (ak′ro-dont) [acro- + Gr. *odous* tooth] having the teeth attached to the upper surface of the jaw rather than encased in a socket, a condition seen in many lizards.

acrodynia (ak″ro-din′e-ah) [acro- + Gr. *odynē* pain + *-ia*] a disease of infancy and early childhood characterized by pain and swelling in, and pink coloration of, the fingers and toes, and by listlessness, irritability, failure to thrive, generalized inconstant rashes, profuse perspiration, photophobia, loss of teeth, and sometimes scarlet coloration of cheeks and tip of nose; repeated ingestion of or contact with mercury is the cause of most, if not all, cases, and individual sensitivity may also be a factor. Called also *erythredema polyneuropathy* and *pink disease*. **rat a.,** a condition in rats, dogs, and pigs due to deficiency of pyridoxine, and marked by swelling and necrosis of the paws, the tips of ears and nose, and the lips.

acrodysplasia (ak″ro-dis-pla′se-ah) acrocephalosyndactyly.

acroedema (ak″ro-ĕ-de′mah) [acro- + *edema*] (*obs.*) permanent edema of the hand or foot.

acroesthesia (ak″ro-es-the′ze-ah) [acro- + Gr. *aisthēsis* sensation + *-ia*] 1. increased sensitiveness. 2. pain in the extremities.

acrognosis (ak″rog-no′sis) [acro- + Gr. *gnōsis* knowledge] sensory recognition of the limbs and of the different portions of each limb in relation to each other; limb knowledge.

acrohypothermy (ak″ro-hi′po-ther′me) [acro- + Gr. *hypo* under + *thermē* heat] abnormal coldness of the hands and feet.

acrokeratosis (ak″ro-ker″ah-to′sis) a condition involving the skin of the extremities, with the appearance of horny growths. **paraneoplastic a.,** Bazex's syndrome. **a. verrucifor′mis,** a genodermatosis inherited as an autosomal dominant trait, characterized by the occurrence on the dorsal aspects of the hands and feet, elbows, knees, and insteps of numerous closely grouped verrucous papules, and sometimes associated with the presence of diffuse hyperkeratosis of the palms and soles. Acrokeratosis verruciformis and keratosis follicularis frequently occur together.

acrokinesia (ak″ro-ki-ne′ze-ah)   acrocinesis.

acrolein (ak-ro′le-in) [L. *acer* acrid + *oleum* oil] a volatile acrid liquid, CH₂:CHCHO, from the decomposition of glycerin; called also *acryaldehyde,* and *allyl aldehyde.*

acromacria (ak″ro-mak′re-ah)   arachnodactyly.

acromastitis (ak″ro-mas-ti′tis) [*acro-* + Gr. *mastos* mamma + *-itis*] inflammation of the nipple.

acromegalia (ak″ro-mĕ-ga′le-ah)   acromegaly.

acromegalic (ak″ro-mĕ-gal′ik)   pertaining to or characterized by acromegaly.

acromegalogigantism (ak″ro-meg″ah-lo-ji′gan-tizm) gigantism and acromegaly due to hypersecretion of the pituitary growth hormone beginning before puberty and continuing into maturity.

acromegaloidism (ak″ro-meg′ah-loid-izm) a bodily condition resembling acromegaly but not due to pituitary disorder.

acromegaly (ak″ro-meg′ah-le) [*acro-* + Gr. *megalē* great] a chronic disease of adults caused by hypersecretion of the pituitary growth hormone and characterized by enlargement of many parts of the skeleton, especially the distal portions—the nose, ears, jaws, fingers, and toes; the converse of acromicria. Called also *Marie's disease.*

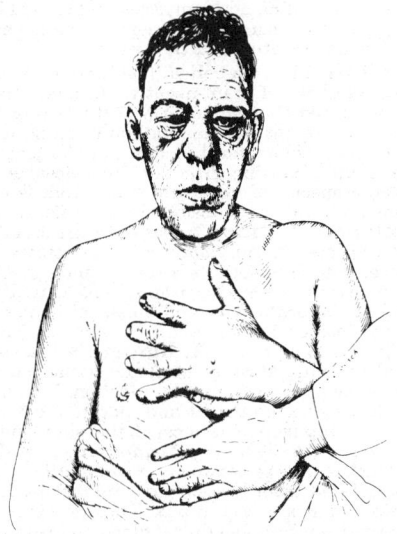

Acromegaly

acromelalgia (ak″ro-mĕ-lal′je-ah)   erythromelalgia.

acromelic (ak″ro-me′lik) [*acro-* + Gr. *melos* limb] pertaining to or affecting the end of a limb.

acrometagenesis (ak″ro-met″ah-jen′ĕ-sis) [*acro-* + Gr. *meta* beyond + *genesis* production] undue growth of the extremities.

acromial (ah-kro′me-al)   pertaining to the acromion.

acromicria (ak″ro-mik′re-ah) [*acro-* + Gr. *mikros* small + *-ia*] a condition characterized by hypoplasia of the extremities of the skeleton—the nose, jaws, fingers, and toes; the converse of acromegaly.

acromikria (ak″ro-mik′re-ah)   acromicria.

acromi(o)- [L. *acromion,* q.v.] a combining form denoting relationship to the acromion.

acromioclavicular (ah-kro″me-o-klah-vik′u-lar) pertaining to the acromion and clavicle, especially to the articulation between the acromion and clavicle. See also *articulatio acromioclavicularis.*

acromiocoracoid (ah-kro″me-o-kor′ah-koid) pertaining to the acromion and the coracoid process; called also *coracoacromial.*

acromiohumeral (ah-kro″me-o-hu′mer-al) pertaining to the acromion and humerus.

acromion (ah-kro′me-on) [*acro-* + Gr. *ōmos* shoulder] [NA] the lateral extension of the spine of the scapula, projecting over the shoulder joint and forming the highest point of the shoulder; called also *acromial process* and *acromion scapulae.*

acromionectomy (ah-kro″me-on-ek′to-me) resection of the distal end of the acromion, done in the treatment of acromioclavicular arthritis.

acromioscapular (ah-kro″me-o-skap′u-lar) pertaining to the acromion and scapula.

acromiothoracic (ah-kro″me-o-tho-ras′ik) pertaining to the acromion and thorax.

acromphalus (ah-krom′fah-lus) [*acro-* + Gr. *omphalos* navel] 1. undue prominence of the navel; sometimes a sign of umbilical hernia. 2. the center of the navel.

acromycosis (ak″ro-mi-ko′sis) (*obs.*) mycosis of the limbs.

acromyotonia (ak″ro-mi-o-to′ne-ah) [*acro-* + Gr. *mys* muscle + *tonos* contraction + *-ia*] contracture of the hand or foot resulting in spastic deformity (Sicard, 1915).

acromyotonus (ak″ro-mi-ot′o-nus)   acromyotonia.

acronarcotic (ak″ro-nar-kot′ik)   both acrid and narcotic.

acroneurosis (ak″ro-nu-ro′sis) [*acro-* + *neurosis*] any neuropathy of the extremities.

acronine (a′kro-nēn) chemical name: 3,12-dihydro-6-methoxy - 3,3,12 - trimethyl - 7*H* - pyrano [2,3 - *c*] acridin -7-one; an antineoplastic agent, C₂₀H₁₉NO₃.

acronym (ak′ro-nim) [*acro-* + Gr. *onoma* name] a word formed by the initial letters of the principal components of a compound term, as laser or maser.

acro-osteolysis (ak″ro-os″te-ol′ĭ-sis) osteolysis involving the distal phalanges of the fingers and toes.

acropachia (ak″ro-pak′e-ah) [*acro-* + Gr. *pachys* thick + *-ia*] a condition seen in dogs, characterized by hyperostosis of the bones of the limbs, later involving other skeletal regions; it may be associated with tumors or tuberculosis.

acropachy (ak′ro-pak″e) [*acro-* + Gr. *pachys* thick] hypertrophic pulmonary osteoarthropathy.

acropachyderma (ak″ro-pak″e-der′mah) [*acro-* + Gr. *pachys* thick + *derma* skin] thickening of the skin over the extremities, as occurs in acromegaly and pachydermoperiostitis. Called also *pachyacria.* **a. with pachyperiostitis,** pachydermoperiostosis.

acroparalysis (ak″ro-pah-ral′ĭ-sis) [*acro-* + *paralysis*] paralysis of the extremities.

acroparesthesia (ak″ro-par″es-the′ze-ah) [*acro-* + *paresthesia*] 1. paresthesia of the tips of the extremities due to nerve compression at any of several levels, or polyneuritis. 2. a disease marked by attacks of tingling, numbness, and stiffness in the extremities, chiefly the fingers, hands, and forearms, sometimes with pain, pallor of the skin, or slight cyanosis. Two forms have been described—the simple form (Schultze's type), which tends to end in acrocyanosis, and the vasomotor or angiospastic form (Nothnagel's type), which may end in recovery or go on to gangrene.

acropathology (ak″ro-pah-thol′o-je) [*acro-* + *pathology*] the pathology of diseases affecting the extremities.

acropathy (ah-krop′ah-the) [*acro-* + Gr. *pathos* disorder] any disease of the extremities.

acropeptide (ak″ro-pep′tīd) a protein fraction obtained by heating protein to above 140° C. in nonaqueous solvents.

acropetal (ah-krop′e-tal) [*acro-* + L. *petere* to seek] rising toward the summit.

acrophobia (ak″ro-fo′be-ah) [Gr. *akron* height, promontory + *phobia*] irrational fear of heights.

acroposthitis (ak″ro-pos-thi′tis) [Gr. *acroposthia* prepuce + *-itis*] inflammation of the prepuce.

acroscleroderma (ak″ro-skle″ro-der′mah)   acrosclerosis.

acrosclerosis (ak″ro-skle-ro′sis) [*acro-* + *sclerosis*] a condition generally regarded as a form of systemic scleroderma that combines the features of Raynaud's disease with scleroderma of the distal parts of the extremities, especially of the digits (sclerodactyly), and of the neck and the face, particularly the nose. Called also *acroscleroderma.*

acrosome (ak′ro-sōm) [*acro-* + Gr. *sōma* body] the caplike, membrane-bound structure derived from Golgi elements found at the anterior portion of the nucleus of a spermatozoon; it contains lysosomal enzymes and a proteolytic enzyme, which are believed to facilitate entry of spermatozoa into ova. Called also *acrosomal cap* and *anterior head cap.* See also *acrosome reaction*, under *reaction*.

acrosphenosyndactylia (ak″ro-sfe″no-sin″dak-til′e-ah) acrocephalosyndactyly.

acrostealgia (ak″ros-te-al′je-ah) [*acro-* + Gr. *osteon* bone + *algos* pain + *-ia*] a painful apophysitis of the bones of the extremities.

acrosyndactyly (ak″ro-sin-dak′tĭ-le) [*acro-* + Gr. *syn* with + *daktylos* finger] fusion of the terminal portion of two or more digits, with clefts or sinuses present between their proximal phalanges.

acroteric (ak″ro-ter′ik) pertaining to the tips or outermost parts.

Acrotheca pedrosoi (ak″ro-the′kah pĕ-dro′soi) *Fonsecaea pedrosoi.*

Acrothesium floccosum (ak″ro-the′se-um flok-ko′sum) *Epidermophyton floccosum.*

acrotic (ah-krot′ik) 1. [Gr. *akros* extreme] affecting the surface. 2. [*a* neg. + Gr. *krotos* beat] pertaining to absence or weakness of the pulse.

acrotism (ak′ro-tizm) [*a* neg. + Gr. *krotos* beat + *-ism*] absence or imperceptibility of the pulse.

acrotrophodynia (ak″ro-trof″o-din′e-ah) [*acro-* + Gr. *trophē* nutrition + *odynē* pain + *-ia*] a trophic disorder with neuritis and paresthesia from exposure of extremities to cold and moisture.

acrotrophoneurosis (ak″ro-trof″o-nu-ro′sis) trophoneurotic disturbance of the extremities.

acrylaldehyde (ak″ril-al′de-hīd) acrolein.

acrylamide (ah-kril′ah-mīd) the crystalline amide of acrylic acid, $CH_2CHCONH_2$.

acrylate (ah-kril′āt) a salt, ester, or conjugate base of acrylic acid.

acrylic (ah-kril′ik) pertaining to polymers of acrylic acid, methacrylic acid or acrylonitrile, as acrylic fibers or acrylic resins.

acrylic acid (ah-kril′ik) 2-propenoic acid, $CH_2=CH-COOH$.

acrylonitrile (ak″rĭ-lo-ni′tril) chemical name: 2-propenenitrile. A compound, $CH_2:CH \cdot CN$, used in the making of plastics and as a pesticide; its vapors are irritant to the respiratory tract and eyes, and may cause systemic poisoning.

A.C.S. American Cancer Society; American Chemical Society; American College of Surgeons.

A.C.S.M. American College of Sports Medicine.

act (akt) a doing, or a thing done; a performance involving motor activity. **Harrison antinarcotic a.,** see under *H.* **reflex a.,** a relatively fixed action or pattern of response performed as a result of the triggering of a reflex arc and usually without involvement of the higher centers.

Actaea (ak-te′ah) [L.; Gr. *aktē* elder-tree] a genus of ranunculaceous plants. **A. odora′ta,** bitter weed, a plant that causes heavy losses of sheep and goats in the Southwest. **A. richardso′ni,** rubber weed which is poisonous to sheep. **A. spica′ta,** red cohosh.

actaplanin (ak″tah-pla′nin) a glycopeptide antibiotic of unknown structure derived from a species of *Actinoplanes,* containing a chlorophenyl group, glucose, mannose rhamnose, and several unknown amino acids; a veterinary growth stimulant.

ACTH adrenocorticotropic hormone; see *corticotropin.*

Acthar (ak′thar) trademark for preparations of corticotropin.

ACTH-RF corticotropin (adrenocorticotropic hormone) releasing factor.

Actidil (ak′tĭ-dil) trademark for a preparation of triprolidine hydrochloride.

Acti-Dione (ak″tĭ-di′ōn) trademark for a preparation of cycloheximide.

actin (ak′tin) a protein of the myofibril, localized in the I band; acting along with myosin particles, it is responsible for the contraction and relaxation of muscle. In the absence of salt, it becomes globular (*G-actin*), and in the presence of potassium chloride and adenosine triphosphate it polymerizes, forming long fibers (F-actin). Cf. *actomyosin* and *myosin.*

Actineliida (ak″tĭ-ne-li′ĭ-dah) an order of mostly planktonic marine protozoa (class Acantharea, superclass Actinopoda) characterized by the presence of a variable number of radial spines.

acting out (ak′ting owt) the expression of unconscious feelings and fantasies in behavior; reacting to present situations as if they were the original situation that gave rise to the feelings and fantasies, i.e., acting out of a transference. Often applied imprecisely to any sort of disapproved impulsive behavior.

actinic (ak-tin′ik) [Gr. *aktis* ray] pertaining to those rays of light beyond the violet end of the spectrum that produce chemical effects.

actinicity (ak″tĭ-nis′ĭ-te) actinism.

actiniform (ak-tin′ĭ-form) [Gr. *aktis* ray] formed like a ray; radiate.

actinine (ak′tĭ-nin) a base occurring in the sea anemone *Actinia equina.*

actinism (ak′tĭ-nizm) [Gr. *aktis* ray] that property of radiant energy which produces chemical changes, as in photography or heliotherapy; called also *actinicity.*

actinium (ak-tin′e-um) [Gr. *aktis* ray] a rare metallic chemical element occurring in the ores of uranium and having radioactive properties; its atomic number is 89, its atomic weight 227, and its symbol Ac.

actin(o)- [Gr. *aktis,* gen. *aktinos* a ray] a combining form denoting relation to a ray, as ray-shaped, or pertaining to some form of radiation.

actinobacillosis (ak″tĭ-no-bas″ĭ-lo′sis) a disease of domestic animals resembling actinomycosis and caused by *Actinobacillus lignieresii,* sometimes seen in man; the bacillus forms radiating structures in the tissues.

Actinobacillus (ak″tĭ-no-bah-sil′lus) [*actino-* + L. *bacillus* small rod] a genus of gram-negative, fermentative nonmotile, coccoid or rod-shaped bacteria of the family Pasteurellaceae, part of the normal mammalian microflora. They are potentially pathogenic for humans and for cattle, sheep, horses, and pigs, causing granulomatous lesions. **A. actinoi′des,** a species of uncertain status that is pathogenic for goats and calves, causing lung lesions. **A. actinomycetemco′mitans,** a species that is found in association with species of *Actinomyces* in actinomycotic lesions and septicemias. Their etiologic role is unclear. Called also *Bacterium actinomycetem comitans.* **A. equu′li,** a species found in the oral cavity and tonsils of horses. It causes suppurative lesions in horses and swine; it also produces endocarditis in the latter. **A. lignière′sii,** a species that is primarily an animal commensal and pathogen, which has also been associated with human infection. It causes granulomatous lesions in the throat and mouth of cattle (wooden tongue) and suppurative lesions of the skin and lungs in sheep. **A. mal′lei,** *Pseudomonas mallei.* **A. pseudomal′lei,** *Pseudomonas pseudomallei.* **A. su′is,** a species isolated from horses, pigs, and cattle. It produces pneumonia and septicemia in pigs. The organisms have also been isolated from human clinical blood and respiratory and wound specimens. **A. whitmor′i,** *Pseudomonas pseudomallei.*

Actinobifida (ak″tĭ-no-bĭ′fĭ-dah) [*actino-* + L. *bifidus* divided] a genus of bacteria of the family Micromonosporaceae, order Actinomycetales, consisting of soil organisms that form a mycelium containing branched hyphae and bearing spores. The type species is *A. dichotomica.*

actinobolin (ak″tĭ-nob′o-lin) a broad-spectrum antibiotic elaborated by *Streptomyces griseoviridus* var. *atrofaciens,* $C_{13}H_{20}N_2O_6$, which exhibits activity against a wide range of bacteria and against various neoplasms, and inhibits cariogenic microorganisms in rats; it is being studied for use in the control of caries in humans.

Actinocephalus (ak″tĭ-no-sef′ah-lus) [*actino-* + Gr. *kephalē* head] a genus of parasitic gregarine protozoa (suborder Septatina, order Eugregarina) found in the gut of insects, characterized by the presence of a sessile epimerite with 8 to 10 finger-like apical processes and biconical spores.

actinochemistry (ak″tĭ-no-kem′is-tre) [*actino-* + *chemistry*] chemistry dealing with action of rays of light; photochemistry.

actinocongestin (ak″tĭ-no-kon-jĕs′tin) congestin.

actinocutitis (ak″tĭ-no-ku-ti′tis) [*actino-* + *cutitis*] radiodermatitis.

actinodaphnine (ak″tĭ-no-daf′nin) a crystalline alkaloid, $C_{18}H_{17}O_4N$, from the bark of *Actinodaphne hookeri.*

actinodermatitis (ak″ti-no-der″mah-ti′tis) cutaneous inflammation due to excessive exposure to sunlight or exposure to x-rays.

actinograph (ak-tin′o-graf) [*actino-* + Gr. *graphein* to write] 1. (*obs.*) roentgenogram. 2. an instrument for recording variations in the actinic effect of the sun's rays.

actinohematin (ak″tĭ-no-hem′ah-tin) a red respiratory pigment occurring in certain sea anemones.

actinology (ak″tĭ-nol′ŏ-je) [*actino-* + *-logy*] 1. the science of photochemistry; the science of the chemical effects of light. 2. the study of radiant energy.

actinolyte, actinolite (ak-tin′o-līt) [*actino-* + Gr. *lytos* soluble, from *lyein* to loosen] any substance that is markedly changed by light.

Actinomadura (ak″tĭ-no-mad′ŭ-rah) [*actino-* + *Madura,* a city in the state of Madras, Republic of India (now named Madurai)] a genus of bacteria of the family Nocardiaceae, order Actinomycetales, consisting of nonacid-fast organisms that form nonfragmenting branched filaments. **A. madu′rae,** a species distributed worldwide in soil, and a common cause of actinomycotic mycetoma; called also *Nocardia madurae.* **A. pelletier′ii,** a species commonly found in Africa, India, and North and South America; it is the cause of actinomycotic mycetoma.

actinometer (ak″tĭ-nom′ĕ-ter) [*actino-* + Gr. *metron* measure] 1. an instrument for measuring the intensity of actinic effects. 2. an apparatus for measuring the penetrating power of actinic rays.

actinometry (ak″tĭ-nom′ĕ-tre) the measurement of the photochemical power of light.

actinomycelial (ak″tĭ-no-mi-se′le-al) 1. pertaining to the mycelium of an actinomyces. 2. actinomycetic.

Actinomyces (ak″tĭ-no-mi′sēz) [*actino-* + Gr. *mykēs* fungus] a genus of bacteria of the family Actinomycetaceae, order Actinomycetales, consisting of gram-positive, asporogenous, irregularly staining organisms that form branched filaments. They are nonacid-fast and nonmotile. **A. asteroi′des,** *Nocardia asteroides.* **A. bo′vis,** a nonacid-fast, facultatively anaerobic species of serologic group B. It is a normal inhabitant of animal mucous membranes, and the specific etiologic agent of actinomycosis (lumpy jaw) in cattle. **A. brasilien′sis,** *Nocardia brasiliensis.* **A. dentocari-o′sus,** *Rothia dentocariosa.* **A. eppinge′ri,** *Nocardia asteroides.* **A. erikson′ii,** *Bifidobacterium eriksonii.* **A. gonidiafor′mis,** *Fusobacterium gonidiaformans.* **A. israe′lii,** a nonacid-fast anaerobic species of serologic group D, parasitic in the mouth and proliferating in necrotic tissue. It is the etiologic agent of human actinomycosis, especially that associated with the use of intrauterine devices, of actinomycotic mycetoma, of periodontal disease, and occasionally of injections in cattle. **A. lu′teus,** *Nocardia lutea.* **A. mur′is, A. mur′is-rat′ti,** *Streptobacillus moniliformis.* **A. naeslun′dii,** an aerobic species of serologic group A. It is a normal inhabitant of the oral cavity and an etiologic agent of human actinomycosis and periodontal disease. **A. necroph′orus,** *Fusobacterium necrophorum.* **A. odontolyt′icus,** a facultatively anaerobic species of serologic group E. It is a natural inhabitant of the human oral cavity and has been found in dental caries. **A. pseudonecroph′orus,** *Fusobacterium necrophorum.* **A. vina′ceus,** *Streptomyces vinaceus.* **A. visco′sus,** a facultative anaerobic species of serologic group F. It is found in the oral cavity of man, hamsters, and rats, and is a cause of dental caries in laboratory animals; pathogenicity for humans has not been established.

actinomyces (ak″tĭ-no-mi′sēz), pl. *actinomyce′tes.* An organism of the genus *Actinomyces.*

Actinomycetaceae (ak″tĭ-no-mi″sĕ-ta′se-e) a family of bacteria, order Actinomycetales, consisting of gram-positive, nonsporulating irregularly shaped rods, which tend to form branched filaments. It contains the genera *Actinomyces, Arachnia, Bacterionema, Bifidobacterium,* and *Rothia.*

Actinomycetales (ak″tĭ-no-mi″sĕ-ta′lēz) an order of bacteria made up of elongated cells that tend to form branching filaments; it includes the families Actinomycetaceae, Actinoplanaceae, Dermatophilaceae, Frankiaceae, Micromonosporaceae, Mycobacteriaceae, Nocardiaceae, and Streptomycetaceae.

actinomycete (ak″tĭ-no-mi′sēt) any organism of the order Actinomycetales.

actinomycetes (ak″tĭ-no-mi-se′tēz) plural of *actinomyces* and *actinomycete.*

actinomycetic (ak″tĭ-no-mi-set′ik) of or caused by actinomyces; of or pertaining to organisms of the order Actinomycetales or diseases caused by such organisms.

actinomycetin (ak″tĭ-no-mi-se′tin) a substance derived from cultures of the actinomycete *Streptomyces albus;* it lyses dead bacteria.

actinomycetoma (ak″tĭ-no-mi″se-to′mah) [*actino-* + *mycetoma*] actinomycotic mycetoma.

actinomycin (ak″tĭ-no-mi′sin) a large, complex family of antibiotics obtained from cultures of various species of *Streptomyces,* which have antibacterial, antifungal, and cytotoxic properties. Actinomycin D (dactinomycin) is used as an antineoplastic agent.

actinomycoma (ak″tĭ-no-mi-ko′mah) [*actinomyces* + *-oma*] a tumor-like reactive lesion due to actinomycetes.

actinomycosis (ak″tĭ-no-mi-ko′sis) [*actino-* + Gr. *mykēs* fungus] an infectious disease caused by *Actinomyces israelii* in man and by *A. bovis* in cattle. It is characterized by indolent inflammatory lesions of the lymph nodes draining the mouth (*cervicofacial area*), by intraperitoneal abscesses, including liver abscess, or by lung abscess due to aspiration, in that order of frequency. The lymphadenitis is characterized by slow, relatively painless enlargement of the lymph nodes (lumpy jaw), with reddening of the overlying skin. Infection of the peritoneal cavity or lung is associated with gradually increasing fever and loss of weight, but few localizing signs. Pus drained from a suppurative lesion sometimes contains dense mycelial clusters in the form of yellowish granules (sulfur granules).

actinomycotic (ak″tĭ-no-mi-kot′ik) pertaining to or affected with actinomycosis.

actinomycotin (ak″tĭ-no-mi′ko-tin) a therapeutic preparation of cultures of *Actinomyces,* used in treating actinomycosis.

Actinomyxia (ak″tĭ-no-mik′se-ah) [*actino-* + Gr. *myxa* mucus] a subclass of parasitic protozoa (class Actinosporea, phylum Myxozoa) having characters of the class. It comprises one order: Actinomyxida.

Actinomyxida (ak″tĭ-no-mik′sĭ-dah) an order of parasitic protozoa (subclass Actinomyxia, class Actinosporea) having characters of the class. *Triactinomyxon* is a representative genus.

actinon (ak′tĭ-non) radon-219.

actinoneuritis (ak″tĭ-no-nu-ri′tis) [*actino-* + *neuritis*] radioneuritis.

actinophage (ak-tin′o-fāj) a virus that causes the lysis of actinomycetes.

Actinophryida (ak″tĭ-no-fre′ĭ-dah) [*actino-* + Gr. *ophrys* brow, rim] an order of naked protozoa (class Heliozoa, superclass Actinopoda) without a centroplast or axoplast but with microtubular stiffening elements present in the axopodia that are usually discernible as axonemes. Some species have flagella or a flagellated stage.

actinophytosis (ak″tĭ-no-fi-to′sis) infection with *Actinomyces* or *Nocardia.*

Actinoplanaceae (ak″tĭ-no-plah-na′se-e) a family of bacteria of the order Actinomycetales, consisting of gram-positive, spore-forming organisms that form a definite mycelium. They occur widely in nature as soil saprophytes. It includes the genera *Actinoplanes, Amorphosporangium, Ampullariella, Dactylosporangium, Kitasatoa, Pilimelia, Planobispora, Planomonospora, Spirillospira,* and *Streptosporangium.*

Actinoplanes (ak″tĭ-no-pla′nēz) [*actino-* + Gr. *planēs* one who wanders] a genus of bacteria of the family Actinoplanaceae, order Actinomycetales, made up of saprophytic forms found on a wide variety of plant material and in soil.

Actinopoda (ak″tĭ-nop′o-dah) [*actino-* + Gr. *pous* foot] a superclass of usually planktonic, often spherical protozoa (subphylum Sarcodina, phylum Sarcomastigophora), characterized chiefly by the presence of axopodia with microtubular stereoplasm. When present, the skeleton is composed of organic matter and silica, silica alone, or strontium sulfate. It comprises four classes: Acantharea, Heliozoa, Phaedarea, and Polycystinea.

actinopraxis (ak″tĭ-no-prak′sis) [*actino-* + Gr. *praxis* doing] (*obs.*) the diagnostic and therapeutic use of the rays of radioactive substances; radiopraxis.

actinoquinol sodium (ak-tin′o-kwĭ-nōl) chemical name: 8-ethoxy-5-quinolinesulfonic acid sodium salt; an ultraviolet screen, $C_{11}H_{10}NNaO_4S$.

actinoscopy (ak″tĭ-nos′ko-pe) [*actino-* + Gr. *skopein* to view] (*obs.*) examination by means of the roentgen ray.

Actinosporea (ak″tĭ-no-spor′e-ah) [*actino-* + *spore*] a class of parasitic protoza (phylum Myxozoa) found in invertebrates, especially annelids, and having spores with three polar capsules, each enclosing a coiled polar tube; a spore membrane with three valves; several to many sporoplasma; and a reduced trophozoite stage; with proliferation occurring mainly during sporogenesis. It comprises one subclass: Actinomyxia.

actinostereoscopy (ak″tĭ-no-ste″re-os′ko-pe) (*obs.*) actinoscopy.

actinotherapeutics (ak″tĭ-no-ther″ah-pu′tiks) actinotherapy.

actinotherapy (ak″tĭ-no-ther′ah-pe) [*actino-* + Gr. *therapeia* treatment] treatment of disease with ultraviolet or actinic rays.

actinotoxin (ak″tĭ-no-tok′sin) a crude poison derived from alcoholic extracts of the tentacles of sea anemones.

action (ak′shun) [L. *actio*] any performance of function or movement either of any part or organ or of the whole body. **ball-valve a.,** the intermittent obstruction caused by a free or partially attached foreign body in a tubular or cavitary structure, as by a foreign body in a bronchus, a stone in a bile duct, or a tumor in the cardiac atrium. **buffer a.,** an action that tends to stabilize an inanimate system or a body function or state, such as pH, blood pressure, [Ca^{++}], etc.; most commonly used to denote the stabilization of pH by acid-base buffers (tampon a.). **calorigenic a.,** 1. specific dynamic action. 2. the total energy released in the body by a food or food constituent. **capillary a.,** the transport of a fluid in a tube, caused by adhesion of the fluid to the tube wall. **contact a.,** contact catalysis. **cumulative a.,** action of increased intensity, as may be evidenced after administration of several doses of a drug due to the accumulation of the drug in the body so that the biological effect is greater than after the first dose. Called also *cumulative effect.* **diastasic a., diastatic a.,** the action of diastase in converting starch into glucose. **disordered a. of heart** (D.A.H.), neurocirculatory asthenia. **reflex a.,** a response resulting from the passage of excitation potential from a receptor to a muscle or gland, over a system of neurons without the necessity of volition. **specific a.,** the action of a drug which is exerted on a certain definite pathogenic organism. **specific dynamic a.,** the increase in metabolism over the basal rate brought about by the ingestion and assimilation of food, varying from 4 to 6 per cent for fats and carbohydrates to 30 per cent for protein. **tampon a.,** buffer a. **thermogenic a.,** the action of a food or drug in increasing the production of heat or the temperature of the body. **trigger a.,** an action that releases energy whose character has no relation to the process which released it. **vitaminoid a.,** an action resembling the action of vitamins.

activate (ak′tĭ-vāt) to render active.

activation (ak″tĭ-va′shun) the act or process of rendering active, as (*a*) in the transformation of pre-enzyme into an active enzyme by the action of a kinase or another pre-enzyme, or gain in the purifying of sewage by means of activated sludge; (*b*) the process by which the central nervous system is stimulated into activity through the mediation of the reticular activating system; (*c*) the deliberate induction of a pattern of electrical activity in the brain, as in the electrocardiographic diagnosis of epilepsy. **lymphocyte a.,** stimulation of lymphocytes by specific antigen or nonspecific mitogens resulting in macromolecular synthesis (RNA, protein, and DNA) and production of lymphokines; it is followed by proliferation and differentiation of the progeny into various effector and memory cells.

activator (ak′tĭ-va″tor) 1. a substance that renders some other substance more active, especially one that combines with an enzyme to increase its catalytic activity. 2. a substance that stimulates the development of a particular structure in the embryo. Cf. *inductor* and *organizer.* 3. functional a. 4. a chemical or other form of energy that activates the initiator of a polymerization reaction. **bow a.,**

a functional activator, the halves of which are connected by a wire bow or safety-pin loop; between the halves of the anterior area, a layer of rubber is attached as a shock absorber and to open the bite in front. Called also *Schwarz a.* **functional a.,** a myofunctional removable orthodontic appliance that acts as a passive transmitter of the force produced by the function of the activated muscle, and applied to the teeth and alveolar processes to effect tooth movement. Called also *Andresen appliance, monoblock a.,* and *monoblock appliance.* **monoblock a.,** a removable orthodontic appliance utilizing muscle forces to achieve therapeutic correction; called also *Andresen appliance* and *functional a.* **plasminogen a.,** a substance that has the ability to activate plasminogen and convert it into plasmin, its active form. **polyclonal a.,** a mitogen that activates lymphocytes of many antigenic specificities, in contrast to an antigen, which only activates cells specific for the antigen. Some polyclonal activators activate T cells; others activate B cells.

active (ak′tiv) characterized by action; not passive; not expectant. **optically a.,** capable of rotating the plane of polarization of a light wave.

activity (ak-tiv′ĭ-te) 1. the state of being active; the ability to produce some effect; the extent of some function or action. 2. a thermodynamic quantity that represents the effective concentration of a solute in a nonideal solution; if concentrations are replaced by activities, the equations for equilibrium constants, electrode potentials, osmotic pressure, boiling point elevation, freezing point depression, and vapor pressures of volatile solutes are converted from approximations that hold only for dilute solutions to exact equations that hold for all concentrations. The activity is equal to the product of the concentration and the activity coefficient, a dimensionless number measuring deviation from nonideality. Symbol a. 3. radioactivity; the number of disintegrations per unit time of a radioactive material, measured in curies or becquerels. Symbol A. 4. optical activity. **enzyme a.,** the catalytic effect exerted by an enzyme, expressed as units per milligram of enzyme (specific activity) or as molecules of substrate transformed per minute per molecule of enzyme (molecular activity). The conventional unit of enzyme activity is the International Unit (IU), equal to one micromole of substrate transformed per minute. A proposed coherent Systeme Internationale (SI) unit is the katal (kat), equal to one mole of substrate transformed per second. **leukemia-associated inhibitory a. (LIA),** the inhibition of normal marrow cells of donors from forming colonies of granulocytes and macrophages, induced *in vitro* by the presence of cell extracts, or of culture media conditioned by cells, from the bone marrow, spleen, or blood of patients with acute leukemia. **nonsuppressible insulin-like a.** (NSILA), insulin-like growth factor(s). **optical a.,** the ability of a chemical compound to rotate the plane of polarization of plane-polarized light. **specific a.,** activity per unit weight of a radioactive material, or the activity of a radioisotope per unit weight of the element (including stable isotopes) present.

actodigin (ak″to-dij′in) chemical name: 3β-(β-D-glucopyranosyloxy)-14,23-dihydroxy-24-nor-5β, 14β-chol-20-(22)-en-21-oic acid γ-lactone; a cardiotonic, $C_{29}H_{44}O_9$.

actomyosin (ak″to-mi′o-sin) a complex of the proteins actin and myosin occurring in muscle. Cf. *actin* and *myosin.* See also *myosin ATPase.*

Actonia (ak-to′ne-ah) a genus of ascomycetous fungi of the order Endomycetales, described as producing creamy patches in the throat resembling diphtheria; it is probably not a valid genus.

Actrapid (ak-trap′id) trademark for preparations of insulin injection (regular insulin).

actual (ak′chu-al) [L. *actualis*] real rather than potential.

actuary (ak′chu-a″re) a person whose business is the calculation of premiums and risks in insurance.

acu- (ak′u) [L *acus* needle] a combining form denoting relationship to a needle.

Acuaria spiralis (ak″u-a′re-ah spi-ra′lis) a filarioid parasite in the proventriculus and esophagus of fowls.

acuity (ah-ku′ĭ-te) [L. *acuitas* sharpness] clarity or clearness, especially of the vision. **Vernier a.,** displacement threshold; see under *threshold.*

aculeate (ah-ku′le-āt) [L. *aculeatus* thorny] covered with sharp points; pointed.

acuminate (ah-ku′mĭ-nāt) [L. *acuminatus*] sharp pointed.

acupoint (ak′u-point) a specific site of needle insertion along a body meridian in acupuncture.

acupressure (ak′u-presh″er) [*acu*- + L. *pressio* or *pressura* pressure] compression of a bleeding vessel by inserting needles into adjacent tissue.

acupuncture (ak′u-pungk″cher) [*acu*- + L. *punctura* a prick] the Chinese practice of insertion of needles into specific exterior body locations to relieve pain, to induce surgical anesthesia, and for therapeutic purposes.

acus (a′kus) [L.] a needle or needle-like process.

acusection (ak′u-sek″shun) cutting by means of the electrosurgical needle.

acusector (ak′u-sek″tor) [*acu*- + L. *sectere* to cut] an electric needle used like a scalpel for incising tissues.

acute (ah-kūt′) [L. *acutus* sharp] 1. sharp; poignant. 2. having a short and relatively severe course.

acyanotic (ah-si″ah-not′ik) characterized by absence of cyanosis.

acyclia (ah-si′kle-ah) arrest of circulation of body fluids.

acyclic (a-si′klik) 1. in chemistry, having an open-chain structure; aliphatic. 2. occurring independently of a cycle, as of the menstrual cycle.

acyclovir (a-si′klo-vir) a synthetic acyclic purine nucleoside with selective antiviral activity against herpes simplex virus (types 1 and 2, varicella-zoster virus, Epstein-Barr virus, and cytomegalovirus). It is used in the treatment of genital and mucocutaneous herpesvirus infections in certain patients, both immunocompromised and nonimmunocompromised.

acyl (as′il) an organic radical derived from an organic acid by removal of the hydroxyl group.

Acylanid (as″il-an′id) trademark for a preparation of acetyldigitoxin.

acylase (as′ĭ-lās) amidase (def. 2).

acylation (as″ĕ-la′shun) the introduction of an acid radical into the molecule of a chemical compound.

acylcholine acylhydrolase (as″il-ko′lin as″il-hi′dro-lās) cholinesterase.

acyl-CoA (as″il-ko′a) acyl coenzyme A.

acyl-CoA desaturase (a′sil de-să′choor-ās) [EC 1.14.99.5] an enzyme activity of the oxidoreductase class that catalyzes the reaction: stearoyl CoA + O_2 + NAD(P)H oleoyl CoA + $2H_2$ O + NAD(P)$^+$. It is a complex in the endoplasmic reticulum involving a flavoprotein (FAD), cytochrome b_5, and an NACH or NADPH cytochrome b_5 reductase. Also called *stearoyl-CoA desaturase.*

acyl coenzyme A (as″il, a″sil, ko-en′zīm) a thiol ester of a carboxylic acid, particularly a long-chain fatty acid, and coenzyme A. Its formation is the first step in fatty acid oxidation, leading to the sequential production of two-carbon groups and progressively shorter acyl coenzyme A compounds until the entire chain is degraded. Abbreviated acyl CoA.

acylsphingosine deacylase (a″sil-sfing′go-sēn de-a′sil-ās) [EC 3.5.1.23] an enzyme of the hydrolase class that catalyzes the reaction *N*-acylsphingosine + H_2O = sphingosine + a fatty acid anion. A genetic deficiency of the enzyme, transmitted as an autosomal recessive trait, results in accumulation of ceramides and gangliosides (Farber disease). Called also *ceramidase.*

acyltransferase (as″il, a″sil, trans′fer-ās) [EC 2.3] one of a subclass of the transferase class that catalyze the transfer of an acyl group from a donor (often the corresponding acyl coenzyme A derivative) to an acceptor compound. Many form esters or amides. Called also *transacylase.*

acystia (ah-sis′te-ah) [*a* neg. + Gr. *kystis* bladder] congenital absence of the bladder.

acystinervia (ah-sis″tĕ-ner′ve-ah) [*a* neg. + Gr. *kystis* bladder + L. *nervus* nerve + *-ia*] defective nervous tone in the bladder.

acystineuria (ah-sis″te-nu′re-ah) acystinervia.

AD diphenylchlorarsine; anodal duration.

A.D. abbreviation for L. *au′ris dex′tra,* right ear.

ad [L. *ad* to] used in writing prescriptions to indicate that a substance (usually a diluent) be added up to a certain amount.

ad- [L. *ad* to] a prefix meaning to or toward, addition to, nearness, or intensification.

-ad 1. [L. *ad* to] an adverbial suffix meaning toward, as in cephalad, caudad. 2. [Gr. *-as,* gen. *-ados*] a suffix denoting a group, as in triad, or derivation from or connection with.

A.D.A. American Dental Association; American Diabetes Association; American Dietetic Association.

ADA adenosine deaminase.

adactylia (ah″dak-til′e-ah) adactyly.

adactylism (a-dak′tĭ-lizm) adactyly.

adactylous (a-dak′tĭ-lus) pertaining to adactyly; lacking digits on the hand or foot.

adactyly (a-dak′tĭ-le) [*a* neg. + Gr. *daktylos* finger] a developmental anomaly characterized by the absence of digits on the hand or foot.

adamantine (ad″ah-man′tin) pertaining to the enamel of the teeth.

adamantinocarcinoma (ad″ah-man″tĭ-no-kar″-sĭ-no′mah) (*obs.*) ameloblastic sarcoma.

adamantinoma (ad″ah-man″tĭ-no′mah) ameloblastoma. **pituitary a.,** craniopharyngioma. **a. polycys′ticum,** an adamantinoma (ameloblastoma) that has undergone cystic degeneration.

adamantoblast (ad″ah-man′to-blast) [Gr. *adamas* a hard substance + *blastos* germ] ameloblast.

adamantoblastoma (ad″ah-man″to-blas-to′mah) ameloblastoma.

adamantoma (ad″ah-man-to′mah) ameloblastoma.

adamas (ad′ah-mas) [Gr. "unconquerable"] anything that is fixed or unalterable. **a. den′tis,** the enamel of the teeth.

Adami's theory (ad-am′ēz) [John George *Adami,* Canadian pathologist, 1862–1926] see under *theory.*

Adamkiewicz demilunes (ah-dam-ke′viks) [Albert *Adamkiewicz,* Polish pathologist, 1850–1921] see under *demilune.*

Adams' operation, saw (ad′amz) 1. [William *Adams,* English surgeon, 1810–1900] see under *operation,* defs. 1, 2, and 3, and under *saw.* 2. [Sir William *Adams,* British surgeon, 1783–1827] see under *operation,* def. 5.

Adams-Stokes disease (syncope, syndrome) [Robert *Adams,* Irish physician, 1791–1875; William *Stokes,* Irish physician, 1804–1878] see under *disease.*

adamsite (ad′amz-īt) diphenylaminearsine chloride.

Adansonia (ad″an-so′ne-ah) [after Michel *Adanson,* French naturalist, 1727–1806] a genus of trees in the Bombacaceae family. *A. digita′ta* is the baobab, a huge tree of Africa, found also in India. In Africa, the young leaves and seeds are eaten as food and the pulp is widely used for its diaphoretic properties.

adansonian (ad″an-son′ne-an) named for Michel *Adanson;* see *numerical taxonomy,* under *taxonomy.*

adaptation (ad″ap-ta′shun) [L. *adaptare* to fit] 1. the adjustment of an organism to its environment, or the process by which it enhances such fitness. 2. the normal ability of the eye to adjust itself to variations in the intensity of light; the adjustment to such variations. 3. the decline in the frequency of firing of a neuron, particularly of a receptor, under conditions of constant stimulation. 4. in dentistry, (*a*) the proper fitting of a denture, (*b*) the degree of proximity and interlocking of restorative material to a tooth preparation, (*c*) the exact adjustment of bands to teeth. 5. in microbiology, the adjustment of bacterial physiology to a new environment; see *genetic a.* and *phenotypic a.* **auditory a.,** a decrease in auditory sensitivity during auditory stimulation as a result of the stimulation. **color a.,** 1. fading of hue and dulling of brightness of visual perceptions with prolonged stimulation. 2. adjustment of vision to degree of brightness or color tone of illumination indoors or out; includes *dark a.* **dark a.,** the adaptation of the eye to vision in the dark or in reduced illumination (night vision), with build-up of rhodopsin in the retinal rods; called also *scotopic a.* **enzymatic a.,** inducible enzyme synthesis; see under *synthesis.* See also *phenotypic a.* **genetic a.,** the natural selection of the progeny of a mutant better suited to a new environment; especially seen in the development of bacterial strains resistant to certain antibiotics and drugs. **light a.,** adaptation of the eye to vision in the sunlight or in bright illumination (photopia), with reduction in the concentration of the photosensitive pigments of the eye; called also *photopic a.* **phenotypic a.,** a change in the structural and physiological properties of an organism in response to a genetic mutation or to a change in environment. Especially in microbiology, phenotypic adaptation refers to the utilization of new nutrients by induced enzyme formation, the requirement for new growth factors resulting from genetic mutation, or a change in cell surface components (peptidoglycan, capsule, pili, flagella) resulting from environment or genetic alterations. **photopic a.,** light a. **retinal a.,** the adjustment of the photoreceptor cell of the eye to the surrounding illumination. **scotopic a.,** dark a.

adapter (ah-dap′ter) a device by which different parts of an apparatus or instrument are connected.

adaptive (ah-dap′tiv) being capable of adaptation.

adaptometer (ad″ap-tom′ĕ-ter) [*adaptation* + *-meter*] an instrument for measuring the time required for retinal adaptation: i.e., for regeneration of the visual purple. It is used to help detect night blindness, vitamin A deficiency, and retinitis pigmentosa. **color a.,** an instrument using colored and neutral filters and control of illuminant to demonstrate adaptation of eye to color or light.

adaxial (ad-ak′se-al) located alongside of, or directed toward, the axis.

ADCC antibody-dependent cell-mediated cytotoxicity.

add. abbreviation for L. *ad′de*, add, or *adde′tur*, let there be added; used in writing prescriptions.

adde (ad′e) [L.] add.

adder (ad′er) 1. *Vipera berus.* 2. any of many venomous snakes of the family Viperidae, such as the puff adder and the European viper. See table accompanying *snake.* **death a.,** an extremely venomous elapid snake, *Acanthophis antarcticus* of Australia and New Guinea, with a short, stout body and a tail with a spine at the tip. **puff a.,** an extremely venomous, brightly colored, viperine snake, *Bitis arientans,* of Africa and Arabia; when annoyed it inflates its stubby body and hisses loudly.

addict (ad′ikt) a person who cannot resist a habit, especially the use of drugs or alcohol, for physiological or psychological reasons.

addiction (ah-dik′shun) the state of being given up to some habit, especially strong dependence on a drug. **alcohol a.,** alcoholism in which tolerance or withdrawal is present. **drug a.,** a state of heavy dependence on a drug, defined by some authorities as a state of physical dependence characterized by tolerance or withdrawal and by others in a wider sense that includes emotional dependence, i.e., compulsive or pathological drug use, also referred to as abuse or habituation. **polysurgical a.,** Munchausen syndrome.

addiment (ad′ĭ-ment) (*obs.*) complement.

Addis count, test [Thomas *Addis,* San Francisco physician, 1881–1949] see under *count.*

addisin (ad′ĭ-sin) a substance present in the gastric juice that has stimulating power on bone-marrow formation; such an extract from the gastric juice of the hog is used in pernicious anemia.

Addison's anemia, disease (ad′-ĭ-sonz) [Thomas *Addison,* English physician, 1793–1860; he was a colleague of Bright at Guy's Hospital] see *pernicious anemia,* under *anemia;* see *circumscribed scleroderma,* under *scleroderma;* and see under *disease.*

Addison's planes, point (ad′ĭ-sonz) [Christopher *Addison,* English anatomist, 1869–1951] see under *plane* and *point.*

addisonian (ad″dĭ-so′ne-an) named for Thomas *Addison;* see pernicious *anemia,* under *anemia,* and see under *disease.*

addisonism (ad′ĭ-son-izm″) a group of symptoms associated with tuberculosis, consisting of pigmentation and debility, resembling those of Addison's disease.

additive (ad′ĭ-tiv) 1. characterized by addition; see also under *effect.* 2. a substance, as a flavoring agent, preservative, or vitamin, added to another substance to improve its appearance, increase its nutritional value, etc.

adducent (ah-du′sent) performing adduction.

adduct (ah-dukt′) [L. *adducere* to draw toward] 1. to draw toward the median plane or (in the digits) toward the axial line of a limb. 2. a chemical addition product.

adduction (ah-duk′shun) the act of adducting or the state of being adducted.

adductor (ah-duk′tor) [L.] that which adducts; see *Table of Musculi.*

Adelea (ah-del′e-ah) [Gr. *adēlos* unseen] a genus of coccidian protozoa (suborder Adeleina, order Eucoccidiida) parasitic in the intestinal epithelium of arthropods, characterized by the development of sporocysts in a thin-walled oocyst.

Adeleina (ad″ĕ-le′ĭ-nah) a suborder of homoxenous or heteroxenous protozoa (order Eucoccidiida, subclass Coccidia) parasitic in the intestinal epithelium and associated glands of invertebrates, characterized by syzygy during development that usually involves a macrogamete and microgamont, with the latter producing one to four sporozoites enclosed in an envelope. Representative genera include *Adelea, Haemogregarina, Hepatozoon,* and *Klossiella.*

adelomorphic (ah-del″o-mor′fik) adelomorphous.

adelomorphous (ah-del″o-mor′fus) [Gr. *adēlos* not evident + *morphē* form] not having a clearly defined form; see under *cell.*

adenalgia (ad″ĕ-nal′je-ah) [aden- + Gr. *algos* pain + *-ia*] pain in a gland; called also *adenodynia.*

adenase (ad′ĕ-nās) adenine deaminase.

adendric (ah-den′drik) adendritic.

adendritic (ah″den-drit′ik) [a neg. + Gr. *dendron* tree] lacking dendrites.

adenectomy (ad″ĕ-nek′to-me) [aden- + Gr. *ektomē* excision] surgical removal of a gland.

adenectopia (ad″ĕ-nek-to′pe-ah) [aden- + Gr. *ektopos* displaced + *-ia*] malposition or displacement of a gland.

adenia (ah-de′ne-ah) chronic great enlargement of the lymphatic glands; see also *lymphoma* and *pseudoleukemia.*

adenic (ah-de′nik) pertaining to or resembling a gland.

adeniform (ah-den′ĭ-form) [aden- + L. *forma* shape] resembling a gland, especially in shape.

adenine (ad′ĕ-nēn) a white crystalline base, 6-aminopurine, $C_5H_5N_5$, found in various animal and vegetable tissues as one of the purine base constituents of DNA and RNA. It is one of the decomposition products of nuclein and may be found in the urine. Adenine is nonpoisonous, and occurs in the form of pearly crystals. **a. arabinoside,** vidarabine. **a. hypoxanthine,** a leukomaine, $C_5H_5N_5 + C_4H_4N_4O$, a compound of adenine and hypoxanthine. **a. nucleotide,** adenylic a. **a. sulfate,** white crystals, $(C_5H_5N_5)_2 \cdot H_2SO_4$, formerly used in nucleotide therapy in agranulocytosis.

adenine deaminase (ad′ĕ-nīn, ad′ĕ-nēn, de-am′ĭ-nās) [EC 3.5.4.2] an enzyme of the hydrolase class that catalyzes the reaction adenine + H_2O = hypoxanthine + NH_3. The enzyme is found in microorgansims and invertebrates but not in mammals. Called also *adenase.*

adenine phosphoribosyl transferase (ad′ĕ-nēn fos″-fo-ri′bo-sil trans′fer-ās) [EC 2.4.2.7] an enzyme of the transferase class that catalyzes the reaction adenine + 5-phospho-α-D-ribose 1-diphosphate = AMP + pyrophosphate. The enzyme is responsible for salvage of adenine within the cell. Deficiency of the enzyme, an autosomal recessive trait, causes infant colic, hematuria, and urinary calculi of 2,8-dihydroxyadenine.

adenine phosphoribosyl transferase (APRT) deficiency an autosomal recessive disorder involving the purine salvage enzyme APRT; clinical signs range from none to urolithiasis (causing colic, hematuria, urinary tract infection, and dysuria) to acute renal failure and permanent kidney damage.

adenitis (ad″ĕ-ni′tis) inflammation of a gland. Cf. *acinitis.* **cervical a.,** a condition characterized by enlarged, inflamed, and tender lymph nodes of the neck; seen in certain infectious diseases of children, such as acute infections of the throat. **mesenteric a.,** mesenteric lymphadenitis. **phlegmonous a.,** inflammation of a gland and the surrounding connective tissue; called also *adenophlegmon.*

Adenium (ah-de′ne-um) a genus of African plants of the family Aponcynaceae which are used for arrow poisons; they contain cardioactive glycosides (e.g., somalin) which are close in structure and action to the digitalis glycosides.

adenization (ad″ĕ-ni-za′shun) the assumption by other tissue of an abnormal glandlike appearance; adenoid change.

aden(o) [Gr. *adēn*, gen. *adenos* gland] a combining form denoting relationship to a gland or glands.

adenoacanthoma (ad″ĕ-no-ak″an-tho′mah) an adenocarcinoma in which some or the majority of the cells exhibit squamous differentiation; called also *adenocancroid*.

adenoameloblastoma (ad″ĕ-no-ah-mel″o-blas-to′mah) an odontogenic tumor characterized by the formation of ductlike structures in place of or in addition to a typical ameloblastic pattern.

adenoangiosarcoma (ad″ĕ-no-an″je-o-sar-ko′mah) (*obs.*) an angiosarcoma involving gland structures.

adenoblast (ad′ĕ-no-blast″) [*adeno-* + Gr. *blastos* germ] an embryonic cell that gives rise to glandular tissue.

adenocancroid (ad″ĕ-no-kang′kroid) adenoacanthoma.

adenocarcinoma (ad″ĕ-no-kar″sĭ-no′mah) carcinoma derived from glandular tissue or in which the tumor cells form recognizable glandular structures; adenocarcinomas may be classified according to the predominant pattern of cell arrangement, as papillary, alveolar, etc., or according to a particular product of the cells, as mucinous adenocarcinoma. **acinar a., acinous a.,** alveolar a. **alveolar a.,** adenocarcinoma composed of cells arranged in the form of alveoli. **follicular a.,** one in which the cells are arranged in the form of follicles, usually of thyroid origin. **a. of kidney,** renal cell carcinoma. **mucinous a.,** mucinous carcinoma. **papillary a., polypoid a.,** an adenocarcinoma in which the tumor elements are arranged as finger-like processes or as a solid spherical nodule projecting from an epithelial surface.

adenocele (ad′ĕ-no-sēl″) [*adeno-* + Gr. *kēlē* tumor] an adenomatous cystic tumor.

adenocellulitis (ad″ĕ-no-sel″u-li′tis) inflammation of a gland and the tissue around it.

adenochondroma (ad″ĕ-no-kon-dro′mah) a tumor containing both adenomatous and chondromatous elements, as in the mixed tumor of salivary gland; called also *chondroadenoma*.

adenochondrosarcoma (ad″ĕ-no-kon″dro-sar-ko′mah) (*obs.*) a tumor containing the elements of adenoma, chondroma, and sarcoma.

adenocyst (ad′ĕ-no-sist″) [*adeno-* + Gr. *kystis* bladder] adenocystoma.

adenocystoma (ad″ĕ-no-sis-to′mah) an adenoma in which there is cyst formation. **papillary a. lymphomato′sum,** a rare cystic tumor containing epithelial and lymphoid tissues found in the regions of the submaxillary and parotid glands; called also *Warthin's tumor* and *adenolymphoma*.

adenocyte (ad′ĕ-no-sīt″) [*adeno-* + Gr. *kytos* hollow vessel] a mature secretory cell of a gland.

adenodynia (ad″ĕ-no-din′e-ah) [*adeno-* + Gr. *odynē* pain + *-ia*] pain in a gland.

adenoepithelioma (ad″ĕ-no-ep″ĭ-the″le-o′mah) a tumor composed of glandular and epithelial elements.

adenofibroma (ad″ĕ-no-fi-bro′mah) a tumor composed of connective tissue containing glandular structures. **a. edemato′des,** a tumor composed of glandular and connective tissue elements in which there is marked edema of the stroma, as in nasal polyp.

adenofibrosis (ad″ĕ-no-fi-bro′sis) fibroid change in a gland.

adenogenous (ad″ĕ-noj′ĕ-nus) [*adeno-* + Gr. *gennan* to produce] originating from glandular tissue.

adenographic (ad″ĕ-no-graf′ik) pertaining to adenography.

adenography (ad″ĕ-nog′rah-fe) [*adeno-* + Gr. *graphein* to write] roentgenography of a gland or glands.

adenohypophyseal (ad″ĕ-no-hi″po-fiz′e-al) adenohypophysial.

adenohypophysectomy (ad″ĕ-no-hi-pof″ĭ-sek′to-me) ablation of the glandular portion (the adenohypophysis) of the hypophysis.

adenohypophysial (ad″ĕ-no-hi″po-fiz′e-al) pertaining to the adenohypophysis.

adenohypophysis (ad″ĕ-no-hi-pof′ĭ-sis) [*adeno-* + *hypophysis*] [NA] the anterior (glandular) lobe of the pituitary gland (hypophysis), as distinguished from the posterior (neural) lobe (neurohypophysis). Called also *lobus anterior*

hypophysis [NA alternative]. See *pituitary gland*, under *gland*.

adenoid (ad′ĕ-noid) [*aden-* + Gr. *eidos* form] 1. resembling a gland. 2. in the plural, lymphoid tissue that normally exists in the nasopharynx of children and is known as the pharyngeal tonsil. Also, a popular term for hypertrophy of this tissue. 3. pertaining to adenoids.

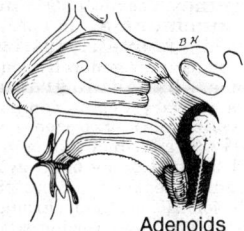

Adenoids

adenoidectomy (ad″ĕ-noid-ek′to-me) [*adenoid* + Gr. *ektomē* excision] excision of the adenoids.

adenoidism (ad′ĕ-noid-izm) the symptom-complex which results from the presence of greatly enlarged adenoids.

adenoiditis (ad″ĕ-noid-i′tis) inflammation of the adenoid tissue of the nasopharynx.

adenoleiomyofibroma (ad″ĕ-no-li″o-mi″o-fi-bro′mah) a leiomyofibroma containing adenomatous elements.

adenolipoma (ad″ĕ-no-lĭ-po′mah) a tumor composed of both glandular and fatty tissue elements.

adenolipomatosis (ad″ĕ-no-lip″o-mah-to′sis) a condition characterized by the development of multiple adenolipomas.

adenologaditis (ad″ĕ-no-log″ah-di′tis) [*adeno-* + Gr. *logades* whites of the eyes + *-itis*] 1. ophthalmia neonatorum. 2. inflammation of the glands of the conjunctiva.

adenolymphitis (ad″ĕ-no-lim-fi′tis) lymphadenitis.

adenolymphocele (ad″ĕ-no-lim′fo-sēl) [*adeno-* + *lymphocele*] lymphadenocele.

adenolymphoma (ad″ĕ-no-lim-fo′mah) papillary adenocystoma lymphomatosum (Warthin's tumor) of salivary glands.

adenoma (ad″ĕ-no′mah) [*adeno-* + *-oma*] a benign epithelial tumor in which the cells form recognizable glandular structures or in which the cells are clearly derived from glandular epithelium. **acidophilic a.,** a tumor, usually found in the anterior lobe of the pituitary gland, whose cells stain with acid dyes; such pituitary tumors may give rise to excessive secretion of growth hormone, resulting in gigantism or acromegaly. A specific type of acidophilic adenoma, involving the lactotrophic cells, may give rise to nonpuerperal galactorrhea. **a. adamanti′num,** ameloblastoma. **a. alveola′re,** an adenoma whose cells are arranged like those of an alveolar gland. **basophil a., basophilic a.,** a small tumor of the anterior lobe of the pituitary gland whose cells stain with basic dyes and may give rise to excessive secretion of adrenocorticotropic hormone (ACTH), resulting in Cushing's syndrome. **bronchial a's,** adenomas situated in the submucosal tissues of large bronchi; they have a glandular structure and are thought to be derived from the mucous glands of the bronchi or from the ducts of those glands. Sometimes composed of well-differentiated cells and usually circumscribed, these tumors have two histologic forms: carcinoid and cylindroma. Although termed "adenomas," these tumors are now recognized as being of low-grade malignancy. **carcinoid a. of bronchus,** carcinoid tumor of bronchus; see under *tumor*. **chief cell a.,** adenoma of the parathyroid gland composed of solid masses of small chief cells similar to those seen in the normal gland. **chromophobe a., chromophobic a.,** a tumor of the anterior lobe of the pituitary gland whose cells do not stain readily with either acid or basic dyes and whose presence may be associated with hypopituitarism; although classically these adenomas have been said to be composed of sparsely granulated or degranulated (nonfunctioning) cells, some contain functioning cells and may be associated with a hyperpituitary state, e.g., acromegaly or Cushing's syndrome. **cortical a's,** minute adenomas in the cortex of the kidney, arising from the renal tubules. **a. des′truens** (*obs.*), an invasive, destructive adenocarcinoma of the stomach. **a. endometrioi′des ova′rii,** ovarian endometriosis. **eo-**

sinophil a., a tumor of eosinophilic cells of the anterior lobe of the pituitary gland whose presence is associated with acromegaly and gigantism. **a. fibro′sum,** fibroadenoma. **follicular a.,** adenoma of the thyroid in which the cells are arranged in the form of follicles. **a. gelatino′ sum,** colloid goiter. **a. hidradenoi′des,** hidradenoma. **Hürthle cell a.,** see under *tumor.* **islet a., langerhansian a.,** an islet cell adenoma of the pancreas. **a's of kidney,** cortical a's. **malignant a.,** adenocarcinoma. **mucinous a.,** an epithelial tumor whose cells produce mucin. **a. ova′rii testicula′re,** a Sertoli cell tumor of the ovary, now generally regarded as a variant of arrhenoblastoma. **oxyphilic granular cell a.,** a benign adenoma of salivary glands composed of acidophilic granular cells; called also *oncocytoma* and *pyknocytoma.* **papillary cystic a.,** a form of adenoma in which the alveoli are distended by fluid or by outgrowths of tissue. **pituitary a.,** a benign neoplasm of the pituitary gland; see *acidophilic a., basophilic a.,* and *chromophobe a.* **pleomorphic a.,** a benign, slow-growing tumor of the salivary gland, occurring as a small, painless, firm nodule, usually of the parotid gland, but also found in any major or accessory salivary gland anywhere in the oral cavity. It is most often seen in women in the fifth decade. Histologically, the tumor presents a variety of cells: cuboidal, columnar, and squamous cells, showing all forms of epithelial growth. **racemose a.,** an adenoma whose structure resembles that of a racemose gland. **sebaceous a., a. seba′ceum,** nevoid hyperplasia of sebaceous glands, forming multiple yellow papules or nodules of the face (Balzer type); a cutaneous malformation or hamartoma of the face involving blood vessels and connective tissue associated with the tuberous sclerosis complex (Pringle type). In the Pringle type the term adenoma sebaceum is a misnomer since the sebaceous glands are rarely involved. Called also *Pringle's disease.* **a. sudorip′arum,** adenoma of the sweat glands; called also *spiradenoma* and *hidradenoma.* **tubular a.,** a Sertoli cell tumor. **a. tubula′re testicula′re ova′rii,** a Sertoli cell tumor of the ovary, now generally recognized as a variant of arrhenoblastoma; called also *adenoma ovarii testiculare.* **villous a.,** a large soft papillary polyp on the mucosa of the large intestine.

adenomalacia (ad″ĕ-no-mah-la′she-ah) [*adeno-* + Gr. *malakia* softness] abnormal softening of a gland.

adenomatoid (ad″ĕ-no′mah-toid) resembling adenoma.

adenomatosis (ad″ĕ-no-mah-to′sis) 1. a condition characterized by development of numerous adenomatous growths. 2. a contagious neoplastic viral disease of adult sheep and goats, caused by bovid herpesvirus, with adenomatous proliferation in the alveoli and small bronchioles. Called also *jaagsiekte* and *lunger disease.* **multiple endocrine a.,** multiple endocrine neoplasia. **a. o′ris,** enlargement of the mucous glands of the lip without secretion or inflammation. **pluriglandular a.,** multiple endocrine neoplasia. **polyendocrine a.,** multiple endocrine neoplasia. **pulmonary a.,** 1. alveolar cell carcinoma. 2. a chronic progressive pneumonia of sheep, probably of viral origin, with adenomatous proliferation in the alveoli and small bronchioles. Called also *jaagsiekte* and *lunger disease.*

adenomatous (ad″ĕ-nom′ah-tus) pertaining to adenoma or to nodular hyperplasia of a gland.

adenomegaly (ad″ĕ-no-meg′ah-le) enlargement of the glands.

adenomere (ad′ĕ-no-mēr″) [*adeno-* + Gr. *meros* part] the blind terminal portion of a developing gland, becoming the functional portion of the organ.

adenomyoepithelioma (ad″ĕ-no-mi″o-ep″ĭ-the-le-o′mah) adenoid cystic carcinoma. **a. of stomach,** malformation of the gastric glands or Brunner's glands.

adenomyofibroma (ad″ĕ-no-mi″o-fi-bro′mah) a fibroma containing adenomatous and myomatous tissue.

adenomyoma (ad″ĕ-no-mi-o′mah) [*adeno-* + Gr. *mys* muscle + *-oma*] see *adenomyosis.* **a. psammopapilla′re,** a multiple papillary tumor in the broad ligament, described by Pick.

adenomyomatosis (ad″ĕ-no-mi″o-mah-to′sis) the formation of multiple adenomyomatous nodules in the parauterine tissues or in the uterus.

adenomyomatous (ad″ĕ-no-mi-o′mah-tus) pertaining to or resembling adenomyoma.

adenomyometritis (ad″ĕ-no-mi″o-mĕ-tri′tis) adenomyosis.

adenomyosarcoma (ad″ĕ-no-mi″o-sar-ko′mah) a mixed mesodermal tumor in which striated muscle cells are one component. **embryonal a.,** Wilms' tumor.

adenomyosis (ad″ĕ-no-mi-o′sis) a benign condition characterized by ingrowth of the endometrium into the uterine musculature, sometimes associated with an overgrowth of the latter. If the lesion forms a circumscribed tumor-like nodule, it is called *adenomyoma.* Called also *endometriosis interna* or *uterina, adenomyosis uteri,* and *adenomyometritis.* **a. exter′na,** endometriosis. **stromal a.,** stromatosis. **a. subbasa′lis,** a bandlike, usually diffuse and superficial invasion of the myometrium by epithelial elements, accompanied by small clusters of endometrial stromal cells. **a. tu′bae,** 1. an old term for salpingitis isthmica nodosa. 2. the growth of the endometrium into the lumen of the uterine tube from the uterus, replacing the endosalpinx. **a. u′teri,** adenomyosis.

adenomyxoma (ad″ĕ-no-mik-so′mah) (*obs.*) a tumor composed of both glandular and mucous elements.

adenomyxosarcoma (ad″ĕ-no-mik″so-sar-ko′mah) (*obs.*) a sarcoma containing both glandular and mucous elements.

adenoncus (ad″ĕ-nong′kus) [*adeno-* + Gr. *onkos* weight] enlargement of a gland.

adenoneural (ad″ĕ-no-nu′ral) pertaining to a gland and a nerve.

adenopathy (ad″ĕ-nop′ah-the) [*adeno-* + Gr. *pathos* disease] enlargement of the glands, especially of the lymphatic glands.

adenopharyngitis (ad″ĕ-no-far″in-ji′tis) [*adeno-* + Gr. *pharynx* pharynx + *-itis*] inflammation of the adenoids and pharynx, usually involving the tonsils.

adenophlegmon (ad″ĕ-no-fleg′mon) [*adeno-* + *phlegmon*] phlegmonous adenitis.

adenophthalmia (ad″ĕ-nof-thal′me-ah) [*adeno-* + Gr. *ophthalmos* eye + *-ia*] inflammation of the meibomian glands.

adenopituicyte (ad″ĕ-no-pĭ-tu′ĭ-sīt) see *pituicyte.*

adenosarcoma (ad″ĕ-no-sar-ko′mah) a mixed tumor composed of sarcomatous and glandular elements, as Wilms' tumor. **embryonal a.,** Wilms' tumor.

adenosclerosis (ad″ĕ-no-skle-ro′sis) [*adeno-* + Gr. *sklērōsis* hardening] the hardening of a gland.

adenosine (ah-den′o-sēn) a nucleoside, adenine β-D-ribofuranoside. Symbol A. **cyclic a. monophosphate (cyclic AMP, cAMP, 3′, 5′-AMP),** a cyclic nucleotide, adenosine 3′, 5′-cyclic monophosphate, that serves as an intracellular "second messenger" mediating the action of many peptide or amino acid–derived hormones, including catecholamines (at β receptors), histamine (at H_2 receptors), glucagon, ACTH (adrenocorticotropic hormone), ADH (antidiuretic hormone), LH (luteinizing hormone), FSH (follicle-stimulating hormone), PTH (parathyroid hormone), calcitonin, gastrin, secretin, TSH (thyroid stimulating hormone) and TRH (TSH releasing hormone). The hormone, "the first messenger," binds to a specific receptor on cell membrane of target cells. This activates the enzyme adenylate cyclase, which produces cyclic AMP from ATP. Cyclic AMP binds to protein kinases inducing the phosphorylation of various enzymes, converting them from an inactive to an active form or vice versa. Cyclic AMP has a transient activity because it is rapidly degraded by a phophodiesterase. **a. 3′:5′-cyclic phosphate,** a cyclic nucleotide participating in the activities of many hormones, including catecholamines, ACTH, vasopressin, etc. Because this compound is formed from ATP by the action of adenyl cyclase which in turn is stimulated by the interaction of the aforementioned hormones with the plasma membrane of target cells, it has been called the "second messenger" in a mechanism of hormone action. Called also *cyclic AMP.* **a. diphosphate (ADP),** a nucleotide, adenosine 5′-pyrophosphate, involved in energy metabolism; it is produced by hydrolysis of ATP and converted back to ATP by the processes of oxidative phosphorylation and substrate-level phosphorylation. **a. monophosphate (AMP),** a nucleotide, adenosine 5′-phosphate, involved in energy metabolism; it is produced by hydrolysis of ATP and converted to ADP by adenylate kinase. Called also *adenylic acid.* **a. phosphate,** any of the three interconvertible compounds in which adenosine is attached through its ribose group to one (a. monophosphate), two (a.

diphosphate), or three (a. triphosphate) phosphoric acid molecules. **a. 3′-phosphate,** see *adenylic acid,* under *acid.* **a. 5′-phosphate,** see *adenylic acid,* under *acid.* **a. triphosphate (ATP),** a nucleotide, adenosine 5′-triphosphate, involved in energy metabolism and required for RNA synthesis; it occurs in all cells and is used to store energy in the form of high-energy phosphate bonds. Hydrolysis of ATP to ADP and inorganic phosphate cleaves one high-energy bond; hydrolysis of ATP to AMP and inorganic pyrophosphate cleaves two, because inorganic pyrophosphate is immediately cleaved by inorganic pyrophosphatase. The free energy derived from hydrolysis of ATP is used to drive metabolic reactions including the synthesis of nucleic acids and proteins, to move molecules against concentration gradients (active transport), and to produce mechanical motion (contraction of myofibrils and microtubules).

adenosine deaminase (ah-den′o-sēn de-am′ĭ-nās) [EC 3.5.4.4] an enzyme of the hydrolase class that catalyzes the reaction adenosine + H_2O = inosine + NH_3. The reaction is a part of the purine salvage mechanism. A deficiency of this enzyme, transmitted as an autosomal recessive trait, has been found in many individuals with severe combined immunodeficiency syndrome. Abbreviated ADA.

adenosine kinase (ah-den′o-sēn ki′nās) [EC 2.7.1.20] an enzyme of the transferase class that catalyzes the reaction ATP + adenosine = ADP + AMP. The reaction is part of the purine salvage mechanism.

adenosinetriphosphatase (ah-den″o-sin-tri-fos′fah-tās) [EC 3.6.1.3] an enzyme of the hydrolase class that catalyzes the reaction ATP + H_2O = ADP + orthophosphate. The reaction is a result of the concerted action of proteins using ATP to drive processes such as muscle contraction, maintenance of concentration gradients, membrane transport, and regulation of ion concentrations. Isolated component proteins, such as myosin, or damaged organelles, may exhibit the activity *in vitro,* as such. Called also *ATPase.* See also *myosin, Na⁺, K⁺-ATPase, Ca²⁺, Mg²⁺-ATPase.*

adenosis (ad″ĕ-no′sis) 1. any disease of the glands. 2. the abnormal development or formation of gland tissue. **blunt duct a.,** a form of mammary dysplasia characterized by dominance of the proliferation of the epithelial parenchyma; it is often accompanied by fibrosis and cystic disease of the breast. **a. vagi′nae,** the presence in the vagina of multiple ectopic areas of folded endocervical mucosa.

S-**adenosylmethionine** (ah-den″o-sil-mĕ-thi′o-nēn) a reaction product of ATP and methionine in which the S atom of methionine is bound to the ribose of adenosine; it serves as a methyl donor in transmethylation reactions.

adenotome (ad′ĕ-no-tōm″) [adeno- + Gr. *tomē* cutting] an instrument for excision of the adenoids.

adenotonsillectomy (ad″ĕ-no-ton″sil-lek′to-me) removal of the adenoids and tonsils.

adenous (ad′ĕ-nus) pertaining to a gland.

adenoviral (ad″ĕ-no-vi′ral) pertaining to or caused by adenoviruses.

adenovirus (ad″ĕ-no-vi′rus) one of a group of viruses found in all parts of the world, causing disease of the upper respiratory tract and conjunctivae, and also present in latent infections in normal persons. Some 31 differentiable serotypes have been described and given numbers. Types 1, 2, and 5 have been recovered from tonsils and adenoids of persons not ill with respiratory disease, as well as from patients with febrile respiratory infections; types 3, 4, 7, 14, and 21 have been isolated from patients with acute respiratory disease. Adenovirus type 3 is the specific etiologic agent of pharyngoconjunctival fever, and adenovirus type 8 is thought to be the specific cause of epidemic keratoconjunctivitis. In addition to the human adenovirus types, there are simian, bovine, avian, canine, and murine types. Many adenoviruses induce malignancy in certain species.

adenyl (ad′ĕ-nil) a chemical radical resulting from the formal loss of an OH group attached to phosphorus from adenosine-5′-monophosphoric acid (5′-AMP).

adenylate (ah-den′ĭ-lāt) an ionized form of adenosine monophosphate (AMP).

adenylate cyclase (ah-den′ĭ-lāt si′klās) [EC 4.6.1.1] an enzyme of the lyase class that catalyzes the reaction ATP = 3′,5′ – cyclic AMP + pyrophosphate. The enzyme occurs in plasma cell membranes and is activated by certain hormones

(epinephrine, vasopressin, glucagon, and corticotropin). The resultant cyclic AMP serves as an important metabolic regulator. Called also *adenyl cyclase, adenylyl cyclase.*

adenylate deaminase (ah-den′ĭ-lāt de-am′ĭ-nās) AMP deaminase.

adenylate kinase (ah-den′ĭ-lāt ki′nās) [EC 2.7.4.3] an enzyme of the transferase class that catalyzes the reaction ADP + ADP = ATP + AMP, thus regenerating ATP from 2 moles of ADP. The enzyme occurs predominantly in muscle and provides a means of using all of the energy from ATP for muscle contraction. The reaction makes AMP concentration a sensitive indicator of depletion of the high-energy phosphate pool, since [AMP] ∝ [ADP]². Called also *AMP kinase.*

adenyl cyclase (ad″ĕ-nil si′klās) adenylate cyclase.

adenylic acid (ad″ĕ-nil′ic) adenosine monophosphate.

adenylic acid deaminase (ad″ĕ-nil′ik as′id de-am′ĭ-nās) AMP deaminase.

adenylosuccinase (ad″ĕ-nil-o-suk′sĭ-nās) adenylosuccinate lyase.

adenylosuccinate lyase (ad″ĕ-nil-o-suk′sĭ-nāt li′ās) [EC 4.3.2.2] an enzyme of the lyase class that catalyzes the reaction adenylosuccinate = fumarate + AMP. The enzyme occurs in the liver where the reaction is a step in purine synthesis; in muscle it is involved in the utilization of energy. Called also *adenylosuccinase.*

adenylpyrophosphatase (ad″ĕ-nil-pi″ro-fos′fah-tās) adenosenetriphosphatase (obs.).

adenylpyrophosphate (ad″ĕ-nil-pi″ro-fos′fāt) adenosine triphosphate.

adenylyl (ad′ĕ-nĭ-lil) the radical formed by removal of OH from the phosphate group of adenosine monophosphate.

adenylyltransferase (ad″ĕ-nĭ-lil-trans′fer-ās) one of the nucleotidyltransferases [EC 2.7.7] that catalyzes the transfer of an adenylyl residue from one compound to another.

adeps (ad′eps), gen. *ad′ipis* [L.] lard; the purified omental fat of the hog, used in the preparation of ointments. **a. anseri′nus,** goose grease. **a. benzoina′tus,** benzoinated lard. **a. la′nae,** anhydrous lanolin. **a. la′nae hydro′sus,** lanolin. **a. ovil′lus,** sheep lard, or tallow. **a. por′ci,** hog lard. **a. re′nis,** the fatty capsule of the kidney. **a. suil′lus,** hog lard.

adequacy (ad′ĕ-kwah-se) the state of being sufficient for a specific purpose. **velopharyngeal a.,** sufficient functional closure of the velum against the postpharyngeal wall so that air and hence sound cannot enter the nasopharyngeal and nasal cavities.

adermia (ah-der′me-ah) [a neg. + Gr. *derma* skin + -ia] congenital defect or absence of the skin.

adermine (ah-der′min) pyridoxine; vitamin B₆.

adermogenesis (ah-der″mo-jen′ĕ-sis) [a neg. + Gr. *derma* skin + *genesis* production] imperfect development of the skin.

Ad grat. acid. abbreviation for L. *ad gra′tum acidita′tem,* to an agreeable sourness, an obsolete instruction in pharmacy.

ADH antidiuretic hormone; see *vasopressin.*

Adhatoda (ad-hat′o-dah) a plant genus of the Acanthaceae family. *A. vasica,* known as the Malabar nut tree, is used in India for its antispasmodic and expectorant properties.

adhere (ad-hēr′) to cling together; to become fastened.

adherence (ad-hēr′ens) the act or quality of sticking to something. **immune a.,** the adherence of antigen-antibody complexes or cells coated with antibody or complement to cells bearing complement receptors or Fc receptors. The agglutination reaction between antigen-antibody complexes or antibody coated cells and indicator cells, usually human erythrocytes, bearing complement receptors is used as a detector system in complement fixation tests (immune adherence hemagglutination assay).

adhesin (ad-he′zin) lectin.

adhesio (ad-he′ze-o), pl. *adhesio′nes* [L. "clinging together"] a connecting band or structure. **a. interthalam′ica** [NA], a mass of gray matter connecting the thalami across the midline of the third ventricle; it develops as a secondary adhesion and is often absent. Called also *intermediate mass* and *massa intermedia.*

adhesion (ad-he′zhun) [L. *adhaesio,* from *adhaerere* to stick to] 1. the property of remaining in close proximity, as that resulting from the physical attraction of molecules to a substance, or the molecular attraction existing between the surfaces of contacting bodies. 2. the stable joining of parts to each other, which may occur abnormally. 3. a fibrous band or structure by which parts abnormally adhere. **amniotic a's,** fibrous adhesions from the amnion to the fetus. **attic a's** (*obs.*), adhesions about the gallbladder and pyloric region. **primary a.,** healing by first intention. **secondary a.,** healing by second intention. **sublabial a.,** abnormal union of the sublabial mucosa of the upper lip to the alveolar process; usually present in cleft lip. **traumatic uterine a's,** adhesions of the uterus, most often in the cervical canal, frequently in the uterine cavity, and sometimes in both the cervix and the corpus, which are usually caused by curettage; cervical adhesions cause amenorrhea (see *Asherman's syndrome,* under *syndrome*), whereas corporeal adhesions usually are asymptomatic.

adhesiotomy (ad-he″ze-ot′o-me) the cutting or division of adhesions.

adhesive (ad-he′siv) 1. sticky; tenacious. 2. a substance that causes close adherence of adjoining surfaces. **dental a.,** see under *sealant.* **denture a.,** a compound, in powder or paste form, used to stabilize dentures in the mouth.

adhesiveness (ad-he′siv-nes) the property of remaining adherent. **platelet a.,** the physical property of platelets by which they stick to a variety of materials in vivo and in vitro, but more specifically this phenomenon as it occurs in the initial formation of a clot and in the maintenance of hemostasis.

Adhib. abbreviation for L. *adhiben′dus,* to be administered.

adiabatic (ah-di″ah-bat′ik) conducted without the evolution or absorption of heat.

adiactinic (ah-di″ak-tin′ik) [*a* neg. + Gr. *dia* through + *aktis* ray] not permitting the passage of actinic rays.

adiadochocinesia (ah-di″ah-do″ko-si-ne′se-ah) adiadochokinesia.

adiadochocinesis (ah-di″ah-do″ko-si-ne′sis) adiadochokinesia.

adiadochokinesia (ah-di″ah-do″ko-kine′se-ah) [*a* neg. + Gr. *diadochos* succeeding + *kinesis* motion + *-ia*] inability to perform rapid alternating movements. Cf. *diadochokinesia.*

adiadochokinesis (ah-di″ah-do″ko-ki-ne′sis) adiadochokinesia.

adiadokokinesia (ah-di″ah-do″ko-ki-ne′se-ah) adiadochokinesia.

adiadokokinesis (ah-di″ah-do″ko-ki-ne′sis) adiadochokinesia.

Adiantum (ad″e-an′tum) [*a* neg. + Gr. *dianein* to moisten] a genus of ferns of the family Polypodiaceae, popularly called maidenhair. *A. pedatum* (North America, eastern Asia) has been used as an expectorant and demulcent.

adiaphoria (ah-di″ah-fo′re-ah) [Gr. "indifference"] nonresponse to stimuli as a result of previous exposure to similar stimuli; see also *refractory period,* under *period.*

adiaspiromycosis (ad″i-ah-spi″ro-mi-ko′sis) a pulmonary disease of many species of rodents throughout the world and rarely of man. It is caused by the inhalation of spores produced by the saprophytic soil fungus *Emmonsia parva* or *E. crescens,* and marked by the presence of huge spherules (adiaspores) without endospores in the lungs. The condition is often confused with the tissue phase of *Coccidioides immitis.* Called also *haplomycosis.*

adiaspore (ad′i-ah-spor) a spore produced by the soil fungi *Emmonsia parva* and *E. crescens,* which, after inhalation into the lungs, enlarges to form a huge spherule without endospores.

adiathermance (ah-di″ah-ther′mans) adiathermancy.

adiathermancy (ah-di″ah-ther′man-se) [*a* neg. + Gr. *dia* through + *thermansis* heating] the condition of being impervious to heat waves.

adicillin (ad″i-sil′in) chemical name: (4-amino-4-carboxybutyl)penicillin. A cephalosporin that is less active against gram-positive bacteria than penicillin G but more active against gram-negative organisms and is highly active against *Neisseria;* it has been used in the treatment of typhoid fever and gonorrhea. Called also *cephalosporin N* and *penicillin N.*

Adie's pupil, syndrome (a′dez) [William John *Adie,* British neurologist, 1886–1935] see *tonic pupil,* under *pupil,* and see under *syndrome.*

adiemorrhysis (ah-di″e-mor′i-sis) [*a* neg. + Gr. *dia* through + *haima* blood + *rhysis* flow] stoppage of circulation of blood.

adient (ad′e-ent) tending toward the source of stimulation; positive. Cf. *abient.*

adipectomy (ad″i-pek′to-me) [L. *adeps* + Gr. *ektomē* excision] lipectomy.

adiphenine hydrochloride (ad″i-fen′ēn) chemical name; α-phenyl-2-(diethylamino)ethyl ester hydrochloride. An antispasmodic anticholinergic, $C_{20}H_{25}NO_2 \cdot HCl$, used orally as a smooth muscle relaxant in the treatment of hypermotility and spasm of the genitourinary and gastrointestinal tracts.

adipic (ah-dip′ik) [L. *adeps* fat] adipose.

adipic acid (ah-dip′ik) trivial name for hexanedioic acid, $HOOC(CH_2)_4 \ COOH$.

adip(o)- [L. *adeps,* q.v.] a combining form denoting relationship to fat.

adipocele (ad′i-po-sēl″) [*adipo-* + Gr. *kēlē* hernia] a hernia containing fat or fatty tissue, as an epiplocele.

adipocellular (ad″i-po-sel′u-lar) composed of connective tissue and fat.

adipoceratous (ad″i-po-ser′ah-tus) pertaining to or resembling adipocere.

adipocere (ad′i-po-sēr″) [*adipo-* + L. *cera* wax] a peculiar waxy substance formed during the decomposition of animal bodies, and seen especially in human bodies buried in moist places; it consists principally of insoluble salts of fatty acids. Called also *grave wax* and *corpse* or *grave fat.*

adipocyte (ad′i-po-sīt″) a fat cell; see under *cell.*

adipofibroma (ad″i-po-fi-bro′mah), pl. *adipofibro′mas.* A lipoma containing fibrous tissue component.

adipogenesis (ad″i-po-jen′e-sis) the formation of fat.

adipogenic (ad″i-po-jen′ik) [*adipo-* + Gr. *gennan* to produce] producing fat or fatness.

adipogenous (ad″i-poj′e-nus) adipogenic.

adipohepatic (ad″i-po-he-pat′ik) pertaining to or marked by fatty degeneration of the liver.

adipoid (ad′i-poid) [*adipo-* + Gr. *eidos* form] lipoid, def. 1.

adipokinesis (ad″i-po-ki-ne′sis) the mobilization of fat in the body, often with the liberation of free fatty acids into the blood plasma; see also *lipolytic hormones,* under *hormone.*

adipokinetic (ad″i-po-ki-net′ik) pertaining to, characterized by, or promoting adipokinesis.

adipokinin (ad″i-po-ki′nin) a hypothetical hormone of the anterior lobe of the pituitary gland, probably the anterior pituitary extract containing what is now known as β-lipotropin.

adipolysis (ad″i-pol′i-sis) [*adipo-* + Gr. *lysis* dissolution] lipolysis.

adipolytic (ad″i-po-lit′ik) lipolytic.

adipoma (ad″i-po′mah) (*obs.*) lipoma.

adipometer (ad″i-pom′e-ter) an instrument for measuring the thickness of the skin fold, as a means of determining the presence of obesity.

adiponecrosis (ad″i-po-ne-kro′sis) necrosis of fatty tissue in the body. **a. subcuta′nea neonato′rum,** subcutaneous fat induration in newborn and young infants; called also *subcutaneous fat necrosis* and *pseudosclerema.*

adipopectic (ad″i-po-pek′tik) pertaining to, characterized by, or promoting adipopexis.

adipopexia (ad″i-po-pek′se-ah) adipopexis.

adipopexic (ad″i-po-pek′sik) adipopectic.

adipopexis (ad″i-po-pek′sis) [*adipo-* + Gr. *pēxis* fixation] the fixation or storing of fats.

adiposalgia (ad″i-pōs-al′je-ah) [*adipo-* + Gr. *algos* pain + *-ia*] a neuropathic state in which there are painful areas of subcutaneous fat.

adipose (ad′i-pōs) [L. *adiposus* fatty] 1. of a fatty nature; fatty; fat. 2. the fat present in the cells of adipose tissue.

adiposis (ad″i-po′sis) [L. *adeps* fat + *-osis*] 1. obesity or corpulence; an excessive accumulation of fat in the body. 2. fatty change of an organ or tissue. **a. cerebra′lis,** cerebral adiposity. **a. doloro′sa,** a disease accompanied by painful localized fatty swellings and by various nerve lesions. The disease is usually seen in women, and may cause death from pulmonary complications. Called also *Dercum's disease.* **a. hepat′ica,** fatty change of the liver. **a. tubero′sa sim′plex,** a disorder resembling adiposis dolorosa, marked by development in the subcutaneous tissue of fatty masses which are sometimes painful to pressure; called also *Anders' disease.* **a. universa′lis,** a deposit of fat generally throughout the body, including the internal organs.

adipositas (ad″ĭ-pos′ĭ-tas) [L.] fatness. **a. cerebra′lis,** cerebral adiposity. **a. cor′dis,** fat heart, def. 2. **a. ex vac′uo,** fatty atrophy.

adipositis (ad″ĭ-po-si′tis) panniculitis.

adiposity (ad″ĭ-pos′ĭ-te) the state of being fat; fatness; obesity. See *adiposogenital dystrophy,* under *dystrophy.* **cerebral a.,** fatness due to cerebral disease, especially disease of the hypothalamus, as in adiposogenital dystrophy. **pituitary a.,** obesity formerly believed to be due to pituitary insufficiency but actually due to involvement of the diencephalon.

adiposuria (ad″ĭ-po-su′re-ah) [*adipo-* + *-uria*] the presence of fat in the urine; lipuria, or lipiduria.

adipsa (ah-dip′sah) remedies to allay thirst; foods which do not produce thirst.

adipsia (ah-dip′se-ah) [*a* neg. + Gr. *dipsa* thirst + *-ia*] absence of thirst, or abnormal avoidance of drinking.

adipsous (ah-dip′sus) quenching thirst, as certain fruits.

adipsy (ah-dip′se) adipsia.

aditus (ad′ĭ-tus), pl. *ad′itus* [L.] [NA] a general term for the entrance or approach to an organ or part. **a. ad an′-trum** [NA], an opening between the epitympanum and the mastoid antrum. **a. ad pel′vis,** the pelvic inlet. **a. laryn′gis** [NA], the aperture by which the pharynx communicates with the larynx; called also *aperture of larynx.* **a. or′bitae** [NA], the opening to the orbit in the cranium; called also *orbital aperture, orbital opening,* and *anterior opening of orbital cavity.* **a. vagi′nae,** ostium vaginae.

adjunct (ad′junkt) an accessory or auxiliary agent or measure.

adjunctive (ad-junk′tiv) assisting or aiding.

adjustment (ah-just′ment) 1. the act or process of modification of physical parts made in response to changing conditions. 2. in psychology, the relative degree of harmony between an individual's needs and the requirements of the environment. 3. a modification made in a denture after its completion and insertion in the mouth. 4. the mechanism for raising and lowering the tube of a microscope to bring the object being examined into focus. 5. in chiropractic, manipulation of the spine, said to restore normal nerve function. **occlusal a.,** selective grinding of occlusal surfaces of the teeth to eliminate premature contacts and occlusal interferences. Called also *occlusal equilibration.* See also *milling-in.*

adjuvant (aj′ĕ-vant, ad-joo′vant) [L. *adjuvans* aiding] 1. assisting, or aiding. 2. a substance which aids another, such as an auxiliary remedy; in immunology, nonspecific stimulator (e.g., BCG vaccine) of the immune response. **A. 65,** trademark for a water-in-oil emulsion containing antigen in peanut oil with Arlacel A and aluminum monostearate as the emulsifying agent. **Freund's a.,** a water-in-oil emulsion incorporating antigen, in the aqueous phase, into lightweight paraffin oil with the aid of an emulsifying agent. On injection, this mixture (*Freund's incomplete a.*) induces strong persistent antibody formation. The addition of killed, dried mycobacteria, e.g., *Mycobacterium butyricum,* to the oil phase (*Freund's complete a.*) elicits cell-mediated immunity (delayed hypersensitivity), as well as humoral antibody formation. **mycobacterial a.,** Freund's complete a.; see *Freund's a.*

adjuvanticity (aj″ĕ-van-tis′ĭ-te, ad-joo″van-tis′ĭ-te) the ability to modify the immune response.

Adler's test (ad′lerz) [Oscar *Adler,* German physician, 1879–1932, and his brother Rudolph, 1882–1952] benzidine test; see *Table of Tests.*

Adler's theory (ad′lerz) [Alfred *Adler,* Vienna psychiatrist, 1870–1937] see under *theory.*

ad lib. abbreviation for L. *ad lib′itum,* at pleasure.

adlumidine (ad-loo′mi-din) a crystalline alkaloid, $C_{19}H_{16}O_6N$, from *Adlumia fungosa,* a species of herbaceous ferns.

adlumine (ad-loo′min) a crystalline alkaloid, $C_{21}H_{21}NO_6$, from *Adlu′mia fungosa,* a species of herbaceous ferns.

admedial (ad-me′de-al) situated near the median plane.

admedian (ad-me′de-an) toward the median plane, or midline of the body.

adminicula (ad″mĭ-nik′u-lah) [L.] plural of *adminiculum.*

adminiculum (ad″mĭ-nik′u-lum), pl. *adminic′ula* [L.] a prop or support. **a. lin′eae al′bae** [NA], the expansion of fibers extending from the superior pubic ligament to the posterior surface of the linea alba.

admittance (ad-mit′ans) the reciprocal of impedance, the peak current divided by the peak voltage in an alternating current circuit; the unit of admittance is the reciprocal ohm (Ω^{-1}) or mho. Symbol A.

admov. abbreviation for L. *ad′move, admovea′tur,* add, let there be added.

ad nauseam (ad-naw′se-am) [L.] to the extent of producing nausea.

adnerval (ad-ner′val) 1. situated near a nerve. 2. toward a nerve, said of an electric current which passes through muscle toward the entrance point of a nerve.

adneural (ad-nu′ral) [*ad-* + Gr. *neuron* nerve] adnerval.

adnexa (ad-nek′sah) [L., pl] appendages or adjunct parts; see also *appendage.* **a. mastoi′dea** [NA], the structures in the mastoid, or posterior, wall of the middle ear (*auris media*), including the mastoid antrum and its aditus and the mastoid air cells. **a. o′culi,** the eyelids, lacrimal apparatus, and other appendages of the eye. **a. u′teri,** the uterine appendages: the ovaries, uterine tubes, and ligaments of the uterus.

adnexal (ad-nek′sal) pertaining to adnexa, especially the adnexa uteri.

adnexectomy (ad″nek-sek′to-me) [*adnexa* + Gr. *ektomē* excision] excision or removal of the adnexa.

adnexitis (ad″nek-si′tis) inflammation of the adnexa uteri.

adnexogenesis (ad-nek″so-jen′ĕ-sis) [L. *adnexa* + Gr. *genesis* production] embryonic development of the adnexa or accessory structures.

adnexorganogenic (ad-neks″or-gah-no-jen′ik) giving rise to or originating in the adnexa uteri.

adolescence (ad″o-les′ens) [L. *adolescentia*] the period of life beginning with the appearance of secondary sex characters and terminating with the cessation of somatic growth, roughly from 11 to 19 years of age; cf. *puberty.*

adolescent (ad″o-les′ent) 1. pertaining to adolescence. 2. an individual during the period of adolescence.

adonidin (ah-don′ĭ-din) a poisonous glycoside, $C_{24}H_{42}O_9$, from *Adonis vernalis,* not unlike digitalin in its effects; formerly used as a cardiac stimulant.

adonin (ah-do′nin) a glucoside, $C_{20}H_{40}O_9$, from *Adonis amurensis,* a plant of Asia.

Adonis (ah-do′nis) [L.] a genus of poisonous ranunculaceous plants, native to Europe, Asia, and Africa. *A. aestiva′lis* and *A. verna′lis* were formerly used as cardiac stimulants.

adonite (ad′o-nit) adonitol.

adonitol (ah-don′ĭ-tol) a pentahydric alcohol found in *Adonis vernalis;* by oxidation it yields ribose.

adoral (ad-o′ral) [L. *ad* near + *os, oris* mouth] toward or near the mouth.

ADP adenosine diphosphate.

Ad pond. om. abbreviation for L. *ad pon′dus om′nium,* to the weight of the whole.

adrenal (ah-dre′nal) [L. *ad* near + *ren* kidney] 1. situated near the kidney. 2. an adrenal gland. **Marchand's a's,** accessory adrenal bodies in the broad ligament.

adrenalectomize (ah-dre″nal-ek′to-mīz) to excise one or both adrenal glands.

adrenalectomy (ah-dre″nal-ek′to-me) [*adrenal* + Gr. *ektomē* excision] excision of one or both adrenal glands; suprarenalectomy.

Adrenalin (ah-dren′ah-lin) trademark for preparations of epinephrine.

adrenaline (ah-dren′ah-lēn) the official British Pharmacopoeia name for epinephrine. **a. acid tartrate,** epinephrine bitartrate.

adrenalinemia (ah-dren″ah-lin-e′me-ah) [*adrenalin* + *-emia*] the presence of epinephrine in the blood.

adrenalinogenesis (ah-dren″ah-lin-o-jen′ĕ-sis) the formation of epinephrine.

adrenalinuria (ah-dren″ah-lin-u′re-ah) the presence of epinephrine in the urine.

adrenalism (ah-dren′al-izm) ill health due to adrenal dysfunction. Cf. *dysadrenalism.*

adrenalitis (ah-dre″nal-i′tis) inflammation of the adrenal glands.

adrenalone (ah-dren′ah-lōn) chemical name: 1-(3,4-dihydroxyphenyl)-2-(methylamino)ethanone. An adrenergic, C_9-$H_{11}NO_3$, obtained by oxidation of an epinephrine derivative; it has vasoconstrictor activity.

adrenalopathy (ah-dre″nal-op′ah-the) [*adrenal* + Gr. *pathos* disease] any disease of the adrenal glands.

adrenalotropic (ah-dren″ah-lo-trop′ik) [*adrenal* + Gr. *tropos* a turning] having a special affinity for the adrenal glands; adrenal-stimulating.

adrenarche (ad″ren-ar′ke) [*adrenal* + Gr. *archē* beginning] augmentation of adrenal cortical secretion, involving especially androgens, a physiologic change that occurs at approximately the age of eight years in both sexes.

adrenergic (ad″ren-er′jik) 1. activated by, characteristic of, or secreting epinephrine or substances with similar activity; the term is applied to those nerve fibers that liberate norepinephrine at a synapse when a nerve impulse passes, i.e., the sympathetic fibers. See also under *receptor.* 2. an agent that produces such an effect. Called also *sympathomimetic.* Cf. *cholinergic.*

adrenic (ah-dren′ik) pertaining to the adrenal glands.

adrenin (ah-dre′nin) epinephrine.

adrenine (ah-dre′nin) epinephrine.

adrenitis (ad″re-ni′tis) adrenalitis.

adren(o)- [L. *ad* near + *ren* kidney] a combining form denoting relationship to the adrenal gland.

adrenoceptive (ah-dre″no-sep′tiv) pertaining to the sites on effector organs that are acted upon by adrenergic transmitters.

adrenoceptor (ah-dre″no-sep′tor) adrenergic receptor; see under *receptor.*

adrenochrome (ad-re′no-krōm″) chemical name: 2,3-dihydro-3-hydroxy-1-methyl-1*H*-indole-5,6-dione. A red oxidation product of epinephrine, $C_9H_9NO_3$, which possesses hemostatic properties due to its effect on capillary permeability, and has been used as an experimental psychomimetic. It is used in the form of its stable derivative *carbazochrome salicylate.*

adrenocortical (ad-re″no-kor′te-kal) pertaining to or arising from the cortex of the adrenal gland.

adrenocorticohyperplasia (ah-dre″no-kor″tĭ-ko-hi″perpla″ze-ah) adrenal cortical hyperplasia.

adrenocorticomimetic (ad-re″no-kor″te-ko-mi-met′-ik) producing effects similar to those of hormones of the cortex of the adrenal glands.

adrenocorticotrophic (ad-re″no-kor″te-ko-trof′ik) corticotropic.

adrenocorticotrophin (ad-re″no-kor″te-ko-trof′in) corticotropin.

adrenocorticotropic (ad-re″no-kor″te-ko-trop′ik) corticotropic.

adrenocorticotropin (ad-re″no-kor″te-ko-trop′in) corticotropin.

adrenodoxin (ah-dre″no-dok′sin) an iron-sulfide protein of the adrenal cortex that serves as an electron carrier in the biosynthesis of adrenal steroids.

adrenogenic (ad-ren″o-jen′ik) caused by adrenocortical or adrenal medullary activity.

adrenogenous (ad″ren-oj′ĕ-nus) [*adreno-* + Gr. *gennan* to produce] produced or arising in the adrenals.

adrenoglomerulotropin (ah-dre″no-glo-mer″u-lo-tro′pin) a hormone of unspecified origin alleged to stimulate the production of aldosterone by the adrenal cortex.

adrenogram (ad-ren′o-gram) a roentgenogram of the adrenal glands.

adrenokinetic (ad-re″no-kĭ-net′ik) [*adreno-* + Gr. *kinētikos* moving] stimulating the adrenal gland.

adrenoleukodystrophy (ah-dre″no-loo″ko-dis′tro-fe) a genetic disease of childhood marked by diffuse abnormality of the cerebral white matter and adrenal atrophy. It is characterized by mental deterioration progressing to dementia and by aphasia, apraxia, dysarthria, and loss of vision. Clinical adrenal insufficiency occurs in about a third of the patients, but almost all show abnormal adrenal functioning when tested. It is transmitted as an X-linked recessive trait.

adrenolutin (ah-dre″no-lu′tin) chemical name: 1-methyl-1*H*-indole-3,5,6-triol; degradation product of epinephrine, $C_9H_9NO_3$.

adrenolytic (ad″ren-o-lit′ik) [*adreno-* + Gr. *lysis* a loosening] inhibiting the action of adrenergic nerves; inhibiting the response to epinephrine.

adrenomedullotropic (ad-re″no-med″u-lo-trop′ik) having a stimulatory influence on the adrenal medulla.

adrenomegaly (ad-ren″o-meg′ah-le) [*adreno-* + Gr. *megaleia* bigness] enlargement of one or both of the adrenal glands.

adrenomimetic (ah-dre″no-mi-met′ik) having actions similar to those of adrenergic compounds; sympathomimetic.

adrenopathy (ad″ren-op′ah-the) [*adreno-* + Gr. *pathos* disease] adrenalopathy.

adrenopause (ad-ren′o-pawz) cessation or suppression of function of the adrenal glands.

adrenoprival (ad-ren′o-pri″val) pertaining to or characterized by deprivation of the adrenal glands, as a result of their removal or suppression of their function.

adrenoreceptor (ah-dre″no-re-sep′tor) adrenergic receptor; see under *receptor.*

Adrenosem (ah-dren′o-sem) trademark for preparations of carbazochrome salicylate.

adrenostatic (ad-re″no-stat′ik) 1. inhibiting the activity of the adrenal glands. 2. an agent that inhibits the activity of the adrenal glands.

adrenosterone (ad″re-no′ster-ōn″) androst-4-ene-3,11,77-trione, a crystalline androgenic steroid, $C_{19}H_{24}O_3$, isolated from the adrenal cortex.

adrenotoxin (ad-ren″o-tok′sin) any substance that is toxic to the adrenals.

adrenotrophic (ad-ren″o-trof′ik) [*adreno-* + Gr. *trophē* nutrition] adrenotropic.

adrenotrophin (ad-ren″o-trof′in) corticotropin.

adrenotropic (ad-ren″o-trop′ik) [*adreno-* + Gr. *tropos* a turning] having specific affinity for or growth-promoting or hormonal secretory influence on the adrenal glands; suprarenotropic.

adrenotropin (ad-ren″o-trop′in) corticotropin.

Adriamycin (a″dre-ah-mi′sin) [from "Adriatic" + *mycin*] trademark for preparations of doxorubicin hydrochloride.

Adrian (a′dre-an) **of Cambridge** Baron (Edgar Douglas Adrian) English physiologist, 1889–1977; co-winner, with Sir Charles Scott Sherrington, of the Nobel prize for medicine or physiology in 1932 for their work on the function of the neuron.

adromia (ah-dro′me-ah) [*a* neg. + Gr. *dromos* a running + *-ia*] absence of conduction in nerve of muscle.

Adroyd (ad′roid) trademark for a preparation of oxymetholone.

Adrucil (a′dru-sil) trademark of a preparation of fluorouracil for injection.

adrue (ad-ru′a) the *Cyperus articulatus,* a grasslike plant of the West Indies, with an aromatic tonic, antiemetic, and anthelmintic root.

ADS antidiuretic substance; see *vasopressin.*

adsorb (ad-sorb′) to attract and retain other material on the surface.

adsorbate (ad-sor′bāt) a substance taken up on a surface by adsorption.

adsorbent (ad-sor′bent) 1. pertaining to or characterized by adsorption. 2. an agent that attracts other materials or particles to its surface.

adsorption (ad-sorp′shun) [L. *ad* to + *sorbere* to suck] the attachment of one substance to the surface of another; the concentration of a gas or a substance in solution in a liquid on a surface in contact with the gas or liquid, resulting in a relatively high concentration of the gas or solution at the surface. Cf. *absorption.* **agglutinin a.,** the taking up by bacteria suspended in diluted antiserum of those agglutinins specific for that microorganism. **immune a.,** the use of antigen as a specific adsorbent for antibody or the use of antibody or antiserum as a specific adsorbent for antigen; the antigen-antibody complex is removed by filtration or centrifugation.

adsternal (ad-ster′nal) toward or near the sternum.

adst. feb. abbreviation for L. *adstan′te feb′re*, while fever is present; cf. *abs. feb.*

adterminal (ad-ter′mĭ-nal) passing toward the end of a muscle; said of an electric current.

adtorsion (ad-tor′shun) intorsion.

Ad 2 vic. abbreviation of L. *ad du′as vi′ces*, at two times, for two doses.

adult (ah-dult′) [L. *adultus* grown up] 1. having attained full growth or maturity. 2. a living organism which has attained full growth or maturity.

adulterant (ah-dul′ter-ant″) a substance used as an addition to another substance for sophistication or adulteration.

adulteration (ah-dul″ter-a′shun) addition of an impure, cheap, or unnecessary ingredient to cheat, cheapen, or falsify a preparation; in legal terminology, incorrect labeling, including dosage not in accordance with the label.

adumbration (ah″dum-bra′shun) a geometric lack of sharpness; an inherent property of the focal spot which causes the production of double images. In radiology, the giving forth of a shadow.

Adv. abbreviation for L. *adver′sum*, against.

advance (ad-vans′) [Fr. *avancer*] to perform the operation of advancement.

advancement (ad-vans′ment) surgical detachment, as of a muscle or tendon, followed by reattachment at an advanced point; chiefly an operation for strabismus. The round ligaments of the uterus have sometimes been advanced for retrodisplacement. **capsular a.,** the artificial attachment of a part of a vagina bulbi (Tenon's capsule) in such a way as to draw forward the insertion of an ocular muscle.

adventitia (ad″ven-tish′e-ah) [L. *adventicious* from without] outermost; denoting the layer of loose connective tissue forming the outermost coating of an organ. See *tunica adventitia.*

adventitial (ad″ven-tish′al) pertaining to the tunica adventitia.

adventitious (ad″ven-tish′us) [L. *ad* to + *venire* to come] 1. accidental or acquired; not natural or hereditary. 2. found out of the normal or usual place.

adynamia (ah″di-na′me-ah) [*a* neg. + Gr. *dynamis* might + *-ia*] lack or loss of the normal or vital powers; asthenia. **a. episo′dica heredita′ria,** periodic paralysis II.

adynamic (ad″i-nam′ik) characterized by adynamia; asthenic.

A.E. abbreviation for Ger. *antitoxineinheit* (antitoxic unit).

ae- for words beginning thus, see also those beginning e-.

Aeby's muscle, plane (a′bēz) [Christopher Theodore *Aeby*, Swiss anatomist, 1835–1885] see *musculus depressor labii inferioris*, and see under *plane*.

aec- for words beginning thus, see words beginning ec-.

aeciospore (e′se-o-spōr″) [Gr. *aikia* injury + *sporas* seed] a yellow, thin-walled, single-celled, binucleate spore of the wheat rust fungus formed in chainlike series within an aecium, produced in the spring on the leaves of barberry plants.

aecium (e′se-um), pl. *ae′cia* [Gr. *aikia* injury] 1. a cuplike structure formed on certain plants by wheat rust fungi, containing aeciospores. 2. a fruiting body of a fungus that bursts through the epidermis of the host.

Aedes (a-e′dēz) [Gr. *aēdēs* unpleasant] a genus of culicine mosquitoes with broad appressed scales on the head and scutellum. The palpi in the female are short and sparsely tufted and have three segments of equal length; in the male, the palpi are long and tufted. In addition to the vectors listed below, the following species are annoying because of their bites: *A. aldrichi, A. communis, A. excrucians, A. punctor, A. stimulans,* and *A. vexans.* Also *Aëdes.* See *mosquito.* **A. aegyp′ti,** the tiger mosquito, which breeds near houses and transmits urban yellow fever and dengue; it may also transmit filariasis and encephalitis. **A. africa′nus,** an arboreal mosquito that attacks monkeys and is a vector of the yellow fever virus over much of Central Africa. It also carries the Zika virus. **A. albopic′tus,** a species that transmits yellow fever, equine encephalomyelitis, and dengue. **A. cine′reus,** a species occurring in certain parts of the United States which transmits equine encephalomyelitis. **A. flaves′cens,** a species of the Pacific Islands which transmits filariasis. **A. ingram′i,** a species found in the pool from which Uganda S virus was isolated in 1947. **A. leucocelae′nus,** a South American species that transmits jungle yellow fever. **A. polynesien′sis,** a species of the South Pacific islands which is a vector of filaria and dengue. **A. pseudoscutella′ris,** a species of the Pacific Islands which is a vector of filaria. **A. scapula′ris,** a vector of the Cache Valley virus in Trinidad. **A. simp′soni,** a vector of jungle yellow fever in Africa. **A. sollic′itans,** the common salt-marsh mosquito of the Atlantic and Gulf coasts; it may transmit equine encephalomyelitis. **A. spenc′erii,** a species of mosquito found on the Saskatchewan prairies. **A. taeniorhyn′chus,** a species which transmits dengue in Florida. **A. to′goi,** a species of Japan that serves as a vector of *Brugia malayi*, which causes filariasis malayi. **A. varipal′pus,** a species found along the Pacific coast.

aedoeocephalus (ēd″e-o-sef′ah-lus) [Gr. *aidoia* genitals + *kephalē* head] a monster with no mouth, a nose like a penis, and but one orbit.

Aeg. abbreviation for L. *aeger, aegra*, the patient.

Aegyptianella (e-jip″she-ah-nel′ah) [named for *Egypt*, where the organism was first described in 1929] a genus of bacteria of the family Anaplasmataceae, order Rickettsiales, occurring as a parasite in wild and domestic birds. **A. pullo′rum,** a species found in the blood of fowls. Called also *Balfour's bodies.*

aelurophobia (e-loo″ro-fo′be-ah) [Gr. *ailouros* cat + *phobia*] ailurophobia.

aequator (e-kwa′tor) [L. "equalizer"] equator.

aequum (e′kwum) [L. "equal"] Pirquet's term for the amount of food required to maintain weight under a given condition of activity.

aer- see *aero-.*

aerasthenia (a″er-as-the′ne-ah) [*aer-* + *asthenia*] aeroneurosis.

aerated (a′er-āt″ed) [L. *aeratus*] 1. charged with air. 2. charged with carbon dioxide. 3. oxygenated.

aeration (a″er-a′shun) 1. the exchange of carbon dioxide for oxygen by the blood in the lungs. 2. the charging of a liquid with air or gas.

aeremia (a″er-e′me-ah) [*aer-* + Gr. *haima* blood + *-ia*] aeroembolism; decompression sickness (bends).

aerendocardia (a″er-en″do-kar′de-ah) [*aer-* + Gr. *endon* in + *kardia* heart] (*obs.*) the presence of gas or air within the heart.

aerenterectasia (a″er-en″ter-ek-ta′ze-ah) [*aer-* + Gr. *enteron* intestine + *ektasis* distention + *-ia*] (*obs.*) distention of the intestines with air or gas.

aerial (a-e′re-al) pertaining to the air.

aeriferous (a″er-if′er-us) [*aer-* + L. *ferre* to bear] conveying air, as the bronchi.

aeriform (a-er′ĭ-form) [*aer-* + L. *forma* form] like the air; gaseous.

aero- [Gr. *aēr* air] a combining form denoting relationship to air or gas.

aeroasthenia (a″er-o-as-the′ne-ah) aeroneurosis.

Aerobacter (a″er-o-bak′ter) [*aero-* + Gr. *baktron* a rod] in former systems of classification, a genus of bacteria of the family Enterobacteriaceae, consisting of gram-negative, facultatively anaerobic, motile rods; individual species have been assigned to the genera *Enterobacter* and *Klebsiella*. **A. aerog′enes,** *Enterobacter aerogenes.* **A. cloa′cae,** *Enterobacter cloacae.*

aerobe (a′er-ōb) [*aero-* + Gr. *bios* life] a microorganism that can live and grow in the presence of free oxygen. **facultative a's,** microorganisms that are able to live under either aerobic or anaerobic conditions. **obligate a's,** microorganisms that require molecular oxygen for growth.

aerobic (a-er-o′bik) 1. having molecular oxygen present. 2. growing, living, or occurring in the presence of molecular oxygen. 3. requiring oxygen for respiration.

aerobiology (a″er-o-bi-ol′o-je) [*aero-* + *biology*] that branch of biology which deals with the distribution of living organisms by the air, either the exterior or outdoor air (extramural a.) or the indoor air (intramural a.).

aerobiosis (a″er-o-bi-o′sis) [*aero-* + Gr. *biosis* way of life] life in the presence of molecular oxygen.

aerobiotic (a″er-o-bi-ot′ik) pertaining to aerobiosis.

aerocele (a′er-o-sēl″) [*aero-* + Gr. *kēlē* tumor] a tumor formed by air filling an adventitious pouch, such as laryngo-cele and tracheocele. **epidural a.,** a collection of air between the dura mater and the wall of the spinal column. **intracranial a.,** traumatic pneumocephalus.

Aerococcus (a″er-o-kok′us) a genus of aerobic, gram-positive cocci of the family Streptococcaceae. **A. vir′idans,** a species indistinguishable from *Gaffkya homari*, which may be pathogenic for lobsters, and has been found in infections of the urinary tract and in endocarditis in humans.

aerocolpos (a″e-ro-kol′pos) [*aero-* + Gr. *kolpos* bosom or fold] distention of the vagina with gas.

aerocystography (a″er-o-sis-tog′rah-fe) roentgenography of the bladder after it has been injected with air; called also *pneumocystography*.

aerocystoscope (a″er-o-sis′to-skōp) aerourethroscope.

aerocystoscopy (a″er-o-sis-tos′ko-pe) [*aero-* + Gr. *kystis* bladder + *skopein* to inspect] examination of the bladder with the aerourethroscope.

aerodermectasia (a″er-o-der″mek-ta′ze-ah) [*aero-* + Gr. *derma* skin + *ektasis* extension + *-ia*] subcutaneous emphysema; it may be spontaneous, traumatic, or surgical in origin.

aerodontalgia (a″er-o-don-tal′je-ah) [*aero-* + Gr. *odous* tooth + *algos* pain] toothache experienced at lowered atmospheric pressures, as in aircraft flight or in a decompression chamber, caused by the expansion of air in the maxillary sinuses. Called also *aero-odontalgia* and *aero-odontodynia*.

aerodontics (a″er-o-don′tiks) that branch of dentistry which is concerned with effects on the teeth of high altitude flying.

aerodynamics (a″er-o-di-nam′iks) [*aero-* + Gr. *dynamis* might] the science of air and gases in motion.

aeroembolism (a″er-o-em′bo-lizm) embolism due to air; it may occur in surgery of head, neck, and heart, induced abortion, and severe decompression sickness.

aeroemphysema (a″er-o-em″fĭ-ze′mah) pulmonary emphysema and edema with collection of nitrogen bubbles in the tissues of the lung; due to excessively rapid atmospheric decompression.

aerogastria (a″er-o-gas′tre-ah) the presence of gas in the stomach; stomach bubble. See also *magenblase*. **blocked a.,** retention of air in the stomach due to spasm of the esophagus.

aerogel (a′er-o-jel″) a solid formed by replacing the liquid of a gel with a gas.

aerogen (a′er-o-jen″) an aerogenic, or gas-producing, bacterium.

aerogenesis (a″er-o-jen′ĕ-sis) [*aero-* + Gr. *genesis* production] gas production.

aerogenic (a″er-o-jen′ik) producing gas; said of bacteria that liberate free gaseous products.

aerogenous (a″er-oj′ĕ-nus) aerogenic.

aerogram (a′er-o-gram″) [*aero-* + Gr. *gramma* mark] a roentgenogram of an organ after it has been injected with air; called also *pneumogram*.

aerohydrotherapy (a″er-o-hi″dro-ther′ah-pe) [*aero-* + Gr. *hydōr* water + *therapeia* treatment] (*obs.*) the therapeutic use of air and water.

aeroionotherapy (a″er-o-i″o-no-ther′ah-pe) [*aero-* + *ionotherapy*] treatment of respiratory conditions by the inhalation of air with altered electrical charges.

aeromedicine (a″er-o-med′ĕ-sin) aviation medicine.

aerometer (a″er-om′ĕ-ter) [*aero-* + Gr. *metron* measure] an instrument for weighing air or for estimating the density of air.

Aeromonas (a″er-o-mo′nas) [*aero-* + Gr. *monas* unit] a genus of gram-negative, facultatively anaerobic, rod-shaped bacteria of the family Vibrionaceae, consisting of small organisms with polar flagella, found in salt and fresh water, sewage, and soil. They cause disease in humans, amphibians,

fish, and reptiles. **A. hydroph′ila,** a species that causes "red leg disease" in frogs. In humans, the organism is a cause of cellulitis, wound infections, acute diarrheal disease, septicemia, and urinary tract infections. Called also *Proteus hydrophilus* and *Proteus melanovogenes*. **A. puncta′ta,** a species that is a possible pathogen of frogs. **A. sal-monic′ida,** the etiologic agent of furunculosis in salmon and other fish. It has not been recovered from human specimens.

aeroneurosis (a″er-o-nu-ro′sis) [*aero-* + *neurosis*] (*obs.*) neurosis or neurasthenia in aviators, formerly supposed to be a specific syndrome caused by flying.

aero-odontalgia (a″er-o-o″don-tal′je-ah) aerodontalgia.

aero-odontodynia (a″er-o-o-don″to-din′e-ah) aerodontalgia.

aero-otitis (a″er-o-o-ti′tis) [*aero-* + *otitis*] barotitis.

aeropathy (a″er-op′ah-the) [*aero-* + Gr. *pathos* disease] any disease due to change in atmospheric pressure, such as decompression sickness or air sickness.

aeropause (a′er-o-paws″) the region between the stratosphere and outer space, where to all practical purposes the atmosphere does not exist.

aeroperitoneum (a″er-o-per″ĭ-to-ne′um) [*aero-* + *peritoneum*] pneumoperitoneum.

aeroperitonia (a″er-o-per″ĭ-to′ne-ah) pneumoperitoneum.

aerophagia (a″er-o-fa′je-ah) [*aero-* + Gr. *phagein* to eat] excessive swallowing of air, usually an unconscious process associated with anxiety, resulting in abdominal distention or belching, often interpreted by the patient as signs of a physical disorder.

aerophagy (a″er-of′ah-je) aerophagia.

aerophil (a′er-o-fil″) [*aero-* + Gr. *philein* to love] an aerophilic organism.

aerophilic (a″er-o-fil′ik) requiring air for proper growth; aerobic.

aerophilous (a″er-of′ĭ-lus) aerophilic.

aerophobia (a″er-o-fo′be-ah) [*aero-* + *phobia*] irrational fear of drafts or fresh air, often connected with the idea of harmful airborne influences.

aeropiesotherapy (a″er-o-pi-e″so-ther′ah-pe) [*aero-* + Gr. *piesis* pressure + *therapy*] the therapeutic use of compressed or rarefied air.

aeroplankton (a″er-o-plank′ton) the organisms (bacteria, pollen, etc.) present in the air.

Aeroplast (ār′o-plast″) trademark for a preparation of vibesate.

aeroplethysmograph (a″er-o-plĕ-thiz′mo-graf) [*aero-* + Gr. *plēthysmos* enlargement + *graphein* to record] an apparatus for measuring respiratory volumes by recording changes in body volume; see also *plethysmograph*.

Aeroseb-Dex (ār′o-serb-deks′) trademark for preparations of dexamethasone.

aerosialophagy (a″er-o-si″ah-lof′ah-je) sialoaerophagy.

aerosinusitis (a″er-o-si″nus-i′tis) barosinusitis.

aerosis (a″er-o′sis) the production of gas in the tissues or organs of the body.

aerosol (a′er-o-sol″) 1. a colloid system in which the continuous phase (dispersion medium) is a gas, e.g., fog. 2. a bactericidal solution which can be finely atomized for the purpose of sterilizing the air of a room. 3. a solution of a drug which can be atomized into a fine mist for inhalation therapy.

aerosolization (a″er-o-sol″ĭ-za′shun) the process of dispersing in a fine mist.

aerosolology (a″er-o-sol-ol′o-je) the scientific study of aerosol therapy.

Aerosporin (a″er-o-spo′rin) trademark for a preparation of polymyxin B sulfate.

aerostatics (a″er-o-stat′iks) [*aero-* + Gr. *statikos* causing to stand] the science of gases in equilibrium.

aerotaxis (a″er-o-tak′sis) [*aero-* + Gr. *taxis* arrangement] a movement of an organism in response to the presence of molecular oxygen.

aerotherapeutics (a″er-o-ther″ah-pu′tiks) [*aero-* + Gr. *therapeia* treatment] (*obs.*) the use of air in the treatment of diseases.

aerotherapy (a″er-o-ther′ah-pe) (*obs.*) aerotherapeutics.

aerothermotherapy (a″er-o-ther″mo-ther′ah-pe) [*aero-* + Gr. *thermē* heat + *therapeia* treatment] (*obs.*) treatment with currents of hot air.

aerotitis (a″er-o-ti′tis) barotitis.

aerotolerant (a″er-o-tol′er-ant) able to survive or to grow slowly in an aerobic environment; said of certain anaerobic microorganisms.

aerotonometer (a″er-o-to-nom′ĕ-ter) [*aero-* + Gr. *tonos* tension + *metron* measure] an instrument for measuring the partial pressure of the gases in the blood.

aerotropism (a″er-ot′ro-pizm) [*aero-* + Gr. *tropos* a turning] movement of an organism toward (*positive a.*) or away from (*negative a.*) a supply of air.

aerotympanal (a″er-o-tim′pah-nal) [*aero-* + L. *tympanum* drum] pertaining to atmospheric pressure (air) and the middle ear.

aerourethroscope (a″er-o-u-re′thro-skōp″) [*aero-* + *urethroscope*] a urethroscope by which the urethra is dilated with air before inspection; called also *aerocystoscope.*

aerourethroscopy (a″er-o-u″re-thros′ko-pe) the use of the aerourethroscope.

aes-, aet- for words beginning thus, see also those beginning *es-, et-.*

aesculapian (es″ku-la′pe-an) 1. pertaining to Aesculapius, the god of medicine, or to the art of medicine. 2. a physician.

Aesculapius (es″ku-la′pe-us) [L., from Gr. *Asklēpios*] the mythical god or deified hero of healing; also known as *Asclepios.* See also *Asclepiad, asclepion, Hygeia,* and *Panacea,* and under *staff.*

aesculin (es′ku-lin) esculin.

Aesculus (es′ku-lus) a genus of trees, species of which contain a coumarin type of glycoside, esculin, which has been held responsible for their veterinary toxicity. The bark and seeds of *A. hippocastanum,* the horse chestnut, were formerly used in treatment of rheumatism and malaria and as an anticoagulant. *A. glabrus* is popularly known as *buckeye* (q.v.).

aesthesi(o)- for words beginning thus, see those beginning *esthesio-.*

aesthetic (es-thet′ik) esthetic.

aesthetics (es-thet′iks) esthetics.

aet. abbreviation for L. *ae′tas,* age.

Aethusa (e-thoo′sah) a genus of umbelliferous plants, one species of which, *A. cynapium* L. (fool's parsley), has a reputation for human toxicity. The fruit contains a volatile alkaloid, cynapine, purported to be related to coniine.

Aëtius (a-e′she-us) (or **Aetios**) **of Amida** (or **Antiochenus**) (502–575) a Byzantine Greek writer and physician to the Emperor Justinian; his *Tetrabiblion* gives details of the works of Rufus (of Ephesus), Leonides, Soranus, and Philumenus, and good accounts of diseases of the eye, ear, nose, and throat, and also of technical procedures (e.g., tonsillectomy, urethrotomy, and the treatment of hemorrhoids).

A.F.C.R. American Federation for Clinical Research.

afebrile (a-feb′ril) without fever.

afetal (ah-fe′tal) without a fetus.

affect (af′fekt) the external expression of emotion attached to ideas or mental representations of objects; cf. *mood.* **blunted a.,** severe reduction in the intensity of affect; a common symptom of schizophrenic disorders. **flat a.,** lack of signs expressing affect.

affection (ah-fek′shun) 1. a state of emotion or feeling. 2. affliction. **celiac a.,** the infant form of nontropical sprue (q.v.).

affective (ah-fek′tiv) pertaining to affect.

affectivity (af″ek-tiv′ĭ-te) subject to affective stimuli.

affectomotor (ah-fek″to-mo′tor) [*affect* + *motor*] characterized by elevated mood and hyperactivity, as in mania.

affenspalte (af′en-spahl″te) [Ger. "ape fissure"] Reidinger's term for sulcus lunatus.

afferent (af′er-ent) [L. *ad* to + *ferre* to carry] centripetal; esodic; conveying toward a center, as an afferent nerve.

afferentia (af″er-en′she-ah) [L.] 1. any afferent vessels, whether blood or lymph vessels. 2. the lymph vessels in general.

affinin (af′ĭ-nin) a lipid amide obtained from *Heliopsis longipes* (A. Gray) Blake, Compositae. It has insecticidal and local anesthetic properties. The plant is used in Mexico as a dental analgesic.

affinity (ah-fin′ĭ-te) [L. *affinitas* relationship] 1. inherent likeness or relationship. 2. a special attraction for a specific element, organ, or structure. 3. chemical affinity; the force that binds atoms in molecules; the tendency of substances to combine by chemical reaction. 4. the strength of noncovalent chemical binding between two substances as measured by the dissociation constant of the complex. 5. in immunology, a thermodynamic expression of the strength of interaction between a single antigen-binding site and a single antigenic determinant (and thus of the stereochemical compatibility between them), most accurately applied to interactions among simple, uniform antigenic determinants such as haptens. Expressed as the association constant (K liters mole^{-1}), which, owing to the hetergeneity of affinities in a population of antibody molecules of a given specificity, actually represents an average value (mean intrinsic association constant). Cf. *avidity.* 6. the reciprocal of the dissociation constant. Symbol A.

afflux (af′luks) [L. *affluxus, affluxio*] the rush of blood or liquid to a part.

affluxion (ah-fluk′shun) afflux.

affusion (ah-fu′zhun) [L. *affusio*] the pouring of water upon a part or upon the body for reducing fever; now rarely done. See *ablution.*

afibrinogenemia (ah-fi″brin-o-jĕ-ne′me-ah) deficiency or, more literally, absence of fibrinogen (coagulation factor I) in the blood. **congenital a.,** an uncommon hemorrhagic coagulation disorder, probably transmitted by an autosomal recessive gene, and characterized by complete incoagulability of the blood.

aflatoxicosis (af″lah-tok″sĭ-ko′sis) a form of mycotoxicosis affecting turkeys and other farm animals fed on ground nut meal contaminated with the molds *Aspergillus flavus* and related species, which produce aflatoxin; widespread epidemics with high mortality rates have been reported from all parts of the world. Called also *x disease.*

aflatoxin (af″lah-tok′sin) a toxic factor, $C_{17}H_{12}O_6$, produced by *Aspergillus flavus* and *A. parasiticus,* molds contaminating ground nut seedlings. It is responsible for deaths of fowl and other farm animals (aflatoxicosis) fed with infected ground nut meal. In experimental animals, aflatoxin causes liver necrosis, bile duct proliferation, and cirrhosis and, on prolonged administration, leads to hepatocellular carcinoma and cholangiocarcinoma. It has also been implicated as a cause of human hepatic carcinoma.

AFP alpha-fetoprotein.

Afrin (af′rin) trademark for a preparation of oxymetazoline hydrochloride.

A.F.S. American Fertility Society.

afteraction (af″ter-ak′shun) an effect occurring after cessation of the causative stimulus, such as the negative variation of the electric current continuing for a short time in a tetanized muscle.

afterbirth (af′ter-berth″) the placenta and membranes, delivered from the uterus after the birth of the child.

afterbrain (af′ter-brān″) metencephalon.

aftercare (af′ter-kār) the care and treatment of a convalescent patient, especially one who has undergone surgery; called also *aftertreatment.*

aftercataract, after-cataract (af″ter-kat′ah-rakt) see under *cataract.*

aftercurrent (af″ter-kur′ent) a current produced in a muscle and nerve after cessation of an electric current that has been flowing through it.

afterdischarge (af″ter-dis′charj) the portion of the response to stimulation in a sensory nerve which persists after the stimulus has ceased.

aftergilding (af″ter-gild′ing) the histologic application of gold salts to nerve tissue after fixation and hardening.

afterimage (af′ter-im″ij) a visual impression persisting briefly after cessation of the stimuli causing the original image. In a *positive* afterimage the brights, darks, and colors remain unchanged; in a *negative* afterimage the brights and darks are reversed, and the colors are complementary; called also *accidental* or *negative image,* and *aftervision.*

afterimpression (af″ter-im-presh′un) aftersensation.

aftermovement (af″ter-mōōv′ment) spontaneous elevation of the arm by idiomuscular contraction after benumbing it by powerful pressure against a rigid object; called also *Kohnstamm's phenomenon.*

afterpains (af′ter-pānz″) the cramplike pains felt after the birth of the child, due to the contractions of the uterus.

afterperception (af″ter-per-sep′shun) the perception of a sensation after the stimulus producing it has ceased.

afterpotential (af″ter-po-ten′shal) see under *potential.*

aftersensation (af″ter-sen-sa′shun) a sensation lasting after the stimulus that produced it has been removed; called also *afterimpression.*

afterstain (af′ter-stān″) (*obs.*) counterstain.

aftertaste (af′ter-tāst″) a taste continuing after the substance producing it has been removed.

aftertreatment (af″ter-trēt′ment) aftercare.

aftervision (af″ter-vizh′un) afterimage.

aftosa (af-to′sah) [Sp.] foot-and-mouth disease.

afunction (a-funk′shun) loss of function.

AG atrial gallop.

Ag chemical symbol for *silver* (L. *argentum*); abbreviation for *antigen.*

A.G.A. American Gastroenterological Association.

agalactia (ah″gah-lak′she-ah) [*a* neg. + Gr. *gala* milk + *-ia*] absence or failure of the secretion of milk; called also *agalactosis.* **contagious a.,** a contagious disease of goats and sometimes of sheep, caused by mycoplasma, a pleuropneumonia-like organism. The disease occurs principally in parts of southern Europe and North Africa, affecting both females and males; it is marked by lesions of the eyes and joints and in the mammary glands of females.

agalactosis (ah-gal″ak-to′sis) agalactia.

agalactosuria (ah-gal″ak-to-su′re-ah) [*a* neg. + *galactose* + Gr. *ouron* urine + *-ia*] absence of galactose from the urine.

agalactous (ah″gah-lak′tus) 1. suppressing the secretion of milk. 2. not nursed; artificially fed.

agalorrhea (ah-gal″o-re′ah) [*a* neg. + Gr. *gala* milk + *rhoia* flow] absence or arrest of the flow of milk.

agamete (ag′ah-mēt) [*a* neg. + Gr. *gamos* marriage] the product of asexual multiple fission in protozoa.

agammaglobulinemia (a-gam″ah-glob″u-lĭ-ne′me-ah) [*a*-neg. + *gamma globulin* + *-emia*] absence of all classes of immunoglobulins in the blood. Cf. *hypogammaglobulinemia* and *dysgammaglobulinemia.* See *immunodeficiency.* **acquired a.,** see under *hypogammaglobulinemia.* **Bruton's a.,** X-linked a. **common variable a.,** see under *immunodeficiency.* **congenital a.,** see under *hypogammaglobulinemia.* **lymphopenic a.,** severe combined immunodeficiency. **Swiss type a.,** see *severe combined immunodeficiency,* under *immunodeficiency.* **X-linked a., X-linked infantile a.,** a primary immunodeficiency disorder with X-linked recessive inheritance characterized by absence of circulating B lymphocytes, absence of plasma cells and germinal centers in lymphoid tissues, and very low levels of circulating immunoglobulins. Infants with the disorder are well during the first 6–9 months of life because of the presence transplacentally acquired maternal immunoglobulin. They then acquire repeated severe bacterial infections with highly virulent, encapsulated, extracellular organisms, e.g., staphylococci, streptococci, pneumococci, and *Haemophilus influenzae,* which must be controlled by antibiotic prophylaxis and immune globulin replacement therapy. Response to most viral infections and live vaccines is normal; there is increased susceptibility to hepatitis virus and enterovirus infection. The pathogenic defect appears to be a failure of pre-B cells to differentiate into mature B cells. Called also *Bruton's agammaglobulinemia* or *disease, X-linked infantile hypogammaglobulinemia,* and *congenital agammaglobulinemia,* or *hypogammaglobulinemia.*

agam(o)- [Gr. *agamos* unmarried] a combining form meaning asexual.

Agamococcidiida (ah-gam″o-kok″sĭ-de′ĭ-dah) [*a* neg. + Gr. *gamos* marriage + *kokkus* berry] an order of parasitic protozoa (subclass Coccidia, class Sporozoea), the life cycle of which involves sporogony only.

agamocytogeny (ah-gam″o-si-toj′ĕ-ne) schizogony.

Agamodistomum (ag″ah-mo-dis′to-mum) a genus of immature trematodes whose sexual organs are undeveloped and whose relationship to adult types has not been determined. **A. ophthalmo′bium,** an immature trematode parasite reported to have been found in the crystalline lens of the human eye.

Agamofilaria (ah-gam″o-fi-la′re-ah) a name given to filarial worms which are known only in immature stages and which cannot be assigned to any known genus or species.

agamogenesis (ag″ah-mo-jen′ĕ-sis) [*a* neg. + Gr. *gamos* marriage + *genesis* production] schizogony.

agamogenetic (ag″ah-mo-jĕ-net′ik) reproducing asexually.

agamogony (ag″ah-mog′ŏ-ne) [*a* neg. + Gr. *gamos* marriage + *gonos* offspring] schizogony.

Agamomermis culicis (ag″ah-mo-mer′mis ku′lĭ-sis) a mermithid nematode parasitic in the mosquito.

Agamonema (ag″ah-mo-ne′mah) a genus of immature and unidentified nematodes, whose relationship to adult types has not yet been determined.

Agamonematodum migrans (ag″ah-mo-ne″mah-to′dum mi′grans) a name once applied to the nematode larva which causes creeping eruption in the southern United States. See *Ancylostoma.*

agamont (ag′ah-mont) [*a* neg. + Gr. *gamos* marriage + *on* being] schizont.

agamous (ag′ah-mus) 1. asexual. 2. having no recognizable sexual organs.

aganglionic (a-gang″gle-on′ik) pertaining to or characterized by the absence of ganglion cells.

aganglionosis (ah-gang″gle-on-o′sis) [*a*- neg. + *ganglion* + *-osis*] congenital absence of parasympathetic ganglion cells, as in congenital megacolon.

agar (ahg′ar) [NF] a complex sulfated polymer of galactose units, extracted from *Gelidium cartilagineum, Gracilaria confervoides,* and related red algae. It is a mucilaginous substance having the property of melting at 100° C. and solidifying into a gel at 40° C. It is not digested by most bacteria and is used as a gel in the preparation of solid culture media for microorganisms, as a bulk laxative, in making emulsions, and as a supporting medium for immunodiffusion and immunoelectrophoresis. See *Table of Culture Media* for specific agars.

agar-agar (ag″ar-ag′ar) [Singhalese] referring to certain edible seaweeds; agar.

Agarbacterium (ag″ar-bak-te′re-um) in former systems of classification, a genus of bacteria made up of the organisms now classified in the genus *Flavobacterium.*

agaric (ah-gar′ik) [Gr. *agarikon* a sort of tree fungus] 1. any mushroom, more especially any species of *Agaricus.* 2. the tinder or punk prepared from dried mushrooms. **fly a.,** a poisonous species, *Amanita muscaria.* **larch a., purging a.,** a preparation obtained from *Polyporus officinalis,* a spongy mass growing on several species of trees; formerly used as an anhidrotic. **surgeons' a.,** a preparation obtained from *Polyporus officinalis,* which grows on several species of trees; used as a hemostatic. **white a.,** larch a.

agaric acid (ah-gar′ik; ag′ah-rik) agaricic acid.

Agaricales (ah-gar″ĭ-ka′lēz) an order of basidiomycetous fungi of the series Hymenomycetes, subclass Homobasidiomycetidae, made up of the mushrooms, including the genera *Agaricus* and *Amanita.*

agaricic acid (ag″ah-ris′ik) a resinous acid from white agaric, *Polysporus officinalis,* which is responsible for its anhidrotic action.

Agaricus (ah-gar′ĭ-kus) a genus of mushrooms. See also *agaric,* and *agaric acid,* under *acid.* **A. campes′tris,** the common edible, or field, mushroom. **A. musca′rius,** *Amanita muscaria.*

agastria (ah-gas′tre-ah) absence of the stomach.

agastric (ah-gas′trik) [*a* neg. + Gr. *gastēr* stomach] having no alimentary canal.

Agathinus (ag″ah-thi′nus) **of Sparta** (1st century A.D.) a Greek physician who was a pupil of Athenaeus and, like his master, a pneumatist.

Agave (ah-ga′ve) [L.; Gr. *agauē* noble] a genus of amaryllidaceous plants with many species possessing spiny-margined leaves and tall candelabra-shaped inflorescences. Some species serve as a source of an alcoholic beverage. The fresh juice of *A. americana* L. is purgative and diuretic, and has been used as an abortifacient. Several species contain saponins.

AGCT Army General Classification Test.

age (āj) 1. the duration of individual existence measured in units of time. 2. the measure of some individual attribute in terms of the chronological age of an average normal individual showing the same degree of proficiency, e.g., achievement age. 3. to undergo change as the result of the passage of time. **achievement a.,** a measure of achievement expressed in terms of the chronological age of an average child showing the same degree of attainment. **anatomical a.,** age expressed in terms of the chronological age of the average individual showing the same body development. **Binet a.,** mental age as determined by Binet's test. **bone a.,** osseous development shown roentgenographically, stated in terms of the chronological age at which the development is ordinarily attained. **chronological a.,** the age of a person expressed in terms of the period elapsed from the time of birth. **coital a.,** the age of a conceptus defined by the time elapsed since the coitus that led to fertilization. **developmental a.,** age estimated from the degree of anatomical development. In psychology, the age of an individual as determined by the degree of his emotional, mental, anatomical, and physiologic maturation. **emotional a.,** the age of an individual expressed in terms of the chronological age of an average normal individual showing the same degree of emotional maturity. **fertilization a.,** conceptus age defined by the time elapsed since fertilization. **functional a.,** the combined expression of the chronological, emotional, mental, and physiological ages of an individual. **gestational a.,** age of conceptus or pregnancy. In human clinical practice, pregnancy is timed from onset of the last normal menstruation. Elsewhere the onset may be timed from estrus, coitus, artificial insemination, vaginal plug formation, fertilization, or implantation. **menstrual a.,** conceptus age defined by the time elapsed since the onset of the mother's last normal menstruation. **mental a.,** the score achieved by a person in an intelligence test, expressed in terms of the chronological age of an average normal individual showing the same degree of attainment. **physical a., physiological a.,** the age of an individual expressed in terms of the chronological age of a normal individual showing the same degree of anatomical and physiological development. **postovulatory a.,** conceptus age defined by the time elapsed since release of the oocyte from the ovary.

agenesia (ah″jĕ-ne′se-ah) agenesis. **a. cortica′lis,** congenital failure of development of the cortical cells, especially the pyramidal cells, of the brain, resulting in infantile cerebral paralysis and idiocy.

agenesis (ah-jen′ĕ-sis) [*a* neg. + Gr. *genesis* production] 1. absence of an organ; frequently used to designate such absence resulting from failure of appearance of the primordium of an organ in embryonic development. Cf. *aplasia.* 2. sterility or impotence. **callosal a.,** defect of the callosal structures of the brain. **gonadal a.,** complete failure of gonadal development; see *Turner's syndrome,* under *syndrome.* **nuclear a.,** Möbius' syndrome. **ovarian a.,** failure of development of the ovaries; see *Turner's syndrome,* under *syndrome.* **sacral a.,** see *caudal regression syndrome,* under *syndrome.*

agenitalism (ah-jen′ĭ-tal-izm) absence of the genitalia, or a condition due to lack of the internal secretion of the testes or ovaries.

agenized (a′jĕn-izd″) treated with nitrogen trichloride for bleaching purposes, as flour.

agenosomia (ah-jen″o-so′me-ah) congenital absence or rudimentary development of the genitals and eventration of the lower part of the abdomen.

agenosomus (ah-jen″o-so′mus) [*a* neg. + Gr. *gennan* to beget + *sōma* body] a monster exhibiting agenosomia.

agent (a′jent) [L. *agens* acting] any power, principle, or substance capable of producing an effect, whether physical, chemical, or biological. **activating a.,** one of two factors present in adult tissues which, when administered to embryos, interact to induce regional development; when administered alone, this factor induces archencephalic development. Called also *dorsalizing* or *neuralizing a.* Cf. *caudalizing a.* **adrenergic blocking a.,** a compound that selectively inhibits response to sympathetic impulses and to catecholamines and other adrenergic amines. See *alpha-adrenergic blocking a., beta-adrenergic blocking a.,* and *adrenergic neuron blocking a.* **adrenergic neuron blocking a.,** one that inhibits the release of norepinephrine from postganglionic adrenergic nerve endings. **alkylating a.,** a highly reactive chemical compound capable of forming covalent linkages with various nucleophilic groups in proteins and nucleic acids, e.g., phosphate, amino, sulfhydryl, hydroxyl, carboxyl groups, and the nitrogen atoms in the heterocyclic rings of histidine and the purine and pyrimidine bases of DNA and RNA. Five major classes of alkylating agents are used as antineoplastic or immunosuppressive agents: nitrogen mustards (mechlorethamine, cyclophosphamide); ethylenimine derivatives (thiotepa); alkyl sulfonates (busulfan); nitrosoureas (carmustine, lomustine, streptozocin); and triazines (dacarbazine). The major biological effects of alkylating agents are produced by attack on DNA causing cross-linking of DNA strands, chain scission, or removal of bases. Bifunctional agents, which can form cross links and block DNA replication are primarily cytotoxic; monofunctional agents are more mutagenic and carcinogenic. Alkylating agents are not cell-cycle specific; however, cell killing occurs primarily in rapidly proliferating tissues in which there is insufficient time between mitoses for DNA repair systems to reverse the effects of the agent. Hematopoietic, reproductive, and epithelial tissues are particularly sensitive to alkylating agents; depression of blood cell counts, amenorrhea or impaired spermatogenesis, damage to the intestinal mucosa, and alopecia occur in varying degrees. **alpha-adrenergic blocking a.,** one that blocks the alpha receptor sites of effector organs to the effects of catecholamines. **beta-adrenergic blocking a.,** an agent that blocks the beta receptor sites of effector organs to the effects of catecholamines. **Bittner a.,** mouse mammary tumor virus. **blocking a.,** an agent that inhibits the response of effector organs to neural impulses of the autonomic nervous system; it may be an adrenergic or cholinergic blocking agent. **caudalizing a.,** one of two factors present in adult tissues which, when administered to embryos, interact to induce regional development; when administered alone, this factor induces only mesodermal development. Called also *mesodermalizing* or *transforming a.* Cf. *activating a.* **chelating a.,** 1. a compound that combines with metal ions by means of two or more coordinating positions to form stable ring structures, e.g., heme. 2. a substance used to reduce the concentration of free metal ion in solution by complexing it. Called also *metal complexing a.* **chimpanzee coryza a.,** respiratory syncytial virus. **cholinergic blocking a.,** one that blocks or inactivates acetylcholine. **clearing a.,** an agent used in staining technique for fixed cells, which has the same refractive index as that of protein particles. **delta a.,** hepatitis delta virus. **dorsalizing a.,** activating a. **Eaton a.,** *Mycoplasma pneumoniae.* **fixing a's,** agents, such as formalin, alcohol, acids, salts of heavy metals, or mixtures of these, that precipitate the proteins of cells or tissues and render them insoluble. **ganglionic blocking a.,** one that blocks nerve impulses at autonomic ganglionic synapses. **Gordon a.,** a substance present in certain human and animal tissues which produces characteristic clinical symptoms and pathological changes on intracerebral injection into rabbits and guinea pigs. **levigating a.,** a material used for moistening a solid before reducing it to a powder. **mammary tumor a., mouse mammary tumor a.,** mouse mammary tumor virus. **Marcy a.,** a virus causing afebrile diarrhea in man. **mesodermalizing a.,** caudalizing a. **metal complexing a.,** chelating a. **milk a.,** mouse mammary tumor virus. **Norwalk a.,** the causative agent, probably a virus, of an acute infectious gastroenteritis. **A. Orange,** a herbicide and defoliant containing 2,4-D and 2,4,5-T and the contaminant dioxin which is suspected of being carcinogenic and teratogenic. **Pittsburgh pneumonia a.,** *Legionella micdadei.* **progestational a's,** a group of hormones secreted by the corpus luteum and placenta and, in small amounts, by the adrenal cortex, including progesterone, which induce the formation of a secretory endometrium. Agents having progestational activity are also produced synthetically. Called also *gestagens, progestins, progestational hormones,* and *progestogens.* **reducing a.,** a substance capable of donating electrons to another substance, thereby reducing the second substance and itself becoming oxidized. **transforming a.,** a substance that produces transformation in a cell, e.g., a DNA fragment from a bacterial (donor) cell that, when introduced into another bacterial (recipient) cell, is incorporated into the chromosome and produces a permanent, inherited change. **vacuolating a.,** see under *virus.* **wetting a's,** substances that lower the surface tension of water and promote wetting.

ageotropic (ah-je″o-tro′pik) [*a* neg. + Gr. *gēe* earth + *tropikos* turning] not responding to gravity; said of certain plant roots.

AGEPC acetyl glyceryl ether phosphoryl choline; see *platelet activating factor,* under *factor.*

agerasia (ah″jer-a′zee-ah) [*a* neg. + Gr. *gēras* old age] an unusually youthful appearance in a person of advanced years.

ageusia (ah-gu′ze-ah) [*a* neg. + Gr. *geusis* taste] absence of the sense of taste.

ageusic (ah-gu′sik) pertaining to ageusia.

ageustia (ah-gōōs′te-ah) ageusia.

agger (aj′er), pl. **ag′geres** [L.] an eminence; [NA] a general term for such a structure. **a. na′si** [L. "ridge of the nose"] [NA], a ridgelike elevation midway between the anterior extremity of the middle nasal concha and the inner surface of the dorsum of the nose; called also *ridge of nose* and *nasoturbinal concha.* **a. perpendicula′ris,** eminentia fossae triangularis auriculae. **a. val′vae ve′nae,** an elevation of the wall of a vein over the site of a valve.

aggeres (aj′er-ēz) [L.] plural of *agger.*

agglomerated (ah-glom′er-āt″ed) [L. *agglomeratus,* from *ad* together + *glomus* mass] crowded into a mass.

agglutinable (ah-gloo′tĭ-nah-bl) capable of agglutination.

agglutinant (ah-gloo′tĭ-nant) [L. *agglutinans* gluing] 1. promoting union by adhesion. 2. a tenacious or gluey substance which holds parts together during the process of healing.

agglutination (ah-gloo″tĭ-na′shun) [L. *agglutinatio*] 1. the action of an agglutinant substance. 2. the process of union in the healing of a wound. 3. the clumping together in suspension of antigen-bearing cells, microorganisms, or particles in the presence of specific antibodies (agglutinins). Called also *clumping.* **acid a.,** the nonspecific agglutination of microorganisms at relatively low hydrogen ion concentration; it occurs without participation of antibody. **bacteriogenic a.,** clumping of cells due to bacterial action, as in the *Huebener-Thomsen-Friedenreich phenomenon.* See *T agglutinin,* under *agglutinin.* **cold a.,** agglutination with cold agglutinins (q.v.), occurring more efficiently below 37 °C than at 37 °C. **cross a.,** the agglutination of particulate antigen by antibody raised against a different but related antigen; see also *group a.* **group a.,** agglutination—usually to a lower titer—of various members of a group of biologically related organisms or corpuscles by an agglutinin specific for one of that group. For instance, the specific agglutinin of typhoid bacilli may agglutinate other members of the colon-typhoid group, such as *Escherichia coli* and *Salmonella enteritidis.* **H a.,** the agglutination of motile bacteria in the presence of antibody to the heat-labile flagellar antigens. **intravascular a.,** clumping of particulate elements within the blood vessels; used conventionally to denote red blood cell aggregation. **macroscopic a.,** agglutination in which the product of the reaction, the agglutinate, can be observed with the unaided eye. **microscopic a.,** agglutination so done, usually by means of a hanging drop, that the clumping of the microorganisms or corpuscles can be observed with the microscope. **O a.,** the agglutination of bacteria in the presence of antibody to the heat-stable somatic antigen. **passive a.,** agglutination in antiserum of particles owing to adsorbed specific soluble antigen. **platelet a.,** the clumping together of platelets; sometimes used interchangeably with aggregation (q.v.), but probably better reserved for immunological or analogous phenomena. **salt a.,** agglutination that occurs in salt solutions of certain concentrations. **spontaneous a.,** the agglutination of bacteria or other cells in physiologic salt solution due to the lack of sufficient surface polar groups to give stable suspensions in the presence of electrolytes. **Vi a.,** agglutination of bacteria containing Vi antigen on their surface, in the presence of specific agglutinin.

agglutinative (ah-gloo′tĭ-na″tiv) promoting adhesion or agglutination.

agglutinator (ah-gloo′tĭ-na″tor) something which agglutinates; an agglutinin.

agglutinin (ah-gloo′tĭ-nin) antibody which aggregates a particulate antigen, e.g., bacteria, following combination with the homologous antigen in vivo or in vitro. Also, any substance other than antibody, e.g., lectin, that is capable of agglutinating particles. **anti-Rh a.,** an agglutinin not normally present in human plasma but which may be produced in Rh− mothers carrying an Rh+ fetus or after transfusion of Rh+ blood into an Rh− patient. See *blood type.* **chief a.,** major a. **cold a.,** antibody that agglutinates erythrocytes or bacteria more efficiently at temperatures below 37° C than at 37° C. See *cold agglutinin syndrome,* under *syndrome,* and *paroxysmal cold hemoglobinuria,* under *hemoglobinuria.* **complete a.,** see *antibody.* **cross a., cross-reacting a.,** an agglutinin which, although formed in response to one particulate antigen, also has specific action on a different but related antigen. **flagellar a.,** an agglutinin specific for the flagella of a microorganism. **group a.,** an agglutinin which has a specific action on certain organisms or cells, but which will agglutinate other closely related species as well. **H a.,** see under *antigen.* **immune a.,** any agglutinating antibody. **incomplete a.,** see under *antibody.* **leukocyte a.,** an antibody capable of agglutinating leukocytes; leukocyte autoagglutinins and isoagglutinins are associated with a variety of disorders, both with and without frank leukopenia. Called also *leukoagglutinin.* **major a.,** the specific agglutinin present at highest titer in an antiserum. Called also *chief a.* **MG a.,** a specific agglutinin developed against streptococcus MG. **minor a.,** a specific or cross-reacting agglutinin present in an antiserum at lower titer than the major agglutinin. Called also *partial a.* **O a.,** see under *antigen.* **partial a.,** minor a. **platelet a.,** an antibody capable of agglutinating platelets; platelet autoagglutinins and isoagglutinins are associated with a variety of disorders, both with and without frank thrombocytopenia. Called also *thromboagglutinin.* **saline a.,** complete antibody. **somatic a.,** an agglutinin specific for the body of a microorganism. **T a.,** a natural antibody present in normal human sera that causes agglutination of erythrocytes treated with neuraminidase or incubated with neuraminidase-producing bacteria causing exposure of the T antigen. **warm a.,** an agglutinin more reactive at 37° C than at lower temperatures.

agglutinogen (ag″loo-tin′o-jen) 1. any substance which, acting as an antigen, stimulates the production of agglutinin. 2. the particulate antigen used in conducting agglutination tests.

agglutinogenic (ah-gloo″tĭ-no-jen′ik) pertaining to the production of agglutinin; producing agglutinin.

agglutinophilic (ah-gloo″tĭ-no-fil′ik) agglutinating readily.

agglutogenic (ah-gloo″to-jen′ik) agglutinogenic.

aggred. feb. abbreviation for L. *aggredien′te feb′re,* while the fever is coming on.

Aggregata (ag″rĕ-ga′tah) [L. *aggregare* to add to] a genus of coccidian protozoa (suborder Eimeriina, order Eucoccidiidah), the life cycle of which involves schizogony in a crustacean and sporogony and gametogony in a cephalopod.

aggregate (ag′re-gāt) [L. *aggregatus,* from *ad* to + *grex* flock] 1. to crowd or cluster together. 2. crowded or clustered together. 3. a mass or assemblage.

aggregation (ag″re-ga′shun) 1. massing of materials together as in clumping. 2. a clumped mass of material. **familial a.,** a concentration of cases of a disease in families; the occurrence of more cases of a given disorder in close relatives of a person with the disorder than in control families. **platelet a.,** a clumping together of platelets induced in vitro, and probably in vivo, by a number of agents, such as ADP, thrombin, and collagen, as part of a sequential mechanism leading to the initiation and formation of a thrombus or hemostatic plug.

aggregen (ag′rĕ-jen) [L. *aggregare* to collect together + Gk. *gennan* to produce] an organized mass of mammalian cells growing in agitated culture, resembling an aggregate in having a continuous layer of peripheral cells forming a smooth surface, but differing from it in having the capacity to fragment to form daughter aggregens.

aggregometer (ag″grĕ-gom′ĕ-ter) an instrument that detects changes in optical density of plasma (or solution) caused by platelet (or particle) clustering.

aggregometry (ag″grĕ-gom′ĕ-tre) the measurement of platelet aggregation by means of an aggregometer.

aggressin (ah-gres′in) any of a postulated group of non-toxic substances produced by pathogenic bacteria that inhibit the mechanisms of host resistance.

aggression (ah-gresh′un) [L. *aggressus,* from *ad* to + *gradi* to step] a form of behavior which leads to self-assertion; it may arise from innate drives and/or a response to frustration; it may be manifested by destructive and attacking behavior, by covert attitudes of hostility and obstructionism, or by a healthy self-expressive drive to mastery.

AgI chemical symbol for *silver iodide.*

aging (āj′ing) the gradual changes in the structure of any organism that occur with the passage of time, that do not result from disease or other gross accidents, and that eventually lead to the increased probability of death as the individual grows older. Cf. *senescence.*

agitation (aj″u-ta′shun) a state of anxiety accompanied by motor restlessness.

agitographia (aj″e-to-graf′e-ah) [L. *agitare* to hurry + Gr. *graphein* to write + *-ia*] excessive rapidity of writing with unconscious omission of words or parts of words; it is usually associated with agitophasia.

agitolalia (aj″e-to-la′le-ah) agitophasia.

agitophasia (aj″e-to-fa′ze-ah) [L. *agitare* to hurry + Gr. *phasis* speech + *-ia*] excessive rapidity of speech in which words or syllables are unconsciously omitted or imperfectly uttered; called also *agitolalia.*

Agit. vas. abbreviation for L. *agita′to va′se,* the vial being shaken.

Agkistrodon (ag-kis′tro-don) [Gr. *agkistron* fishhook + *odous* tooth] a genus of venomous serpents of the family Crotalidae. *A. contor′trix* is the copperhead and *A. pisciv′orus,* the water moccasin of North America. Called also *Ancistrodon.* See table accompanying *snake.*

aglomerular (ah″glo-mer′u-lar) having no glomeruli; said of a kidney in which the glomeruli have been absorbed or in which they have never formed (as in some fishes).

aglossia (ah-glos′e-ah) [*a* neg. + Gr. *glōssa* tongue + *-ia*] congenital absence of the tongue.

aglossostomia (ah″glos-o-sto′me-ah) [*a* neg. + Gr. *glōssa* tongue + *stoma* mouth + *-ia*] a developmental anomaly characterized by absence of the tongue and mouth opening.

aglucon, aglucone (ă-gloo′kon, ă-gloo′kōn) 1. the non-sugar portion of a glycoside molecule. 2. aglycon.

aglutition (ag-loo-tish′un) inability to swallow.

aglycemia (ah″gli-se′me-ah) [*a* neg. + Gr. *glykys* sweet + *haima* blood + *-ia*] virtually total absence of sugar from the blood. Cf. *hyperglycemia* and *hypoglycemia.*

aglycon, aglycone (ă-gli′kon, ă-gli′kōn) the noncarbohydrate group of a glycoside molecule; called also *genin.*

aglycosuric (ah-gli″ko-su′rik) free from glycosuria.

agmatology (ag″mah-tol′o-je) [Gr. *agmos* fracture + *-logy*] the sum of what is known regarding fractures.

agminated (ag′min-āt″ed) [L. *agmen* a group] clustered.

agnate (ag′nāt) in Scottish law, the nearest relative on the father's side of one adjudged insane, and appointed guardian of the same.

Agnatha (ăg′na-tha) [*a* neg. + Gr. *gnathos* jaw] the jawless fishes; a class of vertebrates including lampreys, hagfishes, and many extinct forms.

agnathia (ag-na′the-ah) [*a* neg. + Gr. *gnathos* jaw + *-ia*] a developmental anomaly characterized by total or virtual absence of the lower jaw.

agnathous (ag-na′thus) pertaining to or affected with agnathia.

agnathus (ag-na′thus) a fetus exhibiting agnathia.

agnea (ag-ne′ah) a condition in which objects are not recognized.

AgNO₃ chemical symbol for *silver nitrate.*

agnogenic (ag″no-jen′ik) [Gr. *agnōs* unknown, obscure + *genesis* origin] of unknown origin or etiology.

agnosia (ag-no′ze-ah) [*a* neg. + Gr. *gnōsis* perception] loss of the power to recognize the import of sensory stimuli; the varieties correspond with the several senses and are distinguished as *auditory, visual, olfactory, gustatory,* and *tactile.* **acoustic a., auditory a.,** inability to recognize the signifi-

cance of sounds. **body-image a.,** autotopagnosia. **finger a.,** loss of ability to indicate one's own or another's fingers. **ideational a.,** loss of the special associations which make up the idea of an object from its component ideas. **tactile a.,** inability to recognize familiar objects by touch or feel. **time a.,** loss of comprehension of the succession and duration of events. **visual a.,** inability to recognize familiar objects by sight.

agnosterol (ag-nos′ter-ol″) polyunsaturated sterol, C₃₀H₄₈O, present in wool fat.

agnus castus (ag′nus kas′tus) [L. "chaste lamb"] the chaste-tree, *Vi′tex ag′nus-cas′tus;* the herb and fruit were used for centuries as an anaphrodisiac and symbol of chastity.

Ag₂O chemical symbol for *silver oxide.*

agofollin (ah-gof′o-lin) estradiol.

-agogue [Gr. *agōgos* leading, inducing] a word termination meaning an agent which leads or induces.

agomphiasis (ag″om-fi′ah-sis) [*a* neg. + Gr. *gomphios* molar + *-ia*] anodontia.

agomphious (ah-gom′fe-us) without teeth.

agomphosis (ag″om-fo′sis) agomphiasis.

agonad (ah-go′nad) [*a* neg. + *gonad*] 1. an individual without gonads. 2. pertaining to such an individual.

agonadal (ah-go′ah-dal) having no sex glands; due to absence of sex glands.

agonadism (ah-go′nah-dizm) the condition of being without sex glands.

agonal (ag′o-nal) 1. pertaining to the death agony; occurring at the moment of or just before death. 2. pertaining to terminal infection.

agoniadin (ag″o-ni′ah-din) a glycoside from *Plume′ria suc′cuba,* a genus of tropical American shrubs.

agonist (ag′o-nist) in anatomy, a prime mover. In pharmacology, a drug that has affinity for and stimulates physiologic activity at cell receptors normally stimulated by naturally occurring substances.

agony (ag′o-ne) [Gr. *agōnia*] 1. severe pain or extreme suffering. 2. the death struggle.

agoraphobia (ag″o-rah-fo′be-ah) [Gr. *agora* marketplace + *phobia*] [DSM III-R] intense, irrational fear of open spaces. Agoraphobia is a complex phobic disorder characterized by marked fear of being alone or of being in public places where escape would be difficult or help might be unavailable if something alarming were to happen and by avoidance of such situations to a degree that severely limits normal activities, e.g., an agoraphobic may remain at home unless in the company of a friend or relative; in some cases anticipation of exposure to the public situation brings on panic attacks.

agouti (ah-goo′te) 1. a rodent of the genus *Dasyprocta,* about the size of a rabbit, found in tropical America. 2. a term used in genetics to indicate the natural wild color pattern of the hair of certain mammals.

-agra [Gr. *agra* a catching, seizure] a word termination denoting a seizure of acute pain.

agraffe (ah-graf′) [Fr.] a clamplike instrument for maintaining the edges of a wound in apposition.

agrammatica (ag″rah-mat′e-kah) agrammatism.

agrammatism (ah-gram′ah-tizm″) [Gr. *agrammatos* unlettered] inability to speak grammatically because of brain injury or disease.

agrammatologia (ah-gram″ah-to-lo′je-ah) agrammatism.

agranulocyte (ah-gran′u-lo-sīt″) a nongranular leukocyte.

agranulocytosis (ah-gran″u-lo-si-to′sis) a symptom complex characterized by marked decrease in the number of granulocytes and by lesions of the throat and other mucous membranes, of the gastrointestinal tract, and of the skin; called also *granulocytopenia* and *Schultz's disease.* **infantile genetic a.,** an autosomal recessive disorder characterized by the early onset of recurrent, severe pyogenic infections, especially of the skin and lung, total absence of neutrophils in the blood or presence in reduced numbers, absolute monocytosis and eosinophilia, markedly decreased numbers of mature neutrophilic precursors in the bone marrow, and early death. Called also *Kostmann's syndrome.* **infectious feline a.,** panleukopenia.

agranuloplastic (ah-gran″u-lo-plas′tik) [*a* neg. + *granule* +

Gr. *plassein* to form] forming nongranular cells only; not forming granular cells.

agraphia (ah-graf′e-ah) [*a* neg. + Gr. *graphein* to write + *-ia*] inability to express thoughts in writing, due to a lesion of the cerebral cortex. **absolute a.,** loss of the power to write even single letters. **acoustic a.,** loss of the power of writing from dictation. **a. amnemon′ica,** agraphia in which letters and words can be written, but not so arranged as to express any idea. **a. atac′tica,** absolute a. **cerebral a.,** mental a. **jargon a.,** agraphia in which the patient can write, but forms only senseless combinations of letters. **literal a.,** inability to write letters of the alphabet. **mental a.,** agraphia due to inability to put thought into phrases. **motor a.,** inability to write because of lack of motor coordination. **musical a.,** loss of the power to write musical symbols. **optic a.,** inability to copy written or printed words, but with ability to write from dictation. **verbal a.,** ability to write single letters, with loss of ability to combine them into words.

agraphic (ah-graf′ik) pertaining to, affected with, or of the nature of agraphia.

Agriolimax (ag″re-o-li′maks″) a genus of slugs. **A. lae′vis,** a species that serves as an intermediate host of *Angiostrongylus cantonensis,* which transmits eosinophilic meningitis.

Agrobacterium (ag″ro-bak-te′re-um) [Gr. *agros* field + *bacterium*] a genus of bacteria of the family Rhizobiaceae, made up of small, gram-negative, aerobic, flagellated rods, found in soil or in the roots or stems of plants. Most species produce hypertrophy (galls) on plant stems. **A. radiobac′ter,** a nonpathogenic species isolated occasionally from clinical specimens.

Agropyron (ag″ro-pi′ron) a genus of grasses, including *A. repens* (L.) Beauv. (Gramineae), couch grass; see *triticum.*

Agropyrum (ag″ro-pi′rum) triticum.

Agrostemma githa′go (ag″ro-stem′ah gith-a′go) corn cockle, *Lychnis githago,* a plant whose seeds may cause poisoning (githagism).

agrypnocoma (ah-grip″no-ko′mah) wakeful coma; lethargy with wakefulness and muttering delirium.

agrypnode (ah-grip′nōd) agrypnotic.

agrypnotic (ah″grip-not′ik) [Gr. *agrypnotikos*] promoting wakefulness.

A.G.S. American Geriatrics Society.

Ag₂SO₄ chemical symbol for *silver sulfate.*

AGT antiglobulin test.

AGTH adrenoglomerulotropin.

ague (a′gu) [Fr. *aigu* sharp] 1. malarial fever, or any other severe recurrent symptom of malarial origin. 2. a chill. **brass-founders′ a.,** a disease of brass-founders, caused by inhalation of zinc fumes.

A.G.V. aniline gentian violet.

agyria (ah-ji′re-ah) [*a* neg. + Gr. *gyros* ring + *-ia*] a malformation in which the convolutions of the cerebral cortex are not normally developed and the brain is usually small; called also *lissencephaly.*

agyric (ah-ji′rik) 1. pertaining to or characterized by agyria. 2. having no gyri.

ah symbol for *hyperopic astigmatism.*

A.H.A. American Heart Association; American Hospital Association.

ahaptoglobinemia (a-hap″to-glo″bĭ-ne′me-ah) the presence of little or no haptoglobin in the blood serum.

AHF antihemophilic factor (blood coagulation Factor VIII, see under *factor*).

AHG antihemophilic globulin (blood coagulation Factor VIII, see under *factor*).

A.H.P. Assistant House Physician.

A.H.S. Assistant House Surgeon.

A.I. anaphylatoxin inhibitor; aortic incompetence; aortic insufficiency; apical impulse; artificial insemination.

A.I.C. Association des Infirmières Canadiennes.

Aicardi syndrome (ĕ-kar′de) [J. *Aicardi,* French neurologist, 20th century] see under *syndrome.*

aichmophobia (āk″mo-fo′be-ah) [Gr. *aichmē* spearpoint + phobia] irrational fear of sharp-pointed objects, often connected with the fear that one might use the object to stab someone.

aid (ād) help or assistance; by extension, applied to any device by which a function can be improved or augmented, as a hearing aid. **first a.,** the initial emergency care and treatment of an injured or ill person before definitive medical and surgical management can be secured. **hearing a.,** a device which amplifies sound to help persons with hearing loss. **pharmaceutic a., pharmaceutical a.,** see under *necessity.* **speech a.,** an appliance used to improve an individual's speech, or therapy which is designed to promote the improvement of speech. **speech a., prosthetic,** an appliance which is used to close a cleft in the hard or soft palate, or both, or to restore other tissue necessary to the production of vocal sounds.

A.I.D. donor insemination.

AIDS acquired immunodeficiency syndrome.

A.I.H. American Institute of Homeopathy; homologous insemination.

A.I.H.A. American Industrial Hygiene Association; autoimmune hemolytic anemia.

Ailanthus (a-lan′thus) [L. from Malacca name] a genus of simarubaceous trees; the bark of *A. glandulosa* (tree of heaven) is purgative, tonic, and anthelmintic, and contains a bitter principle (ailanthin), glycosides, and a saponin.

Ailantus (a-lan′tus) *Ailanthus.*

AILD angioimmunoblastic lymphadenopathy with dysproteinemia.

ailment (āl′ment) any disease or affection of the body, usually referring to slight or mild disorder.

ailurophobia (i-lu″ro-fo′be-ah) [Gr. *ailouros* cat + *phobia*] irrational fear of cats.

ainhum (ān′hum, i′num, or [Portuguese] īn-yoom′) [African "to saw"] a disease affecting the toes, especially the fifth toe, and sometimes the fingers, seen chiefly in black adult males in Africa, in which a linear constriction around the affected digit leads to spontaneous amputation of the distal part of the digit. Called also *dactylolysis spontanea.*

air (ār) [L. *aer;* Gr. *aēr*] the gaseous mixture which makes up the earth's atmosphere; it is an odorless, colorless gas, consisting of about 1 part by volume of oxygen and 4 parts of nitrogen, the proportion varying somewhat according to conditions. It also contains a small amount of carbon dioxide, ammonia, argon, nitrites, and organic matter. **alkaline a.** (*obs.*), free ammonia. **alveolar a.,** see under *gas.* **complemental a., complementary a.** (*obs.*), inspiratory capacity. **functional residual a.** (*obs.*), functional residual capacity; see under *capacity.* **liquid a.,** air liquefied by great pressure; on evaporation it produces intense cold. Liquid air has been used to produce local anesthesia and in the treatment of neuralgia and herpes zoster, and as a source of oxygen for medical use. **reserve a.** (*obs.*), see *expiratory* and *inspiratory reserve volume,* under *volume.* **residual a.,** see under *volume.* **stationary a.** (*obs.*), functional residual capacity. **supplemental a.** (*obs.*), expiratory reserve volume; see under *volume.* **tidal a.,** see under *volume.* **venous alveolar a.,** alveolar air in CO₂ equilibrium with mixed venous blood.

airborne (ār′born) suspended in, transported by, or spread by air, as an infectious disease or a pathogen; see under *infection.*

Airbrasive (ār′bra-siv) trademark for (*a*) an instrument for preparing a cavity in a tooth or removing deposits from teeth by application of silicon carbide or aluminum oxide by air blast; (*b*) the abrasive cutting powder used with the instrument.

airsacculitis (ār″sak-u-li′tis) inflammation of the air sacs in birds.

airway (ār′wa) 1. the route for passage of air into and out of the lungs. 2. a tubular device for securing unobstructed passage of air into and out of the lungs during general anesthesia or on occasions when the patient is not ventilating properly. **esophageal obturator a.,** a hollow tube inserted into the esophagus to maintain airway patency in unconscious persons and to permit positive-pressure ventilation through the face mask connected to the tube. **nasopharyngeal a.,** a hollow tube inserted into a nostril and directed along the floor of the nose to the nasopharynx to prevent the tongue from blocking off passage of air in unconscious persons. **oropharyngeal a.,** a hollow tube inserted into the mouth and back of the throat to prevent the tongue from blocking off passage of air in unconscious persons.

A.I.U.M. American Institute of Ultrasound in Medicine.

Ajellomyces (ah″jĕ-lo-mi′sēz) a genus of ascomycetous perfect fungi of the family Gymnoascaceae, order Eurotiales. *A. dermatitidis,* the perfect stage of *Blastomyces dermatitidis,* is the etiologic agent of North American blastomycosis.

ak- for words beginning thus, see also words beginning *ac-.*

akaryocyte (ah-kar′e-o-sit″) [*a* neg. + Gr. *karyon* kernel + *kytos* hollow vessel] a non-nucleated cell, e.g., an erythrocyte.

akaryomastigont (a-kar″e-o-mas′tĭ-gont) [*a* neg. + *karyo-* + *mastigont*] a condition characteristic of certain flagellate protozoa in which the mastigont system is not associated with a nucleus. Cf. *karyomastigont.*

akaryota (ah-kar″e-o′tah) akaryocyte.

akaryote (ah-kar′e-ōt) [*a* neg. + Gr. *karyon* kernel] akaryocyte.

akatamathesia (ah-kat″ah-mah-the′zhe-ah) [*a* neg. + Gr. *katamathēsis* understanding] inability to understand.

akatanoesis (ah-kat″ah-no′ĕ-sis) [*a* neg. + Gr. *katanoein* to understand] inability to understand oneself (Heveroch, 1914).

akathisia (ak″ah-thiz′e-ah) [*a-* neg. + Gr. *kathisis* a sitting down + *-ia*] 1. a condition of motor restlessness in which there is a feeling of muscular quivering, an urge to move about constantly, and an inability to sit still, a common extrapyramidal side effect of neuroleptic drugs. 2. an inability to sit down because of intense anxiety at the thought of doing so.

akee (ah′ke) native Jamaican name for the fruit of the tree *Blighia sapida,* Kon. Sapindaceae. The seeds contain the toxic principles hypoglycine A and B, and the aril of the unripe fruit contains hypoglycine A. The whitish, ripe aril is cooked and consumed as a delicacy. Ingestion of unripe fruit causes Jamaican vomiting sickness.

Åkerlund deformity (ek′er-loond) [Åke Olof *Akerlund,* Swedish roentgenologist, 1885–1958] see under *deformity.*

akinesia (ah″ki-ne′ze-ah) [*a* neg. + Gr. *kinēsis* motion + *-ia*] 1. absence or poverty of movements. 2. the temporary paralysis of a muscle by the injection of procaine. **a. al′gera,** a form of conversion hysteria in which the symptom is generalized pain associated with movement of any kind. **a. amnes′tica,** immobility from disuse of muscles. **O′Brien a.,** paralysis of the orbicularis oculi muscle produced by injection of an anesthetic solution directly over the orbital branch of the seventh nerve as it emerges from behind the ear and extends toward the orbital region along the ramus of the jaw, permitting better exposure of the bulb of the eye. **reflex a.,** loss of reflex movement.

akinesis (ah″ki-ne′sis) akinesia.

akinesthesia (ah-kin″es-the′zhe-ah) absence of kinesthesia; absence of the perception of movement.

akinetic (ah″ki-net′ik) 1. pertaining to, characterized by, or causing akinesia. 2. amitotic.

Akineton (a″ki-ne′ton) trademark for preparations of biperiden.

akiyami (ah″ke-yah′me) nanukayami.

aklomide (ak′lo-mīd) chemical name: 2-chloro-4-nitrobenzamide. A substance, $C_7H_5ClN_2O_3$, used as a coccidiostatic agent in poultry.

Akokanthera (ak″o-kan-the′rah) *Acocanthera.*

akoria (ah-ko′re-ah) acoria.

Akrinol (ak′rin-ol) trademark for a preparation of acrisorcin.

Akureyri disease (ah-ku′ra-re) [*Akureyri,* a town in northern Iceland] benign myalgic encephalomyelitis.

Al chemical symbol for *aluminum.*

-al 1. [from *aldehyde*] a suffix used in forming the names of chemical compounds, indicating presence of the aldehyde group, —CHO, as chloral. 2. [L. *-alis* adjective-forming suffix] an adjective-forming suffix meaning pertaining to or characterized by, as *arterial, diarrheal;* also a noun-forming suffix denoting an act or a process, as *denial.*

ALA α-aminolevulinic acid.

Ala alanine.

ala (a′lah), pl. *a′lae* [L. "wing"] [NA] a general term for a winglike structure or process; called also *wing.* **a. al′ba media′lis,** area vestibularis. **a. au′ris,** auricula. **a. cerebel′li,** a. lobuli centralis. **a. cine′rea,** trigonum nervi vagi. **a. cris′tae gal′li** [NA], a small winglike process on the anterior part of the crista galli of the ethmoid bone; called also *frontal hamulus, hamulus frontalis,* and *processus alaris ossis ethmoidalis.* **a. il′ii,** a. ossis ilii. **a′lae lin′gulae cerebel′li,** vincula lingulae cerebelli. **a. lob′uli centra′lis cerebel′li** [NA], the lateral hemispheric extension of the central lobule in the cranial lobe of the cerebellum; called also *a. cerebelli.* **a. mag′na os′sis sphenoida′lis, a. ma′jor os′sis sphenoida′lis** [NA], great (major) wing of sphenoid bone: a large wing-shaped process arising from either side of the body of the sphenoid bone; its cerebral surface forms the anterior part of the floor of the middle cranial fossa, and its orbital surface forms the chief part of the lateral wall of the orbit. Called also *a. temporalis ossis sphenoidalis, lateral wing of sphenoid bone,* and *alisphenoid bone.* **a. mi′nor os′sis sphenoida′lis** [NA], small wing of sphenoid bone: the thin triangular plate of bone that extends horizontally and laterally from either side of the anterior part of the body of the sphenoid bone; it articulates with the frontal bone and helps form the roof of the orbit and the floor of the anterior cranial fossa. Called also *a. orbitalis* and *a. parva ossis sphenoidalis.* **a. na′si** [NA], wing of nose: the flaring cartilaginous expansion forming the outer side of each naris. **a. orbita′lis,** a. minor. **a. os′sis il′ii** [NA], a. os′sis il′ium, the expanded superior portion of the ilium which forms the lateral boundary of the greater pelvis. **a. par′va os′sis sphenoida′lis,** a. minor ossis sphenoidalis. **a. pon′tis,** tenia ventriculi quarti. **a. sacra′lis** [NA], **a. sa′cri, a. of sacrum,** the upper surface of the lateral part of the sacrum. **a. tempora′lis os′sis sphenoida′lis,** a. major ossis sphenoidalis. **a. vespertilio′nis** ["bat's wing"], mesosalpinx. **a. of vomer, a. vo′meris** [NA], wing of vomer: one of the two lateral expansions on the superior border of the vomer, coming into contact with the sphenoidal process of the palatine bone and the vaginal process of the medial pterygoid plate.

alacrima (a-lak′rĭ-mah) [*a* neg. + L. *lacrima* tear] marked deficiency or absence of secretion of tears. The hereditary form is autosomal dominant and is characterized by deficient lacrimation from infancy, punctate corneal epithelial erosions, hypoplasia of the lacrimal gland, and anosmia. Alacrima also occurs in association with dysautonomia, anhidrotic ectodermal dysplasia, and adnexal abnormalities, or as an isolated congenital defect.

alactasia (ah-lak-ta′se-ah) malabsorption of lactose due to deficiency of lactase; it is a genetically determined condition in which lactose is not absorbed from the intestine, but is degraded in the large intestine and excreted in the feces as lactic acid, glucose, and galactose. It is very rare in infants of any race, but is common in nonwhite adults.

alae (a′le) [L.] plural of *ala.*

Alajouanine's syndrome (al′ah-zhoo-ah-nēnz′) [T. *Alajouanine,* French neurologist, 20th century] see under *syndrome.*

alalia (ah-la′le-ah) [*a* neg. + Gr. *lalein* to speak + *-ia*] lack of ability to talk; see also *aphasia.* **a. coph′ica,** deaf-mutism. **a. organ′ica,** alalia due to organic disease. **a. physiolo′gica,** deaf-mutism. **a. prolonga′ta,** delayed speech.

alalic (ah-lal′ik) pertaining to, affected with, or of the nature of alalia.

alamecin (al-ah-me′sin) an antibiotic substance produced by *Trichoderma viride.*

Alangium lamarckii (ah-lan′je-um lah-mark′e-e) an East Indian plant whose root is emetic, antipyretic, diuretic, and purgative. *A. salviifolium* is much used in Indian medicine as an emetic substitute for ipecac.

alanine (al′ah-nēn) a natural amino acid occurring in two forms: alpha-alanine, $CH_3CH(NH_2) \cdot COOH$, 2-aminopropionic acid, and beta-alanine, $CH_2NH_2 \cdot CH_2COOH$, 3-aminopropionic acid.

alanine aminotransferase (al′ah-nēn ah-me″no-trans′fer-ās) [EC 2.6.1.2] an enzyme of the transferase class that catalyzes the reaction L-alanine + 2-ketoglutarate = pyruvate + L-glutamate. The reaction transfers nitrogen for excretion or for incorporation into other compounds. The enzyme is found in serum and body tissues, especially in the liver. The activity in the serum is greatly increased in cases of liver disease; high levels occur also in infectious mononucleosis. Called also *alanine transaminase, glutamic-pyruvic transaminase.* Abbreviated ALT, GPT.

β-alaninemia (al″ah-nēn-e′me-ah) hyper-beta-alaninemia·

alanine transaminase (al′ah-nēn trans-am′ĭ-nās) alanine aminotransferase.

β-alanine transaminase (al′ah-nēn trans-am′ĭ-nās) aminobutyrate aminotransferase.

Alanson's amputation [Edward *Alanson,* British surgeon, 1747–1823] see under *amputation.*

alantin (ah-lan′tin) inulin.

alanyl (al′ah-nil) the acyl radical of alanine.

alanyl-leucine (al″ah-nil-loo′sin) a dipeptide, $CH_3 \cdot CH-(NH_2) \cdot CO \cdot NH(COOH) \cdot CH \cdot CH_2 \cdot CH(CH_3)_2$.

alar (a′lar) [L. *alaris*] pertaining to an ala, or wing.

alastrim (ah-las′trim) variola minor.

alate (a′lāt) [L. *alatus* winged] having wings; winged.

alba (al′bah), gen. and plural *al′bae* [L., feminine of *albus*] white; used as an adjective in names of certain anatomical tissues or structures, as substantia alba, and of certain diseases, as pityriasis alba.

Albalon (al′bah-lon) trademark for preparations of naphazoline hydrochloride.

Albamycin (al′bah-mi″sin) trademark for preparations of novobiocin.

Albarrán's disease, gland, tubules (al″bar-anz′) [Joaquin *Albarrán* y Domínguez, Cuban surgeon in Paris, 1860–1912] see *colibacilluria,* and under *gland,* and *tubule.*

albedo (al-be′do) [L.] whiteness. **a. re′tinae,** edema of the retina.

Albee's operation (awl′bēz) [Fred. Houdlett *Albee,* New York surgeon, 1876–1945] see under *operation.*

albendazole (al-ben′dah-zōl) a benzimidazole related to thiabendazole and used as an anthelmintic in veterinary medicine.

Albers-Schönberg disease [Heinrich Ernst *Albers-Schönberg,* Hamburg roentgenologist, 1865–1921] osteopetrosis.

Albert's diphtheria stain (al′bertz) [Henry *Albert,* American physician, 1878–1930] see *Table of Stains.*

Albert's operation, suture [Eduard *Albert,* Austrian surgeon, 1841–1900] see under *operation* and *suture.*

Albertini's treatment (al-ber-tēn′ēz) [Ippolito Francesco *Albertini,* Italian physician, 1662–1738] see under *treatment.*

albicans (al′bĭ-kanz), gen. *albican′tis,* pl. *albican′tia* [L., from *albus* white] white; see *corpus albicans.*

albiduria (al″bĭ-du′re-ah) [L. *albidus* whitish + Gr. *ouron* urine + *-ia*] the discharge of white or pale urine.

albidus (al′bĭ-dus) [L., from *albus* white] whitish.

Albini's nodules (al-be′nēz) [Giuseppe *Albini,* Italian physiologist, 1827–1911] see under *nodule.*

albinism (al′bĭ-nizm) [Port. *albino,* from L. *albus* white + *-ism*] 1. the general term for a number of inborn aminoacidopathies affecting the pigment cell (melanocyte) system of the eye and skin and causing hypomelanosis or amelanosis of the eye, skin, and hair. 2. tyrosinase-negative (ty-neg) oculocutaneous a. **localized a.,** piebaldism. **ocular a. (OA),** albinism in which pigment of the hair and skin is normal or only slightly diluted; ocular abnormalities vary with the type of OA, with the X-linked Nettleship type as the classic. **ocular a., autosomal recessive (AROA),** a severe form of OA in which both males and females are as severely affected as are hemizygous males with X-linked OA. **ocular a., Forsius-Eriksson type,** Forsius-Eriksson syndrome. **ocular a., X-linked (Nettleship) (XOAN),** the classic type of OA; hemizygous males are affected with reduced pigmentation of the irides, nystagmus, head nodding and tilting, photophobia, decreased visual acuity of varying degree, and strabismus; the pupillary reflex is present; the fundus is depigmented; and the choroidal vessels stand out. Heterozygous females show translucent irides and a mosaic of pigmentation in the fundus due to lyonization and may also show nystagmus and photophobia. Called also *OA1* and *Nettleship-Falls type ocular a.*

oculocutaneous a. (OCA), a human albinism occurring in ten types all distinguished in their incidence and genetic, biochemical, and clinical characteristics but having in common varying degrees of decreased melanotic pigment of the skin, hair, and eyes, hypoplastic foveas, photophobia, nystagmus, and decreased visual acuity. The ten types are: *tyrosinase-negative (ty-neg) oculocutaneous albinism* (q.v.); *tyrosinase-positive (ty-pos) oculocutaneous albinism* (q.v.); *the Hermansky-Pudlak syndrome* (*HPS*) (q.v.); the *Chédiak-Higashi syndrome* (*CHS*) (q.v.); the *Cross syndrome* (q.v.); *brown oc·locutaneous albinism; rufous albinism* (called also *xanthism); autosomal dominant oculocutaneous albinism; black locks, oculocutaneous albinism and deafness of the sensorineural type* (called also *BADS syndrome* q.v.); and *yellow mutant* (*ym*) *oculocutaneous albinism* (called also *Amish* or *xanthous albinism*). **partial a.,** piebaldism. **tyrosinase-negative (ty-neg) oculocutaneous a.,** a recessive disorder affecting 1 of 39,000 Caucasians and 1 of 18,000 Blacks. The phenotype, characterized by absence of pigment in hair, skin, and eyes, does not vary with race or age. Signs include white hair throughout life, skin that is pink and highly susceptible to neoplasias, absence of pigmented nevi or freckles, gray to blue eyes, prominent red reflexes from the fundi, severe nystagmus, photophobia, and reduced visual acuity (most patients are legally blind). Called also *a., a.I, complete perfect a.,* and *ATN.* **tyrosinase-positive (ty-pos) oculocutaneous a.,** a recessive disorder affecting 1 of 37,000 Caucasians and 1 of 15,000 Blacks. Phenotypes, characterized by reduced, but usually visible, pigmentation in hair, skin, and eyes, vary with race and age. Onset of pigment formation is delayed, pigment accumulates with age, and intensity of accumulation depends on race; hence all ty-pos infants resemble ty-neg infants, and ty-pos adult Blacks may be darker than normal blonde Caucasians. The presence of pigmented nevi distinguishes ty-pos and ty-neg Caucasians. Called also *a-II, albinoidism,* and *complete imperfect a.*

albinismus (al″bĭ-niz′mus) [L.] albinism. **a. circumscrip′tus,** piebaldism.

albino (al-bi′no) an individual affected with albinism.

albinoidism (al-bĭ-noid′izm) [*albinism* + *-oid* + *-ism*] 1. ocular or oculocutaneous hypopigmentation differing from albinism by the absence of hypoplastic foveas, nystagmus, photophobia, and, usually, decreased visual acuity. 2. tyrosinase-positive oculocutaneous albinism. **oculocutaneous a.,** an autosomal dominant hypomelanosis of the skin and hair with rare association of nystagmus, photophobia, and markedly decreased visual acuity. It is a mildly expressed form of tyrosinase-positive oculocutaneous albinism. **punctate oculocutaneous a.,** a rare autosomal dominant trait marked by blond hair, mildly defective visual acuity (20/30), dilated pupils, and anisocoria.

albinotic (al″bĭ-not′ik) pertaining to or characterized by albinism.

albinuria (al″bĭ-nu′re-ah) albiduria.

Albinus' muscle (al-bi′nus) [Bernard Siegfried *Albinus,* anatomist and surgeon in Leyden, 1697–1770] 1. musculus risorius. 2. musculus scalenus medius.

Albrecht's bone (al′brektz) [Karl Martin Paul *Albrecht,* German anatomist, 1851–1894] basiotic bone.

Albright's syndrome (awl′brīts) [Fuller *Albright,* Boston physician, 1900–1969] see under *syndrome.*

Albucasis (al″boo-kas′is) [L., from Ar. Abū-L-Qāsim, 936 –1013] the most famous Arabic writer on surgery; the surgical part of his encyclopedic *Altrasrif* greatly influenced medieval European medicine. Known also as *Abulcasis* and *Abulkasim.*

albuginea (al″bu-jin′e-ah) [L. from *albus* white] a tough whitish layer of fibrous tissue investing a part, especially a dense white membrane forming the immediate covering of the testicle; called also *tunica albuginea testis* [NA]. **a. o′culi,** the sclera. **a. ova′rii,** the outer layer, or tunica, of the ovary. **a. pe′nis,** the outer envelope of the corpora cavernosa.

albugineotomy (al″bu-jin″e-ot′o-me) [*albuginea* + Gr. *tomē* a cutting] incision of the tunica albuginea of the testis.

albugineous (al″bu-jin′e-us) [L. *albugineus*] pertaining to or resembling a tough whitish layer of fibrous tissue (tunica albuginea testis).

albuginitis (al″bu-jĭ-ni′tis) inflammation of any one of the albugineous tissues or tunics.

albukalin (al″bu-ka′lin) a substance, $C_8H_{16}N_2O_6$, found in leukemic blood.

albumen (al-bu′men) [L., from *albus* white] 1. egg white. 2. albumin.

albumimeter (al″bu-mim′ĕ-ter) albuminimeter.

albumin (al-bu′min) [*albumen* + -*in*] 1. any protein that is soluble in water and moderately concentrated salt solutions and is coagulable by heat. 2. serum albumin; the major plasma protein (approximately 60 per cent of the total), which is responsible for much of the plasma colloidal osmotic pressure and serves as a transport protein carrying large organic anions, such as fatty acids, bilirubin, and many drugs, and also carrying certain hormones, such as cortisol and thyroxine, when their specific binding globulins are saturated. Albumin is synthesized in the liver. Low serum levels occur in protein malnutrition, active inflammation and serious hepatic and renal disease. **a. A,** the normal type of human serum albumin, as opposed to electrophoretic variants. **acid a.,** albumin altered by the action of an acid. **alkali a.,** any albumin which has been treated with an alkali. **blood a.,** serum a; see *albumin.* **derived a.,** any albumin denatured by chemical action, as albuminate. **egg a.,** a glycoprotein that constitutes 20 per cent of the white of hens' eggs; called also *ovalbumin.* **a. human** [USP], a preparation of albumin fractionated from whole blood, serum, or plasma of healthy human donors; used as a plasma volume expander for emergency treatment of shock or hemorrhage; it has also been used to correct hypoalbuminemia of nephrotic syndrome or cirrhosis. **iodinated I 125 serum a.,** iodinated I 125 albumin injection; see under *injection.* **iodinated I 131 serum a.,** iodinated I 131 albumin injection; see under *injection.* **native a.,** an albumin in its natural state, i.e., not denatured. **radioiodinated (¹²⁵I) serum a. (human),** iodinated I 125 albumin injection; see under *injection.* **radioiodinated (¹³¹I) serum a. (human),** iodinated I 131 albumin injection; see under *injection.* **serum a.,** see *albumin.* **technetium Tc 99m aggregated a.,** see under *technetium.* **vegetable a.,** any albumin of vegetable origin.

Albuminar (al-bu′mĭ-nar) trademark for preparations of albumin human.

albuminate (al-bu′mĭ-nāt″) albumin denatured by a base or an acid, characterized by solubility in dilute acids or alkalis and by being insoluble in dilute salt solutions, water, or alcohol; called also *derived albumin* and *derived protein.*

albuminaturia (al-bu″mĭ-na-tu′re-ah) [*albuminate* + *urine*] proteinuria in which there is an excess of albuminates in the urine.

albuminemia (al-bu″mĭ-ne′me-ah) [*albumin* + Gr. *haima* blood + -*ia*] the presence of albumin in the blood plasma or serum; proteinemia.

albuminimeter (al-bu″mĭ-nim′ĕ-ter) [*albumin* + *meter*] an instrument used in determining the proportion of albumin present, as in the urine.

albuminimetry (al-bu″mĭ-nim′ĕ-tre) the determination of the proportion of albumin present.

albuminocholia (al-bu″mĭ-no-ko′le-ah) [*albumin* + Gr. *cholē* bile + -*ia*] the presence of albumin in the bile.

albuminocytological (al-bu″mĭ-no-si″to-loj′ĭ-k'l) pertaining to the level of protein as albumin in relation to number of cells present in cerebrospinal fluid.

albuminoid (al-bu′mĭ-noid″) [*albumin* + Gr. *eidos* form] 1. resembling albumin. 2. fibrous protein. 3. a scleroprotein.

albuminolysis (al-bu″mĭ-nol′ĭ-sis) the splitting up of albumins.

albuminometer (al-bu″mĭ-nom′ĕ-ter) albuminimeter.

albuminoptysis (al″bu-mĭ-nop′tĭ-sis) [*albumin* + Gr. *ptyein* to spit] presence of albumin in the sputum.

albuminoreaction (al-bu″mĭ-no-re-ak′shun) the reaction of the sputum to tests for albumin; the presence of albumin (positive reaction) is indicative of pulmonary inflammation.

albuminorrhea (al-bu″mĭ-no-re′ah) [*albumin* + Gr. *rhoia* flow] excessive excretion of albumins.

albuminous (al-bu′mĭ-nus) containing, charged with, or of the nature of an albumin.

albuminuretic (al-bu″mĭ-nu-ret′ik) [*albumin* + Gr. *ourētikos* diuretic] 1. pertaining to, characterized by, or promoting albuminuria. 2. an agent that promotes albuminuria.

albuminuria (al″bu-mĭ-nu′re-ah) [*albumin* + Gr. *ouron* urine + -*ia*] presence in the urine of serum albumin; see *proteinuria.* **Bamberger's hematogenic a.,** that which occurs during the latter periods of severe anemia.

albuminuric (al″bu-mĭ-nu′rik) proteinuric.

albumoscope (al-bu′mo-skōp″) [*albumin* + Gr. *skopein* to view] an instrument for determining the presence and amount of albumin in the urine.

Albuspan (al′bu-span) trademark for preparations of albumin human.

Albutein (al′bu-tēn) trademark for preparations of albumin human.

albuterol (al-bu′ter-ōl) chemical name: α¹-[(*tert*-butylamino)methyl]-4-hydroxy-*m*-xylene-α,α′-diol; a β-adrenergic stimulant, $C_{13}H_{21}NO_3$, used as a bronchodilator. Called also *salbutamol.* **a. sulfate,** the sulfate salt of albuterol, $(C_{13}H_{21}NO_3) \cdot H_2SO_4$, having the same actions and uses as the base.

Alcaine (al′kān) trademark for a preparation of proparacaine hydrochloride.

Alcaligenes (al″kah-lij′ĕ-nēz) [Arabic *al-qualy* potash + Gr. *gennan* to produce] a widespread genus of gram-negative, aerobic, rod-shaped, alkaline-producing bacteria of uncertain affiliation, found in the intestines of vertebrates and as part of the normal skin flora, and occasionally the cause of opportunistic infections. **A. dentri′ficans,** a species isolated from a variety of clinical specimens. **A. faeca′lis,** a species isolated from hospital environments and from blood, sputum, and urine specimens. It is a cause of nosocomial septicemia in immunocompromised patients, generally arising from contaminated hemodialysis or intravenous fluids. Called also *A. odorans* and *Bacterium faecalis alcaligenes.* **A. odo′rans,** *A. faecalis.*

alcapton (al-kap′ton) alkapton body; see under *body.*

alcaptonuria (al-kap″to-nu′re-ah) alkaptonuria.

alcaptonuric (al-kap″to-nu′rik) alkaptonuric.

alchemy (al′kĕ-me) the supposed art of transmutation of baser metals into gold; also chemical magic.

alclofenac (al-klo′fen-ak) a phenylacetic acid derivative with analgesic, antipyretic, and anti-inflammatory properties, used to treat rheumatoid arthritis.

Alcmaeon (alk-me′on) **of Crotona** (c. 500 B.C.) a physician, younger contemporary and student of Pythagoras. Alcmaeon described bodily states as an interplay of opposites: health is an *isonomy* of hot and cold, wet and dry, etc.; disease, a *monarchy* of one of these qualities; thus he was one of the precursors of humoralism. Alcmaeon considered the brain to be the seat of sensation and thought, performed the first known human dissections, distinguished veins from arteries, discovered "passages" from the eye to the brain, and was the first observer of the development of a chick embryo in an incubated egg. See also *Empedocles of Acragas.*

Alcock's canal (al′koks) [Benjamin *Alcock,* Professor of Anatomy, Queen's College, Cork, from 1849 to 1855; born 1801, date of death in America unknown] canalis pudendalis.

alcogel (al′ko-jel) a gel that has alcohol as its dispersion medium.

alcohol (al′ko-hol) [Arabic *al-kohl* powder of antimony] 1. chemical name: ethanol. A transparent, colorless, mobile, volatile liquid, C_2H_5OH, miscible with water, ether, and chloroform, obtained by fermentation of carbohydrates with yeast. Called also *ethyl alcohol.* 2. [USP] a preparation containing not less than 92.3 per cent and not more than 93.8 per cent by weight, corresponding to not less than 94.9 per cent and not more than 96.0 per cent by volume, at 15.56° C., of C_2H_5OH; used as a topical anti-infective and solvent. 3. any of a class of organic compounds formed from the hydrocarbons by the substitution of one or more hydroxyl groups for an equal number of hydrogen atoms; the term is extended to various substitution products which are neutral in reaction and which contain one or more of the alcohol groups. They are distinguished as *monohydric, dihydric, trihydric,* etc., depending on the number of hydroxyl groups present. Alcohols may be classified as *primary, secondary,* or *tertiary* according to whether the hydroxyl group is attached to a carbon atom that is covalently bonded to one, two, or three other carbon atoms. **absolute a.**, dehydrated a. **amyl a.**, a colorless oily liquid, $C_5H_{11}OH$, with characteristic odor; miscible with alcohol, ether, and chloroform and slightly soluble in water. **amyl a., tertiary**, amylene hydrate. **anisyl a.**, an alcohol, *p*-methoxybenzyl alcohol, $CH_3O \cdot C_6H_4 \cdot OH$, in pungent shining prisms. **aromatic a.**, any of the phenols. **azeotropic isopropyl a.** [USP], a preparation containing 91 to 93 per cent of isopropyl alcohol by volume, and the remainder consisting of water. **batyl a.**, the monooctadecyl ether of glycerol, CH_2-$OHCHOHCH_2O(CH_2)_{17}CH_3$; 3-(octadecyloxy)-1,2-propanediol. An isolate from shark liver oils and from yellow bone marrow, now synthesized. Has been used for bracken fern (*Pteridium aquilinum* (L.) Kuhn; Polypodiaceae) poisoning in cattle. **benzyl a.** [NF], a clear colorless oily liquid, C_6-$H_5 \cdot CH_2 \cdot OH$, occurring in balsam of Peru, tolu balsam, and styrax; used as a bacteriostatic in solutions for injection. It is also applied topically as a local anesthetic. Called also *phenylcarbinol* and *phenylmethanol*. **bornyl a.**, Borneo camphor. **butyl a.**, a clear liquid, C_4H_9OH, from the molasses of beets; four isomeric forms are known. **camphyl a.**, borneol. **carnaubyl a.**, a constituent, $CH_3(CH_2)_{23}$-OH, of carnauba wax and of wool fat. **ceryl a.**, a fatty alcohol, $CH_3(CH_2)_{24}CH_2OH$, from Chinese wool; called also *cerotin*. **cetyl a.** [NF], a fatty alcohol, $CH_3(CH_2)_{14}CH_2OH$, from spermaceti; used as an emulsifying and stiffening agent. Called also *ethal*. **cinnamyl a.**, chemical name: 3-phenyl-2-propen-1-ol. It is obtained from storax and balsam of Peru. **dehydrated a.** [USP], an extremely hygroscopic, transparent, colorless, volatile liquid with characteristic odor and burning taste, containing not less than 99.5 per cent by volume of C_2H_5OH; called also *absolute a.* **denatured a.**, alcohol which has been rendered unfit for beverage or medicinal purposes by addition of methanol or acetone, but which may still be used for industrial purposes or as a solvent. **deodorized a.**, one that contains 92.5 per cent of absolute alcohol and is free from fusel oil (amyl alcohol) and organic impurities. **dihydric a.**, an alcohol containing two hydroxyl groups. **diluted a.** [NF], a mixture of alcohol and water containing 41 to 42 per cent by weight, or 48.4 to 49.5 per cent by volume, at 15.56° C., of C_2H_5OH; used as a solvent. **ethyl a.**, alcohol. **fatty a.**, any hydroxide of a hydrocarbon derived from the paraffin series. **glyceryl a., glycyl a.**, glycerin. **isoamyl a.**, amyl a. **isobutyl a.**, chemical name: (2-methyl-1-propanol). A clear colorless liquid, $(CH_3)_2CHCH_2OH$, with a characteristic odor; miscible with alcohol and with ether; called also *isobutanol*. **isopropyl a.** [USP], chemical name: 2-propanol. A clear colorless liquid, $CH_3CH(OH)CH_3$, an isomer of propyl alcohol and a homologue of ethyl alcohol. It is miscible with water, alcohol, ether, and chloroform; used as a solvent and as a basis for isopropyl rubbing alcohol (q.v.). Called also *avantin* and *dimethyl carbinol*, and *isopropanol*. **isopropyl rubbing a.** [USP], a preparation containing between 68 and 72 per cent isopropyl alcohol in water, used as a rubefacient. Formerly called *isopropyl alcohol rubbing compound.* **ketone a.**, an alcohol which contains the ketone (carbonyl) group. **lanolin a's** [NF], a mixture of aliphatic alcohols, triterpenoid alcohols, and sterols, obtained by hydrolysis of lanolin and containing not less than 30 per cent cholesterol. **methyl a.**, methanol. **monohydric a.**, an alcohol containing only one hydroxyl group. **nicotinyl a.**, a vasodilator with properties similar to those of nicotinic acid, used in peripheral vascular disorders. Called also *nicotinic a.* **palmityl a.**, cetyl a. **pantothenyl a.**, 1. panthenol. 2. dexpanthenol. **phenylethyl a.** [USP], chemical name: 2-phenylethanol. A colorless liquid, $C_8H_{10}O$, with a roselike odor and a sharp, burning taste; used as a bacteriostatic for drug solutions. Called also *benzyl carbonol.* **polyglucosic a.**, an alcohol having the formula $C_{6n}H_{10n} + 2O_{5n}$. **polyvinyl a.** [USP], a water-soluble synthetic resin, represented by the formula $(C_2H_4O)_n$, in which *n* varies between 500 and 5000; used as a viscosity-increasing agent in pharmaceutical preparations and as a pharmaceutic necessity for ophthalmic solution dosage forms. **primary a.**, an alcohol containing the monovalent carbinol group, —CH_2OH. **n-propyl a.**, chemical name: 1-propanol. A clear colorless liquid with an alcohol-like odor, $CH_3 \cdot CH_2 \cdot CH_2OH$, miscible with water and most organic solvents; used as a solvent for resins. **rubbing a.** [USP], a preparation of acetone, methyl isobutyl ketone, and 68.5 to 71.5 per cent ethyl

alcohol; used as a rubefacient. **secondary a.**, an alcohol containing the divalent group =CHOH. **stearyl a.**, a solid alcohol [$CH_3(CH_2)_{16}CH_2OH$], prepared from stearic acid by catalytic hydrogenation; a pharmacological preparation [NF], containing not less than 90 per cent of stearyl alcohol, the remainder consisting chiefly of cetyl alcohol, is used as an ingredient of hydrophilic ointment, hydrophilic petrolatum, and polyethylene glycol ointment. **sugar a.**, a polyhydric alcohol having no more than one hydroxy group attached to each carbon atom formed by the reduction of the carbonyl group of a sugar to a hydroxy group. **tertiary a.**, an alcohol containing the trivalent group, ≡COH. **tribromoethyl a.**, tribromoethanol. **trihydric a.**, an alcohol containing three hydroxyl groups. **unsaturated a.**, alcohol that is derived from unsaturated hydrocarbons (alkenes, or olefins). **wood a.**, methanol.

alcohol dehydrogenase (al'ko-hol de-hi'dro-jen-ās) [EC 1.1.1.1] an enzyme of the oxidoreductase class that catalyzes the reaction alcohol + NAD^+ = aldehyde or ketone + NADH. The reaction is the first step in the metabolism of alcohols by the liver. Called also *acetaldehyde reductase*. Abbreviated AD and ADH.

alcoholemia (al″ko-hol-e′me-ah) [*alcohol* + Gr. *haima* blood + *-ia*] the presence of alcohol in the blood.

alcoholic (al″ko-hol′ik) [L. *alcoholicus*] 1. pertaining to or containing alcohol. 2. a person suffering from alcoholism (q.v.).

alcoholism (al′ko-hol-izm) a disorder characterized by a pathological pattern of alcohol use that causes a serious impairment in social or occupational functioning. In DSM III-R this is termed alcohol abuse or, if tolerance or withdrawal is present, alcohol dependence. **acute a.**, (*obs.*), alcohol intoxication; simple drunkenness. **chronic a.**, (*obs.*) alcoholism.

alcoholization (al″ko-hol″i-za′shun) treatment by application or injection of alcohol.

alcoholize (al′ko-hol-īz″) 1. to treat with alcohol. 2. to transform into alcohol.

alcoholuria (al″ko-hol-u′re-ah) the presence of alcohol in the urine.

alcoholysis (al″ko-hol′ĭ-sis) [*alcohol* + Gr. *lysis* dissolution] a process analogous to hydrolysis, but in which alcohol takes the place of water.

alcosol (al′ko-sol) a sol in which the dispersion medium is alcohol.

alcuronium chloride (al-kūr-o′nĭ-um) a non-depolarising skeletal muscle relaxant with effects like those of tubocurarine chloride.

Aldactazide (al-dak′tah-zīd) trademark for a preparation of spironolactone with hydrochlorothiazide.

Aldactone (al-dak′tōn) trademark for a preparation of spironolactone.

aldehyde (al′dĕ-hīd) [*alcohol* + L. *de* away from + *hydrogen*] 1. any one of a large class of organic compounds containing the group —CHO, that is, with the carbonyl group, C=O, occurring at the end of the carbon chain. 2. acetaldehyde. **cinnamic a.**, a colorless aldehyde, C_6H_5-(CH)$_2$CHO, obtained from oil of cinnamon, and used in flavors and perfumes. **cumic a.**, an aromatic volatile oil, para-isopropylbenzaldehyde, $C_3H_7 \cdot C_6H_4 \cdot CHO$, from several essential oils. **glyceric a., glycerin a.**, one of the allomeric forms of triose; it is the $CH_2OH \cdot CHOH \cdot CHO$, a reference substance for the stereochemical classification of the simple sugars. **glycolic a.**, see *diose*. **keto a.**, an aldehyde that contains the keto group CO and CHO. **salicylic a.**, a fragrant colorless liquid, $C_6H_4OH \cdot CHO$, soluble in water, from volatile oil of shrubs of the genus *Spiraea;* called also *salicylaldehyde*. **trichloracetic a.**, chloral.

aldehyde dehydrogenase (NAD⁺) (al′dĕ-hīd de-hi′-dro-jen-ās) [EC 1.2.1.3] an enzyme of the oxidoreductase class that catalyzes acid anion + NADH = aldehyde + NAD^+ + H_2O, the oxidation of various aldehydes (including the conversion of acetic aldehyde to acetic acid). Called also *acetaldehyde dehydrogenase*.

aldehyde-lyase (al′dĕ-hīd-li′ās) [EC 4.1.2] an enzyme of the lyase class that catalyzes cleavage of a C—C bond in a molecule containing a hydroxyl group and a carbonyl group to form two smaller molecules, each being an aldehyde or a ketone. Called also *aldolase*.

aldehyde oxidase (al′dĕ-hīd ok′sĭ-dās) [EC 1.2.3.1] an enzyme of the oxidoreductase class that catalyzes the reaction aldehyde + H_2O + O_2 = acid + superoxide. It is a flavohemoprotein containing molybdenum. The enzyme is found in liver tissue and catalyzes the oxidation of acetaldehyde, quinoline, and pyridines.

aldin (al′din) an aldehyde base.

Aldinamide (al-din′ah-mīd) trademark for preparations of pyrazinamide.

aldobionic acid (al″do-bi-on′ik as′id) a disaccharide containing a uronic acid as one of its component sugars and occurring in various plant gums and certain pathogenic organisms; it can be formed by the hydrolysis of the specific polysaccharide of type 3 *Streptococcus pneumoniae*.

Aldochlor (al′do-klor) trademark for preparations of methyldopa and chlorothiazide.

aldohexose (al″do-hek′sōs) a hexose that is an aldehyde derivative; any of a class of sugars that contain six carbon atoms and an aldehyde group, as glucose or mannose.

aldolase (al′do-lās) 1. an aldehyde-lyase. 2. fructose-bis-phosphate aldolase.

Aldomet (al′do-met) trademark for a preparation of methyldopa.

aldopentose (al″do-pen′tōs) any of a class of sugars that contain five carbon atoms and an aldehyde group, as arabinose.

Aldoril (al′do-ril) trademark for preparations of methyldopa and hydrochlorothiazide.

aldose (al′dōs) a sugar containing an aldehyde group, —CHO.

aldose 1-epimerase (al′dōs ĕ-pim′er-ās) [EC 5.1.3.3] an enzyme of the isomerase class that catalyzes interconversion of the α- and β- forms of glucose, galactose, lactose, and maltose. Commonly called *mutarotase*.

aldoside (al′do-sīd) a glycoside that on hydrolysis yields an aldose sugar.

aldosterone (al′do-ster-ōn″, al-dos′ter-ōn) the main mineralocorticoid hormone secreted by the adrenal cortex, the principal biological activity of which is the regulation of electrolyte and water balance by promoting the renal retention of sodium (and therefore of water) and the excretion of potassium; the retention of fluid induces an increase in plasma volume, edema, and hypertension. The secretion of aldosterone is stimulated by angiotensin II.

aldosteronism (al″do-ster′ŏn-izm″) an abnormality of electrolyte metabolism caused by excessive secretion of aldosterone; called also *hyperaldosteronism*. **primary a.,** that arising from oversecretion of aldosterone by an adrenal cortical adenoma, characterized typically by hypokalemia, alkalosis, muscular weakness, polyuria, polydipsia, and hypertension. Called also *Conn's syndrome*. **pseudoprimary a.,** that caused by bilateral adrenal hyperplasia and having the same signs and symptoms as primary aldosteronism. **secondary a.,** that due to extra-adrenal stimulation of aldosterone secretion; it is commonly associated with edematous states, as in nephrotic syndrome, hepatic cirrhosis, heart failure, and accelerated (malignant) hypertension.

aldosteronogenesis (al″do-ster-o-no-jen′e-sis) the production of aldosterone by the adrenal cortex.

aldosteronoma (al″do-ster″on-o′mah) an aldosterone-secreting tumor of the adrenal cortex.

aldosteronopenia (al″do-ster-o-no-pe′ne-ah) hypoaldosteronism.

aldosteronuria (al″do-ster″ōn-u′re-ah) the presence of excessive aldosterone in the urine.

aldotetrose (al″do-tet′rōs) an aldehyde sugar containing four atoms of carbon.

aldoxime (al-dok′sīm) a compound formed by the union of an aldehyde with hydroxylamine.

Aldrich mixture (awl′drich) [Robert Henry *Aldrich*, American surgeon, born 1902] see under *mixture*.

Aldrich syndrome (awl′drich) [Robert A. *Aldrich*, American pediatrician, born 1917] Wiskott-Aldrich syndrome.

Aldrich-Mees lines (al′drich-mēz) [C.J. *Aldrich*; R.A. *Mees*, Dutch scientist, 20th century] Mees' lines.

aldrin (al′drin) chemical name: 1,2,3,4,10,10-hexachloro-1,4,4a,5,8,8a-hexahydro-1,4:8-dimethanonaphthalene. A chlorinated naphthalene derivative, $C_{12}H_8Cl_6$, used as an insecticide.

alecithal (ah-les′ĭ-thal) [*a* neg. + Gr. *lekithos* yolk] without yolk; applied to eggs with very little yolk. See under *ovum*.

Alectorobius talaje the tick *Ornithodoros talaje*.

alembic (ah-lem′bik) [Arabic *al-imbīq*, the still, from Gr. *ambix* cup] a retort with a removable cap formerly used by chemists.

alembroth (ah-lem′broth) a compound, $(NH_4Cl)_2HgCl_2$ + $2H_2O$, of mercuric and ammonium chlorides, formerly used as an antiseptic dressing.

alemmal (ah-lem′al) [*a* neg. + Gr. *lemma* husk] (*obs.*) having no neurilemma; said of a nerve fiber.

Aletris farinosa L. (Liliaceae) (al′ĕ-tris fah-rĭ-nōs′ah) a perennial herb indigenous to eastern North America, used medicinally by the Catawba Indians. The dried roots (colic root, or unicorn root) are used as a diuretic and uterine tonic; cold-water leaf infusion is used for colic and stomach ailments. It contains starch and diosgenin.

aleukemia (ah″lu-ke′me-ah) [*a* neg. + Gr. *leukos* white + *haima* blood + *-ia*] 1. absence or deficiency of leukocytes in the blood. 2. aleukemic leukemia.

aleukemic (ah″lu-ke′mik) marked by aleukemia; see under *leukemia*.

aleukia (ah-lu′ke-ah) [*a* neg. + Gr. *leukos* white + *-ia*] absence of leukocytes from the blood; leukopenia. **alimentary toxic a.,** a form of mycotoxicosis associated with the ingestion of grain that has overwintered in the field; causative agents include members of the genera *Fusarium, Cladosporium, Alternaria, Penicillium, Mucor, Piptocephalis, Trichoderma, Rhizopus, Trichothecium, Thammidium, Verticillium,* and *Actinomyces*. Abbreviated ATA. **a. hemorrha′gica,** an accessory or auxiliary term which actually refers to the condition of aplastic anemia (see under *anemia*).

aleukocytic (ah-lu″ko-sit′ik) showing no leukocytes.

aleukocytosis (ah-lu″ko-si-to′sis) [*a* neg. + *leukocyte* + *-osis*] deficiency in the proportion of white cells in the blood; leukopenia.

aleuriospore (ah-lu′re-o-spōr) [Gr. *aleuron* flour + *spore*] a terminal or lateral, asexual spore similar to a conidium except that it is not shed (not deciduous), being released only by dissolution of its attachment to the mycelium.

Aleurisma (al″u-riz′mah) *Chrysosporium*.

Aleurobius farinae (ah-lu-ro′bĭ-us fah-ri′ne) *Tyroglyphus farinae*.

Aleuronat (ah-lu′ro-nat″) trademark for a brand of wheat flour from which most of the starch has been removed; used by diabetics.

aleurone (ah-lōōr′ōn″, al′yah-rōn″) 1. the protein granule of globulins and peptones found in ripe seeds. 2. the outer layer of the endosperm in gluten-rich cereal grains.

aleuronoid (ah-lu′ro-noid″) resembling flour.

Alexander (al″ek-san′der) **of Tralles** (c. 525–605) a Byzantine Greek physician and compiler who practiced in Rome; his writings were mainly on pathology and the treatment of internal diseases and included descriptions of intestinal parasites and vermifuges. Also known as *Alexander Trallianus*.

Alexander's operation (al″ek-zan′derz) [William *Alexander*, Liverpool surgeon, 1844–1919] see under *operation*.

Alexander's disease (al″ek-zen′derz) [W. Stewart *Alexander*, English pathologist, 20th century] see under *disease*.

Alexander-Adams operation (al″ek-zan′der-ad′amz) [William *Alexander*; James Alexander *Adams*, gynecologist in Glasgow, 1857–1930] see *Alexander's operation*, under *operation*.

alexeteric (ah-lek″sĕ-ter′ik) [Gr. *alexētēr* defender] effective against infection or poison.

alexia (ah-lek′se-ah) [*a* neg. + Gr. *lexis* word + *-ia*] a form of receptive aphasia in which there is loss of the ability to understand written language as a result of a cerebral lesion; called also *aphemesthesia, optical alexia, visual amnesia, visual aphasia,* and *word blindness*. **cortical a.,** a form of sensory aphasia due to lesions of the left gyrus angularis. **motor a.,** alexia in which the patient understands what he sees written or printed, but cannot read it aloud. **musi-**

cal a., loss of the ability to read music; music blindness. **optical a.,** alexia. **subcortical a.,** a form due to interruption of the connection between the optic center and the gyrus angularis.

alexic (ah-lek'sik) pertaining to alexia.

alexidine (ah-leks'ĭ-dēn) chemical name: N,N''-bis(2-ethylhexyl)-3,12-diimino-2,4,11,13-tetraazatetradecanediimidamide; an antibacterial, $C_{26}H_{56}N_{10}$.

alexin (ah-lek'sin) [Gr. alexein to ward off] (obs.) complement.

alexinic (al''ek-sin'ik) pertaining to or having the properties of an alexin.

alexipharmac (ah-lek''se-far'mak)[Gr. alexein to ward off + pharmakon poison] 1. warding off the ill effects of a poison. 2. an antidote or remedy for poisoning.

alexithymia (ah-leks''ĭ-thi'me-ah)[a neg. + Gr. lexis word + Gr. thymos mind + ia] inability to verbalize one's emotions.

alexocyte (ah-lek'so-sīt'') [Gr. alexein to ward off + kytos hollow vessel] a cell of the animal organism secreting alexins; the term was formerly applied to eosinophil cells.

aleydigism (ah-li'dig-izm'') absence of androgen secretion of the interstitial cells of Leydig.

Alezzandrini's syndrome (al''ĕ-zan-dre'nēz) [A.S. Alezzandrini, Argentine ophthalmologist, 20th century] see under syndrome.

Alflorone (al'flo-rōn) trademark for preparations of fludrocortisone.

ALG antilymphocyte globulin.

alga (al'gah) any individual organism of the algae.

algae (al'je) [L., pl., "seaweeds"] a group of cryptogamous plants, in which the body is unicellular or consists of a thallus; it includes the seaweed and many unicellular fresh-water plants, most of which contain chlorophyll. Algae account for about 90 per cent of the earth's photosynthetic activity. **blue-green a.,** Cyanobacteria.

algal (al'gal) of, pertaining to, or caused by algae.

alganesthesia (al-gan''es-the'ze-ah) [Gr. algos pain + anesthesia] analgesia.

algaroba (al''gah-ro'bah) the finely pulverized meal of the dried ripe fruit (St. John's bread, or carob fruit) of Ceratonia siliqua L., Leguminosae. It contains albuminous proteins, carbohydrates, and small amounts of fat and crude fiber, and is used in pharmaceutical formulations as an adsorbent and demulcent in treatment of diarrhea.

alge- see algesi(o)-.

algedonic (al''je-don'ik) [alge- + Gr. hēdonē pleasure] characterized by or relating to pleasure and pain.

algefacient (al''je-fa'shent) [L. algere to be cold + faciens making] cooling; refrigerant.

algeldrate (al-jel'drāt) nonreactive, powdered, hydrated aluminum hydroxide; an antacid, $AlH_3O_3 \cdot xH_2O$.

algesia (al-je'ze-ah) sensitiveness to pain; hyperesthesia.

algesic (al-je'zik) painful.

algesichronometer (al-je''ze-kro-nom'ĕ-ter) [algesi- + Gr. chronos time + metron measure] an instrument for recording the time required to produce a painful impression.

algesimeter (al''je-sim'ĕ-ter) [algesi + Gr. metron measure] an instrument used in measuring the sensitiveness to pain as produced by pricking with a sharp point. **Björnström's a.,** an apparatus for determining the sensitiveness of the skin. **Boas' a.,** an instrument for determining the sensitiveness over the epigastrium.

algesimetry (al''jĕ-sim'ĕ-tre) the measurement of sensitiveness to pain; called also algesiometry.

algesi(o)-, alge-, algi(o)-, alg(o)- [Gr. algēsis sense of pain; Gr. algos pain] combining forms denoting relationship to pain.

algesiogenic (al-je''ze-o-jen'ik) [algesi- + Gr. gennan to produce] producing pain.

algesiometer (al-je''ze-om'ĕ-ter) algesimeter.

algesthesia (al''jes-the'ze-ah) pain sensibility; algesthesis.

algesthesis (al''jes-the'sis)[algesi- + Gr. aisthēsis perception] the perception of pain; any painful sensation.

algestone acetophenide (al-jes'tōn) a progestin with actions similar to those of progesterone.

algetic (al-jet'ik) painful.

-algia [Gr. algos pain + -ia] a word termination denoting a painful condition.

algicide (al'jĭ-sīd) [algae + L. caedere to kill] a substance which is destructive to algae.

algid (al'jid) [L. algidus] chilly or cold, def. 1.

algin (al'jin) sodium alginate, a purified carbohydrate (sodium mannuronate) extracted from brown algae species and used as a stabilizing colloid in numerous pharmaceuticals, cosmetics, and foods.

alginate (al'jĭ-nāt) a salt of alginic acid, which is extracted from marine kelp. Calcium, sodium, and ammonium alginates have been used as foam, clot, or gauze for absorbable surgical dressings. Soluble alginates, such as sodium, potassium, and magnesium alginates, form a viscous sol which can be changed into a gel by a chemical reaction with compounds such as calcium sulfate, a property which makes them useful as materials for taking dental impressions.

alginic acid (al-jin'ik) an acid polysaccharide obtained from seaweed, used for thickening, emulsifying, and stabilizing foods and drugs.

Alginomonas (al''jĭ-no-mo'nas) in former systems of classification, a genus of bacteria made up of organisms now assigned to the genus Pseudomonas.

alginuresis (al''jin-u-re'sis) [Gr. algos pain + ourēsis urination] painful urination.

algi(o)- see algesi(o)-.

algiomotor (al''je-o-mo'tor) producing painful movements, such as spasm or dysperistalsis.

algiomuscular (al''je-o-mus'ku-lar) causing painful muscular movements.

algiovascular (al''je-o-vas'ku-lar) pertaining to vascular action resulting from painful stimulation.

alg(o)- see algesi(o)-.

algodystrophy (al''go-dis'tro-fe) [algo- + dystrophy] a combination of pain and dystrophic changes in bone, as in Sudeck's atrophy.

algogenesia (al''go-jĕ-ne'ze-ah) [algo- + Gr. gennan to produce] the production of pain.

algogenesis (al''go-jen'ĕ-sis) algogenesia.

algogenic (al-go-jen'ik) 1. [algo- + Gr. gennan to produce] causing pain. 2. [L. algor cold + Gr. gennan to produce] producing cold.

algolagnia (al''go-lag'ne-ah) [algo- + Gr. lagneia lust] any psychosexual disorder associated with the derivation of pleasure from experiencing or inflicting physical or psychological pain. **active a.,** sadism. **passive a.,** masochism.

algologist (al-gol'o-jist) 1. one who specializes in algology. 2. phycologist.

algology (al-gol'o-je) 1. [algo- + -logy] the discipline that deals with the study of pain. 2. [alga + -logy] phycology.

algomenorrhea (al''go-men-o-re'ah) [algo- + menorrhea] (obs.) dysmenorrhea.

algometer (al-gom'ĕ-ter) [algo- + Gr. metron measure] an instrument for testing sensitivity to painful stimuli. **pressure a.,** an instrument for measuring sensitivity to pressure.

algometry (al-gom'ĕ-tre) the measurement of sensitivity to painful stimuli, as with an algometer.

algophilia (al''go-fil'e-ah) (obs.) masochism.

algophobia (al''go-fo'be-ah) [algo- + phobia] exaggerated, irrational fear of pain.

algopsychalia (al''go-si-ka'le-ah) [algo- + Gr. psychē soul] psychalgia (def. 1).

algorithm (al'go-rith'm) a mechanical procedure for solving a certain type of mathematical problem; a step-by-step method of solving a problem, as in making a diagnosis.

algoscopy (al-gos'ko-pe) [L. algor cold + Gr. skopein to view] (obs.) cryoscopy.

algosis (al-go'sis) the presence of algae or fungi in a part of the body.

algospasm (al'go-spazm) [algo- + spasm] painful spasm or cramp.

algovascular (al''go-vas'ku-lar) algiovascular.

Ali Abbas (ah'le ah'bas)) [L. Haly Abbas, from Ar. Ali

ibn-al-*Abbās*, al Majūsi, 930–994] a Persian physician whose *Al-Maliki*(*Liber Regius*, "Royal Book") was the leading medical text for 100 years, when it was superseded by Aricenna's *Canon*. Also known as *Haly Abbas*.

Alibert's disease (al-e-berz′) [Jean Louis Marc *Alibert*, French dermatologist, 1768–1837] see *mycosis fungoides*.

alible (al′ĭ-b'l) [L. *alibilis*] nutritive; assimilable as a food.

alicyclic (al″ĭ-sik′lik) having the properties of both aliphatic and cyclic substances.

Alidase (al′ĭ-dās) trademark for a preparation of hyaluronidase for injection.

alienation (āl″yen-a′shun) [L *alienatio,* from *alienus* strange, foreign] 1. estrangement from society; feelings of being an outsider, foreigner, or outcast. 2. estrangement from one's self; feelings of unreality or depersonalization. 3. alienation of affect; isolation of ideas from feelings, avoidance of emotional situations, and other efforts to estrange one's self from one's feelings. 4. (*obs.*) insanity or mental derangement.

alienia (ah″li-e′ne-ah) [*a* neg. + L. *lien* spleen] absence of the spleen.

alienist (āl′yen-ist) [Fr. *aliéniste,* from *aliéné* insane, from *L. alienatus* estranged] (*obs.*) a psychiatrist.

ali-esterase (al″ĭ-es′ter-ās) carboxylesterase.

aliflurane (al″ĭ-floo′rān) chemical name: 1-chloro-1,2,2,3-tetrafluoro-3-methoxy-cyclopropane; an inhalation anesthetic, $C_4H_3ClF_4O$.

aliform (al′ĭ-form) [L. *ala* wing + *forma* shape] shaped like a wing.

alignment (ah-līn′ment) [Fr. *aligner* to put in a straight line] 1. the act of arranging in a line; the state of being arranged in a line. 2. bringing natural or artificial teeth into line, so that they form the two regular parabolic curves of the dental arches and reestablish a harmonious relationship with the supporting structures and with the opposite dentition. Spelled also *alinement*.

aliment (al′ĕ-ment) [L. *alimentum*] food or nutritive material.

alimentary (al″ĕ-men′tar-e) pertaining to food or nutritive material, or to the organs of digestion.

alimentation (al″ĕ-men-ta′shun) the act of giving or receiving nutriment. **artificial a.,** the giving of food or nourishment to persons who cannot take it in the usual way. **forced a.,** 1. the feeding of a person against his will. 2. the giving of more food to a person than his appetite calls for. **parenteral a.,** administration of nutriment intravenously. **rectal a.,** the administration of concentrated nourishment by instillation into the rectum. **total parenteral a.,** the intravenous administration of the total nutrient requirements of the patient with gastrointestinal dysfunction, accomplished via a central venous catheter, usually inserted in the superior vena cava via a subclavian vein. Called also *parenteral hyperalimentation* and *total parenteral nutrition*.

alimentology (al″ĕ-men-tol′o-je) the science of nutrition.

alimentotherapy (al″ĕ-men″to-ther′ah-pe) [*aliment* + Gr. *therapeia* treatment] dietetic treatment; treatment by systematic feeding.

alinasal (al″e-na′sal) pertaining to the ala nasi.

alinement (ah-līn′ment) alignment.

alinjection (al″in-jek′shun) (*obs.*) repeated injection of alcohol for preserving anatomic specimens.

aliphatic (al″ĕ-fat′ik) [Gr. *aleiphar, aleiphatos* oil] pertaining to an oil; a term applied to the "open-chain" or fatty series of hydrocarbons.

alipogenic (a-lip″o-jen′ik) not lipogenic; not forming fat.

alipoidic (a″lip-oi′dik) free from lipoids.

alipotropic (al″lip-o-trop′ik) having no influence on the metabolism of fat.

aliquorrhea (al″i-kwo-re′ah) hypoliquorrhea.

aliquot (al′ĕ-kwot) the part of a number which will divide it without a remainder; e.g., 2 is an aliquot of 6. By extension, any portion that bears a known quantitative relationship to a whole or to other portions of the same whole, as an aliquot portion of a solution; a sample of a whole taken to determine the quantitative composition of the whole.

alismin (ah-lis′min) an extractive from *Alisma plantago,* or water plantain.

alisphenoid (al-e-sfe′noid) [*ala* + *sphenoid*] 1. pertaining to the greater wing of the sphenoid. 2. a cartilage of the fetal chondrocranium on either side of the basisphenoid; later in development it forms the greater part of the greater wing of the sphenoid.

alizarin (ah-liz′ah-rin) [Arabic *ala sara* extract] a red crystalline dye, 1,2-dihydroxyanthraquinone, $C_6H_4(CO)_2C_6H_2$-$(OH)_2$ prepared synthetically or obtained from madder; its compounds are used as indicators. **a. monosulfonate,** a. red; see under *red.* **a. No. 6,** purpurin (def. 2). **a. red,** see under *red.* **a. yellow, a. yellow g.,** see under *yellow.*

alizarinopurpurin (al″ĭ-zar″ĭ-no-pur′pu-rin) purpurin (def. 2).

alkalemia (al″kah-le′me-ah) [*alkali* + Gr. *haima* blood + -*ia*] increased pH or decreased hydrogen ion concentration of the blood.

alkalescence (al″kah-les′ens) slight or incipient alkalinity.

alkalescent (al″kah-les′ent) having a tendency to alkalinity.

alkali (al′kah-li) [Arabic *al-qalīy* potash] any of a class of compounds which form soluble soaps with fatty acids, turn red litmus blue, and form soluble carbonates. Essentially the hydroxides of cesium, lithium, potassium, rubidium, and sodium, they include also the carbonates of these metals and of ammonia. **caustic a.,** any solid hydroxide of a fixed alkali. **fixed a.,** any of the alkalis except ammonium. **volatile a.,** ammonia, NH_3; also ammonium hydroxide.

alkalify (al-kal′e-fi) to make alkaline.

Alkaligenes (al″kah-lij′e-nēz) *Alcaligenes.*

alkaligenous (al″kah-lij′ĕ-nus) yielding an alkali.

alkalimeter (al″kah-lim′ĕ-ter) [*alkali* + *meter*] an instrument for measuring the alkali contained in any mixture.

alkalimetry (al″kah-lim′ĕ-tre) the measurement of the alkalis present in any substance. **Engel's a.,** a method of determining the alkalinity of the blood by titrating a diluted specimen with normal tartaric acid solution until it reddens litmus paper; the amount of tartaric solution necessary to produce the result indicates the degree of alkalinity of the blood.

alkaline (al′kah-līn, -lin) [L. *alkalinus*] having the reactions of an alkali.

alkaline phosphatase (al′kah-līn, -lin fos′fah-tās) [EC 3.1.3.1] an enzyme of the hydrolase class that catalyzes the reaction orthophosphoric monoester + H_2O = alcohol + orthophosphate, with optimal activity at pH 9.5–10.5. A divalent cation such as zinc, manganese, magnesium, or cobalt is required as an activator. Differing forms of the enzyme occur in a variety of normal and malignant tissues; many are poorly characterized. The activity in serum is useful in the clinical diagnosis of many illnesses, with markedly increased levels being found in bone diseases, bone regeneration, hepatic obstruction, and hepatitis. A genetic deficiency of the bone enzyme, transmitted as an autosomal recessive trait, causes hypophosphatasia. Called also *phosphomonoesterase.* Abbreviated ALP. **leucocyte a.p.,** alkaline phosphatase found in the cytoplasmic granules of leukocytes. The enzyme activity is lowered in chronic myelogenous leukemia and other conditions. Abbreviated LAP.

alkalinity (al″kah-lin′ĭ-te) the fact or quality of being alkaline.

alkalinization (al″kah-lin″ĭ-za′shun) alkalization.

alkalinize (al′kah-lin-iz″) alkalize.

alkalinuria (al″kah-lin-u′re-ah) [*alkaline* + *urine*] an alkaline condition of the urine.

alkalitherapy (al″kah-li-ther′ah-pe) treatment by alkalis; the administration of large amounts of alkali in the treatment of peptic ulcer and hyperchlorhydria.

alkalization (al″kah-li-za′shun) the act of making alkaline.

alkalize (al′kah-līz) to render alkaline.

alkalizer (al′kah-līz′er) an agent that neutralizes acids or causes alkalinization.

alkalogenic (al″kah-lo-jen′ik) producing alkalinity.

alkaloid (al′kah-loid″) [*alkali* + -*oid*] one of a large group of nitrogenous basic substances found in plants. They are usually very bitter and many are pharmacologically active.

Examples are atropine, caffeine, coniine, morphine, nicotine, quinine, strychnine. The term is also applied to synthetic substances (*artificial a's*) which have structures similar to plant alkaloids, such as procaine. **animal a.,** 1. a ptomaine. 2. a leukomaine. **vinca a's,** alkaloids produced by the common periwinkle plant (*Vinca rosea*); two, vincristine and vinblastine, are used as antineoplastic agents.

alkalometry (al″kah-lom′ĕ-tre) [*alkaloid* + *-metry*] the dosimetric administration of alkaloids.

alkalosis (al″kah-lo′sis) a pathologic condition resulting from accumulation of base, or from loss of acid without comparable loss of base in the body fluids, and characterized by decrease in hydrogen ion concentration (increase in pH). Cf. *acidosis.* **altitude a.,** increased alkalinity in blood and tissues due to exposure to high altitudes. **compensated a.,** a condition in which compensatory mechanisms have returned the pH toward normal; see *metabolic a., conpensated,* and *respiratory a., compensated.* **hypokalemic a.,** a variety of metabolic alkalosis associated with a low serum potassium level; retention of alkali or loss of acid occurs in the extracellular (but not intracellular) fluid compartment, although the pH of the intracellular fluid may be below normal. It may be caused by hypertrophy and hypoplasia of the juxtaglomerular cells, as in Bartter's syndrome. **metabolic a.,** a disturbance in which the acid-base status of the body shifts toward the alkaline side because of retention of base or loss of noncarbonic, or fixed (nonvolatile), acids. **metabolic a., compensated,** a state of alkalosis in which the pH of the blood has been returned toward normal by respiratory compensation. **respiratory a.,** a state due to excess loss of carbon dioxide from the body. **respiratory a., compensated,** a respiratory alkalosis in which the pH of the blood has been returned toward normal through retention of acid or excretion of base by renal mechanisms.

alkalotherapy (al″kah-lo-ther′ah-pe) alkalitherapy.

alkalotic (al″kah-lot′ik) pertaining to or characterized by alkalosis.

alkaluria (al″kah-lu′re-ah) the presence of an alkali in the urine.

alkamine (al′kah-min) an alcohol which contains an amine group.

alkane (al′kān) a saturated hydrocarbon of the methane series, one in which all carbon atoms are joined by single bonds; called also *paraffin.*

alkanet (al′kă-net) the reddish dye-containing root of *Alkanna tinctoria* Tausch, Boraginaceae; formerly used as an astringent, but now mainly as a colorant for candies, cosmetics, and wines. It contains alkannin (the dye principle) and tannin.

alkannin (al′kah-nin) a red powder, the coloring ingredient of alkanet; used as a colorant and, in the form of alkannin paper as an indicator alkalis turn the paper blue, acids red.

alkapton (al-kap′tōn) [*alk*ali + Gr. *haptō* to fasten or bind to] see *alkapton bodies,* under *body.*

alkaptonuria (al″kap-to-nu′re-ah) [*alkaptone* + *-uria*] an inborn aminoacidopathy due to defective homogentisate 1,2-dioxygenase; accumulation of homogentisic acid leads to homogentisic aciduria (the urine darkens on standing or alkalinization), ochronosis, and arthritis. Called also *homogentisic acid oxidase deficiency.* **spontaneous a.,** a hereditary and congenital anomaly of the metabolism of tyrosine with excretion in the urine of homogentisic acid.

alkaptonuric (al-kap″to-nu′rik) pertaining to, characterized by, or causing alkaptonuria; by extension, sometimes used as a noun to designate an individual with alkaptonuria.

alkatriene (al″kah-tri′ēn) an unsaturated aliphatic hydrocarbon containing three double bonds.

alkavervir (al″kah-ver′vir) a yellow powdery mixture of alkaloids obtained from selective extraction of *Veratrum viride;* it is used orally as a vasodilator in the treatment of hypertension.

alkene (al′kēn) an unsaturated aliphatic hydrocarbon containing one double bond; olefin.

Alkeran (al-ker′an) trademark for a preparation of melphalan.

alkyl (al′kil) the radical which results when an aliphatic hydrocarbon loses one hydrogen atom.

alkylamine (al″kil-ah′mēn) an amine containing an alkyl radical.

alkylate (al′kĭ-lāt) to treat with an alkylating agent.

alkylation (al″kĭ-la′shun) the substitution of an alkyl group for an active hydrogen atom in an organic compound.

alkylogen (al-kil′o-jen) an alkyl ester of any of the halogen acids, e.g., ethyl chloride.

alkyne (al′kīn) an unsaturated hydrocarbon containing a triple bond between two carbon atoms; the alkynes are members of the acetylene series.

allachesthesia (al″ah-kes-the′ze-ah) [Gr. *allachē* elsewhere + *aisthēsis* perception + *-ia*] allesthesia. **optical a.,** visual allesthesia.

allantiasis (al″an-ti′ah-sis) [*allanto-* + *-iasis*] sausage poisoning; poisoning from sausages containing the toxins of *Clostridium botulinum.* See *botulism.*

allant(o)- [Gr. *allas,* gen. *allantos* sausage] a combining form denoting relationship to a sausage or to the allantois.

allantochorion (ah-lan″to-ko′re-on) a compound membrane formed by fusion of the allantois and chorion.

allantogenesis (al″an-to-jen′ĕ-sis) the formation and development of the allantois.

allantoic (al″an-to′ik) pertaining to the allantois.

allantoid (ah-lan′toid) [*allanto-* + Gr. *eidos* form] 1. resembling the allantois. 2. sausage shaped.

allantoidean (al″an-toi′de-an) 1. pertaining to the allantois. 2. any animal with an allantois during its embryonic development; in the plural, *amniotes* is the more usual term.

allantoidoangiopagous (al″an-toi″do-an″je-op′ah-gus) [*allanto-* + Gr. *angeion* vessel + *pagos* thing fixed] joined by the vessels of the umbilical cord; see under *twin.*

allantoidoangiopagus (al″an-toi″do-an″je-op′ah-gus) twin fetuses joined by the vessels of the umbilical cord; allantoidoangiopagous twins. Called also *omphaloangiopagus.*

allantoin (ah-lan′to-in) chemical name: 5-ureidohydantoin. A white crystallizable substance, $C_4H_6N_4O_3$, the diureide of glyoxylic acid, found in allantoic fluid, fetal urine, and many plants, and as a urinary excretion product of purine metabolism in most mammals but not in man or the higher apes. It is produced synthetically by the oxidation of uric acid, and was once used to encourage epithelial formation in wounds and ulcers and in osteomyelitis. It is the active substance in maggot treatment, being secreted by the maggots as a product of purine metabolism.

allantoinuria (ah-lan″to-in-u′re-ah) the presence of allantoin in the urine.

allantois (ah-lan′to-is) [Gr. *allantos* sausage + *eidos* form] an initially tubular ventral diverticulum of the hindgut of embryos of reptiles, birds, and mammals. In reptiles and birds, it expands to a large sac for storing urine and, after fusing with the chorion which lines the shell, provides for gas exchange. The allantois is prominent in some mammals (carnivores, ungulates); in others, including man, it is vestigial except that its blood vessels give rise to those of the umbilical cord. See illustration under *amnion.*

allantotoxicon (ah-lan″to-tok′se-kon) [*allanto-* + Gr. *toxikon* poison] a hypothetical poison formerly supposed to cause allantiasis.

allel (ah-lēl′) allele.

allele (ah-lēl′) any alternative form of a gene that can occupy a particular chromosomal locus. In humans and other diploid organisms there are two alleles, one on each chromosome of a homologous pair. See also *Mendel's laws,* under *law* and *multiple a's.* **multiple a's,** a series of more than two alleles. **silent a.,** see under *gene.*

allelic (ah-le′lik) pertaining to alleles; produced by alternative genes.

allelism (al′e-lizm) the existence of alleles, or their relationship to one another.

allel(o)- [Gr. *allēlōn* of one another] a combining form denoting relationship to another.

allelocatalysis (ah-le″lo-kah-tal′ĭ-sis) [*allelo-* + *catalysis*] the once held theory of mutual stimulation of cells to growth, or stimulation of growth in a bacterial culture by the addition to it of other cells of the same type.

allelocatalytic (ah-le″lo-kat-ah-lit′ik) catalyzing each other; causing or marked by allelocatalysis.

allelochemics (al-le″lo-kem′iks) chemical interactions between species, involving release of active chemical substances, such as scents, pheromones, and toxins.

allelotaxis (ah-le″lo-tak′sis) [*allelo-* + Gr. *taxis* arrangement] the development of an organ from several embryonic structures.

allelotaxy (ah-le′lo-tak″se) allelotaxis.

Allemann's syndrome (al′manz) [Richard *Allemann,* Swiss physician, 1893–1958] see under *syndrome.*

Allen's fossa [Harrison *Allen,* Philadelphia anatomist, 1841–1897] see under *fossa.*

Allen's paradoxic law, treatment [Frederick Madison *Allen,* American physician, 1879–1964] see under *law* and *treatment.*

Allen's test (al′enz) [Edgar V. *Allen,* American physician, born 1900] see under *tests.*

Allen-Doisy test, unit (al′en doi′se) [Edgar *Allen,* American anatomist, 1892–1943; Edward Adelbert *Doisy,* American biochemist, born 1893] see under *test,* and see *mouse unit* and *rat unit,* under *unit.*

allergen (al′er-jen) [*allergy* + *-gen*] an antigenic substance capable of producing immediate-type hypersensitivity (allergy). **pollen a.,** any protein antigen of weed, tree, or grass pollens capable of causing allergic asthma or rhinitis; pollen allergen extracts are used in skin testing for pollen sensitivity and in immunotherapy (desensitization) for pollen allergy.

allergenic (al″er-jen′ik) acting as an allergen; inducing allergy.

allergic (ah-ler′jik) pertaining to, caused by, affected with, or of the nature of allergy.

allergist (al′er-jist) a physician who specializes in the diagnosis and treatment of allergic conditions.

allergization (al″er-jĭ-za′shun) active sensitization or the introduction of allergens into the body.

allergize (al′er-jīz) to subject to sensitization; to make allergic.

allergoid (al′er-goid) an allergen rendered less allergenic but not less antigenic (formation of IgE but not of IgG blocking antibody is decreased) by formalin or glutaraldehyde treatment.

allergological (al″er-go-loj′ĭ-kal) pertaining to allergology.

allergologist (al″er-gol′o-jist) one who specializes in allergology.

allergology (al″er-gol′o-je) the branch of medicine devoted to the study of allergy, its etiology, diagnosis, and treatment.

allergosis (al″er-go′sis), pl. *allergo′ses.* Any allergic disease.

allergy (al′er-je) [Gr. *allos* other + *ergon* work] 1. a state of hypersensitivity induced by exposure to a particular antigen (allergen) resulting in harmful immunologic reactions on subsequent exposures; the term is usually used to refer to hypersensitivity to an environmental antigen (atopic allergy or contact dermatitis) or to drug allergy; the original meaning, now obsolete, included all states of altered immunologic reactivity, immunity as well as hypersensitivity. Gell and Coombs used the term "allergic reaction" to mean any harmful immunologic reaction causing tissue injury (see *Gell and Coombs classification,* under *classification*). 2. The medical specialty dealing with diagnosis and treatment of allergic disorders. **atopic a.,** atopy (def. 2). **bacterial a.,** hypersensitivity to a bacterial antigen, e.g., delayed-type hypersensitivity to *Mycobacterium tuberculosis.* **bronchial a.,** see *asthma.* **cold a.,** any condition in which signs and symptoms of allergy are produced by exposure to cold, e.g., cold urticaria. **contact a.,** see under *hypersensitivity.* **delayed a.,** see under *hypersensitivity.* **drug a.,** an allergic reaction occurring as the result of unusual sensitivity to a drug. **food a., gastrointestinal a.,** allergy produced by ingested antigens, such as food or drugs; strawberries, milk, and eggs are the most common offenders. The organ affected usually is the skin. **hereditary a.,** atopy (def. 2). **immediate a.,** see under *hypersensitivity.* **latent a.,** allergy which is not manifested by symptoms but which may be detected by tests. **physical a.,** any condition in which signs and symptoms of allergy are produced by exposure to cold (cold urticaria or angioedema), heat (cholin-

ergic urticaria), or light (photosensitivity). **pollen a.,** hay fever. **polyvalent a.,** a simultaneous allergic response to several allergens. **spontaneous a.,** atopy (def. 2).

Allescheria (al″es-ke′re-ah) a genus of ascomycetous fungi of the family Eurotiaceae, order Eurotiales, representing the perfect (sexual) stage of *Monosporium.* **A. boy′dii,** a species of fungi, commonly isolated from maduromycosis and other human infection; its imperfect (asexual) stage is *Monosporium apiospermum.*

allesthesia (al″es-the′ze-ah) [Gr. *allos* other + *aisthēsis* perception + *-ia*] a condition in which a sensation, as of pain or touch, is experienced at a point remote from that at which the stimulus is applied or occurs, as in allochiria. **visual a.,** a condition in which visual images are transposed from one half of the visual field to the other, either vertically or horizontally; called also *optical allachesthesia.*

allethrin (al′ĕ-thrin) a synthetic analogue of the natural insecticides cinerin, jasmolin, and pyrethrin, used as an insecticide.

alliaceous (al″e-a′shus) pertaining to or resembling the smell of garlic; pertaining to the genus *Allium.*

alliance (ah-li′ans) a union formed for the furtherance of interests of the members; an agreement to cooperate for specific purposes. **therapeutic a.,** a conscious contractual relationship between therapist and patient in which each agrees to work together to help the patient with his problems. **working a.,** in group therapy, the collaboration between the group as a whole and each patient to promote the mental health and emotional maturation of the members.

alligation (al″ĭ-ga′shun) the process of finding the cost of a mixture of known quantities of ingredients, each of known value, or of determining the quantities of solutions of various strengths to be used to form a mixture of a particular strength.

Allis's inhaler, sign (al′is-iz) [Oscar Huntington *Allis,* Philadelphia surgeon, 1833–1921] see under *inhaler* and *sign.*

alliteration (ah-lit″er-a′shun) [L. *ad* to + *litera* letter] a dysphrasia in which the patient uses words containing the same consonant sounds.

allithiamine (al″ĭ-thi′ah min) any of several analogues of thiamine that are easily absorbed from the intestinal tract.

Allium (al′e-um) [L. "garlic"] a genus of liliaceous plants, including the garlic and onion. Garlic contains a sulfur ester derivative known as allicin, which has antimicrobial activity. It is a common home remedy among various European ethnic groups as an antitussive, antiseptic, rubefacient, diaphoretic, toothache and earache remedy, vermifuge, and as an aid in nervous conditions.

all(o)- [Gr. *allos* other] a combining form denoting a condition differing from the normal, or reversal, or referring to another.

alloalbumin (al″o-al-bu′min) any genetic variant of albumin.

alloantibody (al″o-an′-tĭ-bod″e) isoantibody.

alloantigen (al″o-an′tĭ-jen) isoantigen.

allobar (al′o-bar) [*allo-* + Gr. *baros* weight] a form of a chemical element having an atomic weight different from that of the naturally occurring form.

allobarbital (al″o-bar′bĭ-tal) chemical name: 5,5-di-2-propenyl-2,4,6(1*H*,3*H*,5*H*)pyrimidinetrione. An intermediate in long-acting barbiturate, $C_{10}H_{12}N_2O_3$, occurring as a white, crystalline powder; used orally as a sedative and hypnotic, and orally in combination with acetaminophen or with acetaminophen and codeine as an analgesic. Formerly called *diallylbarbituric acid.*

allobiosis (al″o-bi-o′sis) [*allo-* + Gr. *bios* life] the condition of altered reactivity which an organism manifests under changed environmental or physiologic conditions.

allocentric (al″o-sen′trik) focused on the thoughts and feelings of others; not egocentric.

allocheiria (al″o-ki′re-ah) allochiria.

allochesthesia (al″o-kes-the′ze-ah) allesthesia.

allochezia (al″o-ke′ze-ah) [*allo-* + Gr. *chezein* to defecate] (*obs.*) 1. the discharge of nonfecal matter by the anus. 2. the discharge of feces by an abnormal passage.

allochiral (al″o-ki′ral) [*allo-* + Gr. *cheir* hand] pertaining to allochiria.

allochiria (al″o-ki′re-ah) [allo- + Gr. cheir hand + -ia] a condition in which, if one extremity is stimulated, the sensation is referred to the opposite side (Obersteiner).

allochroic (al″o-kro′ik) changeable in color, a term generally applied to minerals.

allochroism (al″o-kro′izm) [allo- + Gr. chroa color + -ism] change or variation in color, as in certain minerals.

allochromacy (al″o-kro′mah-se) the formation of other coloring agents from a dye that is unstable in solution.

allochromasia (al″o-kro-ma′ze-ah) change in color of the hair or skin.

allocinesia (al″o-si-ne′ze-ah) [allo- + Gr. kinēsis motion + -ia] a condition in which the patient performs a movement on the side of the body opposite to that directed.

allocolloid (al″o-kol′oid) [allo- + colloid] a colloid in which a single element in its allotropic forms makes up the colloid system.

allocortex (al″o-kor′teks) [allo- + L. cortex bark, rind, shell] the older, original part of the cerebral cortex, comprising the archeocortex and the paleocortex. Cf. neocortex.

allocrine (al′o-krin) [allo- + Gr. krīnein to separate] heterocrine.

Allodermanyssus (al″o-der″mah-nis′sus) a genus of blood-sucking mites. **A. sanguin′eus,** a species that parasitizes mice and is a vector of Rickettsia akari, the causative agent of rickettsialpox.

allodesmism (al″o-des′mizm) [allo- + Gr. desmos bond] allomerism based on a difference in the bonds uniting the atoms.

allodynia (al″o-din′e-ah) [allo- + Gr. odynē pain] pain resulting from a non-noxious stimulus to normal skin.

alloeroticism (al″o-ĕ-rot′ĭ-sizm) sexual feeling directed to another person; cf. autoeroticism.

alloerotism (al″o-er′o-tizm) [allo- + erotism] alloeroticism.

alloesthesia (al″o-es-the′ze-ah) allesthesia.

allogamy (al-log′ah-me) [allo- + Gr. gamos marriage] cross fertilization.

allogeneic (al″o-jĕ-ne′ik) 1. having cell types that are antigenically distinct. 2. in transplantation biology, denoting individuals (or tissues) that are of the same species but antigenically distinct. Called also homologous. NOTE: In contrast, syngeneic (or isogeneic) refers to individuals having identical genotypes, and xenogeneic to individuals of different species, which by definition have different genotypes.

allogenic (al″o-jen′ik) allogeneic.

allogotrophia (al″o-go-tro′fe-ah) nourishment of one part of the body at the expense of another part.

allograft (al′o-graft) a graft of tissue between individuals of the same species but of disparate genotype; called also allogeneic graft and homograft.

Allogromiina (al″lo-gro-mi′ĭ-nah) [allo- + L. groma pole] a suborder of protozoa (order Foraminifera, class Granuloreticulosea) having a membranous or tectinous test with ferruginous or, rarely, small quantities of agglutinated material.

allogroup (al′o-grōōp) an allotype linkage group, especially of allotypes for the four IgG subclasses, which are closely linked and inherited as a unit.

alloimmune (al″o-im-mūn′) specifically immune to an allogeneic antigen.

alloisomerism (al″o-i-som′er-izm) isomerism which does not appear in the formula.

allokeratoplasty (al″o-ker′ah-to-plas″te) [allo- + keratoplasty] repair of the cornea by the use of foreign material.

allokinesis (al″o-ki-ne′sis) movement that is not performed voluntarily but is produced passively or occurs reflexly.

allokinetic (al″o-ki-net′ik) [allo- + Gr. kinēsis movement] pertaining to or characterized by allokinesis.

allolactose (al″o-lak′tōs) a disaccharide, isomeric with lactose, occurring in milk.

allolalia (al″o-la′le-ah) [allo- + Gr. lalein to speak + -ia] any defect of speech of central origin.

allomerism (ah-lom′er-izm) [allo- + Gr. meros part] change of chemical constitution without change in the crystalline form. Cf. allomorphism.

allometric (al′o-met′rik) [allo- + Gr. metron measure] denoting the disproportionate growth of organs or parts of an organism; pertaining to allometry.

allometron (al″o-met′ron) [allo- + Gr. metron measure] an evolutionary change in bodily form or proportion as expressed in measurements and indices.

allometry (al-lom′ĕ-tre) the measurement of changing shape of an organism with increase in size, i.e., the determination of the relationship of two varying dimensions, usually linear.

Allomonas (al″o-mo′nas) [allo- + Gr. monas unit, from monos single] a proposed genus of facultatively anaerobic, gram-negative, rod-shaped bacteria of uncertain affiliation, found in freshwater reservoirs, sewage, and fecal samples. The type species is A. ente′rica.

allomorphism (al″o-mor′fizm) [allo- + Gr. morphē form] change of crystalline form without change in chemical constitution. Cf. allomerism.

allonomous (al-lon′o-mus) [allo- + Gr. nomos law] regulated by stimuli from the outside.

allopath (al′o-path) a term sometimes applied to a practitioner of allopathy.

allopathic (al″o-path′ik) pertaining to or characteristic of allopathy.

allopathist (al-lop′ah-thist) allopath.

allopathy (al-lop′ah-the) [allo- + Gr. pathos disease] a term applied to that system of therapeutics in which diseases are treated by producing a condition incompatible with or antagonistic to the condition to be cured or alleviated. Called also heteropathy. Cf. homeopathy.

allophanamide (al-o-fan-am′id) biuret.

allophanate (alo-fan′āt) a salt of allophanic acid.

allophanic acid (al″o-fan′ik) urea carbonic acid (N-carboxyurea, H₂NCONHCOOH), which does not occur as the free acid but only in salts or compounds; its amide (allophanamide) is biuret.

allophasis (al-lof′ah-sis) [allo- + Gr. phasis speech] incoherent speech; delirium.

allophenic (al″o-fe′nik) [allo- + Gr. phainein to show] of or relating to single individuals originating from more than one conceptus; having orderly coexistence of cells with different phenotypes ascribable to known allelic genotypic differences; mosaic.

allophore (al′o-fōr) erythrophore.

allophthalmia (al″of-thal′me-ah) heterophthalmia.

alloplasia (al″o-pla′ze-ah) [allo- + Gr. plasis formation + -ia] heteroplasia.

alloplasmatic (al″o-plaz-mat′ik) [allo- + Gr. plassein to form] formed by differentiation from the cytoplasm.

alloplast (al′o-plast) an inert foreign body used for implantation into tissue.

alloplastic (al″o-plas′tik) [allo- + Gr. plassein to form] pertaining to or characterized by alloplasty; pertaining to an alloplast.

alloplasty (al′o-plas-te) [allo- + -plasty] adaptation by alteration of the external environment (alloplastic change). Cf. autoplasty.

allopregnane (al″o-preg′nān) see pregnane.

allopregnanediol (al″o-preg″nān-di′ol) an isomer of pregnanediol occurring in female urine.

allopsychic (al″o-si′kik) [allo- + Gr. psychē soul] pertaining to the mind in its relation to the external world.

allopurinol (al″o-pūr′ĭ-nōl) [USP] an isomer of hypoxanthine; used in the treatment of hyperuricemia of gout and that secondary to blood dyscrasias or cancer chemotherapy. Both allopurinol and its primary metabolite, oxypurinol, are potent inhibitors of xanthine oxidase and reduce serum levels and urinary excretion of uric acid.

allorhythmia (al″o-rith′me-ah) [allo- + Gr. rhythmos rhythm + -ia] irregularity in the rhythm of the heart beat or pulse that recurs in a regular fashion.

allorhythmic (al″o-rith′mik) affected with or of the nature of allorhythmia.

all or none the fact, discovered by Bowditch (1871), that the heart muscle, under whatever stimulus, will contract to the fullest extent or not at all. In the heart, stimulation of any single atrial or ventricular muscle fiber causes the action potential to travel over the entire atrial or ventricular mass, or not to travel at all. In other muscles and in nerves, this principle is limited to individual fibers; i.e., stimulation of a fiber causes an action potential to travel over the entire fiber, or not to travel at all. Called also *all-or-none law*.

allorphine (al′lor-fēn) nalorphine.

allose (al′ōs) a sugar, $C_6H_{12}O_6$, isomeric with glucose.

allosensitization (al″o-sen″sĭ-ti-za′shun) sensitization to alloantigens (isoantigens), as to Rh antigens during pregnancy (see *Rh isoimmunization*). Called also *isosensitization*.

allosome (al′o-sōm) [*allo-* + Gr. *sōma* body] 1. (*obs.*) a sex chromosome; see under *chromosome*. 2. a foreign constituent of the cytoplasm of a cell which has entered from the outside. **paired a.,** a diplosome.

allosteric (al″o-ster′ik) pertaining to allosterism.

allosterism (al′o-ster″ism) the condition in which the binding of a compound to a subunit of an enzyme or other protein molecule (e.g., hemoglobin) at a site (allosteric site) other than the functional binding site changes the conformation of the protein.

allostery (al″o-ste′re) allosterism.

allotherm (al′o-therm″) [*allo-* + Gr. *thermē* heat] 1. poikilotherm. 2. heterotherm.

allotope (al′o-tōp) a site on the constant or nonvarying portion of an antibody molecule that can be recognized by a combining site of other antibodies. Cf. *idiotope*.

allotopia (al″o-to′pe-ah) dystopia.

allotopic (al″o-top′ik) dystopic.

allotoxin (al″o-tok′sin) [*allo-* + *toxin*] any substance formed by tissue change within the body which serves as a defense against toxins by neutralizing their poisonous properties.

allotransplantation (al″o-trans″plan-ta′shun) [*allo-* + *transplantation*] transplantation of tissue from one individual into the body of another member of the same species but of a different genotype from the donor.

allotri(o)- [Gr. *allotrios* strange] a combining form meaning strange or foreign.

allotriodontia (ah-lot″re-o-don′she-ah) [*allotrio-* + Gr. *odous* tooth + *-ia*] 1. the transplantation of teeth from one individual into the mouth of another. 2. the existence of teeth in abnormal places, as in dermoid tumors.

allotriogeustia (ah-lot″re-o-gu′ste-ah) [*allotrio-* + Gr. *geusis* taste + *-ia*] a perverted condition of the sense of taste.

allotriolith (al″o-tri′o-lith) [*allotrio-* + Gr. *lithos* stone] a calculus in an abnormal situation, or one composed of unusual materials.

allotriophagy (ah-lot″re-of′ah-je) [*allotrio-* + Gr. *phagein* to eat] (*obs.*) pica.

allotriosmia (al″o-tri-os′me-ah) heterosmia.

allotriuria (ah-lot″re-u′re-ah) [*allotrio-* + Gr. *ouron* urine + *-ia*] a strange or perverted condition of the urine.

allotrope (al′o-trōp) an allotropic form.

allotrophic (al″o-trof′ik) rendered non-nutritious by the process of digestion.

allotropic (al″o-trop′ik) 1. exhibiting allotropism. 2. preoccupied with the ideas, actions, and feelings of others; said of a personality that is inclined to be preoccupied by others rather than oneself; not self-centered.

allotropism (ah-lot′ro-pizm) [*allo-* + Gr. *tropos* a turning] 1. the existence of a substance in two or more distinct forms (allotropic forms) with distinct physical properties, e.g., graphite and diamond, allotropic forms of carbon. 2. a tropism between different structures, e.g., between spermatozoa and ova (Roux).

allotropy (ah-lot′ro-pe) allotropism.

allotrylic (al″o-tril′ik) [*allotrio-* + Gr. *hylē* matter] produced by the presence of a foreign body or principle.

allotype (al′o-tīp) any of several allelic variants of a protein that are characterized by antigenic differences (allotypic markers), especially allelic variants of immunoglobulin heavy and light chains. Cf. *isotype* and *idiotype*. **Am a′s,** [for alpha chain marker] allotypes of human α2 chains (IgA2 heavy chains); two markers designated A2m(1) and A2m(2) have been identified. **Gm a′s,** [for gamma chain marker] allotypes of human γ chains (IgG heavy chains); 25 markers designated Gm(1) through Gm(25) have been identified. Each

marker occurs only in certain specific IgG subclasses. A specific allotype (allelic γ chain) may have more than one marker. **Inv a′s,** Km a′s. **Km a′s,** [for kappa chain marker] allotypes of human κ light chains; three markers designated Km(1), Km(2), and Km(3) have been identified. Km(2) always occurs with Km(1), thus the possible serotypes are Km(1), Km(1,2) and Km(3). Called also Inv *a′s*, Inv(1)–(3). **Oz a.,** an allotypic antigenic marker on the lambda chain of human immunoglobulins, equivalent to the Km allotypes on kappa light chains.

allotypic (al″o-tip′ik) characterized by allotypes.

allotypy (al″o-ti′pe) [*allo-* + Gr. *typos* type] the genetically controlled property, in proteins, of existing in antigenically distinguishable forms in different members of the same species, i.e., as serum protein isoantigens (not yet distinguishable by chemical or physiochemical means); the condition of being an allotype.

alloxan (al′ok-san) a reddish, crystalline substance, mesoxalyl urea, $CO \cdot NH \cdot CO:NH \cdot CO$, an oxidized product of uric

$$\underbrace{\qquad\qquad}_{CO}$$

acid. It tends to destroy the islet cells of the pancreas, thus producing diabetes. It has been obtained from the mucus of the intestine in diarrhea and has been used in nutrition experiments and as an antineoplastic agent.

alloxantin (al″ok-san′tin) a crystalline derivative of alloxan and dialuric acid, $[CO(NH \cdot CO)_2C(OH)—]_2$, obtained by reduction.

alloxazine (ah-lok′sah-zēn) a heterocyclic compound, $C_{10}H_6N_4O_2$, an isomer of isoalloxazine, which is the basic structure of riboflavin.

alloxuremia (al″ok-su-re′me-ah) [*alloxur* + Gr. *haima* blood + *-ia*] the presence of purine bases in the blood, causing a form of intoxication.

alloxuria (al″ok-su′re-ah) [*alloxur* + Gr. *ouron* urine + *-ia*] the presence of purine bases in the urine.

alloxuric (al″ok-su′rik) pertaining to or characterized by alloxuria.

alloy (al′loi) [Fr. *aloyer* to mix metals] a mixture of two or more metals or metalloids that are mutually soluble in the molten condition; distinguished as binary, ternary, quaternary, etc., depending on the number of metals in the mixture. An alloy may also be classified on the basis of its behavior when solidified. **amalgam a.,** an alloy, composed chiefly of silver, tin, and copper, that is mixed with mercury to form dental amalgam; it is prepared by melting its components and casting it in an ingot that is afterward cut into small particles (filings), or it may be produced in the form of spheres.

alloyage (ah-loi′ij) the combining of metals into alloys.

allspice (awl′spīs) pimenta.

all-*trans* retinal see *retinal* (def. 2).

allyl (al′il) [L. *allium* garlic + Gr. *hylē* matter] a univalent organic group, $CH_2:CH \cdot CH_2$. **a. aldehyde,** acrolein. **a. isothiocyanate,** chemical name: 3-isothiocyanato-1-propene. Volatile oil of mustard, C_3H_5NCS, used as a counterirritant in ointments and plasters and in the preparation of flavors; it is also used in the manufacture of war gas. **a. sulfocarbamide, a. thiocarbamide, a. thiourea,** thiosinamine. **a. tribromide,** a colorless or yellowish liquid, $C_3H_5Br_3$, formerly used as an antispasmodic and anodyne.

allylamine (al″il-am′in) a caustic liquid with an ammoniacal odor, 3-aminopropylene, $CH_2:CH \cdot CH_2 \cdot NH_2$, used in the manufacture of mercurial diuretics.

allylguaiacol (al″lil-gwi′ah-kol) eugenol.

allysine (a-li′sēn) $CO \cdot CHNH_2 \cdot (CH_2)_3 \cdot CHO$, a product of the oxidative deamination of lysine, formed by the action of lysyl oxidase. It is an intermediate in the formation of cross-linkages in collagens.

almadrate sulfate (al′mah-drāt) aluminum magnesium hydroxide oxide sulfate hydrate; an antacid, $Al_4H_6Mg_2O_{14} \cdot S \cdot xH_2O$.

Almeida's disease (al-ma-ēd′ahz) [Floriano Paulo de *Almeida*, Brazilian physician born 1898] paracoccidioidomycosis.

almond (ah′mund) [Fr. *amande*, from L. *amygdala* almond] the fruit of *Prunus amygdalus* Batsch. (*P. communis* L.), almond tree, seeds of the sweet variety (var. *dulcis*) being edible. **bitter a.,** the fruit of *P. amygdalus* var. *amara,* whose seeds are inedible but which contains a volatile oil and amygdalin. On maceration and distillation, the seeds yield bitter almond oil, which contains about 80 per cent benzaldehyde and 2–4 per cent hydrocyanic acid. Used in low doses in various cough mixtures, in liqueurs, and in perfumery. **sweet a.,** the fruit of *P. amygdalus* var. *dulcis.*

almoner (al′mo-ner) a person who dispenses alms. **hospital a.,** *Brit.,* a person trained in dispensing the social service funds of a hospital, and in administering social service work.

Al₂O₃ aluminum oxide.

alochia (ah-lo′ke-ah) [L.; *a* neg. + Gr. *lochia* lochia] absence of the lochia.

Aloe (al′o) [L. *alöe;* Gr. *aloē̆*] a large genus of succulent South African plants of the Liliaceae family. The dried juice of several species (e.g., *A. barbadensis, A. ferox, A. perryi*) contains purgative principles. Aloe may also refer to the fragrant wood of *Aquilaria agallocha* (East Indian tree) of the family Thymelaeaceae.

aloe (al′o) [USP] the dried juice of the leaves of various species of liliaceous plants of the genus *Aloe,* which has purgative properties; it is now used only as an ingredient of *compound benzoin tincture.*

aloe-emodin (al′o-em′o-din) chemical name: 1,8-dihydroxy-3-(hydroxymethyl)-9,10-antracenedione. A compound having cathartic principles, occurring in the free state and as a glycoside in rhubarb, senna leaves, and in various species of *Aloe.*

aloetic (al″o-et′ik) [L. *aloeticus*] pertaining to or containing aloe.

alogia (ah-lo′je-ah) [*a* neg. + Gr. *logos* word + -*ia*] inability to speak, due to a central lesion.

Al(OH)₃ aluminum hydroxide.

aloin (al′o-in) chemical name: 10-glucopyranosyl-1,8-dihydroxy-3-(hydroxymethyl)-9(10*H*)-anthracenone. A mixture of active principles, chiefly barbaloin, $C_{21}H_{22}O_9$, extracted from aloes; used as a purgative to relieve temporary constipation and/or atonic chronic constipation.

alopecia (al″o-pe′she-ah) [Gr. *alōpekia* a disease in which the hair falls out] baldness; absence of the hair from skin areas where it is normally present. **androgenetic a.,** a. areata. **a. area′ta,** a microscopically inflammatory, usually reversible, patchy loss of hair, occurring in sharply defined areas and usually involving the beard or scalp. Called also *androgenetic a., a. circumscripta,* and *pelade.* See also *ophiasis.* **cicatricial a., a. cicatrisa′ta,** an irreversible loss of hair associated with scarring, usually occurring on the scalp. See also *pseudopalade.* **a. circumscrip′ta,** a. areata. **congenital a., a. congenita′lis,** congenital absence of the scalp hair, which may occur alone or be part of a more widespread disorder. **drug a., drug-induced a.,** transient hair loss caused by administration of certain drugs, such as heparin, antimitotics (e.g., cyclophosphamide, methotrexate, and colchicine), and thallium (formerly used in the treatment of tinea capitis). **male pattern a.,** a progressive, diffuse, symmetrical loss of scalp hair, beginning with characteristic frontal recession and leaving ultimately only a sparse peripheral rim of scalp hair; the condition usually starts in the late twenties or early thirties and is androgen dependent, said to be caused by an autosomal dominant gene of variable expressivity. Called also *common male baldness* and *hereditary a.* **moth-eaten a.,** a syphilitic alopecia involving the scalp and beard and occurring in small, irregular scattered patches, resulting in a moth-eaten appearance. **a. mucino′sa,** follicular mucinosis. **postpartum a.,** telogen effluvium occurring shortly after parturition. **premature a.,** male pattern baldness occurring in young men in their early twenties or before. **pressure a.,** traumatic alopecia due to persistent pressure on the scalp, as may be seen in babies lying on their backs and in adults after prolonged surgical procedures or in ill persons after prolonged bed rest. **psychogenic a.,** telogen effluvium due to severe and acute emotional stress, which is believed to be of the alopecia areata type. Called also *stress a.* **radiation a., radiation-induced a.,** transient hair loss following exposure to ionizing radiation. **a. seborrhe′ica,** alopecia associated with excessive oiliness of the scalp, dandruff, and other signs of seborrheic dermatitis. **stress a.,** psychogenic a. **syphilitic a., a. syphilit′ica,** alopecia involving the eyebrows, beard, and scalp in secondary syphilis.

See also *moth-eaten a.* **a. tota′lis,** complete loss of hair from the entire scalp, resulting from progression of alopecia areata. **traction a.,** traumatic alopecia due to continuous or prolonged traction on the hair, as applied in certain styles of hair dressing or in the habit of twisting the hair. **traumatic a.,** telogen effluvium due to injury to the hair follicle, as by rubbing, traction, or chemical agent, and limited to the areas thus traumatized. **traumatic marginal a.,** traction alopecia occurring along the scalp margin. **a. universa′lis,** loss of hair over the entire body, resulting from progression of alopecia areata. **x-ray a.,** loss of hair after exposure to roentgen radiation, the extent and permanence of which are dependent on the field and dosage; called also *roentgen a.*

alopecic (al″o-pe′sik) pertaining to or characterized by alopecia.

aloxanthin (al″ok-san′thin) a yellow principle, $C_{15}H_{10}O_6$, derivable from aloes by the action of potassium dichromate.

aloxiprin (al-ok′sĭ-prin) chemical name: 2-(acetyloxy)benzoic acid polymer with aluminum hydroxide. A polymeric condensation product of aluminum hydroxide and aspirin, $Al_3O_2[C_6H_4(OOCCH_3)COO]_5$, used as an analgesic.

alpha (al′fah) [A, α] the first letter of the Greek alphabet.

alpha-amylose (al″fah-am′ĭ-lōs) the linear component of starch, usually amylose.

alpha₁-antitrypsin (al″fa-an″te-trip′sin) a plasma protein (an α_1-globulin, molecular weight 45000) produced in the liver, which inhibits the activity of trypsin and other proteolytic enzymes. Deficiency of this protein is associated with development of emphysema. Also written α_1-antitrypsin.

Alpha Chymar (al′fah ki′mar) trademark for a preparation of chymotrypsin.

alpha-dinitrophenol (al″fah-di-ni″tro-fe′nol) see under *dinitrophenol.*

alphadione (al″fah-di′ōn) a steroid anesthetic, a combination of two steroids (3α-hydroxy-5α-pregnane-11,20-dione and 21-acetoxy-3α-hydroxy-5α-pregnane-11,20-dione) which are structurally similar to progesterone. It has a wide margin of safety between anesthetic dose and lethal dose.

Alphadrol (al′fah-drol) trademark for a preparation of fluprednisolone.

alpha-estradiol (al″fah-es″trah-di′ol) see *estradiol.*

alpha-fetoprotein (al″fah-fe″to-pro′te-in) a plasma protein, mol. wt. 70,000, with alpha₁ electrophoretic mobility, produced by the fetal liver, yolk sac, and gastrointestinal tract; serum levels decline markedly by the age of one year but are again elevated in most hepatocellular carcinomas and teratocarcinomas and embryonal cell carcinomas of the testes, ovary, and extragonadal sites; elevated levels may also be seen in benign liver disease, such as cirrhosis and viral hepatitis. The two principal uses are in monitoring the response of hepatomas and germ cell neoplasms to treatment and in antenatal diagnosis of neural tube defects (indicated by elevated amniotic fluid alpha-fetoprotein levels). Abbreviated AFP.

alpha globulin see under *globulin.*

alpha-lipoprotein (lip″o-pro′te-in) high-density lipoprotein.

alpha-lobeline (al″fah-lob′e-lin) see *lobeline.*

alphalytic (al″fah-lit′ik) blocking the α-adrenergic receptors of the sympathetic nervous system; also, an agent that so acts.

alpha₂-macroglobulin (mak″ro-glob′u-lin) a 725,000-dalton tetrameric plasma protein that inhibits a wide variety of proteolytic enzymes including trypsin, plasmin, thrombin, kallikrein, and alpha-chymotrypsin. It is the second most important plasma protease inhibitor after alpha₁-antitrypsin. Also written α_2-macroglobulin.

alphamimetic (al″fah-mi-met′ik) stimulating or mimicking the stimulation of the α-adrenergic receptors of the sympathetic nervous system; also, an agent that so acts.

alphanaphthol (al″fah-naf′thol) a form of naphthol occurring as a white or pinkish crystalline compound, soluble in alcohol, ether, and hot water and slightly soluble in cold water; used in the manufacture of dyes, intermediates, and perfumes, and in microscopy.

alphaprodine hydrochloride (al″fah-pro′dēn) [USP] chemical name: *cis*-(+)-13-dimethyl-4-phenyl-4-piperidinol propanoate (ester) hydrochloride. A white, crystalline powder, $C_{16}H_{23}NO_2 \cdot HCl$, used intravenously or subcutaneously as a narcotic analgesic in conditions requiring rapid and brief analgesia.

alpha-tocopherol (al″fah-to-kof′er-ol) see under *tocopherol.*

alpha-tropeine (al″fah-tro′pe-in) a substance derivable from scopolamine and hyoscine.

alphitomorphous (al″fit-o-mor′fus) [Gr. *alphiton* barleymeal + *morphē* form] having a mealy appearance; said of certain fungous parasites of plants.

alprazolam (al-pra′zo-lam) a benzodiazepine with the same general properties as diazepam, used as a tranquilizer.

alprenolol hydrochloride (al-pren′o-lol) chemical name: 1-[(1-methylethyl)amino]-3-[2-(2-propenyl)phenyl]-2-propanol hydrochloride; a beta-adrenergic blocking agent, $C_{15}H_{23}NO_2HCl$, having the same actions as propranolol (q.v.).

alprostadil (al-pros′tah-dil) a prostaglandin of the E series used for the temporary maintenance of the ductus arteriosus in the treatment of congenital heart disease. Called also *prostaglandin* E_1.

alrestatin sodium (al′rĕ-stat″in) an enzyme inhibitor (aldose reductase).

ALS antilymphocyte serum.

alseroxylon (al″ser-ok′sĭ-lon) a purified extract of *Rauwolfia serpentina,* containing reserpine and other amorphous alkaloids, occurring as a reddish brown amorphous powder; used orally as an antihypertensive and sedative.

alstonine (awl′stŏ-nēn) an alkaloid obtained from several apocynaceous plants, e.g., *Alstonia constricta* F. Muell., *Rauwolfia* species, *Catharanthus roseus* G. Don, etc. The bark of several species of *Alstonia* has been used for its tonic, astringent, antiperiodic, and antipyretic properties.

Alström's syndrome (al′strumz) [Carl Henry *Alström,* Swedish geneticist] see under *syndrome.*

Alt. dieb. abbreviation for L. *alter′nis die′bus,* every other day.

alter (awl′ter) to castrate, as housepets or livestock.

alterant (awl′ter-ant) alterative.

alterative (awl′ter-a″tiv) [L. *alterare* to change] an obsolete term originally used for drugs said to re-establish healthy functions of the system.

alteregoism (awl″ter-e′go-izm) interest and sympathy only for persons who are in the same situation as one's self.

alternans (awl-ter′nanz) [L.] alternating or alternation, as in pulsus alternans (alternating strength of the pulse). **electrical a.,** alternating variations in the amplitude of electrocardiographic waves. **a. of the heart,** alternating strength in the heart beat or pulse. **pulsus a.,** the presence of alteration of intensity of heat sounds, indicating left ventricular failure.

Alternaria (awl″ter-na′re-ah) a genus of dematiacious Fungi Imperfecti of the order Moniliales, having dark-colored conidia somewhat resembling *Trichophyton;* it causes several diseases of plants and has been reported in diseases of the lungs and in skin infection in man, and is also a common allergen in human bronchial asthma.

alternariatoxicosis (awl″ter-nar″ĭ-ah-tok-sĭ-ko′sis) a form of mycotoxicosis caused by members of the genus *Alternaria.*

alternating (awl″ter-nāt″ing) occurring in regular succession; alternately direct and reversed.

alternation (awl″ter-na′shun) [L. *alternatio*] interrupted occurrence, being interspersed with different or opposite events. **cardiac a.,** a condition in which, during sphygmoscopy, every other beat is weak at 2 to 10 mm. Hg below the systolic level.

Alteromonas (awl″ter-o-mo′nas) [L. *alter* other + Gr. *monas* unit, from *monos* single] a genus of gram-negative, aerobic, straight or curved, rod-shaped bacteria of uncertain affiliation, motile with a single flagellum, found in coastal and open sea waters. The type species is *A. macleo′dii.* **A. putrefa′ciens,** *Pseudomonas putrefaciens.*

Althaea (al-the′ah) [L.] a genus of malvaceous plants; the root and leaves of *A. officinalis* (marshmallow) contain sugar, pectin, and mucilage and are used as a demulcent and poultice.

althea (al-the′ah) the dried root of *Althaea officinalis,* or

marshmallow root; a decoction was once used as a demulcent, and the boiled root as a poultice.

althiazide (al-thi′ah-zīd) a thiazide diuretic used to treat hypertension.

Alt. hor. abbreviation for L. *alter′nis ho′ris,* every other hour.

Altmann's fluid, granule, theory (ahlt′manz) [Richard *Altmann,* German histologist, 1852–1900] see under *fluid* and *theory,* and see *mitochondrion.*

Altmann-Gersh method (ahlt′man gersh) [Richard *Altmann;* Isidore *Gersh,* American anatomist, born 1907] see under *method.*

altofrequent (al″to-fre′quent) [L. *altus* high + *frequent*] marked by high frequency; see *high-frequency current,* under *current.*

altricious (al-trish′us) requiring a long period of nursing care.

altrose (al′trōs) a sugar, $C_6H_{12}O_6$, isomeric with glucose.

Alu-Cap (al′u-kap) trademark for a preparation of dried aluminum hydroxide gel.

Aludrine (ah-lu′drin) trademark for a preparation of isoproterenol.

Aludrox (al-u′droks) trademark for a preparation of alumina and magnesia.

alum (al′um) [L. *alumen*] 1. [USP] an odorless, colorless, crystalline substance, with local astringent and styptic properties and sweetish taste, and soluble in water, but insoluble in alcohol; it is either potassium alum, $AlK(SO_4)_2 + 12H_2O$, or ammonium alum, $AlNH_4(SO_4)_2 + 12H_2O$. Used as a topical application. 2. a generic term for any member of a class of double sulfates formed on the type of the foregoing compounds. 3. any member of a class of double aluminum-containing compounds. **ammonium a.,** see *alum,* def. 1. **burnt a.,** exsiccated a. **chrome a.,** chromium and potassium sulfate; a violet pigment. **concentrated a.,** aluminum sulfate, incorrectly called an alum. **dried a.,** exsiccated a. **exsiccated a.,** a white odorless powder, with a sweetish, astringent taste, either exsiccated ammonium alum, $AlNH_4(SO_4)_2$, or exsiccated potassium alum, $AlK(SO_4)_2$, and containing at least 96.5 per cent of the labeled product. Called also *burnt* or *dried a.,* and *alumen exsiccatum.* **iron a.,** iron and potassium sulfate. **potassium a.,** see *alum,* def. 1.

alumen (ah-loo′men), gen. *alu′minis* [L.] alum. **a. exsicca′tum,** exsiccated alum.

alumina (ah-loo′mi-nah) aluminum oxide. **a. and magnesia** [USP], a preparation containing 90 to 110 per cent of the labeled amounts of aluminum hydroxide and magnesium hydroxide; used as an antacid in tablet form.

aluminated (ah-loo′mi-nāt″ed) charged with alum.

aluminium (al″u-min′e-um) [L.] aluminum.

Aluminoid (ah-loo′mĭ-noid) trademark for preparations of aluminum hydroxide gel for use in gastric ulcers and hyperacidity.

aluminosis (ah-loo″mĭ-no′sis) a form of pneumoconiosis due to the presence of aluminum-bearing dust in the lungs; called also *a. pulmonum.*

aluminum (ah-loo′mĭ-num) an extremely light, whitish, lustrous, metallic element, obtainable from bauxite or clay: specific gravity, 2.699; atomic weight, 26.982; atomic number, 13; symbol, Al. It is very malleable and ductile, and is used for the manufacture of instruments in dentistry for the fabrication of dentures, obturators, and other prosthetic devices, and as a base for artificial dentures. The aluminum of the pharmacopeia is a fine, free-flowing, silvery powder, free from gritty or discolored particles. Aluminum compounds are used chiefly for their antacid and astringent properties. **a. acetate,** a compound, $C_6H_9AlO_6$, used in solution as an astringent and antiseptic; called also *eston.* **a. aminoacetate,** dihydroxyaluminum aminoacetate. **a. ammonium sulfate,** ammonium alum. **a. carbonate, basic,** an aluminum hydroxide–aluminum carbonate complex, available only in the form of *basic aluminum carbonate gel* (see under *gel*). **a. chlorhydrex,** a topical astringent, reportedly consisting of a coordination complex of basic aluminum chloride and propylene glycol or polyethylene glycol in which the water molecules normally coordinated to the aluminum in aluminum chlorohydrate have been displaced by the glycol, resulting in a relatively less polar complex of low water content. **a. chloride** [USP], a white or yellowish white, deliquescent powder, $AlCl_3 \cdot 6H_2O$, used as a local astringent in a 10 to 25 per cent solution applied topically to the skin. It is also used as a topical antiseptic and in many deodorant preparations to diminish sweating. **a. glycinate,** dihydroxyaluminum aminoacetate. **a. hydrate,** a. hydroxide. **a. hydroxide** [USP], a white, bulky, amorphous powder, $Al(OH)_3$, used as a gastric antacid in the form of *aluminum hydroxide gel* or *dried aluminum hydroxide gel* (see under *gel*). **a. hydroxide, colloidal,** aluminum hydroxide gel. **a. monostearate** [NF], a combination of aluminum with variable proportions of stearic acid and palmitic acid; used in preparation of a suspension of procaine penicillin G. **a. nicotinate,** chemical name: 3-pyridinecarboxylic acid aluminum salt. A complex consisting of aluminum nicotinate, aluminum hydroxide, and nicotinic acid; used chiefly as an anticholesterolemic, antilipoproteinemic, and peripheral vasodilator, administered orally. **a. oxide,** a compound, Al_2O_3, occurring naturally as corundum and in hydrated form as bauxite, that is the raw material in aluminum production; impure crystalline forms include emery, ruby, and sapphire. Very fine grains are used in the production of abrasives, refractories, ceramics, catalysts, laboratory wares, and fluxes, and in chromatography. **a. penicillin,** see under *penicillin*. **a. phosphate,** a white infusible powder, $AlPO_4$, used with calcium sulfate and sodium silicate in dental cements, and as a gastric antacid in the form of aluminum phosphate gel (see under *gel*). **a. potassium sulfate,** potassium alum. **a. subacetate** [USP], a yellow liquid prepared by the interaction of aluminum sulfate, acetic acid, and precipitated calcium carbonate, and used as an astringent wash when diluted with 20 to 40 volumes of water. **a. sulfate** [USP], an odorless white, crystalline powder, with a sweet taste, $Al_2(SO_4)_3 + 18H_2O$, that is astringent and antiperspirant. Incorrectly called *concentrated alum*.

alundum (ah-lun'dum) electrically fused alumina, used in making laboratory appliances which are to be subjected to intense heat.

Alupent (al'u-pent) trademark for preparations of metaproterenol sulfate.

Alurate (al'ūr-āt) trademark for a preparation of aprobarbital.

Alv. adst. abbreviation for L. *al'vo adstric'ta,* when the bowels are constipated.

Alv. deject. abbreviation for L. *al'vi dejectio'nes,* alvine dejections.

alvei (al've-i) [L.] genitive and plural of *alveus*.

alveobronchiolitis (al″ve-o-brong″ke-o-li'tis) inflammation of the bronchioles and alveoli of the lungs.

alveolalgia (al″ve-o-lal'je-ah) [*alveolus* + *-algia*] pain occurring in the dental alveolus, sometimes observed after tooth extraction. See also *dry socket,* under *socket*.

alveolar (al-ve'o-lar) [L. *alveolaris*] pertaining to an alveolus.

alveolate (al-ve'o-lāt) marked by honeycomb-like pits; called also *faveolate*.

alveolectomy (al″ve-o-lek'to-me) [*alveolus* + Gr. *ektomē* excision] subtotal or complete excision of the alveolar process of the maxilla or mandible.

alveoli (al-ve'o-li) plural of *alveolus*.

alveolitis (al″ve-o-li'tis) inflammation of an alveolus. Called also *odontobothritis*. **allergic a., extrinsic allergic a.,** hypersensitivity pneumonitis; a respiratory hypersensitivity reaction to repeated inspiration of organic particles, most often in an occupational setting, with onset about 4 to 8 hours after exposure to the allergen. There is fever, fatigue, chills, unproductive cough, tachycardia, and tachypnea. In the chronic form there is interstitial fibrosis with collagenous thickening of the alveolar septa. The disorder includes farmer's lung, bagassosis, pigeon breeder's lung, etc. **fibrosing a.,** idiopathic pulmonary fibrosis. **a. sic'ca doloro'sa,** dry socket.

alveol(o)- [L. *alveolus, q.v.*] a combining form denoting relationship to an alveolus, especially a dental alveolus.

alveolocapillary (al-ve″o-lo-kap'ĭ-lār″e) pertaining to the pulmonary alveoli and capillaries.

alveoloclasia (al-ve″o-lo-kla'ze-ah) [*alveolo-* + Gr. *klasis* breaking] destruction of the dental alveolus; see *marginal periodontitis,* under *periodontitis*.

alveolodental (al-ve″o-lo-den'tal) pertaining to a tooth and its alveolus.

alveololabial (al-ve″o-lo-la'be-al) pertaining to the alveolar processes and the lips.

alveololabialis (al-ve″o-lo-la″be-a'lis) musculus buccinator.

alveololingual (al-ve″o-lo-ling'gwal) pertaining to the alveolar processes and the tongue.

alveolomerotomy (al-ve″o-lo″mě-rot'o-me) [*alveolo-* + *mero-¹* + *tomy*] excision of part of the alveolar process.

alveolonasal (al-ve″o-lo-na'sal) pertaining to the alveolar point and the nasion.

alveolopalatal (al-ve″o-lo-pal'ah-tal) pertaining to the alveolar process and palate.

alveoloplasty (al-ve'o-lo-plas″te) [*alveolo-* + *-plasty*] conservative contouring of the alveolar process, in preparation for immediate or future denture construction. **interradicular a., intraseptal a.,** the surgical removal of the interradicular bone and collapsing of the cortical plates on each other to achieve an acceptable or more desirable contour.

alveolotomy (al″ve-o-lot'o-me) [*alveolo-* + *-tomy*] incision into a dental alveolus; see also *alveolectomy*.

alveolus (al-ve'o-lus), gen. and pl. *alve'oli* [L., dim. of *alveus* hollow] a general term used in anatomical nomenclature to designate a small saclike dilatation; see also *acinus*. **dental a.,** one of the cavities or sockets in the alveolar process of the mandible or maxilla, in which the roots of the teeth are held by fibers of the periodontal ligament. Called also *alveolar cavities* and *tooth sockets*. See also *alveoli dentales mandibulae* and *alveoli dentales maxillae*. **alve'oli denta'les mandib'ulae** [NA], dental alveoli of the mandible: the cavities or sockets in the alveolar process of the mandible in which the roots of the teeth are held by the periodontal ligament. **alve'oli denta'les maxil'lae** [NA], dental alveoli of the maxilla: the cavities or sockets in the alveolar process of the maxilla in which the roots of the teeth are held by the periodontal ligament. **alve'oli pulmo'nis** [NA], small polyhedral outpouchings along the walls of the alveolar sacs and alveolar ducts through the walls of which gas exchange takes place between alveolar gas and pulmonary capillary blood; called also *pulmonary alveoli, a. pulmonum, Malpighi's vesicles, vesiculae pulmonales,* and *pulmonary vesicles*. **alveoli pulmo'num,** alveoli pulmonis.

alverine citrate (al'vě-rēn) an anticholinergic used as a smooth muscle relaxant in disorders of the gastro-intestinal and genito-urinary tracts.

alveus (al've-us), gen. and pl. *al'vei* [L.] a trough or a canal. **a. commu'nis,** utriculus, def. 2. **a. hippocam'pi** [NA], **a. of hippocampus,** the thin layer of white matter that covers the ventricular surface of the hippocampus.

Alvodine (al'vo-din) trademark for preparations of piminodine esylate.

alymphia (ah-lim'fe-ah) [*a* neg. + L. *lympha* lymph] deficiency or absence of the lymph.

alymphocytosis (ah-lim″fo-si-to'sis) complete or nearly complete absence of lymphocytes from the blood; lymphopenia.

alymphoplasia (ah″lim-fo-pla'ze-ah) failure of development of lymphoid tissue. **thymic a.,** severe combined immunodeficiency.

alymphopotent (ah-lim″fo-po'tent) [*a* neg. + *lymphoid* + L. *potens* able] incapable of producing lymphocytes or lymphoid cells.

Alysiella (ah-le″se-el'ah) [Gr. *alysion* small chain] a genus of gliding bacteria of the family Simonsiellaceae, order Cytophagales, found in the oral cavities of animals, made up of cells forming flat filaments with blunt ends. The genus contains the species *A. filifor'mis*.

Alzheimer's disease (dementia), etc. (altz'hi-merz) [Alois *Alzheimer,* German neurologist, 1864–1915] see *presenile dementia,* under *dementia,* and see under *cell, disease,* and *stain*.

A.M. abbreviation for L. *artium magister,* Master of Arts.

Am 1. chemical symbol for *americium*. 2. see under *allotype*.

am symbol for *myopic astigmatism, meterangle,* and *ametropia.*

A.M.A. Aerospace Medical Association; American Medical Association; Australian Medical Association.

ama (a′mah), pl. *a′mae* [L.] an enlargement of a semicircular canal of the internal ear at the end opposite the ampulla.

amacratic (am″ah-krat′ik) amasthenic.

amacrinal (am″ah-kri′nal) of the nature of amacrines.

amacrine (am′ah-krin) [*a* neg. + Gr. *makros* long + *is, inos* fiber] 1. having no long processes. 2. amacrine cell; see under *cell.*

amadinone acetate (ah-mad′ĭ-nōn) chemical name: 17-(acetyloxy)-6-chloronorpregna-4,6-diene-3,20-dione acetate; a progestin, $C_{22}H_{27}ClO_4$.

amakrine (am′ah-krin) amacrine.

AMAL Aero-Medical Acceleration Laboratory.

amalgam (ah-mal′gam) [Gr. *malagma* poultice or soft mass] an alloy in which mercury is one of the components; dental amalgam is a soft silvery paste when freshly prepared, which hardens into a solid mass. **dental a.,** an amalgam containing mercury, silver, tin, copper, and possibly zinc, which is prepared by mixing mercury with amalgam alloy to form a silvery, soft paste for condensation into the prepared cavity where it hardens to form a dental restoration. **retrograde a.,** see under *filling.*

amalgamable (ah-mal′gah-mah-b'l) capable of forming an amalgam with mercury.

amalgamate (ah-mal′gah-māt″) to unite a metal in an alloy with mercury; to form an amalgam.

amalgamation (ah-mal″gah-ma′shun) 1. the formation of an amalgam. 2. trituration.

amalgamator (ah-mal′gah-ma″tor) triturator.

amandin (am′an-din) a globulin from the almond nut.

Amanita (am″ah-ni′tah) [Gr. *amanitai* a sort of fungus] a genus of mushrooms of the family Agaricaceae, several species of which are poisonous. *A. phalloi′des* (destroying angel, death cup) contains a hemolysin and a mixture of peptide toxins (e.g., phalloidin) which are protoplasmic poisons. These cause irreversible damage in cardiac musculature, liver, and kidney cells after 24 hours. Mortality ranges from 50 to 90 per cent. *A. musca′ria* (fly agaric) contains muscarine and ibotenic acid. The latter is psychotropic. Ingestion of this species causes intoxication (drunkenness) and ultimate loss of consciousness. Other species are also toxic; some are edible.

amanitine (ah-mă-ni′tin) a poisonous alkaloid from fly agaric; also a poisonous glycoside from the various mushrooms, especially from *Amanita phalloides.*

amanitotoxin (ah-man″ĭ-to-tok′sin) *Amanita* toxin.

amantadine hydrochloride (ah-man′tah-dēn) [USP] chemical name: tricyclo[3.3.1.1³·⁷]decan-1-amine hydrochloride. An antiviral compound, $C_{10}H_{17}N \cdot HCl$, occurring as a white or nearly white crystalline powder; used in the prophylaxis and management of type A influenza and, because it augments the release of dopamine, as an antidyskinetic in the treatment of parkinsonism.

amara (ah-ma′rah) [L., pl.] (*obs.*) bitters, def. 2.

Amaranthus (am″ah-ran′thus) [L., from Gr. *amarantos* unfading] a genus of herbs of the family Amarantaceae, several species of which have various medical and food uses. Some species of the western United States are a problem in causing hay fevers. A source of the dye called amaranth, now prepared synthetically.

amaranth (am′ah-ranth) a dark, red-brown powder, $C_{10}H_6(SO_2 \cdot ONa) \cdot N:N \cdot C_{10}H_4(SO_2 \cdot ONa) \cdot OH$, once used as a coloring agent in food, cosmetics, and drugs.

amarine (am′ah-rin) [L. *amarus* bitter] a poisonous crystalline base, $C_6H_5 \cdot CH \cdot NH \cdot C:(C_6H_5)N \cdot CH \cdot C_6H_5$, triphenyl dihydroglyoxaline, from oil of bitter almonds, and also prepared artificially.

amaroid (am′ah-roid) a bitter principle.

amaroidal (am-ah-roi′dal) somewhat bitter; also resembling a bitter in properties.

amarthritis (am″ar-thri′tis) [Gr. *hama* together + *arthron* joint + *-itis*] inflammation of several joints at the same time; polyarthritis.

amasesis (am″ah-se′sis) [*a* neg. + Gr. *masēsis* chewing] inability to chew food.

amasthenic (am″as-then′ik) [Gr. *hama* together + *sthenos* strength] bringing the rays of light into one focus; said of a lens.

amastia (am-mas′te-ah) [*a* neg. + Gr. *mastos* breast] congenital absence of the mammae; sometimes applied to masculine breast characteristics in an adult female. Called also *amazia.*

amastigote (ah-mas′tĭ-gōt) [*a* neg. + Gr. *mastix* whip] any of the bodies representing the morphologic (leishmanial) stage in the life cycle of all trypanosomatid protozoa resembling the typical adult form of members of the genus *Leishmania,* in which the oval or round cell has a nucleus, kinetoplast, and basal body but lacks a free-flowing flagellum, the flagellum being either very short or entirely absent. Called also *Leishman-Donovan body.* Cf. *choanomastigote, epimastigote, opisthomastigote, promastigote,* and *trypomastigote.*

amathophobia (ah-math″o-fo′be-ah) [Gr. *amathos* sand + *phobia*] irrational dread of dust.

amatol (am′ah-tol) a war explosive, being a mixture of trinitrotoluene and ammonium nitrate; moderately toxic by ingestion, inhalation, and absorption through the skin; highly irritating.

amaurosis (am″aw-ro′sis) [L. from Gr. *amaurōsis* darkening] blindness (Hippocrates), especially blindness occurring without apparent lesion of the eye, as from disease of the optic nerve, spine, or brain. Cf. *amblyopia.* **cat's eye a.,** blindness of one eye, with bright reflection from the pupil, as from the tapetum of a cat (Beer); often indicative of retinoblastoma. **central a., a. centra′lis,** amaurosis due to disease of the central nervous system. **cerebral a.,** that which is due to cerebral or brain disease. **a. conge′nita, a. conge′nita of Leber, congenital a.,** a characteristic and rare type of blindness transmitted as an autosomal recessive trait, occurring at or shortly after birth and associated with an atypical form of diffuse pigmentation and commonly with optic atrophy and attenuation of the retinal vessels. **diabetic a.,** loss of vision due to diabetes mellitus. **a. fu′gax,** a transient episode of monocular blindness, or partial blindness, lasting ten minutes or less. **intoxication a.,** toxic amblyopia. **Leber's congenital a.,** a. congenita. **a. partia′lis fu′gax,** sudden transitory partial blindness. **reflex a.,** that which is caused by the reflex action of a remote irritation. **saburral a.,** that which occurs in an attack of acute gastritis. **toxic a.,** toxic amblyopia. **uremic a.,** loss of vision due to uremia.

amaurotic (am″aw-rot′ik) pertaining to, or of the nature of, amaurosis.

amazia (ah-ma′ze-ah) [*a* neg. + Gr. *mazos* breast + *-ia*] amastia.

amb- see *ambi-.*

ambenonium chloride (am″be-no′ne-um) [USP] chemical name: *N,N′*-[(1,2-dioxo-1,2-ethanediyl)bis-(imino-2,1-ethanediyl)]bis[2-chloro-*N,N*-diethylbenzenemethanaminium] dichloride. A cholinergic, $C_{28}H_{42}Cl_4N_4O_2$, occurring as a white powder; used in the treatment of myasthenia gravis to treat the symptoms of muscular weakness and fatigue, administered orally.

amber (am′ber) a yellowish fossil resin, the gum of several species of coniferous trees, found in the alluvial deposits of northeastern Germany.

Amberg's line (am′bergz) [Emil *Amberg,* Detroit otologist, 1868–1948] see under *line.*

ambergris (am′ber-gris) [L. *ambra grisea* gray amber] a grayish waxy mass of material ejected from the intestinal tract of the sperm whale, *Physeter catodon,* and made up of cholesterol and varying amounts of fatty oil, benzoic acid, ambrein, and other materials. Used as a fixative in perfumery.

ambi-, amb-. [L.] an inseparable prefix meaning on both sides.

ambidexterity (am″bĭ-dek-ster′ĭ-te) the ability to perform acts requiring manual skill with either hand, some ordinarily being performed with one and some with the other.

ambidextrality (am″bĭ-dek-stral′ĭ-te) ambidexterity.

ambidextrism (am″bĭ-deks′trizm) ambidexterity.

ambidextrous (am″bǐ-dek′strus)   pertaining to or characterized by ambidexterity.

ambient (am′be-ent) [L. *ambire* to surround]   surrounding; encompassing; prevailing.

ambilateral (am″bǐ-lat′er-al) [*ambi-* + L. *latus* side]   pertaining to or affecting both the right and the left side.

ambilevosity (am″bǐ-lě-vos′ǐ-te)   the inability to perform acts requiring manual skill with either hand.

ambilevous (am″bǐ-le′vus) [*ambi-* + L. *laevus* left-handed]   pertaining to or characterized by ambilevosity.

Ambilhar (am′bil-har)   trademark for preparations of niridazole.

ambiopia (am″be-o′pe-ah) [L.]   diplopia.

ambisexual (am″bǐ-seks′u-al)   denoting sexual characteristics common to both sexes, e.g., pubic hair. Cf. *bisexual.*

ambisinister (am″bǐ-sin′is-ter) [*ambi-* + L. *sinister* left]   ambilevous.

ambisinistrous (am″bǐ-sǐ-nis′trus)   ambilevous.

ambivalence (am-biv′ah-lens) [*ambi-* + L. *valentia* strength, power]   the simultaneous existence of conflicting attitudes, emotions, ideas, or wishes toward the same object.

ambivalent (am-biv′ah-lent)   characterized by or pertaining to ambivalence.

ambiversion (am″bǐ-ver′zhun)   a balance of introversion and extroversion.

ambivert (am′bǐ-vert)   a person who is intermediate between an extrovert and an introvert.

ambly- [Gr. *amblys* dull]   a combining form denoting dullness.

amblyaphia (am-ble-a′fe-ah) [*ambly-* + Gr. *haphe* touch + *-ia*]   bluntness or dullness of the sense of touch.

amblychromasia (am″ble-kro-ma′ze-ah)   the condition of staining faintly or of having little chromatin.

amblychromatic (am″ble-kro-mat′ik) [*ambly-* + Gr. *chrōma* color]   feebly staining.

amblygeustia (am″ble-gu′ste-ah) [*ambly-* + Gr. *geusis* taste + *-ia*]   dullness of the sense of taste.

Amblyomma (am″ble-om′ah) [*ambly-* + Gr. *omma* eye]   a genus of ticks. **A. america′num,** the Lone Star tick of the southern United States, particularly Texas and Louisiana; it is a vector of Rocky Mountain spotted fever. **A. cajennen′se,** a particularly obnoxious species of tropical America; it transmits Rocky Mountain spotted fever. **A. hebrae′um,** the bont tick, an African species which transmits the rickettsial disease of sheep, goats, and cattle known as "heartwater" as well as South African tick-bite fever of man. **A. macula′tum,** a species found on the Gulf Coast. **A. ova′le,** a tropical tick of dogs and tapirs. **A. tubercula′tum,** a species found in Florida. **A. variega′tum,** a species which, like *A. hebraeum,* transmits heartwater; it also transmits the virus causing Nairobi sheep disease.

amblyope (am′ble-ōp)   a person with amblyopia.

amblyopia (am″ble-o′pe-ah) [*ambly-* + *-opia*]   impairment of vision without detectable organic lesion of the eye. Cf. *amaurosis.* **alcoholic a.,** nutritional amblyopia; toxic amblyopia. **arsenic a.,** disturbance of vision due to the use of arsenic. **color a.,** impairment of color vision, caused by toxic or other influences. **a. ex anop′sia,** that which results from long disuse. **nocturnal a.,** abnormal dimness of vision at night. **nutritional a.,** central or cecocentral scotomata due to poor nutrition; seen in alcoholics and patients with severe nutritional deprivation or vitamin B_{12} deficiency, as in pernicious anemia. Complete recovery is possible with good diet and B vitamins; prolonged deficiency results in permanent loss of central vision. **quinine a.,** amblyopia following large doses of quinine; thought to be due to anemia of the retina. **reflex a.,** that which results from peripheral irritation. **strabismic a.,** amblyopia resulting from suppression of vision in one eye to avoid diplopia. **tobacco a.,** nutritional or toxic a. **toxic a.,** amblyopia due to poisoning, as from tobacco or alcohol. **traumatic a.,** amblyopia due to injury. **uremic a.,** impairment of vision due to uremia.

amblyoscope (am′ble-o-skōp) [*amblyopia* + *-scope*]   a hand-held reflecting stereoscope that presents to the two eyes two separate target images through two angled tubes. The angle between the two tubes can be adjusted horizontally and vertically; thus one can measure convergence and divergence, measure or train binocular vision, or stimulate vision in an amblyopic eye. **major a.,** a large, table-mounted amblyoscope that has greater freedom for adjustment than a simple amblyoscope has and in which targets and intensities of illumination can be varied.

Amblyospora (am″ble-os′por-ah) [*ambly-* + *spore*]   a genus of parasitic protozoa (suborder Pansporoblastina, order Microsporida) pathogenic in mosquitoes.

Amblystoma (am-blis′to-mah)   *Ambystoma.*

ambo (am′bo)   ambon.

ambo- [L. *ambo* both]   a combining form signifying both, or on both sides.

amboceptor (am″bo-sep′tor) [*ambo-* + L. *capere* to take]   Ehrlich's term for complement-fixing antibody, which he thought had two receptors, one for antigen, one for complement; now used colloquially to denote the anti–sheep red blood cell antibody used in complement fixation tests.

ambomycin (am″bo-mi′sin)   an antibiotic substance with antineoplastic properties produced by *Streptomyces ambofaciens;* formerly called *duazomycin C.*

ambon (am′bon)   the ring of fibrocartilage forming the edge of the sockets in which the heads of long bones are lodged.

ambosexual (am″bo-seks′u-al) [*ambo-* + *sexual*]   ambisexual.

ambrain (am-bra′in)   ambrin.

ambrein (am-bre′in)   ambrin.

ambrin (am′brin)   a white crystalline tricyclic terpenoid, $C_{30}H_{49}O_2$, resembling cholesterol, found in ambergris and derived metabolically from squalene.

Ambrine (am′brēn)   trademark for preparations of paraffin, rosin, and wax; formerly used as a dressing in the treatment of extensive burns and in rheumatic disorders, introduced by Barthe de Sandfort (1913).

Ambrosia (am-bro′zhe-ah) [L. and Gr., from Gr. *ambrotos* immortal]   a genus of annual weeds which produce quantities of windborne pollen and so cause much hay fever. *A. artemisiaefo′lia* is the common or small ragweed; *A. trif′ida* is the giant ragweed.

ambrosin (am-bro′sin)   (*obs.*) a substance contained in the pollen of ragweed (*Ambrosia*).

ambrosterol (am-bros′tě-rol)   a phytosterol, $C_{20}H_{34}O$ with a melting point of 147° to 149° C. found in the pollen of ragweed (*Ambrosia*).

ambruticin (am″broo-ti′sin)   chemical name: 6-[2-[2-[5-(6-ethyl-3,6-dihydro-5-methyl-2*H*-pyran-2-yl)-3-methyl-1,4-hexadienyl]-3-methycyclopropyl]ethenyl]tetrahydro-4,5-dihydroxy-2*H*-pyran-2-acetic acid; an antifungal antibiotic derived from *Polyangium cellulosum* subspecies *fulvum,* $C_{28}H_{42}O_6$.

ambulance (am′bu-lans) [Fr.]   a vehicle for conveying the sick or injured, and equipped with apparatus for rendering emergency treatment.

ambulant (am′bu-lant) [L. *ambulans* walking]   walking or able to walk.

ambulation (am″bu-la′shun)   the act of walking.

ambulatory (am′bu-lah-to″re)   ambulant.

ambuphylline (am-bu′fil-ēn)   a theophylline derivative with the same uses as aminophylline as a diuretic and smooth muscle relaxant.

ambustion (am-bust′yun)   a burn or scald.

ambutoxate hydrochloride (am-bu-toks′āt)   chemical name: 2-(diethylamino)ethyl 4-amino-2-butoxybenzoate hydrochloride; a spinal anesthetic. Called also *ambucaine.*

Ambystoma (am-bis′to-mah)   a genus of salamanders used for experimental purposes; called also *amblystoma.* See *axolotl.*

amcinafal (am-sin′ah-fal)   chemical name: 9-fluoro-11β,21-dihydroxy-16α,17-[(1-ethylpropylidene)bis(oxy)]pregna-1,4-diene-2,3-dione; an anti-inflammatory, $C_{26}H_{35}FO_6$.

amcinafide (am-sin′ah-fīd)   chemical name: (*R*)-9-fluoro-11β,21-dihydroxy-16α,17-[(1-phenylethylidine)bis(oxy)]pregna-1,4-diene-3,20-dione; an anti-inflammatory, $C_{26}H_{35}FO_6$.

amcinonide (am-sin′o-nīd) [USP]   a fluorinated corticosteroid applied topically for eczematoid conditions.

amdinocillin (am-de′no-sil″in)   a semisynthetic penicillin,

$C_{15}H_{23}N_3O_3S$, effective against many gram-negative bacteria and used in the treatment of urinary tract infections; administered intravenously or intramuscularly. Called also *mecillinam.*

ameba (ah-me′bah), pl. *ame′bae* [L., from Gr. *amoibē* change] any organism or cell capable of ameboid change or movement of the body by cytoplasmic extrusions (pseudopodia), especially a sarcodine protozoan of the superclass Rhizopoda.

ameban (ah-me′ban) carbarsone.

amebiasis (am″e-bi′ah-sis) the state of being infected with amebae, especially with *Entamoeba histolytica.* Although free-living protozoa such as *Acanthamoeba, Hartmannella,* and *Naegleria* are potential human pathogens, the term amebiasis is usually restricted to infection with *E. histolytica.* **a. cu′tis,** cutaneous manifestation of amebiasis usually manifested as painful ulcers with distinct undermined borders surrounded by erythematous rims, principally seen in patients with active intestinal or hepatic disease, which may occur as a result of direct extension of amebic bowel disease to adjacent skin areas following surgery; direct extension of a hepatic abscess, spontaneously after a surgical procedure; or direct implantation of trophozoites on the skin, with or without preexisting skin lesions. **hepatic a.,** amebic hepatitis. **intestinal a.,** amebic dysentery. **pulmonary a.,** amebic infection in the thoracic space, secondary to intestinal amebiasis and usually associated with amebic liver abscesses; it may affect the pleura, the diaphragm, the lung, and/or the bronchi.

amebic (ah-me′bik) pertaining to or of the nature of an ameba.

amebicidal (ah-me″bĭ-si′dal) destructive to amebae.

amebicide (ah-me′bĭ-sid) [*ameba* + L. *caedere* to kill] an agent which is destructive to amebae.

amebiform (ah-me′bĭ-form) shaped like or resembling an ameba.

ameb(i)(o)- [L., from Gr. *amoibē* change] a combining form denoting a relationship to an ameba. See also words beginning *amoeb(i)(o)-.*

amebiosis (am″e-bi-o′sis) amebiasis.

amebism (am′e-bizm) 1. ameboid movement. 2. invasion of the system with amebae.

amebocyte (ah-me′bo-sīt″) [*ameba* + Gr. *kytos* hollow vessel] an ameba-like cell found in coelomic fluid, blood (leukocytes), or other tissues of almost all animals.

amebodiastase (ah-me″bo-di′as-tās) amebadiastase.

ameboflagellate (ah-me″bo-flaj′ĕ-lāt) [*amebo-* + *flagellate*] a microorganism having both an ameboid and a flagellate stage in its life cycle; said of certain protozoa.

ameboid (ah-me′boid) [*ameba* + Gr. *eidos* form] resembling an ameba in form or in movements.

ameboididity (am″e-boi-did′ĭ-te) (*obs.*) ameboidism.

ameboidism (ah-me′boid-izm) a type of motility characteristic of amebae and certain other cells, occurring as a result of protrusion of pseudopods.

ameboma (am″e-bo′mah) a tumor-like mass produced by localized inflammation due to amebiasis.

amebula (ah-me′bu-lah) [dim. of *ameba*] 1. the small ameboid daughter cell occurring following reproduction in certain rhizopod amebae. 2. the motile ameboid stage of a spore prior to aggregation in certain protozoa or on germination of the spore in others. Also written *amoebula.*

ameburia (am″ĕ-bu′re-ah) [*ameba* + Gr. *ouron* urine + *-ia*] the discharge or presence of amebae in the urine.

amedalin hydrochloride (ah-me′dah-lin) chemical name: 1,3-dihydro-3-methyl-3-[3-(methylamino)-propyl]-1-phenyl-2*H*- indol-2-one monohydrochloride; an antidepressant, $C_{19}H_{22}N_2O \cdot HCl$.

ameiosis (a″mi-o′sis) aberrant meiosis in which only an equational division occurs, as in parthenogenesis.

AMEL Aero-Medical Equipment Laboratory.

amelanosis (ah-mel″ah-no′sis) [*a* neg. + *melanosis*] complete lack of melanin in the tissues. Cf. *depigmentation, hypomelanosis,* and *hypopigmentation.*

amelia (ah-me′le-ah) [*a* neg. + Gr. *melos* limb + *-ia*] congenital absence of a limb or limbs; cf. *phocomelia.*

amelification (ah-mel″ĭ-fi-ka′shun) [Old Fr. *amel* enamel + L. *facere* to make] the development of enamel cells into enamel.

amelioration (ah-mēl″yo-ra′shun) [L. *ad* to + *melior* better] improvement, as of the condition of a patient.

amel(o)- [Middle English *amel* enamel, from Old Fr. *esmal*] a combining form denoting enamel.

ameloblast (ah-mel′o-blast″) [Old Fr. *amel* enamel + Gr. *blastos* germ] a cylindrical epithelial cell in the innermost layer of the enamel organ which takes part in the elaboration of the enamel prism. The ameloblasts cover the dental papilla. Called also *adamantoblast, ganoblast, enamel builder,* and *enameloblast.*

ameloblastoma (ah-mel″o-blas-to′mah) a true neoplasm of tissue of the type characteristic of the enamel organ, but which does not undergo differentiation to the point of enamel formation; called also *adamantinoma.* **melanotic a.,** melanotic neuroectodermal tumor. **pigmented a.,** melanotic neuroectodermal tumor. **pituitary a.,** craniopharyngioma.

amelodentinal (am″ĕ-lo-den′tĭ-nal) pertaining to the enamel and dentin of a tooth.

amelogenesis (ah″mel-o-jen′ĕ-sis) [*amelo-* + *genesis*] the elaboration of dental enamel by ameloblasts. **a. imperfec′ta,** an autosomal dominant or X-linked disorder in which there is faulty development of the dental enamel owing to agenesis, hypoplasia, or hypocalcification of the enamel. It is marked by enamel that is very thin and friable and frequently stained in various shades of brown. Called also *hereditary brown enamel.* See also *enamel hypoplasia,* under *hypoplasia,* and *enamel hypocalcification,* under *hypocalcification.*

amelogenic (am″ĕ-lo-jen′ik) forming enamel; pertaining to amelogenesis.

amelogenin (am″ĕ-lo-jen′in) any of several proteins secreted by ameloblasts and forming the organic matrix of tooth enamel.

amelus (am′ĕ-lus) an individual exhibiting amelia.

amenia (ah-me′ne-ah) [*a* neg. + *menses* + *-ia*] amenorrhea.

amenorrhea (ah-men″o-re′ah) [*a* neg. + Gr. *mēn* month + *rhoia* flow] absence or abnormal stoppage of the menses; called also *amenia.* **dietary a.,** cessation of menstruation accompanying loss of weight due to dietary restriction, the loss of weight and of appetite being less extreme than in anorexia nervosa and unassociated with psychological problems. Called also *nutritional a.* **dysponderal a.,** amenorrhea associated with disorder of weight, such as obesity or extreme underweight. **hypothalamic a.,** amenorrhea associated with disorders of the hypothalamus. **lactation a.,** absence of the menses incidental to lactation. **nutritional a.,** dietary a. **ovarian a.,** amenorrhea resulting from deficiency of ovarian hormones. **physiologic a.,** absence of menses not due to organic disorder, usually occurring in pregnancy. **pituitary a.,** absence of the menses owing to pituitary deficiency. **premenopausal a.,** physiologic decrease of menstruation during establishment of the climacterium. **primary a.,** failure of menstruation to occur at puberty. **relative a.,** menstrual flow which is less than normal for the individual; called also *oligomenorrhea.* **secondary a.,** cessation of menstruation after it has once been established at puberty. **traumatic a.,** amenorrhea due to blockage of the cervical canal by adhesions, most often a result of curettage, as in Asherman's syndrome.

amenorrheal (ah-men-o-re′al) pertaining to amenorrhea.

amensalism (a-men′sal-izm) symbiosis in which one population (or individual) is adversely affected and the other is unaffected.

amentia (ah-men′she-ah) [L. *a* away + *mens* mind + *-ia*] 1. (*obs.*) profound mental retardation. 2. the terminal stage of degenerative dementia. **phenylpyruvic a.** (*obs.*), the mental retardation resulting from untreated phenylketonuria.

Americaine (ah-mer′ĭ-kān″) trademark for preparations of benzocaine.

American Type Culture Collection (ATCC) an organization established in Rockville, MD, as a depository for reference cultures. It maintains and distributes authentic reference strains of algae, bacteria, fungi, and protozoa, bacteriophages and viruses, and cell lines of animal tissues.

americium (am″ĕ-ris′e-um) the chemical element of atomic number 95, atomic weight 243, symbol Am, obtained by cyclotron bombardment of uranium and plutonium.

amerism (am′er-izm) [*a* neg. + Gr. *meros* part] the quality of not splitting into segments or fragments.

ameristic (am″er-is′tik) [*a* neg. + Gr. *meristos* divided] not split into segments.

Ames test (āmz) [Bruce *Ames*, American biochemist, born 1928] see under *tests*.

ametabolon (ah″mĕ-tab′o-lon) an animal that develops without undergoing metamorphosis.

ametabolous (ā″mĕ-tab′o-lus) not undergoing metamorphosis.

ametachromophil (ah″met-ah-kro′mo-fil) orthochromophil.

ametaneutrophil (ah-met-ah-nu′tro-fil) orthochromophil.

amethocaine hydrochloride (ah-meth′o-kān) tetracaine hydrochloride.

amethopterin (ah-meth-op′ter-in) methotrexate.

ametria (ah-me′tre-ah) [*a* neg. + Gr. *mētra* uterus] congenital absence of the uterus.

ametrometer (am″ĕ-trom′ĕ-ter) [*ametropia* + Gr. *metron* measure] an instrument for measuring the degree of ametropia.

ametropia (am″ĕ-tro′pe-ah) [Gr. *ametros* disproportionate + *-opia*] discrepancy between the size and refractive powers of the eye, such that images are not brought to a proper focus on the retina; consequently hypermetropia, myopia, or astigmatism are produced. See illustration at *refraction.* **axial a.,** ametropia due to lengthening of the eyeball along the optic axis. **curvature a.,** ametropia due to variations in the curvature of the surface of the eye. **index a.,** ametropia due to alterations in the refractive index media of the eye. **position a.,** ametropia due to faulty position of the crystalline lens. **refractive a.,** ametropia due to fault in the dioptric system of the eye.

ametropic (am″ĕ-trop′ik) affected with or pertaining to ametropia.

amfenac sodium (am′fĕ-nak) chemical name: 2-amino-3-benzoylbenzeneacetic acid sodium salt monohydrate; an anti-inflammatory, $C_{15}H_{12}NNaO_3H_2O$.

amfonelic acid (am-fo-ne′lik) a central nervous system stimulant.

Amh mixed astigmatism with myopia predominating.

AMI acute myocardial infarction.

amianthoid (am″e-an′thoid) [Gr. *amianthos* asbestos + *eidos* form] having the appearance of asbestos; a term applied to certain fibers seen in degenerated costal and laryngeal cartilage.

amibiarson (am″ĭ-bĭ-ar′sōn) carbarsone.

Amicar (am′ĭ-kar) trademark for a preparation of aminocaproic acid.

amichloral (am″ĭ-klor′al) chemical name: 6-*O*-[2,2,2-trichloro-1-hydroxyethyl)-α-D-glucopyranose polymer with α-D-glucopyranose; a food additive for use in veterinary medicine, $(C_8H_{11}Cl_3O_6)_x(C_8H_{10}O_5)_y$.

Amici's disk, line, striae (ah-me′chēz) [Giovanni Battista *Amici*, Italian physicist, 1784–1863] see *Z band,* under *band,* and see under *stria.*

amicrobic (ah″mi-kro′bik) [*a* neg. + *microbe*] not caused by microbes.

amicroscopic (ah-mi″kro-skop′ik) too small to be observed by use of the microscope.

amicula (ah-mik′u-lah) [L.] plural of *amiculum.*

amiculum (ah-mik′u-lum), pl. *amic′ula* [L.] 1. a coat or covering. 2. a. olivare. **a. oliva′re** [NA], **a. of olive,** a capsule of myelinated fibers that surrounds the caudal olivary nucleus; called also *amiculum.*

amidapsone (ah″me-dap′sōn) chemical name: [4-[(4-aminophenyl)sulfonyl]phenyl]urea; an antiviral for use in poultry, $C_{13}H_{13}N_3O_3S$.

amidase (am′ĭ-dās) [EC 3.5.1.4] an enzyme that catalyzes the reaction monocarboxylic acid amide + H_2O = monocarboxylate + NH_3.

amide (am′īd) [*ammonia* + *-ide*] an organic compound derived from ammonia by substituting an acyl radical for

hydrogen, or from an acid by replacing the —OH group by —NH_2. **niacin a., nicotinic acid a.,** niacinamide.

amide synthetase (am″īd sin′thĕ-tās) [EC 6.3.1] one of a sub-subclass of enzymes of the ligase class that catalyze the formation of amide bonds.

amidin (am′ĭ-din) [Fr. *amidon* starch] amylose, def. 2.

amidine (am′ĭ-din) any compound containing the monovalent group ·C(:NH)·NH_2. **insoluble a., tegumentary a.,** amylopectin.

amidine-lyase (am′ĭ-dēn-li′ās) [EC 4.3.2] a sub-subclass of enzymes of the lyase class that catalyze the cleavage of a carbon-nitrogen bond in compounds such as adenylosuccinate and argininosuccinate.

amidinotransferase (am-ĭ-dēn″o-, ah″mĭ-din″o-trans′fer-ās) [EC 2.1.4] a sub-subclass of enzymes of the transferase class that catalyze the transfer of an amidino group from one compound to another.

amido- a prefix indicating the presence of the radical NH_2 along with the radical CO.

amidoazotoluene (am″ĕ-do-a″zo-tol′u-ēn) a reddish brown powder, $CH_3·C_6H_4·N_2·C_6H_3·CH_2·NH_2$, derived from scarlet red; used in an 8 per cent ointment to stimulate the growth of epithelium.

amidobenzene (am″ĕ-do-ben′zēn) aniline.

amidogen (am′ĭ-do-jen″) the hypothetic radical, NH_2, found in amido compounds.

amidohexose (am″ĭ-do-hek′sōs) a hexose combined with the amido group NH_2.

amidohydrolase (am″ĭ-do-hi′dro-lās) [EC 3.5.1-2] the systematic name for enzymes of the hydrolase class that catalyze the hydrolysis of C—N bonds in linear or cyclic amide compounds. Called also *deamidase.*

amido-ligase (am′ĭ-do-li′gās) [EC 6.3.5] a sub-subclass of enzymes of the ligase class that catalyze the transfer of the amide nitrogen from glutamine to an acceptor molecule, driven by the concomitant hydrolysis of ATP to ADP or AMP and forming an amide or amidine group on the acceptor.

amidopyrine (am″ĭ-do-pi′rēn) aminopyrine.

Amidostomum (am″ĭ-dos′to-mum) a genus of roundworms. **A. an′seris,** a roundworm parasitic in the mucous membrane of the intestinal tract of ducks and geese.

amidoxime (am-ĭ-dok′sīm) any of a class of compounds formed from the amidines by substituting hydroxyl for a hydrogen atom of the amido group.

amidulin (ah-mid′u-lin) the granulose of starch freed from its envelope of amylose by the action of hydrochloric acid; called also *soluble starch.*

Amigen (am′ĭ-jen) trademark for a protein hydrolysate preparation for intravenous injection.

amikacin sulfate (am″ĭ-ka′sin) [USP] chemical name: (S)-*O*-3-amino-3-deoxy-α-D-glucopyranosyl-(1 → 6)-*O*-[6-amino-6-deoxy-α-D-glucopyranosyl(1→4)]-*N*¹-(4-amino-2-hydroxy-1-oxobutyl)-2-deoxy-D-streptamine sulfate (1:1) salt. A semisynthetic aminoglycoside antibiotic derived from kanamycin, $C_{22}H_{43}N_5O_{13}·2H_2SO_4$, effective against gram-negative bacteria including *Pseudomonas, Providencia, Klebsiella-Enterobacter-Serratia, Acinetobacter,* and *Proteus* species, and *Escherichia coli* and *Citrobacter freundii,* and some gram-positive organisms, including penicillinase- and non-penicillinase-producing staphylococci; used in the treatment of a wide range of infections due to susceptible organisms, administered intramuscularly and intravenously.

Amikin (am′ĭ-kin) trademark for a preparation of amikacin sulfate.

amiloride (ah-mil′o-rīd) a potassium-sparing diuretic; used as *amiloride hydrochloride* [USP] in the treatment of edema and, usually in combination with hydrochlorothiazide, in the treatment of hypertension.

amimia (ah-mim′e-ah) [*a* neg. + Gr. *mimos* mimic + *-ia*] loss of the power of expression by the use of signs or gestures. **amnesic a.,** a condition in which gestures can be made, but their meaning cannot be remembered.

aminacrine hydrochloride (am-in-ak′rin) chemical name: 9-aminoacridine monohydrochloride. An antiseptic dye, $C_{13}H_{10}N_2·HCl$, occurring as a pale yellow, crystalline powder, which is effective against many gram-negative and gram-positive bacteria; used as a topical anti-infective, mainly in the treatment of infected wounds. Called also *aminoacridine hydrochloride.*

aminarsone (am-in-ar′sōn) carbarsone.

amine (ah-mēn′; am′in) an organic compound containing nitrogen; any member of a group of chemical compounds formed from ammonia by replacement of one or more of the hydrogen atoms by organic (hydrocarbon) radicals. The amines are distinguished as *primary, secondary,* and *tertiary,* according to whether one, two, or three hydrogen atoms are replaced. The amines include allylamine, amylamine, ethylamine, methylamine, phenylamine, propylamine, and many other compounds. **biogenic a′s,** amines arising by biosynthesis that play a role in neural functioning, e.g., norepinephrine, serotonin, dopamine, and acetylcholine; called also *bioamines.* **catechol a.,** catecholamine. **methyl dimethoxy methyl phenyl ethyl a.,** a long-acting hallucinogenic substance. Abbreviated DMP. **vasoactive a.'s,** amines that cause vasodilation and increase small vessel permeability, e.g., histamine and serotonin.

amine oxidase (copper-containing) (ah-mēn′ok′sĭ-dās) [EC 1.4.3.6] an enzyme of the oxidoreductase class that catalyzes the reaction $RCH_2NH_2 + H_2O + O_2 = RCHO + NH_3 + H_2O_2$. The enzyme is a copper protein and may contain pyridoxal phosphate. It acts upon primary monoamines and diamines, including histamine. Called also *diamine oxidase.*

amine oxidase (flavin-containing) (ah-mēn′ok′sĭ-dās) [EC 1.4.3.4] an enzyme of the oxidoreductase class that catalyzes the reaction $RCHNH_2 + H_2O + O_2 =$ aldehyde $+ NH_3 + H_2O_2$. The enzyme is a flavoprotein acting on primary, secondary, and tertiary amines, including serotonin, norepinephrine, epinephrine, and dopamine. Called also *monoamine oxidase (MAO).* See also under *inhibitor.*

aminitrozole (am′ĭ-ni′tro-zōl) nithiamide.

amino (ah-me′no, am′ĭ-no) the monovalent chemical group —NH_2. As a prefix (amino-) it indicates the presence in a compound of the group —NH_2.

aminoacetic acid (ah-me′no-ah-se′tik) [USP] systematic chemical name and nonproprietary drug name for glycine; used in irrigating solutions.

amino acid (ah-me′no) any organic compound containing an amino (—NH_2) and a carboxyl (—COOH) group. The 20 α-amino acids listed in the accompanying table are the amino acids from which proteins are synthesized by formation of peptide bonds during ribosomal translation of messenger RNA; all except glycine, which is not optically active, have the *L* configuration. Other amino acids occurring in proteins, such as hydroxyprolene in collagen, are formed by posttranslational enzymatic modification of amino acid residues in polypeptide chains. There are also several important amino acids, such as the neurotransmitter γ-aminobutyric acid, that have no relation to proteins. Abbreviated AA. **α-a. a.,** one in which the amino and carboxyl groups are both attached to the same carbon atom. **ω-a. a.,** one having the amino and carboxyl groups attached to opposite ends of a carbon chain. **essential a. a's,** the nine α-amino acids required for protein synthesis that cannot be synthesized by humans and must be obtained in the diet: histidine, isoleucine, leucine, lysine, methionine, phenylalanine, threonine, tryptophan, and valine. **nonessential a.a's,** the eleven α-amino acids required for protein synthesis that are synthesized by humans and are not specifically required in the diet.

aminoacidemia (ah-me′no-, am′ĭ-no-as′ĭ-de′me-ah) [*amino acid* + Gr. *haima* blood + *-ia*] an excess of amino acids in the blood.

aminoacidopathy (am′ĭ-no-as′ĭ-dop′ah-the) any of a group of disorders due to a defect in an enzymatic step in the metabolic pathway of one or more amino acids or in a protein mediator necessary for transport of certain amino acids into or out of cells.

D-amino-acid oxidase (ah-me′no-as′id ok′sĭ-das) [EC 1.4.3.3] an enzyme of the oxidoreductase class that catalyzes the reaction D-amino acid $+ H_2O + O_2 = $ 2-keto acid anion $+ NH_3 + H_2O_2$. It is a flavoprotein found in the cytoplasm of kidney, brain, and liver; its metabolic role is unclear.

L-amino-acid oxidase (ah-me′no as′id ok′sĭ-dās) [EC 1.4.3.2] an enzyme of the oxidoreductase class that catalyzes the reaction L-amino acid $+ H_2O + O_2 = $ 2-oxo acid $+ NH_3 + H_2O_2$. It is a flavoprotein, present in liver and kidney and found in snake venom. It acts on all naturally occurring monocarboxylic L-amino acids except serine and threonine. The mammalian enzymes also attack 2-hydroxy acids; their function is unclear.

aminoaciduria (ah-me′no-, am′ĭ-no-as′ĭ-du′re-ah) [*amino acid* + Gr. *ouron* urine + *-ia*] an excess of amino acids in the urine; called also *acidaminuria.*

aminoacridine hydrochloride (am′ĭ-no-ak′rĭ-din) aminacrine hydrochloride.

aminoacyl (ah-me′no-as′il) an acyl radical of an amino acid, e.g., alanyl, glycyl, etc. **a.-tRNA,** an amino acid residue joined by an ester linkage to the 2′ or 3′ hydroxyl group of the terminal adenosine residue of a transfer RNA (see also *translation*).

aminoacylase (am′ĭ-no-as′ĭ-lās) [EC 3.5.1.14] an enzyme of the hydrolase class that catalyzes the reaction *N*-acyl-amino acid $+ H_2O = $ fatty acid anion $+$ amino acid. It occurs in the kidney and acts on a variety of substrates, including hippuric acid and benzamide; it also hydrolyzes dehydropeptides.

aminoacyl histidine dipeptidase (ah-me′no-a′sil his′-tĭ-dēn di-pep′tĭ-das) [EC 3.4.13.3] an enzyme of the hydrolase class that catalyzes the reaction carnosine (or other aminoacyl-L-histidine dipeptide) $+ H_2O = $ β-alanine (or other amino acid) $+$ L-histidine. Genetic defect in the enzyme, transmitted as an autosomal recessive trait, causes carnosinemia. Called also *carnosinase.*

aminoacyltransferase (ah-me′no-a′sil-trans′fer-ās) [EC 2.3.2] a sub-subclass of enzymes of the transferase class that catalyze the transfer of an aminoacyl group from one molecule to another with formation of an ester or an amide linkage.

aminoacyl-tRNA synthetase (ah-me′no-a′sil sin′thĕ-tās) [EC 6.1.1] a sub-subclass of enzymes of the ligase class that catalyze the reaction amino acid $+$ tRNA $+$ ATP $=$ aminoacyl-tRNA $+$ AMP $+$ PP$_1$. The enzymes are amino acid–activating enzymes, and each is highly specific for one amino acid and for any tRNA corresponding to that amino acid. Individual enzymes are known by the name of the amino acid acted on, e.g., alanyl-tRNA synthetase and aspartyl-tRNA synthetase.

o-aminoazotoluene (ah-me′no-, am′ĭ-no-az′′o-tol′u-ēn) chemical name: methyl-4-[(2-methylphenyl)azo]benzeneamine; a red crystalline solid, $CH_3 \cdot C_6H_4 \cdot N_2 \cdot C_6H_3(CH_3)NH_2$, that is actively carcinogenic.

aminobenzene (ah-me′′no-, am′′ĭ-no-ben′zēn) aniline.

p-aminobenzoic acid (PABA) (ah-me′′no-ben-zo′ik) [USP] a substance required for the synthesis of folic acid by many organisms. PABA is included in the B vitamin complex, although it is not an essential nutrient for humans. PABA also absorbs ultraviolet light and is used as *aminobenzoic acid* [USP] as a topical sunscreen.

γ-aminobutyrate (ah-me′′no-bu′tĭ-rāt) the conjugate base of aminobutyric acid.

aminobutyrate aminotransferase (ah-me′′no-bu′-tĭ- rāt ah-me′′no-trans′fer-ās) [EC 2.6.1.19] an enzyme of the transferase class that catalyzes the reaction 4-aminobutyrate $+$ 2-ketoglutarate $=$ succinate semialdehyde $+$ L-glutamate. This reaction occurs predominantly in the neurons of the brain. The enzyme also acts on β-alanine to produce melonic semialdehyde. A congenital deficiency of the enzyme, transmitted as an autosomal recessive trait, causes hyperbeta-alaninemia. Called also *β-alanine α-ketoglutarate transaminase, β-alanine-oxoglutarate aminotransferase,* and *β-alanine transaminase.*

γ-aminobutyric acid (ah-me′′no-bu-tēr′ik) GABA; an ω-amino acid that serves as the principal inhibitory neurotransmitter in the brain.

ε-aminocaproic acid (ah-me′′no-kah-pro′ik) an ω-amino acid that inhibits plasminogen activator substances and, to a lesser degree, plasmin; used as *aminocaproic acid* [USP] for treatment of acute bleeding syndromes due to excessive fibrinolysis.

aminodinitrophenol (am′′ĭ-no-di-ni′′tro-fe′nol) dinitroaminophenol.

2-aminoethanol (am′′ĭ-no-eth′ah-nol) ethanolamine.

aminoform (ah-min′o-form) methenamine.

aminoglutethimide (ah-me′′no-, am′′ĭ-no-gloo-teth′ĭ-mīd) chemical name: 3-(4-aminophenyl)-3-ethyl-2,6-piperidide-

AMINO ACIDS

THE 20 α-AMINO ACIDS SPECIFIED BY THE GENETIC CODE

NAME	SYMBOLS*		STRUCTURAL FORMULA
Alanine	Ala	A	$HOOC-\overset{NH_2}{\underset{|}{CH}}-CH_3$
Arginine	Arg	R	$HOOC-\overset{NH_2}{\underset{|}{CH}}-CH_2-CH_2-CH_2-NH-\overset{NH}{\underset{|}{\underset{NH_2}{C}}}$
Asparagine	Asn	N	$HOOC-\overset{NH_2}{\underset{|}{CH}}-CH_2-\overset{O}{\overset{\|}{C}}-NH_2$
Aspartic Acid	Asp	D	$HOOC-\overset{NH_2}{\underset{|}{CH}}-CH_2-COOH$
Cysteine	Cys	C	$HOOC-\overset{NH_2}{\underset{|}{CH}}-CH_2-SH$
Glutamic Acid	Glu	E	$HOOC-\overset{NH_2}{\underset{|}{CH}}-CH_2-CH_2-COOH$
Glutamine	Gln	Q	$HOOC-\overset{NH_2}{\underset{|}{CH}}-CH_2-CH_2-\overset{O}{\overset{\|}{C}}-NH_2$
Glycine	Gly	G	$HOOC-\overset{NH_2}{\underset{|}{CH}}-H$
Histidine	His	H	$HOOC-\overset{NH_2}{\underset{|}{CH}}-CH_2$ (imidazole ring)
Isoleucine	Ile	I	$HOOC-\overset{NH_2}{\underset{|}{CH}}-\overset{CH_3}{\underset{|}{CH}}-CH_2-CH_3$
Leucine	Leu	L	$HOOC-\overset{NH_2}{\underset{|}{CH}}-CH_2-\overset{CH_3}{\underset{|}{CH}}-CH_2$
Lysine	Lys	K	$HOOC-\overset{NH_2}{\underset{|}{CH}}-CH_2-CH_2-CH_2-CH_2-NH_2$
Methionine	Met	M	$HOOC-\overset{NH_2}{\underset{|}{CH}}-CH_2-CH_2-S-CH_3$
Phenylalanine	Phe	F	$HOOC-\overset{NH_2}{\underset{|}{CH}}-CH_2$ (phenyl ring)
Proline	Pro	P	$HOOC$ (pyrrolidine ring)
Serine	Ser	S	$HOOC-\overset{NH_2}{\underset{|}{CH}}-CH_2-OH$
Threonine	Thr	T	$HOOC-\overset{NH_2}{\underset{|}{CH}}-\overset{OH}{\underset{|}{CH}}-CH_3$
Tryptophan	Trp	W	$HOOC-\overset{NH_2}{\underset{|}{CH}}-CH_2$ (indole ring)
Tyrosine	Tyr	Y	$HOOC-\overset{NH_2}{\underset{|}{CH}}-CH_2$ (phenol ring)$-OH$
Valine	Val	V	$HOOC-\overset{NH_2}{\underset{|}{CH}}-\overset{CH_3}{\underset{|}{CH}}-CH_3$

*The three-letter and single-letter symbols that are used in presenting the sequence of a polypeptide or protein, e.g., Gly-Phe-Tyr. By convention, the N-terminal is shown at the left, the C-terminal at the right. For emphasis, the same formula may be written as H-Gly-Phe-Tyr-OH.

dione. A glutethimide derivative, $C_{13}H_{16}N_2O_2$, formerly used as an anticonvulsant in epilepsy. It inhibits adrenal cortical secretion, and has been used experimentally in the treatment of secondary hyperaldosteronism, edema, adrenal and ectopic ACTH-secreting tumors, and metastatic breast cancer.

aminoglycoside (am″ĭ-no-gli′ko-sīd) 1. a chemical compound containing an aminocyclitol ring and one or more amino sugars. 2. any of a group of aminoglycoside bacterial antibiotics (e.g., amikacin, gentamicin, streptomycin) derived from various species of *Streptomyces* or produced synthetically. Aminoglycoside antibiotics inhibit protein synthesis by binding with the 30S ribosomal subunit.

aminogram (am-i′no-gram) a graphic representation of the pattern of amino acids present in a substance as determined quantitatively.

aminoheterocyclic (am″ĭ-no-het″er-o-sik′lik) having a closed chain or ring formation which includes the —NH₂ group.

aminohippurate (am″ĭ-no-hip′u-rāt) a salt of aminohippuric acid.

p-aminohippurate (ah-me″no-, am″ĭ-no-hip′u-rāt) a salt or the conjugate base of *p*-aminohippuric acid. **a. sodium** [USP], the sodium salt of aminohippuric acid, $C_9H_9N_2NaO_3$, which is injected intravenously for the measurement of effective renal plasma flow and determination of the functional capacity of the tubular excretory mechanism.

aminohippuric acid (ah-me″no-, am″ĭ-no-hip-u′rik) [USP] the glycine conjugate of para-aminobenzoic acid; its sodium salt (aminohippurate sodium) is used to measure the effective renal plasma flow and to determine the functional capacity of the tubular excretory mechanism. Called also *para-aminohippuric acid*, and *PAH* or *PAHA*.

p-aminohippuric acid (PAH) (ah-me′no-, am″ĭ-no-hĭpūr′ik) the glycine amide of *p*-aminobenzoic acid. PAH is rapidly excreted primarily by renal tubular secretion. The clearance of PAH, *aminohippuric acid* [USP] or *aminohippurate sodium* [USP], administered by continuous infusion is considered the definitive measurement of effective renal plasma flow (ERPF).

aminohydrolase (ah-me″no-hi′dro-lās) deaminase.

aminohydroxybenzoic acid (ah-me″no-, am′′ĭ-no-hidrok″se-ben-zo′ik) a group of chemotherapeutic agents used in the treatment of infections with acid-fast bacilli.

aminolevulinate (ah-me″no-lev′u-lin′āt) the conjugate base of δ-aminolevulinic acid.

aminolevulinate dehydratase (ah-me″no-lev″u-lin′āt de-hi′drah-tās) porphobilinogen synthase.

5-aminolevulinate synthase (ah-me″no-lev″u-lin′āt sin′thās) [EC 2.3.1.37] an enzyme of the transferase class that catalyzes the reaction succinyl-CoA + glycine = 5-aminolevulinate + CoA + CO₂. It is a pyridoxal-phosphate protein. The reaction is the first step of the heme biosynthetic pathway. Called also *δ-aminolevulinate synthase*.

δ-aminolevulinic acid (ah-me″no-lev″u-lin′ik) ALA; an intermediate in the synthesis of heme, produced from succinyl-CoA and glycine. Two molecules of ALA are condensed to form porphobilinogen. Blood and urinary ALA levels are increased in lead poisoning.

aminolipid (ah-me″no-, am″ĭ-no-lip′id) any of a class of fatty substances containing amino nitrogen and fatty acids.

aminolipin (ah-me″no-, am″ĭ-no-li′pin) aminolipid.

aminolysis (am″ĭ-nol′ĭ-sis) [*amine* + Gr. *lysis* dissolution] reaction with an amine, resulting in the addition of (or substitution by) an imino group, —NH—.

aminometradine (ah-me″no-, am″ĭ-no-met′rah-dēn) chemical name: 6-amino-3-ethyl-1-(2-propenyl)-2,4(1*H*,3*H*)-pyrimidinedione; a nonmercurial diuretic for oral administration, $C_9H_{13}N_3O_2$.

aminometramide (ah-me″no-, am″ĭ-no-met′rah-mīd) aminometradine.

aminonitrogen (ah-me″no-, am″ĭ-no-ni′tro-jen) see under *nitrogen*.

aminonitrothiazole (am″ĭ-no-ni″tro-thi′ah-zōl) chemical name: 2-amino-5-nitrothiazole. A greenish-yellow to orange-yellow fluffy powder, $C_3H_3N_3O_2S$, used in the treatment and prevention of blackhead in turkeys.

aminopentamide sulfate (ah-me″no-, am″ĭ-no-pen′tahmīd) chemical name: α-[2-(dimethylamino)propyl]-α-phe-nylbenzeneacetamide sulfate; an anticholinergic, $C_{19}H_{24}N_2$-OH_2SO_4, with atropine-like action.

aminopeptidase (ah-me″no-, am″ĭ-no-pep′tĭ-dās) [EC 3.4.11] any of a number of enzymes of the hydrolase class that catalyze hydrolysis of the terminal peptide bond at the amino end of an oligopeptide, thus releasing the terminal amino acid. Those in the brush border or in the interior cytoplasm of the intestinal mucosa are important in protein digestion. Individual aminopeptidases have different specificities.

aminopeptidase (cytosol) (ah-me″no, am″ĭ-no-pep′tĭd-ās) cytosol aminopeptidase.

aminopherase (am″ĭ-nof′er-ās) aminotransferase.

aminophylline (ah-me″no-fil′in) [USP] chemical name: 3,7-dihydro-1,3-dimethyl-1*H*-purine-2,6-dione compound with 1,2-ethanediamine. A salt of theophylline, $C_{16}H_{24}N_{10}O_4$, occurring as white or slightly yellowish granules or powder. Aminophylline is a smooth muscle relaxant and is used chiefly for its bronchodilator effect in such diseases as asthma, bronchitis, and emphysema; administered orally, rectally, or intravenously. It also may be used for its myocardial stimulant and coronary vasodilator actions, diuretic action, and respiratory center stimulant effect. Called also *theophylline ethylenediamine*.

aminopolypeptidase (ah-me″no-, am″ĭ-no-pol″e-pep′tĭ-dās) aminopeptidase.

aminopterin (am″ĭ-nop″ter-in) 4-aminofolic acid, a folic acid antagonist formerly used as an antineoplastic, now replaced by methotrexate.

aminopteroylglutamic acid (am-ĭ-nop″ter-o-il-gloo′tah-mik) aminopterin.

aminopurine (ah-me″no-, am″ĭ-no-pu′rin) a purine that is a component of nucleic acid and the nucleotides; the aminopurines include adenine and guanine.

aminopyrine (ah-me″no-, am″ĭ-no-pi′rin) chemical name: 4-(dimethylamino)-1,2-dihydro-1,5-dimethyl-2-phenyl-3*H*-pyrazol-3-one. A pyrazole derivative, $C_{13}H_{17}N_3O$, an effective analgesic and antipyretic, but seldom used because it has been associated with fatal agranulocytosis. Called also *aminophenazone* [INN]; formerly called *amidopyrine*.

aminorex (ah-min′o-reks) chemical name: 4,5-dihydro-5-phenyl-2-oxazoline; a sympathomimetic anorexic, $C_9H_{10}N_2O$.

aminosaccharide (ah-me″no-, am″ĭ-no-sak′ah-rīd) a sugar in which the OH group has been replaced by an amino group, —NH₂.

aminosalicylate (am″ĭ-no-sah-lis′ah-lāt) any salt of aminosalicylic acid. The USP preparations, *aminosalicylate calcium*, *aminosalicylate potassium*, and *aminosalicylate sodium*, are used as tuberculostatic antibacterials.

p-aminosalicylate (ah-me″no-sah-lis′ah-lāt) a salt of *p*-aminosalicylic acid.

p-aminosalicylic acid (ah-me″no-sal-ĭ-sil′ik) PAS; an analogue of p-aminobenzoic acid (PABA) that inhibits folic acid synthesis in *Mycobacterium tuberculosis* and is bacteriostatic, inhibiting growth and multiplication of the tubercle bacillus; available as *aminosalicylic acid* [USP], *aminosalicylate calcium* [USP], *aminosalicylate potassium* [USP], and *aminosalicylate sodium* [USP].

aminosidine sulfate (am″ĭ-no-si′din) paromomycin sulfate.

aminosis (am″ĭ-no′sis) the pathologic production of amino acids in the body.

Aminosol (ah-me′no-sol) trademark for an amino acid preparation for intravenous injection.

aminostiburia (ah-me″no-, am″ĭ-no-sti-bu′re-ah) the glycoside of urea stibamine.

aminosuria (ah-me″no-, am″ĭ-no-su′re-ah) [*amine* + *-uria*] an excess of amines in the urine.

Aminosyn (ah-me′no-sin) trademark for a crystalline amino acid solution for intravenous administration; it contains a mixture of essential and nonessential amino acids but no peptides.

aminothiazole (ah-me″no-, am″ĭ-no-thi′ah-zol) chemical name: 2-thiazylamine. A sulfonamide compound, $NH_2 \cdot C \cdot N \cdot CH \colon CH \cdot S$, that has been used in the treatment of hyperthyroidism.

aminotransferase (ah-me″no-, am″ĭ-no-trans′fer-ās) [EC 2.6.1] a sub-subclass of enzymes of the transferase class that catalyze the transfer of an amino group from a donor (generally an amino acid) to an acceptor (generally α2-keto acid). Most of these enzymes are pyridoxal-phosphate-proteins. Called also *transaminase*.

aminotrate (am″ĭ-no-trāt″) the generic name for compounds composed of proteins and vitamins, used as a dietary food supplement. **a. phosphate,** trolnitrate phosphate.

aminuria (am″ĭ-nu′re-ah) an excess of amines in the urine.

amiodarone (ah-me′o-dah-rōn″) a cardiac vasodilator and antiarrhythmic agent.

Amipaque (am′ĭ-pāk) trademark for metrizamide.

amiphenazole hydrochloride (am″ĭ-fen′ah-zōl) chemical name: 2,4-diamino-5-phenylthiazole monohydrochloride; a respiratory stimulant, $C_9H_9N_3S \cdot HCl$, which acts as an antagonist to morphine and other narcotics.

amiquinsin hydrochloride (am″ĭ-kwin′sin) chemical name: 4-amino-6,7-dimethoxyquinoline hydrochloride monohydrate; an antihypertensive agent, $C_{11}H_{12}N_2O_2 \cdot HCl \cdot H_2O$.

amisometradine (am-i″so-met′rah-dēn) chemical name: 6-amino-3-methyl-1-(2-methyl-2-propenyl)-2,4(1H,3H)-pyrimidine-dione. A white crystalline powder, $C_9H_{13}N_3O_2$, used as an oral diuretic.

amithiozone (am″ĭ-thi′ŏ-zōn) thiacetazone.

amitosis (am″ĭ-to′sis) [a neg. + Gr. *mitos* thread + *-osis*] direct cell division; cell division by simple cleavage of the nucleus without the formation of spireme (mitotic) spindle figure or chromosomes. Called also *holoschisis*.

amitotic (am″ĭ-tot′ik) of the nature of amitosis; not occurring by mitosis; called also *akinetic*.

amitriptyline hydrochloride (am″ĭ-trip′tĭ-lēn) [USP] chemical name: 3-(10,11-dihydro-5H-dibenzo[a,d]cyclohepten-5-ylidene)-*cyclohepten-5-ylidene*)-N,N-dimethyl-1-propanamine hydrochloride. An antidepressant, $C_{20}H_{23}N \cdot HCl$, occurring as a white or practically white, crystalline powder; administered orally or intramuscularly.

ammeter (am′me-ter) [ampere + Gr. *metron* measure] an instrument calibrated to read in amperes or subdivisions of amperes the strength of a current flowing in a circuit.

Ammi (am′me) a genus of umbelliferous plants. *A. visna′ga* grows in Mediterranean countries and has been used in the treatment of urethral spasm and renal colic. Fruits of this species contain khellin. **A. ma′jus** (L.) Lam. Khella. (Umbelliferae), a species found in Mediterranean countries that is a source of methoxsalen.

ammoaciduria (am″o-as″ĭ-du′re-ah) an excess of ammonia and amino acids in the urine.

Ammon's filaments, fissure, operation (am′unz) [Friedrich August von *Ammon*, ophthalmologist and pathologist in Dresden, 1799–1861] see under *filament, fissure,* and *operation*.

Ammon's horn (am′unz) [*Ammon*, a ram-headed god of the Egyptians] hippocampus.

ammonemia (ah″mo-ne′me-ah) hyperammonemia.

ammonia (ah-mo′ne-ah) [named from Jupiter *Ammon*, near whose temple in Libya it was formerly obtained] a colorless alkaline gas, NH_3, of a penetrating odor and soluble in water, forming ammonia water; called also *volatile alkali*. **a. hemate,** a compound of ammonia and hematein, used as a violet-black stain for microscopic specimens.

ammoniac (ah-mo′ne-ak) [L. *ammoniacum*] a fetid gum-resin, stimulant and expectorant, from a Persian umbelliferous plant, *Dorema ammoniacum*, used in bronchitis and asthma. Ammoniac plaster and plaster of ammoniac and mercury are used as counterirritants in pleurisy and rheumatism.

ammoniacal (am″o-ni′ah-kal) containing ammonia or treated with excess ammonia.

ammonia lyase (ah-mo′ne ah-li′ās) [EC 4.3.1] a sub-subclass of enzymes of the lyase class that catalyze the formation of a C≡C bond in a molecule by liberation of ammonia, e.g., histidine ammonia-lyase.

ammoniate (ah-mo′ne-āt) 1. to treat or to combine with ammonia. 2. the product of combination with ammonia.

ammoniemia (ah-mo″ne-e′me-ah) hyperammonemia.

ammonification (ah-mo″nĭ-fi-ka′shun) the formation of ammonia by the action of bacteria on proteins.

ammonirrhea (am″o-nĭ-re′ah) [*ammonia* + *-rrhea*] the excretion of ammonia in the urine or sweat.

ammonium (ah-mo′ne-um) the hypothetical radical, NH_4; it forms salts analogous to those of the alkaline metals. **a. acetate,** a crystal compound with an acetous odor, NH_4-$C_2H_3O_2$, formerly used as a diaphoretic; in veterinary medicine it is used as a diuretic, diaphoretic, antipyretic, and as a vehicle. **a. alum,** see *alum*, def. 1. **a. benzoate,** a white crystalline salt, $C_6H_5 \cdot CO \cdot ONH_4$, stimulant and diuretic. **a. bromide,** a sedative, NH_4Br, occurring as colorless crystals or a yellowish white crystalline powder; used occasionally in treatment of grand mal seizures. See also *bromides*. **a. carbonate** [NF], a mixture of ammonium bicarbonate and ammonium carbamate in varying proportions, used as a source of ammonia and as an expectorant. It is also used as an ingredient of aromatic ammonia spirit and of smelling salts. Called also *sal volatilis* or *volatile*. **a. chloride** [USP], a systemic acidifying agent and diuretic administered orally or by intravenous infusion. It also has been used as an expectorant. Called also *a. muriate*. **ferric a. citrate, brown,** a preparation containing 16.5 to 18.5 per cent iron, about 9 per cent ammonia, and about 65 per cent hydrated citric acid; formerly used in treatment of iron deficiency anemia. Called also *iron and ammonium citrate*. **ferric a. citrate, green,** a preparation containing 14.5 to 16 per cent iron, about 7.5 per cent ammonia, and about 75 per cent hydrated citric acid; formerly used in treatment of iron deficiency anemia. **a. ferric sulfate, ferric a. sulfate,** pale violet crystals, $FeNH_4(SO_4)_2 \cdot 12H_2O$, very soluble in water, used as a reagent. It has also been used as an astringent, styptic, and an *in vitro* diagnostic aid in phenylketonuria. **a. ferric tartrate, ferric a. tartrate,** reddish brown transparent scales used as a hematinic in iron deficiency anemia; called also *iron and ammonium tartrate*. **a. ferrous sulfate, ferrous a. sulfate,** pale bluish green crystals or granules, $(NH_4)_2(SO_4)_2 \cdot 6H_2O$, soluble in water, used as a reagent. **a. hypophosphite,** white powder or colorless crystals, $NH_4H_2PO_2$, formerly used as an expectorant. **a. ichthyolate,** a reddish brown viscous fluid used like ichthammol. **a. ichthyosulfonate,** ichthammol. **a. iodide,** an odorless compound, NH_4I, occurring as minute, colorless, cubic crystals or as a white granular powder, with a sharp salty taste; formerly used as an expectorant. **a. mandelate,** the ammonium salt of mandelic acid, $C_8H_{11}NO_3$, used orally as a urinary anti-infective. **a. muriate,** a. chloride. **a. nitrate,** a colorless crystalline or white granular compound, NH_4NO_3, readily soluble in water and soluble in 20 parts of alcohol. Used in making nitrous oxide gas; formerly used as a diuretic and urine acidifier. **a. oxalate,** $(NH_4)_2C_2O_4 + H_2O$; used as a test solution. **a. persulfate,** a colorless crystalline substance, $(NH_4)_2S_2O_8$; formerly used as a deodorant and disinfectant. **a. phosphate,** a compound occurring in colorless translucent prisms, $(NH_4)_2HPO_4$ and $NH_4H_2PO_4$; formerly used in gout and rheumatism. **a. purpurate,** murexide. **a. rhodanilate,** a reagent for proline; it is $NH_4[Cr(CNS)_4(C_6H_4 \cdot NH_2)_2]$. **a. salicylate,** an odorless compound, $C_7H_5NH_4O_3$, occurring as colorless lustrous prisms or plates, or as a faintly pink crystalline powder; formerly used as an analgesic. **a. sulfoichthyolate,** ichthammol. **a. valerate,** a sedative, $CH_3(CH_2)_3$-$COONH_4$.

ammoniuria (ah-mo″ne-u′re-ah) [*ammonia* + *-uria*] an excess of ammonia in the urine.

ammonolysis (am″o-nol′ĭ-sis) a process analogous to hydrolysis, but in which ammonia takes the place of water, resulting in attachment of (or replacement by) an amino group, NH_2.

ammonotelic (ah-mo″no-tel′ik) [*ammonia* + Gr. *telikos* belonging to the completion, or end] having ammonia as the chief excretory product of nitrogen metabolism, as in fresh-water fishes.

Ammospermophilus (am″mo-sper-mof′ĭ-lus) a genus (or subgenus) of desert ground squirrels of western North America. **A. leucu′rus,** the desert antelope ground squirrel, which is a natural host of the plague-transmitting flea, *Thrassis francisi*.

ammotherapy (am″o-ther′ah-pe) [Gr. *ammos* sand + *therapeia* healing] (*obs.*) treatment of disease by the sand bath.

amnalgesia (am″nal-je′ze-ah) [*amn*esia + *algesia*] a technique by which all pain and memory of a potentially painful procedure are abolished, involving the use of drugs or, for minor procedures, hypnosis.

amnemonic (am″ne-mon′ik) [*a* neg. + Gr. *mnēmē* a remembrance, record] (*obs.*) pertaining to, characterized by, or causing loss of memory.

amnesia (am-ne′ze-ah) [Gr. *amnēsia* forgetfulness] lack or loss of memory; inability to remember past experiences. **anterograde a.,** impairment of memory for events occurring after the onset of amnesia; inability to form new memories. Cf. *retrograde a.* **auditory a.,** word deafness. **Broca's a.,** inability to remember spoken words. **circumscribed a.,** loss of memory for all events during a circumscribed period of time. Called also *localized a.* **continuous a.,** loss of memory for all events after a certain time continuing up to the present. **emotional a.,** amnesia which is primarily emotional in origin, as in certain hysterical or dissociative states following intolerable emotional stress. **episodic a.,** amnesia for a particular episode or a small area of experience. **generalized a.,** loss of memory encompassing the individual's entire life. **infantile a.,** the usual inability to recall the events of infancy and early childhood. **lacunar a.,** partial loss of memory; amnesia for certain isolated experiences. **localized a.,** 1. circumscribed a. 2. lacunar a. **olfactory a.,** loss of memory for smell. **organic a.,** amnesia due to organic lesions; see *amnestic syndrome,* under *syndrome.* **postconcussional a.,** amnesia resulting from a concussion of the brain. **posthypnotic a.,** a directed forgetfulness of the subject for experiences undergone while he was in the hypnotic state. **post-traumatic a.,** amnesia resulting from concussion or other head trauma. Called also *traumatic a.* See *amnestic syndrome,* under *syndrome.* **psychogenic a.,** [DSM III-R], a dissociative disorder characterized by a sudden loss of memory for important personal information, usually circumscribed or selective amnesia, rarely generalized or continuous amnesia, and which is not due to an organic mental disorder; the amnesia may follow severe psychological stress or may be an unconscious response to internal conflicts or an intolerable life situation; complete recovery of memory almost always occurs. **retrograde a.,** inability to recall events that occurred before the actual onset of amnesia; loss of memories of past events. Cf. *anterograde a.* **selective a.,** loss of memory for a group of related events but not for other events occurring during the same period of time. **tactile a.,** astereognosis. **transient global a.,** an episode of short-term memory loss, usually nonrecurrent, and lasting a few hours, without other signs or symptoms of neurological impairment; the cause is unknown but may involve an ischemic or epileptic attack. **traumatic a.,** post-traumatic a. **verbal a.,** loss of memory for words. **visual a.,** alexia.

amnesiac (am-ne′se-ak) a person affected with amnesia.

amnesic (am-ne′sik) affected with or characterized by amnesia.

amnestic (am-nes′tik) 1. amnesic. 2. causing amnesia.

Amnestrogen (am-nes′tro-jen) trademark for a preparation of esterified estrogens.

amni(o)- [*amnion,* q.v.] a combining form denoting relationship to the amnion.

amniocele (am′ne-o-sēl) omphalocele.

amniocentesis (am″ne-o-sen-te′sis) percutaneous transabdominal puncture of the uterus to obtain amniotic fluid.

amniochorial (am″ne-o-ko′re-al) pertaining to the amnion and chorion.

Amniocolidae (am″ne-o-kol′ĭ-de) Hydrobiidae.

amniocyte (am′ne-o-sīt) a cell of fetal origin obtained in an amniotic fluid specimen.

amniogenesis (am″ne-o-jen′ĕ-sis) [*amnio-* + Gr. *genesis* formation] the development of the amnion.

amniography (am″ne-og′rah-fe) [*amnio-* + Gr. *graphein* to record] roentgenography of the gravid uterus after injection of opaque media into the amniotic fluid, outlining the amniotic cavity and fetus.

amnion (am′ne-on) [Gr. "bowl"; "membrane enveloping the fetus"] the thin but tough extraembryonic membrane of reptiles, birds, and mammals that lines the chorion and contains the fetus and the amniotic fluid around it; in mammals it is derived from trophoblast by folding or splitting. **a. nodo′sum,** multiple focal lesions of the amnion, consisting of masses of adherent amniotic squamae partially invaded by amniotic mesoderm; a nodular condition of the fetal surface of the amniotic membrane.

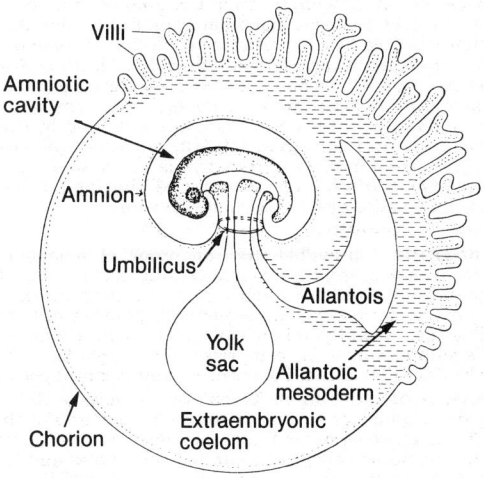

Amnion, chorion, and other embryonic membranes surrounding the embryo of a placental mammal.

amnionic (am″ne-on′ik) amniotic.

amnionitis (am″ne-o-ni′tis) inflammation of the amnion.

Amnioplastin (am-ne-o-plas′tin) trademark for the dried and sterilized amnionic membrane applied to prevent adhesions after craniotomy.

amniorrhea (am″ne-o-re′ah) [*amnion* + Gr. *rhoia* flow] the escape of the amniotic fluid, or liquor amnii.

amniorrhexis (am″ne-o-rek′sis) [*amnion* + Gr. *rhēxis* rupture] rupture of the amnion.

amnioscope (am′ne-o-skōp″) an endoscope that, by introduction into the cervical canal, permits direct visualization of the fetus and the amniotic fluid.

amnioscopy (am″ne-os′ko-pe) direct observation of the fetus and the color and amount of the amniotic fluid by means of a specially designed endoscope inserted through the uterine cervix.

Amniota (am-ne-o′tah) a major group of vertebrates comprising those which develop an amnion, including reptiles, birds, and mammals; opposed to Anamniota.

amniote (am′ne-ōt) any animal or group belonging to the Amniota.

amniotic (am″ne-ot′ik) pertaining to or developing an amnion.

Amniotin (am-ni′o-tin) trademark for estrogens derived from the urine of pregnant mares.

amniotome (am′ne-o-tōm″) [*amnion* + Gr. *tomē* a cutting] an instrument for cutting the fetal membranes.

amniotomy (am″ne-ot′o-me) [*amnion* + Gr. *tomē* a cutting] deliberate rupture of the fetal membranes to induce labor.

amobarbital (am″o-bar′bĭ-tal) [USP] chemical name: 5-ethyl-5-(methylbutyl)-2,4,6(1H,3H,5H)-pyrimidinetrione. An intermediate-acting barbiturate, $C_{11}H_{18}N_2O_3$, occurring as a white, crystalline powder; used orally as a sedative and hypnotic. Called also *amylobarbitone* and *isoamylethylbarbituric acid.* **a. sodium** [USP], the monosodium salt of ammobarbital, $C_{11}H_{17}N_2NaO_3$, occurring as a white, friable, granular powder; administered orally, intravenously, and intramuscularly as a hypnotic and sedative.

amodiaquine hydrochloride (am″o-di′ah-kwin) [USP] chemical name: 4-[(7-chloro-4-quinolinyl)amino]-2-[(diethylamino)-methyl]-phenol dihydrochloride dihydrate. An antimalarial, $C_{20}H_{22}ClN_3O \cdot 2HCl \cdot 2H_2O$, occurring as a yellow, crystalline powder, whose activity is limited to the asexual erythrocytic forms of plasmodia; administered orally.

amoeb-, amoebi-, amoebo- [L., from Gr. *amoibē* change] a combining form denoting relationship to an ameba. See also words beginning *ameb(i)(o)-.*

Amoeba (ah-me′bah) [L. from Gr. *amoibē* change] a genus of ameboid protozoa (suborder Tubulina, order Amoebida), characterized by the presence of a vesicular nucleus, usually one contractile vacuole, and lobopodia. Most are free living. Those parasitic in humans and once included in this genus have been assigned to other genera. **A. pro′teus,** a species found in fresh water and widely studied in the laboratory. **A. uri′nae granula′ta,** an ameba-like cell found in the urine in cases of infective jaundice with proteinuria. **A. verruco′sa,** an ameba-like cell having a large knobby nucleus and a deeply staining nucleolus.

amoeba (ah-me′bah) ameba.

Amoebida (ah-me′bid-ah) an order of ameboid, largely freshwater protozoa (subclass Gymnamoebia, class Lobosea) containing all of the amebae parasitic in animals, including humans, most of which are nonpathogenic or only mildly so. They are typically uninucleate and have mitochondria but no flagellate stage. It comprises five suborders: Tubulina, Thecina, Flabellina, Conopodina, and Acanthopodina.

Amoebobacter (ah-me″bo-bak′ter) [*ameba* + Gr. *baktron* a rod] a genus of aquatic phototrophic bacteria of the family Chromatiaceae, order Rhodospirillales, consisting of spherical nonmotile cells that contain gas vacuoles and fix carbon dioxide in the presence of hydrogen sulfide. Cell suspensions are pink to purple. The type species is *A. ro′seus.*

Amoebotaenia (ah-me″bo-te′ne-ah) a tapeworm parasitic in chickens.

amoebula (ah-me′bu-lah) [dim. of *amoeba*] amebula.

amok (ah-mok′) [Malay "furious attack"] a culture-specific syndrome seen almost exclusively in the Malay people consisting of a sudden, unprovoked outburst of indiscriminate homicidal fury (running amuck). Spelled also *amuck.*

Amomum (ah-mo′mum) [L.; Gr. *amōmon*] a genus of perennial herbs of the ginger family native to tropical Asia; its seeds are used as a substitute for cardamom (q.v.).

amopyroquin hydrochloride (am-o-pi′ro-kwin) chemical name: 4-[(7-chloro-4-quinolyl)amino]-α-1-pyrrolidinyl-*o*-cresol dihydrochloride; an antimalarial drug.

amorph (ah′morf) see *silent gene,* under *gene.*

amorpha (ah-mor′fah) [*a* neg. + Gr. *morphē* form] diseases that evince no definite structural changes.

amorphia (ah-mor′fe-ah) [*a* neg. + Gr. *morphē* form + *-ia*] the fact or quality of being amorphous.

amorphism (ah-mor′fizm) amorphia.

Amorphosporangium (a-mor″fo-spo-ran′je-um) [Gr. *amorphos* without form + *spora* spore + *angeion* vessel] a genus of soil bacteria of the family Actinoplanaceae, order Actinomycetales, consisting of cells bearing irregular, lobed sporangia. The type species is *A. auran′ticolor.*

amorphous (ah-mor′fus) [*a* neg. + Gr. *morphē* form] having no definite form; shapeless; having no specific orientation of atoms; in pharmacy, not crystallized.

amorphus (ah-mor′fus) [*a* neg. + Gr. *morphē* form] a shapeless monster.

Amoss' sign (a′mos) [Harold Lindsay *Amoss,* American physician, 1886–1956] see under *sign.*

amotio (ah-mo′she-o), gen. *amotinonis,* pl. *amotiones* [L., from *amovēre* to move away from] a removing. **a. re′tinae,** detachment of the retina.

amoxapine (ah-moks′ah-pēn) chemical name: 2-chloro-11-(1-piperazinyl)dibenz[*b,f*] [1,4]oxazepine; an antidepressant, $C_{17}H_{16}ClN_3O$.

amoxicillin (ah-moks″ĭ-sil′in) [USP] a semisynthetic derivative of ampicillin, $C_{16}H_{19}N_3O_5S$, effective against a broad spectrum of gram-positive and gram-negative bacteria; used especially in the treatment of infections due to susceptible strains of *Haemophilus influenzae, Escherichia coli, Proteus mirabilis, Neisseria gonorrhoeae,* streptococci (including *S. faecalis* and *S. pneumoniae*), and nonpenicillinase-producing staphylococci. It is administered orally.

Amoxil (ah-moks′il) trademark for a preparation of amoxicillin.

AMP adenosine monophosphate. **cyclic AMP,** adenosine 3′:5′-cyclic phosphate.

amp. ampere.

AMP deaminase (de-am′ĭ-nās) [EC 3.5.4.6] an enzyme of the hydrolase class that catalyzes the reaction $AMP + H_2O$ = inosine monophosphate + NH_3. Isoenzyme A (myoadeny-late deaminase) is present in large amounts in muscle tissue and is a major source of ammonium ions during muscle contraction. Genetic deficiency of this isoenzyme, an autosomal recessive trait, is characterized by muscle fatigue following exercise. Two additional isoenzymes have been identified; isoenzyme B, found in liver, kidney and testes, and isoenzyme C, found in heart muscle. Called also *adenylic acid deaminase* and *adenylate deaminase.*

amperage (am′per-ij) the strength of an electric current expressed in amperes or milliamperes.

ampere (am′pēr) [André M. *Ampère,* 1775–1836] the unit of electric current: in SI, the amount of current that carries a charge of 1 coulomb through a conductor in 1 second; in the MKS system, the current produced by 1 volt acting through a resistance of 1 ohm. The international ampere is the unvarying electrical current which, when passed through a solution of silver nitrate in accordance with certain specifications, deposits silver at the rate of 0.001118 gm. per second. Abbreviated a. or amp.

ampheclexis (am″fĕ-klek′sis) [Gr. *amphi* on both sides + *eklexis* selection] sexual selection on the part of both male and female.

Amphedroxyn (am″fĕ-drok′sin) trademark for a preparation of methamphetamine.

amphetamine (am-fet′ah-min) 1. chemical name: (±)-α-methylphenethylamine. Racemic amphetamine; a sympathomimetic amine, $C_9H_{13}N$, occurring as a colorless mobile liquid; has a stimulating effect on both the central and peripheral nervous systems. It relaxes both systolic and diastolic blood pressure and bronchial muscle, contracts the sphincter of the urinary bladder, and depresses the appetite. Abuse of this drug and its salts may lead to dependence, characterized by strong psychic dependence, to marked tolerance, and to mild physical dependence associated with tachycardia, increased blood pressure, restlessness, irritability, insomnia, personality changes, and in the severe form of chronic intoxication, psychosis similar to schizophrenia. Abrupt withdrawal can cause severe fatigue, mental depression, and abnormalities in the electroencephalogram. 2. [pl.] a group of closely related compounds having similar actions, including both racemic amphetamine and its salts, dextroamphetamine, and methamphetamine. **a. phosphate,** a white, crystalline powder, $C_9H_{16}NO_4P$, having the same actions and uses as the sulfate salt; administered orally and parenterally. **a. sulfate** [USP], a white, crystalline powder, $C_{18}N_{28}N_2H_2O_4S$, having the same actions as the base, used chiefly for its central stimulant effects in the treatment of mental depression, psychopathic states, narcolepsy, hyperkinetic behavior disorders in children, and exogenous obesity; administered orally. **a. sulfate, dextro,** dextroamphetamine.

amph(i)- [Gr. *amphi* on both sides] a prefix meaning on both sides; around or about; double.

amphiarkyochrome (am″fe-ar′ke-o-krōm″) [*amphi-* + Gr. *arkys* net + *chrōma* color] a nerve cell, the stainable portion of whose body is a pale network, of which the nodal points are joined by a readily and intensely stainable network.

amphiarthrodial (am″fe-ar-thro′de-al) pertaining to amphiarthrosis.

amphiarthrosis (am″fe-ar-thro′sis) [*amphi-* + Gr. *arthrōsis* joint] a form of articulation permitting little motion, the apposed surfaces of bone being connected by fibrocartilage; called also *junctura cartilaginea* [NA].

amphiaster (am″fe-as″ter) [*amphi-* + Gr. *astēr* star] the figure of achromatin fibers formed in karyokinesis, consisting of two asters joined by a spindle; called also *diaster.*

Amphibia (am-fib′e-ah) [*amphi-* + Gr. *bios* life] a class of vertebrate animals that breathe by means of gills in the larval state, but after metamorphosis generally breathe by means of lungs; it includes frogs, toads, newts, and salamanders.

amphibious (am-fib′e-us) [see *Amphibia*] capable of living both on land and in water.

amphiblastic (am″fe-blas′tik) [*amphi-* + Gr. *blastos* germ] denoting the complete but unequal cleavage of a telolecithal egg.

amphiblastula (am″fe-blas′tu-lah) [*amphi-* + *blastula*] a blastula with unequal blastomeres.

amphibolia (am″fe-bo′le-ah) [Gr. *amphibolia* uncertainty] (*obs.*) a term used to describe the course of an untreatable febrile disease at a stage before its outcome was clear.

amphibolic (am″fe-bol′ik) uncertain; vacillating; of doubtful prognosis; see under *stage.*

amphicarcinogenic (am″fe-kar″sĭ-no-jen′ik) tending, optionally, to increase or to decrease carcinogenic activity.

amphicelous (am″fe-se′lus) [*amphi-* + Gr. *koilos* hollow] concave at both ends; a term usually applied to the hollow-ended vertebral centra of certain cold-blooded vertebrates.

amphicentric (am″fe-sen′trik) [*amphi-* + Gr. *kentron* center] beginning and ending in the same vessel, as a branch of a rete mirabile.

amphichroic (am″fe-kro′ik) [*amphi-* + Gr. *chrōma* color] exhibiting two colors; affecting both red and blue litmus.

amphichromatic (am″fe-kro-mat′ik) amphichroic.

amphicreatine (am″fe-kre′ah-tin) [*amphi-* + *creatine*] a leukomaine, $C_9H_{19}N_7O_4$, from muscle, occurring in the form of opaque yellowish white crystals.

amphicreatinine (am″fe-kre-at′ĭ-nin) [*amphi-* + *creatinine*] a poisonous leukomaine, $C_9H_{19}N_4O_4$, from muscle.

amphicroic (am″fe-kro′ik) [*amphi-* + Gr. *krouein* to test] amphichroic.

amphicyte (am′fe-sīt) [*amphi-* + Gr. *kytos* hollow vessel] a satellite cell, def. 1.

amphicytula (am″fe-sit′u-lah) [*amphi-* + *cytula*] a fertilized telolecithal ovum.

amphidiarthrosis (am″fe-di″ar-thro′sis) [*amphi-* + *diarthrosis*] a joint having the nature of both a ginglymus and arthrodia, as the articulation of the lower jaw.

amphigastrula (am″fe-gas′tru-lah) [*amphi-* + *gastrula*] a gastrula composed of cells unequal in size in its upper and lower hemispheres.

amphigenetic (am″fe-jĕ-net′ik) produced by means of both sexes, as *amphigenetic* reproduction.

amphigonadism (am″fe-gon′ah-dizm) possession of both ovarian and testicular tissue; true hermaphroditism.

amphigony (am-fig′o-ne) sexual reproduction.

amphikaryon (am″fe-kar′e-on) [*amphi-* + Gr. *karyon* kernel] a diploid nucleus.

amphileukemic (am″fe-lu-ke′mik) [*amphi-* + *leukemic*] showing leukemic changes which vary in degree with the changes in the organ.

Amphimerus (am-fim′er-us) a genus of trematodes. *A. nover′ca* is a biliary-duct parasite of dogs and foxes and occasionally of hogs and man. *A. pseudofelin′eus* infects cats and coyotes in the central United States.

amphimorula (am″fe-mor′u-lah) [*amphi-* + *morula*] the morula resulting from unequal cleavage, the cells of the two hemispheres being of unequal size.

amphinucleus (am″fe-nu′kle-us) [*amphi-* + *nucleus*] a nucleus that consists of a single body made of spindle fibers and centrosome, around which the chromatin is massed; it is the ordinary form of protozoan nucleus. Called also *centronucleus.*

Amphioxus (am″fe-ok′sus) a primitive fishlike marine chordate, considered similar to the ancestor of the vertebrates.

amphipath (am′fe-path) a molecule showing amphipathic properties.

amphipathic (am″fe-path′ik) of or relating to molecules containing groups with characteristically different properties, e.g., both hydrophilic and hydrophobic properties.

amphipyrenin (am″fe-pi′re-nin) [*amphi-* + Gr. *pyrēn* stone of a fruit] the substance of the nuclear membrane of a cell.

Amphistoma, Amphistomum (am-fis′to-mah, am-fis′to-mum) [*amphi-* + Gr. *stoma* mouth] a genus of parasitic trematode worms, many species of which have been reassigned to other genera. **A. con′icum,** *Paramphistomum cervi.* **A. hom′inis,** *Gastrodiscoides hominis.* **A. wat-so′ni,** *Watsonius watsoni.*

amphistome (am-fis′tōm) a fluke having the ventral sucker near the posterior end, usually found in the rumen or intestine of herbivorous mammals. The genera *Paramphistomum* and *Watsonius* include most of the medically important amphistomes.

amphistomiasis (am″fe-sto-mi′ah-sis) the condition of being infected with trematodes of the genus *Amphistoma* or of the family Paramphistomidae.

amphitene (am″fĕ-tēn) zygotene.

amphitheater (am″fe-the′ah-ter) an operating room or lecture room with seats arranged in tiers for students or spectators.

amphitrichous (am-fit′rĕ-kus) [*amphi-* + Gr. *thrix* hair] having a single flagellum, or a single tuft of flagella, at each end; said of a bacterial cell. See *flagellum.*

amphitypy (am-fit′ĭ-pe) the condition of showing both types.

ampho- [Gr. *amphō* both] a prefix meaning both.

amphochromatophil (am″fo-kro-mat′o-fil) 1. amphophil. 2. amphophilic.

amphochromophil (am″fo-kro′mo-fil) [*ampho-* + Gr. *chrōma* color + *philein* to love] 1. amphophil. 2. amphophilic.

amphocyte (am′fo-sīt) an amphophilic cell.

amphodiplopia (am″fo-dĭ-plo′pe-ah) [*ampho-* + *diplopia*] double vision in both eyes.

amphogenic (am″fo-jen′ik) [*ampho-* + Gr. *gennan* to produce] producing offspring of both sexes.

Amphojel (am′fo-jel) trademark for a preparation of aluminum hydroxide gel.

ampholyte (am′fo-līt) [*ampho-* + *electrolyte*] an amphoteric electrolyte.

amphomycin (am-fo-mi′sin) an antibiotic substance produced by *Streptomyces canus.*

amphophil (am′fo-fil) 1. a cell that stains readily with acid or basic dyes; an amphophilic cell. Called also *amphochromatophil* and *amphochromophil.* 2. amphophilic.

amphophile (am′fo-fīl″) denoting cells of the adenohypophysis that are thought to be actively secreting: the lightly granulated acidophils and basophils.

amphophilic (am-fo-fil′ik) [*ampho-* + Gr. *philein* to love] stainable with either acid or basic dyes. **a.-basophils,** staining with both acid and basic stains, but having a greater affinity for basic ones. **gram-a.,** tending to stain both positive and negative with Gram stain. **a.-oxyphil,** staining with both acid and basic dyes, but having a greater affinity for the acid ones.

amphophilous (am-fof′i-lus) amphophilic.

amphoric (am-for′ik) [L. *amphoricus,* from L. *amphora,* Gr. *amphoreus* jar] pertaining to a bottle; resembling the sound made by blowing across the mouth of a bottle, particularly such a sound resulting from percussion or a breath sound heard over a cavity in the lung.

amphoricity (am″fo-ris′ĭ-te) the condition of giving off amphoric sounds on percussion or auscultation.

amphoriloquy (am″fo-ril′o-kwe) [L. *amphora* jar + *loqui* to speak] the production of amphoric sounds in speaking.

amphorophony (am″fo-rof′o-ne) [Gr. *amphoreus* jar + *phonē* voice] an amphoric sound of the voice.

amphoteric (am-fo-ter′ik) [Gr. *amphoteros* pertaining to both] having opposite characters; capable of acting either as an acid or as a base; combining with both acids and bases; affecting both red and blue litmus.

amphotericin B (am″fo-ter′ĭ-sin) [USP] one of two antifungal antibiotics, the other designated amphotericin A (not used clinically), derived from a strain of *Streptomyces nodosus,* $C_{47}H_{73}NO_{17}$; administered by intravenous infusion in the treatment of systemic fungal infections, such as aspergillosis, histoplasmosis, cryptococcosis, coccidioidomycosis, etc. It may also be applied topically to the skin in lotion or cream in the treatment of candidiasis and related infections.

amphotericity (am″fo-ter-is′ĭ-te) amphoterism.

amphoterism (am-fo′ter-izm) the condition or quality of possessing both basic and acid properties.

amphoterodiplopia (am-fot″er-o-dĭ-plo′pe-ah) [Gr. *amphoteros* both + *diplopia*] amphodiplopia.

amphoterous (am-fot′er-us) amphoteric.

amphotony (am-fot′o-ne) [*ampho-* + Gr. *tonos* tension] a condition in which both sympathicotonia and vagotony are said to exist; hypertonia of the entire sympathetic nervous system.

ampicillin (amp″ĭ-sil′in) [USP] chemical name: [2S-[2α,5α-6β(S*)]][(aminophenylacetyl) amino]-3,3-dimethyl-

7-oxo-4-thia-1-azabicyclo[3.2.0]heptane-2-carboxylic acid. A semisynthetic, acid-resistant penicillin, $C_{16}H_{19}N_3O_4S$, occurring as a white, crystalline powder, effective orally against many gram-negative and gram-positive bacteria; used mainly in the treatment of infections of the urinary tract and urinary system, and in chronic bronchial infections, especially those due to susceptible strains of *Shigella, Salmonella, Escherichia coli, Haemophilus influenzae, Proteus mirabilis,* and *Neisseria gonorrhoeae.* **a. sodium** [USP], **sodium a.,** the monosodium salt of ampicillin, $C_{16}H_{18}N_3NaO_4S$, having the same actions and uses as the base; administered intramuscularly or intravenously.

AMP kinase (ki′nās) adenylate kinase.

amplexation (am″plek-sa′shun) [L. *amplexus* embrace] treatment of fractured clavicle by an apparatus which fixes the shoulder and embraces the chest and neck.

amplexus (am-plek′sus) [L.] an embrace, as in the sexual clasping of the female by the male frog; see *pseudocopulation.*

amplification (am″plĭ-fĭ-ka′shun) [L. *amplifica′tio*] the process of making larger, as the increase of an auditory or visual stimulus, as a means of improving its perception. **image a.,** amplification of an image by means of an electron-image or electron multiplier tube.

amplifier (am′plĕ-fi″er) an electronic device that increases the strength of an input signal, or an apparatus for increasing the magnification of a microscope.

amplitude (am′plĕ-tūd) [L. *amplitudo*] largeness or fullness; wideness or breadth of range or extent. **a. of accommodation,** range of accommodation; see under *range.* **a. of convergence,** the difference in the power required to turn the eyes from their far point to their near point of convergence.

ampoule (am′pūl) ampule.

amprotropine phosphate (am″pro-tro′pēn) chemical name: α-(hydroxymethyl)benzeneacetic acid 3-(diethylamino)-2,2-dimethylpropyl ester phosphate. An anticholinergic, $C_{18}H_{32}NO_7$, occurring as a white, crystalline powder, which has been used as a spasmolytic to depress gastrointestinal motility.

ampul (am′pūl) ampule.

ampule (am′pūl) [Fr. *ampoule*] a small glass or plastic container capable of being sealed so as to preserve its contents in a sterile condition; used principally for containing sterile parenteral solutions.

ampulla (am-pul′lah), gen. and pl. *ampul′lae* [L. "a jug"] a general term used in anatomical nomenclature to designate a flasklike dilatation of a tubular structure. **anterior membranaceous a.,** a. membranacea anterior. **a. canali′culi lacrima′lis** [NA], ampulla of lacrimal canaliculus: a dilatation of a lacrimal canaliculus just before it opens into the lacrimal sac; called also *a. ductus lacrimalis.* **a. chy′li,** cisterna chyli. **a. duc′tus deferen′tis** [NA], the enlarged and tortuous distal end of the ductus deferens; called also *Henle's a.* and *a. of vas deferens.* **a. duc′tus lacrima′lis,** a. canaliculi lacrimalis. **duodenal a., a. duode′ni** [NA], duodenal cap: the superior part of the duodenum, as seen radiographically after a barium meal. A true duodenal ampulla is seen in some domestic mammals. **Henle′s a.,** a. ductus deferentis. **hepatopancreatic a., a. hepatopancreat′ica** [NA], the dilatation formed by junction of the common bile and the pancreatic ducts proximal to their opening into the lumen of the duodenum; called also *a. of Vater.* **a. of lacrimal canaliculus,** a. canaliculi lacrimalis. **ampul′lae lactif′erae,** sinus lactiferi. **lateral membranaceous a.,** a. membranacea lateralis. **Lieberkühn′s a.,** the termination of a lacteal in an intestinal villus. **ampul′lae membrana′ceae** [NA], membranaceous ampullae: the dilatations at one end of each of the three membranous semicircular ducts, each named according to the duct of which it forms a part. **a. membrana′cea ante′rior** [NA], anterior membranaceous ampulla: the dilatation at the end of the anterior membranous semicircular duct. **a. membrana′cea latera′lis** [NA], lateral membranaceous ampulla: the dilatation at the end of the lateral membranous semicircular duct. **a. membrana′cea poste′rior** [NA], posterior membranaceous ampulla: the dilatation at the end of the posterior membranous semicircular duct. **ampul′lae os′seae** [NA], osseous ampullae: the dilatations at one of the ends of the bony semicircular canals, each named according to the canal of which it forms a part, and

lodging the correspondingly named ampulla of a semicircular duct. **a. os′sea ante′rior** [NA], the dilatation at one end of the anterior semicircular canal; see *ampullae osseae.* **a. os′sea latera′lis** [NA], the dilatation at one end of the lateral semicircular canal; see *ampullae osseae.* **a. os′sea poste′rior** [NA], the dilatation at one end of the posterior semicircular canal; see *ampullae osseae.* **phrenic a.,** the dilatation at the lower end of the esophagus. **posterior membranaceous a.,** a. membranacea posterior. **rectal a., a. rec′ti** [NA], the dilated portion of the rectum just proximal to the anal canal. **a. of Thoma,** one of the small terminal expansions of an interlobar artery in the pulp of the spleen. **a. tu′bae uteri′nae** [NA], a. of uterine tube: the thin-walled, almost muscle-free, midregion of the uterine tube; its mucosa is greatly plicated. **a. of uterine tube,** a. tubae uterinae. **a. of vas deferens,** a. ductus deferentis. **a. of Vater,** a. hepatopancreatica.

ampullae (am-pul′e) [L.] plural of *ampulla.*

ampullar (am-pul′ar) pertaining to an ampulla, especially to the ampulla hepatopancreatica.

Ampullariella (am″pul-la″re-el′ah) [L., dim. of *ampullarius* bottlemaker] a genus of soil bacteria of the family Actinoplanaceae, order Actinomycelales, consisting of cells bearing bottle- or flask-shaped sporangia. The type species is *A. regular′is.*

ampullary (am′pu-la″re) ampullar.

ampullate (am-pul′āt) flask shaped.

ampullitis (am″pul-li′tis) inflammation of an ampulla, especially of the ampulla ductus deferentis.

ampullula (am-pul′u-lah) [L.] any minute ampulla, like many of those of the lymphatic and lacteal vessels.

amputation (am″pu-ta′shun) [L. *amputare* to cut off, or to prune] the removal of a limb or other appendage or outgrowth of the body. **above-knee (A-K) a.,** amputation of the leg in which the femur is divided in the supracondylar region, at midthigh, or high on the thigh. **Alanson′s a.,** circular amputation, the stump being shaped like a hollow cone. **Alouette′s a.,** amputation at the hip, with a semicircular outer flap to the great trochanter and a large internal flap from within outward; called also *Alouette's operation.* **amniotic a.,** the alleged amputation of a fetal limb by a band of amnion. **aperiosteal a.,** amputation with complete removal of the periosteum from the end of the stump of the bone; called also *Bunge's a.* **Béclard′s a.,** amputation at the hip joint by cutting the posterior flap first. **below-knee (B-K) a.,** amputation of the lower leg in which the bone division is done a few centimeters distal to the tibial tuberosity. **Bier′s a.,** osteoplastic amputation of the leg with a bone flap cut out of the tibia and fibula above the stump; called also *Bier's operation.* **Bunge′s a.,** aperiosteal a. **Callander′s a.,** a tendoplastic amputation at the knee joint with long anterior and posterior flaps, the patella being removed to leave a fossa for the end of the divided femur. **Carden′s a.,** a single-flap operation, cutting through the femur just above the knee. **central a.,** one in which the scar is situated at or near the center of the stump. **chop a.,** amputation by a circular cut through the parts without the formation of a flap. **Chopart′s a.,** amputation of the foot, with the calcaneus, talus, and other parts of the tarsus being retained; called also *mediotarsal a.* **cinematic a., cineplastic a.,** kineplasty. **circular a.,** one performed by means of a single flap and by a circular cut in a direction vertical to the long axis of a limb. **closed a.,** one in which flaps are made from the skin and subcutaneous tissue and sutured over the end of the bone; called also *flap a.* **coat-sleeve a.,** a circular amputation, with a single skin flap made very long, the end being closed with a tape. **congenital a.,** the alleged amputation of a fetal limb *in utero* by a constricting band; called also *intrauterine a.* and *natural a.* **a. in contiguity,** an amputation at a joint. **a. in continuity,** an amputation elsewhere than at a joint. **cutaneous a.,** amputation in which the flaps are composed entirely of skin. **Dieffenbach′s a.,** see under *operation,* def. 1. **double-flap a.,** one in which two flaps are formed. **Dupuytren′s a.,** amputation of the arm at the shoulder joint; called also *Lisfranc's a.* **eccentric a.,** one in which the scar is not at the center of the stump. **elliptic a.,** one in which the cut has an elliptic outline on account of the oblique direction of the incision. **Farabeuf′s a.,** amputation of the leg, with a large external flap. **flap a.,** closed a. **flapless**

a., guillotine a. **forequarter a.,** interscapulothoracic a. **Gritti's a.,** amputation of the leg through the knee, using the patella as an osteoplastic flap over the end of the femur. **Gritti-Stokes a.,** a modification of Gritti's amputation, using an oval anterior flap; called also *Stoke's a.* or *operation.* **guillotine a.,** rapid amputation of a limb by a circular sweep of the knife and a cut of the saw, the entire cross-section being left open for dressing; done when primary closure of the stump is contraindicated, owing to the possibility of recurrent or developing infection. Called also *flapless a.* and *open a.* **Guyon's a.,** amputation above the malleoli. **Hancock's a.,** a modification of Pirogoff's amputation, a part of the astragalus (talus) being retained in the flap, the lower surface being sawed off, and the cut surface of the calcaneus being brought into contact with it; called also *Hancock's operation.* **Hey's a.,** disarticulation of the metatarsus from the tarsus, with removal of a part of the medial cuneiform bone; called also *Hey's operation.* **hindquarter a.,** interilioabdominal a. **interilioabdominal a., interinnominoabdominal a.,** amputation of an entire lower limb, including the whole or part of the hip bone; called also *hindquarter a.* **interpelviabdominal a.,** amputation of the thigh with excision of the lateral half of the pelvis; called also *Jaboulay's a.* or *operation.* **interscapulothoracic a.,** amputation of the upper extremity, including the scapula and the clavicle; called also *forequarter a.* **intrauterine a.,** congenital a. **Jaboulay's a.,** interpelviabdominal a. **kineplastic a.,** kineplasty. **Kirk's a.,** a tendoplastic amputation just above the femoral condyles, the tendon of the quadriceps femoris muscle being sutured over the end of the divided femur. **Langenbeck's a.,** amputation in which the flaps are cut from without inward. **Larrey's a.,** a method of disarticulation of the humerus at the shoulder joint by an incision extending from the acromion about three inches down the arm, splitting the deltoid muscle, and from this point going around the arm to the center of the axilla; called also *Larrey's operation.* **Le Fort's a.,** a modification of Pirogoff's amputation in which the calcaneus is sawed through horizontally instead of vertically. **linear a.,** amputation by a simple straight division of all the tissues. **Lisfranc's a.,** 1. Dupuytren's a. 2. a division of the foot between the tarsus and the metatarsus. **Mackenzie's a.,** amputation like that of Syme except that the flap is taken from the inner side of the ankle. **Maisonneuve's a.,** amputation by breaking the bone, followed by cutting of the soft parts. **major a.,** amputation of a leg above the ankle or of an arm above the wrist. **Malgaigne's a.,** subastragalar a. **mediotarsal a.,** Chopart's a. **minor a.,** amputation of a small part, as of a finger or toe. **mixed a.,** that which is performed by a combination of the circular and flap methods. **musculocutaneous a.,** one in which the flap consists of muscle and skin. **natural a.,** congenital a. **oblique a.,** oval a. **open a.,** guillotine a. **osteoplastic a.,** one in which the two severed surfaces of bone are brought into contact so as to unite. **oval a.,** one in which the incision consists of two reversed spirals; called also *oblique a.* and *loxotomy.* **periosteoplastic a.,** subperiosteal a. **phalangophalangeal a.,** amputation of a digit at a phalangeal joint. **Pirogoff's a.,** amputation of the foot at the ankle, part of the calcaneus being left in the lower end of the stump. **pulp a.,** pulpotomy. **racket a.,** one in which there is a single longitudinal incision continuous below with a spiral incision on each side of the limb. **rectangular a.,** one with a long and a short rectangular skin flap, as in Teale's amputation. **Ricard's a.,** intertibiocalcaneal disarticulation, astragalectomy, and the placing of the calcaneus in the tibiofibular mortise. **root a.,** excision of one root of a multirooted tooth, or two roots of upper molars; amputation of the root of a single-rooted tooth is called *apicoectomy,* and that of two roots of a two-rooted mandibular tooth is *hemisectomy.* Called also *radiectomy* and *radisectomy.* **spontaneous a.,** loss of a part which occurs without surgical intervention, as in leprosy, diabetes mellitus, and Buerger's disease. **Stokes' a.,** Gritti-Stokes a. **subastragalar a.,** amputation of the foot, leaving the astragalus (talus) in the lower end of the stump; called also *Malgaigne's a.* **subperiosteal a.,** one in which the cut end of the bone is covered with a flap of periosteum; called also *periosteoplastic a.* **Syme's a.,** amputation of the foot at the ankle joint with removal of both malleoli; called also *Syme's operation.* **Teale's a.,** amputation with preservation of a long rectangular flap of muscle and integument on

one side of the limb and a short rectangular flap on the other. **a. by transfixion,** one performed by thrusting a long knife through the limb and cutting the flaps from within outward. **traumatic a.,** amputation of a part by accidental injury. **Tripier's a.,** one like Chopart's, except that a part of the tarsus is removed. **Vladimiroff-Mikulicz a.,** osteoplastic resection of the foot with incision of the calcaneus and talus.

amputee (am″pu-te′) a person who has had one or more limbs amputated.

A.M.R.A. American Medical Record Association.

amrinone (am′rǐ-nōn) chemical name: 5-amino-[3,4′-bipyridin]-6(1*H*)-one; an oral cardiotonic, $C_{10}H_9N_3O$.

A.M.R.L. Aerospace Medical Research Laboratories.

A.M.S. American Meteorological Society.

ams. *amount of a substance.*

A.M.S.A. American Medical Student Association.

Amsler's chart, marker (ahm′zlerz) [Marc *Amsler,* Swiss ophthalmologist, 1891–1968] see under *chart* and *marker.*

Amsustain (am′sus-tān) trademark for a preparation of dextroamphetamine.

amu atomic mass unit.

amuck (ah-muk′) [Malay *amok*] 1. amok. 2. (*colloq.*) wild, frenzied, or uncontrollable.

amusia (ah-mu′ze-ah) [Gr. *amousia* want of harmony] inability to produce (*motor a.*) or to comprehend (*sensory a., tone deafness*) musical sounds (Knoblunch). **instrumental a.,** that in which the patient has lost the power of playing a musical instrument. **vocal motor a.,** that in which the patient cannot sing in tune.

Amussat's operation (am″oo-sahz′) [Jean Zuléma *Amussat,* French surgeon, 1796–1856] see under *operation.*

A.M.W.A. American Medical Women's Association; American Medical Writers' Association.

amychophobia (ah-mi″ko-fo′be-ah) [Gr. *amychē* a scratch + *phobia*] irrational fear of being scratched, as by the claws of a cat.

amyctic (ah-mik′tik) caustic or irritating.

amyelencephalia (ah-mi″el-en-seh-fa′le-ah) [*a* neg. + Gr. *myelos* marrow + *enkephalos* brain + *-ia*] congenital absence of both brain and spinal cord.

amyelencephalus (ah-mi″el-en-sef′ah-lus) a monster exhibiting amyelencephalia.

amyelia (ah″mi-e′le-ah) [*a* neg. + Gr. *myelos* marrow + *-ia*] congenital absence of spinal cord.

amyelic (ah″mi-el′ik) having no spinal cord.

amyelinic (ah-mi″ě-lin′ik) without myelin; having no medullary sheath.

amyelonic (ah-mi″ě-lon′ik) [*a* neg. + Gr. *myelos* marrow] 1. having no spinal cord. 2. having no bone marrow.

amyelotrophy (ah-mi″ě-lot′ro-fe) [*a* neg. + Gr. *myelos* marrow + *trophē* nourishment] atrophy of the spinal cord.

amyelus (ah-mi′e-lus) [*a* neg. + Gr. *myelos* marrow] a monster exhibiting amyelia.

amygdala (ah-mig′dah-lah) [Gr. *amygdalē* almond] a term used in anatomical nomenclature to designate an almond-shaped structure; often used alone to refer to the corpus amygdaloideum (see under *corpus*). **a. accesso′ria, accessory a.,** tonsilla lingualis. **a. ama′ra,** the bitter almond; see *almond.* **a. of cerebellum,** tonsilla cerebelli. **a. dul′cis,** the sweet almond of many varieties; see *almond.*

amygdalase (ah-mig′dah-lās) β-glucosidase.

amygdalic acid (ah-mig′dah-lik) mandelic acid.

amygdalin (ah-mig′dah-lin) chemical name: (*R*)-α-[(6-*O*-β-glucopyranosyl-β-D-glucopyranosyl) oxy] benzeneacetonitrile. A cyanogenetic glycoside, $C_6H_5CH(CN)\cdot O\cdot C_{12}H_{21}O_{10}$, characteristically found in seeds and other plant parts of members of the Rosaceae family, e.g., almonds. It is split by the enzyme emulsin into glucose, benzaldehyde, and hydrocyanic acid. The term is sometimes used interchangeably with *Laetrile.*

amygdaline (ah-mig′dah-lin″) [L. *amygdalinus*] 1. like an almond. 2. pertaining to a tonsil; tonsillar.

amygdal(o)- [Gr. *amygdalē* almond] a combining form denoting relationship to an almond-shaped structure or to the tonsil.

amygdaloid (ah-mig′dah-loid) [*amygdalo-* + Gr. *eidos* form] resembling an almond, or tonsil.

amygdalophenin (ah-mig″dah-lof′ĕ-nin) salicyl phenetidin, $C_6H_4(OC_2H_5)NH \cdot OC \cdot CH(OH)C_6H_5$.

amygdalose (ah-mig′dah-los) a disaccharide from amygdalin; it splits into two molecules of dextrose.

amyl (am′il) [Gr. *amylon* starch] the univalent radical, C_5-H_{11}. **a. acetate,** a colorless limpid liquid, the acetic acid ester of amyl alcohol, $CH_3 \cdot CO \cdot OC_5H_{11}$; it has the odor of bananas and is called *banana oil.* **a. chloride,** the colorless liquid, $C_5H_{11}Cl$, used as a solvent; formerly used as an anesthetic. **a. nitrite** [USP], a flammable, clear, yellowish liquid, $C_5H_{11}NO_2$, with a peculiar, ethereal, fruity odor, which is volatile at low temperatures; it is a vasodilator, administered by inhalation to relieve pain of anginal syndrome (angina pectoris, angina of effort) and of biliary colic, to relieve asthmatic paroxysms, to control convulsions, and in cyanide poisoning. Called also *isoamyl nitrite.* **a. salicylate,** a compound, $C_5H_{11} \cdot O_2C \cdot C_6H_4 \cdot OH$, formerly used locally as an analgesic.

amylaceous (am″ĭ-la′she-us) [L. *amylaceus*] starchy; containing starch; of the nature of starch.

amylase (am′ĭ-lās) an enzyme of the hydrolase class that catalyzes the hydrolysis of 1,4-α-glucosidic linkages in polysaccharides. α**-a.** [EC 3.2.1.1], an enzyme of the hydrolase class that catalyzes the hydrolysis of inner 1,4-α-D glucosidic linkages in polysaccharides containing three or more glucose residues, resulting in a mixture of linear and branched oligosaccharides. The enzyme is secreted by the salivary gland and pancreas of mammals. Called also *diastase, endo-amylase, glycogenase* and *ptyalin.* β**-a.** [EC 3.2.1.2], an enzyme of the hydrolase class that catalyzes the hydrolysis of 1,4-α-D-glycosidic linkages in polysaccharides to remove maltose units from the nonreducing ends of the chain. The enzyme occurs in plants and bacteria. Called also *diastase* and *exo-amylase.* γ **-a.,** glucan 1,4-α-glucosidase. **endo-a.,** one that attacks 1,4-α-D-glucosidic linkages in a random manner. See α*-amylase.* **exo-a.,** one that attacks 1,4-α-D-glycosidic linkages only from the non-reducing outer ends of the polysaccharide, releasing either maltose or β-D-glucose. See β- and γ*-amylase.* **pancreatic a.,** the α-amylase of the pancreas. **salivary a.,** α-amylase occurring in the saliva.

amylasuria (am″ĭ-lās-u′re-ah) an excess of amylase in the urine, a sign of pancreatitis.

Amylcaine Hydrochloride (am″il-kān hi″dro-klo′rīd) trademark for a preparation of naepaine.

amylemia (am″ĭ-le′me-ah) [Gr. *amylon* starch + *haima* blood + *-ia*] an excess of starch in the blood.

amylene (am′ĭ-lēn) chemical name: 2-methyl-2-butene. A flammable liquid hydrocarbon of five isomeric forms, C_5H_{10}, practically insoluble in water and miscible with alcohol and ether. It is an unsafe anesthetic. **a. chloral,** an oily colorless liquid, composed of chloral and amylene hydrate; formerly used as a hypnotic. **a. hydrate** [NF], chemical name: 2-methyl-2-butanol. A clear colorless liquid, with camphoraceous odor, $C_2H_5 \cdot C(CH_3)_2OH$; miscible with alcohol, chloroform, ether, and glycerin, it is used as a solvent in pharmaceutical preparations and also as an ingredient of *tribromoethanol solution* and as a hypnotic. Called also *a. alcohol.*

amylic (ah-mil′ik) [L. *amylicus*] pertaining to amyl.

amylin (am′ĭ-lin) amylopectin.

amylism (am′ĭ-lizm) poisoning by amylene hydrate.

amyl(o)- [Gr. *amylon* starch] a combining form denoting relationship to starch.

amylobarbitone (am″ĭ-lo-bar′bĭ-tōn) amobarbital.

amylocellulose (am″ĭ-lo-sel′u-lōs) amylose, def. 2.

amyloclastic (am″ĭ-lo-klas′tik) [*amylo-* + Gr. *klastikos* breaking up] digesting or splitting up starch.

amylocoagulase (am″ĭ-lo-ko-ag′u-lās) a ferment occurring in cereals which coagulates soluble starch.

amylodextrin (am″ĭ-lo-deks′trin) a compound colored yellow by iodine, formed during the change of starch into sugar.

amylodyspepsia (am″ĭ-lo-dis-pep′se-ah) [*amylo-* + *dyspepsia*] inability to digest starch-containing foods.

amylogen (ah-mil′o-jen) amylose, def. 2.

amylogenesis (am″ĭ-lo-jen′ĕ-sis) [*amylo-* + Gr. *gennan* to produce] the formation of starch.

amylogenic (am″ĭ-lo-jen′ik) producing starch.

amylo-1,6-glucosidase (am″ĭ-lo-gloo-ko′sĭ-dās, gloo-ko-sīd′ās) [EC 3.2.1.33] an enzyme of the hydrolase class that catalyzes the hydrolysis of interior 1,6-α-D-glucoside linkages at points of branching in chains of 1,4-linked α-D-glucose residues. In mammals it also has a 4-glucanotransferase site that transfer triglucoside residues to short chains, which can then be attacked by phosphorylase. The net result is the breakdown of glycogen to free glucose and glucose 1-phosphate. The enzyme occurs in muscle and liver. A genetic deficiency of the enzyme, carried as an autosomal recessive trait, results in glycogen storage disease III. Called also *debranching enzyme (glycogen).*

amylo-1,6-glucosidase deficiency glycogen storage disease, type III.

amylohemicellulose (am″ĭ-lo-hem″e-sel′u-lōs) a polysaccharide found in the cell wall of plants; it is much like the amylose of starch in that it is insoluble in water and stains blue with iodine.

amylohydrolysis (am″ĭ-lo-hi-drol′ĭ-sis) hydrolysis of starch; amylolysis.

amyloid (am′ĭ-loid) [*amylo-* + Gr. *-oid* form] 1. resembling starch; characterized by starchlike staining properties. 2. a substance produced by the action of sulfuric acid on cellulose, which gives a blue color when treated with iodine. 3. the pathologic extracellular proteinaceous substance deposited in amyloidosis. It is a waxy, amorphous, eosinophilic, hyaline-like material that exhibits a green birefringence under polarized light when stained with Congo red. Amyloid deposits are composed primarily of straight, nonbranching fibrils having a diameter of 7.5–10 nm and indefinite length aggregated in bundles or interlocked in a feltlike meshwork; each fibril is composed of identical polypeptide chains arranged in stacked antiparallel β-pleated sheets. There are two major biochemical types of amyloid protein: *amyloid light chain (AL) protein,* occurring in primary amyloidosis, is homologous to the variable region of either κ or λ immunoglobulin light chains; *amyloid A (AA) protein,* occurring in secondary amyloidosis, is antigenically related to a high-molecular-weight acute phase reactant, termed the *serum amyloid A (SAA) protein.* Other types occur in heredofamilial and localized amyloidosis.

amyloidosis (am″ĭ-loi-do′sis) [*amyloid-* + *-osis*] a group of conditions of diverse etiologies characterized by the accumulation of insoluble fibrillar proteins (amyloid) in various organs and tissues of the body such that vital function is compromised. The associated disease states may be inflammatory, hereditary, or neoplastic, and the deposition can be local or generalized or systemic. The most widely used classification is based on the chemistry of the amyloid fibrils and includes immunocyte-derived (primary or AL) and reactive systemic (secondary or AA) forms. Amyloidosis associated with multiple myeloma has been considered to be in a separate category because the pattern of tissue involvement resembles that of the primary type but the amyloidosis is secondary to a known cause. Also, since the hereditary forms of amyloidosis have their own distinctive pattern of organ involvement, they may constitute a separate, heterogenetic group. **AA a.,** reactive systemic a. **a. of aging,** senile a. **AL a.,** immunocyte-derived a. **cutaneous a.,** amyloidosis localized to the skin and usually associated with pruritus, which may be a characteristic of primary disease or occur in secondary amyloidosis. See *lichen a., macular a.,* and *nodular a.* **familial a.,** hereditary a. **hereditary a., heredofamilial a.,** a group of amyloidoses, usually found in limited geographic areas, and characterized by widespread tissue involvement indistinguishable from the reactive systemic form and by the presence of fibrillar proteins of the AA type. Most of these disorders have an autosomal dominant mode of inheritance, the exception being familial Mediterranean fever, which is an autosomal recessive condition. Based on the principal sites of amyloid deposition, it is classified in the following major subtypes: neuropathies, nephropathies, cardiopathies, and miscellaneous. Called also *AA a.* and *familial a.* **idiopathic a.,** primary a. **immunocyte-derived a.,** that in which the deposited fibrillar material is usually of the AL type and is most often systemic or generalized in distribution. It is a primary type of amyloidosis, usually involving the heart, tongue, carpal ligaments, peripheral nerves, gastrointestinal tract, and skin. Called also *AL a., light chain–related a.* and *primary a.* **immunocytic a.,** systemic amyloidosis in which the amyloid is composed of the AL protein derived from immunoglobulin light chains; this category includes amyloidosis associated with multiple myeloma and other plasma cell dyscrasias and primary amyloidosis. **lichen a.,** the most common form of cutaneous amyloidosis, characterized by the symmetrical distribution over the extensor surfaces of the lower extremities, thighs, dorsal feet, and lower back of translucent, yellow to brown, dome-shaped, discrete pruritic papules; the chest, shoulders, and skin of the abdominal walls may be involved later. Called also *lichen amyloidosus*. **light chain–related a.,** immunocyte-derived a. **macular a.,** cutaneous amyloidosis manifested by ill-defined, sometimes pruritic grayish brown macules distributed on the upper back, breasts, buttocks, arms, ankles, and thighs. **nodular a.,** a form of localized amyloidosis in which single or multiple, amyloid-containing nodular or tumefactive masses are found most often in the lung, urinary bladder, larynx, tongue, conjunctiva, and skin, especially that of the extremities, trunk, genitals, and face. **primary a.,** that in which no obvious predisposing condition is associated. The term is sometimes used synonymously with *immunocyte-derived amyloidosis*. Called also *idiopathic i.* See *immunocytic a.* **reactive systemic a.,** that in which the deposited fibrillar material is of the AA type, and occurs secondary to a chronic infectious process (e.g., tuberculosis and osteomyelitis) or a chronic noninfectious inflammatory disease (e.g., rheumatoid arthritis). It may also occur in association with certain nonlymphoid tumors and some nonimmunoglobulin-producing lymphomas, the two most common being renal cell carcinoma and Hodgkin's disease. See also *secondary a.* **secondary a.,** that occurring in association with or following a chronic inflammatory, infectious or noninfectious, disease. The term is sometimes used synonymously with *reactive systemic amyloidosis*. **senile a.,** that seen in the elderly and usually involving the heart, brain, pancreas, and spleen. Called also *a. of aging*.

amylolysis (am″ĭ-lol′ĭ-sis) [*amylo-* + Gr. *lysis* solution] the digestion and disintegration of starch, or its conversion into sugar; called also *amylohydrolysis*.

amylolytic (am″ĭ-lo-lit′ik) pertaining to, characterized by, or promoting amylolysis.

amylopectin (am″ĭ-lo-pek′tin) the insoluble constituent of starch; it stains violet red with iodine and forms a paste with hot water. The soluble constituent of starch is amylose. Called also *alpha-amylose, amylin, insoluble* or *tegumentary amidine,* and *starch cellulose.*

amylopectinosis (am″ĭ-lo-pek″tĭ-no′sis) glycogen storage disease, type IV; see under *disease.*

amylophagia (am″ĭ-lo-fa′je-ah) [*amylo-* + Gr. *phagein* to eat] starch eating; an abnormal craving for starch.

amyloplast (ah-mil′o-plast″) [*amylo-* + Gr. *plassein* to form] a starch-forming vegetable leuko-plastid.

amyloplastic (am″ĭ-lo-plas′tik) forming starch.

amylorrhea (am″ĭ-lo-re′ah) [*amylo-* + Gr. *rhoia* flow] the presence of an abnormal amount of starch in the stools.

amylorrhexis (am″ĭ-lo-rek′sis) [*amylo-* + Gr. *rhēxis* a breaking] the enzymatic hydrolysis of starch.

amylose (am′ĭ-lōs) 1. any carbohydrate of the starch group; a polysaccharide. 2. the soluble constituent of starch; it stains blue with iodine and does not form a paste with hot water. The other constituent is amylopectin. Called also *amidin, amylocellulose, amylogen,* and *granulose.* **alpha-a.** amylopectin.

amylosis (am″ĭ-lo′sis) amyloidosis.

amylosuria (am″ĭ-lo-su′re-ah) the presence of amylose in the urine.

amylosynthesis (am″ĭ-lo-sin′the-sis) the synthesis of starch from sugar.

amylo-1:4,1:6-transglucosidase (am″ĭ-lo-trans″gloo-kōs′ĭ-dās) 1,4-α-glucan branching enzyme.

amylo-1:4,1:6-transglucosidase deficiency glycogen storage disease, type IV.

Amylsine Hydrochloride (am′il-sin hi″dro-klo′-rīd) trademark for a preparation of naepaine.

amylum (am′ĭ-lum) [L.; Gr. *amylon*] starch. **a. ioda′tum,** iodized starch.

amyluria (am″ĭ-lu′re-ah) [*amylo-* + Gr. *ouron* urine + *-ia*] an excess of starch in the urine.

amyoesthesis (ah-mi″o-es-the′sis) [*a* neg. + Gr. *mys* muscle + *aisthēsis* sensation] the lack of muscle sense.

amyoplasia (ah-mi″o-pla′ze-ah) [*a* neg. + Gr. *mys* muscle + *plassein* to form] lack of muscle formation. **a. con-gen′ita,** a generalized lack of muscular development and growth, with contracture and deformity at most of the joints; called *congenital multiple arthrogryposis* and *arthrogryposis multiplex congenita.*

amyostasia (ah-mi″o-sta′ze-ah) [*a* neg. + Gr. *mys* muscle + *stasis* a standing still] a tremor of the muscles, seen especially in locomotor ataxia.

amyostatic (ah-mi″o-stat′ik) marked by amyostasia or muscular tremors.

amyosthenia (ah-mi″os-the′ne-ah) [*a* neg. + Gr. *mys* muscle + *sthenos* strength] muscular weakness.

amyosthenic (ah-mi″os-then′ik) pertaining to, characterized by, or causing amyosthenia.

amyotaxia (ah-mi″o-tak′se-ah) ataxia.

amyotaxy (ah-mi′o-tak′se) [*a* neg. + Gr. *mys* muscle + *tassein* to arrange] ataxia.

amyotonia (a″mi-o-to′ne-ah; ah-mi″o-to′ne-ah) [*a* neg. + Gr. *mys* muscle + *tonos* tension + *-ia*] atonic condition of the musculature of the body; called also *myatonia* and *myatony.* **a. congen′ita** (Oppenheim, 1900), a vague term denoting any of several rare congenital diseases of children marked by general hypotonia of the muscles; called also *congenital atonic pseudoparalysis, myatonia congenita,* and *Oppenheim's disease.*

amyotrophia (ah-mi″o-tro′fe-ah) [*a* neg. + Gr. *mys* muscle + *trophē* nourishment + *-ia*] amyotrophy. **neuralgic a.,** neuralgic amyotrophy. **a. spina′lis progressi′va,** progressive muscular atrophy.

amyotrophic (ah-mi″o-trof′ik) pertaining to or characterized by amyotrophy.

amyotrophy (ah″mi-ot′ro-fe) atrophy of muscle tissue. **diabetic a.,** progressive asymmetrical weakening and wasting of muscles accompanied by aching or stabbing pain, usually limited to the muscles of the pelvic girdle and thigh, and associated with uncontrolled diabetes. **neuralgic a.,** a condition characterized by pain across the shoulder and upper arm, with atrophy and paralysis of the muscles of the shoulder girdle.

amyous (am′e-us) [*a* neg. + Gr. *mys* muscle] deficient in muscular tissue.

amyrol (am′ĭ-rol) two isomeric principles, $C_5H_{26}O$, from sandalwood oil.

Amytal (am′ĭ-tal) trademark for amobarbital.

amyxia (ah-mik′se-ah) [*a* neg. + Gr. *myxa* mucus + *-ia*] absence of mucus.

amyxorrhea (ah-mik″so-re′ah) [*a* neg. + Gr. *myxa* mucus + *rhoia* flow] absence of mucus secretion. **a. gas′trica,** deficiency of mucus in the gastric secretion.

An chemical symbol for *actinon.*

An. anode; anodal.

an- 1. the form of *a-* neg. used before a vowel or *h;* see *a-* (def. 1). 2. the form of the prefix *ana-* used before a vowel or *h;* see *ana-.*

A.N.A. American Nurses' Association.

ANA antinuclear antibodies.

ana (an′ah) [Gr.] so much of each; usually written āā.

ana-, an- [Gr. *ana* up, back, again] a prefix meaning upward, excessive, or again.

anabasine (ah-nab′ah-sin) an alkaloid, $C_5H_4N \cdot C_5H_{10}N$, from the plant *Anabasis aphylla*, which closely resembles nicotine; it is used as an insecticide.

anabasis (ah-nab′ah-sis) [Gr. "ascent"] the stage of increase in a disease.

anabatic (an″ah-bat′ik) [Gr. *anabatikos*] 1. increasing or growing more intense. 2. pertaining to or characterized by anabasis.

Anabena (ah-nab′ĕ-nah) a genus of blue-green algae which sometimes impart an objectionable odor to a water supply.

anabiosis (an″ah-bi-o′sis) [Gr. *anabiōsis* a reviving] restoration of vital processes after their apparent cessation.

anabiotic (an″ah-bi-ot′ik) apparently lifeless, but still capable of living.

anabolism (ah-nab′o-lizm″) [Gr. *anabolē* a throwing up] any constructive metabolic process by which organisms convert substances into other components of the organism's chemical architecture.

anabolite (ah-nab′o-līt″) any product of anabolism or of a constructive metabolic process.

anacamptic (an″ah-kamp′tik) pertaining to reflection, as of sound or light.

anacamptometer (an″ah-kamp-tom′ĕ-ter) [Gr. *anakampsis* reflection + *metron* measure] an instrument for measuring the reflexes (Duprat, 1886).

Anacardium (an″ah-kar′de-um) [L.; *ana-* + Gr. *kardia* heart] a genus of tropical trees with a poisonous juice. *A. occidentale*, the cashew tree, affords the cashew nut and a useful gum, as well as anacardic acid.

anacardol (an″ah-kar′dol) a constituent, 3-pentadecadienylphenol, $C_{15}H_{27} \cdot C_6H_4OH$, of cashew nut shell liquid; it causes reactions in persons sensitive to poison ivy.

anacatadidymus (an″ah-kat″ah-did′ĭ-mus) anakatadidymus.

anacatesthesia (an″ah-kat″es-the′ze-ah) anakatesthesia.

anachoresis (an″ah-ko-re′sis) [Gr. *anachōrēsis* a retreating] the preferential collection or deposits of particles at a certain site, as of bacteria or of metals which have localized out of the blood stream in areas of inflammation; called also *anachoretic effect*.

anachoretic (an″ah-ko-ret′ik) pertaining to, characterized by, or resulting from anachoresis.

anachoric (an″ah-ko′rik) anachoretic.

anachronobiology (an″ah-kron″o-bi-ol′o-je) a term suggested to denote the study of the constructive effects (growth, development, and maturation) of time on a living system. Cf. *catachronobiology*.

anacidity (an″ah-sid′ĭ-te) [*an* neg. + *acidity*] lack of normal acidity. **gastric a.,** achlorhydria.

anaclasis (ah-nak′lah-sis) [Gr. *anaklasis* reflection] 1. reflection or refraction of light. 2. reflex action. 3. refracture. 4. forcible flexion of a limb; the breaking up of an ankylosis.

anaclisis (an″ah-kli′sis) [*ana-* + Gr. *klinein* to lean] physical and emotional dependence on another for protection and gratification; used to refer to the normal dependence of an infant on its mother or to excessive leaning on others for emotional support in an older individual.

anaclitic (an″ah-klit′ik) pertaining to anaclisis; exhibiting excessive emotional dependency.

anacmesis (an-ak′me-sis) anakmesis.

anacobra (an″ah-ko′brah) cobra venom treated with formaldehyde and heat.

anacousia (an″ah-ku′ze-ah) anakusis.

anacrotic (an″ah-krot′ik) pertaining to or characterized by anacrotism.

anacrotism (ah-nak′ro-tizm) [*ana-* + Gr. *krotos* beat + *-ism*] an anomaly of the pulse evidenced by the presence of a prominent notch on the ascending limb of the pulse tracing.

anacusis (an″ah-ku′sis) anakusis.

anadenia (an″ah-de′ne-ah) [*an* neg. + Gr. *adēn* gland + *-ia*] (*obs.*) 1. absence of glands. 2. insufficiency of glandular function. **a. ventric′uli,** absence or destruction of the glands of the stomach.

anadidymus (an″ah-did′ĭ-mus) [*ana-* + Gr. *didymos* twin] a twin monster, divided below but single toward the cephalic pole (monstra duplicia anadidyma—Förster); called also *duplicitas inferior* and *duplicitas posterior*.

anadipsia (an″ah-dip′se-ah) [*ana-* + Gr. *dipsa* thirst + *-ia*] intense thirst.

anadrenalism (an″ah-dre′nal-izm) absence or failure of adrenal function.

anadrenia (an″ah-dre′ne-ah) anadrenalism.

Anadrol (an′ah-drol) trademark for a preparation of oxymetholone.

anaerobe (an-a′er-ōb) [*an* neg. + Gr. *aēr* air + *bios* life] a microorganism that lives and grows in the complete, or almost complete, absence of molecular oxygen. **facultative a's,** microorganisms which are able to grow under either anaerobic or aerobic conditions. **obligate a's,** microorganisms that can grow only in the complete absence of

molecular oxygen; some are killed by oxygen. **spore-forming a.,** see *Clostridium* and *Desulfotomaculum*.

anaerobian (an″a-er-o′be-an) (*obs.*) 1. living without air. 2. an anaerobe.

anaerobic (an″a-er-o′bik) 1. lacking molecular oxygen. 2. growing, living, or occurring in the absence of molecular oxygen; pertaining to an anaerobe.

anaerobion (an″a-er-o′be-on), pl. *anaero′bia*. Former term for anaerobe.

anaerobiosis (an-a″er-o-bi-o′sis) [*an* neg. + Gr. *aēr* air + *biosis* way of life] life only in the absence of molecular oxygen; called also *anoxybiosis*.

Anaerobiospirillum (ah″nah-ro″be-o-spi-ril′um) [*an-* neg. +*aero-* + *bio-* + *spirillum*] a genus of gram-negative, anaerobic, helical, rod-shaped bacteria of the family Bacteroidaceae, motile with bipolar flagella, found in the throats and colons of dogs. The single species is *A. succiniciprodu′cens*.

anaerobiotic (an-a″er-o-bi-ot′ik) (*obs.*) anaerobic.

anaerogenic (an-a″er-o-jen′ik) [*an* neg. + Gr. *aēr* air + *gennan* to produce] 1. producing little or no gas. 2. suppressing the formation of gas by the gas-producing bacteria.

Anaeroplasma (an-a″er-o-plaz′mah) a genus of bacteria of the order Mycoplasmatales, found in the rumens of cattle and sheep.

anaeroplasty (an-a′er-o-plas″te) [*an* neg. + Gr. *aēr* air + *plassein* to form] exclusion of air from wounds as a method of treatment.

anaerosis (an″a-er-o′sis) [*an* neg. + Gr. *aēr* air + *-osis*] interruption of the respiratory function, especially in the newborn.

Anaerovibrio (ah″nah-ro-vib′re-o) [*an-* neg. + *aero-* + *vibrio*] a genus of gram-negative, anaerobic, slightly curved rod-shaped bacteria of the family Bacteroidaceae, made up of organisms that are motile with a single polar flagellum. They occur in the rumen of sheep and cattle. The single species is *A. lipoly′tica*.

anagen (an′ah-jen) the phase of the hair cycle during which synthesis of hair takes place.

Anagnostakis' operation (ah-nag″nos-ta′kis) [Andreas *Anagnostakis*, Greek ophthalmologist, 1826–1897] see under *operation*.

anagocytic (an-ag′o-si′tik) retarding or inhibiting the growth of cells.

anagoge (an′ah-go′je) anagogy.

anagogic (an″ah-goj′ik) [*ana-* + Gr. *agogē* leading] pertaining to the moral, uplifting, progressive strivings of the unconscious.

anagogy (an″ah-go′je) psychic material that has an idealistic quality.

anagotoxic (an-ag″o-tok′sik) acting antagonistically to toxin; counteracting toxic action.

anakatadidymus (an″ah-kat″ah-did′ĭ-mus) [*ana-* + Gr. *kata* down + *didymos* twin] a twin monster separate above and below, but united in the middle (monstra duplicia anakatadidyma— Förster).

anakatesthesia (an″ah-kat″es-the′ze-ah) [*ana-* + Gr. *kata* down + *aisthēsis* perception + *-ia*] a hovering feeling or sensation.

anakhre (an-ak′er) goundou.

anakmesis (an-ak′me-sis) [*an* neg. + Gr. *akmēnos* full grown] arrest of maturation; specifically, increase of early granular cells (stem cells) in the marrow with lack of further maturation, as observed in the marrow in agranulocytosis.

anakusis (an″ah-koo′sis) [*an* neg. + Gr. *akouein* to hear] total deafness.

anal (a′nal) [L. *analis*] pertaining to the anus.

analbuminemia (an″al-bu″mĭ-ne′me-ah) a state characterized by deficiency or absence of albumins in the blood serum.

analeptic (an″ah-lep′tik) [Gr. *analepsis* a repairing] a drug which acts as a restorative, such as caffeine, amphetamine, pentylenetetrazol, etc.

analgesia (an″al-je′ze-ah) [*an* neg. + Gr. *algēsis* pain + *-ia*] absence of sensibility to pain; absence of pain on noxious stimulation; designating particularly the relief of pain without loss of consciousness; called also *alganesthesia*. **a. al′gera,** spontaneous pain in a denervated part; pain in an

area or region which is anesthetic; called also *a. dolorosa.*
audio a., audioanalgesia. **continuous caudal a.,** the relief of the pain of labor and childbirth by the continuous bathing of the sacral and lumbar plexuses within the epidural space by the injection of an anesthetic solution. This method is used also in general surgery to block the pain pathways below the navel. Called also *continuous caudal anesthesia.* **a. doloro′sa,** a. algera. **epidural a.,** analgesia induced by introduction of the analgesic agent into the epidural space of the vertebral canal. **infiltration a.,** paralysis of the nerve endings at the site of operation by subcutaneous injection of an anesthetic. **narcolocal a.,** local analgesia preceded by premedication. **paretic a.,** loss of the sense of pain accompanied by partial paralysis. **permeation a.,** surface a. **relative a.,** in dental anesthesia, a maintained level of conscious-sedation, short of general anesthesia, in which the pain threshold is elevated, usually induced by inhalation of nitrous oxide and oxygen. **surface a.,** local analgesia produced by an anesthetic applied to the surface of such mucous membranes as those of the eye, nose, throat, larynx, and urethra; called also *permeation a.*

analgesic (an″al-je′zik) 1. relieving pain. 2. not sensitive as to pain. 3. an agent that alleviates pain without causing loss of consciousness.

Analgesine (an″al-je′sin) trademark for a preparation of antipyrine.

analgetic (an″al-jet′ik) analgesic.

analgia (an-al′je-ah) [*an* neg. + Gr. *algos* pain + *-ia*] absence of sensibility to pain.

analgic (an-al′jik) insensible to pain.

anality (a-nal′ĭ-te) the psychic organization of all the sensations, impulses, and personality traits derived from the anal stage (q.v.) of psychosexual development.

anallergic (an″ah-ler′jik) not allergic; not causing anaphylaxis or hypersensitivity.

analog (an′ah-log) [shortening of *analogue*] 1. pertaining to electronic equipment in which data are represented by electrical signals or physical magnitudes having continuously varying values. Cf. *digital* (def. 3). 2. analogue (def. 2.).

analogous (ah-nal′o-gus) [Gr. *analogos* according to a due ratio, conformable, proportionate] resembling or similar in some respects, as in function or appearance, but not in origin or development; cf. *homologous,* def. 1.

analogue (an′ah-log) 1. a part or organ having the same function as another, but of a different evolutionary origin; cf. *homologue* (def. 1). 2. a chemical compound with a structure similar to that of another but differing from it in respect to a certain component; it may have a similar or opposite action metabolically. Cf. *homologue* (def. 2). **folic acid a.,** a structural analogue of folic acid; see *folic acid antagonist* under *antagonist.* **homologous a.,** a part that is similar to another in both function and structure. **metabolic a.,** a closely similar compound which tends to replace an essential metabolite. **purine a.,** a structural analogue of one of the purine bases (purine, adenine, or guanine): 6-mercaptopurine and 6-thioguanine are used as antineoplastics, azathioprine as an immunosuppressive; the antiviral agent vidarabine (adenine arabinoside) is an analogue of the adenine nucleoside adenosine. **pyrimidine a.,** a structural analogue of one of the pyrimidine bases (cytosine, thymine, or uracil): 5-fluorouracil and cytarabine (cytosine arabinoside), analogue of the cytosine nucleotide deoxycytidine, are important antineoplastic agents. **substrate a.,** a substance with a structure similar to the natural substrate of an enzyme and which, because of this similarity, in some cases inhibits the action of the enzyme, as in competitive inhibition.

analogy (ah-nal′o-je) [Gr. *analogia* equality of ratios, proportion] the quality of being analogous; resemblance or similarity in function or appearance, but not in origin or development.

analphalipoproteinemia (an-al″fah-lip″o-pro″te-in-e′me-ah) Tangier disease; see *familial lipoprotein deficiency.*

analysand (ah-nal′ĭ-sand) one who is being psychoanalyzed.

analysis (ah-nal′ĭ-sis), pl. *anal′yses* [*ana-* + Gr. *lysis* dissolution] 1. separation into component parts or elements; the act of determining the component parts of a substance. 2. psychoanalysis. **activation a.,** a quantitative determination of the presence of certain types of nuclei in a sample by transmuting them into radioactive nuclei and analyzing the emanating radiation. **bite a.,** occlusal a. **blood gas a.,** the determination of oxygen and carbon dioxide concentrations and the pH of the blood by laboratory tests; the following measurements may be made: Po_2, partial pressure of oxygen in arterial blood; Pco_2, partial pressure of carbon dioxide in arterial blood; So_2, percent saturation of hemoglobin with oxygen in arterial blood; the total CO_2 content of (venous) plasma; and the pH. **bradycinetic a.,** cineradiographic study of motor activity. **cephalometric a.,** measurement of the head, using the vector quantities distance and direction, based on the tracing of the x-ray photograph of the living head, usually in the lateral view. **character a.,** psychoanalytic treatment of a character disorder (personality disorder). **chromatographic a.,** chromatography. **colorimetric a.,** analysis by means of the various color tests. **densimetric a.,** analysis by ascertaining the specific gravity of a solution and estimating the amount of matter dissolved. **Downs′ a.,** radiographic cephalometric criteria developed by Downs as an aid in orthodontic diagnosis. **ego a.,** in a psychoanalytic treatment, the analysis of the defense mechanisms employed by the ego and superego against unacceptable unconscious impulses. **end-group a.,** evaluation of the degree of linearity and branching of polysaccharide by determination of the number of end groups; determination of the amino- and carboxyl-terminal amino acids of a protein permitting an evaluation of the number of peptide chains per molecule as well as the state of purity of the protein. **gasometric a.,** the measurement of the different components of a gaseous mixture. **gravimetric a.,** quantitative a. **group a.,** group therapy in which interpretation is given to the patients and insight is evoked. **occlusal a.,** an analysis of the contact of the teeth in centric relation and during excursions of the mandible to determine if occlusal dysfunction is present. Called also *bite a.* **organic a.,** the analysis of animal and vegetable tissues. **polariscopic a.,** analysis by means of the polariscope. **proximate a.,** the determination of the simpler constituents of a substance. **qualitative a., qualitive a.,** the determination of the nature of the constituents of a compound or a mixture of compounds. **quantitative a., quantitive a.,** the determination of the proportionate quantities of the constituents of a compound. **radiochemical a.,** direct or indirect identification or determination of the content of specific elements in a substance through measurement of the disintegration rates of radionuclides. **sequential a.,** a statistical technique in which the sample size is not fixed in advance, rather, sampling is stopped as soon as significant results are observed. The criteria for stopping the trials at each sample size are set so that the overall probability (for all sample sizes) of accepting a specified alternative hypothesis is held to a preset level. Cf. *hypothesis t.* **spectroscopic a., spectrum a.,** analysis by means of determining the wave length(s) at which electromagnetic energy is absorbed by a sample. **transactional a.,** a type of psychotherapy based on an understanding of the interactions (transactions) between patient and therapist and between patient and others in his environment. **ultimate a.,** the determination of the ultimate elements of a compound. **a. of variance (ANOVA),** a statistical hypothesis test for comparison of the means of multiple random variables to assess the influence of certain factors on the means, or for the assessment of whether certain factors associated with a variable contribute to the variance. The variables are assumed to have normal distributions with identical (but unknown) variances. The total sum of squares of the deviations of the variables from their grand mean (the summed products of the sample sizes and sample means divided by the total of the sample sizes) is divided (analyzed) into two components, one being the sum of squares of several linear combinations of the deviations (which measure the effects being tested) and the other being the remainder of the total—hence the name of the procedure. Under the null hypothesis that the tested effects do not exist, independent estimates of the unknown variance can be derived from the two components. If the ratio of the two estimates is large by comparison with the F-distribution, the null hypothesis is rejected and the effects are reported as significant. **vector a.,** analysis of a moving force to determine both its magnitude and its direction, e.g., analysis of the scalar electrocardiogram to determine the magnitude and direction of the electromotive force for one complete cycle of the heart. **volumetric a.,** quantitative analysis by measuring volumes of liquids.

analysor (an′ah-li″zor) analyzer.

analyst (an′ah-list) 1. one who performs analysis. 2. psychoanalyst.

analyte (an′ah-līt) a substance undergoing analysis.

analytic (an″ah-lit′ik) pertaining to analysis.

analyzer (an′ah-li″zer) 1. a Nicol prism attached to a polarizing apparatus which extinguishes the ray of polarized light. 2. Pavlov's name for a specialized part of the nervous system which controls the reactions of the organism to changing external conditions. 3. a nervous receptor together with its central connections, by means of which sensitivity to stimulations is differentiated. **amino acid a.,** an analytical instrument that separates, identifies, and measures quantities of amino acids and related compounds. **amino acid sequence a.,** an instrument for determining protein components in plasma, useful in blood-lipid evaluation. **blood gas a.,** an instrument for measuring partial pressures of oxygen, carbon dioxide, carbon monoxide, and nitrogen in blood. **breath a.,** an instrument for determining the volume and composition of respired gases; some types are specifically designed for detecting alcohol in the breath. **image a.,** an instrument that counts, measures and classifies cells and images viewed on microscopes, photographs, transparencies, etc. **oxygen gas a.,** an instrument for measuring the oxygen content of a gaseous mixture, or dissolved oxygen in a liquid, or saturation of blood hemoglobin with O_2 or partial pressure of O_2 in blood. **voice a.,** an electronic instrument for printing out waveforms corresponding to vocal characteristics, as an aid in identifying voice and speech problems or a particular speaker.

Aname (an′ah-me) a genus comprising the venomous "bird spiders" of the family Theraphosidae.

Anamirta cocculus L. Wight & Arn. (Menispermaceae) (an″ah-mer′tah kok′u-lus) a species of East Indian woody vines whose dried berries or fruit, cocculus indicus, yield picrotoxin. Called also *A. paniculata.*

anamirtin (an″ah-mer′tin) an oily glyceride, $C_{19}H_{24}O_{10}$, from the dried berries or fruit of *Anamirta cocculus.*

anamnesis (an″am-ne′sis) [Gr. *anamnēsis* a recalling] 1. recollection. 2. a medical or psychiatric patient history, as opposed to catamnesis (follow-up). 3. immunologic memory.

anamnestic (an″am-nes′tik) pertaining to anamnesis.

Anamniota (an″am-ne-o′tah) [*an* priv. + Gr. *amnion*] a major group of vertebrates comprising those which develop no amnion, including fishes and amphibians; opposed to Amniota.

anamniote (an-am′ne-ōt″) any animal or group belonging to the Anamniota.

anamniotic (an″am-ne-ot′ik) [*an* neg. + *amnion*] having no amnion.

anamorphosis (an″ah-mor-fo′sis) [*ana-* + Gr. *morphē* form] an ascending progression or change of form in the evolution of a group of animals or plants.

ananabasia (an-an″ah-ba′se-ah) [*an* neg. + Gr. *anabasis* ascent + *-ia*] (*obs.*) inability to ascend high places.

ananaphylaxis (an-an″ah-fī-lak′sis) antianaphylaxis.

Ananase (an′ah-nās) trademark for a preparation of bromelains.

ananastasia (an-an″as-ta′se-ah) [*an* neg. + Gr. *anastasis* a standing up + *-ia*] inability to stand up or to rise from a sitting posture.

anancastic (an″an-kas′tik) [Gr. *anankastos* forced] obsessive-compulsive.

anandia (an-an′de-ah) aphemia.

anangioid (an-an′je-oid) [*an* neg. + Gr. *angeion* vessel + *eidos* form] seemingly without blood vessels.

anapepsia (an″ah-pep′se-ah) complete absence of pepsin from the stomach secretion.

anaphase (an′ah-fāz) [*ana-* + Gr. *phasis* phase] that stage in meiosis and mitosis, following the metaphase, in which the centromeres divide and the chromatids lined up on the spindle begin to move apart toward the poles of the spindle to form the daughter chromosomes. See also *meiosis* and *mitosis.* **flabby a.,** a mitotic phase in which the gel is disoriented and separation of the doubled chromosomes fails to occur, owing to interference with spindle formation caused by cell poisoning.

anaphia (an-a′fe-ah) [*an* neg. + Gr. *haphē* touch + *-ia*] lack or loss of the sense of touch.

anaphoresis (an″ah-fo-re′sis) the passage of charged particles toward the positive pole (anode) in electrophoresis.

anaphoria (an″ah-fo′re-ah) [*ana-* + Gr. *pherein* to bear + *-ia*] a tendency for the visual axes of both eyes to divert above the horizontal plane.

anaphrodisia (an″af-ro-diz′e-ah) [*an* neg. + Gr. *Aphroditē* Venus + *-ia*] (*obs.*) lack of sexual desire.

anaphrodisiac (an″af-ro-diz′e-ak) 1. repressing sexual desire. 2. a drug or medicine that allays sexual desire.

anaphylactic (an″ah-fī-lak′tik) pertaining to anaphylaxis.

anaphylactin (an″ah-fī-lak′tin) the antibody in anaphylaxis, now identified as IgE. Called also *reaginic* or *cytophilic antibody.*

anaphylactogen (an″ah-fī-lak′to-jen) an antigen capable of inducing anaphylaxis.

anaphylactogenesis (an″ah-fī-lak″to-jen′ĕ-sis) the production of anaphylaxis.

anaphylactogenic (an″ah-fī-lak″to-jen′ik) producing anaphylaxis.

anaphylactoid (an″ah-fī-lak′toid) resembling anaphylaxis.

anaphylatoxin (an″ah-fī″lah-tok′sin) a substance produced by complement activation that causes the release of histamine and other mediators of immediate hypersensitivity from basophils and mast cells, thereby producing signs and symptoms of immediate hypersensitivity (anaphylaxis) without involvement of IgE. The anaphylatoxins are low-molecular-weight complement cleavage products, C3a, C4a, and C5a, which bind to specific receptors on mast cells and basophils; C4a has comparatively weak anaphylatoxin activity; C5a is also a chemotactic factor for granulocytes and macrophages.

anaphylaxin (an″ah-fī-lak′sin) anaphylactin.

anaphylaxis (an″ah-fī-lak′sis) [*ana-* + Gr. *phylaxis* protection] 1. systemic or generalized anaphylaxis, anaphylactic shock; a manifestation of immediate hypersensitivity (q.v.) in which exposure of a sensitized individual to a specific antigen or hapten results in life-threatening respiratory distress, usually followed by vascular collapse and shock and accompanied by urticaria, pruritus, and angioedema. Common agents causing anaphylaxis include Hymenoptera venom, pollen extracts, certain foods, horse and rabbit sera, heterologous enzymes and hormones, and certain drugs, such as penicillin and lidocaine. 2. a general term originally applied to the situation in which exposure to a toxin resulted not in development of immunity (prophylaxis) but in hypersensitivity. The term was extended to include all cases of systemic anaphylaxis in response to foreign antigens and also to include a variety of experimental models, e.g., passive cutaneous anaphylaxis. Anaphylaxis has now been subsumed under the more general concept of immediate (Type I) hypersensitivity. **active a.,** the anaphylactic state produced in an individual by the injection of a foreign immunogen; distinguished from passive anaphylaxis. **aggregate a.,** an anaphylactic reaction initiated by the formation of large amounts of antigen-antibody complexes upon injection of the antigen. The complexes activate complement, producing anaphylatoxins (C3a and C5a) that trigger the release of mediators of immediate hypersensitivity from basophils and mast cells. **antiserum a.,** passive anaphylaxis. **generalized a.,** see *anaphylaxis.* **inverse a.,** 1. anaphylaxis in which the shocking agent is antibody (anaphylactin) rather than antigen (anaphylactogen). 2. anaphylactic shock produced by a single intravenous injection into guinea pigs of Forssman antibody which interacts with Forssman antigen in their tissues. Called also *reverse anaphylaxis.* **local a.,** anaphylaxis confined to a limited area, e.g., passive cutaneous anaphylaxis. **passive a.,** anaphylaxis occurring in a normal individual as a result of the injection of the serum of a previously sensitized individual; called also *antiserum a.* **passive cutaneous a. (PCA),** a passively transferred local anaphylactic reaction used in the study of reaginic antibodies; the skin of an animal is sensitized by intradermal injection of serum from a sensitized animal, and after a 24- to 72-hour latent period the antigen and Evans blue dye are injected intravenously. Reaction of the antigen with skin-fixed antibody causes the release of histamine, which increases vascular permeability, permits leakage of the albumin-bound dye, and produces a blue spot at the site of the intradermal injection. **reverse a.,** anaphylaxis following the injection of antigen succeeded by the injection of antiserum; also local reactions from the union of circulating antibodies with antigen fixed by tissue cells. **systemic a.,** see *anaphylaxis.*

anaphylotoxin (an″ah-fi″lo-tok′sin)   anaphylatoxin.

anaplasia (an″ah-pla′ze-ah) [Gr. *ana* backward + *plassein* to form]   a loss of differentiation of cells (dedifferentiation) and of their orientation to one another and to their axial framework and blood vessels, a characteristic of tumor tissue. **monophasic a.,** reversion of a cell form to embryonic type, as in cancer formation. **polyphasic a.,** change of a cell into a cell of more complex character.

Anaplasma (an″ah-plaz′mah) [Gr. *anaplasma* something without form]   a genus of bacteria of the family Anaplasmataceae, order Rickettsiales. It includes two species that are the etiologic agents of anaplasmosis in cattle and deer (*A. margina′le*) and sheep (*A. o′vis*).

Anaplasmataceae (an″ah-plaz″mah-ta′se-e)   a family of bacteria of the order Rickettsiales, made up of microorganisms parasitic in red blood cells or free in the plasma of various vertebrates, in which they appear as reddish violet bodies when stained with Giemsa stain. They are naturally parasitic in ruminants and transmitted by arthropods, causing disease in cattle, deer, birds, and cats but not in humans. The family includes the genera *Aegyptianella, Anaplasma, Eperthrozoon,* and *Haemobartonella.*

anaplasmodastat (an″ah-plaz-mo′dah-stat″)   any of a group of chemical agents for control of anaplasmosis in animals.

anaplasmosis (an″ah-plaz-mo′sis)   a disease of cattle and related ruminants marked by high temperature, anemia, and icterus, and caused by *Anaplasma marginale,* which is transmitted by ticks and other blood-sucking arthropods. In sheep, the disease is caused by *Anaplasma ovis.* Called also *gallsickness.*

anaplastia (an″ah-plas′te-ah)   anaplasia.

anaplastic (an″ah-plas′tik) [*ana-* + Gr. *plassein* to form]   characterized by anaplasia or reversed development; said of cells.

anaplerosis (an″ah-ple-ro′sis) [Gr. "filling up, restoration"]   1. the repair or replacement of lost or defective parts.   2. an enzymatic reaction in intermediary metabolism that restores the concentration of a crucial intermediate that has been depleted in cellular function.

anaplerotic (an″ah-plĕ-rot′ik)   describing a reaction or suite of reactions involved in anaplerosis.

anapnograph (an-ap′no-graf) [Gr. *anapnoē* respiration + *graphein* to record]   (*obs.*) a device once used to register the speed and pressure of the respired air current; replaced by the pneumotachygraph.

anapnometer (an″ap-nom′ĕ-ter) [Gr. *anapnoē* respiration + *metron* measure]   (*obs.*) a spirometer.

anapnotherapy (an″ap-no-ther′ah-pe) [Gr. *anapnein* to inhale + *therapeia* treatment]   treatment by inhalation of gas, as in resuscitation.

anapophysis (an″ah-pof′ĭ-sis) [*ana-* + Gr. *apophysis* process of a bone]   an accessory vertebral process, especially an accessory process of a thoracic or lumbar vertebra.

Anaprox (an′ah-proks)   trademark for preparations of naproxen sodium.

anaptic (an-ap′tik) [*an* neg. + Gr. *haphē* touch]   marked by anaphia.

anarithmia (an″ah-rith′me-ah) [*an* neg. + Gr. *arithmos* number]   inability to count, due to a central lesion.

anarrhexis (an″ah-rek′sis) [*ana-* + Gr. *rhēxis* fracture]   the operation of refracturing a bone.

anarthria (an-ar′thre-ah) [*an* neg. + Gr. *arthroun* to articulate + *-ia*]   severe dysarthria resulting in speechlessness.

anasarca (an″ah-sar′kah) [*ana-* + Gr. *sarx* flesh]   generalized massive edema.

anasarcous (an″ah-sar′kus)   affected with or of the nature of anasarca.

anascitic (an″ah-sit′ik)   without ascites.

anastalsis (an″ah-stal′sis) [*ana-* + Gr. *stalsis* contraction]   reversed peristalsis.

anastaltic (an″ah-stal′tik) [Gr. *anastaltikos* contracting]   1. astringent   2. a styptic medicine.

anastigmatic (an″ah-stig-mat′ik)   not astigmatic; corrected for astigmatism.

anastomose (ah-nas′to-mōs)   1. to connect with one another by anastomosis, as arteries and veins.   2. to create a connection between two formerly separate structures.

anastomosis (ah-nas″to-mo′sis), pl. *anastomo′ses* [Gr. *anastomōsis* opening, outlet]   1. a connection between two vessels.   2. an opening created by surgical, traumatic, or pathological means between two normally separate spaces or organs.   **antiperistaltic a.,** enterostomy in which the intestinal segments are so joined that the directions of the peristaltic waves in the two conjoined portions are opposed.   **a. arteriolovenula′ris** [NA], a vessel that directly interconnects an artery and a vein and that acts as a shunt to bypass the capillary bed. Called also *a. arteriovenosa* [NA alternative].   **a. arteriolovenula′ris sim′plex,** - NA alternative for *a. arteriovenosa simplex.*   **a. arterioveno′sa,** NA alternative for *a. arteriolovenularis.*   **a. arterioveno′sa glomerifor′mis** [NA], glomeriform arteriovenous a.: a specialized arteriovenous shunt occurring most abundantly in the skin of the hands and feet (especially the digital pads and nail beds) and also of the nose and ears, which in addition to helping regulate blood flow is concerned with temperature regulation and conservation. Called also *a. arteriolovenularis glomeriformis* [NA alternative], *glandula glomiformis, glomiform gland, glomeriform arteriovenular a., glomus,* and *glomus body.* See also *glomus tumor,* under *tumor.*   **a. arterioveno′sa sim′plex** [NA], simple arteriovenus a.: a vessel that directly interconnects an artery and a vein, acting as a shunt to bypass the capillary bed. Called also *a. arteriolovenularis simplex* [NA alternative] and *simple arteriovenular a.*   **arteriovenous a.,** a communication surgically created between an artery and a vein.   **arteriovenous a., glomeriform,** a. arteriovenosa glomeriformis.   **arteriovenous a., simple,** a. arteriovenosa simplex.   **arteriovenular a., glomeriform,** a. arteriovenosa glomeriformis.   **arteriovenular a., simple,** a. arteriovenosa simplex.   **a. arteriolovenula′ris glomerifor′mis,** NA alternative for *a. arteriovenosa glomeriformis.*   **Braun's a.,** formation of an anastomosis between the afferent and efferent intestinal loops just distal to a gastroenteric stoma to prevent vicious cycling of gastric and duodenal contents.   **Clado's a.,** the anastomosis between the appendicular and ovarian arteries in the appendiculo-ovarian ligament.   **crucial a.,** an arterial anastomosis in the proximal part of the thigh, formed by the anastomotic branch of the sciatic, the internal circumflex, the first perforating, and the transverse portion of the external circumflex.   **Galen's a.,** the anastomosis between the superior and inferior laryngeal nerves.   **heterocladic a.,** an anastomosis between branches of different arteries.   **homocladic a.,** an anastomosis between branches of the same artery.   **Hyrtl's a.,** see *Hyrtl's loop,* under *loop.*   **ileorectal a.,** surgical anastomosis of the ileum and rectum after total colectomy, as is often done in treatment of ulcerative colitis.   **intestinal a.,** the establishment of a communication between two portions of the intestinal tract.   **isoperistaltic a.,** enterostomy in which the intestinal segments are so joined that the peristaltic waves in the two conjoined portions progress in the same direction.   **portosystemic a.,** anastomosis between the portal and systemic venous circulation.   **postcostal a.,** a longitudinal linkage of the seven highest intersegmental arteries in the embryo that gives rise to the vertebral artery.   **precapillary a.,** anastomosis between small arteries just before they become capillaries.   **precostal a.,** a longitudinal anastomosis of intersegmental arteries in the embryo that gives rise to the thyrocervical and costocervical trunks.   **pyeloileocutaneous a.,** direct connection of the renal pelvis to an isolated loop of the ileum, which is then anchored to the abdominal wall at the stoma, to drain exteriorly.   **a. of Riolan,** anastomosis of the superior and inferior mesenteric arteries.   **Roux-en-Y a.,** any Y-shaped anastomosis in which the small intestine is included; after division of the small intestine segment, the distal end is implanted into another organ, such as the stomach or esophagus, and the proximal end into the small intestine below the anastomosis to provide drainage without reflux. **stirrup a.,** an arterial branch joining the dorsalis

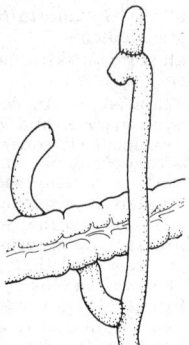

Roux-en-Y anastomosis.

pedis with the external plantar artery. **Sucquet-Hoyer a.,** segmentum arteriale anastomosis arteriovenae glomeriformis. **terminoterminal a.,** surgical anastomosis between the peripheral end of an artery and the central end of the corresponding vein and between the central end of the artery and the terminal end of the vein. **transureteroureteral a.,** the operation of connecting one ureter to the ureter on the opposite side. **ureteroileocutaneous a.,** connection of the transected ureter to an isolated loop of the ileum, which is then anchored to the abdominal wall at the stoma, to drain exteriorly. **ureteroureteral a.,** the operation of joining portions of the same ureter.

anastomotic (ah-nas″to-mot′ik) pertaining to or of the nature of an anastomosis.

anastral (an-as′tral) [*an* neg. + Gr. *astēr* star] lacking, or pertaining to the lack of, an aster; used in reference to a mitotic figure.

anastrophic (an″ah-strof′ik) [Gr. *anastrophē* a turning back, reversal] capable of being inactivated and then reactivated; said of certain proteinases.

anat. anatomy; anatomical.

anatherapeusis (an″ah-ther″ah-pu′sis) [Gr. *ana* upward + *therapeusis*] treatment by increasing doses.

anatomic (an″ah-tom′ik) anatomical.

anatomical (an″ah-tom′ĭ-kal) pertaining to anatomy, or to the structure of the organism.

anatomicomedical (an-ah-tom″e-ko-med′ĭ-kal) pertaining to anatomy and medicine or to medical anatomy.

anatomicopathological (an″ah-tom″e-ko-path″o-loj′ĭ-kal) pertaining to pathological anatomy.

anatomicophysiological (an-ah-tom″e-ko-fiz″e-o-loj′ĭ-kal) pertaining to anatomy and physiology.

anatomicosurgical (an-ah-tom″e-ko-ser′jĭ-kal) pertaining to anatomy and surgery.

anatomist (ah-nat′o-mist) a person skilled or learned in anatomy; a specialist in the field of anatomy.

anatomist's snuff-box the hollow at the back of the hand and the base of the thumb, between the tendons of the extensor pollicis longus and extensor pollicis brevis muscles.

anatomopathology (an″ah-to-mo-pah-thol′o-je) the anatomical aspects of pathology.

anatomy (ah-nat′o-me) [*ana-* + Gr. *temnein* to cut] 1. the science of the structure of the animal body and the relation of its parts; it is largely based on dissection, from which it obtains its name. 2. dissection of an organized body. **applied a.,** anatomy as applied to diagnosis and treatment. **artificial a.,** the study of anatomical structure by use of models or other artificial means. **artistic a.,** the study of anatomy as applied to drawing, painting, and sculpture. **clastic a.,** anatomy studied by the aid of models in which various layers can be removed to show the position of organs and parts underneath. **comparative a.,** a comparison of the structure of different animals and plants, one with another. **corrosion a.,** anatomy studied by means of corrosive agents that remove the tissues not intended to be observed. **dental a.,** the study of the structure of the teeth and their correlated parts. **descriptive a.,** the study or description of individual parts of the body; called also *systematic a.* **developmental a.,** the field of embryology concerned with the changes that cells, tissues, organs, and the body as a whole undergo from a germ cell of each parent to the resulting, adult offspring. **general a.,** the study of the structure and composition of the body, and its tissues and fluids in general. **gross a.,** that which deals with structures that can be distinguished with the naked eye; called also *macroscopic a.* **histologic a.,** histology. **homologic a.,** the study of the correlated parts of the body in different animals. **macroscopic a.,** gross a. **medical a.,** anatomy concerned with the study of points connected with the physical examination and localization of internal abnormalities. **microscopic a., minute a.,** histology. **morbid a., pathological a.,** the anatomy of diseased tissues. **physiognomonic a.,** the study of the external expression of the body surface, especially of the face. **physiological a.,** the study of the organs with respect to their normal functions. **plastic a.,** the study of anatomy by the aid of models and manikins, especially those that can be taken apart. **practical a.,** anatomy studied by means of demonstration and dissection. **radiological a.,** the study of the anatomy of organs and tissues based on their visualization on x-ray films. **regional a.,** descriptive anatomy arranged according to the regions of the body. The study of limited portions or regions of the body, and the relationships of their parts. **special a.,** the study of particular organs or parts. **surface a.,** the study of the form and markings of the surface of the body, especially in relation to deeper parts. **surgical a.,** the study of limited portions or regions of the body, with a view to the diagnosis and treatment of surgical conditions. **systematic a.,** descriptive a. **topographic a.,** the study of parts in their relation to surrounding parts. **transcendental a.,** the study of the general design and morphology of the body and the analogies and homologies of its parts. **veterinary a.,** the anatomy of domestic animals. **x-ray a.,** radiological a.

anatoxic (an″ah-tok′sik) pertaining to anatoxin.

anatoxin (an″ah-tok′sin) [*ana-* + *toxin*] toxoid. **diphtheria a., a.-Ramon,** diphtheria toxoid.

anatripsis (an″ah-trip′sis) [Gr. "rubbing"] (*obs.*) therapeutic rubbing or friction massage.

anatriptic (an″ah-trip′tik) [Gr. *anatriptos* rubbed up] 1. pertaining to anatripsis. 2. a medication applied by rubbing.

anatrophic (an″ah-trof′ik) 1. correcting or preventing atrophy. 2. a remedy that prevents waste of the tissues.

anatropia (an″ah-tro′pe-ah) [*ana-* + Gr. *trepein* to turn] upward deviation of the visual axis of one eye when the other eye is fixing.

anatropic (an″ah-trop′ik) pertaining to anatropia; deviating upward.

anavenin (an″ah-ven′in) a venom which has become inactivated by the addition of formaldehyde but which retains its antigenic properties.

anaxon (an-ak′son) [*an* neg. + Gr. *axōn* axis] a term formerly used to describe a nerve cell which appears to lack an axon.

anazolene sodium (an-az′o-lēn) chemical name: 4-[(4-anilino-5-sulfo-1-naphthyl)azo]-5-hydroxy-2,7-naphthalenedisulfonic acid trisodium salt. A reddish black powder, $C_{26}H_{16}N_3Na_3O_{10}S_3$, used as a diagnostic aid in the determination of blood volume and cardiac output; called also *anoxynaphthonate sodium.*

Ancalomicrobium (an-ka″lo-mi-kro′be-um) [Gr. *ankalē* arm + *mikros* small + *bios* life] a genus of appendaged bacteria found in water, made up of gram-negative cells growing singly that produce two to eight prosthecae and reproduce by budding. The type species is *A. adet′um.*

Ancef (an′sef) trademark for a preparation of cefazolin sodium.

anchone (ang-ko′ne) (*obs.*) spasmodic constriction of the throat in hysteria.

anchor (ang′ker) a means by which something is held securely. **endosteal implant a.,** a metal implant in the shape of a ship's anchor, usually made of a chromium-cobalt alloy, being a part of the substructure of an implant denture, which is placed deep into the bone to provide retention for the prosthesis.

anchorage (ang′ker-ij) 1. surgical fixation of a displaced viscus. 2. in operative dentistry, the fixation of fillings or of artificial crowns or bridges. 3. in orthodontics, the nature and degree of resistance to displacement offered by an anatomical unit when used for the purpose of effecting tooth movement. 4. in tissue cell culture, the attachment of proliferating cells to a solid surface. **cervical a.,** an orthodontic anchorage in which the back of the neck is used for resistance through a strap fitted around the neck. **compound a.,** an orthodontic anchorage in which the resistance is obtained from two or more teeth. **extramaxillary a.,** extraoral a. **extraoral a.,** an orthodontic anchorage in which the resistance unit is outside of the oral cavity, the force being transmitted to the teeth by means of headgear attached to the teeth. Called also *extramaxillary a.* **intermaxillary a.,** an orthodontic anchorage in which the resistance units situated in one jaw are used to effect tooth movement in the other jaw. Called also *maxillomandibular a.* **intraoral a.,** an orthodontic anchorage in which the resistance units are all located within the oral cavity. **maxillomandibular a.,** intermaxillary a. **multiple a.,** an orthodontic anchorage in which more than one type of resistance unit is utilized. Called also *reinforced a.* **occipital a.,** an orthodontic anchorage in which the resistance is borne by the top and back of the head, and the force transmitted to the teeth by means of the headgear and heavy elastics connected with attachment on the teeth. **reciprocal a.,** anchorage in which the movement of one or more dental units is balanced against the movement of one or more opposing dental units. Cf. *reciprocal force.* **reinforced a.,** multiple a. **simple a.,** an orthodontic anchorage in which larger teeth or groups of teeth and their location are used to move teeth of lesser size; the resistance to the movement comes solely from resistance to tipping movement of the anchored unit. **stationary a.,** an orthodontic anchorage in which the resistance to the movement of one or more dental units comes from the resistance to bodily movement of the anchorage unit. A questionable concept of anchorage implying that selected teeth remain stable.

anchyl(o)- for words beginning thus, see those beginning *ankyl(o)-.*

ancillary (an′sil-lār″e) [L. *ancillaris* relating to a maid servant] assisting in the performance of a service or the achievement of a result.

ancipital (an-sip′ĭ-tal) [L. *an′ceps* two headed] having two heads or two edges.

Ancistrodon (an-sis′tro-don) *Agkistrodon.*

ancistroid (an-sis′troid) [Gr. *ankistron* fishhook + *-oid*] hook shaped.

Ancobon (an′ko-bon) trademark for a preparation of flucytosine.

anconad (ang′ko-nad) [Gr. *ankōn* elbow + L. *ad* toward] toward the elbow or olecranon.

anconagra (ang″kon-ag′rah) [Gr. *ankōn* elbow + *agra* seizure] gout of the elbow.

anconal (ang′kŏ-nal) anconeal.

anconeal (ang-ko′ne-al) pertaining to the elbow.

anconitis (ang″ko-ni′tis) inflammation of the elbow joint.

anconoid (ang′ko-noid) resembling the elbow.

ancrod (an′krod) a proteinase obtained from the venom of the Malayan pit viper *Agkistrodon rhodostoma,* acting specifically on fibrinogen; used as an anticoagulant in the treatment of retinal vein occlusion and deep vein thrombosis and to prevent postoperative rethrombosis.

ancyl(o)- for words beginning thus, see also words beginning *ankyl(o)-.*

Ancylostoma (an″kĭ-los′to-mah, an″sĭ-los′to-mah) [Gr. *ankylos* crooked + *stoma* mouth] a genus of nematode parasites of the family Ancylostomidae, the Old World hookworms. **A. america′num,** *Necator americanus.* **A. brazilien′se,** a species found in cats and dogs in the southeastern United States, Brazil, and other tropical countries; its larvae may cause creeping eruption in man. **A. cani′num,** the common hookworm of dogs and cats; the larvae of which may cause creeping eruption in man. **A. ceylon′icum,** *A. braziliense.* **A. duodena′le,** the common European or Old World hookworm, a nematode

worm, the male being 10 to 12 mm. ($\frac{1}{3}$ to $\frac{1}{2}$ inch) long and 0.4 mm. ($\frac{1}{60}$ inch) broad, the female somewhat larger; the mature parasites inhabit the small intestine, producing the condition known as ancylostomiasis. Formerly called *Uncinaria duodenalis.*

ancylostomatic (an″kĭ-lo-sto-mat′ik, an″sĭ-lo-sto-mat′ik) caused by *Ancylostoma.*

ancylostome (an-kil′o-stōm, an-sil′o-stōm) 1. an individual of the genus *Ancylostoma.* 2. an individual of the family Ancylostomidae; a hookworm.

ancylostomiasis (an″kĭ-los″to-mi′ah-sis) 1. infection with hookworms of the genus *Ancyclostoma.* 2. hookworm disease.

Ancylostomidae (an″kĭ-lo-sto′mĭ-de, an″sĭ-lo-sto′mĭ-de) a family of phasmid nematodes of the superfamily Strongyloidea, comprising all the hookworms, including the genera *Ancylostoma, Bunostomum, Necator,* and *Uncinaria.*

Ancylostomum (an″kĭ-los-to′mum, an″sĭ-los-to′mum) *Ancylostoma.*

ancyroid (an′sĭ-roid) [Gr. *ankyra* anchor + *oid*] shaped like an anchor or hook.

Anda (an′dah) [Brazilian] a genus of euphorbiaceous trees. *A. as′su* and *A. gome′sii,* of Brazil, afford purgative oils.

Andernach's ossicles (ahn′der-nahks) [Johann Winther von *Andernach,* German physician, 1487–1574] ossa suturarum.

Anders' disease (an′ders) [James Meschter *Anders,* Philadelphia physician, 1854–1936] adiposis tuberosa simplex.

Andersch's ganglion, nerve (an′dersh-ez) [Carolus Samuel *Andersch,* German anatomist of the 18th century] see *ganglion inferius nervi glossopharyngei* and *nervus tympanicus.*

Andersen's disease, syndrome (triad) (an′der-sonz) [Dorothy Hansine *Andersen,* New York pathologist, born 1901] see under *disease* and *syndrome.*

Anderson splint (an′der-son) [Roger *Anderson,* Seattle orthopedic surgeon, 1891–1971] see under *splint.*

Andira (an-di′rah) a genus of tropical leguminous trees. Goa powder (q.v.) and chrysarobin (q.v.) are derived from *A. araro′ba,* of Brazil. Many species afford poisons, and several are anthelmintic.

andirine (an-di′rin) surinamine.

Andrade's indicator (an-drah′dēz) [Eduardo Penny *Andrade,* American bacteriologist, 1872–1906] see under *indicator.*

Andral's decubitus (sign) (an-dralz′) [Gabriel *Andral,* French physician, 1797–1876] see under *decubitus.*

andreioma (an″dre-o′mah) [*andr-* + *-oma*] arrhenoblastoma.

andreoblastoma (an″dre-o-blas-to′mah) arrhenoblastoma.

Andresen appliance (an′drě-sen) [V. *Andresen,* Norwegian orthodontist] see *functional activator,* under *activator.*

andriatrics, andriatry (an″dre-at′riks; an-dri′ah-tre) [Gr. *anēr* man + *iatrikos* healing] (obs.) andrology.

andr(o)- [Gr. *anēr, andros* man] a combining form denoting relationship to the male.

androblastoma (an″dro-blas-to′mah) 1. a rare, benign tumor of the testis that histologically resembles the fetal testis; there are three varieties: diffuse stromal, mixed (stromal and epithelial), and tubular (epithelial). Sertoli cells in the epithelial elements may produce estrogen and cause feminization. Called also *Sertoli cell tumor.* 2. arrhenoblastoma.

androcyte (an′dro-sīt) [*andro-* + Gr. *kytos* hollow vessel] male sex cell, especially an immature stage.

androdedotoxin (an″dro-de″do-tok′sin) a poisonous principle from the leaves of rhododendrons.

androecium (an″dro-e′she-um) stamen.

androgalactozemia (an″dro-gah-lak″to-ze′me-ah) [*andro-* + Gr. *gala* milk + *zēmia* loss] lactation from the male breast.

androgamone (an″dro-gam′ōn) a gamone released by spermatozoa.

androgen (an′dro-jen) [*andro-* + Gr. *gennan* to produce] any substance that conduces to masculinization, such as the testicular hormone; see *androsterone* and *testosterone.*

androgenesis (an″dro-jen′ě-sis) [*andro-* + Gr. *genesis* production] development of an egg which contains only paternal chromosomes.

androgenic (an″dro-jen′ik) producing masculine characteristics.

androgenicity (an″dro-jĕ-nis′ĭ-te) the quality of exerting a masculinizing effect.

androgenization (an″dro-jen-i-za′shun) 1. the state of producing an excess of androgens in the female. 2. normal virilization in the male.

androgenized (an-droj′ĕ-nizd) 1. subjected to the production or presence of an excess of androgen in the female. 2. normally virilized, as in the male.

androgenous (an-droj′ĕ-nus) [andro- + Gr. gennan to beget] pertaining or tending to the production of male rather than female offspring.

androgone (an′dro-gōn) [andro- + Gr. gonos seed] a spermatogenic cell.

androgyne (an′dro-jīn) a female pseudohermaphrodite.

androgynism (an-droj′ĭ-nizm) female pseudohermaphroditism.

androgynoid (an-droj′ĭ-noid) 1. a pseudohermaphrodite. 2. pertaining to female pseudohermaphroditism.

androgynous (an-droj′ĭ-nus) 1. pertaining to or characterized by female pseudohermaphroditism. 2. pertaining to a state of phenotypic ambiguity with respect to sexual characteristics.

androgyny (an-droj′ĭ-ne) 1. female pseudohermaphroditism. 2. a physical state of sexual ambiguity.

android (an′droid) [andro- + Gr. eidos shape] resembling a man; manlike.

androidal (an-droi′dal) android.

andrology (an-drol′o-je) [andro- + -logy] scientific study of the masculine constitution and of the diseases of the male sex; especially the study of diseases of the male organs of generation.

androma (an-dro′mah) [andr- + -oma] arrhenoblastoma.

Andromeda (an-drom′ĕ-dah) [L.] a genus of ericaceous shrubs and trees, some of which afford a poisonous narcotic principle. A. maria′na, A. nit′ida, and A. polifo′lia are among the poisonous species.

andromedotoxin (an-drom″ĕ-do-tok′sin) [Andromeda + toxin] a poisonous crystalline principle, $C_{22}H_{36}O_7$, from various ericaceous plants, such as Kalmia latifolia (mountain laurel) and related species; it is toxic to sheep and other livestock that graze on the plants, causing salivation, nasal discharge, emesis, paralysis, coma, and death.

andromerogon (an″dro-mer′o-gon) [andro- + Gr. meros part + gonē seed] an organism developed from an ovum containing the male pronucleus only, the cells, as a result, containing only the paternal set of chromosomes.

andromerogone (an″dro-mer′o-gōn) andromerogon.

andromerogony (an″dro-mĕ-rog′o-ne) [andro- + Gr. meros a part + gonos procreation] development of a portion of an ovum containing the male pronucleus only, the nucleus of the ovum having been removed before fusion of the male and female pronuclei occurred. Cf. gynomerogony and merogony.

andromimetic (an″dro-mĭ-met′ik) [andro- + Gr. mimētikos imitating] producing male characteristics; having a masculinizing effect; simulating the action of androgen.

andromorphous (an″dro-mor′fus) [andro- + Gr. morphē form] having a masculine appearance.

andropathy (an-drop′ah-the) [andro- + Gr. pathos disease] any disease peculiar to males.

androphile (an′dro-fīl) anthropophilic.

androphilous (an-drof′ĭ-lus) anthropophilic.

Andropogon (an″dro-po′gon) a genus of grasses. A. sor′ghum includes broom corn, kafir corn, and sorghum.

androstane (an′dro-stān) the tetracyclic hydrocarbon nucleus ($C_{19}H_{32}$) from which the androgens are derived.

androstanediol (an″dro-stān′de-ol) an androgen, $C_{19}H_{32}$-O_2.

androstanedione (an″dro-stān′de-ōn) an androgen, C_{19}-$H_{28}O_2$, (3,17-diketo androstane), formed in the testes.

androstanolone (an″dro-stan′o-lōn) an androgen, $C_{19}H_{30}$-O_2, occurring in two isomeric forms; see androsterone.

androstene (an′dro-stēn) a cyclic hydrocarbon, $C_{19}H_{30}$, with one double bond; a steroid occurring in two isomeric

forms forming the nucleus of testosterone and some other androgens.

androstenediol (an″dro-stēn′de-ol) an androgen, $C_{19}H_{30}$-O_2, occurring in two isomeric forms, 3-trans, 17-dihydroxy Δ^5-androstene and 3-cis, 17-dihydroxy Δ^5-androstene.

androstenedione (an″dro-stēn′de-ōn) an androgen, C_{19}-$H_{26}O_2$, 3,17-diketo Δ^4-androstene; an androgenic steroid hormone that is less potent than testosterone, it is secreted by the testis, adrenal cortex, and ovary.

androsterone (an-dros′ter-ōn) a weak androgen excreted in the urine of both men and women. It is 3α-hydroxy-5α-androstan-17-one, $C_{19}H_{30}O_2$. When injected intramuscularly it partly counteracts the effects of castration.

-ane a word termination denoting (1) a saturated open-chain hydrocarbon, C_nH_{2n+2}; (2) an organic compound in which hydrogen has replaced the hydroxyl group.

anecdotal (an″ek-do′tal) [Gr. anekdotos not published] based on descriptions of unmatched individual cases rather than on controlled studies.

anecdysis (an-ek′dĭ-sis) [an neg. + Gr. ekdysis a way out] a long period during the molting cycle of arthropods when there are no signs of either recovery from a molt or preparations for the next molt.

anechoic (an-ĕ-ko′ik) [an neg. + Gr. ēchō a returned sound + -ic] 1. without echoes; said of a chamber for measuring the effects of sound. 2. in ultrasonography, permitting the passage of ultrasound waves without reflecting them back to their source (without giving off echoes). Called also sonolucent.

anectasis (an-ek′tah-sis) [an neg. + Gr. ektasis distention] congenital atelectasis due to developmental immaturity.

Anectine (an-ek′tin) trademark for preparations of succinylcholine chloride.

Anel's operation, probe, syringe [Dominique Anel, French surgeon, 1679–1730] see under operation, probe, and syringe.

anelectrotonic (an″e-lek-tro-ton′ik) pertaining to anelectrotonus.

anelectrotonus (an″e-lek-trot′o-nus) [Gr. ana up + electrotonus] lessened irritability of a nerve in the region of the positive pole or anode during the passage of an electric current.

anemia (ah-ne′me-ah) [Gr. an neg. + haima blood + -ia] a reduction below normal in the number of erythrocytes per cu. mm., in the quantity of hemoglobin, or in the volume of packed red cells per 100 ml. of blood which occurs when the equilibrium between blood loss (through bleeding or destruction) and blood production is disturbed. **achrestic a.,** megaloblastic anemia morphologically resembling pernicious anemia, but with multiple other causes. **achylic a., a. achy′lica,** hypochromic a., idiopathic. **acquired sideroachrestic a.,** refractory sideroblastic a. **acute a.,** a nonspecific term indicating anemia of relatively short duration, as acute hemorrhagic anemia. **Addison's a., Addison-Biermer a., addisonian a.** (obs.), pernicious a. **anhematopoietic a., anhemopoietic a.,** anemia due to defective formation of erythrocytes. **aplastic a.,** a form of anemia generally unresponsive to specific antianemia therapy, often accompanied by granulocytopenia and thrombocytopenia, in which the bone marrow may not necessarily be acellular or hypoplastic but fails to produce adequate numbers of peripheral blood elements. The term actually is all-inclusive and most probably encompasses several clinical syndromes. Called also aregenerative a. and refractory a. **aregenerative a.,** aplastic a. **aregenerative a., chronic congenital,** hypoplastic a., congenital, def. 1. **autoimmune hemolytic a. (AIHA),** a general term covering a large group of anemias involving autoantibodies against red cell antigens. Those due to warm-reactive antibodies, usually IgG but occasionally IgM or IgA, may be idiopathic or secondary to autoimmune diseases, hematologic neoplasms, viral infections, or immunodeficiency diseases, and usually involve sequestration of sensitized erythrocytes by the spleen. Those due to cold-reactive antibodies, usually IgM but occasionally IgG, include cold agglutinin syndrome and paroxysmal cold hemoglobinuria and usually involve complement-dependent intravascular hemolysis or sequestration of erythrocytes by the liver. **Bagdad Spring a.** (obs.) a type of hemolytic anemia most probably due to erythrocyte deficiency of glucose-6-phosphate dehydrogenase. **Bartonella a.,** Oroya fever in man; also occurring in a number of animals, e.g., the dog, as well as in the rat, in which the anemia is latent until splenectomy. **Biermer's a., Biermer-Ehrlich a.** (*obs.*), pernicious a. **Blackfan-Diamond a.,** hypoplastic a., congenital. **cameloid a.,** elliptocytosis. **cattle a.,** a condition caused by infection with *Theileria parva;* East Coast fever. **chlorotic a.,** chlorosis. **congenital hypoplastic a.,** see *hypoplastic a., congenital.* **congenital a. of newborn,** erythroblastosis fetalis. **congenital nonspherocytic hemolytic a.,** see *hemolytic a., congenital nonspherocytic.* **Cooley's a.,** see *β-thalassemia,* under *thalassemia.* **cow's milk a.,** anemia in infants due to lack of iron in a cow's milk diet. **cytogenic a.** (*obs.*), progressive pernicious a. **deficiency a.,** anemia caused by a lack of a specific substance required for normal hemoglobin synthesis and erythrocytic maturation arising by several means, such as malabsorption or poor dietary intake; called also *nutritional a.* **dilution a.,** a condition in which the anemia is more apparent than real, being due to an increased plasma volume rather than to a decreased total circulating red cell mass. **dimorphic a.,** a condition characterized by a dual erythrocyte population, as defined by a double peak of the diameter frequency curve, observed when combined deficiencies of vitamin B_{12} (or analogous substance) and iron exist concurrently in the same patient. It may also occur in persons receiving blood transfusions. **drepanocytic a.** (*obs.*), sickle cell a. **drug-induced immune hemolytic a.,** immune hemolytic anemia induced by drugs, classified by mechanism as *penicillin type,* in which the drug, acting as a hapten bound to the red cell membrane, induces the formation of specific antibodies; *methyldopa type* in which the drug, possibly by inhibition of suppressor T cells, induces the formation of anti-Rh antibodies; or the *stibophen or "innocent bystander" type,* in which circulating drug-antibody immune complexes bind nonspecifically to red cells. The first two types usually involve warm-reactive antibodies and accelerated sequestration of red cells by the reticuloendothelial system; the third usually involves cold-reactive antibodies and complement-dependent intravascular hemolysis. **Edelmann's a.** (*obs.*), a type of chronic infectious anemia. **elliptocytary a., elliptocytotic a.,** elliptocytosis. **equine infectious a.,** a viral disease of equines marked by recurring attacks of malaise with abrupt rises of temperature, and spread through the blood by inoculation, especially by blood-sucking insects. Called also *infectious a. of horses, Vallee's disease,* and *swamp fever.* **erythroblastic a. of childhood,** erythroblastic a., familial; see *β-thalassemia,* under *thalassemia.* **erythronormoblastic a.** (*obs.*), hypochromic a. **essential a.,** primary a. **familial erythroblastic a.,** see *thalassemia.* **Fanconi's a.,** see under *syndrome* (def. 1). **folic acid deficiency a.,** macrocytic anemia due to deficiency of folic acid. **globe cell a.** (*obs.*), hereditary spherocytosis. **glucose-6-phosphate dehydrogenase deficiency a.,** a genetically determined hemolytic anemia caused by a deficiency of this enzyme in erythrocytes which results in hemolysis of the erythrocyte by drugs of certain groups (such as antimalarials, sulfonamides, nitrofurans, antipyretics and analgesics, and sulfones), fava beans, and other agents. Recent studies imply that this predisposition to hemolysis may be expressed in varying degrees and that other biochemical defects, in addition to that involving glucose-6-phosphate dehydrogenase, may also be present in the erythrocytes. **goat's milk a.,** a macrocytic anemia, observed particularly in Germany and Italy, occurring in infants fed exclusively on goat's milk, associated with a megaloblastic bone marrow, thrombocytopenia, leukopenia, hyperbilirubinemia, and hyperferremia. **ground itch a.,** hookworm disease. **Heinz-body a's,** a group of hemolytic syndromes of diverse etiology with the common morphologic characteristic of having one or more Heinz bodies within affected erythrocytes. **hemolytic a.,** see *autoimmune hemolytic a.* and *drug-induced hemolytic a.* **hemolytic a., acquired,** that due to causes other than hereditary factors, including infectious agents, poisons, and physical agents, in which there is premature destruction of red blood cells. **hemolytic a., acute,** a condition characterized by sudden destruction of erythrocytes by hemolysis. **hemolytic a., congenital,** a general term for anemia, present at birth, in which the lifespan of red blood cells is diminished. **hemolytic a., congenital nonspherocytic,** a heterogeneous group of nonspherocytic hereditary anemias in which shortened red cell

survival is associated with erythrocyte membrane defects, multiple intracellular deficiencies, or unstable hemoglobins. **hemolytic a., hereditary nonspherocytic,** a heterogeneous group of congenital hemolytic anemias characterized by absence of spherocytosis, negative antiglobulin tests, and absence of a detectable abnormal hemoglobin. **hemolytic a., immune,** see *autoimmune hemolytic a.* and *drug-induced immune hemolytic a.* **hemolytic a., infectious,** that due to an incompletely compensated decrease in red blood cell survival secondary to infectious agents, including protozoa (e.g., *Plasmodium* in malaria), bacteria, and certain viruses. **hemolytic a., microangiopathic,** hemolytic anemia due to intravascular fragmentation of red blood cells. **hemolytic a., toxic,** that due to toxic agents, including drugs and animal and vegetable poisons. **hemorrhagic a.,** anemia caused by the sudden and acute loss of blood; called also *acute posthemorrhagic a.* **hookworm a.,** hypochromic microcytic anemia resulting from infection with *Ancylostoma* or *Necator.* **hypochromic a.,** a condition characterized by a disproportionate reduction of red cell hemoglobin and an increased area of central pallor in the red cells. **hypochromic a., idiopathic,** iron deficiency a. **hypochromic microcytic a.,** hypochromic anemia in which the red cells are reduced in size and in hemoglobin content. **a. hypochro′mica siderochres′tica heredita′ria,** a hereditary, chronic, refractory sideroblastic anemia affecting males; called also *hereditary sideroachrestic a.* **hypoferric a.** (*obs.*), iron deficiency a. **hypoplastic a.,** a general term indicating a form of anemia due to varying degrees of erythrocytic hypoplasia without leukopenia or thrombocytopenia. **hypoplastic a., congenital,** 1. a progressive anemia of unknown etiology encountered in the first year of life, unaccompanied by leukopenia and thrombocytopenia, unresponsive to hematinics, and often requiring multiple blood transfusions to sustain life; called also *chronic congenital aregenerative anemia, erythrogenesis imperfecta,* and *Blackfan-Diamond a.* and *syndrome.* 2. Fanconi's syndrome, def. 1. **icterohemolytic a.** (*obs.*), hemolytic anemia with jaundice. **idiopathic a.,** primary a. **infectious a. of horses,** equine infectious a. **intertropical a.,** hookworm disease. **iron deficiency a.,** anemia characterized by low or absent iron stores, low serum iron concentration, elevated free erythrocyte porphyrin, low transferrin saturation, elevated transferrin, low serum ferritin, low hemoglobin concentration or hematocrit, and hypochromic microcytic red blood cells. Symptoms may include pallor, angular stomatitis and other oral lesions, gastrointestinal complaints, retinal hemorrhages and exudates, and thinning and brittleness of the nails, occasionally leading to spoon nails (koilonychia). **kennel a.,** a disease of dogs caused by *Ancylostoma caninum.* **Lederer's a.** (*obs.*), an acute hemolytic anemia of short duration and unknown etiology, possibly autoimmune, which, when originally described, further helped to establish the concept of acquired hemolytic anemia as distinct from the congenital spherocytic type. **leukoerythroblastic a.,** leukoerythroblastosis. **macrocytic a.,** a name applied to a category of anemias, of varying etiologies, characterized by larger than normal red cells, absence of the customary central area of pallor, and an increased mean corpuscular volume and mean corpuscular hemoglobin. **macrocytic a., nutritional,** folic acid deficiency a. **macrocytic a., tropical,** a type of nutritional macrocytic anemia occurring in India, China, and the African west coast, resembling pernicious anemia in many respects but without achlorhydria and only erratically responsive to vitamin B_{12}. Folic acid produces marked improvement in most cases. **Mediterranean a.,** see *β-thalassemia,* under *thalassemia.* **megaloblastic a.,** anemia characterized by the presence of megaloblasts in the bone marrow. **megaloblastic a., familial,** a rare familial form of anemia observed in Norwegian and Finnish children, characterized by selective intestinal malabsorption of vitamin B_{12} uninfluenced by intrinsic factor, and associated with proteinuria and structural genitourinary tract anomalies; called also *Imerslund* and *Imerslund-Graesbeck syndrome.* **megalocytic a.,** macrocytic a. **microangiopathic a.,** hemolytic a., microangiopathic. **microcytic a.,** anemia characterized by erythrocytes the majority of which are smaller than normal. **milk a.,** cow's milk a. **miners′ a.,** hookworm disease. **mountain a.,** a form of mountain sickness. **myelopathic a., myelophthisic a.,** leukoerythroblastosis. **a. neonato′rum,** the mildest form of erythroblastosis fetalis in which anemia is the chief manifestation; now replaced by the term erythroblastosis qualified by an adjective indicating the degree of severity. **normochromic a.,** anemia in which the hemoglobin content of the red cells as measured by the MCHC is in the normal range. **normocytic a.,** anemia characterized by a proportionate decrease in the hemoglobin content, the packed red cell volume, and the number of erythrocytes per cubic millimeter of blood. **nutritional a.,** deficiency a. **osteosclerotic a.,** a form of myelophthisis occurring in association with osteosclerosis, as a result of the effect on bone marrow of changes in the bones. **pernicious a.,** a megaloblastic anemia occurring in children but more commonly in later life, characterized by histamine-fast achlorhydria, in which the laboratory and clinical manifestations are based on malabsorption of vitamin B$_{12}$ due to a failure of the gastric mucosa to secrete adequate and potent intrinsic factor. Called also *Addison's* or *addisonian a., Addison-Biermer a., cytogenic a.,* and *malignant a.* **pernicious a., juvenile,** megaloblastic anemia occurring in infancy, childhood, or adolescence, resembling the adult form in its response to vitamin B$_{12}$ but distinguished from it by inconstant histamine-fast achlorhydria. **phenylhydrazine a.,** a hemolytic anemia resulting from ingestion of phenylhydrazine, which most probably is converted to a compound that, by acting as an oxidant, transforms oxyhemoglobin to methemoglobin, and then sulfhemoglobin, and finally produces Heinz-Ehrlich bodies. In certain instances, due to an intracellular deficiency of reduced glutathione, and enzymes such as glucose-6-phosphate dehydrogenase, erythrocytes may be particularly sensitive to this agent. **physiologic a.,** the normocytic, normochromic anemia that occurs in infants at the age of two or three months, owing to normal depression of erythropoiesis and hemoglobin synthesis, probably resulting as an adjustment to the change-over from placental to pulmonary oxygenation. **polar a.,** an anemic condition that occurs during exposure to low temperature; initially microcytic, but subsequently becoming normocytic. The basic mechanism is not defined precisely, but it may be due to loss of circulating erythrocytes secondary to trauma or capillary wall diapedesis, in addition to failure of compensatory bone marrow response. Called also *arctic a.* **posthemorrhagic a., acute,** hemorrhagic a. **posthemorrhagic a. of newborn,** anemia of the newborn due to hemorrhage into the placenta or from umbilical vessels; it may range from mild to severe. **primaquine-sensitive a.,** glucose-6-phosphate dehydrogenase a. **primary a.,** an outmoded concept, since all the anemias are regarded as symptoms, and are therefore "secondary." **a. pseudoleuke′mica infan′tum,** a condition originally described as a specific entity in children under age three, with anisocytosis, poikilocytosis, peripheral red blood cell immaturity, leukocytosis, lymphadenopathy, and hepatosplenomegaly; now considered to be a syndrome produced by many factors such as malnutrition, chronic infection, malabsorption, and hemoglobinopathies. **pure red cell a.,** anemia characterized by absence of red cell precursors in the bone marrow. **pyridoxine-responsive a.,** a form of sideroblastic anemia in which there is a therapeutic response to pyridoxine; it affects predominantly young or middle-aged males. **a. refracto′ria sideroblas′tica,** sideroblastic anemia characterized by failure to respond to hematinics; called also *acquired sideroachrestic a.* **refractory a.,** anemia unresponsive to hematinics. **refractory sideroblastic a.,** a. refractoria sideroblastica. **Runeberg's a.** *(obs.),* a remittent form of pernicious anemia; called also *Runeberg's disease* or *type.* **scorbutic a.,** anemia due to deficiency of ascorbic acid (vitamin C); in naturally occurring human scurvy the anemia is generally normocytic, although in experimentally induced vitamin C deficiency the anemia is of the megaloblastic type. **secondary a.,** a term originally used to distinguish anemia due to antecedent or associated disease from anemia thought to be a fundamental disease of the hematopoietic system (primary anemia); the distinction is obsolete since anemia is now recognized as a symptom and thus is always "secondary." **sickle cell a.,** a hereditary, genetically determined hemolytic anemia, one of the hemoglobinopathies, occurring almost exclusively in Negroes, characterized by arthralgia, acute attacks of abdominal pain, ulcerations of the lower extremities, sickle-shaped erythrocytes in the blood, and, for full clinical expression, the homozygous presence of S hemoglobin in the red blood cells, as defined by hemoglobin electrophoresis. Called also *sickl-*

emia, and *Herrick's a.* See also *sickle cell–thalassemia disease,* under *disease.* **sideroachrestic a.,** sideroblastic a. **sideroblastic a.,** a heterogeneous group of anemias with diverse clinical manifestations and with multiple causes each involving a derangement in the final pathway of heme synthesis, in which iron stores of the reticuloendothelial tissues are almost always increased and bone marrow normoblasts contain iron (sideroblasts). Called also *sideroachrestic a.* **sideropenic a.,** a group of anemias characterized by low levels of iron in the plasma; it includes iron deficiency anemia and the anemias of chronic disorders. **simple achlorhydric a.** *(obs.),* iron deficiency a. **slaty a.,** a term applied to a grayish color of the face in poisoning by acetanilid or silver. **spherocytic a.,** hereditary spherocytosis. **splenic a., a. splenet′ica,** congestive splenomegaly; Banti's disease. **spur-cell a.,** anemia in which the red cells have a bizarre spiculated shape and are destroyed prematurely, primarily in the spleen; it is an acquired form occurring in severe liver disease and represents an abnormality in the cholesterol content of the red-cell membrane. **tropical a.,** hookworm disease. **Von Jaksch's a.,** a. pseudoleukemica infantum.

anemic (ah-ne′mik) pertaining to or characterized by anemia.

anem(o)- [Gr. *anemos* wind] a combining form denoting relationship to wind.

anemometer (an″ĕ-mom′ĕ-ter) [anemo- + Gr. *metron* measure] an instrument for measuring the velocity of air or gas flow.

Anemone (ah-nem′o-ne) a large genus of plants of the family Ranunculaceae, with divided leaves and conspicuous flowers of sepals. They generally contain ranunculin, which converts enzymatically to toxic protoanemonin, a principle held responsible for animal poisoning. Protoanemonin ultimately converts to anemonin, a substituted diacrylic acid dilactone, which has been used as a sedative and antispasmodic. Anemonin is present in *A. pulsatilla* and other species. Several species have been used medicinally.

anemonin (ah-nem′o-nin) the active principle of *Anemone pulsatilla,* a colorless crystalline substance, $C_{10}H_8O_4$, or pulsatilla camphor.

anemonism (ah-nem′o-nizm) poisoning by plants of the genus *Anemone.*

anemonol (ah-nem′o-nol) an exceedingly poisonous volatile oil from various species of *Anemone* and from other ranunculaceous plants.

anemophilous (an″ĕ-mof′ĭ-lus) [anemo- + Gr. *philein* to love] pollinated by the wind; said of certain flowers.

anemophobia (an″ĕ-mo-fo′be-ah) [anemo- + *phobia*] irrational fear of wind or of drafts.

anemotaxis (an″ĕ-mo-tak′sis) [anemo- + Gr. *taxis* arrangement] adjustment with reference to the wind.

anemotrophy (an″ĕ-mot′ro-fe) [an neg. + Gr. *haima* blood + *trophē* nourishment] deficiency of blood nourishment.

anemotropism (an″ĕ-mot′ro-pism) [anemo- + Gr. *tropos* a turning] a turning toward or away from the wind.

anencephalia (an″en-sĕ-fa′le-ah) anencephaly.

anencephalic (an″en-sĕ-fal′ik) exhibiting anencephaly; having no brain.

anencephalous (an″en-sef′ah-lus) having no brain.

anencephalus (an″en-sef′ah-lus) a monster exhibiting anencephaly.

anencephaly (an″en-sef′ah-le) [an neg. + Gr. *enkephalos* brain] congenital absence of the cranial vault, with cerebral hemispheres completely missing or reduced to small masses attached to the base of the skull.

anenterous (an-en′ter-us) [an neg. + Gr. *enteron* intestine] lacking intestines.

anenzymia (an″en-zi′me-ah) [an- neg. + *enzyme* + -ia] a morbid condition resulting from absence of an enzyme normally present in the body. **a. catala′sea,** acatalasia.

anephric (a-nef′rik) being without kidneys.

anephrogenesis (a″nef-ro-jen′ĕ-sis) [a neg. + Gr. *nephros* kidney + *genesis*] congenital absence of kidney tissue.

anepiploic (an-ep′e-plo′ik) devoid of omentum.

anepithymia (an-ep″e-thim′e-ah) loss of any natural appetite.

anerethisia (an-er″ĕ-thiz′e-ah) [*an* neg. + Gr. *erethizein* to excite + *-ia*] deficient irritability.

anergia (an-er′je-ah) anergy.

anergic (an-er′jik) [*an* neg. + Gr. *ergon* work] 1. characterized by abnormal inactivity; inactive. 2. marked by asthenia or lack of energy. 3. pertaining to anergy.

anergy (an′er-je) 1. lack of energy; asthenia. 2. diminished reactivity to specific antigen(s); it may take the form of diminished immediate hypersensitivity or diminished delayed hypersensitivity, or both. **negative a.,** transient reduction in reactivity to allergens in a sensitized individual, occurring as a result of intervening events, such as cachexia. **positive a.,** reduction in reactivity to allergens in a sensitized individual, owing to alterations in the immune response in the course of disease, as in tuberculosis.

aneroid (an′er-oid) [*a* neg. + Gr. *nēros* liquid + *eidos* form] not containing liquid.

anerythroplasia (an″ĕ-rith″ro-pla′ze-ah) [*an* neg. + Gr. *erythros* red + *plassein* to form + *-ia*] absence of erythrocyte formation.

anerythroplastic (an″ĕ-rith″ro-plas′tik) pertaining to or characterized by anerythroplasia.

anerythropoiesis (an″ĕ-rith″ro-poi-e′sis) [*an* neg. + *erythropoiesis*] deficient production of erythrocytes.

anerythroregenerative (an″ĕ-rith″ro-re-jen′er-a″tiv) see *aregenerative.*

anesthecinesia (an-es″the-sĭ-ne′ze-ah) [*an* neg. + Gr. *aisthēsis* perception + *kinēsis* movement + *-ia*] loss of sensibility and motor power.

anesthekinesia (an-es″the-kĭ-ne′ze-ah) anesthecinesia.

anesthesia (an″es-the′ze-ah) [*an* neg. + Gr. *aisthēsis* sensation] loss of feeling or sensation. Although the term is used for loss of tactile sensibility, or of any of the other senses, it is applied especially to loss of the sensation of pain, as it is induced to permit performance of surgery or other painful procedures. **angiospastic a.,** loss of sensibility dependent on spasm of the blood vessels. **balanced a.,** anesthesia which utilizes a combination of drugs, each in an amount sufficient to produce its major or desired effect to the optimum degree and keep its undesirable or unnecessary effects to a minimum. **basal a.,** anesthesia which acts as a basis for further and deeper anesthesia; a state of narcosis produced by preliminary medication so profound that the added inhalation anesthetic necessary to produce surgical anesthesia is greatly reduced. **Bier's local a.,** local anesthesia produced by injection of a 0.5 per cent solution of procaine into the veins of a limb that has been rendered bloodless by elevation and constriction; called also *vein a.* **block a.,** see *regional a.* and *block.* **bulbar a.,** lack of sensation caused by a lesion of the pons. **caudal a.,** anesthesia produced by injection of a local anesthetic into the caudal or sacral canal. **central a.,** lack of sensation caused by disease of the nerve centers. **cerebral a.,** lack of sensation caused by a cerebral lesion. **closed a.,** inhalational anesthesia maintained by the continuous rebreathing of a relatively small amount of the anesthetic gas, normally used with an absorption apparatus for the removal of carbon dioxide. **colonic a.,** anesthesia induced by injection of the anesthetic agent into the rectum and lower colon. **compression a.,** loss of sensation resulting from pressure on a nerve. **conduction a.,** regional a. **continuous caudal a.,** see under *analgesia.* **Corning's a.,** see *spinal a.,* def. 1. **crossed a.,** hemianesthesia cruciata. **dissociated a.,** dissociation a., loss of certain sensations while others remain intact. **doll's head a.,** loss of sensation affecting the head, neck, and upper part of the thorax. **a. doloro′sa,** pain in an area or region that is anesthetic. **electric a.,** anesthesia induced by passage of an electric current. **endobronchial a.,** anesthesia produced by introduction of a gaseous mixture through a slender tube placed in a large bronchus. **endotracheal a.,** anesthesia produced by introduction of a gaseous mixture through a wide-bore tube inserted into the trachea. **epidural a.,** anesthesia produced by injection of the anesthetic agent between the vertebral spines and beneath the ligamentum flavum into the extradural space; called also *peridural a.* **facial a.,** loss of sensation caused by a lesion of the facial nerve. **frost a.,** abolition of feeling or sensation as a result of topical refrigeration produced by a jet of highly volatile liquid. **gauntlet a.,** loss of sensation in the hand and wrist; called also *glove a.* **general a.,** a state of un-

consciousness, produced by anesthetic agents, with absence of pain sensation over the entire body and a greater or lesser degree of muscular relaxation; the drugs producing this state can be administered by inhalation, intravenously, intramuscularly, rectally, or via the gastrointestinal tract. **girdle a.,** loss of sensation in a zone encircling the hips. **glove a.,** gauntlet a. **gustatory a.,** loss of the sense of taste. **Gwathmey's oil-ether a.,** anesthesia produced by introduction into the rectum of a mixture of liquid ether and olive oil. **high pressure a.,** anesthesia produced by controlled application of pressure to a nerve trunk or its branches. **hypnosis a.,** production of insensibility to pain during surgical procedures by means of hypnotism. **hypotensive a.,** anesthesia accompanied by the deliberate lowering of the blood pressure, a procedure said to reduce blood loss. **hypothermic a.,** anesthesia accompanied by the deliberate lowering of the body temperature. **hysterical a.,** loss of tactile sensation occurring as a symptom of conversion hysteria, often recognizable by its lack of correspondence with nerve distributions. **infiltration a.,** the production of local anesthesia by deposition of a local anesthesia solution in the area of small, terminal nerve endings. **inhalation a.,** anesthesia produced by the inhalation of vapors of a volatile liquid or gaseous anesthetic agent. **insufflation a.,** anesthesia produced by blowing a mixture of gases or vapors through a tube introduced into the respiratory tract. **intercostal a.,** anesthesia produced by blocking intercostal nerves with a local anesthetic. **intranasal a.,** local anesthesia produced by insertion into the nasal fossae of pledgets soaked in a solution of an anesthetic agent which is effective after topical application, or by insufflation of a mixture of anesthetic gases or vapors through a tube introduced into the nose. **intraoral a.,** anesthesia produced within the oral cavity by injection, spray, pressure, etc. **intraosseous a.,** a local anesthetic effect produced by the administration of an anesthetic agent directly into the cancellous portion of bone. **intrapulpal a.,** a local anesthetic effect produced by the administration of an anesthetic agent directly into the dental pulp. **intraspinal a.,** spinal a., def. 1. **intravenous a.,** anesthesia produced by introduction of an anesthetic agent into a vein. **Kulenkampff's a.,** anesthesia of the upper extremity produced by injection of a local anesthetic around the brachial plexus. **local a.,** anesthesia confined to one part of the body. **lumbar epidural a.,** anesthesia produced by injection of the anesthetic agent into the epidural space at the second or third lumbar interspace. **Meltzer's a.,** see under *method.* **mental a.,** loss of ability to recognize or identify sensory stimulations. **mixed a.,** anesthesia which is produced by administration of more than one anesthetic agent; see also *balanced a.* **muscular a.,** loss of the muscular sense. **nausea a.,** loss of the sensation of nausea, usually stimulated by noxious and disgusting substances. **nerve blocking a.,** regional a. **olfactory a.,** anosmia. **open a.,** general inhalation anesthesia utilizing a cone; there is no significant rebreathing of expired gases. **paraneural a.,** anesthesia produced by injection of the anesthetic agent around a nerve; called also *paraneural infiltration.* **parasacral a.,** regional anesthesia produced by injection of a local anesthetic around the sacral nerves as they emerge from the sacral foramina. **paravertebral a.,** regional anesthesia produced by injection of a local anesthetic around the spinal nerves at their exit from the spinal column, and outside the spinal dura. **partial a.,** anesthesia with retention of some degree of sensibility. **peridural a.,** epidural a. **perineural a.,** regional anesthesia produced by injection of the anesthetic agent close to the nerve. **peripheral a.,** loss of sensation which is due to changes in the peripheral nerves. **permeation a.,** analgesia of a body surface produced by the application of a local anesthetic, most commonly to mucous membranes; called also *surface a.* **plexus a.,** anesthesia produced by the injection of a local anesthetic around a nerve plexus. **pressure a.,** anesthesia produced by a local anesthetic forced into the tissues by pressure. **rectal a.,** anesthesia induced by introduction of an anesthetic agent into the rectum. **refrigeration a.,** local anesthesia produced by applying a tourniquet and chilling the part to near freezing temperature; called also *crymoanesthesia.* **regional a.,** the production of insensibility of a part by interrupting the sensory nerve conductivity from that region of the body. It may be produced by (1) *field block,* that is, the creation of walls of anesthesia encircling the operative field by means of injections of a local anesthetic; or (2) *nerve block*, that is, injection of the anesthetic agent close to the nerves whose conductivity is to be cut off. Called also *block a.*, *conduction a.*, and *block.* **sacral a.,** anesthesia produced by injection of a local anesthetic into the extradural space of the sacral canal. **saddle block a.,** the production of anesthesia in a region corresponding roughly with the areas of the buttocks, perineum, and inner aspects of the thighs which impinge on the saddle in riding, by introducing the anesthetic agent low in the dural sac. **segmental a.,** loss of sensation caused by lesions of nerve roots. **semiclosed a.,** general inhalation anesthesia in which there is partial rebreathing of the expired gases, with a carbon dioxide absorber in the circuit. **semiopen a.,** general inhalation anesthesia administered by use of an open cone or a partially open circuit; there is partial rebreathing of the expired gases without a carbon dioxide absorber in the circuit. **spinal a.,** 1. anesthesia produced by injection of a local anesthetic into the subarachnoid space around the spinal cord; called also *Corning's a.* or *method, intraspinal a.,* and *subarachnoid a.* 2. loss of sensation due to a spinal lesion. **splanchnic a.,** anesthesia produced by injection of a local anesthetic around the semilunar ganglia. **subarachnoid a.,** spinal a., def. 1. **surface a.,** permeation a. **surgical a.,** that degree of anesthesia at which surgery may safely be performed; ordinarily used to designate such depth of general anesthesia. **tactile a.,** loss or impairment of the sense of touch. **thalamic hyperesthetic a.,** see *thalamic syndrome*, under *syndrome*. **thermal a., thermic a.,** loss of the temperature sense. **topical a.,** anesthesia produced by application of a local anesthetic directly to the area involved, as to the oral mucosa or the cornea. **total a.,** loss of all sensibility in the affected part. **transsacral a.,** spinal anesthesia produced by injection of the anesthetic agent into the sacral canal and about the sacral nerves through each of the posterior sacral foramina. **traumatic a.,** loss of sensation caused by injury to a nerve. **twilight a.,** twilight sleep. **unilateral a.,** hemianesthesia. **vein a.,** Bier's local a. **visceral a.,** loss of visceral sensations.

anesthesimeter (an-es″thĕ-sim′ĕ-ter) [*anesthesia* + Gr. *metron* measure] 1. an instrument to regulate the amount of an anesthetic administered. 2. an instrument for taking the degree of insensitiveness.

Anesthesin (ah-nes′thĕ-sin) trademark for a preparation of benzocaine.

anesthesiologist (an″es-the″ze-ol′o-jist) a physician or dentist specializing in anesthesiology. Cf. *anesthetist.*

anesthesiology (an″es-the″ze-ol′o-je) [*anesthesia* + *-logy*] that branch of medicine which studies anesthesia and anesthetics.

anesthesiophore (an″es-the′ze-o-fōr″) [*anesthesia* + Gr. *phoros* bearing] 1. conveying the anesthetic action. 2. the portion of the molecule of a chemical compound which is responsible for its anesthetic action.

anesthetic (an″es-thet′ik) 1. pertaining to, characterized by, or producing anesthesia. 2. a drug or agent that is used to abolish the sensation of pain. **general a.,** an agent that produces general anesthesia. **local a.,** an agent whose anesthetic action is limited to an area of the body determined by the site of its application; it produces its effect by blocking nerve conduction. **topical a.,** a local anesthetic applied directly to the area to be anesthetized, usually the mucous membranes or the skin.

anesthetist (ah-nes′thĕ-tist) a person, such as a nurse or technician, trained in the administration of anesthetics. Cf. *anesthesiologist.*

anesthetization (ah-nes″thĕ-tĭ-za′shun) the production of insensibility to pain.

anesthetize (ah-nes′thĕ-tīz) to put under the influence of anesthetics.

anesthetometer (an″es-thĕ-tom′ĕ-ter) an apparatus for measuring and mixing anesthetic vapors and gases.

anesthetospasm (an″es-thet′o-spazm) spasm with anesthesia.

anestrum (an-es′trum) anestrus.

anestrus (an-es′trus) a period of sexual inactivity intervening between two estrous cycles.

anethene (an′e-thēn) a hydrocarbon, $C_{10}H_{16}$, from oil of dill.

anethole (an′ĕ-thōl) [NF] chemical name: (*E*)-1-methoxy-

4-(1-propenyl)benzene. A colorless or faintly yellow liquid, $C_{10}H_{12}O$, obtained from anise and fennel oils and other sources, or prepared synthetically; used as a flavoring agent for drugs, and formerly as a carminative and expectorant. Called also *anise camphor.*

Anethum (ah-ne′thum) [L.; Gr. *anēthon*] a genus of plants, including fennel and dill, the source of oil of dill and a source of carvone. The fruit of *A. graveolens* (*Peucedanum graveolens*), or dill, is carminative and stimulant.

anetic (ah-net′ik) relaxing or soothing.

anetiological (an-e″te-o-loj′e-kal) [*an* neg. + *etiologic*] not conforming to etiologic principles.

anetoderma (an″ĕ-to-der′mah) [Gr. *anetos* slack + *derma* skin] localized elastolysis producing circumscribed areas of soft, thin, wrinkled skin that often protrude as small outpouchings. It may be a primary condition, which may or may not be associated with inflammatory lesions, or it may be secondary to some other condition involving the skin, such as syphilis, leprosy, or tuberculosis. Called also *atrophia cutis, atrophia maculata, atrophoderma maculatum,* and *macular atrophy.* See also *atrophoderma.* **Jadassohn's a., Jadassohn-Pellizari a.,** primary anetoderma occurring following an inflammatory or urticarial eruption; the lesions are round or oval erythematous macules that become atrophic, wrinkled, and pale protrusions. It is usually seen in women in their second to fourth decade. Cf. *Schweninger-Buzzi a.* **perifollicular a.,** anetoderma occurring around hair follicles not preceded by folliculitis; it may be caused by an elastase-producing strain of *Staphylococcus epidermidis*, it may be drug induced, or endocrine factors may be involved. Called also *perifollicular elastolysis.* **postinflammatory a.,** a condition usually occurring during infancy characterized by the development of erythematous papules that enlarge to form oval plaques with a cordlike border with a scaly collarette at the inner margin. All areas of the body except the palms and soles may be affected with the face, ears, and neck always being involved; it is followed by laxity of the skin clinically resembling cutis laxa. Called also *postinflammatory elastolysis.* **Schweninger-Buzzi a.,** progressive primary anetoderma without any preceding inflammatory condition, characterized by the abrupt appearance of many bluish white macules, some of which are protuberant, and usually seen in women. Cf. *Jadassohn's a.*

aneugamy (an-u′gah-me) [*an-* neg. + Gr. *eu* well + *gamos* marriage] union of gametes in one or both of which the chromosomes have not been reduced to the normal haploid number, resulting in an abnormal number of chromosomes (aneuploidy) in the zygote.

aneuploid (an′u-ploid) [*an-* + *euploid*] 1. a chromosome number that is not an exact multiple of the normal diploid number. 2. an individual or cell having an aneuploid number of chromosomes.

aneuploidy (an″u-ploi′de) any deviation from an exact multiple of the haploid number of chromosomes, whether fewer (hypoploidy, as in Turner's syndrome) or more (hyperploidy, as in Down's syndrome). Individuals exhibiting aneuploidy are usually abnormal physiologically and morphologically. Cf. *euploidy* and *polyploidy.*

aneurin (ah-nu′rin) [*an* neg. + Gr. *neuron* nerve] thiamine hydrochloride (vitamin B_1).

aneurine hydrochloride (an′u-rin) thiamine hydrochloride.

aneurogenic (a″nu-ro-jen′ik) pertaining to or characterized by absence of formation of nerve fibers.

aneurysm (an′u-rizm) [Gr. *aneurysma* a widening] a sac formed by the dilatation of the wall of an artery, a vein, or the heart. The chief signs of arterial aneurysm are the formation of a pulsating tumor, and often a bruit (*aneurysmal bruit*) heard over the swelling. Sometimes there are symptoms from pressure on contiguous parts. **abdominal a.,** an aneurysm of the abdominal aorta. **ampullary a.,** sacculated a. **a. by anastomosis, a. anastomot′ica** (*obs.*), a dilatation of several arteries which forms a pulsating tumor under the skin. **aortic a.,** aneurysm of the aorta. **aortic sinusal a.,** aneurysm arising in the aortic sinuses of Valsalva; these rare lesions may be either developmental or syphilitic. **arteriovenous a.** (William Hunter, 1761), a communication, sometimes congenital, often traumatic, between an artery and a vein in which the blood flows directly into a neighboring vein (*aneurysmal varix*) or else is carried into such a vein by a connecting sac (*varicose*

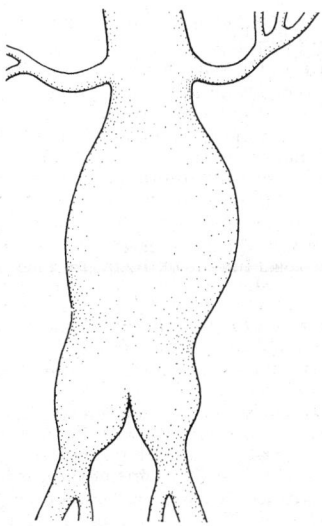

Aneurysm of the abdominal aorta and common iliac arteries.

aneurysm). **arteriovenous pulmonary a.,** arteriove-nous fistula. **atherosclerotic a.,** an aneurysm arising as a result of weakening of the media in severe atherosclero-sis. **axillary a.,** aneurysm of the axillary artery. **bac-terial a.,** see *infected a.* **berry a.,** a small saccular an-eurysm of a cerebral artery, usually at the junction of vessels in the circle of Willis, having a narrow opening into the artery; such aneurysms frequently rupture, causing sub-arachnoid hemorrhage. **brain a.,** berry a. **cardiac a.,** thinning and dilatation of a portion of the wall of the left ventricle, usually consequent to myocardial infarction but rare forms have been described. **cerebral a.,** berry a. **cirsoid a.,** racemose a. **compound a.,** one in which some of the coats are ruptured and others merely dilated; called also *mixed a.* **congenital cerebral a.,** berry a. **Crisp's a.** (*obs.*), aneurysm of the splenic artery. **cylin-droid a.,** the uniform dilatation of a considerable part of an artery; called also *tubular a.* **cystogenic a.** (*obs.*), one formed by the rupture of a cyst into an artery. **dissect-ing a.,** one resulting from hemorrhage that causes longitudi-nal splitting of the arterial wall, producing a tear in the intima and establishing communication with the lumen; it usually affects the thoracic aorta. Called also *aortic dissec-tion, Laennec's disease,* and *Shekelton's a.* **ectatic a.,** one formed by distention of a section of an artery without rupture of any of its coats. **embolic a.,** the most common form of mycotic aneurysm. **embolomycotic a.** (*obs.*), aneurysm due to embolism from some vegetative condition in the heart. **false a.,** one in which the entire wall is injured and the blood is contained by the surrounding tissues, with eventual formation of a sac communicating with the artery (or heart); called also *aneurysmal hematoma, pulsatile hematoma,* and *spurious a.* **fusiform a.,** a spindle-shaped arterial aneu-rysm in which the stretching process affects the entire circumference of the artery; called also *Richet's a.* Cf. *saccular a.* **hernial a.,** one in which the sac is formed by an inner coat projecting through the outer. **infected a.,** aneurysm produced by growth of bacteria (*bacterial a.*) or fungi (*mycotic a.*) in the vessel wall, or infection arising within a preexisting arteriosclerotic aneurysm. Called also *bacterial a.* and *mycotic a.* **innominate a.,** aneurysm of the innominate artery (brachiocephalic trunk). **intracra-nial a.,** any aneurysm situated within the cranium. **lat-eral a.,** one that projects from one side of an artery. **miliary a.,** aneurysm of a minute artery, chiefly intracra-nial or retinal. **mixed a.** (*obs.*), compound a. **mural a.** (*obs.*), aneurysm of the heart wall. **mycotic a.,** see *in-fected a.* **orbital a.,** one situated within the orbit of the eye. **Park's a.,** an arteriovenous aneurysm occurring at the elbow and establishing communication between the brachial artery and the brachial and median basilic veins.

pelvic a., one situated within the pelvis. **Pott's a.,** an aneurysmal varix. **racemose a.,** a condition in which the blood vessels become dilated, lengthened, and tortuous; called also *cirsoid a.* and *diffuse arterial ectasia.* **Ras-mussen's a.,** dilatation of an artery in a tuberculous cavity; its rupture produces hemorrhage. **renal a.,** an aneurysm within the kidney. **Richet's a.,** fusiform a. **Rodri-gues' a.,** a varicose aneurysm with the sac lying contiguous to the artery. **saccular a., sacculated a.,** an eccen-tric, localized distended sac affecting only a part of the circumference of the arterial wall. Cf. *fusiform a.* **ser-pentine a.,** an elongated and varicose senile condition of certain arteries, such as the splenic, iliac, and temporal. **Shekelton's a.,** dissecting a. **spurious a.,** false a. **suprasellar a.,** aneurysm of the internal carotid artery above the sella turcica. **syphilitic a.,** aortic aneurysm occurring in cases of cardiovascular syphilis. **thoracic a.,** one situated within the thorax. **traumatic a.,** an an-eurysm due to injury. **true a.,** an aneurysm in which the sac is formed by the arterial walls one of which, at least, is unbroken. **tubular a.,** cylindroid a. **varicose a.,** an aneurysm in which the artery communicates with contiguous veins by means of an intervening sac. **venous a.,** aneu-rysm of a vein. **ventricular a.,** an aneurysmal dilata-tion of a portion of the wall of the left ventricle or, rarely, a saccular protrusion through it (*false a.* of the heart). **ver-minous a.,** aneurysm of equines caused by strongylid worms; called also *worm a.* **worm a.,** verminous a.

aneurysmal (an″u-riz′mal) pertaining to or resembling an aneurysm.

aneurysmatic (an″u-riz-mat′ik) aneurysmal.

aneurysmectomy (an″u-riz-mek′to-me) [*aneurysm* + Gr. *ektomē* excision] extirpation of an aneurysm by removal of the sac.

aneurysmoplasty (an″u-riz′mo-plas″te) [*aneurysm* + Gr. *plassein* to form] plastic reconstruction of an aneurysmal artery.

aneurysmorrhaphy (an″u-riz-mor′ah-fe) [*aneurysm* + Gr. *rhaphē* suture] the operation of suturing an aneurysm.

aneurysmotomy (an″u-riz-mot′o-me) [*aneurysm* + Gr. *tomē* cut] the operation of incising the sac of an aneurysm.

ANF antinuclear factor; see *antinuclear antibody* (*ANA*), under *antibody*.

angei- for words beginning thus, see those beginning *angi-*.

Angelica (an-jel′e-kah) [L., from Gr. *angelikos* angelic] a genus of umbelliferous plants; the roots and fruit of *A. archangelica* (garden angelica) afford volatile oils, angelic acid (formerly a sedative), and several acids. The plant has carminative, diaphoretic, and diuretic properties.

angeline (an′jĕ-lin) surinamine.

Angelucci's syndrome (an″jĕ-loo′chēz) [Arnaldo *Ange-lucci*, Naples ophthalmologist, 1854–1933] see under *syn-drome.*

Anghelescu's sign (ahn-jĕ-les′kōōz) [Constantin *Anghe-lescu*, Roumanian surgeon, 1869–1948] see under *sign.*

angialgia (an″je-al′je-ah) [*angi-* + Gr. *algos* pain + *-ia*] pain in a blood vessel; called also *angiodynia.*

angiasthenia (an″je-as-the′ne-ah) [*angi-* + a neg. + Gr. *sthe-nos* strength + *-ia*] loss of tone in the vascular system; vascular instability.

angiectasis (an″je-ek′tah-sis) [*angi-* + Gr. *ektasis* dilatation] gross dilatation and often lengthening of a blood vessel.

angiectatic (an″je-ek-tat′ik) pertaining to or character-ized by angiectasis.

angiectomy (an″je-ek′to-me) [*angi-* + Gr. *ektomē* excision] the excision or resection of a vessel.

angiectopia (an″je-ek-to′pe-ah) [*angi-* + Gr. *ek* out + Gr. *topos* place + *-ia*] abnormal position or course of a vessel.

angiitis (an″je-i′tis), pl. *angii′tides* [*angi-* + *-itis*] inflam-mation of a vessel, chiefly of a blood or a lymph vessel; called also *vasculitis.* **allergic granulomatous a.,** a form of systemic necrotizing vasculitis in which there is prominent lung involvement, generally manifested by eosinophilia, granulomatous reactions, and usually severe asthma; if present, cutaneous lesions consist of tender subcutaneous nodules, large ecchymotic plaques, and cutaneous infarcts. Called also *Churg-Strauss syndrome* and *allergic granuloma-tosis.* **consecutive a.,** inflammation of a vessel caused by extension of the inflammation from the neighboring tissues. **leukocytoclastic a.,** hypersensitivity vasculitis. **necrotizing a.,** see under *vasculitis.* **visceral a.,** a term proposed for a group of disorders marked by peculiar lesions of the small arteries, such as periarteritis nodosa, allergic angiitis, and lupus erythematosus disseminatus.

angina (an-ji'nah, an'ji-nah) [L.] spasmodic, choking, or suffocative pain; now used almost exclusively to denote angina pectoris. **abdominal a., a. abdomina'lis, a. abdom'inis,** intestinal a. **a. acu'ta,** simple sore throat. **agranulocytic a.,** agranulocytosis. **benign croupous a.,** pharyngitis herpetica. **Bretonneau's a.,** diphtheria. **a. catarrha'lis,** acute pharyngitis. **a. cor'dis,** a. pectoris. **a. croupo'sa** (*obs.*), pseudomembranous or croupous sore throat. **a. cru'ris,** intermittent claudication. **a. decu'bitus,** cardiac pain occurring in a recumbent position. **a. dyspep'tica,** a condition resembling angina pectoris but due to distention of the stomach with gas. **a. epiglottide'a,** inflammation of the epiglottis. **exudative a.,** croup. **a. follicula'ris,** follicular tonsillitis. **a. gangreno'sa,** gangrenous inflammation of the fauces. Called also *malignant a.* **hippocratic a.,** retropharyngeal abscess. **hysteric a.,** pain simulating angina in a hysterical patient. **intestinal a.,** cramping postprandial abdominal pain caused by ischemia of the smooth muscle of the bowel in patients with mesenteric vascular insufficiency. **a. inver'sa,** a variant form of angina pectoris in which there is elevation, rather than depression, of the RS-T interval of the electrocardiogram. **lacunar a.,** tonsillitis. **a. laryn'gea,** laryngitis. **Ludwig's a.,** a severe form of cellulitis of the submaxillary space and secondary involvement of the sublingual and submental spaces, usually resulting from an infection in the mandibular molar area or a penetrating injury of the floor of the mouth. Elevation of the tongue, difficulty in eating and swallowing, edema of the glottis, fever, rapid breathing, and moderate leukocytosis are the most common symptoms. **malignant a.,** a. gangrenosa. **a. membrana'cea,** croup. **neutropenic a.,** agranulocytosis. **a. nosoco'mii,** pharyngitis ulcerosa. **a. pec'toris,** a paroxysmal thoracic pain, with a feeling of suffocation and impending death, due, most often, to anoxia of the myocardium and precipitated by effort or excitement; has been called *a. cordis, angor pectoris, Elsner's asthma, Heberden's asthma* or *disease, Rougnon-Heberden disease,* and *stenocardia.* **a. pec'toris vasomoto'ria,** a condition marked by precordial pain due to vasomotor disturbance and showing no organic disease of the heart; called also *vasomotor a.* **a. phlegmono'sa,** peritonsillar abscess. **Plaut's a., pseudomembranous a.,** necrotizing ulcerative gingivostomatitis. **preinfarction a.,** status anginosus. **Prinzmetal's a.,** a variant of angina pectoris in which the attacks occur during rest, exercise capacity is well preserved, and attacks are associated electrocardiographically with elevation of the ST-segment. Called also *variant a. pectoris.* **a. rheumat'ica,** pharyngitis associated with rheumatic diathesis. **a. scarlatino'sa,** pharyngitis associated with scarlet fever. **Schultz's a.,** agranulocytosis. **a. sim'plex,** simple sore throat. **a. sine dolo're,** an episode of coronary insufficiency in which no pain is experienced. **a. tonsilla'ris,** peritonsillar abscess. **a. trachea'lis,** croup. **a. ulcero'sa,** pharyngitis ulcerosa. **variant a. pectoris,** Prinzmetal's a. **vasomotor a.,** a. pectoris vasomotoria. **Vincent's a.,** painful membraneous ulceration with edema and hyperemic patches of the oropharynx and throat, caused by spreading of acute necrotizing ulcerative gingivitis.

anginal (an-ji'nal, an'ji-nal) pertaining to or characteristic of angina.

anginiform (an-jin'i-form) resembling angina.

anginoid (an'ji-noid) resembling angina.

anginophobia (an''jin-o-fo'be-ah) [angina + phobia] irrational dread of choking.

anginose (an'ji-nōs) [L. *anginosus*] pertaining to or affected with angina, especially angina pectoris.

anginosis (an''ji-no'sis) a general term for anginal conditions; angina; often used to denote continuing pain; status anginosus.

anginous (an'ji-nus) anginose.

angi(o)- [Gr. *angeion* vessel] a combining form denoting relationship to a vessel, usually a blood vessel.

angioaccess (an''je-o-ak'ses) a site of entry into a blood vessel, as one maintained for recurrent hemodialysis.

angioasthenia (an''je-o-as-the'ne-ah) angiasthenia.

angioataxia (an''je-o-ah-tak'se-ah) [angio- + ataxia] irregular tension of the blood vessels.

angioblast (an'je-o-blast'') [angio- + Gr. *blastos* germ] 1. the mesenchymal tissue of the embryo from which the blood cells and blood vessels differentiate; called also *angioderm.* 2. an individual vessel-forming cell.

angioblastic (an''je-o-blas'tik) pertaining to angioblast.

angioblastoma (an''je-o-blas-to'mah) a term applied to certain blood-vessel tumors of the brain: those arising in the cerebellum (cerebellar angioblastoma) may be cystic and associated with von Hippel-Lindau's disease; also, a blood-vessel tumor arising from the meninges of the brain or spinal cord (angioblastic meningioma).

angiocardiogram (an''je-o-kar'de-o-gram) the film produced by angiocardiography.

angiocardiography (an''je-o-kar''de-og'rah-fe) [angio- + Gr. *kardia* heart + *graphein* to write] roentgenography of the heart and great vessels after introduction of contrast material into a blood vessel or one of the cardiac chambers.

angiocardiokinetic (an''je-o-kar''de-o-ki-net'ik) [angio- + Gr. *kardia* heart + *kinēsis* motion] 1. affecting the motions or movements of the heart and blood vessels. 2. any agent that affects the movements of the heart and vessels.

angiocardiopathy (an''je-o-kar''de-op'ah-the) any disease of the heart and blood vessels.

angiocarditis (an''je-o-kar-di'tis) [angio- + Gr. *kardia* heart + -*itis*] inflammation of the heart and great blood vessels.

angiocavernous (an''je-o-kav'er-nus) of the nature of angioma and cavernoma.

angiocheiloscope (an''je-o-ki'lo-skōp'') [angio- + Gr. *cheilos* lip + *skopein* to view] an instrument for observing blood circulation of the lips under magnification.

angiochondroma (an''je-o-kon-dro'mah) a chondroma about which there is an excessive development of blood vessels.

angioclast (an'je-o-klast'') [angio- + Gr. *klastos* broken] former name for hemostat.

Angiococcus (an''je-o-kok'us) [Gr. *angeion* vessel + *kokkos* berry] in former systems of classification, a genus of bacteria of the family Myxococcaceae, the taxonomic status of which is uncertain. One species has been assigned to the genus *Streptosporangium.*

Angio-Conray (an''je-o-kon'ra) trademark for a preparation of sodium iothalamate.

angiocrine (an'je-o-krīn) [angio- + endocrine] denoting vasomotor disorders of endocrine origin.

angiocrinosis (an''je-o-kri-no'sis) a vasomotor disorder of endocrine origin.

angiocyst (an'je-o-sist'') [angio- + cyst] angioblastic cyst.

angioderm (an'je-o-derm) angioblast, def. 1.

angiodermatitis (an''je-o-der-mah-ti'tis) [angio- + dermatitis] inflammation of the vessels of the skin. Angiodermatitis occurring in association with arteriovenous fistula is known as *pseudo-Kaposi sarcoma.* **disseminated pruritic a.,** itching purpura.

angiodiascopy (an''je-o-di-as'ko-pe) [angio- + Gr. *dia* through + *skopein* to view] direct visual inspection of blood vessels of the extremities, a light being held behind the part.

angiodynia (an''je-o-din'e-ah) [angio- + Gr. *odynē* pain + -*ia*] angialgia.

angiodysplasia (an''je-o-dis-pla'ze-ah) small vascular abnormalities, especially of the intestinal tract.

angiodystrophia (an''je-o-dis-tro'fe-ah) [angio- + dystrophy] defective nutrition of blood vessels. **a. ova'rii,** angiodystrophia of the blood vessels of the ovary.

angiodystrophy (an''je-o-dis'tro-fe) angiodystrophia.

angioectatic (an''je-o-ek-tat'ik) angiectatic.

angioedema (an''je-o-e-de'mah) [angio- + edema] a vascular reaction involving the deep dermis or subcutaneous or submucosal tissues, representing localized edema caused by dilatation and increased permeability of the capillaries, and characterized by development of giant wheals. Hereditary angioedema, transmitted as an autosomal dominant trait, tends to involve more visceral lesions than the sporadic form and is caused by a deficiency or functional impairment of complement component C1 esterase inhibitor (C1INH), resulting in increased levels of several vasoactive mediators of anaphylaxis. *Urticaria* (q.v.) is the same physiologic reaction occurring in the superficial portions of the dermis. Called also *angioneurotic, circumscribed, giant, Milton's, periodic,* or *Quincke's edema; Bannister's, Milton's,* or *Quincke's disease;* and *giant urticaria.* **hereditary a.,** inherited C1 inhibitor (C1 INH) deficiency; an autosomal dominant disorder manifested as recurrent episodes of edema of the skin, upper respiratory tract, and gastrointestinal tract. It may be mediated by such factors as minor trauma, sudden changes in environmental temperature, and sudden emotional stress. There are two variants: one in which no C1 INH is produced, and another in which there are normal serum levels of a nonfunctional C1 INH. The lack of C1 INH causes uncontrolled activation of the classical complement pathway and the production of a kininlike substance (C2 kinin) derived from the attack of C1 on C2 and C4. **vibratory a.,** angioedema due to vibratory stimuli to the skin, occurring as an inherited autosomal dominant disorder, in association with cholinergic urticaria, or after prolonged occupational exposure to vibration.

angioedematous (an″je-o″e-de′mah-tus) pertaining to or characterized by angioedema.

angioelephantiasis (an″je-o-el″ĕ-fan-ti′ah-sis) extensive angiomatous condition of the subcutaneous tissues.

angioendothelioma (an″je-o-en″do-the″le-o′mah) hemangioendothelioma.

angiofibroma (an″je-o-fi-bro′mah) an angioma containing fibrous tissue; called also *telangiectatic fibroma.* **juvenile a.,** nasopharyngeal a. **nasopharyngeal a.,** a tumor of the nasopharynx composed of fibrous connective tissue with abundant endothelium-lined vascular spaces, usually occurring during puberty, most commonly in boys. It is characterized by nasal obstruction which may become total, hyponasality, discomfort in swallowing, auditory tube obstruction and massive epistaxis. Called also *juvenile a.* and *nasopharyngeal fibroangioma.*

angiofollicular (an″je-o-fol-lik′u-lar) pertaining to a lymphoid follicle and its blood vessels.

angiogenesis (an″je-o-jen′ĕ-sis) [*angio-* + *genesis*] the formation of new blood vessels. **tumor a.,** the induction of the growth of blood vessels from surrounding tissue into a solid tumor by a diffusible chemical factor released by the tumor cells.

angiogenic (an″je-o-jen′ik) 1. arising in the vascular system. 2. developing into blood vessels.

angioglioma (an″je-o-gli-o′mah) a very vascular form of glioma.

angiogliomatosis (an″je-o-gli″o-mah-to′sis) a condition marked by the formation of multiple vascular gliomas.

angiogram (an′je-o-gram″) a roentgenogram of blood vessels filled with a contrast medium.

angiogranuloma (an″je-o-gran″u-lo′mah) [*angio-* + *granuloma*] an angioma containing granulation tissue, which represents a vasoproliferative inflammatory response. When the epithelial surface is ulcerated and suppuration is evident, the lesion is referred to as pyogenic granuloma.

angiograph (an′je-o-graf″) [*angio-* + Gr. *graphein* to record] angiogram.

angiography (an″je-og′rah-fe) [*angio-* + Gr. *graphein* to record] 1. the roentgenographic visualization of blood vessels following introduction of contrast material; used as a diagnostic aid in such conditions as cerebrovascular attacks (strokes) and myocardial infarctions. 2. a treatise on the vessels; the study of the vessels. **cerebral a.,** radiography of the vascular system of the brain after injection of contrast material into the arterial blood stream. **coronary a.,** radiographic visualization of the coronary arteries after the introduction of contrast material. **intravenous digital subtraction a.,** a fluoroscopic x-ray imaging technique that uses electronic circuitry that subtracts the background of bone and soft tissue to provide a useful image of vessels after peripheral or central intravenous injection of contrast medium.

angiohemophilia (an″je-o-he″mo-fil′e-ah) von Willebrand's disease.

angiohyalinosis (an″je-o-hi″ah-lĭ-no′sis) [*angio-* + *hyalino-*

sis] hyaline degeneration of the walls of blood vessels. **a. hemorrhag′ica,** a variety characterized by congenital hemorrhage.

angioid (an′je-oid) [*angio-* + Gr. *eidos* form] resembling a blood vessel.

angioinvasive (an″je-o-in-va′siv) tending to invade the walls of blood vessels.

angiokeratoma (an″je-o-ker″ah-to′mah) [*angio-* + *keratoma*] a discrete, pink to red telangiectasia having a tendency to undergo secondary epithelial changes, including acanthosis and hyperkeratosis. An underlying vascular abnormality is present in many cases. Called also *angiokeratosis* and *telangiectatic wart.* **a. circumscrip′tum,** a condition mainly occurring in infancy or early childhood, chiefly in females, characterized by the usually unilateral development of papules and small nodules that may coalesce to form plaques, which are generally localized in a small patch, often with a linear configuration. **a. cor′poris diffu′sum, diffuse a.,** Fabry disease. **a. of Fordyce,** a condition seen in older men in which multiple small, vascular papules that become keratotic occur along the superficial veins of the scrotum and rarely over the penis, inguinal area, or upper thigh. Most cases are associated with a history of some type of venous obstruction. Called also *a. of scrotum.* Similar lesions may occur on the vulva. **a. of Mibelli,** a condition occurring in children or young adults characterized by the symmetrical development on the dorsum of the fingers and toes and elbows and knees of discrete, aggregated, or confluent, soft reddish to purple vascular papules that later become hyperkeratotic. Most cases are associated with a history of chilblains, cold sensitivity, or frost bite. **a. of scrotum,** a. of Fordyce. **solitary a.,** angiokeratoma manifested as a small, bluish black warty papule that occurs most frequently on the lower extremities, usually singly, in childhood and adolescence.

angiokeratosis (an″je-o-ker″ah-to′sis) angiokeratoma.

angiokinesis (an″je-o-kĭ-ne′sis) [*angio-* + Gr. *kinēsis* movement] vascular activity.

angiokinetic (an″je-o-kĭ-net′ik) pertaining to vascular activity; vasomotor.

angioleiomyoma (an″je-o-li″o-mi-o′mah) [*angio-* + *leiomyoma*] a leiomyoma arising from vascular smooth muscle, usually occurring as a solitary nodular, sometimes painful, tumor on the lower extremity in middle-aged women; it is usually more deeply situated than ordinary leiomyoma and is usually subcutaneous. Called also *angiomyoma* and *vascular leiomyoma.*

angioleucitis (an″je-o-lu-si′tis) [*angio-* + Gr. *leukos* white + *-itis*] lymphangitis.

angioleukitis (an″je-o-lu-ki′tis) lymphangitis.

angiolipoleiomyoma (an″je-o-lip″o-li-o-mi-o′mah) see *angiomyolipoma.*

angiolipoma (an″je-o-lĭ-po′mah) a tumor composed of a mixture of adipose tissue and blood vessels.

angiologia (an″je-o-lo′je-ah) angiology; in NA terminology *angiologia* encompasses the nomenclature relating to the heart, arteries, veins, lymphatic system, and spleen.

angiology (an″je-ol′o-je) [*angio-* + Gr. *logos* treatise] the scientific study of the vessels of the body; applied also to the sum of knowledge relating to the blood vessels and lymph vessels.

angiolupoid (an″je-o-loo′poid) [*angio-* + *lupoid*] a distinctive, rare manifestation of cutaneous sarcoidosis localized to the malar region, bridge of the nose, or around the eyes, and consisting of livid blue-red nodular lesions that coalesce to form plaques.

angiolymphangioma (an″je-o-lim-fan″je-o′mah) a mixed angioma in which lymph vessels and blood vessels are involved.

angiolymphitis (an″je-o-lim-fi′tis) lymphangitis.

angiolysis (an″je-ol′ĭ-sis) [*angio-* + Gr. *lysis* dissolution] retrogression or obliteration of blood vessels, such as occurs during embryonic development.

angioma (an″je-o′mah) [*angio-* + *-oma*] a tumor whose cells tend to form blood vessels (*hemangioma*) or lymph vessels (*lymphangioma*); a tumor made up of blood vessels or lymph vessels. **a. arteria′le racemo′sum,** a dilatation and complex intertwining of many new-formed and altered vessels of small caliber with subsequent involvement of normal vessels. **arteriovenous a. of brain,** congenital angioma of the brain, composed of arterial and venous channels with many arteriovenous shunts, and characterized by frequent focal epileptic seizures and progressive impairment of the blood supply, which gives rise to increasing hemiparesis. It is distinguished by an intracranial bruit. **capillary a's,** cherry a's. **a. caverno′sum, cavernous a.,** cavernous hemangioma. **cherry a's,** bright red to purple, smooth dome-shaped lesions representing a telangiectatic vascular disturbance, usually found on the trunk and proximal extremities; they occur in most of the elderly, but the onset may be in early adult life. Called also *capillary a's, De Morgan's spots,* and *senile a's.* **a. cu′tis,** a kind of nevus made up of a network of dilated blood vessels. **fissural a.,** angioma occurring in embryonal fissures of the face, neck, or lips. **hypertrophic a.,** hemangioendothelioma. **a. lymphat′icum,** lymphangioma. **plexiform a.,** ordinary angioma made up of dilated and tortuous capillaries usually located in the skin. **senile a's,** cherry a's. **a. serpigino′sum,** generalized essential telangiectasia characterized by groups of tiny, copper-colored to bright red angiomatous puncta that enlarge by forming new puncta at the periphery with central clearing, which produces annular or serpiginous patterns. The eruption usually occurs on the lower extremities. Called also *Hutchinson's disease.* **simple a.,** a nevus or telangiectasis; a tumor composed of a network of small vessels or of distended capillaries bound together by connective tissue. **spider a.,** vascular spider. **telangiectatic a.,** an angioma made up of dilated blood vessels. **a. veno′sum racemo′sum,** the swellings caused by severe varicosity of superficial veins. **venous a. of brain,** congenital angioma of the brain, composed of abnormal venous arteries and characterized by frequent focal epileptic seizures and progressive hemiparesis.

angiomatosis (an″je-o-mah-to′sis) a diseased state of the vessels with the formation of multiple angiomas. **cerebroretinal a.,** von Hippel-Lindau disease. **encephalofacial a., encephalotrigeminal a.,** Sturge-Weber syndrome. **hepatic a.,** peliosis hepatis. **a. of retina,** von Hippel's disease. **retinocerebral a.,** von Hippel-Lindau disease.

angiomatous (an″je-om′ah-tus) of the nature of angioma.

angiomegaly (an″je-o-meg′ah-le) [angio- + Gr. *megas* large] enlargement of blood vessels; especially a condition of the eyelid marked by great increase in its volume.

angiometer (an″je-om′ĕ-ter) [angio- + Gr. *metron* measure] an instrument once used for measuring the diameter or caliber and the tension of the blood vessels.

angiomyolipoma (an″je-o-mi″o-lĭ-po′mah) a benign tumor containing vascular, adipose, and muscle elements; it occurs most often in the kidney with smooth muscle elements (angiolipoleiomyoma) in association with tuberous sclerosis, and is considered to be a hamartoma.

angiomyoma (an″je-o-mi-o′mah) [angio- + *myoma*] angioleiomyoma.

angiomyosarcoma (an″je-o-mi″o-sar-ko′mah) a tumor made up of elements of angioma, myoma, and sarcoma.

angiomyxoma (an″je-o-mik-so′mah) a chorioangioma in which capillary-like blood vessels are very evident; it may extend into the umbilical cord and often contains myxomatous tissue resembling that in the normal cord.

angionecrosis (an″je-o-nĕ-kro′sis) [angio- + Gr. *nekros* dead + -osis] necrosis of the walls of blood vessels.

angioneoplasm (an″je-o-ne′o-plazm) [angio- + *neoplasm*] a tumor or neoplasm of blood vessels.

angioneuralgia (an″je-o-nu-ral′jĕ-ah) [angio- + *neuralgia*] a condition marked by burning pain in an extremity attended by edema and redness of the part; thought to be an early stage of Raynaud's disease.

angioneurectomy (an″je-o-nu-rek′to-me) [angio- + Gr. *neuron* nerve + *ektomē* excision] excision of vessels and nerves.

angioneuropathic (an″je-o-nu″ro-path′ik) pertaining to or of the nature of an angioneuropathy.

angioneuropathy (an″je-o-nu-rop′ah-the) [angio- + *neuropathy*] any neuropathy affecting primarily the blood vessels; a disorder of the vasomotor system, as angiospasm, angioparalysis, or vasomotor paralysis.

angioneurotic (an″je-o-nu-rot′ik) denoting a neuropathy affecting the vascular system; see under *angioedema.*

angioneurotomy (an″je-o-nu-rot′o-me) [angio- + Gr. *neuron* nerve + *tomē* cutting] the operation of cutting vessels and nerves.

angionoma (an″je-o-no′mah) [angio- + Gr. *nomē* ulcer] ulceration of a blood vessel.

angiopancreatitis (an″je-o-pan″kre-ah-ti′tis) (*obs.*) inflammation of the pancreatic vessels or of the vascular tissue of the pancreas.

angioparalysis (an″je-o-pah-ral′ĭ-sis) [angio- + *paralysis*] vasomotor paralysis.

angioparesis (an″je-o-par′e-sis) [angio- + *paresis*] vasomotor paralysis.

angiopathology (an″je-o-pah-thol′o-je) the pathology of, or the changes seen in, diseases of the blood vessels.

angiopathy (an-je-op′ah-the) [angio- + Gr. *pathos* disease] any disease of the vessels.

angiophakomatosis (an″je-o-fak″o-mah-to′sis) [angio- + Gr. *phakos* lens + -*oma*] von Hippel-Lindau disease.

angioplasty (an″je-o-plas″te) [angio- + Gr. *plassein* to form] an angiographic procedure for elimination of areas of narrowing in blood vessels. **percutaneous transluminal a.,** dilatation of a blood vessel by means of a balloon catheter inserted through the skin and through the lumen of the vessel to the site of the narrowing, where the balloon is inflated to flatten plaque against the artery wall.

angiopoiesis (an″je-o-poi-e′sis) [angio- + Gr. *poiein* to make] the process of vessel formation.

angiopoietic (an″je-o-poi-et′ik) pertaining to or causing angiopoiesis.

angiopressure (an′je-o-presh″ur) the application of pressure to a blood vessel to control hemorrhage.

angioreticuloendothelioma (an″je-o-rĕ-tik″u-lo-en″do-the-le-o′mah) Kaposi's sarcoma.

angioreticuloma (an″je-o-re-tik″u-lo′mah) a hemangioma, especially one of the brain.

angiorrhaphy (an″je-or′ah-fe) [angio- + Gr. *rhaphē* suture] suture of a vessel or vessels. **arteriovenous a.,** the suturing of an artery to a vein, so as to divert the arterial current into the vein.

angiosarcoma (an″je-o-sar-ko′mah) [angio- + *sarcoma*] a hemangiosarcoma. **a. myxomato′des** (*obs.*), an angiosarcoma in which the walls of the vessels are affected with mucous degeneration.

angiosclerosis (an″je-o-skle-ro′sis) [angio- + *sclerosis*] a nonspecific term indicating hardening of the walls of the blood vessels.

angiosclerotic (an″je-o-skle-rot′ik) pertaining to or marked by angiosclerosis.

angioscope (an′je-o-skōp″) [angio- + Gr. *skopein* to view] a microscope for observing capillary blood vessels.

angioscotoma (an″je-o-sko-to′mah) [angio- + *scotoma*] a cecocentral scotoma caused by shadows of the retinal blood vessels.

angioscotometry (an″je-o-sko-tom′ĕ-tre) [angio- + *scotoma* + -*metry*] the plotting or mapping of the scotoma caused by the shadow of retinal blood vessels; used particularly in the diagnosis of glaucoma.

angiospasm (an′je-o-spazm″) [angio- + Gr. *spasmos* spasm] spasmodic contraction of the blood vessels.

angiospastic (an″je-o-spas′tik) of the nature of angiospasm; causing contraction of the blood vessels.

angiosperm (an′je-o-sperm″) [angio- + Gr. *sperma* seed] a true flowering plant; a plant having its seeds in an enclosed ovary.

angiospermin (an″je-o-sper′min) a substance derived from flowering plants and said to have hormone-like properties.

angiostenosis (an″je-o-ste-no′sis) [angio- + *stenosis*] narrowing of the caliber of a vessel.

angiosteosis (an″je-os″te-o′sis) [angio- + Gr. *osteon* bone] ossification or calcification of a vessel.

angiosthenia (an″je-os-the′ne-ah) [angio- + Gr. *sthenos* strength + -*ia*] arterial tension.

angiostomy (an″je-os′to-me) [angio- + Gr. *stomoun* to provide with an opening or mouth] the operation of making an opening into a blood vessel; also, the opening so made.

angiostrongyliasis (an″je-o-stron″jĭ-li′ah-sis) infection with *Angiostrongylus cantonensis.*

Angiostrongylus (an″je-o-stron′jĭ-lus) [Gr. *angeion* vessel + *strongylos* round] a genus of parasitic nematodes of the family Metastrongylidae. **A. cantonen′sis,** the lungworm that parasitizes the domestic rat in Australia and many of the Pacific islands, including Hawaii. Larval development occurs in snails, slugs, and planarians; in rats, the adult worms are found in the bronchioles. Human infection, which is caused by ingestion of larvae in raw snails or slugs or paratenic hosts, such as prawns or freshwater crabs, results in migration of the larval worms to the central nervous system, where they provoke eosinophilic meningitis. **A. vaso′rum,** a species parasitic in the pulmonary arteries of dogs.

angiostrophe (an″je-os′tro-fe) [*angio-* + Gr. *strophē* a twist] the twisting of a vessel to arrest hemorrhage.

angiostrophy (an″je-os′tro-fe) angiostrophe.

angiotelectasis (an″je-o-tĕ-lek′tah-sis), pl. *angiotelec′tases* [*angio-* + Gr. *telos* end + *ektasis* dilatation] dilatation of the minute arteries and veins.

angiotensin (an″je-o-ten′sin) a polypeptide present in the blood and formed by the catalytic action of renin on angiotensinogen in the blood plasma. The decapeptide angiotensin I, the inactive form, is in turn acted upon by a peptidase (converting enzyme), chiefly in the lungs, to form the octapeptide hormone angiotensin II, a powerful vasopressor and a stimulator of aldosterone secretion by the adrenal cortex. By its vasopressor action, it raises blood pressure and diminishes fluid loss in the kidney by restricting flow. Angiotensin II is hydrolyzed to form the heptapeptide angiotensin III, which has lesser vasopressor activity but is more active on the adrenal cortex. **a. amide,** chemical name: 1-L-asparagine-5-L-valineangiotensin II. An amide derivative of angiotensin, $C_{49}H_{70}N_{14}O_{11}$, occurring as a white to slightly off-white, amorphous powder, which is a powerful vasoconstrictor and vasopressor, and is used in the treatment of certain hypotensive states; usually administered by slow intravenous infusion, and sometimes intramuscularly or subcutaneously.

angiotensinase (an″je-o-ten′-sĭ-nās) 1. any of the peptidases in plasma and tissues that inactivate angiotensin. 2. [EC 3.4.99.3] an enzyme of the hydrolase class that inactivates angiotensin II by preferential cleavage of the tyrosine-isoleucine bond.

angiotensin-I converting enzyme (an″je-o-ten′sin) dipeptidyl carboxypeptidase I.

angiotensinogen (an″je-o-ten′sin-o-jen) a serum $α_2$-globulin secreted in the liver which, on hydrolysis by renin, gives rise to angiotensin; formerly called *hypertensinogen.*

angiotome (an′je-o-tōm″) [*angio-* + Gr. *tomē* a cutting] any one of the segments of the vascular system of the embryo; called also *vascular segment* and *intersegment.*

angiotomy (an″je-ot′o-me) [*angio-* + Gr. *tomē* a cutting] the cutting or severing of a blood or lymph vessel.

angiotonase (an″je-o-to′nās) angiotensinase.

angiotonia (an″je-o-to′ne-ah) vasotonia.

angiotonic (an″je-o-ton′ik) [*angio-* + Gr. *tonos* tension] increasing the vascular tension.

angiotonin (an″je-o-to′nin) angiotensin.

angiotribe (an′je-o-trīb″) [*angio-* + Gr. *tribein* to crush] an exceedingly strong forceps in which pressure is applied by means of a screw; the instrument is used to crush tissue containing an artery in order to control hemorrhage from the vessel. Called also *vasotribe.*

angiotripsy (an′je-o-trip″se) production of hemostasis by use of the angiotribe; called also *vasotripsy.*

angiotrophic (an″je-o-trof′ik) [*angio-* + Gr. *trophē* nutrition] pertaining to vascular nutrition.

angitis (an-ji′tis) angiitis.

angle (ang′g'l) [L. *angulus*] 1. the area or point of junction of two intersecting borders or surfaces; see *angulus.* 2. the degree of divergence of two intersecting lines or planes. **a. of aberration,** a. of deviation. **acromial a.,** angulus acromialis. **acromial a. of scapula,** angulus lateralis scapulae. **alpha a.,** that formed by the intersection of the visual line with the optic axis at the nodal point. It is *positive* when the visual axis crosses the cornea on the nasal side of the optic axis, as in most individuals; *negative* when

the visual axis crosses the cornea on the temporal side of the optic axis; and *nil* when the visual axis and the optic axis coincide. **Alsberg's a.,** see *Alsberg's triangle,* under *triangle.* **alveolar a.,** the angle between a line running through a point beneath the nasal spine and the most prominent point of the lower border of the alveolar process of the superior maxilla and the cephalic horizontal (glabella to opisthocranion). **anterior a. of petrous portion of temporal bone,** angulus anterior pyramidis ossis temporalis. **a. of aperture,** the angle between two lines from the focus of a lens to the ends of its diameter. **auriculo-occipital a.,** the angle between lines from the auricular point to the lambda and opisthion. **axial a.,** any angle the formation of which is partially dependent on the axial wall of a tooth cavity preparation, as the axiodistal angle or buccoaxial angle. See table of *Cavity Angles* and illustration of *Tooth Angles.* **axial line a.,** any line angle which is parallel with the long axis of a tooth. For names of various angles see table of *Cavity Angles* and illustration of *Tooth Angles.* **Bennett a.,** the angle formed by the sagittal plane and the path of the advancing condyle during lateral movement of the mandible, as viewed in the horizontal plane. See also *Bennett movement,* under *movement.* **beta a.,** the angle between the radius fixus and a line joining the bregma and hormion. **biorbital a.,** the angle formed by intersection of a posterior extension of the axes of the two orbits. **Broca's a.,** ophryospinal a. **buccal a's,** the angles formed between the buccal surface and the other surfaces of a posterior tooth, or between the buccal wall of a tooth cavity and other walls, named according to the surfaces which participate in their formation. See table of *Cavity Angles* and illustration of *Tooth Angles.* **cardiodiaphragmatic a.,** the angle formed by the junction of the shadows of the heart and diaphragm in posteroanterior roentgenograms of the chest; called also *cardiophrenic a.* **cardiohepatic a.,** the angle formed by the horizontal limit of hepatic dullness with the upright line of cardiac dullness in the fifth right intercostal space, close to the sternal border; called also *Ebstein's a.* **cardiophrenic a.,** cardiodiaphragmatic a. **carrying a.,** the angle formed laterally by the axes of the arm and forearm when the forearm is extended in the anatomical position. **cavity a's,** the angles formed by the junction of two or more walls of a tooth cavity, named according to the walls participating in their formation. See table of *Cavity Angles.* **cavosurface a.,**

CAVITY ANGLES

Line Angles

(Formed by the junction of two walls)

axiodistal	gingivoaxial
axiogingival	labiogingival
axioincisal	linguoaxial
axiolabial	linguodistal
axiolingual	linguogingival
axiomesial	linguomesial
axio-occlusal	linguopulpal
axiopulpal	mesiobuccal
buccoaxial	mesiogingival
buccodistal	mesiolabial
buccogingival	mesiolingual
buccomesial	mesio-occlusal
buccopulpal	mesiopulpal
distobuccal	pulpoaxial
distogingival	pulpodistal
distolabial	pulpolabial
distolingual	pulpolingual
disto-occlusal	pulpomesial
distopulpal	

Point Angles

(Formed by the junction of three walls)

axiodistogingival	distopulpolingual
axiodisto-occlusal	gingivobuccoaxial
axiolabiogingival	gingivolinguoaxial
axiolinguogingival	mesiobuccopulpal
axiomesiogingival	mesiolinguopulpal
axiomesio-occlusal	mesiopulpolabial
distobuccopulpal	mesiopulpolingual
distolinguopulpal	pulpobuccoaxial
distopulpolabial	pulpolinguoaxial

the angle formed by the junction of a wall of a tooth cavity preparation and a surface of the crown of the tooth. **cephalic a.,** various angles of the skull or face. **cephalic-medullary a.,** the angle at which the brain stem meets the base of the brain. **cephalometric a.,** measurement of intersecting anthropometric lines on tracings made of oriented head films in radiologic orthodontic diagnosis.

cerebellopontile a., that between the cerebellum and the pons. chi a., the angle between two lines from the hormion to the staphylion and to the basion, respectively. collodiaphyseal a., the angle formed by the intersection of the long axes of the neck and shaft of the femur. condylar a., the angle between the planes of the basilar clivus and the foramen magnum. a. of convergence, that between the visual axis and the median line when an object is looked at. a. of convexity, a roentgenographic cephalometric measurement formed by connecting the nasion, point A, and pogonion (NAP), which reflects the convexity or concavity of the facial profile. coronary a., angulus frontalis ossis parietalis. costal a., angulus costae. costophrenic a., the angle formed at the junction of the costal and diaphragmatic pleurae. costovertebral a., the angle formed on either side of the vertebral column, between the last rib and the lumbar vertebrae. craniofacial a., the angle between the basifacial and basicranial axes at the middle of the ethmoidosphenoid suture. critical a., the angle of incidence at which a ray of light passing from one medium to another of different density changes from refraction to total reflection; called also *limiting a.* cusp a., 1. the angle made by the slopes of a cusp of a tooth with the plane that passes through the tip of the cusp and that is perpendicular to a line bisecting the cusp, measured mesiodistally or buccolingually. 2. the angle made by the slopes of a cusp with a perpendicular line bisecting the cusp, measured mesiodistally or buccolingually. 3. one half of the included angle between the buccal and lingual or mesial and distal cusp inclines. cusp plane a., the incline of the cusp plane in relation to the plane of occlusion. Daubenton's a., an angle formed by junction of the opisthiobasal and opisthionasial lines; called also *occipital a.* a. of declination, Mikulicz's a. a. of deviation, the angle between a refracted ray and the incident ray prolonged; called also *a. of aberration.* a. of direction, the angle through which the eye must move to bring the image onto the fovea. distal a's, the angles formed between the distal surface and other surfaces of a tooth, or between the distal wall of a tooth cavity and other walls; named according to the surfaces which participate in their formation. See table of *Cavity Angles* and illustration of *Tooth Angles.* Ebstein's a., cardiohepatic a. elevation a., 1. the angle made by the visual plane when moved upward or downward with its normal position. 2. see *Alsberg's triangle,* under *triangle.* epigastric a., the angle made by the xiphoid process with the body of the sternum. ethmocranial a., the angle formed by the plane of the cribriform plate of the ethmoid bone prolonged to meet the basicranial axis; called also *ethmoid angle.* ethmoid a., ethmocranial a. external a. of border of tibia, margo interosseus tibiae. external a. of scapula, angulus lateralis scapulae. facial a., the angle formed by the junction of the Frankfort Horizontal plane and the nasion-pogonion line in the lateral roentgenographic cephalometric tracing. Used to express the degree of retrusion or protrusion of the chin. See also *prognathism* and *retrognathia.* filtration a., angulus iridocornealis. frontal a. of parietal bone, angulus frontalis ossis parietalis. gamma a., the angle formed by junction of the line of fixation and the optic axis at the center of rotation of the eye. gonial a., the angle formed by the intersection of the body of the mandible and the ascending mandibular ramus; an important consideration in prognathic procedures. Called also *angulus mandibulae* [NA]. horizontal a., in dental radiology the angle, measured within a horizontal plane, at which the central ray of the useful beam is projected relative to a vertical plane of reference. a. of incidence, the angle made with the perpendicular by a ray of light which strikes a denser or a rarer medium; see *refraction.* incisal a., one of the angles formed by the junction of the incisal and the mesial or distal surfaces of an anterior tooth; called the *mesial* and the *distal incisal angle,* respectively. incisal guide a., the angle formed with the horizontal plane by drawing a line in the sagittal plane between incisal edges of the maxillary and mandibular central incisors when the teeth are in centric occlusion. incisal mandibular plane a., one of the three angles composing the Tweed triangle, designating the axial inclination of the lower incisor to the mandibular plane in the lateral cephalometric radiograph. a. of inclination, inclinatio pelvis. inferior a. of duodenum, flexura duodeni inferior. inferior a. of parietal bone, anterior, angulus sphenoidalis ossis

parietalis. inferior a. of parietal bone, posterior, angulus mastoideus ossis parietalis. inferior a. of scapula, angulus inferior scapulae. infrasternal a. of thorax, angulus infrasternalis thoracis. inner a. of humerus, margo medialis humeri. internal a. of tibia, margo medialis tibiae. iridial a., iridocorneal a., a. of iris, angulus iridocornealis. Jacquart's a., ophryospinal a. a. of jaw, angulus mandibulae. kappa a., the angle between the pupillary axes. kyphotic a., the superior angle formed by intersection of two lines drawn on the lateral chest roentgenogram, tangential to the anterior borders of the second and eleventh intervertebral spaces, an index of the degree of deformity in thoracic kyphosis. labial a's, the angles formed between the labial surface and other surfaces of an anterior tooth, or between the labial wall of a tooth cavity and other walls; named according to the surfaces participating in their formation. See table of *Cavity Angles* and illustration of *Tooth Angles.* lambda a., the angle between the pupillary axis and the line of sight. lateral a. of border of tibia, margo interosseus tibiae. lateral a. of eye, angulus oculi lateralis. lateral a. of humerus, margo lateralis humeri. lateral a. of scapula, angulus lateralis scapulae. limiting a., critical a. line a., an angle formed by the junction of two planes; used to designate the junction of two surfaces of a tooth, or of two walls of a tooth cavity preparation. Line angles of the posterior teeth include the mesio-occlusal, linguo-occlusal, mesiolingual, distolingual, mesiobuccal, distobuccal, bucco-occlusal and disto-occlusal angles. Those of the anterior teeth include the labioincisal, linguoincisal, mesiolabial, distolabial, mesiolingual, and distolingual angles. See table of *Cavity Angles* and illustration of *Tooth Angles.* lingual a's, the angles formed between the lingual and other surfaces of a tooth, or between the lingual wall of a tooth cavity preparation and other walls; named according to the surfaces which participate in their formation, e.g., the linguopulpal angle is formed at the junction of the lingual and pulpal walls of a cavity preparation. See table of *Cavity Angles* and illustration of *Tooth Angles.* Louis' a., Ludwig's a., angulus sterni. lumbosacral a., sacrovertebral a. a. of mandible, mandibular a., angulus mandibulae. mastoid a. of parietal bone, angulus mastoideus ossis parietalis. maxillary a., the angle between two lines extending from the point of contact of the upper and lower central incisors to the ophryon and the most prominent point of the lower jaw (pogonion). medial a. of eye, angulus oculi medialis. medial a. of humerus, margo medialis humeri. medial a. of scapula, angulus superior scapulae. medial a. of tibia, margo medialis tibiae. mesial a's, the angles formed between the mesial surface and other surfaces of a tooth, or between the mesial wall of a tooth cavity and other walls, named according to the surfaces participating with the mesial in their formation. See table of *Cavity Angles* and illustration of *Tooth Angles.* metafacial a., the angle between the base of the skull and the pterygoid process; called also *Serres' a.* meter a., a unit of convergence of the eye: that amount of convergence required for binocular fixation of an object at 1 meter and using 1 diopter of accommodation. Mikulicz's a., an angle formed by two planes, one passing through the long axis of the epiphysis of the femur and the other through the long axis of the diaphysis; it is normally 130 degrees. Called also *a. of declination.* minimum separabile a., minimum separable a., 1. the smallest angle of separation at which the eye recognizes two points, lines, or objects as being separate. 2. minimum visible a. minimum visible a., minimum visual a., the angle which the minimum separabile subtends at the eye; 60 seconds of arc is usually taken as standard for a normal eye. a. of mouth, angulus oris. a. of Mulder, the angle formed by the intersection of the facial line of Camper and a line from the root of the nose to the spheno-occipital suture. nu a., the angle between the radius fixus and a line joining the hormion and nasion. occipital a., Daubenton's a. occipital a. of parietal bone, angulus occipitalis ossis parietalis. ocular a's, see *angulus oculi lateralis* and *angulus oculi medialis.* olfactive a., the angle formed by the line of the olfactory fossa and the os planum of the sphenoid bone; called also *olfactory a.* olfactory a., olfactive a. ophryospinal a., the angle at the anterior nasal spine between lines from the auricular point and the glabella; called also *Jacquart's a., Topinard's a.,* and *Broca's a.* optic a., vi-

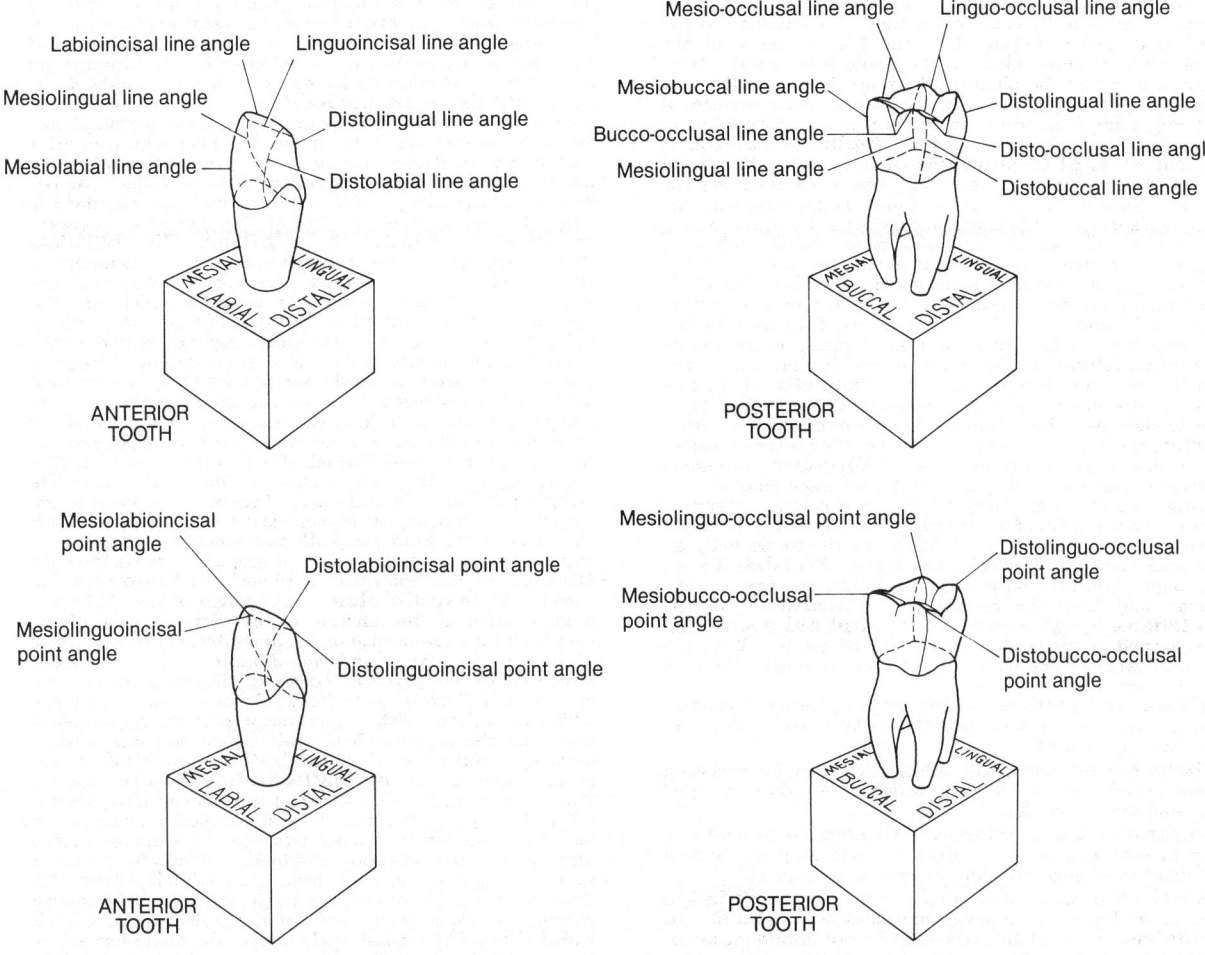

Tooth angles: *Top*, line angles; *Bottom*, point angles.

sual a. **orifacial a.,** one of the facial angles formed by the junction of the Frankfort Horizontal plane with the nasion-pogonion plane. **parietal a.,** the angle formed by junction of lines passing through the extremities of the transverse bizygomatic diameter and the maximum transverse frontal diameter; called also *Quatrefage's a.* **parietal a. of sphenoid bone,** margo parietalis alae majoris. **a. of pelvis,** inclinatio pelvis. **pelvivertebral a.,** inclinatio pelvis. **phrenopericardial a.,** the space or angle between the pericardium and the diaphragm. **Pirogoff's a.,** venous a. **point a.,** any angle formed by the junction of three surfaces of a tooth crown, or three walls of a tooth cavity preparation, named according to the tooth surfaces or the cavity walls participating in its formation. Point angles on the posterior teeth include the mesiolinguo-occlusal, mesiobucco-occlusal, distolinguo-occlusal, and distobucco-occlusal angles. Point angles on the anterior teeth include the mesiolabioincisal, mesiolinguoincisal, distolabioincisal, and distolinguoincisal angles. See table of *Cavity Angles* and illustration of *Tooth Angles*. **a. of polarization,** the angle at which light is most completely polarized. **posterior a. of petrous portion of temporal bone,** angulus posterior pyramidis ossis temporalis. **principal a.,** refracting a. **a. of pubis,** angulus subpubicus. **Quatrefage's a.,** parietal a. **Ranke's a.,** the angle between the horizontal plane of the skull and a line through the center of the maxillary alveolar margin and the center of the nasofrontal suture. **a. of reflection,** that which a reflected ray makes with a line perpendicular to the reflecting surface. **refracting a.,** that between the two refracting faces of a prism; called also *principal a.* **a. of refraction,** the angle between a refracted ray and a line perpendicular to the refracting surface; see *refraction.* **a. of rib,** angulus costae. **rolandic a., a. of Rolando,** the angle formed by junction of the median plane and the central sulcus (fissure of Rolando). **sacrovertebral a.,** the angle formed at the junction of the sacrum with the lowest lumbar vertebra; called also *lumbosacral a.* **Serres' a.,** metafacial a. **sigma a.,** the angle between the radius fixus and a line from the staphylion to the hormion. **somatosplanchnic a.,** the angle formed by junction of the somatic and splanchnic layers of the mesoblast in the embryo. **sphenoid a., sphenoidal a.,** 1. an angle at the top of the sella turcica between lines from the nasal point and from the tip of the rostrum of the sphenoid. 2. the anterior inferior angle of the parietal bone; called also *Welcher's a.* **sphenoidal a. of parietal bone,** angulus sphenoidalis ossis parietalis. **squint a.,** the angle by which the visual line of the squinting eye deviates from a line drawn to the object which should be fixed; called also *squint deviation.* **sternal a.,** angulus sterni. **sternoclavicular a.,** the angle formed by junction of the sternum and clavicle. **a. of sternum,** angulus sterni. **subcostal a.,** angulus infrasternalis thoracis. **subpubic a.,** angulus subpubicus. **subscapular a.,** a transverse depression on the costal or ventral surface of the scapula, where the bone appears bent on itself perpendicular to and passing through the glenoid cavity. **substernal a.,** angulus infrasternalis thoracis. **superior a. of duodenum,** flexura duodeni superior. **superior a. of parietal bone, anterior,** angulus frontalis ossis parietalis. **superior a. of parietal bone, posterior,** angulus occipitalis ossis parietalis. **superior a. of petrous portion of temporal bone,** angulus superior pyramidis ossis temporalis. **superior a. of scapula,** angulus superior scapulae.

a. of Sylvius, the angle formed by junction of the lateral sulcus (fissure of Sylvius) and a line perpendicular to the horizontal plane tangential to the highest point of the hemisphere. **tentorial a.,** the angle between the basicranial axis and the plane of the tentorium. **tooth a's,** the angles formed by the junction of two or more surfaces of a tooth, named according to the surfaces participating in their formation (see illustration). **Topinard's a.,** ophryospinal a. **a. of torsion,** the angle between the axes of any two different portions of long bones. **tuber a.,** the angle formed by junction of two lines, one parallel with the superior surface of the tuber calcanei and the other joining the anterior and posterior articular facets; normally about 30 degrees. **venous a.,** the angle formed by junction of the internal jugular and subclavian veins; called also *Pirogoff's a.* **vertical a.,** in dental radiology the angle, measured within a vertical plane, at which the central ray of the useful beam is projected relative to a horizontal plane of reference. **vesicourethral a.,** the angle formed by junction of the bladder wall and the urethra. **vesicourethral a., anterior,** the angle formed by junction of the anterior wall of the bladder and the urethra. **vesicourethral a., posterior,** the angle formed by junction of the posterior wall of the bladder and the urethra. **a. of Virchow,** the angle between the nasobasilar line and the nasosubnasal line. **visual a.,** the angle formed between two lines extending from the nodal point of the eye to the extremities of the object seen; called also *optic a.* **Vogt's a.,** the angle between the nasobasilar and alveolonasal lines. **Weisbach's a.,** the angle at the alveolar point between lines passing from the basion and from the middle of the frontonasal suture. **Welcher's a.,** sphenoid a., def. 2. **xiphoid a's,** the angles formed by the borders of the xiphoid notch. **Y a.,** the angle between the radius fixus and a line joining the lambda and the inion.

Angle's classification, splint (ang'elz) [Edward Hartley *Angle*, American orthodontist, 1855–1930] see under *malocclusion* and *splint.*

anglicus sudor (ang'le-kus su'dor) the English sweating fever; a deadly pestilential fever which several times ravaged England during the Middle Ages.

angophrasia (ang"go-fra'zhe-ah) [Gr. *anchein* to choke + *phrasis* utterance + *-ia*] a drawing form of speech broken by choking spasms occurring in general paresis.

angor (ang'gor) [L. "a strangling"] angina. **a. a'nimi,** a feeling of life slipping away and impending death. **a. ocula'ris,** a condition marked by fear of imminent blindness and by sudden attacks of mist before the eyes, possibly due to angiospasm of ocular vessels. **a. pec'toris,** angina pectoris.

angstrom (ang'strem) the unit of wavelength of electromagnetic and corpuscular radiations, equal to 10^{-7} mm. Called also *Angström unit.* Symbol Å or A.

Angström's law, unit (awng'strem) [Anders Jonas *Angström,* Swedish physicist, 1814–1874] see under *law,* and see *angstrom.*

Anguillula (ang-gwil'u-lah) [L. "little eel"] a genus of nematode parasites, many species of which have been reassigned to other genera. **A. ace'ti,** *Turbatrix aceti.* **A. intestina'lis, A. stercora'lis,** *Strongyloides stercoralis.*

Anguilluli'na putrefa'ciens (ang-gwil"u-li'nah pu"trĕ-fa'she-enz) *Ditylenchus dipsaci.*

angular (ang'gu-lar) [L. *angula'ris*] sharply bent; having corners or angles.

angulation (ang"gu-la'shun) [L. *angulatus* bent] 1. the formation of a sharp obstructive angle, as in the intestine, the ureter, or similar tubes. 2. deviation from a straight line, as in a badly set bone.

anguli (ang'gu-li) [L.] genitive and plural of *angulus.*

angulus (ang'gu-lus), gen. and pl. an'guli [L.] an angle; used as a general term in anatomical nomenclature to designate a triangular area or the angle of a particular structure or part of the body. **a. acromia'lis** [NA], acromial angle: the easily palpable subcutaneous bony point where the lateral border of the acromion becomes continuous with the spine of the scapula. **a. ante'rior pyram'idis os'sis tempora'lis,** a short area on the petrous part of the temporal bone consisting of two parts: one, adjoined to the squamous part of the bone at the petrosquamous suture; the other, a free part articulating with the great wing of the sphenoid; called also *anterior angle of petrous portion of temporal bone.* **a. cos'tae** [NA], costal angle: a prominent line on the external surface of a rib, a little in front of the tubercle, where the rib is bent in two directions and at the same time twisted on its long axis; called also *angle of rib.* **a. fronta'lis os'sis parieta'lis** [NA], frontal angle of parietal bone: the anterosuperior angle of the parietal bone, which is membranous at birth and forms part of the anterior fontanelle; called also *anterior superior angle of parietal bone* and *coronary angle.* **a. infectio'sus,** perlèche. **a. infe'rior scap'ulae** [NA], inferior angle of scapula: the angle formed by the junction of the medial and lateral borders of the scapula. **a. infrasterna'lis thora'cis** [NA], infrasternal angle of thorax: the angle on the anteroinferior surface of the thorax, the apex of which is the sternoxiphoid junction, and the sides of which are the seventh, eighth, and ninth costal cartilages; it partially delimits two sides of the triangular epigastric region on the ventral body surface; called also *subcostal* or *substernal angle.* **a. i'ridis, a. iridocornea'lis** [NA], iridocorneal angle: a narrow recess between the sclerocorneal junction and the attached margin of the iris, marking the periphery of the anterior chamber of the eye; it is the principal exit site for the aqueous fluid. Called also *filtration angle, iridial angle, angle of iris,* and *angulus iridis.* **a. latera'lis scap'ulae** [NA], lateral angle of scapula: the head of the scapula, which bears the glenoid cavity and articulates with the head of the humerus; called also *acromial* or *external angle of scapula,* and *condyle of scapula.* **a. latera'lis tib'iae, a. Ludovi'ci,** a. sterni. **a. mandib'ulae** [NA], angle of mandible: the angle created at the junction of the posterior edge of the ramus and the lower edge of the mandible; called also *angle of jaw, gonial angle,* and *mandibular angle.* **a. mastoi'deus os'sis parieta'lis** [NA], mastoid angle of parietal bone: the posteroinferior angle of the parietal bone, which articulates with the posterior part of the temporal bone and the occipital bone; called also *posterior inferior angle of parietal bone.* **a. media'lis scap'ulae,** a. superior scapulae. **a. media'lis tib'iae,** margo medialis tibiae. **a. occipita'lis os'sis parieta'lis** [NA], occipital angle of parietal bone: the posterosuperior angle of the parietal bone, which during fetal life participates in the formation of the posterior fontanelle; called also *posterior superior angle of parietal bone.* **a. o'culi latera'lis** [NA], lateral angle of eye: the angle formed by the lateral junction of the superior and inferior eyelids. **a. o'culi media'lis** [NA], medial angle of eye: the angle formed by the medial junction of the superior and inferior eyelids. **a. o'ris** [NA], angle of mouth: the angle formed at either side of the mouth by junction of the upper and the lower lip. **a. parieta'lis os'sis sphenoida'lis,** margo parietalis alae majoris. **a. poste'rior pyram'idis os'sis tempora'lis,** the angle on the petrous portion of the temporal bone that separates the posterior from the inferior surface; called also *posterior angle* or *border of petrous portion of temporal bone.* **a. pu'bis,** a. subpubicus. **a. sphenoida'lis os'sis parieta'lis** [NA], sphenoid angle of parietal bone: the anteroinferior angle of the parietal bone, which articulates with the great wing of the sphenoid bone and the frontal bone; called also *anterior inferior angle of sphenoid bone.* **a. sterna'lis,** NA alternative for *a. sterni.* **a. ster'ni** [NA], sternal angle: the angle formed on the anterior surface of the sternum at the junction of its body and manubrium; called also *a. Ludovici, a. sternalis* [NA alternative], and *Louis'* or *Ludwig's angle.* **a. of stomach,** incisura angularis ventriculi. **a. subpu'bicus** [NA], subpubic angle: the apex of the pubic arch; the angle formed at the point of meeting of the conjoined rami of the ischial and pubic bones of the two sides of the body. Called also *a. pubis, subpubic arch,* and *arch of pelvis.* **a. supe'rior pyram'idis os'sis tempora'lis,** the angle on the internal surface of the petrous portion of the temporal bone that separates its posterior and anterior surfaces. Called also *superior angle of petrous portion of temporal bone* and *superior border of petrous portion of temporal bone.* **a. supe'rior scap'ulae** [NA], superior angle of scapula: the angle made by the superior and medial borders of the scapula; called also *medial angle of scapula* and *a. medialis scapulae.* **a. veno'sus,** the angle at the junction of the internal jugular vein and the subclavian vein.

anhalamine (an-hal'ah-min) a crystalline alkaloid, $C_{11}H_{15}NO_3$, from *Lophophora williamsii.*

anhalonine (an″hah-lo′nin) a crystalline alkaloid, $C_{12}H_{15}$-NO_3, from *Lophophora williamsii,* with the pharmacological properties of mescaline.

Anhalonium lewinii (an″hah-lo′ne-um lu-win′e-e) *Lophophora williamsii.*

anhaphia (an-ha′fe-ah) anaphia.

anhedonia (an″he-do′ne-ah) [*an* neg. + Gr. *hēdonē* pleasure + *-ia*] total loss of feeling of pleasure in acts that normally give pleasure.

anhidrosis (an″hĭ-dro′sis) [*an* neg. + Gr. *hidrōs* sweat + *-osis*] absence or deficiency of sweating. Called also *anidrosis* and *hidroschesis.* See also *hypohidrosis.* **thermogenic a.,** tropical anhidrotic asthenia.

anhidrotic (an″hĭ-drot′ik) 1. pertaining to or characterized by anhidrosis. 2. an agent that reduces, diminishes, or prevents sweating. Called also *anidrotic.*

anhydrase (an-hi′drās) hydro-lyase.

anhydration (an″hi-dra′shun) dehydration.

anhydremia (an″hi-dre′me-ah) [*an* neg. + Gr. *hydōr* water + *haima* blood + *-ia*] deficiency of water in the blood.

anhydride (an-hi′drīd) [*an* neg. + Gr. *hydōr* water] a chemical compound derived from a substance, especially an acid, by the abstraction of a molecule of water. The anhydrides of bases are oxides; those of alcohols are ethers. **abietic acid a.,** a resinous substance, $C_{44}H_{62}O_4$, found in rosin. **acetic a.,** a colorless mobile liquid of a pungent acetic odor, the anhydride of acetic acid $(CH_3CO)_2O$. **arsenous a.,** arsenic trioxide. **carbonic a.,** carbon dioxide. **chromic a.,** chromic acid. **perosmic a.,** osmium tetroxide. **silicic a.,** silica. **sorbitol a.,** sorbitan. **sulfurous a.,** sulfur dioxide. **trimellitic a.,** a low-molecular-weight reactive chemical used in the manufacture of plastics, epoxy resin, coatings, and paints; inhalation of its dust or fumes produces a variety of respiratory symptoms.

anhydrochloric (an″hi-dro-klo′rik) achlorhydric.

anhydrohydroxyprogesterone (an-hi″dro-hi-drok″se-pro-jes′ter-ōn) ethisterone.

anhydromuscarine (an″hi-dro-mus′kah-rin) a synthetic alkaloid, $OH(CH_3)_3N \cdot CH_2CHO$, that has been used in experimental medicine.

Anhydron (an-hi′dron) trademark for a preparation of cyclothiazide.

anhydrosugar (an″hi-dro-shug′ar) a substance produced from cane sugar by heating it under diminished pressure to about 170° C. It does not ferment nor reduce copper solutions, and it has been used as a food in diabetes.

anhydrous (an-hi′drus) [*an* neg. + Gr. *hydōr* water] deprived or destitute of water.

aniacinamidosis (ah-ni″ah-sin-am″ĭ-do′sis) any disorder due to nicotinamide deficiency.

aniacinosis (ah-ni″ah-sĭ-no′sis) nicotinic acid (niacin) deficiency.

Anichkov's (Anitschkow's) myocyte (cell) (ah-nich′-kofs) [Nikolai Nikolaevich *Anichkov,* Russian pathologist, 1885–1964] see under *myocyte.*

anicteric (an″ik-ter′ik) without icterus; not associated with jaundice.

anidean (ah-nid′e-an) pertaining to anideus.

anideus (ah-nid′e-us) [*an* neg. + Gr. *idea* form] holoacardius amorphus. **embryonic a.,** a blastoderm in which no embryonic axis develops.

anidoxime (an″ĭ-doks′ēm) chemical name: 3-(diphenyl-amino)-1-phenyl-1-propanone *O*-[[(4-methylphenyl)amino]-carbonyl]oxime; an analgesic, $C_{21}H_{27}N_3O_3$.

anidrosis (an-ĭ-dro′sis) anhidrosis.

anidrotic (an″ĭ-drot′ik) anhidrotic.

anile (a′nīl) [L. *anus,* old woman] 1. like an old woman. 2. in one's dotage.

anileridine (an″ĭ-ler′ĭ-dēn) [USP] chemical name: 1-[2-(4-aminophenyl)ethyl]-4-phenyl-4-piperidinecarboxylic acid. A synthetic narcotic analgesic, $C_{22}H_{28}N_2O_2$, occurring as a white, crystalline powder, used as the phosphate salt for premedication for general anesthesia in surgery, as a postoperative sedative, and as an obstetric analgesic; administered subcutaneously or intramuscularly. Abuse of this drug may lead to dependence. **a. hydrochloride** [USP], a white or nearly white crystalline powder, $C_{22}H_{28}N_2O_2 \cdot 2HCl$, having the same actions and uses as the base; administered orally.

anilid (an′ĭ-lid) anilide.

anilide (an′ĭ-lid) any compound formed from aromatic amines by substitution of an acyl group for the hydrogen of NH_2.

aniline (an′ĭ-lin) [Arabic *an′nil* indigo, *nīl* blue; L. *nil* indigo] a colorless oily liquid, $C_6H_5NH_2$, from coal tar and from indigo, made commercially by reducing nitrobenzene. It is slightly soluble in water; freely so in ether and alcohol. Combined with other substances, especially chlorine and the chlorates, it forms the aniline colors or dyes that are derived from coal tar. It is an important cause of serious industrial poisoning. The predominant acute toxic effect is methemoglobinemia. Called also *amidobenzene* and *aminobenzene.* See also *anilinism.* **a. sulfate,** a white crystalline substance, $(C_6H_5NH_2)_2H_2SO_4$.

anilingus (a″nĭ-ling′gus) [L. *anus* + *lingere* to lick] sexual stimulation of the anus with the lips or tongue.

anilinism (an′ĭ-lin-izm) a condition produced by exposure to aniline, and marked by methemoglobinemia and aplastic anemia, vertigo, muscular weakness, cyanosis, and digestive derangement.

anilinophil (an-ĭ-lin′o-fil) [*aniline* + Gr. *philein* to love] (*obs.*) an anilinophilous element or structure.

anilinophile (an″ĭ-lin′o-fīl) (*obs.*) 1. anilinophilous. 2. anilinophil.

anilinophilous (an″ĭ-lin-of′ĭ-lus) (*obs.*) staining readily with aniline dyes.

anilism (an′ĭ-lizm) anilinism.

anility (ah-nil′ĭ-te) [L. *anus,* old woman] 1. the state of being like an old woman. 2. senility; dotage.

anilopam hydrochloride (an′il-o-pam″) chemical name: 4-[2-(1,2,4,5-tetrahydro-8-methoxy-2-methyl-3*H*-3-benzazepin-3-yl)ethyl]benzeneamine dihydrochloride; an analgesic, $C_{20}H_{26}N_2O \cdot 2HCl$.

anil-quinoline (an″il-kwin′o-lin) synthetic quinoline prepared from aniline.

anima (an′ĭ-mah) [L., the animating spirit present in any animal] 1. the soul. 2. the active principal of a drug. 3. in jungian psychology, the soul or inner being of a person, as opposed to the *persona,* the social role or facade presented to the world; also used to refer to the feminine aspect of a man's soul, the analogous masculine aspect of a woman's soul being termed the *animus.*

animal (an′ĭ-mal) [L. *animalis,* from *anima* life, breath] 1. a living organism having sensation and the power of voluntary movement and requiring for its existence oxygen and organic food. 2. pertaining to such an organism. **control a.,** see *control,* def. 2. **conventional a.,** an experimental animal that has not been reared under gnotobiotic conditions. **decerebrate a.,** an experimental animal that has been subjected to decerebration; such an animal exhibits rigid extension of the legs, with strong tonic contraction of the extensor muscles and to some extent the flexor muscles. See also *decerebrate,* and see *decerebrate rigidity,* under *rigidity.* **experimental a.,** an animal which is used as a subject of experimental procedures in the laboratory. **Houssay a.,** an experimental animal deprived of both pituitary gland and pancreas. **hyperphagic a.,** an experimental animal in which the cells of the ventromedial nucleus of the hypothalamus have been destroyed, abolishing its awareness of the point at which it should stop eating; excessive eating and savageness characterize such an animal. **Long-Lukens a.,** an experimental animal which has been deprived of the pancreas and adrenal glands. **nuclein a.,** an animal into which a certain amount of nuclein has been injected. **slime a.,** see *Mycetozoida.* **spinal a.,** an animal whose spinal cord has been severed, thus cutting off communication with the brain. **thalamic a.,** an animal in which the brain stem has been transected just above the thalamus.

animalcule (an″ĭ-mal′kūl) [L. *animalculum*] (*obs.*) any minute or microscopic animal organism.

animalculist (an″ĭ-mal′ku-list) a believer in the theory that the undeveloped embryo exists preformed in the spermatozoon; cf. *ovist.*

animality (an″ĭ-mal′ĭ-te) the distinguishing characteristics of animals.

animation (an″ĭ-ma′shun) 1. the state of being alive. 2.

liveliness of spirits. **suspended a.,** a temporary state of apparent death.

animism (an′ĭ-mizm) [L. *anima* soul] 1. the obsolete doctrine that the soul is the source of all organic development. 2. the belief that nonliving objects and phenomena (such as clouds) are inhabited and motivated by a nonphysical agent; it is a characteristic of the thinking of early childhood. 3. the theory that behavior is controlled by an immaterial mind or soul.

animus (an′ĭ-mus) [L., the rational part of the mind; intellect or motivations] 1. ill will or hostility; animosity. 2. in jungian psychology, the masculine aspect of a woman's soul or inner being; see *anima.*

anincretinosis (an-in″kre-tĭ-no′sis) [*an* neg. + *incretion*] (*obs.*) a disorder due to defect or lack of some internal secretion.

anion (an′i-on) [Gr. *ana* up + *iōn* going] an ion carrying a negative charge owing to a surplus of electrons; in an electrochemical cell anions migrate toward the anode.

anionic (an″i-on′ik) pertaining to or containing an anion.

anionotropy (an″e-on-ot′ro-pe) [*anion* + Gr. *tropos* a turning] a type of tautomerism in which the migrating group is a negative ion rather than the more usual hydrogen ion. Cf. *prototropy.*

aniridia (an″ĭ-rid′e-ah) [*an* neg. + *iris*] absence of the iris; a usually bilateral, hereditary anomaly that is rarely complete, a rudimentary stump usually being visible on gonioscopy.

anisakiasis (an″is-sa-ki′ah-sis) infection with the roundworm *Anisakis marina.* Human infection is caused by third-stage larvae eaten in undercooked infected marine fish (e.g., herring); the larvae then burrow into the stomach wall, producing an eosinophilic granulomatous mass. Called also *eosinophilic granuloma.*

Anisakis (an″ĭ-sa′kis) a genus of nematodes that parasitize the stomachs of marine mammals and birds, where they reach the adult stage; the infective third-stage larvae occur in various marine fishes. Man is occasionally infected by ingestion of raw fish containing larvae. See also *anisakiasis.* **A. ma′rina,** a species causing anisakiasis.

anisate (an′ĭ-sāt) a salt of anisic acid.

anischuria (an″is-ku′re-ah) [*an* neg. + Gr. *ischouria* retention of the urine] (*obs.*) incontinence of urine; enuresis.

anise (an′is) [L. *anisum*] the fruit of *Pimpinella anisum,* an umbelliferous plant; it is used as a carminative and expectorant. **Chinese a., Indian a.,** the dried ripe fruit of *Illicium verum,* an Asian tree. It yields anise oil and is used as a stimulant and carminative. **star a.,** the fruit of *Illicium religiosum* (*I. japonicum; I. anisatum*), the Japanese star anise (shikimmi); it is very poisonous due to content of hananomin.

aniseikonia (an″ĭ-si-ko′ne-ah) [Gr. *anisos* unequal + *eikōn* image + *-ia*] a condition in which the ocular image of an object as seen by one eye differs in size and shape from that seen by the other.

aniseikonic (an″ĭ-si-kon′ik) pertaining to or correcting aniseikonia.

anisic acid (ah-nis′ik) *p*-methoxybenzoic acid, an antiseptic compound obtained from anise and fennel.

anisindione (an″is-in-di′ōn) [NF] chemical name: 2-(4-methoxyphenyl)-1*H*-indene-1,3(2*H*)-dione. One of the indanedione anticoagulants, $C_{16}H_{12}O_3$, occurring as a white to creamy white powder; administered orally.

anisine (an′ĭ-sin) a crystalline alkaloid, $C_{22}H_{24}N_2O_3$, from anise; used as a bactericide and wood fungicide.

anis(o)- [Gr. *anisos* unequal, uneven] a combining form meaning unequal or dissimilar.

anisoaccommodation (an-i″so-ah-kom″o-da′shun) a difference in the accommodative capacity of the two eyes.

anisochromasia (an-i″so-kro-ma′ze-ah) [*aniso-* + Gr. *chrōma* color] a condition in which only the peripheral zone of an erythrocyte is colored.

anisochromatic (an-i″so-kro-mat′ik) [*aniso-* + Gr. *chrōma* color] 1. not of the same color throughout. 2. pertaining to solutions used for testing color blindness, containing two pigments which are distinguished by both the normal and the color blind eye. Cf. *pseudoisochromatic.*

anisochromia (an″ĭ-so-kro′me-ah) [*aniso-* + Gr. *chrōma*

color + *-ia*] variation in the color of the erythrocytes due to unequal hemoglobin content.

anisocoria (an-i″so-ko′re-ah) [*aniso-* + Gr. *korē* pupil + *-ia*] inequality in diameter of the pupils.

anisocytosis (an-i″so-si-to′sis) [*aniso-* + Gr. *kytos* hollow vessel + *-osis*] presence in the blood of erythrocytes showing excessive variation in size.

anisodactylous (an-i-so-dak′tĭ-lus) [*aniso-* + Gr. *daktylos* finger] having corresponding digits of unequal length.

anisodactyly (an-i-so-dak′tĭ-le) a condition characterized by having corresponding digits of unequal length.

anisodiametric (an-i″so-di″ah-met′rik) characterized by different dimensions in different diameters.

anisodont (an-i′so-dont) [*anis-* + Gr. *odous* tooth] 1. one who has unequal, asymmetric teeth. 2. an animal having irregular, asymmetric teeth, as in certain reptiles.

anisogamete (an″ĭ-so-gam′ēt) a gamete of different size and structure from the one with which it unites. See *macrogamete* and *microgamete.*

anisogametic (an″ĭ-so-gah-met′ik) characterized by the production of gametes of different size and structure.

anisogamous (an″ĭ-sog′ah-mus) having conjugating elements (gametes) that differ in size and structure.

anisogamy (an″i-sog′ah-me) [*aniso-* + Gr. *gamos* marriage] sexual conjugation in which the gametes differ in structure and size, as in the malarial parasites.

anisoic (an″ĭ-so′ik) pertaining to anise.

anisoiconia (an-i″so-i-ko′ne-ah) aniseikonia.

anisokaryosis (an-i″so-kar″e-o′sis) [*aniso-* + Gr. *karyon* nucleus + *-osis*] inequality in the size of the nuclei of cells.

Anisolobis (an-i″so-lo′bis) a genus of beetles, the earwigs. Nymphs and adults of *A. euborellia* (Lucas) are intermediate hosts of helminth parasites of man and animals.

anisomastia (an-i″so-mas′te-ah) [*aniso-* + Gr. *mastos* breast + *-ia*] inequality in the size of the breasts.

anisomelia (an-i″so-me′le-ah) [*aniso-* + Gr. *melos* limb + *-ia*] inequality between paired limbs.

anisomeric (an-i″so-mer′ik) not isomeric.

anisometrope (an-i″so-met′rōp) a person with anisometropia.

anisometropia (an-i″so-mĕ-tro′pe-ah) [*aniso-* + Gr. *metron* measure + *-opia*] a difference in the refractive power of the two eyes.

anisometropic (an-i″so-mĕ-trop′ik) pertaining to or characterized by anisometropia.

Anisomorpha (an-i″so-mor′fah) a genus of insects. **A. buprestoi′des,** the walking stick; a species of orthopterous insects capable of discharging an irritating fluid.

anisophoria (an″i-so-fo′re-ah) [*aniso-* + *phoria*] a condition in which the balance of the vertical muscles of one eye differs from that of the other eye, so that the visual lines do not lie in the same horizontal plane.

anisopia (an″i-so′pe-ah) [*aniso-* + Gr. *ōps* eye + *-ia*] inequality of vision in the two eyes.

anisopiesis (an-i″so-pi-e′sis) [*aniso-* + Gr. *piesis* pressure] variation or inequality in the blood pressure as registered in different parts of the body.

anisopoikilocytosis (an-i″so-poi″kĭ-lo-si-to′sis) the presence in the blood of erythrocytes of varying sizes and abnormal shapes.

anisorhythmia (an-i″so-rith′me-ah) [*aniso-* + Gr. *rhythmos* rhythm + *-ia*] (*obs.*) irregular heart action marked by lack of synchronism in the rhythm of atria and ventricles.

anisosmotic (an″ĭ-sos-mot′ik) not having the same osmotic pressure or not containing the same effective concentration of osmotically active components.

anisospore (an-i′so-spōr″) [*aniso-* + Gr. *sporos* spore] 1. a sexual spore, the male and female differing in size or shape. 2. an asexual spore produced by a heterosporous organism. See *isospore.*

anisosporous (an-i″sos′po-rus) having anisospores.

anisosthenic (an-i″sos-then′ik) [*aniso-* + Gr. *sthenos* strength] not having equal strength; said of paired muscles.

anisotonic (an-i″so-ton′ik) 1. showing a variation in tonicity or tension. 2. having an osmotic pressure differing from that of a solution with which it is compared.

a., a developmental anomaly consisting of posterior embryotoxon, hypoplasia of iris stroma, and usually glaucoma. See also *anterior chamber cleavage syndrome,* under *syndrome.* **Uhl's a.,** congenital hypoplasia of the myocardium of the right ventricle, resulting in decreased output of the right side of the heart. **Undritz a.,** hereditary hypersegmentation of neutrophils; see under *hypersegmentation.*

anomer (an′o-mer) [Gr. *ana* up + *meros* part] the α or β form of a sugar produced when the possibility of stereoisomerism is available to the reducing carbon atom by the formation of an oxygen-containing ring.

anomeric (an″o-mer′ik) pertaining to an anomer; denoting the reducing carbon atom in an anomer.

anomia (ah-no′me-ah) [*an* neg. + Gr. *onoma* name + *-ia*] loss of the power of naming objects or of recognizing and recalling their names; cf. *nominal aphasia* and *dysnomia.*

anonacein (an″o-na′se-in) an alkaloid of *Hylopia aethiopica* used in Africa as an aphrodisiac.

anonaine (an″o-na′in) an alkaloid, $C_{17}H_{17}O_2N$, from *Annona reticulata.*

anonychia (an″o-nik′e-ah) [*an* neg. + Gr. *onyx* nail + *-ia*] absence of the nail(s).

anonymous (ah-non′ĭ-mus) nameless; innominate.

anoperineal (a″no-per-ĭ-ne′al) pertaining to the anus and perineum.

Anopheles (ah-nof′ĕ-lēz) [Gr. *anōphelēs* hurtful] a genus of mosquitoes characterized by long slender palpi, nearly as long as the proboscis, and by holding the body at an angle with the surface on which it rests while the head and proboscis are in line with the body. Many species are vectors of malaria, and some are vectors of *Wuchereria bancrofti;* called also *Cellia.*

CHIEF MALARIA-CARRYING ANOPHELES SPECIES OF THE WORLD

Modified from Russell et al., *Practical Malariology.*

A. aconitus	A. maculatus maculatus
A. albimanus	A. maculipennis
A. albitarsis	A. mangyanus
A. amictus	A. messeae
A. annularis	A. minimus
A. annulipes annulipes	A. minimus flavirostris
A. aquasalis	A. moucheti moucheti
A. atroparvus	A. moucheti nigeriensis
A. bancroftii	A. multicolor
A. barbirostris barbirostris	A. nili
A. bellator	A. pattoni
A. claviger	A. pharoensis
A. culicifacies	A. philippinensis
A. darlingi	A. pretoriensis
A. farauti	A. pseudopunctipennis
A. fluviatilis	pseudopunctipennis
A. freeborni	A. punctimacula
A. funestus	A. punctulatus
A. gambiae	punctulatus
A. hancocki	A. quadrimaculatus
A. hargreavesi	A. sacharovi
A. hyrcanus nigerrimus	A. sergentii
A. hyrcanus sinensis	A. stephensi stephensi
A. jeyporiensis candidiensis	A. subpictus subpictus
A. jeyporiensis jeyporiensis	A. sundaicus
A. kochi	A. superpictus
A. labranchiae atroparvus	A. umbrosus
A. labranchiae labranchiae	A. varuna
A. leucosphyrus leucosphyrus	A. walkeri
A. lungae	

anophelicide (ah-nof′ĕ-lĭ-sīd″) [*anopheles* + L. *caedere* to kill] destructive to anopheline mosquitoes.

anophelifuge (ah-nof′ĕ-lĭ-fūj) [*anopheles* + L. *fugare* to put to flight] preventing the bite or attack of anopheline mosquitoes.

anopheline (ah-nof′ĭ-lĭn) pertaining to or caused by mosquitoes of the tribe Anophelini.

Anophelini (ah-nof″ĭ-li′ni) a tribe of mosquitoes of the subfamily Culicinae, family Culicidae. It includes the genera *Anopheles, Chagasia,* and *Nyssorphynchus,* and the subgenus *Stethomyia.* Members of the genus *Anopheles* act as carriers of the malarial parasite.

anophelism (ah-nof′ĕ-lizm) infestation of a district with anopheline mosquitoes.

anophoria (an-o-fo′re-ah) [Gr. *anō* upward + Gr. *pherein* to bear] hyperphoria.

anophthalmia (an″of-thal′me-ah) [*an* neg. + Gr. *ophthalmos* eye] a developmental defect characterized by complete absence of the eyes (rare) or by the presence of vestigial eyes.

anophthalmos (an″of-thal′mos) anophthalmia.

anoplasty (a′no-plas″te) [L. *anus* anus + Gr. *plassein* to form] a plastic or restorative operation on the anus.

Anoplocephala (an″op-lo-sef′ah-lah) [Gr. *anoplos* unarmed + Gr. *kephalē* head] a genus of tapeworms of the family Anoplocephalidae, found in horses.

Anoplocephalidae (an″o-plo-sĕ-fal′ĭ-de) a family of medium-sized or large tapeworms of the order Cyclophyllidea, subclass Cestoda, commonly parasitic in various herbivorous animals and man. Genera of medical and veterinary importance are *Anoplocephala, Moniezia, Bertiella,* and *Thysanosoma.*

Anoplura (an″o-plu′rah) [Gr. *anoplos* unarmed + *oura* tail] an order of insects, the sucking lice, characterized by the absence of wings; it includes only two genera of medical interest, *Pediculus* and *Phthirus.* Cf. *Mallophaga.*

anorchia (an-or′ke-ah) anorchism.

anorchid (an-or′kid) [*an* neg. + Gr. *orchis* testis] 1. an individual with no testes in the scrotum. 2. an individual lacking testes.

anorchidic (an″or-kid′ik) 1. pertaining to anorchism; having no testes in the scrotum. 2. having no testes.

anorchidism (an-or′kĭ-dizm″) anorchism.

anorchism (an-or′kizm) congenital absence of the testis, which may occur unilaterally or bilaterally.

anorectal (a″no-rek′tal) pertaining to the anus and rectum or to the junction region between the two.

anorectic (an″o-rek′tik) [Gr. *anorektos* without appetite for] 1. pertaining to anorexia; having no appetite. 2. a substance that diminishes the appetite.

anorectitis (a″no-rek-ti′tis) inflammation of the anorectum.

anorectocolonic (a″no-rek″to-ko-lon′ik) pertaining to the anus, rectum, and colon.

anorectum (a″no-rek′tum) [*anus* + *rectum*] the anus and rectum considered together as a single unit.

anoretic (an″o-ret′ik) anorectic.

anorexia (an″o-rek′se-ah) [Gr. "want of appetite"] lack or loss of the appetite for food. **a. nervo′sa** [DSM III-R], a mental disorder occurring predominantly in females, having onset usually in adolescence, and characterized by refusal to maintain a normal minimal body weight, intense fear of becoming obese that is undiminished by weight loss, disturbance of body image resulting in a feeling of being fat even when extremely emaciated, and amenorrhea (in females). Associated features seen in many cases are denial of the illness and resistance to psychotherapy, markedly decreased interest in sex, eating binges, self-induced vomiting, abuse of laxatives or diuretics, and peculiar behavior connected with food, such as hiding food around the house. Hospitalization to prevent death from starvation is necessary in many cases. Cf. *bulimia.*

anorexiant (an″o-rek′se-ant) anorexigenic.

anorexic (an″o-rek′sik) anorectic.

anorexigenic (an″o-rek″sĭ-jen′ik) [*anorexia* + Gr. *gennan* to produce] 1. producing anorexia, or diminishing the appetite. 2. an agent that produces anorexia, or controls the appetite. Called also *anorexiant.*

anorganic (an″or-gan′ik) denoting tissue (e.g., bone) from which the organic material has been removed.

anorganology (an″or-gan-ol′o-je) the study of nonliving things; abiology.

anorgasmy (an-or-gaz′me) [*an* neg. + *orgasm*] failure to experience orgasm in coitus.

anorthography (an″or-thog′rah-fe) [*an* neg. + Gr. *orthos* straight + *graphein* to write] loss of the power of writing correctly.

anorthopia (an″or-tho′pe-ah) [*an-* neg. + *ortho-* + *-opia*] 1. distorted vision in which straight lines appear as curves or angles, and symmetry is incorrectly perceived. 2. strabismus.

anorthoscope (an-or′tho-skōp″) [*an* neg. + *ortho* + *-scope*] an instrument for combining two disconnected pictures in one perfect visual image.

anoscope (a'no-skōp) [*anus* + Gr. *skopein* to examine] a speculum for examining the anus and lower rectum.

anoscopy (ah-nos'ko-pe) examination of the anus and lower rectum by means of an anoscope.

anosigmoidoscopic (a''no-sig-moi''do-skop'ik) pertaining to anosigmoidoscopy.

anosigmoidoscopy (a''no-sig''moi-dos'ko-pe) [*anus* + *sigmoid* + Gr. *skopein* to examine] endoscopic examination of the anus, rectum, and sigmoid colon.

anosmatic (an''oz-mat'ik) [*an* neg. + Gr. *osmasthai* to smell] having no sense of smell, or only an imperfect sense of smell. Cf. *osmatic*, def. 2.

anosmia (an-oz'me-ah) [*an* neg. + Gr. *osmē* smell + *-ia*] absence of the sense of smell; called also *anosphrasia* and *olfactory anesthesia*. **a. gustato'ria,** the loss of the power to smell foods. **preferential a.,** lack of ability to sense certain odors only. **a. respirato'ria,** loss of smell due to nasal obstruction.

anosmic (an-oz'mik) 1. pertaining to or characterized by anosmia. 2. odorless. Called also *aosmic*.

anosognosia (an-o''so-no'ze-ah) [*a* neg. + Gr. *nosos* disease + *gnosis* knowledge + *-ia*] unawareness or denial of a neurological deficit, such as hemiplegia.

anosphrasia (an''os-fra'ze-ah) [*an* neg. + Gr. *osphrasis* sense of smell] anosmia.

anospinal (a''no-spi'nal) pertaining to the anus and the spinal cord.

anosteoplasia (an-os''te-o-pla'se-ah) [*an* neg. + Gr. *osteon* bone + *plasis* formation + *-ia*] defective bone formation.

anostosis (an''os-to'sis) [*an* neg. + Gr. *osteon* bone + *-osis*] defective development of bone.

anotia (an-o'she-ah) [*an* neg. + Gr. *ous* ear + *-ia*] congenital absence of the external ear(s).

anotropia (an''o-tro'pe-ah) [Gr. *anō* upward + *trepein* to turn] a condition in which the visual axes tend to rise above the object looked at.

anotus (an-o'tus) [*an* neg. + Gr. *ous* ear] an earless fetus.

ANOVA analysis of variance.

anovaginal (a''no-vaj'ĭ-nal) pertaining to the anus and vagina, or communicating with the anal canal and vagina, as an anovaginal fistula.

anovaria (an''o-va're-ah) anovarism.

anovarianism (an''o-va're-an-ism) anovarism.

anovarism (an-o'var-izm) [*an* neg. + *ovary*] absence of the ovaries.

anovesical (a''no-ves'ĭ-kal) [L. *anus* fundament + *vesica* bladder] pertaining to the anus and urinary bladder.

anovular (an-ov'u-lar) not accompanied with the discharge of an ovum.

anovulation (an''ov-u-la'shun) absence of ovulation.

anovulatory (an-ov'u-lah-to''re) anovular.

anovulia (an''ov-u'le-ah) (*obs.*) anovulation.

anovulomenorrhea (an-ov''u-lo-men''o-re'ah) anovular menstruation.

anoxemia (an''ok-se'me-ah) [*an* neg. + *oxygen* + Gr. *haima* blood + *-ia*] reduction of oxygen content of the blood below physiologic levels.

anoxemic (an''ok-se'mik) characterized by or due to a lack of the normal proportion of oxygen in the blood.

anoxia (ah-nok'se-ah) a total lack of oxygen; often used interchangeably with *hypoxia* to mean a reduced supply of oxygen to the tissues. **altitude a.,** high-altitude sickness. **anemic a.,** anoxia resulting from a decrease in amount of hemoglobin or number of erythrocytes in the blood. **anoxic a.,** anoxia resulting from interference with the source of oxygen. **fulminating a.,** a rapid fall in the oxygen content of the blood. **histotoxic a.,** anoxia resulting from disturbance in the tissues that impairs utilization of oxygen. **myocardial a.,** failure of coronary blood flow to keep up with myocardial needs. **a. neonato'rum,** anoxia of the newborn. **stagnant a.,** anoxia resulting from inadequate blood flow through the capillaries with resultant abnormal oxygen extraction and low tissue oxygen tension.

anoxiate (ah-nok'se-āt) to put into a state of anoxia.

anoxic (ah-nok'sik) pertaining to or charcterized by anoxia.

Anoxyphotobacteria (an-ok''se-fo''to-bak-te're-ah) [*an* neg. + *oxygen* + *photo-* + *bacteria*] a class of bacteria of the division Gracilicutes, kingdom Procaryotae, made up of gram-negative anaerobic organisms that derive energy from light (phototrophic metabolism). It includes the purple nonsulfur bacteria (Rhodospirillaceae), the purple sulfur bacteria (Chromatiaceae), and the green sulfur bacteria (Chlorobiaceae).

ANS 1. anterior nasal spine, a cephalometric landmark; the tip of the anterior nasal spine as seen on the x-ray film in norma lateralis. 2. autonomic nervous system.

ansa (an'sah), gen. and pl. *an'sae* [L. "handle"] a general term used in anatomical nomenclature to designate a looplike structure; called also *loop*. **a. cervica'lis** [NA], a nerve loop in the neck that supplies the infrahyoid muscles and that presents a superior root, which connects with the hypoglossal nerve (and actually consists of fibers of the second or first cervical nerve), and an inferior root (nervus descendens cervicalis), which connects with the second and third cervical nerves. Called also *a. hypoglossi*. **a. hypoglos'si,** a. cervicalis. **a. lenticula'ris,** a small fiber tract arising in the globus pallidus of the lenticular nucleus and extending around the medial border of the internal capsule to join and mingle with the fibers of the fasciculus lenticularis, some of which synapse with cells in the *subthalamic* nucleus, nucleus of the prerubral field (field H of Forel), and the zona incerta and others continue to the ventral nuclei of the thalamus. In official anatomical nomenclature [NA], the ansa lenticularis and fasciculus lenticularis are considered together, and are designated *ansa et fasciculus lenticulares*. **an'sae nervo'rum spina'lium** [NA], loops of nerve fibers joining the ventral roots of the spinal nerves. **a. peduncula'ris** [NA], a complex grouping of fibers connecting the amygdaloid nucleus, the piriform area, and the anterior part of the hypothalamus, and various thalamic nuclei. The fiber bundles pass below the internal capsule, a principal bundle being the inferior peduncle of the thalamus. **a. subcla'via** [NA], nerve filaments that pass anterior and posterior to the subclavian artery to form a loop interconnecting the middle and inferior cervical ganglia; called also *a. of Vieussens* and *annulus of Vieussens*. **a. of Vieussens,** a. subclavia. **a. vitelli'na,** an embryonic vein from the yolk sac to the umbilical vein.

ansae (an'se) [L.] genitive and plural of *ansa*.

ansate (an'sāt) [L. *ansatus,* from *ansa* handle] having a handle; loop-shaped.

Ansbacher unit (ahns'bahk-er) [Stefan *Ansbacher,* German-American biologist, born 1905] see under *unit*.

anseriform (an'ser-ĭ-form'') of or belonging to the Anseriformes.

Anseriformes (an''ser-i-form'ēz) the order including ducks, geese, and swans.

anserine (an'ser-in) [L. *anserinus*] 1. pertaining to or like a goose. 2. a basic substance, beta-alanylmethylhistidine, first found in goose muscle, and subsequently in the muscle of many animals, not including man.

ansiform (an'sĭ-form) loop-shaped.

Ansolysen (an''so-li'sen) trademark for preparations of pentolinium tartrate.

Anspor (an'spōr) trademark for a preparation of cephradine.

ant. anterior.

ant- see *anti-*.

Antabuse (an'tah-būs'') trademark for a preparation of disulfiram.

antacid (ant-as'id) [*ant-* + L. *acidus* sour] 1. counteracting acidity. 2. a substance that counteracts or neutralizes acidity, usually of the stomach.

antagonism (an-tag'o-nizm'') [Gr. *antagōnisma* struggle] opposition or contrariety between similar things, as between muscles, medicines, or organisms; cf. *antibiosis*. **bacterial a.,** the antagonistic (inhibiting) effect of one bacterial organism on another by reason of its production of an antibiotic (antibiosis) or by its superior competitive ability to absorb nutrients. **metabolic a.,** interference with the metabolism or function of a given chemical compound by another bearing a close structural resemblance, the similarity in structure being the basis of the interference. For the various forms of such interference, see under *inhibition*.

salt a., the antagonistic action of different salts in maintaining normal permeability of the plasma membrane.

antagonist (an-tag′o-nist) [Gr. *antagōnistēs* an opponent] 1. a muscle whose action is the direct opposite of that of another muscle. 2. a substance that tends to nullify the action of another, as a drug that binds to a cell receptor without eliciting a biological response. 3. a tooth in one jaw that articulates with a tooth in the other jaw. **aldosterone a.,** a compound that blocks the action of aldosterone. A class of diuretics, typified by spironolactone, competes with aldosterone for receptor sites, thus blocking the aldosterone-dependent exchange of sodium and potassium in the distal tubule. **associated a's,** muscles that act on different parts, and by their combined actions move the parts in parallel directions. **competitive a.,** a substance that competes with a substrate or with an enzyme which ordinarily attacks the substrate, thus interfering with usual metabolic activity. The antagonist is usually a substrate analogue. See *antimetabolite.* **direct a's,** muscles that act on the same part, and by their combined actions keep the part at rest. **enzyme a.,** an antimetabolite that interferes with the normal action of an enzyme. See *enzyme inhibition,* under *inhibition.* **folic acid a.,** an antimetabolite of folic acid; those used as chemotherapeutic agents are competitive inhibitors of dihydrofolate reductase: trimethoprim is used as an antibacterial, pyrimethamine as an antimalarial, and methotrexate as an antineoplastic. Called also *antifol* and *antifolate.* **insulin a.,** any of a number of factors, hormones, and antibodies that block the action of insulin, including epinephrine, somatotropin, glucocorticoids, and glucagon (all of which counteract the metabolic effects of insulin), and the more direct-acting factors associated with plasma protein fractions. **metabolic a.,** an antimetabolite that interferes with the utilization of a substance essential in metabolism. **narcotic a.,** an agent that opposes the action of narcotics on the nervous system. **sulfonamide a.,** para-aminobenzoic acid.

antalgesic (ant-al-je′zik) antalgic.

antalgic (ant-al′jik) 1. counteracting or avoiding pain, as a posture or gait assumed so as to lessen pain. 2. analgesic.

antalkaline (ant-al′kah-lĭn″) [ant- + *alkali*] 1. neutralizing alkalinity. 2. an agent that neutralizes alkalis.

antaphrodisiac (ant″af-ro-diz′e-ak) 1. abrogating the sexual instinct. 2. an agent that allays sexual impulses; called also *anterotic.*

antapoplectic (ant″ap-o-plek′tik) [ant- + Gr. *apoplēxia* apoplexy] an agent for alleviating stroke.

antarthritic (ant″ar-thrit′ik) [ant- + Gr. *arthritikos* gouty] 1. alleviating arthritis. 2. an agent that alleviates arthritis.

antasthenic (ant″as-then′ik) [ant- + Gr. *astheneia* weakness] 1. alleviating weakness, or restoring strength. 2. an agent that alleviates weakness and restores strength.

antasthmatic (ant″az-mat′ik) [ant- + Gr. *asthma* asthma] 1. affording relief in asthma. 2. an agent that relieves the spasm of asthma.

antatrophic (ant″ah-trof′ik) correcting or opposing the progress of atrophy.

antazoline (an-taz′o-lēn) chemical name: 4,5-dihydro-*N*-phenyl-*N*-(phenylmethyl)-1*H*-imidazole-2-methanamine. An antihistaminic, $C_{17}H_{19}N_3$. Called also *imidamine.* **a. hydrochloride,** a white or almost white, crystalline powder, $C_{17}H_{20}ClN_3$, used to relieve allergic symptoms and to treat allergic manifestations; administered orally. **a. phosphate** [USP], a white to off-white crystalline powder, $C_{17}H_{19}N_3 \cdot H_2PO_4$, used in a 0.5 per cent solution, applied topically to the eyes in the treatment of allergic conjunctivitis.

ante- [L. *ante* before] a prefix meaning prior to or in front of.

antebrachium (an″te-bra′ke-um) [ante- + L. *brachium* arm] [NA] the part of the upper member of the body, between the elbow and the wrist; called also *antibrachium* and *forearm.*

antecardium (an-te-kar′de-um) [ante- Gr. *kardice* heart] regio epigastrica.

antecedent (an″te-se′dent) [L. *antecedere* to go before, precede] a precursor. **plasma thromboplastin a. (PTA),** Factor XI; see *coagulation factors,* under *factor.*

ante cibum (an′te si′bum) [L.] before meals, usually abbreviated *a.c.* in prescriptions, etc.

antecubital (an″te-ku′bĭ-tal) situated in front of the cubitus, or elbow.

antecurvature (an″te-kur′vah-chur″) [ante- + L. *curvatura* bend] a slight anteflexion.

anteflect (an′te-flekt) to bend forward.

anteflexed (an′te-flekst) in a condition of anteflexion.

anteflexio (an″te-flek′se-o) [L.] anteflexion. **a. u′teri,** anteflexion, def. 2.

anteflexion (an-te-flek′shun) [ante- + L. *flexio* bend] 1. an abnormal forward curvature of an organ or part. 2. the normal forward curvature of the uterus (anteflexio uteri).

antegrade (an′te-grād) anterograde.

antelocation (an″te-lo-ka′shun) [ante- + L. *locatio* placement] the forward displacement of an organ.

ante mortem (an′te mor′tem) [L.] before death.

antenatal (an″te-na′tal) [ante- + L. *natus* born] occurring or formed before birth; prenatal. Cf. *antepartal.*

antenna (an-ten′ah), pl. anten′nae. a feeler of an arthropod; one of the two lateral appendages on the anterior segment of the head of arthropods.

Antepar (an′te-par) trademark for a preparation of piperazine citrate and piperazine phosphate.

antepartal (an″te-par′tal) occurring before parturition, or childbirth, with reference to the mother. Cf. *antenatal.*

ante partum (an′te par′tum) [L.] in obstetrics, before the onset of labor, with reference to the mother.

antepartum (an″te-par′tum) [L.] antepartal.

antephase (an′te-fāz) the portion of interphase immediately preceding mitosis (or meiosis) when energy is being produced and stored for mitosis (or meiosis) and chromosome reproduction is taking place.

antephialtic (ant″ef-e-al′tik) [ant- + Gr. *ephialtēs* nightmare] alleviating or preventing nightmare.

anteposition (an″te-po-zish′un) forward displacement, as of the uterus.

anteprostate (an″te-pros′tāt) [ante- + *prostate*] glandula bulbourethralis.

anteprostatitis (an″te-pros-tah-ti′tis) inflammation of glandula bulbourethralis.

antepyretic (an″te-pi-ret′ik) [ante- + *pyretic*] occurring before the stage of fever.

Antergan (ant′er-gan) trademark for a preparation of phenbenzamine.

antergia (ant-er′je-ah) [ant- + Gr. *ergon* work] antagonism; resistance.

antergic (ant-er′jik) working in opposite directions; a term applied to antagonistic muscles.

antergy (ant′er-je) antergia.

anteriad (an-te′re-ad) toward the anterior surface of the body.

anterior (an-ter′e-or) [L. "before"; neut. *anterius*] situated in front of or in the forward part of an organ, toward the head end of the body; [NA] a term used in reference to the ventral or belly surface of the body.

antero- [L. *anterior* before] a prefix signifying before.

anteroclusion (an″ter-o-kloo′zhun) mesioclusion.

anteroexternal (an″ter-o-eks-ter′nal) situated on the front and to the lateral side; anterolateral (which is preferred).

anterograde (an′ter-o-grād″) [antero- + L. *gredi* to go] moving or extending forward; called also *antegrade.*

anteroinferior (an″ter-o-in-fēr′e-or) situated in front and below.

anterointernal (an″ter-o-in-ter′nal) situated on the front and to the medial side; anteromedial (which is preferred).

anterolateral (an″ter-o-lat′er-al) situated in front and to one side; preferred to *anteroexternal.*

anteromedial (an″ter-o-me′de-al) situated in front and to the medial side; preferred to anterointernal.

anteromedian (an″ter-o-me′de-an) situated in front and toward the median plane.

anteroposterior (an″ter-o-pos-tēr′e-or) from front to

back of the body; in roentgenology it denotes such direction of the beam.

anteroseptal (an″ter-o-sep′tal) situated in front of the atrioventricular septum.

anterosuperior (an″ter-o-su-pēr′e-or) situated in front and above.

anterotic (ant″e-rot′ik) antaphrodisiac.

anteroventral (an″ter-o-ven′tral) situated in front and toward the ventral surface.

anteversion (an″te-ver′zhun) [*ante-* + L. *versio* a turning] the forward tipping or tilting of an organ; displacement in which the organ is tipped forward, but is not bent at an angle, as occurs in anteflexion.

antexed (an-tekst′) bent forward.

antexion (an-tek′shun) an abnormal forward bending, as of the spine.

anthelix (ant′he-liks) [*ant-* + Gr. *helix* coil] [NA] the prominent semicircular ridge seen on the lateral aspect of the auricle of the external ear, anteroinferior to the helix; called also *antihelix*.

anthelminthic (ant″hel-min′thik) anthelmintic.

anthelmintic (ant″hel-min′tik) [*ant-* + Gr. *helmins* worm] 1. destructive to worms. 2. an agent that is destructive to worms.

anthelmycin (an-thel-mi′sin) an antibiotic substance produced by *Streptomyces longissimus*, which has anthelmintic activity.

anthelotic (ant″he-lot′ik) [*ant-* + Gr. *hēlos* nail] 1. effective against corns. 2. a remedy for corns.

Anthemis (an′the-mis) [L.; Gr. *anthemis*] 1. a genus of composite-flowered plants. 2. the flower heads of *A. nobilis*, or common camomile, formerly used for coughs, in spasmodic conditions in infants, and as a stomachic tonic.

anthemorrhagic (ant″hem-o-raj′ik) [*ant-* + *hemorrhage*] antihemorrhagic.

anther (an′ther) [Gr. *anthēros* blooming] the portion of the stamen of flowering plants containing the microsporangia (pollen sacs) in which haploid microspores (pollen grains) are formed.

antheridium (an″ther-id′e-um), pl. *antherid′ia* [L. *anthera* medicine made from flowers + Gr. *idion* a diminutive ending] male organ of a cryptogamic plant in which microgametes are produced. Cf. *archegonium*.

antherozoid (an′ther-o-zoid″) the motile fertilizing cell of certain fungi.

antherpetic (ant″her-pet′ik) curing or preventing herpes.

anthiolimine (an-thi-o′lĭ-mēn) antimony lithium thiomalate.

Anthiomaline (an″thi-o-mal′in) trademark for antimony lithium thiomalate.

anthocyanidin (an″tho-si-an′ĭ-din) a pigment obtained by hydrolysis of anthocyanin.

anthocyanin (an″tho-si′ah-nin) [Gr. *anthos* flower + *kyanos* blue] any of a class of pigments of blue, red, and violet flowers; they are glycosides, yielding anthocyanidin and a sugar on hydrolysis.

anthocyaninemia (an″tho-si″ah-nin-e′me-ah) the presence of anthocyanin in the blood.

anthocyaninuria (an″tho-si″ah-nin-u′re-ah) the presence of anthocyanin in the urine.

Anthomyia (an″tho-mi′yah) a genus of small black houseflies. Two species of medical importance were formerly assigned to this genus. See *Fannia canicularis* and *F. scalaris*.

Anthomyiidae (an″tho-mi′ĭ-de) [Gr. *anthos* flower + *myia* fly] in some systems of classification, a family of the order Diptera; the only genus of medical importance is *Fannia*, the larvae of which may cause both urinary and intestinal myiasis in man.

anthophobia (an″tho-fo′be-ah) [Gr. *anthos* flower + *phobia*] irrational dislike or dread of flowers.

Anthozoa (an″tho-zo′ah) [Gr. *anthos* flower + *zoia* animal] a class of coelenterates with large polyps and no medusa stage; it includes corals.

anthracene (an′thrah-sēn) a colorless hydrocarbon, $C_6H_4(CH)_2C_6H_4$, from coal tar, used in the manufacture of anthracene dyes.

anthracic (an-thras′ik) pertaining to or resembling anthrax.

anthrac(o)- [Gr. *anthrax* charcoal, carbuncle] a combining form denoting relationship to coal or carbon, or to a carbuncle.

anthracoid (an′thrah-koid) [*anthraco-* + Gr. *eidos* form] resembling anthrax or a carbuncle.

anthracometer (an″thrah-kom′ĕ-ter) [*anthraco-* + Gr. *metron* measure] an instrument for measuring the carbon dioxide of the air.

anthraconecrosis (an″thrah-ko-nĕ-kro′sis) [*anthraco-* + Gr. *nekrōsis* death] necrotic transformation of a tissue into a black dry mass.

anthracosilicosis (an″thrah-ko-sil′ĭ-ko′sis) [*anthraco-* + *silicon*] a mixed condition of anthracosis and silicosis.

anthracosis (an-thrah-ko′sis) [*anthraco-* + *-osis*] a usually asymptomatic form of pneumoconiosis caused by deposition of coal dust in the lungs; it is present in most urban dwellers. When the coal dust accumulates in large amounts, it may result in pneumoconiosis of coal workers. **a. lin′guae,** black tongue.

anthracotherapy (an″thrah-ko-ther′ah-pe) [Gr. *anthrax* coal + *therapy*] treatment with charcoal.

anthracotic (an″thrah-kot′ik) pertaining to or affected with anthracosis.

anthracycline (an″thrah-si′klēn) any of several antineoplastic antibiotics, including doxorubicin and daunorubicin, produced by *Streptomyces peucetius*. Daunorubicin is used for acute leukemias; doxorubicin is used for these and also for lymphomas and solid tumors. The use of these drugs is limited by a chronic, cumulative, dose-related toxicity (anthracycline cardiomyopathy or cardiotoxicity) resulting in irreversible congestive heart failure that is unresponsive to digitalis. Nausea and vomiting, alopecia, and bone marrow depression are other major side effects.

Anthra-Derm (an′thrah-derm) trademark for a preparation of anthralin.

anthragallol (an″thrah-gal′ol) chemical name: 1,2,3-trihydrox-9,10-anthracenedione. A product of the interaction of gallic, benzoic, and sulfuric acids, $C_{14}H_8O_5$.

anthralin (an′thrah-lin) [USP] chemical name: 1,8,9-anthracenetriol. A synthetic compound, $C_{14}H_{10}O_3$, occurring as a yellowish brown, crystalline powder; applied topically to the skin in the treatment of dermatophytoses, chronic eczema, alopecia areata, and other skin diseases. Called also *dithranol*.

anthramucin (an″thrah-mu′sin) (*obs.*) anthrax capsule.

anthramycin (an″thrah-mi′sin) (*E*)-3-(5,10,11,11a-tetrahydro-9,11-dihydroxy-8-methyl-5-oxo-1*H*-pyrrolo[2,1-*c*][1,4]benzodiazepin-2-yl)-2-propenamide. An antineoplastic antibiotic, $C_{16}H_{17}N_3O_4$, produced by *Streptomyces refuineus* var. *thermotolerans*.

anthranilic acid (an″thrah-nil′ik) *o*-aminobenzoic acid, a product of tryptophan catabolism.

anthraquinone (an″thrah-kwin′ōn) chemical name: 9,10-anthracenedione. A derivative of anthracene, $C_{14}H_8O_2$; its derivatives, which are found in aloes, cascara sagrada, senna, and rhubarb, have cathartic properties.

anthrarobin (an″thrah-ro′bin) [*anthracene* + *araroba*] chemical name: 1,2,10-anthracenetriol. A yellowish white powder from alizarin, $C_6H_4:C(OH)\cdot CH:C_6H_2(OH)_2$; it is useful in psoriasis and various skin diseases in 10 to 20 per cent ointment, and as a parasiticide.

anthrax (an′thraks) [Gr. "coal," "carbuncle"] an infectious bacterial zoonotic disease usually acquired by ingestion of *Bacillus anthracis* or its spores from infected pastures by herbivores or indirectly from infected carcasses by carnivores. It is transmitted to humans usually by contact with infected animals or their discharges (*agricultural a.*) or with contaminated animal products (*industrial a.*). Anthrax is classified by primary routes of inoculation as: cutaneous, gastrointestinal, and inhalational. Called also *charbon, milzbrand,* and *splenic fever.* **agricultural a.,** see *anthrax.* **cerebral a.,** meningeal a. **cutaneous a.,** the most common type of anthrax in humans, due to inoculation of *Bacillus anthracis* into superficial wounds or abrasions. It occurs in two forms manifested by: (1) a small, painless, pruritic papular lesion (which has been called malignant carbuncle or pustule even though no liquefactive necrosis or pus formation occurs) at the site of inoculation, often with one or more satellite lesions, that enlarges, ulcerates, and becomes crusted with an adherent dense black eschar, which often heals spontaneously, but may progress to a systemic condition and may involve the meninges; and (2) bullae at the site of inoculation that break down to form a necrotic eschar surrounded by massive spreading edema (*malignant edema*) associated with induration, high fever, and severe toxemia. **gastrointestinal a.,** anthrax due to ingestion of poorly cooked meat contaminated with *Bacillus anthracis,* with deposition of spores in the submucosa of the intestinal tract, where they germinate, multiply, and produce toxin, with resultant massive edema that may obstruct the bowel, hemorrhage, and necrosis. Called also *intestinal a.* **industrial a.,** see *anthrax.* **inhalational a.,** a highly fatal form of anthrax due to inhalation of dust containing anthrax spores, which are transported by the alveolar pneumocytes to the regional lymph nodes where they germinate, multiply, and produce toxin, and characterized by hemorrhagic edematous mediastinitis, pleural effusions, dyspnea, cyanosis, stridor, and shock. It is usually an occupational disease, most often affecting those who handle and sort contaminated wools and fleeces. Called also *a. pneumonia, pulmonary a., ragpicker's* or *ragsorter's disease,* and *woolsorter's disease* or *pneumonia.* **intestinal a.,** gastrointestinal a. **malignant a.,** anthrax. **meningeal a.,** a rare, highly fatal form of anthrax resembling typical hemorrhagic meningitis due to hematogenous spread of the anthrax bacillus from a primary focus of infection, and manifested by hemorrhagic cerebrospinal fluid and accompanying neurological signs and symptoms. Called also *cerebral a.* **pulmonary a.,** inhalational a. **symptomatic a.,** blackleg.

anthrop(o)- [Gr. *anthrōpos* man, human being] a combining form denoting a relationship to man, or to a human being.

anthropobiology (an″thro-po-bi-ol′o-je) the biological study of man and the anthropoid apes.

anthropocentric (an″thro-po-sen′trik) [*anthropo-* + Gr. *kentrikos* of or from the center] with a human bias; considering man the center of the universe.

anthropogeny (an″thro-poj′ĕ-ne) [*anthropo-* + Gr. *gennan* to produce] the evolution and development of man.

anthropography (an″thro-pog′rah-fe) [*anthropo-* + Gr. *graphein* to write] that branch of anthropology which deals with the distribution of the varieties of man, as distinguished by physical character, institutions, customs, etc.; cf. *ethnography.*

anthropoid (an′thro-poid) [*anthropo-* + Gr. *eidos* form] resembling man. The anthropoid apes are the tailless apes, including the chimpanzee, gibbon, gorilla, and orangutan.

Anthropoidea (an″thro-poi′de-ah) a suborder of Primates including the monkeys, apes, and man.

anthropokinetics (an″thro-po-ki-net′iks) [*anthropo-* + Gr. *kinētikos* for putting in motion] the study of the total human being in action, with integrated applications from the special fields of the biological and physical sciences, psychology, and sociology.

anthropology (an″thro-pol′o-je) [*anthropo-* + *-ology*] the science that treats of man, his origins, historical and cultural development, and races. **criminal a.,** that branch of anthropology which treats of criminals and crimes. **cultural a.,** that branch of anthropology which treats of man in relation to his fellows and to his environment. **physical a.,** that branch of anthropology which treats of the physical characteristics of man.

anthropometer (an″thro-pom′ĕ-ter) an instrument especially designed for measuring various dimensions of the body.

anthropometric (an″thro-po-met′rik) pertaining to or connected with anthropometry.

anthropometrist (an″thro-pom′ĕ-trist) a person skilled in anthropometry.

anthropometry (an″thro-pom′ĕ-tre) [*anthropo-* + Gr. *metron* measure] the science which deals with the measurement of the size, weight, and proportions of the human body.

anthropomorphism (an″thro-po-mor′fizm) [*anthropo-* + Gr. *morphē* form] the attribution of human form or character to nonhuman objects.

anthroponomy (an″thro-pon′o-me) [*anthropo-* + Gr. *nomos* law] the science that deals with the laws of human development in relation to environment and to other organisms.

anthropopathy (an″thro-pop′ah-the) [*anthropo-* + Gr. *pathos* suffering] the ascription of human emotions to nonhuman subjects.

anthropophilic (an″thro-po-fil′ik) [*anthropo-* + Gr. *philein* to love] preferring human beings to other animals; said of certain mosquitoes. Cf. *anthropozoophilic* and *zoophilic.*

anthropophobia (an″thro-po-fo′be-ah) [*anthropo-* + *phobia*] irrational dread of human society.

anthroposcopy (an″thro-pos′ko-pe) [*anthropo-* + Gr. *skopein* to examine] the judging of the type of body build by inspection rather than by anthropometry.

anthroposophy (an″thro-pos′o-fe) [*anthropo-* + Gr. *sophos* wise] knowledge of the nature of man.

anthropozoophilic (an″thro-po-zo″o-fil′ik) [*anthropo-* + Gr. *zōon* animal + *philein* to love] attracted to both human beings and animals; said of certain mosquitoes. Cf. *anthropophilic* and *zoophilic.*

anthypnotic (ant″hip-not′ik) (*obs.*) antihypnotic.

anthysteric (ant″his-ter′ik) antihysteric.

anti-, ant- (Gr. *anti* against) a prefix signifying counteracting, effective against, opposing, or opposite.

antiabortifacient (an″ti-ah-bor″ti-fa′shent) an agent that prevents abortion or promotes successful gestation.

antiadrenergic (an″ti-ah-dren-er′jik) 1. opposing the effects of impulses conveyed by adrenergic postganglionic fibers of the sympathetic nervous system. 2. an agent that so acts. Called also *sympatholytic.* Cf. *anticholinergic.*

antiagglutinin (an″ti-ah-gloo′ti-nin) a substance that opposes the action of an agglutinin.

antiaggressin (an″ti-ah-gres′in) a substance once thought to be formed in the body by repeated injection of an aggressin, and tending to oppose the action of the aggressin.

antialbumin (an″ti-al-bu′min) a precipitin for albumin.

antiamebic (an″ti-ah-me′bik) 1. destroying or suppressing the growth of amebas. 2. an agent that destroys or suppresses the growth of amebas.

antiamylase (an″ti-am′ĭ-lās) a substance counteracting the action of amylase.

antianaphylaxis (an″ti-an-ah-fi-lak′sis) a condition in which the anaphylaxis reaction is not obtained because of the presence of free antibodies in the blood; the state of desensitization to antigens.

antiandrogen (an″ti-an′dro-jen) any substance capable of inhibiting the biological effects of androgenic hormones.

antianemic (an″ti-ah-ne′mik) 1. counteracting or preventing anemia. 2. an agent that counteracts or prevents anemia.

antianopheline (an″ti-ah-nof′ĕ-lin) directed against anopheline mosquitoes or their larvae.

antiantibody (an″ti-an′ti-bod″e) an antibody directed against antigenic determinants on other antibody (immunoglobulin) molecules.

antiantidote (an″ti-an′ti-dōt″) a substance that counteracts the action of an antidote.

antiantitoxin (an″ti-an′ti-tok′sin) an antibody, formed in immunization with an antitoxin, which counteracts the effect of the latter.

antianxiety (an″te-ang-zi′ĕ-te) reducing anxiety. Antianxiety drugs (called also *anxiolytic drugs* and *minor tranquilizers*) include the benzodiazepines (diazepam and congeners) and a few less widely used nonbenzodiazepines (meprobamate, hydroxyzine).

antiapoplectic (an″ti-ap″o-plek′tik) affording relief in or preventing stroke (apoplexy).

antiarachnolysin (an″ti-ar″ak-nol′ĭ-sin) a substance counteracting spider toxin.

antiarin (an-te′ar-in) a poisonous principle, $C_{14}H_{20}O_5$ + $2H_2O$, from the upas tree, *Antiaris toxicaria;* formerly used as a heart depressant.

Antiaris (an″ti-a′ris) [Javanese *antiar*] a genus of artocarpous trees. *A. toxicaria* (*Bohun upas*), the upas tree of Java, yields a latex used as an arrow poison. The major toxic principle is a digitalis-like cardioactive glycoside, α-antiarin.

antiarrhythmic (an″ti-ah-rith′mik) 1. preventing or alleviating cardiac arrhythmia. 2. an agent that prevents or alleviates cardiac arrhythmia.

antiarsenin (an″ti-ar′sĕ-nin) a nonarsenical substance believed to be developed in the body by immunizing doses of arsenous acid.

antiarthritic (an″tĭ-ar-thrit′ik) antarthritic.

antiasthmatic (an″tĭ-az-mat′ik) antasthmatic.

antiatherogenic (an″tĭ-ath″er-o-jen′ik) combating the formation of atheromatous lesions in arterial walls.

antiautolysin (an″tĭ-aw-tol′ĭ-sin) a substance which opposes the action of autolysin.

antibacterial (an″tĭ-bak-te′re-al) 1. destroying or suppressing the growth or reproduction of bacteria. 2. a substance that destroys bacteria or suppresses their growth or reproduction.

antibechic (an″tĭ-bek′ik) [anti- + Gr. bēchikos suffering from cough] 1. relieving a cough. 2. an agent that relieves cough.

antibiosis (an″tĭ-bi-o′sis) [anti- + Gr. bios life] an association between two organisms that is detrimental to one of them, or between one organism and an antibiotic produced by another.

antibiotic (an″tĭ-bi-ot′ik) [anti- + Gr. bios life] 1. destructive of life. 2. a chemical substance produced by a microorganism which has the capacity, in dilute solutions, to inhibit the growth of or to kill other microorganisms. Antibiotics that are sufficiently nontoxic to the host are used as chemotherapeutic agents in the treatment of infectious diseases of man, animals, and plants. **broad-spectrum a.,** one that is effective against a wide range of bacteria, both gram-positive and gram-negative.

antibiotin (an″tĭ-bi′o-tin) a compound that is antagonistic to biotin; avidin.

antiblastic (an″tĭ-blas′tik) [anti- + Gr. blastos germ] retarding growth or multiplication, as of tumor or bacterial cells.

antibody (an′tĭ-bod″e) an immunoglobulin molecule that has a specific amino acid sequence by virtue of which it interacts only with the antigen that induced its synthesis in cells of the lymphoid series (especially plasma cells), or with antigen closely related to it. Antibodies are classified according to their mode of action as agglutinins, bacteriolysins, hemolysins, opsonins, precipitins, etc. See *immunoglobulin*. **acetylcholine receptor a's,** anti–acetylcholine receptor a's. **anaphylactic a.,** IgE antibody causing anaphylaxis. **anti–acetylcholine receptor (anti-AChR) a's,** circulating autoantibodies against the acetylcholine receptors of the myoneural junction. High titers are demonstrable in about 85 per cent of myasthenia gravis patients; false positives are rare. Called also *acetylcholine receptor a.'s.* **anti-D a.,** antibody directed against the "Rh₀" or "D" antigen of the Rh blood group. **anti-DNA a.,** see *antinuclear a.* **anti–glomerular basement membrane (anti-GEM) a's,** see *anti–glomerular basement membrane antibody disease,* under *disease.* **anti-idiotype a.,** antibody that binds selectively to a specific idiotope. **antimicrosomal a's,** organ-specific autoantibodies directed against a thyroid microsomal antigen, demonstrable in almost all patients with Hashimoto's thyroiditis. **antimitochondrial a's,** circulating antibodies directed against inner mitochondrial membrane antigens seen in almost all patients with primary biliary cirrhosis and rarely in other liver diseases. Called also *mitochondrial a's.* **antinuclear a's (ANA),** antibodies directed against nuclear antigens; ANA against a variety of different antigens are almost invariably found in systemic lupus erythematosus and are frequently found in rheumatoid arthritis, scleroderma (systemic sclerosis), Sjögren's syndrome, and mixed connective tissue disease. ANA may be detected by immunofluorescent staining. Serologic tests are also used to determine antibody titers against specific antigens. **antireceptor a's,** autoantibodies against cell-surface receptors, e.g., those directed against acetylcholine receptors in myasthenia gravis, against TSH receptors in Graves' disease, against insulin receptors in type B insulin resistance with acanthosis nigricans, and against β₂-adrenergic receptors in some patients with allergic disorders. **antithyroglobulin a's,** autoantibodies directed against thyroglobulin, demonstrable in about 50 to 75 per cent of patients with Hashimoto's thyroiditis and in about one-third of patients with other types of thyroiditis, Graves' disease, and thyroid carcinoma. **antithyroid a's,** see *antimicrosomal a's* and *antithyroglobulin a's.* **auto-anti-idiotypic a's,** autologous anti-idiotype antibodies that suppress the immune response in many experimental situations; auto-anti-idiotypic antibodies occur in certain autoimmune disorders. **autologous a.,** self-derived antibody; autoantibody. **bispecific a.,** antibody in which each of two antigen-binding sites is specific for separate antigenic determinants. It is an artificial antibody produced in the laboratory, formed by reassociating half molecules of two different antibody specificities to form a hybrid or bispecific antibody with antigen-binding sites of separate specificities. Called also *hybrid a.* **blocking a.,** any antibody that by combining with an antigen blocks another immunologic reaction with the antigen. In most patients, immunotherapy (hyposensitization or desensitization) for allergic disorders induces IgG blocking antibodies that can bind the allergen and prevent it from binding to cell-fixed IgE, triggering immediate hypersensitivity; it can thus induce partial immunologic tolerance. Blocking antibodies directed against tumor-specific antigens have been suggested as one mechanism allowing tumors to escape immune surveillance. Blocking antibodies can prevent agglutination in serologic tests (see *incomplete a.*) **cell-bound a., cell-fixed a.,** any antibody bound to a cell surface either by its antigen combining sites to cell-surface antigenic determinants or by other sites to specific cell-surface receptors (Fc receptors, IgE receptors). **cold a., cold-reactive a.,** antibody, usually IgM but occasionally IgG, that reacts less efficiently with antigen at 37° C than at lower temperatures. **complement-fixing a.,** antibody that activates complement when reacted with antigen; IgM and IgG (the usual complement-fixing antibodies) fix complement by the classic pathway, whereas IgA fixes complement by the alternative pathway. **complete a.,** antibody capable of agglutinating cells in physiologic saline solution. Called also *saline agglutinin.* Cf. *incomplete a.* **cross-reacting a.,** one that combines with an antigen other than the one that induced its production. **cytophilic a.,** cytotropic a. **cytotoxic a.,** any specific antibody directed against cellular antigens, which when bound to the antigen, activates the complement pathway or activates killer cells, resulting in cell lysis. **cytotropic a.,** antibody that binds to mast cells and basophils at specific receptors; subsequent binding of antigen to the cell-fixed antibody triggers release of mediators of immediate hypersensitivity. Such antibodies produced by the animal itself in response to antigenic challenge or transferred from another animal of the same species (*homocytotropic* or *reaginic antibodies* or *reagin*) are always of the IgE class. In some cases IgG, IgA, or IgM from one species (heterocytotropic antibodies) can sensitize tissues of another species; e.g., rabbit IgG can sensitize guinea pig skin for passive cutaneous anaphylaxis. **duck virus hepatitis yolk a.,** yolk antibody derived from chicken eggs, used for treatment of duck virus hepatitis. **Forssman a.,** heterophile antibody directed against the Forssman antigen. **heteroclitic a.,** antibody produced in response to immunization with one antigen but having a higher affinity for a second antigen that was not present during immunization. **heterocytotropic a.,** see *cytotropic a.* **heterogenetic a.,** heterophile a. **heterogenetic a., heterophile a.,** antibody directed against heterophile antigens. Heterophile sheep erythrocyte agglutinins appear in the serum of patients with infectious mononucleosis (see *Paul-Bunnell test* under *tests*). Called also *heterogenetic a.* **homocytotropic a.,** see *cytotropic a.* **hybrid a.,** bispecific a. **immune a.,** antibody induced by immunization or by transfusion incompatibility, in contrast to the natural antibodies. **incomplete a.,** 1. antibody that binds to erythrocytes or bacteria but does not produce agglutination; the nonagglutinating antibody is detectable with the antiglobulin (Coombs) test. For example, IgG anti-Rh antibodies do not agglutinate erythrocytes in physiologic saline whereas IgM antibodies do (the large IgM molecule can cross-link the erythrocytes at a wider separation so that there is less electrostatic repulsion due to the zeta potential). 2. a univalent antibody fragment, e.g., Fab fragment. **isophil a.,** antibody against red blood cell antigens produced in members of the species from which the red cells originated. **mitochondrial a's,** antimitochondrial a's. **monoclonal a's,** chemically and immunologically homogeneous antibodies produced by hybridomas, used as laboratory reagents in radioimmunoassays, ELISA, and immunofluorescence assays; also used experimentally in cancer immunotherapy. **natural a's,** antibodies present in the serum of normal individuals in the apparent absence of any contact with the specific antigen, probably induced by exposure to cross-reacting antigens. They may result from unknown exposure to naturally occurring antigens, e.g., food or bacterial flora. **neutralizing a.,** see *viral neutralization,* under *neutralization.* **P-K a's,** Prausnitz-Küstner a's. **polyclonal a.,** antibody produced by more than one clone of antibody-synthesizing plasma cells (B-lumphocytes); antibody that is not monoclonal, e.g., that produced by immunizing an animal. **Prausnitz-Küstner a's,** cytotropic IgE antibodies responsible for cutaneous anaphylaxis; see *Prausnitz-Küstner reaction,* under *reaction.* **protective a.,** antibody responsible for immunity to an infectious agent observed in passive immunity. **reaginic a.,** reagin. **Rh a's,** those directed against Rh antigen(s) of human erythrocytes. Not normally present, but may be produced when Rh-negative persons receive Rh-positive blood by transfusion or when an Rh-negative person is pregnant with an Rh-positive fetus. **saline a.,** complete a. **sensitizing a.,** a loosely used term, applied to antibodies that are attached to body cells and that "sensitize" the cells or render them susceptible to destruction by body defenses. **TSH-displacing a. (TDA),** TSH-binding inhibitory immunoglobulins. **warm a., warm-reactive a.,** antibody, usually IgG but occasionally IgM or IgA, that reacts more efficiently with antigen at 37° C than at lower temperatures.

antibrachium (an″tĭ-bra′ke-um) antebrachium.

antibromic (an″tĭ-bro′mik) [*anti-* + Gr. *brōmos* smell] deodorant.

anticachectic (an″tĭ-kah-kek′tik) 1. preventing or relieving cachexia. 2. an agent that prevents or relieves cachexia.

anticalculous (an″tĭ-kal′ku-lus) preventing or alleviating calculus.

anticarcinogen (an″tĭ-kar-sin′o-jen) an agent that counteracts the effect of a carcinogen.

anticarcinogenic (an″tĭ-kar-sin″o-jen′ik) inhibiting or preventing the development of carcinoma.

anticardium (an″tĭ-kar′de-um) [*anti-* + Gr. *kardia* heart] antecardium (epigastrium).

anticariogenic (an″tĭ-kār″e-o-jen′ik) suppressing the development of caries; anticarious.

anticarious (an″tĭ-ka′re-us) anticariogenic.

anticatalyst (an″tĭ-kat′ah-list) a substance that retards the action of a catalyzer by acting on the catalyzer itself.

anticatalyzer (an″tĭ-kat′ah-līz″er) anticatalyst.

anticathexis (an″tĭ-kah-thek′sis) [*anti-* + *cathexis*] in psychoanalysis, the energy required for the ego to maintain repression of unacceptable ideas and impulses.

anticathode (an″tĭ-kath′ōd) the part of a vacuum tube opposite the cathode; the target.

anticephalalgic (an″tĭ-sef-ah-lal′jik) curing or preventing headache.

anticheirotonus (an″tĭ-ki-rot′o-nus) [Gr. *anticheir* thumb + *tonos* tension] spasmodic flexion of the thumb.

antichlorotic (an″tĭ-klo-rot′ik) effective against chlorosis.

anticholelithogenic (an″tĭ-ko″le-lith″o-jen′ik) 1. serving to prevent the formation of gallstones. 2. an agent that so acts.

anticholesteremic (an″tĭ-ko-les″ter-e′mik) 1. promoting a reduction of cholesterol levels in the blood. 2. any agent that promotes a reduction of blood cholesterol levels, e.g., the sitosterols and clofibrate. Called also *anticholesterolemic.*

anticholesterolemic (an″tĭ-ko-les″tĕ-ro-le′mik) anticholesteremic.

anticholinergic (an″tĭ-ko″lin-er′jik) [*anti-* + *cholinergic*] 1. blocking the passage of impulses through the parasympathetic nerves. 2. an agent that blocks the parasympathetic nerves. Called also *parasympatholytic.* Cf. *antiadrenergic.*

anticholinesterase (an″tĭ-ko-lin-es′ter-ās) [*anti-* + *cholinesterase*] a drug that prevents the hydrolysis of acetylcholine by the enzyme acetylcholinesterase, thereby permitting high levels of acetylcholine to accumulate at reactive sites.

antichymosin (an″tĭ-ki′mo-sin) an antibody that prevents the action of rennin on milk.

anticipate (an-tis′ĭ-pāt) [*ante-* + L. *capere* to take] to occur or recur before the regular time; said of a disease or of symptoms. See *anticipation.*

anticipation (an-tis″ĭ-pa′shun) the apparent occurrence of a hereditary disease at a progressively earlier age in successive generations; now considered by most authorities to be an artifact arising from the ease of identification of succeeding cases or because cases of later onset are more likely to be fertile.

anticlinal (an″tĭ-kli′nal) [*anti-* + Gr. *klinein* to slope] sloping in opposite directions, as opposite sides of triangular structures.

anticnemion (an″tik-ne′me-on) [*anti-* + Gr. *knēmē* leg] the shin.

anticoagulant (an″tĭ-ko-ag′u-lant) 1. preventing blood clotting. 2. any substance that prevents blood clotting. Those administered for prophylaxis or treatment of thromboembolic disorders are heparin, which inactivates thrombin and several other clotting factors and which must be administered parenterally, and the oral anticoagulants (warfarin, dicumarol, and congeners), which inhibit the hepatic synthesis of vitamin K–dependent clotting factors. Anticoagulant solutions used for the preservation of stored whole blood and blood fractions are acid citrate dextrose (ACD), citrate phosphate dextrose (CPD), citrate phosphate dextrose-adenine (cPDA-1), and heparin. Anticoagulants used to prevent clotting of blood specimens for laboratory analysis are heparin and several substances that make calcium ions unavailable to the clotting process, including EDTA (ethylenediaminetetraacetic acid), citrate, oxalate, and fluoride. **circulating a.,** a substance present in the blood which inhibits normal blood clotting and thus may cause a hemorrhagic syndrome; it may be directed against a specific coagulation factor and may accompany various hematologic and nonhematologic diseases.

anticoagulative (an″tĭ-ko-ag′u-la″tiv) preventing or opposing coagulation.

anticoagulin (an″tĭ-ko-ag′u-lin) a substance that suppresses, delays, or nullifies the coagulation of blood.

anticodon (an″tĭ-ko′don) a triplet of nucleotides in transfer RNA that is complementary to the codon in messenger RNA which specifies the amino acid.

anticollagenase (an″tĭ-ko-laj′ĭ-nās) an antienzyme that neutralizes the activity of collagenase.

anticomplement (an″tĭ-kom′ple-ment) a substance that opposes or counteracts the action of a complement.

anticomplementary (an″tĭ-kom″plĕ-men′ta-re) capable of reducing or destroying the power of a complement.

anticonceptive (an″tĭ-kon-sep′tiv) contraceptive.

anticoncipiens (an″tĭ-kon-sip′e-enz) a contraceptive agent.

anticonvulsant (an″tĭ-kon-vul′sant) 1. preventing or relieving convulsions. 2. an agent that prevents or relieves convulsions.

anticonvulsive (an″tĭ-kon-vul′siv) anticonvulsant.

anticrotin (an″tĭ-kro′tin) the antitoxin of crotin.

anticurare (an″tĭ-koo-rah′re) an agent that counteracts the action of curare on skeletal muscle.

anticus (an-ti′kus) [L.] anterior.

anticytolysin (an″tĭ-si-tol′ĭ-sin) a substance opposing the action of cytolysin.

anticytotoxin (an″tĭ-si″to-tok′sin) a substance that opposes the action of a cytotoxin.

anti-D antibody against the "D" or "Rh₀" Rh blood group antigen; see *Rh₀(D) immune globulin* under *globulin.*

antidepressant (an″tĭ-de-pres′sant) 1. preventing or relieving depression. 2. an agent that stimulates the mood of a depressed patient, including tricyclic antidepressants and monoamine oxidase inhibitors. **tricyclic a's,** a group of antidepressant drugs that contain three fused rings in their chemical structure and that potentiate the action of catecholamines; they include imipramine, amitriptyline, nortriptyline, protriptyline, desipramine, and doxepin.

antidiabetic (an″tĭ-di″ah-bet′ik) 1. preventing or alleviating diabetes. 2. an agent that prevents or alleviates diabetes.

antidiabetogenic (an″tĭ-di-ah-be″to-jen′ik) 1. preventing the development of diabetes. 2. an agent that prevents the development of diabetes.

antidiarrheal (an″tĭ-di″ah-re′al) 1. counteracting diarrhea. 2. an agent that is effective in combating diarrhea.

antidiarrheic (an″tĭ-di″ah-re′ik) antidiarrheal.

antidinic (an″tĭ-din′ik) [*anti-* + Gr. *dinos* whirl] effective against vertigo.

antidipticum (an″tĭ-dip′te-kum) an agent that lessens thirst.

antidiuresis (an″tĭ-di″u-re′sis) suppression of urinary secretion.

antidiuretic (an″tĭ-di″u-ret′ik) 1. suppressing the rate of urine formation. 2. an agent that suppresses urine formation.

antidotal (an″tĭ-do′tal) serving as an antidote.

antidote (an′tĭ-dōt) [L. *antidotum*, from Gr. *anti* against + *didonai* to give] a remedy for counteracting a poison. **a. against arsenic**, dimercaprol; hydrated oxide of iron with magnesia was once used. **chemical a.,** an antidote that reacts chemically with a poison to form a harmless compound. **Hall a.,** a solution of 7.35 parts potassium iodide and 4 parts quinine hydrochloride in 480 parts water; once used as an antidote for mercuric chloride poisoning. **mechanical a.,** an antidote that prevents the absorption of a poison. **physiologic a.,** an antidote that counteracts the effects of a poison by producing opposing physiologic effects. **"universal" a.,** a mixture of 2 parts activated charcoal, 1 part magnesium oxide, and 1 part tannic acid; given when the exact poison is not known. There is no true "universal" antidote and this mixture is no longer recommended by most authorities; activated charcoal alone is preferred.

antidotic (an″tĭ-dot′ik) antidotal.

antidromic (an″tĭ-drom′ik) [Gr. *antidromein* to run in a contrary direction] conducting impulses in a direction opposite to the normal; said of neurons in the posterior roots of the spinal cord. Evidence suggests, however, that this phenomenon results from ephaptic transmission rather than backward transmission. Cf. *orthodromic*.

antidysenteric (an″tĭ-dis″en-ter′ik) 1. preventing, alleviating, or curing dysentery. 2. an agent that prevents, alleviates, or cures dysentery.

antidysentericum (an″tĭ-dis″en-ter′e-kum) a preparation of myrobalan, pelletierin, extract of rose, extract of pomegranate, and gum arabic.

antiedematous (an″tĭ-e-dem′ah-tus) antiedemic.

antiedemic (an″tĭ-e-dem′ik) 1. preventing or alleviating edema. 2. an agent that prevents or alleviates edema.

antiemetic (an″tĭ-e-met′ik) [*anti-* + Gr. *emetikos* inclined to vomit] 1. preventing or alleviating nausea and vomiting. 2. an agent that prevents or alleviates nausea and vomiting. See also *antinauseant*.

antienzyme (an″tĭ-en′zīm) [*anti-* + *enzyme*] an agent that prevents or retards the action of an enzyme.

antiepileptic (an″tĭ-ep″ĕ-lep′tik) 1. combating epilepsy. 2. an agent that combats epilepsy.

antiepithelial (an″tĭ-ep″ĕ-the′le-al) destructive to epithelial cells.

antierotica (an″tĭ-e-rot′e-kah) drugs which have an anaphrodisiac effect.

antiesterase (an″tĭ-es′ter-ās) an agent that inhibits or counteracts the activity of ester-hydrolyzing enzymes.

antiestrogen (an″te-es′-tro-jen) 1. blocking the action of estrogens. 2. an agent that so acts.

antiestrogenic (an″tĭ-es″tro-jen′ik) counteracting or suppressing estrogenic activity.

antifebrile (an″tĭ-feb′ril) antipyretic.

antifebrin (an″tĭ-feb′rin) acetanilid.

antifertilizin (an″tĭ-fer′tĭ-li″zin) a substance with which fertilizin reacts in agglutinating spermatozoa of certain marine invertebrates.

antifibrillatory (an″tĭ-fib′rĭ-lah-tor″e) 1. preventing or stopping fibrillation of the heart. 2. an agent that prevents or stops fibrillation of the heart.

antifibrinolysin (an″tĭ-fi″brĭ-nol′ĭ-sin) an inhibitor of fibrinolysin.

antifibrinolytic (an″tĭ-fi″brĭ-no-lit′ik) inhibiting fibrinolysis.

antifilarial (an″tĭ-fĭ-la′re-al) 1. effective against filaria. 2. an agent that is effective against filaria.

antiflatulent (an″tĭ-flat′u-lent) 1. relieving or preventing flatulence. 2. an agent that relieves or prevents flatulence.

antiflux (an′tĭ-fluks) a substance that prevents the attachment of solder.

antifol (an′tĭ-fōl) folic acid antagonist.

antifolate (an″tĭ-fo′lāt) folic acid antagonist.

antifungal (an″tĭ-fung′gal) 1. destructive to fungi, or suppressing their reproduction or growth; effective against fungal infections. 2. an agent that is destructive to fungi, suppresses the growth or reproduction of fungi, or is effective against fungal infections.

antigalactic (an″tĭ-gah-lak′tik) [*anti-* + Gr. *gala* milk] 1. diminishing the secretion of milk. 2. an agent that tends to suppress milk secretion.

antigelatinase (an″tĭ-jeh-lat′ĭ-nās) a substance in the serum of animals infected with bacteria which prevents the digestion of gelatin.

antigen (an′tĭ-jen) [*antibody* + Gr. *gennan* to produce] any substance which is capable, under appropriate conditions, of inducing a specific immune response and of reacting with the products of that response, that is, with specific antibody or specifically sensitized T-lymphocytes, or both. Antigens may be soluble substances, such as toxins and foreign proteins, or particulate, such as bacteria and tissue cells; however, only the portion of the protein or polysaccharide molecule known as the antigenic determinant (q.v.) combines with antibody or a specific receptor on a lymphocyte. Abbreviated Ag. **acetone-insoluble a.,** (*obs.*) the alcohol-soluble, acetone-insoluble extract of beef heart used in nontreponemal antigen serologic tests for syphilis; the antigenic component is now known to be cardiolipin. **allogeneic a.,** one occurring in some but not all individuals of the same species, e.g., histocompatibility antigens and human blood group antigens; isoantigen. **Am a's,** see under *allotype*. **Au a., Australia a.,** hepatitis B surface a. **beef heart a.,** (*obs.*) alcoholic extract of beef heart used in nontreponemal antigen serologic tests for syphilis; the antigenic component is now known to be cardiolipin. **blood-group a's,** erythrocyte surface antigens whose antigenic differences determine blood groups. See *blood group* under *B*. **Boivin a.,** O antigen of gram-negative bacteria. **capsular a.,** K a. **carcinoembryonic a. (CEA),** a glycoprotein, mol. wt. 200,000, secreted into the glycocalyx coating the luminal surface of gastrointestinal epithelia. Originally thought to be a specific antigen of the fetal digestive tract and adenocarcinoma of the colon, CEA is now known to occur normally in feces and pancreaticobiliary secretions and to appear in the plasma in a diverse group of neoplastic and non-neoplastic conditions including cancers of the colon, pancreas, stomach, lung, and breast, alcoholic cirrhosis and pancreatitis, inflammatory bowel disease, rectal polyps, and cigarette smoking. The primary use of CEA is in monitoring response to treatment of colorectal cancer. **cholesterinized a.,** (*obs.*) beef heart antigen to which cholesterol has been added. **class I a's,** major histocompatibility antigens found on virtually every cell, human erythrocytes being the only notable exception; they are found on molecules consisting of two noncovalently bound chains. One, a 44,000-dalton polymorphic glycoprotein partially embedded in the cell membrane, is determined by an MHC gene (HLA-A, -B, or -C in humans); the other, β_2-microglobulin, a 12,000-dalton nonpolymorphic protein, is determined by a non-MHC gene. Class I antigens are the classic histocompatibility antigens recognized during graft rejection and are also the antigens involved in MHC restriction (q.v.). **class II a's,** major histocompatibility antigens found only on immunocompetent cells, primarily B lymphocytes and macrophages; they are found on molecules consisting of two noncovalently bound chains, the 34,000-dalton α chain and 29,000-dalton β chain, both glycoproteins partially embedded in the cell membrane and both determined by MHC genes. The human HLA-D, -DR, -DQ, -DT, -MB, -MT, and -Te loci are all associated with antigenic determinants on class II antigen molecules. **class III a's,** a term used to refer to nonhistocompatibility antigens mapping in the major histocompatibility complex, e.g., the complement components C2, C4, and factor B. **common a.,** an antigenic determinant group (epitope) that is present in two or more different antigen molecules and frequently leads to cross-reactions among them. **common acute lymphoblastic leukemia a. (CALLA),** a tumor-associated antigen occurring on lymphoblasts in about 80 per cent of patients with acute lymphoblastic leukemia (ALL) and also in 40-50 per cent of patients with blastic phase chronic myelogenous leukemia (CML). It does not occur on normal lymphoid cells except during fetal development. **common leukocyte a's,** a group of glycoproteins, antigenically similar but of different molecular weights, found on B cells, T cells, thymocytes, and leukopoietic cells. **complete a.,** an antigen which both stimulates the immune response and reacts with the products (e.g., antibody) of that response. **conjugated a.,** antigen produced by coupling a hapten to a protein carrier molecule through covalent bonds; when it induces immunization, the resultant immune response is directed against both the hapten and the carrier. **cross-reacting a.,** 1. one that combines with antibody produced in response to a different but related antigen, owing to similarity of antigenic determinants. 2. identical antigens in two bacterial strains, so that antibody produced against one strain will react with the other. **D a.,** a red cell antigen of the Rh blood group system, important in the development of isoimmunization in Rh-negative persons exposed to the blood of Rh-positive persons. **delta a.,** a 32- to 37-nm RNA particle coated with hepatitis B surface antigen. **E a.,** a red cell antigen of the Rh blood group system. **extractable nuclear a's (ENA),** protein antigens, not containing DNA, that are extractable from cell nuclei in phosphate-buffered saline; anti-ENA antibodies are a component of the antinuclear antibodies occurring in systemic lupus erythematosus and other connective tissue diseases. **febrile a's,** a standard panel of serologic antigens (*Salmonella, Proteus, Francisella tularensis,* and *Brucella*) used in screening patients with unexplained fever. **flagellar a.,** H antigen. **Forssman a.,** a heterogenetic antigen inducing the production of antisheep hemolysin, occurring in various unrelated animals, mainly in the organs but not in the erythrocytes (guinea pig, horse), but sometimes only in the erythrocytes (sheep), and occasionally in both (chicken). In the original and strict sense, the antigen is typified by that found in the guinea pig kidney and characterized by heat stability and solubility in alcohol; the antigenic determinant is polysaccharide in nature. Its antibody is absorbed by tissues containing the antigen, contains no lysin for bovine cells and little or no agglutinin for sheep cells. The term is also used loosely to refer to any antigen producing sheep hemolysin, but antibodies to it are not identical, as they are in the case of the true Forssman (or F) antigen. **Frei a.,** antigen for the Frei test, material prepared from lymphogranuloma venereum organisms grown in chick embryo yolk sacs. **Gm a's,** see under *allotype.* **H a.,** 1. [Ger. *Hauch,* breath (because motile bacteria form a spreading film around colonies resembling that produced by breathing on glass)] bacterial flagellar antigens important in the serological classification of enteric bacilli, especially *Salmonella.* Cf. *O a.* 2. see under *substance.* **H-2 a's,** the major histocompatibility antigens in mice. **hepatitis a., hepatitis-associated a. (HAA),** hepatitis B surface a. **hepatitis B core a. (HBcAg),** a core protein antigen of the hepatitis B virus present inside complete virions (Dane particles) and in free core particles in the nuclei of infected cells; the antigen is not present in the blood of infected individuals, but anti-HBc antibodies appear during the acute infection; they do not protect against reinfection. **hepatitis B e a. (HBeAg),** a core protein antigen of hepatitis B virus present in the blood in some infected individuals. Anti-HBe antibodies appear transiently during convalescence; they do not protect against reinfection. **hepatitis B surface a. (HBsAg),** a coat protein antigen of the hepatitis B virus present on complete virions (Dane particles) and smaller spherical and filamentous particles circulating in the blood of individuals with active or chronic infections. Anti-HBs antibodies appear in the blood in late convalescence and are protective against reinfection. Originally called *Australia (Au) antigen* because it was first found in an Australian aborigine; also formerly called *hepatitis-associated a. (HAA)* and *serum-hepatitis (SH)* a. See *hepatitis B vaccine* under *vaccine.* **heterogeneic a.,** xenogeneic a. **heterogenetic a.,** heterophile a. **heterologous a.,** an antigen that reacts with an antibody that is not the one (the homologous antigen) that induced its formation. **heterophil a., heterophile a.,** any of a group of cross-reacting antigens occurring in several species and having a species distribution that does not correspond to phylogenetic relationships, e.g., Forssman antigen. Called also *heterogenetic a.* **histocompatibility a's,** systems of allelic alloantigens that can stimulate an immune response that leads to transplant rejection when the donor and recipient are mismatched. Called also *transplantation antigens.* See *HLA*

a's. **histocompatibility a's, major,** those in the major histocompatibility complex; HLA antigens in humans and H-2 antigens in mice. **histocompatibility a's, minor,** systems of allelic alloantigens that can cause transplant rejection, but with a long delay (up to 100 days); about 15-30 such systems have been found in mice. **HLA a's,** (*Human Leukocyte Antigens*), histocompatibility antigens governed by genes of the HLA complex (the human major histocompatibility complex), a region on the short arm of chromosome 6 containing several genetic loci, each having multiple alleles. Loci are designated by letters, HLA-A, -B, -C, -DP, -DQ, -DR (there are at least three subloci in the D region), -MB, -MT, and -Te, and alleles at each locus by numbers, e.g., HLA-A1, provisional designations being indicated by "w" (for "workshop"), e.g., HLA-DRw10. The A, B, C, DR, MB, MT, and Te antigens are defined and typed by serologic reactions. The D antigens are defined and typed by one-way mixed lymphocyte culture (MLC) using panels of HLA-D-homozygous typing cells. The SB (for "secondary B cell") antigens are defined and typed by primed lymphocyte typing. See *class I, class II,* and *class III a's.* **homologous a.,** 1. the antigen that induces the formation of an antibody. 2. isoantigen. **H-Y a.,** a minor histocompatibility antigen present in all tissues of normal males and coded for by a structural gene on the short arm of the Y chromosome; it is thought to promote the differentiation of indifferent gonads into testes, thus determining male sex. **Ia a.** [*I* region–associated], class II histocompatibility antigens found on the surface of mouse B cells, macrophages, and accessory cells. They are also found on granulocyte precursors but disappear during maturation. Ia antigens are governed by the Ia genes of the H-2 complex (q.v.). **Inv group a.,** see *Km allotypes,* under *allotype.* **isogeneic a.,** isoantigen. **isophile a.,** isoantigen. **K a.,** [Ger. *Kapsel* capsule] a bacterial capsular antigen, a surface antigen external to the cell wall, such as the *Salmonella* Vi antigens and pneumococcal capsular antigens. **Km a's,** see under *allotype.* **Kveim a.,** a saline suspension of human sarcoid tissue prepared from the spleen or lymph nodes of a patient with active sarcoidosis. **LD a's,** lymphocyte-defined a's. **Ly a's, Lyt a's,** cell-surface markers differentiating subpopulations of murine T lymphocytes: Ly 1, Ly 2, and Ly 3. Most thymocytes and undifferentiated peripheral T cells are Ly $1^+2^+3^+$; helper cells are Ly $1^+2^-3^-$; cytotoxic T cells and suppressor cells are Ly $1^-2^+3^+$. **Lyb a's,** cell-surface markers on murine B lymphocytes: Lyb 1,2,3,4, and 5. Lyb 1,2, and 4 are found on all B cells, Lyb 3 and 5 on a subset of mature B cells. **lymphocyte-defined (LD) a's,** major histocompatibility antigens defined and typed by the mixed lymphocyte reaction (MLR), e.g., HLA-D antigens. **lymphogranuloma venereum a.** [USP], official name for Frei antigen. **M a.,** a type-specific antigen that appears to be located primarily in the cell wall and is associated with virulence of *Streptococcus pyogenes.* **Mitsuda a.,** lepromin. **mumps skin test a.,** [USP], a preparation of killed mumps virus, used in the mumps skin test (q.v.). **nuclear a's,** the components of cell nuclei with which antinuclear antibodies (see under *antibody*) react. **O a.** [Ger. *ohne Hauch* without breath], the lipopolysaccharide-protein somatic antigens of gram-negative bacteria, important in the serological classification of enteric bacilli. See *lipopolysaccharide.* Cf. *H a.* **oncofetal a.,** an antigenic gene product that is expressed during fetal development, partially or completely repressed in adult tissues, and derepressed in some tissues that have undergone neoplastic transformation; oncofetal antigens, e.g., alpha-fetoprotein, carcinoembryonic antigen, and pancreatic oncofetal antigen, are thus useful tumor markers. **organ-specific a.,** any antigen that occurs exclusively in a particular organ and serves to distinguish it from other organs. Two types of organ specificity have been proposed: (1) first-order or tissue specificity is attributed to the presence of an antigen characteristic of a particular organ in a single species; (2) second-order organ specificity is attributed to an antigen characteristic of the same organ in many, even unrelated species. Called also *tissue-specific a.* **Oz a.,** an antigenic marker on the lambda chain of human immunoglobulins, equivalent to Km allotypes on kappa light chains. Together with Kern markers, they delineate three types of human lambda chain. **pancreatic oncofetal a. (POA),** a glycoprotein, mol. wt. 800,000, found in fetal and neoplastic pancreatic tissue but not in that of normal adults; it also occurs at lower levels in the serum of patients with cancer at other sites and some normal adults. **partial a.,** hapten. **pollen a.,** see *pollen allergen,* under *allergen.* **Pr a.,** see *cold agglutinin syndrome* under *syndrome.* **private a's,** 1. antigens of low-frequency blood groups, so called because they occur in only a few kindreds. 2. HLA antigens found only on the gene product of a single allele. 3. a tumor antigen expressed only on a particular type of chemically induced tumor. Cf. *public a's.* **public a's,** 1. antigens of high-frequency blood groups, so called because they occur in the general population at high frequencies. 2. HLA antigens occurring on the products of several allelic genes. Cf. *private a's.* **recall a.,** an antigen to which an individual has previously been sensitized and which is subsequently administered as a challenging dose to elicit a hypersensitivity reaction. **SD a's,** serologically defined a's. **self-a.,** autoantigen. **sequestered a's,** the cellular constituents of tissue (e.g., lens of the eye) sequestered anatomically from the lymphoreticular system during embryonic development and thus thought not to be recognized as "self." Should such tissue be exposed to the lymphoreticular system during adult life, an autoimmune response would be elicited. **sero-defined (SD) a's, serologically defined (SD) a's,** major histocompatibility antigens defined by serologic methods, e.g., HLA-A, HLA-B, and HLA-C antigens. **serum hepatitis a., SH a.,** hepatitis B surface a. **shock a.,** an antigen capable of eliciting anaphylactic shock in a sensitized animal. **Sm a.,** [after a patient, Smith] an uncharacterized nuclear antigen that is a nonhistone acidic protein not complexed with DNA or RNA; anti-Sm antibodies make up a part of the antinuclear antibodies in about one-third of patients with systemic lupus erythematosus, but do not occur in other connective tissue diseases, except mixed connective tissue disease. **somatic a's,** antigens, usually cell surface antigens, of the body of a bacterial cell, in contrast to flagellar or capsular antigens. See *O a.* **species-specific a's,** antigens that are restricted to a single species but occur in all members of that species. **SS-A a.,** see *Sjögren's syndrome* under *syndrome.* **SS-B a.,** see *Sjögren's syndrome* under *syndrome.* **T a.,** 1. tumor antigen; any of several antigens, coded for by the viral genome, associated with transformation of infected cells by certain DNA tumor viruses, e.g., SV 40. 2. any of a series, T1 through T10, of human T lymphocyte cell-surface markers that identify developmental stages and functional subsets (see table at *lymphocyte*). 3. an antigen present on human erythrocytes that is exposed by treatment with neuraminidase or contact with certain bacteria. See *T agglutinin* under *agglutinin.* **Tac a.,** the receptor for interleukin 2. **T-dependent a.,** one that requires the presence of helper T cells to stimulate antibody production by B cells; most antigens are T-dependent. **Thy 1 a., theta (θ) a.,** a cell-surface marker occurring on all murine T lymphocytes. **T-independent a.,** an antigen that can trigger B cells to produce antibodies without the participation of T cells; most are polymers with a simple repeating pattern and are B cell mitogens; only IgM is produced and few memory cells are formed. **tissue-specific a.,** organ-specific a. **TL a.** (Thymus Leukemia), a differentiation antigen, first discovered on thymic leukemia cells, that occurs on thymocytes but not peripheral T cells in some strains of mice. **transplantation a's,** histocompatibility a's. **tumor-associated a.,** any antigen associated with a tumor, including tumor-specific antigens, tissue-specific antigens, oncofetal antigens, and virus-related antigens. **tumor-specific a. (TSA),** any cell-surface antigen of a tumor that does not occur on normal cells of the same origin. **tumor-specific transplantation a. (TSTA),** any of the cell surface histocompatibility antigens of any given tumor that evoke a specific immune response on transplantation to a syngeneic host. **VDRL a.,** an alcohol solution containing 0.03 per cent cardiolipin, 0.99 per cent cholesterol, and enough lecithin to produce standard reactivity. See VDRL test, under *test.* **Vi a.,** a K antigen of *Salmonella typhi* originally thought to be responsible for virulence. **xenogeneic a.,** an antigen common to members of one species but not to members of other species; called also *heterogeneic a.*

antigenemia (an″tĭ-je-ne″me-ah) [*antigen* + *-emia*] the presence of antigen (e.g., hepatitis B antigen) in the blood.

antigenemic (an″tĭ-jen-e′mik) exhibiting antigenemia.

antigenic (an-tĭ-jen′ik) having the properties of an antigen.

antigenicity (an″tĭ-jĕ-nis′ĭ-te) the property of being able

to induce a specific immune response or the degree to which a substance is able to stimulate an immune response. Called also *immunogenicity.*

antiglobulin (an″tĭ-glob′u-lin) an antibody directed against gamma globulin, as used in the Coombs' test.

antiglyoxalase (an″tĭ-gli-ok′sah-lās) a pancreatic substance that inhibits the action of glyoxalase.

antigoitrogenic (an″tĭ-goi″tro-jen′ik) [*anti-* + *goiter* + Gr. *gennan* to produce] preventing or inhibiting the development of goiter.

antigonadotropic (an″tĭ-go″nad-o-tro′pik) inhibiting the gonadotropic hormones.

antigrowth (an′tĭ-grōth) counteracting the growth hormone.

antihallucinatory (an″tĭ-hah-lu′sĭ-nah-to″re) counteracting hallucinogenesis; suppressing hallucinations.

anti-HBc antibody to hepatitis B core antigen (HB$_c$Ag).

anti-HBs antibody to hepatitis B surface antigen (HB$_s$Ag).

antihelix (an″tĭ-he′liks) anthelix.

antihelmintic (an″tĭ-hel-min′tik) anthelmintic.

antihemagglutinin (an″tĭ-hem-ah-gloo′tĭ-nin) a substance whose action is antagonistic to hemagglutinin.

antihemolysin (an″tĭ-he-mol′ĭ-sin) any agent that opposes the action of a hemolysin.

antihemolytic (an″tĭ-he″mo-lit′ik) preventing hemolysis.

antihemophilic (an″tĭ-he″mo-fil′ik) see *coagulation Factor VIII,* under *factor.*

antihemorrhagic (an″tĭ-hem″o-raj′ik) 1. stopping hemorrhage. 2. an agent that prevents or stops hemorrhage.

antiheterolysin (an″tĭ-het″er-ol′ĭ-sin) a substance that counteracts heterolysin.

antihistamine (an″tĭ-his′tah-mēn) a drug that counteracts the action of histamine. The antihistamines are of two types. The conventional ones, as those used in allergies, block the H$_1$ histamine receptors, whereas the others block the H$_2$ receptors. See *histamine.* Called also *antihistaminic.*

antihistaminic (an″tĭ-his-tah-min′ik) 1. counteracting the effect of histamine. 2. antihistamine.

antihormone (an″tĭ-hor′mōn) any substance that opposes the action of a hormone.

antihyaluronidase (an″tĭ-hi-ah-lu-ron′ĭ-dās) an antienzyme that opposes the action of hyaluronidase.

antihypercholesterolemic (an″tĭ-hi″per-ko-les″ter-ol-e′mik) effective in decreasing or preventing an excessively high level of cholesterol in the blood. By extension, sometimes used to designate an agent that exerts such an effect.

antihyperglycemic (an″tĭ-hi″per-gli-se′mik) 1. counteracting high levels of glucose in the blood. 2. an agent that counteracts high levels of glucose in the blood.

antihyperlipoproteinemic (an″tĭ-hi″per-lip″o-pro″te-in-e′mik) 1. promoting a reduction of lipoprotein levels in the blood. 2. an agent that so acts.

antihypertensive (an″tĭ-hi″per-ten′siv) 1. counteracting high blood pressure. 2. an agent that reduces high blood pressure.

antihypnotic (an″tĭ-hip-not′ik) 1. preventing or hindering sleep. 2. an agent that prevents or hinders sleep.

antihypotensive (an″tĭ-hi″po-ten′siv) 1. counteracting low blood pressure. 2. an agent that so acts.

antihysteric (an″tĭ-his-ter′ik) 1. preventing or relieving hysteria. 2. an agent that counteracts hysteria.

anti-icteric (an″tĭ-ik-ter′ik) relieving icterus or jaundice.

anti-idiotype (an″tĭ-id′e-o-tīp) an antibody directed against an idiotypic determinant of another antibody. See *idiotype–anti-idiotype network* under *network.*

anti-infective (an″tĭ-in-fek′tiv) 1. capable of killing infectious agents or of preventing them from spreading and causing infection. 2. an agent that so acts.

anti-inflammatory (an″tĭ-in-flam′ah-to″re) 1. counteracting or suppressing inflammation. 2. an agent that counteracts or suppresses the inflammatory process.

anti-insulin (an″tĭ-in′su-lin) a substance that counteracts the action of insulin.

anti-isolysin (an″tĭ-i-sol′ĭ-sin) a substance that counteracts an isolysin.

antikenotoxin (an″tĭ-ke″no-tok′sin) a substance that inhibits the action of kenotoxin.

antiketogen (an″tĭ-ke′to-jen) a substance that inhibits the formation of ketone bodies.

antiketogenesis (an″tĭ-ke″to-jen′ĕ-sis) inhibition of the formation of ketone bodies.

antiketogenetic (an″tĭ-ke″to-jĕ-net′ik) antiketogenic.

antiketogenic (an″tĭ-ke″to-jen′ik) preventing or inhibiting the formation of ketone bodies.

antiketoplastic (an″tĭ-ke″to-plas′tik) antiketogenic.

antikinase (an″tĭ-ki′nās) an antibody thought to inhibit the action of kinase.

antikinesis (an″tĭ-ki-ne′sis) [anti- + Gr. kinēsis movement] the tendency of organisms to resist and lean in an opposite direction to a dragging rotary force, e.g., on a slowly revolving plane (Dubois, 1898).

antileishmanial (an″tĭ-lesh-ma′ne-al) 1. effective against leishmania. 2. an agent that is effective against leishmania.

antileprotic (an″tĭ-lep-rot′ik) 1. therapeutically effective against leprosy. 2. an agent that is therapeutically effective against leprosy.

antileukocidin (an″tĭ-lu-ko′si-din) a substance that counteracts leukocidin; called also antileukotoxin.

antileukocytic (an″tĭ-lu″ko-sit′ik) destructive to white blood corpuscles (leukocytes).

antileukoprotease (an″tĭ-lu″ko-pro′te-ās) an antienzyme of the blood plasma that inhibits the digestion of protein by leukoprotease.

antileukotoxin (an″tĭ-lu″ko-tok′sin) antileukocidin.

antilewisite (an′tĭ-lu′ĭ-sīt) dimercaprol; also called British antilewisite, or BAL.

antilipemic (an″tĭ-li-pe′mik) 1. counteracting high levels of lipids in the blood. 2. an agent that counteracts high levels of lipids in the blood.

antilipotropic (an″tĭ-lip″o-trop′ik) interfering with the mobilization of fat in the liver.

antilipotropism (an″tĭ-lip-ot′ro-pizm) interference with the mobilization of fat in the liver.

Antilirium (an″tĭ-lir′e-um) trademark for a preparation of physostigmine salicylate.

antilithic (an″tĭ-lith′ik) [anti- + Gr. lithos stone] 1. preventing the formation of stone or calculus. 2. an agent that prevents the formation of stone or calculus.

antilysin (an″tĭ-li′sin) [anti- + lysin] a substance that opposes the action of a lysin.

antilysis (an″tĭ-li′sis) the inhibition or suppression of lysis.

antilytic (an″tĭ-lit′ik) pertaining to antilysis; inhibiting or suppressing lysis.

antimalarial (an″tĭ-mah-la′re-al) 1. therapeutically effective against malaria. 2. an agent that is therapeutically effective against malaria. Called also antipaludian.

antimephitic (an″tĭ-mĕ-fit′ik) preventing or neutralizing mephitic substances.

antimere (an′tĭ-mēr) [anti- + Gr. meros a part] one of the opposite corresponding parts of an organism which are symmetrical with respect to the longitudinal axis of its body; cf. metamere.

antimeristem (an″tĭ-me-ris′tem) a preparation of a fungus, Mucor racemus (var. malignus), isolated from malignant tumors of animals; a supposed antitoxin used against the microorganisms that caused the tumors.

antimesenteric (an″tĭ-mes′en-ter″ik) designating that part of the intestine which is opposite to the site of attachment of the mesentery.

antimetabolite (an″tĭ-mĕ-tab′o-līt) a substance bearing a close structural resemblance to one required for normal physiological functioning, and exerting its effect by interfering with the utilization of the essential metabolite. For various ways in which antimetabolites inhibit metabolic processes, see under inhibition.

antimethemoglobinemic (an″tĭ-met-he″mo-glo″bĭ-ne′mik) 1. effective in reducing the production of methemoglobin; effective in the treatment of methemoglobinemia. 2. an agent that produces such effects.

antimetropia (an″tĭ-mĕ-tro′pe-ah) [anti- + metr- + -opia]

difference in the refractive error of the two eyes, e.g., hyperopia in one eye with myopia in the other.

antimiasmatic (an″tĭ-mi″az-mat′ik) [anti- + Gr. miasma pollution] effective against noxious emanations or exhalations.

antimicrobial (an″tĭ-mi-kro′be-al) 1. killing microorganisms, or suppressing their multiplication or growth. 2. an agent that kills microorganisms or suppresses their multiplication or growth.

antimicrobic (an″tĭ-mi-kro′bik) (obs.) antimicrobial.

antimineralocorticoid (an″tĭ-min″er-al-o-kor′tĭ-koid) a substance that suppresses the secretion or opposes the action of mineralocorticoids.

Antiminth (an′tĭ-minth) trademark for a preparation of pyrantel pamoate.

antimitotic (an″tĭ-mi-tot′ik) inhibiting or preventing mitosis.

antimongoloid (an″tĭ-mon′go-loid) denoting a feature opposite to one characteristic of mongolism, as antimongoloid slant of the palpebral fissures.

antimongolism (an″te-mon′go-lizm) a term applied to the syndromes associated with group chromosome 21 deletions or chromosome 21 monosomy, characterized by antimongoloid obliquity of the palpebral fissures, hypertonia, high-arched palate, micrognathia, and microcephaly, and by mental and growth retardation.

antimonial (an″tĭ-mo′ne-al) pertaining to or containing antimony.

antimonic (an″tĭ-mon′ik) containing antimony in its pentad valency. **a. acid** antimony pentoxide.

antimonid (an″tĭ-mo′nĭd) any binary compound of antimony.

antimonious (an″tĭ-mo′ne-us) containing antimony in its triad valency.

antimonium (an″tĭ-mo′ne-um), gen. antimo′nii [L.] antimony.

antimony (an′tĭ-mo″ne) [L. antimonium or stibium] a crystalline metallic element with a bluish luster, symbol Sb, atomic number 51, atomic weight 121.75, forming various medicinal and poisonous salts. **a. chloride**, a. trichloride. **a. lithium thiomalate**, a compound, $Li_6C_{12}H_9$-$O_{12}SbS_3 \cdot 9H_2O$, which has been used for the same purposes as antimony potassium tartrate, especially in the treatment of schistosomiasis; administered intramuscularly. Called also anthiolimine. **a. pentoxide**, a white or yellowish powder, Sb_2O_5, used in preparation of antimony compounds; called also antimonic acid. **a. potassium tartrate** [USP], a trivalent antimony compound; used as an antischistosomal, especially for treatment of Schistosoma japonicum infections. The mechanism of action is inhibition of phosphofructokinase; the inhibition is greater in the schistosome than in the mammalian host. It was formerly used in other tropical diseases and as a nauseant emetic. Called also tartar emetic. **a. sodium dimercaptosuccinate**, stibocaptate. **a. sodium gluconate**, 1. a pentavalent antimony compound, $C_6H_9Na_2O_9Sb$, used as an antileishmanial, administered intravenously or intramuscularly. 2. a trivalent antimony compound, $C_6H_8NaO_7Sb$, used as an antischistosomal, administered intravenously. Called also sodium stibogluconate, stibogluconate sodium, and sodium antimony gluconate. **a. sodium tartrate**, a trivalent antimony compound, $C_4H_4NaO_7Sb$, having the same actions and uses as the potassium tartrate but more water-soluble and less irritant when injected. Called also Plimmer's a. and sodium antimonyltartrate. **a. sodium thioglycollate**, a trivalent antimony compound, $C_4H_4NaO_4S_2Sb$, which has been used as an antileishmanial and antischistosomal. Called also sodium antimonylthioglycollate. **tartrated a.**, a. potassium tartrate. **a. thioglycollamide**, an organic antimony compound, $Sb(S \cdot CH_2 \cdot CO \cdot NH_2)_3$, the triamide of antimony thioglycollic acid; used in the treatment of granuloma inguinale, kala-azar, and filariasis. **a. trichloride**, very deliquescent, colorless, transparent crystals or crystalline mass, $SbCl_3$, highly soluble in water. **a. trioxide**, a white odorless crystalline powder, Sb_2O_3, used in the preparation of tartar emetic (antimony potassium tartrate).

antimonyl (an-tim′o-nil″) the univalent radical SbO—.

antimuscarinic (an″tĭ-mus′kah-rin″ik) effective against the poisonous activity of muscarine.

antimutagen (an″tĭ-mu′tah-jen) a substance that antagonizes the mutagenic effects of other substances.

antimyasthenic (an″tĭ-mi″as-then′ik) 1. counteracting or relieving muscular weakness in myasthenia gravis. 2. an agent that counteracts or relieves muscular weakness in myasthenia gravis.

antimycobacterial (an″tĭ-mi″ko-bak-te′re-al) 1. effective against mycobacteria. 2. an agent that is effective against mycobacteria.

antimycotic (an″tĭ-mi-kot′ik) suppressing the growth of fungi.

antinarcotic (an″tĭ-nar-kot′ik) counteracting narcotic depression.

antinatriuresis (an″tĭ-na″tre-u-re′sis) inhibition of the excretion of sodium in the urine.

antinauseant (an″tĭ-naw′ze-ant) 1. preventing or relieving nausea. 2. an agent that prevents or relieves nausea. See also *antiemetic*.

antineoplastic (an″tĭ-ne″o-plas′tik) 1. inhibiting or preventing the development of neoplasms; checking the maturation and proliferation of malignant cells. 2. an agent having such properties.

antineoplaston (an″te-ne″o-plas′ton) any of a number of peptides isolated from human urine that inhibit cell division in certain cancer cells but not in normal cells.

antinephritic (an″tĭ-nĕ-frit′ik) counteracting inflammation of the kidneys.

antineuralgic (an″tĭ-nu-ral′jik) counteracting neuralgia.

antineuritic (an″tĭ-nu-rit′ik) counteracting neuritis.

antineurotoxin (an″tĭ-nu″ro-tok′sin) a substance that counteracts a neurotoxin.

antineutrino (an″tĭ-nu-tre′no) the antiparticle of the neutrino.

antineutron (an″tĭ-nu′tron) an elementary particle without a charge and with a mass and spin equal to that of a neutron, but with magnetic moment opposite to that of a neutron; the antiparticle of a neutron.

antiniad (an-tin′e-ad) toward the antinion.

antinial (an-tin′e-al) pertaining to the antinion.

antinion (an-tin′e-on) [*anti-* + Gr. *inion* occiput] the frontal pole of the head; the median frontal point farthest from the inion.

antinuclear (an″tĭ-nu′kle-ar) destructive to or reactive with components of the cell nucleus, as antinuclear antibody.

antiodontalgic (an″tĭ-o″don-tal′jik) relieving toothache.

antioncotic (an″t-ong-kot′ik) [*anti-* + Gr. *onkos* bulk, mass] 1. tending to reduce swelling and effective against tumors. 2. an agent that reduces swelling or suppresses growth of tumors.

antiophidica (an″tĭ-o-fid′ĭ-kah) [*anti-* + Gr. *ophis* snake] remedies that combat the effects of snake bite.

antiopsonin (an″te-op′so-nin) a substance that has an inhibitory influence on opsonins; antitropin.

antiovulatory (an″tĭ-ov′u-lah-to″re) suppressing ovulation.

antioxidant (an″tĭ-ok′sĭ-dant) one of many widely used synthetic or natural substances added to a product to prevent or delay its deterioration by action of oxygen in the air. Rubber, paints, vegetable oils, and prepared foods commonly contain antioxidants.

antioxidase (an″tĭ-ok′sĭ-dās) a substance that impairs oxidase activity.

antioxidation (an″tĭ-ok-sĭ-da′shun) the prevention of oxidation.

antioxygen (an″tĭ-ok′sĭ-jen) antioxidant.

antiparallel (an″te-par′ah-lel) [*anti-* + *parallel*] denoting molecules that are arranged side by side, but in opposite directions. For example, the strands of deoxyribonucleic acid are antiparallel with their 5′-3′ linkages running in opposite directions.

antiparalytic (an″tĭ-par″ah-lit′ik) [*anti-* + *paralysis*] relieving paralysis.

antiparasitic (an″tĭ-par″ah-sit′ik) 1. destructive to parasites. 2. an agent destructive to parasites.

antiparastata (an″tĭ-pah-ras′tah-tah) [*anti-* + Gr. *parastatēs* testis] bulbourethral gland (glandula bulbourethralis [NA]).

antiparasympathomimetic (an″tĭ-par″ah-sim″pah-tho-mĭ-met′ik) producing effects that resemble those of interruption of the parasympathetic nerve supply.

antiparkinsonian (an″tĭ-par″kin-so′ne-an) 1. effective in the treatment of parkinsonism. 2. an agent effective in the treatment of parkinsonism.

antiparticle (an″tĭ-par″tĭ-k′l) either of two particles, one of matter and one of antimatter, that annihilate each other upon collision, as an electron and a positron.

antipedicular (an″tĭ-pĕ-dik′u-lar) effective against *Pediculus* (sucking lice), or in the treatment of pediculosis; antipediculotic.

antipediculotic (an″tĭ-pĕ-dik″u-lot′ik) 1. effective against lice. 2. an agent effective against lice.

antipepsin (an″tĭ-pep′sin) an antienzyme that inhibits the action of pepsin.

antiperiodic (an″tĭ-pe″re-od′ik) preventing periodic recurrence of symptoms, as in malaria.

antiperistalsis (an″tĭ-per″ĭ-stal′sis) reversed peristalsis.

antiperistaltic (an″tĭ-per″ĭ-stal′tik) 1. pertaining to or causing antiperistalsis. 2. diminishing peristaltic action. 3. an agent that diminishes peristaltic action.

antiperspirant (an″tĭ-per′spĭ-rant″) 1. inhibiting or preventing perspiration. 2. an agent that inhibits or prevents perspiration.

antiphagocytic (an″tĭ-fag-o-sit′ik) counteracting or opposing phagocytosis.

antiphlogistic (an″tĭ-flo-jis′tik) 1. counteracting inflammation and fever. 2. an agent that counteracts inflammation and fever.

antiphrynolysin (an″tĭ-frĭ-nol′ĭ-sin) the antivenin for the toxin of toad venom.

antiphthiriac (an″tĭ-ther′e-ak) effective against lice.

antiphthisic (an″tĭ-tiz′ik) checking or relieving pulmonary tuberculosis (phthisis).

antiplasmin (an″tĭ-plaz′min) a substance in the blood that inhibits plasmin.

antiplasmodial (an″tĭ-plaz-mo′de-al) having a destructive action on plasmodia.

antiplastic (an″tĭ-plas′tik) [*anti-* + Gr. *plassein* to form] 1. unfavorable to the healing process. 2. an agent that suppresses formation of the blood or other cells.

antiplatelet (an″tĭ-plāt′let) directed against or destructive to blood platelets.

antipneumococcal (an″tĭ-nu″mo-kok′al) destroying or inhibiting the growth of *Streptococcus pneumoniae*.

antipneumococcic (an″tĭ-nu″mo-kok′sik) antipneumococcal.

antipodagric (an″tĭ-po-dag′rik) effective against gout.

antipodal (an″tĭp′ŏ-dal) occupying opposite positions; diametrically opposed; pertaining to an antipode.

antipode (an″tĭ-pōd) something occupying a directly opposed position. In chemistry, a molecule whose atoms are arranged in a directly opposite manner.

antipolycythemic (an″tĭ-pol″e-si-the′mik) 1. effective against polycythemia. 2. an agent effective against polycythemia.

antiport (an′tĭ-port) a mechanism of coupling the transport of two compounds across a membrane in opposite directions.

antiposia (an″tĭ-po′se-ah) antipathy to drinking.

antiprecipitin (an″tĭ-pre-sip′ĭ-tin) a substance antagonistic in its action to precipitin.

antiprostate (an″tĭ-pros′tāt) the bulbourethral gland (glandula bulbourethralis [NA]).

antiprotease (an″tĭ-pro′te-ās) a substance that checks the proteolytic action of enzymes, as antitryptase.

antiprothrombin (an″tĭ-pro-throm′bin) directed against prothrombin; a general term indicating a type of anticoagulant that acts by retarding the conversion of prothrombin to thrombin, without actually designating the specific means by which this occurs.

antiprotozoal (an″tĭ-pro-to-zo′al) 1. destroying protozoa, or checking their growth or reproduction. 2. an agent that destroys protozoa, or checks their growth or reproduction.

antiprotozoan (an″tĭ-pro″to-zo′an) antiprotozoal.

antipruritic (an″tĭ-proo-rit′ik) 1. relieving or preventing itching. 2. an agent, usually a topical application, that relieves or prevents itching.

antpsoriatic (an″tĭ-so″re-at′ik) 1. effective against psoriasis. 2. an agent effective against psoriasis.

antipsychomotor (an″tĭ-si′ko-mo′tor) suppressing or inhibiting the motor effects of cerebral or psychic activity.

antipsychotic (an″te-si-kot′ik) effective in the treatment of psychosis. Antipsychotic drugs (called also *neuroleptic drugs* and *major tranquilizers*) are a chemically diverse (including phenothiazines, thioxanthenes, butyrophenones, dibenzoxazepines, dibenzodiazepines, and diphenylbutyl-piperidines) but pharmacologically similar class of drugs used to treat schizophrenic, paranoid, schizoaffective, and other psychotic disorders; acute delirium and dementia, and manic episodes (during induction of lithium therapy); to control the movement disorders associated with Huntington's chorea, Gilles de la Tourette's syndrome, and ballismus; and to treat intractable hiccups and severe nausea and vomiting. Antipsychotic agents bind to dopamine, histamine, muscarinic cholinergic, α-adrenergic, and serotonin receptors. Blockade of dopaminergic transmission in various areas is thought to be responsible for their major effects: antipsychotic action by blockade in the mesolimbic and mesocortical areas; extrapyramidal side effects (dystonia, akathisia, parkinsonism, and tardive dyskinesia) by blockade in the basal ganglia; and antiemetic effects by blockade in the chemoreceptor trigger zone of the medulla. Sedation and autonomic side effects (orthostatic hypotension, blurred vision, dry mouth, nasal congestion, and constipation) are caused by blockade of histamine, cholinergic, and adrenergic receptors.

antiputrefactive (an″tĭ-pu″tre-fak′tiv) counteracting putrefaction.

antipyogenic (an″tĭ-pi″o-jen′ik) [*anti-* + Gr. *pyon* pus + *gennan* to produce] preventing or hindering the development of pus.

antipyresis (an″tĭ-pi-re′sis) [*anti-* + Gr. *pyressein* to have a fever] the therapeutic use of antipyretics.

antipyretic (an″tĭ-pi-ret′ik) [*anti-* + Gr. *pyretos* fever] 1. relieving or reducing fever. 2. an agent that relieves or reduces fever. Called also *antifebrile, antithermic,* and *febrifuge.*

antipyrine (an″tĭ-pi′rēn) [USP] a pyrazolone analgesic and antipyretic, now seldom used because it can produce agranulocytosis. **a. camphorate,** an antipyretic compound formerly used in night sweats. **a. mandelate,** a salt, $C_{19}H_{20}N_2O_4$, prepared by fusing antipyrine and mandelic acid.

antipyrotic (an″tĭ-pi-rot′ik) [*anti-* + Gr. *pyrōsis* a burning] 1. therapeutically effective against burns. 2. an agent that is effective in the treatment of burns.

antiradiation (an″tĭ-ra″de-a′shun) capable of counteracting the effects of radiation; effective against radiation injury.

antirennin (an″tĭ-ren′in) an antienzyme formed in the blood serum of animals injected with rennin; it counteracts the rennitic coagulation of milk.

antirheumatic (an″tĭ-ru-mat′ik) [*anti-* + *rheumatic*] 1. relieving or preventing rheumatism. 2. an agent that relieves or prevents rheumatism.

antiricin (an″tĭ-ri′sin) a substance that opposes the action of ricin (e.g., antitoxin produced following the introduction of ricin into the animal body).

antirickettsial (an″tĭ-rĭ-ket′se-al) 1. effective against rickettsiae. 2. an agent that is effective against rickettsiae.

antirobin (an″tĭ-ro′bin) the antitoxin of robin, a poison of the locust tree.

antisaluresis (an″tĭ-sal″u-re′sis) antinatriuresis.

antischistosomal (an″tĭ-shis″to-so′mal) 1. effective against schistosomes. 2. an agent that is destructive to schistosomes.

antiscorbutic (an″tĭ-skor-bu′tik) [*anti-* + *scorbutus*] effective in the prevention or relief of scurvy.

antisecretory (an″tĭ-se-kre′to-re) 1. inhibiting or diminishing secretion; secretoinhibitory. 2. an agent that so acts, as certain drugs that inhibit or diminish gastric secretions.

antisense (an″tĭ-sens′) in molecular genetics, referring to the strand of a double-stranded DNA that is complementary to the sense (q.v.) strand.

antisepsis (an″tĭ-sep′sis) [*anti-* + Gr. *sēpsis* putrefaction] 1. the prevention of sepsis by antiseptic means. 2. any procedure that reduces to a significant degree the microbial flora of skin or mucous membranes. **physiologic a.,** the combination of methods by which the body excludes germs; called also *autoantisepsis.*

antiseptic (an″tĭ-sep′tik) 1. pertaining to asepsis. 2. preventing decay or putrefaction. 3. a substance that inhibits the growth and development of microorganisms without necessarily killing them. Cr. *disinfectant* and *germicide.* **Credé's a.,** silver citrate. **Dakin's a.,** see *diluted sodium hypochlorite solution,* under *solution.* **Lister's a.,** mercury-zinc cyanide.

antiserum (an″tĭ-se′rum) a serum that contains antibody or antibodies; it may be obtained from an animal that has been immunized either by injection of antigen into the body or by infection with microorganisms containing the antigen. Antisera may be monovalent (specific for one antigen) or polyvalent (specific for more than one antigen). **Erysipelothrix rhusiopathiae a.,** an antiserum prepared by hyperimmunization of horses with *E. rhusiopathiae,* used for prevention and treatment of swine erysipelas.

antisialagogue (an″tĭ-si-al′ah-gog) 1. counteracting the formation of saliva. 2. an agent that counteracts any influence that promotes the flow of saliva.

antisialic (an″tĭ-si-al′ik) [*anti-* + Gr. *sialon* saliva] 1. checking the flow of saliva. 2. an agent that checks the secretion of saliva.

antisideric (an″tĭ-sĭ-der′ik) [*anti-* + Gr. *sidēros* iron] incompatible with iron.

antisocial (an″tĭ-so′shal) denoting (1) behavior that violates the rights of others or is criminal or (2) a specific syndrome of personality traits, *antisocial personality disorder* (see under *personality*), that is held to be associated with much antisocial behavior.

antispasmodic (an″tĭ-spaz-mod′ik) 1. relieving spasm, usually of smooth muscle, as in arteries, bronchi, intestine, bile duct, ureters or sphincters, but also of voluntary muscle. Cf. *antispastic.* 2. an agent that relieves spasm. **biliary a.,** an agent that relieves spasm of the biliary duct and sphincter. **bronchial a.,** an agent that relieves bronchial spasm.

antispastic (an″tĭ-spas′tik) antispasmodic with specific reference to skeletal muscle.

antistaphylococcic (an″tĭ-staf″ĭ-lo-kok′sik) killing or suppressing staphylococci.

antistaphylohemolysin (an″tĭ-staf″ĭ-lo-he-mol′ĭ-sin) antistaphylolysin.

antistaphylolysin (an″tĭ-staf-ĭ-lol′ĭ-sin) a substance that opposes the action of staphylolysin.

antisterility (an″tĭ-ste-ril′ĭ-te) combating sterility.

Antistine (an-tis′tin) trademark for preparations of antazoline.

antistreptococcic (an″tĭ-strep″to-kok′sik) 1. effective against streptococci. 2. an agent that is effective against streptococci.

antistreptokinase (an″tĭ-strep″to-ki-nās) an antibody that inhibits streptokinase.

antistreptolysin (an″tĭ-strep-tol′ĭ-sin) an antibody that inhibits streptolysin.

antisudoral (an″tĭ-su′dor-al) antisudorific.

antisudorific (an″tĭ-su″dor-if′ik) [*anti-* + L. *sudor* sweat] 1. inhibiting perspiration. 2. an agent that inhibits perspiration.

antisympathetic (an″tĭ-sim″pah-thet′ik) 1. producing effects that resemble those of interruption of the sympathetic nerve supply. 2. an agent that produces effects resembling those of interruption of the sympathetic nerve supply.

antitemplate (an″tĭ-tem′plāt) a hypothetical substance said to inhibit mitosis of normal cells and, on injury to cells, to diffuse out of the cells to initiate mitosis.

antitetanic (an″tĭ-tĕ-tan′ik) preventing or curing tetanus.

antithenar (an″tĭ-the′nar) [*anti-* + Gr. *thenar* palm, sole] situated opposite to the palm or the sole.

antithermic (an″tĭ-ther′mik) [*anti-* + Gr. *thermē* heat] antipyretic.

antithrombin (an″tĭ-throm′bin) [*anti-* + *thrombin*] a general term for a naturally occurring or therapeutically administered substance (e.g., heparin) that neutralizes the action of thrombin and thus limits or restricts blood coagulation. Six naturally occurring antithrombins have been designated by Roman numerals (I to VI); of these, antithrombins I and III appear to be of major importance. **a. I,** a term referring to the capacity of fibrin to adsorb large amounts of thrombin and thus neutralize (but not inactivate) it. **a. III,** a protein (an α_2-globulin, molecular weight 64,000) of normal plasma and extravascular sites that inactivates thrombin in a time-dependent irreversible reaction and serves as a cofactor of heparin in its anticoagulant activities. Antithrombin III also inhibits certain coagulation factors.

antithromboplastin (an″tĭ-throm″bo-plas′tin) any agent or substance that prevents or interferes with the interaction of the blood coagulation factors as they generate prothrombinase (prothrombin converting principle).

antithrombotic (an″tĭ-throm-bot′ik) preventing or interfering with the formation of thrombi; an agent that so acts.

antithyroid (an″tĭ-thi′roid) counteracting the functioning of the thyroid, especially in its synthesis of thyroid hormone.

antithyrotoxic (an″tĭ-thi″ro-tok′sik) counteracting the toxic effects of excessive internal secretion or exogenous dosage of thyroid and thyroid hormones.

antithyrotropic (an″tĭ-thi″ro-trop′ik) inhibiting the action of the thyrotropic hormone.

antitonic (an″tĭ-ton′ik) reducing tone or tonicity.

antitoxic (an″tĭ-tok′sik) effective against a poison; pertaining to antitoxin.

antitoxigen (an″tĭ-tok′sĭ-jen) antitoxinogen.

antitoxin (an″tĭ-tok′sin) 1. antibody against a toxin. 2. a purified antiserum from animals (usually horses) immunized by injections of a toxin or toxoid, administered as a passive immunizing agent to neutralize a specific bacterial toxin, e.g., botulinus, tetanus, or diphtheria. **botulinal a., botulinum a., botulinus a.,** botulism a. **botulism a.** [USP], an equine antitoxin against the toxins produced by the type A, B, or E strain of *Clostridium botulinum.* Generally trivalent (ABE) antitoxin is used. Called also *botulinal a., botulinum a.,* and *botulinus a.* **bovine a.,** antitoxin containing antibodies derived from the cow instead of from the horse, for use on persons who are hypersensitive to horse serum. **Clostridium perfrigens types C and D a.,** an antitoxin prepared from serum of animals hyperimmunized with toxins of *C. perfrigens* types C and D, administered immediately after birth for prevention of enterotoxemia in calves, lambs, and suckling pigs. **diphtheria a.** [USP], equine antitoxin against the toxin of *Corynebacterium diphtheriae,* used for treatment of diphtheria. **gas gangrene a.,** a polyvalent equine antitoxin against toxins of *Clostridium* species causing gas gangrene, formerly administered for prevention or treatment of gas gangrene. **tetanus a.** [USP], equine antitoxin against the toxins of *Clostridium tetani;* rarely used; tetanus immune globulin is used if available. **tetanus and gas gangrene a's,** a combination of tetanus and gas gangrene antitoxins.

antitoxinogen (an″tĭ-tok-sin′o-jen) [*antitoxin* + *-gen*] an antigen that stimulates the production of antitoxin, i.e., a toxin or toxoid.

antitoxinum (an″tĭ-tok-si′num) [L.] antitoxin.

antitragicus (an″tĭ-traj′ĭ-kus) see *Table of Musculi.*

antitragus (an″tĭ-tra′gus) [*anti-* + *tragus*] [NA] a projection opposite the tragus, bounding the cavum conchae posteroinferiorly and continuous above with the anthelix.

antitreponemal (an″tĭ-trep″o-ne′mal) 1. effective against *Treponema.* 2. an agent that is effective against *Treponema.*

antitrichomonal (an″tĭ-trich″o-mo′nal) 1. effective against *Trichomonas.* 2. an agent that is destructive to *Trichomonas.*

antitrismus (an″tĭ-triz′mus) a spasm that prevents the closure of the mouth.

antitrope (an′tĭ-trōp) [*anti-* + Gr. *trepein* to turn] 1. any organ that forms a symmetrical pair with another.

antitropic (an″tĭ-tro′pic) corresponding, but oppositely oriented, as a right and a left glove.

antitropin (an″tĭ-tro′pin) any substance that opposes the action of tropin; antiopsonin.

antitrypanosomal (an″tĭ-trĭ-pan″o-so′mal) 1. effective

against trypanosomes. 2. a drug for combating trypanosomiasis.

antitrypsic (an″tĭ-trip′sik) antitryptic.

α_1**-antitrypsin** (an″tĭ-trip′sin) alpha₁-antitrypsin.

antitryptase (an″tĭ-trip′tās) a substance that inhibits or counteracts the action of tryptase.

antitryptic (an″tĭ-trip′tik) [*anti-* + *tryptic*] counteracting the activity of trypsin.

antituberculin (an″tĭ-tu-ber′ku-lin) an antibody developed following the injection of tuberculin.

antituberculotic (an″tĭ-tu-ber″ku-lot′ik) 1. therapeutically effective against tuberculosis. 2. an agent that is therapeutically effective against tuberculosis.

antituberculous (an″tĭ-tu-ber″ku-lus) therapeutically effective against tuberculosis.

antitubulin (an″tĭ-too′bu-lin) an agent that prevents the polymerization of tubulin, and thus the formation of microtubules in a cell.

antitumorigenic (an″tĭ-tu″mor-ĭ-jen′ik) counteracting tumor formation.

antitussive (an″tĭ-tus′iv) 1. relieving or preventing cough. 2. an agent that relieves or prevents cough.

antityphoid (an″tĭ-ti′foid) counteracting or preventing typhoid.

antityrosinase (an″tĭ-ti-ro′sĭ-nās) an antienzyme that counteracts tyrosinase.

antiulcerative (an″tĭ-ul′ser-a″tiv) 1. preventing or promoting the healing of ulcers. 2. an agent that so acts.

antiuratic (an″tĭ-u-rat′ik) preventing the deposit of urates.

antivaccinationist (an″tĭ-vak″sĭ-na′shun-ist) a person who is opposed to vaccination.

antivenene (an″tĭ-vĕ-nēn′) [*anti-* + L. *venenum* poison] antivenin.

antivenin (an″tĭ-ven′in) [*anti-* + L. *venenum* poison] a proteinaceous material used in the treatment of poisoning by animal venom. See also *antivenomous serum,* under *serum.* **black widow spider a.,** *Latrodectus mactans* a. **a. (Crotalidae) polyvalent** [USP], a sterile serum containing specific venom-neutralizing globulins, produced by hyperimmunization of horses with the venoms of the fer-de-lance and the Florida, Texas, and tropical rattlesnakes; used as a passive immunizing agent for the treatment of envenomation by most pit vipers throughout the world. **Latrodectus mactans a.,** an antitoxic serum specific in the treatment of black widow spider (*L. mactans*) bites, prepared by immunizing horses against venom of the black widow spider; called also *black widow spider a.* **a. (Micrurus fulvius)** [USP], a sterile, nonpyrogenic preparation derived by drying a frozen solution of specific venom-neutralizing globulins obtained from serum of horses immunized against the venom of Eastern coral snakes (*Micrurus fulvius*). **polyvalent crotaline a.,** a. (Crotalidae) polyvalent.

antivenom (an″tĭ-ven′om) antivenin.

antivenomous (an″tĭ-ven′o-mus) counteracting venom.

antiviral (an″tĭ-vi′ral) 1. destroying viruses or suppressing their replication. 2. an agent that destroys viruses or suppresses their replication.

antivirotic (an″tĭ-vi-rot′ik) 1. antiviral. 2. an agent that destroys viruses or checks their growth or multiplication.

antivitamer (an″tĭ-vi′tah-mer) a substance that inactivates a vitamer.

antivitamin (an″tĭ-vi′tah-min) a substance that inactivates a vitamin.

antivivisection (an″tĭ-viv″ĭ-sek′shun) opposition to vivisection.

antivivisectionist (an″tĭ-viv″ĭ-sek′shun-ist) an individual opposed to vivisection.

antixenic (an″tĭ-ze′nik) [*anti-* + Gr. *xenos* strange or foreign] pertaining to the reaction of living tissue to any foreign substance.

antixerophthalmic (an″tĭ-ze″rof-thal′mik) counteracting xerophthalmia.

antixerotic (an″tĭ-ze-rot′ik) counteracting or preventing xerosis.

antizyme (an′tĭ-zīm) a protein whose synthesis is induced by a product of an enzyme reaction and which combines with and inhibits the action of that enzyme.

antizymohexase (an″tĭ-zi′mo-hek′sās)   an antienzyme that counteracts zymohexase.

antizymotic (an″tĭ-zĭ-mot′ik)   inhibiting or suppressing the action of enzymes.

antodontalgic (an″to-don-tal′jik)   antiodontalgic.

Anton's symptom (syndrome) (an′tonz) [Gabriel *Anton*, German neuropsychiatrist, 1858–1933]   see under *symptom*.

antophthalmic (ant″of-thal′mik)   relieving ophthalmia.

antorphine (an-tor′fēn)   nalorphine.

antra (an′trah) [L.]   plural of *antrum*.

antracele (an′trah-sēl)   antrocele.

antral (an′tral)   of or pertaining to an antrum.

antrectomy (an-trek′to-me) [*antrum* + Gr. *ektomē* excision]   surgical excision of an antrum, as resection of the pyloric antrum of the stomach.

Antrenyl (an′trĕ-nil)   trademark for a preparation of oxyphenonium.

Antricola (an-trik′ŏ-lah)   a genus of soft ticks that infest birds; several species feed on bats.

antritis (an-tri′tis)   inflammation of an antrum, chiefly the maxillary antrum.

antr(o)- [L. *antrum*, q.v.]   a combining form denoting relationship to an antrum, or sinus; often used with specific reference to the maxillary antrum, or sinus.

antroatticotomy (an″tro-at″ĭ-kot′o-me)   atticoantrotomy.

antrobuccal (an″tro-buk′kal)   pertaining to or communicating with the maxillary antrum (sinus) and (oral) buccal cavity, as an antrobuccal fistula.

antrocele (an′tro-sēl) [*antro-* + Gr. *kēlē* tumor]   a cystic accumulation of fluid in the maxillary antrum (sinus).

antroduodenectomy (an″tro-du″o-de-nek′to-me)   surgical removal of the pyloric antrum and adjacent portion of the duodenum, formerly done in the treatment of duodenal ulcer.

antrodynia (an″tro-din′e-ah) [*antro-* + Gr. *odynē* pain]   pain in an antrum.

antronalgia (an″tro-nal′je-ah) [*antro-* + *-algia*]   pain in the maxillary antrum.

antronasal (an″tro-na′zal)   pertaining to the maxillary antrum and the nose.

antrophore (an′tro-fōr) [*antro-* + Gr. *pherein* to bear]   a form of soluble medicated bougie.

antrophose (an′tro-fōz) [*antro-* + *phose*]   a phose originating in the central ocular mechanism.

antropyloric (an″tro-pĭ-lor′ik)   pertaining to or affecting the pyloric part of the stomach, including its antrum.

antroscope (an′tro-skōp″) [*antro-* + Gr. *skopein* to examine]   an instrument for illuminating and examining the maxillary antrum.

antroscopy (an-tros′ko-pe)   the use of the antroscope; inspection of an antrum.

antrostomy (an-tros′to-me) [*antro-* + Gr. *stomoun* to provide with an opening, or mouth]   the operation of making an opening into an antrum for purposes of drainage.

antrotome (an′tro-tōm)   an instrument for performing antrotomy.

antrotomy (an-trot′o-me) [*antro-* + Gr. *tomē* cut]   the cutting open of an antrum.

antrotympanic (an″tro-tim-pan′ik)   pertaining to the mastoid antrum and the tympanic cavity.

antrotympanitis (an″tro-tim″pah-ni′tis) [*antro-* + *tympanitis*]   inflammation of the mastoid antrum and of the middle ear.

antrum (an′trum), pl. *an′trums* or *an′tra* [L.; Gr. *antron* cave]   a cavity or chamber; used as a general term in anatomical nomenclature, especially to designate a cavity or chamber within a bone. **a. au′ris**, meatus acusticus externus. **cardiac a., a. cardi′acum**, the short conical portion of the esophagus below the diaphragm, its base being continuous with the cardiac orifice of the stomach. **ethmoid a., a. ethmoida′le**, bulla ethmoidalis ossis ethmoidalis. **frontal a.**, sinus frontalis. **gastric a.**, a. pylori. **a. of Highmore, a. highmo′ri**, sinus maxillaris. **Malacarne's a.** (*obs.*), substantia perforata posterior. **mas-**

toid a., a. mastoi′deum [NA], an air space in the mastoid portion of the temporal bone, communicating with the tympanic cavity and the mastoid cells; called also *a. tympanicum, tympanic a.*, and *mastoid cavity*. **a. maxilla′re, maxillary a.**, sinus maxillaris. **a. pylo′ri, pyloric a., a. pylor′icum** [NA], the dilated portion of the pyloric part of the stomach, between the body of the stomach and the pyloric canal; called also *a. of Willis* and *gastric a.* **tympanic a., a. tympan′icum**, a. mastoideum. **a. of Willis**, a. pyloricum.

Antrypol (an′trĭ-pol)   trademark for a preparation of suramin sodium.

ANTU   a powerful rodenticide, alphanaphthyl thiourea, that produces massive pulmonary edema and pleural effusion in rats.

Anturane (an′choo-rān)   trademark for a preparation of sulfinpyrazone.

Antyllus (an-til′us) 2nd or 3rd century A.D.)   a noted Greek surgeon of antiquity, a Pneumatist, whose treatment of aneurysms by ligation above and below remained standard practice until the time of John Hunter (18th century). He also made contributions to plastic surgery, ophthalmology, and public health. His writings remain only in fragments, and in the works of others (particularly Oribasius).

anuclear (ah-nu′kle-ar)   having no nuclei; said of cells, such as erythrocytes, which have lost their nuclei.

anucleated (a-nu′kle-āt″ed)   denucleated.

ANUG   acute necrotizing ulcerative gingivitis.

anuloplasty (an″u-lo-plas′te) [*anulus* + *-plasty*]   annuloplasty.

anulus (an′u-lus), gen. and pl. *an′uli* [L., from *anus* ring]   1. a ring or a ringlike or circular structure. 2. NA alternative for annulus. **a. fibro′sus dis′ci intervertebra′lis** [NA], the circumferential ringlike portion of an intervertebral disk, composed of fibrocartilage and fibrous tissue; called also *annulus fibrosus fibrocartilaginis intervertebralis* and *fibrous ring of intervertebral disk*. **a. inguina′lis profun′dus**, see *annulus inguinalis profundus*. **a. inguina′lis superficia′lis**, see *annulus inguinalis superficialis*.

Anura (ah-nu′rah)   the order of frogs and toads.

anuran (ah-nu′ran)   any member of Anura.

anuresis (an″u-re′sis)   1. retention of urine in the bladder. 2. anuria.

anuretic (an-u-ret′ik)   pertaining to or characterized by anuresis.

anuria (ah-nu′re-ah) [*an* neg. + Gr. *ouron* urine + *-ia*]   complete suppression of urinary secretion by the kidneys; called also *anuresis*. **angioneurotic a.**, anuria occurring in cortical necrosis of the kidney. **calculous a.**, anuria caused by a renal calculus. **obstructive a.**, failure of urinary excretion due to a blockage, as by a calculus, in the urinary passages. **postrenal a.**, anuria resulting from obstruction of the ureters. **prerenal a.**, cessation of renal secretion of urine resulting from fall of blood pressure below the level necessary to maintain adequate filtration pressure in the glomeruli. **renal a.**, failure of urinary secretion by the kidney in the presence of adequate filtration pressure in the glomeruli and patency of the ureters. **suppressive a.**, failure of secretion of urine in the kidneys.

anuric (ah-nu′rik)   pertaining to or characterized by anuria.

anurous (ah-nu′rus) [*an* neg. + Gr. *oura* tail]   without a tail.

anus (a′nus), gen. *a′ni*, pl. *a′nus* [L. "ring," "circle"]   the distal or terminal orifice of the alimentary canal. **artificial a.**, an opening from the bowel formed by the creation of a colostomy. **ectopic a.**, imperforate a. **imperforate a.**, persistence of the anal membrane, so that the anus is closed. The defect is not always complete; sometimes a narrow opening permits the passage of the bowel contents. When completely imperforate, the anus is seen as a dimple (the proctodeal pit) in the skin of the perineum. The latter condition is often associated with atresia of the lower rectum. **preternatural a.**, an anus situated at some unusual or abnormal place. **a. of Rusconi**, the blastopore. **a. vesica′lis**, anomalous opening of the rectum into the bladder, the anus being imperforate. **a. vestibula′ris,**

anomalous opening of the rectum on the vulva, the anus being imperforate. **vulvovaginal a.,** a. vestibularis.

anusitis (a-nus-i′tis) inflammation of the anus.

anvil (an′vil) incus.

anxietas (ang-zi′ĕ-tas) [L.] a nervous restlessness; anxiety. **a. tibia′rum,** restless legs syndrome.

anxiety (ang-zi′ĕ-te) the unpleasant emotional state consisting of psychophysiological responses to anticipation of unreal or imagined danger, ostensibly resulting from unrecognized intrapsychic conflict. Physiological concomitants include increased heart rate, altered respiration rate, sweating, trembling, weakness, and fatigue; psychological concomitants include feelings of impending danger, powerlessness, apprehension, and tension. Cf. *fear.* **castration a.,** that due to a fantasized loss of or injury to the genitals. **free-floating a.,** severe, generalized anxiety having no apparent connection to any specific object, situation, or idea. **separation a.,** see under *disorder.*

anxiolytic (ang″zi-o-lit′ik) 1. reducing anxiety. 2. an anxiolytic or antianxiety agent; see *antianxiety.*

anydremia (an″ĭ-dre′me-ah) [*an* neg. + Gr. *hydōr* water + *haima* blood + *-ia*] anhydremia.

AO anodal opening; opening of the atrioventricular valves.

A.O.A. American Optometric Association; American Orthopsychiatric Association; American Osteopathic Association.

AOC anodal opening contraction.

AOCl anodal opening clonus.

A.O.M.A. American Occupational Medical Association.

AOO anodal opening odor.

AOP anodal opening picture.

aorta (a-or′tah), pl. *aor′tas, aor′tae* [L.; Gr. *aortē*] the main trunk from which the systemic arterial system proceeds [NA]. It arises from the left ventricle of the heart; passes upward (*pars ascendens aortae*), bends over (*arcus aortae*), passes down through the thorax (*pars thoracica aortae*) and through the abdomen to about the level of the fourth lumbar vertebra (*pars abdominalis aortae*), where it divides into the two common iliac arteries. Called also *arteria a.* and *arteria maxima Galeni.* See *Table of Arteriae.* **abdominal a., a. abdomina′lis,** NA alternative for *pars abdominalis aortae.* **a. ascen′dens, ascending a.,** NA alternative for *pars ascendens aortae.* **a. descen′dens, descending a.,** NA alternative for *pars descendens aortae.* **dextropositioned a.,** a congenital anomaly resulting from increased rotation of the lower end of the bulbar septum, bringing the aorta farther to the right. It is seen in tetralogy of Fallot. **overriding a.,** a congenital anomaly occurring in tetralogy of Fallot, in which the aorta is displaced to the right so that it appears to arise from both ventricles and straddles the ventricular septal defect. **palpable a.,** one which, on account of a thin retracted abdominal wall, is easily palpable. **primitive a.,** either of two main vascular trunks before fusion into a single aorta in the early embryo. **a. sacrococcyg′ea,** arteria sacralis mediana. **a. thoraca′lis, thoracic a.,** pars thoracica aortae. **a. thorac′ica,** NA alternative for *pars thoracica aortae.* **ventral a.,** a single short vascular segment that, in fishes, in some amphibians, and in the embryo of higher vertebrates, connects the heart with the aortic arches. In mammalian development, it becomes continuous with the aortic arch.

aortae (a-or′te) [L.] genitive and plural of *aorta.*

aortal (a-or′tal) aortic.

aortalgia (a″or-tal′je-ah) [*aorta* + Gr. *algos* pain] pain in the region of the aorta.

aortectomy (a″or-tek′to-me) [*aorta* + Gr. *ektomē* excision] excision of part of the aorta.

aortic (a-or′tik) of or pertaining to the aorta.

aorticopulmonary (a-or″tĭ-ko-pul′mo-ner″e) pertaining to or lying between the aorta and pulmonary artery.

aorticorenal (a-or″te-ko-re′nal) pertaining to the aorta and the kidneys.

aortitis (a″or-ti′tis) [*aorta* + *-itis*] inflammation of the aorta. **Döhle-Heller a.,** syphilitic a. **luetic a.,** syphilitic a. **nummular a.,** aortitis with white circular patches on the inner coat of the vessel. **rheumatic a.,** inflammation of the aorta due to rheumatism, which may progress to patchy fibrosis. **syphilitic a., a. sy-**

philit′ica, aortitis caused by syphilis; its complications include insufficiency of the aortic valve, stenosis or occlusion of the coronary orifices, and aortic aneurysm. Called also *Döhle-Heller a., Heller-Döhle disease,* and *luetic a.*

aortocoronary (a-or″to-kor′ŏ-na-re) pertaining to or communicating with the aorta and coronary arteries.

aortogram (a-or′to-gram″) the roentgenographic record resulting from aortography.

aortography (a″or-tog′rah-fe) [*aorta* + Gr. *graphein* to write] roentgenography of the aorta after the intravascular injection of an opaque medium. **retrograde a.,** roentgenography of the aorta after passage of a catheter through a peripheral artery to the aorta and the rapid injection of a radiopaque substance. **translumbar a.,** roentgenography of the aorta after injection of a radiopaque medium into it through a needle inserted into the lumbar area at about the level of the 12th thoracic vertebra.

aortopathy (a″or-top′ah-the) [*aorta* + Gr. *pathos* disease] any disease of the aorta.

aortorrhaphy (a″or-tor′ah-fe) [*aorta* + Gr. *rhaphē* suture] suture of the aorta.

aortosclerosis (a-or″to-skle-ro′sis) sclerosis of the aorta.

aortotomy (a″or-tot′o-me) [*aorta* + Gr. *tomē* a cutting] incision of the aorta.

AOS anodal opening sound.

aosmic (a-oz′mik) anosmic.

A.O.T.A. American Occupational Therapy Association.

AP anterior pituitary (gland); angina pectoris; anteroposterior; arterial pressure.

ap- see *apo-.*

A.P.A. American Pharmaceutical Association; American Podiatric Association; American Psychiatric Association; American Psychological Association.

apaconitine (ap″ah-kon′ĭ-tin) [*ap-* + *aconitine*] a poisonous base derived from aconitine.

apallesthesia (ah-pal″es-the′ze-ah) pallanesthesia.

Apamide (ap′ah-mīd) trademark for a preparation of acetaminophen.

apancrea (ah-pan′kre-ah) absence of the pancreas.

apancreatic (ah-pan″kre-at′ik) due to absence of the pancreas.

Apansporoblastina (a″pan-spor″o-blas-ti′nah) [*a* neg. + *pansporoblast*] a suborder of parasitic protozoa (order Microsporida, class Microsporea) in which a pansporoblastic membrane is usually absent, being vestigial when present, and never persisting as a sporophorous vesicle; the sporoblast is most often dinucleate. Representative genera include *Encephalitozoon, Glugea,* and *Nosema.*

aparalytic (ah-par″ah-lit′ik) without paralysis.

aparathyreosis (ah-par″ah-thi-re-o′sis) aparathyrosis.

aparathyroidism (ah-par″ah-thi′roid-izm) aparathyrosis.

aparathyrosis (ah-par″ah-thi-ro′sis) absence or deficiency of the parathyroid glands.

aparthrosis (ap″ar-thro′sis) [Gr. *aparthrōsis*] junctura synovialis.

apastia (ah-pas′te-ah) [Gr. "fasting"] abstention from food, as a neurologic symptom.

apastic (ah-pas′tik) pertaining to or characterized by apastia.

apathetic (ap″ah-thet′ik) indifferent; undemonstrative.

apathism (ap′ah-thizm) the state of being slow in responding to stimuli.

apathy (ap′ah-the) [Gr. *apatheia*] lack of feeling or emotion; indifference.

apatite (ap′ah-tīt) a calcium phosphate of the composition $Ca_5(PO_4)_3OH$, one of the two mineral constituents of bones and teeth (the other being $CaCO_3$). Apatite is soluble in acids of soft drinks and in carbohydrate fermentation, but its OH^- ion is readily exchanged for F^- ion from some fluorides, and the resulting fluoro- apatite is not susceptible to acid decay.

apazone (ap′ah-zōn) a pyrazolone derivative having antiinflammatory, analgesic, antipyretic, uricosuric effects; used for treatment of rheumatoid arthritis and osteoarthritis. Called also *azapropazone* [INN, BAN].

APC 1. abbreviation for *acetylsalicylic acid, phenacetin,* and *caffeine*, available in capsule or tablet form; antipyretic and analgesic. 2. atrial premature contraction.

APE anterior pituitary extract.

apeidosis (ap″i-do′sis) [*ap-* + Gr. *eidos* form] progressive disappearance of characteristic form in either the histologic or clinical aspect of a disease.

apellous (a-pel′us) [*a* neg. + L. *pellis* skin] 1. skinless; not covered with skin; not cicatrized (said of a wound). 2. having no prepuce.

apepsia (ah-pep′se-ah) [*a* neg. + Gr. *peptein* to digest] (*obs.*) cessation or failure of the digestive functions.

apepsinia (ah″pep-sin′e-ah) (*obs.*) total absence or lack of secretion of pepsinogen by the stomach.

aperient (ah-pe′re-ent) [L. *aperiens* opening] a mild or gentle purgative; called also *aperitive* and *laxative.*

aperiodic (ah″pe-ri-od′ik) having no definite period; said of membranes that have no definite periods of vibration of their own, but are free to take up any vibrations imparted to them.

aperistalsis (ah″per-ĭ-stal′sis) [*a* neg. + *peristalsis*] absence of peristaltic action.

aperitive (ah-per′ĭ-tiv) 1. stimulating the appetite. 2. aperient.

Apert's disease (syndrome) (ah-parz′) [Eugène *Apert*, French pediatrician, 1868–1940] acrocephalosyndactyly.

Apert-Crouzon disease (ah-par′kroo-zon′) [Eugène *Apert*; Octave *Crouzon*, French neurologist, 1874–1938] see under *disease.*

apertognathia (ah-per″tog-na′the-ah) open bite.

apertometer (ap″er-tom′ĕ-ter) an apparatus for measuring the angle of aperture of microscopical objectives.

apertura (ap″er-tu′rah), gen. and pl. *apertu′rae* [L., from *aperire* to open] a general term used in anatomical nomenclature to designate an opening. **a. exter′na aqueduc′tus vestib′uli** [NA], external aperture of aqueduct of vestibule: the external opening for the aqueduct of the vestibule, located on the posterior surface of the petrous part of the temporal bone, lateral to the opening for the internal acoustic meatus; called also *fissure of aqueduct of vestibule.* **a. exter′na canalic′uli coch′leae** [NA], external aperture of canaliculus of cochlea: the external opening of the cochlear canaliculus on the margin of the jugular foramen in the temporal bone. **a. infe′rior canalic′uli tympan′ici,** inferior aperture of tympanic canaliculus: the lower opening of the tympanic canaliculus on the inferior surface of the petrous portion of the temporal bone; called also *external aperture of tympanic canaliculus.* **a. latera′lis ventric′uli quar′ti** [NA], an opening at the end of each lateral recess of the fourth ventricle by which the ventricular cavity communicates with the subarachnoid space; called also *lateral aperture of fourth ventricle, foramen of Luschka,* and *foramen of Key and Retzius.* **a. media′lis ventric′uli quar′ti,** a. mediana ventriculi quarti. **a. media′na ventric′uli quar′ti** [NA], a deficiency in the lower portion of the roof of the fourth ventricle through which the ventricular cavity communicates with the subarachnoid space; called also *a. medialis ventriculi quarti, median aperture of fourth ventricle,* and *foramen of Magendie.* **a. nasa′lis ante′rior,** NA alternative for *a. piriformis.* **a. pel′vis infe′rior** [NA], **a. pel′vis [mino′ris] infe′rior,** the inferior, very irregular aperture of the minor pelvis, bounded by the coccyx, the sacrotuberous ligaments, part of the ischium, the sides of the pubic arch, and the pubic symphysis; called also *exitus pelvis* and *inferior aperture of minor pelvis.* **a. pel′vis supe′rior** [NA], **a. pel′vis [mino′ris] supe′rior,** the superior aperture of the minor pelvis, bounded by the crest and pecten of the pubic bones, the arcuate lines of the ilia, and the anterior margin of the base of the sacrum; called also *superior aperture of minor pelvis.* **a. pirifor′mis** [NA], piriform aperture: the anterior nasal opening in the skull; called also *anterior nasal aperture* and *a. nasalis anterior* [NA alternative]. **a. si′nus fronta′lis** [NA], aperture of frontal sinus: the external opening of the frontal sinus into the nasal cavity. **a. si′nus sphenoida′lis** [NA], aperture of sphenoid sinus: a round opening just above the superior nasal concha, interconnecting the sphenoid sinus and nasal cavity; called also *sphenoidal ostium.* **a. supe′rior canalic′uli tympan′ici,** superior aperture of tympanic canaliculus: the upper opening of the tympanic canaliculus in the temporal bone, leading to

the tympanum; called also *internal aperture of tympanic canaliculus.* **apertu′rae supe′rior et infe′rior fos′sae axilla′ris,** superior and inferior apertures of axillary fossa: the openings of the axillary fossa into the axillary region; the superior is between the clavicle, scapula, and first rib and the inferior is covered by the axillary fascia. **a. thora′cis infe′rior** [NA], inferior aperture of thorax: the irregular opening at the inferior part of the thorax bounded by the twelfth thoracic vertebra, the twelfth ribs, and the curving edge of the costal cartilages as they meet the sternum; called also *inferior thoracic aperture.* **a. thora′cis supe′rior** [NA], superior aperture of thorax: the elliptical opening at the summit of the thorax, bounded by the first thoracic vertebra, the first ribs and cartilage, and the upper margin of the manubrium sterni; called also *superior thoracic aperture.* **a. tympan′ica canalic′uli chor′dae tym′pani** [NA], tympanic aperture of canaliculus of chorda tympani: the opening through which the chorda tympani enters the tympanic cavity.

aperturae (ap″er-tu′re) [L.] genitive and plural of *apertura.*

aperture (ap′er-chur) [L. *apertura*, q.v.] 1. an opening, or orifice; see also *apertura.* 2. the diameter of a microscope objective lens or the (adjustable) diameter of the iris diaphragm of a camera lens. **angle of a., angular a.,** the angle formed at a luminous point between the most divergent rays that are capable of passing through the objective of a microscope; called also *a. of lens.* **cloacal a.,** the posterior opening on the body surface of the cloaca in vertebrates such as birds, reptiles, fish, and amphibians. Called also *vent.* **external a. of aqueduct of vestibule,** apertura externa aqueductus vestibuli. **external a. of canaliculus of cochlea,** apertura externa canaliculi cochleae. **external a. of tympanic canaliculus,** apertura inferior canaliculi tympanici. **a. of frontal sinus,** apertura sinus frontalis. **a. of glottis,** rima glottidis. **inferior a. of minor pelvis,** apertura pelvis inferior. **inferior a. of thorax,** apertura thoracis inferior. **inferior a. of tympanic canaliculus,** apertura inferior canaliculi tympanici. **internal a. of tympanic canaliculus,** apertura superior canaliculi tympanici. **a. of larynx,** aditus laryngis. **lateral a. of fourth ventricle,** apertura lateralis ventriculi quarti. **a. of lens,** angle of a. **median a. of fourth ventricle,** apertura mediana ventriculi quarti. **nasal a., anterior,** apertura piriformis. **numerical a.,** a measure of the efficiency of a microscope objective, being the product of the sine of one-half the angle of the aperture times the lowest refractive index of any medium between the objective and specimen; usually abbreviated N.A. **orbital a.,** aditus orbitae. **piriform a.,** apertura piriformis. **a. of sphenoid sinus,** apertura sinus sphenoidalis. **spinal a.,** foramen vertebrale. **spurious a. of facial canal,** hiatus canalis nervi petrosi majoris. **spurious a. of fallopian canal,** hiatus canalis nervi petrosi majoris. **superior and inferior a's of axillary fossa,** aperturae superior et inferior fossae axillaris. **superior a. of minor pelvis,** apertura pelvis superior. **superior a. of thorax,** apertura thoracis superior. **superior a. of tympanic canaliculus,** apertura superior canaliculi tympanici. **thoracic a., inferior,** apertura thoracis inferior. **thoracic a., superior,** apertura thoracis superior. **tympanic a. of canaliculus of chorda tympani,** apertura tympanica canaliculi chordae tympani.

apex (a′peks), pl. *apexes* or *a′pices* [L.] 1. a general term used in anatomical nomenclature to designate the top of a body, organ, or part, or the pointed extremity of a conical structure; called also *tip.* 2. the point of greatest activity, or the point of greatest response to any type of stimulation, such as electrical stimulation of a muscle. **a. of arytenoid cartilage,** a. cartilaginis arytenoideae. **a. auric′ulae** [NA], a pointed protrusion sometimes observed on the upper border of the ear; called also *darwinian a.* **a. of bladder,** a. vesicae urinariae. **a. cap′itis fib′ulae** [NA], a process pointing upward on the posterior surface of the head of the fibula, giving attachment to the arcuate popliteal ligament of the knee joint and part of the biceps tendon; called also *a. of head of fibula.* **a. cartilag′inis arytenoi′deae** [NA], apex of arytenoid cartilage: the upper part of the arytenoid cartilage, which bends posteriorly and medially and connects with the corniculate cartilage. **a. cor′dis** [NA], apex of the heart: the blunt rounded extremity of the heart formed by the left ventricle; it is directed ventrally, inferiorly, and to the left. **a. cor′nus dorsa′lis medul′lae spina′lis** [NA] apex of dorsal horn of spinal cord: the extremity of the dorsal horn, or column, of the spinal cord which is capped by the substantia gelatinosa; called also *a. of posterior horn of spinal cord* and *a. cornus posterioris medullae spinalis* [NA alternative]. **a. cor′nus posterio′ris medul′lae spina′lis,** NA alternative for *a. cornus dorsalis medullae spinalis.* **a. cus′pidis** [NA], the apex of the cusp of a tooth. **darwinian a.,** a. auriculae. **a. of dorsal horn of spinal cord,** a. cornus dorsalis medullae spinalis. **a. of head of fibula,** a. capitis fibulae. **a. of heart,** a. cordis. **a. lin′guae** [NA], the most distal portion of the tongue; called also *a. of tongue.* **a. of lung,** a. pulmonis. **a. na′si** [NA], the most distal portion of the nose. **a. os′sis sa′cri** [NA], apex of the sacrum: the caudal end of the body of the fifth sacral vertebra, which articulates with the coccyx. **a. par′tis petro′sae os′sis tempora′lis** [NA], apex of petrous portion of temporal bone: the truncated portion of the petrous part of the temporal bone that is directed anteriorly and medially and ends at the medial opening of the carotid canal. **a. of patella, a. patel′lae** [NA], the inferiorly directed blunt point of the patella, to which the patellar ligament is attached. **a. of petrous portion of temporal bone,** a. partis petrosae ossis temporalis. **a. of posterior horn of spinal cord,** a. cornus dorsalis medullae spinalis. **a. prosta′tae** [NA], **a. of prostate gland,** the lower portion of the prostate, located just above the urogenital diaphragm. **a. pulmo′nis** [NA], apex of the lung: the rounded upper extremity of either lung, extending upward as high as the first thoracic vertebra. **a. rad′icis den′tis** [NA], **root a.,** the terminal end of the root of a tooth. **a. of sacrum,** a. ossis sacri. **a. of tongue,** a. linguae. **a. vesi′cae urina′riae** [NA], apex of bladder: the site of junction of the superior and inferolateral surfaces of the urinary bladder, from which the middle umbilical ligament (urachus) extends to the umbilicus; called also *fundus of bladder, vertex vesicae urinariae,* and *fundus* or *vertex of urinary bladder.*

apexcardiogram (a″peks-kar′de-o-gram) the graphic record obtained by apexcardiography.

apexcardiography (a″peks-kar″de-og′rah-fe) a method of graphically recording the pulsations of the precordium in the region of the cardiac apex.

APF animal protein factor.

Apgar score (scale) (ap′gar) [Virginia *Apgar,* American anesthesiologist, 1909–1974] see under *score.*

A.P.H.A. American Public Health Association.

A.Ph.A. American Pharmaceutical Association.

aphacia (ah-fa′se-ah) aphakia.

aphacic (ah-fa′sik) aphakic.

aphagia (ah-fa′je-ah) [*a* neg. + Gr. *phagein* to eat + -*ia*] abstention from eating. **a. al′gera,** refusal of a person to take food because it gives pain.

aphagopraxia (ah-fa″go-prak′se-ah) loss of the ability to swallow.

aphakia (ah-fa′ke-ah) [*a* neg. + *phak-* + -*ia*] absence of the lens of the eye; it may occur congenitally or from trauma, but is most commonly caused by extraction of a cataract.

aphakic (ah-fa′kik) pertaining to aphakia.

aphalangia (ah″fah-lan′je-ah) [*a*-neg. + *phalanx* + -*ia*] a developmental anomaly characterized by absence of a digit or of one or more phalanges of a finger or toe.

Aphanozoa (af″ah-no-zo′ah) [Gr. *aphanēs* invisible + *zōon* animal] ultramicroscopic organisms.

aphasia (ah-fa′ze-ah) [*a* neg. + Gr. *phasis* speech] defect or loss of the power of expression by speech, writing, or signs, or of comprehending spoken or written language, due to injury or disease of the brain centers. For types of aphasia not given below, see *agrammatism, anomia, paragrammatism,* and *paraphasia.* **acoustic a.,** auditory a. **ageusic a.,** loss of power to express words relating to the sense of taste. **amnemonic a.,** forgetfulness of words, with consequent aphasia; called also *a. lethica.* **amnesic a., amnestic a.,** anomic a. **anomic a.,** fluent aphasia in which comprehension and repetition are both preserved; called also *amnestic a.* **anosmic a.,** inability to express in words sensations of smell. **associative a.,** aphasia due to a disturbance of connection between the parts comprising the central structure. **ataxic a.,** expressive a. **auditory a.,** aphasia due to disease of the hearing center of the brain; word deafness. **Broca's a.,** expressive a. **central a.,** global a. **combined a.,** aphasia of two or more forms occurring concomitantly in the same person. **commissural a.,** aphasia due to a lesion in the insula interrupting the path between the motor and sensory speech centers; called also *frontolenticular a.* and *lenticular a.* **complete a.,** aphasia due to lesion of all the speech centers, producing inability to communicate with others in any way. **conduction a.,** fluent aphasia in which there is normal comprehension of spoken language but words are repeated incorrectly. **cortical a.,** global a. **expressive a.,** aphasia in which there is impairment of the ability to speak and write, due to a lesion of the cortical center. The patient understands written and spoken words, and knows what he wants to say, but cannot utter the words. Called also *ataxic a., Broca's a., motor a., frontocortical a.,* and *verbal a.* **expressive-receptive a.,** global a. **fluent a.,** aphasia in which speech is well articulated and grammatically correct but is lacking in content. **frontocortical a.,** expressive a. **frontolenticular a.,** commissural a. **functional a.,** aphasia resulting from hysteria or severe hysterical disorder. **gibberish a.,** jargon a. **global a.,** aphasia which involves all the functions which go to make up speech or communication; called also *central a., cortical a., expressive-receptive a.,* and *pictorial a.* **graphomotor a.,** aphasia in which the person cannot express himself in writing. **Grashey's a.,** aphasia due to lessened duration of sensory impressions, causing disturbance of perception and association, without lack of function of the centers or conductivity of the tracts; it is seen in acute diseases and concussion of the brain. **impressive a.,** sensory a. **intellectual a.,** true a. **jargon a.,** a form of receptive aphasia with utterance of meaningless phrases; called also *gibberish a.* **Kussmaul's a.,** voluntary refraining from speech, as in the insane. **lenticular a.,** commissural a. **a. leth′ica,** amnemonic a. **Lichtheim's a.,** a form of aphasia in which spontaneous speech is lost but the ability to repeat words is retained. **mixed a.,** global a. **motor a.,** expressive a. **nominal a.,** aphasia marked by the defective use of names of objects; cf. *anomia* and *dysnomia.* **nonfluent a.,** aphasia in which little speech is produced, and is uttered slowly, with great effort and poor articulation; it is due to a lesion in Broca's area. **optic a.,** inability to name objects seen, due to interruption of the connection between the speech and visual centers. **parieto-occipital a.,** combined alexia and apraxia. **pathematic a.,** aphasia due to passion or fright. **pictorial a.,** global a. **psychosensory a.,** receptive a. **receptive a.,** inability to understand written, spoken, or tactile speech symbols, due to disease of the auditory and visual word centers, as in word blindness; called also *impression a., sensory a., temporoparietal a.,* and *Wernicke's a.* **semantic a.,** aphasia characterized by a lack of recognition of the full significance of words and phrases or by loss of memory for words. **sensory a.,** receptive a. **subcortical a.,** aphasia due to a lesion interrupting impulses toward the afferent tracts that proceed to the auditory speech center. **syntactical a.,** aphasia characterized by inability to arrange words properly, so that the patient talks jargon. **tactile a.,** inability to name objects which are felt. **temporoparietal a.,** receptive a. **total a.,** global a. **transcortical a.,** aphasia caused by a lesion of a pathway between the speech center and other cortical centers. **true a.,** aphasia due to lesion of any one of the speech centers; called also *intellectual a.* **verbal a.,** expressive a. **visual a.,** alexia. **Wernicke's a.,** receptive a.

aphasiac (ah-fa′ze-ak) aphasic, def. 2.

aphasic (ah-fa′zik) 1. pertaining to or affected with aphasia. 2. a person affected with aphasia.

aphasiology (a-fa″ze-ol′o-je) the scientific study of aphasia and the specific neurologic lesions producing it.

aphasmid (a-faz′mid) [*a* neg. + *phasmid*] a nematode belonging to the subclass Aphasmidia. Cf. *phasmid.*

Aphasmidia (a-faz-mid′e-ah) a subclass of Nematoda comprising those organisms which do not possess phasmids, and including the superfamilies Trichuroidea, Mermithoidea, and Dioctophymoidea.

apheliotropism (ap″he-le-ot′ro-pizm) negative heliotropism.

aphemesthesia (ah″fe-mes-the′ze-ah) [*a* neg. + Gr. *phēmē* voice + *aisthēsis* perception] alexia.

aphemia (ah-fe′me-ah) [*a* neg. + Gr. *phēmē* voice] loss of the power of speech, due to a central lesion; see *expressive aphasia,* under *aphasia.* Called also *anandia.*

aphemic (ah-fem′ik) pertaining to or characterized by aphemia.

aphephobia (af″e-fo′be-ah) [Gr. *haphē* touch + *phobia*] haphephobia.

apheresis (ah-fĕ-re′sis) [Gr. *aphairesis* removal] any procedure in which blood is withdrawn from a donor, a portion (plasma, leukocytes, platelets, etc.) is separated and retained, and the remainder is retransfused into the donor. It includes leukapheresis, thrombocytapheresis, etc. Called also *pheresis.*

apheter (af′ĕ-ter) [Gr. *aphienai* to dissolve] a supposed material that gives to inogen the stimulus that decomposes it, and thus causes muscular contraction.

aphonia (ah-fo′ne-ah) [*a* neg. + Gr. *phōnē* voice] loss of voice. **a. cleric′rum,** see under *dysphonia.* **hysteric a.,** loss of speech due to hysteria. **a. paralyt′ica,** aphonia due to paralysis or disease of the laryngeal nerves. **spastic a.,** interference with the voice caused by muscular spasm.

aphonic (ah-fon′ik) 1. pertaining to or affected with aphonia. 2. without audible voice.

aphonogelia (ah″fo-no-je′le-ah) [*a* neg. + Gr. *phōnē* voice + *gelōs* laughter] inability to laugh aloud.

aphose (ah-fōz′) [*a* neg. + Gr. *phōs* light] any phose or subjective visual sensation due to absence or interruption of light.

aphosphagenic (ah-fos″fah-jen′ik) due to deficiency of phosphorus.

aphosphorosis (ah-fos″fo-ro′sis) a morbid condition caused by a deficiency of phosphorus in the diet.

aphotesthesia (a″fot-es-the′ze-ah) [*a* neg. + Gr. *phōs* light + *aisthēsis* perception] reduced sensitivity of the retina to light resulting from excessive exposure to rays of the sun.

aphotic (ah-fot′ik) without light; totally dark.

aphrasia (ah-fra′ze-ah) [*a* neg. + Gr. *phrasis* utterance] inability to speak or to understand words arranged as phrases.

aphrodisia (af″ro-diz′e-ah) [Gr. *aphrodisia* sexual pleasures] sexual excitement.

aphrodisiac (af″ro-diz′e-ak) 1. exciting the libido. 2. any drug that arouses the sexual instinct.

aphrodisiomania (af″ro-diz″e-o-ma′ne-ah) (*obs.*) erotomania.

aphtha (af′thah), pl. *aph′thae* [L.; Gr. "thrush"] a small ulcer, such as the small oval or round ulcer(s) covered with a grayish exudate and surrounded by a red halo characteristic of recurrent aphthous stomatitis. **Bednar's aphthae,** symmetric excoriation of the hard palate over the pterygoid plates in infants; thought to be due to pressure of the nipple against the palate during nursing, or to sucking of the tongue or foreign objects. **contagious aphthae, epizootic aphthae,** foot-and-mouth disease of cattle. **epizootic aphthae,** foot-and-mouth disease. **malignant aphthae** (*obs.*), foot-and-mouth disease of cattle. **Mikulicz's aphthae,** periadenitis mucosa necrotica recurrens. **recurring scarring aphthae,** periadenitis mucosa necrotica recurrens.

aphthae (af′the) [L.] 1. plural of *aphtha.* 2. recurrent aphthous stomatitis.

aphthoid (af′thoid) [Gr. *aphtha* thrush + *eidos* form] 1. resembling thrush; thrushlike. 2. an exanthema resembling that of thrush.

aphthongia (af-thon′je-ah) [*a* neg. + Gr. *phthongos* sound] aphasia due to spasm of the speech muscles.

aphthosis (af-tho′sis) any condition marked by aphthae.

aphthous (af′thus) pertaining to, characterized by, or affected with aphthae.

aphylactic (a″fi-lak′tik) pertaining to or characterized by aphylaxis.

aphylaxis (a″fi-lak′sis) absence of phylaxis.

apical (ap′ĭ-kal) pertaining to or located at the apex.

apicectomy (a″pĭ-sek′to-me) [*apic-* + *-ectomy*] excision of the apex of the petrous portion of the temporal bone.

apices (ap′ĭ-sēz) [L.] plural of *apex.*

apicitis (a″pe-si′tis) [*apic-* + *-itis*] inflammation of an apex, as the apex of a tooth, the apex of the lung, or the apex of the petrous portion of the temporal bone (petrositis).

apic(o)- [L. *apex* top, summit] a prefix denoting a relationship to the top, as of an organ or other structure.

Apicocomplexa (a″pĭ-ko-kom-plek′sah) [*apico-* + *complex*] a phylum of uninucleate, parasitic tissue-dwelling protozoa characterized by the presence of an apical complex; a micropore(s) is generally present at some stage of development. Flagella and cilia are absent in the adult stage; many mature apicocomplexans glide by means of ultrastructural ridges and fibers on the body surface. They typically reproduce asexually by means of multiple fission, forming merozoites or schizoites, or by endodyogeny, or sexually by syngamy. It comprises two classes: Perkinsea and Sporozoea. Called also *Sporozoa.*

apicocomplexan (a″pĭ-ko-kom-plek′san) 1. any protozoan of the subphylum Apicocomplexa. 2. pertaining or relating to protozoa of the subphylum Apicocomplexa.

apicoectomy (a″pĭ-ko-ek′to-me) [*apico-* + *-ectomy*] excision of the apical portion of a tooth through an opening made in the overlying labial, buccal, or palatal alveolar bone; called also *root resection.* Cf. *hemisectomy.*

apicolysis (a″pĕ-kol′ĭ-sis) [*apico-* + *lysis*] the operation of causing the apex of the lung to collapse; formerly used in treatment of tuberculosis.

apicostomy (a″pĕ-kos′to-me) dental trephination.

apicotomy (a″pe-kot′o-me) puncture of the apex of the petrous portion of the temporal bone.

apii (a′pe-i) genitive of *apium.* **a. fruc′tus,** see under *Apium.*

A.P.I.M. abbreviation for *Association Professionnelle Internationale des Médecins,* an international body which deals with the conduct of medical practice from the economic point of view.

apinealism (ah-pin′e-al-izm) the effects allegedly produced by removal of the pineal body.

apiotherapy (a″pe-o-ther′ah-pe) treatment with bee venom.

apiphobia (a″pĕ-fo′be-ah) [L. *apis* bee + *phobia*] irrational fear of bees.

apisination (a″pis-ĭ-na′shun) [L. *apis* bee] poisoning by the sting of bees.

apitoxin (a″pĕ-tok′sin) the toxic protein constituent of bee venom.

apituitarism (ah″pĭ-tu′ĭ-tar-izm″) 1. hypopituitarism. 2. congenital absence of the pituitary, as in anencephaly.

Apium (a′pe-um) [L.] a genus of umbelliferous plants, including celery; celery seed (*apii fructus*), the ripe fruit of *A. graveolens,* has been used as a diuretic and antispasmodic.

A.P.L. trademark for a preparation of human chorionic gonadotropin.

aplacental (a″plah-sen′tal) [*a* neg. + *placenta*] having no placenta.

aplanatic (ap″lah-nat′ik) [*a* neg. + Gr. *planan* to wander] pertaining to aplanatism.

aplanatism (ah-plan′ah-tizm) freedom from spherical aberration and coma; said of a lens.

aplasia (ah-pla′zhe-ah) [*a* neg. + Gr. *plassein* to form] lack of development of an organ or tissue, or of the cellular products from an organ or tissue. Cf. *agenesis* and *hypoplasia.* **a. axia′lis extracortica′lis conge′nita,** Pelizaeus-Merzbacher disease. **a. cu′tis congen′ita,** localized failure of development of skin, most commonly of the scalp, less frequently of the trunk and limbs. The defects are usually covered by a thin translucent membrane or scar tissue, or may be raw, ulcerated, or covered by granulation tissue. **hereditary retinal a.,** amaurosis congenita. **nuclear a.,** Möbius' syndrome. **a. of ovary,** gonadal dysgenesis. **pure red cell a.,** severe normochromic, normocytic anemia, reticulocytosis, and erythroblastopenia in otherwise normal bone marrow. It occurs as a *chronic* form, either primary or secondary to immune disorders, or an *acute* form, which is self-limited and associated with drugs or infection. **retinal a.,** retinal dysplasia, defs. 1 and 2. **thymic a.,** absence of the thymus gland, as in DiGeorge's syndrome. **thymic-parathyroid a.,** DiGeorge's syndrome.

aplasmic (ah-plaz′mik)   containing no protoplasm or sarcoplasm.

aplastic (ah-plas′tik) [*a* neg. + Gr. *plassein* to form]   pertaining to or characterized by aplasia; anatomically undeveloped from the primordium or from the stem cell.

Aplectana (ah-plek′tah-nah)   a genus of nematodes parasitic in the intestinal tract of amphibians and reptiles.

apleuria (ah-plu′re-ah) [*a*- neg. + *pleur*- + -*ia*.]   absence of ribs.

apnea (ap-ne′ah) [*a* neg. + Gr. *pnoia* breath]   1. cessation of breathing.   2. asphyxia.   **deglutition a.,** a temporary arrest of the activity of the respiratory nerve center during an act of swallowing.   **initial a.,** a condition in which an infant fails to establish sustained respiration within two minutes of delivery.   **late a.,** cessation of respiration in an infant for more than 60 seconds after spontaneous breathing has been established and sustained.   **a. neonato′rum,** failure of the newborn infant to initiate pulmonary ventilation.   **sleep a.,** transient attacks of failure of automatic control of respiration, resulting in alveolar hypoventilation, which becomes more pronounced during sleep. It may result in acidosis and in vasoconstriction of pulmonary arterioles, producing pulmonary arterial hypertension.   **traumatic a.,** cessation of pulmonary ventilation following physical injury.

apneic (ap′ne ik)   pertaining or relating to apnea or affected with apnea.

apneumatic (ap″nu-mat′ik)   1. free from air.   2. done with the exclusion of air.

apneumatosis (ap″nu-mah-to′sis) [*a* neg. + Gr. *pneumatōsis* inflation]   congenital atelectasis of the lungs.

apneumia (ap-nu′me-ah) [*a* neg. + Gr. *pneumōn* lung]   congenital absence of the lungs.

apneusis (ap-nu′sis)   a condition marked by maintained inspiratory activity unrelieved by expiration, each inspiration being long and cramplike; it follows excision of the upper portion of the pons (pneumotaxic center).

apneustic (ap-nu′stik)   pertaining to or characterized by apneusis.

apo-, ap- [Gr. *apo* from]   a prefix denoting separation or derivation from.

apoatropine (ap″o-ah′tro-pēn)   chemical name: *endo-α*-methylenebenzeneacetic acid 8-methyl-8-azabicyclo [3.2.1] oct-3-yl ester. An antispasmodic alkaloid, $C_{17}H_{21}NO_2$, derived from belladonna.

apocamnosis (ap″o-kam-no′sis)   apokamnosis.

apocenosis (ap″o-sĕ-no′sis)   an increased flow of blood or other body fluid.

apochromat (ap″o-kro-mat′) [*apo-* + *chromatic* aberration]   an apochromatic objective; see under *objective*.

apochromatic (ap″o-kro-mat′ik)   free from chromatic and spherical aberration; see under *objective*.

apocope (ah-pok′o-pe) [Gr. *apokopē*]   a cutting off; amputation.

apocoptic (ap″o-kop′tik)   resulting from or pertaining to an amputation.

apocrine (ap′o-krin) [Gr. *apokrinesthai* to be secreted]   denoting that type of glandular secretion in which the free end or apical portion of the secreting cell is cast off along with the secretory products that have accumulated therein.

apocrinitis (ap″o-krin-i′tis) [*apo-* + Gr. *krinein* to separate]   hidradenitis suppurativa.

apocrustic (ap″o-krus′tik)   1. astringent and repellent.   2. an astringent and repellent agent.

apocynin (ah-pos′ĕ-nin)   see *Apocynum*.

Apocynum (ah-pos′ĕ-num)   a genus of poisonous North American apocynaceous plants noted for their digitalis-like cardioactive principles, e.g., *A. androsaemifolium* L. (dogbane, wild or milk ipecac, rheumatism weed) and *A. cannabinum* L. (Canadian hemp, black Indian hemp). Both contain apocynin, formerly used like digitalis.

apodal (ah-po′dal)   having no feet.

Apodemus (ap″o-de′mus)   a genus of Old World field mice. **A. sylvat′icus,** the wood mouse, a species that serves as a reservoir of *Leptospira grippotyphosa*.

apodia (ah-po′de-ah) [*a* neg. + *pod*- + -*ia*]   a developmental anomaly characterized by absence of one or both of the feet.

apoenzyme (ap″o-en′zīm)   the protein component of an enzyme that is separable from the prosthetic group (cofactor or coenzyme) but that requires the presence of the prosthetic group to form the functioning compound (holoenzyme).

apoferritin (ap″o-fer′ĭ-tin)   a colorless protein, with a molecular weight of 460,000, occurring in the mucosal cells of the small intestine, forming a compound with iron called ferritin, which has been implicated in the regulation of iron absorption in the gastrointestinal tract.

apogamia, apogamy (ap″o-gam′e-ah; ah-pog′ah-me) [*apo-* + Gr. *gamein* to wed]   1. reproduction without conjugation of gametes and usually without meiosis, as in certain seed plants.   2. parthenogenesis.

apogee (ap′o-je)   the state of greatest severity of a disease.

apokamnosis (ap″o-kam-no′sis)   abnormal liability to fatigue in myasthenia; a feeling of tiredness, numbness, and heaviness in a limb motion.

apolar (ah-po′lar) [*a* neg. + Gr. *polos* pole]   not having poles or processes.

apolegamic (ap″o-leh-gam′ik) [Gr. *apolegein* to pick out + *gamos* marriage]   pertaining to selection, especially sexual selection.

apolegamy (ap″o-leg′ah-me)   selection, especially sexual selection in breeding.

apolipoprotein (ah″po-lip′o-pro′te-in)   any of the protein constituents of lipoproteins; grouped by function in four classes A, B, C, and E (the former apo D is now apo A-III). The A apoproteins, apo A-I, -II, -III, and -IV, occur primarily in HDL and in lesser amounts in chylomicrons; apo A-I is the activator of lecithin-cholesterol acyltransferase (LCAT), which forms cholesteryl esters in HDL. The B apoproteins are recognized by specific cell-surface receptors that mediate endocytosis of lipoprotein particles; B-100 on VLDL, IDL, and LDL is recognized by LDL receptors on liver and extrahepatic cells; B-48 on chylomicrons is recognized by chylomicron remnant receptors on liver cells. The C apoproteins, apo C-I, -II, and -III, occur in VLDL, HDL, and chylomicrons; apo C-II activates lipoprotein lipase, which hydrolyzes triglycerides for transfer from VLDL and chylomicrons to tissues. Apo E occurs in all classes of lipoproteins; it may be involved in the conversion of VLDL to IDL and its clearance from the circulation.

apolipoprotein C-II (apo C-II) deficiency, familial, familial hyperlipoproteinemia, types I and V, due to defective apolipoprotein C-II, a necessary cofactor for lipoprotein lipase activation.

Apollonia (ap″o-lo′ne-ah)   a Christian martyr and the patron saint of dentistry; her teeth were knocked out, and then she was burned alive in 249. Her feast day is February 9.

apomixia, apomixis (ap″o-mik′se-ah; ap″o-mik′sis) [*apo-* + Gr. *mixis* a mingling]   1. asexual reproduction in a species normally reproducing sexually, as in certain seed plants.   2. apogamia.

apomorphine (ap″o-mor′fin) [*apo-* + *morphine*]   a crystalline alkaloid, $C_{17}H_{17}NO_2$, derived from morphine by the abstraction of a molecule of water; it is administered intravenously to induce instantaneous vomiting and was formerly used as an expectorant.   **a. hydrochloride** [USP], a grayish crystalline compound, $C_{17}H_{17}NO_2 \cdot HCl \cdot \frac{1}{2}H_2O$, a potent and prompt emetic.

aponeurectomy (ap″o-nu-rek′to-me) [*aponeurosis* + Gr. *ektomē* excision]   excision of the aponeurosis of a muscle.

aponeurology (ap″o-nu-rol′o-je) [*aponeurosis* + -*logy*]   the sum of knowledge regarding aponeuroses and fasciae.

aponeurorrhaphy (ap″o-nu-ror′ah-fe) [*aponeurosis* + Gr. *rhaphē* suture]   suture of an aponeurosis; fasciorrhaphy.

aponeuroses (ap″o-nu-ro′sēz)   plural of *aponeurosis*.

aponeurosis (ap″o-nu-ro′sis), pl. *aponeuro′ses* [Gr. *aponeurōsis*] [NA]   1. a white, flattened or ribbon-like tendinous expansion, serving mainly to connect a muscle with the parts that it moves.   2. a term formerly applied to certain fasciae.   **abdominal a.,** the conjoined tendons of the oblique and transverse muscles on the abdomen.   **bicipital a.,** a. musculi bicipitis brachii.   **a. bicipita′lis,** NA alternative for *a. musculi bicipitis brachii*.   **clavicoracoaxillary a.,** fascia clavipectoralis.   **crural a.,** fascia cruris.   **Denonvilliers' a.,** septum rectovesicale.   **epicranial a.,** galea aponeurotica.   **falciform a. of rectus abdominis muscle,** falx inguinalis.   **femoral a.,**

fascia lata femoris. **a. of insertion,** the connection of a muscle with the part or parts that it moves. **interchondral aponeuroses, internal** (obs.), see *membrana intercostalis interna.* **intercostal aponeuroses, external,** see *membrana intercostalis externa.* **intercostal aponeuroses, internal,** see *membrana intercostalis interna.* **a. lin′guae** [NA], **lingual a.,** the connective tissue framework of the tongue, supporting and giving attachment to the intrinsic and extrinsic muscles; composed of the connective tissue layer of the tunica mucosa, the lingual septum, and the posterior transverse expansion of the septum which attaches to the hyoid bone. **a. mus′culi bicip′itis bra′chii** [NA], an expansion of the tendon of the biceps brachii muscle by which it is attached to the fascia of the forearm and to the ulna; called also *a. bicipitalis* [NA alternative] *bicipital a.* or *fascia,* and *lacertus fibrosus, semilunar fascia,* and *fibrous fasciculus of biceps muscle.* **a. of occipitofrontal muscle,** galea aponeurotica. **a. palatina** [NA], **palatine a.,** a fibrous sheet in the anterior part of the soft palate, derived mainly from the tendons of the two tensor muscles, giving attachment to the musculus uvulae and to the palatopharyngeus and levator veli palatini muscles. **palmar a., a. palma′ris** [NA], bundles of fibrous tissue radiating toward the bases of the fingers from the tendon of the palmaris longus muscle; called also *volar fascia.* **pharyngeal a., a. pharyn′gis, pharyngobasilar a., a. pharyngobasila′ris,** fascia pharyngobasilaris. **plantar a., a. planta′ris** [NA], bands of fibrous tissue radiating toward the bases of the toes from the medial process of the tuber calcanei; called also *plantar fascia.* **Sibson's a.,** membrana suprapleuralis. **subscapular a.,** a fascia attached to the circumference of the subscapular fossa. **a. of superior surface of levator ani muscle,** fascia diaphragmatis pelvis superior. **supraspinous a.,** a dense fascia that partly envelops the supraspinous muscle. **temporal a.,** fascia temporalis. **vertebral a.,** fascia thoracolumbalis. **a. of Zinn,** see *fibrae zonulares.*

aponeurositis (ap″o-nu-ro-si′tis) [*aponeurosis* + *-itis*] inflammation of an aponeurosis.

aponeurotic (ap″o-nu-rot′ik) pertaining to or of the nature of an aponeurosis.

aponeurotome (ap″o-nu′ro-tōm) a knife for cutting aponeuroses.

aponeurotomy (ap″o-nu-rot′o-me) [*aponeurosis* + Gr. *tomē* a cut] surgical cutting of an aponeurosis.

aponia (ah-po′ne-ah) [Gr.] (obs.) freedom from pain.

aponic (ah-po′nik) relieving pain or fatigue.

Aponomma (ap″o-nom′ah) a genus of ticks infesting tropical reptiles of the Old World.

apophlegmatic (ap″o-fleg-mat′ik) causing a discharge of mucus; expectorant.

apophysary (ah-pof′ĭ-za-re) apophyseal.

apophyseal (ap″o-fiz′e-al) pertaining to or of the nature of an apophysis.

apophyseopathy (ap″o-fiz-e-op′ah-the) [*apophysis* + Gr. *pathos* disease] disease of an apophysis, particularly Osgood-Schlatter disease.

apophyses (ah-pof′ĭ-sēz) plural of *apophysis.*

apophysial (ap″o-fiz′e-al) apophyseal.

apophysiary (ap″o-fiz′e-a″re) apophyseal.

apophysis (ah-pof′ĭ-sis), pl. *apoph′yses* [Gr. "an offshoot"] [NA] any outgrowth or swelling, especially a bony outgrowth that has never been entirely separated from the bone of which it forms a part, such as a process, tubercle, or tuberosity. **basilar a.,** pars basilaris ossis occipitalis. **cerebral a., a. cer′ebri,** pineal body. **genial a.,** spina mentalis. **a. of Ingrassias,** ala minor ossis sphenoidalis. **a. lenticula′ris in′cudis,** processus lenticularis incudis. **odontoid a.,** dens axis. **a. os′sium,** epiphysis. **pterygoid a.,** processus pterygoideus ossis sphenoidalis. **a. of Rau, a. ravia′na, a. raw′ii,** processus anterior mallei.

apophysitis (ah-pof″ĭ-zi′tis) inflammation of an apophysis, especially a disorder of the foot caused by disease of the epiphysis of the calcaneus. **a. tibia′lis adolescen′tium,** Osgood-Schlatter disease.

apoplasmatic (ap″o-plaz-mat′ik) pertaining to substances that are produced by cells and form a constituent part of the

tissues of an organism, such as fibers of connective tissue or the matrix of bone and cartilage.

apoplectic (ap″o-plek′tik) [Gr. *apoplēktikos*] pertaining to, caused by, or affected with apoplexy.

apoplectiform (ap-o-plek′tĕ-form) resembling apoplexy.

apoplectoid (ap″o-plek′toid) resembling apoplexy.

apoplexia (ap″o-plek′se-ah) [L.] apoplexy. **a. u′teri,** sudden uterine hemorrhage, due to arterial degeneration or hemorrhagic infarct.

apoplexy (ap′o-plek″se) [Gr. *apoplēxia*] 1. an apoplectic stroke; sudden neurologic impairment due to a cerebrovascular disorder, limited by some to intracranial hemorrhage, extended by others to include occlusive cerebrovascular lesions. See *stroke syndrome,* under *syndrome.* 2. copious extravasation of blood within any organ. **abdominal a.,** spontaneous intraperitoneal hemorrhage due to rupture of an intra-abdominal blood vessel, independent of any trauma to the abdomen. **adrenal a.,** a morbid condition resulting from massive hemorrhage into the adrenal glands, occurring in Waterhouse-Friderichsen syndrome. **asthenic a.,** stroke syndrome resulting from debility. **bulbar a.,** hemorrhage into the substance of the pons; called also *pontile a.* or *pontine a.* **capillary a.,** stroke syndrome resulting from the rupture of capillary vessels. **cerebellar a.,** hemorrhage into the cerebellum. **cerebral a.,** cerebral hemorrhage. **delayed a.,** cerebral hemorrhage which comes on several days after the receipt of the injury. **embolic a.,** stroke syndrome due to stopping of a cerebral artery by an embolus. **fulminating a.,** cerebral hemorrhage in which the patient suddenly falls and quickly becomes unconscious. **heat a.,** heat stroke. **ingravescent a.,** progressive paralysis due to the slow leakage of blood from a ruptured vessel. **neonatal a.,** stroke syndrome in newborn infants. **ovarian a.,** extensive extravasation of blood into the ovary. **pancreatic a.,** extensive hemorrhage of the pancreas; seen in cardiac failure and portal hypertension. **parturient a.,** milk fever, def. 3. **pituitary a.,** sudden massive degeneration with hemorrhagic necrosis of the pituitary gland, associated with pituitary tumor, signaled by abrupt headache, followed by loss of sight, diplopia, drowsiness, and confusion, or coma. **placental a.,** hemorrhage into a separated placenta with formation of a hematoma between the placenta and uterine wall. **pontile a., pontine a.,** bulbar a. **Raymond's a.,** a type of ingravescent apoplexy marked by paresthesia of the hand on the side which later becomes paralyzed; called also *Raymond's type of a.* **renal a.,** a morbid condition resulting from rupture of an intrarenal blood vessel. **spinal a.,** bleeding or hemorrhage into the substance of the spinal cord. **thrombotic a.,** stroke syndrome due to thrombosis of a cerebral artery. **traumatic late a.,** cerebral hemorrhage following trauma and appearing several days or weeks after the accident. **uteroplacental a.,** Couvelaire's term for a severe uterine condition seen in some cases of separation of the placenta, in which the uterine musculature is disrupted and infiltrated with blood.

apoprotein (ap″o-pro′te-in) the protein moiety of a conjugated protein or protein complex. See also *apolipoprotein.*

apoptosis (ap″o-to′sis) [Gr. "a falling off," from *apo* off + *ptosis* fall] fragmentation of a cell into membrane-bound particles that are then eliminated by phagocytosis.

aporepressor (ap″o-re-pres′or) in genetic theory, a product of regulator genes, of unknown structure, which combines with low-molecular weight corepressor to form the complete repressor, which specifically represses the activity of certain structural genes.

aposia (ah-po′ze-ah) [*a* neg. + Gr. *posis* drinking + *-ia*] (obs.) absence of drinking, or reluctance to ingest fluids.

apositia (ap″o-sish′e-ah) [*apo-* + Gr. *sitos* food + *-ia*] (obs.) aversion to food.

apositic (ap″o-sit′ik) (obs.) pertaining to, characterized by, or causing apositia.

aposome (ap′o-sōm) [*apo-* + Gr. *sōma* body] an inclusion within the cytoplasm that has been made by the activity of the cell itself.

apostasis (ah-pos′tah-sis) [Gr.] the end or crisis of an attack of disease.

aposthia (ah-pos′the-ah) [*a* neg. + Gr. *posthē* foreskin + *-ia*] congenital absence of the prepuce.

Apostomatida (ap″o-sto-mah′tĭ-dah) an order of ciliate

protozoa (superorder Apostomatidea, subclass Hypostomatia) having characters of the superorder. It comprises three suborders: Apostomatina, Astomatophorina, and Pilisuctorina.

Apostomatidea (ap″o-sto″mah-tid′e-um) [*apo-* + Gr. *stomatos* mouth] a superorder of ciliate protozoa (subclass Hypostomatia, class Kinetofragminophorea), the life cycle of which is polymorphic, sometimes involving alternation of hosts, most species being associated with marine crustaceans. They are characterized by the presence of an inconspicuous cytosome (it may be absent in certain stages), a glandular complex (rosette) typically situated near the oral area, and in mature forms, spiraled and often widely spaced somatic ciliature. It comprises one order: Apostomatida.

Apostomatina (ap″o-sto-mah′tĭ-mah) a suborder of ciliate protozoa (order Apostomatida, superorder Apostomatidea) comprising mostly marine crustacean hosts although a few species are associated with polychetes or freshwater crustaceans, characterized by the presence of a cytostome, typically with a rosette, during both immature and mature stages of the life cycle.

apothecary (ah-poth′ĕ-ka″re) [Gr. *apothēke* storehouse] pharmacist. **surgeon a.,** in Great Britain, a practitioner who has passed the examinations required of a surgeon and of an apothecary.

apothecium (ap″o-the′se-um) an open or expanded fruiting body whose asci are contained on its exposed surface. Cf. *cleistothecium, gymnothecium,* and *perithecium.*

apothem (ap′o-them) [*apo-* + Gr. *thema* deposit] a dark deposit that sometimes appears in vegetable infusions and decoctions exposed to the air.

apotheme (ap′o-thēm) apothem.

apotropaic (ap″o-tro-pa′ik) [Gr. *apotropaios* averting evil] prophylactic, in the sense of averting evil influence (in Greek medicine).

apozem, apozema, apozeme (ap′o-zem, ap-oz′e-mah, ap′o-zēm) [Gr. *apozema* decoction, from *apo-* away + *zein* to boil] a medicinal or medicated decoction.

apparatus (ap″ah-ra′tus), pl. *apparatus* or *apparatuses* [L., from *ad* to + *parare* to make ready] an arrangement of a number of parts acting together in the performance of some special function; used in anatomical nomenclature to designate a number of structures or organs which act together in serving some particular function. **Abbe-Zeiss a.,** Thoma-Zeiss counting chamber. **absorption a.,** an apparatus used in gas analysis by means of which the sample to be examined is absorbed and its quantity thus estimated. **Barcroft's a.,** a differential manometer for studying small samples of blood or other tissues. **Beckmann's a.,** an apparatus for determining the molecular weight of a substance by dissolving the substance in a pure liquid and observing either the depression of the freezing point or the elevation of the boiling point of the liquid produced by the dissolved substance. **biliary a.,** the parts concerned in the formation, conduction, and storage of bile, including the secreting cells of the liver, bile ducts, and gallbladder. **central a.,** the dynamic organ of the cell that participates in mitosis; it consists of a centrosome, a centrosphere, and an astrosphere. **chromidial a.,** the chromatin staining material of the cytoplasm of a cell, occurring in the form of granules, rods, strands, and networks. **ciliary a.,** corpus ciliare. **cytopharyngeal a.,** a cytopharynx with walls supported by nematodesmata; see *cyrtos* and *rhabdos.* **a. derivato′rius,** the direct opening of small arteries into small veins without intervention of capillaries, as in phalanges and erectile tissues. **Desault's a.,** Desault's bandage. **digestive a., a. digesto′rius** [NA], the organs associated with the ingestion and digestion of food, including the mouth and associated structures, pharynx, and components of the digestive tube, as well as the associated organs and glands; called also *systema digestorius* [NA alternative]. **Finsen's a.,** Finsen's lamp; see under *lamp.* **genitourinary a.,** a. urogenitalis. **Golgi a.,** see under *complex.* **a. of Golgi-Rezzonico** (*obs.*), spiral filaments seen in the incisures of the myelin sheath, probably artifacts. **a. of Goormaghtigh,** juxtaglomerular cells. **Haldane a.,** see under *chamber.* **Hodgen's a.,** see under *splint.* **Jaquet's a.,** a recording apparatus for venous and cardiac impulses. **Junker a.,** see under *inhaler.* **juxtaglomerular a.,** a collective term for the juxtaglomerular cells in a nephron; see under *cell.* **Kirschner's a.,** Kirsch-

ner's wire. **lacrimal a., a. lacrima′lis** [NA], the system concerned with the secretion and circulation of the tears and the normal fluid of the conjunctival sac; it consists of the lacrimal gland and ducts, and associated structures. See Plate accompanying *eye.* **a. ligamento′sus col′li,** membrana tectoria. **masticatory a.,** the organs and structures involved in mastication, including the teeth and jaws and their supporting structures, temporomandibular joints, mandibular muscles, accessory facial muscles, tongue, lips, cheeks, and oral mucosa together with their innervation. Called also *organs of mastication* and *masticatory system.* **parabasal a.,** the structure comprising the parabasal body and the fibril or thread that connects it to the basal body. **a. of Perroncito,** a mass of fibrils in the form of spirals and networks with newly formed axons which develop in the cut stump of a nerve during regeneration; called also *Perroncito's spirals.* **pilosebaceous a.,** the complex consisting of a hair follicle and its sebaceous gland, and the erector pili muscle. **a. respirato′rius** [NA], **respiratory a.,** the tubular and cavernous organs and structures by means of which pulmonary ventilation and gas exchange between ambient air and the blood are brought about. The chief organs involved are the nose, larynx, trachea, bronchi, bronchioles, and lungs. See Plate 46. Called also *respiratory system* and *systema respiratorium.* **Sayre's a.,** an apparatus for suspending a patient during the application of a plaster-of-Paris jacket. **Soxhlet's a.,** an apparatus by which fatty or lipid constituents can be extracted from solid matter by repeated treatment with distilled solvent. **spindle a.,** see *spindle,* def. 1. **steadiness a.,** see *spindle.* **subneural a.,** evenly spaced, ribbon-like lamellae, formed by infolding of the sarcolemma lining the primary synaptic cleft, and projecting into the underlying sarcoplasm of muscle; the clefts between the lamellae are known as *secondary synaptic clefts.* **sucker a.,** sucker foot; see under *foot.* **a. suspenso′rius len′tis,** zonula ciliaris. **Taylor's a.,** see under *splint.* **a. of Timofeew,** a terminal nervous globular network within a lamellar corpuscle. **Tiselius a.,** an apparatus for the electrophoretic separation of the proteins of blood serum, plasma, and other body fluids. **urogenital a., a. urogenita′lis** [NA], the organs concerned in the production and excretion of urine, together with the organs of reproduction; see Plate L, under *system.* Called also *genitourinary a., genitourinary* or *urogenital system,* and *systema urogenitale.* **vasomotor a.,** the neuromuscular mechanism controlling the constriction and dilation of blood vessels and thus the amount of blood supplied to a part. **Waldenberg's a.,** an apparatus for exhausting or compressing air which is inhaled by the patient or into which the patient exhales. **Wangensteen's a.,** see under *tube.* **Warburg a.,** a device for measuring the quantity of gas liberated or consumed by respiring tissue slices enclosed in a chamber which is attached to a manometer and immersed in water at constant temperature. **Zander a.,** a group of machines designed for exercise of various parts of the body; rarely employed today.

appearance (ah-pēr′ans) [L. *apparere* to be visible] the visible manifestation of the characteristics of an object or entity.

appendage (ah-pen′dij) a thing or part appended; limb. See also *adnexa* and *appendix.* **atrial a., auricular a.,** auricula atrii. **cecal a.,** appendix vermiformis. **a. of epididymis,** appendix epididymidis. **epiploic a's,** appendices epiploicae. **a's of the eye,** the lids, eyebrows, lacrimal apparatus, and conjunctiva; called also *adnexa oculi.* **a's of the fetus,** the trophoblast derivatives or extraembryonic membranes, including the umbilical cord, amnion, and chorion (placenta). **fibrous a. of liver,** appendix fibrosa hepatis. **ovarian a.,** the parovarium. **a's of the skin,** the hair, nails, sebaceous glands, sweat glands, and mammary glands. **testicular a., a. of the testis,** appendix testis. **uterine a's,** the ligaments of the uterus, and the oviducts and the ovaries; called also *adnexa uteri.* **a. of ventricle of larynx,** sacculus laryngis. **vermicular a.,** appendix vermiformis. **vesicular a's of epoophoron,** appendices vesiculosae epoöphorontis.

appendagitis (ah-pen″dah-ji′tis) inflammation of an appendage, particularly of the epiploic appendages. **epiploic a.,** inflammation of one or more of the epiploic appendages of the colon, characterized by pain and tenderness over the affected area.

appendectomy (ap″en-dek′to-me) surgical removal of the

vermiform appendix. **auricular a.,** excision of the auricula atrii.

appendical (ah-pen′de-kal) appendiceal.

appendiceal (ap-en-dis′e-al) pertaining to an appendix.

appendicectomy (ah-pen″dĭ-sek′to-me) [*appendix* + Gr. *ektomē* excision] appendectomy.

appendices (ah-pen′dĭ-sēz) [L.] plural of *appendix*.

appendicitis (ah-pen″dĭ-si′tis) inflammation of the vermiform appendix. **actinomycotic a.,** that caused by *Actinomyces israeli*. **acute a.,** appendicitis of acute onset requiring surgical intervention and usually characterized by pain in the right lower abdominal quadrant with local and referred rebound tenderness, overlying muscle spasm, and cutaneous hyperesthesia. Periumbilical, colicky pain at the onset may be due to obstruction of the appendix by a fecalith. Fever and polymorphonuclear leukocytosis result from the localized infection. Symptoms and signs may be modified by the location of the appendix, by adhesive bands, or by kinking. **amebic a.,** appendicitis caused by infection with *Entamoeba histolytica*. **chronic a.,** 1. appendicitis characterized by fibrotic thickening of the wall of the organ due to previous acute inflammation. 2. a term formerly applied to chronic or recurrent pain in the appendiceal area in the absence of evidence of acute inflammation. **a. by contiguity,** appendicitis caused by infection from neighboring tissues. **foreign-body a.,** appendicitis, usually obstructive, due to a foreign body in the lumen. **fulminating a.,** appendicitis marked by sudden onset and rapid, fatal termination. **gangrenous a.,** appendicitis complicated by gangrene of the organ, owing to interference with the blood supply. **a. granulo′sa,** appendicitis developing on a disease of the mucous membrane which is marked by formation of granulation tissue between the gland tubules (Riedel). **helminthic a.,** verminous appendicitis. **left-sided a.,** 1. diverticulitis; so called because the symptoms resemble those of appendicitis, and the descending (or left) colon is the usual site of involvement. 2. left-sided appendicitis associated with situs inversus. **lumbar a.,** a type of appendicitis in which the appendix is posterior, lying against the peritoneum behind or below the cecum. **a. oblit′erans,** appendicitis with sclerosis and shrinking of the submucous tissue and plastic peritonitis, causing obliteration of the lumen of the appendix; called also *protective a*. **obstructive a.,** a common form of appendicitis attended by obstruction of the lumen of the appendix, usually by a fecalith. **perforating a., perforative a.,** appendicitis with perforation of the organ. **protective a.,** a. obliterans. **purulent a.,** suppurative a. **recurrent a.,** that characterized by recurrent attacks of acute appendicitis. **relapsing a.,** recurrence of appendiceal inflammation after improvement; recurrent appendicitis. **segmental a.,** inflammation confined to a segment of the appendix; it may be proximal, central, or distal. **skip a.,** appendicitis in which two or more areas of focal inflammation are separated by normal appendiceal tissue. **stercoral a.,** appendicitis in which a fecal concretion is the assumed cause. **subperitoneal a.,** appendicitis in which the appendix is buried under the peritoneum instead of being free in the peritoneal cavity. **suppurative a.,** purulent infiltration of the walls of the appendix; called also *purulent a*. **traumatic a.,** appendicitis caused by external trauma. **verminous a.,** appendicitis due to the presence of a worm in the appendix.

appendic(o)- [L. *appendix*, q.v., gen. *appendicis*] a combining form denoting relation to an appendix, especially to the vermiform appendix.

appendicocecostomy (ah-pen″dĭ-ko-se-kos′to-me) the formation of an abnormal opening between the appendix and cecum, usually by surgical means; also, the orifice so established.

appendicocele (ah-pen′dĭ-ko-sēl″) hernia containing the vermiform appendix.

appendicoenterostomy (ah-pen″dĭ-ko″en-ter-os′to-me) the formation of an anastomosis between the vermiform appendix and the intestine.

appendicolithiasis (ah-pen″dĭ-ko″lĭ-thi′ah-sis) [*appendix* + *lithiasis*] a condition marked by concretions in the vermiform appendix.

appendicolysis (ah-pen″dĭ-ko′lĭ-sis) [*appendix* + Gr. *lysis* dissolution] the surgical division of adhesions about the appendix.

appendicopathia (ah-pen″dĭ-ko-path′e-ah) (*obs.*) appendicopathy. **a. oxyu′rica,** disease of the vermiform appendix caused by *Oxyuris*.

appendicopathy (ah-pen″dĭ-kop′ah-the) [*appendix* + Gr. *pathos* disease] any diseased condition of the vermiform appendix.

appendicostomy (ah-pen″dĭ-kos′to-me) [*appendix* + Gr. *stomoun* to provide with an opening, or mouth] surgical creation of an opening from the surface of the abdominal wall into the vermiform appendix for the purpose of irrigating or draining the large bowel.

appendicular (ap″en-dik′u-lar) 1. pertaining to the vermiform appendix. 2. pertaining to an appendage.

appendix (ah-pen′diks), pl. *appendixes, appen′dices* [L. from *appendere* to hang upon] a general term used in anatomical nomenclature to designate a supplementary, accessory, or dependent part attached to a main structure; called also *appendage*. Frequently used alone to refer to the *appendix vermiformis* [NA], or *vermiform appendix* of the colon. **auricular a.,** auricula atrii. **cecal a.,** a. vermiformis. **ensiform a.,** processus xiphoideus. **a. epidid′ymidis** [NA], **a. of epididymis,** a remnant of the mesonephros sometimes situated on the head of the epididymis; called also *appendage of epididymis*. **epiploic appendices, appen′dices epiplo′icae** [NA], peritoneum-covered tabs of fat, 2 to 10 cm. long, attached in rows along the tenia of the colon; called also *appendices omentales* [NA alternative] and *omental appendices*. **a. fibro′sa hep′atis** [NA], **fibrous a. of liver,** a fibrous band at the left extremity of the liver, being the atrophied remnant of formerly more extensive liver tissue. **Morgagni's a.,** see *a. testis* and *appendices vesiculosae epoöphorontis*. **omental appendices,** appendices epiploicae. **appen′dices omenta′les,** NA alternative for *appendices epiploicae*. **a. tes′tis** [NA], the remnant of the müllerian duct (ductus paramesonephricus) on the upper end of the testis; called also *hydatid of Morgagni, morgagnian cyst, sessile hydatid,* and *testicular appendage*. **a. of ventricle of larynx, a. ventricularyn′gis,** sacculus laryngis. **a. vermic′ularis, vermiform a.,** a. vermiformis. **a. vermifor′mis** [NA], vermiform appendix: a wormlike diverticulum of the cecum, varying in length from 3 to 6 inches, and measuring about 1/3 inch in diameter. **appen′dices vesiculo′sae epoöph′ori,** appendices vesiculosae epoöphorontis. **appen′dices vesiculo′sae epoöphoron′tis** [NA], small pedunculated structures attached to the uterine tubes near their fimbriated end, being remnants of the mesonephric ducts; called also *a. morgagnii, appendices vesiculosae epoöphori, hydatids of Morgagni, Morgagni's a., morgagnian cyst,* and *vesicular appendages of epoöphoron*. **xiphoid a.,** processus xiphoideus.

appendolithiasis (ah-pen″do-lĭ-thi′ah-sis) appendicolithiasis.

apperception (ap″er-sep′shun) [L. *ad* to + *percipere* to perceive] conscious perception and appreciation; the power of receiving, appreciating, and interpreting sensory impressions.

apperceptive (ap″er-sep′tiv) pertaining to apperception.

appersonation (ah-per″so-na′shun) appersonification.

appersonification (ap″er-son″ĭ-fi-ka′shun) unconscious identification with another person or delusional belief that one is another person.

appestat (ap′pĕ-stat) [appetite + Gr. *statoe* standing] the brain center (probably in the hypothalamus) concerned with controlling the amount of food intake.

appetite (ap′ĕ-tīt) [L. *appetere* to desire] a natural longing or desire, especially the natural and recurring desire for food.

appetition (ap″ĕ-tish′un) [L. *ad* toward + *petere* to seek] the directing of desire toward a definite purpose or object.

appetitive (ap-pet′ĭ-tiv″) characterized by approach, or exciting approach behavior; said of stimuli or behavior. Cf. *aversive*.

applanation (ap″lah-na′shun) [L. *applanatio*] undue flatness, as of the cornea.

applanometer (ap″lah-nom′ĕ-ter) applanation tonometer.

apple (ap″l) the edible fruit of the rosaceous tree, *Pyrus malus* L. (= *Malus sylvestris* Mill); also the tree itself. Apple seeds are known to be cyanogenetic, and ingestion of large quantities has proven fatal to man. Dried apples in powdered form are used as an antidiarrheal. **Adam's a.,** prominentia laryngea. **bitter a.,** colocynth. **Indian a., May a.,** podophyllum. **thorn a.,** stramonium.

appliance (ah-pli′ans) 1. a device, apparatus, or instrument for performing or facilitating the performance of a particular function. 2. in dentistry, a general term referring to various devices used to provide a function or therapeutic effect, e.g., dental prostheses, obturators, or orthodontic appliances. **Andresen a.,** functional activator. **Begg a.,** an orthodontic appliance consisting of a light wire and brackets permitting the tipping of tooth crowns, horizontal buccal tubes on the appliance anchor molars to prevent their tipping, and elastics. See also *Begg technique,* under *technique.* **Bimler a.,** a removable orthodontic appliance believed to stimulate reflex muscle activity, which in turn produces the desired tooth movement. Called also *Bimler stimulator.* **craniofacial a.,** a device used to immobilize and/or reduce mandibular or midfacial fractures. **Crozat a.,** a removable orthodontic appliance, usually made of a precious metal, used to align teeth during orthodontic therapy. Called *crozat* and *Walker a.* **Denholz a.,** an orthodontic appliance consisting of a wire assembly containing a vestibular acrylic screen and open coil spring segments that fit over the wire arch. **edgewise a.,** a fixed, multiunit orthodontic appliance using a rectangular labial arch wire ligated to brackets cemented to individual teeth or to bands encircling the teeth. So called because the bracket is machined so that the rectangular arch wire is inserted with its long cross section horizontal instead of vertical as in the ribbon arch bracket. Called also *edgewise attachment.* **expansion plate a.,** any orthodontic appliance equipped with an expansion plate. Called also *split plate a.* **extraoral a.,** an orthodontic appliance using a resistance unit outside of the oral cavity; see under *anchorage.* **fixed a.,** an appliance that is cemented to the teeth or attached by means of an adhesive material. Called also *permanent a.* **Frankel a.,** function corrector. **habit-breaking a.,** an orthodontic appliance designed to correct faulty habits, such as finger-sucking, tongue-thrusting, infantile swallowing. **Hawley a.,** see under *retainer.* **Jackson a.,** a removable orthodontic appliance retained in position by crib-shaped wires, bent to follow the outline of the buccal and lingual contours of the bicuspid and molar teeth, and united by cross wires lying in the occlusal embrasures. Called also *Jackson crib.* **Johnson twin wire a.,** twin wire a. **jumping-the-bite a.,** Kingsley a. **Kesling a.,** an occlusal splint made of soft acrylic resin or latex rubber that fits over the occlusal and incisal surfaces of the teeth; it is designed to hold the mandible in a certain relationship to the maxilla to treat bruxism. **Kingsley a.,** an active plate appliance having a bite plate with an inclined anterior plane to move the mandible forward by jumping the bite. Called also *jumping-the-bite a., jumping-the-bite plate,* and *Kingsley plate.* **labiolingual a.,** an orthodontic appliance for intermaxillary therapy, consisting of a maxillary labial arch introduced into horizontal buccal tubes attached to the anchor bands and lingual arches of the same diameter fitted into vertical or horizontal tubes fastened to the lingual side of the anchor bands. **monoblock a.,** functional activator. **orthodontic a.,** a device, either fixed to the teeth or removable, that applies force to the teeth and their supporting structures to produce changes in the relationship of the teeth to each other and to control their growth and development. Used in orthodontic therapy to move the teeth into esthetically desirable positions and physiologic alignment within the dental arch and into proper relationship with the opposing dentition and in the treatment of fractures and injuries of the maxilla to stabilize or immobilize the teeth and jaws. Called also *braces.* **permanent a.,** fixed a. **prosthetic a.,** a device affixed to or implanted in the body, designed to take the place, or perform the function, of a missing body part, such as an artificial arm or leg, or a complete or partial denture. **removable a.,** any orthodontic appliance that the patient is able to insert and remove from the mouth. **ribbon arch a.,** an orthodontic appliance consisting of a flattened wire inserted into a special bracket against the labial and buccal surfaces of the teeth; usually done to move the teeth laterally. Called also *ribbon arch.* **Schwarz a.,** a removable orthodontic appliance with a tissue-borne anchorage and appurtenances of wire for tooth movement. **split plate a.,** expansion plate a. **twin wire a.,** an orthodontic appliance using fixed lingual arches and a labial arch consisting of a pair of round wires attached to brackets on the anterior teeth. Called also

Johnson twin wire a. and *twin wire.* **universal a.,** an orthodontic appliance that combines the edgewise and ribbon arch techniques, affording precise control of individual teeth in all planes of space; it consists of bands or brackets or both for all the teeth in both arches. **Walker a.,** Crozat a.

applicator (ap′lĭ-ka″tor) an instrument for making local applications. **sonic a.,** an electromechanical transducer used in the local application of sound for therapeutic purposes, as in the treatment of muscular ailments.

appliqué (ap″lĭ-ka′) see under *form.*

apposition (ap″o-zish′un) [L. *appositio*] the placing of things in juxtaposition or proximity; specifically, the deposition of successive layers upon those already present, as in cell walls. Called also *juxtaposition.*

apprehension (ap″re-hen′shun) 1. perception and understanding. 2. anticipatory fear or anxiety.

approach (ah-prōch′) surgical approach; the specific anatomic dissection by which an organ or part is exposed in surgery. **Risdon a.,** a surgical method of exposing the ascending ramus of the mandible by means of an incision made below and behind the angle of the mandible, for treatment of fractures, e.g., condylar fractures, or for reconstructive surgery.

approximal (ah-prok′sĭ-mal) situated close together.

approximate (ah-prok′sĭ-māt″) 1. to bring close together, or into apposition. 2. approximal.

approximation (ah-prok″sĭ-ma′shun) the act or process of bringing closer together or into apposition. **successive a.,** shaping.

apractic (ah-prak′tik) pertaining to or characterized by apraxia.

apramycin (ap″rah-mi′sin) an antibacterial antibiotic, $C_{21}H_{41}N_5O_{11}$, produced by *Streptomyces tenebrarius.*

apraxia (ah-prak′se-ah) [Gr. "a not acting," "want of success"] loss of ability to carry out familiar, purposeful movements in the absence of paralysis or other motor or sensory impairment, especially inability to make proper use of an object. **akinetic a.,** loss of ability to carry out spontaneous movement. **amnestic a.,** loss of ability to carry out a movement on command as a result of inability to remember the command, although ability to perform the movement is present. **Bruns' a. of gait,** apraxia in which the patient walks with a broad-based gait, taking short steps with the feet placed flat on the ground and with a tendency to retropulsion. **classic a.,** ideokinetic a. **constructional a.,** a type of motor incapacity characterized by lack of ability to copy simple drawings or to reproduce patterns created with building blocks or matchsticks. **cortical a.,** motor a. **ideational a.,** sensory a. **ideokinetic a., ideomotor a.,** a form due to an interruption between the ideation center and the center for the limb; in it, simple movements can be performed but not complicated ones. Called also *limb-kinetic a.* and *transcortical a.* **innervation a.,** motor a. **Liepmann's a.,** inability to perform coordinated movements of the limbs, without actual paralysis. **limb-kinetic a.,** ideokinetic a. **motor a.,** loss of ability to make proper use of an object, although its proper nature is recognized; called also *cortical* or *innervation a.* **sensory a.,** loss of ability to make proper use of an object, due to lack of perception of its proper nature and purpose; called also *ideational a.* **transcortical a.,** ideokinetic a.

apraxic (ah-prak′sik) apractic.

Apresazide (ah-pres′ah-zīd) trademark for preparations of hydralazine with hydrochlorothiazide.

Apresoline (ah-pres′o-lēn) trademark for preparations of hydralazine.

aprindine (ah-prin′dēn) chemical name: N a-(2,3-dihydro-1H-inden-2-yl)- N′, N′-diethyl-N-phenyl-1,3-propandiamine; a cardiac depressant, $C_{22}H_{30}N_2$, which has been used as an antirrhythmic. **a. hydrochloride,** the monohydrochloride salt of aprindine, $C_{22}H_{30}N_2 \cdot HCl$, having the same actions and uses as the base.

aprobarbital (ap″ro-bar′bĭ-tal) chemical name: 5-(1-methylethyl)-5-(2-propenyl)-2,4,6(1H,3H,5H)-pyrimidinetrione. An intermediate-acting barbiturate, $C_{10}H_{14}N_2O_3$, occurring as a fine, white, crystalline powder; used as a sedative and hypnotic, administered orally. Abuse of this drug may lead to dependence.

Aprocta (ah-prok′tah) a genus of filarial organisms. *A. mi-*

cro-analis and *A. semenova* infest the orbital and nasal cavities of birds.

aproctia (ah-prok′she-ah) [*a* neg. + Gr. *prōktos* anus] congenital absence or imperforation of the anus.

apron (a′prun) a piece of clothing worn as a protection for the body in front. **Hottentot a., pudendal a.,** artificially or abnormally elongated nymphae.

aprosexia (ap″ro-sek′se-ah) [*a* neg. + Gr. *prosechein* to heed] (*obs.*) inability to maintain attention.

aprosody (a-pros′o-de) absence of the normal variations in stress, pitch, and rhythm of speech.

aprosopia (ap″ro-so′pe-ah) [*a* neg. + Gr. *prosōpon* face] partial or complete congenital absence of structures of the face.

aprosopus (ah-pro′so-pus) a monster exhibiting aprosopia.

aprotic (a-pro′tik) denoting a substance that does not possess dissociable protons.

aprotinin (ah-pro-ti′nin) a polypeptide, obtained from animal organs, which inhibits proteinase and kallikrein; it has been used in the treatment of pancreatitis.

A.P.S. American Physiological Society.

apselaphesia (ap″sel-ah-fe′ze-ah) [*a* neg. + Gr. *psēlaphēsis* touch] diminution of the sense of touch.

apsithyria (ap″sĭ-thi′re-ah) [*a* neg. + Gr. *psithyros* whispering + *ia*] (*obs.*) hysterical loss of speech and even of the ability to whisper.

apsychia (ah-si′ke-ah) [*a* neg. + Gr. *psyche* soul + -*ia*] 1. loss or lack of consciousness. 2. a faint or swoon.

A.P.T.A. American Physical Therapy Association.

apterous (ap′ter-us) [*a* neg. + Gr. *pteron* wing] wingless.

Apterygiformes (ap″tĕ-rij″ĭ-form′ēz) the order of kiwis, flightless birds with vestigial wings.

aptitude (ap′tĭ-tūd) natural ability and skill in certain lines of endeavor.

aptyalia, aptyalism (ap″ti-a′le-ah, ap-ti′ah-lizm) [*a* neg. + Gr. *ptyalizein* to spit] deficiency or absence of the saliva; xerostomia; asialia.

APUD [*a*mine *p*recursor *u*ptake (and) *d*ecarboxylation] see under *cell*.

apudoma (ah″pud-o′mah) any tumor composed of APUD cells.

apulmonism (ah-pul′mo-nizm) [*a* neg. + L. *pulmo* lung] a developmental anomaly characterized by pulmonary agenesis.

apus (a′pus) [*a* neg. + Gr. *pous* foot] an individual exhibiting apodia.

apyetous (ah-pi′ĕ-tus) [*a* neg. + Gr. *pyon* pus] showing no pus; not suppurating.

apyknomorphous (ah-pik″no-mor′fus) [*a* neg. + Gr. *pyknos* compact + *morphē* form] not pyknomorphous; not having the stainable cell elements compactly placed—said of certain nerve cells.

apyogenous (ah″pi-oj′ĕ-nus) not caused by pus.

apyous (ah-pi′us) [*a* neg. + Gr. *pyon* pus] having no pus; nonpurulent.

apyrene (ah′pi-rēn) [*a* neg. + Gr. *pyrēn* fruit stone, nucleus] having no nucleus or nuclear material.

apyretic (ah″pi-ret′ik) [*a* neg. + *pyretic*] having no fever; afebrile.

apyrexia (ah″pi-rek′se-ah) [*a* neg. + *pyrexia*] the absence or intermission of fever.

apyrexial (ah″pi-rek′se-al) pertaining to apyrexia, or to the stage of intermission of a fever.

apyrogenic (ah-pi″ro-jen′ik) [*a* neg. + Gr. *pyr* fever + *gennan* to produce] not producing fever.

A.Q. achievement quotient.

Aq. Abbreviation for L. *a′qua,* water. **Aq. dest.,** L. *a′qua destilla′ta,* distilled water. **Aq. pur.,** L. *a′qua pu′ra,* pure water. **Aq. tep.,** L. *a′qua tep′ida,* tepid water.

aqua (ah′kwah, ak′wah), gen. and pl. *a′quae* [L.] water. See also *aromatic water* and various other forms listed under *water.* **a. am′nii,** amniotic fluid. **a. ani′si,** anise water. **a. aromat′ica,** aromatic water. **a. astric′ta,** frozen water. **a. bul′liens,** boiling water. **a. cal′cis,** calcium hydroxide solution. **a. cam′phorae,** camphor water. **a. chlorofor′mi,** chloroform water. **a. cin-**

namo′mi, cinnamon water. **a. commu′nis,** ordinary water. **a. destilla′ta,** distilled water. **a. destilla′ta steril′is,** sterile distilled water. **a. fer′vens,** hot water. **a. foenic′uli,** fennel water. **a. for′tis,** a solution of nitric acid. **a. gaulthe′ria,** wintergreen water. **a. hamamel′idis,** hamamelis water. **a. labyrin′thi** (*obs.*), the clear fluid in the labyrinth of the ear. **a. men′thae piperi′tae,** peppermint water. **a. men′thae vir′idis,** spearmint water. **a. o′culi,** the aqueous humor or fluid of the eye. **a. pericar′dii,** the pericardial fluid. **a. pro injectio′ne,** water for injection. **a. pu′ra,** pure water. **a. re′gia,** a mixture of one part concentrated nitric acid to three or four parts concentrated hydrochloric acid; it is able to dissolve gold and platinum. **a. ro′sae,** rose water. **a. ro′sae for′tior,** stronger rose water. **a. sterilisa′ta,** sterilized water. **a. tep′ida,** warm water. **a. vi′tae,** brandy.

Aquacare (ah′kwah-kār) trademark for preparations of urea.

aquae (ak′we, ah′kwe) [L.] genitive and plural of *aqua.*

aquaeductus (ak″we-duk′tus), gen. and pl. *aquaeduc′tus* [L.] aqueductus.

AquaMEPHYTON (ak″wah-mef′ĭ-ton) trademark for a preparation of phytonadione.

aquaphobia (ak″wah-fo′be-ah) [*aqua-* + *phobia*] irrational fear of water, i.e., of swimming or of being near water where one might fall in and drown.

aquapuncture (ak′wah-pungk″chur) [L. *aqua* water + *puncture*] the subcutaneous injection of water.

Aquaspirillum (ah″kwah-spi-ril′um; ak″wah-spi-ril′um) [*aqua* + *spirillum*] a genus of rigid, generally helical, gram-negative bacteria that are aerobic or microaerophilic and motile with polar flagella; they are found in stagnant, freshwater environments and are considered to be nonpathogenic for humans and animals. The type species is *A. ser′pens.*

Aquatag (ah′kwah-tag) trademark for a preparation of benzthiazide.

Aquatensen (ak″wah-ten′sen) trademark for a preparation of methyclothiazide.

aquatic (ah-kwat′tik) inhabiting or frequenting water.

aqueduct (ak′we-dukt″) a passage or channel in a body structure or organ; see also *aqueductus.* **cerebral a.,** aqueductus mesencephali. **a. of cochlea,** aqueductus cochleae. **a. of Cotunnius,** 1. aqueductus vestibuli. 2. canaliculus cochleae. **fallopian a., a. of Fallopius,** canalis facialis. **a. of mesencephalon,** aqueductus mesencephali. **a. of midbrain,** aqueductus mesencephali. **a. of Sylvius,** aqueductus mesencephali. **ventricular a.,** aqueductus cerebri. **a. of vestibule,** 1. aqueductus vestibuli. 2. ductus endolymphaticus.

aqueductus (ak″we-duk′tus) [L., from *aqua* water + *ductus* canal] [NA] a passage or channel in a body structure or organ, especially a channel for the conduction of fluid; called also *aqueduct* and *aquaeductus.* **a. cer′ebri,** NA alternative for *a. mesencephali.* **a. coch′leae** [NA], aqueduct of cochlea: a small channel that connects the scala tympani with the subarachnoid space; called also *ductus perilymphatici, ductus perilymphaticus,* and *perilymphatic duct.* **a. endolymphat′icus,** ductus endolymphaticus. **a. mesenceph′ali** [NA], aqueduct of mesencephalon: the narrow channel in the mesencephalon that connects the third and fourth ventricles; called also *aqueduct of Sylvius, a. cerebri* [NA alternative], *cerebral aqueduct,* and *iter of Sylvius.* **a. vestib′uli** [NA], aqueduct of vestibule: 1. a small canal extending from the vestibule of the inner ear to open onto the posterior surface of the petrous part of the temporal bone. It lodges the endolymphatic duct and an arteriole and a venule. Called also *aqueduct of Cotunnius.* 2. ductus endolymphaticus.

aqueous (a′kwe-us) 1. watery; prepared with water. 2. the aqueous humor of the eye; see under *humor.*

Aquex trademark for a preparation of clopamide.

aquiparous (ak-wip′ah-rus) [L. *aqua* water + *parere* to produce] producing water or a watery secretion.

aquula (ak′woo-lah), gen. and pl. *a′quulae* [L., dim. of *aqua* water] a little stream. **a. auditi′va exter′na** (*obs.*), perilymph. **a. auditi′va inter′na** (*obs.*), endolymph. **a. cotun′nii,** a. **labyrin′thi exter′na** (*obs.*), perilymph. **a. labyrin′thi inter′na** (*obs.*), a. **labyrin′thi membrana′cei** (*obs.*), endolymph.

AR alarm reaction; aortic regurgitation; artificial respiration.

Ar chemical symbol for *argon*.

ara-A adenine arabinoside; see *vidarabine*.

araban (ar'ah-ban) a pentosan, $(C_5H_{10}O_5)_n$, found in various gums and pectins, consisting of a mixture of anhydrides of l-arabinose.

arabate (ar'ah-bāt) a salt of arabic acid.

arabic acid (ār'ah-bik) arabin.

arabin (ar'ah-bin) an amorphous carbohydrate, $(C_5H_{10}O_5)_2$ $+ H_2O$, from gum arabic, soluble in water; called also *arabic acid*.

arabinose (ah-rab'ĭ-nōs) gum sugar; a crystalline aldopentose, $CH_2OH(CHOH)_3CHO$, obtained from vegetable gums by acid hydrolysis and sometimes found in urine. *d*-Arabinose is a constituent of aloin; *l*-arabinose is the gum sugar.

arabinosis (ah-rab''ĭ-no'sis) poisoning by arabinose, which may produce nephrosis.

arabinosuria (ah-rab''ĭ-no-su're-ah) the presence of arabinose in the urine.

arabinosylcytosine (ah-rab''ĭ-no-sil-si'to-sēn) cytarabine.

arabinulose (ar''ah-bin'u-lōs) a ketopentose.

arabite (ar'ah-bīt) a sweet crystalline principle, $C_5H_{12}O_5$, derivable from arabinose by the action of sodium amalgam.

arabitol (ah-rab'ĭ-tol) an alcohol, $CH_2OH(CHOH)_3CH_2OH$, formed by the reduction of arabinose.

arabopyranose (ar''ah-bo-pi'rah-nōs) arabinose.

ara-C cytosine arabinoside; see *cytarabine*.

arachic acid (ah-rak'ik) arachidic acid.

arachidate (ah-rak'ĭ-dāt) eicosanoate: the ionic form of arachidic acid, $C_{20}H_{40}O_2$, a naturally occurring fatty acid.

arachidic (ar''ah-kid'ik) [L. *arachis* peanut] caused by peanut kernels, as arachidic bronchitis following accidental inhalation of a peanut.

arachidic acid (ar''ah-kid'ik) $CH_3(CH_2)_{18}COOH$, a saturated straight-chain fatty acid containing twenty carbons. It is found in vegetable and fish oils. Called also *eicosanoic acid*, *icosanoic acid*.

arachidonate 5-lipoxygenase (ah-rak'ĭ-don''āt lĭ-pok'-sĕ-jĕ-nās) [EC 1.13.11.34] an enzyme of the oxidoreductase class that catalyzes the reaction arachidonate $+ O_2 = (S)$-5-hydroperoxyarachidonate. The reaction occurs in leukocytes. It is the first step of the lipoxygenase pathway for conversion of arachidonic acid to leukotrienes (A_4, B_4, C_4, D_4, E_4). Called also *lipoxygenase*.

arachidonate 12-lipoxygenase (ah-rak'ĭ-don''āt lĭ-pok'-sĕ-jĕ-nās) [EC 1.13.11.31] an enzyme of the oxidoreductase class that catalyzes the reaction arachidonate $+ O_2 = (S)$-12-hydroperoxyarachidonate. The reaction occurs primarily in platelets. It is the first step of the lipoxygenase pathway for conversion of arachidonic acid to the leukotriene 12-hydroxyeicosatetraenoate (12-HETE). Called also *lipoxygenase*.

arachidonic acid (ah''rah-kĭ-don'ik) $CH_3(CH_2)_4(CH{:}CH{\cdot\cdot}CH_2)_4(CH_2)_2COOH$, 5,8,11,14-eicosatetraenoic acid, an unsaturated fatty acid essential for human nutrition. It occurs in animal fats and is also formed by biosynthesis from dietary linoleic acid. It is a precursor in the biosynthesis of leukotrienes, prostaglandins, and thromboxanes.

arachnephobia (ah-rak''ne-fo'be-ah) arachnophobia.

Arachnia (ah-rak'ne-ah) [Gr. *arachnion* a cobweb] a genus of bacteria of the family Actinomycetaceae, order Actinomycetales. The organisms are gram-positive, anaerobic or microaerophilic, nonsporulating, branched, diphtheroid rods that form thin branching filaments but no mycelia. **A. propion'ica,** a species that is a normal inhabitant of the body cavities and skin of humans and other mammals. It causes human actinomycosis and periodontal disease and infections in cattle.

arachnid (ah-rak'nid) any member of the class Arachnida.

Arachnida (ah-rak'nĭ-dah) [Gr. *arachnē* spider] a class of the Arthropoda, including the spiders, ticks, mites, and scorpions.

arachnidism (ah-rak'nĭ-dizm) the condition produced by the bite of a venomous spider; spider envenomation. Called also *araneism*.

arachnitis (ar''ak-ni'tis) [*arachno-* + *-itis*] arachnoiditis.

arachn(o)- [Gr. *arachnē* spider] a combining form denoting relationship to the arachnoid membrane or to a spider.

arachnodactylia (ah-rak''no-dak-til'e-ah) arachnodactyly.

arachnodactyly (ah-rak''no-dak'tĭ-le) [*arachno-* + Gr. *daktylos* finger] a condition characterized by abnormal length and slenderness of the fingers and toes; called also *acromacria, dolichostenomelia,* and *spider finger*. Sometimes used in the past as a synonym for *Marfan's syndrome*. **contractural a., congenital, (CCA),** a form of hereditary bone dysplasia; see under *dysplasia*.

arachnogastria (ah-rak''no-gas'tre-ah) [*arachno-* + Gr. *gastēr* stomach + *-ia*] the prominent network of veins on the protuberant abdomen caused by ascites, especially in hepatic cirrhosis.

arachnoid (ah-rak'noid) 1. resembling a spider's web. 2. arachnoidea. **a. of brain, cranial a.,** arachnoidea mater encephali. **spinal a., a. of spinal cord,** arachnoidea mater spinalis.

arachnoidal (ar''ak-noi'dal) or of pertaining to the arachnoid.

arachnoidea (ar''ak-noi'de-ah), pl. *arachnoi'deae* [Gr. *arachnoeidēs* like a cobweb] [NA] a delicate membrane interposed between the dura mater and the pia mater, being separated from the pia mater by the subarachnoid space. **a. enceph'ali, a. ma'ter enceph'ali** [NA], the arachnoidea covering the brain; called also *arachnoid of brain* and *cranial arachnoid*. **a. spina'lis, a. ma'ter spina'lis** [NA], spinal arachnoid: the arachnoidea covering the spinal cord; called also *arachnoid of spinal cord*.

arachnoideae (ar''ak-noi'de-e) genitive and plural of *arachnoidea*.

arachnoidism (ah-rak'noi-dizm'') the condition produced by the bite of venomous spiders.

arachnoiditis (ah-rak''noid-i'tis) [*arachnoid* + *-itis*] inflammation of the arachnoidea; called also *arachnitis*. **chronic adhesive a.,** thickening and adhesions of the leptomeninges in the brain or spinal cord, resulting from previous meningitis, other disease processes, or trauma; the signs and symptoms vary with extent and location.

arachnolysin (ar''ak-nol'ĭ-sin) [*arachno-* + *lysin*] the active hemolytic principle of spider venom.

arachnophobia (ah-rak''no-fo'be-ah) [*arachno-* + *phobia*] irrational fear of spiders.

arachnopia (ar''ak-no'pe-ah) [*arachno-* + *pia*] (obs.) the pia-arachnoid.

arachnorhinitis (ah-rak''no-ri-ni'tis) [*arachno-* + *rhinitis*] disease of the nasal passages caused by the presence of a spider.

arack (ah-rak') arrack.

Aradidae (ah-rad'ĭ-de) a family of broad flat bugs which inhabit crevices under bark and similar sites; some species bite man, but are of no medical importance.

Aralen (ār'ah-len) trademark for a preparation of chloroquine.

Aralia (ah-ra'le-ah) [L.] a genus of aromatic and diaphoretic plants, including spikenard or pettymorrel (*A. racemosa*), dwarf elder (*A. hispida*), and other plants used in domestic medicine. Volatile oil appears to be the active constituent. It is one of the ingredients of compound white pine syrup. Called also *spice berry*.

aralia (ah-ra'le-ah) the dried rhizome and roots of *Aralia racemosa;* an ingredient of compound white pine syrup.

aralkyl (ah-ral'kil) an aryl derived from an alkyl radical.

Aramine (ār'ah-min) trademark for a preparation of metaraminol.

Aran's law (ar-ahnz') [François Amilcar *Aran*, French physician, 1817–1861] see under *law*.

Aran-Duchenne muscular atrophy (disease) (ar-ahn'doo-shen') [François Amilcar *Aran;* Guillaume Benjamin Amand *Duchenne*, French neurologist, 1806–1875] spinal muscular atrophy; see under *atrophy*.

Araneae (ah-rān'e-e) an order of the Arachnida comprising the spiders; it is divided into the suborders Labidognatha and Orthognatha.

Araneida (ar''ah-ne'ĭ-dah) Araneae.

araneism (ah-ra'ne-izm)   spider envenomation.

araneous (ah-ra'ne-us) [L. *araneum* cobweb]   like a cob-web.

Arantius' bodies, etc. (ah-ran'she-us) [Julius Caesar *Arantius* (Italian *Aranzi*), an Italian anatomist and physician, 1530–1589]   see under *body, canal, duct, ligament, nodule,* and *ventricle.*

Aranzi   see *Arantius.*

araphia (ah-ra'fe-ah)   dysraphia.

araroba (ar''ah-ro'bah) [Brazilian]   1. *Andira.*   2. Goa powder.

arbaprostil (ar''bah-prost'il)   chemical name: (5Z,11α,13E, 15R)-11, 15-dihydroxy-15-methyl-9-oxo-prosta-5, 13-diene-1-oic acid; a synthetic 15-methyl analogue of dinoprostone, a prostaglandin of the E type, $C_{21}H_{34}O_5$; its esters have been used orally to reduce gastric secretion in the treatment of gastric ulcer and intramuscularly for termination of pregnancy.

Arber (ar'ber), Werner. Swiss microbiologist, born 1929; co-winner, with Daniel Nathans and Hamilton Othanel Smith, of the Nobel prize for medicine or physiology in 1978 for his work on restriction enzymes.

arbor (ar'bor), pl. *arbo'res* [L.]   a treelike structure or part; a structure or system resembling a tree with its branches. **a. bronchia'lis** [NA], bronchial tree: the bronchi and their branching structures. **a. medulla'ris ver'mis,** a. vitae cerebelli. **a. vi'tae,** *Thuja occidentalis,* or white cedar, a tree of the family Cupressaceae, native to eastern North America. Oil from the leaves is used as an expectorant, antirheumatic, and emmenagogue, and externally as a counterirritant and for dermatological diseases. **a. vi'tae cerebel'li** [NA], the treelike outline of white substance seen in a median section of the cerebellum; called also *a. medullaris vermis, a. vitae of vermis, medullary body of vermis, corpus medullare vermis,* and *arborescent white substance of cerebellum.* **a. vi'tae u'teri,** plicae palmatae. **a. vi'tae of vermis,** a. vitae cerebelli.

arboreal (ar-bo're-al)   pertaining to trees; inhabiting or attached to trees.

arbores (ar-bo'rēz) [L.]   plural of *arbor.*

arborescent (ar''bo-res'ent) [L. *arborescens*]   branching like a tree.

arborization (ar''bor-ĭ-za'shun)   1. the branching termination of certain nerve cell processes.   2. a form of the termination of a nerve fiber when in contact with a muscle fiber.   3. the treelike appearance of capillary vessels in inflamed conditions.

arboroid (ar'bo-roid) [L. *arbor* a tree]   branching like a tree.

arborvirus (ar''bor-vi'rus)   former term for *arbovirus.*

arboviral (ar''bo-vi'ral)   pertaining to or caused by arboviruses.

arbovirus (ar'' bo-vi' rus) [from *arthropod-borne* + virus]   any of a group of viruses, including the causative agents of yellow fever, viral encephalitides, and certain febrile infections, which are transmitted to man by various mosquitoes and ticks; those transmitted by ticks are often considered in a separate category (tickborne viruses).

arbutin (ar'bu-tin) [L. *Arbutus*]   see *Arbutus.*

Arbutus (ar-bu'tus) [L.]   a genus of ericaceous trees and shrubs which contain arbutin, a hydroquinone glycoside that has been used for its diuretic and urinary antiseptic properties. **A. u'va-ur'si,** *Arctostaphylos uva-ursi.*

ARC   American Red Cross; anomalous retinal correspondence; AIDS-related complex.

arc (ark) [L. *arcus* bow]   a structure or projected path having a curved or bowlike outline; by extension, a visible electrical discharge generally taking the outline of an arc. In neurophysiology, the pathway of neural reactions. **auricular a., binauricular a.,** a measurement from the center of one auditory meatus to that of the other. **bregmato-lambdoid a.,** the arc extending along the course of the sagittal suture from the bregma to the lambda. **carbon a.,** an electrical discharge between carbon electrodes that gives off an intense white light. **mercury a.,** an electric discharge between electrodes in mercury vapor in a vacuum tube which gives off light rich in ultraviolet rays. **naso-bregmatic a.,** the arc extending from the nasion to the bregma. **naso-occipital a.,** the arc extending from the

nasion to the most inferior part of the external occipital protuberance. **neural a.,** a series of two or more neurons connecting certain receptors and effectors, and constituting the pathway for neural reactions and reflexes; called also *sensorimotor a.* **nuclear a.,** vortex lentis. **reflex a.,** the neural arc utilized in a reflex action; an impulse travels

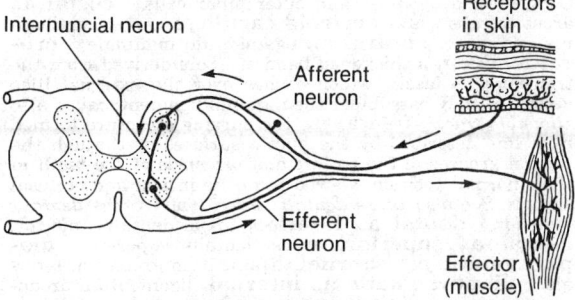

Three-neuron reflex arc.

centrally over afferent fibers to a nerve center, and the response outward to an effector organ or part over efferent fibers. **sensorimotor a.,** neural a. **tungsten a.,** see under *lamp.*

arcade (ar-kād')   an anatomical structure composed of a series of arches. **arterial a's,** a series of anastomosing arterial arches as in the intestinal branches of the superior mesenteric artery. **Flint's a.,** an arteriovenous arch at the base of the renal pyramids.

arcanum (ar-ka'num) [L. "secret"]   a secret medicine or nostrum.

arcate (ar'kāt)   arcuate.

Arcella (ar-sel'ah) [L., dim. of *arcus* box, chest]   a genus of ameboid protozoa (order Arcellinida, subclass Testacealobosia) characterized by the presence of a few slender lobopodia and a transparent test to which the body of the organism is attached by numerous strands of ectoplasm.

Arcellinida (ar''sĕ-lin'ĭ-dah)   an order of free-living protozoa (subclass Testacealobosia, class Lobosia) comprising those amebas enclosed in a test, tectum, or other external membrane that is composed of either organic or inorganic material or both and has a definite aperture through which pseudopodia (lobopodia or filopodia) can be extruded. Representative genera include *Arcella* and *Difflugia.* Called also *Testacea* and *Testacida.*

arch (arch) [L. *arcus* bow]   a structure with a curved or bowlike outline; see also *arcus.* **abdominothoracic a.,** the lower boundary of the front of the thorax. **alveolar a.,** an arch formed by the ridge of the alveolar process of the mandible or maxilla; see *arcus alveolaris mandibulae* and *arcus alveolaris maxillae.* **anterior a. of atlas,** arcus anterior atlantis. **a. of aorta,** arcus aortae. **aortic a's,** paired vessels arching from the ventral to the dorsal aorta through the branchial arches of fishes and amniote embryos. In mammalian development, arches 1 and 2 disappear; arch 3 joins the common to the internal carotid; the left arch 4 remains as the arch of the definitive aorta while the right arch 4 joins the aorta to the subclavian artery; arch 5 disappears; and the ventral halves of arch 6 form the pulmonary arteries while the connections to the dorsal aorta are lost, although the left half, or ductus arteriosus, serves until birth. **arterial a's of kidney,** arteriae arcuatae renis. **axillary a.,** a muscular slip occasionally arising from the cranial border of the latissimus dorsi muscle, crossing the axilla ventral to the axillary vessels and nerves, and joining the under surface of the tendon of the pectoralis major, the coracobrachialis, or the fascia of the biceps brachii muscle. **a. of azygos vein,** arcus venae azygou. **basal a.,** apical base. **branchial a's,** paired arched columns that bear the gills in lower aquatic vertebrates and that, in the embryos of higher vertebrates, appear in comparable form before subsequent modification into structures of the ear and neck. Each arch contains a cartilaginous bar, consisting of right and left halves. The first arch (*mandibular a.*) differentiates into the sphenomandibular and anterior malleolar ligaments, malleus, and incus, the second (*hyoid a.*) into the styloid process, stylohyoid ligament, lesser cornu of the hyoid bone, and cranial part of the hyoid body, the third into the greater cornu of the hyoid bone and the caudal part of its body, and the fourth and fifth into certain laryngeal cartilages. Called also *pharyngeal a's* and *visceral a's.* **carpal a., anterior,** an arch formed by anastomosis of the anterior carpal branches of the radial and ulnar arteries. **carpal a., dorsal, carpal a., posterior,** rete carpi dorsale. **a's of Corti,** a series of arches in the organ of Corti formed by inner and outer pillar cells. **costal a.,** arcus costalis. **a. of cricoid cartilage,** arcus cartilaginis cricoideae. **crural a.,** ligamentum inguinale. **crural a., deep,** a thickened band of fibers derived from the transversalis fascia, which arches over the external iliac vessels as they pass under the inguinal ligament; called also *iliopubic tract.* **dental a.,** the curving structure formed by a line described by the buccal surfaces or through the central grooves of the molars and bicuspids of the teeth in their normal position, viewed from the incisal and occlusal aspects. See also *arcus dentalis inferior* and *arcus dentalis superior.* **dental a., inferior,** arcus dentalis inferior. **dental a., superior,** arcus dentalis superior. **diaphragmatic a., external,** ligamentum arcuatum laterale. **diaphragmatic a., internal,** ligamentum arcuatum mediale. **digital venous a's,** arcus venosi digitales. **dorsal venous a. of foot,** arcus venosus dorsalis pedis. **double aortic a.,** a congenital anomaly in which the aorta divides into two branches which embrace the trachea and esophagus and reunite to form the descending aorta. **epiphyseal a.,** the embryonic structure in the roof of the third ventricle from which the pineal body develops. **femoral a., superficial,** ligamentum inguinale. **fibrous a. of soleus muscle,** arcus tendineus musculi solei. **a's of foot,** see *arcus pedis longitudinalis* and *arcus pedis transversalis.* **glossopalatine a.,** arcus palatoglossus. **Haller's a's,** see *ligamentum arcuatum laterale* and *ligamentum arcuatum mediale.* **hemal a.,** the arch formed by the body, pedicles, and transverse processes of a vertebra, a pair of ribs and their costal cartilages, and the sternum; the sum of all such arches forming the thoracic cage. **hyoid a.,** the second branchial arch; see *branchial a's.* **inguinal a.,** ligamentum inguinale. **jugular venous a.,** arcus venosus juguli. **Langer's axillary a.,** axillary a. **lingual a.,** a wire appliance made to conform to the lingual aspect of the dental arch; used to promote or to prevent movement of the teeth in orthodontic therapy. **lingual a., fixed,** a space-retaining appliance consisting of an arch wire designed to fit the lingual surface of the teeth, and soldered to metal crowns or orthodontic bands. Called also *stationary lingual a.* **lingual a., passive,** an orthodontic appliance for maintaining space and preserving arch length when bilateral primary molars are prematurely lost. **lingual a., stationary,** fixed lingual a. **longitudinal a. of foot,** arcus pedis longitudinalis. **lumbocostal a., external, of diaphragm,** ligamentum arcuatum laterale. **lumbocostal a., internal, of diaphragm,** ligamentum arcuatum mediale. **lumbocostal a., lateral, of Haller,** ligamentum arcuatum laterale. **lumbocostal a., medial, of Haller,** ligamentum arcuatum mediale. **malar a.,** arcus zygomaticus. **mandibular a.,** 1. the first branchial arch; see *branchial a's.* 2. arcus dentalis inferior. **maxillary a.,** 1. palatal a. 2. arcus dentalis superior. **nasal a.,** the arch formed by the nasal bones and by the nasal processes of the maxilla. **neural a. of vertebra,** arcus vertebrae. **open pubic a.,** a congenital anomaly in which the pubic arch is not fused, the bodies of the pubic bones being spread apart. **oral a.,** see *palatal a.* **orbital a. of frontal bone,** margo supraorbitalis ossis frontalis. **palatal a.,** the arch formed by the roof of the mouth from the teeth on one side of the maxilla to the teeth on the other or, if the teeth are missing, from the residual dental arch on one side to that on the other. Called also *maxillary a., palatomaxillary a.,* and *oral a.* **palatine a., anterior,** arcus palatoglossus. **palatine a., posterior,** arcus palatopharyngeus. **palatoglossal a.,** arcus palatoglossus. **palatomaxillary a.,** palatal a. **palatopharyngeal a.,** arcus palatopharyngeus. **palmar arterial a., deep,** arcus palmaris profundus. **palmar arterial a., superficial,** arcus palmaris superficialis. **palmar venous a., deep,** arcus venosus palmaris profundus. **palmar venous a., superficial,** arcus venosus palmaris superficialis. **palpebral a., inferior,** arcus palpebralis inferior. **palpebral a., superior,** arcus palpebralis superior. **paraphyseal a.,** the embryonic structure in the roof of the third ventricle of vertebrates from which the paraphysis develops.

a. of pelvis, angulus subpubicus. **pharyngeal a's,** branchial a's. **pharyngoepiglottic a.,** arcus palatopharyngeus. **pharyngopalatine a.,** arcus palatopharyngeus. **plantar a.,** see *arcus plantaris profundus, arcus plantaris superficialis,* and *arcus plantaris venosus.* **plantar a., deep, plantar arterial a.,** arcus plantaris profundus. **plantar venous a.,** arcus venosus plantaris. **popliteal a.,** ligamentum popliteum arcuatum. **postaural a's,** branchial a's. **posterior a. of atlas,** arcus posterior atlantis. **pubic a., a. of pubis,** arcus pubis. **pulmonary a's,** the most caudal of the aortic arches, which become the pulmonary arteries. **residual a., residual dental a.,** the curved contour of the ridge remaining after tooth removal. **ribbon a.,** see under *appliance.* **a. of ribs,** arcus costalis. **right aortic a.,** a congenital anomaly in which the aorta is displaced to the right and passes behind the esophagus, thus forming a vascular ring that may cause compression of the trachea and esophagus. **Riolan's a.,** the arch formed by the mesentery of the transverse colon. **Shenton's a.,** Shenton's line. **subpubic a.,** angulus subpubicus. **superciliary a.,** arcus superciliaris. **supraorbital a. of frontal bone,** margo supraorbitalis ossis frontalis. **tarsal a's,** see *arcus palpebralis inferior* and *arcus palpebralis superior.* **tendinous a.,** arcus tendineus. **tendinous a. of diaphragm, external,** ligamentum arcuatum laterale. **tendinous a. of diaphragm, internal,** ligamentum arcuatum mediale. **tendinous a. of levator ani muscle,** arcus tendineus musculi levatoris ani. **tendinous a. of lumbodorsal fascia,** ligamentum lumbocostale. **tendinous a. of pelvic fascia,** arcus tendineus fasciae pelvis. **tendinous a. of soleus muscle,** arcus tendineus musculi solei. **a. of thoracic duct,** see *ductus thoracicus.* **thyrohyoid a.,** the third pharyngeal arch, which becomes represented by the greater cornu of the hyoid bone. **transverse a. of foot,** arcus pedis transversalis. **Treitz's a.,** an arch composed of the left superior colic artery and the inferior mesenteric vein; it lies between the ascending portion of the duodenum and the inner edge of the left kidney. **venous a's of kidney,** venae arcuatae renis. **a. of vertebra, vertebral a.,** arcus vertebrae. **visceral a's,** branchial a's. **volar venous a., deep,** arcus venosus palmaris profundus. **volar venous a., superficial,** arcus venosus palmaris superficialis. **V-shaped a.,** a dental arch which narrows and comes to a point at the lingual junction of the maxillary central incisors. **Zimmermann's a.,** an inconstant, rudimentary arch of the embryo, supposed to explain the origin of certain occasionally occurring vessels between the fourth aortic and the pulmonary arch. **zygomatic a.,** arcus zygomaticus.

arch- See *archi-.*

Archaebacteria (ar″ke-bak-te′re-ah) Archaeobacteria.

archae(o)- see *archi-.*

Archaeobacteria (ar″keo-bak-te′re-ah) [*archeo + bacteria*] a group of bacteria made up of the methanogenic bacteria (Methanobacteriaceae), the extreme halophilic bacteria (Halobacteriaceae), and the thermoacidophilic bacteria (*Sulfolobus, Thermoplasma*). These organisms differ from other bacteria in the sequence of ribosomal RNA, in the absence of muramic acid in their cell walls, and in the lack of glyceryl esters in cell lipids. They appear to be remnants of a primitive group of organisms that were capable of synthesizing organic compounds before evolution of the photosynthetic mechanism. Called also *Archaebacteria.*

archaeocerebellum (ar″ke-o-ser″ĕ-bel′um) [*archaeo-* + L. *cerebellum,* dim. of *cerebrum* brain] [NA] the phylogenetically old part of the cerebellum; namely, the flocculonodular node and the lingula, which are principally supplied by vestibulocochlear fibers; the lingula also receives spinocerebellar fibers. Called also *archicerebellum* and *vestibulocerebellum,* and spelled also *archeocerebellum* [NA alternative]. Cf. *neocerebellum* and *palaeocerebellum.*

archaeocortex (ar″ke-o-kor′teks) [*archaeo-* + L. *cortex* bark, rind, shell] [NA] that portion of the cerebral cortex that, with the palaeocortex, develops in association with the olfactory system, and which is phylogenetically older than the neocortex and lacks its layered structure. The embryonic archaeocortex corresponds to the cortex of the dentate gyrus and hippocampus in mature mammals. Called also *archicortex, archipallium,* and *heterotypical* or *olfactory cortex,* and spelled also *archeocortex* [NA alternative].

archaeus (ar-ke′us) Paracelsus' term for the vital principle, the living force in the body or the animate universe.

Archagathus (ark-ag′ah-thus) the first Greek physician
to practice in Rome (219 B.C.), according to Pliny. At first
known as "the wound-curer" (*Vulnerarius*), because of his
surgical exploits he was later termed "the executioner"
(*Carnifex*).

archaic (ar-ka′ik) [Gr. *archaios* ancient] very ancient; pertaining to early evolutionary stages.

archamphiaster (ark-am′fe-as″ter) [*arch-* + Gr. *amphi*
around + *astēr* star] the primitive amphiaster associated
with the formation of polar bodies.

Archangelica (ar″kan-jel′e-kah) [L. from Gr. *archangelikos*
archangelic] a genus of umbelliferous plants. See *angelica*.

Archangiaceae (ark-an″je-a′se-e) a family of gliding bacteria of the order Myxobacterales, found in soils, made up of
tapered cells that produce microcysts. It contains the genus
Archangium.

Archangium (ark-an′je-um) [*arche-* + Gr. *angeion* vessel]
a genus of gliding bacteria of the family Archangiaceae, order
Myxobacterales, found in soil. The type species is *A. ge′phyra*.

arche- see *archi-*.

archebiosis (ar″ke-bi-o′sis) [*arche-* + Gr. *biōsis* way of life]
the spontaneous generation of organisms, a concept proved to
be false; called also *archegenesis, archigenesis,* or *archegony*.

archecentric (ar″kĕ-sen′trik) [*arche-* + *centric*] denoting
a primitive type of structure from which the other types in
the members of the group are derived.

archegenesis (ar″kĕ-jen′ĕ-sis) [*arche-* + Gr. *genesis* repro-
duction] archebiosis.

archegonium (ar″kĕ-go′ne-um) [*arche-* + Gr. *gonos* off-
spring] the female organ of a cryptogamic plant taking
part in the formation of sexually produced spores; cf.
antheridium.

archegony (ar-keg′o-ne) [*arche-* + Gr. *gonē* seed] archebiosis.

archencephalon (ar″ken-sef′ah-lon) [*arche-* + Gr. *enkephalos* brain] the primitive brain, anterior to the end of
the notochord, from which the midbrain and the forebrain
are developed.

archenteron (ar-ken′ter-on) [*arche-* + Gr. *enteron* intestine]
the primitive digestive cavity of those embryonic forms whose
blastula becomes a gastrula by invagination; called also
archigaster, coelenteron, gastrocoele, and *primitive gut*.

archeo- see *archi-*.

archeocerebellum (ar″ke-o-ser″ĕ-bel′um) [*archeo-* + L. *cerebellum*, dim. of *cerebrum* brain] NA alternative spelling
of *archaeocerebellum*.

archeocinetic (ar″ke-o-si-net′ik) archeokinetic.

archeocortex (ar″ke-o-kor′teks) [*archeo-* + L. *cortex* bark,
rind, shell] NA alternative spelling for *archaeocortex*.

archeokinetic (ar″ke-o-ki-net′ik) [Gr. *archaios* ancient +
kinēsis motion] a term applied to the primitive type of
motor nerve mechanism, as seen in the peripheral and
ganglionic nervous systems; cf. *neokinetic* and *paleokinetic*.

archespore (ar′kĕ-spor) [*arche-* + Gr. *sporos* seed] the
mass of cells that give rise to spore mother cells; called also
archesporium and *archispore*.

archesporium (ar″kĕ-spo′re-um) archespore.

archetype (ar″kĕ-tīp) [*arche-* + Gr. *typos* type] an ideal,
original, or standard type or form.

archi-, arch-, archae(o), arche(o)- [Gr. *arche, arch(i)-,*
related to *archē,* beginning, *archos* leader, *archein* to begin,
to rule] 1. a combining form denoting chief or leader. 2. a
combining form denoting first, beginning, or original.

archiblast (ar′kĭ-blast) [*archi-* + Gr. *blastos* germ] 1. the
components of an ovum that actively form the embryo, as
distinguished from the yolk. 2. His' term for the fundamental part of the blastodermic layers as distinguished from
the parablast or peripheral portion of the mesoderm.

archiblastic (ar″kĭ-blas′tik) derived from or pertaining to
the archiblast.

archicarp (ar′kĭ-karp) the group of cells, including the ascogonium, that give rise to the fruiting body of ascomycetous
fungi. Cf. *ascocarp*. See also *ascogonium*.

archicenter (ar″kĭ-sen′ter) [*archi-* + Gr. *kentron* sharp point]

an archetype; an organ or organism that is the primitive form
from which another organ or organism is descended.

archicentric (ar-kĭ-sen′trik) pertaining to an archicenter.

archicerebellum (ar″kĭ-ser″ĕ-bel′um) [*archi-* + *cerebellum*]
archaeocerebellum.

archicortex (ar″kĭ-kor′teks) archaeocortex.

archicyte (ar′kĭ-sīt) [*archi-* + Gr. *kytos* hollow vessel] zygote.

archicytula (ar″kĭ-sit′u-lah) [*archi-* + Gr. *kytos* hollow ves-
sel] a fertilized ovum in the stage in which the nucleus is
first discernible.

archigaster (ar′kĭ-gas″ter) [*archi-* + Gr. *gastēr* belly]
archenteron.

archigastrula (ar″kĭ-gas′troo-lah) [*archi-* + *gastrula*] the
gastrula in its most primitive form of development.

Archigenes (ar-kij′ĕ-nēz) **of Apamea** (c. 53 to c. 117) a
Greek physician, a pupil of Agathinus, an Eclectic influenced
by Pneumatist theories. He practiced at Rome and wrote
several works, including observations on amputation and
ligation, some portions of which are preserved. Galen's theory
of pulse was taken from Archigenes'.

archigenesis (ar-kĭ-jen′ĕ-sis) archebiosis.

Archigregarinida (ar″ke-greg″ah-ri′nĭ-dah) [*archi-* + L.
gregarius crowding together] an order of parasitic protozoa (subclass Gregarinia, class Sporozoea), having an apparently primitive life cycle characteristically including merogony, gametogony, and sporogony and aseptate gamonts;
found in annelids, sipunculids, hemichordates, and ascidians.

archikaryon (ar″kĭ-kar′e-on) [*archi-* + Gr. *karyon* kernel]
the nucleus of a fertilized ovum.

archil (ar′kil) the lichen *Roccella tinctoria;* also, a violet
coloring matter from this and other lichens, employed as an
indicator dye for litmus paper: alkalies give a blue color, and
acids a red color.

archimorula (ar-kĭ-mor′u-lah) [*archi-* + *morula*] a mass
of cells arising from the division of the archicytula and
preceding the archigastrula.

archinephron (ar″kĭ-nef′ron) [*archi-* + Gr. *nephros* kidney]
a unit of the pronephros.

archineuron (ar″kĭ-nu′ron) [*archi-* + Gr. *neuron* nerve]
the neuron at which an efferent impulse starts (Waldeyer).

archipallial (ar″kĭ-pal′e-al) pertaining to the archipallium.

archipallium (ar″kĭ-pal′e-um) [*archi-* + L. *pallium* cloak]
archaeocortex.

archiplasm (ar′kĭ-plazm″) [*archi-* + Gr. *plasma* something
formed] (*obs.*) Boveri's name for the material of the spindle fibers and astral rays. This material was thought to exist
during the entire cell cycle but to become visible after
aggregation at mitosis.

archispore (ar′kĭ-spor) archespore.

Archistomatina (ar″ke-sto″mah-ti′nah) [*archi-* + Gr. *stoma*
mouth] a suborder of commensal ciliate protozoa (order
Protostomatida, subclass Gymnostomatia) found principally
in equids, and characterized by the presence of an apical
cytostome and the simplest type of circumoral infraciliature,
i.e., closely packed kinetosomes, and somatic ciliature mostly
occurring in tufts or bands; no toxicysts are present.

archistome (ar′kĭ-stōm) [*archi-* + Gr. *stoma* mouth] blastopore.

archistriatum (ar″ke-stri-a′tum) [*archi-* + *striatum*] the
primitive corpus striatum, represented in man by the corpus
amygdaloideum.

architectonic (ar″ke-tek-ton′ik) 1. pertaining to architectural pattern. 2. the structure or construction of, as architectonic structure of the brain.

arch(o)- [Gr. *archos* rectum] (*obs.*) a combining form formerly used to denote relationship to the rectum or anus.

archocystosyrinx (ar″ko-sis″to-sir′inks) [*archo-* + Gr. *kystis* bladder + *syrinx* pipe] fistula of the anus and bladder.

archoptosis (ar″ko-to′sis) [*archo-* + Gr. *ptōsis* fall] (*obs.*)
prolapse of the lower rectum through the anal canal.

archorrhagia (ar″ko-ra′je-ah) [*archo-* + Gr. *rhēgnynai* to
burst forth + *-ia*] (*obs.*) hemorrhage from the rectum.

archorrhea (ar″ko-re′ah) [*archo-* + Gr. *rhoia* flow] (*obs.*) a
liquid discharge from the rectum.

archosyrinx (ar″ko-sir′inks) [*archo-* + Gr. *syrinx* pipe] (*obs.*) 1. fistula in ano. 2. a rectal syringe.

archusia (ar-ku′se-ah) a hypothetical substance once thought to be necessary for cell growth.

arciform (ar′sĭ-form) [L. *arcus* bow + *forma* shape] bow-shaped; arcuate.

arctation (ark-ta′shun) [L. *arctatio*] contracture or narrowing of any canal or opening.

Arctostaphylos uva-ursi (ark″to-staf′ĭ-los u′vah-ur′si) the bearberry shrub of the family Ericaceae. The fruits are edible, and the leaves are used medicinally as an astringent, diuretic tea. It contains arbutin (see *Arbutus*). Called also *Arbutus uva-ursi* L.

arcual (ar′ku-al) [L. *arcualis*] pertaining to an arch.

arcualia (ar′ku-a′le-ah) nodules of cartilage in the continuous mesenchymal sheath in close apposition to the external surface of the notochord in vertebrate embryos.

arcuate (ar′ku-āt) [L. *arcuatus* bow shaped] shaped like an arc; arranged in arches.

arcuation (ark-u-a′shun) [L. *arcuatio*] curvature; especially an abnormal curvature.

arcus (ar′kus), pl. *ar′cus* [L. "a bow"] an arch; a general term used in anatomical nomenclature to designate any structure having a curved or bowlike outline. **a. adipo′sus,** a. corneae. **a. alveola′ris mandib′ulae** [NA], alveolar arch of mandible: the superior free border of the alveolar process of the mandible. Called also *alveolar border* or *alveolar limbus of mandible,* and *limbus alveolaris mandibulae.* **a. alveola′ris maxil′lae** [NA], alveolar arch of maxilla: the inferior free border of the alveolar process of the maxilla; called also *alveolar border* or *alveolar limbus of maxilla,* and *limbus alveolaris maxillae.* **a. ante′rior atlan′tis,** anterior arch of atlas: the more slender portion joining the lateral masses of the atlas ventrally, constituting about one-fifth of the entire circumference of the atlas. **a. aor′tae** [NA], arch of the aorta: the continuation of the ascending aorta, giving rise to the brachiocephalic trunk, and the left common carotid and left subclavian arteries; it continues as the thoracic aorta (aorta thoracica). **a. cartilag′inis cricoi′deae** [NA], arch of cricoid cartilage: the slender anterior portion of the cricoid cartilage. **a. cor′neae, a. cornea′lis,** a white or gray opaque ring in the corneal margin, present at birth, or appearing later in life, and becoming quite frequent in those over 50; it results from cholesterol deposits in or hyalinosis of the corneal stroma and may be associated with ocular defects or with familial hyperlipidemia. Called also *a. adiposus, a. juvenilis, a. lipoides corneae,* and *a. senilis.* **a. costa′lis** [NA], **a. costa′rum,** costal arch: the anterior portion of the apertura thoracis inferior, consisting of the costal cartilages of ribs 7 to 10, inclusive; called also *arch of ribs.* **a. denta′lis infe′rior** [NA], inferior dental arch: the portion of the dental arch formed by the teeth of the mandible. Called also *mandibular arch.* **a. denta′lis supe′rior** [NA], superior dental arch: the portion of the dental arch formed by the teeth of the maxilla. Called also *maxillary arch.* **a. dorsa′lis pe′dis,** arteria arcuata pedis. **a. duc′tus thora′cici** [NA], the arch of the thoracic duct; see *ductus thoracicus.* **a. glossopalati′nus,** a. palatoglossus. **a. iliopectin′eus** [NA], the fascial partition that separates the lacuna musculorum and the lacuna vasorum; called also *fascia iliopectinea.* **a. inguina′lis,** NA alternative for *ligamentum inguinale.* **a. juveni′lis,** 1. a. corneae. 2. Axenfeld's anomaly. **a. lipoi′des cor′neae,** a. corneae. **a. lipoi′des myrin′gis,** a ring of degeneration in the tympanic membrane of the aged. **a. lumbocosta′lis latera′lis,** ligamentum arcuatum laterale. **a. lumbocosta′lis media′lis,** ligamentum arcuatum mediale. **a. palati′ni,** see *a. palatoglossus* and *a. palatopharyngeus.* **a. palatoglos′sus** [NA], palatoglossal arch: the anterior of the two folds of mucous membrane on either side of the oropharynx, connected with the soft palate and enclosing the palatoglossal muscle; called also *a. glossopalatinus, glossopalatine arch, anterior palatine arch,* and *anterior column* or *pillar of fauces.* **a. palatopharyn′geus** [NA], palatopharyngeal arch: the posterior of the two folds of mucous membrane on each side of the oropharynx, connected with the soft palate and enclosing the palatopharyngeal muscle; called also *a. pharyngopalatinus, pharyngopalatine* or *pharyngoepiglottic arch, posterior palatine arch,* and *posterior column* or *pillar of fauces.* **a. palma′ris profun′dus**

[NA], deep palmar arterial arch: an arch formed by the terminal part of the radial artery and its anastomosis with the deep branch of the ulnar, and extending from the base of the metacarpal bone of the little finger to the proximal end of the first interosseous space; it gives off palmar metacarpal arteries and perforating branches. Called also *a. volaris profundus.* **a. palma′ris superficia′lis** [NA], superficial palmar arterial arch: an arch formed by the terminal part of the ulnar artery and its anastomosis with the superficial palmar branch of the radial, giving rise to the palmar digital arteries and supplying blood to the palmar aspect of the hands and fingers. Called also *a. volaris superficialis.* **a. palpebra′les,** see *a. palpebralis inferior* and *a. palpebralis superior.* **a. palpebra′lis infe′rior** [NA], inferior palpebral arch: an arch derived from the medial palpebral artery, supplying the lower lid of the eye; called also *a. tarseus inferior.* **a. palpebra′lis supe′rior** [NA], superior palpebral arch: an arch derived from the medial palpebral artery, supplying the upper lid of the eye; called also *a. tarseus superior.* **a. parieto-occipita′lis,** the curved convolution formed by the backward continuation into the occipital lobe of the superior postcentral sulcus. **a. pe′dis longitudina′lis** [NA], the longitudinal arch of the foot, comprising the pars medialis and the pars lateralis. **a. pe′dis transversa′lis** [NA], transverse arch of foot: the metatarsal arch of the foot, formed by the navicular, cuneiform, cuboid, and the five metatarsal bones. **a. pharyngopalati′nus,** a. palatopharyngeus. **a. planta′ris,** a. plantaris profundus. **a. planta′ris profun′dus** [NA], deep plantar arch: the deep arterial arch in the foot, formed by the anastomosis of the lateral plantar artery with the deep plantar branch of the dorsal artery of the foot, and giving off the plantar metatarsal arteries. Called also *plantar arch, plantar arterial arch,* and *arcus plantaris.* **a. poste′rior atlan′tis** [NA], posterior arch of atlas: the slender portion joining the lateral masses of the atlas dorsally, constituting about two-fifths of the entire circumference of the atlas. **a. pu′bicus,** NA alternative for *a. pubis.* **a. pu′bis** [NA], pubic arch: the arch formed by the conjoined rami of the ischial and pubic bones of the two sides of the body. Called also *a. pubicus* [NA alternative]. **a. senil′is,** a. corneae. **a. supercilia′ris** [NA], superciliary arch: a smooth elevation arching upward and laterally from the glabella, a little above the margin of the orbit. **a. tar′seus infe′rior,** a. palpebralis inferior. **a. tar′seus supe′rior,** a. palpebralis superior. **a. tendin′eus** [NA], tendinous arch: a linear thickening of fascia over some part of a muscle, such as that over the soleus or the obturator internus. **a. tendin′eus fas′ciae pel′vis** [NA], tendinous arch of pelvic fascia: a thickening of the superior fascia, extending from the ischial spine to the posterior part of the body of the pubis. **a. tendin′eus mus′culi levato′ris a′ni** [NA], tendinous arch of levator ani muscle: a linear thickening of the fascia over the levator ani muscle. **a. tendin′eus mus′culi so′lei** [NA], tendinous arch of soleus muscle: an aponeurotic band in the front part of the soleus muscle, extending from a tubercle on the neck of the fibula to the soleal line of the tibia. **a. ve′nae azy′gou** [NA], arch of azygos vein: an arch formed by the azygos vein above the root of the right lung. **a. veno′si digita′les,** digital venous arches: communicating branches of veins across the backs of the fingers at their bases. **a. veno′sus dorsa′lis pe′dis** [NA], dorsal venous arch of foot: a transverse venous arch across the dorsum of the foot near the bases of the metatarsal bones. **a. veno′sus jug′uli** [NA], jugular venous arch: a transverse connecting trunk between the anterior jugular veins of either side. **a. veno′sus palma′ris profun′dus** [NA], deep palmar venous arch: a venous arch accompanying the deep palmar arterial arch; called also *a. volaris venosus profundus.* **a. veno′sus palma′ris superficia′lis** [NA], superficial palmar venous arch: a venous arch accompanying the superficial palmar arterial arch; called also *a. volaris venosus superficialis.* **a. veno′sus planta′ris** [NA], plantar venous arch: the deep venous arch that accompanies the arterial plantar arch. **a. ver′tebrae** [NA], vertebral arch: the bony arch composed of the laminae and pedicles of a vertebra; called also *a. vertebralis* [NA alternative], *arch of vertebra,* and *neural arch of vertebra.* **a. vertebra′lis,** NA alternative for *a. vertebrae.* **a. vola′ris profun′dus,** a. palmaris profundus. **a. vola′ris superficia′lis,** a. palmaris superficialis. **a. vola′ris veno′sus profun′dus,** a. venosus palmaris profundus. **a. vola′-**

ris veno′sus superficia′lis, a. venosus palmaris superficialis. **a. zygomat′icus** [NA], zygomatic arch: the arch formed by the articulation of the broad temporal process of the zygomatic bone and the slender zygomatic process of the temporal bone, giving attachment to the masseter muscle and serving as a line of demarcation between the temporal and infratemporal fossae; called also *malar arch.*

ARD acute respiratory disease (of any undefined form).

ardanesthesia (ar″dan-es-the′ze-ah) [L. *ardor* heat + *anesthesia*] thermanesthesia.

ardent (ar′dent) [L. *ardere* to glow] 1. hot or feverish. 2. characterized by eager desire.

ardor (ar′dor) [L.] 1. intense heat. 2. eager desire. **a. uri′nae,** a scalding sensation during the passage of urine. **a. ventric′uli** (*obs.*), pyrosis or heartburn.

Arduen′na (ar″du-en′nah) *Ascarops.*

area (a′re-ah), pl. *a′reae* or *areas* [L.] a limited space; a general term used in anatomical nomenclature to designate a specific surface or functional region. See also *region.* **acoustic a., a. acus′tica,** a. vestibularis. **alisphenoid a.,** the surface of the great wing of the sphenoid bone. **a. amygdaloi′dea ante′rior** [NA], anterior amygdaloid area: a poorly differentiated transition zone in the corticomedial part of the amygdaloid body, through which the nuclei are continuous with adjacent areas. **anterior amygdaloid a.,** a. amygdaloidea anterior. **aortic a.,** the area on the chest over the inner end of the right second costal cartilage. **association a′s,** areas of the cerebral cortex (excluding the primary areas) that are connected with each other and with the neothalamus by numerous fibers passing through the corpus callosum and the white matter of the hemispheres; these areas are responsible for the higher mental and emotional processes, including memory, learning, etc. **auditory a.,** a. vestibularis. **axial a.,** an area on a limb in which there is a hiatus in the numerical sequence of the spinal nerves in their cutaneous distribution. **Bamberger's a.,** an area of cardiac dullness in the left intercostal region, suggestive of pericardial effusion. **bare a. of liver,** a. nuda hepatis. **basal seat a.,** denture-bearing area. **B-dependent a.,** thymus-independent a. **Betz cell a.,** motor a. **Broca's motor speech a.,** an area comprising parts of the opercular and triangular portions of the inferior frontal gyrus; injury to this area may result in motor aphasia. **Broca's parolfactory a.,** a. subcallosa. **Brodmann's a′s,** areas of the cerebral cortex distinguished by differences in the arrangement of their six cellular layers and identified by numbering each area. **catchment a.,** the geographical area that a specialized health care facility is responsible for serving. **a. centra′lis,** macula retinae; see under *macula.* **cingulate a.,** the area comprising the cingulate gyrus and isthmus. **a. coch′leae** [NA], the anterior part of the inferior portion of the fundus of the internal acoustic meatus, near the base of the cochlea; called also *cochlear a. of internal acoustic meatus.* **cochlear a. of internal acoustic meatus,** a. cochleae. **Cohnheim's a′s,** dark, polygonal areas of myofibrils seen on cross-section of a poorly fixed muscle fiber. **contact a.,** 1. any area at which two bodies or materials touch. Called also *contact surface.* See also *proximal surface,* def. 2, under *surface.* 2. facies contactus dentis. **cribriform a. of renal papilla,** a. cribrosa papillae renalis. **a. cribro′sa me′dia,** a. vestibularis inferior. **a. cribro′sa papil′lae rena′lis** [NA], cribriform area of renal papilla: the tip of a pyramid of a kidney, which is perforated by 10–25 openings for the papillary ducts. **a. cribro′sa supe′rior,** a. vestibularis superior. **a. of critical definition,** that part of an optic image within which the detail is clear. **denture-bearing a., denture foundation a., denture-supporting a.,** the surface of the oral tissues (residual alveolar ridge) that supports a denture. Called also *basal seat a.* and *stress-bearing a.* **dermatomic a.,** dermatome. **dorsal hypothalamic a.,** regio hypothalamica dorsalis. **embryonic a.,** embryonic disk. **excitable a.,** a motor area in the cerebral cortex. **excitomotor a.,** motor a. **eye a.,** the area comprising the frontal eye fields of the cortex in the frontal lobe, which are concerned with the control of eye movements. **a. of facial nerve,** a. nervi facialis. **Flechsig's a′s** (*obs.*), three areas—anterior, lateral, and posterior—on each lateral half of the sections of the medulla oblongata, marked out by the fibers of the vagus and hypoglossal nerves. **a's of Forel,** see under *field.* **gastric a's, a′reae gas′-**

tricae, the several areas on organs adjacent to the stomach by which the organs make contact with the stomach. **germinal a., a. germinati′va,** embryonic disk. **glove a.,** that area—fingers, hand, and wrist—ordinarily covered by a glove, which sometimes coincides with the distribution of anesthesia in cases of polyneuropathy. **hypoglossal a., a. hypoglos′si,** the portion of the mouth beneath the tongue. **hypothalamic a., lateral,** a. hypothalamica lateralis. **a. hypothalam′ica dorsa′lis,** NA alternative for *regio hypothalamica dorsalis.* **a. hypothalam′ica latera′lis** [NA], an area in the intermediate hypothalamic region, lateral to the fornix and the mamillothalamic fasciculus. **impression a.,** the surface of the oral structures recorded in an impression. **insular a.,** the cortex of the insula. **intercondylar a′s of tibia,** see *a. intercondylaris anterior tibiae* and *a. intercondylaris posterior tibiae.* **a. intercondyla′ris ante′rior tib′iae** [NA], the broad area between the superior articular surfaces of the tibia; called also *anterior intercondylar a., fossa intercondyloidea anterior tibiae, anterior intercondylar fossa of tibia,* and *patellar fossa of tibia.* **a. intercondyla′ris poste′rior tib′iae** [NA], a deep notch separating the condyles on the posterior surface of the tibia; called also *posterior intercondylar a., fossa intercondyloidea posterior tibiae, posterior intercondylar fossa of tibia,* and *popliteal fossa of tibia.* **interglobular a′s,** the areas of dentin lying between the calcoglobules. **Kiesselbach's a.,** an area on the anterior part of the nasal septum above the intermaxillary bone, which is richly supplied with blood vessels and is a common site of nosebleed; called also *Little's a.* **Krönig's a.** (*obs.*), Krönig's field. **Laimer-Haeckerman a.,** the region of the lower pharynx and upper esophagus, where diverticula most frequently develop. **language a.,** any center of the cortex, usually in the dominant hemisphere, controlling the understanding or use of language. **Little's a.,** Kiesselbach's a. **a. luna′ta** (*obs.*), the posterior semilunar lobule of the cerebellar hemisphere situated rostral to the postlunate (postclival) fissure. **a. martegia′ni,** a slightly enlarged space at the optic disk, marking the beginning of the hyaloid canal. **a. medullovasculo′sa,** a median elongated area of vascular granulation-like tissue in rachischisis. **mesobranchial a.,** the pharyngeal floor, between the pharyngeal arches and pouches of each side. **mirror a.,** the reflecting surface of the cornea and lens when illuminated through the slit lamp. **motor a.,** that area of the cerebral cortex which, upon application of brief electrical stimuli, shows the lowest threshold and shortest latency for the production of muscle movement. Called also *Betz cell a., excitomotor a., precentral a., psychomotor a.,* and *rolandic a.* **a. ner′vi facia′lis** [NA], area of facial nerve: the part of the fundus of the internal acoustic meatus where the facial nerve enters the facial canal. **a. nu′da hep′atis** [NA], bare area of liver: the superior surface of the liver, adjacent to the diaphragm, that lacks a peritoneal covering; its boundaries are formed by the hepatic coronary ligament proper and the triangular ligaments. **Obersteiner-Redlich a.** (*obs.*), the constricted area at the point where a posterior nerve root enters the spinal cord. **olfactory a.,** 1. a general area, including the olfactory bulb, tract, and trigone, the anterior portion of the gyrus cinguli, and the uncus. 2. substantia perforata rostralis. **a. opa′ca,** the outer part of the embryonic disk, as seen in the bird egg. **Panum's a′s,** fusional areas on the retina. **parolfactory a. of Broca,** a. subcallosa. **a. pellu′cida,** the central clear part of the embryonic disk, as seen in the bird egg. **a. perfora′ta,** substantia perforata (perforated space). **peristriate a.,** an area of the occipital cortex nearly surrounding the striate (visual) cortex. **piriform a.,** an area in the rhinencephalon comprising the lateral olfactory process or gyrus, the limen insulae, the uncus, and at least part of the parahippocampal gyrus; in some species it is pear-shaped. Called also *piriform lobe.* **postcentral a.,** the sensory area just posterior to the central sulcus of the cerebral hemisphere, the primary receptive area for general sensations; called also *postrolandic a.* and *somesthetic cortex.* **post dam a.,** posterior palatal seal a. **posterior hypothalamic a.,** see *hypothalamic a's.* **posterior palatal seal a.,** the soft tissues along the junction of the hard and soft palates on which pressure can be applied by a denture to aid in its retention; called also *post dam a.* **a. postre′ma,** a small tongue-shaped area on the lateral wall of the fourth ventricle, between the funiculus separans and the tuberculum gracile, in which the blood-brain barrier may be modified. **postrolandic a.,** postcentral a. **precentral a.,** motor a. **prefrontal a.,** the cortex of the frontal lobe immediately in front of the premotor cortex, concerned chiefly with associative functions. **premotor a.,** the motor cortex of the frontal lobe immediately in front of the precentral gyrus. **preoptic a., a preop′tica** [NA], several groups of cells in the median plane immediately below the rostral commissure of the telencephalon that are functionally related to the hypothalamus; called also *preoptic region.* **pressure a.,** an area which is subjected to excessive pressure, with consequent displacement of tissue. **pretectal a., a. pretecta′lis** [NA], an area at the junction of the mesencephalon and diencephalon, extending from a position dorsolateral to the commissure of the epithalamus toward the cranial colliculus, within which is situated the pretectal nucleus; called also *pretectal region.* **primary a's,** areas of the cerebral cortex comprising the motor and sensory regions. Cf. *association a's.* **primary receptive a.,** the area of cerebral cortex which receives the thalamic projections of the primary sensory modalities, such as vision, hearing, touch, etc. **projection a's,** those areas of the cerebral cortex that receive the most direct projection of the sensory systems of the body. **psychomotor a.,** motor a. **a. pterygoi′dea** (*obs.*), the part of the ansiform lobule of the cerebellar hemisphere immediately behind the great horizontal (postpterygoid) fissure. **pyriform a.,** piriform a. **receptive a.,** primary receptive a. **relief a.,** the portion of the surface of the mouth upon which pressures or forces are reduced or eliminated in prosthodontic therapy. See also *relief,* def. 3. **rest a.,** the prepared surface of a tooth or fixed restoration into which the rest fits, giving support to a removable partial denture. Called also *rest seat.* **rolandic a.,** motor a. **rugae a.,** the portion of the mouth in which rugae are found; called also *rugae zone.* **saddle a.,** the edentulous portion of the dental arch upon which a fixed or removable prosthesis rests. **sensorimotor a.,** the cortex of the pre- and postcentral gyri—the motor area and the primary receptive area for general sensations, respectively. **sensory a.,** primary receptive a. **septal a.,** the area on either cerebral hemisphere comprising the parolfactory area of Broca (area subcallosa) and the corresponding half of the septum pellucidum; the area has olfactory, hypothalamic, and hippocampal connections. **silent a.,** an area of the brain in which pathologic conditions may occur without producing symptoms. **somatic sensory a., somatosensory a.,** the cortical projection area in the postcentral gyrus for information initiated by stimulation of receptors in the skin, joints, muscles, and viscera; it is involved in conscious perception of somatic sensation. Called also *somesthetic a.* **somesthetic a.,** somatosensory a. **stress-bearing a.,** 1. the portion of the mouth capable of providing support for a denture. 2. surfaces of oral structures which resist forces, strains, or pressures brought upon them during function. 3. denture-bearing a. **a. stria′ta,** striate cortex. **strip a.,** a strip of cortex between the motor and premotor areas thought to be suppressor in function. **a. subcallo′sa** [NA], **subcallosal a.,** a small area of cortex on the medial surface of each cerebral hemisphere, immediately in front of the gyrus subcallosus; called also *parolfactory a. of Broca.* **supplementary a's,** small motor and sensory areas of the cerebral cortex in addition to the primary areas. **supporting a.,** 1. the surface of the mouth available for support of a denture. 2. those areas of the maxillary and mandibular edentulous ridges which are considered best suited to carry the forces of mastication when the dentures are in function. **suppressor a's,** cortical areas whose activation suppresses or prevents movement. **T-dependent a.,** thymus-dependent a. **thymus-dependent a.,** any of the areas of the peripheral lymphoid organs populated by T lymphocytes, e.g., the periarteriolar lymphatic sheath in the spleen, the paracortex in lymph nodes, and the parafollicular areas of gut-associated lymphoid tissue. Called also *paracortex, T-dependent a.,* and *tertiary cortex.* **thymus-independent a.,** any of the areas of the peripheral lymphoid organs populated by B lymphocytes, e.g., the lymph nodules (lymphoid follicles) of the spleen, lymph nodes, and gut-associated lymphoid tissue. Called also *B-dependent a.* and *T-independent a.* **T-independent a.,** thymus-independent a. **trigger a.,** an area the stimulation of which may cause physiologic or pathologic changes in another area. **vagus a.,** the area on the floor of the fourth ventricle in which the vagus nerve has its origin (trigonum nervi vagi

[NA]). **a. vasculo′sa,** that part of the area opaca where the blood vessels are first seen, as in the bird egg. **vestibular a.,** a rounded triangular elevation lateral to foveae of the fourth ventricle over which pass the striae medullares; it extends into the lateral recess, where it forms the *auditory,* or *acoustic, tubercle.* **vestibular a., inferior, of internal acoustic meatus,** a. vestibularis inferior. **vestibular a., superior, of internal acoustic meatus,** a. vestibularis superior. **a. vestibula′ris infe′rior** [NA], the lower portion of the fundus of the internal acoustic meatus; called also *inferior vestibular a. of internal acoustic meatus* and *a. cribrosa media.* **a. vestibula′ris supe′rior** [NA], the upper portion of the fundus of the internal acoustic meatus; called also *superior vestibular a. of internal acoustic meatus* and *a. cribrosa superior.* **visual a.,** the striate and peristriate cortex of the occipital lobe. **visuopsychic a.,** the area of the cerebral cortex concerned in the interpretation of visual sensations. **visuosensory a.,** cortical projection area for information initiated by stimulation of the retina area surrounding the calcarine fissure; the area involved in conscious perception of visual information. **a. vitelli′na,** the yolk area beyond the area vasculosa in meroblastic eggs. **vocal a.,** the part of the glottis between the vocal cords. **Wernicke's a.,** originally a term denoting a speech center on the posterior part of the superior temporal gyrus, now used to include the supramarginal and angular gyri as well; called also *Wernicke's center, field,* or *zone.*

areata, areatus (ar″e-a′tah; ar″e-a′tus) occurring in patches, as alopecia areata.

Areca (ar′ĕ-kah) [L.; East Indian] a genus of palm trees, chiefly Asiatic. *A. catechu* L., Palmaceae affords betel nut and an inferior catechu (see *areca*).

areca (ar′e-kah) the dried ripe seed of *Areca catechu* L., Palmaceae, a palm native to the East Indies. It is a common masticatory throughout Asia and India, and contains the alkaloid arecoline and astringent tannins; it has parasympathomimetic and anthelmintic properties. Called also *betel nut* and *pinang.*

arecoline (ah-rek′o-lēn) a cholinomimetic alkaloid obtained from areta (betel nut) having both muscarinic and nicotinic effects; no longer used medicinally. **a. hydrobromide,** a cholinergic, $C_8H_3NO_2 \cdot HBr$, occurring as a white, crystalline powder, having actions similar to those of pilocarpine; it was formerly used in the treatment of glaucoma. Now used as a cathartic and anthelmintic in veterinary medicine.

areflexia (ah″re-flek′se-ah) [*a* neg. + *reflex* + *-ia*] absence of the reflexes.

aregenerative (ah″re-jen′er-a″tiv) characterized by absence of regeneration; applied especially to blood cells in aplastic anemia.

arenaceous (ar″ĕ-na′se-us) sandy; gritty.

arenation (ar″ĕ-na′shun) [L. *arena* sand] (*obs.*) ammotherapy.

Arenaviridae (ah″re-nah-vi′rĭ-de) a family of viruses comprising the arenaviruses (genus *Arenavirus*).

arenavirus (ah″re-nah-vi′rus) [L. *arenaceus* sandy + *virus*] any of a group of viruses made up of pleomorphic virions, from 50 to 300 nm. in diameter, having four large and one to three small segments of single-stranded RNA and having ribosomes within the virions that give a sandy appearance. It includes the lymphocytic choriomeningitis virus, the American hemorrhagic fever viruses (Amapari, Junin, Latino, Machupo, Parana, Pichinde, Tacaribe, and Tamiami viruses), and the Lassa fever virus. Rodents are the common hosts of these viruses. The term (*Arenavirus*) is also used as the genus name (of the family Arenaviridae) of the group.

arenoid (ar′ĕ-noid) [L. *arena* sand + Gr. *eidos* form] resembling sand.

areola (ah-re′o-lah), pl. *are′olae* [L., dim. of *area* space] 1. any minute space or interstice in a tissue. 2. a circular area of a different color, surrounding a central point, as such an area surrounding a pustule or vesicle, or the part of the iris surrounding the pupil of the eye, or the area surrounding the nipple of the breast. **Chaussier's a.,** the areola of induration of a malignant pustule. **a. mam′mae** [NA], **a. of mammary gland,** the darkened ring surrounding the nipple of a breast. **a. of nipple,** a. mammae. **a. papilla′ris,** a. mammae. **second a.,** a ring which, during pregnancy, surrounds the areola mammae. **umbilical a.,** a pigmented patch that sometimes surrounds the navel.

areolae (ah-re′o-le) [L.] genitive and plural of *areola*.

areolar (ah-re′o-lar) pertaining to or containing areolae; containing minute interspaces.

areolitis (ar″e-o-li′tis) inflammation of the areola of the breast.

areometer (ar″e-om′ĕ-ter) [Gr. *araios* thin + *metron* measure] a hydrometer.

areometric (ar″e-o-met′rik) pertaining to hydrometry.

areometry (ar″e-om′ĕ-tre) hydrometry.

Aretaeus (ar-ĕ-te′us) **of Cappadocia** (c. 81 to c. 138) a Greek physician, contemporary of Galen; he was an Eclectic, but influenced by Pneumatist theories. Aretaeus wrote works on acute and chronic diseases. His clinical descriptions (e.g., of diabetes, pleurisy, tetanus) are outstanding and firmly established upon Archigenes' work.

Arey's rule (ār′ēz) [Leslie Brainerd *Arey*, American anatomist, born 1891] see under *rule*.

Arfonad (ar′fon-ad) trademark for a preparation of trimethaphan camsylate.

Arg arginine.

arg. abbreviation for L. *argen′tum*, silver.

argamblyopia (ar″gam-ble-o′pe-ah) [Gr. *argos* idle + *amblyopia*] amblyopia due to long disuse of the eye.

Argand burner [Aimé *Argand*, Swiss physicist, 1755–1803] see under *burner*.

Argas (ar′gas) a genus of ticks. **A. america′nus,** *A. persicus.* **A. brump′ti,** a species found in Africa whose bite causes local inflammation in man. **A. minia′tus,** *A. persicus.* **A. per′sicus,** a cosmopolitan tick, the tampan or tampan tick, one of the most important parasites of poultry, which sucks the blood of fowls, producing a weak condition of flocks, with great economic losses. In Iran, Egypt, India, Australia, and Brazil, it acts as the carrier of fowl spirochetosis. Called also *A. americanus* and *A. minatus,* and *miana bug.* **A. reflex′us,** an ectoparasite of pigeons and other roosting birds, which frequently attacks man and may cause a cutaneous inflammatory lesion.

Argasidae (ar-gas′ĭ-de) a family of the superfamily Ixodoidea, comprising the soft ticks, distinguished from the hard-bodied ticks (Ixodidae) by absence of the scutum. The genera are *Argas, Otobius, Antricola,* and *Ornithodoros.*

argema (ar′je-mah) a white ulcer of the cornea.

Argemona mexicana (ar-jem′ŏ-nah meks″ĭ-kan′ah) a papaverous plant, the prickly poppy, the seeds of which contain a toxic oil; see *epidemic dropsy,* under *dropsy.*

argentaffin (ar-jen′tah-fin) [L. *argentum* silver + *affinis* having affinity for] having an affinity for silver and chromium salts; said of tissues. See also under *cell.*

argentaffinoma (ar″jen-taf″ĭ-no′mah) carcinoid; a tumor of the gastroenteric tract formed from the argentaffin cells (Kultschitzky's cells) found in the enteric canal; such tumors elaborate a variety of catecholamines that produce the symptom complex called carcinoid syndrome. Cf. *enterochromaffin gland.* **a. of bronchus,** carcinoid tumor of the bronchus, highly vascular tumors of the bronchus similar to argentaffinoma of the gastrointestinal tract.

argentation (ar″jen-ta′shun) [L. *argentum* silver] staining with a silver salt.

argenti (ar-jen′ti) genitive of *argentum.* **a. io′didum colloida′le,** colloidal silver iodide. **a. ni′tras,** silver nitrate.

argentic (ar-jen′tik) containing silver.

argentoproteinum (ar-jen″to-pro″te-i′num) silver protein; see under *silver.*

argentum (ar-jen′tum), gen. *argen′ti* [L.] silver. **a. protein′icum for′te,** strong silver protein; see under *silver.* **a. protein′icum mi′te,** mild silver protein; see under *silver.*

argilla (ar-jil′lah) kaolin.

argillaceous (ar″jĭ-la′shus) composed of clay.

arginase (ar′jĭ-nās) [EC 3.5.3.1] an enzyme of the hydrolase class that catalyzes the reaction L-arginine + H_2O = L-ornithine + urea. The enzyme also hydrolyzes canavanine. It is a Mn^{2+}-bound protein, found principally in the liver. The

reaction is part of the urea cycle. A deficiency of the enzyme, transmitted as an autosomal recessive trait, results in argininemia.

arginase deficiency, a genetic aminoacidopathy involving the biosynthesis of urea; arginine is elevated in blood and urine and may cause secondary cystinuria; orotic aciduria is common, but hyperammonemia is rare. Clinical signs include psychomotor retardation, hepatomegaly, and scalp discoloration. Called also *argininemia* and *hyperargininemia.*

arginine (ar′jĭ-nin) chemical name: 2-amino-5-guanidovaleric acid. An amino acid, $C_8H_{14}N_4O_2$, produced by the hydrolysis or digestion of proteins. It is one of the hexone bases (Schulze and Steiger, 1886), and it supplies the amidine group for the synthesis of creatine. Arginine is also formed by the transfer of a nitrogen atom from aspartate to citrulline in the urea cycle. It then gives off urea, to form ornithine. **a. glutamate,** the L(+)-arginine salt, $C_{11}H_{23}N_5O_6$, of L(+)-glutamic acid, used intravenously as an adjunct in the management of ammonia intoxication due to hepatic failure; called also *glutargin.* **a. hydrochloride** [USP], the L(+)-arginine salt of hydrochloric acid, used intravenously as an adjunct in the management of conditions in which there is an excess of ammonia in the blood. **a. monohydrochloride,** a salt of arginine sometimes used in place of ammonium chloride to potentiate mercurial diuretics in refractory heart failure. **suberyl a.,** a compound that functions in the bufotoxins as glucose does in the glucosides; it is $COOH(CH_2)_6CONHCO{:}NH(CH_2)_3CH(NH_2)COOH.$

arginine carboxypeptidase (ar′jĭ-nēn kar-bok″se-pep′tid-ās) [EC 3.4.17.3] an enzyme of the hydrolase class that catalyzes the removal of the C-terminal arginine residue from bradykinin. It is found in plasma.

argininemia (ar″jĭ-nin-e′me-ah) arginase deficiency.

argininosuccinase (ar″jĭ-ne-no-suk′sĭ-nās) argininosuccinate lyase.

argininosuccinate (ar″jĭ-nĭ-no-suk′sĭ-nāt) a compound formed by the condensation of aspartic acid and citrulline, which is an intermediate in the urea cycle.

argininosuccinate lyase (ar-jĭ-ne″no-suk′sin-āt li′ās) [EC 4.3.2.1] an enzyme of the lyase class that catalyzes the reaction L-arginosuccinate = fumarate + L-arginine. The reaction is part of the urea cycle in the liver. A genetic defect in the enzyme results in argininosuccinicaciduria. Called also *argininosuccinase.*

argininosuccinate lyase (ASAL, ASL) deficiency, a genetic aminoacidopathy involving the biosynthesis of urea; there are three clinical types (neonatal, subacute, and delayed onset); clinical findings, which vary widely in severity, include mental retardation, seizures, ataxia, hepatomegaly, and friable hair (trichorrhexis nodosa); citrullinemia may also be present. Called also *argininosuccinase (ASase) d.* and *argininosuccinic aciduria.*

argininosuccinate synthetase (ar-jĭ-ne″no-suk′sin-āt sin′thĕ-tās) [EC 6.3.4.5] an enzyme of the ligase (synthetase) class that catalyzes the reaction ATP + L-citrulline + L-aspartate = AMP + pyrophosphate + L-argininosuccinate. The reaction is a part of the urea cycle in the liver. A genetic defect in the enzyme results in citrullinemia.

argininosuccinate (ASA) synthetase (ASAS, ASS) deficiency, a genetic aminoacidopathy involving the biosynthesis of urea; it occurs in three clinical types (neonatal, subacute, and late onset); the characteristic finding is citrullinemia, with or without hyperammonemia and orotic aciduria. Called also *citrullinemia, citrullinuria.*

argininosuccinic acid (ar″jĭ-nĭ-no-suk-sin′ik) a metabolic intermediate in the urea cycle (q.v.).

argininosuccinicacidemia (ar″jĭ-nĭ″no-suk-sin″ik-as″ĭ-de′me-ah) the presence in the blood of argininosuccinic acid.

argininosuccinicaciduria (ar″jĭ-nĭ″no-suk-sin″ik-as″ĭ-du′re-ah) argininosuccinic lyase deficiency.

arginyl (ar′jĭ-nil) the acyl radical of arginine.

argipressin (ar″jĕ-pres′in) chemical name: 8-α-arginine vasopressin. Vasopressin containing arginine, as that from most mammals, including man. See also *lypressin.*

argon (ar′gon) [Gr. *argos* inert] a chemical element, atomic number 18, discovered in the atmosphere in 1895. One of the inert gases, its symbol is Ar and its atomic weight 39.948.

Argyll Robertson pupil (sign) (ar-gīl′ rob′ert-son) [Douglas Moray Cooper Lamb *Argyll Robertson,* Scottish physician, 1837–1909] see under *pupil.*

argyremia (ar″jĭ-re′me-ah) [Gr. *argyros* silver + *haima* blood + *-ia*] the presence of silver or silver salts in the blood.

argyria (ar-jir′e-ah) a permanent ashen-gray discoloration of the skin, conjunctiva, and internal organs that results from long-continued use of silver salts. Called also *argyrosis.*
a. nasa′lis, argyric discoloration of the nasal mucosa.

argyriasis (ar″jĭ-ri′ah-sis) argyria.

argyric (ar-ji′rik) pertaining to or caused by silver; pertaining to argyria.

argyrism (ar′jĭ-rizm) argyria.

Argyrol (ar′jĭ-rol) trademark for mild silver protein; see under *silver.*

argyrophil (ar-ji′ro-fil) [Gr. *argyros* silver + *philein* to love] capable of binding silver salts, which may subsequently be reduced by light or by a reducing agent to give a black deposit of silver; said of tissues.

argyrosis (ar″jĭ-ro′sis) [Gr. *argyros* silver] argyria.

arhigosis (ah″rĭ-go′sis) [*a* neg. + Gr. *rhigos* cold] inability to perceive cold; absence of the cold sense.

arhinencephalia (ah″rin-en″se-fa′le-ah) [*a* neg. + *rhinencephalon*] congenital absence of the rhinencephalon.

arhinia (ah-rin′e-ah) [*a* neg. + Gr. *rhis* nose + *-ia*] congenital absence of the nose.

arhythmia (ah-rith′me-ah) arrhythmia.

Arias-Stella reaction [Javier *Arias-Stella,* Peruvian pathologist, born 1924] see under *reaction.*

ariboflavinosis (a-ri″bo-fla″vĭ-no′sis) [*a* neg. + *riboflavin* + *-osis*] deficiency of riboflavin in the diet. It produces a syndrome chiefly marked by cheilosis or cheilitis, angular stomatitis, glossitis associated with a purplish red or magenta-colored tongue that may show fissures, corneal vascularization, dyssebacia, and anemia.

aril (ar′il) [L. *arillus* dried grape] an accessory covering or appendage of seeds.

arildone (ar′il-dōn) chemical name: 4-[6-(2-chloro-4-methoxyphenoxy)hexyl]-3,5-heptanedione; an antiviral agent, $C_{20}H_{29}ClO_4$.

arillode (ar′ĭ-lōd) an appendage of certain seeds attached to the micropyle or raphe.

aristin (ah-ris′tin) a crystalline principle from various species of *Aristolochia.*

Aristocort (ah-ris′to-cort) trademark for preparations of triamcinolone and its derivatives.

Aristogel (ah-ris′to-jel) trademark for a preparation of triamcinolone acetonide.

aristogenesis (ah-ris″to-jen′ĕ-sis) [Gr. *aristos* best + *genesis* generation] the gradual continuous adaptive genoplastic origin of new and better organic mechanisms.

aristogenics (ah-ris″to-jen′iks) [Gr. *aristos* best + *gennan* to produce] improvement of the race through promotion of optimal mating between individuals possessing superior characteristics.

Aristolochia (ah-ris″to-lo′ke-ah) [L.; Gr. *aristos* best + *lochia* lochia] a genus of shrubs and herbs of many species, often actively medicinal; see *serpentaria.* A. *reticulata* Nutt. (Texas snakeroot) and A. *serpentaria* L. (Virginia snakeroot) are the source (dried rhizome and roots) of serpentaria, an aromatic bitter. The plants contain aristolochic acid, a phenanthrene-carboxylic acid derivative, the major aromatic bitter principle. It is toxic to experimental animals in sufficient dosage, causing cardiac and respiratory arrest.

aristolochic acid (ah-ris″to-lo′kik) the major bitter aromatic principle of herbs of the genus *Aristolochia* and related species, called also aristolochine.

aristolochine (ah-ris-tol′o-chēn) aristolochic acid.

Aristospan (ah-ris′to-span) trademark for preparations of triamcinolone hexacetonide.

Aristotle (ar′is-tot′l) [384–322 B.C.] Greek philosopher, student of Plato. As a physical scientist, Aristotle stressed direct observation and induction; in biology his teleology is still accepted by vitalists. His studies included comparative anatomy and physiology, embryology, and ethology. Very unfortunately, Aristotle adopted Empedocles' theory of the heart's being the center of intelligence, and also the theory of the four elements and the four qualities (cf. *humoralism*).

Aristotle's anomaly (ar′ĭ-stot-elz) [A Greek philosopher, 384–322 B.C.] see under *anomaly.*

arithmomania (ah-rith″mo-ma′ne-ah) [Gr. *arithmos* number + *mania*] compulsive counting, as paces when walking, steps in a staircase, etc., a common symptom in obsessive-compulsive disorder.

Arizona (ar″ĭ-zo′nah) see *Salmonella arizona.*

arkyochrome (ar′ke-o-krōm) [Gr. *arkys* net + *chrōma* color] any nerve cell in which the chromatic substance arranges itself in the form of a network. Cf. *gyrochrome, perichrome,* and *stichochrome.*

arkyostichochrome (ar″ke-o-stik′o-krōm) [Gr. *arkys* net + *stichos* row + *chrōma* color] any nerve cell that is both an arkyochrome and a stichochrome.

Arlacel A (ar′lah-sel) trademark for an emulsifying agent used for stabilizing water-in-oil emulsion adjuvants, mainly consisting of mannide mono-oleate.

Arlidin (ar′lĭ-din) trademark for preparations of nylidrin hydrochloride.

Arlt's recess, sinus, trachoma (arltz) [Carl Ferdinand Ritter von *Arlt,* ophthalmologist in Vienna, 1812–1887] see under *resess* and *trachoma,* and see *sinus of Maier.*

arm (arm) [A.S. *earm*] 1. the part of the upper extremity between the shoulder joint and elbow, as distinguished from the forearm; popularly, the upper extremity from shoulder to hand. See also *brachium.* 2. a slender part or extension, usually having mobility and independent function, that projects from a main structure. 3. an extension or projection by which a removable partial denture is retained in position in the mouth. 4. chromosome a. **bar clasp a.,** a clasp arm that serves as an extracoronal retainer, originating from the denture base, a major or minor connector, or the framework of a denture, traverses soft tissue, approaches the tooth undercut area from a gingival direction, and terminates in a retentive undercut lying gingival to the height of contour. **bird a.,** a wasted condition of the forearm due to atrophy of the muscles. **chromosome a.,** either of the two segments of the chromosome separated by the centromere; the symbol p indicates the short arm and q the long arm. **circumferential clasp a.,** a clasp arm that originates above the height of contour, traverses part of the suprabulge portion of the tooth, approaches the tooth undercut from an occlusal direction, and terminates in a retentive undercut lying gingival to the height of contour. **glass a.,** a painful condition of the upper arm due to an injury to the long tendon of the biceps muscle or to the tendon of the supraspinatus muscle, at times resulting in subdeltoid bursitis. **golf a.,** a form of neuritis seen in golf players after excessive exercise. **lawn tennis a.,** tennis elbow. **reciprocal a.,** a clasp arm located in such a manner as to reciprocate any force arising from an opposing clasp arm on the same tooth. **retention a., retentive a.,** a rigid clasp that engages the infrabulge area at the terminal end of the arm. **stabilizing a.,** a rigid clasp arm that contacts the tooth at or occlusal to the surveyed height of contour.

armadillo (ar″mah-dil′o) one of a group of burrowing mammals belonging to the order Edentata and possessing horny shields on the dorsal surface of the body; one species in South America is a reservoir for *Trypanosoma cruzi.*

armamentarium (ar″mah-men-tā′re-um) [L.] the equipment of a practitioner or institution, including books, instruments, medicines, and surgical appliances.

Armanni-Ebstein cells [Luciano *Armanni,* Italian pathologist, 1839–1903; Wilhelm *Ebstein,* German internist, 1836–1912] see under *cell.*

armarium (ar-ma′re-um) [L.] armamentarium.

armature (ar′mah-chūr) [L. *armatura* a defensive apparatus] 1. the iron bar or keeper across the open end of a horseshoe magnet. 2. a protective organ or structure.

Armigeres (ar-mij′er-ēz) a genus of mosquitoes. **A. obtur′bans,** a mosquito which transmits dengue in Japan.

Armillifer (ar-mil′lĭ-fer) a genus of endoparasitic animals of the family Porocephalidae, order Porocephalida. **A. armilla′tus,** a species whose adult members are found in the lungs and trachea of the python (*Python sebae* and *P. regius*) and whose larvae occur in the internal organs of monkeys and lions and occasionally of man in Africa. Called also *Porocephalus armillatus* and *P. constrictus.* **A. monilifor′mis,** a species whose larvae are parasitic in man in China, the Philippines, and other Asian islands.

Armophorina (ar″mo-fo-ri′nah, ar″mof-o-ri′nah) [L. *arma* armor + Gr. *phoros* bearing] a suborder of small, polysaprobic, ciliate protozoa (order Heterotrichina, subclass Spirotricha), characterized by an adoral zone of membranelles encircling the body, spiraling posteriad, accompanied by a ciliary stripe, and an antapically situated cytostome; a rigid pellice with one or two posterior spines; and the only other somatic ciliature occurring in a caudal tuft and several anterior cirri.

armpit (arm′pit) fossa axillaris.

Arnaldus de Villanova see *Arnold of Villanova.*

Arndt's law, Arndt-Schulz law [Rudolf *Arndt,* German psychiatrist, 1835–1900; Hugo *Schulz,* German pharmacologist, 1853–1932] see under *law.*

Arneth count (classification, formula, index) (ar-net′) [Joseph *Arneth,* German physician, 1873–1955] see under *count.*

Arnica (ar′nĕ-kah) [L.] a genus of composite-flowered plants, known also as *leopard's bane, wolf's bane,* and *mountain tobacco.* The dried flowerheads of *A. montana* contain a volatile oil, arnicin, aristerol, and anthoxanthine, tannin, and resin. Used topically as a tincture for contusions, sprains, and superficial wounds, and as a counterirritant.

arnica (ar′nĭ-kah) the dried flowerheads of *Arnica montana.* Called also *wolf's bane* and *leopard's bane.*

Arnold (ar′nold) **of Villanova,** or **Arnaldus de Villanova** (c. 1235 to c. 1312) a celebrated Catalan physician who wrote extensively on medicine, alchemy, and religion and who translated Avicenna's writings on the heart from Arabic into Latin.

Arnold's bodies [Julius *Arnold,* German pathologist, 1835–1915] see under *body.*

Arnold's canal, etc. [Philipp Friedrich *Arnold,* German anatomist, 1803–1890] see under *canal, fold, ligament, nerve, substance,* and *syndrome.*

Arnold-Chiari deformity (malformation, syndrome) [Julius *Arnold;* Hans *Chiari,* German pathologist, 1851–1916] see under *deformity.*

arnotto (ar-not′o) annotto.

aroma (ah-ro′mah) [Gr. *arōma* spice] fragrance or odor, especially that of a spice or medicine or of articles of food or drink.

aromatase (ah-ro′mah-tās) an enzyme complex that catalyzes the conversion of testosterone to estradiol.

aromatic (ar″o-mat′ik) [L. *aromaticus;* Gr. *arōmatikos*] 1. having a spicy odor. 2. in organic chemistry, denoting a compound containing a ring system stabilized by a closed circle of conjugated double bonds or nonbonding electron pairs, e.g., benzene, naphthalene.

aromatization (ah-ro″mah-tĭ-za′shun) chemical conversion to an aromatic form.

aromine (ah-ro′min) a fragrant alkaloid from urine containing benzene derivatives.

arousal (ah-row′sal) a state of responsiveness to sensory stimulation; called also *activation, vigilance,* and *wakefulness.*

arprinocid (ar-pri′no-sid) chemical name: 9-[(2-chloro-6-fluorophenyl)methyl]-9*H*-purin-6-amine; a coccidiostat, $C_{12}H_9ClFN_5$.

arrachement (ar″ash-mahwn′) [Fr. "extraction"] extraction of a membranous cataract by pulling out the capsule through a corneal incision.

arrack (ar′rak) an alcoholic liquor distilled from fermented dates, rice, the sap of palms, mahua flowers, etc.

arrangement (ah-rānj′ment) the disposal or positioning of parts. **anterior tooth a.,** the arrangement of anterior teeth for esthetic or phonetic effects. **tooth a.,** 1. the positioning of teeth on a denture for specific purposes. 2. the setting of teeth on temporary bases.

arrector (ah-rek′tor), pl. *arrecto′res* [L.] raising, or that which raises. **a. pi′li,** pl. **arrecto′res pilo′rum** [L. "raisers of the hair"], minute smooth muscles of the skin, attached to the connective tissue sheath of the hair follicles, the contraction of which causes the hair to stand erect and produces the appearance called cutis anserina, or goose flesh.

arrectores (ar″rek-to′rez) [L.] plural of *arrector.*

arrest (ah-rest) stoppage; the act of stopping. **cardiac a.,** sudden cessation of cardiac function, with disappearance of arterial blood pressure, connoting either ventricular fibrillation or ventricular standstill. **deep transverse a.,** the condition during delivery in which the occiput of the fetus turns and stops in the transverse diameter of the pelvis. **developmental a.,** a temporary or permanent cessation of the process of development. **epiphyseal a.,** interruption of growth at the epiphysis of a bone by diaphyseal-epiphyseal fusion. **heart a.,** cardiac a. **maturation a.,** interruption of the process of development before it is complete; applied especially to failure of maturation of granulocytes, with myeloblasts and promyelocytes constituting the dominant bone marrow elements. **sinus a.,** a pause in cardiac rhythm due to a momentary failure of the sinus node to initiate an impulse; called also *sinus standstill.*

arrested (ah-rest′ed) detained; stopped. In obstetrics, the head of the child is said to be arrested when it is *detained,* but not *impacted,* in the pelvic cavity.

arrhaphia (ah-ra′fe-ah) [*a-* neg. + *-rhaphy*] status dysrhaphius.

Arrhenius' equation, formula, theory (doctrine) (ah-re′ne-us) [Svante August *Arrhenius,* Swedish chemist, 1859–1927] see under *equation, formula,* and *theory.*

arrheno- [Gr. *arrhēn* male] a combining form meaning male.

arrhenoblastoma (ah-re″no-blas-to′mah) [*arrheno-* + Gr. *blastos* germ + *-oma*] a neoplasm of the ovary, arising from the ovarian stroma, mimicking to a greater or lesser extent derivatives of the sex cord mesenchyme of the testis, and sometimes causing defeminization and virilization. Called also *andreioma, andreoblastoma, androma, arrhenoma,* and *Sertoli-Leydig cell tumor.*

arrhenogenic (ar″ĕ-no-jen′ik) [*arrheno* + Gr. *gennan* to produce] producing only male offspring.

arrhenokaryon (ar″ĕ-no-kar′e-on) an organism that is produced by androgenesis.

arrhenoma (ar″ĕ-no′mah) arrhenoblastoma.

arrhenoplasm (ah-re′no-plazm) [*arrheno-* + *plasm*] the male element of idioplasm.

arrhenotocia (ar″ĕ-no-to′se-a) arrhenotoky.

arrhenotoky (ar″ĕ-not′o-ke) [*arrheno-* + Gr. *tokos* birth] the production of males only by a virgin mother, as in the unfertilized queen bee.

arrhigosis (ah″rĭ-go′sis) arigosis.

arrhinencephalia (ah″rin-en″se-fa′le-ah) arhinencephalia.

arrhinia (ah-rin′e-ah) arhinia.

arrhythmia (ah-rith′me-ah) [*a* neg. + Gr. *rhythmos* rhythm] any variation from the normal rhythm of the heart beat, including sinus arrhythmia, premature beat, heart block, atrial fibrillation, atrial flutter, pulsus alternans, and paroxysmal tachycardia. **continuous a.,** irregularity in the force, quality, and sequence of the pulse beat, continuing as a permanent phenomenon; called also *perpetual a.* **juvenile a.,** sinus arrhythmia occuring in children. **nodal a.,** nodal rhythm; see under *rhythm.* **perpetual a.,** continuous a. **phasic a.,** sinus a. **respiratory a.,** sinus a. **sinus a.,** the physiologic cyclic variation in heart rate related to vagal impulses to the sinoatrial node; it occurs commonly in children (juvenile a.) and in the aged, and requires no treatment. Called also *phasic a.* and *respiratory a.*

arrhythmic (ah-rith′mik) [*a* neg. + Gr. *rhythmos* rhythm] characterized by absence of rhythm.

arrhythmogenic (ah-rith″mo-jen′ik) [*a* neg. + Gr. *rhythmos* rhythm + *gennan* to produce] producing or promoting arrhythmia.

arrhythmokinesis (ah-rith″mo-kĭ-ne′sis) [*a* neg. + Gr. *rhythmos* rhythm + *kinēsis* movement] defective ability to perform voluntary successive movement of a definite rhythm.

arrowroot (ar′o-root) a starch prepared from the rhizome of *Maranta arundinacea* L., Marantaceae, a plant native to northern South America and the West Indies and now extensively cultivated in almost all tropical countries. It is a prominent constituent of infant, geriatric, and convalescent diets.

Arroyo's sign (ar-ro′yōz) [Carlos F. *Arroyo,* American physician, 1892–1928] asthenocoria.

A.R.R.S. American Roentgen Ray Society.

arsambide (ar-sam'bĭd) carbarsone.

arsenate (ar'sĕ-nāt) any salt of arsenic acid. **ferric a.,** a brownish yellow powder, $4Fe_2O_3 \cdot 5H_2O$, used in anemia; called also *iron arsenite*. **ferrous a.,** a green amorphous powder, $Fe_3(AsO_4)_2 \cdot 6H_2O$, insoluble in water; formerly used in chronic skin conditions and now employed as an insecticide. Called also *iron arsenate*.

arseniasis (ar″sĕ-ni′ah-sis) chronic arsenical poisoning.

arsenic[1] (ar'sĕ-nik) [L. *arsenicum, arsenium,* or *arsenum;* from Gr. *arsēn* strong] 1. a medicinal and poisonous element; it is a brittle, lustrous, grayish solid, with a garlicky odor. Symbol, As; atomic number, 33; atomic weight, 74.922; specific gravity, 5.73. See also under *poisoning.* 2. arsenic trioxide. **a. chloride,** a. trichloride. **a. disulfide,** a poisonous compound, As_2S_2, used as a pigment, in fireworks, in shot manufacture, and in the leather industry; called also *red arsenic sulfide* and *realgar.* **fuming liquid a.,** a. trichloride. **a. iodide,** a red crystalline compound, AsI_3, once used in coryza and skin diseases. **red a. sulfide,** a. disulfide. **a. trichloride,** a very poisonous fuming liquid, $AsCl_3$, which readily liberates highly irritant hydrochloric acid; it is used in war gas and as an intermediate for organic chemicals. **a. trioxide,** white arsenic, a white or glassy compound, As_2O_3, with a sweetish taste and erythropoietic effect; taken in repeated small doses in Alpine countries to increase hemoglobin, resulting in increased working capacity and a ruddy complexion. Formerly used in treatment of skin and hematologic disorders. Called also *arsenous acid, arsenous anhydride,* and *flowers of arsenic.* **a. trisulfide,** a poisonous substance, As_2S_3, occurring in nature as the mineral orpiment; used as a pigment and sometimes as a medicine. Called also *a. yellow* and *auripigment.* **white a.,** a. trioxide. **a. yellow,** a. trisulfide.

arsenic[2] (ar-sen'ik) pertaining to or containing arsenic in a pentavalent state.

arsenic acid (ar-sen′ic) the hydrate, H_3AsO_4, of arsenic pentoxide, which is itself also referred to as arsenic acid.

arsenical (ar-sen′ĭ-kal) [L. *arsenicalis*] 1. pertaining to or containing arsenic. 2. a drug containing arsenic.

arsenicalism (ar-sen′ĕ-kal″izm) chronic arsenical poisoning.

arsenicophagy (ar″sen-ĭ-kof′ah-je) [*arsenic* Gr. *phagein* to eat] the eating of arsenic.

arsenicum (ar-sen′ĕ-kum) [L.] arsenic.

arsenide (ar'sĕ-nīd) any compound of arsenic with another element, in which arsenic is the negative element.

arsenious (ar-sen′e-us) arsenous; pertaining to arsenic in a trivalent state.

arsenism (ar'sen-izm) chronic arsenic poisoning.

arsenite (ar'sĕ-nīt) any salt of arsenous acid.

arsenium (ar-se′ne-um) [L.] the element arsenic.

arsenization (ar″sen-ĭ-za′shun) treatment with arsenic.

arseno- (ar'sĕ-no) a prefix indicating the chemical group —As: As—.

arsenobenzene (ar″sĕ-no-ben′zĕn) a general term for the various arsphenamine compounds used in the treatment of spirochetal diseases.

arsenoblast (ar-sen′o-blast) [Gr. *arsēn* male + *blastos* germ] the male element of a zygote; a male pronucleus.

arsenoceptor (ar-sen′o-sep″tor) a supposed receptor in cells for arsenic.

arsenophagy (ar″sĕ-nof′ah-je) arsenicophagy.

arsenotherapy (ar″sĕ-no-ther′ah-pe) [*arsenic* + Gr. *therapeia* treatment] treatment of disease by the use of arsenic and arsenical preparations.

arsenous (ar'sĕ-nus) containing arsenic in its lower or triad valency.

arsenous acid (ar-sen′us) the hydrate, H_3AsO_3, of arsenic trioxide, which is itself also referred to as arsenous acid.

arsenoxide (ar″sen-ok′sīd) oxophenarsine.

arsenum (ar-se′num) [L.] arsenic.

arsine (ar'sin) any member of a peculiar group of volatile arsenical bases, formed when arsenous acid is brought in contact with albuminous substances. The typical arsine is AsH_3, arsenous hydride or arseniuretted hydrogen, a very poisonous gas, and some of its compounds have been used in warfare. It causes hemolysis, jaundice, gastroenteritis, and nephritis.

arsinic acid (ar-sin′ik) an organic compound containing the —As(OH)₂ functional group.

arsonic acid (ar-son′ik) an organic compound containing the —AsO(OH)₂ functional group.

arsonium (ar-so′ne-um) the univalent radical or ion, AsH_4, which acts in combination like the ammonium ion, NH_4.

arsphenamine (ars-fen′ah-min) chemical name: 4,4′-(1,2-diarsenediyl)bis[2-aminophenol]dihydrochloride. A yellow hygroscopic powder, $[OH \cdot C_6H_3 (NH_2 \cdot HCl) \cdot As:]_2$, introduced as the first specific for the treatment of syphilis, yaws, and other spirillum infections but later virtually replaced in medicine, first by arsenoxide and then by penicillin. It rapidly oxidizes on exposure to air, and is, therefore, put up in hermetically sealed capsules. The substance is converted, immediately before injection, into an unstable sodium salt by the addition of sodium hydroxide solution. Called also *salvarsan* (Germany), *arsenobenzol* (France), *diarsenol* (Canada), *arsaminol* (Japan), *606, Ehrlich-Hata* or *Hata's preparation,* and *magic bullet.* **silver a.,** sodium salt of silver diaminodihydroxyarsenobenzene; it occurs as a brownish-black powder containing about 19 per cent arsenic and 12 to 14 per cent silver; formerly used in the treatment of the neurologic complications in syphilis. Called also *argentum arsphenamina* and *silver salvarsan.* **sodium a.,** a bright yellow powder, the sodium salt of arsphenamine, $C_{12}H_{10}As_2 N_2Na_2O_2$, unstable in air and freely soluble in water; formerly used in the treatment of syphilis. Called also *sodiarsphenamine.* **a. sulfoxylate,** a condensation product of arsphenamine and sodium formaldehyde bisulfite, $[NaO \cdot SO_2 \cdot CH \cdot NH(OH) C_6H_4As]_2$.

arsthinol (ars′thĭ-nol) chemical name: *N*-[2-hydroxy-5-[4-(hydroxymethyl)-1,3,2-dithiarsolan-2-yl] phenyl] acetamide. An antiprotozoal agent, $C_{11}H_{14}AsNO_3S_2$, effective in amebiasis and yaws; administered orally.

ART Accredited Record Technician; automated reagin test.

Artane (ar′tān) trademark for preparations of trihexyphenidyl.

artefact (ar′te-fakt) artifact.

Artemisia (ar″tĕ-mis′e-ah) [L.; Gr. *artemisia* from *Artemis* Diana] a genus of composite-flowered plants, including *A. abrot'anum* (southernwood), *A. absin'thium* (wormwood), and *A. marit'ima (A. pauciflora),* from which santonin is derived. The oil of *A. absinthium* was formerly used in the preparation of the alcoholic beverage, absinthe, but because it contains neurotoxic agents (l-thujone and d-isothujone), its use has been discontinued. Absinthin is the active bitter principle.

arteralgia (ar″ter-al′je-ah) pain emanating from an artery, such as headache from an inflamed temporal artery.

arterectomy (ar″tĕ-rek′to-me) arteriectomy.

arterenol (ar″tĕ-re′nol) norepinephrine.

arteria (ar-te′re-ah), pl. *arte'riae* [L.; Gr. *artēria*] a general term used in anatomical nomenclature to designate any vessel carrying blood away from the heart. For names and description of specific vessels, see *Table of Arteriae.* See also *artery.* **a. luso'ria,** an abnormally situated retroesophageal vessel, usually the subclavian artery from the aortic arch, which may cause symptoms by compression of the esophagus, the trachea, or a nerve.

arteriae (ar-te′re-e) [L.] plural of *arteria.*

arterial (ar-te′re-al) pertaining to an artery or to the arteries.

arterialization (ar-te″re-al-i-za′shun) (*obs.*) the change of venous into arterial blood; the provision or supplying of oxygenated instead of venous blood.

arteriarctia (ar″tĕ-re-ark′she-ah) [*artery* + L. *arctare* to contract] (*obs.*) contraction of an artery; narrowing of the caliber of an artery.

arteriectasia (ar″tĕ-re-ek-ta′ze-ah) arteriectasis.

arteriectasis (ar″tĕ-re-ek′tah-sis) [*artery* + Gr. *ektasis* dilatation] dilatation and, usually, lengthening of an artery.

arteriectomy (ar″tĕ-re-ek′to-me) [*artery* + Gr. *ektomē* excision] excision of a portion of an artery.

arteriectopia (ar″tĕ-re-ek-to′pe-ah) [*artery* + Gr. *ektopos* out of place] displacement of an artery from its normal location.

TABLE OF ARTERIAE

Descriptions of vessels are given on NA terms, and include anglicized names of specific arteries. Although each artery is identified by its origin, branches, and distribution, it should be borne in mind that there are variations in the point of origin, that only named branches are listed, and that only the more noteworthy structures are given in the distribution.

a. aceta′buli, ramus acetabularis arteriae obturatoriae.

arte′riae alveola′res superio′res anterio′res [NA], anterior superior alveolar arteries: *origin,* infraorbital artery; *branches,* dental and peridental rami; *distribution,* incisors and canine regions of upper jaw, maxillary sinus. Called also *anterior dental arteries.*

a. alveola′ris infe′rior [NA], inferior alveolar artery: *origin,* maxillary artery; *branches,* dental, peridental, mental, and mylohyoid rami; *distribution,* lower jaw, lower lip, and chin. Called also *inferior dental artery* and *mandibular artery.*

a. alveola′ris supe′rior poste′rior [NA], posterior superior alveolar artery: *origin,* maxillary artery; *branches,* dental and peridental rami; *distribution,* molar and premolar regions of upper jaw, maxillary sinus. Called also *superior dental artery.*

a. angula′ris [NA], angular artery: *origin,* facial artery; *branches,* none; *distribution,* lacrimal sac, lower eyelid, nose.

a. anon′yma, truncus brachiocephalicus.

a. aor′ta, aorta.

a. appendicula′ris [NA], appendicular artery: *origin,* ileocolic artery; *branches,* none; *distribution,* vermiform appendix. Called also *vermiform artery.*

arte′riae arcifor′mes re′nis, arteriae arcuatae renis.

a. arcua′ta pe′dis [NA], arcuate artery of foot: *origin,* dorsal artery of foot; *branches,* deep plantar branch and dorsal metatarsal artery; *distribution,* foot, toes. Called also *arcus dorsalis pedis.*

arte′riae arcua′tae re′nis [NA], arcuate arteries of kidney: *origin,* interlobar artery; *branches,* interlobular artery and arteriolae rectae; *distribution,* parenchyma of kidney. Called also *arteriae arciformes renis* and *arterial arches of kidney.*

a. ascen′dens ileocol′ica, ramus colicus arteriae ileocolicae.

a. auditi′va inter′na, a. labyrinthi.

arte′riae auricula′res anterio′res, rami auriculares anteriores arteriae temporalis superficialis.

a. auricula′ris poste′rior [NA], posterior auricular artery: *origin,* external carotid; *branches,* auricular and occipital rami, stylomastoid artery; *distribution,* middle ear, mastoid cells, auricle, parotid gland, digastric and other muscles.

a. auricula′ris profun′da [NA], deep auricular artery: *origin,* maxillary artery; *branches,* none; *distribution,* skin of auditory canal, tympanic membrane, temporomandibular joint.

a. axilla′ris [NA], axillary artery: *origin,* continuation of subclavian artery; *branches,* subscapular rami, and supreme thoracic, thoracoacromial, lateral thoracic, subscapular, and anterior and posterior circumflex humeral arteries; *distribution,* upper limb, axilla, chest, shoulder.

arte′riae azy′goi vagi′nae, NA alternative for *rami vaginales arteriae uterinae.*

a. basila′ris [NA], basilar artery: *origin,* from junction of right and left vertebral arteries; *branches,* pontine branches, and anterior inferior cerebellar, labyrinthine, superior cerebellar, and posterior cerebral arteries; *distribution,* brain stem, internal ear, cerebellum, posterior cerebrum.

a. brachia′lis [NA], brachial artery: *origin,* continuation of axillary artery; *branches,* superficial brachial, deep brachial, nutrient of humerus, superior ulnar collateral, inferior ulnar collateral, radial, and ulnar arteries; *distribution,* shoulder, arm, forearm, hand.

a. brachia′lis superficia′lis [NA], superficial brachial artery: a name given to a vessel that arises from high bifurcation of the brachial artery and assumes a more superficial course than usual.

arte′riae bronchia′les, rami bronchiales aortae thoracicae.

a. bucca′lis [NA], buccal artery: *origin,* maxillary artery; *branches,* none; *distribution,* buccinator muscle, mucous membrane of mouth. Called also *a. buccinatoria* and *buccinator artery.*

a. buccinato′ria, a. buccalis.

a. bul′bi pe′nis [NA], artery of bulb of penis: *origin,* internal pudendal artery; *branches,* none; *distribution,* bulbourethral gland, bulb of penis. Called also *a. bulbi urethrae* and *bulbourethral artery.*

a. bul′bi ure′thrae, a. bulbi penis.

a. bul′bi vestib′uli vagi′nae [NA], artery of bulb of vestibule of vagina: *origin,* internal pudendal artery; *branches,* none; *distribution,* vestibular bulb, greater vestibular glands.

a. caeca′lis ante′rior [NA], anterior cecal artery: *origin,* ileocolic; *branches,* none; *distribution,* cecum.

a. caeca′lis poste′rior [NA], posterior cecal artery: *origin,* ileocolic; *branches,* none; *distribution,* cecum.

a. callosomargina′lis [NA], callosomarginal artery: *origin,* postcommunical part of anterior cerebral artery; *branches,* anteromedial frontal, intermediomedial frontal, posteromedial frontal, and singular branches; *distribution,* medial and superlateral surfaces of cerebral hemisphere.

a. cana′lis pterygoi′dei [NA], artery of pterygoid canal: *origin,* maxillary artery; *branches,* pterygoid; *distribution,* roof of pharynx, auditory tube. Called also *vidian artery.*

arte′riae caroticotympan′icae, [NA], caroticotympanic arteries: branches of the petrous part of the internal carotid artery that supply the tympanic cavity; called also *rami caroticotympanici arteriae carot′idis internae.*

a. carot′is commu′nis [NA], common carotid artery: *origin,* brachiocephalic trunk (right), aortic arch (left); *branches,* external and internal carotids; *distribution,* see *a. carotis externa* and *a. carotis interna.* Called also *cephalic artery.*

a. carot′is exter′na [NA], external carotid artery: *origin,* common carotid; *branches,* superior thyroid, ascending pharyngeal, lingual, facial, sternocleidomastoid, occipital, posterior auricular, superficial temporal, maxillary; *distribution,* neck, face, skull. Called also *facial artery.*

a. carot′is inter′na [NA], internal carotid artery: *origin,* common carotid; *branches,* caroticotympanic, ophthalmic, posterior communicating, anterior choroid, anterior cerebral, and middle cerebral arteries; *distribution,* middle ear, brain, pituitary gland, orbit, choroid plexus. It is divided into four parts: cervical, petrous, cavernous, and cerebral.

a. cau′dae pancre′atis [NA], *origin,* splenic; *branches and distribution,* supplies branches to tail of pancreas, and accessory spleen (if present).

arte′riae centra′les anterolatera′les [NA], anterolateral central arteries: *origin,* sphenoidal part of middle cerebral artery; *branches,* two sets of branches, medial and lateral; *distribution,* anterior lenticular and caudate nuclei and internal capsule of brain. Called also *arteriae thalmostriatae anterolaterales* [NA alternative], *anterolateral thalamostriate arteries,* and *striate arteries.*

arte′riae centra′les anteromedia′les [NA], anteromedial central arteries: *origin,* precommunical part of anterior cerebral artery; *branches,* none; *distribution,* anterior and medial corpus striatum. Called also *arteriae thalamostriatae anteromediales* [NA alternative] and *anteromedial thalamostriate arteries.*

arte′riae centra′les posterolatera′les [NA], posterolateral central arteries: *origin,* postcommunical part of posterior cerebral artery; *branches,* none; *distribution,* cerebral peduncle, posterior thalamus, colliculi, pineal and medial geniculate bodies.

arte′riae centra′les posteromedia′les [NA] posteromedial central arteries: *origin,* precommunical part of posterior cerebral artery; *branches,* none; *distribution,* anterior thalamus, lateral wall of third ventricle, and globus pallidus of lentiform nucleus.

a. centra′lis brev′is [NA], short central artery: a branch from the precommunical part of the anterior cerebral artery.

a. centra′lis lon′ga [NA], long central artery: a branch of the precommunical part of the anterior cerebral artery; called also *a. recurrens* [NA alternative].

a. centra′lis ret′inae [NA], central artery of retina: *origin,* ophthalmic artery; *branches,* none; *distribution,* retina. Called also *Zinn's artery.*

a. cerebel′li infe′rior ante′rior, a. inferior anterior cerebelli.

a. cerebel′li infe′rior poste′rior, a. inferior posterior cerebelli.

a. cerebel′li supe′rior [NA], superior cerebellar artery: *origin,* basilar artery; *branches,* none; *distribution,* upper cerebellum, midbrain, pineal body, choroid plexus of third ventricle.

a. cer′ebri ante′rior [NA], anterior cerebral artery: *origin,* internal carotid artery; *branches* (precommunical part) anteromedial central arteries, long and short central arteries, anterior communicating artery, anteromedial central branch, and (postcommunical part) medial frontobasal, callosomarginal (anteromedial, interomedial, posteromedial, and cingular branches), paracentral, precuneal, and parieto-occipital arteries; *distribution,* orbital, frontal, and parietal cortex, corpus callosum, diencephalon, corpus striatum, internal capsule, and choroid plexus of lateral ventricle.

a. cer′ebri me′dia [NA], middle cerebral artery: *origin,* internal carotid; *branches* (sphenoidal part) anterolateral central artery (medial and lateral branches), (insular part) insular artery, lateral frontobasilar artery, anterior, intermediate, posterior temporal arteries, and (terminal, or cortical, part) arteries of central, precentral, and postcentral sulcus, anterior and posterior parietal arteries, artery of angular gyri; *distribution,* orbital, frontal, parietal, and temporal cortex, corpus striatum, internal capsule. Called also *sylvian artery.*

a. cer′ebri poste′rior [NA], posterior cerebral artery: *origin,* terminal bifurcation of basilar artery; *branches* (precommunical part) posteromedial central arteries, (postcommunical part) posterolateral central arteries, and thalamic, medial and lateral posterior choroidal, and peduncular branches, and (terminal, or cortical, part) lateral occipital artery (anterior, medial intermediate and posterior temporal branches) and medial occipital artery (dorsal corpus callosum, parietal, parieto-occipital, calcarine, and occipitotemporal branches); *distribution,* occipital and temporal cortex, diencephalon, midbrain, choroid plexus of lateral and third ventricles, and visual area of cerebral cortex and other structures associated with the visual pathway.

a. cervica′lis ascen′dens [NA], ascending cervical artery: *origin,* inferior thyroid artery; *branches,* spinal rami; *distribution,* muscles of neck, vertebrae, vertebral canal.

a. cervica′lis profun′da [NA], deep cervical artery: *origin,* costocervical trunk; *branches,* none; *distribution,* deep neck muscles.

a. cervica′lis superficia′lis, NA alternative for *ramus superficialis arteriae transversae colli.*

arte′riae cervicovagina′les, several large branches of the uterine artery given off at the side of the uterus at the level of the cervix, to supply the vagina.

a. chorioi′dea, a. choroidea anterior.

a. choroi′dea ante′rior [NA], anterior choroidal artery: *origin,* internal carotid or middle cerebral artery; *branches,* many small branches; *distribution,* interior of brain, including choroid plexus of lateral ventricle and adjacent parts. Called also *a. chorioidea.*

arte′riae cilia′res anterio′res [NA], anterior ciliary arteries: *origin,* ophthalmic and lacrimal arteries; *branches,* episcleral and anterior conjunctival arteries; *distribution,* iris, conjunctiva.

arte′riae cilia′res posterio′res bre′ves [NA], short (posterior) ciliary arteries: *origin,* ophthalmic artery; *branches,* none; *distribution,* choroid coat of eye.

arte′riae cilia′res posterio′res lon′gae [NA], long (posterior) ciliary arteries: *origin,* ophthalmic artery; *branches,* none; *distribution,* iris, ciliary process.

a. circumflex′a ante′rior hu′meri [NA], anterior circumflex humeral artery: *origin,* axillary artery; *branches,* none; *distribution,* shoulder joint and head of humerus, long tendon of biceps, tendon of pectoralis major muscle. Called also *a. circumflexa humeri anterior.*

a. circumflex′a fem′oris latera′lis [NA], lateral circumflex femoral artery: *origin,* deep femoral artery; *branches,* ascending, descending, and transverse branches; *distribution,* hip joint, thigh muscles.

a. circumflex′a fem′oris media′lis [NA], medial circumflex femoral artery: *origin,* deep femoral artery; *branches,* deep, ascending, transverse, and acetabular branches; *distribution,* hip joint, thigh muscles.

a. circumflex′a hu′meri ante′rior, a. circumflexa anterior humeri.

a. circumflex′a hu′meri poste′rior, a. circumflexa posterior humeri.

a. circumflex′a il′ium profun′da [NA], deep circumflex iliac artery: *origin,* external iliac artery; *branches,* ascending branches; *distribution,* iliac region, abdominal wall, groin. Called also *external epigastric artery.*

a. circumflex′a il′ium superficia′lis [NA], superficial circumflex iliac artery: *origin,* femoral artery; *branches,* none; *distribution,* groin, abdominal wall.

a. circumflex′a poste′rior hu′meri [NA], posterior circumflex humeral artery: *origin,* axillary artery; *branches;* none;

distribution, deltoideus, shoulder joint, teres minor and triceps muscles. Called also *a. circumflexa humeri posterior.*

a. circumflex′a scap′ulae [NA], circumflex artery of scapula: *origin,* subscapular artery; *branches,* none; *distribution,* inferolateral muscles of the scapula.

a. clitor′idis, artery of clitoris.

a. col′ica dex′tra [NA], right colic artery: *origin,* superior mesenteric artery; *branches,* none; *distribution,* ascending colon.

a. col′ica me′dia [NA], middle colic artery: *origin,* superior mesenteric artery; *branches,* none; *distribution,* transverse colon. Called also *accessory superior colic artery.*

a. col′ica sinis′tra [NA], left colic artery: *origin,* inferior mesenteric; *branches,* none; *distribution,* descending colon.

a. collatera′lis me′dia [NA], middle collateral artery: *origin,* deep brachial artery; *branches,* none; *distribution,* triceps muscle, elbow joint.

a. collatera′lis radia′lis [NA], radial collateral artery: *origin,* deep brachial artery; *branches,* none; *distribution,* brachioradialis and brachialis muscles.

a. collatera′lis ulna′ris infe′rior [NA], inferior ulnar collateral artery: *origin,* brachial artery; *branches,* none; *distribution,* arm muscles at back of elbow.

a. collatera′lis ulna′ris supe′rior [NA], superior ulnar collateral artery: *origin,* brachial artery; *branches,* none; *distribution,* elbow joint, triceps muscle.

a. com′itans ner′vi ischia′dici [NA], accompanying artery of ischiatic nerve: *origin,* inferior gluteal artery; *branches,* none; *distribution,* accompanies sciatic nerve. Called also *sciatic artery.*

a. com′itans ner′vi media′ni [NA], accompanying artery of median nerve: *origin,* anterior interosseous artery; *branches,* none; *distribution,* median nerve, muscles of front of forearm. Called also *a. mediana* and *median artery.*

a. commu′nicans ante′rior cer′ebri [NA], anterior communicating artery of cerebrum: *origin,* precommunical part of anterior cerebral artery; *branches,* none; *distribution,* establishes connection between the anterior cerebral arteries.

a. commu′nicans poste′rior cer′ebri [NA], posterior communicating artery of cerebrum: establishes connection between internal carotid and posterior cerebral arteries; *branches,* to the optic chiasm, oculomotor nerve, thalamus, hypothalamus, and tail of caudate nucleus.

arte′riae conjunctiva′les anterio′res [NA], anterior conjunctival arteries: *origin,* anterior ciliary; *branches,* none; *distribution,* conjunctiva.

arte′riae conjunctiva′les posterio′res [NA], posterior conjunctival arteries: *origin,* medial palpebral artery; *branches,* none; *distribution,* caruncula lacrimalis, conjunctiva.

a. corona′ria [cor′dis] dex′tra, a. coronaria dextra.

a. corona′ria dex′tra [NA], right coronary artery of heart: *origin,* right aortic sinus; *branches,* posterior interventricular; *distribution,* right ventricle, right atrium. Formerly called *right auricular artery.*

a. corona′ria [cor′dis] sinis′tra, a. coronaria sinistra.

a. corona′ria sinis′tra [NA], left coronary artery of heart: *origin,* left aortic sinus; *branches,* anterior interventricular and circumflex rami; *distribution,* left ventricle, left atrium. Formerly called *left auricular artery.*

a. cremaster′ica [NA], cremasteric artery: *origin,* inferior epigastric; *branches,* none; *distribution,* cremaster muscle, coverings of spermatic cord. Called also *a. spermatica externa* and *external spermatic artery.*

a. cys′tica [NA], cystic artery: *origin,* right branch of proper hepatic artery; *branches,* none; *distribution,* gallbladder.

a. deferentia′lis, a. ductus deferentis.

a. descen′dens genicula′ris [NA], descending genicular artery: *origin,* femoral artery; *branches,* saphenous, articular; *distribution,* knee joint, upper and medial leg. Called also *a. genus descendens.*

arte′riae digita′les dorsa′les ma′nus [NA], dorsal digital arteries of hand: *origin,* dorsal metacarpal arteries; *branches,* none; *distribution,* dorsum of fingers.

arte′riae digita′les dorsa′les pe′dis [NA], dorsal digital arteries of foot: *origin,* dorsal metatarsal arteries; *branches,* none; *distribution,* dorsum of toes.

arte′riae digita′les palma′res commu′nes [NA], common palmar digital arteries: *origin,* superficial volar arch; *branches,* proper palmar digital arteries; *distribution,* fingers. Called also *arteriae digitales volares communis, common volar digital arteries,* and *ulnar metacarpal arteries.*

arte′riae digita′les palma′res pro′priae [NA], proper palmar digital arteries: *origin,* common palmar digital arteries; *branches*, none; *distribution*, fingers. Called also *arteriae digitales volares propriae, collateral digital arteries,* and *proper volar digital arteries.*

arte′riae digita′les planta′res commu′nes [NA], common plantar digital arteries: *origin*, plantar metatarsal arteries; *branches*, proper plantar digital arteries; *distribution*, toes.

arte′riae digita′les planta′res pro′priae [NA], proper plantar digital arteries: *origin*, common plantar digital arteries; *branches*, none; *distribution*, toes.

arte′riae digita′les vola′res commu′nes, arteriae digitales palmares communes.

arte′riae digita′les vola′res pro′priae, arteriae digitales palmares propriae.

a. dorsa′lis clitor′idis [NA], dorsal artery of clitoris: *origin*, internal pudendal artery; *branches*, none; *distribution*, clitoris.

a. dorsa′lis na′si [NA], dorsal artery of nose: *origin*, ophthalmic artery; *branches*, lacrimal; *distribution*, dorsum of nose. Called also *a. nasi externa* [NA alternative].

a. dorsa′lis pe′dis [NA], dorsal artery of foot: *origin*, continuation of anterior tibial; *branches*, lateral and medial tarsal, arcuate, and deep plantar arteries; *distribution*, foot, toes.

a. dorsa′lis pe′nis [NA], dorsal artery of penis: *origin*, internal pudendal artery; *branches*, none; *distribution*, glans, corona, prepuce.

a. dorsa′lis scapula′ris [NA], dorsal scapular artery: *origin*, second or third part of subclavian artery, or may be the deep branch of transverse cervical artery (*ramus profundus arteriae transversae cervicis*); *branches*, none; *distribution*, rhomboid, latissimus dorsi, and trapezius muscles. Called also *a. scapularis dorsalis* [NA alternative].

a. duc′tus deferen′tis [NA], artery of ductus deferens, deferential artery: *origin*, umbilical artery; *branches*, ureteral artery; *distribution*, ureter, ductus deferens, seminal vesicles, testes. Called also *a. deferentialis.*

a. epigas′trica infe′rior [NA], inferior epigastric artery: *origin*, external iliac; *branches*, pubic branch, cremasteric artery, a. of round ligament of uterus; *distribution*, abdominal wall.

a. epigas′trica superficia′lis [NA], superficial epigastric artery: *origin*, femoral; *branches*, none; *distribution*, abdominal wall, groin.

a. epigas′trica supe′rior [NA], superior epigastric artery: *origin*, internal thoracic artery; *branches*, none; *distribution*, abdominal wall, diaphragm.

arte′riae episclera′les [NA], episcleral arteries: *origin*, anterior ciliary artery; *branches*, none; *distribution*, iris, ciliary process.

a. ethmoida′lis ante′rior [NA], anterior ethmoidal artery: *origin*, ophthalmic artery; *branches*, anterior meningeal, anterior septal, and anterior lateral nasal rami; *distribution*, dura mater, nose, frontal sinus, anterior ethmoidal cells.

a. ethmoida′lis poste′rior [NA], posterior ethmoidal artery: *origin*, ophthalmic artery; *branches*, none; *distribution*, posterior ethmoidal cells, dura mater, nose.

a. facia′lis [NA], facial artery: *origin*, external carotid; *branches*, ascending palatine, tonsillar, submental, inferior labial, superior labial, septal, lateral nasal, angular, glandular; *distribution*, face, tonsil, palate, submandibular gland. Called also *a. maxillaris externa* or *external maxillary artery.*

a. femora′lis [NA], femoral artery: *origin*, continuation of external iliac; *branches*, superficial epigastric, superficial circumflex iliac, external pudendal, deep femoral, descending geniculate; *distribution*, lower abdominal wall, external genitalia, lower extremity. NOTE: Vascular surgeons refer to the portion of the femoral artery proximal to the branching of the deep femoral as the *common femoral a.*, and to its continuation as the *superficial femoral a.* In this classification, the descending geniculate artery is a branch of the superficial femoral artery.

a. fibula′ris, [NA], fibular artery: *origin*, posterior tibial artery; *branches*, perforating, communicating, calcaneal, and lateral and medial malleolar branches, and calcaneal rate; *distribution*, outside and back of ankle, deep calf muscles. Called also *a. peronea* [NA alternative] and *peroneal artery.*

a. fronta′lis, a. supratrochlearis.

a. frontobasa′lis latera′lis [NA], lateral frontobasal artery: *origin*, insular part of middle cerebral artery; *branches*, none; *distribution*, cortex of lateroinferior frontal lobe. Called also *ramus orbitofrontalis medialis arteriae cerebri mediae* [NA alternative].

a. frontobasa′lis media′lis [NA], medial frontobasal artery: *origin*, postcommunical part of anterior cerebral artery; *branches*, none; *distribution*, medioinferior cortex of frontal lobe. Called also *ramus orbitofrontalis medialis arteriae cerebri anterioris* [NA alternative].

arte′riae gas′tricae bre′ves [NA], short gastric arteries: *origin*, splenic; *branches*, none; *distribution*, upper part of stomach.

a. gas′trica dex′tra [NA], right gastric artery: *origin*, common hepatic artery; *branches*, none; *distribution*, lesser curvature of stomach. Called also *right coronary artery of stomach* and *pyloric artery.*

a. gas′trica poste′rior [NA], posterior gastric artery: *origin*, splenic artery; *branches*, none; *distribution*, posterior gastric wall.

a. gas′trica sinis′tra [NA], left gastric artery: *origin*, celiac; *branches*, esophageal; *distribution*, esophagus, lesser curvature of stomach. Called also *left coronary artery of stomach.*

a. gastroduodena′lis [NA], gastroduodenal artery: *origin*, common hepatic artery; *branches*, supraduodenal and posterior superior pancreaticoduodenal arteries; *distribution*, stomach, duodenum, pancreas, greater omentum.

a. gastroepiplo′ica dex′tra, NA alternative for *a. gastro-omentalis dextra.*

a. gastroepiplo′ica sinis′tra, NA alternative for *a. gastro-omentalis sinistra.*

a. gastro-omenta′lis dex′tra [NA], right gastro-omental artery: *origin*, gastroduodenal artery; *branches*, gastric, omental; *distribution*, stomach, greater omentum. Called also *a. gastroepiploica dextra* [NA alternative] and *right inferior gastric artery.*

a. gastro-omenta′lis sinis′tra [NA], left gastro-omental artery: *origin*, splenic artery; *branches*, gastric, omental; *distribution*, stomach, greater omentum. Called also *a. gastroepiploica sinistra,* [NA alternative] and *left inferior gastric artery.*

a. ge′nus descen′dens, a. descendens genicularis.

a. ge′nus infe′rior latera′lis, a. inferior lateralis genus.

a. ge′nus infe′rior media′lis, a. inferior medialis genus.

a. ge′nus me′dia, a. media genus.

a. ge′nus supe′rior latera′lis, a. superior lateralis genus.

a. ge′nus supe′rior media′lis, a. superior medialis genus.

a. glu′taea infe′rior, a. glutea inferior.

a. glu′taea supe′rior, a. glutea superior.

a. glu′tea infe′rior [NA], inferior gluteal artery: *origin*, internal iliac; *branches*, sciatic; *distribution*, buttock, back of thigh. Called also *a. glutaea inferior.*

a. glu′tea supe′rior [NA], superior gluteal artery: *origin*, internal iliac artery; *branches*, superficial and deep branches; *distribution*, buttocks. Called also *a. glutaea superior.*

a. gy′ri angula′ris [NA], artery of angular gyrus: *origin*, terminal part of middle cerebral artery; *branches*, none; *distribution*, temporal, parietal, and occipital lobes.

a. haemorrhoida′lis infe′rior, a. rectalis inferior.

a. haemorrhoida′lis me′dia, a. rectalis media.

a. haemorrhoida′lis supe′rior, a. rectalis superior.

arte′riae helici′nae pe′nis [NA], helicine arteries of penis: helicine arteries arising from the vessels of the penis, whose engorgement causes erection of the organ. Called also *arteries of Mueller.*

a. hepat′ica, a. hepatica communis.

a. hepat′ica commu′nis [NA], common hepatic artery: *origin*, celiac trunk; *branches*, right gastric, gastroduodenal, hepatic proper; *distribution*, stomach, pancreas, duodenum, liver, gallbladder, greater omentum. Called also *a. hepatica.*

a. hepat′ica pro′pria [NA], proper hepatic artery: *origin*, common hepatic artery; *branches*, right and left branches; *distribution*, liver, gallbladder. Called also *hepatic funiculus of Rauber.*

a. hyaloi′dea [NA], hyaloid artery: a fetal vessel that continues forward from the central retinal artery through the vitreous body to supply the lens; it normally is not present after birth.

a. hypogas′trica, a. iliaca interna.

a. hypophysia′lis infe′rior [NA], inferior hypophyseal artery: a small branch from the cerebral part of the internal carotid artery that supplies the pituitary gland.

a. hypophysia′lis supe′rior [NA], superior hypophyseal artery: a small branch from the cerebral part of the internal carotid artery that supplies the pituitary gland.

arte′riae il′eae, arteriae ilei.

arte′riae il′ei [NA], ileal arteries: *origin,* superior mesenteric; *branches,* none; *distribution,* ileum. Called also *a. ileae.*

a. ileoco′lica [NA], ileocolic artery: *origin,* superior mesenteric; *branches,* anterior and posterior cecal and appendicular arteries and colic (ascending) and ileal rami; *distribution,* ileum, cecum, vermiform appendix, ascending colon. Called also *inferior right colic artery.*

a. ili′aca commu′nis [NA], common iliac artery: *origin,* abdominal aorta; *branches,* internal and external iliac; *distribution,* pelvis, abdominal wall, lower limb.

a. ili′aca exter′na [NA], external iliac artery: *origin,* common iliac; *branches,* inferior epigastric, deep circumflex iliac; *distribution,* abdominal wall, external genitalia, lower limb. Called also *anterior iliac artery.*

a. ili′aca inter′na [NA], internal iliac artery: *origin,* continuation of common iliac; *branches,* iliolumbar, obturator, superior gluteal, inferior gluteal, umbilical, inferior vesical, uterine, middle rectal, and internal pudendal arteries; *distribution,* wall and viscera of pelvis, buttock, reproductive organs, medial aspect of thigh. Called also *a. hypogastrica, hypogastric artery,* and *posterior pelvic artery.*

a. iliolumba′lis [NA], iliolumbar artery: *origin,* internal iliac; *branches,* iliac and lumbar branches, lateral sacral arteries; *distribution,* pelvic muscles and bones, fifth lumbar segment, sacrum. Called also *small iliac artery.*

a. infe′rior ante′rior cerebel′li [NA], anterior inferior cerebellar artery: *origin,* basilar artery; *branches,* posterior, spinal (usually) and labyrinthine (usually) arteries; *distribution,* anteroinferior part of cerebellum, lower and lateral parts of pons and sometimes upper part of medulla oblongata. Called also *a. cerebelli inferior anterior.*

a. infe′rior latera′lis ge′nus [NA], lateral inferior genicular artery: *origin,* popliteal artery; *branches,* none; *distribution,* knee joint. Called also *a. genus inferior lateralis.*

a. infe′rior media′lis ge′nus [NA], medial inferior genicular artery: *origin,* popliteal artery; *branches,* none; *distribution,* knee joint. Called also *a. genus inferior medialis.*

a. infe′rior poste′rior cerebel′li [NA], posterior inferior cerebellar artery: *origin,* vertebral artery; *branches,* medial and lateral; *distribution,* lower cerebellum, medulla, choroid plexus of fourth ventricle. Called also *a. cerebelli inferior posterior.*

a. infraorbita′lis [NA], infraorbital artery: *origin,* maxillary artery; *branches,* anterior superior alveolar; *distribution,* maxilla, maxillary sinus, upper teeth, lower lid, cheek, nose.

a. innomina′ta, truncus brachiocephalicus.

arte′riae insula′res [NA], insular arteries: *origin,* insular part of middle cerebral artery; *branches,* none; *distribution,* cortex of insula.

arte′riae intercosta′les posterio′res [NA], nine pairs of posterior intercostal arteries (III–XI): *origin,* thoracic aorta; *branches,* dorsal, spinal, lateral and medial cutaneous, collateral, and lateral mammary; *distribution,* thoracic wall.

a. intercosta′lis poste′rior pri′ma [NA], first posterior intercostal artery: *origin,* highest intercostal artery; *branches,* dorsal and spinal branches; *distribution,* upper thoracic wall.

a. intercosta′lis poste′rior secun′da [NA], second posterior intercostal artery: *origin,* highest intercostal artery; *branches,* dorsal and spinal branches; *distribution,* upper thoracic wall.

a. intercosta′lis supre′ma [NA], highest intercostal artery: *origin,* costocervical trunk; *branches,* first and second posterior intercostal arteries; *distribution,* upper thoracic wall. Called also *superior intercostal artery.*

arte′riae interlobula′res hep′atis [NA], interlobular arteries of liver: arteries originating from the right or left branch of the proper hepatic artery, and passing between the lobules of the liver.

arte′riae interlobula′res re′nis [NA], interlobular arteries of kidney: arteries originating from the arcuate arteries of the kidney and distributed to the renal glomeruli. Called also *radiate arteries of kidney.*

a. interos′sea ante′rior [NA], anterior interosseous artery: *origin,* posterior or common interosseous artery; *branches,* median artery; *distribution,* deep parts of front of forearm. Called also *a. interossea volaris* or *volar interosseous artery.*

a. interos′sea commu′nis [NA], common interosseous artery: *origin,* ulnar artery; *branches,* anterior and posterior interosseous arteries; *distribution,* antecubital fossa.

a. interos′sea dorsa′lis, a. interossea posterior.

a. interos′sea poste′rior [NA], posterior interosseous artery: *origin,* common interosseous artery; *branches,* recurrent

interosseous; *distribution,* deep parts of back of forearm. Called also *a. interossea dorsalis* and *dorsal* or *posterior interosseous artery of forearm.*

a. interos′sea recur′rens [NA], recurrent interosseous artery: *origin,* posterior interosseous or common interosseous artery; *branches,* none; *distribution,* back of elbow joint.

a. interos′sea vola′ris, a. interossea anterior.

arte′riae intestina′les, intestinal arteries: the arteries arising from the superior mesenteric, and supplying the intestines, including the pancreaticoduodenal, jejunal, ileal, ileocolic, and colic arteries.

arte′riae jejuna′les [NA], jejunal arteries: *origin,* superior mesenteric; *branches,* none; *distribution,* jejunum.

arte′riae labia′les anterio′res vul′vae, rami labiales anteriores arteriae femoralis.

a. labia′lis infe′rior [NA], inferior labial artery: *origin,* facial artery; *branches,* none; *distribution,* lower lip.

arte′riae labia′les posterio′res vul′vae, rami labiales posteriores arteriae pudendae internae.

a. labia′lis supe′rior [NA], superior labial artery: *origin,* facial artery; *branches,* septal and alar; *distribution,* upper lip, nose.

a. labyrin′thi [NA], artery of labyrinth, labyrinthine artery: *origin,* basilar or anterior inferior cerebellar artery; *branches,* vestibular and cochlear rami; *distribution,* through the internal acoustic meatus to the internal ear. Called also *a. auditiva interna, internal auditory artery,* and *ramus meatus acustici interni arteriae basilaris* [NA alternative].

a. lacrima′lis [NA], lacrimal artery: *origin,* ophthalmic artery; *branches,* lateral palpebral arteries and recurrent meningeal; *distribution,* lacrimal gland, upper and lower eyelids, conjunctiva.

a. laryn′gea infe′rior [NA], inferior laryngeal artery: *origin,* inferior thyroid artery; *branches,* none; *distribution,* larynx, trachea, esophagus.

a. laryn′gea supe′rior [NA], superior laryngeal artery: *origin,* superior thyroid artery; *branches,* none; *distribution,* larynx.

a. liena′lis, NA alternative for *a. splenica.*

a. ligamen′ti ter′etis u′teri [NA], artery of round ligament of uterus: *origin,* inferior epigastric artery; *branches,* none; *distribution,* round ligament of uterus.

a. lingua′lis [NA], lingual artery: *origin,* external carotid; *branches,* suprahyoid, sublingual, dorsal lingual, deep lingual; *distribution,* tongue, sublingual gland, tonsil, epiglottis.

a. lo′bi cauda′ti [NA], either of two branches, one from the right and one from the left hepatic artery, supplying twigs to the caudate lobe of the liver.

arte′riae lumba′les [NA], lumbar arteries: *origin,* abdominal aorta; *branches,* dorsal and spinal branches; *distribution,* posterior abdominal wall, renal capsule.

a. lumba′lis i′ma [NA], lowest lumbar artery: *origin,* middle sacral; *branches,* none; *distribution,* sacrum, gluteus maximus muscle. Called also *fifth lumbar artery.*

a. malleola′ris ante′rior latera′lis [NA], lateral anterior malleolar artery: *origin,* anterior tibial artery; *branches,* none; *distribution,* ankle joint.

a. malleola′ris ante′rior media′lis [NA], medial anterior malleolar artery: *origin,* anterior tibial artery; *branches,* none; *distribution,* ankle joint.

a. mammar′ia inter′na, a. thoracica interna.

a. masseter′ica [NA], masseteric artery: *origin,* maxillary artery; *branches,* none; *distribution,* masseter muscle.

a. maxilla′ris [NA], maxillary artery: *origin,* external carotid artery; *branches,* pterygoid rami, and deep auricular, anterior tympanic, inferior alveolar, middle meningeal, masseteric, deep temporal, buccal, posterior superior alveolar, infraorbital, descending palatine, sphenopalatine, and the artery of the pterygoid canal; *distribution,* both jaws, teeth, muscles of mastication, ear, meninges, nose, nasal sinus, palate. Called also *a. maxillaris interna, internal maxillary artery,* and *deep facial artery.*

a. maxilla′ris exter′na, a. facialis.

a. maxilla′ris inter′na, a. maxillaris.

a. max′ima Gale′ni, aorta.

a. me′dia ge′nus [NA], middle genicular artery: *origin,* popliteal artery; *branches,* none; *distribution,* knee joint, cruciate ligaments, patellar synovial and alar folds. Called also *a. genus media.*

a. media′na, a. comitans nervi mediani.

arte′riae mediastina′les anterio′res, rami mediastinales arteriae thoracicae internae.

a. menin′gea ante′rior, ramus meningeus anterior arteriae ethmoidalis anterioris.

a. menin′gea me′dia [NA], middle meningeal artery: *origin,* maxillary artery; *branches,* frontal, parietal, and lacrimal anastomotic, accessory meningeal, and petrosal rami, and the superior tympanic artery; *distribution,* cranial bones, dura mater.

a. menin′gea poste′rior [NA], posterior meningeal artery: *origin,* ascending pharyngeal; *branches,* none; *distribution,* bones, dura mater of posterior cranial fossa.

a. menta′lis, ramus mentalis arteriae alveolaris inferioris.

arte′riae mesencephal′icae [NA], mesencephalic arteries: *origin,* basilar artery; *branches,* none; *distribution:* cerebral peduncle.

a. mesenter′ica infe′rior [NA], inferior mesenteric artery: *origin,* abdominal aorta; *branches,* left colic, sigmoid, and superior rectal arteries; *distribution,* descending colon, rectum.

a. mesenter′ica supe′rior [NA], superior mesenteric artery: *origin,* abdominal aorta; *branches,* inferior pancreaticoduodenal, jejunal, ileal, ileocolic, right colic, and middle colic arteries; *distribution,* small intestine, proximal half of colon.

arte′riae metacarpa′les dorsa′les [NA], **arte′riae metacar′peae dorsa′les,** dorsal metacarpal arteries: *origin,* dorsal carpal rete and radial artery; *branches,* dorsal digital arteries; *distribution,* dorsum of fingers.

arte′riae metacarpa′les palma′res [NA], **arte′riae metacar′peae palma′res,** palmar metacarpal arteries: *origin,* deep palmar arch; *branches,* none; *distribution,* deep parts of metatarsus. Called also *arteriae metacarpeae volares, volar metacarpal arteries,* and *palmar intermetacarpal arteries.*

arte′riae metatarsa′les dorsa′les [NA], **arte′riae metatar′seae dorsa′les,** dorsal metatarsal arteries: *origin,* arcuate artery of foot; *branches,* dorsal digital arteries; *distribution,* foot, toes.

arte′riae metatarsa′les planta′res [NA], **arte′riae metatar′seae planta′res,** plantar metatarsal arteries: *origin,* plantar arch; *branches,* perforating branches, common and proper plantar digital arteries; *distribution,* toes. Called also *common digital arteries of foot.*

arte′riae muscula′res arte′riae lacrima′lis [NA], the muscular branches of the lacrimal artery, consisting of a superior group and an inferior group that gives origin to the anterior ciliary arteries.

a. musculophren′ica [NA], musculophrenic artery: *origin,* internal thoracic artery; *branches,* none; *distribution,* diaphragm, abdominal and thoracic walls.

arte′riae nasa′les posterio′res, latera′les [NA], posterior lateral nasal arteries: *origin,* sphenopalatine artery; *branches,* none; *distribution,* frontal, maxillary, ethmoidal, and sphenoidal sinuses.

a. na′si exter′na, NA alternative for *a. dorsalis nasi.*

a. nutri′cia [NA] nutrient artery: any artery that supplies the marrow, or medulla, of a long bone; called also *a. nutriens* [NA alternative] and *medullary artery.* See also *nutrient vessels,* under *vessel.*

a. nutri′cia fib′ulae [NA], nutrient artery of fibula: *origin,* fibular artery; *branches,* none; *distribution,* fibula. Called also *a. nutriens fibulae* [NA alternative].

a. nutri′cia tib′iae [NA], nutrient artery of tibia: *origin,* posterior tibial artery; *branches,* none; *distribution,* tibia. Called also *a. nutriens tibiae* [NA alternative].

arte′riae nutri′ciae fem′oris [NA], nutrient arteries of femur: *origin,* third perforating artery; *branches,* none; *distribution,* femur. Called also *arteriae nutrientes femoris* [NA alternative].

arte′riae nutri′ciae hu′meri [NA], nutrient arteries of humerus: *origin,* brachial and deep brachial arteries; *branches,* none; *distribution,* humerus. Called also *arteriae nutrientes humeri* [NA alternative].

a. nu′triens fib′ulae, NA alternative for *a. nutricia fibulae.*

a. nu′triens tib′iae, NA alternative for *a. nutricia tibiae.*

arte′riae nutrien′tes fem′oris, NA alternative for *arteriae nutriciae femoris.*

arte′riae nutrien′tes hu′meri, NA alternative for *arteriae nutriciae humeri.*

a. obturato′ria [NA], obturator artery: *origin,* internal iliac; *branches,* pubic, acetabular, anterior, and posterior branches; *distribution,* pelvic muscles, hip joint.

a. obturato′ria accesso′ria [NA], accessory obturator artery, a name given to the obturator artery when it arises from the inferior epigastric instead of the internal iliac artery.

a. occipita′lis [NA], occipital artery: *origin,* external carotid; *branches,* auricular, meningeal, mastoid, descending, occipital, and sternocleidomastoid rami; *distribution,* muscles of neck and scalp, meninges, mastoid cells.

a. occipita′lis latera′lis [NA], lateral occipital artery: *origin,* terminal, or cortical, part of posterior cerebral artery; *branches,* lateral occipital artery and anterior temporal, middle intermediate temporal and posterior temporal branches; *distribution,* anterior, medial, intermediate, and posterior parts of temporal lobe.

a. occipita′lis media′lis [NA], middle occipital artery: *origin,* terminal, or cortical, part of posterior cerebral artery; *branches,* dorsal corpus callosum, parietal, parieto-occipital, calcarine, and occipitotemporal branches; *distribution,* dorsum of corpus callosum, precuneus, cuneus, lingual gyrus, and posterior part of lateral surface of occipital lobe.

a. ophthal′mica [NA], ophthalmic artery: *origin,* internal carotid; *branches,* lacrimal, supraorbital, central artery of retina, ciliary, posterior and anterior ethmoidal, palpebral, supratrochlear, dorsal nasal; *distribution,* eye, orbit, adjacent facial structures.

a. ova′rica [NA], ovarian artery: *origin,* abdominal aorta; *branches,* ureteral, tubal; *distribution,* ureter, ovary, uterine tube. Called also *tubo-ovarian artery* or *aortic uterine artery.*

a. palati′na ascen′dens [NA], ascending palatine artery: *origin,* facial artery; *branches,* none; *distribution,* soft palate, wall of pharynx, tonsil, auditory tube.

a. palati′na descen′dens [NA], descending palatine artery: *origin,* maxillary artery; *branches,* greater and lesser palatine arteries; *distribution,* soft palate, hard palate, tonsil.

a. palati′na ma′jor [NA], greater palatine artery: *origin,* descending palatine; *branches,* none; *distribution,* hard palate.

arte′riae palati′nae mino′res [NA], lesser palatine arteries: *origin,* descending palatine; *branches,* none; *distribution,* soft palate, tonsil.

arte′riae palpebra′les latera′les [NA], lateral palpebral arteries: *origin,* lacrimal artery; *branches,* none; *distribution,* eyelids, conjunctiva.

arte′riae palpebra′les media′les [NA], medial palpebral arteries: *origin,* ophthalmic artery; *branches,* posterior conjunctival; *distribution,* eyelids.

a. pancreat′ica dorsa′lis [NA], dorsal pancreatic artery: *origin,* splenic; *branches,* inferior pancreatic; *distribution,* neck and body of pancreas.

a. pancreat′ica infe′rior [NA], inferior pancreatic artery: *origin,* dorsal pancreatic; *branches,* none; *distribution,* body and tail of pancreas.

a. pancreat′ica mag′na [NA], great pancreatic artery: *origin,* splenic; *branches and distribution,* right and left branches anastomose with other pancreatic arteries.

arte′riae pancreaticoduodena′les infe′riores [NA], inferior pancreaticoduodenal arteries: *origin,* superior mesenteric artery; *branches,* anterior, posterior; *distribution,* pancreas, duodenum. Called also *duodenal arteries.*

a. pancreaticoduodena′lis supe′rior ante′rior [NA], anterior superior pancreaticoduodenal artery: *origin,* gastroduodenal artery; *branches,* pancreatic and duodenal; *distribution,* pancreas and duodenum.

a. pancreaticoduodena′lis supe′rior poste′rior [NA], posterior superior pancreaticoduodenal artery: *origin,* gastroduodenal artery; *branches,* pancreatic and duodenal; *distribution,* pancreas, duodenum.

a. paracentra′lis [NA], paracentral artery: *origin,* postcommunical part of anterior cerebral artery; *branches,* none; *distribution,* cerebral cortex and medial central sulcus.

arte′riae parieta′les ante′rior et poste′rior [NA], anterior and posterior parietal arteries: *origin,* terminal part of middle cerebral artery; *branches,* anterior and posterior branches; *distribution,* anterior parietal lobe and posterior temporal lobe.

a. parieto-occipita′lis [NA], parieto-occipital artery: *origin,* postcommunical part of the anterior cerebral artery; *branches,* none; *distribution,* parietal lobe and sometimes occipital lobe.

arte′riae perforan′tes [NA], perforating arteries: *origin,* branches (usually three) of the deep femoral artery that perforate the insertion of the adductor magnus to reach the back of the thigh; *branches,* nutrient arteries; *distribution,* adductor, hamstring, and gluteal muscles, and femur.

a. pericallo′sa, NA alternative for *pars postcommunicalis arteriae cerebri anterioris.*

a. pericardiacophren′ica [NA], pericardiacophrenic artery: *origin,* internal thoracic artery; *branches,* none; *distri-*

bution, pericardium, diaphragm, pleura. Called also *superior phrenic artery.*

a. perinea'lis [NA], perineal artery: *origin*, internal pudendal artery; *branches*, none; *distribution*, perineum, skin of external genitalia. Called also *a. perinei.*

a. perine'i, a. perinealis.

a. pero'nea, NA alternative for *a. fibularis.*

a. pharyn'gea ascen'dens [NA], ascending pharyngeal artery: *origin*, external carotid; *branches*, posterior meningeal, pharyngeal, and inferior tympanic; *distribution*, pharynx, soft palate, ear, meninges.

arte'riae phren'icae infe'riores [NA], inferior phrenic arteries: *origin*, abdominal aorta; *branches*, superior suprarenal; *distribution*, diaphragm, suprarenal gland. Called also *great phrenic arteries* and *diaphragmatic arteries.*

arte'riae phren'icae superio'res [NA], superior phrenic arteries: *origin*, thoracic aorta; *branches*, none; *distribution*, upper surface of vertebral portion of diaphragm. Called also *superior diaphragmatic arteries.*

a. planta'ris latera'lis [NA], lateral plantar artery: *origin*, posterior tibial artery; *branches*, plantar arch, and plantar metatarsal arteries; *distribution*, sole of foot and toes. Called also *external plantar artery.*

a. planta'ris media'lis [NA], medial plantar artery: *origin*, posterior tibial artery; *branches*, deep and superficial branches; *distribution*, sole of the foot and toes.

a. planta'ris profun'dus [NA], deep plantar artery: *origin*, dorsal artery of foot; *branches*, none; *distribution*, sole of foot to help form plantar arch. Called also *ramus plantaris profundus arteriae dorsalis pedis.*

arte'riae pon'tis [NA], pontine arteries: *origin*, basilar artery; *branches*, none; *distribution*, pons and adjacent areas of brain. Called also *rami ad pontem arteriae basilaris.*

a. poplit'ea [NA], popliteal artery: *origin*, continuation of femoral artery; *branches*, lateral and medial superior genicular, middle genicular, sural, lateral and medial inferior genicular, anterior and posterior tibial arteries, and the genicular articular and the patellar rete; *distribution*, knee, calf.

a. precunea'lis [NA], precuneal artery: *origin*, postcommunical part of the anterior cerebral artery; *branches*, none; *distribution*, inferior precuneus.

a. prin'ceps pol'licis [NA], principal artery of thumb: *origin*, radial artery; *branches*, radial of index finger; *distribution*, each side and palmar aspect of thumb.

a. profun'da bra'chii [NA], deep brachial artery: *origin*, brachial artery; *branches*, deltoid ramus, nutrient artery, medial and radial collateral arteries; *distribution*, humerus, muscles and skin of arm.

a. profun'da clitor'idis [NA], deep artery of clitoris: *origin*, internal pudendal artery; *branches*, none; *distribution*, clitoris.

a. profun'da fem'oris [NA], deep femoral artery: *origin*, femoral artery; *branches*, medial and lateral circumflex arteries of thigh, perforating arteries; *distribution*, thigh muscles, hip joint, gluteal muscles, femur.

a. profun'da lin'guae [NA], deep lingual artery: *origin*, lingual artery; *branches*, none; *distribution*, tongue. Called also *ranine artery.*

a. profun'da pe'nis [NA], deep artery of penis: *origin*, internal pudendal artery; *branches*, none; *distribution*, corpus cavernosum penis.

arte'riae puden'dae exter'nae [NA], external pudendal arteries: *origin*, femoral artery; *branches*, anterior scrotal or anterior labial and inguinal branches; *distribution*, external genitalia, upper medial thigh.

a. puden'da inter'na [NA], internal pudendal artery: *origin*, internal iliac artery; *branches*, posterior scrotal or posterior labial branches and inferior rectal, perineal, urethral arteries, artery of bulb of penis or vestibule, deep artery of penis or clitoris, dorsal artery of penis or clitoris; *distribution*, external genitalia, anal canal, perineum.

a. pulmona'lis, truncus pulmonalis.

a. pulmona'lis dex'tra [NA], right pulmonary artery: *origin*, pulmonary trunk; *branches*, *of superior lobe:* apical, anterior ascending and descending, posterior ascending and descending, *of medial lobe:* medial and lateral, *of inferior lobe:* anterior basal, lateral basal, medial basal; posterior basal; *distribution*, right lung.

a. pulmona'lis sinis'tra [NA], left pulmonary artery: *origin*, pulmonary trunk; *branches*, *of superior lobe:* apical, ascending and descending, posterior, lingular (inferior and superior), *of inferior lobe:* superior, anterior basal, lateral basal, medial basal, posterior basal; *distribution*, left lung.

a. radia'lis [NA], radial artery: *origin*, brachial artery; *branches*, palmar carpal, superficial palmar and dorsal carpal rami, recurrent radial artery, principal artery of thumb, deep palmar arch; *distribution*, forearm, wrist, hand.

a. radia'lis in'dicis [NA], radial artery of index finger: *origin*, principal artery of thumb; *branches*, none; *distribution*, index finger. Called also *a. volaris indicis radialis* and *volar radial artery of index finger.*

a. recta'lis infe'rior [NA], inferior rectal artery: *origin*, internal pudendal artery; *branches*, none; *distribution*, rectum, anal canal. Called also *a. haemorrhoidalis inferior* and *inferior hemorrhoidal artery.*

a. recta'lis me'dia [NA], middle rectal artery: *origin*, internal iliac artery; *branches*, vaginal; *distribution*, rectum, prostate, seminal vesicles, vagina. Called also *a. haemorrhoidalis media* and *middle hemorrhoidal artery.*

a. recta'lis supe'rior [NA], superior rectal artery: *origin*, inferior mesenteric artery; *branches*, none; *distribution*, rectum. Called also *a. haemorrhoidalis superior* and *superior hemorrhoidal artery.*

a. recur'rens, NA alternative for *a. centralis longa.*

a. recur'rens radia'lis [NA], radial recurrent artery: *origin*, radial artery; *branches*, none; *distribution*, brachioradialis, brachialis, elbow region.

a. recur'rens tibia'lis ante'rior [NA], anterior tibial recurrent artery: *origin*, anterior tibial artery; *branches*, none; *distribution*, tibialis anterior, extensor digitorum longus, knee joint, contiguous fascia and skin.

a. recur'rens tibia'lis poste'rior [NA], posterior tibial recurrent artery: *origin*, anterior tibial artery; *branches*, none; *distribution*, knee.

a. recur'rens ulna'ris [NA], ulnar recurrent artery: *origin*, ulnar artery; *branches*, anterior and posterior; *distribution*, elbow joint region.

arte'riae recurren'tes ulna'res, see *a. recurrens ulnaris.*

arte'riae rena'les NA alternative for *arteriae renis.*

a. rena'lis [NA], renal artery: *origin*, abdominal aorta; *branches*, ureteral branches, inferior suprarenal artery; *distribution*, kidney, suprarenal gland, ureter. Called also *emulgent artery.*

arte'riae re'nis [NA], renal arteries: the arteries of the kidney, including the interlobar, arcuate, and interlobular arteries, and arteriolae rectae. Called also *arteriae renales* [NA alternative].

arte'riae retroduodena'les [NA], retroduodenal arteries: *origin*, first branch of gastroduodenal; *branches*, none; *distribution*, bile duct, duodenum, head of pancreas.

arte'riae sacra'les latera'les [NA], lateral sacral arteries: *origin*, iliolumbar artery; *branches*, spinal branches; *distribution*, structures about coccyx and sacrum.

a. sacra'lis latera'lis, see *rami spinales arteriarum sacralium lateralium.*

a. sacra'lis me'dia, a. sacralis mediana.

a. sacra'lis media'na [NA], median sacral artery: *origin*, continuation of abdominal aorta; *branches*, lowest lumbar artery; *distribution*, sacrum, coccyx, rectum. Called also *a. sacralis media, aorta sacrococcygea,* and *caudal, coccygeal,* or *sacrococcygeal artery.*

a. scapula'ris descen'dens, ramus profundus arteriae transversae cervicis.

a. scapula'ris dorsa'lis, 1. NA alternative for *arteria dorsalis scapularis.* 2. NA alternative for *ramus profundus arteriae transversae cervicis.*

arte'riae scrota'les anterio'res, rami scrotales anteriores arteriae femoralis.

arte'riae scrota'les posterio'res, rami scrotales posteriores arteriae pudendae internae.

a. segmen'ti anterio'ris [NA], anterior segmental artery: *origin*, right hepatic; *branches*, none; *distribution*, anterior segment of right lobe of liver.

a. segmen'ti anterio'ris inferio'ris [NA], anterior inferior segmental artery: *origin*, anterior branch of renal artery; *branches*, none; *distribution*, anterior inferior segment of kidney.

a. segmen'ti anterio'ris superio'ris [NA], anterior superior segmental artery: *origin*, anterior branch of renal artery; *branches*, none; *distribution*, anterior superior segment of kidney.

a. segmen'ti inferio'ris [NA], inferior segmental artery: *origin*, anterior branch of renal artery; *branches*, none; *distribution*, inferior segment of kidney.

a. segmen'ti latera'lis [NA], lateral segmental artery: *origin,* left branch of common hepatic artery; *branches,* none; *distribution,* lateral segment of left lobe of liver.

a. segmen'ti media'lis [NA], medial segmental artery: *origin,* left branch of common hepatic artery; *branches,* none; *distribution,* medial segment of left lobe of liver.

a. segmen'ti posterio'ris [NA], posterior segmental artery: 1. *origin,* right hepatic; *branches,* none; *distribution,* posterior segment of right lobe of liver. 2. *origin,* posterior branch of renal artery; *branches;* none; *distribution,* posterior segment of kidney.

a. segmen'ti superio'ris [NA], superior segmental artery: *origin,* anterior branch of renal artery; *branches,* none; *distribution,* superior segment of kidney.

arte'riae sigmoi'deae [NA], sigmoid arteries: *origin,* inferior mesenteric artery; *branches,* none; *distribution,* sigmoid colon.

a. spermat'ica exter'na, a. cremasterica.

a. sphenopalati'na [NA], sphenopalatine artery: *origin,* maxillary artery; *branches,* posterior lateral nasal artery and posterior septal rami; *distribution,* structures adjoining nasal cavity, the nasopharynx. Called also *nasopalatine artery.*

a. spina'lis ante'rior [NA], anterior spinal artery: *origin,* intracranial part of vertebral artery; *branches,* none; *distribution,* spinal cord.

a. spina'lis poste'rior [NA], posterior spinal artery: *origin,* anterior inferior cerebellar artery (usually); *branches,* none; *distribution,* spinal cord.

a. sple'nica [NA], splenic artery: *origin,* celiac trunk; *branches,* pancreatic and splenic branches, left gastro-omental, and short gastric arteries; *distribution,* spleen, pancreas, stomach, greater omentum. Called also *a. lienalis* [NA alternative].

a. sternocleidomastoi'dea, see *rami sternocleidomastoidei arteriae occipitalis.*

a. stylomastoi'dea [NA], stylomastoid artery: *origin,* posterior auricular; *branches,* mastoid and stapedial rami, posterior tympanic artery; *distribution,* tympanic cavity walls, mastoid cells, stapedius muscle.

a. subcla'via [NA], subclavian artery: *origin,* brachiocephalic trunk (right), arch of aorta (left); *branches,* vertebral, internal thoracic arteries, thyrocervical and costocervical trunks; *distribution,* neck, thoracic wall, spinal cord, brain, meninges, upper limb.

a. subcosta'lis [NA], subcostal artery: *origin,* thoracic aorta; *branches,* dorsal and spinal branches; *distribution,* upper posterior abdominal wall.

a. sublingua'lis [NA], sublingual artery: *origin,* lingual artery; *branches,* none; *distribution,* sublingual gland.

a. submenta'lis [NA], submental artery: *origin,* facial artery; *branches,* none; *distribution,* tissues under chin.

a. subscapula'ris [NA], subscapular artery: *origin,* axillary artery; *branches,* thoracodorsal and circumflex scapular arteries; *distribution,* scapular and shoulder region.

a. sul'ci centra'lis [NA], artery of central sulcus: *origin,* terminal part of middle cerebral artery; *branches,* none: *distribution,* cortex on either side of central sulcus.

a. sul'ci postcentra'lis [NA], artery of postcentral sulcus: *origin,* terminal part of middle cerebral artery; *branches,* none; *distribution,* cortex on either side of postcentral sulcus.

a. sul'ci precentra'lis [NA], artery of precentral sulcus: *origin,* terminal part of middle cerebral artery; *branches,* none; *distribution,* cortex on either side of precentral sulcus.

a. supe'rior latera'lis ge'nus [NA], lateral superior genicular artery: *origin,* popliteal artery; *branches,* none; *distribution,* knee joint, femur, patella, contiguous muscles. Called also *a. genus superior lateralis.*

a. supe'rior media'lis ge'nus [NA], medial superior genicular artery: *origin,* popliteal artery; *branches,* none; *distribution,* knee joint, femur, patella, contiguous muscles. Called also *a. genus superior medialis.*

a. supraduodena'lis [NA], supraduodenal artery: *origin,* gastroduodenal; *branches,* duodenal; *distribution,* superior first part of duodenum.

a. supraorbita'lis [NA], supraorbital artery: *origin,* ophthalmic artery; *branches,* none; *distribution,* forehead, upper muscles of orbit, upper eyelid, frontal sinus.

arte'riae suprarena'les superio'res [NA], superior suprarenal arteries: *origin,* inferior phrenic artery; *branches,* none; *distribution,* suprarenal gland.

a. suprarena'lis infe'rior [NA], inferior suprarenal artery: *origin,* renal artery; *branches,* none; *distribution,* suprarenal gland. Called also *inferior capsular artery.*

a. suprarena'lis me'dia [NA], middle suprarenal artery: *origin,* abdominal aorta; *branches,* none; *distribution,* suprarenal gland. Called also *middle capsular artery* and *aortic suprarenal artery.*

a. suprascapula'ris [NA], suprascapular artery: *origin,* thyrocervical trunk; *branches,* acromial branch; *distribution,* clavicular, deltoid, and scapular regions. Called also *a. transversa scapulae* and *transverse scapular artery.*

a. supratrochlea'ris [NA], supratrochlear artery: *origin,* ophthalmic artery; *branches,* none; *distribution,* anterior scalp. Called also *a. frontalis* and *frontal artery.*

arte'riae sura'les [NA], sural arteries: *origin,* popliteal artery; *branches,* none; *distribution,* popliteal space, calf.

arte'riae tarsa'les media'les [NA], **arte'riae tar'seae media'les,** medial tarsal arteries: *origin,* dorsal artery of foot; *branches,* none; *distribution,* side of foot.

a. tarsa'lis latera'lis [NA], **a. tar'sea latera'lis,** lateral tarsal artery: *origin,* dorsal artery of foot; *branches,* none; *distribution,* tarsus.

a. tempora'lis ante'rior [NA], anterior temporal artery: *origin,* insular part of middle cerebral artery; *branches,* none; *distribution,* cortex of anterior temporal lobe.

a. tempora'lis me'dia arte'riae tempora'lis superficia'lis [NA], middle temporal artery of superficial temporal artery: *origin,* superficial temporal artery; *branches,* none; *distribution* temporal region.

a. tempora'lis me'dia par'tis insula'ris ante'riae cer'ebri me'diae [NA], middle temporal artery of insular part of middle cerebral artery: *origin,* insular part of middle cerebral artery; *branches,* none; *distribution,* cortex of temporal lobe between anterior and posterior arteries.

a. tempora'lis poste'rior [NA] posterior temporal artery: *origin,* insular part of middle cerebral artery; *branches,* none; *distribution,* cortex of posterior temporal lobe.

a. tempora'lis profun'da ante'rior [NA], anterior deep temporal artery: *origin,* maxillary artery; *branches,* to zygomatic bone and greater wing of sphenoid bone; *distribution,* temporal muscle, and anastomoses with middle temporal artery.

a. tempora'lis profun'da poste'rior [NA], posterior deep temporal artery: *origin,* maxillary artery; *branches,* none; *distribution,* temporal muscle, and anastomoses with middle temporal artery.

a. tempora'lis superficia'lis [NA], superficial temporal artery: *origin,* external carotid; *branches,* parotid, auricular, and occipital rami, transverse facial, zygomatico-orbital, and middle temporal arteries; *distribution,* parotid and temporal regions.

a. testicula'ris [NA], testicular artery: *origin,* abdominal aorta; *branches,* ureteral, epididymal; *distribution,* ureter, epididymis, testis. Called also *funicular artery.*

arte'riae thalamostria'tae anterolatera'les, NA alternative for *arteriae centrales anterolaterales.*

arte'riae thalamostria'tae anteromedia'les, NA alternative for *arteriae centrales anteromediales.*

a. thora'cica inter'na [NA], internal thoracic artery: *origin,* subclavian artery; *branches,* mediastinal, thymic, bronchial, tracheal, sternal, perforating, medial mammary, lateral costal, and anterior intercostal branches, pericardiacophrenic, musculophrenic, and superior epigastric arteries; *distribution,* anterior thoracic wall, mediastinal structures, diaphragm. Called also *a. mammaria interna* and *internal mammary artery.*

a. thora'cica latera'lis [NA], lateral thoracic artery: *origin,* axillary artery; *branches,* mammary branches; *distribution,* pectoral muscles, mammary gland. Called also *external mammary artery.*

a. thora'cica supre'ma [NA], highest thoracic artery: *origin,* axillary artery; *branches,* none; *distribution,* axillary aspect of chest wall.

a. thoracoacromia'lis [NA], thoracoacromial artery: *origin,* axillary artery; *branches,* clavicular, pectoral, deltoid, acromial rami; *distribution,* deltoid, clavicular, and thoracic regions. Called also *thoracic axis.*

a. thoracodorsa'lis [NA], thoracodorsal artery: *origin,* subscapular artery; *branches,* none; *distribution,* subscapular and teretes muscles.

arte'riae thy'micae, rami thymici arteriae thoracicae internae.

a. thyreoi'dea i'ma, a. thyroidea ima.

a. thyreoi'dea infe'rior, a. thyroidea inferior.

a. thyreoi'dea supe'rior, a. thyroidea superior.

a. thyroi'dea i'ma [NA], lowest thyroid artery: *origin,* arch of aorta, brachiocephalic trunk or right common carotid;

branches, none; *distribution*, thyroid gland. Called also *a. thyreoidea ima* and *Neubauer's artery*.

a. thyroi'dea infe'rior [NA], inferior thyroid artery: *origin*, thyrocervical trunk; *branches*, pharyngeal, esophageal, and tracheal rami, inferior laryngeal and ascending cervical arteries; *distribution*, thyroid gland and adjacent structures. Called also *a. thyreoidea inferior*.

a. thyroi'dea supe'rior [NA], superior thyroid artery: *origin*, external carotid artery; *branches*, hyoid, sternocleido-mastoid, superior laryngeal, cricothyroid, muscular, and anterior, posterior, and lateral glandular branches; *distribution*, thyroid gland and adjacent structures. Called also *a. thyreoidea superior*.

a. tibia'lis ante'rior [NA], anterior tibial artery: *origin*, popliteal artery; *branches*, posterior and anterior tibial recurrent, and lateral and medial anterior malleolar arteries, lateral and medial malleolar retes; *distribution*, leg, ankle, foot.

a. tibia'lis poste'rior [NA], posterior tibial artery: *origin*, popliteal artery; *branches*, fibular circumflex branch, peroneal, medial plantar, and lateral plantar arteries; *distribution*, leg, foot.

a. transver'sa cer'vicis [NA], **a. transver'sa col'li**, transverse cervical artery: *origin*, subclavian artery; *branches*, deep and superficial rami; *distribution*, root of neck, muscles of scapula.

a. transver'sa facie'i [NA], transverse facial artery: *origin*, superficial temporal artery; *branches*, none; *distribution*, parotid region.

a. transver'sa scap'ulae, a. suprascapularis.

a. tympan'ica ante'rior [NA], anterior tympanic artery: *origin*, maxillary artery; *branches*, none; *distribution*, tympanic cavity.

a. tympan'ica infe'rior [NA], inferior tympanic artery: *origin*, ascending pharyngeal; *branches*, none; *distribution*, tympanic cavity.

a. tympan'ica poste'rior [NA], posterior tympanic artery: *origin*, stylomastoid artery; *branches*, none; *distribution*, tympanic cavity.

a. tympan'ica supe'rior [NA], superior tympanic artery: *origin*, middle meningeal artery; *branches*, none; *distribution*, tympanic cavity.

a. ulna'ris [NA], ulnar artery: *origin*, brachial artery; *branches*, palmar carpal, dorsal carpal, and deep palmar rami, ulnar recurrent and common interosseous arteries, superficial palmar arch; *distribution*, forearm, wrist, hand.

a. umbilica'lis [NA], umbilical artery: *origin*, internal iliac artery; *branches*, deferential, superior vesical arteries; *distribution*, ductus deferens, seminal vesicles, testes, urinary bladder, ureter.

a. urethra'lis [NA], urethral artery: *origin*, internal pudendal artery; *branches*, none; *distribution*, urethra.

a. uteri'na [NA], uterine artery: *origin*, internal iliac artery; *branches*, ovarian and tubal rami, vaginal artery; *distribution*, uterus, vagina, round ligament of uterus, uterine tube, ovary. Called also *fallopian artery*.

a. vagina'lis [NA], vaginal artery: *origin*, uterine artery; *branches*, none; *distribution*, vagina, fundus of bladder.

a. vertebra'lis [NA], vertebral artery: *origin*, subclavian artery; *branches*, *transverse, or cervical, part:* spinal and muscular rami; *intracranial part:* anterior spinal artery and posterior inferior cerebellar artery and its branches; *distribution*, muscles of neck, vertebrae, spinal cord, cerebellum, interior of cerebrum.

arte'riae vesica'les superio'res [NA], superior vesical arteries: *origin*, umbilical artery; *branches*, none; *distribution*, bladder, urachus, ureter.

a. vesica'lis infe'rior [NA], inferior vesical artery: *origin*, internal iliac; *branches*, prostatic; *distribution*, bladder, prostate, seminal vesicles, lower ureter.

a. vola'ris in'dicis radia'lis, a. radialis indicis.

a. zygomatico-orbita'lis [NA], zygomatico-orbital artery: *origin*, superficial temporal; *branches*, none; *distribution*, lateral side of orbit.

---

arteri(o)- [L. *arteria*, q.v.] a combining form denoting relationship to an artery or arteries.

arteriocapillary (ar-te″re-o-kap′ĭ-la″re) pertaining to the arteries and the capillaries.

arteriodilating (ar-te″re-o-di′lāt-ing) increasing the caliber of the arteries, particularly of arterioles.

arteriogenesis (ar-te″re-o-jen′ĕ-sis) [*artery* + Gr. *genesis* production] the formation of arteries.

arteriogram (ar-te′re-o-gram″) [*artery* + Gr. *gramma* a writing] 1. a roentgenogram of an artery after injection of a radiopaque medium. 2. (*obs.*) a sphygmographic tracing of the arterial pulse.

arteriograph (ar-te′re-o-graf) a film produced by arteriography.

arteriography (ar″te-re-og′rah-fe) [*artery* + Gr. *graphein* to write] roentgenography of arteries after injection of radiopaque material into the blood stream. **catheter a.,** radiography of vessels after introduction of contrast material through a catheter inserted into an artery. **selective a.,** radiography of a specific vessel which is opacified by a medium introduced directly into it, usually via a catheter.

arteriola (ar-te″re-o′lah), pl. *arterio'lae* [L., dim. of *arteria*] arteriole: a minute arterial branch, especially [NA] one just proximal to a capillary. **a. glomerula'ris af'ferens** [NA], afferent arteriole of glomerulus: a branch of an interlobular artery that goes to a renal glomerulus; called also *afferent vessel of glomerulus* and *vas afferens glomeruli* [NA alternative]. **a. glomerula'ris ef'ferens** [NA], arteriole of glomerulus: an arteriole that arises from a renal glomerulus; breaking up into capillaries to supply renal tubules; called also *afferent vessel of glomerulus* and *vas efferens glomeruli* [NA alternative]. **a. macula'ris infe'rior** [NA], inferior macular arteriole: the inferior arteriole supplying the macula retinae. **a. macula'ris supe'rior** [NA], superior macular arteriole: the superior arteriole supplying the macula retinae. **a. media'lis ret'inae** [NA], medial arteriole of retina: the small branch supplying blood to the central region of the retina. **a. nasa'lis ret'inae infe'rior** [NA], inferior nasal arteriole of retina: a small branch of the central artery of the retina supplying the inferior nasal region of the retina. **a. nasa'lis ret'inae supe'rior** [NA], superior nasal arteriole of retina: a small branch of the central artery of the retina, supplying the superior nasal region of the retina. **arterio'lae rec'tae re'nis** [NA], branches of the arcuate arteries of the kidney arising from the efferent glomerular arterioles, and passing down to the renal pyramids; called also *straight arteries*, or *arterioles, of the kidney* and *vasa recta*. [NA alternative]. Also sometimes called *arteriolae rectae spuriae* or *false straight arterioles* of the kidney to distinguish them from straight direct branches from the arcuate and interlobular arteries that are called *arteriolae rectae vera* or *true straight arterioles* of the kidney. **arterio'lae rec'tae spu'riae**, see *arteriolae rectae renis*. **arterio'lae rec'tae ve'ra**, see *arteriolae rectae renis*. **a. tempora'lis ret'inae infe'rior** [NA], inferior temporal arteriole of retina: a branch of the central artery of the retina, supplying the inferior temporal region of the retina. **a. tempora'lis ret'inae supe'rior** [NA], superior temporal arteriole of retina: a branch of the central artery of the retina, supplying the superior temporal region of the retina.

arteriolae (ar-te″re-o′le) [L.] genitive and plural of arteriola.

arteriolar (ar″te-re′o-lar) pertaining to or resembling arterioles.

arteriole (ar-te′re-ōl) [L. *arteriola*] a minute arterial branch, especially one just proximal to a capillary; called also *arteriola* [NA]. **afferent a. of glomerulus,** arteriola glomerularis afferens. **efferent a. of glomerulus,** arteriola glomerularis efferens. **ellipsoid a's,** sheathed arteries. **a glomerula'ris ef'ferens** [NA], efferent arteriole of glomerulus: an arteriole that arises from a renal glomerulus, breaking up into capillaries to supply renal tubules; called also *efferent vessel of glomerulus* and *vas efferens glomeruli* [NA alternative]. **Isaacs-Ludwig a.,** an arteriolar twig that sometimes branches from the afferent glomerular arteriole of the kidney to communicate directly with the tubular capillary plexus. **macular a., inferior,** arteriola macularis inferior. **macular a., superior,** arteriola macularis superior. **medial a. of retina,** arteriola medialis retinae. **nasal a. of retina, inferior,** arteriola nasalis retinae inferior. **nasal a. of retina, superior,** arteriola nasalis retinae superior. **postglomerular a.,** efferent glomerular a. **precapillary a's,** arterial capillaries. **preglomerular a.,** afferent glomerular a. **sheathed a's,** see under *artery.* **straight a's of kidney,** arteriolae rectae renis. **straight a's of kidney, false,** see *arteriolae rectae renis.* **straight a's of kidney, true,** see *arteriolae rectae renis.* **temporal a. of retina, inferior,** arteriola temporalis retinae inferior. **temporal a. of retina, superior,** arteriola temporalis retinae superior.

arteriolith (ar-te're-o-lith″) [*artery* + Gr. *lithos* stone] a chalky concretion in an artery.

arteriolitis (ar-tēr″ĭ-o-li'tis) inflammation of the arterioles.

arteriology (ar-te″re-ol'o-je) [*artery* + *-logy*] the sum of what is known regarding the arteries; the science or study of the arteries.

arteriolonecrosis (ar-te″re-o″lo-ne-kro'sis) necrosis of arterioles, as may be seen in nephrosclerosis; called also *arteriolar necrosis.*

arteriolosclerosis (ar-te″re-o″lo-skle-ro'sis) sclerosis and thickening of the walls of the smaller arteries (arterioles). *Hyaline arteriolosclerosis,* in which there is homogeneous pink hyaline thickening of the arteriolar walls, is associated with benign nephrosclerosis. *Hyperplastic arteriolosclerosis,* in which there is a concentric thickening with progressive narrowing of the lumina, may be associated with malignant hypertension, nephrosclerosis, and scleroderma.

arteriolosclerotic (ar-te″re-o″lo-skle-rot'ik) pertaining to or characterized by arteriolosclerosis.

arteriomalacia (ar-te″re-o-mah-la'she-ah) [*artery* + Gr. *malakia* softness] (obs.) abnormal softness of the arterial coats.

arteriometer (ar″te-re-om'ĕ-ter) [*artery* + Gr. *metron* measure] (obs.) an apparatus used for measuring any changes in the caliber of a pulsating artery.

arteriomotor (ar-te″re-o-mo'tor) pertaining to or causing change in the caliber of an artery.

arteriomyomatosis (ar-te″re-o-mi″o-mah-to'sis) a growth of irregular muscular fibers in the walls of an artery causing thickening of the walls.

arterionecrosis (ar-te″re-o-ne-kro'sis) necrosis of an artery or of arteries.

arteriopalmus (ar-te″re-o-pal'mus) (obs.) palpitation or throbbing of an artery.

arteriopathy (ar″te-re-op'ah-the) [*artery* + Gr. *pathos* disease] any arterial disease. **hypertensive a.,** widespread involvement, chiefly of arterioles and small arteries, associated with arterial hypertension and characterized primarily by hypertrophy and thickening of the media.

arterioplasty (ar-te″re-o-plas'te) [*artery* + Gr. *plassein* to form] surgical repair or reconstruction of an artery.

arteriopressor (ar-te″re-o-pres'or) producing increased blood pressure in the arteries.

arteriorenal (ar-te″re-o-re'nal) pertaining to the arteries of the kidney.

arteriorrhagia (ar-te″re-o-ra'je-ah) (obs.) arterial hemorrhage.

arteriorrhaphy (ar-te″re-or'ah-fe) [*artery* + Gr. *rhaphē* suture] suture of an artery.

arteriorrhexis (ar-te″re-o-rek'sis) [*artery* + Gr. *rhēxis* rupture] rupture of an artery.

arteriosclerosis (ar-te″re-o-skle-ro'sis) [*artery* + Gr. *sklēros* hard] a group of diseases characterized by thickening and loss of elasticity of arterial walls; it comprises three distinct forms: atherosclerosis, Mönckeberg's arteriosclerosis, and arteriolosclerosis. **cerebral a.,** arteriosclerosis of the arteries of the brain. **coronary a.,** arteriosclerosis (atherosclerosis) of the coronary arteries. **hyaline a.,** a homogeneous hyaline thickening of the walls of arterioles with consequent narrowing of the lumina. **hypertensive a.,** arteriosclerosis intensified by hypertension. **infantile a.,** see *infantile arteritis,* under *arteritis.* **intimal a.,** arteriosclerosis in which the major changes affect the intima of the arteries. **medial a.,** a condition of large and medium-sized arteries, with primary destruction of the muscle and elastic fibers of the medial coat, which are replaced by fibrous tissue; sometimes there are deposits of calcium (akin to Mönckeberg's arteriosclerosis). **Mönckeberg's a.,** medial arteriosclerosis with extensive deposits of calcium in the media of the artery; called also *Mönckeberg's calcification, degeneration, sclerosis,* or *medial calcific sclerosis.* **nodose a., nodular a.** (obs.), disease of the arteries marked by the formation of fibrous nodes or plaques in the lining membrane of the arteries. **a. oblit'erans,** arteriosclerosis in which proliferation of the intima of small vessels has caused complete obliteration of the lumen of the artery. **peripheral a.,** arteriosclerosis of the extremities. **presenile a.,** physiological arteriosclerosis occurring at an unusually early age and without apparent cause. **senile a.,** arteriosclerosis that accompanies old age, but is not specifically age related.

arteriosclerotic (ar-te″re-o-skle-rot'ik) pertaining to or affected with arteriosclerosis.

arteriosity (ar-te″re-os'ĭ-te) the condition or quality of being arterial.

arteriospasm (ar-te're-o-spazm″) spasm of an artery.

arteriospastic (ar-te″re-o-spas'tik) pertaining to, characterized by, or causing arteriospasm.

arteriostenosis (ar-te″re-o-ste-no'sis) [*artery* + Gr. *stenos* narrow] the narrowing or diminution of the caliber of an artery.

arteriosteogenesis (ar-te″re-os″te-o-jen'ĕ-sis) [*artery* + Gr. *osteon* bone + *gennan* to produce] calcification of an artery.

arteriostosis (ar-te″re-os-to'sis) [*artery* + Gr. *osteon* bone + *-osis*] ossification of an artery.

arteriostrepsis (ar-te″re-o-strep'sis) [*artery* + Gr. *streptos* twisted] the twisting of an artery for the arrest of hemorrhage.

arteriotomy (ar″te-re-ot'o-me) [*artery* + Gr. *tomē* cut] incision of an artery.

arteriotony (ar-te″re-ot'o-ne) [*artery* + Gr. *tonos* tension] the intra-arterial tension of the blood; blood pressure.

arteriotrepsis (ar-te″re-o-trep'sis) arteriostrepsis.

arterious (ar-te're-us) pertaining to the arteries; arterial.

arteriovenous (ar-te″re-o-ve'nus) both arterial and venous; pertaining to or affecting an artery and a vein.

arteritides (ar″tĕ-rit'ĭ-dēz) plural of *arteritis.*

arteritis (ar″tĕ-ri'tis), pl. *arterit'ides* [*artery* + *-itis*] inflammation of an artery; cf. *endarteritis* and *periarteritis.* **brachiocephalic a., a. brachiocephal'ica,** pulseless disease. **coronary a.,** inflammation of the coronary arteries. **cranial a.,** temporal a. **a. defor'mans** (obs.), chronic endarteritis with calcareous infiltration. **equine viral a.,** a frequently fatal viral disease of horses affecting especially the smaller arteries, with hemorrhagic enteritis, abdominal pain and diarrhea, and pulmonary edema. Abortion is common in affected mares. **giant cell a.,** temporal a. **Horton's a.,** temporal a. **a. hyperplas'tica** (obs.), arteritis with the formation of new connective tissue. **infantile a.,** diffuse arteritis in infants and children, rarely with atherosclerotic processes. **localized visceral a.,** allergic vasculitis. **a. nodo'sa,** periarteritis nodosa, def. 1. **a. oblit'erans,** endarteritis obliterans. **rheumatic a.,** generalized inflammation of arterioles and arterial capillaries occurring in rheumatic fever. **syphilitic a.,** a late manifestation of syphilis characterized by intimal proliferation and degeneration of the medial coat, usually involving the ascending aorta, aortic arch, and pulmonary artery, which may lead to aneurysm. **Takayasu's a.,** pulseless disease. **temporal a.,** a chronic vascular disease of unknown origin, most common in the carotid arterial system but also occurring in other large and small systemic arteries, characterized by proliferative inflammation, often with giant cells and granulomas, and by headache, difficulty in chewing, weakness, weight loss, fever, and symptoms of sepsis, with a markedly increased erythrocyte sedimentation rate and leukocytosis. Ocular involvement, ranging from diplopia to complete blindness, occurs in about half the subjects. The disease occurs exclusively in older persons, and is often associated with polymyalgia rheumatica. Called also *cranial a., giant cell a.,* and *Horton's arteritis, disease,* or *syndrome.* **tuberculous a.,** endarteritis obliterans in those arteries intimately involved in a tubercular focus. **a. umbilica′lis,** septic inflammation of the umbilical artery in newborn infants. **a. verruco′sa** (*obs.*), arteritis marked by finger-like projections from the wall into the lumen of the blood vessel.

artery (ar′ter-e) [L. *arteria;* Gr. *artēria,* from *aēr* air + *tērein* to keep, because the arteries were supposed by the ancients to contain air, or from Gr. *aeirein* to lift or attach] a vessel through which the blood passes away from the heart to the various parts of the body; called also *arteria* [NA]. The wall of an artery consists typically of an outer coat (tunica adventitia), a middle coat (tunica media), and an inner coat (tunica intima). **accompanying a. of ischiadic**

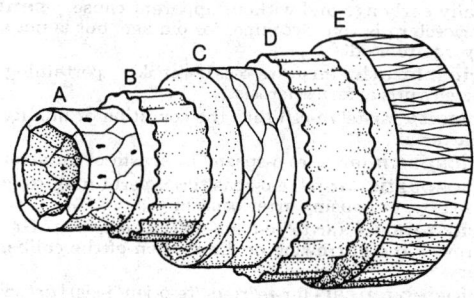

Representation of arterial coats: A, tunica intima; B, internal elastic lamina; C, tunica media; D, external elastic lamina; E, tunica adventitia.

nerve, arteria comitans nervi ischiadici. **accompanying a. of median nerve,** arteria comitans nervi mediani. **acetabular a.,** 1. ramus acetabularis arteriae circumflexae femoris medialis. 2. ramus acetabularis arteriae obturatoriae. **adipose a's of kidney,** rami capsulares arteriae renis. **afferent a. of glomerulus,** vas afferens glomeruli. **alveolar a., inferior,** arteria alveolaris inferior. **alveolar a's, superior, anterior,** arteriae alveolares superiores anteriores. **alveolar a., superior, posterior,** arteria alveolaris superior posterior. **anastomotic atrial a.,** ramus atrialis anastomoticus arteriae coronariae sinistrae. **angular a.,** arteria angularis. **a. of angular gyrus,** arteria gyri angularis. **appendicular a.,** arteria appendicularis. **arcuate a. of foot,** arteria arcuata pedis. **arcuate a's of kidney,** arteriae arcuatae renis. **articular a., proper, of little head of fibula,** ramus circumflexus fibulae arteriae tibialis posterioris. **atrial anastomotic a.,** ramus atrialis anastomoticus arteriae coronariae sinistrae. **atrioventricular nodal a.,** see *ramus nodi atrioventricularis arteriae coronariae dextrae.* **auditory a., internal,** arteria labyrinthi. **auricular a's, anterior,** rami auriculares anteriores arteriae temporalis superficialis. **auricular a., deep,** arteria auricularis profunda. **auricular a., left,** arteria coronaria sinistra. **auricular a., posterior,** arteria auricularis posterior. **auricular a., right,** arteria coronaria dextra. **axillary a.,** arteria axillaris. **azygos a's of vagina,** rami vaginales arteriae uterinae. **basilar a.,** arteria basilaris. **brachial a.,** arteria brachialis. **brachial a., deep,** arteria profunda brachii. **brachial a., superficial,** arteria brachialis superficialis. **brachiocephalic a.,** truncus brachiocephalicus. **bronchial a's,** rami bronchiales aortae thoracicae. **bronchial a's, anterior,** rami bronchiales arteriae thoracicae internae. **buccal a.,** arteria buccalis. **buccinator a.,** arteria buccalis. **bulbourethral a.,** arteria bulbi penis. **a. of bulb of penis,** arteria bulbi penis. **a. of bulb of vestibule of vagina,** arteria bulbi vestibuli vaginae.

capsular a., inferior, arteria suprarenalis inferior. **capsular a., middle,** arteria suprarenalis media. **caroticotympanic a's,** arteriae caroticotympanicae. **carotid a., common,** arteria carotis communis. **carotid a., external,** arteria carotis externa. **carotid a., internal,** arteria carotis interna. **caudal a.,** arteria sacralis mediana. **cecal a., anterior,** arteria caecalis anterior. **cecal a., posterior,** arteria caecalis posterior. **central a's, anterolateral,** arteriae centrales anterolaterales. **central a's, anteromedial,** arteriae centrales anteromediales. **central a's, posterolateral,** arteriae centrales posterolaterales. **central a. of retina,** arteria centralis retinae. **central a's of spleen,** branches of the splenic artery after they leave the trabeculae; their tunica adventitia is replaced by a cylindrical lymphoid sheath and they pass through the aggregations of lymphatic nodules and branch out to terminate as splenic penicilli. **a. of central sulcus,** arteria sulci centralis. **cephalic a.,** arteria carotis communis. **cerebellar a., inferior, anterior,** arteria inferior anterior cerebelli. **cerebellar a., inferior, posterior,** arteria inferior posterior cerebelli. **cerebellar a., superior,** arteria cerebelli superior. **cerebral a's,** arteriae cerebri. **cerebral a., anterior,** arteria cerebri anterior. **a. of cerebral hemorrhage,** any of the medial or lateral branches of the anterolateral central branches (arteries) of the middle cerebral artery, which are common sites of cerebral hemorrhage; called *lenticulostriate a.* **cerebral a., middle,** arteria cerebri media. **cerebral a., posterior,** arteria cerebri posterior. **a's of cerebrum,** arteriae cerebri. **cervical a., ascending,** arteria cervicalis ascendens. **cervical a., deep,** a. cervicalis profunda. **cervical a., descending, deep,** see *rami occipitales arteriae occipitalis.* **cervical a., superficial,** ramus superficialis arteriae transversae colli. **cervical a., transverse,** arteria transversa cervicis. **choroid a., anterior, choroidal a., anterior,** arteria choroidea anterior. **ciliary a's, anterior,** arteriae ciliares anteriores. **ciliary a's, long,** arteriae ciliares posteriores longae. **ciliary a's, posterior, long,** arteriae ciliares posteriores longae. **ciliary a's, posterior, short,** arteriae ciliares posteriores breves. **ciliary a's, short,** arteriae ciliares posteriores breves. **circumflex a., deep, internal,** ramus profundus arteriae circumflexae femoris medialis. **circumflex a., femoral, lateral,** arteria circumflexa femoris lateralis. **circumflex a., femoral, medial,** arteria circumflexa femoris medialis. **circumflex a., humeral, anterior,** arteria circumflexa anterior humeri. **circumflex a., humeral, posterior,** arteria circumflexa posterior humeri. **circumflex a., iliac, deep,** arteria circumflexa ilium profunda. **circumflex a., iliac, superficial,** arteria circumflexa ilium superficialis. **circumflex a. of scapula,** arteria circumflexa scapulae. **a. of clitoris, deep,** arteria profunda clitoridis. **a. of clitoris, dorsal,** arteria dorsalis clitoridis. **coccygeal a.,** arteria sacralis mediana. **cochlear a.,** ramus cochlearis arteriae labyrinthi. **Cohnheim's a.,** terminal a. **colic a., left,** arteria colica sinistra. **colic a., middle,** arteria colica media. **colic a., right,** arteria colica dextra. **colic a., right, inferior,** arteria ileocolica. **colic a., superior, accessory,** arteria colica media. **collateral a., middle,** arteria collateralis media. **collateral a., radial,** arteria collateralis radialis. **collateral a., ulnar, inferior,** arteria collateralis ulnaris inferior. **collateral a., ulnar, superior,** arteria collateralis ulnaris superior. **communicating a., anterior, of cerebrum,** arteria communicans anterior cerebri. **communicating a., posterior, of cerebrum,** arteria communicans posterior cerebri. **conal a., conus a.,** see *ramus coni arteriosi arteriae coronariae dextrae* and *ramus coni arteriosi arteriae coronariae sinistrae.* **conducting a's,** large arterial trunks, characterized by their large size and elasticity, such as the aorta, subclavian, and common carotid, and the brachiocephalic and pulmonary trunks. **conjunctival a's, anterior,** arteriae conjunctivales anteriores. **conjunctival a's, posterior** arteriae conjunctivales posteriores. **conus a., left,** ramus coni arteriosi arteriae coronariae sinistrae. **conus a., right, conus a., third,** ramus coni arteriosi arteriae coronariae dextrae. **copper-wire a's,** retinal arteries on which the bright line of reflex is exaggerated; seen in arteriosclerosis. **cork-screw a's,** small arteries in the macular region of the eye that appear markedly tortuous. **coronary a., descending, poste-**

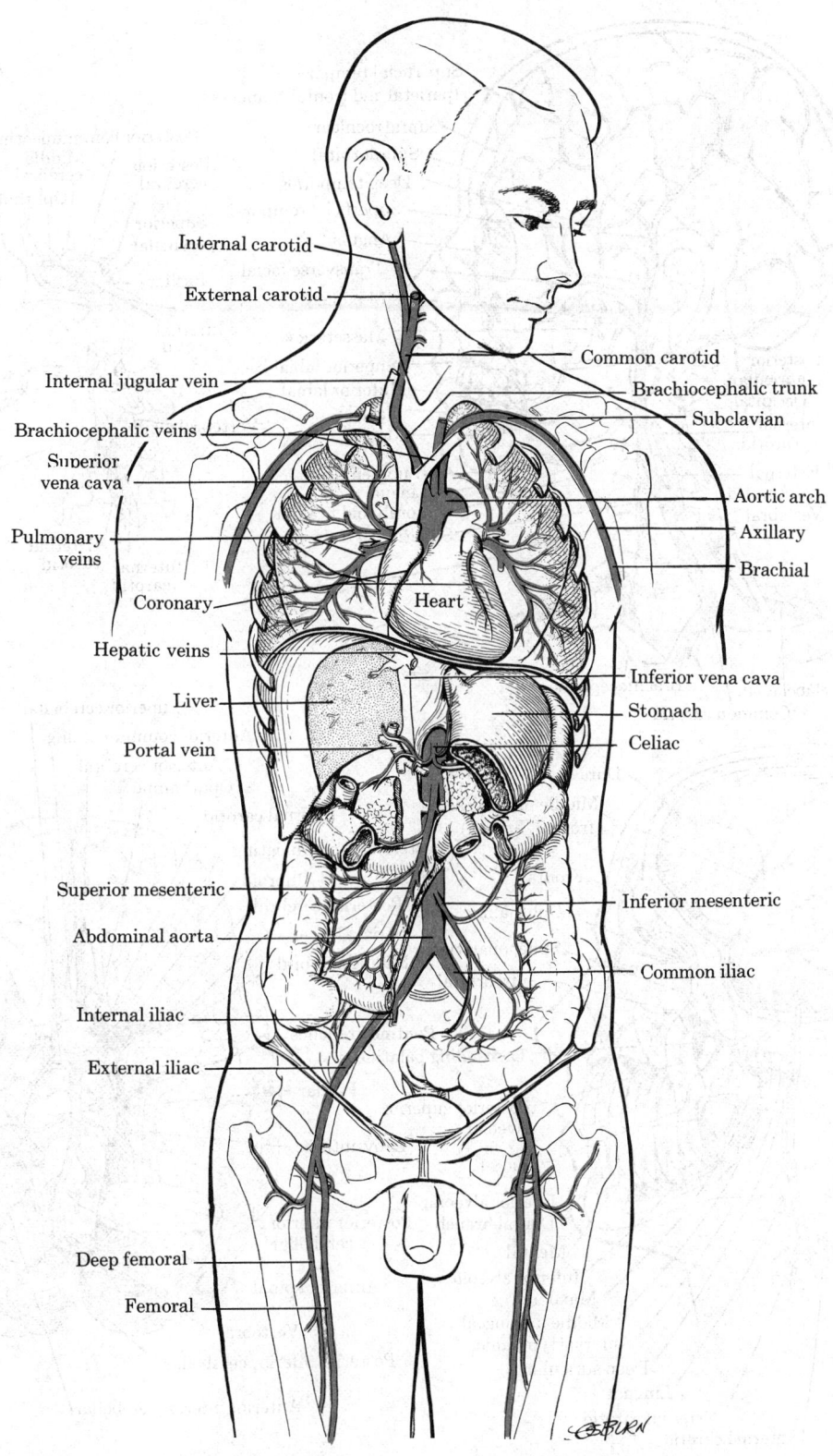

Internal carotid

External carotid

Internal jugular vein

Brachiocephalic veins

Superior
vena cava

Pulmonary
veins

Coronary

Hepatic veins

Liver

Portal vein

Superior mesenteric

Abdominal aorta

Internal iliac

External iliac

Deep femoral

Femoral

Common carotid

Brachiocephalic trunk

Subclavian

Aortic arch

Axillary

Brachial

Heart

Inferior vena cava

Stomach

Celiac

Inferior mesenteric

Common iliac

PLATE 2 —PRINCIPAL ARTERIES OF THE BODY AND THE PULMONARY VEINS

139

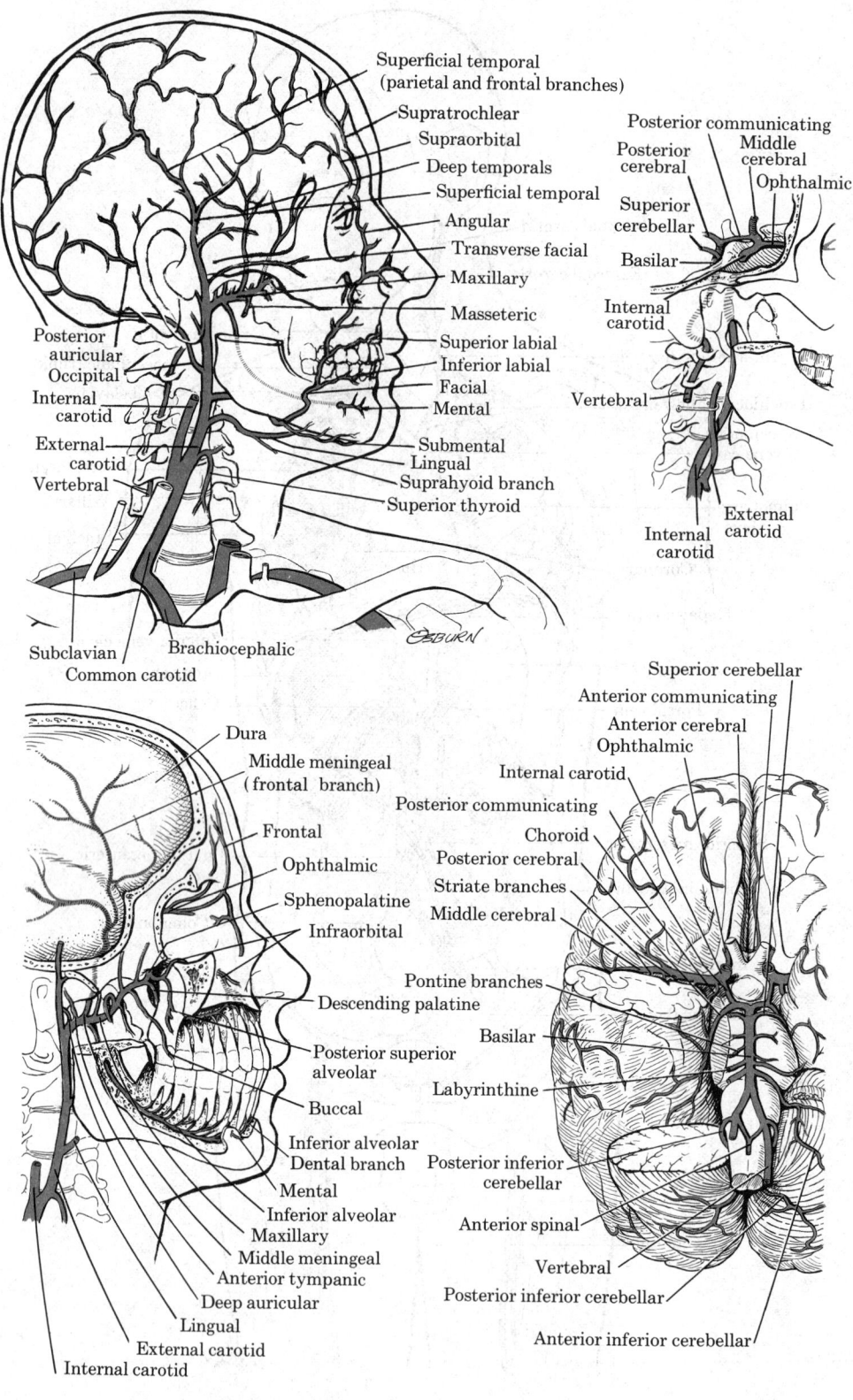

Superficial temporal
(parietal and frontal branches)

Supratrochlear

Supraorbital

Deep temporals

Superficial temporal

Angular

Transverse facial

Maxillary

Masseteric

Superior labial

Inferior labial

Facial

Mental

Submental

Lingual

Suprahyoid branch

Superior thyroid

Posterior
auricular

Occipital

Internal
carotid

External
carotid

Vertebral

Subclavian

Brachiocephalic

Common carotid

Posterior communicating

Posterior
cerebral

Middle
cerebral

Ophthalmic

Superior
cerebellar

Basilar

Internal
carotid

Vertebral

External
carotid

Internal
carotid

Dura

Middle meningeal
(frontal branch)

Frontal

Ophthalmic

Sphenopalatine

Infraorbital

Descending palatine

Posterior superior
alveolar

Buccal

Inferior alveolar
Dental branch

Mental

Inferior alveolar

Maxillary

Middle meningeal

Anterior tympanic

Deep auricular

Lingual

External carotid

Internal carotid

Superior cerebellar

Anterior communicating

Anterior cerebral
Ophthalmic

Internal carotid

Posterior communicating

Choroid

Posterior cerebral

Striate branches

Middle cerebral

Pontine branches

Basilar

Labyrinthine

Posterior inferior
cerebellar

Anterior spinal

Vertebral

Posterior inferior cerebellar

Anterior inferior cerebellar

PLATE 3 —ARTERIES OF THE HEAD, NECK, AND BASE OF THE BRAIN

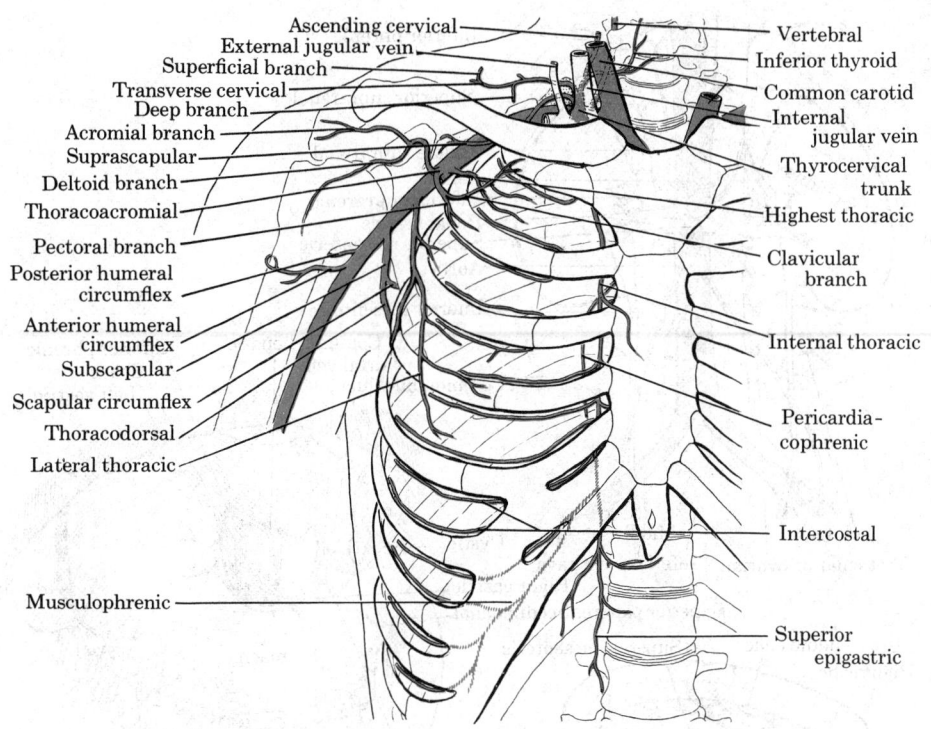

Ascending cervical
External jugular vein
Superficial branch
Transverse cervical
Deep branch
Acromial branch
Suprascapular
Deltoid branch
Thoracoacromial
Pectoral branch
Posterior humeral circumflex
Anterior humeral circumflex
Subscapular
Scapular circumflex
Thoracodorsal
Lateral thoracic

Musculophrenic

Vertebral
Inferior thyroid
Common carotid
Internal jugular vein
Thyrocervical trunk
Highest thoracic
Clavicular branch
Internal thoracic
Pericardia-cophrenic
Intercostal
Superior epigastric

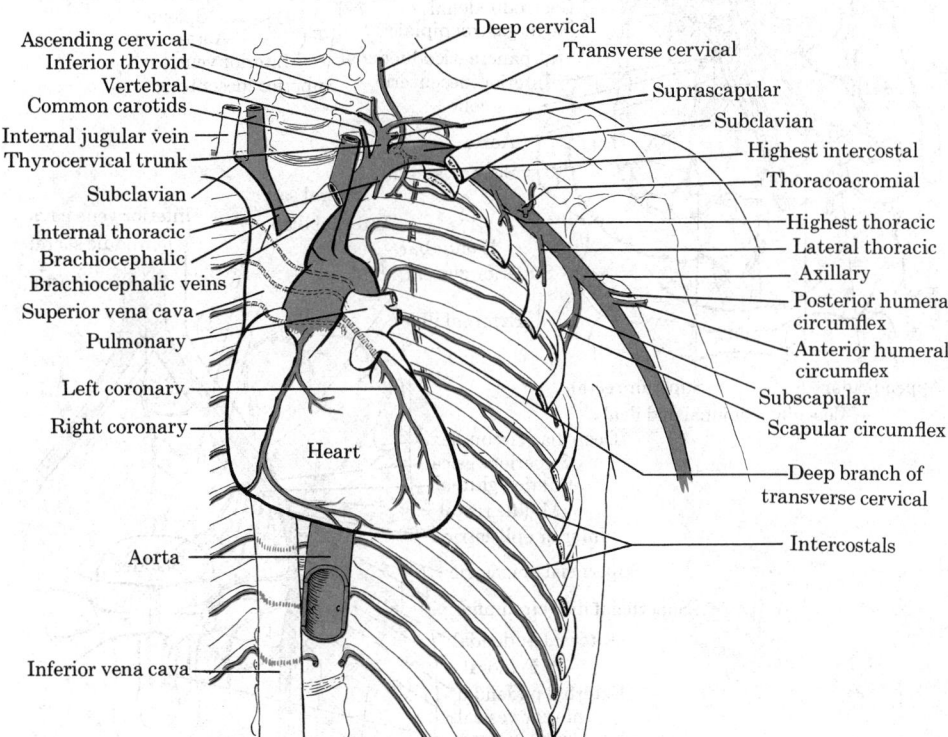

Ascending cervical
Inferior thyroid
Vertebral
Common carotids
Internal jugular vein
Thyrocervical trunk
Subclavian
Internal thoracic
Brachiocephalic
Brachiocephalic veins
Superior vena cava
Pulmonary
Left coronary
Right coronary
Heart
Aorta
Inferior vena cava

Deep cervical
Transverse cervical
Suprascapular
Subclavian
Highest intercostal
Thoracoacromial
Highest thoracic
Lateral thoracic
Axillary
Posterior humeral circumflex
Anterior humeral circumflex
Subscapular
Scapular circumflex
Deep branch of transverse cervical
Intercostals

PLATE 4 —ARTERIES OF THE THORAX AND AXILLA

141

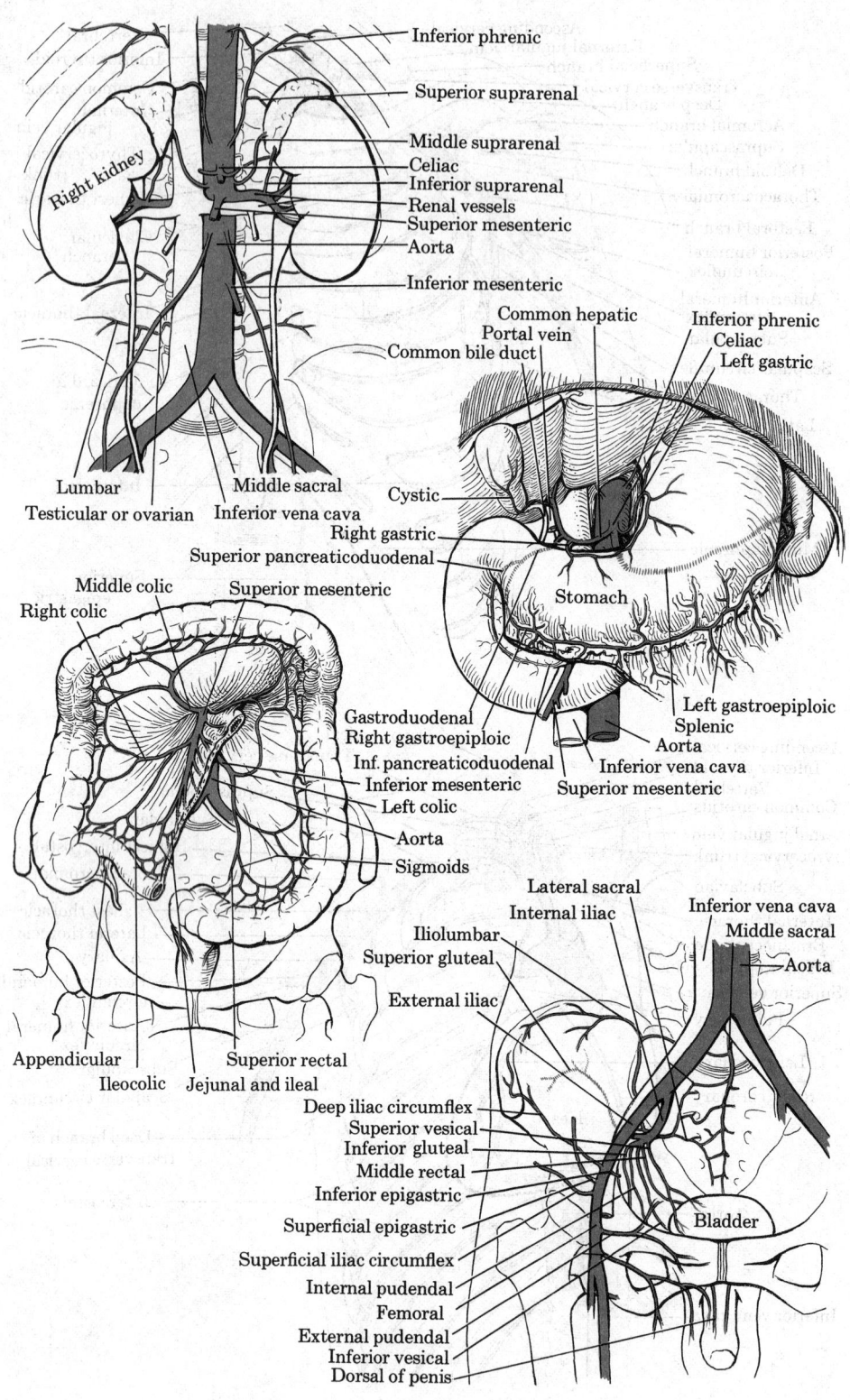

Inferior phrenic
Superior suprarenal
Middle suprarenal
Celiac
Inferior suprarenal
Renal vessels
Superior mesenteric
Aorta
Inferior mesenteric
Right kidney
Lumbar
Middle sacral
Testicular or ovarian
Inferior vena cava

Common hepatic
Portal vein
Common bile duct
Inferior phrenic
Celiac
Left gastric
Cystic
Right gastric
Superior pancreaticoduodenal
Stomach
Left gastroepiploic
Splenic
Aorta
Inferior vena cava
Superior mesenteric

Middle colic
Right colic
Superior mesenteric
Gastroduodenal
Right gastroepiploic
Inf. pancreaticoduodenal
Inferior mesenteric
Left colic
Aorta
Sigmoids
Appendicular
Ileocolic
Superior rectal
Jejunal and ileal

Lateral sacral
Internal iliac
Inferior vena cava
Middle sacral
Iliolumbar
Superior gluteal
Aorta
External iliac
Deep iliac circumflex
Superior vesical
Inferior gluteal
Middle rectal
Inferior epigastric
Superficial epigastric
Bladder
Superficial iliac circumflex
Internal pudendal
Femoral
External pudendal
Inferior vesical
Dorsal of penis

PLATE 5 —ARTERIES OF THE ABDOMEN AND PELVIS

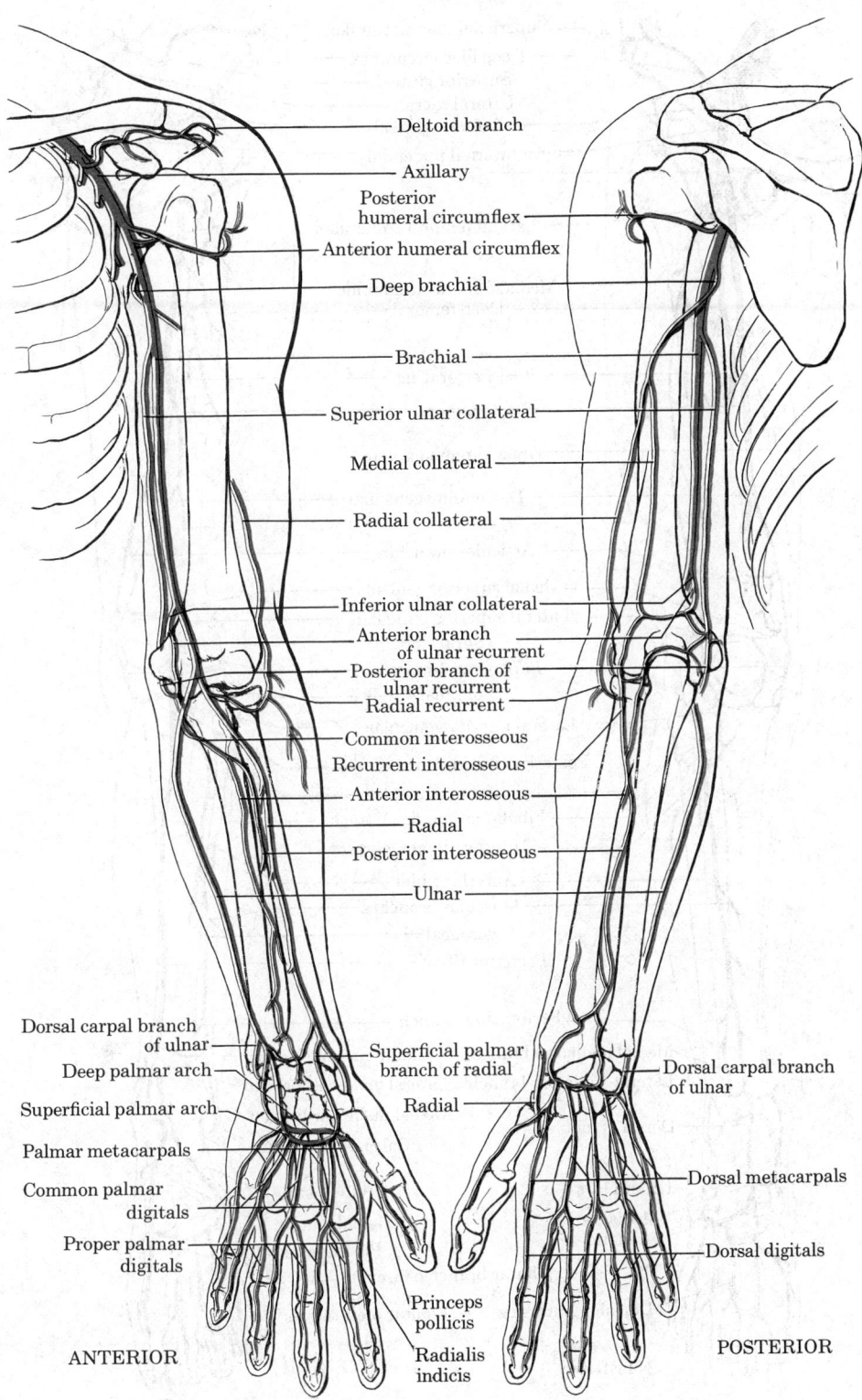

Deltoid branch

Axillary

Posterior humeral circumflex

Anterior humeral circumflex

Deep brachial

Brachial

Superior ulnar collateral

Medial collateral

Radial collateral

Inferior ulnar collateral

Anterior branch of ulnar recurrent

Posterior branch of ulnar recurrent

Radial recurrent

Common interosseous

Recurrent interosseous

Anterior interosseous

Radial

Posterior interosseous

Ulnar

Dorsal carpal branch of ulnar

Deep palmar arch

Superficial palmar arch

Palmar metacarpals

Common palmar digitals

Proper palmar digitals

Superficial palmar branch of radial

Radial

Dorsal carpal branch of ulnar

Dorsal metacarpals

Dorsal digitals

Princeps pollicis

Radialis indicis

ANTERIOR

POSTERIOR

PLATE 6 — ARTERIES OF THE UPPER EXTREMITY

143

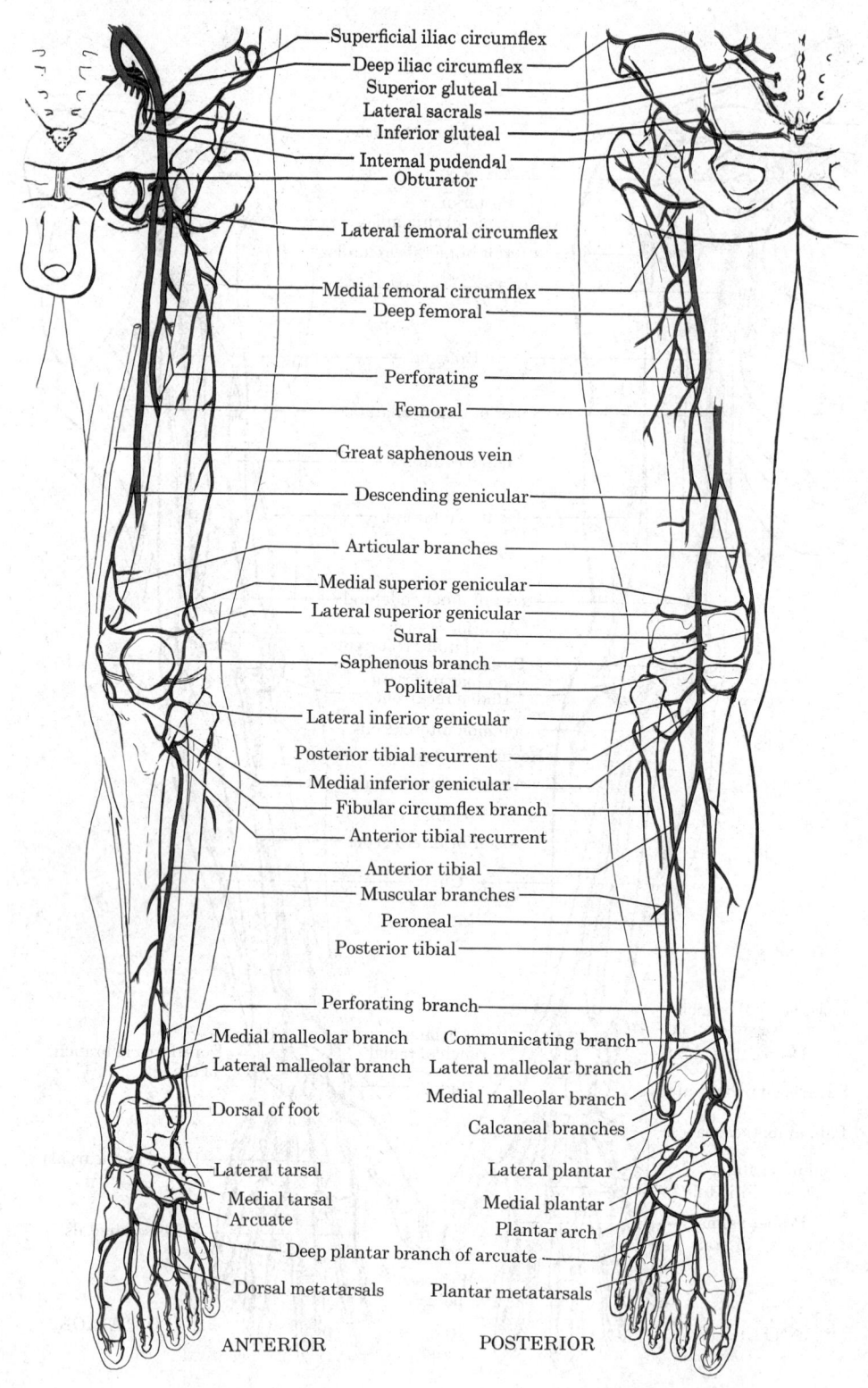

Superficial iliac circumflex
Deep iliac circumflex
Superior gluteal
Lateral sacrals
Inferior gluteal
Internal pudendal
Obturator
Lateral femoral circumflex

Medial femoral circumflex
Deep femoral

Perforating
Femoral

Great saphenous vein

Descending genicular

Articular branches

Medial superior genicular
Lateral superior genicular
Sural
Saphenous branch
Popliteal
Lateral inferior genicular

Posterior tibial recurrent
Medial inferior genicular
Fibular circumflex branch
Anterior tibial recurrent

Anterior tibial
Muscular branches
Peroneal
Posterior tibial

Perforating branch
Medial malleolar branch   Communicating branch
Lateral malleolar branch   Lateral malleolar branch
                             Medial malleolar branch
Dorsal of foot   Calcaneal branches

Lateral tarsal   Lateral plantar
Medial tarsal   Medial plantar
Arcuate   Plantar arch
Deep plantar branch of arcuate
Dorsal metatarsals   Plantar metatarsals

ANTERIOR   POSTERIOR

PLATE 7 —ARTERIES OF THE LOWER EXTREMITY

144

rior, ramus interventricularis posterior. **coronary a., left, of heart,** arteria coronaria sinistra. **coronary a., left, of stomach,** arteria gastrica sinistra. **coronary a., right, of heart,** arteria coronaria dextra. **coronary a., right, of stomach,** arteria gastrica dextra. **cremasteric a.,** arteria cremasterica. **cricothyroid a.,** ramus cricothyroideus arteriae thyroideae superioris. **cystic a.,** arteria cystica. **deferential a.,** arteria ductus deferentis. **deltoid a.,** ramus deltoideus arteriae thoracoacromialis. **dental a's, anterior,** arteriae alveolares superiores anteriores. **dental a., inferior,** arteria alveolaris inferior. **dental a., posterior,** arteria alveolaris superior posterior. **diaphragmatic a's,** arteriae phrenicae inferiores. **diaphragmatic a's, superior,** arteriae phrenicae superiores. **digital a's, collateral,** arteriae digitales palmares propriae. **digital a's of foot, dorsal,** arteriae digitales dorsales pedis. **digital a's of hand, dorsal,** arteriae digitales dorsales manus. **digital a's, palmar, common,** arteriae digitales palmares communes. **digital a's, palmar, proper,** arteriae digitales palmares propriae. **digital a's, plantar, common,** arteriae digitales plantares communes. **digital a's, plantar, proper,** arteriae digitales plantares propriae. **digital a's, volar, common,** arteriae digitales palmares communes. **digital a's, volar, proper,** arteriae digitales palmares propriae. **distributing a's,** most of the arteries except the conducting arteries; of muscular type, they extend from the large vessels to the arterioles. **dorsal a. of clitoris,** arteria dorsalis clitoridis. **dorsal a. of foot,** arteria dorsalis pedis. **dorsal a. of nose,** arteria dorsalis nasi. **dorsal a. of penis,** arteria dorsalis penis. **a. of ductus deferens,** arteria ductus deferentis. **duodenal a's,** arteriae pancreaticoduodenales inferiores. **efferent a. of glomerulus,** vas efferens glomeruli. **elastic a's,** conducting a's. **emulgent a.,** arteria renalis. **end a.,** one which undergoes progressive branching without development of channels connecting with other arteries, so that if occluded it cannot supply sufficient blood to the tissue depending on it. **epigastric a., external,** arteria circumflexa ilium profunda. **epigastric a., inferior,** arteria epigastrica inferior. **epigastric a., superficial,** arteria epigastrica superficialis. **epigastric a., superior,** arteria epigastrica superior. **episcleral a's,** arteriae episclerales. **esophageal a's, inferior,** rami esophagei arteriae gastricae sinistrae. **ethmoidal a., anterior,** arteria ethmoidalis anterior. **ethmoidal a., posterior,** arteria ethmoidalis posterior. **facial a.,** 1. arteria facialis. 2. arteria carotis externa. **facial a., deep,** arteria maxillaris. **facial a., transverse,** arteria transversa faciei. **fallopian a.,** arteria uterina. **femoral a.,** arteria femoralis. **femoral a., common,** see *arteria femoralis*. **femoral a., deep,** arteria profunda femoris. **femoral a., superficial,** see *arteria femoralis*. **fibular a.,** arteria fibularis. **a. of foot, dorsal,** arteria dorsalis pedis. **frontal a.,** arteria supratrochlearis. **frontobasal a., lateral,** arteria frontobasalis lateralis. **funicular a.,** arteria testicularis. **gastric a., left,** arteria gastrica sinistra. **gastric a., left inferior,** arteria gastro-omentalis sinistra. **gastric a., posterior,** arteria gastrica posterior. **gastric a., right,** arteria gastrica dextra. **gastric a., right inferior,** arteria gastro-omentalis dextra. **gastric a's, short,** arteriae gastricae breves. **gastroduodenal a.,** arteria gastroduodenalis. **gastroepiploic a., left,** arteria gastro-omentalis sinistra. **gastroepiploic a., right,** arteria gastro-omentalis dextra. **gastro-omental a., left,** arteria gastro-omentalis sinistra. **gastro-omental a., right,** arteria gastro-omentalis dextra. **genicular a., descending,** arteria descendens genicularis. **genicular a., inferior, lateral,** arteria inferior lateralis genus. **genicular a., inferior, medial,** arteria inferior mediales genus. **genicular a., middle,** arteria media genus. **genicular a., superior, lateral,** arteria superior lateralis genus. **genicular a., superior, medial,** arteria superior medialis genus. **a. of glomerulus,** vas afferens glomeruli. **gluteal a., inferior,** arteria glutea inferior. **gluteal a., superior,** arteria glutea superior. **hardening of a's,** arteriosclerosis. **helicine a's,** small arteries that possess on one side, throughout their length, a band of thickened intima in which longitudinal muscle fibers are embedded. They follow a convoluted or curled course and open directly into cavernous sinuses instead of capillaries; they play a dominant role in erection of erectile tissue.

helicine a's of penis, 1. arteriae helicinae penis. 2. rami helicini arteriae uterinae. **hemorrhoidal a., inferior,** arteria rectalis inferior. **hemorrhoidal a., middle,** arteria rectalis media. **hemorrhoidal a., superior,** arteria rectalis superior. **hepatic a., common,** arteria hepatica communis. **hepatic a., proper,** arteria hepatica propria. **hyaloid a.,** arteria hyaloidea. **a's of hybrid type,** a term denoting the short transitional regions where arteries of the mixed or elastic (conducting) type pass into arteries of the muscular (distributing) type. **hyoid a.,** ramus suprahyoideus arteriae lingualis. **hypogastric a.,** arteria iliaca interna. **hypophysial a., inferior,** arteria hypophysialis inferior. **hypophysial a., superior,** arteria hypophysialis superior. **ileal a's,** arteriae ilei. **ileocolic a.,** arteria ileocolica. **ileocolic a., ascending,** ramus colicus arteriae ileocolicae. **iliac a., anterior,** arteria iliaca externa. **iliac a., common,** arteria iliaca communis. **iliac a., external,** arteria iliaca externa. **iliac a., internal,** arteria iliaca interna. **iliac a., small,** arteria iliolumbalis. **iliolumbar a.,** arteria iliolumbalis. **infracostal a.,** ramus costalis lateralis arteriae thoracicae internae. **infraorbital a.,** arteria infraorbitalis. **inguinal a's,** rami inguinales arteriae femoralis. **innominate a.,** truncus brachiocephalicus. **insular a's,** arteriae insulares. **intercostal a's, anterior,** rami intercostales anteriores arteriae thoracicae internae. **intercostal a., first posterior,** arterial intercostalis posterior prima. **intercostal a., highest,** arteria intercostalis suprema. **intercostal a's, posterior,** arteriae intercostales posteriores. **intercostal a., second posterior,** arteria intercostalis posterior secunda. **intercostal a., superior,** arteria intercostalis suprema. **interlobar a's of kidney,** arteriae interlobares renis. **interlobular a's of kidney,** arteriae interlobulares renis. **interlobular a's of liver,** arteriae interlobulares hepatis. **intermediate atrial a., left,** ramus atrialis intermedius rami circumflexi arteriae coronariae sinistrae. **intermediate atrial a., right,** ramus atrialis intermedius arteriae coronariae dextrae. **intermetacarpal a's, palmar,** arteriae metacarpales palmares. **interosseous a., anterior,** arteria interossea anterior. **interosseous a., common,** arteria interossea communis. **interosseous a., dorsal, of forearm,** arteria interossea posterior. **interosseous a., posterior, of forearm,** arteria interossea posterior. **interosseous a., recurrent,** arteria interossea recurrens. **interosseous a., volar,** arteria interossea anterior. **intersegmental a's,** paired dorsal branches of the embryonic aorta, originally going to the spinal cord but later mainly to the neck, back, and body wall. **interventricular a., anterior,** ramus interventricularis anterior. **interventricular septal a's, anterior,** rami interventriculares septales rami interventricularis anterioris arteriae coronariae sinistrae. **interventricular septal a's, posterior,** rami interventriculares septales rami interventricularis posterioris arteriae coronariae dextrae. **intestinal a's,** arteriae intestinales. **jejunal a's,** arteriae jejunales. **labial a's, anterior, of vulva,** rami labiales anteriores arteriae femoralis. **labial a., inferior,** arteria labialis inferior. **labial a's, posterior, of vulva,** rami labiales posteriores arteriae pudendae internae. **labial a., superior,** arteria labialis superior. **a. of labyrinth, labyrinthine a.,** arteria labyrinthi. **lacrimal a.,** arteria lacrimalis. **laryngeal a., inferior,** arteria laryngea inferior. **laryngeal a., superior,** arteria laryngea superior. **lenticulostriate a.,** a. of cerebral hemorrhage. **lingual a.,** arteria lingualis. **lingual a., deep,** arteria profunda linguae. **lumbar a's,** arteriae lumbales. **lumbar a., fifth, lumbar a., lowest,** arteria lumbalis ima. **malleolar a., anterior, lateral,** arteria malleolaris anterior lateralis. **malleolar a., anterior, medial,** arteria malleolaris anterior medialis. **malleolar a., posterior, lateral,** see *rami malleolares laterales arteriae peroneae*. **malleolar a., posterior, medial,** see *rami malleolares mediales arteriae peroneae*. **mammary a., external,** 1. arteria thoracica lateralis. 2. see *rami mammarii laterales arteriae thoracicae lateralis*. **mammary a., internal,** arteria thoracica interna. **mandibular a.,** arteria alveolaris inferior. **marginal a. (of Drummond),** a long channel running parallel to the large intestine, from the cecum to the sigmoid colon, formed by branches from the superior and inferior mesenteric arteries and giving rise to straight arteries that supply the intestinal wall. **mar-**

ginal a., left, ramus marginalis sinister. **marginal a., right**, ramus marginalis dexter. **masseteric a.**, arteria masseterica. **mastoid a's**, rami mastoidei arteriae auricularis posterioris. **maxillary a.**, arteria maxillaris. **maxillary a., external**, arteria facialis. **maxillary a., internal**, arteria maxillaris. **medial a. of foot, superficial**, ramus superficialis arteriae plantaris medialis. **medial frontobasal a.**, arteria frontobasalis medialis. **median a.**, arteria comitans nervi mediani. **mediastinal a's, anterior**, rami mediastinales arteriae thoracicae internae. **mediastinal a's, posterior**, rami mediastinales aortae thoracicae. **medullary a.**, arteria nutricia. **meningeal a., accessory**, ramus meningeus accessorius arteriae meningeae mediae. **meningeal a., anterior**, ramus meningeus anterior arteriae ethmoidalis anterioris. **meningeal a., middle**, arteria meningea media. **meningeal a., posterior**, 1. arteria meningea posteria. 2. ramus meningeus arteriae vertebralis. **mental a.**, ramus mentalis arteriae alveolaris inferioris. **mesencephalic a's**, arteriae mesencephalicae. **mesenteric a., inferior**, arteria mesenterica inferior. **mesenteric a., superior**, arteria mesenterica superior. **metacarpal a's, dorsal**, 1. arteriae metacarpales dorsales. 2. see *ramus carpalis dorsalis*. **metacarpal a's, palmar**, arteriae metacarpales palmares. **metacarpal a's, ulnar**, arteriae digitales palmares communes. **metacarpal a., volar, deep**, ramus palmaris profundus arteriae ulnaris. **metatarsal a's, dorsal**, arteriae metatarsales dorsales. **metatarsal a's, plantar**, arteriae metatarsales plantares. **a's of mixed type**, arteries having elastic (conducting) and muscular (distributing) elements. **a's of Mueller**, arteriae helicinae penis. **muscular a's**, distributing a's. **musculophrenic a.**, arteria musculophrenica. **mylohyoid a.**, ramus mylohyoideus arteriae alveolaris inferioris. **myomastoid a.**, ramus occipitalis arteriae auricularis posterioris. **nasal a., dorsal, nasal a., external**, arteria dorsalis nasi. **nasal a's, lateral posterior**, arteriae nasales posteriores laterales. **nasopalatine a.**, arteria sphenopalatina. **Neubauer's a.**, arteria thyroidea ima. **nodal a.**, see *ramus nodi sinuatrialis arteriae coronariae dextrae*. **a. of nose, dorsal**, arteria dorsalis nasi. **nutrient a.**, arteria nutricia. **nutrient a's of femur**, arteriae nutriciae femoris. **nutrient a. of fibula**, arteria nutricia fibulae. **nutrient a's of humerus**, arteriae nutriciae humeri. **nutrient a's of kidney**, rami capsulares arteriae renis. **nutrient a. of tibia**, arteria nutricia tibiae. **obturator a.**, arteria obturatoria. **obturator a., accessory**, arteria obturatoria accessoria. **occipital a.**, arteria occipitalis. **occipital a., lateral**, arteria occipitalis lateralis. **occipital a., middle**, arteria occipitalis medialis. **ophthalmic a.**, arteria ophthalmica. **ovarian a.**, arteria ovarica. **palatine a., ascending**, arteria palatina ascendens. **palatine a., descending**, arteria palatina descendens. **palatine a., greater**, arteria palatina major. **palatine a., lesser**, arteriae palatinae minores. **palpebral a's, lateral**, arteriae palpebrales laterales. **palpebral a's, medial**, arteriae palpebrales mediales. **pancreatic a., dorsal**, arteria pancreatica dorsalis. **pancreatic a., great**, arteria pancreatica magna. **pancreatic a., inferior**, arteria pancreatica inferior. **pancreaticoduodenal a., anterior superior**, arteria pancreaticoduodenalis superior anterior. **pancreaticoduodenal a's, inferior**, arteriae pancreaticoduodenales inferiores. **pancreaticoduodenal a., posterior superior**, arteria pancreaticoduodenalis superior posterior. **paracentral a.**, arteria paracentralis. **parietal a's, anterior and posterior**, arteriae parietales anterior et posterior. **pelvic a., posterior**, arteria iliaca interna. **a. of penis, deep**, arteria profunda penis. **a. of penis, dorsal**, arteria dorsalis penis. **perforating a's**, arteriae perforantes. **pericallosal a.**, pars postcommunicalis arteriae cerebri anterioris. **pericardiac a's, posterior**, rami pericardiaci aortae thoracicae. **pericardiacophrenic a.**, arteria pericardiacophrenica. **perineal a.**, arteria perinealis. **peroneal a.**, arteria fibularis. **peroneal a., perforating**, ramus perforans arteriae fibularis. **pharyngeal a., ascending**, arteria pharyngea ascendens. **phrenic a's, great**, arteriae phrenicae inferiores. **phrenic a's, inferior**, arteriae phrenicae inferiores. **phrenic a., superior**, 1. arteria pericardiacophrenica. 2. see *arteriae phrenicae superiores*. **plantar a., deep**, a. plantaris profundus. **plantar a.,**

external, arteria plantaris lateralis. **plantar a., lateral**, arteria plantaris lateralis. **plantar a., medial**, arteria plantaris medialis. **pontine a's**, arteriae pontis. **popliteal a.**, arteria poplitea. **a. of postcentral sulcus**, arteria sulci postcentralis. **a. of precentral sulcus**, a. sulci precentralis. **precuneal a.**, arteria precunealis. **principal a. of thumb**, arteria princeps pollicis. **pterygoid a's**, rami pterygoidei. **a. of pterygoid canal**, arteria canalis pterygoidei. **pubic a.**, ramus pubicus arteriae epigastricae inferioris. **pudendal a's, external**, arteriae pudendae externae. **pudendal a., internal**, arteria pudenda interna. **pulmonary a.**, truncus pulmonalis. **pulmonary a., left**, arteria pulmonalis sinistra. **pulmonary a., right**, arteria pulmonalis dextra. **a. of the pulp**, a name given the first portion of a brushlike group of blood vessels in the spleen. **pyloric a.**, arteria gastrica dextra. **quadriceps a. of femur**, ramus descendens arteriae circumflexae femoris lateralis. **radial a.**, arteria radialis. **radial a., collateral**, arteria collateralis radialis. **radial a. of index finger**, arteria radialis indicis. **radial a., volar, of index finger**, arteria radialis indicis. **radiate a's of kidney**, arteriae interlobulares renis. **radicular a's**, rami spinales arteriae vertebralis. **ranine a.**, arteria profunda linguae. **rectal a., inferior**, arteria rectalis inferior. **rectal a., middle**, arteria rectalis media. **rectal a., superior**, arteria rectalis superior. **recurrent a.**, arteria centralis longa. **recurrent a., radial**, arteria recurrens radialis. **recurrent a., tibial, anterior**, arteria recurrens tibialis anterior. **recurrent a., tibial, posterior**, arteria recurrens tibialis posterior. **recurrent a., ulnar**, arteria recurrens ulnaris. **renal a.**, arteria renalis. **renal a's**, arteriae renis. **retrocostal a.**, ramus costalis lateralis arteriae thoracicae internae. **retroduodenal a's**, arteriae retroduodenales. **revehent a's**, vas efferens glomeruli. **a. of round ligament of uterus**, arteria ligamenti teretis uteri. **sacral a's, lateral**, arteriae sacrales laterales. **sacral a., median**, arteria sacralis mediana. **sacrococcygeal a.**, arteria sacralis mediana. **scapular a., descending**, ramus profundus arteriae transversae cervicis. **scapular a., dorsal**, 1. arteria dorsalis scapularis. 2. ramus profundus arteriae transversae cervicis. **scapular a., transverse**, arteria suprascapularis. **sciatic a.**, arteria comitans nervi ischiadici. **scrotal a's, anterior**, rami scrotales anteriores arteriae femoralis. **scrotal a's, posterior**, rami scrotales posteriores arteriae pudendae internae. **segmental a., anterior**, arteria segmenti anterioris. **segmental a., anterior inferior**, arteria segmenti anterioris inferioris. **segmental a., anterior superior**, arteria segmenti anterioris superioris. **segmental a., inferior**, arteria segmenti inferioris. **segmental a., lateral**, arteria segmenti lateralis. **segmental a., medial**, arteria segmenti medialis. **segmental a., posterior**, arteria segmenti posterioris. **segmental a., superior**, arteria segmenti superioris. **septal a's, anterior**, rami interventriculares septales rami interventricularis anterioris arteriae coronariae sinistrae. **septal a's, posterior**, rami interventriculares septales rami interventricularis. **sheathed a's**, arterial branches having spindle-shaped thickenings in their walls (Schweigger-Seidel sheaths) and forming the penicilli of the spleen; called also *ellipsoid* or *sheathed arterioles*. **short central a.**, arteria centralis brevis. **sigmoid a's**, arteriae sigmoideae. **sinoatrial nodal a., sinuatrial nodal a., sinus node a.**, see *ramus nodi sinuatrialis arteriae coronariae dextrae*. **spermatic a., external**, arteria cremasterica. **spermatic a., internal**, arteria testicularis. **sphenopalatine a.**, arteria sphenopalatina. **spinal a's**, rami spinales arteriae vertebralis. **spinal a., anterior**, arteria spinalis anterior. **spinal a., posterior**, arteria spinalis posterior. **splenic a.**, arteria splenica. **sternal a's, posterior**, rami sternales arteriae thoracicae internae. **sternocleidomastoid a.**, see *rami sternocleidomastoidei arteriae occipitalis*. **sternocleidomastoid a., superior**, ramus sternocleidomastoideus arteriae thyroideae superioris. **straight a's of kidney**, arteriolae rectae renis. **striate a's**, arteriae centrales anterolaterales. **striate a's, lateral**, rami laterales arteriarum centralium anterolateralium. **striate a's, medial**, rami mediales arteriarum centralium anteromedialium. **stylomastoid a.**, arteria stylomastoidea. **subclavian a.**, arteria subclavia. **subcostal a.**, 1. arteria subcostalis. 2. ramus costalis lateralis arteriae thoracicae internae. **sublingual a.**, arteria sublingualis. **submental a.**, arteria submentalis. **subscapular a.**, arteria subscapularis. **supraduodenal a.**, arteria supraduodenalis. **supraorbital a.**, arteria supraorbitalis. **suprarenal a., aortic**, arteria suprarenalis media. **suprarenal a., inferior**, arteria suprarenalis inferior. **suprarenal a., middle**, arteria suprarenalis media. **suprarenal a's, superior**, arteriae suprarenales superiores. **suprascapular a.**, arteria suprascapularis. **supratrochlear a.**, arteria supratrochlearis. **sural a's**, arteriae surales. **sylvian a.**, arteria cerebri media. **tarsal a., lateral**, arteria tarsalis lateralis. **tarsal a's, medial**, arteriae tarsalis mediales. **temporal a., anterior**, arteria temporalis anterior. **temporal a's, deep**, see *arteria temporalis profunda anterior* and *arteria temporalis profunda posterior*. **temporal a., deep, anterior**, arteria temporalis profunda anterior. **temporal a., deep, posterior**, arteria temporalis profunda posterior. **temporal a., middle**, 1. arteria temporalis media arteriae temporalis superficialis. 2. arteria temporalis media partis insularis arteriae cerebri mediae. **temporal a., posterior**, arteria temporalis posterior. **temporal a., superficial**, arteria temporalis superficialis. **terminal a.**, an artery that does not divide into branches, but is directly continuous with capillaries; called also *Cohnheim's a.* **testicular a.**, arteria testicularis. **thalamostriate a's, anterolateral**, arteriae centrales anterolaterales. **thalmostriate a's, anteromedial**, arteriae centrales anteromediales. **thoracic a., highest**, arteria thoracica suprema. **thoracic a., internal**, arteria thoracica interna. **thoracic a., lateral**, arteria thoracica lateralis. **thoracicoacromial a.**, arteria thoracoacromialis. **thoracodorsal a.**, arteria thoracodorsalis. **thymic a's**, rami thymici arteriae thoracicae internae. **thyroid a., inferior**, arteria thyroidea. **thyroid a., inferior, of Cruveilhier**, ramus cricothyroideus arteriae thyroideae superioris. **thyroid a., lowest**, arteria thyroidea ima. **thyroid a., superior**, arteria thyroidea superior. **tibial a., anterior**, arteria tibialis anterior. **tibial a., posterior**, arteria tibialis posterior. **a. of tongue, dorsal**, see *rami dorsales linguae arteriae lingualis*. **tonsillar a.**, ramus tonsillaris arteriae facialis. **transverse cervical a.**, arteria transversa cervicis. **transverse a. of face**, arteria transversa faciei. **transverse a. of neck**, arteria transversa cervicis. **tubo-ovarian a.**, arteria ovarica. **tympanic a., anterior**, arteria tympanica anterior. **tympanic a., inferior**, arteria tympanica inferior. **tympanic a., posterior**, arteria tympanica posterior. **tympanic a., superior**, arteria tympanica superior. **ulnar a.**, arteria ulnaris. **ulnar collateral a., inferior**, arteria collateralis ulnaris inferior. **ulnar collateral a., superior**, arteria collateralis ulnaris superior. **umbilical a.**, arteria umbilicalis. **urethral a.**, arteria urethralis. **uterine a.**, arteria uterina. **uterine a., aortic**, arteria ovarica. **vaginal a.**, arteria vaginalis. **venous a's**, venae pulmonales. **vermiform a.**, arteria appendicularis. **vertebral a.**, arteria vertebralis. **vesical a., inferior**, arteria vesicalis inferior. **vesical a's, superior**, arteriae vesicales superiores. **vestibular a's**, rami vestibulares arteriae labyrinthi. **vidian a.**, arteria canalis pterygoidei. **a. of Zinn**, arteria centralis retinae. **zygomatico-orbital a.**, arteria zygomatico-orbitalis.

Arthracanthida (ar″thrah-kan′thĭ-dah) [*arthr-* + Gr. *akantha* thorn, prickle] an order of marine protozoa (class Acantharea, superclass Actinopoda) usually characterized by the presence of 20 radial spines joined at the cell center by apposition of the bases and by a capsular membrane closely lining the central cell mass. In some species the bases of the spines have lateral wings, while others do not. It comprises two suborders: Sphaenacanthina and Phyllacanthina.

arthragra (ar-thrag′rah) [*arthr-* + Gr. *agra* seizure] a gouty seizure in a joint or in the joints.

arthral (ar′thral) pertaining to a joint.

arthralgia (ar-thral′je-ah) [*arthr-* + *-algia*] pain in a joint. **a. saturni′na**, arthralgia of lead poisoning.

arthralgic (ar-thral′jik) pertaining to arthralgia; affected with arthralgia.

arthrectomy (ar-threk′to-me) [*arthr-* + Gr. *ektomē* excision] the excision of a joint.

arthrempyesis (ar″threm-pi-e′sis) [*arthr-* + Gr. *empyēsis* suppuration] suppuration in a joint.

arthresthesia (ar″thres-the′ze-ah) [*arthr-* + Gr. *aisthēsis* perception] joint sensibility; the perception of joint motions.

arthrifuge (ar′thrĭ-fūj) [*arthritis* + L. *fugare* to put to flight] a cure for gout.

arthritic (ar-thrit′ik) 1. pertaining to or affected with gout or arthritis. 2. a person affected with arthritis.

arthritide (ar′thrĭ-tīd) any skin eruption of arthritic or gouty origin.

arthritides (ar-thrit′ĭ-dēz) plural of *arthritis*.

arthritis (ar-thri′tis), pl. *arthrit′ides* [Gr. *arthron* joint + *-itis*] rheumatism in which the inflammatory lesions are confined to the joints. **acute a.**, arthritis marked by pain, heat, redness, and swelling, due to inflammation, infection, or trauma. **acute gouty a.**, acute arthritis associated with gout. **acute rheumatic a.**, rheumatic fever. **acute suppurative a.**, inflammation of a joint by pus-forming organisms. **atrophic a.**, rheumatoid a. **bacterial a.**, infectious arthritis, usually acute, characterized by inflammation of synovial membranes with purulent effusion into a joint(s), most often due to *Staphylococcus aureus*, *Streptococcus pyogenes*, *Streptococcus pneumoniae*, and *Neisseria gonorrhoeae*, but other bacteria may be involved, and usually caused by hematogenous spread from a primary site of infection although joints may also become infected by direct inoculation or local extension. Called also *pyoarthritis*, *septic a.*, and *suppurative a.* **Bekhterev's a.**, rheumatoid spondylitis. **blennorrhagic a.**, gonococcal a. **chronic inflammatory a.**, rheumatoid a. **chronic villous a.**, a form of rheumatoid arthritis due to villous outgrowths from the synovial membranes, which cause impairment of function and crepitation; called also *dry joint*. **climactic a.**, menopausal a. **cricoarytenoid a.**, inflammation of the cricoarytenoid joint in rheumatoid arthritis; causing laryngeal stridor. **a. defor′mans**, rheumatoid a. **degenerative a.**, osteoarthritis. **exudative a.**, arthritis with exudate into or about the joint. **fungal a., a. fungo′sa**, mycotic a. **gonococcal a., gonorrheal a.**, bacterial arthritis occurring secondary to gonorrhea, often characterized by migratory polyarthritis that usually involves one and sometimes two joints, and commonly associated with erythematous skin lesions. Called also *blennorrhagic a.* **gouty a.**, arthritis due to gout; called also *uratic a.* **hemophilic a.**, bleeding into the joint cavities. **hypertrophic a.**, osteoarthritis. **infectious a.**, arthritis caused by bacteria, rickettsiae, mycoplasmas, viruses, fungi, or parasites. **juvenile a., juvenile chronic a., juvenile rheumatoid a.**, arthritis in one or more joints persisting at least 6 weeks in a child in whom alternative diagnoses have been excluded. **Lyme a.**, see under *disease*. **menopausal a.**, a condition sometimes seen in women at the menopause, due to ovarian hormonal deficiency and marked by pain in the small joints, shoulders, elbows, or knees; called also *arthropathia ovaripriva* and *climactic a.* **a. mu′tilans**, a severe deforming polyarthritis with gross bone and cartilage destruction, usually an atypical variant of rheumatoid arthritis. **mycotic a.**, infectious arthritis occurring secondary to any invasive mycosis, such as coccidioidomycosis, blastomycosis, histoplasmosis, actinomycosis, candidiasis, and sporotrichosis, usually by extension from adjacent bone, and having manifestations similar to those of tuberculous arthritis. Called also *fungal a.* and *a. fungosa.* **navicular a.**, inflammation of the navicular bursa and the cartilage covering the navicular bone of the foot of a horse. **neuropathic a.**, neuropathic arthropathy. **a. nodo′sa**, 1. rheumatoid a. 2. gout. **a. pau′perum**, 1. rheumatoid a. 2. poor man's gout. **proliferative a.**, rheumatoid a. **psoriatic a.**, a syndrome in which psoriasis occurs in association with inflammatory arthritis, which often involves the interphalangeal joints; rheumatoid factor is usually not present in the sera of affected individuals. Called also *arthritic psoriasis, psoriasis arthropathica*, and *p. arthropica.* **rheumatoid a.**, a chronic systemic disease primarily of the joints, usually polyarticular, marked by inflammatory changes in the synovial membranes and articular structures and by atrophy and rarefaction of the bones. In late stages deformity and ankylosis develop. The cause is unknown, but autoimmune mechanisms and virus infection have been postulated. Called also *atrophic a., a. deformans, a. nodosa, a. pauperum, chronic* *inflammatory a., proliferative a., arthronosos deformans, arthrosis deformans,* and *rheumatic gout.* **rheumatoid a., juvenile,** rheumatoid arthritis of children, with swelling, tenderness, and pain involving one or more joints, leading to impaired growth and development, limitation of movement, and ankylosis and flexion contractures of the joints. It is frequently accompanied by systemic manifestations which may include spiking fever, transient rash on the trunk and extremities, hepatosplenomegaly, generalized lymphadenopathy, and anemia. Called also *Still's disease.* **rheumatoid a. of spine,** rheumatoid spondylitis. **septic a.,** bacterial a. **a. sic′ca,** arthritis without exudation into a joint cavity. **suppurative a.,** bacterial a. **syphilitic a.,** a rare form of bacterial arthritis occurring as a manifestation of primary, secondary, or tertiary syphilis; see also *neuropathic arthropathy,* under *arthropathy; Clutton joint,* under *joint;* and *Parrot's pseudoparalysis,* under *pseudoparalysis.* **tuberculous a.,** bacterial arthritis occurring secondary to tuberculosis; it usually affects a single joint and is characterized by chronic inflammation with effusion and destruction of contiguous bone. **uratic a.,** gouty a. **a. urethrit′ica,** Reiter's syndrome. **venereal a.,** Reiter's syndrome. **vertebral a.,** inflammation involving the intervertebral disks, secondary to joint involvement. **viral a.,** infectious arthritis, usually polyarticular and self-limited, associated with a viral disease, such as rubella, mumps, infectious mononucleosis, varicella, hepatitis B, and arboviral or adenoviral infection.

arthr(o)- [Gr. *arthron* joint] a combining form denoting some relationship to a joint or joints.

Arthrobacter (ar″thro-bak′ter) [Gr. *arthron* a joint + *baktron* a rod] a genus of coryneform bacteria, consisting of pleomorphic, gram-variable organisms found in soil.

arthrobacterium (ar″thro-bak-te′re-um) [*arthro-* + *bacterium*] a bacterium of the genus *Arthrobacter.*

Arthrobotrys (ar″thro-bo′tris) a genus of imperfect fungi of the family Moniliaceae, order Moniliales, some of which infect and destroy nematodes.

arthrocele (ar′thro-sel) [*arthro-* + Gr. *kēlē* tumor] a swollen joint.

arthrocentesis (ar″thro-sen-te′sis) puncture and aspiration of a joint.

arthrochalasis (ar″thro-kal′ah-sis) [*arthro-* + Gr. *chalasis* relaxation] abnormal relaxation or flaccidity of a joint. **a. mul′tiplex congen′ita,** overflaccidity of multiple joints, not associated with hyperelasticity of the skin.

arthrochondritis (ar″thro-kon-dri′tis) [*arthro-* + *chondritis*] inflammation of the cartilage of a joint.

arthroclasia (ar″thro-kla′ze-ah) [*arthro-* + Gr. *klaein* to break] the surgical breaking down of an ankylosis in order to secure free movement in a joint.

arthroclisis (ar″thro-kli′sis) arthrokleisis.

Arthroderma (ar″thro-der′mah) a genus of ascomycetous fungi (family Gymnoascaceae, order Eurotiales) in which the hyphae around the gymnothecium are dichotomously branched, with deep constrictions of the cells to give a dumbbell shape. It contains the perfect (sexual) stages of imperfect fungi of the genus *Trichophyton.*

arthrodesia (ar″thro-de′se-ah) arthrodesis.

arthrodesis (ar″thro-de′sis) [*arthro-* + Gr. *desis* binding] the surgical fixation of a joint by a procedure designed to accomplish fusion of the joint surfaces by promoting the proliferation of bone cells; called also *artificial ankylosis.* **Moberg a.,** fusion of a finger joint with a small squared bone peg. **triple a.,** fusion of the subtalar, calcaneocuboid, and talonavicular joints, to provide lateral stability to the paralyzed foot.

arthrodia (ar-thro′de-ah) [Gr. *arthrōdia* a particular kind of articulation] articulatio plana [NA].

arthrodial (ar-thro′de-al) of the nature of an arthrodia.

arthrodynia (ar″thro-din′e-ah) [*arthro-* + *odynē* pain] pain in a joint.

arthrodysplasia (ar″thro-dis-pla′ze-ah) [*arthro-* + *dysplasia*] a hereditary condition marked by deformity of various joints.

arthroempyesis (ar″thro-em″pi-e′sis) [*arthro-* + Gr. *empyēsis* suppuration] suppuration within a joint.

arthroendoscopy (ar″thro-en-dos′ko-pe) arthroscopy.

arthroereisis (ar″thro-ĕ-ri′sis) [*arthro-* + Gr. *ereisis* a raising

up] operative limiting of the motion in a joint that is abnormally mobile from paralysis.

arthrogenous (ar-throj′ĕ-nus) [*arthro-* + Gr. *gennan* to produce] formed as a separate joint, as arthrogenous spore.

arthrogram (ar′thro-gram) a roentgenographic record after introduction of opaque contrast material into a joint.

Arthrographis (ar-throg′rah-fis) a genus of imperfect fungi of uncertain classification, tentatively placed in the family Dermaticeae, order Moniliales. **A. langero′ni,** a species of fungi reported to produce an onychomycosis in man and a benign dermatomycosis in animals. The term is no longer considered valid.

arthrography (ar-throg′rah-fe) [*arthro-* + Gr. *graphein* to write] roentgenography of a joint after injection of opaque contrast material. **air a.,** pneumoarthrography.

arthrogryposis (ar″thro-grĭ-po′sis) [*arthro-* + Gr. *grypōsis* a crooking] 1. persistent flexure or contracture of a joint. tetanoid spasm. **congenital multiple a., a. mul′tiplex conge′nita,** a syndrome characterized by congenital immobility of most of the joints, fixed in various postures, with lack of muscle development and growth.

arthrokatadysis (ar″thro-kah-tad′ĭ-sis) [*arthro-* + Gr. *katadysis* a falling down] a sinking in or subsidence of the floor of the acetabulum with protrusion of the femoral head through it (intrapelvic protrusion) resulting in limitation of movement of the hip joint; called also *Otto's disease.*

arthrokleisis (ar″thro-kli′sis) [*arthro-* + Gr. *kleisis* closure] ankylosis of a joint, or the production of such ankylosis.

arthrolith (ar′thro-lith) [*arthro-* + Gr. *lithos* stone] a calculous deposit in a joint; cf. *arthrophyte* and *joint mouse.*

arthrolithiasis (ar″thro-lĭ-thi′ah-sis) gout.

arthrologia (ar″thro-lo′je-ah) arthrology; in NA terminology *arthrologia* encompasses the nomenclature relating to the articulations (joints) and ligaments. Formerly called *syndesmologia.*

arthrology (ar-throl′o-je) [*arthro-* + *-logy*] the scientific study of the joints and ligaments; also applied to the body of knowledge relating thereto. Called also *syndesmology.*

arthrolysis (ar-throl′ĭ-sis) [*arthro-* + Gr. *lysis* dissolution] the operative loosening of adhesions in an ankylosed joint.

arthromeningitis (ar″thro-men″in-ji′tis) [*arthro-* + Gr. *mēninx* membrane + *-itis*] synovitis.

arthrometer (ar-throm′ĕ-ter) [*arthro-* + Gr. *metron* measure] an instrument for measuring the angles of movements of joints.

arthrometry (ar-throm′ĕ-tre) the measurement of the range of mobility of joints.

Arthromitaceae (ar″thro-mi-ta′se-e) in former systems of classification, a family of bacteria of the order Caryophanales, including the genera *Arthromitus* and *Coleomitus.*

Arthromitus (ar-throm′ĭ-tus) [*arthro-* + Gr. *mitos* thread] a genus of spore-forming, filamentous bacteria of uncertain taxonomic position, which was formerly classified in the family Arthromitaceae, found in the intestinal walls of insects, tadpoles, and crustaceans.

arthroncus (ar-throng′kus) [*arthro-* + Gr. *onkos* mass] swelling of a joint.

arthroneuralgia (ar″thro-nu-ral′je-ah) [*arthro-* + *neuralgia*] pain arising in or around a joint.

arthronosos (ar″thro-no′sos) [*arthro-* + Gr. *nosos* disease] a disease of the joints. **a. defor′mans,** rheumatoid arthritis.

arthro-onychodysplasia (ar″thro-on″ĭ-ko-dis-pla′zhah) onycho-osteodysplasia.

arthro-ophthalmopathy (ar″thro-of-thal-mop′ah-the) an association of degenerative joint disease and eye disease. **hereditary progressive a.,** a hereditary disorder consisting of myopia, progressing to retinal detachment and blindness, and premature degenerative changes in the joints; it is transmitted as an autosomal dominant trait.

Arthropan (ar′thro-pan) trademark for a preparation of choline salicylate.

arthropathia (ar″thro-path′e-ah) [L.] arthropathy. **a. ovaripri′va,** menopausal arthritis. **a. psoriat′ica,** a disease of the joints seen in persons suffering from psoriasis; it resembles rheumatoid arthritis.

arthropathic (ar″thro-path′ik) pertaining to or characterized by arthropathy.

arthropathology (ar″thro-pah-thol′o-je) [arthro- + pathology] the study of the structural and functional changes produced in the joints by disease.

arthropathy (ar-throp′ah-the) [arthro- + Gr. pathos disease] any joint disease. **Charcot's a.,** neuropathic a. **chondrocalcific a.,** progressive polyarthritis with joint swelling and bony enlargement, most commonly in the small joints of the hand but also affecting other joints, characterized roentgenographically by narrowing of the joint space with subchondral erosions and sclerosis and frequently chondrocalcinosis. **inflammatory a.,** a disease of a joint of inflammatory origin. **neurogenic a.,** neuropathic a. **neuropathic a.,** chronic progressive degeneration of the stress-bearing portion of a joint, with bizarre hypertrophic changes at the periphery. It is probably a complication of a variety of neurologic disorders, particularly tabes dorsalis, involving loss of sensation, which leads to relaxation of supporting structures and chronic instability of the joint. Called also *Charcot's a.*, *neurogenic a.*, *Charcot's disease* or *joint*, and *neuropathic arthritis*. **osteopulmonary a.,** clubbing of the fingers and toes, enlargement and swelling of the ends of the long bones associated with cardiac and pulmonary disease. **psoriatic a.,** see under *arthritis*. **static a.,** a disturbance in a joint of the extremity secondary to a disturbance in some other joint of the same extremity, as one in the knee joint secondary to one in the hip joint. **syphilitic a.,** see under *arthritis*. **tabetic a.,** neuropathic arthropathy (q.v.) occurring in patients with tabes dorsalis.

arthrophyma (ar″thro-fi′mah) [arthro- + Gr. phyma swelling] the swelling of a joint.

arthrophyte (ar′thro-fit) [arthro- + Gr. phyton plant] an abnormal growth in a joint cavity; cf. *arthrolith* and *joint mouse*.

arthroplastic (ar″thro-plas′tik) pertaining to arthroplasty.

arthroplasty (ar′thro-plas″te) [arthro- + Gr. plassein to form] plastic surgery of a joint or of joints; the formation of movable joints. **gap a.,** surgical correction of dental ankylosis by creating a space between the ankylosed part and the portion to be made moveable. **interposition a.,** surgical correction of ankylosis of the temporomandibular joint by separating the immobile fragment from the mobilized fragment and interposing a substance, such as fascia, cartilage, metal, or plastic, between them. **intracapsular temporomandibular joint a.,** operative recontouring of the articular surface of the mandibular condyle without the removal of the articular disk.

arthropneumography (ar″thro-nu-mog′rah-fe) arthropneumoroentgenography.

arthropneumoroentgenography (ar″thro-nu″mo-rentgen-og′rah-fe) [arthro- + Gr. pneuma air + roentgenography] roentgenography of a joint after injection into it of air, oxygen, or carbon dioxide.

arthropod (ar′thro-pod) an animal belonging to the Arthropoda.

Arthropoda (ar-throp′o-dah) [arthro- + Gr. pous foot] a phylum of the animal kingdom composed of organisms having a hard, jointed exoskeleton and paired, jointed legs, and including, among other classes, the Arachnida and Insecta, many species of which are important medically as parasites or as vectors of organisms capable of causing disease in man.

arthropodan (ar-throp′o-dan) arthropodous.

arthropodic (ar″thro-po′dic) arthropodous.

arthropodous (ar-throp′o-dus) pertaining to or caused by arthropods.

arthropyosis (ar″thro-pi-o′sis) [arthro- + Gr. pyōsis suppuration] the formation of pus in a joint cavity.

arthrorheumatism (ar″thro-roo′mah-tizm) [arthro- + rheumatism] inflammation within a joint.

arthrorisis (ar″thro-ri′sis) arthroereisis.

arthroscintigram (ar″thro-sin′tĭ-gram) a scintiscan of a joint.

arthroscintigraphy (ar″thro-sin-tig′rah-fe) scintigraphy of a joint.

arthrosclerosis (ar″thro-skle-ro′sis) [arthro- + sklērōsis hardening] stiffening or hardening of the joints.

arthroscope (ar′thro-skōp) [arthro- + Gr. skopein to exam-

ine] an endoscope for examining the interior of a joint and for carrying out diagnostic and therapeutic procedures within the joint.

arthroscopy (ar-thros′ko-pe) examination of the interior of a joint with an arthroscope.

arthrosis (ar-thro′sis) 1. [Gr. arthrōsis a jointing] a joint or articulation. 2. [arthro- + -osis] a disease of a joint. **a. defor′mans,** rheumatoid arthritis.

arthrospore (ar′thro-spōr) [arthro- + Gr. sporos seed] an asexual fungal spore formed by hyphal segmentation.

arthrosteitis (ar″thros-te-i′tis) [arthro- + Gr. osteon bone + -itis] inflammation of the bony structures of a joint.

arthrostomy (ar-thros′to-me) [arthro- + Gr. stomoun to provide with a mouth, or opening] surgical creation of an opening into a joint, as for the purpose of drainage.

arthrosynovitis (ar″thro-sin″o-vi′tis) [arthro- + synovitis] inflammation of the synovial membrane of a joint.

arthrotome (ar′thro-tōm) [arthro- + Gr. tomē cut] a knife for incising a joint.

arthrotomy (ar-throt′o-me) [arthro- + Gr. tomē cut] surgical incision of a joint.

arthrotropic (ar″thro-trop′ik) [arthro- + Gr. tropos a turning] having an affinity for or tending to settle in the joints.

arthroxerosis (ar″thro-ze-ro′sis) [arthro- + Gr. xēros dry + -osis] chronic osteoarthritis.

arthroxesis (ar-throk′sĕ-sis) [arthro- + Gr. xesis scraping] the scraping of diseased tissue from an articular surface.

Arthus reaction (phenomenon), Arthus-type reaction (ar-toos′) [Nicolas-Maurice Arthus, French physiologist, 1862–1945] see under *reaction*.

article (ar′te-kl) [L. articulus a little joint] an interarticular segment; one of the portions or segments forming a jointed series.

articular (ar-tik′u-lar) [L. articularis] of or pertaining to a joint.

articulare (ar-tik′u-la′re) a craniometric landmark used in roentgenographic cephalometry, being the point of intersection of the posterior margin of the ascending ramus of the mandible and the shadow of the cranial base, as seen on the lateral x-ray of the head. Called also *point Ar*.

articulate (ar-tik′u-lāt) [L. articulatus jointed] 1. divided into or united by joints. 2. enunciated in words and sentences. 3. to divide into or to unite so as to form a joint. 4. in dentistry, to adjust or place the teeth in their proper relation to each other in making an artificial denture.

articulated (ar-tik′u-lāt″ed) connected by movable joints; consisting of separate segments so joined as to be movable on each other.

articulatio (ar-tik″u-la′she-o), pl. articulatio′nes [L.] an articulation: a place of junction between two discrete objects; used in anatomical nomenclature [NA] to designate the place of union or junction between two or more bones of the skeleton, indicated by the modifying term. Also used in the plural as a general term to indicate such joints. Called also *joint*, *junctura ossium*, and *osseous joint*. **a. acromioclavicula′ris** [NA], acromioclavicular articulation: the joint formed by the acromion of the scapula and the acromial extremity of the clavicle; called also *scapuloclavicular articulation* or *joint*. **a. atlanto-axia′lis latera′lis,** lateral atlantoaxial articulation: one of a pair of joints, one on either side of the body, formed by the inferior articular surface of the atlas and the superior surface of the axis. **a. atlanto-axia′lis media′na** [NA], medial atlantoaxial articulation: a single joint formed by the two articular facets of the dens of the axis, one in relation with the articular facet on the anterior arch of the atlas, the other in relation with the transverse ligament of the atlas. **a. atlantoepistroph′ica,** see *a. atlantoaxialis lateralis* and *a. atlantoaxialis mediana*. **a. atlanto-occipita′lis** [NA], atlanto-occipital articulation: one of two joints, each formed by a superior articular pit of the atlas and a condyle of the occipital bone; called also *craniovertebral*, *occipital*, or *occipitoatlantal articulation*, and *Cruveilhier's joint*. **a. bicondyla′ris** [NA], bicondylar articulation: a condylar joint with a meniscus between the articular surfaces, as in the temporomandibular joint; called also *bicondylar joint*. **a. calcaneocuboi′dea** [NA], calcaneocuboid articulation: one formed between the cuboidal articular surface of the calcaneus and the cuboid bone. **a. cap′itis cos′tae** [NA], one of the two types of articulations between ribs and vertebrae: the articulation of the head of the rib with the bodies of two vertebrae. Called also *articulation of head of rib, articulationes capitulorum costarum*, and *capitular* or *costocentral articulation*. Cf. *a. costotransversaria*. **a. cap′itis hu′meri**, a. humeri. **articulatio′nes capitulo′rum costa′rum**, see *a. capitis costae*. **articulatio′nes car′pi** [NA], carpal articulations: any of the joints that connect the carpal bones together, comprising: the joints between each row, distal and proximal (*articulationes intercarpales*); the joint between the distal and proximal rows (*a. mediocarpalis*); and the joint formed by the pisiform and triquetal bones. (*a. ossis pisiformis*). Called also *carpal bones*. **articulatio′nes carpometacarpa′les** [NA], **articulatio′nes carpometacar′peae**, carpometacarpal articulations: joints formed by the trapezial, trapezoid, capitate, and hamate bones together with the bases of the four medial metacarpal bones; called also *metacarpocarpal articulations*. **a. carpometacarpa′lis pol′licis** [NA], **carpometacar′pea pol′licis**, the joint formed by the first metacarpal and the trapezial bones; called also *carpometacarpal articulation of thumb* and *first carpometacarpal articulation*. **articulatio′nes cartilagin′eae** [NA], cartilaginous joints: joints in which the union of the bony elements is by intervening cartilage, the two types of cartilaginous joints are synchondrosis and symphysis. Called also *juncturae cartilagineae*. **articulatio′nes cin′guli mem′bri inferio′ris** [NA], the articulations of the girdle of the inferior member, i.e., the sacroiliac articulation and the symphysis pubica; called also *juncturae cinguli membri inferioris*. **articulatio′nes cin′guli mem′bri superio′ris** [NA] the articulations of the girdle of the superior member, i.e., the acromioclavicular and sternoclavicular articulations; called also *juncturae cinguli membri superioris*. **a. cochlea′ris**, a form of hinge joint that permits some lateral motion. **a. compos′ita** [NA], composite articulation: a type of synovial joint in which more than two bones are involved; called also *compound articulation* and *compound* or *composite joint*. **a. condyla′ris**, NA alternative for *a. ellipsoidea*. **a. condyla′ris inver′sa**, a. sellaris. **articulatio′nes costochondra′les** [NA], costochondral articulations: articulations between the lateral extremity of each costal cartilage and the sternal ends of the ribs. **a. costotransversa′ria** [NA], costotransverse articulation: one of the two types of articulations between ribs and vertebrae: the articulation of the tubercle of the rib with the transverse process of a vertebra. This is lacking for the eleventh and twelfth ribs. Called also *articulation of tubercle of rib*. Cf. *a. capitis costae*. **articulatio′nes costovertebra′les** [NA], costovertebral articulations: the articulations between the ribs and vertebrae, of which there are two types: a. capitis costae and a. costotransversaria. **a. cotyl′ica**, NA alternative for *a. spheroidea*. **a. cox′ae** [NA], articulation of hip: the joint formed between the head of the femur and the acetabulum of the hip bone; called also *coxofemoral articulation of Buisson, femoral articulation*, and *hip joint*; loosely called *hip*. **a. cricoarytenoi′dea** [NA], cricoarytenoid articulation: the synovial joint between the upper border of the cricoid cartilage and the base of the arytenoid cartilage. **a. cricothyroi′dea** [NA], the articulation between the lateral aspect of the cricoid cartilage and the inferior horn of the thyroid cartilage. **a. crurotala′ris**, a. talocruralis. **a. cu′biti** [NA], cubital articulation: the joint between the arm and forearm, comprising the humeroulnar, humeroradial, and proximal radioulnar articulations; called also *cubital articulation, articulation of elbow*, and *elbow joint*. **a. cuneocuboi′dea** [NA], cuneocuboid articulation: the synovial joint between the lateral cuneiform bone and the cuboid bone. **a. cuneonavicula′ris** [NA], cuneonavicular articulation: the joint between the anterior surface of the navicular bone and the proximal ends of the three cuneiform bones. **a. dentoalveola′ris**, gomphosis. **a. ellipsoi′dea** [NA], ellipsoidal articulation: a modification of the ball-and-socket type of synovial joint in which the articular surfaces are ellipsoid rather than spheroid; owing to the arrangement of the muscles and ligaments around the joint, all movements are permitted except rotation about a vertical axis. Called also *a. condylaris* [NA alternative], *condylarthrosis, condylar articulation*, and *condylar, condyloid*, or *ellipsoidal joint*. **articulatio′nes fibro′sae** [NA], fibrous joints: joints in which the union of their bony elements is by continuous intervening fibrous tissue, which makes little

motion possible; the three types of fibrous joints are sutura, syndesmosis, and gomphosis. Called also *juncturae ossium, synarthrodes*, and *synarthrodial joints*. **a. ge′nu, a. ge′nus** [NA], articulation of knee: the compound joint formed between the articular surface of the patella, the condyles and patellar surface of the femur, and the superior articular surface of the tibia; called also *knee joint*. **a. hu′meri** [NA], articulation of shoulder: the joint formed by the head of the humerus and the glenoid cavity of the scapula; called also *a. capitis humeri, articulation of head of humerus, articulation of humerus*, and *shoulder joint*. **a. humeroradia′lis** [NA], humeroradial articulation: the joint between the humerus and the radius; called also *brachioradial articulation*. **a. humero-ulna′ris** [NA], humeroulnar articulation: the joint between the humerus and the ulna; called also *brachioulnar articulation*. **a. incudomallea′ris** [NA], incudomalleolar articulation: the junction of the incus and the malleus. **a. incudomalleola′ris**, a. incudomallearis **a. incudostape′dia** [NA], incudostapedial articulation: the junction of the incus and the stapes. **articulatio′nes intercarpa′les** [NA], **articulatio′nes intercar′peae**, intercarpal articulations: the joints between the bones, within each row, distal and proximal, of carpal bones. Called also *intercarpal joints*. See also *articulationes carpi*. **articulatio′nes interchondra′les** [NA], interchondral articulations: the unions, on either side, between the costal cartilages of the upper false ribs, usually ribs seven through ten; called also *intercostal articulations*. **articulatio′nes intercuneifor′mes** [NA], intercuneiform articulations: the synovial joints between the cuneiform bones. **articulatio′nes intermetacarpa′les** [NA], **articulatio′nes intermetacar′peae**, intermetacarpal articulations: the joints formed between the adjoining bases of the second, third, fourth, and fifth metacarpal bones; called also *articulations of metacarpal bones*. **articulatio′nes intermetatarsa′les** [NA], **articulatio′nes intermetatar′seae**, intermetatarsal articulations: the joints formed between the adjoining bases of the five metatarsal bones; called also *articulations of metatarsal bones*. **articulatio′nes interphalangea′les ma′nus** [NA], **articulatio′nes interphalan′geae ma′nus**, interphalangeal articulations of hand: the hinge joints between the phalangeal articulations of the hand. Called also *interphalangeal articulations of digits of hand* and *interphalangeal articulations of fingers*. **articulatio′nes interphalangea′les pe′dis** [NA], **articulatio′nes interphalan′geae pe′dis**, interphalangeal articulations of foot: the hinge joints between the phalangeal articulations of the foot. Called also *interphalangeal articulations of digits of foot* and *interphalangeal articulations of toes*. **articulatio′nes intertar′seae** [NA], intertarsal articulations: the articulations between the various tarsal bones. **a. lumbosacra′lis** [NA], lumbosacral articulation: the articulation between the sacrum and the lumbar vertebrae; called also *junctura lumbosacralis*. **a. mandibula′ris**, a. temporomandibularis. **articulatio′nes ma′nus** [NA], articulations of hand: the joints of the hand, including those of the wrist and the intercarpal, carpometacarpal, intermetacarpal, metacarpophalangeal, and interphalangeal articulations. **a. mediocarpa′lis** [NA], **a. mediocar′pea**, mediocarpal articulation: the joint between the two rows, distal and proximal, of carpal bones. Called also *mediocarpal joint*. See also *articulationes carpi*. **articulatio′nes mem′bri inferio′ris li′beri** [NA], the articulations of the free inferior member, i.e., of the thigh, leg, and foot; called also *juncturae membri inferioris liberi*. **articulatio′nes mem′bri superio′ris li′beri** [NA], the articulations of the free superior member, i.e., of the arm, forearm, and hand; called also *juncturae membri superioris liberi*. **articulatio′nes metacarpophalangea′les** [NA], **articulatio′nes metacarpophalan′geae**, metacarpophalangeal articulations: joints formed between the heads of the five metacarpal bones and the bases of the corresponding proximal phalanges. **articulatio′nes metatarsophalangea′les** [NA], **articulatio′nes metatarsophalan′geae**, metatarsophalangeal articulations: the joints formed between the heads of the five metatarsal bones and the bases of the corresponding proximal phalanges. **articulatio′nes ossiculo′rum audi′tus** [NA], articulations of auditory ossicles, including *a. incudomallearis* and *a. incudostapedia*. **a. os′sis pisifor′mis** [NA], articulation of pisiform bone: the carpal joint formed by the pisiform and triquetral bones. **a.**

ovoida′lis, a. sellaris. **articulatio′nes pe′dis** [NA], articulations of foot: the joints of the foot, including the talocrural, intertarsal, tarsometatarsal, metatarsophalangeal, and interphalangeal articulations. **a. pla′na** [NA], plane articulation: a type of synovial joint in which the opposed surfaces are flat or only slightly curved; it permits only simple gliding movement, in any direction, within narrow limits imposed by ligaments. Called also *arthrodia, gliding articulation, plane* or *gliding joint,* and *arthrodial joint.* **a. radiocarpa′lis** [NA], **a. radiocar′pea,** radiocarpal articulation: a condylar joint formed by the radius and the articular disk with the scaphoid, lunate, and triquetral bones; called also *brachiocarpal joint, wrist,* and *wrist joint.* **a. radio-ulna′ris,** NA alternative for *syndesmosis radio-ulnaris.* **a. radio-ulna′ris dista′lis** [NA], distal radioulnar articulation: the joint formed by the head of the ulna and the ulnar notch of the radius; called also *inferior radioulnar* (or *cubitoradial*) *articulation.* **a. radio-ulna′ris proxima′lis** [NA], proximal radioulnar articulation: the proximal of the two joints between the radius and the ulna; it enters into pronation and supination of the forearm. Called also *superior radioulnar* (or *cubitoradial*) *articulation.* **a. sacrococcyg′ea** [NA], sacrococcygeal articulation: the articulation between the coccyx and sacrum; called also *junctura sacrococcygea, sacrococcygeal symphysis,* and *symphysis sacrococcygea.* **a. sacroili′aca** [NA], sacroiliac articulation: the joint formed between the auricular surfaces of the sacrum and ilium; called also *sacroiliac symphysis,* and *ileosacral articulation.* **a. sella′ris** [NA], a type of synovial joint in which the articular surface of one bone is concave in one direction and convex in the direction at right angles to the first (concavoconvex), and the articular surface of the second bone is reciprocally convexoconcave; movement is permitted along two main axes at right angles to each other. Called also *a. condylaris inversa, a. ovoidalis, ovoid articulation, saddle articulation,* and *saddle* or *sellar joint.* **a. sim′plex** [NA], simple articulation: a type of synovial joint in which only two bones are involved; called also *simple joint.* **a. sphaeroi′dea,** a. spheroidea. **a. spheroi′dea** [NA], spheroidal articulation: a type of synovial joint in which a spheroidal surface on one bone ("ball") moves within a concavity ("socket") on the other bone; it is the most moveable type of joint. Called also *a. cotylica, a. sphaeroidea, ball-and-socket articulation* or *joint, spheroidal joint, multiapial* or *polyaxial joint,* and *enarthrodial joint.* **a. sternoclavicula′ris** [NA], sternoclavicular articulation: the joint formed by the sternal extremity of the clavicle, the clavicular notch of the manubrium of the sternum, and the first costal cartilage. **articulatio′nes sternocosta′les** [NA], sternocostal articulations: the joints between the costal notches of the sternum and the medial ends of the costal cartilages of the upper seven ribs; called also *costosternal* or *chondrosternal articulations.* **a. subtala′ris** [NA], subtalar articulation: the joint formed between the posterior calcaneal articular surface of the talus and the posterior articular surface of the calcaneus; called also *a. talocalcanea.* **articulatio′nes synovia′les** [NA], synovial articulations: specialized joints permitting more or less free movement, the union of the bony elements being surrounded by an articular capsule enclosing a cavity lined by synovial membrane; called also *diarthrodial joints, diarthroses, juncturae synoviales,* and *synovial joints.* See illustration under *joint.* **articulatio′nes synovia′les cra′nii** [NA] the synovial articulations of the cranium, including the temporomandibular, atlanto-occipital, and median and lateral atlantoaxial articulations. **a. talocalca′nea,** a. subtalaris. **a. talocalcaneonavicula′ris** [NA], talocalcaneonavicular articulation: a joint formed by the head of the talus, the anterior articular surface of the calcaneus, the plantar calcaneonavicular ligament, and the posterior surface of the navicular bone. **a. talocrura′lis** [NA], talocrural articulation: the ankle joint, formed by the inferior articular and malleolar articular surfaces of the tibia, the malleolar articular surface of the fibula, and the medial malleolar, lateral malleolar, and superior surfaces of the talus; called also *a. crurotalaris, crurotalar articulation,* and *talocrural, ankle,* and *talotibiofibular joint.* **a. talonavicula′ris,** talonavicular articulation: the junction between the talus and navicular bone. **a. tar′si trans ver′sa** [NA], transverse tarsal articulation: a joint comprising the articulation of the calcaneus and the cuboid bone and the articulation of the talus and the navicular bone. Called also *a. tarsi transversa* [*Choparti*], *transverse tarsal joint,*

and *Chopart's articulation* or *joint.* **articulatio′nes tarsometatarsa′les** [NA], **articulatio′nes tarsometatar′seae,** tarsometatarsal articulations: joints formed by the cuneiform and cuboid bones together with the bases of the metatarsal bones; called also *Lisfranc's joints.* **a. temporomandibula′ris** [NA], temporomandibular articulation: a bicondylar joint formed by the head of the mandible and the mandibular fossa, and the articular tubercle of the temporal bone; called also *a. mandibularis, temporomaxillary articulation,* and *mandibular articulation.* **articulationes tho′racis** [NA] the articulations of the thorax, including those between the heads of the ribs and the bodies of two adjacent vertebrae and the costovertebral, costotransverse, sternocostal, costochondral, and interchondral articulation. **a. tibiofibula′ris,** 1. [NA], superior tibiofibular articulation: a plane joint between the lateral condyle of the tibia and the head of the fibula. 2. NA alternative for *syndesmosis tibiofibularis* (distal or inferior tibiofibular articulation). **a. trochoi′dea** [NA], trochoidal articulation: a type of synovial joint that allows a rotary motion in but one plane; a pivot-like process turns within a ring, or a ring turns on a pivot. Called also *pivot articulation* or *joint.* **articulatio′nes vertebra′les** [NA], the articulations of the vertebrae, including the zygapophyseal, lumbosacral, and sacrococcygeal. **articulatio′nes zygapophysia′les** [NA], zygapophyseal articulations: the articulations between the articular processes of the vertebrae (zygapophyses); called also *juncturae zygapophyseales.*

articulation (ar-tik″u-la′shun) [L. *articulatio*] 1. the place of union or junction between two or more bones of the skeleton; see also *articulatio.* 2. the enunciation of words and sentences. 3. in dentistry: (*a*) the contact relationship of the occlusal surfaces of the teeth while in action; (*b*) the arrangement of artificial teeth so as to accommodate the various positions of the mouth and to serve the purpose of the natural teeth which they are to replace. **acromioclavicular a.,** articulatio acromioclavicularis. **articulator a.,** the use of a mechanical device that simulates the movements of the temporomandibular joint, permitting the orientation of casts in a manner duplicating or simulating various positions or movements of the mandible. **atlantoaxial a., lateral,** articulatio atlantoaxialis lateralis. **atlantoaxial a., medial,** articulatio atlantoaxialis mediana. **atlantoepistrophic a.,** see *articulatio atlantoaxialis lateralis* and *articulatio atlantoaxialis mediana.* **atlantooccipital a.,** articulatio atlanto-occipitalis. **a's of auditory ossicles,** articulationes ossiculorum auditus. **balanced a.,** the simultaneous contact between the upper and lower teeth as they glide over each other when the mandible is moved from centric relation to the various eccentric relations and back to centric relation again. **ball-and-socket a.,** articulatio spheroidea. **bicondylar a.,** articulatio bicondylaris. **brachiocarpal a.,** articulatio radiocarpalis. **brachioradial a.,** articulatio humeroradialis. **brachioulnar a.,** articulatio humeroulnaris. **calcaneocuboid a.,** articulatio calcaneocuboidea. **capitular a.,** articulatio capitis costae. **carpal a's,** 1. articulationes carpi. 2. see *articulationes intercarpales.* **carpometacarpal a's,** articulationes carpometacarpales. **carpometacarpal a., first, carpometacarpal a. of thumb,** articulatio carpometacarpalis pollicis. **chondrosternal a's,** articulationes sternocostales. **Chopart's a.,** articulatio tarsi transversa. **composite a.,** articulatio composita. **compound a.,** articulatio composita. **condylar a.,** articulatio ellipsoidea. **confluent a.,** a manner of speaking in which the syllables are run together. **costocentral a.,** articulatio capitis costae. **costosternal a's,** articulationes sternocostales. **costotransverse a.,** articulatio costotransversaria. **costovertebral a's,** articulationes costovertebrales. **coxofemoral a. of Buisson,** articulatio coxae. **cranioverterbral a.,** articulatio atlanto-occipitalis. **cricoarytenoid a.,** articulatio cricoarytenoidea. **cricothyroid a.,** articulatio cricothyroidea. **crurotalar a.,** articulatio crurotalaris. **cubital a.,** articulatio cubiti. **cubitoradial a., inferior,** articulatio radio-ulnaris distalis. **cubitoradial a., superior,** articulatio radio-ulnaris proximalis. **cuneocuboid a.,** articulatio cuneocuboidea. **cuneonavicular a.,** articulatio cuneonavicularis. **dentoalveolar a.,** gomphosis. **a's of digits of foot,** articulationes interphalangeae pedis. **a's of digits of hand,** articulationes interphalangeae manus. **a. of elbow,** articulatio cubiti. **ellipsoidal a.,** articulatio ellipsoidea. **femoral a.,** articulatio coxae. **fibrous a's,** articulationes fibrosae. **gliding a.,** articulatio plana. **a's of hand,** articulationes manus. **a. of head of humerus,** a. humeri. **a. of head of rib,** articulatio capitis costae. **a. of hip,** articulatio coxae. **humeroradial a.,** articulatio humeroradialis. **humeroulnar a.,** articulatio humero-ulnaris. **a. of humerus,** articulatio humeri. **iliosacral a.,** articulatio sacroiliaca. **incudomalleolar a.,** articulatio incudomallearis. **incudostapedial a.,** articulatio incudostapedia. **intercarpal a's,** 1. articulationes intercarpales. 2. See *articulationes carpi.* **interchondral a's,** articulationes interchondrales. **intercostal a's,** articulationes interchondrales. **intercuneiform a's,** articulationes intercuneiformes. **intermetacarpal a's,** articulationes intermetacarpales. **intermetatarsal a's,** articulationes intermetatarsales. **interphalangeal a's of fingers,** articulationes interphalangeales manus. **interphalangeal a's of foot,** articulationes interphalangeales pedis. **interphalangeal a's of hand,** articulationes interphalangeales manus. **interphalangeal a's of toes,** articulationes interphalangeales pedis. **intertarsal a's,** articulationes intertarsales. **a. of knee,** articulatio genus. **lumbosacral a.,** articulatio lumbosacralis. **mandibular a.,** articulatio temporomandibularis. **manubriosternal a.,** see *symphysis manubriosternalis* and *synchondrosis manubriosternalis.* **maxillary a.,** articulatio temporomandibularis. **mediocarpal a.,** articulatio mediocarpalis. **a's of metacarpal bones,** articulationes intermetacarpales. **metacarpocarpal a's,** articulationes carpometacarpales. **metacarpophalangeal a's,** articulationes metacarpophalangeales. **a's of metatarsal bones,** articulationes intermetatarsales. **metatarsophalangeal a's,** articulationes metatarsophalangeales. **occipito-atlantal a.,** **occipital a.,** articulatio atlanto-occipitalis. **ovoid a.,** articulatio sellaris. **petrooccipital a.,** synchondrosis petrooccipitalis. **phalangeal a's,** see *articulationes interphalangeae manus* and *articulationes interphalangeae pedis.* **a. of pisiform bone,** articulatio ossis pisiformis. **pisocuneiform a.,** articulatio ossis pisiformis. **pivot a.,** articulatio trochoidea. **plane a.,** articulatio plana. **a. of pubis,** symphysis pubica. **radiocarpal a.,** articulatio radiocarpalis. **radioulnar a.,** syndesmosis radioulnaris. **radioulnar a., distal, radioulnar a., inferior,** articulatio radio-ulnaris distalis. **radioulnar a., proximal, radioulnar a., superior,** articulatio radio-ulnaris proximalis. **sacrococcygeal a.,** articulatio sacrococcygea. **sacroiliac a.,** articulatio sacroiliaca. **saddle a.,** articulatio sellaris. **scapuloclavicular a.,** articulatio acromioclavicularis. **a. of shoulder,** articulatio humeri. **simple a.,** articulatio simplex. **spheroidal a.,** articulatio spheroidea. **sternoclavicular a.,** articulatio sternoclavicularis. **sternocostal a's,** articulationes sternocostales. **subtalar a.,** articulatio subtalaris. **synovial a's,** articulationes synoviales. **synovial a's of cranium,** articulatio synoviales cranii. **talocalcaneonavicular a.,** articulatio talocalcaneonavicularis. **talocrural a.,** articulatio talocruralis. **talonavicular a.,** articulatio talonavicularis. **tarsometatarsal a's,** articulationes tarsometatarsales. **temporomandibular a.,** articulatio temporomandibularis. **temporomaxillary a.,** articulatio temporomandibularis. **a's of thorax,** articulationes thoracis. **tibiofibular a's,** either of the articulations between the tibia and the fibula; see *articulatio tibiofibularis,* def. 1 (superior tibiofibular a.) and *syndesmosis tibiofibularis* (inferior tibiofibular a.) **a's of toes,** articulationes interphalangeae pedis. **transverse tarsal a.,** articulatio tarsi transversa. **trochoidal a.,** articulatio trochoidea. **a. of tubercle of rib,** articulatio costotransversaria. **zygapophyseal a's,** articulationes zygapophysiales.

articulationes (ar-tik″u-la″she-o′nēz) [L.] plural of *articulatio.*

articulator (ar-tik′u-la″tor) 1. a device for effecting a jointlike union. 2. dental a. **adjustable a.,** 1. a dental articulator which may be adjusted to permit movement of the casts into recorded eccentric relationships. 2. a dental articulator capable of adjustment to more than one eccentric position. **dental a.,** a mechanical device representing the temporomandibular joint and jaws for simulating jaw movements, to which maxillary and mandibular dental casts may be attached. It is used for the mounting of dental casts for diagnosis, treatment planning, and patient presentation; fabrications of occlusal surfaces for dental restorations; and arrangement of teeth for complete and partial dentures. Dental articulators are classified in four basic groups: Those of *Class I* accept a single interocclusal record and vertical motion may or may not be possible; those of *Class II* permit horizontal and vertical motion but do not orient the motion to the temporomandibular joint through a face-bow transfer; those of *Class III* simulate condylar pathways by using an average or mechanical equivalent for all or part of the motion and allow orientation of the casts to the temporomandibular joint through a face-bow transfer; and those of *Class IV* accept three-dimensional dynamic registrations and allow orientation of the casts to the temporomandibular joint through a face-bow transfer.

articulatory (ar-tik′u-la″to-re) pertaining to utterance.

articulo (ar-tik′u-lo) [L., ablative of *articulus,* q.v.] at the moment or crisis of. **a. mor′tis,** at the moment or point of death.

articulus (ar-tik′u-lus), pl. *articuli* [L.] a joint.

artifact (ar′tĭ-fakt) [L. *ars* art + *factum* made] any artificial product. In histology or microscopy, any structure or feature that has been introduced by processing a tissue. In radiology, a substance or structure not naturally present in living tissue, but of which an authentic image appears in a radiograph.

artifactitious (ar′tĭ-fak-tish′us) having the character of an artifact.

artificial (ar″tĭ-fish′al) [L. *ars* art + *facere* to make] made by art; not natural or pathological.

Artiodactyla (ar″te-o-dak′tĭ-lah) [Gr. *artios* even + *daktylos* finger] an order of ungulates, having an even number of toes, including ruminants, pigs, deer, and antelopes. Cf. *Perissodactyla.*

artiodactylous (ar″te-o-dak′tĭ-lus) having an even number of digits on a hand or foot; pertaining to Artiodactyla.

Artyfechinostomum (ar″te-fek″ĭ-nos′to-mum) *Paryphostomum.* **A. sufrar′tyfex,** *Paryphostomum sufrartyfex.*

arucase (ah′ru-kās) an extract of *Calea pinnatifida* (R. Br.) Less. (aruca plant) of the family Compositae; it has been used in the management of intestinal amebiasis.

Arum (a′rum) a genus of plants. *A. dracontium* is highly poisonous; *A. maculatum* furnishes sago.

Arvin (ar′vin) a purified fraction of the venom of the Malayan pit viper, used as an anticoagulant in thromboembolic disorders.

A.R.V.O. Association for Research in Vision and Ophthalmology.

aryepiglottic (ar″e-ep″ĭ-glot′ik) arytenoepiglottic.

aryepiglotticus (ar″e-ep″ĭ-glot′ĭ-kus) see *Table of Musculi.*

aryepiglottidean (ar″e-ep″ĭ-glo-tid′e-an) arytenoepiglottic.

aryl- (ar′il) a chemical prefix indicating a radical belonging to the aromatic series.

arylamine (ar″il-ah-mēn′, ar″il-am′in) any of a group of amines in which one or more of the hydrogen atoms are replaced by aromatic groups.

arylaminopeptidase (ar″il-ah-me″no-pep′tĭ-dās) cytosol aminopeptidase.

arylarsonic acid (ār″il-ar-son′ik) an arsonic acid in which the —AsO(OH)$_2$ functional group is bonded to an aryl radical.

arylesterase (ar″il-es′ter-ās) [EC 3.1.1.2] an enzyme of the hydrolase class that catalyzes the reaction aryl acetate + H$_2$O = a phenol + acetate. It occurs in normal serum and acts on many phenolic esters. Called also *aryl-ester hydrolase.*

aryl-ester hydrolase (ar′il es′ter hi′dro-lās) arylesterase.

arylformamidase (ar″il-form-am′ĭ-dās) [EC 3.5.1.9] an enzyme of the hydrolase class that catalyzes the reaction N-formyl-L-kynurenine + H$_2$O = formate + L-kynurenine, a reaction in the catabolism of tryptophan. The enzyme also acts on other formyl aromatic amines. Called also *formylkynurenine hydrolase.*

aryl 4-hydroxylase (ar″il hi-drok′sĭ-lās) [EC 1.14.14.1] unspecific monooxygenase.

arylsulfatase (ar″il-sul′fah-tās) [EC 3.1.6.1] a group of enzymes of the hydrolase class that catalyze the hydrolysis of sulfate esters: an alkyl or atyl sulfate + H_2O = an alcohol or phenol + sulfate. Three isozymes are known: types A and B are found in the lysosomes and type C in the microsomes of the cell. A deficiency of one or more isozymes has been associated with metachromatic leukodystrophy and mucopolysaccharidosis VI. Arylsulfatase A is stored in granules of mammalian mast cells and basophils. In antibody-medicated anaphylactic reactions, secretion of the enzyme is a primary mediator of shock. The presence of arylsulfatase in certain species of *Mycobacterium*, especially the rapid growers, is used as a means of identification.

arylsulfatase B (ARSB) deficiency Maroteaux-Lamy syndrome.

arytenoepiglottic (ar-it″ĕ-no-ep″ĭ-glot′ik) [Gr. *arytaina* ladle + *epiglottis*] pertaining to the arytenoid cartilage and to the epiglottis.

arytenoid (ar″ĕ-te′noid) [Gr. *arytaina* ladle + *eidos* form] shaped like a jug or pitcher, as arytenoid cartilage.

arytenoidectomy (ar″ĕ-te″noid-ek′to-me) [*arytenoid* + Gr. *ektomē* excision] surgical removal of an arytenoid cartilage.

arytenoideus (ar″ĕ-te-noi′de-us) [L.] see *musculus arytenoideus obliquus* and *transversus*.

arytenoiditis (ar-it″ĕ-noi-di′tis) inflammation of the arytenoid cartilage or muscles.

arytenoidopexy (ar″ĭ-tĕ-noi′do-pek″se) [*arytenoid* + Gr. *pēxis* fixation] surgical fixation of arytenoid cartilage or muscle.

AS aortic stenosis; arteriosclerosis.

A.S. abbreviation for L. *au′ris sinis′tra*, left ear.

As chemical symbol for *arsenic*.

As. astigmatism.

ASA 1. argininosuccinic acid. 2. acetylsalicylic acid.

A.S.A. 1. American Society of Anesthesiologists; American Standards Association; American Surgical Association. 2. trademark for a preparation of aspirin.

asacria (ah-sa′kre-ah) congenital absence of the sacrum.

asafetida (as″ah-fet′ĭ-dah) the oleo-gum-resin obtained from the roots of *Ferula asafoetida* L. and other related species of Umbelliferae. The main odorous principle is isobutylpropanyldisulfide. Used in India, Iran, etc., as a condiment and food flavoring, and has been used as an animal repellent in veterinary medicine to prevent bandage chewing, and as a carminative, expectorant, and antispasmodic both in humans and animals.

asaphia (ah-sa′fe-ah) [Gr. *asapheia*] indistinctness of utterance.

asaron (as′ah-ron) see *Asarum*.

Asarum (as′ah-rum) [Gr. *asaron*] a genus of the family Aristolochiaceae. *A. europaeum* L. yields a camphor-like aromatic principle known as asaron. *A. canadense* L. (Indian ginger, Canadian snakeroot, wild ginger) yields from its dried roots and rhizomes an acrid resin, methyl eugenol, and an aromatic volatile oil. Both species have been used as aromatics.

A.S.A.S. American Society of Abdominal Surgeons.

A.S.B. American Society of Bacteriologists.

asbestiform (as-bes′tĭ-form) having a fibrous structure like asbestos.

asbestos (as-bes′tos) [Gr. *asbestos* unquenchable] a fibrous, incombustible, magnesium and calcium silicate, used as thermal insulation; its dust causes asbestosis.

asbestosis (as″bĕ-sto′sis) [*asbestos* + *-osis*] a form of lung disease (pneumoconiosis) caused by inhaling fibers of asbestos and marked by interstitial fibrosis of the lung varying in extent from minor involvement of the basal areas to extensive scarring; it is associated with pleural mesothelioma and bronchogenic carcinoma. Called also *amianthosis*.

A-scan see *scan*, def. 2.

ascariasis (as″kah-ri′ah-sis) [*ascaris* + *-iasis*] infection by the roundworm *Ascaris lumbricoides*, which is found in the small intestine, causing colicky pains and diarrhea, especially in children. On ingestion, the larvae migrate from the intestine to the lungs, where they cause a pneumonitis, and then to the trachea, esophagus, and intestine, where they mature. If adult worms are present in sufficient number they may cause intestinal obstruction.

ascaricidal (as-kar″ĭ-si′dal) destructive to intestinal parasites of the genus *Ascaris*.

ascaricide (as-kar″ĭ-sid) [Gr. *askaris* ascaris + L. *caedere* to kill] an agent that destroys worms of the genus *Ascaris*.

ascarid (as′kah-rid) any member of the superfamily Ascaridoidea.

ascarides (as-kar′ĭ-dēz) plural of *ascaris*.

Ascaridia (as″kah-rid′e-ah) a genus of nematode parasites of the superfamily Ascaridoidea. **A. gal′li**, a species parasitic in the large intestine of chickens. **A. linea′ta**, a nematode parasite in the small intestine of fowls, the common roundworm of chickens in the United States.

ascaridiasis (as″kar-ĭ-di′ah-sis) ascariasis.

Ascaridoidea (as″kah-rĭ-doi′de-ah) a superfamily of phasmid nematodes, including the genera *Ascaridia*, *Ascaris*, *Toxocara*, and *Toxascaris*.

ascaridole (ah-skar″ĭ-dōl″) chemical name: 1,4-peroxido-*p*-menthene-2. The major constituent of oil of chenopodium or American wormseed (*Chenopodium ambrosioides*, L., Chenopodiaceae). The oil was once used as an anthelmintic.

ascaridosis (as-kar-ĭ-do′sis) ascariasis.

ascariosis (as-kar-e-o′sis) ascariasis.

Ascaris (as′kah-ris) [L.; Gr. *askaris*] a genus of large intestinal nematode parasites of the superfamily Ascaridoidea. **A. ala′ta, A. ca′nis**, see *Toxocara canis*. **A. e′qui, A. equo′rum**, *Parascaris equorum*. **A. lumbrico-i′des**, the eelworm or roundworm, a common worm resembling the earthworm; it is found in the small intestine, causing colicky pains and diarrhea, especially in children (see *ascariasis*). **A. margina′ta**, see *Toxocara canis*. **A. megaloceph′ ala**, *A. equorum*. **A. o′vis**, a name given to immature specimens of *A. lumbricoides*, occasionally found in sheep and cattle. **A. su′is, A. suil′la, A. su′um**, a name given to *A. lumbricoides* found in swine. **A. vermicula′ris**, see *Enterobius vermicularis*. **A. vitulo′rum**, a species found in cattle and the Indian buffalo.

ascaris (as-kah-ris), pl. *ascar′ides*. a worm of the genus *Ascaris*.

Ascarops (as′kah-rops) a genus of parasitic nematodes; formerly called *Arduenna*. **A. strongyli′na**, a small red blood-sucking species found in the stomach of pigs.

ascending (ah-send′ing) having an upward course.

ascensus (ah-sen′sus) [L., from *ascendere* to go up] a going up; ascent. **a. u′teri**, an abnormally high position of the uterus.

ascertainment (ah″ser-tān′ment) in genetic studies, the method by which persons with a trait or disease are selected or found by an investigator. **complete a.,** the method in which families for study are selected through affected parents, and all their offspring are included. **incomplete a.,** ascertainment in which only those sibships with at least one affected sib are identified; this is far more common than complete ascertainment. **multiple a.,** a type of incomplete ascertainment in which some sibships are counted more than once because they have more than one affected member; multiplex families (those with more than one affected member) have a higher chance of being ascertained than simplex families. **single a.,** a type of incomplete ascertainment in which there is no chance that any one sibship will be ascertained more than once; thus there is only one proband in each sibship, and the change that a sibship will be ascertained is proportional to the number of its affected members. **truncate a.,** a type of incomplete ascertainment in which any sibship in which there is no affected member is not ascertained.

Ascetospora (as″ke-tos′por-ah) [Gr. *asketos* curiously wrought + *spore*] a phylum of cytozoic, celozoic, and histozoic protozoa parasitic principally in aquatic invertebrates, some of which are pathogenic, characterized by the presence of a multicellular spore with one or more sporoplasms without polar capsules or tubes. It comprises two classes: Stellatosporea and Paramyxea.

A.S.C.H. American Society of Clinical Hypnosis.

Asch's operation, splint [Morris Joseph *Asch*, American laryngologist, 1833–1902] see under forceps, operation, and splint.

aschelminth (ask′hel-minth) any worm of the phylum Aschelminthes.

Aschelminthes (ask″hel-minth′ēz) a phylum of unsegmented, bilaterally symmetrical, pseudocoelomate, mostly vermiform animals whose bodies are almost entirely covered with a cuticle, and possess a complete digestive tract lacking definite muscular walls. It includes the classes Gastrotricha, Kinorhyncha, Nematoda, Nematomorpha, and Rotifera.

Ascher's negative glass-rod phenomenon, positive glass-rod phenomenon, syndrome [Karl Wolfgang *Ascher*, Cincinnati ophthalmologist born in Prague, 1887–1971] see *blood-influx phenomenon* and *aqueous-influx phenomenon*, under *phenomenon*, and under *syndrome*.

Ascherson's membrane, vesicles (ash′er-sunz) [Ferdinand Moritz *Ascherson*, German physician, 1798–1879] see under *membrane* and *vesicle*.

Aschheim-Zondek hormone, test (ash′him-tson′dek) [Selmar *Aschheim*, German gynecologist, 1878–1965; Bernhardt *Zondek*, German gynecologist, 1891–1966] see *luteinizing hormone*, under *hormone*, and see under *test*.

aschistodactylia (ah-skis′to-dak-til′e-ah) syndactyly.

Aschner's phenomenon (test), reflex, sign (ash′-nerz) [Bernhard *Aschner*, Austrian gynecologist, 1883–1960] see under *phenomenon*, and see *oculocardiac reflex*, under *reflex*.

Aschoff's bodies (nodules), cell, node (ash′ofs) [Karl Albert Ludwig *Aschoff*, German pathologist, 1866–1942] see under *body* and *cell*, and see *nodus atrioventricularis*.

Aschoff-Tawara node (ash′of-tah-war′ah) [Karl Albert Ludwig *Aschoff* ; Sunao *Tawara*, Japanese pathologist, 1873–1952] nodus atrioventricularis.

A.S.C.I. American Society for Clinical Investigation.

asci (as′i) plural of *ascus*.

ascites (ah-si′tēz) [L.; Gr. *askitēs*, from *askos* bag] effusion and accumulation of serous fluid in the abdominal cavity; called also *abdominal* or *peritoneal dropsy, hydroperitonia,* and *hydrops abdominis.* **a. adipo′sus,** a variety characterized by a milky appearance of the contained fluid, due to the presence of cells that have undergone fatty degeneration; called also *fatty* or *milky a.* **bile a.,** choleperitoneum. **bloody a.,** hemorrhagic a. **chyliform a., a. chylo′sus, chylous a.,** the presence of chyle in the peritoneal cavity as a result of anomalies, injuries, or obstruction of the thoracic duct. **exudative a.,** ascites in which the fluid in the peritoneal cavity is an exudate. **fatty a.,** a. adiposus. **hemorrhagic a.,** that in which the fluid is mixed with blood. **hydremic a.,** that which is associated with, or due to, a watery state of the blood, as in severe malnutrition. **milky a.,** a. adiposus. **a. prae′cox,** ascites that develops prior to edema in constrictive pericarditis. **preagonal a.,** a flow of serum into the peritoneal cavity just before death. **pseudochylous a.,** ascites in which the contained fluid resembles chyle in appearance, but does not contain fatty matter. **transudative a.,** ascites in which the fluid in the peritoneal cavity is a transudate.

ascitic (ah-sit′ik) pertaining to or characterized by ascites.

ascitogenous (as″ĭ-toj′ĕ-nus) causing ascites.

asclepia (as-kle′pe-ah) plural of *asclepion*.

Asclepiades (as″kle-pi′ah-dēz) **of Bithynia** (124 to c. 40 B.C.) a Greek physician born in Prusa in Bithynia (southwest coast of the Black Sea), studied at Alexandria, taught and practiced at Rome after 91 B.C. An Epicurean, he opposed humoralism and introduced into medicine Democritus' atomic theory, according to which inharmonious or irregular movement of atoms causes disease, which one cures by restoring harmony. Asclepiades' methods included diet, friction, bathing, exercise, emetics, and blood-letting. His influence continued (through the Methodical School, founded by his students) till Galen began to practice in A.D. 164. Asclepiades established humane treatment for the mentally ill and made Greek medicine honorable at Rome through his own good character. See also *Democritus*.

Asclepias (as-kle′pe-as) [L.] the milkweeds or swallowworts, a genus of herbs most species of which are generally recognized as poisonous to animals, while some have medicinal qualities; e.g., *A. tuberosa* L. (pleurisy root) has been used as an emetic, diaphoretic, laxative, and expectorant. They contain asclepiadin, volatile oils, and toxic resins.

asclepion (as-kle′pe-on), pl. *asclepia* [Gr. *Asklēpieion* temple of Asklepios (Aesculapius)] one of the early Greek temples of healing, the most celebrated of which were at Cos, Epidaurus, Cnidus, and Pergamos. Greek temple medicine

flourished during the time of Hippocrates (late 5th century B.C.), but was quite independent of his school. See also *Aesculapius* and *Asclepiad*.

Asclepios (as-klep′e-os) Aesculapius.

A.S.C.L.T. American Society of Clinical Laboratory Technicians.

A.S.C.O. American Society of Clinical Oncology; American Society of Contemporary Ophthalmology.

Ascobolus (as-kob′ŏ-lus) a genus of ascomycetous fungi (family Pezizaceae, order Pezizales) used in genetic studies of crossing over.

ascocarp (as′ko-karp) [Gr. *askos* bag + *karpos* fruit] the developed sporophore (fruiting body) in ascomycetous fungi, including the asci and ascospores. Cf. *archicarp*.

Ascocotyle (as″ko-ko′tĭ-le) a genus of nematode parasites. **A. pithecophagic′ola,** a nematode parasite in the monkey-eating eagle in the Philippines.

ascogonium (as″ko-go′ne-um) the receiving (female) organ in ascomycetous fungi which, after fertilization, gives rise to ascogenous hyphae and later to asci and ascospores. Called also *carpogonium* and, in British usage, *archicarp*.

Ascomycetae (as″ko-mi′sĕ-te) Ascomycetes.

ascomycete (as-ko′mi-sēt) any individual fungus of the Ascomycetes.

Ascomycetes (as″ko-mi-se′tēz) [Gr. *askos* bag + *mykēs* fungus] a class of perfect fungi of the division Eumycetes, the individual members of which form ascospores. The class consists of the yeasts, mildews, and cheese, jelly, and fruit molds, and includes the subclasses Hemiascomycetidae, Euascomycetidae, and Loculoascomycetidae. Called also *Ascomycetae* and *sac fungus.*

ascomycetous (as″ko-mi-se′tus) of or pertaining to the Ascomycetes.

ascorbate (as-kor′bāt) a compound or derivative of ascorbic acid.

ascorbemia (as″kor-be′me-ah) the presence of ascorbic acid in the blood.

ascorbic acid (as-skor′bik) vitamin C; a water-soluble vitamin found in many fruits and vegetables. Ascorbic acid is required for the optimal function of a number of enzymes; deficiency causes scurvy and poor wound repair. Called also *cevitamic acid.*

ascorburia (as-kor-bu′re-ah) the presence of ascorbic acid in the urine.

ascorbyl palmitate (as-kor′bil) [NF] chemical name: 6-hexadecanoate L-ascorbic acid. An antioxidant, $C_{22}H_{38}O_7$, occurring as a white to yellowish white powder; used as a preservative in pharmaceutical preparations.

ascospore (as′ko-spōr) [Gr. *askos* bag + *sporos* seed] a sexual spore formed within a special sac, or ascus, as in ascomycetous fungi. See *spore*.

A.S.C.P. American Society of Clinical Pathologists.

ascus (as′kus), pl. *as′ci* [Gr. *askos* a bag] the sporangium or spore case of certain lichens and fungi, consisting of a single terminal cell. See *spore*.

-ase (ās) a word termination used in forming the names of enzymes, ordinarily affixed to a stem that indicates the substrate, the type of reaction catalyzed, or a combination of these factors.

asecretory (ah-se′kre-to″re) without secretion.

Aselli's pancreas (glands) (ah-sel′ēz) [Gasparo *Aselli* (or Gaspare *Asellio,* or Gaspar *Asellius*), Italian anatomist, 1581–1626] see under *pancreas.*

Asellio, Asellius see *Aselli.*

asemantic (a-sĕ-man′tik) [*a* neg. + Gr. *sēmantikos* significant] being or pertaining to a molecule that is not produced by an organism and so is not influenced by the presence in the organism of semantides (q.v.).

asemasia (as″ĕ-ma′ze-ah) [*a* neg. + Gr. *sēmasia* the giving of a signal] aphasia in which there is lack or loss of the power of communication by words or by signals.

asemia (ah-se′me-ah) [*a* neg. + Gr. *sēma* sign + *-ia*] aphasia with inability to employ or to understand either speech or signs, due to a central lesion. **a. graph′ica,** inability either to write (agraphia) or to understand (dyslexia) writing, due to a central lesion. **a. mim′ica,** inability to understand or to perform any action expressive of thought or emotion. **a. verba′lis,** inability to make use of or to understand words.

asepsis (a-sep′sis) [*a* neg. + Gr. *sēpesthai* to decay] 1. freedom from infection. 2. the prevention of contact with microorganisms.

Aseptatina (a″sep-tah-ti′nah) [*a* neg. + *septum*] a suborder of parasitic protozoa (order Eugregarinida, subclass Gregarinia) in which syzygy and gametocysts occur, and the gamont is composed of a single chamber; some species produce a mucron. Representative genera include *Monocystis* and *Selenidium.* See also *Acephalina.*

aseptic (a-sep′tik) [*a* neg. + Gr. *sēpsis* decay] free from infection or septic material; sterile. **a.-antiseptic,** both aseptic and antiseptic.

asepticism (a-sep′tĭ-sizm) the principles and practices of aseptic surgery.

asetake (as″e-tak′e) a poisonous Japanese fungus of the genus *Hebeloma.*

asexual (a-seks′u-al) having no sex; not sexual; not pertaining to sex. Called also *agamic* or *agamous.*

asexuality (a″seks-u-al′ĭ-te) the state of being asexual; absence of sexual interests.

ASF a synthetic resin composed of aniline, formaldehyde, and sulfur, used for mounting microscopic objects.

A.S.G.E. American Society for Gastrointestinal Endoscopy.

A.S.H. American Society of Hematology.

ash (ash) 1. the incombustible residue remaining after any process of incineration. 2. any tree or species of the genus *Fraxinus. F. ornus* and others afford mannitol. The bark of many species is astringent and antiperiodic.

A.S.H.A. American School Health Association; American Speech and Hearing Association.

Asherson's syndrome (ash′er-sunz) [N. *Asherson,* English physician, 20th century] see under *syndrome.*

A.S.H.P. American Society of Hospital Pharmacists.

asialia (a″si-a′le-ah) [*a* neg. + Gr. *sialon* spittle] absence or deficiency of the secretion of the saliva; aptyalism; xerostomia.

asialo (a-si′ah-lo) [*a* neg. + *sialo*] lacking a sialic acid group, as do certain sphingolipids.

asiaticoside (a″zhe-at′ĭ-ko-sīd″) a steroidal glycoside of a trisaccharide and asiatic acid, which is the active principle of the umbelliferous plant *Centella asiatica* L. The compound has been used for various dermatological conditions, including wounds and burns.

asiderosis (ah″sid-er-o′sis) [*a* neg. + Gr. *sidēros* iron] abnormal decrease of the iron reserve of the body.

A.S.I.I. American Science Information Institute.

A.S.I.M. American Society of Internal Medicine.

Asimina (ah-sim′ĭ-nah) [L., from its Algonkian name] a genus of North American trees and shrubs of the family Annonaceae. *A. triloba* (L.) Dunal is the papaw or pawpaw; see *papaw,* def. 2. *A. reticulata* is used to make Seminole tea, used by Seminole Indians in Florida for kidney problems.

asiminine (ah-sim′ĭ-nin) an alkaloid from the seeds of *Asimina triloba.*

-asis [Gr.] a word termination denoting an action, process or condition; see also *-sis.*

asitia (ah-sish′e-ah) [*a* neg. + Gr. *sitos* food] a loathing for food.

asjike (ahs-ji′ke) beriberi.

Asklepios (as-klep′e-os) [Gr. *Asklēpios* son of Apollo and Coronis, tutelary god of medicine] see *Aesculapius.*

ASL antistreptolysin.

Aslanvitol (as-lan-vi′tol) [named for Anna *Asland,* Romanian physiologist, who discovered it] a drug containing procaine hydrochloride, purported to increase longevity by restoring chemical balances in the brain so that its regulatory functions, such as those governing glandular activities, are made more effective.

A.S.M. American Society for Microbiology.

Asn asparagine.

As₂O₃ arsenic trioxide.

ASO arteriosclerosis obliterans.

asoma (a-so′mah), pl. *aso′mata* [*a* neg. + Gr. *sōma* body] a monster with an imperfect head and the merest rudiments of a trunk.

asomatophyte (a-so′mah-to-fīt″) [*a* neg. + Gr. *sōma* body + *phyton* plant] a plant in which there is no distinction between body and reproductive cells.

Asopia (ah-so′pe-ah) a genus of pyralid moths. *A. farinalis,* the meal moth, or worm, acts as the intermediate host of *Hymenolepis diminuta.*

A.S.P. American Society of Parasitologists.

Asp aspartic acid.

aspalasoma (as″pal-ah-so′mah) [Gr. *aspalax* the mole + *sōma* body] a monster with lateral or median abdominal eventration and other deformities.

asparaginase (as-par′ah-jin-ās″) [EC 3.5.1.1] an enzyme of the hydrolase class that catalyzes the reaction L-asparagine + H_2O = L-aspartate + NH_3. This reaction occurs in normal mammalian and bacterial cells. The enzyme, prepared from bacterial sources, is used clinically in the treatment of childhood leukemia.

asparagine (as-par′ah-jēn, as-par′ah-jin) [Gr. *asparagos* asparagus] chemical name: α-aminosuccinic acid. A nonessential amino acid, $C_4H_8N_2O_3$, which is the β-amide of aspartic acid. It is found in most plants, and has diuretic properties. It is used as a culture medium for certain bacteria.

asparaginyl (ah-spār′ah-jin″il) the acyl radical of asparagine.

Asparagus (ah-spar′ah-gus) [L.; Gr. *asparagos*] a genus of liliaceous plants; the root of *A. officinalis* is a mild diuretic. It is claimed by some that methylmercaptan is excreted in urine after ingestion of the vegetable. Others feel that the odoriferous material is asparagine-aminosuccinic acid monoamide.

aspartame (ah-spar′tām) chemical name: *N*-L-α-aspartyl-L-phenylalanine methyl ester. An artificial sweetener, $C_{14}H_{18}N_2O_5$, which is about 200 times as sweet as sucrose and has potential as a low-calorie sweetener.

aspartate (ah-spahr′tāt) a salt of aspartic acid, or aspartic acid in dissociated form.

aspartate aminotransferase (ah-spar′tāt ah-me″no-trans′fer-ās) [EC 2.6.1.1] an enzyme of the transferase class that catalyzes the reaction L-aspartate + 2-ketoglutarate = oxaloacetate + L-glutamate. The enzyme is a pyridoxal phosphate protein. In the liver the reaction transfers excess metabolic nitrogen into aspartate for disposal in the urea cycle. The enzyme occurs also in the cytoplasm and mitochondria of most cells and is released into the blood in tissue damage. Elevation in serum aspartate aminotransferase (SGOT) activity is used as a diagnostic test. Called also *aspartate transaminase* and *glutamic-oxaloacetic transaminase* (GOT). Abbreviated AST.

aspartate carbamoyl transferase (as-par′tāt car-bam′o-il trans′fer-ās) [EC 2.1.3.2] an enzyme that catalyzes the reaction carbamoyl phosphate + L-aspartate = N-carbamoyl-L-aspartate + orthophosphate as part of pyrimidine biosynthesis.

aspartate transaminase (as-par′tāt trans-am′ĭ-nās) aspartate aminotransferase.

asparthione (as-par′thi-ōn″) a tripeptide analogous to glutathione but containing aspartic acid in place of glutamic acid.

aspartic acid (ah-spar′tik) a nonessential amino acid (q.v.) occurring in proteins. Symbols Asp and D.

aspartic proteinase (ah-spar′tik pro′tēn-ās″) [EC 3.4.23] a sub-subclass of enzymes of the hydrolase class that catalyze the hydrolysis of peptide bonds and have a pH optimum below 5.

aspartocin (ah-spar′to-sin) an antibacterial substance produced by *Streptomyces griseus.*

aspartyl (ah-spar′til) the acyl radical of aspartic acid.

β-aspartyl-N-acetylglucosaminidase (as-par′til as″ĕ-til-gloo-kōs″ah-min′ĭ-dās) [EC 3.2.2.11] an enzyme of the hydrolase class that catalyzes the reaction N^1-β1-β-aspartyl-N^2-acetyl-D-glucosaminylamine + H_2O = N-acetyl-D-glucosamine + L-asparagine. It is a lysosomal enzyme involved in the degradation of glycoproteins. Genetic deficiency of the enzyme, an autosomal recessive trait, causes aspartylglycosaminuria. Called also *aspartylglycosaminidase.*

aspartylglycosaminidase (as-par″til-gli-kōs″ah-min′ĭ-dās) β-aspartyl-N-acetylglucosaminidase.

aspartylglycosaminuria (as-par″til-gli′kōs-ah-mĭ-nu′re-ah) a genetic disease, one of the mucolipidoses, transmitted as an autosomal recessive trait, and caused by a deficiency of the enzyme β-aspartyl-N-acetylglucosaminidase. The disorder, found primarily in individuals of Finnish descent, is characterized by excretion of abnormal metabolites, mental retardation, and coarse features, accompanied by diarrhea and frequent infections.

aspecific (ah″spĕ-sif′ik) nonspecific; not caused by a specific organism.

aspect (as′pekt) [L. *aspectus*, from *aspicere* to look toward] 1. that part of a surface facing in any designated direction. 2. the look or appearance. **dorsal a.,** the surface of a body as viewed from the back (human anatomy) or, for quadrupeds, from above (veterinary anatomy). **ventral a.,** the surface of a body as viewed from the front (human anatomy) or from below (veterinary anatomy).

aspergillar (as″per-jil′ar) pertaining to or caused by *Aspergillus*.

aspergilli (as″per-jil′i) plural of *aspergillus*.

aspergillic acid (as″per-gil′ik) an antibiotic substance isolated from *Aspergillus flavus*.

aspergillin (as″per-jil′in) a black antibiotic substance, from the spore of various species of *Aspergillus;* formerly called *vegetable hematin.*

aspergilloma (as″per-jil-o′mah) a tumor-like granulomatous mass formed by colonization of the fungus *Aspergillus* in a bronchus or pulmonary cavity; the organism may disseminate through the blood stream to the brain, heart, and kidneys. Called also *fungus ball.*

aspergillomycosis (as″per-jil″o-mi-ko′sis) aspergillosis.

aspergillosis (as″per-jil-o′sis) a diseased condition caused by species of *Aspergillus* and marked by inflammatory granulomatous lesions in the skin, ear, orbit, nasal sinuses, lungs, and sometimes in the bones and meninges; called also *aspergillomycosis.* **aural a.,** see *otomycosis.* **bronchopneumonic a.,** infection of the bronchi and lungs by *Aspergillus;* see *aspergilloma.* **pulmonary a.,** infection of the lungs with *Aspergillus.*

aspergillotoxicosis (as″per-jil″o-tok″sĭ-ko′sis) aspergillustoxicosis.

Aspergillus (as″per-jil′us) [L. *aspergere* to scatter] a genus of imperfect fungi of the family Moniliaceae. When found, the perfect, or sexual, stage is classified with the ascomycetous fungi in the family Eurotiaceae, order Eurotiales. It includes several of the common molds and some that are opportunistic pathogens. It is characterized by elongated conidiophores thickly set with chains of basipetally formed conidia. See Plate under *mold.* **A. auricula′ris,** a mold of uncertain classification, found in the cerumen of the ear. **A. bar′-bae,** a species of uncertain classification that has been found in mycosis of the beard. **A. clava′tus,** a species occurring in soils and manure; its cultures produce the antibacterial substance patulin. **A. concen′tricus,** a species formerly considered to be the cause of tinea imbricata, now known to be caused by *Trichophyton concentricum.* **A. cook′ei,** *A. mucoroides.* **A. fisher′ii,** a thermophilic soil fungus. **A. fla′vus,** a mold found on corn, peanuts, and grain; it produces aflatoxin (q.v.). **A. fumiga′tus,** a thermotolerant fungus growing in soils and manure. It has been found in infections of the ear, nose, lungs, and other organs of humans and animals, and is considered to be a primary pathogen of birds. Its cultures produce various antibiotics, such as fumagillin and helvolic acid. Formerly called *A. gliocladium* and *Eurotium malignum.* **A. gigan′teus,** a species from which gigantic acid is obtained. **A. glau′cus,** a group of species of bluish molds common on dry and decaying vegetation and rarely occurring in otomycosis or other human infectious processes. **A. gliocla′dium,** former name for the species that furnishes the antibiotic gliotoxin; now called *A. fumigatus.* **A. mucoroi′des,** a species of uncertain classification, probably of the *A. glaucus* group, reported in lung tissue; called also *A. cookei.* **A. nid′ulans,** a species common in soil and occasionally isolated from onychomycosis and rarely from maduromycosis and other disease processes. **A. ni′ger,** a species common in soil and often isolated from otomycosis; it may produce a severe and very persistent infection. **A.**

ochra′ceus, the species that ferments the coffee berry and produces the characteristic and desirable odor. **A. parasit′icus,** a mold found on ground nut seedlings that elaborates aflatoxin (q.v.). **A. pic′tor,** a formerly recognized species, probably identical with *A. versicolor,* once thought to cause pinta, a treponeme disease. **A. re′pens,** a species found in the external auditory canal, where it may produce a false membrane. Its perfect stage is *Eurotium repens.* **A. ter′reus,** a species occasionally associated with infection of the bronchi and lungs; see *aspergilloma.* **A. versi′color,** a species of common soil saprophytes often isolated from dried salted beef; see also *A. pictor.*

aspergillus (as″per-jil′us), pl. *aspergil′li.* An individual of the genus *Aspergillus.*

aspergillustoxicosis (as″per-jil″us-tok″sĭ-ko′sis) a form of mycotoxicosis caused by a member of the genus *Aspergillus.*

asperkinase (ah-sper-ki′nās) a proteolytic enzyme elaborated by *Aspergillus oryzae.*

aspermatism (ah-sper′mah-tizm) aspermia.

aspermatogenesis (ah-sper″mah-to-jen′ĕ-sis) absence of development of spermatozoa.

aspermia (ah-sper′me-ah) [*a* neg. + Gr. *sperma* seed + *-ia*] failure of formation or emission of semen.

A.S.P.E.T. American Society for Pharmacology and Experimental Therapeutics.

asphyctic (as-fik′tik) pertaining to, or affected with, asphyxia.

asphyctous (as-fik′tus) asphyctic.

asphygmia (as-fig′me-ah) temporary disappearance of the pulse.

asphyxia (as-fik′se-ah) [Gr. "a stopping of the pulse"] a condition due to lack of oxygen in respired air, resulting in impending or actual cessation of apparent life. **blue a.,** a. livida. **a. carbon′ica,** suffocation from the inhalation of coal gas, water gas, or carbon monoxide. **a. cyanot′ica,** a. livida. **fetal a.,** asphyxia in utero due to anoxia caused by premature placental separation (abruptio placentae), injudicious use of anesthetics, etc. **a. liv′ida,** asphyxia in which the skin is cyanotic from the lack of oxygen in the blood; called also *blue a.* and *a. cyanotica.* **local a.,** Raynaud's disease (def. 2); see under *disease.* **a. neonato′rum,** respiratory failure in the newborn; see also *respiratory distress syndrome,* under *syndrome.* **a. pal′lida,** asphyxia attended with paleness of the skin; called also *white a.* **secondary a.,** asphyxia recurring after apparent recovery from suffocation. **traumatic a.,** asphyxia occurring as a result of sudden or severe compression of the thorax or upper abdomen, or both; called also *traumatic apnea.* **white a.,** a. pallida.

asphyxial (as-fik′se-al) characterized by or pertaining to asphyxia.

asphyxiant (as-fik′se-ant) a substance capable of producing asphyxia.

asphyxiate (as-fik′se-āt) to put into a state of asphyxia.

asphyxiation (as-fik″se-a′shun) suffocation.

Aspidium (as-pid′e-um) [L.; Gr. *aspidion* little shield] a group of ferns called male shield ferns and male ferns which yield an oleoresin (see under *oleoresin*).

aspidium (as-pid′e-um) the rhizome and stipes of filix mas (male fern), yielding not less than 1.5 per cent of crude filicin. It is a violent poison and is highly irritant to the gastrointestinal tract when taken internally. See also *aspidium oleoresin,* under *oleoresin.*

aspidosperma (as″pĭ-do-sper′mah) the dried bark of *Aspidosperma quebracho-blanco* Schlecht., a tree of the family Apocynaceae. It contains several alkaloids, the main one being aspidospermine. It has been used to control parasitic worms in soil. Medically, it has been used in asthma and dyspnea as a respiratory stimulant.

aspidospermine (as″pĭ-do-sper′mēn) an alkaloid, $C_{22}H_{30}N_2O_2$, from aspidosperma (q.v.).

aspirate (as′pĭ-rāt) 1. to treat by aspiration. 2. the substance or material obtained by aspiration. 3. a consonantal sound in which some part of the respiratory tract is constricted, the nasal cavity shut off, and the breath makes a whistling noise.

aspiration (as″pĭ-ra′shun) [L. *ad* to + *spirare* to breathe] 1. the act of inhaling. 2. the removal of fluids or gases from a cavity by the application of suction. **meconium a.,** aspiration of meconium by the fetus or newborn, which may result in atelectasis, emphysema, or pneumonia. **vacuum a.,** removal of the uterine contents by application of a vacuum using a hollow curet or a cannula introduced into the uterus.

aspirator (as″pĭ-ra′tor) an apparatus used for removal by suction of fluids or gases contained within a cavity.

aspirin (as′pĭ-rin) [USP] acetylsalicylic acid, a drug having anti-inflammatory, analgesic, and antipyretic effects; it is the prototype of the nonsteroidal anti-inflammatory agents whose mechanism of action is inhibition of prostaglandin synthesis; used for relief of pain and fever, for treatment of rheumatoid arthritis and osteoarthritis, and for antiplatelet therapy to reduce the risk of recurrent transient ischemic attacks or of cerebrovascular accident.

asplenia (a-sple′ne-ah) absence of the spleen. **functional a.,** impaired reticuloendothelial function of the spleen, as in children with sickle-cell anemia.

asplenic (a-splen′ik) pertaining to asplenia; caused by absence of the spleen.

asporogenic (as″po-ro-jen′ik) [a neg. + sporogenic] not producing spores; not reproduced by spores.

asporogenous (as″po-roj′ĕ-nus) asporogenic.

asporous (ah-spo′rus) [a neg. + Gr. sporos seed] having no true spores; applied to microorganisms.

A.S.R.T. American Society of Radiologic Technologists.

A.S.S. anterior superior spine.

assay (as-sa′) determination of the amount of a particular constituent of a mixture, or of the biological or pharmacological potency of a drug. **biological a.,** bioassay. **blastogenesis a.,** see lymphocyte proliferation test under tests. **cell-mediated lympholysis (CML) a.,** see under lympholysis. **CH₅₀ a.,** a functional assay of total complement activity that measures the capacity of serial dilutions of serum to lyse a standard preparation of sheep red blood cells coated with antisheep erythrocyte antibody. The reciprocal of the dilution of serum that lyses 50 per cent of the erythrocytes is reported as the whole complement titer in CH_{50} units per milliliter of serum. Called also total or whole complement a. or hemolytic complement a. **complement a., hemolytic, complement a., total, complement a., whole, CH_{50} a. E rosette a.,** an assay for human T lymphocytes based on the existence of a specific receptor on T cells for a sheep red blood cell membrane antigen. Peripheral blood lymphocytes are incubated with sheep red cells. T cells are surrounded by a ring of red cells—an E (erythrocyte) rosette—and are counted using a hemacytometer. **EAC rosette a.,** an assay for human B lymphocytes using complement receptors, a B cell marker. Peripheral blood cells are mixed with ox red blood cells, IgM antierythrocyte antibody, and complement deficient in C5 (to prevent cell lysis). The antibody-and-complement-coated erythrocytes (EAC) form rosettes with B cells, which are counted using a hemocytometer. **enzyme-linked immunosorbent a.,** see ELISA. **four-point a.,** an assay based on a mixture of two doses of test material and two doses of standard material. **hemagglutination inhibition (HI,HAI) a.,** see under tests. **hemolytic plaque a.,** a quantitative assay that counts antibody-producing cells. Lymphocytes sensitized against sheep erythrocytes (SRBCs) are plated in agar with SRBCs. After incubation complement is added; this lyses SRBCs, leaving a clear circular plaque around each cell that produced antibody against SRBC. The plaques are counted and reported as the number of plaque-forming cells (PFCs, pfc). Called also Jerne plaque a. **immune a.,** immunoassay. **immune adherence hemagglutination a. (IAHA),** see immune adherence, under adherence. **immunoradiometric a.,** a variant of radioimmunoassay in which the antigen being measured reacts directly with radiolabeled antibody. **Jerne plaque a.,** hemolytic plaque a. **lymphocyte proliferation a.,** see under tests. **microbiological a.,** assay by the use of microorganisms. **microcytotoxicity a.,** the standard method of typing serologically defined HLA antigens (HLA-A, -B, and -C antigens). Multiple typing sera are placed in wells of a microtiter plate and peripheral blood lymphocytes and complement are added to each well. The pattern of lysed cells indicates the HLA phenotype. **microhemagglutination a.—Treponema pallidum (MHA-TP),** a Treponema pallidum hemagglutination assay using microtechniques. **mixed**

lymphocyte culture (MLC) a., see under culture. **radioligand a.,** a general term for any assay procedure utilizing radioisotopic labeling and biologically specific binding of reagents, e.g., radioimmunoassay, competitive binding assay, and radioreceptor assay. **radioreceptor a.,** a radioligand assay in which a radiolabelled hormone is used to measure the concentration of specific cellular receptors for the hormone in tissue specimens, an example being radioassay of estrogen receptors in breast tissue. **Raji cell a.,** an assay for immune complexes using the Raji lymphoblastoid cell line (see Raji cell, under cell). **stem cell a.,** a test for determining the effectiveness of particular drugs against human cancer, in which human tumor cell suspensions are first incubated with various drugs and then suspended in agar and plated over a layer of agar at the bottom of the plate. Effectiveness of the drugs is determined by counting the number of colonies that grow in comparison with the number of colonies on control plates. **Treponema pallidum hemagglutination a. (TPHA),** a treponemal antigen serologic test for syphilis using tanned sheep red blood cells coated with antigen from the Nichol's strain of T. pallidum and patient serum absorbed with an extract of Reiter treponemes to remove nonspecific antibodies. It is similar in sensitivity and specificity to the FTA-ABS test except that it is less sensitive in detecting primary syphilis.

Assézat's triangle (ah-se-zahz′) [Jules Assézat, French anthropologist, 1832–1876] facial triangle.

assident (as′ĭ-dent) generally but not always accompanying a disease.

assimilable (ah-sim′ĭ-lah-bl) susceptible of being assimilated.

assimilation (ah-sim″ĭ-la′shun) [L. assimilatio, from ad to + similare to make like] 1. the transformation of food into living tissue; anabolism. 2. in psychology, the absorption of new experiences into the existing psychological make-up.

assistant (ah-sis′tant) one who aids or helps another; an auxiliary. **physician a., physician's a.,** see under physician.

Assmann's focus (tuberculous infiltrate) [Herbert Assmann, German internist, 1882–1950] see under focus.

association (ah-so″se-a′shun) [L. associatio, from ad to + socius a fellow] 1. in neurology, correlation involving a high degree of modifiability and also consciousness; see association areas, under area. 2. in genetics the occurrence together of two or more phenotypic characteristics more often than would be expected by change. To be distinguished from linkage (q.v.). 3. in dysmorphology, the nonrandom occurrence in two or more individuals of multiple anomalies not known to be a polytopic field defect, sequence, or syndrome. **clang a.,** see clanging. **dream a's,** emotions or thoughts associated with previous dreams, as developed by the patient in psychoanalysis. **free a.,** a psychoanalytical method in which the patient is encouraged to describe the association of thoughts and emotions as they arise spontaneously during the analysis.

assortment (ah-sort′ment) the random distribution of different combinations of the parental chromosomes to the gametes. As a result, each gamete normally possesses one genome (set of 23 chromosomes) including one chromosome of each type. The genes on the chromosome also assort independently unless they are linked. Called also independent a.

assurin (as′u-rin) a diaminodiphosphatide, $C_{46}H_{94}N_2P_2O_9$, said to occur in the brain substance.

Ast. astigmatism.

astacene (as′tah-sēn) astacin.

astacin (as′tah-sin) a carotenoid pigment, $C_{40}H_{48}O_4$, obtained from the shells of various crustaceans, where it occurs partly protein-bound and partly esterified.

astasia (as-ta′zhe-ah) [a neg. + Gr. stasis stand] motor incoordination with inability to stand. **a.-abasia,** motor incoordination with an inability to stand or walk despite normal ability to move the legs when sitting or lying down, a form of hysterical ataxia. Called also abasia-astasia.

astatic (as-tat′ik) pertaining to astasia.

astatine (as′tah-tin) [Gr. astatos unstable] the radioactive element of atomic number 85, atomic weight 210, symbol At. It is prepared by alpha particle bombardment of bismuth on the cyclotron. It has a half-life of 75 hours and may be of use in the treatment of hyperthyroidism.

astaxanthin (as″tah-zan′thin) a red carotenoid pigment, $C_{40}H_{52}O_4$, constituent of the green chromoprotein from the eggs of crayfish.

asteatodes (as″te-ah-to′dēz) asteatosis.

asteatosis (as″te-ah-to′sis) [a neg. + Gr. *stear* tallow + -*osis*] any disease characterized by such persistent fine dry scaling of the skin surface as to suggest scantiness or absence of the sebaceous secretion. Called also *asteatodes*. See also *chapping; winter itch*, under *itch;* and *xerotic eczema*, under *eczema*.

aster (as′ter) [L.; Gr. *astēr* star] a structure seen in a cell during the prophase of mitosis, composed of a system of microtubules arranged in astral rays around the centrosome; called also *astrosphere, cytaster*, and *kinosphere*. **sperm a.**, the centriole, with astral rays, that precedes the male pronucleus during fertilization.

astereocognosy (ah-ste″re-o-kog′nŏ-se) astereognosis.

astereognosis (ah-ster″e-og-no′sis) [a neg. + Gr. *stereos* solid + *gnōsis* recognition] loss of power to recognize objects or to appreciate their form by touching or feeling them; called also *tactile amnesia*.

asterion (as-te′re-on), pl. *aste′ria* [Gr. "starred"] [NA] the point on the surface of the skull where the lambdoid, parietomastoid, and occipitomastoid sutures meet.

asterixis (as″ter-ik′sis) [a neg. + Gr. *stērixis* a fixed position] a motor disturbance marked by intermittent lapse of an assumed posture, as a result of intermittency of the sustained contraction of groups of muscles, a characteristic of hepatic coma but observed also in numerous other conditions; called also *liver flap* and *flapping tremor*.

asternal (a-ster′nal) 1. not joined to the sternum. 2. pertaining to asternia; lacking a sternum.

asternia (ah-ster′ne-ah) [a neg. + Gr. *sternon* sternum + -*ia*] congenital absence of the sternum.

Asterococcus (as″ter-o-kok′us) in former systems of classification, a genus of bacteria of the order Mycoplasmatales, the organisms of which have been assigned to the genera *Acholeplasma* and *Mycoplasma*.

asteroid (as′ter-oid) [Gr. *astēr* star + *eidos* form] star-shaped; resembling the aster.

Asterol (as′ter-ol) trademark for preparations of diamthazole dihydrochloride.

asterubin (as″te-roo′bin) a basic substance, NH:C(NH.-$CH_2 \cdot SO_2OH) \cdot N(CH_3)_2$, that has been isolated from the starfish.

Asth. asthenopia.

asthenia (as-the′ne-ah) [Gr. *asthenēs* without strength + -*ia*] lack or loss of strength and energy; weakness. **myalgic a.**, a condition in which the general symptoms are a sensation of general fatigue and muscular pains. **neurocirculatory a.**, a syndrome characterized by palpitations, dyspnea, a sense of fatigue, fear of effort, and discomfort brought on by exercise or even slight effort; considered by most authorities to be a particular presentation of anxiety neurosis (anxiety state), the physical symptoms being attributed to autonomic responses to anxiety or to hyperventilation. Called also *DaCosta's syndrome, disordered action of the heart, effort syndrome, functional cardiovascular disease*, and *irritable heart* or *soldier's heart*. **periodic a.**, a condition marked by periodically returning attacks of marked asthenia. **tropical anhidrotic a.**, a rare condition occurring under conditions of heat stress, in which miliaria profunda causes extensive occlusion of the sweat ducts, producing anhidrosis and heat retention that may lead to weakness, dyspnea, tachycardia, elevation of body temperature, and collapse. Called also *sweat retention syndrome* and *thermogenic anhidrosis*.

asthenic (as-then′ik) pertaining to or characterized by asthenia.

asthen(o)- [Gr. *asthenēs* weak, from *a-* neg. + *sthenos* strength] a combining form denoting lack of strength or weakness.

asthenobiosis (as-the″no-bi-o′sis) [*asthenia* + Gr. *bios* life + -*osis*] a condition of reduced biologic activity resembling hibernation or estivation but not directly related to or dependent on temperature or humidity.

asthenocoria (as-the″no-ko′re-ah) [*asthenia* + Gr. *korē* pupil + -*ia*] a condition in which the pupillary light reflex is sluggish; seen in hypoadrenalism. Called also *Arroyo's sign*.

asthenope (as′then-ōp) a person affected with asthenopia.

asthenophobia (as″thĕ-no-fo′be-ah) [*asthenia* + *phobia*] (*obs.*) irrational fear of being weak.

asthenopia (as″thĕ-no′pe-ah) [*asthenia* + -*opia*] weakness or easy fatigue of the visual organs, attended by pain in the eyes, headache, dimness of vision, etc. Previously a diagnostic term; now used mainly as a descriptive term. **accommodative a.**, asthenopia due to strain of the ciliary muscle. **hysterical a.**, functional asthenopia due to neurosis or psychosis. **muscular a.**, that which is due to weakness of the external ocular muscles. **nervous a.**, 1. hysterical a. 2. that due to organic nervous disease. **neurasthenic a.**, 1. that due to neurasthenia after an organic disease; called also *retinal a.* 2. hysterical a. **retinal a.**, neurasthenic a., def. 1. **tarsal a.**, asthenopia due to irregular astigmatism produced by the pressure of the lids on the cornea.

asthenopic (as″thĕ-nop′ik) characterized by asthenopia.

asthenospermia (as″thĕ-no-sper′me-ah) [*asthenia* + Gr. *sperma* seed + -*ia*] reduction in the vitality of spermatozoa.

asthenoxia (as″then-ok′se-ah) [*asthenia* + *oxygen*] lack of power to oxidize waste products.

asthma (az′mah) [Gr. *asthma* panting] a condition marked by recurrent attacks of paroxysmal dyspnea, with wheezing due to spasmodic contraction of the bronchi. Some cases of asthma are allergic manifestations in sensitized persons (*bronchial allergy*); others are provoked by a variety of factors, including vigorous exercise, irritant particles, psychologic stresses, etc. **abdominal a.**, asthma due to upward pressure on the diaphragm. **allergic a.**, bronchial asthma due to allergy; called also *atopic a.* **alveolar a.**, that which is characterized by dilatation of the alveoli of the lungs. **atopic a.**, allergic asthma. **bacterial a.**, asthma due to bacterial infection. **bronchial a.**, see *asthma*. **bronchitic a.**, asthmatic disorder accompanying bronchitis. **cardiac a.**, paroxysmal dyspnea that occurs in association with heart disease, such as left ventricular failure; called also *cardiasthma*. **cat a.**, asthma brought on by inhalation of cat dander by a sensitized person. **catarrhal a.**, bronchitic a. **a. convulsi′vum**, bronchial a. **cotton-dust a.**, byssinosis. **cutaneous a.**, reflex asthma believed to be caused by some irritation of the skin. **diisocyanate a.**, isocyanate a. **dust a.**, asthma caused by inhalation of dust. **Elsner's a.**, angina pectoris. **emphysematous a.**, emphysema of the lungs attended with asthmatic paroxysms. **essential a.**, asthma of unknown or inapparent cause; called also *true a.* **extrinsic a.**, asthma caused by some factor in the environment, usually allergic asthma. **food a.**, asthma brought on by ingestion of certain foods to which the person is allergic. **grinders' a.**, asthmatic symptoms related to the inhalation of fine particles set free in the grinding of metals. **Heberden's a.**, angina pectoris. **horse a.**, a form of allergic asthma in which the attacks are brought on by the presence of horses or of horse products. **humid a.**, asthma with profuse expectoration. **infective a.**, asthma due to infection. **intrinsic a.**, asthma attributed to pathophysiologic disturbances and not to environmental factors. **isocyanate a.**, bronchial asthma caused by allergy to toluene diisocyanate and similar materials. **Kopp's a.**, laryngismus stridulus. **Millar's a.**, laryngismus stridulus. **millers' a.**, a condition of the lungs found in millers, caused by the inhalation of cereal dusts. **miners' a.**, asthma associated with anthracosis. **nasal a.**, asthma caused by a disease of the nose. **nervous a.**, essential asthma, usually associated with emotional disturbances. **pollen a.**, hay fever. **potters' a.**, asthmatic symptoms associated with the pneumoconiosis of workers in the ceramic industries. **reflex a.**, asthma attributed to some reflex action. **Rostan's a.**, cardiac a. **sexual a.**, asthma resulting from sexual intercourse. **spasmodic a.**, bronchial a. **steam-fitters' a.**, asthmatic symptoms associated with asbestosis. **stone a.**, asthmatic symptoms due to broncholithiasis. **stripper's a.**, asthmatic symptoms associated with byssinosis. **symptomatic a.**, asthma that is secondary to some other physical condition. **thymic a.**, an alleged condition occurring usually in children, associated with enlargement of the thymus, paroxysmal attacks of asthma, and a tendency to sudden death. **true a.**, essential asthma. **Wichmann's a.**, laryngismus stridulus.

asthmatic (az-mat′ik) [L. *asthmaticus*] pertaining to or affected with asthma.

asthmatiform (az-mat′ĭ-form) resembling asthma.

asthmogenic (az″mo-jen′ik) 1. causing asthma. 2. a substance capable of causing asthma.

Astiban (as′tĭ-ban) trademark for preparations of stibocaptate.

Asticcacaulis (as-stik″ah-kaw′lis) [a neg. + A. S. *sticca* stick + Gr. *kaulos* a staff] a genus of appendaged bacteria found in soils, made up of rod-shaped cells that typically produce one or more appendages and reproduce by asymmetrical fission. The type species is *A. excen′tricus.*

astigmagraph (ah-stig′mah-graf) [*astigma*tism + *-graph*] an instrument for demonstrating astigmatism.

astigmatic (as″tig-mat′ik) pertaining to or affected with astigmatism.

astigmatism (ah-stig′mah-tizm) [a- neg. + Gr. *stigma* point] unequal curvature of the refractive surfaces of the eye; hence a point source of light cannot be brought to a point focus on the retina but is spread over a more or less diffuse area. This results from the radius of curvature in one plane being longer or shorter than the radius at right angles to it. **acquired**

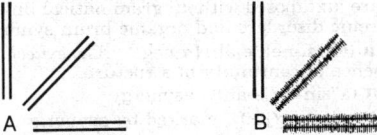

Astigmatism: the appearance of lines as seen by (A) the normal eye and (B) the astigmatic eye.

a., that due to some disease or injury of the eye. **a. against the rule,** that in which the greatest refraction takes place along the horizontal meridian; called also *inverse a.* **compound a.,** that which is complicated in all meridians by hypermetropia or myopia. **congenital a.,** that which exists at birth. **corneal a.,** that due to irregularity in the curvature or refracting power of the cornea. **direct a.,** a. with the rule. **hypermetropic a., compound, hyperopic a., compound,** astigmatism in which all meridians are hyperopic, both principal meridians having their foci behind the retina. **hypermetropic a., hyperopic a.,** that which complicates hyperopia. **hyperopic a., simple,** astigmatism in which one meridian, usually the vertical, is emmetropic and the horizontal meridian is hyperopic. The focus of the vertical meridian is not in the retina; that of the horizontal is behind the retina; horizontal lines appear distinct. **inverse a.,** a. against the rule. **irregular a.,** astigmatism in which the curvature in different parts of the same meridian of the eye varies or in which successive meridians differ irregularly in refraction, the image produced being an irregular area. **lenticular a.,** that which is due to some irregularity or abnormality of the lens. **mixed a.,** that in which one principal meridian is myopic and the other hyperopic. **myopic a.,** that which complicates myopia. **myopic a., compound,** astigmatism in which all meridians are myopic, both principal meridians having their foci in front of the retina; vertical lines are usually more distinct. **myopic a., simple,** astigmatism in which the focus of one meridian is situated on the retina, while that of the other lies in front of the retina; vertical lines appear distinct. **oblique a.,** astigmatism in which the direction of the principal meridians approaches 45° and 135°. **physiological a.,** the slight astigmatism possessed by nearly all eyes and causing the twinkling sensation when distant points of light are viewed. **regular a.,** astigmatism in which the refractive power of the eye shows a uniform increase or decrease from one meridian to the other, being practically constant in each meridian; the image produced is regular in shape, either a line, an oval, or a circle. See also *Sturm's conoid,* under *conoid.* **a. with the rule,** that wherein the meridian in which the greatest refraction takes place is vertical or nearly so; called also *direct a.*

astigmatometer (as″tig-mah-tom′ĕ-ter) [*astigma*tism + *-meter*] an instrument used in measuring astigmatism.

astigmatometry (ah-stig″mah-tom′ĕ-tre) [*astigma*tism + *-metry*] the measurement of astigmatism; the use of the astigmatometer. Called also *astigmometry.*

astigmatoscope (as″tig-mat′o-skōp) [*astigma*tism + Gr. *sko-*

pein to inspect] an instrument for discovering and measuring astigmatism.

astigmatoscopy (ah-stig″mah-tos′ko-pe) the use of the astigmatoscope.

astigmia (ah-stig′me-ah) [a- neg. + Gr. *stigma* a point + *ia*] astigmatism.

astigmic (ah-stig′mik) astigmatic.

astigmometer (as″tig-mom′ĕ-ter) astigmatometer.

astigmometry (as″tig-mom′ĕ-tre) astigmatometry.

astigmoscope (as-tig′mo-skōp) astigmatoscope.

astigmoscopy (ah-stig″mos′ko-pe) astigmatoscopy.

Astomatida (a″sto-mah-ti′dah) [a neg. + Gr. *stoma* mouth] an order of usually large or long, uniformly ciliated, endoparasitic protozoa (subclass Hymenostomatia, class Oligohymenophorea) without a cytostome or a cytoproct, and characterized by the presence of a complex infraciliary endoskeleton and often elaborate holdfast organs (hooks, spines, or sucker) situated at the anterior end of the body. They are found in soil, freshwater, and marine habitats.

Astomatophorina (ah-sto″mah-to-fo-ri′nah, ah-sto″mah-tof′o-ri″nah) [a neg. + Gr. *stoma* mouth + *phoros* bearing] a suborder of ciliate protozoa (order Apostomatida, superorder Apostomatidea), some species of which are found in the coelomic fluid of amphipods and isopods, others in organs of the squid and octopus. They are characterized by the absence of a cytostome, with only the remnants of oral ciliature being present, and an often elongate, vermiform body that exhibits marked thigmotactism.

astomatous (as-tom′ah-tus) [a neg. + Gr. *stoma* mouth] having no mouth, as certain ciliates.

astomia (ah-sto′me-ah) [a neg. + Gr. *stoma* mouth] congenital absence of the mouth.

astomus (ah-sto′mus) a fetus without a mouth opening.

Astrafer (as′trah-fer) trademark for a preparation of dextriferron.

astragalar (as-trag′ah-lar) pertaining to the astragalus (talus).

astragalectomy (as″trag-ah-lek′to-me) [*astragalus* + Gr. *ektomē* excision] excision of the astragalus (talus).

astragalocalcanean (as-trag″ah-lo-kal-ka′ne-an) pertaining to the astragalus (talus) and the calcaneus.

astragalocrural (as-trag″ah-lo-kroo′ral) relating to the astragalus (talus) and the leg.

astragaloscaphoid (as-trag″ah-lo-skaf′oid) pertaining to the astragalus (talus) and the scaphoid (navicular) bone.

astragalotibial (as-trag″ah-lo-tib′e-al) pertaining to the astragalus (talus) and the tibia.

Astragalus (ah-strag′ah-lus) a genus of leguminous plants or many species. *A. gummifer* and other oriental species afford tragacanth; others are poisonous. *A. mollissimus,* of the United States (one of the plants called loco), is poisonous, and its active principle is mydriatic.

astragalus (ah-strag′ah-lus) [L.; Gr. *astragalos* ball of the ankle joint or dice] the talus, def. 1.

astral (as′tral) of or relating to an aster.

astraphobia (as″tra-fo′be-ah) [Gr. *astrapē* lightning + *phobia*] irrational fear of thunder and lightning.

astrapophobia (as″trah-po-fo′be-ah) astraphobia.

astriction (ah-strik′shun) [L. *astringere* to constrict] 1. the action of an astringent. 2. (*obs.*) constipation.

astringe (ah-strinj′) to act as an astringent.

astringent (ah-strin′jent) [L. *astringens,* from *ad* to + *stringere* to bind] 1. causing contraction, usually locally after topical application. 2. an agent which has an astringent action.

astro- [Gr. *astron* star] a combining form denoting relationship to a star, or to an aster.

astroblast (as′tro-blast) [*astro-* + Gr. *blastos* germ] a cell that develops into an astrocyte.

astroblastoma (as″tro-blas-to′mah) an astrocytoma of Grade II, composed of cells with abundant cytoplasm and two or three nuclei.

astrocele (as′tro-sēl) astrocoele.

astrocinetic (as″tro-si-net′ik) astrokinetic.

astrocoele (as′tro-sēl) [*astro-* + Gr. *koilos* hollow] the clear space within the astrosphere of a cell in which the centrosome lies.

astrocyte (as′tro-sīt) [astro- + Gr. *kytos* hollow vessel] a neuroglial cell of ectodermal origin, characterized by fibrous, protoplasmic, or plasmatofibrous processes. Collectively, such cells are called *astroglia*. **fibrous a's,** astrocytes found mainly in the white matter of the brain, having long, thin, infrequently branched cytoplasmic processes containing numerous fibrillar structures. **gemistocytic a.,** gemistocyte. **plasmatofibrous a's,** astrocytes found at the junction of the gray and white matter of the brain; the cytoplasmic processes extending into the white matter are fibrous and those extending into the gray matter are protoplasmic. **protoplasmic a's,** astrocytes found mainly in the gray matter of the brain, having many branching, thick cytoplasmic processes.

astrocytoma (as′′tro-si-to′mah) a tumor composed of astrocytes; such tumors have been classified in order of increasing malignancy as: *Grade I,* consisting of fibrillary or protoplasmic astrocytes; *Grade II* (see *astroblastoma*); and *Grades III* and *IV* (see *glioblastoma multiforme*). **anaplastic a.,** glioblastoma multiforme. **a. fibrilla′re,** an astrocytoma composed of astrocytes which produce fibrillary or neuroglial fibers. **gemistocytic a.,** an astrocytoma in which the cytoplasm of the tumor cells is swollen, homogeneously hyaline, and acidophilic in appearance. **pilocytic a.,** a variant of the fibrillary type of astrocytoma in which the fibrils are arranged in parallel rows. **a. protoplasmat′icum,** a tumor composed of protoplasmic astrocytes.

astrocytosis (as′′tro-si-to′sis) the proliferation of astrocytes owing to the destruction of nearby neurons during a hypoxic or hypoglycemic episode.

astroglia (as-trog′le-ah) [astro- + *neuroglia*] the astrocytes considered as tissue; see *macroglia*.

astroid (as′troid) [astro- + Gr. *eidos* form] 1. star-shaped. 2. (obs.) a structure of the neuroglia formed by a felted mass of fibers.

astrokinetic (as′′tro-ki-net′ik) [astro- + Gr. *kinēsis* motion] pertaining to the movements of the centrosome.

astroma (as-tro′mah) (obs.) astrocytoma.

astrophobia (as′′tro-fo′be-ah) [astro- + *phobia*] (obs.) fear of the stars and celestial space.

astrophorous (as-trof′o-rus) [astro- + Gr. *phoros* bearing] having star-shaped processes.

astroplankton (as′′tro-plank′ton) [Gr. *astron* star + *planktos* wandering] hypothetical living material drifting in outer space.

astropyle (as′′tro-pīl) [astro- + Gr. *pylē* gate] the main opening in the capsular membrane of certain marine planktonic protozoa. See also *parapyle*.

astrosphere (as′tro-sfēr) [astro- + Gr. *sphaira* sphere] 1. the central mass of an aster, exclusive of the rays. 2. aster.

astrostatic (as′′tro-stat′ik) [astro- + Gr. *statikos* standing] pertaining to the centrosome in its resting condition.

astyclinic (as′′tĕ-klin′ik) [Gr. *asty* city + *klinē* bed] a city or municipal hospital, dispensary, or clinic.

asulfurosis (ah-sul-fu-ro′sis) a condition due to lack of sulfur in the body.

asyllabia (ah′′sil-la′be-ah) a condition in which letters are recognized by the patient, but he is unable to form them into syllables.

asylum (ah-si′lum) [L.] a place of refuge and shelter, as an institution of the past for the support and care of helpless and deprived individuals, such as the mentally deficient, emotionally disturbed, or the blind.

asymbolia (ah-sim-bo′le-ah) [a neg. + Gr. *symbolon* symbol + -*ia*] loss of power to comprehend symbolic things, as words, figures, gestures, signs, etc. (Wernicke). **pain a.,** absence of psychic reaction to pain sensations; it may be congenital or result from brain lesion, particularly of the supramarginal gyrus of the dominant parietal lobe.

asymboly (ah-sim′bo-le) asymbolia.

asymmetrical (a′′sim-met′rĭ-kal) characterized by or pertaining to asymmetry.

asymmetry (a-sim′ĕ-tre) [a neg. + Gr. *symmetria* symmetry] lack or absence of symmetry; dissimilarity in corresponding parts or organs on opposite sides of the body which are normally alike. In chemistry, lack of symmetry in the special arrangements of the atoms and radicals within the molecule

or crystal. **chromatic a.,** difference in color in the irides of the two eyes. **encephalic a.,** a condition in which the two sides of the brain are not the same size.

asymphytous (ah-sim′fĭ-tus) separate or distinct; not grown together.

asymptomatic (a′′simp′′to-mat′ik) showing or causing no symptoms.

asynapsis (ah-sĭ-nap′sis) [a neg. + Gr. *synapsis* conjunction] the failure of homologous chromosomes to pair during meiosis.

asynchronism (a-sin′kro-nizm) [a neg. + *synchronism*] the occurrence at distinct times of events normally synchronous; disturbance of coordination.

asynchrony (a-sin′kro-ne) asynchronism.

asynclitism (ah-sin′klĭ-tizm) [a neg. + *synclitism*] 1. oblique presentation of the fetal head in labor. 2. asynchronous maturation of the nucleus and cytoplasm of blood cells. **anterior a.,** Nägele's obliquity. **posterior a.,** Litzmann's obliquity.

asyndesis (ah-sin′dĕ-sis) [a neg. + Gr. *syn* together + *desis* binding] a pattern of language in which words and phrases are juxtaposed without grammatical linkage; seen in schizophrenic disorders and organic brain syndromes.

asynechia (ah′′sĭ-nek′e-ah) [a neg. + Gr. *synecheia* continuity] absence of continuity of structure.

asynergia (a′′sin-er′je-ah) asynergy.

asynergic (a′′sin-er′jik) marked by asynergy.

asynergy (a-sin′er-je) [a neg. + Gr. *synergia* cooperation] lack of coordination among parts or organs normally acting in harmony. In neurology, disturbance of that proper association in the contraction of muscles which assures that the different components of an act follow in proper sequence, at the proper moment, and are of the proper degree, so that the act is executed accurately. **truncal a.,** see under *ataxia*.

asynovia (a′′sin-o′ve-ah) deficiency of the synovial secretion.

asyntaxia (ah′′sin-tak′se-ah) [Gr. "want of arrangement"] lack of proper and orderly embryonic development. **a. dorsa′lis,** failure of the neural groove to close in the developing embryo.

asystole (ah-sis′to-le) [a neg. + *systole*] cardiac standstill or arrest—absence of a heartbeat; called also *Beau's syndrome.*

asystolia (ah′′sis-to′le-ah) asystole.

asystolic (ah′′sis-tol′ik) characterized by asystole.

A.T. 10 dihydrotachysterol.

At chemical symbol for *astatine*.

ATA alimentary toxic aleukia; see under *aleukia*.

Atabrine (ah′tah-brin) trademark for a preparation of quinacrine hydrochloride.

atactic (ah-tak′tik) [Gr. *ataktos* irregular] lacking coordination; irregular; pertaining to or characterized by ataxia.

atactiform (ah-tak′tĭ-form) resembling ataxia.

ataractic (at′′ah-rak′tik) [Gr. *ataraktos* without disturbance; quiet] 1. pertaining to or capable of producing ataraxia. 2. ataractic agent; a tranquilizer.

ataralgesia (at′′ar-al-je′ze-ah) [Gr. *ataraktos* without trouble + -*algesia*] a method of combined sedation and analgesia designed to abolish the mental distress and pain attendant on surgical procedures, with the patient remaining conscious and alert.

Atarax (ah′tah-raks) trademark for preparations of hydroxyzine hydrochloride.

ataraxia (at′′ah-rak′se-ah) [Gr. "impassiveness," "calmness"] serenity, calmness, peace of mind.

ataraxic (at′′ah-rak′sik) ataractic.

ataraxy (at′′ah-rak′se) ataraxia.

atavic (at′ah-vik) atavistic.

atavism (at′ah-vizm) [L. *atavus* grandfather] the apparent inheritance of a characteristic from remote rather than from immediate ancestors, due to a chance recombination of genes or to unusual environmental conditions favorable to their expression in the embryo. Called also *reversion*.

atavistic (at-ah-vis′tik) characterized by atavism.

ataxaphasia (ah-tak′′sah-fa′ze-ah) ataxiaphasia.

ataxia (ah-tak′se-ah) [Gr., from *a* negative + *taxis* order] failure of muscular coordination; irregularity of muscular action. **acute a.,** ataxia of sudden onset. **acute cerebellar a.,** cerebellar ataxia, usually unilateral, associated with infectious disease, tumor, or trauma, resulting in marked hypotonia of muscles on the affected side, asynergy, and assumption of a characteristic posture. **alcoholic a.,** a condition resembling tabes dorsalis, due to loss of proprioception in chronic alcoholism. **autonomic a.,** defective coordination between the sympathetic and parasympathetic nervous systems. **central a.,** ataxia due to lesion of the centers controlling coordination. **cerebellar a.,** ataxia due to disease of the cerebellum. **cerebral a.,** ataxia due to disease of the cerebrum. **a. cor'dis** (obs.), atrial fibrillation. **enzootic a.,** congenital locomotor ataxia of lambs, thought to be associated with copper deficiency; called also *swayback*. **family a.,** Friedreich's a. **Fergusson and Critchley's a.,** a hereditary ataxia resembling multiple sclerosis found in only a few families and with onset between the ages of 30 and 45. **Friedreich's a.,** Friedreich's disease: an autosomal recessive disease, usually beginning in childhood or youth, with sclerosis of the dorsal and lateral columns of the spinal cord. It is attended by ataxia, speech impairment, lateral curvature of the spinal column, and peculiar swaying and irregular movements, with paralysis of the muscles, especially of the lower extremities. It is often associated with hypertrophic cardiomyopathy. Called also *hereditary a., family a.,* and *Friedreich's tabes.* **frontal a.,** disturbance of equilibrium occurring in tumor of the frontal lobe. **hereditary a.,** Friedreich's a. **hysterical a.,** ataxia recognizable as a conversion symptom; see *astasia-abasia,* under *astasia.* **intrapsychic a.,** the separation of ideas and effect seen in schizophrenic disorders; inappropriateness of affect. **kinetic a.,** motor a. **labyrinthic a.,** vestibular a. **Leyden's a.,** pseudotabes. **locomotor a.,** tabes dorsalis. **Marie's a.,** hereditary cerebellar a. **motor a.,** inability to control the coordinate movements of the muscles; called also *kinetic a.* **ocular a.,** nystagmus. **Sanger Brown a.,** a hereditary spinocerebellar degeneration, characterized by onset between 11 and 45 years of age, by ataxia beginning in the legs and spreading to the arms and face and affecting the deglutitive and speech muscles, by oculomotor paresis, and by optic atrophy. **sensory a.,** ataxia due to loss of proprioception (joint position sensation) between the motor cortex and peripheral nerves, resulting in poorly judged movements, the incoordination becoming aggravated when the eyes are closed. **spinal a.,** that which is due to disease of the spinal cord. **spinocerebellar a.,** any hereditary ataxia with cerebellar malfunction resulting in clinical manifestation. **a.-telangiectasia,** a complex hereditary disorder, transmitted as an autosomal recessive trait, characterized by cerebellar ataxia and nystagmus, oculocutaneous telangiectasia, variable degrees of humoral and cellular immunodeficiency with recurrent sinopulmonary bacterial infections, and an increased incidence of lymphoreticular malignancies. There is an increased sensitivity to ionizing radiation caused by a defect in DNA repair. Gonadal hypoplasia, insulin resistance and hyperglycemia, liver function abnormalities, and elevated levels of alpha-fetoprotein and carcinoembryonic antigen are also seen in some patients. Called also *Louis-Bar syndrome.* **thermal a.,** a condition characterized by great and paradoxic fluctuations of the temperature of the body. **truncal a.,** ataxia affecting the muscles of the trunk. **vasomotor a.** (obs.), paralysis or spasm of blood vessels due to some derangement of vasomotor nerves or centers. **vestibular a.,** incoordination due to vestibular disease; called also *labyrinthine a.*

ataxiadynamia (ah-tak″se-ah-di-na′me-ah) ataxoadynamia.

ataxiagram (ah-tak′se-ah-gram″) [*ataxia* + Gr. *gramma* a writing] a tracing drawn by an ataxic patient; also the record made by an ataxiagraph.

ataxiagraph (ah-tak′se-ah-graf″) [*ataxia* + Gr. *graphein* to write] an apparatus used in ascertaining the extent of ataxia by measuring the amount of swaying of the body when standing erect and with the eyes closed.

ataxiameter (ah-tak″se-am′ĕ-ter) [*ataxia* + Gr. *metron* measure] an apparatus for measuring ataxia.

ataxiamnesic (ah-tak″se-am-ne′sik) characterized by both ataxia and amnesia.

ataxiaphasia (ah-tak″se-ah-fa′ze-ah) [*ataxia* + Gr. *aphasia*] a condition characterized by inability to arrange words into sentences.

ataxic (ah-tak′sik) atactic.

ataxiophemia (ah-tak″se-o-fe′me-ah) ataxophemia.

ataxiophobia (ah-tak″se-o-fo′be-ah) ataxophobia.

ataxoadynamia (ah-tak″so-ad′ĕ-na′me-ah) (obs.) ataxia associated with marked weakness.

ataxophemia (ah-tak″so-fe′me-ah) [Gr. *ataxia* disorder + *phēmē* speech] lack of coordination of the speech muscles.

ataxophobia (ah-tak″so-fo′be-ah) [Gr. *ataxia* disorder + *phobia*] irrational dread of disorder.

ataxy (ah-tak′se) ataxia.

ATCC American Type Culture Collection.

-ate (āt) [L. *-atus,* past participial ending of verbs ending in *-are*] 1. a word termination forming a participial noun, as the object of the process indicated by the root to which it is affixed, e.g., *hemolysate,* something hemolyzed; *homogenate,* something homogenized; *injectate,* something injected. Also forming adjectives, signifying possession of the quality indicated by the root, e.g., *dentate* and *corticate;* and verbs, signifying performance of the action indicated by the root, e.g., *decussate* and *pulsate.* 2. in chemistry, a suffix replacing the suffix *-ic* and the word *acid* in forming the names of anions, salts, and esters, e.g., acetic acid, acetate ion, sodium acetate, methyl acetate. Cf. *-ite.*

atelectasis (at″e-lek′tah-sis) [Gr. *atelēs* imperfect + *ektasis* expansion] 1. incomplete expansion of a lung or a portion of a lung, occurring congenitally as a primary or secondary condition, or as an acquired condition. 2. airlessness of a lung that had once been expanded. 3. collapse of a lung. **absorption a., acquired a.,** that produced by any factor, e.g., secretions, foreign body, tumor, abnormal external pressure, etc., which completely obstructs the airway, preventing intake of air into the alveolar sacs and permitting absorption of air into the bloodstream. Called also *obstructive a., reabsorption a.,* and *secondary a.* **compression a.,** acquired atelectasis due to abnormal external pressure on the lung. **congenital a.,** that present at birth or shortly thereafter; it may occur as a primary condition (see *primary a.)* or secondary to some other congenital disorder (see *secondary a.).* **initial a.,** primary a. **lobar a.,** that affecting only a lobe of the lung; called also *segmental a.* **lobular a.,** that affecting a lobule of the lung; called also *patchy a.* **obstructive a.,** absorption a. **patchy a.,** lobular a. **primary a.,** congenital atelectasis, common among premature infants, in which there is failure of initial alveolar expansion, due to pulmonary immaturity or to inadequacy of respiratory effort that may be a result of weakness of respiratory muscles, severe illness, softness of thoracic cage, brain damage with injury to the respiratory center, or oversedation. Called also *initial a.* **relaxation a.,** absorption atelectasis due to bronchial collapse resulting from large amounts of air or fluid in the pleural cavity, as in pneumothorax or pleural effusion. **resorption a.,** absorption a. **secondary a.,** 1. absorption atelectasis occurring at birth or in the newborn period, in which the pulmonary alveoli collapse after initial expansion by air; it is due to obstruction of the airway which prevents further entrance of air or to prevention of air from remaining in the alveoli by increased surfaces forces, occurring as a result of inhalation of amniotic debris or mucous plugs, deficiency of pulmonary surfactant, obstruction by congenital abnormalities, or abnormal external pressure upon the lung. 2. absorption a. **segmental a.,** lobar a.

atelectatic (at″ĕ-lek-tat′ik) pertaining to or characterized by atelectasis.

ateleiosis (ah-te″le-o′sis) [*a* neg. + Gr. *teleios* complete] a term formerly used for hypophysial infantilism.

atelencephalia (ah-tel″en-sĕ-fa′le-ah) [Gr. *ateleia* incompleteness + *enkephalos* brain + *-ia*] congenital imperfect development of the brain.

atelia (ah-te′le-ah) [Gr. *ateleia* incompleteness] imperfect or incomplete development.

ateliosis (ah-te″le-o′sis) ateleiosis.

ateliotic (ah-te″le-ot′ik) pertaining to or characterized by atelia.

atel(o)- [Gr. *atelēs* incomplete] a combining form meaning imperfect or incomplete.

atelocardia (at″ĕ-lo-kar′de-ah) [atelo- + Gr. *kardia* heart] congenitally incomplete development of the heart.

atelocephalous (at″ĕ-lo-sef′ah-lus) [atelo- + Gr. *kephalē* head] having an incomplete head.

atelocephaly (at″ĕ-lo-sef′ah-le) imperfect development of the skull.

atelocheilia (at″ĕ-lo-ki′le-ah) [atelo- + Gr. *cheilos* lip + -ia] a congenitally incomplete development of a lip.

atelocheiria (at″ĕ-lo-ki′re-ah) [atelo- + Gr. *cheir* hand + -ia] congenitally incomplete development of the hand.

ateloencephalia (at″ĕ-lo-en″sĕ-fa′le-ah) atelencephalia.

ateloglossia (at″ĕ-lo-glos′e-ah) [atelo- + Gr. *glōssa* tongue + -ia] congenitally incomplete development of the tongue.

atelognathia (at″ĕ-log-na′the-ah) [atelo- + Gr. *gnathos* jaw + -ia] congenitally incomplete development of the jaw.

atelomyelia (at″ĕ-lo-mi-e′le-ah) [atelo- + Gr. *myelos* marrow + -ia] congenitally incomplete development of the spinal cord.

atelopidtoxin (a-tel-op″id-tok′sin) a potent dialyzable toxin derived from the skin of frogs of the genus *Atelopus*, of Central and South America. The LD$_{50}$ in mice is 16 μg/kg. Its chemical and pharmacological nature has not been fully defined.

atelopodia (at″ĕ-lo-po′de-ah) [atelo- + Gr. *pous* foot + -ia] congenitally incomplete development of the foot.

ateloprosopia (at″ĕ-lo-pro-so′pe-ah) [atelo- + Gr. *prosōpon* face + -ia] congenitally incomplete development of the face.

atelorachidia (at″ĕ-lo-rah-kid′e-ah) [atelo- + Gr. *rhachis* spine + -ia] congenitally incomplete development of the vertebral column.

Atelosaccharomyces (at″ĕ-lo-sak″ah-ro-mi′sēz) former name for *Cryptococcus*.

atelostomia (at″ĕ-lo-sto′me-ah) [atelo- + Gr. *stoma* mouth + -ia] congenitally incomplete development of the mouth.

atenolol (ah-ten′o-lōl) chemical name: 4-[2-hydroxy-3-[(1-methylethyl)amino]propoxyl]benzeneacetamide; an antiadrenergic (β-receptor), $C_{14}H_{22}N_2O_3$.

ATG antithymocyte globulin.

Athalamida (a″thah-lam′ĭ-dah) [a neg. + Gr. *thalamos* inner chamber] an order of naked ameboid protozoa (class Granuloreticulosea, superclass Rhizopoda). *Biomyxa* is a representative genus.

athalposis (ah″thal-po′sis) [a neg. + Gr. *thalpos* warmth + -osis] inability to perceive warmth.

athelia (ah-the′le-ah) [a neg. + Gr. *thēlē* nipple + -ia] congenital absence of the nipple(s).

Athenaeus (ath″ĕ-ne′us) a Greek physician born in Attalia, Asia Minor, who practiced in Rome under the Emperors Claudius and Nero (A.D. 41-68). He considered medicine part of general education, followed Aristotle's physiology, added pneuma ("breath," "spirit") to the four elements as the fifth and founded the Pneumatist School. His school, speculative, not practical or empirical, explained health and sickness in terms of good and bad temperaments.

athermal (ah-ther′mal) [a neg. + Gr. *thermē* heat] not warm; said of springs the water of which is below 15° C.

athermancy (ah-ther′man-se) the state of being athermanous.

athermanous (ah-ther′mah-nus) [a neg. + Gr. *thermē* heat] absorbing heat rays and not permitting them to pass.

athermic (ah-ther′mik) [a neg. + Gr. *thermē* heat] without fever or rise of temperature; apyretic; afebrile.

athermosystaltic (ah-ther″mo-sis-tal′tik) [a neg. + Gr. *thermē* heat + Gr. *systaltikos* drawing together] not contracting under the action of cold or heat; said of skeletal muscle.

ather(o)- [Gr. *athērē* gruel] a combining form denoting fatty degeneration, or relationship to an atheroma.

atheroembolism (ath″er-o-em′bo-lizm) embolism due to blockage of a blood vessel by an atheroembolus.

atheroembolus (ath″er-o-em′bo-lus), pl. *atheroem'boli*. An embolus composed of cholesterol or its esters (typically lodging in small arteries) or of fragments of atheromatous plaques.

atherogenesis (ath″er-o-jen′ĕ-sis) the formation of atheromatous lesions in the arterial intima.

atherogenic (ath″er-o-jen′ik) conducive to or causing atherogenesis.

atheroma (ath″er-o′mah) [Gr. *athērē* gruel + -oma] a mass of plaque of degenerated, thickened arterial intima occurring in atherosclerosis.

atheromatosis (ath″er-o″mah-to′sis) a diffuse atheromatous disease of the arteries.

atheromatous (ath″er-o′mah-tus) affected with or of the nature of atheroma.

atheronecrosis (ath″er-o″ne-kro′sis) (obs.) the necrosis or degeneration accompanying atherosclerosis.

atherosclerosis (ath″er-o″skle-ro′sis) an extremely common form of arteriosclerosis in which deposits of yellowish plaques (atheromas) containing cholesterol, lipoid material, and lipophages are formed within the intima and inner media of large and medium-sized arteries. **a. oblit′erans,** arteriosclerosis obliterans.

atherosis (ath″er-o′sis) (obs.) atherosclerosis.

athetoid (ath′ĕ-toid) [Gr. *athetos* not fixed + *eidos* form] resembling or affected with athetosis.

athetosic (ath″ĕ-to′sik) athetotic.

athetosis (ath″ĕ-to′sis) [Gr. *athetos* not fixed + -osis] a derangement marked by ceaseless occurrence of slow, sinuous, writhing movements, especially severe in the hands, and performed involuntarily; it may occur after hemiplegia, and is then known as *posthemiplegic chorea*. Called also *mobile spasm*. **double a., double congenital a.,** congenital

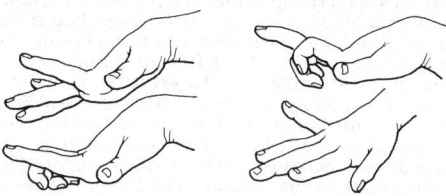

Positions of fingers in movements of athetosis.

bilateral athetosis due to birth trauma, which may occur in association with spastic paraplegia, as in *Vogt's syndrome* and *Little's disease*. **pupillary a.,** hippus.

athetotic (ath″e-tot′ik) pertaining to athetosis.

athiaminosis (ah-thi″ah-mĭ-no′sis) thiamine deficiency.

Athiorhodaceae (a″thi-o-ro-da′se-e) Rhodospirillaceae.

athomin (ath′o-min) a bactericidal principle isolated from the root bark of the "horseradish" tree, *Moringa pterygosperma* Gaertn., Moringaceae, used in India as an antiemetic and in the clinical management of cholera. Called also *GL 54*.

athrepsia (ah-threp′se-ah) [a neg. + Gr. *threpsis* nutrition] 1. marasmus. 2. Ehrlich's term for immunity to tumor inoculation due to a supposed lack of the special nutritive material necessary for tumor growth.

athrepsy (ath′rep-se) athrepsia.

athreptic (ah-threp′tik) pertaining to or characterized by athrepsia.

athrocytosis (ath″ro-si-to′sis) absorption of macromolecules from the lumen of the renal tubules by renal tubular cells by means of a process similar to phagocytosis.

athrophagocytosis (ath″ro-fag″o-si-to′sis) non-nutritive phagocytosis; phagocytosis of inert particles, as the removal of injected carbon particles.

athymia (ah-thim′e-ah) 1. [Gr. "lack of spirit"] (obs.) absence of feeling or emotion; depression or melancholia. 2. [a- neg. + *thymus*] absence of the thymus gland.

athymism (ah-thi′mizm) absence of the thymus or the condition induced by absence or removal of the thymus.

athymismus (ah″thi-mis′mus) athymism.

athyrea (ah-thi′re-ah) 1. hypothyroidism. 2. absence of the thyroid gland.

athyreosis (ah-thi″re-o′sis) [a neg. + *thyreoid* thyroid + -osis] athyrosis.

athyreotic (ah-thi″re-ot′ik) athyrotic.

athyria (ah-thi′re-ah) 1. a condition resulting from absence of the thyroid gland. 2. hypothyroidism.

athyroidation (ah-thi″roi-da′shun) hypothyroidism.

athyroidemia (ah-thi″roi-de′me-ah) [a neg. + thyroid + Gr. haima blood + -ia] absence of thyroid hormone from the blood.

athyroidism (ah-thi′roid-izm) hypothyroidism.

athyroidosis (ah-thi″roi-do′sis) hypothyroidism.

athyrosis (ah″thī-ro′sis) 1. hypothyroidism. 2. absence of the thyroid gland.

athyrotic (ah″thi-rot′ik) pertaining to or characterized by hypothyroidism or by absence of the thyroid gland.

Athysanus (ah-this′ah-nus) a genus of blood-sucking flies of Algeria.

atite (at′īt) a substance in milk that reduces nitrate to nitrite.

atlant(o)- [Gr. atlas, q.v., gen. atlantos] a combining form denoting relationship to the atlas.

atlantad (at-lan′tad) toward the atlas.

atlantal (at-lan′tal) pertaining to the atlas.

atlantoaxial (at-lan″to-ak′se-al) pertaining to the atlas and the axis.

atlantodidymus (at-lan″to-did′ĭ-mus) a monster with one body and two heads.

atlantomastoid (at-lan″to-mas′toid) pertaining to the atlas and the mastoid process.

atlanto-odontoid (at-lan″to-o-don′toid) pertaining to the atlas and the odontoid process of the axis.

atlas (at′las) [Gr. Atlas the Greek god who bears up the pillars of Heaven] 1. [NA], the first cervical vertebra, which articulates above with the occipital bone and below with the axis. 2. a collection of illustrations on one subject, such as anatomy, blood and bone marrow, brain, cardiac disease.

atloaxoid (at″lo-ak′soid) pertaining to the atlas and the axis.

atlodidymus (at″lo-did′ĭ-mus) [atlas + Gr. didymos twin] atlantodidymus.

atloido-occipital (at-loi″do-ok-sip′ĭ-tal) pertaining to the atlas and the occiput.

atmiatrics (at″me-at′riks) [atmo- + Gr. iatrikos healing] treatment by medicated vapors (P. Niemeyer).

atmiatry (at-mi′ah-tre) atmiatrics.

atm atmosphere.

atm(o)- [Gr. atmos steam or vapor] a combining form denoting relationship to steam or vapor.

atmograph (at′mo-graf) [atmo- + Gr. graphein to record] an instrument for recording respiratory movements.

atmolysis (at-mol′ĭ-sis) [atmo- + Gr. lysis loosing] 1. the separation of mixed gases by passing through a porous plate, the more diffusible passing through first. 2. the disintegration of organic tissue by the fumes of volatile fluids, such as benzine, ether, alcohol, etc.

atmometer (at-mom′ĕ-ter) [atmo- + Gr. metron measure] an instrument for measuring exhaled vapors, or the amount of water exhaled by evaporation in a given time, in order to ascertain the humidity of the atmosphere.

atmosphere (at′mos-fēr) [atmo- + Gr. sphaira sphere] 1. the entire gaseous envelope surrounding the earth, including the troposphere, tropopause, and stratosphere. 2. the unit of pressure equal to exactly 101325 pascals, the pressure exerted by the earth's atmosphere at sea level, approximately 760 mm Hg. Symbol, atm.

atmospheric (at″mos-fer′ik) of or pertaining to the atmosphere.

atmotherapy (at″mo-ther′ah-pe) [atmo- + Gr. therapeia treatment] 1. treatment by medicated vapors. 2. treatment by methodic reduction of respiration.

at. no. atomic number.

atocia (ah-to′se-ah) [a neg. + Gr. tokos birth] sterility in the female.

atolide (ah′to-līd) chemical name: 2-amino-4′-(diethylamino)-o-benzotoluidide; an anticonvulsant, $C_{18}H_{23}N_3O$.

atom (at′om) [Gr. atomos indivisible; a- + tomos from temnein to cut] any one of the ultimate particles of a molecule or of any matter. An atom is the smallest particle of an element that is capable of entering into a chemical reaction. The atom consists of a minute central nucleus, in which practically all of the mass of the atom is concentrated, and of surrounding electrons. The nucleus is positively charged; the amount of the charge corresponds to the atomic number of the atom. See Table of Elements, under element. In a neutral atom the surrounding negative electrons are equal in number to the positive charges on the nucleus. The number and arrangement of these electrons determine all the properties of the atom except its atomic weight and its radioactivity. **activated a.,** 1. an ionized atom. 2. an atom in which some of the orbital electrons have been driven out into larger and less stable orbits; the atom is thus prepared to release its stored energy as these electrons return to their normal and stable orbits. Called also excited a. **asymmetric carbon a.,** a carbon atom with four different substituents. Such a molecule does not have a mirror plane passing through the asymmetric atom, and thus may be optically active. **Bohr a.,** the conception of a nuclear atom in which the orbital electrons are able to occupy only certain orbits, these orbits being determined by quantum limitations. **excited a.,** activated atom. **ionized a.,** an atom from which one or more of the outer or valence electrons have been removed, or to which one or more electrons have been added (hence positive and negative ions). **nuclear a.,** the conception or theory of the atom as composed of a small central nucleus surrounded by orbital electrons; called also Rutherford a. For table of the atoms see under element. **recoil a., rest a.,** the portion of an atom from which an alpha particle or other subatomic particle has been given off; this remaining part recoils with a velocity inversely proportional to its mass. **Rutherford a.,** nuclear a. **stripped a.,** an atom from which the orbital electrons have more or less completely removed. **tagged a.,** one which has been made radioactive, so that its course in the body may be checked; see radioactive tracer, under tracer.

atomic (ah-tom′ik) of or pertaining to an atom.

atomism (at′om-izm) Democritus' doctrine that the physical or the physical and nonphysical universe is composed of simple, indivisible (atomos) particles in a void.

atomization (at″om-ĭ-za′shun) the act or process of breaking a liquid up into spray.

atomizer (at′om-īz″er) an instrument for throwing a jet of spray.

atonia (ah-to′ne-ah) atony. **choreatic a.,** deficient muscular tonicity often seen in chorea.

atonic (ah-ton′ik) lacking normal tone or strength; pertaining to or characterized by atony.

atonicity (at″o-nis′ĭ-te) the quality or condition of being without normal tone or strength.

atony (at′o-ne) [L. atonia, from a neg. + Gr. tonos tension] lack of normal tone or strength. **primary ureteral a.,** megaloureter.

atopen (at′o-pen) the allergen involved in an atopic disorder.

atopic (ah-top′ik, a-top′ik) [a neg. + Gr. topos place] 1. ectopic. 2. pertaining to an atopen or to atopy; allergic.

atopognosia (ah-top″og-no′ze-ah) [a neg. + Gr. topos place + gnōsis knowledge + -ia] loss of power of correctly locating a sensation.

atopognosis (ah-top″og-no′sis) atopognosia.

atopomenorrhea (at″ŏ-po-men-o-re′ah) [a neg. + Gr. topos place + men month + rhoia flow] (obs.) vicarious menstruation.

atopy (at′o-pe) [Gr. atopos out of place] 1. a genetic predisposition toward the development of immediate (type I) hypersensitivity reactions against common environmental antigens (atopic allergy), occurring in 10 per cent of the general population, 50 per cent of those with one affected parent, and 75 per cent of those with two affected parents. The most common clinical manifestation is allergic rhinitis; bronchial asthma, atopic dermatitis, and food allergy occur less frequently. The form exhibited may vary over time and may differ from that exhibited by the parents. 2. atopic allergy.

atoxic (ah-tok′sik) [a neg. + Gr. toxikon poison] not poisonous; not due to a poison.

atoxigenic (a-tok″sĭ-jen′ik) not producing or elaborating toxins.

ATP adenosine triphosphate.

ATPase adenosinetriphosphatase.

ATP-cobalamin adenosyltransferase (ko-bal′ah-mēn ah-den″o-sil-trans′fer-ās) cob(1)alamin adenosyltransferase.

atrabiliary (at″rah-bil′e-ă-re) [L. *atra bilis* black bile] (*obs.*) melancholic.

Atractaspis (ah-trak-tas′pis) a genus of African vipers whose bite is toxic to man.

atransferrinemia (a-trans″fer-ĭ-ne′me-ah) absence from the circulating blood of iron-binding protein (transferrin).

atraumatic (a″traw-mat′ik) [*a* neg. + Gr. *traumatikos* of or for wounds] not inflicting or causing damage or injury.

Atrax (a′traks) a genus of tarantula-like spiders (funnel-web spiders) of Australia belonging to the family Dipluridae. The venom of *A. robustus, A. formidabilis* (tree funnel-web spider), and six other species is harmful to man; *A. robustus* has caused several deaths.

atremia (ah-tre′me-ah) [*a* neg. + Gr. *tremein* to tremble] 1. absence of tremor. 2. hysterical inability to walk.

atrepsy (at′rep-se) [*a* neg. + Gr. *threpsis* nutrition] athrepsia (def. 1).

atreptic (ah-trep′tik) athreptic.

atresia (ah-tre′ze-ah) [*a* neg. + Gr. *trēsis* a hole + *-ia*] congenital absence or closure of a normal body orifice or tubular organ; as esophageal and pulmonary atrial a.; called also *clausura*. **anal a., a. a′ni,** imperforate anus. **aortic a.,** absence or closure of the aortic root orifice, a rare congenital anomaly in which the left ventricle is hypoplastic or nonfunctioning, oxygenated blood passing from the left into the right atrium through a septal defect, and the mixed venous and arterial blood passing from the pulmonary artery to the aorta by way of a patent ductus. **aural a.,** absence or closure of the external auditory canal. **biliary a.,** obliteration or hypoplasia of one or more components of the bile ducts due to arrested fetal development, resulting in persistent jaundice and liver damage ranging from biliary stasis to biliary cirrhosis, with splenomegaly as portal hypertension progresses. **choanal a.,** congenital bony or membranous occlusion of one or both choanae, due to failure of the embryonic bucconasal membrane to rupture. **duodenal a.,** congenital absence or occlusion of a portion of the duodenum, characterized by vomiting a few hours after birth, cessation of bowel movements after one to three days, and usually distention of the epigastrium. It is often associated with Down's syndrome. **esophageal a.,** congenital lack of continuity of the esophagus, commonly associated with tracheoesophageal fistula and characterized by excessive salivation, gagging, vomiting when fed, cyanosis, and dyspnea. **follicular a., a. follic′uli,** the degeneration and resorption of an ovarian follicle before it reaches maturity and ruptures. **intestinal a.,** congenital obstruction of the intestine at any level, most commonly of the ileum, due to lack of continuity of the lumen; symptoms vary with the site of obstruction. **a. i′ridis,** closure of the pupillary opening. **mitral a.,** congenital obliteration of the mitral valve orifice; it is associated with hyperplastic left-heart syndrome or transposition of the great vessels. **prepyloric a.,** congenital membranous obstruction of the gastric outlet, characterized by vomiting of gastric contents only. **pulmonary a.,** congenital severe narrowing of the opening between the pulmonary artery and the right ventricle, characterized by cardiomegaly, reduced pulmonary vascularity, and right ventricular atrophy. It is usually associated with tetralogy of Fallot, transposition of the great vessels, or other cardiovascular anomalies. **tricuspid a.,** absence of the orifice between the right atrium and ventricle, circulation being made possible by the presence of an atrial septal defect, blood passing from the right to the left atrium and thence to the left ventricle and aorta. Classification by type is made according to the presence or absence of transposition of the great vessels and of pulmonary stenosis.

atresic (ah-tre′zik) atretic.

atretic (ah-tret′ik) [Gr. *atrētos* not perforated] without an opening; pertaining to or characterized by atresia.

atret(o)- [Gr. *atrētos* not perforated] a combining form denoting absence of a normal opening; imperforate or closed.

atretoblepharia (ah-tre″to-blĕ-fa′re-ah) [*atreto-* + Gr. *blepharon* eyelid + *-ia*] symblepharon.

atretocephalus (ah-tre″to-sef′ah-lus) [*atreto-* + Gr. *kephalē* head] a monster lacking the orifices normally present in the head.

atretocormus (ah-tre″to-kor′mus) [*atreto-* + Gr. *kormos* trunk] a fetus or infant having one of the body openings imperforate.

atretocystia (ah-tre″to-sis′te-ah) [*atreto-* + Gr. *kystis* bladder + *-ia*] lack of the normal opening from the bladder.

atretogastria (ah-tre″to-gas′tre-ah) [*atreto-* + Gr. *gastēr* stomach + *-ia*] lack of the normal opening into the stomach.

atretolemia (ah-tre″to-le′me-ah) [*atreto-* + Gr. *laimos* gullet + *-ia*] lack of the normal opening into the larynx or the esophagus.

atretometria (ah-tre″to-me′tre-ah) [*atreto-* + Gr. *mētra* uterus + *-ia*] lack of the normal opening into the uterus.

atretopsia (ah″tre-top′se-ah) atresia iridis; see under *atresia*.

atretorrhinia (ah-tre″to-rin′e-ah) [*atreto-* + Gr. *rhis* nose + *-ia*] absence of the normal opening into the nose.

atretostomia (ah-tre″to-sto′me-ah) [*atreto-* + Gr. *stoma* mouth + *-ia*] lack of the normal opening into the oral cavity.

atreturethria (ah-tre″tu-re′thre-ah) [*atreto-* + Gr. *ourēthra* urethra + *-ia*] lack of the normal urethral opening.

atria (a′tre-ah) [L.] plural of *atrium*.

atrial (a′tre-al) pertaining to an atrium.

atrichosis (at″rĭ-ko′sis) alopecia.

atrichous (ah-trik′us) [*a* neg. + Gr. *thrix* hair] 1. having no flagella; said of bacteria. 2. having no hair.

atri(o)- [L. *atrium,* q.v.] a combining form denoting relationship to an atrium of the heart.

atriocommissuropexy (a″tre-o-kom″ĭ-su′ro-pek″se) [*atrio-* + *commissure* + *-pexy*] repair of the mitral valve with sutures passed from the ventricle through the valve leaflets and the atrial wall, for correction of mitral insufficiency.

atriomegaly (a″tre-o-meg′ah-le) [*atrio-* + Gr. *megaleios* magnitude] abnormal dilatation or enlargement of an atrium of the heart.

atrionector (at″re-o-nek′tor) [*atrio-* + L. *nector* connector] the sinoatrial node.

atriopeptigen (a″tre-o-pep′tĭ-jen) the 126-amino-acid prohormone of atriopeptin, stored in the perinuclear granules of cardiac atrial myocytes.

atriopeptin (a″tre-o-pep′tin) a peptide hormone secreted by specific cells of the cardiac atrium that promotes the renal loss of fluid and electrolytes.

atrioseptopexy (a″tre-o-sep″to-pek′se) [*atrio-* + *septum* + Gr. *pēxis* a fixing, putting together] surgical repair of a defect in the interatrial septum.

atrioseptoplasty (a″tre-o-sep″to-plas′te) plastic repair of the interatrial septum.

atriotomy (a″tre-ot′o-me) [*atrio-* + Gr. *tomē* a cutting] surgical incision of an atrium of the heart.

atrioventricular (a″tre-o-ven-trik′u-lar) pertaining to an atrium of the heart and to a ventricle.

atrioventricularis communis (a″tre-o-ven-trik″u-la′ris kŏ-mu′nis) a congenital cardiac anomaly in which the endocardial cushions fail to fuse, the ostium primum persists, the atrioventricular canal is undivided, a single atrioventricular valve has anterior and posterior cusps, and there is a defect of the membranous interventricular septum. Called also *persistent common atrioventricular canal.*

atriplicism (ah-trip′lĭ-sizm) poisoning produced by eating a kind of spinach, *Atriplex littoralis.*

atrium (a′tre-um), pl. *a′tria* [L.; Gr. *atrion* hall] a chamber; used in anatomical nomenclature to designate a chamber affording entrance to another structure or organ. Usually used alone to designate an atrium of the heart (a. cordis). **common a.,** the single atrium found in a form of three-chambered heart. **a. cor′dis** [NA], one of the pair of smaller cavities of the heart, with thin muscular walls, from which the blood passes to the ventricles; see *a. dextrum* and *a. sinistrum.* **a. dex′trum** [NA], right atrium: the atrium of the right side of the heart; it receives blood from the superior and the inferior vena cava, and delivers it to the right ventricle. **a. glot′tidis, a. of glottis,** vestibulum laryngis. **a. laryn′gis, a. of larynx,** vestibulum laryngis. **left a.,** a. sinistrum. **a. mea′tus me′dii** [NA], a. of middle meatus of nose: a depression in front of the middle nasal meatus, between the agger nasi and the middle nasal concha. **a. pulmona′le, pulmonary a.,** atrium sinistrum. **right a.,** a. dextrum. **a. sinis′trum** [NA], left atrium: the atrium of the left side of the heart; it receives blood from the pulmonary veins, and delivers it to the left ventricle. Called also *a. pulmonale* and *pulmonary a.* **a. vagi'nae,** vestibulum vaginae.

Atromid-S (at'ro-mid) trademark for a preparation of clofibrate.

Atropa (at'ro-pah) [Gr. *Atropos* "undeviating," one of the Fates] a genus of solanaceous plants, from which various alkaloids are derived, including atropine, hyoscyamine, and scopolamine, which generally possess anticholinergic properties. The genus includes *A. belladonna* and *A. belladonna* var. *acuminata.* See *belladonna.*

atrophedema (ah-trof'ĕ-de'mah) angioneurotic edema.

atrophia (ah-tro'fe-ah) [L.; Gr., from *a* neg. + Gr. *trophē* nourishment] atrophy. **a. bulbo'rum heredita'ria,** Norrie's disease. **a. cer'ebri seni'lis sim'plex,** senile dementia in which there is marked atrophy of the brain associated with conspicuous loss of neurons and abundant lipochrome in those that survive. **a. choroi'deae et re'tinae,** atrophy of the choroid and retina, formerly associated with night blindness. **a. cu'tis,** atrophoderma. **a. cu'tis seni'lis,** senile atrophy of skin. **a. doloro'sa,** atrophy of the eyeball accompanied by violent attacks of pain. **a. infan'tum** (*obs.*), tabes mesenterica. **a. maculo'sa,** anetoderma. **a. mesenter'ica** (*obs.*), tabes mesenterica. **a. musculo'rum lipomato'sa,** pseudohypertrophic muscular dystrophy. **a. seni'lis,** senile atrophy. **a. testic'uli,** wasting of the testis.

atrophic (ah-trof'ik) pertaining to or characterized by atrophy.

atrophie (at-ro-fe') [Fr.] atrophy. **a. blanche** (blahnsh) [Fr. "white atrophy"], a condition characterized by ivory-white, smooth, atrophic scar tissue with telangiectasia within a hyperpigmented areola, usually occurring on the ankles of middle-aged women. **a. noire** (nwahr) [Fr. "black atrophy"], a condition characterized by ulcers surrounded by areas of blue-black pigmentation on the ankles, the pigmentation occurring after recurrent attacks of dermatitis with ulceration.

atrophied (at'ro-fēd) marked by atrophy; shrunken.

atroph(o)- [Gr. *atrophia* want of nourishment] a combining form pertaining to atrophy.

atrophoderma (at"ro-fo-der'mah) [*atropho-* + Gr. *derma* skin] atrophy of the skin or of any part of it. Called also *atrophia cutis* and *atrophodermia.* See also *anetoderma.* **a. biotrip'ticum,** senile atrophy of skin. **idiopathic a. of Pasini and Pierini,** see *a. of Pasini and Pierini.* **a. macula'tum,** anetoderma. **a. neurit'icum,** glossy skin. **a. of Pasini and Pierini,** a condition most commonly occurring on the trunk, especially the back, of young women, characterized by the development of soft, bluish brown to violaceous atrophic plaques with central induration that resemble the lesions of the late stages of morphea. The etiology is unknown, and it usually resolves spontaneously after months or years. Two types have been suggested: one idiopathic and one closely related to or the same as morphea. **a. pigmento'sum** (*obs.*), xeroderma pigmentosum. **a. reticula'tum symmet'ricum facie'i,** folliculitis ulerythematosa reticulata. **a. seni'le,** senile atrophy of skin. **a. vermicula'ris,** atrophodermia vermiculata.

atrophodermatosis (at-ro"fo-der-mah-to'sis) any skin disease having cutaneous atrophy as a prominent symptom.

atrophodermia (at"ro-fo-der'me-ah) [*a-* + *tropho-* + *derm-* + *-ia*] atrophoderma. **a. vermicula'ta,** a group of genodermatoses chiefly characterized by inflammation and later by a reticulated honeycomb- or wormlike follicular atrophy, often accompanied by erythema and follicular plugging, which are transmitted as an autosomal recessive trait, and are usually seen in children and young adults. The lesions are usually confined to the cheeks (*folliculitis ulerythematosa reticulata*) but they may primarily involve the forehead and eyebrow region (*ulerythema orphryogenes*) and from there may spread to the scalp. Called also *atrophoderma reticularis.*

atrophy (at'ro-fe) [L., Gr. *atrophia*] 1. a wasting away; a diminution in the size of a cell, tissue, organ, or part. See also *atrophia* and *atrophie.* 2. to undergo atrophy, or to cause atrophy. **acute yellow a.,** massive hepatic necrosis. **Aran-Duchenne muscular a.,** spinal muscular a. **arthritic a.,** wasting of the muscles and bone that surround a joint, due to injury or to constitutional disease. **black**

a., atrophie noire. **blue a.,** a blue pigmentation that sometimes follows self-injection of drugs by individuals addicted to their use. **bone a.,** resorption of bone evident both in external form and in internal density. Cf. *osteoporosis.* **brown a.,** atrophy in which the affected viscus assumes a brownish hue, due to intracellular accumulation of lipofuscin; it is seen chiefly in the heart, liver, and spleen of the aged. **Charcot-Marie a., Charcot-Marie-Tooth a.,** progressive neuropathic (peroneal) muscular a. **circumscribed cerebral a.,** Pick's disease, def. 1. **compensatory a.,** atrophy, particularly of an endocrine organ, following excessive exogenous supply of its normal secretion or excessive secretion by its paired organ. **compression a.,** atrophy of a part due to constant pressure. **concentric a.,** atrophy of a hollow organ in which its cavity is contracted. **convolutional a.,** Pick's disease, def. 1. **correlated a.,** the wasting of a part following the destruction or removal of a correlated part. **corticostriatospinal a.,** Creutzfeldt-Jakob syndrome. **Cruveilhier's a.,** spinal muscular atrophy. **degenerative a.,** the wasting of a part due to a degeneration of its cells. **Dejerine-Sottas type of a.,** progressive hypertrophic interstitial neuropathy. **Dejerine-Thomas a.,** olivopontocerebellar a. **denervated muscle a.,** muscular atrophy resulting from severance of the motor nerve supplying the muscle. **a. of disuse,** wasting caused by lack of normal exercise of a part. **Duchenne-Aran muscular a.,** spinal muscular a. **eccentric a.,** atrophy of a hollow organ in which the size of the cavity is increased. **Eichhorst's a.,** the femorotibial form of progressive muscular atrophy with contraction of the toes; called also *Eichhorst's type.* **endocrine a.,** atrophy in organs that are dependent upon endocrine stimulation for the maintenance of their normal structure, occurring when their tropic hormone stimulation diminishes or is absent. **endometrial a.,** atrophy of the endometrium occurring physiologically at menopause or pathologically before menopause, and accompanied by absence of menstrual flow and shrinkage of the uterus. **Erb's a.,** pseudohypertrophic muscular dystrophy. **exhaustion a.,** atrophy of an endocrine organ presumably caused by prolonged overwork of that organ. **facial a.,** progressive unilateral facial a. **facioscapulohumeral muscular a.,** Landouzy-Dejerine dystrophy. **fatty a.,** fatty infiltration following atrophy of the tissue elements of a part; called also *adipositas ex vacuo.* **Fazio-Londe a.,** progressive bulbar paralysis in children; see *bulbar paralysis,* under *paralysis.* **gastric a.,** a condition in which the thickness of the mucosa of the stomach is greatly reduced, with complete or almost complete disappearance of the gastric and pyloric glands and their replacement by simple mucus-secreting epithelium and by extensive intestinal metaplasia. **granular a. of kidney,** chronic interstitial inflammation of the kidney producing compression and atrophy of the parenchyma. **gray a.,** secondary optic a. **gyrate a. of choroid and retina,** an autosomal recessive form of tapetoretinal degeneration marked by ring-shaped areas of thinning in the periphery of the fundus which enlarge and become confluent, resulting in tunnel vision; night blindness and other disturbances of vision follow. **healed yellow a.,** postnecrotic cirrhosis. **hemifacial a.,** atrophy of one side of the face. **hemilingual a.,** atrophy of one side of the tongue. **Hoffmann's a.,** Werdnig-Hoffmann paralysis. **Hunt's a.,** neuropathic atrophy of the small muscles of the hand unattended by sensory disturbance. **idiopathic muscular a.,** progressive muscular dystrophy. **infantile a.,** marasmus. **inflammatory a.,** atrophy of the functioning part of an organ caused by overgrowth of the fibrous elements from inflammation. **interstitial a.,** absorption of the mineral matter of bones, so that only the reticulated portion remains. **a. of iris, essential,** a progressive disease of unknown etiology, marked by patchy degeneration and disappearance of the iris stroma followed by loss of epithelium and formation of holes in the iris; it is associated with severe glaucoma. **ischemic muscular a.,** Volkmann's contracture. **juvenile muscular a.,** pseudohypertrophic muscular dystrophy. **lactation a.,** hyperinvolution of the uterus which may follow prolonged lactation. **Landouzy-Dejerine a.,** Landouzy-Dejerine dystrophy. **leaping a.,** progressive muscular atrophy beginning in the hand and extending to the shoulder without affecting the muscles of the arm. **Leber's optic a.,** a hereditary disorder of males characterized by bilateral progressive optic atrophy, with onset usually at about the age of twenty. It is thought to be an X-linked trait. **linear a.,** striae atrophicae. **lobar a.,** Pick's disease, def. 1. **macular a.,** anetoderma. **muscular a.,** a wasting of muscle tissue; there are many kinds and causes. See also *spinal muscular a.* **myelopathic muscular a.,** muscular atrophy due to lesion of the spinal cord, as in spinal muscular atrophy. **myopathic a.,** muscular atrophy due to disease of the muscle tissue. **neural a.,** neuropathic a. **neuritic muscular a.,** neuropathic a. **neuropathic a.,** atrophy of muscular tissue due to disease of the peripheral nervous system; called also *neural a.* **neurotic a.,** neuropathic a. **neurotrophic a.,** atrophy attributed to destruction of the peripheral neurons that maintain the nutrition of a tissue. **numeric a.,** atrophy due to diminution in the number of the constituent elements of a tissue, as well as shrinkage of those that remain. **olivopontocerebellar a.,** atrophy affecting the cerebellar cortex, the middle peduncles, and the inferior olivary bodies. **optic a.,** atrophy of the optic disk resulting from degeneration of the nerve fibers of the optic nerve and optic tract. **optic a., primary,** a form in which the optic disk is characterized by sharp margins, enlarged physiologic cup, enhanced visibility of the lamina cribrosa, and a white color. **optic a., secondary,** a form in which the optic disk is characterized by blurred margins, poor visibility of the lamina cribrosa, filling-in of the physiologic cup, and gray-white glial tissue on its surface and along its blood vessels; called also *gray a.* **pallidal a.,** juvenile paralysis agitans (of Hunt); see under *paralysis.* **Parrot's a. of the newborn,** primary infantile atrophy or marasmus. **pathologic a.,** a decrease in the size of tissues or organs beyond the range of normal variability. **periodontal a.,** reduction of the size of the alveolar process, associated with recession of the gingiva with subsequent exposure of the root surface. **peroneal a.,** progressive neuropathic (peroneal) muscular a. **physiologic a.,** atrophy which affects certain organs in all individuals as part of the normal aging process. **pigmentary a.,** wasting marked by the deposit of pigment in the atrophied cells. **postmenopausal a.,** atrophy of various tissues, such as the genital mucosa, occurring after menopause. **post-traumatic a. of bone,** post-traumatic osteoporosis. **pressure a.,** decrease in the size of a tissue cell caused by excessive pressure. **progressive choroidal a.,** choroideremia. **progressive muscular a.,** spinal muscular a. **progressive neural muscular a., progressive neuromuscular a.,** progressive neuropathic (peroneal) muscular a. **progressive neuropathic (peroneal) muscular a.,** a hereditary form of muscular atrophy, beginning in the muscles supplied by the peroneal nerves, progressing slowly to involve the muscles of the hands and arms. Called also *peroneal a., Charcot-Marie-Tooth a.* or *disease, Charcot-Marie type, Tooth type,* and *progressive neural muscular (neuromuscular) a.* **progressive spinal muscular a.,** spinal muscular a. **progressive unilateral facial a.,** an affection attended by progressive wasting of the skin, tissues, and bone, often of the muscles of one side of the face. **pseudohypertrophic muscular a.,** pseudohypertrophic muscular dystrophy. **pulp a.,** a degenerative process of the dental pulp, characterized by a diminution in size and wasting away of pulpal cells, usually associated with an interference with nutrition. Called also *atrophic pulp degeneration.* **red a.,** atrophy, mainly of the liver, due to chronic congestion from valvular heart disease. **reversionary a.,** anaplasia. **rheumatic a.,** atrophy of muscles after an attack of rheumatism. **segmental dissoriation with brachial muscular a.,** see syringomelia. **senile a.,** the natural atrophy of tissues and organs occurring with advancing age. Called also *atrophia senilis.* Cf. *senile degeneration.* **senile a. of skin,** the mild atrophic changes in the epidermis and dermis that occur naturally with aging. Called also *atrophia cutis senilis, atrophoderma biotripticum,* and *atrophoderma senile.* See also *actinic elastosis,* under *elastosis.* **serous a.,** atrophy with the effusion of a serous fluid into the wasted tissues; wasting of fat. **simple a.,** atrophy due to a shrinkage in size of individual cells. **spinal muscular a.,** a progressive degenerative disease of the motor cells of the spinal cord. Beginning usually in the small muscles of the hands, but in some cases (scapulohumeral type) in those of the upper arm and shoulder, the atrophy progresses slowly to the muscles of the lower extremity. Called also *Aran-Duchenne muscular a., Aran-Duchenne disease, Duchenne-Aran muscular a., Duchenne-Aran disease, Cruveilhier's disease, Duchenne's dis-*

ease, and *progressive spinal muscular a.* **subacute a. of liver, subchronic a. of liver,** subacute hepatic necrosis. **Sudeck's a.,** post-traumatic osteoporosis. **Tooth's a.,** progressive neuropathic (peroneal) muscular atrophy. **toxic a.,** atrophy of an organ in the course of infectious diseases. **trophoneurotic a.,** atrophy due to disease of the nerves or of a center supplying a part. **unilateral facial a.,** progressive unilateral facial a. **vascular a.,** progressive loss of substance in cells and organs when the blood supply to that organ or tissue becomes reduced below a critical level. **Vulpian's a.,** scapulohumeral type of spinal muscular atrophy. **Werdnig-Hoffmann a.,** see under *paralysis.* **Werdnig-Hoffmann spinal muscular a.,** a progressive, infantile, autosomal recessive form of muscular dystrophy, usually occurring in siblings rather than in successive generations, and resulting from degeneration of the anterior horn cells of the spinal cord. It is marked by early onset (usually at about six months of age, but sometimes in fetal life), hypotonia and wasting of the muscles, complete flaccid paralysis, and death, usually in early life. Called also *Werdnig-Hoffmann disease.* **white a.,** 1. atrophy of a nerve, leaving only white connective tissue. 2. atrophie blanche. **yellow a.,** acute yellow a. **Zimmerlin's a.,** a hereditary form of progressive muscular atrophy, beginning in the upper part of the body; called also *Zimmerlin's type.*

atropine (at′ro-pēn) [USP] chemical name: *endo*-(+)-α-(hydroxymethyl)benzeneacetic acid 8-methyl-8-azabicyclo [3.2.1]oct-3-yl ester. An alkaloid, $C_{17}H_{23}NO_3$, derived from species of belladonna, hyoscyamus, or strammonium, or produced synthetically, and occurring as white crystals, usually needle-like, or as a white, crystalline powder. Atropine is an anticholinergic and is used chiefly as an antispasmodic to relax smooth muscles; to relieve the tremor and rigidity of parkinsonism; to increase the heart rate by blocking the vagus nerve; as an antidote for various toxic and anticholinesterase agents; and as an antisecretory, mydriatic, and cycloplegic. **a. methonitrate, a. methylnitrate,** methylatropine nitrate. **a. oxide hydrochloride,** a salt of atropine, having the same actions as atropine. **a. sulfate** [USP], colorless crystals or white, crystalline powder, $(C_{17}H_{23}NO_3)_2 \cdot H_2SO_4 \cdot H_2O$, having the same actions as the base; administered parenterally and orally as an anticholinergic, intravenously as a cholinesterase inhibitor, and applied topically to the conjunctiva as a cycloplegic and mydriatic.

atropinic (at″ro-pin′ik) having actions similar to atropine, that is, antagonizing the muscarinic effects of acetylcholine.

atropinism (at′ro-pin-izm) poisoning caused by ingestion of atropine or belladonna or parts or preparations of any of the plants from which the drugs are derived; the symptoms include excessive dryness of the mouth and throat, dilation of the pupils, fever, rapid pulse, flushing of the face, confusion, mania, and hallucinations, and sometimes a skin rash.

atropinization (at-ro″pin-i-za′shun) subjection to the influence of atropine.

atropism (at′ro-pizm) atropinism.

Atropisol (at′ro-pĭ-sol) trademark for preparations of atropine sulfate.

A.T.S. American Thoracic Society; antitetanic serum.

attachment (ah-tach′ment) 1. the state of being fixed or attached. 2. a connection by which one thing is attached to another. 3. a device for retention and stabilization of a dental prothesis. **edgewise a.,** see under *appliance.* **epithelial a. (of Gottlieb),** a band or wedge of epithelium, the external surface of which adheres to the crown and the internal surface of the lamina propria of the free gingiva, and forming a peripheral cuff that seals the periodontal tissue and protects it from foreign material in the oral cavity. **extracoronal a.,** a precision attachment in which the retaining mechanism is outside the crown of an abutment tooth or restoration. **friction a., internal a.,** intracoronal a. **intracoronal a.,** a precision attachment with a cryptlike unit or slot (female part) built entirely into the crown and an insert or flange (male part) that extends from the prosthesis proper and fits into the slot when the denture is attached to the crown; the flange may be retained by friction between the parallel surfaces of the male and female parts together, or it may be augmented by mechanical locks, screws, or adjustable latches. Called also *friction a., internal a., key-and-keyway a., parallel a., precision a., slotted a.* **key-and-keyway a.,**

parallel a., intracoronal a. **orthodontic a.,** see *bracket* (def. 2). **precision a.,** 1. a device using a precision rest (q.v.) to attach fixed or removable partial dentures to the crown of an abutment tooth or a restoration. One type is the intracoronal attachment and the other is the extracoronal attachment. Called also *precision anchorage.* See also *extracoronal a., intracoronal a.,* and *semiprecision a.* 2. intracoronal a. **semiprecision a.,** attachment of a denture to an abutment tooth or a restoration by a semiprecision rest, (q.v.), sometimes supplemented by a spring-loaded plunger or clip, fitting into a rest seat on the lateral surface of a crown, which is especially deepened to provide added retention. **slotted a.,** intracoronal a.

attack (ah-tak′) an episode or onset of illness. **anxiety a.,** panic a. **panic a.,** an episode of acute intense anxiety, the essential feature of panic disorder (q.v.); panic attacks may also occur in agoraphobia and other phobias and in somatization disorder, schizophrenic disorders, and major depression. Called also *anxiety a.* **transient ischemic a. (TIA),** a brief attack (from a few minutes to hours) of cerebral dysfunction of vascular origin, with no persistent neurological deficit; TIAs are most commonly associated with occlusive vascular disease, especially in the distribution of the carotid and vertebral-basilar systems. **vagal a.,** vasovagal a. **vasovagal a.,** a transient vascular and neurogenic reaction marked by pallor, nausea, sweating, bradycardia, and rapid fall in arterial blood pressure which, when below a critical level, results in loss of consciousness and characteristic electroencephalographic changes. It is most often evoked by emotional stress associated with fear or pain. Called also *vasovagal* or *vasodepressor syncope,* and *Gower's syndrome.*

attar (at′ar) [Persian "essence"] any essential or volatile oil of vegetable origin. **a. of roses,** rose oil.

attention (ah-ten′shun) 1. selective awareness of a part or aspect of the environment. 2. selective responsiveness to one class of stimuli.

attenuant (ah-ten′u-ant) 1. causing thinness, as of the blood. 2. a medicine that thins the blood.

attenuate (ah-ten′u-āt) [L. *attenuare* to thin] 1. to render thin. 2. to render less virulent; see *attenuation,* def. 2.

attenuation (ah-ten″u-a′shun) [L. *attenuatio,* from *ad* to + *tenuis* thin] 1. the act of thinning or weakening. 2. the reduction of the virulence of a pathogenic organism, usually by adaptation to another host or to a different culture medium. 3. the process by which a beam of radiation is reduced in energy when passed through tissue or other material. Cf. *adsorption,* def. 3.

Attenuvax (ah-ten′u-vaks) trademark for a preparation of live attenuated measles virus vaccine.

attic (at′ik) [L. *atticus*] the superior part of the tympanic cavity, above the level of the tympanic membrane; called also *recessus epitympanicus* [NA], *epitympanum,* and *attic of middle ear.*

atticitis (at″ĭ-ki′tis) inflammation of the attic.

atticoantrotomy (at″ĭ-ko-an-trot′o-me) the operation of opening the mastoid antrum and the attic of the middle ear; called also *antroatticotomy.*

atticomastoid (at″ĭ-ko-mas′toid) pertaining to the attic and the mastoid process of the temporal bone.

atticotomy (at″ĭ-kot′o-me) [*attic* + Gr. *temnein* to cut] the surgical opening of the attic. **transmeatal a.,** removal through the external auditory meatus of the outer wall of the attic.

attitude (at′ĭ-tūd) [L. *attitudo* posture] 1. a posture or position of the body. In obstetrics, the relation of the various parts of the fetal body to one another, the normal attitude being one of moderate flexion of all the joints, with the back curved forward, the head slightly bent on the chest, and the arms and legs free to move in all natural directions (habitus). 2. a tendency to respond positively or negatively to other individuals, institutions, or programs of activity. **a. of combat** [Fr. *attitude de combat*], the stiff defensive position of the corpse of one burned to death in a conflagration. **deflexion a.,** the condition early in labor in which the fetal head lies over the pelvic inlet, the large fontanel is lower than the small one or is even with the root of the nose, and the eyes are palpable. **discobolus a.,** a position resembling that of a discus thrower, caused by stimulation of the semicircular canals. **forced a.,** an abnormal position or attitude due

to some disease, such as is seen in meningitis or as the result of contractures.

atto- [Danish *atten* eighteen] a combining form used in naming units of measurement to indicate one-quintillionth (10^{-18}) of the unit designated by the root with which it is combined. Symbol, a.

attollens (ah-tol′enz) [L.] lifting up. **a. au′rem** (obs.), musculus auricularis superior.

attractant (ah-trak′tant) [L. *attrahere* to draw toward] a substance that exerts an attracting influence, such as one used to attract insect or animal pests to traps or to poisons.

attraction (ah-trak′shun) [L. *attractus* past participle of *attrahere* to draw together] 1. the process of drawing one body toward another. 2. a condition in which the teeth or other maxillary and mandibular structures are higher than normal position, thereby causing shortening of the face. Cf. *abstraction,* def. 2. **a. of affinity,** chemical a. **capillary a.,** the force that attracts the particles of a fluid into and along the caliber of a tube. **chemical a.,** the tendency of atoms of one element to unite with those of another; called also *a. of affinity.* **electric a.,** the tendency of bodies bearing opposite electric charges to move toward each other. **magnetic a.,** the tendency of bodies possessing circulating electric currents to move toward each other.

attrahens (at′rah-henz) [L.] drawing toward. **a. au′rem** (obs.), musculus auricularis anterior.

attraxin (ah-trak′sin) Fischer's name for supposed specific bodies existing in solutions which, when the solution is injected into the tissues, exert a chemotactic influence on the epithelial cells.

attrition (ah-trish′un) [L. *attritio* a rubbing against] the physiologic wearing away of a substance or structure (such as the teeth) in the course of normal use.

at. vol. atomic volume.

At. wt. atomic weight.

atypia (a-tip′e-ah) the condition of being irregular or not conforming to type.

atypical (a-tip′ĭ-kal) [*a* neg. + Gr. *typos* type or model] irregular; not conformable to the type; in microbiology, applied specifically to strains of unusual type.

atypism (a-tip′izm) atypia.

A.U. Angström unit; aures unitas (both ears together) or auris uterque (each ear).

Au chemical symbol for *gold* (L. *au′rum*); abbreviation for Australian antigen (see under *antigen*).

A.U.A. American Urological Association.

Au-antigenemia (an″tĭ-jĕ-ne′me-ah) hepatitis B antigenemia.

Aub-Dubois table (awb-doo-bois′) [Joseph Charles *Aub,* Boston physician, 1890–1973; Eugene Floyd *Dubois,* New York physician, 1882–1953] see under *table.*

Aubert's phenomenon (o-bārz′) [Hermann *Aubert,* German physiologist, 1826–1892] see under *phenomenon.*

Auchmeromyia (awk″mer-o-mi′yah) a genus of flies of the family Calliphoridae. **A. lute′ola,** a fly of the Congo and Nigeria having a blood-sucking larva known as the Congo floor maggot; called also *Musca luteola.*

audile (aw′dĭl) pertaining to hearing; understanding or recalling most readily what has been heard. Cf. *visile.*

audi(o)- [L. *audire* to hear] a combining form denoting relationship to hearing.

audioanalgesia (aw″de-o-an″al-je′ze-ah) alleged reduction or abolition of pain accomplished by listening, through a stereophonic head set, to recorded music to which may be added a background sound, so-called "white noise."

audiogenic (aw″de-o-jen′ik) produced by sound.

audiogram (aw′de-o-gram″) [L. *audire* to hear + Gr. *gramma* a writing] a record of the thresholds of hearing of an individual for various sound frequencies. **cortical a.,** a graphic representation of the result of cortical audiometry.

audiologist (aw″de-ol′o-jist) a person skilled in audiology, including the rehabilitation of those whose impaired hearing cannot be improved by medical or surgical means.

audiology (aw″de-ol′o-je) [L. *audire* to hear + *-logy*] the science of hearing, particularly the study of impaired hearing that cannot be improved by medication or surgical therapy.

audiometer (aw″de-om′ĕ-ter) [L. *audire* to hear + Gr. *metron* measure] an electronic device that produces acoustic stimuli of known frequency and intensity for the measurement of hearing. **evoked response a.,** an instrument that detects response to sound stimuli by changes in the electroencephalogram.

audiometric (aw″de-o-met′rik) pertaining to the measurement of hearing, as by means of an audiometer.

audiometrician (aw″de-o-mĕ-trish′an) a technician specializing in the measurement of hearing ability (audiometry).

audiometry (aw″de-om′ĕ-tre) measurement of hearing, as by means of an audiometer. **Békésy a.,** audiometry in which the patient, by pressing a signal button, traces his monaural thresholds for pure tones: the intensity of the tone decreases as long as the button is depressed and increases when it is released. Both continuous and interrupted tones are used. **cortical a.,** an objective method of determining auditory acuity by recording and averaging electric potentials evoked from the cortex of the brain in response to stimulation by pure tones. **electrocochleographic a.,** measurement of electrical potentials from the middle ear or external auditory canal (cochlear microphonics and eighth nerve action potentials) in response to acoustic stimuli. **electrodermal a.,** audiometry in which the subject is conditioned by harmless electric shock to pure tones; thereafter he anticipates a shock when he hears a pure tone, the anticipation resulting in a brief electrodermal response, which is recorded. The lowest intensity at which the response is elicited is taken to be his hearing threshold. **localization a.,** a technique for measuring the capacity to locate the source of a pure tone received binaurally in a sound field. **pure tone a.,** audiometry utilizing pure tones that are relatively free of noise and overtones. **speech a.,** that in which the threshold of speech perception (speech reception threshold) in decibels and the ability to understand speech (speech discrimination) are measured.

audiovisual (aw″de-o-vizh′u-al) simultaneously stimulating, or pertaining to simultaneous stimulation of, the senses of both hearing and sight.

audition (aw-dish′un) [L. *auditio*] the act of hearing; ability to hear. **chromatic a., a. colorée,** a sensation of color produced by sound; a variety of chromesthesia. **gustatory a.,** a condition in which certain sounds call up a sensation of taste.

auditive (aw′dĭ-tiv) a person in whom the prime sense is hearing.

auditognosis (aw″dĭ-tog-no′sis) [L. *auditio* hearing + Gr. *gnōsis* knowledge] the sense by which sounds are understood and interpreted.

auditory (aw′dĭ-to″re) [L. *auditorius*] pertaining to the sense of hearing.

Audouin's microsporon (ow-doo-anz′) [Jean-Victor *Audouin*, Parisian physician, 1797–1841] *Microsporum audouini.*

Auenbrugger's sign (ow-en-broog′erz) [Leopold Elder von *Auenbrugger*, Austrian physician, 1722–1809] see under *sign.*

Auer's bodies (ow′erz) [John *Auer*, American physician, 1875–1948] see under *body.*

Auerbach's ganglion, plexus (ow′er-bahks) [Leopold *Auerbach*, German anatomist, 1828–1897] see under *ganglion*, and see *plexus myentericus.*

Aufrecht's sign (owf′rekhts) [Emanual *Aufrecht*, German physician, 1844–1933] see under *sign.*

augmentor (awg-men′tor) 1. increasing; a term applied to nerves or nerve cells concerned in increasing the size and force of heart contractions. 2. a substance supposed to increase the action of an auxetic.

augnathus (awg-na′thus) [Gr. *au* again + *gnathos* jaw] a monster with a double lower jaw.

Aujeszky's disease (aw-jes′kēz) [Aladár *Aujeszky*, Hungarian physician, 1869–1933] pseudorabies.

aula (aw′lah) [L.; Gr. *aulē* hall] 1. (*obs.*) the anterior end of the third ventricle of the cerebrum. 2. the red erythematous areola formed about the periphery of the vesicle of the vaccination lesion.

auliplexus (aw-lĕ-plek′sus) [*aula* + *plexus*] (*obs.*) a part of the choroid plexus within the aula (def. 1).

aulix (aw′liks) [L. "furrow"] (*obs.*) sulcus hypothalamicus.

aura (aw′rah), pl. *au′rae* [L. "breath"] a subjective sensa-

tion or motor phenomenon that precedes and marks the onset of a paroxysmal attack, such as an epileptic attack (Galen). **a. asthmat′ica,** premonitory symptoms preceding an attack of bronchial asthma. **auditory a.,** an auditory sensation that sometimes precedes an attack of epilepsy. **electric a.,** a breezy sensation experienced on the receipt of a discharge of static electricity. **epigastric a.,** an uncomfortable sensation in the epigastrium that sometimes precedes an epileptic attack. **epileptic a.,** a sensation that sometimes gives warning of an approaching attack of epilepsy. **a. hyster′ica,** an aura like that preceding an epileptic attack sometimes experienced by hysterical patients. **intellectual a.,** a dreamy condition that sometimes precedes an attack of epilepsy; called also *reminiscent a.* **kinesthetic a.,** a sensation of movement of some part of the body, with or without such actual movement. **motor a.,** movement that precedes an epileptic attack. **a. procursi′va,** a spell of running that precedes an epileptic attack. **reminiscent a.,** intellectual a.

aural (aw′ral) 1. [L. *auris*, q.v.] pertaining to or perceived by the ear, as an aural stimulus. 2. [L. *aura*, q.v.] pertaining to or of the nature of an aura.

auranofin (aw-rān′o-fin) chemical name: (2,3,4,6-tetra-*O*-acetyl-1-thio-β-D-glucopyranosato-*S*) (triethylphosphine)-gold; an antirheumatic, $C_{20}H_{34}AuO_9PS$.

aurantia (aw-ran′she-ah) an orange coal tar stain, the ammonium salt of hexanitrodiphenylamine, $C_6H_2(NO_2)_3 \cdot N:C_6H_2(NO_2)_2 \cdot N \cdot O \cdot O \cdot NH_4$; used in staining mitochondria.

aurantiamarin (aw-ran″te-am′ah-rin) a glycoside from orange peel.

aurantiasis (aw″ran-ti′ah-sis) [L. *aurantium* orange + *-iasis*] carotenemia.

Aurelia (aw-rel′ĭ-ah) a genus of large discophorous jellyfish found in Atlantic, Indian, and Pacific waters; nematocysts of many of the larger forms can penetrate the human skin and produce intense pain.

Aureobasidium (aw-re″o-bah-sid′ĭ-um) a genus of imperfect fungi of the family Dematiaceae, order Moniliales, which produce black yeastlike cells; called also *Pullularia.* **A. pul′lulans,** a common soil organism and contaminant; called also *Pullularia pullans.*

aureolin (aw-re′o-lin) a yellow dye.

Aureomycin (aw″re-o-mi′sin) trademark for preparations of crystalline chlortetracycline hydrochloride.

aures (aw′rēz) [L.] plural of *auris.*

auri- [L. *auris* ear] a combining form denoting relationship to the ear.

auriasis (aw-ri′ah-sis) chrysiasis, def. 1.

auric (aw′rik) pertaining to or containing gold.

auricle (aw′rĕ-kl) [L. *auricula* a little ear] 1. the portion of the external ear not contained within the head; the pinna, or flap of the ear. Called also *auricula.* 2. auricula atrii. The term *auricle* was formerly used to designate an atrium of the heart. **cervical a.,** a flap of skin and yellow cartilage sometimes seen on the side of the neck at the external opening of a persistent branchial cleft. **left a. of heart,** auricula atrii sinistri. **right a. of heart,** auricula atrii dextri.

auricula (aw-rik′u-lah), pl. *auric′ulae* [L., dim. of *auris*] a little ear; the NA term for the portion of the external ear not contained within the head; the pinna, or flap of the ear. Called also *ala auris* and *auricle.* Applied also to the ear-shaped appendage of either atrium of the heart (*auricula atrii*), and formerly used as a synonym for the atrium (*atrium cordis*). **a. a′trii** [NA], the ear-shaped appendage of either atrium of the heart; called also *atrial appendage.* **a. a′trii dex′tri** [NA], the ear-shaped appendage of the right atrium of the heart. **a. a′trii sinis′tri** [NA], the ear-shaped appendage of the left atrium of the heart. **a. cor′dis,** a. atrii. **a. dex′tra cor′dis,** a. atrii dextri. **a. sinis′tra cor′dis,** a. atrii sinistri.

auriculae (aw-rik′u-le) [L.] genitive and plural of *auricula.*

auricular (aw-rik′u-lar) [L. *auricularis*] pertaining to an auricle or to the ear, and, formerly, to an atrium of the heart.

auriculare (aw-rik″u-la′re) [L. *auricularis* pertaining to the ear] a craniometric point at the top of the opening of the external auditory meatus.

auricularis (aw″rik-u-la′ris) [L.] pertaining to the ear; auricular.

auriculocranial (aw-rik″u-lo-kra′ne-al) pertaining to an ear and the cranium.

auriculotemporal (aw-rik″u-lo-tem′pŏ-ral) pertaining to an ear and the temporal region.

auriculotherapy (aw-rik″u-lo-ther′ah-pe) electrical stimulation of the outer ear for the relief of pain.

auriculoventricular (aw-rik″u-lo-ven-trik′u-lar) a former term for atrioventricular.

aurid (aw′rid) [L. *aurum* gold] a skin eruption produced by the systemic administration of gold salts.

auriform (aw′rĭ-form) ear-shaped.

aurin (aw′rin) chemical name: 4-[bis(*p*-hydroxyphenyl)methylene]-2,5-cyclohexadien-1-one. A triphenylmethane derivative, $C_{19}H_{14}O_3$, occurring as deep red masses with a greenish metallic luster; used as an indicator and dye intermediate. Called also *pararosolic acid, rosolic acid,* and *corallin.*

aurinarium (aw″ri-na′re-um) a medicated suppository for insertion onto the external auditory meatus.

aurinasal (aw″rĭ-na′zal) pertaining to the ear and the nose.

auripigment (aw″rĭ-pig′ment) arsenic trisulfide.

auris (aw′ris), pl. *au′res* [L.] [NA] the ear; the organ of hearing. See Plate 15. **a. exter′na** [NA], external ear: the portion of the auditory organ comprising the auricle and the external acoustic meatus. **a. inter′na** [NA], internal ear: the labyrinth, comprising the vestibule, cochlea, and semicircular canals; called also *inner ear.* **a. me′dia** [NA], middle ear: the cavity in the temporal bone comprising the cavitas tympanica, adnexa mastoidea, and tuba auditiva. Formerly, the terms *auris media* and *cavitas tympanica* (*cavum tympani*) were regarded as being synonymous.

auriscope (aw′rĭ-skōp) [L. *auris* ear + Gr. *skopein* to examine] a form of otoscope.

aurist (aw′rist) a specialist in ear diseases.

auristics (aw-ris′tiks) [L. *auris* ear] the art of treating diseases of the ear.

aurochromoderma (aw″ro-kro″mo-der′mah) [L. *aurum* gold + Gr. *chrōma* color + Gr. *derma* skin] a permanent greenish-blue staining of the skin due to injection of certain gold compounds.

aurotherapy (aw″ro-ther′ah-pe) chrysotherapy.

aurothioglucose (aw″ro-thi″o-gloo′kōs) [USP] chemical name: (1-thio-D-glucopyranosato)gold. A monovalent gold salt, $C_6H_{11}AuO_5S$, used in the treatment of early active rheumatoid arthritis not controlled by nonsteroidal anti-inflammatory agents, rest, and physical therapy.

aurothiomalate disodium (aw″ro-thi″o-ma′lāt) gold sodium thiomalate.

aurum (aw′rum) [L.] gold.

auscult (aws-kult′) auscultate.

auscultate (aws′kul-tāt) [L. *auscultare* to listen to] to examine by listening, usually to the sounds of the thoracic or abdominal viscera, with or without a stethoscope.

auscultation (aws″kul-ta′shun) the act of listening for sounds within the body, chiefly for ascertaining the condition of the lungs, heart, pleura, abdomen and other organs, and for the detection of pregnancy. **direct a., immediate a.,** auscultation performed without the stethoscope. **Korányi's a.,** auscultatory percussion done by tapping with one forefinger the second joint of the other forefinger applied perpendicularly to the part; called also *Korányi's percussion.* **mediate a.** (Laennec, 1819), auscultation performed by the aid of an instrument (stethoscope) interposed between the ear and the part being examined. **obstetric a.,** auscultation in pregnancy for the study of the sounds of the fetal heart.

auscultatory (aws-kul′tah-to″re) of or pertaining to auscultation.

auscultoplectrum (aws-kul″to-plek′trum) an instrument for use both in auscultation and percussion.

auscultoscope (aws-kul′to-skōp) phonendoscope.

Austin Flint murmur, respiration (aws′tin flint) [*Austin Flint*, American physiologist, 1812–1886] see *Flint's murmur*, under *murmur*, and *cavernous respiration*, under *respiration.*

Australorbis (aws″trah-lor′bis) *Biomphalaria.*

autacoid (aw′tah-koid) [aut- + Gr. *akos* remedy] a term once proposed to replace the term *hormone* and recently suggested as a general term for various physiologically active, endogenous substances (histamine, serotonin, angiotensin, prostaglandins, etc.) that do not yet fit into existing functional classifications.

autarcesis (awt-ar′se-sis) [aut- + Gr. *arkein* to ward off] (*obs.*) the power to resist infection by the normal activity of the body cells as distinguished from immunity of the antibody type.

autarcetic (awt-ar-set′ik) pertaining to autarcesis.

autechoscope (aw-tek′o-skōp) [aut- + Gr. *ēchos* sound + Gr. *skopein* to examine] an instrument for auscultating one's own body.

autecic (aw-te′sik) autoecious.

autecious (aw-te′shus) autoecious.

autecology (aw″te-kol′o-je) [aut- + *ecology*] the ecology of an organism as an individual; cf. *synecology.*

autemesia (aw″tĕ-me′se-ah) [aut- + Gr. *emesis* vomiting] functional or idiopathic vomiting.

autism (aw′tizm) [Gr. *autos* self + -*ism*] 1. autistic thinking; preoccupation with inner thoughts, daydreams, fantasies, delusions, and hallucinations; egocentric, subjective thinking lacking objectivity and connection with reality. The self often predominates to the total exclusion of that which is not self. Used interchangeably with *dereism*, although differing in emphasis. 2. autistic disorder. **akinetic a.,** coma vigil. **early infantile a., infantile a.,** autistic disorder. **infantile a.,** see *autistic disorder*, under *disorder.*

autistic (aw-tis′tik) characterized by or pertaining to autism.

aut(o)- [Gr. *autos* self] a prefix denoting relationship to self.

autoactivation (aw″to-ak″tĭ-va′shun) the activation of a gland by its own secretion.

autoagglutination (aw″to-ah-gloo″tĭ-na′shun) 1. clumping or agglutination of an individual's cells by his own serum, as in autohemagglutination. 2. nonspecific clumping or agglutination of particulate antigens (e.g., bacteria) that does not involve antibody; an important cause of error in bacterial agglutination tests.

autoagglutinin (aw″to-ah-gloo″tĭ-nin) an autologous serum factor with the property of agglutinating the individual's own cellular elements.

autoallergic (aw′to-ah-ler′jik) pertaining to or characterized by autoallergy.

autoallergy (aw″to-al′er-je) autoimmunity.

autoamputation (aw″to-am″pu-ta′shun) the spontaneous detachment from the body and elimination of an appendage or of an abnormal growth, such as a polyp.

autoanalysis (aw″to-ah-nal′ĭ-sis) psychoanalysis of oneself; investigation of one's own psychic components.

autoanamnesis (aw″to-an″am-ne′sis) a history obtained from the patient himself.

autoanaphylaxis (aw″to-an″ah-fĭ-lak′sis) (*obs.*) autoimmunity.

autoantibody (aw″to-an′tĭ-bod″e) an antibody directed against a self antigen, i.e., against a normal tissue constituent. An antibody (immunoglobulin) formed in response to, and reacting against, one of the individual's own normal antigenic endogenous body constituents.

autoanticomplement (aw″to-an″tĭ-kom′ple-ment) an anticomplement formed in the body against its own complement.

autoantigen (aw″to-an″tĭ-jen) an antigen that, despite being a normal tissue constituent, is the target of a humoral or cell-mediated immune response, as in autoimmune disease. Called also *self antigen.*

autoantisepsis (aw″to-an″tĭ-sep′sis) physiological antisepsis.

autoantitoxin (aw″to-an″tĭ-tok′sin) [auto- + *antitoxin*] antitoxin produced by the animal itself, as opposed to exogenous antitoxin.

autoaudible (aw″to-aw′dĭ-bl) audible to one's self; said of heart sounds.

autobacteriophage (aw″to-bak-te′re-o-fāj) bacteriophage derived from the patient under treatment.

autobiotic (aw″to-bi-ot′ik) any of a group of substances produced by cells and controlling the behavior of the producing cells.

autoblast (aw′to-blast) an independent solitary bioblast; a microorganism.

autobody (aw′to-bod″e) an antibody that both carries an idiotypic determinant that is stereochemically similar to the epitope on the antigen against which the antibody was originally directed and at the same time expresses a binding site for the antigen; autobodies therefore have the potential for self-aggregation.

autocatalysis (aw″to-kah-tal′ĭ-sis) a catalytic reaction that gradually accelerates in velocity because some of the products of the reaction themselves act as catalytic agents.

autocatalyst (aw″to-kat′ah-list) an element participating in autocatalysis.

autocatalytic (aw″to-kat-ah-lit′ik) pertaining to, characterized by, or producing autocatalysis.

autocatharsis (aw″to-kah-thar′sis) psychiatric treatment by encouraging the patient to write down his thoughts, feelings, and experiences and thus rid himself of disturbing emotions.

autocatheterism (aw″to-kath′ĕ-ter-izm) [auto- + catheterism] the passage of the catheter by the patient himself.

autocholecystectomy (aw″to-ko″le-sis-tek′to-me) [auto- + cholecystectomy] invagination of the gallbladder into the intestine, with final separation and expulsion of the organ.

autochthonous (aw-tok′tho-nus) [Gr. autochthōn sprung from the land itself] 1. found in the place of formation; not removed to a new site. 2. denoting a tissue graft to a new site on the same individual. Cf. heterochthonous.

autocinesis (aw″to-si-ne′sis) [auto- + Gr. kinēsis motion] autokinesis.

autoclasia (aw″to-kla′ze-ah) [auto- + Gr. klasis breaking] (obs.) a self-perpetuating destructive process in which an autoimmune reaction causes breakdown of tissue, liberating more antigen, which in turn elicits the formation of more autoantibody, and so on.

autoclasis (aw-tok′lah-sis) [auto- + Gr. klasis breaking] destruction of a part by influences developed within itself.

autoclave (aw′to-klāv) [auto- + L. clavis key] an apparatus for effecting sterilization by steam under pressure; it is fitted with a gauge that automatically regulates the pressure, and therefore the degree of heat to which the contents are subjected.

Autoclip (aw′to-klip) trademark for a stainless steel surgical clip for wound closing inserted by means of a mechanical applicator that automatically feeds a series of clips.

autocondensation (aw″to-kon-den-sa′shun) (obs.) application of high-frequency currents to the entire body for therapeutic purposes in which the patient constitutes one plate of a condenser. Rarely employed today.

autoconduction (aw″to-kon-duk′shun) a method of applying high-frequency currents by electromagnetic induction in which the patient placed inside a large solenoid constitutes the secondary of a transformer. Though not employed in the U.S., this procedure is still used in treatment of psychoses in the U.S.S.R.

autocystoplasty (aw″to-sis′to-plas″te) a plastic operation on the bladder using grafts from the patient's body.

autocytolysin (aw″to-si-tol′ĭ-sin) autolysin.

autocytolysis (aw″to-si-tol′ĭ-sis) autolysis.

autocytolytic (aw″to-si″to-lit′ik) autolytic.

autocytotoxin (aw″to-si″to-tok′sin) a cytotoxin for the cells of the body in which it is formed.

autodermic (aw″to-der′mik) [auto- + Gr. derma skin] of the patient's own skin; a term applied to skin grafts. See dermatoautoplasty and autograft.

autodestruction (aw″to-de-struk′shun) self-destruction, specifically that which certain enzymes undergo in solution.

autodigestion (aw″to-di-jes′chun) self-digestion; autolysis; applied especially to the digestion of the walls of the stomach and contiguous structures after death.

autodrainage (aw″to-drān′ij) drainage of an abscess or cavity by diversion of the fluid into a different channel or viscus within the patient's own body; this may be accomplished by surgery or may occur spontaneously.

autoecholalia (aw″to-ek″o-la′le-ah) [auto- + echolalia] parrot-like repetition of words and phrases initially uttered by the patient himself; seen in catatonic schizophrenia and in certain cerebral degenerative disorders.

autoecic (aw-te′sik) [auto- + Gr. oikos house] autoecious.

autoecious (aw″to-e′shus) [auto- + Gr. oikos house] pertaining to or denoting parasitic fungi that pass through their entire developmental cycle upon the same host. Cf. heteroecious.

autoeczematization (aw″to-ek-zem″ah-tĭ-za′shun) the spread, at first locally, and later more generally, of lesions from an originally circumscribed focus of eczema.

autoerotic (aw″to-e-rot′ik) pertaining to autoeroticism.

autoeroticism (aw″to-ĕ-rot′ĭ-sizm) sexual feeling directed toward oneself; cf. heteroeroticism.

autoerotism (aw″to-er′o-tizm) autoeroticism.

autoerythrophagocytosis (aw″to-ĕ-rith″ro-fag″o-si-to′sis) [auto- + erythrocyte + phagocytosis] phagocytosis of erythrocytes by autologous phagocytic cells (e.g., neutrophils, monocytes).

autofluorescence (aw″to-floo″o-res′ens) fluorescence in tissues produced by substances normally present in the tissues. Cf. secondary fluorescence, under fluorescence.

autofluoroscope (aw″to-floo′o-ro-skōp″) a type of scintillation camera that utilizes in its detector sodium iodide crystals packed in an array especially suited to the study of small tumors in large organs.

autofundoscope (aw″to-fun′do-skōp) [auto- + fundus + -scope] an instrument that makes use of the fact that by observing an illuminated blank space through a pin-perforated card, one can see faint images of the retinal vessels of one's own eyes.

autofundoscopy (aw″to-fun-dos′ko-pe) examination with the autofundoscope.

autogamous (aw-tog′ah-mus) characterized by self-fertilization.

autogamy (aw-tog′ah-me) [auto- + Gr. gamos marriage] 1. self-fertilization; fertilization within a cell itself by union of two chromatin masses derived from the same primary nucleus; called also automixis and syngamic nuclear union. Cf. endogamy (def. 1) and exogamy (def. 1). 2. a special case of syngamy in which the gametes are sister cells, resulting from the division of a single mother cell.

autogeneic (aw″to-jen-e′ik) autogenous; pertaining to an autograft.

autogenesis (aw″to-jen′ĕ-sis) [auto- + Gr. genesis production] self-generation; origination within the organism.

autogenetic (aw″to-jĕ-net′ik) pertaining to autogenesis.

autogenous (aw-toj′ĕ-nus) [auto- + genesis] self-generated, self-produced, autologous, endogenous; originating within an organism itself, as an autograft.

autograft (aw′to-graft) a graft of tissue derived from another site in or on the body of the organism receiving it; called also autologous or autochthonous graft, and autoplast.

autografting (aw″to-graft′ing) autotransplantation.

autogram (aw′to-gram) [auto- + Gr. gramma mark] a mark forming on the skin following pressure by a blunt instrument.

autohemagglutination (aw″to-hem″ah-gloo″tĭ-na′shun) agglutination of autologous erythrocytes.

autohemagglutinin (aw″to-hem-ah-gloo′tĭ-nin) a hemagglutinin that causes the clumping or agglutination of autologous erythrocytes.

autohemolysin (aw″to-he-mol′ĭ-sin) autoantibody causing complement-dependent lysis of autologous erythrocytes.

autohemolysis (aw″to-he-mol′ĭ-sis) hemolysis of the blood cells of a person by his own serum.

autohemolytic (aw″to-he″mo-lit′ik) pertaining to autohemolysis.

autohemotherapy (aw″to-he″mo-ther′ah-pe) [auto- + Gr. haima blood + therapeia treatment] treatment by reinjection of the individual's own blood.

autohemotransfusion (aw″to-he″mo-trans-fu′zhun) the withdrawal of a small amount of venous blood and reinjection directly into the same individual.

autohistoradiograph (aw″to-his″to-ra′de-o-graf) autoradiograph.

autohypnosis (aw″to-hip-no′sis) the act or process of hypnotizing oneself.

autohypnotic (aw″to-hip-not′ik) pertaining to autohypnosis.

autoimmune (aw″to-ĭ-mūn′) pertaining to autoimmunity.

autoimmunity (aw″to-ĭ-mu′nĭ-te) a condition characterized by a specific humoral or cell-mediated immune response against constituents of the body's own tissues (self antigens or autoantigens). See also *autoimmune disease.*

autoimmunization (aw″to-im″u-ni-za′shun) the induction in an individual of an immune response to its own tissue constituents, which may lead to pathological sequelae, *i.e.*, to autoimmune disease. Called also *autosensitization.* See also *autoantibody.*

autoinfection (aw″to-in-fek′shun) [*auto-* + *infection*] infection by an agent already present in the body, often the transferral of an agent from one part of the body to another.

autoinfusion (aw″to-in-fu′zhun) [*auto-* + *infusion*] the forcing of the blood toward the heart by bandaging the extremities, compression of the abdominal aorta, etc.

autoinoculable (aw″to-in-ok′u-lah-bl) [*auto-* + *inoculable*] susceptible of being inoculated with microorganisms from one's own body.

autoinoculation (aw″to-in-ok′u-la″shun) [*auto-* + *inoculation*] inoculation with microorganisms from one's own body.

autointerference (aw″to-in″ter-fer′ens) interference with the replication of a virus by an intact, attenuated, or inactivated virus of the same kind.

autointoxicant (aw″to-in-tok′sĭ-kant) a poison generated within the system.

autointoxication (aw″to-in-tok″sĭ-ka′shun) [*auto-* + *intoxication*] intoxication by some poison generated within the body.

autoisolysin (aw″to-i-sol′ĭ-sin) autoantibody that causes complement-dependent lysis of cells in the individual from which it was obtained, as well as those of other animals of the same species.

autokeratoplasty (aw″to-ker′ah-to-plas″te) [*auto-* + *keratoplasty*] corneal grafting with tissue from the patient's other eye.

autokinesis (aw″to-ki-ne′sis) [*auto-* + Gr. *kinēsis* motion] voluntary motion. **visible light a.,** see *autokinetic visible light phenomenon,* under *phenomenon.*

autokinetic (aw″to-ki-net′ik) having the power of voluntary motion.

autolavage (aw″to-lah-vahzh′) [*auto-* + *lavage*] lavage performed on one's self or on one's own stomach.

autolesion (aw″to-le′zhun) a self-inflicted injury.

autoleukoagglutinin (aw″to-loo″ko-ah-gloo′tĭ-nin) an antibody capable of agglutinating leukocytes of the same individual in which it is generated.

autologous (aw-tol′o-gus) [*auto-* + Gr. *logos* relation] autogenous; related to self; originating within an organism itself, as an autograft or autotransfusion.

autolysate (aw-tol′ĭ-sāt) a substance or substances produced by autolysis.

autolysin (aw-tol′ĭ-sin) autoantibody causing complement-dependent lysis of autologous cells; called also *autocytolysin.*

autolysis (aw-tol′ĭ-sis) [*auto-* + Gr. *lysis* dissolution] 1. the spontaneous disintegration of tissues or of cells by the action of their own autogenous enzymes, such as occurs after death and in some pathological conditions; called also *autodigestion, self-digestion,* and *autoproteolysis.* 2. the destruction of cells of the body by its own serum; called also *autocytolysis.* **postmortem a.,** enzymatic self-digestion of cells or tissues after death.

autolysosome (aw″to-li′so-sōm) a vacuolar element of the lysosome system of cells to which hydrolases have been added by fusion with lysosomes.

autolytic (aw-to-lit′ik) pertaining to or causing autolysis; autocytolytic.

autolyze (aw′to-līz) to undergo or to cause to undergo autolysis.

automatic (aw″to-mat′ik) [Gr. *automatos* self-acting] 1. spontaneous or involuntary; done by no act of the will. 2. self-moving; self-regulating.

automatin (aw-tom′ah-tin) an extract of bovine heart muscle formerly used in circulatory disorders.

automatism (aw-tom′ah-tizm) [Gr. *automatismos* self-action] aimless and apparently undirected behavior that is not under conscious control and is performed without conscious knowledge; seen in psychomotor epilepsy, catatonic schizophrenia, psychogenic fugue, and other conditions. Called also *automatic behavior.* **ambulatory a.,** a condition in which the patient walks about and performs acts mechanically and without consciousness of what he is doing. **command a.,** the performance of suggested acts without exercise of critical judgment; seen in catatonic schizophrenia and in the hypnotic state.

automatograph (aw″to-mat′o-graf) [Gr. *automatismos* self-action + *graphein* to write] an instrument for recording involuntary movements.

Autom′eris i′o the io moth that produces dermatitis (io-moth dermatitis) by means of irritant hairs on its larva.

automixis (aw″to-mik′sis) [*auto-* + Gr. *mixis* mixture] autogamy, def. 1.

automysophobia (aw″to-mi″so-fo′be-ah) [*auto-* + *mysophobia*] irrational fear of being unclean or smelling bad.

autonephrectomy (aw″to-nĕ-frek′to-me) [*auto-* + Gr. *nephros* kidney + Gr. *ektomē* excision] obliteration of a kidney as the result of disease.

autonephrotoxin (aw″to-nef″ro-tok′sin) a substance toxic to the cells of the kidney of the body in which it is formed.

autonomic (aw″to-nom′ik) self-controlling; functionally independent. See *autonomic nervous system,* under *system.*

autonomotropic (aw″to-nom-o-trop′ik) [*autonomic* + Gr. *tropos* a turning] having an affinity for the autonomic nervous system.

autonomous (aw-ton′o-mus) pertaining to or characterized by autonomy.

autonomy (aw-ton′o-me) [*auto-* + Gr. *nomos* law] the state of functioning independently, without extraneous influence.

auto-ophthalmoscope (aw″to-of-thal′mo-skōp) [*auto-* + *ophthalmoscope*] an ophthalmoscope for examining one's own eyes.

auto-ophthalmoscopy (aw″to-of-thal-mos′ko-pe) the use of the auto-ophthalmoscope.

auto-oxidation (aw″to-ok′sĭ-da′shun) the phenomenon of combining directly with oxygen at ordinary temperatures, without catalysis.

autopath (aw′to-path) a person who has allergic symptoms because of a sensitive autonomic nervous system.

autopathography (aw″to-pah-thog′rah-fe) [*auto-* + Gr. *pathos* disease + *graphein* to write] a written description of one's own disease.

autopathy (aw-top′ah-the) [*auto-* + Gr. *pathos* disease] a disease without apparent external causation; idiopathic disease.

autophagia (aw″to-fa′je-ah) [*auto-* + Gr. *phagein* to eat + *-ia*] 1. the biting or eating of one's own flesh. 2. nutrition of the body by the consumption of its own tissues. 3. autophagy.

autophagosome (aw″to-fag′o-sōm) [*auto-* + *phagosome*] an intracytoplasmic vacuole containing elements of the cell's own cytoplasm; it fuses with a lysosome, subjecting its contents to enzymatic digestion. Called also *autophagic vesicle, autosome,* and *cytolysosome.*

autophagy (aw-tof′ah-je) 1. the segregation of part of the cell's own cytoplasmic material within a membrane and its digestion after fusion of the segregated vacuole with a lysosome. Cf. *heterophagy.* 2. autophagia.

autopharmacologic (aw″to-fahr″mah-ko-loj′ik) pertaining to substances (e.g., hormones) produced in the body that have pharmacologic activities.

autopharmacology (aw″to-far″mah-kol′o-je) the chemical regulation of bodily function by the natural constituents of the body tissues.

autophil (aw′to-fil) a person with a tendency to allergic manifestations because of a sensitive autonomic nervous system.

autophilia (aw″to-fil′e-ah) [*auto-* + Gr. *philein* to love] (*obs.*) narcissism.

autophobia (aw″to-fo′be-ah) [*auto-* + *phobia*] irrational dread of one's self, of being alone.

autophonometry (aw″to-fo-nom′ĕ-tre) [*auto-* + Gr. *phōne* voice + *metron* measure] the application of a vibrating tuning fork to the body of a patient for the purpose of having him describe the sensations that it produces.

autophthalmoscope (aw″tof-thal′mo-skōp) auto-oph-thalmoscope.

autophyte (aw′to-fīt) [*auto-* + Gr. *phyton* plant] a plant that does not depend on organized food material, but derives its nourishment directly from inorganic matter. Cf. *saprophyte*.

autoplast (aw′to-plast) an autograft.

autoplastic (aw″to-plas′tik) pertaining to autoplasty.

autoplasty (aw′to-plas″te) [*auto-* + *-plasty*] 1. the replacement or reconstruction of diseased or injured parts by tissue taken from another part of the patient's own body. 2. adaption by changing one's self (autoplastic change) rather than changing the external environment. Cf. *alloplasty*. **peritoneal a.,** peritonization.

autopodium (aw″to-po′de-um) see *limb* (def. 1).

autopoisonous (aw″to-poi′zun-us) poisonous to the organism by which it is formed.

autopolymer (aw″to-pol′ĭ-mer) a material that polymerizes without the use of heat, but on the addition of an activator and a catalyst.

autopolymerization (aw″to-pol″ĭ-mer″i-za′shun) polymerization occurring without the use of heat but as a chemical reaction following the addition of an activator and a catalyst.

autoproteolysis (aw″to-pro-te-ol′ĭ-sis) autolysis, def. 1.

autoprothrombin (aw″to-pro-throm′bin) Seegers' term for an activation product of prothrombin. **a. I,** Factor VII; see *coagulation factors*, under *factor*. **a. II,** Factor IX; see *coagulation factors*, under *factor*. **a. C,** Factor X; see under *coagulation factors*, under *factor*.

autoprotolysis (aw″to-pro-tol′ĭ-sis) self-ionization involving proton transfer.

autopsia (aw-top′se-ah) autopsy.

autopsy (aw′top-se) [*auto-* + Gr. *opsis* view] the postmortem examination of a body, including the internal organs and structures after dissection, so as to determine the cause of death or the nature of pathological changes. Called also *necropsy*.

autopsychic (aw″to-si′kik) [*auto-* + Gr. *psyche* soul] pertaining to one's own mind or to self-consciousness.

autopsychorhythmia (aw″to-si-ko-rith′me-ah) [*auto-* + Gr. *psyche* soul + Gr. *rhythmos* rhythm] pathological rhythmic activity of the brain.

autoradiogram (aw″to-ra′de-o-gram) an autoradiograph.

autoradiograph (aw″to-ra′de-o-graf) a radiograph of an object or tissue made by recording the radiation emitted by radioactive material within it, especially after the purposeful introduction of radioactive material.

autoradiography (aw″to-ra″de-og′rah-fe) the making of a radiograph of an object or tissue by recording on a photographic plate the radiation emitted by weakly emitting radioactive material within the object; the technique has been used widely for studying DNA synthesis and location within cells, with tritium-labeled precursors (like thymidine) as the radioactive marker.

autoregulation (aw″to-reg″u-la′shun) the control of certain phenomena by factors inherent in a situation, usually restricted to circulatory physiology; specifically (1) the intrinsic tendency of an organ or tissue to maintain constant blood flow despite changes in arterial pressure, (2) the adjustment of blood flow through an organ in order to provide for its metabolic needs, and (3) (*obs.*) the factors tending to maintain a constant blood pressure. **heterometric a.,** those intrinsic mechanisms controlling the strength of ventricular contractions that depend on the length of myocardial fibers at the end of diastole. **homeometric a.,** those intrinsic mechanisms controlling the strength of ventricular contractions that are independent of the length of myocardial fibers at the end of diastole.

autoreinfusion (aw″to-re″in-fu′zhun) intravenous infusion of a patient's own blood or serum which has escaped into the pleural or peritoneal cavities, usually because of trauma or spontaneous rupture of a major vessel.

autosensitization (aw″to-sen″sĭ-ti-za′shun) sensitization toward one's own tissues; see *autoimmunization*. **erythrocyte a.,** painful bruising syndrome.

autosensitized (aw″to-sen′sĭ-tīzd) rendered hypersensitive to one's own serum or tissues; see *autoimmunization*.

autosepticemia (aw″to-sep″tĭ-se′me-ah) septicemia due to poisons developed within the body.

autoserous (aw″to-se′rus) pertaining to autoserum.

autoserum (aw″to-se′rum) [*auto-* + *serum*] a serum administered to the patient from whom it was derived.

autosexing (aw″to-seks′ing) in avian genetics, the deliberate breeding of an early-appearing sex-linked phenotype to distinguish male from female chicks.

autosite (aw′to-sīt) [*auto-* + Gr. *sitos* food] the larger, more nearly normal component of asymmetrical conjoined twins, to which the parasite is attached as a dependent growth.

autositic (aw″to-sit′ik) pertaining to or of the nature of an autosite.

autosmia (aw-tos′me-ah) [*auto-* + Gr. *osme* smell] the smelling of one's own bodily odor.

autosomal (aw″to-so′mal) pertaining to an autosome.

autosomatognosis (aw″to-so″mah-tog-no′sis) [*auto-* + Gr. *sōma* body + *gnosis* recognition] the feeling that a part of the body that has been removed, as by amputation, is still present. See *phantom limb*, under *limb*.

autosomatognostic (aw″to-so″mah-tog-nos′tik) pertaining to autosomatognosis.

autosome (aw′to-sōm) [*auto-* + Gr. *sōma* body] 1. any ordinary paired chromosome alike in males and females, as distinguished from sex chromosomes; in man there are 22 pairs of autosomes. 2. autophagosome.

autospermotoxin (aw″to-sper″mo-tok′sin) a substance capable of agglutinating the spermatozoa of the animal in which they are formed.

autosplenectomy (aw″to-sple-nek′to-me) the almost complete disappearance of the spleen through progressive fibrosis and shrinkage, such as may occur in sickle cell anemia.

autospray (aw′to-spra) an apparatus for spraying, to be used by the patient himself.

autosterilization (aw″to-ster″ĭ-li-za′shun) a supposed tendency of certain viruses (e.g., poliovirus) to disappear from the tissues after a short time; a concept found to be erroneous.

autostimulation (aw″to-stim′u-la′shun) stimulation of an animal with antigenic material originating from its own tissues.

autosuggestibility (aw″to-sug-jes″tĭ-bil′ĭ-te) a peculiar mental state with loss of will, in which suggestion becomes easy.

autosuggestion (aw″to-sug-jes′chun) [*auto-* + *suggestion*] self-suggestion; the process by which a person induces in himself an uncritical acceptance of an idea, belief, or opinion.

autosynnoia (aw″to-sin-noi′ah) [*auto-* + Gr. *synnoia* meditation] (*obs.*) complete self-absorption; autistic thinking.

autosynthesis (aw″to-sin′thĕ-sis) self-reproduction.

autotemnous (aw″to-tem′nus) [*auto-* + Gr. *temnein* to cut] capable of spontaneous division.

autotherapy (aw″to-ther′ah-pe) [*auto-* + Gr. *therapeia* treatment] 1. the spontaneous cure of disease. 2. self-cure. 3. treatment of disease by filtrates from the patient's own secretions.

autothromboagglutinin (aw″to-throm″bo-ah-gloo′tĭ-nin) a platelet autoagglutinin.

autotomographic (aw″to-tom″o-graf′ik) pertaining to autotomography.

autotomography (aw″to-to-mog′rah-fe) a method of body-section roentgenography involving movement of the patient instead of the x-ray tube.

autotomy (aw-tot′o-me) [*auto-* + Gr. *tome* cut] 1. self-division; fission. 2. the spontaneous shedding of an appendage, as in some invertebrates.

autotopagnosia (aw″to-top″ag-no′se-ah) [*auto-* + Gr. *topos* place + *a* neg. + *gnōsis* knowledge] inability to localize or orient correctly different parts of the body; body-image agnosia.

autotoxemia (aw″to-tok-se′me-ah) autotoxicosis.

autotoxic (aw″to-tok′sik) [auto- + Gr. toxikon poison] pertaining to autointoxication.

autotoxicosis (aw″to-tok″sĭ-ko′sis) [auto- + Gr. toxikon poison + -osis] poisoning by material generated within the body; called also autotoxemia.

autotoxin (aw″to-tok′sin) any pathogenic principle developed within the body from tissue metamorphosis.

autotoxis (aw″to-tok′sis) autotoxicosis.

autotransfusion (aw″to-trans-fu′zhun) reinfusion of blood or blood products derived from the patient's own circulation. **intraoperative a.,** the collection, processing, and reinfusion of a patient's blood shed from a wound or body cavity during surgery. **postoperative a.,** the collection, processing, and reinfusion of the patient's blood shed from the mediastinum following open heart or chest surgery or from the chest following traumatic hemothorax.

autotransplant (aw″to-trans′plant) autograft.

autotransplantation (aw″to-trans″plan-ta′shun) the operation of taking a piece of tissue from one part of a subject and inserting it in another part of the same individual; called also autografting.

autotrepanation (aw″to-trep″ah-na′shun) erosion of the skull by a brain tumor.

autotroph (aw′to-trōf) an autotrophic organism. **facultative a.,** an organism, especially a bacterium, having a metabolism that is either autotrophic or heterotrophic and thus is capable of growth on either inorganic or organic media. **obligate a.,** a microorganism that can exist only by autotrophic means.

autotrophic (aw″to-trof′ik) [auto- + Gr. trophē nutrition] self-sustaining; said of a type of nutrition in which organisms are capable of synthesizing organic molecules as nutritive substances. Cf. heterotrophic.

autotrophy (aw-tot′ro-fe) the state of being autotrophic; autotrophic nutrition.

autovaccination (aw″to-vak″sĭ-na′shun) 1. treatment of a patient with autovaccine. 2. treatment of a patient by causing liberation of antigenic products from some invading microorganism or diseased tissue and thus bringing about the formation of antibodies.

autovaccine (aw″to-vak′sēn) a bacterial vaccine prepared from cultures of organisms isolated from the patient's own secretions or tissues.

autovaccinia (aw″to-vak-sin′e-ah) [auto- + vaccinia] a vaccinial reaction appearing on an area of the body other than at the primary site of smallpox vaccination as a result of transference of vaccinia virus by scratching.

autovaccinotherapy (aw″to-vak″sĭ-no-ther′ah-pe) autovaccination.

autoxemia (aw″tok-se′me-ah) autotoxicosis.

autoxidation (aw″tok-sĭ-da′shun) spontaneous oxidation of a substance that is in direct contact with oxygen.

autoxidizable (aw-tok″sĭ-dīz′ah-bl) spontaneously oxidizable.

autozygous (aw″to-zi′gus) homozygous by virtue of parental descent from a common ancestor.

auxanogram (awks-an′o-gram) the plate culture in auxanography.

auxanographic (awks″an-o-graf′ik) pertaining to auxanography.

auxanography (awks″an-og′rah-fe) [Gr. auxanein to increase + graphein to write] determination of the most suitable medium for a microbe by placing drops of various solutions on a plate containing a poor medium; the microbe will develop the strongest colonies on the spot that contains the best medium.

auxesis (awk-se′sis) [Gr. auxēsis] increase in the size of an organism; often used specifically to designate increase in volume of an organism as a result of growth of its individual cells, without increase in their number.

auxetic (awk-set′ik) [Gr. auxētikos growing] 1. pertaining to auxesis. 2. a substance that stimulates auxesis.

auxiliary (awk-sil′e-a″re) [L. auxiliaris] 1. affording aid. 2. that which affords aid. **torquing a.,** an accessory arch

wire used to apply torsion on a tooth in any of the three planes of space; used in orthodontic therapy.

auxiliomotor (awk-sil″e-o-mo′tor) aiding or stimulating motion.

auxilytic (awk-sĭ-lit′ik) [Gr. auxein to increase + lysis] increasing the lytic or destructive power.

auximone (awk′sĭ-mōn) [Gr. auxein to increase + hormone] a hypothetical substance, akin to vitamin, that favors growth in plants.

auxin (awk′sin) [Gr. auxē increase] a phytohormone (plant hormone) from sprouts of plants and from human urine that promotes growth in plant cells and tissues by elongation rather than by multiplication of cells; there are two forms, auxin A, a cyclopentene derivative of trihydroxy valeric acid, $C_{18}H_{32}O_5$, and auxin B, which is heteroauxin.

auxiometer (awk″se-om′ĕ-ter) [Gr. auxein to increase + metron measure] 1. an apparatus for measuring the magnifying powers of lenses; called also auxometer. 2. a dynamometer.

aux(o)- [Gr. auxē increase] a combining form denoting relationship to growth, or to stimulation or acceleration.

auxoaction (awk″so-ak′shun) the accelerating or stimulating action of a substance.

auxocardia (awk″so-kar′de-ah) [auxo- + Gr. kardia heart] (obs.) 1. diastole. 2. enlargement of the heart.

auxochrome (awk″so-krōm) [auxo- + Gr. chrōma color] a chemical group which, if introduced into a chromogen, will convert the latter into a dye.

auxochromous (awk″so-kro′mus) pertaining to an auxochrome.

auxocyte (awk′so-sīt) [auxo- + Gr. kytos hollow vessel] an oocyte, spermatocyte, or sporocyte in the early stages of its development; called also gonotokont.

auxodrome (awk′so-drōm) [Gr. auxē growth + dromos a course] the course of growth as plotted on a Wetzel grid.

auxoflore (awk′so-flōr) a substance that increases the intensity of fluorescence of a compound. Cf. bathoflore.

auxoflur (awk′so-floor) auxoflore.

auxogluc (awk′so-glook) [auxo- + Gr. glykys sweet] a tasteless atom with which a glucophore combines to form a compound that has a sweet taste.

auxohormone (awk″so-hor′mōn) [auxo- + hormone] a vitamin.

auxology (awk-sol′o-je) (obs.) auxanology.

auxometer (awks-om′ĕ-ter) auxiometer, def. 1.

auxometric (awks″o-met′rik) pertaining or relating to auxometry.

auxometry (awks-om′ĕ-tre) [Gr. auxein to increase + metry] measurement of rate of growth.

auxoneurotropic (awk″so-nu″ro-trop′ik) [auxo- + neurotropic] increasing or strengthening the neurotropic properties of any substance.

auxospireme (awk″so-spi′rēm) the spireme of an auxocyte during the growth cycle.

auxospore (awk′so-spōr) a rejuvenescent cell of certain diatoms formed in response to a diminution in the size of the organism as a result of repeated cell divisions; it sheds the cell walls, enlarges, and then forms new, larger walls.

auxotonic (awk″so-ton′ik) [auxo- + Gr. tonos tension] contracting against increasing resistance.

auxotox (awk′so-toks) a chemical group that causes a compound to be toxic.

auxotroph (awk′so-trōf) an auxotrophic organism.

auxotrophic (awk″so-trof′ik) [auxo- + Gr. trophē nutrition] 1. requiring a growth factor that is not required by the parental or prototype strain; said of microbial mutants. 2. requiring specific organic growth factors in addition to the carbon source present in a minimal medium.

auxotype (awk′so-tīp) [auxo- + type] the type of an individual strain of Neisseria gonorrhoeae as determined by its nutritional requirements.

AV, A-V, atrioventricular; arteriovenous.

Av. average; avoirdupois.

avalvular (ah-val′vu-lar) having no valves.

avantin (av′an-tin) isopropyl alcohol.

avascular (ah-vas′ku-lar) [*a* neg. + *vascular*] not supplied with blood vessels.

avascularization (ah-vas″ku-lar-i-za′shun) the diversion of blood from tissues; it may be accomplished by ligating vessels or by applying tight elastic bandages.

Avellis's syndrome (paralysis) (av-el′ēz) [Georg *Avellis*, German laryngologist, 1864–1916] see under *syndrome.*

Avena (ah-ve′nah) [L.] a genus of grasses. The grains of *A. sativa* constitute the oats of commerce, a nutritive and edible cereal.

avenin (ah-ve′nin) an albuminoid obtained from *Avena sativa,* or oats, said to be identical with gluten casein; called also *plant casein* and *legumin.*

avenolith (ah-ve′no-lith) [L. *avena* oats + Gr. *lithos* stone] an intestinal calculus or enterolith formed around a grain of oats.

Aventyl (ah-ven′til) trademark for a preparation of nortriptyline hydrochloride.

Avenzoar (av″en-zo′ar) (1113–1162) [from Ar. *Abū Marwan Abdal-Malik ibn Abū al-Ala Zuhr,* c. 1091 to c. 1162] an Arab physician born in Seville, Spain; he was the teacher of Averroes. His surviving works deal with therapeutics, hygiene, and diet. Also known as *Abumeron* and *Ibn Zuhr.*

Averroes (av-er′o-ēz) [L., from Ar. Abul-Walīd Muhammad ibn-Ahmad *Ibn-Rushd,* 1126–1198] the last and greatest of the Arab physicians and philosophers of the West, born in Cordova, Spain. His *Kitab-al-Kullyat* or *Colliget* ("Book of Universals") tried to establish a system of medicine on neo-Platonic modifications of Aristotle. Also known as the *Ibn Rushd.*

aversive (ah-ver′siv) characterized by or giving rise to avoidance; noxious. Cf. *appetitive.*

Avertin (ah-ver′tin) trademark for a preparation of tribromoethanol.

avian (a′ve-an) [L. *avis* bird] of or pertaining to birds.

Avicenna (av″ĭ-sen′ah) [L., from Ar. AbūAli al-Husayn ibn Abdallah *ibn Sinā,* 979–1037] the greatest Arab physician and philosopher of the East, born in Persia. His *Canon* is one of the most famous medical books ever written and was the standard text in Europe through the 17th century. He completely expounded the entire corpus of speculative and practical medicine according to Hippocrates, Aristotle, and Galen and systematically compiled all of Graeco-Arabic medicine. Called also *Ibn Sina.*

avidin (av′ĭ-din) a specific protein in egg albumin that interacts with biotin to render it unavailable to an animal, thus producing the syndrome known as biotin deficiency. See also *biotin.*

avidity (ah-vid′ĭ-te) 1. the strength of an acid or a base. 2. the strength of binding between antibody and a complex antigen. Since the antigen has more than one determinant and many of the determinants differ from one another, avidity expresses the overall interaction between antigen and antibody; it is, however greater than the sum of the affinities for the single determinants, since the effective multivalency of the antigen gives rise to a cooperative "bonus" effect. Often represented by constant K_a (the value of the association constant for the reaction Ab +Ag ⇄ AbAg). Avidity is a function of the techniques used in its measurement and can only be expressed in arbitrary units. Cf. *affinity.*

avifauna (a″vĭ-faw′nah) the bird life present in or characteristic of a given region or locality.

avirulence (a-vir′u-lens) lack of virulence; lack of competence of an infectious agent to produce pathologic effects.

avirulent (a-vir′u-lent) not virulent.

avitaminosis (a-vi″tah-mĭ-no′sis) hypovitaminosis.

avitaminotic (a-vi″tah-mĭ-not′ik) pertaining to or characterized by avitaminosis.

avivement (ah-vēv-mon′) [Fr.] the refreshing of the edges of a wound by surgical procedure.

Avlosulfon (av-lo-sul′fon) trademark for a preparation of dapsone.

A.V.M.A. American Veterinary Medical Association.

Avogadro's law, number (constant) (av-o-gad′rōz) [Amedeo *Avogadro,* Italian physicist, 1776–1856] see under *law* and *number.*

avogram (av′o-gram) one septillionth (10^{-24}) of a gram, or one picopicogram (ppg); so named from Avogadro's number, 6.0220×10^{23}. The mass of a molecule in avograms is therefore 1.66 times its conventional molecular weight.

avoidance (ah-void′ans) a conscious or unconscious defense mechanism consisting of refusal to encounter situations, activities, or objects that would produce anxiety or conflict.

avoidant (ah-void′ant) moving away from; negatively oriented.

avoirdupois (av″er-dŭ-poiz′) see under *weight,* and see *Table of Weights and Measures.*

avoparcin (av-o-par′sin) a glycopeptide antibiotic derived from *Streptomyces candidus;* an antibacterial.

avulsion (ah-vul′shun) [L. *avulsio,* from *a-* away + *vellere* to pull] the ripping or tearing away of a part. **nerve a.,** the operation of tearing a nerve by traction. **phrenic a.,** extraction of a piece of the phrenic nerve through an incision at the base of the neck; formerly done in pulmonary tuberculosis to paralyze the corresponding side of the diaphragm in order to secure rest of the lung.

awu atomic weight unit; see *atomic mass unit,* under *unit.*

ax. axis.

Axelrod (ak′s′l-rod) Julius. American biochemist and pharmacologist, born 1912; co-winner, with Ulf Svante von Euler and Sir Bernard Katz, of the Nobel prize for medicine or physiology in 1970 for research on the chemical aspects of nerve impulse transmission.

Axenfeld's anomaly, syndrome (ak′sen-felts″) [Theodor *Axenfeld,* German ophthalmologist, 1867– 1930] see under *anomaly* and *syndrome.*

Axenfeld-Morax see *Morax-Axenfeld.*

axenic (a-zen′ik) [*a* neg. + Gr. *xenos* a guestfriend, stranger] not contaminated by or associated with any foreign organisms; used in reference to pure cultures of microorganisms or to germ-free animals. Cf. *gnotobiotic.*

axes (ak′sēz) [L.] plural of *axis.*

axial (ak′se-al) of or pertaining to the axis of a structure or part, as the long axis of a tooth.

axiation (ak″se-a′shun) the establishment of an axis, or the development of polarity, in an ovum, embryo, organ, or other body structure.

axifugal (ak-sif′u-gal) [L. *axis* axis + *fugere* to flee] directed away from an axon or axis.

axilemma (ak″si-lem′ah) [*axis* + Gr. *lemma* husk] axolemma.

axilla (ak-sil′ah), gen. and pl. *axil′lae* [L.] fossa axillaris.

axillae (ak-sil′e) [L.] genitive and plural of *axilla.*

axillary (ak′sĭ-lar′e) pertaining to the axilla.

axi(o)- [L. *axis,* q.v.] a combining form denoting relationship to an axis. In dentistry, it is used in special reference to the long axis of a tooth, as in the names of cavity angles. See specific terms.

axiobuccal (ak″se-o-buk′al) pertaining to or formed by the axial and buccal walls of a tooth cavity.

axiobuccocervical (ak-se-o-buk″o-ser′vĭ-kal) pertaining to or formed by the axial, buccal, and cervical walls of a tooth cavity.

axiobuccogingival (ak″se-o-buk″o-jin′jĭ-val) pertaining to or formed by the axial, buccal, and gingival walls of a tooth cavity.

axiobuccolingual (ak″se-o-buk″o-ling′gwal) pertaining to or formed by the long axis and the buccal and lingual surfaces of a posterior tooth.

axiocervical (ak″se-o-ser′vĭ-kal) pertaining to or formed by the axial and cervical walls of a tooth cavity.

axiodistal (ak″se-o-dis′tal) pertaining to or formed by the axial and distal walls of a tooth cavity.

axiodistocervical (ak″se-o-dis″to-ser′vĭ-kal) pertaining to or formed by the axial, distal, and cervical walls of a tooth cavity.

axiodistogingival (ak″se-o-dis″to-jin′jĭ-val) pertaining to or formed by the axial, distal, and gingival walls of a tooth cavity.

axiodistoincisal (ak″se-o-dis″to-in-si′zal) pertaining to or formed by the axial, distal, and incisal walls of a tooth cavity.

axiodisto-occlusal (ak″se-o-dis″to-ŏ-kloo′zal) pertaining to or formed by the axial, distal, and occlusal walls of a tooth cavity.

axiogingival (ak″se-o-jin′jĭ-val) pertaining to or formed by the axial and gingival walls of a tooth cavity.

axioincisal (ak″se-o-in-si′zal) pertaining to or formed by the axial and incisal walls of a tooth cavity.

axiolabial (ak″se-o-la′be-al) pertaining to or formed by the axial and labial walls of a tooth cavity.

axiolabiogingival (ak″se-o-la″be-o-jin′jĭ-val) pertaining to or formed by the axial, labial, and gingival walls of a tooth cavity.

axiolabiolingual (ak″se-o-la″be-o-ling′gwal) pertaining to the long axis and the labial and lingual surfaces of an anterior tooth.

axiolingual (ak″se-o-ling′gwal) pertaining to or formed by the axial and lingual walls of a tooth cavity.

axiolinguocervical (ak″se-o-ling″gwo-ser′vĭ-kal) pertaining to or formed by the axial, lingual, and cervical walls of a tooth cavity.

axiolinguogingival (ak″se-o-ling″gwo-jin′jĭ-val) pertaining to or formed by the axial, lingual, and gingival walls of a tooth cavity.

axiolinguo-occlusal (ak″se-o-ling″gwo-ŏ-kloo′sal) pertaining to or formed by the axial, lingual, and occlusal walls of a tooth cavity.

axiomesial (ak″se-o-me′ze-al) pertaining to or formed by the axial and mesial walls of a tooth cavity.

axiomesiocervical (ak″se-o-me′ze-o-ser′vĭ-kal) pertaining to or formed by the axial, mesial, and cervical walls of a tooth cavity.

axiomesiodistal (ak″se-o-me″ze-o-dis′tal) pertaining to the long axis and the mesial and distal surfaces of a tooth.

axiomesiogingival (ak″se-o-me″ze-o-jin′jĭ-val) pertaining to or formed by the axial, mesial, and gingival walls of a tooth cavity.

axiomesioincisal (ak″se-o-me″ze-o-in-si′zal) pertaining to or formed by the axial, mesial, and incisal walls of a tooth cavity.

axiomesio-occlusal (ak″se-o-me″ze-o-ŏ-kloo′zal) pertaining to or formed by the axial, mesial, and occlusal walls of a tooth cavity.

axion (ak-se′on) (obs.) the brain and spinal cord.

axio-occlusal (ak″se-o-ŏ-kloo′zal) pertaining to or formed by the axial and occlusal walls of a tooth cavity.

axiopodium (ak″se-o-po′de-um) axopodium.

axiopulpal (ak″se-o-pul′pal) pertaining to or formed by the axial and pulpal walls of a tooth cavity.

axipetal (ak-sip′ĕ-tal) [L. axis axis + petere to seek] directed toward an axon or axis.

axis (ak′sis), pl. ax′es [L.; Gr. axōn axle] 1. a line about which a revolving body turns or about which a structure would turn if it did revolve; a line around which specified parts of the body are arranged. Used as a general term in NA terminology. 2. [NA] the second cervical vertebra; called also epistropheus, odontoid vertebra, and vertebra dentata. 3. one of the reference lines in a coordinate system. In a two-dimensional coordinate system there are two axes, one horizontal (designated the x-axis), and the other intersecting it (designated the y-axis). Cf. abscissa and ordinate. **arterial a., costocervical,** truncus costocervicalis. **basibregmatic a.,** a vertical line from the basion to the bregma; the maximum height of the cranium. **basicranial a.,** a line from the basion to the gonion. **basifacial a.,** a line joining the gonion and the subnasal point; called also facial a. **binauricular a.,** a line joining the two auricular points. **brain a.** (obs.), brain stem; see under B. **a. bul′bi exter′nus** [NA], an imaginary line that passes from the anterior to the posterior pole of the eyeball; called also external axis of eye and axis oculi externa. **a. bul′bi inter′nus** [NA], an imaginary line in the eyeball, passing from the anterior pole to a point on the anterior surface of the retina just deep to the posterior pole; called also internal axis of eye and axis oculi interna. **celiac a.,** truncus celiacus. **cell a.,** an imaginary line connecting the proximal and distal sides of a cell or passing through the centrosome and nucleus of a cell. **cephalocaudal a.,** the long axis of the body. **cerebrospinal a.** (obs.), the central nervous system. **condylar a.,** an imaginary line passing through the two mandibular condyles around which the mandible may rotate during a part of the opening movement of the jaw; called also condyle chord. **conjugate a.** (obs.), the conjugate diame-

ter of the pelvis; see under diameter. **craniofacial a.,** the axis of the bones at the base of the skull, including the mesethmoid, presphenoid, basisphenoid, and basioccipital bones. **dorsoventral a.,** any line in the median plane at right angles to the long axis of the body. **Downs Y a.,** Y a. **electrical a. of heart,** the resultant of the electromotive forces within the heart at any instant. **embryonic a.,** an imaginary line from the head end to the tail end of an embryo or, before that, the line of elongation of the primitive streak and groove. **encephalomyelonic a., encephalospinal a.** (obs.), the central nervous system. **external a. of eye,** a. bulbi externus. **facial a.,** basifacial a. **frontal a.,** an imaginary line running from right to left through the center of the eyeball. **a. of heart,** an imaginary line passing through the center of the base of the heart and the apex. **hinge a.,** the imaginary line connecting the mandibular condyles around which the mandible can rotate without translatory movement; called also mandibular a. **internal a. of eye,** a. bulbi internus. **a. of lens, a. len′tis** [NA], an imaginary line joining the anterior and posterior poles of the lens of the eye. **long a. of body,** the imaginary straight line projected on the median plane through the neck, thorax, abdomen, and pelvis about which the weights of the torso are most symmetrically distributed. **mandibular a.,** hinge a. **neural a.,** the central nervous system. **a. o′culi exter′na,** a. bulbi externus. **a. o′culi inter′na,** a. bulbi internus. **opening a.,** an imaginary line passing through the mandibular condyles around which the condyles may rotate during opening and closing movements of the mandible. **optic a.,** 1. axis opticus. 2. optical axis. 3. the hypothetical straight line that passes through the centers of curvature of the front and back surfaces of a simple lens; a light ray coinciding with this line will pass through the lens undeviated. **a. op′tica,** a. opticus. **optical a.,** the line formed by the coinciding principal axes of elements composing an optical system, being the continuous line passing through the centers of curvature of the optical surfaces of those elements; called also principal a. **a. op′ticus** [NA], optic axis: an imaginary line passing from the midpoint of the visual field to the fovea centralis of the macula; called also a. optica, sagittal a. of eye, and visual a. **a. pel′vis** [NA], **a. of pelvis,** an imaginary curved line drawn through the minor pelvis at right angles to the plane of the superior aperture, the plane of the cavity, and the plane of the inferior aperture at their central points. **a. of preparation,** the path taken by a dental restoration as it slides on or off the preparation. **principal a.,** optical a. **pupillary a.,** the imaginary line perpendicular to the cornea that passes through the center of the pupil of entrance. **renal a.,** an imaginary straight line extending through the upper and lower poles of the kidney or, radiographically, through the most inferior and superior calices of the kidney; when projected superiorly, it intersects the thoracic spine. **sagittal a. of eye,** a. opticus. **secondary a.,** an imaginary line passing through the optical center of a lens. **thoracic a.,** arteria thoracoacromialis. **thyroid a.,** truncus thyrocervicalis. **vertical a. of eye,** an imaginary line connecting the extreme upper and lower points of the eyeball. **visual a.,** a. opticus. **Y a.,** the angle of an imaginary line connecting the sella turcica and the gnathion related to the Frankfort horizontal plane; it is an indicator of downward and forward growth of the mandible.

axis cylinder (ak″sis-sil′in-der) [axis + cylinder] axon, def. 2.

ax(o)- [Gr. axōn axle, axis] a combining form denoting relationship to an axis, or to an axon.

axoaxonic (ak″so-ak-son′ik) [axo- + axon] referring to a synapse between the axon of one neuron and the axon of another.

axodendritic (ak″so-den-drit′ik) [axo- + Gr. dendron tree] referring to a synapse between the axon of one neuron and dendrites of another; see synapse.

axofugal (ak-sof′u-gal) axifugal.

axograph (ak′so-graf) an apparatus for recording axes in kymographic tracings.

axoid (ak′soid) pertaining to the axis or second cervical vertebra.

axoidean (ak-soi′de-an) axoid.

axolemma (ak-so-lem′ah) [axo- + Gr. eilēma sheath] the

surface membrane of an axon; called also *Mauthner's membrane* or *sheath*.

axolotl (ak′so-lot′l) a larval salamander of the genus *Ambystoma;* used in experiments with thyroid feeding.

axolysis (ak-sol′ĭ-sis) [*axo-* + Gr. *lysis* dissolution] degeneration and breaking up of the axon of a nerve cell.

axometer (ak-som′ĕ-ter) [*axis* + *-meter*] an instrument for measuring an axis, especially an instrument for adjusting a pair of spectacles with respect to the optic axes of the eyes.

axon (ak′son) [Gr. *axōn* axle, axis] 1. the axis of the body; the vertebral column (columna vertebralis [NA]). 2. that process of a neuron by which impulses travel away from the cell body; at the terminal arborization of the axon, the impulses are transmitted to other nerve cells or to effector organs. In the peripheral nervous system, the larger (myelinated) axons are surrounded by a myelin sheath, formed by concentric layers of plasma membrane of the Schwann cell, individual Schwann cells being separated by gaps called nodes of Ranvier. In the central nervous system, the function of the Schwann cell is supplied by oligodendrocytes. Called also *axis cylinder*. **giant a.,** an axon of certain invertebrates, e.g., the squid, whose size (500 to 700 microns) has facilitated physiological studies of cell membrane excitation. **naked a.,** an axon which has no myelin sheath. **unmyelinated a.,** naked a.

axonal (ak′so-nal) pertaining to or affecting an axon.

axonapraxia (ak″son-ah-prak′se-ah) neurapraxia.

axone (ak′sōn) axon.

axoneme (ak′so-nēm) [*axo-* + Gr. *nēma* thread] 1. the axial thread of the chromosome in which is located the axial combination of genes. 2. the central core of a cilium or flagellum, consisting of a central pair of filaments surrounded by nine other pairs; called also *axial filament*.

axonometer (ak″so-nom′ĕ-ter) axometer.

axonotmesis (ak″son-ot-me′sis) [*axo-* + Gr. *tmēsis* a cutting apart] nerve injury characterized by disruption of the axon and myelin sheath but with preservation of the connective tissue fragments, resulting in degeneration of the axon distal to the injury site; regeneration of the axon is spontaneous and of good quality. Cf. *neurapraxia* and *neurotmesis.*

axopetal (ak-sop′ĕ-tal) axipetal.

axophage (ak′so-fāj) [*axo-* + Gr. *phagein* to eat] a neuroglial cell occurring in excavations in the myelin in myelitis.

axoplasm (ak′so-plazm) [*axo-* + Gr. *plasma* plasma] the cytoplasm of an axon.

axoplasmic (ak″so-plas′mik) pertaining to the axoplasm.

axopodia (ak″so-po′de-ah) plural of *axopodium.*

axopodium (ak″so-po′de-um), pl. *axopo′dia* [*axo-* + Gr. *pous* foot] a long and slender, semipermanent type of locomotor pseudopodium that has a central axial filament composed of a bundle of microtubules. Called also *axiopodium.* Cf. *filapodium, lobopodium,* and *reticulopodium.*

axosomatic (ak′so-so-mat′ik) [*axo-* + Gr. *sōma* body] referring to a synapse between the axon of one neuron and the cell body of another.

axospongium (ak″so-spun′je-um) [*axo-* + *spongium*] the meshwork structure making up the substance of the axon of a nerve cell.

axostyle (ak′so-stīl) [*axo-* + Gr. *stylos* pillar] a filamentous or hyaline-supporting structure passing through the longitudinal axis of certain flagellate protozoa, such as trichomonads, and sometimes extending beyond the posterior end of the organism. Its enlarged capitulum may give rise to or be covered by a pelta.

Ayala's quotient (equation, index) [A. G. *Ayala*, Italian neurologist, 1878–1943] see under *quotient.*

ayapana (ah″yah-pah′nah) the leaves of *Eupato′rium tripliner′ve*, a plant growing in many tropical countries; used as an aromatic, stomachic, diaphoretic, and stimulant, and as a household remedy for many conditions in various hot regions.

Ayer's test (ārz) [James Bourne *Ayer*, Boston neurologist, born 1882] see under *test.*

Ayer-Tobey test (ār-to′be) [J. B. *Ayer*; George L. *Tobey*, Jr., Boston otolaryngologist, 1881–1947] Tobey-Ayer test; see under *test.*

Ayerza's disease, syndrome (ah-yer′thaz) [Abel *Ayerza*,

Buenos Aires physician, 1861–1918] see under *disease* and *syndrome.*

Az. azote, French for nitrogen.

azabon (a′zah-bon) chemical name: 4-(3-azobicyclo [3.2.2]non-3-ylsulfonyl)benzenamine; a central nervous system stimulant, $C_{14}H_{20}N_2O_2S$.

azaclorzine hydrochloride (a″zah-klor′zēn) chemical name: 2-chloro-10- [3-(hexahydropyrrolo[1,2-*a*] pyrazin-2-(1*H*)-yl)-1-oxopropyl]-10*H*-phenothiazine dihydrochloride; a coronary vasodilator, $C_{22}H_{24}ClN_3OS \cdot 2HCl$.

azacosterol hydrochloride (ah″zah-kos′ter-ōl) a hypocholesterolemic agent and avian chemosterilant.

azacyclonol (a″zah-si′klo-nol) chemical name: α,α-diphenyl-4-piperidinemethanol. The gamma isomer of pipradrol, $C_{18}H_{21}NO$, occurring as small white odorless crystals; used in the hydrochloride form as a tranquilizer in the treatment of schizophrenia. Called also *gamma-pipradrol.*

5-azacytidine (a″zah-si′tĭ-dēn) chemical name: 5-azacytidine-4-amino-1-ribofuranosyl-1,3,5-triazin-2(1*H*)-one. A cytidine analogue, $C_8H_{12}N_4O_5$, that can be incorporated into RNA and DNA; unlike cytidine it cannot be 5-methylated, a process that is important in gene regulation and post-transcriptional processing of RNA; 5-azacytidine is an investigational antineoplastic agent used for treatment of acute granulocytic leukemia; it has also been shown to have the ability to turn on genes normally expressed only during fetal development (e.g., genes for fetal hemoglobin).

azaguanine (az″ah-gwan′in) a mitotic poison, which resembles the purine guanine, but is actually incorporated into nucleic acids and acts to block nucleic acid synthesis by competitive inhibition.

azamethonium bromide (a″zah-mĕ-tho′ne-um) chemical name: 2,2′-(methylimino)bis[*N*-ethyl-*N*,*N*-dimethylethanaminium]dibromide. A ganglionic blocking agent, $C_{13}H_{33}Br_2N_3$, which has been used as an antihypertensive agent.

azanator maleate (a′zah-na″tor) chemical name: 5-(1-methyl-4-piperidinylidene)-5*H*-[1]benzopyrano[2,3-*b*]pyridine(*Z*)-2-butenedioate(1:1); a bronchodilator, $C_{18}H_{18}N_2O \cdot \cdot C_4H_4O_4$.

azanidazole (a″zah-nid′ah-zōl) chemical name: (*E*)-4-[2-(1-methyl-5-nitro-1*H*-imidazol-2-yl)ethenyl]-2-pyrimidinamine; an antiprotozoal, $C_{10}H_{10}N_6O_2$.

azapetine phosphate (a″zah-pet′ēn) chemical name: 6,7-dihydro-6,7-dihydro-6-(2-propenyl)-5*H*-dibenz[*c,e*]azepine phosphate. An α-adrenergic blocking agent, $C_{17}H_{20}NO_4P$, occurring as white crystalline powder; used as a vasodilator in peripheral vascular disease in which vasospasm is prominent, administered orally.

azapropazone (ah″zah-pro′pah-zōn) [INN, BAN] apazone.

azaribine (a″zah-ri′bēn) 2′,3′,5′-triacetyl-6-azauridine, the prodrug of the uridine metabolite 6-azauridine (AzU), which is metabolically activated to the monophosphate nucleotide (AzUMP), an inhibitor of de novo pyrimidine synthesis. Azaribine is investigational; potential indications are treatment of severe, disabling psoriasis, mycosis fungoides, and polycythemia vera.

azaserine (a″zah-ser′ēn) chemical name: L-serine diazoacetate (ester). An antifungal antibiotic, $C_5H_7N_3O_4$, produced by *Streptomyces* species or by synthesis; it is a glutamine antagonist, inhibiting the synthesis of purine, and has been used as an antineoplastic agent.

azastene (a′zah-stēn) chemical name: 4,4,17-trimethylandrosta-2,5-dieno[2,3-*d*]isoxazol-17β-ol; a contraceptive, $C_{23}H_{33}NO_2$.

azatadine maleate (ah-zat′ah-dēn) chemical name: 6,11-dihydro-11-(1-methyl-4-piperidylidene)-5*H*-benzol [5,6]cyclohepta[1,2-*b*]pyridine maleate (1:2); an antihistaminic, $C_{20}H_{22}N_2 \cdot 2C_4H_4O_4$, used in the treatment of perennial and seasonal allergic rhinitis and chronic urticaria, administered orally.

azathioprine (a″zah-thi′o-prēn) the imidazolyl derivative of 6-mercaptopurine, its active metabolite; used as an immunosuppressive agent for prevention of transplant rejection in renal transplantation and also (investigationally) for treatment of autoimmune diseases such as rheumatoid arthritis, idiopathic thrombocytopenic purpura, autoimmune hemolytic anemias, and systemic lupus erythematosus. Available as *azathioprine* [USP] and *azathioprine sodium* [USP]. **a.**

sodium, the sodium salt of azathioprine, suitable for injection; used for the same purposes as the base.

6-azauridine (a″zah-u′rĭ-dēn) chemical name: 2-β-D-ribofuranoxyl-1,2,4-triazine-3,5(2H,4H)-dione; an antimetabolite, the triazine analogue of uridine, $C_8H_{11}N_3O_6$, which particularly affects neoplastic cells; it has been used in the treatment of acute leukemias.

azedarach (ah-zed′ă-rak″) a common name for *Melia azedarach* L. (Meliaceae) (the chinaberry tree; umbrella tree; pride of China). Its seeds are used for beads and rosaries, and the bark of roots for its anthelmintic properties. Leaf juice is used as a diuretic and emmenagogue. In the United States, it is considered a poisonous plant for humans and animals, the toxicity being felt to reside in the resinous fraction of fruit pulp. Its pharmacological actions include severe local irritation, nervous symptoms, cardioactivity, and dyspnea.

azelaic acid (az″ĕ-la′ik) trivial name for nonanedioic acid, $HOOC(CH_2)_7COOH$, an oxidation product of oleic acid occurring in rancid fats.

azeotropic (a″ze-o-trop′ik) pertaining to or characterized by azeotropy.

azeotropy (a″ze-ot′ro-pe) [*a* neg. + Gr. *zein* to boil + *tropē* a turn, or turning] the absence of any change in the composition of a mixture of substances when it is boiled under a given pressure.

azepindole (a″zĕ-pin′dōl) chemical name: 2,3,4,5-tetrahydro- 1H-[1,4]diazepino[1,2-*a*]indole; an antidepressant, C_{12}-$H_{14}N_2$.

azid, azide (az′id) a compound that contains the group N_3.

azidothymidine (AZT) (az″ĭ-do-thi′mĭ-dēn) a synthetic thymidine analog that inhibits the human immunodeficiency virus that causes acquired immune deficiency syndrome.

azipramine (ah-zip′rah-mēn) chemical name: 6,7-dihydro-N-methyl-N-(phenylmethyl)-indolo[1,7-*ab*][1]benzazepine-1-ethanamine monohydrochloride; an antidepressant, $C_{26}H_{26}N_2 \cdot HCl$.

azlocillin (az″lo-sil′in) an antibiotic derivative of penicillin, $C_{20}H_{23}N_5O_6S$.

azo- a prefix indicating the presence of the group —N:N—, as in azobenzene.

azoamyly (a-zo-am′ĭ-le) [*a* neg. + Gr. *zōon* animal + *amylon* starch] inability of the hepatic cells to store up a normal amount of glycogen.

Azobacter (a-zo-bak′ter) (*obs.*) azotobacter.

azobenzene (az″o-ben′zēn) [*azote* + *benzene*] an orange-red crystalline product, $C_6H_5N:N \cdot C_6H_5$, of the reduction of nitrobenzene, soluble in alcohol and ether, but only sparingly so in water; it is the parent substance of azo dyes and some pH indicators.

azocarmine (az″o-kar′min) either azocarmine G or azocarmine B, red basic dyes used in certain staining procedures.

azoic (ah-zo′ik) [*a* neg. + Gr. *zōe* life] destitute of living organisms.

azoimide (az″o-im′īd) 1. the group:

$$-N{<}{\overset{\textstyle N}{\underset{\textstyle N}{\|}}}$$

2. a protoplasmic poison, hydrazoic acid, N_3H, resembling hydrocyanic acid in its action, made by heating hydrogen chloride with sodium nitrate. It is highly explosive. Called also *triazoic acid* and *hydronitric acid*.

azole (az′ōl) 1. a derivative of a five-membered ring containing nitrogen and either oxygen, sulfur, or an additional nitrogen atom, as well as carbon atoms. 2. pyrrole.

Azolid (az′o-lid) trademark for preparations of phenylbutazone.

azolimine (ah-zo′lĭ-mēn) chemical name: 2-imino-3-methyl-1-phenyl-4-imidazolidinone; a potassium-sparing diuretic, $C_{10}H_{11}N_3O$.

azolitmin (az″o-lit′min) a coloring principle, $C_7H_7NO_4$, from litmus; it is used as a pH indicator, being red at a pH of 4.5 and blue at 8.3.

Azomonas (a″zo-mo′nas) [Fr. *azote* nitrogen + Gr *monas* unit] a genus of gram-negative, aerobic, ovoid to coccoid bacteria of the family Azotobacteriaceae, found in soil and water, made up of sometimes capsulated cells that fix nitrogen. The type species is *A. agilis*.

azomycin (a″zo-mi′sin) chemical name: 2-nitroimidazole. An antibiotic, $C_3H_3N_3O_2$, produced by a species of *Streptomyces*.

azoospermatism (a-zo″o-sper′mah-tizm) azoospermia.

azoospermia (a-zo″o-sper′me-ah) [*a* neg. + *zoosperm*] absence of spermatozoa in the semen, or failure of formation of spermatozoa.

azopigment (a″zo-pig′ment) a purple derivative of bile pigment containing an azo (—N=N—) linkage; formed by reacting bile pigments with diazotizing agents.

azoprotein (az″o-pro′te-in) a protein some constituents of which have been diazotized.

Azorean disease (a-zor′e-an) [*Azores* Islands] see under *disease*.

Azospirillum (a″zo-spi-ri′lum) [*azo-* + *spirillum*] a genus of aerobic or microaerophilic, motile, gram-negative or gram-variable bacteria that are curved or sometimes straight; they are found in soil and are sometimes capable of nitrogen fixation. The type species is *A. lipoferum*.

azosulfamide (az″o-sul′fah-mīd) chemical name: 6-(acetyl- amino) -3-[[4-(aminosufonyl)phenyl]azo] - 4-hydroxy-2,7-naphthalenedisulfonic acid. An antibacterial compound, C_{18}-$H_{14}N_4Na_2O_{10}S$, occurring as a reddish-brown powder; it was one of the forerunners of the sulfonamide drugs.

azote (az′ōt) [*a* neg. + Gr. *zōe* life] nitrogen.

azotemia (az″o-te′me-ah) [*azote* + Gr. *haima* blood + *-ia*] an excess of urea or other nitrogenous compounds in the blood. **extrarenal a.,** prerenal or postrenal a. **postrenal a.,** azotemia due to obstruction of the urinary tract. **prerenal a.,** azotemia resulting from inadequate perfusion of the kidneys, as in hypovolemic shock or congestive heart failure. **renal a.,** azotemia due to reduced glomerular filtration resulting from acute or chronic renal disease.

azotemic (az″o-te′mik) pertaining to or characterized by azotemia.

azotenesis (az″o-tĕ-ne′sis) any disease due to an excess of nitrogenous substances in the system.

azothermia (az″o-ther′me-ah) [*azote* + Gr. *thermē* heat] temperature increase produced by nitrogenous matter in the blood.

azotification (az-o″tĭ-fi-ka′shun) the fixation of atmospheric nitrogen.

azotize (az′o-tīz) to combine or charge with nitrogen.

Azotobacter (ah-zo″to-bak′ter) [Fr. *azote* nitrogen + Gr. *baktron* a rod] a genus of gram-negative, aerobic bacteria of the family Azotobacteraceae, found chiefly in soil and water, made up of ovoid to coccoid cells that fix nitrogen. The type species is *A. chroococ′cum.* Called also *Azotomonas.*

Azotobacteraceae (ah-zo″to-bak″tĕ-ra′se-e) a family of gram-negative, aerobic, rod-shaped bacteria, found in water, soil, and certain plants. They are free-living, nitrogen-fixing organisms, capable of fixing atmospheric nitrogen in the presence of carbohydrate or other sources of energy. The family includes the genera *Azomonas* and *Azotobacter.*

azotometer (az″o-tom′ĕ-ter) [*azote* + Gr. *metron* measure] an instrument for measuring the proportion of nitrogen compounds in a solution.

Azotomonas (az″o-to-mo′nas) *Azotobacter.*

azotomycin (ah-zo″to-mi′sin) an antibiotic substance with antineoplastic properties produced by *Streptomyces ambofaciens;* formerly called *duazomycin B.*

azotorrhea (az″o-to-re′ah) [*azote* + Gr. *rhoia* flow] excessive loss of nitrogen in the feces.

azoturia (az″o-tu′re-ah) [*azote* + Gr. *ouron* urine] 1. an excess of urea or other nitrogen compounds in the urine. 2. a disease of horses marked by a sudden attack of perspiration and paralysis of the hind quarters and by the passing of light red to dark brown urine. It occurs in horses that, after being engaged in continuous work, are rested and well fed for a few days and then returned to work.

azoturic (az″o-tu′rik) pertaining to azoturia or the urinary excretion of nitrogen.

azoxybenzene (az″ok-se-ben-zēn′) a pale yellow product, $C_6H_5 \cdot N \cdot (\cdot O)N \cdot C_6H_5$, of the reduction of nitrobenzene.

azoxy compound (az-ok′se) a compound which contains the group

$$O{<}{\overset{\textstyle N-}{\underset{\textstyle N-}{|}}}$$

AZT azidothymidine.

azulene (az′u-lēn) a blue crystalline hydrocarbon, $C_{10}H_8$, with an odor similar to that of naphthalene, obtained from certain volatile oils, such as oil of cubebs.

Azulfidine (a-zul′fĭ-dēn) trademark for a preparation of sulfasalazine.

azure (azh′-ūr) any of the partially methylated homologues of the series of basic dyes extending from thionine to methylene blue, or to certain mixtures of members of this series. They are metachromatic, and are used in many important staining procedures. **a. A,** asymmetrical dimethylthionine, $(CH_3)_2N\cdot C_6H_3(SN)C_6H_3\cdot NH_2\cdot Cl$. **a. B,** trimethylthionin, $(CH_3)_2N\cdot C_6H_3(SN)C_6H_3\cdot N(CH_3)\cdot Cl$. **a. C,** monomethylthionine chloride, $(CH_3)N\cdot C_6H_3(SN)C_6H_3$-$NH_2\cdot Cl$. **a. I,** azure B. **a. II,** a mixture of equal parts of azure I and methylene blue. **methylene a.,** azure B.

azuresin (azh″u-rez′in) a complex combination of azure A dye and carbacrylic cationic exchange resin, used as a diagnostic aid in detection of gastric secretion.

azurophil (azh-u′ro-fil) [*azure* + Gr. *philein* to love] an element or cell that stains well with blue aniline dyes.

azurophile (azh′u-ro-fīl) 1. azurophil. 2. azurophilic.

azurophilia (azh″u-ro-fil′e-ah) a condition in which the blood contains cells having azurophil granulations.

azurophilic (azh″u-ro-fil′ik) staining well with blue aniline dyes; pertaining to or characterized by azurophilia.

azygogram (az′ĭ-go-gram) the roentgenographic record obtained by azygography.

azygography (az″ĭ-gog′rah-fe) roentgenography of the azygous venous system following its opacification with radiographic contrast material; usually employed for evaluation of abnormal tumor masses in the mediastinum, as evidenced by extrinsic pressure upon, or complete obstruction of, the visualized azygous vein.

azygos (az′ĭ-gos) [*a* neg. + Gr. *zygon* yoke or pair] 1. unpaired. 2. any unpaired part, such as the azygos vein.

azygosperm (ah-zi′go-sperm″) [*a* neg. + Gr. *zygon* yoke or pair + *sperma* seed] azygospore.

azygospore (ah-zi′go-spōr″) [*a* neg. + Gr. *zygon* yoke or pair + *sporos* seed] a spore developed directly from a gamete without conjugation; called also *azygosperm*.

azygous (az′ĭ-gus) having no fellow; unpaired.

azymia (ah-zim′e-ah) [*a* neg. + Gr. *zymē* ferment] absence of an enzyme.

B

B symbol for *bel* and chemical symbol for *boron*. See also *point B*, under *point*.

b 1. symbol for *barn*. 2. symbol for *base*, used in designating lengths of nucleic acid sequence, e.g., 7 kb–a sequence of 7 kilobases (7,000 nucleotides long).

β beta, the second letter of the Greek alphabet; symbol for the β chain of hemoglobin.

β- a prefix designating (1) an anomer of a carbohydrate, e.g., β-D-glucose; (2) a plasma protein migrating with the β band (subdivided into the $β_1$ and $β_2$ bands) in protein electrophoresis, e.g., β-lipoprotein; (3) a substituent group of a steroid that projects above the plane of the ring, e.g., cholest-5-en-3-β-ol (cholesterol); (4) the second carbon atom in the chain starting with the one attached to the principal functional group, e.g., β-ketobutyric acid [see note at α-]; and (5) one of a group of compounds with the same trivial name, e.g., β-tocopherol.

Ba chemical symbol for *barium*.

B.A. Bachelor of Arts.

Babbitt metal (bab′it) [Isaac *Babbitt*, American inventor, 1799–1862] see under *metal*.

Babcock's operation (bab′koks) [William Wayne *Babcock*, Philadelphia surgeon, 1872–1963] see under *operation*.

Babès' treatment, tubercles (bah′bāz) [Victor *Babès*, Roumanian bacteriologist, 1854–1926] see under *treatment* and *tubercle*.

Babès-Ernst granules (bodies) (bah′bāz-ernst) [Victor *Babès;* Paul *Ernst*, German pathologist, 1859–1937] metachromatic granules.

Babesia (bah-be′ze-ah) [Victor *Babès*] a genus of hematozoan protozoa (order Piroplasmida, subclass Piroplasmia) occurring as single or paired intraerythrocytic parasites of various vertebrates, causing diseases in domestic and wild animals and humans and transmitted by ticks, in which a sexual multiplicative cycle occurs. Certain species have been reported to cause a malaria-like disease in both healthy and splenectomized individuals. Formerly called *Babesiella, Nuttallia*, and *Piroplasma*. See also *babesiosis*. **B. argenti′na,** an etiologic agent of bovine babesiosis in Central and South America, transmitted by *Boophilus microplus*, and in Australia, transmitted by *B. microplus* and *B. australis*. **B. bigem′ina,** an etiologic agent of bovine babesiosis in Central and South America, certain regions in Europe, North, Central, and South Africa, the Middle East, the West Indies, and formerly the southern United States, which is transmitted by various ticks, especially *Boophilus annulatus* and *B. microplus*. **B. bo′vis,** a species found in some of the same regions but not always together with *B. begemina*, being the major cause of bovine babesiosis in Europe and the USSR; ticks of *Boophilus* spp. are the chief vectors but in some areas *Ixodes* ticks are vectors. **B. cabal′li,** a species causing biliary fever of horses in Africa, and the Soviet Union, transmitted by ticks of the genera *Anocentor, Dermacentor, Hyalomma,* and *Rhipicephalus*. **B. ca′nis,** an etiologic agent of canine babesiosis in the domestic dog, wolf, and certain jackals, transmitted by *Rhipicephalus sanguineus, Haemophilus leachi, Hyalomma plumbeum,* and *Dermacentor* spp., and occurring worldwide. **B. ca′ti,** an etiologic agent of feline babesiosis in the domestic cat and Indian wildcat, occurring in India; the vector is unknown. **B. diver′gens,** an etiologic agent of bovine babesiosis in temperate regions of northern, western, and central Europe and perhaps Asia, transmitted chiefly by the ticks *Ixodes ricinus* and *Haemophysalis punctata*. **B. e′qui,** a species causing biliary fever of horses in the eastern part of the Soviet Union, Italy, Africa, India, and Brazil, transmitted by ticks of the genera *Dermacentor, Rhipicephalus,* and *Hyalomma;* called also *Nuttallia equi*. **B. fe′lis,** an etiologic agent of feline babesiosis in the domestic cat, Sudanese wildcat, puma, and leopard in the Sudan and South Africa; the vector is unknown. **B. gibso′ni,** an etiologic agent of canine babesiosis in the domestic dog, jackal, wolf, and fox, and also infecting the mongoose, ferret, and badger, transmitted by the ticks *Haemophysalis bispinosa* and *Rhipicephalus sanguineus*, and occurring in India, Sri Lanka, Malaysia, Korea, Egypt, Japan, and the United States. **B. herpailu′ri,** an etiologic agent of feline babesiosis in the jaguarundi in South America and Africa; the vector is unknown. **B. ma′jor,** an etiologic agent of bovine babesiosis, transmitted by the tick *Boocephilus calcaratus*, and occurring in North Africa, Europe, and the USSR. **B. micro′ti,** a parasite of rodents causing babesiosis in both healthy and splenectomized humans in North America; usually transmitted by the tick *Ixodes dammini* but transmission by means of blood transfusion has been reported. **B. mota′si,** a species infecting sheep and goats in parts of Europe, the Middle East, Indochina, Northern Africa, and the USSR, transmitted by the ticks *Rhipicephalus bursa, Dermacentor silvarum,* and *Haemophysalis punctata*. **B. o′vis,** a species infecting sheep and goats in the tropics and in southern Europe, the USSR, and the Middle East, transmitted by the ticks *Rhipicephalus bursa* and *Ixodes persulcatus*. **B. panther′ae,** an etiologic agent of feline babesiosis in the leopard in Kenya; the vector is unknown. **B. perronci′toi,** a species causing swine babesiosis in Africa; the vector is unknown. **B. trautman′ni,** a species causing swine babesiosis in Europe, Asia, Africa, and Central and South America; transmitted by the tick *Rhipicephalus sanguineus*. **B. voge′li,** an etiologic agent of canine babesiosis in the domestic dog, transmitted by the tick *Rhipicephalus sanguineus*, and occurring in Asia and Africa.

babesiasis (bah″bĕ-si′ah-sis) 1. the chronic, asymptomatic form of infection with protozoa of the genus *Babesia;* cf. *babesiosis.* 2. babesiosis.

Babesiella (bah-be″ze-el′ah) *Babesia.*

babesiosis (bah-be″ze-o′sis) a group of tickborne diseases due to infection with protozoa of the genus *Babesia,* occurring in both wild and domestic animals such as cattle, horses, sheep, goats, swine, cats, and dogs. Most cases are associated with anemia, hemoglobinuria, and hemoglobinemia. Human infection causes a malaria-like fever, chills, sweats, myalgia, nausea and vomiting, hemolytic anemia, and splenomegaly. Babesiosis is a classic zoonotic disease in which man is infected incidentally. Called also *babesiasis* and *piroplasmosis.* **bovine b.,** infection of cattle by *Babesia bigemina,* which was once endemic in the southern United States (*Texas fever, Texas cattle fever, redwater fever*) but has been largely eliminated by eradicating its tick vector in that region, *Boophilus annulatus.* The acute phase is manifested by fever, hemoglobinuria, anemia, icterus, and splenomegaly. *Babesia bovis, B. divergens, B. argentina,* and other *Babesia* spp. cause bovine babesiosis in various parts of the world, each employing one or more tick vectors, e.g., *Boophilus microplus, Haemophysalis* spp., and *Rhipicephalus* spp. **canine b.,** infection of dogs and other canines with *Babesia canis, B. gibsoni,* or *B. vogeli,* transmitted by various ticks, the most common being *Rhipicephalus sanguineus,* and characterized in the acute phase by depression, weakness, loss of appetite, pallor of the mucous membranes, icterus, fever, and splenomegaly. The acute form is usually fatal. Called also *biliary fever of dogs* and *malignant jaundice of dogs.* **equine b.,** infection of horses and other equines with *Babesia caballi* and *B. equi,* transmitted by various species of ticks of the genera *Dermacentor, Hyalomma,* and *Rhipicephalus,* and characterized by high fever, immobility, icterus, gastrointestinal disturbances, rapid emaciation, and dependent edema. Called also *biliary fever of horses* and *equine biliary fever.* **feline b.,** infection of cats and other felines with *Babesia cati, B. felis, B. herpailuri,* or *B. pantherae,* the vectors of which are unknown. It is characterized by loss of appetite, lethargy, weakness, rough coat, and pale mucous membranes. **ovine b.,** infection in sheep and goats with *Babesia motasi* or *B. ovis;* the former is transmitted by *Rhipicephalus bursa, Dermacentor silvarum,* and *Haemophysalis punctata,* and the latter by *Rhipicephalus bursa* and *Ixodes persulcatus.* **porcine b.,** swine b. **swine b.,** infection of swine with *Babesia trautmanni* or *B. perroncitoi;* the former occurs in Europe, Asia, Africa, and Central and South America and is transmitted by *Rhipicephalus sanguineus,* and the latter occurs in Africa but its vector is unknown. Called also *porcine b.*

Babinski's law, etc. (bah-bin′skēz) [Joseph François Felix *Babinski,* physician in Paris, 1857–1932] see under *law, phenomenon, reflex, sign,* and *syndrome.*

Babinski-Fröhlich syndrome (bah-bin′ske-fra′lik) [J.F.F. *Babinski;* Alfred *Fröhlich,* Vienna neurologist, 1871–1953] adiposogenital dystrophy.

Babinski-Nageotte syndrome (bah-bin′ske-nazh-yot′) [J.F.F. *Babinski;* Jean *Nageotte,* Paris pathologist, 1866–1948] see under *syndrome.*

Babinski-Vaquez syndrome (bah-bin′ske-vak-a′) [J.F.F. *Babinski;* Louis Henri *Vaquez,* French physician, 1860–1936] Babinski syndrome.

baby (ba′be) an infant; a child not yet able to walk. **blue b.,** an infant born with cyanosis due to a congenital heart lesion or to congenital atelectasis. **collodion b.,** an infant born encased in a tight membrane resembling collodion or parchment, which is subsequently shed, occasionally leaving normal-appearing skin (*lamellar exfoliation,* or *desquamation, of the newborn*). It is usually a primary manifestation of various forms of ichthyosis, most often the lamellar type.

bacampicillin hydrochloride (bah-kam″pi-sil′in) chemical name: 6-[(aminophenylacetyl)amino]-3,3-dimethyl-7-oxo-4-thia-1-azabicyclo[3.2.0]heptane-2-carboxylic acid 1-[(ethoxycarbonyl)oxy]ethyl ester monohydrochloride; an antibacterial, $C_{21}H_{27}N_3O_7S \cdot HCl$.

bacca (bak′ah), gen. and pl. *bac′cae* [L.] a berry.

baccate (bak′āt) resembling a berry.

Baccelli's mixture, sign (bak-chel′ēz) [Guido *Baccelli,* Italian physician, 1832–1916] see under *mixture,* and see *aphonic pectoriloquy,* under *pectoriloquy.*

bacciform (bak′si-form) [L. *bacca* berry + *forma* shape] berry-shaped.

Bachmann's bundle [Jean George *Bachmann,* American physiologist, 1877–1959] see under *bundle.*

Baciguent (bas′i-gwent) trademark for preparations of bacitracin.

Bacillaceae (bas″il-la′se-e) a family of bacteria made up of endospore-forming rods and cocci. The mostly gram-positive organisms are usually soil saprophytes, but a few are insect or animal parasites and may produce disease. It includes five genera: *Bacillus, Clostridium, Desulfotomaculum, Sporolactobacillus,* and *Sporosarcina;* the first two contain important human pathogens.

bacillary (bas′i-la″re) pertaining to bacilli or to rodlike forms.

bacillemia (bas″i-le′me-ah) [*bacillus* + Gr. *haima* blood] the presence of bacilli in the blood.

bacilli (bah-sil′i) [L.] plural of *bacillus.*

bacilli-, bacill(o)- [L. *bacillus,* q.v.] a combining form denoting relationship to a bacillus or to bacilli.

bacilliferous (bah″sil-lif′er-us) bearing or carrying bacilli.

bacilliform (bah-sil′i-form) [*bacillus* + L. *forma* form] having the appearance of a bacillus; rod-shaped.

bacillin (bah-sil′in) an antibiotic substance isolated from strains of *Bacillus subtilis.*

bacill(o)- see *bacilli-.*

bacilluria (bas″i-lu′re-ah) [*bacillus* + *-uria*] the presence of bacilli in the urine.

Bacillus (bah-sil′lus) [L. "little rod"] a genus of bacteria of the family Bacillaceae, including large aerobic or facultatively anaerobic, spore-forming, rod-shaped cells, the great majority of which are gram-positive and motile. The genus is separated into 48 species, of which three are pathogenic, or potentially pathogenic, and the remainder are saprophytic soil forms. Many organisms historically called *Bacillus* are now classified in other genera. **B. aerog′enes capsula′tus,** *Clostridium perfringens.* **B. al′vei,** the etiologic agent of European foulbrood of honeybees. **B. an′thracis,** the causative agent of anthrax in lower animals and humans. Virulence is associated with the production of capsules and a potent exotoxin. **anthrax b.,** *Bacillus anthracis.* **B. botuli′nus,** *Clostridium botulinum.* **B. bre′vis,** an organism that is the source of the antibiotics gramicidin and tyrocidin. **B. bronchisep′ticus,** *Bordetella bronchiseptica.* **B. cer′eus,** a sometimes motile, aerobic or facultatively anaerobic spore-forming species that is a common soil saprophyte. It causes food poisoning by the formation of an enterotoxin in contaminated foods. **B. co′li,** *Escherichia coli.* **B. dysente′riae,** *Shigella dysenteriae.* **enteric b.,** a bacillus belonging to the family Enterobacteriaceae. **B. enterit′idis,** *Salmonella enteritidis.* **B. faeca′lis alcalig′enes,** *Alcaligenes faecalis.* **B. fra′gilis,** *Bacteroides fragilis.* **B. fusifor′mis,** *Fusobacterium nucleatum.* **B. lar′vae,** the specific etiologic agent of American foulbrood of honeybees, not pathogenic for man. **legionnaire's b.,** *Legionella pneumophila.* **B. lep′rae,** *Mycobacterium leprae.* **B. mal′lei,** *Pseudomonas mallei.* **B. megate′rium,** a widely distributed saprophytic soil form, commonly occurring as a laboratory contaminant. **B. necroph′orus,** *Fusobacterium necrophorum.* **B. oedemat′iens,** *Clostridium novyi.* **B. oedem′atis malig′ni No. II,** *Clostridium novyi.* **B. pneumo′niae,** *Klebsiella pneumoniae.* **B. polymyx′a,** a saprophytic soil and water microorganism that produces the antibiotic polymyxin. **B. pseudomal′lei,** *Pseudomonas pseudomallei.* **B. pyocya′neus,** *Pseudomonas aeruginosa.* **B. stearothemoph′ilus,** a thermophilic species that produces very resistant spores and is capable of growth at 65° C. It is used to test for autoclave quality control. **B. sub′tilis,** a common saprophytic soil and water form, often occurring as a laboratory contaminant and occasionally causing conjunctivitis in humans. It produces the antibiotic bacitracin. **B. tet′ani,** *Clostridium tetani.* **B. ty′phi,** **B. typho′sus,** *Salmonella typhi.* **B. welch′ii,** *Clostridium perfringens.*

bacillus (bah-sil′us), pl. *bacil′li* [L.] 1. an organism of the genus *Bacillus.* 2. any rod-shaped bacterium. **Bang's b.,** *Brucella abortus.* **Battey b.,** *Mycobacterium intracellulare.* **Boas-Oppler b.,** a microorganism, probably a species of *Lactobacillus,* first found in the gastric juice of patients with stomach carcinoma. Called also *lactobacillus of Boas-Oppler*. **Bordet-Gengou b.,** *Bordetella pertussis*. **butter b.,** *Clostridium butyricum*. **Calmette-Guérin b.,** an organism of the strain *Mycobacterium bovis*, rendered completely avirulent by cultivation for many years on bile-glycero-potato medium. The strain, commonly called BCG, is used for immunization of humans against tuberculosis and in cancer chemotherapy. **Chauveau's b.,** *Clostridium chauvoei*. **colon b.,** *Escherichia coli*. **coliform bacilli,** gram-negative bacilli found in the intestinal tract that resemble *Escherichia coli*, particularly in the fermentation of lactose with gas. The term generally is used to refer to the genera *Citrobacter, Escherichia, Edwardsiella, Enterobacter, Klebsiella,* and *Serratia*. **DF-2 b.** [*dysgonic fermenter*], a gram-negative aerobic bacillus that forms purplish colonies on heart-infusion agar containing 5 per cent sheep's or rabbit's blood and incubated in an atmosphere of 10 per cent carbon dioxide; bacilli fail to grow on MacConkey agar and are catalase-positive and oxidase-positive. Organisms can be isolated from the oral and nasal secretions of healthy dogs and, following a dog bite, may cause an infection whose manifestations include cellulitis, bacteremia, purulent meningitis, endocarditis, peripheral gangrene, malar purpura, and the Waterhouse-Friderichsen syndrome. Death may occur. The infection tends to be more severe in asplenic patients. **diphtheria b.,** *Corynebacterium diphtheriae*. **Döderlein's b.,** one of the gram-positive rods commonly found in vaginal secretions that may consist of mixtures of *Lactobacillus acidophilus, L. casei, L. cellobiosisus, L. fermentum,* or *Leuconostoc mesenteroides*. Said by some to be identical with *Lactobacillus acidophilus*. **Ducrey's b.,** *Haemophilus ducreyi*. **dysentery bacilli,** gram-negative, non–spore-forming rods causing dysentery in man; see *Shigella*. **Escherich's b.,** *Escherichia coli*. **Flexner's b.,** *Shigella flexneri*. **Friedländer's b.,** *Klebsiella pneumoniae*. **fusiform b.,** fusobacterium. **Gärtner's b.,** *Salmonella enteritidis*. **Ghon-Sachs b.,** *Clostridium septicum*. **glanders b.,** *Pseudomonas mallei*. **Hansen's b.,** *Mycobacterium leprae*. **Hofmann's b.,** *Corynebacterium pseudodiphtheriticum*. **hog cholera b.,** *Salmonella choleraesuis*. **Johne's b.,** *Mycobacterium paratuberculosis*. **Klebs-Löffler b.,** *Corynebacterium diphtheriae*. **Koch-Weeks b.,** *Haemophilus aegyptius*. **lepra b., leprosy b.,** *Mycobacterium leprae*. **Morax-Axenfeld b.,** *Moraxella (Moraxella) lacunata*. **Morgan's b.,** *Proteus morgani*. **Newcastle-Manchester b.,** *Shigella flexneri* type 6, Boyd 88. **paracolon bacilli,** microorganisms commonly found in the intestinal flora, distinguished by delayed (5–21 days) fermentation of lactose. Organisms of this type belong to the genera *Escherichia, Citrobacter,* or *Klebsiella*. **Pfeiffer's b.,** *Haemophilus influenzae*. **Preisz-Nocard b.,** *Corynebacterium pseudotuberculosis*. **rhinoscleroma b.,** *Klebsiella pneumoniae* subsp. *rhinoscleromatis*. **Schmitz's b.,** *Shigella dysenteriae* type 2. **Schmorl's b.,** *Fusobacterium necrophorum*. **Shiga b.,** *Shigella dysenteriae* type 1. **smegma b.,** *Mycobacterium smegmatis*. **Sonne-Duval b.,** *Shigella sonnei*. **Stanley b.,** a serotype of *Salmonella enteritidis* isolated from patients with food poisoning in Stanley, England. **Strong's b.,** *Shigella flexneri*. **swine rotlauf b.,** *Erysipelothrix rhusiopathiae*. **tetanus b.,** *Clostridium tetani*. **timothy b.,** *Mycobacterium phlei*. **tubercle b.,** *Mycobacterium tuberculosis*. **typhoid b.,** *Salmonella typhi*. **vole b.,** *Mycobacterium microti*. **Weeks' b.,** *Haemophilus aegyptius*. **Welch's b.,** *Clostridium perfringens*. **Whitmore's b.,** *Pseudomonas pseudomallei*.

bacitracin (bas″ĭ-tra′sin) [USP] an antibacterial polypeptide produced by the growth of a gram-positive, spore-forming organism belonging to the *licheniformis* group of *Bacillus subtilis,* occurring as a white to pale buff powder. It is effective against many gram-positive bacteria, such as staphylococci, streptococci, and pneumococci, and some gram-negative bacteria, such as gonococci and meningococci. It is applied topically to the skin or conjunctiva or administered by intramuscular injection in the treatment of infections caused by susceptible organisms. **b. zinc** [USP], the zinc salt of bacitracin, occurring as a white to a pale tan powder; used for topical application to the skin.

back (bak) the posterior part of the trunk from the neck to the pelvis; called also *dorsum* [NA]. **flat b.,** a back that appears flat as a result of a decrease of normal lumbar

lordosis and normal thoracic kyphosis. **functional b.,** a condition of fatigue and defective balance marked by more or less continuous lumbar or dorsal pain. **hollow b.,** see *lordosis*. **hump b., hunch b.,** kyphosis. **poker b.,** rheumatoid spondylitis. **saddle b.,** see *lordosis*.

backalgia (bak-al′je-ah) back pain not explained on the basis of structural abnormality or disease process.

backbone (back′bōn) the vertebral column, forming a continuous, comparatively rigid structure in the midline of the back; see *columna vertebralis* [NA].

backcross (bak′kros) in experimental genetics, a mating between a heterozygote and a homozygote. **double b.,** the mating between a double heterozygote and a homozygote.

backflow (bak′flo) the flowing of a current in a direction the reverse of that normally taken; regurgitation. **pyelovenous b.,** the drainage of fluid from the pelvis of the kidney into the venous system under certain conditions of back pressure.

backing (bak′ing) in dentistry, the piece of metal that supports a porcelain or resin facing on a fixed or removable partial denture. **alloy b.,** one made of an alloy instead of pure platinum or gold.

backknee (bak′ne) genu recurvatum.

back-raking (bak-rāk′ing) extraction of impacted feces from the rectum of an animal.

backscatter (bak′skat-er) in radiology, radiation deflected by scattering processes at angles greater than 90 degrees to the original direction of the beam of radiation; see *scatter,* and see also *scattered rays,* under *ray*.

BaCl₂ barium chloride.

baclofen (bak′lo-fen) chemical name: 4-amino-3-(4-chlorophenyl)butanoic acid. A muscle relaxant, $C_{10}H_{12}ClNO_2$, which is an analogue of gamma-aminobutyric acid; administered orally in the treatment of spasticity in multiple sclerosis and other disorders of the spinal cord.

BACON a regimen of bleomycin, Adriamycin (doxorubicin), CCNU (lomustine), Oncovin (vincristine), and nitrogen mustard (mechlorethamine), used in cancer chemotherapy.

BACOP a regimen of bleomycin, Adriamycin (doxorubicin), cyclophosphamide, Oncovin (vincristine), and prednisone, used in cancer chemotherapy.

Bact. *Bacterium*.

-bacter [L. *bacterium,* q.v.] a word termination denoting a bacterium.

bacteremia (bak″ter-e′me-ah) [Gr. *baktērion* little rod + *haima* blood] the presence of bacteria in the blood.

Bacteria (bak-te′re-ah) in former systems of classification, a division of the kingdom Procaryotae, including all prokaryotic organisms except the blue-green algae (Cyanobacteria). See also *Procaryotae*.

bacteria (bak-te′re-ah) [L.] plural of *bacterium*.

Bacteriaceae (bak″te-re-a′se-e) in former systems of classification, a name given to a family of bacteria.

bacterial (bak-te′re-al) pertaining to or caused by bacteria.

bactericidal (bak-tēr″ĭ-si′dal) [*bacterium* + L. *caedere* to kill] destructive to bacteria.

bactericide (bak-tēr′ĭ-sīd) an agent that destroys bacteria. **specific b.,** bacteriolysin.

bactericidin (bak″ter-rĭ-si′din) a substance that leads to the death of bacteria; such substances include both antibody and certain nonantibody components in the serum.

bacterid (bak″ter-id) [Gr. *baktērion* little rod + *-id*] an id reaction associated with a bacterial infection. **pustular b.,** a chronic relapsing cutaneous eruption consisting of vesicles or pustules frequently localized to the palms and soles, which generally occurs in association with a focal infection elsewhere in the body.

bacteridium (bak″ter-id′e-um), pl. *bacterid′ia*. A former generic name for certain bacilli.

bacteriemia (bak-tēr″e-e′me-ah) bacteremia.

bacteriform (bak-tēr′ĕ-form) resembling a bacterium in form.

bacterin (bak′ter-in) bacterial vaccine. **Bordetella bronchiseptica b.,** a suspension of inactivated and adsorbed *Bordetella bronchiseptica,* used for prevention of atrophic rhinitis of swine due to *B. bronchiseptica*. **Clo-**

stridium chauvoei-septicum b.-t., see under *bacterin-toxoid.* **Clostridium haemolyticum b.**, a chemically killed culture of *C. haemolyticum,* used for prevention of bacillary hemoglobinuria (redwater disease) in cattle, sheep, and goats. **Erysipelothrix rhusiopathiae b.**, a formalin-killed, adsorbed culture of *E. rhusiopathiae,* used for immunization of swine against erysipelas. **Haemophilus gallinarum b.**, a chemically inactivated and adsorbed suspension of *H. gallinarum,* used for immunization of chickens against infectious coryza. **Leptospira canicola-grippotyphosa-harjo-icterohaemorrhagiae-pomona b.**, chemically inactivated, adsorbed whole cultures of *L. canicola, L. grippotyphosa, L. harjo, L. icterohemorrhagiae,* and *L. pomona,* used for immunization of cattle against leptospirosis. **P. multocida b.**, 1. chemically killed, adsorbed whole culture of *P. multocida* bovine and porcine isolates, used for prevention of pasturellosis in cattle, sheep, goats, and swine. 2. chemically killed, emulsified whole culture of *P. multocida* avian isolates, used for prevention of fowl cholera in chickens and turkeys. **Pasturella haemolytica-multocida b.**, an inactivated and adsorbed whole culture of *P. haemolytica* and *P. multocida,* used for prevention of pasturellosis in cattle and sheep. **Salmonella dublin-typhimurium b.**, a formalin-inactivated, adsorbed suspension of *S. dublin* and *S. typhimurium,* used for prevention of salmonellosis in cattle. **Staphylococcus aureus b.**, a formalin-inactivated, adsorbed lysed culture of *S. aureus,* used for prevention of *S. aureus* infection in cattle. **Streptococcus equi b.**, a chemically killed, adsorbed suspension of *S. equi,* used for prevention of strangles in horses. **Vibrio fetus b.**, a chemically inactivated, adsorbed whole culture of *Campylobacter*(*Vibrio*) *fetus,* used for immunization of heifers and cows (*C. fetus* subspecies *fetus*) or of ewes (*C. fetus* subspecies *intestinalis* or *jejuni*) for prevention of infertility and abortion due to *C. fetus* infection (bovine or ovine genital campylobacteriosis).

bacterin-toxoid (bak'ter-in tok'soid) an active immunizing agent prepared from chemically inactivated bacterial cultures containing both killed bacteria and inactivated toxin. **Clostridium botulinum type C b.-t.**, a chemically killed, alum-adsorbed culture of *C. botulinum,* type C, used for prevention of type C botulism in mink. **Clostridium chauvoei-septicum b.-t.**, a chemically killed culture of *C. chauvoei* and *C. septicum,* used for prevention of blackleg and malignant edema in cattle, horses, sheep, and goats. **Clostridium novyi-sordelli b.-t.**, a chemically inactivated suspension of *C. novyi* and *C. sordelli,* used for immunization of cattle and sheep against diseases caused by these organisms (e.g., black disease, bighead). **Clostridium perfringens b.-t.**, a chemically killed culture of *C. perfringens* type C and/or type D organisms, used for prevention of enterotoxemia caused by these strains in sheep and cattle.

bacteri(o)- [L. *bacterium,* q.v.] a combining form denoting relationship to bacteria.

bacteriochlorophyll (bak-te''re-o-klo'ro-fil) any of a group of pigments (designated bacteriochlorophyll *a, b, c, d,* or *e*) occurring in bacteria and functioning in anaerobic photosynthesis.

bacteriocidin (bak-te''re-o-si'din) bactericidin.

bacteriocin (bak-te're-o-sin) a protein substance, e.g., colicin or staphylococcin, released by certain bacteria that kills but does not lyse closely related strains of bacteria. Specific bacteriocins attach to specific receptors on cell walls and induce specific metabolic block, e.g., cessation of nucleic acid or protein synthesis of oxidative phosphorylation.

bacteriocinogen (bak-te''re-o-sin''o-jen) a bacterial plasmid that controls the synthesis of bacteriocin.

bacteriocinogenic (bak-te''re-o-sin''o-jen'ik) giving rise to bacteriocin.

bacterioclasis (bak-te''re-ok'lah-sis) [*bacteria* + Gr. *klasis* breaking] bacteriolysis.

bacteriofluorescin (bak-te''re-o-floo-o-res'in) a fluorescent dye produced by *Pseudomonas aeruginosa.*

bacteriogenic (bak-te''re-o-jen'ik) caused by bacteria.

bacteriogenous (bak-te''re-oj'ĕ-nus) bacteriogenic.

bacterioid (bak-te're-oid) [Gr. *baktērion* little rod + *eidos* form] 1. resembling the bacteria. 2. a structure resembling a bacterium.

bacteriologic, bacteriological (bak-te''re-o-loj'ik, bak-te''re-o-loj'ĭ-k'l) pertaining to bacteriology.

bacteriologist (bak-te''re-ol'o-jist) an expert in bacteriology.

bacteriology (bak-te''re-ol'o-je) [*bacteria* + *-logy*] the science that treats of bacteria. Cf. *microbiology.* **clinical diagnostic b.**, the science and practice of collecting specimens from persons or the environment, examining them for bacteria or evidence of bacterial infection, and evaluating the results. **medical b.**, that branch of bacteriology that deals chiefly with bacteria causing human disease. **pathological b.**, that branch of bacteriology which treats chiefly of the effects produced upon the animal body by the presence of bacteria and their toxins. **public health b.**, that branch of bacteriology that deals with the spread and prevention of bacterial disease. **sanitary b.**, bacteriology that deals chiefly with disease prevention based upon sanitation in food and water supplies and distribution, and upon disposal of sewage. **systematic b.**, that branch of bacteriology that studies the classification and relationship of bacteria (taxonomy).

bacteriolysin (bak-te''re-ol'ĭ-sin) an antibacterial antibody that produces lysis of bacterial cells.

bacteriolysis (bak-te''re-ol'ĭ-sis) [*bacteria* + Gr. *lysis* dissolution] disruption of the structural integrity of a bacterial cell resulting in release of the cell contents.

bacteriolytic (bak-te''re-o-lit'ik) pertaining to, characterized by, or promoting the dissolution or destruction of bacteria.

Bacterionema (bak-te''re-o-ne'mah) [*bacterium* + Gr. *nēma* thread] a genus of bacteria of the family Actinomycetaceae, order Actinomycetales, occurring as facultative anaerobic, gram-positive, pleomorphic organisms, comprising nonseptate and septate filaments and bacilli. **B. matrucho'tii**, a species found in the oral cavity of man and other primates, particularly in dental calculus and plaque.

bacterio-opsonin (bak-te''re-o-op-so'nin) an opsonin that acts on bacteria.

bacteriopexia (bak-te''re-o-pek'se-ah) bacteriopexy.

bacteriopexy (bak-te''re-o-pek'se) [*bacteria* + Gr. *pēxis* fixation] the immobilization of bacteria by histiocytes or other phagocytes.

bacteriophage (bak-te're-o-fāj'') [*bacteria* + Gr. *phagein* to eat] a virus that lyses bacteria; see *bacterial virus,* under *virus.* **temperate b.**, a bacteriophage whose genetic material (prophage) becomes an intimate part of the bacterial cell, persisting through many cell division cycles. The affected bacterial cell is known as a *lysogenic bacterium* (q.v.).

bacteriophagia (bak-te''re-o-fa'je-ah) lysis of bacteria by a bacteriophage.

bacteriophagic (bak-te''re-o-faj'ik) [*bacteria* + Gr. *phagein* to eat] pertaining to, characterized by, or producing bacteriophagia.

bacteriophagology (bak-te''re-o-fah-gol'o-je) the study of bacteriophage.

bacterioph'agum intestina'le (bak-te''re-of'ah-gum in-tes''tĭ-na'le) (*obs.*) bacteriophage.

bacteriophagy (bak-te''re-of'ah-je) bacteriophagia.

bacteriophytoma (bak-te''re-o-fi-to'mah) a tumor-like, reactive lesion caused by bacteria.

bacterioplasmin (bak-te''re-o-plaz'min) plasmin produced by bacteria.

bacterioprecipitin (bak-te''re-o-pre-sip'ĭ-tin) a precipitin formed in the body in response to bacterial antigens.

bacterioprotein (bak-te''re-o-pro'te-in) any protein of bacterial origin.

bacteriopsonic (bak-te''re-op-son'ik) exerting an opsonic effect on bacteria.

bacteriopsonin (bak-te''re-op'so-nin) an antibody that interacts with bacteria to render them more susceptible to ingestion by phagocytic cells than they otherwise would be.

bacteriopurpurin (bak-te''re-o-pur'pu-rin) [*bacteria* + L. *purpur* purple] a light purple pigment produced by certain bacteria.

bacteriorhodopsin (bak-te''re-o-ro-dop'sin) [*bacteria* + Gr. *rhodon* rose + *opsis* vision] a purple pigment, similar to rhodopsin, occurring in the cell membrane of bacteria of the genus *Halobacterium*, which converts sunlight directly into electrochemical energy.

bacteriosis (bak-te″re-o′sis)   any bacterial disease.

bacteriospermia (bak-te″re-o-sper′me-ah)   the presence of bacteria in the semen.

bacteriostasis (bak-te″re-os′tah-sis) [*bacteria* + Gr. *stasis* stoppage]   the inhibition of growth, but not the killing, of bacteria by chemicals or biologic materials.

bacteriostat (bak-te′re-o-stat″)   an agent that inhibits the growth of bacteria.

bacteriostatic (bak-te″re-o-stat′ik)   1. inhibiting the growth or multiplication of bacteria.   2. an agent that inhibits the growth or multiplication of bacteria.

bacteriotherapy (bak-te″re-o-ther′ah-pe) [*bacteria* + *therapy*]   treatment of disease by the introduction of bacteria into the system.

bacteriotoxemia (bak-te″re-o-tok-se′me-ah)   the presence of bacterial toxins in the blood.

bacteriotoxic (bak-te″re-o-tok′sik)   toxic to bacteria.

bacteriotoxin (bak-te″re-o-tok′sin) [*bacteria* + *toxin*]   any toxin produced by or toxic to bacteria.

bacteriotropic (bak-te″re-o-trop′ik) [*bacteria* + Gr. *tropos* a turning]   turning toward or changing bacteria; bacteriopsonic.

bacteriotropin (bak-te″re-ot′ro-pin)   bacteriopsonin.

bacteritic (bak″ter-it′ik)   caused by or characterized by bacteria.

Bacterium (bak-te′re-um) [L.; Gr. *baktērion* little rod]   in former systems of classification, a genus of bacteria made up of non–spore-forming, rod-shaped bacteria, not necessarily closely related, that were not fitted into other formally defined genera.   **B. actinomyce′tem co′mitans,** *Actinobacillus actinomycetemcomitans.*   **B. aerog′enes,** *Enterobacter aerogenes.*   **B. aerugino′sum,** *Pseudomonas aeruginosa.*   **B. chol′erae su′is,** *Salmonella choleraesuis.*   **B. cloa′cae,** *Enterobacter cloacae.*   **B. co′li, B. co′li commu′ne,** *Escherichia coli.*   **B. dysente′riae,** *Shigella dysenteriae.*   **B. faeca′lis alcalig′enes,** *Alcaligenes faecalis.*   **B. pes′tis,** *Yersinia pestis.*   **B. son′nei,** *Shigella sonnei.*   **B. tularen′se,** *Francisella tularensis.*

bacterium (bak-te′re-um), pl. *bacte′ria* [L.; Gr. *baktērion* little rod]   in general, any of the unicellular prokaryotic microorganisms that commonly multiply by cell division (fission) and whose cell is typically contained within a cell wall. They may be aerobic or anaerobic, motile or nonmotile, and may be free-living, saprophytic, parasitic, or even pathogenic, the last causing disease in plants or animals. See also *Bacteria.*   **acid-fast b.,** one that retains stains by dyes (e.g., carbolfuchsin or auramine) so tenaciously that it is not decolorized by 5 per cent mineral acids, especially *Mycobacterium* species and *Nocardia.*   **autotrophic b.,** one that has no organic nutritional requirements; none are pathogenic.   **beaded b.,** one having deeply staining granules equally spaced along the rod.   **bifid b.,** one that has a branched rod- or cleft-shaped cell, especially *Bifidobacterium.*   **blue-green b.,** see *Cyanobacteria.*   **Chauveau's b.,** *Clostridium chauvoei.*   **chemoautotrophic b.,** one that is autotrophic and obtains energy by the oxidation of inorganic compounds of iron, nitrogen, sulfur, or hydrogen; none are pathogenic.   **chemoheterotrophic b.,** one that is heterotrophic and obtains energy by the oxidation of organic compounds by mechanisms closely similar to those existing in higher animals.   **chromo b., chromogenic b.,** one that produces pigment.   **coliform b.,** one of the facultative gram-negative, rod-shaped bacteria that are normal inhabitants of the intestinal tract of humans and animals. See *Citrobacter, Edwardsiella, Enterobacter, Escherichia, Klebsiella,* and *Serratia.*   **coryneform bacteria,** a group of bacteria that are morphologically similar to the organisms of the genus *Corynebacterium;* corynebacteria. Called also *coryneform group.*   **Dar es Salaam b.,** *Salmonella salamae.*   **denitrifying b.,** one that is able to reduce nitrates to nitrites, ammonia, or nitrogen gas.   **gram-negative b.,** see under *G.*   **gram-postive b.,** see under *G.*   **hemophilic b.,** one that has a nutritional affinity for constituents of blood or whose growth is stimulated by blood-enriched media.   **heterotrophic b.,** one that requires organic compounds of carbon and nitrogen as sources of energy or as essential parts of the cell.   **higher**

bacteria, a term used to denote filamentous bacteria (e.g., Actinomycetales) that seem to be intermediate between bacteria and fungi.   **hydrogen b.,** a facultative chemoautotrophic microorganism that respires by the oxidation of hydrogen to water, using various organic compounds as carbon and energy sources. Hydrogen bacteria are included in the genera *Pseudomonas* (*P. facilis, P. ruhlandii, P. saccharophila*), *Alcaligenes* (*A. eutrophus, A. paradoxus*), *Paracoccus* (*P. denitrificans*), and *Nocardia* (*N. opaca*).   **iron b.,** an autotrophic microorganism that oxidizes iron from the ferrous to the ferric state, including some of the sheathed bacteria (*Clonothrix, Aenothrix, Leptothrix, Lieskeela, Sphaerotilus*) and the budding bacteria (*Gallionella*).   **lysogenic b.,** one that harbors in its genome the genetic material (prophage) of a temperate bacteriophage and thus reproduces the bacteriophage in cell division; occasionally the prophage develops into the mature form, replicates, lyses the bacterial cell, and is free to infect other cells.   **mesophilic b.,** one whose optimal temperature for growth is in a midrange (30° to 45° C., 86° to 113° F.) that includes the temperature of the human body.   **nitrifying b.,** a soil bacterium of the family Nitrobacteraceae that oxidizes ammonia to nitrites (*Nitrobacter, Nitrococcus, Nitrospina*) or nitrites to nitrates (*Nitrosococcus, Nitrosolobus, Nitrosomonas*).   **nodule bacteria,** bacteria which by their growth in specific nodules on the roots of plants (legumes) tend to bring about fixation of atmospheric nitrogen.   **nonsulfur b., purple,** a photosynthetic, heterotrophic, microaerophilic bacterium of the family Rhodospirillaceae. Purple nonsulfur bacteria reduce CO_2 and oxidize sulfide or thiosulfate but not elemental sulfur in the presence of the pigment bacteriochlorophyll *a.*   **parasitic b.,** one that is dependent on a living host for its nutrition.   **pathogenic b.,** one capable of causing disease.   **photoautotrophic b.,** one that is autotrophic capable of deriving energy from light.   **photoheterotrophic b.,** one that is heterotrophic capable of deriving energy from light.   **photosynthetic b.,** one that contains pigments such as bacteriochlorphylls and carotenoids enabling the organism to conduct photosynthesis and assimilate carbon dioxide, with or without the production of oxygen; the process depends on the presence of oxidizable electron donors such as water and reduced sulfur compounds. See also *Cyanobacteria* and *Rhodospirillales.*   **phototrophic bacteria,** Photobacteria.   **psychrophilic b.,** one whose optimum temperature for growth is 15° to 20° C. (59° to 68° F.).   **purple b.,** a photosynthetic bacterium that reduces CO_2 in the presence of sulfur compounds. Purple bacteria are classified in the family Chromatiaceae (purple sulfur bacteria) and Rhodospirillaceae (purple nonsulfur bacteria).   **pyogenic b.,** one that produces suppuration when it infects an organism.   **pyrogenetic b.,** one that produces fever when it infects an organism.   **rough b.,** a variant form of a bacterium characterized by dry, wrinkled colonies on solid media. See *smooth-rough variation,* under *variation.*   **saprophytic b.,** one that lives in decaying organic matter.   **smooth b.,** one characterized by smooth, glossy colonies on solid media. See *smooth-rough variation,* under *variation.*   **sulfur b.,** a bacterium that oxidizes hydrogen sulfide, sulfur, or thiosulfate. Sulfur bacteria include the photosynthetic purple bacteria (Chromatiaceae), filamentous gliding organisms (*Beggiatoa, Thioploca, Thiothrix*), unicellular gliding organisms (*Achromatium*), and gram-negative chemolithotrophic sulfur oxidizers (*Macromonas, Sulfolobus, Thiobacillus, Thiobacterium, Thiospira, Thiovulum*).   **sulfur b., purple,** a photosynthetic autotrophic anaerobic bacterium of the family Chromatiaceae. Purple sulfur bacteria reduce carbon dioxide and oxidize sulfides and elemental sulfur in the presence of the pigment bacteriochlorophyll *a* or *b.*   **thermophilic b.,** one that grows best at temperature above 40° C. (104° F.) with an optimal range of 50° to 70° C. (122° to 158° F.).   **toxigenic b., toxinogenic b.,** one that produces a toxin.   **water b.,** a gram-negative bacterium capable of rapid growth in all types of water and producing pyrogenic infections, especially in immunocompromised hospital patients, occurring as a contaminant in hemodialysis fluids and in flood waters. The most common water bacteria are species of *Achromobacter, Acinetobacter, Aeromonas, Flavobacterium,* and *Pseudomonas.*

bacteriuria (bak-te″re-u′re-ah) [*bacteria* + Gr. *ouron* urine + *-ia*]   the presence of bacteria in the urine.

bacteriuric (bak-te″re-u′rik)   pertaining to bacteriuria.

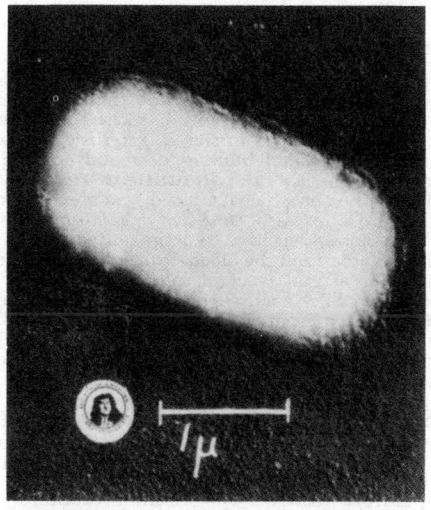

Escherichia coli. (Hedén and Wyckoff, S.A.B.
LS-290.)

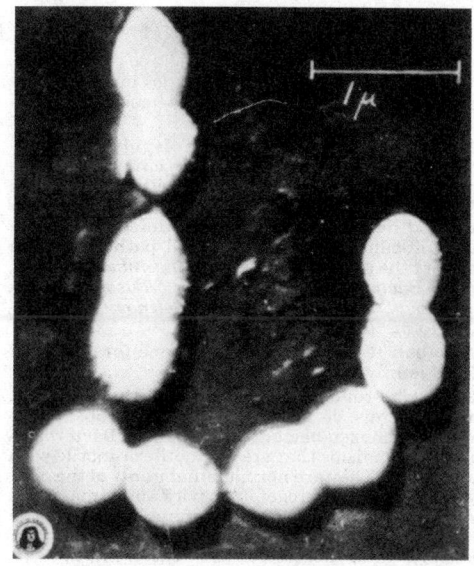

Streptococcus pneumoniae, type 2.
(Williams, S.A.B. LS-162.)

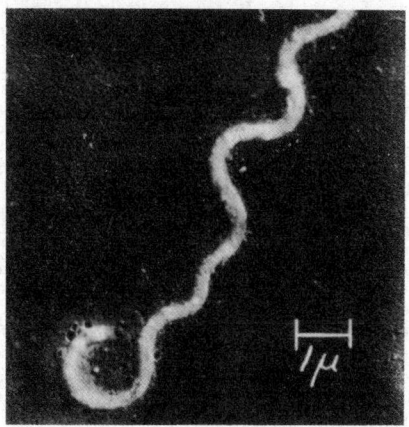

Borrelia vincentii. (Hampp, Scott, and
Wyckoff, S.A.B. LS-248.)

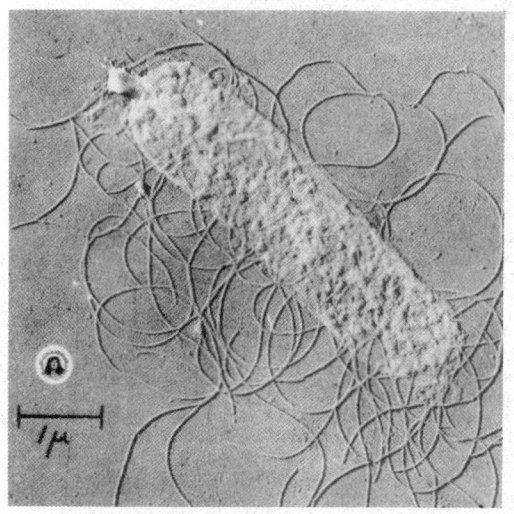

Proteus vulgaris. (Robinow and van Iterson, S.A.B.
LS-260.)

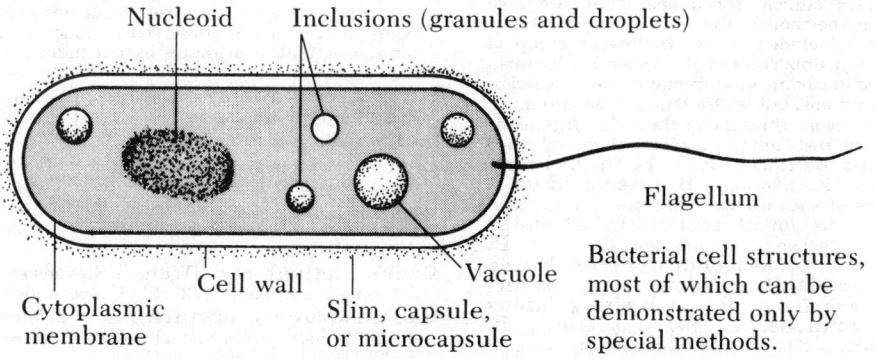

Nucleoid   Inclusions (granules and droplets)

Flagellum

Cell wall

Cytoplasmic
membrane

Slim, capsule,
or microcapsule

Vacuole

Bacterial cell structures,
most of which can be
demonstrated only by
special methods.

**PLATE 8 —ELECTRON MICROGRAPHS OF VARIOUS BACTERIA,
AND DIAGRAM SHOWING STRUCTURES OF
A TYPICAL BACTERIAL CELL**

bacteroid (bak'tĕ-roid) [*bacteria* + Gr. *eidos* form] 1. resembling a bacterium. 2. a structurally modified bacterium.

Bacteroidaceae (bak"tĕ-roi-da'se-e) a family of gram-negative, obligately anaerobic bacteria, occurring as nonsporogenous rods, nonmotile or motile with peritrichous flagella. The organisms occur naturally in cavities of man and animals, and have been isolated from infections. Some species are significant human and animal pathogens. The family consists of the genera *Acetivibrio, Angerobiospirillum, Angerovibrio, Bacteroides, Butyrivibrio, Fusobacterium, Lachnospira, Leptotrichia, Pectinatus, Selenomonas, Succinimonas, Succinivibrio,* and *Wolinella.*

Bacteroideae (bak"tĕ-roi'de-e) former name for a tribe of bacteria of the family Bacteroidaceae.

Bacteroides (bak"tĕ-roi'dēz) [Gr. *baktērion* little rod + Gr. *eidos* form] a genus of gram-negative, anaerobic, non-spore-forming, rod-shaped bacteria of the family Bacteroidaceae, made up of organisms that are nonmotile or motile with peritrichous flagella. They are normal inhabitants of the oral, respiratory, intestinal, and urogenital cavities of humans and animals, and may constitute the predominant bacteria of the normal human colon. Some species are potential pathogens, causing possibly fatal abscesses and bacteremias. **B. asaccharolyt'icus,** a bile-sensitive, pigmented species that does not ferment sugars. The organisms are part of the normal flora of the mucous membranes. They are also important pathogens, causing infections of the head, neck, and other parts of the body. Called also *B. melaninogenicus* subsp. *asaccharolyticus.* **B. bi'vius,** a bile-sensitive, nonpigmented species that is moderately fermentative, found in the female genital tract and in the oral cavity, and occasionally isolated from breast abscesses. **B. capillo'sus,** a weakly fermentative, bile-sensitive, nonpigmented species isolated from cysts, wounds, and feces of humans and the intestinal tract of animals. **B. clostridiifor'mis,** *Clostridium clostridiiforme.* **B. corro'dens,** a former species including facultative organisms that are now assigned to the species *Eikenella corrodens* and anaerobic, urease-positive strains that are assigned to the species *B. ureolyticus.* **B. di'siens,** a bile-sensitive, nonpigmented, weakly fermentative species found in infections of the oral cavity and the female genital tract, and as part of the normal vaginal flora. **B. distaso'nis,** one of the most common species isolated from human feces, which is similar to *B. fragilis* except that it does not ferment amylopectin, amylose, or fucose. **B. egger'thii,** a bile-resistant saccharolytic species found in human feces, and occasionally isolated from clinical specimens, that is similar to *B. fragilis* except that it does not ferment sucrose. **B. fra'gilis,** 1. a species name given to a group of closely related bile-resistant, saccharolytic organisms comprising all the former subspecies of *B. fragilis* (*fragilis, distasonis, ovatus, thetaiotaomicron, vulgatus*), which are now considered to be separate species, and a few other species, e.g., *B. uniformis.* Collectively, the organisms constitute the numerically dominant species found in the human intestine and are the most commonly encountered anaerobic bacteria in clinical specimens. They are also present normally in the mouth, throat, and vaginal tract. 2. one of the species included in the *B. fragilis* group of bacteria. It is the most important of the anaerobic bacteria causing human infection, being most frequently implicated in intra-abdominal infections, but is also found in bacteremias, abscesses, and other lesions throughout the body. Organisms in this species are more resistant to antibiotics than any other anaerobe. Called also *Bacillus fragili.* **B. funduliifor'-mis,** *Fusobacterium necrophorum.* **B. interme'dius,** a weakly fermentative species isolated from the human gingival crevice and various clinical specimens. Called also *B. melaninogenicus* subsp. *intermedius.* **B. melaninoge'nicus** subsp. **asaccharolyt'icus,** *B. asaccharolyticus.* **B. melaninoge'nicus** subsp. **interme'dius,** *B. intermedius.* **B. melaninoge'nicus** subsp. **melaninoge'nicus,** *B. melaninogenicus.* **B. melaninoge'nicus,** a bile-sensitive saccharolytic coccoid species that produces a black hematin pigment, part of the normal flora of the mucous membranes. It is also an important pathogen in oral, lung, and brain abscesses and occurs in other mixed infections. Called also *Ristella melaninogenica.* **B. nodo'sus,** a species that causes foot rot in sheep. **B. ochra'ceus,** *Capnocytophaga ochraceus.* **B. ora'lis,** a bile-sensitive, nonpigmented, strongly fermen-

tative species found principally in the gingival sulcus, which is occasionally associated with infections of the oral cavity and the respiratory and genital tracts. **B. ova'tus,** one of the species included in the *B. fragilis* group of bacteria, isolated from normal human feces and occasionally from clinical specimens. **B. pneumosin'tes,** a species isolated from the nasopharynx, blood, and abscesses of the lung and brain. Called also *Dialister pneumosintes.* **B. praeacu'tus,** a bile-sensitive, nonpigmented, nonfermentative species isolated from the blood, from gangrenous lesions, and from the intestinal tract of infants and adults. **B. putre'dinis,** a bile-sensitive, nonpigmented, nonfermentative species isolated from abdominal and rectal abscesses and from feces of humans, from soil, and from sheep foot rot. **B. rumini'cola,** a bile-sensitive, nonpigmented, strongly fermentative species isolated from the rumens of cattle, sheep, and elk, and from human abscesses and feces. **B. rumini'cola** subsp. **bre'vis,** a subspecies that does not require heme for growth; isolated from human sources. **B. rumini'cola** subsp. **rumini'cola,** a subspecies that requires heme for growth; isolated from cattle and pigs. **B. splanch'nicus,** a bile-resistant, saccharolytic species isolated from human feces, the vagina, and occasionally from abdominal infections, which is similar to *B. fragilis* except that it does not ferment sucrose. **B. thetaiotaom'i-cron,** one of the species included in the *B. fragilis* group of bacteria. Except for *B. fragilis,* it is the most important anaerobe causing human infection. *B. thetaiotaomicron,* with *B. vulgatus,* is the organism most frequently isolated from fecal specimens, and it is frequently found in other human clinical specimens. **B. unifor'mis,** one of the species included in the *B. fragilis* group of bacteria, occurring as part of the normal flora in human and swine feces, and isolated from various human clinical specimens. **B. ureolyt'i-cus,** a bile-sensitive, nonpigmented, nonfermentative species that is urease positive, isolated from infections of the respiratory and intestinal tracts and from various clinical specimens. See also *B. corrodens.* **B. vulga'tus,** one of the species included in the *B. fragilis* group of bacteria. *B. vulgatus,* with *B. thetaiotaomicron,* is the organism most frequently isolated from fecal specimens, and it has occasionally been isolated from human infections.

bacteroides (bak"tĕ-roi'dēz) any bacterium of the genus *Bacteroides.*

bacteroidosis (bak"te-roi-do'sis) infection with organisms of the genus *Bacteroides.*

bacteruria (bak"te-ru're-ah) bacteriuria.

Bactocill (bak'to-sil) trademark for a preparation of oxacillin sodium.

Bactoscilla (bak"tos-sil'ah) a genus of gliding bacteria of uncertain status, related to the family Beggiatoaceae.

baculovirus (bak"u-lo-vi'rus) any of a group of morphologically similar, ether- and heat-labile DNA viruses, which infect various insects, producing granular inclusion capsules in the cells; called also *granulosis virus.*

baculum (bak'u-lum) [L. "a stick, staff"] a heterotopic bone developed in the fibrous septum between the corpora cavernosa and above the urethra, forming the skeleton of the penis in all insectivores, bats, rodents, carnivores, and pinnipeds, and in primates except man; called also *os penis* and *os priapi.*

Badal's operation (bah-dahlz') [Antoine Jules *Badal,* French ophthalmologist, 1840–1929] see under *operation.*

badge (baj) see *film badge.*

Baelz's disease (bāltz'es) [Erwin von *Baelz,* German physician, 1849–1913] see cheilitis glandularis.

Baer's cavity, law, vesicle (bārz) [Karl Ernst von *Baer* (Ber), Russian anatomist, 1792–1876] see under *cavity, law,* and *vesicle.*

Baer's method (bārz) [William Stevenson *Baer,* American orthopedic surgeon, 1872–1931] see under *method.*

Baerensprung's erythrasma (bār'en-sproongs) [Friedrich Wilhelm Felix von *Baerensprung,* German physician, 1822–1864] see under *erythrasma.*

Bäfverstedt's syndrome (ba'fūr-shtets) [Bo Erik *Bäfverstedt,* Swedish physician, born 1905] lymphocytoma cutis.

bag (bag) a sac or pouch. **Barnes' b.,** a water-filled rubber bag for dilating the cervix uteri; called also *Barnes' dilator.* **Bunyan b.,** a bag of light waterproof material for covering wet dressings. **Champetier de Ribes' b.,**

a conic water-filled bag of silk or rubber for dilating the cervix uteri. **colostomy b.,** a receptacle worn over the stoma to receive the fecal discharge from a colostomy. **Douglas b.,** a receptacle for the collection of expired air, permitting measurement of respiratory gases. **Hagner b.,** an inflatable rubber bag to be used by traction through the urethra to prevent hemorrhage following prostatectomy. **ice b.,** a bag filled with ice, for applying cold to the body. **ileostomy b.,** any of various plastic or latex bags for the collection of urine or fecal material following ileostomy or the establishment of an ileal bladder; a flange or similar device fits closely about the ileal stoma and the bag is cemented to the skin or strapped to the body. **Lyster b.,** a rubber-lined bag with faucets and with straps for slinging; used for the water supply in temporary camps. **micturition b.,** a receptacle for urine used by ambulatory patients with urinary incontinence. **nuclear b.,** the central portion of the central or equatorial segment of intrafusal fibers of muscle; it is usually devoid of obvious cross striations and contains an accumulation of 40 to 50 spherical nuclei, which completely fill and often slightly distend the fiber. **Perry b.,** an ileostomy bag with a small latex cuff reinforced by a plastic disk which fits snugly around a protruding stoma; the cuff is held down by a large plastic ring to which a belt is attached. **Petersen's b.,** an inflatable rubber bag inserted into the rectum so as to elevate the bladder in the operation of suprapubic cystotomy. **Pilcher b.,** a modification of the Hagner bag which provides urethral drainage as well as hemostasis. **Politzer's b.,** a soft bag of rubber for inflating the middle ear. **testicular b.,** scrotum. **Voorhees' b.,** a rubber bag that can be inflated with water; formerly used for dilating the cervix uteri. **b. of waters,** the membranes that enclose the amniotic fluid of the fetus. **Whitmore b.,** an ileostomy bag with a malleable flange and a valvular device for urine drainage at the lower end of the bag.

bagasscosis (bag″as-ko′sis) bagassosis.

bagassosis (bag″ah-so′sis) a respiratory disorder due to the inhalation of the dust of bagasse, the waste of sugar cane after the sugar has been extracted.

Baillarger's bands, lines, sign, striae, stripes (bi-yar-zhāz′) [Jules Gabriel François *Baillarger*, French psychiatrist, 1809–1890] see *stria laminae granularis interna corticis cerebri* and *stria laminae pyramidalis interna corticis cerebri*, and see under *sign*.

Bainbridge reflex (bān′brij) [Francis Arthur *Bainbridge*, English physiologist, 1874–1921] see under *reflex*.

bake (bāk) to expose to high temperature at low humidity, as in the hardening of porcelain.

Baker's cyst (ba′kerz) [William Morrant *Baker*, British surgeon, 1839–1896] see under *cyst*.

Baker's velum (ba′kerz) [Henry A. *Baker*, Boston surgeon] see under *velum*.

bakkola (bak′o-lah) a fungus obtained from birch trees in Finland, used in folk medicine in the form of a decoction containing a chrysarobin-like principle or chrysophanic acid, in the treatment of cancer.

BAL [*British antilewisite*] dimercaprol.

balance (bal′ans) [L. *bilanx*] 1. an instrument for weighing. 2. the harmonious adjustment of parts; the harmonious performance of functions. **acid-base b.,** a condition in which the net rate of acid or alkali production by the body is balanced by the net rate of acid or alkali excretion from the body, resulting in a stable concentration of H^+ (hydrogen ions) in the body fluids. **analytical b.,** a laboratory balance sensitive to variations of the order of 0.05 to 0.1 mg. **calcium b.,** the balance between the calcium intake and its output through the body excretions. **fluid b.,** the state of the body in relation to ingestion and excretion of water and electrolytes; called also *water b.* **genic b.,** the ratio of male-determining to female-determining genes in the chromosome assortment as the determiner of sex. **microchemical b.,** a laboratory balance sensitive to variations of the order of 0.001 mg. **nitrogen b.,** the state of the body in regard to ingestion and excretion of nitrogen. In *negative nitrogen balance* the amount of nitrogen excreted is greater than the quantity ingested; in *positive nitrogen balance* the amount excreted is smaller than the amount ingested. **occlusal b.,** balanced occlusion. **semimicro b.,** a balance sensitive to variations of 0.01 mg. **torsion b.,** 1. a weighing balance in which the scale beam is supported by

metallic ribbons that act by torsion. 2. an electrometer that acts by the twisting of a single fiber of the web of a silkworm. **water b.,** fluid b.

balanic (bah-lan′ik) pertaining to the glans penis or glans clitoridis.

balanitis (bal″ah-ni′tis) [*balano-* + *-itis*] inflammation of the glans penis; it is usually associated with phimosis. **amebic b.,** a variety caused by *Entamoeba histolytica.* **b. circina′ta,** a variety attributed to the presence of spirochetes. **b. circumscrip′ta plasmacellula′ris,** a benign erythroplasia histologically characterized by plasma cell infiltration of the dermis, and clinically by persistent inflammation, usually involving the inner surface of the prepuce and glans penis and associated with the development of a single erythematous, moist, shiny lesion. Called also *b. plasmocellularis, balanoposthitis circumscripta plasmocellularis, chronic circumscribed plasmocytic balanoposthitis, plasma cell b.,* and *Zoon's erythroplasia.* Cf. *plasma cell vulvitis.* **b. diabet′ica,** a variety caused by the irritation of the urine in diabetes. **erosive b.,** balanitis due to mixed microbial infection that progresses to gangrenous ulcerations of the penis similar to the lesions seen in noma of oral tissues. **Follmann's b.,** a serous balanitis and posthitis without induration. **b. gangraeno′sa, gangrenous b.,** a rapidly destructive infection producing erosion of the glans penis and often destruction of the entire external genitals; the infection is believed to be due to a spirochete. Called also *balanoposthomycosis* and *Corbus' disease.* **phagedenic b.,** gangrenous b. **plasma cell b., b. plasmacellula′ris,** b. circumscripta plasmacellularis. **plasma cell b., b. plasmocellula′re,** b. circumscripta plasmacellularis. **b. xerot′ica oblit′erans,** a manifestation of lichen sclerosus et atrophicus involving the prepuce and glans penis, sometimes resulting in stricture of the urethral meatus.

balan(o)- [Gr. *balanos* acorn] a combining form indicating relationship to the glans penis or to the glans clitoridis.

balanocele (bal′ah-no-sēl″) [*balano-* + Gr. *kēlē* hernia] protrusion of the glans penis through a rupture of the prepuce.

balanochlamyditis (bal″ah-no-klam″e-di′tis) [*balano-* + Gr. *chlamys* hood + *-itis*] (*obs.*) inflammation of the glans clitoridis and hood.

balanoplasty (bal′ah-no-plas″te) [*balano-* + Gr. *plassein* to form] plastic surgery of the glans penis.

balanoposthitis (bal″ah-no-pos-thi′tis) [*balano-* + Gr. *posthē* prepuce + *-itis*] inflammation of the glans penis and prepuce. **chronic circumscribed plasmocytic b., b. chron′ica circumscrip′ta plasmocellula′ris,** balanitis circumscripta plasmacellularis. **enzootic b.,** disease of uncertain etiology, affecting sheep in Australia and New Zealand, marked by spreading ulceration of the glans penis and prepuce and severe swelling and distention of the sheath; called also *pizzle rot* and *sheath rot.* **specific gangrenous and ulcerative b.,** an acute inflammatory disease of the glans penis and opposed surface of the prepuce, marked by ulcerations and sometimes by gangrene, with a flow of odorous pus, and caused by a spirochete; called also *fourth venereal disease.*

balanoposthomycosis (bal″ah-no-pos″tho-mi-ko′sis) gangrenous balanitis.

balanopreputial (bal″ah-no-pre-pu′she-al) pertaining to the glans penis and the prepuce.

balanorrhagia (bal″ah-no-ra′je-ah) [*balano-* + Gr. *rhēgnynai* to break] balanitis with free discharge of pus.

Balanosporida (bal″ah-no-spor′ĭ-dah) [*balano-* + *spore*] an order of parasitic protozoa (class Stellatosporea, phylum Ascetospora) having spores with one sporoplasm and a spore wall interrupted by an anterior orifice that is covered externally by an operculum or internally by a diaphragm. Representative genera include *Haplosporidium, Minchinia,* and *Urosporidium.*

balantidiasis (bal″an-tĭ-di′ah-sis) infection by protozoan parasites of the genus *Balantidium;* in man, *B. coli* may cause diarrhea and dysentery, with ulceration of the colon mucosa.

balantidiosis (bal″an-tid-e-o′sis) balantidiasis.

Balantidium (bal″an-tid′e-um) [Gr. *balantidion* little bag] a genus of ciliate protozoa (suborder Trichostomatina, order Trichostomatida) including many species found in the intestines of vertebrates and invertebrates. **B. co′li** the largest protozoan and the only ciliate parasite of humans (see *balantidiasis*), which is also found in pigs and monkeys; it may measure 30 to 150 μm long by 25 to 120 μm wide. **B. su′is,** a nonpathogenic species found in pigs considered by some to be identical with *B. coli* and by others to be a separate species.

balantidosis (bal″an-tĭ-do′sis) balantidiasis.

balanus (bal′ah-nus) the glans penis.

balata (bal′ah-tah) the inspissated juice or latex of *Mimusops globosa,* a tree of tropical America; used much like gutta-percha.

Balbiani's body, nucleus (bahl-be-ah′nēz) [Edouard Gérard *Balbiani,* French embryologist, 1823–1899] yolk nucleus.

baldness (bawld′nes) alopecia, especially absence of hair from the scalp. **common male b.,** male pattern alopecia; thinning or absence of hair from around the vertex of the scalp, and recession of the frontal scalp margin on each side of the forehead, forming the so-called "professor angles."

Baldy's operation (bawl′dēz) [John Montgomery *Baldy,* American gynecologist, 1860–1934] see *Webster's operation,* under *operation.*

Baldy-Webster operation (bawl′de-web′ster) [John Montgomery *Baldy;* John Clarence *Webster,* American gynecologist, 1863–1950] see *Webster's operation,* under *operation.*

Balkan frame, splint (bawl′kan) see under *frame* and *splint.*

ball (bawl) a more or less spherical mass. **chondrin b.,** one of the ball-like masses in hyaline cartilage, consisting of cells surrounded by a capsule of basoph lic matrix. **fatty b. of Bichat,** sucking pad (corpus adiposum buccae [NA]). **food b.,** phytobezoar. **fungus b.,** aspergilloma. **hair b.,** trichobezoar. **Marchi b′s,** ellipsoid or ovoid segments of myelin produced by degeneration, staining brown by Marchi methods. **oat hair b.,** a trichobezoar formed in the stomach of the horse from the fine hairs within the outer husk of the oat grain and other materials. **pleural fibrin b′s,** fibrin bodies in the pleural space. **wool b.,** a trichobezoar containing wool fibers and other substances.

Ball's valve (bawlz) [Sir Charles Bent *Ball,* Irish surgeon, 1851–1916] see *valvula anales.*

Ballance's sign (bal′an-siz) [Sir Charles Alfred *Ballance,* British surgeon, 1856–1936] see under *sign.*

Baller-Gerold syndrome (bal′er jer′old) [F. *Baller;* M. *Gerold*] see under *syndrome.*

Ballet's sign (bal-āz′) [Gilbert *Ballet,* French neurologist, 1853–1916] see under *sign.*

ballism (bal′izm) ballismus.

ballismus (bah-liz′mus) [Gr. *ballismos* a jumping about, dancing] violent flinging movements caused by contractions of the proximal limb muscles as a result of destruction of the subthalamic nucleus of Luysii or its fiber connections, sometimes affecting only one side of the body (hemiballismus). Called also *ballism.*

ballistic (bah-lis′tik) 1. jerking or twitching; pertaining to or characterized by ballismus. 2. pertaining to or caused by projectiles.

ballistics (bah-lis′tiks) [Gr. *ballein* to throw] the scientific study of the motion of projectiles in flight. **wound b.,** the scientific study of the speed and direction of missiles (bullets and other projectiles) in relation to the injuries they produce.

ballistocardiogram (bah-lis″to-kar′de-o-gram″) the tracing made by a ballistocardiograph; abbreviated *BCG.*

ballistocardiograph (bah-lis″to-kar′de-o-graf″) an apparatus for recording the movements of the body caused by the heartbeat, used to determine the degree of elasticity or atheroma of the aorta, and, more rarely, to calculate cardiac output.

ballistocardiography (bah-lis″to-kar″de-og′rah-fe) the graphic recording, by means of a ballistocardiograph, of the recoil movements of an animal body which result from motion of its heart and blood.

balloon (bah-lōōn′) 1. a sac that can be inserted into a body cavity or tube and distended with air or gas. 2. to distend with air or gas; to inflate. **Shea-Anthony antral b.,** sinus b. **sinus b.,** a hollow rubber structure, expandable with either liquid or air, used to support depressed

fractures of the walls of the maxillary sinus; called also *Shea-Anthony antral balloon.* The balloon of a Foley catheter is frequently used for this purpose.

ballooning (bah-lōōn′ing) distending any cavity of the body with air or gas for therapeutic purposes.

ballotable (bah-lot′ah-bl) capable of showing ballottement.

ballottement (bah-lot′ment) [Fr. "a tossing about"] a palpatory maneuver to test for a floating object. The term is applied especially to a maneuver for detecting the existence of pregnancy by pushing up the head or breech of a fetus by fingers inserted into the vagina, so as to cause the fetus to rise and fall again like a heavy body in water. **abdominal**

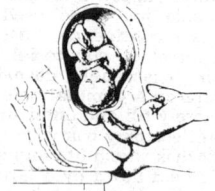

Ballottement

b., indirect b., that which is effected by the finger applied to the abdominal wall. **renal b.,** palpation of the kidney by pressing one hand into the abdominal wall while the other hand makes quick thrusts forward from behind so as to throw the kidney against the anterior hand.

balm (bahm) [Fr. *baume*] 1. a healing or soothing medicine. 2. a plant of the genus *Melis′sa,* especially *M. officina′lis;* it is carminative and aromatic. 3. b. of Gilead. 4. balsam. **blue b.,** *Melissa.* **b. of Gilead,** 1. a liquid oleoresin from *Abies balsamea* (L.) Mill., the balsam fir of North America, which was once used in the treatment of diseases of the urinary tract. 2. the buds of the poplar tree *Populus candicans* Aiton (Salicaceae), which contain volatile oils and resins; used as a stimulating expectorant in cough syrups. 3. Mecca balsam. Called also *balsam of Gilead.* **lemon b.,** *Melissa.* **mountain b.,** *Eriodictyon.* **sweet b.,** *Melissa.*

Balme's cough (bahlmz) [Paul Jean *Balme,* French physician, born 1857] see under *cough.*

balneology (bal″ne-ol′o-je) [L. *balneum* bath + *-logy*] the science of baths and their therapeutic uses.

balneotherapeutics (bal″ne-o-ther-ah-pu′tiks) balneotherapy.

balneotherapy (bal″ne-o-ther′ah-pe) [L. *balneum* bath + Gr. *therapeia* treatment] the treatment of disease by baths.

balneum (bal′ne-um), pl. *bal′nea* [L.] a bath, def. 1. **b. are′nae,** a sand bath; also *ammotherapy.* **b. lac′teum,** milk bath. **b. pneumat′icum,** air bath.

Balopticon (bal-op′te-kon) [Gr. *ballein* to throw + *optikos* pertaining to sight] trademark for a projection apparatus for throwing an enlarged image on a screen.

balsam (bawl′sam) [L. *balsamum;* Gr. *balsamon*] 1. a semifluid, resinous, and fragrant liquid of vegetable origin, usually trees, which is often composed chiefly of resins, volatile oils, and various esters. 2. balm. **Canada b.,** a liquid oleoresin from *Abies balsamea* (L.) Mill. (Pinaceae), the balsam fir of North America, containing volatile oils, chiefly *l*-pinene, and over 70 per cent resins; a microscopic medium. **b. of copaiba,** copaiba. **friars′ b.,** compound benzoin tincture. **b. of Gilead,** see under *balm.* **gurjun b.,** an oleoresin from *Dipterocarpus alatus* Roxb. (Dipterocarpaceae) and other species of *Dipterocarpus* growing in East India; an adulterant of copaiba. **Holland b.,** juniper tar. **Mecca b.,** a light-colored, mobile to viscid liquid with an aromatic odor; it is the resinous juice of *Commiphora opobalsamum,* a small evergreen of the Red Sea region. It is still used as a medicine and cosmetic in eastern countries. **b. of Peru,** peruvian b. **peruvian b.** [NF], a dark brown viscid liquid obtained from *Myroxylon pereirae* Klotzsch (Leguminosae) used as a local protectant and as a rubefacient, applied topically to the skin in ointment or alcohol solution. Called also *b. of Peru.* **St. Thomas' b.,** a resinous juice obtained from the tree, *Santiriopsis balsamifera,* grown on the island of St. Thomas. **silver b.,** juniper tar. **b. of sulfur,** a preparation made by boiling sulfur in linseed or olive oil. **tolu b.** [USP], a balsam obtained from *Myroxylon balsamum*, used as an ingredient of compound benzoin tincture and as an expectorant. **Turlington's b., Wade's b.,** compound benzoin tincture.

balsamo (bal′sah-mo) [Sp.] balsam. **b. de tolu′,** tolu balsam. **b. del Peru′,** peruvian balsam.

Balsamodendron (bal″sah-mo-den′dron) [L.; Gr. *balsamon* balsam + *dendron* tree] a genus of old world amyridaceous trees of many species, producing bdellium and other balsamic drugs.

balsamum (bal′sah-mum) [L.] balsam. **b. peruvia′num,** peruvian balsam.

Balser's fatty necrosis (bahl′zerz) [Wilhelm August *Balser*, German physician of the 19th century] see under *necrosis*.

balteum (bal′te-um) [L.] belt or girdle. **b. vene′reum,** Venus' girdle.

Baltimore (bal′tĭ-mor) David. American biologist, born 1938; co-winner, with Renato Dulbecco and Howard Temin, of the Nobel prize in medicine and physiology for 1975, for discoveries concerning the interaction between tumor viruses and the genetic material of host cells and the role of reverse transcriptase.

Bamberger's albuminuria, etc. (bahm′ber-gerz) [Heinrich von *Bamberger*, Austrian physician, 1822–1888] see under *albuminuria, disease,* and *sign.*

Bamberger-Marie disease [Eugen *Bamberger*, Austrian physician, 1858–1921; Pierre *Marie*, French physician, 1853–1940] hypertrophic pulmonary osteoarthropathy.

bambermycins (bam″ber-mi′sinz) an antibacterial antibiotic complex containing mainly moenomycin A and C, produced by *Streptomyces bambergiensis, S. ederensis, S. geysiriensis,* and *S. ghansensis,* and related strains, or the same substance produced by other means; used as a feed additive in foodstuffs for pigs, poultry, and calves and in veterinary supplements.

bamboo brier (bam-boo′ bri′er) the root of species of *Smilax,* of the United States, used as a food by Indians.

bamnidazole (bam-nid′ah-zōl) chemical name: 2-methyl-5-nitro-1*H*-imidazol-1-ethanol carbamate (ester); an antiprotozoal effective against *Trichomonas,* $C_7H_{10}N_4O_4$.

BAN British Approved Name, an official nonproprietary name approved by the British Pharmacopoeia Commission.

Bancroft's filariasis (ban′krofts) [Joseph *Bancroft,* English physician in Australia, 1836–1894] see under *filariasis.*

bancroftosis (ban″krof-to′sis) infection with *Wuchereria bancrofti.*

band (band) 1. an object or appliance that confines or restricts while allowing a limited or desired degree of movement. 2. a strip that holds together or binds two or more separate objects. 3. a strip of thin metal, formed into a hoop, to encircle horizontally the crown of a natural tooth or its root. 4. an elongated area with parallel or roughly parallel borders that is distinct from the surrounding surface by its color, texture, or other characteristics. See *chromosome b.* **A b.,** the dark-staining zone of a sarcomere, whose center is traversed by the paler H band, which in turn contains the darker M band; called also *A disk, Q disk, anisotropic disk,* and *transverse disk.* **absorption b's,** dark bands in the spectrum due to absorption of light by the medium (a solid, a liquid, or a gas) through which the light has passed. Cf. *absorption lines,* under *line.* **amniotic b.,** a fibrous band passing from fetus to amnion. **anchor b.,** orthodontic b. **anogenital b.,** a fetal fillet that is the rudiment of the perineum. **anterior b. of colon,** tenia libera. **atrioventricular b.,** bundle of His. **auriculoventricular b.,** atrioventricular b. **axis b.,** the primitive streak. **b's of Baillarger,** see *stria laminae granularis interna corticis cerebri* and *stria laminae pyramidalis interna corticis cerebri.* **b. of Broca, Broca's diagonal b.,** stria diagonalis (Broca). **Büngner's b's,** bands of syncytium formed by the union of sheath cells during the regeneration of peripheral nerves; called also *Ledbänder.* **C b., C-b.,** see *chromosome b.,* and *C banding,* under *banding.* **chromosome b.,** any of the alternating dark and light or fluorescent transverse bands produced on chromosomes by differential staining; named according to the procedure used, i.e., C band, G band, Q band, and R band. See *chromosome banding,* under *banding.* **Clado's b.,** the suspensory ligament of the ovary covered with peritoneum. **clamp b.,**

an orthodontic band held in place with a screw nut. **coagulation b.,** the band formed in Weltmann's coagulation test. **b's of colon, longitudinal,** taeniae coli. **contoured b.,** an orthodontic band shaped to the contour of the tooth. **coronary b.,** a band of vascular tissue at the upper edge of the wall of the hoof which is concerned in the secretion of the wall; called also *coronary cushion, coronary ring, cutidure,* or *cutiduris.* **dentate b.,** gyrus dentatus, def. 1. **diagonal b. of Broca,** stria diagonalis (Broca). **elastic b.,** see *elastic,* def. 2. **free b. of colon,** taenia libera. **furrowed b.,** a strip of cortex that connects the tonsil of the hemisphere of the cerebellum to the uvula of the vermis. **G b., G-b.,** see *chromosome b.,* and *chromosome banding,* under *banding.* **b's of Gennari,** see under *line.* **Giacomini's b.,** the grayish band constituting the anterior extension of the gyrus dentatus of the hippocampus over the inferior surface of the uncus. **H b.,** a relatively pale zone sometimes seen traversing the center of the A band of fibrils of striated muscle; called also *Hensen's* or *Engelmann's disk.* **Hall b.,** an intrauterine contraceptive device of surgical stainless steel, measuring $\frac{11}{16}$ inch in diameter and consisting of three flat circular members $\frac{1}{16}$ inch wide and $\frac{1}{1000}$ inch thick, located within the lumen of an open coiled spring. **Harris' b.,** anomalous peritoneal folds which extend from the gallbladder to the inferior surface of the liver to the proximal duodenum, sometimes traversing the mesocolon near the hepatic flexure. **Henle's b.,** fibers from the anterior aponeurosis of the transversus abdominis muscle extending behind the rectus below the arcuate line. **His' b.,** see under *bundle.* **horny b.** (obs.), the anterior part of the stria terminalis; called also *b. of Tarinus.* **b's of Hunter-Schreger,** lines of Schreger. **I b.,** the band or disk within a striated muscle fibril that appears as a light region under the light microscope and as a dark region under polarized light; it contains the proteins actin, troponin, and tropomyosin. Called also *isotropic disk* and *J disk.* **iliotibial b.,** tractus iliotibialis. **Lane's b's,** adhesions between tight loops of the terminal ileum which may extend as ligamentous bands to the right iliac fossa. See also *Lane's kink,* under *kink.* **Leonardo's b.,** a term proposed by Sudhoff for the band of Reil, first delineated by Leonardo da Vinci. **limbic b's,** a superior and an inferior muscular band developed in the right atrium of the fetal heart that become the basis of Lower's tubercle and the sinus septum. **M b.,** the narrow dark band in the center of the H band of the sarcomere; called also *M disk, Hensen's line,* and *mesophragma.* Cf. *Z band.* **Maissiat's b.,** tractus iliotibialis. **Matas' b.,** an aluminum band for temporarily occluding large blood vessels in order to test the condition of the collateral circulation. **matrix b.,** a cylindrical copper or, more commonly, stainless steel band or a short tube with a special clamp or holder filled with a softened impression compound and seated over a tooth, allowing the compound to flow into the prepared cavity, used in obtaining impressions of single teeth that contain prepared cavities. Also used in the placement and contouring of certain restorative materials, e.g., resin and glass ionomer cement, and to form the fourth wall of a class II cavity preparation during the condensation of an amalgam restoration. **Meckel's b.,** a part of the anterior ligament fastening the malleus to the wall of the tympanum. **mesocolic b.,** taenia mesocolica. **moderator b.,** trabecula septomarginalis. **molar b.,** an orthodontic band applied to a molar tooth; a bracket is attached to the band to hold the arch wire of the appliance. **N-b.,** a band produced on a chromosome by the N-staining method; see *Table of Stains and Staining Methods,* under *stain.* **omental b.,** taenia omentalis. **orthodontic b.,** a band fitted over a tooth to anchor a fixed orthodontic appliance. Called also *anchor b.* **Parham b.,** a metallic ribbon used to fix a fractured long bone by encircling the bone at the site of the fracture. **perioplic b.,** the band of secretor cells at the upper border of the hoof of animals; it secretes the periople. **periosteal b.,** see under *collar.* **phonatory b's,** the vocal cords, or an artificial substitute for them. **Q b., Q-b.,** see *chromosome b.,* and *chromosome banding,* under *banding.* **R b., R-b.,** see *chromosome b.,* and *chromosome banding,* under *banding.* **b. of Reil,** 1. a muscular fillet extending across the right ventricle of the heart, now regarded as forming one of the terminal parts of the moderator band; see *bundle of His.* 2. (obs.) see under *ribbon.* **b. of Remak,** axon. **retention b.,** musculus suspensorius duodeni. **b's of Schreger,** see under *line.* **Sebileau's b's** (obs.), three thickenings in the membrana suprapleuralis. **Simonart's b's,** Simonart's threads; see under *thread*. **Soret b.,** the absorption band of porphyrins at 400–410 nm. **b. of Tarinus,** horny b. **Vicq d'Azyr's b.,** a thin stripe of fine myelinated fibers in Brodmann's external granular layer; sometimes called stripe of Kaes, and often incorrectly defined as the outer line of Baillarger. **Z b.,** a thin membrane seen on longitudinal section as a dark line in the center of the I band; the distance between successive Z bands serves to delimit the sarcomeres of striated muscle. Called also *Z disk* or *line, Amici's disk, Dobie's line* or *layer, intermediate disk, Krause's membrane, telophragma,* and *thin disk.* See *inophragma* and cf. *M b.* **zinc b.,** Z b. **zonular b.,** zona orbicularis articulationis coxae.

bandage (ban′dij) 1. a strip or roll of gauze or other material for wrapping or binding any part of the body. 2. to cover by wrapping with a strip of gauze or other material. See also *dressing* and *strapping.* **Ace b.,** trademark for a bandage of woven elastic material. **Barton's b.,** a figure-of-8 bandage supporting the lower jaw below and in front. **Borsch's b.,** an eye bandage covering both the diseased and the healthy eye. **Buller's b.,** see under *shield.* **capeline b.,** a bandage applied like a cap or hood to the head or shoulder or to an amputation stump. **circular b.,** a bandage applied in circular turns, usually about a limb. **compression b.,** a bandage by which pressure is applied to a limb to prevent edema. **crucial b.,** T bandage. **demigauntlet b.,** a bandage that covers the hand but leaves the fingers exposed. **Desault's b.,** a bandage binding the elbow to the side, with a pad in the axilla, for fractured clavicle; called also *Desault's apparatus.* **elastic b.,** a bandage of elastic material applied to an area to exert continuous pressure upon it. **Esmarch's b.,** a rubber bandage applied around a part from distal to proximal in order to expel blood from it; the limb is often elevated as the elastic pressure is applied. **figure-of-8 b.,** a bandage in which the turns cross each other like the figure eight (8). **four-tailed b.,** one with each end cut into two strips of equal width, which are used to secure the center portion under or over the jaw or other prominence. **gauntlet b.,** a bandage that covers the hand and fingers like a glove. **gauze b.,** a continuous strip of tightly rolled absorbent gauze in various widths and lengths. **Gibney b.,** strips of ½-inch adhesive overlapped along the sides and back of the foot and leg to hold the foot in slight varus position and leave the dorsum of the foot and anterior aspect of the leg exposed; called also *Gibney's strapping.* **hammock b.,** a bandage for retaining dressings on the head; it consists of a broad strip placed over the dressing, brought down over the ears, and held in place by a circular bandage around the head. **immobilizing b.,** a bandage for partially immobilizing a part. **many-tailed b.,** a wide bandage with each end cut into several strips of equal width which may be overlapped as the bandage is applied, usually to the abdomen or chest. See *scultetus b.* **Martin's b.,** a roller bandage of thin elastic rubber. **oblique b.,** a bandage applied obliquely up a limb without reverses. Cf. *reversed b.* **plaster b.,** a bandage stiffened with a paste of plaster of Paris, which sets and becomes very hard. **pressure b.,** a bandage for applying pressure. **recurrent b.,** one used on a distal stump, such as a finger, toe, or amputation stump, that is turned lengthwise to cover the end of the stump and is secured in place by circular turns. **reversed b.,** one applied to a limb in such a way that the roll is inverted or half-turned at each revolution, so as to make it fit smoothly the varying dimensions of the limb. **roller b.,** a tightly rolled, circular bandage of varying widths and materials, often commercially prepared. **scultetus b.,** a many-tailed bandage applied with the tails overlapping each other and held in position by safety pins; see illustration. **spica b.,** a figure-of-8 bandage with turns that cross one another regularly like the letter V, usually applied to anatomical areas of quite different dimensions, as the pelvis and thigh or the thorax and arm. See illustration. **spiral b.,** a roller bandage applied spirally around a limb. **spiral reverse b.,** a spiral bandage applied with reverse turns in order to fit more snugly the varying contours and dimensions of a limb. **suspensory b.,** a bandage for supporting the scrotum. **T b.,** a bandage shaped like the letter T; called also *crucial b.* and *Heliodorus' b.* **triangular b.,** a triangle of cloth used as a sling or bandage. **Velpeau's b.,** a bandage to support the arm and provide immobilization of the elbow and shoulder; it is useful in supporting the upper extremity in severe injuries involving

the shoulder girdle and upper end of humerus. **Y b.,** a bandage shaped like the letter Y.

bandaletta (ban″dah-let′tah) [L., from Fr. dim. of *bande* bond, tie, link] 1. a small band. 2. a small bandlike anatomical structure. **b. diagona′lis (Broca),** stria diagonalis (Broca).

bandicoot (ban′de-kōot) an Indian rodent, *Nesokia bengalensis,* which is a reservoir of *Spirillum minus,* the causative organism of rat-bite fever; it also harbors *Coxiella burneti,* which may be transmitted by the bandicoot tick, *Haemaphysalis humerosa.*

banding (band′ing) 1. the act of encircling and binding with a thin strip of material. 2. any of several techniques of staining chromosomes so that a characteristic pattern of transverse dark and light bands becomes visible; see *chromosome b.* **C b., C-b., centromeric b.,** differential staining of chromosomes to elicit chromosome bands, using a method that specifically stains the regions of the chromosomes that contain constitutive heterochromatin (C bands), particularly the pericentromeric areas, secondary constrictions of chromosomes 1, 9, and 16, and the distal segment of the long arm of the Y chromosome; the method consists of a denaturation and renaturation technique involving treatment of the chromosomes with acid, alkali, or heat before Giemsa staining. **chromosome b.,** the use of various physical and cytochemical preparations with differential staining techniques, which allows visualization of differentially stained regions of a chromosome as a continuous series of light and dark bands specific for the chromosome and species, thus permitting definitive identification and delineation of all the chromosomes and chromosomal segments of humans and many other organisms. Named according to the staining technique used, see *C b., G b., Q b.,* and *R b.* **G b., G-b., Giemsa b.,** differential staining of chromosomes to elicit chromosome bands (G bands), consisting of pretreatment with a salt solution or with proteolytic enzymes (usually trypsin or pronase) before staining with Giemsa solution. The same banding pattern may be obtained with other agents. **high-resolution b.,** a banding technique in which cultured cells are blocked in the S phase of the cell cycle; the block is then released, and the culture is harvested when the greatest number of cells is in late prophase or prometaphase, revealing 800-1400 bands rather than the 200 seen in metaphase preparations. Used to detect precise breakpoints or small structural alterations. Called also *prophase b.* **prophase b.,** high-resolution b. **pulmonary artery b.,** an operation to provide constriction of the pulmonary artery with a band to reduce pulmonary blood flow and relieve congestive heart failure in children with congenital heart defects that produce left to right shunts between ventricles or the great arteries. **Q b., Q-b., quinacrine b.,** differential staining of chromosomes to elicit chromosome bands (Q bands), consisting of examination of the chromosomes by fluorescence microscopy after they have been stained with quinacrine mustard or quinacrine hydrochloride. **R b., R-b., reverse b.,** differential staining of chromosomes to elicit chromosome bands (R bands), consisting of pretreatment with hot alkali before staining; the banding pattern shown is the reverse of that of G and Q banding—positively stained R bands are G and Q negative and vice versa. **tooth b.,** the technique of cementing stainless steel bands to the teeth to hold orthodontic attachments in position.

Bandl's ring (ban′dl) [Ludwig *Bandl,* German obstetrician, 1842–1892] *pathologic retraction ring;* see *retraction ring,* under *ring.*

bane (bān) a poison. **leopard's b., wolf's b.,** see *arnica.*

banewort (bān′wort) belladonna leaf.

bang (bang) bhang.

Bang's bacillus, disease, test (bangz) [Bernhard Laurits Frederik *Bang,* Danish physician, 1848–1932] see *Brucella abortus,* and under *disease* and *tests.*

Bang's method (bangz) [Ivar Christian *Bang,* Swedish physiological chemist, 1869–1918] see under *method.*

banian (ban′yan) the *Ficus bengalensis* (L.), an East Indian fig tree; its seeds and bark are tonic, antifebrile, and diuretic.

banisterine (ban-is′ter-in) an alkaloid from *Banisteria caapi,* a woody vine of South America; it has hallucinogenic properties.

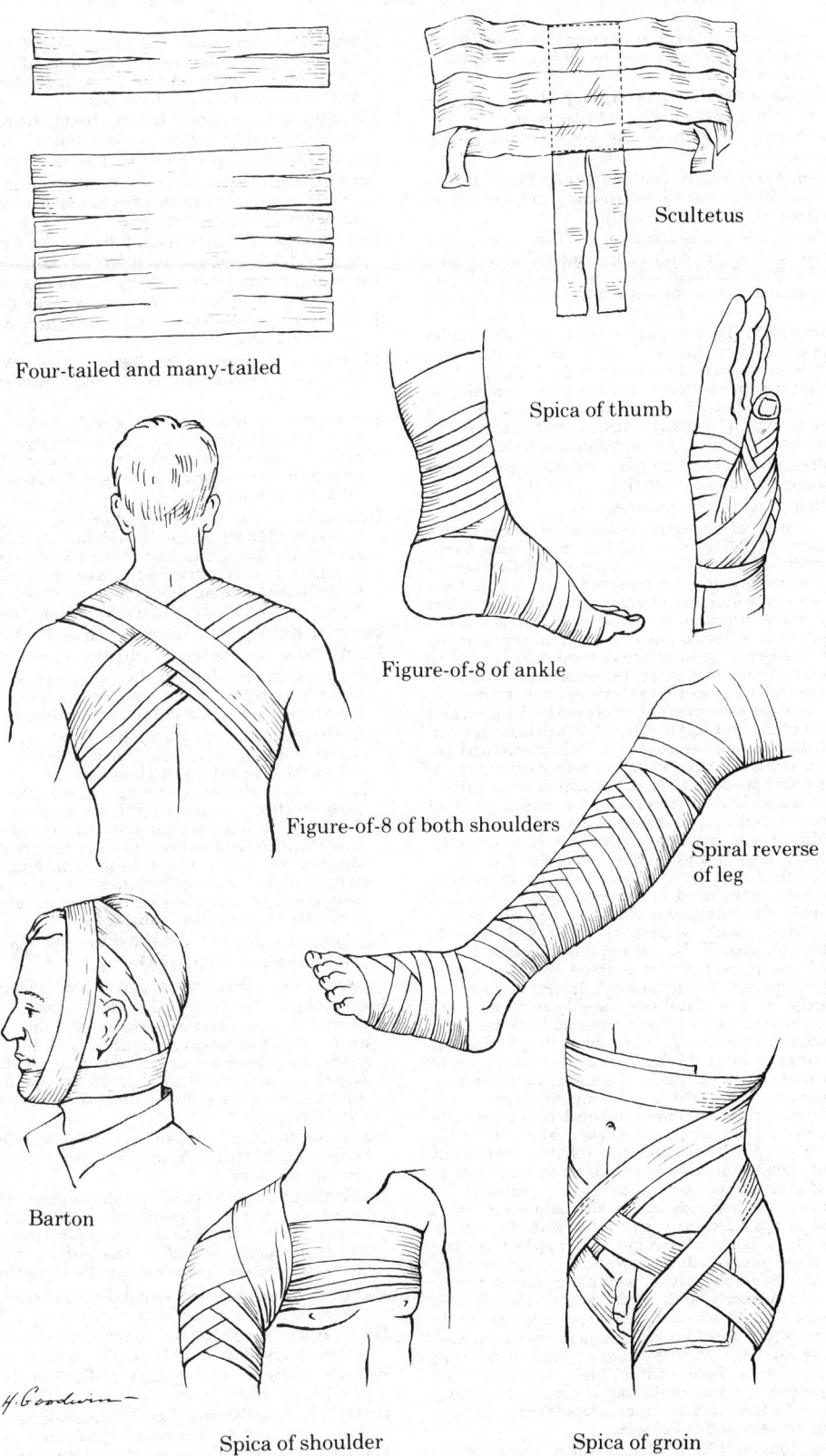

Four-tailed and many-tailed

Scultetus

Spica of thumb

Figure-of-8 of ankle

Figure-of-8 of both shoulders

Spiral reverse
of leg

Barton

H. Goodwin

Spica of shoulder

Spica of groin

PLATE 9 — VARIOUS TYPES OF BANDAGE

189

bank (bangk) a stored supply of human material or tissues for future use by other individuals, as *blood b., bone b., eye b., human-milk b., skin b.,* etc.

Bannister's disease (ban'nis-terz) [Henry Martyn *Bannister,* Chicago physician, 1844–1920] angioedema.

Banthine (ban'thīn) trademark for preparations of methantheline bromide.

Banti's disease, syndrome (ban'tēz) [Guido *Banti,* Italian pathologist, 1852–1925] see under *disease,* and see *congestive splenomegaly,* under *splenomegaly.*

Banting (ban'ting), Sir Frederick Grant. Canadian physician, 1891–1941; co-winner, with John James Richard Macleod, of the Nobel prize for medicine or physiology in 1923 for their isolation, with Charles Herbert Best, of insulin from the pancreas.

Baptisia (bap-tiz'e-ah) [L.; Gr. *baptizein* to dip in or under water] a genus of leguminous plants. **B. leucan'tha** Torr. and Gray, a species, known as wild indigo, which contains quinolizidine alkaloids and has caused poisoning in horses and cows. **B. tincto'ria** R. Br., a species of herbs of North America, which contains cytisine; used as a dye. The dried root has been used as a cathartic and emetic.

baptisin (bap'tĭ-zin) a glycoside from *Baptisia tinctoria,* a brownish powder, soluble in alcohol.

baptitoxine (bap-tĭ-tok'sin) cytisine.

bar (bahr) 1. a unit of pressure, being a pressure of 10^6 dyne/cm²; 1 bar = 0.987 atm or 10^5 Pa; called also *barye.* 2. a metal segment of greater length than width that serves to connect two or more parts of a removable partial denture. 3. the upper part of the gums of a horse, between the grinders and the tusks, which bears no teeth. 4. that portion of the wall of a horse's hoof reflected posteriorly at an acute angle. **arch b.,** any of several types of heavy wire bars shaped to the outer circumference of the dental arch and extending from one side to the other so that intervening teeth may be attached to it; used for treatment of fractures of the jaws and for stabilization of injured teeth. **b. of bladder,** interureteric ridge (*plica interureterica* [NA]). **chromatoid b.,** see under *body,* def. 1. **connector b.,** a connector unit of a removable partial denture that is fabricated as parallel-, round-, or oval-sided bars and serves to connect parts of dentures, splint or connect abutments, connect and splint crowns, or splint teeth that have received root therapy. Called also *connecting b.* and *minor connector.* Cf. *major connector.* **Erich arch b.,** an arch bar made of soft, readily contoured metal, used for intermaxillary fixation. **hyoid b's,** a pair of cartilaginous plates forming the second visceral arch, from which a part of the hyoid bone is developed. **Kazanjian T b.,** an appliance useful in reconstruction of the lip and jaw; it is fixed with an acrylic prosthesis to provide soft tissue support during reconstruction. **Kennedy b.,** 1. a metal bar, usually resting on the lingual surfaces of teeth, that aids in their stabilization and acts as an indirect retainer. 2. continuous clasp. **labial b.,** a major connector located labial to the dental arch, and joining two or more bilateral parts of a mandibular removable partial denture. **lingual b.,** continuous clasp. **median b.,** a fibrotic formation across the neck of the prostate gland, causing obstruction of the urethra. **Mercier's b.,** interureteric ridge (*plica interureterica* [NA]). **occlusal rest b.,** a minor connector used to attach an occlusal rest to a major part of a removable partial denture. **palatal b.,** a major connector that extends across the palate and joins two or more parts of a maxillary removable partial denture. **Passavant's b.,** a horizontal ridge that appears on the posterior wall of the pharynx during swallowing, produced by contraction of the palatopharyngeal sphincter; it also occurs during speech in persons with cleft palate. Called also *pharyngeal ridge* and *Passavant's cushion, pad,* or *ridge.* **sternal b.,** one of the paired cartilaginous bars in the embryo that unite to form the sternum. **terminal b's,** zones where epithelial cells contact one another, once thought to represent an accumulation of dense cementing substance, but with the electron microscope shown to be a junctional complex (see under *complex*).

Bar's incision (bahrz) [Paul *Bar,* French obstetrician, 1853–1945] see under *incision.*

baragnosis (bar''-ag-no'sis) [Gr. *baros* weight + *a* neg. + *gnōsis* knowledge] absence of the power to recognize weight.

Bárány (bah'rah-ne), Robert. Austrian physician, 1876–1936; winner of the Nobel prize for medicine or physiology in 1914 for his work on the physiology and pathology of the vestibular apparatus of the ear.

Bárány's symptom (sign, test), pointing test (bah'rah-nēz) [Robert *Bárány*] see under *symptom* and *tests.*

barba (bar'bah) [L. "the beard"] [NA] the beard.

barbaloin (bar'bah-loin) an anthraquinone pentoside that occurs in various species of *Aloe* and is mainly responsible for their purgative properties.

barbaralalia (bar''bar-ah-la'le-ah) a form of dyslalia that is shown when speaking a foreign language.

barbasco (bar-bas'ko) tropical plants, *Jacquinia paramensis* and *Paullinia pinnata;* used as fish poisons.

barbeiro (bar-ba'ro) [Port.] Brazilian name for *Panstrongylus megistus.*

Barber's psoriasis (bar'berz) [Harold Wordsworth *Barber,* English dermatologist, born 1886] localized pustular psoriasis.

barberry (bar'ber-e) the shrub *Berberis vulgaris* and its fruit, which is the source of a yellow dye. The chief constituents are resins and the alkaloid berberine. Its berries are used as preservatives, and the bark of the stems and roots is used as a bitter tonic.

barbital (bar'bĭ-tal) chemical name: 5,5-diethyl-2,4,6(1*H,3H,5H*)-pyrimidinetrione. A long-acting barbiturate, $C_8H_{12}N_2O_3$, the first of the barbiturate series; used as a hypnotic and sedative, administered orally. **b. sodium, b. soluble,** the soluble monosodium salt of barbital, $C_8H_{11}N_2NaO_3$, having the same actions and uses as the base.

barbitalism (bar'bĭ-tal-izm) (*obs.*) Barbituism.

barbitone (bar'bĭ-tōn) a British name for barbital.

barbituism (bar-bit'u-izm) (*obs.*) a condition caused by the use of barbital or its derivatives and marked by chill, headache, fever, and cutaneous eruptions.

barbiturate (bar''bi-tūr'at; bar-bich'oorit) any of a class of sedative-hypnotic agents derived from barbituric acid or thiobarbituric acid and classified into long-, intermediate-, short-, and ultrashort-acting classes. The ultrashort-acting barbiturates, e.g. thiopental, are used as intravenous anesthetics. The long-acting barbiturate phenobarbital is an important anticonvulsant used in the treatment of epilepsy. Many other barbiturates were widely used as sedatives or hypnotics, but benzodiazepines have replaced them in most uses. Some of these have a high potential for abuse and are Schedule II controlled substances.

barbituric acid (bar''bi-tūr'ik) the parent compound of the barbiturates $C_4H_4N_2O_3$.

barbiturism (bar-bit'u-rizm) (*obs.*) barbituism.

barbotage (bar''bo-tahzh') [Fr. *barboter* to dabble] repeated injection and withdrawal of fluid, as in gastric lavage, or the administration of an anesthetic into the subarachnoid space by alternate injection of a small amount of the anesthetic and withdrawal of a small quantity of cerebrospinal fluid into the syringe, until the anesthetic is completely administered.

barbula (bar'bu-lah, gen. and pl. *bar'bulae.*) [L.] a little beard. **b. hir'ci,** 1. axillary hair (hirci [NA]). 2. tufts of hair in the ears.

Barbulanympha (bar''bu-lah-nim'fah) [L. *barbula* little beard + *nympha*] a genus of multiflagellated, cellulose-digesting, parasitic protozoa (suborder Trichonymphina, order Hypermastigida) found in the gut of the woodroach, and characterized by the presence of two anterior tufts of flagella.

Barcoo disease, rot (bar-koo') [*Barcoo,* a river in South Australia] see *desert sore,* under *sore.*

Barcroft's apparatus (bar'krofts) [Sir Joseph *Barcroft,* British physiologist, 1872–1947] see under *apparatus.*

Bard's sign (bardz') [Louis *Bard,* French physician, 1857–1930] see under *sign.*

Bard-Pic syndrome [Louis *Bard;* Adrien *Pic,* French physician, 1862–1944] see under *syndrome.*

Bardet-Biedl syndrome (bar-da' be'del) [Georges *Bardet,* French physician, born 1885] Laurence-Biedl syndrome.

baresthesia (bar''es-the'ze-ah) [Gr. *baros* weight + *aisthēsis* perception + *-ia*] sensibility for weight or pressure; pressure sense.

baresthesiometer (bar″es-the″ze-om′ĕ-ter) [Gr. *baros* weight + *aisthēsis* perception + *metron* measure] an instrument for determining sensitiveness as to weight or pressure.

Bargen's streptococcus (bar′genz) [Jacob Arnold *Bargen*, California physician, born 1894] see *Streptococcus bovis.*

bariatrics (bar″e-at′riks) [Gr. *baros* weight + *iatrikē* medicine, surgery] a field of medicine encompassing the study of overweight, its causes, prevention, and treatment.

baritosis (bar-ĭ-to′sis) pneumoconiosis due to inhalation of barite or barium dust.

barium (ba′re-um), gen. *ba′rii* [L.; Gr. *baros* weight] a pale yellowish, metallic element belonging to the alkaline earths, whose acid-soluble salts are poisonous; its atomic number is 56; atomic weight 137.34; symbol, Ba. **b. arsenate,** a salt, $Ba_3(AsO_4)_2$, formerly used in tuberculosis and in skin diseases. **b. bromide,** a compound, $BaBr_2 + 2H_2O$, formerly used as a heart tonic and in aneurysm and scrofula. **b. carbonate,** a poisonous salt, $BaCO_3$, formerly used in medicine; now employed in preparing the chloride, etc. **b. chloride,** a compound, $BaCl_2 + 2H_2O$, a cardiac stimulant; formerly used in sclerosis of the nervous tissues and in heart block and aneurysm. **b. cyanoplatinate,** a substance, $BaPt(CN)_4 \cdot 4H_2O$, used for coating the screen of the fluoroscope; called also *b. platinocyanide.* **b. hydrate, b. hydroxide,** $Ba(OH)_2$, a crystalline soluble base employed as a test for sulfates. **b. oxide,** white to yellowish white powder, BaO, used for drying gases; called also *baryta.* **b. platinocyanide,** b. cyanoplatinate. **b. sulfate,** a bulky, fine, white powder without odor or taste, and free from grittiness, $BaSO_4$, used as a contrast medium in roentgenography of the digestive tract. Called also *synthetic baryta* and *blanc fixe.* **b. sulfide,** a heavy, grayish white or pale yellow, poisonous powder, BaS, sometimes used in veterinary medicine as a depilatory for preoperative preparation.

bariumize (bār′e-um-īz) (*obs.*) to treat with barium.

bark (bark) [L. *cortex*] the rind or outer cortical cover of the woody parts of a plant, tree, or shrub; called also *cascara.* **bearberry b.,** cascara sagrada. **bitter b.,** the dried bark of *Alstonia constricta,* a tree of New South Wales and Queensland. **buck-thorn b.,** the dried bark of *Rhamnus frangula.* **butternut b.,** the dried inner bark of the root of *Juglans cinerea.* **calisaya b.,** cinchona. **casca b.,** the bark of *Erythrophloeum guineense;* called also *Mancona b.* **chittem b.,** cascara sagrada. **cinchona b.,** cinchona. **cotton root b.,** the air dried bark of roots of various species of *Gossypium;* formerly used as an oxytocic. Called also *gossypii radicis cortex.* **cramp b.,** the dried bark of *Viburnum opulus.* **cuprea b.,** the bark of *Remijia purdieana* or *R. pedunculata.* **dita b.,** the dried bark of *Alstonia scholaris,* a tree of India and the Philippines. **dogwood b.,** 1. cascara sagrada. 2. see *Cornus.* **elm b.,** the dried inner bark of *Ulmus fulva.* **Jesuits' b.,** cinchona. **Mancona b.,** casca b. **Persian b.,** cascara sagrada. **Peruvian b.,** cinchona. **Purshiana b.,** cascara sagrada. **quebracho b.,** bark derived from a large evergreen tree of the genus *Aspidosperma,* indigenous to various parts of South America. **quillay b.,** quillaia. **sacred b.,** cascara sagrada. **seven b's,** *Hydrangea.* **soap b., soap tree b.,** quillaia. **white oak b.,** the dried inner bark of *Quercus alba.* **wild black cherry b.,** wild cherry; see under *cherry.*

Barkan's operation (bar′kanz) [Otto *Barkan,* San Francisco ophthalmologist, 1887–1958] goniotomy.

barley (bar′le) the annual grasses, *Hordeum vulgare, H. distichon,* etc.; also their seed, a cereal grain. Used for malting and distillation and to some extent as a food substance. Boiled barley water has demulcent properties and has been used as a home remedy in the management of infant diarrhea. **pearl b.,** decorticated polished barley grain.

Barlow's disease (bar′lōz) [Sir Thomas *Barlow,* physician in London, 1845–1945] infantile scurvy.

Barlow syndrome (bar′lo) [John B. *Barlow,* 20th century South African cardiologist] see *mitral valve prolapse syndrome,* under *syndrome.*

barn (barn) [jocular "big as a barn"] a unit of area equal to 10^{-24} square centimeter, used in measuring nuclear scattering cross sections. Symbol b.

Barnes's bag (dilator), curve (barn′zes) [Robert *Barnes,* English obstetrician, 1817–1907] see under *bag* and *curve.*

bar(o)- [Gr. *baros* weight] a combining form denoting relationship to weight or pressure.

baroagnosis (bar″o-ag-no′sis) baragnosis.

baroceptor (bar″o-sep′tor) baroreceptor.

baroelectroesthesiometer (bar″o-e-lek″tro-es-the″ze-om′ĕ-ter) [*baro-* + *electric* + Gr. *aisthēsis* perception + *metron* measure] an instrument to measure the amount of pressure at the time electric sensibility to tingling or pain is felt.

barognosis (bar″og-no′sis) [*baro-* + Gr. *gnōsis* knowledge] conscious perception of weight; the faculty by which weight is recognized; weight knowledge.

baromacrometer (bar″o-mah-krom′ĕ-ter) [*baro-* + Gr. *makros* long + *metron* measure] an instrument for measuring and weighing newborn infants.

baro-otitis (bar″o-o-ti′tis) barotitis. **b. me′dia,** barotitis media.

baropacer (bar″o-pās′er) an electronic unit implanted in the necks of dogs for continuous stimulation of the carotid sinuses.

barophilic (bar″o-fil′ik) [*baro-* + Gr. *philein* to love] growing best under high atmospheric pressure; said of bacterial cells.

baroreceptor (bar″o-re-sep′tor) a sensory nerve ending that is stimulated by changes in pressure, as those in the walls of blood vessels; called also *baroceptor.*

baroscope (bar′ŏ-skōp) [*baro-* + Gr. *skopein* to examine] an instrument used in the quantitative determination of urea.

barosinusitis (bar″o-si″nu-si′tis) inflammation of one or more paranasal sinuses (usually the frontal sinus) due to difference in pressure between the surrounding atmosphere and the air within the sinus cavity; severe localized pain is the predominant symptom. It occurs on ascent or descent in an aircraft to or from high altitude, in the absence of free communication between the sinus and the atmosphere. Called also *aerosinusitis* and *sinus barotrauma.*

barospirator (bar″o-spi′ra-tor) [*baro-* + L. *spirare* to breathe] a machine for producing artificial respiration by means of variations in the air pressure in a closed chamber.

barotaxis (bar″o-tak′sis) [*baro-* + Gr. *taxis* arrangement] stimulation of living matter by change of the pressure relations under which it exists; see also *barotropism.*

barotitis (bar″o-ti′tis) a morbid condition of the ear produced by exposure to differing atmospheric pressures. **b. me′dia,** traumatic inflammation of the middle ear caused by a difference in pressure between the surrounding atmosphere and air in the middle ear space, marked by otalgia, tinnitus, hearing loss, and, occasionally, vertigo. It occurs in descent of aircraft from high altitude. Called also *aerotitis media* and *otitic barotrauma.*

barotrauma (bar″o-traw′mah) [*baro-* + Gr. *trauma* wound] injury caused by pressure: specifically injury of the cartilaginous walls of the eustachian tube and the ear drum due to the difference between atmospheric and intratympanic pressures. **otitic b.,** barotitis media. **sinus b.,** barosinusitis.

barotropism (bar-ot′ro-prizm) [*baro-* + Gr. *tropos* a turning] a relatively stereotyped response, often a movement, to pressure stimuli.

Barr body (bahr) [Murray Llewellyn *Barr,* Canadian anatomist, born 1908] sex chromatin.

Barraquer's disease (bar-rak-erz′) [Roviralta José Antonio *Barraquer,* Spanish physician] see *partial lipodystrophy,* under *lipodystrophy.*

Barraquer's method, operation (bar-rak-erz′) [Ignacio *Barraquer,* Spanish ophthalmologist, 1884–1965] phacoerysis.

Barré-Guillain syndrome (bar-ra′ ge-yan′) acute febrile polyneuritis.

barren (bar′en) sterile; unfruitful.

barrier (bār′e-er) an obstruction. **blood-air b., blood-gas b.,** alveolocapillary membrane. **blood-aqueous b.,** the anatomical mechanism that prevents exchange of materials between the chambers of the eye and the blood. **blood-brain b., blood-cerebral b.,** the barrier separating the blood from the parenchyma of the central nervous system. Presumably it consists of the walls of the capillaries of the central nervous system and the surrounding glial membranes (glial end-feet). Abbreviated *BBB.* **blood-cerebrospinal fluid b.,** blood-brain b. **blood-testis b.,** a barrier separating the blood from the seminiferous tubules, consisting of special junctional complexes between adjacent Sertoli cells near the base of the seminiferous epithelium. **blood-thymus b.,** a barrier in the thymus which excludes certain substances, possibly constituted by the interposition of a sheet of epithelial cell processes around the periphery of the lobules and between the lymphocytes and the perivascular connective tissue. **filtration b.,** the structures separating the blood in the glomerular capillaries and capsular space of the renal corpuscle, consisting of the fenestrated epithelium, the basal lamina, and the slit pores between the pedicels of the podocytes. **gastric mucosal b.,** a physiological property of the gastric mucosa rendering the epithelium relatively impermeable to ions. Its function is impaired by aspirin, organic acids, and bile salts, and in patients subjected to severe trauma or shock. Back diffusion of acid from the gastric lumen may cause mucosal erosion or ulceration. **hematoencephalic b.,** blood-brain b. **histohematic connective tissue b.,** the barrier between the blood and the dependent parenchymal tissue through which diffusion of nutrients and gases takes place. **placental b.,** the placental separation of fetal from maternal blood and bloodborne materials of greater than molecular size. **protective b.,** an intervening shield of radiation-absorbing material such as lead, concrete, or plastic whose atomic number and thickness are specifically sufficient to give adequate body protection against ionizing radiation of various types. **protective b's, primary,** barriers sufficient to reduce a primary beam of radiation to a permissible exposure rate. **protective b's, secondary,** barriers sufficient to reduce stray or scattered radiation to a permissible exposure rate. **radiation b.,** protective b.

barsati (bar-sat-e′) cutaneous habronemiasis.

Bart's syndrome (bartz) [B. J. *Bart*] see under *syndrome.*

Barth's hernia (barths) [Jean Baptiste Philippe *Barth,* German physician, 1806–1877] see under *hernia.*

Bartholin's duct, gland (bar′to-linz) [Caspar Thomèson *Bartholin,* Jr., Danish anatomist, 1655–1738] see *ductus sublingualis major* and *glandula vestibularis major.*

bartholinitis (bar″to-lin-i′tis) inflammation of Bartholin's ducts.

Barton's bandage, fracture, operation (bar′tunz) [John Rhea *Barton,* Philadelphia surgeon, 1794–1871] see under *bandage, fracture,* and *operation.*

Bartonella (bar″to-nel′lah) [A. L. *Barton,* Peruvian physician, 1871–1950] a genus of bacteria of the family Bartonellaceae, order Rickettsiales, made up of gram-negative cells in chains found in fixed tissue cells and in or on erythrocytes. The organism occurs in humans, sometimes asymptomatically, and in arthropod vectors. **B. bacillifor′mis,** a species of small aerobic coccobacilli transmitted to humans by the sandfly *Phlebotomus verrucarum;* it is the etiologic agent of Carrión's disease (Oroya fever and verruga peruana).

Bartonellaceae (bar″to-nel-la′se-e) a family of bacteria of the order Rickettsiales, made up of small rod-shaped, coccoid, or ring- or disk-shaped, filamentous and beaded organisms, usually measuring less than 3μ, occurring as pathogenic parasites in the erythrocytes of man and other animals. It includes the genera *Bartonella* and *Grahamella.*

bartonelliasis (bar″to-nel-li′ah-sis) bartonellosis.

bartonellosis (bar″to-nel-lo′sis) infection with *Bartonella bacilliformis,* transmitted by sandflies of the genus *Phlebotomus,* especially *P. verrucarum,* found only in certain Andean valleys in Peru, Ecuador, and Colombia, and occurring in two distinct stages. The first stage (*Oroya fever*) is an acute, highly fatal, febrile illness associated with severe hemolytic anemia. The second stage (*hemorrhagic pian, Peruvian wart, verruca peruana, verruca peruviana, verruga peruana*) is manifested by a chronic, benign skin eruption of hemangioma-like macules surrounded by hyperpigmented borders. Called also *bartonelliasis* and *Carrión's disease.*

Bartter's syndrome (bar′terz) [Frederic Crosby *Bartter,* American internist, 1914–1983] see under *syndrome.*

Baruch's law, sign (bar′ooks) [Simon *Baruch,* physician in New York, 1840–1921] see under *law* and *sign.*

baruria (bah-roo′re-ah) [Gr. *baros* weight + *ouron* urine + *-ia*] the passage of urine of a high specific gravity.

bary- [Gr. *barys* heavy] a combining form meaning heavy or difficult.

barye (bar′e) bar, def. 1.

baryesthesia (bar″ĭ-esthe′ze-ah) baresthesia.

baryglossia (bar″ĭ-glos′e-ah) [*bary-* + Gr. *glōssa* tongue + *-ia*] thick, slow utterance of speech.

barylalia (bar″ĭ-la′le-ah) [*bary-* + Gr. *lalia* speech] thick, indistinct speech due to imperfect articulation.

baryphonia (bar″ĭ-fo′ne-ah) [*bary-* + Gr. *phōnē* voice + *-ia*] a thick, heavy quality of voice.

baryta (bah-ri′tah) any of several compounds of barium, including calcinated baryta (barium oxide) and caustic baryta (barium hydroxide). **synthetic b.,** barium sulfate.

barytosis (bar″ĭ-to′sis) baritosis.

basad (ba′sad) toward a base or basal aspect.

basal (ba′sal) pertaining to or situated near a base.

Basaljel (ba′sal-jel) trademark for basic aluminum carbonate gel.

basaloid (ba′sah-loid) resembling basal cells of the skin; see under *carcinoma.*

basaloma (ba″sah-lo′mah) basal cell carcinoma.

base (bās) [L., Gr., *basis*] 1. the lowest part or foundation of anything; see also *basis.* 2. the main ingredient of a compound. 3. in chemistry, the nonacid part of a salt; a substance that combines with acids to form salts; a substance that dissociates to give hydroxide ions in aqueous solutions; a substance whose molecule or ion can combine with a proton (hydrogen ion); a substance capable of donating a pair of electrons (to an acid) for the formation of a coordinate covalent bond. 4. a unit of a removable prosthesis that supports the supplied tooth and any intermediary material and in turn receives support from the tissue of the basal seat. **acidifiable b.,** a chemical substance that will unite with water to form an acid. **acrylic resin b.,** a denture base made of an acrylic resin. **alloxur b's, alloxuric b's,** purine b's. **animal b.,** a ptomaine or leukomaine. **apical b.,** that portion of the jaws giving support to the teeth; called also *basal arch.* **cement b.,** a layer of insulating, sometimes medicated dental cement placed in the deep portions of a cavity preparation to protect the pulp, reduce the bulk of the metallic restoration, or eliminate undercuts in tapered preparation. **conjugate b.,** a chemical species that is formed from its conjugate acid by removal of a proton; e.g., acetate (CH_3COO) is the conjugate base of acetic acid (CH_3COOH). **b. of cranium,** see *basis cranii externa* and *basis cranii interna.* **denture b.,** that part of a denture, made either of metal or resin or a combination of both materials, that supports the supplied teeth and receives support from the abutment teeth, the residual alveolar ridge, or both. See also *denture base saddle,* under *saddle.* **denture b., tinted,** a denture base which simulates the coloring and shading of natural oral tissues. **b. of dorsal horn of spinal cord,** basis cornus dorsalis medullae spinalis. **film b.,** a thin, flexible, transparent sheet of cellulose acetate or similar material which carries the radiation and light-sensitive emulsion of x-ray or photographic films. **b. of heart,** basis cordis. **hexone b's,** di-aminomonocarboxylic acids formed by the hydrolysis of proteins, and containing six atoms of carbon; they include arginine, lysine, and histidine. Called also *histone b's* and *diaminoacids.* **histone b's,** hexone b's. **Lewis b.,** an electron-pair donor, e.g., ammonia and halide ion. **b. of lung,** basis pulmonis. **metal b.,** a metallic portion of a denture base forming a part or all of the basal surface of the denture, which serves as the attachment for the plastic (resin) part of the denture base and the teeth. **nitrogenous b.,** an aromatic, nitrogen-containing molecule that serves as a proton acceptor, e.g., purine or pyrimidine. **nuclein b's, nucleinic b's,** purine b's. **ointment b.,** a vehicle for medicinal substances intended for external application to the body. **plastic b.,** a denture or baseplate made of a plastic material. **b. of posterior horn of spinal cord,** basis cornus dorsalis medullae spinalis. **b. of prostate,** basis prostatae. **purine b's,** a group of chemical compounds of which purine is the base, including 6-oxypurine (hypoxanthine), 2,6-dioxypurine (xanthine); 6-aminopurine (adenine); 2-amino-6-oxypurine (guanine); 2,6,8-trioxypurine (uric acid); 3,7-dimethyl xanthine (theobromine). Called also *nuclein* or *nucleinic* b's, and *xanthine* b's. **pyrimidine b's**, a group of chemical compounds of which pyrimidine is the base, including 2,4-dioxy-pyrimidine (uracil), 2,4-dioxy-5-methylpyrimidine (thymine), and 2-oxy-4-aminopyrimidine (cytosine), which are common constituents of nucleic acids. **record b.**, baseplate. **Schreiner's b.**, spermine. **shellac b's**, resinous materials adapted to maxillary or mandibular casts to form baseplates. **b. of stapes**, footplate. **temporary b.**, baseplate. **tinted denture b.**, a denture base which simulates the coloring and shading of natural oral tissues. **tooth-borne b.**, the base of a partial denture which is supported by the abutment teeth and not by the tissues beneath it. **trial b.**, baseplate. **xanthine b's**, purine b's.

basedoid (baz'ĕ-doid) a condition resembling Basedow's (Graves') disease, but without thyrotoxicosis.

Basedow's disease, triad (baz'ĕ-dōz) [Carl Adolph von *Basedow*, German physician, 1799–1854] see *Graves' disease*, under *disease*, and *Merseburg triad*, under *triad*.

basedowiform (baz''ĕ-do'ĭ-form) resembling Basedow's (Graves') disease.

baseline (bās'līn) an observation or value that represents the normal background level of a measurable quantity, used for comparison with values representing response to experimental intervention or an environmental stimulus, usually implying that the baseline and response values refer to the same individual or system.

baseplate (bās'plāt) 1. a temporary preformed shape fabricated of shellac, wax, or acrylic resin, representing the base of a denture and used for making maxillomandibular (jaw) relation records, for arranging artificial teeth, or for trial placement in the mouth. Called also *record base, temporary base*, and *trial base*. Written also *base plate*. 2. Hutch's term for the tissue circumferential to and somewhat eccentric to the urethral orifice which, it is postulated, may act as a floor during the filling of the bladder and assume a cone-shape during micturition to allow the proximal urethra to fill. **gutta-percha b.**, gutta-percha combined with fillers and coloring materials, rolled into sheets; used for temporary restorations, filling root canals, and separating teeth. **stabilized b.**, a baseplate lined with a plastic or other suitable material to improve its adaptation and stability.

bases (ba'sēz) [L.] plural of *basis*.

bas-fond (bah-fon') [Fr.] a fundus, especially that of the urinary bladder.

Basham's mixture (Bash'amz) [William Richard *Basham*, English physician, 1804–1877] iron and ammonium acetate solution; see under *solution*.

basial (ba'se-al) pertaining to the basion.

basialis (ba''se-a'lis) [L.] basial; used in the NA terminology as denoting relationship to a base or to the basion.

basialveolar (ba''se-al-ve'o-lar) extending from the basion to the alveolar point.

basiarachnitis (ba''se-ar''ak-ni'tis) inflammation of the basal part of the arachnoid; called also *basiarachnoiditis*.

basiarachnoiditis (ba''se-ah-rak''noi-di'tis) basiarachnitis.

basic (ba'sik) 1. pertaining to or having the properties of a base. 2. capable of neutralizing acids.

basicaryoplastin (ba''se-kar''e-o-plas'tin) [*basi-* + Gr. *karyon* kernel + *plassein* to form] the basophil paraplastin of the cell nucleus.

basichromatin (ba''se-kro'mah-tin) the basophil portion of the chromatin of the cell nucleus.

basichromiole (ba''se-kro'me-ōl) [*basophil* + *chromiole*] one of the basophil particles forming the chromatin of the cell nucleus.

basicity (bah-sis'ĭ-te) 1. the quality of being a base, or basic. 2. the combining power of an acid; it is measured by the number of hydrogen atoms replaceable by a base.

basicranial (ba''se-kra'ne-al) [*basi-* + Gr. *kranion* cranium] pertaining to the base of the skull.

basicytoparaplastin (ba''se-si''to-par''ah-plas'tin) the basophil paraplastin of the cytoplasm.

basidia (bah-sid'e-ah) plural of *basidium*.

Basidiobolus (bah-sid''ĭ-ob'o-lus) a genus of phycomycetous fungi of the family Entomophthoraceae, order Entomophthorales. **B. haptospo'rus**, the etiologic agent

of subcutaneous phycomycosis; called also *B. meristosporus*. **B. meristospo'rus**, B. haptosporus.

basidiocarp (bah-sid'ĕ-o-karp'') the basidium-producing large fruiting body, the mushroom, composed of masses of intertwined hyphal elements, which is characteristic of the majority of the Basidiomycetes.

Basidiomycetes (bah-sid''e-o-mi-se'tēz) a class of perfect fungi of the division Eumycetes, the club fungi, in which the spores are borne on club-shaped organs (basidia); it includes the subclasses Heterobasidiomycetidae and Homobasidiomycetidae.

basidiomycetous (ba''sid-i-o-mi-se'tus) of or pertaining to fungi of the class Basidiomycetes.

basidiospore (bah-sid'e-o-spōr) a spore formed on a basidium. See *Basidiomycetes* and *spore*.

basidium (bah-sid'e-um), pl. *basid'ia* [Gr. *basis* base] the clublike organ of the fungal class Basidiomycetes which, following karyogamy and meiosis, bears the basidiospore. See *spore*.

basifacial (ba-se-fa'shal) [L. *basis* base + *facies* face] pertaining to the lower part of the face.

basigenous (bah-sij'ĕ-nus) capable of forming a chemical base.

basihyal (ba''se-hi'al) basihyoid.

basihyoid (ba''se-hi'oid) the body of the hyoid bone; in certain of the lower animals, either of the two lateral bones that are its homologues; called also *basihyal*, and *corpus ossis hyoidei*.

basil (ba'sil) [Gr. *basilikon*, neuter of *basilikos* royal] any aromatic plant of the genus *Ocimum*, especially *O. basilicum*; a condiment with carminative properties. Called also *sweet b*.

basilad (bas'ĭ-lad) toward the basilar aspect.

basilar (bas'ĭ-lar) [L. *basilaris*, from *basis* base] pertaining to a base or basal part.

basilaris (bas''ĭ-la'ris) [L.] situated at the base. **b. cra'nii**, a composite of the numerous bones which serve the brain as a supportive floor and form the axis of the whole skull.

basilateral (ba''se-lat'er-al) both basilar and lateral.

basilemma (ba''se-lem'ah) [*basi-* + Gr. *lemma* husk] basement membrane.

basilic (bah-sil'ik) [L. *basilicus*; Gr. *basilikos* royal] important or prominent.

basilicon (bah-sil'ĭ-kon) [Gr. *basilikos* royal] a once popular name for various ointments, and especially for resin cerate.

basin (ba'sn) the pelvis.

basinasial (ba''se-na'ze-al) pertaining to the basion and the nasion.

basio- see *basi-*.

basi(o)-, bas(o)- [Gr. *basis*] a combining form denoting relationship to a base or foundation, to the basion, or to a chemical base.

basioccipital (ba''se-ok-sip'ĭ-tal) pertaining to the basilar process of the occipital bone.

basioglossus (ba''se-o-glos'us) [*basio-* + Gr. *glōssa* tongue] the part of the hyoglossus muscle that is attached to the base of the hyoid bone.

basion (ba'se-on) [Gr. *basis* base] [NA] a craniometric landmark located at the midpoint of the anterior border of the foramen magnum in the midsagittal plane. Called also *point Ba*.

basiotic (ba''se-ot'ik) [*basi-* + Gr. *ous* ear] see under *bone*.

basiparachromatin (ba''se-par''ah-kro'mah-tin) basicaryoplastin.

basiparaplastin (ba''se-par''ah-plas'tin) the basophil portion of the paraplastin.

basipetal (ba-sip'ĕ-tal) [*basi-* + L. *petere* to seek] descending toward the base; developing in the direction of the base, as a spore.

basiphilic (ba''se-fil'ik) basophilic.

basirhinal (ba''se-ri'nal) [*basi-* + Gr. *rhis* nose] pertaining to the base of the brain and to the nose.

basis (ba'sis), pl. *bases* [L.; Gr.] the lower, basic, or fundamental part of an object; [NA] a general term designating the base of a structure or organ, or the part opposite to or distinguished from the apex. **b. cartilag'inis**

arytenoi'deae [NA], base of arytenoid cartilage: the triangular inferior part of the arytenoid cartilage, which bears the articular surface. **b. cer'ebri,** facies inferior cerebri. **b. coch'leae** [NA], base of cochlea: the posterior of the cochlea, which rests upon the internal acoustic meatus. **b. cor'dis** [NA], base of heart: a poorly delimited region of the heart, formed, in general, by the atria and the area occupied by the roots of the great vessels. It lies opposite the middle thoracic vertebrae, its exact position varying with heart action, and is directed superiorly, posteriorly, and to the right. **b. cor'nus dorsa'lis medul'lae spina'lis** [NA], base of dorsal horn of spinal cord: the portion of the dorsal horn, or column, of gray substance in the spinal cord that is continuous with the intermediate gray region; called also *b. cornus posterioris medullae spinalis* [NA alternative] and *base of posterior horn of spinal cord*. **b. cor'nus posterio'ris medul'lae spina'lis,** NA alternative for *b. cornus dorsalis medullae spinalis*. **b. cra'nii exter'na** [NA], external base of cranium: the outer surface of the inferior region of the skull. **b. cra'nii inter'na** [NA], internal base of cranium: the inner surface of the inferior region of the skull, constituting the floor of the cranial cavity. **b. enceph'ali,** facies inferior cerebri. **b. glan'dulae suprarena'lis,** facies renalis glandulae suprarenalis. **b. mandib'ulae** [NA], base of mandible: the lower margin of the body of the mandible; called also *inferior border of mandible*. **b. metacarpa'lis** [NA], the base of a metacarpal bone, being the proximal end of each metacarpal, which articulates with a carpal(s) and with adjacent metacarpals. Called also *b. ossis metacarpalis*. **b. metatarsa'lis** [NA], the base of the metatarsal bone, being the wedge-shaped proximal end of each metatarsal, which articulates with bone(s) of the tarsus and with adjacent metatarsals. Called also *b. ossis metatarsalis*. **b. modi'oli** [NA], base of modiolus: the broad part of the modiolus situated near the lateral part of the internal acoustic meatus. **b. na'si,** the portion of the nose opposite to the apex. **b. os'sis metacarpa'lis,** b. metacarpalis. **b. os'sis metatarsa'lis,** b. metatarsalis. **b. os'sis sa'cri** [NA], base of the sacral bone: the cranial surface of the sacrum; its lateral portions consist of the alae of the sacrum, and its middle portion is the upper surface of the body of the first sacral vertebra that articulates with the fifth lumbar vertebra. Called also *base of sacrum*. **b. patel'lae** [NA], base of patella: the superior border of the patella, to which the tendon of the quadriceps femoris muscle is attached; called also *superior border of patella*. **b. pedun'culi cer'ebri** [NA], the large bundle of nerve fiber tracts forming the ventral part of the cerebral peduncles, which consists of corticospinal, corticonuclear, corticopontine, parietotemporopontine, and frontopontine fibers descending from the cerebral cortex and terminating in the pons and spinal cord. Called also *crus cerebri*. **b. phalan'gis digito'rum ma'nus** [NA], base of phalanx of fingers: the proximal end of each phalanx of the fingers; called also *proximal extremity of phalanx of finger*. **b. phalan'gis digito'rum pe'dis** [NA], base of phalanx of toes: the proximal end of each phalanx of the toes; called also *proximal extremity of phalanx of toe*. **b. prosta'tae** [NA], base of prostate: the broad upper part of the prostate, in contact with the lower surface of the urinary bladder. **b. pulmo'nis** [NA], base of lung: the portion of each lung that is directed toward the diaphragm. **b. pyram'idis rena'lis** [NA], base of renal pyramid: the part of a renal pyramid that is directed away from the renal sinus. **b. scap'ulae,** a name applied to both the vertebral and the axillary borders of the scapula (margo medialis and margo lateralis). **b. sta'pedis** [NA], base of stapes: the oval plate of bone on the stapes that fits into the fenestra vestibuli.

basisphenoid (ba″se-sfe′noid) an embryonic bone that becomes the back part of the body of the sphenoid.

basisylvian (ba″se-sil′ve-an) [*basi-* + *sylvian*] (*obs.*) pertaining to the basilar part of the sylvian fissure (sulcus lateralis).

basitemporal (ba″se-tem′po-ral) [*basi-* + *temporal*] pertaining to the lower part of the temporal bone.

basivertebral (ba″se-ver′te-bral) [*basi-* + L. *vertebra* joint] pertaining to the body of a vertebra.

basket (bas′ket) a basket cell or any basket-shaped structure. **Alzheimer's b's,** neurofibrillary tangles. **cytopharyngeal b.,** cyrtos. **fiber b's,** fine fibers extending

from the external limiting membrane of the retina to surround the adjacent portions of the rods and cones.

Basle Nomina Anatomica (bah′zl no′mĭ-nah an-ah-tom′ĭ-kah) the official body of anatomical nomenclature prepared by a group of German anatomists with some help from anatomists in other countries, and presented for final criticism at the annual meeting of the German Anatomic Society held in Basle, Switzerland in 1895. Abbreviated BNA. It has been superseded by *Nomina Anatomica*.

BaSO₄ barium sulfate.

bas(o)- see *basi(o)-*.

basocyte (ba′so-sīt) (*obs.*) a basophilic cell or leukocyte.

basocytopenia (ba″so-si″to-pe′ne-ah) [*basocyte* + Gr. *penia* poverty] (*obs.*) basophilic leukopenia.

basocytosis (ba″so-si-to′sis) (*obs.*) 1. basophilic leukocytosis. 2. basophilia, def. 1.

basoerythrocyte (ba″so-ĕ-rith′ro-sīt) (*obs.*) an erythrocyte containing basophilic granules.

basoerythrocytosis (ba″so-ĕ-rith″ro-si-to′sis) (*obs.*) basophilia, def. 1.

basograph (ba′so-graf) [Gr. *basis* a walking + *graphein* to write] an instrument for recording abnormalities of gait.

basolateral (ba″so-lat′er-al) pertaining to the base and sides.

basometachromophil (ba″so-met″ah-kro′mo-fil) [*basic* + Gr. *meta* beyond + *chrōma* color + *philein* to love] staining with basic dyes to a color different from that of surrounding substances.

Basommatophora (ba-som″mah-tof′o-rah) a suborder of mostly freshwater snails (order Pulmonata, subclass Euthyneura, class Gastropoda); two families of medical importance are Planorbidae and Lymnaeidae.

basopenia (ba″so-pe′ne-ah) (*obs.*) basophilic leukopenia.

basophil (ba′so-fil) [Gr. *basis* base + *philein* to love] 1. a structure, cell, or other histologic element staining readily with basic dyes. 2. a granular leukocyte with an irregularly shaped, relatively pale-staining nucleus that is partially constricted into two lobes, and with cytoplasm that contains coarse, bluish-black granules of variable size. Basophils contain vasoactive amines, e.g., histamine and serotonin, which are released on appropriate stimulation; called also *basophilic leukocytes*. 3. a beta cell of the adenohypophysis; see also *gonadotroph* (def. 1) and *thyrotroph*. 4. basophilic. **beta b.,** thyrotroph. **Crooke-Russell b's,** the basophils in Crooke's hyaline degeneration; see under *degeneration*. **delta b.,** gonadotroph, def. 1.

basophile (ba′so-fīl) basophilic.

basophilia (ba″so-fil′e-ah) 1. the reaction of relatively immature erythrocytes to basic dyes whereby the stained cells appear blue, gray, or grayish-blue (diffuse basophilia), or bluish granules appear (punctate basophilia or stippling). 2. an abnormal increase in the blood of basophilic erythrocytes; called also *basocytosis* and *basoerythrocytosis*. 3. basophilic leukocytosis.

basophilic (ba-so-fil′ik) staining readily with basic dyes.

basophilism (ba-sof′ĭ-lizm) abnormal increase of basophil cells. **Cushing's b., pituitary b.,** Cushing's syndrome (def. 1); see under *syndrome*.

basophilous (ba-sof′ĭ-lus) basophilic.

basoplasm (ba′so-plazm″) cytoplasm that stains with basic dyes.

Basset's operation (bas-sāz′) [Antoine *Basset*, French surgeon, 1882–1951] see under *operation*.

Bassini's operation (bah-se′nēz) [Edoardo *Bassini*, surgeon in Padua, 1844–1924] see under *operation*.

bassorin (bas′o-rin) a principal constituent of tragacanth gum, made up of a complex of polymethoxylated acids (bassoric acid) which swell in water to form an irreversible gel; used as a pharmaceutical adjuvant.

basswood (bas′wood) the wood of the Linden tree, *Tilia americana* L. (Tiliaceae). Long used in American folk medicine as a decoction of the wood, bark, or flowers for bile and liver disorders.

bastard (bas′tard) [Old Fr.] 1. an illegitimate person; one born out of wedlock. 2. illegitimate. 3. of inferior quality; not genuine.

Bastedo's rule (bas-te′dōz) [Walter Arthur *Bastedo*, physician in New York, 1873–1952] see under *rule*.

Bastian-Bruns law (sign) (bas'chan-broonz') [Henry Charlton *Bastian*, British neurologist, 1837–1915; Ludwig *Bruns*, neurologist in Hanover, 1856–1916] see under *law*.

basylous (bas'ĭ-lus) acting as a base in chemical composition.

bath (bath) 1. a conductive or convective medium, as water, vapor, sand, or mud, with which the body is laved or in which the body is wholly or partly immersed for therapeutic or cleansing purposes; called also *balneum*. 2. the application of a conductive or convective medium to the body for therapeutic or cleansing purposes. 3. a piece of equipment or scientific apparatus in which a body or object may be immersed. **acid b.,** one of water medicated with a mineral acid. **air b.,** the therapeutic exposure of the body to air, which is usually warm; called also *balneum pneumaticum*. **alcohol b.,** the laving of the body with dilute alcohol; it is defervescent and stimulant. **alkaline b.,** the washing of a patient in a weak solution of an alkaline carbonate; useful in skin diseases. **alum b.,** the use of alum water as a bathing medium. **antipyretic b.,** a bath given to reduce fever. **antiseptic b.,** a bath containing an antiseptic. **aromatic b.,** a medicated bath in which the water is scented with a decoction of aromatic plants or volatile oils. **astringent b.,** a bath in a liquid containing tannic acid, alum, or other astringent. **borax b.,** one in water medicated with glycerin and borax. **bran b.,** an emollient bath of water in which bran has been boiled. **Brand b.** (1861), a cold bath of short duration in which the water is at 68° F., and during which the patient is gently massaged. **bubble b.,** a bath in which the water has been filled with bubbles produced by mechanical or chemical means. **cabinet b.,** a hot-air bath or a radiant heat bath in which the patient is enclosed in a special cabinet. **camphor b.,** a bath given in an atmosphere containing the vapor of camphor. **carbon dioxide b.,** a water bath impregnated with carbon dioxide, such as the Nauheim bath. **Charcot's b.** (*obs.*), a bath taken by standing in ankle-deep hot water and sponging the body locally with cold water. **cold b.,** one in which cold water is used at a temperature of less than 65° F. **colloid b.,** a bath containing gelatin, bran, starch, or similar substances. **continuous b.,** a bath of flowing water. **contrast b.,** immersion of a part of the body alternately in hot and in cold water. **cool b.,** one in water from 65° to 75° F. **creosote b.,** a bath containing creosote and glycerin; used in scaly skin diseases. **douche b.,** the application of water to the body from a jet spray. **drip-sheet b.,** see *drip sheet*, under *sheet*. **earth b.,** the placing of a patient in a mass of earth or of sand, usually warmed. **emollient b.,** a bath in an emollient liquid, like a decoction of bran. **Finnish b.,** a sweat bath given in an enclosed, steamy room. Hyperemia of the skin is increased by beating with twigs, and the bath is followed by a cold plunge. **Finsen b.,** a general irradiation of the patient's body with ultraviolet rays. **foam b.,** a bath of foam produced by blowing air or oxygen through the water to which a foam-forming substance (saponin) has been added. **full b.,** one in which the patient's body is fully immersed in the water. **gas-bubble b.,** a bath of water containing gases in such quantities that gas bubbles are set free and ascend to the surface of the water, as in carbon dioxide and oxygen baths. **gelatin b.,** an emollient bath in a thin warm solution of gelatin. **glycerin b.,** a warm emollient bath in water containing glycerin and gum acacia. **graduated b.,** one in which the temperature of the water is gradually modified. **grease b.,** a scrubbing of the body with some greasy preparation (petrolatum, lanolin). **Greville b.** (*obs.*), an electric hot-air bath. **half b.,** a bath of the hips and lower part of the body. **herb b.,** one which contains a decoction of aromatic herbs. **hip b.,** sitz b. **hot b.,** one in water from 98° to 104° F. **hot-air b.,** one in air or vapor from 100° to 130° F. **hyperthermal b.,** a hot bath in which the water is above 104° F. **immersion b.,** one in which the body of the patient is immersed. **iron b.,** one in water which contains iron sulfate. **kinetotherapeutic b.,** a bath providing facilities for underwater exercise. **light b.,** exposure of all or part of the body to light rays, either of the sun or from an apparatus. **linseed b.,** a bath to which has been added the mucilage extracted from linseed. **lukewarm b.,** a neutral bath in which the water is between 92° and 97° F. **medicated b.,** a bath variously charged with medicinal substances. **milk b.,** one taken in milk; called also *balneum lacteum*.

moor b., a mud bath containing earth from a moor or waste land. **mud b.,** application of wet sticky earth to the body, or immersion of the body in such material. **Nauheim b.,** a bath in which the patient is immersed in warm carbonated water. **needle b.,** a shower bath in which the water is projected in a fine, needle-like spray. **oil b.,** one taken in warm olive oil, sometimes variously medicated. **oxygen b.,** a bath impregnated with oxygen. See *gas-bubble b.* **pack b.,** see *pack*. **paraffin b.,** wax b. **peat b.,** a mud bath utilizing partially carbonized vegetable matter. **sand b.,** 1. the immersion of the body in dry, heated sand. 2. the covering of the body with the damp sand of the seashore. Called also *balneum arenae*. **sauna b.,** a sweat bath given in an enclosed, steamy room, usually followed by a cold shower. See *Finnish b.* **Schott b.,** see *Schott's treatment*, under *treatment*. **sea b., sea-water b.,** a bath in water from the sea; usually warm. **sedative b.,** a warm bath in which the patient's body is immersed, usually for several hours, to reduce agitated behavior. **sheet b.,** the applications of wet sheets to the body. **sitz b.,** a bath in which the patient sits in the tub, the hips and buttocks being immersed; called also *hip b.* **sponge b.,** one in which the patient's body is not immersed in water but is rubbed with a wet cloth or sponge. **stimulating b.,** a bath containing tonic, astringent, or aromatic substances. **sweat b.,** any bath given to promote sweating. **tepid b.,** one in water from 75° to 92° F. **vapor b.,** exposure of the body to steam. **warm b.,** one taken in water from 92° to 97° F. **water b.,** a vessel containing water for immersing bodies or for immersing liquid-containing vessels that are to be heated or cooled, or are to be held at a given temperature. **wax b.,** the application of heated liquid wax to a part of the body, the wax being permitted to solidify; also the immersion of a part of the body in heated liquid wax maintained at a constant temperature. Called also *paraffin b.* **whirlpool b.,** a variously sized tank in which the body or an extremity can be submerged as the heated water is mechanically agitated.

bathesthesia (bath"es-the'ze-ah) bathyesthesia.

bathmotropic (bath"mo-trop'ik) [Gr. *bathmos* threshold + *tropos* a turning] influencing the response of tissue to stimuli. **negatively b.,** lessening response to stimuli. **positively b.,** increasing response to stimuli.

bathmotropism (bath-mot'ro-pizm) influence on the excitability of muscular tissue.

bath(o)- see *bathy-*.

bathochrome (bath'o-krōm) an atom or group whose introduction into a compound shifts the compound's absorption peak to a longer wavelength; cf. *hypsochrome*.

bathochromy (bath"o-kro'me) a shift of the absorption band toward lower frequencies (longer wavelengths) with deepening of color from yellow to red to black.

bathoflore (bath'o-flōr) [*batho-* + *fluorescence*] a substance that decreases the intensity of fluorescence of a parent compound; cf. *auxoflore*.

bathomorphic (bath"o-mor'fik) having a deep or myopic eye.

bathrocephaly (bath"ro-sef'ah-le) [Gr. *bathron* a step + *kephalē* head] a developmental anomaly characterized by a steplike posterior projection of the skull, caused by excessive bone formation at the lambdoid suture.

bathy-, bath(o)- [Gr. *bathys* deep, *bathos* depth] a combining form meaning deep, or denoting relationship to depth.

bathyanesthesia (bath"e-an"es-the'ze-ah) [*bathy-* + *anesthesia*] loss of deep sensibility.

bathycardia (bath"e-kar'de-ah) [*bathy-* + Gr. *kardia* heart] a low position of the heart due to anatomical conditions and not to disease.

bathyesthesia (bath"e-es-the'ze-ah) [*bathy-* + Gr. *aisthēsis* perception] deep sensibility; the sensibility in the parts of the body beneath the surface, such as muscle sensibility and joint sensibility.

bathyhyperesthesia (bath"e-hi"per-es-the'ze-ah) [*bathy-* + *hyperesthesia*] increased sensitiveness of deep structures of the body.

bathyhypesthesia (bath"e-hip"es-the'ze-ah) [*bathy-* + *hypesthesia*] decreased sensitiveness of the deep structures of the body.

bathypnea (bath"e-ne'ah) [*bathy-* + Gr. *pnoia* breath] deep breathing.

batonet (ba-to-net′) pseudochromosome.

battery (bat′er-e) 1. a set or series of cells which afford an electric current. 2. any set, series, or grouping of similar things, as a battery of tests.

Battey bacilli (bat′e) [*Battey*, a tuberculosis hospital in Rome, Georgia, where many strains of these mycobacteria were first recognized] see under *bacillus.*

batteyin (bat′e-in) [*Battey* bacillus] a product prepared from Battey bacilli (Group III of the unclassified mycobacteria), comparable to tuberculin, used in a cutaneous test of hypersensitivity.

Battle's operation, sign (bat′t′lz) [William Henry *Battle*, London surgeon, 1855–1936] see under *operation* and *sign.*

Battley's sedative (bat′lēz) [Richard *Battley*, English chemist, 1770–1856] see under *sedative.*

Baudelocque's diameter (line) (bo-dloks′) [Jean Louis *Baudelocque*, French obstetrician, 1746–1810] see under *diameter.*

Bauhin's gland, valve (bo′anz) [Gaspard (Caspar) *Bauhin*, Swiss anatomist, 1560–1624] see *glandulae linguales anteriores* and *valva ileocecalis.*

Baumé's scale (bo-māz′) [Antoine *Baumé*, French chemist, 1728–1804] see under *scale.*

Baumès' symptom (bo-mez′) [Jean Baptiste Timothée *Baumès*, French physician, 1756–1828] see under *sign.*

bay (ba) a recess or inlet. **lacrimal b.,** lacus lacrimalis.

bayberry (ba′ber-e) 1. the fruit of *Laurus nobilis*, the European laurel. 2. the wax myrtle, *Myrica cerifera*, and its berry. 3. the tree, *Pimenta afficinalis*, and its fruit.

Bayer 205 (ba′er) suramin sodium.

Bayes' theorem (bāz) [Thomas *Bayes*, British mathematician, 1702–1761] see under *theorem*, and see *bayesian statistics*, under *statistics.*

Bayle's disease (bālz) [Antoine Laurent Jesse *Bayle*, French physician, 1799–1858] paralytic dementia.

Bayle's granulations (bālz) [Gaspard Laurent *Bayle*, French physician, 1774–1816] see under *granulation.*

Baynton's bandage (bān′tonz) [Thomas *Baynton*, English surgeon, 1761–1820] see under *bandage.*

Bazin's disease (bah-zaz′) [Antoine Pierre Ernest *Bazin*, French dermatologist, 1807–1878] see *erythema induratum.*

B.B.B. blood-brain barrier; see under *barrier.*

B.B.T. basal body temperature.

$\beta 1C, \beta_1 C$ C3; see *complement.*

BCAA branched chain amino acid.

B-CAVe a regimen of bleomycin, CCNU (lomustine), and vinblastine, used in cancer chemotherapy.

BCDF B cell differentiation factors.

BCF basophil chemotactic factor.

BCG bacille Calmette-Guérin (see *BCG vaccine*, under *vaccine*); bicolor guaiac test (see under *tests*); ballistocardiogram.

BCGF B cell growth factors.

BCNU carmustine.

b.d. abbreviation for L. *bis di′e*, twice a day.

B.D.A. British Dental Association.

Bdella (del′ah) [Gr. "leech"] a genus of mites. **B. cardina′lis,** a species that is parasitic on other insects.

bdellium (del′e-um) [L.; Gr. *bdellion*] the fragrant gum-resin of several species of *Commiphora* trees; used as an adulterant of myrrh because of its similar appearance and aromatic properties.

Bdellovibrio (del″o-vib′re-o) [Gr. *bdella* leech + *vibrio*] a genus of small, aerobic, motile, vibrioid, gram-negative bacteria that are obligate parasites on other gram-negative bacteria, replicating between the cell wall and the plasma membrane of the host bacterium; they are found worldwide in soil and fresh and marine waters. The type species is *B. bacteriovorus.*

bdellovibrio (del″o-vib′re-o) any microorganism of the genus *Bdellovibrio.*

B-DOPA a regimen of bleomycin, dacarbazine, Oncovin (vincristine), prednisone, and Adriamycin (doxorubicin), used in cancer chemotherapy.

B.D.S. Bachelor of Dental Surgery.

B.D.Sc. Bachelor of Dental Science.

Be chemical symbol for *beryllium.*

$\beta 1E, \beta_1 E$ C4; see *complement.*

bead (bēd) a small spherical structure or mass. **rachitic b's,** a series of palpable or visible prominences at the points where the ribs join their cartilages; seen in certain cases of rickets.

beaded (bēd′ed) having the appearance of a string of beads.

Beadle (be′d′l), George Wells. American biochemist, born 1903; co-winner, with Edward Lawrie Tatum and Joshua Lederberg, of the Nobel prize for medicine or physiology in 1958 for work on the bread mold *Neurospora crassa*, showing that genes control a cell's production of enzymes and therefore the chemistry of the cell.

beaker (bēk′er) a form of glass cup, usually with a lip for pouring, used by chemists and pharmacists.

Beale's ganglion cells (bēlz) [Lionel Smith *Beale*, British physician, 1828–1906] see under *cell.*

beam (bēm) 1. a unidirectional, or approximately unidirectional, emission of electromagnetic radiation or particles. 2. any slender structure of a denture or orthodontic appliance designed to provide support to the structure and subjected to lateral stresses, such as a dental bar or an orthodontic arch wire whose curvature changes under load. **cantilever b.,** a beam that is supported by one fixed support at only one of its ends. **continuous b.,** a beam that continues over three or more supports; those supports not at the beam ends being equally free supports. **primary b.,** useful b. **restrained b.,** one that has two or more supports; at least one of which permits some freedom of rotation to the point of support. **simple b.,** a straight beam that has two supports, one at either end. **useful b.,** in radiology, that part of the primary radiation which is permitted to emerge from the tubehead assembly of an x-ray machine, as limited by the tubehead aperture or port and accessory collimating devices.

beamtherapy (bēm-ther′ah-pe) see *beam therapy*, under *therapy*, and *chromotherapy*, def. 2.

bean (bēn) any of the seeds contained in pods of various leguminous plants. **broad b.,** Vicia faba. **Calabar b.,** the poisonous seed of the tropical West African leguminous plant *Physostigma venenosum*; it is the source of physostigmine and has been used by natives in ordeal trials. Called also ordeal b. **castor b.,** the seed of the castor oil plant, *Ricinus communis*, which affords castor oil. **ordeal b.,** Calabar b. **St. Ignatius' b.,** the poisonous seed of the tropical tree *Strychnos ignatii;* it contains strychnine and brucine.

beard (bērd) the heavy hair growing on the lower part of a man's face, normally appearing after puberty as a secondary sex characteristic; called also *barba* [NA].

Beard's disease (bērdz) [George Miller *Beard*, American psychiatrist, 1839–1883] neurasthenia.

bearing (bār′ing) a supporting surface or point. **central b.,** application of forces between the maxillae and mandible at a single point as near as possible to the center of the supporting areas of the upper and lower jaws, for the purpose of distributing closing forces evenly throughout the areas of the supporting structures during the registration and recording of maxillomandibular (jaw) relations and during the correction of occlusal errors.

bearing down (bār′ing down) 1. a feeling of weight in the pelvis occurring in certain diseases. 2. the expulsive effort of a woman in labor.

Bearn-Kunkel-Slater syndrome (bern-kung′kel-sla′ter) [Alexander Gordon *Bearn*, English-born American physician, born 1923; Henry George *Kunkel*, American physician, born 1916; and Robert James *Slater*, Canadian-born American pediatrician, born 1923] lupoid hepatitis.

bearwood (bār′wood) cascara sagrada.

beat (bēt) a throb or pulsation, as of the heart or of an artery; see also *pulse.* **apex b.,** the pulsation of the heart felt over its apex normally in the fifth left intercostal space, 8 or 9 cm. from the midline. **capture b's,** occasional ventricular responses to a sinus impulse that reaches the atrioventricular node in a nonrefractory phase. **ciliary b.,** the rhythmic, coordinated contraction of cilia of cells in a two-step process involving intraciliary excitation followed by interciliary conduction. **dropped b.,** absence of a single ventricular contraction. **ectopic b.,** a heart beat originating at some point other than the sinus node. **escaped b's,** heart beats that follow an abnormally long pause. **forced b.,** an extrasystole produced by artificial stimulation of the heart. **fusion b.,** in electrocardiography, the complex resulting when an ectopic ventricular beat coincides with normal conduction to the ventricle; the complex has features of both the normal and the ectopic beat. **premature b.,** extrasystole. **reciprocal b's,** an additional ventricular contraction induced when the ventricle is activated significantly before the sinus impulse reaches the atria, so that the impulse, after effecting an atrial contraction, may retrace its path to induce another ventricular contraction.

Beau's disease, lines, syndrome (bōz) [Joseph Honoré Simon *Beau*, French physician, 1806–1865] see *cardiac insufficiency*, under *insufficiency;* see under *line*, and see *asystole*.

Beauveria (bo-vēr′e-ah) a genus of imperfect fungi of the family Moniliaceae, order Moniliales. *B. bassia′na* causes muscardine in silkworms, and *B. tenel′la* causes a disease of the larvae of beetles; formerly called *Botrytis bassiana* and *Botrytis tenella*, respectively.

bebeerine (be-be′rēn) an alkaloid, $C_{36}H_{38}N_2O_6$, obtained from the bark of *Nectandra rodioei* Hook and the root of *Chondodendron microphyllum* (Eichl.) Moldenke (menispermaceae), and related species; it has been used as a tonic in malaria. Called also *chondodendrine* and *pelosine*.

bebeeru (be-be′roo) the greenheart tree, *Nectandra rodioei* Hook (Lauraceae), of tropical America; its bark, which contains bebeerine, has been used as a tonic in malaria.

becanthone hydrochloride (bĕ-kan′thŏn) chemical name: 1-[[2-[ethyl(2-ethylpropyl)amino]ethyl]amino]-4-methylthioxanthen-9-one monohydrochloride; an antischistosomal agent, $C_{22}H_{28}N_2O_2S \cdot HCl$.

Beccari process (bĕ-kah′re) [Giuseppe *Beccari*, physician in Florence] see under *process*.

bechic (bek′ik) [L. *bechicus*, from Gr. *bēx* cough] pertaining to cough.

Bechterew see *Bekhterev*.

Beck's gastrostomy (beks) [Carl *Beck*, American surgeon, 1856–1911] see under *gastrostomy*.

Beck's triad (beks) [Claude Schaeffer *Beck*, Cleveland surgeon, born 1894] see under *triad*.

Becker's nevus (bek′erz) [Samuel William *Becker*, American physician, born 1894] see under *nevus*.

Becker's phenomenon (sign), test (bek′erz) [Otto Heinrich Enoch *Becker*, German oculist, 1828–1890] see under *phenomenon* and *tests*.

Beckmann's apparatus (bek′manz) [Ernst Otto *Beckmann*, Berlin chemist, 1853–1923] see under *apparatus*.

Beckwith-Wiedemann syndrome (bek′with wēd′ĕ-man) [John Bruce *Beckwith*, American pediatric pathologist, born 1933; Hans Rudolf *Wiedemann*, German pediatrician, born 1915] see under *syndrome*.

Béclard's amputation, etc. (ba-klahrz′) [Pierre Augustin *Béclard*, French anatomist, 1785–1825] see under *amputation, hernia, nucleus,* and *triangle*.

beclomethasone dipropionate (bek″lo-meth′ah-sōn) [USP] chemical name: 9-chloro-11β-hydroxy-16β-methylpregna-1,4-diene-3,20-dione. A glucocorticoid, $C_{28}H_{37}ClO_7$, administered by aerosol inhalation to patients who require chronic treatment with corticosteroids for control of bronchial asthma symptoms. It has also been used topically in the treatment of glucocorticoid-responsive skin diseases.

Becquerel's rays (bek-relz′) [Antoine Henri *Becquerel*, French physicist, 1852–1908; co-winner, with M. S. Curie and P. Curie, of the Nobel prize in physics for 1903, for studies on spontaneous radioactivity] see under *ray*, and see *becquerel*.

becquerel (bek-rel′) [Antoine Henri *Becquerel*] a unit of radioactivity, defined as that of quantity of a radioactive nuclide whose rate of spontaneous nuclear transformation is one decay per second ($1s^{-1}$); 1 curie equals 3.7×10^{10} becquerels; 1 microcurie equals 37 kilobecquerels. Abbreviated Bq.

bed (bed) 1. a supporting structure or tissue. 2. a couch or support for the body during sleep. **air b.,** an airtight, inflatable mattress. **capillary b.,** the total combined mass of capillaries forming a large reservoir which may be more or less completely filled with blood. **CircOlectric b.,** trademark for a revolving circular bed which induces constant pressure alteration. **fracture b.,** a bed for the use of patients with broken bones. **Gatch b.,** a bed fitted with joints beneath the hips and knees of the patient, allowing him to be raised to a half-sitting position and be so maintained by elevating his knees to prevent his sliding toward the footboard. **hydrostatic b.,** a water bed. **Klondike b.,** a bed arranged for outdoor sleeping so that the patient is protected from drafts. **metabolic b.,** a bed so arranged that all the feces and urine of the patient are saved; the amount of excreta compared with the intake gives an indication of the metabolism in the body. **nail b.,** matrix unguis. **Sanders b.,** a powered, rocking bed, used in the treatment of chronic occlusive arterial disease to improve circulation. **sawdust b.,** a bed made from sawdust which is used to prevent bed sores. **water b.,** a rubber mattress filled with water; used to prevent bed sores by distributing the patient's weight; called also *Arnott's b.*

bedbug (bed′bug) a bug of the family Cimicidae, genus *Cimex. C. lectularius*, of temperate regions, and *C. rotundatus* (*hemipterus*), of the tropics, are flattened, oval, reddish insects which inhabit houses, furniture and neglected beds and feed on man, usually at night.

bedlam (bed′lam) [Middle English *bedlem, bethlem*, the popular pronunciation of St Mary of *Bethlehem* Hospital, London, which had mental patients by 1403] 1. an institution for patients with mental illness. 2. bedlamism.

bedlamism (bed′lam-izm) a state of wild tumult; bedlam.

Bednar's aphtha (bed′narz) [Alois *Bednar*, physician in Vienna, 1816–1888] see under *aphtha*.

bedpan (bed′pan) a vessel for receiving the urinary and fecal discharges of a patient unable to leave his bed.

Bedsonia (bed-so′ne-ah) *Chlamydia*.

bedsore (bed-sor) decubitus ulcer.

beef (bēf) the meat of an adult bull, steer, ox, or cow. **b., iron, and wine,** a preparation of beef extract, ferric ammonium citrate, and other ingredients in sherry wine; formerly used as a hematinic agent.

beer (bēr) the fermented infusion of malted barley and hops.

Beer's collyrium, knife, operation (ba′erz) [Georg Joseph *Beer*, German ophthalmologist, 1763–1821] see under *collyrium, knife,* and *operation*.

beerwort (bēr′wert) an infusion of malt in water intended to be converted into beer; it is sometimes used for the cultivation of yeasts and molds.

beeswax (bēz′waks) wax derived from the honeycomb of *Apis mellifera;* see *yellow wax*, under *wax*. **bleached b.,** see *white wax*, under *wax*. **unbleached b.,** see *yellow wax*, under *wax*.

Beevor's sign (be′vorz) [Charles Edward *Beevor*, British neurologist, 1854–1908] see under *sign*.

Begg's appliance, technique (begz) [Peter Raymond *Begg*, Australian orthodontist, born 1898] see under *appliance* and *technique*.

Beggiatoa (bej″je-ah-to′ah) [named for F. S. *Beggiato*] a genus of gliding bacteria of the family Beggiatoaceae, order Cytophagales, made up of colorless cells in unattached filaments that deposit sulfur granules in the presence of hydrogen sulfide. The type species is *B. al′ba*.

Beggiatoaceae (bej″je-ah-to-a′se-e) a family of gliding bacteria of the order Cytophagales, made up of colorless filaments containing cells in chains that show flexing motion. They are free-living organisms found in water and sometimes forming sulfur granules in the presence of hydrogen sulfide. It includes the genera *Beggiatoa, Thioploca,* and *Vitreoscilla*.

Beggiatoales (bej″je-ah-to-a′lēz) in former systems of classification, an order of gliding bacteria, which are now included in the order Cytophagales.

begma (beg′mah) [Gr. *bēgma* phlegm] 1. a cough. 2. the material evacuated from the lungs by coughing (sputum).

behavior (be-hāv′yor) deportment or conduct; any or all of a person's total activity, especially that which can be externally observed. **automatic b.,** automatism. **invariable b.,** activity whose character is determined by innate structure, such as reflex action. **operant b.,** see under *conditioning*. **respondent b.,** see *conditioning*.

variable b., behavior that is modifiable by individual experience.

behaviorism (be-hāv′yor-izm) a school of psychology founded by John B. Watson that regards as the subject matter of psychology only overt actions capable of direct observation and measurement and ignores unobservable mental events such as ideas and emotions.

behaviorist (be-hāv′yor-ist) a psychologist who is a disciple of behaviorism.

behenic acid (be-hen′ik) trivial name for the 22-carbon saturated fatty acid docosanoic acid, present in oil of black mustard and other plant seed oils.

Behçet's syndrome (disease) (ba′sets) [Hulusi *Behçet,* dermatologist, Istanbul, Turkey, 1889–1948] see under *syndrome.*

Béhier-Hardy sign (symptom) (ba′he-a har′de) [Louis Jules *Béhier,* French physician, 1813–1876; Louis Phillipe Alfred *Hardy,* French physician, 1811–1893] see under *sign.*

Behla's bodies (ba′lahs) [Robert Franz *Behla,* German physician, 1850–1921] Plimmer's bodies.

Behring (ba′ring), Emil Adolf von. German physician and bacteriologist, 1854–1917; winner of the first Nobel prize for medicine or physiology in 1901 for his demonstration of immunization against diphtheria and tetanus by injections of antitoxins.

Behring's law (ba′ringz) [Emil Adolf von *Behring*] see under *law.*

BEI butanol-extractable iodine.

Beigel's disease (bi′gelz) [Hermann *Beigel,* German physician, 1830–1879] piedra.

Beijerinckea (bi″jer-ink′e-ah) [M. W. *Beijerinck,* Dutch microbiologist, 1851–1931] a genus of gram-negative, aerobic, rod-shaped bacteria of uncertain affiliation found in tropical soil and water, made up of slime-producing cells that fix nitrogen. The type species is *B. in′dica.*

beikost (bi′kōst) [Ger.] solid and semisolid baby foods, i.e., those other than milk or formula feedings.

bejel (bej′el) [Ar. *bajlah*] nonvenereal syphilis (q.v.) occurring in the Middle East, the Balkans, Central Asia, and Africa.

Békésy (ba′ka-she), Georg von. Hungarian-born American physicist, 1899–1972; winner of the Nobel prize for medicine or physiology in 1961 for his discoveries concerning the physical mechanisms of stimulation within the cochlea.

Bekhterev's (Bechterew's) arthritis, etc. (bek- ter′yevs) [Vladimir Mikhailovich *Bekhterev,* Russian neurologist, 1857–1927] see under *arthritis, disease, layer, nucleus, reaction, reflex, symptom,* and *tests.*

Bekhterev-Mendel reflex (bek-ter′yev-men′del) [V. M. *Bekhterev;* Kurt *Mendel,* German neurologist, 1857–1927] Mendel-Bekhterev reflex.

bel (bel) [Alexander Graham *Bell,* American inventor, 1847–1922] a unit of relative power intensity used for acoustic or electric power, defined as the base 10 logarithm of the ratio of the measured power to some reference power level. A change of one bel is a tenfold power increase. Measurements are usually expressed in decibels (q.v.). Symbol B.

belching (belch′ing) eructation; the noisy voiding of gas from the stomach through the mouth.

belemnoid (be-lem′noid) [Gr. *belemnon* dart + *eidos* form] 1. dart-shaped. 2. the styloid process of the ulna or of the temporal bone.

Bell's law, nerve, palsy (paralysis), phenomenon [Sir Charles *Bell,* Scottish physiologist in London, 1774–1842] see nervus thoracicus longus, and see under *law, palsy,* and *phenomenon.*

Bell's mania [Luther Vose *Bell,* American physician, 1806–1862] acute delirium.

Bell's muscle [John *Bell,* Scottish surgeon and anatomist, 1763–1820] see under *muscle.*

Bell's treatment [William Blair *Bell,* British gynecologist, 1871–1936] see under *treatment.*

Bell-Magendie law (bel′ma-jen′de) [Sir Charles *Bell;* François *Magendie,* French physiologist, 1783–1855] Bell's law.

belladonna (bel″ah-don′ah) [Ital. "fair lady"] the *Atropa belladonna* L. (Solanaceae), or deadly nightshade, a perennial plant indigenous to central and southern Europe and cultivated in North America, containing various anticholinergic alkaloids (e.g., atropine, hyoscyamine, belladonnine, scopolamine, etc.), some of which are produced during the extraction process. Called also *banewort, death's herb,* and *dwale. Belladonna leaf* [USP], consisting of the dried leaves and fruiting tops of *A. belladonna* or *A. belladonna* var. *acuminata,* is used in the preparation of standardized dosage forms; see under *extract* and *tincture.* The root has also been used.

belladonnine (bel″ah-don′nēn) chemical name: 1,2,3,4-tetrahydro-1-phenyl-1,4-naphthalenedicarboxylic acid bis(8-methyl-8-azobicyclo[3.2.1]oct-3-yl)ester. An alkaloid, $C_{34}H_{42}N_2O_4$, derived from belladonna and related solanaceous plants, produced during the process of extraction.

bellaradine (bel-ar′ah-din) cuscohygrine.

Bellini's ducts (tubules), ligament (bel-e′nēz) [Lorenzo *Bellini,* Italian anatomist, 1643–1704] see *tubuli renales recti,* and see under *ligament.*

Bellocq's cannula (sound, tube) (bel-oks′) [Jean Jacques *Bellocq,* French surgeon, 1732–1807] see under *cannula.*

belly (bel′e) 1. the abdomen. 2. the fleshy, contractile part of a muscle; called also *venter musculi* [NA]. **anterior b. of digastric muscle,** venter anterior musculi digastrici. **drum b.,** tympanitic abdomen. **frontal b. of occipitofrontal muscle,** venter occipitalis musculi occipitofrontalis. **occipital b. of occipitofrontal muscle,** venter occipitalis musculi occipitofrontalis. **posterior b. of digastric muscle,** venter posterior musculi digastrici. **prune b.,** see under *syndrome.* **swollen b.,** tympanites in animals. **wooden b.,** abdominal rigidity.

belonephobia (bel″o-nĕ-fo′be-ah) [Gr. *belonē* needle + *phobia*] irrational fear of pins and needles.

belonoid (bel′o-noid) [Gr. *belonē* needle + *-oid*] needle-shaped; styloid.

belonoskiascopy (bel″o-no-ski-as′ko-pe) [Gr. *belonē* needle + *skia* shadow + *-scopy*] a subjective type of retinoscopy in which refractive error is determined by eliminating the perceived shadow of a needle passing in front of the eye fixating on a distant point of light; called also *velonoskiascopy.*

beloxamide (bel-oks′ah-mīd) chemical name: *N*-(benzyloxy)-*N*-(3-phenylpropyl)acetamide; an anticholesteremic agent, $C_{18}H_{21}NO_2$.

Belsey Mark IV operation (bel′se) [Ronald *Belsey,* English surgeon, 20th century] see under *operation.*

belt (belt) an encircling band worn about the waist or abdomen; called also *balteum.* Cf. *girdle.*

bemegride (bem′ĕ-grīd) chemical name: 4-ethyl-4-methyl-2,6-piperidinedione. An analeptic drug, $C_8H_{13}NO_2$, which has been used in the treatment of barbiturate poisoning.

bemidone (bem′ĭ-dōn) chemical name: ethyl 4-(*m*-hydroxyphenyl)-1-methylisonipecotate. A crystal compound, $C_{15}H_{21}NO_3$, soluble in water; formerly used as a narcotic and analgesic.

Benacerraf (ba-nah-ser-rahf′) Baruj. Venezuelan-born American pathologist, born 1920; co-winner, with Jean Baptiste Gabriel Dausset and George Davis Snell, of the Nobel prize for medicine or physiology in 1980 for their work on the major histocompatibility complex and the genetic control of immune responses.

benactyzine hydrochloride (ben-ak′tĭ-zēn) chemical name: α-hydroxy-α-phenylbenzeneacetic acid 2-(diethylamino)ethyl ester hydrochloride. An anticholinergic, $C_{20}H_{26}ClNO_3$, occurring as a white, crystalline powder, which has the ability to increase the emotional threshold of outside influences and to block the thought processes; used as a tranquilizer, administered orally.

Benadryl (ben′ah-dril) trademark for preparations of diphenhydramine hydrochloride.

benapryzine hydrochloride (ben-ah-pri′zēn) chemical name: 2(ethylpropylamino)ethyl benzilate hydrochloride; an anticholinergic, $C_{21}H_{27}NO_3 \cdot HCl$.

Bence Jones protein, etc. [Henry *Bence Jones,* English physician, 1814–1873] see under *cylinder, protein, proteinuria,* and *reaction.*

bend (bend) a flexure or curve; a flexed or curved part. **first order b's,** adjustments made in a labial arch wire, incorporating offsets in the horizontal plane, which are usually made in the areas of the cuspids and premolar and molar teeth, accommodating differences in thickness in the labiolingual or buccolingual diameters of the teeth. **head b.**, cephalic flexure. **neck b.**, cervical flexure. **second order b's**, bends in the vertical plane of an arch wire. **third order b's**, bends in an arch wire to maintain or produce torsion of a tooth. **V b's**, V-shaped bends incorporated in an arch wire, usually placed mesial or distal to the cuspids to improve the axial relationship of teeth. **varolian b.**, the third cerebral flexure in the developing fetus.

bendazac (ben′dah-zak) chemical name: [(1-benzyl-1*H*-indazol-3-yl)oxy]acetic acid; an anti-inflammatory agent, $C_{16}H_{14}N_2O_3$.

bendrofluazide (ben″dro-floo′ah-zīd) bendroflumethiazide.

bendroflumethiazide (ben″dro-floo″mĕ-thi′ah-zīd) [USP] a thiazide diuretic; used for treatment of hypertension and edema.

bends (bendz) pain in the limbs and abdomen occurring as a result of rapid reduction of air pressure; see *decompression sickness*, under *sickness*.

Bendylate (ben′dĭ-lāt) trademark for preparations of diphenhydramine hydrochloride.

bene (be′ne) [L.] well.

beneceptor (ben′e-sep-tor) [L. *bene* well + *ceptor*] a rarely used term for a receptor that transmits stimuli of a beneficial character. Cf. *nociceptor* and *ceptor*, def. 2.

Beneckea (be-nek′e-ah) in former systems of classification, a genus of bacteria, species of which have now been assigned to the genus *Vibrio*.

Benedict's test (ben′e-dikts) [Stanley Rossiter *Benedict*, American physiological chemist, 1884–1936] see under *tests*.

Benedikt's syndrome (ben′e-dikts) [Moritz *Benedikt*, Austrian physician, 1835–1920] see under *syndrome*.

Benemid (ben′ĕ-mid) trademark for probenecid.

benign (be-nīn′) [L. *benignus*] not malignant; not recurrent; favorable for recovery.

benignant (be-nig′nant) benign.

Béniqué's sound (ba-ne-kāz′) [Pierre Jules *Béniqué*, French physician, 1806–1851] see under *sound*.

Benisone (ben′ĭ-sōn) trademark for preparations of betamethasone benzoate.

benjamin (ben′jah-min) benzoin, def. 1.

Bennet's corpuscles (ben′ets) [James Henry *Bennet*, English obstetrician, 1816–1891] see *Nunn's gorged corpuscles* and *Drysdale's corpuscles*, under *corpuscle*.

Bennett's disease (ben′ets) [John Hughes *Bennett*, English physician, 1812–1875] leukemia.

Bennett's fracture (ben′ets) [Edward Hallaran *Bennett*, Irish surgeon, 1837–1907] see under *fracture*.

Benoquin (ben′o-kwin) trademark for preparations of monobenzone.

benorterone (bĕ-nor′ter-ōn) an antiandrogen.

benoxaprofen (ben-oks″ah-pro′fen) chemical name: 2-(4-chlorophenyl)-α-methyl-5-benzoxazoleacetic acid; an anti-inflammatory and analgesic, $C_{16}H_{12}ClNO_3$.

benoxinate hydrochloride (ben-ok′sĭ-nāt) [USP] chemical name: 4-amino-3-butoxybenzoic acid 2-(diethylamino)ethyl ester monohydrochloride. A local anesthetic, $C_{17}H_{28}N_2O_3 \cdot HCl$, occurring as white crystals or as a white, crystalline powder; used in ophthalmology, applied topically to the conjunctiva.

Benoxyl (ben-ok′sil) trademark for preparations of benzoyl peroxide.

benserazide (ben-ser′ah-zīd) chemical name: 2-[(2,3,4-trihydroxyphenyl)-methyl]hydrazide DL serine; a decarboxylase inhibitor, $C_{10}H_{15}N_3O_5$.

Benson's disease (ben′sunz) [Alfred Hugh *Benson*, Irish ophthalmologist, 1852–1912] asteroid hyalosis.

bentazepam (ben-taz′ĕ-pam) chemical name: 1,3,6,7,8,9-hexahydro-5-phenyl-2*H*-[1]benzothieno[2,3-*e*]-1,4-diazepin-2-one; a tranquilizer, $C_{17}H_{16}N_2OS$.

benthos (ben′thos) [Gr. *benthos* bottom of the sea] the flora and fauna of the bottom of oceans.

bentiromide (ben-tēr′o-mīd) a compound, $C_{23}H_{20}N_2O_5$, containing *p*-aminobenzoic acid; used in a noninvasive screening test for pancreatic exocrine insufficiency and to monitor therapy with pancreatic supplements.

bentonite (ben′ton-īt) [NF] a native, colloidal, hydrated aluminum silicate, which on the addition of water swells to produce a slippery paste; its chief pharmaceutical use is as a suspending agent, and it has also been used as a bulk laxative.

Bentyl (ben′til) trademark for preparations of dicyclomine hydrochloride.

benzaldehyde (ben-zal′dĕ-hīd) [NF] artificial essential oil of almond; used as a flavoring agent in orally administered medicaments.

benzalin (ben′zah-lin) nigrosin.

benzalkonium chloride (ben″zal-ko′ne-um) [NF] a mixture of alkylbenzyl dimethylammonium chlorides of the general formula, $[C_6H_5CH_2N(CH_3)_2R]Cl$. A rapidly acting surface disinfectant and detergent, occurring as a white or yellowish white, thick gel or gelatinous pieces, which is active against both gram-negative and gram-positive bacteria and certain viruses, fungi, yeasts, and protozoa; applied topically to the skin and mucous membranes. It is also used as an antimicrobial preservative in ophthalmic solution.

benzamine (ben′zah-mēn) eucaine.

benzanthracene (ben-zan′thrah-sēn) one of a group of hydrocarbons some of which have carcinogenic properties.

benzazoline hydrochloride (benz-az′o-lēn) tolazoline hydrochloride.

benzbromarone (benz-bro′mah-rōn) a potent uricosuric agent that blocks tubular reabsorption of uric acid; used in the treatment of hyperuricemia of gout.

benzcurine iodide (benz′ku-rēn) gallamine triethiodide.

Benzedrex (ben′zĕ-dreks) trademark for a propylhexedrine inhaler.

Benzedrine (ben′zĕ-drēn) trademark for preparations of amphetamine sulfate.

benzene (ben′zēn) a colorless volatile liquid hydrocarbon, C_6H_6, obtained mainly as a by-product in the destructive distillation of coal, along with coal tar, etc. It has an aromatic odor, and burns with a light-giving flame. It dissolves sulfur, phosphorus, iodine, and organic compounds. The fumes may cause fatal poisoning. It was formerly used as a pulmonary antiseptic in influenza, etc., as a teniacide, externally as a parasiticide, and has been suggested in leukemias. Called also *benzol*. **dimethyl b.**, xylene. **b. hexachloride**, chemical name: 1,2,3,4,5,6-hexachlorocyclohexane. A compound, $C_6H_6Cl_6$, prepared by chlorination of benzene in actinic light, consisting of five isomers, the gamma isomer being a powerful insecticide; see also *gamma benzene hexachloride*. Called also *hexachlorocyclohexane*. **methyl b.**, toluene.

benzenoid (ben′zĕ-noid) a compound having a structure related to benzene or other compounds of aromatic character.

benzestrofol (ben-zes′tro-fōl) estradiol benzoate.

benzestrol (ben-zes′trol) [USP] chemical name: 4,4′-(1,2-diethyl-3-methyl-1,3-propanediyl)bisphenol. A synthetic estrogen, $C_{20}H_{26}O_2$, occurring as a white, crystalline powder; administered orally. Called also *octoxollin*.

benzethonium chloride (ben″zĕ-tho′ne-um) [USP] chemical name: *N,N*-dimethyl-*N*-[2-[2-[4-(1,1,3,3-tetra-methylbutyl)phenoxy]ethoxy]ethyl]benzene - methanaminium chloride. A synthetic quatenary ammonium compound, $C_{27}H_{42}ClNO_2$, occurring as white crystals; used as a local anti-infective applied topically as a solution, and as a preservative in pharmaceutical preparations. It is also used in various concentrations for cleaning eating and cooking utensils, as a disinfectant in laundering, to control algal growth in swimming pools, and as an environmental deodorant.

benzhexol hydrochloride (benz-hek′sol) trihexyphenidyl hydrochloride.

benzhydramine hydrochloride (benz-hi′drah-mēn) diphenhydramine hydrochloride.

benzidine (ben′zĭ-din) a colorless, crystalline compound, para-diaminodiphenyl, $(NH_2 \cdot C_6H_4 \cdot C_6H_4 \cdot NH_2)$, formed by the action of acids on hydrazobenzene; used as a test for blood.

benzilonium bromide (benz″il-o′ne-um) chemical name: 1,1-diethyl-3-[(hydroxydiphenylacetyl)oxy]pyrrolidinium bromide; an anticholinergic, $C_{22}H_{28}BrNO_3$, used in the treatment of peptic ulcer and functional gastrointestinal disorders.

benzimidazole (ben"zim-ĭ-da′zōl) a compound, $C_7H_6N_2$, which is toxic to yeast and animals in the absence of its homologous compounds, adenine and guanine. It is also a naturally occurring analog of vitamin B_{12}.

benzin, benzine (ben′zin) [L. *benzinum*] petroleum benzin. **petroleum b., purified b.,** a purified distillate from petroleum consisting of hydrocarbons chiefly of the methane series (mainly pentanes and hexanes), which occurs as a clear, colorless, volatile liquid with a strong ethereal odor; it is highly flammable and may be explosive if the vapors mix with air and are ignited. It is used as a solvent for organic compounds. Called also *benzin* or *benzine, petroleum ether,* and *naphtha.*

benzoate (ben′zo-āt) a salt of benzoic acid.

benzoated (ben′zo-āt-ed) containing or combined with benzoic acid.

benzocaine (ben′zo-kān) [USP] chemical name: 4-aminobenzoic acid ethyl ester. A local anesthetic, $C_9H_{11}NO_2$, occurring as small, white crystals or as a white crystalline powder; applied topically to the skin and mucous membranes.

benzodepa (ben"zo-dep′ah) chemical name: [bis(1-aziridinyl)phosphenyl]carbamic acid phenylmethyl ester. An antineoplastic, $C_{12}H_{16}N_3O_3P$.

benzodiazepine (ben"zo-di-az′ĕ-pēn) any of a group of minor tranquilizers, including chlordiazepoxide, clorazepate, diazepam, flurazepam, oxazepam, etc., having a common molecular structure and similar pharmacological activities, such as antianxiety, muscle relaxing, and sedative and hypnotic effects.

benzodioxan (ben"zo-di-oks′an) a class of α-adrenergic blocking agents, the most important member of which is piperoxan.

benzogynestryl (ben"zo-gi-nes′tril) estradiol benzoate.

benzoic acid (ben-zo′ik) benzenecarboxylic acid, C_6H_5-COOH, a compound widely used as a food preservative to prevent the growth of bacteria and fungi. Benzoic acid is conjugated to glycine in the liver and excreted as hippuric acid. *Benzoic acid* [USP] is a component of *benzoic and salicylic acids ointment* [USP] a topical antifungal agent. Called also *flores benzoini* and *flowers of benzoin.*

benzoic aldehyde (ben-zo′ik) benzaldehyde.

benzoin (ben′zoin) 1. [USP] a balsamic resin with an aromatic odor and taste, which is obtained from *Styrax benzoin* or *S. paralleloneurus* (known as *Sumatra b.*), or from *S. tonkinensis* or other species of *Styrax* (known as *Siam b.*); the former is composed of reddish brown, reddish gray, or grayish brown masses, and the latter of yellowish brown to rusty brown masses. It is used as a topical protectant, and as a topical antiseptic, irritant expectorant, and as an inhalant in respiratory tract inflammation. Called also *benjamin, gum benjamin,* and *gum b.* 2. chemical name: α-hydroxy-α-phenylacetophenone. A white crystalline compound, $C_{14}H_{12}$-O_2, prepared by condensation of benzaldehyde in potassium cyanide solution; called also *benzoylphenylcarbinol.*

benzol (ben′zol) benzene.

benzolism (ben′zo-lizm) poisoning by benzene or its vapor.

benzomethamine (ben"zo-meth′ah-mēn) chemical name: *N*-diethylaminoethyl-*N′*-methylbenzilamide; formerly used to produce parasympathetic blockade and to reduce the secretion of hydrochloric acid in the stomach.

benzonatate (ben-zo′nah-tāt) [USP] chemical name: 2,5,8,11,14,17,20,23,26-nonaoxaoctacos-28-yl ester benzoic acid. An antitussive, $C_{30}H_{53}NO_{11}$, occurring as a clear, pale yellow, viscous liquid, administered orally.

benzononatine (ben-zo″no-na′tin) benzonatate.

Benzopropyl (ben"zo-pro′pil) trademark for a preparation of amydricaine.

benzopurpurine (ben"zo-pur′pu-rin) any one of a series of azo-dyes of a scarlet color, used especially as a contrast stain with hematoxylin and other blue stains. **b. B,** an indicator with a pH range of 2.0 to 4.0.

1,2-benzopyran (ben"zo-pir′an) 1,2-chromene.

benzo[*a*]pyrene (ben"zo-pi′rēn) 3,4-benzpyrene; a highly carcinogenic polycyclic aromatic hydrocarbon occurring as a product of incomplete combustion of carbonaceous materials. It is a procarcinogen that requires metabolic activation to exert a mutagenic effect.

benzopyrronium bromide (ben"zo-pēr-o′ne-um) chemical name: 3-hydroxy-1,1-dimethylpyrrolidinium bromide benzilate; an anticholinergic, $C_{20}H_{24}BrNO_3$.

benzotherapy (ben"zo-ther′ah-pe) treatment with benzoates, especially the treatment of pulmonary abscess by intravenous injection of sodium benzoate.

benzothiadiazide, benzothiadiazine (ben"zo-thi″ah-di′ah-zīd; ben"zo-thi″ah-di′ah-zēn) thiazide.

benzoxiquine (ben-zoks′ĭ-kwin″) chemical name: 8-quinolinol benzoate (ester); a disinfectant, $C_{16}H_{11}NO_2$.

benzoyl (ben′zo-il) the radical, $C_6H_5 \cdot CO$, of benzoic acid and of an extensive series of compounds. **b. peroxide, b. peroxide, hydrous** [USP], a crystalline substance formed by the action of sodium peroxide on benzoyl chloride, used to initiate free radical reactions and to induce skin peeling so as to promote evacuation of comedones in acne vulgaris.

benzoylglycine (ben"zol-gli′sin) hippuric acid.

benzoylpas calcium (ben"zo-il′paz) [USP] chemical name: 4-(benzoylamino)-2-hydroxybenzoic acid calcium salt (2:1) pentahydrate. An antibacterial, $C_{28}H_{20}CaN_2O_8 \cdot 5H_2O$, occurring as a white to cream-colored powder; used as an oral tuberculostatic.

benzoylphenylcarbinol (ben"zol-fen′il-kar′bĭ-nol) benzoin, def. 2.

benzphetamine hydrochloride (benz-fet′ah-mēn) chemical name: *N,α*-dimethyl-*N*-(phenylmethyl)benzeneethanamine hydrochloride. A sympathomimetic amine, C_{17}-$H_{21}N \cdot HCl$, related to amphetamine, occurring as an odorless, white to off-white, crystalline powder; used as an oral anorexiant in the control of exogenous obesity.

benzpiperylon (benz"pĭ-per′ĭ-lōn) chemical name: 4-benzyl-1-(1-methyl-4-piperidyl)-3-phenyl-3-pyrazolin-5-one. A substance, $C_{22}H_{25}N_3O$, used in the treatment of connective tissue disorders.

3,4-benzpyrene (benz-pi′rēn) benzo[*a*]pyrene.

benzpyrinium bromide (benz"pi-rin′e-um) chemical name: 3-[[(dimethylamino)-carbonyl]oxy]-1-(phenylmethyl) pyridinium bromide. A cholinergic, $C_{15}H_{17}BrN_2O_3$, having anticholinesterase actions similar to those of neostigmine.

benzpyrrole (benz-pir′ol) indole.

benzquinamide (benz-kwin′ah-mīd) chemical name: 2-(acetyloxy)-*N,N*-diethyl-1,3,4,6,7,11b-hexahydro-9,10-dimethoxy-2*H*-benzo[*a*]quinolizine-3-carboxamide. A compound, $C_{22}H_{32}N_2O_5$, used intramuscularly or intravenously as an antiemetic; it also has antihistaminic and mild anticholinergic and sedative action.

benzthiazide (benz-thi′ah-zīd) [USP] chemical name: 6-chloro-3-[[(phenyl-methyl)thio]methyl]-2*H*-1,2,4-benzothiadiazine-7-sulfonamide 1,1-dioxide. An orally effective diuretic and antihypertensive agent, $C_{15}H_{14}ClN_3O_4S_3$, occurring as a white, crystalline powder.

benztropine mesylate (benz′tro-pēn) [USP] chemical name: *endo*-3-(diphenylmethoxy)-8-azabicyclo[3.2.1]octane methanesulfonate. A drug, $C_{21}H_{25}NO \cdot CH_4O_3S$, occurring as a white, crystalline powder, having anticholinergic, antihistaminic, and local anesthetic actions; used as an antiparkinsonian agent, administered intramuscularly, intravenously, and orally.

benzurestat (ben-zur′ĕ-stat) chemical name: 4-chloro-*N*-[2-(hydroxyamino)-2-oxoethyl]benzamide; an enzyme (urease) inhibitor, $C_9H_9ClN_2O_3$.

benzydroflumethiazide (ben-zid″ro-floo-mĕ-thi′ah-zīd) bendroflumethiazide.

benzyl (ben′zil) the hydrocarbon radical, C_7H_7 or $C_6H_5 \cdot$-CH_2, of benzyl alcohol and various other compounds. **b. benzoate** [USP], a clear, colorless oily liquid, $C_{14}H_{12}O_2$; used as a pharmaceutic necessity in the preparation of dimercaprol for injection and applied topically to the skin as a scabicide. **b. bromide,** a war gas, $C_6H_5CH_2Br$, causing lacrimation and irritation of the skin; called also *cylite.* **b. carbinol,** phenyl ethyl alcohol, a constituent of oil of rose, possessing anesthetic properties. **b. fumarate,** a white crystalline substance, $C_6H_5CH_2 \cdot OOC \cdot CH:CH:COO$-$CH_2C_6H_5$, containing 63.6 per cent of benzyl. **b. mandelate,** the benzyl ester of mandelic acid; formerly used as an antispasmodic on smooth muscle fiber, as in high blood pressure. **b. succinate,** the dibenzyl ester of succinic acid, $(C_6H_5 \cdot CH_2 \cdot O \cdot CO \cdot CH_2)_2$; formerly used as an antispasmodic to nonstriated muscle.

benzylidene (ben-zil′ĭ-dēn)   a hydrocarbon radical, C_6H_5CH:.

p-benzyloxyphenol (ben″zil-ok″se-fe′nol)   monobenzone.

benzylpenicillin (ben″zil-pen-ĭ-sil′in)   penicillin G; see under *penicillin*. **b. potassium,** penicillin G potassium; see under *penicillin*. **b. procaine,** penicillin G procaine; see under *penicillin*. **b. sodium,** penicillin G sodium; see under *penicillin*.

bephenium (bĕ-fe′ne-um)   an anthelmintic effective against intestinal nematodes, especially hookworms (*Ancylostoma duodenale* and *Necator americanus*) and some other roundworms (*Ascaris lumbricoides* and *Strongyloides stercoralis*); used as *bephenium hydroxynaphthoate* [USP] (called also *bephenium embonate*). It is a cholinergic agonist that causes the worms to relax and be expelled.

Bérard's ligament (ba-rarz′) [Auguste *Bérard*, French surgeon, 1802–1846]   see under *ligament*.

Béraud's valve (ba-rōz′) [Bruno Jean Jacques *Béraud*, French surgeon, 1825–1865]   see under *valve*.

berberine (ber′ber-ēn)   an alkaloid obtained from *Hydrastis canadensis* L. (Berberidaceae), *Berberis* species, and other members of this family; used variously as an antimalarial, carminative, and febrifuge, and externally in dressings for indolent ulcers.

Berberis (ber′ber-is) [L.]   a genus of berberidaceous shrubs, the barberries, which contain berberine.

bereavement (bĕ-rēv′ment)   a deprivation causing grief and desolation, especially the death or loss of a loved one. The period of grief and mourning following a bereavement often resembles clinical depression. See also *mourning*.

bergamot (ber′gah-mot) [L. *bergamium*]   1. the tree, *Citrus bergamia;* also its orange-like fruit, whose rind affords the fragrant oil of bergamot.   2. a popular name for various fragrant labiate plants, such as *Mentha citrata* and *Monarda fistulosa.*

Berger's method, operation (bār-zhāz′) [Paul *Berger*, French surgeon, 1845–1908]   see under *method* and *operation*.

Berger's paresthesia (ber′gerz) [Oskar *Berger*, neurologist in Breslau, 1845–1908]   see under *paresthesia*.

Berger rhythm (ber′ger) [Hans *Berger*, Jena neurologist, 1873–1941]   alpha rhythm; see under *rhythm*.

Berger's sign (symptom) (ber′gerz) [Émile *Berger*, Austrian ophthalmologist, 1855–1926]   see under *sign*.

Bergeron's chorea (disease) (berzh′ronz) [Étienne Jules *Bergeron*, French physician, 1817–1900]   see under *chorea*.

Bergey's classification (ber′gēz) [David Hendricks *Bergey*, American bacteriologist, 1860–1937]   see under *classification*.

Bergman's sign (berg′manz) [Harry *Bergman*, American urologist, born 1912]   see under *sign*.

Bergmann's cells, cords, fibers (berg′manz) [Gottlieb Heinrich *Bergmann*, German physician, died 1861]   see *striae acusticae*, and see under *cell* and *fiber*.

Bergonié treatment (method) (bār-go-nya′) [Jean Alban *Bergonié*, French physician, 1857–1925]   see under *treatment*.

Bergonié-Tribondeau law (bār-go-nya′tre-bon-do′) [J. A. *Bergonié;* Louis *Tribondeau*, French naval physician, 1872–1918]   see under *law*.

Bergström (berk′strām), Sune.   Swedish biochemist, born 1916; co-winner, with Bengt Ingemar Samuelsson and John Robert Vane, of the Nobel prize for medicine or physiology in 1982, for their discoveries of prostaglandins and related substances.

beriberi (ber″e-ber′e) [Singhalese, "I cannot," signifying that the person is too ill to do anything]   a disease caused by a deficiency of thiamine (vitamin B_1) and characterized by polyneuritis, cardiac pathology, and edema. The epidemic form is found primarily in areas in which white (polished) rice is the staple food, as in Japan, China, the Philippines, India, and other countries of Southeast Asia. **atrophic b.,** dry b. **cerebral b.,** Wernicke-Korsakoff syndrome. **dry b.,** a form of beriberi in which flaccid paralysis, muscular atrophy, and areflexia are the prominent signs; cardiac enlargement and tachycardia may be present. Called also

atrophic b. and *paralytic b.*   **infantile b.,** a disease of breast-fed infants whose mothers have thiamine deficiency; it is characterized by diminished urine secretion, progressive edema, and often by acute cardiac failure, which may terminate in sudden death. Vomiting, aphonia, opisthotonos, and convulsions may occur.   **paralytic b.,** dry b.   **ship b.,** a disease resembling tropical beriberi, seen on Norwegian ships, but with edema a more prominent symptom than neuritis.   **wet b.,** a form marked by cardiac failure and edema, but without extensive nervous system involvement.

beriberic (ber″e-ber′ik)   pertaining to or of the nature of beriberi.

Berke operation (berk) [Raynold N. *Berke*, American ophthalmologist, born 1901]   see under *operation*.

Berkefeld filter (ber′ke-feld) [Wilhelm *Berkefeld*, manufacturer, 1836–1897]   see under *filter*.

berkelium (berk′le-um) [named for *Berkeley*, California, where it was produced]   an element of atomic number 97, atomic weight 247, symbol Bk, produced by bombardment of the isotope of americium of atomic weight 241 by helium ions; half-life $4\frac{1}{2}$ hours.

Berlin's disease, edema (ber′linz) [Rudolf *Berlin*, German oculist, 1833–1897]   commotio retinae.

Bernard's canal, etc. (ber-narz′) [Claude *Bernard*, French physiologist, 1813–1878]   see under *canal, duct, layer, puncture,* and *syndrome*.

Bernard-Horner syndrome (ber-nar′hor′ner) [Claude *Bernard;* Johann Friedrich *Horner*, Swiss ophthalmologist, 1831–1886]   Horner's syndrome.

Bernard-Soulier disease (syndrome) (ber-nar′ sool-ya′) [Jean *Bernard*, French hematologist, born 1907; Jean-Pierre *Soulier*, French hematologist, born 1915]   see under *disease*.

Bernays' sponge (ber′nāz) [Augustus Charles *Bernays*, American surgeon, 1854–1907]   see under *sponge*.

Bernhardt's disease, paresthesia (bern′harts) [Martin *Bernhardt*, German neurologist, 1844–1915]   meralgia paresthetica.

Bernhardt-Roth disease, syndrome [Martin *Bernhardt;* Vladimir K. *Roth*, Russian neurologist, 1848–1916]   meralgia paresthetica.

Bernheimer's fibers (bern′hi-merz) [Stefan *Bernheimer*, Austrian ophthalmologist, 1861–1918]   see under *fiber*.

Bernoulli distribution, trial (ber-noo′le, ber-noo-e′) [Jakob *Bernoulli*, Swiss mathematician, 1654–1705]   see under *distribution* and *trial*.

berry (ber′e)   a small fruit with a succulent pericarp. **bear b.,** *Uva ursi.* **buckthorn b.,** *Rhamnus catharctica.* **elder b.,** *Sambucus.* **fish b.,** cocculus indicus. **horse nettle b.,** *Solanum.* **Indian b.,** cocculus indicus. **juniper b.,** juniper. **saw palmetto b.,** *Serenoa.* **spice b.,** aralia.

Berry's ligament (ber′ēz) [Sir James *Berry*, Canadian surgeon, 1860–1946]   ligamentum thyroideum laterale.

Bertiella (ber″te-el′lah)   a genus of tapeworms of the family Anoplocephalidae. **B. sat′yri, B. stu′deri,** a tapeworm found occasionally in man and in the higher apes in Mauritius, India, Africa, Borneo, the West Indies, and the Philippines.

bertielliasis (ber″te-el-li′ah-sis)   infection with *Bertiella*.

Bertin's bones (ossicles), column, ligament (ber′tinz) [Exupère Joseph *Bertin*, French anatomist, 1712–1781]   see *concha sphenoidalis, columnae renales,* and *ligamentum iliofemorale.*

Berubigen (be-roo′bĭ-jen)   trademark for preparations of cyanocobalamin.

berylliosis (ber-il″e-o′sis) [*beryllium* + *-osis*]   beryllium poisoning, usually involving the lungs and less often the skin, subcutaneous tissues, lymph nodes, liver, and other structures. Beryllium fumes, its oxide and salts, and finely divided dust all may cause a tissue reaction when inhaled or implanted in the skin. The *acute form* is basically a toxic or allergic pneumonitis sometimes accompanied by rhinitis, pharyngitis, and tracheobronchitis. The more common *chronic form* is characterized by the development of granulomas and a diffuse interstitial inflammatory reaction; the clinical and pathological findings may be indistinguishable from those of sarcoidosis.

beryllium (ber-il′le-um) [Gr. *bēryllos* beryl] a metallic element of atomic number 4, atomic weight 9.012, symbol Be.

berythromycin (bĕ-rith″ro-mi′sin) chemical name: 12-deoxyerythromycin; an antiamebic and antibacterial, C_{37}-$H_{67}NO_{12}$. Called also *erythromycin B*.

besiclometer (bes″ĭ-klom′ĕ-ter) [Fr. *besides* spectacles + *-meter*] an instrument for measuring the forehead to ascertain the proper width of spectacle frames.

Besnier's prurigo (ba-nyāz′) [Ernest *Besnier*, Paris dermatologist, 1831– 1909] see *atopic dermatitis*, under *dermatitis*, and *prurigo gestationis* of Besnier.

Besnier-Boeck disease (ba-nya′bek) [Ernest *Besnier;* Caesar P. M. *Boeck*, Norwegian dermatologist and syphilologist in Christiana, 1845–1917] sarcoidosis.

Besnoitia (bes-noi′te-ah) a genus of coccidian protozoa (suborder Eimeriina, order Eucoccidiida), the oocysts of which resemble those of *Toxoplasma*. Formerly called also *Globidium*. **B. bennet′ti**, a species causing besnoitiosis in horses. **B. besnoi′ti**, a species causing besnoitiosis in cattle; viscerotropic strains have been found in the impala and blue wildebeest. **B. darlin′gi**, a species found in lizards. **B. jelliso′ni**, a species found in rodents and opossums. **B. taran′di**, a species found in reindeer.

besnoitiosis (bes-noi″te-o′sis) a protozoal disease of cattle, horses, sheep, goats, and other herbivorous animals, due to sporozoan parasites of the genus *Besnoitia*, transmitted mechanically by certain biting flies or by ingestion of oocysts of the etiologic agent shed in the feces of the cat, the definitive host. The organisms localize in the skin, blood vessels, mucous membranes of the upper respiratory tract, and subcutaneous and other tissues, where they eventually form characteristic thick-walled cysts. Other symptoms include fever, anasarca, loss of appetite, photophobia, rhinitis, sclerodermatitis, and alopecia of varying severity. Formerly called globidiosis.

Best (best), Charles Herbert. A Canadian physiologist, born in Maine 1899; discovered histaminase and was associated with Sir Frederick Banting and John James Macleod in the discovery of insulin in 1922.

bestiality (bes-te-al′ĭ-te) [L. *bestia* beast] sexual connection with an animal.

besylate (bes′ĭ-lāt) USAN contraction for benzenesulfonate.

Beta (be′tah) [L.] a genus of plants to which the beet belongs. *B. vulga′ris* L. is the sugar beet, a commercial source of sugar (sucrose).

beta (ba′tah) [B, β] the second letter of the Greek alphabet, β.

Betabacterium (ba″tah-bak-te′re-um) [L. *beta* beet + Gr. *baktērion* little rod] in former systems of classification, a genus of bacteria made up of organisms now assigned to the genus *Lactobacillus*.

Beta-Chlor (ba′tah-klōr) trademark for a preparation of chloral betaine.

beta-cholestanol (ba″tah-ko-les′tah-nol) see under *cholestanol*.

betacism (ba′tah-sizm) [Gr. *bēta* the second letter of the Greek alphabet] the excessive use of the *b* sound in speaking.

Betadine (ba′tah-dīn) trademark for preparations of povidone-iodine.

beta-estradiol (ba″tah-es″trah-di′ol) see *estradiol*.

beta globulin (ba″tah-glob′u-lin) see under *globulin*. **pregnancy-specific b.**, a beta globulin secreted by the placenta; its function is unknown.

betahistine hydrochloride (ba″tah-his′tēn) chemical name: *N*-methyl-2-pyridineethanamine dihydrochloride. A compound, $C_8H_{12}N_2 \cdot 2HCl$, occurring as a white or creamy white, crystalline powder, which has histamine-like action; used orally as a vasodilator to reduce the frequency of the episodes of vertigo in some patients with Ménière's disease, especially those having a high frequency of such episodes.

beta-hydroxybutyric acid (be″tah-hi-drok′se-bu′tĭ-rik) beta-oxybutyric a.

betaine (ba′tah-ēn) chemical name: 1-carboxy-*N,N,N*-trimethylmethanaminium hydroxide inner salt. An oxidation product of choline, $C_5H_{11}NO_2$, which is a transmethylating intermediate in metabolism, and has been shown to have lipotropic activity. Betaine was first found in the sugar beet

and was later shown to be present in many other plants and in animals. It is produced synthetically, and has been used in the treatment of muscular weakness and degeneration. The term has also been used to designate any of a class of trimethyl derivatives of amino acids, e.g., carnitine, or, more generally, the internal salts of quaternary ammonium bases. Called also *lycine* and *oxyneurine*. **b. hydrochloride**, the hydrochloride salt of betaine, $C_5H_{12}ClNO$, which on hydrolysis yields hydrochloric acid; used as a gastric acidifier. It has been used as a lipotropic agent in the treatment of fatty infiltration of the liver.

beta-ketobutyric acid (be″tah-ke″to-bu′tĭ-rik) acetoacetic a.

beta-lactose (ba″tah-lak′tōs) a disaccharide isomeric with lactose, obtained by allowing a solution of lactose to crystallize above 93° C.; it is more soluble and sweeter than lactose.

Betalin (ba′tah-lin) trademark for preparations containing components of the vitamin B complex. *Betalin Complex* is a sterile solution of synthetic B complex factors in sterile distilled water. *Betalin Complex F.C.* consists of synthetic vitamin B factors and synthetic ascorbic acid in sterile distilled water. *Betalin S* is a synthetic preparation of thiamine hydrochloride. *Betalin 12 crystalline* is a sterile isotonic solution of crystalline cyanocobalamin.

beta-lipoprotein (lip″o-pro′te-in) low-density lipoprotein.

beta-lysin (ba″tah li′sin) [so-called to distinguish it from antibodies, "alpha lysins"] a heat-stable cationic protein released by platelets during coagulation that is bactericidal for gram-positive bacteria with the exception of streptococci. Written also *beta lysin*.

betamethasone (ba″tah-meth′ah-sōn) [NF] a synthetic glucocorticoid, occurring as a white to creamy white, crystalline powder, which is the most active of the anti-inflammatory steroids; administered orally or applied to the skin. **b. acetate** [USP], an ester of betamethasone, $C_{24}H_{31}FO_6$, occurring as a white to creamy white powder, having the same actions as the base; used in combination with betamethasone sodium phosphate for intramuscular, intra-articular, intrasynovial, or intralesional injection. **b. benzoate** [USP], the 17-benzoate ester of betamethasone, $C_{28}H_{33}$-FO_6, having the same actions as the base; applied topically to the skin. **b. dipropionate** [USP], the 17,21-dipropionate ester of betamethasone, $C_{28}H_{37}FO_7$, having the same uses as the base; applied topically to the skin. **b. sodium phosphate** [USP], the disodium salt of the 21-phosphate ester of betamethasone, $C_{22}H_{28}FNa_2O_8P$, occurring as a white to almost white powder, having the same actions as the base; used in combination with betamethasone acetate for intramuscular, intra-articular, intrasynovial, or intralesional injection. **b. valerate** [USP], the 17-valerate ester of betamethasone, $C_{27}H_{37}FO_6$, occurring as a white or almost white powder, having the same actions as the base; applied topically to the skin.

betamicin sulfate (ba″tah-mi′sin) chemical name: *O*-6-amino-6-deoxy-α-D-glucopyranosyl-(1→4)-*O*-[3-deoxy-4-*C*-methyl-3-(methylamino)β-L-arabinopyranosyl-(1→6)]-2-deoxy-D-streptamine sulfate; an antibacterial, $C_{19}H_{38}N_4O_{10} \cdot xH_2$-$SO_4$.

beta₂-microglobulin (mi″kro-glob′u-lin) a small (mol. wt. 12,000), nonpolymorphic protein, homologous to the C3 domain of IgG, that is one subunit of class I major histocompatibility antigens.

betanaphthol (ba″tah-naf′thol) a form of naphthol, C_{10}-H_8O, occurring as a colorless or pale-buff crystalline compound having the odor of carbolic acid. Formerly used locally as a counterirritant in alopecia and as an anthelmintic; now used as a topical antiseptic, especially in fungal infections. Called also *isonaphthol*.

beta-naphtholsulfonic acid (be″tah-naf″tho-sul-fon′ik) white pearly scales tinged with red, $OH \cdot C_{10}H_8SO_2 \cdot OH$, used as a test for albumin in the urine; it is a toxic drug that causes profound narcotism and symptoms resembling diabetic coma and is not used as a medication.

betanaphthyl (ba″tah-naf′thil) the combining group, C_{10}-H_8, of betanaphthol. **b. benzoate**, betanaphthol benzoate. **b. salicylate**, betanaphthol salicylate.

betanin (be′tah-nin) the red pigment of the root of the beet.

beta-oxybutyric acid (be″tah-ok″se-bu′tĭ-rik) an acid, $CH_3CHOH \cdot CH_2COOH$, one of the ketone bodies, occurring in the urine in diabetic ketoacidosis and in starvation due to incomplete fatty acid oxidation; called also *beta-hydroxybutyric a.*

Betapar (ba′tah par) trademark for a preparation of meprednisone.

Betapen-VK (ba′tah-pen) trademark for a preparation of penicillin V potassium.

Betaprone (ba′tah-prōn) trademark for a preparation of propiolactone.

betapropiolactone (ba″tah-pro″pe-o-lak′tōn) propiolactone.

betaquinine (ba″tah-kwin′in) quinidine.

betatron (ba′tah-tron) an apparatus for accelerating electrons to millions of electron volts by means of magnetic induction.

Betaxin (be-tak′sin) trademark for preparations of thiamine hydrochloride.

betazole hydrochloride (ba′tah-zōl) [USP] chemical name: 1*H*-pyrazole-3-ethanamine dihydrochloride. A histamine analogue, $C_5H_9N_3 \cdot 2HCl$, occurring as a white, crystalline powder, which stimulates gastric secretion of hydrochloric acid; used in diagnostic tests of gastric secretion, administered intramuscularly or subcutaneously. Called also *gastramine hydrochloride.*

bête (bet) [Fr.] beast. **b. rouge** (bet-roozh′) [Fr. "red beast"], chigger.

betel (be′t'l) [Tamil *vettilei*] an East Indian masticatory, consisting of a piece of betel nut rolled up with lime in a betel leaf; it is tonic, astringent, and stimulant. **b. leaf,** the leaf of *Piper betle;* formerly used as a masticatory and topically as a counterirritant. The oil was used internally for cough and for diphtheria. **b. nut,** the dried ripe seed of *Areca catechu,* a palm tree of South Asia; formerly used as an anthelmintic in veterinary medicine. Called also *areca.*

bethanechol (be-than′ĕ-kōl) a cholinergic agonist, carbamyl-β-methylcholine, that is not hydrolyzed by acetylcholinesterase or pseudocholinesterase and has primarily muscarinic effects; used to stimulate smooth muscle contraction of the gastrointestinal tract and urinary bladder in cases of postoperative or neurogenic atony and retention. Available as *bethanechol chloride* [USP].

bethanechol chloride (be-tha′nĕ-kol) [USP] chemical name: 2-[(aminocarbonyl)oxy]-*N,N,N*-trimethyl-1-propanaminium chloride. A cholinergic, $C_7H_{17}ClN_2O_2$, occurring as colorless or white crystals or as a white crystalline powder; used in the treatment of gastric retention following vagotomy, postoperative urinary retention, postoperative abdominal distention, and in other conditions in which stimulation of the parasympathetic nervous system is desirable; it is administered orally or subcutaneously.

bethanidine sulfate (be-than′i-dēn) chemical name: *N,N*-dimethyl-*N*-(phenylmethyl)guanidine sulfate (2:1). An adrenergic neuron-blocking agent, $C_{10}H_{15}N_3 \cdot \frac{1}{2}H_2SO_4$, used in the treatment of essential hypertension, particularly in the malignant phase.

Bethea's sign (method) (bĕ-tha′ez) [Oscar Walter *Bethea,* New Orleans physician, 1878–1963] see under *sign.*

Betonica (be-ton′i-kah) [L.] a genus of labiate plants. *B. officinalis,* wood betony, was formerly used in medicine: the tops are astringent and aromatic; the root, emetic and cathartic.

Betula (bet′u-lah) [L.] a genus of trees: the birches. **B. al′ba** (white birch), the source of a bark from which rectified birch tar oil is derived; used as an expectorant in various cough syrup formulations, and formerly in certain skin diseases. **B. len′ta** (black birch), a tree whose bark is an important commercial source of methyl salicylate. Now used mainly as a flavoring oil for confections and soda beverages.

betweenbrain (be-twēn′brān) diencephalon (interbrain).

Betz's cells, cell area (bet′zes) [Vladimir Aleksandrovich *Betz,* Russian anatomist, 1834–1894] see under *cell,* and see *psychomotor area,* under *area.*

BeV, Bev billion electron volts, now largely replaced by the term *giga electron volt* (GeV).

Bevan's incision, operation (bev′anz) [Arthur Dean *Bevan,* American surgeon, 1861–1943] see under *incision* and *operation.*

Bevan Lewis cells (bev′an loo′is) [William *Bevan Lewis,* English physiologist, 1847–1929] see under *cell.*

bevel (bev′el) 1. a slanting edge. 2. to produce a slanting of the enamel margins of a tooth cavity.

Bevidox (bev′i-doks) trademark for a solution of vitamin B_{12}; see *cyanocobalamin.*

bezoar (be′zōr) [Persian] a concretion of various character sometimes found in the stomach or intestines of man or other animals. They may belong to one of three types: trichobezoar (hair), phytobezoar (fruit and vegetable fibers), or trichophytobezoar (a mixture of hair, and fruit and vegetable fibers).

Bezold's abscess, etc. (ba′zoltz) [Friedrich *Bezold,* otologist in Munich, 1842–1908] see under *abscess, mastoiditis, perforation, sign,* and *triad.*

Bezold's ganglion (ba′zoltz) [Albert von *Bezold,* German physiologist, 1836–1868] see under *ganglion.*

BF blastogenic factor; see *lymphocyte mitogenic factor,* under *factor.*

β1F, β₁F C5; see *complement.*

BFP biologic false-positive; see under *false-positive.*

BFU-E burst-forming unit—erythroid, the earliest red cell precursor presently detectable in *in vitro* culture, where it has a high requirement for erythropoietin; so named because its growth is composed of subcolonies which give the appearance of a burst.

β1H, β₁H factor H; see *complement.*

bhang (bang) [Hindi] the Asian Indian name for a mixture of the dried leaves and young stems of uncultivated *Cannabis sativa* L. (Cannabaceae), usually ingested as a decoction with milk, sugar, and water, or sometimes smoked or chewed. See *cannabis.*

Bi chemical symbol for *bismuth.*

bi- [L. *bi-,* from *bis* twice] a prefix meaning two, twice, or double. In chemistry, it denotes the presence of a component in twice the proportion of the other component or in twice the usual proportion, or a double radical; except that in bicarbonate, bisulfate, and bitartrate, the prefix *di-* is preferred. Before vowels it appears as *bin-.*

Bial's reagent, test (be′alz) [Manfred *Bial,* German physician, 1870–1908] see under *reagent* and *tests.*

bialamicol hydrochloride (bi″ah-lam′i-kōl) chemical name: 3,3′-bis[(diethylamino)methyl]-5,5′-di-2-propenyl-1,1′-biphenyl]-4-4′-diol dihydrochloride. An antiamebic agent, $C_{28}H_{40}N_2O_2 \cdot 2HCl$, administered orally. Formerly called *biallylamicol.*

biallylamicol (bi-al″il-am′i-kol) former name for bialamicol hydrochloride.

Bianchi's nodules, valve (be-ang′kēz) [Giovanni Battista *Bianchi,* Italian anatomist, 1681–1761] see *noduli valvularum aortae,* and *valve.*

Bianchi's syndrome (be-ang′kēz) [Leonardo *Bianchi,* Italian psychiatrist, 1848–1927] see under *syndrome.*

biarticular (bi″ar-tik′u-lar) pertaining to two joints.

biarticulate (bi″ar-tik′u-lāt) having two joints.

bias (bi′as) 1. (in a measurement process) systematic error. 2. (of a statistical estimator) the difference between the expected value of the estimator and the true parameter value.

biasteric (bi″as-ter′ik) pertaining to the two asteria, especially to the shortest distance between them (biasteric width).

biauricular (bi″aw-rik′u-lar) pertaining to the two auricles of the ears.

Bib. abbreviation for L. *bi′be,* drink.

bib (bib) the remaining fragment of an erythrocyte in which the crescentic gametocyte of *Plasmodium falciparum* is developing in malaria.

bibasic (bi-ba′sik) doubly basic; having two hydrogen atoms that may react with bases. Cf. *dibasic.*

bibeveled (bi′bev-eld) having a slanting surface on two sides, as some dental instruments; hatchet-edged.

Bibliofilm (bib′le-o-film) a negative microfilm of material for a library. It is a trademark registered by Science Service with the idea that it would be applied only to the product of Bibliofilm Services, Incorporated, under the proposed Documentation Institute.

bibliotherapy (bib″le-o-ther′ah-pe) [Gr. *biblion* book + *therapeia* treatment] the reading of books for treatment of mental disorders or for mental health.

bibulous (bib′u-lus) [L. *bibulus,* from *bibere* to drink] 1.

absorbent or spongy. 2. having the property of absorbing moisture. Cf. *hygroscopic.*

bicameral (bi-kam′er-al) [*bi-* + L. *camera* chamber] having two chambers.

bicapsular (bi-kap′su-lar) [*bi-* two + L. *capsula* a capsule] having two capsules, as an articular capsule.

bicarbonate (bi-kar′bo-nāt) any salt containing the HCO₃⁻ anion. **blood b.,** the bicarbonate of the blood, an index of the alkali reserve. **plasma b.,** blood b. **b. of soda,** sodium bicarbonate.

bicarbonatemia (bi-kar″bo-nāt-e′me-ah) hyperbicarbonatemia.

bicardiogram (bi-kar′de-o-gram″) (*obs.*) a curve in an electrocardiogram indicating the composite effect of the right and left atria.

bicaudal (bi-kaw′dal) [*bi-* + L. *cauda* tail] having two tails.

bicaudate (bi-kaw′dāt) bicaudal.

bicellular (bi-sel′u-lar) made up of two cells, or having two cells.

bicephalus (bi-sef′ah-lus) dicephalus.

biceps (bi′seps) [*bi-* + L. *caput* head] a muscle having two heads. **b. bra′chii, b. fem′oris,** see *Table of Musculi.*

Bichat's canal, etc. (be-shaz′) [Marie François Xavier *Bichat,* an eminent French anatomist and physiologist, 1771–1802, founder of scientific histology and pathological anatomy] see under *canal, fissure, foramen, ligament, membrane,* and *tunic.*

bichloride (bi-klo′rīd) any chloride that contains two equivalents of chlorine.

bichromate (bi-kro′māt) dichromate.

Bicillin (bi′sĭ-lin) trademark for a preparation of penicillin G benzathine.

bicipital (bi-sip′ĭ-tal) 1. having two heads. 2. pertaining to a biceps muscle.

BiCNU trademark for preparations of carmustine.

biconcave (bi-kon′kāv) [*bi-* + L. *concavus* hollow] having two concave surfaces, as the opposite sides of a structure.

biconvex (bi-kon′veks) having two convex surfaces, as the opposite sides of a structure.

bicornate (bi-kor′nāt) bicornuate.

bicornuate (bi-kor′nu-āt) [*bi-* + L. *cornutus* horned] having two horns or having horn-shaped branches, as the uterus of most mammals.

bicoronal (bi″ko-ro′ne-al) pertaining to the two coronas, one radiating from each internal capsule of the brain.

bicorporate (bi-kor′pŏ-rāt) [*bi-* + L. *corpus* body] having two bodies.

bicuspid (bi-kus′pid) [*bi-* + L. *cuspis* point] 1. having two cusps or points. 2. a bicuspid valve. 3. a premolar tooth (*dens premolaris* [NA]).

bicuspidal (bi-kus′pĭ-dal) 1. pertaining to a bicuspid tooth (premolar tooth). 2. having two cusps.

bicuspidate (bi-kus′pĭ-dāt) having two cusps.

bicuspoid (bi-kus′poid) a figure in space resembling a bicuspid tooth (premolar tooth) and representing the space traversed in all its movements by a point in one jaw in relation to the other jaw.

b.i.d. abbreviation for L. *bis in di′e,* twice a day.

Bidder's ganglia, organ [Heinrich Friedrich *Bidder,* German anatomist, 1810–1894] see under *ganglion* and *organ.*

bidental (bi-den′tal) [*bi-* + L. *dens* tooth] having, pertaining to, or affecting two teeth.

bidentate (bi-den′tāt) having two teeth or toothlike structures.

bidermoma (bi″der-mo′mah) [*bi-* + Gr. *derma* skin + *-oma*] a variety of teratoma composed of cells and tissues derived from two germ layers.

biduous (bid′u-us) lasting for two days, as a fever.

Biederman's sign (be′der-manz) [Joseph Bear *Biederman,* Cincinnati physician, born 1907] see under *sign.*

Biedert's cream mixture (be′derts) [Philipp *Biedert,* pediatrician in Strasburg, 1847–1916] see under *mixture.*

Biedl's disease, syndrome (be′dlz) [Artur *Biedl,* Austrian physician, 1869–1933] Laurence-Moon-Biedl syndrome.

Bielschowsky's method (be″el-show′skēz) [Max *Bielschowsky,* German neuropathologist, 1869–1940] see *Table of Stains and Staining Methods.*

Bielschowsky-Jansky disease (bel-shov′ski yahn′ski) [M. *Bielschowsky;* Ján *Jansky,* Czech psychiatrist, 1873–1921] late infantile form of cerebral sphingolipidosis; see under *sphingolipidosis.*

Bier's amputation, anesthesia (bērz) [August Karl Gustav *Bier,* surgeon in Berlin, 1861–1949] see under *amputation* and *anesthesia.*

Biermer's anemia (disease), sign (bēr′merz) [Anton *Biermer,* German physician, 1827–1892] see *pernicious anemia,* under *anemia,* and see under *sign.*

Biernacki's sign (byēr-naht′skēz) [Edmund *Biernacki,* Polish physician, 1866–1911] see under *sign.*

Biesiadecki's fossa (bya-syah-det′skēz) [Alfred von *Biesiadecki,* Polish physician, 1839–1888] iliacosubfascial fossa.

bifid, bifidus (bi′fid, bif′ĭ-dus) [L.] cleft into two parts or branches.

Bifidobacterium (bi″fid-o-bak-te′re-um) [L. *bifidus* cleft + Gr. *baktērion* little rod] a genus of gram-positive, anaerobic bacteria of the family Actinomycetaceae, order Actinomycetales. The organisms occur as irregularly staining rods of bifurcated Y and V forms and club or spatulate shapes. **B. adolescen′tis,** a species isolated from human feces, the appendix, the vagina, dental caries, and abscesses. **B. bi′fidum,** a species found in the alimentary tract and in the stools of breast- and bottle-fed infants and in human adults. Called also *Lactobacillus bifidum.* **B. cornu′tum,** *Eubacterium lentum.* **B. erikson′ii,** a species that has been isolated from the feces and from subcutaneous and pulmonary lesions of humans. Called also *Actinomyces eriksonii.* **B. infant′is,** a species that is the predominant bifidobacterium found in the feces of breast-fed infants.

bifidobacterium (bi″fid-o-bak-te′re-um), pl. *bifidobacte′ria.* any bacterium of the genus *Bifidobacterium.*

bifocal (bi-fo′kal) 1. having two foci. 2. pertaining to the compound spectacle, which contains a smaller lens for near vision placed below the center of the larger lens, which is for distant vision. 3. (pl.) bifocal glasses.

biforate (bi-fo′rāt) [*bi-* + L. *fora* opening] having two foramina or openings.

biformyl (bi-for′mil) glyoxal.

bifurcate (bi-fur′kāt) [L. *bifurcatus,* from *bi-* + *furca* fork] forked; divided into two branches.

bifurcatio (bi″fur-ka′she-o), pl. *bifurcatio′nes* [L.] the site of division of a single structure into two. **b. aor′tae** [NA], **b. aor′tica,** bifurcation of aorta: the site of division of the abdominal aorta divides, on the left side of the body of the fourth lumbar vertebra, into the right and left common iliac arteries. **b. carot′idis** [NA], carotid bifurcation: the site where the common carotid artery divides into the external carotid artery and internal carotid artery, usually marked by a dilatation, the carotid sinus. **b. tra′cheae** [NA], bifurcation of trachea: the site of division of the trachea into the right and left main bronchi. **b. trun′ci pulmona′lis** [NA], bifurcation of pulmonary trunk: the site of the division of the pulmonary trunk into right and left pulmonary arteries.

bifurcation (bi″fur-ka′shun) [L. *bifurcatio,* from *bi-* + *furca* fork] 1. division into two branches. 2. the site where a single structure divides into two. **b. of aorta,** bifurcatio aortae. **carotid b.,** bifurcatio carotidis. **b. of pulmonary trunk,** bifurcatio trunci pulmonalis. **b. of trachea,** bifurcatio tracheae.

bifurcationes (bi″fur-ka″she-o′nēz) [L.] plural of *bifurcatio.*

Bigelow's ligament, operation, septum (big′ĕ-lōz) [Henry Jacob *Bigelow,* Boston surgeon, 1818–1890] see *ligamenta iliofemorale,* see *litholapaxy,* and see under *septum.*

bigemina (bi-jem′ĭ-nah) 1. plural of *bigeminum.* 2. a bigeminal pulse.

bigeminal (bi-jem′ĭ-nal) occurring in twos; twin.

bigeminum (bi-jem′ĭ-num), pl. *bigem′ina* [L. "twin"] either one of the corpora bigemina of the fetus or of a bird; the fetal bigemina become the corpora quadrigemina (colliculi).

bigeminy (bi-jem′ĭ-ne) the condition of occurring in pairs; especially the occurrence of two beats of the pulse in rapid succession; see *bigeminal pulse,* under *pulse.* **nodal b.,** a form of arrhythmia consisting of nodal extrasystoles followed by nodal automatic beats.

bigerminal (bi-jer′mĭ-nal) pertaining to two germs or ova.

bighead (big′hed) 1. bulging of the skull bones of an animal, due to osteomalacia. 2. an acute infectious disease of young rams due to *Clostridium novyi*, which enters the tissues through head wounds acquired in fighting; it is characterized by intense edematous swelling of the head, face, and neck; called also *swelled head*. 3. photosensitivity in white-faced sheep, occurring after the ingestion of certain plants, characterized by thickening and pendulous swelling of the face and ears. 4. hydrocephalus in mink.

bigjaw (big′jaw) actinomycosis in cattle.

bigleg (big′leg) lymphangitis of a horse's leg.

bigonial (bi-go′ne-al) connecting the two gonions.

bilabe (bi′lāb) [*bi-* + L. *labium* lip] an instrument for taking small calculi from the bladder through the urethra.

bilaminar (bi-lam′ĭ-nar) [*bi-* + L. *lamina* layer] having or pertaining to two layers, as the basement membrane that comprises the basal lamina and the reticular lamina.

Bilarcil (bil-ar′sil) trademark for preparations of metrifonate.

bilateral (bi-lat′er-al) [*bi-* + L. *latus* side] having two sides, or pertaining to both sides.

bilateralism (bi-lat′er-al-izm) bilateral symmetry.

bile (bīl) [L. *bilis*] a fluid secreted by the liver and poured into the small intestine via the bile ducts. Important constituents are conjugated bile salts, cholesterol, phospholipid, bilirubin diglucuronide, and electrolytes. Bile is alkaline due to its bicarbonate content, golden brown to greenish yellow in color, and has a bitter taste. Hepatic bile (see *A b.*) secreted by the liver, is concentrated in the gallbladder. Its formation depends on active secretion by liver cells into the bile canaliculi. Excretion of bile salts by liver cells and secretion of bicarbonate rich fluid by ductular cells in response to secretin are the major factors which normally determine the volume of secretion. Conjugated bile salts and phospholipid normally dissolve cholesterol in a mixed micellar solution. In the upper small intestine, bile is in part responsible for alkalinizing the intestinal content, and conjugated bile salts play an essential role in fat absorption by dissolving the products of fat digestion (fatty acids and monoglycerides) in water soluble micelles. Called also *gall*. **A b.,** bile from the common bile duct; samples are obtained by use of a duodenal tube before gallbladder stimulation. It usually contains 20–200 mg. of bilirubin per 100 ml. **B b.,** bile from the gallbladder; samples are obtained by use of a duodenal tube after gallbladder contraction stimulation, usually with magnesium sulfate. It may occur despite absence of the gallbladder and contains up to 1 gram of bilirubin per 100 ml. **C b.,** hepatic bile; it is obtained from a duodenal drainage tube after the gallbladder has been emptied. **cystic b., gallbladder b.,** the bile that is held for some time in the gallbladder before moving into the intestine. **limy b.,** bile containing an increased amount of calcium, usually as the carbonate but sometimes as the phosphate or bilirubinate. It varies in consistency from a thick, milky fluid to a putty, gel, or solid. It is usually suspended in a thin, more watery bile. Called also *milk of calcium b.* **milk of calcium b.,** limy b. **ox b.,** the fresh bile of the ox, a brownish green to dark green viscous fluid; the extract is used as a choleretic. Called also *fel bovis* and *oxgall*. **Platner's crystallized b.,** a crystalline substance obtained by the action of ether in an alcoholic extract of bile. **white b.,** the colorless liquid containing mucoproteins and calcium salts sometimes found in the gallbladder in obstructions above the entrance of the cystic duct. Its accumulation in the distended biliary tract is called *hydrops*.

Bilharzia (bil-har′ze-ah) [Theodor Maximilian *Bilharz*, German physician, 1825–1862] *Schistosoma*.

bilharzial (bil-har′ze-al) pertaining to or caused by *Schistosoma* (*Bilharzia*).

bilharziasis (bil″har-zi′ah-sis) schistosomiasis.

bilharzic (bil-har′zik) bilharzial.

bilharzioma (bil-har″ze-o′mah) a tumor in the skin or mucous membrane caused by a schistosome.

bilharziosis (bil-har″ze-o′sis) schistosomiasis.

bili- [L. *bilis* bile] a combining form denoting relationship to the bile.

biliary (bil′e-a-re) pertaining to the bile, to the bile ducts, or to the gallbladder.

biliation (bil″e-a′shun) the secretion of bile.

bilicyanin (bil″ĭ-si′ah-nin) [*bili-* + L. *cyaneus* blue] a blue pigment derivable from biliverdin by oxidation; called also *cholecyanin* and *cholocyanin*.

bilidigestive (bil″e-di-jes′tiv) pertaining to the gallbladder and digestive tract.

biliflavin (bil″ĭ-fla′vin) [*bili-* + L. *flavus* yellow] a yellow pigment obtainable from biliverdin.

bilifulvin (bil″ĭ-ful′vin) [*bili-* + L. *fulvus* tawny] an impure bilirubin of a tawny color; also a tawny pigment from extract of ox bile; not normally found in healthy human bile.

bilifuscin (bil″ĭ-fus′in) [*bili-* + L. *fuscus* brown] a pigment from human bile and gallstones.

biligenesis (bil″ĭ-jen′ĕ-sis) the production or formation of bile.

biligenetic (bil″ĭ-jĕ-net′ik) 1. pertaining to biligenesis. 2. biligenic.

biligenic (bil″ĭ-jen′ik) [*bili-* + Gr. *gennan* to produce] producing bile.

biligulate (bi-lig′u-lāt) [*bi-* + L. *ligula* little tongue] having two tonguelike structures.

bilihumin (bil″ĭ-hu′min) [*bili-* + L. *humus* earth] an insoluble pigment of gallstones.

bilin (bi′lin) [L. *bilis* bile] collective name for yellow bile pigments including i-urobilin, stercobilin, and d-urobilin, formed by spontaneous oxidation of the central methyene group of corresponding bilinogen; they are generated in the final steps of bilirubin catabolism.

bilious (bil′yus) [L. *biliosus*] characterized by bile, by excess of bile, or by biliousness.

biliousness (bil′yus-nes) a symptom complex comprising nausea, abdominal discomfort, headache, and constipation, formerly attributed to excessive secretion of bile.

biliprasin (bil″ĭ-pra′sin) [*bili-* + Gr. *prasinos* green] a green pigment from gallstones.

bilipurpurin (bil″ĭ-pur′pu-rin) [*bili-* + L. *purpur* purple] a purple pigment, $C_{34}H_{36}O_6N_4$, occurring in the bile of ruminants; derived from chlorophyll.

bilirachia (bil″ĭ-ra′ke-ah) the presence of bile pigments in the spinal fluid.

bilirhachia (bil″ĭ-ra′ke-ah) [*bili-* + Gr. *rhachis* spine + *-ia*] the presence of bile pigments in the spinal fluid.

bilirubin (bil″ĭ-roo′bin) [*bili-* + L. *ruber* red] a bile pigment; it is a breakdown product of heme mainly formed from the degradation of erythrocyte hemoglobin in reticuloendothelial cells, but also formed by breakdown of other heme pigments, e.g., cytochromes. Bilirubin normally circulates in plasma as a complex with albumin, and is taken up by the liver cells and conjugated to form bilirubin diglucuronide, which is the water-soluble pigment excreted in bile. In patients with cholestasis conjugated bilirubin (bilirubin diglucuronide) accumulates in the blood and tissues and is excreted in the urine; unconjugated bilirubin is not excreted in the urine. High concentrations of bilirubin may result in jaundice. **direct b., conjugated b.,** bilirubin that has been taken up by the liver cells and conjugated to form the water-soluble bilirubin diglucuronide. **indirect b.,** unconjugated bilirubin. **unconjugated b.,** the lipid-soluble form of bilirubin that circulates in loose association with the plasma proteins; called also *indirect b.*

bilirubinate (bil″ĭ-roo′bĭ-nāt) a salt of bilirubin.

bilirubinemia (bil″ĭ-roo-bĭ-ne′me-ah) [*bilirubin* + Gr. *haima* blood + *-ia*] the presence of bilirubin in the blood; see *hyperbilirubinemia*.

bilirubinic (bil″ĭ-roo-bin′ik) pertaining to bilirubin.

bilirubin UDP-glucuronyltransferase (bil″e-roo′bin gloo-ku′ron-il-trans″fer-ās) glucuronosyltransferase.

bilirubinuria (bil″ĭ-roo-bĭ-nu′re-ah) presence of bilirubin in the urine.

bilis (bi′lis) [L.] bile. **b. bovi′na, b. buba′ta,** ox bile extract; see under *extract*.

bilitherapy (bil″ĭ-ther′ah-pe) (*obs.*) treatment with bile or bile salts.

biliuria (bil″ĭ-u′re-ah) [*bili-* + *-uria*] the presence of bile pigments in the urine.

biliverdin (bil″ĭ-ver′din) [*bili-* + L. *viridis* green] a green pigment, $C_{33}H_{34}O_6N_4$, the initial bile pigment from catabolism of hemoglobin, converted to bilirubin by reduction of a methene bridge; it may arise from air oxidation of bilirubin. Called also *biliverdinic acid* and *dehydrobilirubin*.

biliverdinate (bil″ĭ-ver′dĭ-nāt) a salt of biliverdin.

bilixanthin, bilixanthine (bil″ĭ-zan′thin) [*bili-* + Gr. *xanthos* yellow] choletelin.

Billroth's cords, disease, etc. (bil′rōts) [Christian Albert Theodor *Billroth*, surgeon in Vienna, 1829–1894] see under *cord, disease, operation,* and *strand.*

bilobate (bi-lo′bāt) [*bi-* + L. *lobus* lobe] having two lobes.

bilobular (bi-lob′u-lar) having two lobules.

bilobulate (bi-lob′u-lāt) bilobular.

bilocular (bi-lok′u-lar) [*bi-* + L. *loculus* cell] having two compartments.

biloculate (bi-lok′u-lāt) bilocular.

biloma (bi′lo-mah) an encapsulated collection of bile in the peritoneal cavity.

Bilopaque (bil′o-pāk) trademark for a preparation of tyropanoate sodium.

bilophodont (bi-lof′ŏ-dont) [*bi-* + Gr. *lophos* ridge + *odous* tooth] having molariform teeth with two ridges on them; applied to certain mammals, e.g., the kangaroo.

Biltricide (bil′tri-sid) trademark for a preparation of praziquantel.

Bimana (bim′ah-nah) [*bi-* + L. *manus* hand] a name sometimes applied to a category of mammals distinguished by possessing hands of character differing from that of the feet, and made up of man alone.

bimanual (bi-man′u-al) [*bi-* + L. *manualis* of the hand] with both hands; performed by both hands.

bimastoid (bi-mas′toid) pertaining to both mastoid processes.

bimaxillary (bi-mak′sĭ-ler″e) pertaining to or affecting both jaws.

bimethoxycaine lactate (bi″mĕ-thoks′ĭ-kān) lactic acid compound with 2,2′-dimethoxy-α-α′-dimethyldiphenethylamine (1:1); a local anesthetic.

Bimler's appliance (bim′lerz) [H. P. *Bimler*] see under *appliance.*

bimodal (bi-mo′dal) having two modes; of a graph, having two maxima.

bimolecular (bi″mo-lek′u-lar) relating to or formed from two molecules.

bin- see *bi-.*

binangle (bin′ang-g′l) having two angles; a dental instrument having two angulations in the shank connecting the handle, or shaft, with the working portion of the instrument, known as the blade, or nib.

binary (bi′na-re) [L. *binarius* of two] made up of two elements or of two equal parts; denoting a number system with a base of two.

binaural (bi-naw′ral, bin-aw′ral) [L. *bini* two + *auris* ear] pertaining to both ears.

binauricular (bin″aw-rik′u-lar) [L. *bini* two + *auricula* little ear] pertaining to both auricles of the ears.

bind (bīnd) 1. to wrap with a binder or bandage. 2. to form a weak, reversible chemical bond, e.g., antigen to antibody or hormone to receptor. 3. a predicament or dilemma. **double b.,** a situation in which one person receives conflicting messages from another and in which response to either message or recognition of the conflict or withdrawal is met with rejection or disapproval; a concept developed by Gregory Bateson and thought to be a characteristic mode of interaction in some families of schizophrenics.

binder (bīnd′er) an abdominal girdle or bandage, especially one applied after childbirth to support the relaxed abdominal walls.

binegative (bi-neg′ah-tiv) having two negative charges, especially in ions such as SO_4^{--}.

Binet's test (be-nāz′) [Alfred *Binet,* French physiologist, 1857– 1911] see under *tests.*

Binet-Simon test (be-na′ se-mon′) [Alfred *Binet;* Théodore *Simon,* French physician, 1873–1961] Binet's test.

Bing's test (bingz) [Albert *Bing,* German otologist, 1844–1922] see under *tests.*

biniramycin (bin-ēr-ah-mi′sin) an antibacterial substance produced by a variant of *Streptomyces bikiniensis.*

binocular (bin-ok′u-lar) [L. *bini* two + *oculus* eye] 1. pertaining to both eyes. 2. having two eyepieces, as in a microscope.

binomial (bi-no′me-al) [*bi-* + L. *nomen* name] 1. composed of two names, as the scientific names of organisms formed by combination of genus and species names (binomial nomenclature). 2. a mathematical expression consisting of two terms connected by a plus or a minus sign; see *binomial coefficient* and *distribution,* under *coefficient* and *distribution.*

binophthalmoscope (bin″of-thal′mo-skōp) [L. *bini* two + *ophthalmoscope*] an ophthalmoscope for examining both fundi of the patient at one time.

binoscope (bin′o-skōp) [L. *bini* two + *-scope*] an instrument for inducing binocular vision in squint by presenting one object in the central part of the field of vision, the peripheral parts of the field being screened out.

binotic (bin-ot′ik) [L. *bini* two + Gr. *ous* ear] pertaining to both ears.

binovular (bin-ov′u-lar) [L. *bini* two + *ovum* an egg] pertaining to or derived from two distinct ova.

Binswanger's dementia (encephalitis) (bins′wang-er) [Otto *Binswanger,* German neurologist, 1852–1929] see under *dementia.*

binuclear (bi-nu′kle-ar) [*bi-* + L. *nucleus* nut] having two nuclei.

binucleate (bi-nu′kle-āt) binuclear.

binucleation (bi″nu-kle-a′shun) the formation of two nuclei within a cell through division of the nucleus without division of the cytoplasm.

binucleolate (bi-nu-kle′o-lāt) [*bi-* + L. *nucleolus*] having two nucleoli.

bio- [Gr. *bios* life] combining form denoting relationship to life, or to living organisms.

bioacoustics (bi″o-ah-koo′stiks) the science dealing with the communicating sounds made by animals.

bioactive (bi″o-ak′tiv) having an effect on or eliciting a response from living tissue.

bioaeration (bi″o-a″er-a′shun) a modification of the activated sludge method of purifying sewage.

bioamine (bi″o-am′ēn) biogenic amine.

bioaminergic (bi″o-am″in-er′jik) of or pertaining to neurons that secrete biogenic amines.

bioassay (bi″o-as-sa′) [*bio-* + *assay*] determination of the active power of a sample of a drug by noting its effect on a live animal or an isolated organ preparation, as compared with the effect of a standard preparation; called also *biological assay.*

bioastronautics (bi″o-as′tro-naw-tiks) the science concerned with study of the effects of space and interplanetary travel on living organisms.

bioavailability (bi″o-ah-vāl″ah-bil′ĭ-te) the degree to which a drug or other substance becomes available to the target tissue after administration.

bioblast (bi′o-blast) [*bio-* + Gr. *blastos* germ] 1. mitochondrion. 2. elementary unit of protoplasmic structure; Altmann's granule.

biocatalyst (bi″o-kat′ah-list) enzyme.

biocenosis (bi″o-se-no′sis) [*bio-* + Gr. *koinos* common] the relation of diverse organisms that live in association.

biocenotic (bi″o-se-not′ik) characterized by biocenosis.

biochemistry (bi″o-kem′is-tre) [*bio-* + *chemistry*] the chemistry of living organisms and of vital processes; physiological chemistry.

biochemorphic (bi″o-ke-mor′fik) pertaining to biochemorphology.

biochemorphology (bi″o-ke-mor-fol′o-je) the study of the relationship between chemical constitution and biological action.

biocidal (bi″o-si′dal) pertaining to that which kills living organisms.

bioclimatics (bi″o-kli-mat′iks) bioclimatology.

bioclimatologist (bi″o-kli″mah-tol′ŏ-jist) an individual skilled in bioclimatology.

bioclimatology (bi″o-kli″mah-tol′o-je) [*bio-* + *climatology*] the science devoted to the study of effects on living organisms of conditions of the natural environment (rainfall, daylight, temperature, humidity, air movement) prevailing in specific regions of the earth. See also *biometeorology*.

(BiO)₂CO₂   subcarbonate of bismuth.

biocoenosis (bi″o-se-no′sis)   biocenosis.

biocolloid (bi″o-kol′oid) [*bio-* + *colloid*]   a colloid from animal, plant, or microbial tissue.

biocompatible (bi″o-kom-pat′ĭ-b'l)   being harmonious with life; not having toxic or injurious effects on biological function.

biocompatibility (bi″o-kom-pat″ĭ-bil′ĭ-te)   the quality of being biocompatible.

biocybernetics (bi″o-si″ber-net′iks)   the science of communications and control in animals.

biocycle (bi″o-si′k'l) [*bio-* + Gr. *kyklos* cycle]   the rhythmic repetition of certain phenomena observed in living organisms.

biodegradable (bi″-o-de-grād′ah-b'l)   susceptible of decomposition by natural biological processes, as by the action of bacteria, plants, animals, etc.

biodegradation (bi″o-deg′rah-da′shun)   the series of processes by which living systems render chemicals less noxious to the environment.

biodetritus (bi″o-de-tri′tus)   detritus derived from the disintegration and decomposition of once-living organisms; further designated as phytodetritus or zoodetritus, depending on whether the original organism was vegetal or animal.

biodynamics (bi″o-di-nam′iks) [*bio-* + Gr. *dynamis* might]   the scientific study of the nature and determinants of all organismic (including human) behavior.

bioelectricity (bi″o-e″lek-tris′ĭ-te)   the electrical phenomena that appear in living tissues, as that generated by muscle and nerve tissue.

bioelectronics (bi″o-e″lek-tron′iks)   the study of the role of intermolecular transfer of electrons in biological regulation and defense.

bioelement (bi″o-el′e-ment)   any chemical element that is a component of living tissue.

bioenergetics (bi″o-en″er-jet′iks)   the study of the energy transformations in living organisms.

bioequivalence (bi″o-e-kwiv′ah-lens)   the quality of being bioequivalent.

bioequivalent (bi″o-e-kwiv′ah-lent)   having the same strength and similar bioavailability in the same dosage form as another specimen of a given drug substance.

biofeedback (bi″o-fēd′bak)   the process of furnishing an individual information, usually in an auditory or visual mode, on the state of one or more physiological variables such as heart rate, blood pressure, or skin temperature; such a procedure often enables the individual to gain some voluntary control over the physiologic variable being sampled. **alpha b.**, a procedure in which a person is presented with continuous information, usually auditory, on the state of his brain-wave pattern, with the intent of increasing the percentage of alpha activity; this is done with the expectation that it will be associated with a state of relaxation and peaceful wakefulness. Called also *alpha feedback*.

bioflavonoid (bi″o-fla′vo-noid)   a generic term for a group of compounds that are widely distributed in plants and that are concerned with maintenance of a normal state of walls of small blood vessels. See *flavonoid*.

biogen (bi′o-jen) [*bio-* + Gr. *gennan* to produce]   one of several labile proteins supposedly representing the ultimate molecular basis of life.

biogenesis (bi″o-jen′ĕ-sis) [*bio-* + Gr. *genesis* origin]   Thomas Huxley's theory, opposed to spontaneous generation, that living matter always arises by the agency of preexisting living matter; see also *panspermy*. 2. recapitulation; see under *theory*.

biogenetic (bi″o-jĕ-net′ik)   pertaining to biogenesis.

biogenic (bi″o-jen′ik)   having origins in biological processes, as a biogenic amine.

biogenous (bi-oj′ĕ-nus)   originating from life or producing life.

biogeochemistry (bi″o-je″o-kem′is-tre) [*bio-* + Gr. *gē* earth + *chemistry*]   the study of interactions between the biosphere and its mineral environment, e.g., the study of the effect of living organisms on the weathering of rocks and of the concentration of elements by living systems.

biogeography (bi″o-je-og′rah-fe)   the scientific study of geographic distribution of living organisms.

biograph (bi′o-graf)   1. an instrument for analyzing and rendering visible the movements of animals; used in diagnosis of certain nervous diseases. 2. spirograph.

biohazard (bi′o-haz″ard)   a potentially dangerous infectious agent such as may be found in a clinical microbiology laboratory or used in experimental studies on genetic recombination.

biohydraulic (bi″o-hī-draw′lik) [*bio-* + Gr. *hydōr* water]   pertaining to the action of water and solutions in living tissue.

bioimplant (bi″o-im′plant)   denoting a prosthesis made of biosynthetic material.

biokinetics (bi″o-ki-net′iks) [*bio-* + Gr. *kinētikos* of or for putting in motion]   the science of the movements within developing organisms.

biologic, biological (bi-o-loj′ik; bi-o-loj′ĕ-kal)   pertaining to biology.

biologicals (bi-o-loj′ĭ-kalz)   medicinal preparations made from living organisms and their products, including serums, vaccines, antigens, antitoxins, etc.

biologist (bi-ol′ŏ-jist)   an expert in biology.

biologos (bi-ol′ŏ-gos) [*bio-* + Gr. *logos* reason]   the intelligent power displayed in organic activities.

biology (bi-ol′ŏ-je) [*bio-* + *-logy*]   the science that deals with the phenomena of life and living organisms in general. **molecular b.**, the study of molecular structures and events underlying biological processes, including the relation between genes and the functional characteristics they determine. **radiation b.**, the scientific study of effects of ionizing radiation on living organisms.

bioluminescence (bi″o-loo″mĭ-nes′ens)   chemoluminescence occurring in living cells, especially the emission of light as a result of cellular oxidation of a heat-stable substrate (luciferin) in the presence of a heat-sensitive enzyme (luciferase).

biolysis (bi-ol′ĭ-sis)   chemical decomposition of organic matter by the action of living organisms.

biolytic (bi-o-lit′ik) [*bio-* + Gr. *lytikos* loosening]   1. pertaining to or characterized by biolysis. 2. destructive to life.

biomass (bi′o-mass)   the entire assemblage of living organisms, both animal and vegetable, of a particular region, considered collectively.

biomaterial (bi″o-mah-te′re-al)   any substance (other than a drug), synthetic or natural, that can be used as a system or part of a system that treats, augments, or replaces any tissue, organ, or function of the body.

biomathematics (bi″o-math″ĕ-mat′iks) [*bio-* + *mathematics*]   the application of mathematics to biology and medicine.

biome (bi′ōm) [Gr. *bios* life + *-ome* (-oma) mass]   the recognizable community unit of a given region, produced by interaction of climatic factors, biota, and substrate, usually designated according to the characteristic adult or climax vegetation, as tundra, coniferous forest or taiga, deciduous forest, grassland, and the like.

biomechanics (bi″o-mĕ-kan′iks) [*bio-* + *mechanics*]   the application of mechanical laws to living structures, specifically to the locomotor systems of the human body. See also *bionics*. **dental b.**, the relationship between the biologic behavior of oral structures and the physical influence of a dental restoration or appliance. Called also *dental biophysics*.

biomedical (bi″o-med′ĭ-kal)   biological and medical; pertaining to the application of the natural sciences (biology, biochemistry, biophysics, etc.) to the study of medicine.

biomedicine (bi″o-med′ĭ-sin)   clinical medicine based on the principles of the natural sciences (biology, biochemistry, biophysics, etc.).

biomembrane (bi″o-mem′brān)   any membrane, e.g., cell membrane, of an organism.

biomembranous (bi″o-mem′brah-nus)   of or pertaining to a biomembrane.

biometeorologist (bi″o-me″te-or-ol′ŏ-jist)   an individual skilled in biometeorology.

biometeorology (bi″o-me″te-or-ol′ŏ-je) [*bio-* + Gr. *meteōros* raised from off the ground + *logos* treatise] that branch of ecology which deals with the effects on living organisms of the extraorganic aspects of the physical environment (such as temperature, humidity, barometric pressure, rate of air flow, and air ionization). It considers not only the natural atmosphere but also artificially created atmospheres such as those to be found in buildings and shelters, and in closed ecological systems, such as satellites and submarines.

biometer (bi-om′ĕ-ter) [*bio-* + Gr. *metron* measure] an apparatus by which extremely minute quantities of carbon dioxide can be measured; used in measuring the carbon dioxide given off from functioning tissue.

biometrician (bi″o-mě-trish′an) a specialist in biometry.

biometrics (bi-o-met′riks) biometry.

biometry (bi-om′ě-tre) [*bio-* + Gr. *metron* measure] 1. the science of the application of statistics in biology, medicine, and agriculture. 2. in life insurance, the calculation of the expectation of life.

biomicroscope (bi″o-mi′krŏ-skōp) a microscope for examining living tissue in the body. **slit-lamp b.,** see *slit lamp,* under *lamp.*

biomicroscopy (bi″o-mi-kros′ko-pe) [*bio-* + *microscopy*] 1. microscopic examination of living tissue in the body. 2. examination of the cornea or the lens by a combination of slit lamp and corneal microscope.

biomolecule (bi″o-mol′ě-kūl) a molecule produced by a living cell, as a protein, carbohydrate, or lipid.

biomotor (bi″o-mo′tor) an apparatus for producing artificial respiration.

Biomphalaria (bi-om″fah-la′re-ah) a genus of planorbid snails, species of which are intermediate hosts of *Schistosoma mansoni;* called also *Australorbis.*

bion (bi′on) [Gr. *bioun* a living being] an individual living organism.

bionecrosis (bi″o-ne-kro′sis) necrobiosis.

bionergy (bi-on′er-je) [*bion* + Gr. *ergon* work] life force; the force exercised in the living organism.

bionics (bi-on′iks) the science concerned with study of the functions, characteristics, and phenomena found in the living world and application of the knowledge gained to new devices and techniques in the world of machines. See also *biomechanics.*

bionomics (bi″o-nom′iks) [*bio-* + Gr. *nomos* law] the study of the relations of organisms to their environment; ecology.

bionomy (bi-on′ŏ-me) [*bio-* + Gr. *nomos* law] the sum of knowledge regarding the laws of life.

bionucleonics (bi″o-nu″kle-on′iks) the study of the biological applications of radioactive and rare stable isotopes.

bio-osmotic (bi″o-oz-mot′ik) [*bio-* + *osmotic*] a term applied to osmotic pressure phenomena in living organisms.

biophagism (bi-of′ah-jizm) [*bio-* + Gr. *phagein* to eat] the eating or absorption of living matter.

biophagous (bi-of′ah-gus) feeding on living matter.

biophagy (bi-of′ah-je) biophagism.

biophotometer (bi″o-fo-tom′ě-ter) [*bio-* + *photo-* + *-meter*] an instrument for measuring the adaptation of the eye to dark as an indication of vitamin A deficiency.

biophysical (bi-o-fiz′ĭ-kal) pertaining to biophysics.

biophysics (bi-o-fiz′iks) [*bio-* + *physics*] the science dealing with the application of physical methods and theories to biological problems. **dental b.,** see under *biomechanics.*

biophysiography (bi″o-fiz-e-og′rah-fe) [*bio-* + *physiography*] structural or descriptive biology.

biophysiology (bi″o-fiz-e-ol′ŏ-je) [*bio-* + Gr. *physis* nature + *-logy*] that part of biology which includes organogeny, morphology, and physiology.

bioplasia (bi-o-pla′ze-ah) [*bio-* + Gr. *plassein* to form] the storing up of food energy in the form of growth.

bioplasm (bi′o-plazm) [*bio-* + Gr. *plasma* anything molded] 1. protoplasm. 2. the more essential or vital part of cytoplasm, contrasted with the *hyaloplasm.* Called also *plasmogen.*

bioplasmic (bi-o-plaz′mik) of or pertaining to bioplasm.

bioplast (bi′o-plast) 1. an independently existing mass of living matter. 2. an ameboid cell.

biopoiesis (bi″o-poi-e′sis) [*bio-* + Gr. *poiein* to make] the origin of life from inorganic matter.

biopolymer (bi″o-pol′ĭ-mer) a polymer formed in a living organism, as a polypeptide formed from amino acids (monomers).

bioprosthesis (bi″o-pros-the′sis) [*bio-* + *prosthesis*] a prosthesis made of biological material.

biopsy (bi′ŏp-se) [*bio-* + Gr. *opsis* vision] the removal and examination, usually microscopic, of tissue from the living body, performed to establish precise diagnosis. **aspiration b.,** biopsy in which the tissue is obtained by the aspiration of suction through a needle attached to a syringe. **bite b.,** the instrumental removal of a fragment of tissue. **brush b.,** biopsy in which cells or tissue is obtained by manipulating tiny brushes against the tissue or lesion in question (e.g., through a bronchoscope) at the desired site. **chorionic villus b.,** see under *sampling.* **cone b.,** biopsy in which an inverted cone of tissue is excised, as from the uterine cervix. **cytological b.,** a procedure in which cells are obtained by various methods for pathological examinations, as by irrigation of hollow viscera. **endoscopic b.,** removal of tissue by appropriate instruments introduced through an endoscope. **excisional b.,** biopsy of tissue removed by excision; biopsy of an entire lesion, including a significant margin of contiguous normal-appearing tissue. **exploratory b.,** exploration combined with biopsy to determine the type and extent of neoplasms, both deep and superficial. **incisional b.,** biopsy of a selected portion of a lesion and, if possible, of adjacent normal-appearing tissue. **needle b.,** biopsy in which tissue from deep within the body is obtained by insertion through the skin of a specifically designed needle that detaches tissue with an inner needle so that it can be brought to the surface in its lumen. **percutaneous b.,** biopsy in which tissue is obtained by a needle inserted through the skin. **punch b.,** biopsy in which tissue is obtained by a punch. **sternal b.,** biopsy of bone marrow of the sternum; done by puncture or trephining. **surface b.,** biopsy of cells scraped from the surface of suspicious or obvious lesions, most commonly employed in examination for cancer of the cervix.

biopsychic (bi″o-si′kik) pertaining to mental phenomena in their relation to the living organism.

biopsychology (bi″o-si-kol′o-je) psychobiology.

biopterin (bi-op′ter-in) a naturally occurring pteridine, 2-amino-4-hydroxy-6-(1,2-dihydroxypropyl) pteridine.

bioptic (bi-op′tik) pertaining to or dependent on biopsy.

bioptome (bi′op-tōm″) a cutting instrument for taking biopsy specimens.

biopyoculture (bi″o-pi′o-kul″tūr) [*bio-* + Gr. *pyon* pus + *culture*] a culture made from pus whose cells are alive.

biorational (bi″o-rash′un-al) based on biological principles; having an effect by natural means; said, for example, of such pesticidal agents as viruses, bacteria, protozoa, fungi, or naturally occurring biochemicals.

biorbital (bi-or′bĭ-tal) pertaining to both orbits.

bioreversible (bi″o-re-ver′sĭ-b'l) capable of being changed back to the original biologically active chemical form by processes within the organism; said of drugs.

biorgan (bi′or-gan) a physiological organ, as distinguished from a morphological organ, or *idorgan.*

biorheology (bi″o-re-ol′o-je) the study of the deformation and flow of matter in living systems and in materials directly derived from them.

biorhythm (bi′o-rithm) the cyclic occurrence of physiological events, as a circadian rhythm.

bioroentgenography (bi″o-rent″gen-og′rah-fe) [*bio-* + *roentgenography*] the making of kinematographic x-ray pictures.

bios (bi′os) [Gr. "life"] any one of a group of growth factors for single-celled organisms such as yeast. Bios occurs in yeast, leaves of plants, bran, and the outer covering of seeds, and is probably a mixture of B vitamins and pantothenic acid. **b. I,** inositol. **b. II,** biotin.

bioscience (bi″o-si′ens) the study of biology wherein all the sciences (physics, chemistry, etc.) are applied.

biose (bi′ōs) a sugar containing two carbon atoms.

biosis (bi-o′sis) [Gr. *bios* life] vitality, or life.

biosmosis (bi″os-mo′sis) osmosis through a living membrane.

biospectrometry (bi″o-spek-trom′ĕ-tre) measurement by a spectroscope of the quantity of a substance in living tissue.

biospectroscopy (bi″o-spek-tros′ko-pe) examination of living tissue with the spectroscope.

biosphere (bi′ŏ-sfēr) 1. that part of the universe in which living organisms are known to exist, comprising the atmosphere, hydrosphere, and lithosphere. 2. the sphere of action between an organism and its environment.

biostatics (bi″ŏ-stat′iks) [bio- + Gr. statikos causing to stand] the science of the structure of organisms in relation to their function.

biostatistician (bi″o-stat″is-tish′in) a specialist in biostatistics.

biostatistics (bi″o-stah-tis′tiks) biometry.

biostereometrics (bi″o-ste″re-o-met′riks) analysis of the spatial and spatial-temporal characteristics of biological form and function by means of three-dimensional mapping of the body.

biosynthesis (bi″o-sin′thĕ-sis) the building up of a chemical compound in the physiologic processes of a living organism.

biosynthetic (bi″o-sin-thet′ik) pertaining to or characterized by biosynthesis.

Biot's respiration (breathing, sign) (be-ōz′) [Camille Biot, French physician of 19th century] see under respiration.

biota (bi-o′tah) [Gr. bios life] all the living organisms of a particular area; the combined flora and fauna of a region.

biotaxis (bi″o-tak′sis) [bio- + Gr. taxis arrangement] the selecting and arranging powers of living cells.

biotaxy (bi″o-tak′se) 1. biotaxis. 2. taxonomy.

biotelemetry (bi″o-tel-em′ĕ-tre) the recording and measuring of certain vital phenomena of living organisms that are situated at a distance from the measuring device.

biothesiometer (bi″o-the″se-om′ĕ-ter) an instrument for measuring the vibratory-perception threshold.

biotic (bi-ot′ik) 1. pertaining to life or living matter. 2. pertaining to the biota.

biotics (bi-ot′iks) [Gr. biōtikos living] the functions and qualities peculiar to living organisms, or the sum of knowledge regarding these qualities.

biotin (bi′o-tin) a colorless crystalline compound, 2′-keto-3,4-imidazolido-2-tetrahydrothiophene-δ-n-valeric acid, $CH_2 \cdot CH \cdot NH \cdot CO \cdot NH \cdot CH \cdot (CH_2)_4 \cdot COOH$, identical with vitamin H and coenzyme R; it is a ubiquitous member of the vitamin B complex required by or occurring in all forms of life tested. Deficiency of biotin has been produced in humans and experimental animals fed uncooked egg white, such deficiency being due to the avidin present in the egg white, which renders the biotin of the diet unavailable. Manifestations of biotin deficiency in experimental animals include paralysis, usually of the hindquarters (cows, dogs, rats), dermatitis (rats, pigs, fowl), alopecia (mice, pigs, monkeys), and graying of brown and black fur (mice, monkeys). *Alpha b.* is the product isolated from egg yolk; *beta b.* is that isolated from liver. Called also *bios II.* Cf. *avidin.*

biotomy (bi-ot′ŏ-me) [bio- + Gr. tomē a cutting] 1. the study of animal and plant structure by dissection. 2. vivisection.

biotoxication (bi″o-tok″sĭ-ka′shun) an intoxication resulting from a plant or animal poison (biotoxin).

biotoxicology (bi″o-tok″sĭ-kol′o-je) [bio- + Gr. toxikon poison + -logy] the science of poisons produced by living things, their cause, detection, and their effects, and of the treatment of conditions produced by them.

biotoxin (bi″o-tok′sin) any poisonous substance produced by and derived from a living organism, either plant or animal.

biotransformation (bi″o-trans″for-ma′shun) the series of chemical alterations of a compound (e.g., a drug) which occur within the body, as by enzymatic activity.

biotrepy (bi-ot′rĕ-pe) the study of the body by means of its reactions to chemical substances.

biotype (bi′o-tīp) 1. a group of individuals possessing the same genotype. 2. a variant strain of a bacterial species, differing in identifiable physiologic characteristics.

biotypology (bi″o-ti-pol′o-je) the study of anthropological types with their constitutional variations, inadequacies, etc.

biovular (bi-ov′u-lar) binovular.

biparasitic (bi″par-ah-sit′ik) living parasitically upon a parasite; hyperparasitic.

biparental (bi″pah-ren′tal) derived from two parents, male and female.

biparietal (bi″pah-ri′ĕ-tal) pertaining to the two parietal eminences or bones.

biparous (bip′ah-rus) [bi- + L. parere to produce] producing two ova or offspring at one time.

bipartite (bi-par′tīt) [L. bipartitus] having two parts or divisions, as the uterus of most mammals.

biped (bi′ped) [bi- + L. pes foot] 1. having two feet. 2. an animal with two feet.

bipedal (bip′ĕ-dal) [bi- + L. pes foot] having or pertaining to both feet.

bipenniform (bi-pen′ĭ-form) doubly feather-shaped; said of muscles whose fibers are arranged on each side of a tendon, like the barbs on the shaft of a feather.

biperforate (bi-per′fŏ-rāt) [bi- + L. perforatus bored through] having two perforations.

biperiden (bi-per′ĭ-den) [USP] chemical name: α-bicyclo-[2.2.1]hept-5-en-2-yl-α-phenyl-1-piperidenepropanol. A synthetic anticholinergic, $C_{21}H_{29}NO$, occurring as a white, crystalline powder, having antisecretory, spasmolytic, and mydriatic actions. It is used, in the form of the hydrochloride or lactate salts, as an antiparkinsonian agent, and is also useful in the treatment of drug-induced extrapyramidal reactions. **b. hydrochloride** [USP], the hydrochloride of biperiden, $C_{21}H_{29}NO \cdot HCl$, administered orally. **b. lactate** [NF], the lactate of biperiden, $C_{21}H_{29}NO \cdot C_3H_6O_3$, administered intramuscularly and intravenously.

biphenamine hydrochloride (bi-fen′ah-mēn) chemical name: 2-(diethylamino)ethyl 2-hydroxy-3-biphenylcarboxylate hydrochloride; an antibacterial, antifungal, and topical anesthetic, $C_{19}H_{23}NO_3 \cdot HCl$.

biphenyl (bi-fe′nil) diphenyl. **polychlorinated b. (PCB),** any of a group of substances in which chlorine replaces hydrogen in biphenyl and which are toxic and accumulate in animal tissues; it is used as a heat-transfer agent and as an insulator in electrical equipment.

bipolar (bi-po′lar) 1. having two poles; having processes at both poles. 2. a bipolar neuron. 3. pertaining to both poles. 4. denoting bacterial staining confined to the poles (ends) of the organism. 5. pertaining to mood disorders in which both manic and depressive episodes occur.

Bipolarina (bi″po-lah-ri′nah) [bi- + polar] a suborder of parasitic protozoa (order Bivalvulida, class Myxosporea) characterized by the presence of spores with polar capsules at opposite ends of the spore or with widely divergent polar capsules located in a sutural plane or zone. Representative genera include *Myxidium* and *Sphaeromyxa.*

bipositive (bi-poz′ĭ-tiv) having two positive charges, as in Ca^{++}.

bipotential (bi″po-ten′shal) pertaining to or characterized by bipotentiality.

bipotentiality (bi″po-ten″she-al′ĭ-te) [bi- + L. potentia power] possession of the power of developing or acting in either of two possible ways. **b. of the gonad,** the capability of an undifferentiated gonad to develop into either an ovary or a testis.

biramous (bi-ra′mus) [bi- + L. ramus branch] consisting of or possessing two branches.

Bird's formula, treatment (birdz) [Golding Bird, English physician, 1814–1854] see under formula and treatment.

Bird's sign (birdz) [Samuel Dougan Bird, Australian physician, 1832–1904] see under sign.

bird-arm (bird′arm) a forearm that is greatly reduced in size as the result of atrophy of the muscles.

bird-leg (bird′leg) a leg that is greatly reduced in size as the result of atrophy of the muscles.

bird-lime (bird′līm) [bird + L. limus slime] a viscous or gummy substance of various origin, used for catching small birds; some kinds were used formerly in dressing wounds and sores.

birefractive (bi″re-frak′tiv) doubly refractive.

birefringence (bi″re-frin′jens) the quality of transmitting light unequally in different directions; double refraction. In biological materials, it indicates an ordering of the molecules, e.g., they may be oriented to one another much as in a crystal. **crystalline b.,** birefringence occurring in systems in which the bonds between molecules or ions have a regular asymmetrical arrangement; it is independent of the refractive index of the medium. **flow b.,** that exhibited only when the substance is in solution and flowing; e.g., it is seen in solutions of long thin molecules, such as nucleoproteins. **form b.,** that produced by regular orientation of submicroscopic asymmetrical particles in a substance or object, differing in refractive index from the surrounding medium; it is the most common form occurring in organisms. **intrinsic b.,** crystalline b. **strain b.,** birefringence observed occasionally in isotropic structures when subjected to tension or pressure; it occurs in muscle and in embryonic tissues. **streaming b.,** flow b.

birefringent (bi″re-frin′jent) [*bi-* + L. *refringere* to break up] doubly refractive.

Birkett's hernia (ber′kets) [John *Birkett,* English surgeon, 1815–1904] synovial hernia.

Birnberg bow (bern′berg) [Charles H. *Birnberg,* American obstetrician and gynecologist, born 1900] see under *bow.*

birth (birth) the act or process of being born. **complete b.,** the complete separation of the infant from the maternal body (after cutting of the umbilical cord). **cross b.,** labor with the fetus lying transversely in the uterus. **dead b.,** birth of a fetus which, during or before birth, has lost all signs of antenatal life, including heart beat, pulsation, and movement. **head b.,** a birth in which the head presents. **multiple b.,** the birth of two or more offspring produced in the same gestation period, the frequency of birth of viable offspring after such multiple pregnancy having been computed as follows: twins, 1 in 80; triplets, 1 in 6400 (80 × 80); quadruplets, 1 in 512,000 (80 × 80 × 80); etc. (Hellin's law). **post-term b.,** birth of a post-mature, or over-term, infant. **premature b.,** birth of a premature infant.

birthmark (berth′mark) any congenital blemish or spot on the skin, usually visible at birth or shortly after, such as certain nevi or a cutaneous mole.

bis- [L. *bis* twice] a prefix meaning two or twice.

bisacodyl (bis-ak′o-dil; bis″ah-ko′dil) [USP] chemical name: 4,4′-(2-pyridinylmethylene)bisphenol diacetate (ester). A cathartic, $C_{22}H_{19}NO_4$, occurring as a white to off-white, crystalline powder; administered orally or by rectal suppository. **b. tannex,** a water-soluble complex of bisacodyl and tannic acid; a cathartic.

bisacromial (bis″ah-kro′me-al) pertaining to the two acromial processes.

bisaxillary (bis-ak′sĭ-lar″e) pertaining to both axillae.

Bischoff's test (bish′ofs) [Carl Adam *Bischoff,* German chemist, 1855–1908] see under *tests.*

biscuit (bis′ket) dental porcelain that has undergone the first firing and has assumed a surface texture like that of a cookie. **hard b.,** dental porcelain during firing and after shrinking but before vitrification; shrinkage is complete and porosity is slight. Called also *high bisque.* **medium b.,** dental porcelain during firing at the stage where there has been complete cohesion of the powder particles and definite shrinkage, but there is still some porosity. Called also *medium bisque.* **soft b.,** dental porcelain during firing while it undergoes stiffening but before shrinkage has begun; the porcelain is rigid but very porous. Called also *low bisque.*

biscuiting (bis′ket-ing) the first baking of porcelain paste, by which biscuit is formed.

bisection (bi-sek′shun) [*bi-* + L. *sectio* a cut] division into two parts by cutting.

biseptate (bi-sep′tāt) [*bi-* + L. *septum* partition] divided into two parts by a septum.

bisexual (bi-sek′shoo-al) [*bi-* + L. *sexus* sex] 1. of or pertaining to bisexuality. Cf. *ambisexual* and *unisexual.* 2. an individual exhibiting bisexuality.

bisexuality (bi-seks″u-al′ĭ-te) 1. true hermaphroditism; the condition of having gonads of both sexes. 2. loosely, having phenotypic or behavioral characteristics of both sexes. 3. sexual attraction to persons of both sexes; exhibition of both homosexual and heterosexual behavior. 4. existence of the psychological qualities of both sexes, both masculinity and femininity, in the same person.

bisferious (bis-fe′re-us) [L. *bis* twice + *ferire* to beat] having two beats; usually refers to a widely notched arterial pulse, sometimes palpable.

Bishop's sphygmoscope (bish′ups) [Louis Faugères *Bishop,* American physician, 1864–1941] see under *sphygmoscope.*

bishydroxycoumarin (bis″hi-drok″se-koo′mah-rin) [USP] dicumarol.

bisiliac (bi-sil′e-ak) [L. *bis* twice + *iliac*] pertaining to both iliac bones or to any two corresponding points on the two iliac bones.

bis in die (bis in de′a) [L.] twice a day; abbreviated b.d. or b.i.d.

bismuth (biz′muth) [L. *bismuthum*] a silver-white metal; atomic number 83; atomic weight 208.980; symbol Bi: its salts have been used in inflammatory diseases of the stomach and intestine, and in the treatment of syphilis. Since the introduction of antibiotics, treatment with bismuth has declined. **b. albuminate,** a white or grayish insoluble powder formerly used for intestinal and gastric cramps. **b. and ammonium citrate,** a white crystalline compound formerly used as an astringent in intestinal irritation. **b. arsanilate,** a compound, $NH_2C_6H_4 \cdot AsO$, formerly used in the treatment of syphilis. **b. benzoate,** a whitish tasteless powder, $Bi(C_6H_5CO_2)_3Bi(OH)_3$, formerly used as an external and internal antiseptic. **b. betanaphthol,** a light brown insoluble aromatic powder, $(C_{10}H_7 \cdot O)_3 \cdot Bi \cdot 3H_2O$, formerly used as an intestinal astringent and antiseptic. **b. borophenate,** a compound formerly used as an antiseptic dusting powder. **b. carbonate, basic,** b. subcarbonate. **b. cerium salicylate,** a bismuth salt in the form of a pinkish, insoluble powder, formerly used in enteritis, diarrhea, etc. **b. chrysophanate,** an amorphous yellow powder, $(C_{15}H_9O_4)_3Bi_2O_3$, resulting from the mixture of chrysarobin and bismuth hydroxide; formerly used in skin diseases. **b. citrate,** an amorphous powder, $BiC_6H_5O_7$, used in pharmacy and in the preparation of other bismuth remedies. **b. ethyl camphorate,** a bismuth preparation, $(C_{12}H_{19}O_4)_3Bi$, containing 23.5 per cent of bismuth; formerly used as an antisyphilitic. **b. glycollylarsanilate,** glycobiarsol. **b. magma,** milk of bismuth. **b. nitrate,** $Bi(NO_3)_3 \cdot 5H_2O$, formerly used in diarrhea. **b. oxybromide,** an impalpable yellowish powder, BiOBr, to be given in a tragacanth emulsion; formerly used in nervous dyspepsia. **b. oxychloride,** a white powder, sometimes known as pearl white, BiOCl, formerly used as a local antiseptic. **b. oxyiodide,** a brownish-red powder, BiOI, formerly used as a local antiseptic. **b. oxyiodopyrogallate,** a fine, yellowish-red powder, $C_6H_2(OH)_2 \cdot O \cdot Bi$-(OH)I, formerly used as a surgical antiseptic powder. **b. permanganate,** a black bulky powder, $Bi(MnO_4)_3$, formerly used as an antiseptic dusting powder. **b. phosphate,** a white odorless powder, $BiPO_4$, formerly used as an intestinal antiseptic. **b. and potassium tartrate,** a white odorless powder, $C_4H_2O_9Bi_3K \cdot 4H_2O$, formerly used intramuscularly in syphilis. **b. pyrogallate,** a yellow powder, $C_6H_3 \cdot OH \cdot O \cdot O \cdot BiOH$, formerly used as an internal and external antiseptic. **b. salicylate,** a white, tasteless, and insoluble powder formerly used as an intestinal antiseptic. **b. sodium tartrate,** a compound, $BiNa(C_4H_4O_6)_2$, formerly used in the treatment of syphilis. **b. sodium triglycollamate,** double salt of sodium bismuthyl triglycollamate and disodium triglycollamate; formerly used for lupus erythematosus and chronic syphilis. **b. subcarbonate,** a white to yellowish white powder, $(BiO)_2CO_3 \cdot H_2O$, yielding at least 90 per cent Bi_2O_3; it is used as a topical protectant to relieve skin irritations, and it has been used internally as an antacid and astringent. Called also *basic bismuth carbonate.* **b. subgallate,** a basic salt, Bi-$(OH)_2 \cdot C_7H_5O_5$, which on drying yields 52 to 57 per cent of bismuth trioxide; formerly used as an astringent and protective in the treatment of ulcerative colitis, dysentery, and diarrhea. **b. subnitrate** [USP], a basic salt, $BiO \cdot NO_3 \cdot H_2O$, which on ignition yields not less than 71 per cent of bismuth trioxide, occurring as a white, slightly hygroscopic powder; used as a pharmaceutic necessity, and formerly as an antacid, antiseptic, and radiopaque medium. Called also *b. white* and *Spanish white.* **b. subsalicylate,** a basic salt, $C_7H_5BiO_4$, which on ignition yields 62 to 66 per cent bismuth trioxide; it has been given orally in the treatment of enteritis and intramuscularly in the treatment of syphilis, lupus erythematosus, and necrotizing ulcerative gingivitis. **b. tannate,** a compound formed by the action of tannic acid on bismuth hydroxide; formerly used as an astringent in diarrhea. **b. tribromphenate,** a yellow powder, C_{18}-$H_6BiBr_9O_3$, formerly used as a topical antiseptic. **b. white,** b. subnitrate.

bismuthia (biz-mu'the-ah) blue discoloration of the skin and mucous membranes as the result of the administration of bismuth compounds.

bismuthism (biz'muth-izm) bismuthosis.

bismuthosis (biz"mu-tho'sis) chronic bismuth poisoning, characterized by anuria, stomatitis, dermatitis, and diarrhea.

bisobrin lactate (bis'o-brin) chemical name: *meso*-1,1'-tetramethylenebis[1,2,3,4-tetrahydro-6,7-dimethoxyisoquinoline] dilactate; a fibrinolytic agent, $C_{26}H_{36}N_2O_4 \cdot 2C_3H_6O_3$.

2,3-bisphosphoglycerate (bis-fos"fo-glis'er-āt) a salt or ester of bisphosphoglyceric acid; it is contained in red blood cells, where it plays a role in liberating oxygen from hemoglobin in the peripheral circulation. It is also an intermediate in the conversion of 3-phosphoglycerate to 2-phosphoglycerate. Called also *2,3-diphosphoglycerate*.

bisphosphoglycerate mutase (bis-fos"fo-glis'er-at-mu'tās) [EC 5.4.2.4] an enzyme of the transferase class that catalyzes the reaction 3-phospho-D-glyceroyl phosphate = 2,3-bisphospho-D-glycerate. The reaction, which requires Mg^+ as a cofactor, regulates the formation of 2,3-bisphosphoglycerate. A deficiency of the enzyme, an autosomal recessive trait, results in hemolytic anemia.

bisphosphoglycerate phosphatase (bis-fos"fo-glis"er-āt fos'fah-tās) [EC 3.1.3.13] an enzyme of the hydrolase class that catalyzes the reaction 2,3-bisphospho-D-glycerate + H_2O = 3-phospho-D-glycerate + orthophosphate. The reaction is one of the control mechanisms regulating the affinity of hemoglobin for oxygen.

bisphosphoglyceromutase (bis-fos"fo-glis"er-o-mu'tās) bisphosphoglycerate mutase.

bispore (bi'spōr) one of two asexual spores produced by the red algae.

bisque (bisk) [Fr.] biscuit. **high b., low b., medium b.,** see under *bisque.*

bistephanic (bi"stĕ-fan'ik) pertaining to the two stephanions, especially to the shortest distance between them (bistephanic width).

Biston betularia (bis'ton be-tu-la're-ah) the peppered moth, used in the study of industrial melanism.

bistort (bis'tort) [L. *bis* twice + *tortus* twisted] the plant, *Polygonum bistorta;* its root [L. *bistortae radix*] contains tannins and has mild astringent and tonic properties.

bistoury (bis'too-re) [Fr. *bistouri*] a long, narrow surgical knife, straight or curved, used for incising abscesses and enlarging sinuses, fistulas, etc.

bistratal (bi-stra'tal) [*bi-* + L. *stratum* layer] disposed in two layers.

bisulfate (bi-sul'fāt) an acid sulfate (not to be confused with *disulfate*).

bisulfide (bi-sul'fīd) disulfide.

bisulfite (bi-sul'fīt) an acid sulfite.

bitartrate (bi-tar'trāt) any salt containing the anion $C_4H_5O_6^-$ derived from the diacid tartaric acid ($C_4H_6O_6$).

bite (bīt) 1. the forcible closure of the lower against the upper teeth. 2. the measure of force exerted in the closure of the teeth. 3. a record of the relationship of upper and lower teeth, in occlusion, obtained by biting into a mass of modeling substance. 4. the part of an artificial tooth on the lingual side between the shoulder and the incisal edge of the tooth. 5. a wound or puncture made by the teeth or other parts of the mouth. 6. a morsel of food. **balanced b.,** balanced occlusion. **check b.,** a thin sheet of wax or a modeling compound placed between the teeth in centric, eccentric, lateral, or protrusive occlusion, and pressed to their buccal or labial surfaces after the jaws have been closed; used to check dental occlusion in the articulator in properly aligning study models. Written also *check-bite.* **closed b.,** malocclusion with decreased occlusal vertical dimension and an abnormal overbite in which the mandible protudes. Called also *deep b., closed-bite malocclusion,* and *deep overbite.* **cross b.,** crossbite. **deep b.,** closed b. **edge-to-edge b., end-to-end b.,** see under *occlusion.* **open b.,** a condition marked by failure of certain opposing teeth to establish occlusal contact when the jaws are closed. Called also *apertognathia, nonocclusion,* and *open-bite occlusion.*

over b., overbite. **scissors b.,** total lingual crossbite of the mandible, with the mandibular teeth completely contained within the maxillary dental arch in habitual occlusion. **underhung b.,** a characteristic of mandibular prognathism in which the incisal edges of the mandibular anterior teeth extend labially to the incisal edges of the maxillary anterior teeth when the jaws are in habitual occlusion. **wax b.,** an impression, made simultaneously, of both the upper and the lower jaw, by having the subject bite on a double layer of soft baseplate wax. **X-b.,** crossbite.

bite-block (bīt'blok) occlusion rim.

bitegage (bīt'gāj) a device used in prosthetic dentistry as an aid in securing proper occlusion of the maxillary and mandibular teeth.

bitelock (bīt'lok) occlusion rim.

bitemporal (bi-tem'po-ral) pertaining to both temples or temporal bones.

biteplane (bit'plān) an orthodontic removable appliance, made of acrylic resin, covering all the maxillary teeth, and kept in place by orthodontic wrought wire clasps and labial wires; used in the diagnosis and treatment of pain of the temporomandibular joint and adjacent muscles. Written also *bite plane.*

biteplate (bīt'plāt) bite plate.

biterminal (bi-ter'min-al) performed by using two terminals of an alternating current.

bite-wing (bīt'wing) a central tab or wing of a dental x-ray film, which is held between the upper and lower teeth during radiography of oral structures. See also under *film* and *radiograph.*

bithionol (bǐ-thi'o-nol) chemical name: 2,2'-thiobis(4,6-dichlorophenol). A bacteriostatic agent, $C_{12}H_6Cl_4O_2S$, especially effective against gram-positive cocci; formerly used in the formulation of surgical soap compositions. Called also *TBP.*

Bithynia (bǐ-thin'ĕ-ah) a genus of snails, species of which are the intermediate hosts of *Opisthorchis.* **B. longicor'nus,** *Alocinma longicornis.*

Bitis (bi'tis) a genus of venomous, brightly colored, thick-bodied, viperine snakes, possessing heart-shaped heads; it includes the puff adder (*B. arientans*), Gaboon viper (*B. gabonica*), and rhinoceros viper (*B. nasicornis*). See table accompanying *snake.*

bitolterol (bi-tōl'ter-ōl) chemical name: 4-methylbenzoic acid 4-[2-[(1,1-dimethylethyl)amino]-1-hydroxyethyl]-1,2-phenylene ester; a beta-adrenergic bronchodilator administered as an aerosol in the treatment of asthma.

Bitot's spots (patches) (be'tōz) [Pierre A. *Bitot,* Bordeaux physician, 1822–1888] see under *spot.*

bitrochanteric (bi"tro-kan-ter'ik) pertaining to both trochanters on one femur or to both greater trochanters.

bitter (bit'er) 1. having an austere and unpalatable taste, like that of quinine. 2. [pl.] a medicinal agent that has a bitter taste; used as a tonic, alterative, or appetizer. Called also *amara.* **aromatic b's,** bitter vegetable drugs that have an aromatic quality. **simple b's,** any drug with a bitter taste that has no general influence upon the system except through its action upon the stomach or intestine. **styptic b's,** bitter drugs with a markedly astringent quality. **Swedish b's,** compound tincture of aloes.

bitterling (bit'er-ling) see *bitterling test,* under *tests.*

bitters (bit'erz) a popular name for various alcoholic medicines and drinks; see under *bitter.*

Bittorf's reaction (bit'orfs) [Alexander *Bittorf,* German physician, 1876–1949] see under *reaction.*

bitumen (bǐ-tu'men) [L.] any one of various natural and artificial dry petroleum products. **sulfonated b.,** ichthammol.

bituminosis (bi"tu-mǐ-no'sis) a form of pneumoconiosis due to the dust from soft coal.

biurate (bi'u-rāt) an acid urate; a monobasic salt of uric acid.

biuret (bi'u-ret) [L. *bis* twice + *urea*] a derivative of urea, $H_2NCO \cdot NH \cdot CO \cdot NH_2$, equivalent to two molecules of urea less one of ammonia; called also *allophanamide.* See also under *tests.*

bivalence (biv'ah-lens) [*bi-* + L. *valens* powerful] the property of an atom of certain chemical elements of forming chemical bonds with two other atoms or groups.

bivalent (bi-va′lent) 1. divalent. 2. the structure formed by a pair of homologous chromosomes joined by synapsis along their length during the zygotene and pachytene stages of the first meiotic prophase. After each of the paired chromosomes separates into two sister chromatids during the pachytene stage, this structure is then called a *tetrad*.

bivalve (bi′valv) [*bi-* + L. *valva* valve] having two valves, as the shells of such mollusks as clams.

Bivalvia (bi-val′ve-ah) [*bi-* + L. *valva* valve + *-ia*] Pelecypoda.

Bivalvulida (bi″val-vu′lĭ-dah) [*bi-* + *valve*] an order of parasitic protozoa (class Myxosporea, phylum Myxozoa), the spores of which have two valves. It comprises three suborders: Bipolarina, Eurysporina, and Platysporina.

biventer (bi′ven-ter) [*bi-* + L. *venter* belly] a part or organ (as a muscle) with two bellies. **b. cer′vicis,** musculus spinalis capitis.

biventral (bi-ven′tral) 1. having two bellies. 2. musculus digastricus.

biventricular (bi″ven-trik′u-lar) pertaining to or affecting both ventricles of the heart.

bivitelline (bi″vi-tel′in) having two yolks.

bixin (bik′sin) [L. *Bixa* a plant genus] an orange-red color or stain, $C_{25}H_{30}O_4$, from annotto.

bizygomatic (bi″zi-go-mat′ik) [*bi-* + Gr. *zygōma* zygoma] pertaining to the two most prominent points on the two zygomatic arches. See also *bizygomatic breadth,* under *breadth.*

Bizzozero's cells, corpuscles, platelets (bit-sot′ ser-ōz) [Giulio *Bizzozero*, Italian physician, 1846–1901] platelets.

Bjerrum's scotoma (sign) (byer′oomz) [Jannik Petersen *Bjerrum*, Danish ophthalmologist, 1851–1920] see under *scotoma.*

Bjerrum's screen (byer′oomz) [J. *Bjerrum*, Danish ophthalmologist, 1827–1892] tangent screen.

Bk chemical symbol for *berkelium.*

black (blak) reflecting no light or true color; of the darkest hue. **animal b., bone-b.,** animal charcoal. **indulin b.,** nigrosin. **ivory b.,** animal charcoal. **lamp b.,** finely divided carbon deposited from the smoky flame of burning oils, rosin, etc. **Paris b.,** animal charcoal.

Blackfan-Diamond anemia (syndrome) (blak′fan di′ah-mond) [Kenneth D. *Blackfan*, American pediatrician, 1883–1941; Louis Klein *Diamond*, American pediatrician, born 1902] see *hypoplastic anemia, congenital,* under *anemia.*

Black's formula (blaks) [J. A. *Black*, English army surgeon] see under *formula.*

Blackberg and Wanger's test (blak′berg, wang′gerz) [Solon Nathaniel *Blackberg*, Chicago physician, 1897–1962; J. O. *Wanger*] see under *tests.*

black haw (blak haw) see *Viburnum prunifolium* L. (Caprifoliaceae), a North American medicinal plant.

blackhead (blak′hed) 1. a comedo. 2. a disease of turkeys; see *histomoniasis of turkeys.*

blackleg (blak′leg) an acute anaerobic bacterial disease of cattle and sheep producing crepitant swelling in the musculature, caused by *Clostridium chauvoei.* Called also *symptomatic anthrax, blackquarter,* and *quarter evil.*

blackout (blak′owt) a condition characterized by failure of vision and momentary unconsciousness, due to diminished circulation to the brain.

blackquarter (blak kwor′ter) blackleg.

blacksnake (blak′snāk) usually *Pseudechis porphyriacus,* a large, semiaquatic, venomous, elapid snake of Australia, whose body is black on top and red underneath. See table accompanying *snake.* Also, *Coluber constrictor,* the American blacksnake or black racer.

blacktongue (blak-tung′) pellagra in dogs.

bladder (blad′der) [L. *vesica, cystis;* Gr. *kystis*] a membranous sac, such as one serving as receptacle for a secretion; often used alone to designate the urinary bladder. Called also *vesica.* **allantoic b.,** a membranous sac formed in amphibians as an outgrowth of the cloaca for the storage of urine. **atonic b.,** a condition marked by a dilated, poorly contracting urinary bladder without evidence of a lesion of the central nervous system. **atonic neurogenic b.,** neurogenic bladder due to destruction of the sensory nerve fibers from the bladder to the spinal cord, marked by the absence of control of bladder functions and of the desire to void, overdistention of the bladder, and an abnormal amount of residual urine; it is most frequently associated with tabes dorsalis (*tabetic b.*) and pernicious anemia, but may be seen in association with other diseases. Called also *paralytic b.* and *sensory paralytic b.* **automatic b.,** neurogenic bladder due to complete transection of the spinal cord above the sacral segments, marked by complete loss of micturition reflexes and bladder sensation, violent involuntary voiding, and an abnormal amount of residual urine. Called also *cord b., reflex b.,* and *spastic b.* **autonomic b.,** autonomous b. **autonomous b.,** neurogenic bladder due to a lesion in the sacral portion of the spinal cord that interrupts the reflex arc which controls the bladder. The lesion may be in the cauda equina, conus medullaris, sacral roots, or pelvic nerve. It is marked by loss of normal bladder sensation and reflex activity, inability to initiate urination normally, and incontinence. Called also *denervated b.* and *nonreflex b.* **chyle b.,** cisterna chyli. **cord b.,** automatic b. **denervated b.,** autonomous b. **double b.,** reduplication of the bladder. **fasciculated b.,** a bladder which, from hypertrophy of the muscular coat, is ridged on its inner surface. **gall b.,** see *gallbladder.* **irritable b.,** a state of the bladder marked by increased frequency of contraction with associated desire to urinate. **motor paralytic b.,** neurogenic bladder due to impairment of the motor neurons or nerves controlling the bladder. The *acute* form is marked by painful distention and inability to initiate micturition, the *chronic* form by difficulty in initiating micturition, straining, decrease in size and force of stream, interrupted stream, and recurrent infection of the urinary tract. **nervous b.,** a colloquial term for a functional condition characterized by a constant desire to urinate without the power to do so completely. **neurogenic b.,** any condition of dysfunction of the urinary bladder caused by a lesion of the central or peripheral nervous system, as *atonic neurogenic b., automatic b., autonomous b., motor paralytic b.,* and *uninhibited neurogenic b.* **nonreflex b.,** autonomous b. **paralytic b.,** atonic neurogenic b. **reflex b.,** automatic b. **sacculated b.,** a bladder with pouches between the hypertrophied muscular fibers. **sensory paralytic b.,** atonic neurogenic b. **spastic b.,** automatic b. **string b.,** a term sometimes erroneously used as a synonym for cord bladder; see *automatic b.* **tabetic b.,** see *atonic neurogenic b.* **uninhibited neurogenic b.,** neurogenic bladder due to a lesion in the region of the upper motor neurons with subtotal interruption of the corticospinal pathways, marked by urgency, frequent involuntary voiding, and small-volume threshold of activity. **urinary b.,** the musculomembranous sac, situated in the anterior part of the pelvic cavity, that serves as a reservoir for urine, which it receives through the ureters and discharges through the urethra. Called also *vesica urinaria* [NA].

Blainville's ear (blah′vēlz) [Henri Marie Ducrotay de *Blainville,* French zoologist, 1777–1850] see under *ear.*

Blake's disk (blākz) [Clarence John *Blake,* Boston otologist, 1843–1919] see under *disk.*

Blalock-Hanlon operation (bla′lok han′lon) [Alfred *Blalock,* American surgeon, 1899–1964; C. Rollins *Hanlon,* American surgeon, born 1915] see under *operation.*

Blalock-Taussig operation (bla′lok taw′sig) [Alfred *Blalock;* Helen Brooke *Taussig,* American pediatrician, 1898–1986] see under *operation.*

blanc (blaw) [Fr.] white. **b. fixe,** barium sulfate.

Blancophor (blank′o-fōr) trademark for optical whitening agents (blankophores) chemically related to the sulfonamides, which produce brightness by absorbing invisible ultraviolet light and reflecting it as visible blue light. They are added to detergents, paper, and textiles, and may produce phototoxic effects, e.g., phototoxic dermatitis; they may also produce allergic contact sensitization.

bland (bland) [L. *blandus*] mild or soothing.

Blandin's glands (blah-daz′) [Philippe Frédéric *Blandin,* French surgeon, 1798–1849] see *glandulae linguales anteriores* and *ganglion submandibulares.*

Blandlube (bland′lūb) trademark for a preparation of mineral oil.

blankophore (blank′o-fōr) see *Blancophor.*

Blasius' duct (blah′se-ooz) [Gerhard *Blasius* (Blaes), Dutch anatomist of the 17th century] ductus parotideus.

Blaskovics operation (blas′ko-vitz) [Laszlo de Blaskovics, Hungarian ophthalmologist, 1869–1938] see under *operation*.

blast (blast) [Gr. *blastos* germ] 1. an immature stage in cellular development before appearance of the definitive characteristics of the cell; used also as a word termination, as in adamantoblast, hematoblast, neuroblast, etc. See *blasto-*. 2. [Anglo-Saxon *blaest* blast] the wave of air pressure (*air concussion*) produced by the detonation of a high-explosive bomb, shell, or other explosion. A wave of high-pressure velocity (shock wave) is created and this is followed by one of negative decreased velocity, exerting a suction-like action. Blast causes pulmonary concussion and hemorrhage (*lung blast, blast chest*), laceration of other thoracic and abdominal viscera, ruptured ear drums, and minor effects in the central nervous system. **immersion b.,** internal injury to seamen in the water caused by explosion of a depth bomb near them.

blastema (blas-te′mah) [Gr. *blastēma* shoot] 1. the primitive substance from which cells are formed. 2. a group of cells that give rise to a new individual, in asexual reproduction, or to an organ or part, in either normal development or in regeneration.

blastemic (blas-tem′ik) pertaining to the blastema.

blastid (blas′tid) the site indicative of an organizing nucleus in a fertilized ovum.

blastide (blas′tīd) blastid.

blastin (blas′tin) a substance that stimulates or increases cell proliferation; a substance providing alimentation for cells.

blast(o)- [Gr. *blastos* shoot, germ] a combining form denoting relationship to a bud or budding, particularly to an early embryonic stage, as to a primitive or formative element, cell, or layer.

Blastobacter (blas″to-bak′ter) [*blasto-* + Gr. *baktron* a rod] a genus of budding bacteria found in fresh waters, made up of rod-, wedge-, or club-shaped cells attached in a rosette formation. The type species is *B. henri′ci*.

Blastocaulis (blas″to-kaw′lis) *Planctomyces*.

blastocele (blas′to-sēl) blastocoele.

blastocelic (blas″to-se′lik) blastocoelic.

blastochyle (blas′to-kīl) [*blasto-* + Gr. *chylos* juice] the fluid contained in the blastocoele.

blastocoele (blas′to-sēl) [*blasto-* + Gr. *koilos* hollow] the fluid-filled cavity of the mass of cells (blastula) produced by cleavage of a fertilized ovum; see illustration under *blastula*. Sometimes spelled *blastocoel*. Called also *cleavage, segmentation,* or *subgerminal cavity*.

blastocoelic (blas″to-se′lik) pertaining to the blastocoele.

Blastocrithidia (blas″to-krĭ-thid′e-ah) [*blasto-* + Gr. *krithē* barleycorn] a genus of protozoa (suborder Trypanosomatina, order Kinetoplastida) parasitic in arthropods and other invertebrates, which pass through epimastigote, amastigote, and presumably promastigote developmental stages in their life cycle.

blastocyst (blas′to-sist) [*blasto-* + Gr. *kystis* bladder] the mammalian conceptus in the post-morula stage; it is like a blastula in having a fluid-filled cavity, unlike it in having the surface layer not exclusively embryoblast but mainly or entirely trophoblast, in having an eccentric embryoblast, and in not being limited to one germ layer.

Blastocystis (blas″to-sis′tis) a genus of yeasts of uncertain classification. **B. hom′inis,** microorganism appearing as a spherical cystic structure, 5 to 15µ in diameter, frequently found in human feces.

blastocyte (blas′to-sīt) [*blasto-* + Gr. *kytos* hollow vessel] an embryonic cell that has not yet become differentiated.

blastocytoma (blas″to-si-to′mah) blastoma.

Blastodendrion (blas″to-den′dre-on) (obs.) *Candida*.

blastodendriosis (blas″to-den′dre-o′sis) candidiasis.

blastoderm (blas′to-derm) [*blasto-* + Gr. *derma* skin] collectively, the mass of cells produced by cleavage of a fertilized ovum, forming the hollow sphere of the blastula, or the cellular cap above a floor of segmented yolk in the discoblastula of telolecithal eggs; see illustration under *blastula*. Called also *germinal membrane,* or *membrana germinativa*.

bilaminar b., the stage of development in which the embryo is represented by two primary layers: the ectoderm and the entoderm. See *gastrula*. **embryonic b.,** the region of the blastoderm forming the embryo proper. **extraembryonic b.,** the region of the blastoderm forming membranes rather than the embryo proper. **trilaminar b.,** the stage of development in which the embryo is represented by the three primary layers: the ectoderm, the mesoderm, and the entoderm.

blastodermal (blas″to-der′mal) pertaining to or derived from the blastoderm.

blastodermic (blas″to-der′mik) blastodermal.

blastodisc (blas′to-disk) [*blasto-* + Gr. *diskos* disk] the convex structure formed by the blastomeres at the animal pole of an ovum undergoing incomplete cleavage.

blastogenesis (blas″to-jen′ĕ-sis) 1. the development of an individual from a blastema, that is, by asexual reproduction. 2. transmission of inherited characters by the germ plasm. 3. the morphological transformation of small lymphocytes into larger cells resembling blast cells, occurring on exposure to phytohemagglutinin or to antigens to which the donor is immunized.

blastogenetic (blas″to-jĕ-net′ik) blastogenic.

blastogenic (blas″to-jen′ik) originating in the germ or germ cell; pertaining to or characterized by blastogenesis.

blastogeny (blas-toj′ĕ-ne) [*blasto-* + Gr. *genesis* production] the germ history of an organism or species.

Blastogregarinina (blas″to-greg″ah-ri′nĭ-nah) [*blasto-* + L. *gregarius* crowding together] a suborder of parasitic protozoa (order Eugregarinida, subclass Gregarinia) comprising marine polychetes, and characterized by gamonts that undergo gametogony while attached to the intestine, with anisogamous budding of gamonts; syzygy does not occur and gametocysts are absent. The gamont is aseptate with a mucron for attachment to the host's tissues.

blastokinin (blas″to-ki′nin) a globulin found in the uterine lumen of some mammals near the time of blastocyst implantation; called also *uteroglobulin*.

blastolysis (blas-tol′ĭ-sis) [*blasto-* + Gr. *lysis* dissolution] destruction or splitting up of germ substance.

blastolytic (blas″to-lit′ik) pertaining to, characterized by, or producing blastolysis.

blastoma (blas-to′mah), pl. *blasto′mas* or *blasto′mata* [*blasto-* + *-oma*] a neoplasm composed of embryonic cells derived from the blastema of an organ or tissue; called also *blastocytoma*. **pluricentric b.,** a blastoma that arises from a number of scattered cells or groups of cells. **unicentric b.,** a blastoma arising from one cell or from a single group of cells.

blastomatoid (blas-to′mah-toid) [*blastoma* + Gr. *eidos* form] resembling blastomas.

blastomatosis (blas″to-mah-to′sis) the formation of blastomas; tumor formation.

blastomatous (blas-to′mah-tus) pertaining to or of the nature of blastoma.

blastomere (blas′to-mēr) [*blasto-* + Gr. *meros* a part] one of the cells produced by cleavage of a fertilized ovum; called also *segmentation sphere* and *cleavage cell*.

blastomerotomy (blas″to-mēr-ot′o-me) [*blastomere* + Gr. *tomē* a cut] destruction of a blastomere or of blastomeres; called also *blastotomy*.

blastomogenic (blas″to-mo-jen′ik) producing or tending to produce new growths or tumors.

blastomogenous (blas″to-moj′ĕ-nus) blastomogenic.

Blastomyces (blas″to-mi′sēz) [*blasto-* + Gr. *mykēs* fungus] a genus of thermal dimorphic imperfect fungi of the family Moniliaceae, order Moniliales, which grow as mycelial forms at room temperature and as yeastlike forms at body temperature. The term is applied to the yeasts pathogenic for man and animals. **B. brasilien′sis,** *Paracoccidioides brasiliensis*. **B. coccidioi′des,** former name for *Coccidioides immitis*. **B. dermatit′idis,** the etiologic agent of North American blastomycosis; its perfect, or sexual, stage is known as *Ajellomyces dermatitidis*. Formerly called *Cryptococcus gilchristi* and *Endomyces capsulatus, E. epidermatidis,* and *E. epidermidis*. **B. farcimino′sus,** former name for *Histoplasma farciminosus*.

blastomyces (blas″to-mi′sēz), pl. *blastomyce′tes*. A fungus of the genus *Blastomyces*.

blastomycete (blas″to-mi′sēt) any organism of the genus *Blastomyces;* also, any yeastlike organism.

blastomycetes (blas″to-mi-se′tēz) plural of *blastomyces* and *blastomycete.*

blastomycin (blas″to-mi′sin) a skin test antigen prepared from *Blastomyces dermatitidis* organisms, of no diagnostic or prognostic value and seldom used.

Blastomycoides immitis (blas″to-mi-koi′dēz im-mi′tis) former name for *Coccidioides immitis.*

blastomycosis (blas″to-mi-ko′sis) 1. infection caused by organisms of the genus *Blastomyces.* 2. a general term for any infection caused by a yeastlike organism. **Brazilian b.,** paracoccidioidomycosis. **cutaneous b.,** see *North American b.* **European b.,** infection caused by *Cryptococcus neoformans,* especially the cutaneous form of cryptococcosis (q.v.). **keloidal b.,** an infection caused by *Loboa loboi,* characterized by the appearance of red, smooth, hard cutaneous nodules which, histologically, have the appearance of a keloid. Called also *Lobo's disease.* **North American b.,** an infection usually acquired through the pulmonary route, caused by *Blastomyces dermatitidis,* and marked by suppurating tumors in the skin (*cutaneous b.*) or by lesions in the lungs, bones, subcutaneous tissues, liver, spleen, and kidneys (*systemic b.*). Called also *Gilchrist's disease* and *Chicago disease.* **South American b.,** paracoccidioidomycosis. **systemic b.,** see *North American b.*

blastoneuropore (blas″to-nu′ro-pōr) [*blasto-* + Gr. *neuron* nerve + *poros* opening] in certain embryos, a temporary aperture formed by the coalescence of the blastopore and neuropore.

blastophthoria (blas″tof-tho′re-ah) [*blasto-* + Gr. *phthora* corruption] degeneration of the germ cells.

blastophthoric (blas″tof-tho′rik) pertaining to, characterized by, or producing blastophthoria.

blastophyllum (blas″to-fil′um) [*blasto-* + Gr. *phyllon* leaf] a primitive germ layer.

blastophyly (blas-tof′ĭ-le) [*blasto-* + Gr. *phylē* tribe] the tribal history, or arrangement, of organisms.

blastopore (blas″to-pōr) [*blasto-* + Gr. *poros* opening] the opening of the archenteron to the exterior of the embryo, at the gastrula stage; called also *archistome, protostoma,* and *anus of Rusconi.*

blastosphere (blas″to-sfēr) [*blasto-* + Gr. *sphaira* sphere] blastula.

blastospore (blas″to-spōr) [*blasto-* + *spore*] a spore formed by budding, as in yeast.

blastostroma (blas″to-stro′mah) that part of the egg which takes an active part in the formation of the blastoderm.

blastotomy (blas-tot′o-me) blastomerotomy.

blastozooid (blas″to-zo′oid) [*blasto-* + Gr. *zōo-eidēs* like an animal] an individual developed as a result of asexual reproduction. Cf. *oozooid.*

blastula (blas′tu-lah), pl. *blas′tulae* [L.] the usually spherical structure produced by cleavage of a fertilized ovum, consisting of a single layer of cells (blastoderm) surrounding a fluid-filled cavity (blastocoele); called also *blastosphere.* See also *discoblastula.*

blastulae (blas′tu-le) [L.] plural of *blastula.*

blastular (blas′tu-lar) pertaining to the blastula.

blastulation (blas″tu-la′shun) conversion of morula to blastula by development of a central cavity (blastocoele or cleavage cavity).

Blatta (blat′ah) [L.] a genus of insects—the cockroaches. The dried insects exert diuretic action, but are no longer used in medicine. They may act as the intermediate host of *Raillietina madagascariensis* and *Gongylonema scutatum.* B. (*Blatella*) *germanica,* the German roach, now widely distributed, is called the Croton bug. It is light brown in color and small in size. *B. orientalis,* the black beetle, is a common European species.

Blattabacterium (blat″ah-bak-te′re-um) [L. *blatta* cockroach + *bacterium*] a genus of nonpathogenic bacteria of uncertain affiliation made up of straight or curved, rod-shaped organisms found as endosymbionts in cockroaches.

bleaching (blēch′ing) the act or process of removing stains or color by chemical means. **coronal b.,** the use of a

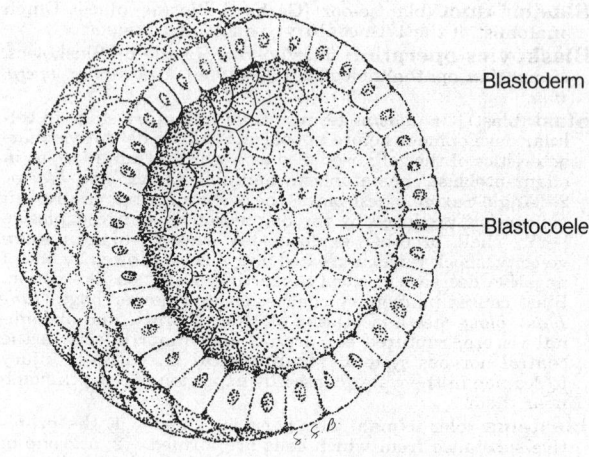

Section of a blastula.

chemical agent, usually but not necessarily in combination with heat, to remove discolorations from the crown of a pulpless tooth.

bleb (bleb) bulla.

bleeder (blēd′er) 1. one who bleeds freely or is subject to hemorrhagic diathesis. 2. any blood vessel cut during a surgical procedure that requires clamping, cautery, or ligature. 3. one who lets blood; a phlebotomist.

bleeding (blēd′ing) 1. the escape of blood from an injured vessel. 2. the letting of blood; phlebotomy. **functional b.,** bleeding from the uterus when no organic lesions are present. **implantation b.,** bleeding occurring at the time of implantation of the fertilized ovum in the decidua, being due to leakage of blood into the uterine lumen from disrupted blood vessels about the implantation site. Cf. *placentation b.* **occult b.,** escape of such a small amount of blood that it can be detected only by chemical test or by examination with the microscope or spectroscope. **placentation b.,** bleeding occurring from the uterus during the early weeks of pregnancy, when the maternal blood vessels are being eroded. Cf. *implantation b.* **summer b.,** dermatorrhagia parasitica.

blennadenitis (blen″ad-ĕ-ni′tis) [*blenn-* + Gr. *adēn* gland + *-itis*] inflammation of mucous glands.

blennaphrosin (blen-af′ro-sin) a preparation of a double salt of potassium nitrate and methenamine with extract of kava-kava; formerly used in gonorrhea and cystitis.

blennemesis (blen-em′ĕ-sis) [*blenn-* + Gr. *emesis* vomiting] the vomiting of mucus.

blenn(o)- [Gr. *blenna* mucus] a combining form denoting relationship to mucus.

blennogenic (blen″no-jen′ik) [*blenno-* + Gr. *gennan* to produce] muciparous.

blennogenous (blen-noj′ĕ-nus) muciparous.

blennoid (blen′noid) [*blenn-* + Gr. *eidos* form] mucoid, def. 1.

blennorrhagia (blen″no-ra′je-ah) [*blenno-* + Gr. *rhēgnynai* to break forth] 1. any excessive discharge of mucus; blennorrhea. 2. former name for *gonorrhea.*

blennorrhagic (blen″no-raj′ik) pertaining to or of the nature of blennorrhagia.

blennorrhea (blen″no-re′ah) [*blenno-* + Gr. *rhoia* flow] 1. a free discharge from the mucous surfaces, especially a gonorrheal discharge from the urethra or vagina. 2. former name for *gonorrhea.* **inclusion b.,** see under *conjunctivitis.* **b. neonato′rum,** ophthalmia neonatorum. **Stoerk's b.,** blennorrhea with profuse chronic suppuration producing hypertrophy of the mucosa of the nose, pharynx, and larynx.

blennorrheal (blen″no-re′al) pertaining to or of the nature of blennorrhea.

blennostasis (blen-nos′tah-sis) [*blenno-* + Gr. *stasis* standing] the suppression of an abnormal mucous discharge, or the correction of an excessive one.

blennostatic (blen″no-stat′ik) [*blenno-* + Gr. *histanai* to halt] 1. pertaining to blennostasis. 2. mucostatic, def. 1.

blennothorax (blen″no-tho′raks) [*blenno-* + Gr. *thōrax* chest] an accumulation of mucus in the chest.

blennuria (blen-nu′re-ah) [*blenn-* + Gr. *ouron* urine] the existence of mucus in the urine.

Blenoxane (blen-oks′ān) trademark for a preparation of bleomycin sulfate.

bleomycin (ble″o-mi′sin) any of a mixture of glycopeptide antibiotics produced by a strain of *Streptomyces verticillus,* designated A₁ to A₆, A₂′, and B₁ to B₆, that bind to DNA causing chain scission and removal of purine and pyrimidine bases, resulting in inhibition of DNA synthesis and, to a lesser extent, RNA and protein synthesis and also accumulation of cells in the G₂ phase of the cell cycle. The drug used clinically is a mixture consisting primarily of bleomycins A₂ and B₂; it is used as an antineoplastic in combination chemotherapy regimens for treatment of squamous cell carcinomas of the head and neck, testicular carcinoma, Hodgkin's disease and non-Hodgkin's lymphomas, and uterine cervix carcinoma. Major side effects are a dose-related, occasionally fatal pneumonitis and pulmonary fibrosis and severe skin reactions; nausea and vomiting and fever are also common reactions. Available as *bleomycin sulfate* [USP]. **b. sulfate,** a mixture of the sulfate salts of the components of bleomycin, especially that of bleomycin A₂. *Sterile bleomycin sulfate* [USP] is used alone or in conjunction with other chemotherapeutic agents in the palliative treatment of squamous cell carcinoma of the head and neck, Hodgkin's disease and other lymphomas, and testicular tumors; administered intravenously, intramuscularly, intra-arterially, or subcutaneously.

Bleph (blef) trademark for preparations of sulfacetamide sodium.

blepharadenitis (blef″ar-ad″ĕ-ni′tis) [*blephar-* + Gr. *adēn* gland + *-itis*] inflammation of the meibomian glands; called also *blepharoadenitis.*

blepharal (blef′ah-ral) pertaining to the eyelids.

blepharectomy (blef″ah-rek′to-me) [*blephar-* + *ectomy*] excision of a lesion of the eyelids.

blepharelosis (blef″ah-rel-o′sis) [*blephar-* + Gr. *eilein* to roll] entropion.

blepharism (blef′ah-rizm) [L. *blepharismus;* Gr. *blepharizein* to wink] spasm of the eyelids; continuous blinking.

blepharitis (blef″ah-ri′tis) [*blephar-* + *-itis*] inflammation of the eyelids. **b. angula′ris,** blepharitis ulcerosa affecting the medial commissure (angle) and blocking the punctum lacrimalis. **b. cilia′ris, b. margina′lis,** a chronic inflammation of the hair follicles and sebaceous gland openings of the margins of the eyelids; called also *blear eye, lippa,* and *lippitude.* **nonulcerative b.,** blepharitis often associated with seborrhea of the scalp, brows, and skin behind the ears, marked by greasy scaling of the margins of the lids, scales around the lashes, hyperemia, and thickening; called also *seborrheic b.* and *squamous seborrheic b.* **seborrheic b.,** nonulcerative b. **b. squamo′sa,** a marginal blepharitis in which the edges of the lids are covered with scales. **squamous seborrheic b.,** nonulcerative b. **b. ulcero′sa,** an ulcerous form of marginal blepharitis.

blephar(o)- [Gr. *blepharon* eyelid] a combining form denoting relationship to an eyelid.

blepharoadenitis (blef″ah-ro-ad″ĕ-ni′tis) blepharadenitis.

blepharoadenoma (blef″ah-ro-ad″ĕ-no′mah) adenoma of the eyelid.

blepharoatheroma (blef″ah-ro-ath″er-o′mah) an encysted tumor or sebaceous cyst of an eyelid.

blepharochalasis (blef″ah-ro-kal′ah-sis) [*blepharo-* + Gr. *chalasis* relaxation] relaxation of the skin of the eyelid, due to atrophy of the intercellular tissue; called also *dermatolysis palpebrarum.*

blepharochromidrosis (blef″ah-ro-kro-mĭ-dro′sis) [*blepharo-* + Gr. *chrōma* color + Gr. *hidrōs* sweat + *-osis*] excretion of a sweat containing pigment from the eyelids, usually of a bluish shade.

blepharoclonus (blef″ah-rok′lo-nus) [*blepharo-* + *clonus*] clonic spasm of the orbicularis oculi muscle, appearing as an increased winking of the eye.

blepharoconjunctivitis (blef″ah-ro-kon-junk″tĭ-vi′tis) inflammation of the eyelids and conjunctiva.

Blepharocorynthina (blef″ah-ro-ko″rin-thi′nah) [*blepharo-* + Gr. *koryntheus* basket] a suborder of ciliate protozoa (order Trichostomatida, subclass Vestibuliferia) found in herbivorous mammals, especially horses, and characterized by a marked reduction in somatic ciliature and apically by a retractable oral area, prominent frontal lobe, and a distinctive corkscrew-like process.

blepharodiastasis (blef″ah-ro-di-as′tah-sis) [*blepharo-* + Gr. *diastasis* separation] excessive separation of the eyelids, or inability to close them completely, causing the fissure to be very wide.

blepharoncus (blef″ah-rong′kus) [*blepharo-* + Gr. *onkos* bulk, mass] a tumor on the eyelid.

blepharopachynsis (blef″ah-ro-pak-in′sis) [*blepharo-* + Gr. *pachynsis* thickening] abnormal thickening of an eyelid.

blepharophimosis (blef″ah-ro-fĭ-mo′sis) [*blepharo-* + Gr. *phimōsis* a muzzling] abnormal narrowness of the palpebral fissures in the horizontal direction, caused by lateral displacement of the inner canthi.

blepharoplast (blef′ah-ro-plast″) [*blepharo-* + Gr. *plassein* to form] basal body.

blepharoplasty (blef′ah-ro-plas″te) plastic surgery of the eyelids.

blepharoplegia (blef″ah-ro-ple′je-ah) [*blepharo-* + Gr. *plēgē* stroke] paralysis of an eyelid or of both muscles of the eyelid.

blepharoptosis (blef″ah-ro-to′sis) [*blepharo-* + Gr. *ptōsis* a fall] drooping of an upper eyelid due to paralysis; ptosis.

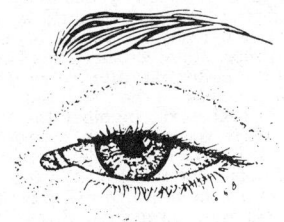

Blepharoptosis.

blepharopyorrhea (blef″ah-ro-pi-ŏ-re′ah) [*blepharo-* + Gr. *pyon* pus + *rhoia* flow] purulent ophthalmia.

blepharorrhaphy (blef″ah-ror′ah-fe) [*blepharo-* + *-rrhaphy*] the operation of suturing the eyelids together; tarsorrhaphy.

blepharospasm (blef′ah-ro-spazm″) [*blepharo-* + *spasm*] tonic spasm of the orbicularis oculi muscle, producing more or less complete closure of the eyelids. **essential b.,** blepharospasm that is present when there is no abnormality of the eye, or trigeminal (fifth cranial) nerve. **symptomatic b.,** blepharospasm occurring in association with a lesion of the eye or of the trigeminal (fifth cranial) nerve.

blepharosphincterectomy (blef″ah-ro-sfingk″ter-ek′to-me) [*blepharo-* + *sphincter* + *ectomy*] excision of some of the fibers of the orbicularis muscle, together with overlying skin, to relieve pressure of the eyelid on the cornea in blepharospasm.

blepharostat (blef′ah-ro-stat″) [*blepharo-* + Gr. *histanai* to cause to stand] an instrument for holding the eyelids and keeping them apart during surgical operations on the eye.

blepharostenosis (blef″ah-ro-stĕ-no′sis) blepharophimosis.

blepharosynechia (blef″ah-ro-sĭ-ne′ke-ah) [*blepharo-* + Gr. *synecheia* a holding together] the growing together or adhesion of the eyelids.

blepharotomy (blef″ah-rot′o-me) [*blepharo-* + *-tomy*] surgical incision of an eyelid; tarsotomy.

Blessig's cysts (spaces, lacunae), groove (bles′sigz) [Robert *Blessig,* German physician, 1830–1878] see under *cyst* and *groove.*

blight (blīt) any fungal disease of plants.

blind (blīnd) [A.S. *blind*] not having the sense of sight; see *blindness.*

blindgut (blīnd'gut) caecum (def. 2).

blindness (blīnd'nes) lack or loss of ability to see; lack of perception of visual stimuli, due to disorder of the organs of sight or to lesions in certain areas of the brain; see also *amaurosis.* **amnesic color b.,** inability to recognize or to name a hue, although it is correctly perceived. **blue b.,** imperfect perception of the blue spectrum; see *tritanopia.* **blue-yellow b.,** imperfect perception of blue and yellow tints; see *tetartanopia,* def. 2. **Bright's b.,** former term for dimness or complete loss of sight occurring in uremia, without lesion of the retina or optic disk. **color b.,** a term colloquially and incorrectly applied to any deviation from normal perception of hues; see *deuteranopia, protanopia, tetartanopia,* and *tritanopia.* **concussion b.,** functional blindness due to violent explosions, as by high explosive shells, bombs, etc. **cortical b.,** blindness due to a lesion of the cortical visual center. **cortical psychic b.,** loss of optic memory image and of spatial orientation due to lesion of the optic lobe. **day b.,** hemeralopia. **eclipse b.,** partial or total loss of central vision caused by a burn on the macula from direct fixation on the sun or from viewing a partial solar eclipse without proper protective lenses. **electric-light b.,** temporary impairment of vision due to exposure to ultraviolet rays. Photophobia, blepharospasm, redness of the eye, and swelling of the conjunctiva are the symptoms, which usually occur several hours after exposure. **epidemic b.,** a form of avian leukosis with blindness and misshapen pupil or irregular depigmentation of the iris in one or both eyes. **flight b.,** amaurosis fugax caused by high centrifugal forces encountered in aviation. **functional b.,** inability to see because of conversion hysteria; it occurs without disorder of the organs of sight. **green b.,** imperfect perception of green tints; see *deuteranopia.* **hysterical b.,** functional b. **legal b.,** blindness as defined by law; in most states of the United States, maximal visual acuity of the better eye, after correction, of 20/200 or less, with a total diameter of the visual field in that eye of 20 degrees or less. **letter b.,** inability to recognize individual letters. **mind b.,** psychic b. **moon b.,** periodic ophthalmia. **night b.,** nyctalopia. **note b.,** inability to read musical notes, due to a lesion of the central nervous system. **object b.,** inability to recognize the nature and purpose of objects seen. **psychic b.,** inability to recognize the nature of the source of visual stimuli, because of some lesion of the brain; called also *mind b.* and *soul b.* **red b.,** imperfect perception of red tints; see *protanopia.* **red-green b.,** imperfect perception of red and green tints. **river b.,** blindness caused by onchocerciasis. **snow b.,** dimness of vision, usually temporary, due to the glare of the sun upon snow. **soul b.,** psychic b. **syllabic b.,** inability to recognize syllables. **taste b.,** inability to perceive certain gustatory stimuli, some substances producing no sensation of taste. **text b.,** alexia. **total b.,** complete absence of light perception. **twilight b.,** aknephascopia. **word b.,** alexia. **yellow b.,** tritanopia.

blister (blis'ter) [L. *vesicula*] a vesicle, especially a bulla. **blood b.,** a vesicle having bloody contents; it may be caused by a pinch or bruise, but is often due to persistent friction. **fever b.,** herpes febrilis. **water b.,** one with clear watery contents.

bloat (blōt) 1. tympany of the stomach or cecum. 2. enteritis in young rabbits, accompanied by gaseous distention of the abdomen.

Blocadren (blo'kah-dren) trademark for a preparation of timolol maleate.

Bloch (blok), Konrad. German-born American biochemist born 1912; co-winner, with Feodor Lynen, of the Nobel prize for medicine or physiology in 1964, for investigations in biosynthesis and metabolism of cholesterol and fatty acids.

Bloch's scale (bloks) [Marcel *Bloch,* French pathologist, 1885– 1925] see under *scale.*

Bloch-Sulzberger syndrome (blok-sulz-berg'er) [Bruno *Bloch,* Swiss dermatologist, 1878–1933; Marion Baldur *Sulzberger,* American dermatologist, born 1895] incontinentia pigmenti.

block (blok) 1. an obstruction or stoppage. 2. regional anesthesia; see under *anesthesia.* **adrenergic b.,** see under *blockade.* **air b.,** interference with the normal inflation and deflation of the lungs and with the pulmonary blood flow, produced by the leakage of air from the pulmonary alveoli into the interstitial tissue of the lung (interstitial emphysema) and into the mediastinum (mediastinal emphysema). **alveolar-capillary b.,** interference in the normal diffusion of gases across the membrane between the alveolar spaces and the pulmonary capillaries. **arborization b.,** a gross intraventricular conduction defect in the distal ramifications of the bundle branches. **bundle-branch b.,** see under *heart block.* **caudal b.,** anesthesia produced by injection of a local anesthetic into the caudal or sacral canal. **comparator b.,** see *comparator.* **cryogenic b.,** local cooling of tissue. **dynamic b.,** spinal subarachnoid b. **ear b.,** trauma of the middle ear and the resulting inflammation and pain in compressed-air workers in which the eustachian tube is not patulous; called also *tubal b.* **epidural b.,** anesthesia produced by injection of the anesthetic agent between the vertebral spines and beneath the ligamentum flavum into the extradural space. **field b.,** regional anesthesia obtained by blocking conduction in nerves with chemical or physical agents. **heart b.,** see *heart block,* under *H.* **intercostal b., intercostal nerve b.,** anesthesia produced by blocking intercostal nerves with a local anesthic. **intranasal b.,** local anesthesia produced by insertion into the nasal fossae of pledgets soaked in a solution of an anesthetic agent that is effective after topical application, or by insufflation of a mixture of anesthetic gases or vapors through a tube introduced into the nose. **intraspinal b.,** subarachnoid b. **mental b.,** see *blocking* (def. 2). **metabolic b.,** the blockade of a biosynthetic pathway caused by a genetic enzyme deficiency or by inhibition of an enzyme by a drug or other substance. **methadone b.,** see *narcotic blockade,* under *blockade.* **Mobitz b.,** dropped beat. **nerve b.,** regional anesthesia secured by making extraneural or paraneural injections of anesthetics in close proximity to the nerve whose conductivity is to be cut off. **paracervical b.,** anesthesia of the inferior hypogastric plexus and ganglia produced by injection of the local anesthetic into the lateral fornices of the vagina; called also *uterosacral b.* **paraneural b.,** anesthesia produced by injection of the anesthetic agent around a nerve. **parasacral b.,** regional anesthesia produced by injection of a local anesthetic around the sacral nerves as they emerge from the sacral foramina. **paravertebral b.,** infiltration of the cervicothoracic (stellate) ganglion with procaine hydrochloride; performed for stroke, tachycardia, etc. **peri-infarction b.,** the association of myocardial infarction with surrounding intraventricular conduction disturbance other than left or right bundle-branch block. **perineural b.,** regional anesthesia produced by injection of the anesthetic agent close to the nerve. **presacral b.,** anesthesia produced by injection of the local anesthetic into the sacral nerves on the anterior aspect of the sacrum. **pudendal b.,** anesthesia produced by blocking the pudendal nerves, accomplished by injection of the local anesthetic into the tuberosity of the ischium. **sacral b.,** anesthesia produced by injection of a local anesthetic into the extradural space of the spinal canal. **saddle b.,** the production of anesthesia in a region corresponding roughly with the areas of the buttocks, perineum, and inner aspects of the thighs which impinge on the saddle in riding, by introducing the anesthetic agent low in the dural sac. **sinoatrial b., sinoauricular b.,** a disturbance in which the atrial response is delayed or omitted because of partial or complete interference with the propagation of impulses from the sinoatrial node to the atria. **sinus b.,** 1. pain in the paranasal sinuses due to air being trapped in them in decompression sickness. 2. sinoatrial b. **spinal b.,** subarachnoid b. **spinal subarachnoid b.,** a condition in which the flow of cerebrospinal fluid is interfered with by an obstruction in the spinal canal; called also *dynamic b.* **splanchnic b.,** anesthesia produced by blocking the splanchnic nerves and the celiac ganglia; it is accomplished by injection of the anesthetic agent into the retroperitoneal tissues in the immediate vicinity of the celiac or solar plexuses. **stellate b.,** the analgesic blocking of the stellate (cervicothoracic) ganglion. **subarachnoid b.,** anesthesia produced by the injection of a local anesthetic into the subarachnoid space around the spinal cord; called also *intraspinal b.* and *spinal b.* **sympathetic b.,** blocking of the sympathetic trunk by paravertebral infiltration with an anesthetic agent. **transsacral b.,** anesthesia produced by injection of the anesthetic agent into the sacral canal and about the sacral nerves through each of the posterior sacral foramina. **tubal b.,** ear b. **uterosacral b.,** paracervical b. **vagal b., vagus nerve b.,** blocking of vagal impulses obtained by injection of a solution of local anesthetic into the vagus nerve at its exit from the skull. **ventricular b.,** obstruction to the flow of cerebrospinal fluid within the ventricular system or through the exit foramina (foramina of Magendie and Luschka) by which the ventricles communicate with the subarachnoid space; it results in obstructive hydrocephalus. **Wenckebach b.,** partial heart block in which the ventricular rhythm is irregular, partly because of the changing P-R interval and partly because of dropped beats.

blockade (blok-ād′) 1. receptor blockade, the blocking of the effect of a hormone or neurotransmitter at a cell-surface receptor by a pharmacologic antagonist bound to the receptor. 2. in histochemistry, a chemical reaction that by modifying certain chemical groups blocks a specific staining method. **adrenergic b.,** selective inhibition of the response to sympathetic impulses and to catecholamines and other adrenergic amines at either the alpha or beta receptor sites of the effector organ or at the postganglionic adrenergic neuron. **adrenergic neuron b.,** see *adrenergic b.* **alpha-adrenergic b., alpha-b.,** see *adrenergic b.* **beta-adrenergic b., beta-b.,** see *adrenergic b.* **cholinergic b.,** selective inhibition of cholinergic nerve impulses at autonomic ganglionic synapses, at postganglionic parasympathetic effectors, or the neuromuscular junction. **narcotic b.,** inhibition of the euphoric effects of narcotic drugs by the use of other drugs, such as methadone, in the treatment of addiction. **neuromuscular b.,** a failure in neuromuscular transmission that can be induced by a variety of disturbances at the myoneural junction. **renal b.,** obstructive uropathy with involvement of the genitourinary system distal to the collecting tubules; blockade of individual nephrons or nephron groups and the resultant anuria. **virus b.,** interference by a virus with the action of another virus; attenuated virus of a disease has been used to inhibit the multiplication of an active virus. Called also *virus interference* and *cell blockade.*

blockage (blok′ij) the process of blocking or obstructing; the condition of being blocked or obstructed. **tendon b.,** fixation of a tendon by a Kirschner wire to bone or tendon sheath to relieve tension and prevent retraction.

Blockain (blok′ān) trademark for a preparation of propoxycaine hydrochloride.

blocker (blok′er) something that blocks or obstructs passage, activity, etc. **α-b.,** a drug that induces adrenergic blockade at α-adrenergic receptors. **β-b.,** a drug that induces adrenergic blockade at either β_1- or β_2-adrenergic receptors or at both. **calcium channel b.,** one of a group of drugs that inhibit the entry of calcium into cells or inhibit the mobilization of calcium from intracellular stores, resulting in slowing of atrioventricular and sinoatrial conduction and relaxation of arterial smooth and cardiac muscle; used in the treatment of angina, cardiac arrhythmias, and hypertension.

blocking (blok′ing) 1. interfering with afferent nerve impulses; see *regional anesthesia,* under *anesthesia.* 2. thought blocking or thought deprivation; sudden cessation of the train of thought that occurs when a repressed painful thought is approached. 3. casting of tissue blocks in an embedding medium such as paraffin wax so that sections can be cut with a microtome. **adrenergic b.,** see under *blockade.* **thought b.,** see *blocking* (def. 2).

blockout (blok′owt) elimination in a master cast of undesirable undercut areas, including all areas that would offer interference to the placement of the denture framework and those not crossed by a rigid part of the denture, accomplished by filling in areas to be blocked out with suitable materials. See also *relief,* def. 4.

Blocq's disease (bloks) [Paul Oscar *Blocq,* French physician, 1860–1896] astasia-abasia.

Blondlot rays (blond-lo′) [Prosper René *Blondlot,* French physicist, 1849–1930] n rays.

blood (blud) [L. *sanguis, cruor;* Gr. *haima*] the fluid that circulates through the heart, arteries, capillaries, and veins, carrying nutriment and oxygen to the body cells; called also *haema* [NA], *hema* [NA alternative], and *sanguis.* It consists of a pale yellow liquid, the *plasma,* containing the microscopically visible formed elements of the blood: the erythrocytes, or red blood corpuscles; the leukocytes, or white blood corpuscles; and the thrombocytes, or blood platelets. **arterial b.,** oxygenated blood, found in the pulmonary veins, the left chambers of the heart, and the systemic arteries; it is bright red in color. **cord b.,** blood contained within the umbilical vessels at the time of delivery of the infant. **defibrinated b.,** whole blood from which fibrin was separated during the clotting process. **laky b.,** blood containing at least some lysed erythrocytes. **occult b.,** blood present in such small quantities that it can be detected only by chemical tests of suspected material, or by microscopic or spectroscopic examination. **peripheral b.,** blood obtained from acral areas, or from the circulation remote from the heart, as from earlobe, fingertip, or heel pad (in a child), or from the antecubital vein; the blood in the systemic circulation. **sludged b.,** blood in which the red cells have become aggregated into masses; it occurs particularly in the smaller blood vessels, where the velocity of blood flow is diminished. **venous b.,** deoxygenated blood, found in the systemic veins, the right chambers of the heart, and the pulmonary arteries; it is dark red in color. **whole b.,** blood from which none of the elements have been removed. *Whole blood* [USP] or *whole human blood* is blood that has been drawn from a selected donor under strict aseptic conditions, containing citrate ion or heparin as an anticoagulant, and used as a blood replenisher.

blood bank (blud bangk) see *bank.*

Bloodgood's disease (blud′goodz) [Joseph Colt *Bloodgood,* Baltimore surgeon, 1866–1935] cystic disease of the breast; see under *disease.*

blood group (blud′ groōp) 1. an erythrocytic allotype (or phenotype) defined by one or more cellular antigenic structural groupings under the control of allelic genes. Erythrocytic antigenic determinants irregularly incite allotypic and sometimes xenotypic immune responses. Blood groups, especially for man, are identified by agglutination supported by specific human or animal antisera and by lectins extracted from certain plants. Bovine blood group reactions, however, are usually lytic. An abbreviated classification of human blood groups is given in the accompanying table. 2. any characteristic, function, or trait of a cellular or fluid component of blood, considered as the expression (phenotype or allotype) of the actions and interactions of dominant genes, and useful in medicolegal and other studies of human inheritance. Such characteristics include the antigenic groupings of erythrocytes, leukocytes, platelets, and plasma proteins. Called also *blood type.* **ABO b. g.,** the major human blood type system, which depends on the presence or absence of two antigenic structures, A and B. The gene for A is responsible for synthesis of *N*-acetyl-α-D-galactosaminyl transferase, whereas that for B is responsible for α-D-galactosyl transferase. Either A or B is created when one of these hexasaccharides is positioned by a specific transferase in $1 \rightarrow 3$ linkage to the β-D-galactose of an H-active oligosaccharide. Type O occurs when neither transferase is present or, very rarely (Bombay type), when H does not exist. When both transferases are present, type AB results. Differences in degree of transferase activity are determined at the same locus: weak transferase gives rise to weak antigens (A_2, A_3 A_x, B_3 B_x). Similar oligosaccharides, especially in bacterial cell walls, immunize persons lacking A or B so that their serum contains anti-A or anti-B activity. A and B antigens are on the mucopolysaccharides of secretors; persons with dominant genes have H-active mucoids. A and B are largely glycolipids in the red cell membrane. **Auberger b. g.,** Au^a, related to the Lutheran blood group. **Cartwright b. g.,** erythrocytic antigens Yt^a and Yt^b. **Diego b. g.,** the blood group antigens Di^a and Di^b, determined by allelic genes. Di^a is most frequent in South American Indians, Japanese, and Chinese. **Dombrock b. g.,** an erythrocytic antigen commonest in whites (65 per cent) but not rare elsewhere. **Duffy b. g.,** a blood group consisting principally of the antigens Fy^a and Fy^b, determined by allelic genes. Amorphic genes are common in blacks. **high frequency b. g.,** erythrocytic antigens found in over 99 per cent of individuals; hence, also known as *public antigens.* **I b. g.,** that involving receptors of most cold reactive hemagglutinins; it is best expressed on cells of almost all normal adults, but is strongest on cord blood cells. **Kell b. g.,** multiple red cell antigens, especially three pairs of alternates, determined by complex genes at one locus, including an amorph; also regulated by the X chromosome, it is associated with sex-linked chronic granulomatous disease. One antigen, K6, is more frequent in

HUMAN BLOOD GROUP SYSTEMS AND ERYTHROCYTIC ANTIGENIC DETERMINANTS

Antigenic determinants are systematized according to observed and assumed independent assortment of their responsible genes. Within many systems, alleles are responsible for differing combinations of antigenic determinants.

BLOOD GROUP SYSTEM	ANTIGENIC DETERMINANTS*
ABO	A, A₁, B
H	H
I	I, i, Iᵀ, Iᴰ, Iᶠ
MN	M, N, S, s, U, Clᵃ, Far, He, Hill, Hu, M `, Mᶜ, Mᵉ, M₁, Miᵃ, Mtᵃ, Mur, M`, Nyᵃ, Riᵃ, Sᴮ, Sj, Stᵃ, Sul, Tm, Uᴮ, Vr, Vw, N `, Z
P	P1, P2 (Tjᵃ), P3 (Pᴷ)
Rh	Rh1 (D, Rhₒ), Rh2 (C, rhʼ), Rh3 (E, rhʼʼ), Rh4 (c, hrʼ), Rh5 (e, hrʼʼ), Rh6 (f, ce, hr), Rh7 (Ce, rhᵢ), Rh8 (Cˣ, rhᵛ), Rh9 (Cˣ, rhˣ), Rh10 (V, ceˢ, hrᵛ), Rh11 (Eˣ, rhˣ²), Rh12 (G, rhᴳ), Rh13 (Rhᴬ), Rh14 (Rhᴮ), Rh15 (Rhᶜ), Rh16 (Rhᴰ), Rh17 (Hrₒ), Rh18 (Hr), Rh19 (hrˢ), Rh20 (VS, eˢ), Rh21 (Cᴳ), Rh22 (CE), Rh23 (Dʷ), Rh24 (Eᵀ), Rh26, Rh27 (cE), Rh28 (hrᴴ), Rh29 (RH), Rh30 (Goᵃ), Rh31 (hrᴮ), Rh32, Rh33
Lutheran	Luᵃ (Lu1), Luᵇ (Lu2), Luᵃᵇ (Lu3), Lu4, Lu5, Lu6, Lu7, Lu8, Lu9, Lu10, Lu11, Lu12, Lu13, Lu14 (Swᵃ)
Kell	K1 (K), K2 (k), K3 (Kpᵃ), K4 (Kpᵇ), K5 (Ku), K6 (Jsᵃ), K7 (Jsᵇ), K8 (kw), K9 (KL), K10 (Ulᵃ), K11, K12, K13, K14, K15, K16
Lewis	Leᵃ (Le1), Leᵇ (Le2), Leˣ (Leᵃᵇ, Le3), Mag (Le4), Leᶜ (Le5), Leᵈ
Duffy	Fyᵃ (Fy1), Fyᵇ (Fy2), Fyᵃᵇ (Fy3), Fy4
Kidd	Jkᵃ (Jk1), Jkᵇ (Jk2), Jkᵃᵇ (Jk3)
Cartwright	Ytᵃ, Ytᵇ
Xg	Xgᵃ
Dombrock	Doᵃ, Doᵇ
Auberger	Auᵃ
Cost-Sterling	Csᵃ, Ykᵃ
Wright	Wrᵃ, Wrᵇ
Diego	Diᵃ, Diᵇ
Vel	Vel 1, Vel 2
Sciana	Sm, Buᵃ
Bg	Bgᵃ, Bgᵇ, Bgᶜ, Ho, Ho-like, Ot, Sto, DBG (similar to HL-A7 of lymphocytes)
Gerbich	Ge1, Ge2, Ge3 (anti-Gel = M.Y.; anti-Ge1,2 = Ge; anti-Ge1,2,3 = Yus)
Coltan	Coᵃ, Coᵇ
Stoltzfus	Sfᵃ

Low-incidence antigenic determinants not thus far associated with a blood group system:

Beᵃ, Bec, Bi, Big Charles, Bpᵃ, Bxᵃ, By, Cad, Chrᵃ, Coates, Craig, Dahl, Donaviesky, Driver, Duch, Evans, Evelyn, Fin, Fuerhart, Gfᵃ, Gilbraith, Good, Green, Hands, Heibel, Hil, Htᵃ, Jeᵃ, Jnᵃ, Job, Kam, Ken, Kosis, Lev, Lwᵃ, McCall, Man, Mar, Moᵃ, Nij, Orr, Ptᵃ, Rdᵃ, Reid, Rm, Skjelbred, Thᵃ, Toᵃ, Trᵃ, Ven, Wb, Weeks, Wu, Yhᵃ, Za, 754

High-incidence antigenic determinants not thus far associated with a blood group system:

Anᵃ, Atᵃ, Bou, Bra, Car, Chido (Gursha), Cip, Dp, El, Enᵃ, Fuj, Gnᵃ Goᵇ, Gyᵃ, Hen, Hy, Joᵃ, Jr, Kelly, Knops, Lan, MZ443, Ola, Pea Savior, Sch, Sdᵃ, Simon, Ters, Todd, Vennera, Wil, Winbourne

Antigenic determinants that depend on gene interactions:

ABO/I	IH, IA, IB, iH
P/I	IP1, IP2(ITjᵃ), IᵀP1, iP1
Lewis/I	ILeᵇʰ
Lewis/ABO	A,Leᵇ
P/ABO	Luke
Xor/Duffy	Fy5
Rh/LW	Rh25 (LW)

*Symbols within parentheses are those of alternative nomenclatures.
(Compiled by Dr. Fred H. Allen, Jr.)

---

blacks. **Kidd b. g.,** a group consisting principally of Jkᵃ and Jkᵇ antigens, determined by allelic genes; amorphic genes are commonest in Orientals. **Lewis b. g.,** a blood group determined by plasma glycolipids which adhere to erythrocytic surfaces. It is based on dominant independent *Le* genes, but interacts with the H precursor oligosaccharides of A and B. Whereas *le/le* provides the "double negative" blood type Le (a–b–), *Le* without H gives rise to Leᵃ, i.e., blood type Le (a+b–) and with H gives rise to LeᵇH, i.e., blood type Le(a–b+). **low frequency b. g.,** erythrocytic antigens found in fewer than 1 per cent of individuals; also known as *private antigens.* **Lutheran b. g.,** a complex system somewhat resembling the Kell group in having pairs of alternative antigens and amorphic genes, but also subject to a dominant independently segregating repressor. **MN b. g.,** a complex system (MNSs) consisting principally of two pairs of antigens determined by closely linked genes (cross-

overs have been observed, but rarely). M and N, determined by allelic genes, depend on sialic (neuraminic) acid residues. S and s are also determined by allelic genes, and an amorphic gene is common in blacks when another antigen (U) is missing. The system also includes numerous low frequency antigens. **P b. g.,** a system originally consisting of only P (now P1) but found to include P2 (Tjᵃ), a very high frequency antigen, and P3 (Pᴷ), a very low frequency antigen. P1 is most common in blacks (90 per cent), less common in Caucasians (75 per cent) and least common in Orientals (30 per cent). **Rh b. g.,** the most complex of all human blood groups because the genes differ by determining a different number of the 33 antigens thus far described, and do so with remarkably different quality. Blacks show the greatest degree of diversity, Orientals the least. The major antigen, Rh1 (RhₒD), is highly immunogenic and, before the development of passive immunization prophylaxis, was responsible for serious hemolytic disease of the newborn. Two other pairs of alternative antigens are inherited with or without Rh1; these are Rh21 (rh^G, C^G) and Rh4 (hr', c), and Rh3 (rh'', E) and Rh5 (hr'', e). The commonest groups of antigens are $R^{1,-3,-21}$ (in Caucasians), $R^{1,-3,-21}$ (in blacks), $R^{1,-3,21}$ (in Orientals and Caucasians), and $R^{1,3,-21}$ (in Orientals and Caucasians). Another antigen Rh10 (hr^v, V) is common in blacks.

bloodless (blud′les) 1. deprived of blood; anemic or exsanguinate. 2. performed with little or no loss of blood.

blood plasma (blud plaz′mah) the liquid portion of the blood in which the particulate components are suspended; see *blood*.

blood pressure (blud presh′ur) see under *pressure*.

bloodroot (blud′rōōt) sanguinaria.

blood serum (blud se′rum) the clear liquid that separates from the blood when it is allowed to clot completely. It is therefore blood plasma from which fibrinogen has been removed in the process of clotting. **glycerin b. s.,** blood serum containing glycerin; called also *glycerin culture medium*. **Löffler′s b. s.,** see *Loeffler coagulated serum m.* in Table of Culture Media.

blood stream, bloodstream (blud′strēm) the blood flowing through the circulatory system in the living body.

blood type (blud′ tīp) see *blood group*.

bloom (blōōm) a surface texture on a colony of microorganisms that appears velvety or powdery owing to aerial projections of hyphae.

Bloom′s syndrome (blōōmz) [David *Bloom*, American dermatologist, born 1892] see under *syndrome*.

blotch (bloch) a blemish or spot.

Blount′s disease (blunts) [W. P. *Blount*, American orthopedic surgeon, born 1900] tibia vara; see under *tibia*.

blowpipe (blo′pīp) a tube through which a current of air or other gas is forced upon a flame to concentrate and intensify the heat.

blue (blōō) 1. one of the principal colors of the spectrum, the color of the sky. 2. having the color of the clear sky. 3. a dye that is blue in color. **alcian b.,** a copper-containing dye for staining acid mucopolysaccharides; it may be combined with periodic acid–Schiff reagent. **alizarin b.,** a blue dyestuff derived from anthracene. **alkali b.,** a dye, sodium triphenylrosaniline monosulfate; called also *isamine b.* **aniline b.,** a mixture of the trisulfonates of triphenyl rosaniline and of diphenyl rosaniline; also known variously as *anthracene b., China b., marine b., soluble b.* (*3M* or *2R*), and *water b.* **aniline b., W. S.,** a mixture of the sulfonation products of mixtures of phenylated rosaniline and pararosaniline, soluble in water. **anthracene b.,** alizarin b. **azidine b., 3 B.,** trypan b. **benzamine b., 3 B.,** trypan b. **benzo b.,** trypan b. **Berlin b.,** Prussian b. **Borrel′s b.,** a silver oxide stain for spirochetes. **brilliant b., C.,** brilliant cresyl b. **brilliant cresyl b.,** an oxazin dye, usually C$_{15}$H$_{16}$N$_3$OCl, used in staining blood; called also *C. brilliant b.* and *cresyl b., R. N* or *B. B. S.* **bromchlorphenol b.,** an indicator, dibrom-dichlor-phenol-sulfonphthalein, (C$_6$H$_2$ClBrOH)$_2$·C$_6$H$_4$·SO$_2$ONa. **bromophenol b.,** a dye, tetrabromophenolsulfonphthalein, used as an indicator in determining hydrogen ion concentration, being yellow at pH 3 and blue at pH 4.6. **bromothymol b.,** a dye, dibromothymolsulfonphthalein, used as an indicator in determining hydrogen ion concentration; it has a pH range of 6.0 to 7.6, being yellow at 6.0 and blue at 7.6. **china b.,** aniline b. **chlorazol b., 3 B.,** trypan b. **Congo b., 3 B.,** trypan b. **cresyl b., 2 R. N.** or **B. B. S.,** brilliant cresyl b. **cyanol b.,** a bright blue acid coal tar color related to triphenylmethane. **diamine b.,** trypan b. **dianil b., H. 3 G.,** trypan b. **Evans b.,** a green, bluish green, or brown odorless powder, C$_{34}$H$_{24}$N$_6$Na$_4$O$_{14}$S$_4$, injected intravenously in determining blood volume; called also *T-1824.* **Helvetia b.,** methyl b. **indigo b.,** indigotin. **indigo b., soluble,** indigotin disulfonate sodium. **indophenol b.,** the blue pigment produced in the Nadi reaction and in the indophenol test; it is (CH$_3$)$_2$N·C$_6$H$_4$·N:C$_{10}$H$_6$:O. **isamine b.,** alkali b. **Kühne′s methylene b.,** a mixture of methylene blue and dehydrated alcohol in phenol solution. **Löffler′s methylene b.,** a mixture of methylene blue and alcohol in aqueous solution of potassium hydroxide. **marine b.,** aniline b. **methyl b.,** a dark blue powder, sodium triphenyl-para-rosaniline sulfonate, formerly used as an antiseptic.

Called also *Helvetia b.* **methylene b.** [USP], 3,7-bis-(dimethylamino)phenazothionium chloride. Dark green crystals or crystalline powder having a bronze-like luster, C$_{16}$H$_{18}$-ClN$_3$S·3H$_2$O, used as a stain and as an indicator; also used in treatment of methemoglobinemia. Called also *Swiss b.* and *methylthionine chloride.* **methylene b., N. N.,** new methylene blue, N. **methylene b., O.,** toluidine blue, O. **naphthamine b., 3 B. X.,** trypan b. **new methylene b., N.,** C$_2$H$_5$·NH(CH$_3$)C$_6$H$_2$(SN)C$_6$H$_2$(CH$_3$)N(C$_2$H$_5$)HCl. Called also *methylene blue, N. N.* **Niagara b., 3 B.,** trypan b. **Nile b., A., Nile b. sulfate,** an oxazin dye which stains fatty acids blue; it is (C$_2$H$_5$)$_2$N·C$_6$H$_3$(ON)C$_{10}$H$_5$··NH$_2$·(SO$_4$)$_\frac{1}{2}$. **polychrome methylene b.,** a mixture of methylene green, methylene azure, methylene violet, and methylene blue. **Prussian b.,** an amorphous blue powder, Fe$_4$[Fe(CN)$_6$]$_3$; called also *Berlin b.* **pyrrole b.,** C$_4$-H$_4$N·C[C$_6$H$_4$·N(CH$_3$)$_2$]$_2$. **quinaldine b.,** chemical name: 1-ethyl-2-[3-(1-ethyl-2(1*H*) quinolylidene) propenyl] quinolinium chloride. A bright blue-green stain, C$_{25}$H$_{25}$ClN$_2$, used in the cytodiagnosis of ruptured fetal membranes. **soluble b., 3 M.** or **2 R.,** aniline b. **spirit b.,** a mixture of diphenylrosaniline, C$_6$H$_5$·NHCl·C$_6$H$_4$·C[C$_6$H$_3$(CH$_3$)NH$_2$]C$_6$-H$_4$·NH·C$_6$H$_5$, and triphenylrosaniline, C$_6$H$_5$·NHCl·C$_6$H$_4$C[C$_6$H$_4$(CH$_3$)NH·C$_6$H$_5$] C$_6$H$_4$·NH·C$_6$H$_5$. **Swiss b.,** methylene b. **thymol b.,** an indicator, thymolsulfonphthalein, with an acid pH range of 1.2 to 2.8, being red at 1.2 and yellow at 2.8, and an alkaline pH range of 8.0 to 9.6, being yellow at 8.0 and blue at 9.6. **toluidine b., toluidine b., O,** the chloride salt or zinc chloride double salt of aminodimethylaminotoluphenazthionium chloride; useful as a stain for demonstrating basophilic and metachromatic substances. Called also *methylene blue, O.* **trypan b.,** an acid, azo dye that has been used in vital staining and as a remedy in protozoan infections; it is the sodium salt of toluidin-diazo-diamino-naphthol-disulfonic acid, [CH$_3$·C$_6$H$_3$·N:N··C$_{10}$H$_3$(NH$_2$)(SO$_2$·ONa)$_2$·OH]$_2$. Variously known as *azidine b., 3 B; benzamine b., 3 B; benzo b.; chlorazol b.; Congo b., 3 B; diamine b.; dianil b., H. 3G.; naphthamine b., 3 B. X.;* and *Niagara b., 3 B. X.* **Victoria b.,** a triphenylmethane dye with bacteriostatic properties; it is a phenyltetramethyl-triaminotriphenylmethane chloride, C$_6$H$_5$·NH(Cl)C$_6$H$_4$:C[C$_6$H$_4$·N(CH$_3$)$_2$]$_2$Cl. **b. vitriol,** cupric sulfate. **water b.,** aniline b.

bluensomycin (blu″en-so-mi′sin) an antibiotic substance obtained from cultures of *Streptomyces bluensis,* or the same substance produced by other means.

bluestone (blu′stōn) cupric sulfate.

bluetongue (bloo′tung) a viral disease of sheep, cattle, goats, and wild ruminants, transmitted by biting flies of the genus *Culicoides;* the etiologic agent, the bluetongue virus, is an orbivirus; clinical manifestations include fever and inflammation, and ulceration and necrosis of the tongue, lips, and dental pads.

Blum′s syndrome (bloomz) [Paul *Blum*, Strasbourg physician, 1878–1933] hypochloremic azotemia.

Blumberg (blum′berg), Baruch Samuel. American physician, born 1925; co-winner, with Daniel Carleton Gajdusek, of the Nobel prize for medicine or physiology in 1976 for their discoveries of new mechanisms for the origin and dissemination of infectious diseases, specifically hepatitis B virus.

Blumberg′s sign (blum′bergz) [Jacob Moritz *Blumberg,* surgeon and gynecologist in Berlin, and later in London, 1873–1955] see under *sign*.

Blumenau′s nucleus (bloo′men-owz) [Leonid Wassiljewitsch *Blumenau,* Russian neurologist, 1862–1931] see under *nucleus*.

Blumenbach′s clivus, plane, process (bloo′men-bahks) [Johann Friedrich *Blumenbach,* German physiologist, 1752–1840] see *clivus* and *processus uncinatus ossis ethmoidalis,* and see under *plane*.

Blumenthal′s disease (bloo′men-tahlz) [Ferdinand *Blumenthal,* German physician, born 1870] erythroleukemia.

blunthook (blunt′hook) an instrument used mainly in embryotomy.

blush (blush) sudden, brief erythema of the face and neck, resulting from vascular dilatation due to emotion or heat.

Blutene (bloo′tēn) trademark for a preparation of tolonium.

B.M.A. British Medical Association.

B.M.R. basal metabolic rate.

B.M.S.   Bachelor of Medical Science.

BNA   abbreviation for *Basle Nomina Anatomica*, the anatomical terminology accepted at Basel, Switzerland, in 1895; superseded by *Nomina Anatomica*.

B.O.A.   British Orthopaedic Association.

board (bord)   1. a long flat piece of wood or other material. 2. a group of administrators or experts serving a special function.   **angle b.,** in dental radiology, a device used to facilitate the establishment of reproducible angular relationships between a patient's head and the plane of an x-ray film.

Boas' algesimeter, etc. (bo′az) [Ismar Isidor *Boas,* physician in Berlin, 1858–1938] see under *algesimeter, point, test,* and *test meal.*

Boas-Oppler bacillus (bo′az op′ler) [Ismar Isidor *Boas;* Bruno *Oppler,* German physician of the 19th century] see under *bacillus.*

Bochdalek's duct, foramen (gap, sinus), ganglion (pseudoganglion), hernia, valve (bok′dal-eks) [Vincent Alexander *Bochdalek,* anatomist in Prague, 1801–1883] see *ductus thyroglossalis, hiatus pleuroperitonealis,* and *plexus dentalis superior,* and see under *hernia* and *valve.*

Bock's ganglion, nerve (boks) [August Carl *Bock,* German anatomist, 1782–1833] see *carotid ganglion,* under *ganglion,* and see *rami pharyngei nervi vagi,* under *ramus.*

Bockhart's impetigo (bok′harts) [Max *Bockhart,* German physician of the nineteenth century] see under *impetigo.*

Bodansky unit (bo-dan′ske) [Aaron *Bodansky,* American biochemist, 1887–1961] see under *unit.*

bodenplatte (bo″den-plaht′tĕ) [Ger.]   floor plate.

Bodo (bo′do)   a genus of ovoid but plastic, free-living, anaerobic or microaerophilic, biflagellate protozoa (suborder Bodonina, order Kinetoplastida), commonly found in sea and fresh water and in stagnant and sewage-polluted water, or they may be coprozoic; they feed on bacteria. The genus comprises numerous species, none of which are human pathogens.

Bodonina (bo″do-ni′nah)   a suborder of typically biflagellate protozoa, with one flagellum directed anteriorly and the other posteriorly, parasitic or free-living (order Kinetoplastida, class Zoomastigophorea), usually with a DNA-containing adbasal kinetoplast, which is often large, or with the DNA arranged in several discrete bodies or dispersed throughout the mitochondrion. Representative genera include *Bodo* and *Cryptobia.*

body (bod′e)   1. the trunk, or animal frame, with its organs. 2. a cadaver or corpse.   3. the largest and most important part of any organ; see also *corpus* and *soma.*   4. any mass or collection of material.   **acetone b's,** ketone b's.   **adipose b. of cheek,** corpus adiposum buccae.   **adipose b. of ischiorectal fossa,** corpus adiposum fossae ischiorectalis.   **adipose b. of orbit,** corpus adiposum orbitae.   **adrenal b.,** adrenal gland.   **alkapton b's,** a class of substances with an affinity for alkali, found in the urine and causing the condition known as alkaptonuria; the compound commonly found, and most commonly referred to by the term, is homogentisic acid.   **Amato b's,** irregular, pale-staining, blue cytoplasmic clumps, occurring in neutrophils of patients with various infectious diseases, such as diphtheria, scarlet fever, and pneumonia, and probably identical with Döhle bodies.   **amygdaloid b.,** corpus amygdaloideum.   **amylaceous b's, amyloid b's,** corpora amylacea.   **anococcygeal b.,** ligamentum anococcygeum.   **aortic b.,** any of the small bodies whose structure is similar to the structure of carotid bodies. Aortic bodies occur near the arch of the aorta, the ductus arteriosus, and the right subclavian arteries, and are supplied by branches of the vagus nerve. They are believed to function as chemoreceptors. Called also *aortic glomus, glomus aorticum,* and *vagal body.*   **apical b.,** acrosome.   **b's of Arantius,** nodules of aortic valve; see *noduli valvularum semilunarium.*   **Arnold's b's** (*obs.*), small pieces of erythrocytes in the blood, or red cell shadows.   **asbestos b's, asbestosis b's,** golden yellow bodies of various shapes formed by the deposition of calcium and iron salts and proteins on a spicule of asbestos, occurring in the sputum, lung secretion, and feces of patients with asbestosis. Cf. *ferruginous b's.*   **Aschoff b's,** submiliary collections of cells and leukocytes in the interstitial tissues of the heart in rheumatic myocarditis; called also *Aschoff's nodules.*   **asteroid b.,** an irregularly star-shaped inclusion body found in the giant cells in sarcoidosis

and also found in numerous other diseases.   **Auer b's,** finely granular, lamellar bodies having acid-phosphatase activity; they are found in the cytoplasm of myeloblasts, myelocytes, monoblasts, and granular histiocytes, and rarely in plasma cells, but are absent in lymphoblasts or lymphocytes. Their presence is virtually pathognomonic of leukemia.   **Babès-Ernst b.,** metachromatic granule.   **Balbiani's b.,** yolk nucleus.   **Balfour b's,** *Aegyptianella pullorum.*   **bamboo b.,** asbestos b's.   **Barr b.,** sex chromatin.   **basal b.,** one of the cylindrical cytoplasmic bodies structurally resembling the centriole, from which it originates, located on the subsurface of flagellate protozoa and giving rise to the axoneme. Basal bodies are connected together in longitudinal rows by bundles of fibrils called kinetodesmata. Called also *basal granule, blepharoplast,* and *kinetosome.* See also *kinetoplast* and *parabasal b.*   **Behla's b's,** Plimmer's b's.   **Bence Jones b's,** Bence Jones protein; see under *protein.*   **bigeminal b's** (*obs.*), superior and inferior colliculi.   **Bollinger's b's,** inclusion bodies found in all tissue cells in fowlpox; called also *Bollinger's granules.* Cf. *Borrel b's.*   **Borrel b's,** minute granules composing the Bollinger bodies of fowlpox.   **Bracht-Wächter b's,** non-specific inflammatory foci of lymphocytic and mononuclear cells in the myocardium, observed in bacterial endocarditis.   **brassy b.,** a dark, shrunken blood corpuscle seen in malaria.   **Cabot's ring b's,** lines in the form of loops or figures of eight, possibly remnants of the nuclear membrane, seen in stained erythrocytes in severe anemias; they are stained red with the Wright-Leishman stain and blue with eosinate of methylthionine chlorides.   **Call-Exner b's,** the accumulations of densely staining material that appear among granulosa cells in maturing ovarian follicles and that may be intracellular precursors of follicular fluid; also seen in ovarian tumors of granulosal origin.   **cancer b's,** see *Plimmer's b's,* and *Russell b's.*   **carotid b.,** glomus caroticum.   **cavernous b. of clitoris,** corpus cavernosum clitoridis.   **cavernous b. of penis,** corpus cavernosum penis.   **cell b.,** that portion of a cell which contains the nucleus, independent of any such projections as an axon or dendrites which the cell may have.   **central b.,** the structures at the center of the aster during mitosis.   **central fibrous b. of heart,** trigonum fibrosum dextrum cordis.   **b. of cerebellum,** corpus cerebelli.   **chromaffin b.,** paraganglion.   **chromatin b's,** chromatinic b's.   **chromatinic b.,** the genetic material of bacteria. See nucleoid (def. 3).   **chromatoid b.,** 1. one of the dense accumulations of RNA found in the cysts of certain amebae (e.g., *Entamoeba* species), manifested as a deeply staining rodlike body. Called also *chromatoid bar.* 2. a dense chromatoid mass near the distal centriole of a spermatozoon, from which the so-called ring centriole seemingly arises.   **chromophilous b's,** Nissl b's.   **ciliary b.,** corpus ciliare.   **coccoid x b's,** minute bodies found in the blood in psittacosis.   **coccygeal b.,** glomus coccygeum.   **colostrum b's,** colostrum corpuscles.   **Councilman b's,** acidophilic round bodies of hepatocellular origin seen in viral hepatitis, yellow fever, and other hepatic diseases; called also *Councilman's lesions.*   **crystalloid b.,** a body near the nuclei of the cells of the seminiferous tubules.   **cytoid b's,** globular, shiny white structures resembling cell nuclei in size and shape, appearing in degenerated retinal nerve fibers; seen histologically in cotton-wool spots.   **Deetjen's b's,** blood platelets.   **demilune b.,** achromocyte.   **dense b's,** small regions of increased density in the sarcoplasm of skeletal muscles to which myofilaments seem to attach; cf. *attachment plaques,* under *plaque.*   **denticulate b.** (*obs.*), gyrus dentatus.   **Döhle's b's, Döhle's inclusion b's,** discrete, round or oval, blue-staining inclusions seen in the periphery of the cytoplasm of neutrophils, consisting mainly of RNA derived from rough endoplasmic reticulum, found in association with many infections, burns, aplastic anemia, uncomplicated pregnancy, and after administration of toxic agents. Similar structures, which are often larger and more prominent, are present in granulocytes other than neutrophils in the May-Hegglin anomaly. Called also *leukocyte inclusions.*   **Donné's b's,** colostrum corpuscles.   **Donovan's b.,** *Calymmatobacterium granulomatis.*   **Dutcher b.,** an intranuclear invagination of immunoglobulin-containing cytoplasm found in neoplastic plasmacytoid lymphocytes and plasma cells.   **Ehrlich's hemoglobinemic b's** (*obs.*), dark bodies, occurring in the center of degenerated red cells but which do not represent true red cell inclusions.   **elementary b.,** 1. a blood platelet. 2. an inclusion body.

Elschnig b's, clear grapelike clusters formed by proliferation of epithelial cells after extracapsular extraction of a cataractous lens; called also *Elschnig's pearls.* **epithelial b.,** parathyroid gland. **ferruginous b's,** structures similar to asbestos bodies, composed of a central mineral filament coated with a protein-iron complex. **fibrin b's of pleura,** movable or adherent, round, homogeneous, sharply demarcated opacities near the base of the pleural cavity, which may occur secondary to pleural effusion, pneumothorax, or hemopneumothorax; called also *pleural fibrin balls.* **filling b's,** fullkörper. **foreign b.,** a mass or particle of material that is not normal to the place where it is found. **b. of fornix,** corpus fornicis. **fruiting b.,** a specialized structure, as an apothecium, which produces spores; see Plate accompanying *mold.* **fuchsin b's,** Russell's b's. **b. of gallbladder,** corpus vesicae biliaris. **gamma-Favre b's,** small intracytoplasmic inclusion bodies found in lymphogranuloma venereum. **gastric b.,** corpus gastricum. **geniculate b.,** see *corpus geniculatum laterale* and *corpus geniculatum mediale.* **Giannuzzi's b's,** crescents of Giannuzzi. **glomus b.,** anastomosis arteriovenosa glomeriformis. **Golgi b.,** see under *complex.* **Gordon's elementary b.,** a particle originally thought to be the viral cause of Hodgkin's disease, but later shown to be obtainable from any tissue containing eosinophils or involved with this neoplasm; called also *Gordon's encephalopathic agent.* **Guarnieri's b's,** inclusion bodies in the cells of the affected tissues in smallpox and vaccinia, regarded as caused by the reaction of the cell to the virus of the disease; called also *Guarnieri's corpuscles.* **habenular b.,** habenula, def. 2. **Halberstaedter-Prowazek b's,** trachoma b's. **Harting b's,** deposits of calcium (calcospherites) in the cerebral capillaries. **Hassall's b's,** Hassall's corpuscles. **Hassall-Henle b's,** see under *wart.* **Heinz b's, Heinz-Ehrlich b's,** coccoid inclusion bodies resulting from oxidative injury to and precipitation of hemoglobin, seen in the presence of certain abnormal hemoglobins (HHb H, Köln, etc.) and erythrocytes with enzyme deficiencies. Refractile in fresh blood smears, they are not visible when stained with Romanowsky dyes but may be stained supravitally. Called also *Heinz granules.* See also *Heinz-body anemia.* **Hensen's b.,** a rounded modified Golgi net under the cuticle of an outer hair cell of the organum spirale. **Herring b's,** hyaline or colloid masses scattered throughout the pars nervosa of the pituitary gland. **b. of Highmore,** mediastinum testis. **Howell's b's,** Howell-Jolly b's. **Howell-Jolly b's,** smooth, round remnants of nuclear chromatin seen in erythrocytes in megaloblastic anemia, hemolytic anemia, and after splenectomy. Called also *Howell's b's* and *Jolly's b's.* **hyaline b's,** drusen. **hyaloid b.,** vitreous body (corpus vitreum [NA]). **immune b.,** antibody. **inclusion b's,** round, oval, or irregular-shaped bodies occurring in the cytoplasm and nuclei of cells of the body, as in disease caused by filtrable virus infection such as rabies, smallpox, herpes, etc.; called also *elementary b's* and *intranuclear inclusions.* **infrapatellar fatty b.,** corpus adiposum infrapatellare. **infundibular b.,** posterior lobe of the pituitary gland (lobus posterior hypophyseos [NA]). **inner b's,** round bodies seen in erythrocytes after certain stainings, such as Ehrlich's hemoglobinemic bodies, Heinz-Ehrlich bodies, and Schmauch's bodies. **intermediate b. of Flemming,** a small bridge of acidophil material connecting the two daughter cells for a time at the end of mitosis. **interrenal b.,** an elongated organ that lies between the kidneys in elasmobranch fishes and that corresponds to the adrenal medulla in mammals. **intravertebral b.,** corpus vertebrae. **Jaworski b's,** see under *corpuscle.* **Joest's b's,** intranuclear inclusion bodies found in the brain of animals with Borna disease. **Jolly's b's,** Howell-Jolly b's. **jugulotympanic b.,** tympanic b. **juxtarestiform b.,** a structure connecting the lateral vestibular nucleus with the nucleus fastigii and conveying vestibular impulses. **ketone b's,** the substances β-hydroxybutyric acid, acetoacetic acid, and acetone, which are produced by fatty acid and carbohydrate metabolism in the liver in approximately a 78:20:2 ratio. Acetoacetate is produced from acetyl-CoA; most is enzymatically converted to β-ketobutyrate, but a small amount is spontaneously decarboxylated to acetone. The ketone bodies can be used as fuels by muscle and brain tissue. In starvation and uncontrolled diabetes mellitus, large quantities are produced causing metabolic acidosis and elevated blood and urine levels of all three ketone bodies. **Kur-**

loff's b's, bodies seen in the large mononuclear leukocytes of guinea pigs and related rodents. Observations with the electron microscope indicate that they probably result from intracellular secretion or from a sequestering and concentration of a serum molecular component. **Lafora's b's,** intracytoplasmic inclusions consisting of a complex of glycoprotein and acid mucopolysaccharide; widespread deposits of these bodies are found in myoclonus epilepsy. **Lallemand's b's, Lallemand-Trousseau b's,** Bence Jones cylinders. **L.C.L. b's,** minute coccoid bodies found in tissue infected with psittacosis; called also *Levinthal-Coles-Lillie b's.* **Leishman-Donovan b.,** amastigote. **lenticular b.** (*obs.*), nucleus lentiformis. **Levinthal-Coles-Lillie b's,** L.C.L. b's. **Lewy b's,** concentrically laminated, round bodies found in vacuoles in the cytoplasm of some of the neurons of the midbrain in paralysis agitans. **Lieutaud's b.,** trigonum vesicae. **Lindner's initial b's,** cytoplasmic elementary bodies, resembling those in trachomatous epithelia, found in inclusion conjunctivitis of newborns. **Lipschütz b's,** intranuclear inclusion bodies found in the lesions of herpes simplex, both in the epithelial cells of the primary skin lesion (skin or cornea) and in the affected nerve cells. **Lostorfer's b's,** Lostorfer's corpuscles. **Luschka's b.,** glomus coccygeum. **Luys' b.,** nucleus subthalamicus. **lyssa b's,** red staining masses somewhat resembling Negri bodies but less sharply defined and with less internal structure. **Mallory's b's,** 1. hyaline endoplasmic reticulum within hepatocytes in nutritional cirrhosis. 2. bodies in the lymph spaces and epidermal cells in scarlet fever. **malpighian b's of kidney,** corpuscula renis. **malpighian b's of spleen,** folliculi lymphatici splenici. **mamillary b., mammillary b.,** corpus mamillare. **Marchal b's,** cell inclusion bodies observed in ectromelia. **Masson b's,** the cellular components that fill the pulmonary alveoli and alveolar ducts in rheumatic pneumonia; they are possibly the equivalent of modified Aschoff bodies. **medullary b. of cerebellum,** corpus medullare cerebelli. **medullary b. of vermis,** arbor vitae cerebelli. **melon-seed b.,** any of a class of small fibrous masses sometimes occurring in the joints and in cysts of the tendon sheaths. **metachromatic b's,** metachromatic granules. **Michaelis-Gutmann b's,** bodies found in the lesion of malacoplakia of the bladder. **mitochondrial b.,** a fused colony of mitochondria found in the spermatids of insects. **molluscum b's,** large homogeneous intracytoplasmic inclusions found in the stratum granulosum and stratum corneum in molluscum contagiosum, which contain replicating virions and cellular debris. **Mooser b's,** bodies resembling rickettsiae, seen in the epithelial cells of the tunica vaginalis exudate in some forms of typhus. **Mörner's b.,** nucleoalbumin. **Mott b's,** clear globules present in the cytoplasm of plasma cells in multiple myeloma. **multilamellar b.,** any of the osmiophilic, lipid-rich, layered bodies found in the type II alveolar cells of the lung; called also *cytosome.* **multivesicular b.,** a secondary lysosome manifested as a spherical, membrane-bound vacuole, containing numerous small vesicles in a matrix that exhibits acid phosphatase activity. **Negri b's,** oval or round inclusion bodies, seen in the cytoplasm and sometimes in the processes of nerve cells of rabid animals after death; their presence is considered conclusive proof of rabies. **Neill-Mooser b.,** large mononuclear cells filled with rickettsiae, seen in the inflammatory exudate of the scrotal swelling of laboratory animals infected with murine typhus. See also under *reaction.* **nigroid b.,** granula iridica of the equine or bovine iris. **Nissl b's,** large granular basophilic bodies found in the cytoplasm of neurons, composed of rough endoplasmic reticulum and free polyribosomes; called also *chromophilous b's, tigroid b's, chromophil corpuscles* or *substance,* and *chromatic granules.* **Nothnagel's b's,** oval or round bodies, plain or striated, from 15 to 60 μ in diameter, sometimes found in the stools of persons who eat meat. **no-threshold b's,** no-threshold substances. **Odland b.,** keratinosome. **Oken's b's,** mesonephros. **olivary b.,** oliva. **onion b's,** epithelial pearls. **oryzoid b's,** rice b's. **pacchionian b's,** granulationes arachnoideales. **pampiniform b.,** epoöphoron. **Pappenheimer b's,** basophilic iron-containing granules observed in various types of erythrocytes. **para-aortic b's,** corpora paraaortica; see also *paraganglion.* **parabasal b.,** a cytoplasmic body of various appearance, structure, and function closely associated with the nucleus, kinetoplast, and basal body in certain parasitic flagellate protozoa; it is usually connected to the basal body by a fibril or thread, which together are known as the *parabasal apparatus*. More than one such structure may be present in each organism. Some authorities consider the parabasal body to be the Golgi complex of these cells. **paranuclear b.,** centrosome. **paraphyseal b.,** paraphysis (def. 1). **pararenal b., pararenal fatty b.,** corpus adiposum pararenale. **paraterminal b.,** gyrus paraterminalis. **parathyroid b.,** a parathyroid gland. **parietal b.,** epiphyseal eye. **parolivary b's,** accessory olivary nuclei; see *nucleus olivaris accessorius dorsalis* and *medialis.* **Paschen b's,** inclusion bodies in the cells of the tissues in variola and vaccinia; they are infective but whether they are the infective agents or mechanical carriers of the invisible virus is not known. Called also *Paschen's corpuscles* or *granules.* **pearly b's,** epithelial pearls. **perineal b.,** centrum tendineum perinei. **pheochrome b.,** paraganglion. **Pick b's,** filamentous intracytoplasmic inclusions seen in neurons in Pick's disease (def. 1). **pineal b.,** 1. a small, somewhat flattened, cone-shaped body (*corpus pineale* [NA]) in the epithalamus, lying above the superior colliculi and below the splenium of the corpus callosum. Arising embryologically from the ependyma of the third ventricle of the brain and consisting of cords of pinealocytes supported by interstitial cells, it is the site of synthesis of melatonin, which inhibits gonad development and influences estrus in mammals and produces lightening of the dermal pigmentation in amphibians by stimulating the aggregation of melanosomes into melanophores. Its hormonal function in human physiology is not firmly established. Melatonin secretion is diminished during exposure to environmental light; the pineal body synthesizes and releases melatonin in response to norepinephrine, whose rate of release declines when light activates retinal photoreceptors. Called also *epiphysis cerebri, glandula pinealis* [NA alternative], and *pineal gland.* 2. the posterior eyelike structure arising from the median of the dorsal wall of the thalamus in some lower vertebrates. See also *epiphyseal eye,* under *eye.* **pituitary b.,** pituitary gland. **Plimmer's b's,** small round capsulated bodies found in cancer, and thought by the discoverer to be the parasite causing the disease; called also *Behla's b's* and *cancer b's.* **polar b's,** 1. the small abortive cells with a haploid chromosome complement, consisting of a tiny piece of cytoplasm and a nucleus, resulting from unequal division of the primary oocyte (*first polar b.*) and, if fertilization occurs, of the secondary oocyte (*second polar b.*); the polar body appears as a speck at the animal pole of the egg. 2. metachromatic granules located at one or both ends of a bacterial cell. **postbranchial b's,** ultimobranchial b's. **presegmenting b's,** malarial parasites (*Plasmodium*) before they undergo segmentation. **Prowazek's b's,** 1. trachoma bodies. 2. extremely small inclusion bodies found in the material from smallpox pustules and in cowpox vaccine and regarded by Prowazek as the cause of the disease. **Prowazek-Greeff b's,** trachoma b's. **psammoma b.,** a spherical, concentrically laminated mass of calcareous material, usually of microscopic size; such bodies occur in both benign and malignant epithelial and connective-tissue tumors, and are sometimes associated with chronic inflammation. **pseudolutein b.,** corpus atretica. **purine b's,** purine bases. **pyknotic b's,** bodies in the mucus of stools in amebiasis; they are the nuclear remains of tissue cells and leukocytes. **quadrigeminal b's,** corpora quadrigemina. **Reilly b's,** large, coarse granulations found in the leukocytes in Hurler's syndrome. **Renaut's b's,** pale granules in the degenerating nerve fibers in muscular dystrophy. **residual b.,** 1. a secondary lysosome that has completed its digestive processes but retains indigestible or very slowly digestible material. 2. residuum, def. 2. **residual b. of Regnaud,** an anucleate mass consisting of fine granules, lipid droplets, and degenerating organelles, cast off after the completion of regional differentiation of the tail during spermiogenesis. **restiform b.,** pedunculus cerebellaris caudalis. **b. of Retzius,** a protoplasmic mass containing pigment granules at the lower end of a hair cell of the organum spirale. **rice b's,** small bodies resembling grains of rice which form in the tendons of joints and in the fluid of hygroma; called also *oryzoid b's,* and *corpora oryzoidea.* **Rosenmüller's b.,** epoöphoron. **Ross's b's,** spherical copper-colored bodies showing dark granulations and sometimes having ameboid movements; seen in the blood and tissue fluids in syphilis. **Russell b's,** globular

plasma cell inclusions, mucoprotein in nature, containing surface gamma globulin, and representing aggregates of immunoglobulins synthesized by the cell; called also *cancer b's* and *fuchsin b's.* **sand b's,** acervulus. **Sandström's b's,** parathyroid glands. **Schaumann's b's,** the red or brown, nodular, shell-like lesions of sarcoidosis. **Schmorl b.,** a portion of the nucleus pulposus that has protruded into an adjoining vertebra. **Seidelin b's,** a name once applied to structures observed in the red cells in yellow fever, believed by the discoverer to be the cause of the disease. **semilunar b's,** crescents of Giannuzzi. **spongy b. of male urethra,** corpus spongiosum penis. **spongy b. of penis,** corpus cavernosum penis. **Stieda b.,** an ultrastructural organelle located at the polar region of the sporocyst of certain coccidia, appearing as a knoblike structure or representing a plug occluding a hole in the sporocyst, the breakdown of which allows excystation of the sporozoites. **b. of stomach,** corpus gastricum. **striate b.,** corpus striatum. **supracardial b's,** aortic paraganglia. **suprarenal b.,** adrenal gland. **Symington's b.,** ligamentum anococcygeum. **telobranchial b's,** ultimobranchial b's. **threshold b's,** threshold substances. **thyroid b.,** thyroid gland (glandula thyroidea [NA]). **tigroid b's,** Nissl b's. **Todd b's,** eosinophilic structures formed in the cytoplasm of the red cells of certain amphibians. **Torres-Teixeira b's,** inclusion bodies found in the cells in variola minor. **trachoma b's,** inclusion bodies found in clusters in the cytoplasm of the epithelial cells from the conjunctiva of trachomatous eye; called also *Halberstaedter-Prowazek b's, Prowazek's b's,* and *Prowazek-Greeff b's.* **trapezoid b.,** corpus trapezoideum. **Trousseau-Lallemand b's,** Bence Jones cylinders. **tympanic b.,** an ovoid body occurring in the adventitia of the upper part of the superior bulb of the internal jugular vein; its structure and presumably its function are similar to those of the glomus caroticum (carotid body). Called also *glomus jugulare, jugular glomus,* and *jugulotympanic body.* See also *glomus jugulare tumor,* under *tumor.* **ultimobranchial b's,** embryonic derivatives of the fifth pharyngeal pouches, which migrate along with the parathyroid glands and are incorporated in the thyroid gland; in submammalian vertebrates they remain as discrete masses in the neck or mediastinum throughout adult life. The parafollicular cells of these bodies produce calcitonin. Called also *postbranchial b's* and *telobranchial b's.* **vagal b.,** aortic b. **vermiform b's,** peculiar sinuous invaginations of the plasma membrane of Kupffer cells of the liver, having a central linear density between parallel membranes and a faint transverse striation; similar structures are seen in macrophages of certain organs and in the Langerhans cells of the epidermis. **Verocay b's,** small groups of fibrils surrounded by rows of palisaded nuclei, seen in schwannomas. **vitelline b.,** yolk nucleus. **vitreous b.,** the transparent gel that fills the inner portion of the eyeball between the lens and the retina; called also *corpus vitreum* [NA], *hyaloid b., humor cristallinus,* and *crystalline* or *vitreous humor.* **watchglass b.,** see under *organelle.* **Winkler's b.,** spherical bodies seen in the lesions of syphilis. **wolffian b.,** mesonephros. **xanthine b's,** purine bases. **yellow b. of ovary,** corpus luteum. **zebra b.,** concentric, laminated, figure-like, cytoplasmic inclusions of Schwann cells, occurring singly or in clusters as a result of degeneration phenomena. **Zuckerkandl's b's,** paraganglia found along the course of the aorta near its bifurcation.

body rocking (bod′e rok′ing)   a rhythmic backward and forward motion in a sitting position.

body snatching (bod′e snach′ing)   the illegal procural of dead bodies, especially the robbing of a grave of a recently buried corpse.

Boeck's disease, sarcoid (beks) [Caesar P. M. *Boeck,* Norwegian dermatologist and syphilologist, 1845–1917]   sarcoidosis.

Boerhaave's syndrome (boor′hahv-ēz) [Hermann *Boerhaave,* Dutch physician, 1668–1738]   see under *syndrome.*

Boettcher (bet′sher)   see *Böttcher.*

Boettger   see *Böttger.*

Bogros' space (bōg-rōz′) [Annet Jean *Bogros,* French anatomist, 1786–1823]   see under *space.*

Bohr effect (bor) [Christian *Bohr,* Scandinavian physiologist, 1855–1911]   see under *effect.*

Bohun upas (bo'hun u'pas)   the poison tree of Java, *Antiaris toxicaria*.

boil (boil)   furuncle.   **Aleppo b., Bagdad b., Biskra b.,** the Old World form of cutaneous leishmaniasis.   **blind b.,** a boil that does not develop a white or yellow "head" at its apex through which pus may be discharged; an abscess.   **Delhi b.,** cutaneous leishmaniasis.   **gum b.,** parulis.   **Jericho b.,** the Old World form of cutaneous leishmaniasis.   **Oriental b.,** the Old World form of cutaneous leishmaniasis.   **shoe b.,** capped elbow in the horse.

Bol.   abbreviation for L. *bo'lus*, pill.

bolasterone (bōl-ah'ster-ōn)   chemical name: 17β-hydroxy-7α,17-dimethylandrost-4-en-3-one; an anabolic agent, $C_{21}H_{32}O_2$.

boldenone undecylenate (bōl'dĕ-nōn)   chemical name: 17β-hydroxyandrosta-1,4-dien-3-one 10-undecenoate; an anabolic agent, $C_{30}H_{44}O_3$.

boldine (bol-dēn')   an alkaloid from *Peumus* (*Boldu*) *boldus* Molina (Monimiaceae), which possesses diuretic properties.

boldo (bol'do) [L. *boldus, boldoa*]   the leaves and stems of *Peumus* (*Boldu*) *boldus* Molina (Monimiaceae), a Chilean evergreen shrub. Once official in the U.S. National Formulary (1936) and still common in numerous over-the-counter remedies in Canada and other countries, it contains over 15 alkaloids and is used variously as a choleretic, diuretic, stomachic, sedative, and anthelmintic.

boldoa (bol'do-ah) [L.]   boldo.

boldoin (bol'do-in)   a glycoside obtainable from boldo.

bolenol (bōl'ĕ-nōl)   chemical name: 19-nor-17α-pregn-5-en-17-ol; an anabolic agent, $C_{20}H_{32}O$.

Boletus (bo-le'tus) [L.; Gr. *bōlitēs*]   a genus of basidiomycetous Hymenomycetes, some of which are edible and others poisonous.   **B. sata'nas,** a species that causes mycetismus gastrointestinalis.

Bolk's retardation theory [Louis *Bolk*, Dutch anatomist, 1866–1930]   see under *theory*.

Bollinger's bodies, granules (bol'in-gerz) [Otto von *Bollinger*, German pathologist, 1843–1909]   see under *body* and *granule*.

bolometer (bo-lom'ĕ-ter) [Gr. *bolē* a throw, a ray + *metron* measure]   1. an instrument for measuring the force of the heart beat.   2. an instrument for measuring minute changes in heat radiated by an object, such as a portion of the human body.

bolus (bo'lus) [L.; Gr. *bolos* lump]   1. a rounded mass of food or a pharmaceutical preparation ready to swallow, or such a mass passing through the gastrointestinal tract.   2. a concentrated mass of pharmaceutical preparation given intravenously for diagnostic purposes, e.g., an opaque contrast medium or radioactive isotope.   3. a mass of scattering material, such as wax, paraffin, bags of water, or a rice-flour mixture, placed between the radiation source and the skin so as to achieve precalculated isodose pattern in the tissue irradiated.   **b. al'ba,** kaolin.   **alimentary b.,** the mass of food in the oropharynx or the esophagus, comprising one swallow.

bomb (bom)   a heavy metal-shielded apparatus containing a quantity of radium or other radioactive element for use in clinical teleradiation therapy.

bombard (bom-bard')   to expose the whole body or a specific tissue target to the action of ionizing radiation.

bombesin (bom'bĕ-sin)   a tetradecapeptide first isolated from the skin of certain frogs; on infusion into dogs, it stimulates gastric acid secretion, gallbladder contraction, pancreatic secretion, and relaxation of the choledochoduodenal junction; a pressor substance, it is present in the brain tissue and gut of man and is classified as a neuropeptide.

bombicesterol (bom''be-ses'ter-ol)   a sterol obtained from the chrysalis of the silkworm and from sponges.

bombykol (bom'bĭ-kol)   a pheromone secreted by silkworms that serves as a sex attractant; it is a 16-carbon alcohol with two double bonds.

Bombyx mori (bom'biks mor'i)   the commercial silkworm, used extensively in experimental genetics.

bond (bond)   1. the linkage between two atoms or radicals of a chemical compound.   2. a mark used to indicate the number and attachment of the valences of an atom in constitutional formulas; it is represented by a pair of dots or a line between the atoms, e.g., H—O—H, H—C≡C—H or

H:O:H, H:C:::C:H.   **coordinate covalent b.,** a covalent bond in which one of the bonded atoms furnishes both of the shared electrons.   **covalent b.,** a chemical bond between two atoms or radicals formed by the sharing of a pair (single bond), 2 pairs (double bond), or 3 pairs of electrons (triple bond).   **disulfide b.,** a strong covalent bond, —S—S—, important in linking polypeptide chains in proteins, the linkage arising as a result of the oxidation of the sulfhydryl (SH) groups of two molecules of cysteine; called also *disulfide bridge*.   **energy-rich b.,** high-energy b.   **glycosidic b's,** the bonds between the monosaccharide components of a polysaccharide.   **high-energy b.,** a chemical bond the hydrolysis of which yields high levels of free energy; such bonds involve phosphate (high-energy phosphate b.) or sulfur (high-energy sulfur b.) or other mixed anhydride types of chemical structure.   **high-energy phosphate b.,** an energy-rich phosphate linkage present in adenosine triphosphate, phosphocreatine, and certain other intermediates of carbohydrate metabolism. On hydrolysis at pH 7 it yields about 8000 calories per mole, in contrast to the 3000 calories of the ester phosphate bond. This energy can be transferred, stored, or used in metabolic processes, such as the synthesis of glycogen from glucose, or in the supply of energy for muscle activity.   **high-energy sulfur b.,** an energy-rich sulfur linkage, the most important of which occurs in the acetyl-CoA molecule, the main source of energy for fatty acid biosynthesis.   **hydrogen b.,** a weak, primarily electrostatic, bond between a hydrogen atom bound to a highly electronegative element (such as oxygen or nitrogen) in a given molecule, or part of a molecule, and a second highly electronegative atom in another molecule or in a different part of the same molecule. The hydrogen bond is generally represented by three dots, e.g., X—H···Y, where X and Y are electronegative atoms.   **hydrophobic b.,** a linkage resulting from the tendency of nonpolar molecules (or their side chains) to aggregate in an aqueous environment because of their mutual repulsion of solvent.   **ionic b.,** a chemical bond in which electrons are transferred from one atom (e.g., sodium) to another (e.g., chlorine) so that one bears a positive and the other a negative charge, the attraction between these opposite charges forming the bond.   **pair b.,** in ethology, the more or less permanent relationship between a male and a female for the purposes of mating and rearing the young.   **peptide b.,** the ·CO·NH· bond formed between the carboxyl group of one amino acid and the amino group of another; it is an amide linkage joining amino acids to form peptides.   **Van der Waals b.,** a weak chemical bond arising from a nonspecific attractive force originating when two atoms are close to one another; this weak binding is only effective when several atoms of one molecule are bound to several atoms in another molecule.

bonding (bond'ing)   joining together securely with an adhesive substance, such as glue or cement.   **tooth b.,** the technique of fixing orthodontic brackets and other attachments directly to the enamel surface with orthodontic adhesives.

bone (bōn) [L. *os;* Gr. *osteon*]   1. the hard form of connective tissue that constitutes the majority of the skeleton of most vertebrates; it consists of an organic component (the cells and matrix) and an inorganic, or mineral, component; the matrix contains a framework of collagenous fibers and is impregnated with the mineral component, chiefly calcium phosphate (85 per cent) and calcium carbonate (10 per cent), which imparts the quality of rigidity to bone. Called also *osseous tissue*.   2. any distinct piece of the osseous framework, or skeleton, of the body; called also *os*. See Plate accompanying *skeleton*.   **accessory b.,** an occasionally occurring bone or ossicle adjoining one of the bones of the carpus or of the tarsus; recognized in the roentgenogram.   **acetabular b.,** acetabulum.   **acromial b.,** acromion.   **alar b.,** os sphenoidale.   **Albers-Schönberg marble b's,** osteopetrosis.   **Albrecht's b.,** basiotic b.   **alisphenoid b.,** ala major ossis sphenoidalis.   **alveolar b.,** the thin layer of bone making up the bony processes of the maxilla and mandible, and surrounding and containing the teeth; it is pierced by many small openings through which blood vessels, lymphatics, and nerve fibers pass. See also *alveolar process*.   **ankle b.,** talus, def. 1.   **astragaloid b.,** talus, def. 1.   **astragaloscaphoid b.,** Pirie's b.   **back b.,** see *backbone*.   **basal b.,** the relatively fixed and unchangeable framework of the mandible and maxilla, which limits the extent to which teeth can be moved in the alveolar or supporting bone if the occlusion is to remain stable. **basi-hyal b.,** the body of the hyoid bone. **basilar b.,** basioc-cipital b. **basioccipital b.,** a bone developing from a separate ossification center in the fetus, which becomes the basilar part of the occipital bone; called also *basilar b.* **basiotic b.,** a small bone of the fetus between the basisphe-noid and the basioccipital bones; called also *Albrecht's b.* **basisphenoid b.,** an embryonic bone that becomes the back part of the body of the sphenoid. **Bertin's b.,** con-cha sphenoidalis. **breast b.,** sternum. **bregmatic b.,** parietal b. **brittle b's,** osteogenesis imperfecta. **bun-dle b.,** one of the two types of bones comprising the alveolar bone, so called because of the continuation into it of the principal fibers of the periodontal ligament. Large amounts of more calcified cementing substance render bundle bone more resistant to x-rays than surrounding bones; therefore it appears on dental radiographs as a thin radiopaque line (hence the synonym *lamina dura*). Called also *lamellated b.* **calcaneal b.,** calcaneus. **calf b.,** fibula. **cancel-lated b., cancellous b.,** substantia spongiosa ossium. **cannon b.,** a bone in the limb of hoofed animals, extending from the fetlock to the knee or hock joint. **capitate b.,** os capitatum. **carpal b's,** the eight bones of the wrist; see *ossa carpi* [NA]. **carpal b., central,** os centrale. **carpal b., first,** os trapezium. **carpal b., fourth,** os hamatum. **carpal b., great,** os capitatum. **carpal b., intermediate,** os lunatum. **carpal b., radial,** os sca-phoideum. **carpal b., second,** os trapezoideum. **car-pal b., third,** os capitatum. **carpal b., ulnar,** os tri-quetrum. **cartilage b.,** any bone that develops within cartilage, in contrast to membrane bone, ossification taking place within a cartilage model; called also *endochondral b., replacement b.,* and *substitution b.* **cavalry b.,** rider's b. **central b.,** os centrale. **chalky b's,** osteopetrosis. **cheek b.,** os zygomaticum. **chevron b.,** the ∨-shaped hemal arches of the third, fourth, and fifth coccygeal vertebrae of a dog. **coccygeal b.,** os coccygis. **coffin b.,** the third or distal phalanx of the foot of a horse; called also *pedal b.* and *os pedis.* **collar b.,** clavicula. **com-pact b.,** substantia compacta ossium. **coronary b.,** the small pastern bone of the horse. **cortical b.,** the com-pact bone of the shaft of a bone that surrounds the medullary cavity. **costal b.,** os costale. **cranial b's, b's of cra-nium,** the bones that constitute the cranial part of the skull, including the occipital, sphenoid, temporal, parietal, frontal, ethmoid, lacrimal and nasal bones, the inferior nasal concha, and vomer; called also *ossa cranii* [NA]. See also *facial b's.* **cribriform b.,** os ethmoidale. **cuboid b.,** os cuboi-deum. **cuneiform b. of carpus,** os triquetrum. **cu-neiform b., external,** os cuneiforme laterale. **cunei-form b., first,** os cuneiforme mediale. **cuneiform b., intermediate,** os cuneiforme intermedium. **cunei-form b., internal,** os cuneiforme mediale. **cuneiform b., lateral,** os cuneiforme laterale. **cuneiform b., me-dial,** os cuneiforme mediale. **cuneiform b., middle,** os cuneiforme intermedium. **cuneiform b., second,** os cuneiforme intermedium. **cuneiform b., third,** os cuneiforme laterale. **dermal b.,** a bone developed by ossification in the skin. **b's of digits of foot,** ossa digitorum pedis. **b's of digits of hand,** ossa digitorum manus. **ear b's,** auditory ossicles. **ectethmoid b's,** the lateral masses of the ethmoid bone. **ectocuneiform b.,** os cuneiforme laterale. **endo-chondral b.,** cartilage b. **entocuneiform b.,** os cune-iforme mediale. **epactal b's,** ossa suturalia. **epactal b., proper,** os interparietale. **ethmoid b.,** os ethmoi-dale. **exercise b.,** a bone developed in a muscle, tendon, or fascia, as a result of excessive exercise. **exoccipital b.,** one of the two lateral portions of the occipital bone, devel-oping, from separate centers of ossification, into the portions that bear the condyles. **b's of face, facial b's,** the bones that constitute the facial part of the skull, including the hyoid, palatine, and zygomatic bones, the mandible, and the maxilla; called also *ossa faciei* [NA]. The facial bones are considered by many to include the lacrimal and nasal bones, the inferior nasal concha, and the vomer, but not the hyoid bone. **femoral b.,** femur, def. 1. **fibular b.,** fibula. **b's of fingers,** ossa digitorum manus. **flank b.,** ilium (os ilium [NA]). **flat b.,** one whose thickness is slight, sometimes consisting of only a thin layer of compact bone, or of two layers with intervening spongy bone and marrow; usually bent or curved, rather than flat. Called also *os planum* [NA]. **frontal b.,** os frontale. **funny b.,** the region of the median condyle of the humerus where it is crossed by the ulnar nerve. **hamate b.,** os hamatum. **haunch b.,** os coxae. **heel b.,** calcaneus. **hip b.,** os coxae. **humeral b.,** humerus. **hyoid b.,** a horse-shoe-shaped bone situated at the base of the tongue, just above the thyroid cartilage; called also *os hyoideum* [NA], *lingual b.,* and *tongue b.* **iliac b.,** os ilii. **incarial b.,** os interparietale. **incisive b.,** os incisivum. **innomi-nate b.,** os coxae. **intermediate b.,** os lunatum. **in-terparietal b.,** os interparietale. **intrachondrial b.,** osseous tissue occurring in cartilage matrix which has undergone calcification; consistently found in patches within the middle layer of the otic capsule. **irregular b.,** os ir-regulare. **ischial b.,** os ischii. **ivory b's,** osteopetrosis. **jaw b., lower,** mandibula. **jaw b., upper,** maxilla. **jugal b.,** os zygomaticum. **lacrimal b.,** a thin scalelike bone at the anterior part of the medial wall of the orbit, articulating with the frontal and ethmoidal bones and the maxilla and inferior nasal concha; called also *os lacrimale* [NA] and *os unguis.* **lamellated b.,** one of the two types of bone comprising the alveolar bone, with some lamellae roughly parallel with the marrow spaces and others forming haversian systems. Cf. *bundle b.* **lenticular b. of hand, lentiform b.,** os pisiforme. **lingual b.,** hyoid b. (os hyoideum [NA]). **long b.,** a bone that has a longitudi-nal axis of considerable length, consisting of a shaft (the diaphysis) and an expanded portion (the epiphysis) at each end that is usually articular; any of the long bones of the limbs. Called also *os longum* [NA]. **lunate b.,** os luna-tum. **malar b.,** os zygomaticum. **marble b's,** osteope-trosis. **mastoid b.,** pars mastoidea ossis temporalis. **maxillary b.,** maxilla. **maxillary b., inferior,** man-dibula. **maxillary b., superior,** maxilla. **maxillo-turbinal b.,** concha nasalis inferior. **membrane b.,** any bone that develops within a connective tissue membrane, in contrast to cartilage bone. **mesocuneiform b.,** os cu-neiforme intermedium. **metacarpal b's,** the five cylin-drical bones of the hand; see *ossa metacarpi* [NA]. **meta-carpal b., middle, metacarpal b., third,** os metacar-pale tertium. **metatarsal b's,** the five bones forming the skeleton of the metatarsus; see *ossa metatarsi* [NA]. **multangular b., accessory,** os centrale. **multangu-lar b., larger,** os trapezium. **multangular b., smaller,** os trapezoideum. **nasal b.,** either of the two small oblong bones that together form the bridge of the nose; called also *os nasale* [NA]. **navicular b. of foot,** os na-viculare. **navicular b. of hand,** os scaphoideum. **nonlamellated b.,** woven b. **occipital b.,** a single trapezoid-shaped bone situated at the posterior and inferior part of the cranium; see *os occipitale* [NA]. **odontoid b.,** dens axis. **orbital b.,** os zygomaticum. **orbitosphe-noidal b.,** ala minor ossis sphenoidalis. **palate b.,** pala-tine b. **palatine b.,** one of the two irregularly shaped bones forming the posterior part of the hard palate, the lateral wall of the nasal fossa between the medial pterygoid plate and the maxilla, and the posterior part of the floor of the orbit. Called also *os palatinum* [NA] and *palate b.* **pa-rietal b.,** one of the two quadrilateral bones forming part of the superior and lateral surfaces of the skull, and joining each other in the midline at the sagittal suture; called also *os parietale* [NA] and *bregmatic b.* **pastern b.,** either of two bones of the horse's foot: *large pastern b.,* the first phalanx of a horse's foot; *small pastern b.,* the second phalanx of a horse's foot. **pedal b.,** coffin b. **pelvic b.,** os coxae. **perios-teal b.,** bone that is developed directly from and beneath the periosteum. **petrosal b., petrous b.,** pars petrosa ossis temporalis. **phalangeal b's of foot,** ossa digitorum pedis. **phalangeal b's of hand,** ossa digitorum manus. **Pirie's b.,** an occasionally occurring ossicle found above the head of the talus; called also *astragaloscaphoid b.* **pisi-form b.,** os pisiforme. **pneumatic b.,** one that contains air-filled cavities or sinuses; called also *os pneumaticum* [NA]. **postsphenoidal b.,** the posterior portion of the sphenoid bone. **postulnar b.,** os pisiforme. **prefrontal b.,** pars nasalis ossis frontalis. **prefrontal b. of von Bar-deleben,** processus frontalis maxillae. **preinterparie-tal b.,** a wormian bone sometimes observed, detached from the anterior part of the interparietal bone. **premaxil-lary b.,** premaxilla. **presphenoidal b.,** the anterior portion of the sphenoid bone that develops separately and unites with the posterior portion (postsphenoidal bone) between the seventh and eighth months of intrauterine life. **primitive b.,** woven b. **pterygoid b.,** processus ptery-goideus ossis sphenoidalis. **pubic b.,** the anterior inferior part of the hip bone (os coxae) on either side; see *os pubis* [NA]. **pyramidal b.,** os triquetrum. **radial b.,** radius, def. 2. **replacement b.,** cartilage b. **resurrection b.,** sacrum (os sacrum [NA]). **rider's b.,** a localized ossification of the inner aspect of the lower end of the tendon of the adductor muscle of the thigh (adductor tubercle), sometimes seen in horseback riders; called also *cavalry b.* **Riolan's b's,** small bones resembling wormian bones, sometimes found in the suture between the occipital bone and the petrous portion of the temporal bone. **rudimentary b.,** a bone that has only partially developed. **sacral b.,** os sacrum. **scaphoid b.,** os scaphoideum. **scaphoid b. of foot,** os naviculare. **scaphoid b. of hand,** os scaphoideum. **scapular b.,** scapula. **semilunar b.,** os lunatum. **sesamoid b's,** numerous ovoid nodular bones, often small, usually found embedded within a tendon or joint capsule, principally in the hands and feet (*ossa sesamoidea manus* and *ossa sesamoidea pedis,* respectively); two sesamoid bones, the fabella and patella, are associated with the knee. **sesamoid b's of foot,** ossa sesamoidea pedis. **sesamoid b's of hand,** ossa sesamoidea manus. **shin b.,** tibia. **short b.,** one whose main dimensions are approximately equal, e.g., one of the bones of the carpus or tarsus; called also *os breve* [NA]. **b's of skull,** ossa cranii. **solid b.,** substantia compacta ossium. **sphenoid b.,** a single, irregular, wedge-shaped bone at the base of the skull, which forms a part of the floor of the anterior, middle, and posterior cranial fossae; called also *os sphenoidale* [NA] and *alar b.* **sphenoturbinal b.,** concha sphenoidalis. **splint b's,** the reduced second and fourth metacarpal and metatarsal bones of the Equidae. **spoke b.,** radius, def. 2. **spongy b.,** substantia spongiosa ossium. **spongy b., inferior,** concha nasalis inferior. **spongy b., superior,** concha nasalis superior. **squamo-occipital b.,** the squamous portion of the fetal occipital bone, including the supraoccipital and interparietal bones. **squamous b.,** pars squamosa ossis temporalis. **stifle b.,** the patella of the horse. **stirrup b.,** stapes. **substitution b.,** cartilage b. **supernumerary b.,** a bone occurring in addition to the normal one, as a vertebra or a rib (cervical rib). **suprainterparietal b.,** a wormian bone sometimes occurring at the posterior part of the sagittal suture. **supraoccipital b.,** a bone developing from a separate ossification center in the fetus, which becomes the squamous part of the occipital bone below the superior nuchal line. **suprapharyngeal b.,** os sphenoidale. **suprasternal b's,** ossa suprasternalia. **sutural b's,** ossa suturalia. **tarsal b's,** the seven bones of the ankle; see *ossa tarsi* [NA]. **tarsal b., first,** os cuneiforme mediale. **tarsal b., second,** os cuneiforme intermedium. **tarsal b., third,** os cuneiforme laterale. **temporal b.,** one of the two irregular bones forming part of the lateral surfaces and base of the skull, and containing the organs of hearing; called also *os temporale* [NA]. **thigh b.,** femur, def. 1. **thoracic b's,** ossa thoracis. **b's of toes,** ossa digitorum pedis. **tongue b.,** os hyoideum. **trapezium b.,** os trapezium. **trapezium b., lesser,** os trapezoideum. **trapezium b. of Lyser,** os trapezoideum. **trapezoid b.,** os trapezoideum. **trapezoid b. of Henle,** processus pterygoideus ossis sphenoidalis. **trapezoid b. of Lyser,** os trapezium. **triangular b.,** os triquetrum. **triangular b. of tarsus,** os trigonum tarsi. **triquetral b.,** os triquetrum. **turbinate b., highest,** concha nasalis suprema. **turbinate b., inferior,** concha nasalis inferior. **turbinate b., middle,** concha nasalis media. **turbinate b., superior,** concha nasalis superior. **turbinate b., supreme,** concha nasalis suprema. **tympanic b.,** pars tympanica ossis temporalis. **ulnar b.,** ulna. **unciform b., uncinate b.,** os hamatum. **vesalian b.,** os vesalianum pedis. **vomer b.,** vomer. **whettle b's,** vertebrae thoracicae. **wormian b's,** ossa suturalia. **woven b.,** bony tissue found in the embryo and young children and in various pathologic conditions in adults, in which the bone fails to show the oriented arrangement of collagen fibers characteristic of lamellated bone; called also *nonlamellated b.* and *primitive b.* **xiphoid b.,** sternum. **zygomatic b.,** the triangular bone of the cheek; see *os zygomaticum.*

bonelet (bōn′let) a small bone, or ossicle.

Bonhoeffer's symptom (bon′hef-erz) [Karl *Bonhoeffer,* psychiatrist in Berlin, 1868–1948] see under *symptom.*

Bonine (bo′nēn) trademark for preparations of meclizine hydrochloride.

Bonnet's capsule, sign (bo-nāz′) [Amédée *Bonnet,* French surgeon, 1809–1858] the capsule enclosing the posterior part of the eyeball. See *vagina bulbi,* and under *sign.*

Bonnier's syndrome (bon-e-āz) [Pierre *Bonnier,* French physician, 1861–1918] see under *syndrome.*

Bonwill crown, triangle (bon′wil) [William Gibson Arlington *Bonwill,* American dentist, 1833–1899] see under *crown* and *triangle.*

book-lung (bŏŏk′lung) see under *lung.*

Böök's syndrome (bāk) [Jan Arvid *Böök,* Swedish geneticist, born 1915] PHC syndrome.

boomslang (boom′slang) a venomous, colubrid, arboreal snake, *Dispholidus typus,* of South Africa. See table accompanying *snake.*

Boophilus (bo-off′ĭ-lus) [Gr. *bous* ox + *philein* to love] a genus of blood-sucking, ixodid cattle ticks comprising many species that are vectors of bovine anaplasmosis and babesiosis, including *B. annulatus,* the vector of *Bahesia begimina, B. microplus,* the vector of *Babesia bovis, B. calcaratus,* the vector of *Babesia major,* and *B. decoloratus,* the vector of *Anaplasma marginale.*

Booponus (bo-op′o-nus) [Gr. *bous* ox + *ponos* pain] a fly of the Philippines whose larvae (foot maggots) cause lameness in cattle and goats.

booster (bōōst′er) see under *dose.*

boot (bōōt) an encasement for the foot; a protective casing or sheath. **Gibney's b.,** an adhesive tape support used in treatment of sprains and other painful conditions of the ankle, the tape being applied in a basketweave fashion with strips placed alternately under the sole of the foot and around the back of the leg. **Unna's paste b.,** a dressing for varicose ulcers, consisting of a paste made from gelatin, zinc oxide, and glycerin, which is applied to the entire leg, then covered with a spiral bandage, this in turn being given a coat of the paste; the process is repeated until satisfactory rigidity is attained.

boracic acid (bŏ-ras′ik) boric acid.

borate (bo′rāt) any salt of boric acid.

borated (bo′rāt-ed) combined with or containing borax or boric acid.

borax (bo′raks), gen. *bora′cis* [L. from Arabic; Persian *būrah*] sodium borate.

borborygmus (bor″bo-rig′mus), pl. *borboryg′mi* [L.] a rumbling noise caused by the propulsion of gas through the intestines.

border (bor′der) a bounding line, edge, or surface. For names of borders of various anatomical structures not included here, see entries under *margo.* **b. of acetabulum,** limbus acetabuli. **alveolar b. of mandible,** arcus alveolaris mandibulae. **alveolar b. of maxilla,** arcus alveolaris maxillae. **brush b.,** a specialization of the free surface of a cell, consisting of minute cylindrical processes (microvilli) that greatly increase the surface area; noted especially on the cells of the proximal convolution in a renal tubule and on the intestinal epithelium of vertebrates. Called also *striated b.* **denture b.,** 1. the limit, boundary, or circumferential margin of a denture base. 2. the margin of the denture base at the junction of the polished surface with the impression (tissue) surface. 3. the extreme edges of a denture base at the buccolabial, lingual, and posterior limits. 4. the extreme margins of a denture base. Called also *denture edge.* **external b. of tibia,** facies lateralis tibiae. **inferior b. of mandible,** basis mandibulae. **orbital b. of sphenoid bone,** facies orbitalis alae majoris. **b. of oval fossa,** limbus fossae ovalis. **posterior b. of petrous portion of temporal bone,** angulus posterior pyramidis ossis temporalis. **posterointernal b. of fibula,** crista medialis fibulae. **striated b.,** brush b. **superior b. of patella,** basis patellae. **superior b. of petrous portion of temporal bone,** angulus superior pyramidis ossis temporalis. **vermilion b.,** the exposed red portion of the upper or lower lip.

borderline (bor′der-līn) in psychiatry, "on the borderline" between neurosis and psychosis. See under *personality.*

Bordet (bor-da′), Jules Jean Baptiste Vincent. Belgian bacteriologist and serologist, 1870–1961; winner of the Nobel prize for medicine or physiology in 1919 for his work in immunology.

Bordet-Gengou agar (culture medium), bacillus,

phenomenon (reaction) (bor-da′-zhaw-goo′) [Jules Jean Baptiste Vincent *Bordet*; Octave *Gengou*, French bacteriologist, 1875–1957] see *Table of Culture Media*, and see *Bordetella pertussis* and *complement fixation*.

Bordetella (bor″dĕ-tel′lah) [Jules Jean Baptiste Vincent *Bordet*] a genus of gram-negative aerobic, minute coccobacilli of uncertain affiliation. It is made up of organisms that are parasites and pathogens of the respiratory tract of humans and lower animals and produce a dermonecrotic toxin. **B. bronchisep′tica,** a species resembling *B. pertussis* morphologically, culturally, and antigenically except that *B. bronchiseptica* is motile and grows sparsely on nutrient agar; it is a frequent cause of bronchopneumonia in guinea pigs and other rodents, swine, dogs, and lower primates. Called also *Bacillus bronchisepticus, Brucella bronchiseptica,* and *Hemophilus bronchisepticus.* **B. parapertus′sis,** a species immunologically related to *B. pertussis,* from which it can be distinguished by the readiness with which *B. parapertussis* grows on simple culture media. It occasionally causes classic pertussis and an acute respiratory infection clinically indistinguishable from mild or moderate pertussis (*parapertussis*). Called also *Haemophilus parapertussis.* **B. pertus′sis,** the usual causative agent of pertussis (whooping cough) in humans, found only in the human respiratory tract. Virulent strains are encapsulated with smooth colonies (Phase I); prolonged laboratory culture produces loss of surface K antigens and altered colonial morphology (Phases II, III, and IV) progressing to obviously rough strains that are avirulent. Called also *Bordet-Gengou bacillus, Haemophilus pertussis,* and *Pseudomonas pertucinogens* (Phase IV).

boric acid (bor′ik) a mild acid used as an acidifying agent and in buffer solutions; it is also a weak germicide used on intact skin, mucous membranes, and cornea; accidental ingestion may cause fatal poisoning. Called also *boracic acid.*

borism (bo′rizm) poisoning by a boron compound.

borjom (bor′jom) a natural mineral water from Caucasia.

Borna disease [*Borna,* a district in Saxony where an epidemic occurred] see under *disease.*

borneol (bor′ne-ol) chemical name: *endo*-1,7,7-trimethylbicyclo[2.2.1]heptan-2-ol. A terpene alcohol, $C_{10}H_{18}O$, found in the Borneo camphor tree (*Dryobalanops aromatica*) and many other plants, or prepared synthetically, and used, chiefly in the form of its esters, in the manufacture of perfume and incense. Called also *Borneo camphor, bornyl alcohol,* and *camphyl alcohol.* **b. acetate,** see under *bornyl.*

Bornholm disease (born′hōm) [named from the Danish island, *Bornholm*] epidemic pleurodynia.

bornyl (bor′nil) a univalent radical of borneol. **b. acetate,** an ester of borneol found in the oil of *Rosmarinus officinalis* and many other oils, and used as a flavoring agent and in the manufacture of perfume; called also *borneol acetate.* **b. alcohol,** borneol. **b. chloride,** chemical name: *endo*-2-chlorol-7,7-trimethylbicyclo[2.2.1]heptane. A compound, $C_{10}H_{17}Cl$, prepared from pinene, the chief constituent of turpentine oil, by the action of hydrochloric acid, in the process of producing synthetic camphor. Called also *artificial camphor, pinene hydrochloride,* and *turpentine camphor.*

boroglyceride (bo″ro-glis′er-īd) boroglycerin.

boroglycerin (bo″ro-glis′er-in) a compound ($C_3H_5BO_3$) prepared by heating 2 parts of boric acid and 3 parts of glycerin; formerly used as an antiseptic. **b. glycerite,** a preparation of boric acid and glycerin, containing between 47.5 and 52.5 per cent of boroglycerin; formerly used as an antibacterial. Called also *glyceritum boroglycerini* and *glycerol boroglycerite.*

boroglycerol (bo″ro-glis′e⁻-ol) boroglycerin.

boron (bo′ron) [L. *borium*] a nonmetallic element occurring in the form of crystals and as a powder. It is the base of borax and boric acid: symbol B, atomic number 5, specific gravity 2.54, atomic weight 10.811. **b. carbide,** a compound, B_4C, slightly harder than silicon carbide (q.v.), obtained by heating boron at very high temperature to effect its union with carbon; used as a neutron absorber in nuclear reactors, and as an abrasive agent in industry and dentistry.

Borrelia (bŏ-rel′e ah) [after Amédée *Borrel,* French bacteriologist in Strasbourg, 1867–1936] a genus of bacteria of the family Spirochaetaceae, order Spirochaetales, made up of gram-negative, anaerobic, helical cells up to 1μ wide by 20μ long, with coarse, shallow, irregular coils surrounding a central fibrillar substance. The organisms are parasitic, living on mucous membranes, and are the cause of relapsing fever in humans and animals. **B. anseri′na,** the etiologic agent of avian borreliosis, transmitted by species of the tick *Argas,* which occurs worldwide in wild and domestic fowl. It is not pathogenic for humans. **B. ber′bera,** *B. recurrentis.* **B. bucca′lis,** *Treponema buccale.* **B. burgdor′feri,** the causative agent of Lyme disease, transmitted by the tick *Ixodes dammini.* **B. car′teri,** *B. recurrentis.* **B. caucas′ica,** an etiologic agent of relapsing fever in the Caucasus, transmitted by the tick *Ornithodoros verrucosus* from a reservoir of infection in field mice. **B. crocidu′rae,** an etiologic agent of relapsing fever in humans in North Africa, transmitted by the tick *Ornithodoros erraticus sonrai,* which is carried by small rodents. **B. dipodil′li,** a species of uncertain status that is an etiologic agent of North African tickborne relapsing fever, transmitted by the tick *Ornithodoros erraticus sonrai,* which is carried by small rodents. **B. dutto′nii,** an etiologic agent of endemic relapsing fever in Central and South Africa, carried by the tick *Ornithodoros moubata,* which transmits the microorganism from human to human in its saliva. Called also *B. hochii* and *Dutton's spirochete.* **B. herm′sii,** an etiologic agent of endemic relapsing fever in western North America, transmitted by the tick *Ornithodoros hermsii,* which is transported by chipmunks and tree squirrels. **B. hispan′ica,** the etiologic agent of endemic relapsing fever in the Iberian peninsula and Northwest Africa, transmitted by the large tick *Ornithodoros erraticus,* which lives on rodents, reptiles, and amphibians; the organism is transmitted as the tick is feeding. **B. ko′chii,** *B. duttonii.* **B. latysche′wii,** the etiologic agent of a type of relapsing fever in Iran and Central Asia, transmitted by the tick *Ornithodoros tartakovskyi,* which is carried by rodents and reptiles. **B. mazzot′tii,** the etiologic agent of relapsing fever in the southern United States, Mexico, and Central and South America, transmitted by the tick *Ornithodoros talaje,* which is carried by rodents, armadillos, and monkeys. **B. merione′si,** a species of uncertain status that is an etiologic agent of North African tickborne relapsing fever and is transmitted by *Ornithodoros erraticus sonrai,* which is carried by small rodents. **B. micro′ti,** a species that causes North African tickborne relapsing fever. It is transmitted by *Ornithodoros erraticus sonrai,* which is carried by small rodents. **B. neotropica′lis,** *B. venezuelensis.* **B. no′vyi,** *B. recurrentis.* **B. obermey′eri,** *B. recurrentis.* **B. par′keri,** an etiologic agent of endemic relapsing fever in the western United States. Burrowing rodents, such as ground squirrels, carry the tick vector, *Ornithodoros parkeri,* which transmits the organism in its bite. **B. per′sica,** an etiologic agent of endemic relapsing fever in Asia and Africa. The organism is transmitted in the bite of the tick vector *Ornithodoros tholozani,* which is carried by rodents living in caves, stables, and burrows. **B. recurren′tis,** the causative agent of worldwide epidemic louseborne relapsing fever, transmitted by the human body louse, *Pediculus humanus.* The organism is spread by rubbing infected hemolymph of lice into the skin, as in scratching. The organism produces successive antigenic mutants that cause the clinical relapses. Called also *B. berbera, B. carteri, B. novyi,* and *B. obermeyeri.* **B. theile′ri** an etiologic agent of tickborne spirochetosis in cattle, horses, and sheep in South Africa and Australia, transmitted by species of *Rhipicephalus* and *Boophilus.* **B. turica′tae,** an etiologic agent of endemic relapsing fever in southwestern United States and Mexico. The organism is transmitted by the bite of the tick *Ornithodoros turicata,* which is carried by rodents and reptiles. **B. venezuelen′sis,** an etiologic agent of relapsing fever in Central and South America, transmitted by the tick *Ornithodoros rudis,* which is carried by monkeys and rodents. Called also *B. neotropicalis.* **B. vincen′tii,** *Treponema vincentii.*

borreliosis (bŏ-rel″e-o′sis) infection with spirochetes of the genus *Borrelia.*

Borsieri's sign (line) (bor″se-er′ēz) [Giovanni Battista *Borsieri* de Kanilfeld, French physician, 1725–1785] see under *line.*

Borthen's operation (bor′tenz) [Johan *Borthen,* Norwegian ophthalmologist] iridotasis.

Bose's hook (bo′sez) [Heinrich *Bose,* German surgeon, 1840–1900] see under *hook.*

boss (bos) a rounded eminence, as on the surface of a bone or tumor. **parietal b's,** sharp prominences on each side of the parietal bones.

bosselated (bos′ĕ-lāt-ed) [Fr. *bosseler*] marked or covered with bosses.

bosselation (bos″ĕ-la′shun) 1. a small eminence; one of a set of bosses. 2. the condition or fact of being bosselated; the process of becoming bosselated.

Bostock's catarrh (disease) (bos′toks) [John *Bostock*, English physician, 1773–1846] hay fever.

Boston's sign (bos′tonz) [L. Napoleon *Boston*, American physician, 1871–1931] see under *sign.*

bot (bot) the larva of botflies, which may be parasitic in the stomach of animals and sometimes in that of man. **sheep nose b.,** the larva of *Oestrus ovis,* which is frequently found in the nasal passages of sheep.

Botallo's duct, foramen, ligament [Leonardo *Botallo,* Italian surgeon in Paris, born 1530] see *ductus arteriosus, foramen ovale cordis,* and *ligamentum arteriosum.*

botanic (bo-tan′ik) 1. pertaining to or derived from plants; of the vegetable kingdom. 2. pertaining to botany.

botany (bot′ah-ne) [L. *botanica* from Gr. *botanē* herb] the science of plants or of the vegetable kingdom. **medical b.,** the botany of plants used in medicine.

botfly (bot′fli) an insect of the order Diptera, family Oestridae, whose larvae are parasitic in animals, especially horses and sheep. The genera include *Oestrus, Gasterophilus, Dermatobia,* and *Cuterebra.*

bothridium (both-rid′e-um) one of the four leaf-like suckers symmetrically placed around the anterior end of the scolex of a tetraphyllidean cestode; called also *phyllidea.*

bothriocephaliasis (both″re-o-sef″ah-li′ah-sis) diphyllobothriasis.

Bothriocephalus (both″re-o-sef″ah-lus) [Gr. *bothrion* pit + *kephalē* head] *diphyllobothrium.*

bothrium (both′re-um) [Gr. *bothrion* pit] a sucker in the form of a groove such as is seen on either side of the head of *Diphyllobothrium latum.*

bothropik (both-rop′ik) pertaining to, characteristic of, or derived from snakes of the genus *Bothrops.*

Bothrops (both-rops) [Gr. *bothros* pit + *ōps* eye] a genus of South American serpents. *B. atrox* is the fer-de-lance and *B. jararaca* is the jararaca (q.v.). See table accompanying *snake.*

botogenin (bot-o-je′nin) a steroid sapogenin, $C_{27}H_{40}O_4$, derived from *Dioscorea mexicana,* which is a precursor in a patented process for the partial synthesis of steroid hormones.

botryoid (bot′re-oid) [Gr. *botrys* bunch of grapes + *eidos* form] resembling a bunch of grapes.

botryomycosis (bot″re-o-mi-ko′sis) [Gr. *botrys* bunch of grapes + *mykēs* fungus + *-osis*] a chronic purulent granulomatous bacterial infection usually caused by *Staphylococcus aureus,* originally thought to be due to fungi called "botryomycetes," characterized by lesions containing sulfur granules composed of a central mass of bacteria surrounded by a capsule, and histologically resembling actinomycosis or mycetoma. Human infection is usually localized to the skin but may involve other organs such as the viscera and lymph nodes, especially in debilitated patients; infection in domestic animals most often occurs as chronic, localized or spreading abscesses of the skin.

botryomycotic (bot″re-o-mi-kot′ik) pertaining to or affected with botryomycosis.

botrytimycosis (bo-tri″te-mi-ko′sis) infection with fungi of the genus *Botrytis.*

Botrytis (bo-tri′tis) a genus of fungi of the family Moniliaceae, order Moniliales, including the common gray mold and some plant pathogens, which causes onion rot, peony blight, and turnip fire. **B. bassia′na,** *Beauveria bassiana.* **B. tenel′la,** *Beauveria tenella.*

bots (bots) a name given the diseased condition in horses and other animals, attributed to the presence of larvae of botflies of various genera.

Böttcher's cells, crystals (bet′sherz) [Arthur *Böttcher,* German anatomist, 1831–1889] see under *cell* and *crystals.*

bottle (bot′l) a hollow narrow-necked vessel of glass or other material, used in laboratory procedures or for other

purposes. **Castaneda b.,** a biphasic bottle containing both broth and a solid agar slant; used in the cultivation of fastidious organisms from blood. **Junker b.,** see under *inhaler.* **Spritz b.,** a wash bottle for laboratory use. **wash b.,** 1. a flexible squeeze-bottle with delivery tube, or a bottle having two tubes through the cork, so arranged that blowing into one will force a stream of liquid from the other; used in washing chemical materials. 2. a bottle containing some washing fluid, through which gases are passed for the purpose of freeing them from impurities. **Woulfe's b.,** a three-necked bottle used for washing gases or for saturating liquids with a gas.

botuliform (boch′oo-in-form) [L. *botulus* sausage + *forma* shape] sausage-shaped.

botulin (boch′oo-lin) [L. *botulus* sausage] a highly active neurotoxin sometimes found in imperfectly preserved or canned meats and vegetables; it is produced by *Clostridium botulinum* and is peculiar in that it resists the action of the gastric juice. The toxin occurs in six antigenically distinct forms, A, B, C, D, E, and F. Called also *botulinum toxin.* See *botulism.*

botulinal (boh″oo-li′nal) pertaining to *Clostridium botulinum* or to its toxin (botulin).

botulinogenic (boch′oo-lin″o-jen′ik) [*botulin* + Gr. *gennan* to produce] producing or containing botulin.

botulism (boch′oo-lizm) [L. *botulus* sausage] a type of food poisoning caused by a neurotoxin (botulin) produced by the growth of *Clostridium botulinum* in improperly canned or preserved foods. It is characterized by vomiting, abdominal pain, difficulty of vision, nervous symptoms of central origin, disturbances of secretion, motor disturbances, dryness of the mouth and pharynx, dyspepsia, a barking cough, mydriasis, and ptosis. In adults, botulism is typically caused by the ingestion of preformed toxin; in some cases, however, it results from the production of toxin in the gastrointestinal tract by ingested organisms (cf. *infant b.*). Botulism is the broader term; *allantiasis* refers only to sausage poisoning. **infant b.,** that affecting infants, typically 4 to 26 weeks of age, marked by constipation, lethargy, hypotonia, and feeding difficulty; it may lead to respiratory insufficiency. It results from toxin produced in the gut by ingested organisms, rather than from preformed toxins. **wound b.,** botulism resulting from infection of a wound with *Clostridium botulinum;* it is marked by the same symptoms as the foodborne form except for the absence of gastrointestinal symptoms.

botulismotoxin (boch′ŏŏ-liz″mo-tok′sin) botulin.

bouba (boo′bah) yaws.

Bouchard's coefficient, disease, nodes (nodules), sign (boo-sharz′) [Charles Jacques *Bouchard,* French physician, 1837–1915] see under *coefficient, disease, node,* and *sign.*

Bouchardat's test, treatment (boo-shar-dahz′) [Apollinaire *Bouchardat,* French chemist, 1806–1886] see under *tests* and *treatment.*

bouche (boosh′) [Fr.] mouth. **b. de tapir** (de tah-pēr′), tapir mouth.

Bouchut's respiration, tubes (boo-shooz′) [Jean Antoine Eugène *Bouchut,* French physician, 1818–1891] see under *respiration* and *tube.*

bougie (boo-zhe′) [Fr. "wax candle"] a slender, flexible, hollow or solid, cylindrical instrument for introduction into the urethra or other tubular organ, usually for the purpose of calibrating or dilating constricted areas. **b. à boule** (ah-bool′) [Fr.], bulbous b. **acorn-tipped b.,** a bulbous bougie with a tip shaped like an acorn. **bulbous b.,** one with a bulb-shaped tip; called also *bougie à boule.* **caustic b.,** one that has a piece of silver nitrate or other caustic agent attached to its end; used as a portcaustic. **conic b.,** one with a cone-shaped tip. **cylindrical b.,** one with a round or circular section. **dilating b.,** a bougie whose diameter can be increased by turning a screw; commonly used for dilating a stricture of the urethra. **elastic b.,** one made of rubber or other elastic material. **elbowed b.,** one with an elbow or sharp, beaklike bend, near the tip. **filiform b.,** one of very slender caliber; often used for the gentle exploration of strictures or sinus tracts of small diameter with multiple false passages. **fusiform b.,** one with a belly or expansion in its shaft. **Hurst's b's,** a series of mercury-filled tubes of graded diameter for dilating the cardioesophageal region. **Maloney b's,** a series sim-

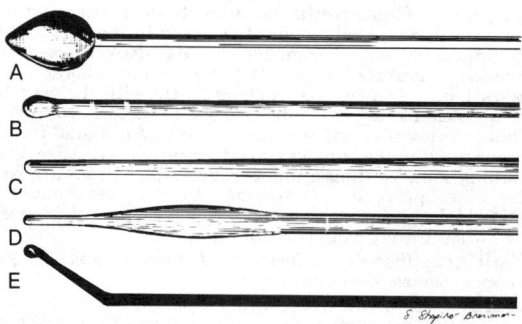

Bougies: *A*, Otis bougie à boule; *B*, olive-tipped bougie; *C*, Garceau bougie; *D*, Braasch bulbous bougie; *E*, filiform bougie.

ilar to Hurst's bougies but having cone-shaped tips. **olive-tipped b.,** a bulbous bougie with a tip shaped like an olive. **rosary b.,** a beaded bougie for use in a strictured urethra. **wax-tipped b.,** a long, slender, flexible bougie with a wax tip for passage into the ureter through the cystoscope to confirm the diagnosis of ureteral calculus. **whip b.,** one with a filiform point and a stem of gradually increasing caliber.

bougienage (boo-zhe-nahzh′) the passage of a bougie through a tubular structure or organ, to increase its caliber, as in the treatment of stricture of the esophagus.

bouginage (boo-zhe-nahzh′) bougienage.

Bouillaud's disease, sign, syndrome (boo-e-yōz′) [Jean Baptiste *Bouillaud,* French physician, 1796–1881] see *rheumatic endocarditis,* under *endocarditis,* and see under *sign* and *syndrome.*

bouillon (boo-e-yaw′) [Fr.] a broth or soup prepared from the flesh of animals; used in food preparations and as a bacteriological culture medium. In the latter use, it is generally called *broth;* see Table of Culture Media for specific broths.

Bouin's fluid (solution) (bwahz′) [Paul *Bouin,* French anatomist, 1870–1962] see under *fluid.*

boulimia (boo-lim′e-ah) bulimia.

bound (bownd) 1. restrained or confined; not free. 2. held in chemical combination.

bouquet (boo-ka′) [Fr.] a structure suggesting resemblance to a bunch of flowers, as a cluster of vessels, nerves, or fibers, or the polarized stage of synapsis at the start of meiosis.

Bourgery's ligament (boor′jer-ēz) [Marc Jean *Bourgery,* French anatomist and surgeon, 1797–1849] ligamentum popliteum obliquum.

Bourneville's disease (boor′ne-vēz) [Désiré-Magloire *Bourneville,* French neurologist, 1840–1909] sclerosis tuberosa.

bout (bout) an attack or episode of illness.

bouton (boo-taw′) [Fr.] button. **b's terminaux′,** synaptic end-feet.

boutonneuse (boo-ton-uhz′) [Fr. "pimply"] boutonneuse fever.

Bouveret's disease (syndrome) (boo-ver-āz′) [Léon *Bouveret,* French physician, 1850–1929] see *paroxysmal tachycardia,* under *tachycardia*

Bovet (bo′vet), Daniel. Swiss-born Italian pharmacologist, born 1907; winner of the Nobel prize for medicine or physiology for 1957 for developing antihistamines and muscle relaxants.

Bovimyces pleuropneumoniae (bo″vĕ-mi′sēz ploor″o-nu-mo′ne-e) *Mycoplasma mycoides.*

bovine (bo′vīn) [L. *bos, bovis* ox, bullock, cow] pertaining to, characteristic of, or derived from the ox (cattle).

bow (bo) a bow-shaped device. **Birnberg b.,** an intrauterine contraceptive device consisting of polyethylene molded in a rod and shaped in the outline of two isosceles triangles of equal size placed apex to apex, one containing a nylon tail to facilitate removal of the appliance. **Logan b.,** an appliance used to prevent tension on sutures after surgical repair of cleft lip.

Bowditch's law (bow′dich-ez) [Henry Pickering *Bowditch,*

Boston physiologist, 1840–1911] see *all-or-none,* under *A;* see under *law;* and see *treppe.*

bowel (bow′el) [Fr. *boyau*] the intestine.

bowenoid (bo′en-oid) anaplastic; said of the neoplastic cells derived from the epidermis, which constitute lesions of intraepidermal squamous cell carcinoma (Bowen's disease).

Bowen's disease (precancerous dermatosis) (bo′enz) [John Templeton *Bowen,* American dermatologist, 1857 –1941] see under *disease.*

bowie (bo′e) a disease resembling rickets, which affects unweaned lambs in New Zealand.

bowleg (bo′leg) an outward curvature of one or both legs near the knee; genu varum. **nonrachitic b.,** tibia vara.

Bowman's capsule, etc. (bo′manz) [Sir William *Bowman,* an English physician, 1816–1892] see under *capsule, lamina, muscle, probe, theory,* and *tube.*

box (boks) a rectangular structure. **anatomical snuff-b.,** a triangular depression on the dorsum of the wrist at its radial border formed between the tendon of the extensor pollicis longus medially and the tendons of the extensor pollicis brevis and abductor pollicis longus laterally, formed when the thumb is abducted and extended. **CAT b.,** in genetics, a conserved, non-coding "promotor" sequence about 80 bp upstream from the start of transcription of a gene. See also *Hogness b.* **Hogness b.,** in genetics, a conserved, non-coding "promoter" sequence about 30 bp upstream from the start of transcription of a gene. See also *CAT b.* Called also *TATA b.* **Skinner b.,** an experimental enclosure for testing animal conditioning, in which the subject animal performs (e.g., presses a bar or lever) to obtain a reward. **TATA b.,** Hogness b. **Yerkes discrimination b.,** a maze with a series of doors, used in the laboratory in studies of visual discrimination in animals; opening of the proper door produces a reward, but opening of the wrong door produces an electric stimulus.

boxing (bok′sing) in the fabrication of dental restorations and appliances, the building up of vertical walls of wax or other suitable material to form a box around a dental impression into which the freshly mixed plaster or stone is poured; done to produce the desired size and form of the base of the cast and to preserve certain landmarks of the impression.

box-note (boks′nōt) a hollow sound heard in percussing the chest in emphysema.

Boyer's bursa, cyst (bwah-yāz′) [Alexis de *Boyer,* French surgeon, 1757–1833] see under *bursa* and *cyst.*

Boyle's law (boilz) [Robert *Boyle,* British physicist, 1627– 1691] see under *law.*

Bozeman's catheter, operation, position, speculum (bōz′manz) [Nathan *Bozeman,* American surgeon, 1825–1905] see under *catheter, position,* and *speculum,* and see *hysterocytocleisis.*

Bozeman-Fritsch catheter (bōz′man-fritsh) [Nathan *Bozeman;* Heinrich *Fritsch,* German gynecologist, 1844– 1915] Bozeman's catheter.

Bozzolo's sign (bot′tso-lōz) [Camillo *Bozzolo,* Italian physician, 1845–1920] see under *sign.*

B.P. 1. blood pressure. 2. British Pharmacopoeia, a publication of the General Medical Council, describing and establishing standards for medicines, preparations, materials, and articles used in the practice of medicine, surgery, or midwifery.

b.p. *boiling point.*

bp abbreviation for *base pair.*

B.P.A. British Paediatric Association.

B. Ph. British Pharmacopoeia.

Bq abbreviation for *becquerel.*

Br chemical symbol for *bromine.*

brace (brās) 1. a device that holds parts together or in place. 2. an orthopedic appliance (orthosis) used to support, align, or hold parts of the body in position. 3. (pl.) an orthodontic appliance (see under *appliance*). **Blount b.,** a distraction brace consisting of a molded pelvic band with anterior and posterior metal bars connecting to chin or throat piece and occipital hold; used in scoliosis. **Fisher b.,** a skeletal brace with axillary holds and a corset front. **Goldthwait b.,** a skeletal brace of three padded, leather-covered metal strips, the uppermost fitting above the nipple line and the lowest encircling the pelvis. **Jewett b.,** a skeletal brace with pads as corrective pressure points at the sternal notch, above the pubis, and in the lumbar lordosis. **Jones b.,** one consisting of two vertical parallel bars that join a wider horizontal bar at the bottom, held in place by shoulder straps, an abdominal support, and groin straps, leaving the chest free. **McKee b.,** a skeletal brace with a lumbar pad; used to support the lumbar spine and prevent flexion. **Milwaukee b.,** a distraction brace with a molded pelvic belt that fits above the upper edge of the iliac crest, joined to a turnbuckle that extends the length of the spine to an occipital hold with a throat mold; used in scoliosis and ankylosing spondylitis. **Taylor b.,** see under *splint*.

bracelet (brās′let) a small encircling band, denoting, in the plural, transverse markings across the palmar surface of the skin of the wrists. **Nageotte's b's,** bands covered with circular spines on the axons at the level of the nodes of Ranvier.

brachia (bra′ke-ah) [L.] plural of *brachium*.

brachial (bra′ke-al) [L. *brachialis*, from *brachium* arm] pertaining to the arm.

brachialgia (bra″ke-al′je-ah) [Gr. *brachiōn* arm + *-algia*] pain in the arm or arms. **b. stat′ica paresthet′ica,** painful paresthesias in the arm and hand during sleep due to compression of the blood vessels; called also *Wartenberg's disease*.

brachiation (bra″ke-a′shun) [L. *brachium* + *-ation* suffix implying action] locomotion in a position of suspension by means of the hands and arms, as exhibited by monkeys when swinging from branch to branch.

brachi(o)- [L. *brachium*, q.v.] a combining form denoting arm.

brachiocephalic (brak″e-o-sĕ-fal′ik) [Gr. *brachiōn* arm + *kephalē* head] pertaining to the arm and head.

brachiocrural (brak″e-o-kroo′ral) [L. *brachium* arm + *crus* leg] pertaining to the arm and leg.

brachiocubital (brak″e-o-ku′bĭ-tal) [L. *brachium* arm + *cubitus* elbow] pertaining to the arm and elbow or forearm.

brachiocyllosis (brak″e-o-sĭ-lo′sis) [Gr. *brachiōn* arm + *kyllōsis* a crooking] brachiocyrtosis.

brachiocyrtosis (brak″e-o-ser-to′sis) [Gr. *brachiōn* arm + *kyrtos* bent] crookedness of the arm.

brachiofaciolingual (brak″e-o-fa″she-o-ling′gwal) pertaining to or affecting the arm, the face, and the tongue.

brachiogram (brak′e-o-gram) (*obs.*) a tracing of the pulse beat at the brachial artery.

brachiotomy (bra″ke-ot′o-me) [Gr. *brachiōn* arm + *tomē* a cut] (*obs.*) the surgical or obstetrical cutting or removal of an arm.

brachium (bra′ke-um), pl. *bra′chia* [L.; Gr. *brachiōn*] [NA] 1. the arm; specifically the arm from shoulder to elbow. 2. a general term used to designate an armlike process or structure. **b. of caudal colliculus, b. collic′uli cauda′lis** [NA] brachium of caudal colliculus: fibers from the lateral lemniscus that pass deep to the caudal colliculus and run forward to terminate in the medial geniculate body; called also *b. of inferior colliculus, b. colliculi inferioris* [NA alternative], and *b. quadrigeminum inferius*. **b. collic′uli crania′lis,** b. colliculi rostralis. **b. collic′uli inferio′ris,** NA alternative for *b. colliculi caudalis*. **b. collic′uli rostra′lis** [NA], fibers ascending ventrolaterally from the lateral aspect of the rostral colliculus of the mesencephalon, conveying fibers from the retina and the optic radiation to the cranial colliculus; called also *b. of cranial colliculus, b. colliculi cranialis, b. colliculi superioris* [NA alternative], *b. of superior colliculus,* and *b. quadrigeminum superius*. **b. collic′uli superio′ris,** NA alternative for *b. colliculi rostralis*. **b. of cranial colliculus,** b. colliculi rostralis. **b. of inferior colliculus,** b. colliculi inferioris. **b. op′ticum,** one of the processes extending from the corpora quadrigemina to the optic thalamus. **b. quadrigem′inum infe′rius,** b. colliculi caudalis. **b. quadrigem′inum supe′rius,** b. colliculi rostralis. **b. of rostral colliculus,** b. colliculi rostralis. **b. of superior colliculus,** b. colliculi rostralis.

Bracht's maneuver (brokts) [Erich Franz *Bracht*, German gynecologist and obstetrician, born 1882] see under *maneuver*.

Bracht-Wächter lesion (brokt-vek′ter) [Erich Franz Eugen *Bracht*, German pathologist, born 1882; Hermann Julius Gustav *Wächter* German physician, born 1878] see under *lesion*.

brachy- [Gr. *brachys* short] a combining form meaning short.

Brachyarcus (bra″ke-ar′kus) [*brachy-* + L. *arcus* bow] a genus of nonmotile, gram-negative, curved bacteria found in lakes, made up of anaerobic or microaerophilic bow-shaped rods. The type species is *B. thioph′ilus*.

brachybasia (brak″e-ba′se-ah) [*brachy-* + Gr. *basis* walking] a slow, shuffling, short-stepped gait, as seen in double hemiplegia.

brachycardia (brak″e-kar′de-ah) bradycardia.

brachycephalia (brak″e-se-fa′le-ah) brachycephaly.

brachycephalic (brak″e-se-fal′ik) pertaining to or characterized by brachycephaly. Called also *brachycephalous* and *eurycephalic*. See also *brachycranic*.

brachycephalism (brak″e-sef′ah-lizm) brachycephaly.

brachycephalous (brak″e-sef′ah-lus) brachycephalic.

brachycephaly (brak″e-sef′ah-le) [*brachy-* + Gr. *kephalē* head] having a comparatively short head, with a cephalic index of 81.0 to 85.4, a characteristic of American Indians, Malayans, and Burmese.

brachycheilia (brak″e-ki′le-ah) [*brachy-* + Gr. *cheilos* lip + *-ia*] abnormal shortness of the lip.

brachychily (brak-ik′ĭ-le) brachycheilia.

brachychronic (brak″e-kron′ik) [Gr. *brachychronios* of short duration] acute; said of a disease (Rabagliati).

brachycnemic (brak″e-ne′mik) brachyknemic.

brachycranial (brak″e-kra′ne-al) brachycranic.

brachycranic (brak″e-kra′nik) [*brachy-* + L.; Gr. *kranion* skull] having a comparatively short head, with a cranial index of 80.0 to 84.9. Called also *brachycranial* and *eurycranic*. See also *brachycephalic*.

brachydactyly (brak″e-dak′tĭ-le) [*brachy-* + Gr. *daktylos* finger] abnormal shortness of the fingers and toes.

brachyesophagus (brak″e-ĕ-sof′ah-gus) [*brachy-* + *esophagus*] abnormal shortness of the esophagus.

brachyfacial (brak″e-fa′shal) [*brachy-* + *facial*] having a comparatively low, broad face, with a facial index of 90 or less. Called also *brachyprosopic*.

brachygnathia (brak-ig-na′the-ah) [*brachy-* + Gr. *gnathos* jaw + *-ia*] abnormal shortness of the lower jaw.

brachygnathous (brah-kig′nah-thus) having an unusually short lower jaw.

brachykerkic (brak″e-ker′kik) [*brachy-* + Gr. *kerkis* the radius of the arm] having a short radius, with a radiohumeral index less than 75.

brachyknemic (brak″e-ne′mik) [*brachy-* + Gr. *knēmē* shin] having short legs, with the tibiofemoral index of 82 or less; also spelled *brachycnemic*.

brachymetacarpalism (brak″e-met″ah-kar′pal-izm) brachymetacarpia.

brachymetacarpia (brak″e-met″ah-kar′pe-ah) [*brachy-* + *metacarpus* + *-ia*] abnormal shortness of the metacarpal bones.

brachymetapody (brak″e-mĕ-tap′o-de) [*brachy-* + *meta-* (def. 2) + *pod-* + *-ia*] abnormal shortness of some of the metacarpal or metatarsal bones.

brachymetatarsia (brak″e-met″ah-tar′se-ah) [*brachy-* + *metatarsus* + *-ia*] abnormal shortness of the metatarsal bones.

brachymorphic (brak″e-mor′fik) [*brachy-* + Gr. *morphē* form] built along lines that are shorter and broader than those of the normal figure; called also *brachytypical* and *brevilineal*.

brachyphalangia (brak″e-fah-lan′je-ah) [*brachy-* + *phalanx*] abnormal shortness of one or more of the phalanges of a finger or toe.

brachyskelous (brak″e-ske′lus) [*brachy-* + Gr. *skelos* leg] abnormal shortness of one or both legs.

brachystaphyline (brak″e-staf′ĭ-līn) [*brachy-* + Gr. *staphylē* uvula] pertaining to or characterized by a short, wide palate, with a palatal index of 85.0 or more.

brachystasis (brah-kis′tah-sis) [*brachy-* + *stasis*] a state in which a muscle fiber is relatively decreased in length, and resists stretch; it contracts and relaxes, manifesting the same tension after contraction as before.

brachytherapy (brak″e-ther′ah-pe) in radiotherapy, treatment with ionizing radiation whose source is applied to the surface of the body or is located a short distance from the body area being treated; cf. *teletherapy.*

brachytypical (brak″e-tip′e-k'l) brachymorphic.

brachyuranic (brak″e-u-ran′ik) having a narrow maxilla, with a maxilloalveolar index of 115.0 or more.

bracing (brās′ing) 1. holding parts together or in place. 2. making something rigid or steady. 3. resistance to horizontal components of masticatory force.

bracken (brak′en) a fern, *Pteridium aquilinum* (L.) Kuhn (Polypodiaceae), of worldwide distribution noted as a poisonous plant in veterinary medicine. In monogastric animals, the plant produces severe intoxication due to enzymatic destruction of thiamine by a thiaminase present in the plant. In ruminants, the poisoning is apparently due to a dialyzable, small molecule which causes bone marrow hypoplasia, leading to death.

bracket (brak′it) 1. a support projecting from the main structure. 2. orthodontic b., a small metal attachment soldered or welded to an orthodontic band or cemented directly to the teeth, serving to fasten the arch wire to the band or tooth. Called also *orthodontic attachment.* See also *orthodontic appliance,* under *appliance.*

bract (brakt) a small modified leaf in a flower cluster.

Bradford frame (brad′ford) [Edward Hickling *Bradford,* Boston orthopedic surgeon, 1848–1926] see under *frame.*

bradshot (brad′shot) braxy.

bradsot (brad′sot) braxy.

brady- [Gr. *bradys* slow] a combining form meaning slow.

bradyacusia (brad″e-ah-ku′se-ah) [*brady-* + Gr. *akouein* to hear] dullness of hearing.

bradyarrhythmia (brad″e-ah-rith′me-ah) [*brady-* + *a* neg. + Gr. *rhythmos* rhythm] bradycardia associated with an irregularity in the heart rhythm.

bradyarthria (brad″e-ar′thre-ah) [*brady-* + Gr. *arthroun* to utter distinctly] bradylalia.

bradyauxesis (brad″e-awk-se′sis) [*brady-* + Gr. *auxēsis* increase] a form of heterauxesis in which the part grows more slowly than the whole.

Bradybaena (brad″e-be′nah) a genus of snails that serve as hosts to *Dicrocoelium dentriticum.*

bradycardia (brad″e-kar′de-ah) [*brady-* + Gr. *kardia* heart] slowness of the heart beat, as evidenced by slowing of the pulse rate to less than 60. **Branham's b.,** see under *sign.* **cardiomuscular b.** (*obs.*), that caused by disease of the muscle of the heart. **central b.,** bradycardia dependent on disease of the central nervous system. **essential b.,** bradycardia occurring without discoverable cause. **nodal b.,** bradycardia in which the stimulus of the heart's contraction arises in the atrioventricular node or main bundle. **postinfective b.,** bradycardia occurring after infectious disease. **sinoatrial b.,** sinus b. **sinus b.,** a slow sinus rhythm, with a heart rate less than 60. **vagal b.,** bradycardia due to increased vagal tone.

bradycardiac (brad″e-kar′de-ak) 1. pertaining to, characterized by, or causing bradycardia. 2. an agent that acts to slow the pulse.

bradycardic (brad″e-kar′dik) bradycardiac.

bradycinesia (brad″e-sĭ-ne′ze-ah) bradykinesia.

bradycrotic (brad″e-krot′ik) [*brady-* + Gr. *krotos* pulsation] pertaining to, characterized by, or inducing slowness of pulse.

bradydiastalsis (brad″e-di″ah-stal′sis) (*obs.*) slow or delayed bowel movement.

bradydiastole (brad″e-di-as′to-le) [*brady-* + *diastole*] abnormal prolongation of the diastole.

bradyecoia (brad″e-e-koi′ah) [Gr. *bradyēkoos* slow of hearing] partial deafness.

bradyesthesia (brad″e-es-the′ze-ah) [*brady-* + Gr. *aisthēsis* perception] slowness or dullness of perception.

bradygenesis (brad″e-jen′ĕ-sis) [*brady-* + *genesis*] the lengthening of certain stages in embryonic development.

bradyglossia (brad″e-glos′e-ah) [Gr. *bradyglōssos* slow of speech] abnormal slowness of utterance.

bradykinesia (brad″e-kĭ-ne′se-ah) [*brady-* + Gr. *kinēsis*

movement] abnormal slowness of movement; sluggishness of physical and mental responses.

bradykinetic (brad″e-kĭ-net′ik) [*brady-* + Gr. *kinēsis* motion] 1. characterized by or performed by slow movement. 2. denoting a method of showing the details of motor action by motion pictures taken very rapidly and shown very slowly.

bradykinin (brad″e-ki′nin) [*brady-* + Gr. *kinein* motion] a nonapeptide (Arg-Pro-Pro-Gly-Phe-Ser-Pro-Phe-Arg) produced by activation of the kinin system in a variety of inflammatory conditions. It is an extremely potent vasodilator; it also increases vascular permeability, stimulates pain receptors, and causes contraction of a variety of extravascular smooth muscles. The name refers to the slowly developing contraction produced in isolated guinea pig ileum. Bradykinin is produced by the action of plasma kallikrein on HMW (high-molecular-weight) kininogen, a plasma α_2-globulin, and destroyed by several kininases in the lungs and other tissues. Two other kinins Lys-bradykinin (called also kallidin) and Met-Lys-bradykinin are produced by other kallikreins.

bradylalia (brad″e-la′le-ah) [*brady-* + Gr. *lalein* to talk] abnormally slow utterance of words due to a brain lesion; called also *bradyarthria* and *bradyphasia.*

bradylexia (brad″e-lek′se-ah) [*brady-* + Gr. *lexis* word] abnormal slowness in reading, due neither to defect of intelligence or of vision nor to ignorance of the alphabet.

bradylogia (brad″e-lo′je-ah) [Gr.] abnormal slowness of speech due to slowness of thinking, as in a mental disorder.

bradymenorrhea (brad″e-men″o-re′ah) [*brady-* + *menorrhea*] menstruation marked by long duration.

bradyphagia (brad″e-fa′je-ah) [*brady-* + Gr. *phagein* to eat] abnormal slowness in eating.

bradyphasia (brad″e-fa′ze-ah) [*brady-* + Gr. *phasis* speech] bradylalia.

bradyphemia (brad″e-fe′me-ah) [*brady-* + Gr. *phēmē* speech] slowness of speech.

bradyphrasia (brad″e-fra′ze-ah) [*brady-* + Gr. *phrasis* utterance] slowness of speech due to mental disorder.

bradyphrenia (brad″e-fre′ne-ah) [*brady-* + Gr. *phrēn* mind] a condition marked by extreme fatigability of initiative, interest, and psychomotor activity resulting from epidemic encephalitis.

bradypnea (brad″e-ne′ah) [*brady-* + Gr. *pnoia* breath] abnormal slowness of breathing.

bradypragia (brad″e-pra′je-ah) [*brady-* + Gr. *prattein* to act] slowness of action.

Bradyrhizobium (bra″de-ri-zo′be-um) [Gr. *bradus* slow + L. *rhizobium* root living] a genus of gram-negative, aerobic, pleomorphic, rod-shaped bacteria of the family Rhizobiaceae, consisting of nitrogen-fixing endosymbionts, which are found in the root nodules of leguminous plants. The type species is *B. japon′icum.*

bradyrhythmia (brad″e-rith′me-ah) [*brady-* + Gr. *rhythmos* rhythm] bradycardia.

bradyspermatism (brad″e-sper′mah-tizm) [*brady-* + Gr. *sperma* semen] abnormally slow ejaculation of semen.

bradysphygmia (brad″e-sfig′me-ah) [*brady-* + Gr. *sphygmos* pulse] bradycardia.

bradystalsis (brad″e-stal′sis) [*brady-* + (*peri-*)*stalsis*] abnormal slowness of peristalsis.

bradytachycardia (brad″e-tak″e-kar′de-ah) [*brady-* + Gr. *tachys* swift + *kardia* heart] alternating attacks of bradycardia and tachycardia, as may occur in sick sinus syndrome.

bradyteleocinesia (brad″e-tel″e-o-si-ne′ze-ah) bradyteleokinesis.

bradyteleokinesis (brad″e-tel″e-o-kĭ-ne′sis) [*brady-* + Gr. *telein* to complete + *kinēsis* movement] a defect of motor coordination in which a movement is slowed or stopped prior to reaching its goal.

bradytocia (brad″e-to′se-ah) [*brady-* + Gr. *tokos* birth] lingering or slow parturition.

bradytrophia (brad″e-tro′fe-ah) a condition characterized by slow-acting nutritive processes.

bradytrophic (brad″e-trof′ik) [*brady-* + Gr. *trophē* nutrition] having slow-acting nutritive processes.

bradyuria (brad″e-u′re-ah) [*brady-* + Gr. *ouron* urine] abnormally slow passage of urine.

bradyzoite (bra″de-zo′īt) [*brady-* + *zōon* animal] a small, comma-shaped form of *Toxoplasma gondii,* found in clusters enclosed by an irregular wall (*pseudocyst*) in the tissues, chiefly muscles and the brain, in chronic (latent) toxoplasmosis; considered to be the slow-growing form. Cf. *tachyzoite*.

braidism (brād′izm) [after James *Braid*] hypnotism.

Braid's strabismus (brādz) [James *Braid*, English surgeon 1795–1860] see under *strabismus*.

Brailey's operation (bra′lēz) [William Arthur *Brailey*, English ophthalmologist, 1845–1915] see under *operation*.

braille (brāl) [Louis *Braille*, a French teacher of the blind, 1809–1852] a system of writing and printing for the blind by means of tangible points or dots.

brain (brān) [Anglo-Saxon *braegen*] that part of the central nervous system contained within the cranium, comprising the prosencephalon, mesencephalon, and rhombencephalon; it is derived (developed) from the anterior part of the embryonic neural tube. Called also *encephalon* [NA]. See also *cerebrum*. **new b.,** neencephalon (neoencephalon). **old b.,** paleencephalon (paleoencephalon). **olfactory b., smell b.,** rhinencephalon, def. 1. **respirator b.,** the brain after clinical brain death but while vital functions are being artificially maintained; it is characterized by marked autolysis and necrosis. **'tween b.,** diencephalon (interbrain). **water b.,** gid. **wet b.,** an edematous condition of the brain; see *brain edema*, under *edema*.

Brain's reflex (brānz) [Walter Russell *Brain*, British neurologist, 1895–1966] see under *reflex*.

brain stem (brān′stem) the stemlike portion of the brain connecting the cerebral hemispheres with the spinal cord and comprising the pons, medulla oblongata, and mesencephalon; the diencephalon is considered part of the brain stem by some. Called also *encephalic trunk* and *truncus encephalicus* [NA].

brainwashing (brān′wash-ing) any systematic effort aimed at instilling certain attitudes and beliefs in a person against his will, usually beliefs in conflict with his prior beliefs and knowledge. It initially referred to political indoctrination of prisoners of war and political prisoners.

brake (brāk) a mechanism for arresting or inhibiting an activity. **duodenal b.,** a mechanism lodged largely in the duodenum that inhibits gastric secretion and motility.

bran (bran) the meal derived from the epidermis or outer covering of a cereal grain.

branch (branch) a division or offshoot from a main stem, especially of blood vessels, nerves, or lymphatics; for specific anatomical structures, see under *ramus*. **left bundle b.,** crus sinistrum fasciculi atrioventricularis. **right bundle b.,** crus dextrum fasciculi atrioventricularis.

branched-chain α-**keto acid decarboxylase** branched chain α-ketoacid dehydrogenase.

branched-chain α-**keto acid dehydrogenase** a multienzyme complex composed of 2-ketoisovalerate dehydrogenase (lipoamide), dihydrolipoamide dehydrogenase (NAD), and a dihydrolipoamide acyltransferase. It contains thiamine pyrophosphate, lipoate, and FAD and requires NAD and coenzyme A as cofactors. The complex catalyzes the oxidative decarboxylation of the branched chain amino acids leucine, isoleucine, and valine. A defect in one of the components of the complex causes maple syrup urine disease (see under *disease*).

brancher deficiency glycogen storage disease, type IV.

brancher enzyme, branching enzyme 1,4-α-glucan branching enzyme.

branchia (brang′ke-ah) [Gr. *branchia* gills] the gills of fishes and of others of the lower vertebrates; represented in the human fetus by the branchial arches, separated by clefts.

branchial (brang′ke-al) pertaining to or resembling the gills of a fish or the derivatives of homologous parts in higher forms.

branchiogenic (brang″ke-o-jen′ik) gill-forming; forming a branchial arch.

branchiogenous (brang″ke-oj′ĕ-nus) [*branchia* + Gr. *gennan* to produce] formed from a branchial cleft or arch.

branchioma (brang″ke-o′mah) a tumor derived from branchial epithelium or branchial rests.

branchiomere (brang′ke-o-mēr″) a segment of the splanchnic mesoderm from which the branchial arches are developed.

branchiomeric (brang″ke-o-mer′ik) pertaining to the branchiomeres or branchial arches.

branchiomerism (brang″ke-om′er-izm) [*branchia-* + Gr. *meros* part] metamerism based on the serial repetition of the branchial arches.

Branchiostoma (brang″ke-o-sto′mah) [*branchia* + Gr. *stoma* mouth] *Amphioxus*.

Brand bath (brahnt) [Ernst *Brand*, German physician, 1827–1897] see under *bath*.

brandy (bran′de) the potable alcoholic distillate of fermented juices of various fruits, e.g., grapes, apples, cherries, peaches, etc., containing 48 to 54 per cent ethanol; used medically as a stomachic, tonic, peripheral vasodilator, and sedative.

Branham's sign (bradycardia) (bran′hamz) [H. H. *Branham*, American surgeon of 19th century] see under *sign*.

Branhamella (bran″hah-mel′ah) [Sara Elizabeth *Branham*, American bacteriologist, born 1888] *Moraxella* (*Branhamella*). **B. catarrha′lis,** *Moraxella* (*Branhamella*) *catarrhalis*.

brash (brash) heartburn. **water b.,** heartburn with regurgitation of sour fluid or almost tasteless saliva into the mouth. **weaning b.,** diarrhea in an infant when put on food other than its mother's milk.

Brassica (bras′e-kah) [L.] a genus of cruciferous plants to which the cabbage, turnip, mustard, and related species belong. *B. al′ba* (L.) Rabenh. (*Sinapis alba* L.) is white mustard, and *B. ni′gra* (L.) Koch. is black mustard. When the seeds of these plants are crushed and moistened, volatile oils are liberated. See *mustard* and *oil of mustard*.

brassidic acid (brah-sid′ik) trivial name for the 22-carbon unsaturated fatty acid *trans*-13-docosenoic acid.

Braun's anastomosis (brawnz) [Heinrich *Braun*, German surgeon, 1847–1911] see under *anastomosis*.

Braun's canal (brawnz) [Carl von *Braun*, Viennese obstetrician, 1822–1891] neurenteric canal; see under *canal*.

Braun's hook (brawnz) [Gustav *Braun*, Austrian gynecologist, 1829–1911] see under *hook*.

Braune's canal (brawn′ez) [Christian Wilhelm *Braune*, German anatomist, 1831–1892] see under *canal*.

Braxton Hicks contraction (sign), version (braks′ton hiks) [John *Braxton Hicks*, English gynecologist, 1823–1897] see under *contraction* and *version*.

braxy (brak′se) a disease of sheep caused by *Clostridium septicum*, and marked by hemorrhagic abomasitis, with hemorrhage into the peritoneal cavity, by abdominal pain, and, usually, by diarrhea and high fever.

brayera (bra-ye′rah) the dried panicles of the pistillate flowers of *Hagenia abyssinica* J. F. Gmel., having medical and veterinary use as a vermifuge and teniacide, respectively.

brazilin (brah-zil′in) a yellow crystalline substance obtained from the bark of *Biancea sappan* and other redwood trees; it is very similar to hematoxylin and oxidizes to a bright red dye, brazilein.

breadth (bredth) the distance measured horizontally from side to side; see also under *diameter*. **b. of accommodation,** range of accommodation. **bizygomatic b.,** the distance between the most laterally situated points (zygia) on the zygomatic arches.

break (brāk) 1. to interrupt the continuity, or an interruption in the continuity of a structure, especially a bone. See *fracture*. 2. the interruption of an electric circuit, as distinguished from the make. **chromatid b.,** interruption of the continuity of a chromatid, the portions immediately proximal and distal to the site may then become out of alignment.

breast (brest) the anterior aspect of the chest, often applied especially to the modified cutaneous glandular structure it bears; see *mamma* [NA]. **caked b.,** stagnation mastitis. **chicken b.,** pigeon b. **Cooper's irritable b.,** neuralgia of the breast. **funnel b.,** funnel chest. **irritable b.,** Cooper's irritable b. **pigeon b.,** a condition of the chest in which the sternum is prominent, due to obstruction to infantile respiration or to rickets; called also *chicken b.*, *keeled chest*, *pectus carinatum*, and *pectus gallinatum*. **proemial b.,** that condition of the female breast which is a prelude to pathologic changes. **shoe-makers' b.,** sinking in of the sternum in shoe-makers, produced by the pressure of tools against the lower part of the sternum and

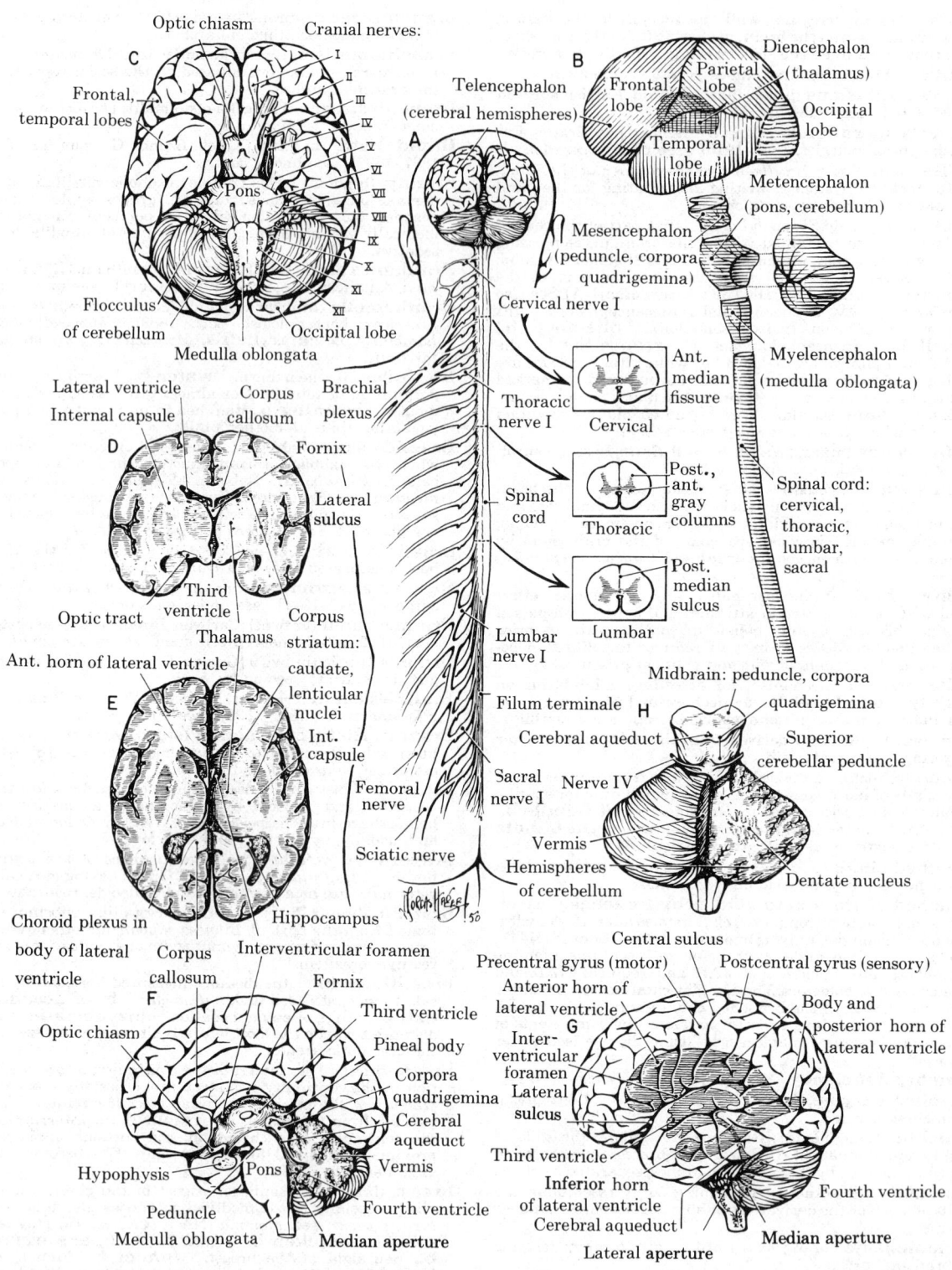

Optic chiasm

Cranial nerves:

C

Frontal, temporal lobes

Pons

Flocculus of cerebellum

Medulla oblongata

Occipital lobe

Telencephalon (cerebral hemispheres)

A

Cervical nerve I

Thoracic nerve I

Brachial plexus

Spinal cord

Lumbar nerve I

Filum terminale

Femoral nerve

Sacral nerve I

Sciatic nerve

B

Frontal lobe

Parietal lobe

Diencephalon (thalamus)

Temporal lobe

Occipital lobe

Metencephalon (pons, cerebellum)

Mesencephalon (peduncle, corpora quadrigemina)

Myelencephalon (medulla oblongata)

Spinal cord: cervical, thoracic, lumbar, sacral

Ant. median fissure

Cervical

Post., ant. gray columns

Thoracic

Post. median sulcus

Lumbar

Lateral ventricle

Internal capsule

Corpus callosum

D

Fornix

Lateral sulcus

Optic tract

Third ventricle

Corpus striatum: caudate, lenticular nuclei

Thalamus

Ant. horn of lateral ventricle

E

Int. capsule

Choroid plexus in body of lateral ventricle

Corpus callosum

Hippocampus

Interventricular foramen

F

Fornix

Optic chiasm

Third ventricle

Pineal body

Corpora quadrigemina

Cerebral aqueduct

Hypophysis

Pons

Vermis

Peduncle

Fourth ventricle

Medulla oblongata

Median aperture

Midbrain: peduncle, corpora quadrigemina

H

Cerebral aqueduct

Nerve IV

Superior cerebellar peduncle

Vermis

Hemispheres of cerebellum

Dentate nucleus

Central sulcus

Precentral gyrus (motor)

Postcentral gyrus (sensory)

Anterior horn of lateral ventricle

Inter-ventricular foramen

Lateral sulcus

Third ventricle

G

Body and posterior horn of lateral ventricle

Inferior horn of lateral ventricle

Cerebral aqueduct

Lateral aperture

Fourth ventricle

Median aperture

PLATE 10 — VARIOUS ASPECTS AND SECTIONS OF BRAIN AND SPINAL CORD

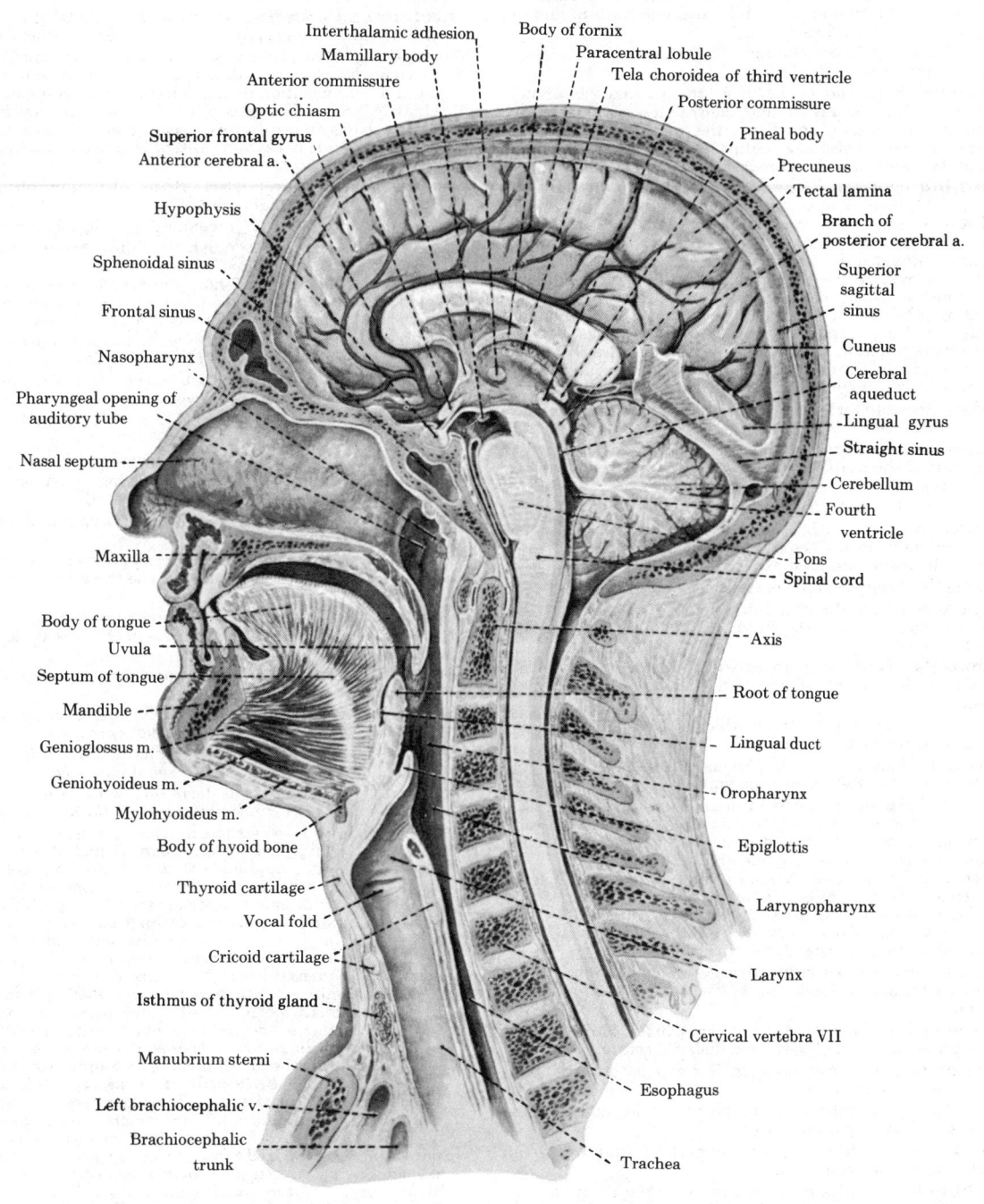

Interthalamic adhesion
Mamillary body
Anterior commissure
Optic chiasm
Superior frontal gyrus
Anterior cerebral a.
Hypophysis
Sphenoidal sinus
Frontal sinus
Nasopharynx
Pharyngeal opening of
auditory tube
Nasal septum
Maxilla
Body of tongue
Uvula
Septum of tongue
Mandible
Genioglossus m.
Geniohyoideus m.
Mylohyoideus m.
Body of hyoid bone
Thyroid cartilage
Vocal fold
Cricoid cartilage
Isthmus of thyroid gland
Manubrium sterni
Left brachiocephalic v.
Brachiocephalic
trunk

Body of fornix
Paracentral lobule
Tela choroidea of third ventricle
Posterior commissure
Pineal body
Precuneus
Tectal lamina
Branch of
posterior cerebral a.
Superior
sagittal
sinus
Cuneus
Cerebral
aqueduct
Lingual gyrus
Straight sinus
Cerebellum
Fourth
ventricle
Pons
Spinal cord
Axis
Root of tongue
Lingual duct
Oropharynx
Epiglottis
Laryngopharynx
Larynx
Cervical vertebra VII
Esophagus
Trachea

**PLATE 11 — HEMISECTION OF THE HEAD AND NECK, SHOWING VARIOUS PARTS OF
THE BRAIN IN RELATION TO OTHER STRUCTURES**

the xiphoid cartilage. **shotty b.,** cystic disease of the breast; see under *disease.* **thrush b.,** the speckled appearance of the myocardium under the endocardium in fatty degeneration of the heart.

breast-feeding (brest′ fēd′ing) the nursing of an infant at the mother's breast.

breath (breth) [L. *spiritus halitus*] the air taken in and expelled by the expansion and contraction of the thorax. **bad b.,** halitosis. **lead b.,** the metallic odor of the breath in lead poisoning; called also *halitus saturninus.* **liver b.,** fetor hepaticus (hepatic fetor).

breathing (brēth′ing) the alternate inspiration and expiration of air into and out of the lungs; see *respiration.* **Biot's b.,** see under *respiration.* **bronchial b.,** vesicular breath sounds. **frog b., glossopharyngeal b.,** respiration unaided by the primary or ordinary accessory muscles of respiration, the air being "swallowed" rapidly into the lungs by use of the tongue and muscles of the pharynx; used by patients with chronic muscle paralysis to augment their breathing. **intermittent positive pressure b.,** the active inflation of the lungs during inspiration under positive pressure from a cycling valve; abbreviated IPPB. **periodic b.,** Cheyne-Stokes respiration.

Breda's disease (bra′dahz) [Achille *Breda,* Italian dermatologist, 1850–1933] yaws.

bredouillement (bra-dwe-maw′) a speech defect in which only part of the word is pronounced, due to extreme rapidity of utterance.

breech (brēch) buttocks (nates [NA]).

bregma (breg′mah) [Gr. "front of the head"] [NA] the point on the surface of the skull at the junction of the coronal and sagittal sutures; used as a craniometric landmark.

bregmatic (breg-mat′ik) pertaining to the bregma.

bregmatodymia (breg″mah-to-dim′e-ah) [*bregma* + Gr. *didymos* twin + *-ia*] the state of conjoined twins fused at the bregmas.

Brehmer's treatment (method) (bra′merz) [Hermann *Brehmer,* German physician, 1826–1889] see under *treatment.*

brei (bri) [Ger. "pulp"] tissue that has been ground to a pulp; a homogenate.

Breisky's disease (bri′skēz) [August *Breisky,* German gynecologist, 1832–1889] kraurosis vulvae.

bremsstrahlung (brem′strah-lung) [Ger. "braking radiation"] 1. the continuous spectrum of electromagnetic radiation produced by the rapid deceleration of a fast-moving charged particle (such as an electron or beta particle) in the electric field of another charged particle (usually a nucleus). Called also *braking radiation, white radiation* (by analogy to the continuous optical spectrum obtained from white light), and *continuous x-ray spectrum.* 2. the deceleration of a charged particle that produces this radiation.

Brennemann's syndrome (bren′e-manz) [Joseph *Brennemann,* Chicago pediatrician, 1872–1944] see under *syndrome.*

Brenner's formula (test) (bren′erz) [Rudolf *Brenner,* German physician, 1821–1884] see under *formula.*

Brenner tumor [Fritz *Brenner,* German pathologist, born 1877] see under *tumor.*

brenz- [Ger.] a prefix meaning burnt; for words beginning thus, see those beginning *pyro-.*

brephic (bref′ik) [Gr. *brephos* embryo] pertaining to an early stage of development.

breph(o)- [Gr. *brephos* embryo, newborn infant] a combining form denoting relationship to the embryo or fetus, or to the newborn infant.

brephoplastic (bref″o-plas′tik) [*brepho-* + Gr. *plassein* to form] formed from embryonic tissue or during embryonic life.

brephopolysarcia (bref″o-pol″e-sar′se-ah) [*brepho-* + *polysarcia*] (*obs.*) excessive fleshiness in an infant.

brephotrophic (bref″o-trof′ik) [*brepho-* + Gr. *trophē* nutrition] pertaining to the nourishment of infants.

Breschet's canals, hiatus, sinus, veins (brĕ-shāz′) [Gilbert *Breschet,* French anatomist, 1784-1845] see *canales diploici, helicotrema, sinus sphenoparietalis,* and *venae diploicae.*

Brethine (breth′ēn) trademark for preparations of terbutaline sulfate.

Bretonneau's angina, disease (bret-o-nōz′) [Pierre Fidèle *Bretonneau,* French physician, 1778–1862] diphtheria.

bretylium tosylate (brĕ-til′e-um) chemical name: 2-bromo-*N*-ethyl-*N,N*-dimethylbenzenemethanaminium 4-methylbenzenesulfonate. An adrenergic blocking agent, $C_{18}H_{24}BrNO_3S$, occurring as a white, crystalline powder; originally used as an antihypertensive agent, it is now used as an antiarrhythmic in certain cases of ventricular tachycardia or fibrillation.

Breus mole (broys) [Carl *Breus,* Austrian obstetrician, 1852–1914] see under *mole.*

brevi- [L. *brevis* short] a combining form meaning short.

Brevibacterium (brev″e-bak-te′re-um) [*brevi-* + Gr. *baktērion* little rod] a genus of coryneform bacteria of uncertain status, consisting of short, unbranched rods found in salt and fresh water, dairy products, and decomposing material of many types. Many are of industrial importance.

brevicollis (brev″ĕ-kol′is) [*brevi-* + L. *collum* neck] shortness of the neck; see *dystrophia brevicollis.*

breviductor (brev″ĕ-duk′tor) [*brevi-* + L. *ductor* leader] (*obs.*) musculus adductor brevis.

breviflexor (brev″ĕ-flek′sor) [*brevi-* + L. *flexor* bender] a short flexor muscle.

brevilineal (brev″ĕ-lin′e-al) brachymorphic.

breviradiate (brev″ĕ-ra′de-āt) having short processes; a term applied to one type of neuroglia cells.

Brevital (brev′ĭ-tal) trademark for a preparation of methohexital sodium.

brevium (bre′ve-um) a name formerly given to a supposed isotope of tantalum now known to be the element protactinium.

Brewer's infarcts, point (broo′erz) [George Emerson *Brewer,* New York surgeon, 1861–1939] see under *infarct* and *point.*

Bricanyl (brik′ah-nil) trademark for preparations of terbutaline sulfate.

Bricker's operation (brik′erz) [Eugene M. *Bricker,* American surgeon, born 1908] see under *operation.*

Brickner's sign (brik′nerz) [Richard Max *Brickner,* New York neurologist, born 1896] see under *sign.*

brickpox (brik′poks) a form of swine erysipelas (Ger. *Backsteinblattern*) caused by *Erysipelothrix insidiosa.*

bridge (brij) 1. a structure that connects two distant points, including parts of an organ. Called also *pons.* 2. a prosthetic dental appliance that replaces lost teeth, being supported and held in position by attachments to adjacent teeth; the term is usually restricted to a fixed partial denture. 3. intercellular b. **arteriolovenular b.,** the main and largest capillary connecting an arteriole and a venule; it retains some muscle elements and is rarely completely collapsed. **cantilever b.,** a fixed partial denture in which the pontic is cantilevered, i.e., retained only on one side by the abutment tooth. Called also *extension b.* **cell b's,** see *intercellular b.* and *protoplasmic b.* **conjugative b.,** in bacterial conjugation, a connection formed between two bacterial cells by the attachment of an F pilus from an F⁺ cell to an F⁻ cell. **cytoplasmic b.,** 1. protoplasmic b. 2. intercellular b. **dentin b.,** a scarlike deposit of reparative dentin or other calcific substance which reseals exposed pulp or which forms across the excised surface of pulp after pulpotomy. **disulfide b.,** see under *bond.* **extension b.,** one having an artificial tooth attached beyond the point of anchorage of the tooth; sometimes called *cantilever b.* **fixed b.,** a fixed partial denture. **fixed-fixed b.,** fixed b. with rigid connectors. **fixed-movable b.,** fixed b. with rigid and nonrigid connectors. **fixed b. with rigid connectors,** a fixed partial denture in which all components are rigidly soldered or cast in one piece. Called also *fixed-fixed b.* **fixed b. with rigid and nonrigid connectors,** a fixed partial denture consisting of a major retainer attached to a pontic and supplied with a dovetail, and a minor retainer supplied with a slot into which the dovetail of the pontic fits; it provides some stress-breaking by allowing some movement. Called also *fixed-movable b.* **Gaskell's b.,** bundle of His. **intercellular b.,** a structure seen especially in the prickle cell layer of the epidermis, formed by the meeting of short cytoplasmic projections from the cell surface of adjacent cells. The structure was formerly thought to constitute a bridge for cytoplasmic continuity between cells, but it has been demonstrated that the processes make contact at a desmosome (q.v.); hence each cell is independent. Called also *cytoplasmic b.* **b. of the nose,** the upper portion of the external nose formed by the junction of the nasal bones. **protoplasmic b.,** a strand of protoplasm connecting two secondary spermatocytes, occurring as a result of incomplete cytokinesis; called also *cytoplasmic b.* **removable b.,** partial removable denture. **salt b.,** 1. an inverted-U–shaped tube filled with a gel, usually composed of agar, water, and potassium chloride, used to separate two chemically incompatible solutions in an electrochemical cell. 2. a chemical bond between a nitrogen atom, carrying a positive charge, and an oxygen atom, carrying a negative charge. **stationary b.,** a fixed partial denture. **ureteric b.,** Bell's muscle. **b. of Varolius,** pons, def. 2.

bridgework (brij′werk) a partial denture retained by attachments other than clasps. **fixed b.,** a partial denture retained by crowns or inlays cemented to the natural teeth. **removable b.,** a partial denture retained by attachments which permit its removal.

bridle (bri′d'l) 1. a frenum. 2. a loop or filament that crosses the lumen of a passage or the surface of an ulcer.

bridou (bre-doo′) perlèche.

Brieger's cachexia reaction, test (bre′gerz) [Ludwig *Brieger,* physician in Berlin, 1849–1919] see *cachexia reaction,* under *reaction,* and see under *tests.*

Bright's blindness, disease, eye (brīts) [Richard *Bright,* English physician, 1789–1858] see under *blindness, disease,* and *eye.*

brightic (bri′tik) 1. affected with glomerulonephritis (Bright's disease). 2. a person with glomerulonephritis.

brightism (brīt′izm) acute or chronic nephritis.

Brill's disease (brilz) [Nathan Edwin *Brill,* American physician, 1860–1925] Brill-Zinsser disease.

Brill-Symmers disease [Nathan Edwin *Brill;* Douglas *Symmers,* American physician, 1879–1952] nodular lymphoma.

Brill-Zinsser disease (bril′zin′ser) [Nathan Edwin *Brill;* Hans *Zinsser,* American bacteriologist, 1878–1940] see under *disease.*

brim (brim) the edge of the superior strait of the true pelvis; apertura pelvis superior.

Brinell hardness number (brin-el′) [Johann August *Brinell,* Swedish engineer, 1849–1925] see under *number.*

brinolase (bri′no-lās) a fibrinolytic enzyme produced by the fungus *Aspergillus oryzae.*

Brinton's disease (brin′tonz) [William *Brinton,* English physician, 1823–1867] linitis plastica.

Brion-Kayser disease (bre-on′ ki′zer) [Albert *Brion,* physician in Strasburg, born 1874; Heinrich *Kayser,* German physician, 1876–1940] paratyphoid.

Briquet's syndrome (bre-kāz′) [Paul *Briquet,* French physician, 1796–1881] see under *syndrome.*

brisement (brēz-maw′) [Fr. "crushing"] the breaking up or tearing of anything, as of an ankylosis. **b. forcé,** the forcible breaking up or tearing of a bony ankylosis.

Brissaud's dwarf, infantilism, reflex, scoliosis (bre-sōz′) [Edouard *Brissaud,* French physician, 1852–1909] see under *dwarf;* see *infantile myxedema,* under *myxedema;* see under *reflex;* and see *sciatic scoliosis,* under *scoliosis.*

Brissaud-Sicard syndrome (bre-so′-se-kar′) [Edouard *Brissaud;* Jean Athanase *Sicard,* Paris neurologist, 1872–1929] see under *syndrome.*

Bristacycline (bris″tah-si′klēn) trademark for a preparation of tetracycline hydrochloride.

Bristamin (bris′tah-min) trademark for a preparation of phenyltoloxamine.

broach (brōch) 1. an elongated, tapered and serrated cutting tool for shaping and enlarging holes. 2. barbed b.; root canal b. **barbed b.,** a thin, flexible, hand-operated or engine-driven endodontic instrument, usually tapered with a series of sharply pointed barbs along the operative head; used for engaging and removing the dental pulp and other substances intact from the root canal or pulp chamber. **pathfinder b.,** root canal probe. **root canal b.,** a broach, usually barbed, used for removing the soft tissue

contents of the root canal; see *barbed b.* **smooth b.,** root canal probe.

Broadbent's sign (brod′bentz) [Sir William Henry *Broadbent,* English physician, 1835–1907] see under *sign.*

Broca's amnesia, etc. (bro′kahz) [Pierre Paul *Broca,* celebrated French anatomist, anthropologist, and surgeon, 1824–1880] see under *amnesia, aphasia, area, band, center, convolution, fissure, formula, gyrus, plane, point, pouch,* and *region.*

Brockenbrough's sign (brok′en-browz) [Edwin C. *Brockenbrough,* American surgeon, born 1930] see under *sign.*

Brock's infundibulectomy, operation, syndrome (broks) [Sir Russell Claude *Brock,* British surgeon, born 1903] see under *infundibulectomy;* see *transventricular closed valvotomy,* under *valvotomy;* and see *middle lobe syndrome,* under *syndrome.*

Brödel's white line (brü′del) [Max *Brödel,* Baltimore medical artist, 1870–1941] see under *line.*

Broders' index (classification) (bro′derz) [Albert Compton *Broders,* American pathologist, 1885–1964] see under *index.*

Brodie's abscess, disease, knee (bro′dēz) [Sir Benjamin Collins *Brodie,* English surgeon, 1783–1862] see under *abscess, disease,* and *knee.*

Brodie's ligament (bro′dēz) [J. Gordon *Brodie,* Edinburgh anatomist, 1786–1818] transverse humeral ligament.

Brodmann's area [Korbinian *Brodmann,* German neurologist, 1868–1918] see under *area.*

Broesike's fossa (bre′ze-kēz) [Gustav *Broesike,* German anatomist, born 1853] see *parajejunal fossa,* under *fossa.*

brofoxine (bro-foks′ēn) chemical name: 6-bromo-1,4-dihydro-4,4-dimethyl-2*H*-3,1-benzoxazin-2-one; a tranquilizer, $C_{10}H_{10}BrNO_2$.

broken wind (bro′ken wind) heaves.

bromated (bro′māt-ed) brominated.

bromatherapy (bro″mah-ther′ah-pe) bromatotherapy.

bromatology (bro″mah-tol′o-je) [Gr. *brōma* food + *-logy*] the science of foods and dietetics.

bromatotherapy (bro″mah-to-ther′ah-pe) [Gr. *brōma* food + *therapeia* treatment] the use of food in treating disease; called also *bromatherapy.*

bromatotoxin, bromatotoxismus (bro″mah-to- tok′sin; bro″mah-to-tok-sis′mus) [Gr. *brōma* food + *toxin*] the poison formed in food by fermentation, etc.

bromatoxism (bro-mah-tok′sizm) [Gr. *brōma* food + *toxikon* poison] food poisoning.

bromazepam (bro-mah′zĕ-pam) chemical name: 7-bromo-1,3-dihydro-5- (2-pyridyl) -2*H*-1,4-benzodiazepin- 2-one; a minor tranquilizer, $C_{14}H_{10}BrN_3O$, with actions similar to those of diazepam.

bromelain (bro′mĕ-lān) [EC 3.4.22.4] an enzyme of the hydrolase class that catalyzes the hydrolysis of alanine, glycine, lysine, and tyrosine peptide bonds in protein molecules. It is derived from the pineapple plant, *Ananas sativus.* Bromelain causes the clotting of milk, and is used as an anti-inflammatory agent, for tenderizing meat, for preparing protein hydrolysates, and for chill-proofing beef. Used in immunology to render red cells agglutinable by incomplete antibody. Called also *bromelin.*

bromelin (bro-mel′in) bromelain.

bromethol (bro-meth′ol) tribromoethanol solution.

bromhexine hydrochloride (brom-heks′ēn) chemical name: 2-amino-3,5-dibromo-*N*-cyclohexyl-*N*-methylbenzenemethanamine monohydrochloride; an expectorant and mucolytic, $C_{14}H_{20}Br_2N_2 \cdot HCl$.

bromhidrosis (bro″mĭ-dro′sis) [Gr. *brōmos* stench + *hidrōs* sweat] axillary (apocrine) sweat which has become foul-smelling as a result of its bacterial decomposition.

bromic (bro′mik) pertaining to or containing pentavalent bromine, as in bromic acid, $HBrO_3$.

bromide (bro′mīd) any binary compound of bromine in which the bromine carries a negative charge (Br⁻); specifically a salt (or organic ester) of hydrobromic acid (H⁺Br⁻). Bromides produce depression of the central nervous system, and were once widely used for their sedative effect. Because overdosage causes serious mental disturbances they are now used seldomly, except occasionally in grand mal seizures. See also *brominism.*

bromidrosis (bro″mĭ-dro′sis) bromhidrosis.

brominated (bro″mĭ-nāt′ed) combined with or containing bromine; bromated; brominized.

bromine (bro′mēn; bro′min) [L. *bromium, brominium, bromum;* Gr. *brōmos* stench] a reddish-brown liquid element, symbol Br, giving off suffocating vapors. Its atomic number is 35; atomic weight, 79.909. See also *bromide* and *brominism.*

brominism (bro′min-izm) bromism.

brominized (bro′min-īzd) brominated.

bromism (bro′mizm) [*bromide* + -ism] chronic bromide intoxication, once a common problem, now rare, caused by chronic ingestion of proprietary bromide preparations; it is characterized by mental dullness, deficient memory, slurred speech, drowsiness, tremors, and ataxia. Skin eruptions of various forms are common. In most cases bromism also produces an organic mental disorder, which may be a delirium, a hallucinosis, or a transitory psychotic state resembling paranoid schizophrenia. Called also *brominism.*

bromisovalum (brōm″i-so-val′um) chemical name: *N*-(aminocarbonyl)-2-bromo-3-methylbutanamide. A sedative and hypnotic, $C_6H_{11}BrN_2O_2$, occurring as white, needle-shaped or scale-like crystals; administered orally.

bromization (bro″mi-za′shun) impregnation with bromides or bromine; the administration of large doses of bromides.

bromized (bro′mīzd) under the influence of bromides.

brom(o)- [Gr. *brōmos* stench] a combining form meaning foul-smelling, or, in chemical terms, indicating the presence of bromine.

bromobenzene (bro″mo-ben′zēn) a colorless liquid, C_6H_5-Br, with a pleasant, characteristic odor, obtained by bromination of benzene in the presence of iron.

bromochlorotrifluoroethane (bro″mo-klo″ro-tri-floo-o″ro-eth′ān) halothane.

bromocriptine (bro″mo-krip′tēn) 2-bromo-α-ergocryptine, a dopamine agonist, an ergot alkaloid used to suppress prolactin secretion and thereby to inhibit lactation and stimulate ovulation in galactorrhea-amenorrhea syndrome and hypogonadism; it is also used in the treatment of Parkinson's disease. It raises serum growth hormone levels in normal persons, but lowers them in those with acromegaly.

5-bromodeoxyuridine (bro″mo-de-ok-se-u′rĭ-din) a thymidine analogue causing breakage in chromosomal regions rich in heterochromatin.

bromoderma (bro″mo-der′mah) [*bromine* + Gr. *derma* skin] a skin eruption due to the use of bromides.

bromodiphenhydramine hydrochloride (bro″mo-di″fen-hi′drah-mēn) [USP] chemical name: 2-[(4-bromophenyl)phenylmethoxy]-*N,N*-dimethylethanamine hydrochloride. An antihistaminic, $C_{17}H_{20}BrNO \cdot HCl$, occurring as a white to pale buff, crystalline powder; administered orally.

bromoiodism (bro″mo-i′o-dizm) poisoning with bromine and iodine or their compounds.

bromomania (bro″mo-ma′ne-ah) [*bromo-* + mania] (*obs.*) an organic mental disorder produced by chronic bromide intoxication; see *bromism.*

bromomenorrhea (bro″mo-men-o-re′ah) [Gr. *brōmos* stench + *mēn* month + *rhoia* flow] the discharge of menses characterized by an offensive odor.

bromopnea (brōm″op-ne′ah) [Gr. *brōmos* stench + *pnoia* breath] halitosis.

5-bromouracil (bro″mo-u′rah-sil) a pyrimidine analogue with mutagenic properties.

bromoxanide (bro-moks′ah-nīd) chemical name: *N*-[4-bromo-2- (trifluoromethyl) phenyl] - 3 - (1,1-dimethylethyl) -2- hydroxy-6- methyl-5-nitrobenzamide; an anthelmintic, $C_{19}H_{18}BrF_3N_2O_4$.

bromperidol (brom-per′ĭ-dōl) chemical name: 4-[4-(4-bromophenyl)-4-hydroxy-1-piperidinyl]-1-butanone; a tranquilizer, $C_{21}H_{23}BrFNO_2$.

brompheniramine (brōm″fen-ir′ah-mēn) chemical name: γ-(4-bromophenyl)-*N,N*-dimethyl-2-pyridinepropanamine. The bromine analogue of chlorpheniramine, $C_{16}H_{19}BrN_2$, an antihistaminic drug. **b. maleate** [USP], the maleate salt of brompheniramine, $C_{16}H_{19}BrN_2 \cdot C_4H_4O_4$, occurring as white crystalline powder; administered orally or by intramuscular, subcutaneous, or intravenous injection for

therapy and prophylaxis of conditions in which antihistamines may be effective.

bromphenol (brōm-fe′nol) one of a series of brominized phenols, sometimes found in the precipitates of tested urine.

Bromsulphalein (brom-sul′fah-lin) trademark for a preparation of sulfobromophthalein sodium. Abbreviated BSP.

bromum (brō′mum) [L.] bromine.

Bromural (brōm-u′ral) trademark for preparations of bromisovalum.

bromurated (brōm′u-rāt″ed) containing bromine or bromine salts; brominated.

bromuret (brōm′u-ret) a bromide.

bronchadenitis (brong″kad-ĕ-ni′tis) [Gr. *bronchia* bronchia + *adēn* gland + *-itis*] inflammation of the bronchial glands.

bronchi (brong′ki) [L.] 1. genitive and plural of *bronchus.* 2. [NA] the bronchial tree and the bronchial lobes and segments considered together.

bronchia (brong′ke-ah) [L.] plural of *bronchium.*

bronchial (brong′ke-al) [L. *bronchialis*] pertaining to one or more bronchi.

bronchiarctia (brong″ke-ark′she-ah) [*bronchus* + L. *arctare* to constrict] bronchostenosis.

bronchiectasia (brong″ke-ek-ta′ze-ah) bronchiectasis.

bronchiectasic (brong″ke-ek-ta′zik) bronchiectatic.

bronchiectasis (brong″ke-ek′tah-sis) [*bronchus* + Gr. *ektasis* dilatation] chronic dilatation of the bronchi marked by fetid breath and paroxysmal coughing, with the expectoration of mucopurulent matter. It may affect the tube uniformly (*cylindric b.*), or occur in irregular pockets (*sacculated b.*), or the dilated tubes may have terminal bulbous enlargements (*fusiform b.*). **capillary b.,** dilatation of the bronchioles. **cystic b.,** bronchiectasis in which the dilatations of the bronchi are spherical. **dry b.,** that in which the infection is episodic and may be attended by hemoptysis, the cough being nonproductive during quiescent periods. **follicular b.,** bronchiectasis in which the lymphoid tissue in the affected regions becomes greatly enlarged and, by projecting into the bronchial lumen, may seriously distort and partially obstruct the bronchus.

bronchiectatic (brong″ke-ek-tat′ik) pertaining to or characterized by bronchiectasis.

bronchiloquy (brong-kil′o-kwe) [*bronchus* + L. *loqui* to speak] a high-pitched pectoriloquy due to a consolidated lung.

bronchiocele (brong′ke-o-sēl) [*bronchiole* + Gr. *kēlē* tumor] a dilatation or swelling of a branch smaller than a bronchus.

bronchiocrisis (brong″ke-o-kri′sis) bronchial crisis; see under *crisis.*

bronchiogenic (brong″ke-o-jen′ik) bronchogenic.

bronchiole (brong′ke-ōl) [L. *bronchiolus*] one of the finer (1 mm. or less) subdivisions of the branched bronchial tree, differing from the bronchi in having no cartilage plates and having cuboidal epithelial cells. Called also *bronchiolus.* **alveolar b.,** respiratory b. **lobular b.,** terminal b. **respiratory b.,** the final branch of a bronchiole; a subdivision of a terminal bronchiole, it has alveolar outcroppings and itself divides into several alveolar ducts. Called also *alveolar b.* **terminal b.,** the last portion of a bronchiole whose sole function is gas conduction; it subdivides into respiratory bronchioles. Called also *lobular b.*

bronchiolectasis (brong″ke-o-lek′tah-sis) [*bronchiole* + Gr. *ektasis* dilatation] dilatation of the bronchioles.

bronchioli (brong-ki′o-li) [L.] genitive and plural of *bronchiolus.*

bronchiolitis (brong″ke-o-li′tis) bronchopneumonia. **acute obliterating b.,** cirrhosis of the lung due to induration of the walls of the bronchioles. **b. exudati′va** (Curschman), inflammation of the bronchioles, with exudation of Curschmann's spirals and grayish, tenacious sputum; often associated with asthma. **b. fibro′sa oblit′erans,** bronchiolitis marked by ingrowth of connective tissue from the wall of the terminal bronchi with occlusion of their lumina. **vesicular b.,** bronchopneumonia.

bronchiolus (brong-ki′o-lus), pl. *bronchi′oli* [L.] [NA] bronchiole: one of the finer subdivisions of the branched bronchial tree; see *bronchiole.* **bronchi′oli re-**

spirato′rii [NA], respiratory bronchioles: the final branches of the bronchioles, into which the alveolar ducts open; see *respiratory bronchiole*, under *bronchiole*.

bronchiospasm (brong″ke-o-spazm″) bronchospasm.

bronchiostenosis (brong″ke-o-stĕ-no′sis) bronchostenosis.

bronchisepticin (brong″ke-sep′tĭ-sin) an antigen prepared from *Brucella bronchiseptica;* used in the skin test for canine distemper.

bronchismus (brong-kis′mus) bronchospasm.

bronchitic (brong-kit′ik) [L. *bronchiticus*] pertaining to, affected with, or of the nature of bronchitis.

bronchitis (brong-ki′tis) [*bronchus* + *-itis*] inflammation of one or more bronchi. **acute b.,** a bronchitic attack with a short and more or less severe course. It is due to exposure to cold, to the breathing of irritant substances, and to acute infection. It is marked by fever, pain in the chest, especially on coughing, dyspnea, and cough. **acute laryngotracheal b.,** a form of nondiphtheritic croup, clinically resembling diphtheria, except that there is no membrane; it mainly affects boys during the first year of life, usually in the winter. **arachidic b.,** bronchitis caused by the presence of a peanut kernel in a bronchus. **capillary b.,** bronchopneumonia. **Castellani's b.,** bronchospirochetosis. **catarrhal b.,** a form of acute bronchitis with a profuse mucopurulent discharge. **cheesy b.,** a form accompanying some cases of tuberculosis of the lung, in which the alveoli are filled with cells that undergo a cheesy degeneration (caseous necrosis). **chronic b.,** a long-continued form, often with a more or less marked tendency to recurrence after stages of quiescence. It is due to repeated attacks of acute bronchitis or to chronic general diseases; characterized by attacks of coughing, by expectoration, either scanty or profuse, and by secondary changes in the lung tissue. **croupous b.,** bronchitis characterized by violent cough and paroxysms of dyspnea, in which casts of the bronchial tubes are expectorated with Charcot-Leyden crystals and eosinophil cells. Variously known as *exudative, fibrinous, membranous, plastic,* and *pseudomembranous bronchitis.* **dry b.,** a form with a scanty secretion of tough sputum. **ether b.,** that due to the irritation of ether. **exudative b.,** croupous b. **fibrinous b.,** croupous b. **hemorrhagic b.,** bronchospirochetosis. **infectious asthmatic b.,** a syndrome marked by the development of symptoms of bronchospasm following respiratory tract infections in persons with asthma; also, asthma of bacterial origin. **infectious avian b.,** an acute, highly contagious, respiratory viral disease of chickens characterized by tracheal rales, coughing, sneezing, nasal discharge, and a drop in egg production. **mechanic b.,** a variety caused by the inhalation of dust or of solid particles. **membranous b.,** croupous b. **b. obliterans,** a form in which the smaller bronchi become filled with nodules made up of fibrinous exudate. **parasitic b.,** hoose. **phthinoid b.,** tuberculous bronchitis with purulent expectoration. **plastic b.,** croupous b. **productive b.,** bronchitis associated with a productive cough. **pseudomembranous b.,** croupous b. **putrid b.,** a form of chronic bronchitis in which the sputum is very offensive. **secondary b.,** that which occurs either as a complication of some acute disease, such as a local expression of some constitutional disorder. **staphylococcus b.,** bronchitis caused by staphylococci. **streptococcal b.,** bronchitis caused by streptococci. **suffocative b.,** suffocation produced by excessive secreting and exudates in acute bronchopneumonia. **verminous b.,** hoose. **vesicular b.,** that in which the inflammation extends into the alveoli, which are sometimes visible under the pleura as whitish-yellow granulations like millet seeds.

bronchium (brong′ke-um), pl. *bron′chia* [L.] one of the subdivisions of a bronchus, smaller than the bronchus and larger than the bronchioles.

bronch(o)- [L. *bronchus,* q.v.] a combining form denoting relationship to the bronchi.

bronchoadenitis (brong″ko-ad″e-ni′tis) bronchadenitis.

bronchoalveolar (brong″ko-al-ve′o-lar) pertaining to a bronchus and alveoli; called also *bronchovesicular.*

bronchoalveolitis (brong″ko-al″ve-o-li′tis) bronchopneumonia.

bronchoaspergillosis (brong″ko-as″per-jil-lo′sis) bronchial disease resulting from infection with *Aspergillus.*

bronchoblastomycosis (brong″ko-blas″to-mi-ko′sis) North American blastomycosis of the pulmonary type; see under *blastomycosis.*

bronchoblennorrhea (brong″ko-blen″o-re′ah) chronic bronchitis in which the sputum is copious, thin, and mucopurulent.

bronchocandidiasis (brong″ko-kan″dĭ-di′ah-sis) candidiasis of the respiratory tract. It has been reported in two forms: an afebrile *mild form* manifested as chronic bronchitis with dyspnea and cough, and a usually fatal *severe form* that resembles tuberculosis. Called also *bronchomoniliasis* and *broncho-oidiosis.*

bronchocavernous (brong″ko-kav′er-nus) both bronchial and cavitary.

bronchocele (brong′ko-sēl) [*bronchus* + Gr. *kēlē* tumor] a localized dilatation of a bronchus.

bronchoconstriction (brong″ko-kon-strik′shun) the act or process of decreasing the caliber of a bronchus; bronchostenosis.

bronchoconstrictor (brong″ko-kon-strik′tor) 1. constricting or narrowing the lumina of the air passages of the lungs. 2. an agent that causes narrowing of the lumina of the air passages of the lungs.

bronchodilatation (brong″ko-dil-ah-ta′shun) a dilated state of a bronchus, or the site at which a bronchus is dilated.

bronchodilation (brong″ko-di-la′shun) the act or process of increasing the caliber of a bronchus.

bronchodilator (brong″ko-di-la′tor) 1. dilating or expanding the lumina of air passages of the lungs. 2. an agent that causes expansion of the lumina of the air passages of the lungs.

bronchoegophony (brong″ko-e-gof′o-ne) egobronchophony.

bronchoesophageal (brong″ko-ĕ-sof″ah-je′al) pertaining to or communicating with a bronchus and the esophagus, as a bronchoesophageal fistula.

bronchoesophagology (brong″ko-ĕ-sof-ah-gol′o-je) that branch of medicine which deals with the tracheobronchial tree and the esophagus.

bronchoesophagoscopy (brong″ko-ĕ-sof-ah-gos′ko-pe) the instrumental examination of the bronchi and esophagus.

bronchofiberscope (brong″ko-fi′ber-skōp) a flexible bronchoscope utilizing fiberoptics.

bronchofiberscopy (brong″ko-fi-ber′sko-pe) bronchofibroscopy.

bronchofibroscopy (brong″ko-fi-bros′ko-pe) examination of the bronchi through a bronchofiberscope.

bronchogenic (brong-ko-jen′ik) originating in a bronchus.

bronchogram (brong′ko-gram) the roentgenogram obtained by bronchography. **air b.,** a radiographic shadow of an air-filled bronchus running through an airless lung; applied also to any tapering, branching radiolucency in an opacified lung that corresponds in size and distribution to (and is assumed to be) a part of the bronchial tree.

bronchographic (brong″ko-graf′ik) pertaining to or obtained by bronchography.

bronchography (brong-kog′rah-fe) [*bronchus* + Gr. *graphein* to write] roentgenography of the lung after the instillation of an opaque medium in a bronchus.

broncholith (brong′ko-lith) [*bronchus* + Gr. *lithos* stone] lung calculus.

broncholithiasis (brong″ko-lĭ-thi′ah-sis) a condition in which calculi (broncholiths) are present within the lumen of the tracheobronchial tree.

bronchologic (brong″ko-loj′ik) pertaining to bronchology.

bronchology (brong-kol′o-je) the study and treatment of diseases of the tracheobronchial tree.

bronchomalacia (brong″ko-mah-la′she-ah) a deficiency in the cartilaginous wall of the trachea or a bronchus that may lead to atelectasis or obstructive emphysema; it may be congenital or acquired.

bronchomoniliasis (brong″ko-mo-nĭ-li′ah-sis) bronchocandidiasis.

bronchomotor (brong″ko-mo′tor) affecting the caliber of the bronchi.

bronchomucotropic (brong″ko-mu″ko-trop′ik) augmenting secretion by the respiratory mucosa.

bronchomycosis (brong″ko-mi-ko′sis) [*bronchus* + Gr. *mykēs* fungus] any bronchial disorder due to fungi, particularly infection of the lungs caused by *Candida albicans.*

bronchonocardiosis (brong″ko-no-kar″de-o′sis) nocardial infection of the bronchi.

broncho-oidiosis (brong″ko-o-id″e-o′sis) bronchocandidiasis.

bronchopancreatic (brong″ko-pan″kre-at′ik) communicating with a bronchus and the pancreas, as a bronchopancreatic fistula.

bronchopathy (brong-kop′ah-the) [*bronchus* + Gr. *pathos* disease] any disease of the air passages of the lungs.

bronchophony (brong-kof′o-ne) [*bronchus* + Gr. *phōnē* voice] the sound of the voice as heard through the stethoscope applied over a healthy large bronchus. Heard elsewhere, it indicates solidification of the lung tissue. **pectoriloquous b.,** a bronchophony with an accompaniment of pectoriloquy. **sniffling b.,** that which is accompanied with a sniffing sound, as of air drawn through the nose. **whispered b.,** that which is heard while the patient is whispering.

bronchoplasty (brong′ko-plas″te) [*bronchus* + Gr. *plassein* to mold] plastic surgery of a bronchus.

bronchoplegia (brong″ko-ple′je-ah) paralysis of the muscles of the walls of the bronchial tubes.

bronchopleural (brong″ko-ploor′al) pertaining to a bronchus and the pleura, or communicating with a bronchus and the pleural cavity, as a bronchopleural fistula.

bronchopleuropneumonia (brong″ko-plu″ro-nu-mo′ne-ah) pneumonia complicated by bronchitis and pleurisy.

bronchopneumonia (brong″ko-nu-mo′ne-ah) [*bronchus* + *pneumonia*] a name given to an inflammation of the lungs which usually begins in the terminal bronchioles. These become clogged with a mucopurulent exudate forming consolidated patches in adjacent lobules. The disease is frequently secondary in character, following infections of the upper respiratory tract, specific infectious fevers, and debilitating diseases. In infants and debilitated persons of any age it may occur as a primary affection. Called also *bronchial pneumonia, bronchiolitis, bronchoalveolitis, bronchopneumonitis, catarrhal pneumonia, lobular pneumonia, capillary bronchitis* and *vesicular bronchiolitis.* **postoperative b.,** bronchopneumonia following surgical operations, particularly those on the abdomen. The cause is related to the inhalation of irritant vapors during anesthesia and the inhalation of infected material from the mouth or nose during the temporary depression of the cough reflex. **subacute b.,** bronchopneumonia that is more indolent than usual. **virus b.,** pneumonia caused by viral infection.

bronchopneumonic (brong″ko-nu-mon′ik) pertaining to, affected with, or caused by bronchopneumonia.

bronchopneumonitis (brong″ko-nu″mo-ni′tis) bronchopneumonia.

bronchopneumopathy (brong″ko-nu-mop′ah-the) disease of the bronchi and lung tissue.

bronchopulmonary (brong″ko-pul′mo-ner″e) pertaining to the lungs and their air passages; both bronchial and pulmonary.

bronchoradiography (brong″ko-ra-de-og′rah-fe) radiographic visualization of the bronchial tree.

bronchorrhagia (brong″ko-ra′je-ah) [*bronchus* + Gr. *rhēgnynai* to burst forth] hemorrhage from the bronchi.

bronchorrhaphy (brong-kor′ah-fe) [*bronchus* + Gr. *rhaphē* suture] suture of a bronchus.

bronchorrhea (brong-ko-re′ah) [*bronchus* + Gr. *rhoia* flow] excessive discharge of mucus from the air passages of the lungs.

bronchoscope (brong′ko-skōp) an instrument for inspecting the interior of the tracheobronchial tree and carrying out endobronchial diagnostic and therapeutic maneuvers, such as taking specimens for culture and biopsy and removing foreign bodies. **fiberoptic b.,** bronchofiberscope.

bronchoscopic (brong″ko-skop′ik) pertaining to bronchoscopy or to the bronchoscope.

bronchoscopy (brong-kos′ko-pe) [*bronchus* + Gr. *skopein* to examine] examination of the bronchi through a bronchoscope. **fiberoptic b.,** bronchofibroscopy.

bronchosinusitis (brong″ko-si″nus-i′tis) coexisting infection of the paranasal sinuses and the lower respiratory passages.

bronchospasm (brong′ko-spazm) spasmodic contraction of the smooth muscle of the bronchi, as occurs in asthma.

bronchospirochetosis (brong″ko-spi″ro-ke-to′sis) an infectious disease caused by the presence in the bronchi of the *Spirochaeta bronchialis* and marked by chronic bronchitis attended by the spitting of blood; called also *Castellani's bronchitis* or *disease,* and *hemorrhagic bronchitis.*

bronchospirography (brong″ko-spi-rog′rah-fe) the recording of bronchospirometry results.

bronchospirometer (brong″ko-spi-rom′ĕ-ter) an instrument used in bronchospirometry.

bronchospirometry (brong″ko-spi-rom′ĕ-tre) determination of the vital capacity, oxygen intake, and carbon dioxide excretion of a single lung, or simultaneous measurements of the function of each lung separately. **differential b.,** measurement of the function of each lung separately.

bronchostaxis (brong″ko-stak′sis) bleeding from the bronchial wall.

bronchostenosis (brong″ko-ste-no′sis) [*bronchus* + Gr. *stenōsis* a narrowing] stricture or cicatricial diminution of the caliber of a bronchial tube; called also *bronchiarctia* and *bronchoconstriction.*

bronchostomy (brong-kos′to-me) [*bronchus* + Gr. *stomoun* to provide with a mouth, or opening] the surgical creation of an opening into a bronchus.

bronchotome (brong′ko-tōm) a cutting instrument used in performing bronchotomy.

bronchotomy (brong-kot′o-me) [*bronchus* + Gr. *tomē* a cutting] surgical incision of a bronchus.

bronchotracheal (brong″ko-tra′ke-al) pertaining to the bronchi and trachea; tracheobronchial.

bronchovesicular (brong″ko-ve-sik′u-lar) bronchoalveolar.

bronchus (brong′kus), pl. *bron′chi* [L.; Gr. *bronchos* windpipe] any of the larger air passages of the lungs, having an outer fibrous coat with irregularly placed plates of hyaline cartilage, an interlacing network of smooth muscle, and a mucous membrane of columnar ciliated epithelial cells. **apical b.,** b. segmentalis apicalis. **cardiac b.,** b. segmentalis basalis medialis. **eparterial b.,** ramus bronchialis eparterialis. **hyparterial bronchi,** rami bronchiales hyparteriales. **lingular b., inferior,** b. lingularis inferior. **lingular b., superior,** b. lingularis superior. **lobar bronchi, bron′chi loba′res** [NA], passages arising from the primary bronchi and passing to the lobes of the right and left lungs. There are three right lobar bronchi (*b. lobaris superior dexter, b. lobaris medius dexter, b. lobaris inferior dexter*) and two left lobar bronchi (*b. lobaris superior sinister* and *b. lobaris inferior sinister*), which divide into the lobar segments. **primary bronchi, right and left,** bronchi principales dexter/sinister [NA]. **bron′chi principa′les dexter/sinis′ter** [NA] right and left primary bronchi: the two main branches into which the trachea divides, each passing to the respective lung. **secondary bronchi,** subdivisions of the primary bronchi, including the lobar and segmental bronchi. **segmental b., anterior,** b. segmentalis anterior. **segmental b., anterior basal,** b. segmentalis basalis anterior. **segmental b., apical,** b. segmentalis apicalis. **segmental b., apicoposterior,** b. segmentalis apicoposterior. **segmental bronchi, bron′chi segmenta′les** [NA], air passages arising from the lobar bronchi and passing to the different segments of the two lungs, where they further subdivide into smaller and smaller passages (bronchioles). Roman numerals are used to designate the segmental bronchi. The *bronchus lobaris superior dexter* has three segments: *b. segmentalis spicalis* (b. I), *b. segmentalis posterior* (b. II), and *b. segmentalis anterior* (b. III); the *b. lobaris medius dexter* has two segments: *b. segmentalis lateralis* (b. IV), and *b. segmentalis medialis* (b. V); the *b. lobaris inferior dexter* has five segments: *b. segmentalis apicalis* (b. VI) [alternative *b. segmentalis superior*], *b. segmentalis basalis medialis* (b. VII

) [alternative *b. segmentalis cardiacus*], *b. segmentalis basalis anterior* (b. VIII), *b. segmentalis lateralis* (b. IX), and *b. segmentalis posterior* (b. X); the *b. lobaris superior sinister* has four segments: *b. segmentalis apicoposterior* (b. I & II), *b segmentalis anterior* (b. III), *b. lingularis superior* (b. IV), and *b. lingularis inferior* (b. V); the *b. lobaris inferior sinister* has five segments: *b. segmentalis apicalis* (b. VI) [alternative *b. segmentalis superior*], *b. segmentalis basalis medialis* (b. VII), [alternative *b. segmentalis cardiacus*], *b. segmentalis basalis anterior* (b. VIII), *b. segmentalis basalis lateralis* (b. IX), and *b. segmentalis basalis posterior* (b. X). See the Plate of Pulmonary Segments. **segmental b., cardiac,** b. segmentalis basalis medialis. . **segmental b., lateral,** b. segmentalis lateralis. **segmental b., lateral basal,** b. segmentalis basalis lateralis. **segmental b., medial,** b. segmentalis medialis. **segmental b., medial basal,** b. segmentalis basalis medialis. **segmental b., posterior,** b. segmentalis posterior. **segmental b., posterior basal,** b. segmentalis basalis posterior. **segmental b., superior,** the apical segment of either the right inferior lobar bronchus or of the left inferior lobar bronchus. **stem b.,** the continuation of the primary bronchus of the embryo, from which branches are given off to the lobes of the lungs. **tracheal b.,** an ectopic or supernumerary bronchus, extending directly from the trachea to the apical segment of the upper lobe of the right lung, occurring normally in some animals but as a congenital anomaly in man.

brontophobia (bron″to-fo′be-ah) [Gr. *brontē* thunder + *phobia*] irrational fear of thunder; astraphobia.

Brooke's disease, tumor (brooks) [Henry Ambrose Grundy *Brooke*, English (Manchester) dermatologist, 1854–1919] see *keratosis follicularis multiplex*, and *trichoepithelioma papillosum multiplex*.

Brophy's operation (bro′fēz) [Truman William *Brophy*, American oral surgeon, 1848–1928] see under *operation*.

brosse (bros) [Fr. *brush*] a brushlike organelle of cilia seen on the anterodorsal surface of certain ciliate protozoa, such as those of the suborder Prorodontina; its function is unknown.

broth (broth) 1. a thin soup prepared by boiling meat or vegetables. 2. a liquid culture medium for the cultivation of microorganisms; see *Table of Culture Media* for specific broths.

brow (brow) the forehead, or either lateral half of it. **olympian b., olympic b.,** the prominent forehead seen in congenital syphilis.

brown (brown) a dusky, reddish yellow color. **aniline b., Bismarck b.,** a basic aniline dye, phenylene-diazo-metaphenylene-diamine, $C_6H_4[N_2C_6H_3(NH)_2]_2$, much used as a stain and counterstain in histology; called also *Manchester b.* and *phenylene b.* **Manchester b., phenylene b.,** aniline b.

Brown (brown), Michael Stuart. American physician, born 1941; co-winner, with Joseph Leonard Goldstein, of the Nobel prize for medicine or physiology in 1985 for their discoveries about the regulation of cholesterol metabolism and the treatment of diseases caused by abnormally high levels of cholesterol in the blood.

Brown-Séquard's paralysis, etc. (brown′ sa-karz′) [Charles Edouard *Brown-Séquard*, French physiologist, 1817–1894] see under *paralysis, syndrome,* and *treatment*.

Browne operation (brown) [Sir Denis *Browne*, London surgeon, born 1892] see under *operation*.

brownian movement (brow′ne-an) [Robert *Brown*, English botanist, 1773–1858] see under *movement*.

Browning's vein (brown′ingz) [William *Browning*, Brooklyn anatomist, 1855–1941] see under *vein*.

Broxolin (brok′so-lin) trademark for a preparation of glycobiarsol.

B.R.S. British Roentgen Society.

Bruce's tract (broos′ez) [Alexander *Bruce*, Edinburgh anatomist, 1854–1911] fasciculus septomarginalis.

Brucella (broo-sel′lah) [Sir David *Bruce*, English physician, 1855–1931] a genus of gram-negative, aerobic coccobacilli or short, rod-shaped bacteria of uncertain affiliation, made up of nonmotile cells that require biotin, niacin, thiamine, and sometimes serum for growth. The organisms are animal parasites and pathogens, causing brucellosis (undulant fever), transmissible to humans through contact with infected tissue

or dairy products. **B. abor′tus,** the commonest cause of brucellosis (undulant fever) in man; it is the causative agent of infectious abortion of cattle, which constitutes the animal reservoir of infection; called also *Bang's bacillus.* **B. bronchisep′tica,** *Bordetella bronchiseptica.* **B. ca′nis,** a species that causes generalized lymphadenitis and splenitis in dogs. Early fetal death or abortion is seen in many infected females, and epididymitis, scrotal dermatitis, and testicular atrophy are seen in infected males. Human infection is manifested by symptoms that resemble those of an upper respiratory viral infection. **B. meliten′sis,** a species found in healthy and diseased goats and sheep; it is pathogenic for humans, causing brucellosis. **B. neoto′mae,** a species found in the wood rat of the western United States; not known to be pathogenic for humans. **B. o′vis,** a species pathogenic for sheep, causing ram epididymitis; not known to cause disease in humans. **B. rangif′eri taran′di,** *B. suis.* **B. su′is,** a species found primarily in pigs but also in rabbits and reindeer; it is highly pathogenic for humans, causing brucellosis. **B. tularen′sis,** *Francisella tularensis.*

brucella (broo-sel′ah) an individual organism of the genus *Brucella.*

Brucellaceae (broo″sel-la′se-e) in former systems of classification, a family of gram-negative aerobic cocci and rod-shaped bacteria. It included the genera *Actinobacillus, Bordetella, Brucella, Calymmatobacterium, Haemophilus, Moraxella, Noguchia,* and *Pasteurella.*

brucellar (broo-sel′ar) pertaining to or caused by *Brucella.*

brucellin (broo-sel′in) a preparation from pooled cultures of the three species of *Brucella,* used in the diagnosis of brucellosis.

brucellosis (broo″sĕ-lo′sis) [Sir David *Bruce,* Edinburgh anatomist, 1854–1931] a generalized infection of humans involving primarily the reticuloendothelial system, caused by species of *Brucella,* namely, *B. melitensis, B. abortus, B. suis,* and *B. canis,* transmitted by direct or indirect contact with the natural animal reservoirs, including cattle, sheep, goats, swine, deer, and rabbits, or their infected products or tissue, characterized by fever, sweating, weakness, malaise, and weight loss. Called also *febris melitensis, febris undulans, Malta fever, Mediterranean fever,* and *undulant fever.*

Bruch's glands (brooks) [Karl Wilhelm Ludwig *Bruch,* German anatomist, 1819–1884] see under *gland,* and see *complexus basalis choroideae.*

brucine (broo′sin) [from *Brucea,* a genus of shrubs named for J. *Bruce,* 1730–1794] chemical name: 2,3-dimethoxystrychnidin. A poisonous alkaloid, $C_{23}H_{26}N_2O_4$, from *Strychnos ignatii* and *S. nux-vomica,* which resembles strychnine in its action, but is less poisonous. One of the principal constituents of nux vomica and ignatia, it was formerly used in the same manner as strychnine (q.v.).

Bruck's disease (brooks) [Alfred *Bruck,* German physician, born 1865] see under *disease.*

Bruck's test (brooks) [Carl *Bruck,* German dermatologist, 1879–1944] see under *tests.*

Brücke's lines, etc. (bre′kez) [Ernst Wilhelm von *Brücke,* Austrian physiologist, 1819–1892] see under *line, muscle, reagent, test,* and *tunic.*

Brudzinski's sign (reflex) (brood-zin′skēz) [Józef *Brudzinski,* Polish physician, 1874–1917] see under *sign.*

Brugia (bruj′ē-ah) a genus of filarial worms once considered to be members of the genus *Wuchereria.* **B. ma′layi,** a species causing human filariasis and elephantiasis throughout Southeast Asia, the China Sea, and eastern India; it is similar to, and often found in association with, *Wuchereria bancrofti.* Called also *Wuchereria malayi* and *Brug's filaria.* **B. pahan′gi,** a species found in man, cats, tigers, and other wild and domestic animals in Malaya; in man, it may produce the symptoms of tropical eosinophilia.

bruise (brooz) a superficial injury produced by impact without laceration; a contusion. **stone b.,** a painful bruise, especially of the bare feet of children.

bruissement (brwēs-maw′) [Fr.] a purring tremor; see under *tremor.*

bruit (brwe, broot) [Fr.] a sound or murmur heard in auscultation, especially an abnormal one. **aneurysmal b.,** a blowing sound heard over an aneurysm. **b. d'airain** (brwe da-ră′) [Fr. "sound of brass"], a clear ringing musical note sometimes heard on percussion over a pneumothorax cavity. **b. de bois** (brwe duh bwah′) [Fr. "sound of wood"], a dull wooden nonmusical note sometimes heard on percussion over a pneumothorax cavity. **b. de canon** (brwe duh kah-naw′) [Fr. "sound of cannon"], an abnormally loud first heart sound, heard intermittently in complete heart block. **b. de choc** (brwe duh shawk′) [Fr. "sound of impact"], the second cardiac sound, accompanied by a sound of impact, such as is heard over an aneurysm of the aorta. **b. de clapotement** (brwe duh klah-pōt-maw′) [Fr. "sound of rippling"], a splashing sound indicative of dilatation of the stomach when pressure is made on the wall of the abdomen. **b. de claquement** (brwe duh klak′-maw) [Fr. "sound of clapping"], a snapping sound caused by the sudden contact of parts. **b. de craquement** (brwe duh krak-maw′) [Fr. "a sound of crackling"], a crackling pericardial or pleural bruit. **b. de cuir neuf** (brwe duh kwēr nuf) [Fr. "sound of new leather"], a creaking noise; usually a sign of pericarditis or pleurisy. **b. de diable** (brwe duh de-ahbl′) [Fr. "humming top"], a buzzing venous murmur in anemia; see *venous hum,* under *hum.* **b. de drapeau** (brwe duh drah-po′) [Fr. "sound of a flag"], a flapping rustle heard in croup and laryngitis, and sometimes in nasal polyp. **b. de froissement** (brwe duh frwahs-maw′) [Fr. "sound of clashing"], a clashing noise of various origin. **b. de frolement** (brwe duh frol-maw′) [Fr. "sound of rustling"], a rustling murmur from pericardial or pleural friction. **b. de frottement** (brwe duh frot-maw′) [Fr. "sound of friction"], a rubbing sound of various origin. **b. de galop** (brwe duh gah-lo′) [Fr. "sound of galloping"], triple heart sounds in gallop cadence. **b. de grelot** (brwe duh gruh-lo′) [Fr. "sound of a rattle"], a rattling sound usually caused by the presence of a foreign body in the respiratory passages. **b. de Leudet** (brwe duh led-a′), Leudet's tinnitus. **b. de lime** (brwe duh lēm) [Fr. "sound of a file"], a filing cardiac sound. **b. de moulin** (brwe duh moo-lă′) [Fr. "sound of a mill"], a splashing or waterwheel sound synchronous with systole, sometimes audible at some distance from the patient, variously attributed to cardiac, pericardiac, or mediastinal causes. **b. de parchemin** (brwe duh parsh-maw′) [Fr. "sound of parchment"], a sound as of two pieces of parchment rubbed together, of valvular cardiac origin. **b. de piaulement** (brwe duh pyōl-maw′) [Fr. "sound of whining"], a cardiac murmur like the mewing of a cat. **b. de pot fêlé** (brwe duh po fĕ-la′) [Fr. "cracked-pot sound"], a sound heard in percussion over cavities of the chest. **b. de rape** (brwe duh rahp) [Fr. "sound of a grater"], a rasping, cardiac, valvular murmur. **b. de rappel** (brwe duh rah-pel′) [Fr. "sound of drum beating to arms"], a sound as of a drum; a delayed mitral murmur. **b. de Roger** (brwe duh ro-zha′), a loud long systolic murmur heard in the third interspace to the left of the sternum, characteristic of a small ventricular septal defect. Called also *Roger's bruit* or *murmur.* **b. de scie** (brwe duh se) [Fr. "sound of a saw"], a cardiac murmur resembling the sound of a saw. **b. de soufflet** (brwe duh soo-fla′) [Fr. "sound of a bellows"] see *souffle.* **b. de tabourka** (brwe duh tah-bōōr′kah), timbre métallique. **b. de tambour** (brwe duh tahm-bor′) [Fr. "sound of drum"], a ringing sound heard in syphilitic aortic regurgitation. **false b.,** one due to pressure by the stethoscope, or derived from the circulation in the ear of the auscultator. **Leudet's b.,** see under *tinnitus.* **b. placentaire** (brwe pla″sawn-tār′) [Fr. "placental sound"], placental souffle. **Roger's b.,** b. de Roger. **b. skodique** (brwe skaw-dēk′), skodaic resonance. **systolic b.,** a noise (heard on auscultation) occurring with the systole of the heart. **Verstraeten's b.,** an abnormal sound heard in auscultation over the lower border of the liver in cachectic patients.

Brunn's membrane, epithelial nests (brōōnz) [Albert von *Brunn,* German anatomist, 1849–1895] see under *membrane* and *nest.*

Brunner's glands (brun′erz) [Johann Conrad *Brunner,* Swiss anatomist, 1653–1727] glandulae duodenales.

Bruns' disease (brunz′ez) [John Dickson *Bruns,* New Orleans physician, 1836–1883] pneumopaludism.

Bruns' syndrome (sign) (brōōnz) [Ludwig *Bruns,* neurologist in Hanover, 1858–1916] see under *syndrome.*

Brunschwig's operation (brōōn′swigz) [Alexander *Brunschwig,* American surgeon, 1901–1969] pancreatoduodenectomy.

Brunsting's syndrome (broon′stings) [Louis A. *Brunsting,* Sr., American dermatologist, born 1900] see under *syndrome.*

brush (brush) tufts of bristles, hair, or other flexible materials set into a handle. **Haidinger's b.,** two conical brushlike images with apexes touching, seen on looking through a Nicol prism; used in determining visual function. **b's of Ruffini,** a form of nerve ending occurring in the papillae of the skin in the form of densely interlaced branches; called also *terminal cylinders* and *organ of Ruffini.* **stomach b.,** a brush used to cleanse and stimulate the mucous lining of the stomach.

Bruton's agammaglobulinemia, disease (broo-tunz) [Ogden C. *Bruton,* American pediatrician, born 1908] see *X-linked agammaglobulinemia,* under *agammaglobulinemia.*

brux (bruks) to grind the teeth rhythmically or spasmodically; cf. *bruxism.*

bruxism (bruk′sizm) [Gr. *brychein* to gnash the teeth] an oral habit consisting of involuntary rhythmic or spasmodic nonfunctional gnashing, grinding, and clenching of teeth in other than chewing movements of the mandible, usually performed during sleep, which may lead to occlusal trauma. Causes are believed to be related to repressed aggression, emotional tension, anger, fear, and frustration. See also *bruxomania* and *clenching.* **centric b.,** bruxism characterized by clenching in centric occlusion. Called also *clamping habit* and *clenching habit.*

bruxomania (bruk″so-ma′ne-ah) [Gr. *brychein* + *mania*] bruxism occurring in the daytime, usually performed unconsciously.

Bryant's line, traction (bri′ants) [Thomas *Bryant,* English surgeon, 1828–1914] see under *line* and *traction.*

Bryce-Teacher ovum [Thomas Hastie *Bryce,* Scottish anatomist, 1862–1946; John Hammond *Teacher,* Scottish pathologist, 1869–1930] see under *ovum.*

Bryobia (bri-o′be-a) a genus of spider mites. **B. praetio′sa,** the clover, or spinning, mite; a spider mite found on clover, which may greatly annoy man.

bryonia (bri-o′ne-ah) [L.; Gr. *bryōnia*] the air-dried root of *Bryonia alba* L. or other related species (Cucurbitaceae). It contains several glycosides, including bryonin and bryonidin. Formerly used both medically and in veterinary practice as a drastic and irritant purgative.

B.S. Bachelor of Surgery; Bachelor of Science; breath sounds; blood sugar.

BSA body surface area.

B-scan see *scan,* def. 2.

BSP Bromsulphalein.

B.T.U., B.Th.U British thermal unit.

bubo (bu′bo) [L. from Gr. *boubōn* groin] a tender, enlarged, and inflamed lymph node, particularly in the axilla or groin, due to such infections as plague, syphilis, gonorrhea, lymphogranuloma venereum, and tuberculosis. **bullet b.,** the characteristic hard bubo of primary syphilis. **chancroidal b.,** a suppurating form accompanying or following chancroid; called also *virulent b.* **climatic b.,** lymphogranuloma venereum. **malignant b.,** the bubo of bubonic plague. **primary b.,** a bubo which is due to venereal exposure but which is not preceded by any visible lesion; called also *bubon d'emblée.* **syphilitic b.,** nontender, nonfluctuant, firm regional lymphadenopathy that follows the chancre of syphilis. **tropical b.,** lymphogranuloma venereum. **virulent b.,** chancroidal b.

bubon (bu-baw′) [Fr.] bubo. **b. d'emblée** (bu-baw″-dah-bla′) [Fr. "at the first onset"], primary bubo.

bubonic (bu-bon′ik) [L. *bubonicus*] characterized by or pertaining to buboes; see also under *plague.*

bubonocele (bu-bon′o-sēl) [Gr. *boubōn* groin + *kēlē* tumor] inguinal or femoral hernia forming a swelling in the groin.

bubonulus (bu-bon′u-lus) [L. "a small bubo"] a nodule or abscess along a lymphatic vessel, especially one on the dorsum of the penis (Nisbet's chancre).

bucainide maleate (bu-ka′nīd) chemical name: 1-hexyl-4- [[methylpropyl] imino] phenylmethyl]-piperazine (Z)-2-butenedioate (1:2); a cardiac depressant with antiarrhythmic action, $C_{21}H_{35}N_3 \cdot 2C_4H_4O_4$.

bucardia (bu-kar′de-ah) [Gr. *bous* ox + *kardia* heart] cor bovinum.

bucca (buk′ah) [L.] [NA] the fleshy portion of the side of the face; the cheek. Called also *mala* [NA alternative]. **b. ca′vi o′ris** [NA], the fleshy portion of the side of the oral cavity, which is continuous with the commissure of the lips.

buccal (buk′al) [L. *buccalis*, from *bucca* cheek] pertaining to or directed toward the cheek. In dental anatomy, used to refer to the buccal surface of a tooth; see *buccal surface*, under *surface*. Cf. *labial*.

buccally (buk′ah-le) toward the cheek.

buccinator (buk′sĭ-na″tor) [L. "trumpeter"] see *Table of Musculi*.

bucc(o)- [L. *bucca* cheek] a combining form denoting relationship to the cheek.

buccoaxial (buk″ko-ak′se-al) pertaining to or formed by the buccal and axial walls of a tooth cavity preparation.

buccoaxiocervical (buk″ko-ak″se-o-ser′vĭ-kal) buccoaxiogingival.

buccoaxiogingival (buk″ko-ak″se-o-jin′jĭ-val) pertaining to or formed by the buccal, axial, and gingival walls of a tooth cavity; called also *buccoaxiocervical*.

buccocervical (buk″o-ser′vĭ-kal) 1. pertaining to the cheek and neck. 2. pertaining to the buccal surface of the neck of a posterior tooth. 3. buccogingival.

buccoclusal (buk″o-kloo′sal) 1. pertaining to buccocclusion. 2. bucco-occlusal.

buccoclusion (buk″o-kloo′zhun) malocclusion in which the dental arch or a quadrant or group of teeth is buccal to the normal.

buccodistal (buk″ko-dis′tal) distobuccal.

buccogingival (buk″ko-jin′jĭ-val) 1. pertaining to the cheek and gingiva. 2. pertaining to or formed by the buccal and gingival walls of a tooth cavity preparation.

buccoglossopharyngitis (buk″ko-glos′o-far″in-ji′tis) inflammation involving the cheek, tongue, and pharynx. **b. sic′ca,** inflammation and dryness of the buccal mucosa, tongue, and pharynx. Cf. *Sjögren's syndrome*, under *syndrome*.

buccolabial (buk″o-la′be-al) pertaining to the cheek and lip.

buccolingual (buk″o-ling′gwal) 1. pertaining to the cheek and tongue. 2. pertaining to the buccal and lingual surfaces of a posterior tooth.

buccolingually (buk″o-ling′gwah-le) from the cheek toward the tongue.

buccomaxillary (buk″o-mak′sĭ-ler″e) 1. pertaining to the cheek and maxilla. 2. communicating with the buccal cavity and the maxillary sinus, as a buccomaxillary fistula.

buccomesial (buk″o-me′ze-al) pertaining to or formed by the buccal and mesial surfaces of a tooth, or the buccal and mesial walls of a tooth cavity.

bucco-occlusal (buk″o-ŏ-kloo′zal) pertaining to or formed by the buccal and occlusal surfaces of a tooth.

buccopharyngeal (buk″o-fah-rin′je-al) pertaining to the mouth and pharynx.

buccoplacement (buk′o-plās″ment) displacement of a tooth toward the cheek.

buccopulpal (buk″o-pul′pal) pertaining to or formed by the buccal and pulpal walls of a tooth cavity.

buccostomy (buk-kos′to-me) the surgical creation of permanent buccal fistulae to prevent wind-sucking in horses.

buccoversion (buk″o-ver′zhun) the position of a tooth which lies buccally to the line of occlusion.

buccula (buk′ŭ-lah) [L. "a little cheek"] (*obs.*) a redundant fold under the chin, commonly called a double chin.

Bucephalus (bu-sef′ah-lus) a genus of trematodes. **B. papillo′sus,** a trematode parasitic in the stomach and intestines of fresh-water fish.

buchu (bu′ku) the name of several species of *Barosma* (Rutaceae), which contain urinary antiseptic and diuretic volatile oils.

Buck's extension, fascia, operation (buks) [Gurdon *Buck,* American surgeon, 1807–1877] see under *extension, fascia,* and *operation*.

buckeye (buk′i) a popular designation for *Aesculus glabra* and other trees and shrubs of the same genus. The fruit of trees in this genus are toxic to livestock due to a glycoside, esculin.

buckling (buk′ling) the process or an instance of becoming crumpled or warped. **scleral b.,** a technique for repair of detachment of the retina, in which indentations or infoldings of the sclera are made over the tears in the retina so as to promote adherence of the retina to the choroid.

Bucky diaphragm, rays (buk′e) [Gustav P. *Bucky,* German roentgenologist in America, 1880–1963] see under *diaphragm,* and see *grenz rays,* under *ray*.

buclizine hydrochloride (bu′klĭ-zēn) chemical name: 1-[(4-chlorophenyl) phenylmethyl]-4- [[4-(1,1-dimethylethyl) phenyl] methyl] piperazine dihydrochloride. An antihistamine, $C_{28}H_{33}ClN_2 \cdot 2HCl$, used mainly as an antinauseant in the management of motion sickness; administered orally.

bucrylate (bu′krĭ-lāt) chemical name: isobutyl 2-cyanoacrylate; a tissue adhesive, $C_8H_{11}NO_2$.

bud (bud) any small part of the embryo or adult metazoon more or less resembling the bud of a plant and presumed to have potential for growth and differentiation. **bronchial b.,** an outgrowth from the stem bronchus giving rise to the air passages of its respective pulmonary lobe. **end b.,** the remnant of the primitive knot, from which arises the caudal portion of the trunk; called also *tail b.* **gustatory b.,** taste b. **limb b.,** a swelling on the trunk of the embryo that becomes a limb. **liver b.,** a diverticulum from the foregut that gives rise to the liver and its ducts. **lung b.,** an outgrowth from the foregut that gives rise to the trachea, bronchi, and all the branchings that form a tracheobronchial tree. **metanephric b.,** ureteric b. **periosteal b.,** vascular connective tissue from the periosteum growing through apertures in the periosteal bone collar into the cartilaginous matrix of the primary center of ossification. **tail b.,** 1. the primordium of the caudal appendage. 2. end bud. **taste b.,** one of the minute terminal organs of the gustatory nerve that contain the receptor surfaces for the sense of taste. See also *caliculus gustatorius* [NA]. **tooth b.,** a knoblike tooth primordium developing into an enamel organ surrounded by a dental sac and encasing the dental papilla. See also under *germ*. **ureteric b.,** an outgrowth of the mesonephric duct that gives rise to all but the nephrons of the permanent kidney; called also *metanephric b.* **b. of urethra,** bulbus penis. **vascular b.,** an outgrowth of an existing vessel from which a new blood vessel arises. **wing b.,** a swelling on the trunk of an avian embryo that gives rise to a wing.

Budd's cirrhosis (disease), jaundice (budz) [George *Budd,* London physician, 1808–1882] see under *cirrhosis* and see *massive hepatic necrosis,* under *necrosis*.

Budd-Chiari syndrome (disease) (bud′ke-ar′e) [George *Budd;* Hans *Chiari,* Austrian pathologist, 1851–1916] see under *syndrome*.

buddeized milk (boo′de-īzd) [E. *Budde,* Danish sanitary engineer, born 1871] see under *milk*.

budding (bud′ing) 1. gemmation; a form of asexual reproduction in which the body divides into two unequal parts, the larger part being considered the parent and the smaller one the bud. 2. the process by which a new blood vessel arises from a preexisting vessel.

Budge's center (bood′gēz) [Julius Ludwig *Budge,* German physiologist, 1811–1888] 1. the ciliospinal center. 2. the genital center.

budgerigar, budgie (buj′er-e-gar″; buj′e) [Australian name] a species of parakeet, *Melopsittacus undulatus,* used for experimental work in psittacosis, and also popular as cage pets; called also *shell parakeet*.

Budin's joint, rule (boo-daz′) [Pierre-Constant *Budin,* Paris gynecologist, 1846–1907] see under *joint* and *rule*.

BUDR 5-bromodeoxyuridine.

Buerger's disease, symptom (ber′gerz) [Leo *Buerger,* physician in New York, 1879–1943] see *thromboangiitis obliterans* and under *symptom*.

Buergi's theory (ber′gēz) [Emil *Buergi,* Swiss pharmacologist, born 1872] see under *theory*.

büffelseuche (bif′el-zoi″kĕ) [Ger.] pasteurellosis of the buffalo.

buffer (buf′er) 1. a chemical system that prevents change in the concentration of another chemical substance, e.g., proton donor and acceptor systems serve as buffers preventing marked changes in hydrogen ion concentration (pH). 2. a physical or physiological system that tends to maintain constancy, e.g., reflexes regulating blood pressure. **bicar-**

bonate b., a buffer system composed of bicarbonate ions and dissolved carbon dioxide; in the body, this system is an important factor in determining the pH of the blood as the concentration of bicarbonate ions is regulated by the kidneys and of carbon dioxide by the respiratory system. **cacodylate b.,** one containing an organic arsenical salt, used in preparing fixatives for electron microscopy. **phosphate b.,** a buffer system composed of acid phosphate and sodium or potassium salts, e.g., monosodium and disodium acid phosphate; in the body, it is important in regulating the pH of the renal tubular fluids. **protein b.,** a buffer system involving proton donor and proton acceptor groups of the amino acid residues of proteins. **TRIS b.,** see *tromethamine.* **veronal b.,** a barbital buffer commonly used in the preparation of fixatives for electron microscopy.

buffering (buf'er-ing) the action produced by a buffer.

bufilcon A (bu-fil'kon) a contact lens material (hydrophobic).

bufin (bu'fin) a white secretion obtained by stimulating the parotid gland of certain species of toads by electricity; it has a physiologic action similar to that of digitalis but is not used in Western medicine.

Bufo (bu'fo) [L. "toad"] a genus of toads, species of which have been extensively studied by population geneticists.

buformin (bu-for'min) chemical name: *N*-butylimidocarbonimidic diamide; an oral hypoglycemic agent, $C_6H_{15}N_5$.

bufotalin (bu-fo-tal'in) a poisonous principal, $C_{26}H_{36}O_6$, present in the skin and saliva of the common European toad, *Bufo vulgaris.*

bufotenin (bu-fo'tĕ-nin) a specific basic pressor principle, 5-hydroxy indole ethyl dimethyl amine, $OH \cdot C_8H_5N \cdot CH_2 \cdot CH_2 \cdot N(CH_3)_2$, prepared from the skin glands of the toad, *Bufo bufo bufo.* It is used as a hallucinogenic in experimental medicine.

bufotherapy (bu''fo-ther'ah-pe) [L. *bufo* toad + *therapy*] the use of toad toxins in the treatment of disease.

bufotoxin (bu''fo-tok'sin) any toxin derived from the skin of toads.

bug (bug) an insect of the order Hemiptera. **assassin b.,** see *Reduviidae.* **barley b.,** *Acarus hordei.* **blister b.,** *Lytta vesicatoria.* **blue b.,** *Argas persicus.* **cone-nose b.,** see *Reduviidae.* **croton b.,** *Blatta (Blatella) germanica.* **harvest b.,** chigger. **hematophagous b.,** a bug that lives on blood, such as the bedbug. **kissing b.,** see *Reduviidae.* **Malay b.,** see *Reduviidae.* **miana b.,** *Argas persicus.* **red b.,** chigger. **wheat b.,** *Pyemotes.*

Buhl's disease, desquamative pneumonia (būlz) [Ludwig von *Buhl,* German pathologist, 1816–1880] see under *disease* and *pneumonia.*

buiatrics (bu''e-at'riks) [Gr. *bous* ox, cow + *iatrikos* surgery, medicine] the treatment of diseases of cattle.

Buist's method (būsts) [Robert C. *Buist,* Scotch obstetrician, 1860–1939] see *artificial respiration,* under *respiration.*

bulb (bulb) [L. *bul'bus;* Gr. *bolbos*] 1. a rounded mass, or enlargement. 2. (*obs.*) *medulla oblongata.* **b. of aorta,** bulbus aortae. **auditory b.,** the membranous labyrinth and cochlea. **b. of corpus spongiosum,** bulbus penis. **duodenal b.,** pars superior duodeni. **end b.,** 1. an ovoid or spheroid body located at the termination of a nerve fiber, and dispersed in the skin, mucous membranes, muscles, joints, and connective tissue of the internal organs. End-bulbs show a wide diversity, from simple end knobs to complex sensory end organs with connective tissue sheaths. For descriptions of specific types, see under *corpusculum.* 2. one of the end-feet. **end b's of Krause,** corpuscula bulboidea; see under *corpusculum.* **b. of eye,** bulbus oculi. **gustatory b.,** taste bud (caliculus gustatorius). **b. of hair,** bulbus pili. **b. of heart,** bulbus cordis. **b. of jugular vein, inferior,** bulbus inferior venae jugularis. **b. of jugular vein, superior,** bulbus superior venae jugularis. **b's of Krause,** corpuscula bulboidea; see under *corpusculum.* **b. of occipital horn of lateral ventricle,** bulbus cornus occipitalis ventriculi lateralis. **olfactory b.,** bulbus olfactorius. **b. of ovary,** a bulb formed by the interweaving of veins with the bundles of involuntary muscle within the mesovarium; called also *Rouget's b.* **b. of penis,** bulbus penis. **b. of posterior horn of lateral ventricle,** bulbus cornus occipitalis ventriculi lateralis. **Rouget's b.,** b. of ovary. **sinova-**

ginal b., one of paired sacculations of the urogenital sinus, forming the lowermost part of the vagina. **taste b.,** taste bud (caliculus gustatorius). **terminal b's of Krause,** corpuscula bulboidea; see under *corpusculum.* **b. of urethra,** bulbus penis. **vaginal b.,** 1. a solid end of a paramesonephric duct in the embryo. 2. bulbus vestibuli vaginae. **b. of vestibule of vagina, vestibulovaginal b.,** bulbus vestibuli vaginae.

bulbar (bul'bar) pertaining to a bulb; pertaining to or involving the medulla oblongata, as bulbar paralysis.

bulbi (bul'bi) [L.] genitive and plural of *bulbus.*

bulbiform (bul'bĭ-form) bulb-shaped.

bulbitis (bul-bi'tis) inflammation of the bulb of the penis.

bulboatrial (bul''bo-a'tre-al) pertaining to the bulbus cordis and atrium.

bulbocapnine (bul''bo-kap'nin) an alkaloid, $C_{19}H_{19}NO_4$, derived from the roots of *Corydalis bulbosa* DC. or *C. cava* (L.) Schweigg. & Korte (Fumariaceae) (*Capnoides cavum*). It has an inhibitory effect on the reflex and motor activities of striated muscle, and has been used in the treatment of muscular tremors and vestibular nystagmus. See also under *experiment.*

bulbocavernosus (bul''bo-kav''er-no'sus) musculus bulbospongiosus.

bulbogastrone (bul''bo-gas'trōn) a polypeptide secreted by the duodenal bulb when the bulb is acidified; it inhibits gastric acid secretion in dogs.

bulboid (bul'boid) bulb-shaped.

bulbopontine (bul''bo-pon'tin) a term once applied to that portion of the brain made up of the pons and the region of the medulla oblongata situated dorsad to it.

bulbospongiosus (bul''bo-spon''je-o'sus) see Table of *Musculi.*

bulbourethral (bul''bo-u-re'thral) pertaining to the bulb of the urethra (bulbus penis [NA]).

bulbous (bul'bus) having the form or nature of a bulb; bearing or arising from a bulb.

bulbus (bul'bus), gen. and pl. *bul'bi* [L.] 1. a rounded mass or enlargement. 2. NA alternative for *medulla oblongata.* **b. aor'tae** [NA], bulb of aorta: the enlargement of the aorta at its point of origin from the heart, where the bulges of the aortic sinuses occur. **b. arterio'sus,** b. cordis. **b. carot'icus,** carotid sinus. **b. cor'dis,** the foremost of the three parts of the primitive heart of the embryo; called also *bulb of heart* and *bulbus arteriosus.* **b. cor'nus occipita'lis ventric'uli latera'lis** [NA] bulb of occipital horn of lateral ventricle: an eminence in the upper part of the medial wall of the occipital horn of the lateral ventricle, above the calcar avis, produced by the splenial fibers of the forceps frontalis as they pass posteriorly into the occipital lobe; called also *b. cornus posterioris ventriculi lateralis* [NA alternative] and *bulb of posterior horn of lateral ventricle.* **b. cor'nus posterio'ris ventric'uli latera'lis,** NA alternative for b. cornus occipitalis ventriculi lateralis. **b. cor'nus occipita'lis ventric'uli latera'lis** [NA] bulb of occipital horn of lateral ventricle: an eminence in the upper part of the medial wall of the occipital horn of the lateral ventricle, above the calcar avis, produced by the splenial fibers of the forceps frontalis as they pass posteriorly into the occipital lobe; called also *b. cornus posterioris ventriculi lateralis* [NA alternative] and *bulb of posterior horn of lateral ventricle.* **b. cor'poris spongio'si,** b. penis. **b. infe'rior ve'nae jugula'ris** [NA], inferior bulb of jugular vein: a dilatation of the internal jugular vein just before it joins the brachiocephalic vein; called also *b. venae jugularis inferior.* **b. o'culi** [NA], the bulb, or globe, of the eye; called also *eyeball* and *bulb of eye.* See under *eye.* **b. olfacto'rius** [NA], olfactory bulb; the bulblike expansion of the olfactory tract on the under surface of the frontal lobe of each cerebral hemisphere; the olfactory nerves enter it. Called also *Morgagni's tubercle.* **b. pe'nis** [NA], bulb of penis: the enlarged proximal part of the corpus spongiosum found between the two crura of the penis; called also *b. corporis spongiosi* and *b. urethrae.* **b. pi'li** [NA], bulb of hair: the bulbous expansion at the proximal end of a hair, in which the hair shaft is generated. **b. supe'rior ve'nae jugula'ris** [NA], superior bulb of jugular vein: a dilatation at the beginning of the internal jugular vein; called also *b. venae jugularis superior* and *Heister's diverticulum.* **b. ure'thrae,** b. penis. **b. ve'nae jugula'ris in-**

fe′rior, b. inferior venae jugularis. **b. ve′nae jugula′-ris supe′rior,** b. superior venae jugularis. **b. vestib′-uli vagi′nae** [NA], bulb of vestibule of vagina: a body consisting of paired elongated masses of erectile tissue, one on either side of the vaginal opening, united anteriorly by a narrow median band that passes along the lower surface of the clitoris.

bulesis (bu-le′sis) [Gr. *boulēsis*] the will, or an act of the will.

bulimia (bu-lim′e-ah) [L.; Gr. *bous* ox + *limos* hunger] 1. a mental disorder occurring predominantly in females, with onset usually in adolescence or early adulthood, characterized by episodes of binge eating that continue until terminated by abdominal pain, sleep, or self-induced vomiting, by awareness that the binges are abnormal; by fear of not being able to stop eating voluntarily; and by self-deprecation and depressed mood following the binges. The binges usually alternate with periods of normal eating or fasting. It differs from anorexia nervosa, in which bulimic episodes may occur, in that there is no extreme weight loss in bulimia. 2. (*obs.*) abnormally increased appetite; hyperorexia. **b. nervo′sa** [DSM III-R], bulimia.

bulimic (bu-lim′ik) pertaining to or affected with bulimia.

Buliminae (bu-lim′ĭ-ne) a subfamily of snails (family Hydrobiidae, order Mesogastropoda) that includes the medically important genera *Bulimus, Alocinma,* and *Parafossarulus.*

Bulimus (bu-li′mus) a genus of small fresh-water snails. **B. fuchsia′nus,** the chief intermediate host of the human liver flukes *Clonorchis* and *Opisthorchis;* it is commonly found in southern China. **B. leach′ii,** a species found in northern Europe and the northwestern United States, which ingests the eggs of *Opisthorchis felineus* and in whose body the eggs hatch.

Bulinus (bu-li′nus) a genus of snails, several species of which are the intermediate hosts of *Schistosoma haematobium* and *Opisthorchis.*

bulkage (bulk′ij) material that will increase the bulk of the intestinal contents and consequently stimulate peristalsis.

Bull. abbreviation for L. *bul′liat,* let it boil.

bulla (bul′ah), pl. *bul′lae* [L.] 1. a large vesicle, more than 5 mm. in circumference, containing serous or seropurulent fluid. Called also *bleb* and *blister.* 2. an anatomical structure having a bulla-like configuration or appearance. **emphysematous b.,** any space of more than 1 centimeter in diameter in distended areas of the emphysematous lung. **ethmoid b.,** see *b. ethmoidalis cavi nasi* and *b. ethmoidalis ossis ethmoidalis.* **b. ethmoida′lis ca′vi na′si** [NA], ethmoidal bulla of nasal cavity: the large ethmoid air cell lodged in the bulla ethmoidalis ossis ethmoidalis. **b. ethmoida′lis os′sis ethmoida′lis** [NA], ethmoidal bulla of ethmoidal bone: a rounded projection of the ethmoid bone into the lateral wall of the middle nasal meatus just below the middle nasal concha, enclosing a large ethmoid air cell; called also *antrum ethmoidale* and *ethmoid antrum.* **b. mastoi′dea,** a large air cell in the mastoid of lower animals. **b. os′sea,** the dilated part of the bony external meatus of the ear.

bullae (bul′e) plural of *bulla.*

bullate (bul′āt) [L. *bullatus*] 1. characterized by the presence of bullae. 2. inflated.

bullation (bul-la′shun) [L. *bullatio*] 1. the condition characterized by the presence of bullae. 2. the state of being inflated.

Buller's shield (bandage) (bul′erz) [Frank *Buller,* Canadian ophthalmologic surgeon, 1844–1905] see under *shield.*

bullneck (bul′nek) bull neck; see under *neck.*

bullosis (bul-lo′sis) the production of, or a condition characterized by, bullous lesions. **diabetic b.,** a condition in which bullae appear spontaneously, usually on the ankles and feet, in some uncontrolled diabetics.

bullous (bul′us) pertaining to or characterized by bullae.

bumblefoot (bum′bel-foot) inflammation of the ball of the foot of fowls, usually caused by staphylococcus.

bumetanide (bu-met′ah-nīd) a high-ceiling diuretic.

Buminate (bu′mĭ-nāt) trademark for preparations of human albumin.

Bumke's pupil (boom′kez) [Oswald Conrad Edward *Bumke,* German neurologist, 1877–1950] see under *pupil.*

bumps (bumpz) a symptom of the primary form of coccidioidomycosis (q.v.); called also *desert* or *valley bumps.*

BUN blood urea nitrogen; see *urea nitrogen.*

bunamidine hydrochloride (bu-nah′mĭ-dēn) chemical name: *N,N*-dibutyl-4-(hexyloxy)-1-naphthamidine monohydrochloride; an anthelmintic, $C_{25}H_{38}N_2O \cdot HCl$.

bunamiodyl (bu″nah-mi′o-dil) chemical name: 2-[[2,4,6-triiodo-3-[(1-oxobutyl)amino]phenyl]methylene]butanoic acid monosodium salt. A radiopaque medium, $C_{15}H_{16}I_3NO_3$, used in roentgenography of the biliary tract. Called also *buniodyl.*

bundle (bun′d'l) a collection of fibers or strands, as of muscle fibers, or a fasciculus or band of nerve fibers. **aberrant b's,** collections of pyramidal fibers leaving the corticonuclear tract at successive levels of the brain stem, and giving off fibers to the motor nuclei of the cranial nerves. **atrioventricular b., a-v. b.,** b. of His. **Bachmann's b.,** a transverse band of muscle fibers extending between the bases of the right and left auricles of the heart in dogs. **basis b's,** fasciculi proprii; see under *fasciculus.* **Bruce's b.,** cornucommissural b. **cornucommissural b.,** a name once given the fasciculus proprius on the surface of the posterior column and posterior commissure of the spinal cord. **forebrain b., medial,** a complex group of fibers arising from the basal olfactory regions, the periamygdaloid region, and the septal nuclei, and passing to the lateral hypothalamus; some fibers continue into the midbrain tegmentum and are relayed to the autonomic and visceral nuclei of the brain stem. **fundamental b's of spinal cord, ground b's, of spinal cord,** fasciculi proprii medullae spinalis. **Helweg's b.,** tractus olivospinalis. **b. of His,** a small band of atypical cardiac muscle fibers that originates in the atrioventricular node in the interatrial septum, passes through the atrioventricular junction, and then runs beneath the endocardium of the right ventricle on the membranous part of the interventricular septum. It divides at the upper end of the muscular part of the interventricular septum into right and left branches which descend in the septal wall of the right and left ventricle, respectively, to be distributed to those two chambers. This bundle propagates the atrial contraction rhythm to the ventricles, and its interruption produces heart block. Called also *fasciculus atrioventricularis* [NA], *atrioventricular* or *a-v b., Kent-His b., b. of Stanley Kent, His' band, Gaskell's bridge,* and *ventriculonector.* **Keith's b.,** a bundle of fibers in the wall of the right atrium, between the openings of the venae cavae; called also *sinoatrial b.* **Kent's b.,** a muscular bundle in the heart of several mammalian species (sometimes in man), forming a direct connection between the atrial and ventricular walls. **Kent-His b.,** b. of His. **longitudinal medial b.,** fasciculus longitudinalis medialis. **main b.,** the portion of the bundle of His between the atrioventricular node and the division into right and left branches; see *b. of His.* **medial forebrain b.,** fasciculus prosencephalicus medialis. **Meynert's b.,** tractus habenulo-interpeduncularis. **Monakow's b.,** tractus rubrospinalis. **muscle b.,** one of the primary longitudinal subdivisions of a muscle, made up of muscle fibers and separated from other bundles by fascial septa or perimysium. **olivocochlear b. of Rasmussen,** a bundle of fibers originating in the superior olivary complex and usually terminating in the cochlea of the opposite side; called also *b. of Oort* and *b. of Rasmussen.* **b. of Oort,** olivocochlear b. of Rasmussen. **posterior longitudinal b.,** fasciculus longitudinalis medialis. **predorsal b.** (*obs.*), tectospinal tract. **b. of Rasmussen,** olivocochlear b. of Rasmussen. **Schultze's b.,** interfascicular fasciculus. **Schutz's b.,** fasciculus longitudinalis dorsalis. **sinoatrial b.,** Keith's b. **solitary b.,** tractus solitarius medullae oblongatae. **b. of Stanley Kent,** b. of His. **thalamomamillary b.,** fasciculus mamillothalamicus. **Thorel's b.,** a bundle of muscle fibers in the human heart, connecting the sinoatrial and atrioventricular nodes, and passing around the mouth of the inferior vena cava. **transverse b's of palmar aponeurosis,** fasciculi transversi aponeurosis palmaris; see under *fasciculus.* **Türck's b.,** tractus temporopontinus. **b. of Vicq d'Azyr,** fasciculus mamillothalamicus. **Weissmann's b.,** the bundle of striated muscle fibers of a neuromuscular spindle.

bundle branch (bun′d'l branch) a branch of the bundle of His.

bungarotoxin (bung″gah-ro-tok′sin) a strong neurotoxin from the venom of kraits (*Bungarus*); three electrophoretic fractions, α-, β-, and γ-bungarotoxin, have been identified. α-Bungarotoxin, the chief fraction, binds irreversibly with acetylcholine receptors, producing neuromuscular block.

Bungarus (bung′gah-rus) a genus of venomous elapid snakes found in India; the krait. See table accompanying *snake*.

Bunge's amputation (boong′gez) [Richard *Bunge*, German surgeon, born 1870] aperiosteal amputation.

Bunge's law (boong′gez) [Gustav von *Bunge*, physiologist at Basel, 1844–1920] see under *law*.

Bunge's spoon (boong′gez) [Paul *Bunge*, German ophthalmologist, 1853–1926] see under *spoon*.

bungeye (bung′i) a condition caused by infestation of the eye of horses with *Habronema*, and marked by small worm-containing granulomas in the conjunctiva; called also *blue-eye*.

Büngner's bands (cell cordons) (bing′nerz) [Otto von *Büngner*, German neurologist, 1858–1905] see under *band*.

buniodyl (bu-ni′o-dil) bunamiodyl.

bunion (bun′yun) [L. *bunio*; Gr. *bounion* turnip] abnormal prominence of the inner aspect of the first metatarsal head, accompanied by bursal formation and resulting in a lateral or valgus displacement of the great toe. **tailor's b.,** bunionette.

bunionectomy (bun-yun-ek′to-me) [bunion + Gr. *ektomē* excision] excision of an abnormal prominence on the mesial aspect of the first metatarsal head.

bunionette (bun-yun-et′) enlargement of the lateral aspect of the fifth metatarsal head; called also *tailor's bunion*.

bunodont (bu′no-dont) [Gr. *bounos* hill + *odous* tooth] having cheek teeth with low rounded cusps on the occlusal surface of the crown, as in mammals with mixed diet, such as swine, many rodents, and man.

bunolol hydrochloride (bu′no-lōl) chemical name: 5-[3-[(1,1-dimethylethyl)amino]-2-hydroxypropoxy]-3-4-dihydro-1(2*H*)naphthalenone hydrochloride; a beta-adrenergic blocking agent, $C_{17}H_{25}NO_3 \cdot HCl$, having the same actions as propranolol (q.v.).

bunolophodont (bu″no-lo′fo-dont) [Gr. *bounos* hill + *lophos* ridge + *odous* tooth] having cheek teeth with both rounded cusps and transverse ridges on the occlusal surface of the crown, as in some kangaroos.

bunoselenodont (bu″no-sĕ-le′no-dont) [Gr. *bounos* hill + *selēnē* moon + *odous* tooth] having cheek teeth with both rounded cusps and crescentic ridges on the occlusal surface of the crown.

Bunostomum (bu″no-sto′mum) a genus of hookworms of the family Ancylostomidae that parasitize cattle, sheep, and other ruminants; called also *Monodontus*.

Bunsen burner, coefficient (bun′sen) [Robert Wilhelm Eberhard von *Bunsen*, German chemist, 1811–1899] see under *burner* and *coefficient*.

buphthalmia (būf-thal′me-ah) buphthalmos; hydrophthalmos.

buphthalmos (buf-thal′mos) [Gr. *bous* ox + *ophthalmos* eye] enlargement and distention of the fibrous coats of the eye; hydrophthalmos; infantile glaucoma. Called also *megophthalmos*.

buphthalmus (būf-thal′mus) buphthalmos; hydrophthalmos.

bupicomide (bu-pik′o-mīd) chemical name: 5-butyl-2-pyridinecarboxamide; an antihypertensive, $C_{10}H_{14}N_2O$.

bupivacaine hydrochloride (bu-piv′ah-kān) chemical name: *dl*-1-butyl-2′-6′-pipecoloxylidide hydrochloride. A local anesthetic, $C_{18}H_{28}N_2O \cdot HCl$, occurring as a white crystalline powder; used for peripheral nerve block, infiltration, and sympathetic, caudal, or epidural block.

buprenorphine hydrochloride (bu″pre-nor′fēn) chemical name: 17-(cyclopropylmethyl)-α-(1,1-dimethylethyl)-4,5α-epoxy-18,19-dihydro-3-hydroxy-6-methoxy-α-methyl-6,14-ethenomorphinan-7α(*S*)-methanol hydrochloride; a synthetic derivative of thebaine, $C_{29}H_{41}NO_4 \cdot HCl$, used as an analgesic.

bupropion hydrochloride (bu-pro′pe-on) chemical name: (±)-1-(3-chlorophenyl)-2-[(1,1-dimethylethyl) amino]-1-propanone hydrochloride; an antidepressant, $C_{13}H_{18}ClNO \cdot HCl$.

bur (ber) a rotary dental instrument made of steel or tungsten carbide, employing cutting heads of various shapes, held and revolved in a handpiece, and deriving power from the dental electric motor or air power; used to remove carious material from within decayed teeth, reduce decayed or fractured hard tissues, form the design of the cavity preparation, and finish and polish the teeth and restorations. Called also *drill*.

Burdach's columns, etc. (boor′daks) [Karl Friedrich *Burdach*, German physiologist, 1776–1847] see under *columns, fasciculus, fiber, fissure, nucleus,* and *tract*.

buret, burette (bu-ret′) a graduated glass tube used in volumetric chemistry to deliver a measured amount of liquid.

Burghart's symptom (sign) (boorg′harts) [Hans Gerny *Burghart*, German physician, 1862–1932] see under *symptom*.

burimamide (bu-rim′ah-mīd) an antagonist to histamine, competing for the histamine₂ receptor site on cells.

burn (bern) injury to tissues caused by contact with dry heat (fire), moist heat (steam or hot liquid), chemicals (e.g., corrosive substances), electricity (current or lightening), friction, or radiant and electromagnetic energy. Burns of the first degree show redness; of the second degree, vesication; of the third degree, necrosis through the entire skin. Burns of the first and second degree are known as partial-thickness burns, those of the third degree as full-thickness burns. **brush b.,** a wound caused by violent rubbing or friction, as by a rope pulled through the hands; called also *friction b*. **chemical b.,** irritant dermatitis caused by various caustic substances, such as acids, disinfectants, and alkalis. **contact b.,** an electric burn produced by contact with electric current. **electric b., electrical b.,** see *flash b*. and *contact b*. **flash b.,** a thermal lesion produced by a very brief exposure to radiant heat of high intensity, as in an explosion or a sudden discharge of electricity. **friction b.,** brush b. **radiation b.,** a burn caused by exposure to x-ray, radium, sunlight, atomic, or any other type of radiant energy. **sun b.,** sunburn. **thermal b.,** injury due to contact with flame, hot objects, or hot liquids, as distinguished from chemical and electric burns. **x-ray b.,** a lesion caused by exposure to x-rays.

burner (ber′ner) the part of a lamp, stove, or furnace from which the flame issues. **Argand b.,** a burner for oil or gas, with an inner tube for supplying air to the flame. **Bunsen b.,** a gas burner in which the gas is mixed with air before ignition, in order to give complete oxidation.

Burnet (bur-net′), Sir Frank Macfarlane. Australian physician and virologist, 1899–1985; co-winner, with Peter B. Medawar, of the Nobel prize in medicine and physiology for 1960, for the discovery of acquired immunological tolerance and for the conceptual framework of immunology in the clonal selection theory.

Burnett's disinfecting fluid (solution) (bur′nets) [Sir William *Burnett*, English surgeon, 1779–1861] see under *fluid*.

burnisher (ber′nish-er) a dental instrument with a blade or nib with a beveled edge used for smoothing out roughness at the margin of a restoration and the enamel.

burnishing (ber′nish-ing) 1. condensation and polishing under the sliding pressure of a smooth hard instrument, as in finishing the surface of a gold filling. 2. adaptation of a thin, annealed sheet metal by means of a burnisher, as in forming a band about a tooth root or in fitting a matrix for porcelain.

Burns' ligament, space (bernz) [Allan *Burns*, Scottish anatomist, 1781–1813] see *margo falciformis hiatus saphenus* and *fossa jugularis*, def. 1.

Burow's operation, solution, vein (boor′ovz) [Karl August *Burow*, surgeon in Königsberg, 1809–1874] see under *operation* and *vein*, and see *aluminum acetate solution*, under *solution*.

burquism (burk′izm) [V. B. *Burg*, French neurologist, 1823–1884] a system of metallotherapy.

burr (bur) bur.

bursa (ber′sah), pl. *bur′sae* [L.; Gr. "a wine skin"] a sac or saclike cavity filled with a viscid fluid and situated at places in the tissues at which friction would otherwise develop. **b. of Achilles (tendon),** b. tendinis calcanei. **acro-**

mial b., b. subdeltoidea. **adventitious b.,** an abnormal cyst due to friction or some other mechanical cause, and containing synovial fluid; called also *supernumerary b.* **anconeal b.,** b. subcutanea olecrani. **anconeal b. of triceps muscle,** b. subtendinea musculi tricipitis brachii. **b. anseri'na** [NA], **anserine b.,** a bursa between the tendons of the sartorius, gracilis, and semitendinosus muscles, and the tibial collateral ligament; called also *anterior genual b.* **bicipital b., bicipitofibular b.,** b. subtendinea musculi bicipitis femoris inferior. **bicipitoradial b., b. bicipitoradia'lis** [NA], a bursa between the radial tuberosity and the biceps tendon; called also *b. mucosa radialis.* **Boyer's b.,** one situated beneath the hyoid bone. **Brodie's b.,** b. subtendinea musculi gastrocnemii medialis. **calcaneal b.,** b. tendinis calcanei. **calcaneal b., subcutaneous,** b. subcutanea calcanea. **b. of calcaneal tendon,** b. tendinis calcanei. **Calori's b.,** a bursa situated between the trachea and the arch of the aorta. **b. copula'trix,** an appendage at the posterior end of the male of certain nematodes. **coracobrachial b.,** b. musculi coracobrachialis. **coracoid b.,** b. subtendinea musculi subscapularis. **b. cubita'lis interos'sea** [NA], **cubitoradial b.,** a bursa between the ulna, the biceps tendon, and nearby muscles; called also *interosseous cubital b.* and *ulnoradial b.* **deltoid b.,** b. subacromialis. **b.-equivalent,** analogous to the bursa of Fabricius; see *B lymphocyte,* under *lymphocyte,* and *bursa-equivalent tissue,* under *tissue.* **b. of Fabricius,** a lymphoid organ of birds that, like the thymus, develops as an epithelial outpouching of the gut but near the cloaca rather than the foregut; it atrophies at 5 or 6 months of age, persisting as a fibrous remnant in sexually mature birds; before involution it is the site of maturation of B lymphocytes (q.v.). **fibular b.,** b. subtendinea musculi bicipitis femoris inferior. **Fleischmann's b.,** one beneath the tongue. **b. of flexor carpi radialis muscle,** vagina synovialis tendinis musculi flexoris carpi radialis. **gastrocnemiosemimembranous b.,** b. musculi semimembranosi. **genual b., anterior,** b. anserina. **genual b., external inferior,** b. subtendinea musculi bicipitis femoris inferior. **genual bursae, internal superior,** bursae subtendineae musculi sartorii. **genual b., posterior,** b. musculi semimembranosi. **bur'sae glutaeofemora'les** bursae intermusculares musculorum gluteorum. **gluteal b.,** one situated beneath the gluteus maximus muscle. **gluteal intermuscular bursae,** bursae intermusculares musculorum gluteorum. **gluteofascial bursae,** bursae intermusculares musculorum gluteorum. **gluteofemoral bursae,** bursae intermusculares musculorum gluteorum. **gluteotuberosal b.,** b. ischiadica musculi glutei maximi. **His b.,** the dilatation at the end of the archenteron. **humeral b.,** 1. b. subacromialis. 2. b. subtendinea musculi gastrocnemii lateralis. **hyoid b.,** b. subcutanea prominentiae laryngealis. **iliac b., subtendinous, b. ili'aca subtendin'ea,** b. subtendinea iliaca. **b. iliopectine'a** [NA], **iliopectineal b.,** a bursa between the iliopsoas tendon and the iliopectineal eminence; called also *subiliac b.* and *ileopubic vesicular b.* **b. of iliopsoas muscle,** b. subtendinea iliaca. **inferior b. of biceps femoris muscle,** b. subtendinea musculi bicipitis femoris inferior. **infracardiac b.,** the cranial end of a coelomic recess of the embryo, extending upward between the esophagus and right lung bud; frequently persisting in the adult. **infracondyloid b., external,** recessus subpopliteus. **infragenual b.,** infrapatellaris profunda. **infrahyoid b., b. infrahyoi'dea** [NA], a bursa sometimes present below the hyoid bone at the attachment of the sternohyoid muscle. **infrapatellar b.,** b. subtendinea prepatellaris. **infrapatellar b., deep,** b. infrapatellaris profunda. **infrapatellar b., subcutaneous,** b. subcutanea infrapatellaris. **infrapatellar b., superficial inferior,** b. subcutanea tuberositatis tibiae. **b. infrapatella'ris profun'da** [NA], a bursa between the patellar ligament and the tibia. Called also *deep infrapatellar b., infragenual b., subpatellar b.,* and *subligamentous b.* **b. infrapatella'ris subcuta'nea,** b. subcutanea infrapatellaris. **bur'sae intermuscula'res musculo'rum gluteo'rum** [NA], intermuscular gluteal bursae: several sacs that surround the tendon attaching the gluteus maximus to the femur; called also *bursae glutaeofemorales, gluteofascial bursae,* and *gluteofemoral bursae.* **interosseous cubital b.,** b. cubitalis interossea. **intertubercular b.,** vagina synovialis intertubercularis. **b. intratendin'ea ole-**

cra'ni [NA], intratendinous bursa of olecranon: a bursa within the triceps tendon near its insertion; called also *intratendinous supra-anconeal b.* and *Monro's b.* **ischiadic b.,** b. ischiadica musculi obturatorii interni. **b. ischiad'ica mus'culi glu'tei max'imi** [NA], ischial bursa of gluteus maximus muscle: a bursa between the ischial tuberosity and the gluteus maximus; b. called also *b. sciatica musculi glutei maximi* [NA alternative], *gluteotuberosal b.,* and *sciatic b. of gluteus maximus muscle.* **b. ischiad'ica mus'culi obturato'rii inter'ni** [NA], ischial bursa of internal obturator muscle: a bursa between the tendon of the obturator internus muscle and the lesser sciatic notch; called also *b. sciatica musculi obturatorii interni* [NA alternative], *ischiadic b., b. musculi obturatoris interni, sciatic b. of obturator internus muscle,* and *tuberoischiadic b.* **ischial b. of gluteus maximus muscle,** b. ischiadica musculi glutei maximi. **ischial b. of internal obturator muscle,** b. ischiadica musculi obturatorii interni. **lateral b. of gastrocnemius muscle,** b. subtendinea musculi gastrocnemii lateralis. **b. of latissimus dorsi muscle,** subtendinea musculi latissimi dorsi. **Luschka's b.,** b. pharyngea. **medial b. of gastrocnemius muscle,** b. subtendinea musculi gastrocnemii medialis. **Monro's b.,** b. intratendinea olecrani. **b. muco'sa,** b. synovialis. **b. muco'sa submuscula'ris,** b. synovialis submuscularis. **mucous b.,** b. synovialis. **multilocular b.,** one which is subdivided into several compartments. **b. mus'culi bicip'itis fem'oris infe'rior,** b. subtendinea musculi bicipitis femoris inferior. **b. mus'culi bicip'itis fem'oris supe'rior** [NA], superior bursa of biceps femoris muscle: a bursa between the long head of the biceps, the semitendinosus, the tendon of the semimembranosus, and the ischial tuberosity; called also *subtendinous b.* **b. mus'culi coracobrachia'lis** [NA], a bursa between the coracobrachialis and subscapularus muscles and the coracoid process; called also *coracobrachial b.* and *subcoracoid b.* **b. mus'culi extenso'ris car'pi radia'lis bre'vis** [NA], a bursa between the tendon and the base of the third metacarpal bone. **b. mus'culi gastrocne'mii latera'lis,** b. subtendinea musculi gastrocnemii lateralis. **b. mus'culi gastrocne'mii media'lis,** b. subtendinea musculi gastrocnemii medialis. **b. mus'culi infraspina'ti,** b. subtendinea musculi infraspinati. **b. mus'culi latis'simi dor'si,** b. subtendinea musculi latissimi dorsi. **b. mus'culi obturato'ris inter'ni,** see *b. ischiadica musculi obturatorii interni* and *b. subtendinea musculi obturatorii interni.* **b. mus'culi pirifor'mis** [NA], bursa of piriform muscle: a bursa between the piriformis tendon, the superior gemellus muscle, and the femur; called also *piriform b.* **b. mus'culi poplite'i,** recessus subpopliteus. **b. mus'culi sarto'rii pro'pria** see *bursae subtendineae musculi sartorii.* **b. mus'culi semimembrano'si** [NA], bursa of semimembranosus muscle: a bursa between the semimembranosus muscle and the medial head of the gastrocnemius. Called also *gastrocnemiosemimembranous b., posterior genual b., retrocondyloid b., semimembranosagastrocnemial b.,* and *semimembranous b.* **b. mus'culi sternohyoi'dei,** see *b. infrahyoidea* and *b. retrohyoidea.* **b. mus'culi subscapula'ris,** b. subtendinea musculi subscapularis. **b. mus'culi tenso'ris ve'li pala'ti** [NA], bursa of tensor veli palatini muscle: a bursa between the hamular process of the sphenoid bone and the tendon of the tensor veli palatini. **b. mus'culi tere'tis majo'ris,** b. subtendinea musculi teretis majoris. **b. mus'culi thyreohyoi'dei,** a bursa under the thyrohyoid muscle. **b. of olecranon,** b. subcutanea olecrani. **omental b., b. omenta'lis** [NA], a serous peritoneal cavity situated behind the stomach, the lesser omentum, and part of the liver and in front of the pancreas and duodenum. It communicates with the general peritoneal cavity (greater sac) through the epiploic foramen and sometimes is continuous with the cavity of the greater omentum. Called also *lesser peritoneal cavity.* **ovarian b., b. ova'rica,** the peritoneal fossa in which the ovary is situated. **patellar b., deep,** b. subtendinea prepatellaris. **patellar b., middle,** b. subfascialis prepatellaris. **patellar b., prespinous,** b. subcutanea tuberositatis tibiae. **patellar b., subcutaneous,** b. subcutanea prepatellaris. **peroneal b., common,** vagina synovialis musculorum peroneorum communis. **b. pharyn'gea** [NA], **pharyngeal b.,** an inconstant blind sac located above the pharyngeal tonsil in the midline of the posterior wall of the nasopharynx; it represents persistence of an embryonic communication between the anterior tip of the notochord and the roof of the pharynx. Called also *Luschka's b., Tornwaldt's b.* and *Tornwaldt's cyst.* **b. of piriform muscle,** b. musculi piriformis. **popliteal b., b. of popliteal muscle,** recessus subpopliteus. **postcalcaneal b.,** b. subcutanea calcanea. **postcalcaneal b., deep,** b. tendinis calcanei. **postgenual b., external,** b. subtendinea musculi gastrocnemii lateralis. **b. praepatella′ris subcuta′nea,** b. subcutanea prepatellaris. **b. praepatella′ris subfascia′lis,** b. subfascialis prepatellaris. **b. praepatella′ris subtendin′ea,** b. subtendinea prepatellaris. **prepatellar b., middle,** b. subfascialis prepatellaris. **prepatellar b., subcutaneous,** b. subcutanea prepatellaris. **prepatellar b., subfascial,** b. subfascialis prepatellaris. **prepatellar b., subtendinous,** b. subtendinea prepatellaris. **bur′sae prepatella′res,** see *b. subcutanea prepatellaris, b. subfascialis prepatellaris,* and *b. subtendinea prepatellaris.* **b. prepatella′ris profun′da, b. prepatella′ris subaponeurot′ica,** b. subtendinea prepatellaris. **pretibial b.,** b. subcutanea tuberositatis tibiae. **bur′sae pro′priae mus′culi sarto′rii,** bursae subtendineae musculi sartorii. **pyriform b.,** b. musculi piriformis. **b. of quadratus femoris muscle,** b. subtendinea iliaca. **retrocondyloid b.,** b. musculi semimembranosi. **retroepicondyloid b., lateral, deep,** b. subtendinea musculi gastrocnemii lateralis. **retrohyoid b., b. retrohyoi′dea** [NA], a bursa sometimes present behind the hyoid bone at the attachment of the sternohyoid muscle. **retromammary b.,** a well-defined loose areolar tissue between the deep layer of superficial fascia on the posterior aspect of the breast, and the deep fascia covering the pectoralis major and other muscles of the chest wall. **sciatic b. of gluteus maximus muscle,** b. ischiadica musculi glutei maximi. **sciatic b. of obturator internus muscle,** b. ischiadica musculi obturatorii interni. **b. scia′tica mus′culi glu′tei max′imi,** NA alternative for *b. ischiadica musculi glutei maximi.* **b. scia′tica mus′culi obturato′rii inter′ni,** NA alternative for *b. ischiadica musculi obturatorii interni.* **semimembranosogastrocnemial b., semimembranous b.,** b. of semimembranosus muscle. **semitendinous b.,** b. musculi bicipitis femoris superior. **sternohyoid b., b. sternohyoi′dea,** see *b. infrahyoidea* and *b. retrohyoidea.* **subachilleal b.,** b. tendinis calcanei. **subacromial b., b. subacromia′lis** [NA], one between the acromion and the insertion of the supraspinatus muscle, extending between the deltoid and the greater tubercle of the humerus; called also *deltoid b.* and *humeral b.* **subcalcaneal b.,** b. subcutanea calcanea. **subclavian b.,** an inconstant bursa between the fibers of the rhomboid ligament. **subcoracoid b.,** 1. bursa musculi coracobrachialis. 2. bursa subtendinea musculi subscapularis. **subcrural b.,** b. suprapatellaris. **b. subcuta′nea** [NA], **subcutaneous b., subcutaneous synovial b.,** a synovial sac found beneath the skin; called also *b. synovialis subcutanea.* **b. subcuta′nea acromia′lis** [NA], a bursa between the acromion and the overlying skin; called also *subcutaneous acromial b.* **b. subcuta′nea calca′nea** [NA], subcutaneous calcaneal bursa: a bursa between the calcaneus and the skin on the sole of the foot; called also *postcalcaneal b.,* and *subcalcaneal b.* **b. subcuta′nea infrapatella′ris** [NA], subcutaneous infrapatellar bursa: a bursa between the upper end of the patellar ligament and the skin; called also *b. infrapatellaris subcutanea, subpatellar b.,* and *superficial b. of knee.* **b. subcuta′nea malle′oli latera′lis** [NA], subcutaneous bursa of lateral malleolus: a bursa between the lateral malleolus and the skin. **b. subcuta′nea malle′oli media′lis** [NA], subcutaneous bursa of medial malleolus: a bursa between the medial malleolus and the skin. **b. subcuta′nea olecra′ni** [NA], subcutaneous bursa of olecranon: a bursa between the olecranon process and the skin; called also *anconeal b.* and *superficial b. of olecranon.* **b. subcuta′nea prepatella′ris** [NA], subcutaneous prepatellar bursa: a bursa between the patella and the skin; called also *b. prepatellaris subcutanea.* **b. subcuta′nea prominen′tiae laryngea′lis** [NA], subcutaneous bursa of prominence of larynx: a bursa over the anterior prominence of the thyroid cartilage of the larynx, under the skin; called also *hyoid b., subhyoid b.,* and *thyrohyoid b.* **b. subcuta′nea tuberosita′tis tib′iae** [NA], subcutaneous bursa of tuberosity of tibia: a bursa between the tibial tuberosity and the skin; called also *patellar b., prespinous b.,*

pretibial b., and *superficial inferior infrapatellar b.* **subcutaneous acromial b.,** b. subcutanea acromialis. **subcutaneous b. of lateral malleolus,** b. subcutanea malleoli lateralis. **subcutaneous b. of medial malleolus,** b. subcutanea malleoli medialis. **subcutaneous b. of olecranon,** b. subcutanea olecrani. **subcutaneous b. of prominence of larynx,** b. subcutanea promentiae laryngeaalis. **subcutaneous b. of tuberosity of tibia,** b. subcutanea tuberositatis tibiae. **subdeltoid b., b. subdeltoi′dea** [NA], a bursa between the deltoid and the shoulder joint capsule, usually connected to the subacromial bursa; called also *acromial b.* **subfascial b., subfascial synovial b.,** b. subfascialis. **b. subfascia′lis** [NA], subfascial bursa: synovial sac found beneath a fascial layer; called also *b. synovialis subfascialis* and *subfascial synovial b.* **b. subfascia′lis prepatella′ris** [NA], subfascial prepatellar bursa: a bursa between the front of the patella and the investing fascia of the knee; called also *b. praepatellaris subfascialis, middle patellar* (or *prepatellar*) *b.* **subhyoid b.,** b. subcutanea prominentiae laryngeaalis. **subiliac b.,** 1. b. iliopectinea. 2. b. subtendinea iliaca. **subligamentous b.,** b. infrapatellaris profunda. **submuscular b., submuscular synovial b.,** b. submuscularis. **b. submuscula′ris** [NA], submuscular bursa: a synovial sac found beneath a muscle; called also *b. synovialis* and *submuscular synovial b.* **subpatellar b.,** 1. b. infrapatellaris profunda. 2. b. subcutanea infrapatellaris. **b. subtendin′ea** [NA], subtendinous bursa: a synovial sac found between tendons and bone, tendons and ligaments, and one tendon and another. Called also *b. synovialis subtendinea* and *subtendinous synovial b.* **b. subtendin′ea ili′aca** [NA], subtendinous iliac bursa: a bursa between the iliopsoas tendon and the lesser trochanter; called also *b. iliaca subtendinea, b. of quadratus femoris muscle, b. of iliopsoas muscle,* and *subiliac b.* **b. subtendin′ea mus′culi bicip′itis fem′oris infe′rior** [NA], inferior subtendinous bursa of bicipitis femoris muscle: a bursa between the tendon of the biceps femoris muscle and the fibular collateral ligament of the knee joint; called also *bicipital b., biciptofibular b., fibular b., external inferior genual b.,* and *b. musculi bicipitus femoris inferior.* **b. subtendin′ea mus′culi gastrocne′mii latera′lis** [NA], a bursa between the tendon of the lateral head of the gastrocnemius muscle and the joint capsule; called also *b. musculi gastrocnemii lateralis, subtendinous b. of lateral head of gastrocnemius muscle, humeral b., lateral b. of gastrocnemius muscle, external postgenual b.,* and *deep lateral retroepicondyloid b.* **b. subtendin′ea mus′culi gastrocne′mii media′lis** [NA], a bursa between the tendon of the medial head of the gastrocnemius, the condyle of the femur, and the joint capsule; called also *b. musculi gastrocnemii medialis, subtendinous b. of medial head of gastrocnemius muscle, Brodie's b., internal supracondyloid b., medial b. of gastrocnemius muscle,* and *medial supracondyloid b.* **b. subtendin′ea mus′culi infraspina′ti** [NA], subtendinous bursa of infraspinatus muscle: a bursa between the tendon of the infraspinatus and the joint capsule or the greater tubercle; called also *b. musculi infraspinati.* **b. subtendin′ea mus′culi latis′simi dor′si** [NA], a bursa between the tendons of the latissimus dorsi and teres major muscles; called also *b. musculi latissimi dorsi* and *b. of latissimus dorsi muscle.* **b. subtendin′ea mus′culi obturato′rii inter′ni** [NA], subtendinous bursa of internal obturator muscle: a bursa beneath the tendon of the obturator internus muscle; called also *b. musculi obturatoris interni.* **bur′sae subtendin′eae mus′culi sarto′rii** [NA], subtendinous bursae of sartorius muscle: bursae between the tendons of the sartorius, semitendinosus, and gracilis muscles; called also *internal superior genual bursae, b. musculi sartorii propria,* and *bursae propriae musculi sartorii.* **b. subtendin′ea mus′culi subscapula′ris** [NA], subtendinous bursa of subscapularis muscle: a bursa between the tendon of the subscapularis muscle and the glenoid border of the scapula; called also *b. musculi subscapularis, coracoid b.,* and *subcoracoid b.* **b. subtendin′ea mus′culi tere′tis majo′ris** [NA], subtendinous bursa of teres major muscle: a bursa deep to the tendon of insertion of the teres major muscle; called also *b. musculi teretis majoris.* **b. subtendin′ea mus′culi tibia′lis anteri′o′ris** [NA], subtendinous bursa of anterior tibial muscle: a bursa between the tibialis anterior and the medial surface of the medial cuneiform bone. **b. subtendin′ea mus′culi tibia′lis posterio′ris** [NA], subtendinous bursa of posterior tibial muscle: a bursa between the tibialis posterior and the navicular bone. **b. subtendin′ea mus′culi trape′zii** [NA], a bursa between the trapezius and the medial end of the spine of the scapula. **b. subtendin′ea mus′culi tricip′itis bra′chii** [NA], **b. subtendin′ea olecra′ni,** an inconstant sac between the triceps tendon, the olecranon, and the dorsal ligament of the elbow; called also *anconeal b. of triceps muscle.* **b. subtendin′ea prepatella′ris** [NA], subtendinous prepatellar bursa: a bursa sometimes present between the quadriceps tendon and the patellar periosteum; called also *b. prepatellaris subtendinea, deep patellar b., infrapatellar b., b. prepatellaris profunda* or *subaponeurotica,* and *subcutaneous patellar b.* **subtendinous b. of anterior tibial muscle,** b. subtendinea musculi tibialis anterioris. **subtendinous b. of biceps femoris muscle, inferior,** b. subtendinea musculi bicipitis femoris inferior. **subtendinous b. of infraspinatus muscle,** b. subtendinea musculi infraspinati. **subtendinous b. of internal obturator muscle,** b. subtendinea musculi obturatorii interni. **subtendinous b. of lateral head of gastrocnemius muscle,** b. subtendinea musculi gastrocnemii lateralis. **subtendinous b. of medial head of gastrocnemius muscle,** b. subtendinea musculi gastrocnemii medialis. **subtendinous b. of obturator internus muscle,** b. subtendinea musculi obturatorii interni. **subtendinous b. of posterior tibial muscle,** b. subtendinea musculi tibialis posterioris. **subtendinous bursae of sartorius muscle,** bursae subtendineae musculi sartorii. **subtendinous b. of subscapularis muscle,** b. subtendinea musculi subscapularis. **subtendinous b., subtendinous synovial b.,** b. subtendinea. **subtendinous b. of teres major muscle,** b. subtendinea musculi teretis majoris. **superficial b. of knee,** b. subcutanea infrapatellaris. **superficial b. of olecranon,** b. subcutanea olecrani. **superior b. of biceps femoris muscle,** b. musculi bicipitis femoris superior. **supernumerary b.,** adventitious b. **supra-anconeal b., intratendinous b.,** b. intratendinea olecrani. **supracondyloid b., internal, supracondyloid b., medial,** b. subtendinea musculi gastrocnemii medialis. **supragenual b., suprapatellar b.,** b. suprapatellaris. **b. suprapatella′ris** [NA], suprapatellar bursa: a bursa between the distal end of the femur and the quadriceps tendon; called also *supragenual b.* and *subcrural b.* **synovial b.,** b. synovialis. **synovial b. of trochlea,** vagina tendinis musculi obliqui superioris. **b. synovia′lis** [NA], synovial bursa: a closed synovial sac interposed between surfaces which glide upon each other; it may be simple or multilocular in structure, and subcutaneous, submuscular, subfascial, or subtendinous in location; called also *b. mucosa* and *mucous b.* **b. synovia′lis subcuta′nea,** b. subcutanea. **b. synovia′lis subfascia′lis,** b. subfascialis. **b. synovia′lis submuscula′ris,** b. submuscularis. **b. synovia′lis subtendin′ea,** b. subtendinea. **b. ten′dinis Achil′lis,** b. tendinis calcanei. **b. ten′dinis calca′nei** [NA], bursa of calcaneal tendon: a bursa between the calcaneal tendon and the back of the calcaneus; called also *b. of Achilles (tendon), calcaneal b., deep postcalcaneal b., subachilleal b.,* and *b. tendinis Achillis.* **b. of tendon of Achilles,** b. tendinis calcanei. **b. of tensor veli palatini muscle,** b. musculi tensoris veli palati. **b. of testes,** scrotum. **thyrohyoid b.,** b. subcutanea prominentiae laryngeaalis. **thyrohyoid b., anterior,** see *b. infrahyoidea* and *b. retrohyoidea.* **Tornwaldt's b.,** b. pharyngea. **trochanteric b., subcutaneous,** b. trochanterica subcutanea. **trochanteric b. of gluteus maximus muscle,** b. trochanterica musculi glutei maximi. **trochanteric bursae of gluteus medius muscle,** bursae trochantericae musculi glutei medii. **trochanteric b. of gluteus minimus muscle,** b. trochanterica musculi glutei minimi. **b. trochanter′ica mus′culi glu′taei me′dii ante′rior,** see *bursae trochantericae musculi glutei medii.* **b. trochanter′ica mus′culi glu′taei me′dii poste′rior,** see *bursae trochantericae musculi glutei medii.* **b. trochanter′ica mus′culi glu′tei max′imi** [NA], trochanteric bursa of gluteus maximus muscle: a bursa between the fascial tendon of the gluteus maximus, the posterolateral surface of the greater trochanter, and the vastus lateralis muscle. **bur′sae trochanter′icae mus′culi glu′tei me′dii** [NA], trochanteric bursae of gluteus medius muscle: bursae between the gluteus medius and the lateral surface of the greater trochanter, and

sometimes between the tendons of the gluteus medius and the piriformis. **b. trochanter′ica mus′culi glu′tei min′imi** [NA], trochanteric bursa of gluteus minimus muscle: a bursa between the edge of the gluteus minimus and the greater trochanter. **b. trochanter′ica subcuta′nea** [NA], subcutaneous trochanteric bursa: a bursa between the greater trochanter of the femur and the skin. **trochlear synovial b.,** vagina synovialis musculi obliqui superioris. **tuberoischiadic b.,** b. ischiadica musculi obturatorii interni. **ulnoradial b.,** b. cubitalis interossea. **vesicular b., ileopubic,** b. iliopectinea. **vesicular b. of sternohyoideus muscle,** see *b. infrahyoidea* and *b. retrohyoidea.*

bursae (ber′se) [L.] genitive and plural of *bursa.*

bursal (ber′sal) [L. *bursalis*] of or pertaining to a bursa.

bursalogy (ber-sal′o-je) [*bursa* + *-logy*] the sum of knowledge regarding the bursae.

Bursata (ber-sa′tah) a term sometimes used to designate those Nematoda which have a bursa copulatrix.

bursatti, bursautee (ber-sat′e, ber-sawt′e) cutaneous habronemiasis.

bursectomy (ber-sek′to-me) [*bursa* + Gr. *ektomē* excision] excision of a bursa.

bursicon (bur′sĭ-kon) an insect hormone appearing in the blood after molting, which is required for the tanning and hardening of new cuticle.

bursitis (ber-si′tis) inflammation of a bursa, occasionally accompanied by a calcific deposit in the underlying supraspinatus tendon; the most common site is the subdeltoid bursa. **Achilles b.,** achillobursitis. **adhesive b.,** see under *capsulitis.* **calcific b.,** see under *tendinitis.* **Duplay's b.** (*obs.*), inflammation of the subacromial or subdeltoid bursa; see *calcific tendinitis,* under *tendinitis.* **ischiogluteal b.,** inflammation of the bursa over the ischial tuberosity, characterized by sudden onset of excruciating pain over the center of the buttock and down the back of the leg. **olecranon b.,** inflammation and enlargement of the bursa over the olecranon; called also *miners' elbow.* **omental b.,** peritonitis localized to the omental bursa (lesser sac). **pharyngeal b.,** Tornwaldt's b. **popliteal b.,** a swelling behind the knee, caused by escape of synovial fluid which then becomes enclosed in a sac or membrane; called also *Baker's cyst* and *synovial cyst of the popliteal space.* **prepatellar b.,** inflammation of the bursa in front of the patella, with fluid accumulating within it; called also *housemaid's knee.* **radiohumeral b.,** tennis elbow. **retrocalcaneal b.,** achillodynia. **scapulohumeral b.,** calcific tendinitis. **subacromial b.,** see *calcific tendinitis,* under *tendinitis.* **subdeltoid b.,** see *calcific tendinitis,* under *tendinitis.* **superficial calcaneal b.,** achillobursitis. **Thornwaldt's b., Tornwaldt's b.,** chronic inflammation of the pharyngeal bursa, attended with formation of a pus-containing cyst, and nasopharyngeal stenosis; called also *pharyngeal b.,* and *Tornwaldt's disease.*

bursolith (ber′so-lith) [*bursa* + Gr. *lithos* stone] a calculus or concretion in a bursa.

bursopathy (ber-sop′ah-the) [*bursa* + Gr. *pathos* disease] any disease of a bursa.

bursotomy (ber-sot′o-me) [*bursa* + Gr. *tomē* a cutting] incision of a bursa.

burst (berst) a sudden, intense increase or outbreak. **metabolic b.,** respiratory b. **respiratory b.,** a sequence of four metabolic events that occur during oxidative killing of ingested microorganisms by granulocytes and mononuclear phagocytes, consisting of (1) an increase in oxygen consumption, (2) formation of superoxide anion, (3) formation of hydrogen peroxide, and (4) activation of the hexose monophosphate shunt. Molecular oxygen is converted to superoxide by NADPH oxidase and NADH oxidase. Superoxide is converted to hydrogen peroxide by superoxide dismutase. Hydrogen peroxide is utilized in myeloperoxidase-dependent bacterial killing, and both superoxide and hydrogen peroxide are spontaneously converted to other toxic metabolites, e.g., singlet oxygen and hydroxyl radicals. The hexose monophosphate shunt regenerates NADPH.

bursula (ber′su-lah) [L.] a small bag or pouch.

Burton's line (sign) (ber′tunz) [Henry *Burton,* British physician, 1799–1849] see *lead line,* under *line.*

Buschke's disease, scleredema (boōsh′kez) [Abraham

Buschke, German dermatologist, 1868–1943] see *cryptococcosis* and *scleredema.*

Buschke-Löwenstein's tumor (bōōsh′kĕz-la′ven-stīnz) [Abraham *Buschke;* Ludwig W. *Löwenstein*] see under *tumor.*

Buschke-Ollendorff syndrome (bōōsh′ke-o′len-dorf) [Abraham *Buschke;* Helene *Ollendorff,* German dermatologist, 20th century] dermatofibrosis lenticularis disseminata.

bushmaster (bush′mas-ter) a large venomous pit viper, *Lachesis muta,* of the Amazon region of South America. See table accompanying *snake.*

buspirone hydrochloride (bu-spi′rŏn) chemical name: 8-[4- [4 -(2-pyrimidinyl)- 1 -piperazinyl]butyl]- 8 - azaspiro[4, 5]decane- 7,9-dione; a tranquilizer, $C_{21}H_{31}N_5O_2 \cdot HCl$.

Busquet's disease (bōōs-kāz′) [P. *Busquet,* French physician] see under *disease.*

Busse-Buschke disease [Otto *Busse,* German physician, 1867–1922; Abraham *Buschke,* German dermatologist, 1868–1943] cryptococcosis.

busulfan (bu-sul′fan) [USP] a bifunctional cytotoxic alkylating agent, 1,4-butanediol dimethanesulfonate, an antineoplastic agent unrelated to the nitrogen mustards; used primarily for treatment of chronic granulocytic leukemia and also polycythemia vera and myeloid metaplasia; the major side effect is bone marrow depression.

But. abbreviation for L. *bu′tyrum,* butter.

butabarbital sodium (bu-tah-bar′bĭ-tal) [USP] chemical name: 5-ethyl-5-(1-methylpropyl)-2,4-6(1*H,3H,5H*)pyrimidinetrione monosodium salt. A barbituric acid derivative, $C_{10}H_{15}N_2NaO_3$, occurring as a white powder; used as a sedative and hypnotic, administered orally.

butacaine sulfate (bu″tah-kān′ sul′fāt) [USP] chemical name: 3-(dibutylamino)-1-propanol 4-aminobenzoate sulfate. A local anesthetic, $(C_{18}H_{30}N_2O_2)_2 \cdot H_2SO_4$, occurring as a white to practically white, crystalline powder; used to produce topical anesthesia in the eye or in the mouth.

butaclamol hydrochloride (bu″tah-kla′mōl) chemical name: (+)- 3α-(1,1-dimethylethyl)-2,3,4,4aα,8,9,13bβ,14-octahydro-1*H*-benzo[6,7]cyclohepta[1,2,3-de]pyrido[2,1-α]isoquinolin hydrochloride; a tranquilizer, $C_{25}H_{31}NO \cdot HCl$.

butadiazamide (bu″tah-di-az′ah-mīd) chemical name: *N*-(5-butyl-1,3,4-thiadiazol-2-yl)-*p*-chlorobenzenesulfonamide; a hypoglycemic agent, $C_{12}H_{14}ClN_3O_2S_2$.

butalbital (bu-tal′bĭ-tal) [USP] chemical name: 5-(2-methylpropyl)-5-(2-propenyl)-2,4,6(1*H,3H,5H*)-pyrimidinetrione. An intermediate-acting barbiturate, occurring as a white, crystalline powder, $C_{11}H_{16}N_2O_3$; administered orally.

butallylonal (bu-tah-lil′o-nal) chemical name: 5-(2-bromo-2-propenyl)-5-(1-methylpropyl)-2,4,6(1*H,3H,5H*) pyrimidinetrione. An intermediate-acting barbiturate, $C_{11}H_{15}Br-N_2O_3$, used as a hypnotic.

butamben (bu-tam′ben) [USP] chemical name: 4-aminobenzoic acid butyl ester. A local anesthetic, $C_{11}H_{15}NO_2$, occurring as a white, crystalline powder; applied topically in the treatment of painful skin conditions and pain associated with hemorrhoids or anal fissure. Called also *butyl aminobenzoate.*

butamirate citrate (bu″tah-mi′rāt) chemical name: α-ethyl-2-[2-(diethylamino)ethoxy]ethyl ester benzeneacetic acid 2-hydroxy-1,2,3-propanetricarboxylate (1:1); an antitussive, $C_{18}H_{29}NO_3 \cdot C_6H_8O_7$.

butamisole hydrochloride (bu-tam′ĭ-sōl) chemical name: (−)- 2 - methyl-*N*-[3-(2,3,5,6-tetrahydroimidazo[2,1-*b*] thiazol-6-yl)- phenyl]propanamide monohydrochloride; a veterinary anthelmintic, $C_{15}H_{19}N_3OS \cdot HCl$.

butamoxane hydrochloride (bu-tah-moks′ān) chemical name: *N*-butyl-1,4-benzodioxan-2-methylamine hydrochloride; a tranquilizer, $C_{13}H_{19}NO_2 \cdot HCl$.

butane (bu′tān) *n*-butane; an aliphatic hydrocarbon of the methane series, C_4H_{10}, from petroleum, occurring as a colorless flammable gas with a characteristic odor. **normal b.,** $CH_3—(CH_2)_2CH_3$.

butanoic acid (bu″tah-no′ik) *n*-butyric acid.

butaperazine (bu-tah-per′ah-zēn) chemical name: 1-[10-[3-(4-methyl-1-piperazinyl)propyl]10*H*-phenothiazin-2-yl]-1-butanone. A phenothiazide derivative, $C_{24}H_{31}N_3OS$, used as an antipsychotic drug in the treatment of acute and chronic schizophrenia; administered orally. **b. maleate,** the ma-

leate ester of butaperazine, $C_{24}H_{31}N_3OS \cdot 2C_4H_4O_4$, having the same actions and uses as the base.

Butazolidin (bu″tah-zol′ĭ-din) trademark for preparations of phenylbutazone.

Butcher's saw (booch′erz) [Richard George Herbert *Butcher,* Irish surgeon, 1819–1891] see under *saw.*

Butesin (bu-te′sin) trademark for a preparation of butyl aminobenzoate.

butethal (bu′tĕ-thal) chemical name: 5-butyl-5-ethyl-2,4,6-(1*H,3H,5H*)pyrimidinetrione. An intermediate-acting barbiturate, $C_{10}H_{16}N_2O_3$, used as a sedative; administered orally.

butethamine hydrochloride (bu-teth′ah-mēn) chemical name: 2-[(2-methylpropyl)amino]ethanol 4-aminobenzoate (ester) hydrochloride. A local anesthetic, $C_{13}H_{20}N_2O_2 \cdot HCl$, occurring as small, white crystals or white, crystalline powder; used for nerve block anesthesia in dentistry.

Buthus (bu′thus) a genus of scorpions. **B. carolinia′-nus,** a species occurring in the southern United States. **B. quinquestria′tus,** a dangerous species occurring in Egypt.

butirosin sulfate (bu-tĕr′o-sin) an aminoglycoside antibiotic complex, $C_{21}H_{41}N_5O_{12} \cdot 2H_2SO_4 \cdot 2H_2O$, obtained from certain strains of *Bacillus circulans,* consisting of butirosins A and B; an antibacterial.

Butisol sodium (bu′tĭ-sol) trademark for preparations of sodium butabarbital.

butonate (bu′to-nāt) chemical name: butanoic acid 2,2,2-trichloro-1-(dimethoxyphosphinyl)ethyl ester; an insecticide and anthelminthic that is a potent cholinesterase inhibitor, $C_8H_{14}Cl_3O_5P$.

butoprozine hydrochloride (bu″to-pro′zēn) chemical name: [4-[3-(dibutylamino)propoxy]phenyl](2-ethyl-3-indolizinyl)methanone monohydrochloride; an antiarrhythmic cardiac depressant and antianginal, $C_{28}H_{38}N_2O_2 \cdot HCl$.

butopyronoxyl (bu″to-pi″ro-nok′sil) chemical name: 3,4-dihydro-2,2-dimethyl-4-oxo-2*H*-pyran carboxylic acid butyl ester. An insect repellent effective against ticks, $C_{12}H_{18}O_4$, occurring as a yellow to pale reddish brown liquid.

butorphanol (bu-tor′fah-nōl) chemical name: 17-(cyclobutylmethyl)morphinan-3,14-diol; a synthetic opioid, $C_{21}H_{29}NO_2$, having analgesic and antitussive properties. **b. tartrate,** the tartrate salt of butorphanol, $C_{21}H_{29}NO_2 \cdot C_4H_6O_6$, administered intramuscularly as an analgesic.

butoxamine hydrochloride (bu-toks′ah-mēn) chemical name: α-[1-[(1,1-dimethylethyl)amino]ethyl]-2,5-dimethoxybenzenemethanol. A beta-adrenergic blocking agent, $C_{15}H_{25}NO_3 \cdot HCl$.

butriptyline hydrochloride (bu-trip′tĭ-lēn) chemical name: (+)-10,11-dihydro-*N,N,β*-trimethyl-5*H*-dibenzo[*a, d*]cycloheptene-5-propylamine hydrochloride; an antidepressant, $C_{21}H_{27}N \cdot HCl$.

Bütschli's nuclear spindle (bitsh′lēz) [Otto *Bütschli,* German zoologist, 1848–1920] see *spindle,* def. 1.

butt (but) to bring the surfaces of two distinct objects squarely or directly into contact with each other.

butter (but′er) [L. *butyrum;* Gr. *boutyron*] the oily mass procured by churning cream. **b. of antimony,** antimony trichloride. **b. of arsenic,** arsenic trichloride. **cacao b., cocoa b.,** [NF], the fat obtained from the roasted seed of *Theobroma cacao;* used as a suppository base, and has been used for its emollient properties in cosmetics and is sometimes used to soften and protect the skin. Called also *theobroma oil.* **b. of tin,** stannic chloride. **b. of zinc,** zinc chloride.

butterfly (but′er-fli) 1. a mass of absorbent cotton with wing-shaped appendages, used mainly in uterine surgery. 2. a small piece of adhesive tape with broad, wing-shaped ends by means of which the edges of a superficial wound may be approximated. 3. a pattern formed by a skin eruption across the nose and adjacent areas of the cheeks, as in systemic lupus erythematosus, seborrheic dermatitis, and rosacea. Called also *butterfly rash.*

Buttiauxella (but″e-awk-sel′ah) a genus of gram-negative, facultatively anaerobic, rod-shaped bacteria of the family Enterobacteriaceae. The organisms belong to Enteric Groups 63 and 64, and are sucrose negative. The type species is *B. agres′tis.*

buttock (but′ok) one of the gluteal prominences; called also *clunis* or *breech* and, in the plural, *nates.*

button (but′n) 1. a knoblike elevation or structure. 2. a small appliance shaped like a spool or disk and used in surgery for the construction of intestinal anastomosis. **bromide b.,** a verrucous cutaneous lesion occurring as a result of sensitivity to bromides. **dog b.,** nux vomica. **iodide b.,** a verrucous cutaneous lesion occurring as a result of sensitivity to iodides. **Jaboulay b.,** a device for performing lateral intestinal anastomosis without the aid of sutures, consisting of two button-like cylinders of metal that are fitted together on the screw and key-ring principle through a small intestinal opening. **mescal b's,** transverse slices of the flowering heads of the Mexican dumpling cactus, *Lophophora williamsii* or mescal, whose major active principle is mescaline; used in divinatory and religious ceremonies by North American Indians. **Murphy's b.,** a device for joining the ends of a divided intestine so that union may take place. It consists of two short metal cylinders of different diameter, each having a collar at one end; the collars are sutured to the divided ends, and the narrower cylinder is locked into its mate. **Oriental b.,** cutaneous leishmaniasis. **peritoneal b.,** a short flanged glass tube for insertion between the peritoneal cavity and a subcutaneous pocket through which peritoneal transudate may be drained. **quaker b.,** nux vomica. **terminal b's,** see *end-feet.*

buttonhole (but′n-hōl) 1. a short straight incision into a cavity or organ. 2. an abnormal narrowing of the caliber of a structure. **mitral b.,** an advanced state of stenosis of the mitral orifice of the heart, adhesion and shortening of the cusps having produced a narrow slit-like orifice.

butyl (bu′til) a hydrocarbon radical, C_4H_9 or $CH_3 \cdot CH_2 \cdot CH_2 \cdot CH_2^-$. **b. acetate,** a liquid compound, $C_6H_{12}O_2$, used in the manufacture of lacquer, artificial leather, photographic film, plastics, and safety glass; it is an irritant which may cause conjunctivitis, and is narcotic in high concentrations. **b. aminobenzoate** [NF], chemical name, *n*-butyl *p*-aminobenzoate. A white, odorless, tasteless crystalline powder, $C_{11}H_{15}NO_2$, soluble in dilute acids, alcohol, ether, and chloroform; used as a local anesthetic. Called also *butamben.* **b. chloride,** chemical name: 1-chlorobutane. A clear colorless volatile liquid, C_4H_9Cl, miscible with dehydrated alcohol and with ether; used as a veterinary anthelmintic. **b. formate,** an industrial solvent, $CH_3 \cdot (CH_2)_3COOH$, the vapors of which are powerfully lacrimatory and suffocating. **b. hydride,** a hydrocarbon, C_4H_{10}, from petroleum; its vapor is an unsafe anesthetic.

butylene (bu′ti-lēn) a gaseous hydrocarbon, C_4H_8.

butylmercaptan (bu″til-mer-kap′tan) a thioalcohol, thiobutyl alcohol, $CH_3 \cdot CH_2 \cdot CH_2CH_2SH$, the active principle of the odoriferous secretion of the skunk.

butylparaben (bu-til-par′ah-ben) [NF] chemical name: 4-hydroxybenzoic acid butyl ester. An antifungal agent, $C_{11}H_{14}O_3$, occurring as small, colorless crystals or white powder, used as a pharmaceutic preservative.

Butyn (bu′tin) trademark for a preparation of butacaine sulfate.

butyr(o)- [L. *butyrum* butter] a combining form denoting relationship to butter, or to butyric acid.

butyraceous (bu″ti-ra′she-us) of a buttery consistency.

butyrate (bu′ti-rāt) a salt of butyric acid.

butyric (bu-tir′ik) derived from butter, as butyric acid.

butyric acid (bu-tēr′ik) 1. any 4-carbon carboxylic acid, either *n*-butyric acid or isobutyric acid. 2. *n*-butyric acid, $CH_3(CH_2)_2COOH$, occurring in rancid butter and sweat and also, in esterified form, in much animal fat. Systematic name: *butanoic acid.*

butyrin (bu′ti-rin) a triglyceride of butyric acid existing in butter, $C_3H_5(C_4H_7O_2)_3$, a liquid fat with an acrid, bitter taste; called also *tributyrin.*

butyrine (bu′ti-rin) an amino acid derivative of butyric acid; it is α-amino butyric acid.

Butyrivibrio (bu-ti″re-vib′re-o) [L. *butyricus* butyric + *vibrio*] a genus of gram-negative, non–spore-forming, anaerobic bacteria of the family Bacteroidaceae, found in the rumen contents of animals, and consisting of motile curved rods that may be in chains or filaments. The type species is *B. fibrosol′vens.*

butyroid (bu′ti-roid) [*butyr-* + Gr. *eidos* form] resembling or having the consistency of butter.

butyromel (bu-tir′o-mel) fresh, unsalted butter, 2 parts, and honey, 1 part: a substitute for cod liver oil.

butyrometer (bu″ti-rom′ĕ-ter) [*butyr-* + Gr. *metron* measure] an apparatus for estimating the proportion of butter fat in milk; called also *butyroscope.*

butyrophenone (bu″ti-ro-fe′nōn) any of a class of structurally related antipsychotic agents; the prototype is haloperidol.

butyroscope (bu-ti′ro-skōp) [*butyr-* + Gr. *skopein* to examine] butyrometer.

butyrous (bu′ti-rus) like butter; having a butter-like appearance.

bypass (bi′pas) an auxiliary flow; a shunt. **aortocoronary b.,** a section of saphenous vein grafted between the aorta and a coronary artery distal to an obstructive lesion in the latter. Called also *coronary artery b.* **aortoiliac b.,** insertion of a vascular prosthesis from the abdominal aorta to the femoral artery to bypass intervening atherosclerotic segments. **aortorenal b.,** insertion of a section of saphenous vein, hypogastric artery, or suitable substitute between the aorta and renal artery to bypass occluded or stenotic segments. **cardiopulmonary b.,** diversion of the flow of blood to the heart directly to the aorta, via a pump oxygenator, avoiding both the heart and the lungs; a form of extracorporeal circulation used in heart surgery. **coronary b., coronary artery b.,** aortocoronary b. **femoropopliteal b.,** insertion of a vascular prosthesis from the femoral to the popliteal artery to bypass occluded, narrowed, or injured segments. **gastric b.,** gastrojejunostomy in which the stomach is transected high on the body, the proximal remnant being joined to a loop of jejunum in end-to-side anastomosis. **intestinal b.,** resection of the intestine, with anastomosis of the proximal to the distal portion, as in jejunoileostomy. **jejunal b., jejunoileal b.,** surgical anastomosis of the proximal part of the jejunum to the distal part of the ileum so as to bypass much of the small intestine and reduce intestinal absorption. **left heart b.,** diversion of the flow of blood from the pulmonary veins directly to the aorta, avoiding the left atrium and the left ventricle. **partial b.,** the deviation of only a portion of blood flowing through an artery. **partial ileal b.,** anastomosis of the proximal end of the transected ileum to the cecum, the bypass of the portion of the small intestine resulting in decreased intestinal absorption of and increased fecal excretion of cholesterol; sometimes used in treatment of hyperlipidemia and in weight reduction. **right heart b.,** diversion of the flow of blood from the entrance of the right atrium directly to the pulmonary arteries, avoiding the right atrium and right ventricle.

by-product (bi-prod′ukt) a secondary product obtained during the manufacture of a primary product.

byssaceous (bis-sa′she-us) [Gr. *byssos* flax] composed of fine flaxlike threads.

byssinosis (bis″ĭ-no′sis) [Gr. *byssos* flax + *-osis*] a pulmonary disease occurring among cotton textile workers and preparers of flax and soft hemp, due to inhalation of textile dust. The acute form is marked by tightness of the chest, wheezing, and cough on return to work after a brief absence (Monday dyspnea). The chronic form, occurring after years of exposure, is marked by permanent dyspnea. It is probably due to smooth muscle contraction resulting from histamine release induced by chemicals in the dust. Called also *brown lung, cotton-dust* or *stripper's asthma, cotton-mill fever,* and *Monday fever.*

byssinotic (bis″ĭ-not′ik) 1. pertaining to byssinosis. 2. one affected with byssinosis.

byssocausis (bis″o-kaw′sis) [Gr. *byssos* flax + *kausis* burning] moxibustion.

byssoid (bis′oid) [Gr. *byssos* flax + *eidos* form] made up of a fringe, the filaments of which are unequal in length.

byssophthisis (bis″o-thi′sis) [Gr. *byssos* flax + *phthisis* consumption] (obs.) byssinosis.

byssus (bis′us), pl. *bys′suses* or *bys′si* [L., from Gr. *byssos* flax] lint, charpie, or cotton.

bystander (bi′stan-der) that which is only incidentally involved in a process. **innocent b.,** a term referring to drug-induced hemolytic anemias or thrombocytopenias in which drug-specific antibodies react with the drug to form circulating immune complexes, which then nonspecifically

adhere to erythrocytes, platelets, and other cells, causing complement-dependent lysis.

C

C chemical symbol for *carbon;* symbol for cervical vertebrae (C-1 through C-7); complement (the complement components are numbered C1 through C9; activated components are denoted by small letters, e.g., C5a and C5b); *coulomb;* and *cytosine* or *cytidine* (in nucleic acids).

C symbol for *capacitance, compliance* (subscripts denote the structure: C_L lung compliance, C_T thoracic compliance, and C_{LT} total lung-thorax compliance); *clearance* (subscripts denote the substance: C_n inulin clearance, C_{cr} creatinine clearance, etc.); and *heat capacity* (C_P at constant pressure, C_v at constant volume).

°C symbol for degree Celsius (centigrade).

C. cathode (or cathodal); Celsius or centigrade; congius (gallon); closure; contraction; color sense; cylinder; cervical (in vertebral formulas); clonus; clearance (in kidney function tests).

c symbol for *molar concentration, specific heat capacity* (C_P at constant pressure, C_v at constant volume), and the velocity of light in a vacuum.

c contact; *centi-;* former symbol for curie, replaced by Ci.

C′ former symbol for *complement;* replaced by *C*.

χ chi, the twenty-second letter of the Greek alphabet.

χ² chi-squared; see under *distribution* and *tests*.

CA chronological age; Croup-associated (virus); cardiac arrest; coronary artery.

Ca Chemical symbol for *calcium*.

ca. abbreviation for L. *circa* about.

cabinet (kab′ĭ-net) a small closet, or place of enclosure. **Sauerbruch's c.** (*obs.*), a cabinet within which the air pressure can be increased or diminished; used in early operations on the chest, the patient's head being outside the cabinet, and his body and the surgeon within it.

Cabot's ring bodies (kab′ots) [Richard Clarke *Cabot,* Boston physician, 1868–1939] see under *body*.

cabufocon A (kab″u-fo′kon) chemical name: cellulose acetate butanoate; either of two hydrophobic contact lens materials, designated A or B.

cacaerometer (kak″a-er-om′ĕ-ter) [*cac-* + Gr. *aēr* air + *metron* measure] an instrument for measuring the impurity of air.

cacao (kah-ka′o) 1. cocoa. 2. *Theobroma cacao.* 3. the seeds of *T. cacao*.

cacation (kak-a′shun) defecation.

cacatory (kak′ah-to″re) marked by severe diarrhea.

cacesthenic (kak″es-then′ik) having defective sense organs.

cachectic (kah-kek′tik) pertaining to or characterized by cachexia.

cachectin (kah-kek′tin) a hormonelike protein produced by macrophages that releases fat and reduces the concentration of enzymes required for the production and storage of fat. It can also induce shock when bacterial endotoxins cause its release. It is the same substance as tumor necrosis factor.

cachet (kah-sha′) [Fr.] a disk-shaped wafer or capsule for enclosing a dose of medicine.

cachexia (kah-kek′se-ah) [*cac-* + Gr. *hexis* habit + *-ia*] a profound and marked state of constitutional disorder; general ill health and malnutrition. **cancerous c.,** the weak, emaciated condition seen in cases of malignant tumor. **c. exophthal′mica,** Graves' disease. **fluoric c.,** that seen in fluorosis. **hypophyseal c.,** see *panhypopituitarism.* **c. hypophysiopri′va,** the train of symptoms resulting from total deprivation of function of the pituitary gland, including phthisis, loss of sexual function, atrophy of the pituitary target glands, bradycardia, hypothermia, apathy, and coma. **lymphatic c.,** pseudoleukemia. **malarial c.,** a group of physical signs of a chronic nature that result from antecedent attacks of severe malaria; the principal signs are anemia, sallow skin, yellow sclera, splenomeg-

aly, hepatomegaly, and, in children, retardation of body growth and puberty. **c. mercuria′lis,** that seen in chronic mercurial poisoning. **pituitary c.,** see *panhypopituitarism.* **saturnine c.,** that seen in chronic lead poisoning. **c. suprarena′lis,** Addison's disease. **uremic c.,** cachexia associated with other systemic symptoms of advanced renal failure. **verminous c.** (*obs.*), the condition of anemia and debility which accompanies infection with worms, especially *Ancylostoma*.

cachexy (kah-kek′se) cachexia.

cachinnation (kak″ĭ-na′shun) [L. *cachinnare* to laugh aloud] immoderate, loud, and inappropriate laughter; commonly seen in disorganized schizophrenia.

CaCl₂ calcium chloride.

CaCl(OCl) chlorinated lime.

CaCO₃ calcium carbonate.

CaC₂O₄ calcium oxalate.

cac(o)- [Gr. *kakos* bad] a combining form meaning bad, or ill.

cacodemonomania (kak″o-de″mon-o-ma′ne-ah) a condition marked by delusions of being possessed by evil spirits.

cacodyl (kak′o-dil) [*caco-* + Gr. *ozein* to smell + *hylē* matter] tetramethylbiarsine, a colorless liquid, $(CH_3)_2As—As(CH_3)_2$, with an offensive odor; it gives off a poisonous vapor and is inflammable when exposed to air. **c. cyanide,** a white powder, $(CH_3)_2AsCN$, which, when exposed to the air, gives off an extremely poisonous vapor. **c. hydride,** a colorless liquid, $(CH_3)_2AsH$, with a strong, garlicky odor; on exposure to air, it gives off a poisonous vapor and ignites spontaneously. Symptoms of poisoning are the same as those of arsenic poisoning.

cacodylate (kak′o-dil-āt) a salt of cacodylic acid; the cacodylates were once used in skin diseases, tuberculosis, malaria, and other conditions.

cacodylic acid (kak″o-dil′ik) dimethyl arsinic acid, $(CH_3)_2AsO_2H$.

cacoethic (kak″o-e′thik) ill-conditioned; malignant.

cacogenesis (kak″o-jen′ĕ-sis) [*caco-* + Gr. *genesis* production] defective development.

cacogenic (kak″o-jen′ik) 1. having a tendency toward racial deterioration through bad sexual selection. 2. pertaining to cacogenesis.

cacogenics (kak″o-jen′iks) [*caco-* + Gr. *gennan* to generate] deterioration of the physical and moral properties of a race resulting from the mating and propagation of inferior individuals.

cacogeusia (kak″o-ju′se-ah) [*caco-* + Gr. *geusis* taste] a sensation of bad taste not related to the ingestion of specific substances.

cacomelia (kak″o-me′le-ah) [*caco-* + Gr. *melos* limb] congenital deformity of a limb.

cacoplastic (kak″o-plas′tik) [*caco-* + Gr. *plastikos* forming] susceptible of only an imperfect formation.

cacorhythmic (kak″o-rith′mik) [*caco-* + Gr. *rhythmos* rhythm] marked by irregularity of rhythm.

cacosmia (kak-oz′me-ah) [*caco-* + Gr. *osmē* smell] a sensation of bad smell not related to exposure to a specific odor.

cacothenic (kak″o-then′ik) pertaining to cacothenics.

cacothenics (kak″o-then′iks) [Gr. *kakothēnein* to be in a bad state] deterioration of a race resulting from deleterious influences in the environment.

cacotrophy (kak-ot′ro-fe) [*caco-* + Gr. *trophē* nourishment] malnutrition; impaired or disordered nourishment.

cactinomycin (kak″tin-o-mi′sin) a highly toxic antibiotic of the actinomycin group, actinomycin C, produced by *Streptomyces chrysomallus,* consisting of a mixture of actinomycins C_2 and C_3 and dactinomycin (actinomycin D); formerly used as an antineoplastic.

cacumen (kak-u′men), pl. *cacu′mina* [L. "summit"] (*obs.*) 1. the top or apex of an organ. 2. the top and uppermost branchlets of a plant. 3. culmen.

cacuminal (kak-u′mĭ-nal) pertaining to the cacumen.

cadaver (kah-dav′er) [L., from *cadere*, to fall, to perish] a dead body; corpse; generally applied to a human body preserved for anatomical study, when it is commonly referred to as a subject.

cadaveric (kah-dav′er-ik) of or pertaining to a cadaver.

cadaverine (kah-dav′er-in) [L. *cadaver* corpse] a foul-smelling nitrogenous base, pentamethylenediamine, produced by decarboxylation of lysine. It is produced in decaying protein material by the action of bacteria, particularly species of *Vibrio*.

cadaverous (kah-dav′er-us) resembling a cadaver.

caddis (kad′is) see under *fly*.

cadmiosis (kad″me-o′sis) pneumoconiosis due to inhalation of and tissue reaction to cadmium dust.

cadmium (kad′me-um) [Gr. *kadmia* earth] a bivalent metal, not unlike tin in appearance and properties; symbol, Cd; atomic number, 48; atomic weight, 112.40. Its salts are poisonous. **c. anthranilate,** a salt of anthranilic acid (o-aminobenzoic acid) used as an ascaricide in swine. **c. bromide,** a poisonous substance, $CdBr_2$, used in photography, process engraving, and lithography; when swallowed it causes increased salivation, choking, abdominal pain, diarrhea, and tenesmus. **c. iodide,** a compound, CdI_2, formerly used as a nematocide. **c. oleate,** a preparation formerly used in various skin diseases. **c. salicylate,** a salt, $(C_6H_4(OH)CO_2)_2Cd + H_2O$, in fine, white, tabular crystals, or in an amorphous powder, formerly used as an antiseptic. **c. sulfate,** a salt, $CdSO_4$, weak solutions of which were formerly used as astringents in eye, ear, and urethral inflammations. **c. sulfide,** a light yellow or orange powder, CdS, used in 1 per cent suspension in treatment of seborrheic dermatitis of the scalp.

caduca (kah-du′kah) the decidua (membranae deciduae [NA]).

caduceus (kah-doo′se-us) [L., from Doric Gr. *karykeion*, herald's staff] the winged staff of Hermes or Mercury, the messenger of the gods, with two snakes winding around it. Used as a medical symbol and as the emblem of the Medical Corps, U.S. Army. The official symbol of the medical profession is the staff of Aesculapius.

caducous (kah-du′kus) [L. *cadere* to fall] falling off; deciduous.

cae- for words beginning thus, see also those beginning *ce-*.

caecum (se′kum) [L.] 1. a blind pouch or cul-de-sac. 2. [NA] the first part of the large intestine, forming a dilated pouch into which open the ileum, colon, and appendix vermiformis; spelled also *cecum* [NA alternative]. Called also *blindgut, blind intestine,* and *intestinum caecum.* **cupular c. of cochlear duct, c. cupula′re duc′tus cochlea′ris** [NA], the closed blind apical end of the cochlear duct. **vestibular c. of cochlear duct, c. vestibula′re duc′tus cochlea′ris** [NA], a small blind outpouching at the vestibular end of the cochlear duct.

caecus (se′kus) [L. "blind"] a blind pouch. **c. mi′nor ventric′uli,** the cardiac part of the stomach (pars cardiaca ventriculi [NA]).

Caedibacter (se″dĭ-bak′ter) [L. *caedes* slaughter + Gr. *baktron* a rod] a genus of bacteria of uncertain affiliation that are parasites of paramecia.

caen(o)- see *cen(o)-* (def. 1).

caeruleus (ser-roo′le-us) [L. "dark blue," "azure," probably from *caelum* sky] blue; azure; cerulean. Written also *coeruleus* (q.v.).

caesarean (se-za′re-an) see *cesarean section,* under *section.*

caesium (se′ze-um) cesium.

CaF₂ calcium fluoride.

caffeine (kah-fēn′, kaf′fe-in) [L. *caffeina*] [USP] chemical name: 1,3,7-trimethyl-3,7-dihydro-1*H*-purine-2,6-dione. An odorless, bitter, white powder, $C_8H_{10}N_4O_2$, one of the xanthines (q.v.), soluble in water and alcohol, and obtainable from coffee, tea, guarana, and maté. Caffeine stimulates the central nervous system, mainly affecting the cerebrum; has a diuretic effect on the kidneys; stimulates striated muscle; and has a group of effects on the cardiovascular system. It is used as a central and respiratory stimulant and for the relief of headache; administered orally. A combination of caffeine and sodium benzoate in water for injection is administered parenterally. Called also *guaranine* and *methyltheobromine.* See also *caffeinism.* **c. borocitrate,** a white soluble powder having sedative and antiseptic effects; no longer used in medicine. **c. chloral,** a soluble crystalline combination of caffeine and chloral, $C_8H_{10}N_4O_2$—CCl_3COH, formerly used as an analgesic. **c. citrate, citrated c.,** a preparation of equal parts of caffeine and citric acid, used for the same purposes as caffeine; administered orally. **c. hydrobromide,** colorless, efflorescent crystals, formerly used as a diuretic. **c. nitrate,** a salt in yellowish, needle-like crystals. **c. phthalate,** a sedative and antiseptic; no longer used in medicine. **c. and sodium benzoate,** see *caffeine.* **c. triiodide,** a compound in dark-green prisms, $(C_8H_{10}N_4O_2I_2 \cdot HI_2) + 3H_2O$, formerly used as an iodine substitute. **c. valerianate,** a former remedy for whooping cough and hysteric vomiting.

caffeinism (kaf′ēn-izm, kaf′e-in-izm″) a morbid condition resulting from ingestion of excessive amounts of caffeine. The manifestations include insomnia, restlessness, excitement, tachycardia, tremors, and diuresis.

Caffey's disease (kaf′fēz) [John *Caffey,* American pediatrician, 1895–1966] infantile cortical hyperostosis.

cage (kāj) a box or enclosure. **population c.,** an enclosure in which populations of *Drosophila* can be isolated through many generations. **thoracic c.,** compages thoracis.

CaH₂O₂ calcium hydroxide.

cain(o)- see *cen(o)-* (def. 1).

Cajal see *Ramón y Cajal.*

Cajal's cells, interstitial nucleus, stain (ka-halz′) [Santiago Ramón y *Cajal*] see under *cell,* see *nucleus interstitialis,* under *nucleus,* and see *Table of Stains.*

cajeputol (kaj′e-pu-tol) eucalyptol.

Cal large calorie (kilocalorie).

cal calorie.

calage (kah-lahzh′) [Fr.] propping with pillows to immobilize the viscera and thus relieve seasickness.

calamine (kal′ah-mīn) [USP] a mild astringent and protectant, consisting of zinc oxide with a small proportion of ferric oxide, and occurring as a fine, pink powder; applied topically in the treatment of skin diseases.

calamus (kal′ah-mus) [L.] 1. a reedlike structure. 2. the plant *Acorus calamus* L. (Araceae), and its aromatic rhizome; it is used as a flavoring agent and insect repellent, and was formerly used as a carminative and vermifuge. **c. scripto′rius,** the lowest portion of the floor of the fourth ventricle, shaped like a pen and situated between the restiform bodies.

calcaneal (kal-ka′ne-al) pertaining to the calcaneus.

calcanean (kal-ka′ne-an) calcaneal.

calcaneitis (kal-ka″ne-i′tis) inflammation of the calcaneus.

calcane(o)- [L. *calcaneus,* q.v.] a combining form denoting relationship to the calcaneus.

calcaneoapophysitis (kal-ka″ne-o-ah-pof″ĕ-zi′tis) an affection of the posterior part of the calcaneus marked by pain at the point of insertion of the Achilles tendon, with swelling of the soft parts.

calcaneoastragaloid (kal-ka″ne-o-ah-strag′ah-loid) pertaining to the calcaneus and astragalus.

calcaneocavus (kal-ka″ne-o-ka′vus) clubfoot in which talipes calcaneus is combined with talipes cavus.

calcaneocuboid (kal-ka″ne-o-ku′boid) pertaining to the calcaneus and cuboid bone.

calcaneodynia (kal-ka″ne-o-din′e-ah) pain in the heel, or calcaneus.

calcaneofibular (kal-ka″ne-o-fib′u-lar) pertaining to the calcaneus and the fibula.

calcaneonavicular (kal-ka″ne-o-nah-vik′u-lar) pertaining to the calcaneus and navicular bone.

calcaneoplantar (kal-ka″ne-o-plan′tar) pertaining to the calcaneus and the sole of the foot.

calcaneoscaphoid (kal-ka″ne-o-ska′foid) calcaneonavicular.

calcaneotibial (kal-ka″ne-o-tib′e-al) pertaining to the calcaneus and the tibia.

calcaneovalgocavus (kal-ka″ne-o-val″go-ka′vus) clubfoot in which talipes calcaneus, talipes valgus, and talipes cavus are combined.

calcaneum (kal-ka′ne-um), pl. *calca′nea* [L.] calcaneus.

calcaneus (kal-ka′ne-us), pl. *calca′nei* [L.] 1. [NA] the irregular quadrangular bone at the back of the tarsus; called also *calcaneal bone, calcaneum, heel bone, os calcis,* and *os tarsi fibulare.* 2. talipes calcaneus.

calcanodynia (kal″kah-no-din′e-ah) calcaneodynia.

calcar (kal′kar) [L. "spur"] a spur, or a structure resembling a spur. **c. a′vis** [NA], an eminence on the medial wall of the occipital horn of the lateral ventricle, below the bulb of the occipital horn, produced by lateral extension of the calcarine sulcus. **c. femora′le,** the plate of strong tissue which strengthens the neck of the femur. **c. pe′dis,** the heel.

calcarea (kal-ka′re-ah) [L.] calcium oxide or hydroxide. **c. chlora′ta,** chlorinated lime, a disinfectant and bleaching agent. **c. hy′drica,** a solution of calcium hydroxide; liquor calcis, or lime water. **c. phosphor′ica,** precipitated calcium phosphate. **c. us′ta,** quicklime or caustic lime; calcium oxide or unslaked lime.

calcareous (kal-ka′re-us) [L. *calcarius*] pertaining to or containing lime or calcium; chalky.

calcarine (kal′kar-in) [L. *calcarius* spur-shaped] 1. spur-shaped. 2. pertaining to the calcar.

calcariuria (kal-ka″re-u′re-ah) [L *calcarius* containing lime + Gr. *ouron* urine + *-ia*] the presence of lime salts in the urine.

calcaroid (kal′kar-oid) resembling calcium; a term given to certain deposits in cerebral tissue which resemble calcification but do not give a specific reaction for calcium.

calcemia (kal-se′me-ah) [*calcium* + Gr. *haima* blood + *-ia*] hypercalcemia.

calci-, calc(o)- [L. *calx,* gen. *calcis* lime] a combining form relationship to calcium or calcium salts.

calcibilia (kal″sĭ-bil′e-ah) the presence of calcium in the bile.

Calcibind (kal′sĭ-bīnd) trademark for a preparation of sodium cellulose phosphate.

calcic (kal′sik) of or pertaining to lime or to calcium.

calcicosilicosis (kal″sĭ-ko-sil″ĭ-ko′sis) a variety of pneumoconiosis due to the inhalation of mineral dust containing silica and lime.

calcicosis (kal″sĭ-ko′sis) [L. *calx* lime] a morbid condition of the lung resulting from the inhalation of marble dust.

calcidiol (kal″sĭ-di′ol) 25-hydroxycholecalciferol.

calcifames (kal-sif′ah-mēz) calcium hunger; see under *hunger.*

calcifediol (kal″sif-ĕ-di′ōl) 25-hydroxycholecalciferol.

calciferol (kal-sif′er-ol) 1. see *vitamin D,* under *vitamin.* 2. ergocalciferol.

calcific (kal-sif′ik) forming lime.

calcification (kal″sĭ-fĭ-ka′shun) [*calcium* + L. *facere* to make] the process by which organic tissue becomes hardened by a deposit of calcium salts within its substance. **dystrophic c.,** the deposition of calcium in abnormal tissue, such as scar tissue or atherosclerotic plaques, but without abnormalities of blood calcium. **metastatic c.,** the deposition of calcium in tissues as a result of abnormalities in calcium and phosphate levels in the blood and tissue fluids. **Mönckeberg's c.,** see under *arteriosclerosis.*

calcigerous (kal-sij′er-us) [*calcium* + L. *gerere* to bear] producing or carrying calcium salts.

Calcimar (kal′sĭ-mar) trademark for a preparation of salmon calcitonin, available for clinical use.

calcimeter (kal-sim′ĕ-ter) [*calcium* + Gr. *metron* measure] an instrument for estimating the amount of calcium present, as in the blood.

calcination (kal″sĭ-na′shun) [L. *calcinare* to char] the process of reducing to a dry powder by heat.

calcine (kal′sin) to reduce to a dry powder by heat.

calcinosis (kal″sĭ-no′sis) a condition marked by the deposition of calcium salts in various tissues of the body; called also *exudative calcifying fasciitis* and *calcium gout.* **c.**

circumscrip′ta, localized deposition of calcium in small nodules in subcutaneous tissues or muscle, usually in systemic scleroderma or dermatomyositis. **c. cu′tis,** a condition marked by deposits of calcium salts in the skin in the form of nodules or plaques. **c. interstitia′lis,** a disorder of calcium metabolism marked by abnormal deposits of calcium in the connective tissues. **c. intervertebra′lis,** deposit of calcium in one or more intervertebral disks; called also *chondritis intervertebralis calcanea* and *Verse's disease.* **tumoral c.,** development of large periarticular masses about the shoulder, elbow, and hip, marked by symptoms such as sciatica due to pressure on adjacent nerves. It is of unknown etiology, with onset usually in the first or second decade of life. **c. universa′lis,** widespread deposition of calcium salts in the dermis, panniculus, and muscles, in the form of nodules or plaques, most often in children, principally girls, with dermatomyositis.

calciokinesis (kal″se-o-ki-ne′sis) mobilization of calcium stored in the body.

calciokinetic (kal″se-o-ki-net′ik) pertaining to or causing calciokinesis.

calciorrhachia (kal″se-o-ra′ke-ah) [*calcium* + Gr. *rhachis* spine + *-ia*] the presence of calcium in the spinal fluid.

calcipectic (kal″sĭ-pek′tik) pertaining to, characterized by, or causing calcipexy.

calcipenia (kal″sĭ-pe′ne-ah) [*calcium* + Gr. *penia* poverty] deficiency of calcium.

calcipenic (kal″sĭ-pe′nik) pertaining to or characterized by calcipenia.

calcipexic (kal″sĭ-pek′sik) calcipectic.

calcipexis (kal″sĭ-pek′sis) calcipexy.

calcipexy (kal′sĭ-pek″se) [*calcium* + Gr. *pēxis* fixation] fixation of calcium in the tissues of the organism.

calciphilia (kal″sĭ-fil′e-ah) [*calcium* + Gr. *philein* to love] a tendency to absorb lime salts from the blood and thus to become calcified.

calciphylactic (kal″sĭ-fi-lak′tik) pertaining to or characterized by calciphylaxis.

calciphylaxis (kal″sĭ-fi-lak′sis) the formation of calcified tissue in response to administration of a challenging agent subsequent to induction of a hypersensitive state. **systemic c.,** the generalized appearance of calcifications in internal organs or tissues, occurring in response to intravenous or intraperitoneal injection of the challenging agent. **topical s.,** the formation of a circumscribed area of calcification in response to subcutaneous injection of the challenging agent.

calciprivia (kal″sĭ-priv′e-ah) [*calcium* + L. *privus* without + *-ia*] deprivation or loss of calcium.

calciprivic (kal″sĭ-priv′ik) pertaining to or characterized by calciprivia.

calcipyelitis (kal″sĭ-pi-ĕ-li′tis) calculous pyelitis.

calcitonin (kal″sĭ-to′nin) a 32-amino-acid polypeptide hormone elaborated by the parafollicular cells of the thyroid gland in response to hypercalcemia; it lowers plasma calcium and phosphate levels, inhibits bone resorption, and acts as an antagonist to parathyroid hormone. It is secreted in lower vertebrates by the ultimobranchial glands. It is used in the treatment of severe hypercalcemia and Paget's disease of bone. Called also *thyrocalcitonin.*

calcitriol (kal″sĭ-tri′ol) 1,25-dihydroxycholecalciferol.

calcium (kal′se-um), gen. *cal′cii* [L. *calx* lime] a silvery yellow metal, the basic element of lime. Symbol, Ca; atomic number, 20; atomic weight, 40.08. It is found in nearly all organized tissues, being the most abundant mineral in the body. In combination with phosphorus it forms calcium phosphate, the dense, hard material of the teeth and bones. It is an essential dietary element, a constant blood calcium level being essential for the maintenance of the normal heartbeat, and for the normal functioning of nerves and muscles. It also plays a role in multiple phases of blood coagulation (in which it is called *coagulation factor IV*) and in many enzymatic processes. **c. acetate,** a resolvent, $Ca(C_2H_3O_2)_2$. **c. benzamidosalicylate,** benzoylpas calcium. **c. benzoate,** a compound, $Ca(C_6H_5CO_2)_2 + 3H_2O$, formerly used in nephritis. **c. bromide,** an odorless white deliquescent granular salt, $CaBr_2$, formerly used as a sedative and anticonvulsant. **c. carbide,** grayish black lumps or crystals, CaC_2, which yield acetylene on decomposition by water. **c. carbimide,** 1. c. cyanamide. 2. c. carbimide, citrated. **c. carbimide, citrated,** a mixture containing calcium cyanamide and citric acid; an antialcoholic. See also *c. cyanamide*. **c. carbonate,** a compound, $CaCO_3$, occurring naturally in bones, shells, etc. It is used chiefly as an antacid in its native form, in a prepared form (see *prepared chalk*, under *chalk*), and in a precipitated form (see *c. carbonate, precipitated*). **c. carbonate, precipitated** [USP], an odorless, tasteless, fine white crystalline powder, $CaCO_3$, used as an antacid; called also *precipitated chalk*. **c. caseinate,** a nutrient preparation of casein and calcium. **c. chloride** [USP], a salt, $CaCl_2 2H_2O$, occurring as white, hard fragments or granules. It is used as a calcium replenisher, administered intravenously, and has been used as an acid-producing diuretic and urinary acidifier and to control bleeding in such conditions as purpura, intestinal bleeding, and small multiple hemorrhages. It is also a specific antidote for magnesium poisoning, administered intravenously. **c. creosotate,** a mixture of the calcium constituents of creosote, formerly used as a disinfectant and antiseptic. **c. cyanamide,** a compound, $CaCN_2$, obtained by the interaction of nitrogen and calcium carbide in an electric furnace, which inhibits one or more of the enzymes required for oxidation of acetaldehyde formed from alcohol; used as a fertilizer, defoliant, herbicide, pesticide, and anthelmintic for swine. Because the drinking of alcohol after inhalation or ingestion of calcium cyanamide produces very unpleasant symptoms (see *mal rouge*), it has been considered as a basis for treating alcholism; a mixture of calcium cyanamide and citric acid (*citrated c. carbimide*) has been used for this purpose. Called also *c. carbimide* and, sometimes, *cyanamide*. **c. cyclamate,** cyclamate calcium. **c. disodium edathamil, c. disodium edetate,** edetate calcium disodium. **c. Disodium Versenate,** trademark for edetate calcium disodium. **c. EDTA,** edetate calcium disodium. **c. fluoride,** a compound, CaF_2, occurring in the bones and teeth. **c. glubionate,** chemical name: (4-O-β-D-galactopyranosyl-D-gluconato-O^1)(D-gluconato-O^1)calcium monohydrate. A calcium replenisher, $C_{18}H_{32}CaO_{19}H_2O$, administered orally. **c. gluconate,** a calcium salt of gluconic acid, $C_{12}H_{22}CaO_{14}$, occurring as odorless, tasteless, white crystalline granules or powder. It is used as a calcium replenisher, administered intravenously or orally, and has been used to decrease capillary permeability in various conditions. It is an oral antidote for fluoride or oxalic acid poisoning. **c. glycerophosphate,** the calcium salt of glycerophosphoric acid, $C_3H_7CaO_6P$; it has been used as a calcium and phosphorus dietary supplement and as a pharmaceutic necessity. **c. hydroxide** [USP], a salt, $Ca(OH)_2$, occurring as a white powder; used in solution as a topical astringent. **c. hypophosphite,** an odorless bitter compound, $Ca(PH_2O_2)_2$, occurring in colorless, transparent, monoclinic prisms, as small lustrous scales, or as a white crystalline powder; formerly used in conditions of impaired nutrition or vigor. **c. iodate,** a compound, $Ca(IO_3)_2 + 6H_2O$, formerly used as an antiseptic. **c. iodide,** a hygroscopic compound, CaI_2, formerly used as an expectorant. **c. iodobehenate,** a white or yellowish powder, $(C_{21}H_{42}ICOO)_2Ca$, containing at least 23.5 per cent of iodine; formerly used as an antigoitrogenic. **c. iodostearate,** a cream-colored odorless powder, $C_{36}H_{68}CaIO_4$, formerly used in the treatment of colloid goiter. **c. lactate** [USP], chemical name: 2-hydroxypropanoic acid calcium salt. A calcium replenisher, $C_6H_{10}CaO_6 \cdot x H_2O$, occurring as white granules or powder; administered orally in the treatment of calcium deficiency. **c. levulinate** [USP], chemical name: 4-oxo-pentanoic acid calcium salt. A calcium replenisher, $C_{10}H_{14}CaO_6 \cdot 2H_2O$, occurring as a white, crystalline or amorphous powder; administered parenterally in the treatment of calcium deficiency. **c. mandelate,** the calcium salt of mandelic acid, $C_{16}H_{14}CaO_6$, used orally as a urinary anti-infective. **c. oxalate,** a typical compound, CaC_2O_4, occurring in the urine as crystals and in certain calculi. **c. oxide,** a corrosively alkaline and caustic earth, CaO, used for absorbing carbon dioxide from air, and industrially as a cheap alkali and as a base for mortar; called also *calcarea usta, calx, lime,* and *quicklime*. **c. pantothenate** [USP], chemical name: *N*-(2,4,-dihydroxy-3,3-dimethyl-1-oxobutyl)-β-alanine calcium salt. The calcium salt of the dextrorotatory isomer of pantothenic acid, $C_{18}H_{32}CaN_2O_{10}$, the B-complex vitamin, occurring as a white powder; used, usually in combination with other B vitamins, as a nutritional supplement. See also *racemic c. pantothenate*. **c.**

pantothenate, racemic [USP], a mixture of the calcium salts of the dextrorotatory and levorotatory isomers of pantothenic acid, with a physiological activity about half that of calcium pantothenate. **c. permanganate,** a crystalline salt, $Ca(MnO_4)_2 + 5H_2O$, formerly used as an antiseptic. **c. phenolsulfonate,** c. sulfocarbolate. **c. phosphate,** any of three salts containing calcium and the phosphate radical (PO_4); see *c. phosphate, dibasic, monobasic,* and *tribasic*. **c. phosphate, dibasic** [USP], an odorless, tasteless, white powder, $CaHPO_4 \cdot 2H_2O$, used as a calcium supplement and as a base in preparation of tablets; called also *dicalcium phosphate*. **c. phosphate, monobasic,** colorless shining scales or powder, $CaH_4(PO_4)_2$, used in fertilizers, baking powders, and wheat flours, and as a mineral supplement in foods and feeds. Called also *c. superphosphate*. **c. phosphate, tribasic** [NF], an odorless, tasteless, white powder, $Ca_3(PO_4)_2$, used as a calcium supplement; it is also used as an antacid and as a laxative. **c. polycarbophil,** a calcium salt of a loosely cross-linked, hydrophilic resin of the polycarboxylic type; a cathartic. **c. propionate,** the calcium salt of propionic acid, $C_6H_{10}CaO_4$, which has antifungal properties; used alone or in combination with sodium propionate or other agents as a preservative to inhibit mold production in bakery and milk products, other foods, tobacco, and pharmaceuticals and as a topical antifungal in the treatment of various mycoses. **radioactive c.,** radiocalcium. **c. stearate** [NF], chemical name: octadecanoic acid calcium salt. A compound of calcium with organic acids obtained from fats, $C_{36}H_{70}CaO_4$, occurring as a fine, white to yellow white, bulky powder; used as a tablet lubricant. **c. sulfate** [NF], an abundant natural product, CaO_4S, found in nature as anhydrite, and occurring in a hydrated form known as gypsum; when gypsum is calcined it forms *plaster of Paris*. Dried calcium sulfate dihydrate is used as a tablet diluent. **c. sulfide,** a compound, CaS. **c. sulfite,** a compound, $CaSO_3$, resulting from the extraction of sulfur dioxide, by calcium hydroxide, from air or flue gas. **c. sulfocarbolate,** a white crystalline substance, $Ca(C_6H_5-SO_4)_2 + 6H_2O$, soluble in water. **c. superphosphate,** monobasic c. phosphate. **c. trisodium pentetate,** pentetate calcium trisodium.

calciumedetate sodium (kal″se-um-ed′ĕ-tāt) edetate calcium disodium.

calcium-magnesium adenosine triphosphate (ah-den″o-sin-tri-fos′fah-tās) a complex in the sarcoplasmic reticulum catalyzing the uptake of calcium ions and release of magnesium ions driven by hydrolysis of ATP to ADP and orthophosphate.

calciuria (kal″sĭ-u′re-ah) the presence of calcium in the urine.

calc(o)- see *calci-*.

calcoglobulin (kal″ko-glob′u-lin) the form of globulin that occurs in calcifying tissue.

calcospherite (kal″ko-sfēr′it) one of the small globular bodies formed during the process of calcification, by chemical union between the calcium particles and the albuminous organic matter of the intercellular substance. These particles coalesce to form calcoglobulin.

calculary (kal′ku-la-re) pertaining to a calculus.

calculi (kal′ku-li) plural of *calculus*.

calculogenesis (kal″ku-lo-jen′ĕ-sis) the formation of calculi.

calculosis (kal″ku-lo′sis) lithiasis.

calculous (kal′ku-lus) pertaining to, of the nature of, or affected with calculus.

calculus (kal′ku-lus), pl. *cal′culi* [L. "pebble"] an abnormal concretion occurring within the animal body and usually composed of mineral salts. **alternating c.,** a urinary calculus made up of successive layers of different composition; called also *combination c*. **alvine c.,** a concretion in the intestine formed by hardening of portions of the fecal contents. **articular c.,** a deposit in a joint; it is usually composed of sodium urate, sometimes of calcium urate. Called also *joint c., calculous concretion,* and *chalk stone*. **biliary calculi,** gallstones (cholelithiasis) composed almost entirely of the excessive blood pigment liberated by hemolysis, with calcium deposits in bone. **bronchial c.,** lung c. **calcium oxalate c.,** a hard, rough calculus composed of calcium oxalate. **cholesterol c.,** a calculus formed of cholesterol; called also *metabolic c.* and *metabolic stone*.

combination c., alternating c. **cystine c.,** a soft variety of urinary calculus composed of cystine. **decubitus c.,** a calculus formed in the urinary tract as a result of long immobilization. **dental c.,** a hard, stonelike concretion, varying in color from creamy yellow to black, that forms on the teeth or dental prostheses through calcification of dental plaque. According to location, there are two general types: *supragingival c.* and *subgingival c.* Called also *odontolith, tartar,* and *dental tophus.* **encysted c.,** a urinary calculus enclosed in a sac developed from the wall of the bladder; called also *pocketed c.* **fibrin c.,** urinary calculi formed largely from fibrinogen in blood. **fusible c.,** a calculus formed of a mixture of calcium phosphate and triple phosphates which fuses to a black, enamel-like mass when tested under the blowpipe. **gastric c.,** gastrolith. **gonecystic c.,** calculus of a seminal vesicle. **hemic c.,** a calculus developed from a blood clot. **hemp seed c.,** a small, smooth, pale urinary calculus of calcium oxalate of the size and shape of a hemp seed. **hepatic c.,** a gallstone formed in the intrahepatic bile ducts. **indigo c.,** calculus formed by oxidation of the indican of the urine. **intestinal c.,** enterolith. **joint c.,** articular c. **lacrimal c.,** one in a lacrimal gland or duct; dacryolith. **lacteal c.,** mammary c. **lung c.,** a concretion formed in the bronchi by accretion about an inorganic nucleus, or from calcified portions of lung tissue or adjacent lymph nodes; called also *lung stone* and *broncholith.* **mammary c.,** a concretion in one of the lactiferous ducts; called also *lacteal c.* **matrix c.,** a yellowish white to light tan urinary calculus with the consistency of putty, containing calcium salts but composed chiefly of an organic matrix consisting of a mucoprotein and a sulfated mucopolysaccharide. **metabolic c.,** cholesterol c. **mulberry c.,** a hard, smooth urinary calculus of calcium oxalate, so called from its shape. **nasal c.,** rhinolith. **nephritic c.,** renal c. (*obs.*), **ovarian c.,** an enlarged and calcified corpus luteum. **oxalate c.,** a hard urinary calculus of calcium oxalate. Some are covered with minute sharp spines that may abrade the renal pelvic epithelium; others are smooth (see *mulberry c.*). **pancreatic c.,** a concretion formed in the pancreatic duct from calcium carbonate with other salts and organic materials. **phosphate c., phosphatic c.,** a renal calculus composed of calcium oxalate and ammonium urate; it may be hard, soft, or friable, and so large that it may fill the pelvis and calices. **pocketed c.,** encysted c. **preputial c.,** postholith. **prostatic c.,** a concretion formed in the prostate, chiefly of calcium carbonate and phosphate. **renal c.,** a calculus occurring in the kidney; called also *nephritic c.* **renal c., primary,** one formed in an apparently healthy urinary tract, usually composed of oxalates or urates. **renal c., secondary,** one associated with infection and obstruction, usually composed of ammonium magnesium phosphate. **salivary c.,** 1. sialolith. 2. supragingival c. **serumal c.,** subgingival c., so called because it is supposed to result from exudation of serum. **shellac c.,** a gastrolith caused by drinking shellac varnish. **spermatic c.,** a concretion in a seminal vesicle. **staghorn c.,** a calculus of the renal pelvis usually extending into multiple calices. **stomachic c.,** a bezoar or other concretion in the stomach; a gastrolith. **struvite c.,** a urinary calculus composed of very pure ammoniomagnesium phosphate, forming the hard crystals known to mineralogists as struvite. **subgingival c.,** calculus located below the crest of the marginal gingiva, usually in periodontal pockets. Called also *serumal c.* **submorphous c.,** a calculus made up of molecules of a crystalline salt, together with molecules of the colloid matter in which the salt is contained. **supragingival c.,** calculus covering the coronal surface of the tooth to the crest of the gingival margin. Called also *salivary c.* **tonsillar c.,** a calcareous concretion in a tonsil. **urate c.,** a calculus composed of urates, usually smooth, round, and yellow-brown, occurring chiefly in newborn or young infants. **urethral c.,** calculus of the urethra with symptoms varying according to sex and the site of lodgment. **uric acid c.,** hard, yellow or reddish-yellow calculi formed from uric acid. **urinary c.,** a calculus in any part of the urinary tract; it is *vesical* when lodged in the bladder (stone, gravel), and *renal* when in the pelvis of the kidney. **urostealith c.,** a urinary calculus formed of fatty matter. **uterine c.,** an intrauterine concretion formed mainly by the calcification of a tumor; called also *womb stone.* **vesical c.,** a form found in the urinary bladder; called also *bladder stone* and *cystolith.* **vesicoprostatic c.,** a prostatic calculus extending into the

bladder. **xanthic c.,** a urinary calculus composed mainly of xanthine.

Caldani's ligament (kal-dah′nēz) [Leopoldo Marcantonio *Caldani,* Italian anatomist, 1725–1813] see under *ligament.*

Caldwell-Luc operation (kald′wel-luk′) [George W. *Caldwell,* American physician, 1834–1918; Henry *Luc,* French laryngologist, 1855–1925] see under *operation.*

Caldwell-Moloy classification [William Edgar *Caldwell,* American obstetrician, 1880–1943; Howard Carman *Moloy,* American obstetrician, 1903–1953] classification of female pelves as gynecoid, android, anthropoid, and platypelloid; see under *classification.*

Calef. abbreviation for L. *calefactus,* warmed, or for L. *calefac,* make warm.

calefacient (kal″e-fa′shent) [L. *calidus* warm + *facere* to make] 1. warming; causing a sensation of warmth. 2. an agent that causes a sensation of warmth.

Calendula (kah-len′du-lah) [L.] a genus of composite-flowered plants. The dried florets of *C. officinalis,* pot marigold, are stimulant and resolvent, and were once used externally for inflammatory lesions of the skin and mucous membranes.

calf (kaf) [L. *sura*] the fleshy mass formed chiefly by the gastrocnemius muscle at the back of the leg (below the knee). Called also *sura* [NA].

caliber (kal′ĭ-ber) [Fr. *calibre* the bore of a gun] the diameter of a canal or tube.

calibration (kal′ĭ-bra′shun) 1. determination of the accuracy of an instrument, usually by measurement of its variation from a standard, to ascertain necessary correction factors. 2. measurement of the caliber of a tube.

caliceal (kal″ĭ-se′al) pertaining to or affecting a calix.

calicectasis (kal″ĭ-sek′tah-sis) dilatation of a calix of a kidney.

calicectomy (kal″ĭ-sek′to-me) excision of a calix of a kidney.

calices (ka′lĭ-sēz) [L.] plural of *calix.*

calicine (kal′ĭ-sēn) related to or resembling a calix.

calicivirus (kal″ĭ-sĭ-vi′rus) a subgroup of picornaviruses, including the virus of vesicular exanthem.

caliculi (kah-lik′u-li) genitive and plural of *caliculus.*

caliculus (kah-lik′u-lus), gen. and pl. *calic′uli* [L., dim. of *calix*] a small cup or cup-shaped structure. **c. gustato′rius** [NA], one of the minute, barrel-shaped terminal organs of the gustatory nerve, situated around the bases of the circumvallate papillae of the tongue, each consisting of a group of spindle-shaped cells made up of outer supporting cells and inner sense cells. Called also *taste bud* or *bulb, gustatory bud* or *bulb,* and *Schwalbe's corpuscle.* **c. ophthal′micus** [NA], an indentation of the distal wall of the optic vesicle, brought about by rapid marginal growth and producing a double-layered cup, attached to the diencephalon by a tubular stalk. Called also *ocular cup, ophthalmic cup,* and *optic cup.*

caliectasis (ka″lĭ-ek′tah-sis) [*calix* + Gr. *ektasis* dilatation] caliectasis.

caliectomy (ka″lĭ-ek′to-me) [*calix* + Gr. *ektomē* excision] calicectomy.

californium (kal″ĭ-for′ne-um) [named from *California* (University and state), where it was first produced] chemical element of atomic number 98, atomic weight 249, symbol Cf, produced by irradiation of the isotope of curium of atomic weight 242 with helium ions; half-life 45 minutes.

calipers (kal′ĭ-perz) [from *caliber*] compasses with bent or curved legs used for measuring the thickness or diameter of a solid. **skinfold c.,** an instrument designed for measuring the thickness of folds of skin gathered at various areas of the body; used in studies of nutritional status and of physical constitution.

calisthenics (kal″is-then′iks) [Gr. *kalos* beautiful + *sthenos* strength] a system of light gymnastics for promoting strength and grace of carriage.

calix (ka′liks), pl. *cal′ices* [L.] a cup-shaped organ or cavity. **renal calices,** calices renales. **renal calices, greater,** calices renales majores. **renal calices, major,** calices renales majores. **renal calices, minor,** calices renales minores. **cal′ices rena′les** [NA], renal calices: any one of the recesses of the pelvis of the kidney which enclose the pyramids; called also *calyces renales* and *infundibula of kidney.* **cal′ices rena′les majo′res** [NA], major renal calices: the two or more larger subdivisions of the renal pelvis, into which the minor calices open; called also *calyces renales majores* and *greater renal calices.* **cal′ices rena′les mino′res** [NA], minor renal calices: a varying number of smaller subdivisions of the renal pelvis which enclose the pyramids, and open into the major calices; called also *calyces renales minores.*

CALLA common acute lymphoblastic leukemia antigen.

Callander's amputation (kal′an-derz) [C. Latimer *Callander,* San Francisco surgeon, 1892–1947] see under *amputation.*

Callaway's test (kal′ah-wāz) [Thomas *Callaway,* English physician, 1791–1848] see under *tests.*

Calleja's islets (islands) (kal-ya′hahz) [Camilo *Calleja y Sanchez,* Spanish anatomist, died 1913] see under *islet.*

callicrein (kal″ik-re′in) kallikrein.

Calliphora (kah-lif′o-rah) [Gr. *kallos* beauty + *phoros* bearing] a genus of scavenger flies of the family Calliphoridae, the blow flies or bluebottle flies, which deposit their eggs in decaying matter, on wounds, or in the openings of the body. **C. vomito′ria,** the common blow fly or bluebottle fly,

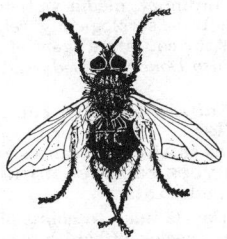

Calliphora vomitoria.

whose larvae may invade the nasal fossae or produce intestinal myiasis. Other species are *C. azurea, C. erythrocephala,* and *C. lionensis.*

Calliphoridae (kal″lĭ-for′ĭ-de) a family of medium-sized to large flies of the order Diptera, including the genera *Auchmeromyia, Calliphora* (type genus), *Cordylobia, Cochliomyia, Chrysomyia, Lucilia, Phaenicia,* and *Phormia;* all species may serve as vectors of pathogens and may also produce myiasis in man.

Callison's fluid (kal′ĭ-sunz) [James S. *Callison,* American physician, born 1873] see under *fluid.*

Callitroga (kal″lĭ-tro′gah) *Cochliomyia.*

callosal (kah-lo′sal) pertaining to the corpus callosum.

callositas (kah-los′ĭ-tas) [L.] a callus.

callosity (kah-los′ĭ-te) [L. *callositas,* from *callus*] a callus.

callosomarginal (kah-lo″so-mar′jĭ-nal) pertaining to the callosal and marginal gyri.

callosum (kah-lo′sum) corpus callosum.

callous (kal′us) hard; like callus.

callus (kal′us) [L.] 1. localized hyperplasia of the horny layer of the epidermis due to pressure or friction. Called also *callosity.* See also *hyperkeratosis* (def. 1), *keratoderma, keratoma* (def. 1), *keratosis, tyloma,* and *tylosis.* 2. an unorganized meshwork of woven bone developed on the pattern of the original fibrin clot, which is formed following fracture of a bone and is normally ultimately replaced by hard adult bone; called also *bony c.* 3. a mass of plant tissue formed over a wound or at the base of a cutting. **bony c.,** see callus (def. 2). **central c.,** a provisional callus formed within the medullary cavity of a fractured bone; it arises from the cells covering the endosteal and trabecular surfaces near the fracture. Called also *inner c., medullary c.,* and *myelogenous c.* **definitive c.,** the exudate formed between the fractured ends of the bone, which is permanent and becomes changed into true bone; called also *intermediate c.* and *permanent c.* **ensheathing c.,** provisional callus forming a sheath about the ends of the fragments of a fractured bone. **external c.,** the collar of callus formed by the periosteum in a long bone. **inner c.,** central c. **intermediate c.,** definitive c. **internal c., medullary c., myelogenous c.,** central c. **permanent c.,** definitive c. **provisional c., temporary c.,** callus

formed within the medullary cavity and about the ends of a broken bone, and which is absorbed as the repair is completed.

calmative (kal′mah-tiv, kahm′ah-tiv) 1. sedative; allaying excitement. 2. an agent that allays excitement or has a sedative effect.

Calmette's test (conjunctival reaction, ophthalmic reaction), vaccine (kal-metz′) [Albert Léon Charles *Calmette,* French bacteriologist, 1863–1933] see under *tests,* and see *BCG vaccine,* under *vaccine.*

calmodulin (kal-mod′u-lin) a calcium-binding protein present in all nucleated cells, thought to be an essential mediator of most calcium-sensitive cellular processes.

Calobata (kah-lo′bah-tah) a genus of South American flies whose larvae sometimes occur in the human intestine.

calomel (kal′o-mel) [L. *calomelas;* Gr. *kalos* fair + *melas* black] chemical name: mercurous chloride. A heavy, white, odorless, impalpable powder, HgCl, insoluble in water, alcohol, ether, and cold dilute acids; rarely used today as a cathartic. **vegetable c.,** podophyllum.

calor (ka′lor) [L.] heat; one of the cardinal signs of inflammation. **c. febri′lis,** the heat of fever. **c. fer′vens,** an intense heat. **c. inna′tus,** the normal or natural heat of the body. **c. inter′nus,** the heat of the interior of the body. **c. mor′dax, c. mor′dicans,** 1. biting or stinging heat. 2. the hot, burning, reddish-colored skin occurring in scarlet fever.

caloradiance (kal″o-ra′de-ans) the radiation or rays which lie between 250 and 55,000 millimicrons, such as the rays from the sun, carbon arcs, incandescent rods and filaments, and hot black bodies.

calorescence (kal″o-res′ens) the conversion of nonluminous into luminous heat rays.

Calori's bursa (kah-lo′rēz) [Luigi *Calori,* Italian anatomist, 1807–1896] see under *bursa.*

calori- [L. *calor,* gen. *caloris* heat] a combining form denoting relationship to heat.

caloric (kah-lo′rik) pertaining to heat or to calories.

caloricity (kal″o-ris′ĭ-te) the power of the animal body of developing and maintaining heat.

calorie (kal′o-re) [Fr.; L. *calor* heat] any of several units of heat defined as the amount of heat required to raise the temperature of 1 kilogram of water 1 degree Celsius at a specified temperature. The calorie used in chemistry and biochemistry is equal to exactly 4.184 joules. Symbol cal. NOTE: There was formerly a distinction made between the "small calorie," defined above and the "large calorie" written Calorie with a capital "C" and abbreviated Cal, which was equal to 1000 calories or one kilocalorie. The use of the large calorie survives only in nutrition, where calorie, now usually written with a small "c," means kilocalorie when specifying the energy content of foods. **gram c.,** small c. **I.T. c., International Table c.,** a unit of heat, equivalent to 4.1868 joules. **large c.,** the calorie used in metabolic studies, being the amount of heat required to raise the temperature of 1 kilogram of water 1 degree Celsius (centigrade), specifically from 14.5° to 15.5° C. at a pressure of 1 atmosphere; abbreviated kg.-cal. Called also *kilocalorie.* Also used to express the fuel or energy value of food. **mean c.,** one one-hundredth of the amount of heat required to raise the temperature of 1 gram of water from 0 to 100° C. **small c.,** the amount of heat required to raise the temperature of 1 gram of water 1 degree Celsius (centigrade), specifically from 14.5° to 15.5° C. at a pressure of 1 atomosphere; abbreviated g.-cal. Called also *gram c.* and *standard c.* **standard c.,** small c. **thermochemical c.,** a unit of heat, equivalent to 4.184 joules.

calorifacient (kah-lor″ĭ-fa′shent) [L. *calor* heat + *facere* to make] producing heat; said of certain foods.

calorific (kal″o-rif′ik) [L. *calor* heat + *facere* to make] producing heat.

calorigenetic (kah-lor″ĭ-jĕ-net′ik) calorigenic.

calorigenic (kah-lor″ĭ-jen′ik) [L. *calor* heat + Gr. *gennan* to produce] producing heat or energy; increasing heat or energy production; increasing the consumption of oxygen.

calorimeter (kal″o-rim′ĕ-ter) [L. *calor* heat + Gr. *metron* measure] an instrument for measuring the amount of heat exchanged in any system. In physiology, an apparatus for measuring the amount of heat produced by an individual.

bomb c., an apparatus for measuring the potential energy of food, a weighed amount of the food being placed on a platinum dish inside a hollow steel container (bomb) filled with pure oxygen. The heat produced by its combustion is absorbed by a known quantity of water in which the container is immersed, permitting its measurement. **compensating c.,** an apparatus in which the object to be tested, such as a developing chick in an egg, is placed at one junction of a thermocouple and an electrical resistance at the other. From the amount of current that must pass through the resistance to keep both junctions at the same temperature (as shown by lack of current in the thermocouple circuit), it is possible to calculate the amount of heat generated in the object being tested. **respiration c.,** an apparatus for the measurement of the gaseous exchange between a living organism and the atmosphere surrounding it and the simultaneous measurement of the amount of heat produced by that organism.

calorimetric (kah-lor″ĭ-met′rik) pertaining to or performed by calorimetry.

calorimetry (kal″o-rim′ĕ-tre) [L. *calor* heat + Gr. *metron* measure] measurement of the amounts of heat absorbed or given out. **direct c.,** measurement of the amount of heat produced by a subject enclosed within a small chamber. **indirect c.,** measurement of the amount of heat produced by a subject by determination of the amount of oxygen consumed and the quantity of nitrogen and carbon dioxide eliminated.

caloriscope (kah-lor′ĭ-skōp) an instrument for showing the caloric values of mixtures for infant feedings.

caloritropic (kah-lor″ĭ-trop′ik) [L. *calor* heat + Gr. *tropos* a turning] thermotropic.

calory (kal′o-re) pl. *calories.* Calorie.

Calot's triangle (kah-lōz′) [Jean-François *Calot,* French surgeon, 1861–1944] see under *triangle.*

calotte (kah-lot′) [Fr. "cap"] a part shaped like a skull cap. In ophthalmology, a cap-shaped specimen removed from the eyeball for histopathologic examination.

calsequestrin (kal″sĕ-kwes′trin) [*cal*cium + *sequester* + *-in* a chemical suffix] a calcium-binding protein rich in carboxylate side chains, occurring on the inner membrane surface of the sarcoplasmic reticulum; it serves to chelate and store calcium ions.

Calurin (kal″u-rin) trademark for a preparation of carbaspirin calcium.

calusterone (kal-u′ster-ōn) chemical name: (7β-17β)-17-hydroxy-7,17-dimethylandrost-4-en-3-one; an antineoplastic agent, $C_{21}H_{32}O_2$, formerly used for palliation of inoperable or metastatic breast carcinoma in postmenopausal women.

calutron (kal′u-tron) an apparatus for separating the isotopes of uranium.

calvacin (kal′vah-sin) an antineoplastic substance derived from the fungus *Calvatia gigantea.*

calvaria (kal-va′re-ah) [L.] [NA] the domelike superior portion of the cranium, composed of the superior portions of the frontal, parietal, and occipital bones; called also *calvarium, concha of cranium,* and *skullcap.*

calvarial (kal-va′re-al) pertaining to the calvaria.

calvarium (kal-va′re-um) the calvaria.

Calvatia (kal-va′she-ah) a genus of basidiomycetous fungi of the order Lycoperdales, series Gasteromycetes. **C. gigan′tea,** the giant puffball, the source of calvacin.

Calvé-Perthes disease (kal-va′per-tās) [Jacques *Calvé,* French orthopedist, 1875–1954; Georg Clemens *Perthes,* German surgeon, 1869–1927] osteochondrosis of the capitular epiphysis of the femur; see under *osteochondrosis.*

Calvin cycle (kal′vin) [Melvin *Calvin,* American chemist, born 1911; winner of the Nobel prize in chemistry for 1961 for development of techniques to determine the chemical reactions of plant carbon dioxide assimilation] see under *cycle.*

calvities (kal-vish′e-ēz) [L.] baldness; see *alopecia.*

calx (kalks) [L.] 1. lime or chalk. 2. NA alternative for regio calcanea. 3. any residue obtained by calcination. 4. lime or calcium oxide, CaO; quicklime: alkaline, caustic, and escharotic. **c. chlora′ta, c. chlorina′ta,** chlorinated lime. **c. sulfura′ta,** a mixture of at least 60 per cent of calcium sulfide with a variable proportion of calcium sulfate and carbon. It is used in skin and pustular diseases, and as a depilatory. Called also *sulfurated lime.*

calyceal (kal″ĭ-se′al) caliceal.

calycectasis (kal″ĭ-sek′tah-sis) calicectasis.

calycectomy (kal″ĭ-sek′to-me) calicectomy.

calyces (kal′ĭ-sēz) plural of *calyx.*

calycine (kal′ĭ-sin) calicine.

calycle (kal′ĭ-kl) a caliculus.

calyculi (kah-lik′u-li) [L.] caliculi.

calyculus (kah-lik′u-lus), gen. and pl. *calyc′uli* [L., dim. of Gr. *kalyx* cup of a flower] caliculus. **c. gustato′rius,** caliculus gustatorius. **c. ophthal′micus,** caliculus ophthalmicus.

calymma (kah-lim′ah) [Gr. *kalymma* covering] the highly vacuolated cortical layer of cytoplasm surrounding the central capsule of certain protozoa of the superclass Actinopoda, such as radiolarians, and separated from but continuous with the intracapsular cytoplasm by means of a perforated membrane.

Calymmatobacterium (kah-lim″ah-to-bak-te′re-um) [Gr. *kalymma* a hood or veil + *bacterium*] a genus of facultatively anaerobic, gram-negative, rod-shaped, capsulated bacteria, characteristically found as intracellular organisms in the cytoplasm of large mononuclear phagocytes, all of which are human pathogens. **C. granulo′matis,** a species that is not viable on ordinary media but cultivable on fresh egg-yolk medium. It is serologically related to *Klebsiella pneumoniae* and is the causative agent of human granuloma inguinale. Called also *Donovan's body* and *Donovania granulomatis.*

calyx (ka′liks), pl. *cal′yces* [Gr. *kalyx* cup of a flower] calix. **cal′yces rena′les,** calices renales; see under *calix.* **cal′yces rena′les majo′res,** calices renales majores; see under *calix.* **cal′yces rena′les mino′res,** calices renales minores; see under *calix.*

Camallanus (kam″ah-la′nus) a genus of nematodes of the order Spiraroidea, species of which are parasites in the intestines of fishes, reptiles, and amphibians.

Cambaroides (kam″bah-roi′dēz) a genus of crayfish which harbor the metacercariae of *Paragonimus.*

cambendazole (kam-ben′dah-zōl) chemical name: [2-(4-thiazolyl)-1*H*-benzimidazol-5-yl]cambamic acid; an anthelmintic, $C_{14}H_{14}N_4O_2S$.

cambium (kam′be-um) [L. "exchange"] 1. the loose cellular inner layer of the periosteal tissue in the intramembranous ossification of bone. 2. a layer of cells beneath the bark of woody plants.

cambogia (kam-bo′je-ah) [L.] gamboge.

camelpox (kam′el-poks) an eruptive disease of camels due to a poxvirus.

camera (kam′er-ah), pl. *cameras* or *cam′erae* [L. "chamber"] 1. a box, chamber, or compartment. 2. any enclosed space or ventricle. **c. ante′rior bul′bi** [NA], anterior chamber of eye: that portion of the aqueous-containing space between the cornea and the lens which is bounded in front by the cornea and part of the sclera, and behind by the iris, part of the ciliary body, and that part of the lens which presents through the pupil. Called also *c. oculi anterior.* **c. lu′cida,** an optical device utilizing a prism or mirrors so arranged as to throw the reflected image of an object upon paper, thus permitting its outlines to be traced with a pencil. **c. obscu′ra,** a combined box, lens, and screen, used for viewing, tracing, or making photographs. **c. o′culi,** either one of the chambers of the eye. **c. o′culi ante′rior,** c. anterior bulbi. **c. o′culi poste′rior,** c. posterior bulbi. **c. poste′rior bul′bi** [NA], posterior chamber of the eye: that portion of the aqueous-containing space between the cornea and the lens which is bounded in front by the iris, and behind by the lens and suspensory ligament; called also *c. oculi posterior.* **recording c.,** photokymograph. **scintillation c.,** an electronic instrument that produces photographs or cathode-ray tube images of the gamma ray or positron emissions from organs containing tracer compounds. **c. vi′trea bul′bi** [NA], vitreous chamber.

camerae (kam′er-e) [L.] plural of *camera.*

Camerer's law (kam′er-erz) [Johann Friedrich Wilhelm *Camerer,* German pediatrician, 1842–1910] see under *law.*

camisole (kam′ĭ-sōl) [Fr.] straitjacket.

Cammann's stethoscope (kam'anz) [George Philip *Cammann*, American physician, 1804–1863] a binaural stethoscope.

Camoquin (kam'o-kwin) trademark for a preparation of amodiaquine hydrochloride.

CAMP a regimen of cyclophosphamide, Adriamycin (doxorubicin), methotrexate, and procarbazine, used in cancer chemotherapy.

cAMP adenosine 3′:5′-cyclic phosphate; cyclic AMP.

campanula (kam-pan'u-lah) [L. *campana* a bell] a bell-shaped organ or part. **c. hal'leri,** the swollen end of the falciform process in the eye of fish.

Campbell's ligament (kam'belz) [William Francis *Campbell*, American surgeon, 1867–1926] the suspensory ligament of the axilla.

campeachy, campechy (kam-pe'che) *Haematoxylon.*

Camper's angle, fascia, ligament (kam'perz) [Pieter *Camper*, Dutch physician, 1722–1789] see *facial angle* and *maxillary angle*, under *angle*; see *diaphragma urogenitale*; and see under *fascia*.

campesterol (kam-pes'ter-ol) a sterol, $C_{28}H_{48}O$, from rape seed oil, soy bean oil, and wheat germ oil; it is isomeric with ergastanol.

camphene (kam-fēn') chemical name: 2,2-dimethyl-3-methylenebicyclo[2.2.1]heptane. A terpene, $C_{10}H_{16}$, found in many essential oils or prepared synthetically from pinene in the process of producing synthetic camphor.

camphol (kam'fol) Borneo camphor.

camphor (kam'for, kam'fer) [L. *camphora*; Gr. *kamphora*] 1. [USP] chemical name: 1,7,7-trimethylbicyclo[2.2.1]heptane-2-one. A ketone, $C_{10}H_{16}O$, obtained from the wood of *Cinnamomum camphora*, an evergreen tree native to eastern Asia, or produced synthetically (see *synthetic c.*), and occurring as colorless or white crystals, granules, or crystalline masses or as colorless to white, translucent, tough masses, with a penetrating characteristic odor and a pungent, aromatic taste. It is applied topically to the skin as an antipruritic and anti-infective and is used as a pharmaceutical necessity in certain pharmaceutic preparations. Called also *gum c.* 2. any compound having characteristics similar to those of camphor. **anise c.,** anethole. **artificial c.,** bornyl chloride. **Borneo c.,** 1. the dextrorotatory form of borneol. 2. borneol. **monobromated c.,** that in which one hydrogen atom has been replaced by one bromine atom; formerly used as a sedative. **peppermint c.,** natural menthol. **synthetic c.,** a camphor produced from pinene, the principal constituent of turpentine. **thyme c.,** thymol. **turpentine c.,** bornyl chloride.

camphora (kam-fo'rah) [L.] camphor.

camphoraceous (kam″fo-ra'shus) having characteristics resembling those of camphor.

camphorated (kam'fo-rāt″ed) [L. *camphoratus*] containing or tinctured with camphor.

camphoric acid (kam-for'ik) a dicarboxylic acid formed by oxidation of camphor, formerly used as a respiratory stimulant.

camphorism (kam'for-izm) poisoning by camphor; the condition is marked by convulsions, coma, and gastritis.

campimeter (kam-pim'ĕ-ter) [L. *campus* field + *-meter*] an apparatus for mapping the central portion of the visual field on a flat surface.

campimetry (kam-pim'ĕ-tre) the determination of the presence of defects in the central portion of the visual field by use of the campimeter.

campospasm (kam'po-spazm) [Gr. *kampē* a bending + *spasm*] camptocormia.

campotomy (kam-pot'o-me) [L. *campi* fields (of Forel) + Gr. *tomē* a cutting] the stereotaxic surgical technique of producing a lesion in Forel's fields, beneath the thalamus, for correction of tremor in Parkinson's disease.

camptocormia (kamp″to-kor'me-ah) [Gr. *kamptos* bent + *kormos* trunk + *-ia*] a static deformity consisting of forward flexion of the trunk; called also *camptospasm.*

camptocormy (kamp″to-kor'me) camptocormia.

camptodactylia (kamp″to-dak-til'e-ah) camptodactyly.

camptodactylism (kamp″to-dak'til-izm) camptodactyly.

camptodactyly (kamp″to-dak'tĭ-le) [Gr. *kamptos* bent +

daktylos finger] permanent and irreducible flexion of one or more fingers (Landouzy).

camptomelia (kamp″to-me'le-ah) [Gr. *kamptos* bent + *melos* limb + *-ia*] bending of the limbs, producing permanent bowing or curving of the affected part; see also *camptomelic syndrome*, under *syndrome.*

camptomelic (kamp″to-me'lik) pertaining to camptomelia; see also under *syndrome.*

camptospasm (kamp'to-spazm) camptocormia.

Campylobacter (kam″pĭ-lo-bak'ter) [Gr. *kampylos* curved + *baktron* a rod] a genus of curved or spiral rod-shaped bacteria made up of gram-negative microaerophilic to anaerobic cells that are motile with polar flagella. The organisms are found in the oral cavity, intestinal tract, and reproductive organs of humans and animals. Some species are pathogenic, causing enteritis and systemic disease in humans and abortion in cattle and sheep. **C. cinae'di,** a species that causes proctitis and diarrhea in homosexual men. **C. co'li,** a species that causes diarrhea in humans. **C. feca'lis,** a nonpathogenic species isolated from sheep feces and the reproductive organs of cattle. **C. fennel'liae,** a species that causes proctitis and diarrhea in homosexual men. **C. fe'tus,** a microaerophilis species occurring as several subspecies. Called also *Vibrio fetus.* **C. fe'tus** subsp. **fe'tus,** a subspecies that causes abortion and infertility in cattle. It is an occasional human pathogen, capable of causing systemic infection in immunocompromised hosts. **C. fe'tus** subsp. **intestina'lis,** *C. fetus* subsp. *fetus.* **C. fe'tus** subsp. **jeju'ni,** *C. jejuni.* **C. fe'tus** subsp. **venera'lis,** a subspecies that causes abortion and infertility in cattle. **C. hyointestina'lis,** a species that causes ileitis in swine. **C. jeju'ni,** a subspecies that is a common cause of acute bacterial gastroenteritis in humans and infectious abortion in sheep, which is also found as a commensal in swine, cattle, cats, and chickens. Called also *Vibrio coli* and *Vibrio jejuni.* **C. pylo'ri,** a species that causes gastritis and pyloric ulcers in humans. **C. sputo'rum,** a nonpathogenic, microaerophilic to anaerobic species occurring as three subspecies. **C. sputo'rum** subsp. **bub'ulus,** a subspecies found in the genital tracts of sheep and cattle. **C. sputo'rum 'subsp. muco'salis,** a subspecies found in the intestinal mucosa and the oral cavity of pigs. **C. sputo'rum** subsp. **sputo'rum,** a subspecies found in the human oral cavity.

campylobacteriosis (kam″pĭ-lo-bak″te-re-o'sis) infection with organisms of the genus *Campylobacter.* **bovine genital c.,** a venereal disease of cattle caused by *Campylobacter* (*Vibrio*) *fetus* subspecies *fetus;* characterized by infertility and early embryonic death. Called also *bovine genital vibrosis.* **ovine genital c.,** an infectious disease of sheep caused by *Campylobacter* (*Vibrio*) *fetus* subspecies *intestinalis* and *jejuni,* characterized by abortion, and transmitted orally. Called also *ovine genital vibriosis.*

camsylate (kam'sĭ-lāt) USAN contraction for camphorsulfonate.

Canada-Cronkhite syndrome (kan'ah-dah-krong'kīt) [Wilma Jeanne *Canada,* American radiologist; Leonard W. *Cronkhite,* Jr., American internist, born 1919] see under *syndrome.*

canal (kah-nal') a relatively narrow tubular passage or channel; see also *canalis.* **abdominal c.,** canalis inguinalis. **accessory palatine c's,** canales palatini minores. **adductor c.,** canalis adductorius. **Alcock's c.,** canalis pudendalis. **alimentary c.,** digestive tract. **alisphenoid c.,** a canal in the alisphenoid bone which in many animals transmits the internal carotid artery. **alveolar c's,** see *canalis mandibulae* and *canales alveolares maxillae.* **alveolar c., anterior; alveolar c. of maxilla; alveolar c., posterior,** see *canales alveolares maxillae.* **anal c.,** the terminal portion of the alimentary canal, extending from the rectum to its distal opening; called also *canalis analis* [NA]. **arachnoid c.** (obs.), cisterna venae magnae cerebri. **c. of Arantius,** ductus venosus. **archenteric c.,** neurenteric c. **archinephric c.,** pronephric duct. **Arnold's c.,** a channel in the petrous portion of the temporal bone for passage of the auricular branch of the vagus nerve. **arterial c.,** ductus arteriosus. **atrioventricular c.,** the common canal connecting the primitive atrium and ventricle. It sometimes persists as a congenital anomaly, as a result of failure of closure of the gap between the interatrial and interventricular septa due to arrest in development of the endocardial cushions. **auditory c., external,** meatus acusticus externus. **auditory c., internal,** meatus acusticus internus. **basipharyngeal c.,** canalis vomerovaginalis. **Bichat's c.,** cisterna venae magnae cerebri. **biliary c's, interlobular,** ductuli interlobulares. **biliary c's, intralobular,** small passages for conducting the bile within the substance of the lobules of the liver (ductuli biliferi [NA]). **birth c.,** the canal through which the fetus passes in birth, comprising the cervix uteri, vagina, and vulva; called also *obstetric c.* and *parturient c.* **blastoporic c.,** neurenteric c. **bony c's of ear,** see entries beginning *canalis semicircularis.* **Braun's c.,** neurenteric c. **Braune's c.** (*obs.*), the uterine cavity and vagina, after complete dilation of the os of the cervix in labor. **Breschet's c's,** canales diploici. **calciferous c's,** canals containing lime salts in cartilage that is undergoing calcification. **caroticotympanic c's,** canaliculi caroticotympanici. **carotid c.,** canalis caroticus. **carpal c.,** canalis carpi. **c's of cartilage,** canals in an ossifying cartilage during its stage of vascularization. **central c. of modiolus,** see *canales longitudinales modioli.* **central c. of spinal cord,** canalis centralis medullae spinalis. **central c. of Stilling, central c. of vitreous,** canalis hyaloideus. **cerebrospinal c.,** the primitive cavity of the brain and spinal cord. **cervical c. of uterus,** canalis cervicis uteri. **chordal c.,** notochordal c. **c. of chorda tympani,** canaliculus chordae tympani. **ciliary c's,** spatia anguli iridocornealis. **Civinini's c.,** canaliculus chordae tympani. **Cloquet's c.,** canalis hyaloideus. **cochlear c.,** ductus cochlearis. **condylar c., condyloid c.,** canalis condylaris. **condyloid c., anterior,** canalis hypoglossalis. **connecting c.,** the arched or coiled part of a uriniferous tubule, joining it to a collecting tubule. **c. of Corti,** inner tunnel. **c. of Cotunnius,** the aqueductus vestibuli and canaliculus cochleae considered as a continuous passage. **craniopharyngeal c.,** an occasional passage through the sphenoid bone, opening into the sella turcica. **crural c.,** canalis femoralis. **crural c. of Henle,** canalis adductorius. **c. of Cuvier,** ductus venosus. **dental c., inferior,** canalis mandibulae. **dental c's, posterior,** 1. see *canales alveolares maxillae.* 2. foramina alveolaria maxillae. **dentinal c's,** canaliculi dentales. **digestive c.,** see under *tract.* **diploic c's,** canales diploici. **Dorello's c.,** an opening sometimes found in the temporal bone through which the abducens nerve and inferior petrosal sinus together enter the cavernous sinus. **entodermal c.,** the primitive gut or alimentary canal (canalis alimentarius [NA]). **c. of epididymis,** ductus epididymidis. **ethmoid c., anterior,** a passage in the frontal and ethmoid bones for the nasal branch of the ophthalmic nerve and anterior ethmoid vessels. **ethmoid c., posterior,** foramen ethmoidale posterius. **eustachian c.,** tuba auditiva. **eustachian c., osseous,** canalis musculotubarius. **facial c., c. for facial nerve,** canalis facialis. **fallopian c.,** canalis facialis. **femoral c.,** canalis femoralis. **Ferrein's c.,** rivus lacrimalis. **flexor c.,** canalis carpi. **ganglionic c.,** canalis spiralis modioli. **Gartner's c.,** ductus epoöphorontis longitudinalis. **gastric c.,** canalis gastricus. **genital c.,** any canal for the passage of ova or for copulatory use; called also *genital duct.* **gubernacular c's,** four small openings in young crania, one behind each incisor tooth. **c. of Guidi,** canalis pterygoideus. **gynecophoral c., gynecophorous c.,** the ventral slit in which the male schistosome carries the female. **hair c.,** an epidermal canal through which a hair grows in order to erupt. **Hannover's c.,** a potential space existing between the anterior and posterior portions of the suspensory ligament of the lens. **haversian c.,** one of the freely anastomosing channels of the haversian system in compact bone. Called also *canalis nutricius ossis* [NA], *haversian space, nutrient c. of bone,* and *plasmatic c.* **hemal c.,** the space within the hemal arch. **Henle's c's,** Henle's loops. **Hensen's c.,** ductus reuniens. **c's of Hering,** openings through which the bile canaliculi communicate with the terminal branches of the bile duct system, the cholangioles; distinguished by their walls, which consist of parenchymal liver cells on one side and cells of the ductules (cholangioles) on the other. **hernial c.,** that through which a hernia passes. **Hirschfeld's c's,** interdental c's. **His c.,** ductus thyroglossalis. **Holmgren-Golgi c's,** minute canals in the cytoplasm of cells, particularly of nerve cells, forming a complex apparatus throughout the cytoplasm; called also

intracytoplasmic c's. **c. of Hovius,** one of a series of connections between the venae vorticosae in certain mammals. **Huguier's c.,** iter chordae anterius. **Hunter's c.,** canalis adductorius. **Huschke's c.,** a passage formed by union of the tubercles of the tympanic ring (anulus tympanicus); it commonly disappears during the years of childhood. **hyaloid c.,** canalis hyaloideus. **hypoglossal c.,** canalis hypoglossalis. **iliac c.,** lacuna musculorum. **incisive c.,** canalis incisivus. **infraorbital c.,** canalis infraorbitalis. **inguinal c.,** canalis inguinalis. **intercellular c's,** interfacial c's. **interdental c's,** channels in the alveolar process of the mandible, between the roots of the medial and lateral incisors, for the passage of anastomosing blood vessels between the sublingual and inferior dental arteries; called also *Hirschfeld's c's.* **interfacial c's,** a labyrinthine system of expanded intercellular spaces between desmosomes; called also *intercellular c's.* **intersacral c's,** foramina intervertebralia ossis sacri. **intestinal c.,** the intestine; that part of the alimentary canal which lies between the pylorus and the anus. **intracytoplasmic c's,** Holmgren-Golgi c's. **Jacobson's c., c. for Jacobson's nerve,** canaliculus tympani. **Kovalevsky's c.,** neurenteric c. **lacrimal c.,** canalis nasolacrimalis. **Laurer's c.,** a passage in trematode worms extending from the ovarian duct to the dorsal surface of the body. **longitudinal c's of modiolus,** canales longitudinales modioli. **Löwenberg's c.,** the part of the ductus cochlearis above the membrane of Corti. **mandibular c.,** canalis mandibulae. **maxillary c., superior,** foramen rotundum ossis sphenoidalis. **medullary c.,** 1. cavitas medullaris. 2. canalis vertebralis. **c's of modiolus,** see *canalis spiralis modioli* and *canales longitudinales modioli.* **Müller's c.,** ductus paramesonephricus. **musculotubal c.,** canalis musculotubarius. **nasal c., nasolacrimal c.,** canalis nasolacrimalis. **nasopalatine c.,** canalis incisivus. **neural c.,** canalis vertebralis. **neurenteric c. (of Kovalevsky),** a passage, in the embryo, from the posterior part of the neural tube into the archenteron; called also *Braun's c., archenteric c.,* and *blastoporic c.* **notochordal c.,** a tunnel extending from the primitive pit into the notochordal process of the embryo; called also *chordal c.* **c. of Nuck,** processus vaginalis peritonei. **nutrient c. of bone,** haversian c., or canalis nutricius ossis. **obstetric c.,** birth c. **obturator c.,** canalis obturatorius. **obturator c. of pubic bone,** sulcus obturatorius ossis pubis. **c. of Oken,** ductus mesonephricus. **olfactory c.,** the nasal fossae at an early stage of their embryonic development. **omphalomesenteric c.,** yolk stalk. **optic c.,** canalis opticus. **orbital c's,** foramina ethmoidalia. **orbital c., anterior internal,** foramen ethmoidale anterius. **orbital c., posterior internal,** foramen ethmoidale posterius. **palatine c's, accessory,** canales palatini minores. **palatine c., anterior,** 1. canalis incisivus. 2. foramen incisivum. **palatine c's, lesser, palatine c's, posterior,** canales palatini minores. **palatomaxillary c.,** 1. canalis palatinus major. 2. see *foramen palatinum majus.* **palatovaginal c.,** canalis palatovaginalis. **paraurethral c's of male urethra,** ductus paraurethrales urethrae masculinae. **parturient c.,** birth c. **pelvic c.,** the passage from the superior to the inferior strait of the pelvis. **perivascular c.,** a lymph space about a blood vessel. **persistent common atrioventricular c.,** atrioventricularis communis. **Petit's c.,** spatia zonularia. **pharyngeal c.,** canalis palatovaginalis. **plasmatic c.,** haversian c. **pleural c's,** a pair of passages in the embryo, connecting the primitive pericardial and peritoneal cavities. **portal c.,** a space within the capsule of Glisson and liver substance, containing branches of the portal vein, of the hepatic artery, and of the hepatic duct. **pterygoid c.,** canalis pterygoideus. **pterygopalatine c.,** 1. canalis palatinus major. 2. canalis palatovaginalis. **pudendal c.,** canalis pudendalis. **pulmoaortic c.,** ductus arteriosus. **pulp c.,** canalis radicis dentis. **pyloric c.,** canalis pyloricus. **c's of Recklinghausen,** small lymph spaces in the connective tissue. **recurrent c.,** canalis pterygoideus. **Reichert's c.,** ductus reuniens. **c's of Rivinus,** ductus sublinguales minores. **root c.,** canalis radicis dentis. **root c., accessory,** a lateral branching of the main root canal, usually occurring in the apical third of the root. **Rosenthal's c.,** canalis spiralis modioli. **sacculocochlear c.,** a passage connecting the sacculus and the cochlea. **sacculoutric-**

ular c., ductus utriculosaccularis. **sacral c.,** canalis sacralis. **Santorini's c.,** ductus pancreaticus accessorius. **Schlemm's c.,** a branching, circumferential vessel lying in the internal scleral sulcus, a major component of the drainage pathway for aqueous humor; called also *sinus venosus sclerae* [NA]. **scleral c., scleroticochoroidal c.,** the channel in the choroid and sclera of the eye through which the optic nerve passes; see also *lamina cribrosa sclerae*. **semicircular c's,** three long canals of the bony labyrinth of the ear. See *canales semicircularis ossei* [NA]. **semicircular c., anterior,** canalis semicircularis anterior. **semicircular c., horizontal,** canalis semicircularis lateralis. **semicircular c., lateral,** canalis semicircularis lateralis. **semicircular c's, membranous,** see *ductus semicircularis anterior, ductus semicircularis lateralis,* and *ductus semicircularis posterior.* **semicircular c., posterior,** canalis semicircularis posterior. **seminal c.,** a passage for the transmission of semen, or of spermatozoa. **serous c.,** a minute lymph space. **sheathing c.,** the passage from the peritoneal cavity to the tunica vaginalis testis. **Sondermann's c's,** conical extensions of the lumen of Schlemm's canal sometimes observed in the inner wall of the canal. **spermatic c.,** the canalis inguinalis in the male, providing for passage of the spermatic cord. **sphenopalatine c.,** 1. canalis palatovaginalis. 2. canalis palatinus major. **sphenopharyngeal c.,** canalis palatovaginalis. **spinal c.,** canalis vertebralis. **spinal medullary c.** (*obs.*), canalis centralis medullae spinalis. **spiral c. of cochlea,** canalis spiralis cochleae. **spiral c. of modiolus,** canalis spiralis modioli. **spiroid c.,** canalis facialis. **c. of Steno, Stensen's c.,** parotid duct (ductus parotideus [NA]). **c. of Stilling,** canalis hyaloideus. **c. of stomach,** canalis gastricus. **subsartorial c.,** canalis adductorius. **Sucquet-Hoyer c.,** segmentum arteriale anastomosis arteriovenae glomeriformis. **supraciliary c.,** a small opening sometimes present near the supraorbital notch, which transmits a nutrient artery and a branch of the supraorbital nerve to the frontal sinus. **supraoptic c.,** a minute canal which is the anterior continuation of the optic recess above the optic chiasma. **supraorbital c.,** incisura frontalis. **tarsal c.,** sinus tarsi. **c. for tensor tympani muscle,** semicanalis musculi tensoris tympani. **Theile's c.,** a space formed by reflection of the pericardium on the aorta and the pulmonary artery. **Tourtual's c.,** canalis palatinus major. **tubal c.,** semicanalis tubae auditivae. **tubotympanic c.,** the inner division of the first branchial cleft in the fetus, from which the auditory tube and middle ear cavity are derived. **tympanic c. of cochlea,** scala tympani. **umbilical c.,** annulus umbilicalis. **urogenital c's,** that portion of the urogenital sinus used jointly by the müllerian and mesonephric ducts. **uterine c.,** the cavity of the uterus. **uterocervical c.,** canalis cervicis uteri. **utriculosaccular c.,** ductus utriculosaccularis. **vaginal c.,** the space within the vagina; called also *vulvouterine c.* **Van Hoorne's c.,** thoracic duct (ductus thoracicus [NA]). **vector c.** (*obs.*), a channel for the passage of ova; an oviduct, def. 1. **ventricular c.,** canalis gastricus. **Verneuil's c's,** collateral vessels of a venous trunk. **vertebral c.,** canalis vertebralis. **vestibular c.,** scala vestibuli. **vidian c.,** canalis pterygoideus. **Volkmann's c's,** passages other than haversian canals, for the passage of blood vessels through bone. **vomerine c.,** canalis vomerovaginalis. **vomerobasilar c., lateral inferior,** canalis palatovaginalis. **vomerobasilar c., lateral superior,** canalis vomerovaginalis. **vomerorostral c.,** canalis vomerorostralis. **vomerovaginal c.,** canalis vomerovaginalis. **vulvar c.,** vestibulum vaginae. **vulvouterine c.,** vaginal c. **c. of Wirsung,** ductus pancreaticus. **zygomaticofacial c.,** foramen zygomaticofaciale. **zygomaticotemporal c.,** foramen zygomaticotemporale.

canales (kah-na'lēz) [L.] plural of *canalis*.

canalicular (kan″ah-lik'u-lar) resembling or pertaining to a canaliculus.

canaliculi (kan″ah-lik'u-li) [L.] plural of *canaliculus*.

canaliculitis (kan″ah-lik'u-li′tis) [L. *canaliculus*, from *canalis* channel + *-itis* inflammation] inflammation of the lacrimal ducts.

canaliculization (kan″ah-lik'u-li-za′shun) the development of canaliculi, as in bone.

canaliculorhinostomy (kan″ah-lik″u-lo-ri-nos'to-me) dacryocystorhinostomy.

canaliculus (kan″ah-lik'u-lus), pl. *canalic'uli* [L. dim. of *canalis*] [NA] an extremely narrow tubular passage or channel; used as a general term in anatomical nomenclature for various small channels. **apical c.,** any of the numerous tubular invaginations arising from the clefts between the microvilli of the proximal convoluted tubule of the kidney and extending downward into the apical cytoplasm. **bile canaliculi, biliary canaliculi,** fine tubular canals running between liver cells, throughout the parenchyma, usually occurring singly between each adjacent pair of cells, and forming a three-dimensional network of polyhedral meshes, with a single cell in each mesh. Called also *bile capillaries*. **bone canaliculi,** branching tubular passages radiating like wheel spokes from each bone lacuna to connect with the canaliculi of adjacent lacunae, and with the haversian canal. **caroticotympanic canaliculi, canalic'uli caroticotympan'ici** [NA], caroticotympanic canals: tiny passages in the temporal bone interconnecting the carotid canal and the tympanic cavity, and carrying communicating twigs between the internal carotid and tympanic plexuses; called also *caroticotympanic foramina.* **c. of chorda tympani, c. chor′dae tym′pani** [NA], a small canal that opens off the facial canal just before its termination, transmitting the chorda tympani nerve into the tympanic cavity; called also *canal of chorda tympani, canalis chordae tympani,* and *Civinini's canal.* **c. of cochlea, c. coch′leae** [NA], a small canal in the petrous part of the temporal bone that interconnects the scala tympani of the inner ear with the subarachnoid cavity; it houses the perilymphatic duct and a small vein. Called also *aqueduct of Cotunnius.* **dental canaliculi, canalic'uli denta′les** [NA], dentinal canals: minute channels in dentin, extending from the pulp cavity to the cementum and enamel. Called also *dental* or *dentinal tubules.* **haversian c.,** any one of a system of minute channels in compact bone connected with each haversian canal. **incisor c.,** ductus incisivus. **innominate c., c. innomina′tus,** 1. sulcus nervi petrosi minoris. 2. foramen venosum. **c. innomina′tus of Arnold,** foramen petrosum. **intercellular c.,** one located between adjacent cells, such as one of the secretory capillaries, or canaliculi, of the gastric parietal cells. **intracellular canaliculi of parietal cells,** a system of canaliculi that seem to be intracellular, but are formed by deep invaginations of the surface of the gastric parietal cells rather than extending into the cytoplasm of the cell. **c. lacrima′lis** [NA], the short passage in an eyelid, beginning at the punctum, that leads from the lacrimal lake to the lacrimal sac; called also *lacrimal duct* and *ductus lacrimalis.* **c. laqueifor′mis,** Henle's loops. **mastoid c., mastoid c. for Arnold's nerve,** c. mastoideus. **c. mastoi′deus** [NA], a minute passage beginning in the lateral wall of the jugular fossa of the temporal bone and passing into the temporal bone. The tympanic branch of the vagus nerve passes through it to exit via the tympanomastoid fissure. Called also *mastoid c. (for Arnold's nerve).* **c. petro′sus, petrous c.,** sulcus nervi petrosi minoris. **pseudobile c.,** one of the dark-staining columns of cells from the bile ducts seen in the portal area of the liver in cirrhosis. **secretory c.,** see under *capillary.* **Thiersch's c.,** one of the small channels in newly formed repair tissue through which the nutritive fluids circulate. **tympanic c., tympanic c. for Jacobson's nerve,** c. tympanicus. **c. tympan′icus** [NA], a small opening on the inferior surface of the petrous part of the temporal bone in the floor of the petrosal fossa; it transmits the tympanic branch of the glossopharyngeal nerve and a small artery. Called also *Jacobson's canal, canal for Jacobson's nerve,* and *tympanic canaliculus (for Jacobson's nerve).*

canalis (kah-na'lis), pl. *cana′les* [L.] [NA] a general term for a relatively narrow tubular passage or channel; called also *canal.* **c. adducto′rius** [NA], adductor canal: an intramuscular interval on the medial aspect of the middle third of the thigh, which contains the femoral vessels and the saphenous nerve. The lateral wall is formed by the vastus medialis, the posterior wall by the adductor longus and adductor magnus, the roof by a layer of fascia, and it is covered by the sartorius. Called also *crural canal of Henle, Hunter's canal, subsartorial canal,* and *canalis subsartorialis.* **c. alimenta′rius,** digestive tract. **cana′les alveola′res,** see *canales alveolares maxillae* and *c. mandibulae.* **cana′les alveola′res maxil′lae** [NA], alveolar canals of maxilla: several canals in the maxilla for the passage of the posterior superior alveolar vessels and nerves, each canal beginning on the infratemporal surface of the maxilla at an alveolar foramen; called also *posterior dental canals.* **c. ana'lis** [NA], anal canal: the terminal portion of the alimentary canal, extending from the rectum to the anus; called also *pars analis recti.* **c. basipharyn'geus,** canalis vomerovaginalis. **c. carot'icus** [NA], carotid canal: a passage in the petrous portion of the temporal bone, beginning on the inferior surface just anterior to the jugular foramen, and running anteromedially for about 2 cm.; it is seen interiorly in the floor of the middle cranial fossa, where it meets the carotid sulcus on the body of the sphenoid bone. It houses the internal carotid artery. **cana'les paraurethra'les ure'thrae masculi'nae,** NA alternative for *ductus paraurethrales urethrae masculinae.* **c. carpa'lis,** NA alternative for *c. carpi.* **c. car'pi** [NA], carpal canal: an osseofibrous tunnel for passage of the tendons of the flexor muscles of the hand and digits, formed by the flexor retinaculum as it roofs over the concavity of the carpus on the palmar surface; called also *c. carpalis* [NA alternative], *carpal tunnel,* and *flexor canal.* **c. centra'lis medul'lae spina'lis** [NA], central canal of spinal cord: a small canal extending throughout the length of the spinal cord, lined by ependymal cells. Above, it continues into the medulla oblongata, where it opens into the fourth ventricle. **c. cerv'icis u'teri** [NA], cervical canal of uterus: the part of the uterine cavity that lies within the cervix. **c. chor'dae tym'pani,** canaliculus chordae tympani. **c. con-dyla'ris** [NA], condylar canal: an opening sometimes present in the floor of the condylar fossa for the transmission of a vein from the transverse sinus; called also *c. condyloideus, condyloid canal,* and *posterior condyloid foramen.* **c. con-dyloi'deus,** canalis condylaris. **cana'les diplo'ici** [NA], diploic canals: bony canals in the cranial bones, located in the spongy bone between the compact tables and providing for passage of the veins of the diploë; called also *canales diploici* [*Brescheti*] and *Breschet's canals.* **c. facia'lis** [NA], **c. fascia'lis** [**Fallo'pii**], facial canal: a canal in the temporal bone for the facial nerve, beginning in the internal acoustic meatus and passing anterolaterally dorsal to the vestibule of the inner ear for about 2 mm. Turning sharply backward at the genu of the facial canal, it runs along the medial wall of the tympanic cavity, then turns inferiorly and reaches the exterior of the petrous part of the bone at the stylomastoid foramen. Called also *canal for facial nerve, fallopian aqueduct* or *canal, aqueduct of Fallopius,* and *spiroid canal.* **c. femora'lis** [NA], femoral canal: the cone-shaped medial part of the femoral sheath lateral to the base of the lacunar ligament; called also *crural canal.* **c. gas'tricus** [NA], gastric canal: the longitudinal grooved channel formed by the more or less regular ridges along the lesser curvature of the stomach; called also *canal of stomach, magenstrasse, ventricular canal, c. ventricularis* [NA alternative], and *c. ventriculi.* **c. hyaloi'deus** [NA], hyaloid canal: a passage running from in front of the optic disk to the lens of the eye; in the fetus it transmits the hyaloid artery. Called also *central canal of Stilling, central canal of vitreous,* and *Cloquet's canal.* **c. hypoglossa'lis** [NA], hypoglossal canal: an opening in the lateral part of the occipital bone at the base of the condyle, which transmits the hypoglossal nerve and a branch of the posterior meningeal artery; called also *anterior condyloid canal,* and *anterior condyloid foramen.* **c. incisi'vus** [NA], incisive canal: one of the small canals opening into the incisive fossa of the hard palate, and transmitting small vessels and nerves from the floor of the nose into the front part of the roof of the mouth; called also *anterior palatine canal,* or *groove, nasopalatine canal,* and *foramen of Stensen.* **c. infraorbita'lis** [NA], infraorbital canal: a passage beneath the orbital surface of the maxilla, continuous posteriorly with the infraorbital sulcus, and opening anteriorly on the anterior surface of the body of the maxilla in the infraorbital foramen. It contains the infraorbital vessels and nerve. **c. inguina'lis** [NA], inguinal canal: the passage superficial to the deep inguinal ring for transmission of the spermatic cord in the male and the round ligament in the female; called also *abdominal canal.* **cana'les longitudina'les modi'oli** [NA], longitudinal canals of modiolus: short tunnels in the modiolus that transmit blood vessels and nerves. **c. mandib'ulae** [NA], mandibular canal: a canal that traverses the ramus and body of the mandible between the mandibular and mental foramina, transmitting the inferior alveolar vessels and nerve; called also *inferior dental canal.* **c. mus-culotuba'rius** [NA], musculotubal canal: the combined

canals of the auditory tube and the tensor tympani muscle in the temporal bone; called also *osseous eustachian canal.* **c. nasolacrima'lis** [NA], nasolacrimal canal: a canal formed by the lacrimal sulcus of the maxilla, lacrimal bone, and inferior nasal concha; it contains the nasolacrimal duct. Called also *lacrimal canal,* and *nasal canal.* **c. nu-tri'cius os'sis, c. nu'triens os'sis,** nutrient canal of bone: one of the freely anastomosing channels of the haversian system of compact bone, which contain blood vessels, lymph vessels, and nerves; called also *haversian canal* and *haversian space.* **c. obturato'rius** [NA], obturator canal: an opening within the obturator membrane for the passage of the obturator vessels and nerve; its boundaries are the edge of the obturator membrane, together with the obturator groove of the pubic bone. **c. op'ticus** [NA], optic canal: one of the paired openings in the sphenoid bone where the small wings are attached to the body of the bone at the apex of the orbit; each canal transmits one of the optic nerves and the ophthalmic artery of that side. Called also *foramen opticum ossis sphenoidalis* and *optic foramen of sphenoid bone.* **cana'les palati'ni,** canales palatini minores. **c. palati'nus ma'jor** [NA], great palatine canal: a passage in the sphenoid and palatine bones for the greater palatine vessels and nerve; called also *c. pterygopala-tinus, palatomaxillary canal, pterygopalatine canal, spheno-palatine canal,* and *Tourtual's canal.* **cana'les palati'ni mino'res** [NA], lesser palatine canals: openings in the palatine bone that branch off the great palatine canal to carry the lesser and middle palatine nerves and vessels to the roof of the mouth. Called also *canales palatini,* and *accessory* or *posterior palatine canals.* **c. palatovagina'-lis** [NA], palatovaginal canal: a narrow canal located in the roof of the nasal cavity between the inferior surface of the body of the sphenoid bone and the sphenoidal process of the palatine bone; it opens posteriorly into the nasal cavity and anteriorly into the pterygopalatine fossa. Called also *c. pharyngeus, pharyngeal canal, pterygopalatine canal, spheno-palatine canal, sphenopharyngeal canal,* and *lateral inferior vomerobasilar canal.* **c. pharyn'geus,** canalis palatovaginalis. **c. pterygoi'deus** [NA], pterygoid canal: a horizontally running canal that passes forward through the base of the medial pterygoid plate of the sphenoid bone to open into the posterior wall of the pter-gopalatine fossa just medial and inferior to the foramen rotundum; it transmits the pterygoid vessels and nerves. Called also *c. pterygoideus* [*Vidii*], *canal of Guidi, recurrent canal,* and *vidian canal.* **c. pterygopalati'nus,** *c. palatinus major.* **c. pudenda'lis** [NA], pudendal canal: the tunnel in the special fascial sheath through which the pudendal vessels and nerve pass; it is intimately related to the obturator fascia. Called also *Alcock's canal.* **c. pylor'i-cus** [NA], pyloric canal: the short, narrow part of the stomach extending from the gastroduodenal junction to the pyloric antrum. **c. rad'icis den'tis** [NA], root canal: the portion of the dental pulp cavity in the root of a tooth, extending from the pulp chamber to the apical foramen; more than one canal may be present in a single root, two commonly being present in the mesial root of the mandibular first molar. Called also *pulp canal.* **c. reu'niens,** ductus reu-niens. **c. sacra'lis** [NA], sacral canal: the continuation of the vertebral canal through the sacrum. **c. semicir-cula'ris ante'rior** [NA], anterior semicircular canal: the anterior of the osseous semicircular canals, lodging the ductus semicircularis anterior. Called also *c. semicircularis superior.* See *canales semicirculares ossei.* **c. semicir-cula'ris latera'lis** [NA], lateral semicircular canal: the lateral of the semicircular canals, lodging the ductus semicir-cularis lateralis; called also *horizontal semicircular canal.* See *canales semicirculares ossei.* **cana'les semicircu-lar'es os'sei** [NA], three long canals of the bony labyrinth of the ear (lateral, anterior, and posterior), forming loops and opening into the vestibule by five openings. They lodge the semicircular ducts (ductus semicirculares [NA]) of the mem-branous labyrinth. Called also *semicircular canals.* **c. semicircula'ris poste'rior** [NA], posterior semicircular canal: the posterior of the semicircular canals, lodging the ductus semicircularis posterior; see *canales semicirculares ossei.* **c. semicircula'ris supe'rior,** *c.* semicircularis anterior. **c. spina'lis,** *c.* vertebralis. **c. spira'lis co-ch'leae** [NA], spiral canal of cochlea: a winding tube that makes two and one-half turns about the modiolus of the cochlea; it is divided into two compartments, scala tympani and scala vestibuli, by the lamina spiralis. Called also *cochlear duct.* **c. spira′lis modio′li** [NA], spiral canal of modiolus: a canal following the course of the bony spiral lamina of the cochlea and containing the spiral ganglion of the cochlear division of the vestibulocochlear nerve. Called also *ganglionic canal* and *Rosenthal's canal.* **c. subsartoria′lis,** c. adductorius. **c. ventricula′ris,** NA alternative for *c. gastricus.* **c. ventric′uli,** c. gastricus. **c. vertebra′lis** [NA], vertebral canal: the canal formed by the foramina in the successive vertebrae, which encloses the spinal cord and meninges; called also *c. spinalis, medullary canal, neural canal,* and *spinal canal.* **c. vomerorostra′lis** [NA], vomerorostral canal: a canal located between the vomer and sphenoidal rostrum. **c. vomerovagina′lis** [NA], vomerovaginal canal: an inconstant opening formed by the articulating margins of the ala of the vomer and the body of the sphenoid bone; called also *c. basipharyngeus, basipharyngeal canal, lateral superior vomerobasilar canal,* and *vomerine canal.*

canalization (kan″al-i-za′shun) 1. the formation of canals, natural or pathologic. 2. the surgical establishment of canals for drainage. 3. the formation of new canals or paths, especially blood vessels, through an obstruction, such as a clot. 4. in psychology, the formation in the central nervous system of new pathways by the repeated passage of nerve impulses.

canaloplasty (kah-nal′o-plas″te) plastic reconstruction of a passage, as of the external auditory meatus.

canarypox (kah-na′re-poks) an eruptive disease of canaries due to a poxvirus.

Canavalia (kan″ah-val′ĭ-ah) a genus of leguminous plants, the Jack bean, native to the West Indies but widely cultivated as a source of food for humans and livestock. *C. ensifor′mis* D.C. and other species are the source of canavalin and concanavallin.

canavalin (kan″ah-val′in) an antibacterial substance isolated from the meal of the Jack bean (*Canavalia ensiformis* D.C., and other species of *Canavalia*).

canavanase (kan-av′ah-nās) arginase.

canavanine (kan-av′ĭ-nin) 2-amino-4-(guanidino-oxy)-butyric acid isolated from soy bean meal; it is $NH_2 \cdot C(:NH) \cdot NH \cdot O \cdot CH_2 \cdot CH_2 \cdot CH(NH_2) \cdot COOH$.

cancellated (kan′sel-lāt-ed) having a lattice-like structure; cancellous.

cancelli (kan-sel′i) [L.] plural of *cancellus.*

cancellous (kan′sĕ-lus) of a reticular, spongy, or lattice-like structure; said mainly of bony tissue.

cancellus (kan-sel′us), pl. *cancel′li* [L. "a lattice"] [NA] any structure arranged like a lattice.

cancer (kan′ser) [L. "crab"] a cellular tumor the natural course of which is fatal. Cancer cells, unlike benign tumor cells, exhibit the properties of invasion and metastasis and are highly anaplastic. Cancers are divided into two broad categories of carcinoma and sarcoma. **acinar c., acinous c.,** alveolar adenocarcinoma. **adenoid c.,** a malignant tumor made up of or containing cylindrical tubes lined with epithelium. **c. à deux** [Fr. "cancer in two"], cancer attacking simultaneously or consecutively two persons who live together. **alveolar c.,** see under *adenocarcinoma.* **aniline c.,** cancer due to aniline dyes, occurring among those who work in dye factories and dyeing establishments. **apinoid c.,** scirrhous c. **areolar c.** (*obs.*), mucinous carcinoma. **c. atroph′icans,** scirrhous cancer surrounded by sclerosed and atrophied tissue. **betel c., buyo cheek c. black c.,** malignant melanoma. **boring c.,** epithelioma of the skin of the face. **branchiogenous c.,** cancer originating in the superior cervical triangle, and supposed to be derived from a relic of an embryonal branchial cleft. **Butter's c.,** carcinoma of the hepatic flexure of the colon. **buyo cheek c.,** cancer of the cheek seen in natives of the Philippine Islands from chewing buyo leaf or betel; called also *betel c.* **cellular c.,** medullary carcinoma. **cerebriform c.,** medullary carcinoma. **chimney-sweeps′ c.,** carcinoma of the scrotum due to soot poisoning; called also *soot c.* **chondroid c.,** scirrhous carcinoma with a cartilage-like texture. **claypipe c.,** carcinoma of the lip due to irritation caused by a pipe stem. **colloid c.,** mucinous carcinoma. **contact c.,** cancer developing in a part of the body in contact with a previously existing cancer. **corset c.,** cancer en cuirasse. **cystic c.,** carcinoma that has undergone cystic degeneration.

dendritic c., papillary carcinoma. **dermoid c.** (*obs.*), squamous cell carcinoma. **duct c.,** carcinoma arising from the epithelium of a duct. **dye workers' c.,** carcinoma of the urinary bladder frequently observed among workers in aniline dyes. **encephaloid c.,** medullary carcinoma. **c. en cuirasse,** a carcinoma about the skin of the thorax; called also *corset c.* and *jacket c.* **endothelial c.,** endothelioma. **epidermal c.,** malignant epithelioma of the skin. **epithelial c.,** carcinoma. **fungous c.** (*obs.*), fungus haematodes. **glandular c.,** adenocarcinoma. **green c.,** chloroma. **hard c.,** scirrhous carcinoma. **hematoid c.** (*obs.*), fungus haematodes. **c. in si′tu,** carcinoma in situ. **jacket c.,** c. en cuirasse. **kang c., kangri c.,** epithelioma in the thigh or abdomen affecting Indian and Chinese natives, and attributed to irritation from the kang (heated brick oven) or from the kangri (fire basket). **latent c.,** microscopic carcinomas of the prostate discovered, in the absence of any clinical manifestations, in the course of histological examination. **medullary c.,** see under *carcinoma.* **melanotic c.,** malignant melanoma. **mule-spinners' c.,** a form of epithelioma affecting mule spinners in the cotton-spinning industry. **occult c.,** a small prostatic carcinoma that gives rise to clinically evident distant metastases before it is itself clinically detectable. **paraffin c.,** a malignant growth occurring in those who work in paraffin. **pitch-workers' c.,** epithelioma of the face, neck, and scrotum seen in those who work in pitch. **retrograde c.,** a dormant atrophied malignant growth. **rodent c.,** rodent ulcer. **roentgenologist's c.,** cancer affecting the hands of those who work with roentgen rays. **scirrhous c.,** see under *carcinoma.* **soft c.,** medullary carcinoma. **solanoid c.,** (*obs.*), scirrhous carcinoma. **soot c.,** chimney-sweeps' c. **spindle cell c.,** a rare type of carcinoma affecting older persons, in which spindle-cell growth predominates, often associated with giant-cell cancer. These tumors may arise from any epithelial surface, but are most often found in sites that usually produce squamous or transitional cell carcinomas. **tar c.,** carcinoma caused by inflammatory irritation of fumes of tar or by the irritating effect of tar on the skin. **tubular c.,** an adenocarcinoma in which the cells are arranged in the form of tubules. **villous duct c.,** carcinoma with a villous growth pattern arising from the wall of a cyst.

canceremia (kan″ser-e′me-ah) the presence of cancer cells in the blood.

cancericidal (kan″ser-ĭ-si′dal) [*cancer* + L. *caedere* to kill] destructive to cancer or malignant cells.

cancerigenic (kan″ser-ĭ-jen′ik) giving rise to a malignant tumor.

cancerin (kan′ser-in) a white crystalline ptomaine, $C_8H_5NO_3$, from the urine in carcinoma.

cancerism (kan′ser-izm) the cancerous diathesis, i.e., the tendency to the development of malignant disease.

cancerocidal (kan″ser-o-si′dal) cancericidal.

cancerogenic (kan″ser-o-jen′ik) cancerigenic.

cancerophobia (kan″ser-o-fo′be-ah) cancerphobia.

cancerous (kan′ser-us) of the nature of or pertaining to cancer.

cancerphobia (kan″ser-fo′be-ah) irrational fear of cancer.

cancer-ulcer (kan′ser-ul′ser) carcinomatous ulceration.

cancriform (kang′krĭ-form) resembling a cancer.

cancroid (kang′kroid) [*cancer* + Gr. *eidos* form] 1. resembling cancer. 2. a skin cancer of a moderate degree of malignancy.

cancrum (kang′krum) [L.] canker. **c. na′si,** gangrenous rhinitis of children. **c. o′ris,** noma (def. 1). **c. puden′di,** gangrenous erosion of the genitalia; see *erosive balanitis,* under *balanitis,* and *erosive vulvitis,* under *vulvitis.*

candela (kan-del′ah) [L. *candēla* candle] the SI unit of luminous intensity equal to one-sixtieth of the luminous intensity per square centimeter of a blackbody radiating at the temperature of the freezing point of platinum. Called also *candle, new candle,* and *standard candle.* Abbreviated cd.

Candeptin (kan-dep′tin) trademark for preparations of candicidin.

candicidin (kan″dĭ-si′din) [USP] an antifungal antibiotic produced by a strain of *Streptomyces griseus;* it is especially effective against *Candida albicans*, and is administered intravaginally in the treatment of vaginal candidiasis.

Candida (kan'dĭ-dah) [L. *candidus* glowing white] a genus of yeastlike imperfect fungi of the family Cryptococcaceae, order Moniliales, characterized by producing yeast cells, mycelia, pseudomycelia, and blastospores. It is commonly part of the normal flora of the skin, mouth, intestinal tract, and vagina, but can cause a variety of infections, including candidiasis, onychomycosis, tinea corporis, tinea pedis, vaginitis, and thrush. *C. albicans* is the usual pathogen, but *C. tropicalis* may also cause infection. Other species are *C. guilliermondi* and *C. krusei*. Called also *Monilia* and *Oidium*, and, formerly, *Blastodendrion*, and *Castellania*. **C. al'bicans,** the most frequent agent of candidiasis. **C. mesenter'ica,** a species which causes fermentation in fruit acids; called also *Saccharomyces mesentericus*. **C. parapsilo'sis,** a species of limited pathogenicity but particularly associated with endocarditis, paronychia, and otitis externa. **C. tropica'lis,** a species that is an occasional cause of candidiasis. **C. vin'i,** a species from fermenting liquors and diabetic urine, in which it produces a slight fermentation seen as cylindrical, oval, or elliptical cells, forming branched chains; called also *Saccharomyces mycoderma*.

candidal (kan'dĭ-dal) pertaining to or caused by *Candida*.

candidemia (kan"dĭ-de'me-ah) the presence in the blood of fungi of the genus *Candida*, usually resulting from candidal endocarditis or systemic candidiasis.

candidiasis (kan"dĭ-di'ah-sis) infection with a fungus of the genus *Candida*. It is usually a superficial infection of the moist cutaneous areas of the body, and is generally caused by *C. albicans*; it most commonly involves the skin (dermatocandidiasis), oral mucous membranes (thrush, def. 1), respiratory tract (bronchocandidiasis), and vagina (vaginitis). Rarely there is a systemic infection or endocarditis. Called also *moniliasis, candidosis, oidomycosis, and, formerly, blastodendriosis*. **cutaneous c.,** candidiasis of the skin, which may be manifested as eczema-like lesions of the interdigital spaces, perlèche, or chronic paronychia; called also *dermatocandidiasis*. **endocardial c.,** mycotic endocarditis caused by various species of *Candida*.

candidid (kan'dĭ-did) a secondary skin eruption that is the expression of hypersensitivity to infection with *Candida* elsewhere on the body; called also *moniliid*.

candidin (kan'dĭ-din) a skin test antigen derived from *Candida albicans*, used in testing for the development of delayed-type hypersensitivity to constituents of the microorganism.

candidosis (kan-dĭ-do'sis) candidiasis.

candiduria (kan"did-u're-ah) the presence of *Candida* organisms in the urine.

candle (kan'd'l) 1. a mass of wax or similar substance, usually cylindrical in shape, with a wick for burning, to furnish illumination or heat. 2. a cylindrical mass of material used as a filter in microbiology. 3. candela. **foot c.,** see under F. **meter c.,** see *lux*. **new c., standard c.,** candela.

candlefish (kan'd'l fish) a marine fish, *Thaleichthys pacificus*, of the smelt family, yielding a fixed oil with properties similar to those of cod liver oil.

candol (kan'dol) a dry malt extract.

cane (kān) a wooden stick or metal rod used for support in walking. **adjustable c.,** a cane whose length can be easily altered. **English c.,** a supporting device consisting of a single upright with a hand rest at right angles to it; an extension piece above the hand rest, attached at an angle of about 125 degrees to the upright and bent away from the body, has a holder at the top which fits around the forearm, permitting the weight of the body to be supported on the hand and back of the forearms. **quadripod c.,** one adapted for increased stability by forking to provide a four-legged rectangular base of support. **tripod c.,** one similar to a quadripod cane except that it forks to provide a three-legged, triangular base of support.

canescent (kah-nes'ent) [L. *canus* gray] 1. becoming white or grayish. 2. in biology, having grayish or whitish hairs or down; hoary.

canine (ka'nīn) [L. *canis* a dog, hound] 1. of, pertaining to, or like that which belongs to a dog. 2. a canine tooth; see under *tooth*.

caninus (ka-ni'nus) musculus levator anguli oris.

canities (kah-nish'e-ēz) [L.] diffuse grayness or whiteness of the scalp hair, especially as associated with aging. Cf. *poliosis*.

canker (kang'ker) 1. ulceration, chiefly of the mouth and lips. 2. disease of the keratogenous membrane in horses, beginning at the frog and extending to the sole and wall, marked by a loss of function of the horn-secreting cells and the discharge of a serous exudate in place of normal horn. 3. inflammation of the lining of the external ear in dogs and cats. Called also *cancrum*.

canna (kan'ah) [L.] a reed, or cane. **c. ma'jor,** the tibia. **c. mi'nor,** the fibula.

cannabidiol (kan"ah-bĭ-di'ōl) a nonpsychoactive diphenol, $C_{21}H_{30}O_2$, isolated from cannabis.

cannabinoid (kan-ab'ĭ-noid) any of the principles of *Cannabis*, including tetrahydrocannabinol, cannabinol, and cannabidiol.

cannabinol (kah-nab'ĭ-nol) a nonpsychoactive constituent, $C_{21}H_{26}O_2$, of resinous exudates of *Cannabis sativa* L.; its tetrahydro derivatives are active principles.

cannabis (kan'ah-bis) [Gr. *kannabis* hemp] the dried flowering tops of hemp plants, *Cannabis sativa* L. (Cannabaceae), which contain the euphoric principles Δ^1-3,4-*trans* and Δ^6-3,4-*trans* tetrahydrocannabinol, as well as cannabinol and cannabidiol. It is classified as a hallucinogenic and is prepared as bhang, ganja, hashish, and marihuana. See also *cannabism*.

cannabism (kan'ah-bizm) (*obs.*) cannabis intoxication or cannabis abuse.

cannibalism (kan'ĭ-bal-izm) the eating of one's own kind.

Cannizzaro's reaction (kan"e-zah'rōz) [Stanislao *Cannizzaro*, chemist in Rome, 1826–1910] see under *reaction*.

Cannon's ring (point) (kan'unz) [Walter Bradford *Cannon*, Boston physiologist, 1871–1945, the first to adapt x-ray techniques to the study of digestive function] see under *ring*.

cannula (kan'u-lah) [L. dim. of *canna* "reed"] a tube for insertion into a duct or cavity; during insertion its lumen is usually occupied by a trocar. **perfusion c.,** a double tube for running a continuous flow of liquid into and out of an organ. **washout c.,** a cannula attached to a manometer and inserted into a blood vessel so that the connection between the artery and the manometer can be irrigated in long observations.

cannulate (kan'u-lāt) to introduce a cannula, which may be left in place.

cannulation (kan"u-la'shun) the insertion of a cannula.

cannulization (kan"u-li-za'shun) cannulation.

canon (kan'un) [L. "rule"] a working rule or formula for use in scientific procedure.

canrenoate potassium (kan-ren'o-āt) chemical name: 17-hydroxy-3-oxo-17α-pregna-4,6-diene-21-carboxylic acid monopotassium salt; an aldosterone antagonist, $C_{22}H_{29}KO_4$.

canrenone (kan-ren'ōn) chemical name: 17-hydroxy-3-oxo-17α-pregna-4,6-diene-21-carboxylic acid γ-lactone. An aldosterone antagonist, $C_{22}H_{28}O_3$; called also *phanurane*.

cant (kant) an inclination or slope. **c. of mandible,** the angle formed by the intersection of the mandibular (gonion-gnathion) plane with the sella-nasion or Frankfort plane.

canthal (kan'thal) pertaining to a canthus.

canthariasis (kan"thah-ri'ah-sis) [Gr. *kantharos* beetle] infection by beetles as endoparasites in the body of a mammal, following ingestion of larval or adult forms.

cantharidal (kan-thar'ĭ-dal) containing or pertaining to cantharides.

cantharidate (kan-thar'ĭ-dāt) any salt of cantharidic acid.

cantharides (kan-thar'ĭ-dēz) [L.] the dried Spanish fly, *Lytta (Cantharis) vesicatoria*, sometimes called "blister bug." Cantharides were once applied externally as a powerful rubefacient and blistering agent and given internally as a diuretic and aphrodisiac.

cantharidic acid (kan"thah-rid'ik) a dibasic acid formed when cantharidin dissolves in water.

cantharidin (kan-thar'ĭ-din) the most important active principle of cantharides; it is the lactone of cantharidic acid, $C_{10}H_{12}O_4$, occurs in crystalline form, has a bitter taste, and produces blistering of the skin.

cantharidism (kan-thar′ĭ-dizm)   a morbid condition resulting from the misuse of cantharides.

Cantharis (kan′thah-ris) [L.; Gr. *kantharos* beetle]   *Lytta.* **C. vesicato′ria,** *Lytta vesicatoria.*

canthectomy (kan-thek′to-me) [*canth-* + *ectomy*]   surgical removal of a canthus.

canthi (kan′thi) [L.]   plural of *canthus.*

canthitis (kan-thi′tis)   inflammation of a canthus or of the canthi.

canth(o)- [Gr. *kanthos*]   a combining form denoting relationship to the canthus.

cantholysis (kan-thol′ĭ-sis) [*cantho-* + *lysis*]   surgical division of the canthus of an eye or of a canthal ligament.

canthoplasty (kan′tho-plas″te) [*cantho-* + Gr. *plassein* to form]   plastic surgery of the medial and/or lateral canthus, especially section of the lateral canthus to lengthen the palpebral fissure; also the surgical restoration of a defective canthus.

canthorrhaphy (kan-thor′ah-fe) [*cantho-* + *-rrhaphy*]   the suturing of the palpebral fissure at either canthus.

canthotomy (kan-thot′o-me) [*cantho-* + *-tomy*]   surgical division of the outer canthus.

canthus (kan′thus), pl. *can′thi* [L.; Gr. *kanthos*]   the angle at either end of the fissure between the eyelids; the canthi are distinguished as outer or temporal, inner or nasal.

Cantil (kan′til)   trademark for a preparation of mepenzolate bromide.

Cantor tube (kan′tor) [Meyer O. *Cantor,* American physician, born 1907]   see under *tube.*

cantus galli (kan′tus gal′li) [L. "cock-crowing"]   laryngismus stridulus.

canula (kan′u-lah)   cannula.

CaO   calcium oxide.

Ca(OH)₂   calcium hydroxide.

caoutchouc (koo′chōōk) [Fr.]   gum-elastic or India rubber; the concrete juice of various trees and plants, such as *Siphonia elastica.* It is a hydrocarbon, $C_{20}H_{32}$, soluble in chloroform, ether, and carbon disulfide. Called also *elastica.*

C.A.P.   College of American Pathologists.

Cap.   abbreviation for L. *ca′piat,* let him take.

cap (kap)   1. a protective covering for the head or for a similar structure.   2. colloquial term for an artificial crown. **acrosomal c.,** acrosome. **bishop's c.,** pars superior duodeni. **5′ c.e.c.,** a structure consisting of a 7-methyl-guanosine (m⁷G) residue attached backwards (i.e., 5′ to 5′) by a triphosphate linkage to the 5′ end of primary mRNA transcripts in eukaryotes: In addition, the first and, in some cases, second nucleotide of the mRNA are methylated at the 2′ position of the ribose residue. The 5′ cap protects the mRNA from attack by 5′ exonucleases and also functions in the recognition of the mRNA by ribosomes. **cradle c.,** crusta lactea. **duodenal c.,** see under *ampulla.* **dutch c.,** a contraceptive cervical diaphragm. **enamel c.,** a caplike structure of the enamel organ, developed during the third month of fetal development, and composed of an outer layer and an inner enamel layer; between the two layers are looser ectodermal cells that become the stellate reticulum. Called also *germinal c.* **germinal c.,** enamel c. **head c.,** the double-layed caplike structure over the upper two-thirds of the acrosome of a spermatozoon, consisting of the collapsed acrosomal vesicle. **head c., anterior,** acrosome. **knee c.,** patella. **metanephric c's,** masses of metanephric blastema that adhere to the primordial pelvis of the kidney and to its ampullary dilatations. **phrygian c.,** the cholecystographic appearance of the gallbladder showing kinking between the body and the fundus, in which the fundus is fixed and folded. **polar c.,** a chromophilic, saclike organelle occurring beneath the spore wall in the polar region of microsporidian protozoa. Called also *polar capsule.* **postnuclear c.,** a broad band encircling the postacrosomal region of the nucleus of a spermatozoon. **pyloric c.,** pars superior duodeni. **root c.,** a thimble-shaped group of cells forming a protective covering over the apical meristem in the tip of a plant root. **skull c.,** calvaria. **c. of Zinn,** a prominence of the pulmonary arc in the left upper portion of the cardiac silhouette, usually seen in posteroanterior roentgenograms in cases of patent ductus arteriosus, and representing the dilated pulmonary artery.

capacitance (kah-pas′ĭ-tans)   1. the property of being able to store an electric charge.   2. the ratio of the charge stored by a capacitor to the voltage across the capacitor. Symbol *C.* Formerly called *capacity.* **membrane c.,** the electrical capacitance of a cell membrane, as of an axon or muscle fiber.

capacitation (kah-pas″ĭ-ta′shun)   the process by which spermatozoa become capable of fertilizing an ovum after it reaches the ampullary portion of the uterine tube.

capacitor (kah-pas′ĭ-tor)   a device for holding and storing charges of electricity.

capacity (kah-pas′ĭ-te) [L. *capacitas,* from *capere* to take]   1. power or ability to hold, retain, or contain, or the ability to absorb.   2. an expression of the measurement of material that may be held or contained.   3. capacitance.   4. mental ability to receive, accomplish, endure, or understand. **cranial c.,** an expression of the amount of space within the cranium. **diffusing c., diffusion c.,** the ability of the alveolocapillary membrane to transfer gas: a reflection of the thinness and area of the alveolocapillary membrane. It is the amount of gas transferred per minute from the alveolar gas to the pulmonary capillary blood divided by the mean pressure gradient of the gas between the alveolar gas and the capillary blood; unit, ml/min/torr (or mm Hg). Symbol, D. **functional residual c.,** the amount of air remaining at the end of normal quiet respiration; abbreviated FRC. See accompanying illustration. **heat c.,** the amount of heat absorbed in raising a quantity of a substance one degree Celsius at a specified temperature. Symbol C (C_p at constant pressure, C_v at constant volume). **inspiratory c.,** the volume of gas that can be taken into the lungs on a full inspiration, starting from the resting inspiratory position; it is equal to the tidal volume plus the inspiratory reserve volume. Abbreviated IC. See accompanying illustration. **maximal breathing c.,** the greatest volume of gas that can be breathed per minute by voluntary effort; abbreviated MBC. **maximal tubular excretory c.,** see *tubular maximum,* under *maximum.* **molar heat c.,** the amount of heat absorbed in raising one mole of a substance one degree celsius at a specified temperature. **respiratory c.,** the ability of the blood to absorb oxygen from the lungs and carbon dioxide from the tissues. **specific heat c.,** the amount of heat absorbed in raising one gram of a substance one degree Celsius at a specified temperature. Symbol c (c_p at constant pressure, c_v at constant volume). **thermal c.,** the amount of heat absorbed by a body in being raised from 15° to 16° C. in temperature; called also *heat c.* **total lung c.,** the volume of gas contained in the lungs at the end of a maximal inspiration; abbreviated TLC. See accompanying illustration. **virus neutralizing c.,** the ability of a serum to inhibit the

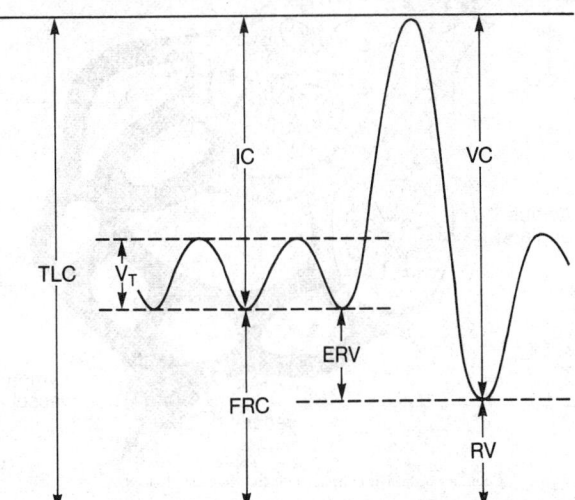

Subdivisions of total lung capacity: *TLC,* total lung capacity; *V,* tidal volume; *IC,* inspiratory capacity; *FRC,* functional residual capacity; *ERV,* expiratory reserve volume; *VC,* vital capacity; *RV,* residual volume.

infectivity of a virus. **vital c.,** the volume of gas that can be expelled from the lungs from a position of full inspiration, with no limit to the duration of expiration; it is equal to the inspiratory capacity plus the expiratory reserve volume. See accompanying illustration.

Capastat (kap′ah-stat)   trademark for a preparation of capreomycin sulfate.

capelet (kap′e-let) [L. *capelletum*]   a swelling on the point of a horse's hock or on its elbow; called also *capulet*.

capeline (kap′ĕ-lin) [Fr.]   a cap-shaped bandage for the head or for the stump of an amputated limb.

Capgras syndrome (kap′grah) [Jean Marie Joseph *Capgras*, French psychiatrist, 1873–1950]   see under *syndrome*.

capillarectasia (kap″ĭ-lār″ek-ta′se-ah) [*capillary* + Gr. *ektasis* distention]   dilatation of capillaries.

Capillaria (kap″ĭ-la′re-ah)   a genus of nematodes of the superfamily Trichuroidea; called also *Hepaticola* and *Trichosoma*.   **C. contor′ta,** a roundworm parasitic in domestic fowls; called also *Trichosoma contortum*.   **C. hepat′ica,** a species parasitic in the liver tissue of rats and of a wide variety of other mammals; a few human infections have been reported.   **C. philippinen′sis,** a parasite of the human intestine in Luzon, causing severe diarrhea, malabsorption, and high mortality.

capillariasis (kap″ĭ-lah-ri′ah-sis)   infection with nematodes of the genus *Capillaria*, especially *C. philippinensis*.

capillariomotor (kap″ĭ-lār″e-o-mo′tor)   pertaining to the functional activity of the capillaries.

capillarioscopy (kap″ĭ-lār″e-os′ko-pe)   capillaroscopy.

capillaritis (kap″ĭ-lār-i′tis)   inflammation of the capillaries.

capillarity (kap″ĭ-lār′ĭ-te)   the action by which the surface of a liquid where it is in contact with a solid, as in capillary tubes, is elevated or depressed.

capillaropathy (kap″ĭ-lār-op′ah-the) [*capillary* + Gr. *pathos* disease]   any disease of the capillaries.

capillaroscopy (kap″ĭ-lār-os′ko-pe) [*capillary* + Gr. *skopein* to examine]   diagnostic examination of the capillaries with the microscope.

capillary (kap′ĭ-lār″e) [L. *capillaris* hair-like]   1. pertaining to or resembling a hair.   2. any one of the minute vessels that connect the arterioles and venules, forming a network in nearly all parts of the body. Their walls act as semipermeable membranes for the interchange of various substances, including fluids, between the blood and tissue fluid; called also *vas capillare* [NA].   3. vas lymphocapillare.   **arterial c's,**

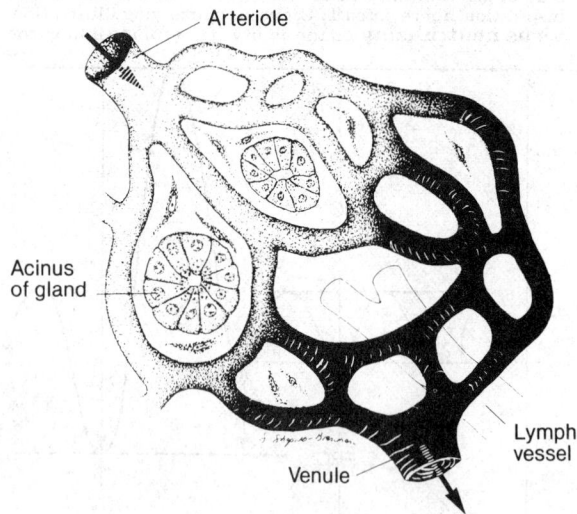

Capillary bed. Lighter areas indicate oxygenated blood.

minute vessels lacking a continuous muscular coat, intermediate in structure and location between arterioles and capillaries; called also *precapillaries, precapillary arterioles,* and *metarterioles*.   **bile c's,** 1. bile canaliculi.   2. a term sometimes used to designate the cholangioles.   **continuous c's,** one of the two major types of capillaries found in

muscle, skin, lung, central nervous system, and other tissues, characterized by the presence of an uninterrupted endothelium and a continuous basal lamina, and by fine filaments and numerous pinocytotic vesicles. Cf. *fenestrated c's*.   **erythrocytic c's,** capillaries of the bone marrow of early life which seem to produce erythrocytes.   **fenestrated c's,** one of the two major types of capillaries, found in the intestinal mucosa, renal glomeruli, pancreas, endocrine glands, and other tissues, and characterized by the presence of circular fenestrae or pores that penetrate the endothelium; these pores may be closed by a very thin diaphragm. Cf. *continuous c's*.   **glomerular c.,** any of the capillaries of a renal glomerulus.   **lymph c., lymphatic c.,** vas lymphocapillare.   **Meigs' c's,** capillaries in the myocardium.   **secretory c's,** any of the extremely fine intercellular canaliculi situated between adjacent gland cells, such as the gastric parietal cells, being formed by the apposition of grooves in the surfaces of the cells, and opening into the gland's lumen.   **sheathed c's,** see under *artery*.   **sinusoidal c.,** vas sinusoideum.   **venous c's,** minute vessels lacking a muscular coat, intermediate in structure and location between venules and capillaries; called also *postcapillaries* and *postcapillary venules*.

capilli (kah-pil′li) [L.]   plural of *capillus*.

capillitium (kap″ĭ-lish′e-um) [L. "head of hair"]   a filamentous structure that interlaces among the spores in the fruiting bodies of certain bacteria (Myxobacterales), protozoa (Eumycetozoa), and fungi (Gasteromycetas).

capillomotor (kap″ĭ-lo-mo′tor)   capillariomotor.

capillus (kah-pil′lus), pl. *capil′li* [L.]   a hair; used in the plural, in anatomical terminology, especially to designate the aggregate of hair on the scalp.

capistration (kap″ĭ-stra′shun) [L. *capistratus* masked]   phimosis.

capita (kap′ĭ-tah) [L.]   plural of *caput*.

capital (kap′ĭ-tal)   1. of the highest importance; involving danger to life.   2. of or pertaining to the head of the femur.

capitate (kap′ĭ-tāt) [L. *caput* head]   head-shaped.

capitation (kap″ĭ-ta′shun)   the annual fee paid to a physician or group of physicians by each participant in a health plan.

capitatum (kap″ĭ-ta′tum) [L. "having a head"]   the capitate bone, or os capitatum [NA].

capitellum (kap″ĭ-tel′um) [L. dim. of *caput* head]   capitulum humeri.

capitonnage (kap″ĭ-to-nahzh′) [Fr.]   the surgical closure of a cyst cavity by applying sutures in such a way as to cause approximation of the opposing surfaces.

capitopedal (kap″ĭ-to-ped′al)   pertaining to the head and foot.

Capitrol (kap′ĭ-trol)   trademark for a preparation of chloroxine.

capitula (kah-pit′u-lah) [L.]   plural of *capitulum*.

capitular (kah-pit′u-lar)   pertaining to a capitulum or head of a bone.

capitulum (kah-pit′u-lum), pl. *capit′ula* [L. dim. of *caput*]   1. a general term for a little head, or a small eminence on a bone by which it articulates with another bone; in NA applied only to the distal end of the humerus, since that bone already possesses a head (caput).   2. a bulbous, knoblike, or enlarged terminal protuberance of a body or part, such as: (*a*) the movable head zone bearing the mouth parts of an acarine (called also *gnathosoma*); (*b*) the calcareous framework enclosing the mantle and body of a barnacle; (*c*) the end of an insect's antennae; (*d*) the proximal ends of the nematodesmata of certain ciliate protozoa of the superclass Hyperstomatia, which may be prominent and toothlike; or (*e*) the anterior end of the axostyle of certain zooflagellates, containing the nucleus of the organism.   **c. cos′tae,** caput costae.   **c. fib′ulae,** caput fibulae.   **c. hu′meri** [NA], **c. of humerus,** an eminence on the distal end of the lateral epicondyle of the humerus for articulation with the head of the radius; called also *capitellum* and *little* or *radial head of humerus*.   **c. mal′lei,** caput mallei.   **c. [proces′sus condyloi′dei] mandib′ulae,** caput mandibulae.   **c. ra′dii,** caput radii.   **c. sta′pedis,** caput stapedis.   **c. ul′nae,** caput ulnae.

Capla (kap′lah)   trademark for a preparation of mebutamate.

capneic (kap′ne-ik) [Gr. *kapnos* smoke] increased carbon dioxide in the atmosphere.

capn(o)- [Gr. *kapnos* smoke] a combining form signifying a sooty or smoky appearance.

Capnocytophaga (kap″no-si-tof′ah-gah) [*capno-* + Gr. *kytos* cell + *phagein* to eat] a genus of gram-negative, facultatively anaerobic, rod-shaped or fusiform bacteria of uncertain affiliation, which occur in normal and diseased sites of the human oral cavity. It has also been associated with systemic disease in debilitated persons. It includes the species *C. gingivalis*, *C. ochraceus* (called also *Bacteroides ochraceus*), and *C. sputigena*.

capnohepatography (kap″no-hep″ah-tog′rah-fe) radiography of the liver after intravenous injection of carbon dioxide gas.

capnophilic (kap-no-fil′ik) [Gr. *kapnos* smoke + *philein* to love] growing best in the presence of carbon dioxide; said of bacteria.

Ca₃(PO₄)₂ $Ca_3(PO_4)_2$ tribasic calcium phosphate.

capobenate sodium (kap-o-ben′āt) chemical name: 6-[(3,4,5-trimethoxybenzoyl) amino]hexanoic acid monosodium salt. The monosodium salt of capobenic acid, $C_{16}H_{22}NNaO_6$, having cardiac depressant activity; used as an antiarrhythmic.

capobenic acid (kap-oh-ben′ik) a vasodilator used in the treatment and prevention of myocardial infarction.

capon (ka′pon) a castrated domestic fowl.

caponize (ka′pon-īz) to castrate, especially male domestic fowl.

capotement (kah-pōt-maw′) [Fr.] a splashing sound heard in the dilated stomach.

cappie (kap′e) a disease of young sheep characterized by thinning of the bones of the scalp, possibly due to phosphorus-deficient diet.

capping (kap′ing) 1. the provision of a protective or obstructive covering. 2. the movement of cell surface antigens into a small region (cap) on the cell surface owing to the cross linking of antigens by specific antibody. 3. in restorative dental procedures: (*a*) covering of tooth cusps weakened by caries with a protective metal overlay; see *cusp restoration,* under *restoration;* (*b*) colloquial term for replacement of the crown of a natural tooth with an artificial crown (cap). **pulp c.,** covering of an exposed or nearly exposed pulp with a dressing or cement to protect the pulp against further injury and to provide an environment for healing and repair processes. In *direct capping,* the dressing is placed directly over the pulp at the site of exposure. In *indirect capping,* it is placed over a thin partition of remaining dentin, which if removed, might expose the dental pulp.

caprate (kap′rāt) any salt of capric acid.

capreolary (kap′re-o-la″re) capreolate.

capreolate (kap′re-o-lāt) tendril shaped, like the spermatic vessels.

capreomycin (kap″re-o-mi′sin) a polypeptide antibiotic produced by *Streptomyces capreolus*, which is active against human strains of *Mycobacterium tuberculosis* and has four microbiologically active components. **c. sulfate, sterile** [USP], the disulfate salt of capreomycin, occurring as a white to practically white, amorphous powder; used as a tuberculostatic, administered intramuscularly.

capric acid (kap′rik) trivial name for the 10-carbon, straight chain, saturated fatty acid; systematic name: *decanoic acid*.

caprillic (kah-pril′ik) [L. *caper* goat] goatlike; said of sounds resembling the bleating of a goat.

capriloquism (kah-pril′o-kwizm) [L. *caper* goat + *loqui* to speak] egophony.

caprin (kap′rin) any one of the caprates of glycerin (glycerol) especially the glyceryl tricaprate, or tricaprin, C_3H_5-[$CH_3(CH_2)_8COO]_3$, from ordinary butter.

caprine (kap′rin) [L. *caper* goat] 1. pertaining to or derived from a goat. 2. norleucine.

Capripoxvirus (kap″ri-poks′vi-rus) a genus of the family Poxviridae, subfamily Chordopoxvirinae, which includes the sheep pox virus, goat pox virus, and lumpy skin disease virus.

caprizant (kap′ri-zant) [L. *caprizans,* from *caper* a goat] leaping or bounding (like a goat); said of the pulse.

caproate (kap′ro-āt) 1. any salt of caproic acid. 2. USAN contraction for hexanoate.

caproic acid (kah-pro′ik) trivial name for the 6-carbon, straight chain, saturated fatty acid; systematic name: *hexanoic acid*.

caproin (kah-pro′in) any caproate of glycerin (glycerol) especially the tricaproate, $C_3H_5(C_6H_{13}O_2)_3$; it occurs in butter.

caprone (kap′rōn) a volatile oil, di-*n*-amylketone 6-undecanone, $CH_3(CH_2)_4 \cdot CO(CH_2)_4 \cdot CH_3$, from butter.

caproyl (kap-ro′il) the hydrocarbon radical, C_6H_{13}; hexyl.

caproylamine (kap″ro-il-am′in) n-hexylamine.

caprylate (kap′ri-lāt) any salt of caprylic acid.

caprylic acid (kah-pril′ik) trivial name for the 8-carbon, straight-chain, saturated fatty acid; systematic name: *octanoic acid*.

caprylin (kap′ri-lin) any caprylate of glycerin (glycerol) especially the tricaprylate, $C_3H_5(C_7H_{15}CO_2)_3$.

capsaicin (kap-sa′ĭ-sin) the pungent active principle in capsicum.

Capsebon (kap′se-bon) trademark for a suspension of cadmium sulfide.

Capsicum (kap′sĭ-kum) [L.] a genus of solanaceous plants of various species, including the cayenne or red pepper.

capsicum (kap′sĭ-kum) the dried fruit of various species of *Capsicum*, used as an irritant and carminative. It is known in commerce as African chillies (*C. frutescens*), tabasco pepper (*C. annum* var. *conoidis*), Louisiana long pepper (*C. annum* var. *longum*), and Louisiana sport pepper (a hybrid).

capsid (kap′sid) [L. *capsa* a box] the shell of protein that protects the nucleic acid of a virus; it may have helical or cubic symmetry and is composed of structural units, or capsomers. According to the number of subunits possessed by capsomers, they are called dimers (2), trimers (3), pentamers (5), or hexamers (6).

capsitis (kap-si′tis) inflammation of the capsule of the crystalline lens.

capsomer (kap′so-mer) [L. *capsa* a box + Gr. *meros* part] the morphological unit of the capsid of a virus.

capsomere (kap′so-mēr) capsomer.

capsotomy (kap-sot′o-me) capsulotomy.

Capsul. abbreviation for L. *cap′sula,* capsule.

capsula (kap′su-lah), pl. *cap′sulae* [L. "a small box"] [NA] a general term for a cartilaginous, fatty, fibrous, or membranous structure enveloping another structure, organ, or part; called also *capsule.* **c. adipo′sa,** a capsule consisting principally of fat. **c. adipo′sa re′nis** [NA], adipose capsule of kidney: the investment of perirenal fat surrounding the fibrous capsule of the kidney and continuous at the hilus with the fat in the renal sinus; called also *fatty capsule of kidney* and *perinephric* or *perirenal fat.* **c. articula′ris** [NA], articular capsule: the sac-like envelope which encloses the cavity of a synovial joint by attaching to the circumference of the articular end of each involved bone; it consists of a fibrous membrane and a synovial membrane. Called also *joint* or *synovial capsule.* **c. articula′ris acromioclavicula′ris** [NA], acromioclavicular articular capsule: a ligamentous sac surrounding the acromioclavicular joint. **c. articula′ris articulatio′nis tar′si transver′sae** [NA], a ligamentous sac surrounding the transverse tarsal joint. **c. articula′ris articulatio′nis temporomandibula′ris** [NA], a ligamentous sac surrounding the temporomandibular joint; called also *c. articularis mandibulae* and *capsule of temporomandibular joint.* **c. articula′ris articulatio′num vertebra′rum** [NA], capsule of vertebral articulations: one of the bands of tissue, partly white fibrous and partly yellow elastic, that unite the articular processes of adjacent vertebrae. **c. articula′ris atlantoaxia′lis latera′lis** [NA], atlantoaxial articular capsule: a ligamentous sac surrounding the lateral atlantoaxial joint; called also (pl.) *capsulae articulares atlantoepistrophicae.* **cap′sulae articula′res atlantoepistro′phicae,** see *c. articularis atlantoaxialis lateralis.* **c. articula′ris atlantooccipita′lis** [NA], capsule of atlantooccipital articulation: one of a pair of distinct ligamentous bands, each of which is attached at one end to the lateral mass of the atlas and at the other end to the margins of an occipital condyle. **c. articula′ris calcaneocuboi′dea** [NA], capsule of calcaneocuboidal joint: a ligamentous sac surrounding the calcaneocuboidal joint. **c. articula′ris capi′tis cos′-**

tae [NA], articular capsule of head of rib: a ligamentous sac surrounding the articulation of the head of a rib; called also *capsulae articulares capituli costae.* **cap′sulae ar-ticula′res capit′uli cos′tae,** see *c. articularis capitis costae.* **cap′sulae articula′res carpometacar′peae** [NA], capsules of carpometacarpal joints: ligamentous sacs surrounding the carpometacarpal joints; they are continuous with the capsules of the intercarpal joints. **c. articula′-ris carpometacar′pea pol′licis** [NA], capsule of carpo-metacarpal articulation of thumb: a ligamentous sac sur-rounding the carpometacarpal joint of the thumb. **c. ar-ticula′ris costotransversa′ria** [NA], capsule of costo-transverse joint: a ligamentous sac surrounding the costotransverse articulation. **c. articula′ris cox′ae** [NA], capsule of hip joint: a large, strong ligamentous sac surrounding the hip joint. **c. articula′ris cricoarytenoi′dea** [NA], cricoarytenoid articular cap-sule: the fibrous and synovial layers enclosing the cricoaryt-enoid joint; called also *c. articularis cricoarytaenoidea.* **c. articula′ris cricothyroi′dea** [NA], the capsule of the cricothyroid joint; called also *c. articularis cricothyreoidea.* **c. articula′ris cu′biti** [NA], articular capsule of elbow: the capsule formed around the cubital articulation by its various ligaments. **cap′sulae articula′res digito′-rum man′us,** capsulae articulares interphalangearum manus. **cap′sulae articula′res digito′rum pe′dis,** capsulae articulares interphalangearum pedis. **c. ar-ticula′ris ge′nus** [NA], capsule of knee joint: the loose, thin, but strong sac enclosing the knee joint; called also *c. articularis genu.* **c. articula′ris hu′meri** [NA], articu-lar capsule of humerus: a ligamentous sac surrounding the shoulder joint. **cap′sulae articula′res inter-metacar′peae** [NA], capsules of intermetacarpal joints: ligamentous sacs that surround the intermetacarpal joints; they are continuous with the capsules of the carpometacarpal joints. **cap′sulae articula′res intermetatar′seae** [NA], capsules of intermetatarsal joints: the capsules around the four joints between the bases of the metatarsal bones. **cap′sulae articula′res interphalangea′rum man′us** [NA], capsules of interphalangeal joints of hand: incomplete ligamentous sacs surrounding the interphalan-geal joints of the hand; called also *capsulae articulares digitorum manus.* **cap′sulae articula′res inter-phalangea′rum pe′dis** [NA], capsules of interphalan-geal joints of foot: the capsules surrounding the interphalan-geal articulations of the toes; called also *capsulae articulares digitorum pedis.* **c. articula′ris mandib′ulae,** c. arti-cularis articulationis temporomandibularis. **c. articula′-ris man′us** [NA], a loose ligamentous sac surrounding the radiocarpal joint and the intercarpal joints together; called also *capsule of radiocarpal joint.* **cap′sulae ar-ticula′res metacarpophalan′geae** [NA], capsules of metacarpophalangeal joints: ligamentous sacs that surround the metacarpophalangeal joints. **cap′sulae ar-ticula′res metatarsophalan′geae** [NA], capsules of metatarsophalangeal joints: the five capsules surrounding the metatarsophalangeal articulations. **c. articula′ris os′sis pisifor′mis** [NA], articular capsule of pisiform bone: a thin, loose ligamentous sac surrounding the joint of the pisiform bone. **c. articula′ris radioulna′ris dis-ta′lis** [NA], distal radioulnar articular capsule: a loose liga-mentous sac surrounding the distal radioulnar joint. **c. articula′ris sternoclavicula′ris** [NA], capsule of ster-noclavicular joint: a ligamentous sac surrounding the sterno-clavicular joint. **c. articula′ris sternocosta′lis** [NA], sternocostal articular capsule: the ligamentous sac that surrounds a sternocostal joint. **c. articula′ris talocal-ca′nea** [NA], a loose ligamentous sac surrounding the sub-talar joint; called also *capsule of subtalar joint.* **c. ar-ticula′ris talocrura′lis** [NA], a thin ligamentous sac surrounding the ankle joint; called also *capsule of ankle joint.* **c. articula′ris talonavicula′ris,** a capsule surrounding the talonavicular joint. **cap′sulae articula′res tar-sometatar′seae** [NA], capsules of tarsometatarsal joints: the three capsules that surround the joints between the metatarsal and cuneiform bones. **c. articula′ris tibi-ofibula′ris** [NA], capsule of tibiofibular joint: a fibrous sac enclosing the tibiofibular articulation. **c. bul′bi,** vagina bulbi. **c. cor′dis,** pericardium. **c. exter′na** [NA], ex-ternal capsule: the thin layer of white substance that separates the lateral part of the lentiform nucleus (putamen) from the claustrum. **c. extre′ma** [NA], the white matter between the claustrum and the cortex of the insula. **c. fi-**

bro′sa, a capsule consisting largely of fibrous elements. **c. fibro′sa glan′dulae thyroi′deae** [NA], fibrous cap-sule of thyroid gland: a connective tissue coat intimately adherent to the underlying gland; called also *c. glandulae thyroideae.* **c. fibro′sa [Glisso′ni], c. fibro′sa hep′atis,** c. fibrosa perivascularis. **c. fibro′sa peri-vascula′ris** [NA], perivascular fibrous capsule: the connec-tive tissue sheath that accompanies the vessels and ducts through the hepatic portal. It is continuous with the fibrous coat. Called also *c. fibrosa hepatis, fibrous capsule of liver, Glisson's capsule, hepatobiliary capsule,* and *c. fibrosa [Glis-soni].* **c. fibro′sa re′nis** [NA], fibrous capsule of kid-ney: the connective tissue investment of the kidney, which continues through the hilus to line the renal sinus; called also *tunica fibrosa renis.* **c. gan′glii** [NA], capsule of gan-glion: the laminated connective tissue capsule surrounding a neural ganglion and continuous with epineurium of its associated nerve root. **c. glan′dulae thyroi′deae,** c. fibrosa glandulae thyroideae. **c. glomer′uli** [NA], cap-sule of glomerulus: the double-walled globular dilatation that forms the beginning of a uriniferous tubule of the kidney and surrounds the glomerulus; it consists of an inner, or visceral, layer (*capsular epithelium*) and an outer, or parietal, layer (*glomerular epithelium*); called also *Bowman's, glomerular, malpighian,* and *müllerian capsule.* **c. inter′na** [NA], in-ternal capsule: a fanlike mass of white fibers that separates the lentiform nucleus laterally from the head of the caudate nucleus, the dorsal thalamus, and the tail of the caudate nucleus medially; it consists of an anterior limb, a genu, and a posterior limb consisting of three parts, thalamolenticular, sublenticular, and retrolenticular. The internal capsule carries both afferent and efferent fibers of the cerebral cortex. **c. len′tis** [NA], capsule of lens: the elastic enve-lope covering the lens of the eye and fusing with the fibers of the ciliary zonule; called also *crystalline capsule* and *phaco-cyst.* **c. nu′clei denta′ti,** a layer formed by fibers pass-ing to and from the dentate nucleus. **cap′sulae nu′clei lentifor′mis,** see *c. externa* and *c. interna.* **c. pan-crea′tis,** capsule of pancreas: a thin sheath of areolar tissue that invests the pancreas (but does not form a definite capsule), the septa of which extend into the gland and divide it into lobules. **c. prosta′tica** [NA], capsule of prostate: the fibroelastic capsule, containing an extensive plexus of veins, that surrounds the prostate. **cap′sulae re′nis,** see *c. adiposa renis* and *c. fibrosa renis.* **c. sero′sa lie′nis,** tunica serosa lienis. **c. tonsilla′ris** [NA], ton-sillar capsule: a fibrous capsule covering the lateral surface of the palatine tonsils and separating them from the underly-ing connective tissue.

capsulae (kap′su-le) [L.] plural of *capsula.*

capsular (kap′su-lar) pertaining to a capsule.

capsulation (kap″su-la′shun) the enclosure of a medicine in a capsule.

capsule (kap′sūl) [L. *capsula* a little box] 1. a structure in which something is enclosed, such as a hard or a soft, soluble container of a suitable substance, for enclosing a dose of medicine. 2. an anatomical structure enclosing an organ or body part; see *capsula.* **adherent c.,** an investing struc-ture that is not readily separated from the organ or substance contained within it. **adipose c.,** one consisting largely of fat. **adrenal c.,** adrenal gland (glandula suprarenalis [NA]). **adrenal c′s, accessory,** accessory adrenal glands (glandulae suprarenales accessoriae [NA]). **articu-lar c.,** the sac-like envelope which encloses the cavity of a synovial joint; see *capsula articularis,* and for names of capsules of particular joints see other entries beginning *capsula articularis,* under *capsula.* Called also *joint c.* and *synovial c.* **articular c., fibrous,** membrana fibrosa capsulae articularis. **auditory c.,** the cartilaginous cap-sule of the embryo that develops into the bony labyrinth of the inner ear. **bacterial c.,** an envelope of gel surround-ing a bacterial cell, usually polysaccharide but sometimes polypeptide in nature, which is associated with the virulence of pathogenic bacteria. **biopsy c.,** a device which may be passed into the intestine for the purpose of securing speci-mens of the mucosa for examination under the microscope. **Bonnet's c.,** vagina bulbi. **Bowman's c.,** capsula glo-meruli. **c's of the brain,** layers of white matter in the cerebrum; see *capsula externa* and *capsula interna.* **brood c's,** capsular projections from the internal mem-brane of hydatid cysts, from which the scoleces arise. **cartilage c.,** a basophilic zone of cartilage matrix bordering on a lacuna and its enclosed cartilage cell. **central c.**, a structure seen in certain protozoa of the superclass Actinopoda, such as radiolarians, that encloses the central nucleated core of cytoplasm and is surrounded by a membrane perforated to permit communication with the outer cortex (*calymma*). **Crosby c.**, an instrument used to obtain intestinal material for biopsy, consisting of a cylindrical capsule containing a knife which is spring-activated and triggered by suction. **crystalline c.**, capsula lentis. **decavitamin c.** [USP], a capsule containing not less than 1.2 mg. of vitamin A, 10 μg. of vitamin D, 70 mg. of ascorbic acid, 10 mg. of calcium pantothenate, 1 μg. of cyanocobalamin, 50 μg. of folic acid, 20 mg. of niacinamide, 2 mg. of pyridoxine hydrochloride, 2 mg. of riboflavin, 2 mg. of thiamine hydrochloride or its equivalent as thiamine mononitrate, and a suitable form of alpha tocopherol. It is used as a dietary supplement. **external c.**, capsula externa. **extreme c.**, capsula extrema. **fatty c. of kidney**, capsula adiposa renis. **fibrous c.**, one composed chiefly of fibrous elements. **fibrous c. of corpora cavernosa of penis**, tunica albuginea corporum cavernosorum penis. **fibrous c. of graafian follicle**, tunica externa thecae folliculi. **fibrous c. of kidney**, capsula fibrosa renis. **fibrous c. of liver**, capsula fibrosa perivascularis. **fibrous c. of spleen**, tunica fibrosa lienis. **fibrous c. of testis**, tunica albuginea testis. **fibrous c. of thyroid gland**, capsula fibrosa glandulae thyroideae. **c. of ganglion**, capsula ganglii. **Gerota's c.**, fascia renalis. **Glisson's c.**, capsula fibrosa perivascularis. **glomerular c.**, **c. of glomerulus**, capsula glomeruli. **Hearson's c.** (*obs.*), a thermostatic chamber for regulating the temperature in incubators. **c. of heart**, pericardium. **hepatobiliary c.**, capsula fibrosa perivascularis. **hexavitamin c.** [NF], a capsule containing not less than 1.5 mg. of vitamin A, 10 μg. of vitamin D, 75 mg. of ascorbic acid, 2 mg. of thiamine hydrochloride or an equivalent amount of thiamine mononitrate, 3 mg. of riboflavine, and 20 mg. of niacinamide; used as a dietary supplement. **internal c.**, capsula interna. **joint c.**, articular c.; see also under *capsula articularis*. **c. of lens**, capsula lentis. **malpighian c.**, capsula glomeruli. **Müller c.**, **müllerian c.**, capsula glomeruli. **ocular c.**, vagina bulbi. **optic c.**, the embryonic structure from which the sclera is developed. **otic c.**, the skeletal element enclosing the inner ear mechanism. In the human embryo, it develops as cartilage at various ossification centers and becomes completely bony and unified at about the twenty-third week of fetal life. **c. of pancreas**, capsula pancreatis. **pelvioprostatic c.**, fascia prostatae. **perinephric c.**, see *capsula adiposa renis* and *capsula fibrosa renis*. **periotic c.**, the tissue surrounding the otic sac in the embryo. **polar c.**, 1. any of the thick-walled vesicles seen in the spores of certain protozoa and containing the polar filament. 2. see under *cap.* **c. of prostate**, capsula prostatica. **radiotelemetering c.**, telemetering c. **renal c.**, see *capsula adiposa renis* and *capsula fibrosa renis*. **serous c. of spleen**, tunica serosa lienis. **sodium iodide** ¹³¹I **c's**, capsules containing radioactive iodine as sodium iodide, used in tests of thyroid disease and in the suppression of thyroid function. **suprarenal c.**, adrenal gland (glandula suprarenalis [NA]). **synovial c.**, articular c. (capsula articularis [NA]). **telemetering c.**, a small radio transmitter encased in a capsule the size of an ordinary drug capsule that can be swallowed or otherwise inserted in the body to give information about conditions (pressure, temperature, pH, etc.) within an organ; called also *radio pill*. **Tenon's c.**, vagina bulbi. **tonsillar c.**, capsula tonsillaris. **triasyn B c's**, capsules containing thiamine, riboflavin, and nicotinamide, used as a vitamin supplement.

capsulectomy (kap″su-lek′to-me) [*capsule* + *-ectomy*] excision of a capsule, especially a joint capsule or the capsule of the lens. **renal c.**, excision of the capsule of the kidney.

capsulitis (kap″su-li′tis) the inflammation of a capsule, as that of the lens, joint, liver, or labyrinth. **adhesive c.**, adhesive inflammation between the joint capsule and the peripheral articular cartilage of the shoulder with obliteration of the subdeltoid bursa, characterized by painful shoulder of gradual onset, with increasing pain, stiffness, and limitation of motion. Called also *adhesive bursitis, peritendinitis*, or *tendinitis, frozen shoulder*, and *periarthritis of shoulder*. **hepatic c.**, perihepatitis.

capsulolenticular (kap″su-lo-len-tik′u-lar) pertaining to the lens of the eye and its capsule.

capsuloma (kap″su-lo′mah) a capsular or subcapsular tumor of the kidney.

capsuloplasty (kap′su-lo-plas″te) [*capsule* + Gr. *plassein* to form] a plastic operation on a joint capsule.

capsulorrhaphy (kap″su-lor′ah-fe) [*capsule* + Gr. *raphē* suture] suturing of a capsule, especially a joint capsule.

capsulotome (kap-su′lo-tōm) [*capsule* + *-tome*] a cutting instrument used for incising the capsules of the lens.

capsulotomy (kap″su-lot′o-me) [*capsule* + *-tomy*] the incision of a capsule, especially of that of the eye, as in cataract operation, or that of a joint. **renal c.**, incision of a renal capsule.

captamine hydrochloride (kap′tah-mēn) chemical name: 2-(dimethylamino)ethanethiol hydrochloride; a depigmenting agent, $C_4H_{11}NS \cdot HCl$.

captodiame hydrochloride (kap-to-di′am) captodiamine hydrochloride.

captodiamine hydrochloride (kap″to-di′ah-mēn) chemical name: 2[[[4-(butylthio)phenyl]phenylmethyl]thio]-*N,N*-dimethylethamine hydrochloride. A tranquilizer and muscle relaxant, $C_{21}H_{29}NS_2HCl$, used as a sedative. Called also *captodiame hydrochloride*.

captopril (kap′to-pril) a drug that inhibits the activity of angiotensin-converting enzymes, thus preventing the conversion of angiotensin I to the active form, angiotensin II; used as an antihypertensive agent.

capulet (kap′u-let) capelet.

capuride (kap′ur-īd) chemical name: *N*-(aminocarbonyl)-2-ethylmethylpentamide; a hypnotic, $C_9H_{18}N_2O_2$.

caput (kap′ut), pl. *cap′ita* [L. "head"] [NA] 1. the superior extremity of the body, comprising the cranium and face, and containing the brain, the organs of special sense, and the first organs of the digestive system; the head. 2. a general term applied to the expanded or chief extremity of an organ or part. **c. angula′re mus′culi quadra′ti la′bii superio′ris**, musculus levator labii superioris alaeque nasi. **c. bre′ve mus′culi bicip′itis bra′chii** [NA], the short head of the biceps brachii muscle, arising from the apex of the coracoid process; called also *medial head of biceps brachii muscle, short head of coracoradialis muscle*, and *coracoradialis*. **c. bre′ve mus′culi bicip′itis fem′oris** [NA], the short head of the biceps femoris muscle, arising from the linea aspera femoris. **c. cor′nus dorsa′lis medul′lae spina′lis** [NA], head of dorsal horn of spinal cord: the oval or fusiform portion of the dorsal horn, or column, of gray substance in the spinal cord between the constricted portion (neck) and the apex of the horn; called also *c. cornus posterioris medullae spinalis* [NA alternative] and *head of posterior horn of spinal cord*. **c. cor′nus posterio′ris medul′lae spina′lis**, NA alternative for *c. cornus dorsalis medullae spinalis*. **c. cos′tae** [NA], head of rib: the posterior end of a rib, which articulates with the body of a vertebra; called also *capitulum costae*. **c. distor′tum**, torticollis. **c. epididym′idis** [NA], head of epididymis: the upper part of the epididymis, in which are found the straight and coiled portions of the efferent ductules of the testis; called also *globus major epididymidis*. **c. fem′oris** [NA], head of femur: the proximal end of the femur, articulating with the hip bone. **c. fib′ulae** [NA], head of fibula: the proximal extremity of the fibula; called also *capitulum fibulae*. **c. gallinag′inis** [L. "woodcock's head"], colliculus seminalis. **c. humera′le mus′culi flexo′ris car′pi ulna′ris** [NA], the humeral head of the flexor carpi ulnaris muscle, arising from the medial epicondyle of the humerus. **c. humera′le mus′culi flexo′ris digito′rum subli′mis**, c. humero-ulnare musculi flexoris digitorum superficialis. **c. humera′le mus′culi pronato′ris tere′tis** [NA], the humeral head of the pronator teres muscle arising from the medial epicondyle of the humerus. **c. humera′lis**, c. humeri. **c. hu′meri** [NA], head of humerus: the proximal end of the humerus, which articulates with the glenoid cavity of the scapula; called also *c. humeralis*. **c. humero-ulna′re mus′culi flexo′ris digito′rum superficia′lis** [NA], the humero-ulnar head of the flexor digitorum superficialis muscle, arising from the medial epicondyle of the humerus and coronoid process of ulna; called also *c. humerale musculi flexoris digitorum sublimis* and *humeral head of flexor* *digitorum sublimis muscle.* **c. infraorbita′le mus′culi quadra′ti la′bii superio′ris,** musculus levator labii superioris. **c. latera′le mus′culi gastrocne′mii** [NA], the lateral head of the gastrocnemius muscle, arising from the lateral condyle and posterior surface of the femur, and the capsule of the knee joint; called also *lateral gastrocnemius muscle.* **c. latera′le mus′culi tricip′itis bra′chii** [NA], the lateral head of the triceps brachii muscle, arising from the posterior surface of the humerus, the lateral border of the humerus, and the lateral intermuscular septum; called also *great* or *second head of triceps brachii muscle,* and *lateral* or *short anconeus muscle.* **c. lie′nis,** extremitas posterior lienis. **c. lon′gum mus′culi bicip′itis bra′chii** [NA], the long head of the biceps brachii muscle, arising from the upper border of the glenoid cavity; called also *interarticular ligament of articulation of humerus.* **c. lon′gum mus′culi bicip′itis fem′oris** [NA], the long head of the biceps femoris muscle, arising from the ischial tuberosity. **c. lon′gum musculi tricip′itis bra′chii** [NA], the long head of the triceps brachii muscle, arising from the infraglenoid tubercle of the scapula; called also *first, middle,* or *scapular head of triceps brachii muscle.* **c. mal′lei** [NA], head of malleus: the upper portion of the malleus, which articulates with the incus; called also *capitulum mallei.* **c. mandib′ulae** [NA], head of mandible: the articular surface of the condyloid process of the mandible; called also *capitulum* [*processus condyloidei*] *mandibulae* and *head of condyloid process of mandible.* **c. media′le mus′culi gastrocne′mii** [NA], the medial head of the gastrocnemius muscle, arising from the medial condyle of the femur and the capsule of the knee joint; called also *medial gastrocnemius muscle.* **c. media′le mus′culi tricip′itis bra′chii** [NA], the medial head of the triceps brachii muscle, arising from the posterior surface of the humerus below the radial groove, the medial border of the humerus, and the medial intermuscular septum; called also *medial anconeus muscle* and *deep* or *short head of triceps brachii muscle.* **c. medu′sae,** Medusa's head: dilated cutaneous veins around the umbilicus, seen mainly in the newborn and in patients suffering with cirrhosis of the liver; so called because the veins resemble the head of the snake-haired Gorgon, Medusa. Called also *cirsomphalos.* **c. metacarpa′lis** [NA], the head of a metacarpal bone, being the distal extremity of each metacarpal, which articulates with the base of a proximal digit. Called also *c. ossis metacarpalis* and *condyle of metacarpal.* **c. metatarsa′lis** [NA], the head of a metatarsal bone, being the distal extremity of each metatarsal, which articulates with the base of a digit. Called also *c. ossis metatarsalis.* **c. mus′culi** [NA], head of muscle: the end of a muscle at the site of its attachment to a bone or other fixed structure (origin). **c. natifor′me,** a head in rickets in which the eminences of the frontal and parietal bones form elevations separated by depressions which mark the lines of the cranial sutures; called also *hot cross bun head.* **c. nu′clei cauda′ti** [NA], head of caudate nucleus: the largest and most anterior part of the caudate nucleus, which bulges into the anterior horn of the lateral ventricle. **c. obli′quum mus′culi adducto′ris hal′lucis** [NA], the oblique head of the adductor hallucis muscle, originating from the bases of the second, third, and fourth metatarsal bones, and the sheath of the peroneus longus muscle; called also *great* or *long head of adductor hallucis muscle.* **c. obli′quum mus′culi adducto′ris pol′licis** [NA], the oblique head of the adductor pollicis muscle, arising from the capitate and trapezoid bones and the base of the second metacarpals. **c. os′sis metacarpa′lis,** c. metacarpalis. **c. os′sis metatarsa′lis,** c. metatarsalis. **c. pancre′atis** [NA], head of pancreas: the discoidal mass forming the enlarged right extremity of the pancreas, lying in a flexure of the duodenum. **c. pe′nis,** glans penis. **c. phalan′gis digito′rum ma′nus** [NA], head of phalanx of fingers: the distal articular surface of each of the proximal and middle phalanges of the fingers; called also *trochlea phalangis digitorum manus.* [NA alternative]. **c. phalan′gis digito′rum pe′dis** [NA], head of phalanx of toes: the distal articular extremity of each of the proximal and middle phalanges of the toes; called also *trochlea phalangis digitorum pedis.* **c. pla′num,** a flattened head occurring with osteochondritis deformans juvenilis. **c. proge′neum,** prognathism. **c. quadra′tum,** an abnormally shaped head, sometimes occurring with rickets. **c. radia′le mus′culi flexo′ris digito′rum superficia′lis** [NA], the radial head of the flexor digitorum superficialis muscle,

arising from the oblique line and anterior border of the radius. **c. ra′dii** [NA], head of radius: the disk on the proximal end of the radius that articulates with the capitulum of the humerus and the radial notch of the ulna; called also *capitulum radii.* **c. rec′tum mus′culi rec′ti fem′oris** [NA], the straight or anterior head of the rectus femoris muscle, arising from the anteroinferior iliac spine, which fuses with the reflected or posterior head and continues down into the belly of the muscle. **c. reflex′um mus′culi rec′ti fem′oris** [NA], the reflected or posterior head of the rectus femoris muscle, arising from a groove above the rim of the acetabulum, which fuses with the straight or anterior head and continues down into the belly of the muscle. **c. stape′dis** [NA], the head of the stapes, which articulates with the incus; called also *capitulum stapedis.* **c. succeda′neum,** edema occurring in and under the fetal scalp during labor. **c. ta′li** [NA], head of talus: the rounded anterior end of the talus; called also *head of astragalus.* **c. transver′sum mus′culi adducto′ris hal′lucis** [NA], the transverse head of the adductor hallucis muscle, arising from the capsules of the metatarso-phalangeal joints of the third, fourth, and fifth toes. **c. transver′sum mus′culi adducto′ris pol′licis** [NA], the transverse head of the adductor pollicis muscle arising from the lower two thirds of the anterior surface of the third metacarpal. **c. ul′nae** [NA], head of ulna: the articular surface of the distal extremity of the ulna; called also *capitulum ulnae.* **c. ulna′re mus′culi flexo′ris car′pi ulna′ris** [NA], the ulnar head of the flexor carpi ulnaris muscle, arising from the olecranon, and the adjacent part of the ulna. **c. ulna′re mus′culi pronato′ris ter′etis** [NA], the ulnar head of the pronator teres muscle, arising from the coronoid process of the ulna; called also *coronoid head of pronator teres muscle.* **c. zygomat′icum mus′culi quadra′ti la′bii superio′ris,** musculus zygomaticus minor.

C.A.R. Canadian Association of Radiologists.

Carabelli cusp (sign, tubercle) (kah-rah-bel′e) [Georg C. *Carabelli,* dentist in Vienna, 1787–1842] see under *cusp.*

caramel (kar′ah-mel, kahr′mel) [NF] a concentrated solution of the product obtained by heating sugar or glucose until the sweet taste is destroyed and a uniform dark brown mass results; used as a coloring agent for pharmaceuticals and foods.

caramiphen (kah-ram′ĭ-fen) chemical name: 1-phenylcyclopentanecarboxylic acid 2-(dimethylamino)ethyl; an anticholinergic with actions similar to but weaker than those of atropine (q.v.). **c. edisylate, c. ethanedisulfonate,** an ester of caramiphen, $C_{38}H_{60}N_2O_{10}S_2$, with the anticholinergic effects of the base; used as an antitussive, administered orally. **c. hydrochloride,** an ester of caramiphen, $C_{18}H_{28}ClNO_2$, with the anticholinergic effects of the base; used mainly in the treatment of Parkinson's disease and parkinsonism, administered orally.

carat (kar′at) 1. a measure of the fineness of gold, pure gold being 24 carats. 2. a unit of weight of precious stones, being 205.5 milligrams or $3\frac{1}{6}$ grains troy.

carate (kah-rah′ta) pinta.

caraway (kar′ah-wa) [NF] the dried ripe fruit of the umbelliferous plant *Carum carvi* of Europe and central and western Asia; its brown mericarps have an aromatic odor and taste and are used as a flavoring agent for pharmaceuticals.

carbachol (kar′bah-kōl) [USP] a cholinergic agonist, carbamylcholine chloride, that is not hydrolyzed by acetylcholinesterase or pseudocholinesterase; formerly used to stimulate gastrointestinal tract and urinary bladder smooth muscle contraction, it is now used primarily as a miotic.

carbadox (kar′bah-doks) chemical name: 2-(2-quinoxalinylmethylene)hydrazine carboxylic acid methyl ester N^1,N^4-dioxide; an antibacterial, $C_{11}H_{10}N_4O_4$, used in veterinary medicine.

carbamate (kar′bah-māt) any ester of carbamic acid. **ethyl c.,** urethan.

carbamazepine (kar-bah-maz′ĕ-pēn) chemical name: 5H-dibenz[b,f]azepin-5-carboxamide. An anticonvulsant and analgesic, $C_{15}H_{12}N_2O$, occurring as a white to off-white powder; used in the treatment of pain associated with trigeminal neuralgia and in epilepsy manifested by certain types of seizures, administered orally.

carbamic acid (kar-bam′ik) a compound, H_2NCOOH,

that exists only in the form of salts or esters (carbamates), amides (carbamides), and other derivatives (its acyl radical, H_2NCO-, is carbamoyl).

carbamide (kar-bam′ĭd) urea.

carbaminohemoglobin (kar-bam″ĭ-no-he″mo-glo′bin) a chemical combination of carbon dioxide with hemoglobin, CO_2HHb, being one of the forms in which carbon dioxide exists in the blood.

carbamoyl (kar′bah-moil) the radical NH_2CO. Called also *carbamyl.*

carbamoyl-phosphate synthase (ammonia) (kar-bam′o-il) [EC 6.3.4.16] an enzyme of the ligase (synthetase) class that catalyzes the reaction $2ATP + NH_3 + CO_2 + H_2O = 2ADP + $ orthophosphate $+$ carbamoyl phosphate. It occurs primarily in liver mitochondria. The reaction is the first committed step in urea synthesis through the urea cycle. A deficiency of the enzyme, an autosomal recessive trait, results in hyperammonemia (type 2).

carbamoyl phosphate synthetase (CAPS) deficiency (kar-bam′o-il fos′fāt sin′thĕ-tās) a genetic aminoacidopathy involving the biosynthesis of urea; characteristic symptoms include pronounced hyperammonemia with no orotic aciduria, protein intolerance, and neurologic disorders during the neonatal period. Called also *congenital hyperammonemia type I.*

carbamoyl-phosphate synthetase (glutamine-hydrolyzing) (gloo″tah-min hi′dro-līz-ing) [EC 6.3.5.5] an enzyme activity of the ligase (synthetase) class that catalyzes the reaction $2\ ATP + $ glutamine $+ CO_2 + H_2O = 2ADP + $ orthophosphate $+$ glutamate $+$ carbamoyl phosphate. The synthetase activity takes place in the cytosol, is inhibited by UTP, and is the first step in the synthesis of pyrimidine nucleotides.

carbamoyltransferase (kar-bam′o-il-trans′fer-ās) [EC 2.1.3] one of a sub-subclass of enzymes of the transferase class that catalyze the transfer of a carbamoyl group from a donor compound to an acceptor compound, e.g., ornithine carbamoyltransferase. Called also *transcarbamoylase.*

carbamyl (kar′bah-mil) carbamoyl.

carbamylcholine chloride (kar″bah-mil-ko′lēn klo′rīd) carbachol.

carbantel lauryl sulfate (kar′ban-tel) chemical name: *N*- [[(4-chlorophenyl)amino]carbonyl]pentanimidamide compound with dodecyl hydrogen sulfate (1:1); an anthelmintic, $C_{12}H_{16}ClN_3O \cdot C_{12}H_{26}O_4S$.

carbaril (kar′bah-ril) chemical name: 1-naphthalenol methylcarbamate; an insecticide and parasiticide, $C_{12}H_{11}NO_2$. Called also *carbaryl.*

carbarsone (kar′bar-sōn) [USP] chemical name: [4-[(aminocarbonyl)amino]phenyl]arsonic acid. A pentavalent organic arsenical, $C_7H_9AsN_2O_4$, occurring as a white powder; used as an antiamebic, administered orally or in a retention enema. It is also administered orally in the treatment of balantiasis and intravaginally in vaginitis due to *Trichomonas vaginalis.*

carbaryl (kar′bah-ril) carbaril.

carbaspirin calcium (karb-as′pĭ-rin) chemical name: 2-(acetyloxy)benzoic acid calcium salt compound with urea (1:1); an analgesic, $C_{19}H_{18}CaN_2O_9$, which also has antipyretic properties, and has been used like aspirin.

carbazide (kar′bah-zīd) a urea derivative, carbodiazide, $CO(N_3)_2$, in which both the amide groups of urea have been replaced by hydrazine residues.

carbazochrome salicylate (kar-baz′o-krōm) chemical name: 2-hydroxybenzoic acid monosodium salt compound with 2-(1,2,3,5-tetrahydro-3-hydroxy-1-methyl-5-oxo-6*H*-indol-6-ylidene)- hydrazinecarboxamide (1:1). A complex of adrenochrome monosemicarbazone with sodium salicylate, $C_{17}H_{17}N_4NaO_6$, occurring as an orange-red crystallized powder; used as a hemostatic to control capillary bleeding and to prevent capillary permeability, administered orally or intramuscularly.

carbazocine (kar-bah′zo-sēn) chemical name: *cis*--14-(cyclopropylmethyl) - 1,2,3,4,4a,5,6,11 - octahydro - 5,11b-iminoethano-11b*H*-benzo[H-benzo[*a*]carbazole; an analgesic, $C_{22}H_{28}N_2$.

carbazotate (kar-baz′o-tāt) any salt of picric acid; a picrate.

carbenicillin (kar″ben-ĭ-sil′in) chemical name: *N*-(2-car-

boxy-3,3-dimethyl-7-oxo-4-thia-1-azabicyclo[3·2·0]hept-6-yl)- -2-phenylmalonamic acid. A semisynthetic penicillin, $C_{17}H_{18}N_2O_6S$, effective against gram-negative bacteria, such as susceptible strains of *Pseudomonas aeruginosa*, indole-positive *Proteus* species, certain strains of *Escherichia coli*, and *Haemophilus influenzae*; it also inhibits the growth of some gram-positive pathogens. Called also *carfecillin.* **c. disodium,** the disodium salt of carbenicillin, $C_{17}H_{16}N_2Na_2O_6S$, occurring as a white to off-white, crystalline powder, and having the same actions as the base; administered intramuscularly or intravenously in severe systemic infections and septicemia, urinary and genitourinary tract infections, acute and chronic respiratory infections, and soft-tissue infections. A sterile preparation is prepared in conformance with USP standards. Called also *c. sodium.* **c. indanyl sodium** [USP], the sodium salt of the indanyl ester of carbenicillin disodium, $C_{26}H_{25}N_2NaO_6S$, having the same actions as the base; administered orally in the treatment of upper and lower urinary tract infections due to susceptible strains of *Pseudomonas* species, *Proteus* species, *Escherichia coli, Enterobacter*, and enterococci. Called also *carindacillin sodium.* **c. phenyl sodium,** the sodium salt of the phenyl ester of carbenicillin disodium, $C_{23}H_2N_2NaO_6S$, which has been used for the same purposes as carbenicillin indanyl sodium. Called also *carfecillin sodium.* **c. potassium,** the potassium salt of carbenicillin, $C_{17}H_{17}KN_2O_6S$. **c. sodium,** c. disodium.

carbenoxolone sodium (kar″ben-oks′o-lōn) chemical name: 3-(3-carboxy-1-oxopropoxy)-11-oxo-olean-12-en-29-oic acid disodium salt. A derivative of glycyrrhizin, $C_{34}H_{48}Na_2O_7$, having marked anti-inflammatory actions and aldosterone-like activity; used in the treatment of gastric ulcer.

carbetapentane citrate (kar-ba″tah-pen′tān) chemical name: 1-phenylcyclopentanecarboxylic acid 2-(2-diethylaminoethoxy)ethyl citrate. An antitussive agent, $C_{20}H_{31}NO_3 \cdot C_6H_8O_7$, with mild atropine-like antisecretory activity; used in the treatment of cough associated with upper respiratory infections, administered orally.

carbethyl salicylate (kar-beth′il) chemical name: salicylic ethyl ester carbonate. It is used as an analgesic and antiarthritic.

carbhemoglobin (karb″he-mo-glo′bin) carbaminohemoglobin.

carbide (kar′bīd) a compound of carbon with an element or radical. **metallic c.,** a compound of carbon with a transition metal, as in Fe_3C (as distinguished from a salt-like carbide, such as CaC_2).

carbidopa (kar″bĭ-do′pah) [USP] chemical name: (*S*)-α-hydrazino-3,4-dihydroxy-α-methylbenzenepropranoic acid. An inhibitor, $C_{10}H_{14}N_2O_4 \cdot H_2O$, of the decarboxylation of peripheral levodopa to dopamine, which does not penetrate the central nervous system. When given with levodopa, carbidopa produces higher brain concentrations of dopamine with lower doses of levodopa, thus lessening the side effects seen with higher doses. It is used orally, in combination with levodopa, as an antiparkinsonian agent, and has been used in the treatment of Lesch-Nyhan syndrome and Gilles de la Tourette syndrome.

carbimazole (kar-bi′mah-zōl) chemical name: carbonothioic acid *O*-ethylS-(1-methyl-1*H*-imidazol-2-yl) ester. An inhibitor of thyroid hormone synthesis occurring as a white or creamy white, crystalline powder; administered orally in the treatment of hyperthyroidism.

carbinol (kar′bĭ-nol) 1. methanol. 2. any aromatic or fatty alcohol formed by substituting one, two, or three hydrocarbon groups for hydrogen in methanol. **acetylmethyl c.,** a keto-isomer of aldol, $CH_3 \cdot CHOH \cdot CO \cdot CH_3$, which is formed from glucose by certain bacteria and which is detected in a broth culture of bacteria by the Voges-Proskauer reaction. **dimethyl c.,** isopropyl alcohol.

carbinoxamine maleate (kar″bin-ok′sah-mēn) [USP] chemical name: 2-[(4-chlorophenyl)-2-pyridinylmethoxy]-*N*,*N*-dimethylethanamine (*Z*)-2-butenedioate. A potent antihistaminic, $C_{16}H_{19}ClN_2O \cdot C_4H_4O_4$, occurring as a white, crystalline powder; used in the treatment of allergic disorders, administered orally.

carbo (kar′bo) [L.] charcoal. **c. activa′tus,** activated charcoal. **c. anima′lis,** a variety prepared from bones and other animal matter; a decolorizing agent. **c. anima′lis purifica′tus,** purified animal charcoal. **c.**

lig'ni, wood charcoal, a deodorant, adsorbent, and disinfectant.

Carbocaine (kar″bo-kān) trademark for preparations of mepivacaine hydrochloride.

carbocholine (kar″bo-ko′lēn) carbachol.

carbocromen hydrochloride (kar″bo-kro′mēn) chromonar hydrochloride.

carbocyclic (kar″bo-si′klik) having or pertaining to a closed chain or ring formation which includes only carbon atoms; said of chemical compounds.

carbocysteine (kar″bo-sis-te′in) chemical name: S-(carboxymethyl)cysteine; a mucolytic, $C_5H_9NO_4S$.

carbodiimide (kar″bo-di-im′id) a derivative of urea, NH:C:NH.

carbogaseous (kar″bo-gas′e-us) charged with carbon dioxide gas.

carbogen (kar′bo-jen) a mixture of oxygen with 5 per cent carbon dioxide.

carbohemia (kar″bo-he′me-ah) [*carbon* dioxide + Gr. *haima* blood + *-ia*] the presence of excess carbon dioxide in the blood.

carbohemoglobin (kar″bo-he-mo-glo′bin) carbaminohemoglobin.

carbohydrase (kar″bo-hi′drās) any enzyme that catalyzes the hydrolysis of a carbohydrate, producing oligosaccharides or simple sugars.

carbohydrate (kar″bo-hi′drāt) an aldehyde or ketone derivative of a polyhydric alcohol, particularly of the pentahydric and hexahydric alcohols. They are so named because the hydrogen and oxygen are usually in the proportion to form water, $(CH_2O)_n$. The most important carbohydrates are the starches, sugars, celluloses, and gums. They are classified into mono-, di-, tri-, poly- and heterosaccharides. **reserve c's,** carbohydrates that can be stored in the plant or animal in the form of high molecular weight, hydrolyzable compounds such as starch or glycogen.

carbohydraturia (kar″bo-hi′drah-tu′re-ah) excess of carbohydrates in the urine.

carbohydrogenic (kar″bo-hi″dro-jen′ik) producing carbohydrates.

carbolate (kar′bo-lāt) 1. phenolate. 2. to charge with carbolic acid.

carbolfuchsin (kar″bol-fook′sin) see *Table of Stains*, and see under *solution*.

carbolic acid (kar-bol′ik) trivial name for phenol (1).

carbolism (kar′bol-izm) phenol poisoning.

carbolize (kar′bol-īz) to treat with phenol.

carboluria (kar″bo-lu′re-ah) [*carbolic* + Gr. *ouron* urine + *-ia*] the presence of phenol in the urine.

carbolxylene (kar″bol-zi′lēn) a mixure of 1 part carbolic acid and 3 parts xylene, used for clearing microscopical sections.

carbomer, carbomer 934 P (kar′bo-mer) [NF] a polymer of acrylic acid, cross-linked with a polyfunctional agent; used as an emulsifying agent and as a suspending agent in pharmaceutical preparations.

carbometer (kar-bom′ĕ-ter) (*obs.*) carbonometer.

carbometry (kar-bom′ĕ-tre) (*obs.*) carbonometry.

carbon (kar′bon) [L. *carbo*, coal, charcoal] 1. a nonmetallic tetrad element, found nearly pure in the diamond, and approximately pure in charcoal, graphite, and anthracite; symbol, C; atomic number, 6; atomic weight, 12.011. 2. an electrode made of carbon shell in which medicaments may be enclosed. ^{13}C, a natural isotope of carbon, of atomic mass 13, used as a tracer in chemical reactions in living tissue. ^{14}C, a radioactive isotope of carbon, of atomic mass 14, used in cancer and metabolic research. **c. dioxide,** an odorless, colorless gas, CO_2, resulting from the oxidation of carbon. It is formed in the tissues and eliminated by the lungs. CO_2 and the carbonates assist in maintaining the neutrality of the tissues and fluids of the body. Inhalations of carbon dioxide, containing not less than 99 percent by volume of CO_2 [USP], mixed with air or oxygen, are used to stimulate respiration. Solid carbon dioxide (*Dry Ice* or *carbon dioxide snow*) has been used as an escharotic to destroy certain skin lesions. **c. disulfide,** a colorless, flammable, poisonous liquid, CS_2, used as a solvent; it is a counterirritant and has local anesthetic properties but is not used as such. **c.**

monoxide, a colorless poisonous gas, CO, formed by burning carbon or organic fuels with a scanty supply of oxygen; it causes asphyxiation by combining irreversibly with the blood hemoglobin. **c. oxysulfide,** a colorless gas, COS, uniting with air to form an explosive mixture. **radioactive c.,** radiocarbon. **c. tetrachloride** [NF], a clear, colorless, volatile liquid, CCl_4, used as a solvent in pharmaceutical preparations. Inhalation of its vapors can depress central nervous system activity and cause degeneration of the liver and kidneys. Called also *perchlormethane* and *tetrachlormethane*. **c. trichloride,** a white solid, hexachloroethane, C_2Cl_6; it is a stimulant and has local anesthetic properties but is not used as such.

carbonate (kar′bon-āt) any salt of carbonic acid. **ferrous c.,** a compound, $FeCO_3$, used in iron deficiency anemia; called also *iron carbonate*.

carbonate dehydratase (kar′bon-āt de-hi′drah-tās) [EC 4.2.1.1] an enzyme of the lyase class that catalyzes the reaction $H_2CO_3 = CO_2 + H_2O$. It is a zinc protein occurring in kidney tubule cells and in red blood cells. The reaction catalyzes the equilibration of dissolved carbon dioxide and carbonic acid, thus making possible the rapid movement of carbon dioxide from tissues to blood to alveolar air. Called also *carbonic anhydrase*.

carbonemia (kar″bon-e′me-ah) carbohemia.

carbonic acid (kar-bon′ik) the chemical species H_2CO_3, which exists in chemical equilibrium with dissolved carbon dioxide in water; its dissociated forms are the bicarbonate (HCO_3^-) and carbonate (CO_3^{3-}) ions. In the blood the predominant species are HCO_3 and dissolved CO_2 in approximately a 20:1 ratio. The conversion of CO_2 to H_2CO_3 is catalyzed by the enzyme carbonic anhydrase.

carbonic anhydrase (kar-bon′ik an-hi′drās) carbonate dehydratase.

carbonize (kar′bo-nīz) to char or to convert into charcoal.

carbonometer (kar″bo-nom′ĕ-ter) (*obs.*) an apparatus for performing carbonometry.

carbonometry (kar″bo-nom′ĕ-tre) [*carbon* + Gr. *metron* measure] (*obs.*) measurement of the amount of carbon dioxide exhaled with the breath.

carbonuria (kar″bo-nu′re-ah) [*carbon* + Gr. *ouron* urine + *-ia*] the presence of carbon dioxide or other carbon compounds in the urine. **dysoxidative c.,** pathologic increase of carbon compounds in the urine due to deficient oxidation.

carbonyl (kar′bo-nil) [*carbon* + Gr. *hylē* matter] the organic radical, C:O, occurring in compounds such as aldehydes, ketones, carboxylic acids, and esters. **c. chloride,** phosgene.

carboprost (kar′bo-prost) chemical name: (5z)-9α,11α,15-trihydroxy-15S-methyl-prosta-5,13E-dien-1-oic acid. A synthetic 15-methyl analogue of dinoprost, a prostaglandin of the F type, $C_{21}H_{36}O_5$; it has been used as an oxytocic for termination of pregnancy and missed abortion, administered intramuscularly. **c. methyl,** the methyl ester of carboprost, $C_{22}H_{38}O_5$, having the same actions and similar uses as the base; administered in vaginal suppositories or in an intravaginal device. **c. tromethamine,** an oxytocic compound of carboprost and 2-amino-2-(hydroxymethyl)-1,3-propanediol (1:1), $C_{21}H_{36}O_5 \cdot C_4H_{11}NO_3$.

Carborundum (kar″bo-run′dum) trademark for a compound of carbon and silicon, silicon carbide, SiC, a substance which ranks next to the diamond in hardness; used as an abrasive and as a refractory.

Carbowax (kar′bo-waks) trademark for a series of polyethylene glycols; used in compounding water-soluble ointment vehicles.

γ-carboxyglutamate (kar-bok″se-gloo′tah-māt) a salt or dissociated form of carboxyglutamic acid; see under *acid*.

carboxyhemoglobin (kar-bok″se-he″mo-glo′bin) hemoglobin combined with carbon monoxide, which occupies the sites on the hemoglobin molecule that normally bind with oxygen and which is not readily displaced from the molecule; exposure to carbon monoxide thus results in cellular anoxia.

carboxyhemoglobinemia (kar-bok″se-he″mo-glo″bin-e′me-ah) the presence of carboxyhemoglobin in the blood.

carboxyl (kar-bok′sil) the monovalent radical, —COOH, occurring in those organic acids termed carboxylic acids.

carboxyl (acid) proteinase (kar-bok′sil pro′tēn-ās″) aspartic proteinase.

carboxylase (kar-bok′sĭ-lās) an enzyme that catalyzes the addition of a molecule of carbon dioxide to another compound to form a carboxyl group. The carboxylases include some carboxy-lyases [EC 4.1.1] and those ligases, usually biotinyl-proteins, that cleave ATP to drive the reaction [EC 6.4.1]. **amino acid c.,** an enzyme in many bacteria that catalyzes the removal of CO_2 from amino acids, thus producing amines. **multiple c. deficiency (MCD),** a genetic aminoacidopathy leading to impaired function of biotin-dependent enzymes and to accumulation of propionate and β-methylcrotonylglycine. Clinical signs include developmental retardation, diffuse erythematous rash, alopecia, and ketoacidosis. Called also *holocarboxylase synthetase d.*

carboxylate (kar-boks′ĭ-lāt) any salt, ester, or conjugate base of a carboxylic acid.

carboxylation (kar-bok″sĭ-la′shun) the addition of carbon dioxide or bicarbonate to from a carboxyl group, as to pyruvate to form oxaloacetate.

carboxylesterase (kar-bok″sil-es′ter-ās) [EC 3.1.1.1] an enzyme of the hydrolase class that catalyzes the reaction carboxylic ester + H_2O = alcohol + carboxylic acid anion. It has a wide specificity, acting on glycerol esters of short-chain fatty acids, esters of dibasic acids, monohydric alcohols, and of vitamin A.

carboxylic ester hydrolase (kar″bok-sil′ik es′ter hi′dro-lās) carboxylesterase.

carboxyltransferase (kar-bok″sil-trans′fer-ās) [EC 2.1.3] one of a sub-subclass of enzymes of the transferase class that catalyze the transfer of a carboxyl group from a donor compound to an acceptor compound. Called also *transcarboxylase.*

carboxy-lyase (kar-bok′se-li′ās) [EC 4.1.1] a sub-subclass of enzymes of the lyase class that catalyze the addition or removal of a carboxyl group to or from a compound; it includes the carboxylases and decarboxylases.

carboxymethylcellulose sodium (kar-bok″se-meth″il-sel′u-lōs) [USP] the sodium salt of a polycarboxymethyl ether of cellulose; used as a suspending agent, tablet excipient, and viscosity-increasing agent in pharmaceutical preparations, and administered orally as a cathartic.

carboxymyoglobin (kar-bok″se-mi″o-glo′bin) a compound formed from myoglobin on exposure to carbon monoxide, with formation of a covalent bond with oxygen and without change of the charge of the ferrous state.

carboxypeptidase (kar-bok″se-pep′tĭ-dās) [EC 3.4.16-17] any of two sub-subclasses of enzymes of the hydrolase class that cleave a C-terminal amino acid residue from a peptide or polypeptide. **metallo c.** [EC 3.4.17] one that requires a divalent cation such as zinc or cobalt for activity. **serine c.** [EC 3.4.16], one containing a diisopropyl fluorophosphate-sensitive serine in the catalytic site, and having a pH optimum in the acid range. See also *serine carboxypeptidase.*

carboxypeptidase A (kar-bok″se-pep′tĭ-dās) [EC 3.4.17.1] an enzyme of the hydrolase class that catalyzes the reaction peptidyl-L-amino acid + H_2O = peptide + L amino acid, releasing carboxy-terminal amino acid residues with the exception of C arginine, lysine, and proline. It is a zinc-metalloenzyme found in pancreatic juice.

carboxypeptidase B (kar-bok″se-pep′tĭ-dās) [EC 3.4.17.2] an enzyme of the hydrolase class that catalyzes the reaction peptidyl-L-lysine (-L-arginine) + H_2O = peptide L-lysine (or L-arginine). It is a zinc-metalloenzyme found in pancreatic juice.

carboxypeptidase N (kar-bok″se-pep′tĭ-dās) arginine carboxypeptidase.

carboxypolypeptidase (kar-bok″se-pol″e-pep′tĭ-dās) 1. carboxypeptidase. 2. carboxypeptidase A.

carbromal (kar-bro′mal) chemical name: *N*-(aminocarbonyl)-2-bromo-2-ethylbutaneamide. A sedative with weak hypnotic activity, $C_7H_{13}BrN_2O$, occurring as a white, crystalline powder; administered orally.

carbuncle (kar′bung-kl) [L. *carbunculus* little coal] a necrotizing infection of skin and subcutaneous tissue composed of a cluster of boils (furuncles), usually due to *Staphylococcus aureus*, with multiple formed or incipient drainage sinuses. **malignant c.,** see *cutaneous anthrax,* under *anthrax.* **renal c.,** a massive localized parenchymal suppuration con-

sequent to bacterial metastasis, following localized vascular thrombosis or infarction of the kidney.

carbuncular (kar-bung′ku-lar) resembling or of the nature of a carbuncle.

carbunculoid (kar-bung′ku-loid) resembling a carbuncle.

carbunculosis (kar-bung″ku-lo′sis) a condition marked by the development of carbuncles.

carbutamide (kar-bu′tah-mīd) chemical name: 1-butyl-3-sulfanilylurea; a hypoglycemic agent, $C_{11}H_{17}N_3O_3S$.

carbuterol hydrochloride (kar-bu′ter-ōl) chemical name: [5-[2-[(1,1-dimethylethyl)amino]-1-hydroxyethyl]-2-hydroxyphenyl]urea monohydrochloride. An adrenergic, $C_{13}H_{21}N_3O_3 \cdot HCl$, which has been used as a bronchodilator, administered by inhalation.

carcass (kar′kas) [Fr. *carcasse*] a dead body; generally applied to other than a human body.

Carcassonne's ligament, perineal ligament (kar-kah-sonz′) [Bernard Gauderic *Carcassonne,* French surgeon, born 1728] see *ligamentum puboprostaticum* and *ligamentum transversum perinei.*

carceag (kar′se-ag) a disease of sheep in the Balkan States caused by *Babesia (Piroplasma) ovis* and transmitted by the tick *Rhipicephalus bursa.*

carciag (kar′se-ag) carceag.

carcinelcosis (kar″sin-el-ko′sis) [Gr. *karkinos* cancer + *helkōsis* ulceration] (*obs.*) malignant ulceration.

carcinemia (kar″sin-e′me-ah) [*carcinoma* + Gr. *haima* blood + *-ia*] cancerous cachexia.

carcin(o)- [Gk. *karkinos* a crab] a combining form meaning relationship to carcinoma.

carcinogen (kar-sin′o-jen) any cancer-producing substance.

carcinogenesis (kar″sĭ-no-jen′ĕ-sis) [Gr. *karkinos* cancer + *genesis* production] the production of carcinoma.

carcinogenic (kar″sĭ-no-jen′ik) producing carcinoma.

carcinogenicity (kar″sĭ-no-jĕ-nis′ĭ-te) the power, ability, or tendency to produce carcinoma.

carcinoid (kar′sĭ-noid) a yellow circumscribed tumor occurring in the small intestine, appendix, stomach, or colon; argentaffinoma (q.v.). See also under *syndrome.*

carcinology (kar″sĭ-nol′o-je) (*obs.*) oncology.

carcinolysin (kar″sĭ-nol′ĭ-sin) [*carcinoma* + Gr. *lysis* dissolution] a ferment derived from a Chinese variety of pine called "haisung." It has been given subcutaneously or intramuscularly for cancer.

carcinolysis (kar″sĭ-nol′ĭ-sis) destruction of carcinoma cells, as by perfusion of an antineoplastic agent through the vessels of the body segment in which the growth occurs.

carcinolytic (kar″sĭ-no-lit′ik) [*carcinoma* + Gr. *lytikos* destroying] pertaining to, characterized by, or causing carcinolysis.

carcinoma (kar″sĭ-no′mah), pl. *carcinomas* or *carcino′mata* [Gr. *karkinōma* from *karkinos* crab, cancer] a malignant new growth made up of epithelial cells tending to infiltrate the surrounding tissues and give rise to metastases. **acinar c., acinous c.,** alveolar adenocarcinoma. **adenocystic c.,** adenoid cystic c. **adenoid cystic c.,** carcinoma characterized by bands or cylinders of hyalinized or mucinous stroma separating or surrounded by nests or cords of small epithelial cells. When the cylinders occur within masses of epithelial cells, they give the tissue a perforated, sievelike, or cribriform appearance. Such tumors occur in the mammary glands, the mucous glands of the upper and lower respiratory tract, and the salivary glands. They are malignant but slow-growing, and tend to spread locally via the nerves. Called also *adenocystic c., adenomyoepithelioma, cribriform c.,* and *cylindroma.* NOTE: Certain unrelated tumors may have a cylindromatous or adenoid cystic pattern, e.g., cutaneous cylindroma, ameloblastoma, and a type of basal cell carcinoma of the skin. **c. adenomato′sum,** adenocarcinoma. **c. of adrenal cortex,** malignant tumors of adrenal cortical cells that may cause endocrine disorders such as Cushing's syndrome and adrenogenital syndrome. **alveolar c.,** alveolar adenocarcinoma. **alveolar cell c.,** carcinoma of the lung marked clinically by severe cough with voluminous expectoration and histologically by distinctive, tall, columnar to cuboidal epithelial cells that line up along the alveolar septa, project into the alveolar spaces in numerous branching papillary formations, and may contain mucinous secretion; called also *bronchiolar c., alveolar cell tumor*, and *pulmonary adenomatosis*. **basal cell c., c. basocellula're,** an epithelial tumor that seldom metastasizes but has potentialities for local invasion and destruction. Clinically, it is divided into types: nodular, cicatricial, morphaic, and erythematoid (pagetoid). Called also *basaloma* and *hair matrix c.* **basaloid c.,** a rare transitional-cell carcinoma of the anus, resembling basal cell carcinoma of the skin. **basosquamous cell c.,** carcinoma that histologically exhibits both basal and squamous elements. **bronchioalveolar c., bronchiolar c.,** alveolar cell c. **bronchiolar c.,** alveolar cell c. **bronchogenic c.,** carcinoma of the lung, so called because it arises from the epithelium of the bronchial tree. **cerebriform c.,** medullary c. **cholangiocellular c.,** primary carcinoma of the liver originating in bile duct cells, called also *cholangioma* and *cholangiocarcinoma*. **chorionic c.,** choriocarcinoma. **colloid c.,** mucinous c. **comedo c.,** comedocarcinoma. **corpus c.,** carcinoma of the body of the uterus. **cribriform c.,** adenoid cystic c. **c. en cuirasse,** a rare carcinoma infiltrating the entire skin of the anterior chest wall and frequently breaking it down. **c. cuta'neum,** malignant epithelioma of the skin. **cylindrical c., cylindrical cell c.,** carcinoma in which the cells are cylindrical or nearly so. **duct c.,** carcinoma of any duct. **c. du'rum** (*obs.*), scirrhous c. **embryonal c.,** 1. a highly malignant, primitive form of carcinoma, probably of germinal cell or teratomatous derivation, usually arising in a gonad and rarely in other sites. 2. (*obs.*) seminoma. **encephaloid c.** (*obs.*), medullary c. **epidermoid c.,** carcinoma in which the cells tend to differentiate in the same way that the cells of the epidermis do; that is, they tend to form prickle cells and undergo cornification. **c. epithelia'le adenoi'des,** adenoid basal cell c. **exophytic c.,** a malignant epithelial neoplasm with marked outward growth like a wart or papilloma. **c. ex ul'cere** (*obs.*), carcinomatous degeneration of a benign ulcer. **c. fibro'sum,** scirrhous c. **gelatiniform c.,** mucinous c. **gelatinous c.,** colloid c. **giant cell c.,** carcinoma containing many giant cells. **c. gigantocellula're,** carcinoma containing many giant cells. **glandular c.,** adenocarcinoma. **granulosa cell c.,** see under *tumor*. **hair-matrix c.,** basal cell c. **hematoid c.** (*obs.*), a highly vascular carcinoma. **hepatocellular c.,** primary carcinoma of the liver cells; called also *hepatoma, malignant hepatoma*, and *hepatocarcinoma*. **Hürthle cell c.,** see under *tumor*. **hyaline c.** (*obs.*), mucinous c. **hypernephroid c.,** renal cell c. **infantile embryonal c.,** mesonephroma (type 2). **c. in si'tu,** a neoplastic entity wherein the tumor cells are confined to the epithelium of origin, without invasion of the basement membrane; popularly applied to such cells in the uterine cervix. Called also *cancer in situ* and *preinvasive c.* **intraepidermal c.,** carcinoma confined within the epidermis, the basal layer of the epidermis not being penetrated by the proliferating cells; Bowen's disease. **intraepithelial c.,** c. in situ. **Krompecher's c.,** rodent ulcer. **Kulchitzky-cell c.,** carcinoid tumor of the small or large intestine. **large-cell c.,** a bronchogenic tumor of undifferentiated (anaplastic) cells of large size. **lenticular c., c. lenticula're,** scirrhous carcinoma of the skin with the formation of flattened papules and nodules which run together, forming fungoid masses. **lipomatous c.,** (*obs.*), carcinoma with fatty degeneration. **lymphoepithelial c.,** lymphoepithelioma. **c. medulla're, medullary c.,** carcinoma composed mainly of epithelial elements with little or no stroma. **melanotic c.,** malignant melanoma. **c. mol'le,** medullary c. **mucinous c.,** adenocarcinoma producing mucin in significant amounts. **c. mucip'arum,** mucinous c. **c. mucocellula're,** Krukenberg's tumor. **mucoepidermoid c.,** a malignant epithelial tumor of glandular tissue, especially the salivary glands, characterized by acini with mucus-producing cells and by the presence of malignant squamous elements. **c. muco'sum, mucous c.,** mucinous c. **c. myxomato'des,** carcinoma in which the stroma has undergone myxomatous degeneration. **nasopharyngeal c.,** a malignant tumor arising in the epithelial lining of the space behind the nose (the nasopharynx) and occurring at high frequency in southern China. The Epstein-Barr virus has been implicated as a causative agent. **oat cell c.,** a small-cell c. **c. ossif'icans, osteoid c.,** carcinoma in which there is osteoid or

osseous metaplasia of the stroma. **papillary c.,** carcinoma in which there are papillary excrescences. **periportal c.,** carcinoma of the liver, extending along and around the portal vessels. **preinvasive c.,** c. in situ. **prickle cell c.,** squamous cell c. **pultaceous c.** (*obs.*), comedocarcinoma. **renal cell c. of kidney,** carcinoma of the renal parenchyma usually occurring in middle age or later and composed of tubular cells in varying arrangements; symptoms depend on extent of invasion. Called also *adenocarcinoma of kidney* and *hypernephroid carcinoma*. **reserve cell c.,** oat cell c. **c. sarcomato'des** (*obs.*), spindle cell c. **schneiderian c.,** a neoplasm of the mucosa of the nose and the paranasal sinuses. **scirrhous c.,** carcinoma with a hard structure owing to the formation of dense connective tissue in the stroma. **c. scro'ti,** carcinoma of the scrotum. **signet-ring cell c.,** a highly malignant, mucus-secreting tumor in which the mucus-secreting cells are anaplastic and appear rounded, with the nucleus displaced to one side by a globule of mucus in the cytoplasm. **c. sim'plex,** an undifferentiated carcinoma. **small-cell c.,** a radiosensitive tumor composed of small, oval, undifferentiated cells that are intensely hematoxyphilic and typically bronchogenic. Called also *oat-cell c.* **solanoid c.** (*obs.*), scirrhous c. **spheroidal cell c.,** c. simplex. **spindle cell c.,** squamous cell carcinoma marked by fusiform development of rapidly proliferating cells. **c. spongio'sum,** medullary c. **squamous c., squamous cell c.,** carcinoma developed from squamous epithelium, and having cuboid cells. **string c.,** a carcinoma of the large intestine, most commonly the ascending or transverse colon, giving it the appearance of being bound tightly by a string. **c. telangiectat'icum, c. telangiecto'des,** carcinoma involving the cutaneous capillaries and producing telangiectatic changes. **transitional cell c.,** a malignant tumor arising from a transitional type of stratified epithelium, usually affecting the urinary bladder. **c. tubero'sum, tuberous c.,** scirrhous carcinoma of the skin with the formation of nodular projections. **verrucous c.,** a variety of epidermoid carcinoma that has a predilection for the buccal mucosa but also affects other oral soft tissue, the larynx, and the genitals. It is a slow-growing, somewhat invasive, exophytic neoplasm, either papillary or verrucous in appearance. **c. villo'sum,** carcinoma in which the cells are arranged in a villous pattern.

carcinomata (kar″sĭ-no′mah-tah) plural of *carcinoma*.

carcinomatoid (kar″sĭ-nom′ah-toid) resembling carcinoma.

carcinomatophobia (kar″sĭ-no″mah-to-fo′be-ah) cancerphobia.

carcinomatosis (kar″sĭ-no-mah-to′sis) the condition of widespread dissemination of cancer throughout the body; called also *carcinosis*.

carcinomatous (kar″sĭ-nom′ah-tus) pertaining to or of the nature of cancer; malignant.

carcinomelcosis (kar″sĭ-no-mel-ko′sis) [*carcinoma* + Gr. *helkōsis* ulceration] (*obs.*) an ulcerated carcinoma.

carcinophilia (kar″sĭ-no-fil′e-ah) [*carcinoma* + Gr. *philein* to love] special affinity for cancerous tissue.

carcinophilic (kar″sĭ-no-fil′ik) having an affinity for cancerous tissue.

carcinophobia (kar″sĭ-no-fo′be-ah) [*carcinoma* + *phobia*] cancerphobia.

carcinosarcoma (kar″sĭ-no-sar-ko′mah) a malignant tumor composed of carcinomatous and sarcomatous tissues. **embryonal c.,** Wilms' tumor.

carcinosis (kar″sĭ-no′sis) carcinomatosis. **miliary c.,** carcinomatosis marked by development of numerous nodules resembling miliary tubercles. **c. pleu'rae,** secondary cancer of the pleura in which the membrane is studded with nodules. **pulmonary c.,** alveolar cell carcinoma.

carcinostatic (kar″sĭ-no-stat′ik) tending to check the growth of carcinoma.

carcinous (kar′sĭ-nus) carcinomatous.

cardamom (kar′dah-mom) [L. *cardamomum*; Gr. *kardamōmon*] the fruit of *Elettaria cardamomum* of the ginger family, a perennial herb native to tropical Asia; its seed is used as a flavoring agent, and has been used as a carminative. Also, the fruit of herbs of the same family, e.g., that of *Amomum*.

Cardarelli's sign (symptom) (kar-dar-el′ēz) [Antonio *Cardarelli*, Italian physician, 1831–1927] see under *sign.*

cardelmycin (kar-del-mi′sin) novobiocin.

Carden's amputation (kar′denz) [Henry Douglas *Carden*, English surgeon, died 1872] see under *amputation.*

cardia (kar′de-ah) [Gr. *kardia* heart] 1. ostium cardiacum. 2. pars cardiaca gastris.

cardiac (kar′de-ak) [L. *cardiacus*, from Gr. *kardiakos*] 1. pertaining to the heart. 2. a cordial, or restorative medicine. 3. a person with a heart disorder. 4. pertaining to the orifice (*ostium cardiacum*) between the esophagus and the part of the stomach immediately adjacent to and surrounding the orifice (*pars cardiaca gastris*).

cardialgia (kar″de-al′je-ah) [*cardia-* + *-algia*] 1. (*obs.*) an uneasy or painful sensation in the anterior chest or upper abdomen; heartburn. 2. cardiodynia.

cardianeuria (kar″de-ah-nu′re-ah) [*cardia-* + Gr. *aneuros* without nerves + *-ia*] (*obs.*) deficiency of tone in the heart.

cardiant (kar′de-ant) a drug or agent stimulating the heart.

cardiasthenia (kar″de-as-the′ne-ah) [*cardia-* + Gr. *astheneia* weakness] weakness of the heart.

cardiasthma (kar-de-as′mah) cardiac asthma.

cardiataxia (kar″de-ah-tak′se-ah) [*cardia-* + *ataxia*] (*obs.*) incoordination in the movements of the heart.

cardiectasis (kar″de-ek′tah-sis) [*cardia-* + Gr. *ektasis* dilatation] dilatation of the heart.

cardiectomized (kar″de-ek′tŏ-mīzd) having the heart removed, as a cardiectomized animal.

cardiectomy (kar″de-ek′tŏ-me) [*cardia-* + Gr. *ektomē* excision] excision of the cardiac portion of the stomach.

Cardilate (kar′dĭ-lāt) trademark for a preparation of erythrityl tetranitrate.

cardinal (kar′dĭ-nal) [L. *cardinalis*, from *cardo* a hinge] of primary or preeminent importance.

cardi(o)- [Gr. *kardia* heart] a combining form denoting relationship to the heart or to the cardiac orifice or portion of the stomach.

cardioaccelerator (kar″de-o-ak-sel′er-a-tor) 1. quickening the heart action. 2. an agent that accelerates the heart action.

cardioactive (kar″de-o-ak′tiv) having an effect upon the heart.

cardioangiography (kar″de-o-an″je-og′rah-fe) angiocardiography.

cardioangiology (kar″de-o-an″je-ol′o-je) [*cardio-* + Gr. *angeion* vessel + *-logy*] the medical specialty which deals with the heart and blood vessels.

cardioaortic (kar″de-o-a-or′tik) pertaining to the heart and the aorta.

cardioarterial (kar″de-o-ar-te′re-al) pertaining to the heart and the arteries.

Cardiobacterium (kar″de-o-bak-te′re-um) [*cardio-* + *bacterium*] a genus of gram-negative, facultatively anaerobic, fermentative, rod-shaped bacteria, part of the normal flora of the nose and throat, and also isolated from blood. **C. ho′minis,** a species that is part of the normal flora of the nose and pharynx, and also an etiologic agent of endocarditis.

cardiocairograph (kar″de-o-ki′ro-graf) [*cardio-* + Gr. *kairos* time + *graphein* to write.] a technique by means of which roentgenograms of the heart can be made at any chosen phase of its cycle.

cardiocele (kar′de-o-sēl″) [*cardio-* + Gr. *kēlē* tumor] protrusion of the heart through a fissure of the diaphragm or through a wound.

cardiocentesis (kar″de-o-sen-te′sis) [*cardio-* + Gr. *kentēsis* puncture] surgical puncture or incision of the heart.

cardiochalasia (kar″de-o-kah-la′ze-ah) [*cardio-* + Gr. *chalasis* relaxation + *-ia*] relaxation or incompetence of sphincter action of the cardiac orifice of the stomach.

cardiocinetic (kar″de-o-sĭ-net′ik) cardiokinetic.

cardiocirculatory (kar″de-o-ser′ku-lah-tor′e) pertaining to blood flow through the heart and vascular system.

cardiocirrhosis (kar″de-o-sir-ro′sis) [*cardio-* + *cirrhosis*] cirrhosis of the liver complicating heart disease with recurrent intractable congestive heart failure; cardiac cirrhosis. See *Hutinel's disease*, under *disease.*

cardiodiaphragmatic (kar″de-o-di″ah-frag-mat′ik) pertaining to the heart and diaphragm.

cardiodilatin (kar″de-o-di′lah-tin) [*cardio-* + *dilation*] one of two polypeptide hormones, the other being cardionatrin, secreted by the atrial granules in cardiac muscle, it acts upon vascular smooth muscle, producing relaxation and vasodilation, and is involved in the control of blood pressure.

cardiodilator (kar″de-o-di′la-tor) an instrument for dilating the cardia in cardiospasm or stricture.

cardionatrin (kar″de-o-na′trin) [*cardio-* + L. *natrium* sodium] one of two polypeptide hormones, the other being cardiodilatin, secreted by the atrial granules in cardiac muscle, it has potent diuretic and natriuretic effects, and is involved in the control of sodium excretion by the body. Called also *atrial natriuretic factor.*

cardiodiosis (kar″de-o-di-o′sis) the dilatation of the cardiac end of the stomach.

cardiodynamics (kar″de-o-di-nam′iks) [*cardio-* + *dynamics*] the science of the motions and forces involved in the heart's action.

cardiodynia (kar″de-o-din′e-ah) [*cardio-* + Gr. *odynē* pain] pain in the heart.

cardioesophageal (kar″de-o-ĕ-sof″ah-je′al) pertaining to the cardia of the stomach and the esophagus, as the cardioesophageal junction or sphincter.

cardiogenesis (kar″de-o-jen′e-sis) [*cardio-* + Gr. *gennan* to produce] the development of the heart in the embryo.

cardiogenic (kar″de-o-jen′ik) [*cardio-* + Gr. *gennan* to produce] 1. originating in the heart; caused by abnormal function of the heart. 2. pertaining to cardiogenesis.

Cardiografin (kar″de-o-gra′fin) trademark for meglumine diatrizoate.

cardiogram (kar′de-o-gram″) [*cardio-* + Gr. *gramma* a writing] a tracing of a cardiac event made by means of the cardiograph. **apex c.,** a graphic record, in the form of a simple displacement curve, of the thrust of the apex of the heart as manifested on the surface of the body. **esophageal c.,** a tracing of the contractions of the left atrium made by registering the pulsations in the esophagus. **negative c.,** a cardiogram in which the curve falls below the abscissa instead of rising above it. **precordial c.,** kinetocardiogram. **vector c.,** vectorcardiogram.

cardiograph (kar′de-o-graf″) [*cardio-* + Gr. *graphein* to write] an instrument designed to record some element of the heartbeat.

cardiographic (kar″de-o-graf′ik) pertaining to cardiography.

cardiography (kar″de-og′rah-fe) the technique of graphically recording some physical or functional aspects of the heart. See also *ballistocardiography, echocardiography, electrocardiography, electrokymography, kinetocardiography, phonocardiography, roentgen kymography, vibrocardiography*, etc. **apex c.,** the graphic recording of low-frequency pulsations at the anterior chest wall over the apex of the heart. **ultrasonic c.,** echocardiography. **vector c.,** vectorcardiography.

Cardio-Green (kar′de-o-grēn) trademark for a preparation of indocyanine green.

cardiohepatic (kar″de-o-hĕ-pat′ik) pertaining to the heart and the liver.

cardiohepatomegaly (kar″de-o-hep″ah-to-meg′ah-le) enlargement of the heart and liver.

cardioid (kar′de-oid) heartlike; resembling a heart.

cardioinhibitor (kar″de-o-in-hib′ĭ-ter) an agent which restrains the heart's action.

cardioinhibitory (kar″de-o-in-hib′ĭ-to-re) restraining or inhibiting the movements of the heart.

cardiokinetic (kar″de-o-ki-net′ik) 1. stimulating the action of the heart. 2. an agent that stimulates action of the heart.

cardiokymographic (kar″de-o-ki″mo-graf′ik) pertaining to cardiokymography.

cardiokymography (kar″de-o-ki-mog′rah-fe) the recording of the motion of the heart by means of the electrokymograph.

cardiolipin (kar″de-o-lip′in) [*cardio-* + Gr. *lipos* fat] 1,3-

diphosphatidylglycerol, a phospholipid occurring primarily in mitochondrial inner membranes and in bacterial plasma membranes. Cardiolipin is the main antigenic component of Wassermann-type antigens used in nontreponemal serologic tests for syphilis.

cardiologist (kar-de-ol′o-jist) a physician skilled in the diagnosis and treatment of heart disease.

cardiology (kar-de-ol′o-je) [cardio- + -logy] the study of the heart and its functions.

cardiolysis (kar″de-ol′ĭ-sis) [cardio- + Gr. lysis loosening] an operation of freeing the heart and pericardium in adhesive mediastinopericarditis; it is done by resecting the ribs and the sternum over the pericardium.

cardiomalacia (kar″de-o-mah-la′she-ah) [cardio- + Gr. malakia softness] morbid softening of the muscular substance of the heart.

cardiomegalia (kar″de-o-mĕ-ga′le-ah) cardiomegaly. **c. glycogen′ica circumscrip′ta,** glycogenic cardiomegaly. **c. glycogen′ica diffu′sa,** glycogen storage disease, type II; see under disease.

cardiomegaly (kar″de-o-meg′ah-le) [cardio- + Gr. megas large] cardiac hypertrophy. **glycogenic c.,** a morbid condition characterized by enlargement of the heart, with localized deposits of glycogen in the heart muscle; called also cardiomegalia glycogenica circumscripta.

cardiomelanosis (kar″de-o-mel″ah-no′sis) melanosis of the heart.

cardiometer (kar″de-om′ĕ-ter) [cardio- + Gr. metron measure] an instrument used in estimating the power of the heart's action.

cardiometry (kar″de-om′ĕ-tre) the estimation of the force of the heart's action.

cardiomotility (kar″de-o-mo-til′ĭ-te) the movements of the heart; the motility of the heart.

cardiomyoliposis (kar″de-o-mi″o-li-po′sis) [cardio- + Gr. mys muscle + lipos fat] fatty degeneration of the heart muscle.

cardiomyopathy (kar″de-o-mi-op′ah-the) [cardio- + Gr. mys muscle + pathos disease] a general diagnostic term designating primary myocardial disease, often of obscure or unknown etiology. **alcoholic c.,** a congestive cardiomyopathy resulting in cardiac enlargement and low cardiac output, occurring in chronic alcoholics; the heart disease in beriberi (thiamine deficiency) is also associated with alcoholism. **congestive c.,** a syndrome characterized by cardiac enlargement, especially of the left ventricle, myocardial dysfunction, and congestive heart failure. **infiltrative c.,** myocardial disease resulting from deposition in the heart tissue of abnormal substances, as may occur in amyloidosis, hemochromatosis, etc. **peripartum c.,** cardiac enlargement and congestive heart failure of unknown cause beginning in the last month of gestation or the first few months after delivery. **postpartum c.,** cardiac enlargement and congestive heart failure of unknown cause occurring in a mother during the first few months after delivery of a child. **primary c.,** that in which the basic pathological process involves the myocardium itself and not other cardiac structures and in which the cause is unknown and not part of a disease affecting other organs. **restrictive c.,** a form in which the ventricular walls are excessively rigid, impeding ventricular filling; it is marked by abnormal diastolic function but by normal or nearly normal systolic function. **secondary c.,** any form that is due to another cardiovascular disorder (e.g., hypertension) or is a manifestation of systemic disease (e.g., sarcoidosis).

cardiomyopexy (kar″de-o-mi′o-pek″se) [cardio- + Gr. mys muscle + pēxis fixation] surgical removal of the epicardium and application of a pedicled flap of adjacent muscle to the denuded myocardium and pericardium; formerly used as a means of supplying collateral circulation to the heart.

cardiomyotomy (kar″de-o-mi-ot′ŏ-me) [cardio- + Gr. mys muscle + tomē a cutting] esophagocardiomyotomy.

cardionecrosis (kar″de-o-nĕ-kro′sis) necrosis or gangrene of the heart.

cardionector (kar″de-o-nek′ter) [cardio- + L. nector joiner] systema conducens cordis.

cardionephric (kar″de-o-nef′rik) pertaining to the heart and the kidney.

cardioneural (kar″de-o-nu′ral) pertaining to the heart and nervous system.

cardioneurosis (kar″de-o-nu-ro′sis) [cardio- + neurosis] neurocirculatory asthenia.

cardio-omentopexy (kar″de-o-o-men′to-pek″se) the operation of suturing a portion of the omentum to the heart, the omentum having been drawn through an incision in the diaphragm; formerly used as a means of supplying collateral circulation to the heart.

cardiopaludism (kar″de-o-pal′u-dizm) heart disease due to malaria, marked by gallop rhythm in the tricuspid area, intermittent heart action, dilatation of the right heart, and reduplication of the diastolic sound.

cardiopath (kar′de-o-path) a person with heart disease.

cardiopathia (kar″de-o-path′e-ah) cardiopathy.

cardiopathic (kar″de-o-path′ik) pertaining to or marked by disease of the heart.

cardiopathy (kar″de-op′ah-the) [cardio- + Gr. pathos disease] any disorder or disease of the heart. In addition to heart disease of inflammatory origin, there are arteriosclerotic cardiopathy, due to arteriosclerosis; fatty cardiopathy, due to growth of fatty tissue; hypertensive cardiopathy, due to high blood pressure; nephropathic cardiopathy, due to kidney disease; thyrotoxic cardiopathy, due to thyroid intoxication; toxic cardiopathy, due to the effect of some toxin; and valvular cardiopathy, due to faulty valve action. **infarctoid c.,** a heart condition with symptoms resembling those of myocardial infarction.

cardiopericardiopexy (kar″de-o-per″ĭ-kar′de-o-pek-se) [cardio- + pericardium + Gr. pēxis fixation] the operative establishment of adhesive pericarditis; formerly used to increase blood flow to the heart.

cardiopericarditis (kar″de-o-per″ĭ-kar-di′tis) [cardio- + pericarditis] inflammation of both the heart and the pericardium.

cardiophobia (kar″de-o-fo′be-ah) [cardio- + phobia] irrational dread of heart disease.

cardiophrenia (kar″de-o-fre′ne-ah) phrenocardia.

cardioplasty (kar′de-o-plas″te) [cardio- + Gr. plassein to form] esophagogastroplasty.

cardioplegia (kar″de-o-ple′je-ah) [cardio- + Gr. plēgē stroke + -ia] arrest of contraction of the myocardium, as may be induced by the use of chemical compounds or of cold (cryocardioplegia) in the performance of surgery upon the heart.

cardioplegic (kar″de-o-plej′ik) pertaining to cardioplegia.

cardiopneumatic (kar″de-o-nu-mat′ik) [cardio- + Gr. pneuma breath] of or pertaining to the heart and respiration.

cardiopneumograph (kar″de-o-nu′mo-graf) [cardio- + Gr. pneuma breath + graphein to record] an apparatus that registers cardiopneumatic movements.

cardiopneumonopexy (kar″de-o-nu-mon′o-pek″se) an operation formerly used to provide collateral blood supply to the heart muscle by various methods of connecting the heart with the left lung, including production of vascular adhesions through the use of mechanical abrasion or chemical irritants.

cardioptosia (kar″de-op-to′se-ah) cardioptosis.

cardioptosis (kar″de-op′tŏ-sis) [cardio- + Gr. ptōsis falling] downward displacement of the heart; called also Wenckebach's disease.

cardiopulmonary (kar″de-o-pul′mo-ner-e) pertaining to the heart and lungs.

cardiopuncture (kar″de-o-punk′cher) cardiocentesis.

cardiopyloric (kar″de-o-pi-lor′ik) pertaining to the cardia (ostium cardiacum [NA]) and the pylorus.

Cardioquin (kar′de-o-kwin″) trademark for a preparation of quinidine polygalacturonate.

cardiorenal (kar″de-o-re′nal) pertaining to the heart and the kidney.

cardiorrhaphy (kar″de-or′ah-fe) [cardio- + Gr. raphē suture] the operation of suturing the heart muscle.

cardiorrhexis (kar″de-o-rek′sis) [cardio- + Gr. rhēxis rupture] rupture of the heart.

cardiosclerosis (kar″de-o-skle-ro′sis) [cardio- + Gr. sklēros hard] fibrous induration of the heart.

cardioscope (kar′de-o-skōp″) [cardio- + Gr. skopein to examine] an instrument once used for inspecting the interior of the heart and for manipulation within the heart.

cardioselective (kar″de-o-sĕ-lek′tiv) having greater activity on heart tissue than on other tissue.

cardiospasm (kar′de-o-spazm″) achalasia of the esophagus; see under *achalasia.*

cardiosphygmogram (kar″de-o-sfig′mŏ-gram) a tracing made by the cardiosphygmograph.

cardiosphygmograph (kar″de-o-sfig′mŏ-graf) a combination of the cardiograph and sphygmograph for recording the movements of the heart and an arterial pulse.

cardiosplenopexy (kar″de-o-splen′o-pek″se) suture of splenic parenchyma to the denuded surface of the heart, formerly used as a method of revascularization of the myocardium.

cardiosymphysis (kar″de-o-sim′fĭ-sis) [*cardio-* + Gr. *symphysis* growing together] (*obs.*) a condition in which the heart has become fixed to the chest by combined adhesion of the visceral and parietal pericardia to each other and by adhesion of the parietal pericardium to the mediastinal structures.

cardiotachometer (kar″de-o-tah-kom′ĕ-ter) [*cardio-* + Gr. *tachos* speed + *metron* measure] the instrument used in cardiotachometry.

cardiotachometry (kar″de-o-tah-kom′ĕ-tre) continuous recording of the heart rate for long periods of time.

cardiotherapy (kar″de-o-ther′ah-pe) [*cardio-* + Gr. *therapeia* treatment] the treatment of heart diseases.

cardiothyrotoxicosis (kar″de-o-thi″ro-tok″se-ko′sis) hyperthyroidism with cardiac involvement.

cardiotocograph (kar″de-o-to′ko-graf) the instrument used in cardiotocography.

cardiotocography (kar″de-o-to-kog′rah-fe) [*cardio-* + Gr. *tokos* childbirth + *graphein* to write] the monitoring of the fetal heart rate and uterine contractions, as during delivery. Also spelled *cardiotokography.*

cardiotokography (kar″de-o-to-kog′rah-fe) cardiotocography.

cardiotomy (kar″de-o-ot′ŏ-me) [*cardio-* + Gr. *tome* a cutting] 1. surgical incision of the heart for repair of cardiac defects. 2. incision into the cardiac end of the stomach or the cardiac orifice.

cardiotonic (kar″de-o-ton′ik) 1. having a tonic effect on the heart. 2. an agent that has a tonic effect on the heart.

cardiotopometry (kar″de-o-to-pom′ĕ-tre) [*cardio-* + Gr. *topos* place + *metron* measure] measurement of the area of cardiac dullness.

cardiotoxic (kar″de-o-tok′sik) having a poisonous or deleterious effect upon the heart.

cardiovalvular (kar″de-o-val′vu-lar) pertaining to the valves of the heart.

cardiovalvulitis (kar″de-o-val″vu-li′tis) inflammation of the valves of the heart.

cardiovalvulotome (kar″de-o-val′vu-lo-tōm″) [*cardio-* + L. *valvula* valve + Gr. *tome* cut] an instrument for performing cardiovalvulotomy.

cardiovalvulotomy (kar″de-o-val″vu-lot′o-me) [*cardio-* + L. *valvula* valve + Gr. *tome* a cutting] the operation of incising a cardiac valve, or of excising a portion of it, done for the relief of stenosis.

cardiovascular (kar″de-o-vas′ku-lar) pertaining to the heart and blood vessels.

cardiovascular-renal (kar″de-o-vas′ku-lar-re′nal) pertaining to the heart, blood vessels, and kidney.

cardiovasology (kar″de-o-vas-ol′o-je) cardioangiology.

cardioversion (kar″de-o-ver′zhun) the restoration of normal rhythm of the heart by electrical shock.

cardioverter (kar′-de-o-ver″ter) an energy-storage capacitor-discharge type of condenser which is discharged with an inductance; it delivers a direct-current shock which restores normal rhythm of the heart.

carditis (kar-di′tis) [*cardio-* + *-itis*] inflammation of the heart. **rheumatic c.,** cardiac involvement in rheumatic fever, which when severe may be manifested by congestive heart failure, progressive cardiac enlargement, pericarditis, and significant murmurs. **streptococcal c.,** carditis occurring as a result of streptococcal sore throat. **verru-**

cous c., a nonbacterial endocarditis marked by a continuous chain of wartlike vegetations near the line of closure of the cusps of the mitral and tricuspid valves; seen in lupus erythematosus and occasionally in scleroderma, thrombotic purpura, and other collagen diseases.

carfecillin sodium (kar″fĕ-sil′in) carbenicillin phenyl sodium.

carfentanil citrate (kar-fen′tah-nil) chemical name: 4-[(1-oxopropyl) phenyl amino]-1-(2-phenylethyl)-4-piperidine carboxylic acid methyl ester 2-hydroxy 1,2,3-propanetricarboxylate (1:1); an analgesic and narcotic, $C_{24}H_{30}N_2O_3 \cdot C_6H_8O_7$.

caricous (kar′ĭ-kus) [L. *carica* fig] shaped like or resembling a fig.

caries (ka′re-ēz, kar′ēz) [L. "rottenness"] 1. the molecular decay or death of a bone, in which it becomes softened, discolored, and porous. It produces a chronic inflammation of the periosteum and surrounding tissues, and forms a cold abscess filled with a cheesy, fetid, puslike liquid, which generally burrows through the soft parts until it opens externally by a sinus or fistula. 2. dental c. **backward c.,** dental caries that progresses backward from the dentino-enamel junction into the enamel; called also *internal c.* **cemental c.,** dental caries that involves the cementum of a tooth. **central c.,** a chronic abscess in the interior of a bone. **dental c.,** localized destruction of calcified tissue initiated on the tooth surface by decalcification of the enamel of the teeth, followed by enzymatic lysis of organic structures, leading to cavity formation that, if left unchecked, penetrates the enamel and dentin and may reach the pulp. Several theories on etiology have been proposed: The *acidogenic theory,* according to which acids produced by bacteria cause decalcification and softening of the residue; the *proteolytic theory,* according to which microorganisms destroy enamel protein; and the *proteolysis-chelation theory,* according to which keratolytic microorganisms cause formation of chelates, which in turn cause decalcification. Classified by Greene Vardiman Black into five groups on the basis of similarity of treatment required. (See table for Classification of Dental Caries, to which a sixth group is sometimes added.) Called also *tooth decay.* See also *cavity.* **dental c., pri-**

BLACK'S CLASSIFICATION OF DENTAL CARIES

Class I: Cavities occurring in pit and fissure defects in occlusal surfaces of bicuspids and molars, lingual surfaces of upper incisors, and facial and lingual grooves sometimes found on occlusal surfaces of molar teeth.
Class II: Cavities in proximal surfaces of bicuspids and molars.
Class III: Cavities in proximal surfaces of incisors and cuspids not requiring removal of incisal angle.
Class IV: Cavities in proximal surfaces of incisors and cuspids that require removal of incisal angle.
Class V: Cavities in gingival third of labial, or lingual, or buccal surfaces.
Class VI: Cavities in incisal edges and smooth surfaces of teeth above the height of contour. (NOTE: not a true Black classification.)

---

mary, dental caries in which the lesion constitutes the initial attack on the tooth surface. **dental c., secondary,** dental caries occurring around the edges and under restorations. **dentinal c.,** dental caries that spreads along the dentinoenamel junction and involves dentinal tubules, eventually reaching the pulp. **dry c.,** a form of tuberculous caries of the joints and ends of bones; called also *c. sicca.* **enamel c.,** dental caries that involves the enamel of a tooth. **c. fungo′sa,** a form of tuberculosis of a bone. **internal c.,** backward c. **lateral c.,** dental caries that extends laterally at the dentinoenamel junction. **necrotic c.,** a disease in which pieces of bone lie in a suppurating cavity. **pit c.,** dental caries originating in pits or fissures, usually of the occlusal surfaces of molars and premolars or on the lingual surfaces of the maxillary incisors, typically occurring as a deep cavity with a narrow point of penetration. Called also *fissure c.* **c. sic′ca,** dry c. **spinal c.,** tuberculotic osteitis of the vertebrae and of the intervertebral cartilages.

carina (kah-ri′nah), pl. *cari′nae* [L. "keel"] a ridgelike structure. **c. for′nicis,** a ridge on the under surface of the fornix. **c. of trachea, c. tra′cheae** [NA], a projection of the lowest tracheal cartilage, forming a prominent semilunar ridge running anteroposteriorly between the orifices of the two bronchi. **urethral c. of vagina, c. urethra′lis vagi′nae** [NA], the column of rugae in the lower part of the anterior wall of the vagina, immediately beneath the urethra.

carinae (kah-ri'ne) [L.] genitive and plural of *carina*.

carinate (kar'ĭ-nāt) [L. *carina* a keel] keel shaped; having a keel-like process.

carination (kar"ĭ-na'shun) a ridged condition of a part.

carindacillin sodium (kar"in-dah-sil'in) carbenicillin indanyl sodium.

cariogenesis (kār"e-o-jen'ĕ-sis) development of caries.

cariogenic (kār"e-o-jen'ik) [*caries* + Gr. *gennan* to produce] conducive to the production of caries.

cariogenicity (kār"e-o-jĕ-nis'ĭ-te) the quality of being conducive to the production of caries.

cariology (kar"e-ol'o-je) 1. [*cario-* +-*logy*] the study of cariogenesis and its prevention. 2. karyology.

cariosity (kar"e-os'ĭ-te) the quality of being carious.

carious (ka're-us) [L. *cariosus*] affected with or of the nature of caries.

carisoprodol (kar"i-so-pro'dol) chemical name: (1-methylethyl)carbamic acid-2-[[(aminocarbonyl)oxy]methyl]-2-methylpentyl ester. A centrally acting skeletal muscle relaxant, $C_{12}H_{24}N_2O_4$, occurring as a white, crystalline powder; used for the symptomatic management of acute, painful musculoskeletal disorders, administered orally. Called also *isopropyl meprobamate*.

Carleton's spots (karl'tonz) [Bukk G. *Carleton*, American physician, 1856–1914] see under *spot*.

carmalum (kar-mal'um) a stain composed of carmine, alum, and water.

carmantadine (kar-man'tah-dēn) chemical name: 1-tricyclo-[3.3.1.1^{3,7}]dec-1-yl-azetidinecarboxylic acid; an antiparkinsonian agent, $C_{14}H_{21}NO_2$.

carminative (kar-min'ah-tiv) [L. *carminare* to card, to cleanse, from *carmen*, a card for wool] 1. relieving flatulence. 2. a medicine that relieves flatulence and assuages pain.

carmine (kar'min) a red coloring matter derived from cochineal by the addition of alum and used as a histologic stain; called also *carminum* and *coccinellin*. **alizarin c.,** alizarin red. **indigo c.,** indigotin disulfonate sodium. **lithium c.,** vital stain for macrophages. **Schneider's c.,** a saturated solution of carmine in concentrated acetic acid.

carminic acid (kar-min'ik) an aromatic acid that is the essential constituent of the dye carmine.

carminophil (kar-min'o-fil) [*carmine* + Gr. *philein* to love] 1. easily stainable with carmine. 2. a cell or other element that readily takes a stain from carmine. 3. one of the acidophils, or alpha cells (*mammotropes*), of the adenohypophysis staining readily with azocarmine; called also *epsilon acidophil*.

carminum (kar-mi'num) carmine.

carmustine (kar-mus'tēn) a cytotoxic alkylating agent of the nitrosourea group, used as an antineoplastic primarily against brain tumors, multiple myeloma, colorectal carcinoma, and Hodgkin's disease and non-Hodgkin's lymphomas.

carneous (kar'ne-us) [L. *carneus*, from *caro* flesh] fleshy.

carnidazole (kar-nid'ah-zōl) chemical name: [2-(2-methyl-5-nitro-1*H*-imidazol-1-yl)ethyl]carbamothioic acid *O*-methyl ester; an antiprotozoal, $C_8H_{12}N_4O_3S$.

carnification (kar"nĭ-fĭ-ka'shun) [L. *caro* flesh + *facere* to make] the change of tissue, such as that of the lungs, into a substance resembling flesh.

carnitine (kar'nĭ-tēn) a naturally occurring amino acid, $C_7H_{15}NO_3$, required for mitochondrial oxidation of long-chain fatty acids; it is a betaine derivative found in skeletal muscle and liver, which acts as a carrier of acyl groups (fatty acids) across the mitochondrial membrane to the matrix, where they combine with coenzyme A to form acyl CoA. It has been used as an investigational antithyroid and antiangina agent.

carnitine palmitoyl transferase (kar'nĭ-tēn pal"mĭ-to"il-trans'fer-ās) [EC 2.3.1.21] an enzyme of the transferase class that catalyzes the reaction palmitoyl-CoA + L-carnitine = CoA + L-palmitoyl carnitine. The reaction is part of the mechanism for transport of acyl groups across the inner membrane of mitochondria. Deficiency of the enzyme is a cause of defective fatty acid oxidation.

Carnivora (kar-niv'ŏ-rah) [L. *caro* flesh + *vorare* to devour] an order of mammals that are primarily carnivorous, with teeth adapted for flesh eating, a simple stomach, and a short intestine.

carnivore (kar'nĭ-vōr) an animal that eats flesh, especially members of the order Carnivora.

carnivorous (kar-niv'o-rus) eating or subsisting on flesh.

carnosinase (kar'no-sĭ-nās) aminoacyl-histidine dipeptidase.

carnosinase deficiency an autosomal recessive aminoacidopathy of carnosine metabolism, causing myoclonic seizures, severe mental retardation, and spasticity; called also *carnosinemia* and *hyper-beta carnosinemia*.

carnosine (kar'no-sin) chemical name: β-alanylhistidine. A dipeptide, $C_9H_{14}N_4O_2$, composed of beta-alanine and histidine, found in skeletal muscle of vertebrates.

carnosinemia (kar"no-sĭ-ne'me-ah) carnosinase deficiency.

carnosinuria (kar"no-sĭ-nu're-ah) an aminoaciduria characterized by excess of carnosine in the urine; occurs in carnosinemia or may be dietary in origin, especially in young children.

carnosity (kar-nos'ĭ-te) [L. *carnositas* fleshiness] any abnormal fleshy excrescence.

Carnot's test (kar'nōz) [Paul *Carnot*, French physician, 1869–1957] see under *tests*.

carnutine (kar-nu'tin) a ptomaine found in muscle tissue.

caro (ka'ro), pl. *car'nes* [L.] flesh or muscular tissue. **c. quadra'ta ma'nus,** musculus palmaris brevis. **c. quadra'ta syl'vii,** musculus quadratus plantae.

Caroli's disease (kar'o-lēz) [Jacques *Caroli*, French physician, born 1902] see under *disease*.

carota (kah-ro'tah), pl. *caro'tae* [L.] carrot.

carotene (kar'o-tēn) [L., *carota* carrot] one of four isomeric pigments (α-, β-, γ-, and δ-carotene), having colors from violet to red-yellow to yellow, found in many dark green, leafy, and yellow vegetables (e.g., collards, turnips, carrots, sweet potatoes, and squash), and yellow fruit (e.g., apricots, oranges, peaches, and cantaloupes). They are fat-soluble, unsaturated aliphatic hydrocarbons that are converted to vitamin A in animals by an enzyme in the intestinal wall and the liver. β-Carotene is the major precursor (provitamin) of vitamin A in humans. Called also *carotin*. **beta c.,** chemical name: β,β-carotene; an ultraviolet screen, $C_{40}H_{56}$.

β-carotene 15,15'-dioxygenase [EC 1.13.11.21] an enzyme of the oxidoreductase class that catalyzes the reaction β-carotene + O_2 = 2 retinal. It occurs in the intestinal mucosa.

carotenemia (kar"o-te-ne'me-ah) [*carotene* + Gr. *haima* blood + -*ia*] presence of excessive carotene in the blood; occurring as a result of the excessive ingestion of carotene-containing foods or of synthetic β-carotene, and sometimes producing yellowing of the skin (see *carotenoderma*). Carotenemia may also occur in diabetes mellitus, which has been ascribed to both hyperlipemia and to failure of the liver to convert carotene to vitamin A. It may also be seen in hypothyroidism, one reason of which being that it is believed that the presence of thyroid hormone is necessary for the conversion of carotene to vitamin A. Called also *carotenosis*, *carotinemia*, *carotinosis*, and *xanthemia*.

carotenoderma (kar-ot'en-o-der'mah) [*carotene* + *derma*] yellowness of the skin due to carotenemia, which clinically resembles jaundice except that the sclerae are spared. The palms and soles and behind the ears are the areas of the skin usually most strongly stained. Called also *carotenodermia*.

carotenodermia (kah-rot"ĕ-no-der'me-ah) carotenoderma.

carotenoid (kah-rot'ĕ-noid) 1. any group of pigments, yellow to deep red in color, chemically consisting of tetraterpene (polyisoprene) hydrocarbons. Carotenoids are synthesized in plants (giving color to the tomato and carrot, for example) and in certain animal tissues. They concentrate in animal fat when eaten (where they are called *lipochromes*). Examples are β-carotene, lycopene, and xanthophyll. 2. marked by a yellow color.

carotenosis (kar"o-te-no'sis) carotenemia.

carotic (kah-rot'ik) [Gr. *karos* deep sleep] pertaining to or of the nature of carus, or stupor.

caroticotympanic (kah-rot″ĭ-ko-tim-pan′ik) pertaining to the carotid canal and the tympanum.

carotid (kah-rot′id) [Gr. *karōtis* from *karos* deep sleep] relating to the principal artery of the neck (arteria carotis communis); see also under *body, sinus,* etc.

carotidynia (kah-rot″ĭ-din′e-ah) carotodynia.

carotin (kar′o-tin) carotene.

carotinemia (kar″o-tin-e′me-ah) carotenemia.

carotinosis (kar″o-tĭ-no′sis) carotenemia.

carotodynia (kah-rot″o-din′e-ah) [*carotid* + Gr. *odynē* pain] tenderness along the course of the common carotid artery.

caroxazone (kah-roks′ah-zōn) chemical name: 2-oxo-2*H*-1,3-benzoxazine-3(4*H*)-acetamide; an antidepressant, $C_{10}H_{10}N_2O_3$.

carp (karp) a fruiting body of a fungus.

carpal (kar′pal) [L. *carpalis*] of or pertaining to the carpus, or wrist.

carpale (kar-pa′le) a carpal bone.

carpectomy (kar-pek′to-me) [*carpus* + Gr. *ektomē* excision] excision of a carpal bone.

carpel (kar′pel) a one-celled pistil, or one of the members composing a compound pistil or seed vessel.

carphenazine maleate (kar-fen′ah-zēn) [USP] chemical name: 1-[10-[3-[4-(2-hydroxyethyl)1-piperazinyl]propyl]-10*H*-phenothiazin-2-yl]-1-propanone(Z)-2-butenedioate (1:2). A phenothiazine antipsychotic agent, $C_{24}H_{31}N_3O_2S \cdot 2C_4H_4O_4$, occurring as a yellow, finely divided powder; used in the treatment of acute or chronic schizophrenic reactions in hospitalized patients, administered orally.

carphologia (kar″fo-lo′je-ah) carphology.

carphology (kar-fol′o-je) [Gr. *karphologein* to pick bits of wool off a person's coat] the involuntary picking at the bedclothes seen in grave fevers and in conditions of great exhaustion; called also *carphologia* and *crocidismus.*

carpitis (kar-pi′tis) inflammation of the synovial membranes of the bones of the carpal joint of domestic animals, producing swelling, pain, and lameness.

carpocarpal (kar″po-kar′pal) pertaining to two parts of the carpus, especially to the articulations between carpal bones.

Carpoglyphus (kar″po-gli′fus) a genus of mites. **C. passula′rum,** a tyroglyphid mite that infests dried fruit, causing dermatitis in those who handle the infested fruit.

carpogonium (kar″po-go′ne-um) ascogonium; more specifically the female sex organ in members of the order Erysiphales, class Ascomycetes.

carpometacarpal (kar″po-met″ah-kar′pal) pertaining to the carpus and metacarpus.

carpopedal (kar″po-pe′dal) [*carpus* + L. *pes, pedalis* foot] pertaining to or affecting the carpus and the foot, as carpopedal spasm.

carpophalangeal (kar″po-fah-lan′je-al) pertaining to the carpus and the phalanges.

carpoptosis (kar″pop-to′sis) [*carpus* + *ptosis*] wristdrop.

carpospore (kar′po-spōr) a diploid spore in the red algae which, by germination, produces tetraspores.

carprofen (kar-pro′fen) chemical name: (±)-6-chloro-α-methylcarbazole-2-acetic acid; an anti-inflammatory, $C_{15}H_{12}ClNO_2$.

Carpue's operation, rhinoplasty (kar′pūz) [Joseph Constantine *Carpue,* English surgeon, 1764–1846] Indian rhinoplasty.

Carpule (kar′pūl) trademark for a glass, rubber-stoppered cartridge containing local anesthetic solutions, fitted in a special syringe for hypodermic injection.

carpus (kar′pus) [L., from Gr. *karpos*] the joint between the arm and hand, the wrist, made up of eight bones; see *ossa carpi,* and names of specific bones. Also, the part of the hand between the forearm and metacarpus. The term is also applied to the corresponding forelimb joint in quadrupeds. **c. cur′vus,** Madelung's deformity.

Carr-Price test [Francis Howard *Carr,* British chemist, born 1874; E. A. *Price* English biochemist, 20th century] see under *tests.*

carrageen, carragheen (kar′ah-gēn) the dried and bleached plant *Chondrus crispus* (L.) Stackhouse, or *Gigartina mammillosa* (Goodenough and Woodward) J. Aghardt,

(Gigartinaceae). It contains a valuable polysaccharide widely used as a gel, thickening agent, and emulsifier. It also has demulcent properties.

carrageenan, carragheenin (kar″ah-ge′nan) a colloidal extractive derived from various species of red marine algae (*Chondrus, Eucheuma, Gigartina,* etc.), composed of a mixture of sodium, potassium, calcium, and magnesium salts of an acid sulfate of a galactose-containing polysaccharide. Used chiefly as a suspending agent in foods, pharmaceuticals, cosmetics, etc.

carreau (kar-ro′) [Fr.] (*obs.*) enlargement and hardening of the abdomen caused by disease of the peritoneum and abdominal walls.

Carrel (kah-rel′), Alexis. French surgeon residing in the United States, 1873–1944; winner of the Nobel prize for medicine or physiology in 1912 for his work in suturing blood vessels, transfusion, and organ transplants.

Carrel's method, treatment, tube (kar-elz′) [Alexis *Carrel*] see under *method, treatment,* and *tube.*

Carrel-Dakin fluid, treatment [Alexis *Carrel;* Henry Drysdale *Dakin,* American chemist, 1880–1952] see *diluted sodium hypochorite solution,* under *solution,* and see under *treatment.*

carrier (kar′e-er) 1. an individual who harbors the specific organisms of a disease without manifest symptoms and is capable of transmitting the infection; the condition of such an individual is referred to as the *carrier state.* 2. electron carrier; a chemical substance that can accept one or more electrons and then donate them to another substance (being reduced and then reoxidized). 3. an instrument or apparatus for carrying something. 4. in genetics, an individual who is heterozygous for a recessive gene and thus does not express the recessive phenotype but can transmit it to offspring. Only females can be carriers of X-linked recessive traits. 5. a substance that carries a radioisotopic or other label, as in a tracer study. A second isotope mixed with a particular isotope is also referred to as a carrier; see *carrier-free.* 6. a transport protein that carries specific substances, e.g., in the blood or across cell membranes. 7. in immunology, a macromolecular substance to which a hapten is coupled in order to produce an immune response against the hapten; immune responses being usually produced only against large molecules capable of simultaneously binding both B cells and helper T cells. Called also *schlepper.* **amalgam c.,** an instrument for carrying freshly mixed amalgam to the prepared cavity. **electron c.,** carrier, def. 2. **foil c.,** see under passer. **gametocyte c.,** in malaria, a person who has gametocytes in his blood stream and so can infect *Anopheles* mosquitoes that feed on him and thus transmit malaria. **lentulo paste c.,** lentulo. **paste c.,** lentulo.

carrier-free (kar′e-er-fre) a term denoting a radioisotope of an element in pure form, i.e., essentially undiluted with a stable isotope carrier.

Carrión's disease (kar-e-onz′) [Daniel A. *Carrión,* (1850–1885), a student in Peru who inoculated himself and died of the disease] bartonellosis.

carrot (kar′ut) [L. *carota*] the umbelliferous plant, *Daucus carota;* its seed is diuretic and stimulant.

cart (kart) a wheeled vehicle for conveying patients or equipment and supplies in a hospital. **crash c.,** resuscitation c. **dressing c.,** one containing all the supplies and equipment that may be necessary for changing dressings of surgical or injured patients. **resuscitation c.,** one containing all the equipment necessary for initiating emergency resuscitation.

cartazolate (kar-taz′o-lāt) chemical name: 4-(butylamino)-1-ethyl-1*H*-pyrazolo[3,4-*b*]pyridine-5-carboxylic acid ethyl ester; an antidepressant, $C_{15}H_{22}N_4O_2$.

carteolol hydrochloride (kar′te-o-lōl) chemical name: 5-[3-[(1,1-dimethylethyl)amino]-2-hydroxypropoxy]-3,4-dihydro-2(1*H*)-quinolinone monohydrochloride; an antiadrenergic (β-receptor), $C_{16}H_{24}N_2O_3 \cdot HCl$.

cartilage (kar′tĭ-lij) [L. *cartilago*] a specialized, fibrous connective tissue, forming most of the temporary skeleton of the embryo, providing a model in which most of the bones develop, and constituting an important part of the growth mechanism of the organism. It exists in several types, the most important of which are hyaline cartilage, elastic cartilage, and fibrocartilage. Also used as a general term to designate a mass of such tissue in a particular site in the body. See *cartilago*. **accessory c's of nose,** cartilagines alares minores. **c. of acoustic meatus,** cartilago meatus acustici. **alar c., greater,** cartilago alaris major. **alar c's, lesser,** cartilagines alares minores. **annular c.,** cartilago cricoidea. **aortic c.,** the second costal cartilage on the right side. **arthrodial c.,** articular c. **articular c.,** a thin layer of cartilage, usually hyaline, on the articular surface of bones in synovial joints. Called also *cartilago articularis* [NA], *arthrodial c., diarthrodial c., investing c.,* and *obducent c.* **arytenoid c.,** cartilago arytenoidea. **c. of auditory tube,** cartilago tubae auditivae. **c. of auricle, auricular c.,** cartilago auriculae. **branchial c.,** one of the rods of cartilage in the branchial arches of the embryo. **calcified c.,** cartilage in which granules of calcium phosphate and calcium carbonate have been deposited in the interstitial substance. **cariniform c.,** the cartilaginous prolongation at the anterior end of the sternum of a horse. **cellular c.,** a variety composed almost entirely of cells, with little interstitial substance; called also *parenchymatous c.* **ciliary c's,** see *tarsus inferior palpebrae* and *tarsus superior palpebrae.* **circumferential c.,** labrum glenoidale. **conchal c.,** cartilago auriculae. **connecting c.,** cartilage connecting the surfaces of an immovable joint; called also *interosseous c.* **corniculate c.,** cartilago corniculata. **costal c.,** cartilago costalis. **costal c., interarticular,** ligamentum sternocostale intraarticulare. **cricoid c.,** cartilago cricoidea. **cuneiform c.,** cartilago cuneiformis. **dentinal c.,** the substance remaining after the lime salts of dentin have been dissolved in an acid. **diarthrodial c.,** articular c. **elastic c.,** a substance that is more opaque, flexible, and elastic than hyaline cartilage, and is further distinguished by its yellow color. The interstitial substance is penetrated in all directions by frequently branching fibers which give all the reactions for elastin. Called also *reticular c.* and *yellow c.* **ensiform c.,** processus xiphoideus. **epactal c's,** cartilagines nasales accessoriae. **epiglottic c.,** cartilago epiglottica. **epiphyseal c.,** cartilago epiphysialis. **eustachian c.,** cartilago tubae auditivae. **falciform c's,** see *meniscus lateralis articulationis genus* and *meniscus medialis articulationis genus.* **floating c.,** a detached piece of cartilage, usually from the articular surface of the medial condyle and femur, but also from the patella or lateral condyle of the femur. **gingival c.,** the tissue covering the loculus which contains an unerupted tooth. **guttural c.,** cartilago arytenoidea. **hyaline c.,** a flexible, somewhat elastic, semitransparent substance with an opalescent bluish tint, composed of a basophilic, fibril-containing inter-

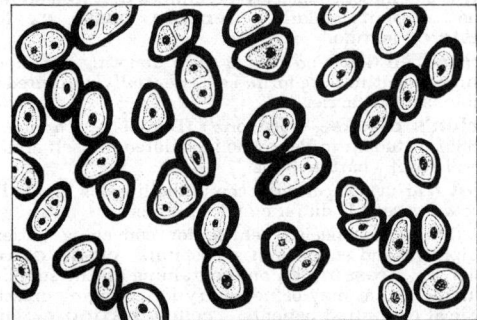

Hyaline cartilage. The matrix nearest the chondrocytes is intensely staining; although the matrix appears homogenous, collagen fibrils may be visualized by polarized light or electron microscopy.

stitial substance with cavities in which the chondrocytes occur; called also *chondroid.* **inferior c. of nose,** cartilago alaris major. **innominate c.,** cartilago cricoidea. **interarticular c.,** 1. ligamentum longitudinale posterius. 2. an interarticular disk. **interarticular c. of little head of rib,** ligamentum capitis costae intraarticulare. **interosseous c.,** connecting c. **intervertebral c's,** disci intervertebrales. **intrathyroid c.,** a cartilage connecting the alae of the thyroid cartilage in early life. **investing c.,** articular c. **Jacobson's c.,** cartilago vomeronasalis. **laryngeal c's,** cartilagines laryngis. **laryngeal c. of Luschka,** cartilago sesamoidea ligamenti

vocalis. **lateral c's,** in the horse, the cartilages from the end of the third phalanx to the heel of the hoof. **lateral c. of nose,** cartilago nasi lateralis. **Luschka's c.,** cartilago sesamoidea ligamenti vocalis. **mandibular c.,** Meckel's c. **meatal c.,** cartilago meatus acustici. **Meckel's c.,** the cartilaginous bar (in the embryo) into which the mesenchymal core of the mandibular process of the first mandibular arch is converted; from it or its sheath, the sphenomandibular ligament, the anterior malleolar ligament, the malleus, and the incus develop. Called also *mandibular c., tympanomandibular c.,* and *Meckel's rod.* **minor c's,** cartilagines nasales accessoriae. **mucronate c.,** processus xiphoideus. **nasal c's,** cartilagines nasi. **nasal c's, accessory,** cartilagines nasales accessoriae. **nasal c., lateral,** cartilago nasi lateralis. **c. of nasal septum,** cartilago septi nasi. **c's of nose,** cartilagines nasi. **obducent c.,** articular c. **ossifying c.,** temporary c. **palpebral c's,** see *tarsus inferior palpebrae* and *tarsus superior palpebrae.* **parachordal c's,** the two cartilages at the sides of the occipital part of the notochord of the embryo. **parenchymatous c.,** cellular c. **periotic c.,** an oval mass on the upper surface of the fetal chondrocranium investing the inner ear. **permanent c.,** cartilage that does not normally become ossified. **posterior cricoarytenoid c.,** ligamenta cricoarytenoideum posterius. **precursory c.,** temporary c. **pulmonary c.,** the third costal cartilage on the left side. **pyramidal c.,** cartilago arytenoidea. **Reichert's c's,** cartilaginous bars in the lateral side of the embryonic tympanum from which develop the styloid processes, the stylohyoid ligaments, and the lesser cornua of the hyoid bone. **reticular c.,** elastic c. **Santorini's c.,** cartilago corniculata. **scutiform c.,** cartilago thyroidea. **semilunar c. of knee joint, external,** meniscus lateralis articulationis genus. **semilunar c. of knee joint, internal,** meniscus medialis articulationis genus. **septal c. of nose,** cartilago septi nasi. **sesamoid c. of larynx,** cartilago triticea. **sesamoid c's of nose,** cartilagines nasales accessoriae. **sesamoid c. of vocal ligament,** cartilago sesamoidea ligamenti vocalis. **sigmoid c's,** see *meniscus lateralis articulationis genus* and *meniscus medialis articulationis genus.* **slipping rib c.,** loosening and deformity of the costal cartilages, causing painful symptoms. **sternal c.,** cartilago costalis. **stratified c.,** fibrocartilage. **subvomerine c's,** cartilago vomeronasalis. **supra-arytenoid c.,** cartilago corniculata. **tarsal c's,** see *tarsus inferior palpebrae* and *tarsus superior palpebrae.* **temporary c.,** any cartilage that is being replaced by bone or that is normally destined to be replaced by bone; called also *ossifying c.* and *precursory c.* **tendon c.,** a form of embryonic cartilage by which tendons and bones are united. **thyroid c.,** cartilago thyroidea. **tracheal c's,** cartilagines tracheales. **triangular c. of nose,** cartilago nasi lateralis. **triquetral c., triquetrous c.,** 1. cartilago arytenoidea. 2. discus articularis articulationis radioulnaris distalis. **triticeal c., triticeous c.,** cartilago triticea. **tubal c.,** cartilago tubae auditivae. **tympanomandibular c.,** Meckel's c. **vomeronasal c.,** cartilago vomeronasalis. **Weitbrecht's c.,** discus articularis articulationis acromioclavicularis. **Wrisberg's c.,** cartilago cuneiformis. **xiphoid c.,** processus xiphoideus. **Y c.,** a Y-shaped cartilage in the acetabulum, joining the ilium, ischium, and pubes. **yellow c.,** elastic c.

cartilagin (kar′tĭ-laj″in) a protein found in cartilage, which is changed by boiling into chondrin; called also *chondrigen.*

cartilagines (kar″tĭ-laj′ĭ-nēz) [L.] plural of *cartilago.*

cartilaginification (kar″tĭ-lah-jin″ĭ-fĭ-ka′shun) conversion into cartilage.

cartilaginiform (kar″tĭ-lah-jin′ĭ-form) resembling cartilage; called also *cartilaginoid.*

cartilaginoid (kar″tĭ-laj′ĭ-noid) cartilaginiform.

cartilaginous (kar″tĭ-laj′ĭ-nus) consisting of or of the nature of cartilage.

cartilago (kar-tĭ-lah′go), pl. *cartilag′ines* [L.] a specialized, fibrous connective tissue; see *cartilage.* Used in anatomical nomenclature to designate a mass of such tissue in a particular site in the body. **c. ala′ris ma′jor** [NA], greater alar cartilage: either of two thin, curved cartilages, one on either side at the apex of the nose, each of which possesses a lateral and a medial crus; called also *inferior*

cartilage of nose. **cartilag′ines ala′res mino′res** [NA], lesser alar cartilages: various small cartilages located in the fibrous tissue of the alae nasi; called also *accessory cartilages of nose.* **c. articula′ris** [NA], articular cartilage: a thin layer of cartilage, usually hyaline, on the articular surface of bones in synovial joints; called also *arthrodial, diarthrodial, investing,* and *obducent cartilage.* **c. arytenoi′dea** [NA], arytenoid cartilage: one of the paired, pitcher-shaped cartilages of the back of the larynx at the upper border of the cricoid cartilage; called also *c. arytaenoidea* and *c. triquetra,* and *guttural, pyramidal, triquetral,* and *triquetrous cartilage.* **c. auric′ulae** [NA], cartilage of auricle: the internal plate of elastic cartilage which is found in the external ear; called also *auricular* and *conchal cartilage.* **c. cornicula′ta** [NA], corniculate cartilage: a small nodule of cartilage at the apex of each arytenoid cartilage; called also *c. corniculata [Santorini], c. santorini, Santorini's* and *supra-arytenoid cartilage, corniculum,* and *corpus santoriana.* **c. cornicula′ta [Santori′ni],** c. corniculata. **c. costa′lis** [NA], costal cartilage: a bar of hyaline cartilage by which the ventral extremity of a rib is attached to the sternum in the case of the true ribs, or to the superiorly adjacent ribs in the case of the upper false ribs; called also *sternal cartilage.* **c. cricoi′dea** [NA], cricoid cartilage: a ringlike cartilage forming the lower and back part of the larynx; called also *annular* or *innominate cartilage.* **c. cuneifor′mis** [NA], cuneiform cartilage: either of the paired cartilages, one on either side in the aryepiglottic fold; called also *c. cuneiformis [Wrisbergi], c. wrisbergi,* and *Wrisberg's cartilage.* **c. cuneifor′mis [Wrisber′gi],** c. cuneiformis. **c. ensifor′mis,** processus xiphoideus. **c. epiglot′tica** [NA], epiglottic cartilage: the plate of cartilage that constitutes the central part of the epiglottis. **c. epiphysia′lis** [NA], epiphyseal cartilage: the disk or plate of cartilage interposed between the epiphysis and the shaft of the bone during the period of growth; by its growth the bone increases in length. Called also *epiphyseal disk* or *plate* and *growth disk* or *plate.* **cartilag′ines falca′tae,** see *meniscus lateralis articulationis genus* and *meniscus medialis articulationis genus.* **c. jacobso′ni,** c. vomeronasalis. **cartilag′ines laryn′gis** [NA], laryngeal cartilages: cartilages of the larynx, including the cricoid, thyroid, and epiglottic, and two each of arytenoid, corniculate, and cuneiform cartilages. **c. mea′tus acus′tici** [NA], cartilage of acoustic meatus: the trough-shaped cartilage of the cartilaginous part of the external acoustic meatus; called also *meatal cartilage.* **cartilag′ines nasa′les accesso′riae** [NA], accessory nasal cartilages: one or more small cartilages on either side of the nose between the greater alar and lateral nasal cartilages; called also *cartilagines sesamoideae nasi, epactal* or *minor cartilages,* and *sesamoid cartilages of nose.* **cartilag′ines na′si** [NA], nasal cartilages: the cartilages of the nose, including the lateral nasal, greater and lesser alar, nasal septal, vomeronasal, and the accessory nasal cartilages. **c. na′si latera′lis** [NA], lateral nasal cartilage: a lateral expansion of the septal cartilage on either side of the nose just inferior to the nasal bone; called also *lateral* or *triangular cartilage of nose.* **c. santori′ni,** c. corniculata. **c. sep′ti na′si** [NA], cartilage of nasal septum: the hyaline cartilage forming the framework of the cartilaginous part of the nasal septum, and including the lateral nasal cartilages; called also *septal cartilage of nose.* **c. sesamoi′dea laryn′gis, Luschka,** c. sesamoidea ligamenti vocalis. **c. sesamoi′dea ligamen′ti voca′lis** [NA], sesamoid cartilage of vocal ligament: a small cartilage occasionally found within the vocal ligaments; called also *laryngeal cartilage of Luschka,* and *Luschka's cartilage.* **cartilag′ines sesamoi′deae na′si,** cartilagines nasales accessoriae. **c. thyroi′dea** [NA], thyroid cartilage: the largest cartilage of the larynx, with two broad, posteriorly diverging laminae and two pairs of horns, superior and inferior, that extend from the posterior borders of the laminae; called also *c. thyreoidea* and *scutiform cartilage.* **cartilag′ines trachea′les** [NA], tracheal cartilages: the 16 to 20 incomplete rings which, held together and enclosed by a strong, elastic, fibrous membrane, constitute the wall of the trachea. **c. triquet′ra,** 1. cartilago arytenoidea. 2. discus articularis articulationis radioulnaris distalis. **c. tritic′ea** [NA], triticeal cartilage: a small cartilage in the thyrohyoid ligament. Called also *sesamoid cartilage, corpusculum triticeum,* and *corpus triticeum.* **c. tu′bae auditi′vae** [NA], cartilage of auditory tube: the cartilage on the inferomedial surface of the temporal bone that supports the walls of the cartilaginous portion of the auditory tube; called also *tubal* or *eustachian cartilage.* **c. vomeronasa′lis** [NA], vomeronasal cartilage: either of the two narrow, longitudinal strips of cartilage, one lying on either side of the anterior portion of the lower margin of the septal cartilage; called also *c. vomeronasalis [Jacobsoni], c. jacobsoni,* and *Jacobson's* or *subvomerine cartilage.* **c. vomeronasa′lis [Jacobso′ni],** c. vomeronasalis. **c. wrisbergi,** c. cuneiformis.

cartilagotropic (kar″tĭ-lag-o-trop′ik) [L. *cartilago* cartilage + Gr. *tropos* a turning] having affinity for cartilage.

caruncle (kar′ung-kl) a small fleshy eminence, whether normal or abnormal; called also *caruncula* [NA]. **amniotic c's,** small epithelial amniotic growths occasionally found at the placental insertion of the umbilical cord, the fold of amnion, or Schultze's fold, carrying the vitelline duct. **hymenal c's,** carunculae hymenales. **lacrimal c.,** caruncula lacrimalis. **major c. of Santorini,** papilla duodeni major. **Morgagni's c., morgagnian c.,** lobus medius prostatae. **myrtiform c's,** carunculae hymenales. **sublingual c.,** caruncula sublingualis. **urethral c.,** a small, polypoid, deep red growth on the mucous membrane of the urinary meatus in women.

caruncula (kah-rung′ku-lah), pl. *carun′culae* [L. dim. of *caro* flesh] [NA] a small fleshy eminence; called also *caruncle.* **carun′culae hymena′les** [NA], hymenal caruncles: small elevations of the mucous membrane encircling the vaginal orifice, being relics of the torn hymen; called also *carunculae myrtiformis.* **c. lacrima′lis** [NA], lacrimal caruncle: the red eminence at the medial angle of the eye. **c. mammilla′ris** (obs.), trigonum olfactorium. **carun′culae myrtifor′mes,** carunculae hymenales. **c. saliva′ris,** c. sublingualis. **c. sublingua′lis** [NA], an eminence on each side of the frenulum of the tongue, at the apex of which are the openings of the major sublingual duct and the submandibular duct. Called also *c. salivaris* and *sublingual caruncle.*

carunculae (kah-rung′ku-le) [L.] plural of *caruncula.*

Carus' curve (circle) (kah′rus) [Karl Gustav *Carus,* German obstetrician, 1789–1869] see under *curve.*

Carvallo sign (kar-vah′yō) [J.M. Rivero-*Carvallo,* Mexican cardiologist, 20th century] see under *sign.*

carver (kar′ver) a knife or other instrument used for carving or fashioning an object by cutting, such as one used for shaping artificial teeth and dental restorations.

carvone (kar′vōn) chemical name: *p*-mentha-6,8-dien-2-one. A terpene ketone, $C_3H_5 \cdot C_6H_6O_6 \cdot CH_3$, found in many volatile oils, such as caraway oil, oil of dill, and spearmint oil.

cary(o)- [Gr. *karyon* nucleus, or nut] a combining form denoting relationship to a nucleus; see also words beginning *karyo-.*

Caryophanaceae (kar″e-o-fah-na′se-e) in former systems of classification, a family of bacteria containing the genera *Caryophanon, Lineola,* and *Simonsiella.*

Caryophanales (kar″e-o-fah-na′lēz) in former systems of classification, an order of bacteria made up of the families Arthomitaceae, Caryophanaceae, and Oscillospiraceae.

Caryophanon (ka″re-o′fah-non) [*caryo-* + Gr. *phanus* bright] a genus of bacteria of uncertain affiliation, consisting of gram-positive, asporogenous, rod-shaped organisms found in cow dung.

caryophil (kar′e-o-fil) staining easily with thiazinammonium stains.

Carysomyia (kar″ĭ-so-mi′yah) *Chrysomyia.*

carzenide (kar′zĕ-nīd) chemical name: *p*-sulfamoylbenzoic acid; a carbonic anhydrase inhibitor, $C_7H_7NO_4S$.

Casal's necklace (kah-salz′) [Gaspar *Casal,* Spanish physician, 1679–1759] see under *necklace.*

casanthranol (kah-san′thrah-nōl) a purified mixture of the anthranol glycosides derived from *Cascara sagrada*; a cathartic.

cascade (kas-kād′) a series of steps or stages (as of a physiological process) which, once initiated continues to the final step by virtue of each step being triggered by the preceding one, sometimes with cumulative effect. **electron c.,** the passage of electrons during oxidative phosphorylation from a large negative (reducing) potential through a series of cytochromes to a positive (oxidizing) potential.

cascara (kas-kār′ah) [Sp.] bark. **c. amar′ga** [Sp. "bit-

ter bark"], the bark of *Sweetia panamensis* Benth. (Leguminosae), a tree of tropical America; it is alterative and tonic.
c. sagra'da [Sp. "sacred bark"] [USP], the dried bark of *Rhamnus purshiana* DC. (Rhamnaceae), a shrub of the Pacific states of the United States, used as a cathartic; called also *bearberry bark, chittem bark, dogwood bark, Persian bark,* and *Purshiana bark.* Its laxative principles are glycosidal anthraquinones, e.g., emodin and barbaloin.

case (kās) 1. a particular instance of disease, as a *case* of leukemia; sometimes used incorrectly to designate the patient with the disease. 2. a term sometimes used incorrectly in dentistry to designate a flask, denture, casting, or the like. **borderline c.,** an instance of a disease in which the symptoms resemble those of a recognized condition but are not typical of it. **index c.,** the case of the original patient (propositus, or proband), which provides the stimulus for study of other members of the family, to ascertain a possible genetic factor in causation of the presenting condition. In epidemiology of contagious disease, the first case of a disease, as opposed to subsequent cases. **trial c.,** a box containing convex and concave spherical, and convex and concave cylindrical lenses, arranged in pairs, a trial spectacle frame, and various other devices used in testing vision.

caseation (ka″se-a′shun) [L. *caseus* cheese] 1. the precipitation of casein. 2. a form of necrosis in which the tissue is changed into a dry, amorphous mass resembling cheese.

casebook (kās-book) a book in which a physician enters the records of his cases.

case history (kās his-to′re) the collected data concerning an individual, his family, and environment, including his medical history and any other information that may be useful in analyzing and diagnosing his condition or for instructional purposes.

casein (ka′se-in, ka′sēn, ka-sēn′) [L. *caseus* cheese] a phosphoprotein, the principal protein of milk, the basis of curd and of cheese. It is precipitated from milk as a white amorphous substance by dilute acids, and redissolves on the addition of alkalis or of excess acid. Rennin (and other milk-clotting enzymes) influence the hydrolysis of casein to soluble paracasein, which in the presence of calcium (Ca^{++}) is converted to an insoluble curd (insoluble paracasein or calcium paracaseinate). Casein, usually in the form of its calcium, potassium, or sodium salts, is added to other ingredients of the diet to increase its protein content. NOTE: In British nomenclature, casein is called *caseinogen,* and paracasein is called *casein.* **c.-calcium,** calcium caseinate. **gluten c.,** a casein-like substance in the seeds of various cereal plants; glutin. **c.-sodium,** a nutrient preparation of casein and sodium hydroxide. **vegetable c.,** a protein resembling casein, e.g., wheat gluten.

caseinate (ka′se-ah-nāt″, ka-se′nāt) 1. any salt of casein. 2. a combination of casein and a metal.

caseinogen (ka″se-in′o-jen) [*casein* + Gr. *gennan* to produce] the British term for casein.

caseinogenate (ka″se-in′o-jĕ-nāt) a salt of caseinogen.

caseogenous (ka″se-oj′ĕ-nus) producing caseation; conversion into cheese (casein).

caseous (ka′se-us) resembling cheese or curd; cheesy.

caseum (ka′se-um) [L. "cheese"] cellular debris of a cheese-like consistency, produced as a result of caseation.

caseworm (kās′werm) echinococcus.

CaSO₄ calcium sulfate.

Casoni's intradermal test (reaction) (kah-so′nēz) [Tommaso *Casoni,* Italian physician, 1880–1933] see under *tests.*

cassava (kah-sah′vah) [Sp. *casabe*] a shrub of the genus *Manihot,* especially *M. esculenta* Crantz (Euphorbiaceae), and their starchy root products. The roots contain hydrogen cyanide, which is removed during processing to obtain starch. The starch is used in foods (soups, breads, tapioca) and glues.

Casselberry's position (kas′el-ber-e) [William Evans *Casselberry,* American laryngologist, 1859–1916] see under *position.*

Casser's (Casserio's, Casserius') fontanelle, etc. (kah′serz) [Giulio *Casserio,* Italian anatomist, 1556– 1616] see under *fontanelle, ligament,* and *muscle.*

casserian (kah-se′re-an) named for Giulio Casserio, as casserian fontanelle.

cassette (kah-set′) [Fr. "a little box"] 1. a lightproof hous-

ing for x-ray film, containing front and back intensifying screens between which the film is placed; it is usually backed with lead to prevent backscatter. 2. a magazine for film or magnetic tape.

Cassia (kash′e-ah) [L.; Gr. *kasia*] a genus of leguminous trees, shrubs, and herbs, found in the warmer regions of the world. *C. acutifo'lia* Del., native to Africa and cultivated in India, and *C. angustifo'lia* Vahl., native to Arabia, afford Alexandria senna and Tinnevelly senna, respectively.

cast (kast) 1. a negative copy or likeness of an object, a solid reproduction of an enclosed space, such as a mold of a hollow organ (e.g., a renal tubule, bronchiole), formed of effused plastic matter and extruded from the body, such as a urinary cast. 2. an accurate reproduction or a replica of an object or part produced in a plastic material that has taken form in an impression or mold. 3. to form an object in a mold. 4. a rigid dressing, molded to the body while pliable, and hardening as it dries, to give firm support. 5. dental c.; a positive reproduction of the maxillary or mandibular arch or a portion thereof made from an impression of that arch. Called also *model.* 6. strabismus. **bacterial c.,** a uri-

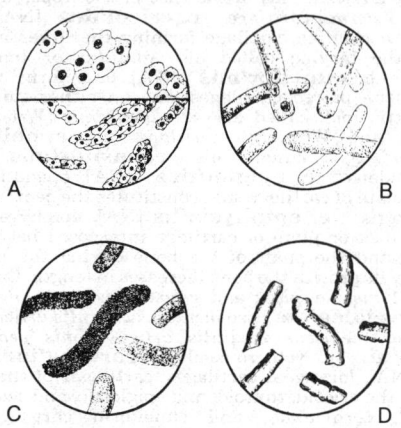

Casts. *A,* Squamous epithelium from urine *(top)* and epithelial casts *(bottom). B,* Hyaline casts. *C,* Granular casts. *D,* Waxy casts.

nary cast made up of bacteria or containing a large number of bacteria. **blood c.,** a urinary cast that bears blood cells on its surface. **coma c.,** a urinary cast containing strongly refracting granules; said to indicate oncoming coma in diabetes. Called also *Külz's c.* or *cylinder.* **decidual c.,** the mass of degenerating or necrotic decidua discharged from the uterus at the time of rupture of an ectopic pregnancy. **dental c.,** see *cast,* def. 5. **diagnostic c.,** a positive reproduction of the maxillary and/or mandibular arches, usually made from gypsum, and used for study and treatment planning. Called also *preextraction c., preoperative c.,* and *study c.* **epithelial c.,** a urinary cast made up of columnar renal epithelium or of round cells. **false c.,** pseudocast. **fatty c.,** any cast made up of material loaded with fat globules. **fibrinous c.,** a cast resembling a waxy cast, but having a distinctly yellow color like beeswax; often seen in acute nephritis. **gnathostatic c.,** a cast of the teeth trimmed so that the occlusal plane is in its normal position in the mouth when the cast is set on a plane surface; used in orthodontic diagnosis. **granular c.,** a dark colored urinary cast of a granular or cell-like substance, it being a degenerated form of a hyaline or waxy cast. **hair c.,** 1. trichobezoar. 2. (usually pl.) a hair disorder marked by the presence of discrete, white, shiny, freely movable keratinous tubular structures, about 3 to 5 mm. long, encircling the hair shafts within 1 to 3 cm. of the scalp surface, which are formed by retention and desquamation of segments of the internal root sheath. They may be mistaken for nits. **hanging c.,** one applied to the arm in fracture of the shaft of the humerus and suspended by a sling looped around the neck. **hemoglobin c.,** an irregular, dark, granular cast composed of disintegrated red blood corpuscles. **hyaline c.,** a nearly transparent urinary cast made up of homogeneous protein, but slightly refractive. **investment c.,** refractory c. **Külz's c.,** coma c. **leukocyte c.,** a hyaline cast in which leukocytes are incorporated; called also *pus c.*

master c., a facsimile of oral structures, including the prepared tooth surfaces, residual ridge areas, and/or other parts of the dental arch, reproduced from an impression from which a prosthesis is to be fabricated. **mucous c.,** cylindroid, def. 2. **preextraction c., preoperative c.,** diagnostic c. **pus c.,** leukocyte cast. **quarter c.,** a cut in the quarter of a horse's hoof. **red cell c.,** hyaline cast in which red cells are incorporated. **refractory c.,** one made of heat-resistant materials that will withstand high temperatures without disintegrating and that, when used in partial denture casting, has expansion to compensate for metal shrinkage. Called also *investment c.* **renal c.,** urinary c. **spiral c.,** a urinary cast having a spiral or twisted shape. **spurious c., spurious tube c.,** cylindroid, def. 2. **study c.,** diagnostic c. **tube c.,** urinary c. **urate c.,** an agglomeration of urates on a shred of fibrin or other substance. **urinary c.,** a cast formed from gelled protein precipitated in the renal tubules and molded to the tubular lumen; pieces of these casts break off and are washed out with the urine. Urinary casts may be classified as granular, hyaline, epithelial, etc. Called also *renal c., tube c.,* and *urinary cylinder.* **waxy c.,** a urinary cast made up of a highly refractive, translucent, amyloid substance.

Castanea (kas-ta'ne-ah) [L.; Gr. *kastanea*] a genus of trees, the chestnuts. *C. dentata* (Marsh.) Borkh. (Fagaceae) is the American chestnut. Its wood and leaves contain 6–11 per cent tannin. It has been used as an astringent and in pertussis. The leaves and buds may be poisonous to livestock if consumed in sufficient quantities. The nut is edible.

Castellani's bronchitis (disease), paint, test (kas-tel-an'ēz) [Aldo *Castellani*] see *bronchospirochetosis,* and see under *paint* and *tests.*

Castellani-Low symptom [Aldo *Castellani;* George Carmichael *Low,* English physician, 1872–1952] see under *symptom.*

Castellania (kas-tel-a'ne-ah) [Aldo *Castellani*] (obs.) *Candida.*

casting (kast'ing) 1. any object formed by the solidification of plastic material, such as a gypsum product or molten metal, poured into an impression or mold, or the act of forming such an object, e.g., the fabrication of a metallic dental restoration or appliance, or a metallic dental restoration or appliance fabricated by such a process. 2. a metallic dental restoration made to fit a cavity preparation and retained to or luted into it with a cementing medium. **vacuum c.,** the pouring of plastic material into an impression or mold, under conditions of lowered atmospheric pressure, the end of the mold distal to the ingate is subjected to a vacuum, allowing atmospheric pressure to force the casting material into the mold.

Castle's factors (kas'elz) [William Bosworth *Castle,* American physician, born 1897] 1. intrinsic factor. 2. cyanocobalamin (extrinsic factor).

castrate (kas'trāt) 1. to deprive of the gonads, rendering the individual incapable of reproduction. In the male, to geld or emasculate; in the female, to spay. 2. an individual that has been rendered incapable of reproduction by removal or destruction of the gonads.

castration (kas-tra'shun) [L. *castratio*] removal of the gonads, or their destruction as by radiation or parasites. **female c.,** bilateral oophorectomy, or spaying. **male c.,** bilateral orchiectomy. **parasitic c.,** defective sexual development due to infestation with parasites in early life.

castroid (kas'troid) eunuchoid.

casual (kaz'u-al) [L. *casualis*] 1. pertaining to accidental injuries or to accidents. 2. an occupant of a casual bed in a hospital.

casualty (kaz'u-al-te) 1. an accident; an accidental wound; death or disablement from an accident; also the person so injured or killed. 2. in the armed forces, one missing from his unit as a result of death, injury, illness, capture, because his whereabouts are unknown, or other reasons.

casuistics (kaz"u-is'tiks) the recording and study of cases of disease.

CAT computerized axial tomography.

cat (kat) any member of the family Felidae (lions, leopards, wildcats, etc.), especially the domesticated cat, *Felis catus.* **calico c.,** a cat with fur of three colors: black, white, and orange. Most are female; affected males are sterile, having extra X chromosomes (XXY, XXXY, etc.). **tortoise-shell c.,** calico c.

cata- [Gr. *kata* down] a prefix signifying down, lower, under, against, along with, very; see also words beginning *kata-.*

catabasial (kat-ah-ba'ze-al) [*cata-* + *basion*] having the basion lower than the opisthion; said of certain skulls.

catabasis (kah-tab'ah-sis) [*cata-* + Gr. *bainein* to go] the stage of decline of a disease.

catabatic (kat-ah-bat'ik) pertaining to the decline of a disease; abating.

catabiosis (kat"ah-bi-o'sis) [Gr. *katabiōsis* a passing life] the normal senescence of cells.

catabiotic (kat"ah-bi-ot'ik) 1. pertaining to or characterized by catabiosis. 2. dissipated or used up in the performance of function; said of the energy obtained from food.

catabolic (kat"ah-bol'ik) pertaining to or of the nature of catabolism.

catabolin (kah-tab'o-lin) catabolite.

catabolism (kah-tab'o-lizm) [Gr. *katabolē* a throwing down] any destructive metabolic process by which organisms convert substances into excreted compounds. **antibody c.,** the rapid degradation (shortened half-life) of foreign gamma globulin in the body.

catabolite (kah-tab'o-līt) any product of catabolism.

catabolize (kah-tab'ŏ-liz) to subject to catabolism; to undergo catabolism.

catachronobiology (kat"ah-kron"o-bi-ol'o-je) a term suggested to denote the study of the deleterious effects of time on a living system. Cf. *anachronobiology.*

catacrotic (kat"ah-krot'ik) pertaining to or characterized by catacrotism.

catacrotism (kah-tak'ro-tizm) [*cata-* + Gr. *krotos* beat] an anomaly of the pulse evidenced by appearance of a small additional wave or notch in the descending limb of the pulse tracing.

catadicrotic (kat"ah-di-krot'ik) pertaining to or characterized by catadicrotism.

catadicrotism (kat"ah-di'kro-tizm) [*cata-* + Gr. *dis* twice + *krotos* beat] an anomaly of the pulse evidenced by appearance of two small additional waves or notches in the descending limb of the pulse tracing.

catadidymus (kat"ah-did'ĭ-mus) katadidymus.

catadioptric (kat"ah-di-op'trik) deflecting and reflecting light at the same time.

catagen (kat'ah-jen) the brief portion of the hair growth cycle in which growth (anagen) stops and resting (telogen) starts.

catagenesis (kat"ah-jen'ĕ-sis) [*cata-* + Gr. *genesis* production] involution or retrogression.

catagenetic (kat"ah-jĕ-net'ik) pertaining to catagenesis.

catagmatic (kat"ag-mat'ik) [Gr. *katagma* fracture] having the power of consolidating a broken bone.

catalase (kat'ah-lās) [EC 1.11.1.6] an enzyme of the oxidoreductase class that catalyzes the reaction $H_2O_2 + H_2O_2 = O_2 + 2H_2O$. It is found in almost all cells except certain obligate anaerobic and lactic acid bacteria. Genetic deficiency of the enzyme, an autosomal recessive trait, results in acatalasia.

catalepsy (kat'ah-lep"se) [Gr. *katalēpsis*] the condition of maintaining whatever body posture one is placed in; a symptom seen in severe cases of catatonic schizophrenia. Called also *cerea flexibilitas* and *waxy flexibility.*

cataleptic (kat"ah-lep'tik) 1. pertaining to, characterized by, or inducing catalepsy. 2. a person affected with catalepsy.

cataleptiform (kat"ah-lep'tĭ-form) resembling catalepsy.

cataleptoid (kat"ah-lep'toid) cataleptiform.

catalogia (kat"ah-lo'je-ah) verbigeration.

Catalpa (kah-tal'pah) a genus of bignoniaceous trees. *C. bignonioides* Walt. and *C. speciosa* Warder., of the United States, afford seeds formerly used in asthma.

catalysis (kah-tal'ĭ-sis) [Gr. *katalysis* dissolution] increase in the velocity of a chemical reaction or process produced by the presence of a substance that is not consumed in the net chemical reaction or process; *negative catalysis* denotes the slowing down or inhibition of a reaction or process by the presence of such a substance. **contact c., heteroge-**

neous c., catalysis produced by the adsorbing power of contact surfaces; e.g., catalysis caused by colloidal platinum. **surface c.,** catalysis in which the reacting substances are adsorbed onto the surface of the catalyst and there react. Cf. *contact c.*

catalyst (kat′ah-list) any substance that brings about catalysis; called also *accelerant.* **negative c.,** a catalyst that retards the velocity of a reaction.

catalytic (kat″ah-lit′ik) [Gr. *katalyein* to dissolve] 1. causing or pertaining to an alterative effect; causing catalysis. 2. an alterative or specific medicine.

catalyzator (kat″ah-lĭ-za′tor) catalyst.

catalyze (kat′ah-līz) to cause or produce catalysis.

catalyzer (kat′ah-līz″er) catalyst.

catamenia (kat″ah-me′ne-ah) [Gr. *katamēnia*] the monthly uterine discharge; menstruation, or the menses.

catamenial (kat″ah-me′ne-al) pertaining to the menses or to menstruation.

catamenogenic (kat″ah-men″o-jen′ik) inducing menstruation.

catamnesis (kat″am-ne′sis) the follow-up history of a patient after he is discharged from treatment or a hospital.

catamnestic (kat″am-nes′tik) pertaining to catamnesis.

catapasm (kat′ah-pazm) [Gr. *katapasma*] a dusting powder applied to an injured surface.

cataphasia (kat″ah-fa′ze-ah) [cata- + Gr. *phasis* speech] verbigeration.

cataphora (kah-taf′o-rah) [Gr. *kataphora*] lethargy with intervals of imperfect waking; called also *coma somnolentium.*

cataphoresis (kat″ah-fo-re′sis) [cata- + Gr. *phorēsis* bearing] the passage of charged particles toward the negative pole (cathode) in electrophoresis.

cataphoretic (kat″ah-fo-ret′ik) of, or pertaining to, cataphoresis.

cataphoria (kat″ah-fo′re-ah) [cata- + Gr. *pherein* to bear] a permanent downward turning of the visual axes of both eyes after the visual fusional stimuli have been eliminated.

cataphoric (kat″ah-for′ik) pertaining to cataphoresis or to cataphora.

cataphylaxis (kat″ah-fĭ-lak′sis) [cata- + Gr. *phylaxis* a guarding] (*obs.*) 1. the movement of leukocytes and antibodies to the site of an infection. 2. a breaking down of the body's natural defense to infection.

cataplasia (kat″ah-pla′se-ah) [cata- + Gr. *plassein* to form] retrograde metamorphosis, a form of atrophy in which the tissues revert to earlier and more embryonic conditions.

cataplasis (kat-ap′lah-sis) cataplasia.

cataplasm (kat′ah-plazm) [L. *cataplasma;* Gr. *kataplasma*] a poultice or soft external application, often medicated. **kaolin c.,** a poultice prepared with kaolin, boric acid, and glycerin; called also *cataplasma kaolini.*

cataplasma (kat″ah-plaz′mah) [L.; Gr. *kataplasma*] cataplasm. **c. fermen′ti,** a poultice containing yeast. **c. kaoli′ni,** kaolin cataplasm.

cataplectic (kat″ah-plek′tik) 1. pertaining to or characterized by cataplexy. 2. coming on suddenly and overwhelmingly.

cataplexis (kat′ah-plek″sis) [Gr.] cataplexy.

cataplexy (kat′ah-plek-se) a condition in which there are abrupt attacks of muscular weakness and hypotonia triggered by an emotional stimulus such as mirth, anger, fear, or surprise. It is often associated with narcolepsy.

catapophysis (kat″ah-pof′ĭ-sis) a process, or projection, of bone or of brain matter.

Catapres (kat″ah-pres) trademark for a preparation of clonidine hydrochloride.

cataract (kat′ah-rakt) [L. *cataracta,* from Gr. *katarraktēs* waterfall, floodgate, portcullis (perhaps because an ocular opacity and a portcullis are obstructions)] an opacity, partial or complete, of one or both eyes, on or in the lens or capsule, especially an opacity impairing vision or causing blindness. The many kinds of cataract are classified by their morphology (size, shape, location) or etiology (cause and time of occurrence). **after-c.,** a recurrent capsular cataract; any membrane in the pupillary area after performance of a procedure for extraction or absorption of the lens. **ami-**

noaciduria c., capsular thickening occurring in aminoaciduria, homocystinuria, and oculocerebrorenal syndrome. **atopic c.,** cataract sometimes occurring in the third decade in those with longstanding atopic dermatitis. **axial fusiform c.,** anterior and posterior polar cataracts joined with threadlike opacities extending axially through the lens; called also *spindle c.* **black c.,** black or dark-colored opacity occurring in senile nuclear sclerotic cataract. **blue c., blue dot c.,** 1. a small, round developmental opacity that appears white, brown, or blue; it is common in the periphery of the cortex and occasionally moves into the axial zone of the lens. Called also *cerulean c., punctate c.,* and *cataracta cerulea.* 2. coronary cataract. **brown c., brunescent c.,** senile cataract appearing as a brown opacity. **calcareous c.,** dystrophic calcium salt deposits in the subcapsular and cortical areas of the lens. **capsular c.,** capsular thickening occurring in heat cataracts and oculocerebrorenal syndrome. **cerulean c.,** 1. blue c. 2. coronary c. **complete c.,** total c. **complicated c.,** secondary c. **congenital c.,** 1. a general term for common, usually bilateral opacities present at birth; they may be mild or severe and may or may not impair vision, depending upon their size, location, and density. From 35 to 50 per cent of all congenital cataracts are sporadic and of unknown cause; another 25 per cent are inherited, usually as autosomal dominant traits; the remaining 25 to 40 percent may be the result of intrauterine infection, drug-induced toxicity, ionizing radiation, trauma, prematurity, and chromosomal, endocrine, metabolic, and systemic disorders. Congenital cataracts are often associated with low birth weight, central nervous system abnormalities, mental retardation, convulsions, and cerebral palsy. 2. developmental cataract. **contusion c.,** one due to shock or to injury of the eyeball. **coralliform c.,** a developmental, sutural opacity radiating axially forward and outward from the lens and ending in ampullae behind the capsule. **coronary c.,** 1. a white punctate or flakelike opacity around the periphery of the lens, forming a ring or crown. Coronary cataracts is transmitted by dominant inheritance and may be present in 25 per cent of the general population. 2. blue cataract. **cortical c.,** 1. developmental punctate opacity common in the cortex and present in most lenses. The cataract is white or cerulean, increases in number with age, but rarely affects vision. 2. cuneiform cataract. **cuneiform c.,** the most common senile cataract, consisting of white, wedgelike opacities distributed like spokes around the periphery of the cortex. **cupuliform c.,** a posterior subcapsular cortical opacity seen as brown, saucer-shaped granules or cysts. It is centrally located and therefore seriously impairs vision very quickly. Cupuliform cataracts occur in 60- to 80-year-olds, but earlier appearance may be an inherited trait. **dermatogenic c.,** syndermatotic c. **developmental c.,** small, very common opacities occurring in youth as a result of a congenitally caused defect (e.g., heredity, malnutrition, toxicity, inflammation). The number of developmental cataracts increases with age, but they rarely impair vision. Called also *evolutionary c.* **diabetic c.,** a rare, usually bilateral, opacity shaped like a snowflake, affecting the anterior and posterior cortices of young diabetics. The opacification can be reversed when the blood glucose is brought under control, but usually the opacity progresses rapidly to a mature cataract. **duplication c.,** a disk-shaped cortical opacity forming in layers under capsular cataracts with clear zones between the layers. **electric c.,** opacification that may occur after electric shock, especially to the head. Anterior subcapsular cataracts may form and develop within days after a severe shock; slowly developing or stationary opacities may follow a shock not on the head. **embryonal nuclear c.,** an opacity confined to the embryonic nucleus of the lens. It is an autosomal dominant trait, is often bilateral, has a powdery appearance, and seldom affects vision. Called also *cataracta centralis pulverulenta.* **embryopathic c.,** a congenital opacity caused by intrauterine infection, e.g., rubella, syphilis, or toxoplasmosis. **evolutionary c.,** developmental c. **galactosemic c.,** a cataract commonly observed in infants with galactosemia. The opacities look like oil droplets, are bilateral, and are zonular or nuclear. **glassblowers′ c.,** heat c. **glaucomatous c.,** a patchy anterior subcapsular opacity following an attack of acute glaucoma; called also *glaukomflecken.* **heat c.,** posterior subcapsular opacity caused by chronic exposure to infrared radiation. **heterochromic c.,** a secondary, posterior cortical cataract symptomatic of heterochromic cyclitis; failing vision is often the first symptom. **hypermature c.,** a cataract with a swollen, milky cortex, the result of autolysis of the lens fibers of a mature cataract. **hypocalcemic c.,** punctate, sometimes cerulean, opacities, initially subcapsular, becoming lamellar, occurring with infantile tetany, hypoparathyroidism, or rickets. **immature c., incipient c.,** an incomplete cataract; the lens is only slightly opaque and the cortex clear. **intumescent c.,** a mature cataract that progresses; the lens becomes swollen from the osmotic effect of degenerated lens protein, and this may lead to secondary angle closure (acute) glaucoma. **juvenile c.,** a cataract in a child under nine years old; such cataracts are usually congenital or traumatic. **lamellar c.,** a concentric opacity, broad or narrow, usually consisting of powdery white dots, affecting one lamella or zonule of an otherwise clear lens. Lamellar cataracts are the most common congenital cataracts (about 50 per cent), and their causes include hypocalcemia, hypoglycemia, galactosemia, and rubella. Called also *zonular c.* **mature c.,** a cataract that produces swelling and opacity of the entire lens. Most cataracts are removed before maturity. **membranous c.,** a cataract formed of a collapsed, flattened capsule with little or no cortex or epithelium. **metabolic c.,** an opacity due to an endocrine or biochemical disorder. **morgagnian c.,** a mature cataract in which most of the cortex has become opaque and liquefied, so that the nucleus moves freely within the lens. **nuclear c.,** 1. embryonal nuclear c. 2. senile nuclear sclerotic c. **nutritional deficiency c.** subcapsular opacity observed in patients with anorexia nervosa and in alcoholics. **overripe c.,** hypermature c. **polar c.,** an anterior or posterior subcapsular opacity, usually disk-shaped; the anterior cataract is the more common; the posterior reduces visual acuity more often. **postinflammatory c.,** a secondary cataract due to inflammation. **c's of prematurity,** clusters of vacuoles of unknown cause in the Y-shaped sutures of the lens in about 3 per cent of premature newborns; usually the cataracts disappear spontaneously within a month. **presenile c.,** a subcapsular senile cataract in a person under 40. **primary c.,** a cataract developing independently of any other disease. **punctate c.,** 1. blue c. 2. coronary c. **pyramidal c.,** a conoid anterior polar cataract with its apex pointing forward. **radiation c.,** a subcapsular opacity caused by ionizing radiation such as x-rays, gamma rays, and neutrons, and by nonionizing radiation such as infrared (heat) rays, ultraviolet waves, microwaves, and laser radiation. **ringform congenital c.,** a very rare opacity in which the lens nucleus is absent, and only a doughnut-shaped remnant of lens is left. **ripe c.,** mature cataract. **rubella c.,** a congenital nuclear cataract caused by maternal rubella during the first trimester of pregnancy. **secondary c.,** a cataract, usually posterior subcapsular, arising from (1) disease, especially iridocyclitis; (2) degeneration such as chronic glaucoma or retinal detachment; (3) surgery, particularly glaucoma filtering or retinal reattachment. Also called *complicated c.* **senile c.,** the most common kind of cataract, of unknown cause, painless, and developing without any traumatic, ocular, systemic, or congenital disorder. Senile cataracts are associated solely with aging, some degree of cataract being normal in persons over 50. Of the several kinds of senile cataract, 70 per cent form in the cortical area of the lens, 25 per cent in the nuclear, and 5 per cent in the subcapsular. **senile nuclear sclerotic c.,** an increasing hardening of the nucleus, with the opacity appearing brown or black and the lens becoming inelastic and unable to accommodate; the opacity is usually bilateral, begins between ages 50 and 60, and progresses slowly. **snowflake c., snowstorm c.,** a cataract that has the appearance of numerous grayish or bluish-white flaky opacities, frequently seen in young diabetics. **Soemmering's ring c.,** see under *ring.* **spindle c.,** axial fusiform c. **subcapsular c.,** an opacity situated beneath the anterior or posterior capsule of the lens. **sunflower c.,** a brightly colored, usually red anterior capsular opacity with a sunflower pattern that occurs in patients with Wilson's disease and hypercupremia; it has little effect on vision and clears after treatment with penicillamine. **supranuclear c.,** an opacity in the deep cortex of the lens, just above the nucleus. **sutural c.,** a congenital opacity of the lens affecting the Y-shaped sutures of the fetal membrane; it usually does not affect vision. **syndermatotic c.,** an inherited, usually bilateral opacity associated with cutaneous disease and occurring in youth; called also *dermatogenic c.* **thermal c.,** heat c. **total c.,** an opacity of all the fibers of the lens; called also *complete c.* **toxic c.,** an opacity caused by exposure to a drug or other toxic substance, such as miotics, antimiotics, corticosteroids, metals, nitro compounds, and substituted hydrocarbons. **traumatic c.,** a cataract resulting from injury to the eye, either immediately after injury (e.g., from perforation of the capsule) or years later (e.g., from concussion of the lens without a rupture of the capsule). **zonular c.,** lamellar c.

cataracta (kat″ah-rak′tah) [L.] cataract. **c. brunes′-cens,** brown cataract. **c. caeru′lea,** blue cataract. **c. centralis pulverulenta,** embryonal nuclear cataract. **c. complica′ta,** secondary cataract. **c. ni′gra,** black cataract.

cataractogenic (kat″ah-rak″to-jen′ik) tending to induce the formation of cataracts.

cataractous (kat″ah-rak′tus) of the nature of or affected with cataract.

cataria (kah-ta′re-ah) [L. "catnip"] the leaves and tops of *Nepeta cataria* L. (Labi), or catnip, a labiate plant; used as a carminative and mild nerve stimulant. Feline species are attracted to and fondle the plant because of its aromatic oils, which contain nepetalactone.

catarrh (kah-tahr′) [L. *catarrhus*, from Gr. *katarrhein* to flow down] inflammation of a mucous membrane, with a free discharge (Hippocrates); especially such inflammation of the air passages of the head and throat. **atrophic c.,** chronic rhinitis with wasting of mucous and submucous tissues. **autumnal c.,** hay fever. **Bostock's c.,** hay fever. **hypertrophic c.,** chronic catarrh that results in irregular, and sometimes papillary, thickening of the mucous and the submucous tissues. **Laënnec's c.,** a kind of asthmatic bronchitis, with viscous, pearly expectoration. **malignant c. of cattle,** a virus disease of cattle characterized by exudative inflammation of the mucous membranes, corneal opacities, and enlargement of the lymphatic glands. **postnasal c.,** chronic rhinopharyngitis. **sinus c.,** a disorder of the lymph nodes characterized by dilatation of the sinuses accompanied by some proliferation of the littoral cells, which become swollen and detach themselves from the wall of the sinuses to lie free in the lumen. **suffocative c.,** asthma. **vernal c.,** see under *conjunctivitis.*

catarrhal (kah-tahr′al) of the nature of or pertaining to catarrh.

Catarrhina (kat″ah-ri′nah) [*cata-* + Gr. *rhis* nose] Cercopithecoidea.

catarrhine (kat′ah-rīn) 1. pertaining to the superfamily Catarrhina. 2. characterized by nostrils that are close together and directed downward.

catastalsis (kat″ah-stal′sis) [*cata-* + Gr. *stalsis* contraction] (*obs.*) a downward moving wave of contraction without a preceding wave of inhibition occurring in the digestive tube.

catastaltic (kat″ah-stal′tik) [Gr. *katastaltikos*] 1. inhibitory; restraining. 2. an agent that tends to restrain or check any process.

catastatic (kat″ah-stat′ik) of the nature of or pertaining to a catastate.

catathermometer (kat″ah-ther-mom′ĕ-ter) katathermometer.

catathymia (kat″ah-thi′me-ah) in psychoanalysis, the existence in the unconscious of elements sufficiently affect laden to produce effects in consciousness.

catathymic (kat″ah-thi′mik) pertaining to catathymia.

catatonia (kat-ah-to′ne-ah) [*cata-* + Gr. *tonos* tension + *-ia*] catatonic schizophrenia.

catatonic (kat″ah-ton′ik) 1. see under *schizophrenia.* 2. an individual affected with *catatonic schizophrenia.*

catatricrotic (kat″ah-tri-krot′ik) pertaining to or characterized by catatricrotism.

catatricrotism (kat″ah-tri′kro-tizm) [*cata-* + Gr. *treis* three + *krotos* beat] an anomaly of the pulse evidenced by appearance of three small additional waves or notches in the descending limb of the pulse tracing.

catechin (kat′ĕ-kin) chemical name: *trans*-2-(3,4-dihydroxyphenyl)- 3, 4- dihydro- 2*H*-1- benzopyan- 3, 5, 7-triol. A crystalline astringent principle, $C_{15}H_{14}O_6 4H_2O$, from catechu (e.g., *Acacia catechu* Willd., Leguminosae and gambier, *Uncaria gambier* [Hunter] Roxb., Rubiaceae). Called also *catechol* and *catechuic acid.*

catechol (kat′ĕ-kol) 1. catechin. 2. pyrocatechol.

catecholamine (kat″ĕ-kol′ah-mēn, kat″ĕ-kol′ah-min) one of a group of similar compounds having a sympathomimetic action, the aromatic portion of whose molecule is catechol, and the aliphatic portion an amine. Such compounds include dopamine, norepinephrine, and epinephrine.

catecholaminergic (kat″e-kol-am″in-er′jik) activated by or secreting catecholamines.

catechol oxidase (kat′ĕ-kol ok′si-dās) [EC 1.10.3.1] an enzyme of the oxidoreductase class that catalyzes the reaction 2 catechol + O_2 = 2 1,2-benzoquinone + $2H_2O$. It is a complex of copper-containing proteins that act also upon substituted catechols, including tyrosine. Called also *diphenol oxidase, polyphenol oxidase*. Cf. *monophenol monooxygenase (tyrosinase)*.

catechu (kat′ĕ-ku) 1. a powerfully astringent extract from the heartwood of *Acacia catechu* Willd., Leguminosae, the chief constituents of which are catechin, quercetin, and catechutannic acid; formerly used as an antidiarrheal agent. Called also *black c.* 2. gambir. **pale c.,** gambir.

catechuic acid (kat″e-ku′ik) catechin.

catelectrotonus (kat″e-lek-trot′o-nus) [*cata-* + *electrotonus*] increase of irritability of a nerve or muscle near the cathode during passage of an electric current.

Catenabacterium (kat″ĕ-nah-bak-te′re-um) [L. *catena* chain + *bacterium*] in former systems of classification, a genus of bacteria of the family Lactobacillaceae, made up of nonsporulating, anaerobic, gram-positive, rod-shaped organisms. These organisms are now assigned to the genera *Eubacterium* and *Lactobacillus*.

catenating (kat′e-nāt″ing) [L. *catena* a chain] forming part of a chain or complex of symptoms.

catenoid (kat′e-noid) [L. *catena* chain] arranged like a chain or resembling a chain.

catenulate (kah-ten′u-lāt) catenoid.

catgut (kat′gut) an absorbable sterile strand obtained from collagen derived from healthy mammals, originally prepared from the submucous layer of the intestines of sheep; used as a surgical ligature. **chromic c., chromicized c.,** catgut sterilized and impregnated with chromium trioxide to prolong its tensile strength in tissues. **I.K.I. c.,** catgut treated with a solution of 1 part of iodine in 100 parts of a potassium iodide solution; called also *iodine c.* **iodine c.,** I.K.I. c. **iodochromic c.,** catgut treated with a solution of iodine, potassium, iodide, and potassium dichromate. **silverized c.,** catgut impregnated with silver to give it increased strength and resisting qualities.

Cath. abbreviation for L. *cathar′ticus*, cathartic.

Catha (kath′ah) a genus of plants. **C. ed′ulis** Forsk. (Celastraceae), a shrub or tree native to tropical East Africa, whose leaves are chewed or brewed into a tea and consumed for its central nervous system stimulating properties. The active principle is D-norpseudoephedrine.

cathaeresis (kah-thēr′e-sis) catheresis.

catharometer (kath″ah-rom′ĕ-ter) an instrument for measuring the thermal conductivity of air by the rate of heat loss from a heated platinum wire.

catharsis (kah-thar′sis) [Gr. *katharsis* a cleansing] 1. a cleansing or purgation. 2. in psychiatry, release of ideas, thoughts, and repressed material from the unconscious, accompanied by an emotional response and relief.

cathartic (kah-thar′tik) [Gr. *kathartikos*] 1. causing evacuation of the bowels. 2. an agent that causes evacuation of the bowels by increasing bulk, stimulating peristaltic action, etc. Called also *purgative* (q.v.), *coprogogue*, and *eccoprotic*. 3. producing catharsis. **bulk c.,** one that stimulates evacuation of the bowel by increasing the bulk of the feces. **lubricant c.,** one that acts by softening the feces and reducing friction between them and the intestinal wall. **saline c.,** one that increases fluidity of the intestinal contents by retention of water by osmotic forces, and indirectly increases motor activity. **stimulant c.,** one that directly increases motor activity of the intestinal tract.

cathectic (kah-thek′tik) pertaining to cathexis.

Cathelin's method, segregator (kat-laz′) [Fernand *Cathelin*, Paris urologist, 1873–1945] see under *method* and *segregator*.

cathemoglobin (kath″em-o-glo′bin) a substance produced

by oxidizing hemochromogen; it consists of oxidized heme and denatured globin.

cathepsin (kah-thep′sin) one of a number of enzymes of the hydrolase class that catalyze the hydrolysis of peptide bonds. Most cathepsins are lysosomal endopeptidases with an acidic optimum pH. **c. A,** a serine carboxypeptidase. **c. B₁** [EC 3.4.22.1], a thiol-proteinase. **c. B₂** [EC 3.4.16.1], a serine carboxypeptidase. **c. C,** dipeptidyl peptidase I. **c. D** [EC 3.4.23.5], a carboxyl proteinase. **c. E,** cathepsin D. **c. G** [EC 3.4.21.20], a serine proteinase. **c. L** [EC 3.4.22.15], a thiol proteinase.

catheresis (kah-thēr′e-sis) [Gr. *kathairesis* a reduction] 1. weakness caused by medicine. 2. a mild action.

catheretic (kath″ĕ-ret′ik) 1. mildly caustic. 2. weakening or prostrating.

catheter (kath′ĕ-ter) [Gr. *kathetēr*] a tubular, flexible, surgical instrument for withdrawing fluids from (or introducing fluids into) a cavity of the body, especially one for introduction into the bladder through the urethra for the withdrawal of urine. **acorn-tipped c.,** one used in ureteropyelography to occlude the ureteral orifice and prevent backflow from the ureter during and following the injection of an opaque medium. **angiographic c.,** a catheter through which a contrast medium is injected for visualization of the vascular system of an organ. Such catheters may have pre-formed ends to facilitate selective locating (as in a renal or coronary vessel) from a remote entry site. They may be named according to the site of entry and destination, as *femoral-renal, brachial-coronary*, etc. **bicoudate c., c. bicoudé,** an elbowed catheter with two bends. **Bozeman's c., Bozeman-Fritsch c.,** a double-current uterine catheter; called also *Fritsch's c.* **Braasch bulb c.,** a bulb-tipped catheter used for dilation and determination of the inner diameter of the ureter. **cardiac c.,** a long, fine catheter especially designed for passage, usually through a peripheral blood vessel, into the chambers of the heart under roentgenologic control. **central venous c.,** a catheter introduced via a large (jugular, subclavian, etc.) vein into the superior vena cava or right atrium for the purposes of administering parenteral fluids (as in hyperalimentation) or medications or for measurement of central venous pressure. **conical c.,** a catheter with a cone-shaped tip designed to dilate the ureter. **c. coudé,** an elbowed c. **c. à demeure,** indwelling c. **de Pezzer c.,** a self-retaining catheter having a bulbous extremity. **double-current c.,** a catheter having two channels; one for injection and one for removal of fluid. **Drew-Smythe c.,** an instrument used for the artificial rupture of the amniotic membranes to induce labor. **elbowed c.,** one with a sharp bend near the beak; used principally in cases of enlarged prostate. Called also *c. coudé*. **eustachian c.,** an instrument for inflating the eustachian tube, used in treating some diseases of the middle ear. **female c.,** a short catheter for passage through the female urethra. **filiform-tipped c.,** a catheter used to dilate tight urethral strictures and to bypass obstructions due to angulations or calculi in the ureter. **Foley c.,** an indwelling catheter retained in the bladder by a balloon inflated with air or liquid. **Fritsch's c.,** Bozeman-Fritsch c. **Garceau's c.,** conical c. **Gouley's c.,** a solid, curved steel instrument, grooved on its inferior surface so that it can be passed over a guide through a urethral stricture. **indwelling c.,** a catheter that is held in position in the urethra. **Malecot c.,** a two- or four-winged catheter for use in the female bladder. **Nélaton's c.,** a catheter of soft rubber. **olive-tip c.,** a ureteral catheter with an olive-shaped end, used to dilate a constricted ureteral orifice; larger sizes are also utilized for dilating urethral strictures or for calibrating the diameter of such strictures. **Pezzer's c.,** see *de Pezzer c.* **Phillips' c.,** a urethral catheter with a woven filiform guide. **prostatic c.,** a catheter having a short angular tip for passing an enlarged prostate. **Robinson c.,** a straight catheter with two to six openings to allow drainage, especially useful in the presence of blood clots which may occlude one or more openings. **self-retaining c.,** a catheter constructed to be retained in the bladder and urethra. **spiral-tip c.,** a catheter with an off-center filiform tip. **Swan-Ganz c.,** a soft, flow-directed catheter with a balloon at the tip for measuring pulmonary arterial pressures; it is introduced into the venous system (via the basilic, internal jugular, or subclavian vein) and is guided by blood flow into the superior vena cava, the right atrium and ventricle, and into the pulmonary artery. **toposcopic c.,** a miniature catheter that can pass through narrow, tortuous vessels to convey chemotherapy directly to brain tumors. **tracheal c.,** an instrument for removing mucus from the trachea by application of suction. **two-way c.,** a double-lumen catheter to provide both irrigation and drainage. **vertebrated c.,** a catheter made in small sections fitted together so as to be flexible. **whistle-tip c.,** a catheter with a terminal opening as well as a lateral one. **winged c.,** a catheter with winglike projections on the end to retain it in the bladder.

catheterization (kath″ĕ-ter-i-za′shun) the employment or passage of a catheter. **cardiac c.,** passage of a small catheter through a vein in an arm or leg or the neck and into the heart, permitting the securing of blood samples, determination of intracardiac pressure, and detection of cardiac anomalies. **hepatic vein c.,** passage of a cardiac catheter through an arm vein, right atrium, inferior vena cava, and hepatic vein, into a small hepatic venule, for recording of intrahepatic venous pressures. **retrourethral c.,** passage through the urethra of a catheter first introduced through an incision into the bladder, and then passed through the internal urethral orifice.

catheterize (kath′ĕ-ter-īz) to introduce a catheter within a body cavity; usually used to designate the passage of a catheter into the bladder for the drainage of urine.

catheterostat (kath-e′ter-o-stat) a holder for containing and sterilizing catheters.

cathetometer (kath″ĕ-tom′ĕ-ter) an instrument for aiding in the reading of thermometers, burets, etc.

cathexis (kah-thek′sis) [Gr. *kathexis*] in psychoanalysis, conscious or unconscious investment of psychic energy in a person, idea, or object.

cathisophobia (kath″ĭ-so-fo′be-ah) [Gr. *kathizein* to sit down + *phobein* to be affrighted by + *ia*] akathisia.

cathode (kath′ōd) [Gr. *kata* down + *hodos* way] 1. in an electrochemical cell, the electrode at which reduction occurs, i.e., the negative electrode in an electrolytic cell and the positive electrode in a voltaic cell. 2. the negative electrode of devices such as electron tubes, x-ray tubes, and electrophoresis cells. Cf. *anode.*

cathodic (kah-thŏd′ik) pertaining to or emanating from a cathode.

catholicon (kah-thol′ĭ-kon) [Gr. *katholikos* general] a panacea or universal medicine.

catholyte (kath′o-līt) that portion of an electrolyte that adjoins the cathode.

Cathomycin (kath′o-mi″sin) trademark for preparations of novobiocin.

cation (kat′i-on) [Gr. *kata* down + *iōn* going] an ion carrying a positive charge owing to a deficiency of electrons; in an electrochemical cell cations migrate toward the cathode.

cationic (kat″ĭ-on′ik) pertaining to or containing a cation.

cationogen (kat″ĭ-on′o-jen) a compound that may become or may liberate a cation in the body.

catlin (kat′lin) a long, straight, sharp-pointed, double-edged knife used in amputations.

catling (kat′ling) catlin.

catoptric (kah-top′trik) [Gr. *katoptrikos* in a mirror] pertaining to a reflected image, or to reflected light.

catoptrics (kah-top′triks) that branch of physics which treats of reflected light.

catoptroscope (kah-top′tro-skōp) [Gr. *katoptron* mirror + -*scope*] an instrument for examining objects by reflected light.

Cattani's serum (kah-tan′ez) [Giuseppina *Cattani*, Italian pathologist, 1859–1915] see under *serum.*

cauda (kaw′dah), pl. *cau′dae* [L.] [NA] a tail, or tail-like appendage; in anatomical nomenclature, a general term for a structure resembling such an appendage. **c. cor′poris stria′ti,** c. nuclei caudati. **c. epididym′idis** [NA], tail of epididymis: the lower part of the epididymis, where the ductus epididymidis is continuous with the ductus deferens; called also *globus minor epididymidis.* **c. equi′na** [NA], the collection of spinal roots that descend from the lower part of the spinal cord and occupy the vertebral canal below the cord; their appearance resembles the tail of a horse. **c. he′licis** [NA], the termination of the posterior margin of the cartilage of the helix. **c. nu′clei cauda′ti** [NA],

tail of caudate nucleus: the part of the caudate nucleus that tapers off from the body, curves around in the roof of the inferior horn of the lateral ventricle, and extends rostrally as far as the amygdaloid nucleus; called also *c. corporis striati.* **c. pancre′atis** [NA], tail of pancreas: the left extremity of the pancreas, usually in contact with the medial aspect of the spleen and the junction of the transverse and descending colon.

caudad (kaw′dad) directed toward the tail; opposite to craniad or cephalad.

caudae (kaw′de) [L.] genitive and plural of *cauda.*

caudal (kaw′dal) 1. pertaining to a cauda. 2. denoting a position more toward the cauda, or tail, than some specified point of reference; same as inferior, in human anatomy. See *caudalis.*

caudalis (kaw-da′lis) pertaining to the cauda (tail), or to the inferior end of the body; [NA] a term used to denote relationship to the caudal or inferior extremity of an organ or part.

caudalward (kaw′dal-ward) toward the caudal end; in a direction away from the head.

caudate (kaw′dāt) [L. *caudatus*] having a tail.

caudatolenticular (kaw-da″to-len-tik′u-lar) pertaining to the caudate and lenticular nuclei of the striatum.

caudatum (kaw-da′tum) [L.] the nucleus caudatus.

caudectomy (kaw-dek′to-me) the surgical removal of all or part of the tail, as of a dog.

caudocephalad (kaw-do-sef′ah-lad) [L. *cauda* tail + Gr. *kephalē* head + L. *ad* toward] 1. proceeding in a direction from the tail toward the head. 2. in both a caudal and a cephalic direction.

caul (kawl) 1. a piece of amnion that sometimes envelops a child's head at birth; pileus. Called also *cowl.* 2. the omentum, usually used to designate the greater omentum.

Caulk's punch [John Roberts *Caulk*, St. Louis urologist, 1881–1938] see under *punch.*

Caulobacter (kaw″lo-bak′ter) [Gr. *kaulos* stalk + *baktron* a rod] a genus of appendaged bacteria found in soil and fresh water containing organic matter, made up of rod-shaped, fusiform, or vibrioid cells that typically produce a stalk extending from one pole and reproduce by asymmetrical cell fission. The type species is *C. vibrioi′des.*

Caulococcus (kaw″lo-kok′us) [Gr. *kaulos* stalk + *coccus* berry] a genus of budding bacteria of uncertain status, found in mud and the bottom waters of lakes, made up of coccoid cells sometimes connected by fine threads. They contain manganese and iron deposits. The type species is *C. manganifer.*

caumesthesia (kaw″mes-the′ze-ah) [Gr. *kauma* burn + *aisthēsis* perception] a condition in which, with a low temperature, the patient experiences a sense of burning heat.

causal (kaw′zal) pertaining to a cause; directed against a cause.

causalgia (kaw-zal′je-ah) [Gr. *kausos* heat + -*algia*] a burning pain, often accompanied by trophic skin changes, due to injury of a peripheral nerve.

causative (kawz′ah-tiv) effective or responsible as a cause or agent.

cause (kawz) [L. *causa*] that which brings about any condition or produces any effect. **constitutional c.,** one acting within the body that is not restricted to a specific site, but is systemic or has a genetic basis. **exciting c.,** one that leads directly to a specific condition. **immediate c.,** a cause that is operative at the beginning of the specific effect; called also *precipitating c.* **local c.,** one that is not general or constitutional, but is confined to the site where the effect is produced. **precipitating c.,** immediate c. **predisposing c.,** anything that renders a person more liable to a specific condition without actually producing it. **primary c.,** the principal factor contributing to the production of a specific result. **proximate c.,** that which immediately precedes and produces an effect. **remote c.,** any cause that does not immediately precede and produce a specific condition; a predisposing, secondary, or ultimate cause. **secondary c.,** one that is supplemental to the primary cause. **specific c.,** one that produces a special or specific effect. **ultimate c.,** the earliest factor, in point of time, that has contributed to production of a specific result.

caustic (kaws'tik) [L. *causticus;* Gr. *kaustikos*] 1. burning or corrosive; destructive to living tissues. 2. having a burning taste. 3. an escharotic or corrosive agent. Called also *cauterant.* **Churchill's iodine c.,** a caustic solution of iodine and potassium iodide in water. **Filhos's c.,** 5 parts of potassium hydroxide and 1 part of calcium oxide. **Landolfi's c.,** a compound containing chlorides of antimony, bromine, gold, and zinc. **Lugol's c.,** 1 part each of iodine and potassium iodide dissolved in 2 parts of water. **lunar c.,** toughened silver nitrate. **mitigated c.,** silver nitrate diluted with potassium nitrate. **Plunket's c.,** a caustic paste made of 60 parts of arsenic, 100 of sulfur, and 480 each of *Ranunculus acris* and *R. flammula.* **Rousselot's c.,** a caustic containing red mercuric sulfide, burnt sponge, and arsenic trioxide. **Vienna c.,** caustic potash with lime. **zinc c.,** a mixture of 1 part of zinc chloride and 3 parts of flour.

causticize (kaws'tĭ-sīz) to render caustic.

cauterant (kaw'ter-ant) 1. any caustic material or application. 2. caustic.

cauterization (kaw"ter-i-za'shun) the destruction of tissue with a hot instrument, an electric current, or a caustic substance.

cautery (kaw'ter-e) [L. *cauterium;* Gr. *kautērion*] 1. the application of a caustic substance, a hot instrument, an electric current, or other agent to destroy tissue. 2. a caustic substance or hot instrument used in cauterization. **actual c.,** the application of an agent that actually burns tissue. **button c.,** an iron disk with a handle, formerly used as a cautery. **chemical c.,** chemocautery. **cold c.,** cryocautery. **electric c., galvanic c.,** see *galvanocautery.* **gas c.,** cauterization by means of a specially controlled jet of burning gas. **potential c.,** cauterization by an escharotic without applying heat; called also *virtual c.* **virtual c.,** potential c.

cava (ka'vah) [L.] 1. plural of *cavum.* 2. a vena cava.

caval (ka'val) pertaining to a vena cava.

cavascope (kav'ah-skōp) [L. *cavum* hollow + Gr. *skopein* to examine] an instrument for illuminating and examining a cavity.

cave (kāv) [L. *cavum*] a small enclosed space within the body or an organ; see under *cavity* and *cavum.*

caveola (ka-ve-o'lah), pl. *caveo'lae* [L.] a small pit, depression, or invagination, such as any of the minute pits or incuppings of the cell membrane formed during pinocytosis, which close and then pinch off to form small, free, fluid-filled vesicles (pinosomes) in the cytoplasm. Called also *c. intracellularis* and *plasmalemmal vesicle.*

cavern (kav'ern) a pathologic cavity, such as occurs in the lung in tuberculosis. **c's of corpora cavernosa of penis,** cavernae corporum cavernosorum penis. **c's of corpus spongiosum,** cavernae corporis spongiosi. **Schnabel's c's,** glaucomatous optic atrophy with elevated intraocular pressure.

caverna (ka-ver'nah), pl. *caver'nae* [L.] [NA] a general term used to designate a cavity. **caver'nae cor'poris spongio'si** [NA], caverns of corpus spongiosum: the dilatable spaces within the corpus spongiosum of the penis, which fill with blood and become distended with erection. **caver'nae corpo'rum cavernoso'rum pe'nis** [NA], caverns of corpora cavernosa of penis: the dilatable spaces within the corpora cavernosa of the penis, which fill with blood and become distended with erection.

caverniloquy (kav"er-nil'o-kwe) [L. *caverna* cavity + *loqui* to speak] the low-pitched pectoriloquy indicative of a pulmonary cavity.

cavernitis (kav"er-ni'tis) inflammation of the corpora cavernosa or corpus spongiosum of the penis. **fibrous c.,** Peyronie's disease.

cavernoscope (kav'er-no-skōp") an instrument for viewing any cavity, as one inserted through an intercostal space into the pleural cavity.

cavernoscopy (kav"er-nos'ko-pe) the inspection of a cavity with the aid of a cavernoscope.

cavernositis (kav"er-no-si'tis) cavernitis.

cavernostomy (kav"er-nos'to-me) operative incision into a cavity.

cavernous (kav'er-nus) [L. *cavernosus*] containing caverns or hollow spaces.

Cavia (ka've-ah) a genus of small South American rodents. **C. coba'ya,** the guinea pig.

cavilla (kah-vil'ah) os sphenoidale.

cavitary (kav'ĭ-ta"re) 1. characterized by the presence of a cavity or cavities. 2. any entozoon with a body space or alimentary canal.

cavitas (kav'ĭ-tas), pl. *cavita'tes* [L., from *cavus* hollow] [NA] a hollow space or depression; called also *cavum* [NA alternative]. **c. abdomina'lis,** abdominal cavity: the body cavity located between the diaphragm above and the pelvis below; called also *abdominal region* and *regio abdominalis.* **c. articula'ris** [NA], articular cavity: the minute space of a synovial joint, enclosed by the synovial membrane and articular cartilages. **c. con'chae,** cavity of concha: the inferior part of the concha of the auricle, which leads into the external acoustic meatus; called also *innominate fossa of auricle.* **c. corona'lis** [NA], pulp chamber: the portion of the dental (pulp) cavity located in the tooth crown, occupied by the dental pulp. **c. cra'nii** [NA], cranial cavity: the space enclosed by the bones of the cranium. **c. den'tis** [NA], dental cavity: the natural cavity in the central portion of a tooth occupied by the dental pulp, which is divided into the pulp chamber (*c. coronalis*) and the root canal (*canalis radicis dentis*); called also *c. pulparis* [NA alternative], *nerve cavity,* and *pulp cavity.* **c. epidura'lis** [NA], epidural cavity: the space between the dura mater and the walls of the vertebral canal, containing venous plexuses and fibrous and alveolar tissue; called also *epidural space.* **c. glenoida'lis** [NA], glenoid cavity: a depression in the lateral angle of the scapula for articulation with the humerus; called also *glenoid fossa of scapula.* **c. infraglot'tica** [NA], infraglottic cavity: the most inferior part of the laryngeal cavity, extending from the rima glottidis above to the cavity of the trachea below. **c. laryn'gis** [NA], laryngeal cavity: the space enclosed by the walls of the larynx. **c. medulla'ris** [NA], medullary cavity: the space in the diaphysis of a long bone containing the marrow; called also *marrow cavity, medullary canal,* and *medullary space.* **c. na'si** [NA], nasal cavity: the proximal portion of the passages of the respiratory system, extending from the nares to the pharynx; it is divided into left and right halves by the nasal septum and is separated from the oral cavity by the hard palate. **c. o'ris** [NA], oral cavity: the cavity of the mouth and associated structures, including the cheek, palate, oral mucosa, the glands whose ducts open into the cavity, the teeth, and the tongue. **c. o'ris exter'na,** vestibulum oris. **c. o'ris pro'pria** [NA], oral cavity proper: the part of the oral cavity internal to the teeth. **c. pel'vis** [NA], pelvic cavity: the space within the walls of the pelvis. Called also *cavum pelvis.* **c. pericardia'lis** [NA], pericardial cavity: the potential space between the parietal layer and the visceral layer (epicardium) of the serous pericardium. **c. peritonea'lis** [NA], peritoneal cavity: the potential space of capillary thinness between the parietal and the visceral peritoneum, which is normally empty except for a thin serous fluid that keeps the surfaces moist. Called also *greater peritoneal cavity.* **c. pharyn'gis** [NA], pharyngeal cavity: the space enclosed by the walls of the pharynx. **c. pleura'lis** [NA], pleural cavity: the potential space between the parietal and visceral pleurae. **c. pulpa'ris,** NA alternative for *c. dentis.* **c. sep'ti pellu'cidi** [NA], cavity of septum pellucidum: the median cleft between the two laminae of the septum pellucidum; called also *Duncan's* or *Vieussens's ventricle, fifth ventricle, first ventricle of cerebrum, pseudocele* or *pseudocoele, pseudoventricle,* and *ventricle of Arantius* or *Sylvius.* **c. subarachnoidea'lis** [NA], subarachnoid cavity: the space between the arachnoidea and the pia mater, containing cerebrospinal fluid and bridged by delicate trabeculae; called also *subarachnoid space.* **c. thora'cis** [NA], the thoracic cavity: the portion of the body cavity situated between the neck and the respiratory diaphragm; called also *pectoral cavity.* **c. tympan'ica** [NA], tympanic cavity: the major portion of the middle ear (auris media), consisting of a narrow air-filled cavity in the temporal bone that contains the auditory ossicles and communicates with the mastoid air cells and the mastoid antrum by means of the aditus and the nasopharynx by means of the auditory tube. The middle ear and the tympanic cavity were formerly regarded as being synonymous. Called also *drum, eardrum,* and *tympanum.* **c. u'teri** [NA], uterine cavity: the flattened space within the uterus, communicating on either side at the cornu with the uterine tubes and below with the vagina.

cavitates (kav″ĭ-ta′tēz) [L.] plural of *cavitas*.

cavitation (kav″ĭ-ta′shun) 1. the formation of cavities, as in pulmonary tuberculosis. 2. a cavity.

cavitis (ka-vi′tis) inflammation of a vena cava.

cavity (kav′ĭ-te) [L. *cavitas*] 1. a hollow place or space, or a potential space, within the body or in one of its organs; it may be normal or pathological. See also *cavitas* and *cavum*. 2. the lesion, or area of destruction in a tooth, produced by dental caries; classified as simple, compound, or complex, according to the number of surfaces involved. See also *dental caries*, under *caries*. 3. prepared c. **abdominal c.**, cavitas abdominalis. **absorption c's**, cavities in developing compact bone due to osteoclastic erosion, usually occurring in the areas laid down first. **alveolar c's**, dental alveoli. **amniotic c.**, the closed sac between the embryo and the amnion, containing the amniotic fluid. **articular c.**, cavitas articulare. **Baer's c.**, the cleavage cavity beneath the blastoderm. **body c.**, a visceral cavity, such as the thoracic, abdominal, or pelvic cavity. **bony c. of nose**, cavum nasi osseum. **buccal c.**, 1. that portion of the oral cavity bounded on one side by the teeth and gingivae (or the residual alveolar ridges), and on the other by the cheeks. 2. a carious lesion beginning on the buccal surface of a posterior tooth. 3. oral c. See *cavitas oris*. 4. a preoral chamber seen in higher ciliate protozoa, manifested as an indentation or pouch containing compound ciliary organelles and leading to the cytostomal-cytopharyngeal complex. Called also *peristome*. **cleavage c.**, the cavity of the blastula; blastocoele. **complex c.**, a carious lesion that involves three or more surfaces of a tooth in its prepared state. **compound c.**, a carious lesion that involves two surfaces of a tooth. **c. of concha**, cavitas conchae. **cotyloid c.**, acetabulum. **cranial c.**, cavitas cranii. **dental c.**, 1. see *cavity* (def. 2), and see under *caries*. 2. cavitas dentis. **distal c.**, a carious lesion beginning on the distal surface of a tooth. **epidural c.**, cavitas epiduralis. **faucial c.**, cavitas pharyngis. **fibrotic c's**, cavities of the lung in tuberculosis composed of tuberculous granulation tissue surrounded by scar tissue, often the source from which the disease spreads to other pulmonary segments. **fissure c.**, a carious lesion beginning in a fissure of a tooth. See *pit caries*, under *caries*. **gastrovascular c.**, the body cavity of a coelenterate, which opens to the outside at one end to form a mouth; called also *coelenteron*. **glandular c.**, a hollow sac formed by invagination of the epithelial sheath in the developing multicellular gland. **glenoid c.**, cavitas glenoidalis. **head c.**, modified somites that in lower vertebrates give rise to the extrinsic eye muscles. **hemal c.**, hemocoelom. **incisal c.**, a carious lesion beginning on the incisal surface of an anterior tooth. **infraglottic c.**, cavitas infraglottica. **ischiorectal c.**, fossa ischiorectalis. **labial c.**, a carious lesion beginning on the labial surface of an anterior tooth. **laryngeal c.**, cavitas laryngis. **laryngopharyngeal c.**, the laryngopharynx (pars laryngea pharyngis [NA]). **lingual c.**, a carious lesion beginning on the lingual surface of a tooth. **lymph c's**, the larger lymph spaces and cisterns of the body. **marrow c.**, cavitas medullaris. **mastoid c.**, antrum mastoideum. **Meckel's c.**, cavum trigeminale. **mediastinal c., anterior**, mediastinum anterius. **mediastinal c., middle**, mediastinum medium. **mediastinal c., posterior**, mediastinum posterius. **mediastinal c., superior**, mediastinum superius. **medullary c.**, cavitas medullaris. **mesial c.**, a carious lesion beginning on the mesial surface of a tooth. **nasal c.**, cavitas nasi. **nerve c.**, cavitas dentis. **occlusal c.**, a carious lesion beginning on the occlusal surface of a posterior tooth. **oral c.**, cavitas oris. **oral c., external**, vestibulum oris. **oral c., proper**, cavitas oris propria. **orbital c.**, orbita. **pectoral c.**, cavitas pectoris. **pelvic c.**, cavitas pelvis. **pericardial c.**, cavitas pericardialis. **peritoneal c.**, cavitas peritonealis. **peritoneal c., greater**, cavitas peritonealis. **peritoneal c., lesser**, bursa omentalis. **pharyngeal c.**, cavitas pharyngis. **pharyngolaryngeal c.**, the laryngopharynx (pars laryngea pharyngis [NA]). **pharyngonasal c.**, the nasopharynx (pars nasalis pharyngis [NA]). **pharyngo-oral c.**, the oropharynx (pars oralis pharyngis [NA]). **pit c.**, a carious lesion beginning in a pit of a tooth. See *pit caries*, under *caries*. **pleural c.**, cavitas pleuralis. **pleuroperitoneal c.**, the temporarily continuous coelomic cavity in the embryo that will later be partitioned by the developing diaphragm. **popliteal c.**,

fossa poplitea. **prepared c.**, one that is produced in a tooth to support and retain the filling material and protect the tooth structure remaining after removal of all carious tissue. See also *cavity preparation*, under *preparation*. **proximal c.**, a carious lesion beginning on a proximal (the mesial or distal) surface of a tooth. **pulp c.**, cavitas dentis. **rectoischiadic c.**, fossa ischiorectalis. **Retzius's c.**, spatium retropubicum. **Rosenmüller's c.**, recessus pharyngeus. **segmentation c.**, the blastocoele. **c. of septum pellucidum**, cavitas septi pellucidi. **serous c.**, a celomic cavity, like that enclosed by the pericardium, peritoneum, or pleura, not communicating with the outside of the body, and whose lining membrane secretes a serous fluid. **sigmoid c. of radius**, incisura ulnaris radii. **sigmoid c. of ulna, greater**, incisura trochlearis ulnae. **sigmoid c. of ulna, lesser**, incisura radialis ulnae. **simple c.**, a carious lesion that involves only one surface of a tooth in its preparation, designated according to the surface involved as buccal, distal, incisal, labial, lingual, mesial, or occlusal. **somatic c.**, the intraembryonic portion of the coelom. **somite c.**, myocoele. **splanchnic c.**, visceral c. **subarachnoid c.**, cavitas subarachnoidealis. **subdural c.**, spatium subdurale. **tension c's**, cavities of the lung in which the air pressure is greater than that of the atmosphere. Radiologically, they appear as large, spherical, thin-walled defects indicative of productive inflammatory reaction in the bronchus that drains the cavity or of partial stenosis due to peribronchial fibrosis. **thoracic c.**, cavitas thoracis. **trigeminal c.**, cavum trigeminale. **tympanic c.**, cavitas tympanicum. **uterine c.**, cavitas uteri. **visceral c.**, one of the cavities of the body containing organs, such as the thoracic, abdominal, or pelvic cavity; called also *splanchnic* c. **yolk c.**, the space between the germ disk and the yolk of the developing ovum of some animals; called also *subgerminal* c.

cavography (ka-vog′rah-fe) venacavography.

cavosurface (ka′vo-sur″fis) the surface of a cavity, as of a tooth.

cavovalgus (ka″vo-val′gus) see *talipes cavovalgus*.

cavum (ka′vum), pl. *ca′va* [L.] 1. a cavity or space. 2. NA alternative for *cavitas*. **c. meck′elii**, c. trigeminale. **c. mediastina′le ante′rius**, mediastinum anterius. **c. mediastina′le poste′rius**, mediastinum posterius. **c. o′ris exter′num**, vestibulum oris. **c. rectoischiad′icum**, fossa ischiorectalis. **c. ret′zii**, spatium retropubicum. **c. subdura′le**, spatium subdurale. **c. trigemina′le** [NA], trigeminal cavity: the small outpocketing of the dura mater surrounding the ganglion and divisions of the trigeminal nerve, and located at the end of the petrous portion of the temporal bone, which contains the trigeminal ganglion; called also c. *meckelii* and *Meckel's cavity*. **c. ver′gae**, Verga's ventricle.

cavus (kav′us) [L. "hollow"] see *talipes cavus*.

cavy (ka′ve) a small rodent of the family Caviidae, the best known representative of which is the guinea pig (*Cavia cobaya*).

Caytine (ka′tēn) trademark for a preparation of protokylol hydrochloride.

Cb chemical symbol for *columbium*, now called *niobium*.

C3b INA C3b inactivator; see *complement*.

C.B. abbreviation for L. *Chirur′giae Baccalau′reus*, Bachelor of Surgery.

c.b.c. complete blood count.

CBF cerebral blood flow.

CBG corticosteroid-binding globulin; see *transcortin*.

CBS chronic brain syndrome.

C.C. chief complaint.

cc. cubic centimeter.

CCA 1. chimpanzee coryza agent (respiratory syncytial virus). 2. congenital contractural arachnodactyly; see *hereditary bone dysplasia*, under *dysplasia*.

CCAT conglutinating complement absorption test.

C. C. 914 a thioarsenite, *p*-carbamido-phenyl-bis (carboxymethyl-mercapto) arsine, used in treatment of intestinal amebiasis.

C. C. 1037 a thioarsenite, *p*-carbamido-phenyl-bis (2-carboxyphenyl-mercapto) arsine, used in intestinal amebiasis.

CCC cathodal closure contraction.

CCF crystal-induced chemotactic factor.

CCCl cathodal closure clonus.

CCK cholecystokinin.

CCK-179 the methanesulfonate salts of equal parts of dihydroergocornine, dihydroergocristine, and dihydroergocryptine, used as an antihypertensive and as a vasodilator in the treatment of peripheral vascular diseases.

CCl₄ carbon tetrachloride.

CCl₃·CHO chloral.

CCl₃·CH(OH)₂ chloral hydrate.

c.cm. cubic centimeter.

CCNU lomustine. **methyl CCNU, MeCCNU** semustine.

CCU coronary care unit.

C.D. abbreviation for L. *conjugata diagonalis*, the diagonal conjugate diameter of the pelvic inlet, and for *curative dose*.

C.D.₅₀ median curative dose; a dose that abolishes symptoms in 50 per cent of the test subjects.

Cd 1. chemical symbol for *cadmium*. 2. abbreviation for *caudal* or *coccygeal*; used in vertebral formulas.

cd candela.

CDC Centers for Disease Control.

CDC/AIDS see *acquired immune deficiency syndrome*.

cdf cumulative distribution function.

cDNA complementary DNA or copy DNA; synthetic DNA transcribed from a specific RNA through the reaction of the enzyme reverse transcriptase.

CDP cytidine diphosphate.

Ce chemical symbol for *cerium*.

CEA carcinoembryonic antigen.

ceasmic (se-as′mik) [Gr. *keasma* chip] characterized by the persistence after birth of embryonic fissures.

cebocephalus (se″bo-sef′ah-lus) a monster exhibiting cebocephaly.

cebocephaly (se″bo-sef′ah-le) [Gr. *kebos* monkey + *kephalē* head] a developmental anomaly characterized by a monkey-like head, the nose being defective and the eyes close together.

ceca (se′kah) [L.] plural of *cecum*.

cecal (se′kal) [L. *caecalis*] 1. ending in a blind passage. 2. pertaining to the cecum.

cecectomy (se-sek′to-me) [*cecum* + Gr. *ektomē* excision] surgical removal of the cecum.

Cecil's operation (se′silz) [Arthur Bond *Cecil*, Los Angeles surgeon, born 1885] see under *operation*.

cecitis (se-si′tis) inflammation of the cecum.

cec(o)- [L. *cecum*, q.v.] a combining form denoting relation to the cecum.

cecocele (se′ko-sēl) a hernia containing part of the cecum.

cecocentral (se″ko-sen′tral) centrocecal.

cecocolic (se″ko-kol′ik) pertaining to the cecum and the colon.

cecocolon (se″ko-ko′lon) the cecum and colon considered as a unit.

cecocolopexy (se″ko-ko′lo-pek″se) an operation for fixing the cecum and ascending colon to the abdominal wall.

cecocolostomy (se″ko-ko-los′to-me) the surgical creation of an anastomosis between the cecum and the colon; also, the anastomosis so constructed. Called also *colocecostomy*.

cecofixation (se″ko-fik-sa′shun) cecopexy.

cecoileostomy (se″ko-il″e-os′to-me) [*cecum* + *ileum* + Gr. *stomoun* to provide with a mouth, or opening] ileocecostomy.

Cecon (se′kon) trademark for preparations of ascorbic acid.

cecopexy (se′ko-pek′se) [*cecum* + Gr. *pēxis* fixation] fixation or suspension of the cecum to correct excessive mobility of the organ; called also *cecofixation*.

cecoplication (se″ko-pli-ka′shun) [*cecum* + L. *plica* fold] plication of the cecal wall to correct ptosis or dilatation of the organ.

cecorrhaphy (se-kor′ah-fe) [*cecum* + Gr. *rhaphē* suture.] suture or repair of the cecum.

cecosigmoidostomy (se″ko-sig″moi-dos′to-me) formation of an artificial opening between the cecum and sigmoid,

usually by surgical procedure; also, the opening so constructed.

cecostomy (se-kos′to-me) [*cecum* + Gr. *stomoun* to provide with a mouth, or opening] the surgical creation of an artificial opening or fistula into the cecum; also, the opening so constructed.

cecotomy (se-kot′o-me) [*cecum* + Gr. *tomē* a cutting] the operation of cutting into the cecum.

cecum (se′kum) [L. *caecum* blind, blind gut] 1. any blind pouch or cul-de-sac. 2. NA alternative for *caecum*. **gastric ceca** outpocketings of the midgut, of uncertain function, seen in many insects. **high c.,** a cecum situated higher up in the abdomen than normal. **mobile c., c. mo′bile,** abnormal mobility of the cecum and lower portion of the ascending colon, caused by incomplete rotation or faulty fixation of the cecum in embryonic development.

Cedecea (se-de′se-a) [named for Centers for *Disease Control*, Atlanta, Georgia] a genus of gram-negative, facultatively anaerobic, rod-shaped bacteria of the family Enterobacteriaceae, isolated primarily from clinical specimens of the human respiratory tract, and a possible opportunistic pathogen. The type species is *C. da′visae*.

Cedilanid (se″di-lan′id) trademark for a preparation of lanatoside C.

Cedilanid-D trademark for a preparation of deslanoside.

Cediopsylla (se″de-o-sil′ah) a genus of fleas, including some of the rabbit fleas.

CeeNU trademark for preparations of lomustine.

cefaclor (sef′ah-klor) chemical name: [6R-[6α,7β(R*)]]-7-[(amino-phenylacetyl)amino]-3-chloro-8-oxo-5-thia-1-azabicyclo[4.2.0]oct-2-ene-2-carboxylic acid; a semisynthetic ceph-alosporin antibiotic, $C_{15}H_{14}ClN_3O_4S$.

cefadroxil (sef″ah-droks′il) [USP] chemical name: [6R-[6α,7β(R*)]]-7-[[amino(4-hydroxyphenyl)acetyl]amino]-3-methyl-8-oxo-5-thia-1-azabicyclo[4.2.0]oct-2-ene-2-carboxylic acid; a semisynthetic cephalosporin antibiotic, $C_{16}H_{17}N_3O_5S$.

Cefadyl (sef′ah-dil) trademark for a preparation of cephapirin sodium.

cefamandole (sef″ah-man′dōl) chemical name: [6R-[6α,7β(R*)]]-7-[(hydroxyphenylacetyl)amino]-3-[[(1-methyl-1H-tetrazol-5-yl)thio]methyl-8-oxo-5-thia-1-azabicyclo[4.2.0]oct-2-ene-2-carboxylic acid; a semisynthetic cephalosporin antibiotic, $C_{18}H_{18}N_6O_5S_2$. **c. nafate,** the monosodium salt of cefamandole, $C_{19}H_{17}N_6NaO_6S_2$.

cefaparole (sef′ah-pah-rōl″) chemical name: [6R-[6α,7β(R*)]]-7-[[amino(4-hydroxyphenyl)acetyl]amino]-3-[[(5-methyl-1-3,4-thiadiazol-2-yl)thio]methyl]-8-oxo-5-thio-1-azabicyclo[4.2.0]oct-2-ene-2-carboxylic acid; a semisynthetic cephalosporin antibiotic, $C_{19}H_{19}N_5O_5S_3$.

cefatrizine (sef″ah-tri′zēn) chemical name: [6R-[6α,7β-(R*)]]-7-[[amino(4-hydroxyphenyl)acetyl]amino]-8-oxo-3-[(1H-1,2,3-triazol-4-ylthio)methyl]-5-thia-1-azabicyclo[4.2.0]oct-2-ene-2-carboxylic acid; a semisynthetic cephalosporin antibiotic, $C_{18}H_{18}N_6O_5S_2$.

cefazaflur sodium (se-faz′ah-flor) chemical name: (6R-trans)-[[(1-methyl-1H-tetrazol-5-yl)thio]methyl]-8-oxo-7[[[(trifluoromethyl)thio]acetyl]amino]-5-thia-1-azabicyclo-[4.2.0]oct-2-ene-2-carboxylic acid monosodium salt; a semisynthetic cephalosporin antibiotic, $C_{13}H_{12}F_3N_6NaO_4S_3$.

cefazolin (se-faz′o-lin) chemical name: (6R-trans)-3-[[(5-methyl-1,3,4-thiadiazol-2-yl)thio]methyl]-8-oxo-7-[[(1H-tetrazol-1-yl)acetyl]-amino]-5-thia-azabicyclo[4.2.0]oct-2-ene-2-carboxylic acid. A semisynthetic analogue, $C_{14}H_{14}N_8S_3$, of the natural antibiotic cephalosporin C, effective against a wide range of gram-negative and gram-positive bacteria. **c. sodium,** the monosodium salt of cepazolin, $C_{14}H_{13}N_8NaO_4S_3$, having the same actions as the base; used in the treatment of infections of the respiratory tract, genitourinary tract, skin, soft tissues, bones, joints, and blood due to sensitive pathogens, administered intramuscularly and intravenously. It is available for therapeutic use as *sterile cefazolin sodium* [USP].

ceforanide (se-for′ah-nīd) chemical name: (6R-trans)-7-[[[2-(aminomethyl)phenyl]acetyl]amino]-3-[[[1-(carboxymethyl)-1H tetrazol-5-yl]thio]methyl]-8-oxo-5-thio-1-azabicyclo[4.2.0]oct-2-2-carboxylic acid; an antibacterial, $C_{20}H_{21}N_7O_6S_2$.

cefotaxime (sef″o-tak′sēm) a semisynthetic broad-spectrum cephalosporin antibiotic effective against many organisms that have become resistant to penicillin, cephalosporin, and aminoglycoside antibiotics.

cefotaxime sodium (sef″oh-taks′ēm) [USP] a third-generation cephalosporin used as an antibacterial.

cefoxitin (sĕ-foks′ĭ-tin) chemical name: (6R-cis)-3-[[(aminocarbonyl)oxy]methyl]-7-methoxy-8-oxo-7-[(2-thienylacetyl)-amino]-5-thia-1-azabicyclo[4.2.0]oct-2-ene-2-carboxylic acid. A semisynthetic derivative of cephamycin C, an analogue of the cephalosporin antibiotic cephalothin, especially effective against gram-negative organisms, with strong resistance to degradation by β-lactamase.

ceftazidime (sef′ta-zĭ-dēm) a cephalosporin derivative with high activity against *Pseudomonas* spp.

ceftizoxime sodium (sef″tĭ-zoks′ēm) a third-generation cephalosporin used as an antibacterial.

ceftriaxone sodium (sef-tri′ah-zōn) a semisynthetic cephalosporin antibacterial.

Cel. Celsius (thermometric scale).

cel (sel) a unit of velocity, being the velocity of 1 cm. per second.

celarium (sĕ-la′re-um) mesothelium.

Celbenin (sel′bĕ-nin) trademark for preparations of sodium methicillin.

-cele (sēl) 1. [Gr. *kēlē* hernia] a word termination denoting relationship to a tumor or swelling. 2. [Gr. *koilia* cavity] a word termination denoting relationship to a cavity; see also words spelled -*coele*.

celenteron (se-len′ter-on) 1. archenteron. 2. gastrovascular cavity.

Celestone (se-les′tōn) trademark for preparations of betamethasone.

celiac (se′le-ak) [Gr. *koilia* belly] pertaining to the abdomen.

celiectomy (se″le-ek′to-me) [celi- + Gr. *ektomē* excision] surgical removal of an abdominal organ.

celi(o)- [Gr. *koilia* belly] a combining form denoting relationship to the abdomen. For words beginning thus, see also words beginning cel(o)- and coel(o)-.

celiocentesis (se″le-o-sen-te′sis) [celio- + Gr. *kentēsis* puncture] puncture into the abdominal cavity, usually for the withdrawal of fluid.

celiocolpotomy (se″le-o-kol-pot′o-me) [celio- + Gr. *kolpos* vagina + *tomē* a cutting] incision into the abdomen through the vaginal wall.

celioenterotomy (se″le-o-en″ter-ot′o-me) [celio- + *enterotomy*] incision through the abdominal wall into the intestine.

celiogastrotomy (se″le-o-gas-trot′o-me) [celio- + *gastrotomy*] incision through the abdominal wall into the stomach.

celiohysterectomy (se″le-o-his″ter-ek′to-me) [celio- + *hysterectomy*] 1. excision of the uterus through an abdominal incision. 2. cesarean hysterectomy.

celioma (se-le-o′mah) [celio- + -*oma*] a tumor of the abdomen, especially mesothelioma of the peritoneum.

celiomyomectomy (se″le-o-mi″o-mek′to-me) [celio- + *myomectomy*] surgical removal of a uterine myoma (leiomyoma) performed through an abdominal incision.

celiomyomotomy (se″le-o-mi″o-mot′o-me) [celio- + *myomotomy*] incision into a muscular organ or tumor through the abdominal wall.

celiomyositis (se″le-o-mi″o-si′tis) [celio- + *myositis*] inflammation of the abdominal muscles.

celioncus (se″le-on′kus) (obs.) celioma.

celioparacentesis (se″le-o-par″ah-sen-te′sis) [celio- + *paracentesis*] paracentesis of the abdominal cavity, usually with a trocar or needle.

celiopathy (se″le-op′ah-the) [celio- + Gr. *pathos* disease] any abdominal disease.

celiophyma (se″le-o-fi′mah) (obs.) celioma.

celiorrhaphy (se″le-or′ah-fe) [celio- + Gr. *rhaphē* suture] suture of the abdominal wall.

celiosalpingectomy (se″le-o-sal″pin-jek′to-me) [celio- + *salpingectomy*] excision of a uterine tube through an abdominal incision.

celiosalpingotomy (se″le-o-sal″pin-got′o-me) incision of a uterine tube through an incision in the abdominal wall.

celioscope (se′le-o-skōp″) [celio- + Gr. *skopein* to examine] an endoscope for examining the abdominal cavity.

celioscopy (se″le-os′ko-pe) examination of the abdominal cavity through a celioscope.

celiothelioma (se″le-o-the″le-o′mah) (obs.) mesothelioma of the peritoneum.

celiotomy (se″le-ot′o-me) [celio- + Gr. *tomē* a cutting] surgical incision into the abdominal cavity. **vaginal c.,** incision into the abdominal cavity through the vagina. **ventral c.,** incision into the abdominal cavity through the abdominal wall.

celitis (se-li′tis) any abdominal inflammation.

cell (sel) [L. *cella* compartment] 1. any one of the minute protoplasmic masses that make up organized tissue, consisting of a nucleus which is surrounded by cytoplasm which contains the various organelles and is enclosed in the cell or plasma membrane. A cell is the fundamental, structural, and functional unit of living organisms. See accompanying illustration. In some of the lower forms of life, e.g., bacteria, a morphological nucleus is absent, although nucleoproteins (and genes) are present. 2. a small, more or less closed space. **A c.,** 1. alpha c. 2. amacrine c. **Abbé-Zeiss counting c.,** see *Thoma-Zeiss counting chamber,* under *chamber.* **absorptive c., intestinal,** one of the cells of the intestinal epithelium, having a brush border made up of many closely packed parallel microvilli, and believed to be associated with absorption, particularly of macromolecules. **accessory c's,** cells, predominantly of the monocyte-macrophage lineage, that cooperate with B and T lymphocytes in the generation of the immune response. **acid c.,** parietal c. **acidophilic c.,** a cell having an affinity for acid dyes; called also *acidocyte.* See also *acidophil.* **acinar c., acinous c.,** any of the cells lining an acinus, especially applied to the zymogen-secreting cells of the pancreatic acini. **acoustic hair c.,** any one of the cells provided with cilia that serve as sensory receptors in the organ of Corti; called also *auditory c.* **adelomorphous c.** (obs.), chief c. (def. 1). **adipose c.,** a fat cell. **adventitial c's,** macrophages that occur along the walls of blood vessels; called also *Marchand's c's* and *perithelial c's.* **agger nasi c's,** the cells of the anterior part of the ethmoid crest. **air c.,** one containing air, such as an alveolus of the lungs (alveolus pulmonis) or one of the air-containing cells of the auditory tube (cellulae pneumaticae tubae auditivae). **albuminous c.,** serous c. **algoid c's,** cells resembling algae, seen in cases of chronic diarrhea. **alpha c's,** 1. cells situated in the periphery of the pancreatic islets, which secrete glucagon. 2. the acidophils of the adenohypophysis; see also *carminophil* and *orangeophil.* Called also *A c's.* **alveolar c.,** any cell of the walls of the pulmonary alveoli. Often restricted to the cells of the alveolar epithelium (type I and type II alveolar cells) and alveolar phagocytes. **alveolar c's, type I,** the flattened cells of the alveolar epithelium, distinguished by their greatly attenuated cytoplasm and paucity of organelles; called also *membranous pneumonocytes* and *squamous* or *small alveolar cells.* **alveolar c's, type II,** pleomorphic cells of the pulmonary alveolar epithelium that secrete surfactant and are distinguished by abundant cytoplasm containing numerous lipid-rich multilamellar bodies; called also *granular pneumonocytes* and *great or large alveolar cells.* **Alzheimer's c's,** 1. giant astrocytes with large, prominent nuclei found in the brain in hepatolenticular degeneration and hepatic coma. 2. degenerated astrocytes. **amacrine c's,** five types of retinal neurons that seem to lack large axons, having only processes that resemble dendrites. Called also *A c's.* **ameboid c.,** any cell that is able to change its form and move about. See *migratory c.* and *wandering c.* **amine precursor uptake and decarboxylation c's,** APUD c's. **amphophilic c.,** one that stains readily with either acid or basic dyes; called also *amphocyte, amphophil, amphochromatophil,* and *amphochromaphil.* **Anichkov's (Anitschkow's) c.,** see *Anichkov's myocyte,* under *myocyte.* **antigen-presenting c's,** a group of dendritic cells arising in the bone marrow and migrating to other body sites, the function of which seems to be the retention of antigens on their surfaces for presentation to the lymphocytes, thereby inducing an immune response. The group includes follicular dendritic cells, interdigitating cells, veil cells, and Langerhans cells. **antigen-reactive c's,** 1. T lymphocytes that rapidly proliferate in response to challenge by antigen. 2. antigen-sensitive c's. **antigen-sensitive c's,** small lym-

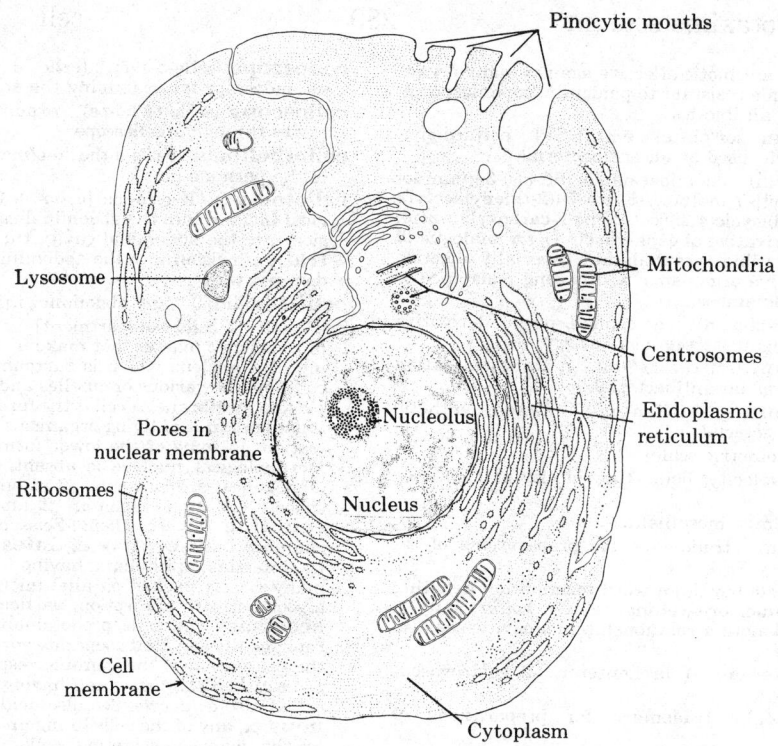

Pinocytic mouths

Lysosome

Mitochondria

Centrosomes

Pores in
nuclear membrane

Nucleolus

Endoplasmic
reticulum

Ribosomes

Nucleus

Cell
membrane

Cytoplasm

TYPICAL ANIMAL CELL

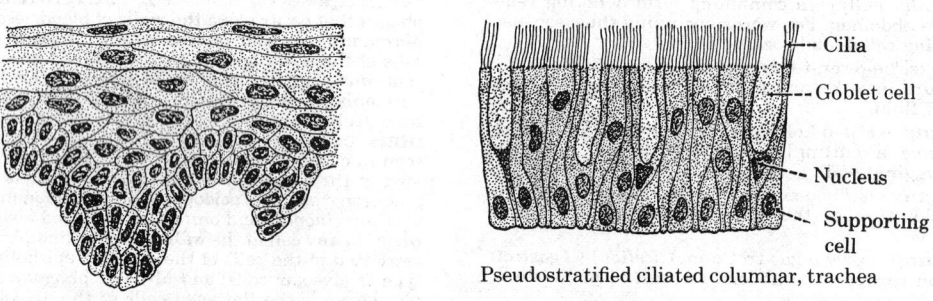

Stratified squamous, esophagus

Cilia

Goblet cell

Nucleus

Supporting
cell

Pseudostratified ciliated columnar, trachea

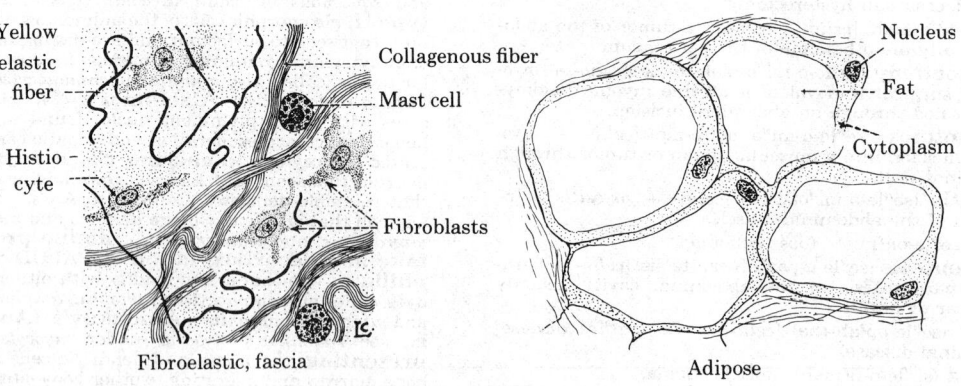

Yellow
elastic
fiber

Collagenous fiber

Mast cell

Histio-
cyte

Fibroblasts

Fibroelastic, fascia

Nucleus

Fat

Cytoplasm

Adipose

VARIOUS TYPES OF EPITHELIAL CELL

Plate 12 — THE CELL: CELL STRUCTURES AND EPITHELIAL CELL TYPES

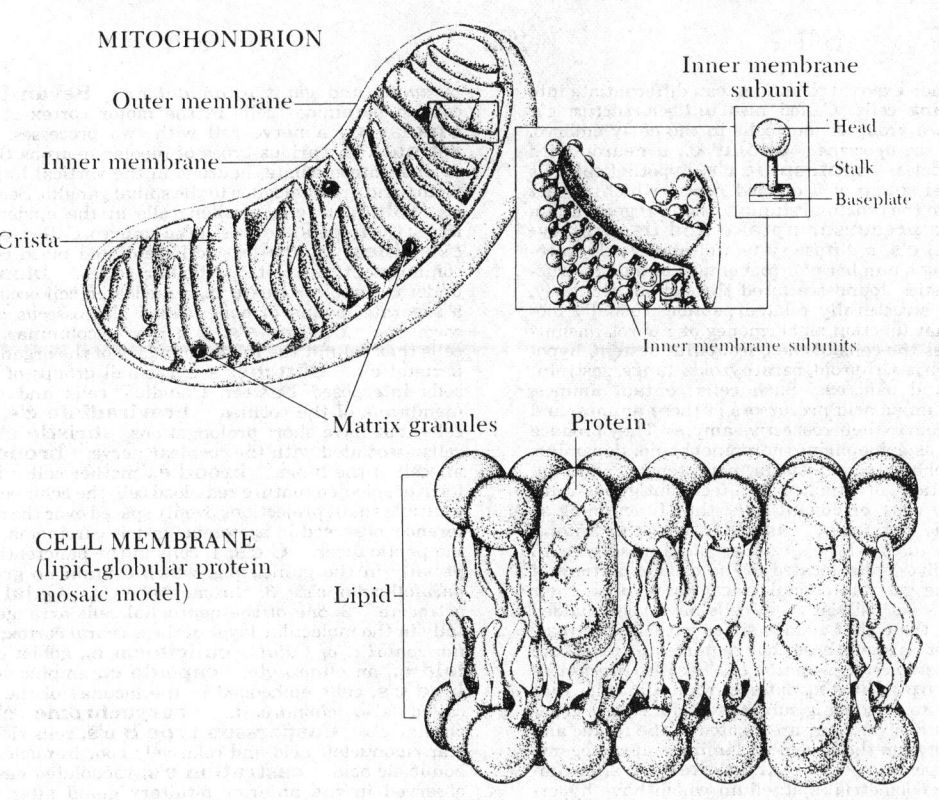

MITOCHONDRION

Outer membrane

Inner membrane

Crista

Matrix granules

Inner membrane subunit

Head

Stalk

Baseplate

Inner membrane subunits

CELL MEMBRANE
(lipid-globular protein mosaic model)

Protein

Lipid

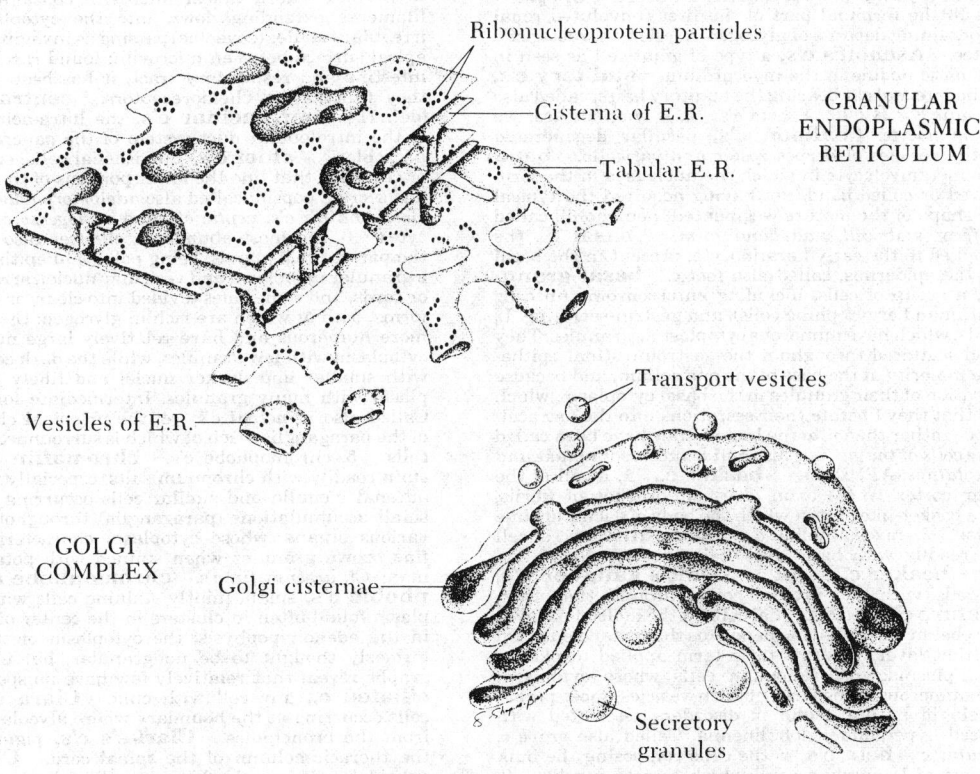

Ribonucleoprotein particles

Cisterna of E.R.

Tabular E.R.

GRANULAR ENDOPLASMIC RETICULUM

Vesicles of E.R.

Transport vesicles

GOLGI COMPLEX

Golgi cisternae

Secretory granules

Plate 13 — CELL ORGANELLES AND CELL MEMBRANE

phocytes that when exposed to antigen can differentiate into antibody-producing cells. Called also *antigen-reactive c's.* **antipodal c's,** a group of four cells in the early embryo. **apocrine c's,** see *apocrine.* **apolar c.,** a neuron with no processes or poles. **apotrophic c's,** hypothetical cells in the peripheral stump of a divided nerve, which attract young axons from the proximal stump to aid in regeneration. **APUD [amine precursor uptake and decarboxylation system] c's,** a diffuse system of apparently unrelated cells sharing a number of cytochemical and ultrastructural characteristics, found scattered throughout the body, that synthesizes structurally related peptides (usually biogenic amines) that function as hormones or neurotransmitters, and includes the cells of the chromaffin system, hypothalamus, hypophysis, thyroid, parathyroids, lungs, gastrointestinal tract, and pancreas. Such cells contain amines, concentrate the amino acid precursors of these amines, and decarboxylate them to their respective amines. They produce substances such as epinephrine, norepinephrine, dopamine, serotonin, enkephalin, somatostatin, neurotensin, and substance P, the actions of which may affect contiguous cells, nearby groups of cells, or distant cells, thus functioning as local or systemic hormones. **argentaffin c's,** enterochromaffin cells (q.v.) whose granules stain readily with chromium and silver salts, located in the basilar portions of the glands of the gastrointestinal tract. Based upon their staining reactions with silver, these cells have been divided into two groups: those that reduce silver without pretreatment (*argentaffin c's*), and those that require prior exposure to a reducing substance (*argyrophilic c's*). See also *argentaffinoma.* **argyrophilic c's,** enterochromaffin cells that require exposure to a reducing substance before their granules will react with silver; they are located in the fundic and pyloric glands between the basement lamina and zymogenic cells. See also *argentaffin c's.* **Arias-Stella c's,** columnar cells in the endometrial epithelium which have hyperchromatic enlarged nuclei and which appear to be associated with chorionic tissue in an intrauterine or extrauterine site. **arkyochrome c.,** a neuron in which the Nissl bodies are arranged in a network. **Armanni-Ebstein c's,** epithelial cells in the terminal part of the first convoluted renal tubule containing deposits of glycogen: a lesion characteristic of diabetes. **Aschoff's c's,** a type of giant cell as seen in the rheumatic nodule in the myocardium. **auditory c's,** cells in the internal ear bearing the auditory hairs; called also *acoustic hair c.* **B c's,** 1. beta c's. 2. B lymphocytes; see under *lymphocyte.* **balloon c's,** peculiar degenerated cells in the vesicles of herpes zoster and varicella. **band c.,** a late metamyelocyte in which the nucleus is in the form of a curved or coiled band, not having acquired the typical lobulate shape of the mature (segmented) neutrophil; called also *staff* or *stab cell,* and *band form.* **basal c.,** the name applied to the early keratinocyte, present in the basal layer of the epidermis; called also *foot c.* **basal granular c's,** a group of cells, including enterochromaffin cells (argentaffin and argyrophilic cells), and gastrin-secreting, L, and S cells, which have numerous cytoplasmic granules. They are found scattered throughout the gastrointestinal epithelium, the majority at the base of the epithelium, and because of the location of their granules in the basal cytoplasm, which suggests that they liberate their secretions into the extracellular space rather than into the lumen, they have been called *endocrine cells of the gut.* See also *amine precursor uptake and decarboxylation (APUD) c's.* **basket c.,** 1. a cell of the cerebellar cortex whose axon gives off brushes of fibrils, forming a basket-like nest in which the body of each Purkinje cell rests. 2. myoepithelial c. **basophilic c.,** a cell staining readily with basic dyes; called also *basocyte* and *basophil.* **beaker c.,** goblet c. **Beale's ganglion c's,** bipolar cells with one process coiled around the other. **Bergmann's c's,** peculiar glial cells in the molecular layer of the cerebellar cortex having dendrites that extend outward through that layer. **berry c.,** a term applied to plasma cells and plasmacytoid reticulum cells whose cytoplasm contains numerous transparent bluish vesicles, most probably protein in nature; found in disorders associated with pronounced hypergammaglobulinemia. Called also *grape c.* and *morular c.* **beta c's,** 1. the cells composing the bulk of the islets of Langerhans and which secrete insulin. 2. the basophilic cells of the adenohypophysis; see also *gonadotrope* (def. 3) and *thyrotrope* (def. 2). Called also *B c's.* **Betz's c's,** large pyramidal ganglion cells found in the internal pyramidal layer of the cerebral cortex; called also *giant*

pyramids and *giant pyramidal c's.* **Bevan-Lewis c's,** certain pyramidal cells in the motor cortex of the brain. **bipolar c.,** a nerve cell with two processes. **bipolar retinal c's,** various types of bipolar neurons that are the second, intermediate, neurons in the vertical linkage of the retina and are analogous to the spinal ganglia. See also *visual c's.* **bladder c's,** swollen cells in the epidermis of the tips of the fingers and toes of the embryo. Called also *Zander's c's.* **blast c.,** the least differentiated blood cell without commitment as to its particular series. **blood c's,** see under *corpuscle.* **bone c.,** a nucleated cell occupying each a separate lacuna of bone; called also *osseous c.* and *bone corpuscle.* **border c's,** 1. a row of columnar supporting cells that delimit the inner boundary of the organ of Corti. 2. parietal c's. **Böttcher's c's,** small groups of polyhedral cells interposed between Claudius' cells and the basilar membrane of the cochlea. **breviradiate c's,** neuroglial cells that have short prolongations. **bristle c's,** the hair cells associated with the cochlear nerve. **bronchic c.,** an air cell of the lungs. **brood c.,** mother cell. **burr c.,** a form of spiculed mature red blood cell, the echinocyte, having multiple small projections evenly spaced over the cell circumference; observed in azotemia, gastric carcinoma, and bleeding peptic ulcer. **C c's,** 1. cells in the pancreatic islets, especially in the guinea pig, which contain no granules. 2. parafollicular c's. 3. chromophobe c's. **Cajal c.,** 1. an astrocyte. 2. one of the neuroglial cells arranged horizontally in the molecular layer of the cerebral cortex; called also *horizontal c. of Cajal.* **caliciform c.,** goblet c. **cameloid c.,** an elliptocyte. **capsule c.,** amphicyte. **cartilage c's,** cells embedded in the lacunae of the cartilages; called also *chondrocyte.* **caryochrome c's,** karyochrome c's. **Caspersson type B c's,** cells rich in nucleolar ribonucleic acid and relatively poor in nuclear deoxyribonucleic acid. **castration c's,** vacuolated basophil cells observed in the anterior pituitary gland after castration. **caudate c's,** neuroglial cells of the gray matter having several streaming prolongations like the tail of a comet; called also *cometal c's.* **caveolated c's,** epithelial cells with thick, short, apical microvilli containing bundles of filaments extending down into the cytoplasm and with irregular tubules (caveolae) passing as invaginations from the apical surface between microvilli; found rarely in the small intestine and respiratory tract, it has been suggested that they function as chemoreceptors. **central c.,** chief c's (def. 1). **centroacinar c's,** the intra-acinar beginnings of the intralobular duct system of the pancreas. **chalice c.,** goblet c. **chief c's,** 1. epithelial cells, either columnar or cuboidal, that line the lower portions of the gastric glands and secrete pepsin; called also *adelomorphous c's, central c's, Heidenhain's c's, peptic c's,* and *zymogenic c's.* 2. pinealocytes. 3. the most abundant cells (see also *oxyphil c's*) of the parathyroid glands, being polygonal epithelial cells with a granular cytoplasm and vesicular nuclei, arranged in plates or cords, and sometimes divided into clear, or light, and dark forms, both of which are rich in glycogen: the clear cells are more numerous and have relatively large nuclei and clear cytoplasm with few granules, while the dark cells are smaller with smaller and darker nuclei and finely granular cytoplasm with many granules. Intermediate forms also exist. Called also *principal c's.* 4. the principal chromaffin cells of the paraganglia, each of which is surrounded by supporting cells. 5. chromophobe c's. **chromaffin c's,** cells that stain readily with chromium salts, especially the cells of the adrenal medulla and similar cells occurring in widespread small accumulations (paraganglia) throughout the body in various organs, whose cytoplasm characteristically shows fine brown granules when stained with potassium bichromate. Cf. *argentaffin c's.* **chromophobe c's, chromophobic c's,** small, faintly staining cells with scanty cytoplasm found often in clusters in the center of the cell cords in the adenohypophysis; the cytoplasm of these cells was formerly thought to be nongranular, but electron micrographs reveal that relatively few have no specific granules. **ciliated c.,** any cell with cilia. **Clara c's,** unciliated cells occurring at the boundary where alveolar ducts branch from the bronchioles. **Clarke's c's,** pigmented cells in the thoracic column of the spinal cord. **Claudius' c's,** cuboidal cells, which along with Böttcher's cells, form the floor of the external spiral sulcus, external to the organ of Corti. **clear c's,** cells with empty-appearing cytoplasm. **cleavage c.,** any one of the cells derived from the fertilized ovum by mitosis; a blastomere. **clump c's,** round, thick, pigmented cells seen in the sphincter muscle of the iris. **collenchyma c's,** elongated living cells with walls thickened in the corners, which compose the collenchyma of plants. Cf. *schlerenchyma c's.* **columnar c.,** an elongate epithelial cell. **cometal c's,** caudate c's. **commissural c's,** heteromeral c's. **committed c.,** a lymphocyte which, after contact with antigen, is obligated to follow an individual course of development. In the bone marrow, these arise from pluripotential stem cells and themselves form precursor lines for various blood cells. **compound granule c.,** microglia. **cone c.,** retinal cone. **connective tissue c's,** a general name for the cellular elements of the fibrous and nonfibrous components of the various forms of connective tissue. **contractile fiber c's,** the spindle-shaped and nucleated cells which, collected into bundles, make up unstriated or smooth muscle. **contrasuppressor c's,** suppressor cells that augment the immune response by suppressing the activity of other suppressor cells. **corneal c.,** a modified connective tissue cell occupying each corneal space. **c's of Corti,** the cells of the organ of Corti. **corticotroph-lipotroph c.,** corticotroph. **counting c.,** see under *chamber.* **cover c.,** any cell that covers and protects other cells, especially any long epithelial cell of the outer layer of the taste buds; called also *encasing c.* **crescent c's,** crescents of Giannuzzi. **cribrate c.,** a cell whose walls are perforated with numerous sievelike pores. **Crooke's c's,** the pituitary basophils of Crooke's hyaline degeneration; see under *degeneration.* **cuboid c.,** an epithelial cell of which the transverse and vertical diameters are approximately equal. **Custer c's,** cells with long delicate protoplasmic processes replacing the lymphoid tissue of lymph nodes in reticuloendothelial disease. **cylindric c.,** columnar c. **cytotoxic T c's,** cytotoxic T lymphocytes. **D c's,** delta c's. **daughter c.,** any cell formed by the division of a mother cell. **Davidoff's c's,** Paneth's c's. **decidual c's,** connective-tissue cells of the uterine mucous membrane, enlarged and specialized during pregnancy. **Deiters' c's,** 1. the outer phalangeal cells of the organ of Corti; see under *supporting c's.* 2. neuroglial cells. **delomorphous c's** *(obs.),* parietal c's. **delta c's,** 1. cells in the islets of Langerhans filled with small blue-staining secretory granules, which contain somatostatin. 2. gonadotrophs. Called also *D c's.* **demilune c's,** crescents of Giannuzzi. **dendritic c's,** 1. a heterogeneous group of nonphagocytic lymph node constituents comprising follicular dendritic cells of the germinal centers, interdigitating cells of the deep cortex, and veil cells of the afferent lymph and lymphatic sinuses, all of which have an irregular shape with numerous branching processes and an inconspicuous complement of cell organelles. 2. follicular dendritic c's. **dendritic c's, follicular,** antigen-presenting cells found in the germinal centers of the lymph nodes, and having the property of retaining for long periods of time antigen-antibody complexes in the labyrinth of clefts bounded by their surface processes. Called also *dendritic c's.* **dentin c.,** odontoblast. **dome c's,** the large cells that compose the epitrichium of the fetus. **Dorothy Reed c's,** Reed-Sternberg c's. **Downey c's,** atypical lymphocytes of three types invariably present in infectious mononucleosis. Type I is a mature cell with a kidney-shaped or lobulated nucleus with vacuolated, basophilic foamy cytoplasm; type II cells contain plasmacytoid nuclei with less vacuolated and basophilic cytoplasm; type III has a finer chromatin pattern and one or two nucleoli. **dust c's,** alveolar macrophages. **effector c.,** 1. a cell that becomes active in response to stimulation. 2. in immunology, a differentiated lymphocyte that carries out some part of the immune response, e.g., antibody production, lymphokine production, or helper, suppressor, or killer fuction. Cf. *memory c.* **electrochemical c.,** an apparatus consisting of two half-cells, each containing a solution in which an electrode is placed, connected by a salt bridge or semipermeable membrane. A voltaic cell is one in which chemical reactions occurring at the electrodes supply a voltage to an external circuit; an electrolytic cell is one in which an applied voltage drives the reactions occurring at the electrodes in the opposite direction from that in which they proceed spontaneously. **electrolytic c.,** an electrochemical cell (q.v.) to which voltage is applied to drive chemical reactions. **elementary c's, embryonic c's,** blastomere. **emigrated c.,** a leukocyte that has passed through the wall of a blood vessel into the neighboring tissue. **enamel c.,** ameloblast. **encasing c.,** cover c. **endo-**

crine c's of gut, basal granular c's. **endothelioid c's,** large protoplasmic cells frequently seen in disease of the blood-making organs and believed by some to be derived from the endothelial lining of the blood vessels and lymph vessels. **enterochromaffin c's,** a group of basal granular cells (q.v.) whose granules stain readily with silver and chromium salts, and which are sites of synthesis and storage of serotonin (5-hydroxytryptamine); included in the group are *argentaffin cells* and *agyrophilic cells.* **ependymal c's,** the cells of the ependyma; called also *ependymocytes.* **epidermic c's,** the cells of the epidermis. **epithelial c's,** cells that cover the surface of the body and line its cavities. **epithelioid c's,** 1. large polyhedral cells of connective tissue origin. 2. highly phagocytic, modified macrophages, resembling epithelial cells, having large, pale and vesicular nuclei with abundant, eosinophilic cytoplasm, which are characteristic of granulomatous inflammation; they may coalesce to form multinucleate giant cells. 3. pinealocytes. **erythroid c's,** blood cells of the erythrocytic series. **ethmoidal c's, bony,** cellulae ethmoidales osseae. **eukaryotic c.,** a cell with a true nucleus; see *eukaryote.* **F c.,** 1. in bacterial genetics, a cell with an inheritable mating type. The F$^+$ (male donor) carries the F (fertility) plasmid, while the F$^-$ cell (female recipient) lacks this factor. 2. PP c. **fat c.,** a connective tissue cell specialized for the synthesis and storage of fat; such cells are bloated with globules of triglycerides, the nucleus being displaced to one side and the cytoplasm seen as a thin line around the fat droplet. Called also *adipose c., adipocyte,* and *lipocyte.* **fat-storing c's of liver,** lipid-accumulating, stellate cells located in the perisinusoidal space of the liver. **fatty granule c.,** microglia containing fat. **Ferrata's c.,** hemohistioblast. **fiber c.,** any elongated and linear cell. **flagellate c.,** any cell having a flagellum, usually motile. **floor c's,** the cells of the floor of the arch of Corti. **foam c's,** 1. cells with a peculiar vacuolated appearance due to the presence of complex lipoids; such cells are seen notably in xanthoma and have, therefore, been termed *xanthoma c's.* Called also *lattice c's.* 2. Mikulicz's c's. **follicle c's, follicular c's,** cells located in the epithelium of follicles, e.g., the cells of the thyroid follicles and ovarian follicles. Called also *follicular epithelial c's.* **follicular epithelial c's,** follicle c's. **foot c's,** 1. basal cells. 2. Sertoli's cells. **foreign body giant c's,** giant cells, resembling Langhans' giant cells, having clusters of nuclei scattered in an irregular pattern throughout the cytoplasm, formed by coalescence and fusion of macrophages, with only a rare internal nuclear division, characteristic of granulomatous inflammation induced by inoculation or implantation of exogenous materials in dermis or subcutaneous tissue. **formative c.,** a cell of the inner cell mass of the conceptus, a blastomere destined to form a part of the embryo, as distinct from a trophoblast cell. **Foulis' c's,** large nucleated epithelial cells seen in fluids from malignant ovarian cysts. **Fuller c.,** electromotive force cell resembling the Grenet cell, but employing amalgamated zinc and copper electrodes. **fusiform c.,** spindle c. **G c's,** granular enterochromaffin cells in the mucosa of the pyloric part of the stomach, which are the source of gastrin. **galvanic c.,** voltaic c. **gametoid c's,** carcinoma cells resembling reproductive cells (gametes). **gamma c's of hypophysis,** chromophobic c's. **ganglion c.,** 1. a form of large nerve cell characteristic of ganglia; called also *gangliocyte.* 2. any of those retinal cells that are the third, last, neurons in the vertical linkage of the retina and are analogous to the relays in the spinal cord and brain stem. At least six types of ganglion cells have been classified according to their dendritic patterns. See also *visual c.* **Gaucher's c.,** a large and distinctive cell characteristic of Gaucher's disease, with one or more eccentrically placed nuclei and with fine wavy kerasin fibrils running parallel to the long axis of the cell, imparting a wrinkled, tissue-paper appearance to the gray or bluish opaque cytoplasm. **Gegenbaur's c.,** osteoblast. **germ c's,** the cells of an organism whose function it is to reproduce the kind, i.e., an ovum or spermatozoon, or an immature stage of either, called also *initial c's* and *sexual c's.* **germ c., primordial,** the earliest recognizable precursor in the embryo of an ovum or spermatozoon. **germinal c.,** a cell capable of dividing and differentiating. **ghost c.,** 1. a keratinized denucleated cell with an unstained, shadowy center where the nucleus had been. 2. an erythroclast. Called also *shadow c.* **c's of Giannuzzi,** see under *crescent.* **giant c.,** 1. any very large cell, such as the megakaryocyte of bone marrow. 2. any of the very large, multinucleate, modified macrophages, which may be formed by coalescence of epithelioid cells or by nuclear division without cytoplasmic division of monocytes, e.g., those characteristic of granulomatous inflammation (*Langhans' giant c's*) and those that form around large foreign bodies (*foreign body giant c's*). **giant pyramidal c's,** Betz's c's. **Gierke's c's,** small, deeply staining nerve cells that constitute the chief cells of the substantia gelatinosa. **gitter c.,** microglia. **Gley's c's,** large glandular cells in the interstitial tissue of the testicle. **glia c.,** a cell of the neuroglia. **glitter c's,** polymorphonuclear leukocytes that stain a pale blue with gentian-violet-safranin and contain granules in the cytoplasm that exhibit brownian movement; their presence in urine may indicate pyelonephritis. **glomerular c.,** glomus c., def. 1. **glomus c.,** 1. any of the moderately large specific epithelioid cells (type I) of the carotid body (see *glomus caroticum*) containing abundant cytoplasm and membrane-bound, electron-dense granules and having a few dentritic processes; they are richly supplied with nerve endings and are surrounded by cells without cytoplasmic granules (type II). Called also *glomerular c.* 2. any of the modified smooth muscle cells with uniform nuclei, pale-staining cytoplasm, and indistinct margins that surround the arterial segment of a glomeriform arteriovenous anastomosis, which are richly innervated by fibers of the autonomic nervous system. **goblet c.,** a unicellular mucous gland found in the epithelium of various mucous membranes, especially that of the respiratory passages and intestines. Droplets of mucigen collect in the upper part of the cell and distend it, while the basal end remains slender, and the cell assumes the shape of a goblet. Called also *beaker c., caliciform c.,* and *chalice c.* See also *ptyocrinous.* **Golgi's c's,** see under *neuron.* **gonadotroph c.,** gonadotroph. **gonadotropic c.,** gonadotrope, def. 3. **Goormaghtigh c's,** juxtaglomerular c's. **granular c.,** the name applied to a keratinocyte in the stratum granulosum of the epidermis, when it has become flattened and rhomboidal in shape and contains a dense collection of variously sized darkly staining granules, before it dies and desquamates. **granule c's,** diminutive stellate cells found chiefly in the granular layers of the cerebral and cerebellar cortices. **granulosa c's,** cells surrounding the vesicular ovarian follicle and forming the stratum granulosum and cumulus oophorus; after ovulation they are transformed into lutein cells. **granulosa-lutein c's,** lutien cells of the corpus luteum derived from granulosa cells. **grape c.,** berry c. **gustatory c's,** the taste cells. **gyrochrome c.,** see *gyrochrome.* **hair c's,** neuroepithelial cells with hairlike processes (kinocilia or stereocilia, or both) found in the organ of Corti, ampullar crest, and utricle and saccule of the inner ear; the hair cells receive afferent and efferent fibers of the cochlear nerve (organ of Corti) or the vestibular nerve. **hairy c.,** any of the abnormal large cells found in the blood in hairy-cell leukemia, having a round or oval nucleus, gray-blue cytoplasm, moderately clumped nuclear chromatin, small or not visible nucleoli, and numerous irregular cytoplasmic villi that give the cell a flagellated or hairy appearance. Called also *tricholeukocyte.* **Hammar's myoid c's,** myoid c's (def. 2). **heart-disease c's, heart-failure c's, heart-lesion c's,** macrophages containing granules of iron, found in the pulmonary alveoli and sputum in congestive heart failure. **hecatomeral c's,** cells of gray matter of the spinal cord whose axis cylinder processes divide and send one branch into the white substance of the same side of the cord and another into the anterolateral columns of the other side. **heckle c.,** prickle c. **Heidenhain's c's,** the chief cells and parietal cells of the gastric glands. **HeLa c's,** cells of the first continuously cultured carcinoma strain, descended from a human cervical carcinoma; used in the study of life processes, including viruses, at the cell level. **helmet c.,** an abnormal red cell form resembling a helmet, seen in hemolytic anemia. **helper c's,** differentiated T lymphocytes whose cooperation (help) is required for the production of antibody against most (T-dependent) antigens. B cell activation requires recognition of the antigenic determinant against which specific antibody is produced by antigen receptors on a B cell, recognition of some other antigenic determinant by antigen receptors on a helper cell, and a signal passed from the helper cell to the B cell, probably requiring direct cell-to-cell contact. Murine helper cells are marked by the Ly-1 antigen, human helper cells by the T4 antigen. See *lymphocyte.* **Henle's c's** (*obs.*), large granu-

lar nucleated cells in the seminiferous tubules. **Hensen's c's,** tall supporting cells arranged in rows adjacent to the last row of outer phalangeal cells, constituting the outer border of the organ of Corti. **hepatic c's,** the polyhedral epithelial cells that constitute the substance of an acinus of the liver; called also *liver c's.* **heteromeral c's,** nerve cells of the gray matter of the spinal cord whose axon processes pass to the white matter of the opposite side; called also *commissural c's.* **hilus c's,** groups of large epithelioid cells closely associated with vascular spaces and unmyelinated nerve fibers in the hilus of the ovary and the adjacent mesovarium; they seem to be histologically and functionally related to the Leydig cells of the testis. **Hodgkin's c's,** Reed-Sternberg c's. **Hofbauer c's,** large, globular cells filled with vacuoles and large spherical nuclei, which are found in the chorionic villi of the early placenta; they are probably macrophages. **homozygous typing c's (HTC),** cells homozygous for a known HLA-D specificity; panels of HTC of all established HLA-D types are used to determine the HLA-D type of unknown cells using one-way mixed lymphocyte reactions. **horizontal c.,** a retinal neuron; there are two types, and their functions are unclear. Each cell has a multipolar soma in the internal nuclear layer and one long neurite and several short ones. All the neurites serve as both axons and dendrites, extending along and ramifying within the internal nuclear layer. The long neurite synapses in the outer plexiform layer with both pedicles and spherules; the short neurites synapse either with pedicles or with spherules. Called also *H c.* **horizontal c. of Cajal,** Cajal's c. **horn c's,** 1. epithelial cells that have lost their protoplasm, have sharp edges, and look horny. 2. any ganglion cell of the horns of the spinal cord. **Hortega c.,** microglia. **Hürthle c's,** large eosinophilic cells sometimes found in the thyroid gland; they seem to be parathyroid rests included by chance in thyroid tissue. See also *Hürthle cell tumor*, under *tumor.* **hyperchromatic c.,** one that stains more intensely than is typical of its cell type. **I-c.,** see mucolipidosis II. **immunologically competent c.,** immunocyte. **incasing c's,** a single layer of fusiform cells around the gustatory cells of the tongue. **indifferent c.,** a cell that has no characteristic structure, or that is not an essential part of the tissue in which it is found. **inflammatory c.,** a cell (neutrophil, macrophage, etc.) participating in the inflammatory response to a foreign substance. **initial c's,** germ c's. **integrator c.,** interneuron. **intercalary c's,** dark, rodlike structures between the other (secretory and nonsecretory) cells of the endosalpinx, which may be emptied secretory cells; called also *peg c's.* **intercapillary c's,** mesangial c's. **interdental c's,** cells found in the spiral limbus between the dentes acustici, which secrete the tectorial membrane of the cochlear duct. **interdigitating c's,** antigen-presenting cells found in the thymus-dependent (parafollicular) areas of the deep cortex of lymph nodes and spleen and having numerous surface processes that interdigitate with adjacent lymphocytes; the surface of these cells contain an Ia antigen of the major histocompatibility complex that causes T cells to cluster. **interfollicular c's,** Hürthle c's. **interstitial c's,** 1. Leydig's c's. 2. masses of large epithelioid, lipid-containing cells in the ovarian stroma, believed to have a secretory function, derived from the theca interna of atretic ovarian follicles, and thus, in humans, more numerous during the first year of life when atresia is commonest. In women, they are either absent or poorly represented, but in some lower mammals, especially rodents, they are more prominent; see also *interstitial gland* (def. 2), under *gland.* 3. cells with elongated nuclei and long cytoplasmic processes, found in the perivascular areas and between the cords of pinealocytes in the pineal body, and regarded by some to be glial elements. 4. nerve cells with finely vacuolated protoplasm and short, branching processes that interlace with other processes to form an irregular feltwork in the enteric plexuses, submucosa, and interior of the villi of the intestinal tract. 5. fat-storing c's of liver. **islet c's,** cells composing the islets of Langerhans; see *islets of Langerhans.* **juvenile c.,** Schilling's name for a polymorphonuclear leukocyte in which the nuclear element is a single fragment no longer containing a definite nucleolus; called also *young form* and *metamyelocyte.* **juxtaglomerular c's,** specialized cells containing secretory granules, located in the tunica media of the afferent glomerular arterioles; they are receptors thought to stimulate secretion of the adrenal hormone aldosterone and to play a major role in renal autoregulation. Called also *apparatus of Goormagh-tigh*, *Goormaghtigh c's*, *juxtaglomerular apparatus*, *sentinel c's*, *periarterial pad*, and *polkissen*. **K c's,** 1. killer cells; cells mediating antibody-dependent cell-mediated cytotoxicity (ADCC). They are small lymphocytes without T or B cell surface markers. K cells recognize IgG antibody coating the target cell by means of Fc receptors. Lysis of the target cell is extracellular, requires direct cell-to-cell contact, and does not involve complement. 2. cells located predominantly in the midzone of the duodenal and jejunal mucosa that synthesize gastric inhibitory polypeptide. **karyochrome c's,** cells of the chromatophil substance of neurons that contain much chromatin in the nucleus and a small amount of cytoplasm. **killer c's,** 1. K c's. 2. cytotoxic T lymphocytes; see under *lymphocyte*. **killer T c's,** cytotoxic T lymphocytes; see under *lymphocyte*. **Kulchitsky's c's,** argentaffin cells situated between the cells that line the glands of Lieberkühn of the intestine. **Kupffer's c's,** large star-shaped or pyramidal cells with a large oval nucleus and a small prominent nucleolus. These intensely phagocytic cells line the walls of the sinusoids of the liver and form a part of the reticuloendothelial system (q.v.). Called also *stellate c's of liver* and *von Kupffer's c's*. **L c's,** 1. cells from a strain (C3H) of mouse fibroblasts grown in tissue culture for many years; employed for their ability to support replication of many types of viruses. 2. argyrophilic basal granular cells with large cytoplasmic granules in the mucosa of the upper intestine; because of the resemblance of their ultrastructure to that of the alpha cells of the islets of Langerhans, they are believed by some to synthesize and secrete a glucagon-like hyperglycemic substance, enteroglucagon; called also *large granule c's*. **lacrimoethmoid c's,** the ethmoid cells situated under the lacrimal bone. **lactotroph c.,** lactotroph. **lactotropic c.,** mammotrope. **lacunar c.,** a variant of the Reed-Sternberg cell, typically having a single nucleus surrounded by an ample, pale-staining cytoplasm enclosed in a sharply defined cell membrane; it is primarily associated with nodular sclerosing Hodgkin's disease. **Langerhans c's,** 1. stellate dendritic cells, which appear clear on light microscopy, having an indented nucleus, and characteristic inclusions (*Birbeck granules*), but lacking tonofilaments, desmosomes, and melanosomes, found principally in the stratum spinosum of the epidermis; similar cells have been identified in other stratified epithelia, including those of the lymph nodes, spleen, and thymus. They are believed to be antigen-presenting cells because they have surface markers characteristic of macrophages and monocytes, thus being involved in certain immune responses. 2. stellate dendritic cells found in the corneal epithelium. **Langhans' c's,** 1. polyhedral epithelial cells constituting cytotrophoblast (Langhans' layer). 2. Langhans' giant c's. **Langhans' giant c's,** giant cells, resembling foreign body giant cells, having their nuclei arranged in a complete circle or in a horseshoe-shaped pattern at the periphery of the cells, characteristically seen in granulomatous inflammations, as occur in tuberculosis, syphilis, sarcoidosis, and deep fungal infections. **large granule c's,** L c's (def. 2). **LE c.,** see under *tests*. **Leishman's chrome c's,** basophil granular leukocytes occurring in black water fever. **lepra c.,** a histiocyte in a leprous nodule that has been converted by the action of lepra bacilli into a sac containing degenerated protoplasm and bacilli; called also *Virchow's c*. **Leydig's c's,** 1. clusters of epithelioid cells constituting the endocrine tissue of the testis, which elaborate androgens, chiefly testosterone; called also *interstitial c's* or *interstitial c's of Leydig*, and *interstitial glands*. 2. mucous cells that do not pour their secretion out over the surface of the epithelium. **light c's,** parafollicular c's. **littoral c's,** flattened cells lining the walls of lymph or blood sinuses. **liver c's,** hepatic c's. **Loevit c.** (*obs.*), erythroblast. **longiradiate c's,** neuroglial cells having long prolongations. **luteal c's, lutein c's,** the plump, pale-staining, polyhedral cells of the corpus luteum; they include the granulosa lutein cells and the theca lutein cells. **lymph c.,** lymphocyte. **lymphadenoma c's,** Reed-Sternberg c's. **lymphoid c.,** cells of the immune system that react specifically with antigen and elaborate specific cell products; they comprise the lymphocytes and plasma cells. **malpighian c.,** keratinocyte. **Marchand's c.,** adventitial c. **marginal c's,** crescents of Giannuzzi. **Marié-Davy c.,** an electromotive force cell with a carbon collecting plate, the fluid, depolarizer, and amalgamator being a paste of mercuric or mercurous sulfate and water. **marrow c.,** any one of the

immature blood cells that develop in the bone marrow; called also *myeloid c*. **Martinotti's c's,** fusiform cells with ascending axon processes in the layers of the cerebral cortex, especially in the multiform layer and also in the internal pyramidal layer. **mast c.,** a connective tissue cell whose specific physiologic function remains unknown; capable of elaborating basophilic, metachromatic cytoplasmic granules that contain histamine, heparin, and, in certain species, such as the rat and mouse, serotonin; called also *mastocyte* and *labrocyte*. **mastoid c's,** cellulae mastoideae. **matrix c's,** flat cells found in the lobules of sebaceous glands; they undergo a rather abrupt transformation into the pale, foamy-looking, fat-containing cells of the alveoli. **Mauthner's c.,** a large cell in the metencephalon of fishes and amphibians that gives rise to Mauthner's fiber. **megaspore mother c.,** any of the diploid cells developed in the megasporangium of plants which divide by meiosis to produce four haploid daughter cells (megaspores), usually only one of which survives to become a megagametophyte, or female gametophyte. **memory c's,** T and B lymphocytes that mediate immunologic memory (q.v.); believed to retain information that permits a subsequent challenge to be followed by a more rapid efficient immunologic reaction on subsequent exposures to an antigen than occurred on first exposure. **Merkel's c's, Merkel-Ranvier c's,** 1. clear cells in the basal layer of the epidermis that contain catecholamine granules and resemble melanocytes. 2. menisci tactus. **Merkel tactile c.,** menisci tactus. **mesangial c's,** cells found in the mesangium, the connective tissue stalk in the glomerular capsule of the kidney. **mesenchymal c's,** the pluripotential cells constituting the mesenchymae. **mesothelial c's,** flattened epithelial cells of mesenchymal origin that line the serous cavities. **metallophil c's,** cells in which the cytoplasm has a great affinity for metal salts; these are cells of the reticuloendothelial system, and also a series of related cells that are not selectively stained by vital staining. **Meynert's c's,** solitary pyramidal cells in the cerebral cortex about the calcarine fissure. **microspore mother c.,** any of the diploid cells with large nuclei developed in the microsporangium of plants which divide by meiosis to produce four haploid microspores. **migratory c's,** ameboid cells found in blood and tissue spaces. See also *wandering c*. **Mikulicz's c's,** the cells in rhinoscleroma that contain the bacillus of the disease; called also *foam c's*. **mitral c's,** the pyramidal cells forming one of the layers of the olfactory bulb. **Mooser c.,** a large mononuclear (serosal) cell with numerous rickettsiae in the cytoplasm, observed in inflammatory exudate in murine typhus; called also *Neill-Mooser bodies*. **morular c.,** berry c. **mossy c.,** 1. protoplasmic astrocyte. 2. any of the cells of the oligodendroglia or of the microglia. **mother c.,** a cell that divides so as to form new or daughter cells; called also *brood c.* and *parent c*. **motor c.,** an efferent neuron, especially one of the cells of the spinal cord that has its axon continued into a motor nerve fiber. **Mott c.,** a plasma cell in which Russell bodies have formed in scleroma. **mouth c's,** squamous cells detached from the epithelium lining the oropharynx, found in the sputum. **mucoalbuminous c's, mucoserous c's,** trophochrome c's. **mucous c's,** cells that secrete mucus or mucin. **mucous neck c's,** cells found in the necks of gastric glands; they fill the spaces between the parietal cells and are filled with pale transparent granules. **mulberry c.,** 1. a vacuolated plasma cell; see also *berry c.* 2. a rounded cell, with centrally placed nuclei and coarse cytoplasmic vacuoles near the outer border, developing at the periphery of a retrogressing corpus luteum. **c's of Müller,** see under *fiber*. **muscle c.,** any contractile cell peculiar to muscle. Smooth muscle cells are elongated spindle-shaped cells containing a single nucleus and longitudinally arranged myofibrils. For cardiac and skeletal muscle cells, see *muscle fiber*, under *fiber*. **mycosis c.,** one of the numerous atypical lymphoid cells with hyperchromatic, markedly convoluted nuclei, derived from T cells predominantly of the helper/inducer phenotype, which may be found singly in the epidermis or in small collections forming Pautrier's microabscesses in mycosis fungoides. **myeloid c.,** marrow c. **myeloma c.,** a cell found in bone marrow and occasionally in peripheral blood of patients with multiple myeloma. In the more anaplastic forms, the cell is large, has abundant blue-staining cytoplasm with no perinuclear pallor, and has one or more moderately large and vesicular nuclei that may be centrally or eccentrically placed and may contain nucleoli. In better differentiated tumors, the cell is smaller and, except for the finer chromatic structure, greatly resembles a plasmacyte. **myoepithelial c's,** modified smooth muscle cells, contractile in nature, believed to be of ectodermal origin, located around the secretory units of certain glands (salivary, mammary, sweat, and lacrimal glands) between the gland cells and basement membrane, having long dendritic interweaving cytoplasmic processes, and containing myofilaments. It is assumed that contraction of these cells functions to help express secretion from the gland. Called also *basket c's.* **myoepithelioid c's,** juxtaglomerular c's; so called because they appear to be highly modified smooth muscle cells. **myoid c's,** 1. cells found in the seminiferous tubules of common laboratory rodents, which cytologically resemble smooth muscle and are presumed to be contractile and to be responsible for the rhythmic shallow contractions of the seminiferous tubules of these species; called also *peritubular contractile c's.* 2. striated muscle cells found in the thymus of nonmammalian vertebrates, especially reptiles and birds, and rarely in mammals; called also *Hammar's myoid c's.* **myointimal c.,** a smooth muscle cell occurring in the intima of an artery. **Nageotte's c's,** cells of the cerebrospinal fluid that become greatly increased in number in disease. **nerve c.,** a neuron, with its processes, collaterals, and terminations, regarded as a structural unit of the nervous system. See *neuron.* **Neumann's c's** (obs.), nucleated red cells in the bone marrow developing into erythrocytes. **neuroepithelial c's,** neuroglia c's. **neuroglia c's, neuroglial c's,** the cells of the supportive tissue of the central nervous system (neuroglia); these non-neural cells are of three kinds: astrocytes (macroglia), oligodendrocytes, and microglia. Called also *Deiters' c's* and *neuroepithelial c's.* See Plate accompanying *nerve.* **neuromuscular c.,** a form of cell chiefly or always seen in the lower animals, of which the outer part receives stimuli and the inner part is contractile. **neutrophilic c.,** a cell, particularly a leukocyte, stainable by neutral dyes; called also *neutrophil.* **nevus c.,** a polymorphic, melanin-containing cell variously postulated to be a normal mature melanocyte or a modified one, or to be derived from a Schwann cell or an embryonal nevoblast. Such cells occur in aggregations, or nests (*theques*), in the epidermis and reach the dermis by a kind of centripetal extrusion (*abtropfung*), and are the main constituents of nevocytic nevi. Called also *nevocyte.* **niche c.,** septal c. **Niemann-Pick c's,** round, oval, or polyhedral cells present in the bone marrow and spleen in Niemann-Pick disease; they have foamy, lipid-containing cytoplasm, in the form of sphingomyelin, which gives a positive reaction with Sudan III and other fat stains. Called also *Pick's c's.* **NK c's,** natural killer cells; cells capable of mediating cytotoxic reactions without prior sensitization against the target. NK cells are small lymphocytes without B or T cell surface markers that originate in the bone marrow and develop fully in the absence of the thymus; their cytotoxic activity is not antibody-dependent. NK cells can lyse a wide variety of tumor cells and other cell types and are probably important in natural resistance to tumors. Interferon augments NK cell activity. See *lymphocyte.* **noble c's,** the differentiated cells of the organs and tissues of the body. **normal c.,** any cell found naturally in any part or organ free from disease. **nucleated c.,** any cell having a nucleus. **nucleated red c., nucleated red blood c.,** any of the immature forms of a red blood cell, as a normoblast. **null c's,** lymphocytes that lack the surface markers for B or T cells (surface immunoglobulin or the pan-T antigen); K cells and NK cells. **nurse c's, nursing c's,** Sertoli's c's. **oat c's, oat-shaped c's,** cells shaped like oat grains, seen in some kinds of carcinoma; also a characteristic of erythrocytes in sickle cell anemia. **olfactory c's,** a set of specialized and nucleated fusiform cells of the mucous membrane of the nose embedded among the epithelial cells; called also *Schultze's c's.* **osseous c.,** a bone cell. **osteoprogenitor c's,** relatively undifferentiated cells found on or near all of the free surfaces of bone, which, under certain circumstances, undergo division and transform into osteoblasts or coalesce to give rise to osteoclasts. **owl's eye c's,** desquamated renal epithelial cells. **oxyntic c's,** parietal c's. **oxyphil c's, oxyphilic c's,** acidophilic cells found, along with the more numerous chief cells, in the parathyroid glands; they increase in number with age, have small dark nuclei and abundant finely granular cytoplasm, and are larger and have many more mitochondria than the chief cells. **packed human blood c's** [USP], **packed red blood c's (hu-**

man), whole blood from which plasma has been removed; used therapeutically in blood transfusions. **Paget's c., pagetoid c.,** a large, irregularly shaped, pale anaplastic tumor cell with vacuolated cytoplasm and a vesicular nucleus that tends to be hyperchromatic, usually surrounded by a clear zone, and occurring singly or in small clusters in the epidermis in Paget's disease of the breast and in extramammary Paget's disease. **palatine c's,** those parts of ethmoid cells that are extended into the palatine bone. **palisade c's** a compact layer of cylindrical chloroplast-bearing cells located in the mesophyll layer of a leaf, and so arranged that their long axes are at right angles to the epidermal surface of the leaf. **Paneth's c's,** narrow, pyramidal, or columnar epithelial cells with a round or oval nucleus close to the base of the cell, occurring in the fundus of the crypts of Lieberkühn; they contain large secretory granules that may contain peptidase. Called also *Davidoff's c's.* **parafollicular c's,** ovoid cells with an irregular nucleus and many brown or black cytoplasmic granules, which are located along with the principal cells of the thyroid follicles, in the follicular epithelium and interfollicular spaces, and which elaborate the polypeptide hormone calcitonin. They arise during embryonic life from the fifth pharyngeal pouches and are incorporated in the thyroid gland in mammals, but form discrete epithelial cell masses (*ultimobranchial bodies*) in submammalian vertebrates. Called also *C c's* and *light c's.* **paraluteal c's, paralutein c's,** theca-lutein c's. **parenchymal hepatic c's, parenchymal liver c's,** hepatic c's. **parent c.,** mother c. **parietal c's,** large spheroidal or pyramidal cells that are the source of gastric hydrochloric acid and are the site of intrinsic factor production; they are found scattered along the walls of the gastric glands, with their tapered ends pushed between the chief cells. Called also *acid c's, border c's, Heidenhain's c's, oxyntic c's,* and *delomorphous c's.* **pathologic c.,** any cell that results from a disease process or that belongs to or arises from a pathogenic microorganism. **pavement c's,** the flat cells composing pavement epithelium. **pediculated c's,** neuroglial cells that possess a pedicle implanted into a capillary wall. **peg c's,** intercalary c's. **peptic c's,** a name sometimes given to the chief cells of the stomach. **pericapillary c's,** perithelium. **pericellular c's,** neuroglial cells that surround a neuron. **perithelial c.,** adventitial c. **peritubular contractile c's,** myoid c's, def. 1. **perivascular c's,** cells accumulated around the outside of small blood vessels. **pessary c.,** a markedly hypochromic erythrocyte in which the hemoglobin is present merely as a narrow circumferential rim. **phalangeal c's,** elongated supporting cells of the organ of Corti with bases that rest on the basilar membrane adjacent to the pillar cells; the *inner* ones are arranged in a row on the inner surface of the inner pillar cells and surround the inner hair cells; the *outer* ones (*c's of Deiters*) support the outer hair cells. **pheochrome c's,** cells of the medulla of the adrenal gland that stain dark with chromium salts. **photoautotrophic c's,** green plant cells. **photoreceptor c's,** visual c's. **physaliferous c's,** spheroidal nucleated cells, containing glycogen or mucin, characteristic of chordoma. **Pick's c's,** Niemann-Pick c's. **pigment c.,** any cell containing pigment granules. **pillar c's,** elongated supporting cells in a double row (*inner* and *outer pillar c's*) in the organ of Corti, having their heads joined and their bases resting on the basilar membrane widely separated so as to form a tunnel (*inner tunnel* or *canal of Corti*) that extends the length of the cochlea. Called also *Corti's rods.* **pineal c.,** pinealocyte. **plasma c's,** terminally differentiated cells of the B lymphocyte lineage that produce antibodies; they are oval or round cells with extensive rough endoplasmic reticulum, a well-developed Golgi apparatus, and a round nucleus having a characteristic "cartwheel" heterochromatin pattern. Called also *plasmacytes.* **pneumatic c's,** the cell-like structures of the petrous bone. **PNH c's,** erythrocytes seen in paroxysmal nocturnal hemoglobinuria, classified as normal or normal-like cells (PNH I cells), a group of abnormal cells requiring about one-fourth as much complement as normal cells for an equal amount of lysis (PNH II cells), and a group of abnormal cells requiring one-fifteenth as much complement (PNH III cells). **polar c's,** polar bodies, def. 1. **polychromatic c's, polychromatophil c's,** immature erythrocytes staining with both acid and basic stains so that their color is a diffuse mixture of blue-gray and pink. **polyhedral c's,** cells having a polyhedral shape. **polyplastic c.,** a cell made up of various structural elements; also one that passes through various modifications of form. **PP c.**, one of the cells situated in the pancreatic islets and exocrine pancreas that secrete pancreatic polypeptide. **pre-B c's**, the earliest identifiable precursors of B lymphocytes: large, rapidly dividing cells found in the fetal liver and adult bone marrow that lack surface immunoglobulin but contain diffuse cytoplasmic immunoglobulin of the IgM type. **prefollicle c's**, cells encapsulating the germ cells in the fetal ovary. **pregnancy c.**, altered chromophobe cell observed in the anterior pituitary in pregnant women. **pre-T c.**, a T lymphocyte precursor before undergoing induction of the maturation process in the thymus; it lacks the characteristics of a mature T lymphocyte. **prickle c.**, a cell with delicate radiating processes that connect with similar cells; the name applied to one of the dividing keratinocytes present in the stratum germinativum of the epidermis. Called also *heckle c.* **primary c.**, an irreversible (non-rechargeable) electromotive force cell, e.g., the Leclanché cell. **primitive granulosa c's**, prefollicle c's. **primitive wandering c.**, a small mononuclear cell of the embryo that arises from the mesoderm and subsequently by differentiation gives rise to wandering cells of the body (Saxer, Maximow). **primordial germ c's**, the earliest germ cells, originating extragonadally but migrating early in embryonic development. **principal c's**, 1. chief c's, def. 3. 2. the fundamental cells of an organ, which usually have a specific function. **prokaryotic c.**, a cell without a true nucleus; see *prokaryote.* **prolactin c.**, mammotroph. **prop c's**, Purkinje c's. **psychic c's**, the cells of the cerebral cortex. **pulmonary epithelial c's**, extremely thin nonphagocytic squamous cells with flattened nuclei, constituting the outer layer of the aveolar wall in the lungs. **pulpar c's**, the typical cells of the spleen substance. **Purkinje's c's**, large branching neurons in the middle layer of the cortex cerebelli; called also *prop c's* and *Purkinje's corpuscles.* **pyramidal c.**, one of the large multipolar pyramid-shaped ganglion cells of the cerebral cortex which, with their attached fibers, constitute the pyramidal neurons. **RA c.**, ragocyte. **radial c's of Müller**, Müller's fibers. **Raji c's**, one of a cultured human lymphoblastoid cell line, derived from a patient with Burkitt's lymphoma, that possesses receptors for the C1q, C3b, and C3d complement components and can be used for detection of immune complexes. **red c., red blood c.**, one of the elements of the peripheral blood, an erythrocyte. Normally, in humans, the mature form is a non-nucleated, yellowish, biconcave disk, adapted, by virtue of its configuration and its hemoglobin content, to transport oxygen. **Reed c's, Reed-Sternberg c's**, giant histiocytic cells, typically multinucleate, most often binucleate with the two halves of the cell appearing as mirror-images of each other; the nuclei are enclosed in abundant amphophilic cytoplasm and contain prominent nucleoli. The presence of the cells is the common histologic characteristic of Hodgkin's disease. A variant form is the lacunar cell (q.v.). Called also *Dorothy Reed's c's, Reed's c's, Sternberg-Reed's c's, Hodgkin's c's, Sternberg's giant c's,* and *lymphadenoma c's.* **Renshaw c's**, interneurons in the ventromedial region of the ventral horn that make inhibitory connections with the motoneurons. **reserve c's**, cells of the basal or germinal layer of the bronchial epithelium. **residential c.**, a cell that does not wander, especially one of the cells of the substantia propria of the cornea. **resting c.**, a cell that is not undergoing karyokinesis. **resting wandering c.**, a fixed macrophage. **reticular c's**, the cells forming the reticular fibers of connective tissue; those forming the framework of lymph nodes, bone marrow, and spleen are part of the reticuloendothelial system and under appropriate stimulation may differentiate into macrophages. **reticuloendothelial c.**, see *reticuloendothelial c.,* under *system.* **reticulum c.**, reticular c. **rhagiocrine c.**, macrophage. **Rieder's c.**, a myeloblast observed in acute leukemia, having a nucleus with several wide and deep indentations suggesting lobulation, which may represent asynchronism of nuclear and cytoplasmic maturation. **Rindfleisch's c's** (*obs.*), eosinophils. **rod c's**, 1. retinal rods. 2. microglia as observed in chronic diseases of the cerebral cortex and in dementia paralytica, in which the cells are markedly attenuated in form, their processes being confined mainly to the two extremities. 3. littoral c's. **Rohon-Beard c's**, giant ganglion cells in the spinal cord of some vertebrates. **Rolando's c's**, the ganglion cells of Rolando's gelatinous substance. **root c's**, cells of the

nerve roots. **Rouget c's**, contractile cells found upon the walls of capillaries; see *pericyte.* **round c.**, any cell having a spherical shape, especially a lymphocyte. **S c's**, 1. mucoid cells of the adenohypophysis that contain a cysteine-rich protein. 2. basal granular cells found predominantly in the duodenum, which have cytoplasmic granules and which are the source of secretin production; called also *small granule c's.* **Sala's c's**, star-shaped cells of connective tissue in the fibers that form the sensory nerve endings situated in the pericardium. **sarcogenic c's**, the cells that are developed into muscle fiber. **satellite c's**, 1. neurilemmal elements encapsulating a ganglion cell. 2. free nuclei that accumulate around cells in certain diseases. 3. elongated cells that are closely associated with a muscle fiber; they either are flattened against the fiber or occupy shallow depressions in its surface. **scavenger c.**, a cell which absorbs and removes irritant products. **Schultze's c's**, olfactory c's. **Schwann c.**, any of the large nucleated cells whose cell membrane spirally enwraps the axons of myelinated peripheral neurons and is the source of myelin; a single Schwann cell supplies the myelin sheath between two nodes of Ranvier. **sclerenchyma c's**, thick-walled, lignified, usually dead cells, which compose the sclerenchyma of plants. Cf. *collenchyma c's.* **segmented c.**, a mature granulocyte in which the nucleus is divided into definite lobes joined by a filamentous connection, as distinguished from a band cell. **seminal c's**, epithelial cells within the tubuli seminiferi. **seminoma c.**, a large, round to polygonal cell having a round, moderately large nucleus with clumped chromatin in the center of clear abundant cytoplasm and one or more nucleoli, occurring in fairly well-differentiated sheets or cords in classical seminoma of the testis. **sensitized c.**, 1. a cell that has been immunologically activated by an antigen (primed). 2. an antibody-coated cell used in complement fixation tests. **sensory c.**, one of the neurons of the peripheral sense organs. **sentinel c's**, juxtaglomerular c's. **septal c.**, a name applied to alveolar cells occupying angular niches in the alveolar walls. **serous c.**, a cell concerned in the secretion of a watery fluid rich in protein, like the secretory cells of the parotid gland; called also *albuminous c.* **Sertoli's c's**, elongated cells in the tubules of the testes to which the spermatids become attached; they provide support, protection, and, apparently, nutrition until the spermatids become transformed into mature spermatozoa; called also *sustentacular c's, nurse* or *nursing c's, foot c's,* and *trophocytes.* **sexual c's**, germ c's. **Sézary c.**, an abnormal mononuclear cell with a hyperchromic infolded cribriform nucleus and a narrow rim of cytoplasm that may contain vacuoles, occurring in small and large cell variants; it is a characteristic finding in cutaneous T-cell lymphoma and its variants. **shadow c.**, ghost c. **sickle c.**, an erythrocyte shaped like a sickle or crescent, the abnormal shape caused by the presence of varying proportions of hemoglobin S; see *sickle cell anemia,* under *anemia.* **signet-ring c.**,

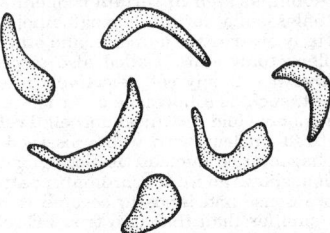

Sickle cells.

one in which the nucleus has been pressed to one side by an accumulation of intracytoplasmic mucin; see *Krukenberg's tumor* under *tumor.* **silver c's**, argentaffin c's. **skeletogenous c.**, an osteoblast. **small granule c's**, S c's, def. 2. **smudge c's**, a name applied to disrupted leukocytes appearing during the course of preparation of peripheral blood smears. **somatic c's**, the cells of the somatoplasm; undifferentiated body cells. **somatotropic c.**, somatotroph. **sperm c.**, a spermatozoon. **spermatogenic c's**, cells that produce sperm; called also *androgones.* **spermatogonial c.**, spermatogonium. **sphenoid c's**, the two large cavities or sinuses of the sphenoid bone; see *sinus sphenoidalis.* **spider c.**, 1. an astrocyte, especially a fibrous astrocyte. 2. a cell occurring in rhabdomyosarcoma; its nucleus, with a narrow rim of cytoplasm, is located in what appears to be a large vacuole, with thread-like processes radiating to the outer cell wall. **spindle c.,** a spindle-shaped cell; called also *fusiform c.* **spur c.,** a form of spiculed mature red blood cell, whose prototype is the acanthocyte of congenital abetalipoproteinemia, characterized by five to ten spiny projections of varying length distributed irregularly over the cell surface. **squamous c.,** a flat, scalelike epithelial cell. **stab c.,** band c. **staff c.,** band c. **star c's,** cells with large vacuoles in their cytoplasm and cytoplasmic bridges; seen in ameloblastoma. **stave c's.,** littoral c's. **stellate c's,** any cell having a star-shaped appearance produced by numerous processes that extend in different directions, such as the Kupffer cells in the liver, astrocytes, and granule cells in the granular layers of the cerebral and cerebellar cortices. **stem c.,** 1. any precursor cell. 2. a blood cell progenitor, or mother cell, having the capacity for both replication and differentiation, and giving rise to various morphologically recognizable precursors of different blood cell lines, such as the proerythrocyte and myeloblast, which cannot self-replicate and must differentiate into more mature daughter cells. **Sternberg's giant c's,** Reed-Sternberg c's. **Sternberg-Reed c's,** Reed-Sternberg c's. **stipple c.,** a red blood cell containing granules of varying size and shape, taking a basic or bluish stain with Wright's stain, as in punctate basophilia. **supporting c's,** cells that serve to provide support and protection and perhaps contribute to the nutrition of principal or other cells of certain organs; such cells are found in the labyrinth of the inner ear, organ of Corti, olfactory epithelium, taste buds, and seminiferous tubules (Sertoli's cells). Called also *sustentacular c's.* **suppressor c's,** differentiated T lymphocytes that suppress antibody synthesis or cell-mediated immunity. They may be activated in response to antigen or to idiotypic determinants present on antibodies and T and B cell antigen receptors and may act either by suppressing the activity of helper cells or by inhibiting the differentiation of activated lymphocytes into effector cells. Murine suppressor cells are marked by the Ly-2 and Ly-3 antigens, human suppressor cells by the T5 and T8 antigens. Cf. *contrasuppressor c's.* **sustentacular c's,** supporting c's. **sympathicotrophic c's,** large epithelioid cells occurring in groups and connected with bundles of nonmyelinated nerve fibers in the hilus of the ovary. **sympathochromaffin c's,** small round cells in the fetal suprarenal gland, the forerunners of the sympathetic and medullary cells. **syncytial c.,** a cell whose cytoplasm is confluent with that of an adjacent cell. **synovial c's,** fibroblasts lying between the cartilaginous fibers in the synovial membrane of joints. **T c's,** T lymphocytes; see under *lymphocyte.* **tactile c.,** corpuscula tactus. **tadpole c's,** cells with an elongated cytoplasmic tail. **target c.,** 1. an abnormally thin erythrocyte which, when stained, shows a dark center and a peripheral ring of hemoglobin, separated by a pale unstained ring containing less hemoglobin, as seen in certain congenital and acquired anemias, thalassemia, certain hemoglobinopathies, liver disease, especially obstructive jaundice, and other disorders, and the postsplenectomy state. Called also *target,* or *"Mexican hat," erythrocyte.* 2. any cell selectively affected by a particular agent, such as a hormone or drug. **tart c.,** a macrophage or monocytoid reticuloendothelial cell that contains a phagocytized nucleus with well preserved nuclear structure; the phagocytized nucleus, as distinguished from an LE cell inclusion, shows an intact chromatin pattern, chromatin that is more dense and tends to become vacuolated, and is frequently smaller than that in a true LE cell. **taste c's,** the interior cells of a taste bud hidden by the cover cells; called also *gustatory c's* and *taste corpuscles.* **tautomeral c's,** cells of the gray matter of the spinal cord whose axons pass into the white substance of the same side of the cord. **T**DTH **c's,** activated T cells producing lymphokines mediating the delayed-type hypersensitivity reaction; most are in the population exhibiting the same surface markers as helper cells. **tegmental c's,** cells that cover any delicate structure. **tendon c's,** flattened tissue cells of connective tissue occurring in rows between the primary bundles of the tendons. **Tγ c's,** T lymphocytes bearing Fc receptors for IgG; they exhibit suppressor cell function. **theca c's,** theca-lutein c's. **theca-lutein c's,** lutein cells derived from the theca interna; called also *paraluteal* or *paralutein c's.* **Thoma-Zeiss counting c.,** see under *chamber.* **thyroidectomy c's,** hypertrophied thyrotrophs found in the anterior pituitary gland after thyroidectomy. **thyrotroph c.,** thyrotroph. **thyrotropic c.,** thyrotrope, def. 2. **Tμ c's,** lymphocytes bearing Fc receptors for IgM; they exhibit helper cell function. **totipotential c.,** an embryonic cell that is capable of developing into any variety of body cells. **touch c.,** corpuscula tactus. **Touton giant c.,** a large vacuolated cell with numerous nuclei surrounding a peripheral rim of foamy cytoplasm; characteristic of such diseases as xanthomas, juvenile xanthogranuloma, and histiocytosis X. **trophochrome c's,** serous cells whose secretory granules give a staining reaction for mucus with mucicarmine; called also *mucoalbiminous c's* and *mucoserous c's.* **tubal air c's,** cellulae pneumaticae tubae auditivae. **Türk's c.,** a nongranular, mononuclear cell displaying morphologic characteristics of both an atypical lymphocyte and a plasma cell, observed in the peripheral blood during severe anemias, chronic infections, and leukemoid reactions; called also *Türk's irritation leukocyte.* **tympanic c's,** cellulae tympanicae. **type I c's,** alveolar c's, type I. **type II c's,** alveolar c's, type II. **Tzanck c.,** a degenerated epithelial cell caused by acantholysis, and found especially in pemphigus. **ultimobranchial c's,** parafollicular c's. **vacuolated c.,** a cell whose protoplasm contains vacuoles. **c's of van Gehuchten,** Golgi neurons of type II, i.e., neurons with short branching processes. **vasofactive c's, vasoformative c's,** cells that join with other cells to form blood vessels. **veil c's, veiled c's,** antigen-presenting cells with numerous surface ruffles or veil-like processes found in the afferent lymph and lymphatic sinuses; they may contain inclusions similar to those characteristic of the Langerhans' cells of the epidermis (Birbeck granules). **ventricular c.,** any of the columnar epithelial cells of the neural tube. **veto c's,** a subset of suppressor cells that are passively recognized by autoreactive cytotoxic T cells that recognize major histocompatibility antigens on the veto cells; this one-way recognition results in the elimination of the autoreactive cytotoxic T cells. **Vignal's c's,** embryonic connective tissue cells secreting myelin and associated with the formation of the axons of nerves in the fetus. **Virchow c's,** lepra c's. **visual c's,** the neuroepithelial portion of the retina; photoreceptor cells that are the first neurons of the vertical linkage of the retina. There are two kinds of visual cells—retinal cones and retinal rods. Each rod or cone has an inner, axonal, process synapsing with one or more horizontal or bipolar retinal cells, has a soma in the outer nuclear layer, and has a photosensitive outer dendritic process that extends toward the pigment epithelium. Called also *photoreceptor c's.* See also *ganglion c.* and *bipolar retinal c.; retinal cone,* under *cone;* and *retinal rod,* under *rod.* **voltaic c.,** an electrochemical cell (q.v.) that serves as a voltage source. Called also *galvanic c.* **von Kupffer's c's,** Kupffer's c's. **wandering c's,** cells capable of ameboid movement, such as free macrophages, lymphocytes, mast cells, and plasma cells. **Warthin-Finkeldey c's,** multinucleate giant cells with intranuclear inclusions, of lymphoreticular origin, seen in various organs, including lymph nodes, tonsil, appendix, and thymus, just prior to or during the prodromal phase of measles. **wasserhelle c's** [Ger.], water-clear c. **water-clear c.,** a large clear cell found in the parathyroid gland; these cells have a ballooned appearance and are especially numerous in adenoma of the gland. Called also *wasserhelle c.* **Wedl c's,** large swollen cells (bladder cells) formed by the capsular epithelium in cataract development. **white c., white blood c.,** leukocyte. **wing c's,** cells in the corneal epithelium with convex anterior surfaces and concave posterior surfaces. **xanthoma c.,** foam c. **Zander's c's,** bladder c's. **zymogenic c's,** chief c's, def. 1.

cella (sel′ah), gen. and pl. *cel′lae* [L.] [NA] an enclosure, or compartment. **c. latera′lis ventric′uli latera′lis** (*obs.*), the lateral part of the lateral ventricle of the brain. **c. me′dia ventric′uli latera′lis** (*obs.*), the central part of the lateral ventricle of the brain; called also *pars centralis.*

cellaburate (sel-ah-bur′āt) chemical name: cellulose acetate butanoate; a plastic filming agent.

cellae (sel′le) [L.] genitive and plural of *cella.*

Cellase 1000 (sel′ās) trademark for a preparation of cellulase, used as a digestant adjunct.

Cellfalcicula (sel″fal-sik′u-lah) a genus of bacteria of uncertain status, which have been assigned conditionally to the genus *Pseudomonas.*

Cellia (sel′e-ah) [Angelo *Celli*, Italian physician, 1857–1914] *Anopheles*.

cellicolous (sel-lik′ŏ-lus) [L. *cella* cell + *colere* to dwell] inhabiting cells.

celliferous (sel-lif′er-us) producing or bearing cells.

celliform (sel′ĭ-form) cell-like.

cellifugal (sel-lif′u-gal) cellulifugal.

cellipetal (sel-lip′e-tal) cellulipetal.

cellobiose (sel″lo-bi′ōs) a disaccharide, $C_{12}H_{22}O_{11}$, formed from cellulose by the action of cellulase; called also *cellose*.

cellobiuronic acid (sel″o-bi″u-ron′ik as′id) 4-β-glucuronosidoglucose, a disaccharide consisting of glucose and glucuronic acid linked at positions 1 and 4, found in the capsular polysaccharides of *Streptococcus pneumoniae*. See also *pneumococcus polysaccharide*, under *polysaccharide*.

cellohexose (sel″o-hek′sōs) a crystalline hexasaccharide, $C_{36}H_{62}O_{31}$, obtained by the hydrolysis of cellulose.

celloidin (sĕ-loi′din) a concentrated preparation of pyroxylin, employed in microscopy for embedding specimens for section cutting.

cellon (sel′on) tetrachlorethane.

cellophane (sel′o-fān) a transparent tissue of regenerated cellulose used as a dialysis membrane and for bandages, compresses, etc.

cellose (sel′ōs) cellobiose.

cellotetrose (sel″o-tet′rōs) a crystalline tetrasaccharide, $C_{24}H_{42}O_{21}$, obtained by the hydrolysis of cellulose.

cellotriose (sel″o-tri′ōs) a crystalline trisaccharide, $C_{18}H_{32}O_{16}$, obtained by the hydrolysis of cellulose.

cellula (sel′u-lah), gen. and pl. *cel′lulae* [L., dim. of *cella*] 1. a small cell; [NA] a general term for a small, more or less enclosed space. 2. in histology, a cell. **cel′lulae ethmoida′les** [NA], ethmoidal cells: air-containing spaces in the ethmoid bone, communicating with the infundibulum ethmoidale and the bulla ethmoidalis; classified, on the basis of their openings, as *sinus* (or *cellulae*) *anteriores, mediae*, and *posteriores*, and collectively forming the sinus ethmoidalis. **cel′lulae len′tis**, fibrae lentis. **cel′lulae mastoi′deae** [NA], mastoid cells: the air spaces of the mastoid process of the temporal bone. **cel′lulae pneumat′icae tu′bae auditi′vae** [NA], air cells in the floor of the auditory tube close to the carotid canal, being similar to the air cells of the mastoid part of the temporal bone; called also *air cells of auditory tube*; *cellulae pneumaticae tubariae*, and *tubal air cells*. **cel′lulae pneumat′icae tuba′riae**, cellulae pneumaticae tubae auditivae. **cel′lulae tympan′icae** [NA], tympanic cells: spaces in the tympanic cavity between the bony projections from the floor, or jugular wall.

cellulae (sel′u-le) [L.] plural of *cellula*.

cellular (sel′u-lar) pertaining to, or made up of, cells.

cellularity (sel″u-lār′ĭ-te) the state of a tissue or other mass as regards the number of constituent cells.

cellule (sel′ūl) [L. *cellula*] a small cell; see also *cellula*. **c. claire**, clear cell.

cellulicidal (sel″u-lis′ĭ-dal) [L. *cellula* cellule + *caedere* to kill] destroying cells.

cellulifugal (sel″u-lif′u-gal) [L. *cellula* cellule + *fugere* to flee] directed away from a cell body.

cellulipetal (sel″u-lip′ĕ-tal) [L. *cellula* cellule + *petere* to seek] directed toward a cell body.

cellulitis (sel″u-li′tis) [*cellule* + *-itis*] an acute, diffuse, spreading, edematous, suppurative inflammation of the deep subcutaneous tissues and sometimes muscle, which may be associated with abscess formation. It is usually caused by infection of an operative or traumatic wound, burn, or other cutaneous lesion by various bacteria, but group A streptococci and *Staphylococcus aureus* are the most common etiologic agents. Cellulitis may also occur in immunocompromised hosts, or it may follow erysipelas. It tends to spread to tissue spaces and cleavage planes owing to bacterial elaboration of large amounts of hyaluronidases that break down polysaccharide ground substance, fibrinolysins that digest fibrin barriers, and lecithinases that destroy cell membranes. Clinical manifestations include an area of edema, warmth, and tenderness with indistinct margins. Cf. *erysipelas* and *phlegmon*, def. 1. **anaerobic c.**, see *clostridial anaerobic c.* and *nonclostridial anaerobic c.* **clostridial anaerobic c.**, cellulitis due to a necrotizing clostridial infection, especially one caused by *Clostridium perfringens*, usually arising in devitalized tissue in a contaminated wound or in otherwise compromised tissues, and characterized by a foul-smelling discharge, widespread gas formation, and frank crepitus. The clinical findings are relatively milder than those seen in true gas gangrene. **dissecting c. of scalp**, perifolliculitis capitis abscedens et suffodiens. **facial c.**, acute cellulitis involving the face, especially the cheek or periorbital or orbital tissues, although other areas such as the neck may be affected, which may be produced by spread of an infection from nearby or distant foci. It is characterized by a bluish or purplish red, tender, poorly demarcated area of indurated cellulitis with an edematous border, and often accompanied by fever, local pain, and bacteremia. *Haemophilus influenzae* type b is the etiologic agent in children under 5 years of age. Group B streptococci and *Streptococcus pneumoniae* have also been shown to cause a clinically similar condition in children. In adults and older children, *Staphylococcus aureus* and group A streptococci are the predominant etiologic agents. **finger c.**, felon. **gangrenous c.**, necrotizing fasciitis. **indurated c.**, a hard, brawny induration of the skin of the lower leg, sometimes painful and disabling, caused by a low-grade inflammation in association with chronic venous insufficiency (see *postphlebitic syndrome*, under *syndrome*), which is seen most often proximal to the internal malleolus but which can affect other areas and even the entire circumference of the leg. Called also *phlebitic induration*. **necrotizing c.**, see under *fasciitis*. **nonclostridial anaerobic c.**, cellulitis usually occurring as a result of microbial synergism between different aerobic and anaerobic bacteria, generally characterized by progressive tissue destruction, which eventually leads to a fatal septicemia caused by the aerobic component, with or without an associated anaerobic bacteremia. **orbital c.**, facial cellulitis usually secondary to sinusitis in children, the four cardinal signs of which are proptosis, lid swelling, chemosis, and impaired ocular motility. Rarely, it can cause blindness and death. **pelvic c.**, parametritis. **periurethral c.**, see under *phlegmon*. **phlegmonous c.**, phlegmon, def. 1. **ulcerative c.**, see under *lymphangitis*.

cellulofibrous (sel″u-lo-fi′brus) partly cellular and partly fibrous.

Cellulomonas (sel″u-lo-mo′nas) [*cellulose* + Gr. *monas* a unit, from *monos* single] a genus of coryneform bacteria, consisting of pleomorphic, gram-variable organisms that attack cellulose and are found in soil.

celluloneuritis (sel″u-lo-nu-ri′tis) inflammation of neurons. **acute anterior c.**, Raymond's name for acute anterior poliomyelitis, polyneuritis, and Landry's paralysis, which he considered one disease.

cellulose (sel′u-lōs) a carbohydrate, $(C_6H_{10}O_5)_n$ the most abundant polysaccharide in nature, being a rigid, unbranched, long-chain polymer of glucose and forming the skeleton of most plant structures and of plant cells; it is a colorless, transparent solid, insoluble in water, alcohol, etc., but soluble in Schweitzer's reagent. **absorbable c.**, oxidized c. **c. acetate phthalate** [NF], a reduction product of phthalic anhydride and a partial acetate ester of cellulose; it is a free-flowing white powder used as a tablet-coating agent. **acid c.**, any combination of cellulose with carboxyl groups, such as pectinic acid; they are mostly gelatinous bodies. **microcrystalline c.** [NF], purified, partially depolymerized cellulose prepared by treating alpha cellulose, obtained as a pulp from fibrous plant material with mineral acids; used as a tablet and capsule diluent. **oxidized c.** [USP], cellulose partially oxidized and with a varying content of carboxylic acid groups, which confers some solubility in dilute alkali; it is insoluble in water. Dried in a vacuum over phosphorus pentoxide, it is used as a local hemostatic. Called also *absorbable c.* and *absorbable cotton*. **starch c.**, a nonlinear glucan polysaccharide obtained from waxy corn; not a true cellulose since it is not a β-glycoside; it is comparatively insoluble and said to be concentrated in the outer portion of starch grain. **tetranitrate c.**, $(C_{12}H_{16}N_4O_{18})_n$, the principle constituent of pyroxylin.

cellulosic acid (sel″u-lo′sik) oxidized cellulose.

cellulosity (sel″u-los′ĭ-te) the condition of being composed of cells.

cellulotoxic (sel″u-lo-tok′sik) 1. toxic to cells. 2. produced by cell toxins.

cellulous (sel′u-lus) made up of cells.

cel(o)- 1. [Gr. *kēlē* tumor] a combining form denoting relationship to a tumor or swelling. 2. [Gr. *koilos* hollow] see *coel(o)*. 3. [Gr. *koilia* belly] see *celi(o)*.

celom (se′lom) coelom.

celomic (se-lom′ik) coelomic.

Celontin (se-lon′tin) trademark for a preparation of methsuximide.

celophlebitis (se″lo-fle-bi′tis) [*celo*- (2) + *phlebitis*] inflammation of a vena cava.

celoschisis (se-los′ki-sis) [*celo*- (2) + *schisis* cleft] congenital fissure of the abdominal wall.

celoscope (sel′o-skōp) celioscope.

celoscopy (se-los′kŏ-pe) celioscopy.

celosomia (se-lo-so′me-ah) [*celo*- (1) + Gr. *sōma* body] a developmental anomaly characterized by eventration, fissure, or absence of the sternum, with hernial protrusion of the viscera.

celosomus (se″lo-so′mus) a fetus exhibiting celosomia; called also *kelosomus*.

celothel (se′lo-thel) mesothelium.

celothelioma (se″lo-the-le-o′mah) mesothelioma.

celothelium (se″lo-the′le-um) mesothelium.

celotomy (se-lot′o-me) herniotomy.

celovirus (sel″o-vi′rus) CELO virus.

celozoic (se″lo-zo′ik) [*celo*- (2) + *zōon* animal] inhabiting the intestinal cavities of the body; said of parasites.

Celsius scale, thermometer (sel′se-us) [Anders *Celsius*, Swedish astronomer, 1701–1744] see under *scale* and *thermometer*.

Celsus (sel′sus) Aulus Cornelius (1st century A.D.) a Roman encyclopedist. Of his many writings, only his *De re medicina* (in eight books) survives; the four classical signs (Celsus' quadrilateral) of inflammation—*calor* (heat), *dolor* (pain), *rubor* (redness), and *tumor* (swelling)—are mentioned in the third book of this work. Celsus was a layman writing for other laymen; his outline of the history of medicine is very important.

cement (se-ment′) [L. *cemen′tum*] 1. a substance that serves to produce solid union between two surfaces. 2. a filling material, such as zinc phosphate, used in dentistry to assist in retaining gold castings in prepared teeth and to insulate the tooth pulp from metallic and other fillings. 3. cementum. **calcium hydroxide c.,** a dental cement that promotes the formation of a protective layer of secondary dentin, which is particularly beneficial in aiding healing of the pulp; used principally for pulp capping and as a thermal insulating base. **dental c.,** any of several bonding substances available in the form of two components that are mixed together immediately before use, setting to a hard mass; used in restorative and orthodontic dental procedures as luting (cementing) agents, as bases, and as restorative materials. Resins and polymers used as restorative materials are usually called restorative resins rather than cements. **glass ionomer c.,** a dental cement of low strength and toughness produced by mixing a powder prepared from a calcium aluminosilicate glass and a liquid prepared from an aqueous solution of prepared polyacrylic acid; used chiefly for small restorations on the proximal surfaces of anterior teeth and for restoration of eroded areas at the gingival margin. **intercellular c.,** a mucilaginous substance that holds cells, and especially epithelial cells, together. **muscle c.,** the myoglia. **nerve c.,** the neuroglia. **polycarboxylate c.,** a dental cement made by mixing a powder consisting chiefly of zinc oxide and an aqueous solution of polyacrylic acid; used as a luting agent for cementing restorations and orthodontic bands or brackets and as a cavity lining. **resin c.,** one of several polymer or monomer/polymer systems, usually containing finely divided inorganic filler particles, used as an insoluble dental luting agent; used in the cementation of orthodontic brackets to etched enamel and the cementation of etched based metal extracoronal retainers to etched enamel. **root canal c.,** see under *sealer*. **silicate c.,** a dental cement made by mixing a buffered phosphoric acid solution with a powder that is a mixture of acid soluble glass prepared by fusing silica, alumina, calcium oxide, and other glass-forming substances, which sets to form

a hard, translucent, porcelain-like solid; used chiefly for temporary and semipermanent restorations of anterior teeth where use of metals might be objectionable. **silicophosphate c.,** a mixture of silicate and zinc phosphate cements, chiefly used as temporary filling material and for cementation of orthodontic bands and cast restorations. **zinc oxide–eugenol c.,** a dental cement made by mixing zinc oxide powder with eugenol liquid and a small amount of water; used chiefly in temporary restorations, thermal insulating bases, and root canal fillings. **zinc phosphate c.,** a dental cement made by mixing a powder that consists chiefly of zinc oxide and magnesium oxide as a modifier with a liquid that is a mixture of phosphoric acid, water, and metallic salts that act as buffering agents; used primarily as a luting agent for fabricated restorations and secondarily in temporary restorations and as a thermal insulating agent.

cementation (se″men-ta′shun) the attachment of anything by the means of cement, such as the use of cement in attaching restorative material to a natural tooth, or the use of an adhesive material to attach bands to the tooth.

cementicle (se-men′ti-k'l) a small, discrete focus of calcified tissue that may or may not represent true cementum, found in the periodontal ligament. **adherent c., attached c.,** one that is firmly connected with the cementum. **free c., interstitial c.,** one that is completely surrounded by connective tissue of the periodontal ligament.

cementification (se-men″ti-fi-ka′shun) cementogenesis.

cementin (se-men′tin) the material that sometimes unites the margins of squamous endothelial cells.

cementitis (se″men-ti′tis) inflammation of the cementum of a tooth.

cement(o)- [L. *cementum*, q.v.] a combining form denoting relationship to the cementum.

cementoblast (sĕ-men′to-blast) [*cementum* + *blast*] a large cell ranging in shape from cuboidal to squamous with a large central nucleus and usually a single nucleolus, which is active in the formation of cementum (cementogenesis).

cementoblastoma (se-men″to-blas-to′mah) an odontogenic fibroma in which the cells are developing into cementoblasts, and there is only a small proportion of calcified tissue; called also *cementifying fibroma*.

cementoclasia (se-men″to-kla′se-ah) [*cementum* + Gr. *klasis* breaking + *-ia*] dissolution and resorption of the cementum of a tooth; usually a complication of trauma or pathologic conditions.

cementoclast (se-men′to-klast″) [*cementum* + Gr. *klasis* a breaking] a cell, cytomorphologically the same as an osteoclast, involved in cementum resorption; the cavities produced by resorption are known as *resorption lacunae*. Called also *odontoclast*.

cementocyte (sĕ-men′to-sīt) [*cementum* + *-cyte*] a cell in the lacunae of cellular cementum, ranging in shape from round to oval or flattened, and exhibiting numerous protoplasmic processes extending from its free surface. Called also *cement cell*.

cementogenesis (se-men″to-jen′ĕ-sis) [*cementum* + Gr. *genesis* formation] the development of the cementum on the root dentin of a tooth; called also *cementification*.

cementoid (sĕ-men′toid) [*cement* + *-oid*] the surface uncalcified layer of the cementum in areas of intact periodontal tissue. Called also *precementum* and *uncalcified cementum*.

cementoma (se″men-to′mah) a mass of cementum lying free at the apex of a tooth, probably a reaction to injury rather than a neoplasm.

cementopathia (se-men′to-path′e-ah) periodontitis or periodontosis resulting from disease or defect of the cementum.

cementoperiostitis (se-men″to-per″e-os-ti′tis) periodontitis, def. 1.

cementosis (se″men-to′sis) hypercementosis.

cementum (se-men′tum) [L.] [NA] the bonelike rigid connective tissue covering the root of a tooth from the cemento-enamel junction to the apex and lining the apex of the root canal; it also serves as an attachment structure for the periodontal ligament, thus assisting in tooth support. Called also *substantia ossea dentis*. **acellular c.,** the cementum without cellular components that covers one-third to one-half of the tooth root adjacent to the cementoenamel junction; it is usually apposed by a layer of cellular cementum. **afi-**

brillar c., a layer of cementum, containing acid mucopolysaccharides and possibly nonfibrillar collagen, that sometimes extends onto the enamel of a tooth at the cemento-enamel junction. **cellular c.,** the cementum covering the apical one-half to two-thirds of the tooth root, which contains cementocytes embedded in the calcified matrix; it is usually apposed by a layer of acellular cementum. **uncalcified c.,** cementoid.

cenadelphus (se″nah-del′fus) [Gr. *koinos* common + *adelphos* brother] a twin monster in which the two components are equally developed.

cenencephalocele (se″nen-sef′ah-lo-sēl) an encephalocele or protrusion of the brain without cystic condition.

cenesthesia (se″nes-the″ze-ah) [Gr. *koinos* common + *aisthēsis* perception] the general feeling or sense of conscious existence; the sense of normal functioning of the organs of the body.

cenesthesic (se″nes-the′sik) pertaining to cenesthesia.

cenesthesiopathy (se″nes-the″ze-op′ah-the) [cenesthesia + Gr. *pathos* disease + -ia] cenesthopathy.

cenesthetic (se″nes-thet′ik) cenesthesic.

cenesthopathy (se″nes-thop′ah-the) a general feeling of discomfort, unease, and lack of wellness not referable to any particular part of the body.

cen(o)- 1. [Gr. *kainos* new, fresh] a combining form denoting new; written also *cain(o)-* and *kain(o)-*. 2. [Gr. *kenos* empty] a combining form denoting empty; written also *caen(o)-* and *ken(o)-*. 3. [Gr. *koinos* shared in common] a combining form denoting relationship to a common feature or characteristic; written also *coen(o)-, coin(o)-,* and *koin(o)-*.

cenobium (se-no′be-um) [Gr. *koinobios* living in communion with others] a colony of independent cells or organisms held together by a common investment.

cenocyte (se′no-sīt) [*ceno-* (3) + Gr. *kytos* hollow vessel] 1. a multinucleate plant cell enclosed within a hollow wall, examples of which are found within the fungi and algae. 2. a multinucleate bit of cytoplasm in which the nuclei are not separated by walls. 3. a multinucleate plant protoplast.

cenogenesis (se″no-jen′ĕ-sis) [*ceno-* (1) + Gr. *genesis* production] the appearance of new features in development, in adaptive response to environmental conditions. Cf. *palingenesis,* def. 2.

Cenolate (sen′o-lāt) trademark for a preparation of ascorbic acid.

cenopsychic (se″no-si′kik) [*ceno-* (1) + Gr. *psychē* soul] of recent appearance in mental development.

cenosis (se-no′sis) [Gr. *kenōsis* an emptying, or emptiness] a morbid discharge.

cenosite (se′no-sīt) coinosite.

cenotic (se-not′ik) pertaining to or characterized by cenosis.

cenotoxin (se″no-tok′sin) kenotoxin.

cenotype (se′nŏ-tīp) [*ceno-* (3) + *type*] the original type from which all forms have arisen.

censor (sen′sor) a term used by Freud to refer to the mental faculty that guards the border between the unconscious and preconscious, preventing unconscious thoughts and wishes from coming into consciousness unless disguised, as in dreams. In Freud's later theory, the actions of the censor (displacement, condensation, symbolism, and repression) are considered defense mechanisms of the ego and superego.

censorship (sen′sor-ship) the operation of the censor.

center (sen′ter) [Gr. *kentron*; L. *centrum*] 1. the middle point of a body. 2. a collection of neurons concerned with performance of a particular function; see also *area.* **accelerating c.,** a center in the brain stem involved in acceleration of the heart; called also *cardioaccelerating c.* **acoustic c.,** auditory c. **anospinal c's,** the centers for contracting the sphincter ani, for relaxing it (defecation center), and for the anal reflex; all are in the lumbar enlargement. **apneustic c.,** a nerve center in the brain stem controlling normal respiration. **auditopsychic c.,** a center dealing with the interpretation of sounds, in the superior temporal gyrus. **auditory c.,** the center for hearing, in the more anterior of the transverse temporal gyri; called also *acoustic c.* **brain c.,** 1. an area of the cerebral cortex having a specialized structure or function. 2. a group of cells in the brain having a special function. See also *specific areas,* under *area.* **Broca's c.,** the speech center.

Budge's c. 1. ciliospinal center. 2. genital center. **cardioaccelerating c.,** accelerating c. **cardioinhibitory c.,** a center in the medulla oblongata that exerts an inhibitory influence on the heart by way of the vagus. Called also *Kronecker's center.* **cardiomotor c.,** Tawara's name for the atrioventricular node, on the theory that the heart's impulse arises there. **cell c.,** centrosome. **cheirokinesthetic c.,** the center in the posterior part of the left second frontal gyrus, controlling movements concerned in writing. **chiral c.,** the center of dissymmetry in a molecule, usually an atom with four different substituents (e.g., a carbon with four single bonds or the nitrogen of a quaternary amine). **c's of chondrification,** dense aggregations of embryonic mesenchymal cells at sites of future cartilage formation; called also *protochondral tissue.* **ciliospinal c.,** a center in the lower cervical and upper dorsal portions of the spinal cord, connected with the dilatation of the pupil; called also *Budge's c.* **community mental health c. (CMHC),** a mental health facility or group of affiliated agencies that provide various psychotherapeutic services to a designated catchment area. **coordination c.,** a nerve center serving the function of coordination. **correlation c.,** a nerve center serving the function of correlation. **cortical c.,** any portion of the cerebral cortex that can be differentiated functionally from its neighbors; such a center is sometimes called area, field, or zone. **coughing c.,** a center in the medulla oblongata, situated above the respiratory center, which controls the act of coughing. **defecation c.,** see *anospinal c.* **deglutition c.,** a nerve center in the medulla oblongata that controls the function of swallowing. **dentary c.,** an ossification center of the mandible, giving origin to the lower border and outer plate. **C's for Disease Control (CDC),** an agency of the U.S. Department of Health and Human Services, with headquarters in Atlanta, Georgia, concerned with all phases of control of communicable, vector-borne, and other occupational diseases. The CDC's responsibilities include epidemiology, surveillance, detection, laboratory science, ecologic investigations, training, and disease control methods for an increasing variety of health problems. Formerly called *Communicable Disease Center* (1946) and *Center for Disease Control* (1970). **dominating c.,** the principal or controlling center of a group having a common function. **ejaculation c.,** the center that controls the erection of the penis and the normal discharge of semen; it is in the lumbar region of the spinal cord, and is itself regulated from the oblongata. Called also *erection c.* **epiotic c.,** the center of ossification that forms the mastoid process. **epiphyseal c.,** secondary c. of ossification. **erection c.,** ejaculation c. **eupraxic c.,** any cerebral center that controls the proper performance of any action or set of actions. **facial c.,** a center for face movements, located in the lower part of the ascending frontal convolution. **Flemming c.,** germinal c. **ganglionic c.,** any mass of gray matter between the lateral ventricles and the decussation of the anterior pyramids, including the thalami, striati, and other basal ganglia. **genital c., genitospinal c.,** the ejaculation center of the male or the parturition center of the female; said to be in the cord, near the second lumbar vertebra. Called also *Budge's c.* **germinal c.,** the area in the center of a lymph nodule containing aggregations of actively proliferating lymphocytes (antibody-forming B-cells); it appears as a spherical mass surrounded by a capsule of elongated cells that is partially invested by a crescentic cap of small lymphocytes. Called also *Flemming c.* and *secondary nodule.* **glossokinesthetic c.,** the center in the posterior part of the left second frontal gyrus that controls movements concerned in articulate speech. **gustatory c.,** the cerebral center supposed to control taste, situated in the cortex of the uncinate convolution; called also *taste c.* **health c.,** 1. a community health organization for creating health work and coordinating the efforts of all health agencies. 2. an educational complex consisting of a medical school and various allied health professional schools. **heat-regulating c's,** thermoregulator c's. **inhibitory c.,** any nerve center that restrains any function or process or controls other centers. **Kerckring's c.,** an ossification center sometimes present in the posterior margin of the foramen magnum at about the sixteenth week of fetal life, which unites with the other squamous parts prior to birth. Called also *Kerckring's ossicle.* **kinetic c.,** the centrospheres of a fertilized ovum. **Kronecker's c.,** cardioinhibitory c. **Kupressoff's c.,** micturition c. **Lumsden's c.,** pneumotaxic c. **medullary c. of cerebel-**

lum, corpus medullare cerebelli. **medullary respiratory c.,** a center in the medulla oblongata that coordinates respiratory movements. **micturition c.,** a center controlling the bladder and inhibiting the tension of the vesical sphincter, situated in the lumbar enlargement; called also *Kupressoff's c.* **motor c.,** any center that originates, controls, inhibits, or maintains a motor impulse. **nerve c.,** a collection of nerve cells in the central nervous system that are associated together in the performance of some particular function. **optic c.,** that point in a lens, or combination of lenses, where all rays that help to form a clear image cross the principal axis; in the eye, about 2 mm. behind the cornea. **ossification c.,** punctum ossificationis. **ossification c., primary,** punctum ossificationis primarium. **ossification c., secondary,** punctum ossificationis secundarium. **oval c., greater** (*obs.*), centrum semi-ovale. **panting c.,** polypneic c. **parenchymatous c.,** a nerve center situated in the substance of a viscus. **phrenic c.,** centrum tendineum. **pneumotaxic c.,** a center in the upper part of the pons that rhythmically inhibits inspiration independently of the vagi; called also *Lumsden's c.* **polypneic c.,** a center in the tuber cinereum that accelerates the rate of breathing. **pteriotic c.,** a center of ossification from which are developed the tegmen tympani and the covering of the lateral semicircular canal. **reaction c.,** germinal c. **rectovesical c.,** a cord reflex center for the rectum and bladder. **reflex c.,** any center in the brain or cord in which a sensory impression is changed into a motor impulse; the reflex centers already discovered are numerous. **respiratory c's,** a series of centers in the medulla and pons which coordinate respiratory movements; they include the pneumotaxic center, apneustic center, and the medullary respiratory center. **rotation c.,** the point or axis about which a body rotates. **semioval c.,** centrum semiovale. **sensory c.,** a center that receives or appreciates a sensory impulse. **Setchenow's (Sechenoff's) c's,** reflex inhibitory centers in the cord and oblongata. **sex-behavior c.,** the ventromedial nucleus of hypothalamus; see under *nucleus.* **speech c.,** a center in the left (or right) inferior frontal gyrus; called also *Broca's c.* **sphenotic c.,** a center of ossification in the sphenoid bone for the lingula. **splenial c.,** one of the ossification centers of the mandible, forming a part of its inner plate. **sudorific c's, sweat c's,** centers in the spinal cord controlling diaphoresis, with a dominant center in the oblongata. **swallowing c.,** deglutition c. **taste c.,** the gustatory center. **tendinous c.,** centrum tendineum. **thermoregulatory c's,** hypothalamic centers regulating the conservation and dissipation of heat. **vasoconstrictor c.,** a center in the medulla oblongata that controls contraction of the blood vessels. **vasodilator c.,** a center in the medulla oblongata for dilating the blood vessels. **vasomotor c's,** centers in the tuber cinereum, oblongata, and cord, believed to regulate the caliber of the blood vessels and to cause their contraction and dilatation. **vesical c., vesicospinal c.,** the micturition center or rectovesical center. **vomiting c.,** a center in the lower central region of the medulla oblongata; its stimulation causes vomiting. **Wernicke's c.,** the central speech center; see under *area.* **word c., auditory,** a center in the left superior transverse temporal gyrus that controls the perception of words that are heard. **word c., visual,** one in the posterior part of the left parietal lobe; it appears to govern the perception of printed or written words.

centesimal (sen-tes′ĭ-mal) [L. *centesimus* hundredth] divided into hundredths or based upon divisions into hundredths.

centesis (sen-te′sis) [Gr. *kentēsis*] perforation or tapping, as with an aspirator, trocar, or needle. Used also as a word termination, affixed to a root indicating the part on which the operation is performed, as *abdominocentesis, thoracocentesis,* and the like.

centi- [L. *centum* one hundred] a combining form denoting (1) one hundredth (10^{-2}) of the unit designated by the root with which it is combined (symbol, c) as in centimeter (cm) or (2) one hundred, as in centipede.

centigrade (sen′tĭ-grād) [L. *centum* hundred + *gradus* a step] consisting of or having 100 gradations (steps or degrees); abbreviated C. See *Celsius* (*centigrade*) *scale,* under *scale.*

centigray (sen′tĭ-grā″) a unit of absorbed radiation dose equal to one hundredth of a gray, or 1 rad; abbreviated cGy.

centiliter (sen′tĭ-le″ter) one hundredth part of a liter (10^{-2} l.), or the equivalent of 0.33815 of a fluid ounce; abbreviated cl.

centimeter (sen′tĭ-me″ter) [Fr. *centimètre*] a unit of length equal to one-hundredth of a meter (10^{-2} m); abbreviated cm. **cubic c.,** a unit of volume equal to that of a cube one centimeter on a side, equal to 1 ml or 10^{-6} m^3. Symbol cm^3. Abbreviated cc. or cu. cm.

centimorgan (sen′tĭ-mor′gan) one-hundredth of a morgan; the unit of distance on a linkage map. The map distance between adjacent loci, expressed in centimorgans, is equal to the recombination frequency, expressed as a percentage. For nonadjacent loci the map distance is greater than the recombination frequency, because recombination frequencies are not additive. Symbol, cM. Called also *map unit.*

centipede (sen′tĭ-pēd) an elongated arthropod of the class Chilopoda characterized by having one pair of legs to each body segment; they may have 15 to 173 pairs of legs. Centipedes paralyze and kill insects and small animals with their poison claws, which are modified legs of the first body segment. A few species are capable of penetrating the skin of man, causing painful bites. See *Scolopendra.*

centipoise (sen′tĭ-poiz) one one-hundredth of a poise.

centistoke (sen′tĭ-stōk) one one-hundreth of a stoke.

centiunit (sen″te-u′nit) one one-hundredth of the conventional unit.

centra (sen′trah) [L.] plural of *centrum.*

centrad (sen′trad) 1. [*centr-* +*-ad*] toward the center or a center, especially toward the center of the body. 2. [L. *centum* hundred +*radian*] a measure of an angle of deviation, being 0.57 degree, or one one-hundredth part of a radian; its symbol is $\triangledown$; called also *prism degree.*

centrage (sen′trāj) the condition in which the centers of the various refracting surfaces of the eye are in the same straight line.

central (sen′tral) situated at or pertaining to a center; not peripheral.

centralis (sen-tra′lis) [NA] a general term denoting a centrally located structure.

centraphose (sen′trah-fōz) any aphose, or sensation of darkness, originating in the optic or visual centers.

centration (sen-tra′shun) the inability to pay attention to more than one salient feature at a time; it is a normal stage in human intellectual development.

centraxonial (sen″trak-so′ne-al) having the axis in a central median line.

centre (sen′ter) center.

centrencephalic (sen″tren-sĕ-fal′ik) pertaining to the center of the encephalon; see under *system.*

centri-, centr(o)- [L. *centrum* center, from Gr. *kentron* sharp point] a combining form denoting relationship to a center, or to a central location.

centric (sen′trik) 1. pertaining to or situated at the center; central. 2. a term sometimes used as a noun to refer to *centric occlusion, centric relation,* or *power centric.* **power c.,** the position of the mandible during a forceful bite. **true c.,** centric relation.

centriciput (sen-tris′ĭ-put) [*center* + L. *caput* head] the central part of the upper surface of the head, located between the occiput and sinciput.

centrifugal (sen-trif′u-gal) [*center* + L. *fugere* to flee] moving away from a center; moving away from the cerebral cortex; efferent or exodic.

centrifugalization (sen-trif″u-gal-ĭ-za′shun) centrifugation.

centrifugate (sen-trif′u-gāt) material subjected to centrifugation.

centrifugation (sen-trif″u-ga′shun) the process of separating the lighter portions of a solution, mixture, or suspension from the heavier portions by centrifugal force; called also *centrifugalization.* **density gradient c.,** ultracentrifugation in a liquid, such as cesium chloride solution, the density of which increases along the lines of centrifugal force, the substances under test seeking their level of density. **differential c.,** that based on the sedimentation coefficient of the substances under investigation; applied to homogenates to derive various subcellular fractions. **isopyknic**

c., that in which the solvent is of the same density as the substance to be isolated.

centrifuge (sen′trĭ-fūj) [*center* + L. *fugere* to flee] 1. a machine by which centrifugation is effected. 2. to subject to centrifugation. **microscope c.,** a high-speed centrifuge with a built-in microscope, permitting a specimen to be viewed under centrifugal force.

centrilobular (sen″trĭ-lob′u-lar) pertaining to the central portion of a lobule.

centriole (sen′trĭ-ōl) either of the two cylindrical organelles located in the centrosome and containing nine triplets of microtubules arrayed around their edges; centrioles migrate to opposite poles of the cell during cell division and serve to organize the spindles. They are capable of independent replication and of migrating to form basal bodies. **anterior c.,** proximal c. **distal c.,** that centriole of a spermatozoon which, after migrating to the cell surface and giving rise to a slender flagellum, returns to a position just caudal to the proximal centriole; called also *posterior c.* **posterior c.,** distal c. **proximal c.,** that centriole of a spermatozoon which migrates to a position in a depression in the wall of the posterior portion of the nucleus, with its axis at right angles to the main axis of the spermatozoon, and from which the axoneme extends; called also *anterior c.* **ring c.,** a dark annular structure at the posterior end of the middle piece of a spermatozoon; it is not a true centriole. Called also *annulus of spermatozoon.*

centripetal (sen-trip′e-tal) [*center* + L. *petere* to seek] moving toward a center; moving toward the cerebral cortex; afferent or esodic.

centr(o)- see *centri-*.

centrocecal (sen″tro-se′kal) pertaining to the central macular area and the blind spot; called also *cecocentral.*

Centrocestus (sen″tro-ses′tus) a genus of flukes. **C. cuspida′tus,** a fluke occurring in the Egyptian kite. *C. cuspidatus* var. *canina* is reported from dogs in Taiwan; it may be the same as *Stamnosoma formosanum.*

centrocinesia (sen″tro-si-ne′se-ah) centrokinesia.

centrocinetic (sen″tro-si-net′ik) centrokinetic.

centrodesmose (sen″tro-des′mōs) the connection between intranuclear centrioles during mitosis in certain protozoa; see *desmose.* Called also *centrodesmus.*

centrodesmus (sen″tro-des′mus) centrodesmose.

Centrohelida (sen″tro-he′lĭ-dah) [*centro-* + Gr. *helios* sun] an order of protozoa (class Heliozoa, superclass Actinopoda) frequently having a skeleton consisting of siliceous plates or spines or of organic spicules. They usually have a centroplast on which axonemes insert, or if the centroplast is absent, a large eccentric nucleus. Some species have flagella or flagellated stages.

centrokinesia (sen″tro-ki-ne′se-ah) [*center* + Gr. *kinēsis* movement] movement originating from central stimulation.

centrokinetic (sen″tro-ki-net′ik) pertaining to, characterized by, or promoting centrokinesia.

centrolecithal (sen″tro-les′ĭ-thal) [*centro-* + Gr. *lekithos* yolk] having the yolk centrally located; see under *ovum.*

centrolobular (sen″tro-lob′u-lar) centrilobular.

centromere (sen′tro-mēr) [*centro-* + Gr. *meros* part] the constricted portion of the chromosome at which the chromatids are joined and by which the chromosome is attached to the spindle during cell division. According to its location, a centromere is said to be metacentric (central), submetacentric (off center), or acrocentric (near one end). Called also *kinetochore* and *primary constriction.*

centromeric (sen″tro-mer′ik) pertaining to or resembling a centromere.

centronucleus (sen″tro-nu′kle-us) amphinucleus.

centro-osteosclerosis (sen″tro-os″te-o-skle-ro′sis) centrosclerosis.

centrophenoxine (sen″tro-fen-oks′ēn) meclofenoxate.

centrophose (sen′tro-fōz) any phose, or sensation of light, originating in the visual centers.

centroplasm (sen′tro-plazm) the substance of the centrosome.

centroplast (sen′tro-plast) a central granule from which the axial filaments of the axopodia of certain heliozoa arise.

centrosclerosis (sen″tro-skle-ro′sis) [*center* + *osteosclerosis*]

the filling of the marrow cavity of a bone with osseous material.

centrosome (sen′tro-sōm) [*centro-* + Gr. *sōma* body] the cell center; the centrosphere together with the two centrioles.

centrosphere (sen′tro-sfēr) [*centro-* + Gr. *sphaira* sphere] 1. a specialized area of condensed cytoplasm that contains the centrioles and plays an important part in mitosis; called also *cytocentrum, microcentrum, attractin sphere,* and *paranuclear body.* 2. centrosome.

centrostaltic (sen″tro-stal′tik) [*centro-* + Gr. *stellein* to send] pertaining to a center of motion.

centrotherapy (sen″tro-ther′ah-pe) externally applied treatment designed to act upon the nerve centers.

centrum (sen′trum), pl. *cen′tra* [L.; Gr. *kentron*] 1. [NA] a center. 2. the body of a vertebra. **c. ossificatio′nis,** punctum ossificationis. **c. ossificatio′nis prima′rium,** punctum ossificationis primarium. **c. ossificatio′nis secunda′rium,** punctum ossificationis secundarium. **c. semiova′le,** semioval center: the white matter of the cerebral hemispheres which underlies the cerebral cortex and which, in horizontal sections superior to the corpus callosum, has a semioval shape; it contains projection, commissural, and association fibers; called also *greater oval center.* **c. tendin′eum** [NA], **c. tendin′eum [diaphrag′matis],** the trefoil-shaped aponeurosis, immediately below the pericardium, onto which the diaphragmatic fibers converge to insert; called also *central tendon of diaphragm, phrenic center,* and *tendinous center.* **c. tendin′eum perine′i** [NA], central tendon of perineum: the fibromuscular mass in the median plane of the perineum where converge and attach the bulbospongiosus and sphincter ani externus muscles, the two levatores ani, and the two deep and the two superficial transverse perineal muscles; called also *corpus perinealis* and *perineal body,* especially in gynecology. **c. ver′tebrae,** corpus vertebrae.

Centruroides (sen″troo-roi′dēz) a genus of subtropical and tropical American scorpions, some of which are poisonous.

Cenurus (sen-u′rus) Coenurus. **C. cerebra′lis,** *Coenurus cerebralis.*

cephacetrile sodium (sef′ah-sĕ-trīl) chemical name: 7-(2-cyanoacetamido)-3-(hydroxymethyl)-8-oxo-5-thia-1-azabicyclo[4.2.0].oct-2-ene-2-carboxylic acid acetate (ester) monosodium salt. An antibiotic, $C_{13}H_{12}N_3NaO_6S$, effective against a wide range of gram-positive and gram-negative bacteria.

Cephaelis (sef′a-e′lis) a genus of tropical shrubs and trees. *C. acuminata* and *C. ipecacuanha* are sources of ipecac (q.v.).

cephalad (sef′ah-lad) [Gr. *kephalē* head] toward the head; opposite to caudad.

cephalalgia (sef′ah-lal′je-ah) [Gr. *kephalalgia*] pain in the head; headache. Called also *cephalgia* and *cephalodynia.* **histamine c.,** former name for migrainous neuralgia. **pharyngotympanic c.,** Legal's disease. **quadrantal c.,** headache affecting one quadrant of the head.

cephaledema (sef″al-ĕ-de′mah) [*cephal-* + Gr. *oidēma* swelling] edema of the head.

cephalematocele (sef″al-ĕ-mat′o-sēl) cephalhematocele.

cephalematoma (sef″al-em″ah-to′mah) cephalhematoma.

cephalexin (sef″ah-lek′sin) [USP] chemical name: [6*R*-[6α,8β(*R**)]]-7-[(aminophenylacetyl)amino]-3-methyl-8-oxo-5-thia-1-azabicyclo[4.2.0]oct-2-ene-2-carboxylic acid monohydrate. A semisynthetic analogue, $C_{16}H_{17}N_3O_4S \cdot H_2O$, of the natural antibiotic cephalosporin C, occurring as a white to off-white, crystalline powder, effective against a wide range of gram-negative and gram-positive bacteria; used in the treatment of infections of the urinary and respiratory tracts and of skin and soft tissues due to sensitive pathogens, administered orally.

cephalgia (sĕ-fal′je-ah) cephalalgia.

cephalhematocele (sef″al-he-mat′o-sēl) [*cephal-* + Gr. *haima* blood + *kēlē* tumor] a bloody tumor under the pericranium, communicating with one or more sinuses of the dura through the cranial bones. **Stromeyer's c.,** a subperiosteal cephalhematocele which communicates with veins and becomes filled with blood during strong expiratory efforts.

cephalhematoma (sef″al-he″mah-to′mah) [*cephal-* + *hematoma*] a subperiosteal hemorrhage limited to the surface of one cranial bone, a usually benign condition seen frequently in the newborn as a result of bone trauma. Called also *cephalohematoma.* **c. defor′mans,** a bulging of the anterior part of the skull due to hyperostosis, osteoporosis, and cavity formation in the bone.

cephalhydrocele (sef″al-hi′dro-sēl) [*cephal-* + *hydrocele*] a serous or watery accumulation under the pericranium. **c. traumat′ica,** Billroth's disease, def. 1.

cephalic (sĕ-fal′ik) [L. *cephalicus;* Gr. *kephalikos*] pertaining to the head, or to the head end of the body.

cephalin (sef′ah-lin) a crude preparation of phospholipids containing primarily phosphatidylserine and phosphatidylethanolamine (which are sometimes called cephalids). Cephalin can induce blood coagulation and has been used in a plasma protein flocculation test (the *cephalin-cholesterol flocculation test*).

Cephalina (sef″ah-li′nah) [Gr. *kephalē* head] Septatina.

cephalitis (sef″ah-li′tis) encephalitis.

cephalization (sef″al-i-za′shun) [Gr. *kephalē* head] 1. the concentration or initiation of the growth tendency at the head end of the embryo. 2. the development of a head; the concentration of nervous tissue and sense organs at the anterior end of the organism.

cephal(o)- [Gr. *kephalē* head] a combining form denoting relationship to the head.

cephalocathartic (sef″ah-lo-kah-thar′tik) [*cephalo-* + Gr. *kathartikos* purgative] cleansing or clearing the head.

cephalocaudad (sef″ah-lo-kaw′dad) 1. proceeding in a direction from the head toward the tail; caudad. 2. in both a cephalic and caudal direction.

cephalocaudal (sef″ah-lo-kaw′dal) [*cephalo-* + L. *cauda* tail] pertaining to the long axis of the body, in a direction from head to tail.

cephalocele (se-fal′o-sēl) [*cephalo-* + Gr. *kēlē* hernia] a protrusion of a part of the cranial contents. **orbital c.,** protrusion of the cranial contents through a defect in the orbital wall, named according to its contents as meningocele, encephalocele, etc.

cephalocentesis (sef″ah-lo-sen-te′sis) [*cephalo-* + Gr. *kentēsis* puncture] the surgical puncture of the head.

cephalochord (sef′ah-lo-kord″) [*cephalo-* + Gr. *chordē* cord] the intracranial portion of the embryonic notochord.

Cephalochordata (sef″ah-lo-kor-da′tah) a subphylum of primitive, small, fishlike chordates in which the notochord extends the entire length of the body; it includes the genus *Amphioxus.*

cephalochordate (sef″ah-lo-kor′dāt) any member of the Cephalochordata.

cephalocyst (sef′ah-lo-sist″) a larval cestode, such as a hydatid cyst.

cephalodactyly (sef″ah-lo-dak′tĭ-le) [*cephalo-* + Gr. *daktylos* a finger or toe] malformation of the head and digits. **Vogt's c.,** acrocephalosyndactyly.

cephalodiprosopus (sef″ah-lo-di-pros′o-pus) [*cephalo-* + Gr. *di-* twice + *prosopus* face] a monster with a partially incomplete head attached to the head proper.

cephalodymia (sef″ah-lo-dim′e-ah) the condition of a cephalodymus.

cephalodymus (sef″ah-lod′ĭ-mus) [*cephalo-* + Gr. *didymos* twin] a twin monster with a single or united head.

cephalodynia (sef″ah-lo-din′e-ah) [*cephalo-* + Gr. *odynē* pain] cephalalgia.

cephalogenesis (sef″ah-lo-jen′ĕ-sis) [*cephalo-* + Gr. *gennan* to produce] the development of the head in the embryo.

cephaloglycin (sef″ah-lo-gli′sin) [USP] chemical name: [6R-[6α,7β(R*)(R*)]]3-[(acetyloxy)methyl]-7-[(aminophenyl-acetyl)amino]-8-oxo-5-thio-1-azabicyclo[4.2.0]oct-2-ene-2-carboxylic acid dihydrate. A semisynthetic analogue, $C_{18}H_{19}N_3O_6S \cdot 2H_2O$, of the natural antibiotic cephalosporin C, occurring as a white to off-white, crystalline powder, effective against a wide range of gram-negative and gram-positive bacteria; used in the treatment of acute and chronic urinary infections due to sensitive pathogens, administered orally.

cephalogram (sef′ah-lo-gram) [*cephalo-* + *-gram*] cephalometric radiograph.

cephalogyric (sef″ah-lo-ji′rik) [*cephalo-* + Gr. *gyros* a turn] pertaining to turning motions of the head.

cephalohematocele (sef″ah-lo-he-mat′o-sēl) cephalhematocele.

cephalohematoma (sef″ah-lo-he″mah-to′mah) cephalhematoma.

cephaloma (sef-ah-lo′mah) (*obs.*) medullary carcinoma.

cephalomelus (sef″ah-lom′ĕ-lus) [*cephalo-* + Gr. *melos* limb] a monster with an accessory limb growing from the head.

cephalomenia (sef″ah-lo-me′ne-ah) [*cephalo-* + Gr. *mēn* month] vicarious menstruation from the head, as in a nasal discharge at the menstrual period.

cephalometer (sef″ah-lom′ĕ-ter) [*cephalo-* + Gr. *metron* measure] an instrument for measuring the head; an orienting device for positioning the head for radiographic examination and measurement.

cephalometry (sef″ah-lom′ĕ-tre) scientific measurement of the dimensions of the head. In dentistry, certain combinations of linear and angular measurements developed from tracing the oriented lateral and frontal radiographic head film are used to assess craniofacial growth and development on a longitudinal basis and to determine the nature of orthodontic treatment response. **fetal c.,** measurement of the fetal skull *in utero* by means of x-ray films or by interpreting the echoes of ultrasonic radiation received from each side of the skull; useful in determining the proper time for elective termination of pregnancy.

cephalomotor (sef″ah-lo-mo′tor) [*cephalo-* + L. *motus* motion] moving the head; pertaining to motions of the head.

Cephalomyia (sef″ah-lo-mi′yah) Oestrus.

cephalonia (sef″ah-lo′ne-ah) a condition in which the head is abnormally large with sclerotic hyperplasia of the brain.

cephalopagus (sef″ah-lop′ah-gus) craniopagus.

cephalopathy (sef″ah-lop′ah-the) [*cephalo-* + Gr. *pathos* disease] any disease of the head.

cephalopelvic (sef″ah-lo-pel′vik) pertaining to the relationship of the fetal head to the maternal pelvis.

cephalopelvimetry (sef″ah-lo-pel-vim′ĕ-tre) pelvicephalometry.

cephalopharyngeus (sef″ah-lo-fah-rin′je-us) musculus constrictor pharyngis superior; see *Table of Musculi.*

cephaloplegia (sef″ah-lo-ple′je-ah) [*cephalo-* + Gr. *plēgē* stroke] paralysis of the muscles about the head and face.

Cephalopoda (sef″ah-lop′ŏ-dah) [*cephalo-* + Gr. *pous* foot] the class of mollusks embracing the octopus, squid, cuttlefish, and nautilus.

cephalorhachidian (sef″ah-lo-rah-kid′e-an) (*obs.*) pertaining to the head and the spinal column.

cephaloridine (sef″ah-lor′ĭ-dēn) chemical name: (6R-trans)-1-[[2-carboxy-8-oxo-7-[(2-thienylacetyl)amino]-5-thia-1-azabicyclo[4.2.0]oct-2-en-3-yl]methyl]pyridinium hydroxide inner salt. A semisynthetic analogue, $C_{19}H_{17}N_3O_4S_2$, of the natural antibiotic cephalosporin C, occurring as a white to off-white crystalline powder, effective against many gram-positive and some gram-negative bacteria; used in the treatment of infections of the bones, joints, skin, soft tissues, and major organ and body systems due to sensitive pathogens, administered intramuscularly or intravenously. Sterile cephaloridine, prepared in conformance with USP specifications, is suitable for parenteral use.

cephalosporin (sef″ah-lo-spōr′in) any of a group of broad-spectrum, relatively penicillinase-resistant antibiotics derived from the fungus *Cephalosporium,* which share the nucleus 7-aminocephalosporanic acid and are structurally related to the penicillins. The cephalosporins available for medicinal use are semisynthetic derivatives of the natural antibiotic *cephalosporin* C. **c. C,** chemical name: 7-(D-5-aminocarboxyvaleramido)-3-(hydroxymethyl)-3-oxo-5-thia-1-azabicyclo [4.2.0] oct-2-ene-2-carboxylic acid acetate. A cephalosporin isolated from *Cephalosporium acremonium,* $C_{16}H_{21}N_3O_8S$, which is the parent compound of a number of semisynthetic antibiotics, including cefazolin sodium, cephalexin, cephaloridine, cephaloglycin, cephalothin, cephapirin, and cephradine, used in the treatment of a wide range of infections due to sensitive gram-positive and gram-negative bacteria. **c. N,** adicillin. **c. P,** an antibacterial steroid, $C_{33}H_{50}O_8$; the crude form contains at least five components (P_1, P_2, P_3, P_4, P_5), P_1 being the major active substance.

cephalosporinase (sef″ah-lo-spōr′in-ās) β-lactamase.

cephalosporiosis (sef″ah-lo-spo″re-o′sis) infection with species of *Cephalosporium* (q.v.).

Cephalosporium (sef″ah-lo-spo′re-um) [*cephalo-* + Gr. *sporos* seed] a genus of soil-inhabiting imperfect fungi of the family Moniliaceae, order Moniliales; some species are the source of the cephalosporins. **C. falcifor′me,** *Acremonium kiliense.* **C. granulo′matis,** a species reported as causing gumma-like lesions in man.

cephalostat (sef′ah-lo-stat″) a head-positioning device used in dental radiology, facial photography, cephalometry, and other procedures requiring exact positioning of the head. See also *gnathostat.*

cephalostyle (sef′ah-lo-stīl″) the cranial end of the notochord.

cephalotetanus (sef″ah-lo-tet′ah-nus) [*cephalo-* + *tetanus*] cephalic tetanus.

cephalothin (sef′ah-lo-thin″) chemical name: (6R-*trans*)-3-[(acetyloxy)methyl]-8-oxo-7-[(2-thienyl)amino]-5-thia-1-azabicyclo[4.2.0]oct-2-ene-2-carboxylic acid. A semisynthetic analogue, $C_{16}H_{16}N_2O_6S_2$, of the natural antibiotic cephalosporin C, effective against a wide range of gram-positive and gram-negative bacteria. **c. sodium** [USP], the monosodium salt of cephalothin, $C_{16}H_{15}N_2NaO_6S_2$, used in the treatment of those infections of the major organ and tissue systems of the body that are due to sensitive pathogens; it is administered parenterally.

cephalothoracic (sef″ah-lo-tho-ras′ik) pertaining to the head and thorax.

cephalothoracopagus (sef″ah-lo-tho″rah-kop′ah-gus) a twin monster united at the head, neck, and thorax. **c. disym′metros,** a cephalothoracopagus fused squarely in the frontal plane and presenting two broad anterior surfaces and two narrow posterior ones, with a common head bearing two faces, each being formed by the right and left halves of the different components. **c. monosym′metros,** a cephalothoracopagus with one complete face formed by a right and a left half of the two components, the other face being only rudimentary.

cephalotome (sef′ah-lo-tōm) an instrument for cutting the fetal head.

cephalotomy (sef-ah-lot′o-me) [*cephalo-* + Gr. *temnein* to cut] 1. the cutting up of the fetal head to facilitate delivery. 2. dissection of the fetal head.

cephalotropic (sef″ah-lo-trop′ik) [*cephalo-* + Gr. *tropos* a turning] having an affinity for brain tissue.

cephamycin (sef″ah-mi′sin) any of a family of naturally occurring antibacterial antibiotics derived from various species of *Streptomyces* or produced semisynthetically, which are resistant to degradation by β-lactamase. Cephamycins A, B, and C have been isolated.

cephapirin (sef-ah-pi′rin) chemical name: [6R-*trans*]-3-[(acetyloxy)methyl]-8-oxo-7-[[(4-pyridinylthio)acetyl]amino]-5-thia-1-azabicyclo-[4.2.0]oct-2-ene-carboxylic acid. A semisynthetic analogue, $C_{17}H_{16}N_3O_5S_2$, of the natural antibiotic cephalosporin C, effective against a wide range of gram-negative and gram-positive bacteria. **c. sodium,** the monosodium salt of cephapirin, $C_{17}H_{16}N_3NaO_6S_2$, used in the treatment of infections of the respiratory and genitourinary tracts, skin, soft tissues, bones, joints, and blood due to sensitive pathogens. It is administered intramuscularly and intravenously. Sterile cephapirin sodium [USP] conforms to FDA regulations concerning antibiotic drugs.

cephradine (sef′rah-dēn) [USP] chemical name: [6R-[6α,7β(R*)]]-7-[(amino-1,4-cyclohexadien-1-ylacetyl)amino]-3-methyl-8-oxo-5-thia-1-azabicyclo[4.2.0]oct-2-ene-carboxylic acid. A semisynthetic analogue, $C_{16}H_{19}N_3O_4S$, of the natural antibiotic cephalosporin C, effective against a wide range of gram-positive and gram-negative bacteria; used in the treatment of infections of the urinary tract, skin, and soft tissues due to sensitive pathogens, administered orally or by intramuscular or intravenous injection.

ceptor (sep′tor) any nervous apparatus that receives external stimuli or impressions and transfers them to the nerve centers. Cf. *beneceptor* and *nociceptor.* **chemical c.,** a ceptor that transforms proper stimuli into electrochemical reactions in the body. **contact c.,** a ceptor that receives stimuli of direct physical contact. **distance c.,** the nervous apparatus through which an individual perceives or is affected by his distant environment. **nerve c.,** ceptor, def. 2.

cera (se′rah) [L.] wax. **c. al′ba,** white wax. **c. fla′va,** yellow wax.

ceraceous (se-ra′shus) [L. *cera* wax] waxlike in appearance.

ceramic (sĕ-ram′ik) 1. of or pertaining to ceramics. 2. a product, such as porcelain, produced by the action of heat on earthy materials, in which silicon and silicates occupy a predominant position. 3. a metal oxide.

ceramics (sĕ-ram′iks) [Gr. *keramos* potters' clay] 1. the modeling and processing of objects made of clay or similar material. 2. objects made of ceramic material. **dental c.,** the employment of porcelain and similar materials in restorative dentistry; called also *ceramodontics.*

ceramidase (ser-am′ĭ-dās) acylsphingosine deacylase.

ceramidase deficiency Farber disease.

ceramide (ser′ah-mīd) any of a group of naturally occurring sphingolipids in which the NH_2 group of sphingosine is acylated with a fatty acyl CoA derivative to form an *N*-acylsphingosine. **galactosyl c.,** cerebroside. **c. glucoside,** the major sphingolipid accumulated in Gaucher's disease; called also *glucocerebroside.* **c. trihexoside,** the major sphingolipid accumulated in Fabry's disease.

ceramide trihexosidase (ser′ah-mīd tri″hek-so′sĭ-dās) α-D-galactosidase A.

ceramide trihexosidase deficiency Fabry disease. **lactosyl c.,** lactosylceramidosis.

ceramodontics (se-ram″o-don′tiks) dental ceramics.

cerasin (ser′ah-sin) a class of gums from cherry, plum, and other trees, containing carbohydrate; they are insoluble in cold water.

cerasine (ser′ah-sīn) a red azo dye, $C_{10}H_7 \cdot N{:}N \cdot C_{10}H_4(SO_2{-}ONa)_2 \cdot OH$, used as a cytoplasmic stain.

cerasus (ser′ah-sus) [L.] cherry, or cherry tree; see *Prunus.*

cerate (se′rāt) [L. *ceratum,* from *cera* wax] a medicinal preparation for external application, made with a basis of fat or wax, or both, intermediate in consistency between an ointment and a plaster. **simple c.,** a mixture of benzoinated lard and white wax, melted together. **Turner's c.,** calamine ointment.

ceratectomy (ser-ah-tek′to-me) keratectomy.

ceratin (ser′ah-tin) keratin.

Ceratomyxa (sĕ-ra″she-o-mik′sah) [Gr. *keratias* horned + *myxa* mucus, slime] a genus of ameboid protozoa (order Protosteliida, sublcass Protosteliia) found on or in decaying wood, presenting as a hornlike gelatinous mass, and characterized by the presence of spores on the surface of the fruiting body.

Ceratium (sĕ-ra′she-um) [Gr. *keration,* dim. of *keras* horn] a genus of plantlike, marine and freshwater protozoa (order Dinoflagellida, class Phytomastigophorea), which like other dinoflagellates, when present in vast numbers, produce discoloration of the water (red tide).

cerat(o)- for words beginning thus, see also those beginning *kerato-.*

ceratocricoid (ser″ah-to-kri′koid) pertaining to the posterior horn of the thyroid cartilage and the cricoid cartilage.

ceratocricoideus (ser″at-to-kri-koi′de-us) see *Table of Musculi.*

ceratohyal (ser″ah-to-hi′al) pertaining to a cornu minus of the hyoid bone.

Ceratomyxa (sĕ-ra″to-mik′sah) [*cerato-* + Gr. *myxa* mucus] a genus of parasitic protozoa (suborder Eurysporina, order Bivalvulida) found in the salmonid fishes and often causing death of the host.

ceratopharyn′geus (ser″at-o-fahr-in′je-us) see *Table of Musculi.*

Ceratophyllus (ser″ah-tof′ĭ-lus) [Gr. *keras* horn + *phyllon* leaf] a genus of fleas, now including only bird fleas, but formerly including those of birds and small mammals. **C. acu′tus,** *Diamanus montanus.* **C. fascia′tus,** *Nosopsyllus fasciatus.* **C. galli′nae,** a species that attacks chickens and man. **C. idahoen′sis,** *Oropsylla idahoensis.* **C. monta′nus,** *Diamanus montanus.* **C. punjaben′sis,** a rat flea of India. **C. silantiew′i,** *Oropsylla silantiewi.* **C. tesquo′rum,** a plague-transmitting flea of ground squirrels in the Russian steppes.

Ceratopogonidae (ser″ah-to-po-gon′ĭ-de) biting midges or sandflies.

ceratum (se-ra′tum) [L.] cerate.

cerberin, cerberine (ser′bĕ-rin) a poisonous alkaloid, $C_{32}H_{48}O_9$, from *Cerbera odallam*, a tree of Asia; a cardiotonic agent.

cercaria (ser-ka′re-ah), pl. *cerca′riae* [Gr. *kerkos* tail] the final free-swimming larval stage of a trematode parasite, consisting of a body and tail. Some cercariae encyst on aquatic vegetation and penetrate the skin of a fish or the tissues of an aquatic arthropod to form encysted metacercariae. Cercariae of schistosomes penetrate directly into the skin of the definitive host without forming metacercariae.

cercaricidal (ser-ka″re-si′dal) destructive to cercariae.

cercarienhullenreaktion (ser-ka″re-en-hul″en-re-ak′-shun) a test for *Schistosoma mansoni*, utilized in measuring the efficiency of chemotherapy against schistosmiasis. When cercariae of *S. mansoni* are placed *in vitro* in contact with sera of monkeys or men infected with *S. mansoni*, a transparent envelope is formed around each cercaria.

cerclage (sār-klahzh′) [Fr. "an encircling"] encircling of a part with a ring or loop, such as encirclement of the incompetent cervix uteri, or the binding together of the ends of a fractured bone with a metal ring or wire loop (tiring).

cerco- [Gr. *kerkos* tail] a combining form denoting a relationship to a tail or to a tail-like structure.

cercocystis (ser″ko-sis′tis) cysticercoid.

cercoid (ser′koid) the last stage in the development of a tapeworm.

cercopithecoid (ser″ko-pith′ĕ-koid) an Old World monkey, having a tail but not using it as a limb.

Cercopithecoidea (ser″ko-pith″ĕ-koid′e-ah) a superfamily of the order Primates (suborder Anthropoidea), characterized by nostrils that are close together and directed downward, including the Old World apes and monkeys, and man; formerly called *Catarrhina*.

Cercosphaera addisoni (ser″ko-sfēr′ah ad″ĭ-so′ni) *Microsporum audouini*.

Cercospora apii (ser″kos′por-ah a′pe-i) a fungus that is a common plant pathogen (celery blight) and that causes cercosporamycosis in man.

Cercosporalla vexans (ser″kos-pŏ-ral′ah vek′sanz) a species of molds of the Fungi Imperfecti, order Moniliales, family Moniliaceae, which has been reported to cause skin eruptions, probably a variant of *Trichophyton mentagrophytes*.

cercus (ser′kus), pl. *cer′ci* [L.; Gr. *kerkos* tail] a bristle-like structure.

cerea flexibil′itas (sēr′e-ah flek″sĭ-bil′ĭ-tas) [L. "waxy flexibility"] the "waxy flexibility" seen in some severe cases of catatonic schizophrenia in which the patient maintains whatever body position he is placed in; called also *catalepsy*.

cereal (se′re-al) [L. *cerealis*] 1. Pertaining to edible grain. 2. any graminaceous plant bearing an edible seed; also the seed or grain of such a plant.

cerebella (ser″ĕ-bel′ah) [L.] plural of *cerebellum*.

cerebellar (ser″ĕ-bel′ar) pertaining to the cerebellum.

cerebellifugal (ser″ĕ-bel-lif′ŭ-gal) [*cerebellum* + L. *fugere* to flee] tending or proceeding from the cerebellum.

cerebellipetal (ser″ĕ-bel-lip′ĕ-tal) [*cerebellum* + L. *petere* to seek] tending or moving toward the cerebellum.

cerebellitis (ser″ĕ-bel-li′tis) inflammation of the cerebellum.

cerebell(o)- [L. *cerebellum*, q.v.] a combining form denoting relationship to the cerebellum.

cerebellofugal (ser″ĕ-bel-lof′ŭ-gal) cerebellifugal.

cerebello-olivary (ser″ĕ-bel″o-ol′ĭ-va-re) conducting or proceeding from the cerebellum to the olivary body.

cerebellopontile (ser″ĕ-bel″o-pon′tēl) conducting or proceeding from the cerebellum to the pons varolii.

cerebellopontine (ser″ĕ-bel″o-pon′tēn) cerebellopontile.

cerebellorubral (ser″ĕ-bel″o-ru′bral) conducting or proceeding from the cerebellum to the red nucleus.

cerebellorubrospinal (ser″ĕ-bel″o-roo″bro-spi′nal) conducting or proceeding from the cerebellum, to the red nucleus, and then to the spinal cord.

cerebellospinal (ser″ĕ-bel″o-spi′nal) conducting or proceeding from the cerebellum to the spinal cord.

cerebellum (ser″ĕ-bel′um) [L. dim. of *cerebrum* brain] [NA] the part of the metencephalon that occupies the posterior cranial fossa behind the brain stem and is concerned in the coordination of movements. It is a fissured mass consisting of a body, comprising a narrow middle strip (the vermis) and two lateral lobes (the hemispheres, connected with the brain stem by three pairs (caudal, middle, and rostral), of peduncles. Functionally, the cerebellum is subdivided into a cranial (anterior) lobe, which is separated from the caudal (posterior or median) lobe by the primary fissure, which is in turn separated from the flocculonodular lobe by the dorsolateral (posterolateral) fissure.

cerebra (ser′e-brah, sĕ-re′brah) [L.] plural of *cerebrum*.

cerebral (ser′ĕ-bral, sĕ-re′bral) pertaining to the cerebrum.

cerebration (ser″ĕ-bra′shun) [L. *cerebratio*] functional activity of the cerebrum; thinking; mental activity.

cerebriform (sĕ-reb′rĭ-form) [L. *cerebrum* brain + *forma* form] resembling the brain or brain substance.

cerebrifugal (ser″ĕ-brif′u-gal) [*cerebrum* + L. *fugere* to flee] conducting or proceeding away from the brain, or cerebrum.

cerebripetal (ser″ĕ-brip′ĕ-tal) [*cerebrum* + L. *petere* to seek] conducting or proceeding toward the brain, or cerebrum.

cerebritis (ser″ĕ-bri′tis) inflammation of the cerebrum. **saturnine c.,** brain inflammation due to lead poisoning.

cerebr(o)- [L. *cerebrum*, q.v.] a combining form denoting relationship to the cerebrum.

cerebrocardiac (ser″ĕ-bro-kar′de-ak) [*cerebrum* + L. *cardia* heart] pertaining to the brain and heart.

cerebrocerebellar (ser″ĕ-bro-ser″ĕ-bel′ar) pertaining to the cerebrum and the cerebellum.

cerebrocuprein (ser″ĕ-bro-ku′pre-in) a copper protein isolated from the human and bovine brain.

cerebrogalactose (ser″ĕ-bro-gah-lak′tos) galactose (of cerebrosides).

cerebrogalactoside (ser″ĕ-bro-gah-lak′to-sīd) cerebroside.

cerebrohyphoid (ser″ĕ-bro-hi′foid) [*cerebrum* + Gr. *hyphē* web + *eidos* form] resembling brain tissue.

cerebroid (ser′ĕ-broid) resembling the brain substance.

cerebrology (ser″ĕ-brol′o-je) [*cerebrum* + *-logy*] the sum of knowledge regarding the brain.

cerebroma (ser″ĕ-bro′mah) any abnormal mass of brain substance.

cerebromacular (ser″ĕ-bro-mak′u-lar) pertaining to or affecting the brain and the macula retinae.

cerebromalacia (ser″ĕ-bro-mah-la′she-ah) [*cerebrum* + Gr. *malakos* soft] abnormal softening of the substance of the cerebrum.

cerebromedullary (ser″ĕ-bro-med′u-la-re) cerebrospinal.

cerebromeningeal (ser″ĕ-bro-mĕ-nin′je-al) pertaining to the brain and its membranes.

cerebromeningitis (ser″ĕ-bro-men″in-ji′tis) meningoencephalitis.

cerebron (ser′ĕ-bron) phrenosin.

cerebronic acid (ser″e-bron′ik) 2-hydroxylignoceric acid, a 2-hydroxy fatty acid found in phrenosin.

cerebro-ocular (ser″e-bro-ok′u-lar) pertaining to the brain and the eye.

cerebropathia (ser″ĕ-bro-path′e-ah) [L.] cerebropathy. **c. psy′chica toxe′mica,** Korsakoff's psychosis.

cerebropathy (ser″ĕ-brop′ah-the) [*cerebrum* + Gr. *pathos* disease] any disorder of the brain.

cerebrophysiology (ser″ĕ-bro-fiz″e-ol′o-je) the physiology of the cerebrum.

cerebropontile (ser″ĕ-bro-pon′til) pertaining to the cerebrum and pons.

cerebrorachidian (ser″ĕ-bro″rah-kid′e-an) cerebrospinal.

cerebrosclerosis (ser″ĕ-bro″skle-ro′sis) [*cerebrum* + *sclerosis*] morbid hardening of the substance of the cerebrum.

cerebrose (ser′e-brōs) galactose (of cerebrosides).

cerebroside (ser′ĕ-bro-sīd″) a general designation of an acid amide of a C_{24}, C_{18}, or C_{16} fatty acid with sphingosine or dihydrosphingosine in glycosidic linkage with galactose or glucose. Kerasin and phrenosin are typical members of this class. It is abundant in membranes of nervous tissue, especially the myelin sheath, and is a major component of the cell coats of higher organisms. Called also *cerebrogalactoside,* *galactocerebroside,* and *glucocerebroside.*

cerebroside β-galactosidase (ser'ĕ-bro-sīd" gah-lak-tōs'ĭ-dās) galactosylceramidase.

cerebroside β-glucosidase (ser-e'bro-sīd" gloo-kōs'ĭ-dās) glucosylceramidase.

cerebroside sulfatase (ser-e'bro-sīd" sul'fah-tās) [EC 3.1.6.8] an enzyme of the hydrolase class that catalyzes the reaction cerebroside 3-sulfate + H_2O = cerebroside + sulfate. Deficiency of the enzyme, an autosomal recessive trait, is one of the causes of metachromatic leukodystrophy.

cerebrosidosis (ser"ĕ-bro"si-do'sis) a lipoidosis in which the fatty accumulation in the body consists largely of kerasin, as in Gaucher's disease.

cerebrosis (ser"ĕ-bro'sis) any disease of the cerebrum.

cerebrospinal (ser"ĕ-bro-spi'nal) pertaining to the brain and spinal cord.

cerebrospinant (ser"ĕ-bro-spi'nant) any medicine or agent that affects the brain and spinal cord.

cerebrostomy (ser"ĕ-bros'to-me) [*cerebrum* + Gr. *stoma* opening] the making of an artificial opening into the cerebrum.

cerebrotendinous (ser"ĕ-bro-ten'dĭ-nus) pertaining to the cerebrum and the tendons.

cerebrotomy (ser"ĕ-brot'o-me) [*cerebrum* + Gr. *temnein* to cut] incision of the brain.

cerebrotonia (ser"ĕ-bro-to'ne-ah) [*cerebro-* + *ton-* + *-ia*] a temperment type characterized by love of privacy, emotional restraint, and intellectual intensity; the behavioral counterpart of ectomorphy.

cerebrovascular (ser"ĕ-bro-vas'ku-lar) pertaining to the blood vessels of the cerebrum, or brain.

cerebrum (ser'ĕ-brum, sĕ-re'brum) [L.] 1. [NA] the main portion of the brain, occupying the upper part of the cranial cavity; its two hemispheres (see *cerebral hemisphere,* under *hemisphere*), united by the corpus callosum, form the largest part of the central nervous system in man. It is derived (developed) from the telencephalon of the embryo. 2. a term sometimes applied to the postembryonic prosencephalon and mesencephalon together or to the entire brain. **c. exsicca'tum,** the gray substance of the brain of calves, freed from fats, dried, and pulverized; used therapeutically in brain and nervous diseases.

cerecloth (sēr'kloth) cloth impregnated with wax and made antiseptic; used in dressings.

Cerenkov radiation (ka'ren-kov) [Pavel Aleksandrovich *Cerenkov,* Russian physicist born 1904] see under *radiation.*

cereoli (se-re'o-li) plural of *cereolus.*

cereolus (se-re'o-lus), pl. *cere'oli* [L., dim. of *cereus* wax taper] a medicated bougie.

cerevisia (ser"ĕ-viz'e-ah), gen. and pl., *cerevis'iae* [L.] beer, ale, porter, or other brewed malt liquor. **cerevis'iae fermen'tum,** brewer's yeast. **cerevis'iae fermen'tum compres'sum,** compressed yeast.

cerevisiae (ser"e-viz'e-e) [L.] genitive and plural singular of *cerevisia.*

cerin (se'rin) cerotic acid.

Cerithidia (ser"ĭ-thid'e-ah) a genus of spiral-shelled snails found in brackish water in tropical and subtropical areas. **C. cing'ulata,** the chief intermediate host of *Heterophyes heterophyes;* it is found in Japan.

cerium (se're-um) [L.] a metallic element: symbol, Ce; atomic number, 58; atomic weight, 140.12. **c. oxalate,** a white, insoluble powder, a mixture of the oxalates of cerium, neodymium, praseodymium, lanthanum, and other elements; sedative, tonic, and nervine; has been used as a sedative and antiemetic.

ceroid (se'roid) an insoluble, acid-fast, sudanophilic, lipid pigment found in the liver, the nervous system, and muscle.

cerolipoid (se"ro-li'poid) a waxy substance existing in plants.

ceroma (se-ro'mah) [Gr. *kērōma* waxy mass] a tumor of tissue that has undergone a waxy degeneration.

ceroplasty (se'ro-plas"te) [L. *cera* wax + Gr. *plassein* to mold] the making of anatomical models in wax.

cerotin (ser'o-tin) ceryl alcohol.

certifiable (ser"tĭ-fi'ah-b'l) capable of being certified; said of infectious diseases, cases of which must by law be reported to public health officers.

Cerubidine (sĕ-roo'bĭ-dēn) trademark for a preparation of daunorubicin.

cerulean (sĕ-roo'le-an) [L. *caeruleus*] blue; azure. Written also *caeruleus* and *coeruleus* (q.v.).

cerulein (sĕ-roo'le-in) a decapeptide amide isolated from the skin of frogs; it is a peptide analogue of cholecystokinin and gastrin; in mammals it is a powerful stimulant of gallbladder contraction.

ceruloplasmin (sĕ-roo"lo-plaz'min) ferroxidase.

cerumen (sĕ-roo'men) [L. from *cera* wax] the waxlike secretion found within the external meatus of the ear; called also *earwax.* **impacted c.,** accumulated cerumen forming a solid mass that adheres to the wall of the external auditory canal. **inspissated c.,** dried earwax in the external canal of the ear.

ceruminal (sĕ-roo'mĭ-nal) of or pertaining to the cerumen.

ceruminolysis (sĕ-roo"mĭ-nol'ĭ-sis) the solution or disintegration of cerumen in the external auditory meatus.

ceruminolytic (sĕ-roo"mĭ-no-lit'ik) 1. pertaining to, characterized by, or promoting ceruminolysis. 2. an agent that dissolves cerumen in the external auditory canal.

ceruminoma (sĕ-roo"mĭ-no'mah) tumor of the ceruminous glands.

ceruminosis (sĕ-roo"mĭ-no'sis) excessive or disordered secretion of cerumen.

ceruminous (sĕ-roo'mĭ-nus) ceruminal.

ceruse (se'rōōs) [L. *cerussa*] the basic carbonate of lead; white lead.

cervical (ser'vĭ-kal) [L. *cervicalis,* from *cervix* neck] pertaining to the neck, or to the neck of any organ or structure.

cervicalis (ser"vĭ-ka'lis) [L.] cervical.

cervicectomy (ser"vĭ-sek'to-me) excision of the cervix uteri; called also *trachelectomy.*

cervicitis (ser"vĭ-si'tis) inflammation of the cervix uteri; called also *trachelitis.* **granulomatous c.,** granulomatous infections of the cervix, including tuberculosis, syphilis, and granuloma inguinale. **traumatic c.,** a nonspecific cervicitis resulting from such procedures as irradiation or cauterization.

cervicoaxillary (ser"vĭ-ko-ak'sĭ-lār-e) pertaining to the neck and axilla.

cervicobrachial (ser"vĭ-ko-bra'ke-al) pertaining to the neck and arm.

cervicobrachialgia (ser"vĭ-ko-brak"e-al'je-ah) pain in the neck radiating to the arm, due to compression of nerve roots of the cervical spinal cord.

cervicobuccal (ser"vĭ-ko-buk'al) buccocervical.

cervicocolpitis (ser"vĭ-ko-kol-pi'tis) inflammation of the cervix uteri and vagina. **c. emphysemato'sa,** colpitis emphysematosa with similar lesions occurring beneath the squamous mucosa of the cervix uteri.

cervicodorsal (ser"vĭ-ko-dor'sal) pertaining to the neck and back.

cervicodynia (ser"vĭ-ko-din'e-ah) [*cervix* + Gr. *odynē* pain] pain in the neck.

cervicofacial (ser"vĭ-ko-fa'she-al) pertaining to the neck and face.

cervicolabial (ser"vĭ-ko-la'be-al) labiocervical.

cervicolingual (ser"vĭ-ko-ling'gwal) linguocervical.

cervico-occipital (ser"vĭ-ko-ok-sip'ĭ-tal) pertaining to the neck and occiput.

cervicoplasty (ser"vĭ-ko-plas'te) [*cervix* + Gr. *plassein* to form] plastic surgery on the neck.

cervicoscapular (ser"vĭ-ko-skap'u-lar) pertaining to the neck and scapula.

cervicothoracic (ser"vĭ-ko-tho-ras'ik) pertaining to the neck and thorax.

cervicovaginitis (ser"vĭ-ko-vaj"ĭ-ni'tis) inflammation involving both the cervix uteri and vagina.

cervicovesical (ser"vĭ-ko-ves'e-kal) pertaining to the cervix uteri and urinary bladder.

Cervilaxin (ser"vĭ-lak'sin) trademark for a preparation of relaxin.

cervimeter (ser-vim′ĕ-ter) [*cervix* + Gr. *metron* measure] an apparatus for measuring the cervix uteri.

cervix (ser′viks), pl. *cer′vices* [L.] neck; [NA] a term denoting the front portion of the collum, or neck (the part connecting the head and trunk), or a constricted part of an organ (e.g., cervix uteri). **c. of axon,** a constricted part of an axon, before the myelin sheath is added. **c. colum′nae posterio′ris medul′lae spina′lis,** NA alternative for *c. cornus dorsalis medullae spinalis.* **c. cor′nus dorsa′lis medul′lae spina′lis** [NA], neck of dorsal horn of spinal cord: the constricted portion of the dorsal horn, or column, of gray matter in the spinal cord between the base of the horn and the head; called also *c. cornus posterioris medullae spinalis* [NA alternative] and *neck of posterior horn of spinal cord.* **c. den′tis,** [NA], the slightly constricted region of union of the crown and the root or roots of a tooth; called also *collum dentis, dental neck,* and *neck of tooth.* **c. glan′dis,** collum glandis penis. **incompetent c.,** one that is abnormally prone to dilate in the second trimester of pregnancy, resulting in premature expulsion of the fetus (middle trimester abortion). **c. mal′lei,** collum mallei. **tapiroid c.,** a uterine cervix with a peculiarly elongated anterior lip. **c. u′teri,** neck of uterus: the lower and narrow end of the uterus, between the isthmus and the ostium uteri. **c. vesi′cae** [NA], a constricted portion of the urinary bladder, formed by the meeting of its inferolateral surfaces proximal to the opening of the urethra.

ceryl (se′ril) a univalent aliphatic, straight-chain hydrocarbon radical having the formula $C_{26}H_{53}$.

c.e.s. central excitatory state; see under *state.*

cesarean (se-sa′re-an) [L. *caesus,* from *caedere* to cut] see under *section.*

cesium (se′ze-um) [L. *caesium,* from *caesius* blue] a rare univalent metallic element with an alkaline oxide; atomic number, 55; atomic weight, 132.905; symbol, Cs. Some of its salts and binary compounds are used like those of potassium.

Cestan-Chenais syndrome (ses-tan′ shĕ-na′) [Raymond *Cestan,* French neurologist, 1872–1934; Louis *Chenais,* French physician, 1872–1950] see under *syndrome.*

Cestan-Raymond syndrome (ses-tan′ ra-maw′) [Raymond *Cestan;* Fulgence *Raymond,* French neurologist, 1844–1910] Raymond-Cestan syndrome.

cesticidal (ses″tĭ-si′dal) destructive to cestodes.

Cestoda (ses-to′dah) a subclass of Cestoidea comprising the true tapeworms, which have a head or scolex, and segments or proglottides. Adult tapeworms are endoparasitic in the alimentary tract and associated ducts of various vertebrate hosts; their larval stages (cysticercus, coenurus, hydatid, sparganum) may be found in various organs or tissues. Of the eleven orders, two—Pseudophyllidea and Cyclophyllidea—contain species that parasitize man and other animals. Called also *Eucestoda.*

Cestodaria (ses-to-da′re-ah) a subclass of tapeworms, the unsegmented tapeworms of the class Cestoidea, which are endoparasitic in the intestines and coelom of various primitive fishes and rarely in reptiles.

cestode (ses′tōd) 1. any tapeworm or platyhelminth of the class Cestoidea, especially those of the subclass Cestoda. 2. cestoid.

cestodiasis (ses″to-di′ah-sis) infection by cestodes.

cestodology (ses″to-dol′o-je) the scientific study of cestodes.

cestoid (ses′toid) [Gr. *kestos* girdle + *eidos* form] resembling a tapeworm.

Cestoidea (ses-toi′de-ah) a class of tapeworms (platyhelminths) characterized by the absence of a mouth and digestive tract and by the presence of a noncuticular layer covering their bodies. It comprises two subclasses: Cestodaria and Cestoda.

cetaben sodium (se′tah-ben) chemical name: 4-(hexadecylamino)benzoic acid sodium salt; an antihyperlipoproteinemic, $C_{23}H_{38}NNaO_2$.

cetaceum (sĕ-ta′se-um) spermaceti.

cetalkonium chloride (set-al-ko′ne-um) chemical name: *N*-hexadecyl-*N,N*-dimethylbenzene methanaminium chloride. A cationic quaternary ammonium surfactant, $C_{25}H_{46}$-ClN, used as a topical anti-infective and disinfectant.

cetanol (se′tah-nol) a solid white alcohol, $C_{16}H_{33}OH$, from sperm oil.

cetiedil citrate (sĕ-ti′ĕ-dil) chemical name: 2-(hexahydro-1*H*-azepin-1-yl) ethyl ester α-cyclohexyl-2-hydroxy-1,2,3-propanetricarboxylate (1:1); a peripheral vasodilator, $C_{20}H_{31}NO_2S \cdot C_6H_8O_7$, which has been used in the treatment of arteritis, Raynaud's disease, and acrocyanosis.

cetocycline hydrochloride (se″to-si′klēn) chemical name: [4*R*-(4α,4aβ,12aβ)]-acetyl-4-amino-4a,12a-dihydro-3,10,11,12a-tetrahydroxy-6,9-dimethyl-1,12(4*H*,5*H*)-naphthacenedione; an antibacterial, $C_{22}H_{21}NO_7 \cdot HCl$.

cetohexazine (se-to-heks′ah-zēn) ketohexazine.

Cetraria (sĕ-tra′re-ah) 1. a genus of lichens. 2. the official name of *C. islandica,* so-called Iceland moss; it is nutritious and useful in lung and bowel affections, and is a source of lichenin.

cetrimide (se′trĭ-mīd) cetrimonium bromide.

cetrimonium bromide (set″rĭ-mo′ne-um) a quaternary ammonium antiseptic and detergent composed of a mixture of tetradecyltrimethylammonium bromide with dodecyl- and hexadecyltrimethyl ammonium bromides, $C_{19}H_{42}BrN$, occurring as a white to creamy white powder; applied topically to the skin to cleanse wounds, as a preoperative disinfectant, and to treat seborrhea of the scalp; solutions are also used to cleanse utensils and to store surgical instruments. Abbreviated CTBA. Called also *cetrimide* and *cetyltrimethylammonium bromide.*

cetyl (se′til) a univalent alcohol radical, $CH_3(CH_2)_{14}CH_2$.

cetylpyridinium chloride (se″til-pi″rĭ-din′e-um) [USP] chemical name: 1-hexadecylpyridinium chloride. A cationic disinfectant, $C_{21}H_{38}ClN \cdot H_2O$, occurring as a white powder; used as a local anti-infective administered sublingually or applied topically to intact skin and mucous membranes, and as a preservative in pharmaceutical preparations.

cetyltrimethylammonium bromide (se″til-meth″il-ah-mo′ne-um) cetrimonium bromide.

Cevalin (se′vah-lin) trademark for preparations of ascorbic acid (vitamin C).

Cevex (se′veks) trademark for a liquid preparation of ascorbic acid (vitamin C).

Ce-Vi-Sol (se′vi-sol) trademark for a preparation of ascorbic acid for calibrated dropper dosage.

cevitamic acid (se-vi-tam′ik) ascorbic acid.

Ceylancyclostoma (se″lan-si-klos′to-mah) *Ancylostoma braziliense.*

ceyssatite (sēs′ah-tīt) [*Ceyssat,* a village of France] a white earth from France, useful as an adsorbent powder in eczema and hyperidrosis, and in preparing ointments and medicated pastes.

CF cardiac failure; Christmas factor (see under *factor*).

C.F. carbolfuchsin; citrovorum factor.

Cf chemical symbol for *californium.*

cf. abbreviation for L. *confer* bring together, compare.

c.f.f. critical fusion frequency (flicker fusion threshold); see under *flicker.*

C.F.T. complement-fixation test; see under *fixation.*

CFU-C colony-forming unit–culture, a granulocytic precursor cell which grows in *in vitro* culture in the presence of appropriate stimulators.

CFU-E colony-forming unit–erythroid, a red cell precursor detectable in *in vitro* culture; it precedes the proerythroblast in development but follows the BFU-E.

CFU-S colony-forming unit–spleen, the pluripotential stem cell which gives rise to the erythroid, granulocytic, and megakaryocytic cell lines; so named because the cell gives rise to colonies of marrow cells in the spleen of irradiated mice.

CG trademark for a preparation of indocyanine green.

CGD chronic granulomatous disease.

cGMP cyclic guanosine monophosphate.

C.G.S., c.g.s. abbreviation for *centimeter-gram-second* system, a system of measurements in which the units are based on the centimeter as the unit of length, the gram as the unit of mass, and the second as the unit of time.

cGy centigray.

C.H. crown-heel (length of fetus).

CH$_{50}$ see *CH$_{50}$ assay,* under *assay.*

CH$_4$ methane.

C_2H_2 acetylene.

C_2H_4 ethylene.

C_6H_6 benzene.

Chabert's disease (shah-bārz′) [Philebert *Chabert*, French veterinarian, 1737–1814] blackleg.

Chabertia (shah-ber′te-ah) a genus of nematodes parasitic in animals. **C. ovi′na**, a species of worms, the large-mouth bowel worm, parasitic in the colon of sheep, goats, and cattle.

Chaddock's reflex (sign) (chad′oks) [Charles Gilbert *Chaddock*, St. Louis neurologist, 1861–1936] see under *reflex*.

chafe (chāf) to irritate the skin, as by the rubbing together of opposing folds.

Chagas' disease (chag′as) [Carlos *Chagas*, physician in Brazil, 1879–1934] see under *disease*.

Chagas-Cruz disease (chag′as-kruz) [Carlos *Chagas*; Oswald *Cruz*, Brazilian physician, 1871–1917] Chagas' disease.

Chagasia (chah-gas′e-ah) [Carlos *Chagas*] a subgenus of *Anopheles* mosquitoes of Central and South America.

chagasic (chah-gas′ik) pertaining to or due to Chagas' disease.

chagoma (chah-go′mah) an erythematous nodule appearing within a few days at the site of inoculation by a reduviid bug of *Trypanosoma cruzi*, the parasite causing Chagas' disease; lymphatic vessels draining the site may become blocked with scar tissue and produce edema of the area.

Chagres fever (chag′res) [named from a river in Panama] see under *fever*.

Chailletia (ka-il-e′she-ah) a genus of trees and shrubs, nearly all tropical. **C. cymo′sa**, a species of South Africa that contains the poison fluoroacetic acid. **C. toxica′ria**, of West Africa, bears poisonous fruit and seeds.

Chain (chān) Ernst Boris. German-born British biochemist, 1906–1979; co-winner, with Sir Alexander Fleming and Sir Howard Walter Florey, of the Nobel prize for medicine or physiology in 1945 for his work on antibacterial substances produced by microorganisms.

chain (chān) a collection of objects linked together in linear fashion, or end to end, as the assemblage of atoms or radicals in a chemical compound, or an assemblage of individual bacterial cells. **branched c.**, an open chain of atoms, usually carbon, with one or more side chains attached to it. **closed c.**, several atoms linked together so as to form a ring, which may be saturated, as in cyclopentane, or

```
          C
          |
        C   C
        ‖   |
  —C—C—C   C—
  |  |  |   ‖   |
              C
              |
 Open chain
        Closed chain
```

aromatic, as in benzene. **food c.**, a sequence of organisms through which energy is transferred from its ultimate source in a plant; each organism eats the preceding and is eaten by the following member in the sequence. **H c., heavy c.**, any of the larger polypeptide chains of antibody molecules, two identical heavy chains occurring (with two identical light chains) in each immunoglobulin monomer. The heavy chains determine the immunoglobulin class and subclass and are designated accordingly: γ, α, μ, ε, and δ, the heavy chains of IgG, IgA, IgM, IgE, and IgD. The subclass may be designated by a number, e.g., γ1, the heavy chain of IgG1. Heavy chains have four homology regions of about 110 amino acid residues: one variable region (V_H) and three constant regions (C_H1, C_H2, C_H3) except for μ and ε chains which have an extra constant region (C_H4). See *immunoglobulin*. **J c.**, [for "joining"] a 15-kilodalton polypeptide occurring in all immunoglobulin polymers, a single J chain occurring in each IgM pentamer and in each IgA dimer, trimer, or tetramer. **kappa c.**, a type of light polypeptide chain of immunoglobulin molecules; see *light c.* **lambda c.**, a type of light polypeptide chain found in immunoglobulin molecules; see *light c.* **lateral c.**, side c. **light c.**, any of the smaller polypeptide chains

of antibody molecules, two identical light chains occurring (with two identical heavy chains) in each immunoglobulin monomer. There are two types, designated κ and λ, both occurring in all immunoglobulin classes (in a ratio of about two κ chains to one λ chain in humans). Light chains have two homology regions of about 110 amino acid residues: one variable region (V_L) and one constant region (C_L). Called also *L c.* See *immunoglobulin*. **nuclear c.**, a longitudinal array of nuclei occurring on an intrafusal fiber of muscle. **open c.**, several atoms united to form an open chain; compounds of this series are related to methane and are also called *fatty, aliphatic, acyclic,* or *paraffin* compounds. **side c.**, a chain of atoms attached to a larger chain or to a ring; called also *lateral c.* **sympathetic c.**, the sympathetic trunk (truncus sympathicus [NA]).

Chalara (kah-lar′ah) a genus of imperfect fungi of the order Moniliales, which causes many diseases of plants, such as oak wilt.

chalasia (kah-la′ze-ah) [Gr. *chalasis* relaxation] relaxation of a bodily opening, such as the cardiac sphincter, which is a cause of vomiting in infants.

chalaza (kah-la′zah) [Gr. "lump"] a spiral band of albumin extending from either end of the yolk of a bird's egg to the shell.

chalazia (kah-la′ze-ah) [Gr.] plural of *chalazion*.

chalazion (kah-la′ze-on), pl. *chala′zia* or *chalazions* [Gr. "small lump"] a small eyelid mass that results from chronic inflammation of a meibomian gland and shows a granulomatous reaction to liberated fat when subjected to histopathological examination; sometimes called *meibomian* or *tarsal cyst.*

chalazodermia (kah-laz″o-der′me-ah) cutis laxa.

chalcitis (kal-si′tis) chalkitis.

chalcone (kal′kōn) [Gr. *chalkos* copper or brass] any one of a group of yellow pigments that are substituted benzalacetophenone derivatives.

chalcosis (kal-ko′sis) [Gr. *chalkos* copper] the presence of copper deposits in the tissues. **c. cor′neae**, deposition of copper in the cornea resulting in a pigmented ring in the deeper layers.

chalicosis (kal-ĭ-ko′sis) [Gr. *chalix* gravel] a disorder of the lungs or bronchioles (chiefly among stone-cutters), due to the inhalation of fine particles of stones; it is a form of pneumoconiosis. Called also *flint disease.*

chalk (chawk) [L. *calx*] a natural calcium carbonate; the amorphous remains of minute marine organisms deposited on the sea bottom and decomposed by the action of acids and heat. Used as a polishing agent in dentistry and frequently as an ingredient in dentifrices. **French c.**, talc. **precipitated c.**, precipitated calcium carbonate. **prepared c.**, native calcium carbonate freed from most of its impurities by elutriation; used as an antacid, and has been used in the treatment of diarrhea and in the preparation of dentifrices.

chalkitis (kal-ki′tis) [Gr. *chalkos* brass] inflammation of the eyes caused by rubbing the eyes after the hands have been used on brass; called also *brassy eye.*

challenge (chal′enj) in immunology, (1) to administer antigen to evoke an immunologic response in a previously sensitized individual, or (2) an instance of so challenging.

chalone (kal′ōn) [Gr. *chalan* to relax] 1. a group of tissue-specific (but not species-specific) water-soluble proteins that are produced within a tissue and that inhibit mitosis of cells of that tissue and whose action is reversible. 2. (obs.) a substance which neutralizes the action of a hormone; inhibitory hormone.

chalonic (kah-lon′ik) of or pertaining to a chalone.

chalybeate (kah-lib′e-āt) [L. *chalybs*; Gr. *chalyps* steel] containing or charged with iron: ferruginous or martial.

chamaecephalic (kam″e-sĕ-fal′ik) pertaining to or characterized by chamaecephaly.

chamaecephaly (kam″e-sef′ah-le) [Gr. *chamai* low + *kephalē* head] the condition of having a low flat head, that is, a cephalic index of 70 or less.

chamaeprosopic (kam″ĕ-pro-sop′ik) pertaining to or characterized by chamaeprosopy.

chamaeprosopy (kam″ĕ-pros′o-pe) [Gr. *chamai* low + *prosōpon* face] the condition of having a low, broad face, i.e., a facial index of 90 or less.

chamber (chām′ber) [L. *camera*; Gr. *kamara*] an enclosed space or antrum. **Abbé-Zeiss counting c.**, Thoma-Zeiss counting c. **acoustic c.**, a soundproof room or enclosure used in measuring hearing. **air-equivalent ionization c.**, in radiology, a chamber in which the materials of the wall and electrodes are such that ionizing radiations produce ionization essentially similar to that in a free-air ionization chamber. **altitude c.**, a vacuum chamber used to simulate the effects of high altitude and low atmospheric pressure. **anterior c. of eye,** that portion of the aqueous-containing space between the cornea and the lens which is bounded in front by the cornea and part of the sclera, and behind by the iris, part of the ciliary body, and that part of the lens which presents through the pupil; called also *camera anterior bulbi* [NA]. **aqueous c.**, that part of the eyeball which is filled with aqueous humor; see *anterior c. of eye* and *posterior c. of eye.* **Boyden c.**, a device consisting of two compartments separated by a micropore filter, used in tests for chemotaxis. Cells are placed in the upper compartment and the chemotactic agent in the lower; if cells are attracted to the agent, they migrate through the pores of the filter. The filter is then stained so that cell migration can be measured. **counting c.**, a microscopic slide with a depression ground to uniform thickness, the base of which is marked in grids, and into which a measured volume of a sample of blood or of a bacterial culture is introduced and covered with a specially fitted cover glass. Cells and formed blood elements in the squares are counted under a microscope; the number of cells per unit volume of original sample is calculated from representative counts. **detonating c.**, a muffler surrounding the discharging balls of a static machine or resonator for deadening the sound of a spark discharge. **diffusion c.**, an apparatus for separating a substance by means of a semipermeable membrane. **c's of eye,** the various spaces in the eyeball; see *anterior c. of eye, posterior c. of eye,* and *vitreous c.* **free-air ionization c.**, an ionization chamber in which the ionization in an accurately defined volume of free air is measured. **Haldane c.**, an air-tight chamber in which animals may be confined for the performance of metabolic studies; called also *Haldane apparatus.* **c's of the heart,** the cavities of the atria and ventricles. **hyperbaric c.**, a compartment in which the air pressure may be raised to more than normal atmospheric pressure; used in treatment of gas gangrene and other anaerobic infections, or other conditions in which a high concentration of oxygen is desirable, and for studying the effects of pressure and decompression in animals and man. **ionization c.**, a device for measuring ionizing radiation by the measurement of the ionization of the gas contained in the chamber. **lethal c.**, a chamber that may be filled with gas, for killing small animals. **posterior c. of eye,** that portion of the aqueous-containing space of the eye which is bounded in front by the iris, and behind by the lens and suspensory ligament; called also *camera posterior bulbi* [NA]. **pulp c.**, cavitas coronalis. **relief c.**, a recess in the impression surface of a denture to reduce or eliminate pressure or force from that area of the mouth. See also *relief,* defs. 3 and 4. **Storm Van Leeuwen c.**, a room that can be kept free of airborne antigens for allergic patients. **thimble c.**, a small, thin-walled ionization chamber, usually with walls of organic material; used as a dosimeter. **Thoma-Zeiss counting c.**, a device consisting of a receptacle in the bottom of a slide for a microscope, with ruled lines dividing the area into minute squares, to facilitate the counting of blood corpuscles or other cells; called also *Abbe-Zeiss counting c.* **tissue-equivalent ionization c.**, an ionization chamber in which the walls, electrodes, and gas are selected to produce ionization essentially equivalent to that which would occur in the tissue under consideration. **vitreous c.**, the space in the eyeball enclosing the vitreous humor, bounded anteriorly by the lens and ciliary body, and posteriorly by the posterior wall of the eyeball; called also *camera vitrea bulbi* [NA]. **Zappert's c.**, a form of counting chamber.

Chamberland filter (shahm-ber-lah′) [Charles Edouard *Chamberland,* French bacteriologist, 1851–1908] see under *filter.*

Chamberlen forceps [Peter (Pierre) *Chamberlen,* English obstetrician, 1560–1631] see under *forceps.*

chamecephalic (kam″ĕ-sĕ-fal′ik) chamaecephalic.

chamecephaly (kam″ĕ-sef′ah-le) chamaecephaly.

chameprosopic (kam″ĕ-pro-sop′ik) chamaeprosopic.

chameprosopy (kam″ĕ-pros′o-pe) chamaeprosopy.

Champetier de Ribes' bag (shahmp-te-a′ de rēbz′) [Camille Louis Antoine *Champetier de Ribes,* French obstetrician, 1848–1935] see under *bag.*

chancre (shang′ker) [Fr. for "canker," a destructive sore, from L. *cancer* crab] 1. the usually painless primary lesion of syphilis, occurring at the site of entry of the infection, typically presenting as a small red papule or crusted erosion that breaks down to become round or oval, indurated, and slightly elevated with an eroded surface that exudes a serous fluid, and gives rise to a nontender nonfluctuant, firm regional lymphadenopathy (bubo); it heals without scarring. Called also *hard c., hard sore, hunterian c.,* and *true c.* 2. any of various primary cutaneous lesions that are seen at the site of inoculation of infection in such diseases as herpes, sporotrichosis, tuberculosis, tularemia, and trypanosomiasis. **hard c., hunterian c.**, chancre, def. 1. **mixed c.**, a skin lesion due to simultaneous infection with *Treponema pallidum* (primary syphilis) and *Haemophilus ducreyi* (chancroid); called also *mixed sore.* **monorecidive c.**, c. redux. **c. re′dux,** the reappearance of a chancre after partial healing as a result of insufficient treatment, accompanied by lymphadenopathy and the presence of numerous spirochetes at the site of the lesion; called also *monorecidive c.* **soft c.**, chancroid. **true c.**, chancre, def. 1. **tuberculous c.**, see *primary inoculation tuberculosis,* under *tuberculosis.*

chancriform (shang′kre-form) resembling a chancre.

chancroid (shang′kroid) [*chancre* + Gr. *eidos* form] a sexually transmitted disease caused by *Haemophilus ducreyi,* characterized by a painful primary ulcer at the site of inoculation, usually on the external genitalia, associated with regional lymphadenitis. Called also *soft chancre, sore,* or *ulcer,* and *chancroid* or *chancroidal ulcer.* See also *mixed chancre,* under *chancre.* **phagedenic c.**, a variety attended by sloughing of the tissues. **serpiginous c.**, a variety which tends to spread in curved lines.

chancroidal (shang-kroi′dal) pertaining to chancroid.

chancrous (shang′krus) of the nature of chancre.

change (chānj) an alteration. **Armanni-Ebstein c.**, see under *lesion.* **Crooke's c's, Crooke-Russell c's,** see *Crooke's hyaline degeneration,* under *degeneration.* **harlequin color c.**, transient reddening of one half of the body longitudinally with simultaneous blanching of the other half; a temporary vasomotor disorder of the newborn.

Ch'ang Shan (chang′ shan) the Chinese name for the root of the shrub *Dichroa febrifuga* Lour. Basak, Aseru (Saxifragaceae), of China, Java, India, and the Philippines. The Chinese have used it for its antiparasitic, emetic, and antipyretic effect in malaria. It contains several isomeric active alkaloids, e.g., febrifugine, isofebrifugine, and α-, β-, and γ-dichroines.

channel (chan′el) [L. *canalis* a water pipe] that through which anything flows; a cut or groove. **blood c's,** narrow passages with no distinct walls, but containing blood; they are found in fresh granulation tissue. **central c.**, a long straight capillary that connects an arteriole to a venule. **lymph c's,** the smaller lymph sinuses; irregular in and about the lymphatic glands and around lymphatic vessels. **perineural c.**, a lymph channel that surrounds a nerve trunk. **thoroughfare c.**, a channel between terminal arterioles and venules, larger than a capillary.

Chantemesse' reaction (shant-mes′) [André *Chantemesse,* French bacteriologist, 1851–1919] see under *reaction.*

Chaoborus (ka″o-bor′us) a genus of non–blood-sucking gnats of the family Culicidae; called also *Corethra.* **C. lacus′tris,** the Clear Lake gnat of California.

Chaos chaos (ka′os ka′os) *Pelomyxa carolinensis.*

Chaoul therapy, tube (showl) [Henri *Chaoul,* Berlin radiologist, 1887–1964] see under *therapy* and *tube.*

chapped (chapt) roughened and cracked, or split open by the cold or frequent wetting, as chapped hands or lips.

character (kar′ak-ter) [Gr. *charaktēr* an engraved or impressed mark or stamp] 1. a quality or attribute indicative of the nature of an object or organism. 2. in genetics, the expression in the phenotype of a gene or group of genes; see also *gene* and *inheritance.* 3. in psychiatry, a term used, especially in the psychoanalytic literature, in much the same way as personality (q.v.). **acquired c.**, a noninheritable modification produced in an animal as a result of its own activities or of environmental influences. **imvic c's,** four important characters in the classification of the coliform organisms: they are indole, methyl-red, Voges-Proskauer, and citrate. **primary sex c's,** those characters of the male and female that are concerned directly in reproduction. **secondary sex c's,** those characters specific to the male or female organism but not directly concerned in reproduction.

characteristic (kar″ak-ter-is′tik)   1. character.   2. typical of an individual or other entity. **demand c's,** cues regarding the purpose of the study or the behavior expected that an experimental subject perceives and responds to.

characterology (kar″ak-ter-ol′o-je)   the study of character and personality.

charas (chahr′as)   ganja.

charbon (shar-baw′) [Fr. "coal"]   anthrax. **c. symptomatique′,** blackleg.

charcoal (char′kōl)   carbon prepared by charring wood or other organic material. **activated c.,** [USP], the residue from the destructive distillation of various organic materials, treated to increase its adsorptive powers; used as a general purpose antidote. Called also *carbo activatus.* **animal c.,** charcoal prepared from bone; called also *animal, ivory,* or *Paris black,* and *bone-black.* **purified animal c.,** charcoal prepared from bone and purified by removal of materials dissolved by hot hydrochloric acid and water; adsorbent and decolorizer.

Charcot's arthropathy, etc. (shar-kōz′) [Jean Martin *Charcot,* French neurologist, 1825–1893]   see under *arthropathy, bath, cirrhosis, disease, fever, foot, gait, joint, syndrome,* and *triad.*

Charcot-Leyden crystals (shar-ko′ li′den) [J. M. *Charcot;* Ernst Victor von *Leyden,* German physician, 1832–1910]   see under *crystal.*

Charcot-Marie atrophy (type) (shar-ko′ mah-re′) [J. M. *Charcot;* Pierre *Marie,* French physician, 1853–1940]   progressive neuropathic (peroneal) muscular atrophy; see under *atrophy.*

Charcot-Marie-Tooth atrophy, disease, type (shar-ko′mah-re′tooth) [J. M. *Charcot;* Pierre *Marie;* Howard Henry *Tooth,* English physician, 1856–1925]   progressive neuropathic (peroneal) muscular atrophy.

Charcot-Neumann crystals (shar-ko′noy′mahn)   see under *crystal.*

charlatan (shar′lah-tan) [Fr.]   a pretender to knowledge or skills that he does not possess; in medicine, a quack.

charlatanism (shar′lah-tan-izm)   the pretension of knowledge and skills that one does not possess; in medicine, quackery.

charlatanry (shar′lah-tan-re)   charlatanism.

Charles' law (sharlz) [Jacques Alexandre César *Charles,* French physicist, 1746–1823]   see under *law.*

charley horse (char′le-hors)   soreness and stiffness in a muscle caused by overstrain or contusion; the term is usually restricted to injuries of the quadriceps muscle.

Charlouis' disease (shar″loo-ēz′) [M. *Charlouis,* Dutch physician in Java, 19th century]   yaws.

Charrière scale (shar″e-ār′) [Joseph Frédéric Benoit *Charrière,* French instrument maker, 1803–1876]   see under *scale.*

Chart.   abbreviation for L. *char′ta,* paper.

chart (chart)   1. a simplified graphic representation of the fluctuation of some variable, as of pulse, temperature, and respiration, or a record of all the clinical data of a particular case.   2. to record graphically the fluctuation of some variable, or to record the clinical data of a particular case. **alignment c.,** nomogram. **Amsler's c's,** a set of charts showing various geometric patterns in black and white, e.g., grids or parallel lines, used for detecting defects of the central visual field. **Guibor's c.,** a chart containing outline pictures for orthoptic training. **reading c.,** a chart bearing material printed in type of gradually increasing sizes; used in testing acuity of near vision. **Reuss' color c's,** charts with colored letters printed on colored backgrounds, used in testing color vision; called also *Reuss' tables.* **Snellen's c.,** see *Snellen's test type,* under *test type.*

charta (kar′tah), pl. *char′tae* [L.; Gr. *chartēs*]   1. paper.   2. a piece of paper, medicated or otherwise. **c. explorato′ria caeru′lea,** blue litmus paper; see under *paper.* **c. ex-**

plorato′ria lu′tea, turmeric paper; paper stained with turmeric for use as a test paper. **c. explorato′ria ru′bra,** red litmus paper; see under *paper.*

chartaceous (kar-ta′shus)   papyraceous.

chartula (kar′tu-lah), pl. *char′tulae* [L. dim. of *charta* paper]   a small piece of paper, as for containing a dose of a medicinal powder.

chasma (kaz′mah) [Gr. "a cleft"]   a yawning; an opening.

chasmatoplasson (kaz-mat′o-plas″on)   plasson in an expanded condition. Cf. *pyknoplasson.*

chasmus (kas′mus) [L., from Gr. *chasma* a cleft]   chasma.

Chassaignac's tubercle (shas″ān-yahks′) [Charles Marie Édouard *Chassaignac,* French surgeon, 1804–1879]   *tuberculum caroticum vertebrae cervicalis IV.*

chaude-pisse (shōd-pēs) [Fr.]   a burning sensation experienced during micturition.

Chauffard's syndrome (sho-farz′) [Anatole Marie Emile *Chauffard,* French physician, 1855–1932]   see under *syndrome.*

Chauffard-Still syndrome (sho-far′stil) [Anatole Marie Emile *Chauffard;* Sir George Frederick *Still,* English physician, 1868–1941]   Chauffard's syndrome.

Chauliac (sho′le-ahk′), Guy de (1300–1368).   An eminent French surgeon who practiced in Avignon. His treatise on surgery (*Chirurgia magna*) was regarded as a standard work until Paré's time.

chaulmoogric acid (chawl-moo′grik)   an unsaturated cyclic fatty acid from chaulmoogra oil.

Chaunacanthida (chawn″ah-kan′thĭ-dah) [Gr. *chaunos* spongy + *akantha* thorn, prickle]   an order of marine protozoa (class Acantharea, superclass Actinopoda) characterized by the presence of 20 radial spines with bases more or less loosely articulated; if present, the capsular membrane is situated far outside of the central cell mass.

Chaussier's areola, line (sho′se-āz′) [François *Chaussier,* Parisian surgeon and anatomist, 1746–1828]   see under *areola* and *line.*

Chauveau's bacillus, bacterium (sho-vōz′) [Auguste *Chauveau,* Paris veterinarian, 1827–1917]   *Clostridium chauvoei.*

Ch.B.   abbreviation for L. *Chirur′giae Baccalau′reus,* Bachelor of Surgery.

C₂H₅Br   ethyl bromide.

C_2H_5Br ethyl bromide.

CHCl₃   chloroform.

$CHCl_3$ chloroform.

C₂H₄Cl₂   ethylene chloride.

$C_2H_4Cl_2$ ethylene chloride.

C₂H₅Cl   ethyl chloride.

C_2H_5Cl ethyl chloride.

C₂H₅CO₂NH₂   ethyl carbamate.

$C_2H_5CO_2NH_2$ ethyl carbamate.

(CH₃·CO)₂O   acetic anhydride.

$(CH_3 \cdot CO)_2O$ acetic anhydride.

CH₃·COOH   acetic acid.

$CH_3 \cdot COOH$ acetic acid.

C₄H₉·COOH   valeric acid.

$C_4H_9 \cdot COOH$ valeric acid.

CHD   coronary heart disease.

Ch.D.   abbreviation for L. *Chirur′giae Doc′tor,* Doctor of Surgery.

ChE   cholinesterase.

Cheadle's disease (che′delz) [Walter Butler *Cheadle,* London pediatrician, 1835–1910]   infantile scurvy.

check-bite (chek′bīt)   check bite; see under *bite.*

checkerboard (chek′er-bōrd)   in genetics, a grid with margins which shows the gametes of each parent (in the margins) and their possible progeny (in the squares); called also *Punnett square.*

cheek (chēk)   a fleshy protuberance, especially the fleshy portion of the side of the face; called also *bucca* [NA]. Also applied to the fleshy mucous-membrane covered side of the oral cavity (bucca cavum oris [NA]). **cleft c.,** facial cleft caused by developmental failure of union between the maxillary and primitive frontonasal processes.

cheesy (che′ze)   caseous, resembling cheese.

cheilectomy (ki-lek′to-me) [*cheil-* + Gr. *ektomē* excision]   1. excision of a lip.   2. the operation of chiseling off the irregular bony edges of a joint cavity that interfere with motion.

cheilectropion (ki″lek-tro′pe-on) [*cheil-* + *ectropion*]   eversion of the lip.

cheilitis (ki-li′tis) [*cheil-* + *-itis*]   inflammation affecting the lips. Spelled also *chilitis.* Cf. *cheilosis.* **actinic c.,**

painful swelling of the lip(s) and development of scaly crust and erosions on the vermilion border after overexposure to sun rays; it may be acute or chronic. Called also *solar c.* **angular c.,** perlèche. **apostematous c.,** see *c. glandularis.* **commissural c.,** cheilitis affecting principally the angles (commissures) of the mouth. See also *perlèche.* **c. exfoliati′va,** persistent exfoliation of the lip caused by inflammation of the mucous membrane, similar to but not identical with dermatitis seborrheica. **c. glandula′ris,** a rare disease in which the lower lip becomes enlarged, firm, and finally everted, exposing the openings of the accessory salivary glands, which are inflamed and dilated, appearing as pinhead-sized red macules on the mucosa; the glands themselves are enlarged and sometimes nodular. The condition may be associated with carcinoma of the lip. It occurs in three basic types: The *simple type* is characterized by multiple painless, pin-head-sized lesions, with central depressions and dilated canals, and may develop into either of the other two types. The *superficial suppurative type* is characterized by painless swelling, induration, crusting, and superficial and deep ulcerations of the lip; called also *Baelz's disease.* The *deep suppurative type* is a basically deep-seated infection, with abscesses and fistulous tracts that eventually form scars; called also *apostematous c., c. glandularis apostematosa,* and *myxadenitis labialis.* **c. glandula′ris apostemato′sa,** see *c. glandularis.* **c. granulomato′sa,** an inflammation of the lips marked by granular papules. **impetiginous c.,** impetigo of the lips. **migrating c.,** perlèche. **solar c.,** actinic c. **c. venena′ta,** that due to a toxic substance.

cheil(o)-, [Gr. *cheilos* lip] a combining form denoting relationship to the lip, or to an edge.

cheiloangioscopy (ki″lo-an″je-os′ko-pe) [*cheilo-* + Gr. *angeion* vessel + *skopein* to examine] microscopical observation of the circulation in the blood vessels of the lip.

cheilocarcinoma (ki″lo-kar″sĭ-no′mah) carcinoma of the lip.

cheilognathopalatoschisis (ki″lo-na″tho-pal″ah-tos′kĭ-sis) cheilognathouranoschisis.

cheilognathoprosoposchisis (ki″lo-na″tho-pros″o-pos′kĭ-sis) [*cheilo-* + Gr. *gnathos* jaw + *prosopon* face + *schisis* cleft] a developmental anomaly characterized by presence of an oblique facial cleft continuing into the lip and upper jaw.

cheilognathoschisis (ki″lo-na-thos′kĭ-sis) [*cheilo-* + Gr. *gnathos* jaw + *schisis* cleft] a developmental anomaly that is characterized by the presence of a cleft in the lip and jaw.

cheilognathouranoschisis (ki″lo-na″tho-u-rah-nos′kĭ-sis) [*cheilo-* + Gr. *gnathos* jaw + *ouranos* palate + *schisis* cleft] a developmental anomaly characterized by the presence of a cleft in the lip, upper jaw, and palate.

cheilophagia (ki″lo-fa′je-ah) [*cheilo-* + Gr. *phagein* to eat] biting of the lips.

cheiloplasty (ki′lo-plas″te) [*cheilo-* + Gr. *plassein* to form] plastic surgery of the lip; labioplasty.

cheilorrhaphy (ki-lor′ah-fe) [*cheilo-* + Gr. *rhaphē* suture] the operation of suturing the lip, as in surgical repair of a congenitally cleft lip.

cheiloschisis (ki-los′kĭ-sis) [*cheilo-* + Gr. *schisis* cleft] cleft lip.

cheilosis (ki-lo′sis) [*cheil-* + *-osis*] a noninflammatory condition of the lips characterized by chapping and fissuring. Cf. *cheilitis.* **angular c.,** perlèche.

cheilostomatoplasty (ki″lo-sto-mat′o-plas″te) [*cheilo-* + Gr. *stoma* mouth + *plassein* to form] plastic restoration of the mouth and lips.

cheilotomy (ki-lot′o-me) [*cheilo-* + Gr. *tomē* a cutting] incision into the lip.

Cheiracanthium (ki″rah-can′the-um) *Chiracanthium.*

Cheiracanthus (ki″rah-kan′thus) *gnathostoma.*

cheiragra (ki-rag′rah) [*cheir-* + Gr. *agra* seizure] gout of the hand, especially tophaceous gout with torsion of the fingers.

cheiralgia (ki-ral′je-ah) pain in the hand. **c. paresthet′ica,** isolated neuritis of the superficial ramus of the radial nerve.

cheirarthritis (ki″rar-thri′tis) [*cheir-* + *arthritis*] inflammation of the joints of the hand and fingers.

cheir(o)- [Gr. *cheir* hand] a combining form denoting relationship to the hand. For words beginning with this root, see also those beginning *chir(o)-.*

cheirobrachialgia (ki″ro-bra″ke-al′je-ah) a syndrome of paresthesia and pain in the arm, hand, and fingers; called also *cheirobrachialgia paresthetica.*

cheirocinesthesia (ki″ro-sin″es-the′ze-ah) cheirokinesthesia.

cheirognomy (ki-rog′no-me) [*cheiro-* + Gr. *gnomōn* judge] the study of the hand as a guide to characteristics of the individual.

cheirognostic (ki″rog-nos′tik) [*cheiro-* + Gr. *gnostikos* knowing] pertaining to or characterized by the ability to distinguish stimuli as originating on the right or the left side of the body.

cheirokinesthesia (ki″ro-kin″es-the′ze-ah) the subjective perception of the movements of the hand, especially in writing.

cheirokinesthetic (ki″ro-kin″es-thet′ik) pertaining to or characterized by cheirokinesthesia.

cheirology (ki-rol′o-je) dactylology.

cheiromegaly (ki-ro-meg′ah-le) abnormal enlargement of the hands.

cheiroplasty (ki′ro-plas″te) [*cheiro-* + Gr. *plassein* to form] plastic surgery on the hand.

cheiropodalgia (ki″ro-po-dal′je-ah) [*cheiro-* + Gr. *pous* foot + *algos* pain] pain in the hands and feet.

cheiropompholyx (ki″ro-pom′fo-liks) [*cheiro-* + Gr. *pompholyx* a bubble] pompholyx.

cheiroscope (ki′ro-skōp) [*cheiro-* + *-scope*] an instrument used in the training of binocular vision, by which the image of a test object seen reflected in a mirror by the sound eye is projected by the other eye to a drawing board, where it is traced with a pencil guided by the hand of the subject.

cheirospasm (ki′ro-spazm) [*cheiro-* + Gr. *spasmos* spasm] spasm of the muscles of the hand.

chelate (ke′lāt) [Gr. *chēlē* claw] to combine with a metal in complexes in which the metal is part of a ring. By extension, a chemical compound in which a metallic ion is sequestered and firmly bound into a ring within the chelating molecule. Chelates are used in chemotherapeutic treatments for metal poisoning.

chelation (ke-la′shun) combination with a metal in complexes in which the metal is part of a ring.

chelen (ke′len) ethyl chloride.

chelicera, (ke-lis′er-ah), pl. chelic′erae [Gr. *chēlē* claw + *keras* horn] a pair of pincer-like head appendages of spiders, scorpions, and other arachnids. In certain arthropods, such as spiders, mites, and scorpions, anterior chelicerae serve as feeding appendages.

Chel-Iron (kēl′i-ron) trademark for preparations of ferrocholinate.

cheloid (ke′loid) keloid.

cheloma (ke-lo′mah) keloid.

chelonian (ke-lo′ne-an) [Gr. *chelōnē* tortoise] pertaining to turtles and tortoises, (order Chelonia).

chemabrasion (kēm-ah-bra′shun) superficial destruction and exfoliation of the epidermis and the upper layer of the dermis by application of a cauterant to the skin; done to remove scars, tattoos, pigmented nevi, etc. Called also *chemexfoliation.* See also *planing.*

chemanesia (kēm″ah-ne′ze-ah) the controlled and reversible amnesia induced by a drug, as in certain anesthesia procedures.

chemexfoliation (kēm′eks-fo′le-a″shun) chemabrasion.

chemi- see *chem(o)-.*

chemiatric (kem″e-at′rik) iatrochemical.

chemiatry (kem′e-ah-tre) iatrochemistry.

chemical (kem′ĭ-kal) 1. of, or pertaining to, chemistry. 2. a substance composed of chemical elements, or obtained by chemical processes.

chemic(o)- see *chem(o)-.*

chemicobiological (kem″ĭ-ko-bi″o-loj′e-kal) biochemical.

chemicocautery (kem″ĭ-ko-kaw′ter-e) chemocautery.

chemicogenesis (kem″ĭ-ko-jen′ĕ-sis) [*chemistry* + Gr. *gene-*

sis production] development of an ovum by chemical stimulation.

chemicophysical (kem″ĭ-ko-fiz′e-kal) pertaining to chemistry and physics; pertaining to physical chemistry.

chemicophysiologic (kem″ĭ-ko-fiz″e-o-loj′ik) pertaining to physiology and chemistry.

chemiluminescense (kem″ĭ-loo″mĭ-nes′ens) chemoluminescence.

chemiosmosis (kem″e-os-mo′sis) chemosmosis.

chemiosmotic (kem″e-o-os-mot′ik) chemosmotic.

chemiotaxis (kem″e-o-tak′sis) chemotaxis.

chemiotherapy (kem″e-o-ther′ah-pe) chemotherapy.

chemism (kem′izm) chemical activity; chemical property or relationship.

chemisorption (kem″ĭ-sorp′shun) the chemical adsorption of one material by another, resulting in the production of a different chemical compound.

chemist (kem′ist) 1. an individual skilled in chemistry. 2. (British) a pharmacist.

chemistry (kem′is-tre) [Gr. *chēmeia*] the science that treats of the elements and atomic relations of matter, and of the various compounds of the elements. **analytical c.,** chemistry that deals with analysis of different elements in a compound. **applied c.,** the application of chemistry to industry and the arts; called also *industrial c.* **biological c.,** biochemistry. **colloid c.,** chemistry dealing with the nature and composition of colloids. **ecological c.,** the study of those chemical compounds synthesized by plants that serve no metabolic purpose but which, by reason of their toxic effect on insects and higher animals, influence a community of interacting plants and animals. **forensic c.,** use of chemical knowledge in the solution of legal problems. **industrial c.,** applied c. **inorganic c.,** that branch of the science of chemistry which deals with compounds that do not occur in the plant or animal worlds; called also *mineral c.* **medical c.,** chemistry as it relates to medicine. **metabolic c.,** biochemistry. **mineral c.,** inorganic c. **organic c.,** that branch of chemistry which deals with compounds that contain carbon. **pharmaceutical c.,** chemistry that deals with the composition and preparation of substances used in treatment of patients or diagnostic studies. **physical c.,** that branch of chemistry which deals with the relationship of chemical and physical properties. **physiological c.,** biochemistry. **structural c.,** chemical study of the structure of molecules. **surface c.,** in the field of catalysis, the study of chemical reactions between the outermost layer of atoms of a solid and molecules brought to the solid surface in the liquid or gaseous state. **synthetic c.,** that branch of chemistry which deals with the building up of chemical compounds from simpler substances or from the elements.

chem(o)- chemi-, chemic(o)- [Gr. *chēmeia* alchemy] a combining form denoting relationship to chemistry, or to a chemical.

chemoattractant (ke″mo-ah-trak′tant) a chemotactic factor that induces positive chemotaxis.

chemoautotroph (ke″mo-aw′to-trōf) a chemoautotrophic microorganism.

chemoautotrophic (ke″mo-aw″to-trōf′ik) [*chemo-* + Gr. *trophē* nutrition] requiring for growth only inorganic compounds with carbon dioxide as the sole source of carbon (autotrophic), and oxidizing inorganic chemical compounds as the source of energy; said of certain bacteria and protozoa. Cf. *photoautotrophic.*

chemobiotic (ke″mo-bi-ot′ik) the combination of a chemotherapeutic agent and an antibiotic, as of one or more of the sulfonamide compounds with penicillin.

chemocautery (ke″mo-kaw′ter-e) destruction of tissue by application of a caustic chemical substance.

chemocephalia (ke″mo-sĕ-fa′le-ah) chamaecephaly.

chemocephaly (ke″mo-sef′ah-le) chamaecephaly.

chemoceptor (ke′mo-sep-tor) chemoreceptor.

chemocoagulation (ke″mo-ko-ag″u-la′shun) coagulation or destruction of tissue by the application of chemicals.

chemodectoma (ke″mo-dek-to′mah) [*chemo-* + *dektos* to be received or accepted + *-oma*] any benign, chromaffin-negative tumor of the chemoreceptor system, such as a tumor of

the carotid, aortic, or tympanic body. Called also *nonchromaffin paraganglioma.*

chemodifferentiation (ke″mo-dif″er-en-she-a′shun) the invisible point of decision which foreruns and controls the actual differentiation of cells into the rudimentary organs of the embryo.

chemodynesis (ke″mo-di′nĕ-sis) the initiation of cytoplasmic streaming in plant cells by chemicals.

chemoheterotroph (ke″mo-het′er-o-trōf″) a chemoheterotrophic organism.

chemoheterotrophic (ke″mo-het″er-o-trōf′ik) heterotrophic; requiring preformed organic compounds as a source of carbon and oxidizing organic compounds as a source of energy.

chemohormonal (ke″mo-hor-mo′nal) pertaining to drugs having hormone activity.

chemoimmunology (ke″mo-im-u-nol′o-je) immunochemistry.

chemokinesis (ke″mo-ki-ne′sis) [*chemo-* + Gr. *kinēsis* motion] increased activity of an organism due to the presence of a chemical substance.

chemokinetic (ke″mo-ki-net′ik) pertaining to or exhibiting chemokinesis.

chemolithotroph (ke″mo-lith′o-trōf) a chemolithotrophic organism.

chemolithotrophic (ke″mo-lith″o-trōf′ik) chemoautotrophic; utilizing carbon dioxide as the sole source of carbon and deriving energy from the oxidation of inorganic compounds.

chemoluminescence (ke″mo-loo″mĭ-nes′ens) luminescence produced by the direct transformation of chemical energy into light energy.

chemolysis (ke-mol′ĭ-sis) [*chemo-* + Gr. *lysis* solution] chemical decomposition.

chemomorphosis (ke″mo-mor-fo′sis) [*chemo-* + Gr. *morphē* form] change of form due to chemical action.

chemonucleolysis (ke″mo-nu″kle-ol′ĭ-sis) [*chemo-* + *nucleo-* + *lysis*] dissolution of the nucleus pulposus of an intervertebral disk by injection of a chemolytic agent, e.g., the enzyme chymopapain; used especially in the treatment of herniation of a disk.

chemo-organotroph (ke″mo-or′gah-no-trōf″) a chemoorganotrophic organism.

chemo-organotrophic (ke″mo-or″gah-no-trōf′ik) heterotrophic; requiring preformed organic compounds as a source of carbon and oxidizing organic compounds as a source of energy; said of bacteria.

chemopallidectomy (ke″mo-pal″ĭ-dek′to-me) [*chemo-* + *pallidum* + *ektomē* excision] destruction of a portion of the globus pallidus by the introduction of a chemical agent.

chemopallidothalamectomy (ke″mo-pal″ĭ-do-thal″-ah-mek′to me) destruction of a portion of the globus pallidus and thalamus by the introduction of a chemical agent.

chemopharmacodynamic (ke″mo-far″mah-ko-di-nam′ik) denoting the relationship between chemical constitution and biologic or pharmacologic activity.

chemophysiology (ke″mo-fiz-i-ol′o-je) biochemistry.

chemoprophylaxis (ke″mo-pro″fi-lak′sis) [*chemo-* + Gr. *prophylax* an advance guard] use of a chemotherapeutic agent as a means of preventing development of a specific disease. **primary c.,** prophylactic use of a chemotherapeutic agent before infection has occurred in an individual. **secondary c.,** prophylactic use of a chemotherapeutic agent in an individual after infection has occurred (with *Mycobacterium tuberculosis,* for example) but before disease has become manifest.

chemopsychiatry (ke″mo-si-ki′ah-tre) the use of drugs in the treatment of mental and emotional disorders; psychopharmacology.

chemoreception (ke″mo-re-sep′shun) [*chemo-* + L. *receptio,* from *recipere* to receive] the process of being sensitive to or perceiving chemical stimuli in the surrounding medium.

chemoreceptor (ke″mo-re-sep′tor) 1. a receptor adapted for excitation by chemical substances, e.g., olfactory and gustatory receptors, or a sense organ, as the carotid body or the aortic (supracardial) bodies, which is sensitive to chemical changes in the blood stream, especially reduced oxygen content, and reflexly increases both respiration and blood pressure. See *receptor.* 2. a supposed group of atoms in cell protoplasm having the power of fixing chemicals, in the same way as bacterial poisons are fixed. Called also *chemoceptor*.

chemoresistance (ke″mo-re-zis′tans) specific resistance acquired by cells to the action of chemicals.

chemosensitive (ke″mo-sen′sĭ-tiv) sensitive to changes in chemical composition.

chemosensory (ke″mo-sen′so-re) relating to the perception of chemical substances, as in odor detection.

chemoserotherapy (ke″mo-se″ro-ther′ah-pe) the treatment of disease with both drugs and serum.

chemosis (ke-mo′sis) [Gr. *chēmōsis*] excessive edema of the ocular conjunctiva.

chemosmosis (ke″mos-mo′sis) chemical action taking place through an intervening membrane.

chemosmotic (ke″mos-mot′ik) pertaining to chemosmosis.

chemosorption (kem″o-sorp′shun) chemisorption.

chemosphere (ke′mo-sfēr) the layer of the upper atmosphere where photochemical reactions become important (30–80 km.).

chemostat (ke′mo-stat) an apparatus in which the environment is so controlled that bacterial populations are maintained in a steady state of continuous cell division in a constant environment.

chemosterilant (ke″mo-ster′ĭ-lant) a chemical compound the ingestion of which causes sterility of an organism; such compounds have been used as a means of controlling various insects and other pests by inducing sterility in the male.

chemosurgery (ke″mo-sur′jer-e) the destruction of tissue by chemical agents; originally applied to chemical fixation of malignant, gangrenous, or infected tissue, with the use of frozen sections to facilitate systematic microscopic control of the extent of ablation.

chemosynthesis (ke″mo-sin′the-sis) [*chemo-* + Gr. *synthesis* putting together] the synthesis of carbohydrate from carbon dioxide and water as a result of the energy derived from chemical reactions, rather than from absorbed light. Such synthesis is carried out by certain bacteria and algae. Cf. *photosynthesis*.

chemosynthetic (ke″mo-sin-thet′ik) pertaining to or characterized by chemosynthesis.

chemotactic (ke″mo-tak′tik) of or pertaining to chemotaxis.

chemotaxin (ke″mo-tak′sin) chemotactic factor.

chemotaxis (ke″mo-tak′sis) [*chemo-* + Gr. *taxis* arrangement] orientation of a cell along a chemical concentration gradient or movement in the direction of the gradient, either toward (positive chemotaxis) or away from (negative chemotaxis) the greater concentration of the substance, referred to as a chemotactic factor, chemotactin, or chemoattractant. Macrophages, neutrophils, eosinophils, and lymphocytes exhibit chemotaxis in response to a wide variety of substances released at sites of inflammatory reactions, including lymphokines, mediators released by basophils and mast cells, bacterial products, and C5a and other activated complement components. Cf. *chemokinesis*.

chemothalamectomy (ke″mo-thal-ah-mek′to-me) destruction of a portion of the thalamus by the introduction of a chemical agent.

chemotherapeutic (ke″mo-ther-ah-pu′tik) pertaining to chemotherapy.

chemotherapeutics (ke″mo-ther-ah-pu′tiks) chemotherapy.

chemotherapy (ke″mo-ther′ah-pe) the treatment of disease by chemical agents; first applied to use of chemicals that affect the causative organism unfavorably but do not harm the patient.

chemotic (ke-mot′ik) 1. pertaining to or affected with chemosis. 2. an agent that increases the production of lymph in the ocular conjunctiva.

chemotroph (ke′mo-trōf) a chemotrophic organism.

chemotrophic (ke″mo-trof′ik) deriving energy from the oxidation of organic (chemo-organotrophic) or inorganic (chemolithotrophic) compounds; said of bacteria. Cf. *phototrophic*.

chemotropic (ke″mo-trop′ik) of or pertaining to chemotropism.

chemotropism (ke-mot′ro-pizm) [*chemo-* + Gr. *tropos* a turning] tropism in response to a chemical stimulus.

chemurgy (kem′er-ge) [*chemo-* + Gr. *ergon* work] chemistry applied to the industrial use of raw organic products, especially agricultural products.

chenic acid (ke′nik) chenodeoxycholic acid.

chenodeoxycholate (ke″no-de-ok″sĭ-ko′lāt) the salt or dissociated form of chenodeoxycholic acid; see under *acid*.

chenodeoxycholic acid (ke″no-de-ok″se-kol′ic) 3α, 7α-dihydroxy-5β-cholan-24-oic acid, the third most abundant acid of human bile; it has gallstone-dissolving properties, probably because it suppresses synthesis of cholesterol by the liver, and is administered for this purpose. Called also *chenic acid* and *chenodiol*.

chenodeoxycholylglycine (ke″no-de-ok″se-ko′lil-gli′sēn) a bile salt, the glycine conjugate of chenodeoxycholic acid; called also *glycochenodeoxycholic acid*.

chenodeoxycholyltaurine (ke″no-de-ok″se-ko′lil-taw′rēn) a bile salt, the taurine conjugate of chenodeoxycholic acid; called also *taurochenodeoxycholic acid*.

chenodiol (ke″no-di′ōl) chenodeoxycholic acid.

Chenopodium (ke″no-po′de-um) a genus of herbs of the temperate regions of the world; see also under *oil*.

chenotherapy (ke″no-ther′ah-pe) treatment with chenodeoxycholic acid, as for dissolution of gallstones.

Cherchevski's (Cherchewski's) disease (sher-shev′skēz) [Mikhail *Cherchevski*, Russian physician] see under *disease*.

Cheron's serum (sha-rawz′) [Jules *Cheron*, French gynecologist, 1837–1900] see under *serum*.

cherry (cher′e) [L. *cerasus*] the name of various rosaceous trees and species of the genus *Prunus*; see *Prunus*. **choke c.,** *Prunus virginiana.* **c. laurel,** an Old World evergreen cherry tree, *Prunus laurocerasus* L. (Rosaceae); the source of a preparation (cherry laurel water) formerly used as an antispasmodic, sedative, and anodyne, and for cough. **rum c.,** *Prunus serotina.* **wild c.,** 1. *Prunus serotina.* 2. [USP] the carefully dried stem bark of *P. serotina*, used in a syrup as a flavored vehicle for drugs; called also *wild black cherry bark*. See also under *syrup*.

cherubism (cher′u-bizm) [*cherub* + *-ism*] hereditary and progressive bilateral swelling at the angle of the mandible, sometimes involving the entire jaw. The swelling imparts a cherubic look to the face, in some cases enhanced by upturning of the eyes. Called also *familial fibrous dysplasia of jaw* and *familial bilateral giant cell tumor*.

chest (chest) the thorax. **alar c.,** flat chest. **barrel c.,** a rounded, bulging chest with abnormal increase in the anteroposterior diameter, showing little movement on respiration; seen in emphysema and in kyphosis. **blast c.,** pulmonary concussion and hemorrhage occurring as the result of injury by a blast. **cobbler's c.,** a chest showing a sinking in at the lower end of the sternum. **flail c.,** one whose wall moves paradoxically with respiration, owing to multiple fractures of the ribs. **flat c.,** deformity of the chest in which it is flattened from front to back; called also *alar c.* and *pterygoid c.* **foveated c.,** funnel chest. **funnel c.,** a chest in which there is funnel-shaped depression in the middle of the anterior thoracic wall, the deepest part being in the sternum; called also *foveated c., funnel breast, pectus excavatum* or *recurvatum, koilosternia, chonechondrosternon,* and *trichterbrust.* **keeled c.,** pigeon breast. **paralytic c.,** a long and narrow chest with emaciation so that the ribs stand out sharply under the skin. **phthinoid c.,** the same as *flat chest;* so called as indicating a tubercular diathesis. **pigeon c.,** pigeon breast. **pterygoid c.,** flat chest. **tetrahedron c.,** a chest that suggests a solid with four sides, each an equilateral triangle, the chest projecting in a peak between the nipples.

chestnut (chest′nut) 1. *Castanea.* 2. one of the masses of horn on the medial surface of the forearm and on the distal part of the medial surface of the tarsus of horses. **horse c.,** *Aesculus.*

Cheyletiella (sha″lĕ-te-el′lah) a genus of nonburrowing mites, some species of which may cause a dermatosis in human beings. **C. bla′kei,** a species infesting the cat. **C. parasitov′orax,** a species infesting the rabbit. **C. yas′guri,** a species infesting the dog.

Cheyne-Stokes asthma, etc. (chān′stōks) [John *Cheyne*, Scottish physician, 1777–1836; William *Stokes*, Irish physician, 1804–1878] see *cardiac asthma,* under *asthma,* and see under *nystagmus, psychosis,* and *respiration.*

CHF congestive heart failure.

CHI₃ iodoform.

chi (ki) [X, χ] the twenty-second letter of the Greek alphabet.

χ chi, the twenty-second letter of the Greek alphabet.

χ² chi-squared; see under *distribution* and *tests*.

C₂H₅I ethyl iodide.

Chiari's network (reticulum), syndrome (disease) (ke-ar′ēz)[Hans von *Chiari*, Austrian pathologist, 1851–1916] see under *network*, and see *Budd-Chiari syndrome*, under *syndrome*.

Chiari-Arnold syndrome (ke-ar′e-ar′nold) [Hans von *Chiari; Julius Arnold*, Austrian pathologist, 1835–1915] Arnold-Chiari deformity.

Chiari-Frommel syndrome (disease) (ke-ar′e-from′el) [Johann Baptist *Chiari*, German obstetrician, 1817–1854; Richard *Frommel*, German gynecologist, 1854–1912] see under *syndrome*.

chiasm (ki′azm) [L., Gr. *chiasma*] a decussation or X-shaped crossing; see *chiasma*. **c. of digits of hand,** chiasma tendinum digitorum manus. **optic c.,** chiasma opticum. **tendinous c. of flexor digitorum sublimis muscle,** chiasma tendinum digitorum manus.

chiasma (ki-as′mah), pl. *chias′mata* [L.; Gr. a cross, crosspiece; from the shape of the letter *chi*, X] 1. a decussation or X-shaped crossing. 2. in genetics, the places where pairs of homologous chromatids remain in contact during late prophase to anaphase of the first meiotic division, indicating where an exchange of homologous segments has taken place between non-sister chromatids by crossing over. 3. in official anatomical nomenclature the crossing of two elements or structures, as the optic nerves. **c. op′ticum** [NA], the optic chiasm: the part of the hypothalamus formed by the decussation, or crossing, of the fibers of the optic nerve from the medial half of each retina; called also *optic decussation* and *decussation of optic nerve*. **c. ten′dinum digito′rum ma′nus** [NA], the crossing of the tendons of the flexor digitorum profundus through the tendons of the flexor digitorum sublimis; called also *chiasm of digits of hand* and *tendinous chiasm of flexor digitorum sublimis muscle*.

chiasmal (ki-az′mal) chiasmatic.

chiasmata (ki-az′mah-tah) [L.] plural of *chiasma*.

chiasmatic (ki-az-mat′ik) resembling a chiasm; crosswise.

chiasmatypy (ki-az′mah-ti″pe) [Gr. *chiasma* a crossing + *type*] crossing over.

chiasmic (ki-az′mik) chiasmatic.

chiasmometer (ki″az-mom′e-ter) chiastometer.

chiastometer (ki″as-tom′ĕ-ter) [Gr. *chiastos* crossed + *metron* measure] an apparatus for measuring any deviation of the optic axes from their normal parallelism; called also *chiasmometer*.

Chiba needle (che′bah) [*Chiba* University in Japan] see under *needle*.

chickenpox (chik′en-poks) varicella: a highly contagious infectious disease due to a herpesvirus, varicella-zoster virus, usually affecting children, spread by direct contact or the respiratory route via droplet nuclei, and characterized by the appearance on the skin and mucous membranes of successive crops of typical pruritic vesicular lesions that are easily broken and become scabbed, and generally accompanied by mild constitutional symptoms. It is relatively benign in children except in those with severe underlying disease, but adult infection may be complicated by pneumonia and encephalitis. See also *herpes zoster*.

chick-pea (chik′pe) the plant *Cicer arietinum* of Southern Europe whose seeds are used as food and may be toxic to certain individuals.

Chievitz's layer, organ (che′wits-ez) [Johan Henrik *Chievitz*, Danish anatomist, 1850–1901] see under *layer* and *organ*.

chigger (chig′er) the six-legged red larva of mites of the family Trombiculidae, which attach to the skin of their hosts, and whose bites produce a wheal, usually accompanied by intense itching and severe dermatitis. The habitat of these mites is tall grass and underbrush. *Eutrombicula alfreddugèsi* is the common chigger of the United States; *E. splendens* is a species found in southeastern localities; and *Trombicula autumnalis* is the chigger of Europe. Some

species in the Asiatic-Pacific region are vectors of the rickettsiae of scrub typhus. Chiggers are to be distinguished from chigoes. Called also *bête rouge, harvest mite, mower's mite, red bug,* and *red mites.*

chigo (chig′o) chigoe.

chigoe (chig′o) the flea, *Tunga* (*Dermatophilus, Sarcopsylla, Pulex*) *penetrans,* of tropical and subtropical America and Africa. The pregnant female flea burrows into the skin of the feet (often beneath the nail), legs, or other part of the body, causing intense irritation and ulceration, and sometimes leading to spontaneous amputation of a digit. Chigoes are to be distinguished from chiggers. Called also *burrowing flea, chigo, jigger,* and *sand flea.*

chikungunya (chik″un-gun′yah) [Swahili "that which bends up"] a self-limited dengue-like disease caused by an alphavirus transmitted chiefly by mosquitoes of the genus Aedes, principally occurring in Southeast Asia and Africa; it has been associated with hemorrhagic fever.

Chilaiditi's sign, syndrome (ke-lah-the′tez) [Demetrios *Chilaiditi,* Austrian-born physician, born 1883] see under *sign* and *syndrome.*

chilblain, chilblains (chil′blān, chil′blānz) [L. *pernio*] a recurrent localized erythema and doughy subcutaneous swelling caused by exposure to cold associated with dampness, and accompanied by pruritus and a burning sensation, usually involving the hands, feet, ears, and face in children, the legs and toes in women, and the hands and fingers in men. Called also *erythema pernio* and *pernio.*

child (chīld) the human young, from infancy to puberty. **preschool c.,** a child between two and six years of age. **school c.,** a child between six and ten to twelve years of age.

childbed (chīld′bed) the puerperal state or period.

childbirth (chīld′birth) the act or process of giving birth to a child; see *labor.*

childhood (chīld′hood) the period of life of the human young generally considered to extend from infancy to puberty.

chilitis (ki-li′tis) cheilitis.

chill (chil) a shivering or shaking; an attack of involuntary contractions of the voluntary muscles, accompanied by a sense of cold and pallor of the skin; called also *ague.* **brass c., brazier's c.,** see *brassfounder's fever.* **creeping c.,** a chilly sensation, without any definite tremor or chattering of the teeth. **nervous c.,** a tremor due to some form of excitement and unaccompanied by alteration of temperature. **shaking c.,** a chill in which there is a definite tremor. **spelter c's,** see under *fever.* **urethral c.,** a chilly sensation, with or without tremor, sometimes following the passage of a catheter. **zinc c.,** spelter's fever.

chil(o)- for words beginning thus, see also words beginning *cheilo-.*

Chilognatha (ki-log′nah-thah) an order of arthropods of the class Diplopoda, superclass Myriapoda, embracing the millipedes.

chilomastigiasis (ki″lo-mas″tĭ-gi′ah-sis) infection with *Chilomastix.*

Chilomastix (ki″lo-mas′tiks) [*chilo-* + Gr. *mastix* whip] a genus of pear- or lemon-shaped parasitic protozoa (order Retortamonadida, class Zoomastigophorea), having three flagella and a single nucleus, beside which the cytostome is located, and found in the intestines of various vertebrates, including humans. All species are considered nonpathogenic or only slightly so, but one species, *C. mesnili,* has been associated with rare cases of watery diarrhea.

chilomastixiasis (ki″lo-mas″tik-si′ah-sis) chilomastigiasis.

Chilopoda (ki-lop′ŏ-dah) [Gr. *cheilos* lip + *pous* foot] a class of the phylum Arthropoda, embracing the centipedes.

chimaera (ki-me′rah) chimera.

chimera (ki-me′rah) [Gr. *chimaira* a mythological fire-spouting monster with a lion's head, goat's body, and serpent's tail] an individual organism whose body contains cell populations derived from different zygotes, of the same or of different species, occurring spontaneously, as in twins (blood group chimeras), or produced artificially, as an organism which develops from combined portions of different embryos, or one in which tissues or cells of another organism have been introduced. Cf. *mosaic.* **heterologous c.,** a chimera in which the foreign cells or tissues are derived from an organism of a different species. **homologous c.,** a chimera in which the foreign cells or tissues are derived from an organism of the same species but of a different genotype. **isologous c.,** a chimera in which the foreign cells or tissues are derived from a different organism of the same genotype, such as an identical twin. **radiation c.,** an organism that survives with immunologic characteristics of host and donor after a bone marrow graft from an antigenically different donor, the host having first been subjected to sublethal whole-body irradiation so that there is no immune response to foreign cells by the donor.

chimerism (ki-mēr′izm) the quality of being a chimera; in genetics, the presence in an individual of cells of different origin, as of blood cells derived from a dizygotic co-twin. Cf. *mosaicism.*

chimpanzee (chim-pan′ze, chim-pan-ze′) an anthropoid ape, *Pan troglodytes,* inhabiting the tropical rain forests of Africa, used for experimental purposes because of its susceptibility to some of the diseases of man and in behavioral studies because of its high level of intelligence.

chin (chin) the anterior prominence of the lower jaw; the mentum [NA]. **galoche c.** (gah-losh′) [Fr. "galosh"], a long pointed chin.

chinacrine (kin′ah-krin) quinacrine.

chincap (chin′kap) an extraoral orthodontic appliance consisting of a caplike device fitted over the chin, which is connected to the headgear by elastics for the purpose of exerting upward and backward force on the mandible in the treatment of prognathism.

chiniofon (kin′e-o-fon) a canary yellow powder, containing 26.5–29.0 per cent iodine, formerly used as an antiprotozoan in amebic dysentery.

chionablepsia (ki″o-nah-blep′se-ah) [Gr. *chiōn* snow + *ablepsia* blindness] snow blindness.

chip (chip) a small piece, as of something broken off. **bone c's,** small pieces of bone, usually cancellous, generally used to fill in bony defects to facilitate recalcification.

Chiracanthium (ki″rah-kan′the-um) a genus of venomous spiders, two species of which, *C. inclu′sum* and *C. diver′sium,* have produced local reactions in man in California and Hawaii, respectively.

chiral (ki′ral) exhibiting chirality.

chirality (ki-ral′ĭ-te) [Gr. *cheir* hand] the property of handedness, of not being superimposable on a mirror image; the handedness of an asymmetric molecule, as specified by its optical rotation or absolute configuration.

chir(o)- [Gr. *cheir* hand] a combining form denoting relationship to the hand; for words beginning thus, see also those beginning *cheir*(o)-.

chirobrachialgia (ki″ro-bra″ke-al′je-ah) cheirobrachialgia.

chirognostic (ki″rog-nos′tik) cheirognostic.

chiromegaly (ki″ro-meg′ah-le) cheiromegaly.

Chironomidae (ki″ro-nom′ĭ-de) a family of the suborder Nematocera, order Diptera, that comprises the true midges.

Chironomus (ki-ron′o-mus) a genus of gnatlike flies noted for their giant chromosomes.

chiroplasty (ki′ro-plas″te) cheiroplasty.

chiropodalgia (ki″ro-po-dal′je-ah) cheiropodalgia.

chiropodical (ki″re-pod′ĭ-kal) pertaining to chiropody (now called *podiatry*).

chiropodist (ki-rop′o-dist) podiatrist.

chiropody (ki-rop′o-de) podiatry.

chiropractic (ki″ro-prak′tik) [*chiro-* + Gr. *prassein* to do] a science of applied neurophysiologic diagnosis based on the theory that health and disease are life processes related to the function of the nervous system: irritation of the nervous system by mechanical, chemical, or psychic factors is the cause of disease; restoration and maintenance of health depend on normal function of the nervous system. Diagnosis is the identification of these noxious irritants and treatment is their removal by the most conservative method.

chiropractor (ki″ro-prak′tor) a practitioner of chiropractic.

chiropraxis (ki″ro-prak′sis) chiropractic.

chiroscope (ki′ro-skōp) cheiroscope.

chirospasm (ki′ro-spazm) cheirospasm.

chirurgenic (ki″rur-jen′ik) [*chirur*gery + Gr. *gennan* to produce] arising as a result of a surgical procedure.

chirurgeon (ki-rur′jun) archaic term for a surgeon.

chirurgery (ki-rur′jer-e) [L. *chirurgia,* from Gr. *cheir* hand + *ergon* work] archaic term for surgery.

chirurgic (ki-rur′jik) archaic term for surgical.

chisel (chis′l) 1. a wedge-like instrument with a cutting edge at the end of the blade. 2. a dental instrument, the cutting edge of which is in line with the center of the handle; used for planing or smoothing a surface, as during cavity preparation. **periodontal c.,** a straight instrument that curves slightly as the blade extends from the shank, the straight cutting edge at the end of the instrument being beveled at a 45° angle. Used chiefly for scaling the proximal surfaces of teeth too closely spaced to permit the use of other scalers. Called also *chisel scaler.*

chi-squared (ki′skwärd) see under *distribution* and *tests.*

chitin (ki′tin) [Gr. *chitōn* tunic] a white, insoluble, horny polysaccharide, $C_{30}H_{50}O_{19}N_4$, the principal constituent of the shells of arthropods and the shards of beetles and found in certain fungi. On hydrolysis it yields a linear homopolymer of β-(1→4)-2-acetamido-2-deoxy-D-glucose (an acetyl glucosamine). Next to cellulose, it is the most abundant natural polysaccharide.

chitinous (kit′ĭ-nus) composed of or of the nature of chitin.

chitobiose (ki″to-bi′ōs) a disaccharide composed of two glucosamine units, obtained by hydrolysis of de-acetylated chitin (chitosan).

chitosan (ki′to-san) a polysaccharide composed of repeating glucosamine units; obtained by de-acetylation of chitin and used in the preparation of chitobiose.

chitose (ki′tōs) a sugar, 2,5-anhydro-D-mannose, $C_6H_{12}O$, formed by the reduction of chitonic acid.

chitotriose (ki″to-tri′ōs) a trisaccharide composed of three glucosamine units; obtained from chitosan by hydrolysis.

chiufa (che-oo′fah) a gangrenous inflammation of the colon and rectum occurring in mountainous regions of South America and South Africa.

chlamydemia (klah-mĭ-de′me-ah) the presence of chlamydiae in the blood.

Chlamydia (klah-mid′e-ah) [Gr. *chlamys* cloak] a genus of bacteria of the family Chlamydiaceae, order Chlamydiales, occurring as gram-negative, coccoid organisms that multiply only within a host cell and have a unique growth cycle (see *Chlamydiaceae*). They are common pathogens of animals and cause a variety of diseases in humans. Called also *PLT group* and, formerly, *Bedsonia, Chlamydozoon,* and *Miyagawanella.* **C. psitta′ci,** a species, various strains of which cause psittacosis in man and psittacine birds and ornithosis in nonpsittacine birds; pneumonitis in cattle, sheep, swine, cats, goats, and horses; epizootic bovine abortion and enzootic abortion of ewes; enteritis of calves; sporadic encephalomyelitis of calves; epizootic chlamydiosis of hares and muskrats; and conjunctivitis of cattle, sheep, and guinea pigs. **C. tracho′matis,** a species occuring predominantly as a human pathogen, causing trachoma, inclusion conjunctivitis (or inclusion blennorrhea), "nonspecific" urethritis, proctitis, mouse pneumonitis, and lymphogranuloma venereum. Called also *TRIC group.*

chlamydia (klah-mid′e-ah), pl. *chlamyd′iae.* Any member of the genus *Chlamydia.*

Chlamydiaceae (klah-mid″e-a′se-e) a family of bacteria of the order Chlamydiales consisting of small coccoid microorganisms that have a unique, obligately intracellular developmental cycle and are incapable of synthesizing ATP. Infection occurs when the small, rigid-walled extracellular form (elementary body) enters the cell and changes into a larger, thin-walled form (initial body) that divides by fission. The daughter cells thus formed reorganize and condense to become elementary bodies that then infect other cells. The organisms are parasites of humans and other vertebrates, capable of producing a variety of diseases. They have also been found in arthropods. The family contains the genus *Chlamydia.*

chlamydiae (klah-mid′e-e) plural of *chlamydia.*

chlamydial (klah-mid′e-al) pertaining to or caused by *Chlamydia.*

Chlamydiales (klah-mid′e-al-ēz) an order of bacteria made up of coccoid, gram-negative, parasitic microorganisms that multiply only within the cytoplasm of vertebrate host cells by a unique developmental cycle. It includes the family Chlamydiaceae.

chlamydiosis (klah-mid″e-o′sis) any infection or disease caused by species of *Chlamydia*.

Chlamydobacteriaceae (klah-mi″do-bak-te″re-a′se-e) in former systems of classification, a family of bacteria made up of the genera *Leptothrix*, *Sphaerotilus*, and *Toxothrix*.

Chlamydobacteriales (klah-mi″do-bak-te″re-a′lēz) in former systems of classification, an order of bacteria made up of nonpigmented filamentous bacteria.

Chlamydodontina (klah-mid″o-don-ti′nah) [Gr. *chlamys* cloak + *odous* tooth] a suborder of ciliate protozoa (order Cyrtophorida, superorder Phyllopharyngidea), characterized by the presence of thigmotactic ciliature on the ventral body surface without a specialized glandlike adhesive organelle, a broad, dorsoventrally flattened body with the ventral surface in contact with the substrate, and a heteromerous macronucleus; they are free living, commensal, or parasitic in freshwater fishes.

Chlamydomonas (klah-mid″do-mo′nas) [Gr. *chlamys* cloak + *monas* unit] a genus of plantlike, biflagellate, solitary protozoa (order Volvocida, class Phytomastigophorea).

chlamydospore (klam′ĭ-do-spōr″) [Gr. *chlamys* cloak + *spore*] a thick-walled intercalary or terminal asexual spore formed by the rounding-up of a cell; it is not shed. See *spore*. Cf. *condium*.

Chlamydozoaceae (klam″ĭ-do″zo-a′se-e) Chlamydiaceae.

Chlamydozoon (klam″ĭ-do-zo′on) *Chlamydia*.

chloasma (klo-az′mah) [Gr. *chloazein* to be green] melasma. **c. hepat′icum,** a term formerly used to refer to circumscribed facial hyperpigmentation resembling melasma that may occur as a cutaneous manifestation of chronic liver disease.

chlophedianol hydrochloride (klo″fĕ-di′ah-nol) chemical name: 2-chloro-α-[(dimethylamino)ethyl]-α-phenylbenzenemethanol hydrochloride. An antitussive agent, $C_{17}H_{20}ClNO \cdot HCl$, occurring as a white, crystalline powder; administered orally.

chloracetic acid (klor″ah-se′tik) chloroacetic acid.

chloracetization (klor-as″e-tĭ-za′shun) the production of local anesthesia by application of equal parts of chloroform and glacial acetic acid; no longer used.

chloracne (klor-ak′ne) an acneiform eruption caused by exposure to chlorine compounds. Called also *chlorine acne*.

chloral (klo′ral) [*chlorine* + *-al*] 1. chemical name: trichloroacetaldehyde. A colorless, oily liquid, $Cl_3C \cdot CHO$, having a pungent, irritating odor, and prepared by the mutual action of alcohol and chlorine. It is used in the manufacture of chloral hydrate and DDT. 2. chloral hydrate. **c. beta-ine,** an adduct formed by the reaction of chloral hydrate with betaine, occurring as a white, crystalline powder, having actions and uses similar to those of chloral hydrate but having the advantage of eliminating undesirable gastrointestinal symptoms sometimes associated with chloral hydrate; administered orally. **butyl c.,** see *butylchloral hydrate*. **c. carmine,** a staining fluid made of carmine, 0.05 gm.; hydrochloric acid, 30 minims; alcohol, 20 cc.; and chloral hydrate, 25 gm. **c. hydrate** [USP], chemical name: 2,2,2-trichloro-1,1-ethanediol. A hypnotic and sedative, $C_2H_3Cl_3O_2$, occurring as colorless, transparent, or white crystals; administered orally.

chloralism (klo′ral-izm) a morbid condition caused by excessive use of chloral.

chloralization (klo″ral-ĭ-za′shun) 1. chloralism. 2. formerly, anesthesia by the use of chloral.

chloralose (klo′rah-lōs) chemical name: 1,2,O-(2,2,2-trichloroethylidene)-α-D-glucofuranose. A compound of chloral and glucose, $C_8H_{11}Cl_3O_6$, which has been used as a hypnotic, but is primarily used as a surgical anesthetic in laboratory animals, rodenticide for mice, and bird repellent on grain. Called also *α-chloralose*.

chlorambucil (klor-am′bu-sil) [USP] a cytotoxic alkylating agent of the nitrogen mustard group, used as an antineoplastic, primarily for treatment of chronic lymphocytic leukemia and Waldenström's macroglobulinemia, and also for Hodgkin's disease, lymphosarcoma, and ovarian

carcinoma; the major side effect is bone marrow depression.

chloramine-T (klo′rah-mēn) chemical name: N-chloro-4-methylbenzenesulfonamide sodium salt. A chlorine derivative, $C_7H_7ClNNaO_2S$, which has been used in solution as a topical antiseptic to irrigate and dress wounds and as a mouthwash, and has been used to sterilize drinking water.

chloramphenicol (klo″ram-fen′ĭ-kol) [USP] chemical name: [R-(R*,R*)]-2,2-dichloro-N-[2-hydroxy-1-(hydroxymethyl)-2-(4- nitrophenyl)ethyl]acetamide. A broad-spectrum antibiotic, $C_{11}H_{12}Cl_2N_2O_5$, originally derived from *Streptomyces venezuelae* and later shown to be elaborated by other spirochetes, and produced synthetically. It occurs as fine, white to grayish white or yellowish white, needle-like crystals or elongated plates, and is effective against rickettsiae, gram-positive and gram-negative bacteria, and certain spirochetes, being used especially in the treatment of typhus and other rickettsial infections and in typhoid, shigellosis, and related enteric diseases; used as an antibacterial, administered orally or applied topically to the conjunctiva, or as an antirickettsial, administered orally. **c. palmitate** [USP], the monopalmitic ester of chloramphenicol, $C_{27}H_{42}Cl_2N_2O_6$, occurring as a fine, white, unctuous, crystalline powder, having the same actions and uses as the base; administered orally. **c. sodium succinate,** the sodium succinate derivative of chloramphenicol, $C_{15}H_{15}Cl_2N_2NaO_8$, occurring as a light yellow powder, having the same actions and uses as the base; administered intravenously. Sterile chloramphenicol sodium [USP] conforms to FDA regulations concerning antibiotic drugs.

chlorate (klo′rāt) any salt of chloric acid.

chlorazanil hydrochloride (klo-rah′zah-nil) chemical name: N-(4-chlorophenyl)-1,3,5-triazine-2,4-diamine monohydrochloride; a diuretic, $C_9H_8ClN_5HCl$.

chlorbutol (klōr-bu′tol) chlorobutanol.

chlorcyclizine hydrochloride (klōr-si′klĭ-zēn) [USP] chemical name: 1-[(4-chlorophenyl)phenylmethyl]-4-methylpiperazine monohydrochloride. An antihistaminic, $C_{18}H_{21}ClN_2 \cdot HCl$, occurring as white, crystalline powder; administered orally.

chlordan (klōr′dan) chlordane.

chlordane (klōr′dan) a poisonous substance of the chlorinated hydrocarbon group, used as an insecticide; human poisoning may occur by percutaneous absorption, ingestion, or inhalation.

chlordantoin (klōr-dan′to-in) chemical name: 5-(1-ethylpentyl)-3-[(trichloromethyl)thio]-2,4-imidazolidinedione. An antifungal agent, $C_{11}H_{17}Cl_3N_2O_2S$, effective against various fungi, including *Candida albicans*; used topically in the treatment of fungal infections of the vulvovaginal region and of the skin.

chlordiazepoxide (klōr″di-az″ĕ-pok′sīd) [USP] chemical name: 7-chloro-N-methyl-5-phenyl-3H-1,4-benzodiazepin-2-amine-4-oxide. One of the benzodiazepine tranquilizers, $C_{16}H_{14}ClN_3O$, occurring as a yellow, crystalline powder; administered orally in the treatment of conditions in which anxiety, tension, and apprehension are prominent symptoms, in acute anxiety, and in chronic alcoholism or alcohol withdrawal. **c. hydrochloride** [USP], the monohydrochloride salt of chlordiazepoxide, $C_{16}H_{21}ClN_2 \cdot HCl$, occurring as a white, or almost white, crystalline powder; used for the same purposes as the base, administered orally, intravenously, or intramuscularly.

chlordimorine hydrochloride (klōr-dim′or-ēn) chemical name: 4-[3-[(3-chloro-4-biphenylyl)oxy]propyl]morpholine hydrochloride; an antifungal agent, $C_{19}H_{22}ClNO_2$.

Chlorella (klo-rel′ah) a genus of fresh-water green algae which are the source of chlorellin and are used in studies of photosynthesis.

chlorellin (klo-rel′in) a bacteriostatic substance derived from fresh water algae of the genus *Chlorella*.

chloremia (klo-re′me-ah) [Gr. *chlōros* green + *haima* blood + *-ia*] 1. chlorosis. 2. hyperchloremia.

chlorenchyma (klo-ren′kĭ-mah) the chlorophyll-bearing tissue of plants.

chloretic (klo-ret′ik) an agent that accelerates the flow of bile.

Chloretone (klo′re-tōn) trademark for a preparation of chlorobutanol.

chlorguanide (klōr-gwan′īd) proguanil.

chlorhexidine (klōr-heks′ĭ-dēn) chemical name: N,N''-bis(4-chlorophenyl)-3,12-diimino-2,4-11,13-tetraazatetradecanediimidamide. An antibacterial, $C_{22}H_{30}Cl_2N_{10}$, effective against a wide variety of gram-negative and gram-positive organisms. **c. acetate,** the diacetate salt of chlorhexidine, $C_{22}H_{30}Cl_2N_{10}O_4 \cdot 2C_2H_4O_2$, occurring as a white, crystalline powder, having the same actions as the base; used mainly as a preservative for eye-drops. **c. gluconate,** the digluconate salt of chlorhexidine, $C_{22}H_{30}Cl_2N_{10} \cdot 2C_6H_{12}O_7$, having the same actions as the base; used as a topical anti-infective for the skin and mucous membranes. **c. hydrochloride,** the dihydrochloride salt of chlorhexidine, $C_{22}H_{30}Cl_2N_{10} \cdot 2HCl$, occurring as a white or almost white, crystalline powder, having the same actions as the base; used as a topical anti-infective for the skin and mucous membranes.

chlorhistechia (klōr″his-tek′e-ah) [chloride + Gr. histos tissue + echein to hold + -ia] the presence of an abnormally large amount of chloride in a tissue.

chlorhydria (klōr-hi′dre-ah) an excess of hydrochloric acid in the stomach.

chloric (klo′rik) [L. chloricus] derived from or containing pentavalent chlorine; a term used to distinguish those compounds which contain a smaller proportion of chlorine than the chlorous compounds, and forming salts known as chlorates.

chloride (klo′rīd) a salt of hydrochloric acid; any binary compound of chlorine in which the latter is the negative element. Formerly called muriate. **acid c.,** a substance formed by substituting chlorine for hydroxyl in an acid molecule. **ferric c.,** orange-yellow or brownish yellow crystalline pieces, $FeCl_3 \cdot 6H_2O$, very soluble in water; used as a reagent and as a diagnostic aid in phenylketonuria; it was formerly used as a hematinic in the treatment of iron deficiency anemias, and has been used as a topical astringent and styptic. Called also iron chloride. **mercuric c.,** mercury bichloride. **mercurous c.,** calomel. **stannous c.,** chemical name: tin chloride ($SnCl_2$) dihydrate; a pharmaceutic aid, $SnCl_2 \cdot 2H_2O$.

chloridimeter (klo″rĭ-dim′ĕ-ter) [chloride + Gr. metron measure] an instrument for measuring the chloride content of the urine or other fluid.

chloridimetry (klo″rĭ-dim′ĕ-tre) the determination of the chloride content of fluids.

chloridion (klo″rid-i′on) negatively ionic chlorine, the anion of hydrochloric acid and the chlorides.

chloridometer (klo″rĭ-dom′ĕ-ter) chloridimeter.

chloridorrhea (klor″ĭd-o-re′ah) diarrhea with an excess of chlorides in the stool.

chloriduria (klo″rĭ-du′re-ah) [chloride + Gr. ouron urine + -ia] excess of chlorides in the urine.

chlorinated (klo′rĭ-nāt″ed) charged with chlorine.

chlorine (klor′ēn, klo′rēn, klo′rĭn) [L. chlorum or chlorinum, from Gr. chlōros green] a yellowish green, gaseous element, of suffocating odor; symbol, Cl; atomic number, 17; atomic weight, 35.453; specific gravity, 1.56. It is a disinfectant, decolorant, and irritant poison. It is used for disinfecting, fumigating, and bleaching, either in an aqueous solution or in the form of chlorinated lime. **c. dioxide,** an oxidizing and germicidal agent, ClO_2, used in the purification of water and for bleaching.

chlorinum (klo-ri′num) [L.] (obs.) chlorine.

chloriodized (klōr-i′o-dīzd) containing chlorine and iodine.

chlorisondamine chloride (klōr″i-son′dah-mēn) chemical name: 4,5,6,7-tetrachloro-1,3-dihydro-2-methyl-2-[2-(trimethylammonio)ethyl]-2H-isoindolium dichloride. An asymmetrical bisquaternary ammonium derivative with ganglionic blocking action, $C_{14}H_{20}Cl_6N_2$, used as an antihypertensive.

chlorite (klo′rīt) any salt of chlorous acid.

chlormadinone acetate (klōr-mah′dĭ-nōn) chemical name: 17-(acetyloxy)-6-chloro-pregna-4,6-diene-3,20-dione. A progestin, $C_{23}H_{29}ClO_4$, formerly used in oral contraceptive products.

chlormerodrin (klōr-mer′o-drin) chemical name: [3-[(aminocarbonyl)amino] - 2 - methoxypropyl]chloromercury. An orally effective mercurial diuretic, $C_5H_{11}ClHgN_2O_2$, occurring as a white powder. **c. Hg 197** [USP], chlormerodrin tagged with radioactive mercury (^{197}Hg); used as a diagnostic

aid in renal function determination, administered intravenously. **c. Hg 203** [NF], chlormerodrin tagged with radioactive mercury (^{203}Hg); used as a diagnostic aid in renal function determination, administered intravenously.

chlormethazanone (klōr″meth-az′ah-nōn) chlormezanone.

chlormethyl (klōr-meth′il) methyl chloride.

chlormezanone (klōr-mez′ah-nōn) chemical name: 2-(4-chlorophenyl)tetrahydro-3-methyl-4H-1,3-thiazin-4-one. A muscle relaxant and tranquilizer, $C_{11}H_{12}ClNO_3S$, occurring as a white, crystalline powder; administered orally.

chlor(o)- [Gr. chlōros green] a combining form meaning green, or denoting the presence of chlorine.

chloroacetic acid (klor″o-ah-se′tik) a strong acid, CH_2Cl-COOH, used as a laboratory reagent.

chloroazodin (klo″ro-a′zo-din) [USP] chemical name: N,N''-dichlorodiazenedicarboximidamide. An antibacterial, $C_2H_4Cl_2N_6$, which has been used as an antiseptic.

Chlorobacteriaceae (klo″ro-bak-te″re-a′se-e) Chlorobiaceae.

Chlorobacterium (klo″ro-bak-te′re-um) [chloro- + bacterium] a complex of green phototrophic bacteria living symbiotically on the surface of protozoa such as amebae and flagellates.

Chlorobiaceae (klo″ro-be-a′se-e) a family of aquatic phototrophic bacteria of the order Rhodospirillales, comprising the green sulfur bacteria. It consists of anaerobic, mostly nonmotile cells that produce brown to green pigments and fix carbon dioxide in the presence of sulfide or sulfur. It contains the genera Chlorobium, Chloropseudomonas, Clathrochloris, Pelodictyon, and Prosthecochlorus. Formerly called Chlorobacteriaceae.

Chlorobium (klo-ro′be-um) [chloro- + Gr. bios life] a genus of aquatic phototrophic bacteria of the family Chlorobiaceae, order Rhodospirillales, consisting of ovoid to rod-shaped nonmotile cells that do not contain gas vacuoles. The organisms fix carbon dioxide in the presence of hydrogen sulfide. Cell suspensions are yellow-green to brown. The type species is C. limi′cola.

chlorobrightism (klo″ro-brīt′izm) chlorosis with albuminuria.

chlorobutanol (klo″ro-bu′tah-nol) [NF] chemical name: 1,1,1-trichloro-2-methyl-2-propanol. Colorless to white crystals, $C_4H_7Cl_3O$, with a camphoraceous odor and taste; used as an antimicrobial preservative in various pharmaceutical solutions, especially injectables. It has been used as a local dental analgesic, hypnotic, antipruritic, sedative, somnifacient, and antiseptic.

Chlorochromatium (klo″ro-kro-ma′te-um) [chloro- + Gr. chroma color] a complex of green phototrophic sulfur bacteria found in mud and stagnant waters containing hydrogen sulfide.

chlorocruorin (klo″ro-kroo′o-rin) a green respiratory pigment occurring in certain marine worms.

chloroerythroblastoma (klo″ro-e-rith″ro-blas-to′mah) a new growth containing the elements of granulocytic sarcoma (chloroma) and erythrocytic sarcoma (erythroblastoma).

chloroethane (klo-ro-eth′ān) ethyl chloride.

chloroform (klor′o-form) trichloromethane, $CHCl_3$, a colorless, volatile liquid with a strong ethereal odor and a sweetish, burning taste, a common laboratory solvent; it is hepatotoxic and nephrotoxic when ingested. It was once widely used as an inhalation anesthetic and analgesic, and as an antitussive, carminative, and counterirritant. **acetone c.,** chlorobutanol.

chloroformism (klo′ro-form″izm) 1. the habitual use of chloroform for its narcotic effect. 2. the anesthetic effect of the vapor of chloroform.

chloroformization (klo″ro-form″i-za′shun) the administration of chloroform.

chloroguanide hydrochloride (klor″o-gwan′īd) proguanil hydrochloride.

chlorolabe (klor′o-lāb) [chloro- + Gr. lambanein to take] name proposed for the pigment in retinal cones that is more sensitive to the green portion of the spectrum than are the other pigments (cyanolabe and erythrolabe).

chloroleukemia (klo″ro-lu-ke′me-ah) chloroma.

chlorolymphosarcoma (klo″ro-lim″fo-sar-ko′mah) chloroma; so called because mononuclear cells in the peripheral blood were thought to be lymphocytes rather than myeloblasts.

chloroma (klo-ro'mah) [*chloro-* + *-oma*] a malignant green-colored tumor arising from myeloid tissue, associated with myelogenous leukemia and occurring anywhere in the body. Besides containing green pigment, which has no clear metabolic role and is principally myeloperoxidase (verdoperoxidase), chloroma tissue demonstrates a bright red fluorescence under ultraviolet light. Called also *green cancer, chloroleukemia, chlorolymphosarcoma,* and *granulocytic sarcoma.*

p -chloromercuribenzoate (klo'' ro-mer'' ku-re-ben'zo-āt) a univalent organic mercury compound that reacts with sulfhydryl groups on proteins, or other molecules, thereby often inhibiting their activities.

chloromethapyriline citrate (klo''ro-meth''ah-pi'ri-lēn) chlorothen citrate.

chlorometry (klo-rom'ĕ-tre) the quantitative determination of chlorine.

chloromonad (klo''ro-mo'nad) [*chloro-* + Gr. *monas* unit, from *monos* single] a protozoan of the order Chloromonadida.

Chloromonadida (klo''ro-mo-nad'ĭ-dah) [*chloro-* + Gr. *monas* unit, from *monos* single] an order of plantlike, biflagellate protozoa (class Phytomastigophorea, subphylum Mastigophorea), most members of which have pale green chromatophores; their metabolic products are fatty oils.

Chloromycetin (klo''ro-mi-se'tin) trademark for preparations of chloramphenicol.

chloromyeloma (klo''ro-mi-ĕ-lo'mah) chloroma attended with growths in the bone marrow.

chloronaphthalene (klo''ro-naf'thah-lēn) any of the products of the chlorination of naphthalene; exposure to such substances may cause halogen acne.

chloropexia (klo''ro-pek'se-ah) the fixation of chlorine in the body tissues.

chlorophane (klo'ro-fān) [*chloro-* + Gr. *phainein* to show] a greenish yellow pigment obtainable from the retina.

p-chlorophenol (klo''ro-fe'nol) parachlorophenol.

chlorophyl (klo'ro-fil) chlorophyll.

chlorophyll (klor'o-fil) [*chloro-* + Gr. *phyllon* leaf] any of a group of green pigments found in all photosynthetic cells that differ from heme pigments in that the central metal atom of the chelate is magnesium (not iron), there is a fused cyclopentanone ring in addition to the four pyrrole rings, and there is a long phytol side chain. Chlorophylls function by absorbing light producing an excited electron, which is passed along a chain of pigment molecules, ultimately resulting in the production of ATP or NADH. Chlorophyll *a* occurs in all organisms exhibiting aerobic photosynthesis (green plants, algae, and cyanobacteria), chlorophyll *b* in higher plants, chlorophylls c_1 and c_2 in diatoms and brown algae, chlorophyll *d* in red algae. Bacteriochlorophylls occur in bacteria exhibiting anaerobic photosynthesis. Preparations of water-soluble chlorophyll salts are applied topically for deodorization of skin lesions and administered orally to deodorize ulcerative lesions and the urine and feces in colostomy, ileostomy, or incontinence.

chlorophyllin (klo'ro-fil-in) any of the water-soluble salts obtained by alkaline hydrolysis of chlorophyll with replacement of the methyl and phytyl ester groups by sodium or potassium.

chloropia (klo-ro'pe-ah) chloropsia.

Chloropidae (klo-rop'ĭ-de) a family of small to minute flies (order Diptera); two medically important genera are *Hippelates* and *Siphunculina.*

chloroplast (klo'ro-plast) [*chloro-* + Gr. *plastos* formed] any one of the chlorophyll-bearing bodies of plant cells; called also *chloroplastid.*

chloroplastid (klo''ro-plas'tid) chloroplast.

chloroprivic (klo''ro-pri'vik) [*chlorine* + L. *privare* to deprive] deprived of chlorides; due to loss of chlorides.

chloroprocaine hydrochloride (klo''ro-pro'kān) [USP] chemical name: 2-(diethylamino)ethyl ester benzoic acid monohydrochloride. A local anesthetic, $C_{17}H_{19}ClN_2O_2 \cdot HCl$, occurring as a white, crystalline powder; used in minor and general surgery for infiltration, field block, and regional nerve block, including caudal and epidural block.

chloroprocaine penicillin (klo''ro-pro'kān) see under *penicillin.*

Chloropseudomonas (klo''ro-soo''do-mo'nas) [*chloro-* + Gr. *pseudēs* false + *monas* unit, from *monos* single] a genus of aquatic phototrophic bacteria of the family Chlorobiaceae, order Rhodospirillales, consisting of rod-shaped, motile cells that do not contain gas vacuoles. The organisms fix carbon dioxide in the presence of hydrogen sulfide. Cell suspensions are yellow to green. The type species is *C. ethyl'ica.*

chloropsia (klo-rop'se-ah) [*chloro-* + *-opsia*] a chromatopsia in which all objects seen appear to have a greenish tinge, a symptom of digitalis poisoning.

Chloroptic (klōr-op'tik) trademark for preparations of chloramphenicol.

chloroquine (klo'ro-kwin) [USP] chemical name: N^4-(7-chloro-4-quinolinyl)-N^1,N^1-diethyl 1,4-pentanediamine. A compound, $C_{18}H_{26}ClN_3$, occurring as a white or slightly yellow, crystalline powder; used as antimalarial in certain forms of malaria and as an antiamebic in extraintestinal amebiasis, administered intramuscularly. **c. phosphate** [USP], the phosphate salt of chloroquine, $C_{18}H_{26}ClN_3 \cdot 2H_3PO_4$, occurring as a white, crystalline powder; used as an antimalarial for the suppression and treatment of certain forms of malaria, as an antiamebic in extraintestinal amebiasis, and as a lupus erythematosus suppressant, administered orally.

chlorosis (klo-ro'sis) a disorder, especially common during the nineteenth century and disappearing abruptly soon thereafter, generally affecting adolescent females, believed to be associated with iron deficiency anemia, and characterized by greenish yellow discoloration of the skin and by hypochromic erythrocytes.

Chlorostigma (klo''ro-stig'mah) a genus of plants, e.g., *C. stuckertianum* (Asclepiadaceae). Its alkaloid, chlorostigmine, has been used to stimulate the secretion of milk during lactation.

chlorostigmine (klōr''o-stig'mēn) a galactopoietic alkaloid from plants of the genus *Chlorostigma.*

chlorothen citrate (klo'ro-then) chemical name: N-[(5-chloro-2-thienyl)methyl]-N,N''-dimethyl-N-2-pyridinyl-1,2-ethanediamine dihydrogen citrate. An antihistaminic, $C_{14}H_{18}ClN_3S \cdot C_6H_8O_7$, occurring as a white, crystalline powder; administered orally.

chlorothenium citrate (klo''ro-then'ĭ-um) chlorothen citrate.

chlorothiazide (klor''o-thi'ah-zīd) [USP] a thiazide diuretic; used for treatment of hypertension and edema; also available as *chlorothiazide sodium* [USP].

chlorothymol (klo''ro-thi'mol) chemical name: 4-chloro-5-methyl-2-(1-methylethyl)phenol; a powerful germicide, $C_{10}H_{13}ClO$, which has been used as a topical antibacterial and fungicide.

chlorotic (klo-rot'ik) pertaining to, or affected with chlorosis.

chlorotrianisene (klo''ro-tri-an'ĭ-sēn) [USP] chemical name: 1,1',1''-(1-chloro-1-ethenyl-2-ylidene)tris-4-methoxybenzene. A synthetic estrogen, $C_{23}H_{21}ClO_3$, occurring as small white crystals or as a crystalline powder; used to suppress lactation in postpartum women, for palliative treatment in inoperable prostatic carcinoma, and for replacement therapy of estrogen deficiency, administered orally.

chlorous (klo'rus) derived from or containing trivalent chlorine, as in chlorous acid, $HClO_2$; a term used to distinguish those compounds which contain a larger proportion of chlorine than the chloric compounds, and forming salts known as chlorites.

chlorous acid (klor'us) a weak inorganic acid, $HClO_2$.

chlorovinyldichloroarsine (klo''ro-vin''il-di-klo''ro-ar'sin) lewisite.

chloroxine (klo-roks'ēn) chemical name: 5,7-dichloro-8-quinolinol. A synthetic antibacterial, $C_9H_5Cl_2NO$; used in the topical treatment of dandruff and seborrheic dermatitis of the scalp.

chloroxylenol (klo''ro-zi'lĕ-nōl) chemical name: 4-chloro-3,5-dimethylphenol. An antibacterial, C_8H_9ClO, which is most active against streptococci; used mainly as a disinfectant for the skin.

chlorphenesin (klōr-fen'ĕ-sin) chemical name: 3-(4-chlorophenoxy)-1,2-propanediol. An antibacterial, antifungal, and antitrichomonal agent, $C_9H_{11}ClO_3$, occurring as white or pale cream-colored crystals or crystalline masses; used in the treatment of tinea pedis and other fungal infections of the skin and in fungal and trichomonal infections of the vagina, applied topically or intravaginally. **c. carbamate,** a skeletal muscle relaxant, $C_{10}H_{12}ClNO_4$ occurring as a white, crystalline powder; used as an adjunct in the short-term treatment of skeletal muscle spasms, such as sprains, strains, and trauma to tendons and ligaments, administered orally.

chlorpheniramine (klōr″fen-ir′ah-mēn) chemical name: γ-(4-chlorophenyl)-N,N-dimethyl-2-pyridinepropanamine. An antihistaminic, $C_{16}H_{19}ClN_2$, derived from pheniramine. **c. maleate** [USP], the maleate salt of chlorpheniramine, $C_{16}H_{19}ClN_2 \cdot C_4H_4O_4$, occurring as a white, crystalline powder; administered orally or by subcutaneous injection for therapy and prophylaxis of conditions in which antihistamines may be effective. Called also *chlorprophenpyridamine maleate.*

chlorphenoxamine hydrochloride (klōr″fen-ok′sah-mēn) [USP] chemical name: 2-[1-(4-chlorophenyl)-1-phenylethoxy]-N,N-dimethylethanamine hydrochloride. An anticholinergic, $C_{18}H_{23}Cl_2NO$, with weak antihistaminic action, occurring as needle-like crystals; used as a skeletal muscle relaxant in the treatment of Parkinson's disease, administered orally.

chlorphentermine hydrochloride (klōr-fen′ter-mēn) chemical name: 4-chloro-α,α-dimethylbenzeneethanamine hydrochloride. A sympathomimetic amine, $C_{10}H_{14}ClN \cdot HCl$, occurring as a white to off-white powder; used as an anorexic agent, administered orally.

chlorpromazine (klōr-pro′mah-zēn) [USP] chemical name: 2-chloro-N,N-dimethyl-10H-phenothiazine-10-propanamine. A phenothiazine derivative, $C_{17}H_{19}ClN_2S$, occurring as a white, crystalline solid; used as an antiemetic and tranquilizer, administered by rectal suppository. **c. hydrochloride** [USP], the hydrochloride of chlorpromazine, occurring as a white, crystalline powder, used orally, intramuscularly, or intravenously as a major tranquilizer.

chlorpropamide (klōr-pro′pah-mīd) [USP] chemical name: 4-chloro-N-[(propylamino)carbonyl]benzenesulfonamide. An orally effective hypoglycemic agent, $C_{10}H_{13}ClN_2O_3S$, occurring as a white, crystalline powder.

chlorprophenpyridamine (klōr″pro-fen-pi-rid′ah-mēn) chlorpheniramine.

chlorprothixene (klōr-pro-thiks′ēn) [USP] chemical name: (Z)-3-(2-chloro-9H-thioxanthen-9-ylidene)-N,N-dimethyl-1-propanamine. A drug, $C_{18}H_{18}ClNS$, occurring as a yellow crystalline powder, having sedative, antiemetic, antihistaminic, anticholinergic, and alpha-adrenergic blocking activity; used to control the symptoms of psychotic disorders, administered orally or by intramuscular injection.

chlorquinaldol (klōr-kwin′al-dol) chemical name: 5,7-dichloro-8-hydroxyquinaldine. A yellow, crystalline powder, $C_{10}H_7Cl_2NO$, insoluble in water; used as a topical keratoplastic, bactericide, and fungicide in dermatoses.

chlortetracycline (klōr″tet-rah-si′klēn) chemical name: 7-chloro-4-dimethylamino-1,4,4a,5,5a,6,11,12a-octahydro-3,6,10,12,12a-pentahydroxy-6-methyl-1,11-dioxo-2-naphthacenecarboxamide. A broad-spectrum antibiotic, $C_{22}H_{23}ClN_2O_8$, elaborated by *Streptomyces aureofaciens;* it was the first of the tetracycline group to be discovered. **c. hydrochloride** [USP], the monohydrochloride salt of chlortetracycline, $C_{22}H_{23}ClN_2O_8 \cdot HCl$, occurring as a yellow crystalline powder; a broad-spectrum antibiotic used as an antibacterial and antiprotozoal, administered orally, by intravenous injection, or applied topically to the conjunctiva.

chlorthalidone (klor-thal′ĭ-dōn) [USP] a diuretic with the same pharmacologic action as that of thiazide diuretics; used for treatment of hypertension and edema.

Chlor-Trimeton (klōr-tri′mĕ-ton) trademark for preparations of chlorpheniramine maleate.

chlorum (klo′rum), gen. *chlo'ri* [L.] chlorine.

chloruresis (klōr″u-re′sis) [*chloride* + Gr. *ourein* to urinate] the excretion of chlorides in the urine.

chloruretic (klōr″u-ret′ik) 1. promoting the excretion of chlorides in the urine. 2. an agent that promotes the excretion of chlorides in the urine.

chloruria (klo-roo′re-ah) [*chloride* + Gr. *ouron* urine + -*ia*] presence of chlorides in the urine.

chlorzoxazone (klōr-zok′sah-zōn) chemical name: 5-chloro-2(3H)-benzoxazolone. A skeletal muscle relaxant, $C_7H_4ClNO_2$, occurring as a white or creamy white, glistening, crystalline powder; used to relieve discomfort of painful musculoskeletal disorders, administered orally.

Ch.M. abbreviation for L. *Chirur'giae Magis'ter,* Master of Surgery.

$C_6H_5NH_2$ aniline.

$C_3H_5(NO_3)_3$ glyceryl trinitrate (nitroglycerin).

$C_5H_4N_4O_3$ uric acid.

$C_5H_{11}NO_2$ amyl nitrite.

C_8H_9NO acetanilid.

$C_9H_9NO_3$ hippuric acid.

$C_6H_2(NO_2)_3OH$ trinitrophenal (picric acid).

CH_2O formaldehyde.

CH_2O_2 formic acid.

CH_4O methyl alcohol.

$C_2H_2O_4$ oxalic acid.

$C_2H_4O_2$ acetic acid.

C_2H_6O ethyl alcohol.

C_3H_6O acetone.

$C_3H_6O_3$ lactic acid.

$C_3H_8O_3$ glycerin.

$C_4H_6O_2$ crotonic acid.

$C_4H_6O_5$ malic acid.

$C_4H_6O_6$ tartaric acid.

$C_4H_8O_2$ butyric acid; isobutyric acid.

$C_4H_{10}O$ ether (ethyl ether).

$C_5H_{10}O_2$ valeric acid.

$C_5H_{12}O$ amyl alcohol.

C_6H_6O phenol.

$C_6H_8O_7$ citric acid.

$(C_6H_{10}O_5)_n$ starch, glycogen, or other hexose polymers.

$C_6H_{12}O_6$ dextrose (d-glucose).

$C_7H_4O_7$ meconic acid.

$C_7H_6O_2$ benzoic acid.

$C_7H_6O_3$ salicylic acid.

$C_7H_6O_5$ gallic acid.

$C_{12}H_{22}O_{11}$ cane sugar.

$C_{15}H_{10}O_4$ chrysophanic acid.

$C_{18}H_{34}O_2$ oleic acid.

$C_{18}H_{36}O_2$ stearic acid.

choana (ko′a-nah), pl. *choa'nae* [L.; Gr. *choanē* funnel] 1. any funnel-shaped cavity or infundibulum. 2. [pl.] [NA] the paired openings between the nasal cavity and the nasopharynx; called also *posterior nares.* **primary c.,** the opening of the embryonic olfactory sac into the mouth. **secondary c.,** the definitive choana after the formation of the palate.

choanae (ko-a′ne) [L.] genitive and plural of *choana.*

choanal (ko′ah-nal) pertaining to a choana.

choano- [L., Gr. *choanē* funnel] a combining form denoting a relationship to a funnel or to a funnellike structure.

choanoid (ko′ah-noid) [Gr. *choanē* funnel + *eidos* form] funnel-shaped.

choanocyte (ko′ah-no″sīt) [*choano-* + Gr. *kytos* hollow vessel] a unique type of cell having a flagellum surrounded by a thin cytoplasmic collar; characteristic of sponges and certain protozoa.

choanoflagellate (ko″ah-no-flaj′ĕ-lāt) [*choano-* + L. *flagellum* whip] any protozoan of the order Choanoflagellida.

Choanoflagellida (ko″ah-no-flah-jel′ĭ-dah) [*choano-* + *flagellum*] an order of flagellate, stalked or free-swimming marine and freshwater protozoa (class Zoomastigophorea, subphylum, Mastigophora) having a single apical flagellum, the proximal part of which is surrounded by a collar-like ring composed of parallel rodlike pseudopodia that filters food particles from the water current produced by motion of the flagellum, and a membranous sheath or basket-like lorica composed of siliceous costae.

choanomastigote (ko″ah-no-mas′tĭ-gōt) [*choano-* + Gr. *mastix* whip] any of the bodies representing the morphologic ("barleycorn") stage in the life cycle of trypanosomatid protozoa of the genus *Crithidia,* in which the kinetoplast and basal body are anterior to the nucleus and the flagellum emerges through a funnel-shaped depression at the anterior end of the cell. Cf. *amastigote, epimastigote, opisthomastigote, promastigote,* and *trypomastigote.*

Choanotaenia (ko-a''no-te'ne-ah) [Gr. *choanē* funnel + *taenia* (def. 2)] a genus of tapeworms. **C. infundib'ulum,** an important tapeworm parasite of both chickens and turkeys.

chocolate (chok'o-lat)[L.*chocolata,* from Mexican *chocolatl*] a dried paste prepared from the kernels of the cacao, *Theobroma cacao,* with sugar and flavoring substances.

C₆H₅OH phenol.

choke (chōk) 1. to interrupt respiration by obstruction or compression, or the condition resulting from such interruption. 2. [pl.] a burning sensation beginning in the substernal region, with increasing uncontrollable urge to cough, and great apprehension and anxiety, leading to vasovagal attack, experienced during decompression. **thoracic c.,** in veterinary medicine, obstruction of the thoracic part of the esophagus with a foreign body. **water c.,** laryngeal spasm caused by fluid entering the larynx and especially by getting between the true and false vocal cords.

cholagogic (ko''lah-goj'ik) stimulating the flow of bile to the duodenum.

cholagogue (ko'lah-gog) [*chol-* + Gr. *agōgos* leading] an agent that stimulates the flow of bile into the duodenum.

cholaic acid (ko-la'ik) cholyltaurine.

cholaligenic (ko-lal''ĭ-jen'ik) [*cholalic* acid + Gr. *gennan* to produce] (*obs.*) forming cholalic (cholic) acid from cholesterol—one of the functions of the liver.

Cholan-DH (ko'lan) trademark for preparations of dehydrocholic acid.

cholaneresis (ko''lah-ner'ĕ-sis) increase in the output or elimination of bile acids, their conjugates, or their salts.

cholangeitis (ko''lan-ji'tis) cholangitis.

cholangiectasis (ko-lan''je-ek'tah-sis) dilatation of a bile duct.

cholangi(o)- [*chol-* + *angi(o)-*] a combining form denoting relationship to a bile duct.

cholangioadenoma (ko-lan''je-o-ad''ĕ-no'mah) a benign adenoma of the liver made up of congeries of small alveoli with distinct lumina, lined by cubical or cylindrical cells resembling those of normal bile ducts.

cholangiocarcinoma (ko-lan''je-o-kar''sĭ-no'mah) cholangiocellular carcinoma.

cholangiocholecystocholedochectomy (ko-lan''ge-o-ko''le-sis''to-ko''le-do-kek'to-me) excision of hepatic duct, common bile duct, and gallbladder.

cholangioenterostomy (ko-lan''je-o-en''ter-os'to-me) [*chol-* + Gr. *angeion* vessel + *enteron* intestine + *stomoun* to provide with an opening, or mouth] surgical anastomosis of a bile duct to the intestine.

cholangiogastrostomy (ko-lan''je-o-gas-tros'to-me) [*chol-* + Gr. *angeion* vessel + *gastēr* stomach + *stomoun* to provide with an opening, or mouth] surgical anastomosis of a bile duct to the stomach.

cholangiogram (ko-lan'je-o-gram'') a roentgenogram of the gallbladder and bile ducts.

cholangiography (ko-lan''je-og'rah-fe)[*chol-* + Gr. *angeion* vessel + *graphein* to write] roentgenography of the biliary ducts after administration or injection of a contrast medium, orally, intravenously, or percutaneously. **fine needle transhepatic c. (FNTC),** transhepatic cholangiography performed by means of a very fine, highly flexible steel needle (skinny needle). **operative c.,** cholangiography performed during a surgical procedure on the gallbladder. **transhepatic c.,** cholangiography after introduction of radiopaque media into the biliary system by percutaneous puncture of a bile duct. See also *endoscopic retrograde cholangiopancreatography,* under *cholangiopancreatography.* **transjugular c.,** cholangiography after catheterization of a hepatic vein via the internal jugular vein in the neck and entry into a bile duct by percutaneous puncture across the wall of the hepatic vein.

cholangiohepatitis (ko-lan''je-o-hep''ah-ti'tis) severe inflammation of the bile passages often associated with liver fluke infestation, which causes obstruction of the bile ducts.

cholangiohepatoma (ko-lan''je-o-hep''ah-to'mah) primary carcinoma of the liver of mixed liver cell and bile-duct cell origin; called also *hepatocholangiocarcinoma.*

cholangiojejunostomy (ko-lan''je-o-jĕ-ju-nos'to-me) surgical anastomosis of a bile duct to the jejunum. **intrahepatic c.,** portoenterostomy.

cholangiolar (ko''lan-je'o-lar) pertaining to a cholangiole.

cholangiole (ko-lan''je-ōl) [*chol-* + Gr. *angeion* vessel + *-ole* diminutive suffix] one of the fine terminal elements of the bile duct system, leaving the portal canal, and pursuing a course at the periphery of a lobule of the liver; called also *bile* or *biliary ductule* and, rarely, *bile capillary.*

cholangiolitis (ko-lan''je-o-li'tis) inflammation of the cholangioles.

cholangioma (ko-lan''je-o'mah) [*chol-* + Gr. *angeion* vessel + *-oma*] cholangiocellular carcinoma.

cholangiopancreatography (ko-lan''je-o-pan''kre-ah-tog'rah-fe) roentgenographic examination of the bile ducts and pancreas after administration of a contrast medium. **endoscopic retrograde c. (ERCP),** a procedure consisting of a combination of retrograde cholangiography and transhepatic cholangiography used to demonstrate all portions of the biliary tree, performed by cannulation of the common bile duct and pancreatic duct through the papilla of Vater by means of a flexible fiberoptic endoscope and retrograde injection of radiopaque contrast media.

cholangiostomy (ko''lan-je-os'to-me) [*chol-* + Gr. *angeion* vessel + *stomoun* to provide with an opening, or mouth] creation of an opening into a bile duct; sometimes used to refer to a fistula into the bile duct.

cholangiotomy (ko''lan-je-ot'o-me)[*chol-* + Gr. *angeion* vessel + *tomē* a cutting] incision into a bile duct.

cholangitis (ko''lan-ji'tis) [*chol-* + Gr. *angeion* vessel + *-itis*] inflammation of a bile duct. **chronic nonsuppurative destructive c.,** primary biliary cirrhosis. **c. len'ta,** chronic infectious cholangitis without gallstones or biliary tract obstruction. **primary sclerosing c.,** a progressive chronic fibrosing inflammation of the bile ducts of unknown cause, occurring most commonly in young men and frequently in association with chronic ulcerative colitis. **progressive nonsuppurative c.,** primary biliary cirrhosis.

cholanic acid (ko-lan'ik) a steroidal acid, 5β-cholan-24-oic acid, which can be considered the parent compound of the bile acids.

cholanopoiesis (ko''lah-no-poi-e'sis) the synthesis of bile acids or of their conjugates and salts by the liver.

cholanopoietic (ko''lah-no''poi-et'ik) 1. pertaining to or promoting cholanopoiesis. 2. an agent that promotes cholanopoiesis.

cholanthrene (ko-lan'thrēn) a pentacyclic hydrocarbon, C₂₀H₁₄, of great carcinogenicity.

cholate (ko'lāt) a salt or ester of cholic acid.

chole- see *chol(o)-.*

cholebilirubin (ko''le-bil''e-ru'bin) a pigment, C₃₂H₅₀O₁₁N₂, differing from bilirubin, occurring in gallbladder bile; it gives a direct reaction to the Van den Bergh test.

Cholebrine (ko'le-brin) trademark for a preparation of iocetamic acid.

cholecalciferol (ko''le-kal-sif'er-ol) [USP] chemical name: activated 5,7-cholestadien-3β-ol. An antirachitic vitamin occurring as white, odorless crystals, C₂₇H₄₄O, soluble in alcohol, chloroform, and fatty oils; it undergoes metabolic conversion before exerting biological effects (see *dihydroxycholecalciferol*). Called also *activated 7-dehydrocholesterol* and *vitamin D₃.*

cholechromopoiesis (ko''le-kro''mo-poi-e'sis) the synthesis of bile pigments.

cholecyanin (ko''le-si'ah-nin) bilicyanin.

cholecyst (ko'le-sist) [*chole-* + Gr. *kystis* bladder] the gallbladder (vesicae biliaris [NA]).

cholecystagogic (ko''le-sis''tah-goj'ik) cholecystokinetic.

cholecystagogue (ko''le-sis'tah-gog) a cholecystokinetic agent.

cholecystalgia (ko''le-sis-tal'je-ah) [*cholecyst* + *-algia*] 1. gallbladder colic due to impaction of a gallstone in the cystic duct. 2. pain due to inflammation of the gallbladder.

cholecystatony (ko''le-sis-tat'o-ne) atony of the gallbladder.

cholecystectasia (ko″le-sis″tek-ta′ze-ah) [*cholecyst* + Gr. *ektasis* distention] distention of the gallbladder.

cholecystectomy (ko″le-sis-tek′to-me) [*cholecyst* + Gr. *ektomē* excision] surgical removal of the gallbladder.

cholecystenteric (ko″le-sis″ten-ter′ik) pertaining to communication between the gallbladder and intestine; called also *cholecystointestinal.*

cholecystenteroanastomosis (ko″le-sis-ten″ter-o-ah-nas″to-mo′sis) cholecystenterostomy.

cholecystenterorrhaphy (ko″le-sis-ten″ter-or′ah-fe) suture of the gallbladder to the small intestine.

cholecystenterostomy (ko″le-sis″ten″ter-os′to-me) [*cholecyst* + Gr. *enteron* bowel + *stomoun* to provide with an opening, or mouth] surgical anastomosis of the gallbladder to the intestine.

cholecystgastrostomy (ko″le-sist-gas-tros′to-me) cholecystogastrostomy.

cholecystic (ko″le-sis′tik) pertaining to the gallbladder.

cholecystis (ko″le-sis′tis) [Gr. *chole* bile, gall + *kystis* bladder] the gallbladder.

cholecystitis (ko″le-sis-ti′tis) [*cholecyst* + -*itis*] inflammation of the gallbladder. **acute c.,** a form usually due to obstruction of the gallbladder outlet, with signs ranging from mild edema and congestion to severe infection with gangrene and perforation. **chronic c.,** inflammation of the gallbladder with relatively mild symptoms persisting over a long period. **c. emphysemato′sa, emphysematous c.,** inflammation of the gallbladder caused by gas-producing organisms, characterized by gas in the gallbladder lumen and frequently infiltrating into the wall of the gallbladder and surrounding tissues; called also *gaseous c.* **follicular c.,** inflammation of the gallbladder in which there is conspicuous formation of lymphoid follicles, which commonly contain germinal centers. **gaseous c.,** emphysematous c. **c. glandula′ris prolif′erans,** a thickening of the wall of the chronically inflamed gallbladder, with formation of crypts which may develop into cysts.

cholecystnephrostomy (ko″le-sist″ne-fros′to-me) cholecystopyelostomy.

cholecystocholangiogram (ko″le-sis″to-ko-lan′je-o-gram) roentgenogram of the gallbladder and bile ducts.

cholecystocolonic (ko″le-sis″to-ko-lon′ik) pertaining to communication between the gallbladder and colon, as cholecystocolonic fistula.

cholecystocolostomy (ko″le-sis″to-ko-los′to-me) surgical anastomosis of the gallbladder to the colon; called also *colocholecystostomy.*

cholecystocolotomy (ko″le-sis″to-ko-lot′o-me) surgical incision of the gallbladder and colon.

cholecystoduodenostomy (ko″le-sis″to-du″o-dĕ-nos′to-me) surgical anastomosis of the gallbladder and the duodenum.

cholecystoenterostomy (ko″le-sis-to-en″ter-os′to-me) cholecystenterostomy.

cholecystogastric (ko″le-sis″to-gas′trik) pertaining to communication between the gallbladder and stomach, as a cholecystogastric fistula.

cholecystogastrostomy (ko″le-sis″to-gas-tros′to-me) surgical anastomosis between the gallbladder and the stomach.

cholecystogogic (ko″le-sis″to-goj′ik) cholecystokinetic.

cholecystogram (ko″le-sis′to-gram) a roentgenogram of the gallbladder.

cholecystography (ko″le-sis-tog′rah-fe) [*cholecyst* + Gr. *graphein* to write] roentgenography of the gallbladder.

cholecystoileostomy (ko″le-sis″to-il″e-os′to-me) surgical anastomosis of the gallbladder and the ileum.

cholecystointestinal (ko″le-sis″to-in-tes′tĭ-nal) cholecystenteric.

cholecystojejunostomy (ko″le-sis″to-jĕ-ju-nos′to-me) surgical anastomosis of the gallbladder and the jejunum.

cholecystokinetic (ko″le-sis″to-ki-net′ik) causing or promoting contraction of the gallbladder.

cholecystokinin (ko″le-sis″to-kin′in) [*cholecyst* + Gr. *kinein* to move] a 33-amino-acid polypeptide hormone secreted by the mucosa of the upper intestine and by the hypothalamus; it stimulates contraction of the gallbladder (with release

of bile) and secretion of pancreatic enzymes. It is synonymous with pancreozymin. Abbreviated CCK.

cholecystolithiasis (ko″le-sis″to-lĭ-thi′ah-sis) [*cholecyst* + *lithiasis*] cholelithiasis.

cholecystolithotripsy (ko″le-sis″to-lith′o-trip″se) [*cholecyst* + *lithotripsy*] the crushing of gallstones within the gallbladder.

cholecystonephrostomy (ko″le-sis″to-ne-fros′to-me) cholecystopyelostomy.

cholecystopathy (ko″le-sis-top′ah-the) [*cholecyst* + Gr. *pathos* disease] any gallbladder disease.

cholecystopexy (ko″le-sis′to-pek″se) [*cholecyst* + Gr. *pēxis* fixation] suspension or fixation of the gallbladder by surgical means.

cholecystoptosis (ko″le-sis″to-to′sis) [*cholecyst* + Gr. *ptōsis* fall] downward or distal displacement of the gallbladder.

cholecystopyelostomy (ko″le-sis″to-pi″ĕ-los′to-me) surgical anastomosis of the gallbladder to the pelvis of the kidney; called also *cholecystonephrostomy.*

cholecystorrhaphy (ko″le-sis-tor′ah-fe) [*cholecyst* + Gr. *rhaphē* suture] suture or repair of the gallbladder.

cholecystosis (ko″le-sis-to′sis) any noninflammatory disease of the gallbladder. **hyperplastic c.,** abnormal increase in cellular structure of the gallbladder.

cholecystostomy (ko″le-sis-tos′to-me) [*cholecyst* + Gr. *stomoun* to provide with an opening, or mouth] the creation of an opening into the gallbladder for drainage.

cholecystotomy (ko″le-sis-tot′o-me) [*cholecyst* + Gr. *tomē* a cutting] surgical incision of the gallbladder; done for exploration, drainage (cholecystostomy), or removal of calculi.

choledochal (ko″lĕ-dok′al) pertaining to the common bile duct.

choledochectomy (kol″ĕ-do-kek′to-me) [*choledochus* + Gr. *ektomē* excision] excision of a portion of the common bile duct.

choledochendysis (kol″ĕ-do-ken′dĭ-sis) [*choledochus* + Gr. *endysis* entrance] choledochotomy.

choledochitis (kol″ĕ-do-ki′tis) inflammation of the common bile duct, or ductus choledochus.

choledoch(o)- [*choledochus*] a combining form denoting relation to the common bile duct.

choledochocele (ko-led′o-ko-sēl) a rare form of congenital cystic dilatation of the common bile duct in which the dilated portion is within the wall of the duct.

choledochocholedochostomy (ko-led″o-ko-kol″ĕ-do-kos′to-me) surgical formation of an anastomosis between two portions of the common bile duct.

choledochoduodenostomy (ko-led″o-ko-du″o-dĕ-nos′to-me) surgical anastomosis of the common bile duct to the duodenum.

choledochoenterostomy (ko-led″o-ko-en″ter-os′to-me) surgical anastomosis of the common bile duct to the intestine.

choledochogastrostomy (ko-led″o-ko-gas-tros′to-me) surgical anastomosis of the common bile duct and the stomach.

choledochogram (ko-led′ŏ-ko-gram″) a roentgenogram of the common bile duct.

choledochography (ko-led″o-kog′rah-fe) [*choledochus* + Gr. *graphein* to write] roentgenography of the common bile duct after the administration of opaque material.

choledochohepatostomy (ko-led″o-ko-hep″ah-tos′to-me) surgical anastomosis of the common bile duct to the hepatic duct.

choledochoileostomy (ko-led″o-ko-il-e-os′to-me) surgical anastomosis of the common bile duct and the ileum.

choledochojejunostomy (ko-led″o-ko-jĕ-ju-nos′to-me) surgical anastomosis of the common bile duct and the jejunum.

choledocholith (ko-led′ŏ-ko-lith″) a calculus in the common bile duct.

choledocholithiasis (ko-led″ŏ-ko-lĭ-thi′ah-sis) the occurrence of calculi in the common bile duct.

choledocholithotomy (ko-led″ŏ-ko-lĭ-thot′o-me) incision of the common bile duct for the removal of stone.

choledocholithotripsy (ko-led″o-ko-lith′o-trip″se) the crushing of a gallstone within the common bile duct.

choledochoplasty (ko-led″o-ko-plas′te)   the performance of a plastic operation on the common bile duct; plastic repair of the duct following injury.

choledochorrhaphy (ko-led″o-kor′ah-fe) [*choledochus* + Gr. *rhaphē* suture]   suture or repair of the common bile duct.

choledochoscope (ko-led′o-ko-skōp″)   an instrument used during surgical exploration for direct inspection of the interior of the common bile duct.

choledochostomy (ko-led″o-kos′to-me) [*choledochus* + Gr. *stomoun* to provide with an opening, or mouth]   surgical formation of an opening into the common bile duct and drainage by catheter or T-tube.

choledochotomy (ko-led″o-kot′o-me) [*choledochus* + Gr. *tomē* a cutting]   incision into the common bile duct for exploration or removal of a calculus; called also *choledochendysis*.

choledochus (ko-led′o-kus) [*chole-* + Gr. *dochos* receptacle]   the ductus choledochus, or common bile duct.

Choledyl (ko-lēd′il)   trademark for a preparation of oxtriphylline.

choleglobin (ko″le-glo′bin)   a compound of globin and an open-ring iron porphyrin, being an intermediate in the formation of bile pigment from the catabolism of hemoglobin.

cholehematin (ko″le-hem′ah-tin)   a red pigment (not a bile pigment) found in the bile of herbivorous animals; it is derived from chlorophyll and is the same as phylloerythrin and bilipurpurine.

cholehemia (ko″le-he′me-ah)   (*obs.*) cholemia.

choleic (ko-le′ik)   pertaining to or derived from the bile; see under *acid*.

cholelith (ko′le-lith) [*chole-* + Gr. *lithos* stone]   a gallstone.

cholelithiasis (ko″le-lĭ-thi′ah-sis) [*chole-* + *lithiasis*]   the presence or formation of gallstones.

cholelithic (ko″le-lith′ik)   pertaining to or caused by gallstones.

cholelithotomy (ko″le-lĭ-thot′o-me)   removal of gallstones through an incision in the gallbladder.

cholelithotripsy (ko″le-lith′o-trip-se) [*cholelith* + Gr. *tribein* to crush]   the crushing of gallstones.

cholelithotrity (ko″le-lĭ-thot′rĭ-te)   cholelithotripsy.

cholemesis (ko-lem′ĕ-sis) [*chole-* + Gr. *emein* to vomit]   vomiting of bile.

cholemia (ko-le′me-ah) [*chole-* + Gr. *haima* blood + *-ia*]   the presence of bile or bile pigments in the blood. **familial c., Gilbert c.,** Gilbert syndrome.

cholemic (ko-le′mik)   pertaining to, marked by, or due to cholemia.

cholemimetry (ko″le-mim′ĕ-tre)   determination of the amount of bile pigment in the blood.

cholepathia (ko″le-path′e-ah) [*chole-* + Gr. *pathos* disease + *-ia*]   a morbid condition of the biliary tract. **c. spas′tica** (*obs.*), a morbid condition of the biliary tract, characterized by spasm of the bile ducts.

choleperitoneum (ko″le-per″ĭ-to-ne′um) [*chole-* + *peritoneum*]   the presence of bile in the peritoneum resulting from rupture of the bile passages; called also *biliary* or *bile peritonitis*, and *choleperitonitis*.

choleperitonitis (ko″le-per″ĭ-to-ni′tis)   choleperitoneum.

cholepoiesis (ko″le-poi-e′sis)   1. the manufacture and secretion by the liver of bile constituents other than water. 2. the manufacture and secretion of bile salts by the liver.

cholepoietic (ko″le-poi-et′ik) [*chole-* + Gr. *poiein* to make]   forming or secreting a constituent peculiar to bile; increasing the secretion of bile without a fall in its specific gravity.

choleprasin (ko″le-pra′sin)   one of the pigments of bile isolated from gallstones.

cholera (kol′er-ah) [Gr., from *cholē* bile]   an acute infectious, sometimes fulminant, enteritis endemic in India and Southeast Asia and periodically spreading to other parts of the world, including the Middle East, Africa, and southern Europe, in epidemics and pandemics. It is caused by a potent enterotoxin (choleragen) elaborated by *Vibrio cholerae*, in the small intestine where it acts on epithelial cells to cause secretion of large quantities of isotonic fluid from the mucosal surface, and marked in the severe, full-blown cases by severe, painless, watery diarrhea with the passing of rice-water stools, which are diagnostic, resulting in massive gastrointestinal fluid loss and saline depletion, acidosis, and shock; effortless vomiting; muscle cramps; and a characteristic faint high-pitched voice. Cholera is spread by feces-contaminated water and food.   **Asiatic c.,** classic cholera; so called because the disease was originally confined to Asia.   **chicken c.,** pasteurellosis in chickens; see *fowl c.*   **dry c.,** c. sicca.   **fowl c.,** hemorrhagic septicemia caused by *Pasteurella multocida* and occurring in all species of domestic fowl, canaries, waterfowl, seagulls, game birds, and birds of prey, all over the world.   **c. gallina′rium,** fowl c.   **hog c.,** an infectious communicable disease of swine occurring in epizootics and caused by a virus; marked by fever, loss of appetite, emaciation, ulceration of the intestines, diarrhea, and ecchymoses in the kidney and on the skin of the ventral surface of the body; called also *swine fever*.   **c. mor′bus,** a once popular name for an acute gastroenteritis, with diarrhea, cramps, and vomiting, occurring in summer or autumn; called also *summer c.* or *summer complaint*.   **pancreatic c.,** Verner-Morrison syndrome.   **c. sic′ca,** a rare type of cholera in which ileus produces pooling of fluid in the gut, associated with profound shock with diarrhea; called also *dry c.*   **summer c.,** c. morbus.

choleragen (kol′er-ah-jen)   the exotoxin produced by the cholera vibrio, which is thought to stimulate electrolyte and water secretion into the small intestine in Asiatic cholera.

choleraic (kol″ĕ-ra′ik)   of, pertaining to, or of the nature of cholera.

choleraphage (kol′er-ah-fāj)   a bacteriophage that infects cholera bacilli.

choleresis (ko-ler′ĕ-sis) [*chole-* + Gr. *hairesis* a taking]   the secretion of bile by the liver by either cholepoiesis or hydrocholeresis.

choleretic (ko″ler-et′ik)   1. stimulating the production of bile by the liver by either cholepoiesis or hydrocholeresis. 2. a choleretic agent.

choleria (ko-ler′e-ah)   an irritable or hostile temperament.

choleric (kol′er-ik) [Gr. *cholerikos*, from *chole* bile]   hottempered, irascible, having the temperament that, according to the humoral theory of the ancient Greeks, is caused by an excess of yellow bile.

choleriform (ko-ler′ĭ-form)   choleroid.

cholerigenic (kol″er-ĭ-jen′ik)   causing cholera.

cholerigenous (kol-er-ij′e-nus)   causing cholera.

choleroid (kol′er-oid) [Gr. *cholera* + *eidos* form]   resembling cholera.

cholescintigram (ko″le-sin′tĭ-gram)   the two-dimensional record, obtained by cholescintigraphy, of the concentration of radionuclide in the biliary system.

cholescintigraphy (kol″ĕ-sin-tig′rah-fe)   scintigraphy of the biliary tract.

cholestane (ko′les-tān)   a saturated steroid hydrocarbon, $C_{27}H_{48}$, with C-18 and C-19 methyl groups and an isooctyl side chain at C-17; obtained by reduction of cholesterol and other C_{27} steroids.

5β-cholestane-3α, 7α, 12α, 25-tetraol 24S-hydroxylase (ko′les-tān tĕ′trah-ol′ hi-drok′sĭ-lās)   an enzyme that catalyzes the conversion of 5β-cholestane-3α, 7α, 12α, 25-tetraol to 5β-cholestane-3α, 7α, 12α, 24S, 25-pentaol. The reaction is part of a pathway of bile acid biosynthesis involving 25-hydroxylation of cholesterol. Deficiency of the enzyme, an autosomal recessive trait, results in cerebrotendinous xanthomatosis. Called also *24-hydroxylase*.

cholestanol (ko-les′tah-nol)   a compound, $C_{27}H_{47}OH$, formed by the reduction of cholesterol. **beta-c.,** an isomer of coprosterol derived from cholesterol by bacterial action and found in the feces; called also *dihydrocholesterol*.

cholestasia (ko″le-sta′ze-ah)   cholestasis.

cholestasis (ko″le-sta′sis) [*chole-* + Gr. *stasis* stoppage]   stoppage or suppression of the flow of bile, having intrahepatic or extrahepatic causes.

cholestatic (ko″le-stat′ik)   pertaining to or characterized by cholestasis.

cholesteatoma (ko″le-ste″ah-to′mah) [*chole-* + *steatoma*]   a cystlike mass, with a lining of stratified squamous epithelium, usually of keratinizing type, filled with desquamating debris frequently including cholesterol. Cholesteatomas occur in the meninges, central nervous system, and bones of the skull, but are most common in the middle ear and mastoid region. **congenital c.,** epidermoidoma. **c. tym′pani,** cholesteatoma associated with chronic infection of the middle ear, formed of the outer desquamating layers of stratified squamous epithelium which has extended inward and upward to line the tympanum, epitympanum, and antrum.

cholesteatomatous (ko″le-ste″ah-to′mah-tus) relating to or of the nature of cholesteatoma.

cholesteatosis (ko″le-ste-ah-to′sis) fatty degeneration due to cholesterol esters.

cholestene (ko′les-tēn) an unsaturated hydrocarbon, $C_{27}H_{46}$, formed by the dehydrogenation of cholestane.

cholesteremia (ko-les″ter-e′me-ah) [cholesterol + Gr. haima blood + -ia] hypercholesterolemia.

cholesterin (ko-les′ter-in) cholesterol.

cholesterinemia (ko-les″ter-in-e′me-ah) hypercholesterolemia.

cholesterinosis (ko-les″ter-ĭ-no′sis) cholesterosis.

cholesterinuria (ko-les″ter-ĭ-nu′re-ah) cholesteroluria.

cholesterogenesis (ko-les″ter-o-jen′ĕ-sis) synthesis of cholesterol.

cholesterohistechia (ko-les″ter-o-his-tek′e-ah) [cholesterol + Gr. histos tissue + echein to hold + -ia] the presence of an abnormally large amount of cholesterol in a tissue.

cholesterohydrothorax (ko-les″ter-o-hi″dro-tho′raks) presence in the thoracic cavity of watery fluid that contains cholesterol crystals.

cholesterol (ko-les′ter-ol) [chole- + Gr. stereos solid] 1. a pearly, fatlike steroid alcohol, $C_{27}H_{45}OH$, crystallizing in the form of leaflets or plates from dilute alcohol, and found in animal fats and oils, in bile, blood, brain tissue, milk, yolk of egg, myelin sheaths of nerve fibers, the liver, kidneys, and adrenal glands. It constitutes a large part of the most frequently occurring type of gallstones and occurs in atheroma of the arteries, in various cysts, and in carcinomatous tissue. Most of the body's cholesterol is synthesized in the liver, but some is absorbed from the diet. It is a precursor of bile acids and is important in the synthesis of steroid hormones. 2. [USP] a commercial preparation of cholesterol used as a pharmaceutic aid. Called also cholesterin.

cholesterol desmolase (kol-es′ter-ol dez″mol-ās) cholesterol monooxygenase (side-chain–cleaving).

cholesterolemia (ko-les″ter-ol-e′me-ah) [cholesterol + Gr. haima blood + -ia] hypercholesterolemia.

cholesteroleresis (ko-les″ter-ol-er′ĕ-sis) increased elimination of cholesterol in the bile.

cholesterolestersturz (ko-les″ter-ol-es′ter-stoorts) [Ger.] decrease in the proportion of esters in the blood cholesterol.

cholesterol monooxygenase (side-chain cleaving) (kol-es′ter-ol mon″o-ok′sĭ-jen-ās) an enzyme of the oxidoreductase class that catalyzes the reaction cholesterol + reduced adrenal ferredoxin + O_2 = pregnenolone + 4-methylpentanal + oxidized adrenal ferredoxin + H_2O. The enzyme is a heme-thiolate protein. The reaction involves three successive monooxygenase reactions with 22-R-hydroxycholesterol and 20S, 22R-dihydroxycholesterol as enzyme-bound intermediates. The reaction occurs in mitochondria and is the first step in the conversion of cholesterol to steroid hormones. Called also cholesterol desmolase and 20,22-desmolase.

cholesterolopoiesis (ko-les″ter-ol″o-poi-e′sis) the synthesis of cholesterol by the liver.

cholesterolosis (ko-les″ter-ol-o′sis) cholesterosis.

cholesterol sulfatase (ko-les″ter-ol sul′fah-tās) steroid sulfatase.

cholesteroluria (ko-les″ter-ol-u′re-ah) [cholesterol + Gr. ouron urine + -ia] the presence of cholesterol in the urine; called also cholesterinuria.

cholesterosis (ko-les″ter-o′sis) a condition in which cholesterol is deposited in tissues in abnormal quantities. Called also cholesterinosis and cholesterolosis. **extracellular c.,** a condition formerly believed to be a variant of erythema elevatum diutinum but now considered to be the same disorder.

choletelin (ko-let′ĕ-lin) [chole- + Gr. telos end] a yellow pigment, $C_{16}H_{18}N_2O_6$, the oxidation product of bilirubin; bilixanthine.

choletherapy (ko″le-ther′ah-pe) [chole- + therapy] treatment by the administration of bile salts.

choleuria (ko″le-u′re-ah) [chole- + Gr. ouron urine + -ia] choluria.

choleverdin (ko″le-ver′din) biliverdin.

cholic acid (ko′lik) a primary bile acid $3\alpha,7\alpha,12\alpha$-trihydroxy-5β-cholanic acid.

choline (ko′lin) hydroxyethyl trimethyl ammonium hydroxide, $CH_2OH \cdot CH_2N^+(CH_3)_3$, derivable from many animal and some vegetable tissues and produced synthetically. Considered to be a vitamin of the B complex, it is the basic constituent of lecithin and prevents the deposition of fat in the liver; the acetic acid ester of choline (acetylcholine) is essential in synaptic transmission of nerve impulses. Choline is also oxidized to form betaine in methionine biosynthesis. Choline readily forms salts, several of which (c. bitartrate, c. chloride, and c. dihydrogen citrate) have been used in medicine as lipotropic agents in the treatment of fatty degeneration and hepatic cirrhosis. **acetyl glyceryl ether phosphoryl c.,** platelet activating factor; see under factor. **c. magnesium trisalicylate,** a combination of choline salicylate and magnesium salicylate, used as an antiarthritic. **phosphatidyl c.,** lecithin. **c. salicylate,** the choline salt of salicylic acid; used as an analgesic, antipyretic, and antirheumatic. **c. theophyllinate,** oxtriphylline.

choline acetylase (ko′lēn ah-set′ĭ-lās) choline acetyltransferase.

choline acetyltransferase (ko′lēn as″ĕ-tēl-trans′fer-ās) [EC 2.3.1.6] an enzyme of the transferase class that catalyzes the reaction acetyl-CoA + choline = CoA + O-acetylcholine. The enzyme occurs in synaptosomes of the autonomic nervous system and skeletal muscle, and in some regions of the central nervous system. Called also choline acetylase. **c. e. I, true c.e.,** acetylcholinesterase.

cholinergic (ko″lin-er′jik) 1. stimulated, activated or transmitted by choline (acetylcholine): a term applied to those nerve fibers which liberate acetylcholine at a synapse when a nerve impulse passes, i.e., the parasympathetic nerve endings. 2. an agent that produces such effects. Called also parasympathomimetic. Cf. adrenergic.

cholinesterase (ko″lin-es′ter-ās) [EC 3.1.1.8] an enzyme of the hydrolase class that catalyzes the reaction acylcholine + H_2O = choline + carboxylic acid anion. It acts on a variety of choline esters. The determination of enzyme activity is useful in the clinical diagnosis of succinylcholine sensitivity and of poisoning by organophosphate insecticides. Called also choline esterase II (unspecific), pseudocholinesterase, and serum cholinesterase. Abbreviated CHS and PCE. Cf. acetylcholinesterase.

cholinoceptive (ko″lin-o-sep′tiv) pertaining to the sites on effector organs that are acted upon by cholinergic transmitters.

cholinoceptor (ko″lin-o-sep′tor) cholinergic receptor; see under receptor.

cholinolytic (ko″lin-o-lit′ik) 1. blocking the action of acetylcholine, or of cholinergic agents. 2. an agent that blocks the action of acetylcholine in cholinergic areas, that is, organs supplied by parasympathetic nerves, and voluntary muscles.

cholinomimetic (ko″lĭ-no-mi-met′ik) having an action similar to that of acetylcholine; parasympathomimetic.

chol(o)-, chole- [Gr cholē bile] a combining form denoting relationship to the bile.

cholochrome (kol′o-krōm) [cholo- + Gr. chrōma color] any biliary pigment.

cholocyanin (kol″o-si′ah-nin) [cholo- + Gr. kyanos blue] bilicyanin.

chologenetic (kol″o-je-net′ik) [cholo- + Gr. gennan to produce] producing bile; cholepoietic.

Cholografin (ko″lo-gra′fin) trademark for preparations of iodipamide.

cholohematin (kol″o-hem′ah-tin) cholehematin, a brown bile pigment.

cholohemothorax (ko″lo-he″mo-tho′raks) [cholo- + Gr. haima blood + thōrax chest] presence of bile and blood in the thorax.

chololith (kol′o-lith) cholelith.

chololithiasis (kol″o-lĭ-thi′ah-sis) cholelithiasis.

chololithic (kol″o-lith′ik) cholelithic.

cholopoiesis (kol″o-poi-e′sis) cholepoiesis.

cholothorax (ko″lo-tho′raks) [cholo- + Gr. thŏrax chest] cholohemothorax.

Choloxin (ko-lok′sin) trademark for a preparation of dextrothyroxine sodium.

choluria (ko-lu′re-ah) [chol- + Gr. ouron urine + -ia] the presence of bile in the urine; discoloration of the urine with bile pigments.

choluric (ko-lur′ik) pertaining to or marked by choluria.

cholylglycine (ko″lil-gli′sēn) a bile salt, the glycine conjugate of cholic acid, called also glycocholic acid.

cholyltaurine (ko″lil-taw′rēn) a bile salt, the taurine conjugate of cholic acid, called also taurocholic acid and cholaic acid.

chondodendrine (kon″do-den′drēn) bebeerine.

Chondodendron (kon″do-den′dron) a genus of climbing menispermaceous shrubs. **C. tomento′sum** Ruiz et Pavon, one of the sources of curare, or South American arrow poison. The major alkaloid is D-tubocurarine, which is used as a skeletal muscle relaxant in surgery, to control convulsion in strychnine toxicity and tetanus, and as a diagnostic aid in myasthenia gravis.

chondral (kon′dral) pertaining to cartilage.

chondralgia (kon-dral′je-ah) chondrodynia.

chondralloplasia (kon″dral-lo-pla′ze-ah) [chondr- + Gr. allos other + plassein to form] dyschondroplasia.

chondrectomy (kon-drek′to-me) [chondr- + Gr. ektomē excision] surgical removal of cartilage.

chondric (kon′drik) cartilaginous; of or relating to cartilage.

Chondrichthyes (kon-drik′thĭ-ēz) [Gr. chondros cartilage + ichthys fish] a class of fishes with cartilaginous skeletons, including sharks, skates, and their allies.

chondrification (kon″drĭ-fĭ-ka′shun) [chondri- + L. facere to make] the formation of cartilage; transformation into cartilage.

chondrigen (kon′drĭ-jen) chondrogen.

chondrin (kon′drin) a protein, resembling gelatin, from cartilage (Johannes Müller, 1837); it is considered to be a mixture of gelatin and mucin.

Chondrina (kon-dri′nah) a genus of snails that serves as a host of Dicrocoelium dendriticum.

chondri(o)- [Gr. chondrion granule] a combining form denoting relationship to a granule.

chondriome (kon′dre-ōm) all of the mitochondria of a cell or organism considered as one structure.

chondriosome (kon′dre-o-sōm″) [chondrio- + Gr. sōma body] mitochondrion.

chondritis (kon-dri′tis) [chondr- + -itis] inflammation of cartilage. **costal c.,** Tietze's syndrome. **c. intervertebra′lis calca′nea,** calcinosis intervertebralis.

chondr(o)- [Gr. chondros cartilage] a combining form denoting relationship to cartilage.

chondroadenoma (kon″dro-ad″ĕ-no′mah) adenochondroma.

chondroangioma (kon″dro-an″je-o′mah) a benign mesenchymoma containing chondromatous and angiomatous elements.

chondroblast (kon′dro-blast) [chondro- + Gr. blastos germ] a cell that arises from the mesenchyma and forms cartilage; called also chondroplast.

chondroblastoma (kon″dro-blas-to′mah) [chondroblast + -oma] a benign tumor composed of cells which arise from chondroblasts or their precursors and which tend to differentiate into cartilage cells; it occurs primarily in the epiphyses of adolescents. **benign c.,** chondroblastoma.

chondrocalcinosis (kon″dro-kal″sĭ-no′sis) [chondro- + L. calx lime + -osis] the presence of calcium salts, especially calcium pyrophosphate, in the cartilaginous structures of one or more joints; when accompanied by attacks of goutlike symptoms, it is known as pseudogout.

chondrocarcinoma (kon″dro-kar″sĭ-no′mah) carcinoma with chondromatous metaplasia.

chondroclast (kon′dro-klast) [chondro- + Gr. klan to break] a giant cell of the class that is believed associated with the absorption of cartilage.

Chondrococcus (kon″dro-kok′us) [chondro- + Gr. kokkos berry] in former systems of classification, a genus of bacteria made up of organisms now assigned to the genera Archangium, Flexibacter, and Myxococcus.

chondrocostal (kon″dro-kos′tal) [chondro- + L. costa rib] of or pertaining to the ribs and costal cartilages.

chondrocranium (kon″dro-kra′ne-um) [chondro- + Gr. kranion head] the cartilaginous skull of the embryo.

chondrocyte (kon′dro-sīt) [chondro- + Gr. kytos hollow vessel] a mature cartilage cell embedded in a lacuna within the cartilage matrix. **isogenous c's,** cartilage cells that make up a single group.

chondrodermatitis (kon″dro-der″mah-ti′tis) an inflammatory process involving cartilage and skin; used almost exclusively to mean chondrodermatitis nodularis chronica helicis. **c. nodula′ris chron′ica hel′icis,** a condition seen principally in middle-aged men marked by the presence of a small painful skin-colored, grayish, or waxy and translucent, firm, scaly, nodular lesion on the helix of the ear, most often the right one; multiple lesions may occur along the rim of the ear. Called also Winkler's disease.

chondrodynia (kon″dro-din′e-ah) [chondro- + Gr. odynē pain] pain in a cartilage.

chondrodysplasia (kon″dro-dis-pla′ze-ah) [chondro- + dysplasia] enchondromatosis. **hereditary deforming c.,** enchondromatosis. **c. puncta′ta,** a heterogeneous group of bone dysplasias, the common characteristic of which is stippling of the epiphyses in infancy. The group includes a severe autosomal recessive form (rhizomelic dwarfism), an autosomal dominant form (Conradi-Hünermann syndrome), and a milder X-linked form. Called also chondrodystrophia calcificans congenita, chondrodystrophia congenita punctata, chondrodystrophia fetalis calcificans, Conradi's disease or syndrome, dysplasia epiphysealis punctata, hypoplastic fetal chondrodystrophy, and stippled epiphyses.

chondrodystrophia (kon″dro-dis-tro′fe-ah) [chondro- + dys- + Gr. trophē nutrition] chondrodystrophy. **c. calcif′icans congen′ita, c. congen′ita puncta′ta, c. feta′lis calcif′icans,** chondrodysplasia punctata.

chondrodystrophy (kon″dro-dis′tro-fe) a morbid condition characterized by abnormal development of cartilage. **familial c.,** hereditary deforming chondrodysplasia. **hereditary deforming c.,** dyschondroplasia. **hyperplastic c.,** chondrodystrophy with excessive growth of the epiphyses. **hypoplastic c.,** chondrodystrophy in which the bone is spongy and the epiphyses are irregularly developed. **hypoplastic fetal c.,** chondrodysplasia punctata. **c. mala′cia,** a form marked by softening of the epiphyseal cartilage.

chondroendothelioma (kon″dro-en″do-the″le-o′mah) a benign mesenchymoma containing chondromatous and endotheliomatous elements.

chondroepiphyseal (kon″dro-ep″ĭ-fiz′e-al) pertaining to the epiphyseal cartilages.

chondroepiphysitis (kon″dro-ep″ĭ-fiz-i′tis) inflammation involving the epiphyseal cartilages.

chondrofibroma (kon″dro-fi-bro′mah) [chondroma + fibroma] a fibroma with cartilaginous elements.

chondrogen (kon′dro-jen) [chondro- + Gr. gennan to produce] a substance regarded as the basis of cartilage and of the corneal tissue: boiling turns it into chondrin.

chondrogenesis (kon″dro-jen′ĕ-sis) [chondro- + Gr. genesis production] the formation of cartilage.

chondrogenic (kon″dro-jen′ik) giving rise to or forming cartilage.

chondroglossus (kon″dro-glos′us) see Table of Musculi.

chondroglucose (kon″dro-glu′kōs) a sugar formed by the action of hydrochloric acid on chondrin from cartilage.

chondrography (kon-drog′rah-fe) [chondro- + Gr. graphein to write] a description or account of the cartilages.

chondroid (kon′droid) resembling cartilage.

chondroitic (kon″dro-it′ik) pertaining to, derived from, or resembling cartilage.

chondroitin sulfate (kon-dro′ĭ-tin) a glycosaminoglycan that predominates in the ground substance of cartilage, bone, and blood vessels but also occurs in other connective tissues. It is a linear chain of about 60 repeating disaccharide units; each contains one residue of D-glucuronic acid (GlcUA) and one of N-acetyl-D-galactosamine (GalNAc) linked by glycosidic bonds that are alternately 1→3 and 1→4, so that the formula for the repeating unit is (1→3)-β-GalNAc-

$(1\rightarrow4)$-β-GlcUA. There are two forms: chondroitin 4-sulfate (chondroitin sulfate A) and chondroitin 6-sulfate (chondroitin sulfate C), in which sulfate groups are esterified to galactosamine at C-4 and C-6, respectively. Chondroitin sulfate B is now called *dermatan sulfate.*

chondroitinsulfatase (kon-droi″tin-sul′fah-tās)   *N*-acetylgalactosamine-6-sulfatase.

chondroitinuria (kon-dro″ĭ-tin-u′re-ah)   the presence of chondroitic acid in the urine.

chondrolipoma (kon″dro-lĭ-po′mah)   a benign mesenchymoma containing lipomatous and cartilaginous elements.

chondrology (kon-drol′o-je) [*chondro-* + *-logy*]   the sum of knowledge in regard to the cartilages.

chondrolysis (kon-drol′ĭ-sis) [*chondro-* + Gr. *lysis* dissolution]   the degeneration of cartilage cells that occurs in the process of intracartilaginous ossification.

chondroma (kon-dro′mah) [*chondro-* + *-oma*]   a tumor or tumor-like growth of cartilage cells. It may remain within the substance of a cartilage or bone (*true chondroma,* or *enchondroma*) or may develop on the surface of a cartilage (*ecchondroma,* or *ecchondrosis*).   **joint c.,** a mass of cartilage in the synovial membrane of a joint; see *synovial chondromatosis.*   **c. sarcomato′sum,** chondrosarcoma.   **synovial c.,** a cartilaginous body formed in a synovial membrane; see under *chondromatosis.*   **true c.,** enchondroma.

chondromalacia (kon″dro-mah-la′she-ah) [*chondro-* + Gr. *malakia* softness]   softening of the articular cartilage, most frequently in the patella.   **c. feta′lis,** a condition in which the limbs of the stillborn fetus are soft and pliable due to softening of the epiphyseal cartilage.   **c. patel′lae,** premature degeneration of the patellar cartilage, the patellar margins being tender so that pain is produced when the patella is pressed against the femur.

chondromatosis (kon″dro-mah-to′sis)   multiple formation of chondromas.   **synovial c.,** a rare condition in which cartilage is formed in the synovial membranes of joints, tendon sheaths, or bursa, by metaplasia of the connective tissue beneath the surface of the membrane. Some metaplastic foci on the surface of the membrane may become sessile, and then pedunculated, and finally become detached, producing a number of loose bodies. Called also *synovial chondrometaplasia.*

chondromatous (kon-drom′ah-tus)   pertaining to or of the nature of cartilage.

chondromere (kon′dro-mēr) [*chondro-* + Gr. *meros* part]   a cartilaginous vertebra of the fetal vertebral column.

chondrometaplasia (kon″dro-met″ah-pla′ze-ah)   a condition characterized by metaplastic activity of the chondroblasts.   **synovial c.,** synovial chondromatosis.   **tenosynovial c.,** synovial chondromatosis affecting the sheath of a tendon.

chondromitome (kon″dro-mi′tōm) [*chondro-* + Gr. *mitos* thread]   the paranucleus.

chondromucin (kon″dro-mu′sin)   a dense homogeneous intercellular substance in cartilage, being a compound of a protein with chondroitic acid; called also *chondromucoid.*

chondromucoid (kon″dro-mu′koid)   chondromucin.

chondromucoprotein (kon″dro-mu″ko-pro′te-in)   the principal constituent of the ground substance of cartilage, a copolymer of a mucoprotein, chondroitin-4-sulfate (chondroitin sulfate A), and chondroitin-6-sulfate (chondroitin sulfate C).

Chondromyces (kon″dro-mi′sēz) [*chondro-* + Gr. *mykēs* fungus]   a genus of gliding bacteria of the family Polyangiaceae, order Myxobacterales, found in soil and dung from herbivores. The type species is *C. croca′tus.*

chondromyoma (kon″dro-mi-o′mah)   a benign mesenchymoma containing myomatous and cartilaginous elements.

chondromyxoma (kon″dro-mik-so′mah)   myxoma containing cartilaginous elements.

chondromyxosarcoma (kon″dro-mik″so-sar-ko′mah)   a malignant mesenchymoma containing sarcomatous and cartilaginous elements.

chondronecrosis (kon″dro-nĕ-kro′sis)   necrosis of cartilage.

chondro-osseous (kon″dro-os′e-us)   composed of cartilage and bone.

chondropathia (kon″dro-path′e-ah)   chondropathy.   **c. tubero′sa,** Tietze's syndrome.

chondropathology (kon″dro-pah-thol′o-je)   the pathology of disease of cartilage.

chondropathy (kon-drop′ah-the) [*chondro-* + Gr. *pathos* disease]   disease of a cartilage.

chondrophyte (kon′dro-fīt) [*chondro-* + Gr. *phyton* a growth]   a cartilaginous growth at the articular extremity of a bone.

chondroplasia (kon″dro-pla′ze-ah)   the formation of cartilage by specialized cells (chondrocytes).   **c. puncta′ta,** dysplasia epiphysealis punctata.

chondroplast (kon′dro-plast) [*chondro-* + Gr. *plassein* to form]   chondroblast.

chondroplastic (kon″dro-plas′tik)   pertaining to plastic operations on cartilage.

chondroplasty (kon′dro-plas″te) [*chondro-* + Gr. *plassein* to form]   plastic surgery on cartilage; repair of lacerated or displaced cartilage.

chondroporosis (kon″dro-po-ro′sis) [*chondro-* + Gr. *poros* a passage]   the formation of spaces or sinuses in the cartilages; it occurs normally during ossification.

chondroproteid (kon″dro-pro′te-id)   chondroprotein.

chondroprotein (kon″dro-pro′te-in)   any of a series of glycoproteins occurring in cartilage, comprising lardacein and chondromucoid; they yield chondroitic acid on decomposition.

chondrosamine (kon-dro′sam-in)   a galactosamine, CH_2-$OH(CHOH)_3CH(NH_2)CHO$, which results from hydrolysis of chondrosin.

chondrosarcoma (kon″dro-sar-ko′mah) [*chondro-* + *sarcoma*]   a malignant tumor derived from cartilage cells or their precursors; called also *chondroma sarcomatosum.*   **central c.,** one developing in the interior of a bone; called also *enchondrosarcoma.*   **mesenchymal c.,** a chondrosarcoma that is multicentric in origin.

chondrosarcomatosis (kon″dro-sar″ko-mah-to′sis)   the formation of multiple chondrosarcomas.

chondrosarcomatous (kon″dro-sar-ko′mah-tus)   pertaining to or of the nature of chondrosarcoma.

chondroseptum (kon″dro-sep′tum) [*chondro-* + *septum*]   the cartilaginous part of the nasal septum.

chondrosin (kon′dro-sin)   a disaccharide, 2-amino-2-deoxy-3-*O*- (β-D-glucopyranurosyl)-D-galactopyranose, $(C_{12}H_{21}NO_{11})$; the most common aldohexuronic acid in nature occurring as a structural unit. It is obtained by hydrolysis of chondroitins and chondroitin sulfates.

chondrosis (kon-dro′sis) [Gr. *chondros* cartilage]   the formation of cartilaginous tissue.

chondroskeleton (kon″dro-skel′ĕ-ton)   1. a cartilaginous skeleton, as in certain fish.   2. that part of the skeleton composed of cartilage.

chondrosome (kon′dro-sōm) [*chondro-* + Gr. *sōma* body]   chondriosome.

chondrosteoma (kon-dros″te-o′mah)   osteochondroma.

chondrosternal (kon″dro-ster′nal)   pertaining to the costal cartilages and the sternum.

chondrosternoplasty (kon″dro-ster′no-plas″te)   surgical correction of funnel chest.

chondrotome (kon′dro-tōm)   an instrument for cutting cartilage.

chondrotomy (kon-drot′o-me) [*chondro-* + Gr. *temnein* to cut]   the dissection or surgical division of cartilage.

Chondrotrichida (kon″dro-trik′ĭ-dah) [*chondro-* + Gr. *trichos* hair]   an order of marine and freshwater ciliate protozoa (superorder Phyllopharyngidea, subclass Hypomastia) found as ectocommensals, chiefly on crustaceans, and occurring variously as vase-shaped, sessile, and sedentary forms. They are characterized by the presence of ciliature on the ventral surface of the body, a cytopharynx without nematodesmata, an adhesive organelle, and a heteromerous macronucleus. It comprises two suborders: Exogemmina and Cryptogemmina.

chondrotrophic (kon″dro-trof′ik) [*chondro-* + Gr. *trophē* nutrition]   having an influence on the formation or growth of cartilage.

chondroxiphoid (kon″dro-zi′foid) [*chondro-* + *xiphoid*] pertaining to the xiphoid process.

chondrus (kon′drus) the dried, sun-bleached plant of the seaweed *Chondrus crispus*; used as a protective agent for the skin; called also *carrageen* or *carragheen*, *Irish moss*, *killeen*, *pearl moss*, and *salt rock moss*.

chonechondrosternon (ko″ne-kon″dro-ster′non) funnel chest.

CHOP a regimen of cyclophosphamide, hydroxydaunomycin (doxorubicin), Oncovin (vincristine), and prednisone, used in cancer chemotherapy.

Chopart's amputation (operation), articulation (joint) (sho-parz′) [François *Chopart*, French surgeon, 1743–1795] see under *amputation*, and see *articulatio tarsi transversa*.

chorangioma (ko-ran″je-o′mah) chorioangioma.

chord (kord) cord. **condyle c.**, condylar axis.

chorda (kor′dah), pl. *chor′dae* [L., from Gr. *chordē* cord] [NA] any cord or sinew. **c. dorsa′lis**, notochord. **c. gubernac′ulum**, gubernacular cord: a portion of the gubernaculum testis or of the round ligament of the uterus that develops in the inguinal crest and adjoining body wall. **c. mag′na**, tendo calcaneus. **c. obli′qua membra′nae interos′seae antebra′chii** [NA], a small ligamentous band extending from the lateral face of the tuberosity of the ulna to the radius a little distal to its tuberosity; called also *oblique cord of elbow joint*, and *Weitbrecht's cord* or *ligament*. **c. spermat′ica**, spermatic cord. **c. spina′lis**, medulla spinalis. **c. tendin′eae cor′dis** [NA], the tendinous cords that connect each cusp of the two atrioventricular valves to appropriate papillary muscles in the heart ventricles. **c. tym′pani** [NA], a nerve originating from the facial nerve (nervus intermedius) and distributed to the submandibular, sublingual, and lingual glands and the anterior two-thirds of the tongue; modality: parasympathetic and special sensory. **c. umbilica′lis**, umbilical cord. **c. voca′lis**, ligamentum vocale. **chor′dae Willis′ii**, dural trabeculae, which are numerous fibrous bands that extend transversely across the inferior angle of the superior sagittal sinus.

chordae (kor′de) [L.] genitive and plural of *chorda*.

chordal (kor′dal) pertaining to any chorda (chiefly used of the notochord).

chorda-mesoderm (kor″dah-mez′o-derm) tissue of the dorsal lip of the blastopore, which gives rise to both notochord and mesoderm.

Chordata (kor-da′tah) [L. *chordatus* having a cord] a phylum of the animal kingdom comprising all animals that have a notochord during some stage of their development. It includes the subphyla Cephalochordata, Urochordata, and Vertebrata.

chordate (kor′dāt) 1. an animal belonging to the phylum Chordata. 2. having a notochord.

chordectomy (kor-dek′to-me) [*chordo-* + Gr. *ektomē* excision] cordectomy.

chordee (kor′de, kor′da) [Fr. *cordée* corded] downward bowing of the penis as a result of a congenital anomaly (hypospadias) or a urethral infection (gonorrhea); called also *gryposis penis*.

chorditis (kor-di′tis) inflammation of a vocal or spermatic cord. **c. canto′rum**, inflammation of the vocal cords in professional singers. **c. fibrino′sa**, acute laryngitis marked by the deposition of fibrin and the formation of erosions on the vocal cords. **c. nodo′sa**, c. tuberosa. **c. tubero′sa**, a condition marked by the formation of a small whitish nodule on one or both vocal cords, occurring in persons who use their voice excessively; called also *c. nodosa*. **c. voca′lis**, inflammation of the vocal cords. **c. voca′lis infe′rior**, chronic subglottic laryngitis.

chord(o)- [L. *chorda*, q.v.] a combining form denoting relationship to a cord.

chordoblastoma (kor″do-blas-to′mah) [*chordo-* + Gr. *blastos* germ + *-oma*] a tumor, the cells of which tend to differentiate into cells like those of the notochord.

chordocarcinoma (kor″do-kar″sĭ-no′mah) chordoma.

chordoepithelioma (kor″do-ep″ĭ-the″le-o′mah) a chordoma.

chordoid (kor′doid) resembling the notochord.

chordoma (kor-do′mah) [*chordo-* + *-oma*] a malignant tumor arising from the embryonic remains of the notochord; called also *chordocarcinoma* and *chordoepithelioma*. Cf. *ecchordosis physaliphora*.

chordopexy (kor′do-pek″se) cordopexy.

chordosarcoma (kor″do-sar-ko′mah) chordoma.

chordoskeleton (kor″do-skel′ĕ-ton) [*chordo-* + *skeleton*] that portion of the bony skeleton which is formed around the notochord.

chordotomy (kor-dot′o-me) [*chordo-* + Gr. *tomē* a cutting] cordotomy.

chorea (ko-re′ah) [L.; Gr. *choreia* dance] the ceaseless occurrence of a wide variety of rapid, highly complex, jerky movements that appear to be well coordinated but are performed involuntarily. **acute c.**, Sydenham's c. **Bergeron's c.**, electric chorea of childhood, characterized by violent rhythmic spasms, but running a benign course. **chronic c.**, **chronic progressive hereditary c.**, Huntington's c. **chronic progressive nonhereditary c.**, senile c. **c. cor′dis**, chorea with great irregularity of the heart's action. **dancing c.**, saltatory chorea. **degenerative c.**, Huntington's c. **diaphragmatic c.**, the utterance of a peculiar cry in cases of painless tic; called also *laryngeal c.* and *Schrötter's c.* **c. dimidia′ta**, hemichorea. **Dubini c.**, an acute, fatal form of electric chorea due to acute infection of the central nervous system; called also *Dubini's disease*. **electric c.**, a variety with violent and sudden movements. See *Bergeron's c.*, *Dubini's c.*, and *Henoch's c.* **c. fes′tinans**, old name for ataxia with festination; paralysis agitans. **fibrillary c.**, fibrillary contractions of various muscles; paramyoclonus. **c. gravida′rum**, Sydenham's chorea occurring in the early months of pregnancy, with or without a previous history of rheumatic disease; it may recur in subsequent pregnancies. **hemilateral c.**, hemichorea. **Henoch's c.**, chronic progressive electric chorea; see also *c. major*. **hereditary c.**, Huntington's c. **Huntington's c.**, a relatively common autosomal dominant disease characterized by chronic progressive chorea and mental deterioration terminating in dementia; the age of onset is variable but usually occurs in the fourth decade of life. Death usually follows within 15 years. Called also *chronic (progressive hereditary) c.*, *degenerative c.*, *hereditary c.*, and *Huntington disease*. **hyoscine c.**, chorea-like movements occurring in acute hyoscine (scopolamine) intoxication. **hysterical c.**, conversion hysteria in which the symptoms are choreiform movements. **juvenile c.**, Sydenham's c. **laryngeal c.**, diaphragmatic c. **limp c.**, chorea associated with extreme weakness; called also *c. mollis*. **malleatory c.**, rhythmic chorea in which the patient performs persistent movements of hammering. **methodic c.**, a variety in which the movements take place at regular intervals. **mimetic c.**, that which is caused by imitation. **c. mi′nor**, Sydenham's c. **c. mol′lis**, limp c. **Morvan's c.** (obs.), fibrillary contractions of the muscles of the calves and posterior part of the thighs, sometimes extending to the trunk, but never affecting the neck and face. **c. noctur′na**, chorea in which the movements continue during sleep. **c. nu′tans**, nodding spasm, or chorea with nodding head movements. **one-sided c.**, hemichorea. **paralytic c.**, chorea in which immobility replaces movement; see *Huntington's c.* **post-hemiplegic c.**, a form that affects the partially paralyzed muscles after hemiplegia; see *athetosis*. **prehemiplegic c.**, choreic movements that may precede an attack of hemiplegia. **saltatory c.**, rhythmic chorea with dancing movements; called also *dancing c.* **Schrötter's c.**, diaphragmatic c. **senile c.**, a benign, usually mild disorder of the elderly, marked by choreiform movements unassociated with mental disturbance. **simple c.**, Sydenham's c. **Sydenham's c.**, an acute, usually self-limited disorder of early life, usually between the ages of five and fifteen, or during pregnancy, and closely linked with rheumatic fever. It is characterized by involuntary movements that gradually become severe, affecting all motor activities including gait, arm movements, and speech. A mild psychic component is usually present. The disorder may be limited to one side of the body (hemichorea) or may take the form of muscular rigidity (paralytic chorea). Called also *St. Vitus' dance*.

choreal (ko′re-al) choreic.

choreatic (ko″re-at′ik) choreic.

choreic (kŏ-re'ik) pertaining to, of the nature of, or characterized by chorea.

choreiform (kŏ-re'ĭ-form) [*chorea* + L. *forma* form] resembling chorea.

choreoathetoid (ko"re-o-ath'ĕ-toid) pertaining to or characterized by choreoathetosis.

choreoathetosis (ko"re-o-ath"ĕ-to'sis) a condition marked by choreic and athetoid movements.

choreoid (ko're-oid) choreiform.

chorial (ko're-al) of or relating to the chorion.

chorioadenoma (ko"re-o-ad"ĕ-no'mah) adenomatous tumor of the chorion. **c. destru'ens,** a form of hydatidiform mole in which molar chorionic villi penetrate into the myometrium and/or parametrium or, rarely, are transported to distant sites, most often the lungs; called also *invasive, metastasizing, or malignant mole.*

chorioallantoic (ko"re-o-al"an-to'ik) pertaining to the chorioallantois.

chorioallantois (ko"re-o-ah-lan'to-is) an extraembryonic structure derived from union of the chorion and allantois which by means of vessels in the associated mesoderm serves in gas exchange. In reptiles and birds, it is a membrane apposed to the egg shell; in many mammals, it forms the placenta.

chorioamnionitis (ko"re-o-am"ne-o-ni'tis) inflammation of fetal membranes.

chorioangiofibroma (ko"re-o-an"je-o-fi-bro'mah) angiofibroma of the chorion.

chorioangioma (ko"re-o-an"je-o'mah) an angiomatous tumor of the chorion.

chorioblastoma (ko"re-o-blas-to'mah) choriocarcinoma.

chorioblastosis (ko"re-o-blas-to'sis) overgrowth of the chorion.

choriocapillaris (ko"re-o-kap"ĭ-la'ris) lamina choroidocapillaris.

choriocarcinoma (ko"re-o-kar"sĭ-no'mah) an epithelial malignancy of trophoblastic cells, formed by the abnormal proliferation of cuboidal and syncytial cells of the placental epithelium, without the production of chorionic villi. Almost all cases arise in the uterus, developing from hydatidiform mole (50 per cent), following abortion (25 per cent), or during normal pregnancy (22 per cent). The remainder occur in ectopic pregnancies and genital (ovarian and testicular) and extragenital teratomas. Called also *chorioblastoma, chorioepithelioma, chorionic carcinoma* or *epithelioma, deciduocellular sarcoma,* and *syncytioma malignum.*

choriocele (ko're-o-sēl) [*chorion* + Gr. *kēlē* hernia] protrusion of the eye through an aperture in the choroid.

chorioepithelioma (ko"re-o-ep"ĭ-the"le-o'mah) choriocarcinoma. **c. malig'num,** choriocarcinoma.

choriogenesis (ko"re-o-jen'ĕ-sis) [*chorio-* + Gr. *genesis* origin] the development of the chorion.

chorioid (ko're-oid) the choroid, def. 1.

chorioidea (ko"re-oi'de-ah) the choroid, def. 1.

chorioid(o)- for words beginning thus, see those beginning *choroid(o)-.*

chorioma (ko"re-o'mah) [*chorion* + *-oma*] any trophoblastic proliferation, benign or malignant.

choriomammotropin (ko"re-o-mam"o-tro'pin) human placental lactogen.

choriomeningitis (ko"re-o-men"in-ji'tis) cerebral meningitis with lymphocytic infiltration of the choroid plexuses. **lymphocytic c.,** a form of viral meningitis usually occurring in adults 20 to 40 years of age during the fall and winter months.

chorion (ko're-on) [Gr. "membrane"] 1. in human embryology, the cellular, outermost extraembryonic membrane, composed of trophoblast lined with mesoderm; it develops villi about 2 weeks after fertilization, is vascularized by allantoic vessels a week later, gives rise to the placenta, and persists until birth. 2. in mammalian embryology, the cellular, outer extraembryonic membrane, not necessarily developing villi. 3. endometrial stroma. 4. in biology, the noncellular membrane covering eggs of various animals, including fish and insects. See illustration under *amnion.* **c. frondo'sum,** the region of the chorion that bears villi; called also *shaggy c.* **c. lae've,** the smooth (nonvillous) and membranous part of the chorion. **primitive c.,** the

chorion from its inception by addition of mesoderm to trophoblast through the stage in which it has many primitive villi. **shaggy c.,** c. frondosum.

chorionepithelioma (ko"re-on-ep"ĭ-the"le-o'-mah) choriocarcinoma.

chorionic (ko"re-on'ik) pertaining to the chorion.

chorioplacental (ko"re-o-plah-sen'tal) pertaining to the chorion and the placenta.

Chorioptes (ko"re-op'tēz) a genus of parasitic mites infesting the skin and hair of domestic animals and causing a sort of mange (*chorioptic acariasis* or *itch*).

chorioretinal (ko"re-o-ret'ĭ-nal) pertaining to the choroid and retina.

chorioretinitis (ko"re-o-ret"ĭ-ni'tis) [*chorion* + *retinitis*] inflammation of the choroid and retina; retinochoroiditis. **c. sclopetaria,** a concussive, nonpenetrating injury characterized by choroidal and retinal rupturing, hemorrhage, fibrosis and retinal destruction, and poor vision; caused by an orbital missile (gunshot). **toxoplasmic c.,** a unilateral or bilateral condition occurring principally as a late sequel of congenital toxoplasmosis, manifested by recurrent episodes of ocular pain and decreased vision with progressive visual loss, and associated with deep, heavily pigmented, necrotic lesions in both the macular and peripheral retina and posterior uveitis. Called also *ocular toxoplasmosis* and *toxoplasmic retinochoroiditis.*

chorioretinopathy (ko"re-o-ret"ĭ-nop'ah-the) [*chorion* + *retinopathy*] a noninflammatory process involving both choroid and retina.

chorista (ko-ris'tah) [Gr. *chōristos* separated] defective development due to, or characterized by, displacement of the primordium.

choristoblastoma (ko-ris"to-blas-to'mah) [Gr. *chōristos* separated + *blastos* germ + *-oma*] choristoma.

choristoma (ko"ris-to'mah) [Gr. *chōristos* separated + *-oma*] a mass of tissue histologically normal for an organ or part of the body other than the site at which it is located; called also *aberrant rest* and *heterotopic tissue.*

choroid (ko'roid) [*chorion* + Gr. *eidos* form] 1. the thin, pigmented, vascular coat of the eye extending from the ora serrata to the optic nerve; it furnishes blood supply to the retina and conducts arteries and nerves to the anterior structures. Called also *chorioid, choroidea* [NA] and *chorioidea.* 2. resembling the chorion or corium.

choroidal (ko-roi'dal) pertaining to the choroid.

choroidea (ko-roi'de-ah) [NA] the choroid, def. 1.

choroidectomy (ko"roi-dek'to-me) surgical removal or destruction of the choroid plexus of the lateral ventricles of the brain.

choroideremia (ko"roi-der-e'me-ah) [*choroid* + Gr. *erēmia* destitution] hereditary primary choroidal degeneration, transmitted as an X-linked trait and beginning in the first decade of life. In males, the earliest symptom is usually night blindness, followed by constricted visual field and eventual blindness as the degeneration of the pigment epithelium of the retina progresses to complete atrophy. In females, it is nonprogressive; usually there is normal vision and often an atypical pigmentary retinopathy. Called also *progressive tapetochoroidal dystrophy.*

choroiditis (ko"roid-i'tis) [*choroid* + *-itis*] uveitis affecting the choroid, the posterior portion of the uveal tract. **acute diffuse serous c.,** 1. a disease of sudden onset in adults, characterized by widespread, yellowish, fundal edema, by retinal detachment with loss of sight, and by later retinal reattachment with probable restoration of sight. 2. Harada's syndrome. **anterior c.,** that in which there are points of inflammation in the peripheral choroid. **areolar c., areolar central c.,** that which starts around or near the macula lutea and progresses toward the periphery. Unlike other forms of choroiditis, the lesions are pigmented at first and then lose their pigmentation. Called also *Förster's c.* and *Förster's disease.* **central c.,** a variety in which the inflammation is in the region of the macula lutea. **diffuse c.,** a widespread, exudative lesion of the choroid. **disseminated c.,** exudative choroiditis with numerous isolated foci of inflammation on the fundus. **Doyne's familial honeycombed c.,** a hereditary degenerative ocular abnormality marked by light-colored patches in the neighborhood of the optic disk and macula; called also *Doyne's familial colloid degeneration* and *Doyne's honeycomb* *degeneration.* **exudative c.,** that which is characterized by scattered patches of an exudate. **focal c.,** a localized choroiditis. **Förster's c.,** areolar c.; called also *Förster disease.* **c. gutta′ta seni′lis,** Tay's c. **juxtapapillary c.,** choroiditis near the optic disk. **macular c.,** choroiditis underlying the macula. **metastatic c.,** a form due to metastasis in pyemia, meningitis, etc. **senile macular exudative c.,** disciform macular degeneration. **c. sero′sa,** glaucoma. **suppurative c.,** that which leads to the formation of pus. **Tay's c.,** degeneration of the choroid marked by irregular yellow spots around the macula lutea, and believed to be due to an atheromatous state of the arteries; seen in advanced life. Called also *c. guttata senilis* and *Tay's disease.*

choroidocyclitis (ko-roi″do-sik-li′tis)   uveitis in the choroid and ciliary processes.

choroidoiritis (ko-roi″do-i-ri′tis)   uveitis in the choroid coat and the iris.

choroidopathy (ko″roi-dop′ah-the) [*choroid* + *-pathy*] 1. choroiditis. 2. choroidosis.

choroidoretinitis (ko-roi″do-ret″ĭ-ni′tis)   chorioretinitis.

chortosterol (kor-tos′ter-ol) [Gr. *chortis* grass] the sterol of grass; also a mixture of sterols found in the feces of the horse, hence *hippocoprosterol.*

Christian's disease (syndrome) (kris′chanz) [Henry Asbury *Christian*, American physician, 1876–1951] Hand-Schüller-Christian disease.

Christian-Weber disease (kris′chan-web′er) [H. A. *Christian;* Frederick Parkes *Weber,* British physician, 1863–1962] relapsing febrile nodular nonsuppurative panniculitis.

Christison's formula (kris′tĭ-sonz) [Sir Robert *Christison,* Scotch physician, 1797–1882] Trapp's formula; see under *formula.*

Christmas disease, factor [*Christmas,* for the name of the first patient with the disease who was studied in detail] see *coagulation Factor IX,* under *factor.*

Christ-Siemens-Touraine syndrome (krist-se′menz-too-rān′) [J. *Christ,* German dentist; Hermann Werner *Siemens,* German dermatologist, born 1891; Henri *Touraine,* French dermatologist, 1883–1961] anhidrotic ectodermal dysplasia.

chromaffin (kro-maf′in) [*chromium-* + L. *affinis* having affinity for] taking up and staining strongly with chromium salts; said of certain cells occurring in the adrenal, coccygeal, and carotid glands, along the sympathetic nerves, and in various organs whose cytoplasmic granules give a brownish reaction with chromium salts. Called also *chromaphil.*

chromaffinity (kro″mah-fin′ĭ-te) the property of staining strongly with chrome salts.

chromaffinoblastoma (kro-maf″ĭ-no-blas-to′mah) (obs.) argentaffinoma.

chromaffinoma (kro″maf-ĭ-no′mah) any tumor containing chromaffin cells. **medullary c.,** pheochromocytoma.

chromaffinopathy (kro″maf-ĭ-nop′ah-the) [*chromaffin* + Gr. *pathos* disease] any disease of the chromaffin system.

chromaphil (kro′mah-fil) [*chrom-* + Gr. *philein* to love] chromaffin.

chromargentaffin (krōm″ar-jen′tah-fin) [*chromium* + L. *argentum* silver + L. *affinis* having affinity for] staining with chromium salts and impregnable with silver; said of certain cells of the mucous membrane of the intestinal tract. Cf. *enterochromaffin gland* and *argentaffinoma.*

chromate (kro′māt) 1. any salt of chromic acid. 2. to subject to the action of a salt of chromic acid.

Chromatiaceae (kro-ma′te-a′se-e) a family of aquatic phototrophic bacteria of the order Rhodospirillales, commonly known as purple sulfur bacteria. It is made up of mostly anaerobic cells that produce purple, orange, and brown pigments and fix carbon dioxide in the presence of elemental sulfur and sulfide. It contains the genera *Amoebobacter, Chromatium, Ectothiorhodospira, Lamprocystis, Thiocapsa, Thiocystis, Thiodictyon, Thiopedia, Thiosarcina,* and *Thiospirillum.*

chromatic (kro-mat′ik) 1. pertaining to color; stainable with dyes. 2. pertaining to chromatin.

chromatid (kro′mah-tid) one of the paired chromosome strands, joined at the centromere, which make up a metaphase chromosome, resulting from chromosome reduplication during the S phase (DNA synthetic phase) of interphase.

nonsister c's, the two chromatids of one homologous chromosome with respect to those of the other homologue. **sister c's,** the two chromatids of a chromosome held together by a centromere; dyads.

chromatin (kro′mah-tin) [Gr. *chrōma* color] the more readily stainable portion of the cell nucleus, forming a network of nuclear fibrils within the achromatin of a cell. It is a deoxyribonucleic acid attached to a protein (primarily histone) structure base and is the carrier of the genes in inheritance. It occurs in two states, euchromatin and heterochromatin, with different staining properties, and during cell division it coils and folds to form the chromosomes. Called also *chromoplasm.* **nucleolar-associated c., nucleolus-associated c.,** heterochromatin containing DNA, situated around, and sometimes extending into, the nucleolus of a cell. **sex c.,** a chromatin mass (Barr body) in the nucleus of interphase cells of most mammalian species, including humans. It represents a single, inactive, condensed X chromosome. See *Lyon hypothesis,* under *hypothesis.*

chromatinic (kro″mah-tin′ik) of or pertaining to the chromatin.

chromatin-negative (kro″mah-tin-neg′ah-tiv) lacking sex chromatin; characteristic of the nuclei of cells in a normal male or in other individuals with only one X chromosome.

chromatin-positive (kro″mah-tin-poz′ĭ-tiv) having sex chromatin (Barr body) in the nuclei of autosomal cells, a characteristic of the normal female or of other individuals with two (or more) X chromosomes.

chromatism (kro′mah-tizm) abnormal pigment deposits.

Chromatium (kro-ma′te-um) [Gr. *chrōma* color] a genus of aquatic phototrophic bacteria of the family Chromatiaceae, order Rhodospirillales, consisting of ovoid to rod-shaped motile cells that do not contain gas vacuoles. The organisms fix carbon dioxide in the presence of hydrogen sulfide. Cell suspensions are orange-brown and pink to purple. The type species is *C. oken′ii.*

chromatize (kro′mah-tīz) to charge with some chromium compound.

chromat(o)- [Gr. *chrōma,* gen. *chrōmatos* color] a combining form denoting relationship to (1) color, or (2) chromatin.

chromatoblast (kro-mat′o-blast) [*chromato-* + Gr. *blastos* germ] a cell that can become a chromatophore, or bearer of pigment.

chromatocinesis (kro″mah-to-si-ne′sis) chromatokinesis.

chromatogenous (kro″mah-toj′ĕ-nus) [*chromato-* + Gr. *gennan* to produce] producing color or coloring matter.

chromatogram (kro-mat′o-gram) [*chromato-* + Gr. *graphein* to record] originally, the pattern of bands of substances separated by column chromatography, so called because the technique was first used to separate plant pigments producing a pattern of colored bands; by extension, a permanent record produced by any form of chromatography, e.g., in paper or thin-layer chromatography, a dried and stained filter paper or plate and, in gas or high-performance liquid chromatography, the chart recorder output.

chromatograph (kro-mat′o-graf) 1. the apparatus used in chromatography. 2. to analyze by chromatography.

chromatographic (kro″mah-to-graf′ik) pertaining to or produced by chromatography.

chromatography (kro″mah-tog′rah-fe) any of a diverse group of techniques used to separate mixtures of substances based on differences in the relative affinities of the substances for two different media, one (the mobile phase) a moving fluid and the other (the stationary phase or sorbent) a porous solid or gel or a liquid coated on a solid support; the speed at which each substance is carried along by the mobile phase depends on its solubility (in a liquid mobile phase) or vapor pressure (in a gas mobile phase) and on its affinity for the sorbent. **adsorption c.,** that in which the stationary phase is a nonspecific adsorbent, such as silica gel, porous polymers, or charcoal. **affinity c.,** that based on a highly specific biologic interaction such as that between antigen and antibody, enzyme and substrate, or receptor and ligand. Any of these substances, covalently linked to an insoluble support or immobilized in a gel, may serve as the sorbent allowing the interacting substance to be isolated from relatively impure samples; often a 1000-fold purification can be achieved in one step. **column c.,** a type of chromatography using a sorbent packed in a column. The sample, dissolved in a solvent, is poured in the top. Some components are retained in the column bound to the sorbent. They are then washed out (eluted) in successive aliquots of the same solvent (more strongly bound components being eluted later) or of different solvents. **gas c. (GC),** a type of automated chromatography in which the sample, dissolved in a solvent, is vaporized and carried by an inert gas through a column packed with a sorbent to any of several types of detector. Each component of the sample, separated from the others by passage through the column, produces a separate peak in the detector output, which is graphed by a chart recorder. The sorbent may be an inert porous solid (*gas-solid c.*) or a nonvolatile liquid coated on a solid support (*gas-liquid c.*). **gas-liquid c. (GLC),** see *gas c.* **gas-solid c. (GSC),** see *gas c.* **gel-filtration c., gel-permeation c.,** that in which the stationary phase consists of gel-forming hydrophilic beads containing pores of an accurately controlled size. As the sample is carried through the gel small molecules are frequently trapped in the pores and delayed while larger molecules pass unimpeded. Sample components are thus separated on the basis of size and shape. Called also *molecular exclusion c.* and *molecular sieve c.* **high-performance liquid c., high-pressure liquid c. (HPLC),** a type of automated chromatography in which the mobile phase is a liquid, which is forced under high pressure through a column packed with a sorbent. As in gas chromatography, a detector at the end of the column coupled to a chart recorder graphs the sample efflux. Various separation methods, including adsorption, gel filtration, ion-exchange, and partition, are used. **ion-exchange c.,** that in which the stationary phase is an ion-exchange resin. The mobile phase is an aqueous buffer solution that determines the degree of ionization of the sample components and thus their affinity for the stationary phase. **liquid-liquid c.,** partition c. **molecular sieve c.,** exclusion c. **paper c.,** a type of chromatography in which the stationary phase is a sheet of special-grade filter paper; it is in all other aspects similar to thin-layer chromatography (q.v.). **partition c.,** that in which the stationary and mobile phases are immiscible liquids and the sample components are separated on the basis of their partition coefficients. Called also *liquid-liquid c.* **thin-layer c. (TLC),** type of chromatography in which the stationary phase is a thin layer of an adsorbent, e.g., silica gel, coated on a rectangular plate and the mobile phase is a solvent mixture. The sample is applied to a small spot on the plate, and then the plate is stood on end with its lower edge in solvent. As the solvent rises by capillary action through the adsorbent, the components of the sample are carried along at different rates and can be visualized as a row of spots after the plate is dried and stained or viewed under ultraviolet light.

chromatoid (kro′mah-toid) having the tinctorial properties of chromatin; see also under *body.*

chromatokinesis (kro″mah-to-ki-ne′sis) [*chromatin* + Gr. *kinēsis* movement] movement of chromatin during the life and division of a cell.

chromatology (kro″mah-tol′o-je) [*chromato-* + *-logy*] the science of colors.

chromatolysis (kro″mah-tol′ĭ-sis) [*chromato-* + Gr. *lysis* dissolution] disintegration of the Nissl (chromophil) bodies of a nerve cell as the result of injury, or of fatigue or exhaustion; a part of the so-called axon reaction.

chromatometer (kro″mah-tom′ĕ-ter) [*chromato-* + *-meter*] an instrument for measuring color or color perception; called also *chromatoptometer, chromometer,* and *chromoptometer.*

chromatopectic (kro″mah-to-pek′tik) chromopectic.

chromatopexis (kro″mah-to-pek′sis) chromopexy.

chromatophagus (kro″mah-tof′ah-gus) [*chromato-* + Gr. *phagein* to devour] destroying pigments.

chromatophil (kro′mah-to-fil″) a cell or element that stains easily.

chromatophile (kro′mah-to-fil″) 1. chromatophil. 2. chromatophilic.

chromatophilia (kro″mah-to-fil′e-ah) [*chromato-* + Gr. *philein* to love + *-ia*] the condition of staining easily.

chromatophilic (kro″mah-to-fil′ik) staining easily.

chromatophilous (kro″mah-tof′ĭ-lus) chromatophilic.

chromatophore (kro″mah-to-fōr″) [*chromato-* + Gr. *pherein* to bear] any pigmentary cell or color-producing plastid, such as those of the cutis or deep layers of the epidermis. Cf. *melanophore.*

chromatophoroma (kro″mah-to-fo-ro′mah) (*obs.*) malignant melanoma.

chromatophoromatosis (kro″mah-to-fo″ro-mah-to′sis) (*obs.*) malignant melanomatosis.

chromatophorotropic (kro″mah-to-fo″ro-trop′ik) having an influence or effect on chromatophores, as the pigmentary effect of melanocyte-stimulating hormone.

chromatoplasm (kro′mah-to-plazm) the colored portions of the protoplasm of a pigmented cell.

chromatopsia (kro″mah-top′se-ah) [*chromato-* + *-opsia*] 1. a visual defect in which colored objects appear unnaturally colored and colorless objects appear tinged with color. The chromatopsias are named for the colors seen: cyanopsia, blue; chloropsia, green; erythropsia, red; xanthopsia, yellow. Chromatopsia may be caused by drugs, disturbance of the optic centers, cataract extraction, or dazzling light. 2. imperfect perception of color; anomalous color vision.

chromatoptometer (kro″mah-top-tom′ĕ-ter) chromatometer.

chromatoptometry (kro″mah-top-tom′ĕ-tre) the testing of the power of discriminating colors.

chromatoscope (kro-mat′to-skōp) [*chromato-* + *-scope*] an instrument used in chromatoscopy (def. 1).

chromatoscopy (kro″mah-tos′kŏ-pe) [*chromato-* + *-scopy*] 1. the testing of color vision. 2. diagnosis of renal function by the color of the urine following the administration of dyes. **gastric c.,** diagnosis of gastric function by the color of the gastric contents; a test for achylia gastrica.

chromatoskiameter (kro″mah-to-ski-am′ĕ-ter) [*chromato-* + *skia-* + *-meter*] chromatometer that uses colored shadows.

chromatotaxis (kro″mah-to-tak′sis) [*chromatin* + Gr. *taxis* arrangement] the attraction or influence of certain substances on the chromatin of a cell nucleus, causing destruction of the chromatin, while the cell body remains intact.

chromatotropism (kro″mah-tot′ro-pizm) [*chromato-* + Gr. *tropos* a turning] an orienting response to a color.

chromaturia (kro″mah-tu′re-ah) [*chromato-* + Gr. *ouron* urine + *-ia*] abnormal coloration of the urine.

-chrome [Gr. *chroma* color] a word termination denoting relationship to color.

1,2-chromene (kro′mēn) a plant pigment, a constituent of oxidized tocopherol; called also *1,2-benzopyran.*

chromesthesia (kro″mes-the′ze-ah) [*chrom-* + Gr. *aisthēsis* perception] the association of imaginary sensations of color with actual sensations of hearing, taste, or smell; see *photism.*

chromhidrosis (kro″mĭ-dro′sis) [*chrom-* + Gr. *hidrōs* sweat] the secretion of colored sweat; called also *chromidrosis.*

chromic acid (kro′mik) the common name for chromium trioxide (CrO_3), although the term strictly refers to the species H_2CrO_4, which exists only in aqueous solution. It is a highly toxic, corrosive, strong oxidizing agent.

chromicize (kro′mĭ-sīz) to treat with a chromium compound.

chromidrosis (kro″mid-ro′sis) chromhidrosis.

chromium (kro′me-um) [L.; Gr. *chrōma* color] a blue-whitish, brittle metal: atomic number, 24; atomic weight, 51.996; specific gravity, 7.1; symbol, Cr; several of its compounds are pigments, and the metal itself is used for weather-resistant plating. Chromium, which plays a role in glucose metabolism, is considered essential in trace amounts in nutrition. **c. trioxide,** chromic acid, see def. 2.

chrom(o)- [Gr. *chrōma* color] a combining form denoting relationship to color.

Chromobacterium (kro″mo-bak-te′re-um) [*chromo-* + *bacterium*] a genus of gram-negative, aerobic or facultatively anaerobic, usually nonpathogenic, rod-shaped bacteria, found in soil and water in tropical countries, characteristically producing violet pigment that is soluble in alcohol but not in water or chloroform. **C. viola′ceum,** a species that may infect humans, causing abscesses, diarrhea, and urinary tract and systemic infections.

chromoblast (kro′mo-blast) [*chromo-* + Gr. *blastos* germ] an embryonic cell that develops into a pigment cell.

chromoblastomycosis (kro″mo-blas″to-mi-ko′sis) chromomycosis.

chromocenter (kro′mo-sen″ter) [*chromo-* + *center* (def. 1)]

1. karyosome. 2. a fused mass of heterochromatin with spokelike extensions of euchromatin, representing the chromosomes in the salivary glands of some insects.

chromocholoscopy (kro″mo-ko-los′ko-pe) [chromo- + Gr. cholē bile + Gr. skopein to examine] testing the biliary function by a pigment excretion test (methylthionine chloride).

chromoclastogenic (kro″mo-klas″to-jen′ik) giving rise to or inducing chromosomal disruption or damage.

chromocystoscopy (kro″mo-sis-tos′ko-pe) [chromo- + cystoscopy] examination of the interior of the bladder after administration of indigo carmine or other dye which is excreted in the urine, for identification and study of the activity of the ureteral orifices; called also chromoureteroscopy and cystochromoscopy.

chromocyte (kro′mo-sīt) [chromo- + Gr. kytos hollow vessel] any colored cell or pigmented corpuscle.

chromodacryorrhea (kro″mo-dak″re-o-re′ah) [chromo- + dacryo- + -rrhea] the shedding of bloody tears.

chromodiagnosis (kro″mo-di″ag-no′sis) [chromo- + diagnosis] 1. diagnosis by change of color. 2. diagnosis of functional derangements by observing the rate at which coloring matters, such as methylthionine chloride, are excreted. 3. diagnostic examination made through colored glass or sheets of colored gelatin.

chromoflavine (kro″mo-fla′vin) acriflavine.

chromogen (kro′mo-jen) 1. a chemical compound, itself without color, that can be transformed into a colored compound, or can react with another material to form a colored compound. 2. a microorganism that produces pigment, e.g., certain strains of Mycobacterium that produce yellow to red colonies. **Porter-Silber c's,** 17-hydroxycorticosteroids, adrenocorticosteroids with a dihydroxyacetone side chain; so called because their concentration in plasma or urine can be determined by the Porter-Silber reaction employing sulfuric acid–phenylhydrazine reagent.

chromogene (kro′mo-jēn) [chromosome + gene] a gene that is located on a chromosome. Cf. plasmagene.

chromogenesis (kro″mo-jen′ĕ-sis) [chromo- + genesis] the formation of pigments or colors, as by bacterial action.

chromogenic (kro″mo-jen′ik) producing a pigment or coloring matter.

chromogranin (kro″mo-gran′in) a soluble protein constituent of the secretory granules of the chromaffin cells of the adrenal medulla.

chromoisomerism (kro″mo-i-som′er-izm) [chromo- + isomerism] isomerism in which the isomers have different colors.

chromolipoid (kro″mo-lip′oid) lipochrome.

chromoma (kro-mo′mah) (obs.) an ulcerated malignant melanoma.

chromomere (kro′mo-mēr) [chromo- + Gr. meros part] 1. any one of the beadlike granules seen in prophase occurring in series along the chromonema of a chromosome; called also idiomere. 2. granulomere.

chromometer (kro-mom′ĕ-ter) 1. chromatometer. 2. colorimeter.

chromomycosis (kro″mo-mi-ko′sis) a chronic fungal infection of the skin, usually beginning at the site of a puncture wound or other trauma and affecting one leg or foot (mossy foot) but sometimes involving other areas of the body, producing wartlike nodules or papillomas that may or may not ulcerate; microscopically, the lesions are characterized by round, brown bodies that reproduce by equatorial splitting and not by budding. The disease occurs sporadically in many areas of the world, and may be caused by Phialophora verrucosa, Fonsecaea pedrosoi, F. compactum, Cladosporium carrionii, and other dematiaceous fungi. Called also chromoblastomycosis.

chromonar hydrochloride (kro′mo-nar) chemical name: [[3-[2-(diethylamino)-ethyl]4-methyl-2-oxo-2H-1-benzopyran-7- yl]oxy]acetic acid ethyl ester hydrochloride; a coronary vasodilator, $C_{20}H_{27}NO_5 \cdot HCl$. Called also carbocromen hydrochloride.

chromone (kro′mōn) [Gr. chrōma color] coumarin.

chromonema (kro″mo-ne′mah), pl. chromone′mata [chromo- + Gr. nēma thread] the coiled central thread of a chromatid, as opposed to the more densely coiled chromomere regions.

chromonemal (kro″mo-ne′mal) of or pertaining to a chromonema.

chromonemata (kro″mo-ne′mah-tah) plural of chromonema.

chromoneme (kro′mo-nēm) chromonema.

chromonucleic acid (kro″mo-nu-kle-ik) deoxyribonucleic acid (DNA).

chromoparic (kro-mo-par′ik) [chromo- + L. parere to produce] producing or giving rise to color; chromogenic.

chromopectic (kro″mo-pek′tik) pertaining to, characterized by, or promoting chromopexy.

chromopexic (kro″mo-pek′sik) chromopectic.

chromopexy (kro′mo-pek″se) [chromo- + Gr. pēxis fixation] the fixation of pigment, a term applied especially to the function of the liver in forming bilirubin.

chromophage (kro′mo-fāj) [chromo- + Gr. phagein to eat] pigmentophage.

chromophane (kro′mo-fān) [chromo- + Gr. phainein to show] a retinal pigment found in some species of animals.

chromophil (kro′mo-fil) [chromo- + Gr. philein to love] any easily stainable cell, structure, or tissue.

chromophile (kro′mo-fīl) 1. chromophil. 2. chromophilic.

chromophilic (kro-mo-fil′ik) readily or easily stained; said especially of certain leukocytes and other histologic elements.

chromophilous (kro-mof′ĭ-lus) chromophilic.

chromophobe (kro′mo-fōb) [chromo- + Gr. phobein to be affrighted by] any cell, structure, or tissue that does not stain readily; applied especially to the nonstaining cells of the anterior hypophysis (pituitary gland).

chromophobia (kro″mo-fo′be-ah) the quality of staining poorly with dyes.

chromophore (kro′mo-fōr) any chemical group whose presence gives a decided color to a compound and which unites with certain other groups (auxochromes) to form dyes; called also color radical.

chromophoric (kro″mo-fōr′ik) [chromo- + Gr. pherein to bear] 1. bearing color; said of chromogenic bacteria when the pigment is a component of the bacterial cell itself. 2. pertaining to a chromophore.

chromophorous (kro-mof′o-rus) chromophoric.

chromophose (kro′mo-fōs) [chromo- + phose] a subjective sensation of a spot of color in the eye.

chromophototherapy (kro″mo-fo″to-ther′ah-pe) [chromo- + Gr. phōs light + therapeia treatment] treatment with colored light.

chromoplasm (kro′mo-plazm) [chromo- + Gr. plasma something formed] chromatin.

chromoplast (kro′mo-plast) chromoplastid.

chromoplastid (kro″mo-plas′tid) [chromo- + plastid] any pigment-producing plastid other than a chloroplast.

chromoprotein (kro″mo-pro′te-in) [chromo- + protein] a colored conjugated protein. Examples are the red hemoglobin of the higher animals, the blue hemocyanin of many lower animals, and the red and blue pigments of seaweeds. Chromoproteins have respiratory functions and are closely related to the green chlorophyll of the higher plants.

chromopsia (kro-mop′se-ah) chromatopsia.

chromoptometer (kro″mop-tom′ĕ-ter) chromatoptometer.

chromoretinography (kro″mo-ret″ĭ-nog′rah-fe) [chromo- + retina + -graphy] color photography of the retina.

chromorhinorrhea (kro″mo-ri″no-re′ah) [chromo- + Gr. rhis nose + Gr. rhoia a flow] the discharge of a pigmented secretion from the nose.

chromosantonin (kro″mo-san′to-nin) yellow santonin; an isomeric form produced when santonin is exposed to sunlight.

chromoscope (kro′mo-skōp) chromatoscope.

chromoscopy (kro-mos′kŏ-pe) chromatoscopy.

chromosomal (kro″mo-so′mal) pertaining to chromosomes.

chromosome (kro′mo-sōm) [chromo- + Gr. sōma body] 1. in animal cells, a structure in the nucleus containing a linear thread of DNA, which transmits genetic information and is

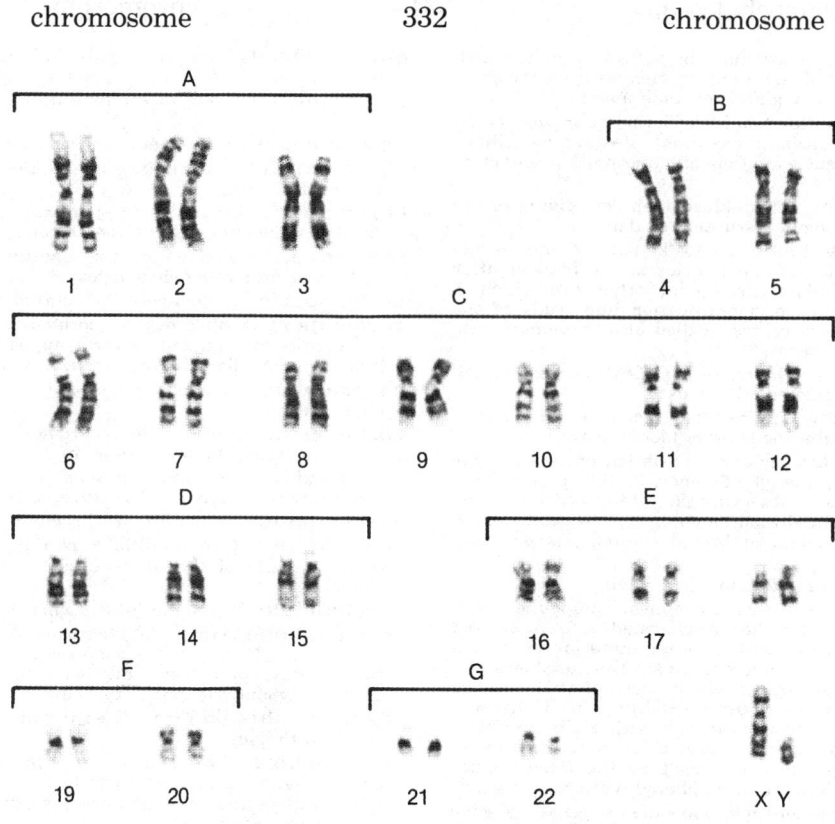

Human male chromosomes with Giemsa banding (Type G banding), arranged as a karyotype.

associated with RNA and histones; during cell division, the material (chromatin) composing the chromosome is compactly coiled, making it visible with appropriate staining and permitting its movement in the cell with minimal entanglement. Each organism of a species normally has a characteristic number of chromosomes in its somatic cells, 46 being the number normally present in man, including the two (XX or XY) which determine the sex of the organism. See *illustration*.   2. in bacterial genetics, a closed circle of double-stranded DNA that contains the genetic material of the cell and is attached to the cell membrane; the bulk of the material forms a compact bacterial nucleus (called also *chromatinic body*).   **accessory c's,** supernumerary c's.   **acentric c.,** a chromosome with no centromere.   **acrocentric c.,** a chromosome with the centromere near one end. In humans such chromosomes have satellited short arms that carry genes for ribosomal RNA.   **B c.,** supernumerary c.   **bivalent c.,** see *bivalent,* def. 2.   **daughter c's,** the name for chromatids when they reach the poles of the cell in the anaphase stage of mitosis.   **dicentric c.,** a structurally abnormal chromosome with two centromeres.   **gametic c.,** single-stranded chromosome of a haploid cell (gamete).   **giant c's,** 1. polytene c's.   2. lampbrush c's.   **heterotypical c's,** see *sex c's.*   **homologous c's,** a matching pair of chromosomes, one from each parent, with the same gene loci in the same order.   **lampbrush c's,** giant chromosomes of the oocytes of many lower animals arranged like a cylindrical brush.   **m-c.,** mitochondrial c.   **metacentric c.,** a chromosome with its centromere in the center and arms of equal length.   **mitochondrial c.,** a single circular chromosome within each mitochondrion, resembling a bacterial chromosome and capable of synthesizing protein since it contains ribosomal RNA, messenger RNA, and transfer RNA. The mitochondrial chromosome carries the genes for 13 proteins and is the basis for extrachromosomal

inheritance (q.v.); some authorities consider it the 25th human chromosome in addition to the 22 autosomes and the X and Y chromosomes.   **nucleolar c's,** those in relation to which the nucleoli reorganize during the telophase of mitosis.   **odd c's,** see *sex c's.*   **Ph¹ c., Philadelphia c.,** an abnormality of chromosome 22, characterized by shortening of its long arms (the missing portion usually translocated to chromosome 9) and present in marrow cells of most patients with chronic myelocytic leukemia.   **polytene c's,** giant bundles of unseparated chromonemata occurring especially in the salivary glands of some insects; called also *giant c's.*   **ring c.,** a chromosome in which both ends have been lost (deletion) and the two broken ends have reunited to form a ring.   **sex c's,** chromosomes that are associated with the determination of sex, in mammals constituting an unequal pair, the X and the Y chromosome.   **small c., m-c.**   **somatic c.,** a chromosome of a diploid (tissue) cell of the body.   **submetacentric c.,** a chromosome with its centromere slightly off-center so that the arms are different in length.   **supernumerary c.,** one or more extra chromosomes found inconstantly in wild populations of certain species of animals; they are not homologous to members of the regular set of chromosomes and apparently exert little influence on the phenotypic effect. Called also *accessory* and *Bc.*   **telocentric c.,** a chromosome with a terminal centromere; not found in humans.   **W c's, Z c's,** the sex chromosomes of certain insects, birds, and fishes, in which the female is heterogametic (i.e., has a W and a Z chromosome) and the males are homogametic (having only Z chromosomes).   **X c.,** the female sex chromosome, being the differential sex chromosome carried by half the male gametes and all female gametes in man and other male-heterogametic species.   **Y c.,** the male sex chromosome, being the differential sex chromosome carried by half the male gametes and none of the female gametes in man and

A–G	Chromosome groups
1–22	Autosome numbers
X, Y	Sex chromosomes
/	Diagonal line separating cell lines in descriptions of mosaicism
?	Identification of chromosome or chromosome structure questionable
+ −	When placed before the chromosome number, these denote addition or loss of a whole chromosome; when placed after the chromosome number, they denote an increase or decrease in length of a chromosome part.
:	Break with no reunion
::	Break with reunion
→	From ... to
ace	Acentric
cen	Centromere
del	Deletion
der	Derivative chromosome
dic	Dicentric
dup	Duplication
end	Endoreduplication
h	Secondary constriction or negatively staining region
i	Isochromosome
ins	Insertion
inv	Inversion
inv ins	Inverted insertion
mar	Marker chromosome
mat	Maternal origin
p	Short arm
pat	Paternal origin
q	Long arm
r	Ring chromosome
rcp	Reciprocal translocation
rec	Recombinant chromosome
rob	Robertsonian translocation
s	Satellite
t	Translocation
ter	Terminal

Repeated symbols denote duplication of chromosome structure.

Symbols for rearrangements are placed before the chromosome number and the rearranged chromosomes are placed in parenthesis, e.g., t(14q21q), r(18).

in some other male-heterogametic species in which the homologue of the X chromosome has been retained.

chromospermism (kro″mo-sper′mizm) [*chromo-* + *sperm*] a colored condition of the sperm.

chromotherapy (kro″mo-ther′ah-pe) [*chromo-* + Gr. *therapeia* treatment] 1. treatment of disease by variously colored lights. 2. the therapeutic use of restricted areas of the spectrum; called also *beamtherapy.*

chromotoxic (kro″mo-tok′sik) [*chromo-* + Gr. *toxikon* poison] destructive to hemoglobin or due to the destruction of hemoglobin.

chromotrichia (kro″mo-trik′e-ah) [*chromo-* + Gr. *thrix* hair + *-ia*] coloration of the hair.

chromotrichial (kro″mo-trik′e-al) pertaining to the coloration of the hair.

chromotropic (kro″mo-trop′ik) [*chromo-* + Gr. *tropikos* turning] turning to or attracting color or pigment.

chromoureteroscopy (kro″mo-u-re″ter-os′ko-pe) chromocystoscopy.

chromourinography (kro″mo-u″rĭ-nog′rah-fe) diagnosis by measuring the intensity of color and the time of appearance in the urine after injection of a dye.

chronic (kron′ik) [L. *chronicus,* from Gr. *chronos* time] persisting over a long period of time.

chronicity (kro-nis′ĭ-te) the quality of being chronic.

chroniosepsis (kron″e-o-sep′sis) a chronic form of sepsis.

chron(o)- [Gr. *chronos* time] a combining form denoting relationship to time.

chronobiologic, chronobiological (kron″o-bi″o-loj′ik; kron″o-bi″o-loj′ĭ-kal) pertaining to chronobiology; relating to the effects of time and biological rhythms on living systems.

chronobiologist (kron″o-bi-ol′o-jist) a specialist in chronobiology.

chronobiology (kron″o-bi-ol′ŏ-je) [*chrono-* + Gr. *bios* life +

-logy] the scientific study of the effect of time on living systems; see *anachronobiology* and *catachronobiology.*

chronognosis (kron″og-no′sis) [*chrono-* + Gr. *gnōsis* knowledge] the subjective appreciation of the passage of time.

chronograph (kron′o-graf) [*chrono-* + Gr. *graphein* to write] an instrument for recording small intervals of time.

chronometry (kro-nom′ĕ-tre) [*chrono-* + Gr. *metrein* to measure] the measurement of time or intervals of time. **mental c.,** the measurement and study of the duration of mental processes.

chronomyometer (kron″o-mi-om′ĕ-ter) an apparatus for measuring chronaxy.

chronophobia (kron″o-fo′be-ah) [*chrono-* + *phobia*] fear of time, or prison neurosis; panic, anxiety, and claustrophobia exhibited by prisoners having difficulty adjusting to a long prison sentence.

chronophotograph (kron″o-fo′to-graf) [*chrono-* + *photograph*] one of a series of photographs of a moving object taken for the purpose of showing successive phases of the motion.

chronoscope (kron′o-skōp) [*chrono-* + Gr. *skopein* to examine] an instrument for measuring minute intervals of time.

chronosphygmograph (kron″o-sfig′mo-graf) Jaquet's instrument for observing the rhythm as well as the character of the pulse.

chronotaraxis (kro-no-tar-ak′sis) [*chrono-* + Gr. *taraxis* confusion] disorientation for time; observed as a transient symptom following thalamic or frontal lobe lesions.

chronotropic (kron″o-trop′ik) [*chrono-* + Gr. *tropikos* turning] affecting the time or rate, as the rate of contraction of the heart.

chronotropism (kro-not′ro-pizm) interference with the regularity of a periodic movement, such as the heart beat.

chrotoplast (kro′to-plast) [Gr. *chrōs* skin + *plassein* to form] a dermal or skin cell.

chrysalis (kris′ah-lis) [L.] the pupa of some insects, especially of a moth or butterfly.

chrysarobin (kris″ah-ro′bin) a brownish to yellow-orange microcrystalline powder consisting of a mixture of the neutral principles extracted from Goa powder; a reduction product of chrysophanic acid, it is used topically in the treatment of psoriasis and other chronic skin disease.

chrysazin (kris′ah-zin) danthron.

chrysiasis (krĭ-si′ah-sis) [*chrys-* + *-iasis*] 1. deposition of gold particles in the tissues as a result of prolonged or excessive parenteral chrysotherapy, which commonly causes adverse reactions consisting primarily of dermatitis, stomatitis, or transient mild proteinuria; more serious toxicity involves the hematopoietic system, liver, kidney, eye (cornea, lens), or other vital organ. Called also *auriasis.* 2. chrysoderma.

chrys(o)- [Gr. *chrysos* gold] a combining form denoting relationship to gold.

chrysoderma (kris″o-der′mah) [*chryso-* + *derma*] a manifestation of chrysiasis presenting as a permanent gray- to lilac-colored pigmentation on the face, eyelids, and other sun-exposed areas of the body. Called also *aurochromoderma* and *chrysiasis.*

chrysomonad (kris″o-mo′nad) [*chryso-* + Gr. *monas* unit, from *monos* single] a protozoan of the order Chrysomonadida.

Chrysomonadida (kris″so-mo-nad′ĭ-dah) [*chryso-* + Gr. *monas* unit, from *monos* single] an order of free-swimming, flagellate, chiefly ameboid, plastic, plantlike, marine and freshwater protozoa (class Phytomastigophorea, subphylum Mastigophora) having two unequal flagella, golden-brown chloroplasts when present, and a cyst wall that is typically siliceous. *Synura* is a representative genus.

Chrysomonadina (kris″o-mon-ah-di′nah) an order of very small, free-swimming, chiefly ameboid protozoa of the class Phytomastigophorea, subphylum Mastigophora, which usually have one or two flagella, and are found in fresh and marine waters. It includes the families Syncryptidae and Ochromonadidae.

Chrysomyia (kris″o-mi′yah) [*chryso-* + Gr. *myia* fly] a genus of flies of the family Calliphoridae, of Africa, Australia, and parts of Asia. **C. al′biceps,** a South African species whose larvae (wool maggots) live in the soiled wool of sheep. **C. bezzia′na,** a species widely distributed in Asia and Africa and frequently found in wounds of man and animals; it may cause severe and disfiguring myiasis in man. Called also *Cochliomyia bezziana.* **C. macella′ria,** *Cochliomyia hominivorax.*

chrysophanic acid, medicinal (kris-o-fan′ik) an incorrect term for chrysarobin.

chrysophoresis (kris″o-fo-re′sis) diffusion of gold particles to various organs of the body after therapeutic administration of preparations of gold, by macrophages and polymorphonuclear leukocytes.

Chrysops (kris′ops) [*chryso-* + Gr. *ōps* eye] a genus of bloodsucking tropical tabanid flies, the grove flies. **C. cecu′tiens,** a species that inflicts bites about the eyes of men and animals. **C. dimidia′ta,** a species of southwestern Africa that is an intermediate host of *Loa loa;* called also *mango* or *mangrove fly.* **C. disca′lis,** a common vector of tularemia in the western part of the United States; called also *deer fly.* **C. sila′cea,** an intermediate host of *Loa loa.*

Chrysosporium (kris-o-spōr′ĭ-um) a genus of imperfect, keratinophilic, soil fungi, related to the dermatophytes; some species have been isolated from dermatophytosis. Formerly called *Aleurisma* and *Glenosporella.*

chrysotherapy (kris″o-ther′ah-pe) [*chryso-* + *therapy*] treatment with gold salts; called also *aurotherapy.*

Chrysozona (kris″o-zo′nah) [*chryso-* + Gr. *zōne* girdle] a genus of tabanid flies. *C. ital′ica* and *C. pluvia′lis* are common in Europe; called also *Hematopota.*

chthonophagia (thon″o-fa′je-ah) [Gr. *chthōn* earth + *phagein* to eat] geophagia.

chthonophagy (thon-of′ah-je) geophagia.

Churg-Strauss syndrome (cherg-strows) [Jacob *Churg,* American pathologist, born 1910; Lotte *Strauss,* American pathologist, born 1913] allergic granulomatous angiitis.

churus (chur′us) ganja.

Chvostek's sign (symptom, test) (vos′teks) [Franz *Chvostek,* Austrian surgeon, 1835–1884] see under *sign.*

Chvostek-Weiss sign (vos′tek-vīs′) [Franz *Chvostek;* Nathan *Weiss,* physician in Vienna, 1851–1883] Chvostek's sign.

chylangioma (ki″lan-je-o′mah) [*chyle* + *angioma*] a tumor made up of intestinal lymph vessels.

chylaqueous (ki-la′kwe-us) [*chyle* + L. *aqua* water] both chylous and watery.

chyle (kīl) [L. *chylus* juice] the milky fluid taken up by the lacteals from the food in the intestine during digestion. It consists of lymph and droplets of triglyceride fat (chylomicrons) in a stable emulsion. It passes into the veins by the thoracic duct, becoming mixed with the blood; called also *chylus* [NA].

chylectasia (ki″lek-ta′se-ah) [*chyle* + Gr. *ektasis* dilatation] dilatation of a chylous vessel; e.g., of a lacteal.

chylemia (ki-le′me-ah) [*chyle* + Gr. *haima* blood + *-ia*] the presence of chyle in the blood.

chylifacient (ki″lĭ-fa′shent) forming chyle.

chylifaction (ki″lĭ-fak′shun) [*chyle* + L. *facere* to make] the formation of chyle; called also *primary assimilation* and *chylopoiesis.*

chylifactive (ki″lĭ-fak′tiv) [*chyle* + L. *facere* to make] chylifacient.

chyliferous (ki-lif′er-us) [*chyle* + L. *ferre* to bear] 1. forming chyle. 2. conveying chyle.

chylification (ki″lĭ-fĭ-ka′shun) [*chyle* + L. *facere* to make] the formation of chyle.

chyliform (ki′lĭ-form) resembling chyle.

chylocele (ki′lo-sēl) [*chyle* + Gr. *kēlē* tumor] elephantiasis scroti. **parasitic c.,** elephantiasis scroti.

chylocyst (ki′lo-sist) [*chyle* + Gr. *kystis* bladder] the cisterna chyli.

chyloderma (ki″lo-der′mah) [*chyle* + Gr. *derma* skin] elephantiasis.

chyloid (ki′loid) resembling chyle.

chylology (ki-lol′o-je) the study of chyle.

chylomediastinum (ki″lo-me″de-as-ti′num) the presence of chyle in the mediastinum.

chylomicrograph (ki″lo-mi′kro-graf) a curve plotted from counts of chylomicrons.

chylomicron (ki″lo-mi′kron), pl. *chylomicrons, chylomi′cra* [*chylo-* + Gr. *mikros* small] a particle of the class of lipoproteins responsible for the transport of exogenous cholesterol and triglycerides from the small intestine to tissues after meals. Chylomicrons are spherical particles with a core of triglycerides surrounded by a monolayer of phospholipids, cholesterol, and apolipoproteins. They have a density of 0.92–0.96 g/ml and a diameter of 75–600 nm and are formed by the intestinal mucosa and carried via the intestinal lacteals and lymphatic system to the bloodstream. In the capillaries of muscle and adipose tissue, the triglycerides are hydrolyzed by endothelial lipoprotein lipase. The resulting particles (chylomicron remnants) depleted of triglycerides and enriched in cholesterol and cholesteryl esters are rapidly cleared by the liver by receptor-mediated endocytosis.

chylomicronemia (ki″lo-mi″kron-e′me-ah) hyperchylomicronemia.

chylopericarditis (ki″lo-per″ĭ-kar-di′tis) pericarditis with effusion of chyle into the pericardial sac.

chylopericardium (ki″lo-per″ĭ-kar′de-um) [*chyle* + *pericardium*] the presence of effused chyle in the pericardium.

chyloperitoneum (ki″lo-per″ĭ-to-ne′um) the presence of effused chyle in the peritoneal cavity.

chylophoric (ki″lo-for′ik) [*chyle* + Gr. *phoros* bearing] conveying chyle.

chylopleura (ki″lo-ploo′rah) chylothorax.

chylopneumothorax (ki″lo-nu″mo-tho′raks) the presence of chyle and air in the pleural cavity.

chylopoiesis (ki″lo-poi-e′sis) [*chyle* + Gr. *poiēsis* formation] chylifaction or chylification.

chylopoietic (ki″lo-poi-et′ik) concerned in the formation of chyle.

chylorrhea (ki″lo-re′ah) 1. discharge of chyle due to rupture of or injury to the thoracic duct. 2. chylous diarrhea, due to rupture of lymphatics in the small intestine.

chylosis (ki-lo′sis) the process of conversion of food into chyle and of absorption of the latter into the tissues.

chylothorax (ki″lo-tho′raks) [*chyle* + Gr. *thōrax* chest] the presence of effused chyle in the thoracic cavity; called also *chylopleura.*

chylous (ki′lus) pertaining to, mingled with, or of the nature of chyle.

chyluria (ki-lu′re-ah) [*chyle* + Gr. *ouron* urine + *-ia*] the presence of chyle in the urine, giving it a milky appearance, due to obstruction anywhere between the intestinal lymphatics and the thoracic duct, which causes rupture of renal lymphatics into the renal tubules. It may occur as a result of obstruction of the retroperitoneal lymphatics in bancroftian filariasis. Called also *galacturia.*

chylus (ki′lus) [L. *juice*] [NA] the milky fluid taken up by the lacteals from the food in the intestine after digestion. See *chyle.*

Chymar (ki′mar) trademark for preparations of chymotrypsin.

chymase (ki′mās) [EC 3.4.21.39] an enzyme of the hydrolase class that catalyzes the hydrolysis of peptide bonds. It is a serine proteinase that cleaves peptide bonds at the carbonyl end of tyrosine, tryptophane, phenylalanine, and leucine. It is found in mast cell granules.

chyme (kīm) [Gr. *chymos* juice] the semifluid, homogeneous, creamy, or gruel-like material produced by gastric digestion of food; called also *chymus.*

Chymex (ki′meks) trademark for a preparation of bentiromide.

chymification (ki″mĭ-fĭ-ka′shun) [*chyme* + L. *facere* to make] the formation of chyme; gastric digestion.

chymopapain (ki″mo-pah-pa′in) [EC 3.4.22.6] an enzyme of the hydrolase class, a thiol proteinase, that catalyzes the hydrolysis of proteins and polypeptides to smaller polypeptides. It resembles papain and occurs also in the latex of the tropical tree *Carica papaya.* The enzyme is used to break down the mucopolysaccharide-protein complexes in the nucleus pulposus of herniated intervertebral disk.

chymorrhea (ki″mo-re′ah) [*chyme* + Gr. *rhoia* flow] a discharge or flow of chyme.

chymosin (ki′mo-sin) [EC 3.4.23.4] an enzyme of the hydrolase class that catalyzes the cleavage of a single bond in soluble casein K to form paracasein, which then reacts with calcium to form an insoluble curd. It is found in the fourth stomach of the calf and other ruminants. A commercial preparation is used for making cheese and rennet custards. Called also *rennin* (not to be confused with *renin*).

chymosinogen (ki″mo-sin′o-jen) prochymosin.

chymotrypsin (ki″mo-trip′sin) 1. [EC 3.4.21.1] an endopeptidase enzyme of the hydrolase class that catalyzes preferentially the cleavage of polypeptides at the carboxyl end of hydrophobic amino acids, especially tyrosine, tryptophan, phenylalanine, and leucine. It is secreted by the pancreas in the form of chymotrypsinogen and is activated by the action of trypsin in the small intestine. Chymotrypsins A and B, of differing molecular size, have similar specificities. 2. [USP] a proteolytic enzyme preparation crystallized from an extract of the pancreas of the ox, *Bos taurus;* used for enzymatic zonulolysis in intracapsular lens extraction. It has also been used to debride necrotic lesions and to reduce inflammation and edema, administered orally, buccally, and intramuscularly.

chymotrypsinogen (ki″mo-trip-sin′o-jen) a crystallizable pre-enzyme occurring in the pancreas and converted to chymotrypsin by trypsin.

chymous (ki′mus) pertaining to chyme.

chymus (ki′mus) chyme.

Chytridiales (ki-trid″ĕ-a′lēz) an order of usually aquatic fungi of the subclass Chytrididiomycetes, class Phycomycetes, most of which are parasites of algae, higher plants, microscopic animals, and fresh-water fungi, although some are saprophytic; they usually have a thallus that is not a true mycelium. It includes the genus *Chytridium.*

Chytridiomycetes (ki-trid′ĕ-o-mi-se′tēz) a subclass of phycomycetous fungi in which the reproductive cells most commonly have one flagellum and the cells walls are composed of chitin; it includes the order Chytridiales.

Chytridium (ki-trid′e-um) a genus of water molds of the order Chytridiales, subclass Chytridiomycetes, which are usually parasitic on plants.

C.I. color index; Colour Index.

Ci curie.

Ciaccio's glands (chah′chōz) [Giuseppe Vincenzo *Ciaccio,* Italian anatomist, 1824–1901] glandulae lacrimales accessoriae.

Ciaccio's method, stain (chah′chōz) [Carmelo *Ciaccio,* Palermo pathologist, 1877–1956] see *Table of Stains.*

Cib. abbreviation for L. *ci′bus,* food.

cibarian (sĭ-ba′re-an) [L. *cibus* food] pertaining to food.

cibisotome (sĭ-bis′o-tōm) cystitome.

cicatrectomy (sik″ah-trek′to-me) excision of a cicatrix.

cicatrices (sĭ-ka′trĭ-sēz, sik″ah-tri′sēz) plural of *cicatrix.*

cicatricial (sik″ah-trish′al) pertaining to or of the nature of a cicatrix.

cicatricotomy (sik″ah-tri-kot′o-me) [*cicatrix* + Gr. *tomē* a cutting] incision of a cicatrix.

cicatrix (sik-a′triks; sik′ah-triks), pl. *cica′trices* [L.] a scar; the new tissue formed in the healing of a wound. **filtering c.,** a cicatrix following glaucoma operation through which the aqueous humor escapes. **hypertrophic c.,** a hard, rigid tumor formed by hypertrophy of the tissue of a cicatrix. **vicious c.,** a cicatrix that causes deformity or impairs the function of an extremity.

cicatrizant (sik-at′rĭ-zant) an agent that promotes cicatrization.

cicatrization (sik″ah-trĭ-za′shun) the formation of a cicatrix or scar.

cicatrize (sik′ah-trīz) to heal by the formation of a scar or cicatrix.

ciclafrine hydrochloride (sik′lah-frēn) chemical name: 3-(1-oxa-4-azaspiro[4.6]undec-2-yl)phenol hydrochloride; an antihypotensive, $C_{15}H_{21}NO_2 \cdot HCl$.

ciclopirox olamine (si″klo-pēr′oks) chemical name: 6-cyclohexyl-1-hydroxy-4-methyl-2-(1*H*)-pyridinone compound with 2- aminoethanol (1:1); an antifungal, $C_{12}H_{17}NO_2 \cdot C_2H_7$-NO.

cicloprofen (si″klo-pro′fen) chemical name: α-methyl-9*H*-fluorene-2-acetic acid; an anti-inflammatory, $C_{16}H_{14}O_2$.

Cicuta (sik′u-tah) a genus of umbelliferous plants, including the water hemlocks, long recognized for their poisonous qualities. **C. macula′ta** L., American water hemlock; its root is very poisonous, containing cicutoxin. **C. viro′sa,** the highly poisonous European water hemlock, which contains cicutoxin.

cicutoxin (sik″u-toks′in) a very poisonous, highly unsaturated higher alcohol from *Cicuta.*

-cide [L. *-cida,* from *caedere* to kill] a word termination denoting a killer or a killing.

Cidex (si′deks) trademark for a preparation of glutaraldehyde.

CIE counterimmunoelectrophoresis.

CIF clonal inhibitory factor.

ciguatera (se″gwah-ta′rah) [Sp. (orig. Taino) *cigua* a poisonous snail + *-era,* Sp. noun suffix] a form of ichthyosarcotoxism, marked by gastrointestinal and neurological symptoms due to ingestion of marine fish (e.g., grouper and snapper) that store the toxin in their tissues; it occurs in tropical and subtropical coastal areas. The term was formerly applied to all types of fish poisoning in the West Indies, where the name originated.

C.I.H. Certificate in Industrial Health.

Ci-hr curie-hour.

cilia (sil′e-ah) [L.] plural of *cilium.*

ciliaris (sil″e-a′ris) [L., from *cilium*] see *Table of Musculi.*

ciliariscope (sil″e-ar′ĭ-skōp) [*ciliary* + *-scope*] an instrument for examining the ciliary region of the eye.

ciliarotomy (sil″e-ar-ot′o-me) [*ciliary* + *-tomy*] surgical division of the ciliary zone for glaucoma.

ciliary (sil′e-er″e) [L. *ciliaris,* from *cilium*] pertaining to or resembling the eyelashes or cilia; used particularly in reference to certain structures in the eye, as the ciliary (ciliaris) muscle, ciliary nerve, ciliary process, and ciliary ring.

Ciliata (sil″e-a′tah) in former systems of classification, a class of ciliophorans comprising those protozoa characterized by the presence of cilia throughout their life cycle.

ciliate (sil′e-āt) 1. having cilia. 2. any protozoan of the phylum Ciliophora; a ciliophoran.

ciliated (sil′e-āt″ed) provided with cilia or with a fringe of hairs.

ciliectomy (sil″e-ek′to-me) [*cili-* + *-ectomy*] 1. excision of a portion of the ciliary body. 2. excision of a portion of the ciliary margin of the eyelid with the roots of the lashes.

ciliogenesis (sil″e-o-jen′ĕ-sis) [*cilio-* + *genesis*] the formation or development of cilia.

Ciliophora (sil″e-of′o-rah) [*cilio-* + Gr. *phoros* bearing] a phylum of protozoa characterized by the presence of cilia or compound ciliary structures as locomotor or food-gathering organelles at some time during their life cycle, a subpellicular infraciliature composed of ciliary basal bodies and kinetodesmata (even when cilia are absent), and two types of nuclei, a macronucleus and a micronucleus (with rare exceptions); a contractile vacuole is typically present. Sexuality involves conjugation, autogamy, and cytogamy. Most ciliophorans are free living, many are commensals of vertebrates and invertebrates, and some are parasites. The phylum comprises three classes: Kinetofragminophorea, Oligohymenophorea, and Polyhymenophorea. Cf. *Opalinata.*

ciliophoran (sil″e-of′o-ran) any protozoan of the phylum Ciliophora; a ciliate.

cilioretinal (sil″e-o-ret′ĭ-nal) pertaining to the retina and the ciliary body.

cilioscleral (sil″e-o-skle′ral) pertaining to the ciliary apparatus and to the sclera.

ciliospinal (sil″e-o-spi′nal) [*cilio-* + *spinal*] pertaining to the ciliary body and the spinal cord; see under *center* and *reflex.*

ciliotomy (sil″e-ot′o-me) [*cilio-* + *tomy*] surgical division of the ciliary nerves.

cilium (sil′e-um), pl. *cil′ia* [L.] 1. an eyelid or its outer edge. 2. [pl.] [NA] the hairs growing on the edges of the eyelids; called also *eyelashes.* 3. a minute vibratile, hairlike process projecting from the free surface of a cell; composed of nine pairs of microtubules arrayed around a central pair, cilia are extensions of basal bodies. They beat rhythmically to move the cell about in its environment or to move fluid or mucous films over its surface. Ciliary movement consists of an *effective stroke*, in which the cilium stiffens and moves forward rapidly, and a *recovery stroke*, in which the cilium becomes flexible and bends. Cilia may all beat simultaneously (*isochronal rhythm*) or successive cilia in each row may start their beat sequentially producing a wavelike movement (*metachronal rhythm*). Cf. *flagellum*. **olfactory cilia,** see under *hair*.

cillo (sil′o) cillosis.

Cillobacterium (sil″lo-bak-te′re-um) in former systems of classification, a genus of bacteria of the family Lactobacillaceae, made up of nonsporulating, anaerobic, gram-positive, rod-shaped organisms. These organisms are now assigned to the genus *Eubacterium*.

cillosis (sil-o′sis) [L. from Fr. *ciller* to wink + *-osis*] a spasmodic quivering of the eyelid; called also *cillo*.

cimbia (sim′be-ah) [L.] a white band running across the ventral surface of the crus cerebri.

cimetidine (si-met′ĭ-dēn) chemical name: N''-cyano-N-methyl-N'-[2-[[(5-methyl-1H-imidazol-4-yl)-methyl]thio]ethyl]guanidine. An antagonist to histamine H_2 receptors, $C_{10}H_{16}N_6S$, which inhibits gastric acid secretion in response to all stimuli, and is effective especially in the treatment of peptic ulcer; administered orally, intravenously, and by intravenous infusion.

Cimex (si′meks) [L. "bug"] a genus of insects, the bedbugs, of the family Cimicidae. **C. boue′ti,** the tropical bedbug of West Africa and South America; called also *Leptocimex boueti*. **C. hemip′terus,** *C. rotundatus*. **C. lectula′rius,** the common bedbug that infests man in temperate areas; called also *Acanthia lectularia*. **C. pilosel′lus,** an American species found in bats. **C. pipistrel′la,** a species that transmits a trypanosome disease of bats. **C. rotunda′tus,** a flattened, oval, reddish bedbug that infests man in the tropics; called also *C. hemipterus*.

cimex (si′meks), pl. *cim′ices* [L.] an individual of the genus *Cimex*; a bedbug.

cimices (sim′ĭ-sēz) plural of *cimex*.

cimicid (si′mĭ-sid) pertaining to insects of the family Cimicidae.

Cimicidae (si-mis′ĭ-de) a family of wingless, blood-sucking, hemipterous insects of the suborder Heteroptera, including the bedbugs and related forms. *Cimex*, *Haematosiphon*, *Leptocimes*, and *Oeciacus* are medically important genera.

Cimicifuga (sim″ĭ-sif′u-gah) [L. *cimex* bug + *fugare* to put to flight] a genus of ranunculaceous plants. The rootlets of *C. racemosa* (L.) Nutt. (black snakeroot or cohosh) are tonic and antispasmodic.

cimicosis (sim″ĭ-ko′sis) itching of the skin due to the bites of *Cimex lectularius* (bedbug).

cinanserin hydrochloride (sin-an′ser-in) chemical name: N-[2-[[3-(dimethyl-amino)propyl]thio]phenyl]-3-phenyl-2-propenamide monohydrochloride. A serotonin antagonist, $C_{20}H_{24}N_2OS \cdot HCl$, which has been used in the treatment of mania and schizophrenia.

cinching (sinch′ing) [Sp. *cincha* girdle] surgical shortening of an ocular muscle by plicating.

Cinchona (sin-ko′nah) [named from a countess of *Chinchon*] a genus of rubiaceous trees, all natives of South America, the source of the medicinally important quinoline alkaloids, quinine, quinidine, cinchonine, and cinchonidine. Mainly used for malaria and as cardiac depressants. The major species used are *C. succirubra* Pavon et Klotzsch and hybrids (red cinchona), *C. calisaya* Weddell, *C. Ledgeriana* (Howard) Moens et Trimen, and hybrids (yellow cinchona).

cinchona (sin-ko′nah) the dried bark of the stem or of the root of various species of *Cinchona*. It is the source of the medicinally important quinoline alkaloids *quinine*, *quinidine*, *cinchonine*, and *cinchonidine*. Cinchona was once widely used as an antimalarial but it has been largely replaced by its alkaloids. Called also *calisaya bark*, *cinchona bark*, *Jesuit's bark*, *Peruvian bark*, and *quinquina*.

cinchonidine (sin-ko′nĭ-dēn) chemical name: (8α,9R)-cinchonan-9-ol. An alkaloid of cinchona, $C_{19}H_{22}N_2O$, used as an antimalarial, chiefly in the form of the sulfate salt; administered orally.

cinchonine (sin′ko-nin) [L. *cinchonina*] chemical name: (9S)-cinchona-9-ol. An alkaloid of cinchona, $C_{19}H_{22}N_2O$, used as an antimalarial, chiefly in the form of the sulfate salt; administered orally.

cinchoninic acid (sing″ko-nin′ik) quinoline 4-carboxylic acid, an oxidation product of cinchona alkaloids.

cinchonism (sin′ko-nizm) the morbid or injurious effect of the injudicious use of cinchona bark or its alkaloids; it is attended by nausea, vomiting, headache, tinnitus aurium, deafness, symptoms of cerebral congestion, vertigo, and visual disturbances.

cinchophen (sin′ko-fen) chemical name: 2-phenyl-quinoline-4-carboxylic acid. An analgesic, antipyretic, and uricosuric agent, $C_{16}H_{11}NO_2$, formerly used in the treatment of gout and acute rheumatic fever. Called also *phenylcinchoninic acid* and *phenylquinoline carboxylic acid*.

cinclisis (sin′klĭ-sis) [Gr. *kinklisis* a wagging] a rapidly repeated movement, such as rapid breathing, or rapid winking.

cine- [Gr. *kinēsis* movement] a combining form denoting relationship to movement.

cineangiocardiography (sin″e-an″je-o-kar″de-og′rah-fe) the photographic recording of fluoroscopic images of the heart and great vessels by motion picture techniques.

cineangiograph (sin″ĕ-an″je-o-graf) a motion picture camera for photographing fluoroscopic images.

cineangiography (sin″e-an″je-og′rah-fe) the photographic recording of fluoroscopic images of the blood vessels by motion picture techniques. **radionuclide c.,** that in which a sample of human serum albumin labeled with a radioisotope (technetium 99) is injected into the peripheral blood and then a scintillation camera records emitted radiation over the chest area, the heart movements being shown on a video tube.

cinedensigraphy (sin″ĕ-den-sig′rah-fe) the recording of movements of internal body structures by means of x-rays and radiosensitive cells.

cinefluorography (sin″ĕ-floo″or-og′rah-fe) cineradiography.

cinemascopia (sin″ĕ-mah-sko′pe-ah) the use of motion picture records for the study of movements of the body.

cinemascopy (sin″ĕ-mas′ko-pe) cinemascopia.

cinematics (sin″ĕ-mat′iks) kinematics.

cinematization (sin″ĕ-mat-ĭ-za′shun) kineplasty.

cinematography (sin″ĕ-mah-tog′rah-fe) cineradiography.

cinematoradiography (sin″ĕ-mah-to-ra″de-og′rah-fe) cineradiography.

cinemicrography (sin″ĕ-mi-krog′rah-fe) the making of moving pictures of a small object through the lens system of a microscope. **time-lapse c.,** the taking of motion pictures of a minute object through a microscope at a slower than normal speed, so that with projection at normal speed the movements of the object appear to occur more rapidly.

cineol (sin′e-ol) eucalyptol.

cinepazet maleate (sin″ĕ-paz′et) chemical name: 4-[1-oxo-3-(3,4,5-trimethoxyphenyl)-2-propenyl]-1-piperazineacetic acid ethyl ester. A coronary vasodilator, $C_{20}H_{28}N_2O_6 \cdot C_4H_4O_4$, which has been used in the treatment of angina of effort.

cinephlebography (sin″ĕ-flĕ-bog′rah-fe) cineradiography of the veins after administration of a contrast medium. In *ascending functional cinephlebography*, the contrast medium is introduced into a vein in the foot and its progress is observed as it courses through the tibial, popliteal, femoral, and iliac veins.

cineplastics (sin″ĕ-plas′tiks) kineplasty.

cineplasty (sin″ĕ-plas″te) kineplasty.

cineradiography (sin″ĕ-ra″de-og′rah-fe) the making of a motion picture record of the successive images appearing on a fluoroscopic screen; called also *cinefluorography*, *cinematography*, *cinematoradiography*, *cineroentgenofluorography*, and *cineroentgenography*.

cinerea (sĭ-ne′re-ah) [L. *cinereus* ashen hued] the gray matter of the nervous system.

cinereal (sĭ-ne′re-al) pertaining to the gray matter of the brain or nervous system.

cineritious (sin″er-ish′us) [L. *cineritius*] ashen gray; of the color of ashes.

cineroentgenofluorography (sin″ĕ-rent″gen-o-floo″or-og′rah-fe) cineradiography.

cineroentgenography (sin″ĕ-rent″gen-og′rah-fe) cineradiography.

cinesalgia (sin″es-al′je-ah) [Gr. *kinēsis* motion + *-algia*] pain in a muscle when it is brought into action.

cinesi- for words beginning thus, see those beginning *kinesi-*.

cinet(o)- for words beginning thus, see those beginning *kinet(o)-*.

cineurography (sin″ĕ-u-rog′rah-fe) cineradiography of the urinary tract.

cingestol (sin-jes′tōl) chemical name: 19-nor-17α-pregn-5-en-20-yn-17-ol; a progestin, $C_{20}H_{28}O$.

cingula (sing′gu-lah) [L.] plural of *cingulum*.

cingule (sin′gūl) cingulum.

cingulectomy (sin″gu-lek′to-me) bilateral extirpation of the anterior half of the gyrus cinguli.

cingulotomy (sing″gu-lot′o-me) the creation, by stereotaxic introduction of electrodes, of lesions in the gyrus cinguli for relief of intractable pain and in treatment of psychiatric disorders and addiction.

cingulum (sin′gu-lum), pl. *cin′gula* [L. "girdle"] 1. [NA] an encircling structure or part; anything that encircles a body. Called also *cingule* and *girdle*. 2. [NA], a bundle of association fibers that partly encircles the corpus callosum not far from the median plane, the fibers of which interrelate the cingulate and hippocampal gyri. 3. the lingual lobe of an anterior tooth, making up the bulk of the cervical third of its lingual surface; called also *basal*, *linguocervical*, and *linguogingival ridge*. **c. hemisphe′rii**, gyrus cinguli. **c. mem′bri inferio′ris** [NA], girdle of inferior member: the encircling bony structure supporting the lower limbs, comprising the two ossa coxae, articulating with each other and with the sacrum, to complete the essentially rigid bony ring; called also *c. pelvicum* and *pelvic girdle*. **c. pel′vicum**, NA alternative for *c. membri inferioris*. **c. mem′bri superio′ris** [NA], girdle of superior member: the encircling bony structure supporting the upper limbs, comprising the clavicles and scapulae, articulating with each other and with the sternum and vertebral column, respectively; called also *c. pectorale* [NA alternative] and *pectoral*, *shoulder*, or *thoracic girdle*. **c. pectora′le**, NA alternative for *c. membri superioris*.

cingulumotomy (sing″gu-lum-ot′o-me) cingulotomy.

C1 INH C1 inhibitor; see *complement*.

cinnamaldehyde (sin-ah-mal′dĕ-hīd) a yellowish oily liquid with a strong odor of cinnamon, C_9H_8O, used as a flavoring agent.

cinnamene (sin′ah-mēn) styrol.

cinnamic (sĭ-nam′ik) of or relating to cinnamon; see under *acid*.

cinnamic acid (sĭ-nam′ik) a fragrant acid, phenylacrylic acid, $C_6H_5CH=CHCOOH$, occurring in cinnamon and balsams and other aromatic resins.

cinnamol (sin′ah-mol) styrol.

Cinnamomum (sin″ah-mo′mum) a genus of evergreen trees native to Asia. The wood of *C. camphora* is the source of camphor and the bark of *C. loureirii* of cinnamon.

cinnamon (sin′ah-mon) [L.; Gr. *kinnamon*] [NF] the dried bark of *Cinnamomum loureirii*, containing, in each 100 gm., not less than 2.5 ml. of volatile oil; used as a flavor in pharmaceutical preparations.

cinnarizine (sĭ-nar′ĭ-zēn) chemical name: 1-(diphenylmethyl)-4-(3-phenyl-2-propenyl)piperazine. An antihistamine, $C_{26}H_{28}N_2$, used chiefly in the treatment of nausea and vertigo associated with labyrinthine disorders and in the prevention and treatment of motion sickness.

cinnopentazone (sin-o-pen′tah-zōn) cintazone.

cinology (sĭ-nol′o-je) kinesiology.

cinometer (sĭ-nom′ĕ-ter) kinesimeter.

cinoplasm (sin′o-plazm) kinoplasm.

cinoxacin (sin-oks′ah-sin) chemical name: 1-ethyl-1,4-dihydro-4-oxo-[1,3]dioxolo[4,5-g]cinnoline-3-carboxylic acid. An antibacterial, $C_{12}H_{10}N_2O_5$, which inhibits most gram-negative organisms.

cinoxate (sin-oks′āt) chemical name: 3-(4-methoxyphenyl)-2-propenoic acid 2-ethoxyethyl ester; an ultraviolet screen, $C_{14}H_{18}O_4$, applied topically to the skin.

cinromide (sin′ro-mīd) chemical name: 3-(3-bromophenyl)-2-propenamide; an anticonvulsive, $C_{11}H_{12}BrNO$.

cintazone (sin′tah-zōn) chemical name: 2-pentyl-6-phenyl-1H-pyrazolo[1,2-a]cinnoline-1,3(2H)-dione; an anti-inflammatory agent, $C_{22}H_{22}N_2O_2$. Called also *cinnopentazone*.

cionectomy (si″o-nek′to-me) [Gr. *kiōn* uvula + *ektomē* excision] excision of the uvula or of a part of it; uvulectomy.

Cionella (si″o-nel′ah) a genus of land snails that serve as hosts of *Dicrocoelium dentriticum*.

Cionellidae (si″o-nel′ĭ-de) a family of garden snails (suborder Stylommatophora, subclass Euthyneura, class Gastropoda) that serve as hosts of *Dicrocoelium dendriticum*.

cionitis (si″o-ni′tis) [Gr. *kiōn* uvula + *-itis*] inflammation of the uvula; uvulitis.

cionoptosis (si″on-op-to′sis) [Gr. *kiōn* uvula + Gr. *ptōsis* a falling] undue elongation of the uvula.

cionorrhaphy (si″ŏ-nor′ah-fe) plastic repair of the uvula.

cionotome (si-on′o-tōm) [Gr. *kiōn* uvula + *tomē* a cutting] a cutting instrument for amputating the uvula; uvulotome.

cionotomy (si″o-not′o-me) [Gr. *kiōn* uvula + *tomē* a cutting] surgical removal of part of the uvula; uvulotomy.

ciprocinonide (sip″ro-si′no-nīd) chemical name: 21-[(cyclopropylcarbonyl)-oxy]-6α,9-difluoro-11β-hydroxy-16α,17-[(1-methylethylidene) bis(oxy)] pregna- 1,4- diene -3,20-dione; an adrenocorticosteroid, $C_{28}H_{34}F_2O_7$.

ciprofibrate (si″pro-fi′brāt) chemical name: 2-[4-(2,2-dichlorocyclopropyl)phenoxy]-2-methylpropanoic acid; an antihyperlipidemic, $C_{13}H_{14}Cl_2O_3$.

circadian (ser″kah-de′an) [L. *circa* about + *dies* a day] pertaining to a period of about 24 hours; applied especially to the rhythmic repetition of certain phenomena in living organisms at about the same time each day (circadian rhythm).

circannual (ser-kan′u-al) [L. *circa* about + *annus* year] occurring every year; applied especially to the rhythmic repetition of certain phenomena (e.g., the flowering of plants) in living organisms at about the same time each year.

circellus (ser-sel′lus) [L., dim. of *circulus*] a small ring, or circle.

circinate (ser′sĭ-nāt) resembling a ring, or circle.

circle (ser′k'l) [L. *circulus*] a round figure, structure, or part. See also *annulus* and *ring*. **arterial c.**, circulus arteriosus. **arterial c. of iris, greater**, circulus arteriosus iridis major. **arterial c. of iris, lesser**, circulus arteriosus iridis minor. **arterial c. of Willis**, circulus arteriosus cerebri. **Berry's c's**, charts with circles on them for testing stereoscopic vision. **c. of Carus**, see under *curve*. **c. of confusion**, a disk representing the image of a theoretical point made by a lens. **defensive c.**, the coexistence of two conditions that tend to have an antagonistic or inhibitory effect on each other. **c. of dispersion**, **c. of dissipation**, the circular space on the retina within which the image of a luminous point is formed. **c. of Haller**, 1. circulus vasculosus nervi optici. 2. (*obs.*) valvula pylori. **c. of Hovius**, an intrascleral circular arrangement of anastomosing ciliary veins anterior to the vorticose veins, not far from the corneoscleral margin, occurring in mammals other than man; called also *circulus venosus hovii*. **Huguier's c.**, the circle formed about the junction of the cervix with the body of the uterus by the uterine arteries. **c. of iris, greater**, annulus iridis major. **c. of iris, lesser**, annulus iridis minor. **Latham's c.**, a circle 2 inches in diameter covering the area of pericardial dullness and situated midway between the left nipple and the lower end of the sternum. **Minsky's c's**, a series of circles used for the graphic recording of eye lesions. **Robinson's c.**, an arterial circle formed by anastomoses between the abdominal aorta, common iliac, hypogastric, uterine, and ovarian arteries. **sensory c.**, an area on the body within which it is impossible to distinguish separately the impressions arising from two sites of stimulation. **vascular c.**, circulus vasculosus. **vascular c. of optic nerve**, circulus vasculosus nervi optici. **Vieth-Müller c.**, see under *horopter*. **c's of Weber**, circles of points on the skin marking the points of tactile sense discrimination. **c. of Willis**, circulus arteriosus cerebri. **c. of Zinn**, circulus vasculosus nervi optici.

circlet (ser′klet) a small circular structure.

circling (ser′kling) movement in a circle, as manifested by animals with listeriosis.

circuit (ser′kit) [L. *circuitus*] the round or course traversed by an electrical current. The circuit is said to be *closed* when it is continuous, so that the current may pass through it; it is *open, broken,* or *interrupted* when it is not continuous and the current cannot pass through it. **gate c.,** gate. **open c.,** a circuit having some break in it so that current is not passing or cannot pass. **reflex c.,** a chain of neurons that function in a reflex act. **short c.,** 1. an unwanted low-resistance connection between two points in an electric circuit. 2. a communication between two portions of intestine, one above and the other below an obstruction.

circular (ser′ku-lar) [L. *circularis*] shaped like a circle; occurring in a circle.

circulation (ser″ku-la′shun) [L. *circulatio*] movement in a regular or circuitous course, as the movement of the blood through the heart and blood vessels. **allantoic c.,** fetal circulation through the umbilical vessels; called also *umbilical c.* **assisted c.,** pumping that aids the natural activity of the heart. **collateral c.,** that which is carried on through secondary channels after obstruction of the principal vessel supplying the part; called also *compensatory c.* **compensatory c.,** collateral c. **coronary c.,** that within the coronary vessels of the heart. **cross c.,** the circulation in a portion of the body of one animal of blood supplied from another animal. **derivative c.,** the passage of blood from arteries to the veins without going through capillaries. **enterohepatic c.,** the recurrent cycle in which bile salts and other substances excreted by the liver pass through the intestinal mucosa and become reabsorbed by the hepatic cells and re-excreted. **extracorporeal c.,** the circulation of blood outside the body, as through a heart-lung apparatus for carbon dioxide–oxygen exchange, or through an artificial kidney for removal of substances usually excreted in the urine. **fetal c.,** that propelled by the fetal heart through the fetus, umbilical cord, and placental villi. **first c.,** primitive c. **fourth c.,** the con-

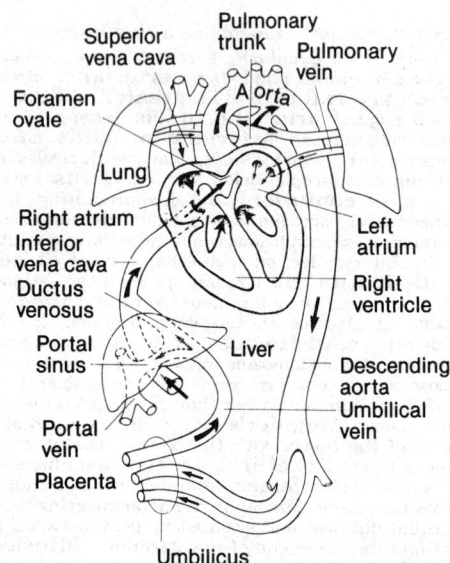

Superior vena cava
Pulmonary trunk
Pulmonary vein
Aorta
Foramen ovale
Lung
Right atrium
Inferior vena cava
Ductus venosus
Portal sinus
Liver
Left atrium
Right ventricle
Descending aorta
Umbilical vein
Portal vein
Placenta
Umbilicus

Schematic diagram of fetal circulation.

tinuous movement of lymphocytes from their sources in all the hematopoietic and connective tissues to the blood passing through all the tissues and organs, then to the lymph nodes, then into the lymph of the thoracic duct, and into the blood again. **greater c.,** systemic c. **hypophyseoportal c.,** that passing from the capillaries of the median eminence of the hypothalamus into the portal vessels to the sinusoids

of the adenohypophysis. **intervillous c.,** the flow of maternal blood through the intervillous space. **lesser c.,** pulmonary c. **lymph c.,** the passage of the lymph through lymph vessels and glands. **omphalomesenteric c.,** vitelline c. **persistent fetal c.,** pulmonary hypertension in the postnatal period secondary to right-to-left shunting of the blood through the foramen ovale and ductus arteriosus. **placental c.,** the fetal circulation; also, the maternal circulation through the intervillous space of the placenta. **portal c.,** the circulation of blood from the capillaries of one organ through larger vessels to the capillaries of another organ, before returning through larger veins back to the heart, especially the passage of the blood from capillaries of the gastrointestinal tract and spleen through capillaries of the liver before entering the hepatic vein. See also *hypophyseoportal c.* **portoumbilical c.,** Cruveilhier-Baumgarten syndrome. **primitive c.,** the earliest circulation by which nutriment and oxygen are conveyed to the embryo; called also *first c.* **pulmonary c.,** that carrying the venous blood from the right ventricle to the lungs, and returning oxygenated blood to the left atrium of the heart; called also *lesser c.* **sinusoidal c.,** that occurring through the sinusoids of various organs. **systemic c.,** the general circulation, carrying oxygenated blood from the left ventricle to various tissues of the body, and returning the venous blood to the right atrium of the heart; called also *greater c.* **thebesian c.,** the circulation of blood through the thebesian veins. **umbilical c.,** allantoic c. **vitelline c.,** the circulation through the blood vessels of the yolk sac; called also *omphalomesenteric c.*

circulatory (ser′ku-lah-to″re) pertaining to the circulation.

circulus (ser′ku-lus), pl. *cir′culi* [L. "a ring"] a circle or circuit, used in anatomical nomenclature to designate such an arrangement, usually of arteries or veins. **c. arterio′sus** [NA], arterial circle: a complete or incomplete circle of anastomosing arteries. **c. arterio′sus cer′ebri** [NA], the important polygonal anastomosis formed by the internal carotid, the anterior and posterior cerebral arteries, the anterior communicating artery, and the posterior communicating arteries; called also *c. arteriosus [Willisi], circle of Willis,* and *c. Willisii.* **c. arterio′sus hal′leri,** c. vasculosus nervi optici. **c. arterio′sus i′ridis ma′jor** [NA], greater arterial circle of the iris: a circle of anastomosing arteries situated in the ciliary body along the ciliary margin of the iris. **c. arterio′sus i′ridis mi′nor** [NA], lesser arterial circle of the iris: a circle of anastomosing arteries in the iris near the pupillary margin. **c. arterio′sus [Willis′i],** c. arteriosus cerebri. **c. articula′ris vasculo′sus** [NA], an arrangement of anastomosing vessels encircling a joint. **c. umbilica′lis,** an arterial plexus in the subperitoneal tissue surrounding the navel. **c. vasculo′sus** [NA], vascular circle: a complete or incomplete circle of anastomosing blood vessels. **c. vasculo′sus ner′vi op′tici** [NA], a circle of arteries in the sclera surrounding the site of entrance of the optic nerve; called also *c. vasculosus nervi optici [Halleri], c. arteriosus halleri, c. zinnii, circle of Haller,* and *circle of Zinn.* **c. veno′sus hal′leri,** plexus venosus areolaris. **c. veno′sus ho′vii,** circle of Hovius. **c. veno′sus rid′leyi,** sinus circularis. **c. willis′ii,** c. arteriosus cerebri. **c. zin′nii,** c. vasculosus nervi optici.

circum- [L.] a prefix signifying around.

circumanal (ser″kum-a′nal) surrounding the anus.

circumarticular (ser″kum-ar-tik′u-lar) around a joint.

circumaxillary (ser″kum-ak′sĭ-lār″e) around the axilla.

circumbulbar (ser″kum-bul′bar) surrounding the eyeball.

circumcallosal (ser″kum-kah-lo′sal) surrounding the corpus callosum.

circumcise (ser′kum-sīz) to perform circumcision.

circumcision (ser″kum-sizh′un) [L. *circumcisio* a cutting around] the removal of all or part of the prepuce, or foreskin. **female c.,** 1. incision of the fold of the skin over the glans clitoridis; called also *clitoridotomy* and *pharaonic c.* 2. infibulation. **pharaonic c.,** female circumcision in which part of the clitoris is excised. Cf. *infibulation.*

circumcorneal (ser″kum-kor′ne-al) around the cornea.

circumcrescent (ser″kum-kres′ent) [*circum-* + L. *crescere* to grow] growing around and over.

circumduction (ser″kum-duk′shun) [L. *circumducere* to draw around] the active or passive circular movement of a limb or of the eye.

circumference (ser-kum′fer-ens) [*circum-* + L. *ferre* to bear] the outer limit or margin of a rounded body. **articular c.**, circumferentia articularis; see specific names under *circumferentia*.

circumferentia (ser-kum″fer-en′she-ah) [L.] circumference. **c. articula′ris,** articular circumference: the rounded surface of a bone which is received into a depression of another bone with which it articulates. **c. articula′ris cap′itis ul′nae** [NA], articular circumference of head of ulna: the semilunar surface of the head of the ulna which articulates with the ulnar notch of the radius; called also *c. articularis capituli ulnae*. **c. articula′ris capit′uli ul′nae,** c. articularis capiti ulnae. **c. articula′ris ra′dii** [NA], the rounded surface of the head or capitulum of the radius which articulates with the radial notch of the ulna; called also *articular circumference of head of radius*.

circumferential (ser″kum-fer-en′shal) pertaining to forming a circumference.

circumflex (ser′kum-fleks) [L. *circumflexus* bent about] curved like a bow.

circumflexus (ser″kum-flek′sus) [L.] bent about; circumflex.

circumgemmal (ser″kum-jem′al) [*circum-* + L. *gemma* bud] surrounding a bud; a term applied to that form of nerve ending in which an end-bud is surrounded by fibrils.

circuminsular (ser″kum-in′su-lar) [*circum-* + L. *insula* island] surrounding, situated, or occurring about the insula.

circumintestinal (ser″kum-in-tes′tĭ-nal) surrounding the intestine.

circumlental (ser″kum-len′tal) situated or occurring around the lens.

circumnuclear (ser″kum-nu′kle-ar) surrounding or occurring near the nucleus.

circumocular (ser″kum-ok′u-lar) surrounding or occurring around the eye.

circumoral (ser″kum-o′ral) [*circum-* + L. *os, oris* mouth] around or near the mouth.

circumorbital (ser″kum-or′bĭ-tal) situated around or occurring near an orbit.

circumpolarization (ser″kum-po″lar-i-za′shun) [*circum-* + *polarization*] the rotation of a ray of polarized light to the right or left; cf. *optical rotation*, under *rotation*.

circumrenal (ser″kum-re′nal) [*circum-* + L. *ren* kidney] situated or occurring near a kidney.

circumscribed (ser′kum-skrībd) [*circum-* + L. *scribere* to write] bounded or limited; confined to a limited space.

circumscriptus (ser″kum-skrip′tus) [L.] circumscribed.

circumstantiality (ser″kum-stan″she-al′ĭ-te) a pattern of speech characterized by delay in getting to the point because of the interpolation of unnecessary, tedious details and irrelevant parenthetical remarks; common in persons with obsessive-compulsive personality traits. Cf. *tangentiality*.

Circumstraint (sir′kum-strānt″) trademark for a device used to hold a baby for circumcision.

circumvallate (ser″kum-val′āt) [*circum-* + L. *vallare* to wall] surrounded by a trench or by a ridge; see *vallate papilla*, under *papilla*.

circumvascular (ser″kum-vas′ku-lar) [*circum-* + L. *vasculum* vessel] situated or occurring about the vessels.

circumvolute (ser″kum-vo′lūt) [*circum-* + L. *volutus* rolled] twisted about.

circumvolutio (ser″kum-vo-lu′she-o) a convolution, or the folding of one object about another. **c. crista′ta,** gyrus fornicatus.

cirrhogenous (sir-roj′ĕ-nus) producing cirrhosis or hardening.

cirrhonosus (sir-ron′o-sus) [Gr. *kirrhos* orange yellow + *nosos* disease] a fetal disease characterized by a golden-yellow staining of the pleura and peritoneum.

cirrhosis (sir-ro′sis) [Gr. *kirrhos* orange-yellow] liver disease characterized pathologically by loss of the normal microscopic lobular architecture, with fibrosis and nodular regeneration; see *c. of the liver*. The term is sometimes used to refer to chronic interstitial inflammation of any organ. **acholangic biliary c.,** a liver ailment affecting children up to 12 years old, due to complete or partial agenesis of the intrahepatic, intralobular bile ducts, with manifestations similar to those in obstructive biliary cirrhosis. **acute juvenile c.,** chronic active hepatitis. **alcoholic c.,** cirrhosis in the alcoholic, attributed by some to associated nutritional deficiency and by others to chronic excessive exposure to alcohol as a hepatotoxin. **atrophic c.,** cirrhosis in which the liver is decreased in size; it may be seen in the alcoholic, but is more common in posthepatitic or postnecrotic cirrhosis. **bacterial c.,** a variety said to be of microbic origin. **biliary c.,** cirrhosis of the liver due to obstruction or infection of the major extra- or intrahepatic bile ducts (except in *primary biliary c.*). It is marked by jaundice, abdominal pain, steatorrhea, and enlargement of the liver and spleen. See *primary* and *secondary biliary c.* **biliary c. of children,** secondary biliary cirrhosis due to congenital atresia of the bile ducts; called also *infantile liver.* See also *Indian childhood c.* **Budd's c.** (*obs.*), chronic hepatic enlargement once thought to be caused by intestinal intoxication. **calculus c.,** secondary biliary cirrhosis caused by the presence of gallstones. **cardiac c.,** fibrosis of the liver, probably following central hemorrhagic necrosis, in association with congestive heart disease. It is characterized by scarring about the central veins of the hepatic lobules. **cardiotuberculous c.** (*obs.*), Hutinel's disease. **Charcot's c.,** primary biliary c. **congestive c.,** cirrhosis resulting from increased hepatic venous pressure or thrombosis; commonly due to congestive heart failure (cardiac c.) or to obstruction of the hepatic vein. **Cruveilhier-Baumgarten c.,** see under *syndrome*. **fatty c.,** cirrhosis in which liver cells are infiltrated with fat (triglyceride), the infiltration usually being due to alcohol ingestion; Laënnec's c. **Hanot's c.,** 1. primary biliary c. 2. secondary biliary c. **hypertrophic c.,** primary biliary c. **Indian childhood c.,** cirrhosis of the liver of unknown etiology occurring in children in India, characterized typically by insidious onset, stunting of growth, hepatomegaly, and a low inconstant fever. In the late stages, portal hypertension with ascites, evidence of collateral circulation, hematemesis, splenomegaly, and edema may be seen. Cf. *veno-occlusive disease of the liver*, under *disease*. **Laënnec's c.,** cirrhosis of the liver closely associated with chronic excessive alcohol ingestion. In the early stages, liver enlargement may reflect fatty infiltration of liver cells (fatty c.), with necrosis and inflammation due to acute alcohol injury; progressive fibrosis extending from portal areas separates uniform small regeneration nodules. See *c. of liver* for symptoms. **c. of liver,** a group of chronic diseases of the liver characterized by loss of normal hepatic lobular architecture with fibrosis, and by destruction of parenchymal cells and their regeneration to form nodules. The disease has a lengthy latent period, usually followed by the sudden appearance of abdominal swelling and pain, hematemesis, dependent edema, or jaundice. In advanced stages, ascites, jaundice, portal hypertension, and central nervous system disorders, which may end in hepatic coma, become prominent. Called also *chronic interstitial hepatitis*. **c. of lung,** see *diffuse interstitial pulmonary fibrosis*, under *fibrosis*. **malarial c.,** cirrhosis associated with malaria; the malaria is probably not an etiologic factor. **c. mam′mae,** chronic interstitial mastitis. **metabolic c.,** cirrhosis of the liver associated with metabolic diseases, such as hemochromatosis, Wilson's disease, glycogen storage disease, galactosemia, and disorders of amino acid metabolism. **multilobular c.,** postnecrotic c. **periportal c.,** postnecrotic c. **pigment c., pigmentary c.,** a condition marked by a slightly to moderately enlarged, chocolate-brown liver, the surface of which is diffusely nodular; it is the characteristic lesion of hemochromatosis. **pipe stem c.,** cirrhosis of the liver characterized by fibrotic scars around the large portal vessels; seen in hepatic schistosomiasis, in which fibrosis surrounds parasites or ova trapped in branches of the portal vein. **portal c.,** Laënnec's c. **posthepatitic c.,** cirrhosis (usually macronodular) resulting as a sequel to acute hepatitis. **postnecrotic c.,** cirrhosis that follows subacute hepatic necrosis due to toxic or viral hepatitis. The reticulin framework of normal lobules collapses and may be replaced by broad bands of fibrous tissue separating regeneration nodules (multilobular liver) of varying size. Called also *multilobar c., periportal c., toxic c.,* and *healed yellow atrophy.* **primary biliary c.,** a rare form of biliary cirrhosis of unknown etiology in which small intrahepatic bile ducts are destroyed while the major intra- and extrahepatic ducts remain patent; 90 per cent of patients are female; most are middle-aged; it is characterized by chronic cholestasis with pruritus, jaundice, hypercholesterolemia and xanthomas, osteomalacia, and, in the later stages, by portal hypertension and liver failure. Almost all patients have circulating antimitochondrial antibodies. **pulmonary c.,** see *diffuse interstitial pulmonary fibrosis,* under *fibrosis.* **secondary biliary c.,** cirrhosis of the liver resulting from chronic bile obstruction due to congenital atresia or stricture. **stasis c.,** a general term for cirrhosis due to obstruction of the outflow of the hepatic vein; see also *cardiac c., veno-occlusive disease,* and *Budd-Chiari syndrome.* **c. of stomach,** linitis plastica. **syphilitic c.,** cirrhosis of the liver due to congenital or tertiary syphilis. **Todd's c.,** primary biliary c. **toxic c.,** postnecrotic c. **unilobular c.,** primary biliary c. **vascular c.,** cirrhosis of the liver following upon obstruction of the hepatic vein, portal vein, or general hepatic circulation.

cirrhotic (sir-rot′ik)   pertaining to or characterized by cirrhosis.

cirri (sir′i)   plural of *cirrus.*

cirrus (sir′us), pl. *cir′ri* [L. "curl"]   any of various slender or filamentous, usually flexible, appendages, such as one of the compound organelles composed of groups of fused cilia seen in certain peritrichious ciliate protozoa that are used for locomotion; an eversible penis seen in flatworms; a finger-like projection of a polychete parapodium; one of the two setose branches of the thoracic legs of barnacles; one of the lateral appendages on the stalk, or aboral base, of a crinoid; or one of the short tentacle-like projections around the mouth of cephalochordates that form a coarse sieve preventing entrance of large particles (e.g., sand) into the mouth.

cirsectomy (ser-sek′to-me) [Gr. *kirsos* varix + *ektomē* excision]   excision of a portion of a varicose vein.

cirsenchysis (ser-sen′kĭ-sis) [Gr. *kirsos* varix + *enchysis* injection]   treatment of varicose veins by injection of a sclerosing solution.

cirs(o)- [Gr. *kirsos* varix]   a combining form denoting relationship to a varix.

cirsocele (ser′so-sēl) [*cirso-* + Gr. *kēlē* tumor]   varicocele.

cirsodesis (ser-sod′ĕ-sis) [*cirso-* + Gr. *desis* ligation]   the ligation of varicose veins.

cirsoid (ser′soid) [*cirso-* + Gr. *eidos* form]   resembling a varix.

cirsomphalos (ser-som′fah-los) [*cirso-* + *omphalos* navel]   a varicose state of the navel; caput medusae.

cirsophthalmia (ser″sof-thal′me-ah) [*cirso-* + Gr. *ophthalmos* eye]   a varicose state of the conjunctival vessels.

cirsotome (ser′so-tōm) [*cirso-* + Gr. *tomē* a cutting]   a cutting instrument for use in operating on varicosities.

cirsotomy (ser-sot′o-me) [*cirso-* + Gr. *temnein* to cut]   incision of varicose veins.

cis (sis) [L. "on this side"]   1. a prefix denoting on this side, on the same side, on the near side. 2. in organic chemistry, having certain atoms or radicals on the same side. 3. in genetics, having the two mutant genes of a pseudoallele on the same chromosome. Cf. *trans.*

cisclomiphene (sis-klo′mĭ-fēn)   enclomiphene.

cismatan (sis′mah-tan)   the seeds of *Cassia absus;* used in Egypt as a cure for ophthalmia.

cisplatin (sis′plah-tin)   chemical name: (*SP-4-2*)diamminedichloroplatinum; a platinum coordination compound, $Cl_2H_6N_2Pt$, used as an antineoplastic agent, primarily for treatment of testicular carcinoma, also for carcinomas of the bladder, ovary, head and neck, and prostate. Major side effects are nausea and vomiting; dose-related, cumulative renal dysfunction; and ototoxicity manifested by tinnitus and high-frequency hearing loss. Former nonproprietary name: *cis-platinum II.*

***cis*-platinum** (sis-plat′ĭ-num)   cisplatin.

11-*cis* retinal   see *retinal.*

cissa (sis′ah) [Gr. *kissa,* var. of *kitta*]   citta.

Cissampelos (sis-am′pĕ-los) [Gr. *kissos* ivy + *ampelos* vine]   a genus of menispermaceous climbing plants. *C. capensis* of Africa, is emetic and purgative. *C. pareira* L. is used by tropical American tribes for snakebites; also used as a diuretic, expectorant, emmenagogue, and febrifuge. It contains pelosine, an alkaloid.

cistern (sis′tern)   a closed space serving as a reservoir for

fluid; see also *cisterna.* **basal c.,** cisterna interpeduncularis. **cerebellomedullary c.,** cisterna cerebellomedullaris. **c. of chiasma, chiasmatic c.,** cisterna chiasmatis. **c. of fossa of Sylvius,** cisterna fossae lateralis cerebri. **great c.,** cisterna cerebellomedullaris. **interpeduncular c.,** cisterna interpeduncularis. **c. of lateral fossa of cerebrum,** cisterna fossae lateralis cerebri. **c. of Pecquet,** cisterna chyli. **posterior c.,** cisterna cerebellomedullaris. **subarachnoidal c's,** cisternae subarachnoideales. **c. of Sylvius,** cisterna fossae lateralis cerebri. **terminal c's,** pairs of transversely oriented channels that are confluent with the sarcotubules, which together with an intermediate T tubule constitute a triad of skeletal muscle. See also *T system,* under *system; T tubule,* under *tubule;* and *triad of skeletal muscle.*

cisterna (sis-ter′nah), pl. *cister′nae* [L.] [NA]   a cistern: a closed space serving as a reservoir for lymph or other body fluid, especially one of the enlarged subarachnoid spaces containing cerebrospinal fluid. **c. am′biens,** one that connects the cisterna venae magnae cerebri with the cisterna interpeduncularis. **c. basa′lis,** c. interpeduncularis. **c. cerebellomedulla′ris** [NA], cerebellomedullary cistern: the enlarged subarachnoid space between the under surface of the cerebellum and the posterior surface of the medulla oblongata, and continuous below with the spinal subarachnoid space. It can be tapped by means of a needle inserted through the posterior atlanto-occipital membrane (cisternal puncture). Called also *c. magna,* and *great* or *posterior cistern.* **c. chiasmat′ica,** c. chiasmatis. **c. chias′matis** [NA], chiasmatic cistern: a subarachnoid space between the optic chiasma and the rostrum of the corpus callosum; called also *cistern of chiasma.* **c. chy′li** [NA], a dilated portion of the thoracic duct at its origin in the lumbar region; it receives several lymph-collecting vessels, including the intestinal, lumbar, and descending intercostal trunks. Called also *ampulla chyli, chylocyst, cistern of Pecquet, receptaculum chyli,* and *receptaculum Pecqueti.* **c. fos′sae latera′lis cer′ebri** [NA], cistern of lateral fossa of cerebrum: the space between the arachnoid and the lateral cerebral fossa; called also *c. fossae lateralis cerebri* [Sylvii], *cistern* or *fossa of Sylvius,* and *c. sulci lateralis.* **c. fos′sae Syl′vii,** c. fossae lateralis cerebri. **c. intercrura′lis profun′da,** c. interpeduncularis. **c. interpeduncula′ris** [NA], interpeduncular cistern: a dilatation of the subarachnoid space between the cerebral peduncles; called also *c. intercruralis profunda,* and *basal cistern.* **c. mag′na,** c. cerebellomedullaris. **perinuclear c.,** the space separating the inner from the outer nuclear membrane; called also *perinuclear space.* **cister′nae subarachnoida′les,** cisternae subarachnoideales. **cister′nae subarachnoidea′les** [NA], subarachnoidal cisterns: localized enlargements of the subarachnoid space, occurring in areas where the dura mater and arachnoid do not closely follow the contour of the brain with its covering pia mater, and serving as reservoirs of cerebrospinal fluid; called also *cisternae subarachnoidales.* **c. sul′ci latera′lis, c. Sylvii,** c. fossae lateralis cerebri. **c. ve′nae mag′nae cer′ebri,** the superior confluent of the subarachnoid space, lying in the angle between the splenium of the corpus callosum and the superior surfaces of the cerebellum and mesencephalon, and containing the great vein of the cerebrum. Called also *Bichat's* or *arachnoid canal.*

cisternae (sis-ter′ne) [L.]   genitive and plural of *cisterna.*

cisternal (sis-ter′nal)   pertaining to a cistern, especially the cisterna cerebellomedullaris.

cisternographic (sis″ter-no-graf′ik)   pertaining to cisternography.

cisternography (sis″ter-nog′rah-fe)   radiography of the basal cistern of the brain after subarachnoid injection of a contrast medium.

cistron (sis′tron) [L. *cis* on this side + *trans* on the other side + Gr. *on* neuter ending]   the smallest unit of genetic material that must be intact to function as a transmitter of genetic information, i.e., to determine the sequence of amino acids of one polypeptide chain. The cistron is identified by the *cis-trans* test. The gene by one definition is identical to the cistron.

Citanest (si′tah-nest)   trademark for preparations of prilocaine hydrochloride.

Citelli's syndrome (che-tel′ēz) [Salvatore *Citelli,* Italian laryngologist, 1875–1947]   see under *syndrome.*

Citellus (si-tel′us) *Spermophilus.*

citrate (sit′rāt) any anionic form of citric acid; any salt or ester of citric acid. **cupric c.,** a bluish green, crystalline powder, $Cu_2C_6H_4O_7$; antiseptic and astringent. **ferric c.,** garnet-red scales or brown granules, $FeC_6H_5O_7 \cdot xH_2O$, used as a reagent; called also *iron citrate.* **c. phosphate dextrose (CPD),** a solution containing citric acid, sodium citrate, sodium biphosphate, and dextrose that is the primary anticoagulant used for preservation of whole blood or red cells for up to 21 days. Called also *anticoagulant citrate phosphate dextrose solution* [USP]. **c. phosphate dextrose adenine (CPDA-1),** an anticoagulant solution, containing citric acid, sodium citrate, sodium biphosphate, dextrose, and adenine, used for the preservation of whole blood and red cells for up to 35 days; it extends red cell survival by providing adenine needed for the maintenance of red cell ATP levels.

citrated (sit′rāt-ed) containing a citrate, especially potassium citrate.

citrate synthase (sit′rāt sin′thās) citrate (si)-synthase.

citrate (si)-synthase (sit′rāt sin′thās) [EC 4.1.3.7] an enzyme of the lyase (synthase) class that catalyzes the reaction acetyl-CoA + H_2O + oxaloacetate = citrate + CoA. This is the initial condensation reaction in the citric (tricarboxylic) acid cycle. Called also *citrate synthase.*

citreoviridin (sī″tre-o-vir′ĭ-din) a toxic compound isolated from the fungus *Penicillium citreoviride,* said to have the empirical formula of $C_{23}H_{30}O_6$.

citric acid (sit′rik) a compound, 2-hydroxy-1,2,3-propane-tricarboxylic acid, $HOOCCH_2COH(COOH)CH_2COOH$, which is an intermediate in the tricarboxylic acid (Krebs) cycle (q.v.) and is obtained from citrus fruits. Citrate chelates calcium ions and prevents blood clotting and is used as an anticoagulant for stored whole blood and red cells and also for blood specimens.

Citrobacter (sit″ro-bak′ter) [L. *citrus* lemon + Gr. baktron a rod] a genus of gram-negative, facultatively anaerobic, rod-shaped bacteria of the family Enterobacteriaceae, made up of motile organisms that are able to use citrate as a sole carbon source. The organisms occur in water, food, feces, and urine. They have been associated with diarrhea and secondary infections in debilitated persons, occasionally causing severe primary septicemia. **C. amalona′ticus,** a species that produces indole, does not ferment adonitol, and is not inhibited by potassium cyanide; found in humans as an opportunistic pathogen. **C. diver′sus,** a species that produces indole, ferments adonitol, and is inhibited by potassium cyanide; it occasionally causes neonatal meningitis. **C. freun′dii** the most commonly isolated species. It does not produce indole or ferment adonitol and is not inhibited by potassium cyanide; found in soil, water, sewage and food, in clinical specimens from normal persons, and as an opportunistic pathogen. **C. interme′dius,** a variant of *C. freundii.* Called also *Escherichia intermedia.*

Citromyces (sit″ro-mi′sēz) [*citric acid* + Gr. *mykes* fungus] a name formerly used for some species of *Penicillium,* especially those which produce citric acid from sugars.

citron (sit′ron) [L. *citrus*] the orange-like tree, *Citrus medica,* and its fruit.

citronella (sit″ron-el′ah) a fragrant grass, *Cymbopogon (Andropogon) nardus* (L.) Rendle, the source of a volatile oil (citronella oil) used in perfumes and insect repellents.

citrophosphate (sit″ro-fos′fāt) a compound of a citrate and a phosphate.

citrulline (sit-rul′lin) alpha-amino delta-carbamido normal valeric acid, $NH_2 \cdot CO \cdot NH \cdot (CH_2)_3 \cdot CH(NH_2) \cdot COOH$; it is formed from ornithine and is itself converted into arginine in the urea cycle.

citrullinemia (sit-rul″in-e′me-ah) argininosuccinate synthetase deficiency.

citrullinuria (sit-rul″in-u′re-ah) argininosuccinate synthetase deficiency.

Citrullus (sĭ-trul′lus) a genus of curcurbitaceous plants, including *C. vulga′ris,* the watermelon, the seeds of which are the source of cucurbital and cucurbocitrin.

Citrus (sit′rus) [L.] a genus of rutaceous trees: *C. aurantifolia,* the lime; *C. aurantium,* the orange; *C. bergamia,* the bergamot; *C. limonum,* the lemon; *C. medica,* the citron; *C. sinensis,* the sweet orange.

citta (sit′ah) [Gr. *kitta*] craving for unusual foods during pregnancy; cravings for starch, sweets, fruits, vegetables, pickles, or raw cereals are common and are sometimes associated with *pica,* eating of nonnutritive substances, such as ice, clay, or chalk.

cittosis (sit-to′sis) citta.

Civatte's poikiloderma (siv-ats′) [Achille *Civatte,* French dermatologist, 1877–1956] see under *poikiloderma.*

Civinini's ligament, process (spine) (che″ve-ne′nēz) [Filippo *Civinini,* Italian anatomist, 1805–1844] see *ligamentum pterygospinale* and *processus pterygospinosus.*

Cl chemical symbol for *chlorine.*

cladiosis (klad″e-o′sis) a fungal disease resembling sporotrichosis, marked by chains of subcutaneous nodules along the forearm, and from which an organism called *Scopulariopsis blochi* was isolated; the organism was later found to be a *Paecilomyces,* and was probably a contaminant. Called also *gummatous lymphangitis.*

Clado's anastomosis, band (klah′dōz) [Spiro *Clado,* French gynecologist, born 1856] see under *anastomosis* and *band.*

Cladonia (klah-do′ne-ah) [Gr. *klados* branch] a genus of lichens. *C. rangiferina,* reindeer moss, was formerly used as a stomachic and pectoral.

Cladorchis watsoni (kla-dor′kis wat-so′ni) *Watsonius watsoni.*

cladosporiosis (klad″o-spo″re-o′sis) a general term for infection with *Cladosporium,* including black degeneration of the brain, chromomycosis, and tinea nigra.

Cladosporium (klad″o-spo′re-um) a genus of dematiacious Fungi Imperfecti of the order Moniliales. *C. herbarum* produces "black spot" on meat in cold storage. It will grow at a temperature of 18° F. (–8° C.). *C. carrionii* is an agent of chromomycosis. *C. werneckii* and *C. mansonii* are agents of tinea nigra. *C. trichoides* and other species cause black degeneration of the brain.

Cladothrix (klad′o-thriks) [Gr. *klados* branch + *thrix* hair] a genus of bacteria made up of organisms now classified in the genera *Actinomyces, Bacterionema, Nocardia, Sphaerotilus,* and *Streptomyces.*

clairvoyance (klār-voi′ans) [Fr.] a form of extrasensory perception in which knowledge of objectives events is acquired without the use of the senses. Cf. *telepathy.*

clamoxyquin hydrochloride (klah-moks′ĭ-kwin) chemical name: 5-chloro-7-[[[3-(diethylamino)propyl]amino]-methyl]-8-quinolinol dihydrochloride; an antiamebic agent, $C_{21}H_{26}ClNO$, which has been used in intestinal amebiasis.

clamp (klamp) 1. any device used to grip, join, compress, or fasten parts. 2. a surgical instrument for effecting compression. See also under *forceps.* **Cope's c.,** a crushing clamp with several hinged segments for use in surgery of the colon and rectum. **cotton roll rubber dam c.,** a rubber dam clamp with a buccal and lingual wing or flange to hold cotton rolls in position in the mouth; useful in the placement of direct gold or other restorative material in subgingival class V cavity preparations. **Crile's c.,** a rubber-shod clamp to secure temporary hemostasis in suture of blood vessels. **Doyen's c.,** a forceps with flexible blades for clamping tissues to control bleeding temporarily during operations on the gastrointestinal tract. **Gant's c.,** a right-angled clamp used in operating on hemorrhoids. **gingival c.,** a clamp for retracting gingival tissues. **Goldblatt's c.,** a clamp for the renal artery to produce experimental hypertension. **Joseph's c.,** a clamp used after a nasal operation to improve the alignment of the mobilized fragments of the bony framework of the nose. **Martel's c.,** a crushing clamp used in resection of the colon. **Mikulicz's c.,** a clamp used for crushing the septum between the proximal and distal segments of the colon after exteriorization. **Payr c.,** a crushing clamp used in resections of the stomach, intestine, and colon. **pedicle c.,** clamp forceps, def. 1; see under *forceps.* **Potts' c.,** an atraumatic clamp used to grasp a blood vessel. **Rankin c.,** a three-bladed clamp for crushing the colon during resection. **rubber dam c.,** a device made of spring metal that is used to retain the rubber dam on a tooth, having beveled jaws that contact the tooth and a bow that connects the jaws. **Sehrt's c.,** a clamp for compressing the aorta or for compressing a limb to arrest hemorrhage; called also *Sehrt's compressor.* **voltage c.,** an electronic technique employing the feedback principle to impose a fixed potential difference across a cell membrane. **Willett c.,** Willett forceps. **Yellen c.,** a special clamp used for circumcision.

clang (klang) a harsh quality of a sound or of the voice.

clanging (klang′ing) a pattern of speech in which sound rather than sense governs word choice, and rhyming and punning (*clang association*) substitute for logic; commonly observed in schizophrenia and manic episodes.

clap (klap) gonorrhea.

clapotage (klap″o-tahzh′) clapotement.

clapotement (klah-pawt-maw′) [Fr.] a splashing sound heard on succussion; called also *clapotage*.

claquement (klak-maw′) [Fr.] a clapping or snapping. **c. d'ouverture,** opening snap.

clarificant (klar-if′ĭ-kant) an agent that clears liquids of turbidity.

clarification (klar″ĭ-fĭ-ka′shun) [L. *clarus* clear + *facere* to make] the clearing of a liquid from turbidity.

clarify (klar′ĭ-fi) [L. *clarificare* to render clear] to clear of turbidity or of suspended matter.

Clark II an irritant poison gas, diphenylcyanoarsine, (C₆H₅)₂AsCN.

Clark's test (klarks) [Guy Wendell *Clark*, American biochemist, born 1887] see under *tests*.

Clark-Collip method (klark-kol′ip) [Earl Perry *Clark*, American biochemist, born 1892; James Bertram *Collip*, Canadian biochemist, 1892–1965] see under *method*.

Clarke's cells, column, nucleus (klarks) [Jacob Augustus Lockhart *Clarke*, English anatomist and physician, 1817–1880] see under *cell*, and see *columna thoracica*.

clasmatocyte (klaz-mat′o-sit) [Gr. *klasma* a piece broken off + *kytos* hollow vessel] Ranvier's name for certain branched cells in connective tissue that allegedly detach portions of their processes as a means of discharging their secretions. As now used the term is equivalent to the cell described under macrophage.

clasmatocytosis (klaz-mat″o-si-to′sis) an excess of clasmatocytes.

clasmatodendrosis (klaz-mat″o-den-dro′sis) [Gr. *klasma* a piece broken off + *dendron*] a breaking up of the protoplasmic expansions of astrocytes.

clasmatosis (klaz″mah-to′sis) [Gr. *klasma* a piece broken off] the breaking off of parts of a cell.

clasmocytoma (klaz″mo-si-to′mah) reticulum cell sarcoma.

clasp (klasp) 1. a device by which something is held. 2. in dentistry, a part of an extracoronal direct retainer that retains and stabilizes the denture by attaching to abutment teeth. **Adams c.,** a modified arrow clasp that utilizes buccal, mesial, and distal proximal undercuts of a tooth for retention. **arrow c., arrowhead c.,** a clasp made by bending a piece of stainless steel wire in the shape of an arrowhead; used to stabilize an orthodontic appliance by holding the teeth in the interproximal areas. **bar c.,** one whose arms are bar-type extensions from major connectors or from within the denture base; the arms approach the point of contact on the tooth in the cervico-occlusal direction. **circumferential c.,** one that encircles more than 180° of a tooth, including opposite angles, and usually contacts the tooth throughout the extent of the clasp, at least one terminal being in the infrabulge area. **continuous c., continuous lingual c.,** one made of two or more stainless steel lingual clasps joined to each other and then joined to a major connector by two or more minor connectors; used to brace lingual upper teeth. Called also *continuous bar retainer, Kennedy bar,* and *lingual bar.* **Crozat c.,** a metal attachment of a removable appliance adapted to the embrasure.

class (klas) 1. a taxonomic category subordinate to a phylum (or subphylum) and superior to an order. 2. in statistics, a group of variables all of which show a particular value or a value falling between certain limits. The *frequencies of class* is the number of variables that it contains.

classic (klas′ik) of first class or rank; standard.

classification (klas″sĭ-fĭ-ka′shun) the systematic arrangement of similar entities on the basis of certain differing characteristics. **adansonian c.,** numerical taxonomy. **Angle's c.,** a classification of dental malocclusion based on the mesiodistal (anteroposterior) position of the mandibular

dental arch and teeth relative to the maxillary dental arch and teeth; see under *malocclusion*. **Arneth's c.,** see under *count*. **Bergey's c.,** a system of classification of bacteria in which the organisms are grouped according to Gram reaction, metabolism, and morphology, with each group being further subdivided into orders, families, genera, and species. **Broders' c.,** see under *index*. **Caldwell-Moloy c.,** classification of female pelves as gynecoid, android, anthropoid, and platypelloid; see under *pelvis*. **Chicago c.,** the classification of human chromosomes adopted by geneticists at Chicago in 1966 for the identification of chromosomal bands and regions and for the location of structural chromosomal abnormalities. See also *Denver c.* and *Paris c.* **Denver c.,** the classification of human chromosomes on the basis of size and centromere position, adopted by geneticists in Denver in 1960. The 23 pairs of chromosomes are arranged into seven groups, labeled A to G, in the order of decreasing length. See also *Chicago c.* **Gell and Coombs c.,** a classification of immune mechanisms of tissue injury, called by Gell and Coombs "allergic reactions," comprising four types: *Type I,* immediate hypersensitivity reactions, mediated by IgE antibody; *Type II,* cytotoxic reactions, mediated by antitissue antibody, including complement-dependent lysis, antibody-dependent cell-mediated cytotoxicity (ACDD), and phagocytosis induced by opsonizing antibody; *Type III,* reactions mediated by immune complexes, including serum sickness, Arthus reactions, and immune complex disorders; and *Type IV* delayed hypersensitivity reactions, mediated by sensitized T lymphocytes either by release of lymphokines or by T-cell–mediated cytotoxicity, including contact dermatitis, allograft rejection, and graft-versus-host disease. Other authorities have added *Type V,* antibody interference with the function of biologically active substances, including autoimmune diseases mediated by antireceptor antibodies and coagulation disorders mediated by antibodies to coagulation factors. **Jansky's c.,** a classification of ABO blood types designated by roman numerals I to IV, corresponding with types O, A, B, and AB, respectively. **Kauffman-White c.,** a scheme for the serologic identification of species of *Salmonella* by classification of their reactions to O, H, and Vi antisera. **Keith-Wagener-Barker c.,** a classification of hypertension and arteriolosclerosis based on retinal changes. Group 1, essential benign hypertension indicated by moderate arteriolar attenuation. Group 2, constant high blood pressure but no apparent effect on health, indicated by more definite arteriolar attenuation with localized constriction. Group 3, hypertension with retinal, renal, cerebral, and other symptoms, indicated by marked attenuation of the arterioles, cotton-wool exudates, and hemorrhages. Group 4, severe hypertension with severe nervous system, visual, and other organ disturbances, indicated by ophthalmoscopic signs of Group 3, with papilledema. **Kennedy c.,** a classification of partially edentulous conditions and partial dentures, based on the location of the edentulous spaces in relation to the remaining teeth. **Lancefield c.,** a serologic classification of the hemolytic streptococci, based on extraction and examination by a precipitin technique of group-specific carbohydrate antigens contained in the cell wall. Groups A through O have been established. **McNeer c.,** a classification of gastric carcinoma as (1) polypoid, (2) ulcerocancerous, (3) ulcerating and infiltrating, and (4) infiltrating. **Migula's c.,** a classification of bacteria drawn up by Migula in 1900. **Moss' c.,** a classification of ABO blood types designated by roman numerals I to IV, corresponding with types AB, A, B, and O, respectively. **New York Heart Association (NYHA) c.,** a functional and therapeutic classification for prescription of physical activity for cardiac patients. Class I (or A): patients with no limitation of activities; they suffer no symptoms from ordinary activities. Class II (or B): patients with slight limitation of activity; they are comfortable at rest or with mild exertion. Class III (or C): patients with marked limitation of activity; they are comfortable only at rest. Class IV (or D): patients who should be at complete rest, confined to bed or chair; any physical activity brings on discomfort. **numerical c.,** see under *taxonomy*. **Paris c.,** a modification made in Paris in 1971 of the Chicago classification of human chromosomes, providing more detailed genetic information; see also *Denver c.* **Runyon c.,** a classification of mycobacteria based on the pigmentation and growth condition of the organisms. See *nontuberculous mycobacteria,* under *mycobacterium*. **Skinner c.,** a method of classifying partially edentulous conditions and partial dentures, based on the location of the edentulous spaces in relation to the remaining teeth.

-clast [Gr. *-klastēs* breaker, from *klan* to break] a word termination denoting that which breaks or destroys.

clastic (klas′tik) [Gr. *klastos* broken] 1. causing or undergoing a division into parts. 2. separable into parts, as an anatomical model.

clastogenic (klas″to-jen′ik) [Gr. *klastos* broken + *-genic*] giving rise to or inducing disruption or breakages, as of chromosomes.

clastothrix (klas′to-thriks) [Gr. *klastos* broken + *thrix* hair] trichorrhexis nodosa.

clathrate (klăth′rāt) [L. *clathare* to provide with a lattice] 1. having the shape or appearance of a lattice. 2. a clathrate compound; also, pertaining or relating to a clathrate compound. See under *compound*.

clathrin (klath′rin) a 180,000-dalton protein that coats the cytoplasmic face of "coated pits" involved in receptor-mediated endocytosis of low-density lipoprotein (LDL), insulin, and other ligands.

Clathrochloris (klath″ro-klo′ris) [L. *clathri* lattice + Gr. *chlōros* green] a genus of aquatic phototrophic bacteria of the family Chlorobiaceae, order Rhodospirillales, consisting of spherical to ovoid nonmotile cells that contain gas vacuoles and fix carbon dioxide in the presence of hydrogen sulfide. Cell suspensions are yellow to green. The type species is *C. sulfur′ica*.

Clathrocystis (klath″ro-sis′tis) a genus name formerly given microorganisms, some of which are now classified in the genus *Lamprocystis*.

Clauberg's test (klaw′bergz) [Karl Wm. *Clauberg*, German bacteriologist, born 1893] see under *test*.

Claude (klawd) Albert. Belgian-born American cytologist, born 1899; co-winner, with Christian René de Duve and George Emil Palade, of the Nobel prize for medicine or physiology in 1974 for their discoveries concerning the structural and functional organization of the cell.

Claude's hyperkinesis sign, syndrome (klawdz) [Henri *Claude*, French psychiatrist, 1869–1945] see under *sign* and *syndrome*.

claudicant (klaw′dĭ-kant) pertaining to or affected by claudication; by extension, sometimes used to denote a patient with intermittent claudication.

claudication (klaw″dĭ-ka′shun) [L. *claudicatio*] limping or lameness. **intermittent c.,** a complex of symptoms characterized by absence of pain or discomfort in a limb when at rest, the commencement of pain, tension, and weakness, after walking is begun, intensification of the condition until walking becomes impossible, and the disappearance of the symptoms after a period of rest. The condition is seen in occlusive arterial diseases of the limbs, such as thromboangiitis obliterans, and in compression of the cauda equina. Called also *Charcot's syndrome* and *angina cruris*. **venous c.,** intermittent claudication caused by venous stasis.

claudicatory (klaw′dĭ-kah-tor′e) pertaining to or marked by claudication.

Claudius' cell (klaw′de-us) [Friedrich Matthias *Claudius*, Austrian anatomist, 1822–1869] see under *cell*.

claustra (klaws′trah) [L.] plural of *claustrum*.

claustral (klaws′tral) pertaining to or of the nature of a claustrum.

claustrophilia (klaws″tro-fil′e-ah) a pathological desire to be shut in, to close all doors, windows, etc.

claustrophobia (klaws″tro-fo′be-ah) [L. *claudere* to shut + *phobia*] irrational fear of being shut in; fear of enclosed spaces, such as elevators and tunnels.

claustrum (klaws′trum), pl. *claus′tra* [L. "a barrier"] [NA] the thin layer of gray matter lateral to the external capsule of the lentiform nucleus, separating the nucleus from the white substance of the insula; it is mainly composed of spindle cells. Called also *claustrum of insula*. **c. gut′turis, c. o′ris,** palatum molle. **c. virgina′le,** hymen.

clausura (klaw-su′rah) [L. "closure"] atresia.

clava (kla′vah) [L. "stick"] tuberculum nuclei gracilis.

clavacin (kla′vah-sin) patulin.

claval (kla′val) pertaining to the clava (tuberculum nuclei gracilis [NA]).

clavate (kla′vāt) [L. *clavatus* club] pertaining to the clava (tuberculum nuclei gracilis [NA]); club-shaped.

Claviceps (klav′ĭ-seps) [L. *clava* club + *caput* head] a genus of parasitic ascomycetous fungi of the family Clavicipitaceae, order Clavicipitales, which infest the seeds of various plants. *C. purpurea* is the source of the common ergot of rye. See *ergot*, def. 1.

Clavicipitaceae (klav″ĭ-sip″ĭ-ta′se-e) a family of fungi of the order Clavicipitales having long cylindrical asci and long filiform ascospores, including the genera *Claviceps* and *Cordyceps*.

Clavicipitales (klav″ĭ-sip″ĭ-ta′lēz) an order of ascomycetous fungi of the series Pyrenomycetes, in which the perithecia are formed in well-developed stroma and the asci have thick caps; it includes the family Clavicipitaceae.

clavicle (klav′ĭ-k'l) the bone articulating with the sternum and scapula; see *clavicula*.

clavicotomy (klav″ĭ-kot′o-me) [clavicle + Gr. *tomē* a cutting] the operation of cutting or dividing the clavicle.

clavicula (klah-vik′u-lah) [L. dim. of *clavis* key] [NA] the clavicle: a bone, curved like the letter *f*, that articulates with the sternum and scapula, forming the anterior portion of the shoulder girdle on either side; called also *collar bone*.

clavicular (klah-vik′u-lar) pertaining to the clavicle.

claviculus (klah-vik′u-lus), pl. *clavic′uli* [L. dim. of *clavus* nail] any one of Sharpey's fibers (a set of fibers that hold together the laminae of a bone).

claviformin (klav″ĭ-for′min) patulin.

clavipectoral (klav″ĭ-pek′to-ral) [L. *clavis* clavicle + *pectus* breast] pertaining to the clavicle and thorax.

clavus (kla′vus), pl. *cla′vi* [L. "nail"] a corn. **c. du′rus,** hard corn. **c. hyster′icus,** a sensation as if a nail were being driven into the head. **c. mol′lis,** soft corn. **c. secali′nus,** ergot, def. 1.

clawfoot (klaw-fut) a high-arched foot with the toes hyperextended at the metatarsophalangeal joint and flexed at the distal joints; called also *gampsodactyly* and *griffe des orteils*.

clawhand (klaw-hand) flexion and atrophy of the hand and fingers; it occurs in lesions of the ulnar nerve, in leprosy, and in syringomyelia. Called also *main en griffe*.

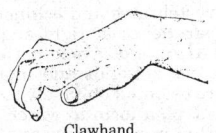

Clawhand.

clay (kla) a native hydrated aluminum silicate, resulting from the decomposition of rocks caused by weathering; various forms of clays have been used in medicine, both externally and internally, since earliest times. **China c.,** kaolin.

clazolam (kla′zo-lam) chemical name: 2-chloro-5,9,10,-14b-tetrahydro-5-methylisoquino[2,1-*d*][1,4]benzodiazepin-6-(7*H*)-one; a minor tranquilizer, $C_{18}H_{17}ClN_2O$.

clazolimine (kla-zo′lĭ-mēn) chemical name: 1-(4-chlorophenyl)-2-imino-3-methyl-4-imidazolidinone; a diuretic, $C_{10}H_{10}ClN_3O$.

Cl₃C·CHO chloral.

clear (klēr) to remove cloudiness from microscopical specimens by the use of a clearing agent.

clearance (klēr′ans) 1. the process of clearing; the rate at which a substance is removed from the blood. 2. a quantitative measure of the rate at which a substance is removed from the blood; the volume of plasma that is completely cleared of the substance per unit time. The renal clearance of a substance is given by the formula: $C = V \times U/P$, where C is the clearance, V the urine volume in ml/min, U the urine concentration of the substance, and P the plasma concentration. Symbol C. 3. the space existing between opposed structures. **p-aminohippurate c.,** the renal clearance of exogenously administered p-aminohippuric acid, accepted as the most accurate measurement of effective renal plasma flow (ERPF). **creatinine c.,** the renal clearance of endogenous creatinine, a commonly used clinical measurement that closely estimates the glomerular filtration rate (GFR). **free water c.,** the net amount of solute-free water moved from the blood to the urine; the difference between the urine volume and the osmolal clearance. **immune c.,** immune elimination. **interocclusal c.,** see under distance. **inulin c.,** the renal clearance of inulin maintained at a constant serum level by continuous infusion, accepted as the most accurate measurement of the glomerular filtration rate (GFR). **occlusal c.,** a condition in which the opposing occlusal surfaces may glide over one another without any interfering projection. **osmolal c.,** the amount of water cleared from the plasma, resulting in urine having the same osmolality as plasma, calculated as urine volume × urine osmolality ÷ plasma osmolality. **plasma iron c.,** plasma iron clearance half-time. **urea c.,** the renal clearance of endogenous urea, an infrequently used clinical measurement of total (both glomerular and tubular) renal function.

clearer (klēr′er) a clearing agent; an agent used in microscopy to remove the cloudiness from a specimen.

cleavage (klēv′ij) the mitotic segmentation of the fertilized ovum, the size of the structure remaining unchanged, as the cleavage cells, or blastomeres, become smaller and smaller with each division. **accessory c.,** peripheral cleavage in telolecithal eggs due to polyspermy. **adequal c.,** a form in which the blastomeres are practically equal in size. **complete c.,** holoblastic c. **determinate c.,** cleavage following a precise pattern, each blastomere having a characteristic and unalterable fate, i.e., each blastomere becoming the precursor of a definite part of the embryo. **discoidal c.,** cleavage limited to the animal pole of highly telolecithal eggs. **equal c.,** a form in which the blastomeres are equal in size. **equatorial c.,** cleavage that occurs in a plane passing through the equator of the egg. **holoblastic c.,** a form in which the entire egg participates in cell division; called also *complete* or *total c.* **incomplete c.,** meroblastic c. **indeterminate c.,** that following a less rigid cleavage pattern, the blastomeres having more developmental possibilities than they usually show, each of which, when isolated, being capable of developing into a normal embryo. **latitudinal c.,** cleavage in planes passing at right angles to the egg axis. **meridional c.,** cleavage in planes passing through the egg axis. **meroblastic c.,** a form in which only the protoplasmic portions of the egg participate; called also *incomplete* or *partial c.* **partial c.,** meroblastic c. **radial c.,** a cleavage pattern characteristic of vertebrates and echinoderms, in which the spindle axes are parallel or at right angles to the polar axis of the egg. **spiral c.,** a cleavage pattern characteristic of such invertebrates as annelids and mollusks, in which the cleavage planes are oriented obliquely to the polar axis of the egg. **superficial c.,** a form in which only the surface region of centrolecithal eggs participate. **total c.,** holoblastic c. **unequal c.,** a form in which the blastomeres about the vegetal pole remain larger in size than those nearer the animal pole.

cleft (kleft) a fissure or elongated opening, especially one occurring in the embryo or derived from a failure of parts to fuse during embryonic development. **anal c.,** crena ani. **branchial c.,** any of the slitlike openings in the gills of fishes, formed between the branchial arches. Also, any of the homologous branchial grooves of the mammalian embryo. **cervical c's,** clefts in the endocervical mucosa. **cholesterol c.,** a cleft in a section of tissue embedded in paraffin, due to the dissolving of cholesterol crystals. **clunial c.,** crena ani. **corneal c.,** see under *fissure*. **facial c.,** the clefts between the embryonic processes that normally unite to form the face. Failure of such union, depending on its site, causes such developmental defects as cleft cheek; cleft lip (harelip); cleft mandible; oblique facial cleft; and transverse facial cleft. **facial c., lateral,** transverse facial cleft extending from the angle of the mouth toward the ear. See also *macrostomia*. **facial c., oblique,** a rare form of facial cleft extending from the lip to the inner canthus of the eye. It may be superficial but usually separates the underlying bone and is associated with cleft lip, cleft palate, or lateral facial cleft. Called also *meloschisis* and *prosopanoschisis*. **facial c., transverse,** lateral facial c. **genital c.,** a depression of the external genital region of the fetus, which develops into the male urethra or the vestibule. **gingival c.,** an area of isolated gingival recession occurring over a dehiscence of the bone covering the root. **gluteal c.,** crena ani. **hyobranchial c.,** the cleft between the hyoid and the next succeeding arch in the developing embryo;

called also *posthyoidean* c. **hyoid c.,** hyomandibular c. **hyomandibular c.,** the cleft between the mandibular and hyoid arches in the developing embryo; called also *hyoid c.* **interdental c.,** diastema. **Lanterman's c's,** incisures of Lanterman. **Larrey's c.,** trigonum sternocostale. **Maurer's c's,** Maurer's dots. **natal c.,** crena ani. **posthyoidean c.,** hyobranchial c. **Schmidt-Lanterman c's,** incisures of Lanterman. **Stillman's c.,** a small apostrophe-shaped or slitlike fissure of the gingiva extending from the gingival margin to a depth of up to 5 to 6 cm. **synaptic c.,** a narrow extracellular cleft between the pre- and postsynaptic cell membranes at the synapse. **visceral c's,** grooves between the branchial (visceral) arches of the embryo. **vulval c.,** rima pudendi.

clegs (klegz) a common name for certain tabanid flies, the horseflies or gadflies.

cleidagra (kli-dag′rah) [*cleid-* + Gr. *agra* seizure] gouty pain in the clavicle.

cleidal (kli′dal) pertaining to or affecting the clavicle.

cleidarthritis (kli″dar-thri′tis) [*cleid-* + Gr. *arthron* joint] gout in the clavicular region.

cleid(o)- [Gr. *kleis*, gen. *kleidos*, key, clavicle] a combining form denoting relationship to the clavicle.

cleidocostal (kli″do-kos′tal) pertaining to the clavicle and the ribs.

cleidocranial (kli″do-kra′ne-al) [*cleido-* + Gr. *kranion* head] pertaining to the clavicle and the head.

cleidoic (kli-do′ik) [Gr. *kleidouchos* holding the keys] isolated from the environment, self-contained, as the ova (eggs) of reptiles, birds, and primitive mammals, which are self-sufficient, having become a closed system, and, except for oxygen intake, developing at the expense of the substances stored inside the egg itself, directly into miniature adults without passing through a larval stage.

cleidomastoid (kli″do-mas′toid) pertaining to the clavicle and the mastoid process.

cleidorrhexis (kli″do-rek′sis) [*cleido-* + Gr. *rhēxsis* rupture] cleidotomy.

cleidotomy (kli-dot′o-me) [*cleido-* + Gr. *tomē* a cutting] surgical division of the clavicle of the fetus in difficult labor, to facilitate passage of the shoulders through the birth canal; called also *cleidorrhexis*.

cleisagra (kli-sag′rah) cleidagra.

cleisiophobia (kli″se-o-fo′be-ah) [Gr. *kleisis* closure + *phobia*] (obs.) claustrophobia.

cleistothecium (klis″to-the′se-um) [Gr. *kleisis* closure + *thēkē* case] the fruiting body, or carp, produced by certain ascomycetes, in which there is no pore for the escape of ascospores, the spores being released after decay of the cleistothecium. Cf. *apothecium, gymnothecium,* and *perithecium*.

cleithrophobia (kli″thro-fo′be-ah) (obs.) claustrophobia.

clemastine (klem′as-tēn) chemical name: (+)-2-[2-[(p-chloro-α-methyl-α-phenylbenzyl)oxy]ethyl]-1-methylpyrrolidine; an antihistaminic, $C_{21}H_{26}ClNO$. **c. fumarate,** a salt of clemastine, $C_{21}H_{26}ClNO \cdot C_4H_4O_4$; an antihistaminic used in the treatment of allergic rhinitis and allergic skin disorders.

Clematis (klem′ah-tis) [Gr. *klēmatis*] a genus of ranunculaceous plants, many of them active poisons.

clemizole (klem′ĭ-zōl) chemical name: 1-[(4-chlorophenyl)methyl]-2-(1-pyrrolidinylmethyl)-1*H*-benzimidazole; an antihistaminic, $C_{19}H_{20}ClN_3$. **c. hydrochloride,** the hydrochloride salt of clemizole, $C_{19}H_{20}ClN_3 \cdot HCl$, used as an antihistaminic in the treatment of skin allergies, food and cosmetic hypersensitivities, and serum sickness; administered orally. **c. penicillin,** see under *penicillin*.

clenching (klench′ing) the clamping and pressing of the jaws and teeth together in centric occlusion, frequently associated with acute nervous tension or physical effort, such as pushing or lifting a heavy object or performing a difficult task. See also *bruxism*.

Cleocin (kle′o-sin) trademark for preparations of clindamycin.

cleoid (kle′oid) [Middle English *cle* claw + *-oid*] a claw-shaped nib used to carve amalgam restorations.

Clethrionomys (kleth″re-on′o-mis) a genus of voles.

C. glario′lus, a species implicated as a reservoir of epidemic hemorrhagic fever.

Clevelandellina (klĕvel″an-del′ĭ-nah) a suborder of endoparasitic, ciliate protozoa (order Heterotrichina, subclass Spirotricha) characterized by the presence of well-developed somatic ciliature, sometimes separated into distinct areas by well-defined suture lines (*systèmes sécants*), and in some species by a dorsoanterior sucker. They are found in the digestive tract of insects and other arthropods or lower vertebrates and occasionally in oligochetes or mollusks. *Nyctotherus* is a representative species.

click (klik) a brief sharp sound; see also *clicking*. **ejection c′s,** see under *sound*. **Ortolani's c.,** see under *sign*. **systolic c′s,** short, dry, clicking heart sounds during systole, indicative of various heart conditions.

clicking (klik′ing) a series of clicks, such as the snapping, cracking, or crepitant noise evident on excursions of the mandibular condyle.

clid(o)- for words beginning thus, see those beginning *cleid(o)-*.

clidinium bromide (klĭ-din′e-um) [USP] chemical name: 3-[(hydroxydiphenylacetyl) oxy]- 1- methyl- 1- azoniabicyclo-[2.2.2]octane bromide. A quaternary ammonium anticholinergic, $C_{22}H_{26}BrNO_3$, with pronounced antispasmodic and antisecretory effects on the gastrointestinal tract, occurring as a white or nearly white, crystalline powder; used as adjunctive therapy in the treatment of peptic ulcer and other gastrointestinal disorders, administered orally.

climacteric (kli-mak′ter-ik, kli″mak-ter′ik) [Gr. *klimaktēr* rung of ladder, critical point in human life] the syndrome of endocrine, somatic, and psychic changes occurring at the termination of the reproductive period in the female (menopause); it may also accompany the normal diminution of sexual activity in the male. Called also *climacterium*.

climacterium (kli″mak-te′re-um) climacteric. **c. prae′-cox,** premature menopause.

climatology (kli″mah-tol′o-je) [Gr. *klima* the supposed slope of the earth from the equator to the pole + *logos* treatise] the science devoted to the study of the conditions of the natural environment (rainfall, daylight, temperature, humidity, air movement) prevailing in specific regions of the earth. **medical c.,** that concerned especially with the effect of climatic factors on man, on his functions and health, and on the treatment of his ills.

climatotherapeutics (kli″mah-to-ther″ah-pu′tiks) climatotherapy.

climatotherapy (kli″mah-to-ther′ah-pe) [*climate* + Gr. *therapeia* treatment] the treatment of disease by means of a favorable climate.

climax (kli′maks) [Gr. *klimax* a ladder, staircase] the acme, or period of greatest intensity, as in the course of a disease (crisis), or in sexual excitement (orgasm).

climograph (kli′mŏ-graf) [*climate* + Gr. *graphein* to write] a diagram representing the effect of climate on man.

clinarthrosis (klin″ar-thro′sis) [Gr. *klinein* to bend + *arthrōsis* a jointing] abnormal deviation in the alignment of the bones at a joint.

clindamycin (klin″dah-mi′sin) chemical name: 2S-*trans*-methyl-7-chloro-6,7,8-trideoxy-6-[[(1-methyl-4-propyl-2-pyrrolidinyl)carbonyl]amino]-1-thio-L-α-D-*galacto*-octopyranoside. A semisynthetic analogue of the natural antibiotic lincomycin from which it is produced by chlorination, $C_{18}H_{33}ClN_2O_5S$; it is effective primarily against gram-positive bacteria. **c. hydrochloride** [USP], the hydrated hydrochloride salt of clindamycin, $C_{18}H_{33}ClN_2O_5S \cdot HCl$, occurring as a white or practically white, crystalline powder; used primarily in the treatment of penicillin-resistant gram-positive infections and in patients allergic to penicillin; administered orally. **c. palmitate hydrochloride** [USP], a water-soluble hydrochloride salt of the ester of clindamycin and palmitic acid, $C_{34}H_{63}ClN_2O_6S \cdot HCl$, occurring as a white to off-white amorphous powder, having the same actions and uses as the hydrochloride salt; it is suitable for the preparation of solutions for oral administration. **c. phosphate** [USP], a water-soluble ester of clindamycin and phosphoric acid, $C_{18}H_{34}ClN_2O_8PS$, occurring as a white to off-white, hygroscopic, crystalline powder, having the same actions and uses as the hydrochloride salt; it is suitable for preparation of parenteral dosage forms, administered intramuscularly or intravenously.

cline (klīn) [Gr. *klinein* to slope] a continuous series of differences in structure or function exhibited by the members of a species along a line extending from one part of their range to another.

clinic (klin′ik) [Gr. *klinikos* pertaining to a bed] 1. a clinical lecture; examination of patients before a class of students; instruction at the bedside. 2. an establishment where patients are admitted for special study and treatment by a group of physicians practicing medicine together. **ambulant c.,** one for patients not confined to the bed. **dry c.,** a clinical lecture with the presentation of case histories but without the presence of the patients described.

clinical (klin′e-k′l) pertaining to a clinic or to the bedside; pertaining to or founded on actual observation and treatment of patients, as distinguished from theoretical or basic sciences.

clinician (klĭ-nish′an) an expert clinical physician and teacher. **nurse c.,** see under *nurse*.

clinicogenetic (klin″ĭ-ko-jĕ-net′ik) pertaining to the clinical manifestations of a chromosomal (genetic) abnormality.

clinicopathologic (klin″e-ko-path″o-loj′ik) pertaining both to the symptoms of disease and to its pathology.

Clinistix (klin′ĭ-stiks) trademark for an enzyme-impregnated strip of plastic used to test for sugar in the urine. The strip is dipped into the urine and results of positive or negative are indicated by the color of the strip.

Clinitest (klin′ĭ-test) trademark for reagent tablets containing copper sulfate, used to test for the presence of sugar in the urine. Ten drops of water and 5 of urine are placed in a test tube. The tablet, which generates heat, is added and the solution is allowed to boil. After a few moments the color of the solution is compared to a color chart.

clinocephalism (kli-no-sef′ah-lizm) clinocephaly.

clinocephaly (kli″no-sef′ah-le) [Gr. *klinein* to bend + *kephalē* head] congenital flatness or concavity of the vertex of the head.

clinodactylism (kli″no-dak′tĭ-lizm) clinodactyly.

clinodactyly (kli″no-dak′tĭ-le) [Gr. *klinein* to bend + *daktylos* finger] permanent lateral or medial deviation or deflection of one or more fingers.

clinography (kli-nog′rah-fe) [Gr. *klinē* bed + *graphein* to write] a system of graphic representations of the temperature, symptoms, and pathologic manifestations exhibited by a patient.

clinoid (kli′noid) [Gr. *klinē* bed + *eidos* form] resembling a bed; bed-shaped, as the clinoid processes. See *processus clinoideus*.

clinology (kli-nol′ŏ-je) [Gr. *klinein* to recline + *-logy*] the science of the retrogression of an animal organism.

clinostatic (kli″no-stat′ik) occurring when the patient lies down.

clinostatism (kli″no-stat″izm) [Gr. *klinē* bed + *stasis* position] a lying-down position of the body.

clinotherapy (kli″no-ther′ah-pe) treatment by keeping the patient in bed.

clioquinol (kli″o-kwin′ol) iodochlorhydroxyquin.

clioxanide (kli-oks′ah-nīd) chemical name: 2-(acetyloxy)-N-(4-chlorophenyl)-3,5-diiodobenzamide; an anthelmintic, $C_{15}H_{10}CII_2NO_3$.

CLIP corticotropin-like intermediate lobe peptide.

clip (klip) a metallic device for approximating the edges of a wound or for the prevention of bleeding from small individual blood vessels.

cliprofen (klĭ-pro′fen) chemical name: 3-chloro-α-methyl-4-(2-thienylcarbonyl)benzeneacetic acid; an anti-inflammatory, $C_{14}H_{11}ClO_3S$.

cliseometer (klis″e-om′ě-ter) [Gr. *klisis* inclination + *metron* measure] an instrument for measuring the angle which the pelvic axis makes with the spinal column.

clisis (kli′sis) [Gr. *klisis* inclination] attraction or inclination.

Clistin (klis′tin) trademark for preparations of carbinoxamine maleate.

clitellum (kli-tel′um) [L. *clitellae* packsaddle] a saddle-like glandular segment in earthworms and leeches that secretes the cocoon in which the eggs are enclosed.

clithrophobia (klith″ro-fo′be-ah) (*obs.*) claustrophobia.

clition (klit′e-on) [Gr. *kleitys* slope, clivus] the midpoint of the anterior border of the clivus.

Clitocybe (kli-tos′ĭ-be) a genus of club fungi of the family Agaricus, order Agaricales. *C. gigan′tea* is the source of clitocybine, *C. nebula′ris* the source of nebularine. The ingestion of *C. illu′dens*, the orange jack-o-lantern mushroom, causes mycetismus gastrointestinalis.

clitocybine (klit″o-si′bin) any one of a group of antibiotic substances obtained from a mushroom, *Clitocybe gigantea*, of the Agaricus family.

clitoral (klit′o-ral, kli′to-ral, klĭ-tor′al) pertaining to the clitoris.

clitorectomy (klit″o-rek′to-me) clitoridectomy.

clitoridauxe (klit′o-rid-awk″se) [*clitoris* + Gr. *auxe* increase] enlargement of the clitoris; clitorism.

clitoridean (klit″o-rid′e-an, kli″to-rid′e-an, klĭ-tor-id′e-an) clitoral.

clitoridectomy (klit″o-rĭ-dek′to-me, kli″to-rĭ-dek′to-me, klĭ-tor″ĭ-dek′to-me) [*clitoris* + Gr. *ektomē* excision] excision of the clitoris; called also *clitorectomy*.

clitoriditis (klit″o-rĭ-di′tis, kli″to-rĭ-di′tis, klĭ-tor″ĭ-di′tis) clitoritis.

clitoridotomy (klit″o-rĭ-dot′o-me, kli″to-rĭ-dot′o-me, klĭ-tor″ĭ-dot′o-me) [*clitoris* + Gr. *tomē* cut] incision of the clitoris; female circumcision.

clitorimegaly (klit″o-rĭ-meg′ah-le, kli″to-rĭ-meg′ah-le) [*clitoris* + Gr. *megalē* great] an enlarged clitoris.

clitoris (klit′o-ris, kli′to-ris, klĭ-tor′is) [Gr. *kleitoris*] a small, elongated, erectile body, situated at the anterior angle of the rima pudendi; homologous with the penis in the male. Called also *coles femininus*.

clitorism (klit′o-rizm, kli′to-rism) 1. hypertrophy of the clitoris. 2. persistent and usually painful erection of the clitoris.

clitoritis (klit″o-ri′tis, kli″to-ri′tis) inflammation of the clitoris.

clitoromegaly (klit″o-ro-meg′ah-le, kli″to-ro-meg′ah-le) clitorimegaly.

clitoroplasty (klit′o-ro-plas″te) plastic surgery of the clitoris.

clitorotomy (klit″o-rot′o-me) [*clitoris* + Gr. *tomē* a cut] surgical incision of the clitoris.

clival (kli′val) pertaining to the clivus.

clivography (kli-vog′rah-fe) radiographic visualization of the clivus, or posterior cranial fossa.

clivus (kli′vus) [L. "slope"] [NA] a bony surface in the posterior cranial fossa, sloping upward from the foramen magnum to the dorsum sellae, the lower part being formed by a portion of the basilar part of the occipital bone (c. ossis occipitalis) and the upper part by a surface of the body of the sphenoid bone (c. ossis sphenoidalis). Called also *c. blumenbachii*. **basilar c.**, **c. basila′ris**, c. ossis occipitalis. **c. blumenbach′ii**, clivus. **c. monticuli**, declive. **c. os′sis occipita′lis**, the lower part of the clivus, formed by the basilar portion of the occipital bone; called also *basilar c.* or *c. basilaris*, and *basilar groove of occipital bone*. **c. os′sis sphenoida′lis**, the upper part of the clivus, formed by a surface of the body of the sphenoid bone; called also *basilar groove of sphenoid bone*.

clo (klo) a unit of measurement, being the insulation provided by man's normal everyday clothing and representing approximately the insulation provided by ¼ in. thickness of wool.

cloaca (klo-a′kah), pl. *cloa′cae* [L. "drain"] 1. in zoology, a common passage for fecal, urinary, and reproductive discharge in most lower vertebrates. 2. in mammalian embryology, the terminal end of the hindgut before division into rectum, bladder, and genital primordia. 3. in pathology, an opening in the involucrum of a necrosed bone. **congenital c.**, persistent c. **ectodermal c.**, that portion of the embryonic cloaca originally external to the cloacal membrane. **entodermal c.**, that portion of the embryonic cloaca originally internal to the cloacal membrane. **persistent c.**, the congenital persistence of a common cavity into which the intestinal, urinary, and reproductive ducts open; called also *congenital c.*

cloacal (klo-a′kal) pertaining to the cloaca.

cloacitis (klo″ah-si′tis) an infectious disease of fowls, marked by ulceration of the cloaca and a chronic discharge.

cloacogenic (klo″ah-ko-jen′ik) originating from the cloaca or from persisting cloacal remnants; said of a group of rare transitional-cell nonkeratinizing epidermoid anal cancers.

clobazam (klo′bah-zam) chemical name: 7-chloro-1-methyl-5-phenyl-1*H*-1,5-benzodiazepine-2,4(3*H*,5*H*)-dione; a minor tranquilizer, $C_{16}H_{13}ClN_2O_2$.

clock (klok) a device by which time may be measured. **biological c.**, the physiologic mechanism that governs the rhythmic occurrence of certain biochemical, physiological, and behavioral phenomena in plants and animals.

clocortolone (klo-kor′to-lōn) chemical name: 9-chloro-6α-fluoro-11β,21-dihydroxy-16α-methylpregna-1,4-diene-3,-20-dione. A glucocorticoid, $C_{22}H_{28}ClFO_4$, available as the 21-acetate, $C_{24}H_{30}ClFO_5$, and as the 21-pivalate, $C_{27}H_{36}Cl$-FO_5, esters.

clodanolene (klo-dan′o-lēn) chemical name: 1-[[[5-(3,4-dichlorophenyl)-2-furanyl]methylene]amino]-2,4-imidazolidinedione; a skeletal muscle relaxant, $C_{14}H_9Cl_2N_3O_3$.

clodazon hydrochloride (klo′dah-zōn) chemical name: 5-chloro-1,3-dihydro-1-[3-(dimethylamino)propyl]-2-*H*-benzimidazol-2-one monohydrochloride monohydrate; an antidepressant, $C_{18}H_{20}ClN_3O \cdot HCl \cdot H_2O$.

clodronic acid (klo-dron′ik) a bone calcium regulator.

clofazimine (klo-fah′zĭ-mēn) chemical name: *N*,5-bis(4-chlorophenyl)-3,5-dihydro-3-[(1-methylethyl)imino]-2-phenazamine; an antibacterial, $C_{27}H_{22}Cl_2N_4$, having leprostatic and tuberculostatic actions.

clofedanol (klo-fed′ah-nōl) chlophedianol.

clofenamic acid (klo″fen-am′ik) a fenamate analgesic, anti-inflammatory agent.

clofibrate (klo-fi′brāt) [USP] chemical name: 2-(4-chlorophenoxy)-2-methylpropanoic acid methyl ester. An antihyperlipidemic agent, $C_{12}H_{15}ClO_3$, occurring as a colorless to pale yellow liquid; used to reduce elevated serum lipids, administered orally.

clogestone acetate (klo-jes′tōn) chemical name: 3β-17-bis(acetyloxy)-6-chloropregna-4,6-dien-20-one; a progestin, $C_{25}H_{33}ClO_5$.

clomacran phosphate (klo′mah-kran) chemical name: 2-chloro-9,10-dihydro-*N*,*N*-dimethyl-9-acridinepropanamine phosphate; a tranquilizer, $C_{18}H_{21}ClN_2 \cdot H_3PO_4$.

Clomid (klo′mid) trademark for a preparation of clomiphene citrate.

clomiphene citrate (klo′mĭ-fēn) [USP] chemical name: 2-[4-(2-chloro-1,2-diphenylethenyl)phenoxy]ethanamine. A synthetic gonad-stimulating principle structurally related to the proestrogen chlorotrianisene, occurring as a white to pale yellow powder and consisting of a mixture of the *cis*- and *trans*-isomers; used to induce ovulation in certain forms of anovulatory infertility, administered orally.

clomipramine hydrochloride (klo-mip′rah-mēn) chemical name: 3-chloro-10,11-dihydro-*N*,*N*-dimethyl-5*H*-dibenz[*bf*]azepine-5-propanamine monohydrochloride; a tricyclic antidepressant, $C_{19}H_{23}ClN_2 \cdot HCl$.

clonal (klōn′al) of or pertaining to a clone.

clonality (klo-nal′ĭ-te) the ability to form clones.

clonazepam (klo-naz′ĕ-pam) chemical name: 5-(o-chlorophenyl)-1,3-dihydro-7-nitro-2*H*-1,4-benzodiazepin-2-one; an anticonvulsant, $C_{15}H_{10}ClN_3O_3$.

clone (klōn) [Gr. *klōn* young shoot or twig] 1. one or a group of genetically identical cells, organisms, or plants derived by vegetative reproduction from a single parent; also, a DNA population derived from a single hybrid DNA molecule (recombinant vector, q.v.) by replication in a eukaryotic or bacterial host cell. 2. used as a verb to denote the establishment of a clone. **forbidden c.**, see *clonal deletion theory*, under *theory*.

clonic (klon′ik) [Gr. *klonos* turmoil] pertaining to or of the nature of clonus.

clonicity (klo-nis′ĭ-te) the condition of being clonic.

clonicotonic (klon″e-ko-ton′ik) both clonic and tonic.

clonidine hydrochloride (klo′nĭ-dēn) chemical name: *N*-(2,6-dichlorophenyl)-4,5-dihydro-1*H*-imidazol-2-amine monohydrochloride. An adrenergic, $C_9H_9Cl_2N_3 \cdot HCl$, used as an antihypertensive; administered orally.

cloning (klo′ning) the formation of a clone. **DNA c.**, in genetics, the production of many identical copies of a specific DNA fragment.

clonism (klon′izm) [Gr. *klonos* turmoil] a succession of clonic spasms.

clonismus (klo-niz′mus) clonism.

clonixeril (klo-niks′er-il) chemical name: 2-[(3-chloro-2-methylphenyl)amino]-2,3-dihydroxypropyl ester; an analgesic, $C_{16}H_{17}ClN_2O_4$.

clonixin (klo-niks′in) chemical name: 2-[(3-chloro-2-methylphenyl)amino]-3-pyridinecarboxylic acid; an analgesic, $C_{13}H_{11}ClN_2O_2$.

clonogenic (klo″no-jen′ik) [*clone* + Gr. *gennan* to produce] giving rise to a clone of cells.

clonograph (klon′o-graf) [*clonus* + Gr. *graphein* to write] an instrument for recording spasmodic movements of parts and tendon reflexes.

Clonopin (klon′o-pin) trademark for a preparation of clonazepam.

clonorchiasis (klo″nor-ki′ah-sis) infection of the biliary passages with the liver fluke *Opisthorchis sinensis,* which may lead to inflammation of the biliary tree, proliferation of the biliary epithelium, progressive portal fibrosis, and sometimes biliary duct carcinoma; extension into the liver parenchyma may lead to fatty changes and cirrhosis.

clonorchiosis (klo-nor″ke-o′sis) clonorchiasis.

Clonorchis sinensis (klo-nor′kis si-nen′sis) [Gr. *klōn* branch + *orchis* testicle] *Opisthorchis sinensis.*

clonospasm (klon′o-spazm) [Gr. *klonos* turmoil + *spasmos* spasm] clonic spasm.

Clonothrix (klo′no-thriks) [Gr. *klōn* branch + *thrix* hair] a genus of sheathed bacteria found in water, made up of colorless cylindrical cells in filaments that may show false branching. Their sheaths are sometimes encrusted with iron or manganese compounds. The type species is *C. fus′ca.*

clonotype (klo′no-tīp) [*clone* + *type*] a particular combination of immunoglobulin heavy and light chains, e.g., that produced by a single clone of plasma cells. A single organism produces a repertoire of about 10^7 to 10^8 clonotypes; a single antigenic determinant may react with 10^3 to 10^4 clonotypes.

clonus (klo′nus) [Gr. *klonos* turmoil] alternate muscular contraction and relaxation in rapid succession. **ankle c.,** a series of abnormal reflex movements of the foot, induced by sudden dorsiflexion of the foot, which causes alternate contraction and relaxation of the triceps surae muscle (gastrocnemius and soleus muscles); called also foot c. **anodal closure c. (ACCl),** clonic muscular contraction occurring at the anode when the electrical circuit is closed. **anodal opening c. (AOCl),** muscular contraction occurring at the anode when the electrical circuit is opened or broken. **cathodal closure c. (CCCl),** clonic muscular contraction occurring at the cathode when the electrical circuit is closed. **cathodal opening c. (COCl),** clonic muscular contraction occurring at the cathode when the electrical circuit is opened or broken. **foot c.,** ankle c. **patellar c.,** rhythmic jerking movement of the patella produced by grasping the patella between the thumb and forefinger and pushing it forcibly toward the foot one or more times; an abnormal reflex with alternate contraction and relaxation of the quadriceps muscle. **toe c.,** abnormal rhythmic movement of the great toe, induced by suddenly extending the first phalanx. **wrist c.,** spasmodic movement of the hand, which is induced by forcibly extending the hand at the wrist.

clopamide (klo-pah′mīd) chemical name: 3-(aminosulfonyl)-4-chloro-*N*-(2,6-dimethyl-1-piperidinyl)benzamide. A diuretic, $C_{14}H_{20}ClN_3O_3S$, used in the treatment of edema associated with various disorders and in hypertension.

Clopane (klo′pān) trademark for preparations of cyclopentamine hydrochloride.

clopenthixol (klo″pen-thiks′ol) chemical name: 4-[3-(2-chloro-9*H*-thioxanthen-9-ylidene)propyl]-1-piperazineethanol. A compound, $C_{22}H_{25}ClN_2OS$, having sedative, tranquilizing, antiemetic, antihistaminic, anticholinergic, and alpha-adrenergic blocking properties; it has been used as a tranquilizer in the treatment of schizophrenia.

clopidol (klo′pĭ-dol) chemical name: 3,5-dichloro-2,6-dimethyl-4-pyridinol; a coccidiostat for poultry, $C_7H_7Cl_2NO$.

clopimozide (klo-pim′o-zīd) chemical name: 1-[1-[4,4-bis-

(4-fluorophenyl)butyl]-4-piperidinyl]-5-chloro-1,3-dihydro-2-*H*-benzimidazol-2-one; a tranquilizer, $C_{28}H_{28}ClF_2N_3O$.

clopirac (klo′pĭ-rak) chemical name: 1-(4-chlorophenyl)-2,5-dimethyl-1*H*-pyrrole-3-acetic acid; an anti-inflammatory, $C_{14}H_{14}ClNO_2$.

cloprednol (klo-pred′nol) chemical name: 6-chloro-11β,17,21-trihydroxypregna-1,4,6-triene-3,20-dione; a glucocorticoid, $C_{21}H_{25}ClO_5$.

cloprostenol (klo-pros′tĕ-nol) chemical name: (±)-(Z)-7-[(1*R**,2*R**,3*R**,5*S**)-2-[(*E*)-(3*R**)-4-(*m*-chlorophenoxy)-3-hydroxy-1-butenyl]-3,5-dihydroxycyclopentyl]-5-heptenoic acid; a prostaglandin, $C_{22}H_{28}ClO_6$. Also available as the sodium salt.

Cloquet's canal, fascia, hernia, ligament, septum (klo-kāz′) [Jules Germain *Cloquet,* French surgeon, 1790–1883] see under *fascia,* and see *canalis hyaloidens, crural hernia, vestigium processus vaginalis,* and *septum femorale.*

Cloquet's ganglion (pseudoganglion) (klo-kāz′) [Hippolyte *Cloquet,* anatomist in Paris, 1787–1840] see under *ganglion.*

clorazepate (klor-az′ĕ-pāt) a benzodiazepate anxiolytic agent; used as clorazepate monopotassium or clorazepate dipotassium. **c. dipotassium,** the dipotassium salt of clorazepic acid, $C_{16}H_{11}ClK_2N_2O_4$, used orally as a minor tranquilizer. **c. monopotassium,** the monopotassium salt of clorazepic acid, $C_{16}H_{10}ClKN_2O_3$; a minor tranquilizer.

clorazepic acid (klor′ah-zep′ik) the free acid of clorazepate.

clorexolone (klo-reks′o-lon) chemical name: 6-chloro-2-cyclohexyl-2,3-dihydro-3-oxo-1*H*-isoindole-5-sulfonamide. A diuretic, $C_{14}H_{11}ClO$, used in the treatment of edema associated with various disorders and in hypertension.

cloroperone hydrochloride (klo″ro-per′on) chemical name: 4-[4-(4-chlorobenzoyl)-1-piperidinyl]-1-(4-fluorophenyl)-1-butanone hydrochloride; a tranquilizer, $C_{22}H_{23}ClFNO_2 \cdot HCl$.

clorophene (klo′ro-fen) chemical name: 4-chloro-2-(phenylmethyl)phenol. A disinfectant, $C_{14}H_{17}ClN_2O_3S$, effective against a wide variety of bacteria and fungi.

Clorpactin XCB (klor-pak′tin) trademark for a preparation of oxychlorosene.

clorprenaline hydrochloride (klor-pren′ah-lēn) chemical name: 2-chloro-α-[[1-methylethyl)amino]methyl]benzenemethanol monohydrochloride monohydrate. An adrenergic, $C_{11}H_{16}ClNO \cdot HCl \cdot H_2O$, used as a bronchodilator.

clortermine hydrochloride (klor-ter′men) chemical name: 2-chloro-α,α-dimethylbenzeneethanamine hydrochloride. An adrenergic, $C_{10}H_{14}ClN \cdot HCl$, used as an oral anorexic in the short-term treatment of exogenous obesity.

closantel (klo′san-tel) chemical name: *N*-[5-chloro-4-[(4-chlorophenyl)-cyanomethyl]-2-methylphenyl]-2-hydroxy-3,5-diiodobenzamide; an anthelmintic, $C_{22}H_{14}Cl_2I_2N_2O_2$.

closiramine aceturate (klo-ser′ah-men) chemical name: 8-chloro-11-[2-(dimethylamino)ethyl]-6,11-dihydro-5*H*-benzo[5,6]cyclohepta[1,2-*b*]pyridine compound with *N*-acetylglycine (1:1); an antihistaminic, $C_{18}H_{21}ClN_2 \cdot C_4H_7NO_3$.

clostridia (klos-trid′e-ah) [L.] plural of *clostridium.*

clostridial (klos-strid′e-al) pertaining to or caused by clostridia.

clostridiopeptidase (klos-trid″e-o-pep′tĭ-dās) see *Clostridium histolyticum collagenase,* under *collagenase.*

Clostridium (klo-strid′e-um) [Gr. *klōster* spindle] a genus of bacteria of the family Bacillaceae, made up of obligate anaerobic or microaerophilic, gram-positive, spore-forming, rod-shaped bacilli, with spores of greater diameter than the vegetative cells. The spores may be central, terminal, or subterminal. One hundred or more species have been differentiated on the basis of physiology, morphology, and toxin formation. Pathogenic species produce destructive exotoxins or enzymes. The organisms occur in soil, in water, and in the intestinal tract of humans and lower animals. **C. acetobutyl′icum,** a species found widely distributed in agricultural soils but not found to be pathogenic. **C. ag′ni,** a name once given type B of *C. perfringens,* which causes dysentery in lambs. **C. bifermen′tans,** a species found widely distributed in nature, occurring commonly in feces, sewage, and soil; it is sometimes associated with cases of gas gangrene. **C. botuli′num,** the agent causing botulism in man, wild ducks, and other waterfowl, limberneck of fowl, certain forms of forage poisoning in cattle and horses in Australia, and lamziekte of cattle in South Africa. It produces a powerful exotoxin that is resistant to proteolytic digestion, and is divided into types A, B, C alpha and beta, D, E, F, and G on the basis of the immunological specificity of the toxin. Formerly called *Bacillus botulinus*. **C. butyr′icum,** a species isolated from the soil, fecal material, and dairy products. **C. cada′veris,** a species found in feces and infections of animals and man. **C. chauvoe′i,** the principal cause of blackleg, or symptomatic anthrax, in cattle and sheep; called also *C. feseri,* and *Chauveau's bacillus* or *bacterium.* **C. clostridiifor′me,** a weakly gram-positive species that is commonly isolated from clinical specimens; called also *Bacteroides clostridiiformis.* **C. dif′ficile,** a species that is part of the normal colon flora in human infants and sometimes in adults. It produces a toxin that causes pseudomembranous enterocolitis in patients receiving antibiotic therapy. **C. fe′seri,** *C. chauvoei.* **C. haemolyt′icum,** a species isolated from the blood and other tissues of cattle dying with bacillary hemoglobinuria, thought by some to be a type of *C. novyi.* **C. histolyt′icum,** a pathogenic species found in wounds and frequently associated with gas gangrene. It is commonly found in soil. **C. innoc′uum,** a species of uncertain pathogenicity, commonly isolated from gas gangrene and other anaerobic infections. **C. kluy′veri,** a species isolated from wetland soil of fresh and salt water, which has been used in studies of microbial synthesis and oxidation of fatty acids. **C. limo′sum,** a toxogenic species found in soil and in a variety of animal infections, sometimes pathogenic for animals. **C. no′vyi,** a species that is an important cause of gas gangrene in humans and a source of infection in lower animals. Three immunological types have been identified, designated A, B, and C. Formerly called *C. oedematiens* and *Bacillus oedematis maligni No. II.* **C. oedemat′iens,** *C. novyi.* **C. ovitox′icus,** a name once given type D of *C. perfringens,* which causes enterotoxemia of sheep. **C. palu′dis,** a name once given type C of *C. perfringens,* which causes struck in sheep. **C. parabotuli′num e′qui,** *C. botulinum.* **C. parabotuli′nus,** *C. botulinum* type C. **c. paraputri′ficum,** a species found in soil and feces. **C. pasteuria′num,** an anaerobic microorganism occurring in soil, which was the first nitrogen-fixing bacterium to be studied in pure culture. **C. pastoria′num,** *C. pasteurianum.* **C. perfrin′gens,** the most common etiologic agent of gas gangrene, differentiable, on the basis of the distribution of 12 different toxins, into several different types: *type A* causes gas gangrene, necrotizing colitis, and food poisoning in humans; *type B* causes lamb dysentery; *type C* causes enteritis necroticans in man and struck in sheep; *type D* causes enterotoxemia in sheep; *type E* causes enterotoxemia in lambs and calves. *C. perfringens* is also a major cause of food poisoning; see *clostridial food poisoning,* under *poisoning.* Called also *C. welchii* and, formerly, *Bacillus capsulatum* or *B. welchii.* **C. ramo′sum,** a species found in human and animal infections and in feces, one of the most commonly isolated clostridia in clinical specimens. **C. sep′ticum,** a toxicogenic species commonly occurring in animal intestines and soil, strikingly pathogenic for various animals but reportedly associated with gaseous infections in humans in only 20 per cent of cases. Six immunological groups have been distinguished. Called also *Vibrio septicus, vibrion septique,* and *Ghon-Sachs bacillus.* **C. sordel′lii,** a species of uncertain pathogenicity, found associated with infections of man and animals. **C. sphenoi′des,** a species found in infected wounds in man. **C. sporog′enes,** a species widely distributed in nature; a harmless saprophyte in pure culture, it is reportedly associated with pathogenic anaerobes in gangrenous infections. **C. subtermina′le**, a species found in soil and wounds. **C. ter′tium,** a species found widely distributed in feces, sewage, and soil, and associated with gas gangrene. **C. tet′ani,** a common inhabitant of soil and human and horse intestines, and the cause of tetanus in humans and domestic animals; its potent exotoxin is made up of two components, a neurotoxin, or tetanospasmin, and a hemolytic toxin, or tetanolysin. Formerly called *Bacillus tetani.* **C. welch′ii,** British name for *C. perfringens.*

clostridium (klo-strid′e-um), pl. *clostrid′ia.* a microorganism belonging to the genus *Clostridium.*

closure (klo′shur) the act of shutting, or of bringing together two parts, one or both of which may be movable. **flask c.,** the bringing together of the two halves or parts of a flask in which a denture base is formed. **flask c., final,** the last closure of a flask before curing the denture-base material packed in the mold. **flask c., trial,** preliminary closure of the flask, to eliminate excess material and to ensure that the mold is completely filled. **velopharyngeal c.,** closure of nasal air escape by the elevation of the soft palate and contraction of the posterior pharyngeal wall.

closylate (klo′sĭ-lāt) USAN contraction for *p*-chlorobenzesulfonate.

clot (klot) a semisolidified mass, as of blood or lymph; called also *coagulum.* **agonal c., agony c.,** a blood clot formed in the heart during the death agony. **antemortem c.,** a blood clot formed in the heart or in a large vessel before death. **blood c.,** a coagulum formed of blood, either in or out of the body. **chicken fat c.,** a blood clot that appears yellow because of the settling out of the erythrocytes before clotting occurred. **currant jelly c.,** a clot of reddish color because of the presence of erythrocytes enmeshed in it. **distal c.,** a clot formed in a blood vessel distal to a ligature. **external c.,** a clot formed outside a blood vessel. **heart c.,** postmortem coagulation within the heart. **internal c.,** a blood clot formed within a blood vessel. **laminated c.,** a blood clot formed by successive deposits, giving it a layered appearance; called also *stratified c.* **marantic c.,** a blood clot formed because of enfeebled circulation and general malnutrition. **muscle c.,** a clot formed by coagulation of muscle plasm. **passive c.,** a clot formed in the sac of an aneurysm through which the blood has stopped circulating. **plastic c.,** a clot formed from the intima of an artery at the point of ligation, permanently obstructing the artery. **postmortem c.,** a blood clot formed in the heart or in a large blood vessel after death. **proximal c.,** a clot formed in a blood vessel proximal to a ligature. **spider-web c.,** the fine fibrin clot that forms when a sample of fluid from a subject with tuberculous meningitis is allowed to stand, especially when it is warmed to 37° C. for a few hours. **stratified c.,** laminated c. **washed c., white c.,** a blood clot composed of fibrin and platelets.

clothiapine (klo-thi′ah-pēn) chemical name: 2-chloro-11-(4-methyl-1-piperazinyl)dibenzo[*b,f*][1,4]thiazepine; a tranquilizer, $C_{18}H_{18}ClN_3S$.

clotrimazole (klo-trim′ah-zōl) [USP] chemical name: 1-[(2-chlorophenyl)diphenylmethyl]-1*H*-imidazole. A broad-spectrum antifungal agent, $C_{22}H_{17}ClN_2$, applied topically to the skin in the treatment of candidiasis and various forms of tinea, and administered intravaginally in the treatment of vulvovaginal candidiasis.

clouding (klowd′ing) loss of clarity. **c. of consciousness,** loss of perception or comprehension of the environment, with loss of ability to respond properly to external stimuli.

Cloudman's melanoma S91 (klowd′manz) [Arthur Mosher *Cloudman,* American zoologist, born 1901] see under *melanoma.*

Clouston's syndrome (klow′stonz) [H. R. *Clouston*] hidrotic ectodermal dysplasia.

clove (klōv) [L. *clavus* a nail or spike] an aromatic spice, the dried flower bud of *Eugenia caryophyllus;* formerly used as a carminative, for the relief of nausea and vomiting, and to stimulate digestion. See also *clove oil,* under *oil.*

cloxacillin sodium (kloks″ah-sil′in) [USP] chemical name: [[[3-(2α-chlorophenyl)-5α-methyl-4-isoxazolyl]carbonyl]amino]-3,3-dimethyl-7-oxo-4-thia-1-azabicyclo[3.2.0]-heptane-2-carboxylic acid monosodium monohydrate. A semisynthetic penicillinase-resistant penicillin, $C_{19}H_{17}ClN_3Na-O_5SH_2O$, occurring as a white, crystalline powder; used primarily in the treatment of infections due to penicillinase-producing staphylococci, administered orally.

cloxyquin (kloks′ĭ-kwin) chemical name: 5-chloro-8-quinolinol; an antibacterial, $C_9H_6ClNO.$

clozapine (klo′zah-pēn) chemical name: 8-chloro-11-(4-methyl-1-piperazinyl)-5-*H*-dibenzo[*b,e*][1,4]diazepine; a sedative, $C_{18}H_{19}ClN_4$.

clubbing (klub′ing) a proliferative change in the soft tissues about the terminal phalanges of the fingers or toes.

clubfoot (klub′foot) a congenitally deformed foot; called also *reel foot.* See *talipes.*

clubhand (klub'hand) a deformity of the hand due to congenital absence of the radius or ulna in which the hand is twisted out of shape or position; called also *talipomanus*. **radial c.,** the most common type of clubhand in which the hand is deflected toward the radial side; when the hand is held in the anatomical position it is known as *manus valga* and when it is held in the opposite direction as *manus vara*. Called also *manus valga*. See also *Madelung deformity*, under *deformity*. **ulnar c.,** clubhand in which the hand is deflected toward the ulnar side; when the hand is held in the anatomical position it is known as *manus vara* and when it is held in the opposite direction as *manus valga*. Called also *manus vara*.

clubroot (klub'root) finger and toe disease.

clump (klump) an aggregation as of bacteria caused by the action of agglutinins (agglutination).

clumping (klump'ing) the aggregation of particles, such as bacteria, into irregular masses.

cluneal (kloo'ne-al) pertaining to the buttocks.

clunis (kloo'nis), pl. *clu'nes* [L.] the buttock; see *nates*.

clupanodonic acid (kloo-pan"o-don'ik) an unsaturated fatty acid, 4,8,12,15,18-docosapentaenoic acid, found in fish oils.

clupeine (kloo'pe-in) [L. *clupea* herring] a protamine obtainable from the spermatozoa of the herring.

cluttering (klut'er-ing) hurried nervous speech, marked by the dropping of syllables.

Clutton's joint (klut'unz) [Henry Hugh *Clutton*, London surgeon, 1850–1909] see under *joint*.

clysis (kli'sis) [Gr. *klysis*] 1. (obs.) the washing out of a body cavity. 2. the administration other than by the oral route of any one of several solutions to replace lost body fluid, supply nutriment, or raise blood pressure. 3. the solution so administered.

clysma (kliz'mah), pl. *clys'mata* [Gr. *klysma*] a clyster, or enema.

Clysodrast (kli'so-drast) trademark for a preparation of bisacodyl tannex.

clyster (klis'ter) [Gr. *klystēr* a syringe] an injection into the rectum; an enema.

clysterize (klis'ter-īz) [L. *clysterizare;* Gr. *klystēr*] to treat with enemas, or with injections into the rectum.

clytocybine (kli"to-si'bēn) clitocybine.

C.M. abbreviation for L. *Chirur'giae Ma'gister*, Master in Surgery.

cM centimorgan.

Cm chemical symbol for *curium*.

cm. centimeter.

cm.² square centimeter.

cm.³ cubic centimeter.

CMA Certified Medical Assistant.

C.M.A. Canadian Medical Association.

CMD cerebromacular degeneration.

CMF a regimen of cyclophosphamide, methotrexate, and 5-fluorouracil, used in cancer chemotherapy.

CMHC community mental health center.

cm H₂O centimeter of water, a unit of pressure equal to that exerted by a column of water at 4°C one millimeter high at mean sea level; officially defined as the pressure exerted by a 1 cm column of fluid with a density of 1 g/cm³ in a gravitational field of 9.80665 m/s², which equals 9.80665 pascals.

CMI cell-mediated immunity.

CML cell-mediated lympholysis.

c.mm. cubic millimeter.

C-MOPP a regimen of cyclophosphamide, mechlorethamine, Oncovin (vincristine), procarbazine, and prednisone, used in cancer chemotherapy.

CMP cytidine monophosphate.

C.M.R. cerebral metabolic rate.

c.m.s. abbreviation for L. *cras ma'ne sumen'dus,* to be taken tomorrow morning.

C.N. abbreviation for L. *cras noc'te*, tomorrow night.

C.N.A. Canadian Nurses' Association.

cnemial (ne'me-al) pertaining to the shin.

Cnemidocoptes (ne"mĭ-do-kop'tēz) *Knemidokoptes*.

cnemis (ne'mis) the lower leg, shin, or tibia.

cnemitis (ne-mi'tis) inflammation of the tibia.

cnemoscoliosis (ne"mo-sko"le-o'sis) [Gr. *knēmē* leg + *skoliōsis* crookedness] a lateral bending of the leg.

Cnidaria (ni-dar'e-ah) [Gr. *knidē* a nettle] a phylum of marine invertebrates that includes sea anemones, hydras, corals, and jellyfish (all of which were formerly assigned to the phylum Coelenterata), plus comb jellies or sea walnuts, characterized by a radially symmetrical body bearing tentacles around the mouth.

cnidarian (ni-dar'e-an) 1. pertaining or belonging to the phylum Cnidaria. 2. an individual of the phylum Cnidaria. See also *coelenterate* (def. 3).

Cnidian (ni'de-an) pertaining to *Cnidos*, a Dorian Greek city on the southwest Asia Minor coast. Cnidos was famous for its temple of healing, its medical school, and its libraries. The Cnidian school stressed thorough diagnosis and classification of diseases (especially pathology) to the extent of ignoring the patient. Cf. *Hippocrates of Cos*.

cnid(o)- [Gr. *knidē* a nettle] a combining form denoting a relationship to a nettle or nettle-like structure.

cnidoblast (ni'dŏ-blast) [*cnido-* + *blast*] the epidermal cells of coelenterates which contain the nematocysts, especially numerous on the tentacles.

cnidocil (ni'dŏ-sil) [*cnido-* + *cil*ium] a bristle-like process at one end of a cnidoblast, which, when stimulated, triggers the discharge of the nematocyst.

Cnidospora (ni"do-spor'ah) [*cnido-* + *spore*] Microspora.

Cnidosporidia (ni"do-spo-rid'e-ah) Microsporida.

C.N.M. Certified Nurse-Midwife; see *nurse-midwife*.

CNOH cyanic acid.

CNS central nervous system.

c.n.s. abbreviation for L. *cras noc'te sumen'dus*, to be taken tomorrow night.

CO carbon monoxide.

CO₂ carbon dioxide.

Co chemical symbol for *cobalt*.

co- see *con-*.

C.O.A. Canadian Orthopaedic Association.

CoA coenzyme A.

coacervate (ko-as'er-vāt) [L. *coacervatus* heaped up] the viscous phase separating from a colloid-containing system in the phenomenon of coacervation.

coacervation (ko-as"er-va'shun) the separation of a mixture of two liquids, one or both of which are colloids, into two phases, one of which (the coacervate) contains the colloidal particles, the other being an aqueous solution, e.g., as when gum arabic is added to gelatin.

Coactin (ko-ak'tin) trademark for a preparation of amdinocillin.

coadaptation (co"ad-ap-ta'shun) [*co-* + L. *adapta're* to adapt] the mutual, correlated, adaptive changes in two interdependent organs.

coadunation (ko"ad-u-na'shun) [L. *co-* together + *ad* to + *u'nus* one] union of dissimilar substances in one mass.

coadunition (ko"ad-u-nish'un) coadunation.

coagglutination (ko"ah-gloo"tĭ-na'shun) the aggregation of particulate antigens combined with agglutinins of more than one specificity.

coagula (ko-ag'u-lah) [L.] plural of *coagulum*.

coagulability (ko-ag"u-lah-bil'ĭ-te) the state of being capable of forming or of being formed into clots.

coagulable (ko-ag'u-lah-b'l) susceptible of being coagulated.

coagulant (ko-ag'u-lant) [L. *coagulans*] 1. promoting, accelerating, or making possible the coagulation of blood. 2. an agent that promotes or accelerates the coagulation of blood.

coagulase (ko-ag'u-lās) a bacterial enzyme that reacts with a cofactor found in blood plasma to catalyze the formation of fibrin from fibrinogen. It is produced by *Staphylococcus aureus* and by *Yersinia pestis*.

coagulate (ko-ag'u-lāt) [L. *coagulare*] 1. to cause to clot. 2. to become clotted.

coagulation (ko-ag"u-la'shun) [L. *coagulatio*] 1. the process of clot formation; see *blood c.* 2. in colloid chemistry, the solidification of a sol into a gelatinous mass; an alteration of a disperse phase or of a dissolved solid which causes the separation of the system into a liquid phase and an insoluble mass called the clot or curd. Coagulation is usually irreversible. 3. in surgery, the disruption of tissue by physical means to form an amorphous residuum, as in electrocoagulation and photocoagulation. **blood c.,** the sequential process by which the multiple coagulation factors of the blood interact, ultimately resulting in the formation of an insoluble fibrin clot; it may be divided into three stages: stage 1, the formation of intrinsic and extrinsic prothrombin converting principle; stage 2, the formation of thrombin; stage 3, the formation of stable fibrin polymers. **diffuse intravascular c., disseminated intravascular c. (DIC),** a disorder characterized by reduction in the elements involved in blood coagulation due to their utilization in widespread blood clotting within the vessels; the activation of the clotting mechanism may arise from any of a number of disorders. In the late stages, it is marked by profuse hemorrhaging. Called also *consumption coagulopathy* and *defibrination syndrome.* **electric c.,** electrocoagulation. **massive c.,** coagulation of the spinal fluid so as to form an almost solid clot; a condition seen in some cases of *Froin's syndrome* in meningomyelitis or tumor of the cord.

coagulative (ko-ag'u-la"tiv) associated with coagulation or promoting a process of coagulation; of the nature of coagulation.

coagulator (ko-ag"u-la'tor) a surgical device that utilizes electrical current or light to stop bleeding.

coagulogram (ko-ag'u-lo-gram") a term used colloquially in clinical hematology to denote a series of laboratory tests measuring the various parameters of hemostasis.

coagulopathy (ko-ag"u-lop'ah-the) any disorder of blood coagulation. **consumption c.,** diffuse intravascular coagulation.

coagulum (ko-ag'u-lum), pl. *coag'ula* [L.] a clot or curd. **closing c.,** Schlusscoagulum.

coalescence (ko-ah-les'ens) [L. *coalescere* to grow together] the fusion or blending of parts.

COAP a regimen of cyclophosphamide, Oncovin (vincristine), ara-C (cytarabine), and prednisone, used in cancer chemotherapy.

coapt (ko-apt') [L. *coaptare*] to approximate, as the edges of a wound or the ends of a fractured bone.

coarctate (ko-ark'tāt) [L. *coarctare* to straighten or tighten] 1. to press close together; contract. 2. pressed together; restrained.

coarctation (ko"ark-ta'shun) [L. *coarctatio,* from *cum* together + *arctare* to make tight] a condition of stricture or contraction. **c. of aorta,** a localized malformation characterized by deformity of the aortic media, causing narrowing, usually severe, of the lumen of the vessel. **c. of aorta, adult type,** a form characterized by a localized constriction at or below the insertion of the ductus arteriosus and distal to the aortic isthmus and left clavian artery, and by a closed ductus and absence of cyanosis. **c. of aorta, infantile type,** a form characterized by diffuse involvement of the aortic isthmus, by association with other anomalies, including a patent ductus, and by cyanosis. **reversed c.,** pulseless disease.

coarse (kōrs) not fine; not microscopical.

coarticulation (ko"ar-tik"u-la'shun) [L. *con* together + *articulare* to join] a synarthrosis.

coat (kōt) [L. *cot'ta* a tunic] a membrane or other structure covering or lining a part or organ; see also *tunic* and *tunica.* **adventitial c.,** tunica adventitia; see terms beginning thus under *tunica.* **adventitious c. of uterine tube,** tela subserosa. **albugineous c.,** tunica albuginea; see terms beginning thus under *tunica.* **buffy c.,** the thin yellowish layer of leukocytes overlying the packed red cells in centrifuged blood; called also *buffy crust* and *leukocytic cream.* **cremasteric c. of testis,** musculus cremaster. **dartos c.,** tunica dartos. **external c. of capsule of graafian follicle,** tunica externa thecae folliculi. **external c. of esophagus,** tunica adventitia esophagi. **external c. of ureter,** tunica adventitia ureteris. **external c. of vessels,** tunica externa vasorum. **external c. of viscera,** tunica adventitia. **extraneous c.,** a cement-like structure, constituting a visible cell wall, in some

animal cells; it generally plays no role in permeability, but has other important functions. **fibrous c.,** tunica fibrosa; see terms beginning thus under *tunica.* **fibrous c. of corpus cavernosum of penis,** tunica albuginea corporum cavernosorum. **fibrous c. of eye,** tunica fibrosa bulbi. **fibrous c. of ovary,** theca folliculi. **fibrous c. of testis,** tunica albuginea testis. **internal c. of capsule of graafian follicle,** tunica interna thecae folliculi. **internal c. of pharynx of Luschka,** tela submucosa pharyngis. **mucous c.,** tunica mucosa; for various specific structures, see terms beginning thus under *tunica.* **mucous c. of tympanic cavity,** tunica mucosa cavitatis tympanici. **muscular c.,** tunica muscularis; see terms beginning thus under *tunica.* **pharyngobasilar c.,** fascia pharyngobasilaris. **proper c.,** tunica propria; see also *lamina propria.* **proper c. of corium, proper c. of dermis,** stratum reticulare dermidis. **proper c. of pharynx,** tela submucosa pharyngis. **proper c. of testis,** tunica albuginea testis. **sclerotic c.,** the sclera. **serous c.,** tunica serosa; see terms beginning thus under *tunica.* **submucous c.,** tela submucosa; see terms beginning thus under *tela.* **subserous c.,** tela subserosa; see terms beginning thus under *tela.* **uveal c.,** uvea; called also *vascular c. of eyeball.* **vaginal c. of testis,** tunica vaginalis testis. **vascular c. of eyeball,** uvea; called also *uveal c.* **vascular c. of pharynx,** tela submucosa pharyngis. **vascular c. of stomach,** tela submucosa ventriculi. **vascular c. of viscera,** tela submucosa. **villous c. of small intestine,** tunica mucosa intestini tenuis. **white c.,** tunica albuginea.

CoA-transferase (ko a trans'fer-ās) [EC 2.8.3.] one of a sub-sub group of enzymes of the transferase class that catalyze the transfer of coenzyme A from one molecule to another.

Coats' disease, retinitis (kōts) [George *Coats,* London ophthalmologist, 1876–1915] exudative retinopathy.

cobalamin (ko-bal'ah-min) the cobalt-containing complex common to all members of the vitamin B_{12} group; frequently used generically to designate any substituted derivative, even cyanocobalamin. **c. concentrate** [USP], a dried, partially purified product resulting from the growth of selected *Streptomyces* cultures, containing in each gram not less than 500 μg. of cobalamin; used as a vitamin B_{12} supplement.

cob(1)alamin adenosyltransferase (ko-bal'ah-min ah-den"o-sil-trans'fer-ās) [EC 2.5.1.17] an enzyme of the transferase class that catalyzes the reaction ATP + cob(1)alamin + H_2 = orthophosphate + pyrophosphate + adenosylcobalamin. The reaction is the final step in the biosynthesis of the coenzyme form of vitamin B_{12}. Deficiency of the enzyme, an autosomal recessive trait, leads to deficient methylmalonyl-CoA mutase and results in methylmalonic acidemia, form cobalamin B.

cobalt (ko'bawlt) [L. *cobaltum*] a metal, atomic number, 27; atomic weight 58.9332; symbol Co; the metal is used in magnetic alloys, and the compounds afford pigments. In animals, a deficiency of this element leads to anemia; an excess of normal dietary requirements leads to erythrocytosis. In the human, although cobalt has been used with limited transient effectiveness to treat the anemia of infection, and renal disease, its sole physiological function, most probably, is as a constituent of vitamin B_{12}. Radioisotopes of cobalt, particularly ^{60}Co, a gamma emitter, are used in experimental biology and medicine and in cancer therapy. **c. salipyrine,** a salicylate of cobalt and antipyrine, forming a pale red powder. **c. 60,** a radioactive isotope of cobalt, ^{60}Co, which has a half-life of 5.27 years, used as a source of radiation in the treatment of malignancies and in industrial radiography.

cobaltosis (ko"bawl-to'sis) pneumoconiosis due to inhalation of and tissue reaction to cobalt dust.

cobaltous (ko-bawl'tus) pertaining to or containing cobalt in its bivalent state.

COBMAM a regimen of cyclophosphamide, Oncovin (vincristine), bleomycin, methotrexate, Adriamycin (doxorubicin), and MeCCNU (semustine), used in cancer chemotherapy.

cobra (ko'brah) any of several extremely poisonous elapid snakes commonly found in Africa, Asia, and India, which are capable of expanding the neck region to form a hood, and have two comparatively short, erect, deep grooved fangs. A serum obtained from animals inoculated with cobra venom is used in counteracting the effects of bites by the cobra. See table accompanying *snake*.   **black-necked c.,** *Naja nigricollis,* a species that usually does not bite but discharges venom by spitting when agitated; the venom is not poisonous but may cause severe irritation or even blindness if it enters the eyes. Called also *spitting c.*   **Indian c.,** a yellowish to dark brown cobra, *Naja tripudians,* characterized by black and white markings that resemble a pair of spectacles on its hood; it sometimes attains a length of 6 feet. Called also *c. de capello* and *Naja naja.*   **king c.,** a very large cobra, *Naja hannah,* sometimes reaching a length of 12 feet.   **spitting c.,** black-necked c.

cobraism (ko'brah-izm)   poisoning by cobra venom.

cobralysin (ko-bral'ĭ-sin)   a hemolytic substance derived from the poison of the cobra.

COBS   abbreviation for *cesarean-obtained barrier-sustained,* a term applied to animals delivered by cesarean section into a germ-free environment and maintained under the same conditions.

cobweb (kob'web) [A.S. abbreviation of *attercop,* poison head, and *web,* from *wefan*]   the web of various kinds of spider; sometimes used as a styptic, in the moxa, and as a domestic remedy: a febrifuge and antispasmodic.

COC   cathodal opening contraction.

coca (ko'kah)   the leaves of *Erythroxylon coca,* a South American plant from which cocaine is obtained; once used as a central nervous system stimulant and still widely used in parts of South America as a euphoriant masticatory.

cocaine (ko'kān; ko-kān') [USP]   chemical name: [1R-(exo,exo)]-3-(benzoyloxy)-8-methyl-8-azabicyclo[3.2.1]octane-2-carboxylic acid methyl ester. A crystalline alkaloid, $C_{17}H_{21}$-NO_4, obtained from leaves of *Erythroxylon coca* (coca leaves) and other species of *Erythroxylon,* or by synthesis from ecgonine or its derivatives; used as a local narcotic anesthetic applied topically to mucous membranes.   **c. hydrochloride** [USP], the hydrochloride salt of cocaine, $C_{17}H_{21}NO_4\cdot$-HCl, occurring as colorless crystals or a white crystalline powder; used as an anesthetic, applied topically to mucous membranes.

cocainism (ko'kah-nizm, ko-kān'izm)   (*obs.*) cocaine intoxication or cocaine abuse.

cocainization (ko''kah-nĭ-za'shun; ko-ka''nĭ-za'shun)   the act of putting under the influence of cocaine.

cocainize (ko'kah-nīz; ko-ka'nīz)   to put under the influence of cocaine.

cocarboxylase (ko''kar-bok'sĭ-lās)   thiamine pyrophosphate.

cocarcinogen (ko-kar'sĭ-no-jen'')   a factor that, in combination with other factors, produces cancer.

cocarcinogenesis (ko-kar''sĭ-no-jen'ĕ-sis)   the development, according to one theory, of cancer only in preconditioned cells and as a result of conditions favorable to its growth.

coccal (kok'al)   resembling or pertaining to cocci.

coccerin (kok'sĕ-rin)   a wax from *Coccus,* the cochineal insect, being an ester of cocceryl alcohol and two acids, 13-keto-n-dotriacontanoic acid and n-triacontanoic acid; used as a biological stain.

cocci (kok'si) [L.]   plural of *coccus.*

Coccidia (kok-sid'e-ah) [Gr. *kokkos* berry]   a subclass of parasitic protozoa (class Sporozoea, phylum Apicocomplexa) found in both vertebrates, including humans, and higher invertebrates. Their life cycle involves merogony, gametogony, and sporogony, and gamonts are usually present, with mature gamonts being small and typically intracellular, without an epimerite or mucron. Syzygy does not usually occur, but if it does, it involves anisogamous gametes. It comprises three orders: Agamococcidiida, Protococcidiida, and Eucocciduida. See also *coccidiosis.*

coccidia (kok-sid'e-ah)   plural of *coccidium.*

coccidial (kok-sid'e-al)   pertaining to coccidia.

coccidian (kok-sid'e-an)   1. pertaining to Coccidia.   2. any individual of the order Coccidia.

coccidioidal (kok-sid''e-oi'dal)   caused by *Coccidioides.*

Coccidioides (kok-sid''e-oi'dēz)   a genus of pathogenic imperfect fungi of the family Moniliaceae, order Moniliales. In soil it grows as a mycelium with arthrospores; in tissue as a

spherule with endospores. *C. im'mitis* (*Blastomyces coccidioides, Blastomycoides immitis*) causes coccidioidomycosis.

coccidioidin (koksid''e-oi'din) [USP]   a skin test antigen prepared from mycelial phase *Coccidioides immitis* organisms. Because most individuals in endemic areas are skin test positive it is not useful in diagnosis. A negative skin test (cutaneous anergy) occurs in many patients with disseminated disease and indicates a poor prognosis. Cf. *spherulin.*

coccidioidoma (kok-sid''e-oi-do'mah)   residual pulmonary granulomatous nodules seen roentgenographically as solid round foci in coccidioidomycosis.

coccidioidomycosis (kok-sid''e-oi''do-mi-ko'sis)   a fungous disease caused by infection with *Coccidioides immitis,* occurring in a primary and a secondary form. Called also *coccidioidal granuloma, Posada's mycosis, Posada-Wernicke disease, California disease,* and *desert fever.* The *primary* form is an acute, benign, self-limited respiratory infection due to inhalation of spores, and varying in severity from that of a common cold to symptoms resembling those accompanying influenza, with pneumonia, cavitation, high fever, and, rarely, erythema nodosum (bumps). Called also *desert rheumatism, San Joaquin Valley fever,* and *valley fever.* The *secondary* form (or *progressive c.*) is a virulent and severe, chronic, progressive, granulomatous disease resulting in involvement of the cutaneous and subcutaneous tissues, viscera, central nervous system, and lungs, with anemia, phlebitis, and various allergic responses. This form may be caused by a new infection or by reactivation of arrested primary disease.   **primary extrapulmonary c.,** coccidioidomycosis in which infection occurs by primary cutaneous inoculation, usually with secondary lymphadenopathy; called also *chancriform syndrome.*

coccidioidosis (kok-sid''e-oi-do'sis)   coccidioidomycosis.

coccidiosis (kok''sid-e-o'sis)   infection by coccidia. In man, the term is applied to the presence of *Isospora hominis* or *I. belli* in the stools; such infection is often asymptomatic, rarely causing a severe watery mucous diarrhea. In mammals, such as cattle, sheep, rabbits, swine, cats, and dogs, especially young animals, coccidiosis causes destruction of the intestinal mucosa, accompanied by diarrhea, intestinal hemorrhage, emaciation, and sometimes fatal dysentery. It is due principally to species of *Eimeria* and *Isospora.* In domesticated mammals, four genera of coccidia are associated with disease: *Eimeria, Tyzzeria, Isospora,* and *Hepatozoon.* Among domesticated animals, coccidial infections cause greatest damage to poultry; *Eimeria* species are highly infective, producing high morbidity and mortality rates, especially in young birds.

coccidiostat (kok-sid'ĭ-o-stat'')   any of a group of chemical agents, e.g., nitrofurazone, nitrophenide, nicarbazin, mixed in feed or drinking water to control coccidiosis in animals.

coccidiostatic (kok-sid''ĭ-o-stat'ik)   1. inhibiting the growth of coccidia.   2. an agent that inhibits the growth of coccidia; see *coccidiostat.*

Coccidium (kok-sid'e-um) [L.; dim. of Gr. *kokkos* berry]   in former systems of classification, a genus of coccidians, the organisms of which have been assigned to other genera. **C. bigem'inum,** *Isospora bigemina.*   **C. cunic'uli,** *Eimeria stiedae.*   **C. ovifor'me,** *Eimeria stiedae.*   **C. tenel'lum,** *Eimeria tenella.*

coccidium (kok-sid'e-um), pl. *coccid'ia.*   Any organism of the order Coccidia.

coccigenic (kok''sĭ-jen'ik)   caused by cocci.

coccillana (kok''sĭ-yah'nah)   cocillana.

coccinella (kok''sĭ-nel'ah)   cochineal.

coccinellin (kok''sĭ-nel'in) [L. *coccinellinum*]   carmine; the coloring principle of cochineal.

cocco- [Gr. *kokkos* berry]   a word element denoting a resemblance to a berry.

coccobacillary (kok''o-bas'ĭ-ler''e)   pertaining to or resembling a coccobacillus.

coccobacilli (kok''o-bah-sil'li)   plural of *coccobacillus.*

Coccobacillus (kok''o-bah-sil'us) [*cocco-* + L. *bacillus* little rod]   in former systems of classification, a genus of bacteria made up of organisms now classified in the genera *Bacteroides, Fusobacterium,* and *Haemophilus.*

coccobacillus (kok''o-bah-sil'us), pl. *coccobacil'li.*   An oval bacterial cell intermediate between the coccus and bacillus forms.

coccobacteria (kok″o-bak-te′re-ah) [Gr. *kokkos* berry + *baktērion* rod] a common name for the spheroid bacteria, or for the various bacterial cocci.

coccode (kok′ōd) a globular granule.

coccogenic (kok′o-jen′ik) coccigenic.

coccogenous (kok-oj′ĕ-nus) [*coccus* + Gr. *gennan* to produce] coccigenic.

coccoid (kok′oid) resembling a coccus; globose.

cocculin (kok′u-lin) picrotoxin.

coccolith (kok′o-lith) [cocco- + Gr. *lithos* stone] the exoskeleton of calcareous platelets formed by certain marine protozoa of the order Prymnesiida.

Coccolithus (kok″o-lith′us) a genus of tiny plantlike, flagellate marine protozoa (order Prymnesiida, class Phytomastigophorea) covered by calcareous platelets (coccoliths).

cocculus (kok′u-lus) [L., dim. of *coccus*] a small berry. **c. in′dicus,** the dried berry or fruit of *Anamirta cocculus,* from which picrotoxin is derived.

Coccus (kok′us) [L.; Gr. *kokkos* berry] a genus of hemipterous insects which are the source of cochineal, kermes, and lac.

coccus (kok′us), pl. **coc′ci** [L.] a spherical bacterial cell, usually slightly less than 1μ in diameter.

coccyalgia (kok″se-al′je-ah) coccygodynia.

coccycephalus (kok″se-sef′ah-lus) [Gr. *kokkyx* cuckoo + *kephalē* head] a monster whose head is beak shaped.

coccydynia (kok″sĕ-din′e-ah) coccygodynia.

coccygalgia (kok″se-gal′je-ah) coccygodynia.

coccygeal (kok-sij′e-al) pertaining to or located in the region of the coccyx.

coccygectomy (kok″se-jek′to-me) [*coccyx* + Gr. *ektomē* excision] excision of the coccyx.

coccygerector (kok″se-je-rek′tor) the ventral sacrococcygeal muscle.

coccygeus (kok-sij′e-us) [L.] pertaining to the coccyx.

coccygodynia (kok″se-go-din′e-ah) [*coccyx* + Gr. *odynē* pain] pain in the coccyx and neighboring region; called also *coccygalgia.*

coccygotomy (kok″se-got′o-me) [*coccyx* + Gr. *tomē* a cutting] freeing the coccyx from its attachments.

coccyodynia (kok″se-o-din′e-ah) coccygodynia.

coccyx (kok′siks) [Gr. *kokkyx* cuckoo, whose bill it is said to resemble] NA alternative for *os coccygis;* the small bone caudad to the sacrum in man, formed by union of four (sometimes five or three) rudimentary vertebrae, and forming the caudal extremity of the vertebral column.

Cochicella (kok″ĭ-sel′ah) a genus of snails that serve as a host of *Dicrocoelium dendriticum.*

cochineal (koch″ĭ-nēl′) the dried female insects, *Coccus cacti,* enclosing the young larvae; formerly used as a coloring agent for pharmaceutical agents. It is the source of carmine and carminic acid.

cochl. abbreviation for L. *cochlea′re,* a spoonful. **cochl. amp.,** L. *cochlea′re am′plum,* a heaping spoonful. **cochl. mag.,** L. *cochlea′re mag′num,* a tablespoonful. **cochl. med.,** L. *cochlea′re me′dium,* a dessertspoonful. **cochl. parv.,** L. *cochlea′re par′vum,* a teaspoonful.

cochlea (kok′le-ah) [L. "snail shell"] 1. anything of a spiral form. 2. [NA] a spirally wound tube, resembling a snail shell, which forms part of the inner ear. Its base lies against the lateral end of the internal acoustic meatus and its apex is directed anterolaterally. It consists of the modiolus, a bony canal, and the osseous spiral lamina, which partially divides the cochlea into the essential organs of hearing, the scala vestibuli and scala tympani; the scalae communicate through the helicotrema. Called also *acoustic labyrinth.* **membranous c.,** ductus cochlearis.

cochlear (kok′le-ar) of or pertaining to the cochlea.

cochleare (kok″le-a′re) [L.] spoon or spoonful. **c. am′plum** [L. "large spoon"], a heaping spoonful. **c. mag′num,** a tablespoon or tablespoonful. **c. me′dium,** a dessertspoon or dessertspoonful. **c. par′vum,** a teaspoon or teaspoonful.

Cochlearia (kok″le-a′re-ah) [L.] a genus of cruciferous plants. *C. armoracia* L. is the common horse radish, used as a condiment and appetite stimulant, and has also been used as a rubifacient and plaster, like mustard, because it contains sinigrin and myrosin, which yield on hydrolysis the counter-

irritant principle allyl isothiocyanate. **C. officina′lis,** a species once used as an antiscorbutic; called also *scurvy grass.*

cochleariform (kok″le-ar′ĭ-form) [L. *cochleare* spoon + *form*] shaped like a spoon.

cochleitis (kok″le-i′tis) inflammation of the cochlea.

cochleotopic (kok″le-o-top′ik) relating to the organization of the auditory pathways and auditory area of the brain.

cochleovestibular (kok″le-o-ves-tib′u-lar) pertaining to the cochlea and vestibule of the ear.

Cochliomyia (kok″le-o-mi′yah) [Gr. *kochlias* snail with a spiral shell + *myia* fly] a genus of flies of the family Calliphoridae. **C. america′na,** *C. hominivorax.* **C. bezzia′na,** *Chrysomyia bezziana.* **C. hominivo′rax,** the screw-worm fly, a bluish green fly that deposits its eggs during the warmest hours of the day on wounds of animals; the larvae, known as screw-worms, after hatching, burrow into the wound and feed on living tissue. Called also *C. americana* and *Chrysomyia macellaria.*

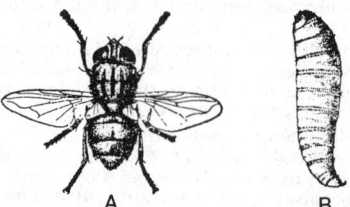

Cochliomyia hominivorax: A, adult; *B,* maggot (x 3).

cochlitis (kok-li′tis) cochleitis.

cocillana (ko″se-yah′nah) the bark of *Guarea rusbyi* (Britt.) Rusby (Meliaceae) used as an emetic, expectorant, and cathartic.

Cockayne's syndrome (disease) (kok-ānz′) [Edward Alfred *Cockayne,* English physician, 1880–1956] see under *syndrome.*

cocktail (kok′tāl) a beverage concocted of various ingredients. **frostbite c.,** a solution of alcohol, procaine, and heparin, in 5 per cent glucose, once recommended in treatment of frostbite. **lytic c.,** a concoction of various drugs used to block the function of the autonomic nervous system at every level, thus inhibiting the homeostatic defense reactions of the organism and producing the state known as artificial hibernation. **McConckey c.,** an emulsion of cod liver oil and tomato juice. **Philadelphia c.,** Rivers′ c. **Rivers′ c.,** a solution of dextrose in isotonic saline solution, with thiamine chloride and insulin added, given by intravenous drip for detoxification in acute alcoholism.

COCl cathodal opening clonus.

cocoa (ko′ko) [NF] a powder prepared from the roasted, cured kernels of the ripe seed of *Theobroma cacao,* which contains caffeine and theobromine; used as a flavor in pharmaceutical preparations. See also *cocoa syrup,* under *syrup.*

coconscious (ko-kon′shus) not in the field of the conscious yet capable under favorable circumstances of being remembered; preconscious.

cocontraction (ko″kon-trak′shun) the mutual coordination of antagonist muscles as of flexors and extensors in maintaining a straight limb.

coconut (ko′ko-nut) the fruit of *Cocos nucifera,* a palm tree whose sap affords palm wine or toddy, while the nut is an important article of food, and supplies great quantities of a valuable oil. See also under *oil.*

Coct. abbreviation for L. *coc′tio,* boiling.

coction (kok′shun) [L. *coctio,* a cooking] 1. the process of boiling. 2. digestion (def. 2).

coctoantigen (kok″to-an′tĭ-jen) an antigen modified by heat treatment.

cocto-immunogen (kok″to-ĭ-mu′no-jen) coctoantigen.

coctolabile (kok″to-la′bil) [L. *coctus* cooked + *labilis* perishable] destroyed or altered by heating to the boiling point of water.

coctoprecipitin (kok″to-pre-sip′ĭ-tin) [L. *coctus* cooked + *precipitin*] a precipitin produced by immunization with a coctoantigen.

coctoprotein (kok″to-pro′te-in) a heated protein.

coctostabile (kok″to-sta′bil) [L. *coctus* cooked + *stabilis* resisting] not altered by heating to the temperature of boiling water.

coctostable (kok″to-sta′b'l) coctostabile.

coculine (kok′u-lēn) sinomenine.

cocultivation (ko″kul-tĭ-va′shun) the culturing of cells (e.g., normal uninfected human cells) with infected or latently infected cells of the same kind.

code (kōd) [L. *codex* something written] 1. a set of rules governing one's conduct. 2. a system by which information can be communicated. **degeneracy of c.,** see under *degeneracy.* **genetic c.,** the manner in which information specifying the sequence of amino acid residues in the polypeptides synthesized by living organisms is encoded in the sequence of nucleotides in their genomes (see accompanying table). See also *codon, transcription,* and *translation.* **triplet c.,** see *triplet* (def. 3).

THE GENETIC CODE

UUU	UCU	UAU	UGU
AAA	AGA	ATA	ACA
phe	ser	tyr	cys
UUC	UCC	UAC	UGC
GAA	GGA	GTA	GCA
phe	ser	tyr	cys
UUA	UCA	UAA	UGA
TAA	TGA	TTA	TCA
leu	ser	*term*	*term*
UUG	UCG	UAG	UGG
CAA	CGA	CTA	CCA
leu	ser	*term*	trp
CUU	CCU	CAU	CGU
AAG	AGG	ATG	ACG
leu	pro	his	arg
CUC	CCC	CAC	CGC
GAG	GGG	GTG	GCG
leu	pro	his	arg
CUA	CCA	CAA	CGA
TAG	TGG	TTG	TCG
leu	pro	gln	arg
CUG	CCG	CAG	CGG
CAG	CGG	CTG	CCG
leu	pro	gln	arg
AUU	ACU	AAU	AGU
AAT	AGT	ATT	ACT
ile	thr	asn	ser
AUC	ACC	AAC	AGC
GAT	GGT	GTT	GCT
ile	thr	asn	ser
AUA	ACA	AAA	AGA
TAT	TGT	TTT	TCT
ile	thr	lys	arg
AUG	ACG	AAG	AGG
CAT	CGT	CTT	CCT
met *(init)*	thr	lys	arg
GUU	GCU	GAU	GGU
AAC	AGC	ATC	ACC
val	ala	asp	gly
GUC	GCC	GAC	GGC
GAC	GGC	GTC	GCC
val	ala	asp	gly
GUA	GCA	GAA	GGA
TAC	TGC	TTC	TCC
val	ala	glu	gly
GUG	GCG	GAG	GGG
CAC	CGC	CTC	CCC
val *(init)*	ala	glu	gly

Each grouping matches a messenger RNA codon *(top),* its complementary DNA codon *(middle),* and the amino acid they specify *(bottom).* U = uracil; C = cytosine; A = adenine; G = guanine; T = thymine; see *amino acid* for amino acid symbols. The codons marked *term* are chain termination codons. Those marked *init* are chain initiation codons which code for methionine (in the cytosol of eukaryotic cells) or *N*-formylmethionine (in mitochondria and prokaryotes) at the beginning of polypeptide chains and for the indicated amino acid (methionine or valine) within polypeptide chains.

codeine (ko′dēn) [L. *codeina*] [USP] chemical name: 7,8-didehydro-4,5α-epoxy-3-methoxy-17-methyl-morphinan-6α-ol monohydrate. A narcotic alkaloid obtained from opium or prepared by methylating morphine, $C_{18}H_{21}NO_3 \cdot H_2O$, occurring as colorless or white crystals or as a white, crystalline powder; used as an analgesic and antitussive, administered orally. Called also *methylmorphine.* **c. phosphate** [USP], the phosphate salt of codeine, $C_{18}H_{21}NO_3 \cdot H_3PO_4 \cdot \frac{1}{2}H_2O$, occurring as fine white, needle-shaped crystals or a white crystalline powder; used as a narcotic analgesic and antitussive; administered subcutaneously. **c. sulfate** [USP], white crystals or white crystalline powder, $(C_{18}H_{21}NO_3)_2 \cdot H_2SO_4 \cdot 3H_2O$; used as a narcotic analgesic, administered orally.

codex (ko′deks), pl. *cod′ices* [L.] an authorized medicinal formulary; especially the French Pharmacopoeia, *Codex medicamentarium.*

Codman's sign, triangle (kod′manz) [Ernest Amory Codman, Boston surgeon, 1869–1940] see under *sign* and *triangle.*

codominance (ko-dom′ĭ-nans) codominant gene.

codominant (ko-dom′ĭ-nant) see under *gene.*

codon (ko′don) a set of three adjacent bases on a single strand of DNA or RNA. Of the 64 different codons, 61 direct the incorporation of a specific amino acid into a polypeptide chain and three signal chain termination (see table of the genetic code). **chain-initiation c's,** the condons, AUG or GUG, occurring at the beginning of mRNA sequences coding for polypeptide chains. There they are recognized by the initiator tRNA, which carries the amino acid methionine (in the cytosol of eukaryotes) or *N*-formyl methionine (in prokaryotes, mitochondria, and chloroplasts). In the middle of a polypeptide chain these codons are recognized by other tRNAs so that AUG directs the incorporation of methionine and GUG of valine. **chain-termination c's,** the three codons UAA, UAG, and UGA that cause termination of the synthesis of a growing polypeptide chain and its release from the ribosome. Called also *nonsense* c's. **nonsense c's,** chain-termination c's.

coe- for words beginning thus, see also words beginning *ce-.*

coefficient (ko″ĕ-fish′ent) 1. a numerical factor multiplying a term in an algebraic equation. 2. a number preceding a formula in a chemical equation, indicating the relative number of molecules of that species entering the reaction. 3. a dimensionless constant characterizing a chemical or physical process. 4. a dimensionless statistical parameter. **absorption c.,** 1. absorptivity. 2. see *linear absorption c.* 3. see *mass absorption c.* **activity c.,** the ratio of the activity (of an electrolyte) as measured by some property, such as the depression of the freezing point of a solution, to the true concentration (molality). It is usually less than 1 and increases as the solution becomes more dilute, approaching unity at infinite dilution, when the attractive forces between oppositely charged ions become negligible. **Ambard's c.,** see under *formula.* **Baumann's c.,** the ratio of the ethereal to the total sulfates in the urine. **binomial c.,** the number of different sets of size k that can be chosen from a set of n objects; denoted $\binom{n}{k}$ or $_nC_k$, and equal to $\dfrac{n!}{k!(n-k)!}$.

So called because it is the coefficient of x^k in the binomial $(1+x)^n$. **biological c.,** the amount of potential energy consumed by the body when at rest. **Bouchard's c.,** 1. the ratio between the amount of urine and the total solids present in the urine. 2. urotoxic coefficient. **Bunsen c.,** the number of milliliters of gas dissolved in a milliliter of liquid at atmospheric pressure (760 mm Hg) and a specified temperature. Symbol, α. Called also *solubility c.* **Chick-Martin c.,** see *Chick-Martin method,* under *method.* **confidence c.,** the probability that a confidence interval will contain the true value of the population parameter. For example, if the confidence coefficient is .95, 95 percent of the confidence intervals so calculated for each of a large number of random samples will contain the parameter (and 5 per cent will not). **correlation c.,** a statistical measure which when squared gives the degree of association between the values of two random variables. Most correlation coefficients are normalized so that they have values between +1 (which indicates perfect correlation) and −1 (which indicates perfect inverse correlation); a value of 0 indicates no correlation. As the absolute value of the correlation coefficient increases, so does the strength of correlation. When not otherwise specified, the product-moment correlation coefficient (r) is meant. **creatinine c.,** the figure obtained by dividing the total of milligrams of creatinine in the day's urine by the body weight expressed in kilograms. **cryoscopic c.,** the comparison of the freezing point depression of an electrolyte with that of an ideal nonelectrolyte of the same concentration (usually 1 molal of each). **c. of demineralization,** the proportion of mineral matter to the total dry residue of the urine; it averages 30 per cent. **dilution c.,** a number that expresses the effectiveness of a disinfectant for a given organism. It is calculated by the equation $tc^n = k$, where t is the time required for killing all organisms, c is the concentration of disinfectant, n is the dilution coefficient, and k is a constant. A low coefficient indicates the disinfectant is effective at a low concentration. **distribution c.,** partition c. **extinction c.,** absorptivity. **Falta's c.,** the percentage of ingested sugar eliminated from the system. **Haines' c.,** see under *formula.* **Häser's c.,** see under *formula.* **homogeneity c.,** in radiology, the ratio of the half-value layer to the second half-value layer; it is unity for radiation in which the photons all originate with the same energy. **hygienic laboratory c.,** phenol c. **c. of inbreeding,** an expression of the probability that an individual has received both alleles of a pair from a single ancestor common to both parents, or of the proportion of loci at which he is homozygous. **isometric c. of lactic acid,** the ratio of the total isometric tension a muscle can produce before fatigue, to the milligrams of lactic acid it produced. **Kendall's rank correlation c.,** Kendall's tau (τ); a nonparametric measure of correlation calculated as follows: a sample of n observations is arranged in ascending order according to the values of one variable; then, looking at the corresponding values of the other variable, the number of observations later in the sequence that exceed each of the observations is counted; finally the sum of the counts is multiplied by 4, divided by $n(n-1)$, and decreased by 1 to give a value ranging between -1 and $+1$. **Lancet c.,** phenol c. **lethal c.,** that concentration of a disinfectant that will kill sporeless bacteria (*inferior lethal c.*) or bacterial spores (*superior lethal c.*) in water at a temperature of 20° to 25° C. in the shortest period of time. **linear absorption c.,** in radiation physics, the fraction of a beam of roentgen rays or gamma rays that is absorbed per unit thickness of the absorber. **linear attenuation c.,** in radiation physics, the fraction of a beam of roentgen rays or gamma rays that is absorbed or scattered per unit thickness of the absorber. **Loebisch's c.,** see under *formula.* **Long's c.,** see under *formula.* **Maillard's c.,** a coefficient expressing the relationship between the urea and the total nitrogen of the urine. **mass absorption c.,** in radiology, the linear absorption coefficient divided by the density of the absorber. **mass attenuation c.,** the linear attenuation coefficient divided by the density of the absorbing material. **osmotic c.,** a factor, φ, which corrects for the deviation in the behavior of a solute in question from ideal behavior defined by the ideal gas equation as applied to osmotic pressure. **c. of partage,** a number indicating the ratio between the amount of an acid absorbed by ether from an aqueous solution of the acid and the amount remaining in solution. Symbol c'. **partition c.,** the ratio in which a given substance distributes itself between two or more different phases; called also *distribution c.* **Pearson's correlation c.,** product-moment correlation c. **phenol c.,** a measure of the bactericidal activity of a chemical compound in relation to phenol. The test is standardized (Rideal-Walker method, U. S. Department of Agriculture method). The coefficient is calculated by dividing the concentration of the test compound at which it kills the test organism in 10 minutes, but not in 5 minutes, by the concentration of phenol that kills the organism under the same conditions. It can be determined in the absence of organic matter, or in the presence of a standard amount of added organic matter. **product-moment c.,** the covariance of two random variables divided by the product of their standard deviations. Symbol r. Called also *Pearson's correlation c.* **c. of relationship,** an expression of the probability that two persons have inherited a certain gene from a common ancestor; or the proportion of all their genes that have been inherited from common ancestors. **Rideal-Walker c.,** see *phenol c.* **sedimentation c.,** the velocity at which a particle sediments in a centrifuge divided by the applied centrifugal field, the result having units of time (velocity divided by acceleration), usually expressed in Svedberg units (S), which equal 10^{-13} second. Sedimentation coefficients are used to characterize the size of macromolecules, e.g., 5.8S rRNA, 22S rRNA; they increase with increasing mass and density and are higher for globular

than for fibrous particles. Called also *sedimentation constant.* **selection c.,** a measure of the disadvantage in survival value of a given genotype as compared with that of a standard genotype in a population. **solubility c.,** Bunsen c. **Spearman's rank correlation c.,** Spearman's rho (ρ); the product-moment correlation coefficient of two variables calculated after ranks have been substituted for actual values. **temperature c.,** a number indicating the effect of temperature upon the velocity constant of a chemical reaction. Cf. *van't Hoff's rule,* under *rule.* **c. of thermal conductivity,** a number indicating the quantity of heat that passes in a unit of time through a unit thickness of a substance when the difference in temperature is 1° C. **c. of thermal expansion,** the change in volume per unit volume of a substance produced by a 1° C. temperature increase. **Trapp's c.,** see under *formula.* **urohemolytic c.,** the smallest degree of dilution necessary to render a specimen of urine hemolytic. **urotoxic c.,** a number expressing the toxicity of the urine; it is the quantity of urotoxic units produced per unit weight and eliminated in unit time. Called also *Bouchard's c.* **c. of variation (CV),** the standard deviation divided by the mean, sometimes multiplied by 100; a dimensionless quantity indicating the relative variability around the mean. **velocity c.,** a number expressing the rate of a reaction; the rate of transformation of a unit mass of a substance in a chemical reaction. **c. of viscosity,** the force necessary to slide tangentially a unit of area of smooth surface at unit velocity on another parallel surface separated from the first surface by a unit layer of viscous substance. **volume c.,** the volume of packed red cells per 100 ml. of blood.

coelarium (se-la′re-um) [L., from Gr. *koilos* a hollow] the membrane that lines the body cavity of the embryo, or coelom; it consists of a parietal layer, the *exocoelarium,* and a visceral layer, the *endocoelarium.* Called also *mesothelium.*

-coele [Gr. *koilia* cavity] a word termination denoting a cavity or space; sometimes spelled *-cele* and *-coel.*

Coelenterata (se-len″ter-a′tah) [Gr. *koilos* hollow + *enteron* intestine] former name for a phylum of marine invertebrates that included sea anemones, hydras, jellyfish, and corals, which are now assigned to the phylum Cnidaria. See also *coelenterate.*

coelenterate (se-len′ter-āt) 1. pertaining or belonging to the phylum Coelenterata. (Cnidaria). 2. an individual of the phylum Coelenterata (Cnidaria); a cnidarian. 3. the cnidarians and ctenophores collectively.

coelenteron (se-len′ter-on) 1. archenteron. 2. gastrovascular cavity.

coeliac (se′le-ak) celiac.

coel(o)- [Gr. *koilos* hollow] a combining form denoting relationship to a cavity or space; sometimes spelled *cel(o)-.*

coeloblastula (se″lo-blas′tu-lah) [*coelo-* + Gr. *blastos* germ] the common type of blastula, consisting of a hollow sphere composed of blastomeres.

coelom (se′lom) [Gr. *koilōma*] the body cavity. In the mammalian embryo, it is situated between the somatopleure and the splanchnopleure; it is both extraembryonic and intraembryonic. From the intraembryonic portion arise the principal cavities of the trunk. Also spelled *celom.* Called also *coeloma* and *somatic cavity.* **extraembryonic c.,** the portion of the coelom external to the embryo, bordered by chorionic mesoderm and the mesoderm of the amnion and yolk sac; it communicates temporarily at the umbilicus with the intraembryonic coelom. Called also *exocoelom.*

coeloma (se-lo′mah) coelom.

coelomate (sēl′o-māt) 1. having a coelom. 2. an individual of the Eucoelomata; eucoelomate.

coelomic (se-lom′ik) pertaining to the coelom.

coelomyarian (se″lo-mi-a′re-an) designating a type of nematode musculature in which the muscle fibers are next to the hypodermis and perpendicular to it; myofibrils extend varying distances up the side of the muscle cell, partially enclosing the sarcoplasm.

coelosomy (se″lo-so′me) a developmental anomaly characterized by protrusion of the viscera from and their presence outside the body cavity.

coelothel (se′lo-thel) [Gr. *koilos* hollow + *thēlē* nipple] mesothelium.

coen(o)- see *cen(o)-* (def. 3).

coenurosis (se″nu-ro′sis) gid.

Coenurus (se-nu′rus) [Gr. *koinos* common + *oura* tail] a genus of certain tapeworm larvae. **C. cerebra′lis,** the larva of the *Multiceps multiceps,* found in the brain of sheep, goats, and other ruminants, and rarely in man.

coenurus (se-nu′rus) the larval stage of tapeworms of the genus *Multiceps,* a semitransparent, fluid-filled, bladder-like organism that contains multiple scoleces attached to the inner surface of its wall and that does not form brood capsules. It develops in various parts of the host body, especially in the central nervous system. Cf. *cystercercus* and *hydatid cyst.*

coenzyme (ko-en′zīm) an organic nonprotein molecule, frequently a phosphorylated derivative of a water-soluble vitamin, that binds with the protein molecule (apoenzyme) to form the active enzyme (holoenzyme). **c. A,** a coenzyme in which phosphopantothenic acid, β-mercaptoethylamine, and adenosine-3′, 5′-bisphosphate are covalently linked. The terminal SH group is enzymatically acylated to form high-energy thiol ester compounds such as the acetyl, acetoacetyl, acetoacetate, and long chain fatty acid (acyl) compounds. These thiol esters play a central role in various metabolic reactions, e.g., the citric (tricarboxylic) acid cycle, the transfer of acetyl groups, and the oxidation of fatty acids. Abbreviated CoA and CoA-SH. See also *acetoacetyl coenzyme A, acetyl coenzyme A, acylcoenzyme A,* and *succinyl coenzyme A.* **c. I,** nicotinamide-adenine dinucleotide (NAD). **c. II,** nicotinamide-adenine dinucleotide phosphate (NADP). **c. Q,** ubiquinone. **c. R,** biotin.

COEPS cortically originating extrapyramidal system: pathways from the cortex to the spinal cord, the major ones being the corticostriatal and corticopallidal, corticothalamic, corticoreticular, and corticopontine pathways.

coeruleus (ser-roo′le-us) [L.] widely accepted variant spelling of the original Latin term *caeruleus* (q.v.), as in locus coeruleus [NA]; cerule.

coeur (ker) [Fr.] heart. **c. en sabot** (ker-on-să-bo′), a heart visible radiographically as having an increased transverse diameter, a convexity in the inferior line, and an elevation and rounded shape of the apex, so that its form suggests vaguely that of a wooden shoe; noted in tetralogy of Fallot.

cofactor (ko′fak-tor) an element or principle, as a coenzyme, with which another must unite in order to function. **platelet c. I,** Factor VIII; see *coagulation factors,* under *factor.* **platelet c. II,** Factor IX; see *coagulation factors,* under *factor.*

coffea (kof′e-ah) [L., from *coffee*] coffee.

coffee (kof′e) [L. *coffea, caffea*] the dried seeds of *Coffea arabica* L. and *C. liberica* (Rubiaceae), trees believed to have originated in Africa, but now growing in nearly all tropical regions: a drink made by decoction or infusion of the dried and roasted ripe seeds is invigorating, tonic, and conservant; useful in chronic asthma, headache, and opium poisoning. The active principles include caffeine in seed, coffee oil, sugars, protein, and numerous volatile flavor oils.

Coffey-Humber treatment [Walter B. *Coffey,* American surgeon, 1868–1944; John D. *Humber,* American surgeon, born 1895] see under *treatment.*

cogener (ko′jĕ-ner) congener.

Cogentin (ko-jen′tin) trademark for preparations of benztropine mesylate.

cognition (kog-nish′un) [L. *cognitio,* from *cognoscere* to know] that operation of the mind by which we become aware of objects of thought or perception; it includes all aspects of perceiving, thinking, and remembering.

cognitive (kog′nĭ-tiv) of, pertaining to, or characterized by cognition.

cohesion (ko-he′zhun) [L. *cohaesio,* from *con* together + *haerere* to stick] the force that causes various particles to unite.

cohesive (ko-he′siv) uniting together, or characterized by cohesion.

Cohn's solution (kōnz) [Ferdinand Julius *Cohn,* German bacteriologist, 1828–1898] see under *solution.*

C₄O₆H₄NaK potassium sodium tartrate.

Cohnheim's areas, etc. (kōn′hīmz) [Julius Friedrich *Cohnheim,* German pathologist, 1839–1884] see under *area, field,* and *theory.*

cohoba (ko-ho′bah) parica.

cohobation (ko″ho-ba′shun) the repeated distilling of a liquid from the same material; redistillation.

cohort (ko′hort) [L. *cohors* one of the ten units making up a Roman legion] 1. in epidemiology, a group of individuals who share a common characteristic, e.g., all of the individuals born in one year (a birth cohort) or a group of individuals entered in a prospective study or a clinical trial. The term always carries the connotation that individuals are observed over a period of time and that summary statistics describe the experience of real individuals rather than mathematical abstractions, e.g., a cohort study or a cohort life table. 2. a taxonomic category approximately equivalent to a division, order, or suborder in various systems of classification.

cohosh (ko-hosh′) a North American (Algonkin) name for various medicinal plants, as *Actaea spicata,* or red cohosh; *Caulophyllum thalictroides,* or blue cohosh; and *Cimicifuga racemosa,* or black cohosh.

coil (koil) [Old Fr. *collier,* from L. *colligere* to gather together] anything wound in a spiral. **random c.,** a term used to refer to any protein secondary structure that does not have a regular repetitive pattern, e.g., α-helix or β-sheet.

coin(o)- see *cen(o)-* (def. 3).

coinosite (koi′no-sīt) [Gr. *koinos* common + *sitos* food] a free or unfixed commensal organism; called also *cenosite.*

coisogeneic (ko-i″so-jĕ-na′ik) of or relating to strains of inbred animals that are constructed to be genetically identical except for a difference at a single genetic locus.

coisogenic (ko-i″so-jen′ik) congenic.

coital (ko′ĭ-tal) pertaining to coitus.

coition (ko-ish′un) coitus.

coitophobia (ko″ĭ-to-fo′be-ah) [*coitus* + *phobia*] irrational fear of coitus.

coitus (ko′ĭ-tus) [L. *coitio* a coming together, meeting] sexual connection per vaginam between male and female. **c. incomple′tus, c. interrup′tus,** coitus in which the penis is withdrawn from the vagina before ejaculation; a widely used but unreliable method of contraception. **c. reserva′tus,** coitus in which ejaculation is intentionally suppressed.

Coix (ko′iks) [L.; Gr. *koix* a palm] a genus of grasses. *C. lacryma,* an Asiatic species, bears large seeds called *Job's tears,* which have been strung as beads for infants' use in teething; said to be anodyne and diuretic.

Col. abbreviation for L. *co′la,* strain.

col (kol) [Fr., from L. *collum* neck] a valley-like depression of the interdental gingiva, which connects the facial and lingual papillae and conforms to the shape of the interproximal contact area.

col- see *con-.*

Colace (ko′lās) trademark for a preparation of docusate sodium.

colamine (ko′lah-min) monoethanolamine.

Colat. abbreviation for L. *cola′tus,* strained.

colation (ko-la′shun) [L. *colatio*] 1. the process of straining or filtration. 2. the product of such a process.

colatorium (kol″ah-to′re-um), pl. *colato′ria* [L., from *colare* to strain] a strainer or colander; a sieve.

colature (ko′lah-tūr) [L. *colatura,* from *colare* to strain] a liquid obtained by straining.

colauxe (ko-lawk′se) [Gr. *kolon* colon + *auxē* increase] (*obs.*) dilatation of the colon.

ColBENEMID (kol-ben′e-mid) trademark for a preparation of probenecid with colchicine.

colchicine (kol′chĭ-sēn) [USP] an alkaloid obtained from *Colchicum* spp.; used in the treatment of gouty arthritis. Colchicine binds to microtubules and is used in the laboratory to arrest cell division by disrupting the mitotic spindle. Its action in gout may be due to inhibition of granulocyte migration into areas of inflammation.

Colchicum (kol′chĭ-kum) a genus of Old World liliaceous herb, the meadow saffron, from whose corm or dried ripe seed colchicine is obtained.

cold (kōld) 1. privation, or relatively low degree, of heat. 2. common cold; a catarrhal disorder of the upper respiratory tract, which may be viral, a mixed infection, or an allergic reaction. It is marked by acute coryza, slight rise in temperature, chilly sensations, and general indisposition. **allergic c.,** hay fever. **common c.,** see *cold,* def. 2. **June c.,** hay fever. **rose c.,** a form of seasonal hay fever caused by the pollen of roses.

coldsore (kōld′sōr) see *herpes simplex.*

Cole's sign (kōlz) [Lewis Gregory *Cole,* American roentgenologist, 1874–1954] see under *sign.*

colectomy (ko-lek′to-me) [*colon* + Gr. *ektomē* excision] excision of a portion of the colon (*partial c.*) or of the whole colon (*complete* or *total c.*).

Coleman-Shaffer diet [Warren *Coleman,* New York physician, 1869–1948; Philip Anderson *Shaffer,* American biochemist, 1881–1960] see under *diet.*

cole(o)- [Gr. *koleos* sheath] a combining form denoting relationship to the vagina, or to a sheath.

Coleomitus (ko″le-o-mi′tus) [*coleo-* + Gr. *mitos* thread] a genus of spore-forming filamentous bacteria of uncertain taxonomic position, which was formerly classified in the family Arthromitaceae.

Coleoptera (kol″e-op′ter-ah) [*coleo-* + Gr. *pteron* wing] an order of insects comprising the beetles.

coles (ko′lēz) [Gr. *kōlē*] the penis. **c. femini′nus,** the clitoris.

Colesiota (ko-le″se-o′tah) [J. D. W. A. *Coles*] a genus (incertae sedis) of bacteria occurring as a single species, *C. conjuncti′vae,* the agent causing infectious ophthalmia of sheep.

colestipol (ko-les′tĭ-pōl) chemical name: tetraethylenepentamine polymer with 1-chloro-2,3-epoxypropane; an antilipemic agent.

Colet. abbreviation for L. *cole′tur,* let it be strained.

Colettsia (ko-let′se-ah) [J. D. W. A. *Coles*] a genus (incertae sedis) of bacteria occurring as a single species, *C. pe′coris,* a parasitic microorganism found in the conjunctiva of domestic animals.

colibacillemia (ko″lĭ-bas-ĭ-le′me-ah) the presence of *Escherichia coli* in the blood.

colibacillosis (ko″lĭ-bas-ĭ-lo′sis) infection with *Escherichia coli.* **c. gravida′rum,** severe infection with *Escherichia coli* during pregnancy.

colibacilluria (ko″lĭ-bas″ĭ-lu′re-ah) presence of *Escherichia coli* in the urine; called also *Albarrán's disease.*

colibacillus (ko″lĭ-bah-sil′us) *Escherichia coli.*

colic (kol′ik) [Gr. *kōlikos*] 1. pertaining to the colon. 2. acute abdominal pain; characteristically, intermittent visceral pain with fluctuations corresponding to smooth muscle peristalsis. **appendicular c.,** vermicular c. **biliary c.,** paroxysms of pain and other severe symptoms due to the passage of gallstones along the bile duct; called also *gallstone* or *hepatic c.,* and *cholecystalgia.* **bilious c.,** abdominal pain accompanied by the vomiting of bile. **copper c.,** a severe colic due to copper poisoning. **Devonshire c.,** lead colic. **endemic c.,** a dangerous form of colic peculiar to hot countries. **flatulent c.,** tympanites. **gallstone c.,** biliary c. **gastric c.,** pain in the stomach. **hepatic c.,** biliary c. **infantile c.,** benign paroxysmal abdominal pain during the first three months of life. **intestinal c.,** colic originating from the small bowel, characteristically periumbilical in location. **lead c.,** colic due to lead poisoning. **menstrual c.,** severe abdominal pain at the menstrual period; dysmenorrhea. **nephric c.,** renal c. **ovarian c.,** ovarian pain. **painters' c.,** lead c. **pancreatic c.,** abdominal pain caused by obstruction of the excretory duct of the pancreas. **Poitou c.,** lead c. **renal c.,** pain produced by thrombosis or dissection of the renal artery, renal infarction, intrarenal mass lesions, the passage of a stone within the collecting system, or thrombosis of the renal vein; called also *nephric c.* **sand c.,** chronic indigestion in horses and cattle due to the presence in the stomach or intestine of sand taken in with food or drink. **saturnine c.,** lead c. **stercoral c.,** intestinal colic due to accumulation of feces. **tubal c.,** painful spasmodic contraction of the fallopian tube. **ureteral c.,** colicky pains due to obstruction of the ureter. **uterine c.,** severe abdominal pain arising in the uterus, usually at the menstrual period. **vermicular c.,** a condition of colic in the vermiform appendix occasioned by a catarrhal inflammation resulting from blocking of the outlet of the appendix; called also *appendicular c.* **verminous c.,** colic due to the pres-

ence of intestinal worms; called also *worm c.* **wind c.,** pain in the bowels due to their distention with air or gas. **worm c.,** verminous c. **zinc c.,** colic resulting from chronic zinc poisoning.

colica (kol′ĭ-kah) [L.] colic. **c. pic′tonum,** lead colic. **c. scorto′rum** (*obs.*), severe colicky pain in the region of the fallopian tubes; seen in salpingitis.

colicin (kol′ĭ-sin) [*coli* (from *Escherichia coli*) + *-cin* (adapted from L. *caedere* to kill)] a bacteriocin secreted by colicinogenic strains of *Escherichia coli* and *Shigella sonnei* that is lethal to closely related bacterial strains. Specific colicins attach to specific receptors on cell membranes and impair systems of electron transport, membrane function, molecular synthesis, or energy production.

colicinogen (kol″ĭ-sin′o-jen) bacteriocinogen; a plasmid in some strains of *Escherichia coli* that induces secretion of the corresponding colicin. Some colicinogens aso serve as sex factors. Called also *colicinogenic (colicin) factor (Cf.).*

colicinogenic (kol″ĭ-sin″o-jen′ik) elaborating colicin; said of strains of *Escherichia coli.*

colicinogeny (kol″ĭ-sin-oj′ĕ-ne) the production of colicin; see *colicinogen.*

colicky (kol′ik-e) pertaining to or affected by colic.

colicoplegia (kol″ĭ-ko-ple′je-ah) [Gr. *kōlikos* colic + *plēgē* stroke] lead colic and lead paralysis together.

colicystitis (ko″lĭ-sis-ti′tis) cystitis dependent upon the presence of *Escherichia coli.*

colicystopyelitis (ko-lĭ-sis″to-pi″e-li′tis) [*colon* + Gr. *kystis* bladder + *pyelos* pelvis] inflammation of the bladder and kidney pelvis due to *Escherichia coli.*

coliform (ko′lĭ-form) [L. *colum* a sieve] 1. a collective term denoting enteric, fermentative gram-negative rods, and sometimes restricted to the lactose-fermenting, gram-negative enteric bacilli, i.e., *Citrobacter, Edwardsiella, Enterobacter, Escherichia, Klebsiella,* and *Serratia.* 2. any organism of that group.

colinearity (ko″lin-e-ar′ĭ-te) the correspondence between the linear sequence of the nucleotide codons, the RNA, and the linear sequence of amino acids in the polypeptide coded for by that sequence; a concept implicit in the original Watson-Crick model of the DNA structure.

colinephritis (ko″lĭ-ne-fri′tis) nephritis due to the presence of *Escherichia coli.*

coliphage (kol′ĭ-fāj) any bacteriophage that infects *Escherichia coli.*

Coliphorina (ko″lĭ-fo-ri′nah) [Gr. *kōlon* member + *phoros* bearing] a suborder of mostly marine ciliate protozoa (order Heterotrichina, subclass Spirotricha) characterized by the presence of an adoral zone of membranelles borne on a pair of prominent peristomial winglike organelles extending out from the lorica-encased body, and uniform, holotrichous ciliation.

coliplication (ko″lĭ-pli-ka′shun) coloplication.

colipuncture (ko′lĭ-punk″tūr) colocentesis.

colistimethate sodium (ko-lis″tĭ-meth′āt) chemical name: colistinmethanesulfonic acid pentasodium. The pentasodium salt of the methanesulfonate derivative of colistin, $C_{58}H_{105}N_{16}Na_5O_{28}S_5$, occurring as a white to slightly yellow, fine powder, having actions and uses similar to those of the base (colistin); administered intramuscularly or intravenously.

colistin (ko-lis′tin) a polypeptide antibiotic of the polymyxin (q.v.) group, produced by the growth of the soil bacterium *Bacillus polymyxa* var. *colistinus,* specifically effective against many gram-negative bacteria, especially *Pseudomonas aeruginosa,* but also useful against others, including *Escherichia coli* and species of *Aerobacter, Klebsiella, Shigella,* and *Brucella; Proteus* species are resistant. **c. sulfate** [USP], the sulfate salt of colistin, occurring as a white to cream-colored, hygroscopic powder; used in the treatment of various systemic, urinary tract, gastrointestinal, ophthalmic, and otic infections due to susceptible gram-negative bacteria, administered orally, parenterally, and topically.

colitides (ko-lit′ĭ-dēz) plural of *colitis.* Inflammatory disorders of the colon considered collectively.

colitis (ko-li′tis) inflammation of the colon. **amebic c.,** see under *dysentery.* **antibiotic-associated c.,** see under *enterocolitis.* **balantidial c.,** colitis due to infestation with *Balantidium coli.* **c. cys′tica profun′da,** a condition marked by mucous retention cysts in the colic submucosa that are characteristic of the healing of chronic lesions of bacillary dysentery. **c. cys′tica superficia′- lis,** a cystic condition of the colic mucous membrane sometimes seen in children with such chronic debilitating disease as leukemia, possibly the result of malnutrition and vitamin deficiency. **granulomatous c.,** transmural colitis with the formation of noncaseating granulomas. **c. gra′vis,** ulcerative c. **ischemic c.,** acute vascular insufficiency of the colon usually involving the portion supplied by the inferior mesenteric artery; symptoms include pain at the left iliac fossa, bloody diarrhea, low-grade fever, abdominal distention, and abdominal tenderness. The classic radiologic sign is thumbprinting due to localized elevation of the mucosa by submucosal hemorrhage or edema. Ulceration may follow. **mucous c.,** former term for *irritable bowel syndrome;* see under *syndrome.* **c. polypo′sa,** ulcerative colitis associated with the formation of pseudopolyps (edematous, inflamed islands of mucosa between areas of ulceration). **pseudomembranous c.,** see under *enterocolitis.* **regional c., segmental c.,** transmural or granulomatous inflammatory disease of the colon; regional enteritis involving the colon. It may be associated with ulceration, strictures, or fistulas. **transmural c.,** inflammation of the full thickness of the bowel, rather than mucosal and submucosal disease, usually with the formation of noncaseating granulomas. It may be confined to the colon, segmentally or diffusely, or may be associated with small bowel disease (regional enteritis). Clinically, it may resemble ulcerative colitis, but the ulceration is often longitudinal or deep, the disease is often segmental, stricture formation is common, and fistulas, particularly in the perineum, are a frequent complication. **c. ulcerati′va, ulcerative c.,** chronic, recurrent ulceration in the colon, chiefly of the mucosa and submucosa, of unknown cause; it is manifested clinically by cramping abdominal pain, rectal bleeding, and loose discharges of blood, pus, and mucus with scanty fecal particles. Complications include hemorrhoids, abscesses, fistulas, perforation of the colon, pseudopolyps, and carcinoma.

colitose (kol′ĭ-tōs) an unusual sugar found in the O-specific chains in the lipopolysaccharides of certain serotypes of *Salmonella* and *Escherichia coli.*

colitoxemia (ko″lĭ-tok-se′me-ah) toxemia due to infection with *Escherichia coli.*

colitoxicosis (ko″lĭ-tok″sĭ-ko′sis) intoxication caused by *Escherichia coli.*

colitoxin (ko″lĭ-tok′sin) a substance contained in *Escherichia coli* that is the cause of colitoxicosis.

coliuria (ko″lĭ-u′re-ah) presence of *Escherichia coli* in the urine.

colla (kol′ah) [L.] plural of *collum.*

collacin (kol′ĭ-sin) degenerate collagenous tissue; collastin.

collagen (kol′ah-jen) [Gr. *kolla* glue + *gennan* to produce] the protein substance of the white fibers (collagenous fibers) of skin, tendon, bone, cartilage, and all other connective tissue; composed of molecules of tropocollagen (q.v.), it is converted into gelatin by boiling. See also under *disease.* **fibrous long-spacing (FLS) c.,** a form of collagen having a periodicity of about 240 nm. instead of the 64 nm. characteristic of the native fibers; found in the trabecular network of the eye and in aging collagen. **segment long-spacing (SLS) c.,** collagen occurring in segments about 240 nm. long instead of in fibers.

collagenase (kol-laj′ĕ-nās) an enzyme that catalyzes the hydrolysis of peptide bonds in collagen. **Clostridium histolyticum c.** [EC 3.4.24.3] an enzyme of the hydrolase class that catalyzes the cleavage of native collagen into small fragments, preferentially attacking the —gly bond in the sequence —Z—Pro—X—Gly—Pro—X. Similar collagenases are produced by various other bacteria. They are extracellular Zn^{2+} enzymes that degrade the collagen framework of muscles, facilitating the spread of gas gangrene by the organisms. Forms with different substrate specificities are known as collagenase I and II or collagenase A and B. Called also *clostridiopeptidase A.* **vertebrate c.** [EC 3.4.24.7] a group of enzymes of the hydrolase class that catalyze the cleavage of native collagen at a glycine-leucine or glycine-isoleucine bond, leaving a large amino-terminal fragment (75%) and a small carboxyl-terminal fragment (25%). They require zinc and occur ubiquitously in animals, being

involved in the degradation of collagen during tissue repair or during embryonic and fetal development.

collagenation (kol-laj″ĕ-na′shun) the appearance of collagen in developing cartilage.

collagenic (kol″ah-jen′ik) 1. collagenous. 2. collagenogenic.

collagenitis (ko-laj′ĕ-ni′tis) inflammatory involvement of collagen fibers in the fiber component of connective tissue, characterized by pain, swelling, low-grade fever, and by increased erythrocyte sedimentation rate.

collagenoblast (kol-laj′ĕ-no-blast) a cell which arises from a fibroblast and which, as it matures, is associated with the production of collagen; it may also, at times, form cartilage and bone by metaplasia. Collagenoblasts are also known as *fibroblasts.*

collagenocyte (kol-laj′ĕ-no-sīt″) a mature collagen-producing cell; see *collagenoblast.*

collagenogenic (kol″lah-jen-o-jen′ik) pertaining to or characterized by the production of collagen; forming collagen or collagen fibers.

collagenolysis (kol″ah-jen-ol′ĭ-sis) dissolution or digestion of collagen.

collagenolytic (kol-laj″ĕ-no-lit′ik) effecting the digestion of collagen.

collagenosis (kol-laj″ĕ-no′sis) collagen disease; see under *disease.*

collagenous (kol-laj′ĕ-nus) pertaining to collagen; forming or producing collagen.

collapse (kŏ-laps′) [L. *collapsus*] 1. a state of extreme prostration and depression, with failure of circulation. 2. abnormal falling in of the walls of any part or organ. **circulatory c.,** shock; circulatory insufficiency without congestive heart failure. **c. of the lung,** an airless or fetal state of all or a part of a lung, as seen in atelectasis from bronchial obstruction and in pneumothorax. **massive c.,** a condition in which an entire lung becomes airless, often due to obstruction of a main bronchus.

collar (kol′ler) an encircling band, generally around the neck. **Casal's c.,** see under *necklace.* **c. of pearls,** syphilitic leukoderma. **periosteal bone c.,** a band of spongy bone that forms around the middle of the diaphysis of early bones. **Spanish c.,** paraphimosis. **c. of Stokes,** an edematous thickening of the neck and soft parts of the thorax associated with dilatation of the veins from the neck to the diaphragm, seen in cases of obstruction of the superior vena cava. **venereal c., c. of Venus,** syphilitic leukoderma.

collarette (kol″er-et′) 1. a narrow rim of loosened keratin overhanging the periphery of a circumscribed skin lesion, attached to the normal surrounding skin, especially in moniliasis and pityriasis rosea. 2. (*obs.*) collar-like dermatitis in pellagra. 3. angular line.

collastin (kŏ-las′tin) degenerate collagenous tissue that stains like normal elastic tissue.

collateral (kŏ-lat′er-al) [L. *con* together + *la′tus* side] 1. secondary or accessory; not direct or immediate. 2. a small side branch, as of a blood vessel or nerve. **Schaffer c's,** branches of the axons of the stratum pyramidale of the hippocampus, some of which end on cells in the stratum oriens, but many of which pass into the stratum moleculare.

collenchyma (ko-leng′kĭ-mah) [Gr. *kolla* glue + *enchyma* infusion] supportive tissue occurring just beneath the epidermis of stems and leaf stalks of plants, composed of elongated living cells with walls thickened in the corner. Cf. *sclerenchyma.*

Colles' fascia, ligament, etc. (kol′ēz) [Abraham *Colles,* an Irish surgeon, 1773–1843] see *fascia diaphragmatis urogenitalis inferior* and *ligamentum inguinale reflexum,* and see under *fracture* and *space.*

Collet's syndrome (kol-lāz′) [Frédéric Justin *Collet,* Lyons laryngologist, born 1870] see under *syndrome.*

Collet-Sicard syndrome (kol-la′-se-kar′) [Frédéric Justin *Collet;* Jean Athanase *Sicard,* Paris neurologist, 1872–1929] Collet's syndrome.

colliculectomy (kŏ-lik″u-lek′to-me) [*colliculus* + Gr. *ektomē* excision] excision of the colliculus seminalis.

colliculi (kŏ-lik′u-li) [L.] genitive and plural of *colliculus.*

colliculitis (kŏ-lik″u-li′tis) inflammation about the colliculus seminalis.

colliculus (kŏ-lik′u-lus), pl. *collic′uli* [L.] a small elevation, or mound. **c. of arytenoid cartilage,** c. cartilaginis arytenoideae. **bulbar c.,** corpus spongiosum penis. **c. cartilag′inis arytenoi′deae** [NA], colliculus of arytenoid cartilage: a small eminence on the anterior margin and anterolateral surface of the arytenoid cartilage; called also *c. cartilaginis arytaenoideae.* **caudal c., c. cauda′lis** [NA], one of the caudal (inferior) pair of rounded eminences in the tectum of the mesencephalon that contains auditory reflex centers; called also *c. inferior* [NA alternative]. **c. cauda′tus,** nucleus caudatus. **cervical c. of female urethra, of Barkow,** crista urethralis femininae. **cranial c., c. crania′lis** (*obs.*), c. superior. **facial c., c. facia′lis** [NA], an elevation of the medial eminence above the medullary striae in the rhomboid fossa, caused by the internal genu of the facial nerve as it loops backward around the abducent nucleus. **inferior c., c. infe′rior,** NA alternative for *c. caudalis.* **rostral c., c. rostra′lis** [NA], one of the rostral (cranial or superior) pair of rounded eminences in the tectum of the mesencephalon that contains visual reflex centers; called also *c. cranialis* and *c. superior* [NA alternative]. **seminal c., c. semina′lis** [NA], a prominent portion of the urethral crest on which are the opening of the prostatic utricle and, on either side of it, the orifices of the ejaculatory ducts; called also *caput gallinaginis, seminal crest, seminal hillock,* and *verumontanum.* **superior c., c. supe′rior,** NA alternative for *c. rostralis.*

colligative (kol′ĭ-ga″tiv) in physical chemistry, depending on the number of molecules present in a given space, rather than on their size, molecular weight or chemical constitution. The colligative properties of solutions are osmotic pressure, boiling point elevation, freezing point depression, and vapor pressure lowering.

collimation (kol″lĭ-ma′shun) making parallel. In microscopy, the process of making light rays parallel; the process of aligning the optical axis of the optical system to the reference mechanical axes or surfaces of the instrument, or the adjustment of two or more optical axes with respect to each other. In radiology, the elimination of the peripheral (more divergent) portion of an x-ray beam by means of metal tubes, cones, or diaphragms interposed in the path of the beam. In nuclear medicine, the use of shielding to reduce the angle of view of a detector.

collimator (kol″ĭ-ma′tor) a diaphragm or system of diaphragms made of an absorbing material, designed to define the dimensions and direction of a beam of radiation.

Collin's osteoclast (kol′inz) [Anatole *Collin,* Parisian instrument maker, 1831–1923] see under *osteoclast.*

Collinsonia (kol″in-so′ne-ah) [after Peter *Collinson,* 1694–1768] a genus of labiate herbs. C. *canadensis,* stoneroot or richweed, is tonic and diuretic.

Collip unit (kol′ip) [James Bertram *Collip,* Canadian biochemist, 1892–1965] see under *unit.*

colliquation (kol″ĭ-kwa′shun) [L. *con* together + *liquare* to melt] liquefactive degeneration of tissue. **ballooning c.,** liquefaction of cell protoplasm attended by edematous swelling. **reticulating c.,** liquefaction of cell protoplasm with the formation of reticulations.

colliquative (kŏ-lik′wah-tiv) [L. *con* together + *liquare* to melt] 1. characterized by an excessive fluid discharge. 2. marked by liquefaction of tissues.

collision (ko-lĭ′zhun) in obstetrics, the contact *in utero* of any parts of one twin with those of the co-twin, so that engagement of either is prevented.

collochemistry (kol″o-kem′is-tre) the chemistry of colloids.

collodiaphyseal (kol″o-di″ah-fiz′e-al) [L. *collum* neck + *diaphysis*] pertaining to the neck and shaft of a long bone, especially the femur.

collodion (ko-lo′de-on) [L. *collodium,* from Gr. *kollōdēs* glutinous] [USP] a clear or slightly opalescent, highly flammable, syrupy liquid compounded of pyroxylin, ether, and alcohol, which dries to a transparent, tenacious film; used as a topical protectant, applied to the skin to close small wounds, abrasions, and cuts, to hold surgical dressings in place, and to keep medications in contact with the skin. **c. elastique,** flexible c. **flexible c.** [USP], a preparation of camphor, castor oil, and collodion, used for the same purposes

as collodion but providing a flexible, contracting film. Called also *c. elastique.* **salicylic acid c.** [USP], a preparation containing between 9.5 and 11.5 per cent salicylic acid in flexible collodion; used as a topical keratolytic for warts and corns.

colloid (kol′oid) [Gr. *kollōdēs* glutinous] 1. glutinous or resembling glue. 2. a state of matter in which the matter is dispersed in or distributed throughout some medium called the dispersion medium. The matter thus dispersed is called the disperse phase of the colloid system. The particles of the disperse phase are larger than an ordinary crystalloid molecule, but are not large enough to settle out under the influence of gravity, and they resist diffusion; they range in size from 1 to 100 nm. or up to 500 or 1000 nm., the range being indefinite and arbitrary. There are two kinds of colloids: *suspension colloids* (suspensoids), in which the disperse phase consists of particles of any insoluble substance, as a metal, and the dispersion medium may be gaseous, liquid, or solid; and *emulsion colloids* (emulsoids), in which the dispersion medium is usually water and the disperse phase consists of highly complex organic substances, such as starch or glue, which absorb much water, swell, and become uniformly distributed throughout the dispersion medium in a manner not well understood. The former tend to be less stable than the latter. Cf. *crystalloid.* 3. the translucent, yellowish, gelatinous substance resulting from colloid degeneration. **amyl c., anodyne c.,** a local anodyne preparation containing ½ ounce each of amyl hydride and absolute alcohol, 1 grain aconitine, 6 grains veratrine, and 2 oz. of collodion. **antimony trisulfide c.,** antimony sulfide (Sb_2S_3), a pharmaceutic aid. **association c.,** a colloid in which the dispersed particles are each made up of many molecules. **bovine c.,** conglutinin. **dispersion c.,** see *colloid,* def. 2. **emulsion c.,** see *colloid,* def. 2. **hydrophilic c.,** emulsion c.; see *colloid,* def. 2. **hydrophobic c.,** suspension c.; see *colloid,* def. 2. **irreversible c.,** a colloid that cannot be dispersed. Cf. *reversible c.* **lyophilic c.,** emulsion c.; see *colloid,* def. 2. **lyophobic c.,** suspension c.; see *colloid,* def. 2. **lyotropic c.,** emulsion c.; see *colloid,* def. 2. **protective c.,** one that is able to prevent the precipitation of another colloid. **reversible c.,** a colloid that can be dispersed after having been precipitated or a gel that can be converted into a sol. **stable c.,** reversible c. **stannous sulfur c.,** a sulfur colloid containing stannous ions formed by reacting sodium thiosulfate with hydrochloric acid, then adding stannous ions; a diagnostic aid (bone, liver, and spleen imaging). **suspension c.,** see *colloid,* def. 2. **thyroid c.,** the colloid found in the acini of the thyroid gland, consisting essentially of thyroglobulin.

colloidal (kŏ-loi′dal) of the nature of a colloid. **c-S,** an iron-oxide preparation used intravenously in severe infections.

colloidin (ko-loi′din) a jelly-like substance, $C_9H_{15}NO_6$, one of the products of colloid degeneration.

colloidoclasis (kŏ-loi″do-kla′sis) colloidoclasia.

colloidophagy (kol″oi-dof′ah-je) [*colloid* + Gr. *phagein* to eat] resorption of colloid by macrophages under the influence of the thyroid-stimulating hormone.

colloxylin (kŏ-lok′sĭ-lin) [Gr. *kolla* glue + *xylinos* woody] pyroxylin.

collum (kol′um), pl. *col′la* [L.] [NA] 1. the neck: the portion of the body connecting the head and trunk; the lower front portion of the collum is called the cervix, and the back is called the nucha. 2. a general term applied to any necklike part of a body structure or organ. **c. anatom′icum hu′meri** [NA], anatomical neck of humerus: the somewhat constricted zone on the humerus just distal to the head, separating the articular surface from the tubercles. **c. chirur′gicum hu′meri** [NA], surgical neck of humerus: the region on the humerus just below the tubercles, where the bone becomes constricted. **c. cos′tae** [NA], neck of rib: the part of a rib extending from the head to the tubercle. **c. den′tis** [NA], cervix dentis. **c. distor′tum,** torticollis. **c. fib′ulae** [NA], neck of the fibula: the portion of the fibula between the head and shaft. **c. follic′uli pi′li,** the narrow portion of a hair follicle between the hair bulb and the opening on the surface of the skin. Called also *neck of hair follicle.* **c. glan′dis pe′nis** [NA], neck of the glans penis: the constricted portion between the corona of the glans penis and the corpora cavernosa; called also *cervix* *glandis.* **c. mal′lei** [NA], neck of malleus: the constricted portion of the malleus below the head; called also *cervix mallei.* **c. mandib′ulae** [NA], neck of mandible: the narrow portion supporting the condyle of the mandible; called also *c. processus condyloidei mandibulae.* **c. os′sis fem′oris** [NA], neck of femur: the heavy column of bone connecting the head of the femur and the shaft. **c. proces′sus condyloi′dei mandib′ulae,** c. mandibulae. **c. ra′dii** [NA], neck of radius: the somewhat constricted portion of the radius just distal to the head. **c. scap′ulae** [NA], neck of scapula: the somewhat constricted part of the scapula that surrounds the lateral angle. **c. ta′li** [NA], neck of talus: the constriction between the head and body of the talus. **c. val′gum,** coxa valga. **c. vesi′cae bilia′ris** [NA], neck of gallbladder: the upper constricted portion of the gallbladder, between the body and the cystic duct; called also *c. vesicae felleae* [NA alternative]. **c. vesi′cae fel′leae,** NA alternative for *c. vesicae biliaris.*

collunaria (kol″u-na′re-ah) [L.] plural of *collunarium.*

collunarium (kol″u-na′re-um), pl. *colluna′ria* [L.] a nasal douche.

Collut. abbreviation for L. *collutorium* (mouth wash).

collutoria (kol″u-to′re-ah) [L.] plural of *collutorium.*

collutorium (kol″u-to′re-um), pl. *colluto′ria* [L.] collutory.

collutory (kol″u-to″re) [L. *collutorium*] a mouthwash or gargle. **Miller′s c.,** a mouth wash containing benzoic acid, tincture of krameria, oil of peppermint.

Collyr. abbreviation for L. *collyr′ium,* an eye wash.

collyria (ko-lir′e-ah) [L.] plural of *collyrium.*

Collyriculum (kol″le-rik′u-lum) a genus of trematode parasites. **c. fa′ba,** a trematode parasite forming subcutaneous cysts in chickens, turkeys, and sparrows.

collyrium (kŏ-lir′e-um), pl. *collyr′ia* [L.; Gr. *kollyrion* eye salve] a lotion for the eyes; an eye wash. **Beer′s c.,** lead acetate, rose water, and spirit of rosemary.

coloboma (kol″o-bo′mah), pl. *colobomas* or *colobo′mata* [L.; Gr. *kolobōma* defect, from *koloboun* to mutilate] an absence or defect of some ocular tissue, usually resulting from malclosure of the fetal intraocular fissure, or sometimes from trauma or disease. Colobomatous anomalies range from a small pit in the optic disk to extensive defects in the iris, ciliary body, choroid, retina, and optic disk. A scotoma is usually present, corresponding to the area of the coloboma. **atypical c′s,** one not originating from the embryonic cleft

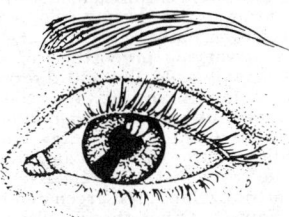

Coloboma of the iris.

nor located in the inferonasal quadrant of the eye; it is usually unilateral. **bridge c.,** a narrow zone of normal fundus between a retinochoroidal coloboma and an optic nerve coloboma. **c. of choroid,** fissure in the choroid, causing a scotoma on the retina, and often associated with defects of the ciliary body and iris. **c. of ciliary body,** a white lesion surrounded by varying pigment and affecting the iris and lens. It is the most frequent congenital defect of the ciliary body and common in trisomy 13. **complete c.,** a typical coloboma when it extends from the pupillary margin to the posterior pole, therefore involving the iris, ciliary body, choroid, retina, and optic disk. **Fuchs′s c.,** a small conus or crescent on the choroid, at the lower edge of the optic disk. **c. of fundus,** retinochoroidal c. **c. i′ridis, c. of iris,** a keyhole-shaped notch in the inferonasal quadrant of the eye; it may also result from an iridectomy. **c. of lens, c. len′tis,** a cleft at the edge of the lens, extending down, with a defect in the zonule of Zinn in the same area. **c. lob′uli,** fissure of the ear lobe, which may occur as a congenital defect, or be acquired. **c. of optic disk, c. of optic nerve,** 1. a coloboma, mild or severe, within or at the optic nerve head. A mild coloboma may be a separate, isolated entity, unilateral, and limited to minor cupping in the optic

disk. A severe coloboma may be part of a bridge coloboma or part of a complete coloboma, or it may enlarge the optic disk two to four times and thus affect the adjacent retina and choroid. Nystagmus, strabismus, severe impairment of vision, microphthalmia, cyclopia, and anencephaly may be present. 2. a defect attributed to the incomplete closure of the fetal fissure of the optic stalk. **c. at optic nerve entrance,** a coloboma of the optic disk that affects only the optic nerve. **c. palpebra′le,** a vertical fissure of an eyelid. **peripapillary c.,** a chorioretinal defect surrounding or extending down from the optic disk. **c. of retina, c. re′tinae,** a congenital fissure of the retina attributed to incomplete closure of the fetal fissure in the optic cup. **retinochoroidal c.,** an absence of retinal and choroidal tissue, usually in the lower fundus, marked by a bright white ectatic zone of exposed sclera extending into and distorting the optic disk. Called also *c. of fundus.* **typical c.,** a defect resulting from incomplete or irregular, or lack of fusion of the lips of the embryonic intraocular fissure by the end of the sixth or seventh week. A typical coloboma is found in the lower nasal quadrant of the eye and is often bilateral. **c. of vitreous,** a notch in the lower border of the vitreous.

colocecostomy (ko″lo-se-kos′to-me) [*colon* + *cecum* + Gr. *stomoun* to provide with an opening, or mouth] cecocolostomy.

colocentesis (ko″lo-sen-te′sis) [*colon* + Gr. *kentēsis* puncture] surgical puncture of the colon for the withdrawal of fluid or gas; called also *colopuncture.*

colocholecystostomy (ko″lo-ko″le-sis-tos′to-me) cholecystostomy.

coloclysis (ko″lo-kli′sis) [*colon* + Gr. *klysis* a drenching] irrigation of the colon.

coloclyster (ko″lo-klis′ter) an enema injected into the colon through the rectum.

colocolostomy (ko″lo-ko-los′to-me) [*colon* + *colostomy*] surgical formation of an anastomosis between two portions of the colon.

colocutaneous (ko″lo-ku-ta′ne-us) pertaining to the colon and skin, or communicating with the colon and the cutaneous surface of the body, as colocutaneous fistula.

colocynth (kol′o-sinth) [L. *colocynthis;* Gr. *kolokynthē*] the dried pulp of the unripe but full-grown fruit of *Citrullus colocynthus;* used as a drastic cathartic. Called also *bitter apple* and *bitter cucumber.*

colocynthidism (kol″o-sin′thĭ-dizm) poisoning by colocynth.

colocynthin (kol″o-sin′thin) a bitter, purgative glycoside, $C_{38}H_{54}O_{13}$, from colocynth.

colocynthis (kol″o-sin′this), gen. *colocyn′thidis* [L.] colocynth.

colodyspepsia (ko″lo-dis-pep′se-ah) dyspepsia due to reflex disturbance set up by the constipated colon.

coloenteritis (ko″lo-en″ter-i′tis) [*colon* + *enteritis*] enterocolitis.

colofixation (ko″lo-fik-sa′shun) fixation or suspension of the colon.

Cologel (kol′o-jel) trademark for a preparation of methylcellulose.

colohepatopexy (ko″lo-hep′ah-to-pek″se) [*colon* + Gr. *hēpar* liver + *pēxis* fixation] fixation of the colon to the liver to prevent the formation of adhesions between the liver and the stomach.

coloileal (ko″lo-il′e-al) ileocolic.

cololysis (ko-lol′ĭ-sis) [*colon* + Gr. *lysis* dissolution] the division of pericolic adhesions.

colometrometer (ko″lo-mĕ-trom′ĕ-ter) an apparatus for measuring the activity of the colon.

colon (ko′lon) [L.; Gr. *kolon*] [NA] that part of the large intestine which extends from the cecum to the rectum; sometimes used inaccurately as a synonym for the entire large intestine. **c. ascen′dens** [NA], **ascending c.,** the portion of the colon between the cecum and the right colic flexure. **c. descen′dens** [NA], **descending c.,** the portion of the colon between the left colic flexure and the sigmoid colon at the pelvic brim; the portion of the descending colon lying in the left iliac fossa is sometimes called the *iliac colon.* **giant c.,** megacolon. **iliac c.,** that part of the descending colon lying in the left iliac fossa and continuous with the sigmoid colon. **irritable c.,** see *irritable bowel* *syndrome,* under *syndrome.* **lead-pipe c.,** a term applied to the radiological appearance of a diseased colon which has become shortened, contracted, and rigid owing to inflammatory fibrosis. In such a colon the normal haustral pattern is lost and function may be impaired. This is usually a consequence of chronic ulcerative or granulomatous colitis. **left c.,** the distal portion of the large intestine, developing embryonically from the hind gut and functioning in the storage and elimination from the body of nonabsorbed residue. **pelvic c.,** sigmoid c. **right c.,** the proximal portion of the large intestine, extending from the ileocecal valve usually to a point proximal to the left colic flexure, developing embryonically from the terminal portion of the midgut and functioning in absorption. **sigmoid c., c. sigmoi′deum** [NA], the S-shaped part of the colon which lies in the pelvis, extending from the pelvic brim to the third segment of the sacrum, and continuous above with the descending (or iliac) colon and below with the rectum; called also *pelvic c.* and *sigmoid flexure.* **spastic c.,** see *irritable bowel syndrome,* under *syndrome.* **transverse c., c. transver′sum** [NA], the portion of the colon that runs transversely across the upper part of the abdomen, from the right to the left colic flexure.

colonalgia (ko″lon-al′je-ah) [*colon* + *-algia*] pain in the colon.

colonic (ko-lon′ik) pertaining to the colon.

colonitis (ko″lo-ni′tis) colitis.

colonization (kol″ŏ-ni-za′shun) innidiation.

Colonna's operation (kŏ-lŏn′ah) [Paul *Colonna,* American orthopedic surgeon, 1892–1966] see under *operation.*

colonopathy (ko″lo-nop′ah-the) [*colon* + Gr. *pathos* disease.] any disease or disorder of the colon.

colonorrhagia (ko″lon-o-ra′je-ah) hemorrhage from the colon.

colonoscope (ko-lon′o-skōp) [*colon* + Gr. *skopein* to examine] an elongated flexible endoscope which permits visual examination of the entire colon; called also *coloscope.*

colonoscopy (ko″lon-os′ko-pe) examination by means of the colonoscope. Called also *coloscopy.*

colony (kol′o-ne) [L. *colonia*] a collection or group of bacteria in a culture derived from the increase of an isolated single organism or group of organisms. **checker c.,** a round, steeply elevated colony with a flat top, resembling the disk used in a game of checkers. It is frequently seen in cultures of *Streptococcus pneumoniae* on blood agar. **D. c.,** dwarf c. **daisy-head c.,** a round gray or black colony with a narrow translucent scalloped border, typically produced by *Corynebacterium diphtheriae* on tellurite blood agar. **daughter c.,** a small bacterial colony formed as a papilla on the surface or in the margin of an older colony. **dwarf c.,** a bacterial colony smaller than normal and containing poorly developed forms; called also *D. colony.* **gregaloid c.,** a transient grouping of protozoa formed by union of previously independent organisms; seen in sarcodines and in the ameboid stages of certain other protozoa. Called also *gregaloid.* **H c.** (Ger. *Hauch* film), a type of bacterial colony that spreads in a thin film over the culture medium. **M. c.,** mucoid c. **motile c.,** one that moves across the surface of the culture plate leaving lines of bacterial cells on the paths of motion, typical of colonies of *Bacillus circulans.* **mucoid c.,** one that is large, dome-shaped, and shiny, containing large quantities of capsular polysaccharide material that may be drawn out in viscous strings by a needle; called also *M. c.* **O c.** (Ger. *ohne Hauch* without film), a bacterial colony that is discrete and compact, as contrasted with an H colony. **R. c., rough c.,** a bacterial colony showing a rough, wrinkled, granular, flattened surface; known as R-type. **S. c., smooth c.,** a bacterial colony showing the smooth, glistening, rounded, regular surface, normally shown by colonies of organisms; known as S-type. **satellite c.,** a bacterial colony that grows more vigorously in the immediate vicinity of a colony of some other organism, as *Hemophilus influenzae* near a colony of staphylococci; called also *bacterial satellite.*

colopathy (ko-lop′ah-the) colonopathy.

colopexia (ko″lo-pek′se-ah) colopexy.

colopexotomy (ko″lo-pek-sot′o-me) [*colon* + Gr. *pēxis* fixation + *tomē* a cutting] incision and fixation of the colon.

colopexy (ko′lo-pek″se) [*colon* + Gr. *pēxis* fixation] fixation or suspension of the colon by surgical means.

colophony (ko-lof′ŏ-ne) [L. *colophonia;* Gr. *Kolophōn* (Colophon) a city of Asia Minor] former name of rosin.

coloplication (ko″lo-pli-ka′shun) [*colon* + L. *plica* fold] the operation of infolding or taking tucks in the wall of the colon in cases of dilatation to shorten or decrease its lumen.

coloproctectomy (ko″lo-prok-tek′to-me) surgical removal of the colon and rectum.

coloproctitis (ko″lo-prok-ti′tis) inflammation of the colon and rectum.

coloproctostomy (ko″lo-prok-tos′to-me) [*colon* + Gr. *prōktos* anus + *stomoun* to provide with an opening, or mouth] colorectostomy.

coloptosis (ko″lop-to′sis) [*colon* + Gr. *ptōsis* fall] downward displacement of the colon, a term based on the outmoded concept that variations in the position of abdominal organs are pathological.

colopuncture (ko′lo-punk″tūr) colocentesis.

Color. abbreviation for L. *colore′tur,* let it be colored.

color (kul′or) [L. *color, colos*] 1. a property of a surface or substance resulting from absorption of certain of the incident light rays and reflection of others falling within the range of wavelengths (roughly 370–760 mμ) adequate to excite the retinal receptors. 2. radiant energy within the range of adequate chromatic stimuli of the retina, that is, between the infrared and ultraviolet. 3. a sensory impression of one of the rainbow hues, excited by stimulation of the retinal receptors, notably the cones, by radiant energy of the appropriate wavelength. **complementary c's,** a pair of colors the sensory mechanisms for which are so linked that when they are mixed on the color wheel they cancel each other out, leaving neutral gray; complementary colors are also associated with each other in after-image and contrast. **confusion c's,** different colors that are likely to be mistakenly matched by individuals with defective color vision (e.g., violet and blue with defect of vision for red); for this reason they are combined in the design on charts used for detecting different types of color vision defects. **contrast c.,** an illusory tinge of complementary hue or brightness induced by a vivid hue or luminance on the area surrounding it in the visual field. **incidental c.,** that seen as an after-image. **metameric c's,** colors that appear identical to the normal eye, but which are the resultants of different combinations of chromatic stimuli or wavelengths. **Munsell's c's,** a set of standardized colors, representing 40 hues in varying degrees of brightness and saturation, identifiable by a simple letter-number formula. **primary c's,** a small number of fundamental colors, usually referred to the retinal receptor cones, mixture of varying proportions of the approximate stimuli of which will yield the 150 discriminable hues of normal human vision. According to (*a*) the Newton theory, the seven rainbow hues: violet, indigo, blue, green, yellow, orange, red; (*b*) the painter and printer: blue (cyan), yellow, red (or magenta); (*c*) the Helmholtzian theory (old school): red, green, blue (or violet); (*d*) the Hering theory: four paired complementary hues, red-green and blue-yellow, plus a black-white pair. (*e*) Other theories list five to seven colors as primaries. **pseudoisochromatic c's,** colors that appear the same to an individual with defective color vision; see *confusion c's.* **pure c.,** a color whose stimulus consists of homogeneous wavelengths, with little or no admixture of other hues. **saturation c.,** one that is high on the chroma or vividness scale, the farthest possible removed from gray.

coloration (kul″er-a′shun) the state of being colored; an arrangement of colors distinguishing a species. **protective c.,** coloration that blends with the background, making the organism less visible to predators. **warning c.,** brilliant, conspicuous coloration of poisonous or unpalatable animals, as a warning to potential predators.

colorectal (ko″lo-rek′tal) pertaining to or affecting the colon and rectum.

colorectitis (ko″lo-rek-ti′tis) coloproctitis.

colorectostomy (ko″lo-rek-tos′to-me) [*colon* + *rectum* + Gr. *stomoun* to provide with an opening, or mouth] formation of an artificial opening between the colon and rectum; called also *coloproctostomy.*

colorectum (kol″o-rek′tum) the colon and rectum considered as a unit.

colorimeter (kul″or-im′ĕ-ter) [*color* + Gr. *metron* measure] an instrument for measuring color differences; especially one for measuring the color of the blood in order to determine the proportion of hemoglobin. Called also *chromometer*. **Duboscq's c.,** an apparatus for measuring concentration by comparing the tint of the substance in question against that of a standard. **titration c.,** a device using colorimetric technique to automatically stop titration at the end point.

colorrhaphy (ko-lor′ah-fe) [*colon* + Gr. *rhaphē* suture] suture or repair of the colon.

colorrhea (ko″lo-re′ah) a discharge of mucus from the colon.

coloscope (kol′o-skōp) colonoscope.

coloscopy (ko-los′ko-pe) colonoscopy.

colosigmoidostomy (ko″lo-sig″moi-dos′to-me) surgical creation of an artificial opening between the sigmoid and the proximal portion of the colon.

colostomy (ko-los′to-me) [*colon* + Gr. *stomoun* to provide with an opening, or mouth] the surgical creation of an opening between the colon and the surface of the body; also used to refer to the opening, or stoma, so created. **dry c.,** colostomy performed in the left half of the colon, the discharge from the stoma consisting of soft or formed fecal residue. **Hartmann's c.,** see under *procedure*. **ileotransverse c.,** surgical anastomosis between the ileum and the transverse colon. **Mikulicz c.,** see under *operation* (def. 5). **wet c.,** colostomy in (*a*) the right half of the colon, the drainage from which is liquid in character, or (*b*) the left half of the colon following anastomosis of the ureters to the sigmoid or descending colon so that urine is also expelled through the same stoma.

colostric (ko-los′trik) pertaining to or occurring in colostrum.

colostrorrhea (ko-los″tro-re′ah) [L. *colostrum* + Gr. *rhoia* flow] spontaneous discharge of colostrum.

colostrous (ko-los′trus) [L. *colostrosus*] containing or filled with colostrum.

colostrum (kŏ-los′trum) [L.] the thin, yellow, milky fluid secreted by the mammary gland a few days before or after parturition. It contains up to 20 per cent protein, predominant among which are immunoglobulins, representing the antibodies found in maternal blood. It contains more minerals and less fat and carbohydrate than does milk. It also contains many colostrum corpuscles and usually will coagulate on boiling due to a large amount of lactalbumin. **c. gravida′rum,** the colostrum secreted before parturition, and especially that secreted during the first few days following delivery. **c. puerpera′rum,** the colostrum secreted after labor.

colotomy (ko-lot′o-me) [*colo-* + Gr. *tomē* a cutting] incision into the colon for removal of a foreign body, polyp, or other benign tumor. Cf. *colostomy*.

colovaginal (ko″lo-vaj′ĕ-nal) pertaining to or communicating with the colon and vagina, as a colovaginal fistula.

colovesical (ko″lo-ves′ĭ-kal) pertaining to or communicating with the colon and urinary bladder, as a colovesical fistula.

colpalgia (kol-pal′je-ah) [*colp-* + *-algia*] vaginodynia.

colpatresia (kol″pah-tre′ze-ah) [*colp-* + *atresia*] atresia or occlusion of the vagina.

colpectasia (kol-pek-ta′se-ah) [*colp-* + Gr. *ektasis* distention + *-ia*] distention or dilatation of the vagina.

colpectasis (kol-pek′tah-sis) colpectasia.

colpectomy (kol-pek′to-me) [*colp-* + Gr. *ektomē* excision] excision of the vagina.

colpeurynter (kol′pu-rin″ter) [*colp-* + Gr. *eurynein* to dilate] metreurynter.

colpeurysis (kol-pu′rĭ-sis) [*colp-* + Gr. *eurynein* to dilate] dilation of the vagina.

colpismus (kol-piz′mus) [Gr. *kolpos* vagina] vaginismus.

colpitis (kol-pi′tis) [*colpo-* + *-itis*] inflammation of the vagina; see also *vaginitis*. **c. emphysemato′sa, emphysematous c.,** vaginitis emphysematosa. **c. mycot′ica,** vaginomycosis.

colp(o)- [Gr. *kolpos* vagina] a combining form denoting relationship to the vagina.

colpocele (kol′po-sēl) [*colpo-* + Gr. *kēlē* hernia] vaginocele.

colpoceliocentesis (kol″po-se″le-o-sen-te′sis) puncture of the abdominal cavity through the vagina, usually the posterior vault.

colpoceliotomy (kol″po-se″le-ot′o-me) [*colpo-* + Gr. *koilia* belly + *tomē* a cutting] incision into the abdomen through the vaginal wall.

colpocleisis (kol″po-kli′sis) [*colpo-* + Gr. *kleisis* closure] surgical closure of the vaginal canal.

colpocystitis (kol″po-sis-ti′tis) [*colpo-* + Gr. *kystis* bladder + *itis*] inflammation of the vagina and of the bladder.

colpocystocele (kol″po-sis′to-sēl) [*colpo-* + Gr. *kystis* bladder + *kēlē* hernia] hernia of the bladder into the vagina, of which the anterior wall becomes prolapsed.

colpocystoplasty (kol″po-sis′to-plas″te) [*colpo-* + Gr. *kystis* bladder + *plassein* to form] plastic operation for the repair of the vesicovaginal wall.

colpocystotomy (kol″po-sis-tot′o-me) [*colpo-* + Gr. *kystis* bladder + *tomē* cutting] incision of the bladder through the vaginal wall.

colpocystoureterocystotomy (kol″po-sis″to-u-re″ter-o-sis-tot′o-me) [*colpo-* + Gr. *kystis* bladder + *ourētēr* ureter + *cystotomy*] the operation of exposing the ureteral orifices by incising the walls of the bladder and the vagina.

colpocytogram (kol″po-si′to-gram) a tabulation of the various types of cells observed in smears taken from the mucous membrane of the vagina.

colpocytology (kol″po-si-tol′o-je) the quantitative and differential study of cells exfoliated from the epithelium of the vagina.

Colpodida (kol-po′dĭ-dah) [Gr. *kolpos* a bosom or fold] an order of mostly free-living, commonly in the soil, ciliate, often reniform protozoa (subclass Vestibuliferia, class Kinetofragminophores).

colpodynia (kol″po-din′e-ah) [*colpo-* + Gr. *odynē* pain] vaginodynia.

colpohyperplasia (kol″po-hi-per-pla′ze-ah) [*colpo-* + *hyperplasia*] excessive growth of the mucous membrane and wall of the vagina. **c. cys′tica,** a variety characterized by the presence of cysts in the mucous membrane. **c. emphysemato′sa,** a variety characterized by the presence of small gas-filled spaces in the mucous membrane.

colpohysterectomy (kol″po-his″ter-ek′to-me) [*colpo-* + *hysterectomy*] (obs.) vaginal hysterectomy.

colpohysterotomy (kol″po-his-ter-ot′o-me) [*colpo-* + *hysterotomy*] (obs.) vaginal hysterotomy.

colpomicroscope (kol″po-mi′kro-skōp) an instrument especially designed for insertion into the vagina, for the microscopic examination of tissues of the cervix in situ; it has higher powers of magnification than the colposcope.

colpomicroscopic (kol″po-mi″kro-skop′ik) pertaining to the colpomicroscope, or to colpomicroscopy.

colpomicroscopy (kol″po-mi-kros′ko-pe) examination of tissues of the cervix in situ with the colpomicroscope.

colpomyomectomy (kol″po-mi″o-mek′to-me) [*colpo-* + *myomectomy*] surgical removal of a uterine myoma (leiomyoma) performed through a vaginal incision.

colpoperineoplasty (kol″po-per″ĭ-ne′o-plas″te) [*colpo-* + Gr. *perinaion* perineum + *plassein* to form] vaginoperineoplasty.

colpoperineorrhaphy (kol″po-per″ĭ-ne-or′ah-fe) [*colpo-* + Gr. *perinaion* perineum + *rhaphē* suture] vaginoperineorrhaphy.

colpopexy (kol′po-pek″se) [*colpo-* + Gr. *pēxis* fixation] suture of the prolapsed vagina to the abdominal wall; vaginofixation.

colpoplasty (kol′po-plas″te) [*colpo-* + Gr. *plassein* to shape] vaginoplasty.

colpopoiesis (kol″po-poi-e′sis) [*colpo-* + Gr. *poiein* to make] the creation of a vagina by plastic surgery.

colpoptosis (kol″po-to′sis) [*colpo-* + Gr. *ptōsis* prolapse] vaginocele.

colporectopexy (kol″po-rek′to-pek″se) [*colpo-* + *rectum* + Gr. *pēxis* fixation] suspension of a prolapsed rectum by suture to the vaginal wall.

colporrhagia (kol″po-ra′je-ah) [*colpo-* + Gr. *rhēgnynai* to burst out] vaginal hemorrhage.

colporrhaphy (kol-por′ah-fe) [*colpo-* + Gr. *rhaphē* suture] 1. the operation of suturing the vagina. 2. the operation of denuding and suturing the vaginal wall for the purpose of narrowing the vagina.

colporrhexis (kol″po-rek′sis) [colpo- + Gr. *rhēxis* rupture] laceration of the vagina.

colposcope (kol′po-skōp) [colpo- + Gr. *skopein* to examine] originally a speculum for examining the vagina; now an instrument inserted into the vagina for examination of the tissues of the vagina and cervix by means of a magnifying lens. Cf. *colpomicroscope*.

colposcopic (kol″po-skop′ik) relating to the colposcope or to colposcopy.

colposcopy (kol-pos′ko-pe) examination of the cervix and vagina by means of the colposcope.

colpospasm (kol′po-spazm) [colpo- + Gr. *spasmos* spasm] vaginal spasm.

colpostat (kol′po-stat) [colpo- + Gr. *statos* standing] an appliance for retaining something, such as radium, in the vagina.

colpostenosis (kol″po-stĕ-no′sis) [colpo- + Gr. *stenōsis* stricture] contraction or narrowing of the vagina.

colpostenotomy (kol″po-stĕ-not′o-me) [colpo- + Gr. *stenōsis* stricture + *tomē* a cutting] a cutting operation for stricture or atresia of the vagina.

colpotomy (kol-pot′o-me) [colpo- + Gr. *tomē* a cutting] incision of the vagina with entry into the cul-de-sac; called also *vaginotomy*. **posterior c.,** culdotomy.

colpoureterocystotomy (kol″po-u-re″ter-o-sis-tot′o-me) [colpo- + *ureter* + *cystotomy*] the exposure of the orifices of the ureters by cutting through the walls of the vagina and bladder.

colpoureterotomy (kol″po-u-re″ter-ot′o-me) incision of the ureter through the vagina, performed for the relief of ureteral stricture.

colpoxerosis (kol″po-ze-ro′sis) [colpo- + Gr. *xēros* dry] abnormal dryness of the vulva and vagina.

colterol mesylate (kōl′tĕ-rōl) chemical name: (±)-4-[2-[(1,1-dimethylethyl)amino]-1-hydroxyethyl] 1,2-benzenediol methanesulfonate (salt); a bronchodilator, $C_{12}H_{19}NO_3 \cdot CH_4O_3S$.

Coluber (kol′u-ber) a genus of nonvenomous snakes (family Colubridae) found in northeastern Asia and North America. *C. constrictor*, is the American blacksnake or black racer.

colubrid (kol′ŭ-brid) 1. any snake of the family Colubridae. 2. of or pertaining to the family Colubridae.

Colubridae (kol-u′brĭ-de) [L. *coluber* serpent] a family of snakes; most of the species are harmless, though the boomslang of South Africa is venomous. See table accompanying *snake*.

columbium (ko-lum′be-um) a former name of the element *niobium*.

columella (kol″u-mel′lah), pl. *columel′lae* [L. "small column," dim. of *columna* column] 1. any of various columnlike anatomical structures. 2. in certain fungi and protozoa, a sterile invagination of the sporangiophore into the fertile area of the sporangium. Called also *columellae*. **c. coch′leae,** modiolus. **c. for′nicis** (*obs.*), columna fornicis. **c. na′si,** the fleshy distal margin of the nasal septum.

columellae (kol″u-mel′e) [L.] genitive and plural of *columella*.

column (kol′um) [L. *colum′na*] an anatomical part in the form of a pillar-like structure, sometimes used specifically for the gray column of the spinal cord; see also *columna*. **c's of abdominal ring,** thickened fibers of the aponeurosis of the external oblique muscle around the superficial abdominal ring. **anal c's,** columnae anales. **anterior c. of fauces,** arcus palatoglossus. **anterior c. of spinal cord,** columna ventralis medullae spinalis. **anterolateral c.,** funiculus lateralis medullae spinalis. **autonomic c. of spinal cord,** columna intermediolateralis medullae spinalis. **c's of Bertin,** columnae renales. **c. of Burdach,** fasciculus cuneatus medullae spinalis. **Clarke's c.** columna thoracica. **dorsal c.,** columna vertebralis. **dorsal gray c.,** nucleus proprius. **dorsal c. of spinal cord,** columna dorsalis medullae spinalis. **enamel c's,** prismata adamantina. **fleshy c's of heart,** trabeculae carneae cordis. **c's of folds of tongue,** papillae foliatae. **fornix c., c. of fornix,** columna fornicis. **fractionating c.,** an apparatus for sep-

arating the volatile constituents of a solution by distillation. **fundamental c.,** fasciculi proprii. **c. of Goll,** fasciculus gracilis medullae spinalis. **Gowers' c.,** tractus spinocerebellaris ventralis. **gray c's,** columnae griseae. **gray c. of spinal cord, anterior,** columna anterior medullae spinalis. **gray c. of spinal cord, lateral,** columna lateralis medullae spinalis. **gray c. of spinal cord, posterior,** columna posterior medullae spinalis. **interomediolateral c. of spinal cord,** columna interomediolateralis medullae spinalis. **c. of Kölliker,** sarcostyle, def. 2. **lateral c. of spinal cord,** columna lateralis medullae spinalis. **c. of Lissauer,** tractus dorsolateralis. **c's of Morgagni,** columnae anales. **muscle c.,** sarcostyle, def. 2. **c. of nose,** septum nasi. **positive c.,** a pinkish stream of light seen when a current of high potential is passed through a tube from which the air has been partly exhausted. **posterior c. of fauces,** arcus palatopharyngeus. **posterior c. of spinal cord,** columna dorsalis medullae spinalis. **posteroexternal c.,** the outer wider portion of the posterior column of the spinal cord. **posteromedian c. of medulla oblongata,** fasciculus gracilis medullae oblongatae. **posteromedian c. of spinal cord,** fasciculus gracilis medullae spinalis. **Rathke's c's,** two cartilages at the anterior end of the notochord. **rectal c's,** columnae anales. **renal c's of Bertin,** columnae renales. **c's of rugae of vagina,** columnae rugarum vaginae. **c. of Sertoli,** an elongated Sertoli cell in the parietal layer of the seminiferous tubules. **spinal c.,** columna vertebralis. **c. of Spitzka-Lissauer,** tractus dorsolateralis. **Stilling's c.,** columna thoracica. **striomotor c.,** an efferent column of the anterior horn of the spinal cord supplying striated muscle. **thoracic c.,** columna thoracica. **Türck's c.,** tractus pyramidalis anterior. **c's of vagina,** columnae rugarum vaginae. **ventral c. of spinal cord,** columna ventralis medullae spinalis. **vertebral c.,** the columnar assemblage of the vertebrae from the cranium through the coccyx; called also *axon, columna vertebralis* [NA], *backbone, spine,* and *dorsal* or *spinal c.*

columna (ko-lum′nah), pl. *colum′nae* [L.] [NA] column: a pillar-like structure; in anatomical nomenclature, used to designate a pillar-like structure or part. **colum′nae ana′les** [NA], **colum′nae a′ni,** anal columns: vertical ridges or folds of mucous membrane at the upper half of the anal canal; called also *columnae rectales* [*Morgagnii*], *rectal columns, columns of Morgagni,* and *mucous folds of rectum*. **c. ante′rior medul′lae spina′lis,** NA alternative for *c. ventralis medullae spinalis*. **c. autonom′ica medul′lae spina′lis,** NA alternative for *c. interomediolateralis medullae spinalis*. **colum′nae berti′ni,** columnae renales. **colum′nae car′neae cor′dis,** trabeculae carneae cordis. **c. dorsa′lis medul′lae spina′lis** [NA], dorsal column of spinal cord: the dorsal portion of the gray substance of the spinal cord, comprising groups of motoneurons extending the whole length of the spinal cord and two groups limited to the thoracic and upper lumbar segments; in transverse section it is seen as a horn (*cornu dorsale medullae spinalis*). Called also *posterior column of spinal cord* and *c. posterior medullae spinalis* [NA alternative]. See also *c. griseae*. **c. for′nicis** [NA], fornix column: either of the two columnar masses of fibers diverging from the anterior end of the body of the fornix to descend into the diencephalon; called also *anterior pillar of fornix, column of fornix,* and *columella fornicis*. **colum′nae gri′seae** [NA], gray columns: the three longitudinally oriented thickenings in the spinal cord (*columnae ventralis, dorsalis,* and *lateralis*), composed of the gray substance, and containing the nerve cell bodies. The columns are commonly referred to as *cornua ventrale, dorsale,* and *laterale,* respectively, because in transverse sections of the spinal cord they have the appearance of horns. **c. interomediolatera′lis medul′lae spina′lis** [NA], interomediolateral column of spinal cord: the column of gray matter the cells of which (interomediolateral nucleus) form the lateral column of the spinal cord; called also *autonomic column of spinal cord* and *c. autonomica medullae spinalis* [NA alternative]. **c. latera′lis medul′lae spina′lis** [NA], lateral column of spinal cord: the lateral portion of the gray matter of the spinal cord, extending from the second thoracic to the first lumbar segment of the spinal cord; in transverse section it is seen as a horn (*cornu laterale medullae spinalis*). Called also *lateral column of spinal cord*. **c. na′si,** septum nasi. **c. poste′rior medul′lae spina′lis,** NA alternative for *c. dorsalis* *medullae spinalis.* **colum′nae recta′les [Morgagn′-ii]**, columnae anales. **colum′nae rena′les** [NA], renal columns: inward extensions of the cortical structure of the kidney, between the renal pyramids; called also columnae renales [*Bertini*], *columnae bertini*, and *renal columns of Bertin.* **colum′nae rena′les [Berti′ni]**, columnae renales. **c. ruga′rum ante′rior vagi′nae** [NA], a well-marked longitudinal ridge on the anterior wall of the vagina. **c. ruga′rum poste′rior vagi′nae** [NA], a well-marked longitudinal ridge on the posterior wall of the vagina. **colum′nae ruga′rum vagi′nae** [NA], columns of rugae of vagina: well-marked longitudinal ridges on either the anterior (c. rugarum anterior vaginae) or posterior (c. rugarum posterior vaginae) wall of the vagina; called also *columns of vagina.* **c. thorac′ica** [NA], thoracic column: a well-defined column of cells in the medial part of the base dorsal gray column of the spinal cord, immediately dorsal to the lateral column, usually extending from the eighth cervical segment caudally to the third or fourth lumbar segment; it gives rise to the ipsilateral dorsal spinocerebellar tract. Called also *Clarke's column* or *nucleus, dorsal nucleus (of Clarke), nucleus dorsalis, nucleus thoracicus* [NA alternative], *Stilling's column* or *nucleus,* and *thoracic nucleus.* **c. ventra′lis medul′lae spina′lis** [NA], ventral column of spinal cord: the ventral portion of the gray substance of the spinal cord, which contains motor neurons that innervate the skeletal muscles of the neck, trunk, and limbs; in transverse section it is seen as a horn (*cornu ventrale medullae spinalis*). Called also *anterior column of spinal cord* and *c. anterior medullae spinalis* [NA alternative]. See also *c. griseae.* **c. vertebra′lis** [NA], the columnar assemblage of the vertebrae from the cranium through the coccyx; called also *axon, vertebral, dorsal,* or *spinal column, backbone,* and *spine.*

columnae (ko-lum′ne) [L.] plural of *columna.*

columnella (kol″um-nel′ah) [L.] columella.

columnization (kol″um-nĭ-za′shun) the supporting of the prolapsed uterus with tampons.

Coly-Mycin M (kol′e-mi″sin) trademark for preparations of colistimethate sodium.

Coly-Mycin S (kol′e-mi″sin) trademark for a preparation of colistin sulfate.

colypeptic (ko″le-pep′tik) kolypeptic.

com- see *con-.*

coma (ko′mah) [L.; Gr. *kōma*] 1. a state of unconsciousness from which the patient cannot be aroused, even by powerful stimulation; called also *exanimation.* 2. the optical aberration produced when an image is received upon a screen which is not exactly at right angles to the line of propagation of the incident light. **agrypnodal c.,** c. vigil. **alcoholic c.,** coma accompanying severe alcoholic intoxication. **alpha c.,** coma in which there are electroencephalographic findings of dominant alpha-wave activity. **apoplectic c.,** the stupor that accompanies stroke. **diabetic c.,** the coma of severe diabetic acidosis. **hepatic c., c. hepat′icum,** coma accompanying hepatic encephalopathy. **hyperosmolar nonketotic c.,** diabetic coma in which the level of ketone bodies is normal, due to hyperosmolarity of extracellular fluid resulting in dehydration of intracellular fluid; often a consequence of overtreatment with hyperosmolar solutions. **irreversible c.,** brain death; see under *death.* **Kussmaul's c.,** the coma and air hunger of diabetic acidosis. **metabolic c.,** the coma accompanying metabolic encephalopathy. **c. somnolen′tium,** cataphora. **uremic c.,** lethargic state due to uremia. **c. vigil,** apparent wakefulness with absent or grossly diminished response to outside stimuli; called also *agrypnodal c.* and *akinetic autism.*

comatose (ko′mah-tōs) pertaining to or affected with coma.

COMB a regimen of cyclophosphamide, Oncovin (vincristine), MeCCNU (semustine), and bleomycin, used in cancer chemotherapy.

Combipres (kom′bĭ-pres) trademark for preparations of clonidine hydrochloride and chlorthalidone.

combustion (kom-bust′yun) [L. *combustio*] rapid oxidation with emission of heat.

comedo (kom′ĕ-do) pl. *comedo′nes.* A plug of keratin and sebum within the dilated orifice of a hair follicle, frequently containing the bacteria *Propionobacterium acnes, Staphylococcus albus,* and *Pityrosporon ovale;* called also *blackhead.* See also *acne vulgaris.*

comedocarcinoma (kŏ-me″do-kar-sĭ-no′mah) an intraductal carcinoma of the breast, the central cells of which are degenerated and easily expressed from the cut surface of the tumor.

comedogenic (kom″ĕ-do-jen′ik) producing comedones.

comedomastitis (kŏ-me″do-mas-ti′tis) mammary duct ectasia.

comes (ko′mēz), pl. *com′ites* [L. *"companion"*] an artery or vein that accompanies a nerve trunk, as arteria comitans nervi ischiadici.

comfimeter (kum-fim′ĕ-ter) an apparatus devised by Leonard Hill to measure the cooling power of the atmosphere at body temperature; it is used as a guide to keeping comfortable conditions in rooms.

comfortization (kum″fort-i-za′shun) the scientific application of physiological principles for the promotion of comfort in potentially stressful situations, as in aircraft design.

comites (kom′ĭ-tēz) plural of *comes.*

commensal (kŏ-men′sal) [L. *com-* together + *mensa* table] 1. living on or within another organism, and deriving benefit without injuring or benefiting the other individual. 2. an organism living on or within another, but not causing injury to the host. See *symbiosis.*

commensalism (kŏ-men′sal-izm″) symbiosis (q.v.) in which one population (or individual) gains from the association and the other is neither harmed nor benefited.

comminuted (kom′ĭ-nūt″ed) [L. *comminutus,* from *com* together + *minuere* to diminish] broken or crushed into small pieces, as a comminuted fracture.

comminution (kom″ĭ-nu′shun) [L. *comminutio*] the act of breaking, or condition of being broken, into small fragments, as of a fractured bone.

Commiphora (kom-if′o-rah) a genus of trees of the East Indies and Africa. *C. molmol* and other species yield myrrh. *C. opobalsamum* Engl. (Burseraceae) yields balsam of Gilead.

commissura (kom″mĭ-su′rah) pl. *commissurae* [L. *"a joining together"*] [NA] commissure: a site of union of corresponding parts; a general term used to designate such a junction of corresponding anatomical structures, frequently, but not always, across the midplane of the body. **c. al′ba medul′lae spina′lis** [NA], the structure formed by fibers crossing from one side of the spinal cord to the other, anterior and posterior to the central canal; called also *white commissure of spinal cord.* **c. ante′rior al′ba medul′lae spina′lis,** the aggregate of fibers crossing from one side of the spinal cord to the other, anterior to the central canal; see *c. alba medullae spinalis* [NA]. **c. ante′rior cer′ebri,** NA alternative for *c. rostralis cerebri.* **c. bulbo′rum,** pars intermedia bulborum vestibuli vaginae. **c. of bulbs of vestibule of vagina,** pars intermedia bulborum vestibuli vaginae. **c. cerebel′li,** pons, def. 2. **c. colliculo′rum cauda′lium** [NA], commissure of caudal colliculi: a band of nerve fibers that connect the two caudal colliculi; called also *c. colliculorum inferiorum* [NA alternative] and *commissure of inferior colliculi.* **c. colliculo′rum crania′lium,** c. colliculorum rostralium. **c. colliculo′rum rostra′lium** [NA], commissure of rostral colliculi: a band of nerve fibers that connect the two cranial colliculi; called also *c. colliculorum cranialium, c. colliculorum superiorum* [NA alternative], and *commissure of superior colliculi.* **c. colliculo′rum superio′rum,** NA alternative for *c. colliculorum rostralium.* **c. epithalam′ica** [NA], commissure of epithalamus: a large fiber bundle that crosses the midline of the epithalamus just dorsal to the point where the cerebral aqueduct opens into the third ventricle; called also *c. posterior cerebri* [NA alternative] and *posterior cerebral commissure.* **c. for′nicis** [NA], commissure of fornix: a band of fibers connecting the hippocampi of the two sides through the body of the fornix; called also *c. hippocampi,* and *hippocampal commissure.* **c. habenula′ris,** NA alternative for *c. habenularum.* **c. habenula′rum** [NA], commissure of habenulae: a band of fibers of the stria medullaris that pass through the habenula of each side to decussate and terminate in the habenula of the other side; called also *habenular commissure* and *c. habenularis* [NA alternative]. **c. hippocam′pi,** c. fornicis. **c. labio′rum ante′rior** [NA], anterior commissure of labia: the junction of the two labia majora anteriorly, at the lower border of the pubic symphysis. **c. labio′rum o′ris** [NA], commissure of lips of mouth: the junction of the upper and lower lips at either side of the mouth. **c. labio′rum poste′rior** [NA], posterior commissure of labia: the apparent junction of the labia majora posteriorly, formed by the forward projection of the tendinous center of the perineum into the pudendal cleft. **c. labio′rum puden′di,** see *c. labiorum anterior* and *c. labiorum posterior.* **c. rostra′lis cer′ebri** [NA], rostral commissure of cerebrum: a bundle of myelinated nerve fibers passing transversely through the lamina terminalis and connecting the parts of the two cerebral hemispheres, and consisting of smaller anterior part and a larger posterior part; called also *anterior commissure of cerebrum* and *c. anterior cerebri* [NA alternative]. **c. mag′na cer′ebri,** corpus callosum. **c. me′dia cer′ebri, c. mol′lis** (obs.), adhesio interthalamica. **c. oliva′rum,** see *fibrae arcuatae internae.* **c. palpebra′rum latera′lis** [NA], the lateral junction of the superior and inferior eyelids; called also *c. palpebrarum temporalis* and *lateral commissure of eyelids.* **c. palpebra′rum media′lis** [NA], the medial junction of the superior and inferior eyelids; called also *c. palpebrarum nasalis* and *medial commissure of eyelids.* **c. palpebra′rum nasa′lis,** c. palpebrarum medialis. **c. palpebra′rum tempora′lis,** c. palpebrarum lateralis. **c. poste′rior cer′ebri,** NA alternative for *c. epithalamica.* **c. rostra′lis cer′ebri** [NA], rostral commissure of cerebrum: a bundle of myelinated nerve fibers passing transversely through the lamina terminalis and connecting the parts of the two cerebral hemispheres, and consisting of smaller anterior part and a larger posterior part; called also *anterior commissure of cerebrum* and *c. anterior cerebri* [NA alternative]. **c. su-praop′tica dorsa′lis** [NA], dorsal supraoptic commissure: the more dorsal fiber bundle that crosses the midline of the brain dorsal to the caudal border of the optic chiasma; see also *supraoptic commissures,* under *commissure.* **c. su-praop′tica ventra′lis** [NA], ventral supraoptic commissure: the more ventral fiber bundle that crosses the midline of the brain dorsal to the caudal border of the optic chiasm; see also *supraoptic commissures,* under *commissure.*

commissurae (kom″ĭ-su′re) [L.] genitive and plural of *commissura.*

commissural (kom-mis′u-ral) pertaining to or acting as a commissure.

commissure (kom′ĭ-shūr) a site of union of corresponding parts; see *commissura.* Used also with specific reference to the sites of junction between adjacent cusps of the valves of the heart. **anterior c. of labia,** commissura labiorum anterior. **c. of caudal colliculi,** commissura colliculorum caudalium. **c. of cerebrum, anterior,** commissura rostralis cerebri. **c. of cerebrum, middle,** adhesio interthalamica. **c. of cerebrum, posterior,** commissura epithalamica. **c. of cerebrum, rostral,** commissura rostralis cerebri. **c. of cranial colliculi,** commissura colliculorum rostralium. **c. of epithalamus,** commissura epithalamica. **c. of eyelids, lateral,** commissura palpebralis lateralis. **c. of eyelids, medial,** commissura palpebrarum medialis. **Forel's c.,** a name once applied to a band that joins the subthalamic nucleus of each side. **c. of fornix,** commissura fornicis. **Ganser's c.,** the anterior supraoptic commissure; see *supraoptic c's.* **gray c.,** substantia grisea intermedia centralis. **Gudden's c.,** the ventral, or inferior, supraoptic commissure; see *supraoptic c's.* **c. of habenulae, habenular c.,** commissura habenularum. **hippocampal c.,** commissura fornicis. **c. of inferior colliculi,** commissura colliculorum caudalium. **interthalamic c.,** adhesio interthalamica. **c. of labia, anterior,** commissura labiorum anterior. **c. of labia, posterior,** commissura labiorum posterior. **laryngeal c.,** the region of junction (anterior or posterior) of the two sides of the larynx. **lateral c. of eyelids,** commissura palpebrarum lateralis. **c. of lips of mouth,** commissura labiorum oris. **medial c. of eyelids,** commissura palpebrarum medialis. **Meynert's c.,** the dorsal, or superior, supraoptic commissure; see *supraoptic c's.* **optic c.** (obs.), chiasma opticum. **posterior c. of labia,** commissura labiorum posterior. **c. of rostral colliculi,** commissura colliculorum rostralium. **c. of superior colliculi,** commissura colliculorum rostralium. **supraoptic c's,** at least three fiber bundles situated dorsal to the optic chiasm, which have been associated with the names of Gudden (ventral or inferior), Meynert (dorsal or superior), and Ganser (anterior), and which have been referred to as commissures but are probably decussa-

tions; their connections in humans is uncertain. Only the dorsal and ventral bundles are recognized in official anatomical nomenclature: see *commissura supraoptica dorsalis* and *commissura supraoptica ventralis.* **supraoptic c., dorsal,** commissura supraoptica dorsalis. **supraoptic c., ventral,** commissura supraoptica dorsalis. **white c. of spinal cord,** commissura alba medullae spinalis. **white c. of spinal cord, lateral,** funiculus lateralis medullae spinalis.

commissurorrhaphy (kom″ĭ-shūr-or′ah-fe) [*commissure* + Gr. *rhaphē* a seam] suture of the component parts of a commissure, to decrease the size of the orifice.

commissurotomy (kom″ĭ-shūr-ot′o-me) [*commissure* + Gr. *tomē* cutting] surgical incision or digital disruption of the component parts of a commissure to increase the size of the orifice; commonly utilized to separate the adherent, thickened leaflets of a stenotic mitral valve.

commitment (kŏ-mit′ment) civil commitment; the legal proceeding by which a person is involuntarily confined to a mental hospital.

commotio (kŏ-mo′she-o) [L. "disturbance"] a concussion; a violent shaking, or the shock which results from it. **c. cer′ebri,** concussion of the brain. **c. re′tinae,** edema around the macular region of the retina, caused by a severe blow to the eyeball, and producing a permanent central scotoma as a result of destruction of the delicate cones in the fovea. Called also *Berlin's disease* or *edema,* and *concussion of the retina.* **c. spina′lis,** concussion of the spine.

communicable (kŏ-mu′nĭ-kah-b'l) capable of being transmitted from one person or species to another, as a communicable disease; contagious. Cf. *infectious.*

communicans (kŏ-mu′nĕ-kanz) [L.] communicating; used in anatomical nomenclature to denote a communicating structure, as a nerve.

communis (kŏ-mu′nis) [L.] common; [NA] a general term denoting a structure serving several branches.

community (kŏ-mu′nĭ-te) a body of individuals living in a defined area or having a common interest or organization. **biotic c.,** an assemblage of populations living in a defined area. **climax c.,** the final, stable, and mature community in a series that appears in succession, which is in equilibrium with the environmental conditions and is composed of a definite group of plant and animal species. The entire sequence of communities is called a *sere* and the individual transitional communities are *seral stages.* **seral c.,** see under *stage.* **therapeutic c.,** a specially structured mental hospital or ward employing group and milieu therapy and encouraging the patient to function within social norms.

Comolli's sign (kom-ol′ēz) [Antonio *Comolli,* Italian pathologist, born 1879] see under *sign.*

Comp. abbreviation for L. *compos′itus,* compound.

compact (kom-pakt′) dense; having a dense structure.

compacta (kom-pak′tah) the more superficial and denser portion of the decidua basalis; stratum compactum.

compaction (kom-pak′shun) a complication of labor in twin births in which there is simultaneous full engagement of the leading fetal poles of both twins, so that the true pelvic cavity is filled and further descent is prevented. Cf. *interlocking.*

compages (kom-pa′jēz) [L.] a joining together or that which is joined together. **c. thora′cis** [NA] the skeletal framework enclosing the thorax, consisting of the thoracic vertebrae and intervertebral disks, the ribs and costal cartilages, and the sternum; called also *thoracic cage, thoracic skeleton,* and *skeleton of thorax.*

comparascope (kom-par′ah-skōp″) a device attached to a microscope for the purpose of comparing two slides.

comparator (kom′pah-ra″tor) a simple colorimeter consisting of a block of wood with holes in which to place the test tubes to be compared, and transverse holes through which to view the colors; called also *comparator block.*

compartment (com-part′ment) a small enclosure within a larger space. **muscular c.,** lacuna musculorum. **vascular c.,** lacuna vasorum.

compartmentalization, compartmentation (kom″-part-men″tah-li-za′shun; kom-part′men-ta′shun) the natural partitioning within cells due to the selectively permeable membranes which enclose each of the separate parts (mitochondria, lysosomes, Golgi complex, etc.), enabling each part to regulate its own contents.

compatibility (kom-pat″ĭ-bil′ĭ-te) [L. *compatibilis* accordant] the quality of being compatible.

compatible (kom-pat′ĭ-b'l) 1. capable of harmonious coexistence; of medications, suitable for simultaneous administration without nullification or aggravation of the effects of either. 2. denoting a donor and recipient of a blood transfusion in which there is no transfusion reaction. 3. histocompatible; denoting a donor and recipient of an organ transplant that is not rejected.

Compazine (kom′pah-zēn) trademark for preparations of prochlorperazine maleate.

compensation (kom″pen-sa′shun) [L. *compensatio*, from *cum* together + *pensare* to weigh] the counterbalancing of any defect of structure or function. In psychology, a conscious process or, more frequently, an unconscious defense mechanism by which a person attempts to make up for real or imagined physical or psychological deficiencies. In cardiology, the maintenance of an adequate blood flow without distressing symptoms, accomplished by such cardiac and circulatory adjustments as tachycardia, cardiac hypertrophy, and increase of blood volume by sodium and water retention. **broken c.,** inability of the heart to maintain sufficient blood flow through the fissures, so that stagnation ensues and symptoms of stasis are produced. **dosage c.,** in genetics, the mechanism by which the effect of the two X chromosomes of the normal female is rendered identical to that of the one X chromosome of the normal male. See *Lyon hypothesis,* under *hypothesis.*

compensatory (kom-pen′sah-to″re) making good a defect or loss; restoring a lost balance.

competence (kom′pĕ-tens) the ability of an organ or part to perform adequately any function required of it. In embryology, the ability of embryonic cells to differentiate into cell types determined by inductors. **embryonic c.,** the ability of embryonic tissue to respond normally to the influence of an inductor. **immunologic c.,** immunocompetence.

competition (kom″pĕ-tish′un) the phenomenon in which two structurally similar molecules "compete" for a single binding site on a third molecule. See *competitive inhibition,* under *inhibition.* **antigenic c.,** an altered response to an immunogen resulting from the simultaneous or close administration of two immunogens: the response to one is normal, while the response to the second is suppressed or diminished.

complaint (kom-plānt′) a symptom, disease, or disorder. **chief c.,** the symptom or group of symptoms about which the patient first consults the doctor; the presenting symptom. **summer c.,** cholera morbus.

complement (kom′plĕ-ment) a term originally used to refer to the heat-labile factor in serum that causes immune cytolysis, the lysis of antibody-coated cells, and now referring to the entire functionally related system comprising at least 20 distinct serum proteins that is the effector not only of immune cytolysis but also of other biologic functions. Complement activation occurs by two different sequences, the classic and alternative pathways. The proteins of the classic pathway are termed "components of complement" and are designated by the symbols C1 through C9. C1 is a calcium-dependent complex of three distinct proteins C1q, C1r, and C1s. The proteins of the alternative pathway (collectively referred to as the properdin system) and complement regulatory proteins are known by semisystematic or trivial names. Fragments resulting from proteolytic cleavage of complement proteins are designated with lower-case-letter suffixes, e.g., C3a. Inactivated fragments may be designated with the suffix "i," e.g., C3bi. Activated components or complexes with biological activity are designated by a bar over the symbol, e.g., C$\overline{1}$ or C$\overline{4b,2a}$. The classic pathway is activated by the binding of C1 to classic pathway activators, primarily antigen-antibody complexes containing IgM, IgG1, IgG2, or IgG3; C1q binds to a single IgM molecule or two adjacent IgG molecules. The alternative pathway can be activated by IgA immune complexes and also by nonimmunologic materials including bacterial endotoxins, microbial polysaccharides, and cell walls. Activation of the classic pathway triggers an enzymatic cascade involving C1, C4, C2, and C3; activation of the alternative pathway triggers a cascade involving C3 and factors B, D, and P. Both result in the cleavage of C5 and the formation of the membrane attack complex. Complement activation also results in the formation of many biologically active complement fragments that act as anaphylatoxins, opsonins, or chemotactic factors. See following table for description of biologically active complement products and complement system enzymes and active complexes. **C$\overline{1s}$:** an enzyme that cleaves C4 into C4a and C4b and C2 into C2a and C2b, generated by cleavage of a peptide bond in C1s when C1 interacts with activators of the classic pathway; it is inhibited by C$\overline{1}$ inhibitor; called also C$\overline{1}$ and C1 esterase. **C2a:** a constituent of C$\overline{4b,2a}$ generated by C1s. **C2 kinin:** a C2 fragment generated by C$\overline{1s}$ having kinin activity not mediated by histamine. **C3a:** an anaphylatoxin generated by C3 convertases. **C3b:** a constituent of the classic pathway C5 convertase and of the alternative pathway C3 and C5 convertases generated by C3 convertases in both pathways and also continuously generated in the circulation in the small amounts required to initiate the alternative pathway; it is inactivated by the action of factor H, factor I, and a proteolytic enzyme, possibly plasmin, producing C3c and C3d. C3b is also an opsonin having receptors on erythrocytes, B lymphocytes, granulocytes, and macrophages. **C3d:** an opsonin generated by inactivation of C3b and having receptors on B lymphocytes and, possibly, macrophages. **C$\overline{3b,Bb}$:** an alternative pathway C3 convertase generated by the interaction of factor B and factor D with C3b deposited on activators of the alternative pathway and thus protected from inactivation by factor I and factor H. **C$\overline{3b,P,Bb}$:** a more stable alternative pathway C3 convertase generated by addition of factor P to C$\overline{3b,Bb}$. **C$\overline{3b_n,Bb}$:** an alternative pathway C5 convertase generated by addition of one or more C3b fragments to C$\overline{3b,Bb}$. **C$\overline{3b_n,P,Bb}$:** a more stable alternative pathway C5 convertase containing factor P. **C4a:** a weak anaphylatoxin generated by C$\overline{1s}$. **C4b:** a constituent of C$\overline{4b,2a}$ generated by C$\overline{1s}$; it is inactivated by the action of C4 binding protein and factor I. C4b is also an opsonin that binds to the same receptors as C3b. **C$\overline{4b,2a}$:** the classic pathway C3 convertase, which cleaves C3 to C3a and C3b, a complex of C4b and C2a formed on cell membrane surfaces in the presence of Mg^{2+}; called also C$\overline{42}$. **C$\overline{4b,2a,3b}$:** the classic pathway C5 convertase, which cleaves C5 to C5a and C5b, a complex formed by attachment of C3b to membrane-bound C$\overline{4b,2a}$; called also C$\overline{423}$. **C5a:** an anaphylatoxin and chemotactic factor for granulocytes and macrophages generated by C5 convertases. **C5b:** a constituent of the membrane attack complex generated by the classic and alternative pathway C5 convertases; it can also be generated by the action of certain serum proteases, e.g., plasmin and trypsin. **C$\overline{5b,6,7}$:** a trimolecular complex of C5b, C6, and C7 that can bind to cell membranes to initiate formation of the membrane attack complex; it can also bind to the S protein forming an inactive complex unable to bind to membranes. C5b,6,7 is also a chemotactic factor for neutrophils. Called also C$\overline{567}$. **C$\overline{5b,6,7,8}$:** a complex generated by binding of C8 to membrane-bound C5b,6,7; it causes a slow leakage of the cell membrane. Called also C$\overline{5678}$. **C$\overline{5b,6,7,8,9}$:** the complete membrane attack complex (cytolytic agent) of the complement system generated by addition of C9 to C5b,6,7,8; this complex has a hydrophilic center that allows the rapid passage of water and ions through the cell membrane causing osmotic lysis of the cell. Called also C$\overline{56789}$.

complemental (kom″plĕ-men′tal) complementary.

complementary (kom″plĕ-men′tă-re) [L. *complere* to fill] supplying a defect, or helping to do so; making complete; accessory.

complementation (kom″ple-men-ta′shun) [L. *complēre* to fill out or up] 1. in genetics, the restoration of wild-type function by two different mutations brought together in the same cell. 2. in virology, the interaction of two defective bacteriophages that results in the replication of both, as occurs in some mixed infections of bacterial cells. **interallelic c.,** intragenic c. **intercistronic c., intergenic c.,** the essentially full restoration of wild-type function in a *cis-trans* test when two mutations are located in two different cistrons (genes). **intracistronic c., intragenic c.,** the partial restoration of function sometimes seen in the *cis-trans* test when the two mutations are located at different sites within the same cistron.

complex (kom′pleks; kom-pleks′) [L. *complexus* woven together, encompassing] 1. complicated; not simple. 2. the sum, combination, or collection of various things or related

CLASSICAL COMPLEMENT ACTIVATION

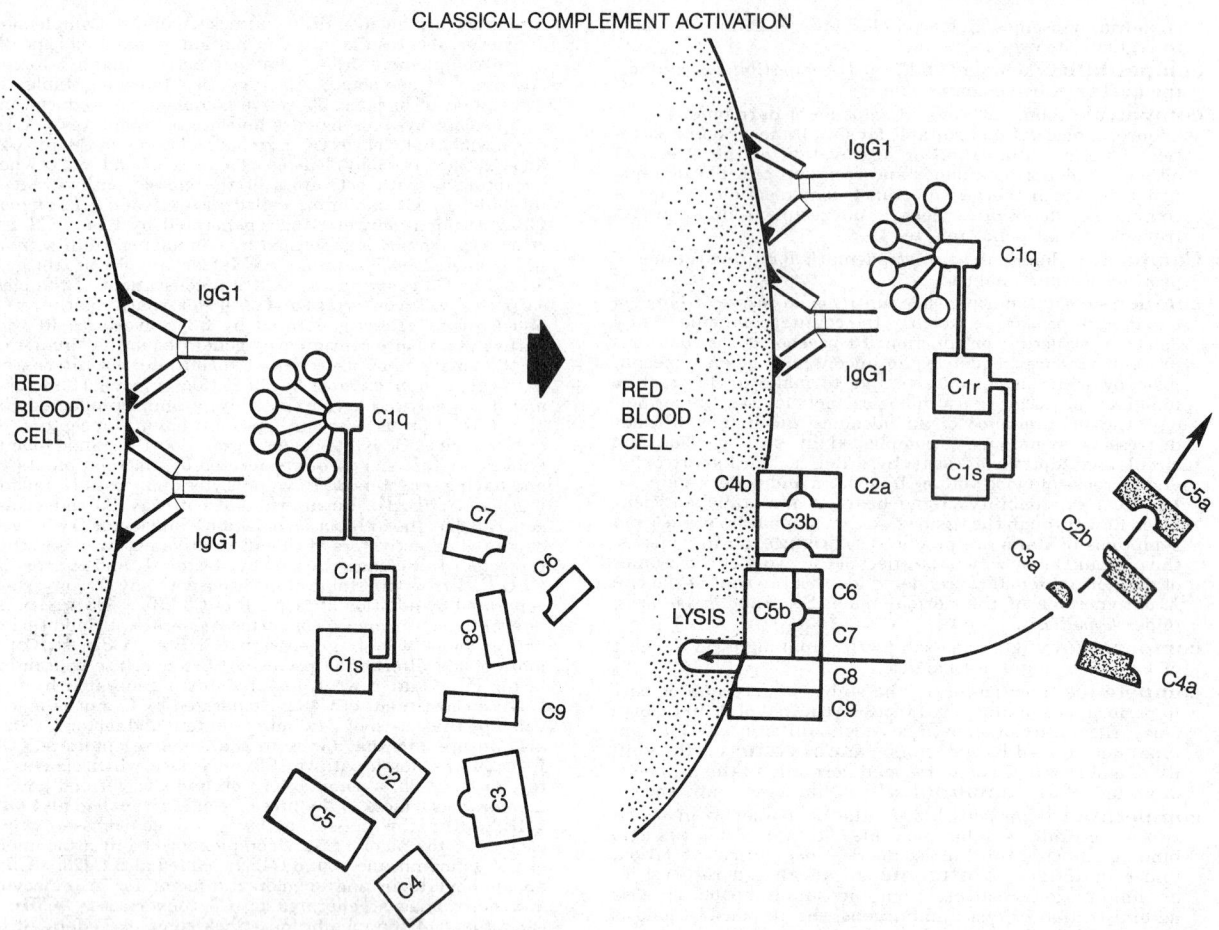

Schematic representation of the classical complement pathway. Two molecules of IgG, termed a "doublet," combine with homologous antigenic determinants on a red blood cell surface and activate the first complement component by interacting with C1q. This is followed by C1r and C1s activation. The reaction sequence of the classical complement pathway is C1,4,2,3,5,6,7,8,9. This biochemical pathway leads to the formation of a "hole" in the cell membrane, resulting in cell swelling and lysis. Although C9 is not essential for lysis, it accelerates the lytic reaction. The alternative or properdin pathway provides a mechanism to mediate the bactericidal and opsonic effects of complement without requiring specific antibody. From the C3 step forward both pathways follow a similar course.

factors, like or unlike; e.g., a complex of symptoms (see *syndrome*). 3. a group of interrelated ideas, mainly unconscious, that have a common emotional tone and strongly influence a person's attitudes and behavior. 4. that portion of an electrocardiographic tracing which represents the systole of an atrium or ventricle. **adrenochrome monosemicarbazone sodium salicylate c.,** carbazochrome salicylate. **AIDS-related c. (ARC),** a complex of signs and symptoms representing a less severe form of human immunodeficiency virus (HIV) infection than classic acquired immune deficiency syndrome, characterized by chronic generalized lymphadenopathy associated with fever, weight loss, prolonged diarrhea, minor opportunistic infections, cytopenias, and T-cell abnormalities associated with AIDS: considered by some authorities to be pre-AIDS, although the proportion of cases that will progress to the full-blown disease is unknown. See also *lymphadenopathy syndrome,* under *syndrome*. **amygdaloid c.,** corpus amygdaloideum. **amyotrophic lateral sclerosis–parkinsonism–dementia c.,** an autosomal dominant disorder occurring among the Chamorro population of Guam and characterized by gradually progressing parkinsonism associated with progressive dementia and amyotrophic lateral sclerosis. **anomalous c.,** a complex that varies from the normal type, as an electrocardiographic complex. **antigen-antibody c.,** the complex formed by the noncovalent binding of an antibody and antigen. Complexes of antibodies belonging to certain immunoglobulin classes may activate complement. Antigen-antibody complexes are medi-

ators of Type III immune responses (Arthus reactions, serum sickness, and immune complex diseases). Called also *immune c.,* particularly in discussing disease processes. **apical c.,** an ultrastructural complex of apical organelles characteristic of apicocomplexan protozoa during some stage of their development, generally consisting of a polar ring(s), a conoid, micronemes, rhoptries, and subpellicular microtubules. It seems to function as a means of attachment to and penetration of host cells. **atrial c.,** the P wave of the electrocardiogram; see *electrocardiogram*. **avian leukosis c.,** see *avian leukosis,* under *leukosis*. **basal c. of choroid,** complexus basalis choroideae. **calcarine c.,** calcar avis. **castration c.,** in psychoanalytic theory, unconscious thoughts and motives stemming from fear of loss of genitals as punishment for forbidden sexual desires. **EAHF c.,** the symptom complex of eczema, asthma, and hay fever. **Eisenmenger c.,** a defect of the interventricular septum with severe pulmonary hypertension, hypertrophy of the right ventricle, and latent or overt cyanosis. **Electra c.,** the female counterpart of the Oedipus complex, a rarely used term since "Oedipus complex" is generally applied to both sexes. (*Greek legend:* the daughter of Agamemnon and Clytemnestra, who incited her brother Orestes to kill their mother and stepfather for having murdered their father.) **factor IX c.** [USP], a sterile, freeze-dried powder consisting of partially purified Factor IX fraction, as well as concentrated Factors II, VII, and X fractions, of venous plasma from healthy human donors. **Ghon c.,** primary c. **Golgi c.,** a complex cuplike structure within cells, made up of several

PROTEINS OF THE COMPLEMENT SYSTEM

NAME	SYNONYMS	ELECTRO-PHORETIC MOBILITY	MOLECULAR WEIGHT	SERUM CONCENTRATION $\mu g/ml$
Classic Pathway				
C1q		γ_2	400,000	65
C1r		β	170,000	35
C1s		α_2	85,000	30
C4	$\beta 1E$	β_1	240,000	350
C2		β_1	117,000	25
C3	$\beta 1C$	β_1	185,000	1400
Alternative Pathway				
C3	Factor A		(see above)	
	Hydrazine-sensitive factor (HSF)			
Factor B	C3 proactivator (C3PA)	β_2	100,000	240
	Glycine-rich β glycoprotein (GBG)			
Factor D	C3 proactivator convertase (C3PAase)	α	25,000	1
	Glycine-rich β glycoproteinase (GBGase)			
Factor P	Properdin	γ	220,000	25
Membrane Attack Mechanism				
C5	$\beta 1F$	β_1	200,000	65
C6		β_1	125,000	55
C7		β_2	120,000	55
C8		γ	150,000	55
C9		α	79,000	60
Regulatory Proteins				
C1 inhibitor (C1 INH)	C1 esterase inhibitor	α_2	105,000	180
C4 binding protein		β	>500,000	250
Factor I	C3b inactivator (C3b INA)	β	90,000	35
	Conglutinogen activating factor (KAF)			
Factor H	$\beta 1H$	β_1	150,000	500
	C3b inactivator accelerator			
S protein	Membrane attack complex inhibitor (MAC INH)	α	80,000	500
Anaphylatoxin inactivator (AI)		α	300,000	trace

elements, each consisting of a number of flattened sacs (cisternae) with associated vacuoles and vesicles. Golgi complexes are membrane sites of the formation of the carbohydrate side chains of glycoproteins and mucopolysaccharides, and of other substances. The secretion vacuoles migrate through the cell membrane and release the glycoproteins and mucopolysaccharides, and thus play a role in internal and external secretion. Cytochemical studies have shown that they are also sites of formation of primary lysosomes and give rise to the acrosome of spermatozoa and the nematocyst of *Hydra.* Called also *Golgi apparatus* and *Golgi body.* **H-2 c.,** the murine major histocompatibility complex. **hapten-carrier c.,** the antigen formed by the coupling of a hapten and a carrier protein. **HLA c.,** the human major histocompatibility complex; see *HLA antigens,* under *antigen.* **immune c.,** antigen-antibody c. **inclusion c's,** compounds in which molecules of one type are enclosed within cavities in the crystalline lattice of another substance. **inferiority c.,** Alfred Adler's concept that everyone is born with a feeling of inferiority stemming from real or imagined organic or psychological deficiency; the manner in which the inferiority is handled determines how a person behaves. **jumped process c.,** dislocation of articular processes of spine. **junctional c.,** the intercellular arrangement between adjacent columnar epithelial cells, consisting of the zonula occludens, the zonula adherens, and the desmosome. **α-ketoglutarate dehydrogenase c.,** a multienzyme complex consisting of at least three distinct enzymes: α-ketoglutarate dehydrogenase [EC 1.2.4.2], dihydrolipoamide succinyltransferase [EC 2.3.1.61], and dihydrolipoamide dehydrogenase [EC 1.8.1.4]. The integrated enzyme complex catalyzes the overall reaction 2-ketoglutarate + CoA-SH + NAD^+ = succinyl coenzyme A + NADH + CO_2. Thiamine diphosphate, lipoic acid, and FAD are required as cofactors. The reaction is an essential part of the citric (tricarboxylic acid) cycle. See also *α-ketoglutarate dehydrogenase complex,* under *complex.* **α-ketoisovalerate dehydrogenase c.,** see *branched chain α-ketoacid dehydrogenase.* **Lutembacher's c.,** see under *syndrome.* **major histocompatibility c. (MHC),** the genes determining the major histocompatibility antigens, in all species a group of closely linked multiallelic genes located in a small region on one chromosome; designated the *HLA complex* in humans and the *H-2 complex* in mice. **membrane attack c.**

(MAC), the pentamolecular complex C5b,6,7,8,9 that is the cytolytic agent of the complement system; see under *complement.* **Meyenburg's c's,** bile duct hamartomas. **Oedipus c.,** in psychoanalytic theory, the feelings and conflicts occurring in a child during the phallic phase of psychosexual development that result from sexual attraction to the opposite-sex parent, including envious, aggressive feelings toward the same-sex parent; these feelings are repressed because of fear of reprisal by the same-sex parent. (*Greek legend:* the son of Jocasta and the Theban king Laius, who, raised by a foster parent, unwittingly killed his father and married his mother. Later when he discovered the true relationship, he blinded himself.) Cf. *Electra complex.* **perihypoglossal c., perihypoglossal nuclear c.,** a group of nerve cells immediately adjacent to the nucleus of the hypoglossal nerve in the gray substance of the medulla oblongata, all of which contain cells with characteristics suggestive of reticular connections; the complex includes the nucleus intercalatus, sublingual nucleus, and nucleus paramedianus dorsalis. Called also *periglossal gray.* **pore c.,** a nuclear pore and its annulus considered together. **primary c.,** 1. the combination of a parenchymal pulmonary lesion (*Ghon focus* or *tubercle*) and a corresponding lymph node focus, occurring in primary tuberculosis, usually in children; it may undergo cellular necrosis and eventually calcify. Similar lesions may also be associated with other mycobacterial infections and with fungal infections such as histoplasmosis and coccidioidomycosis. Called also *Ghon c.* and *Ranke c.* 2. the primary cutaneous lesion at the site of infection in the skin, e.g., chancre in syphilis and tuberculous chancre. **primary inoculation c., primary tuberculous c.,** see under *tuberculosis.* **Ranke c.,** primary c. **sicca c.,** primary Sjögren's syndrome. **symptom c.,** a set of symptoms that occur together; the sum of signs of any morbid state; a syndrome. **synaptonemal c.,** a thick, threadlike structure formed during the zygotene (synaptic) stage of meiosis by the intertwining of two leptotene chromosomes so that they are indistinguishable separately. **ureterotrigonal c.,** ureterovesical junction. **urobilin c.,** a hypothetical substance consisting of a number of urobilinogen molecules linked together, which is the form in which urobilinogen exists in the blood and tissues. **ventricular c's,** the Q, R, S, and T waves of the electrocardiogram, representing ventricular electrical activity.

complexion (kom-plek′shun) [L. *complexio* combination] the color and appearance of the skin of the face.

complexus (kom-plek′sus) [L. "encompassing"] complex. **c. basa′lis choroi′deae** [NA], basal complex of choroid: the transparent inner layer of the choroid, which is in contact with the pigmented layer of the retina. Called also *Bruch's layer* or *membrane, basal lamina of choroid, lamina basalis choroideae* [NA alternative], *l. vitrea,* and *vitreal* or *vitreous lamina.*

compliance (kom-pli′ans) a quality of yielding to pressure or force without disruption, or an expression of the measure of the ability to do so, as an expression of the distensibility of an air- or fluid-filled organ, e.g., the lung or urinary bladder, in terms of unit of volume change per unit of pressure change. Cf. *elastance.*

complicated (kom′plĭ-kāt′ed) [L. *complicare* to infold] involved; associated with other injuries, lesions, or diseases.

complication (kom″plĭ-ka′shun) [L. *complicatio* from *cum* together + *plicare* to fold] 1. a disease or diseases concurrent with another disease. 2. the concurrence of two or more diseases in the same patient.

Compocillin-VK (com″po-sil′in) trademark for a preparation of penicillin V potassium.

component (kom-po′nent) a constituent element or part; specifically in neurology, a series of neurons forming a functional system for conducting the afferent and efferent impulses in the somatic and splanchnic mechanisms of the body. **anterior c.,** Angle's term for "a forward propelling force which is the result of meshing and pounding of the occlusal inclined planes of the teeth and the mesial inclination of the teeth." **complement c's, c's of complement,** see *complement.* **group-specific c.,** vitamin D–binding protein, a serum protein of particular use in anthropological studies because of the great differences in gene frequency in different populations. **M c.,** [*M*yeloma or *M*acroglobulinemia], an increased concentration of a structurally homogenous protein in serum or urine appearing as a sharp spike in the beta or gamma globulin region on protein electrophoresis. The protein is in most cases a monoclonal immunoglobulin, a monoclonal immunoglobulin heavy chain or heavy chain fragment, or a monoclonal immunoglobulin light chain or light chain fragment, either alone or with monoclonal immunoglobulin containing the same light chain. M components are characteristic of plasma cell dyscrasias. **plasma thromboplastin c. (PTC),** Factor IX; see *coagulation factors,* under *factor.* **secretory c. (SC),** a 70,000 dalton glycopeptide occurring in secretory IgA; synthesized not by the plasma cell producing the IgA but added while the IgA is crossing the epithelium; it may protect secretory IgA from proteolytic attack after secretion, or it may play some role in the process of secretion. Secretory component deficiency has been seen in a few patients; there is complete lack of IgA in external secretions although serum IgA is normal. Called also *secretory piece.* **somatic motor c.,** the system of neurons that conduct impulses to the somatic effectors (skeletal muscle) of the body. **somatic sensory c.,** the system of neurons conducting impulses from the somatic receptors. **splanchnic motor c.,** the system of neurons conducting impulses to the splanchnic (visceral) effectors (cardiac muscle, smooth muscle, and glands). **splanchnic sensory c.,** the system of neurons conducting impulses from the splanchnic receptors.

compos mentis (kom′pos men′tis) [L.] sound of mind; sane.

compound (kom-pownd) [L. *componere* to place together] 1. in chemistry, a substance that consists of two or more chemical elements in union. 2. in genetics, a genotype in which there are two different mutant alleles at a locus, or a phenotype produced by such a genotype. Cf. *homozygote, homozygous.* **c. A,** 11-dehydrocorticosterone. **acyclic c.,** an open-chain compound; see under *chain.* **addition c.,** a compound formed by the union of two or more compounds or elements. **aliphatic c.,** an open-chain compound that does not contain multiple bonds; a saturated compound. See under *chain.* **APC c.,** a preparation of acetylsalicylic acid, phenacetin, and caffeine citrate. **aromatic c.,** a closed-chain compound that contains bonds similar to those in benzene; see under *chain.* **c. B,** corticosterone. **benzene c's,** aromatic compounds. **benzoin tincture c.,** see under *tincture.* **binary c.,** a compound whose molecule is composed of atoms of only two elements.

clathrate c's, inclusion complexes in which molecules of one type are trapped within cavities of the crystalline lattice of another substance; called also *clathrates* or *occlusion c's.* **closed-chain c.,** see under *chain.* **coal-tar c.,** a closed-chain compound; see under *chain.* **condensation c.,** a compound that is formed by union of substances with the loss of one or more molecules, usually of low molecular weight, as water or ammonia. **cyclic c.,** a closed-chain compound; see under *chain.* **diazo c.,** a compound containing the group —N₂—. **c. E,** cortisone. **endothermic c.,** one whose formation is attended with absorption of heat. **energy-rich c's,** high-energy c's. **exothermic c.,** one whose formation is attended with loss of heat. **c. F,** cortisol. **fatty c.,** an open-chain compound; see under *chain.* **Grignard c.,** see under *reagent.* **heterocyclic c.,** a chemical substance that contains a ring-shaped nucleus composed of dissimilar elements. **high-energy c's,** a group of pyrophosphates that yield high levels of negative free energies on hydrolysis, and so are basic to the energy supply of living organisms. Among the most important are ATP, acetyl CoA, aminoacyl adenylates, phosphocreatinine, and phosphoenol pyruvate. Called also *energy-rich c's.* **Hurler-Scheie c.,** see under *syndrome.* **inorganic c.,** a compound that contains no carbon. **isocyclic c.,** a chemical substance that contains a ring-shaped nucleus composed of the same elements throughout. **isopropyl alcohol rubbing c.,** a solution containing 70 per cent isopropyl alcohol in water; used as a rubefacient. **Kendall's c. A,** 11-dehydrocorticosterone. **Kendall's c. B,** corticosterone. **Kendall's c. E,** cortisone. **Kendall's c. F,** cortisol. **low-energy c's,** compounds containing phosphate ester or other linkages that yield relatively low levels of negative free energies on hydrolysis, including AMP, glucose-1-phosphate, and glucose-6-phosphate. **nonpolar c's,** compounds in which electrons are shared equally by the two atoms forming a bond and which therefore do not ionize in solution, e.g., the paraffins, olefins, and cyclic compounds. **occlusion c's,** clathrate c's. **open-chain c.,** see under *chain.* **organic c.,** a compound of chemical elements containing carbon atoms. **organometallic c.,** one in which carbon is linked to a metal. **paraffin c.,** an open-chain compound; see under *chain.* **polar c's,** compounds in which the electrons are unequally shared by the two atoms forming the bond and which therefore may act as dipoles or, in some instances, completely ionize. They include the alcohols, water, and ammonia. **quaternary c.,** one composed of four elements. **quaternary ammonium c.,** see *tetraethylammonium.* **ring c.,** see *closed chain,* under *chain.* **saturated c.,** a compound in which the combining capacities of all the elements are satisfied. **substitution c.,** a compound formed by replacement of elements of a molecule by other elements. **ternary c., tertiary c.,** a compound composed of three elements. **unsaturated c.,** a compound in which the combining capacities of all the elements are not satisfied; see *unsaturated,* 2nd def. **Wintersteiner's c. F,** cortisone.

compress (kom′pres) [L. *compressus*] a pad or bolster of folded gauze or other material, applied with pressure; it is sometimes medicated, and may be wet or dry, hot or cold.

compressibility (kom-pres″ĭ-bil′ĭ-te) the volume change per unit of a substance produced by a unit increase in pressure.

compression (kom-presh′un) [L. *compressio* from *comprimere* to squeeze together] 1. the act of pressing together; an action exerted upon a body by an external force which tends to diminish its volume and augment its density. 2. in embryology, the shortening or omission of certain stages during development. **c. of the brain,** a condition in which the brain is compressed by fractures, tumors, blood clots, abscesses, etc. **digital c.,** compression of a blood vessel by the fingers for the purpose of checking hemorrhage. **instrumental c.,** compression of a blood vessel by instruments. **spinal c.,** a condition in which pressure is exerted on the spinal cord, as by a tumor, spinal fracture, etc.; its manifestations, which vary with location and degree of pressure, may include pain, paresthesias, and sensory and motor disturbances.

compressor (kom-pres′or) [L.] any agent by which compression may be achieved. **Deschamps' c.,** an instrument for the direct compression of an artery. **c. na′ris,** the transverse part of the nasal muscle; see *partes transversa* *et alaris musculi nasalis.* **Sehrt's c.,** see under *clamp.* **shot c.,** a forceps for compressing split shot applied to sutures; see also *shotted suture,* under *suture.* **c. ure'-thrae,** musculus sphincter urethrae. **c. vagi'nae,** the bulbospongiosus muscle in the female.

compressorium (kom″pres-o′re-um), pl. *compresso'ria* [L.] a device for making graduated pressure upon objects under microscopic examination.

Compton effect, scattering (komp′ton) [Arthur Holly *Compton,* American physicist, 1892–1962; winner of the Nobel prize in physics for 1927] see under *effect* and *scattering.*

compulsion (kom-pul′shun) 1. a persistent and irresistible impulse to perform an irrational or apparently useless act. 2. a compulsive act or ritual; a repetitive and stereotyped action, such as hand-washing, touching, counting, and checking, that is engaged in for an unknown or unconscious purpose. **repetition c.,** in psychoanalytic theory, the impulse to reenact earlier emotional experiences.

compulsive (kom-pul′siv) 1. pertaining to or characterized by compulsion. 2. perfectionistic, rigid, stubborn, indecisive, preoccupied with work; the personality traits of obsessive-compulsive personality (disorder).

con- [L., from *cum* with] a prefix meaning with or together. It appears as *co-* before a vowel or *h; l* before another *l; m* before *b, m,* or *p;* and *r* before another *r.*

ConA concanavalin A.

conalbumin (kon″al-bu′min) a glucoprotein, formed by the acidification of egg white to pH 3.9, containing 2.1 per cent of mannose and 0.7 per cent of galactose; the noncrystalline part of egg albumin.

conation (ko-na′shun) in psychology, the power that impels to effort of any kind; the conscious tendency to act.

conative (kon′ah-tiv) pertaining to the basic strivings of a person, as expressed in his behavior and actions.

conavanine (kon-ah-van′in) a basic amino acid from soy bean meal, α-amino-γ-guanidinoxybutyric acid.

concameration (kon-kam″er-a′shun) (*obs.*) an arrangement of connecting cavities or chambers.

concanavalin A (kon″kah-nav′ah-lin) [L. *con* with + *canavalin*] a lectin isolated from the jack bean (*Canavalia ensiformis*); it is a hemagglutinin that agglutinates mammalian erythrocytes and a mitogen that stimulates predominantly T lymphocytes. Abbreviated ConA.

concassation (kon″kah-sa′shun) the act of breaking up roots or woods into small pieces in order that their active principles may be more easily extracted by solvents.

concatenate (kon-kat′e-nāt) [L. *con* together + *catena* chain] to fasten or link together, as in a chain.

concatenation (kon-kat″e-na′shun) a series of events or objects occurring together or in sequence.

Concato's disease (kon-kah′tōz) [Luigi Maria *Concato,* Italian physician, 1825–1882] see under *disease.*

concave (kon′kāv) [L. *concavus*] having a rounded, somewhat depressed surface, resembling the hollowed inner surface of a segment of a sphere.

concavity (kon-kav′ĭ-te) [L. *concavitas,* from *con* together + *cavus* hollow] a hollowed-out area on the surface of an organ or other structure.

concavoconcave (kon-ka″vo-kon′kāv) concave on each of two opposite surfaces.

concavoconvex (kon-ka″vo-kon′veks) concave on one surface and convex on the opposite one.

conceive (kon-sēv′) 1. to become pregnant. 2. to take in, grasp, or form in the mind.

concentrate (kon′sen-trāt) [L. *con* together + *centrum* center] 1. to bring to a common center; to gather together at one point. 2. To increase the strength by diminishing the bulk of, as of a liquid; to condense. 3. A drug or other preparation that has been strengthened by the evaporation of its nonactive parts. **liver c.,** a dried, unfractionated product produced from a water extract derived from mammalian liver; used as a hematopoietic. **plant protease c.,** a concentrate of bromelains, proteolytic enzymes derived from pineapple plants; used to reduce inflammation and edema, and to accelerate tissue repair. **vitamin c.,** a concentrated medicinal preparation of a vitamin or vitamins.

concentration (kon″sen-tra′shun) [L. *concentratio*] 1. increase in strength by evaporation. 2. the ratio of the mass or volume of a solute to the mass or volume of the solution or solvent. Cf. *molarity, molality, normality,* and *mol fraction.* **hydrogen ion c.,** the degree of concentration of hydrogen ions in a solution; it is related approximately to the pH of the solution by the equation $(H^+) = 10^{-pH}$. **ionic c.,** the number of moles of an ion that are contained in the unit volume of a solution or in the unit mass of solvent. **limiting isorrheic c. (LIC),** the upper limit of urinary concentration at which a steady state consistent with effective physiologic regulation of solute and water balance can be maintained. **mass c.,** the mass of a constituent substance divided by the volume of the mixture, as milligrams per liter (mg/l), etc. **maximum cell (MC) c.,** the maximum number of microorganisms that can be produced in a given volume of culture medium. **maximum urinary c. (MUC),** the highest attainable concentration of a solute or of the collective solutes of the urine. **minimal bactericidal c. (MBC),** the lowest concentration of a given antibiotic required to kill a specific organism. Called also *minimal lethal c.* **minimal inhibitory c. (MIC),** the lowest concentration of a given antibiotic that inhibits the growth of a specific organism. **minimal isorrheic c. (MIC),** the lower limit of urinary concentration at which a steady state consistent with effective physiologic regulation of solute and water balances can be maintained. **minimal lethal c. (MLC),** minimal bactericidal c. **molar c.,** substance c. **substance c.,** the amount of a constituent substance in moles (millimoles or micromoles) divided by the volume of the mixture, as millimoles per liter (mmol./l.), etc. Called also *molar c.*

concentric (kon-sen′trik) [L. *concentricus,* from *con* together + *centrum* center] having a common center; extending out equally in all directions from a common center.

concept (kon′sept) the image of a thing as held in the mind.

conception (kon-sep′shun) [L. *conceptio*] 1. the onset of pregnancy, marked by implantation of the blastocyst; the formation of a viable zygote. 2. concept.

conceptive (kon-sep′tiv) 1. able to become pregnant. 2. pertaining to conception.

conceptus (kon-sep′tus) [L.] the sum of derivatives of a fertilized ovum at any stage of development from fertilization until birth, including extraembryonic membranes as well as the embryo or fetus.

concha (kong′kah), pl. *con'chae* [L.; Gr. *konchē*] a shell; used in anatomical nomenclature to designate a structure or part that resembles a shell in shape. **c. of auricle, c. auric'ulae** [NA], the hollow of the auricle of the external ear, bounded anteriorly by the tragus and posteriorly by the anthelix. **c. bullo'sa,** a cystic distention of the middle nasal concha, sometimes seen in chronic rhinitis. **c. of cranium,** calvaria. **ethmoidal c., inferior,** c. nasalis media. **ethmoidal c., superior,** c. nasalis superior. **ethmoidal c., supreme,** c. nasalis suprema. **inferior nasal c.,** c. nasalis inferior. **inferior turbinate c.,** c. nasalis inferior. **middle nasal c.,** c. nasalis media. **c. nasa'lis infe'rior** [NA], inferior nasal concha: a thin bony plate with curved margins, articulating with the ethmoid, maxilla, and lacrimal and palatine bones, and forming the lower part of the lateral wall of the nasal cavity, and the mucous membrane covering the plate; called also *inferior spongy* or *turbinate bone* and *maxilloturbinal bone.* **c. nasa'lis me'dia** [NA], middle nasal concha: the lower of two bony plates projecting from the inner wall of the ethmoid labyrinth and separating the superior from the middle meatus of the nose, and the mucous membrane covering the plate; called also *inferior ethmoidal c., middle turbinate bone,* and *ethmoid cornu.* **c. nasa'lis supe'rior** [NA], superior nasal concha: the upper of two bony plates projecting from the inner wall of the ethmoid labyrinth and forming the upper boundary of the superior meatus of the nose, and the mucous membrane covering the plate; called also *superior ethmoidal c.* and *superior turbinate* or *spongy bone.* **c. nasa'lis supre'ma** [NA], supreme nasal concha: a thin bony plate occasionally found projecting from the inner wall of the ethmoid labyrinth above the bony superior nasal concha, and the mucous membrane covering the plate; called also *highest turbinate bone, supreme nasal* or *ethmoidal bone,* and *supreme ethmoidal c.* **nasoturbinal c.,** agger nasi. **sphenoidal c.,** 1. concha sphenoidalis. 2. ala minor ossis sphenoidalis. **c. sphenoida'lis**

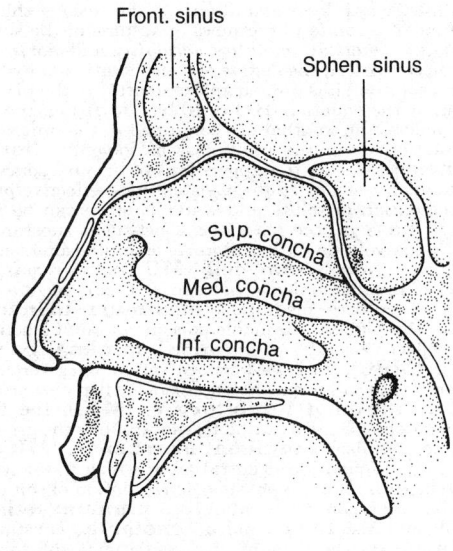

Nasal conchae.

[NA], a thin curved plate of bone at the anterior and lower part of the body of the sphenoid bone, on either side, forming part of the roof of the nasal cavity; called also *sphenoturbinal bone* or *ossicles*, *Bertin's bone* or *ossicles*, and *sphenoidal c.* **superior nasal c.,** c. nasalis superior.

conchae (kong′ke) [L.] genitive and plural of *concha*.

conchiform (kong′kĭ-form) [L. *concha* shell + *forma* shape] shaped like one half of a bivalve shell.

conchiolin (kong-ki′o-lin) [Gr. *konchē* shell] a substance, isomeric with ossein, from the outer surface of shells of mollusks.

conchiolinosteomyelitis (kong-ki″o-lin-os″te-o-mi″ĕ-li′tis) a form of osteomyelitis occurring in pearl workers.

conchitis (kong-ki′tis) an inflammation of a concha.

conchoidal (kong-koi′dal) like a shell.

conchoscope (kong′ko-skōp) [Gr. *konchē* shell + Gr. *skopein* to examine] a speculum for examining the walls of the nasal cavity.

conchotome (kong′ko-tōm) [Gr. *konchē* shell + *tomē* a cutting] an instrument for the surgical removal of the nasal conchae.

conchotomy (kong-kot′o-me) incision of a nasal concha.

Concis. abbreviation for L. *conci′sus*, cut.

conclination (kon″klĭ-na′shun) intorsion.

concoction (kon-kok′shun) [L. *concoctio*] 1. a mixture of medicinal substances usually prepared by the aid of heat. 2. the digestive process.

concomitant (kon-kom′ĭ-tant) [L. *concomitans*, from *cum* together + *comes* companion] accompanying; accessory; joined with another.

concordance (kon-kor′dans) [L. *concordare* to agree] in genetics, the occurrence of a given trait in both members of a twin pair, as opposed to discordance.

concordant (kon-kor′dant) exhibiting concordance.

concrement (kon′kre-ment) [L. *concrementum*] a concretion, especially a calcified tubercle or similar mass.

concrescence (kon-kres′ens) [L. *con-* together + *crescere* to grow] a growing together; a union of parts originally separate. In embryology, the flowing together and piling up of cells. In dentistry, the union of the roots of two approximating teeth by a deposit of cementum.

concrete (kon-krēt′) [L. *concretus*] 1. solid; tangible. 2. a mass of coalesced particles, solidified or hardened after having been more or less fluid.

concretio (kon-kre′she-o) [L.] concretion. **c. cor′dis, c. pericar′dii,** a form of adhesive pericarditis in which the pericardial cavity is obliterated.

concretion (kon-kre′shun) [L. *concretio*, from *cum* together + *crescere* to grow] 1. a calculus or inorganic mass in a natu-ral cavity or in the tissues of an organism. 2. abnormal union of adjacent parts. 3. a process of becoming harder or more solid. **alvine c.,** a bezoar, or calculus, in the stomach or intestine. **calculous c.,** articular calculus. **preputial c.,** a concretion formed beneath a tight foreskin through deposit of urinary salts on the accumulated smegma. **prostatic c's,** rounded and often lamellated masses of amyloid-like material present in many prostatic alveoli. **tophic c.,** tophus, def. 1.

concussion (kon-kush′un) [L. *concussio*] a violent jar or shock, or the condition which results from such an injury. **abdominal c., hydraulic,** abdominal injury produced in persons in the water by violent underwater explosions. **air c.,** see under *blast*, 3rd def. **c. of the brain,** loss of consciousness as the result of a blow to the head. In *mild* concussion there is transient loss of consciousness with possible impairment of the higher mental functions, such as retrograde amnesia and emotional lability. In *severe* concussion there is prolonged unconsciousness with impairment of the functions of the brain stem, such as transient loss of respiratory reflex, vasomotor activity, and dilatation of the pupils. Concussion is sometimes differentiated from contusion in that in the former the injury is functional, whereas in the latter it is organic. **c. of the labyrinth,** deafness with tinnitus, resulting from a blow on or explosion near the ear. **pulmonary c.,** mechanical damage to the lungs produced by an explosion. **c. of the retina,** commotio retinae. **c. of the spinal cord,** transient spinal cord dysfunction due to mechanical injury.

condensation (kon″den-sa′shun) [L. *condensare* to pack close together] 1. the act of rendering or the process of becoming more compact; compression. 2. the packing of dental filling material into a prepared tooth cavity. 3. a mental process in which one symbol stands for a number of components and contains all the emotion associated with them. 4. conversion from the gaseous state to the liquid or solid state; gas liquefaction.

condenser (kon-den′ser) [L. *condensare* to make thick, press close together] 1. a vessel or apparatus for condensing gases or vapors. 2. the lens in a microscope located just above the light source that aligns all available light into one beam. 3. an apparatus by which charges of electricity can be accumulated, consisting of two conducting surfaces separated by a nonconductor. 4. in dentistry, an instrument used to pack a plastic filling material into the prepared cavity of a tooth. **Abbe's c.,** as originally designed, a two-lens condenser combination placed below the stage of a microscope. **automatic c.,** mechanical c. **back-action c.,** one with a U-shaped shank so that the force applied is toward the operator. Called also *reverse c.* **cardioid c.,** a special type of condenser for illuminating a specimen in darkfield microscopy. **darkfield c.,** one with a central stop, permitting production of a hollow cone of light having its apex in the plane of the specimen. **foot c.,** one with a long, angled, foot-shaped nib. **gold c.,** one for compacting gold filling material into the prepared cavity in dental restorations. **mechanical c.,** one equipped with a spring-activated, pneumatic, or electronic mechanism for compacting the restorative material in a prepared tooth cavity through repeated blows. Called also *automatic c.* **paraboloid c.,** a special type of condenser for illuminating a specimen in darkfield microscopy. **reverse c.,** back-action c.

condition (kon-dish′un) to train; to subject to conditioning.

conditioning (kon-dish′un-ing) learning in which a stimulus initially incapable of evoking a certain response acquires the ability to do so by repeated pairing with another stimulus that does elicit the response. **aversive c.,** learning in which punishment is used to associate negative feelings with an undesirable response. **classical c.,** see *conditioning*. **instrumental c.,** learning in which a particular voluntary response is elicited by a stimulus because that response produces consequences which are rewarding to the organism; called also *operant c.* **operant c.,** instrumental c. **respondent c.,** see *conditioning*.

condom (kon′dum) [L. *condus* a receptacle; according to some authorities a corruption of *Condon*, the inventor] a sheath or cover for the penis, worn during coitus to prevent impregnation or infection.

conductance (kon-duk′tans) capacity for conducting or

ability to convey; the unit of electrical conductance is the mho.

conduction (kon-duk′shun) [L. *conductio*] the transfer of sound waves, heat, nervous impulses, or electricity; see also under *system*. **aerial c.**, the passing of sound waves to the ear through the air. **aerotympanal c.**, the conduction of sound to the inner ear through the air and tympanum. **air c.**, the conduction of sound to the inner ear through the auditory canal and middle ear to the inner ear. **anomalous c.**, conduction of the sinus impulse which avoids the delay in passage through the normal atrioventricular node. **antidromic c.**, the conduction of a nerve impulse in a direction contrary to the normal direction, as from the axon toward the dendrites. **avalanche c.**, the conduction of nerve impulses which takes place when the terminals of one neuron come in contact with the bodies of several neurons, resulting in widespread discharge following relatively little input. **bone c.**, the conduction of sound to the inner ear through the bones of the skull; called also *cranial c.*, *osteotympanic c.*, and *tissue c.* **concealed c.**, the conduction of a sinus impulse only part of the way through the conducting pathway of the heart so that a ventricular response is not elicited. **cranial c.**, bone conduction. **decremental c.**, the delay or failure of propagation of an impulse in the normal atrioventricular node resulting from progressive decrease in the rate of the rise and amplitude of the action potential as it spreads through the node. **delayed c.**, a nonspecific term indicating mild degree of atrioventricular heart block with an increase above the normal 0.2 second in the time interval between the atrial and ventricular contractions. **ephaptic c.**, the conduction of a nerve impulse across an ephapse, as opposed to synaptic conduction. **osteotympanic c.**, bone c. **saltatory c.**, the rapid passage of a potential from node (of Ranvier) to node of a myelinated nerve fiber, rather than along the full length of the membrane. **synaptic c.**, the conduction of a nerve impulse across a synapse. **tissue c.**, bone conduction.

conductivity (kon″duk-tiv′ĭ-te) the capacity of a body to conduct a current; when expressed in figures conductivity is the reciprocal of resistance. Gold, silver, and copper are good conductors.

conductor (kon-duk′tor) [L.] 1. a material that possesses conductivity; a substance that transmits electricity. 2. a grooved director for surgical use.

conduit (kon′doo-it) a channel for the passage of fluids. **ileal c.**, the surgical anastomosis of the ureters to one end of a detached segment of ileum, the other end being used to form a stoma on the abdominal wall.

conduplicatio (kon-doo″plĭ-ka′she-o) [L., from *conduplicare* to double] a doubling. **c. cor′poris**, a doubled-up attitude of a fetus in shoulder presentation.

conduplicato corpore (kon-doo″plĭ-kā′to kor′por-e) [L. "with the body doubled up"] spontaneous evolution.

condurangin (kon″du-rang′gin) either of two poisonous glycosides from condurango.

condurango (kon″du-rang′go) [Spanish American] the bark of condurango blanco, *Marsdenia* (*Gonolobus*) *condurango*, a South American asclepiadaceous plant; used as a bitter tonic and stomachic.

Condy's fluid (kon′dēz) [Henry Bollmann *Condy*, English physician, 19th century] see under *fluid*.

condylar (kon′dĭ-lar) pertaining to a condyle.

condylarthrosis (kon″dil-ar-thro′sis) [*condyle* + Gr. *arthrōsis* joint] articulatio ellipsoidea.

condyle (kon′dĭl) [L. *condylus*; Gr. *kondylos* knuckle] a rounded projection on a bone; see *condylus*. **extensor c. of humerus**, epicondylus lateralis humeri. **external c. of femur**, condylus lateralis femoris. **external c. of humerus**, epicondylus lateralis humeri. **external c. of tibia**, condylus lateralis tibiae. **fibular c. of femur**, condylus lateralis femoris. **flexor c. of humerus**, epicondylus medialis humeri. **c. of humerus**, condylus humeri. **internal c. of femur**, condylus medialis femoris. **internal c. of humerus**, epicondylus medialis humeri. **internal c. of tibia**, condylus medialis tibiae. **lateral c. of femur**, condylus lateralis femoris. **lateral c. of humerus**, epicondylus lateralis humeri. **lateral c. of tibia**, condylus lateralis tibiae. **c. of mandible**, processus condylaris mandibulae. **medial c. of femur**, condylus medialis femoris. **medial c. of hu-**

merus, epicondylus medialis humeri. **medial c. of tibia**, condylus medialis tibiae. **occipital c.**, condylus occipitalis. **radial c. of humerus**, epicondylus lateralis humeri. **c. of scapula**, angulus lateralis scapulae. **tibial c. of femur**, condylus medialis femoris. **ulnar c. of humerus**, epicondylus medialis humeri.

condylectomy (kon″dil-ek′to-me) [*condyle* + Gr. *ektomē* excision] excision of a condyle.

condyli (kon′dĭ-li) [L.] genitive and plural of *condylus*.

condylicus (kon-dil′ĭ-kus) pertaining to a condyle; condylar.

condylion (kon-dil′e-on) [Gr. *kondylion* knob] the most lateral point on the surface of the caput mandibulae.

condyloid (kon′dĭ-loid) [*condyle* + Gr. *eidos* form] resembling a condyle or knuckle.

condyloma (kon″dĭ-lo′mah), pl. *condylo′mata* [Gr. *kondylōma*, knuckle or knob] 1. c. acuminatum. 2. rarely, c. latum. 3. in veterinary medicine, hyperplasia of the skin in cloven-hoofed animals, growing between the toes, caused by chronic inflammation. **c. acumina′tum**, a papilloma with a central core of connective tissue in a treelike structure covered with epithelium, usually occurring on the mucous membrane or skin of the external genitals or in the perianal region; although the lesions are usually few in number, they may aggregate to form large cauliflower-like masses. Caused by a virus, it is infectious, and autoinoculable. Called also *acuminate* or *venereal wart, moist* or *mucous papule*, and *verruca acuminata*. **flat c.**, c. latum. **c. la′tum**, a broad and flat syphilitic condyloma located in warm, moist, intertriginous areas, especially about the anus and external genitals; it may become hypertrophic and erode to form a soft, red mass with a moist, weeping surface. Called also *flat c.* **pointed c.**, c. acuminatum.

condylomata (kon″dĭ-lo′mah-tah) [L.] plural of *condyloma*.

condylomatoid (kon″dĭ-lo′mah-toid) resembling a condyloma.

condylomatosis (kon″dĭ-lo″mah-to′sis) the presence of numerous condylomas.

condylomatous (kon″dĭ-lo′mah-tus) of the nature of a condyloma.

condylotomy (kon″dĭ-lot′o-me) [Gr. *kondylos* condyle + *temnein* to cut] surgical incision or division of a condyle or of condyles.

condylus (kon′dĭ-lus), pl. *con′dyli* [L.; Gr. *kondylos* knuckle] [NA] condyle: a rounded projection on a bone, usually for articulation with another. **c. hu′meri** [NA], condyle of humerus: the distal end of the humerus, including the various fossae as well as the trochlea and capitulum. **c. latera′lis fem′oris** [NA], lateral condyle of femur: the lateral of the two surfaces at the distal end of the femur that articulate with the superior surfaces of the head of the tibia; called also *external* or *fibular condyle of femur*. **c. latera′lis hu′meri**, epicondylus lateralis humeri. **c. latera′lis tib′iae** [NA], lateral condyle of tibia: the lateral articular eminence on the proximal end of the tibia; called also *external condyle of tibia*. **c. media′lis fem′oris** [NA], medial condyle of femur: the medial of the two surfaces at the distal end of the femur that articulate with the superior surfaces of the head of the tibia; called also *internal* or *tibial condyle of femur*, and c. tibialis femoris. **c. media′lis hu′meri**, epicondylus medialis humeri. **c. media′lis tib′iae** [NA], medial condyle of tibia: the medial articular eminence on the proximal end of the tibia; called also *internal condyle of tibia*. **c. occipita′lis** [NA], occipital condyle: one of two oval processes on the lateral portions of the occipital bone, on either side of the foramen magnum, for articulation with the atlas. **c. tibia′lis fem′oris**, c. medialis femoris.

cone (kōn) [Gr. *kōnos*; L. *conus*] 1. a solid figure or body with a circular base tapering to a point; specifically, one of the conelike bodies of the retina; called also *conus*. See *retinal c's*. 2. in radiology, a conical or open-ended cylindrical structure attached over the portal of the x-ray tube housing, used as an aid in centering the radiation beam on the target field and as a guide to source-to-film distance; also, often designed to collimate primary and/or scattered radiation, and/or to retain disks for added filtration. 3. in root canal therapy, a solid substance, usually gutta-percha or silver, having a tapered form, and fashioned to conform to the shape of the root canal. **acrosomal c.,** an axial body of the spermatozoon between the acrosomal granule and the nucleus. **antipodal c.,** the cone of rays opposite the spindle fibers of the amphiaster. **arterial c.,** conus arteriosus. **attraction c.,** fertilization c. **bifurcation c.,** the cone-shaped structure at the bifurcation of a dendrite. **cerebellar pressure c.,** a deformity of the brain caused by increased intracranial pressure, which forces the cerebellum downward into the spinal canal. **Dunham's c's,** see under *fan.* **ectoplacental c.,** the thickened trophoblast of the blastocyst in rodents which becomes the fetal portion of the placenta. **elastic c. of larynx,** conus elasticus laryngis. **ether c.,** originally an apparatus to be placed over the face for the administration of ether by inhalation, now used with various anesthetics. **fertilization c.,** a bulging of the cytoplasm in the ovum at the site of contact of a spermatozoon, which gradually engulfs the spermatozoon and then retracts, carrying the spermatozoon inward; called also *attraction c.* **growth c.,** a bulbous enlargement of the growing tip of a nerve axon. **gutta-percha c.,** a plastic, radiopaque cone produced from gutta-percha combined with various other ingredients and available in various standard sizes that conform with the dimensions of root canal reamers and files; used to fill and seal root canals in conjunction with root canal sealer cements. Called also *gutta-percha point.* **Haller's c's,** lobuli epididymidis. **implantation c.,** the cone-shaped insertion of an axon in its neuron. **c. of light,** the triangular reflection of light seen on the membrana tympani; called also *Politzer's c.* and *light reflex.* **long c.,** in dental radiology, a tubular "cone" designed to establish an extended anode-to-skin distance, usually within a range of 10 to 25 cm or more. **medullary c.,** conus medullaris. **ocular c.,** a cone of light in the eye, the base being on the cornea, the apex on the retina; called also *visual c.* **Politzer's c.,** c. of light. **pressure c.,** the area of compression exerted by a mass in the brain, as in uncal or transtentorial herniation. **primitive c.,** the conelike arrangement of the collecting tubules in the kidney. **retinal c.,** a visual cell that serves light and color vision and visual acuity. The synaptic terminal is a broad, flattened pedicle. Outside the fovea the dendritic segments are relatively short and squat with blunt, rounded tips; within the fovea the segments are elongated and narrow and thus resemble rods. There are 6 million to 7 million cones, of which some 10 per cent are concentrated in the fovea, the remainder being fairly uniformly distributed over the rest of the retina. Called also *cone, cone cell,* and *visual cone.* See also *visual cell,* under *cell,* and *retinal rod,* under *rod.* **sarcoplasmic c.,** the conical mass of sarcoplasm at each end of the nucleus of a smooth or cardiac muscle fiber. **short c.,** in dental radiology, a conical or a tubular "cone" having as one of its functions the establishment of an anode-to-skin distance of up to 10 to 25 cm. **silver c.,** see under *point.* **terminal c. of spinal cord,** conus medullaris. **theca interna c.,** a wedge-shaped thickening of the theca interna projecting toward the ovarian surface, found only in growing follicles. **twin c's,** cone cells of the retina in which two cells are blended. **Tyndall c.,** the murky cone of scattered light seen when a colloid is viewed at right angles to the incident beam; it distinguishes colloids from crystalloids. **ureteral c.,** the upper conic part of the ureter; at ordinary rates of urine flow it is filled with urine during the resting phase of the renal pelvis and emptied during activity. **visual c.,** 1. ocular cone. 2. retinal cone.

cone-nose (kōn'nōs) see *Reduviidae.*

Conestron (kon-es'tron) trademark for a preparation of conjugated estrogens.

conexus (cŏ-nek'sus), pl. *conex'us* [L. "connection," from *conectere* to join together] a connecting structure; written also *connexus* (q.v.). **c. intertendin'eus,** NA alternative for *connexus intertendineus.* **c. interthalam'icus,** adhesio interthalamica.

confabulation (kon″fab-u-la'shun) unconscious filling in of gaps in memory with fabricated facts and experiences, commonly seen in organic amnestic syndromes. It differs from lying in that the patient has no intention to deceive and believes the fabricated memories to be real. Called also *fabrication* and *fabulation.*

confectio (kon-fek'she-o) [L.] confection.

confection (kon-fek'shun) [L. *confectio*] a medicated conserve, sweetmeat, or electuary. **Damocrates' c.,** a confection of some thirty ingredients, the chief of which were agaric, frankincense, galbanum, cinnamon, garlic, gentian, ginger, opium, etc. **c. of senna,** a mild laxative containing powdered senna with other ingredients.

confertus (kon-fer'tus) [L.] close together; confluent.

configuration (kon-fig″u-ra'shun) the arrangement of parts of a whole. In chemistry, the spatial arrangement of atoms in a molecule, the property that distinguishes a compound from its stereoisomers. Cf. *constitution.* **cis c.,** in genetics, the condition (coupling) in which two linked mutant genes are on one chromosome and the two equivalent wild-type genes are on the homologous chromosome. Called also *cis position.* Cf. *trans c.* **trans c.,** in genetics, the condition (repulsion) in which one wild-type and one mutant gene are on one chromosome and their corresponding mutant and wild-type alleles are on the homologous chromosome.

confinement (kon-fin'ment) restraint within a specific area; used especially to designate the termination of pregnancy with delivery of the infant; see *labor.*

conflict (kon'flikt) a psychic struggle, often unconscious, arising from the clash of incompatible or opposing impulses, wishes, drives, or external demands. See *extrapsychic c.* and *intrapsychic c.* **approach-approach c.,** conflict resulting from two available goals which are desirable but incompatible. **approach-avoidance c.,** conflict resulting from a single goal having both desirable and undesirable consequences. **avoidance-avoidance c.,** conflict resulting from the desire to avoid two equally distasteful alternatives. **extrapsychic c.,** conflict between a person's wishes or needs and the expectations or desires of others. **intrapersonal c.,** intrapsychic c. **intrapsychic c.,** conflict between incompatible and often unconscious wishes, impulses, needs, thoughts, or demands within one's own mind. Called also *intrapersonal c.*

confluence (kon'floo-ens) [L. *confluens* running together] the meeting of streams; in embryology the flowing of cells, a component process of gastrulation. **c. of sinuses,** confluens sinuum.

confluens (kon'floo-ens) [L., from *confluere* to run together] a place of running together; the meeting of streams. **c. sin'uum** [NA], confluence of sinuses: the dilated point of confluence of the superior sagittal, straight, occipital, and two transverse sinuses of the dura mater, lodged in a depression at one side of the internal occipital protuberance; called also *torcular Herophili.*

confluent (kon'floo-ent) [L. *confluens* running together] becoming merged; not discrete.

confocal (kon-fo'kal) having the same focus.

conformation (kon″for-ma'shun) the particular shape of an entity. In chemistry, the spatial arrangement of atoms in a molecule produced by rotations about single bonds, the property that distinguishes different conformers (conformational isomers) from each other.

conformer (kon'for-mer) any of the group of structures that are produced by rotations about single bonds in a molecule.

confrication (kon″frĭ-ka'shun) [L. *confricatio*] the rubbing of a drug to the consistency of a powder.

confrontation (kon″frun-ta'shun) [L. *con* together + *frons* face] a technique in treating psychological disorders whereby the contradictory statements or actions of a patient are brought directly to his attention.

confusion (kon-fu'zhun) disturbed orientation in regard to time, place, or person, sometimes accompanied by disordered consciousness.

confusional (kon-fu'zhun-al) pertaining to, characterized by, or resulting in confusion.

cong. abbreviation for L. *con'gius,* gallon.

congelation (kon″jĕ-la'shun) [L. *congelatio*] frostbite or freezing.

congenic (kon-jen'ik) [*con-* + L. *genus* race, kind] pertaining to two inbred strains of animals that are genetically identical except at a single locus or a few specified loci so that their known genetic differences are expressed in the same "genetic background." A congenic strain is produced by outbreeding a strain and then eliminating the background genes by many generations of backcrosses while maintaining the desired genetic differences by selection of progeny. Called also *coisogenic.*

congener (kon'jĕ-ner) [L. *con* together + *genus* race] something closely related to another thing, as a member of the same genus, a muscle having the same function as another, or a chemical compound closely related to another in composition and exerting similar or antagonistic effects, or something derived from the same source or stock. Also, a secondary product in alcohol fermentation that helps to determine the composition of the final product.

congeneric (kon″jĕ-ner′ik) pertaining to a congener.

congenerous (kon-jen′er-us) [L. con together + genus race] having a common action or function; derived from the same source. See congener.

congenital (kon-jen′ĭ-tal) [L. congenitus born together] existing at, and usually before, birth; referring to conditions that are present at birth, regardless of their causation. Cf. hereditary.

congested (kon-jest′ed) overloaded, as with blood; in a state of congestion.

congestin (kon-jes′tin) a toxic substance derived from the tentacles of sea anemones which, when injected into dogs, causes intense congestion of the splanchnic vessels, and hemorrhage; originally called actinocongestin. Cf. medusocongestin.

congestion (kon-jest′shun) [L. congestio, from congerere to heap together] excessive or abnormal accumulation of blood in a part. **active c.,** accumulation of blood in a part on account of the dilatation of the lumen of its blood vessels. **functional c.,** increased vascularization and flow of blood to an organ during the performance of its function. **hypostatic c.,** congestion of the lowest part of an organ by reason of the action of gravity when the circulation is much enfeebled. **neuroparalytic c.,** that which results from paralysis of the constrictor fibers of the vasomotor nerves. **neurotonic c.,** that which is due to irritation of the vasodilator nerves. **passive c.,** the congestion of a part due to the obstruction to the escape of blood from the part; called also venous c. **physiologic c.,** increased vascularization and blood flow that occurs during functional activity. **pulmonary c.,** engorgement of the pulmonary vessels, with transudation of fluid into the alveolar and interstitial spaces; it occurs in cardiac disease, infections, and certain injuries. **venous c.,** passive c.

congestive (kon-jes′tiv) pertaining to, characterized by, or resulting in congestion.

congius (kon′je-us) [L.] a gallon; abbreviated c. or cong.

conglobate (kon′glo-bāt) [L. conglobatus] forming a rounded mass or clump; said of certain glands and of a form of acne.

conglobation (kon″glo-ba′shun) the act of forming, or the state of being formed, into a rounded mass.

conglomerate (kon-glom′er-āt) [L. con together + glomerare to heap] heaped together.

conglutin (kon-gloo′tin) a protein from almonds and from seeds of various leguminous plants.

conglutinant (kon-gloo′tĭ-nant) [L. conglutinare to glue together] promoting union, as of the edges of a wound.

conglutinatio (kon-gloo′tĭ-na′she-o) [L. conglutinare to glue together] conglutination. **c. orific′ii exter′ni,** a condition in labor in which the circular fibers around the cervical os will not relax, and the cervix remains closed.

conglutination (kon-gloo′tĭ-na′shun) 1. agglutination by conglutinin or immunoconglutinin of bacteria or erythrocytes in the presence of specific antibody or complements. 2. the abnormal adherence of tissues to each other; adhesion (def. 3).

conglutinin (kon-gloo′tĭ-nin) a nonimmunoglobulin bovine serum protein that aggregates immune complexes with conglutinogen activity (inactivated C3b) in the presence of divalent cations. It has been used as an indicator system, replacing complement fixation, in serologic tests and in the detection of immune complexes. Not to be confused with immunoconglutinin. Called also bovine colloid. **immune c.,** immunoconglutinin.

conglutinogen (kon-gloo′tĭ-no-jen) the capacity of certain immune complexes to react with conglutinin owing to the fixation of the complement component C3 and the subsequent inactivation of C3b by factor I (formerly called conglutinogen-activating factor [KAF]).

congressus (kon-gres′us) [L. "a coming together"] coitus.

CO(NH₂)₂ urea.

coni (ko′ni) [L.] genitive and plural of conus.

conic (kon′ik) conical.

conical (kon′e-kal) cone-shaped.

conidia (ko-nid′e-ah) [L.] plural of conidium.

conidial (ko-nid′e-al) pertaining to or of the nature of conidia; bearing conidia.

conidiophore (ko-nid′e-o-fōr) [L. conidium + Gr. phoros bearing] the branch of the mycelium of a fungus that bears conidia.

Conidiosporales (ko-nid″e-o-spo-ra′lēz) former name for Moniliales.

conidiospore (ko-nid′e-o-spōr) [Gr. konidion a particle of dust + spore] conidium.

conidium (ko-nid′e-um), pl. conid′ia. An asexual fungal spore shed at maturity (deciduous), and formed by splitting off from the summit of a conidiophore; called also exospore. See spore. Cf. aleuriospore and chlamydospore (def. 1).

coniine (co′ne-ēn) a poisonous, liquid alkaloid from Conium maculatum L. (poison hemlock), $C_8H_{17}N$.

coniofibrosis (ko″ne-o-fi-bro′sis) [Gr. konis dust + fibrosis] a form of pneumoconiosis marked by an exuberant growth of connective tissue caused by a specific irritant; it may occur in asbestosis, silicosis, and silicotuberculosis.

coniology (ko-ne-ol′ŏ-je) [Gr. konis dust + -logy] the scientific study of dust, its influence and its effects on plant and animal life.

coniolymphstasis (ko″ne-o-limf′stah-sis) a form of pneumoconiosis caused by dusts that act by blocking the lymphatics.

coniometer (ko″ne-om′ĕ-ter) konometer.

coniophage (ko′ne-o-fāj″) [Gr. konis dust + phagein to eat] a macrophage that ingests dust particles.

coniosis (ko″ne-o′sis) [Gr. konis dust] a disease state caused by the inhalation of dust, such as pneumoconiosis.

Coniosporium (ko″ne-o-spōr′e-um) a genus of saprophytic fungi. C. cortica′le (Cryptostroma corticale), which grows under the bark of certain trees, causes coniosporosis.

coniosporosis (ko″ne-o-spo-ro′sis) a condition characterized by asthmatic symptoms and acute pneumonitis, caused by inhalation of spores of Coniosporium corticale, a fungus which grows under the bark of certain trees; observed in workers engaged in peeling logs.

coniotomy (ko″ne-ot′o-me) cricothyrotomy.

coniotoxicosis (ko″ne-o-tok″sĭ-ko′sis) a form of pneumoconiosis in which the irritants affect the tissues directly.

Conium (ko-ni′um) [L.; Gr. kōneion] a genus of umbelliferous plants, the hemlocks. **C. macula′tum** L., poison hemlock; see hemlock, def. 2.

conization (kon″ĭ-za′shun) the removal of a cone of tissue, as in partial excision of the cervix uteri. **cold c.,** that done with a cold knife, as opposed to electrocautery, to better preserve the histologic elements.

conjugal (kon′ju-gal) [L. con together + jugum a yoke] pertaining to marriage; pertaining to husband and wife.

conjugant (kon′joo-gant) either individual of a pair of organisms or gametes during the process of conjugation; after separation, each is known as an exconjugant.

conjugata (kon″ju-ga′tah) 1. conjugate diameter. 2. diameter conjugata pelvis. **c. anatom′ica,** diameter conjugata pelvis. **c. diagona′lis,** diagonal conjugate diameter. **c. ve′ra,** diameter conjugata pelvis. **c. ve′ra obstet′rica,** obstetric conjugate diameter.

conjugate (kon′ju-gāt) [L. conjugatus yoked together] 1. see under diameter. 2. diameter conjugata pelvis. **anatomic c.,** diameter conjugata pelvis. **diagonal c.,** diagonal conjugate diameter. **external c.,** external conjugate diameter. **obstetric c.,** obstetric conjugate diameter.

conjugation (kon″ju-ga′shun) [L. conjugatio a blending] 1. the act of joining together or the state of being conjugated. 2. a sexual process seen in bacteria, ciliate protozoa, and certain fungi in which nuclear material is exchanged during the temporary fusion of two cells (conjugants). In bacterial genetics a form of sexual reproduction in which a donor bacterium (male) contributes some, or all, of its DNA (in the form of a replicated set) to a recipient (female), which then incorporates differing genetic information into its own chromosome by recombination and passes the recombined set on to its progeny by replication. In *ciliate protozoa*, two conjugants of separate mating types exchange micronuclear material and then separate, each now being a fertilized cell. In certain fungi, the process involves fusion of two gametes, resulting in union of their nuclei and formation of a zygote. 3. in chemistry, the joining together of two compounds to produce another compound, such as the combination of a toxic product with some substance in the body to form a detoxified product, which is then eliminated.

conjunctiva (kon″junk-ti′vah), pl. *conjunctivae* [L.] the delicate membrane that lines the eyelids (*palpebral conjunctiva*) and covers the exposed surface of the sclera (*bulbar* or *ocular conjunctiva*); called also *tunica conjunctiva* [NA].

conjunctival (kon″junk-ti′val) pertaining to the conjunctiva.

conjunctiviplasty (kon-junk′tĭ-vĭ-plas″te) conjunctivoplasty.

conjunctivitis (kon-junk″tĭ-vi′tis) inflammation of the conjunctiva, generally consisting of conjunctival hyperemia associated with a discharge. **actinic c.,** conjunctivitis produced by ultraviolet (actinic) rays, as that of Klieg lights, therapeutic lamps, or acetylene torches. **acute catarrhal c.,** an acute, infectious conjunctivitis associated with cold or catarrh and marked by vivid hyperemia, edema, loss of translucence, and mucous or mucopurulent discharge. Called also *mucopurulent c., simple c.,* and *simple acute c.* **acute contagious c., acute epidemic c.,** a mucopurulent, epidemic conjunctivitis caused by *Haemophilus aegyptius,* occurring in the spring or fall, with the same symptoms as acute catarrhal conjunctivitis. Called also *pinkeye.* **acute hemorrhagic c.,** a highly contagious disease, certain epidemics of which have been associated etiologically with enteroviruses, characterized by subconjunctival hemorrhage varying from minute petechiae to copious, and by sudden swelling of the eyelids and congestion, redness, and pain in the eye. **allergic c., anaphylactic c.,** hay fever. **angular c.,** conjunctivitis with characteristic reddening at the canthi, usually due to Morax-Axenfeld bacillus or *Staphylococcus aureus;* called also *diplobacillary c.* and *Morax-Axenfeld c.* **arc-flash c.,** actinic c. **atopic c.,** allergic conjunctivitis of the immediate type, due to such airborne allergens as pollens, dusts, spores, and animal hair. **atropine c.,** follicular conjunctivitis from continued use of atropine. **blennorrheal c.,** gonorrheal c. **calcareous c.,** c. petrificans. **catarrhal c.,** a mild form characterized by excessive mucous secretion. **chemical c.,** that due to exposure to chemical irritants. **chronic catarrhal c.,** a mild, chronic conjunctivitis with only slight hyperemia and mucous discharge. It may be a sequel to acute catarrhal conjunctivitis, or the result of eyestrain, dust, glare, or ingrown lashes. **croupous c.,** pseudomembranous c. **diphtheritic c.,** membranous conjunctivitis occurring as a primary infection caused by *Corynebacterium diphtheriae* or secondarily to diphtheria of the respiratory tract. **diplobacillary c.,** angular c. **eczematous c.,** phlyctenular c. **Egyptian c.,** trachoma, def. 1. **epidemic c.,** acute contagious c. **follicular c.,** a form characterized by dense localized infiltrations of lymphoid tissue that occur as a response to irritation. **gonococcal c., gonorrheal c.,** a severe form caused by infection with gonococci, marked by greatly swollen conjunctivae and eyelids and by a profuse purulent discharge. The infection is bilateral in newborns, who acquire it from an infected vaginal passage; it is usually unilateral in adults, who acquire it by autoinoculation into the eye of other gonococcal infections, e.g., gonococcal urethritis, either in themselves or in others. Called also *blennorrheal c.* and *gonoblennorrhea.* Cf. *gonorrheal ophthalmia* and *ophthalmia neonatorum,* under *ophthalmia.* **granular c.,** trachoma. **inclusion c.,** conjunctivitis caused by an organism (*Chlamydia trachomatis*) of the psittacosis-lymphogranuloma venereum-trachoma group; it affects primarily newborn infants, beginning as an acute purulent conjunctivitis that leads to papillary hypertrophy of the palpebral conjunctiva. Called also *inclusion blennorrhea* and *swimming pool c.* **infantile purulent c.,** ophthalmia neonatorum. **Koch-Weeks c.,** acute contagious c. **larval c.,** myiasis of the conjunctiva. **lithiasis c.,** c. petrificans. **c. medicamento′sa,** conjunctivitis due to medication. **membranous c.,** severe conjunctivitis marked by the presence of a membrane on the inner surface of the lids formed by the profuse fibrinous exudation from the cul-de-sac, which on attempted removal leaves a raw, bleeding surface; it is

caused by various bacteria, including *Corynebacterium diphtheriae,* streptococci, gonococci, and pneumococci. Cf. *pseudomembranous c.* **meningococcus c.,** conjunctivitis occurring as a complication of epidemic cerebrospinal meningitis. **molluscum c.,** conjunctivitis occurring as a complication of molluscum contagiosum. **Morax-Axenfeld c.,** angular c. **mucopurulent c.,** acute catarrhal c. **necrotic infectious c.,** a unilateral, purulent, necrotic conjunctivitis marked by small, diffuse, elevated, white spots in the palpebral conjunctiva and fornices, with ipsilateral swelling of the preauricular, parotid, and submaxillary lymph glands. Called also *Pascheff's c.* **c. nodo′sa, nodular c.,** ophthalmia nodosa. **Parinaud's c.,** Parinaud's oculoglandular syndrome. **Pascheff's c.,** necrotic infectious c. **c. petri′ficans,** a variety of conjunctivitis marked by the formation of deposits of chalky concretions in the conjunctiva and attended with necrosis; called also *calcareous c., lithiasis c.* and *uratic c.* **phlyctenular c.,** a variety marked by small vesicles or ulcers, each surrounded by a reddened zone; called also *eczematous c.* and *scrofular c.* See also *phlyctenulosis.* **prairie c.,** chronic conjunctivitis marked by white spots on the conjunctiva of the lids. **pseudomembranous c.,** inflammation of the conjunctiva resembling membranous conjunctivitis except that the membrane can be removed without traumatizing the epithelium and in addition to being caused by bacterial infections can also be caused by toxic and allergic factors and various viral infections. Called also *croupous c.* **purulent c.,** acute conjunctivitis caused by bacteria or viruses, particularly gonococci, meningococci, pneumococci, and streptococci, characterized by severe inflammation of the conjunctiva and copious discharge of pus. **scrofular c.,** phlyctenular c. **shipyard c.,** epidemic keratoconjunctivitis. **simple c., simple acute c.,** acute catarrhal c. **spring c.,** vernal c. **swimming pool c.,** inclusion c. **trachomatous c.,** trachoma, def. 1. **tularemic c.,** see *oculoglandular tularemia,* under *tularemia.* **uratic c.,** c. petrificans. **vaccinial c.,** autovaccinia affecting the eye. **vernal c.,** bilateral conjunctivitis of seasonal occurrence, of unknown cause, affecting children, especially boys. Flattened papules and a thick, gelatinous exudate develop on the conjunctivae on the inside of the upper lid; itching and photophobia are present. The condition is usually self-limiting, but it may become severe if corneal vascularization and ulceration develop. Also called *vernal catarrh, spring ophthalmia.* **welder's c.,** actinic c. **Widmark's c.,** congestion of the inferior tarsal conjunctiva, with occasionally slight stippling of the cornea.

conjunctivodacryocystostomy (kon″junk-ti″vo-dak″re-o-sis-tos′to-me) surgical connection of the lacrimal sac directly to the conjunctival sac.

conjunctivoma (kon-junk″tĭ-vo′mah) a tumor of the eyelid made up of conjunctival tissue.

conjunctivoplasty (kon″junk-ti′vo-plas″te) [*conjunctiva* + Gr. *plassein* to form] repair of a defect of the conjunctiva by plastic surgery.

conjunctivorhinostomy (kon″junk-ti″vo-ri-nos′to-me) surgical correction of total lacrimal canalicular obstruction: a dacryocystorhinostomy is done by suturing the posterior flaps, and the lacrimal caruncle is dissected out, preserving the conjunctiva.

Conn's syndrome (konz) [Jerome W. *Conn,* American internist, born 1907] primary hyperaldosteronism.

connatal (kon-na′tal) [L. *con* along with + *natus* birth] occurring at the time of birth; acquired at birth.

connate (kon′nāt) connatal.

connection (kŏ-nek′shun) 1. the act of connecting or state of being connected. 2. anything that connects; a connector. **clamp c.,** a short tubular branch connecting one cell of a hypha to another, formed by fusion during cell division in certain basidiomycetous fungi, and serving in the transfer of the two daughter nuclei of the parent cell to a newly formed cell. **intertendinous c.,** connexus intertendineus.

connector (kŏ-nek′tor) 1. anything serving as a link between two separate objects or units. 2. the portion of a neural arc between the receptor and the effector. 3. the part of a fixed partial denture that unites the retainer and the pontic; it may be rigid or nonrigid. **major c.,** a rigid unit of a removable partial denture, serving as its chassis, which joins the parts of the prosthesis on one side of the dental arch to those on the other side, and to which all other components are attached. Called also *saddle c.* Cf. *connector bar.* **minor c.,** a connecting link between the major connector or base of a partial denture and other units of the prosthesis, such as clasps, indirect retainers, and occlusal rests; called also *connector bar.* **saddle c.,** major c.

Connell's suture (kŏn'elz) [Frank Gregory *Connell,* American surgeon, 1875–1968] see under *suture.*

connexus (kŏ-nek'sus), pl. *connex'us* [L., variant of *conexus,* q.v.] a connecting structure; written also *conexus.* **c. intertendin'eus** [NA], intertendinous connection: narrow bands extending obliquely between the tendons of insertion of the extensor digitorum muscles on the dorsum of the hand. Called also *conexus intertendineus* [NA alternative], *juncturae tendinum,* and *tendinous junctions.*

cono- [Gr. *kōnos cone*] a combining form denoting a relationship to a cone or to a conelike structure.

conoid (ko'noid) [Gr. *kōnoeidēs*] 1. resembling or shaped like a cone. 2. an electron-dense, protrusible, hollow region surrounded by polar rings and composed of spirally coiled microtubules that forms part of the apical complex of apicocomplexan protozoa. **Sturm's c.,** the changing shapes of the diffusion images of a point in various forms of astigmatism; the image may be an ellipse, a circle, or a sharp line.

conomyoidin (ko″no-mi-oi'din) [*cone* + *myoid*] a protoplasmic material within the cones of some retinas that expands and contracts under the influence of light, causing the cones to shift.

conophthalmus (kŏn″of-thal'mus) [*cono-* + *ophthalmus*] staphyloma corneae, def. 1.

Conopodina (ko″no-po-di'nah) [Gr. *kōnos cone*] a suborder of ameboid protozoa (order Amoebida, subclass Gymnamoeba), characterized by the presence of digitiform or mammilliform, usually blunt, normally unbranched subpseudopodia, most commonly produced from a broad hyaline lobe. *Paramoeba* is a representative genus.

Conorhinus (ko″no-ri'nus) [*cono-* + Gr. *rhis nose*] a genus name formerly applied to insects of the family Reduviidae, now placed in the genera *Panstrongylus* and *Triatoma.*

conquinine (kon-kwin'in) quinidine.

Conradi's disease (syndrome) (kon-rah'dēz) [Erich *Conradi,* German physician, born 1882] see *chondrodysplasia punctata.*

Conradi's line (kon-rah'dēz) [Andreas Christian *Conradi,* Norwegian physician, 1809–1869] see under *line.*

Conray (kon'ra) trademark for a preparation of iothalamate meglumine.

Cons. abbreviation for L. *conser'va,* keep.

consanguineous (kon″san-gwin'e-us) related by blood.

consanguinity (kon″san-gwin'ĭ-te) [L. *consanguinitas*] kinship; relationship by blood.

conscience (kon'shens) the nontechnical term for the moral faculty of the mind, corresponding roughly to the psychoanalytic concept of the superego (q.v.), although, unlike the ordinary conception of conscience, the actions of the superego are often unconscious.

conscious (kon'shus) [L. *conscius* aware] 1. having awareness of one's self, acts, and surroundings. 2. the part of the mind that is constantly within awareness, one of the systems of Freud's topographic model of the mind. Cf. *preconscious* and *unconscious.*

consciousness (kon'shus-nes) the state of being conscious, fully alert, aware, and oriented; also, having a clear or intact sensorium. "Disorders of consciousness" are states of disordered attention and apperception in which there is "clouding of consciousness," e.g., confusion or delirium. "Levels of consciousness" refer to clinically differentiable degrees of awareness and alertness; alert wakefulness, lethargy, obtundation, stupor, and coma. **colon c.,** a condition in which the patient is aware of the colon and its activities, because of disturbance of the normal defecation reflex; embracing chronic constipation.

conscious-sedation (kon'shus-se-da'shun) in dental anesthesia, a state of sedation in which the conscious patient is rendered free of fear, apprehension, and anxiety through the use of pharmacological agents.

consensual (kon-sen'shu-al) excited by reflex stimulation; used especially to designate the similar reaction of both pupils to a stimulus applied to only one.

conservative (kon-ser'vah-tiv) [L. *conservare* to preserve] designed to preserve health, restore function, and repair structures by nonradical methods, as conservative surgery. Cf. *radical.*

conserve (kon'serv) [L. *conserva*] a confection, electuary, or medicated sweetmeat.

consolidant (kon-sol'ĭ-dant) [L. *consolidare* to make firm] 1. promoting the healing or union of parts. 2. an agent that promotes the healing or union of parts.

consolidation (kon-sol″ĭ-da'shun) [L. *consolidatio*] solidification; the process of becoming or the condition of being solid, as when the lung becomes firm as air spaces are filled with exudate in pneumonia.

consolute (kon'so-lūt) perfectly miscible.

consonation (kon″so-na'shun) the presence of consonating rales; see under *rale.*

conspecific (kon″spĕ-sif'ik) 1. of or pertaining to the same species. 2. a member of the same species.

constancy (kon'stan-se) the state of being constant. **cell c.,** an extreme example of mosaic development resulting in all individuals in a species having the same number of cells in comparable tissues performing similar functions.

constant (kon'stant) [L. *constans* standing together] 1. not failing; remaining unaltered. 2. a datum, fact, or principle that is not subject to change. **absorption c.,** absorptivity. **association c.,** a measure of the extent of a reversible association between two molecular species; called also *binding c.* **Avogadro's c.,** see under *number.* **binding c.,** association c. **Botzmann's c.,** the gas constant divided by Avogadro's number; 1.38066×10^{-23} joules per kelvin. Symbol, k. **decay c.,** the fraction of the number of atoms of a radionuclide which decay per unit time; symbol λ. Called also *disintegration c.* and *radioactive c.* **dielectric c.,** the dielectric value of any substance compared with air, which is taken as 1. **disintegration c.,** decay c. **dissociation c.,** the equilibrium constant for the dissociation of a weak acid into hydrogen ion and its conjugate base in solution. **equilibrium c.,** for a chemical reaction at equilibrium, the product of the concentrations of the reaction products, each raised to the power equal to the coefficient of the product in the balanced chemical equation for the reaction, divided by the product of the concentrations of the reactants, each raised to the power equal to its coefficient (see formula at *reaction quotient* under *quotient*). Symbol K. **Faraday's c.,** the electric charge of one mole of electrons or one equivalent of ions: 96,493.5 coulombs per mole. Symbol, F. **gas c.,** the proportionality constant in the ideal gas law (q.v.); 8.3144 joules per mole-kelvin or 1.987 calories per mole-kelvin. Symbol R. **gravitational c., c. of gravitation,** the constant of proportionality in the law of gravitation, equal to 6.67×10^{-11} newton m.^{2}/kg.^{2}; symbol G. Called also *Newtonian constant of gravitation.* **Lapicque's c.,** the figure 0.37, used for converting noninductive resistance into direct current equivalents. **Michaelis c.,** a constant representing the substrate concentration at which the velocity of an enzyme reaction is half the maximal velocity; symbol K_m. See also *Michaelis-Menten equation,* under *equation.* **Newtonian c. of gravitation,** gravitational c. **Planck's c., quantum c.,** a constant, h, which represents the ratio of the energy of any quantum of radiation to its frequency; the value of h is 6.625×10^{-27} erg seconds. **radioactive c.,** decay c. **sedimentation c.,** see under *coefficient.*

constipated (kon'stĭ-pāt″ed) affected with constipation.

constipation (kon″stĭ-pa'shun) [L. *constipatio* a crowding together] infrequent or difficult evacuation of the feces. **atonic c.,** constipation due to intestinal atony. **gastrojejunal c.,** constipation due to reflex inhibition from some disease of the gastrointestinal tract. **proctogenous c.,** constipation due to some abnormality of the defecation reflex resulting in failure of fecal masses in the rectum to excite impulses leading to their evacuation. **spastic c.,** constipation marked by spasmodic constriction of a portion of the intestine; seen in neurasthenia and lead poisoning.

constitution (kon″stĭ-tu'shun) [L. *constitutio*] 1. the make-up or functional habit of the body, determined by the genetic, biochemical, and physiologic endowment of the individual, and modified in great measure by environmental factors. Cf. *diathesis, type,* and *genotype.* 2. in chemistry, the atoms making up a molecule and the way they are linked, the property that distinguishes a compound from its structural isomers. Cf. *configuration.* **lymphatic c.,** a condition of hyperplasia of the lymphatic system. **vasoneurotic c.,** a constitution characterized by instability of the vasomotor mechanism.

constitutional (kon″stĭ-tu′shun-al) 1. affecting the whole constitution of the body; not local. 2. pertaining to the constitution.

constriction (kon-strik′shun) [L. *con* together + *stringere* to draw] a constricted part or place; a stricture. **duoden-opyloric c.,** the constriction marking the junction of the stomach and duodenum. **primary c.,** centromere. **Ranvier's c's,** nodes of Ranvier. **secondary c.,** in genetics, the narrowed heterochromatic area of the short arms of acrocentric autosomes by which a satellite is attached.

constrictive (kon-strik′tiv) causing constriction or having a tendency to constriction.

constrictor (kon-strik′tor) [L.] that which constricts, such as a muscle or an instrument by which a part may be constricted. See *Table of Musculi.* **c. isth′mi fau′cium,** musculus palatoglossus. **c. na′ris,** pars transversa musculi nasalis. **c. ure′thrae,** musculus sphincter urethrae. **c. vagi′nae,** the musculus bulbospongiosus in the female.

constructive (kon-struk′tiv) pertaining to any process of construction; in physiology, anabolic.

consult (kon-sult′) [L. *consultus*] to confer with another physician about a case.

consultant (kon-sul′tant) [L. *consultare* to counsel] a physician called in for advice and counsel.

consultation (kon″sul-ta′shun) [L. *consultatio*] a deliberation by two or more physicians with respect to the diagnosis or treatment in any particular case.

consumption (kon-sump′shun) [L. *consumptio* a wasting] 1. the act of consuming, or the process of being consumed. 2. a wasting away of the body; formerly applied especially to tuberculosis of the lungs. **galloping c.,** tuberculosis of the lungs that runs an exceptionally rapid course. **luxus c.,** the ingestion of excess protein which does not form part of the tissues but remains in the body as a reserve supply.

consumptive (kon-sump′tiv) 1. of the nature of or affected with consumption. 2. (*obs.*) a person affected with tuberculosis of the lungs.

Cont. abbreviation for L. *contu′sus,* bruised.

contact (kon′takt) [L. *contactus* a touching together] 1. a mutual touching of two bodies or persons. 2. an individual known to have been sufficiently near to an infected individual to have been exposed to the transfer of infectious material. 3. contactant. **balancing c.,** the contact between the upper and lower occlusal surfaces of the teeth (of the natural or artificial dentition) on the side opposite the working contact. **complete c.,** contact of the entire proximal surface of one tooth with the entire proximal surface of the adjacent tooth. **deflective c.,** deflective occlusal c. **direct c., immediate c.,** transmission of infection from an infected host or reservoir to a susceptible individual by physical contact. **indirect c.,** transmission of infection to a susceptible host by means of formites or a vector or through the air in dust or droplet nuclei (see under *nucleus*); called also *mediate c.* **initial c.,** initial occlusal c. **mediate c.,** indirect c. **occlusal c.,** the contact between the upper and lower teeth when the jaws are closed in habitual occlusion. **occlusal c., deflective,** a form of occlusal interference in which the mandible is diverted from its normal path of closure to central jaw relation or the denture slides or rotates on its basal seat. Called also *deflective c.* and *cuspal interference.* **occlusal c., initial,** the initial normal, noninterfering occlusal contact and intercuspation occurring when the mandibular and maxillary teeth are brought together. In ideal occlusion, it takes place in centric occlusion. Called also *initial c.* **occlusal c., interceptive,** an initial contact of the teeth that stops or deviates from the normal movement of the mandible. **premature c.,** an occlusal contact or interference that occurs before a balanced and stable jaw-to-jaw relationship is reached in either centric relation or centric occlusion, or in the area between the two positions. **proximal c., prox-imate c.,** touching of the proximal surfaces of two adjoining teeth. **weak c.,** contact in which the proximal surface of one tooth barely touches that of the adjacent tooth, enhancing the packing of food between the teeth. **working c.,** the contact between the upper and lower teeth (of the natural

or artificial dentition) on the side toward which the mandible has been moved in mastication.

contactant (kon-tak′tant) an allergen capable of inducing delayed contact-type hypersensitivity of the animal or human epidermis after one or more episodes of contact.

contactologist (kon″tak-tol′o-jist) a craftsman in contactology.

contactology (kon″tak-tol′o-je) the craft of making and fitting contact lenses.

contagion (kon-ta′jun) [L. *contagio* contact, infection] 1. the communication of disease from one individual to another. 2. a contagious disease. **psychic c.,** communication of psychological symptoms through mental influence.

contagiosity (kon-ta″je-os′ĭ-te) the quality of being contagious.

contagious (kon-ta′jus) [L. *contagiosus*] capable of being transmitted from one individual to another, as a contagious disease; communicable. Cf. *infectious.*

contaminant (kon-tam′ĭ-nant) something that causes contamination.

contamination (kon-tam″ĭ-na′shun) [L. *contaminatio,* from *con* together + *tangere* to touch] 1. the presence of any substance or organism that makes a preparation impure. 2. the soiling or pollution by inferior material, as by the introduction of organisms into a wound, or sewage into a stream. 3. the deposition of radioactive material where it is not desired, particularly where its presence may be harmful or constitute a radiation hazard.

content (kon′tent) that which is contained within a thing. **latent c.,** in freudian theory, the hidden and unconscious true meaning of a symbolic representation, such as a dream or fantasy, as opposed to the manifest content. **manifest c.,** in freudian theory, the content of a dream or fantasy as it is experienced and remembered, and in which the latent content is disguised and distorted by displacement, condensation, symbolization, projection, and secondary elaboration.

contiguity (kon″tĭ-gu′ĭ-te) [L. *contiguus* in contact] contact or close proximity; the quality of being contiguous.

contiguous (kon-tig′u-us) [L. *contiguus*] in contact or nearly so.

Contin. abbreviation for L. *continue′tur,* let it be continued.

continence (kon′tĭ-nens) [L. *continentia*] the ability to refrain from yielding to desire, as self-restraint with respect to sexual indulgence. **fecal c.,** the ability to retain the contents of the colon until conditions are proper for defecation. **urinary c.,** the ability to retain the contents of the bladder until conditions are proper for urination.

continent (kon′tĭ-nent) able to refrain from yielding to normal impulses, as sexual desire, or from the urge to defecate or urinate.

continued (kon-tin′ūd) having no remission, intermission, or interruption.

continuity (kon″tĭ-nu′ĭ-te) [L. *continuitas,* uninterrupted succession] the quality of being without interruption or separation.

continuous (kon-tin′u-us) [L. *continuus*] not interrupted; having no interruption.

contour (kon′toor) [Fr.] 1. the normal outline or configuration of the body or of a part. 2. to shape a solid along certain desired lines. **height of c.,** see under *height.*

contoured (kon′toord) having an irregularly undulating outline or surface; said of bacterial colonies.

contouring (kon-toor′ing) the process of forming a contour; shaping. **occlusal c.,** correction by grinding of gross disharmonies of the occlusal tooth forms. See also under *adjustment.*

contra- [L. *contra* against] a prefix signifying against, opposed.

contra-angle (kon″trah-ang′g'l) an angulation by which the working point of a surgical instrument is brought close to the long axis of its shaft; it may involve two, three, or four bends, or angles, in its shank.

contra-aperture (kon″trah-ap′er-chūr) [*contra-* + L. *apertura* opening] a second opening made in an abscess to facilitate the discharge of its contents.

contraception (kon″trah-sep′shun) the prevention of conception or impregnation. **intrauterine c.,** prevention of conception by use of a device inserted in the uterus; see under *device*.

contraceptive (kon″trah-sep′tiv) 1. diminishing the likelihood of, or preventing, conception. 2. an agent that diminishes the likelihood of or prevents conception. **intrauterine c.,** see under *device*. **oral c.,** a hormonal compound taken orally in order to block ovulation and prevent the occurrence of pregnancy.

contract (kon-tract′) [L. *contractus*, from *contrahere* to draw together] 1. to shorten, or reduce in size, as a muscle. 2. to acquire or incur.

contractile (kon-trak′til) [L. *con* together + *trahere* to draw] having the power or tendency to contract in response to a suitable stimulus.

contractility (kon″trak-til′ĭ-te) capacity for becoming short in response to a suitable stimulus. **cardiac c.,** the property of the cardiac muscle cells or tissues to shorten in response to an appropriate stimulus. **galvanic c.,** galvanocontractility. **idiomuscular c.,** a contractility peculiar to wasted or degenerated muscles. **neuromuscular c.,** normal, as distinguished from idiomuscular, contractility.

contraction (kon-trak′shun) [L. *contractus* drawn together] 1. a shortening or reduction in size; in connection with muscles contraction implies shortening and/or development of tension. 2. a morbid or pathologic shortening or shrinkage. 3. abnormal approximation of mandibular and maxillary structures to the median plane. See also distraction, def. 5. **anodal closure c.** (ACC), contraction of the muscles at the anode when the electrical circuit is closed. **anodal opening c.** (AOC), contraction of the muscles at the anode when the electrical circuit is broken. **automatic ventricular c.,** a ventricular contraction caused by an impulse arising in the atrioventricular node; called also *escaped ventricular c.* **Braxton Hicks c's,** light, usually painless, irregular uterine contractions during pregnancy, gradually increasing in intensity and frequency and becoming more rhythmic during the third trimester. **carpopedal c.,** the condition resulting from chronic shortening of the muscles of the fingers, toes, arms, and legs in tetany. **cathodal closure c.** (CCC), contraction of muscles at the cathode when the electrical circuit is closed. **cathodal opening c.** (COC), contraction of the muscles at the cathode when the electrical circuit is opened. **cicatricial c.,** wound c. **clonic c.,** contraction of a muscle alternating with periods of relaxation. **closing c.,** contraction occurring at the point of application of the stimulus when the electrical circuit is closed. **Dupuytren's c.,** Dupuytren's contracture. **escaped ventricular c.,** automatic ventricular c. **fibrillary c's,** abnormal spontaneous contractions occurring successively in different bundles of the fibers of a diseased muscle. **galvanotonic c.,** a sustained muscular contraction produced by a continuous electrical current. **Hicks c's,** Braxton Hicks c's. **hourglass c.,** contraction of an organ (as the stomach or uterus) at or near the middle. **idiomuscular c.,** a contraction produced by direct electrical stimulation of a wasted muscle. **isometric c.,** muscle contraction without appreciable shortening or change in distance between its origin and insertion. **isotonic c.,** muscle contraction without appreciable change in the force of contraction; the distance between the muscle's origin and insertion becomes less. **myotatic c.,** contraction or irritability of a muscle brought into play by sudden passive stretching or by tapping on its tendon. **opening c.,** contraction occurring at the point of application of the stimulus when the electrical circuit is opened. **palmar c.,** Dupuytren's contracture. **paradoxical c.,** the contraction of a muscle caused by the passive approximation of its extremities. **postural c.,** that state of muscular tension and contraction which just suffices to maintain the posture of the body. **premature c.,** extrasystole. **segmentation c.,** see under *movement*. **tetanic c.,** sustained contraction of a muscle without intervals of relaxation; see *tetanus* (def. 2). Called also *tonic c.* **tone c.,** a muscular contraction developing slowly and showing a prolonged phase of relaxation. **tonic c.,** tetanus, def. 2. **twitch c.,** the all-or-none response of muscle cells to a single stimulus. **uterine c.,** contraction of the uterus during labor. **wound c.,** the shrinkage and spontaneous closure of open skin wounds.

contracture (kon-trak′tūr) [L. *contractura*] a condition of fixed high resistance to passive stretch of a muscle, resulting from fibrosis of the tissues supporting the muscles or the joints, or from disorders of the muscle fibers. **Dupuytren's c.,** shortening, thickening, and fibrosis of the palmar fascia, producing a flexion deformity of a finger; sometimes associated with long-standing epilepsy. Applied also to flexion deformity of a toe caused by involvement of the plantar fascia. **ischemic c.,** contracture and degeneration of a muscle due to interference with the circulation from pressure, as by a tight bandage, or from injury or cold. **organic c.,** one that is permanent and continuous. **postpoliomyelitic c.,** any distortion of a joint following an attack of poliomyelitis, due to partial or complete paralysis of one muscle or group of muscles, allowing overuse of an opposing muscle or group of muscles, such as flexion contracture of the knee and paralysis of the quadriceps muscle group. **veratrin c.,** a peculiar type of muscular contraction produced by injecting a muscle with veratrin. **Volkmann's c.,** a contraction of the fingers and sometimes of the wrist, with loss of power, developing rapidly after a severe injury in the region of the elbow joint or improper use of a tourniquet. A similar phenomenon may develop in the distal extremity and involve the foot when similar vascular damage is sustained to the muscles of the leg; called also *ischemic muscular atrophy* and *Volkmann's syndrome.*

contrafissure (kon″trah-fish′ur) a fracture in a part opposite the site of a blow.

contraincision (kon″trah-in-sizh′un) counterincision to promote drainage.

contraindicant (kon″trah-in′dĭ-kant) rendering any particular line of treatment undesirable or improper.

contraindication (kon″trah-in″dĭ-ka′shun) any condition, especially any condition of disease, which renders some particular line of treatment improper or undesirable.

contrainsular (kon″trah-in′su-lar) having an inhibiting influence on pancreatic insular secretion.

contralateral (kon″trah-lat′er-al) [*contra-* + L. *latus* side] situated on, pertaining to, or affecting the opposite side, as opposed to ipsilateral.

contraparetic (kon″trah-pah-ret′ik) 1. counteracting paresis. 2. a preparation useful in the treatment of paresis.

contrasexual (kon″trah-seks′u-al) pertaining to or characteristic of the opposite sex.

contrast (kon′trast) [L. *contra* against + *stare* to stand] the degree to which light and dark areas of an image differ in brightness or in optical density. In radiology, the difference in optical density in a radiograph that results from a difference in radiolucency or penetrability of the subject. **film c.,** contrast inherent in the film. **high c.,** short-scale c. **long-scale c., low c.,** an increased range of grays on a radiograph, which limits visual differentiation to those image densities produced by relatively disparate structural features. **short-scale c.,** a reduced range of grays on a radiograph, which favors visual differentiation of image densities produced by objects or object components with relatively comparable structural features. **subject c.,** contrast resulting from differences in absorption of radiation by various parts of the subject.

contrastimulant (kon″trah-stim′u-lant) [*contra-* + *stimulant*] 1. counteracting or opposing stimulation. 2. a depressant medicine.

contrastimulism (kon″trah-stim′u-lizm) the systematic use of contrastimulant medicines or appliances.

contrastimulus (kon″trah-stim′u-lus) [*contra-* + *stimulus*] a remedy, force, or agent that opposes stimulation.

contrecoup (kon-tr-koo′) [Fr. "counterblow"] injury resulting from a blow on another site, such as a fracture of the skull caused by a blow on the opposite side.

contrectation (kon″trek-ta′shun) [L. *contrectare* to handle] the fondling of a person of the opposite sex.

Cont. rem. abbreviation for L. *continue′tur reme′dium*, let the medicine be continued.

control (kon-trōl′) [Fr. *contrôle* a register] 1. the governing or limitation of certain objects or events. 2. a standard against which experimental observations may be evaluated, as a procedure identical in all respects to the experimental procedure except for absence of the one factor that is being studied. **associative automatic c.,** nerve impulses that arise in the corpus striatum and act upon the final common pathway, and thus upon the muscles. **aversive**

c., in behavior therapy, the use of unpleasant stimuli to change undesirable behavior. **birth c.,** deliberate limitation of childbearing by measures designed to control fertility and to prevent conception; see also *contraception.* **feedback c.,** a physiological control mechanism operating to regulate the metabolic processes of a cell and thus maintain a constant internal environment, in which the accumulation of the product of a reaction leads to a decrease in its rate of production or a deficiency of the product leads to an increase in its rate of production. **idiodynamic c.,** nerve impulses from the cells of the ventral gray column and the motor nuclei of the brain that maintain the muscles in their normal trophic condition. **reflex c.,** control of muscular activity by nerve impulses transmitted to the muscles by one of the reflex arcs by which reflex action is maintained. **Schick test c.** [USP], heat-inactivated diphtheria toxin used as a control in the Schick test. Called formerly *inactivated diagnostic diphtheria toxin.* **sex c.,** regulation of the sex of future offspring by artificial means. **stimulus c.,** any influence exerted by the environment on behavior. **synergic c.,** nerve impulses transmitted to the common pathway from the cerebellum for the regulation of the muscular activity of the synergic units of the body. **tonic c.,** nerve impulses transmitted to the final common pathway through the reflex arc for the maintenance of muscle tone. **vestibuloequilibratory c.,** nerve impulses from the semicircular canals, saccule, and utricle for the maintenance of body equilibrium. **volitional c., voluntary c.,** impulses from the motor area of the cerebral cortex that direct muscular action under the influence of the will.

Controlled Substances Act a federal law enacted in 1970 that regulates the prescribing and dispensing of psychoactive drugs, including narcotics, according to five schedules based on their abuse potential, medical acceptance, and ability to produce dependence; it also establishes a regulatory system for the manufacture, storage, and transport of the drugs in each schedule. Drugs covered by this Act include opium and its derivatives, opiates, hallucinogens, depressants, and stimulants.

contund (kon-tund′) [L. *contundere*] to bruise.

contuse (kon-tūz′) to bruise.

contusion (kon-tu′zhun) [L. *contusio,* from *contundere* to bruise] a bruise; an injury of a part without a break in the skin. **brain c.,** contusion with loss of consciousness as a result of direct trauma to the head, usually associated with fracture of the skull. See also *concussion of the brain.* **contrecoup c.,** a contusion resulting from a blow on one side of the head with damage to the cerebral hemisphere on the opposite side by transmitted force. **c. of spinal cord,** organic injury to the cord due to a blow to the vertebral column, with resultant transient or prolonged dysfunction below the level of the lesion. See also *concussion of spinal cord.*

contusive (kon-tu′siv) producing a bruise.

conular (kon′u-lar) cone-shaped.

Conus (ko′nus) a genus of mollusks, some species of which are able to inflict a poisoned wound.

conus (ko′nus), pl. **co′ni** [L.; Gr. *kōnos*] 1. a cone; [NA] a general term denoting a structure resembling a cone in shape. 2. posterior staphyloma of the myopic eye. **c. arterio′sus** [NA], the anterosuperior portion of the right ventricle of the heart, which is delimited from the rest of the ventricle by the supraventricular crest and which joins the pulmonary trunk, thus forming the outflow tract for blood in the right ventricle. Called also *arterial cone* and *infundibulum (of heart).* **distraction c.,** a crescentic white area at the temporal edge of the papilla of the optic nerve sometimes seen with the ophthalmoscope in myopic eyes. **c. elas′ticus** [NA], elastic cone: the paired lateral portion of the fibroelastic laryngeal membrane, which extends upward in parallel thickenings from the cricoid cartilage to the vocal ligaments. Called also *lateral cricothyroid ligament, cricothyroid* or *cricovocal membrane,* and *membrana cricovocalis* [NA alternative]. The term *conus elasticus* has also been applied to both the entire cricothyroid ligament (i.e., median or anterior and lateral parts) and the median or anterior part of the cricothyroid ligament (*ligamentum cricothyroideum medianum*). **co′ni epididym′idis,** NA alternative for *lobuli epididymidis.* **c. medulla′ris** [NA], medullary cone: the cone-shaped lower end of the spinal cord, at the level of the upper lumbar vertebrae; called also *c. terminalis*

and *terminal cone of spinal cord.* **myopic c.,** posterior staphyloma of the myopic eye. **supertraction c.,** a gray or yellowish ring on the nasal side of the optic papilla sometimes seen with the ophthalmoscope, especially in myopic eyes. **c. termina′lis,** c. medullaris. **co′ni vasculo′si,** lobuli epididymidis.

convalescence (kon″vah-les′ens) [L. *convalescere* to become strong] the stage of recovery following an attack of disease, a surgical operation, or an injury.

convalescent (kon″vah-les′ent) 1. pertaining to or characterized by convalescence. 2. a patient who is recovering from a disease, surgical operation, or injury.

convection (kon-vek′shun) [L. *convectio,* from *convehere* to convey] transmission of heat in liquids or gases by a circulation carried on by the heated particles.

convergence (kon-ver′jens) [L. *convergere* to lean together] 1. in evolution, the development of similar structures or organisms in unrelated taxa. 2. in embryology, the movement of cells from the periphery toward the midline during gastrulation. 3. in ophthalmic physiology, the coordinated inclination of the two lines of sight towards their common point of fixation, or the point of fixation itself. **accommodative c.,** that portion of convergence initiated by the stimulus to accommodation. **amplitude of c.,** see under *amplitude.* **far point of c.,** the point of intersection of the lines of sight at minimum convergence. **fusional c.,** convergence resulting from the attempt to keep the visual stimulus on the fovea of both eyes. **near point of c.,** the point of intersection of the lines of sight at maximum convergence. **negative c.,** outward vergence, or divergence, of the visual axes. **positive c.,** inward deviation of the visual axes. **proximal c.,** convergence induced by the sense of nearness of an object. **tonic c.,** the continuous convergence maintained by the tone of the medial rectus muscle in the primary position.

convergent (kon-ver′jent) [L. *con* together + *vergere* to incline] meeting at or tending toward a common point.

convergiometer (kon-ver″je-om′ĕ-ter) [*convergence* (def. 2) + *-meter*] an instrument for measuring latent strabismus.

Converse method (kon′vers) [John Marquis *Converse,* American plastic surgeon, 1909–1981] see under *method.*

conversion (kon-ver′zhun) [L. *con* with + *versio* turning] 1. an unconscious defense mechanism by which the anxiety that stems from intrapsychic conflict is converted and expressed in a symbolic somatic see also *conversion disorder* under *disorder.*

convertase (kon-ver′tās) an enzyme that converts a substance to its active state. **C3 c.,** an enzyme that splits the complement component C3 to C3a and C3b; the classic pathway C3 convertase is C4b,2a; the alternative pathway C3 convertases are C3b,Bb and C3b,P,Bb; see under *complement.* **C3 proactivator c. (C3PAase),** factor D. **C5 c.,** an enzyme that splits the complement component C5 to C5a and C5b; the classic pathway C5 convertase is C4b,2a,3b; the alternative pathway C5 convertases are C3b$_n$,Bb and C3b$_n$,P,Bd; see under *complement.*

convertin (kon-ver′tin) Factor VII; see *coagulation factors,* under *factor.*

convex (kon′veks) [L. *convexus*] having a rounded, somewhat elevated surface, resembling a segment of the external surface of a sphere.

convexity (kon-vek′si-te) [L. *convexitas*] 1. the condition of being convex. 2. a rounded, somewhat elevated area on the surface of an organ or other structure.

convexobasia (kon-vek″so-ba′se-ah) [*convex* + *base* of the skull] a deformity of the occipital bone, which is bent forward by the spine; seen in osteitis deformans.

convexoconcave (kon-vek″so-kon′kāv) convex on one surface and concave on the other.

convexoconvex (kon-vek″so-kon′veks) convex on each of two opposite surfaces.

convoluted (kon′vo-lūt-ed) [L. *convolutus*] rolled together or coiled.

convolution (kon-vo-lu′shun) [L. *convolutus* rolled together] a tortuous irregularity or elevation caused by a structure being infolded upon itself, as the convolutions of the brain; see also *gyrus.* **Broca's c.,** the inferior frontal gyrus of the left hemisphere of the cerebrum; called also *Broca's gyrus* or *region.* **c's of cerebrum,** gyri cerebri. **Heschl's**

c., the anterior transverse temporal gyrus; see *gyri temporales transversi*, under *gyrus*. **occipitotemporal c.,** gyrus occipitotemporalis lateralis. **Zuckerkandl's c.,** gyrus paraterminalis.

convolutional (kon″vo-lu′shun-al) of or pertaining to a convolution or convolutions.

convolutionary (kon″vo-lu′shun-a-re) convolutional.

convulsant (kon-vul′sant) 1. producing or causing convulsions. 2. an agent that causes convulsions.

convulsibility (kon-vul″sĭ-bil′ĭ-te) capability of being convulsed.

convulsion (con-vul′shun) [L. *convulsio*, from *convellere* to pull together] a violent involuntary contraction or series of contractions of the voluntary muscles. **central c.,** a convulsion not excited by any external cause, but due to a lesion of the central nervous system; called also *essential c.* and *spontaneous c.* **clonic c.,** a convulsion marked by alternating contracting and relaxing of the muscles. **coordinate c.,** a convulsion marked by clonic movements similar to natural, purposeful movements. **crowing c.,** laryngismus stridulus. **epileptiform c.,** any convulsion attended with loss of consciousness. **essential c.,** central c. **febrile c's,** those associated with high fever, occurring in infants and children. **hysterical c., hysteroid c.,** conversion hysteria with symptoms that resemble convulsions. **local c.,** any minor spasm affecting but one muscle or only one part or member. **mimetic c., mimic c.,** facial spasm or tic. **puerperal c.,** involuntary spasms in women just before, during, or just after, childbirth. **salaam c.,** nodding spasm. **spontaneous c.,** central c. **tetanic c.,** a tonic spasm without loss of consciousness; see *tetanus* (def. 2) and *tetany* (def. 1). **tonic c.,** prolonged contraction of the muscles, as a result of an epileptic discharge. **uremic c.,** one due to uremia, or retention in the blood of material that should have been expelled by the kidneys.

convulsivant (kon-vul′sĭ-vant) convulsant.

convulsive (kon-vul′siv) pertaining to, characterized by, or of the nature of convulsion.

Cooley's anemia, disease [Thomas Benton *Cooley*, American pediatrician, 1871–1945] see *thalassemia*.

Coolidge tube (koo′lij) [William David *Coolidge*, American physicist, 1873–1977] see under *tube*.

cooling (kool′ing) the process of reducing the temperature, especially the body temperature of patients and experimental animals. See also *hypothermia*.

Coombs' test (koomz) [R. R. A. *Coombs*, British immunologist, born 1921] see *antiglobulin test*, under *tests*.

Cooper's disease, etc. (koo′perz) [Sir Astley Paston *Cooper*, English surgeon, 1768–1841] see under *breast, disease, fascia, hernia, ligament,* and *testis*.

Cooperia (koo-pe′re-ah) a genus of parasitic nematodes. **C. oncoph′ora, C. pectina′ta, C. puncta′ta,** species of parasitic nematodes sometimes occurring in the small intestine of cattle.

cooperid (koo′per-id) a parasitic nematode of the genus *Cooperia*.

Coopernail's sign (koo′per-nālz) [George Peter *Coopernail*, American physician, born 1876] see under *sign*.

coordinate (ko-or′dĭ-nit) one of a set of numbers that locate a point in space.

coordination (ko-or″dĭ-na′shun) the harmonious functioning of interrelated organs and parts; applied especially to the process of the motor apparatus of the brain which provides for the co-working of particular groups of muscles for the performance of definite adaptive useful responses.

coossification (ko-os″ĭ-fĭ-ka′shun) the action or state of being joined together by ossification.

coossify (ko-os′ĭ-fi) to grow together by ossification.

COP a regimen of cyclophosphamide, Oncovin (vincristine), and prednisone, used in cancer chemotherapy.

copaiba (ko-pi′bah) the resinous juice (balsam) of various leguminous trees of tropical America, especially *Copaifera officinalis* and *C. langsdorffii* Leguminosae; it was formerly used for gonorrhea and chronic inflammation of mucous membranes and as a diaphoretic and expectorant. Called also *balsam of copaiba*.

copal (ko-pal′) [Mex.] the commercial name of many resinous substances of extremely varied origin and character; the original copals came from trees of tropical America, chiefly of the leguminous species *Hymeaea courbaril* L. and various species of *Trachylobium*. It is used in various varnishes and cements and in dentistry for modeling compounds and varnishes for cavities.

coparaffinate (ko-par′ah-fin-āt) a mixture of water-insoluble isoparaffinic acids partially neutralized with isoctyl hydroxybenzyldialkyl amines; used as an anti-infective for the skin.

COP-BLAM a regimen of cyclophosphamide, Oncovin (vincristine), prednisone, bleomycin, Adriamycin (doxorubicin), and Matulane (procarbazine) used in cancer chemotherapy.

COPD chronic obstructive pulmonary disease.

cope (kōp) 1. the upper half of a flask used in the casting art; applied in prosthetic dentistry to the upper or cavity side of a denture flask. 2. coping.

copepod (ko′pĕ-pod) [Gr. *kōpē* oar + *pous* foot] an individual member of Copepoda.

Copepoda (ko-pep′ŏ-dah) [Gr. *kōpē* oar + *pous* foot] a subclass of minute aquatic arthropods (class Crustacea) that are intermediate hosts of *Diphyllobothrium* and *Dracunculus*; ingestion of copepods infected with the early larval stages of *Spirometra mansonoides* may cause human sparganosis.

Copernicia (ko″per-nish′e-ah) a genus of palms, including *C. cerifera* Mart., a South American species, which is the source of carnauba wax.

coping (kōp′ing) a truncated metal cone-shaped cap or a thimble that fits over the prepared natural tooth and serves as an abutment for dentures. Called also *cope*. **transfer c.,** a covering or cap of metal, acrylic resin, or other material, used to position a die in an impression.

copiopia (kop-e-o′pe-ah) [Gr. *kopos* fatigue + *-opia*] eyestrain from overwork or improper use of the eyes.

copodyskinesia (kop″o-dis″ki-ne′ze-ah) [Gr. *kopos* fatigue + *dys-* + *kinēsis* motion] (*obs.*) any difficulty of movement due to fatigue from the habitual performance of some particular action; occupation neurosis.

copolymer (ko-pol′ĭ-mer) a polymer containing monomers of more than one kind.

COPP a regimen of cyclophosphamide, Oncovin (vincristine), procarbazine, and prednisone, used in cancer chemotherapy.

copper (kop′er) [L. *cuprum*; Gr. *Kypros*] a reddish, malleable metal; atomic number, 29; atomic weight, 63.54; symbol Cu, with poisonous salts. Copper is essential in nutrition, being a component of various proteins, including ceruloplasmin, erythrocuprein, cytochrome c oxidase, tyrosinase, etc. Deficiency, which is rare, may result in hypochromic microcytic anemia, neutropenia, and bone changes. **c. abietinate,** a copper salt in green scales, soluble in oil; used as an anthelmintic and vermifuge in veterinary practice. **c. citrate,** see *cupric citrate*, under *citrate*. **c. iodide,** cuprous iodide, CuI. **c. phenolsulfonate,** green prismatic crystals, $(OH \cdot C_6H_4 \cdot SO_2O)_2Cu \cdot 6H_2O$. **c. sulfate,** cupric sulfate; see under *sulfate*.

copperas (kop′er-as) commercial ferrous sulfate, $FeSO_4 \cdot 7H_2O$; disinfectant and deodorizer. See also *ferrous sulfate*, under *ferrous*.

copperhead (kop′er-hed) 1. a venomous snake (a pit viper), *Agkistrodon contortrix*, of the United States, having a brown to copper-colored body with dark bands. 2. a very venomous elapid snake, *Denisonia superba*, of Australia, Tasmania, and the Solomon Islands. See table accompanying *snake*.

copracrasia (kop″rah-kra′se-ah) [Gr. *kopros* dung + *akrasia* want of self control] fecal incontinence.

copragogue (kop′rah-gog) [Gr. *kopros* dung + *agōgos* leading] cathartic.

coprecipitin (ko″pre-sip′ĭ-tin) a precipitin in the same serum with one or more other precipitins.

copremesis (kop-rem′ĕ-sis) [Gr. *kopros* dung + *emesis* vomiting] the vomiting of fecal material.

copr(o)- [Gr. *kopros* dung] a combining form denoting relationship to feces.

coproantibody (kop″ro-an′tĭ-bod′e) an antibody found in the feces, chiefly secretory IgA.

Coprococcus (kop″ro-kok′us) [*copro-* + Gr. *kokkos* berry] a genus of bacteria, made up of gram-positive anaerobic cocci, occasionally isolated from human specimens.

coprodaeum (kop″ro-de′um) [*copro-* + Gr. *hodiaos* on the way] the large dorsal passage in the proximal part of the cloaca in monotremes, into which the intestine opens.

coprodeum (kop″ro-de′um) coprodaeum.

coprolagnia (kop″ro-lag′ne-ah) [*copro-* + Gr. *lagneia* lust] a paraphilia in which sexual excitement is associated with feces or defecation.

coprolalia (kop″ro-la′le-ah) [*copro-* + Gr. *lalia* babble] compulsive, stereotyped use of obscene, "filthy" language, particularly of words relating to feces; seen in some cases of schizophrenia and Gilles de la Tourette's syndrome. Called also *coprophrasia*.

coprolith (kop′ro-lith) [*copro-* + Gr. *lithos* a stone] a hard fecal concretion.

coprology (kop-rol′o-je) [*copro-* + *-logy*] the study of the feces.

coproma (kop-ro′mah) [*copro-* + *-oma*] stercoroma.

Copromastix (kop″ro-mas′tiks) a genus of coprozoic protozoa of the order Polymastigida, class Zoomastigophora, having four equally long anterior flagella and a trailing flagellum. **C. prowazek′i,** a species found in rat and human feces in Brazil.

coprophagia (kop″ro-fa′je-ah) coprophagy.

coprophagous (kop-rof′ah-gus) feeding on dung, or feces.

coprophagy (kop-rof′ah-je) [*copro-* + Gr. *phagein* to eat] the ingestion of dung, or feces.

coprophil (kop′ro-fil) a coprophilic microorganism.

coprophile (kop′ro-fil) 1. coprophil. 2. coprophilic.

coprophilia (kop″ro-fil′e-ah) [*copro-* + Gr. *philia* affection] an absorbing interest in feces or filth.

coprophilic (kop″ro-fil′ik) 1. pertaining to or characterized by coprophilia. 2. living and growing on dung or feces or in feces-polluted water; said of certain bacteria and protozoa.

coprophilous (kop-rof′ĭ-lus) coprophilic.

coprophobia (kop″ro-fo′be-ah) [*copro-* + *phobia*] abnormal repugnance to defecation and to feces.

coprophrasia (kop″ro-fra′ze-ah) coprolalia.

coproporphyria (kop″ro-por-fir′e-ah) the presence of coproporphyrin in the feces. **erythropoietic c.,** an extremely rare erythropoietic porphyria characterized by mild skin photosensitivity and elevated erythrocyte coproporphyrin III levels. **hereditary c.,** a hepatic porphyria transmitted as an autosomal dominant trait characterized biochemically by constant excretion of coproporphyrin III in the feces and intermittent urinary excretion of coproporphyrin, α-aminolevulinic acid (ALA), and porphobilinogen (PBG). The condition is usually asymptomatic, but acute attacks resembling those of acute intermittent porphyria can occur.

coproporphyrin (kop″ro-por′fir-in) the porphyrin (q.v.) produced by oxidation of the methylene bridges in coproporphyrinogen. Coproporphyrin III is excreted in the feces in hereditary coproporphyria.

coproporphyrinogen (kop″ro-por″fĭ-rin′o-jin) a porphyrinogen (q.v.) in which each pyrrole ring has one methyl side chain and one propionate side chain. The type III isomer, formed by decarboxylation of uroporphyrinogen III, is an intermediate in the biosynthesis of heme.

coproporphyrinogen oxidase (kop″ro-por″fĭ-rin′o-jen ok′sĭ-dās) [EC 1.3.3.3] an enzyme of the oxidoreductase class that catalyzes the reaction coproporphyrinogen III + O_2 = protoporphyrinogen-IX + $2CO_2$. It occurs in mitochondria, and the reaction is a part of the pathway of heme biosynthesis. Deficiency of the enzyme, an autosomal dominant trait, results in hereditary coproporphyria.

coproporphyrinuria (kop″ro-por″fir-in-u′re-ah) the presence of coproporphyrin in the urine.

coprostanol (kop″ro-sta′nol) a saturated sterol, $C_{27}H_{48}O$, found in feces, probably reduced from cholesterol; called also *coprosterin* and *coprosterol*.

coprostasis (kop-ros′tah-sis) [*copro-* + Gr. *stasis* stoppage] impaction of the feces in the intestine.

coprostasophobia (kop″ro-sta″so-fo′be-ah) [*coprostasis* + *phobia*] (*obs.*) irrational dread of fecal stasis.

coprosterin (kop″ro-ste′rin) [*copro-* + *sterin*] coprostanol.

coprosterol (kop″ro-ste′rol) coprostanol.

coprozoa (kop″ro-zo′ah) [*copro-* + Gr. *zōon* animal] protozoa which are found in fecal matter outside the body, but which do not inhabit the intestine.

coprozoic (kop″ro-zo′ik) living in fecal material; found in fecal material.

Coptis (kop′tis) [L.] a genus of ranunculaceous plants. C. *tee′ta*, an Asiatic species, is tonic. C. *trifo′lia* (goldthread), of North America, was formerly used as a bitter tonic.

copula (kop′u-lah) [L.] 1. any connecting part or structure. 2. copula linguae. **c. lin′guae,** a median ventral elevation on the embryonic tongue formed by union of the second branchial arches; it represents the future root of the tongue.

copulation (kop″u-la′shun) [L. *copulatio*] sexual union between male and female; coitus.

Coq. abbreviation for L. *co′que,* boil.

Coq. in s. a. abbreviation for L. *co′que in sufficien′te a′qua,* boil in sufficient water.

Coq. s. a. abbreviation for L. *co′que secun′dum ar′tem,* boil properly.

coquille (ko-kēl′) [Fr. "shell"] a glass or lens of uniform thickness shaped like a watch crystal.

cor- see con-.

cor (kor), gen. *cor′dis* [L.] [NA] the muscular organ that maintains the circulation of the blood; see *heart*. **c. adipo′sum,** a heart that has undergone fatty degeneration or that has an accumulation of fat around it; called also *fat, or fatty, heart*. **c. arterio′sum,** the left side of the heart, so called because it contains oxygenated (arterial) blood. **c. bilocula′re,** a congenital anomaly characterized by failure of formation of the atrial and ventricular septums, the heart having only two chambers, a single atrium and a single ventricle, and a common atrioventricular valve. **c. bovi′num** [L. "ox heart"], a greatly enlarged heart due to a hypertrophied left ventricle; called also *c. taurinum* and *bucardia*. **c. dex′trum** [L. "right heart"], the right atrium and ventricle. **c. hirsu′tum,** c. villosum. **c. mo′bile** (*obs.*), an abnormally movable heart. **c. pen′dulum,** a heart so movable that it seems to be hanging by the great blood vessels. **c. pseudotrilocula′re biatria′tum,** a congenital cardiac anomaly in which the heart functions as a three-chambered heart because of tricuspid atresia, the right ventricle being extremely small or rudimentary and the right atrium greatly dilated. Blood passes from the right to the left atrium and thence to the left ventricle and aorta. **c. pulmona′le,** heart disease due to pulmonary hypertension secondary to disease of the lung, or its blood vessels, with hypertrophy of the right ventricle. **c. sinis′trum** [L. "left heart"], the left atrium and ventricle. **c. tauri′num,** c. bovinum. **c. triatria′tum,** a congenital anomaly caused by failure of incorporation of the embryonic common pulmonary vein into the left atrium, the pulmonary veins emptying into an accessory chamber superior to the true left atrium and communicating with it by a small opening, which obstructs pulmonary venous flow, thus simulating mitral stenosis. Called also *triatrial heart*. **c. trilocula′re,** three-chambered heart. **c. trilocular′e biatria′tum,** a congenital anomaly caused by failure of formation of the ventricular septum, the heart having two atria, communicating, by the tricuspid and mitral valves, with a single ventricle. **c. trilocula′re biventricula′re,** a three-chambered heart with one atrium and two ventricles. **c. veno′sum,** the right side of the heart, so called because it contains blood that has given up most of its oxygen (venous blood). **c. villo′sum** [L. "hairy heart"], a roughened state of the pericardium caused by exudate on its surface, occurring in pericarditis; called also *c. hirsutum*.

coracidia (kor″ah-sid′e-ah) [L.] plural of *coracidium*.

coracidium (kor″ah-sid′e-um), pl. *coracidia*. The individual free-swimming or free-crawling, spherical, ciliated embryo of tapeworms of the order Pseudophyllidea.

coracoacromial (kor″ah-ko-ah-kro′me-al) pertaining to the coracoid and acromion processes.

coracoclavicular (kor″ah-ko-klah-vik′u-lar) pertaining to the coracoid process and the clavicle.

coracohumeral (kor″ah-ko-hu′mer-al) pertaining to the coracoid process and the humerus.

coracoid (kor'ah-koid) [Gr. *korakoeidēs* crowlike] 1. like a raven's beak. 2. the coracoid process (processus coracoideus scapulae [NA]).

coracoiditis (kor''ah-koi-di'tis) a painful condition in the region of the scapula and the coracoid process, with deltoid atrophy; attributed to injury of the coracoid process.

coracoradialis (kor''ah-ko-ra''de-a'lis) caput breve musculi bicipitis brachii.

coracoulnaris (kor''ah-ko-ul-na'ris) the fibers of the biceps muscle attached to the fascia of the forearm.

coralliform (ko-ral'ĭ-form) [L. *corallum* coral + *forma* shape] having the form of a coral; branching like a coral.

corallin (kor'ah-lin) aurin. **yellow c.**, the sodium salt of aurin, occurring as yellow masses with a greenish metallic luster, which turns red in solution; called also *corallin yellow*.

coralloid (kor'ah-loid) coralliform.

Coramine (ko'rah-min) trademark for preparations of nikethamide.

corasthma (kor-az'mah) hay fever.

Corbus' disease (kor'bus) [Budd Clarke *Corbus*, American urologist, 1876–1954] balanitis gangrenosa.

cord (kord) [L. *chorda*; Gr. *chordē* string] any long, rounded, flexible structure; see also *chorda*. **Bergmann's c's**, striae medullares ventriculi quarti; see under *stria*. **Billroth's c's**, red pulp c's. **dental c.**, a cordlike mass of cells from which the enamel organ develops. **enamel c.**, a vertical extension of the enamel knot in a developing tooth, connecting the enamel knot with the outer dental epithelium, a temporary structure which disappears before enamel formation begins. **Ferrein's c's**, the inferior, or true, vocal cords (plica vocalis [NA]). **ganglionated c.**, truncus sympathicus. **genital c.**, in the embryo, the midline fused caudal part of the two urogenital ridges, each containing a mesonephric and paramesonephric duct. **gubernacular c.**, chorda gubernaculum. **hepatic c's**, anastomosing plates of hepatic cells radiating outward from the central vein and composing the parenchyma of a hepatic lobule; called also *hepatic cell c's*. **lateral c.**, see *fasciculus lateralis plexus brachialis*, under *fasciculus*. **lumbosacral c.**, truncus lumbosacralis. **lymph c's**, medullary c's (def. 1). **medial c.**, see *fasciculus medialis plexus brachialis*, under *fasciculus*. **medullary c's**, 1. strands of dense lymphoid tissue surrounded by the sinuses of the medulla of a lymph node; called also *lymph c's*. 2. rete c's. **nephrogenic c.**, a longitudinal cord, formed of fused or never separated nephrotome plates, that gives rise to the mesonephric tubule and part of the metanephric tubules. **nerve c.**, any nerve trunk or bundle of nerve fibers. **oblique c. of elbow joint**, chorda obliqua membranae interosseae antebrachii. **ovigerous c's**, rete cords of the primitive ovary that resolve into eggs and their follicles. **Pflüger's c's**, the ovarian tubes. **posterior c.**, see *fasciculus posterior plexus brachialis*, under *fasciculus*. **psalterial c.**, stria vascularis ductus cochlearis. **red pulp c's**, the masses of red pulp of the spleen; called also *Billroth's c's* and *splenic c's*. **rete c's**, strands of primordial cells in the medulla of the embryonic gonads that connect with some of the mesonephric tubules, and from which the rete ovarii or the rete testis develop; called also *medullary c's* and *sex c's*. **scirrhous c.**, chronic fibrous enlargement of the stump of the spermatic cord of a castrated horse caused by bacterial infection, with discharge of pus and sometimes formation of a tumor-like mass with numerous weeping sinuses. **sex c's**, rete c's. **sexual c's**, the seminiferous tubules of the early fetus. **spermatic c.**, the structure that extends from the abdominal inguinal ring to the testis, comprising the ductus deferens, testicular artery, pampiniform plexus, and nerves, as well as various other vessels, enclosed by its various coverings (*tunicae funiculi spermatici*); called also *funiculus spermaticus* [NA], and *chorda spermatica*. **spinal c.**, medulla spinalis. **splenic c's**, red pulp c's. **testis c's**, the rete cords of the embryonic testis. **umbilical c.**, the flexible structure connecting the umbilicus of the embryo and fetus with the placenta and giving passage to the umbilical arteries and vein. In the newborn it measures about 50 cm. in length. First formed during the fifth embryonic week from the allantoic stalk, it contains the omphalomesenteric duct and the allantois. Called also *funiculus umbilicalis* [NA] and *chorda umbilicalis*. **vocal c., false**, a fold of mucous membrane covering muscle in the larynx and separating the ventricle from the vestibule; called also *plica vestibularis* [NA], *plica ventricularis*, *false vocal fold*, and *vestibular fold*.

vocal c., true, a fold of mucous membrane covering the vocalis muscle in the larynx forming the inferior boundary of the ventricle. Called also *plica vocalis* [NA], *vocal fold*, and *Ferrein's c.* **Weitbrecht's c.**, chorda obliqua membranae interosseae antebrachii. **Wilde's c's**, a name once applied to the transverse striae of the corpus callosum (striae transversae corporis callosi [NA]). **Willis' c's**, numerous fibrous bands (dural trabeculae) that extend transversely across the inferior angle of the superior sagittal sinus; called also *chordae Willisii*.

cordal (kor'dal) pertaining to a cord; used specifically in referring to the vocal cord, or the plica vocalis.

cordate (kor'dāt) [L. *cor* heart] heart-shaped.

cordectomy (kor-dek'to-me) [*cord* + Gr. *ektomē* excision] excision of a cord, as a vocal cord.

cordial (kord'yal) [L. *cordialis*] 1. stimulating the heart; invigorating. 2. an aromatized alcoholic liqueur.

cordiale (kor-de-a'le) [L.] cordial.

cordiform (kor'dĭ-form) [L. *cor* heart + *forma* form] heart-shaped.

corditis (kor-di'tis) inflammation of the spermatic cord.

cordopexy (kor'do-pek''se) [*cord* + Gr. *pēxis* fixation] the operation of displacing outward the vocal cord for bilateral vocal cord paralysis.

cordotomy (kor-dot'o-me) 1. section of a vocal cord. 2. interruption of the lateral spinothalamic tract of the spinal cord, usually in the anterolateral quadrant, for relief of intractable pain; it may be done by open surgery or percutaneously by sterotaxic surgery. Also spelled *chordotomy*.

Cordran (kor'dran) trademark for a preparation of flurandrenolide.

Cordyceps (kor'dĭ-seps) a genus of ascomycetous fungi of the family Clavicipitaceae, order Clavicipitales; certain species produce fatal disease of caterpillars. **C. sinen'sis**, a parasite of insect larvae; in Chinese medicine it is reputed to be a drug coagulant; called also *Sphaeria sinensis*.

Cordylobia (kor''dĭ-lo'be-ah) a genus of flies of the family Calliphorida. **C. anthropoph'aga**, a species of flies of Africa the larvae (cayor worms) of which burrow under the skin of man and animals, causing a myiasis; called also *tumbu fly*.

core (kōr) 1. the central part of anything, such as the central mass of necrotic matter in a boil. 2. a bar of iron around which a wire is wound to form an induction coil or electromagnet. 3. cast c. **cast c.**, a metal casting, usually with a post in the root canal, designed to support and retain an artificial crown.

core-, cor(o)- [Gr. *korē* pupil] a combining form denoting relationship to the pupil of the eye; see also words beginning *irid(o)-*.

coreclisis (kōr''e-kli'sis) [*core-* + Gr. *kleisis* closure] iridencleisis.

corectasis (kōr-ek'tah-sis) [*core-* + Gr. *ektasis* a dilatation] dilatation of the pupil.

corectome (kōr-ek'tōm) [*core-* + Gr. *tomē* a cutting] a cutting instrument used in performing iridectomy (corectomy).

corectomedialysis (ko-rek''to-me''de-al'ĭ-sis) [*core-* + *ectomy* + *dialysis*] the operation of forming an artificial pupil by detaching the iris from the ciliary ligament.

corectomy (ko-rek'to-me) [*cor-* + *ectomy*] iridectomy.

corectopia (kōr-ek-to'pe-ah) [*core-* + *ectopia*] abnormal situation of the pupil.

coredialysis (ko''re-di-al'ĭ-sis) [*core-* + *dialysis*] the surgical separation of the external margin of the iris from the ciliary body; called also *iridodialysis*.

corediastasis (ko''re-di-as'tah-sis) [*core-* + Gr. *diastasis* distention] the dilatation or a dilated state of the pupil.

coregonin (ko-reg'o-nin) a protamine obtained from the sperm of the white fish.

corelysis (ko-rel'ĭ-sis) [*core-* + *lysis*] operative destruction of the pupil; especially the surgical detachment of adhesions of the pupillary margin of the iris from the lens.

coremorphosis (kōr''e-mor-fo'sis) [*core-* + *morphosis*] the surgical formation of an artificial pupil.

corenclisis (kōr''en-kli'sis) [*core-* + Gr. *enkleiein* to inclose] iridencleisis.

coreometer (ko″re-om′ĕ-ter) [*core-* + *-meter*] pupillometer.

coreometry (ko″re-om′ĕ-tre) pupillometry.

coreoplasty (ko′re-o-plas″te) [*core-* + *-plasty*] any plastic operation on the iris.

corepressor (ko″re-pres′sor) a small molecule that combines with a protein aporepressor molecule to form an active substance, which then binds to an operator gene and inhibits the synthesis of an enzyme. The mechanism is a negative control in inducible enzyme systems.

corestenoma (ko″re-ste-no′mah) [*core-* + Gr. *stenōma* contraction] an abnormally contracted state of the pupil. **c. conge′nitum,** a congenital condition in which the pupil is partially occluded by excrescences which meet, leaving scattered small openings.

Corethra (ko-re′thrah) *Chaoborus.*

coretomedialysis (ko″re-to-me-dĭ-al′ĭ-sis) corectomedialysis.

coretomy (ko-ret′o-me) iridectomy.

Cori (ko′re) Carl Ferdinand. Czechoslovakian-born American physician and biochemist, 1896–1984; co-winner, with his wife Gerty Theresa Radnitz Cori and Bernardo Alberto Houssay, of the Nobel prize for medicine or physiology in 1947 for their discovery of the catalytic conversion of glycogen to lactic acid.

Cori (ko′re) Gerty Theresa Radnitz. Czechoslovakian-born American physician and biochemist, 1896–1957; co-winner, with her husband Carl Ferdinand Cori and Bernardo Alberto Houssay, of the Nobel prize for medicine or physiology in 1947 for their discovery of the catalytic conversion of glycogen to lactic acid.

Cori cycle, ester (ko′re) [Carl Ferdinand *Cori* and Gerty *Therese Cori*] see *glucose-lactate cycle,* under *cycle,* and see under *glucose-1-phosphate.*

coriaceous (ko-re-a′shus) [L. *corium* leather] resembling leather; leathery, tough; said of bacterial cultures.

coriander (ko″re-an′der) [L. *coriandrum*] the dried ripe fruit of the umbelliferous plant *Coriandrum sativum;* formerly used as a weak carminative and aromatic, but now used as a flavor.

Coriaria (ko-re-a′re-ah) a genus of Old World poisonous coriariaceous plants (shrubs and small trees), containing coriamyrtin; they are also noted for their content of dyes and tannins.

coriin (ko′re-in) a substance formed by treating fibrous connective tissue with alkalis.

corium (ko′re-um) [L. "hide"] NA alternative for *dermis.*

corm (korm) [L. *cormus*] a solid bulblike expansion of a plant stem below the surface of the ground.

Cormack (kor′mak) Allan MacLeod. South African–born American physicist, born 1924; co-winner, with Godfrey Newbold Hounsfield, of the Nobel prize for medicine or physiology in 1979 for their development of computerized axial tomography.

cormethasone acetate (kor-meth′ah-sōn) chemical name: 21-(acetyloxy)-6,6,9-trifluoro-11β, 17-dihydroxy-16α-methylpregna-1,4-diene-3,20-dione; a topical anti-inflammatory, $C_{24}H_{29}F_3O_6$.

corn (korn) [L. *cornu* horn] 1. a horny induration and thickening of the stratum corneum of the skin of the toes, caused by friction and pressure from poorly fitting shoes or hose; it forms a conical mass pointing down into the corium, producing pain and inflammation. There are two kinds: the *hard corn (heloma durum),* usually located on the outside of the little toe or on the upper surfaces of the other toes, and the *soft corn (heloma molle),* found between the toes, most often the fourth and fifth toes, kept softened by moisture. Called also *clavus.* 2. the seeds of a variety of certain cereal grains (*Zea mays* L., Gramineae, used as both animal and human food. Corns yield corn oil, used as a solvent for injections, and corn starch, used as an absorbent and dusting powder. 3. a bruise on the bottom of a horse's foot between the wall of the heel and the bar. **hard c.,** see *corn,* def. 1 **soft c.,** See *corn,* def. 1.

cornea (kor′ne-ah) [L. *corneus* horny] [NA] the transparent structure forming the anterior part of the fibrous tunic of the eye. It consists of five layers: (1) the anterior corneal epithelium, continuous with that of the conjunctiva, (2) the anterior limiting layer (Bowman's membrane), (3) the substantia propria, or stroma, (4) the posterior limiting layer (Descemet's membrane), and (5) the endothelium of the anterior chamber, called also *keratoderma.* **conical c.,** keratoconus. **c. farina′ta,** senile degeneration of the cornea marked by fine dustlike stippling. **flat c.,** the configuration of the cornea when a shallow ocular chamber is present or when the eyeball is atrophic. **c. globo′sa,** megalocornea. **c. gutta′ta,** a degenerative condition of the cornea due to dystrophy of the endothelial cells; called also *dystrophia endothelialis corneae.* **c. opa′ca,** the sclerotic coat of the eye. **c. pla′na,** congenital flatness of the cornea. **sugar-loaf c.** (*obs.*), keratoconus. **c. verticilla′ta,** Fleischer's vortex.

corneal (kor′ne-al) [L. *cornealis*] pertaining to the cornea.

corneitis (kor″ne-i′tis) keratitis.

corneoblepharon (kor″ne-o-blef′ah-ron) [*cornea* + Gr. *blepharon* eyelid] adhesion between the eyelid and cornea.

corneoiritis (kor″ne-o-i-ri′tis) inflammation of the cornea and iris.

corneosclera (kor″ne-o-skle′rah) the cornea and sclera regarded as forming one organ.

corneoscleral (kor″ne-o-skle′ral) affecting or pertaining to both the cornea and the sclera.

corneous (kor′ne-us) [L. *corneus*] hornlike, or horny; consisting of keratin.

corner (kor′ner) the third incisor on either side of each jaw in the horse.

Corner-Allen test, unit [George Washington *Corner,* American anatomist, 1889–1981; Willard Myron *Allen,* American gynecologist, born 1904] see under *tests* and *unit.*

Cornet's forceps (kor′nets) [Georg *Cornet,* German bacteriologist, 1858–1915] a cover glass forceps.

corneum (kor′ne-um) [L. "horny"] see *stratum corneum epidermidis* and *stratum corneum unguis.*

corniculate (kor-nik′u-lāt) shaped like a small horn.

corniculum (kor-nik′u-lum) [L. dim. of *cornu*] cartilago corniculata.

cornification (kor″nĭ-fĭ-ka′shun) [L. *cornu* horn + *facere* to make] 1. conversion into keratin, or horn. 2. conversion of epithelium to the stratified squamous type.

cornified (kor′nĭ-fīd) converted into horny tissue (keratin); keratinized.

Corning's anesthesia (method) (kor′nings) [James Leonard *Corning,* New York neurologist, 1855–1923] see *spinal anesthesia* (def. 1), under *anesthesia.*

cornoid (kor′noid) [L. *cornu* horn + *-oid*] resembling horn; see under *lamella.*

cornu (kor′nu), pl. *cor′nua* [L. "horn"] a hornlike excrescence or projection; used in anatomical nomenclature to designate a structure resembling a horn in shape, especially in section. Called also *horn.* **c. Ammo′nis** [L. "horn of Ammon"], hippocampus. **c. ante′rius medul′lae spina′lis,** NA alternative for *c. ventrale medullae spinalis.* **c. ante′rius ventric′uli latera′lis,** NA alternative for *c. frontale ventriculi lateralis.* **cor′nua cartilag′inis thyroi′deae,** the horns of the thyroid cartilage; see *c. inferius cartilaginis thyroideae* and *c. superius cartilaginis thyroideae.* **c. coccygea′le,** c. coccygeum. **c. coccy′geum** [NA], **c. coccyx,** coccygeal horn: either of the cranial pair of rudimentary articular processes of the coccyx that articulate with the cornua of the sacrum. Called also *c. coccygeale.* **c. cuta′neum,** cutaneous horn. **c. dorsa′le medul′lae spina′lis** [NA], dorsal horn of spinal cord: the horn-shaped configuration presented by the dorsal column of the spinal cord in transverse section; called also *posterior horn of spinal cord* and *c. posterius medullae spinalis* [NA alternative]. See also *columna dorsalis medullae spinalis* and *columna griseae.* **ethmoid c.,** concha nasalis media. **c. fronta′le ventric′uli latera′lis** [NA], frontal horn of lateral ventricle: the part of the lateral ventricle that extends forward from the pars centralis into the frontal lobe; called also *anterior horn of lateral ventricle* and *c. anterius ventriculi lateralis* [NA alternative]. **c. infe′rius cartilag′inis thyroi′deae** [NA], inferior horn of thyroid cartilage: the inferior extension of the posterior border of the thyroid cartilage. **c. infe′rius mar′ginis falcifor′mis** [NA], inferior horn of falciform margin: the distal edge of the falciform margin of the saphenous hiatus, deep to the great saphenous vein. **c. infe′rius ventric′-**

uli latera′lis, NA alternative for *c. temporale ventriculi lateralis.* **c. latera′le medul′lae spina′lis** [NA], lateral horn of spinal cord: the horn-shaped configuration presented by the lateral column of the spinal cord in transverse section. See also *columna griseae* and *columna lateralis medullae spinalis.* **c. ma′jus os′sis hyoi′dei** [NA], greater horn of hyoid bone: a bony projection passing backward and upward from either side of the body of the hyoid bone; called also *lateral horn of hyoid bone.* **c. mi′nus os′sis hyoi′dei** [NA], lesser horn of hyoid bone: a small conical eminence projecting upward on either side of the hyoid bone at the angle of junction between the body and the greater horns; called also *superior horn of hyoid bone.* **c. occipita′le ventric′uli latera′lis** [NA], occipital horn of lateral ventricle: the part of the lateral ventricle that extends backward from the par centralis into the occipital lobe; called also *c. posterius ventriculi lateralis* [NA alternative] and *posterior horn of lateral ventricle.* **cor′nua os′-sis hyoi′dei** [NA], the horns of the hyoid bone; see *c. majus ossis hyoidei* and *c. minus ossis hyoidei.* **c. poste′rius medul′lae spina′lis,** NA alternative for *c. dorsale medullae spinalis.* **c. poste′rius ventric′uli latera′lis,** NA alternative for *c. occipitale ventriculi lateralis.* **sacral c., c. sacra′le** [NA], sacral horn: either of the two hook-shaped processes extending downward from the arch of the last sacral vertebra; called also *coccygeal eminence.* **cor′nua of spinal cord,** the horn-shaped structures seen in transverse section of the spinal cord; see *columna anterior medullae spinalis, columna lateralis medullae spinalis,* and *columna posterior medullae spinalis.* **c. supe′rius cartilag′inis thyroi′deae** [NA], superior horn of thyroid cartilage: the superior extension of the posterior border of the thyroid cartilage. **c. supe′rius mar′ginis falcifor′-mis** [NA], superior horn of falciform margin: the proximal end of the falciform margin of the saphenous hiatus; called also *Scarpa′s ligament.* **c. tempora′le ventric′uli latera′lis** [NA], temporal horn of lateral ventricle: the part of the lateral ventricle that extends downward and forward from the pars centralis behind the thalamus and into the temporal lobe; called also *c. inferius ventriculi lateralis* [NA alternative] and *inferior horn of lateral ventricle.* **c. u′teri dex′trum/sinis′trum** [NA], **c. uteri′num dex′-trum/sinis′trum,** right and left horn of uterus: either of the bluntly rounded superior lateral extremities of the body of the uterus that marks the entrance of the uterine tube. **c. ventra′le medul′lae spina′lis** [NA], ventral horn of spinal cord: the horn-shaped configuration presented by the ventral column of the spinal cord in transverse section; called also *anterior horn of spinal cord* and *c. anterius medullae spinalis* [NA alternative]. See also *columna griseae* and *columna ventralis medullae spinalis.*

cornua (kor′nu-ah) [L.] plural of *cornu.*

cornual (kor′nu-al) pertaining to a cornu or to cornua.

cornuate (kor′nu-āt) cornual.

cornucommissural (kor″nu-kŏ-mis′u-ral) pertaining to a cornu and to a commissure.

cornucopia (kor″nu-ko′pe-ah) [L. *cornu copiae* "horn of plenty"] an extension of the choroid plexus into each of the lateral recesses of the fourth ventricle.

Cornus (kor′nus) [L.] a genus of cornaceous trees and shrubs of both hemispheres; the cornels or dogwoods. The dried root bark of many, especially that of *C. florida,* the common dogwood of North America, was once used as an astringent bitter and tonic.

cor(o)- see *core-.*

corodiastasis (ko″ro-di-as′tah-sis) corediastasis.

corolla (ko-rol′ah) [L. "little crown"] the inner set of leaves of a floral envelope, the individual portions of which are called *petals.*

corona (ko-ro′nah), pl. *coronas,* or *coro′nae* [L.; Gr. *korōnē*] a crown; used in anatomical nomenclature to designate a crownlike eminence or encircling structure. **c. cilia′ris** [NA], ciliary crown: the region on the anterior inner surface of the ciliary body of the eye from which radiate the ciliary processes; called also *pars plicata corporis ciliaris.* **c. cli′nica** [NA], that portion of the tooth above the clinical root, i.e., the portion exposed beyond the gingiva, and thus visible in the oral cavity. Called also *clinical crown* or *extra-alveolar c.* **dental c., c. den′tis** [NA], the upper part of the tooth, which joins the lower part, the root, at the cervix at the cementoenamel junction, and terminates as the grinding surface of molar or premolar teeth or the cutting edge of incisors. Called also *anatomical* or *dental crown.* **c. glan′dis pe′nis** [NA], **c. of glans penis,** the rounded proximal border of the glans penis, separated from the corpora cavernosa penis by the neck of the glans. **c. radia′ta,** 1. [NA] the radiating crown of projection fibers which pass from the internal capsule to every part of the cerebral cortex. 2. an investing layer of radially elongated follicular cells surrounding the zona pellucida of an ovum. **c. ven′eris,** a ring of syphilitic sores around the forehead, sometimes deeply affecting the bones of the head. **Zinn′s c.,** circulus vasculosus nervi optici.

coronad (kor′ŏ-nad) toward the crown of the head or any corona.

coronae (ko-ro′ne) [L.] genitive and plural of *corona.*

coronal (ko-rŏ′nal) [L. *coronalis*] 1. pertaining to the crown of the head or to any corona. 2. situated in the direction of the coronal suture; said of a longitudinal plane or section passing through the body at right angles to the median plane. See under *plane.* Called also *coronalis* [NA].

coronale (kor-o-na′le) 1. the point of the coronal suture at the end of the maximum frontal diameter. 2. the frontal bone (os frontale [NA]).

coronalis (kor″o-na′lis) [L.] coronal; [NA] a term used to denote a structure situated in the direction of the coronal suture.

coronaritis (kor″o-nah-ri′tis) coronary arteritis.

coronary (kor′ŏ-na-re) [L. *corona;* Gr. *korōnē*] encircling in the manner of a crown; a term applied to vessels, nerves, ligaments, etc. The term usually denotes the arteries that supply the heart muscle and, by extension, a pathologic involvement of them.

coronavirus (kor″o-nah-vi′rus) any of a group of morphologically similar, ether-sensitive viruses, probably RNA, causing infectious bronchitis of birds, hepatitis in mice, gastroenteritis in swine, and respiratory infections in humans; called coronaviruses because of their resemblance, under the electron microscope, to a corona or crown.

corone (ko-ro′ne) [L.; Gr. *korōnē* anything hooked or curved] the coronoid process of the mandible (processus coronoideus mandibulae [NA]).

coroner (kor′o-ner) an officer who holds inquests in regard to violent, sudden, or unexplained deaths.

coronet (kor′o-net) the lower part of the pastern of a horse, where the horn joins the skin.

coronion (ko-ro′ne-on) the tip of the coronoid process of the mandible.

coronitis (kor-o-ni′tis) inflammation of the coronary band or cushion of the horse hoof or the claw of cloven-hoofed animals.

coronoid (kor′o-noid) [Gr. *korōnē* anything hooked or curved, a kind of crown + *-oid*] 1. shaped like a crow′s beak. 2. crown-shaped.

coronoidectomy (kor″o-noi-dek′to-me) surgical removal of the coronoid process of the mandible.

coroparelcysis (ko″ro-par-el′sĭ-sis) [*coro-* + Gr. *parelkein* to draw aside] the drawing aside of the pupil in partial corneal opacity in order to bring it under a transparent portion.

coroplasty (ko′ro-plas″te) coreoplasty.

coroscopy (ko-ros′ko-pe) [*coro-* + Gr. *skopein* to examine] retinoscopy.

corotomy (ko-rot′o-me) iridectomy.

corpora (kor′po-rah) [L.] plural of *corpus.*

corporal (kor′po-ral) corporeal.

corporeal (kor-po′re-al) pertaining to the body.

corporic (kor-po′rik) [L. *corpus* body] affecting the body, or corpus, of an organ.

corps (kōr) [Fr., from L. *corpus*] 1. an organized body, or group of individuals. 2. corpus. **medical c.,** the surgeon officers of the army or navy, comprising a surgeon general, medical directors, medical inspectors, surgeons, passed assistant surgeons, and assistant surgeons. **c. ronds,** Darier′s name for round, double-contoured bodies seen in keratosis follicularis.

corpse (korps) [L. *corpus* body] a dead body; used to refer specifically to a human body in the early period after death. Cf. *cadaver.*

corpulency (kor′pu-len″se) [L. *corpulentia*] undue fatness or obesity.

corpus (kor′pus), pl. *cor′pora*, gen. *cor′poris* [L. "body"] a discrete mass of material, as of specialized tissue; used in anatomical nomenclature to designate the entire organism, and applied also to the main portion of an anatomical part, structure, or organ. **c. adipo′sum buc′cae** [NA], adipose body of cheek: an encapsulated mass of fat in the cheek, separated from the subcutaneous fascia by a facial cleft, and situated between the masseter and the external surface of the buccinator muscles; especially well developed in infants and said to aid in sucking. Called also *buccal fat pad, fat pad, sucking cushion*, and *sucking* or *suctorial pad*. **c. adipo′sum fos′sae ischiorecta′lis** [NA], adipose body of the ischiorectal fossa: a pad of fat found in the ischiorectal fossa. **c. adipo′sum infrapatella′re** [NA], infrapatellar fatty body: a mass of fibrous fatty tissue inferior to the patella, in the angle between the deep surface of the patellar ligament and the tibia. **c. adipo′sum or′bitae** [NA], adipose body of orbit: a mass of fatty tissue in the posterior part of the orbit, around the optic nerve, extraocular muscles, and vessels. **c. adipo′sum pararena′le** [NA], pararenal fatty body: a large mass of fat lying dorsal to the renal fascia; called also *paranephric* or *pararenal body* and *paranephric* or *pararenal fat*. **c. al′bicans** (pl. *cor′pora albican′tia*) [NA], white fibrous tissue that replaces the regressing corpus luteum in the human ovary in the latter half of pregnancy, or soon after ovulation when pregnancy does not supervene; called also *c. fibrosum*. **c. alie′num**, a foreign body. **c. amygdaloi′deum** [NA], amygdaloid body: a small, ovoid complex of nuclei partly covered by the pyriform cortex, within the tip of the temporal lobe, anterior to the inferior horn of the lateral ventricle of the brain; it is part of the limbic system and is classified as a part of the basal nuclei. The amygdaloid body is divided into two main groups of nuclei, found in the basolateral and corticomedial parts, and a poorly differentiated transitional region, the anterior amygdaloid area. It has olfactory connections is reciprocally connected to the limbic cortex, and projects fibers to the hippocampus, the septum, the thalamus, and especially to the hypothalamus. Called also *amygdala, amygdaloid complex* or *nucleus*, and *nucleus amygdalae*. **cor′pora amyla′cea** [L. "starchy bodies"], small hyaline masses of degenerate cells found in the prostate, neuroglia, etc. Called also *amylaceous bodies* or *corpuscles, amyloid bodies* or *corpuscles, colloid corpuscles*, and *corpora versicolorata*. **cor′pora aran′tii** [L. "bodies of Arantius"], nodules of aortic valve; see *noduli valvularum semilunarium*. **cor′pora atret′ica**, ovarian follicles that never mature, but undergo degeneration; called also *pseudolutein body*. **cor′pora bigem′ina** (sing. *cor′pus bigem′inum*), corpora quadrigemina. **c. calca′nei**, the body of the calcaneus. **c. callo′sum** [NA], an arched mass of white matter, found in the depths of the longitudinal fissure, composed of transverse fibers connecting the cerebral hemispheres and consisting, from the anterior to the posterior, of rostrum, genu, trunk, and splenium; called also *commissura magna cerebri*. **c. caverno′sum clitor′idis dex′trum/sinis′trum** [NA], cavernous body of clitoris: a column of erectile tissue on either side (right and left), the two fusing to form the body of the clitoris (c. clitoridis). **c. caverno′sum pe′nis** [NA], cavernous body of penis: one of the columns of erectile tissue forming the dorsum and sides of the penis; called also *spongy body of penis*. **c. caverno′sum ure′thrae viril′is**, c. spongiosum penis. **c. cerebel′li** [NA], body of cerebellum: the main portion of the cerebellum, consisting of the two cerebellar hemispheres joined by a median strip, the vermis; see also *cerebellum*. **c. cilia′re** [NA], **c. cilia′ris**, the ciliary body: the thickened part of the vascular tunic of the eye anterior to the ora serrata, connecting the choroid with the iris; it is composed of the corona ciliaris, ciliary processes and folds, the ciliary orbiculus, the ciliary muscle, and a basal lamina. **c. clavic′ulae** [NA], the curved body of the clavicle, extending between the acromial and sternal extremities. **c. clitor′idis** [NA], the main part of the clitoris, formed by the two fused corpora cavernosa, which are embedded anteriorly in the floor of the vestibule of the vagina. **c. coccyg′eum**, glomus coccygeus. **cor′pora alla′ta**, a set of small endocrine glands in the head of insects just behind the brain, which inhibits metamorphosis by secretion of juvenile hormone. **c. cos′tae** [NA], the part of a rib extending between its dorsally placed tubercle and its ventral extremity; called also *shaft of rib*. **c. denta′tum**

cerebel′li, nucleus dentatus. **c. denta′tum oli′vae**, nucleus olivaris. **c. epididym′idis** [NA], the middle part of the epididymis, which is formed by the convolutions of the single ductus epididymidis. **c. fibro′sum**, c. albicans. **c. fib′ulae** [NA], the principal part or shaft of the fibula. **c. fimbria′tum** [L. "fringed body"], a narrow band of white substance bordering the lateral edge of the lower cornu of the lateral ventricle of the cerebrum. **c. fimbria′tum hippocam′pi**, fimbria hippocampi. **cor′pora fla′va** [L. "yellow bodies"], waxy bodies found in the central nervous system and elsewhere, thought to be formed by the transformation of nerve cells. **c. for′nicis** [NA], body of fornix: the middle part of the fornix of the cerebrum, formed by fusion of the two lateral halves under the corpus callosum. **c. gas′tricum** [NA], gastric body: that part of the stomach between the fundus and the pyloric part; called also *body of stomach, c. ventriculare* [NA alternative], and *c. ventriculi*. **c. genicula′tum latera′le** [NA], the lateral geniculate body: an eminence of the metathalamus produced by the underlying lateral geniculate nucleus, just lateral to the medial geniculate body. It relays visual impulses from the optic tract to the calcarine cortex. Called also *optic thalamus*. **c. genicula′tum media′le** [NA], the medial geniculate body: an eminence of the metathalamus produced by the underlying medial geniculate nucleus, just lateral to the superior colliculus. It relays auditory impulses from the lateral lemniscus to the auditory cortex. **c. glan′dulae bulbourethra′lis**, the body of the bulbourethral gland. **c. glan′dulae sudorif′erae** [NA], the coiled secretory part of a sweat gland, found in the deep part of the corium; called also *coil* or *acinus of the sweat gland*. **c. glandula′re prosta′tae**, substantia glandularis prostatae. **c. hemorrhag′icum**, 1. an ovarian follicle containing blood. 2. a corpus luteum containing a blood clot. **c. Highmo′ri, c. highmoria′num** [L. "body of Highmore"], mediastinum testis. **c. hu′meri** [NA], the main part or shaft of the humerus. **c. hypothalam′icum**, nucleus subthalamicus. **c. incu′dis** [NA], the central part of the incus, which contains an excavation in which the head of the malleus articulates. **c. interpeduncula′re**, nucleus interpeduncularis. **c. lin′guae** [NA], the larger anterior part of the tongue, in the floor of the mouth. **c. lu′teum** (pl. *cor′pora lu′tea*) [L. "yellow body"] [NA], a yellow glandular mass in the ovary formed by an ovarian follicle that has matured and discharged its ovum; if the ovum has been impregnated, the corpus luteum increases in size and persists for several months (*true c. luteum, c. luteum of pregnancy, c. luteum graviditatis*); if impregnation has not taken place, the corpus luteum degenerates and shrinks (*false c. luteum, c. luteum of menstruation, c. luteum menstruationis*). The corpus luteum secretes progesterone. Called also *yellow body of ovary*. Cf. *corpus albicans*. **cor′pora lu′tea atret′ica**, corpora lutea in which regressive changes have occurred. **c. Luy′sii**, nucleus subthalamicus. **c. mamilla′re** [NA], the mamillary body: either of the pair of small spherical masses situated close together in the interpeduncular space rostral to the posterior perforated substance in the posterior hypothalamic region, consisting of two main nuclei, lateral and medial, and smaller associated aggregations of gray matter. **c. mam′mae** [NA], the essential mass of the mammary gland, exclusive of the glandular elements, which is thickest beneath the nipple and thinner toward the periphery; see illustration accompanying *mammary gland*, under *gland*. **c. mandib′ulae** [NA], body of mandible: the horizontal horseshoe-shaped portion of the mandible. **c. maxil′lae** [NA], body of maxilla: the large central portion of the maxilla, roughly pyramidal in shape, to which four major processes are connected; it contains the maxillary sinus. **c. medulla′re cerebel′li** [NA], medullary body of cerebellum: the white substance of the cerebellum; called also *center of cerebellum*. **c. medulla′re ver′mis**, arbor vitae cerebelli. **c. metacarpa′lis** [NA], the shaft, or body, of a metacarpal bone. Called also *c. ossis metacarpalis*. **c. nu′clei cauda′ti** [NA], the part of the caudate nucleus lying in the floor of the pars centralis of the lateral ventricle of the brain, extending posteriorly from the head and continuous with the tail. **c. of Oken**, mesonephros. **cor′pora oryzoi′dea** (sing. *cor′pus oryzoi′deum*), rice bodies. **c. os′sis fem′oris** [NA], the main part or shaft of the femur. **c. os′sis hyoi′dei** [NA], body of hyoid bone: the central portion of the hyoid bone to which the large and small horns are attached; called also *basihyal* and *basihyoid*.

c. os'sis il'ii [NA], c. os'sis il'ium, the inferior portion of the ilium, which forms roughly the superior two-fifths of the acetabulum; called also *body of ilium.* c. os'sis is-ch'ii [NA], the thick, irregular, prismatic part of the is-chium. Its superior end participates in the acetabulum, and from its inferior end the ramus of the ischium projects. It incorporates what was formerly called the superior ramus; called also *body of ischium.* c. os'sis metacarpa'lis, c. metacarpalis. c. os'sis metatarsa'lis, c. metatarsalis. c. os'sis pu'bis [NA], body of pubic bone: the irregular mass of the pubic bone that lies alongside the median plane, articulating with the similar portion of the opposite pubic bone. From it extend the superior and inferior rami of the pubic bone. c. os'sis sphenoida'lis [NA], body of sphenoid bone: the central, cuboidal part of the sphenoid bone to which the great wings, small wings, and pterygoid pro-cesses are attached; it contains the sphenoidal sinuses. Called also *c. sphenoidale.* c. pampinifor'me, epoöphoron. c. pancre'atis [NA], body of pancreas: the triangularly prismatic portion of the pancreas, extending from the neck on the right to the tail on the left. cor'pora para-aor'tica [NA], para-aortic bodies: exclaves of glandular cells of sympathetic origin (chromaffin cells) found near the sympathetic ganglia along the aorta in the abdominal cavity; they serve as chemoreceptors responsive to oxygen, carbon dioxide, and hydrogen ion concentration, that help to control respiration. Called also *aortic bodies* and *glomera aortica* [NA alternative]. c. pe'nis [NA], the free part of the penis be-tween the root and the glans, consisting chiefly of the paired corpora cavernosa and the unpaired corpus spongiosum penis; called also *shaft of penis.* c. perinea'lis, centrum tendineum perinei. c. phalan'gis digito'rum ma'nus [NA], the main part or shaft of each phalanx of the fingers. c. phalan'gis digito'rum pe'dis [NA], the main part or shaft of each phalanx of the toes. c. pi-nea'le [NA], the pineal body (see under *body*) or gland, a small, somewhat flattened, cone-shaped body in the epithala-mus, lying above the superior colliculi below the splenium of the corpus callosum. c. pyramida'le medul'lae, pyr-amis medullae oblongatae. cor'pora quadrigem'ina, the cranial and caudal colliculi of the tectum of the mesen-cephalon considered together. c. ra'dii [NA], the main part or shaft of the radius. cor'pora restifor'mia, pe-dunculus cerebellaris caudalis. c. rhomboida'le, nu-cleus dentatus. cor'pora santoria'na, cartilago cor-niculata. c. spongio'sum pe'nis [NA], the column of erectile tissue that forms the urethral surface of the penis, and in which the urethra is found; its distal expansion forms the glans penis. Called also *c. cavernosum urethrae virilis* and *spongy body of male urethra.* c. ster'ni [NA], body of sternum: the second or principal portion of the sternum, located between the manubrium above and the xiphoid process below; called also *gladiolus.* c. stria'tum (pl. *cor'pora stria'ta*) [NA], the striate body: one of the compo-nents of the basal nuclei; specifically, a subcortical mass of gray and white substance in front of and lateral to the thalamus in each cerebral hemisphere. The gray substance of this structure is arranged in two principal masses, the caudate nucleus and the lentiform nucleus; the striate appearance on section of the area being produced by connect-ing bands of gray substance passing from one of these nuclei to the other through the white substance of the internal capsule. c. subthalam'icum, nucleus subthalamicus. c. ta'li [NA], body of talus: the roughly quadrilateral por-tion of the talus, which presents several surfaces for articula-tion with the calcaneus, tibia, and fibula. c. tib'iae [NA], the main part or shaft of the tibia. c. trapezoi'-deum [NA], the trapezoid body: a mass of transverse fibers extending through the central part of the pons and forming a part of the path of the cochlear nerve. c. tritic'eum, cartilago triticea. c. ul'nae [NA], the main part or shaft of the ulna. c. un'guis [NA], nail plate: the large distal, exposed portion of the nail of a digit. c. u'teri [NA], that part of the uterus above the isthmus and below the orifices of the uterine tubes. c. ventricula're, NA al-ternative for *c. gastricum.* c. ventric'uli, c. gastricum. cor'pora versicolora'ta, corpora amylacea. c. ver'tebrae [NA], c. vertebra'le, the body of a vertebra; called also *c. vertebra'lis* [NA alternative], *centrum vertebrae,* and *intravertebral body.* c. vertebra'lis, NA alternative for *c. vertebrae.* c. vesi'cae bilia'ris [NA], body of gall-bladder: the portion of the gallbladder between the fundus and the neck; called also *c. vesicae felleae* [NA alternative].

c. vesi'cae fel'leae, NA alternative for *c. vesicae biliaris.* c. vesi'cae urina'riae [NA], that part of the urinary bladder between the apex and the fundus. c. vi'treum [NA], the vitreous body: the transparent substance that fills the part of the eyeball between the lens and the retina; called also *hyaloid body, crystalline* or *vitreous humor,* and *humor cristallinus.* c. Wolf'fi, mesonephros.

corpuscle (kor'pus'l) any small mass or body; see also *cor-pusculum.* Alzheimer's c's, compound granular corpus-cles in the oligodendroglia of the brain. amylaceous c's, amyloid c's, corpora amylacea. articular c's, corpuscula articularia. axile c., axis c., the central part of a tactile corpuscle. Bennet's large c's, Nunn's gorged c's. Bennet's small c's, Drysdale's c's. blood c's, formed elements of the blood; i.e., erythrocytes and leu-kocytes. blood c., red, erythrocyte. blood c., white, leukocyte. bone c., bone cell. bridge c., desmosome. bulboid c's, corpuscula bulboidea. cartilage c., carti-lage cell. chorea c's, a name given peculiar round hya-line bodies, concentrically laminated and strongly refractile, found in the perivascular sheaths of the vessels of the corpora striata and internal capsule in chorea. chromophil c., Nissl's body. chyle c., a lymphocyte found in chyle. colloid c's, corpora amylacea. colostrum c's, large rounded bodies in colostrum, containing droplets of fat and sometimes a nucleus; they apparently are phagocytic cells of the mammary gland, present for the first two weeks after parturition. Called also *Donné's bodies* or *corpuscles.* con-centric c's, Hassall's c's. corneal c's, star-shaped con-nective tissue cells within the corneal spaces; called also *Toynbee's* and *Virchow's c's.* Dogiel's c., a sensory end-organ found in the mucous membrane of the eyes, nose, mouth, and genitals. Donné's c's, colostrum c's. Drysdale's c's, transparent microscopic cells seen in the fluid of ovarian cysts; called also *Bennet's c's.* dust c's, hemoconia. Eichhorst's c's, a name once given a pecu-liar variety of microcytes seen in pernicious anemia. gen-ital c's, corpuscula genitalia. ghost c., phantom c. Gierke's c's, roundish bodies found in the nervous system, probably identical with Hassall's corpuscles. Gluge's c's, granular corpuscles occurring in diseased nerve tissue. Golgi's c's, encapsulated end-organs found in a tendon at its junction with the muscular fibers, which mediate tension differences to the innervating nerve fibers. Golgi-Maz-zoni c's, tactile corpuscles found in the subcutaneous tissue of the fingertips, resembling pacinian corpuscles, but possess-ing fewer lamellae and a relatively larger cone, and having the contained nerve fibers more extensively branched. Grandry's c's, Grandry-Merkel c's, menisci tactus. Guarnieri's c's, see under *body.* Hassall's c's, spher-ical or ovoid bodies found in the medulla of the thymus, composed of concentric arrays of epithelial cells which contain keratohyalin and bundles of cytoplasmic filaments. Called also *Hassall's bodies, concentric c's, Leber's c's* and *thymus c's.* Herbst's c's, peculiar sensory end-organs in the skin of the bill and in the mucous membrane of the tongue of the duck. Jaworski's c's, spiral mucous bod-ies seen in the secretion of the stomach in hyperchlorhydria. Krause's c's, corpuscula bulboidea. lamellar c's, lamellated c's, corpuscula lamellosa. Leber's c's, Hassall's c's. lingual c., an encapsulated terminal sen-sory nerve ending in a lingual papilla. Lostorfer's c's, granular bodies observed in the blood in syphilis; called also *Lostorfer's c's.* lymph c's, lymphocytes observed in lymph. lymphoid c's, lymphocytes observed in tissues. malpighian c's of kidney, corpuscula renis. malpi-ghian c's of spleen, folliculi lymphatici splenici. Mazzoni's c's, sensory nerve endings resembling Krause's corpuscles. meconium c's, epithelial cells containing many coarse yellow granules, observed in the lower part of the small intestine in a fetus. Meissner's c's, corpus-cula tactus. Merkel's c's, menisci tactus. milk c's, delicate particles of fat suspended in the serum of the milk. mucous c's, bodies resembling leukocytes occurring in mu-cus. nerve c's, the sheath cells lying between the neuri-lemma and the medullary sheath. Norris' c's, decolor-ized erythrocytes. Nunn's gorged c's, epithelial cells found in ovarian cysts that have undergone a high degree of fatty degeneration; called also *Bennet's large c's.* Paci-ni's c's, pacinian c's, lamellated nerve endings (corpus-cula lamellosa) that are concerned in the perception of pressure. Paschen's c's, see under *body.* pessary c., see under *cell.* Purkinje's c's, see under *cell.* pus c., one of the cells of pus, chiefly neutrophilic leukocytes. **Rainey's c.,** any of the uninucleate, crescentic or banana-shaped trophozoites found in sarcocysts in sarcocystosis. **red c.,** erythrocyte. **renal c's,** corpuscula renis. **reticulated c's,** erythrocytes which on proper staining show filamentous reticulations filling a greater part of the cell. **Röhl's marginal c's,** small bodies seen in the margins of erythrocytes of animals after the administration of chemotherapeutic substances. **Ruffini's c's,** lamellated nerve endings (corpuscula lamellosa) that are concerned in the perception of pressure and of warmth. **salivary c.,** a white blood cell that has migrated through the oral epithelium and is mixed in the saliva. **Schwalbe's c.,** caliculus gustatorius. **shadow c.,** phantom c. **splenic c's,** folliculi lymphatici lienales. **tactile c's,** corpuscula tactus. **taste c's,** taste cells. **tendon c's,** flattened cells of connective tissue occurring in rows between the primary bundles of the tendons. **terminal nerve c's,** corpuscula nervosa terminalia. **thymus c's,** Hassall's c's. **Timofeew's c's,** a specialized form of pacinian corpuscle found in the submucosa of the membranous and prostatic portions of the urethra. **touch c's,** corpuscula tactus. **Toynbee's c's,** corneal c's. **Traube's c.,** phantom c. **Tröltsch's c's,** connective tissue spaces lined with flattened endothelial cells, and appearing like corpuscular bodies among the radial fibers of the membrana tympani. **typhic c's,** cells of Peyer's patches that have undergone degeneration in typhoid fever. **Valentin's c's,** small amyloid bodies found in nerve tissue. **Vater's c's, Vater-Pacini c's,** corpuscula lamellosa. **Virchow's c's,** corneal c's. **Wagner's c's,** corpuscula tactus. **Weber's c.,** utriculus prostaticus. **white c.,** leukocyte. **Zimmermann's c.** (*obs.*), achromocyte.

corpuscula (kor-pus′ku-lah) [L.] plural of *corpusculum.*

corpuscular (kor-pus′ku-lar) pertaining to or of the nature of corpuscles.

corpusculum (kor-pus′ku-lum), pl. *corpus′cula* [L. dim. of *corpus*] a small mass or body; used as a general term in anatomical nomenclature to designate certain small discrete masses of specialized tissue, especially of nerve tissue. **corpus′cula articula′ria** [NA], articular corpuscles: encapsulated nerve endings found within joints; called also *corpuscula nervorum articularia.* **corpus′cula bulbifor′mia,** corpuscula bulboidea. **corpus′cula bulboi′dea** [NA], bulboid corpuscles: small encapsulated nerve endings found in the skin, mucous membranes, conjunctiva, and heart, at varying levels; called also *bulbs of Krause, corpuscula bulbiformis,* and *Krause's corpuscles.* **corpus′cula genita′lia** [NA], genital corpuscles: small encapsulated nerve endings occurring in the mucous membrane in the genital region; called also *corpuscula nervorum genitalia.* **corpus′cula lamello′sa** [NA], lamellar or lamellated corpuscles: large encapsulated nerve endings, which are the most complicated of the nerve endings and are found throughout the body. Concerned with the perception of different sensations, various such endings are named for the men who originally described them, e.g., *Pacini's corpuscles* and *Ruffini's corpuscles.* Called also *Vater's* and *Vater-Pacini corpuscles.* **corpus′cula nervo′rum articula′ria,** corpuscula articularia. **corpus′cula nervo′rum genita′lia,** corpuscula genitalia. **corpus′cula nervo′rum termina′lia,** corpuscula nervosa terminalia. **corpus′cula nervo′sa termina′lia** [NA], terminal nerve corpuscles: nerve endings characterized by a fibrous capsule of varying thickness that is continuous with the endoneurium; for different named varieties, see under *corpuscle.* Called also *corpuscula nervorum terminalia* and *encapsulated nerve endings.* **corpus′cula re′nis** [NA], renal corpuscles: bodies forming the beginnings of the nephrons, each consisting of a tuft of capillaries (the glomerulus), surrounded by an expanded portion of the renal tubule (the glomerular capsule); called also *malpighian corpuscles, acinus renalis [malpighii], acinus renis [malpighii], malpighian bodies of kidneys,* and *malpighian* or *renal tufts.* **corpus′cula tac′tus** [NA], tactile corpuscles: medium-sized encapsulated nerve endings found in the skin, most commonly in the palms and soles; called also *tactile* or *touch cells,* and *Meissner's oval, tactile,* or *touch corpuscles.* **c. tritic′eum,** cartilago triticea.

correction (ko-rek′shun) [L. *correctio* straightening out; amendment] a setting right, as the provision of specific lenses for the improvement of vision, or an arbitrary adjustment made in values or devices in performance of experimental procedures.

corrector (kor-rek′tor) something that corrects or sets right. **function c.,** a removable orthodontic appliance utilizing oral and facial muscle forces to move teeth and possibly change the relationship of dental arches; called also *Fränkel appliance.*

correlation (kor″ĕ-la′shun) most generally, the degree to which one phenomenon or random variable is associated with or can be predicted from another. In statistics, correlation usually refers to the degree to which a linear predictive relationship exists between random variables, as measured by a correlation coefficient (q.v.). Correlation may be *positive,* i.e., both variables increase or decrease together, or *negative* or *inverse,* i.e., one variable increases when the other decreases.

correspondence (kor″e-spon′dens) [L. *correspondere* to answer, to correspond] the condition of being in agreement, or conformity. **anomalous retinal c.,** a condition in which disparate points on the retinas of the two eyes come to be associated sensorially; abbreviated A.R.C. **normal retinal c.,** the condition in which corresponding points on the retinas of the two eyes are associated sensorially; abbreviated N.R.C. **retinal c.,** the relation between corresponding points on the retinas of the eyes such that simultaneous stimulation causes the sensation of a single object.

Corrigan's disease, etc. (kor′e-ganz) [Sir Dominic John *Corrigan,* physician in Dublin, 1802–1880] see under *disease, line, pulse, respiration,* and *sign.*

corrigent (kor′ĕ-jent) [L. *corrigens* correcting] 1. amending or rendering milder. 2. any agent that favorably modifies the action of a drug which is too powerful or harsh, or that improves its taste.

corrin (kor′in) a tetrapyrrole ring system resembling the porphyrin ring system of hemoglobin, but in which a pair of the rings is joined directly rather than through a methene bridge, with cobalt being bound to the inner four nitrogen atoms. The cobalamins contain a corrin ring system.

corroid (kor′oid) a compound, such as the cobalamins, containing a corrin ring system.

corrosion (kŏ-ro′zhun) [L. *corrosio*] the slow destruction of the texture or substance of a tissue, as by the action of a corrosive substance.

corrosive (kŏ-ro′siv) [L. *con* with + *rodere* to gnaw] 1. destructive to the texture or substance of the tissues. 2. a substance that destroys the texture or substance of the tissues. Called also *caustic* and *escharotic.*

corrugator (cor′u-ga″tor) [L. *con* together + *ruga* wrinkle] that which wrinkles; a muscle that wrinkles.

corset (kor′set) an orthopedic device that encircles and supports a part, as worn in certain spinal injuries or deformities.

Cort. abbreviation for L. *cor′tex,* bark.

Cortate (kor′tāt) trademark for preparations of desoxycorticosterone acetate.

Cort-Dome (kort′dōm) trademark for preparations of hydrocortisone.

Cortef (kor′tef) trademark for preparations of hydrocortisone.

Cortenema (kor-ten′ĕ-mah) trademark for a preparation of hydrocortisone.

cortex (kor′teks), gen. *cor′ticis,* pl. *cor′tices* [L. "bark, rind, shell"] 1. an external layer, as the bark of a tree, or the rind of a fruit. 2. [NA] the outer layer of an organ or other body structure, as distinguished from the internal substance. **adrenal c.,** the outer, firm, yellowish layer that comprises the larger part of the adrenal (suprarenal) gland, the zona glomerulosa, the zona fasciculata, and the zona reticularis; it secretes, in response to release of corticotropin by the pituitary gland, many steroid hormones, including mineralocorticoids, glucocorticoids, androgens, and progestins (see *adrenal gland,* under *gland*). Called also *cortex glandulae suprarenalis* [NA], *substantia corticalis glandulae suprarenalis,* and *cortical substance of suprarenal gland.* **cerebellar c., c. cerebel′li** [NA], **c. of cerebellum,** the superficial gray matter of the cerebellum; called also *substantia corticalis cerebelli* and *cortical substance of cerebellum.* **cerebral c., c. cere′bri** [NA], **c. of cerebrum,** the thin layer or mantle of gray substance covering the surface of each cerebral hemisphere, folded into gyri that are separated by sulci. It reaches its highest development in man, in whom it is responsible for the higher mental functions, for general movement, for visceral functions, perception, and behavioral reactions, and for the association and integration of these functions. Called also *pallium* [NA alternative]. Many classifications have been suggested: it has been divided into *archeocortex*, *paleocortex*, and *neocortex* (the first two making up the *allocortex*) according to supposed phylogenetic and ontogenetic differences; into areas according to the presence of six cell layers (see *neopallium*) or according to differences in the structure and arrangement of cell and fiber layers; and into functional areas, such as motor, sensory, and association areas. According to official anatomical nomenclature, the cerebral cortex (specifically, the neocortex) has six layers, situated from the surface inward: I, *lamina molecularis;* II, *lamina granularis externa;* III, *lamina pyramidalis externa;* IV, *lamina granularis interna;* V, *lamina pyramidalis interna;* VI, *lamina multiformis.* **c. glan′dulae suprarena′lis** [NA], the outer, firm yellowish layer that comprises the larger part of the suprarenal gland; called also *adrenal cortex* (q.v.), *cortical substance of suprarenal gland,* and *substantia corticalis glandulae suprarenalis.* **heterotypical c.,** archaeocortex. **homotypical c.,** the portion of the cerebral cortex containing all six cell layers; see *neopallium.* **c. of kidney,** renal c. **c. len′tis** [NA], the softer, external part of the lens of the eye; called also *substantia corticalis lentis* and *cortical substance of lens.* **motor c.,** the area of the frontal lobe of the cerebral cortex concerned with primary motor control of the body; Brodmann's area 4. **c. no′di lymphat′ici** [NA], the outer portion of a lymph node, consisting mainly of dense lymphatic tissue and follicles; called also *substantia corticalis lymphoglandulae* and *cortical substance of lymph nodes.* **nonolfactory c.,** neopallium. **olfactory c.,** archaeocortex. **c. ova′rii** [NA], **c. of ovary,** the dense layer of compact stroma forming the peripheral zone around the medulla of the ovary, in which the ovarian follicles are embedded. **piriform c.,** the cortex of the piriform lobe or area. **provisional c.,** the cortex of the fetal adrenal gland that undergoes involution in early fetal life. **renal c., c. re′nis** [NA], cortex of kidney: the outer part of the substance of the kidney, composed mainly of glomeruli and convoluted tubules; called also *substantia corticalis renis* and *cortical substance of kidney.* **somesthetic c.** postcentral area; see under *area.* **striate c.,** the primary visual cortex: the part of the occipital lobe of the cerebral cortex that receives the fibers of the optic radiation from the lateral geniculate body and is the primary receptive area for vision; so called because of the prominent broad line or stria of Gennari. Called also *striate area.* **tertiary c.,** thymus-dependent area. **c. thy′mi, c. of thymus,** the outer part of each lobule of the thymus; it consists chiefly of closely packed lymphocytes (thymocytes) and surrounds the medulla. **visual c.,** the area of the occipital lobe of the cerebral cortex concerned with vision; it consists of the primary visual cortex (Brodmann's area 17; see *striate c.*) and two other areas (Brodmann's areas 18 and 19) whose roles are not as well defined, although area 18 is linked to the opposite hemisphere by the corpus callosum.

cortexone (kor-tek′sōn) (*obs.*) desoxycorticosterone.

Corti's arch, membrane, organ, etc. [Alfonso Corti, Italian anatomist, 1822–1888] see under *arch, canal, cell, fiber, ganglion, rod,* and *tunnel,* and see *membrana tectoria ductus cochlearis* and *organum spirale.*

cortiadrenal (kor″te-ad-re′nal) corticoadrenal.

cortical (kor′tĭ-kal) [L. *corticalis*] pertaining to or of the nature of a cortex or bark.

corticalosteotomy (kor″tĭ-kal-os″te-ot′o-me) osteotomy through the bone cortex at the base of the dentoalveolar segment, which serves to weaken the resistance of the bone to the application of orthodontic forces.

corticate (kor′tĭ-kāt) possessing a cortex or bark.

corticectomy (kor″tĭ-sek′to-me) excision of an area of cerebral cortex (scar or microgyrus) in the treatment of focal epilepsy.

cortices (kor′tĭ-sēz) [L.] plural of *cortex.*

corticifugal (kor″tĭ-sif′u-gal) [*cortex* + L. *fugere* to flee] proceeding, conducting, or moving away from the cortex.

corticipetal (kor″tĭ-sip′e-tal) [*cortex* + L. *petere* to seek] proceeding, conducting, or moving toward the cortex.

cortic(o)- [L. *cortex,* q.v.] a combining form denoting relationship to a cortex.

corticoadrenal (kor″tĭ-ko-ad-re′nal) pertaining to the adrenal cortex.

corticoafferent (kor″tĭ-ko-af′fer-ent) conveying impressions from the lower levels inward and upward to the cerebral cortex; said of certain nerve fibers.

corticoautonomic (kor″tĭ-ko-aw″to-nom′ik) denoting the relationship of autonomic function to definite areas in the cerebral cortex.

corticobulbar (kor″tĭ-ko-bul′bar) pertaining to or connecting the cerebral cortex and the medulla oblongata and/or brain stem.

corticocerebral (kor″tĭ-ko-ser′e-bral) pertaining to the cerebral cortex.

corticodiencephalic (kor″tĭ-ko-di″en-se-fal′ik) pertaining to or connecting the cerebral cortex and the diencephalon.

corticoefferent (kor″tĭ-ko-ef′er-ent) carrying impressions outward and downward from the cerebral cortex; said of certain nerve fibers.

corticofugal (kor″tĭ-kof′u-gal) corticifugal.

corticoid (kor′tĭ-koid) any of the C21 steroids of the adrenal cortex; a corticosteroid (q.v.).

corticomesencephalic (kor″tĭ-ko-mes″en-se-fal′ik) pertaining to or connecting the cerebral cortex and the mesencephalon.

corticopeduncular (kor″tĭ-ko-pe-dung′ku-lar) pertaining to the cortex and the peduncles of the brain.

corticopetal (kor″tĭ-ko-kop′e-tal) corticipetal.

corticopleuritis (kor″tĭ-ko-ploo-ri′tis) inflammation of the visceral pulmonary pleura.

corticopontine (kor″tĭ-ko-pon′tīn) pertaining to or connecting the cerebral cortex and the pons.

corticospinal (kor″tĭ-ko-spi′nal) pertaining to or connecting the cortex of the brain and the spinal cord.

corticosteroid (kor″tĭ-ko-ste′roid) any of the steroids elaborated by the adrenal cortex (excluding the sex hormones of adrenal origin) in response to the release of corticotropin (adrenocorticotropic hormone) by the pituitary gland, to any of the synthetic equivalents of these steroids, or to angiotensin II. They are divided, according to their predominant biological activity, into three major groups: *glucocorticoids,* chiefly influencing carbohydrate, fat, and protein metabolism; *mineralocorticoids,* affecting the regulation of electrolyte and water balance; and *C19 androgens.* Some corticosteroids exhibit both types of activity in varying degrees, and others exert only one type of effect. The corticosteroids are used clinically for hormonal replacement therapy, for suppression of ACTH secretion by the anterior pituitary, as antineoplastic, antiallergic, and anti-inflammatory agents, and to suppress the immune response. Called also *adrenocortical hormone* and *corticoid.*

corticosterone (kor″tĭ-kos′ter-ōn) chemical name: $11\beta,21$-dihydroxypregn-4-ene-3,20-dione. A natural mineralocorticoid with moderate glucocorticoid activity, $C_{21}H_{30}O_4$, possessing life-maintaining properties in adrenalectomized animals and several other activities peculiar to the adrenal cortex. It is similar to 11-deoxycorticosterone, but its life-maintaining and sodium-retaining potencies are less. Called also (*Kendall's*) *compound B.*

corticotensin (kor″tĭ-ko-ten′sin) a low-molecular-weight polypeptide purified from kidney extract that exhibits a vasopressor effect when given intravenously.

corticothalamic (kor″tĭ-ko-thah-lam′ik) pertaining to or connecting the cerebral cortex and the thalamus.

corticotrope (kor′ti-ko-trōp) corticotroph.

corticotroph (kor′ti-ko-trōf) any of the small, irregularly stellate, acidophilic cells of the anterior lobe of the pituitary gland, having small, sparsely distributed secretory granules and secreting ACTH (adrenocorticotropic hormone, corticotropin), which is synthesized as a large prohormone (proopiomelanocortin) containing both ACTH and β-lipotropin (β-LPH). Called also *corticotrope, corticotroph-lipotroph, corticotroph cell,* and *corticotroph-lipotroph cell.*

corticotrophic (kor″tĭ-ko-trof′ik) corticotropic.

corticotroph-lipotroph (kor′tĭ-ko-trof-lip′o-trof) corticotroph.

corticotrophin (kor″tĭ-ko-tro′fin) corticotropin.

corticotropic (kor″tĭ-ko-trop′ik) exerting specific effects upon the cortex of the adrenal gland; called also *adrenocorticotropic.*

corticotropin (kor″tĭ-ko-tro′pin) a 39-amino-acid peptide hormone secreted by the anterior pituitary gland that acts primarily on the adrenal cortex, stimulating its growth and its secretion of corticosteroids. The production of corticotropin is increased during times of stress. A sterile preparation [USP] of the same principle(s) derived from the anterior pituitary of those mammals used for food by man is administered parenterally for diagnostic testing of adrenocortical function. It is used in veterinary medicine in the treatment of ketosis. Called also *adrenocorticotropic hormone (ACTH)* and *adrenocorticotropin.*

cortilymph (kor′tĕ-limf″) [organ of *Corti* + *lymph*] the fluid filling the intercellular spaces of the organ of Corti.

cortin (kor′tin) an obsolete term for and extract from the adrenal cortex containing a mixture of hormones having glucocorticoid and mineralocorticoid activity.

cortisol (kor′tĭ-sol) chemical name: $11\beta,17\alpha,21$-trihydroxy-pregn-4-ene-3,20-dione. The major natural glucocorticoid (q.v.) elaborated by the human adrenal cortex, or hydrocortisone [USP], as it is usually referred to pharmaceutically. See *hydrocortisone* for therapeutic uses. Called also (*Kendall's*) *compound F.*

cortisone (kor′tĭ-sōn) chemical name: $17\alpha,21$-dihydroxy-4-pregnene-3,11,20-trione. A natural glucocorticoid (q.v.), with significant mineralocorticoid properties, $C_{21}H_{28}O_5$; believed to be both a precursor and a metabolite of cortisol (hydrocortisone). The human adrenal cortex secretes only minute amounts of cortisone; the synthetic hormone exerts its pharmaceutical effects through its metabolic conversion to cortisol. **c. acetate** [USP], an ester of cortisone (q.v.), $C_{23}H_{30}O_6$, occurring as a white or practically white, crystalline powder; used as an anti-inflammatory in various conditions, including allergies and the collagen diseases. It is also used as replacement therapy in adrenocortical deficiencies, including Addison's disease and hypopituitarism, administered intramuscularly or orally, and is applied topically to treat steroid-responsive inflammatory conditions of the eye and skin.

cortivazol (kor-tiv′ah-zōl) chemical name: 21-(acetyloxy)-$11\beta,17$-dihydroxy-$6,16\alpha$-dimethyl-2′-phenylpregna-2,4,6-trieno [3,2-c] pyrazol-20-one; a synthetic glucocorticoid, $C_{32}H_{38}$-N_2O_5.

Cortone (kor′tōn) trademark for preparations of cortisone acetate.

Cortril (kor′tril) trademark for preparations of hydrocortisone.

Cortrophin (kor-tro′fin) trademark for preparations of corticotropin.

Cortrosyn (kor′tro-sin) trademark for a preparation of cosyntropin.

corundum (ko-run′dum) naturally occurring aluminum oxide; used in dentistry as an abrasive in grinding wheels and for points mounted on mandrels for the dental engine. See also *emery.*

coruscation (kor″us-ka′shun) [L. *coruscatio* a flash] a glittering sensation, as of flashes of light before the eyes.

Corvisart's disease (kor″ve-sarz′) [Baron Jean Nicolas *Corvisart des Marest*, French physician, 1755–1821] see under *disease.*

corybantiasm (kor″ĕ-ban′te-azm) corybantism.

corybantism (kor″ĕ-ban′tizm) [Gr. *Korybas* a reveller] wild, frenzied, and sleepless delirium.

corydaline (kŏ-rid′ah-lēn) an alkaloid, $C_{22}H_{27}NO_4$, from *Corydalis tuberosa;* a diuretic and tonic.

corydalis (kŏ-rid′ah-lis) [L. from Gr. *korys* helmet] the dried tuber of *Dicentra cucullaria* (L.) Bernh., or of *D. canadensis* (DC.) Walp., Fumariaceae, perennial herbs distributed throughout Ontario to Kentucky and Missouri. Also known as squirrel corn and turkey corn. It contains several isoquinoline type alkaloids, e.g., corydaline, bulbocapnine, corytuberine, etc. Bulbocapnine has been used for various muscle tremors and for vestibular nystagmus. The plant extract was once used as a tonic, antiperiodic, diuretic, and alterative.

corymbiform (ko-rim′bĭ-form) [Gr. *korymbos* the cluster of ivy flower + *form*] clustered; said of lesions grouped around a single, usually larger, lesion, as in tinea versicolor or late secondary syphilis.

corymbose (kor′im-bōs) corymbiform.

corynebacteria (ko-ri″ne-bak-te′re-ah) plural of *corynebacterium.*

Corynebacteriaceae (ko-ri″ne-bak-te″re-a′se-e) in former systems of classification, a family of coryneform bacteria, related to the actinomycetes, consisting of the genera *Arthrobacter, Cellulomonas, Corynebacterium, Erysipelothrix, Listeria,* and *Microbacterium.* For current classification, see the specific genus.

Corynebacterium (ko-ri″ne-bak-te′re-um) [Gr. *korynē* club + *bacterium*] a genus of coryneform bacteria, made up of gram-positive, nonsporulating, nonmotile, straight to slightly curved rods. The catalase-positive organisms are irregularly staining, sometimes granular, and may be arranged in angular and palisade groups. They are widely distributed in nature and include human and animal parasites and pathogens, plant pathogens, and nonpathogens. **C. ac′nes,** *Propionibacterium acnes.* **C. diphthe′riae,** the specific etiologic agent of diphtheria, which also causes skin infections. The organisms are separated according to cultural characteristics into three biotypes: *mitis, intermedius,* and *gravis,* which apparently are not related to pathogenicity. Most strains produce a potent exotoxin. Called also *Klebs-Löffler bacillus.* **C. diphtheroi′des,** *Eubacterium lentum.* **C. e′qui,** a species isolated from pneumonia in foals, the genital tract of mares, aborted equine fetuses, and the lymph glands of swine. It is a possible opportunistic pathogen in humans. **C. genita′lium,** a species associated with genitourinary infections in humans. **C. granulo′sum,** *Propionibacterium granulosum.* **C. haemoly′ticum,** a pathogenic species related to the streptococci and actinomycetes that has been recovered from pharyngitis and skin ulcers in humans. **C. hofman′nii,** *C. pseudodiphtheriticum.* **C. infantisep′ticum,** *Listeria monocytogenes.* **C. kut′scheri,** a species causing latent and overt infections in mice and rats. **C. minutis′simum,** a species of uncertain affiliation that causes erythrasma in humans. **C. murisep′ticum,** a diphtheria-like bacillus producing septicemic disease in mice, but apparently nonpathogenic for other animals. **C. necroph′orum,** *Fusobacterium necrophorum.* **C. o′vis,** *C. pseudotuberculosis.* **C. par′vulum,** *Listeria monocytogenes.* **C. par′vum,** 1. *Propionibacterium acnes.* 2. a heat-killed and formaldehyde-treated preparation of *C. parvum (P. acnes)* administered orally or parenterally as an experimental cancer immunotherapeutic agent, usually in conjunction with conventional chemotherapy. It appears to act by activating macrophages and also seems to depress T cell function. **C. pseudodiphtherit′icum,** a species normally present in the respiratory tract, which closely resembles *C. diphtheriae* but is nontoxigenic; it is sometimes an opportunistic pathogen. Called also *C. hofmannii* and *Hofmann's bacillus.* **C. pseudotuberculo′sis,** a pathogenic toxin-producing species found in lower animals. It causes caseous lymphangitis, abscesses, and chronic purulent infections, especially in sheep and goats, and contagious acne of horses. Occasional human disease may form from contact with infected animals or food. Called also *C. ovis* and *Preisz-Nocard bacillus.* **C. pyog′enes,** a toxicogenic species closely related to group G streptococci. It causes acute pyogenic lesions in cattle, sheep, and pigs, and has been isolated from human pharyngitis and skin lesions. **C. rena′le,** a species that causes cystitis and pyelonephritis in cattle. **C. ten′uis,** a nocardia-like species of uncertain affiliation that is the etiologic agent of trichomycosis axillaris. **C. ul′cerans,** a toxigenic species of uncertain affiliation that causes nasopharyngeal infections in humans and acute mastitis in cattle. **C. vesicula′re,** *Pseudomonas vesicularis.* **C. xero′sis,** an opportunistic pathogenic species found in the conjunctival sac and on the skin and mucous membranes of humans.

corynebacterium (ko-ri″ne-bak-te′re-um), pl. *corynebacteria* [Gr. *korynē* club + *bacterium*] 1. any member of the family Corynebacteriaceae or of the genus *Corynebacterium.* 2. a bacterium that displays coryneform shape during some stage of its development on artificial media. See also *coryneform bacteria,* under *bacterium.* **group JK c.,** a group of pathogenic diphtheroid bacteria cultured from blood, tissue, and wound infections of immunosuppressed patients. **group 3 c.,** *Eubacterium lentum.*

Coryneform (ko-ri″nĕ-form) a group of asporogenous, gram-positive, irregular rod-shaped bacteria containing the genera *Arthrobacter, Cellulomonas, Corynebacterium,* and *Kurthia.*

coryneform (ko-ri′nĕ-form) [Gr. *korynē* club + L. *forma*] club-shaped; see under *bacteria.*

corytuberine (ko″re-tu′ber-ēn) a crystalline alkaloid, C_{19}-$H_{21}NO_4 \cdot 5H_2O$, from commercial corydaline.

coryza (kŏ-ri′zah) [L.; Gr. *koryza*] an acute catarrhal condition of the nasal mucous membrane, with a profuse discharge from the nostrils. **allergic c.,** hay fever. **c. foe′tida,** ozena. **infectious avian c.,** an acute respiratory disease of chickens characterized by nasal discharge, sneezing, and edema of the face, and caused by *Haemophilus gallinarum.* Infection of the lower respiratory tract sometimes occurs. **c. oedemato′sa,** a serous inflammation of the inferior and middle turbinate bones.

coryzavirus (kŏ-ri″zah-vi′rus) one of a group of viral agents isolated from patients with the common cold and believed to be an etiologic agent of the common cold; now called *rhinovirus.*

C.O.S. Canadian Ophthalmological Society.

Coschwitz' duct (kosh′vits) [Georgius Daniel *Coschwitz,* German physician, 1679–1729] see under *duct.*

cosensitize (ko-sen′sĭ-tīz) to sensitize to two or more sensitizing agents.

Cosmegen (kos′mĕ-jen) trademark for a preparation of dactinomycin.

cosmetic (koz-met′ik) [Gr. *kosmētikos*] 1. beautifying the body; tending to preserve, restore, or confer bodily beauty. 2. a beautifying substance or preparation. 3. pertaining to surgical correction of a physical defect.

cosmid (koz′mid) [cohesive end *sito* + plas*mid*] a vector constructed of plasmid DNA packaged in vitro into a phage, useful for cloning large (up to 50 kb) DNA fragments.

costa (kos′tah), gen. and pl. *cos′tae* [L. "rib"] 1. NA alternative for *os costale.* 2. a rodlike structure extending along the base of the undulating membrane in certain flagellate protozoa, such as trichomonads. **c. cervica′lis** [NA], cervical rib: a supernumerary rib arising from a cervical vertebra, usually the seventh. See also *scalenus (cervical rib) syndrome,* under *syndrome.* **c. fluc′tuans,** floating rib: one of the lowest two ribs on either side, whose ventral tips ordinarily have no attachment. **cos′tae fluitan′tes** [NA], floating ribs: the lower two ribs on either side, which ordinarily have no ventral attachment; called also *costae fluctuantes, fluctuating ribs,* and *vertebral ribs.* **c. pri′ma** [NA] the first rib. **cos′tae spu′riae** [NA], the lower five ribs on either side: the ventral tips of the upper three of the five pairs connect with the costal cartilages of the superiorly adjacent ribs; the ventral tips of the lower two pairs ordinarily have no attachment. Called also *false ribs.* **cos′tae ve′rae** [NA], true ribs: the upper seven ribs on either side, which are connected to the sides of the sternum by their costal cartilages. Called also *sternal ribs* and *vertebrosternal ribs.*

costae (kos′te) [L.] genitive and plural of *costa.*

costal (kos′tal) [L. *costalis*] pertaining to a rib or ribs.

costalgia (kos-tal′je-ah) [*costa* + *-algia*] pain in the ribs.

costalis (kos-ta′lis) [L.] costal; used in anatomical nomenclature to denote relationship to a rib.

costatectomy (kos″tah-tek′to-me) costectomy.

costectomy (kos-tek′to-me) [*costa* + Gr. *ektomē* excision] the operation of excising or resecting a rib.

Costen's syndrome (kos′tenz) [James Bray *Costen,* St. Louis otolaryngologist, 1895–1962] temporomandibular dysfunction syndrome.

costicartilage (kos″tĭ-kar′tĭ-lij) [*costa* + *cartilage*] the cartilage of a rib.

costicervical (kos″tĭ-ser′vĭ-kal) pertaining to or connecting the ribs and the neck.

costiferous (kos-tif′er-us) [*costa* + L. *ferre* to carry] bearing a rib, as the thoracic vertebrae of man.

costiform (kos′tĭ-form) shaped like a rib.

costispinal (kos-tĭ-spi′nal) pertaining to or connecting the ribs and spine.

costive (kos′tiv) 1. pertaining to, characterized by, or producing constipation. 2. an agent that depresses intestinal motility.

costiveness (kos′tiv-nes) constipation.

cost(o)- [L. *costa* rib] a combining form denoting relationship to the ribs.

costocentral (kos″to-sen′tral) pertaining to a rib and the centrum (body) of a vertebra.

costocervicalis (kos″to-ser″vĭ-ka′lis) [*costo-* + *cervicalis*] musculus iliocostalis cervicis; see *Table of Musculi.*

costochondral (kos″to-kon′dral) pertaining to a rib and its cartilage.

costoclavicular (kos″to-klah-vik′u-lar) pertaining to the ribs and clavicle.

costocoracoid (kos″to-kor′ah-koid) pertaining to the ribs and coracoid process.

costogenic (kos″to-jen′ik) [*costo-* + Gr. *gennan* to produce] arising from a rib, especially from defect of the marrow of the ribs.

costoinferior (kos″to-in-fe′re-or) pertaining to the lower ribs.

costophrenic (kos″to-fren′ik) pertaining to the ribs and diaphragm.

costopleural (kos″to-plu′ral) pertaining to the ribs and the pleura.

costoscapular (kos″to-skap′u-lar) pertaining to the ribs and the scapula.

costoscapularis (kos″to-skap″u-la′ris) musculus serratus anterior; see *Table of Musculi.*

costosternal (kos″to-ster′nal) pertaining to a rib and to the sternum.

costosternoplasty (kos″to-ster′no-plas″te) surgical repair of funnel chest.

costosuperior (kos″to-su-pe′re-or) pertaining to the upper ribs.

costotome (kos′to-tōm) [*costo-* + Gr. *temnein* to cut] a knife for dividing ribs or costal cartilages.

costotomy (kos-tot′o-me) [*costo-* + Gr. *tomē* a cut] incision or division of a rib or costal cartilage.

costotransverse (kos″to-trans-vers′) lying between the ribs and transverse processes of the vertebrae.

costotransversectomy (kos″to-trans″ver-sek′to-me) excision of a part of a rib with the transverse process of a vertebra.

costovertebral (kos″to-ver′tĕ-bral) pertaining to a rib and a vertebra.

costoxiphoid (kos″to-zi′foid) connecting the ribs and the xiphoid cartilage.

cosyntropin (ko-sin-tro′pin) α^{1-24}-corticotropin: a synthetic corticotropin used in the screening of adrenal insufficiency by plasma cortisol response after intramuscular or intravenous injection.

Cotard's syndrome (ko-tarz′) [Jules *Cotard,* French neurologist, 1840–1889] see under *syndrome.*

cotarnine chloride (ko-tar′nēn) chemical name: 7,8-dihydro-4-methoxy-6-methyl-1,3-dioxolo[4,5-*g*]isoquinolinium chloride. A substance, $C_{12}H_{14}ClNO_3$, prepared by oxidation of noscapine with dilute nitric acid; formerly used as a hemostatic agent.

Cotazym (kot′ah-zīm) trademark for a preparation of pancrelipase.

cothromboplastin (ko-throm″bo-plas′tin) Factor VII; see *coagulation factors,* under *factor.*

cotinine (ko′tĭ-nēn) the major urinary metabolite of nicotine. **c. fumarate,** an antidepressant, $(C_{10}H_{12}N_2O)_2 \cdot C_4H_4O_4$.

co-trimoxazole (ko″tri-moks′ah-zōl) a mixture of trimethoprim and sulfamethoxazole.

Cotte's operation (kots) [Gaston *Cotte,* Lyons surgeon, 1879–1951] see under *operation.*

Cotting's operation (kot′ingz) [Benjamin Eddy *Cotting,* American surgeon, 1812–1898] see under *operation.*

cotton (kot′n) [L. *gossypium*] a textile material derived from the seeds of one or more of the cultivated varieties of

Gossypium. **absorbent c.,** purified c. **collodion c.,** pyroxylin. **gun c.,** pyroxylin. **gun c., soluble,** pyroxylin. **purified c.** [USP], the hair of the seed of cultivated varieties of *Gossypium hirsutum* Linné, or other species of *Gossypium,* freed from impurities, deprived of fatty matter, bleached, and sterilized; used as a surgical dressing. Called also *absorbent cotton,* and *gossypium asepticum, depuratum,* or *purificatum.* **salicylated c.,** purified cotton charged with salicylic acid, an antiseptic dressing. **styptic c.,** cotton impregnated with a styptic solution and dried.

cottonpox (kot′n-poks) variola minor.

cotton-wool (kot′n-wool) raw nonabsorbent cotton, or especially the absorbent form prepared by removing the cottonseed oil.

Cotugno's disease (ko-toon′yoz)[Domenico *Cotugno,* Italian anatomist, 1736–1822] sciatica. See also *Cotunnius.*

Cotunnius' aqueduct, etc. (ko-tun′e-us) [Domenico *Cotugno,* Italian anatomist, 1736–1822] see under *aqueduct, canal, nerve,* and *space.*

coturnism (ko-tur′nizm) food poisoning caused by ingestion of meat of the European migratory quail, genus *Coturnix,* and marked by such symptoms as difficult breathing, impaired speech, nausea, weakness and loss of feeling in the legs, and partial paralysis, and sometimes resulting in death; the causative toxin, which occurs in only some of the quail, is unidentified.

co-twin (ko-twin) a twin; usually applied in twin studies to identify pairs of twins.

cotyledon (kot′ĭ-le′don) [Gr. *kotylēdōn*] 1. the seed leaf of the embryo of a plant. 2. any one of the subdivisions of the uterine surface of a discoidal placenta. 3. one of the tufted areas of a ruminant's placenta.

cotyledontoxin (kot″ĭ-le″don-tok′sin) a toxic, neutral nonalkaloidal, nonglucosidal, non-nitrogenous, amorphous substance obtained from the herbaceous plants *Cotyledon ventricosa* and *C. wallchii.*

Cotylogonimus (kot″ĭ-lo-gon′ĭ-mus) [Gr. *kotylē* cup + *gonimos* productive] *Heterophyes.*

cotyloid (kot′ĭ-loid) [Gr. *kotyloeides* cup shaped] 1. cup-shaped. 2. pertaining to the cotyloid cavity (acetabulum).

cotylopubic (kot″ĭ-lo-pu′bik) relating to the cotyloid cavity (acetabulum) and the os pubis.

cotylosacral (kot″ĭ-lo-sa′kral) relating to the cotyloid cavity (acetabulum) and the sacrum.

cotype (ko-tīp) any strain of microorganisms (of the same taxon), other than a holotype, from the collection of the bacteriologist who originally described the taxon.

couch grass (kowch′ gras) the perennial grass *Agropyrum (Triticum) repens* (L.) Beauv. (Gramineae); its long roots are diuretic and have been used in cystitis, and possess demulcent and antitussive properties.

couching (kowch′ing) [Fr. *coucher* to put to bed] (*obs.*) surgical displacement of the lens in cataract; called also *abaissement, cataractopiesis,* and *depression of cataract.*

cough (kawf) [L. *tussis*] 1. a sudden noisy expulsion of air from the lungs, usually produced to keep the airways of the lungs free of foreign matter; see also under *reflex.* 2. to produce such an expulsion of air. **aneurysmal c.,** a variety of cough associated with aortic aneurysm, and sometimes with paralysis of one vocal cord. **Balme's c.,** cough on lying down, seen in obstruction of the nasopharynx. **barking c.,** the barklike cough of early youth, as in croup. **compression c.,** a deep resonant cough caused by compression of a bronchus; it resembles in character the cough of a dog and is sometimes called *dog c.* **dog c.,** see *compression c.* **dry c.,** one that is not accompanied with expectoration. **ear c.,** a reflex cough caused by disease of the ear, when Arnold's nerve is stimulated. **extrapulmonary c.,** a cough due to causes outside the lungs. **hacking c.,** a short, frequent, shallow, and feeble cough. **mechanical c.,** expulsion of air from the lungs produced by use of an exsufflator, with effects similar to those of a natural cough. **Morton's c.,** a persistent cough in pulmonary tuberculosis which brings on vomiting and thus causes loss of nourishment. **privet c.,** an allergic cough noted in China and attributed to the pollen of privet. **productive c.,** a cough that is effective in removing material from the respiratory tract. **reflex c.,** a cough due to the irritation of some remote organ. **stomach c.,** a cough caused by reflex irritation from stomach disorder. **Sydenham's c.,**

hysterical spasm of the respiratory muscles. **tea taster's c.,** cough in tasters of tea, attributed to inhaling fungi, such as *Candida, Aspergillus,* etc., from tea leaves. **trigeminal c.,** a cough due to irritation of the fibers of the trigeminal nerve distributed to the throat, nose, and external meatus of the ear. **wet c.,** one attended with expectoration. **whooping c.,** pertussis. **winter c.,** chronic bronchitis recurring in the winter.

coulomb (koo′lom) [after Charles Augustin de *Coulomb,* French physicist, 1736–1806] the SI unit of electric charge defined as the charge carried across a surface by a steady current of one ampere in one second. Symbol C.

Coumadin (koo′mah-din) trademark for preparations of sodium warfarin.

coumamycin (koo-mah-mi′sin) coumermycin.

coumaric acid (koo′mah-rik) an acid, $OH \cdot C_6 \cdot H_4 \cdot (CH)_2 \cdot COOH$, from coumarin, readily convertible into salicylic acid.

coumarin (koo′mah-rin) 1. chemical name: $2H$-1-benzopyran-2-one. A principle, $C_9H_6O_2$, with a bitter taste and an odor resembling that of vanilla beans, derived from tonka bean, sweet clover, and other plants, and also prepared synthetically. Coumarin contains a factor, dicumarol (3,3′-methylenebis [4-hydroxy-2H- 1-benzopyran-2-one]), which inhibits the hepatic synthesis of the vitamin K–dependent coagulation factors (prothrombin, Factors VII, IX, and X), and a number of its derivatives are used widely as anticoagulants in the treatment of disorders in which there is excessive or undesirable clotting, such as thrombophlebitis, pulmonary embolism, and certain cardiac conditions. 2. any derivative of coumarin or any synthetic compound with coumarin-like actions.

coumermycin (koo-mer-mi′sin) chemical name: 5-methylpyrrole-2-carboxylic acid, diester with 3,3′-[(3-methylpyrrole 2,4-diyl)bis (carbonylimino)] bis [4-hydroxy-8-methyl-7-[(tetrahydro- 3,4-dihydroxy-5-methoxy-6,6-dimethylpyran-2-yl)oxy]coumarin]; an antibacterial agent, $C_{55}H_{59}N_5$-O_{20}, isolated from *Streptomyces hazeliensis* var. *hazeliensis* and from *S. rishiriensis.*

Councilman's bodies (lesions) (kown′sil-man) [William Thomas *Councilman,* American pathologist, 1854–1933] see under *body.*

count (kownt) [L. *computare* to reckon] a numerical computation or indication. **Addis c.,** the determination of the number of red blood cells, white blood cells, epithelial cells, casts, and the protein content in an aliquot of a twelve-hour urine specimen, used in the diagnosis and management of kidney disease. **Arneth c.,** a method of determining the percentage of neutrophils having the same number (1–5) of nuclear lobes or segments: the normal values (Arneth's formula) are 1 lobe, 5 per cent; 2 lobes, 35 per cent; 3 lobes, 41 per cent; 4 lobes, 17 per cent, 5 lobes, 2 per cent; Arneth's index is the sum of the percentages for 1 and 2 lobes plus half the percentage for 3 lobes. An increase in the percentages with fewer lobes is termed a *shift to the left,* and in the other direction, a *shift to the right.* Called also *neutrophil lobe c.* **blood c.,** determination of the number of formed elements in a measured volume of blood, usually a cubic millimeter (as red blood cell, white blood cell, or platelet count.) **complete blood c.,** a series of tests of the peripheral blood, including the hematocrit (per cent), the amount of hemoglobin (grams per cent), the white cell count (per cubic millimeter), and the proportions of the different white cells as they appear on a blood smear. **differential c.,** a count made by observation, on the stained blood smear, of the proportion of the different types of leukocytes (or other cells), expressed in percentages. **direct platelet c.,** determination of the total number of platelets per cubic millimeter of blood, in a counting chamber, with the use of conventional light or phase microscopy. **filament-nonfilament c.,** determination of the number of juvenile and mature leukocytes, as in the differential blood count. **indirect platelet c.,** calculation of the total number of platelets per cubic millimeter of blood by determining, in a peripheral blood smear, the ratio of platelets to erythrocytes, and computing the number of platelets from the total red cell count. **neutrophil lobe c.,** Arneth c. **Schilling blood c.** (*obs.*), a differential blood count in which the neutrophils are divided into four groups: myelocytes, juvenile cells (or young forms), staff cells, and segmented forms. **staff c.** (*obs.*), Schilling blood c.

counter (kown′ter) an instrument or apparatus by which

numerical value is computed; in radiology, a device for enumerating ionizing events. **Coulter c.,** an automatic instrument used in the enumeration of formed peripheral blood elements, based on the principle that cells are poor electrical conductors compared with saline solution. **Geiger c., Geiger-Müller c.,** a highly sensitive radiation counter that uses a gas-filled tube to indicate the presence of ionizing particles; the type and energy of a particle cannot be determined because the degree of ionization produced is independent of them. **proportional c.,** a gas-filled radiation detection tube in which the pulse produced is proportional to the number of ions formed in the gas by the primary ionizing particle; thus it is possible to discriminate among radiations of different energies or types. **scintillation c.,** an instrument for indicating the emission of ionizing particles, making possible the determination of the concentration of radioactive isotopes in the body or other substance; the radiation is absorbed by a phosphor crystal, which emits minute flashes of light that are detected and amplified by a photomultiplier tube.

counterbalance (kown″ter-bal′ans) counterpoise; offset. **renal c.,** compensatory hypertrophy of a normal kidney or part of a kidney accompanied by the tendency of its diseased mate or part to remain in a relatively atrophic state.

countercurrent (kown′ter-ker″ent) flowing in an opposite direction; see also under *mechanism.*

counterdie (kown′ter-di) the reverse image of a die, usually made of a softer and lower fusing metal than the die.

counterelectrophoresis (kown″ter-e-lek″tro-fo-re′sis) counterimmunoelectrophoresis.

counterextension (kown″ter-eks-ten′shun) countertraction.

counterimmunoelectrophoresis (kown″ter-im″u-no-e-lek″tro-fo-re′sis) one-dimensional double electroimmunodiffusion; a technique in which antibody and antigen are placed in separate wells in an agar plate and driven toward each other by an applied electric field, because the gel is buffered at a pH between the isoelectric points of the antigen and antibody. It is more sensitive and faster than double immunodiffusion and is particularly useful for antigens that diffuse slowly in the gel. Abbreviated CIE. Called also *countercurrent immunoelectrophoresis* and *counterelectrophoresis.*

counterincision (kown″ter-in-sizh′un) a second incision usually made to promote drainage, but occasionally to relieve tension on the edges of a clean wound during closure.

counterinvestment (kown″ter-in-vest′ment) anticathexis.

counterirritant (kown″ter-ir′ĭ-tant) 1. producing a counterirritation. 2. any agent which causes counterirritation.

counterirritation (kown″ter-ir″ĭ-ta′shun) a superficial irritation; an irritation produced in one part of the body and intended to relieve an irritation in another part.

counteropening (kown″ter-o′pen-ing) a second incision made across an earlier one to promote drainage.

counterphobia (kown″ter-fo′be-ah) the seeking out of situations or objects which one fears or has feared, consciously or unconsciously.

counterphobic (kown″ter-fo′bik) pertaining to or characterized by counterphobia.

counterpoison (kown′ter-poi″zn) a poison given to counteract another poison.

counterpulsation (kown″ter-pul-sa′shun) a technique for assisting the circulation and decreasing the work of the heart, by synchronizing the force of an external pumping device with cardiac systole and diastole. **intra-aortic balloon c.,** circulatory support provided by a balloon inserted into the thoracic aorta, which is inflated during diastole (enhancing coronary perfusion pressure) and deflated during systole, resulting in a decrease in afterload and improvement in cardiac function.

counterpuncture (kown′ter-punk″chur) counteropening.

counterstain (kown′ter-stān) a stain applied to render the effects of another stain more discernible.

countertraction (kown′ter-trak″shun) traction opposed to another traction; employed in the reduction of fractures.

countertransference (kown″ter-trans-fer′ens) a transference reaction of a psychoanalyst or other psychotherapist to a patient, i.e., an emotional reaction that is a reflection of

the analyst's own inner needs and conflicts. See *transference.*

coup (koo) [Fr.] stroke. **c. de fouet** (koo-duh-fwa′) [Fr. "stroke of the whip"], rupture of the plantaris muscle accompanied by a sharp disabling pain. **c. de sabre, en c. de sabre** (koo-duh-sahb′, ahn-koo-duh-sahb′) [Fr. "saber stroke"], a linear lesion or scleroderma involving the frontal or frontoparietal area of the forehead and scalp; it is often associated with hemiatrophy of the face. **c. de sang** (koo-duh-sang′), congestion of the brain. **c. de soleil** (koo-duh-sŏ-la′), sunstroke. **c. sur coup** (koo-ser-koo′) ["blow on blow"], the administration of a drug in small doses at short intervals, to secure rapid, complete, or continuous action; abbreviated C.S.C.

couple (kup′l) [L. *copula* a bond] 1. two equal forces operating on an object in parallel but opposite directions. 2. an area of contact between two dissimilar metals, producing a difference in electrical potential.

coupling (kup′ling) 1. in genetics, the occurrence on the same chromosome in a double heterozygote of the two mutant alleles of interest. Cf. *repulsion.* 2. in cardiology, the serial occurrence of a normal heart beat followed closely by a premature beat. **excitation-contraction c.,** the coupling of the action potential to muscle constriction by means of calcium ions which diffuse rapidly into the myofibrils and catalyze the chemical reactions that promote the contractile sliding of actin and myosin filaments. **fixed c.,** coupling in which the premature heart beats follow the preceding normal beats at identical intervals.

courbature (koor′bah-tūr) [Fr.] 1. aching of the muscles. 2. decompression sickness.

Cournand (kōōr′nand), André Frédéric. French-born American physiologist, born 1895; co-winner, with Werner Theodor Otto Forssmann and Dickinson Woodruff Richards, Jr., of the Nobel prize for medicine or physiology in 1956 for the development of cardiac catheterization.

courses (kor′sez) (*obs.*) menses.

Courvoisier's law (sign) (koor-vwah″ze-āz′) [Ludwig Georg *Courvoisier,* Swiss surgeon, 1843–1918] see under *law.*

Courvoisier-Terrier syndrome (koor-vwah″ze-a′-ter-ya′) [L. G. *Courvoisier;* Louis Félix *Terrier,* Paris surgeon, 1837–1908] see under *syndrome.*

Coutard's method (koo-tarz′) [Henri *Coutard,* French radiologist in United States, 1876–1950] see under *method.*

couvade (koo-vad′) a custom of primitive peoples, in which the husband feigns illness during his wife's parturient and puerperal periods.

Couvelaire uterus (koo″vel-ār′) [Alexandre *Couvelaire,* Paris obstetrician, 1873–1948] see *uteroplacental apoplexy,* under *apoplexy.*

couvercle (koo′ver-kl) [Fr.] a blood clot formed outside a vessel.

covalence (ko-vāl′ens) the number of electron pairs an atom can share with other atoms.

covalent (ko-vāl′ent) see under *bond.*

covariance (ko-vār-e-ans) [co- + *variance*] in statistics, a measure of the tendency of two random variables to vary together: the expected value of the product of the deviations of corresponding values of the variables from their respective means.

cover (kov′er) 1. to provide protection against, as by prophylaxis. 2. the prophylaxis so provided.

coverglass (kov′er-glas) a thin glass plate that covers a mounted microscopical object or a culture. Spelled also *cover glass.*

coverslip (kov′er-slip) coverglass.

cowage (kow′aj) 1. a perennial herb, *Mucuna pruriens* DC. (Leguminosae), of the East Indies. 2. the hairs of the cowage pods, which cause severe itching, are used medicinally as a vermifuge, anthelmintic, and counterirritant in admixture with such vehicles as honey. Also used as "itching powders" of joke-shop fame.

Cowden disease (syndrome) (kow′den) [*Cowden,* the family name of the first reported case] see under *disease.*

Cowdria (kow′dre-ah) [Edmund Vincent *Cowdry,* American anatomist and zoologist, 1888–1975] a genus of bacteria of the tribe Ehrlichieae, family Rickettsiaceae, order Rickettsiales, occurring in the cytoplasm of vascular endothelial cells of ruminants. **C. ruminan′tium,** the etiologic agent of heartwater (q.v.) of sheep, goats, and cattle; it is nonpathogenic for man.

cowl (kowl) caul.

Cowper's gland, ligament (kow'perz) [William *Cowper*, English surgeon, 1666–1709] see *bulbourethral gland* and *fascia pectinea*.

cowperian (kow-pe're-an) described by or named in honor of William Cowper.

cowperitis (kow"per-i'tis) inflammation of Cowper's glands (glandula bulbourethralis).

cowpox (kow'poks) a mild, self-limited, eruptive skin disease of milk cows, principally confined to the udder and teats, caused by cowpox virus, with human infection occurring accidentally, e.g., while milking an infected animal; the primary lesions, vesicles, usually appear on the fingers and may rupture and spread to the hands and adjacent areas, and usually heal without scarring. Local edema, lymphangitis, and regional lymphadenitis with or without fever may be associated. Milkers may spread the infection to uninfected cattle. Cowpox is not to be confused with *paravaccinia* (milker's nodes or nodules). Cf. *vaccinia*. The English physician Jenner first demonstrated vaccination in 1798 when he showed that inoculation with material from cowpox lesions conferred immunity against smallpox.

coxa (kok'sah) [L.] [NA] the part of the body lateral to and including the hip joint. Also loosely used to denote the hip joint. **c. adduc'ta, c. flex'a,** c. vara. **c. mag'na,** a condition marked by broadening of the head and neck of the femur. **c. pla'na,** osteochondrosis of the capitular epiphysis of the femur; see under *osteochondrosis.* **c. val'ga,** deformity of the hip in which the angle formed by the axis of the head and the neck of the femur and the axis of its shaft is materially increased. **c. va'ra,** deformity of the hip in which the angle formed by the axis of the head and neck of the femur and the axis of its shaft is materially decreased; called also *c. adducta* and *c. flexa.* **c. va'ra lux'ans,** fissure of the neck of the femur with dislocation of the head developing from coxa vara.

coxalgia (kok-sal'je-ah) [L. *coxa* hip + *-algia*] 1. hip-joint disease. 2. pain in the hip.

coxarthria (koks-ar'thre-ah) coxitis.

coxarthritis (koks"ar-thri'tis) coxitis.

coxarthrocace (koks"ar-throk'ah-se) fungus disease of the hip joint.

coxarthropathy (koks"ar-throp'ah-the) [L. *coxa* hip + Gr. *arthron* joint + *pathos* disease] hip-joint disease.

coxarthrosis (koks-ar-thro'sis) degenerative joint disease or osteoarthritis of the hip joint.

Coxiella (kok"se-el'lah) [Herald Rae *Cox*, American bacteriologist, born 1907] a genus of bacteria of the tribe Rickettsieae, family Rickettsiaceae, order Rickettsiales, occurring as short rods in the vacuoles of host cells. The organisms have been found in various mammals and ticks worldwide, and have been isolated from milk and placentas of infected cattle, sheep, and goats and from the wool of infected sheep. **C. burnet'ii,** the etiologic agent of Q fever, transmitted by *Haemaphysalis, Ixodes, Dermacentor,* and *Amblyomma* ticks. Human infection usually occurs from inhalation of infectious dust and aerosols derived from domestic livestock, and from contaminated wool in textile plants. Called also *Rickettsia burnetii* and *Rickettsia diaporica.*

coxitis (kok-si'tis) inflammation of the hip joint; called also *coxarthritis.* **c. fu'gax,** a transient benign coxitis. **senile c.,** degenerative arthritis of the hip joint.

coxodynia (kok"so-din'e-ah) coxalgia, def. 2.

coxofemoral (kok"so-fem'o-ral) [L. *coxa* hip + *femur* thigh] pertaining to the hip and thigh.

coxotuberculosis (kok"so-tu-ber"ku-lo'sis) [L. *coxa* hip + *tuberculosis*] tuberculous disease of the hip joint.

coxsackievirus (kok-sak'e-vi"rus) [Coxsackie, N.Y., where it was first identified] one of a heterogeneous group of enteroviruses producing, in man, a disease resembling poliomyelitis, but without paralysis; separable into two groups: A, producing degenerative lesions of striated muscle and B, producing leptomeningitis in infant mice. A number of different serotypes have also been identified. Also written *Coxsackie virus.*

cozymase (ko-zi'mās) nicotinamide-adenine dinucleotide (NAD); see under nicotinamide.

C.P. chemically pure; candle power.

cp centipoise.

C3PA C3 proactivator; see *complement.*

C3PAase C3 proactivator convertase; see *complement.*

CPC clinicopathological conference.

CPD citrate phosphate dextrose.

CPDA-1 citrate phosphate dextrose adenine.

C.P.H. Certificate in Public Health.

CPK creatine phosphokinase; see *creatine kinase.*

C. Ped. Certified Pedorthist.

c.p.m. counts per minute, an expression of the particles emitted after administration of a radioactive material such as [131]I.

CPR cardiopulmonary resuscitation.

c.p.s. cycles per second.

CR conditioned response.

C.R. crown-rump; in embryology, the usual axis of measurement of an embryo or fetus.

Cr chemical symbol for *chromium.*

crab (krab) a vernacular term for *Phthirus pubis.*

crack (krak) an incomplete split, break, or fissure. **sand c.,** a crack originating at the ground level in a horse's hoof, sometimes causing lameness. When situated on the inside of the hoof it is termed *quarter c.;* when in the fore part of the hoof it is *toe c.*

crackle (krak'l) a small sharp sound. **pleural c's,** superficial crepitation heard in the early stages of acute fibrinous pleurisy.

cradle (kra'dl) a frame placed over the body of a bed patient for application of heat or cold or for protecting injured parts from contact with the bed clothes. **electric c., heat c.,** a tunnel- or hood-shaped cradle equipped with electric light bulbs, for application of heat to the body of a patient. **ice c.,** a device for lowering a patient's body temperature.

Crafts' test (krafts) [Leo Melville *Crafts,* American neurologist, 1863–1938] see under *tests.*

Craigia (kra'ge-ah) [Charles Franklin *Craig,* U. S. Army surgeon, 1872–1950] *Paramoeba.*

Cramer's splint (krah'merz) [Friedrich *Cramer,* German surgeon, 1847–1903] see under *splint.*

cramp (kramp) a painful spasmodic muscular contraction, especially a tonic spasm. **accessory c.,** spastic torticollis due to a lesion of the accessory nerve. **heat c.,** a form of heat exhaustion in which muscular spasm is attended by pains, dilated pupils, and weak pulse; seen in those who labor in intense heat (stokers, miners, cane-cutters) and lose much water and salt. Called also *Edsall's disease.* **recumbency c's,** cramping of muscles in legs and feet occurring while resting or during light sleep. **stoker's c.,** heat c. **writers' c.,** a muscle cramp in the hand caused by excessive use in writing; called also *graphospasm.*

Crampton's muscle (kramp'tonz) [Sir Philip *Crampton,* Irish surgeon, 1777–1858] see under *muscle.*

Crampton's test (kramp'tonz) [Charles Ward *Crampton,* American physician, born 1877] see under *tests.*

craniad (kra'ne-ad) [L. *cranium* head + *ad* toward] in a cranial direction; toward the anterior (in animals) or superior (in humans) end of the body.

cranial (kra'ne-al) [L. *cranialis*] pertaining to the cranium, or to the anterior (in animals) or superior (in humans) end of the body.

cranialis (kra"ne-a'lis) [L.] pertaining to the cranium, or to the superior end of the body; [NA] a term used to denote relationship to the superior end of the body.

craniamphitomy (kra"ne-am-fit'o-me) [*cranium* + Gr. *amphi* around + *tomē* a cutting] division of the entire circumference of the skull to secure decompression.

Craniata (kra-ne-a'tah) the subphylum of the Chordata containing the species with a true skull and spinal column; the vertebrates.

craniectomy (kra"ne-ek'to-me) [*cranium* + Gr. *ektomē* excision] excision of a part of the skull.

crani(o)- [L. *cranium,* q.v.] a combining form denoting relationship to the cranium or skull.

cranioacromial (kra"ne-o-ah-kro'me-al) pertaining to the cranium and acromion.

cranioaural (kra″ne-o-aw′ral)   pertaining to the cranium and the ear.

craniobuccal (kra′ne-o-buk′al)   pertaining to the head and the mouth.

craniocele (kra′ne-o-sēl″) [cranio- + Gr. kēlē hernia]   a protrusion of any part of the cranial contents through a defect in the skull.

craniocerebral (kra″ne-o-ser′e-bral)   pertaining to the cranium and the cerebrum.

cranioclasis (kra′ne-ok′lah-sis) [cranio- + Gr. klasis fracture]   craniotomy, def. 2.

cranioclast (kra′ne-o-klast″) [cranio- + Gr. klan to break]   an instrument for performing craniotomy (def. 2).

cranioclasty (kra′ne-o-klas″te)   craniotomy, def. 2.

craniodidymus (kra″ne-o-did′ĭ-mus) [cranio- + Gr. didymos twin]   a monster with two heads.

craniofacial (kra″ne-o-fa′shal)   pertaining to the cranium and the face.

craniofenestria (kra″ne-o-fĕ-nes′tre-ah) [cranio- + L. fenestra an opening]   defective development of the bones of the vault of the fetal skull, marked by areas in which no bone is formed.

craniognomy (kra-ne-og′no-me) [cranio- + Gr. gnōmōn an interpreter or judge]   the study of the shape of the head.

craniograph (kra′ne-o-graf″) [cranio- + Gr. graphein to write]   an instrument for outlining the skull.

craniography (kra″ne-og′rah-fe)   the study of the skull by means of photographs, charts, etc.

craniolacunia (kra″ne-o-lah-ku′ne-ah) [cranio- + L. lacuna a hollow + -ia]   defective development of the bones of the vault of the fetal skull marked by depressed areas on the inner surfaces of the bones.

craniology (kra″ne-ol′o-je) [cranio- + -logy]   the scientific study of skulls.

craniomalacia (kra″ne-o-mah-la′she-ah) [cranio- + Gr. malakia softness]   abnormal softness of the skull.

craniomeningocele (kra″ne-o-mĕ-nin′go-sēl) [cranio- + Gr. mēninx membrane + kēlē hernia]   protrusion of cerebral membranes through a defect in the skull.

craniometer (kra″ne-om′ĕ-ter) [cranio- + Gr. metron measure]   an instrument for use in craniometry.

craniometric (kra″ne-o-met′rik)   pertaining to craniometry.

craniometry (kra″ne-om′ĕ-tre) [cranio- + Gr. metrein to measure]   the scientific measurement of the dimensions of the bones of the skull and face.

craniopagus (kra″ne-op′ah-gus) [cranio- + Gr. pagos a thing fixed]   a double monster united by the heads; called also cephalopagus. **c. occipita′lis,** craniopagus in which fusion is in the occipital region. **c. parasit′icus,** craniopagus in which a parasitic head is attached to the head of the autosite. **c. parieta′lis,** craniopagus in which fusion is in the parietal region.

craniopathy (kra″ne-op′ah-the) [cranio- + Gr. pathos disease]   any disease of the skull. **metabolic c.,** a condition characterized by lesions of the calvarium with multiple metabolic changes and marked by headache, obesity, and visual disturbances.

craniopharyngeal (kra″ne-o-fah-rin′je-al)   pertaining to the cranium and the pharynx.

craniopharyngioma (kra″ne-o-fah-rin″je-o′mah)   a tumor arising from cell rests derived from the hypophyseal stalk or Rathke's pouch, frequently associated with increased intracranial pressure, and showing calcium deposits in the capsule or in the tumor proper. Called also craniopharyngeal duct tumor, Rathke's (pouch) tumor, suprasellar cyst, and pituitary adamantinoma or ameloblastoma.

craniophore (kra′ne-o-fōr) [cranio- + Gr. phoros bearing]   a device for holding a skull during measurement of its diameters and angles.

cranioplasty (kra′ne-o-plas″te) [cranio- + Gr. plassein to mold]   any plastic operation on the skull; surgical correction of defects of the skull.

craniopuncture (kra′ne-o-punk″tūr)   puncture of the skull.

craniorachischisis (kra″ne-o-rah-kis′kĭ-sis) [cranio- + Gr.

rhachis spine + schisis fissure]   congenital fissure of the skull and vertebral column.

craniosacral (kra″ne-o-sa′kral)   1. pertaining to the skull and the sacrum.   2. pertaining to the parasympathetic nerves.

cranioschisis (kra″ne-os′kĭ-sis) [cranio- + Gr. schisis fissure]   congenital fissure of the cranium.

craniosclerosis (kra″ne-o-skle-ro′sis) [cranio- + Gr. sklēros hard]   thickening of the bones of the skull.

cranioscopy (kra″ne-os′ko-pe) [cranio- + Gr. skopein to examine]   diagnostic examination of the head.

craniospinal (kra″ne-o-spi′nal)   pertaining to the cranium and the spine.

craniostenosis (kra″ne-o-ste-no′sis) [cranio- + Gr. stenōsis narrowing]   deformity of the skull caused by premature fusion of the cranial sutures, with consequent cessation of growth, the nature of the deformity depending on the sutures involved in the process.

craniostosis (kra″ne-os-to′sis) [cranio- + Gr. osteon bone]   congenital ossification of the cranial sutures.

craniosynostosis (kra″ne-o-sin″os-to′sis)   premature closure of the sutures of the skull.

craniotabes (kra″ne-o-ta′bēz) [cranio- + L. tabes a wasting]   reduction in the mineralization of the skull, with abnormal softness of the bone, usually located in the occipital and parietal bones along the lambdoidal sutures.

craniotome (kra′ne-o-tōm″) [cranio- + Gr. tomē a cutting]   an instrument for use in performing craniotomy.

craniotomy (kra″ne-ot′o-me) [cranio- + Gr. tomē a cut]   1. any operation on the cranium; incision into the cranium.   2. an operation to decrease the size of the head of a dead fetus and facilitate delivery by puncturing the skull and removing its contents; encephalotomy.

craniotonoscopy (kra″ne-o-to-nos′ko-pe) [cranio- + Gr. tonos tone + Gr. skopein to examine]   auscultatory percussion of the head.

craniotopography (kra″ne-o-to-pog′rah-fe) [cranio- + topography]   the study of the relations of the surface of the skull to the various parts of the brain beneath.

craniotrypesis (kra″ne-o-trĭ-pe′sis) [cranio- + Gr. trypēsis a piercing]   trephination of the skull.

craniotympanic (kra″ne-o-tim-pan′ik)   pertaining to the skull and the tympanum.

cranitis (kra-ni′tis)   inflammation of the cranial bones.

cranium (kra′ne-um), pl. cra′nia [L., from Gr. kranion the upper part of the head] [NA]   the skeleton of the head, variously construed as including all of the bones of the head, all of them except the mandible, or the eight bones which form the vault that lodges the brain. See also cranial bones, under bone. **c. bif′idum,** congenital cleft of the cranium. **c. bif′idum occul′tum,** congenital cleft of the cranium without associated abnormality of the brain or meninges, detectable only roentgenographically. **cerebral c., c. cerebra′le,** those portions of the bones of the head that contribute to the brain case. **visceral c., c. viscera′le,** those portions of the bones of the head that form the skeleton of the face; this includes the mandible and hyoid bone.

crapulent, crapulous (krap′u-lent, krap′u-lus) [L. crapulentus, crapulosis drunken]   due to excess in eating or drinking.

crassamentum (kras″ah-men′tum) [L.]   a clot, as of blood.

Crast.   abbreviation for L. cras′tinus, for tomorrow.

crater (kra′ter)   a circular area of depression surrounded by an elevated margin.

crateriform (kra-ter′ĭ-form) [L. crater bowl + forma shape]   depressed or hollowed, like a bowl.

craterization (kra″ter-i-za′shun)   the operation of excising a craterlike piece from a bone.

craunology (kraw-nol′o-je)   crenology.

craunotherapy (kraw″no-ther′ah-pe)   crenotherapy.

cravat (krah-vat′) [Fr. cravate]   a bandage made by folding a triangular piece of cloth from its apex toward the base.

craw-craw (kraw′kraw)   a name for onchocerciasis in West Africa.

crazing (kra′zing)   the appearance of minute cracks on the surface of artificial or natural teeth, porcelain, and resin denture bases.

cream (krēm) the oily or fatty part of milk from which butter is prepared, or a fluid mixture of similar consistency; in pharmaceutical preparations, a semisolid emulsion of the oil-in-water or water-in-oil type, ordinarily used topically. **acrisorcin c.** [USP], acrisorcin in a suitable water-miscible base, containing not less than 90 per cent and not more than 110 per cent of acrisorcin; used as a topical antifungal agent. **benzocaine c.** [USP], a mixture containing 90 to 100 per cent of the labeled amount of benzocaine; used as a local anesthetic, applied topically to the skin and mucous membranes. **betamethasone c.** [USP], a mixture containing 90 to 115 per cent of the labeled amount of betamethasone in a suitable water-miscible base; used topically as an anti-inflammatory glucocorticoid. **betamethasone dipropionate c.** [USP], a mixture containing betamethasone dipropionate equivalent to 90 to 110 of the labeled amount of betamethasone in a suitable cream base; used topically as an anti-inflammatory. **betamethasone valerate c.** [USP], a mixture containing betamethasone valerate equivalent to 95 to 115 per cent of the labeled amount of betamethasone in a suitable cream base; used topically as an anti-inflammatory glucocorticoid. **clotrimazole c.** [USP], a cream containing not less than 90 per cent and not more than 110 per cent of the labeled amount of clotrimazole; used as a topical antifungal agent. **cold c.** [USP], a preparation of spermaceti, white wax, mineral oil, sodium borate, and purified water; used as a topical emollient for minor skin irritations and as a water-in-oil emulsion ointment base. **cortisol acetate c.** [USP], a mixture containing between 90 and 110 per cent of the labeled amount of total steroids in a suitable cream base; used as a topical anti-inflammatory steroid. **crotamiton c.** [USP], a preparation containing 93 to 107 per cent of the labeled amount of crotamiton; used as a scabicide, applied topically to the skin. **cyclomethycaine sulfate c.** [USP], a preparation containing 90 to 110 per cent of the labeled amount of cyclomethycaine sulfate in a suitable cream base; used as a local anesthetic, applied topically. **desoximetasone c.** [USP], a preparation containing between 90 and 110 per cent of the labeled amount of desoximetasone in an emollient cream base; used topically as a corticosteroid anti-inflammatory. **dexamethasone sodium phosphate c.,** a cream containing dexamethasone sodium phosphate equivalent to 90 to 115 per cent of the labeled amount of dexamethasone phosphate; used topically as an anti-inflammatory glucocorticoid. **dibucaine c.** [USP], a mixture containing between 90 and 110 per cent of the labeled amount of dibucaine in a suitable cream base; used topically as a local anesthetic. **dienestrol c.** [USP], a mixture containing between 90 to 110 per cent of the labeled amount of dienestrol in a suitable water-miscible base; used topically for its estrogenic effect in the treatment of postmenopausal and senile vulvovaginitis, atrophic vaginitis, pruritus vulvae due to atrophic changes in the vulval epithelium, dyspareunia associated with atrophic vaginal epithelium, and prior to plastic pelvic surgery in menopausal cases. **dioxybenzone and oxybenzone c.** [USP], a preparation usually containing 3 per cent dioxybenzone and 3 per cent oxybenzone; used as a sunscreening agent, applied topically to the skin. **flumethasone pivalate c.** [USP], a preparation containing not less than 90 per cent and not more than 110 per cent of flumethasone pivalate in a suitable cream base; used topically as an anti-inflammatory glucocorticoid. **fluocinolone acetonide c.** [USP], a cream containing 90 to 110 per cent of the labeled amount of fluocinolone acetonide; used as an anti-inflammatory in steroid-responsive dermatoses, applied topically. **fluocinonide c.** [USP], a preparation containing 90 to 110 per cent of the labeled amount of fluocinonide; used as an anti-inflammatory in steroid-responsive dermatoses, applied topically. **fluorometholone c.** [USP], a cream containing 90 to 110 per cent of the labeled amount of fluorometholone; used topically as an anti-inflammatory in the treatment of steroid-responsive dermatoses. **fluorouracil c.** [USP], a preparation containing 90 to 110 per cent of the labeled amount of fluorouracil; used as an antineoplastic in the treatment of actinic keratoses, applied topically. **flurandrenolide c.** [USP], a cream containing 85 to 115 per cent of the labeled amount of flurandrenolide; used as a topical anti-inflammatory in the treatment of steroid-responsive dermatoses. **gamma benzene hexachloride c.,** lindane c. **gentamicin sulfate c.** [USP], a mixture containing 90 to 135 per cent of gentamicin sulfate, expressed in terms of gentamicin, in a suitable semisolid vehicle; used as a topical antibacterial. **gentian violet c.** [USP], a preparation containing, in each 100 gm., 1.20 to 1.60 gm. of gentian violet, calculated as hexamethylpararosaniline chloride; applied intravaginally in the treatment of vulvovaginal candidiasis. **hydrocortisone c.** [USP], a mixture containing 90 to 110 per cent of the labeled amount of hydrocortisone in a suitable cream base; used topically as an anti-inflammatory in the treatment of steroid-responsive dermatosis. **hydroquinone c.** [USP], a cream containing 94 to 106 per cent of the labeled amount of the hydroquinone; used as a depigmenting agent. **iodochlorhydroxyquin c.** [USP], a mixture containing 90 to 100 per cent of the labeled amount of iodochlorhydroxyquin in a suitable cream base; used as a topical anti-infective in the treatment of a wide range of dermatoses, including all types of eczema. **iodochlorhydroxyquin and hydrocortisone c.** [NF], a preparation containing 90 to 110 per cent of the labeled amounts of iodochlorhydroxyquin and hydrocortisone; used topically for its local anti-infective effect and for the anti-inflammatory and antipruritic activity of glucocorticoids in a wide range of dermatoses. **leukocytic c.,** buffy coat. **lindane c.** [USP], a mixture containing 90 to 100 per cent of the labeled amount of lindane in a suitable cream base; used topically as a pediculicide and scabicide. Called also *gamma benzene hexachloride c.* **mafenide acetate c.** [USP], a preparation containing 90 to 110 per cent of mafenide acetate in terms of the labeled amount of mafenide; used as a topical anti-infective for adjunctive therapy in patients with second and third-degree burns. **methylprednisolone acetate c.** [USP], a mixture containing 90 to 110 per cent of the labeled amount of methylprednisolone acetate in a cream base; used as a topical glucocorticoid. **Moynihan's c.,** a mixture consisting of as much bismuth carbonate in 1:1000 aqueous solution of HgI_2 as will make a thick paste; used as a wound dressing. **neomycin sulfate and dexamethasone sodium phosphate c.,** a preparation containing neomycin sulfate equivalent to 90 to 135 per cent of the labeled amount of neomycin base, and dexamethasone sodium phosphate equivalent to 90 to 115 per cent of the labeled amount of dexamethasone sodium phosphate; used topically for its broad-spectrum antibacterial effects, and for the anti-inflammatory and antipruritic activity of glucocorticoids in a wide range of dermatoses. **nitrofurazone c.** [USP], a mixture containing 95 to 105 per cent of the labeled amount of nitrofurazone in a suitable, emulsified, water-miscible base, used topically as a local anti-infective against a wide variety of gram-negative and gram-positive bacteria in the treatment of many skin lesions, especially second and third degree burns, and to aid healing and prevent infection of skin grafts. **nystatin c.** [USP], a cream containing 90 to 130 per cent of the labeled amount of nystatin, the labeled amount being 100,000 nystatin units per gram of cream. **piperazine estrone sulfate vaginal c.** [USP], a mixture containing 90 to 120 percent of the labeled amount of piperazine estrone sulfate in a suitable cream base; used as an estrogen. **pramoxine hydrochloride c.** [USP], a mixture containing 90 to 110 per cent of the labeled amount of pramoxine hydrochloride in a suitable water-miscible base; used topically as a local anesthetic. **prednisolone c.** [USP], a mixture containing 90 to 110 per cent of the labeled amount of prednisolone in a suitable cream base; used as a topical glucocorticoid. **c. of tartar,** potassium bitartrate. **tetracaine hydrochloride c.** [USP], a mixture containing the equivalent of 1 per cent of tetracaine in a suitable water-miscible base; used as a local anesthetic, applied to the skin. **tolnaftate c.** [USP], a cream containing 90 to 110 per cent of the labeled amount of tolnaftate; used topically as an antifungal in the treatment of various forms of tinea of the skin. **tretinoin c.** [USP], a mixture containing 90 to 130 per cent of the labeled amount of tretinoin; used as a topical keratolytic agent. **triacetin c.,** a cream containing 90 to 110 per cent of the labeled amount of triacetin; used topically as a local antifungal. **triamcinolone acetonide c.** [USP], a mixture containing 90 to 115 per cent of the labeled amount of triamcinolone acetonide in a suitable cream base; used as a topical anti-inflammatory in steroid-responsive dermatoses. **triclobisonium chloride c.,** a cream containing 90 to 110 per cent of the labeled amount of triclobisonium chloride; used intravaginally as a local anti-infective, primarily in the treatment of gynecological infections due to susceptible organisms.

Creamalin (krem'ah-lin) trademark for preparations of aluminum hydroxide gel.

creamometer (kre-mom'ĕ-ter) [cream + Gr. metron measure] an instrument for the determination of the percentage of cream in milk.

crease (krēs) a line or slight linear depression (in anatomical terminology). **ear lobe c.,** a diagonal crease in the ear lobe associated with aging and perhaps a sign of coronary artery disease. **palmar c., flexion c.,** any of the normal grooves across the palm which accommodate flexion of the hand by separating folds of tissue. In certain congenital anomalies, there is only a single transverse (simian) crease. **simian c.,** a single transverse palmar crease formed by fusion of the proximal and distal palmar creases; frequently seen in congenital disorders such as Down's syndrome and rarely in normal persons; called also simian line.

creasote (kre'ah-sōt) creosote.

creatine (kre'ah-tin) [Gr. kreas flesh] N-methyl-guanidinoacetic acid. A crystallizable nitrogenous compound synthesized in the body, phosphorylated creatine (see phosphocreatine) being an important storage form of high-energy phosphate. **c. phosphate,** phosphocreatine.

creatine kinase (kre'ah-tin ki'nās) [EC 2.7.3.2] an enzyme of the transferase class that catalyzes the reaction ATP + creatine = ADP + phosphocreatine. The enzyme is activated by Mg^{2+}. The reaction effectively stores the energy of ATP as phosphocreatine in muscle and brain tissue and holds the muscle concentration of ATP nearly constant during the initiation of exercise. It occurs as three isoenzymes, each having two components composed of M (muscle) and of B (brain) subunits. CK_1 (BB) is found primarily in brain, CK_2 (MB) primarily in cardiac muscle, and CK_3 (MM) primarily in skeletal muscle. Differential determination of isoenzymes is useful for clinical diagnoses. Abbreviated CK.

creatinemia (kre"ah-tĭ-ne'me-ah) [creatin + Gr. haima blood + -ia] excess of creatine in the blood.

creatine phosphokinase (kre'ah-tin fos"fo-ki'nās) creatine kinase.

creatine phosphotransferase (kre'ah-tin fos"fo-trans'fer-ās) creatine kinase.

creatinine (kre-at'ĭ-nin) an anhydride of creatine, being

$$\underset{\underset{CO}{\rule{2.5cm}{0.4pt}}}{NH \cdot C(:NH) \cdot N(CH_3) \cdot CH_2}$$

the end product of creatine metabolism, found in muscle and blood and excreted in the urine.

creatinuria (kre-at'ĭ-nu're-ah) increased concentration of creatine in the urine.

creatorrhea (kre"ah-to-re'ah) [Gr. kreas flesh + rhoia flow] the presence of undigested muscle fibers in the feces.

creatotoxism (kre"ah-to-tok'sism) meat poisoning.

creatoxicon (kre"ah-tok'se-kon) kreotoxicon.

creatoxin (kre"ah-tok'sin) kreotoxin.

crèche (kresh) [Fr.] a day nursery for infants.

Credé's ointment (kra-dāz') [Benno C. Credé, German surgeon, 1847–1929] see under ointment.

Credé's method (maneuver) (kra-dāz') [Karl Sigmund Franz Credé, German gynecologist, 1819–1892] see under method.

CREG cross-reactive group (of HLA antigens).

cremaster (kre-mas'ter) [L.; Gr. kremasthai to suspend] musculus cremaster; see Table of Musculi. **internal c. of Henle,** fibers of the gubernaculum testis, inserted in elements of the fetal spermatic cord.

cremasteric (kre"mas-ter'ik) pertaining to the cremaster.

cremation (kre-ma'shun) [L. crematio a burning] the burning or incineration of dead bodies.

crematorium (kre"mah-to're-um) an establishment for the burning of dead bodies.

cremnocele (krem'no-sēl) vaginolabial hernia.

cremor (kre'mor) [L.] cream. **c. tar'tari** ["cream of tartar"], potassium bitartrate.

crena (kre'nah), pl. cre'nae [L.] [NA] a notch or cleft. **c. a'ni** [NA], the anal cleft; the cleft between the buttocks on which the anus opens. Called also clunial gluteal, or natal

cleft and c. clunium. **c. clu'nium,** c. ani. **c. cor'dis,** sulcus interventricularis anterior.

crenae (kre'ne) [L.] genitive and plural of crena.

crenate, crenated (kre'nāt, kre'nāt-ed) [L. crenatus] scalloped or notched.

crenation (kre-na'shun) the formation of abnormal notching in the edge of an erythrocyte; the notched appearance of an erythrocyte caused by its shrinkage after suspension in a hypertonic solution. Cf. echinosis.

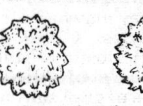

Crenated erythrocytes.

crenilabrin (kren-il-a'brin) a protamine obtained from the sperm of the cunner (fish).

crenocyte (kre'no-sīt) a crenated erythrocyte.

crenocytosis (kre"no-si-to'sis) the presence of crenated erythrocytes in the blood.

crenology (kre-nol'o-je) [Gr. krēnē spring + -logy] the science of therapeutic springs.

crenotherapy (kren"o-ther'ah-pe) [Gr. krēnē spring + therapeia treatment] treatment by water from mineral springs.

Crenothrix (kre'no-thriks) [Gr. krēnē spring + thrix hair] a genus of sheathed bacteria found in water, made up of cylindrical to disk-shaped cells in filaments attached to a substrate. Their sheaths are sometimes encrusted with iron or manganese oxides at the base. The type species is C. polyspo'ra.

Crenotrichaceae (kre"no-trī-ka'se-e) in former systems of classification, a family of bacteria made up of the genera Clonothrix, Crenothrix, and Phragmidiothrix.

crenulation (kren"u-la'shun) crenation.

creophagism, creophagy (kre-of'ah-jism; kre-of'ah-je) [Gr. kreas flesh + phagein to eat] the use of flesh as food.

creosol (kre'o-sol) [creosote + L. oleum oil] chemical name: 2-methoxy-4-methylphenol. A colorless oily liquid, the methyl ether of methyl catechol, $CH_3 \cdot O \cdot C_6H_3(OH)CH_3$, one of the active constituents of creosote.

creosote (kre'o-sōt) a mixture of phenols obtained by distilling wood tar, mainly beech Fagus sylvatica L. (Fagaceae). The liquid is colorless to yellowish, very refractive and oily, and has an empyreumatic odor. It is used externally as an antiseptic and internally in chronic bronchitis as an expectorant. **c. carbonate,** a clear, viscid liquid, a mixture of carbonates of various constituents of creosote, used as an expectorant and antiseptic.

creotoxin (kre"o-tok'sin) kreotoxin.

creotoxism (kre"o-tok'sizm) kreotoxism.

crepitant (krep'ĭ-tant) [L. crepitare to rattle] rattling or crackling.

crepitation (krep"ĭ-ta'shun) [L. crepitare to crackle] 1. a sound like that made by rubbing the hair between the fingers, or like that made by throwing fine salt into a fire. 2. the noise made by rubbing together the ends of a fractured bone.

crepitus (krep'ĭ-tus) [L.] 1. the discharge of flatus from the bowels. 2. crepitation. 3. a crepitant rale. **articular c.,** joint c. **bony c.,** the crackling sound produced by the rubbing together of fragments of fractured bone. **false c.,** joint c. **c. in'dux,** a crepitant rale, or crackling sound, heard in pneumonia at the beginning of the process of solidification of the lung. **joint c.,** the grating sensation caused by the rubbing together of the dry synovial surfaces of joints; called also articular c. **c. re'dux,** crepitus heard in the resolving stage of pneumonia. **silken c.,** a sensation as of two pieces of silk rubbed between the fingers, felt on moving a joint affected with hydrarthrosis.

crepuscular (kre-pus'ku-lar) [L. crepusculum twilight] referring to twilight, as a twilight state; also imperfectly luminous or glimmering.

crescent (kres'ent) [L. crescens] 1. shaped like a new moon. 2. a crescent-shaped structure. **articular c.,** a crescent-shaped articular fibrocartilage. **epithelial c.,** a more or less crescentic mass of epithelial cells between the glomerular tuft and the inside of Bowman's capsule in glomerulonephritis. **c's of Giannuzzi,** crescent-shaped patches of serous cells surrounding the mucous tubules in mixed (mucous and albuminous) glands, and formed by the outnumbered albuminous cells pushed to the blind ends of the terminal portions or into saccular outpocketings. Called also *demilunes of Heidenhain; Giannuzzi's bodies, cells,* or *demilunes; crescent, demilune,* or *marginal cells;* and *semilunar bodies.* **gray c.,** an area on some amphibian eggs from which pigment retreats; it is dorsal and opposite to the point of sperm entry, giving the first visible sign of the dorsoventral axis. **malarial c's,** the gametocytes of *Plasmodium falciparum;* they may be male (microgametocytes) or female (macrogametocytes). Called also *flagellated bodies.* **myopic c.,** a crescentic posterior staphyloma in the fundus of the eye in myopia. **c's of spinal cord** (*obs.*), either of the two lateral bands of gray substance in the spinal cord, each made up of the anterior and posterior horn of the respective side. **sublingual c.,** the crescent-shaped area on the floor of the mouth, formed by the lingual wall of the mandible and the adjacent part of the floor of the mouth.

crescentic (krĕ-sen′tik) resembling a crescent.

cresol (kre′sol) a mixture of isomeric cresols, $CH_3C_6H_4OH$, obtained from coal tar and containing not more than 5 per cent of phenol; it is a poisonous, colorless, or yellowish to brownish yellow, or pinkish liquid, and is a more powerful disinfectant and antiseptic than phenol; used chiefly to sterilize instruments, dishes, utensils, and other inaminate objects. Called also *cresylic acid* and *tricresol.*

cresolphthalein (kre″sol-thal′e-in) an acid-base indicator that is colorless at pH 7.2 and red at 8.8.

cresorcin (kre-sor′sin) chemical name: 2,4-dihydroxytoluene. A crystalline derivative from cresol, $C_7H_8O_2$.

cresorcinol (kre-sor′sin-ol) cresorcin.

cresoxydiol (kres-ok″se-di′ol) mephenesin.

cresoxypropanediol (kres-ok″se-pro-pān′de-ol) mephenesin.

crest (krest) [L. *crista*] a projection or projecting structure, or ridge, especially one surmounting a bone or its border; see also *crista* and *ridge.* **acoustic c.,** crista ampullaris. **acusticofacial c.,** the embryonic cell mass from which develop the ganglia of the seventh and eighth cranial nerves. **ampullar c., ampullary c.,** crista ampullaris. **anterior c. of fibula,** margo anterior fibulae. **anterior c. of tibia,** margo anterior tibiae. **arcuate c. of arytenoid cartilage,** crista arcuata cartilaginis arytenoideae. **basilar c.,** crista basilaris ductus cochlearis. **basilar c. of occipital bone,** tuberculum pharyngeum. **buccinator c.,** crista buccinatoria. **cerebral c's of cranial bone,** juga cerebralia ossium cranii; see under *jugum.* **c. of cochlear window,** crista fenestrae cochleae. **conchal c. of maxilla,** crista conchalis maxillae. **conchal c. of palatine bone,** crista conchalis ossis palatini. **deltoid c.,** tuberositas deltoidea humeri. **dental c.,** the maxillary ridge passing along the alveolar processes of the fetal maxillary bones. **ethmoid c. of maxilla,** crista ethmoidalis maxillae. **ethmoid c. of palatine bone,** crista ethmoidalis ossis palatini. **femoral c.,** linea aspera femoris. **fimbriated c.,** plica fimbriata. **frontal c.,** crista frontalis. **frontal c., external,** linea temporalis ossis frontalis. **frontal c., internal,** crista frontalis. **gingival c.,** the coronal border of the gingiva. **glandular c. of larynx,** ligamentum vestibulare. **gluteal c.,** tuberositas glutea femoris. **c. of greater tubercle of humerus,** crista tuberculi majoris. **c. of hypotrochanteric fossa,** tuberositas glutea femoris. **iliac c.,** crista iliaca. **iliopectineal c. of iliac bone,** linea arcuata ossis ilii. **iliopectineal c. of pelvis,** linea terminalis pelvis. **iliopectineal c. of pubis,** eminentia iliopubica. **c. of ilium,** crista iliaca. **infratemporal c.,** crista infratemporalis. **infundibuloventricular c.,** crista supraventricularis. **inguinal c.,** a prominence on the inguinal body wall in the embryo, participating in the formation of the gubernaculum testis. **interosseous c. of fibula,** margo interosseus fibulae. **interosseous c. of radius,** margo interosseus radii. **interosseous c. of tibia,** margo interosseus tibiae. **interosseous c. of ulna,** margo interosseus ulnae. **intertrochanteric c.,** crista intertrochanterica. **intertrochanteric c., anterior,** linea intertrochanterica. **jugular c. of great wing of sphenoid bone,** margo zygomaticus alae majoris. **lacrimal c., anterior,** crista lacrimalis anterior. **lacrimal c., posterior,** crista lacrimalis posterior. **c.**

of larger tubercle, crista tuberculi majoris. **lateral c. of fibula,** margo posterior fibulae. **c. of lesser tubercle,** crista tuberculi minoris. **c. of little head of rib,** crista capitis costae. **malar c. of great wing of sphenoid bone,** margo zygomaticus alae majoris. **c. of matrix of nail,** cristae matricis unguis. **medial c. of fibula,** crista medialis fibulae. **mental c., external,** protuberantia mentalis. **mitochondrial c's,** complex infoldings in the mitochondrial cavity which originate in a membrane outside the cavity. **nasal c. of maxilla,** crista nasalis maxillae. **nasal c. of palatine bone,** crista nasalis ossis palatini. **c. of neck of rib,** crista colli costae. **neural c.,** a cellular band dorsolateral to the neural tube that gives origin to the cranial and spinal ganglia and many other structures. **obturator c. (anterior),** crista obturatoria. **occipital c., external,** crista occipitalis externa. **occipital c., internal,** eminentia cruciformis. **orbital c.,** margo supraorbitalis ossis frontalis. **palatine c., c. of palatine bone,** crista palatina. **pectineal c. of femur,** linea pectinea femoris. **pharyngeal c. of occipital bone,** tuberculum pharyngeum. **pubic c., c. of pubis,** crista pubica. **radial c.,** margo interosseus radii. **rough c. of femur,** linea aspera femoris. **sacral c.,** crista sacralis mediana. **sacral c., articular,** crista sacralis intermedia. **sacral c., external,** crista sacralis lateralis. **sacral c., intermediate,** crista sacralis intermedia. **sacral c., lateral,** crista sacralis lateralis. **sacral c., medial,** crista sacralis mediana. **seminal c.,** colliculus seminalis. **c. of smaller tubercle,** crista tuberculi minoris. **sphenoidal c.,** crista sphenoidalis. **spinal c. of Rauber,** processus spinosus vertebrarum. **c. of spinous processes of sacrum,** crista sacralis mediana. **spiral c.,** labium limbi vestibulare laminae spiralis. **spiral c. of cochlea,** crista spiralis cochleae. **supinator c., c. of supinator muscle,** crista musculi supinatoris. **supracondylar c. of humerus, lateral,** crista supracondylaris lateralis humeri. **supracondylar c. of humerus, medial,** crista supracondylaris medialis humeri. **supramastoid c.,** crista supramastoidea. **supraventricular c.,** crista supraventricularis. **temporal c. of frontal bone,** linea temporalis ossis frontalis. **terminal c. of right atrium,** crista terminalis atrii dextri. **tibial c.,** margo anterior tibiae. **transverse c. of internal auditory meatus,** crista transversa. **trigeminal c.,** the embryonic cell mass from which the trigeminal ganglion develops. **turbinal c. of maxilla, inferior,** crista conchalis maxillae. **turbinal c. of maxilla, superior,** crista ethmoidalis maxillae. **turbinal c. of palatine bone, inferior,** crista conchalis ossis palatini. **turbinal c. of palatine bone, superior,** crista ethmoidalis ossis palatini. **ulnar c.,** margo interosseus ulnae. **urethral c., female,** crista urethralis femininae. **urethral c., male,** crista urethralis masculinae. **c. of vestibule,** crista vestibuli. **zygomatic c. of great wing of sphenoid bone,** margo zygomaticus alae majoris.

crestomycin sulfate (kres-to-mi′sin) paromomycin sulfate.

cresylic acid (krĕ-sil′ik) cresol.

cretin (kre′tin; kret′in) [Fr.] a person affected with cretinism.

cretinism (kre′tin-izm) a chronic condition due to congenital lack of thyroid secretion, marked by arrested physical and mental development, dystrophy of the bones and soft parts, and lowered basal metabolism. It is the congenital form of this deficiency, while myxedema is the acquired form. Called also *cretinoid idiocy* and *myxedematous infantilism.* **athyreotic c.,** cretinism due to thyroid aplasia or destruction of the thyroid of the fetus *in utero;* called also *sporadic nongoitrous c.* **goitrous c.,** cretinism coexisting with severe hypothyroidism, and characterized by goiter. **spontaneous c., sporadic c.,** cretinism in a person not descended from cretins, and who has not lived in a region where goiter is endemic. **sporadic goitrous c.,** a genetically determined condition in which enlargement of the thyroid gland is associated with deficient biosynthesis of and a consequently reduced supply of circulating thyroid hormone. **sporadic nongoitrous c.,** athyreotic c.

cretinistic (kre″tin-is′tik) pertaining to cretinism.

cretinoid (kre′tin-oid) resembling a cretin; resembling cretinism.

cretinous (kre′tin-us) affected with cretinism.

Creutzfeldt-Jakob disease (syndrome) (kroits′felt-yak′ob) [Hans Gerhard *Creutzfeldt*, German psychiatrist, 1885–1964; Alfons Maria *Jakob*, German psychiatrist, 1884–1931] see under *disease*.

crevice (krev′is) [Fr. *crever* to split] a longitudinal fissure. **gingival c.,** a shallow trough or fissure surrounding the anatomic crown of a tooth; considered by some authorities to be the same as the *gingival sulcus* and by others to be two separate and distinct entities. Called also *subgingival space*.

crevicular (kre-vik′u-lar) pertaining to a crevice, especially the gingival crevice.

CRF corticotropin releasing factor.

crib (krib) 1. any racklike structure. 2. a removable anchorage from an orthodontic appliance. 3. a habit-breaking orthodontic appliance. **clinical c.,** a crib in which an infant is placed for observation. **Jackson c.,** see under *appliance*.

cribbing (krib′ing) a bad habit of some horses in which the animal grasps the manger or other object with the incisor teeth, arches the neck, makes peculiar movements with the head, and swallows quantities of air; called also *windsucking*.

cribra (krib′rah) [L.] plural of *cribrum*.

cribral (krib′ral) pertaining to the cribrum, or sieve-like structure.

cribrate (krib′rāt) [L. *cribratus*] perforated, as a sieve.

cribration (krib-ra′shun) 1. the quality of being cribrate. 2. the process or act of sifting or passing through a sieve, as a drug.

cribriform (krib′rĭ-form) [*cribrum* + L. *forma* form] perforated with small apertures like a sieve.

cribrum (kri′brum), pl. *cri′bra* [L. "sieve"] lamina cribrosa ossis ethmoidalis. **cri′bra orbita′lia of Welcker,** small apertures in the lamina cribrosa ossis ethmoidalis, which give the bone a porous appearance and are thought to transmit veins from the diploë to the orbit.

Cricetus (kri-se′tus) a genus of rodents; see *hamster*.

Crichton-Browne's sign (kri′ton-brownz) [Sir James *Crichton-Browne*, English physician, 1840–1938] see under *sign*.

Crick (krik) Francis Harry Compton. British biologist, born 1916; co-winner, with Maurice Wilkins and James Dewey Watson, of the Nobel prize in medicine and physiology for 1962, for discoveries concerning the molecular structure of nucleic acids and its significance for information transfer in living material.

cricoarytenoid (kri″ko-ar″ĭ-te′noid) pertaining to or extending between the cricoid and arytenoid cartilages.

cricoid (kri′koid) [Gr. *krikos* ring + *eidos* form] 1. resembling a ring; ring shaped. 2. the cricoid cartilage (cartilago cricoidea [NA]).

cricoidectomy (kri″koi-dek′to-me) excision of the cricoid cartilage.

cricoidynia (kri″koi-din′e-ah) [Gr. *krikos* ring + *odynē* pain] pain in the cricoid cartilage.

cricopharyngeal (kri″ko-fah-rin′je-al) pertaining to the cricoid cartilage and the pharynx.

cricothyreotomy (kri″ko-thi″re-ot′o-me) [Gr. *krikos* ring + *thyreos* shield + *tomē* a cutting] incision through the cricoid and thyroid cartilages.

cricothyroid (kri-ko-thi′roid) pertaining to or connecting the cricoid and thyroid cartilages.

cricothyroidotomy (kri″ko-thi″roi-dot′o-me) cricothyrotomy.

cricothyrotomy (kri″ko-thi-rot′o-me) incision through the skin and cricothyroid membrane to secure a patent airway for emergency relief of upper airway obstruction.

cricotomy (kri-kot′o-me) [Gr. *krikos* ring + *tomē* a cutting] incision of the cricoid cartilage.

cricotracheotomy (kri″ko-tra″ke-ot′o-me) incision of the cricoid cartilage and trachea.

cri du chat (kre-du-shah) [Fr. "cat's cry"] see under *syndrome*.

Crile-Matas operation (krīl-mat′as) [George Washington *Crile*, Cleveland surgeon, 1864–1943; Rudolph *Matas*, New Orleans surgeon, 1860–1957] see under *operation*.

criminology (krim″ĭ-nol′o-je) [L. *crimen* crime + *-logy*] the scientific study of crime and criminals.

crines (kri′nēz) [L.] plural of *crinis*.

crinin (krin′in) [Gr. *krinein* to separate] a substance that stimulates glandular secretion.

crinis (kri′nis), pl. *cri′nes* [L.] hair.

crinology (kri-nol′o-je) the scientific study of secretion and secretions.

crinophagy (krin-of′ah-je) [Gr. *krinein* to separate + *phagein* to eat] the intracytoplasmic digestion of the contents (peptides, proteins) of secretory vacuoles, after the vacuoles fuse with lysosomes.

Crinum (kri′num) a genus of amaryllidaceous plants; the root of *C. asiaticum*, of India, has properties like those of squill.

crisis (kri′sis), pl. *cri′ses* [L.; Gr. *krisis*] 1. the turning point of a disease for good or evil; especially, a sudden change, usually for the better, in the course of an acute disease. A disease terminates by crisis when recovery is indicated by a sudden and definite decrease in the intensity of the symptoms. Cf. *lysis* (def. 4). 2. a sudden paroxysmal intensification of symptoms in the course of a disease. **addisonian c., adrenal c.,** the symptoms accompanying an acute onset or worsening of Addison's disease, viz., anorexia, vomiting, abdominal pain, apathy, confusion, extreme weakness, renal loss of sodium and water, and hypotension progressing to shock and, if untreated, death. **anaphylactoid c.,** pseudoanaphylaxis. **aplastic c.,** a transient condition, marked by sudden disappearance of erythroblasts from the bone marrow, developing under various circumstances, including certain hemolytic states and infections. **blast c.,** a sudden, severe change in the course of chronic myelocytic leukemia in which the clinical picture resembles that in acute myelocytic leukemia, with an increase in the proportion of myeloblasts. Recent evidence suggests that in some cases the blast cells may be lymphoblasts. **bronchial c.,** a paroxysm of dyspnea in the course of a case of tabes dorsalis. **cardiac c.,** a severe paroxysm of palpitation of the heart occurring in tabes dorsalis. **catathymic c.,** an isolated, nonrepetitive act of violence that develops as a result of intolerable tension. **celiac c.,** an attack of severe watery diarrhea and vomiting producing dehydration and acidosis, which sometimes occurs in the infantile form of nontropical sprue. **cholinergic c.,** muscular weakness resulting from depolarization block due to overdosage of anticholinesterase agents used for myasthenia gravis; similar to but different from myasthenic crisis. **clitoris c.,** an attack of sexual excitement occurring in women with tabes dorsalis. **deglobulinization c.,** a condition observed in congenital spherocytic anemia, characterized clinically by the acute onset of fever, abdominal pain, and vomiting, associated with reticulocytopenia, leukopenia, thrombocytopenia, and erythroblastopenia. **Dietl's c.,** sudden severe attack of nephralgia or gastric pain, chills, fever, nausea and vomiting, and general collapse; said to be due to partial turning of the kidney upon its pedicle. **false c.,** pseudocrisis. **febrile c.,** an attack of chilliness, fever, and sweating. **gastric c.,** a paroxysm of intense abdominal pain in tabes dorsalis. **genital c. of newborn,** a condition characterized by hyperplasia of the breasts, estrinization of the vaginal mucosa, and sometimes vaginal bleeding, under the influence of transplacentally acquired estrogens. **glaucomatocyclitic c.,** a relatively uncommon, recurrent, unilateral form of secondary open angle glaucoma, lasting one to two weeks, and rarely producing permanent damage to the optic disk or to the outflow facility. It is characterized by high intraocular pressure and marked depression of outflow facility, with minimal inflammatory signs and symptoms. **hepatic c.,** an attack of intense pain in the region of the liver. **identity c.,** a period in the psychosocial development of an individual, usually occurring during adolescence, usually manifested by a loss of the sense of the sameness and historical continuity of one's self, or an inability to accept the role the individual perceives as being expected of him by society. **intestinal c.,** gastric c. **laryngeal c.,** paroxysmal spasm of the larynx in the earlier course of tabes dorsalis. **myasthenic c.,** the sudden development of dyspnea requiring respiratory support in myasthenia gravis; the crisis is usually transient, lasting several days, and accompanied by fever. **nefast c.,** the peculiar onset of severe and unaccountable symptoms in experimental icterogenous spirochetosis. **nephralgic c.,** a paroxysm of pain in the ureter in a case of tabes dorsalis. **nitritoid c.,** a group of symptoms sometimes following the injection of arsphenamine, consisting of redness of the face, dyspnea, a feeling of distress, cough, and precordial pain. The condition is named from its resemblance to the symptoms of amyl nitrite poisoning. **ocular c.,** a sudden attack of intense pain in the eyes, with lacrimation, photophobia, etc. **oculogyric c.,** a crisis occurring in epidemic encephalitis or postencephalitic parkinsonism in which the eyeballs become fixed in one position for minutes or hours. **parkinsonian c.,** a condition sometimes observed in parkinsonism, superficially resembling akinetic mutism or coma vigil, the patient lying stiff and motionless, and making no spontaneous communication. **Pel's c's,** ocular crises in tabes dorsalis. **pharyngeal c.,** a sudden attack occurring in tabes dorsalis, marked by peculiar sensations in the pharynx and involuntary swallowing movements. **rectal c.,** a severe seizure of rectal pain in tabes dorsalis. **renal c.,** an attack of pain resembling renal colic, occurring in tabes. **salt-depletion c.,** salt-losing syndrome. **salt-losing c.,** see under *syndrome.* **tabetic c.,** a painful paroxysm with functional disturbance occurring in the course of tabes dorsalis. **thoracic c.,** an attack of pain resembling angina pectoris, but with spasmodic contracture of the muscles of the chest and arms in tabes dorsalis. **thyroid c., thyrotoxic c.,** a sudden and dangerous increase of the symptoms of thyrotoxicosis. Called also *thyroid* or *thyrotoxic storm.* **vesical c.,** a severe seizure of pain in the bladder in cases of tabes dorsalis. **visceral c.,** a paroxysm of shooting pain in any viscus occurring in a case of tabes dorsalis.

crispation (kris-pa'shun) [L. *crispare* to curl] slight convulsive or spasmodic muscular contractions producing a creeping sensation.

crista (kris'tă), pl. *cris'tae* [L.] [NA] a projection or projecting structure, or ridge, especially one surmounting a bone or its border; called also *crest* and *ridge.* **c. acus'tica,** c. ampullaris. **c. ampulla'ris** [NA], ampullar crest: the most prominent part of a localized thickening of the membrane that lines the ampullae of the semicircular ducts, covered with neuroepithelium containing endings of the vestibular nerve; called also *c. acoustica* or *acoustic crest.* **c. ante'rior fib'ulae,** margo anterior fibulae. **c. ante'rior tib'iae,** margo anterior tibiae. **c. arcua'ta cartilag'inis arytenoi'deae** [NA], arcuate crest of arytenoid cartilage: a ridge on the external surface of the arytenoid cartilage between the triangular pit and the oblong pit. **c. basila'ris duc'tus cochlea'ris** [NA], basilar crest: the triangular eminence on the spiral ligament to which the basilar membrane is attached. **c. buccinato'ria,** buccinator crest: a ridge running from the base of the coronoid process of the mandible to a point near the last molar tooth, giving attachment to the buccinator muscle. **c. cap'itis cos'tae** [NA], **c. capit'uli cos'tae,** crest of head of rib: a horizontal crest dividing the articular surface of the head of the rib into two facets, for articulation with the depression on the bodies of two adjacent vertebrae; called also *crest of little head of rib, cuneiform eminence of head of rib,* and *interarticular ridge of head of rib.* **c. col'li cos'tae** [NA], crest of neck of rib: a crest on the superior border of the neck of a rib, giving attachment to the anterior costotransverse ligament; called also *ridge of neck of rib.* **c. concha'lis maxil'lae** [NA], conchal crest of maxilla: an oblique ridge on the nasal surface of the body of the maxilla, just anterior to the lacrimal sulcus, which articulates with the inferior nasal concha; called also *inferior turbinal crest of maxilla.* **c. concha'lis os'sis palati'ni** [NA], conchal crest of palatine bone: a sharp transverse ridge, near the posterior edge of the palatine bone, which articulates with the inferior concha; called also *inferior turbinal crest of palatine bone.* **cris'tae cu'tis** [NA], ridges of the skin produced by the projecting papillae of the corium on the palm or sole, producing a finger- or foot-print that is characteristic of the individual; called also *dermal ridges.* **c. div'idens,** limbus foraminis ovalis. **c. ethmoida'lis maxil'lae** [NA], ethmoidal crest of maxilla: a low, oblique ridge on the medial surface of the frontal process of the maxilla, which articulates with the middle nasal concha; called also *superior turbinal crest of maxilla.* **c. ethmoida'lis os'sis palati'ni** [NA], ethmoidal crest of palatine bone: a ridge near the upper end of the medial surface of the palatine bone, which articulates with the middle concha; called also *superior*

turbinal crest of palatine bone. **c. falcifor'mis,** c. transversa. **c. fem'oris,** linea aspera femoris. **c. fenes'trae coch'leae** [NA], crest of cochlear window: the ledge of bone that overhangs the cochlear window of the middle ear. **c. fronta'lis** [NA], the frontal crest: a median ridge on the internal surface of the frontal bone, extending upward from the foramen cecum to unite with the sulcus for the superior sagittal sinus; called also *internal frontal crest.* **c. gal'li** [NA], a thick triangular process projecting upward from the cribriform plate of the ethmoid bone; the falx cerebri attaches to it. **c. hel'icis,** crus helicis. **c. ili'aca** [NA], **c. il'ii,** the iliac crest: the thickened, expanded upper border of the ilium; called also *crest of ilium.* **c. infratempora'lis** [NA], infratemporal crest: a crest separating the temporal surface of the great wing of the sphenoid bone into a temporal portion above and an infratemporal portion below. **c. interos'sea fib'ulae,** margo interosseus fibulae. **c. interos'sea ra'dii,** margo interosseus radii. **c. interos'sea tib'iae,** margo interosseus tibiae. **c. interos'sea ul'nae,** margo interosseus ulnae. **c. intertrochanter'ica** [NA], intertrochanteric crest: a prominent ridge running obliquely downward and medialward from the summit of the greater trochanter on the posterior surface of the neck of the femur to the lesser trochanter; called also *intertrochanteric ridge, linea intertrochanterica posterior,* and *posterior intertrochanteric line.* **c. lacrima'lis ante'rior** [NA], anterior lacrimal crest: the lateral margin of the groove on the posterior border of the frontal process of the maxilla. **c. lacrima'lis poste'rior** [NA], posterior lacrimal crest: a vertical ridge dividing the lateral or orbital surface of the lacrimal bone into two parts, and forming one margin of the fossa for the lacrimal sac. **c. latera'lis fib'ulae,** margo posterior fibulae. **c. margina'lis** [NA], marginal ridge: one of the elevated convex crests that form the mesial and distal borders of the occlusal surfaces of posterior teeth and of the lingual surfaces of anterior teeth. **c. ma'tricis un'guis** [NA], crest of matrix of nail: a vascular longitudinal ridge in the nail matrix. **c. media'lis fib'ulae** [NA], medial crest of fibula: the long crest on the posterior surface of the body of the fibula, which separates the origin of the tibialis posterior muscle from that of the flexor hallucis longus muscle; called also *oblique line of fibula* and *posterointernal border of fibula.* **mitochondrial cristae, cris'tae mitochondria'les,** numerous narrow, transverse infoldings of the inner membrane of a mitochondrion. **c. mus'culi supinato'ris** [NA], crest of supinator muscle: a strong ridge forming the posterior margin of the supinator fossa below the radial notch of the ulna, and with it giving attachment to the supinator muscle; called also *supinator crest* or *ridge.* **c. nasa'lis maxil'lae** [NA], nasal crest of maxilla: a ridge, raised along the medial border of the palatine process of the maxilla, with which the vomer articulates. **c. nasa'lis os'sis palati'ni** [NA], nasal crest of palatine bone: a thick ridge projecting upward from the medial part of the horizontal plate of the palatine bone and articulating with the posterior part of the vomer. **c. obturato'ria** [NA], obturator crest: the inferior border of the superior ramus of the os pubis, a strong ridge of bone beginning near the pubic tubercle and extending to the anterior part of the gap in the rim of the acetabulum, forming part of the circumference of the obturator foramen, and giving attachment to the obturator membrane. **c. occipita'lis exter'na** [NA], external occipital crest: a variable crest of bone that sometimes extends from the external occipital protuberance toward the foramen magnum; called also *median* or *middle nuchal line.* **c. occipita'lis inter'na** [NA], internal occipital crest: a median ridge on the internal surface of the occipital bone extending from the midpoint of the cruciform eminence toward the foramen magnum. **c. palati'na** [NA], palatine crest: a transverse crest often seen on the inferior surface of the horizontal plate of the palatine bone a short distance anterior to the posterior border. **c. pu'bica** [NA], pubic crest: the thick, rough, anterior border of the body of the pubic bone. **cris'tae sacra'les articula'res,** see *crista sacralis intermedia.* **c. sacra'lis interme'dia** [NA], intermediate sacral crest: either of two indefinite crests just medial to the dorsal sacral foramina, formed by fusion of the articular processes of the sacral vertebrae; called also *articular sacral crest.* **c. sacra'lis latera'lis** [NA], lateral sacral crest: either of two series of tubercles lateral to the dorsal sacral foramina, representing the transverse processes of the sacral vertebrae; called also *external sacral crest.* **c. sacra′lis me′dia, c. sacra′lis media′na** [NA], medial sacral crest: a median ridge on the dorsal surface of the sacrum, formed by the remnants of the spinous processes of the upper four sacral vertebrae; called also *sacral crest, crest of spinous processes of sacrum,* and *tubercular ridge of sacrum.* **c. sphenoida′lis** [NA], sphenoidal crest: a median ridge on the anterior surface of the body of the sphenoid bone, articulating with the perpendicular plate of the ethmoid. **c. spira′lis,** labium limbi vestibulare laminae spirales. **c. spira′lis coch′leae** [NA], spiral crest of cochlea: the thickened outer or centrifugal portion of the periosteum of the cochlear duct, forming a spiral band to which the basal membrane is attached. Called also *ligamentum spirale cochleae* [NA alternative] and *spiral ligament of cochlea.* **c. supracondyla′ris latera′lis hu′meri** [NA], lateral supracondylar crest of humerus: a prominent curved ridge on the lateral surface of the humerus, giving attachment in front to the brachioradialis and extensor carpi radialis longus muscles; called also *lateral supracondylar ridge of humerus.* **c. supracondyla′ris media′lis hu′meri** [NA], medial supracondylar crest of humerus: a prominent, curved ridge on the medial surface of the humerus, giving attachment to the brachialis muscle in front and to the medial head of the triceps behind; called also *medial supracondylar ridge of humerus.* **c. supramastoi′dea** [NA], supramastoid crest: the superior border of the posterior root of the zygomatic process of the temporal bone. **c. supraventricula′ris** [NA], supraventricular crest: a ridge on the inner surface of the right ventricle of the heart, marking off the conus arteriosus; called also *infundibuloventricular crest.* **c. tempora′lis,** linea temporalis ossis frontalis. **c. termina′lis a′trii dex′tri** [NA], terminal crest of right atrium: a ridge on the internal surface of the right atrium of the heart, located to the right of the orifices of the superior and inferior venae cavae. The pectinate muscles of the right atrium are attached at this crest. It corresponds to a groove on the external surface, the sulcus terminalis. Called also *taenia terminalis.* **c. transver′sa** [NA], transverse crest: a ridge of bone that divides the fundus of the internal acoustic meatus into a superior and an inferior fossa; called also *c. falciformis* and *transverse crest of internal acoustic meatus.* **c. transversa′lis** [NA], transverse ridge: an elevated crest coursing transversely across the occlusal surface of a mandibular premolar to link the apices of the buccal and lingual cusps. It comprises the buccal and lingual cusps and may be an uninterrupted prominence or may be sharply divided at its approximate midpoint by a groove. **c. triangula′ris** [NA], triangular ridge: a ridge that descends from the tips of the cusps of molars and premolars toward the central part of the occlusal surface; so named because the slopes of each side of the ridge resemble two sides of a triangle. See also *oblique ridge* (def. 2), under *ridge,* and *c. transversa′lis.* **c. tuber′culi majo′ris** [NA], crest of greater tubercle (of the humerus): a projection on the greater tubercle of the humerus, forming one lip of the intertubercular groove; called also *crest of larger tubercle, pectoral ridge,* and *external, outer,* or *posterior bicipital ridge.* **c. tuber′culi mino′ris** [NA], crest of lesser tubercle (of the humerus): a projection on the lesser tubercle of the humerus, forming one lip of the intertubercular groove; called also *crest of smaller tubercle,* and *anterior* or *internal bicipital ridge.* **c. tympan′ica,** a ridge on the tympanic ring. **c. ul′nae,** margo interosseus ulnae. **c. urethra′lis femini′nae** [NA], female urethral crest: a prominent longitudinal fold of the mucosa along the posterior wall of the female urethra; called also *c. urethralis muliebris* and *cervical crest of female urethra* (*of Barkow*). **c. urethra′lis masculi′nae** [NA], male urethral crest: a median elevation along the posterior wall of the urethra in the male, lying between the prostatic sinuses; called also *c. urethralis virilis.* **c. urethra′lis mulie′bris,** crista urethralis femininae. **c. urethra′lis vir′ilis,** c. urethralis masculinae. **c. vestib′uli** [NA], crest of vestibule: a ridge between the spherical and elliptical recesses of the vestibule, dividing posteriorly to bound the cochlear recess.

cristae (kris′te) [L.] genitive and plural of *crista.*

cristal (kris′tal) pertaining to a crest or ridge.

Cristispira (kris″tĭ-spi′rah) [L. *crista* crest + Gr. *speira* coil] a genus of bacteria of the family Spirochaetaceae, order Spirochaetales, made up of coarse, flexuous, spiral cells with cross striations and a thin membrane on one side, extending

the whole length of the body; found in the intestinal tracts of mollusks. The type species is *C. pec′tinus.*

Critchett's operation (krich′ets) [George *Critchett,* ophthalmic surgeon, in London, 1817–1882] see under *operation.*

criterion (kri-te′re-on) [Gr. *kritērion* a means for judging] a standard by which something may be judged.

crith (krith) [Gr. *krithē* barleycorn, the smallest weight] the unit of weight for gases, being the weight of a liter of hydrogen gas at 0° C. and pressure equivalent to that of a column of mercury 760 mm. high.

Crithidia (krĭ-thid′e-ah) [Gr. *krithē* barleycorn] a genus of parasitic protozoa (suborder Trypanosomatina, order Kinetoplastida) found in the digestive tract of arthropods and other invertebrates. The adult form is similar to the leptomonads, but the flagellum arises form the kinetoplast just in front of the nucleus, and is attached to the body by an undulating membrane. During their life cycle the organisms pass through choanomastigote (promastigote) and amastigote stages.

crithidia (krĭ-thid′e-ah) 1. any protozoan of the genus *Crithidia.* 2. see *epimastigote.*

crithidial (krĭ-thid′e-al) 1. pertaining to the genus *Crithidia.* 2. denoting a morphologic stage in the life cycle of certain trypanosomid protozoa of the genus *Crithidia;* see *epimastigote.*

critical (krit′ĭ-kl) pertaining to or of the nature of a crisis; in danger of death; in sufficient quantity as to constitute a turning point, as a critical mass or critical concentration.

CRM cross-reacting material; see under *material.*

C.R.N.A. Certified Registered Nurse Anesthetist.

crocein (kro′se-in) any one of a series of bright red stains.

crocidismus (kro″se-diz′mus) [Gr. *krokē* a tuft of wool] carphology.

Crocq's disease (kroks) [Jean B. *Crocq,* Belgian physician, 1868–1925] acrocyanosis.

crofilcon A (kro-fil′kon) a contact lens material (hydrophobic).

Crohn's disease (krōnz) [Burrill Bernard *Crohn,* New York physician, 1884–1983] see under *disease.*

cromoglycate (kro″mo-gli′kāt) a salt of cromoglycic acid; the disodium salt, cromolyn sodium, is used in the treatment of bronchial asthma.

cromoglycic acid (kro″mo-gli′sik) [BAN] cromolyn.

cromolyn (kro′mŏ-lin)) an inhibitor of the release of histamine and other mediators of immediate hypersensitivity from mast cells; used as *cromolyn sodium* [USP] by inhalation for prophylaxis of bronchial asthma. Called also *cromoglycic acid* [BAN]. **c. sodium** [USP], chemical name: 5,5′-[(2-hydroxy- 1, 3- propanediyl) bisoxy)] bis[4- oxo-4H -1 -benzopyran-2-carboxylic acid]disodium salt. The disodium salt of cromoglycic acid, $C_{23}H_{14}Na_2O_{11}$, which interferes with allergic histamine release; administered by inhalation in the prophylactic treatment of bronchial asthmas and rhinitis associated with allergy, and as an ophthalmic solution for prevention and treatment of allergic conjunctivitis.

Cronin method (kro′nin) [Thomas Dillon *Cronin,* American plastic surgeon, born 1906] see under *method.*

Cronkhite-Canada syndrome (krong′kīt-kan′ah-dah) [Leonard W. *Cronkhite,* Jr., American internist, born 1919; Wilma Jeanne *Canada,* American radiologist] see under *syndrome.*

Crooke's changes [Arthur Carleton *Crooke,* British pathologist, born 1905] see *Crooke's hyaline degeneration,* under *degeneration.*

Crookes's space, tube [Sir William *Crookes,* English physicist, 1832–1919] see under *space* and *tube.*

crop (krop) an area specialized for temporary storage of food. In birds, the crop occurs as a dilatation of the esophagus at the base of the neck where food is softened by the uptake of water before digestion begins and then is passed through the proventriculus and into the gizzard. A similar organ is seen in certain invertebrates, such as insects and earthworms.

cropropamide (kro-pro′pah-mīd) chemical name: N-[1-(dimethylcarbamoyl)propyl]-N-propylcrotonamide; an analgesic, $C_{13}H_{24}N_2O_2$. See also *prethcamide.*

cross (kros) 1. any figure or structure in the shape of a cross. 2. any organism produced by crossbreeding; a method of crossbreeding. **phage c.,** a phage (bacteriophage) having genes from two or more parental phages as a result of infection by the parent phages of a single bacterial cell; it is a result of recombination. Also, the process of an instance of the formation of a phage cross. **Ranvier's c's,** dark, cross-shaped markings at the nodes of Ranvier, seen on longitudinal section after staining with silver nitrate. **silver c.,** a crosslike marking seen at the nodes of certain bundles of medullated nerve fibers. **two-factor c.,** recombination involving two genetic markers. **yellow c.,** 2,2'-dichlorodiethyl sulfide.

crossbite (kros′bīt) malocclusion in which the mandibular teeth are in buccal version (or in complete lingual version in posterior segments) to the maxillary teeth, bilaterally, unilaterally, or involving only a pair of opposing teeth, so that opposing occlusal surfaces are not in contact in habitual occlusion. Also written *cross bite* and *X-bite*. **anterior c.,** that in which one or more primary or permanent maxillary incisors are lingual to the mandibular incisors. **buccal c.,** that in which the maxillary molar is buccal to its mandibular antagonist. **lingual c.,** crossbite in which the maxillary or mandibular molar is lingual to its antagonist. **posterior c.,** that in which one or more primary or permanent posterior teeth are locked in an abnormal relation with the opposing teeth of the opposite arch; it may be buccal or lingual crossbite and may be accompanied by a shift of the mandible. **scissors-bite c., telescoping c.,** that in which the mandibular arch is entirely lingual to the maxillary arch.

crossbreeding (kros′brēd-ing) hybridization; the mating of animals or plants of different strains or species.

cross-bridges (kros-brij′ez) in A bands of myofibrils, the intertwining of the thick and the thin filaments to form the dark striations.

crossed (krost) shaped or arranged like a cross; decussating.

cross-eye (kros′i) esotropia.

crossfoot (kros′foot) talipes varus.

crossing over (kros′ing o′ver) the exchanging of genetic material between nonsister chromatids of the paired homologous chromosomes during the pachytene stage of the first meiotic division, resulting in new combinations of genes; called also *chiasmatypy*.

crossmatch (kros′mach) 1. a test of the compatibility of donor and recipient blood performed before transfusion: red cells of the donor are placed in serum of the recipient (major crossmatch) and red cells of the recipient in serum of the donor (minor crossmatch) and antiglobulin is added to increase reactivity; the presence of hemolysis or agglutination indicates incompatibility. 2. pretransplant crossmatch; HLA crossmatch; a test for the presence in the serum of a prospective transplant recipient of cytotoxic antibodies against donor tissue antigens: donor lymphocytes are placed in serum of the recipient; the presence of cytolysis indicates incompatibility and the likelihood of hyperacute graft rejection.

crossmatching (kros-mach′ing) the performance of a crossmatch.

crossover (kros′-over) the result of the reciprocal exchange of genetic material between chromosomes; see *crossing over*.

cross-reactivation (kros″re-ak-tĭ-va′shun) the activation of an inactive virus particle by another active or inactive virus particle in the same cell.

cross-reactivity (kros″re-ak-tiv′ĭ-te) the degree to which an antibody or antigen participates in cross-reactions (see under *reaction*).

cross-sensitization (kros-sen″sĭ-ti-za′shun) sensitization to a substance induced by exposure to another substance having cross-reacting antigens.

crossway (kros′wā) the path by which something crosses; decussation.

crotalid (krot′ah-lid) 1. any snake of the family Crotalidae; a pit viper. 2. of or pertaining to the family Crotalidae.

Crotalidae (kro-tal′ĭ-de) a family of venomous snakes, the pit vipers, characterized by front, movable, hollow fangs, and a depression or pit between the nostril and the eye. It includes the genera *Agkistrodon* (copperhead and water moccasin),

Bothrops (fer-de-lance), *Crotalus* (rattlesnake), *Lachesis* (bushmaster), and *Trimeresurus* (habu). See table accompanying *snake*.

crotalin (kro′tah-lin) a protein found in the venom of rattlesnakes and certain other serpents; formerly used hypodermically in the treatment of epilepsy.

crotaline (krot′ah-lin) crotalid.

crotalism (kro′tal-izm) a disease of animals caused by eating leguminous plants of the genus *Crotalaria*, which are in low bottom land. The disease is characterized by congestion and hemorrhage of the liver and spleen, emaciation, weakness, and stupor. Called also *bottom disease*.

crotalotoxin (kro″tah-lo-tok′sin) a poisonous substance from rattlesnake venom.

Crotalus (krot′ah-ius) [L. from Gr. *krotalon* rattle] a genus of rattlesnakes of the family Crotalidae. *C. horridus* is the common rattlesnake of the eastern United States; *C. adamanteus* is the diamondback rattlesnake of Georgia, Alabama, and Florida; *C. atrox* is the western diamondback rattlesnake of the Southwest and adjacent areas of Mexico; and *C. viridis* is the prairie rattlesnake. See table accompanying *snake*.

crotamine (kro′tah-mēn) a toxic protein occurring in the venom of some *Crotalus* species.

crotamiton (kro″tah-mi′ton) [USP] chemical name: *N*-ethyl-*N*-(2-methylphenyl)-2-butenamide. A scabicide, $C_{13}H_{17}NO$, occurring as a light yellow, oily liquid; applied topically to the skin.

crotaphion (kro-taf′e-on) [Gr. *krotaphos* the temple] a craniometric point at the tip of the great wing of the sphenoid.

crotethamide (kro-teth′ah-mīd) chemical name: *N*-[1-[(dimethylamino)carbonyl]propyl]-*N*-ethyl-2-butenamide; an analgesic, $C_{12}H_{22}N_2O_2$. See also *prethcamide*.

crotin (kro′tin) a poisonous substance (phytotoxin) derived from the seeds of *Croton tiglium*; see *crotonism*.

Croton (kro′ton) [L.; Gr. *krotōn* tick] a genus of euphorbiaceous shrubs, some of which are popular as ornamentals. Certain species are used medically in parts of Mexico and South America, and others, e.g., *C. texensis* (Texas C.) and *C. capitatus*, are poisonous to livestock. *C. eluteria* Benn. is a source of cascarilla bark (tonic and bitter), while *C. tiglium* yields croton oil (see under *oil*), a drastic purgative and counterirritant that can cause pustular eruptions on the skin.

crotonic acid (kro-ton′ik) an unsaturated fatty acid, $CH_3CH=CHCOOH$, found in croton oil.

crotonism (kro′ton-izm) poisoning by croton oil, characterized by burning of the mouth and sometimes emesis, followed by severe watery diarrhea and colic; sometimes accompanied by headache, somnolence, vertigo, prostration, and collapse. Death from circulatory or respiratory failure may occur.

crotoxin (kro-tok′sin) a crystalline neurotoxic principle from the venom of the rattlesnake, *Crotalus terrificus*.

crounotherapy (kroo″no-ther′ah-pe) [Gr. *krounos* spring + *therapeia* treatment] crenotherapy.

croup (kroōp) a condition resulting from acute obstruction of the larynx caused by allergy, foreign body, infection, or new growth, occurring chiefly in infants and children, and characterized by resonant barking cough, hoarseness, and persistent stridor. Called also *angina trachealis, exudative angina,* and *laryngostasis*. **catarrhal c.,** croup accompanied by a catarrhal discharge. **diphtheritic c.,** croup caused by acute laryngeal diphtheria. **false c.,** laryngismus stridulus. **membranous c., pseudomembranous c.,** croup associated with a fibrinous exudate forming a membrane-like deposit, usually caused by *Corynebacterium diphtheriae;* called also *laryngeal diphtheria.* **spasmodic c.,** laryngismus stridulus.

croupous (kroo′pus) of the nature of croup, or attended with an exudation like that of croup.

croupy (kroōp′e) affected with or resembling croup.

Crouzon's disease (kroo-zonz′) [Octave *Crouzon*, French neurologist, 1874–1938] craniofacial dysostosis.

crowding (krowd′ing) the condition in which the teeth are crowded and assume such altered positions as overlapping, displacement in various directions, torsiversion, etc.

crown (krown) [L. *corona*] 1. the topmost part of an organ or other structure, such as the top of the head, or the upper part of a tooth (corona dentis [NA]); see *anatomical c.* and *physiological c.* 2. artificial c. **anatomical c.,** the portion of a tooth that is covered by enamel; see *corona dentis* [NA]. **artificial c.,** a restoration made of metal alone, metal with a veneer of porcelain or resin, or porcelain or resin alone that reproduces the entire surface anatomy of the clinical crown of a tooth; it may be attached to a prepared tooth stump, to one partially rebuilt by a cast metal core alone, or to a cast core and a post, or it may be cemented to the remaining tooth structure. Colloquially called *cap.* **basket c.,** an artificial gold crown fitted over a natural tooth with minimal removal of tissue, so-called because added retention is provided by a thin band of labial metal similar in shape to a basket handle. **bell c.,** a tooth crown whose circumference at the occlusal surface is larger than usual in relation to the size of the circumference at the crown cervix. **Bonwill c.,** an artificial porcelain crown held to the tooth root by means of a threaded metal dowel extending through a hole in the porcelain, and upon which a nut is screwed. **cap c.,** shell c. **celluloid c.,** a temporary crown made of celluloid that facilitates the fabrication of a temporary crown during fixed prosthodontic procedures. **ciliary c.,** corona ciliaris. **clinical c.,** that portion of a tooth which is exposed beyond the gingiva. **collar c.,** an artificial crown attached by a metal ferrule to a natural tooth root. **complete c.,** full c. **dental c.,** corona dentis. **dowel c.,** an artificial crown that replaces the entire coronal portion of a tooth and is retained by a dowel extending into a filled root canal. **extra-alveolar c.,** corona clinica. **full c., full veneer c.,** a dental restoration that completely reproduces the clinical crown of a natural tooth. Called also *complete c.* and *full veneer.* **half-cap c.,** open-face c. **jacket c.,** a porcelain or acrylic resin restoration of the clinical crown of a tooth that usually terminates under the gingiva. **open-face c.,** a gold crown that covers the labial or buccal cervical region in addition to the lingual, proximal, and occlusal surfaces, or the incisal edge of anterior teeth, the buccal or labial surface of the natural crown being left exposed through the opening. Called also *half-cap c.* **overlay c.,** a cast metal artificial crown fitted over a prepared natural crown to support the walls around an inlay that are not strong or thick enough to withstand occlusal stresses, while leaving exposed the labial surface of the natural crown for esthetic purposes. **physiological c.,** the portion of a tooth that is exposed beyond the gingival crevice or the margin of the gum. It may involve all of the part of a tooth covered by enamel (dental c.; see *corona dentis* [NA]) or a portion of it (clinical crown; see *corona clinica* [NA]), and it may also involve a portion of the part not covered by enamel (dental root). **pinledge c.,** an artificial crown retained by means of pins that fit into prepared pinledges in a tooth. **Richmond c.,** an artificial crown consisting of a metal base or cap, which fits the prepared face or a stump of a natural root and carries a post or pivot for insertion into the root canal, and a porcelain facing reinforced with metal backing. **shell c.,** an artificial crown applied like a shell or cap over the remaining natural crown of a tooth; the space between the crown and the shell is filled with cement. Called also *cap c.* **tapered c.,** an artificial crown seated over a tapered abutment so that it may be fitted in place and removed without obstruction. **three-quarter c.,** an artificial crown covering mainly three surfaces of anterior teeth (mesial, distal, and lingual) and four surfaces of posterior teeth (mesial, distal, lingual, and occlusal); used as a retainer for a bridge or as a single unit restoration on a carious fractured tooth. Called also *partial veneer c.* **veneer c., complete,** a restoration of metal, porcelain, or acrylic resin that reproduces the entire surface anatomic form of the clinical crown and fits over a prepared tooth or root. **veneer c., full,** full c. **veneer c., partial,** three-quarter c. **veneered c.,** an artificial crown that bears a thin layer of resin or porcelain on the buccal or labial surface, attached to or bonded to the metal casting; called also *window c.* **window c.,** veneered c.

crowning (krown'ing) that phase in the second stage of labor when a large segment of the fetal scalp is visible at the vaginal orifice, the perineum being distended and the anus opened.

crozat (kro'zat) [G. B. *Crozat*] Crozat appliance.

Crozat appliance, clasp (kro'zat) [G. B. *Crozat*] see under *appliance* and *clasp.*

CRP C-reactive protein; see under *protein.*

CRS Chinese restaurant syndrome.

cruces (kroo'sēz) [L.] plural of *crux.*

crucial (kroo'shal) [L. *crucialis*] 1. (*obs.*) cruciate. 2. severe, searching, and decisive.

cruciate (kroo'she-āt) shaped like a cross.

crucible (kroo'sĭ-bl) [L. *crucibulum*] a vessel for melting refractory substances.

cruciform (kroo'sĭ-form) [*crux* + L. *forma* form] shaped like a cross.

crude (krood) [L. *crudus* raw] raw or unrefined.

crufomate (kroo'fo-māt) chemical name: methylphosphoramidic acid 2-chloro-4-(1,1-dimethylethyl)phenyl methyl ester; a veterinary anthelmintic, $C_{12}H_{19}ClNO_3P$.

cruor (kroo'or), pl. *cruo'res* [L.] a blood clot.

crura (kroo'rah) [L.] plural of *crus.*

crural (kroor'al) pertaining to the leg or to a leglike structure (crus).

crureus (kroo-re'us) musculus vastus intermedius; see *Table of Musculi.*

crus (krus), pl. *cru'ra* [L.] [NA] 1. the leg, from knee to foot. 2. a general term used to designate a leglike part. **ampullary crura of semicircular duct,** crura membranacea ampullaria ductus semicircularis. **ampullary osseous crura,** crura ossea ampullaria. **anterior c. of anterior inguinal ring,** c. mediale anuli inguinalis superficialis. **anterior c. of internal capsule,** c. anterius capsulae internae. **anterior c. of stapes,** c. anterius stapedis. **c. ante'rius cap'sulae inter'nae** [NA], anterior crus of internal capsule: the part of the internal capsule of the brain that separates the caudate and the lentiform nuclei; it contains the anterior thalamic radiations and the frontopalatine tract. Called also *anterior limb of internal capsule* and *pars frontalis capsulae internae.* **c. ante'rius stape'dis** [NA], anterior crus of stapes: the anterior of the two bony limbs in the middle ear that connect the base and head of the stapes; called also *anterior limb of stapes.* **cru'ra anthel'icis** [NA], **crura of anthelix,** the two ridges on the external ear marking the superior termination of the anthelix and bounding the triangular fossa; called also *limbs of anthelix.* **c. bre've incu'dis** [NA], short crus of incus: the backward-projecting process on the incus that is connected to the posterior wall of the tympanic cavity; called also *short limb of incus.* **c. cerebel'li ad pon'tem,** pedunculus cerebellaris medius. **c. cer'ebri,** 1. NA alternative for *pars ventralis pedunculi cerebri.* 2. basis pedunculi cerebri. **c. clitor'idis** [NA], **c. of clitoris,** the continuation of each corpus cavernosum clitoridis, diverging posteriorly to be attached to the pubic arch. **common membranous c. of semicircular duct,** c. membranaceum commune ductus semicircularis. **common osseous c.,** c. osseum commune. **c. commu'ne cana'lis semicircula'ris,** c. osseum commune. **c. dex'trum diaphrag'matis** [NA], right crus of diaphragm; a fibromuscular band arising from the upper three or four lumbar vertebrae, and ascending along with the left crus, to insert into the central tendon of the diaphragm. **c. dex'trum fascic'uli atrioventricula'ris** [NA], the right leg or branch of the atrioventricular bundle, arising from the trunk of the bundle at the superior end of the muscular part of the interventricular septum, and descending to be distributed to the right ventricle of the heart. Called also *right bundle branch.* **crura of diaphragm, cru'ra diaphrag'matis,** see *c. dextrum diaphragmatis* and *c. sinistrum diaphragmatis.* **c. of diaphragm, left,** c. sinistrum diaphragmatis. **c. of diaphragm, right,** c. dextrum diaphragmatis. **external c. of anterior inguinal ring,** c. laterale anuli inguinalis superficialis. **c. fascic'uli atrioventricula'ris dex'trum** [NA], the right branch of the atrioventricular bundle. **c. for'nicis** [NA], **c. of fornix,** either of the two flattened bands of white substance of the brain that are in close contact with the splenium and that unite under the posterior part of the body of the corpus callosum to form the body of the fornix. **c. glan'dis clitor'idis,** frenulum clitoridis. **c. hel'icis** [NA], **c. of helix,** the anterior termination of the helix of the external ear located above the entrance to the external acoustic meatus; called also *crista helicis.* **c. infe'rius an'nuli inguina'lis subcuta'nei,** c. laterale anuli inguinalis superficialis. **internal c. of anterior inguinal ring,** c. mediale anuli inguinalis superficialis. **in-**

ternal c. of greater alar cartilage of nose, c. mediale cartilaginis alaris majoris. **lateral c. of greater alar cartilage,** c. laterale cartilaginis alaris majoris. **lateral c. of superficial inguinal ring,** c. laterale anuli inguinalis superficialis. **c. latera′le an′nuli inguina′lis superficia′lis** [NA], lateral crus of superficial inguinal ring: the part of the superficial inguinal ring that blends with the inguinal ligament as it goes to the pubic tubercle; called also *c. inferius annuli inguinalis subcutanei,* and *external* or *posterior c. of anterior inguinal ring.* **c. latera′le cartilag′inis ala′ris majo′ris** [NA], lateral crus of greater alar cartilage: the part of the greater alar cartilage that curves laterally around the naris and helps maintain its contour. **long c. of incus,** c. longum incudis. **c. lon′-gum in′cudis** [NA], long crus of incus: a process on the incus directed downward and inward, parallel with the manubrium of the malleus; called also *long limb of incus.* **medial c. of external inguinal ring,** ligamentum inguinale reflexum. **medial c. of greater alar cartilage,** c. mediale cartilaginis alaris majoris. **medial c. of superficial inguinal ring,** c. mediale anuli inguinalis superficialis. **c. media′le an′nuli inguina′lis superficia′lis** [NA], medial crus of superficial inguinal ring: the part of the superficial inguinal ring that is attached to the symphysis and that blends with the fundiform ligament of the penis; called also *superior c. of subcutaneous inguinal ring, c. superius annuli inguinalis subcutanei, anterior* or *interior c. of anterior inguinal ring,* and *anterior* or *internal inguinal ligament.* **c. media′le cartilag′inis ala′ris majo′ris** [NA], medial crus of greater alar cartilage: the part of the greater alar cartilage, loosely attached to its fellow of the opposite side, and helping to form the mobile septum of the nose; called also *internal c. of greater alar cartilage.* **cru′ra membrana′cea** [NA], the membranous crura: the two ends of each semicircular duct of the ear, both opening into the utricle. See *crura membranacea ampullaria ductus semi-circularis, c. membranaceum commune ductus semicircularis,* and *c. membranaceum simplex ductus semicircularis.* **cru′ra membrana′cea ampulla′ria duc′tus semicircula′ris** [NA], ampullary membranous crura of semicircular duct: the end of each semicircular duct of the ear, in which the membranous ampulla is situated. **c. membrana′ceum commu′ne duc′tus semicircula′ris** [NA], common membranous crus of semicircular duct: the joined nonampullary ends of the anterior and posterior semicircular duct of the ear. **c. membrana′ceum sim′plex duc′tus semicircula′ris** [NA], simple membranous crus of semicircular duct: the nonampullary end of the lateral semicircular duct of the ear, opening into the utricle. **membranous crura,** crura membranacea. **cru′ra os′sea** [NA], osseous crura: those parts of the bony semicircular canals of the ear that lodge the correspondingly named parts of the membranous crura of the semicircular ducts; see *crura ossea ampullaria, c. osseum commune,* and *c. osseum simplex.* **cru′ra os′sea ampulla′ria** [NA], ampullary osseous crura: the parts of the bony semicircular canals of the ear that lodge the crura membranacea ampullaria ductus semicircularis. **osseous crura,** crura ossea. **c. os′seum commu′ne** [NA], common osseous crus: the part of the bony semicircular canals of the ear that lodges the crus membranaceum commune ductus semicircularis; called also *c. commune canalis semicircularis.* **c. os′seum sim′plex** [NA], simple osseous crus: that part of the bony semicircular canals of the ear that lodges the crus membranaceum simplex ductus semicircularis; called also *c. simplex canalis semicircularis.* **c. pe′nis** [NA], **c. of penis,** the continuation of each corpus cavernosum penis, diverging posteriorly to be attached to the pubic arch. **posterior c. of anterior inguinal ring,** c. laterale anuli inguinalis superficialis. **posterior c. of internal capsule,** c. posterius capsulae internae. **posterior c. of stapes,** c. posterius stapedis. **c. poste′rius cap′sulae inter′nae** [NA], posterior crus of internal capsule: the part of the internal capsule of the brain that separates the thalamus from the lentiform nucleus; it consists of thalamolenticular, sublentiform, and retrolentiform parts. Called also *posterior limb of internal capsule* and *pars occipitalis capsulae internae.* **c. poste′rius stape′dis** [NA], posterior crus of stapes: the posterior of the two bony limbs that connect the base and head of the stapes in the middle ear; called also *posterior limb of stapes.* **short c. of incus,** c. breve incudis. **simple membranous c. of semicircular duct,** c. membranaceum simplex ductus semicircula-

ris. **simple osseous c.,** c. osseum simplex. **c. sim′-plex cana′lis semicircula′ris,** c. osseum simplex. **c. sinis′trum diaphrag′matis** [NA], left crus of diaphragm: a fibromuscular band arising from the upper two or three lumbar vertebrae, and ascending along with the right crus, to insert into the central tendon of the diaphragm. **c. sinis′trum fascic′uli atrioventricula′ris** [NA], the left leg or branch of the atrioventricular bundle, arising from the trunk of the bundle at the superior end of the muscular part of the interventricular septum, and descending to be distributed to the left ventricle of the heart. Called also *left bundle branch.* **superior c. of cerebellum,** pedunculus cerebellaris superior. **superior c. of subcutaneous inguinal ring,** c. mediale anuli inguinalis superficialis. **c. supe′rius an′nuli inguina′lis subcuta′nei,** c. mediale anuli inguinalis superficialis.

crust (krust) [L. *crusta*] a formed outer layer, especially an outer layer of solid matter formed by the drying of a bodily exudate or secretion; called also *scab.* **milk c.,** crusta lactea.

crusta (krus′tah), pl. *crus′tae* [L.] 1. a crust. 2. crus cerebri. **c. lac′tea,** seborrhea of the scalp of nursing infants; called also *cradle cap* and *milk crust.*

Crustacea (krus-ta′she-ah) [L. from *crusta* shell] a large class of arthropods including the lobsters, crabs, shrimps, wood lice, water fleas, and barnacles.

crustaceorubin (krus-ta″se-o-roo′bin) a brown-black pigment (chromoprotein) found in lobster shells and eggs and in certain crabs; called also *zoonerythrin, tetra-erythrin,* and *vitellorubin.*

crustae (krus′te) [L.] genitive and plural of *crusta.*

crustal (krus′tal) pertaining to the crusta.

crustosus (krus-to′sus) [L.] crusted; said of certain lesions of the skin.

crutch (kruch) a device of wood or metal, ordinarily long enough to reach from the armpit to the ground, with a concave surface fitting under the arm and a cross bar for the hand, used for supporting the weight of the body. **Canadian c.,** a crutch consisting of two uprights extending halfway between the elbow and shoulder, with a cross piece for the hand and a curved upper arm part against which the subject leans the upper arm.

Cruveilhier's atrophy (paralysis), disease, joint (kroo-vāl-yāz′) [Jean *Cruveilhier,* French pathologist, 1791–1874; he held the first chair of pathology in the Paris faculty] see *spinal muscular atrophy,* under *atrophy,* see under *disease,* and see *articulatio atlanto-occipitalis.*

Cruveilhier-Baumgarten syndrome (cirrhosis) (kroo-vāl-yā′-baum′gar-ten) [Jean *Cruveilhier;* Paul Clemens von *Baumgarten,* German pathologist, 1848–1928] see under *syndrome.*

crux (kruks), pl. *cru′ces* [L.] cross. **c. of heart,** the intersection of the walls separating the right and left sides and the atrial and ventricular chambers of the heart. **cru′ces pilo′rum** [NA], crosslike figures formed by the pattern of hair growth, the hairs lying in opposite directions.

Cruz's trypanosomiasis (kruz) [Oswaldo *Cruz,* Brazilian physician, 1871–1917] Chagas' disease.

Cruz-Chagas disease (kruz-chag′as) [Oswaldo *Cruz;* Carlos *Chagas,* physician in Brazil, 1879–1934] Chagas' disease.

cry (kri) 1. a sudden loud, involuntary vocal sound. 2. to utter such a sound. 3. weep, def. 1. **arthritic c., articular c.,** night c. **cephalic c.,** a shrill, high-pitched penetrating cry of the newborn suggesting intracranial damage of some severity. **epileptic c.,** a loud scream that often occurs at the onset of an epileptic attack. **hydrocephalic c.,** the loud cry of a patient with acute tuberculous meningitis. **joint c.,** night c. **night c.,** a shrill cry uttered by a child in sleep, often heard in beginning joint disease; called also *arthritic, articular,* or *joint c.*

cryalgesia (kri″al-je′ze-ah) [*cryo-* + Gr. *algēsis* pain] pain due to the application of cold.

cryanesthesia (kri″an-es-the′ze-ah) [*cryo-* + *anesthesia*] loss of the power of perceiving cold.

Cryer's elevator (kri′erz) [Matthew Henry *Cryer,* American surgeon, 1840–1921] see under *elevator.*

cryesthesia (kri″es-the′ze-ah) [*cryo-* + Gr. *aisthēsis* perception] abnormal sensitiveness to cold.

crym(o)- [Gr. *krymos* frost] a combining form denoting relationship to cold.

crymoanesthesia (kri″mo-an-es-the′ze-ah) [*crymo-* + *anesthesia*] refrigeration anesthesia.

crymodynia (kri″mo-din′e-ah) [*crymo-* + Gr. *odynē* pain] rheumatic pain coming on in cold or damp weather.

crymophilic (kri″mo-fil′ik) psychrophilic.

crymophylactic (kri″mo-fi-lak′tik) cryophylactic.

crymotherapeutics (kri″mo-ther″ah-pu′tiks) cryotherapy.

crymotherapy (kri″mo-ther′ah-pe) cryotherapy.

cry(o)- [Gr. *kryos* cold] a combining form denoting relationship to cold.

cryoanalgesia (kri″o-an″al-je′ze-ah) the relief of pain by application of cold by cryoprobe to peripheral nerves.

cryobank (kri′o-bank″) a facility for freezing and preserving semen at low temperatures, usually by immersion in liquid nitrogen at −196.5° C.

cryobiology (kri″o-bi-ol′ŏ-je) [*cryo-* + Gr. *bios* life + *-logy*] the science dealing with the effect of low temperatures on biological systems.

cryocardioplegia (kri″o-kar″de-o-ple′je-ah) cessation of contraction of the myocardium produced by cooling the heart during cardiac surgery.

cryocautery (kri″o-kaw′ter-e) [*cryo-* + *cautery*] cauterization by means of the application of a substance, such as liquid nitrogen or carbon dioxide snow, or an instrument that destroys tissue by freezing; called also *cold cautery*.

cryoextraction (kri″o-eks-trak′shun) the application of low temperature in the removal of a cataractous lens; it is accomplished with an instrument (cryoprobe) whose extremely cold tip forms an adhesion (iceball) with the lens, thus permitting removal of the lens.

cryoextractor (kri″o-eks-trak′tor) [*cryo-* + *extractor*] a cryoprobe used in cryoextraction.

cryofibrinogen (kri″o-fi-brin′o-jen) [*cryo-* + *fibrinogen*] fibrinogen with the abnormal physical property of precipitating in the cold (4° C.) and subsequently redissolving at 37° C.

cryofibrinogenemia (kri″o-fi-brin″o-jen-e′me-ah) the presence of cryofibrinogen in the blood; see *cryofibrinogen*.

cryogammaglobulin (kri″o-gam″ah-glob′u-lin) cryoglobulin.

cryogen (kri′o-jen) [*cryo-* + Gr. *gennan* to produce] a substance used for lowering temperatures.

cryogenic (kri″o-jen′ik) pertaining to or causing the production of low temperatures.

cryoglobulin (kri″o-glob′u-lin) a serum globulin (invariably an immunoglobulin) that precipitates at low temperature (e.g., 4° C) and redissolves at 37° C. Cryoglobulins are classified as *Type I*, monoclonal immunoglobulins; *Type II*, immune complexes involving monoclonal immunoglobulins with antibody activity against polyclonal immunoglobulins; or *Type III*, immune complexes involving polyclonal immunoglobulins; in most cases, these are globulin-antiglobulin immune complexes like type II complexes. Types I and II occur in plasma cell dyscrasias and lymphoproliferative disorders as well as in asymptomatic "essential" cryoglobulinemia. Types II and III occur in autoimmune diseases such as rheumatoid arthritis, systemic lupus erythematosus and Sjögren's syndrome. Type III also occurs in a wide variety of infectious diseases.

cryoglobulinemia (kri″o-glob″u-lin-e′me-ah) the presence of cryoglobulin in the blood, associated with a variety of clinical manifestations including Raynaud's phenomenon, vascular purpura, cold urticaria, necrosis of extremities, bleeding disorders, vasculitis, arthralgia, neurologic manifestations, hepatosplenomegaly, and glomerulonephritis.

cryohydrate (kri″o-hi′drāt) [*cryo-* + *hydrate*] a eutectic mixture, especially one having water as one of its constituents.

cryohypophysectomy (kri″o-hi″po-fiz-ek′to-me) destruction of the hypophysis by the application of cold.

cryometer (kri-om′ĕ-ter) [*cryo-* + Gr. *metron* measure] a thermometer for measuring very low temperatures.

cryopathy (kri-op′ah-the) [*cryo-* + Gr. *pathos* disease] any morbid condition caused by cold.

cryophile (kri′o-fīl″) [*cryo-* + Gr. *philein* love] psychrophile.

cryophilic (kri″o-fil′ik) [*cryo-* + Gr. *philein* to love] psychrophilic.

cryophylactic (kri″o-fi-lak′tik) [*cryo-* + Gr. *phylaxis* a guarding] resistant to very low temperatures; said of bacteria.

cryoprecipitability (kri″o-pre-sip″ĭ-tah-bil′ĭ-te) the quality of being readily precipitated by reduced temperature (cold).

cryoprecipitate (kri″o-pre-sip′ĭ-tāt) [*cryo-* + *precipitate*] any precipitate that results from cooling, as cryoglobulin or antihemophilic factor.

cryoprecipitation (kri″o-pre-sip″ĭ-ta′shun) the precipitation of a substance in solution (e.g., antihemophilic factor in blood plasma) on exposure to lowered temperature.

cryopreservation (kri″o-pres″er-va′shun) [*cryo-* + *preservation*] the maintaining of the viability of excised tissue or organs by storing at very low temperatures.

cryoprobe (kri′o-prōb) an instrument for applying extreme cold to tissue.

cryoprotective (kri″o-pro-tek′tiv) capable of protecting against injury due to freezing, as glycerol protects frozen red blood cells.

cryoprotein (kri″o-pro′te-in) [*cryo-* + *protein*] any blood protein that precipitates on cooling, as cryoglobulin or cryofibrinogen.

cryoscope (kri′o-skōp) an apparatus for performing cryoscopy.

cryoscopical (kri″o-skop′e-kl) pertaining to cryoscopy.

cryoscopy (kri-os′ko-pe) [*cryo-* + Gr. *skopein* to examine] examination of liquids, based on the principle that the freezing point of solutions varies according to the amount and the nature of the substance contained in them in solution.

cryostat (kri′o-stat) [*cryo-* + Gr. *histanai* to halt] 1. a device by which temperature can be maintained at a very low level. 2. in pathology and histology, a chamber containing a microtome for sectioning frozen tissue.

cryosurgery (kri″o-sur′jer-e) destruction of tissue by the application of extreme cold; utilized in some forms of intracranial and cutaneous surgery.

cryothalamectomy (kri″o-thal″ah-mek′to-me) cryothalamotomy.

cryothalamotomy (kri″o-thal″ah-mot′o-me) destruction of a portion of the thalamus by application of extreme cold.

cryotherapy (kri″o-ther′ah-pe) [*cryo-* + Gr. *therapeia* treatment] the therapeutic use of cold.

cryotolerant (kri″o-tol′er-ant) able to withstand unusually low temperatures.

crypt (kript) [L. *crypta*, from Gr. *kryptos* hidden] a blind pit or tube on a free surface; see also *crypta* [NA]. **anal c's,** sinus anales. **bony c.,** the crypt in the developing alveolar bone that becomes the socket of the developing tooth. **dental c.,** tooth c. **enamel c.,** a space bounded by the dental ledges on either side and usually by the enamel organ; it is filled with mesenchyma. **c's of Fuchs,** c's of iris. **c's of Haller,** glandulae preputiales. **c's of iris,** pit-like depressions found in the iris, in the region of the circulus arteriosus minor; called also *c's of Fuchs*. **c's of Lieberkühn,** glandulae intestinales. **c's of Littre,** glandulae preputiales. **Luschka's c's,** deep indentations of the gallbladder mucosa which penetrate into the muscular layer of the organ. **c. of Morgagni,** 1. fossa navicularis urethrae. 2. see *sinus anales*. **mucous c's of duodenum,** glandulae duodenales. **odoriferous c's of prepuce,** glandulae preputiales. **c's of palatine tonsil,** fossulae tonsillares tonsillae palatinae. **c's of pharyngeal tonsil,** fossulae tonsillares tonsillae pharyngeae. **synovial c.,** a pouch in the synovial membrane of a joint. **c's of tongue,** deep, irregular invaginations from the surface of the lingual tonsil. **tonsillar c's,** cryptae tonsillares tonsillae pharyngeae. **tonsillar c's of palatine tonsil,** cryptae tonsillares tonsillae palatinae. **tonsillar c's of pharyngeal tonsil,** cryptae tonsillares tonsillae pharyngeae. **tooth c.,** the depression in the alveolar bone occupied by the tooth germ and the tooth follicle. Called also *dental c.* **c's of Tyson,** glandulae preputiales.

crypta (krip′tah), pl. *cryp′tae* [L.] [NA] a crypt: a blind pit or tube opening on a free surface. **cryp′tae muco′sae,** see *glandula mucosa*. **cryp′tae muco′sae duode′ni,** glandulae duodenales. **cryp′tae odorif′erae, cryp′-**

tae praeputia′les, glandulae preputiales. **cryp′tae tonsilla′res tonsil′lae palati′nae** [NA], tonsillar crypt of palatine tonsils: the blind ends of the tonsillar fossulae on the palatine tonsils; called also *tonsillar crypts*. **cryp′tae tonsilla′res tonsil′lae pharyn′geae** [NA], tonsillar crypts of pharyngeal tonsils: the blind ends of the tonsillar fossulae of the pharyngeal tonsils. **cryp′tae ure′thrae mulie′bris**, glandulae urethrales urethrae femininae.

cryptae (krip′te) [L.] genitive and plural of *crypta*.

cryptanamnesia (kript″an-am-ne′ze-ah) cryptomnesia.

cryptectomy (krip-tek′to-me) [crypt- + Gr. *ektomē* excision] excision or obliteration of a crypt.

cryptenamine (krip-ten′ah-mīn) a mixture of ester alkaloids derived from a nonaqueous extract of *Veratrum viride* Ait. (Liliaceae); it forms a white amorphous powder that possesses antihypertensive properties, and contains several alkaloids, including protoveratrines A and B, neogermitrine, germitrine, germerine, etc. **c. acetates**, a mixture of the acetate salts of cryptenamine, administered intravenously or intramuscularly in the management of eclampsia and hypertensive encephalopathy. **c. tannates**, a mixture of the tannate salts of cryptenamine, administered orally to control moderate to severe hypertension.

cryptesthesia (krip′tes-the′ze-ah) [crypt- + Gr. *aisthēsis* perception] clairvoyance.

cryptic (krip′tik) [Gr. *kryptikos* hidden] concealed, hidden, larval.

cryptitis (krip-ti′tis) inflammation of a crypt. **anal c.**, inflammation of the anal crypts, with pain and tenderness (especially during bowel movements), pruritus, and spasm of the anal sphincter; it may progress to abscess of the crypt.

crypt(o)- [Gr. *kryptos* hidden] a combining form meaning hidden or concealed, or denoting relationship to a crypt.

Cryptobia (krip-to′be-ah) [crypto- + Gr. *bios* life] a genus of parasitic, biflagellate protozoa (suborder Bodonina, order Kinetoplasida) having one free flagellum and the other adherent to the body and forming an undulating membrane; most species are found in the reproductive organs of invertebrates, especially mollusks, but they are also found in the blood and digestive tract of fish. Called also *Trypanoplasma*.

cryptocephalus (krip″to-sef′ah-lus) [crypto- + Gr. *kephalē* head] a monster with an inconspicuous head.

Cryptococcaceae (krip″to-kok-ka′se-e) a family of the Fungi Imperfecti, order Moniliales, the members of which are yeastlike throughout most or all of their life cycle; it includes a number of pathogenic genera, such as *Cryptococcus*, *Candida*, *Geotrichum*, *Trichosporon*, and *Pityrosporon*.

cryptococcosis (krip″to-kok-o′sis) an infection by *Cryptococcus neoformans* which may involve the skin, lungs, or other parts, but has a predilection for the brain and meninges. The cutaneous form is marked by acneiform lesions; called also *European blastomycosis*. The generalized form invades the central nervous system, less often the lungs, liver, spleen and joints. It is fatal if left untreated. Called also *torulosis*, and *Busse-Buschke disease*.

Cryptococcus (krip″to-kok′us) [crypto- + Gr. *kokkos* berry] a genus of asexual yeastlike organisms of the family Cryptococcaceae, which usually have a capsule and do not form pseudomycellium as do the *Candida*. Formerly called *Atelosaccharomyces* and *Torula*. **C. capsula′tus**, former name for *Histoplasma capsulatum*. **C. gilchris′ti**, former name for *Blastomyces dermatitidis*. **C. histolyt′icus**, *C. neoformans*. **C. hom′inis**, *C. neoformans*. **C. meningit′idis**, *C. neoformans*. **C. neofor′mans**, a species causing an infection in humans; see *cryptococcosis*. Formerly called *C. histolytians, hominis*, and *meningitidis*, and *Debaryomyces neoformans hominis* and *Torula histolytica*.

cryptocrystalline (krip″to-kris′tah-līn) [crypto- + *crystalline*] composed of crystals of microscopic size.

Cryptocys′tis trichodec′tis a name erroneously applied to the cysticercoid larval form of the tapeworm *Dipylidium caninum* when it was first discovered in the body cavity of the dog louse, *Trichodectes*.

cryptodeterminant (krip″to-de-ter′min-ant) hidden determinant.

cryptodidymus (krip″to-did′ĭ-mus) [crypto- + Gr. *didymos* twin] a teratism in which one twin is concealed within the body of the other.

cryptoempyema (krip″to-em″pi-e′mah) [crypto- + *empyema*] empyema that is difficult to aspirate, being loculated or interlobar.

cryptogam (krip′to-gam) [crypto- + Gr. *gamos* marriage] any one of the lower plants that have no true flowers, but propagate by spores.

Cryptogemmina (krip″to-jim′ĭ-nah) [crypto- + *gemmare* to bud] a suborder of endocommensal ciliate protozoa (order Chonotrichida, superorder Phyllopharyngidea) found in marine crustaceans. They reproduce by internal budding and have a small, flattened, angular body with spines and a reduced collar.

cryptogenetic (krip″to-jĕ-net′ik) cryptogenic.

cryptogenic (krip″to-jen′ik) [crypto- + Gr. *gennan* to produce] of obscure, doubtful, or unascertainable origin. Cf. *phanerogenic*.

cryptoglioma (krip″to-gli-o′mah) [crypto- + *glioma*] one of the stages in the development of glioma of the retina, marked by shrinking of the eyeball due to cyclitis, which masks the presence of the growth.

cryptoleukemia (krip″to-lu-ke′me-ah) [crypto- + *leukemia*] an archaic term previously applied to a hyperplastic blood process in which there were no abnormal cells in the blood stream.

cryptolith (krip′to-lith) [crypto- + Gr. *lithos* stone] a calculus or concretion in a crypt.

cryptomenorrhea (krip″to-men″o-re′ah) [crypto- + *menorrhea*] a condition in which the symptoms of menstruation are experienced but no external bleeding occurs, as in cases of imperforate hymen.

cryptomere (krip′to-mēr) [crypto- + Gr. *meros* part] a cystic or saclike condition.

cryptomerorachischisis (krip″to-me″ro-rah-kis′kĭ-sis) [crypto- + Gr. *meros* part + *rhachis* spine + *schisis* cleavage] spina bifida occulta.

cryptomnesia (krip″tom-ne′ze-ah) [crypto- + Gr. *mnasthai* to be mindful] the recall of memories not recognized as such but thought to be original creations.

cryptomnesic (krip″tom-ne′sik) pertaining to or characterized by cryptomnesia.

cryptomonad (krip″to-mon′ad) [crypto- + Gr. *monas* unit, from *monos* single] a protozoan of the order Cryptomonanadida.

Cryptomonadida (krip″to-mo-nad′ĭ-dah) an order of plantlike marine and freshwater protozoa (class Phytomastigophorea, subphylum Mastigophora), having two subequal flagella arising subapically in a ventral groove and brown, red, olive-green, blue, or yellow chloroplasts. *Cryptomonas* is a representative genus.

Cryptomonas (krip″to-mo′nas) [crypto- + Gr. *monas* unit, from *monos* single] a genus of elliptical, biflagellate, plantlike freshwater protozoa (order Cryptomonadida, class Phytomastigophorea) having green chromatophores.

cryptoneurous (krip″to-nu′rus) [crypto- + Gr. *neuron* nerve] having no definite or distinct nervous system.

cryptophthalmia (krip″tof-thal′me-ah) cryptophthalmos.

cryptophthalmos (krip″tof-thal′mos) [crypto- + Gr. *ophthalmos* eye] a developmental anomaly in which the skin is continuous over the eyeballs without any indication of the formation of eyelids.

cryptophthalmus (krip″tof-thal′mus) cryptophthalmos.

cryptopine (krip′to-pin) [crypto- + Gr. *opion* opium] a minor alkaloidal constituent, $C_{21}H_{23}NO_5$, of opium, of *Corydalis sempervirens* (L.) Pers., and of *Dicentra* spp. (Fumariaceae).

cryptoplasmic (krip″to-plaz′mik) occurring in a concealed form; said of an infection in which the infecting organism has concealed itself; occult.

cryptopodia (krip″to-po′de-ah) [crypto- + Gr. *pous* foot] a condition characterized by swelling of the lower part of the leg and dorsum of the foot so as to cover all but the soles of the feet.

cryptopyic (krip″to-pi′ik) [crypto- + Gr. *pyon* pus] attended by concealed suppuration.

cryptorchid (krip-tor′kid) [crypto- + Gr. *orchis* testis] pertaining to or characterized by cryptorchidism; by extension, sometimes used to designate an individual exhibiting cryptorchidism.

cryptorchidectomy (krip″tor-kĭ-dek′to-me) [*cryptorchid* + Gr. *ektomē* excision] excision of an undescended testis.

cryptorchidism (krip-tor′kĭ-dizm) a developmental defect characterized by failure of the testes to descend into the scrotum.

cryptorchidopexy (krip-tor″kĭ-do-pek′se) orchiopexy.

cryptorchidy (krip-tor′kĭ-de) cryptorchidism.

cryptorchism (krip-tor′kizm) cryptorchidism.

cryptoscope (krip′to-skōp) [*crypto-* + Gr. *skopein* to examine] a fluoroscope. **Satvioni's c.,** one of the early forms of fluoroscope.

cryptoscopy (krip-tos′ko-pe) fluoroscopy.

cryptosporidiosis (krip″to-spo-rid″e-o′sis) infection with protozoa of the genus *Cryptosporidium*, which may be associated with or contribute to enteric disease in calves, lambs, foals, and piglets. Human infection occurs both in immunocompetent persons, particularly those who work with cattle, in whom it causes a self-limited diarrhea syndrome, and in immunocompromised patients, in whom it is much more serious, being manifested clinically as prolonged debilitating diarrhea, weight loss, fever, and abdominal pain, with occasional spread to the trachea and bronchial tree.

Cryptosporidium (krip″to-spo-rid′e-um) [*crypto-* + *spore*] a genus of minute homoxenous coccidian protozoa (suborder Eimeriina, order Eucoccidiida), characterized by the presence of oocysts with four sporozoites; they are parasitic in the intestinal tracts of many different vertebrates, including reptiles, birds, and mammals and are an uncommon cause of diarrhea in humans. See also *cryptosporidiosis.*

cryptosterol (krip-tos′ter-ol) a triterpenic sterol, $C_{30}H_{50}O$, from yeast; it also occurs in wool fat (see *lanosterol*).

Cryptostroma (krip″to-stro′mah) a genus of fungi. **C. cortica′le,** *Coniosporium corticale.*

cryptotia (krip-to′she-ah) a rare anomaly in which the superior portion of the auricle is buried in the scalp.

cryptotoxic (krip″to-tok′sik) [*crypto-* + *toxic*] having hidden toxic properties; said of a solution normally nontoxic, but which may become toxic when the colloidal balance is disturbed.

cryptoxanthin (krip″to-zan′thin) a yellow carotenoid widely distributed in nature (egg yolk, green grass, yellow corn, etc.), which can be converted into vitamin A in the body.

cryptozoite (krip″to-zo′īt) [*crypto-* + Gr. *zōon* animal] a meront of certain sporozoan protozoa in the exoerythrocytic stage.

cryptozygous (krip-toz′ĭ-gus) [*crypto-* + Gr. *zygon* yoke] having the face no wider than the cranium, so that the zygomatic arches are concealed by the bulging of the cranium when the skull is viewed from above. Cf. *phenozygous.*

Crys. crystal.

crystal (kris′tal) [Gr. *krystallos* ice] a naturally produced angular solid of definite form in which the ultimate units from which it is built up are systematically arranged; they are usually evenly spaced on a regular space lattice. **asthma c's,** Charcot-Leyden c's. **blood c's,** hematoidin crystals in the blood. **Böttcher's c's,** microscopic crystals seen on adding a drop of solution of ammonium phosphate to a drop of prostatic fluid. **Charcot-Leyden c's,** crystalline structures, protein in nature, found wherever eosinophilic leukocytes are undergoing fragmentation, e.g., in the bronchial secretions in bronchial asthma and in stools in some cases of intestinal parasitism. Called also *asthma, leukocytic,* and *Leyden's c's.* **Charcot-Neumann c's,** minute cyrstals of spermine phosphate found in semen and various animal tissues. **coffin lid c's,** peculiar indented crystals of ammoniomagnesium phosphate from alkaline urine; called also *knife rest c's.* **dumbbell c's,** crystals of calcium oxalate occurring in the urine. **ear c.,** statolith, def. 1; see *statoconia.* **hedgehog c's,** a spiny form of uric acid concretions. **knife rest c's,** coffin lid c's. **leukocytic c's, Leyden's c's,** Charcot-Leyden c's. **liquid c's,** certain liquids which manifest some of the optical properties of crystals and the hydrodynamic properties of fluids, e.g., phosphatidyl choline. **Lubarsch's c's,** crystals in the testis resembling sperm crystals. **Platner's c's,** crystals of the salts of the bile acids. **c's of Reinke,** see under *crystalloid.* **rock c.,** quartz; a transparent form of silicon dioxide (silica), SiO_2; used for lenses. **sperm c's, spermin c's,** crystals of spermine phosphate in the semen.

Teichmann's c's, crystals of hemin. **thorn-apple c's,** yellow or reddish brown spheres of ammonium urate which are covered with sharp spicules or prisms, as found in the urine. **Virchow's c's,** yellow or orange crystals of hematoidin sometimes seen in extravasated blood. **whetstone c's,** crystals of xanthine sometimes seen in urine.

crystalbumin (kris″tal-bu′min) 1. an albuminous substance found in an aqueous extract of the crystalline lens. 2. a general term for crystallizable albumins of the type of egg albumin and serum albumin.

crystallin (kris-tal′in) a globulin existing in the crystalline lens of the eye. *Alpha c.* is precipitated by dilute acetic acid; *beta c.* is not.

crystalline (kris′tah-līn) resembling a crystal in nature or clearness.

crystallization (kris″tah-li-za′shun) the formation of crystals; conversion to a crystalline form. **fern-leaf c.,** crystallization of cervical mucus in a fernlike pattern, observable during the first half of the menstrual cycle and said to be most conspicuous at the time of ovulation.

crystallography (kris″tah-log′rah-fe) [*crystal* + Gr. *graphein* to write] the science dealing with the study of crystals. **x-ray c.,** the determination of the three-dimensional structure of molecules by means of diffraction patterns produced by x-rays.

crystalloid (kris′tah-loid) [*crystal* + Gr. *eidos* form] 1. resembling a crystal. 2. a noncolloid substance; a substance which, in solution, passes readily through animal membranes, lowers the freezing point of the solvent containing it, and is generally capable of being crystallized. Cf. *colloid,* def. 1. **Charcot-Böttcher c's,** slender spindle-shaped crystals 10 to 25 μ long, commonly found in Sertoli cells of the human testis but not in other species. **c's of Reinke,** conspicuous, variously shaped, crystal-like structures contained in Leydig cells.

crystalluria (kris-tah-lu′re-ah) the excretion of crystals in the urine, producing renal irritation.

Crysticillin (kris″tĭ-sil′in) trademark for preparations of penicillin G procaine.

Crystodigin (kris″to-dig′in) trademark for preparations of digitoxin.

CS cesarean section; conditioned stimulus.

CS₂ carbon disulfide.

Cs chemical symbol for *cesium.*

C.S.A.A. Child Study Association of America.

C.S.C. coup sur coup.

CSF cerebrospinal fluid; colony-stimulating factor.

C.S.G.B.I. Cardiac Society of Great Britain and Ireland.

C.S.M. cerebrospinal meningitis.

CT computerized tomography.

C.T.A. Canadian Tuberculosis Association.

CTBA cetrimonium bromide.

cteinophyte (ti′no-fīt) [Gr. *kteinein* to kill + *phyton* plant] a fungus that has a destructive influence upon its host; limited to chemical rather than parasitic activity.

cteno- [Gr. *kteis*, gen. *ktenos* comb] a combining form denoting relationship to a comb or comblike structure.

Ctenocephalides (te″no-se-fal′ĭ-dēz) [*cteno-* + Gr. *kephalē* head + *eidos* form, shape] a genus of fleas. **C. ca′nis,** a species frequently found on dogs, which may transmit the dog tapeworm to man; formerly called *Pulex serraticeps.* **C. fe′lis,** a species commonly found parasitic on cats.

Ctenophora (ten-of′o-rah) [*cteno-* + Gr. *pherein* to bear] a phylum of marine invertebrates that includes the comb jellies or sea walnuts, whose bodies consist of two layers of cells enclosing a jelly-like mass; eight rows of cilia, which resemble combs, cover the outer body surface and provide locomotor power.

ctenophore (ten′o-for) 1. pertaining or belonging to the phylum Ctenophora. 2. an individual of the phylum Ctenophora. See also *coelenterate* (def. 3).

Ctenophthalmus (te″nof-thal′mus) [*cteno-* + Gr. *ophthalmos* eye] a genus of fleas. **C. agry′tes,** the European mouse flea.

Ctenopsyllus (te″no-sil′us) (*obs.*) *Leptopsylla.* **C. seg′nis,** *Leptopsylla segnis.*

Ctenus (te′nus) a genus of spiders. *C. ferus* is the South

American wandering spider whose bite causes great pain. In severe cases, weakness and irregularity of the heart beat, breathing difficulty, and temporary blindness may occur; some deaths have occurred in young children.

C-terminal (ter′min-al) the end of the peptide chain carrying the free alpha carboxyl group of the last amino acid, conventionally written to the right.

Ctesias (te′se-as), of Cnidus. (5th century B.C.) a Greek physician and historian, a contemporary of Hippocrates of Cos. Ctesias was a long-time resident at, historian and apologist for, and physician to the royal Persian court.

ctetology (te-tol′ŏ-je) [Gr. *ktētos* acquired + *-logy*] that branch of biology which treats of acquired characters.

CTL cytotoxic lymphocytes; cytotoxic T lymphocytes.

CTP cytidine triphosphate.

Cu chemical symbol for *copper* (L. *cuprum*).

cuajani (kwah-hah′ne) an expectorant preparation from *Prunus occidentalis.*

cubeb (ku′beb) [L. *cubeba;* Arabic *kabāba*] the dried, unripe, almost fully grown fruit of *Piper cubeba* L.f. (Piperaceae), the tailed pepper or Java pepper, found throughout Southern Asia, which contains 10–18 per cent volatile oil, cubebin, resins, fat, and wax. Formerly used to stimulate healing of mucous membranes, and as a diuretic and urinary antiseptic.

cubebin (ku-be′bin) an inactive crystalline principle, $C_{10}H_{10}O_3$, from cubeb; formerly used as a urinary antiseptic.

cubebism (ku′beb-izm) poisoning by cubeb (*Piper cubeba*), characterized by nausea, vomiting, diarrhea, fever with or without skin eruptions, prostration, arthralgia, irritation of the kidneys, soft pulse, loss of consciousness, miosis, delirium, and coma. In severe poisonings, death from respiratory failure may occur.

cubicle (ku′bĭ-k′l) a compartment in a larger area, such as a dormitory or a ward, separated from similar adjoining compartments and from the rest of the room by low partitions.

cubilose (ku′bĭ-lōs) [L. *cubile* nest] a mucilaginous and nutritious principle from the edible nest of the swiftlet, *Collocalia esculenta*, of southern Asia; it is an excretion from the stomach of the bird.

cubit (ku′bit) [L. *cubitus*] a unit of measure, being the distance from the joint between the arm and forearm (elbow) to the tip of the middle finger; ranging, according to various systems of measurement, between 46 and 53 cm.

cubital (ku′bĭ-tal) 1. pertaining to the elbow. 2. pertaining to the ulna or to the forearm.

cubitalis (ku-bĭ-ta′lis) [L.] cubital.

cubitocarpal (ku″bĭ-to-kar′pal) pertaining to the ulna and the carpus.

cubitoradial (ku″bĭ-to-ra′de-al) pertaining to the ulna and the radius.

cubitus (ku′bĭ-tus) [L.] 1. [NA] the bend of the arm; the joint between the arm and forearm; the elbow. 2. the upper limb distal to the humerus: the elbow, forearm, and hand. 3. ulna. **c. val′gus,** deformity of the elbow (judged with the palm facing forward), in which it deviates away from the midline of the body when extended. **c. va′rus,** deformity of the elbow, due to lateral angulation of the joint and accompanied by deviation of the forearm toward the midline of the body when the forearm is extended; called also *gun stock deformity.*

cuboid (ku′boid) [Gr. *kyboeidēs*] 1. resembling a cube. 2. the cuboid bone (os cuboideum [NA]).

cuboidal (ku-boi′dal) resembling a cube.

cu. cm. cubic centimeter.

cucoline (ku′ko-lēn) sinomenine.

cucullaris (ku-ku-la′ris) [L. *cucullus* hood] musculus trapezius; see *Table of Musculi.*

cucumber (ku′kum-ber) [L. *cucumis*] the edible fruit of various species of *Cucumis*, chiefly *C. sativus* L., the seeds of which are diuretic and whose juice is used as an astringent in various cosmetic formulations. **bitter c.,** colocynth.

Cucumis (ku′kum-is) a genus of curcurbitaceous plants which includes several edible species, as well as some which have medicinal properties, e.g., *C. sativus* L., the cucumber (q.v.).

Cucurbita (ku-ker′bĭ-tah) a genus of curcurbitaceous plants, including *C. pepo* L., the pumpkin (q.v.).

cucurbitol (ku-ker′bĭ-tol) a sterol, $C_{24}H_{40}O_4$, obtained from watermelon seeds.

cucurbitula (ku″ker-bit′u-lah) [L. dim. of *cucurbita*, a gourd] a cupping glass. **c. cruen′ta** [L. "bloody cup"], a cupping glass applied to draw blood. **c. sic′ca** [L. "dry cup"], a cupping glass that does not draw blood.

cucurbocitrin (ku″ker-bo-sit′rin) an extract from watermelon seeds; it has been tried in the treatment of hypertension.

cudbear (kud′bār) a red-brown powder, obtained from lichens, such as *Lecanora tartarea*, and used as a coloring matter in pharmacy.

cudding (kud′ing) quidding.

cuff (kuf) a small bandlike structure encircling a part. **musculotendinous c.,** one formed by intermingled muscle and tendon fibers; see *rotator c.* **rotator c.,** a musculotendinous structure about the capsule of the shoulder joint, formed by the inserting fibers of the supraspinatus, infraspinatus, teres minor, and subscapularis muscles, blending with the capsule, and providing mobility and strength to the shoulder joint.

cuffing (kuf′ing) the formation of a cufflike surrounding border, such as collections of leukocytes surrounding blood vessels, noted in certain viral diseases.

Cuignet's method (ke-ēn-yāz′) [Ferdinand Louis Joseph *Cuignet*, French ophthalmologist, born 1823] skiametry.

cuirass (kwe-ras′) [Fr. *cuirasse* breastplate] a covering for the chest. **tabetic c.,** an area of diminished sense of touch encircling the chest of a patient with tabes dorsalis.

Cuj. abbreviation for L. *cu′jus*, of which.

cul-de-sac (kul′dĕ-sahk′) [Fr.] a blind pouch or cecum. **conjunctival c.,** the fold formed by the junction of the palpebral and the ocular conjunctiva. **Douglas' c.,** excavatio recto-uterina. **dural c.,** the terminal portion of the dural sac.

culdocentesis (kul″do-sen-te′sis) [*cul-de-sac* + *centesis*] aspiration of fluid from the rectouterine space by puncture of the apex of the vaginal wall.

culdoscope (kul′do-skōp) an endoscope for performing culdoscopy.

culdoscopy (kul-dos′ko-pe) visual examination of the female pelvic viscera by means of an endoscope introduced into the pelvic cavity through the posterior vaginal fornix.

culdotomy (kul-dot′o-me) [*cul-de-sac* + Gr. *tomē* a cutting] incision into the cul-de-sac (pouch of Douglas); called also *posterior colpotomy.*

Culex (ku′leks) [L. "gnat"] a genus of culicine mosquitoes characterized by short palpi and by holding the body parallel to the surface on which it rests while the head and beak are bent at an angle to the body. Many species occurring throughout the world are vectors of various disease-producing agents. Species include *C. annuliros′tris*, *C. fat′igans*, *C. moles′tus*, *C. pi′piens*, *C. quinquefascia′tus*, *C. tarsa′lis*, and *C. tritaeniorhyn′cus*, among many others.

culicicide (ku-lis′ĭ-sīd) culicide.

Culicidae (ku-lis′ĭ-de) a family of insects of the suborder Nematocerca, order Diptera, including the mosquitoes. There are ten tribes, of which three are of particular medical interest: Anophelini, Culicini, and Megarhinini.

culicidal (ku-lĭ-si′dal) destructive to gnats and mosquitoes.

culicide (ku′lĭ-sīd) [L. *culex* gnat + *caedere* to kill] an agent destructive to gnats and mosquitoes.

culicifuge (ku-lis′ĭ-fūj) [L. *culex* gnat + *fugare* to put to flight] a preparation that repels gnats and mosquitoes.

Culicinae (ku-lĭ-si′ne) a subfamily of the Culicidae, the true mosquitoes, containing the tribes Anophelini, Culicini, and Megarhinini.

culicine (ku′lĭ-sin, ku′lĭ-sīn) 1. a member of the genus *Culex* or related genera. 2. pertaining to, involving, or affecting mosquitoes of the genus *Culex* or related genera.

Culicini (ku-lĭ-si′ni) a tribe of the subfamily Culicinae containing many genera, the most important of which are *Aedes*, *Culex*, *Mansonia*, *Psorophora*, *Theobaldia*, and *Wyeomyia*.

Culicoides (ku-lĭ-koi′dēz) a genus of biting flies of the family Heleidae. *C. aus′teni* and *C. gra′hami* are intermediate hosts of the parasitic roundworm *Mansonella perstans*. *C.*

fu'rens and possibly other species are intermediate hosts of *Mansonella ozzardi*.

Culiseta (ku″lĭ-se′tah) a genus of culicine mosquitoes; formerly called *Theobaldia*. **C. inora′ta,** a vector of the Cache Valley virus in Utah. **C. melanu′ra,** a vector of the viruses causing eastern and western equine encephalitides.

Cullen's sign (kul′enz) [Thomas Stephen *Cullen*, Baltimore surgeon, 1868–1953] see under *sign*.

culling (kul′ing) the process of selective removal. The term is applied to the removal from the circulation, by the spleen, of abnormal erythrocytes, such as those occurring in congenital spherocytosis, or to the selective separation of other elements or organisms.

culmen (kul′men), pl. *cul′mina* [L.] 1. acme or summit. 2. c. cerebelli. **c. cerebel′li** [NA], **c. of cerebellum,** the portion of the rostral lobe of the cerebellum that lies medially between the central lobule and the primary fissure; called also *culmen* and *c. monticuli*. **c. of left lung, c. pulmo′nis sinis′tri,** the nonlingular portion of the superior lobe of the left lung (see *lingula pulmonis sinistri*).

culmina (kul′mĭ-nah) [L.] plural of *culmen*.

Culp ureteropelvioplasty [Ormond Skinner *Culp*, American surgeon, 1910–1977] see under *urethroplasty*.

cult (kult) a system of treating disease based on some special and unscientific theory of disease causation.

cultivation (kul″tĭ-va′shun) [L. *cultivatio*] the propagation of living organisms, applied especially to the propagation of cells in artificial media.

culturable (kul′chur-ah-b'l) capable of being cultured.

cultural (kul′tu-ral) pertaining to a culture.

culture (kul′tūr) [L. *cultura*] 1. the propagation of microorganisms or of living tissue cells in special media conducive to their growth. 2. a growth of microorganisms or other living cells. 3. to induce the propagation of microorganisms or living tissue cells in media conducive to their growth. See also *culture medium*. **asynchronous c.,** one in which cells are randomly distributed with respect to the phase of cell division, as in an ordinary culture of bacteria or animal cells. **attenuated c.,** a culture of pathogenic microorganisms whose virulence is weakened or abolished. **cell c.,** the maintenance or growth of animal cells in vitro, or a culture of such cells. **chorioallantoic c.,** the cultivation of microorganisms, cells, or tissues on the chorioallantois of the developing chick. **continuous flow c.,** the cultivation of bacteria in a continuous flow of fresh medium to maintain bacterial growth in logarithmic phase. **direct c.,** a culture of microorganisms made by direct transfer from a natural source to an artificial medium. **enrichment c.,** one grown on a medium, usually liquid, that has been supplemented to encourage the growth of a given type of organism. **hanging-block c.,** one grown on a block of agar medium fastened to a coverglass, which is then inverted over a hollow slide. **hanging-drop c.,** a culture in which the material to be cultivated is inoculated into a drop of fluid attached to a coverglass, which is inverted over a hollow slide. **mixed c.,** one containing two or more kinds of microorganisms. **mixed lymphocyte c. (MLC),** a type of lymphocyte proliferation test (q.v.) in which lymphocytes from two individuals are cultured together and the proliferative response (mixed lymphocyte reaction) is measured by ^{3}H-labeled thymidine uptake. The test may be performed as a "two-way" MLC in which cells of both individuals can proliferate or as a "one-way" MLC in which the cells of one individual are prevented from responding by treatment with radiation or mitomycin. Three controls are used: cultures of syngeneic pairs, both untreated and radiation- or mitomycin-treated, and a culture of allogeneic irradiated or mitomycin-treated pairs. The primary clinical use of MLC is selection of compatible donors for bone marrow and living-related renal allotransplantation and for typing of HLA-D antigens; it is also used in diagnosis of immunodeficiency diseases. Called also *mixed lymphocyte reaction* (MLR). **needle c.,** stab c. **plate c.,** one grown on a medium, usually agar or gelatin, on a Petri dish. **primary c.,** a cell or tissue culture made by direct transfer from a natural source to an artificial medium. **pure c.,** one containing only one kind of microorganism, without any contaminants. **radioisotopic c.,** a bacterial culture in a medium containing ^{14}C-labeled carbohydrate. Metabolism is detected by the release of $^{14}CO_2$, offering earlier detection of growth than do conventional methods. **roll-tube c.,** one made by inoculating a tube of molten agar medium and rotating it while it is solidifying, the medium being dispersed in a thin layer on the inner surface of the tube. The method is used for making colony counts, particularly of anaerobic bacteria. **secondary c.,** one derived from a primary culture. **selective c.,** one grown on a medium, usually solid, that has been supplemented to encourage the growth of a single species of microorganism. It may also include substances that inhibit the growth of other species. **sensitized c.,** bacterial cells that have been incubated with specific antiserum. **shake c.,** a culture made by inoculating warm liquid agar culture medium in a tube and shaking to distribute contents evenly. Incubation of the resolidified culture allows the development of separated colonies; especially applicable to obligate anaerobes. **slant c.,** one made on a slanting surface of a solidified medium in a tube, the tube being tilted to provide a greater surface area for growth. **slope c.,** slant c. **stab c.,** one in which a tube of solid medium is inoculated by a needle thrust deep into the contents. **stock c.,** a culture of microorganisms maintained in a viable state as a reference strain and subcultured into fresh medium as necessary. **streak c.,** a culture in which the surface of a solid medium is inoculated by drawing across it, in a zigzag fashion, a wire inoculating loop carrying the inoculum. **subculture c.,** one derived from an existing culture. **suspension c.,** a culture in which cells multiply while suspended in a suitable medium. **synchronized c.,** a culture of bacterial or animal cells in which all cells are in the same phase of cell division. **tissue c.,** the maintaining or growing of tissue, organ primordia, or the whole or part of an organ *in vitro* so as to preserve its architecture and/or function. **type c.,** a culture of any species of microorganism usually maintained in a central collection of type or standard cultures.

culture medium (kul′tūr me′de-um) any substance or preparation used for the cultivation of living cells; see *Table of Culture Media*.

TABLE OF CULTURE MEDIA

Abbreviations used in this table are: a.=agar, b.=broth, ba.=base, c.=culture medium, m.=medium.

acetate a., an agar medium containing sodium acetate, sodium chloride, magnesium sulfate, bromothymol blue, and phosphate buffer, used to determine the ability of an organism to utilize acetate as a sole carbon source, especially in the differentiation of *Shigella* and *Escherichia*. Sodium acetate may also be added to citrate agar (Simmons) for culturing nonfermenting gram-negative bacteria.

agar c., one in which agar is used as the solidifying agent.

Amies transport m., an agar medium containing sodium thioglycollate, sodium and potassium chloride, phosphate buffer, calcium chloride, magnesium chloride, and neutral charcoal, used for transport of specimens for anaerobic culture.

antibiotic c. 3 FDA, a broth medium containing peptone, yeast and beef extracts, sodium chloride, glucose, and potassium buffer, used for testing the activity of antibiotic agents against fungi.

antibiotic c. 12 FDA, an agar medium containing peptone, yeast and beef extracts, sodium chloride, and dextrose, used for agar dilution susceptibility tests with antifungal antibiotics. Called also *nystatin assay a*.

beef infusion c., see *infusion m*.

Bennett a., an agar medium containing casein digest, yeast extract, beef extract, and glucose, used as an isolation medium for *Nocardia* and *Streptomyces*.

bile-esculin a. (BEA), an agar medium containing beef extract, peptone, oxgall, ferric citrate, and esculin, sometimes supplemented with horse serum, used for the identification of group D streptococci.

birdseed a., Staib a.

bismuth sulfite (BS) a., an agar culture medium containing beef extract, peptone, glucose, sodium sulfite, bismuth ammonium citrate, and brilliant green, used to isolate *Salmonella* species, especially *S. typhi*, from stool and other clinical specimens. Called also *Wilson-Blair c.*

blood a. (BA), an agar medium containing heart infusion, peptone, and sodium chloride, autoclaved and enriched by the addition of sterile defibrinated blood, used for primary plating and subculturing, especially to determine bacterial hemolysis. The blood used may be sheep (for group A *Streptococcus*), rabbit (for *Haemophilus parahemolyticus*), or horse.

Bordet-Gengou (B-G) a., an agar base containing potato infusion, glycerol, and sodium chloride, enriched with blood, used for the isolation of *Bordetella pertussis* and *B. parapertussis*.

brain-heart infusion (BHIA) m., an agar medium containing calf brain and beef heart infusion, peptone, glucose, and phosphate buffer; sheep blood may also be added. It is used for the cultivation of bacteria, actinomycetes, and fungi. A broth medium without the agar is used for cultivating the pneumococcus for the bile solubility test.

brilliant green (BG) a., a highly selective primary isolation medium containing yeast extract, peptone, lactose, sucrose, sodium chloride, phenol red, and brilliant green in an agar base, used for the culture of salmonellae other than *Salmonella typhi*.

Brucella a., an agar medium containing pancreatic digest of casein, peptic digest of animal tissue, yeast autolysate, and dextrose, for the culture and isolation of *Brucella*. It may be supplemented by the addition of sheep blood and vitamin K_1 solution for the isolation of anaerobic bacteria.

buffered glycerol-saline ba. (Sachs), a broth medium containing sodium chloride, phosphate buffer, phenol red, and glycerol, used to transport and preserve fecal specimen material.

Campylobacter m., an agar medium containing pancreatic casein digest, peptic digest of animal tissues, yeast autolysate, glucose, sodium chloride, and sodium bisulfite, supplemented with sheep erythrocytes, vancomycin, trimethoprim, polymyxin, amphotericin, and cephalothin; used for isolating *Campylobacter* from specimens of fecal origin.

carbohydrate b., a broth medium that contains heart infusion or peptone, sodium chloride, and an indicator supplemented with a single carbohydrate, used to test the ability to ferment various sugars.

Cary-Blair transport m., an agar medium containing thioglycollate, phosphate, and sodium choride, used for the collection and holding of clinical specimens containing gram-negative facultative organisms. The medium may be supplemented with calcium chloride, sodium bisulfite, and resazurin for culture of anaerobes.

casein a., a medium containing dehydrated skim milk and agar, used for differentiation of *Nocardia* and *Streptomyces*.

cetrimide a., an agar medium containing peptone, magnesium chloride, potassium sulfate, cetrimonium hydrochloride (cetrimide), and sometimes glycerol, used for the differentiation of strains of *Pseudomonas*.

charcoal a., a beef heart infusion–peptone culture medium containing soluble starch, yeast extract, and charcoal. The base medium is supplemented with sheep blood and cephalexin for the selective culture of *Bordetella pertussis*.

charcoal-yeast extract (CYE) a., an agar medium containing activated charcoal, L-cysteine, ferric pyrophosphate, and yeast extract, used for the culture of *Legionella*.

charcoal-yeast extract diphasic blood culture m. (CYE-DBCM), a diphasic medium consisting of a lower solid slant containing charcoal and agar, partially covered with a liquid broth containing yeast extract, L-cysteine, and ferric nitrate. It is used for the culture of *Legionella*.

chlamydospore a., an inorganic salt medium containing polysaccharide, biotin, and trypan blue, for the identification of *Candida albicans* by favoring the formation of chlamydospores which are stained blue by the dye.

chocolate a., an agar medium containing casein digest, peptone, cornstarch, sodium chloride, and phosphate buffer; sterile hemoglobin or fresh blood is added and the medium heated until the color is chocolate brown. Other agar media may also be used as the base. It is used for the isolation of fastidious organisms, e.g., *Haemophilus influenzae* and *Neisseria* species.

chopped meat (CM) b., a liquid medium containing chopped meat treated with sodium hydroxide, casein digest,

yeast extract, phosphate buffer, and cysteine; it may also include hemin, vitamin K_1 glucose, and resazurin. It is used for the cultivation of anaerobic bacteria, especially *Clostridium* species.

citrate a. (Simmons), an agar medium containing sodium citrate, sodium chloride, magnesium sulfate, homothymol blue, and phosphate buffer, used to determine the ability of gram-negative bacilli, particularly the Enterobacteriaceae, to utilize citrate as the sole carbon source.

Columbia colistin-nalidixic acid (CNA) a., an agar medium containing peptone, cornstarch, sodium chloride, colistin, nalidixic acid, and sheep blood, used for the selective culture of gram-positive cocci, especially *Proteus* species.

corn meal a., an agar medium containing corn meal infusion, used to stimulate sporulation in the identification of fungi. With the addition of Tween 80 it stimulates the production of chlamydospores by species of *Candida*. It may also be supplemented with dextrose, sucrose, and yeast extract for the general culture of fungi.

cycloserine cefoxitin fructose egg yolk a. (CCFA), an agar medium containing peptone, sodium chloride, magnesium sulfate, fructose, neutral red, and phosphate buffer, supplemented with cycloserine, cefoxitin, and egg yolk, used as a selective medium for *Clostridium difficile*.

cystine-heart a., an agar medium containing beef heart infusion, peptone, glucose, sodium chloride, and L-cystine. The medium is supplemented with hemoglobin for the in vitro conversion of dimorphic hyaline molds.

cystine-tellurite a., an agar medium containing meat infusion, potassium tellurite, cystine, and agar enriched with blood, used for the isolation of *Corynebacterium diphtheriae*.

cystine trypticase a. (CTA), an agar medium containing cystine, pancreatic digest of casein, sodium chloride, sodium sulfite, and phenol red, an aerobic differential medium for the general culture of pathogenic bacteria, including fastidious organisms. It may be supplemented with specific sugars and used to test fermentation reactions in *Neisseria* species.

Czapek-Dox a., an agar medium containing sucrose, sodium nitrate, magnesium sulfate, potassium chloride, ferrous sulfate, and potassium buffer, used for the culture of *Nocardia*, *Streptomyces*, and fungi. Called also *Czapek-Dox c.* and *Czapek solution a.*

Czapek solution a., Czapek-Dox a.

decarboxylase b., a liquid culture medium containing beef extract, peptone, and dextrose, to which is added an amino acid (commonly lysine, arginine, or ornithine), for the determination of the amino acid decarboxylase activity as a differential character of bacteria, especially Enterobacteriaceae.

deoxycholate citrate (Leifson) (LDC) a., an agar medium containing meat infusion, peptone, lactose, sodium and ferric citrates, sodium deoxycholate, and neutral red, used for the primary culture and isolation of *Salmonella* and *Shigella*.

deoxycholate (Leifson) (LD) a., an agar medium containing peptone, lactose, sodium citrate, ferric citrate, sodium chloride, sodium deoxycholate, neutral red, and potassium buffer, used for the isolation of Enterobacteriaceae and differentiation of lactose-fermenting and non–lactose-fermenting species.

differential c., a culture medium, usually solid, that reveals the presence of two or more similar microorganisms by differences in the appearance of their colonies. Such a medium may or may not be selective also.

DNase test a., an agar medium containing deoxyribonucleic acid, peptone, sodium chloride, and toluidine blue, used for differentiating strains of *Serratia*, *Enterobacter*, and *Staphylococcus*.

egg-yolk a. (EYA), an agar medium containing peptone, phosphate buffer, sodium chloride, magnesium sulfate, glucose, and egg-yolk emulsion, used for the culture of *Bacillus anthracis*. When supplemented with hemin or yeast extract it may be used for the culture of *Clostridium* and for the demonstration of lecithinase and lipase activity.

enriched c., a basic medium to which specific nutrients, e.g., serum, blood, and vitamins, have been added to promote the growth of particular organisms.

eosin–methylene blue (EMB) a., an agar medium containing peptone, lactose, eosin Y, methylene blue, and dipotassium phosphate; sucrose may be added. It is used for the primary isolation of species of Enterobacteriaceae.

esculin c., an agar medium containing heart infusion, peptone, sodium chloride, ferric citrate, and esculin, used to differentiate *Escherichia* from *Shigella*.

FDA m., 1. antibiotic c. 3 FDA. 2. antibiotic c. 12 FDA.

Feeley-Gorman (F-G) a., an agar medium containing casein hydrolysate, beef extract, starch, L-cysteine, and ferric pyrophosphate, used for the culture of *Legionella*. A broth culture without the agar is also used for the same purpose.

fermentation m., a basal medium containing no carbohydrate to which is added a single sugar to be tested for fermentability.

Fildes enrichment a., a sterile enzymatic digest of sheep blood added to liquid or solid culture media for the cultivation and isolation of *Haemophilus influenzae* and fastidious streptococci.

Fletcher m., a liquid culture medium containing peptone, and beef extract enriched with 20 per cent fresh pooled rabbit serum, for the isolation, cultivation, and maintenance of *Leptospira*.

gelatin c., a medium containing extract or infusion broth solidified with 12 per cent gelatin, used to determine gelatinase activity in the identification of *Serratia* and *Clostridium*. The medium may be supplemented with thioglycollate for cultivation of *Clostridia* in an aerobic environment.

gram-negative (GN) b., a liquid medium containing peptone, glucose, D-mannitol, sodium citrate, sodium desoxycholate, sodium chloride, and phosphate buffer, used as an enrichment medium for the primary culture of salmonellae and shigellae in fecal specimens.

heart infusion a., an agar medium containing beef heart infusion, peptone, and sodium chloride, used as a base for blood agar and esculin agar.

Hektoen enteric (HE) a., an agar medium containing peptone, bile salts, yeast extract, lactose, sucrose, salicin, sodium chloride, sodium thiosulfate, ferric ammonium citrate, acid fuchsin, and bromthymol blue. It is a selective medium used for the primary isolation and identification of enteric pathogens, especially coliform organisms, salmonellae, and shigellae.

infusion m., a medium containing infusion of fresh meat (commonly veal or beef), peptone, and sodium chloride, used as a liquid medium (broth) or solidified with agar, used for the culture of fastidious bacteria and as a base for enrichment media.

kanamycin-vancomycin blood a. (KVBA), an agar medium containing casein digest, soymeal digest, sodium chloride, yeast extract, sheep blood, L-cystine, vitamin K_1, kanamycin, and vancomycin, used for selective isolation of anaerobes, particularly *Bacteroides*.

kanamycin-vancomycin laked blood (KVLB) a., an agar medium having the same ingredients as kanamycin-vancomycin blood agar except that the blood is laked (hemolyzed) by freezing and thawing. It is used to isolate the *Bacteroides melaninogenicus* group.

Kligler iron a., triple sugar iron agar.

laked blood (LB) a., a solid culture medium containing blood that has been hemolyzed to release hemin.

litmus-milk c., milk culture medium containing sufficient litmus solution to give it a deep lavender color, used to determine lactose fermentation and production of gas in the identification of *Clostridium perfringens*.

Littman a., an agar medium containing peptone, oxgall, dextrose, and crystal violet. Streptomycin may be added to inhibit bacteria, and the medium may be supplemented with birdseed extract. It is used for the isolation and culture of fungi.

Loeffler coagulated serum m., a culture medium containing veal infusion, beef serum, and glucose, solidified by coagulation of the serum, used for the isolation of *Corynebacterium diphtheriae*.

Löwenstein-Jensen c., a solid medium containing asparagine, potato flour, glycerol, magnesium sulfate, malachite green, magnesium citrate, and whole eggs, used for the primary isolation of mycobacteria; the medium is solidified by heat coagulation of the egg.

lysine-iron a. (LIA), an agar medium containing peptone, yeast extract, glucose-, L-lysine, ferric ammonium citrate, sodium thiosulfate, and bromcresol purple, used to determine lysine decarboxylase and lysin deaminase in the Enterobacteriaceae, especially for the genera *Proteus* and *Providencia*.

MacConkey (MC) a., an agar medium containing peptone, lactose bile salts, sodium chloride, neutral red, and crystal violet, used to differentiate lactose fermenters (coliforms) from nonlactose fermenters among the enteric bacilli.

malt extract a., an agar medium containing malt extract, peptone, and dextrose, used for the cultivation of yeasts and molds.

mannitol salt a., an agar medium containing beef extract, peptone, mannitol, phenol red, and 7.5 per cent sodium chloride, used for the selective isolation of pathogenic staphylococci.

Martin-Lester a., Martin-Lewis a., a modification of chocolate agar containing antibiotics, used for the transport and primary isolation of *Neisseria gonorrhoeae* and *N. meningitidis*.

McBride Listeria m., an agar medium containing peptone, beef extract, sodium chloride, glycine anhydride, lithium chloride, and phenylethanol, used for the cultivation of *Listeria*.

meat extract m., one prepared with an extract from meat.

meat infusion m., see *infusion m.*

methylene blue milk c., a liquid medium containing skim milk powder and methylene blue, used in the identification of *Streptococcus*.

methyl red–Voges-Proskauer (MR-VP) b., a broth culture medium containing peptone, glucose, and phosphate, used for the culture of coliform bacteria and differentiation by the methyl red and Voges-Proskauer tests.

Middlebrook 7H10 a., a complex agar medium containing ammonium sulfate, D-glutamic acid, sodium citrate, ferric ammonium phosphate, magnesium sulfate, pyridoxine, biotin, malachite green, and phosphate buffer. OADC enrichment, containing oleic acid, albumin, glucose, and beef catalase, is added. The medium is used for the primary isolation of mycobacteria and for antimicrobial susceptibility testing.

milk c., fresh or dehydrated skim milk used as a culture medium. See also *litmus milk c.* and *methylene blue milk c.*

motility test m., a culture medium containing beef extract and peptone, partially solidified by the inclusion of 0.4 per cent agar, used for the detection of motility of Enterobacteriaceae. A medium containing pancreatic casein digest, yeast extract, sodium chloride, and 0.3 per cent agar is used to determine motility in nonfermenting gram-negative bacteria.

MR-VP b., methyl red–Voges-Proskauer b.

Mueller-Hinton m., an agar medium containing beef infusion, peptone, and starch, used for the primary isolation of *Neisseria gonorrhoeae* and *N. meningitidis*, and for antibiotic and sulfonamide susceptibility testing. A broth medium (MHB), prepared by omitting the agar, is used to determine antibiotic susceptibility by broth dilution testing.

Mueller Hinton-IH a., an agar medium containing beef infusion, casein hydrolysate, starch, hemoglobin and a complex enrichment supplement, used for the culture of *Legionella*.

Mycoplasma isolation c., an agar medium containing beef heart infusion, peptone, sodium chloride, horse serum, yeast extract, and penicillin; thallium acetate and amphotericin B may also be added to reduce bacterial and fungal contamination. A broth culture is made by omitting the agar. It is used for the culture and isolation of mycoplasmas.

nitrate b., nutrient broth containing sodium nitrate, for testing for the bacterial reduction of nitrate to nitrite.

nutrient c., a bacterial culture medium containing beef extract and peptone, used as a liquid medium (nutrient broth) or solidified with agar (nutrient agar, plain agar) for the culture of nonfastidious organisms.

NYC (New York City) m., an agar medium containing protease peptone, cornstarch, phosphate buffer, horse plasma, hemoglobin, glucose, yeast dialysate, vancomycin, colistin, nystatin or amphotericin, and trimethoprim lactate, used as a selective medium for *Neisseria*.

nystatin assay a., antibiotic c. 12 FDA.

oxidation-fermentation (OF) m., an agar medium containing peptone, sodium chloride, bromthymol blue, potassium buffers, and glucose; lactose, mannitol, or sucrose may be used instead of glucose. The medium is used to distinguish oxidative from fermentative utilization of carbohydrates, a characteristic used to differentiate *Acinetobacter*, *Alcaligenes*, and *Pseudomonas* from the Enterobacteriaceae.

peptone–yeast extract–glucose (PYG) m., a liquid medium containing peptone, yeast extract, glucose, resazurin, L-cysteine, and salts, used as a transport medium for anaerobes. It may be supplemented with hemin and vitamin K_1, and used to prepare broth cultures of anaerobes for gas-liquid chromatography.

Petragnani c., a culture medium containing milk, potato flour, potato, whole egg and egg yolk, and malachite green, for the culture of tubercle bacilli; the medium is solidified by heat coagulation of the egg.

phenol red m., a liquid medium containing peptone, sodium chloride, and phenol red, used as a base medium supplemented with various sugars for determining fermentation reactions.

phenylalanine a., an agar medium containing yeast extract, DL-phenylalanine, disodium phosphate, and sodium chloride, used to test for phenylalanine deaminase activity by members of the Enterobacteriaceae, especially species of *Proteus* and *Providencia*.

phenylethyl alcohol (PEA) blood a., an agar medium containing pancreatic digest of casein, papaic digest of soya meal, sodium chloride, and phenylethyl alcohol. Defibrinated blood may be added. It is used for the isolation of gram-positive cocci, especially in a mixed culture containing *Proteus* or other gram-negative bacilli.

potato blood a., Bordet-Gengou a.

potato dextrose a., a culture medium containing potato infusion and dextrose, for culturing and inducing sporulation in molds.

PRAS m., prereduced and anaerobically sterilized media, used for the culture of anaerobes. See *Cary-Blair transport m.* and *peptone-yeast extract glucose m.*

purple broth ba., a broth medium containing peptone, beef extract, sodium chloride, and bromocresol purple, used as a base to which is added a sugar supplement for use in fermentation studies.

rice grain m., a medium containing water and polished white rice that is autoclaved; used for the differentiation of species of *Microspora* and other dermatophytes.

Rogosa selective Lactobacillus (SL) a., a selective culture medium containing tryptone, yeast extract, glucose, arabinose, sucrose, acetate, citrate, and sorbitan monooleate, phosphate buffer, and agar, used in the culture and presumptive identification of lactobacilli.

Sabhi [Sabouraud dextrose and brain heart infusion] a., an agar medium containing brain infusion, heart infusion, gelatin digest, glucose, sodium chloride, peptone, and phosphate buffer; chloramphenicol may be added. It is used for isolating clinically important fungi.

Sabouraud dextrose (SAB) a., an agar medium containing dextrose, peptone, pancreatic digest of casein, and peptic digest of animal tissue; antibiotics may be added. Used for the cultivation and identification of fungi.

Salmonella-Shigella (SS) a., a selective differential culture medium containing beef extract, peptone, lactose, bile salts, sodium and ferric citrates, thiosulfate neutral red, and brilliant green, used for the primary isolation of enteric bacilli, especially *Salmonella* and *Shigella*.

selective c., a liquid or solid culture medium that contains inhibitory substances (antibiotics, dyes, tellurite, bile salts, etc.) that allow the growth of the desired microorganism while inhibiting the growth of contaminants.

selenite b., a liquid medium containing peptone, lactose, phosphate, and sodium selenite, used as an enrichment medium for the isolation of *Salmonella* and *Shigella*.

semisolid c., 1. a culture medium containing 0.3 to 0.5 per cent agar to give it a semisolid consistency; see *motility test medium.* 2. a culture medium containing agar or gelatin that is liquid in the warm state and solid when cooled.

sodium chloride (6.5 per cent) c., a broth medium containing beef heart infusion, peptone, and 6.5 per cent sodium chloride, used for the selective culture of enterococci (especially group D streptococci) and other salt-tolerant organisms. Nutrient broth or soybean-casein digest agar supplemented with 6.5 per cent sodium chloride is also used for *Pseudomonas* and other nonfermenting gram-negative bacteria.

soybean casein digest a., an agar medium containing pancreatic casein digest, papaic soy meal digest, and sodium chloride, used as a general purpose primary isolation medium and as a base for blood agar.

Staib a., an agar medium containing an extract of *Guizottia abyssinica* seeds, creatinine, dextrose, chloramphenicol, and diphenyl, used for the identification of the yeast *Cryptococcus neoformans*. Called also *birdseed a.*

starch a. an agar medium containing peptone, beef extract, sodium chloride, and soluble starch, used for determining hydrolysis of starch. Bromcresol purple may be included for identification of *Haemophilus vaginalis*.

Stuart b., modified, a culture medium containing inorganic salts, asparagine, and glycerol, enriched with rabbit serum and used for the isolation and culture of *Leptospira*.

tellurite taurocholate gelatin a. (TTGA), a selective agar medium containing sodium taurocholate, potassium tellurite, and sodium carbonate, used for the isolation of *Vibrio*.

tetrathionate b., a liquid medium containing peptone, bile salts, calcium carbonate, and sodium thiosulfate, which is converted to tetrathionate by the addition of iodine immediately before use, used as a selective medium for the isolation of *Salmonella* other than *S. typhi*.

Thayer-Martin (TM) a., chocolate agar enriched with vitamins and other supplements, to which is added antibiotic inhibitors (vancomycin, colistin, and nystatin), used for the transport and primary culture of *Neisseria gonorrhoeae* and *N. meningitidis*.

thioglycollate (THIO) b. a liquid medium containing peptone, glucose, sodium chloride, sodium thioglycollate, L-cystine, sodium sulfite, and 0.7 per cent agar, enriched with rabbit serum. It is used as a general utility medium for the growth of both aerobic and anaerobic bacteria. Methylene blue may be added as a redox indicator, and the medium may be enriched with yeast extract, vitamin K₁, and hemin.

thiosulfate citrate bile salts sucrose (TCBS) a., a selective medium containing peptone, yeast extract, citrate, thiosulfate, oxgall, sodium cholate, sucrose, sodium chloride, ferric citrate bromthymol blue, and thymol blue, used for the isolation of *Vibrio cholerae* and *V. parahaemolyticus*.

Tindale's a., a base composed of proteose-peptone, sodium chloride, and agar to which is added as enrichment of bovine serum, L-cystine, sodium thiosulfate, and potassium tellurite; used to detect *Corynebacterium diphtheriae*, which form grayish-black colonies surrounded by a black halo.

Todd-Hewitt b., a liquid medium containing beef heart infusion, peptone, glucose, sodium chloride, sodium bicarbonate, and phosphate buffer, used for growing streptococci for serological grouping.

transport m., a medium used for transport of clinical specimens for bacteriological examination. See *Amies transport m., buffered glycerol-saline ba., Cary-Blain transport m.,* and *peptone yeast extract glucose m.*

triple sugar iron (TSI) a., an agar medium containing peptone, lactose, sucrose, dextrose, ferrous ammonium sulfate, sodium thiosulfate, sodium chloride, and phenol red, used for the preliminary screening of Enterobacteriaceae. Production of hydrogen sulfide causes the formation of black ferrous sulfide along the stab line, gas production causes bubbles in the agar, and fermentation of the sugars is indicated by the amount of acid produced.

trypticase soy b. with agar, a medium containing a trypsin digest of soy meal, peptone, sodium chloride, phosphate buffer, and glucose with 0.1 per cent agar, used for the primary culture of fastidious bacteria, including anaerobes.

tyrosine xanthine a., an agar medium containing nutrient agar and tyrosine or xanthine, used for differentiation of species of aerobic actinomycetes.

urea (Christensen's) a., an agar medium containing peptone or gelatin digest, sodium chloride, dextrose, phenol red, urea, and phosphate buffer, used to detect urease production, especially in enteric bacteria (e.g., species of *Proteus*), *Cryptococcus*, and *Aerobic actinomyces*. See also *urease test b.*

urease test b., a liquid medium containing yeast extract, urea, phenol red, and phosphate buffer, used to determine urease activity in the differentiation of *Proteus* from *Salmonella* and *Shigella* in enteric infections. See also *urea (Christensen's) a.*

veal infusion c., see *infusion m.*

Wilson-Blair c., bismuth-sulfite a.

xylose-lysine-deoxycholate (XLD) a. an agar medium containing xylose, L-lysine, lactose, sucrose, sodium chloride, yeast extract, phenol red, sodium desoxycholate, sodium thiosulfate, and ferric ammonium citrate, used for isolating intestinal pathogens, especially *Shigella* and *Salmonella*.

yeast extract a. an agar medium containing yeast extract and phosphate buffer, used for identification of *Histoplasma capsulatum*, *Blastomyces dermatidis*, and *Coccidiodes immitis*.

---

cumidine (ku′mĭ-din) chemical name: 4-amino-1-isopropylbenzene. A liquid base, C₃H₇·C₆H₄·NH₂, derived from cumic acid.

cu. mm. cubic millimeter.

cumulative (ku′mu-la″tiv) [L. *cumulus* heap] increasing by successive additions, the total being greater than the expected sum of its parts.

cumuli (ku′mu-li) [L.] genitive and plural of *cumulus.*

cumulus (ku′mu-lus), pl. *cu′muli* [L.] a little mound. **c. ooph′orus** [NA], **ovarian c., c. ova′ricus,** a solid mass of follicular cells surrounding the ovum in the side of a developing vesicular ovarian follicle: called also *discus oophorus, ovigerus,* or *proligerus;* and *germ* or *germ-bearing hillock.*

cuneate (ku′ne-āt) [L. *cuneus* wedge] wedge-shaped.

cunei (ku′ne-i) [L.] genitive and plural of *cuneus.*

cuneiform (ku-ne′ĭ-form) [L. *cuneus* wedge + *forma* form] shaped like a wedge.

cuneocuboid (ku″ne-o-ku′boid) pertaining to the cuneiform and cuboid bones.

cuneonavicular (ku″ne-o-nah-vik′u-lar) pertaining to the cuneiform and navicular bones.

cuneoscaphoid (ku″ne-o-skaf′oid) cuneonavicular.

cuneus (ku′ne-us), pl. *cu′nei* [L. "wedge"] a wedge-shaped lobule of the occipital lobe of the cerebrum on its medial aspect, between the parietooccipital and calcarine sulci.

cuniculi (ku-nik′u-li) [L.] genitive and plural of *cuniculus.*

cuniculus (ku-nik′u-lus), pl. *cunic′uli* [L. "rabbit," "rabbit-burrow"] the burrow of an itch mite, *Sarcoptes scabiei,* in the skin.

Cunila (ku-ni′lah) a genus of labiate plants. *C. origanoides* (L.) Butt., of North America (dittany), is the source of a diuretic and diaphoretic tea used by American Indians and early settlers.

cunnilinctus (kun″ĭ-link′tus) cunnilingus.

cunnilingus (kun″ĭ-ling′gus) [L. *cunnus* vulva + *lingere* to lick] oral stimulation of the female genitalia.

cunnus (kun′us) [L.] pudendum femininum.

CuO cupric oxide.

Cu₂O cuprous oxide.

cuorin (ku′o-rin) a mono-aminodiphosphatide lipoid compound isolated from the heart muscle.

cup (kup) 1. a cupping glass. 2. a cup-shaped part or structure. **Diogenes c.,** poculum Diogenis. **dry c.,** a cupping glass applied to the intact skin in order to induce a flow of blood to the area; no longer used. **glaucomatous c.,** a form of ocular disk depression peculiar to glaucoma; called also *glaucomatous excavation.* **Montgomery's c's** (*obs.*), the dilated canals of the tubular glands of the uterus. **optic c.,** 1. physiologic cup. 2. caliculus ophthalmicus. **optic c., ophthalmic c.,** caliculus ophthalmicus. **physiologic c.,** a depression in the center of the optic disk; called also *excavatio disci nervi optici* [NA] and *optic c.* **wet c.,** a cupping glass applied to the incised skin in order to abstract blood; no longer used.

cupola (ku′po-lah) cupula.

cupped (kupt) hollowed out like a cup.

cupping (kup′ing) 1. the application of a cupping glass. 2. the formation of a cup-shaped depression. **pathologic c.,** depression of the optic disk due to disease.

cuprammonia (ku″prah-mo′ne-ah) Schweitzer's reagent.

cupremia (ku-pre′me-ah) [L. *cuprum* copper + Gr. *haima* blood + *-ia*] the presence of copper in the blood.

cupric (ku′prik) containing copper in its divalent form (> Cu), and yielding divalent ions (Cu⁺⁺) in aqueous solution. For cupric compounds, see under the salt, e.g., sulfate.

Cuprimine (kup′rĭ-mēn) trademark for a preparation of penicillamine.

cuprimyxin (kup″rĭ-mik′sin) chemical name: bis(6-methoxy-1-phenazinol-5,10-dioxidato-O^1,O^{10})copper; a veterinary antibacterial and antifungal, $C_{26}H_{18}CuN_4O_8$.

cupriuria (ku″pre-u′re-ah) the presence of copper in the urine.

cuprous (ku′prus) containing copper in its monovalent form (Cu⁺).

cupruresis (ku″proo-re′sis) [L. *cuprum* copper + Gr. *ourēsis* a making water] the urinary excretion of copper.

cupruretic (ku″proo-ret′ik) [L. *cuprum* copper + Gr. *ourētikos* promoting urine] pertaining to or promoting the urinary excretion of copper.

cupula (ku′pu-lah), pl. *cu′pulae* [L.] a small inverted cup or dome-shaped cap over some structure. **c. of ampullary**

crest, c. cristae ampullaris. **c. of cochlea, c. coch′leae** [NA], the rounded or dome-shaped apex of the spiral cochlear duct. **c. cris′tae ampulla′ris** [NA], a cap of viscid, gelatinous fluid over the crista of the ampulla of the ear; in fixed material this cap stains slightly and is thus differentiated from the rest of the ampullar fluid. Called also *c. of ampullary crest.* **c. of pleura, c. pleu′rae,** [NA], **c. pleura′lis,** the domelike roof of the pleural cavity on either side, extending up through the superior aperture of the thorax.

cupulae (ku′pu-le) [L.] genitive and plural of *cupula.*

cupulogram (ku′pu-lo-gram″) the record, in the form of a tracing, made during cupulometry.

cupulolithiasis (ku″pu-lo-lĭ-thi′ah-sis) the presence of calculi in the cupula of the posterior semicircular duct, a cause of benign paroxysmal positional vertigo.

cupulometry (ku″pu-lom′e-tre) a method of testing vestibular function in which subjects are accelerated and decelerated in a rotational chair and the duration of postrotational vertigo and nystagmus are plotted against angular deceleration.

curare (koo-rah′re) [South American] a term applied to a wide variety of highly toxic extracts from numerous botanical sources, including various species of *Strychnos;* used originally as arrow poisons in South America. A form extracted from *Chondodendron tomentosum* has been used for the reduction of spasms in tetanus and in shock treatments, in plastic muscular rigidity, spastic paralysis, and similar conditions, and also as an adjunct to general anesthesia. Cf. *tubocurarine.*

curaremimetic (koo-rah″re-mi-met′ik) having an action similar to that of curare, or producing similar effects.

curari (koo-rah′re) curare.

curariform (ku-ra′rĭ-form) resembling curare.

curarization (ku″rar-i-za′shun) administration of curare until the physiologic effect of the drug is produced.

curative (kūr′ah-tiv) [L. *curare* to take care of] tending to overcome disease and promote recovery.

curb (kurb) a thickening of the metatarsocalcaneal ligament of the horse, causing a swelling at the back of the hock joint and resulting in lameness.

curcumin (kur′ku-min) an orange-yellow, crystalline substance, $C_{21}H_{20}O_6$, which is the coloring principle of turmeric.

curd (kurd) the coagulum of milk, consisting mainly of casein. **alum c.,** a coagulum formed by agitating milk containing a piece of alum. **alum c. of Riverius,** a coagulum prepared with white of an egg and dram of alum.

cure (kūr) [L. *curatio,* from *cura* care] 1. the course of treatment of any disease, or of a special case. 2. the successful treatment of a disease or wound. 3. a system of treating diseases. 4. a medicine effective in treating a disease. 5. the preservation of a product, such as tobacco, meat, or fish. 6. the hardening of a material by the process of curing. 7. a procedure for polymerization of the resinous denture base material. See also *curing.* **rest c.,** (*obs.*), Weir Mitchell treatment. **water c.,** hydropathy.

curet (ku-ret′) [Fr. *curette* scraper] 1. a spoon-shaped instrument for removing material from the wall of a cavity or other surface. 2. to remove growths or other material from the wall of a cavity or other surface with a spoon-shaped instrument. **Hartmann's c.,** an instrument for removing adenoids.

curettage (ku″rĕ-tahzh′) [Fr.] the removal of growths or other material from the wall of a cavity or other surface, as with a curet; called also *curettement.* **apical c.,** periapical c. **gingival c.,** removal with a curet of the inflamed tissue wall of a periodontal pocket, including junctional and pocket epithelium and immediately underlying connective tissue. Called also *subgingival c.* **medical c.,** the induction of bleeding from the endometrium by administration and withdrawal of any progestational agent. **periapical c.,** removal with a curet of diseased pathological soft tissues in the bony crypt surrounding a tooth root apex and smoothing of the apical surface of a tooth without excision of the tooth tip. Called also *apical c.* **subgingival c.,** 1. gingival curettage apical to the epithelial attachment to sever the connective tissue attachment down to the osseous crest without reflection of a flap. 2. gingival c. **suction c.,** vacuum c. **surgical c.,** a flap procedure to excise an inflamed periodontal pocket wall and the connective tissue attachment down to the osseous crest, followed by reattachment of the flap to the teeth. Called also *modified Widman flap.* **ultrasonic c.,** removal of inflamed tissue from the tooth surface and wall of the gingival crevice with an ultrasonic scaler. **vacuum c.,** removal of the uterine contents, after cervical dilation, by means of a hollow curet introduced into the uterus, through which suction is applied. Called also *suction c.* and *vacuum aspiration.*

curette (ku-ret′) [Fr.] curet.

curettement (ku-ret′ment) curettage. **physiologic c.,** enzymatic débridement.

curie (ku′re) [Marie Sklodowska *Curie,* Polish chemist in Paris, 1867–1934, the discoverer of radium, and Pierre *Curie,* 1859–1906, co-winners, with A. H. Becquerel, of the Nobel prize in physics for 1903, for studies on spontaneous radioactivity; Mme. Curie also received the Nobel prize in chemistry in 1911 for discovery and isolation of radium] a unit of radioactivity, defined as the quantity of any radioactive nuclide in which the number of disintegrations per second is 3.700×10^{10}. Abbreviated Ci (formerly c).

Curie's law, therapy (ku′rez) [Pierre *Curie,* French scientist, 1859–1906] see under *law* and *therapy.*

curie-hour (ku′re-owr″) a unit of cumulated radioactivity equal to the presence of 1 curie for 1 hour. Abbreviated Ci-hr.

curietherapy (ku″re-ther′ah-pe) originally, radium or radon therapy; but now applied to therapy given by emanations from any radioactive source.

curing (kūr′ing) a method for promoting and accelerating hardening processes through the use of dampness, heat, cold, or chemical or other agent. **denture c.,** the process by which resinous denture base materials are polymerized or hardened.

curioscopy (ku″re-os′ko-pe) the detection and mapping of objects by means of the nuclear radiations coming from them.

curium (ku′re-um) [Pierre and Marie *Curie*] the chemical element of atomic number 96, atomic weight 247, symbol Cm, obtained by cyclotron bombardment of uranium and plutonium.

curling (kur′ling) shaped like a curl or coil, as the appearance of the esophagus in diffuse esophageal spasm.

Curling's ulcer (kur′lingz) [Thomas Blizard *Curling,* English physician, 1811–1888] see under *ulcer.*

current (kur′ent) [L. *currens* running] 1. anything that flows. 2. the stream of electricity that moves along a conductor. An electric current is due to a difference of potential between two points, this difference being measured in volts. The volume of flow depends on the difference of potential and the resistance to be overcome and is measured in amperes. The quantity of current is measured in coulombs. **abnerval c.,** an electric current passing from a nerve to and through a muscle. **action c.,** the current generated in a cell membrane of a nerve or muscle by the action potential; it serves to depolarize adjacent membrane areas beyond the threshold, thus initiating a repetition of the action potential process along the nerve fiber. Called also *nerve-action c.* **alternating c.,** a current that periodically flows in opposite directions. Abbreviated A.C. **ascending c.,** centripetal c. **axial c.,** the central colored part of the blood current. **centrifugal c.,** an electric current in the body with the positive pole near the nerve center and the negative at the periphery; called also *descending c.* **centripetal c.,** an electric current passing through the body with the positive electrode on the nerve or at the periphery and the negative near the nerve center: called also *ascending c.* **coagulating c.,** an electric current applied by a needle, ball, or other type of electrode to coagulate tissue. **compensating c.,** an electric current for neutralizing the intensity of a muscle current. **d'Arsonval c.,** a high-frequency, low-voltage current of comparatively high amperage. See also *high-frequency c.* **demarcation c.,** c. of injury. **descending c.,** centrifugal c. **De Watteville c.,** a combined galvanic and faradic current. **direct c.,** a current that flows in one direction only. When used medically it is called the galvanic current; this current has distinct and important polarity and marked secondary chemical effects. **electric c.,** the flow of electricity through a conductor. **electrotonic c.,** a current induced in the sheath of a nerve by a current passing through the conducting part of that nerve, or by an action potential in an adjacent nerve. **fulguration c.,** high-frequency current used in destruction of super-

ficial skin lesions. **galvanic c.,** a steady direct current. **high-frequency c.,** an alternating current having a frequency of interruption or change of direction sufficiently high so that tetanic contractions are not set up when it is passed through living contractile tissues; see *d'Arsonval c.* **induced c.,** electricity in a circuit generated by proximity to another current, i.e., by induction. **c. of injury,** the current flowing between pathologically depolarized areas of excitable tissue (as of the heart) and the normally polarized areas, the injury tissue being negative with respect to the normal tissue. Called also *demarcation c.* **Leduc c.,** an interrupted direct current, each pulse of which is approximately of the same current strength and same duration; formerly used as a general anesthetic agent. **Morton's c.** (*obs.*), a type of alternating high-frequency current produced by a static machine; called also *static induced c.* **nerve-action c.,** action c. **Oudin c.,** a high-frequency current of higher voltage than the high-frequency currents used for ordinary diathermy treatment. **saturation c.,** the amount of current in an x-ray tube when the voltage is sufficient to drive all the electrons produced from the cathode filament to the anode as fast as they are produced. **static induced c.,** Morton's c. **surgical c.,** an electric current used to achieve surgical dissection or fulguration. **Tesla's c.** (*obs.*), a high-frequency current of higher voltage than that of the high-frequency currents used for ordinary diathermy treatment, but not so high as that of the Oudin current.

curricula (kur-rik′u-lah) [L.] plural of *curriculum.*

curriculum (kur-rik′u-lum), pl. *curric′ula* [L.] a regular and established course of study.

Curschmann's disease, mask, spiral (koorsh′manz) [Heinrich *Curschmann,* physician in Leipzig, 1846–1910] see *perihepatitis chronica hyperplastica,* and see under *mask* and *spiral.*

curse (kers) an infliction thought to be invoked by a malevolent spirit. **Ondine's c.,** impairment of automatic control of respiration, sometimes due to encephalitis, with voluntary control remaining intact.

Curtius' syndrome (kur′ti-us) [Friedrich *Curtius,* German internist, born 1896] see under *syndrome.*

curtometer (kur-tom′e-ter) (*obs.*) cyrtometer.

curvatura (kur″vah-tu′rah), pl. *curvatu′rae* [L.] [NA] a nonangular deviation from a straight course in a line or surface. **c. gas′trica ma′jor** [NA], greater gastric curvature: the left or lateral and inferior border of the stomach, marking the inferior junction of the anterior and posterior surfaces. Called also *c. ventriculi major* [NA alternative] and *greater curvature of stomach.* **c. gas′trica minor** [NA], lesser gastric curvature: the right or medial border of the stomach, marking the superior junction of the anterior and posterior surfaces. Called also *c. ventriculi minor* [NA alternative] and *lesser curvature of stomach.* **c. ventric′uli ma′jor,** NA alternative for *c. gastrica major.* **c. ventric′uli mi′nor,** NA alternative for *c. gastrica minor.*

curvature (kur′vah-tūr) [L. *curvatura*] deviation from a rectilinear direction. **compensating c.,** see under *curve.* **greater gastric c., greater c. of stomach,** curvatura gastrica major. **lesser gastric c., lesser c. of stomach,** curvatura gastrica minor. **occlusal c.,** curve of occlusion; see under *curve.* **Pott's c.,** abnormal posterior curvature of the vertebral column caused by tuberculous caries. **Spee's c., c. of Spee,** see under *curve.* **spinal c.,** deviation of the spine from its normal direction or position; see *kyphosis, lordosis, scoliosis.*

curve (kurv) [L. *curvum*] a nonangular deviation from a straight course in a line or surface. **alignment c.,** the dental curve determined by a line passing through the center of the teeth and paralleling the dental arch. **anti-Monson c.,** reverse c. **audibility c.,** a plotting of the relationship between frequency and the intensity of sound waves necessary to elicit a sensation. **Barnes's c.,** the segment of a circle whose center is the promontory of the sacrum, the concavity being directed dorsally. **bell-shaped c.,** the curve of the probability density function of the normal distribution (q.v.). **Bragg c.,** a curve showing the increase in intensity of ionization produced by an ionizing particle as it loses velocity and energy; see also *Bragg peak,* under *peak.* **buccal c.,** the portion of the curve of occlusion from the mesial surface of the first premolar to the distal surface of the third molar. **c. of Carus,** the normal axis of the pelvic outlet; called also *circle of Carus*. **compensating c.,** the curve introduced in the construction of artificial dentures to compensate for the opening influence produced by the condylar and incisal guidances during lateral and protrusive mandibular excursive movements. Called also *compensating curvature.* **Damoiseau's c.,** Ellis' line. **dental c.,** c. of occlusion. **dissociation c., oxygen,** oxygen-hemoglobin dissociation c. **dose-effect c., dose-response c.,** a curve indicating the relationship between dose of radiation and the degree of a particular biological effect produced. **dromedary c.,** a temperature or other curve showing two phases of elevation separated by a phase of depression. **dye-dilution c.,** a graph representing the concentration of a fixed dose of a dye (as in the systemic circulation) at specific time intervals; used in studies of cardiac output. **c. of Ellis and Garland,** Ellis' line. **Garland's c.,** Ellis' line. **gaussian c.,** bell-shaped c. **growth c.,** the curve obtained by plotting increase in size or numbers against the elapsed time, as a measure of the growth of a child, or the multiplication of microorganisms. **Harrison's c.,** see under *groove.* **isodose c's,** diagrams delimiting body areas receiving equal quantities of radiation in radiotherapy. **Kaplan-Meier survival c.,** a consistent estimate of the survival curve that can be computed from randomly censored data. At each patient death (or other endpoint) the conditional probability of survival during the interval since the last death is calculated as the number of patients observed to survive beyond that point (i.e., those who have not yet died and have not left the trial for other reasons) divided by the number at risk, which is one more than the numerator. The value of the survival curve at that point is calculated as the product of the conditional probabilities of survival for all of the intervals up to that point. Called also *product-limit estimate.* **labial c.,** that portion of the curve of occlusion between the distal surfaces of the two canine teeth in the dental arch. **logistic c.,** an S-shaped curve that describes population growth under limiting conditions as a function of time; when the population is low, growth begins slowly, then becomes rapid and increases exponentially, finally slowing down and reaching equilibrium as the population reaches the maximum that the environment can support. **Monson c.,** a curve of occlusion conforming to a segment of the surface of a sphere 8 inches in diameter, with its center in the region of the glabella. See also *compensating c.* **muscle c.,** myogram. **normal c., normal c. of distribution,** bell-shaped c. **c. of occlusion,** 1. a curved surface that makes simultaneous contact with major portions of the incisal and occlusal prominences of the existing teeth. 2. the curve of a dentition on which the occlusal surfaces lie. Called also *dental c.* and *occlusal curvature.* **oxygen dissociation c., oxygen-hemoglobin dissociation c., oxyhemoglobin dissociation c.,** a graphic curve representing the normal variation in the amount of oxygen which combines with hemoglobin as a function of the partial pressures of oxygen and carbon dioxide. The dissociation curve is said to shift to the right when less than a normal amount of oxygen is taken up by the blood at a given Po_2, and to shift to the left when more than a normal amount is taken up. Factors influencing the shape of the curve include changes in the blood pH, Pco_2, and temperature, the presence of carbon monoxide, alterations in the constituents of the erythrocytes, and certain disease states. **Price-Jones c.,** a frequency distribution curve of erythrocyte diameters in a peripheral blood smear, estimated visually with the aid of an optical micrometer. **pulse c.,** sphygmogram. **regression c.,** see *regression,* def. 5. **reverse c.,** in excessive wear of the teeth, obliteration of the cusps and formation of either flat or cupped-out occlusal surfaces, associated with reversal of the occlusal plane of the premolar and first and second molar teeth, so that the occlusal surfaces of the mandibular teeth slope facially instead of lingually, and those of the maxillary teeth incline lingually. Called also *anti-Monson c.* **Spee c., c. of Spee,** anatomic curvature of the occlusal alignment of teeth, beginning at the tip of the lower canine, following the buccal cusps of the natural premolars and molars, and continuing to the anterior border of the ramus. Called also *Spee's curvature* and *curvature of Spee.* **survival c.,** a graph of the probability of survival versus time, commonly used to present the results of clinical trials, e.g., a graph of the fraction of patients surviving (until death, relapse, or some other defined endpoint) at each time after a certain therapeutic procedure. **temperature c.,** a graphic tracing showing variations in

body temperature. **tension c's,** lines observed in the arrangement of the cancellous tissue of bones, depending on the directions of tension exerted on the bones. **visibility c.,** a plotting of the relationship between wavelength and the intensity of light necessary to elicit a sensation. **Wunderlich's c.,** the typical variation shown by the temperature in a patient with typhoid fever.

cuscamidine (kus-kam′ĭ-din) a cinchona alkaloid.

cuscamine (kus-kam′in) a cinchona alkaloid.

cuscohygrine (kus-ko-hi′grin) an alkaloid, $C_{13}H_{24}ON_2$, from cusco leaves; called also *belladine.*

Cushing's disease, etc. (koosh′ingz) [Harvey Williams *Cushing,* Boston surgeon, 1869–1939] see under *disease, law, phenomenon,* and *syndrome.*

Cushing's suture (koosh′ingz) [Hayward W. *Cushing,* Boston surgeon, 1854–1934] see under *suture.*

cushingoid (koosh′ing-oid) resembling the features, symptoms, and signs associated with Cushing's syndrome.

cushion (koosh′un) a fleshy, padlike anatomical structure. **coronary c.,** see under *band.* **digital c.,** a wedge-shaped mass of white and elastic fibers, containing fat and cartilage, overlying the frog of a horse's foot. **endocardial c's,** elevations on the atrioventricular canal of the embryonic heart, which later fuse with the free edge of the septum primum to separate the right and left atria. **c. of epiglottis,** 1. petiolus epiglottidis. 2. tuberculum epiglotticum. **eustachian c., c. of eustachian orifice,** torus tubarius. **intimal c's,** longitudinal thickenings of the intima of certain arteries, e.g., the penile arteries, formed by prominent local concentrations of smooth muscle fibers; they serve functionally as valves, controlling blood flow by occluding the lumen of the artery. **Passavant's c.,** see under *bar.* **plantar c.,** a wedge-shaped mass of elastic tissue overlying the frog of a horse's foot. **sucking c.,** corpus adiposum buccae.

cuskohygrine (kus″ko-hi′grin) cuscohygrine.

cusp (kusp) [L. *cuspis* point] a tapering projection; especially one of the triangular segments of a cardiac valve (see under *cuspis*), or a dental cusp (see *cuspis dentalis* [NA]). **aortic c.,** cuspis anterior valvae atrioventricularis sinistrae. **Carabelli c.,** an accessory cusp on the lingual aspect of the mesiolingual cusp of an upper molar, which may be unilateral or bilateral and may vary considerably in size; present in some form in most Caucasians, but virtually never present in those of the Mongoloid race. Called also *Carabelli's tubercle.* **dental c.,** cuspis dentalis. **semilunar c.,** any of the semilunar segments of the aortic valve (having posterior, right, and left cusps) or the pulmonary valve (having anterior, right, and left cusps); called also *valvula semilunaris.*

cuspid (kus′pid) 1. having one cusp or point. 2. a canine tooth.

cuspidate (kus′pĭ-dāt) [L. *cuspidatus*] having a cusp or cusps.

cuspides (kus′pĭ-dēz) [L.] plural of *cuspis.*

cuspis (kus′pis), pl. *cus′pides* [L.] 1. a tapering projection or structure, applied especially to one of the triangular segments of a cardiac valve. 2. c. dentalis. **c. ante′rior val′vae atrioventricula′ris dex′trae** [NA], the anterior of the cusps of the right atrioventricular valve; called also *c. anterior valvulae tricuspidalis.* **c. ante′rior val′vae atrioventricula′ris sinis′trae** [NA], the anterior of the cusps of the left atrioventricular valve; called also *c. anterior valvulae bicuspidalis* and *aortic cusp.* **c. ante′rior val′vulae bicuspida′lis,** c. anterior valvae atrioventricularis sinistrae. **c. ante′rior val′vulae tricuspida′lis,** c. anterior valvae atrioventricularis dextrae. **c. coro′nae,** c. dentalis. **c. denta′lis** [NA], dental cusp: an elevation or mound on the crown of a tooth making up part of the occlusal surface; called also *cuspis coronae* and *dental tubercle.* See also *tuberculum dentale.* **c. media′lis val′vulae tricuspida′lis,** c. septalis valvae atrioventricularis dextrae. **c. poste′rior val′vae atrioventricula′ris dex′trae** [NA], the posterior of the cusps of the right atrioventricular valve; called also *c. posterior valvulae tricuspidalis.* **c. poste′rior val′vae atrioventricula′ris sinis′trae** [NA], the posterior of the cusps of the left atrioventricular valve; called also *c. posterior valvulae bicuspidalis.* **c. poste′rior val′vulae bicuspida′lis,** c. posterior valvae atrioventricularis sinistrae.

c. poste'rior val'vulae tricuspida'lis, c. posterior valvae atrioventricularis dextrae. **c. septa'lis val'vae atrioventricula'ris dex'trae** [NA], the cusp of the right atrioventricular valve which is attached to the membranous interventricular septum; called also *c. medialis valvulae tricuspidalis.*

cutaneous (ku-ta'ne-us) [L. *cutis* skin] pertaining to the skin; dermal; dermic.

cutdown (kut'down) creation of a small, incised opening, especially over a vein (venous cutdown), to facilitate venipuncture and permit the passage of a needle or cannula for the withdrawal of blood or administration of fluids.

Cuterebra (ku-ter-e'brah) a genus of botflies of the family Oestridae (often included in the family Cuterebridae), whose larvae commonly infest rodents.

Cuterebridae (ku"te-reb'rĭ-de) a family of New World batflies (order Diptera), the larvae of which parasitize various mammals, including man.

cuticle (ku'te-kl) [L. *cuticula,* from *cutis* skin] 1. a layer of more or less solid substance which covers the free surface of an epithelial cell. 2. eponychium (def. 1). **dental c.,** cuticula dentis. **enamel c.,** primary c. **primary c.,** a film on the enamel of unerupted teeth, considered to be the final product of degenerating ameloblasts after completion of enamel formation; electron microscopy shows it to consist primarily of ameloblasts of the reduced enamel epithelium attached to the enamel by a basal lamina. Called also *enamel c.* Cf. *cuticula dentis.* **c. of root sheath,** a layer of cells lining the hair follicles. **secondary c.,** cuticula dentis.

cuticula (ku-tik'u-lah), pl. *cutic'ulae* [L. "little skin"] 1. a horny secreted layer. 2. (*obs.*) epidermis. **c. den'tis** [NA], dental cuticle: a film occurring on some teeth on both the enamel and the cementum, external to the primary cuticle, with which it combines, being deposited by the epithelial attachment as it migrates along the tooth and separates from the crown and root. It is not present on cementum to which the periodontal ligament is not attached. Some authorities consider it to be a nonkeratinized product of the epithelial attachment cells, probably contributed by the gingival fluid and saliva; others consider it as a pathologic product of inflamed gingiva, or a conglutinate of erythrocytes. Called also *secondary cuticle* and *Nasmyth's membrane.* Cf. *primary cuticle,* under **cuticle.**

cuticulae (ku-tik'u-le) [L.] genitive and plural of *cuticula.*

cuticulin (ku-tik'u-lin) a lipoprotein containing a large amount of fatty material, which is a constituent of the epicuticle and procuticle of certain arthropods and crustaceans.

cuticulum (ku-tik'u-lum) cuticula. **Flechsig's c.,** a layer of flat cells on the external surface of the neuroglia.

cutidure (ku'tĭ-dūr) coronary band.

cutiduris (ku"tĭ-du'ris) coronary band.

cutin (ku'tin) [L. *cutis* skin] a waxy substance which, combined with cellulose, forms the cuticle of plants.

cutireaction (ku"tĕ-re-ak'shun) [L. *cutis* skin + *reaction*] cutaneous reaction. **von Pirquet c.,** Pirquet reaction.

cutis (ku'tis) [L.] [NA] the skin: the outer protective covering of the body, consisting of the epidermis and dermis, or corium, and resting upon the subcutaneous tissues. **c. anseri'na** [L. "goose skin"], a transitory localized change in the skin surface caused by elevation of the hair follicles as a result of contraction of the arrectores pilorum muscles, a reflection of sympathetic nerve discharge. Called also *goose flesh.* **c. elas'tica,** Ehlers-Danlos syndrome. **c. hyperelas'tica,** Ehlers-Danlos syndrome. **c. lax'a,** a group of connective tissue disorders in which the skin hangs in loose pendulous folds, believed to be associated with decreased elastic tissue formation as well as an abnormality in elastin formation, and usually occurring as a genetic disorder and occasionally in an acquired form. The *congenital form,* which is present at birth or develops during the early months of life, is transmitted as: an autosomal recessive trait, associated with severe complications, including pulmonary and cardiovascular manifestions, diverticula of the urinary and gastrointestinal tracts, and multiple hernias; an autosomal dominant trait, which is essentially benign, being only of cosmetic significance; or an X-linked recessive trait, which is associated with a decrease in the activity of lysyl oxidase, the enzyme responsible for the formation of aldehyde groups, which are essential for collagen cross linkages. The X-linked type is probably identical with Ehlers-Danlos syndrome IX. Affected individuals characteristically have a prematurely aged appearance, hooked nose with everted nostrils, long upper lip, everted lower eyelids, and sagging cheeks. The *acquired form,* which is often preceded by a vague febrile illness, usually presents after puberty but sometimes does not appear until middle age or later. Called also *chalastodermia, chalazodermia, dermatochalasis, dermatochalazia, dermatolysis, dermatomegaly, generalized elastolysis,* and *lax* or *loose skin.* **c. marmora'ta,** a transient form of livedo reticularis occurring as a normal response to cold. Called also *marble skin.* Cf. *livedo reticularis.* **c. rhomboida'lis nu'chae,** actinic elastosis occurring chiefly in men, in which the skin of the nape of the neck becomes thickened, tough, leathery, yellowish in color, and furrowed, acquiring a rhomboidal pattern. **c. ver'ticis gyra'ta,** thickening of the skin of the scalp, most often involving the vertex, and forming folds and furrows resembling sulci and gyri of the brain. It may occur alone or it may be characteristic of another condition, such as pachydermoperiostosis. Called also *gyrate scalp.*

cuvette (ku-vet') [Fr. dim. of *cuve* vat or tub] a glass container, generally possessing well-defined characteristics with regard to dimensions (particularly thickness) and optical properties, and generally used to examine colored and colorless solutions free of turbidity, but also used to examine the light scattering of turbid suspensions, such as bacterial suspensions. Its area of usefulness is determined to a large extent by the chemical composition of the glass: a *silica cuvette* is used for examination of materials in the ultraviolet region of the spectrum; a *Pyrex cuvette* is used for examination of materials in the visible range.

Cuvier's canal, duct (sinus) (koo've-āz) [Georges Léopold Chrétien Frédéric Dagobert, Baron de la *Cuvier,* French naturalist, 1769–1832] see *ductus venosus,* and see under *duct.*

CV cardiovascular; coefficient of variation.

C.V. abbreviation for L. *cras ves'pere,* tomorrow evening, and L. *conjuga'ta ve'ra,* true conjugate diameter of the pelvic inlet.

CVA costovertebral angle; cerebrovascular accident; cardiovascular accident.

CVB a regimen of CCNU (lomustine), vinblastine, and bleomycin, used in cancer chemotherapy.

C.V.O. abbreviation for L. *conjuga'ta ve'ra obstet'rica,* obstetric conjugate diameter of the pelvic inlet.

CVP 1. central venous pressure. 2. a regimen of cyclophosphamide, vincristine, and prednisone, used in cancer chemotherapy.

CVS cardiovascular system.

Cwt. hundredweight.

Cx. cervix; convex.

Cy symbol for *cyanogen.*

cyanamide (si-an'ah-mīd) 1. carbamic acid nitril, $CN \cdot NH_2$ or $NH \cdot C \cdot NH$, the anhydride of urea. 2. calcium cyanamide.

cyanate (si'ah-nāt) a salt of cyanic acid which contains the radical CNO.

cyanhematin (si"an-hem'ah-tin) a compound of cyanogen and hematin.

cyanhemoglobin (si"an-he"mo-glo'bin) the complex of cyanide and hemoglobin.

cyanide (si'ah-nīd) the CN^- anion or a salt containing this ion; all cyanides are extremely toxic; see *cyanide poisoning* under *poisoning.* **mercuric c.,** a colorless, very poisonous salt, $Hg(CN)_2$.

cyanin (si'ah-nin) a coumarin glycoside, $C_{27}H_{30}O_{16}$; its aglycon is cyanidin, and it is used as an indicator with a pH of 7 to 8.

cyanmethemoglobin (si"an-met"he-mo-glo'bin) a tightly bound complex of methemoglobin with the cyanide ion. The standard method of hemoglobinimetry is spectrophotometric determination of cyanmethemoglobin, which is produced quantitatively from oxyhemoglobin, deoxyhemoglobin, carboxyhemoglobin, and methemoglobin, but not sulfhemoglobin, by addition of Drabkin's solution.

cyanmetmyoglobin (si"an-met-mi"o-glo'bin) a compound formed from metmyoglobin by addition of the cyanide ion to yield reduction to the ferrous state.

cyan(o)-, [Gr. *kyanos* blue] a combining form denoting blue.

cyanoalcohol (si″ah-no-al′ko-hol) cyanohydrin.

Cyanobacteria (si″ah-no-bak-te′re-ah) [*cyano-* + *bacteria*] a subgroup of bacteria of the class Oxyphotobacteria, kingdom Procaryotae, comprising the blue-green bacteria, and composed of unicellular or filamentous phototrophic organisms that use water as an electron donor and produce oxygen in the presence of light. Cells are enclosed by a rigid wall containing peptidoglycan, are generally motile, and reproduce by fission. Photopigments include chlorophyll *a* and phycobilin proteins. Cyanobacteria are the only organisms that fix both carbon dioxide (in the presence of light) and nitrogen. Most species are photosynthetic and many are strong nitrogen fixers. These organisms are often used as indicators of eutrophication of lakes and streams. Called also *Cyanophyceae, Schizophyceae,* and formerly *blue-green algae.*

cyanocobalamin (si″ah-no-ko-bal′ah-min) a water-soluble hematopoietic vitamin (vitamin B₁₂), $C_{63}H_{88}CoN_{14}O_{14}P$, found in the liver, fish meal, eggs, and other natural products, or produced from cultures of *Streptomyces griseus*, which combines with intrinsic factor for intestinal absorption and which is needed for maturation of erythrocytes. Absence of intrinsic factor leads to malabsorption of cyanocobalamin and results in pernicious anemia. The official preparation, prepared in accordance with USP specifications, is used in the prophylaxis and treatment of pernicious anemia and other macrocytic anemias, usually administered intramuscularly or subcutaneously. Called also *antipernicious anemia factor, extrinsic factor,* and *LLD factor.* See also *Castle's factor,* under *factor.* **radioactive c.,** cyanocobalamin in which a portion of the molecules contain cobalt of mass number 57 (⁵⁷Co), 58 (⁵⁸Co), or 60 (⁶⁰Co), used as a diagnostic aid in pernicious anemia.

cyanocrystallin (si″ah-no-kris′tal-lin) a blue coloring matter from the integument of decapods.

cyanoform (si-an′o-form) a crystalline substance, CH(CN)₃, formed by the action of potassium cyanide on chloroform.

cyanogen (si-an′o-jen) [*cyano-* + Gr. *gennan* to produce] the radical CN—; also NCCN (dicyanogen dicyan, ethanedinitrile), the latter an exceedingly poisonous gas. Symbol Cy. **c. bromide,** a highly toxic lacrimatory war gas, BrCN. **c. chloride,** a gas, ClCN, used for fumigating houses, ships, etc. It is as lethal for rats and other vermin as hydrocyanic acid, but less dangerous to man, as it also causes lacrimation, which makes it useful as a warning gas in fumigants.

cyanogenesis (si″ah-no-jen′ĕ-sis) [*cyano-* + Gr. *genesis* production] the formation or production of cyanogen or hydrocyanic acid.

cyanogenetic (si″ah-no-jĕ-net′ik) producing cyanogen or hydrocyanic acid.

cyanohydrin (si″ah-no-hi′drin) a compound formed by the addition of hydrocyanic acid to the aldehyde or ketone group; called also *cyanoalcohol.*

cyanolabe (si′ah-no-lāb″) [*cyano-* + Gr. *lambanein* to take] name proposed for the pigment in retinal cones that is more sensitive to the blue range of the spectrum than are the other retinal pigments. Cf. *chlorolabe* and *erythrolabe.*

cyanophil (si-an′o-fil) 1. cyanophilous. 2. a cell or other histologic element readily stainable with blue.

cyanophilous (si″ah-nof′ĭ-lus) [*cyano-* + Gr. *philein* to love] stainable with blue dyes.

cyanophoric (si″ah-no-fōr′ik) yielding hydrocyanic acid; e.g., the glycoside amygdalin yields HCN on hydrolysis.

cyanophose (si′ah-no-fōz) [*cyano-* + Gr. *phōs* light] a blue phose.

Cyanophyceae (si″ah-no-fi′se-e) [*cyano-* + Gr. *phykos* seaweed] Cyanobacteria.

cyanopsia (si″ah-nop′se-ah) [*cyano-* + *-opsia*] a chromatopsia in which all objects appear to have a blue tinge.

cyanopsin (si″ah-nop′sin) [*cyano-* + Gr. *opsis* vision] a visual pigment of bluish tint found in the retinal cones of some animals and important for vision.

cyanose (si′ah-nōs″) [Fr.] cyanosis. **c. tardive′,** tardive cyanosis.

cyanosed (si′ah-nōsd) cyanotic.

cyanosis (si″ah-no′sis) [Gr. *kyanos* blue] a bluish discoloration, applied especially to such discoloration of skin and mucous membranes due to excessive concentration of reduced hemoglobin in the blood. **autotoxic c.,** enterogenous c. **central c.,** cyanosis produced as a result of arterial unsaturation, the aortic blood carrying reduced hemoglobin. **enterogenous c.,** a syndrome due to absorption of nitrites and sulfides from the intestine, principally marked by methemoglobinemia and/or sulfhemoglobinemia associated with cyanosis. It is accompanied by severe enteritis, abdominal pain, constipation or diarrhea, headache, dyspnea, dizziness, syncope, anemia, and, occasionally, digital clubbing and indicanuria. Called also *Stokvis-Talma syndrome, van den Bergh's disease,* and *autotoxic cyanosis.* **false c.,** cyanosis due to the presence of pigment and not to deficient oxygenation of the blood. **hereditary methemoglobinemic c.,** cyanosis caused by a structural variant in the hemoglobin molecule, i.e., one of the M hemoglobins, or by a deficiency of NADH-methemoglobin diaphorase, inherited as an autosomal recessive trait. **c. lie′nis,** passive congestion of the spleen. **peripheral c.,** cyanosis produced as a result of an excessive amount of reduced hemoglobin in the venous blood, caused by extensive oxygen extraction at the capillary level. **pulmonary c.,** central cyanosis caused by poor oxygenation of the blood in the lungs. **c. ret′inae,** distinct cyanosis of the retina, observable in some cases of cyanotic congenital heart disease, patent ductus arteriosus, and other congenital cardiac anomalies. **shunt c.,** central cyanosis caused by mixing of unoxygenated blood with the arterial blood in the heart or great vessels. **tardive c.,** cyanosis in congenital heart disease which appears only after cardiac failure has developed; called also *cyanose tardive.*

cyanotic (si-ah-not′ik) pertaining to or characterized by cyanosis.

Cyantin (si-an′tin) trademark for a preparation of nitrofurantoin.

cyanuria (si″ah-nu′re-ah) the passage of blue urine.

cyanuric acid (si″an-u′rik) a cyclic compound, 2,4,6-trihydroxy-1,3,5-triazine, formed by heating urea.

cyanurin (si″ah-nu′rin) [*cyan-* + Gr. *ouron* urine] indigo blue found in the urine on the addition of a mineral acid to it.

Cyath. abbreviation for L. *cy′athus,* a glassful.

cybernetics (si″ber-net′iks) [Gr. *kybernētēs* helmsman] the science of the processes of communication and control in the animal and in the machine.

CYC cyclophosphamide.

cycasin (si′kah-sin) a toxic principle, methylazoxymethanol β-glucoside, $C_8H_{16}N_2O_7$, from the seeds of *Cycas revoluta* Thumb. and *C. circinalis* L., (Cycadaceae), native to Guam; it is neoplastic to the liver, kidneys, intestine, and lungs after hydrolysis by intestinal bacteria.

cyclacillin (si-klah-sil′in) chemical name: 6-(1-aminocyclohexanecarboxamido) - 3, 3 - dimethyl - 7 - oxo - 4 - thia - 1 - azabicyclo[3.2.0]heptane-2-carboxylic acid; an antibacterial agent, $C_{15}H_{23}N_3O_4S$, effective against a wide range of gram-negative and gram-positive organisms.

Cyclaine (si′klān) trademark for preparations of hexylcaine hydrochloride.

cyclamate (si′klah-māt) any salt of cyclamic acid. Cyclamate calcium and cyclamate sodium were once used widely as non-nutritive sweeteners, but because of an association with bladder tumors in animals they were banned as food additives in the United States in 1969.

Cyclamen (sik′lah-men) [L.] a genus of primulaceous plants. *C. europaeum* L., has an acrid, cathartic root, and is listed as a poisonous plant by European references, although it is a fairly common house plant in the United States.

cyclamic acid (si-klam′ik) the free acid of cyclamate.

cyclamin (sik′lah-min) a glycoside, $C_{20}H_{34}O_{10}$, from *Cyclamen europaeum;* it is strongly purgative and emetic.

Cyclamycin (si′klah-mi″sin) trademark for a preparation of troleandomycin.

cyclandelate (si-klan′dĕ-lāt) chemical name: α-hydroxybenzeneacetic acid 3,3,5-trimethylcyclohexyl ester. An antispasmodic, $C_{17}H_{24}O_3$, with a direct effect on vascular smooth muscle, occurring as a white to pale yellow, crystalline powder; used as a vasodilator mainly in peripheral vascular diseases, administered orally.

cyclarthrodial (sik″lar-thro′de-al) pertaining to a cyclarthrosis.

cyclarthrosis (sik″lar-thro′sis) [Gr. *kyklos* circle + *arthrosis*] a joint that permits rotation.

cyclase (si′klās) an enzyme that catalyzes the formation of a cyclic compound.

cyclazocine (si″klah-zo′sěn) chemical name: 3-(cyclopropylmethyl)-1,2,3,4,5,6-hexahydro -6,11-dimethyl-2,6-methano-benzazocin-8-ol. A narcotic antagonist, $C_{18}H_{25}NO$, which has been used as an analgesic and in the treatment of narcotic dependence.

cycle (si′kl) [Gr. *kyklos* circle] a round or succession of observable phenomena, recurring usually at regular intervals and in the same sequence. **aberrant c.,** one that shows variation in the interval or the sequence of events. **anovulatory c.,** a sexual cycle in which no ovum is discharged. **asexual c.,** generation by budding or division of the parent organism. **biliary c.,** Schiff's biliary c. **Calvin c.,** a dark reaction occurring in photosynthesis in plants in which carbon dioxide is affixed to a five-carbon sugar molecule and subsequently reduced to form other sugars. **carbon c.,** the steps by which carbon (in the form of carbon dioxide) is extracted from the atmosphere by living organisms and ultimately returned to the atmosphere. It comprises a series of interconversions of carbon compounds beginning with the production of carbohydrates by plants during photosynthesis, proceeding through animal consumption, and ending and beginning again in the decomposition of the animal or plant or in the exhalation of carbon dioxide by animals. **cardiac c.,** a complete cardiac movement or heart beat. The period from the beginning of one heart beat to the beginning of the next; the systolic and diastolic movement, with the interval between them. **cell c.,** the cycle of biochemical and morphological events occurring in a reproducing cell population; it consists of: the S *phase,* occurring toward the end of interphase, in which DNA is synthesized; the G_2 *phase,* a relatively quiescent period; the *M phase,* consisting of the four phases of mitosis; and the G_1 *phase* of interphase, which lasts until the S *phase* of the next cycle. **chewing c.,** masticating c. **citrate-pyruvate c.,** the mechanism by which acetyl groups and electrons are moved across the mitochondrial membrane during fatty acid synthesis. **citric acid c.,** tricarboxylic acid c. **Cori c.,** the conversion of glucose residues to lactate in muscles, followed by partial resynthesis of glucose from lactate in the liver and its return to the muscles. **cytoplasmic c.,** that stage in the life of a parasite during which it lives in cytoplasm of the cells of the host. **endogenous c.,** that portion of the life of a parasite which is spent within the body of its host. **estrous c.,** the recurring periods of heat, or estrus, in the adult female of most mammals and the correlated changes in the reproductive tract from one period to the next. See also *metestrus, diestrus,* and *proestrus.* **exogenous c.,** that part of the life of a parasite which is spent outside the body of its definitive host. **forced c.,** a cardiac cycle that is interrupted by a forced beat. **futile c.,** a combination of two or more enzymatic reactions resulting only in the hydrolysis of ATP or other high-energy compound; thermogenesis may result. **gastric c.,** rhythmical alterations in the shape of the stomach due to peristaltic waves. **genesial c.,** the reproductive period of a woman's life. **glucose-lactate c.,** Cori c. **glyoxylate c.,** a metabolic pathway by which certain microorganisms and plants convert fat to carbohydrate, the enzymes of which are contained in microbodies known as *glyoxosomes;* it is a modification of the tricarboxylic acid cycle but differs in that two auxiliary enzymes (isocitratase and malate synthetase) are used and two molecules of acetyl coenzyme A instead of one are required. **gonotrophic c.,** the interval in the life of an insect between the time of feeding to deposition of the ova. **hair c.,** the successive phases in the production of hair, from initiation of its growth to its loss from the follicle, consisting of anagen, catagen, and telogen. **Hodgkin c.,** a regenerative, circular sequence of events between depolarization and permeability to sodium occurring in excitable cells: depolarization increases permeability to sodium, thus increasing the entry of sodium (Na^+) into the cell, and the increased concentration of Na^+ further depolarizes the membrane. **isohydric c.,** the series of chemical reactions in the erythrocyte, in which the uptake of CO_2 and the release of O_2 is accomplished without the production of an excess of hydrogen ions (H^+). **Krebs' c.,** 1. ornithine c.

2. tricarboxylic acid c. **Krebs-Henseleit c.,** ornithine c. **life c.,** the successive events in the life history of an organism; for example, the entire life of a protozoan blood parasite, including the endogenous and exogenous cycles. **mammary c.,** the rhythmic growth of mammary glands after menarche occurring in coordination with the ovarian cycle. **masticating c., masticatory c.,** the complete pathway of the mandible performed in mastication of food. Called also *chewing c.* **menstrual c.,** the period of the regularly recurring physiologic changes in the endometrium, occurring during the reproductive period of human females and a few primates, culminating in partial shedding of the endometrium and some bleeding per vagina (menstruation); see illustration. **mosquito c.,** that period of the life of a malarial parasite that is spent in the body of the mosquito host. **nitrogen c.,** the steps by which nitrogen is extracted from the nitrates of soil and water, incorporated as amino acids and proteins in living organisms, and ultimately reconverted to nitrates: (1) conversion of nitrogen to nitrates by bacteria; (2) the extraction of the nitrates by plants and the building of amino acids and proteins by adding an amino group to the carbon compounds produced in photosynthesis; (3) the ingestion of plants by animals, and (4) the return of nitrogen to the soil in animal excretions or on the death and decomposition of plants and animals. **oogenetic c.,** ovarian c. **ornithine c.,** the cyclic mechanism by which urea is synthesized using ornithine as a carrier. Called also *Krebs c.* and *urea c.* **ovarian c.,** the sequence of physiologic changes in the ovary, including development and rupture of the follicle, discharge of the ovum, and corpus luteum formation and regression; called also *oogenetic c.* **pregnancy c.,** cycle of physiologic changes in reproductive organs during pregnancy. **reproductive c.,** the cycle of physiologic changes occurring in the reproductive organs, from the time of fertilization of the ovum through gestation and parturition. **restored c.,** a cardiac cycle following a returning cycle and taking up the normal rhythm. **returning c.,** a cardiac cycle that begins with an extrasystole. **Schiff's biliary c.,** the cycle in which bile salts in the bile are absorbed by the intestinal villi and are then conveyed back to the liver, where they are used over again; see also *enterohepatic circulation,* under *circulation.* **schizogenic c., schizogenous c.,** the asexual cycle in protozoa during which growth and segmentation occur. **sex c., sexual c.,** 1. the physiologic changes recurring regularly in the genital organs of female mammals when pregnancy does not supervene. 2. the period of sexual reproduction in an organism that also reproduces asexually. **sporogenic c., sporogenous c.,** the sexual cycle in protozoa that is usually passed in another host, often an insect. **tricarboxylic acid c.,** the cyclic metabolic mechanism by which the complete oxidation of the acetyl moiety of acetyl-coenzyme A is effected; see *diagram.* Called also *Krebs' c.* and *citric acid c.* **urea c.,** ornithine c. **uterine c.,** the phenomena occurring in the endometrium during the estrous or menstrual cycle, preparing it for implantation of the blastocyst. **vaginal c.,** the rhythmic alteration occurring in the epithelial lining of the vagina in conjunction with the ovarian cycle.

cyclectomy (sik-lek′to-me) [Gr. *kyklos* circle, ciliary body + *ectomy*] 1. excision of a piece of the ciliary body. 2. excision of a portion of the ciliary border of the eyelid.

cyclencephalus (sik″len-sef′ah-lus) [Gr. *kyklos* circle + *enkephalos* brain] a monster with the cerebral hemispheres blended into one.

cyclic (si′klik, sik′lik) [Gr. *kyklikos*] pertaining to or occurring in a cycle or cycles; the term is applied to chemical compounds that contain a ring of atoms in the nucleus. See *closed chain,* under *chain.*

cyclic AMP cyclic adenosine monophosphate.

cyclic GMP cyclic guanosine monophosphate.

cyclicotomy (sik″le-kot′o-me) cyclotomy.

cyclindole (si-klin′dōl) chemical name: 2,3,4,9-tetrahydro-*N,N*-dimethyl-1*H*-carbazol-3-amine; an antidepressant, $C_{14}H_{18}N_2$.

cyclitis (sik-li′tis) [Gr. *kyklos* ciliary body + *-itis*] inflammation of the ciliary body. **heterochromic c.,** chronic cyclitis producing difference in the color of the two irides, the inflamed eye having the lighter iris. **plastic c.,** cyclitis with exudation of fibrinous matter into the anterior chamber. **pure c.,** inflammation of the ciliary body without involvement of the iris. **purulent c.,** suppuration in the ciliary

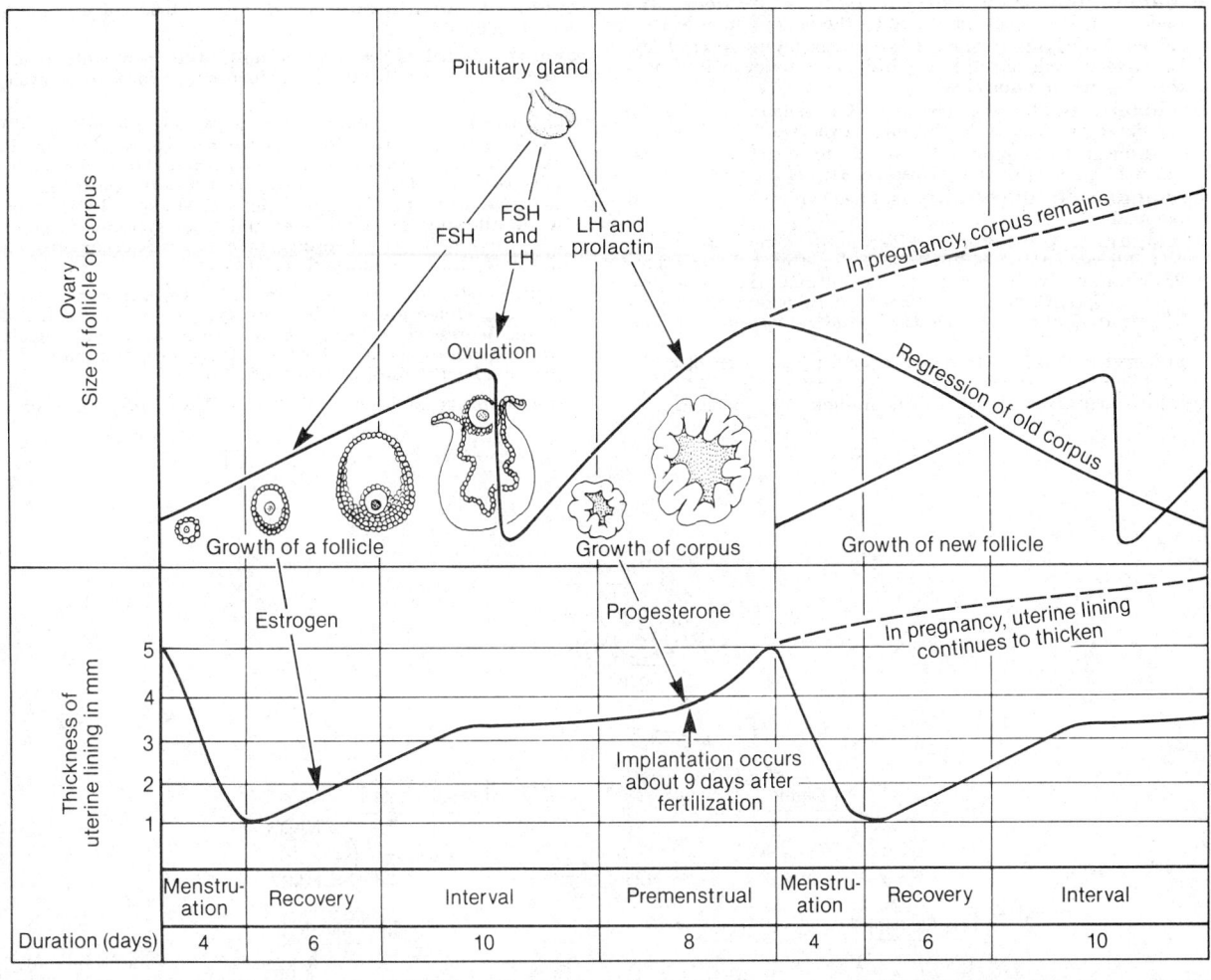

Size of follicle or corpus / Ovary

Thickness of uterine lining in mm

	Menstru-ation	Recovery	Interval	Premenstrual	Menstru-ation	Recovery	Interval
Duration (days)	4	6	10	8	4	6	10

Changes in the menstrual cycle in the human female. Solid lines indicate the course of events when the ovum is not fertilized; dotted lines indicate the course of events when fertilization occurs. Arrows indicate the actions of hormones of the pituitary and the ovary in regulating the cycle.

body; it usually involves the entire uveal tract, constituting endophthalmitis. **serous c.,** simple inflammation of the ciliary body.

cyclizine (si′klĭ-zēn) [USP] chemical name: 1-(diphenyl-methyl)-4-methylpiperazine. An antihistaminic, $C_{18}H_{22}N_2$, occurring as a white, or creamy white, crystalline powder; used in the form of the lactate salt as an antiemetic and antinauseant, especially for the prevention and relief of motion sickness, administered intramuscularly. **c. hy-drochloride** [USP], the monohydrochloride salt of cycli-zine, $C_{18}H_{22}N_2 \cdot HCl$, occurring as a white, crystalline powder or small, colorless crystals, having the same actions and uses as the base; administered orally. **c. lactate,** see *cyclizine*.

cycl(o)- [Gr. *kyklos* circle] a combining form denoting round or recurring; see *cyclic*. Often used with particular reference to the eye, or to the ciliary body of the eye.

cyclobarbital (si″klo-bar′bĭ-tal) chemical name: 5-(1-cy-clohexen-1-yl)-5-ethylbarbituric acid. A short-acting barbitu-rate, $C_{12}H_{16}N_2O_3$, mainly used as a hypnotic; administered orally. **c. calcium,** the calcium salt of cyclobarbital, $C_{24}H_{30}CaN_4O_6$, having actions and uses similar to those of the base; administered orally.

cyclobendazole (si″klo-ben′dah-zōl) chemical name: [5-(cyclopropylcarbonyl)-1*H*-benzimidazol-2-yl]carbamic acid methyl ester; an anthelmintic, $C_{13}H_{13}N_3O_3$.

cyclobenzaprine hydrochloride (si″klo-ben′zah-prēn) [USP] chemical name: 3-(5*H*-dibenzo[*a,d*]cyclohepten-5-ylidene)-*N*, *N*-dimethyl-1-propanamine hydrochloride; a muscle relaxant, $C_{20}H_{21}N \cdot HCl$.

cyclocephalus (si″klo-sef′ah-lus) [*cyclo-* + Gr. *kephalē* head] a cyclops.

cycloceratitis (si″klo-ser″ah-ti′tis) cyclokeratitis.

cyclochoroiditis (si″klo-ko″roid-i′tis) [*cyclo-* + *choroid*] inflammation of the choroid and ciliary body.

cyclocryotherapy (si″klo-kri″o-ther′ah-pe) [*cyclo-* + *cryo-therapy*] freezing of the ciliary body; done in the treat-ment of glaucoma.

cyclocumarol (si″klo-koo′mah-rōl) chemical name: 3,4-di-hydro-2- methoxy- 2- methyl- 4- phenyl- 2*H*, 5*H*-pyrano[3, 2-c] [1]benzopyran-5-one; an anticoagulant, $C_{20}H_{18}O_4$.

cyclodamia (si″klo-da′me-ah) [*cyclo-* + Gr. *damazein* to sub-due] subdued or suppressed accommodation of the eyes.

cyclodialysis (si″klo-di-al′ĭ-sis) [*cyclo-* + *dialysis*] the op-erative formation of a communication between the anterior chamber of the eye and the suprachoroidal space; done in the treatment of glaucoma.

cyclodiathermy (si″klo-di′ah-ther″me) [*cyclo-* + *diathermy*] destruction of a portion of the ciliary body by diathermy; employed as therapy in cases of glaucoma.

cycloduction (si″klo-duk′shun) [*cyclo-* + *duction*] the duction of the eyeball produced by the oblique muscle.

cycloelectrolysis (si″klo-e″lek-trol′ĭ-sis) [*cyclo-* + *electrolysis*] electrolysis of the ciliary body, used to lower intraocular pressure in glaucoma.

cyclogeny (si-kloj′ĕ-ne) [*cyclo-* + Gr. *gennan* to produce] the developmental cycle of a microorganism.

cyclogram (si′klo-gram) a graph or chart of the visual field made with the cycloscope (1st def.).

cycloguanide embonate (si-klo-gwan′īd) cycloguanil pamoate.

cycloguanil pamoate (si-klo-gwan′il) chemical name: 1-(4-chlorophenyl)-1,6-dihydro-6, 6-dimethyl-1,3,5-triazine-2,4-diamine. A metabolite of the antimalarial drug proguanil, $C_{45}H_{44}Cl_2N_{10}O_6$, and itself having potent antimalarial effects. Called also *c. embonate* and *cycloguanide embonate*.

Cyclogyl (si′klo-jil) trademark for a preparation of cyclopentolate hydrochloride.

cyclohexanehexol (si″klo-heks″ān-heks′ōl) inositol.

cyclohexanesulfamic acid (si″klo-hek″sān-sul-fam′ik) cyclamic acid.

cyclohexanol (si″klo-hek′sah-nol) the monohydroxy derivative of the saturated six-carbon-ring hydrocarbon cyclohexane.

cycloheximide (si″klo-heks′ĭ-mīd) chemical name: 3-[2-(3,5-dimethyl- 2- oxocyclohexyl)-2- hydroxyethyl]glutarimide. An antibiotic substance, $C_{15}H_{23}NO_4$, isolated from *Streptomyces griseus*, and used as an agricultural fungicide and in selective media for fungi. It inhibits most saprophytic fungi, while allowing dermatophytes and most systemic fungi to grow, and inhibits nuclear division of karyotic organisms but has no effect on prokaryotic cells (bacteria).

cycloid (si′kloid) characterized by alternating moods of elation and depression. The terms cycloid, cyclothymic, and manic-depressive overlap in meaning, although cycloid would generally be used for the least severe, and manic-depressive for the most severe conditions.

cycloisomerase (si″klo-i-som′er-ās) [EC 5.5.1] one of a

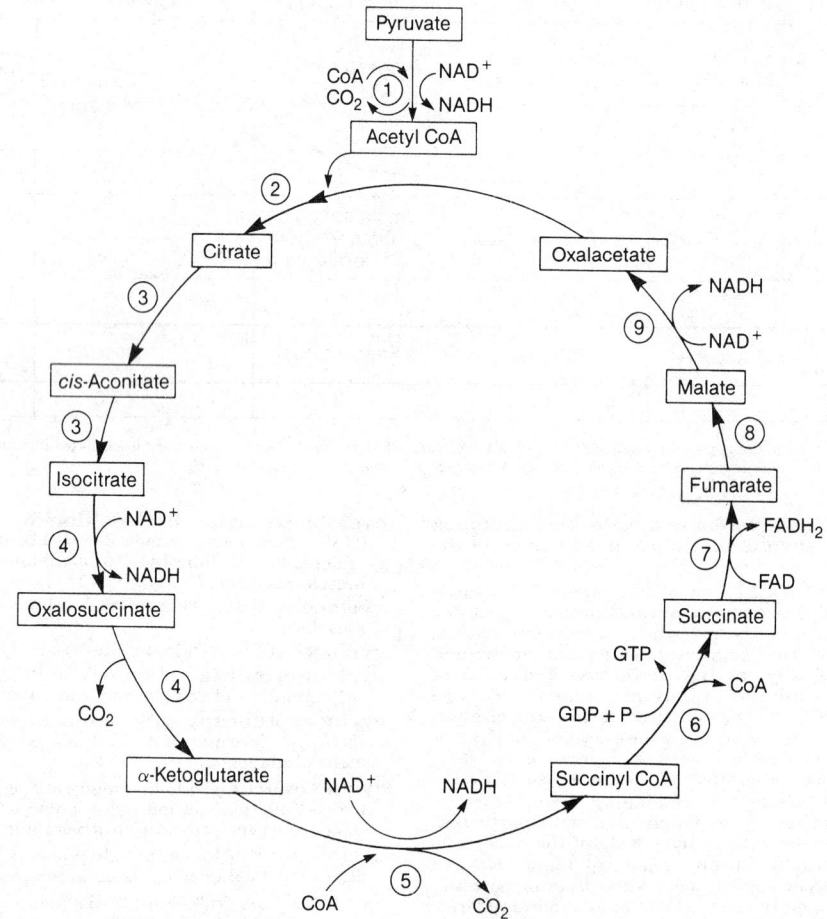

Tricarboxylic acid (Krebs cycle). Diagrammatic representation of reactions by which carbon chains of sugars, fatty acids, and amino acids are metabolized to yield carbon dioxide. Water produced by the cycle and components of the high-energy phosphate pool generated by the associated electron chain are not shown. Key to enzymes (circled numbers): 1 = pyruvate dehydrogenase. 2 = citrate (si)-synthase. 3 = aconitate dehydrogenase. 4 = isocitrate dehydrogenase. 5 = α-ketoglutarate dehydrogenase. 6 = succinyl-CoA ligase (GDP-forming). 7 = succinate dehydrogenase. 8 = fumarate hydratase. 9 = malate dehydrogenase.

sub-subclass of intramolecular lyase enzymes of the isomerase class that catalyze certain rearrangements of a molecule to break or form a ring, e.g., the synthesis of myo-inosital phosphate from glucose 6-phosphate.

cyclokeratitis (si″klo-ker-ah-ti′tis) [cyclo- + keratitis] inflammation of the cornea and ciliary body; called also *Dalrymple's disease.*

cyclo-ligase (si″klo-li′gās) [EC 6.3.3] one of a sub-subclass of enzymes of the ligase (synthetase) class that catalyze the formation of carbon-nitrogen bonds to produce a cyclic compound, driven by the conversion of adenosine triphosphate to adenosine diphosphate.

cyclomastopathy (si″klo-mas-top′ah-the)[cyclo- + Gr. *mastos* breast + *pathos* disease] an affection of the mammae, presenting excessive connective tissue overgrowth or epithelial proliferation or both in response to growth stimuli or as a manifestation of abnormal involution following normal response. Cf. *eccyclomastoma.*

cyclomethycaine sulfate (si″klo-meth′ĭ-kān) [USP] chemical name: 4-(cyclohexyloxy)benzoic acid 3-(2-methyl-1-piperidinyl)propyl ester sulfate (1:1). A local anesthetic, $C_{22}H_{33}NO_3 \cdot H_2SO_4$, occurring as a white, crystalline powder; applied topically to relieve burning, itching, and pain originating in the rectal, vaginal, urethral, or nasal mucous membranes or associated with skin lesions, and also used to facilitate various diagnostic procedures, such as bronchoscopy, sigmoidoscopy, tracheal intubation, etc.

cyclooxygenase (si″klo-ok′sĭ-jĕnās) an activity of prostaglandin endoperoxide synthase (q.v.).

cyclopentamine hydrochloride (si″klo-pen′tah-mēn) [USP] chemical name: N,α-dimethylcyclopentaneethanamine hydrochloride. An adrenergic, $C_9H_{19}N \cdot HCl$, occurring as a white, crystalline powder; used as a vasoconstrictor to reduce nasal congestion, applied topically to the nasal mucous membranes.

cyclopentane (si″klo-pen′tān) a hydrocarbon, C_5H_{10}, in which all five carbon atoms are in a single ring.

cyclopentenophenanthrene (si″klo-pen-tēn″o-fĕ-nan′-thrēn) a polycyclic nucleus present in sterols, bile acids, sex hormones, cardiac poisons, and saponins.

cyclopenthiazide (si″klo-pen-thi′ah-zīd) chemical name: 6-chloro-3-(cyclopentylmethyl)-3,4-dihydro-2H-1,2,4-benzothiadiazine-7-sulfonamide 1,1-dioxide. An orally effective diuretic, $C_{13}H_{18}ClN_3O_4S_2$, used in the treatment of edema associated with various disorders and in hypertension.

cyclopentolate hydrochloride (si″klo-pen′to-lāt) [USP] chemical name: 2-dimethylaminoethyl-1-hydroxy-α-phenyl-cyclopentaneacetate hydrochloride. An anticholinergic, $C_{17}H_{25}NO_3 \cdot HCl$, occurring as a white, crystalline powder; used to produce cycloplegia and mydriasis by instillation into the eye.

cyclophenazine hydrochloride (si″klo-fen′ah-zēn) chemical name: 10-[3-(4-cyclopropyl-1-piperazinyl)propyl]-2-(trifluoromethyl)phenothiazine dihydrochloride; a tranquilizer, $C_{23}H_{26}F_3N_3S \cdot 2HCl$.

cyclophoria (si″klo-fo′re-ah) [cyclo- + phoria] heterophoria in which there is deviation of the eye from the anteroposterior axis in the absence of visual fusional stimuli. See *excyclophoria* and *incyclophoria.* Cf. *cyclotropia.* **accommodative c.,** cyclophoria due to oblique astigmatism. **minus c.,** incyclophoria. **plus c.,** excyclophoria.

cyclophorometer (si″klo-fo-rom′ĕ-ter) [cyclophoria + -meter] an instrument for measuring cyclophoria.

cyclophosphamide (si″klo-fos′fah-mīd) [USP] a cytotoxic alkylating agent of the nitrogen mustard group, used as an antineoplastic, often in combination with other agents, for a wide variety of conditions, including Hodgkin's disease, lymphosarcoma, acute lymphocytic leukemia, Burkitt's lymphoma, carcinoma of the breast, multiple myeloma, chronic lymphocytic leukemia, bronchogenic carcinoma, neuroblastoma, ovarian carcinoma, and carcinoma of the uterine cervix; also used as an immunosuppressive agent to prevent transplant rejection and in the treatment of certain diseases with abnormal immune function. Cyclophosphamide itself is pharmacologically inert; several active metabolites are produced by the microsomal enzyme systems in the liver. Common side effects are nausea and vomiting, bone marrow depression, alopecia, and immunosuppression.

Cyclophyllidea (si″klo-fil-lid′e-ah) an order of tapeworms of the subclass Cestoda, class Cestoidea, comprising seven families that are habitually or accidentally parasitic in man: Taeniidae, Hymenolepididae, Dilepididae, Davaineidae, Anoplocephalidae, Linstowiidae, and Mesocestoididae.

cyclopia (si-klo′pe-ah) [Gr. *kyklos* circle + ōpo eye + -ia] a developmental anomaly characterized by a single orbit, with the globe absent or rudimentary, apparently normal, or duplicated, and the nose absent or present as a tubular appendage located above the orbit.

cyclopin (si′klo-pin) a proteinaceous constituent of *Penicillium cyclopium* that has been shown to inhibit the multiplication of representative members of group A and B arboviruses.

cycloplegia (si″klo-ple′je-ah) [cyclo- + Gr. *plēgē* stroke] paralysis of the ciliary muscle; paralysis of accommodation.

cycloplegic (si″klo-ple′jik) 1. pertaining to, characterized by, or causing cycloplegia. 2. an agent that causes cycloplegia.

cyclopropane (si″klo-pro′pān) [USP] a colorless, flammable gas with a characteristic odor and pungent taste that is an inhalational anesthetic; now little used because of its flammability.

Cyclops (si′klops) a genus of minute crustaceans species of which are hosts to *Dracunculus* and *Diphyllobothrium.*

cyclops (si′klops) [Gr. *kyklōps* one of a race of one-eyed giants] a monster exhibiting cyclopia; called also *cyclocephalus.* **c. hypogna′thus,** a modified cyclops, lacking the typical proboscis, with ears abnormally low, rudimentary mandible, and tiny orifice of the buccal cavity.

cyclose (si′klōs) any of a class of carbohydrates which are polyhydroxy cyclohexanes; they include inositol and phytol.

cycloserine (si″klo-ser′ēn) [USP] a broad-spectrum antibiotic with tuberculostatic activity, produced by growth of *Streptomyces orchidaceus* or obtained by synthesis, occurring as a white to pale yellow, crystalline powder; effective against many gram-negative and gram-positive bacteria, it is used in the treatment of tuberculosis, pulmonary and extrapulmonary, and sometimes in urinary tract infections due to susceptible pathogens, administered orally.

cyclosis (si-klo′sis) [Gr. *kyklōsis* a surrounding, enclosing] movement of the cytoplasm within a cell, without deformation of the cell wall; called also *cytoplasmic* or *protoplasmic streaming.*

cyclospasm (si′klo-spazm) spasm of accommodation of the eyes.

Cyclospasmol (si″klo-spaz′mol) trademark for preparations of cyclandelate.

cyclosporin A (si″klo-spōr′in) cyclosporine.

cyclosporine (si″klo-spōr′in) a cyclic peptide from an extract of soil fungi with immunosuppressant (inhibition of T cell function) and antifungal effects; used to prevent rejection in organ transplant recipients.

cyclostat (si′klŏ-stat) a cylinder of glass in which an experimental animal is rotated about its vertical axis.

cyclotate (si′klo-tāt) USAN contraction for 4-methylbicyclo- [2.2.2]oct-2-ene-1-carboxylate.

cyclotherapy (si″klo-ther′ah-pe) [cyclo- + Gr. *therapeia* treatment] use of the bicycle in treatment.

cyclothiazide (si″klo-thi′ah-zīd) [USP] a thiazide diuretic; used for treatment of hypertension and edema.

cyclothyme (si′klo-thīm) an individual with a cyclothymic personality or exhibiting cyclothymia.

cyclothymia (si″klo-thi′me-ah) [cyclo- + Gr. *thymos* mind] [DSM III-R] a mood disorder characterized by numerous hypomanic and depressive periods with symptoms like those of manic and major depressive episodes but of lesser severity. Called also *affective, cycloid,* or *cyclothymic personality (disorder).*

cyclothymiac (si″klo-thim′e-ak) cyclothymic.

cyclothymic (si″klo-thi′mik) pertaining to or characterized by cyclothymia.

cyclotol (si′klo-tol) a polyhydroxy cyclohexane, such as inositol.

cyclotome (si′klo-tōm) [cyclo- + -tome] a cutting instrument for use in cyclotomy or other operations upon the eye.

cyclotomy (si-klot′o-me) [cyclo- + -tomy] division of or incision of the ciliary muscle.

cyclotron (si'klo-tron) an apparatus for accelerating protons or deuterons to high energies by a combination of a constant magnet and an oscillating electric field.

cyclotropia (si″klo-tro′pe-ah) [cyclo- + tropia] a form of strabismus in which there is permanent cyclophoria of an eye around the anteroposterior axis even in the presence of visual fusional stimuli, resulting in diplopia. Cf. *excyclotropia* and *incyclotropia.*

cycrimine hydrochloride (si′kri-mĭn) [USP] chemical name: α-cyclopentyl-α-phenyl-1-piperidinepropanol hydrochloride. An anticholinergic, $C_{19}H_{29}NO \cdot HCl$, occurring as a white solid; used in the treatment of parkinsonism, administered orally.

cyesiognosis (si-e″se-og-no′sis) [Gr. *kyēsis* conception + *gnōsis* knowledge] (*obs.*) diagnosis of pregnancy.

cyesis (si-e′sis) [Gr. *kyēsis*] pregnancy.

cyestein (si-es′te-in) a skinlike formation sometimes seen on the surface of urine of a pregnant woman.

cyesthein (si-es′the-in) cyestein.

cyl. cylinder; cylindrical lens.

cylicotomy (sil″e-kot′o-me) cyclotomy.

cylinder (sil′in-der) [Gr. *kylindros* a roller] a solid body shaped like a column, especially a cylindrical cast or cylindrical lens. **Bence Jones c's,** cylindrical gelatinous bodies forming the contents of the seminal vesicles; called also *Jones c's,* and *Lallemand's, Lallemand-Trousseau,* or *Trousseau-Lallemand bodies.* **crossed c's,** two cylindrical lenses at right angles to each other. **Külz's c.,** coma cast. **Leydig's c's,** bundles of muscular fibers separated by partitions of protoplasm. **Ruffini's c's,** Ruffini's corpuscles. **terminal c's,** brushes of Ruffini. **urinary c.,** a urinary cast.

cylindrarthrosis (sil″in-drar-thro′sis) [*cylinder* + Gr. *arthrōsis* joint] a joint in which the articular surfaces are cylindrical, as in the proximal radioulnar joint or the odontoid process and atlas.

cylindraxile (sil″in-drak′sil) an axon, def. 2.

cylindrical (sĭ-lin′drĭ-k'l) pertaining to or shaped like a cylinder.

cylindriform (sĭ-lin′drĭ-form) cylindrical.

cylindrocellular (sil″in-dro-sel′u-lar) composed of or containing cylindrical cells.

cylindrodendrite (sil″in-dro-den′drīt) a collateral branch of an axon.

Cylindrogloea (sĭ-lin″dro-gle′ah) [Gr. *kylindros* cylinder + *gloia* gum] a complex of green phototrophic sulfur bacteria related to the family Chlorobiaceae, made up of organisms found in mud and stagnant waters containing hydrogen sulfide.

cylindroid (sil′-in-droid) [Gr. *kylindroeidēs* cylindrical] 1. resembling, or shaped like a cylinder. 2. a cast in the urine, of various origins and of various forms, generally resembling hyaline casts, but differing from the latter in that it tapers to a slender tail which is often twisted or curled upon itself; called also *mucous* or *spurious (tube) cast.*

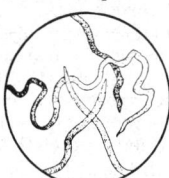

Cylindroids.

cylindroma (sil″in-dro′mah) [*cylinder* + *-oma*] 1. a usually benign tumor of either apocrine or eccrine origin generally arising in early life as single or multiple nodules located on the scalp and less often on the face and extremities, and consisting of cylindrical epithelial masses containing small basophilic and larger pale-staining cells surrounded by pink hyaline sheaths. Multiple lesions, which affect females more often and may completely cover the scalp (hence the descriptive term *turban tumor*), are usually dominantly inherited, and may also be associated with multiple trichoepitheliomas. 2. adenoid cystic carcinoma.

cylindromatous (sil″in-drom′ah-tus) pertaining to or of the nature of cylindroma.

Cylindrothorax (sĭ-lin″dro-tho′raks) a genus of beetles. **C. melanoceph′ala,** a blister beetle of Africa that secretes cantharidin, which if rubbed into the skin causes a severe dermatitis.

cylindruria (sil″in-droo′re-ah) [Gr. *kylindros* cylinder + *ouron* urine + *-ia*] the presence of tube casts in the urine.

cylite (si′līt) benzyl bromide.

cyllosis (sil-lo′sis) [Gr. *kyllōsis*] clubfoot or similar deformity of the foot or leg.

cyllosoma (sil″lo-so′mah) [Gr. *kyllos* lame + *sōma* body] a monster with lower lateral abdominal eventration and absence or imperfect development of the lower limb on the side having the eventration.

cyllosomus (sil″lo-so′mus) cyllosoma.

cymarose (si′mah-rōs) a rare sugar, 2,6-deoxy-3-methoxyaldohexose, $CH_3(CHOH)_2CH(OCH_3)CH_2CHO$, from hydrolysis of various strophanthin glycosides.

cymba (sim′bah), pl. *cym′bae* [L.; Gr. *kymbē*] a boat-shaped structure. **c. con′chae auric′ulae** [NA], the upper part of the concha of the auricle.

cymbiform (sim′bĭ-form) [L. *cymba* boat + L. *forma* form] boat-shaped; scaphoid.

cymb(o)- [Gr. *kymbē*, boat] a combining form meaning boat-shaped.

cymbocephalia (sim″bo-se-fa′le-ah) scaphocephaly.

cymbocephalic (sim″bo-se-fal′ik) [cymbo- + *kephalē* head] scaphocephalic.

cymbocephalous (sim″bo-sef′ah-lus) scaphocephalic.

cymbocephaly (sim″bo-sef′ah-le) scaphocephaly.

cyme (sīm) a form of inflorescence composed of a flat-topped cluster of blossoms.

cymograph (si′mo-graf) kymograph.

cynanche (sĭ-nan′ke) [cyn- + Gr. *anchein* to choke] severe sore throat with threatened suffocation. **c. malig′na,** a gangrenous or putrid sore throat, often diphtheritic or scarlatinal. **c. tonsilla′ris,** peritonsillar abscess.

cynanthropy (sĭ-nan′thro-pe) [cyn- + Gr. *anthrōpos* man] a delusion in which the patient considers himself a dog or behaves like a dog.

cynic (sin′ik) [Gr. *kynikos*] see *risus sardonicus.*

cyn(o)- [Gr. *kyōn* dog] a combining form denoting relationship to a dog, or doglike.

cynocephalic (si″no-se-fal′ik) [cyno- + Gr. *kephalē* head] having a head shaped like that of a dog.

cynodont (si′no-dont) [cyno- + Gr. *odous* tooth] a canine tooth.

cynomolgus (sin-o-mol′gus) a monkey of the genus *Macaca,* especially *M. irus,* used in laboratory research.

Cynomyia (si″no-mi′yah) a genus of blue-bottle flies that deposit their ova in decaying meat and in wounds.

Cynomys (si′no-mis) a genus of prairie dogs species of which harbor plague-transmitting fleas.

cynophobia (si″no-fo′be-ah) [cyno- + *phobia*] irrational fear of dogs.

cyogenic (si″o-jen′ik) [Gr. *kyos* fetus + *gennan* to produce] producing pregnancy.

Cyon's experiment, nerve (se′onz) [Elie de Cyon (Il'ia Faddeevich Tsion), a Russian physiologist, 1842–1912] see under *experiment* and *nerve.*

cyophoria (si″o-fo′re-ah) [Gr. *kyos* fetus + *phoros* bearing] pregnancy.

cyophoric (si″o-for′ik) pertaining to pregnancy.

cyophorin (si-of′o-rin) (*obs.*) kyestein.

cyopin (si′o-pin) [Gr. *kyanos* blue + *pyon* pus] the substance responsible for the color of blue pus.

cyotrophy (si-ot′ro-fe) [Gr. *kyos* fetus + *trophē* nutrition] nutrition of the fetus.

Cyperus (si-pe′rus) [L.; Gr. *kypeiros* rush] a genus of grasslike sedges or rushes. See *adrue.*

cyph(o)- for words beginning thus, see those beginning *kyph(o)-.*

cypionate (sip′e-o-nāt) USAN contraction for cyclopentanepropionate.

cypothrin (si′po-thrin) chemical name: 3,3-dimethylcyano (3 - phenoxyphenyl) methyl ester spiro[cyclopropane-1,1'-[1*H*]-indene]-2-carboxylic acid; a veterinary anthelmintic, $C_{28}H_{23}NO_3$.

cyprazepam (si-prah'zĕ-pam) chemical name: 7-chloro-2-[(cyclopropylmethyl) amino] -5-phenyl-3*H* -1,4-benzodiazepine 4-oxide; a tranquilizer, $C_{19}H_{18}ClN_3O$.

cyprinin (sip'rĭ-nin) a toxic substance derived from the milt of the carp, *Cyprinus carpio.*

cyproheptadine hydrochloride (si"pro-hep'tah-dēn) [USP] chemical name: 4-(5*H*-dibenzo[*a,d*]cyclohepten-5-ylidene)-1-methylpiperidine hydrochloride sesquihydrate. A serotonin and histamine antagonist with anticholinergic and sedative properties, $C_{21}H_{21}N \cdot HCl \cdot 1\frac{1}{2}H_2O$, occurring as a white to slightly yellow, crystalline powder; used as an antihistaminic for relief of symptoms of allergy and as an antipruritic for relief of itching associated with various skin disorders, administered orally.

cyproquinate (si-pro-kwin'āt) chemical name: 6,7-bis(cyclopropylmethoxy)-4-hydroxy-3-quinolinecarboxylic acid ethyl ester; a coccidiostat for poultry, $C_{20}H_{23}NO_5$.

cyproterone acetate (si-pro'ter-ōn) a synthetic antiandrogenic steroid that has been used in the treatment of male sexual disorders.

cyrto- [Gr. *kyrtos* bent] a combining form meaning bent or curved.

cyrtograph (sir'to-graf) [*cyrto-* + Gr. *graphein* to write] a cyrtometer that registers the movements of the chest wall.

cyrtometer (sir-tom'ĕ-ter) [*cyrto-* + *-meter*] a device for use in measuring the curves and curved surfaces of the body.

Cyrtophorida (sir"to-for'ĭ-dah) [*cyrto-* + Gr. *phoros* bearing] an order of dorsoventrally flattened or laterally compressed ciliate protozoa (superorder Phyllopharyngoidea, subclass Hypostomatia) characterized by the presence of three rows of oral ciliature composed of pairs of kinetosomes with inverted polarity; the ventral ciliature is often thigmotactic, and many species have a glandlike adhesive organelle near the posterior end. It comprises three suborders: Chlamydodontina, Dysteriina, and Hypocomatina.

cyrtos (sir'tos) [Gr. *kyrtos* bent] an often curved tubular cytopharyngeal apparatus with walls supported by nematodesmata, characteristic of ciliate protozoa of the subclass Hypostomatia. Called also *cytopharyngeal basket.* Cf. *rhabdos.*

cyrtosis (sir-to'sis) [Gr. *kyrtōsis*] 1. kyphosis. 2. distortion of the bones.

Cys cysteine.

Cys-Cys cystine.

cyst (sist) [Gr. *kystis* sac, bladder] 1. any closed cavity or sac, normal or abnormal, lined by epithelium, and especially one that contains a liquid or semisolid material. 2. a stage in the life cycle of certain parasites, during which they are enclosed within a protective wall; see, for example, *hydatid c., multilocular c.,* and *pseudocyst* (def. 2). **adventitious c.,** pseudocyst (def. 1). **allantoic c.,** urachal c. **alveolar c's,** dilatations of pulmonary alveoli, which may fuse by breakdown of their septa to form large air cysts (pneumatoceles). **alveolar hydatid c.,** a hydatid cyst formed by the larvae of the tapeworm *Echinococcus multilocularis;* see *hydatid disease, alveolar,* under *disease.* **amnionic c.,** cystlike processes containing amniotic fluid resulting from adhesion of amnionic folds. **aneurysmal bone c.,** a solitary lesion of bone that typically causes a bulging of the overlying cortex bearing some resemblance to the saccular protrusion of the aortic wall in aortic aneurysm. **angioblastic c.,** an ingrowth of the mesenchymal tissue having blood-forming power in an embryo. **apical c.,** an epithelium-lined cyst in the bone at the apex of a pulpless tooth. **apoplectic c.,** a cyst formed in a part by extravasation of blood. **arachnoid c.,** a fluid-filled cyst between the layers of the leptomeninges, lined with arachnoid membrane, most commonly occurring in the sylvian fissure; called also *leptomeningeal c.* **atheromatous c.,** keratin cyst, called also *sebaceous cyst.* **Baker's c.,** a swelling behind the knee, caused by escape of synovial fluid which has become enclosed in a sac of membrane; popliteal bursitis; synovial cyst of the popliteal space. **Blessig's c's,** cystic spaces that frequently appear at the periphery of the retina close to the ora serrata without significant effect on vision; called also *Blessig's lacunae, Blessig's spaces, cystoid degeneration,* and *Iwanoff's c's.* **blue dome c.,** a benign retention cyst of the breast containing straw-colored fluid that shows a blue

color when unopened; see *cystic disease of breast,* under *disease.* **Boyer's c.,** a painless and gradual enlargement of the subhyoid bursa. **branchial c., branchial cleft c., branchiogenetic c., branchiogenous c.,** a cyst arising in the lateral aspect of the neck, from epithelial remnants of a branchial cleft, usually located between the second and third branchial arches. **bronchial c's,** bronchogenic c. **bronchogenic c.,** a spherical cyst of bronchial origin lined with bronchial epithelium which may contain secretory elements, generally found in the mediastinum or the lung. It may contain air, and if communication with the trachea or a bronchus exists, may periodically evacuate fluid contents into the air passages, resulting in attacks of voluminous expectoration. Infection will lead to mediastinal or pulmonary abscess. Called also *bronchial c.* **bronchopulmonary c.,** bronchogenic cyst of the lung. **bursal c.,** a cyst derived from a serous bursa. **cervical c.,** a branchial or thyroglossal cyst. **chocolate c.,** one having dark, syrupy contents, resulting from collection of hemosiderin following local hemorrhage, such as sometimes occurs after mastectomy or in the ovary in ovarian endometriosis; called also *endometrial c.* and *Sampson's c.* **choledochal c.,** a congenital cystic dilatation of the common bile duct, which may cause pain in the right upper quadrant, jaundice, fever, or vomiting, or be asymptomatic. **choledochus c.,** a dilatation of the lower end of the common bile duct, usually recognized during childhood. **chyle c.,** an abnormal sac of the mesentery containing chyle. **colloid c.,** a cyst that contains jelly-like material, particularly in the third ventricle. **compound c.,** multilocular c. **corpus luteum c.,** a cyst of the ovary formed by a serous accumulation developed from a corpus luteum. **craniobuccal c.,** a cyst of Rathke's pouch. **craniopharyngeal duct c.,** cysts originating in the vestiges of the craniopharyngeal duct; they are closely related to craniopharyngiomas. **daughter c.,** a small parasitic cyst developed from the wall of a larger one, as from the hydatid cyst of the tapeworm *Echinococcus granulosus;* called also *secondary c.* **dental c.,** one derived from some portion of the odontogenic apparatus. **dentigerous c.,** a fluid-containing odontogenic cyst surrounding the crown of an unerupted tooth, usually involving the crowns of normal permanent teeth. **dermoid c.,** 1. an epidermal cyst, usually present at birth, representing a disorder of embryologic development, generally occurring along lines of embryonic fusion, with middorsal, midventral, and branchial cleft locations, most often involving the head, especially around the eyes, and the neck, and lined with stratified squamous epithelium containing cutaneous appendages, including hair. Called also *dermoid.* 2. a benign teratoma of the ovary, usually found in young women, presumably derived from the ectodermal differentiation of totipotential cells, lined by apparent skin and its associated adnexal structures, and typically filled with a sebaceous caseous material in which is found hair. Called also *benign cystic, cystic,* or *mature teratoma* and *dermoid.* Cf. *malignant teratoma.* **dilatation c.,** a cyst formed by dilation of a previously existing cavity. **distention c.,** a collection of watery fluid in a normal, but distended cavity. **echinococcus c.,** hydatid c. **endometrial c.,** a chocolate cyst, particularly in the ovary, lined with endometrium. **endothelial c.,** a cyst whose sac has an endothelial lining. **enteric c., enterogenous c.,** a cyst of the intestine arising or developing from some fold or pouch along the intestinal tract. Called also *enterocyst* and *enterocystoma.* **ependymal c.,** a circumscribed dilatation of some part of the ependyma. **epidermal c.,** a benign cyst derived from the epidermis or the epithelium of the hair follicle, which is formed by cystic enclosures of epithelium within the dermis that become filled with keratin admixed with variable amounts of lipid-rich debris. The two main types are *epidermal inclusion cyst* and *pilar cyst,* with *dermoid cyst* and *steatocystoma multiplex* being less common variants. Called also *epidermoid c., sebaceous c.,* and *wen.* **epidermal inclusion c.,** a well-circumscribed mobile epidermal cyst occurring on the head, neck, and trunk, formed by keratinizing squamous epithelium with a granular layer, similar to the normal epithelium of the follicular infundibulum. Cf. *pilar c.* **epidermoid c.,** epidermal c. **epithelial c.,** 1. any cyst lined by keratinizing stratified squamous epithelium, found most often in the skin, and including epidermal, pilar, and dermoid cysts, milia, and steatomas. 2. epidermal c. **eruption c.,** a dentigerous cyst presenting as a dilatation of the follicular space about the crown of the erupting deciduous or permanent teeth in children, caused by the accumulation of tissue fluid or blood. **extravasation c.,** a cyst formed by hemorrhage into the tissues. **exudation c.,** a cyst formed by an exudate collected in a closed cavity. **false c.,** an adventitious cyst. **fissural c.,** one arising along a line of fusion of the various embryonic processes; according to location, those of the oral region are classified as median palatal, median anterior maxillary, globulomaxillary, and nasoalveolar. **follicular c.,** one due to the occlusion of the duct of a follicle or small gland; especially a cyst formed by the enlargement of a graafian follicle as a result of accumulated transudate. **ganglionic c.,** subchondral c. **Gartner's c., gartnerian c.,** a cystic tumor developed from Gartner's duct (ductus epoöphoron longitudinalis [NA]). **gas c.,** a small cyst filled with gas, of bacterial origin. **gingival c.,** an odontogenic cyst of the soft tissue of either the free or attached gingiva, presenting as a small, well-circumscribed, painless swelling, sometimes resembling a superficial mucocele. **globulomaxillary c.,** an inclusion cyst of the maxillary bone, located in the globulomaxillary fissure, usually between the lateral incisor and cuspid teeth, which seldom presents any clinical manifestation. **granddaughter c.,** a cyst sometimes seen within a daughter cyst (q.v.). **hemorrhagic c.,** an encapsulated mass of extravasated blood. Called also *sanguineous c.* **hydatid c.,** the larval cyst stage of the tapeworms *Echinococcus granulosus,* and *E. multilocularis,* which contains daughter cysts, each of which contains many scoleces; called also *echinococcus c.* and *hydatid.* See *hydatid disease, unilocular,* under *disease.* **implantation c.,** a cyst formed from a piece of skin that has become implanted into the deep tissues. **incisive canal c.,** median anterior maxillary c. **inclusion c.,** one formed by the inclusion of a small portion of epithelium or mesothelium within connective tissue. **intraepithelial c's,** round or oval cavities which develop in the epithelium of the ureter, bladder, and urethra and contain a peculiar colloid substance. **intraluminal c's,** duplications of the bowel, or retention cysts, which are an infrequent cause of intrinsic obstruction in the newborn. **intrapituitary c's,** Rathke's c's. **involution c.,** mammary duct ectasia. **Iwanoff's c's,** Blessig's c's. **keratinizing c., keratinous c.,** any cyst containing keratinous material; see *epithelial c.* **lacteal c.,** a cyst of the breast due to obstruction of a lactiferous duct; called also *milk c.* **lateral periodontal c.,** a cyst of the lateral periodontal membrane of an erupted tooth, usually occurring in the bicuspid region of the mandible. **leptomeningeal c.,** arachnoid c. **lutein c.,** a cyst of the ovary developed from a corpus luteum. **median anterior maxillary c.,** an inclusion cyst of the maxilla located in or near the incisive canal, which arises from proliferation of epithelial remnants of the nasopalatine duct. Called also *incisive canal c.* and *nasopalatine duct c.* **median mandibular c.,** a rare inclusion cyst occurring in the midline of the mandible, believed to be caused by inclusion of the epithelium trapped in the central groove of the mandibular process, or by cystic degeneration of a supernumerary tooth germ. **median palatal c.,** an inclusion cyst located in the midline of the hard palate between the lateral palatal processes. **meibomian c.,** a cyst of the meibomian gland; called also *chalazion.* **mesenteric c.,** a congenital thin-walled cyst of the abdomen between the leaves of the mesentery, which may be of wolffian or lymphatic duct origin; as it enlarges, it may cause colicky pain and intestinal obstruction. **milk c.,** lacteal c. **morgagnian c.,** see *appendix testis* and *appendices vesiculosae epoöphorontis.* **mother c.,** a cyst enclosing other cysts, as in the cyst stage of *Echinococcus granulosus.* **mucous c.,** a retention cyst that contains mucus. **multilocular c.,** a cyst containing several loculi or spaces; a hydatid cyst composed of many small irregular cavities, which may contain scoleces but generally little fluid, and which tend to enlarge by budding since they have a poorly developed hyaline cuticle, as in *Echinococcus multilocularis;* called also *alveolar c.* **myxoid c.,** a nodular lesion usually overlying a distal interphalangeal finger joint in the dorsolateral or dorsomesial position, consisting of focal mucinous degeneration of the collagen of the dermis; not a true cyst, lacking an epithelial wall, it does not communicate with the underlying synovial space. Called also *synovial c.* and *synovial ganglion.* **Naboth's c's, nabothian c's,** Naboth's follicles. **nasoalveolar c., nasolabial c.,** an inclusion cyst arising from epithelial remnants at the junction of the globular, lateral nasal, and maxillary processes,

which clinically may cause a swelling in the mucolabial fold and in the floor of the nose and superficial erosion of the outer surface of the maxilla. **nasopalatine duct c.,** median anterior maxillary c. **necrotic c.,** a cyst containing necrotic matter. **neural c.,** a cyst or cystlike structure occurring in the central nervous system, as a soapsuds cyst or a porencephalic cyst. **neurenteric c.,** a cyst of the posterior mediastinum containing tissues from the nervous system and other organs, and connecting with the spinal dura mater. **nevoid c.,** an abnormal cyst with vascular walls. **odontogenic c.,** one derived from epithelium, usually containing fluid or semisolid material, which develops during various stages of odontogenesis. Nearly all odontogenic cysts are enclosed within bone. Primordial, dentigerous, periodontal, and gingival cysts are the specific types. **oil c.,** a cyst containing oily matter, due to fatty degeneration of the epithelial lining. **omental c's,** cysts similar in all respects to mesenteric ones except that they are confined to the omentum. **oophoritic c.,** a cyst of the ovary proper. **osseous hydatid c's,** hydatid cysts formed by the larvae of *Echinococcus granulosus* and occurring in bone, which may become weakened and eroded by the exuberant growth. **pancreatic c.,** a retention cyst of the pancreatic duct; called also *pancreatic ranula.* Cf. *pancreatic pseudocyst.* **paranephric c.,** a cyst of the fatty tissue surrounding the kidney. **parapyelitic c's,** apparently congenital cysts of uncertain etiology occurring in the kidney sinus, usually in a small cluster, and causing pelvic compression and local deformity, with pain, hematuria, infection, and pyuria. **parasitic c.,** a cyst formed by the larva of a parasite, such as a hydatid cyst. **parovarian c.,** a cyst of the epoöphoron. **pearl c.,** a cyst or a solid mass of epithelial cells in the iris caused by implantation of an eyelash, cotton, or other foreign particle. **periapical c.,** a periodontal cyst involving the apex of an erupted tooth, frequently a result of infection via the pulp chamber and root canal through carious involvement of the tooth. Called also *radicular c.* **pericardial c.,** a benign tumor containing clear fluid, almost always located immediately adjacent to the pericardium; such cysts must be differentiated from the more serious mediastinal tumors. **perineurial c.,** an outpouching of the perineurial space on the extradural portion of the posterior sacral or coccygeal nerve roots at the junction of the root and ganglion; it may cause low back pain and sciatica. **periodontal c.,** one in the periodontal ligament and adjacent structures, usually at the apex (*periapical c.*), but sometimes along the lateral surfaces of the tooth (*lateral periodontal c.*). **pilar c.,** an epidermal cyst usually occurring as a firm, well-circumscribed, subepidermal nodule, especially on the scalp, and formed by an outer wall of keratinizing epithelium without a granular layer, similar to the normal epithelium of the hair follicle at and distal to the sebaceous duct. Called also *sebaceous c., trichilemmal c.,* and *wen.* Cf. *epidermal inclusion c.* **piliferous c., pilonidal c.,** a hair-containing sacrococcygeal dermoid cyst or sinus which often opens at a postanal dimple. Cf. *coccygeal sinus,* under *sinus.* **placental c.,** a grayish white, disklike cyst of the placenta, resulting from degeneration of trophoblastic cells. **porencephalic c.,** a cyst occurring in the brain substance in porencephaly. **preauricular c., congenital,** a cyst resulting from imperfect fusion of the first and second branchial arches in formation of the auricle, communicating with a pitlike depression just in front of the helix and above the tragus (ear pit). **primordial c.,** a relatively uncommon type of odontogenic cyst that develops through cystic degeneration and liquefaction of the stellate reticulum in an enamel organ before any calcified enamel or dentin has been formed. Such cysts originate from supernumerary teeth, and are found in place of a tooth rather than being associated with one. **proliferous c.,** (*obs.*), multilocular c. **proligerous c.** (*obs.*), cystadenocarcinoma. **pseudomucinous c.,** see under *cystadenoma.* **pyelogenic renal c.,** calyceal diverticulum. **radicular c.,** periapical c. **Rathke's c's,** groups of epithelial cells forming small colloid-filled cysts in the pars intermedia of the pituitary gland. **residual c.,** a periodontal cyst that remains after or develops subsequent to tooth extraction. **retention c.,** one caused by retention of glandular secretion. **Sampson's c.,** chocolate c. **sanguineous c.,** hemorrhagic c. **sarcosporidian c.,** sarcocyst, def. 2. **sebaceous c.,** 1. epidermal c. 2. pilar c. **secondary c.,** a daughter cyst. **secretory c.,** a cyst produced by retention of the normal secretion of a gland. **seminal c.,** a cyst containing semen. **serous c.,** a cyst containing a thin liquid or serum. **soapsuds c's,** cysts that stud the cerebral cortex in cryptococcosis. **solitary bone c.,** a pathologic bone space in the metaphyses of long bones of growing children; of disputed origin, it may be either empty or filled with fluid and have a delicate connective tissue lining. **springwater c.,** pericardial c. **sterile c.,** a true hydatid cyst that fails to produce brood capsules; called also *acephalocyst*. **subchondral c.,** a bone cyst within the fused epiphysis beneath the articular plate; it is lined with a membrane (probably modified synovia) which contains a mucinous material. Called also *ganglionic c*. **sublingual c.,** ranula. **subsynovial c.,** one caused by the distention of a synovial follicle. **suprasellar c.,** craniopharyngioma. **synovial c.,** myxoid c. **Tarlov c.,** perineurial c. **tarry c.,** •1. a corpus luteum cyst resulting from hemorrhage into a corpus luteum. 2. a bloody cyst resulting from endometriosis. **tarsal c.,** a cyst in the tarsus of the lid, also called *chalazion*. **thecal c.,** distention of a sheath of a tendon. **theca-lutein c.,** a cyst of the ovary in which the lutein cells lining the cyst cavity are theca interna cells. **thymic c's,** rare unilocular or multilocular cysts of the upper anterior mediastinum containing tissue resembling that of the thymus; they are congenital in origin. **thyroglossal c., thyrolingual c.,** a cyst in the neck caused by persistence of portions of, or by lack of closure of, the primitive thyroglossal duct. **tissue c.,** see *cyst* (def. 2) and *pseudocyst* (def. 2). **Tornwaldt's c.,** bursa pharyngea. **trichilemmal c.,** pilar c. **true c.,** any cyst that is not a normal structure and not formed by the dilatation of a passage or cavity. **tubular c.,** tubulocyst. **umbilical c.,** vitellointestinal c. **unicameral c.,** unilocular c. **unicameral bone c.,** solitary bone c. **unilocular c.,** a cyst containing but one cavity. Cf. *multilocular c*. **urachal c.,** a form of cystic dilatation of the urachus; called also *allantoic c*. **urinary c.,** a cyst containing urine. **vitellointestinal c.,** a cystlike tumor at the umbilicus, caused by persistence of a portion of the umbilical duct; called also *umbilical c*. **wolffian c.,** a cyst of the broad ligaments of the uterus, regarded as developed from vestiges of the wolffian body (mesonephros).

cystadenocarcinoma (sis-tad″e-no-kar″si-no′mah) carcinoma and cystadenoma.

cystadenoma (sis″tad-e-no′mah) [*cyst-* + *adenoma*] adenoma associated with cystoma. **c. adamanti′num,** ameloblastoma. **mucinous c.,** a multilocular tumor produced by the epithelial cells of the ovary and having mucin-filled cavities; the great majority of these tumors are benign. **papillary c.,** any tumor producing patterns which are both papillary and cystic. **papillary c. lymphomato′sum,** papillary adenocystoma lymphomatosum. **c. par′tim sim′plex par′tim papillif′erum** (*obs.*), papillary cystadenoma. **pseudomucinous c.,** mucinous c.; so called because the cavity contents were thought to be pseudomucin. **serous c.,** a cystic tumor of the ovary, containing thin, clear, yellow serous fluid and varying amounts of solid tissue, with a malignant potential several times greater than that of mucinous cystadenoma.

cystalgia (sis-tal′je-ah) [*cyst-* + *-algia*] pain in the bladder.

cystathionase (sis″tah-thi′o-nas) See *cystathionine γ-lyase* (γ-cystathionase).

cystathionine (sis″tah-thi′o-nin) an unsymmetrical thioether of homocysteine and serine, COOH·CH(NH₂)·CH₂·-CH₂·S·CH₂·CH(NH₂)·COOH, which serves as an intermediate in the transfer of a sulfur atom from methionine to cysteine.

cystathionine γ-lyase (sis″tah-thi′o-nēn gam′ah li′ās) [EC 4.4.1.1] an enzyme of the lyase class that catalyzes the reaction L-cystathionine + H₂O = L-cysteine + NH₃ + 2-ketobutyrate. It is a pyridoxal-phosphate protein. The reaction occurs in the liver and is the step in the catabolism of methionine by which cysteine is synthesized from methionine. A defect in the enzyme, an autosomal recessive trait, results in cystathioninuria. Called also *cystathionase*.

cystathionine β-synthase (sis″tah-thi′o-nēn ba′tah sin′thās) [EC 4.2.1.22] an enzyme of the lyase class that catalyzes the reaction L-serine + L-homocysteine=cystathionine + H₂O. It is a pyridoxal-phosphate protein, found in the mammalian liver. The reaction occurs in the catabolism of methionine. A defect in the enzyme, an autosomal recessive, trait, results in homocystinuria.

cystathioninuria (sis″tah-thi″o-nin-u′re-ah) a hereditary disorder of cystathionine metabolism marked by increased concentrations of cystathionine in the urine, due to deficiency of γ-cystathionase; mental retardation is associated in some instances.

cystatrophia (sis″tah-tro′fe-ah) [*cyst-* + Gr. *atrophia* atrophy] atrophy of the bladder.

cystauchenitis (sis″taw-kĕ-ni′tis) [*cyst-* + Gr. *auchēn* neck + *-itis*] inflammation of the neck of the bladder.

cystauchenotomy (sis″taw-kĕ-not′o-me) [*cyst-* + Gr. *auchēn* neck + *tomē* cut] surgical incision of the neck of the bladder.

cystectasia, cystectasy (sis-tek-ta′ze-ah; sis-tek′tah-se) [*cyst-* + Gr. *ektasis* dilatation] slitting of the membranous portion of the urethra and dilation of the neck of the bladder for the extraction of stone.

cystectomy (sis-tek′to-me) [*cyst-* + Gr. *ektomē* excision] 1. excision of a cyst. 2. resection of the bladder.

cysteic acid (sis-te′ik) an intermediate formed by oxidation of the thiol group of cysteine to a sulfo group, and precursor of taurine.

cysteine (sis-te′in) chemical name: 2-amino-3-mercaptopropionic acid. A sulfur-containing amino acid produced by the enzymatic or acid hydrolysis of proteins. It is easily oxidized to cystine, is sometimes found in the urine, and has limited detoxification properties. Called also *thioaminopropionic acid*. **c. hydrochloride,** a compound suggested for the treatment of cutaneous ulcers.

cysteinyl (sis′tēn-il, sis-te′in-il) the acyl radical of cysteine.

cystelcosis (sis″tel-ko′sis) [*cyst-* + Gr. *helkōsis* ulceration] ulceration of the bladder.

cystencephalus (sis″ten-sef′ah-lus) [*cyst-* + Gr. *enkephalos* brain] a monster with a membranous sac in place of a brain.

cysterethism (sis-ter′e-thizm) [*cyst-* + Gr. *erethismos* irritation] irritability of the bladder.

cysthypersarcosis (sist-hi″per-sar-ko′sis) [*cyst-* + Gr. *hyper* over + *sarkōsis* growth of flesh] a thickening of the muscular coat of the bladder.

cysti- see *cyst(o)-*.

cystic (sis′tik) [Gr. *kystis* bladder] 1. pertaining to a cyst. 2. pertaining to the urinary bladder or to the gallbladder.

cysticerci (sis″tĭ-ser′si) plural of *cysticercus*.

cysticercoid (sis″tĭ-ser′koid) a form of larval tapeworm resembling *Cysticercus*, but having the cyst small, almost devoid of fluid, and provided with a caudal appendage, as in *Hymenolepis*.

cysticercosis (sis″tĭ-ser-ko′sis) infection with cystercerci. In man, it is an infection with the larval forms (*Cysticercus cellulosae*) of *Taenia solium*, which penetrate the intestinal wall and invade such tissues as the subcutaneous tissue, brain, eye, muscle, heart, liver, lung, and peritoneum. Brain involvement may result in epilepsy, increased intracranial pressure, etc.

Cysticercus (sis″tĭ-ser′kus) [Gr. *kystis* bladder + *kerkos* tail] a former genus of larval forms of tapeworms, with such species names as *C. acanthro′trias*, *C. bo′vis* (beef tapeworm), *C. cellulo′sae* (pork tapeworm), *C. fasciola′ris*, *C. o′vis*, and *C. tenuicollis*. **C. bo′vis,** the larva of *Taenia saginata*. **C. cellulo′sae,** the larva of *Taenia solium*; see also *cysticercosis*. **C. o′vis,** the larva of *Taenia ovis*. **C. tenuicol′lis,** the larva of *Taenia hydatigena*.

cysticercus (sis″tĭ-ser′kus), pl *cysticer′ci*. a larval form of tapeworm, consisting of a single scolex enclosed in a bladder-like cyst; cf. *hydatid cyst*, under *cyst*.

cysticolithectomy (sis″tĭ-ko″lĭ-thek′to-me) [Gr. *kystis* bladder + *lithos* stone + *ektomē* excision] removal of a stone from the cystic duct.

cysticolithotripsy (sis″tĭ-ko-lith′o-trip-se) crushing of a calculus within the cystic duct.

cysticorrhaphy (sis″tĭ-kor′ah-fe) [*cystic duct* + *rhaphē* suture] suture or repair of the cystic duct.

cysticotomy (sis″tĭ-kot′o-me) [*cystic duct* + Gr. *tomē* a cutting] incision into the cystic duct.

cystides (sis′tĭ-dēz) plural of *cystis*.

cystid(o)- see *cyst(o)-*.

cystidoceliotomy (sis″tĭ-do-se″le-ot′o-me) cystidolaparotomy.

cystidolaparotomy (sis″tĭ-do-lap″ah-rot′o-me) [*cystido-* + *laparotomy*] incision of the bladder through the abdominal wall.

cystidotrachelotomy (sis″tĭ-do-tra-kel-ot′o-me) [*cystido-* + Gr. *trachēlos* neck + *tomē* a cutting] incision of the neck of the bladder.

cystiferous (sis-tif′er-us) cystigerous.

cystiform (sis′tĭ-form) [*cysti-* + L. *forma* form] having the form or appearance of a cyst.

cystigerous (sis-tij′er-us) [*cysti-* + L. *gerere* to bear] containing cysts.

cystine (sis′tēn, sis′tin) chemical name: 3,3′-dithiobis (2-aminopropanoic acid). An amino acid, $[S \cdot CH_2 \cdot CH(NH_2) \cdot COOH]_2$, produced by the digestion or acid hydrolysis of proteins. It is sometimes found in the urine and in the kidneys in the form of minute hexagonal crystals, frequently forming a cystine calculus in the bladder. Cystine is the chief sulfur-containing compound of the protein molecule, and is readily reduced to two molecules of cysteine (hence, also called *dicysteine*).

cystinemia (sis″tĭ-ne′me-ah) [*cystine* + Gr. *haima* blood + *-ia*] presence of cystine in the blood.

cystinosis (sis″tĭ-no′sis) [*cystine* + *-osis*] lysosomal storage disorders of unknown molecular defect, characterized by widespread deposition of cystine crystals in reticuloendothelial cells. There are three clinical types: the *early onset* or *infantile nephropathic type*, the most common cause of the Fanconi syndrome (def. 2), is marked by vitamin D–resistant rickets, chronic acidosis, polyuria, and dehydration, all resulting from proximal renal tubular dysfunction, and by corneal opacities, growth failure, uremia, and death before ten. The *benign* or *adult nephropathic type* does not affect kidneys or shorten life span, is marked by deposition of cystine in the bone marrow, leukocytes, and corneas, and is diagnosed by ophthalmic examination. The *late onset juvenile* or *adolescent nephropathic type* falls within the two extremes: there are ocular and renal manifestations, but the kidney lesion does not always lead to renal insufficiency. Called also *cystine storage disease* and *Lignac-Fanconi syndrome*.

cystinuria (sis″tĭ-nu′re-ah) [*cystine* + *urine*] a hereditary condition of persistent excessive urinary excretion of cystine and three other dibasic amino acids: lysine, ornithine, and arginine; it is due to impairment of renal transport in tubular reabsorption of these amino acids. The predominant clinical manifestation is the formation of urinary cystine calculi.

cystinuric (sis″tĭ-nu′rik) pertaining to or affected with cystinuria.

cystirrhagia (sis″tĭ-ra′je-ah) cystorrhagia.

cystirrhea (sis″tĭ-re′ah) cystorrhea.

cystis (sis′tis), pl. *cys′tides* [Gr. *kystis*] a pouch or sac; a cyst. **c. fel′lea**, gallbladder.

cystistaxis (sis″tĭ-stak′sis) [*cysti-* + Gr. *staxis* dripping] oozing of blood from the mucous membrane into the bladder.

cystitis (sis-ti′tis) inflammation of the urinary bladder. **allergic c.,** cystitis resulting from some unusual hypersensitivity, characterized by a large number of mononuclear leukocytes and eosinophils in the bladder mucosa and musculature, and in the urinary sediment. **bacterial c.,** bacterial infection of the bladder. **catarrhal c., acute,** cystitis resulting from injury, irritation by foreign bodies, gonorrhea, etc., and marked by burning in the bladder, pain in the urethra, and painful micturition. **c. col′li,** inflammation involving the neck of the bladder. **croupous c.,** diphtheritic c. **cystic c., c. cys′tica,** cystitis with the formation of multiple submucosal cysts in the bladder wall. **diphtheritic c.,** cystitis due to infection by *Corynebacterium diphtheriae*, and characterized by the formation of a false membrane; called also *croupous c.* **c. emphysemato′sa,** an unusual inflammation of the bladder, characterized by the presence of gas-filled vesicles and cysts in the bladder mucosa and musculature. **eosinophilic c.,** cystitis characterized by the presence of large numbers of eosinophils in the urinary sediment. **exfoliative c.,** cystitis with sloughing of the bladder mucosa. **c. follicula′ris,** cystitis in which the mucosa of the bladder is studded with nodules containing lymph follicles. **c. glandula′ris,** cystitis in which the mucosa contains mucin-secreting glands, observed more frequently in cases of exstrophy of the

bladder, and sometimes leading to malignant degeneration. **incrusted c.,** an intense cystitis characterized by deposition of phosphatic or other inorganic salts on the chronically inflamed bladder wall, generally at the site of ulcerations, granulations, or tumors. **interstitial c., chronic,** a condition of the bladder occurring predominantly in women, with an inflammatory lesion, usually in the vertex, and involving the entire thickness of the wall, appearing as a small patch of brownish red mucosa, surrounded by a network of radiating vessels. The lesions, known as Fenwick-Hunner or Hunner ulcers, may heal superficially, and are notoriously difficult to detect. Typically, there is urinary frequency and pain on bladder filling and at the end of micturition. Called also *panmural c.*, *submucous c.*, and *panmural fibrosis of the bladder.* **mechanical c.,** cystitis resulting from irritation by a vesical calculus, manipulation, or a foreign body in the bladder. **panmural c.,** interstitial c., chronic. **c. papillomato′sa,** cystitis characterized by the presence of papillomatous growths on the inflamed mucous membrane. **c. seni′lis femina′rum,** a chronic cystitis occurring in elderly women, marked by abnormal frequency of micturition, with tenesmus and burning. **submucous c.,** interstitial c., chronic.

cystitome (sis′tĭ-tōm) [*cysti-* + *-tome*] an instrument for opening the capsule of the lens of the eye; called also *cibisotome* and *kibisitome.*

cystitomy (sis-tit′o-me) [*cysti-* + *-tomy*] the surgical division of the capsule of the lens; capsulotomy.

cyst(o)-, cysti-, cystido- [Gr. *kystis*, pl. *kystides* a sac or bladder] combining form denoting a relationship to a sac, cyst, or bladder, most frequently used in reference to the urinary bladder.

cystoadenoma (sis″to-ad″e-no′mah) cystadenoma.

Cystobacter (sis″to-bak′ter) [*cysto-* + Gr. *baktron* a rod] a genus of gliding bacteria of the family Cystobacteraceae, order Myxobacterales, found in soil and rabbit dung. The type species is *C. fus′cus.*

Cystobacteraceae (sis″to-bak″ter-a′se-e) a family of gliding bacteria of the order Myxobacterales, made up of tapered, flexible, rod-shaped cells that produce microcysts in sporangia. It contains the genera *Cystobacter*, *Melittangium*, and *Stigmatella.*

cystoblast (sis′to-blast) [*cysto-* + Gr. *blastos* germ] the layer of cells that lines the amniotic cavity of the early embryo on the side of the enveloping layer.

cystocarcinoma (sis″to-kar″sĭ-no′mah) carcinoma associated with cysts.

cystocele (sis′to-sēl) [*cysto-* + Gr. *kēlē* hernia] hernial protrusion of the urinary bladder through the vaginal wall; called also *cystic hernia.*

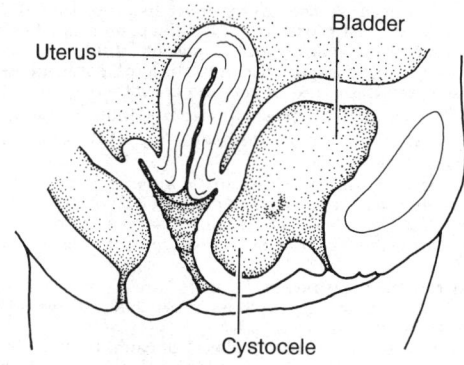

Uterus — Bladder
Cystocele

cystochrome (sis′to-krōm) [*cysto-* + Gr. *chrōma* color] a mixture of indigo carmine and methenamine; used by intramuscular or intravenous injection for the indigo carmine test of renal function.

cystochromoscopy (sis″to-kro-mos′ko-pe) chromocystoscopy.

cystocolostomy (sis″to-ko-los′to-me) [*cysto-* + *colostomy*] the surgical creation of a permanent passage from the bladder to the colon.

Cysto-Conray (sis″to-kon′ra)   trademark for preparations of iothalamate meglumine.

cystodiaphanoscopy (sis″to-di″ah-fah-nos′ko-pe) [*cysto-* + *diaphanoscopy*]   examination within, or transillumination of, the urinary bladder by means of a diaphanoscope.

cystoduodenostomy (sist″o-du-od″e-nos′to-me)   internal drainage of an adjacent cyst into the duodenum.

cystodynia (sis″to-din′e-ah) [*cysto-* + Gr. *odynē* pain]   pain in the urinary bladder.

cystoelytroplasty (sis″to-e-lit′ro-plas″te) [*cysto-* + Gr. *elytron* sheath + *plassein* to form]   surgical repair of vesicovaginal injuries.

cystoenterocele (sis″to-en′ter-o-sēl)   hernia of a portion of the bladder and of the intestine.

cystoepiplocele (sis″to-e-pip′lo-sēl)   hernia of a portion of the bladder and of the omentum.

cystoepithelioma (sis″to-ep″ĭ-the″le-o′mah)   a tumor containing cystic and epitheliomatous elements.

cystofibroma (sis″to-fi-bro′mah) [L.]   fibroma containing cysts.

cystogastrostomy (sis″to-gas-tros′to-me)   internal drainage of an adjacent cyst into the stomach.

Cystografin (sis″to-graf′in)   trademark for a preparation of diatrizoate meglumine.

cystogram (sis′to-gram)   a roentgenogram of the bladder.

cystography (sis-tog′rah-fe) [*cysto-* + Gr. *graphein* to write]   roentgenography of the bladder after injection of the organ with opaque solution.   **delayed c.,** cystography in which film exposures are made at varying intervals up to 30 minutes or longer; useful in the study of urinary reflux.   **voiding c.,** radiography of the bladder while the patient is urinating.

cystoid (sis′toid) [*cysto-* + Gr. *eidos* form]   1. resembling a cyst.   2. a cystlike, circumscribed collection of softened material, differing from a true cyst in having no enclosing capsule.

cystojejunostomy (sis″to-je-ju-nos′to-me)   internal drainage of an adjacent cyst into the jejunum.

cystolith (sis′to-lith) [*cysto-* + Gr. *lithos* stone]   a vesical calculus.

cystolithectomy (sis″to-lĭ-thek′to-me) [*cysto-* + Gr. *lithos* stone + *ektomē* excision]   the removal of a urinary calculus by cutting into the urinary bladder. The term has been used erroneously for excision of a gallstone from the gallbladder.

cystolithiasis (sis″to-lĭ-thi′ah-sis) [*cysto-* + Gr. *lithos* stone]   the development of calculi in the urinary bladder.

cystolithic (sis″to-lith′ik)   pertaining to vesical calculi.

cystolithotomy (sis″to-lĭ-thot′o-me)   cystolithectomy.

cystolutein (sis″to-lu′te-in) [*cysto-* + L. *luteus* yellow]   a yellow pigment from certain ovarian cysts.

cystoma (sis-to′mah) [*cysto-* + *-oma*]   a tumor containing cysts of neoplastic origin; a cystic tumor.   **myxoid c.** (*obs.*), mucinous cystadenoma.   **c. sero′sum sim′plex,** simple cyst of the ovary.

cystomatitis (sis″to-mah-ti′tis)   inflammation of one or more of the cysts of a cystoma.

cystomatous (sis-to′mah-tus)   relating to or containing cystoma.

cystometer (sis-tom′ĕ-ter) [*cysto-* + Gr. *metron* measure]   an instrument for studying the neuromuscular mechanism of the bladder by means of measurements of pressure and capacity.

cystometrogram (sis″to-met′ro-gram)   the tracing recorded by cystometrography.

cystometrography (sis″to-mĕ-trog′rah-fe)   the graphic recording of the pressure exerted at varying degrees of filling of the urinary bladder.

cystometry (sis-tom′ĕ-tre)   the study of bladder efficiency by means of the cystometer.

cystomorphous (sis″to-mor′fus) [*cysto-* + Gr. *morphē* form]   shaped like a cyst or bladder.

cystomyoma (sis″to-mi-o′mah)   (*obs.*) myoma with cystic degeneration.

cystomyxoadenoma (sis″to-mik″so-ad″e-no′mah)   (*obs.*) adenomyoma with cystic degeneration.

cystomyxoma (sis″to-mik-so′mah)   (*obs.*) mucinous cystadenoma.

cystonephrosis (sis″to-nĕ-fro′sis) [*cysto-* + Gr. *nephros* kidney]   cystiform dilatation or enlargement of the kidney.

cystoneuralgia (sis″to-nu-ral′je-ah) [*cysto-* + *neuralgia*]   neuralgia of the bladder.

cystoparalysis (sis″to-pah-ral-ĭ-sis)   cystoplegia.

cystopexy (sis′to-pek″se) [*cysto-* + Gr. *pēxis* fixation]   fixation of the bladder to the abdominal wall in the treatment of cystocele; vesicofixation.

cystophorous (sis-tof′o-rus) [*cysto-* + Gr. *phoros* bearing]   containing cysts.

cystophotography (sis″to-fo-tog′rah-fe)   the photographing of the inside of the bladder.

cystophthisis (sis-tof′thĭ-sis) [*cysto-* + Gr. *phthisis* consumption]   tuberculosis of the bladder.

cystoplasty (sis′to-plas″te) [*cysto-* + Gr. *plassein* to mold]   any plastic or reconstructive operation on the bladder.   **augmentation c.,** enlargement of the bladder by grafting to it a detached segment of intestine (ileum, cecum, or sigmoid).

cystoplegia (sis″to-ple′je-ah) [*cysto-* + Gr. *plēgē* stroke]   paralysis of the bladder; called also *cystoparalysis.*

cystoproctostomy (sis″to-prok-tos′to-me) [*cysto-* + Gr. *proktos* rectum + *stomoun* to provide with an opening, or mouth]   the surgical creation of a communication between the urinary bladder and rectum; called also *cystorectostomy.*

cystoptosis (sis″top-to′sis) [*cysto-* + Gr. *ptōsis* a falling]   prolapse of a part of the inner coat of the bladder into the urethra.

cystopyelitis (sis″to-pi-e-li′tis)   inflammation involving both the urinary bladder and the pelvis of the kidney.

cystopyelography (sis″to-pi″ĕ-log′rah-fe)   roentgenography of the urinary bladder and the pelvis of the kidney.

cystopyelonephritis (sis″to-pi″e-lo-ne-fri′tis) [*cysto-* + Gr. *pyelos* pelvis + *nephros* kidney + *-itis*]   combined cystitis and pyelonephritis.

cystoradiography (sis″to-ra″de-og′rah-fe) [*cysto-* + *radiography*]   radiography of the bladder.

cystorectostomy (sis″to-rek-tos′to-me)   cystoproctostomy.

cystorrhagia (sis″to-ra′je-ah) [*cysto-* + Gr. *rhēgnynai* to burst forth]   hemorrhage from the bladder.

cystorrhaphy (sis-tor′ah-fe) [*cysto-* + Gr. *rhaphē* suture]   the operation of suturing the bladder.

cystorrhea (sis″to-re′ah) [*cysto-* + Gr. *rhoia* flow]   catarrh of the bladder.

cystosarcoma (sis″to-sar-ko′mah)   a variant of mammary fibroadenoma, usually of large size, with an unusually cellular, sarcoma-like stroma; it is locally aggressive, and sometimes metastasizes. Called also *c. phylloides* and *c. phyllodes.*

cystoschisis (sis-tos′kĭ-sis) [*cysto-* + Gr. *schisis* fissure]   fissure of the bladder.

cystosclerosis (sis″to-skle-ro′sis)   a cyst that has undergone sclerosis or fibrosis.

cystoscope (sis′to-skōp″) [*cysto-* + Gr. *skopein* to examine]   an endoscope for visual examination of the bladder.

cystoscopic (sis″to-skop′ik)   pertaining to cystoscopy, or performed with the cystoscope.

cystoscopy (sis-tos′ko-pe)   direct visual examination of the urinary tract with a cystoscope.

cystose (sis′tōs)   resembling or containing a cyst or cysts.

cystospasm (sis′to-spazm) [*cysto-* + Gr. *spasmos* spasm]   spasm of the bladder.

Cystospaz (sis′to-spaz)   trademark for preparations of hyoscyamine.

cystospermitis (sis″to-sper-mi′tis) [*cysto-* + Gr. *sperma* semen]   inflammation of a seminal vesicle.

cystostaxis (sis″to-stak′sis)   cystistaxis.

cystostomy (sis-tos′to-me) [*cysto-* + Gr. *stoma* opening]   the formation of an opening into the bladder.   **tubeless c.,** cutaneous vesicostomy.

cystotome (sis′to-tōm) [*cysto-* + *-tome*]   1. an instrument for incising the bladder.   2. cystitome.

cystotomy (sis-tot′o-me)   surgical incision of the urinary bladder; vesicotomy.   **suprapubic c.,** the operation of cutting into the bladder by an incision just above the pubic symphysis.

cystotrachelotomy (sis″to-tra″kel-ot′o-me) [*cysto-* + Gr. *trachēlos* neck + *tomē* a cut] surgical incision of the neck of the bladder.

cystoureteritis (sis″to-u-re″ter-i′tis) inflammation involving the urinary bladder and ureters.

cystoureterogram (sis″to-u-re′ter-o-gram) a roentgenogram of the urinary bladder and ureters.

cystoureteropyelitis (sis″to-u-re″ter-o-pi″e-li′tis) inflammation involving the urinary bladder, ureter, and pelvis of the kidney.

cystoureteropyelonephritis (sis″to-u-re″ter-o-pi″e-lo-ne-fri′tis) combined inflammation of the bladder, ureter, and pelvis and pyramids of the kidney.

cystourethritis (sis″to-u″re-thri′tis) inflammation of the bladder and urethra.

cystourethrocele (sis″to-u-re′thro-sēl) prolapse of the female urethra and bladder.

cystourethrogram (sis″to-u-re′thro-gram) a roentgenogram of the urinary bladder and urethra.

cystourethrography (sis″to-u-re-throg′rah-fe) roentgenography of the urinary bladder and urethra. **chain c.,** that in which a sterile beaded metal chain is introduced via a modified catheter into the bladder and urethra; used in evaluating anatomical relationships of the bladder and urethra. **voiding c.,** cystourethrography in which radiographs are made before, during, and after voiding.

cystourethroscope (sis″to-u-re′thro-skōp″) an instrument for examining the bladder and posterior urethra.

cystous (sis′tus) cystose.

cystyl (sis′tyl) the divalent acyl radical of cystine.

Cytadren (si′tah-dren) trademark for a preparation of aminoglutethimide.

cytapheresis (sīt″ah-fĕ-re′sis) [*cyt-* + Gr. *aphairesis* removal] a procedure in which cells of one or more kinds (leukocytes, platelets, etc.) are separated from whole blood and retained, the plasma and other formed elements being retransfused into the donor; it includes leukapheresis and thrombocytapheresis.

cytarabine (si-tār′ah-bēn) [USP] a deoxycytidine analogue, cytosine arabinoside (ara-C), that is metabolically activated to the triphosphate nucleotide (ara-CTP), which acts as a competitive inhibitor of DNA polymerase and produces 5 phase–specific cytotoxicity; used as an antineoplastic for induction of remission of acute lymphocytic leukemia and acute myelocytic leukemia in children and adults, generally as part of a combination chemotherapy regimen. Resistance to ara-C can arise by mutations reducing cellular levels of deoxycytidine kinase, which produces ara-CTP, or increasing levels of cytidine deaminase, which inactivates ara-C. Major side effects are nausea and vomiting and bone marrow depression.

cytarme (sit-ar′me) [Gr. *kytos* cell + *armē* union] the flattening of rounded blastomeres at the conclusion of cleavage.

cytaster (si′tas-ter) [Gr. *kytos* hollow vessel + *astēr* star] aster.

Cytauxzoon (si″tawk-zo′on) [*cyt-* + *aux-* + Gr. *zōon* animal] a genus of parasitic protozoa (order Piroplasmida, subclass Piroplasmia) found in African ungulates and in the domestic cat in North America. **C. fe′lis,** a species causing a fatal disease in domestic cats; see *cytauxzoonosis.*

cytauxzoonosis (si″tawk-zo″o-no′sis) a rapidly fatal disease due to infection with protozoa of the genus *Cytauxzoon,* occurring in African ungulates and in domestic cats. The feline infection is caused by *C. felis* and is seen chiefly in cats roaming the wooded areas of the Gulf Coast states of North America. It is clinically characterized by fever, anemia, icterus, anorexia, lethargy, dehydration, and depression, and microscopically by huge reticuloendothelial cells packed with schizonts in the peripheral blood that nearly occlude the lumens of the small and medium-sized veins of the lungs, spleen, and lymph nodes.

-cyte [Gr. *kytos* hollow vessel] a word termination denoting a cell, the type of which is designated by the root to which it is affixed, as *elliptocyte, erythrocyte, leukocyte.*

Cytellin (si-tel′in) trademark for a preparation of sitosterols.

cythemolysis (si″thĕ-mol′ĭ-sis) hemolysis.

cytheromania (sith″er-o-ma′ne-ah) [Gr. *Kythereia* Venus + *mania* madness] nymphomania.

cytidine (si′tĭ-dēn) a nucleoside, cytosine β-D-ribofuranoside. Symbol C. **c. diphosphate (CDP),** a nucleotide, cytidine 5′-pyrophosphate, which serves as a carrier for choline and ethanolamine in phospholipid synthesis. **c. monophosphate (CMP),** a nucleotide, cytidine 5′-phosphate, which serves as a carrier for N-acetylneuraminic acid in glycoprotein synthesis. Called also *cytidylic acid.* **c. triphosphate (CTP),** a nucleotide, cytidine 5′-triphosphate, required for RNA synthesis and for the formation of phosphatidyl choline and phosphatidyl ethanolamine from choline and ethanolamine via the intermediates CDP-choline and CDP-ethanolamine.

cytidine deaminase (si′tĭ-dēn de-am′in-ās) [EC 3.5.4.5] an enzyme of the hydrolase class that catalyzes the reaction cytidine + H_2O = uridine + NH_3. The reaction, occurring in animal tissues and bacteria, is part of the pyrimidine degradation pathway.

cytidylate (si″tĭ-dil′āt) a dissociated form of cytidylic acid.

cytidylic acid (si″tĭ-dil′ik) cytidine monophosphate.

cytidylyl (si″tĭ-dil′il) the radical formed by removal of OH from the phosphate group of cytidine monophosphate.

cytisine (sit′ĭ-sin) [Gr. *kytisos* laburnum] a highly toxic alkaloid, $C_{11}H_{14}N_2O$, from *Cytisus laburnum,* the laburnum tree of Europe, and others of the same genus; formerly used as an antiemetic and antitussive. Called also *baptitoxine, laburnine, sophorine,* and *ulexine.* See also *cytisism.*

cytisism (sit′ĭ-sizm) poisoning by *Cytisus laburnum,* the laburnum tree of Europe, characterized by burning in the mouth and pharynx, thirst, nausea, vomiting, diarrhea, prostration, and irregular pulse; sometimes accompanied by aphasia, visual disturbances, delirium, and unconsciousness. Death from respiratory paralysis may occur.

Cytisus (sit′ĭ-sus) a genus of leguminous trees of Europe, northern Africa, and southern Asia. *C. scopa′rius* (L.) Link., or scotch broom, is the source of scoparin and scoparius. Called also *Sarothamnus.*

cyt(o)- [Gr. *kytos* hollow vessel] a combining form denoting relationship to a cell.

cytoanalyzer (si″to-an″ah-li′zer) an electronic optical apparatus for the detection of malignant cells in smears.

cytoarchitectonic (si″to-ar″kĭ-tek-ton′ik) pertaining to cellular structure or the arrangement of cells in a tissue.

cytoarchitectural (si″to-ar″kĭ-tek′tu-ral) cytoarchitectonic.

cytoarchitecture (si″to-ar′kĭ-tek″tūr) the organization of cells in the structure of an organ or tissue, especially that in the cerebral cortex.

cytobiology (si″to-bi-ol′o-je) [*cyto-* + *biology*] the biology of cells.

cytobiotaxis (si″to-bi-o-tak′sis) [*cyto-* + Gr. *bios* life + *taxis* arrangement] cytoclesis.

cytoblast (si′to-blast) [*cyto-* + Gr. *blastos* germ] Schleiden's name for the cell nucleus.

cytoblastema (si″to-blas-te′mah) [*cyto-* + *blastema*] Schleiden's name for the mother liquid from which cells were said to form.

cytocentrum (si″to-sen′trum) [*cyto-* + Gr. *kentron* center] centrosome.

cytocerastic (si″to-se-ras′tik) cytokerastic.

cytochalasin (si″to-kal′ah-sin) any of a group of fungal metabolites that affect the motility of polymorphonuclear leukocytes. **c. B,** a cytochalasin that causes the disappearance of cytoplasmic microfilaments and inhibits certain cellular processes, e.g., cytokinesis.

cytochemism (si″to-kem′izm) [*cyto-* + *chemism*] chemical activity of cells.

cytochemistry (si″to-kem″is-tre) [*cyto-* + *chemistry*] the study of the locations, structural relationships, and interactions of cellular constituents by means of methods such as electron microscopy, cell fractionation, and immunochemical techniques.

cytochrome (si′to-krōm) [*cyto-* + Gr. *chrōma* color] any electron transfer hemoprotein having a mode of action in which the transfer of a single electron is effected by a reversible valence change of the central iron atom of the heme prosthetic group between the $+2$ and $+3$ oxidation states; classified as cytochromes a in which the heme contains a formyl side chain, cytochromes b, which contain protoheme or a closely similar heme that is not covalently bound to the protein, cytochromes c in which protoheme or other heme is covalently bound to the protein, and cytochromes d in which the iron-tetrapyrrole has fewer conjugated double bonds than the hemes have. Well-known cytochromes have been numbered consecutively within groups and are designated by subscripts (beginning with no subscript), e.g., cytochromes c, c_1, c_2, ... New cytochromes are named according to the wavelength in nanometers of the absorption maximum of the α-band of the iron (II) form in pyridine, e.g., c-555. **c. a_3, aa_3,** c. c oxidase. **c. b,** a cytochrome in the inner mitochondrial membrane that is involved with cytochrome c_1 and an iron-sulfur protein in the transfer of electrons from ubiquinol to cytochrome c in oxidative phosphorylation. **c. b_5,** a cytochrome occurring in the endoplasmic reticulum that acts as an intermediate electron carrier in some reactions catalyzed by mixed function oxidases, e.g., fatty acid desaturation; it activates molecular oxygen for an attack on the substrate. **c. c.,** a cytochrome on the inner mitochondrial membrane that serves as an electron carrier in oxidative phosphorylation. **c. c_1,** a cytochrome in the inner mitochondrial membrane that, with cytochrome b and an iron-sulfur protein, is involved in the transfer of electrons from ubiquinol to cytochrome c in oxidative phosphorylation. **c. P-450, c. P_{450},** trivial name (P for pigment, 450 nm for the absorption maximum of the CO derivative) for a cytochrome occurring in liver endoplasmic reticulum, the renal brush border, and the outer membrane of adrenal mitochondria that serves as an intermediate electron carrier in reactions catalyzed by some monooxygenases, e.g., hydroxylation of steroid hormones and oxidations involved in the detoxification of many drugs; cytochrome P-450 activates molecular oxygen for an attack on the substrate.

cytochrome oxidase (si'to-krōm ok'sĭ-dās) cytochrome c oxidase.

cytochrome c oxidase (si'to-krōm ok'sĭ-dās) [EC 1.9.3.1] an enzyme complex of the inner mitochondrial membrane that catalyzes the reaction 4 ferrocytochrome $c + O_2 = 4$ ferricytochrome $c + 2H_2O$. It contains two distinguishable heme a groups and two Cu^{2+} ions and is associated with the pumping of protons and resultant phosphorylation of ADP to TP. Its reaction is the terminal event in the electron transport scheme by which oxygen is used for fuel combustion. The Fe^{2+} form a has a strong affinity for CO, in the Fe^{3+} form it binds CN^-, S^{2-}, and N_3. The binding of these compounds inactivates the enzyme, a cause of their extreme toxcity for all aerobic organisms. Called also *cytochrome aa_3* and *cytochrome oxidase.*

cytochrome b_5 reductase (si'to-krōm re-duk'tas) [EC 1.6.2.2] an enzyme of the oxidoreductase class that catalyzes the reaction NADH $+ 2$ ferricytochrome $b_5 = $ NAD$^+$ $+ 2$ ferrocytochrome b_5. It is a flavoprotein, tightly bound to the endoplasmic reticulum, probably identical with the NADH-methemoglobin reductase of erythrocytes. The reaction is involved in the desaturation of fatty acids. The enzyme is deficient in the leukocytes and fibroblasts and sometimes in the brain and muscle of patients with hereditary methemoglobinemia. Called also *NADH cytochrome b_5 reductase.*

cytochrome P-450 reductase (si'to-krōm re-duk'tās) NADPH-ferrihemoprotein reductase.

cytochylema (si"to-ki-le'mah) [*cyto-* + Gr. *chylos* juice] hyaloplasm, def. 1.

cytocidal (si"to-si'dal) destructive to cells.

cytocide (si'to-sīd) [*cyto-* + L. *caedere* to kill] an agent that destroys cells.

cytocinesis (si"to-si-ne'sis) cytokinesis.

cytoclasis (si-tok'lah-sis) [*cyto-* + Gr. *klasis* a breaking] the destruction of cells.

cytoclastic (si"to-klas'tik) pertaining to, characterized by, or causing cytoclasis.

cytoclesis (si"to-kle'sis) [*cyto-* + Gr. *klēsis* a call] a form of energy, totally unrelated to electricity, light, heat, or sound, which is generated by living tissues; the vital principle in all living tissues (M. Kelly). The term was first introduced in 1923 by Frederic Wood Jones, who defined it as the influence of body cells on other body cells; the "call of cell to cell." Called also *cytobiotaxis.*

cytocletic (si"to-klet'ik) pertaining to cytoclesis.

cytoctony (si-tok'to-ne) [*cyto-* + Gr. *ktonos* murder] the killing of cells; specifically the killing by viruses of cells in culture.

cytocuprein (si"to-koo'prin) superoxide dismutase.

cytode (si'tōd) [*cyto-* + Gr. *eidos* form] a non-nucleated cell or cell element.

cytodendrite (si"to-den'drīt) [*cyto-* + *dendrite*] dendrite.

cytodesma (si"to-dez'mah) [*cyto-* + Gr. *desma* band] the lamellar or bridgelike tissues binding animal cells together (Studnicka).

cytodiagnosis (si"to-di"ag-no'sis) [*cyto-* + *diagnosis*] diagnosis of disease based on the examination of cells. **exfoliative c.,** the examination of cells that have desquamated from the external or internal surfaces of the body as a means of detecting cancer.

cytodiagnostic (si"to-di"ag-nos'tik) pertaining to or subserving cytodiagnosis.

cytodieresis (si"to-di-er'ĕ-sis) [*cyto-* + Gr. *diairesis* division] cell division, i.e., meiosis or mitosis.

cytodifferentiation (si"to-dif"er-en"she-a'shun) the development of specialized structures and functions in embryonic cells.

cytodistal (si"to-dis'tal) [*cyto-* + *distal*] denoting that part of an axon remote from the cell of origin.

cytoflav (si'to-flav) a phosphoric acid ester of riboflavin, found in the liver and in the heart.

cytoflavin (si"to-fla'vin) a flavin that was first isolated from heart muscle; it is the phosphoric acid ester of riboflavin.

cytogene (si'to-jēn) plasmagene.

cytogenesis (si"to-jen'ĕ-sis) [*cyto-* + Gr. *genesis* origin] the origin and development of cells.

cytogenetical (si"to-jĕ-net'ĕ-kal) pertaining to cytogenetics.

cytogeneticist (si"to-je-net'ĭ-sist) a specialist in cytogenetics.

cytogenetics (si"to-jĕ-net'iks) the branch of genetics devoted to study of the cellular constituents concerned in heredity, that is, the chromosomes. **clinical c.,** the scientific study of the relationship between chromosomal aberrations and pathological conditions.

cytogenic (si-to-jen'ik) 1. pertaining to cytogenesis. 2. forming or producing cells.

cytogenous (si-toj'ĕ-nus) [*cyto-* + Gr. *gennan* to produce] producing cells.

cytogeny (si-toj'ĕ-ne) 1. cytogenesis. 2. cell lineage.

cytoglomerator (si"to-glom"er-a'tor) an apparatus for processing blood before freezing it for storage, and after thawing it.

cytoglucopenia (si"to-gloo"ko-pe'ne-ah) cytoglycopenia.

cytoglycopenia (si"to-gli"ko-pe'ne-ah) [*cyto-* + *glucose* + Gr. *penia* poverty] deficient glucose content of body or blood cells.

cytogony (si-tog'ŏ-ne) [*cyto-* + Gr. *gonos* seed] cytogenic reproduction.

cytohistogenesis (si"to-his"to-jen'ĕ-sis) [*cyto-* + Gr. *histos* web + *genesis* formation] the development of the structure of cells.

cytohistologic (si"to-his"to-loj'ik) involving both cytologic and histologic methods.

cytohistology (si"to-his-tol'o-je) the combination of cytologic and histologic methods.

cytohormone (si"to-hor'mōn) [*cyto-* + *hormone*] a cell hormone.

cytohyaloplasm (si"to-hi'ah-lo-plazm") [*cyto-* + Gr. *hyalos* crystal + *plasma* plasm] the clear substance of cytoplasm.

cytoid (si'toid) [*cyto-* + Gr. *eidos* form] resembling a cell.

cytokalipenia (si"to-kal'ĭ-pe'ne-ah) [*cyto-* + L. *kalium* potassium + Gr. *penia* poverty] deficient potassium content of body or blood cells.

cytokerastic (si"to-kĕ-ras'tik) [*cyto-* + Gr. *kerastos* mixed] pertaining to the development of cells from a lower to a higher order.

cytokine (si"to-kīn) [*cyto-* + Gr. *kinēsis* movement] a generic term for nonantibody proteins released by one cell population (e.g., primed T-lymphocytes) on contact with specific antigen, which act as intercellular mediators, as in the generation of an immune response. Examples include lymphokines and monokines.

cytokinesis (si″to-ki-ne′sis) [*cyto-* + Gr. *kinēsis* motion] the changes that take place in the cytoplasm during cell division; division of the cytoplasm, a process synchronized in eukaryotic cells with nuclear division (mitosis).

cytokinin (si″to-ki′nin) any of a class of phytohormones (N^6-substituted adenines) whose principal functions are the induction of cell division (cytokinesis) and the regulation of differentiation of tissue (organogenesis).

cytolipin H ceramide lactoside.

cytologic (si″to-loj′ik) pertaining to cytology.

cytologist (si-tol′o-jist) a specialist in cytology.

cytology (si-tol′o-je) [*cyto-* + *-logy*] the study of cells, their origin, structure, function, and pathology. **aspiration biopsy c. (ABC)**, the microscopic study of cells obtained from superficial or internal lesions by suction through a fine needle. **exfoliative c.**, microscopic examination of cells desquamated from a body surface or lesion as a means of detecting malignancy and microbiologic changes, to measure hormonal levels, etc. Such cells may be obtained by such procedures as aspiration, washing, smear, and scraping, and the technique may be applied to vaginal secretions, sputum, urine, abdominal fluid, prostatic secretion, etc.

cytolymph (si′to-limf) [*cyto-* + *lymph*] hyaloplasm, def. 1.

cytolysate (si-tol′ĭ-sāt) a preparation of lyzed cells. **blood c.**, hemolysate.

cytolysin (si-tol′ĭ-sin) a substance or antibody that produces dissolution of cells. Cytolysins that have a specific action for certain cells are named accordingly, as *hemolysins*, etc.

cytolysis (si-tol′ĭ-sis) [*cyto-* + Gr. *lysis* dissolution] the dissolution or destruction of cells. **immune c.**, cell lysis produced by antibody with the participation of complement.

cytolysosome (si″to-li′so-sōm) autophagosome.

cytolytic (si″to-lit′ik) pertaining to, characterized by, or causing cytolysis.

cytoma (si-to′mah) [*cyto-* + *-oma*] a cell tumor, as a sarcoma.

cytomegaloviruria (si″to-meg″ah-lo-vi-roo′re-ah) presence in the urine of cytomegaloviruses.

cytomegalovirus (si″to-meg″ah-lo-vi′rus) one of a group of highly host-specific herpesviruses that infect man, monkeys, or rodents, with the production of unique large cells bearing intranuclear inclusions. Depending upon the age and the immune status of the host, cytomegalovirus can cause a variety of clinical syndromes, collectively known as cytomegalic inclusion disease (see under *disease*), although the majority of infections are very mild or subclinical. Called also *salivary gland virus*.

Cytomel (si′to-mel) trademark for a preparation of liothyronine sodium.

cytomere (si′to-mēr) [*cyto-* + Gr. *meros* part] the multinucleate portion of the schizont of certain sporozoa that separates and gives rise to merozoites.

cytometaplasia (si″to-met″ah-pla′ze-ah) [*cyto-* + Gr. *metaplasis* change] alteration in the form or function of a cell.

cytometer (si-tom′ĕ-ter) [*cyto-* + Gr. *metron* measure] a device for counting blood cells, as a hemocytometer.

cytometry (si-tom′ĕ-tre) the counting of blood cells; blood counting.

cytomitome (si″to-mi′tōm) [*cyto-* + Gr. *mitos* thread] a fibril or fibrillary structure in the cytoplasm.

cytomorphology (si″to-mor-fol′o-je) the morphology of cells.

cytomorphosis (si″to-mor-fo′sis) [*cyto-* + Gr. *morphōsis* a shaping] the series of changes through which cells go in the process of formation, development, senescence, etc.

cyton (si′ton) the cell body of a neuron.

cytonecrosis (si″to-nĕ-kro′sis) death of individual cells.

cytopathic (si″to-path′ik) pertaining to or characterized by pathological changes in cells.

cytopathogenesis (si″to-path″o-jen′ĕ-sis) the production of pathological changes in cells.

cytopathogenetic (si″to-path″o-jĕ-net′ik) pertaining to or characterized by cytopathogenesis.

cytopathogenic (si″to-path″o-jen′ik) capable of producing pathological changes in cells.

cytopathogenicity (si″to-path″o-jĕ-nis′ĭ-te) the quality of being capable of producing pathological changes in cells.

cytopathologic, cytopathological (si″to-path″o-loj′ik; si″to-path″o-loj′ĭ-kal) relating to cytopathology; denoting the changes in cells in disease.

cytopathologist (si″to-pah-thol′o-jist) an expert in the study of cells in disease; a cellular pathologist.

cytopathology (si″to-pah-thol′o-je) [*cyto-* + Gr. *pathos* disease + *-logy*] the study of cells in disease; cellular pathology.

cytopenia (si″to-pe′ne-ah) [*cyto-* + Gr. *penia* poverty] deficiency in the cellular elements of the blood.

Cytophaga (si-tof′ah-gah) [*cyto-* + Gr. *phagein* to eat] a genus of gliding bacteria of the family Cytophagaceae found in soil and water, made up of rod-shaped single or filamentous cells that decompose agar, chitin, or cellulose. The type species is *C. hutchinso′nii*.

Cytophagaceae (si″to-fah-ga′se-e) a family of gliding bacteria of the order Cytophagales, made up of rod-shaped single or filamentous cells containing carotenoid pigments. They are saprophytic soil microorganisms, many of which decompose cellulose. The order contains the genera *Cytophaga, Flexibacter, Flexithrix, Herpetosiphon, Saprospira,* and *Sporocytophaga.*

Cytophagales (si″to-fah-ga′lēz) an order of bacteria, found in soil and in fresh and salt water, made up of rod-shaped single and filamentous organisms that are motile by a gliding motion and do not produce fruiting bodies. It consists of the families Beggiatoaceae, Cytophagaceae, Leucotrichaceae, and Simonsiellaceae and the related families Achromatiaceae and Pelonemataceae.

cytophagocytosis (si″to-fag″o-si-to′sis) cytophagy.

cytophagous (si-tof′ah-gus) [*cyto-* + Gr. *phagein* to eat] devouring or consuming cells; said of phagocytes.

cytophagy (si-tof′ah-je) the ingestion of cells by phagocytes.

cytopharynx (si″to-far′inks) [*cyto-* + *pharynx*] a nonciliated gullet-like canal between the cytostome and the endoplasm of ciliate and certain other protozoa. See also *cytopharyngeal apparatus*, under *apparatus*.

cytophil (si′to-fil) an element or substance that has an affinity for cells.

cytophilic (si-to-fil′ik) [*cyto-* + Gr. *philein* to love] having an affinity for cells, as cytophilic antibodies.

cytophotometer (si″to-fo-tom′ĕ-ter) a photometer for measuring localization of organic compounds within cells by measuring the light intensity through selected stained areas of cytoplasm.

cytophotometric (si″to-fo″to-met′rik) pertaining to or accomplished by cytophotometry.

cytophotometry (si″to-fo-tom′ĕ-tre) the study of organic compounds within cells by means of the cytophotometer. Called also *microfluorometry*.

cytophylactic (si″to-fi-lak′tik) pertaining to cytophylaxis.

cytophylaxis (si″to-fi-lak′sis) [*cyto-* + Gr. *phylaxis* a guarding] 1. the protection of cells. 2. increase of cellular activity.

cytophyletic (si″to-fi-let′ik) [*cyto-* + Gr. *phylē* a tribe] pertaining to the genealogy of cells.

cytophysics (si″to-fiz′iks) the physics of cell activity.

cytophysiology (si″to-fiz-e-ol′o-je) [*cyto-* + *physiology*] the physiology of the cell.

cytopigment (si′to-pig′ment) any pigment found in cells.

cytopipette (si″to-pi-pet′) a pipette for taking cytological smears.

cytoplasm (si′to-plazm″) [*cyto-* + Gr. *plasma* plasm] the protoplasm of a cell exclusive of that of the nucleus; it consists of a continuous aqueous solution (cytosol) and the organelles and inclusions suspended in it (phaneroplasm), and is the site of most of the chemical activities of the cell. Cf. *nucleoplasm*.

cytoplasmic (si″to-plaz′mik) pertaining to or contained in the cytoplasm.

cytoplast (si′to-plast) a cell from which the nucleus has been removed and which remains viable for a time.

cytoproct (si′to-prokt) [*cyto-* + Gr. *prōktos* anus] a permanent posterior pore seen in certain ciliates, through which waste egesta can be eliminated. Called also *cytopyge.*

cytoproximal (si′to-prok′sĭ-mal) [*cyto-* + *proximal*] denoting that part of an axon nearer to the cell of origin.

cytopyge (si′to-pig) [*cyto-* + *pygē* rump] cytoproct.

cytoreticulum (si′to-rĕ-tik′u-lum)[*cyto-* + L. *retic′ulum* network] spongioplasm.

cytorrhyctes (si′′to-rik′tēz) [*cyto-* + Gr. *oryssein* to dig] cell inclusions, found in various diseases, which may be specific protozoan pathogens, or they may be manifestations of cell reactions to the parasite causing the disease, or they may be degenerations caused by the disease. See *Siegel's organism,* under *organism.*

Cytosar-U (si′to-sar) trademark for preparations of cytarabine.

cytoscopy (si-tos′ko-pe) [*cyto-* + Gr. *skopein* to examine] examination of cells.

cytosiderin (si′′to-sid′er-in) intracellular pigment due probably to derangement of iron metabolism.

cytosine (si′to-sēn) a base, oxyaminopyrimidine, $C_4H_5N_3O$, a component of nucleic acid. **c. arabinoside,** cytarabine. **5-hydroxymethyl c.,** a pyrimidine that replaces cytosine in the DNA of certain coliphages.

cytoskeletal (si′′to-skel′ĕ-tal) of or pertaining to the cytoskeleton.

cytoskeleton (si′′to-skel′ĕ-ton) a conspicuous internal reinforcement in the cytoplasm of a cell, consisting of tonofibrils, terminal web, or other microfilaments.

cytosol (si′to-sol) the liquid medium of the cytoplasm, i.e., cytoplasm minus organelles and nonmembranous insoluble components.

cytosol aminopeptidase (si′to-sol ah′′me-no-pep′tid-ās) [EC 3.4.11.1] an enzyme of the hydrolase class that catalyzes the reaction aminoacyl-peptide + H_2O = amino acid + peptide. It is a zinc-containing enzyme, active on most L-peptides except those with *N*-terminal lysyl-or arginyl groups. It is found in the cell cytosol of tissues, with high activity in the duodenum, liver, and kidney. Called also *leucine amino-peptidase* (LAP).

cytosolic (si′′to-sol′ik) pertaining to or contained in the cytosol.

cytosome (si′to-sōm) [*cyto-* + Gr. *sōma* body] 1. the body of a cell apart from its nucleus. 2. multilamellar body.

cytospongium (si′′to-spon′je-um) [*cyto-* + Gr. *spongos* sponge] spongioplasm.

cytost (si′tost) [Gr. *kytos* hollow vessel] a specific toxin given off from a cell as a result of injury to it; a specific agent given off from broken-down tissue.

cytostasis (si-tos′tah-sis) [*cyto-* + Gr. *stasis* halt] the closure of capillaries by white blood corpuscles in the early stages of inflammation.

cytostatic (si′′to-stat′ik) [*cyto-* + Gr. *statikos* bringing to a stand-still] 1. suppressing the growth and multiplication of cells. 2. an agent that suppresses cell growth and multiplication.

cytostome (si′to-stōm) [*cyto-* + Gr. *stoma* mouth] the mouth opening of ciliates and certain other protozoa, which opens into the cytopharynx, which in turn opens into the endoplasm.

cytostromatic (si′′to-stro-mat′ik) [*cyto-* + *stroma*] pertaining to the stroma of a cell.

cytotactic (si′′to-tak′tik) pertaining to cytotaxis.

cytotaxigen (si′′to-taks′ĭ-jen) a substance that mediates chemotaxis of cells indirectly by inducing cytotaxin formation; thus antigen-antibody complexes are cytotaxigenic because when added to serum they fix complement, resulting in the liberation of chemotactic factors derived from complement.

cytotaxin (si′′to-taks′in) chemotactic factor.

cytotaxis (si-to-tak′sis) [*cyto-* + Gr. *taxis* arrangement] the movement and arrangement of cells with respect to a specific source of stimulation.

cytothesis (si-toth′ĕ-sis) [*cyto-* + Gr. *thesis* placing] the restitution of injured cells to their normal condition.

cytotoxic (si′′to-tok′sik) pertaining to or exhibiting cytotoxicity.

cytotoxicity (si′′to-tok-sis′ĭ-te) the degree to which an agent possesses a specific destructive action on certain cells or the possession of such action; used particularly in referring to the lysis of cells by immune phenomena and to antineoplastic drugs that selectively kill dividing cells. **antibody-dependent cell-mediated c., antibody-dependent cellular c. (ADCC),** lysis of target cells coated with IgG antibody by several types of effector cells, including K cells, macrophages, and granulocytes; a form of Type II hypersensitivity (see *Gell and Coombs classification,* under *classification*). ADCC involves binding of the effector cell by means of Fc receptors which bind to the Fc portion of the IgG molecule. Lysis of the target cell is extracellular, requires direct cell-to-cell contact, and does not involve complement.

cytotoxin (si′′to-tok′sin) [*cyto-* + *toxin*] a toxin or antibody that has a specific toxic action upon cells of special organs; cytotoxins are named according to the special variety of cell for which they are specific, as *nephrotoxin.*

cytotrophoblast (si′′to-trof′o-blast) [*cyto-* + Gr. *trophē* nutrition + *blastos* germ] the cellular (inner) layer of the trophoblast; called also *Langhans' layer.*

cytotropic (si′′to-trop′ik) [*cyto-* + Gr. *tropos* a turning] attracting cells; possessing an affinity for cells; said especially of antibodies that attach to cell surfaces. See also under *antibody.*

cytotropism (si-tot′ro-pizm) 1. cell movement in response to external stimulation. 2. the tendency of viruses, bacteria, drugs, etc., to exert their effect upon certain cells of the body.

Cytoxan (si-tok′san) trademark for preparations of cyclophosphamide.

cytozoic (si′′to-zo′ik) living within or attached to cells; said of parasites.

cytula (sit′u-lah) the impregnated ovum.

cytuloplasm (sit′u-lo-plazm′′) the combined ovoplasm and spermoplasm in a cytula.

cyturia (sĭ-tu′re-ah) [Gr. *kytos* hollow vessel + *ouron* urine + *-ia*] the presence of cells of any sort in the urine.

CyVADIC a regimen of cyclophosphamide, vincristine, Adriamycin (doxorubicin) and imidazole carboxamide (dacarbazine), used in cancer chemotherapy.

Czermak's spaces (lines) (chār′mahks) [Johann Nepomuk *Czermak,* Bohemian physician, 1828–1873] spatia interglobularia.

Czerny's suture (chār′nēz) [Vincenz *Czerny,* surgeon in Heidelberg, 1842–1916] see under *suture.*

Czerny-Lembert suture (char′ne-lah-bar′) [Vincenz *Czerny;* Antoine *Lembert,* French surgeon, 1802–1851] see under *suture.*

D

D symbol for *debye, deciduous* (in dental formulas), *deuterium, diffusing capacity* (see under *capacity*), *diopter,* and an obsolete unit of vitamin D potency equal to the potency of cod liver oil.

2,4-D a toxic chlorphenoxy herbicide (2,4-dichlorophenoxyacetic acid) that acts as a growth-regulating hormone killing broadleaf plants by overstimulation.

D. abbreviation for L., *dosis,* dose; *da,* give; *detur,* let it be given; *dexter,* right; also for *density, died, distal, dorsal* (in vertebral formulas), and *duration.*

D$_L$ diffusing capacity of the lung D$_{L_{O_2}}$ denotes diffusing capacity for oxygen, D$_{L_{CO}}$, diffusing capacity for carbon monoxide, etc.).

D$_{37}$ the dose necessary to reduce the surviving fraction, as of cells, to e^{-1} or 0.37, where the biological activity declines exponentially as a function of dose.

D- a chemical prefix (small capital D) that specifies the relative configuration of an enantiomer, the mirror image configuration being specified as L-. Carbohydrates are designated as D or L depending on their configuration at the asymmetric carbon atom most distant from the carbonyl functional group; those with the same configuration as D-glyceraldehyde (the arbitrarily chosen standard) are in the D configurational family. Amino acids are designated according to their configuration at the α-carbon (the standard being serine). All of the α-amino acids occurring in proteins have the L configuration; a few D-amino acids occur in short peptides produced by bacteria. For derivatives of glycerol the nomenclature is complicated by the fact that the glycerol chain can be numbered starting at either end. The designation as D or L indicates the configuration at carbon 2 relative to D-glyceraldehyde.

d symbol for *day, deci-, deoxyribose* (in specifying nucleosides, and nucleotides, e.g., A is adenosine, dA is deoxyadenosine) and *diameter.*

d- (de-) [abbreviation for *dextro* (right or clockwise)] a chemical prefix indicating an enantiomer that rotates the plane of polarization of a beam of light in the clockwise direction, the other enantiomer being specified as *l-* (for *levo*). NOTE: The prefixes *d-* and *l-* are now being replaced by (+)- and (–)-, respectively, especially when the prefixes D- and L- are also used, e.g., *l*-fructose is D-(–)-fructose.

δ delta, the fourth letter of the Greek alphabet; symbol for the heavy chain of IgD and the δ chain of hemoglobin.

D.A. developmental age.

dA deoxyadenosine.

da- rarely used symbol for the metric prefix *deka-.*

d'Abano, Pietro see *Peter of Abano.*

Daboia (dah-boi′ah) a genus of snakes. **D. russel′li,** Russell's viper (*Vipera russelli*).

dacarbazine (dah-kar′-bah-zēn) a cytotoxic alkylating agent used as an antineoplastic primarily for treatment of malignant melanoma and in combination chemotherapy for Hodgkin's disease and sarcomas; major side effects are anorexia, nausea and vomiting, and bone marrow depression. Abbreviated DTIC.

d'Acosta see *Acosta.*

DaCosta's syndrome (dah-kah′stahz) [Jacob Mendes *Da-Costa,* American physician, 1833–1900] see *neurocirculatory asthenia,* under *asthenia.*

dacryadenalgia (dak″re-ad-ĕ-nal′je-ah) dacryoadenalgia.

dacryadenitis (dak″re-ad-ĕ-ni′tis) dacryoadenitis.

dacryadenoscirrhus (dak″re-ad″ĕ-no-skir′us) [*dacry-* + Gr. *adēn* gland + *skirrhos* scirrhus] (*obs.*) scirrhous carcinoma of a lacrimal gland.

dacryagogatresia (dak″re-ah-gog″ah-tre′ze-ah) [*dacry-* + Gr. *agōgos* leading + *atresia*] atresia, imperforation, or closure of a lacrimal duct.

dacryagogic (dak″re-ah-goj′ik) pertaining to a dacryagogue.

dacryagogue (dak′re-ah-gog″) [*dacry-* + *-agogue*] 1. an agent that induces a flow of tears. 2. a lacrimal duct.

dacrycystalgia (dak″re-sis-tal′je-ah) dacryocystalgia.

dacrycystitis (dak″re-sis-ti′tis) dacryocystitis.

dacryelcosis (dak″re-el-ko′sis) dacryohelcosis.

dacry(o)- [Gr. *dakryon* tear] a combining form denoting relationship to tears.

dacryoadenalgia (dak″re-o-ad″ĕ-nal′je-ah) [*dacryo-* + *aden-* + *-algia*] pain in a lacrimal gland.

dacryoadenectomy (dak″re-o-ad″ĕ-nek′to-me) [*dacryo-* + *aden-* + *ectomy*] excision of a lacrimal gland.

dacryoadenitis (dak″re-o-ad″ĕ-ni′tis) inflammation of a lacrimal gland.

dacryoblennorrhea (dak″re-o-blen″o-re′ah) [*dacryo-* + *blennorrhea*] mucous discharge from the lacrimal ducts, as in chronic dacryocystitis.

dacryocanaliculitis (dak″re-o-kan″ah-lik″u-li′tis) inflammation of the lacrimal ducts.

dacryocele (dak′re-o-sēl″) dacryocystocele.

dacryocyst (dak′re-o-sist″) [*dacryo-* + *cyst*] the lacrimal sac.

dacryocystalgia (dak″re-o-sis-tal′je-ah) [*dacryocyst* + *-algia*] pain in a lacrimal sac.

dacryocystectasia (dak″re-o-sis″tek-ta′ze-ah) [*dacryocyst* + *ectasia*] dilatation of the lacrimal sac.

dacryocystectomy (dak″re-o-sis-tek′to-me) [*dacryocyst* + *ectomy*] excision of the wall of the lacrimal sac.

dacryocystis (dak″re-o-sis′tis) [*dacryo-* + *cystis*] the lacrimal sac.

dacryocystitis (dak″re-o-sis-ti′tis) inflammation of the lacrimal sac.

dacryocystitome (dak″re-o-sis″tĭ-tōm) [*dacryocyst* + *-tome*] an instrument for incising strictures of the lacrimal duct.

dacryocystoblennorrhea (dak″re-o-sis″to-blen″o-re′ah) [*dacryocyst* + *blennorrhea*] a chronic catarrhal inflammation of the lacrimal sac, with constriction of the lacrimal duct.

dacryocystocele (dak″re-o-sis′to-sēl) [*dacryocyst* + *-cele* (def. 1)] hernial protrusion of the lacrimal sac; called also *dacryocele.*

dacryocystoptosis (dak″re-o-sis″top-to′sis) [*dacryocyst* + *ptosis*] prolapse or downward displacement of the lacrimal sac.

dacryocystorhinostenosis (dak″re-o-sis″to-ri″no-stĕ-no′-sis) narrowing of the duct leading from the lacrimal sac to the nasal cavity.

dacryocystorhinostomy (dak″re-o-sis″to-ri-nos′to-me) [*dacryocyst* + *rhino-* + *-stomy*] surgical creation of a communication between the lacrimal sac and the nasal cavity; called also *dacryorhinocystotomy* and *Toti's operation.*

dacryocystorhinotomy (dak″re-o-sis″to-ri-not′o-me) [*dacryocyst* + *rhino-* + *-tomy*] passage of a probe through the lacrimal sac into the nasal cavity.

dacryocystostenosis (dak″re-o-sis″to-stĕ-no′sis) narrowing of the lacrimal sac.

dacryocystostomy (dak″re-o-sis-tos′to-me) [*dacryocyst* + *-stomy*] surgical creation of a new opening into the lacrimal sac.

dacryocystotome (dak″re-o-sis′to-tōm) a dacryocystitome.

dacryocystotomy (dak″re-o-sis-tot′o-me) [*dacryocyst* + *-tomy*] incision of the lacrimal sac; called also *Ammon's operation.*

dacryogenic (dak″re-o-jen′ik) [*dacryo-* + *-genic*] promoting the secretion of tears.

dacryohelcosis (dak″re-o-hel-ko′sis) [*dacryo-* + *helcosis*] ulceration of the lacrimal sac or lacrimal duct.

dacryohemorrhea (dak″re-o-hem″o-re′ah) [*dacryo-* + *hemo-* + *-rrhea*] the discharge of tears mixed with blood.

dacryolith (dak′re-o-lith″) [*dacryo-* + Gr. *lithos* stone] a concretion in the lacrimal sac or duct.

dacryolithiasis (dak″re-o-lĭ-thi′ah-sis) [*dacryo-* + *lithiasis*] the presence of calculi in the lacrimal sac or duct.

dacryoma (dak″re-o′mah) a tumor-like swelling caused by obstruction of the lacrimal duct.

dacryon (dak′re-on) [Gr. *dakryon* tear] a cranial point at the juncture of the lacrimal and frontal bones, and the maxilla.

dacryops (dak′re-ops) [*dacry-* + Gr. *ōps* eye] 1. a watery state of the eye. 2. distention of a lacrimal duct by contained fluid.

dacryopyorrhea (dak″re-o-pi″o-re′ah) [*dacryo-* + *pyorrhea*] the discharge of tears mixed with pus.

dacryopyosis (dak″re-o-pi-o′sis) [*dacryo-* + *pyosis*] suppuration of the lacrimal sac and duct.

dacryorhinocystotomy (dak″re-o-ri″no-sis-tot′o-me) dacryocystorhinostomy.

dacryorrhea (dak″re-o-re′ah) [*dacryo-* + *-rrhea*] an overabundant flow of tears.

dacryoscintigraphy (dak″re-o-sin-tig′rah-fe) scintigraphy of the lacrimal ducts.

dacryosinusitis (dak″re-o-si″nus-i′tis) inflammation of the lacrimal duct and ethmoid sinus.

dacryosolenitis (dak″re-o-so-lĕ-ni′tis) [dacryo- + Gr. sōlēn duct + -itis] inflammation of a lacrimal duct.

dacryostenosis (dak″re-o-stĕ-no′sis) [dacryo- + stenosis] stricture or narrowing of a lacrimal duct.

dacryosyrinx (dak″re-o-sir′inks) [dacryo- + Gr. syrinx tube] 1. a lacrimal duct (canaliculus lacrimalis [NA]). 2. a lacrimal fistula. 3. a syringe for irrigating the lacrimal ducts.

DACT dactinomycin.

Dactil (dak′til) trademark for preparations of piperiodolate hydrochloride.

dactinomycin (dak″tĭ-no-mi′sin) [USP] an antineoplastic antibiotic (actinomycin D) produced by *Streptomyces pavullus*; it consists of a phenoxazone ring and two cyclic pentapeptide side chains and acts by binding to DNA with the ring intercalated between adjacent guanine-cytosine base pairs resulting in blocking of transcription by RNA polymerase; it is used as an antineoplastic agent for treatment of rhabdomyosarcoma and Wilms' tumor in children and is also effective against Ewing's sarcoma, Kaposi's sarcoma, osteogenic sarcoma and soft tissue sarcomas, testicular carcinoma, and choriocarcinoma. Major side effects are nausea and vomiting, ulceration of the oral mucosa, and bone marrow depression.

dactyl (dak′til) [Gr. *daktylos* a finger] a digit; a finger or toe.

dactylate (dak′tĭ-lāt) possessing finger-like processes.

dactyledema (dak″til-ĕ-de′mah) edema or swelling of the fingers or toes.

dactylion (dak-til′e-on) syndactyly.

dactylitis (dak″tĭ-li′tis) [dactyl- + -itis] inflammation of a finger or toe.

dactyl(o)- [Gr. *daktylos* finger] a combining form denoting relationship to a digit, usually referring to the fingers but sometimes to the toes.

dactylocampsodynia (dak″tĭ-lo-kamp″so-din′e-ah) [dactylo- + Gr. *kampsis* bend + *odynē* pain] painful flexure of the fingers.

dactylogram (dak-til′o-gram) [dactylo- + Gr. *gramma* mark] a fingerprint taken for purposes of identification.

dactylography (dak″tĭ-log′rah-fe) [dactylo- + Gr. *graphein* to write] the study of fingerprints.

dactylogryposis (dak″tĭ-lo-grĭ-po′sis) [dactylo- + Gr. *grypōsis* a hooking] a permanent curving of the fingers.

dactylology (dak″til-ol′o-je) [dactylo- + Gr. *logos* discourse] use of movements of the hands and fingers as a means of communication between individuals; called also *cheirology* and *dactylophasia*.

dactylolysis (dak″tĭ-lol′ĭ-sis) [dactylo- + Gr. *lysis* a loosening] loss or amputation of a digit. **d. spontan′ea,** ainhum.

dactylomegaly (dak″tĭ-lo-meg′ah-le) [dactylo- + Gr. *megaleia* largeness] abnormally large fingers or toes.

dactylophasia (dak″tĭ-lo-fa′ze-ah) [dactylo- + Gr. *phasis* speech] dactylology.

dactyloscopy (dak″tĭ-los′ko-pe) [dactylo- + Gr. *skopein* to examine] examination of fingerprints for purposes of identification.

Dactylosoma (dak″tĭ-lo-so′mah) [dactylo- + Gr. *soma* body] a genus of hematozoic protozoa (order Piroplasmida, subclass Piroplasmia) found in reptiles, amphibians, and fish.

dactylospasm (dak′tĭ-lo-spazm) [dactylo- + Gr. *spasmos* spasm] spasm or cramp of a finger or toe.

Dactylosporangium (dak″til-o-spo-ran′je-um) [Gr. *dactylos* finger + L. *sporangium* spore case] a genus of bacteria of the family Actinoplanaceae, order Actinomycetales, made up of soil organisms forming sporangia in clusters on the surface of a vegetative mycelium. The type species is *D. auranti′acum*.

dactylus (dak′tĭ-lus) [Gr. *daktylos* finger] a digit; a finger or toe.

DADDS diacetyl diaminodiphenylsulfone; see *acedapsone*.

dADP deoxyadenosine diphosphate.

Dagenan (dag′ĕ-nan) trademark for sulfapyridine.

D.A.H. disordered action of the heart. See *neurocirculatory asthenia*, under *asthenia*.

dahlia (dahl′yah) the term for certain unspecified mixtures of methylated and ethylated pararosanilins and rosanilins; C.I.42530. Sometimes used as a basic dye for violet staining. Called also *Hofmann's* or *iodine violet*. **d. B.,** see *gentian violet*, under *violet*.

dahlin (dah′lin) inulin.

Dakin-Carrel method (da′kin-kar-el′) [Henry Drysdale Dakin; Alexis Carrel, French surgeon, 1873–1944] see *Carrel treatment*, under *treatment*.

Dakin's fluid (antiseptic solution) (da′kinz) [Henry Drysdale Dakin, New York chemist, 1880–1952] diluted sodium hypochlorite solution.

dakryon (dak′re-on) dacryon.

Dale (dāl) Sir Henry Hallett. British physiologist and pharmacologist, 1875–1968; co-winner, with Otto Loewi, of the Nobel prize for medicine or physiology in 1936 for their study of acetylcholine as an agent in the chemical transmission of nerve impulses.

Dale's reaction (phenomenon) (dāl) [Sir Henry Hallett Dale] see under *reaction*.

daledalin tosylate (dah-lĕ′dah-lin) chemical name: 3 - methyl - 3 - [3-(methylamino)propyl] - 1 - phenylindoline mono-*p*-toluenesulfonate; an antidepressant, $C_{19}H_{24}N_2 \cdot C_7H_8O_3S$.

Dalmane (dal′mān) trademark for a preparation of flurazepam hydrochloride.

Dalrymple's disease, sign (dal′rim-pelz) [John *Dalrymple*, an English oculist, 1804–1852] see *cyclokeratitis*, and see under *sign*.

dalton (dawl′ton) [John *Dalton*, English chemist and physicist, 1766–1844: the founder of the atomic theory] an arbitrary unit of mass, being $\frac{1}{12}$ the mass of the nuclide of carbon-12, equivalent to 1.657×10^{-24} gm. Called also *atomic mass unit*.

Dalton's law (dawl′tonz) [John *Dalton*] see under *law*.

Dalton-Henry law (dawl′ton hen′re) [John *Dalton*; Joseph *Henry*, American physicist, 1797–1878] see under *law*.

daltonism (dawl′ton-izm) [John *Dalton*] a name applied to defective perception of red and green; deuteranomaly or deuteranopia.

Dam (dahm), Carl Peter Henrik. Danish biochemist, 1895–1976; co-winner, with Edward Adelbert Doisy, of the Nobel prize for medicine or physiology in 1943, for the discovery of vitamin K.

dam (dam) 1. a barrier to obstruct the flow of water or other fluid. 2. a thin sheet of latex used in surgical procedures to separate certain tissues or structures. 3. rubber d. **rubber d.,** a sheet of latex with punched-out holes that is placed over the teeth during dental procedures to isolate the operative field from the rest of the oral cavity.

Damalinia (dam″ah-lin′e-ah) a genus of parasitic insects of the order Mallophaga, the biting lice; several species were formerly classified in the genus *Trichodectes*. *D. bo′vis* infests cattle, *D. cap′re* the goat, *D. e′qui* and *D. pilo′sus* the horse, and *D. herm′si* and *D. o′vis* infest sheep.

damiana (dah″me-ah′nah) the leaves of *Turnera aphrodisiaca* (*T. diffusa*) and *Haplopappus discoideus*, Mexican plants; said to be tonic, analeptic, diuretic, and aphrodisiac. Called also *turnera*.

dammar (dam′ar) a transparent resin of *Dammara orientalis*, *D. alba*, *Hopea micrantha*, *H. splendida*, *Shorea* spp., and other trees; used in varnishes, as a mounting medium in microscopy, and for the preservation of animal and vegetable specimens.

Damoiseau's curve, sign (dam-wah-zōz′) [Louis Hyacinthe Céleste *Damoiseau*, French physician, 1815–1890] see *Ellis's line*, under *line*.

dAMP deoxyadenosine monophosphate.

damp (damp) foul air or noxious gas(es) in a mine. **after-d.,** a gaseous mixture formed in a mine by the explosion of fire damp or dust; it contains nitrogen, carbon dioxide, and usually carbon monoxide. **black d., choke d.,** a nonrespirable atmosphere sometimes formed in a mine by the gradual absorption of the oxygen and the giving off of carbon dioxide by the coal. **cold d.,** foggy vapor charged with carbon dioxide. **fire d.,** light explosive hydrocarbon gases, chiefly methane, CH_4, found in coal mines. **white d.,** carbon monoxide.

damping (damp′ing) the steady diminution of the amplitude of vibration of a specific form of energy, as of electricity or sound waves.

danazol (dah′nah-zōl) [USP] an anterior pituitary suppressant that has been used in the treatment of endometriosis, gynecomastia, fibrocystic mastitis, precocious puberty, and pubertal breast hypertrophy.

dance (dans) movement of a rhythmic, or of an unusual or exaggerated type. **brachial d.,** writhing of tortuous brachial arteries under the skin, sometimes observed in elderly arteriosclerotic patients. **hilar d.,** striking abnormal pulsation of hilar vessels. **hilus d.,** marked pulsations of the hilus shadows of both lungs on roentgen examination; seen in pulmonic regurgitation. **St. Anthony's d., St. Guy's d., St. John's d., St. Vitus' d.,** Sydenham's chorea. **St. Vitus' d. of the voice,** stuttering.

Dancel's treatment (dah-selz′) [Jean François *Dancel*, French physician, born 1804] see under *treatment*.

D and C dilation and curettage (dilation of the cervix and currettage of the uterus).

dander (dan′der) small scales from the hair or feathers of animals, which may be the cause of allergy in sensitive persons.

dandruff (dan′druf) 1. dry scaly material desquamated from the scalp; the term is applied to the excessive scaly material associated with disease, as in seborrheic dermatitis. 2. seborrheic dermatitis of the scalp; called also *pityriasis sicca*.

Dandy-Walker syndrome (deformity) (dan′de-wok′er) [Walter Edward *Dandy*, American surgeon, 1886–1946; Arthur Earl *Walker*, American surgeon, born 1907] see under *syndrome*.

Dane particle (dān) [D. S. *Dane*, British virologist, 20th century] see under *particle*.

daniell (dan′yel) [John Frederick *Daniell*, English scientist, 1790–1845] a unit of electromotive force equal to 1.124 volts.

Danilone (dan′ĭ-lōn) trademark for a preparation of phenindione.

Danlos' syndrome (disease) (dan′los) [Henri Alexandre *Danlos*, French dermatologist, 1844–1912] Ehlers-Danlos syndrome.

DANS 5-dimethylamino-1-naphthalenesulfonic acid. See *dansyl chloride*.

dansyl chloride (dan′sil) [the acyl chloride of DANS] a fluorochrome that emits an apple green fluorescence when excited by ultraviolet light; used as a fluorescent label in immunofluorescence methods and in amino acid analysis.

danthron (dan′thron) [USP] chemical name: 1,8-dihydroxy-9,10-anthracenedione. A cathartic, $C_{14}H_8O_4$, occurring as an orange, crystalline powder; it is administered orally.

dantrolene sodium (dan′tro-lēn) chemical name: 1-[[[5-(4-nitrophenyl)-2-furanyl]methylene]amino] - 2,4 - imidazolidinedione sodium salt tetrahydrate. A skeletal muscle relaxant, $C_{14}H_9N_4NaO$, used as an antispasmodic in conditions such as stroke, multiple sclerosis, and cerebral palsy.

Danysz's phenomenon (effect) (dan′ēz) [Jan *Danysz*, Polish pathologist in Paris, 1860–1928] see under *phenomenon*.

Daphne (daf′ne) [Gr. *daphnē* bay tree] a genus of trees and shrubs. *D. gnidium* and *D. mezereum* L. (Thymelaeaceae), the principal medicinal species, are vesicatory and purgative. Toxic glycosides have caused the plant *D. mezereum* to be listed as poisonous; its attractive berries have poisoned children and livestock. See *mezereum*.

daphnetin (daf-ne′tin) the aglycon of daphnin, $C_9H_6O_4$, 7,8-dihydroxycoumarin.

Daphnia (daf′ne-ah) a genus of fresh-water crustaceans, called water fleas, often used in biological research.

daphnin (daf′nin) glycoside, $C_{15}H_{16}O_9$ + $2H_2O$, from *Daphne mezereum*; 7,8-dihydroxycoumarin-7-β-D-glucoside.

daphnism (daf′nizm) poisoning by species of *Daphne*.

dapsone (dap′sōn) [USP] chemical name: 4,4′-sulfonylbisbenzenamine. An antibacterial, $C_{12}H_{12}N_2O_2S$, occurring as a white or creamy white, crystalline powder. It is the parent compound of a group of sulfonamide-like sulfones, including acedapsone, acetosulfone sodium, glucosulfone sodium, sulfoxone sodium, and solapsone. Dapsone and its derivatives are bacteriostatic for a broad spectrum of gram-negative and gram-positive organisms, including *Mycobacterium tuberculosis* and *M. leprae*, and have suppressive action on *Plasmo-*

dium falciparum. Dapsone is used as a leprostatic, especially in tuberculoid and lepromatous leprosy, as a dermatitis herpetiformis suppressant, and in the prophylaxis of falciparum malaria; administered orally. Called also *diaminodiphenylsulfone* or *DDS*.

Daranide (dar′ah-nīd) trademark for a preparation of dichlorphenamide.

Daraprim (dar′ah-prim) trademark for a preparation of pyrimethamine.

Darbid (dar′bid) trademark for a preparation of isopropamide iodide.

Dare's method (dārz) [Arthur *Dare*, Philadelphia physician, born 1868] see under *method*.

Dar es Salaam bacterium (dahr es sah-lahm′) [*Dar es Salaam*, East Africa, where it was isolated in 1922] *Salmonella salamae*.

Daricon (dar′ĭ-kon) trademark for a preparation of oxyphencyclimine hydrochloride.

Darier's disease, sign (dar′e-āz) [Ferdinand Jean *Darier*, French dermatologist, 1856–1938] see *keratosis follicularis*, and see under *sign*.

Darier-Roussy sarcoid (dar′e-a roo-se′) [F. J. *Darier*; Gustave *Roussy*, French pathologist and neurologist, 1874–1948] see under *sarcoid*.

Darier-White disease (dar′e-a hwīt) [F. J. *Darier*; James Clarke *White*, American dermatologist, 1833–1916] keratosis follicularis.

Darkshevich's fibers, nucleus (dark-sha′vich-ez) [Liverij Osipovich *Darkshevich*, Russian neurologist, 1858–1925] see under *fiber* and *nucleus*.

Darling's disease (dar′lingz) [Samuel Taylor *Darling*, American physician, 1872–1925] histoplasmosis.

darmous (dahr′moos) North African name for fluorine poisoning.

darnel (dar′nel) a rye grass, *Lolium temulentum* L. (Gram.), the seeds of which contain a narcotic poison. Ingestion of flour contaminated with darnel may produce vertigo, staggering, vomiting, visual disturbances, burning pain in the mouth, and prostration.

d'Arsonval current (dar′son-val) [Jacques A. *d'Arsonval*, French physicist, 1851–1940] see under *current*.

Dartal (dar′tal) trademark for a preparation of thiopropazate dihydrochloride.

dartoic (dar-to′ik) of the nature of a dartos; having a slow, involuntary contractility like that of the dartos.

dartoid (dar′toid) resembling the dartos.

dartos (dar′tos) [Gr. "flayed"] 1. musculus dartos, def. 1. 2. tunica dartos, def. 1.

Darvon (dar′von) trademark for a preparation of propoxyphene hydrochloride.

darwinism (dar′wĭ-nizm) [Charles Robert *Darwin*, English naturalist, 1809–1882] the theory of evolution according to which higher organisms have been developed from lower ones through the influence of natural selection.

dasymeter (das-im′ĕ-ter) an instrument for measuring the density of a gas.

Dasypus (das′e-pus) [Gr. *dasypous* a rough foot] a genus of tropical armadillos, species of which are reservoirs of *Trypanosoma cruzi*, including *D. novemcincta*, the nine-banded armadillo.

data (da′tah) [L., plural of *datum*] the material or collection of facts on which a discussion or an inference is based. **censored d.,** in statistics, observations whose values are not completely determined in a study, as, for example, data for patients who drop out of a study before it is complete or patients who have not reached the study's end-point (e.g., relapse or death) when the data are analyzed.

dATP deoxyadenosine triphosphate.

Datura (da-tu′rah) a genus of solanaceous plants, the most famous of which is *D. stramonium* L. Its chief constituents are hyoscyamine and scopolamine, which give the herb anticholinergic properties. The powdered leaf is also incorporated into "asthma powders," which are burned as is or in cigarettes for asthma relief; the smoke carries the alkaloids to the bronchi, causing their relaxation. In large doses, asthma powders may induce intoxication with visual disturbances. **D. me′tel,** a source of scopolamine.

daturine (da-tu′rin) hyoscyamine.

daturism (da-tu′rizm) poisoning caused by plants of the genus *Datura*, which contain several solanaceous alkaloids of the tropane configuration; principal among these are atropine, hyoscyamine, and hyoscine (scopolamine).

Daubenton's angle, plane (line) (do-bon-tonz′) [Louis Jean Marie *Daubenton*, French physician and naturalist, 1716–1800] see under *angle* and *plane*.

daughter (daw′ter) 1. decay product; see under *product*. 2. arising from cell division, as a daughter cell.

daunomycin (daw-no-mi′sin) daunorubicin.

daunorubicin (daw″no-roo′bĭ-sin) an anthracycline (q.v.) antibiotic used as an antineoplastic for treatment of acute lymphocytic leukemia, acute granulocytic leukemia, and acute nonlymphoblastic leukemia. Available as *daunorubicin hydrochloride*. **d. hydrochloride,** the hydrochloride salt of daunorubicin, $C_{27}H_{29}NO_{10} \cdot HCl$, having the same actions as the base; it has been used investigationally in the treatment of acute myelogenous and acute lymphocytic leukemia.

daunosamine (daw-no′sah-mēn) a six-carbon amino sugar found in anthracycline antibiotics.

Dausset (do-sĕ′) Jean Baptiste Gabriel. French physician, born 1916; co-winner, with Baruj Benacerraf and George Davis Snell, of the Nobel prize for medicine or physiology in 1980 for their research on genetically determined structures of the cell surface that regulate immunological reactions. Dausset identified the first HLA (human leukocyte antigen) "MAC."

Davainea (da-va′ne-ah) [Casimir Joseph *Davaine*, French physician, 1812–1882] a genus of tapeworms of the family Davaineidae. **D. proglotti′na,** a species found in fowls.

Davaineidae (da-va-ne′ĭ-de) a family of relatively small tapeworms of the order Cyclophyllidea, subclass Cestoda, which parasitize mammals and birds. *Davainea* and *Raillietina* are medically important genera.

David's disease (dah-vidz′) [Jean Pierre *David*, French surgeon, 1737–1784] tuberculosis of the spine.

Davidoff's (Davidov's) cells (da′vid-ofs) [M. von *Davidoff*, histologist in Munich, d. 1904] Paneth's cells.

Davidsohn differential absorption test (da′vid-son) [Israel Davidsohn, American pathologist, born 1895] Paul-Bunnell-Davidsohn test.

Davidsohn's sign (da′vid-sōnz) [Hermann *Davidsohn*, Prussian physician, 1842–1911] see under *sign*.

Daviel's operation, spoon (dav-e-elz′) [Jacques *Daviel*, French oculist, 1696–1762, the originator of the modern treatment of cataract by extraction of the lens] see under *operation* and *spoon*.

Davis graft (da′vis) [John Staige *Davis*, American surgeon, 1872–1946] a pinch graft.

Dawbarn's sign [Robert Hugh Mackay *Dawbarn*, New York surgeon, 1860–1915] see under *sign*.

dazadrol maleate (da′zah-drōl) chemical name: α-(4-chlorophenyl)-α-(4,5-dihydro-1*H*-imidazol-2-yl)-2-pyridine methanol(Z)-2-butenedioate (1:1) (salt); an antidepressant, $C_{15}H_{14}ClN_3O \cdot C_4H_4O_4$.

dB, db decibel.

DBA dibenzanthracene.

DBE (*obs.*) a synthetic estrogen, $(C_2H_5 \cdot O \cdot C_6H_4)_2C{:}C(Br) \cdot C_6H_5$.

DBI trademark for preparations of phenformin hydrochloride.

D.C. direct current; Doctor of Chiropractic.

D & C dilation and curettage (dilation of the cervix and curettage of the uterus).

dC deoxycytidine.

DCA desoxycorticosterone acetate.

D.Cc. double concave.

dCDP deoxycytidine diphosphate.

D.C.F. *direct centrifugal flotation*; see *Lane method*, under *method*.

D.C.H. Diploma in Child Health.

DCI dichloroisoproterenol.

dCMP deoxycytidine monophosphate.

D.C.O.G. Diploma of the College of Obstetricians and Gynaecologists (British).

dCTP deoxycytidine triphosphate.

D.Cx. double convex.

d.d. abbreviation for L. *de′tur ad,* "let it be given to."

DDD TDE.

o, p′-DDD mitotane.

DDP, *cis*-DDP cisplatin.

DDS diaminodiphenylsulfone; see *dapsone*.

D.D.S. Doctor of Dental Surgery.

D.D.Sc. Doctor of Dental Science.

DDT a moderately toxic chlorinated hydrocarbon pesticide (dichlorodiphenyltrichloroethane), formerly widely used but now banned in the United States except for a few specialized purposes because of the ecological damage it causes.

de- [L. *de* away from, down from] a prefix often denoting negation or privation; it may signify down or away from, cessation, reversal, or removal. It sometimes has an intensive force.

deacetyllanatoside C (de-as″ĕ-til-lah-nat′o-sīd) deslanoside.

deacidification (de″ah-sid″ĭ-fĭ-ka′shun) the act or art of correcting or destroying acidity or of neutralizing an acid.

deactivation (de″ak-tĭ-va′shun) the process of making or becoming inactive, as the removal or loss of radioactivity from a previously radioactive material.

deacylase (de-as′il-ās) a general term for an enzyme of the hydrolase class that catalyzes the hydrolytic cleavage of an acyl group (R–CO–) from an ester compound [EC 3.1] or from an amide compound [EC 3.5].

dead (ded) 1. destitute of life; see also *death*. 2. numb.

deaf (def) lacking the sense of hearing or having profound hearing loss.

deafferentation (de-af″er-en-ta′shun) the elimination or interruption of afferent nerve impulses, as by destruction of the afferent pathway.

deaf-mute (def-mūt′) an individual who is unable to hear or speak; it has been demonstrated that deaf individuals thought to be mute can learn to speak.

deaf-mutism (def-mūt′izm) the absence both of the sense of hearing and of the faculty of speech.

deafness (def′nes) lack of the sense of hearing, or profound hearing loss. Moderate loss of hearing is often called *hearing loss*. See also *hearing loss*, under *H*. **acoustic trauma d.,** that due to blast injury. **Alexander's d.,** see under *hearing loss*. **apoplectiform d.,** Meniere's disease in which the hearing impairment is sudden in onset and fluctuates, and ultimately severe and permanent deafness may occur. **bass d.,** deafness to certain low tones. **boilermakers' d.,** that caused by working in places where the noise level is extremely high. **central d.,** deafness due to causes in the auditory pathways or in the auditory center. **conduction d.,** see under *hearing loss*. **cortical d.,** deafness due to a lesion of cortical brain substance. **functional d.,** apparent deafness without organic lesion. **hysterical d.,** that which may appear or disappear in a hysterical patient without discoverable cause. **labyrinthine d.,** that which is due to disease of the labyrinth. **malarial d.,** that which occurs as a result of malarial poisoning. **Michel's d.,** congenital deafness due to total lack of development of the inner ear. **midbrain d.,** deafness dependent on injury of the fillet tract of the tegmentum. **Mondini's d.,** congenital deafness due to dysgenesis of the organ of Corti, with partial aplasia of the bony and membranous labyrinth and a resultant flattened cochlea. **music d.,** inability to recognize musical notes; amusia. **nerve d., neural d.,** that which is due to a lesion of the auditory nerve or the central neural pathways. **organic d.,** deafness due to defect in the ear or auditory apparatus. **pagetoid d.,** that occurring in osteitis deformans (Paget's disease) of the bones of the skull. **paradoxic d.,** see under *hearing loss*. **perceptive d.,** sensorineural d. **postlingual d.,** deafness acquired after the development of speech. **prelingual d.,** deafness acquired before the development of speech. **Scheibe's d.,** congenital deafness due to aplasia of the saccule and cochlear duct. **sensorineural d.,** deafness due to a lesion in the sensory mechanism (cochlea) of the ear or to a lesion in the acoustic nerve or the central neural pathways or to a combination of such lesions. See also

Rinne test, under *tests*. **tone d.,** sensory amusia. **toxic d.,** deafness caused by the effect of poisons. **vascular d.,** that due to disease of blood vessels of the inner ear. **word d.,** a form of receptive aphasia in which sounds are heard, but convey no meaning to the mind, due to disease of the auditory center of the brain; called also *acoustic* or *auditory aphasia, aphememesthesia, auditory amnesia,* and *logokophosis.*

dealbation (de″al-ba′shun) bleaching.

dealcoholization (de-al″ko-hol-i-za′shun) the removal of alcohol from an object or substance.

deallergization (de-al″er-ji-za′shun) the desensitization of an allergic individual to any particular allergen.

deamidase (de-am′ĭ-dās) amidohydrolase.

deamidation (de-am″ĭ-da′shun) deamidization.

deamidization (de-am″ĭ-di-za′shun) liberation of the ammonia from an amide.

deaminase (de-am′ĭ-nās) [EC 3.5.3.4] one of a sub-subclass of enzymes of the hydrolase class that catalyze the removal of an amino group from amidine compounds with release of ammonia. Called also *aminohydrolase.*

deamination (de-am″ĭ-na′shun) removal of the amino group, —NH₂, from a compound.

deaminization (de-am″ĭ-ni-za′shun) deamination.

Deaner (de′ner) trademark for a preparation of deanol acetamidobenzoate.

deanol acetamidobenzoate (de′ah-nol as″et-am″ĭ-do-ben′zo-āt) chemical name: 4-(acetylamino)benzoic acid compounded with 2-(dimethylamino)ethanol (1:1). A cerebral stimulant with parasympathomimetic activity, $C_{13}H_{20}N_2O_4$, occurring as a white or nearly white, crystalline powder; used as an antidepressant in the treatment of certain behavior and/or learning disorders in children.

deaquation (de″ah-kwa′shun) [L. *de* from + *aqua* water] removal of water from anything; dehydration.

Dearg. pil. (*obs.*) abbreviation for L. *deargen′tur pil′ulae,* let the pills be silvered.

dearterialization (de″ar-te″re-al-i-za′shun) interruption of the supply of oxygenated blood to a part or organ.

dearticulation (de″ar-tik″u-la′shun) dislocation of a joint.

death (deth) the cessation of life; permanent cessation of all vital bodily functions. For legal and medical purposes, the following definition of death has been proposed—the irreversible cessation of all of the following: (1) total cerebral function, (2) spontaneous function of the respiratory system, and (3) spontaneous function of the circulatory system. **apparent d.,** a state of complete interruption of bodily processes from which the patient can be resuscitated. **black d.,** bubonic plague (q.v.) thought to be associated with necrotic purpura and symmetrical gangrene. **brain d.,** irreversible brain damage as manifested by absolute unresponsiveness to all stimuli, absence of all spontaneous muscle activity, including respiration, shivering, etc., and an isoelectric electroencephalogram for 30 minutes, all in the absence of hypothermia or intoxication by central nervous system depressants. Called also *irreversible coma.* **cell d.,** complete degeneration or necrosis of cells. **cot d., crib d.,** sudden infant death syndrome; see under *syndrome.* **fetal d.,** stillbirth; death in utero; failure of the product of conception to show evidence of respiration, heart beat, or definite movement of a voluntary muscle after expulsion from the uterus, with no possibility of resuscitation. **fetal d., early,** fetal death occurring during the first 20 weeks of gestation. **fetal d., intermediate,** fetal death occurring during the twenty-first to twenty-eighth weeks of gestation. **fetal d., late,** fetal death occurring after 28 weeks of gestation. **functional d.,** total, permanent destruction of the central nervous system, with vital functions being sustained by artificial means. **genetic d.,** the failure of a mutation to be passed on to the next generation because of the mutation's damaging phenotypic effects. **liver d.,** death due to failure of hepatic function. **local d.,** death of a part of the body. **molecular d.,** caries, catastasis, or the last stage of a catabolic process. **somatic d.,** cessation of all vital cellular activity. **voodoo d.,** a phenomenon seen among many primitive peoples in which the affected individual dies after transgressing a taboo or becoming convinced that he is bewitched.

Deaur. pil. (*obs.*) abbreviation for L. *deauren′tur pil′ulae,* let the pills be gilded.

Deaver's incision (de′verz) [John Blair *Deaver,* American surgeon, 1855–1931] see under *incision.*

debanding (de-band′ing) the removal of the bands of a fixed orthodontic appliance.

Debaryomyces (de″bar-e-o-mi′sēz) a genus of ascomycetous fungi of the family Saccharomycetaceae. **D. han′sen′ii,** a species which changes sugars into oxalic acid; called also *Saccharomyces hansenii.* **D. hom′inis, D. neofor′mans,** former name for *Cryptococcus neoformans.*

debility (de-bil′ĭ-te) lack or loss of strength.

débouchement (da-bōōsh-maw′) [Fr.] an opening out.

Débove's disease, membrane, treatment (dĕ-bōvz′) [Georges Maurice *Débove,* French physician, 1845–1920] see *splenomegaly,* and see under *membrane* and *treatment.*

debranching enzyme 1. amylo-1,6-glucosidase. 2. isoamylase.

débride (da-brēd′) to remove foreign material and contaminated or devitalized tissue, usually by sharp dissection.

débridement (da-brēd-maw′) [Fr.] the removal of foreign material and devitalized or contaminated tissue from or adjacent to a traumatic or infected lesion until surrounding healthy tissue is exposed. Cf. *épluchage.* **enzymatic d.,** removal of fibrinous or purulent exudate by application of a nontoxic and nonirritating enzyme which is capable of lysing fibrin, denatured collagen, and elastin, but does not destroy normal tissue. **surgical d.,** débridement by mechanical methods, usually sharp dissection.

debris (dĕ-bre′) [Fr.] accumulated fragments; rubbish. **word d.,** sounds made by an aphasic patient in attempting to talk.

Debrisan (dĕ-bri′san) trademark for dextranomer.

debrisoquin sulfate (deb-ris′o-kwin) chemical name: 3,4-dihydro-2(1*H*)-isoquinolinecarboxamidine sulfate; an antihypertensive agent, $C_{10}H_{13}N_3 \cdot \frac{1}{2}H_2SO_4$.

Deb. spis. abbreviation for L. *deb′ita spissitu′dine,* of the proper consistency.

debt (det) something owed. **oxygen d.,** the extra oxygen that must be used in the oxidative energy processes after a period of strenuous exercise to reconvert lactic acid to glucose, and decomposed ATP and creatine phosphate to their original states.

debye (dĕ-bi′) [Peter Joseph Wilhelm *Debye,* Dutch physicist, 1884–1966] a unit of electric dipole moment equal to 10^{-18} statcoulomb-centimeter, used in indicating the dipole moments of molecules. Symbol D.

Dec. abbreviation for L. *decan′ta,* pour off.

deca- [Gr. *deka* ten] a combining form designating ten; used in naming units of measurement to indicate a quantity ten (10^1) times the unit designated by the root with which it is combined. Symbol, dk.

Decaderm (dek′ah-derm) trademark for a preparation of dexamethasone.

Decadron (dek′ah-dron) trademark for preparations of dexamethasone.

Decadron-LA (dek′ah-dron) trademark for preparations of dexamethasone acetate.

Deca-Durabolin (de″ka-dur-ab′o-lin) trademark for a preparation of nandrolone decanoate.

decalcification (de″kal-sĭ-fi-ka′shun) 1. the loss of calcium salts from a bone or tooth. 2. the process of removing calcareous matter.

decalcify (de-kal′sĭ-fi) [L. *de* priv. + *calx* lime] to deprive of calcium salts.

decamethonium (dek″ah-mĕ-tho′ne-um) chemical name: *N,N,N,N′,N′,N′*-hexamethyl-1,10-decanediaminium. A bisquaternary ammonium compound, $C_{16}H_{38}N_2$, structurally analogous to tubocurarine. **d. bromide** [USP], the bromide salt of decamethonium, $C_{16}H_{38}Br_2N_2$, occurring as a white crystalline powder; used as a skeletal muscle relaxant during surgical anesthesia, to aid endotracheal intubation, in obstetrics, and in electroconvulsive therapy, administered intravenously. **d. iodide,** the iodide salt of decamethonium, $C_{16}H_{38}I_2N_2$, which has been used for the same purposes as the bromide salt.

decane (dek′ān) a hydrocarbon, $C_{10}H_{22}$, from paraffin.

decannulation (de-kan″u-la′shun) removal of a cannula, especially of a tracheostomy cannula.

decantation (de″kan-ta′shun) [*de-* + L. *canthus* tire of a wheel] the pouring of a clear supernatant liquid from a sediment.

decapeptide (dek″ah-pep′tīd) a peptide containing ten amino acids.

decapitation (de-kap″ĭ-ta′shun) [*de-* + L. *caput* head] the removal of the head, as of an animal, a fetus, or a bone; beheading.

decapitator (de-kap′ĭ-ta″tor) an instrument for removing the head of a fetus in embryotomy.

Decapoda (de-kah-po′dah) [Gr. *deka* ten + *pous* foot] an order of *Crustacea*, including the crabs, lobsters, shrimps, etc., which have five pairs of legs upon the thorax.

Decapryn (dek′kah-prin) trademark for preparations of doxylamine succinate.

decapsulation (de-kap″su-la′shun) removal of the capsule, especially of the renal capsule.

decarbonization (de-kar″bon-i-za′shun) (*obs.*) the removal of carbon from the blood in the lungs by the substitution of oxygen for carbon dioxide.

decarboxylase (de″kar-bok′sĭ-lās) an enzyme of the lyase class, sub-subclass carboxy-lyase [EC 4.1.1], that catalyzes the removal of a molecule of carbon dioxide from a carboxylic group.

decarboxylation (de″kar-bok″sĭ-la′shun) removal of the carboxyl group.

decavitamin (dek″ah-vi″tah-min) [USP] a combination of vitamins in capsular or tablet form, each of which contains vitamins A and D, ascorbic acid, calcium pantothenate, cyanocobalamin, folic acid, niacinamide, pyridoxine hydrochloride, riboflavin, thiamine hydrochloride, and a suitable form of alpha tocopherol.

decay (de-ka′) [*de-* + L. *cadere* to fall] 1. the gradual decomposition of dead organic matter. 2. the process or stage of decline, as in aging. **beta d.,** disintegration of the nucleus of an unstable radionuclide in which the mass number is unchanged, but the atomic number is increased or decreased by 1, as result of emission of a negatively or positively charged (beta) particle and a neutrino. **radioactive d.,** disintegration of the nucleus of an unstable nuclide by the spontaneous emission of charged particles and/or photons; called also *radioactive disintegration.* **tone d.,** the decrease in threshold sensitivity resulting from the presence of a barely audible continuous sound.

deceleration (de-sel″er-a′shun) decrease in speed or rate.

decenter (de-sen′ter) [*de-* + *center*] in optics, to design or make a lens such that the visual axis does not pass through the optical center of the lens.

decentration (de″sen-tra′shun) the act or process of removing from a center.

deceration (de″se-ra′shun) [*de-* + L. *cera* wax] the removal of paraffin from a tissue section prepared for the microscope.

decerebellation (de-ser″ĕ-bel-la′shun) removal of the cerebellum.

decerebrate (de-ser′ĕ-brāt) 1. to eliminate cerebral function by transecting the brain stem between the superior colliculi and the vestibular nuclei or by ligating the common carotid arteries and the basilar artery at the center of the pons. 2. an animal so prepared. 3. a person with brain damage resulting in neurologic signs similar to those of a decerebrated animal. See also *decerebrate rigidity,* under *rigidity.*

decerebration (de″ser-ĕ-bra′shun) [*de-* + *cerebrum*] the act of decerebrating.

decerebrize (de-ser′ĕ-brīz) to decerebrate (def. 1).

dechloridation (de-klo″rĭ-da′shun) the removal of chloride, or salt.

dechlorination (de-klo″rĭ-na′shun) dechloridation.

dechlorurant (de-klo′roo-rant) an agent that causes dechloruration.

dechloruration (de-klo″roo-ra′shun) diminution of excretion of chlorates in the urine.

decholesterinization (de″ko-les″ter-in-i-za′shun) decholesterolization.

decholesterolization (de″ko-les″ter-ol-i-za′shun) extraction of cholesterol from the blood.

Decholin (de′ko-lin) trademark for preparations of dehydrocholic acid.

deci- [L. *decem* ten] a combining form designating one-tenth; used in naming units of measurement to indicate one-tenth (10⁻¹) of the unit designated by the root with which it is combined. Symbol, d.

decibel (des′ĭ-bel) a unit of relative power intensity equal to one-tenth of a bel, used for electric or acoustic power measurements. The decibel level is ten times the base ten logarithm of the ratio of the measured power to some reference power level. A one decibel change is an increase in the power level by a factor of 1.26, approximately the smallest change in sound level detectable by human ears; a ten decibel (one bel) change multiples the power by a factor of ten and approximately doubles the perceived sound level. In audiometry the reference power level (0 db) corresponds to a root-mean-square sound pressure level of 2×10^{-4} dyn/cm², which is approximately the threshold of hearing for healthy, young persons. Symbol, dB.

decidua (de-sid′u-ah) [L., from *deciduus* falling off] the endometrium of the pregnant uterus, all of which, except the deepest layer, is shed at parturition. Called also *membranae deciduae* [NA], *caduca, decidual* or *deciduous membrane,* and *tunica decidua.* **basal d., d. basa′lis** [NA], the portion of the decidua directly underlying the chorionic vesicle and attached to the myometrium; called also *d. serotina* and *membrana serotina.* **capsular d., d. capsula′ris** [NA], the portion of the decidua directly overlying the chorionic vesicle and facing the uterine cavity; called also *reflex d.* and *d. reflexa.* **menstrual d., d. menstrua′lis,** the hyperemic mucosa of the uterus that is shed during the menstrual period. **parietal d., d. parieta′lis** [NA], the portion of the decidua lining the uterus elsewhere than at the site of attachment of the chorionic vesicle; called also *d. vera.* **reflex d., d. reflex′a,** d. capsularis. **d. seroti′na,** d. basalis. **d. subchoria′lis,** the maternal component of the tissue comprising the closing ring of Winkler-Waldeyer. **true d.,** d. parietalis. **d. tubero′sa papulo′sa,** a cast of the uterine cavity expelled at abortion. **d. ve′ra,** d. parietalis.

decidual (de-sid′u-al) pertaining to the decidua.

deciduate (de-sid′u-āt) characterized by shedding.

deciduation (de-sid″u-a′shun) the shedding of the decidua.

deciduitis (de-sid″u-i′tis) a bacterial disease leading to alterations in the decidua.

deciduoma (de-sid″u-o′mah) [*decidua* + *-oma*] an intrauterine mass containing decidual cells. **Loeb's d.,** a tumor-like structure resembling the maternal placenta, produced in the uteri of guinea pigs by the action of progesterone. **d. malig′num,** choriocarcinoma.

deciduomatosis (de-sid″u-o-mah-to′sis) formation of decidual tissue in the nonpregnant state.

deciduosarcoma (de-sid″u-o-sar-ko′mah) (*obs.*) choriocarcinoma.

deciduosis (de-sid″u-o′sis) the presence of decidual tissue or of tissue resembling the endometrium of pregnancy in an ectopic site.

deciduous (de-sid′u-us) [L. *deciduus,* from *decidere* to fall off] falling off or shed at maturity; the term is used to designate the teeth of the first dentition in animals and man.

decile (des′īl) [L. *decem* ten + *-ile* (by analogy with *quartile*)] any of the nine values that divide the range of a probability distribution into ten equal parts of equal probability, i.e., the 1st, 2nd, 3rd, etc. deciles are the 10th, 20th, 30th, etc. percentiles.

deciliter (des′ĭ-le″ter) one tenth of a liter; 100 milliliters.

decipara (dĕ-sip′ah-rah) [L. *decem* ten + *parere* to produce] a woman who has had ten pregnancies which resulted in viable offspring; also written Para X.

deckplatte (dek′plaht-tĕ) [Ger.] roof plate; see under *plate.*

declination (dek″lĭ-na′shun) [L. *declinare* to decline] deviation from a normally vertical position, as rotation of the eye about its anteroposterior axis so that its vertical meridian lies to the temporal (*positive d.*) or to the nasal side (*negative d.*) of its proper position. Cf. *extorsion* and *intorsion.*

declinator (dek′lĭ-na″tor) an instrument by which parts are retracted during an operation.

decline (de-klīn) 1. the period or stage of the abatement of a disease or paroxysm. 2. a gradual deterioration or wasting away of the physical and mental faculties.

declive (de-klīv′) [Fr. *déclive;* L. *declivis*] [NA] the part of the vermis of the cerebellum just caudal to the primary fissure; called also *d. monticuli cerebelli.*

declivis (de-kli′vis) [L.] declive.

Declomycin (dek′lo-mi″sin) trademark for preparations of demeclocycline.

decoagulant (de″ko-ag′u-lant) 1. reducing the amount of existing coagulants or procoagulants in the blood. 2. a substance which inhibits coagulation of blood by reducing the amount of existing coagulants or procoagulants.

Decoct. abbreviation for L. *decoc′tum,* a decoction.

decoction (de-kok′shun) [L. *decoctum,* from *de* down + *coquere* to boil] 1. the act or process of boiling. 2. a medicine or other substance prepared by boiling. Called also *apozem.* **d. of the woods,** Zittmann's decoction. **Zimmermann's d.,** a cathartic decoction of rhubarb, potassium bitartrate, barley, water, and syrup. **Zittmann's d.,** a decoction of sarsaparilla, calomel, cinnabar, alum, senna, licorice, anise seed, and fennel.

decoctum (de-kok′tum) [L.] a decoction.

decollation (de″kol-la′shun) [*de-* + L. *collum* neck] decapitation, chiefly of a dead fetus.

decoloration (de-kul″or-a′shun) 1. removal of color; bleaching. 2. lack or loss of color.

decolorize (de-kul′or-īz) to free from color; to bleach.

decompensation (de″kom-pen-sa′shun) 1. failure of compensation; cardiac decompensation is marked by dyspnea, venous engorgement, and edema. 2. in psychiatry, failure of defense mechanisms resulting in progressive personality disintegration.

decomplementize (de-kom′ple-men″tīz) to remove complement from.

decomposition (de″kom-po-zish′un) [*de-* + L. *componere* to put together] the separation of compound bodies into their constituent principles by whatever process. **anaerobic d.,** the breakdown of organic compounds in the absence of oxygen. In animals, the process is known as *glycolysis;* in plants and microorganisms, *fermentation.* **d. of movement,** lack of coordination characterized by irregularity in the successive flexion and extension of joints in performing a movement with the limb.

decompression (de″kom-presh′un) the removal of pressure, particularly the slow lessening of pressure on deep-sea divers and caisson workers to prevent the onset of bends, and the reduction of pressure on persons as they ascend to great heights. See also under *sickness.* **abdominal d.,** the removal of pressure from the abdomen during the first stage of labor. **cardiac d.,** d. of heart. **cerebral d.,** removal of a flap of the skull and incision of the dura mater for relief of intracranial pressure. **explosive d.,** decompression more rapid than that corresponding to a rate of ascent greater than 5000 feet per minute. **d. of heart,** pericardiotomy with evacuation of blood or fluid; called also *d. of pericardium.* **Heyns' d.,** a method of abdominal decompression using a partial vacuum. **nerve d.,** relief of pressure on a nerve by surgical removal of the constricting fibrous or bony tissue. **d. of pericardium,** d. of heart. **d. of spinal cord,** relief of pressure on the spinal cord by means of surgery. **suboccipital d.,** cerebral decompression by occipital craniectomy and opening of the dura. **subtemporal d.,** cerebral decompression by removal of a portion of the temporal bone and opening of the dura.

deconditioning (de″kon-dish′un-ing) a change in cardiovascular function after prolonged periods of weightlessness, probably related to a shift of a quantity of blood from the lower limbs to the thorax, resulting in reflex diuresis and a reduction of blood volume.

decongestant (de″kon-jes′tant) 1. tending to reduce congestion or swelling. 2. an agent that reduces congestion or swelling.

decongestive (de″kon-jes′tiv) reducing congestion.

decontamination (de″kon-tam-ĭ-na′shun) the freeing of a person or an object of some contaminating substance such as war gas, radioactive material, etc.

decoquinate (de-ko-kwin′āt) chemical name: 6-(decyloxy)-7-ethoxy-4-hydroxy-3-quinolinecarboxylic acid ethyl ester, a coccidiostat effective against the sporozoan *Eimeria,* $C_{24}H_{35}NO_5$; used in poultry.

decortication (de″kor-tĭ-ka′shun) [*de-* + L. *cortex* bark] 1. the removal of bark, hull, husk, or shell from a plant, seed, or root, as in pharmacy. 2. removal of portions of the cortical substance of a structure or organ, as of the brain, kidney, lung, etc. **chemical d., enzymatic d.,** removal of cortical substance by chemical agents or enzymes. **d. of lung,** removal of constricting visceral pleura to permit the lung to expand. **renal d.,** removal of the capsule of the kidney; decapsulation of the kidney.

decrement (dek′re-ment) [L. *decrementum*] 1. subtraction, or decrease; the amount by which a quantity or value is decreased. 2. the stage of decline of a disease; see *stadium decrementi.*

decrepitate (de-krep′ĭ-tāt) 1. to roast or calcine certain substances (salt, crystals, etc.) until crackling occurs, or until crackling ends. 2. to explode with a crackling noise upon heating, owing to the release of entrapped water as steam.

decrepitation (de-krep″ĭ-ta′shun) the explosion or crackling of certain substances (salt, crystals, etc.) upon heating.

decrudescence (de″kroo-des′ens) diminution or abatement of the intensity of symptoms.

decrustation (de″krus-ta′shun) the detachment of a crust.

dectaflur (dek′tah-floor) chemical name: 9-octadecenylamine hydrofluoride; a dental caries prophylactic, $C_{18}H_{37}\cdot N\cdot HF$.

Decub. abbreviation for L. *decu′bitus,* lying down.

decubation (de″ku-ba′shun) [*de-* + L. *cubare* to lie down] the period in the course of an infectious disease from the disappearance of the symptoms to complete recovery and the end of the infectious period. Cf. *incubation.*

decubital (de-ku′bĭ-tal) pertaining to decubitus (decubitus ulcer).

decubitus (de-ku′bĭ-tus), pl. *decu′bitus* [L. "a lying down"] 1. an act of lying down; also the position assumed in lying down. 2. decubitus ulcer; see under *ulcer.* **d. acu′tus,** a severe decubitus ulcer on a paralyzed side in hemiplegia. **Andral's d.,** decubitus on the sound side; a position assumed in the early stages of pleurisy. **dorsal d.,** lying in the supine position. **lateral d.,** lying on the side; used in radiologic examination, with the x-ray beam directed horizontally; designated right lateral decubitus when the subject lies on his right side and left lateral decubitus when on his left side. **ventral d.,** lying on the stomach.

decumbin (de-kum′bin) a toxic substance obtained from *Penicillium decumbens,* which causes respiratory distress and hemorrhage; the oral LD_{50} for rats is about 275 mg./kg.

decurrent (de-kur′ent) [L. *decurrere* to run down] extending or moving from above downward.

decussate (de-kus′āt) [L. *decussare* to cross in the form of an X] 1. to cross or intersect in the form of the letter X. 2. crossing in the form of the letter X.

decussatio (de″kŭ-sa′she-o), pl. *decussatio′nes* [L.] [NA] decussation; [NA] a general term for the intercrossing of fellow parts or structures in the form of an X. See also *chiasma* and *commissura.* **d. lemnisco′rum medialium** [NA], decussation of medial lemnisci: the region at the caudal end of the medulla oblongata in which the fibers from the nucleus cuneatus and the nucleus gracilis on each side intersect as they cross the midline before ascending as the medial lemniscus. Called also *d. sensoria* [NA alternative] and *decussation of fillet.* **d. moto′ria,** NA alternative for *d. pyramidum.* **d. nervo′rum trochlea′ris, d. nervo′rum trochlea′rium** [NA], decussation of trochlear nerves: the crossing of the fibers of the trochlear nerves in the superior medullary velum. **d. pedunculo′rum cerebella′rium crania′lium** [NA], decussation of cranial cerebellar peduncles: the crossing of the fibers of the cranial cerebellar peduncles within the tegmentum of the mesencephalon; called also *d. pedunculorum cerebellarium superiorum* [NA alternative] and *decussation of superior cerebellar peduncles.* **d. pedunculo′rum cerebella′rium superio′rum,** NA alternative for *d. pedunculorum cerebellarium cranialium.* **d. pyram′idum** [NA], pyramidal decussation: the anterior part of the lower medulla oblongata in which most of the fibers of each pyramid intersect as they cross the midline and descend as the lateral corticospinal tracts. Called also *d. motoria* [NA alternative], *decussation of pyramids*, and *motor decussation*. **d. senso′ria**, NA alternative for *d. lemniscorum medialium*. **decussatio′nes tegmen′ti** [NA], **decussatio′nes tegmento′rum**, decussations of tegmentum: crossing fibers in the midbrain, including the ventral tegmental decussation of the rubrospinal and rubroreticular tracts, and the dorsal tegmental decussation of the tectospinal tract. Called also *tegmental decussations*. **d. trochlea′ris** [NA], trochlear decussation: the crossing of the fibers of the trochlear nerves in the cranial medullary velum; called also *decussation of trochlear nerves* and *d. nervorum trochlearium* [NA alternative].

decussation (de″kŭ-sa′shun) a crossing over; see *decussatio*. **d. of cranial cerebellar peduncles,** decussatio pedunculorum cerebellarium cranialium. **d. of fillet,** decussatio lemniscorum medialium. **Forel's d.,** the ventral tegmental decussation of the rubrospinal and rubroreticular tracts in the mesencephalon. **fountain d. of Meynert,** the dorsal tegmental decussation of the tectospinal tract in the mesencephalon. **d. of medial lemnisci,** decussatio lemniscorum medialium. **motor d.,** decussatio pyramidum. **optic d., d. of optic nerves** (*obs.*), chiasma opticum. **pyramidal d., d. of pyramids,** decussatio pyramidum. **d. of superior cerebellar peduncles,** decussatio pedunculorum cerebellarium cranialium. **tegmental d's, d's of tegmentum,** decussationes tegmenti. **trochlear d., d. of trochlear nerves,** decussatio nervorum trochlearium.

decussationes (de″kŭ-sa″she-o′nēz) [L.] plural of *decussatio*.

dedentition (de″den-tish′un) [*de-* + L. *dens* tooth] the shedding or loss of teeth.

dedifferentiation (de-dif″er-en″she-a′shun) anaplasia.

de d. in d. abbreviation for L. *de di′e in di′em*, from day to day.

dedolation (ded″o-la′shun) 1. a sensation as if the limbs had been bruised. 2. the removal of a thin piece of skin by an oblique cut.

de Duve see *Duve*.

deemanate (de-em′ah-nāt) to deprive of the property of giving off radioactive emanations.

deep (dēp) situated far beneath the surface; not superficial.

de-epicardialization (de″ep-ĭ-kar″dĭ-al-i-za′shun) a surgical procedure formerly used for the relief of intractable angina pectoris, in which epicardial tissue is destroyed by phenolization or the application of other caustic agents to promote the development of collateral circulation.

deet (dēt) diethyltoluamide.

Deetjen's bodies (dāt′yenz) [Hermann *Deetjen*, German physician, 1867–1915] blood platelets.

DEF see under *rate*.

defatigation (de-fat″ĭ-ga′shun) overstrain or fatigue of muscular or nervous tissue.

defatted (de-fat′ed) deprived of fat, as a food.

defaunate (de-fawn′āt) [*de-* + L. *fauna* animal life] to remove or destroy an animal population; sometimes applied to removal of hookworms from the intestinal tract, delousing, etc.

defecation (def″e-ka′shun) [L. *defaecare* to deprive of dregs] 1. the removal of impurities, as chemical defecation. 2. the evacuation of fecal material from the rectum. **fragmentary d.,** the evacuation of small pieces of feces.

defect (de′fekt) an imperfection, failure, or absence. **acquired d.,** a non-genetic imperfection arising secondarily, after birth. **aortic septal d.,** a congenital anomaly in which there is abnormal communication between the ascending aorta and pulmonary artery just above the semilunar valves; called also *aorticopulmonary fenestration, aorticopulmonary septal d.,* and *aorticopulmonary window.* **aorticopulmonary septal d.,** aortic septal d. **atrial septal d's, atrioseptal d's,** congenital cardiac anomalies in which there is persistent patency of the atrial septum due to failure of fusion between either the septum secundum or the septum primum and the endocardial cushions. In *ostium secundum defect* there is a rim of septum all around the defect. In *ostium primum defect,* which is an incomplete form of atrioventricularis communis, there is no septum at the base of the defect, between the mitral and tricuspid valves; it is usually associated with a cleft mitral cusp and occasionally

with a cleft tricuspid valve. **birth d.,** a defect present at birth; the term may refer to a morphological defect (dysmorphism) or to an inborn error of metabolism. **congenital d.,** birth defect; a structural or chemical imperfection present at birth. **cortical d.,** a benign, symptomless, circumscribed rarefaction of cortical bone, detected radiographically; called also *subperiosteal cortical d.* **ectodermal d., congenital,** anhidrotic ectodermal dysplasia. **endocardial cushion d's,** a spectrum of septal defects resulting from imperfect fusion of the endocardial cushions and ranging from persistent ostium primum to persistent common atrioventricular canal; see *atrial septal d's* and *atrioventricularis communis.* **filling d.,** any localized defect in the contour of the stomach, duodenum, or intestine, as seen in the roentgenogram after a barium enema, due to a lesion of the wall projecting into the lumen or to an object in the lumen. **genetic d.,** see under *disease.* **neural-tube d.,** a developmental anomaly resulting in anencephaly or spina bifida. **ostium primum d.,** see *atrial septal d.* **ostium secundum d.,** see *atrial septal d.* **polytropic field d.** a pattern of anomalies derived from the disturbance of a single developmental field. **retention d.,** a defect in the power of recalling or remembering names, numbers, or events. **salt-losing d.,** see under *syndrome.* **septal d.,** a defect in one of the cardiac septa, resulting in an abnormal communication between the opposite chambers of the heart. **subperiosteal cortical d.,** cortical d. **ventricular septal d.,** a congenital cardiac anomaly in which there is persistent patency of the ventricular septum in either the muscular or fibrous portions, most often due to failure of the bulbar septum to completely close the interventricular foramen.

defective (de-fek′tiv) 1. imperfect. 2. a person lacking in some physical, mental, or moral quality.

defeminization (de-fem″ĭ-ni-za′shun) loss of female sexual characteristics.

defense (de-fens′) the practice of, or measures taken to ensure, self-protection. **character d.,** any character trait, e.g., a mannerism, attitude, or affectation, which serves as a defense mechanism. **insanity d.,** a legal concept that a person cannot be convicted of a crime if he lacked criminal responsibility by reason of insanity at the time of commission. See *M'Naghten rule* and *Durham rule,* under *rule,* and *American Law Institute Formulation,* under *formulation.* **muscular d.,** the muscular tension and rigidity which accompanies a localized inflammation (as in appendicitis) or passage of a kidney stone.

deferens (def′er-enz) [L.] deferent; see *ductus deferens.*

deferent (def′er-ent) [L. *deferens* carrying away] conveying anything away, as from a center.

deferentectomy (def″er-en-tek′to-me) vasectomy.

deferential (def″er-en′shal) pertaining to the ductus deferens.

deferentitis (def″er-en-ti′tis) inflammation of the ductus deferens.

deferoxamine (dĕ-fer-oks′ah-mēn) chemical name: *N*′-[5-[[4-[[5-(acetylhydroxyamino) pentyl] amino] -1,4-dioxobutyl]hydroxyamino]pentyl]-*N*-(5-aminopentyl)-*N*-hydroxybutanediamide. A chelating agent, isolated from *Streptomyces pilosus,* $C_{25}H_{48}N_6O_8$, which binds with iron to form a soluble complex. Called also *desferrioxamine.* **d. hydrochloride,** the hydrochloride salt of deferoxamine, $C_{25}H_{48}N_6O_8\cdot$HCl. **d. mesylate,** [USP], the water-soluble mesylate salt of deferoxamine, $C_{25}H_{48}N_6O_8\cdot CH_3SO_3H$, occurring as a white to off-white powder, having the same actions as the base; used as an antidote to iron poisoning, usually administered by intramuscular injection or by intravenous infusion. *Sterile deferoxamine mesylate,* prepared in conformance with USP specifications, is suitable for parenteral use.

defervescence (def″er-ves′ens) [L. *defervescere* to cease boiling] the period of abatement of fever.

defervescent (def″er-ves′ent) 1. causing reduction of fever. 2. an agent that acts to reduce fever.

defibrillation (de-fib″rĭ-la′shun) 1. termination of atrial or ventricular fibrillation, usually by electroshock. 2. separation of the fibers of a tissue by blunt dissection.

defibrillator (de-fib″rĭ-la′tor) [*de-* + *fibrillation*] an electronic apparatus used to counteract atrial or ventricular fibrillation by the application of brief electroshock to the heart, either directly or through electrodes placed on the chest wall.

defibrinated (de-fi′brĭ-nāt″ed) deprived of fibrin.

defibrination (de-fi″brĭ-na′shun) removal of fibrin from the blood; see also under *syndrome*.

deficiency (de-fish′en-se) a lack or defect. For deficiencies of specific enzymes, see under the enzyme name. **debrancher d.,** glycogen storage disease, type III. **17-hydroxylase d.,** see under *syndrome*. **IgA d., isolated, IgA d., selective,** the most common immunodeficiency disorder: deficiency of IgA with normal levels of the other immunoglobulin classes and normal cellular immunity. It is marked by recurrent sinopulmonary infections and an increased incidence of allergy, gastrointestinal disease (celiac disease, ulcerative colitis, Crohn's disease), and autoimmune diseases (rheumatoid arthritis, systemic lupus erythematosus). Many patients have anti-IgA antibodies that can cause severe transfusion reactions. **immune d.,** immunodeficiency. **leukocyte G6PD d.,** an x-linked disorder clinically similar to chronic granulomatous disease (q.v.). **mental d.,** see under *retardation*. **oxygen d.,** anoxemia; hypoxia. **sucrase-α-dextrinase d., intestinal,** disaccharide intolerance I. **sucrase-isomaltase d., congenital,** disaccharide intolerance I. **vitamin d.,** see specific vitamins.

deficit (def′ĭ-sit) a lack or deficiency. **oxygen d.,** see *anoxia, anoxemia,* and *hypoxia.* **pulse d.,** the difference between the heart rate and the pulse rate in atrial fibrillation, resulting from failure of some of the ventricular contractions to produce peripheral pulse waves. **saturation d.,** the difference between the amount of water vapor a given volume of air could contain at a specific temperature and the amount it actually contains.

Definate (def′ĭ-nāt) trademark for a preparation of docusate sodium.

definition (def″ĭ-nish′un) the clear determination of the limits of anything, as of a disease process or a microscopical image. See also *resolution,* def. 2.

definitive (de-fin′ĭ-tiv) established with certainty. In embryology, denoting acquisition of final differentiation or character. In parasitology, denoting the host in which a parasite reaches the sexual stage.

defloration (def″lo-ra′shun) [L. *deflora′tio*] the rupturing of the hymen in sexual intercourse, in vaginal examination, or by manipulation.

deflorescence (def″lo-res′ens) the disappearance of the eruption in any exanthematous disease.

defluvium (de-floo′ve-um) [L., from *defluere* to flow down] defluxio. **postpartum d.,** loss of hair by the mother after delivery. **d. un′guium,** onychomadesis.

defluxio (de-fluk′se-o) [L., from *defluere* flow down] 1. a flowing down. 2. a disappearance.

defluxion (de-fluk′shun) [L. *defluxio*] 1. a sudden disappearance. 2. a copious discharge, as of catarrhal fluid. 3. a falling out, as of the hair.

deformability (de-form″ah-bil′ĭ-te) the ability of cells, such as erythrocytes, to change shape as they pass through narrow spaces, such as the microvasculature.

deformation (de″for-ma′shun) [L. *deformatio* a disfiguring] 1. in dysmorphology, a type of structural defect characterized by the abnormal form or position of a body part, caused by a nondisruptive mechanical force. 2. the process of adapting in shape or form, as the change in shape of erythrocytes as they pass through capillaries.

deforming (de-form′ing) causing or producing deformity.

deformity (de-for′mĭ-te) distortion of any part or general disfigurement of the body; malformation. **Åkerlund d.,** a deformity of the duodenal cap in the radiograph in duodenal ulcer, consisting of an indentation (incisura) in addition to the niche. **Arnold-Chiari d.,** a congenital anomaly in which the cerebellum and medulla oblongata, which is elongated and flattened, protrude down into the spinal canal through the foramen magnum; it may be associated with many other defects, including spina bifida occulta and meningomyelocele. Called also *Arnold-Chiari malformation* or *syndrome*. **boutonnière d.,** a deformity of the finger characterized by flexion of the proximal interphalangeal joint and hyperextension of the distal joint; called also *buttonhole d.* **buttonhole d.,** 1. boutonnière d. 2. see

buttonhole mitral stenosis, under *stenosis*. **crossbar d.,** the stiffening of a segment of the lesser curvature of the stomach, usually due to the healing of a deep penetrating ulcer. **Dandy-Walker d.,** see under *syndrome*. **funnel d.,** a funnel-shaped mitral orifice occurring as a result of fusion and shortening of the chordae tendineae. **gun stock d.,** cubitus varus. **Ilfeld-Holder d.,** prominent scapula with difficulty in raising the arm. **lobster-claw d.,** a developmental anomaly characterized by an abnormal cleft between the central metacarpal bones, the soft tissues of the digits being fused into two masses, one on either side of the cleft. **Madelung's d.,** radial deviation of the hand secondary to overgrowth of the distal ulna or shortening of the radius; called also *carpus curvus*. **recurvatum d.,** a deformity of the proximal interphalangeal joint in which the joint extends when pressure is exerted between the thumb and middle finger. **reduction d.,** congenital absence of a portion or all of a body part, especially the limbs. **rocker-bottom d.,** see under *foot* (def. 1). **rolled edge d.,** a highly characteristic deformity of the aortic valve cusps caused by syphilis. **seal-fin d.,** ulnar deviation of the fingers in rheumatoid arthritis. **silver fork d.,** the peculiar deformity seen in Colles' fracture; see illustration under *fracture*. Called also *Velpeau's deformity*. **Sprengel's d.,** congenital elevation of the scapula, due to failure of descent of the scapula to its normal thoracic position during fetal life. **swan-neck d.,** a finger deformity in which the proximal interphalangeal joint is hyperextended and the distal interphalangeal joint is flexed. **thumb-in-palm d.,** adduction contracture of the thumb. **ulnar drift d.,** a deformity occurring when the proximal phalanx dislocates toward the volar aspect of the metacarpal head and at the same time deviates to the ulnar side of the hand. **Velpeau's d.,** silver fork deformity. **Volkmann's d.,** see under *disease*.

Deg. degeneration; degree.

degassing (de-gas′ing) 1. removal of a gas from a person or an object. 2. treatment of a person or an object subjected to the fumes of gas. 3. the volatilization of foreign matter from the surface of a metal, as in the heat treatment of gold foil in rendering it cohesive; see *anneal,* def. 3.

degeneracy (de-jen′er-ah-se) 1. the state of being degenerate. 2. the process of degenerating. 3. d. of code. **d. of code, code d.,** the presence in the genetic code of more than one codon that may specify for a single amino acid and lead to its insertion into a growing peptide chain.

degenerate 1. (de-jen′er-āt) to change from a higher to a lower type or form. 2. (de-jen′er-it) characterized by degeneration. 3. (de-jen′er-it) a person whose moral or physical state is below the normal.

degeneratio (de-jen″er-a′she-o) [L.] degeneration. **d. mi′cans,** glistening degeneration.

degeneration (de-jen″er-a′shun) [L. *degeneratio*] deterioration; change from a higher to a lower form; especially change of tissue to a lower or less functionally active form. When there is chemical change of the tissue itself, it is *true* degeneration; when the change consists in the deposit of abnormal matter in the tissues, it is *infiltration*. Called also *retrogression*. **Abercrombie's d.,** amyloid d. **adipose d.,** fatty d. **adiposogenital d.,** adiposogenital dystrophy. **albuminoid d., albuminous d.,** cloudy swelling; see under *swelling*. **Alzheimer's neurofibrillary d.,** neurofibrillary tangles. **amyloid d.,** degeneration with the deposit of lardacein in the tissues; it indicates impairment of nutritive function, and is seen in wasting diseases. Also known as *Abercrombie's d., Virchow's d., bacony d., cellulose d., hyaloid d., lardaceous d.,* and *waxy d.* **angiolithic d.,** one characterized by mineral deposits and hyaline changes in the coats of the vessels. **Armanni-Ehrlich's d.,** hyaline degeneration of the epithelial cells of Henle's loops; seen in diabetes. **ascending d.,** wallerian degeneration affecting centripetal nerve fibers and progressing toward the brain or spinal cord. **atheromatous d.,** atheroma. **atrophic pulp d.,** pulp atrophy. **axonal d.,** the reaction of a nerve cell to injury to its axon; it consists of central chromatolysis and eccentricity of the nucleus. **bacony d.,** amyloid d. **basic d., basophilic d.,** basophilia, def. 1. **black d. of brain,** a fungous disease caused by species of *Cladosporium,* especially *C. tricoides,* which is named for its most apparent pathological sign. On tissue section of the brain, multiseptate, brown distorted hyphae are seen. **blastophthoric d.,** blastophthoria.

calcareous d., degeneration with infiltration of calcareous materials into the tissues; called also *earthy d.* **caseous d.,** caseation, def. 2. **cellulose d.,** amyloid d. **cerebromacular d. (CMD), cerebroretinal d.,** 1. degeneration of brain cells and the macula retinae, as in Tay-Sachs disease. 2. any lipidosis with cerebral lesions and degeneration of the retinal macula. 3. any form of amaurotic familial idiocy. **cheesy d.,** caseation, def. 2. **chitinous d.,** amyloid d. **colloid d.,** the assumption by the tissues of a gumlike or gelatinous character; called also *gelatiniform d.* **colloid d. of choroid,** Tay's choroiditis. **comma d.,** progressive degeneration of the nervous matter of the comma tract (interfascicular fasciculus). **congenital macular d.,** an autosomal dominant form of macular degeneration characterized by the presence of a cystlike lesion that in the early stages resembles egg yolk; called also *vitelliform d. of Best, vitelline macular d., Best's macular dystrophy,* and *hereditary vitelliform dystrophy.* **corticostriatal-spinal d.,** Creutzfeldt-Jakob syndrome. **Crooke's hyaline d.,** degeneration of basophils of the pituitary gland, in which they lose their specific granulations and the cytoplasm becomes progressively hyalinized; a constant finding in the presence of elevated plasma corticosteroid levels of any cause, but also occurring in Addison's disease. **cystic d.,** degeneration with the formation of cysts. **cystoid d.,** Blessig's cysts. **descending d.,** wallerian degeneration extending peripherally along nerve fibers. **disciform macular d.,** a form of macular degeneration occurring in persons over 40 years of age, in which sclerosis involving the macula and retina is produced by hemorrhages between Bruch's membrane and the pigment epithelium; called also *macular disciform d., senile exudative macular d., senile macular exudative choroiditis, senile disciform d., Kuhnt-Junius disease, disciform retinitis,* and *central disk-shaped retinopathy.* **Doyne's familial colloid d., Doyne's honeycomb d.,** see under *choroiditis.* **dystrophic d.,** degeneration arising from defective or faulty nutrition. **earthy d.,** calcareous d. **elastoid d.,** amyloid degeneration of the elastic tissue of arteries. **familial colloid d.,** Doyne's familial honeycombed choroiditis. **fascicular d.,** degeneration of paralyzed muscles due to lesion in the motor ganglion cells of the central tube of gray matter of the cord. **fatty d.,** deposit of fat globules in a tissue; called also *adipose d.* **fibrinous d.,** necrosis with deposit of fibrin within the cells of the tissue. **fibroid d.,** degeneration into fibrous tissue. **fibrous d.,** fibrosis. **gelatiniform d.,** colloid d. **glassy d.,** a peculiar change occurring in the heart muscle and other muscles in fevers. **glistening d.,** degeneration of glia tissue characterized by the formation of glistening masses; called also *degeneratio micans* and *Rosenthal's d.* **glycogenic d.,** a form of degeneration in which abnormal amounts of glycogen accumulate in the cells, as in glycogenosis. **Gombault's d.,** progessive hypertrophic interstitial neuropathy. **granulovascular d.,** a condition in which the ganglion cells become filled with vacuoles containing condensed granules of protoplasm. **gray d.,** degeneration of the white substance of the spinal cord, in which it loses myelin and assumes a gray color. **hematohyaloid d.,** a form of hyaline degeneration of thrombi due to conglutination of the red cells or blood platelets. **hemoglobinemic d.,** an archaic term applied to accumulation of hemoglobin in the center of the erythrocyte. **hepatolenticular d.,** Wilson's disease. **Holmes's d.,** primary progressive cerebellar d. **Horn's d.,** degeneration with nuclear proliferation in striated muscles. **hyaline d.,** a regressive cellular change in which the cytoplasm take on a homogeneous glassy eosinophilic appearance. Also used loosely to describe the histologic appearance of tissues. Called also *vitreous d.* and *hyalinosis.* **hyaloid d.,** amyloid d. **hydropic d.,** a variety in which the epithelial cells absorb much water. **lardaceous d.,** amyloid d. **lattice d. of retina,** a frequently bilateral, usually benign asymptomatic condition, characterized by patches of fine gray or white lines that intersect at irregular intervals in the peripheral retina, usually associated with numerous, round, punched-out areas of retinal thinning or retinal holes. **lipoidal d.,** a condition somewhat resembling fatty degeneration or infiltration but in which the extraneous material is lipoid. **macular d.,** degenerative changes in the macula retinae. **macular disciform d.,** disciform macular d. **Mönckeberg's d.,** see under *arteriosclerosis.* **mucinoid d.,** a term used to include both mucoid and colloid degeneration;

called also *mucinous d.* and *myelinic d.* **mucinous d.,** mucous d. **mucoid d.,** degeneration accompanied by deposit of myelin and lecithin in the cells. **mucous d.,** a form in which mucus accumulates in epithelial tissues. **myelinic d.,** mucoid d. **myxomatous d.,** degeneration in which mucus accumulates in connective tissues. **Nissl d.,** degeneration of a nerve cell after division of the nerve fiber supplying it. **olivopontocerebellar d.,** familial cerebellar degeneration occurring in the young or middle aged, characterized by extensive atrophy of the middle cerebellar peduncles and of the ventral surface of the pons, with loss of myelin in the white matter of the cerebellum and of cells in the olivary nuclei, the nuclei pontis, and the Purkinje and granular cell layers of the cerebellum. **pallidal d.,** degeneration of the globus pallidus. **parenchymatous d.,** cloudy swelling. **pigmental d., pigmentary d.,** that in which cells of affected tissue become abnormally pigmented. **polypoid d.,** the development, on a mucous membrane, of polypoid growths. **primary progressive cerebellar d.,** a familial disease marked by motor disorders and due to cerebellar degeneration, occurring in adults between the ages of thirty and forty and progessing slowly to a fatal termination; called also *Holmes' d.* **Quain's d.,** fibrous degeneration of the muscles of the heart. **red d.,** degeneration of a uterine leiomyoma during pregnancy, marked by the formation of soft red areas due to necrosis and edema. **retrograde d.,** axon reaction. **rim d.,** degeneration of the spinal cord affecting the periphery only. **Rosenthal's d.,** glistening d. **sclerotic d.,** a variety of hyaline degeneration affecting connective tissue, especially the intima of arteries. **secondary d.,** wallerian d. **senile d.,** the widespread degenerative changes, principally fibroid and atheromatous, that occur in old age. Cf. *senile atrophy.* **senile disciform d.,** disciform macular d. **senile exudative macular d.,** disciform macular d. **spongy d. of central nervous system, spongy d. of white matter,** a rare, autosomal recessive form of leukodystrophy, characterized by early onset, widespread demyelination and vacuolation of the cerebral white matter that gives rise to a spongy appearance, severe mental retardation, megalocephaly, atony of the neck muscles, spasticity of the arms and legs, and blindness, with death usually occurring at about 18 months of age. Called also *Canavan's disease* and *Canavan-van Bogaert-Bertrand disease.* **subacute combined d. of spinal cord,** degeneration of both the posterior and lateral columns of the spinal cord caused by vitamin B_{12} deficiency; a progressive disease, most often affecting persons over forty years of age, it is usually associated with pernicious anemia. The symptoms include paresthesias, ataxia, unsteadiness of gait, and sometimes emotional disorders. Called also *Lichtheim's disease* or *syndrome, Putnam-Dana syndrome,* and *posterolateral sclerosis.* **trabecular d.,** a change in the walls of the bronchi, which become thin and wasted in respect to the muscular and mucous elements, while the stroma is increased in volume. **transneuronal d.,** atrophy of certain neurons after interruption of afferent axons or death of other neurons to which they send their efferent output. **traumatic d.,** degeneration of a divided nerve up to the nearest node of Ranvier. **Türck's d.,** secondary parenchymatous degeneration of nerve tracts of the cord. **uratic d.,** degeneration marked by the deposit of urates or uric acid. **vacuolar d.,** the formation of vacuoles in the cells of a tissue. **Virchow's d.,** amyloid d. **vitelliform d. of Best, vitelliform macular d., vitelline macular d.,** congenital macular d. **vitreous d.,** hyaline d. **wallerian d.,** fatty degeneration of a nerve fiber which has been severed from its nutritive centers; called also *secondary d.* **waxy d.,** amyloid d. **Wilson's d.,** see under *disease.* **Zenker's d.,** necrosis and hyaline degeneration of striated muscle; called also *Zenker's necrosis.*

degenerative (de-jen′er-a-tiv) of or pertaining to degeneration.

degerm (de-germ′) disinfect.

degloving (de-gluv′ing) intra-oral surgical exposure of the bony mandibular structures, as by rolling the lower lip and vestibular soft tissue over the chin to expose the symphysis. The operation can also be performed in the posterior region if necessary.

Deglut. abbreviation for L. *deglutia′tur,* let it be swallowed.

deglutible (de-gloo′tĭ-bl) capable of being swallowed.

deglutition (deg″loo-tish′un) [L. *deglutitio*] the act of swallowing.

deglutitive (de-gloo′tĭ-tiv) deglutitory.

deglutitory (de-gloo′tĭ-to″re) pertaining to or promoting deglutition.

Degos' disease, syndrome (dĕ-gōz′) [Robert *Degos*, French dermatologist, born 1904] malignant atrophic papulosis.

degradation (deg-rah-da′shun) the reduction of a chemical compound to one less complex, as by splitting off one or more groups.

degranulation (de-gran″u-la′shun) the process of losing granules; said of certain granular cells.

degree (de-gre′) 1. a grade or rank awarded scholars by a college or university. 2. a unit of measure of temperature. 3. a unit of measure of arcs and angles. **d's of freedom,** the number of ways the members of a sample can vary independently; a numerical index of a family of probability distributions that corresponds to the number of independent variables in the definition of each member, e.g., the chi-squared distribution with *n* degrees of freedom is the distribution of the sum of squares of *n* standard normal deviations. **prism d.,** centrad, def. 2.

degrowth (de′grōth) decrease in the mass of living matter because of use of the proteins of the protoplasm to produce energy by the organism.

degustation (de″gus-ta′shun) [L. *degustatio*] the act or function of tasting.

dehab (de′hahb) surra.

dehepatized (de-hep′ah-tīzd) having the liver removed.

Dehio's test (da′he-ōz) [Karl Konstantinovich *Dehio*, Russian physician, 1851–1927] see under tests.

dehiscence (de-his′ens) [L. *dehiscere* to gape] a splitting open. **root d.,** an isolated area in which the root of a tooth is denuded of bone, the denuded area extending from the margin to near the apex; it occurs most commonly on the vestibular than the oral surface, the anterior teeth being affected more often. **wound d.,** separation of the layers of a surgical wound; it may be partial and superficial only, or complete, with disruption of all layers. **Zuckerkandl's d's,** small gaps occasionally seen in the papyraceous layer of the ethmoid bone.

dehumidifier (de″hu-mid′ĭ-fi″er) an apparatus by which the content of moisture in the air is reduced.

dehydrant (de-hi′drant) 1. reducing hydration. 2. an agent that removes or reduces body water.

dehydrase (de-hi′drās) a term formerly applied to both the dehydrogenases and the dehydratases.

dehydratase (de-hi′drah-tās) an enzyme of the lyase class [EC 4.2.1] that catalyzes the removal of water from a compound to form a double bond. Called also *hydro-lyase.*

dehydrate (de-hi′drāt) to remove water from (a compound, the body, etc.).

dehydration (de″hi-dra′shun) [L. *de* away + Gr. *hydōr* water] 1. removal of water from a substance. 2. the condition that results from excessive loss of body water. Called also *anhydration, deaquation,* and *hypohydration.* **absolute d.,** water content below the normal or below a standard amount. **hypernatremic d.,** a condition in which electrolyte losses are disproportionately smaller than water losses. **relative d.,** dehydration resulting from increased osmotic pressure of the body fluids. **voluntary d.,** that resulting when thirst does not stimulate sufficient replacement of water loss.

dehydroandrosterone (de-hi″dro-an-dros′ter-ōn) former name for dehydroepiandrosterone.

dehydroascorbic acid (de-hi″dro-ah-skor′bik) the reversibly oxidized form of ascorbic acid, which has the same vitamin C activity as ascorbic acid when ingested.

dehydrobilirubin (de-hi″dro-bil-ĭ-ru′bin) biliverdin.

dehydrocholaneresis (de-hi″dro-ko″lan-er′ĕ-sis) increase in the output of dehydrocholic acid in the bile.

dehydrocholate (de-hi″dro-ko′lāt) a salt of dehydrocholic acid.

dehydrocholesterol (de-hi″dro-ko-les′ter-ol) a sterol found in the skin which, when properly irradiated, forms vitamin D. **7-d., activated,** cholecalciferol.

dehydrocholic acid (de-hi″dro-ko′lik) [USP] a synthetic bile acid that acts as a hydrocholeretic increasing bile output

to clear the increased bile acid load; bile pigment secretion is not increased; used as a laxative and to produce choleresis after gallbladder surgery or in cholecystography.

11-dehydrocorticosterone (de-hi″dro-kor-tĭ-kos′ter-ōn) chemical name: 21-hydroxypregn-4-ene-3,11,20-trione. A steroid, $C_{21}H_{28}O_4$, from the adrenal cortex, which has a slight effect on protein and carbohydrate metabolism. Also produced synthetically, it is used like cortisone as a glucocorticoid and as an antiallergic agent. Called also *Kendall's compound A.*

dehydrocorydaline (de-hi″dro-kŏ-rid′ah-lin) a yellowish crystalline alkaloid, $C_{22}H_{23}O_4N$, from the roots of species of *Corydalis.*

dehydroepiandrosterone (de-hi″dro-ep″ĭ-an-dros′ter-ōn) an androgen, $C_{19}H_{28}O_2$, occurring in normal human urine and synthesized from cholesterol; it is often present in excessive amounts in body fluids of patients with adrenal virilism. Abbreviated DHEA. Called also *dehydroisoandrosterone* and, formerly, *dehydroandrosterone.*

dehydrogenase (de-hi′dro-jĕ-nās) an enzyme of the oxidoreductase class [EC1] that catalyzes the transfer of hydrogen or electrons from a donor to an acceptor compound. Dehydrogenases are usually designated according to the substrate that is oxidized (hydrogen donor compound).

dehydrogenate (de-hi′dro-jĕ-nāt) to remove hydrogen from.

dehydrogenation (de-hi′dro-jĕ-na′shun) oxidation due to removal of hydrogen by the reaction of a hydrogen acceptor.

dehydroisoandrosterone (de-hi″dro-i″so-an-dro′ster-ōn) dehydroepiandrosterone.

dehydromorphine (de-hi″dro-mor′fin) pseudomorphine.

dehydropeptidase (de-hi″dro-pep′tĭ-dās) aminoacylase.

dehydroretinal (de-hi″dro-ret′ĭ-nal) the aldehyde of dehydroretinol, derived from the visual pigment porphyropsin, found in fresh-water fishes and certain vertebrates and amphibians. Its metabolic role is analogous to that of rhodopsin in other animals. Called also *retinal₂.*

dehydroretinol (de-hi″dro-ret′ĭ-nol) vitamin A₂, the form, $C_{20}H_{28}O$, of vitamin A found in the retina and liver of fresh-water fishes and certain invertebrates and amphibians; it differs from retinol (vitamin A₁) in having one more conjugated double bond and has approximately one-third the biological activity of retinol. Called also *retinol₂.*

dehypnotize (de-hip′no-tīz) to arouse from the hypnoptic state.

deiodination (de-i″o-din-a′shun) the loss or removal of iodine from a compound.

deionization (de-i″on-i-za′shun) the production of a mineral-free state by the removal of ions, especially by use of ion-exchange resins.

deiteral (di′ter-al) pertaining to Deiters' nucleus.

Deiters' cells, etc. (di′terz) [Otto Friedrich Carl *Deiters,* German anatomist, 1834–1863] see under *cell, frame, nucleus, phalanx, process,* and *tract.*

déjà entendu (da-zhah′ on″ton-doo′) [Fr. "already heard"] the feeling that one has heard or perceived something previously although it is in fact new to one's experience.

déjà éprouvé (da-zhah′ a″proo-va′) [Fr. "already tested"] a feeling that something a person has never engaged in has been done.

déjà fait (da-zhah′ fa) [Fr. "already done"] a feeling that what is happening has happened before.

déjà pensé (da-zhah′ pon-sa′) [Fr. "already thought"] a feeling that one has thought the same thoughts before.

déjà raconté (da-zhah′ rak″on-ta′) [Fr. "already told"] an illusory feeling when telling someone about an experience that one had previously related the same experience to the same person or to someone else, when in fact one had not.

déjà vécu (da-zhah′ va-koo′) [Fr. "already lived"] an illusory feeling that a new experience has been previously encountered.

déjà voulu (da-zhah′ voo-loo′) [Fr. "already desired"] a feeling that one has entertained the same desires before.

déjà vu (da-zhah′ voo′) [Fr. "already seen"] an illusion in which a new situation is incorrectly viewed as a repetition of a previous situation.

dejecta (de-jek′tah) excrement.

dejection (de-jek'shun) [L. *dejectio*] 1. a mental state marked by depression and melancholy. 2. discharge of feces; defecation. 3. excrement; feces.

Dejerine's disease, etc. (deh″zher-ēnz') [Joseph Jules *Dejerine*, French neurologist, 1849–1917] see under *disease*, *sign*, *syndrome*, and *type*.

Dejerine-Klumpke paralysis, syndrome (deh″zher-ēn' klump'ke) [Augusta *Dejerine-Klumpke*, French neurologist, 1859–1927] Klumpke's paralysis.

Dejerine-Landouzy dystrophy (type) (deh″zher-ēn' lan-doo'ze) [J. J. *Dejerine*; Louis Théophile Joseph *Landouzy*, French physician, 1845–1917] see *Landouzy-Dejerine dystrophy*, under *dystrophy*.

Dejerine-Lichtheim phenomenon (deh″zher-en' lic-t'him) [J. J. *Dejerine*; Ludwig *Lichtheim*, German physician, 1845–1928] Lichtheim sign.

Dejerine-Roussy syndrome (deh″zher-ēn' roo-se') [J. J. *Dejerine*; Gustav *Roussy*, French pathologist, 1874–1948] thalamic syndrome.

Dejerine-Sottas atrophy, disease, syndrome (deh″zher-ēn' sot'tahz) [J. J. *Dejerine*; Jules *Sottas*, French neurologist, 1866–1943] progressive hypertrophic interstitial neuropathy.

deka- [Gr. *deka* ten] a combining form meaning ten; for words beginning thus, see also those beginning *deca-*.

dekanem (dek'ah-nem) [(obs.) ten nems; abbreviated Dn.

delacrimation (de-lak″rĭ-ma'shun) [L. *delacrimatio* weeping] excessive and abnormal flow of tears.

delactation (de″lak-ta'shun) 1. weaning. 2. the cessation of lactation.

Delafield's fluid, hematoxylin (del'ah-fēldz) [Francis *Delafield*, pathologist in New York, 1841–1915] see under *fluid*, and see *Table of Stains*.

Delalutin (del'ah-lu'tin) trademark for a preparation of hydroxyprogesterone caproate.

delamination (de″lam-ĭ-na'shun) [L. *de* apart + *lamina* plate] separation into layers, as the separation of blastoderm into epiblast and hypoblast during chick embryo development.

Delatestryl (del″ah-tes'tril) trademark for a preparation of testosterone enanthate.

Delbet's sign (del-bāz') [Pierre *Delbet*, French surgeon, 1861–1925] see under *sign*.

Delbrück (del'brik) Max. German-born American biologist, 1906–1981; co-winner, with Alfred Day Hershey and Salvador Edward Luria, of the Nobel prize for medicine or physiology in 1969 for research on the genetic structure of viruses.

de-lead (de-led') to remove lead from a tissue, as from the bones in lead poisoning by the administration of edetate disodium calcium.

Delestrogen (del-es'tro-jen) trademark for a preparation of estradiol valerate.

deleterious (del″ĕ-te're-us) [Gr. *dēlētērios*] hurtful; injurious.

deletion (de-le'shun) [L. *deletio* destruction] in genetics, usually a chromosomal aberration in which a portion of a chromosome is lost. It may also refer to loss of any DNA segment, as in some thalassemia genes and other mutations. **antigenic d.,** loss or masking of antigenic determinants in daughter cells of cells whose parent tissue normally carries them; it may result from neoplastic or other mutational change in the parent tissue or may be due to loss or repression of genetic material from the cell.

delimitation (de-lim″ĭ-ta'shun) [*de-* + L. *limitare* to limit] 1. the process of limiting or of becoming limited. 2. ascertainment of the limits and extent of some diseased tissue or process, or the spread of a disease in a host or a community.

delinquent (de-ling'kwent) 1. failing to do that which is required by law or obligation. 2. a person who neglects a legal obligation. **juvenile d.,** a juvenile offender; an individual who commits a violation of the law within the jurisdiction of the juvenile court system.

deliquescence (del″ĕ-kwes'ens) [L. *deliquescere* to grow moist] the condition of becoming moist or liquefied as a result of the absorption of water from the air.

deliquescent (del″ĕ-kwes'ent) having a tendency to form

an aqueous solution or become liquid by the absorption of moisture from the air.

deliria (de-lir'ĭ-ah) [L.] plural of *delirium*.

deliriant (de-lēr'e-ant) 1. capable of producing delirium. 2. a drug which may produce delirium. 3. a delirious person.

delirifacient (de-lēr″ĭ-fa'she-ent) [L. *delirium* + *facere* to make] 1. capable of causing delirium. 2. a drug which may produce delirium.

delirious (de-lēr'e-us) suffering from delirium.

delirium (de-lēr'e-um), pl. *delir'ia* [*de-* + L. *lira* furrow or track; i.e., "off the track"] [DSM III-R] an acute, reversible organic mental disorder characterized by reduced ability to maintain attention to external stimuli and disorganized thinking as manifested by rambling, irrelevant, or incoherent speech; there are also a reduced level of consciousness, sensory misperceptions, disturbance of the sleep-wakefulness cycle and level of psychomotor activity, disorientation to time, place, or person, and memory impairment. Delirium may be caused by a large number of conditions resulting in derangement of cerebral metabolism, including systemic infection, poisoning, drug intoxication or withdrawal, seizures or head trauma, and metabolic disturbances such as hypoxia, hypoglycemia, fluid, electrolyte, or acid-base imbalances, or hepatic or renal failure. Called also *acute confusional state* and *acute brain syndrome*. **acute d.,** a suddenly appearing and severe delirium lasting only a short time. **d. alcohol'icum,** d. tremens. **alcohol withdrawal d.** [DSM III-R], d. tremens. **d. cor'dis,** atrial fibrillation. **exhaustion d.** (obs.), delirium due to strain or exhaustion from metabolic or nutritional disturbance. **febrile d.,** the delirium of fever. **low d.,** delirium marked by confusion of ideas and slowness of mental action rather than by excitement. **senile d.,** a syndrome occurring in old age, usually of acute onset, and characterized by disorientation, restlessness, insomnia, hallucinations, and aimless wandering, sometimes associated with senile psychosis. **toxic d.,** delirium caused by poisons. **traumatic d.,** that which follows severe head injury; superficially the patient is alert, but there is marked disorientation, memory defect, and confabulation. **d. tre'mens,** delirium caused by cessation or reduction in alcohol consumption, typically in alcoholics with 10 years or more of heavy drinking. Clinical manifestations include autonomic hyperactivity, such as tachycardia, sweating, and hypertension, a coarse, irregular tremor, and delusions, vivid hallucinations, and wild, agitated behavior. The onset is usually 2 or 3 days after cessation of drinking; the delirium and other withdrawal symptoms usually resolve in 3 or 4 days. Called alcohol withdrawal syndrome in DSM III-R.

delitescence (del″ĭ-tes'ens) [L. *delitescere* to lie hidden] 1. sudden disappearance of symptoms or of objective signs of a disease or of a lesion. 2. the period of latency or incubation of a poison or morbific agent.

deliver (de-liv'er) [Fr., from L. *deliberare* to set free] 1. to aid in the process of childbirth. 2. to remove, as the fetus or placenta, or the lens of the eye.

delivery (de-liv'er-e) 1. expulsion or extraction of the child and the after-birth; see also *labor*. 2. removal of a part, as the lens of the eye. **abdominal d.,** delivery of a fetus through an incision made into the intact uterus through the abdominal wall. **breech d.,** delivery of a fetus in breech presentation; see *breech extraction*, under *extraction*. **forceps d.,** extraction of a fetus from the maternal passages by application of forceps to the child's head, without injury to the child or to the mother. **forceps d., high,** forceps delivery in which the forceps is applied to the head before engagement has taken place. **forceps d., low,** forceps delivery in which the forceps is applied when the scalp is or has been visible at the introitus without separating the labia, the skull has reached the pelvic floor, and the sagittal suture is in the anteroposterior diameter of the pelvis; called also *outlet forceps d*. **forceps d., outlet,** forceps d., low. **midforceps d.,** the application of forceps when the fetal head is engaged, but the conditions for outlet (low) forceps delivery have not been met; any forceps delivery requiring artificial rotation. **postmature d.,** delivery of a postmature infant. **postmortem d.,** birth of a fetus after the death of the mother. **premature d.,** birth of a premature infant. **spontaneous d.,** birth of an infant without any mechanical, pharmacologic, or medical assistance.

vaginal d., delivery of an infant through the normal openings of the uterus and vagina.

dell (del′) a slight depression or dimple.

delle (del′eh) the clear area in the center of a stained erythrocyte.

dellen (del′en) [Ger. "dents"] saucer-shaped excavations at the periphery of the cornea, usually on the temporal side, probably caused by insufficiency of the limbal circulation; called also *Fuchs' dimples.*

delling (del′ing) the formation of a slight depression; dimpling.

delmadinone acetate (del-mad′ĭ-nōn) chemical name: 17-(acetyloxy)-6-chloro-pregna-1,4,6-triene-3,20-dione. A progestin, antiandrogen, and antiestrogen, $C_{23}H_{27}ClO_4$, used in veterinary medicine.

delomorphic (del″o-mor′fik) delomorphous.

delomorphous (del″o-mor′fus) [Gr. *dēlos* evident + *morphē* form] having definitely formed and well-defined limits, as a cell or tissue.

delousing (de-lows′ing) the freeing from lice; destruction of lice.

Delphian node (Delphi, a town of ancient Greece, the location of the sanctuary and [Delphian] oracle of Apollo) see under *node.*

delphine (del′fin) delphinine.

delphinine (del′fĭ-nin) a poisonous alkaloid, $C_{33}H_{45}NO_9$, from the seeds of *Delphinium staphisagria;* formerly used for the most part externally to relieve pain in neuralgia, rheumatism, and paralysis. Called also *delphine.*

Delphinium (del-fin′e-um) [L.] a genus of ranunculaceous plants, including *D. consolida,* or larkspur, the seeds of which are diuretic, emmenagogue, and poisonous. The seeds of *D. staphisagria,* or stavesacre, were used for destroying lice. See *staphisagria.*

delphinoidine (del″fĭ-noid′in) an alkaloid from the seeds of *Delphinium staphisagria.*

delphisine (del′fĭ-sin) an alkaloid, isomeric with delphinine, from seeds of *Delphinium staphisagria.*

delta (del′tah) [Δ, δ] 1. the fourth letter of the Greek alphabet. 2. a triangular space. **d. mesoscap′ulae,** the triangular area at the root of the spine of the scapula.

Delta-Cortef (del′tah kor′tef) trademark for a preparation of prednisolone.

deltacortisone (del″tah-kor′tĭ-sōn) prednisone.

Deltalin (del′tah-lin) trademark for a preparation of synthetic vitamin D_2.

Deltasone (del′tah-sōn) trademark for a preparation of prednisone.

deltoid (del′toid) [L. *deltoides* triangular] triangular in outline, as the deltoid muscle.

Deltra (del′trah) trademark for prednisone.

delusion (de-lu′zhun) [L. *delusio,* from *de* from + *ludus* a game] a false belief that is firmly maintained in spite of incontrovertible and obvious proof or evidence to the contrary and in spite of the fact that other members of the culture do not share the belief. **d. of being controlled, d. of control,** the delusion that one's thoughts, feelings, and actions are not one's own but are being imposed by someone else or by some external force. **bizarre d.,** a delusion that is patently absurd and has no possible basis in fact, such as delusions of being controlled or thought broadcasting. **depressive d.,** a delusion that is congruent with a predominant depressed mood, such as a delusion that one is being persecuted because of one's sinfulness or inadequacy, somatic delusions of serious illness, nihilistic delusions, or delusions of poverty. **encapsulated d.,** a delusion that has no significant effect on behavior. **expansive d.,** d. of grandeur. **fragmentary d's,** unconnected delusions not organized around a coherent theme. **d. of grandeur, grandiose d.,** a delusion involving an exaggerated concept of one's importance, power, or knowledge or that one is, or has a special relationship with, a deity or a famous person. **mood-congruent d.,** a delusion occurring as a manifestation of a mood disorder; see also *mood-congruent.* **mood-incongruent d.,** a delusion occurring as a manifestation of a psychotic disorder; see also *mood-congruent.* **d. of negation, nihilistic d.,** a depressive delusion that the self or part of the self, part of the

body, other persons, or the whole world has ceased to exist. **paranoid d's,** delusions of grandeur or delusions of persecution. **d. of persecution, persecutory d.,** a delusion that one is being attacked, harassed, cheated, persecuted, or conspired against. **d. of poverty,** a delusion that one is, or soon will be, bereft of material possessions. **d. of reference,** a delusional conviction that ordinary events, objects, or behaviors of others have an unusual or peculiar meaning specifically for oneself. When less firmly held such beliefs are called *ideas of reference.* **somatic d.,** a delusion that there is some alteration in a bodily organ or its function. **systematized d's,** a group of delusions organized around a common theme.

delusional (de-lu′zhun-al) pertaining to or characterized by delusions.

Delvinal (del′vĭ-nal) trademark for preparations of vinbarbital.

Demansia (de-man′sĭ-ah) a genus of venomous elapid snakes, including the brown snake of Australia and New Guinea. See table accompanying *snake.*

demarcation (de″mar-ka′shun) [L. *demarcare* to limit] the marking off or ascertainment of boundaries. **surface d.,** any dividing line apparent on the surface of a solid body, such as the boundary between living and necrotic tissue.

Demarquay's sign (dem-ar-kāz′) [Jean Nicholas *Demarquay,* a French surgeon, 1811–1875] see under *sign.*

demasculinization (de-mas″ku-lin-i-za′shun) the loss of normal male characters, with testicular atrophy and involution of the prostate.

Dematiaceae (de-mat″ĭ-a′se-e) a family of imperfect fungi of the order Moniliales, producing simple conidiophores, and having dark brown or black conidia, spores, or hyphae. It includes the genera *Acremoniella, Arthrographis, Auerobasidium, Alternaria, Chalara, Cladosporium, Dematium, Fonsecaea, Madurella,* and *Phialophora.*

dematiaceous (de-mat″ĭ-a′shus) of or pertaining to a fungus of the family Dematiaceae.

Dematium (de-ma′she-um) a genus of soil and wood-rotting dematiaceous fungi, species of which have been reported to be isolated from human lesions, but are of questionable significance.

deme (dēm) [Gk. *dēmos* common people] a population of very similar organisms interbreeding in nature and occupying a circumscribed area; called also *genetic population.*

demecarium (dem″ě-kār′e-um) an anticholinesterase agent used topically to produce miosis, reduce intraocular pressure, and potentiate accommodation in the treatment of open-angle glaucoma and in the management of accommodative convergent strabismus. Available as *demecarium bromide* [USP].

demecarium bromide (dem″e-ka′re-um) [USP] chemical name:3,3′-[1,10-decanediylbis[(methylimino)carbonyloxy]] bis[*N,N,N*-trimethylbenzenaminium]dibromide. A potent, long-acting cholinesterase inhibitor, $C_{32}H_{52}Br_2N_4O_4$, occurring as a white or slightly yellow, crystalline powder; applied topically to the conjunctiva in the treatment of glaucoma and convergent strabismus.

demeclocycline (dem″ě-klo-si′klēn) [USP] chemical name: 7- chloro - 4S - (dimethylamino) -1, 4α, 4aα, 5, 5aα, 6β,11,12α-octahydro-3,6,10,12,12a-pentahydroxy-1,11- dioxo-2- naphtha- cenecarboxamide. A broad-spectrum oral antibiotic of the tetracycline group, $C_{21}H_{21}ClN_2O_8$, produced by a mutant strain of *Streptomyces aureofaciens* or semisynthetically, occurring as a yellow, crystalline powder. It also inhibits the effect of antidiuretic hormone on the renal tubules. Called also *demethylchlortetracycline.* **d. hydrochloride** [USP], the monohydrochloride salt of demeclocycline, $C_{21}H_{21}ClN_2O_8 \cdot HCl$, occurring as a yellow, crystalline powder; administered orally. It is also used as a diuretic.

dement (de-ment′) (*obs.*) a person affected with dementia.

demented (de-ment′ed) deprived of reason, mentally deteriorated; affected with dementia.

dementia (de-men′she-ah) [de- + L. *mens* mind] 1. [DSM III] an organic mental disorder characterized by a general loss of intellectual abilities involving impairment of memory, judgment, and abstract thinking as well as changes in personality. It does not include loss of intellectual functioning caused by clouding of consciousness (as in delirium) nor that caused by depression or other functional mental disorder (pseudodementia). Dementia may be caused by a large number of conditions, some reversible and some progressive, that cause widespread cerebral damage or dysfunction. The most common cause is Alzheimer's disease; others are cerebrovascular disease (multi-infarct dementia), central nervous system infection, brain trauma or tumors, pernicious anemia, folic acid deficiency, Wernicke-Korsakoff syndrome, normal-pressure hydrocephalus, and neurological diseases such as Huntington's chorea, multiple sclerosis, and Parkinson's disease. 2. (*obs.*), madness or insanity. **Alzheimer's d.,** see under *disease.* **Binswanger d.,** a degenerative dementia of presenile onset caused by demyelination of the subcortical white matter of the brain accompanying sclerotic changes in the blood vessels supplying it; called also *encephalitis subcorticalis chronica.* **dialysis d.,** a progressive encephalopathy marked by dysarthria with nominal aphasia, dementia, myoclonic jerking, grand mal seizures, and psychosis, occurring in persons undergoing chronic hemodialysis, and probably due to high levels of aluminum in the water used in the dialysis fluid. **epileptic d.,** a progressive mental and intellectual deterioration that occurs in a small fraction of cases of epilepsy; it is thought by some to be caused by neuronal degeneration secondary to circulatory disturbances during seizures. **multi-infarct d.** [DSM III-R], dementia with a stepwise deteriorating course (a series of small strokes) and a "patchy" distribution of neurologic deficits (affecting some functions and not others) caused by cerebrovascular disease. **d. myoclon′ica,** mental deterioration occurring in paramyoclonus multiplex. **paralytic d., d. paralyt′ica,** general paresis. **d. paranoi′des,** (*obs.*), paranoid schizophrenia. **d. prae′cox,** (*obs.*), schizophrenia. **presenile d.,** primary degenerative d. of the Alzheimer type, presenile onset. **primary degenerative d.** of the Alzheimer type (DSM III-R], dementia of insidious onset and gradually progressive course, occurring in almost all cases after the age of 50; classified as *presenile onset* or *senile onset* depending on whether onset is before or after age 65. In most cases there is the characteristic histopathology of Alzheimer's disease (q.v.); in rare cases, that of Pick's disease (q.v.). **d. pugilis′tica,** punch-drunk encephalopathy. **senile d.,** primary degenerative d. of the Alzheimer type, senile onset. **toxic d.** that which is due to excessive use of some poison. **Wernicke's d.,** presbyophrenia.

Demerol (dem′er-ol) trademark for preparations of meperidine (pethidine) hydrochloride.

demethylation (de″meth-ĭ-la′shun) the removal of a methyl group, —CH₃, from a compound.

demethylchlortetracycline (de-meth″il-klōr″tet-rah-si′klēn) demeclocycline.

demi- [Fr. *demi* half, from L. *dimidius*] a prefix meaning half.

demibain (dem′e-bān) [Fr.] sitz bath.

demifacet (dem″e-fas′et) a small plane surface on either of two bones which both articulate with a third bone. **inferior d. for head of rib,** fovea costalis inferior. **superior d. for head of rib,** fovea costalis superior.

demigauntlet (dem-e-gawnt′let) a form of bandage that covers the hand but leaves the fingers exposed.

demilune (dem′e-lūn) 1. a half moon, or crescent. 2. crescentic; crescent shaped. **d's of Adamkiewicz,** crescent-shaped cells beneath the neurilemma of medullated nerve fibers. **d's of Giannuzzi, d's of Heidenhain,** crescents of Giannuzzi.

demimonstrosity (dem″e-mon-stros′ĭ-te) malformation of a part which does not prevent the exercise of its function.

demineralization (de-min″er-al-i-za′shun) excessive elimination of mineral or inorganic salts, as in pulmonary tuberculosis, cancer, and osteomalacia.

demipenniform (dem″e-pen′ĭ-form) feather-shaped as to one of the two margins; said of certain muscles.

Demi-Regroton (dem′ĭ-reg′ro-ton) trademark for preparations of chlorthalidone and reserpine.

Democritus (de-mok′rĭ-tus) **of Abdera** (c. 460 to c. 360 B.C.) a Greek philosopher who was the first to state that everything in nature, including the body and the soul, is made up of atoms of different sizes and shapes, the movements of which are the cause of life and mental activity. Democritus' only influential Greek follower was Epicurus (341–270 B.C.). Their mechanistic, atomistic theory was influential at Alexandria, and the Epicurean school of philosophy corresponds

roughly to the Empiric school of medicine. See also *Asclepiades of Bithynia.*

demodectic (dem-o-dek′tik) pertaining to, or caused by, *Demodex.* See also *mange.*

Demodex (dem′o-deks) [Gr. *dēmos* fat + *dēx* worm] a genus of mites or acarids which cause follicular mange. **D. ca′nis,** the cause of follicular mange in dogs. **D. e′qui,** a species causing mange in horses. **D. folliculo′rum,** the hair follicle mite: a species found in hair follicles of man, and in sebaceous secretions, especially of the face and nose; called also *Acarus folliculorum, face mite,* and *follicle mite.*

Demodicidae (dem″o-dik′ĭ-de) a family of minute follicular mites (order Acarina) that parasitize the skin of various mammals, including man.

demodicidosis (dem″o-dis″ĭ-do′sis) infestation with *Demodex.*

demodicosis (dem″o-dĭ-ko′sis) 1. demodectic mange. 2. demodicidosis.

demogram (de′mo-gram) a graphic representation, in grid form, of the population of a given area according to the time period and the age and sex of the individuals comprising it.

demography (de-mog′rah-fe) [Gr. *dēmos* people + *graphein* to write] the study of mankind collectively, especially of geographical distribution and physical environment. **dynamic d.,** collective physiology of communities, with statistics of births, marriages, deaths, etc. **static d.,** collective anatomy of communities and study of their environment.

demoniac (de-mo′ne-ak) 1. frenzied. 2. possessed by demons, the medieval conception of insanity.

demonophobia (de″mon-o-fo′be-ah) [Gr. *daimōn* demon + *phobia*] irrational fear of demons.

demonstrator (dem′on-stra″tor) [L.] an instructor who teaches individuals or small groups by using dissections or other aids.

De Morgan's spots (de-mor′ganz) [Campbell *De Morgan,* English physician, 1811–1876] cherry angiomas.

demorphinization (de-mor″fin-i-za′shun) treatment of morphine addiction by gradual withdrawal of the drug.

Demours' membrane (da-moorz′) [Pierre *Demours,* French ophthalmologist, 1702–1795] lamina limitans posterior corneae.

demoxepam (dem-oks′ĕ-pam) chemical name: 7-chloro-1,3-dihydro-5-phenyl-2*H*-1,4-benzodiazepin-2-one 4-oxide. A minor tranquilizer, $C_{15}H_{11}ClN_2O_2$, which is an active metabolite of chlordiazepoxide.

demucosation (de″mu-ko-sa′shun) removal of the mucous membrane from a part.

demulcent (de-mul′sent) 1. soothing; bland; allaying the irritation of inflamed or abraded surfaces. 2. a soothing, mucilaginous, or oily medicine or application. Called also *lenitive.*

de Musset see *Musset.*

de Mussy's point (sign) (dŭ-mis-sēz′) [Noel François Odon Guéneau *de Mussy,* French physician, 1813–1885] see under *point.*

demustardization (de-mus″tard-i-za′shun) 1. removal of mustard gas from a person. 2. treatment of a person subjected to the fumes of mustard gas.

demutization (de″mu-ti-za′shun) [*de-* + L. *mutus* mute] the teaching of the deaf to communicate by lip reading or by dactylology.

demyelinate (de-mi′ĕ-lin-āt) to destroy or remove the myelin sheath of a nerve or nerves.

demyelination (de-mi′ĕ-li-na′shun) destruction, removal, or loss of the myelin sheath of a nerve or nerves.

demyelinization (de-mi′ĕ-lin-i-za′shun) demyelination.

denarcotize (de-nar′ko-tīz) to deprive of a narcotic drug in the process of treating addiction.

denasality (de″na-zal′ĭ-te) hyponasality.

denatality (de″na-tal′ĭ-te) decrease in the number of births in proportion to the population.

denatonium benzoate (de-nah-to′nĭ-um) [NF] chemical name: *N*-[2-[(2,6-dimethylphenyl)amino]-2-oxoethyl]-*N,N*-diethylbenzenemethanaminium benzoate. An alcohol denaturant, $C_{28}H_{34}N_2O_3$, occurring as a white, crystalline powder; used as a pharmaceutic aid.

denaturant (de-na′chur-ant) a denaturing agent.

denaturation (de-na″chur-a′shun) the destruction of the usual nature of a substance, as the addition of methanol or acetone to alcohol to render it unfit for drinking, or the change in the physical properties of proteins caused by heat or certain chemicals. **protein d.,** disruption of the configuration (tertiary structure) of a protein, as by heat, change in pH, or other physical or chemical means, resulting in alteration of the physical properties and loss of biological activity of the protein.

denatured (de-na′tūrd) having undergone denaturation.

dendraxon (den-drak′son) [Gr. *dendron* tree + *axon*] a nerve cell whose axon breaks up into terminal filaments almost immediately after leaving the cell. Cf. *inaxon.*

dendric (den′drik) dendritic.

dendriceptor (den′drĭ-sep″tor) one of the sensitive points at the ends of the branching processes of a dendrite, capable of being stimulated by the axon endings of other neurons.

Dendrid (den′drid) trademark for a preparation of idoxuridine.

dendriform (den′drĭ-form) branched, or tree-shaped.

dendrite (den′drīt) [Gr. *dendron* tree] one of the threadlike extensions of the cytoplasm of a neuron (q.v.); in unipolar and bipolar neurons, they resemble axons structurally, but typically, as in multipolar neurons, they branch into treelike processes. Dendrites comprise most of the receptive surface of a neuron. Called also *cytodendrite, dendron, neurodendrite,* and *neurodendron.* Cf. *axon* (def. 2), *collateral* (def. 2), and *telodendron.*

dendritic (den-drit′ik) 1. branched like a tree. 2. pertaining to or possessing dendrites.

dendr(o)- [Gr. *dendron* tree] a combining form denoting relationship to a tree or treelike structure.

dendroarcheology (den″dro-ar″ke-ol′o-ge) dendrochronology.

Dendroaspis (den-dro-as′pis) a genus of extremely venomous elapid snakes of Africa, including the deadly mamba, which are related to cobras but do not have a dilatable hood. See table accompanying *snake.*

Dendrochium (den-dro-ke′um) a genus of imperfect fungi (family Stilbaceae, order Moniliales), including *D. tox′icum,* the etiologic agent of dendrodochiotoxicosis in the U.S.S.R.

dendrochronology (den″dro-kron-ol′o-ge) determination of the age of a tree by observation of the annual growth rings in the trunk.

dendrodendritic (den″dro-den-drit′ik) referring to a synapse between dendrites of two neurons.

dendrodochiotoxicosis (den-dro″do-ke-o-tok″sĭ-ko′sis) an intoxication reported within the U.S.S.R. caused by the fungus *Dendrodochium toxicum.* Mycotoxications of this type are especially common in horses, but may affect humans as well.

dendroid (den′droid) [Gr. *dendron* tree + *eidos* form] branching like a tree or shrub.

dendron (den′dron) [Gr.] a dendrite.

dendrophagocytosis (den″dro-fag″o-si-to′sis) the absorption by microglia cells of broken portions of degenerating astrocytes.

denervate (de-ner′vāt) to deprive of a nerve supply.

denervation (de″ner-va′shun) resection or removal of the nerves to an organ or part.

dengue (deng′e; Spanish, dān-ga) [Sp.] classically, an acute, self-limited (typically 5–7 days′ duration) disease, characterized by fever, prostration, headache, myalgia, rash, lymphadenopathy, and leukopenia, which is caused by four antigenically related but distinct types of the dengue virus. Dengue occurs epidemically and sporadically in India, Japan, West Africa, the eastern Mediterranean area, Southeast Asia, Indonesia, northeastern Australia, Polynesia, the Caribbean, and northern South America. It is transmitted by the bite of infected mosquitoes of the genus *Aedes,* especially *A. aegypti, A. albopictus, A. polynesiensis, A. scutellaris,* and *A. hakanssoni.* Called also *Aden, breakbone, dandy,* and *dengue fever.* **hemorrhagic d.,** a syndrome affecting principally Southeast Asian children, distinguished from classic dengue by hemorrhagic manifestations, including thrombocytopenia and hemoconcentration, and caused by the same four serotypes of dengue virus. WHO's classification according to severity is *grade I,* fever, constitutional symptoms, and positive tourniquet test; *grade II,* grade I plus spontaneous bleeding into skin, gums, gastrointestinal tract, and other sites; *grade III,* grade II plus circulatory failure and agitation; and *grade IV,* profound shock with undetectable blood pressure and pulse. *Dengue shock syndrome* comprises grades III and IV. Called also *Philippine d.* and *Thai hemorrhagic fever.*

denial (dě-ni′al) a defense mechanism in which the existence of unpleasant realities is kept out of conscious awareness. It differs from repression in that the painful subject stems from external rather than internal sources, such as impulses or fantasies.

denidation (den″ĭ-da′shun) [de- + L. *nidus* nest] degeneration and expulsion of the uterine mucous membrane (endometrium) in the menstrual cycle.

Denis Browne splint (den′is brown) [Sir *Denis Browne,* Australian-born English pediatric surgeon, 1892–1967] see under *splint.*

Denis' method (den′is) [Wiley Glover *Denis,* American biochemist, born 1879] see under *method.*

Denisonia (den-ĭ-so′nĭ-ah) a genus of very venomous elapid snakes, including *D. super′ba,* the copperhead of Australia, Tasmania, and the Solomons. See table accompanying *snake.*

denitrification (de-ni″trĭ-fĭ-ka′shun) the setting free of gaseous nitrogen from nitrites and nitrates, as by certain soil bacteria, which results in depletion of nitrogen for plant growth. Denitrification carried out by aquatic bacteria can be beneficial in ridding waste waters of excess nitrates.

denitrifier (de-ni′trĭ-fi″er) a bacterium that causes denitrification.

denitrify (de-ni′trĭ-fi) to remove nitrogen from any substance; see *denitrification.*

denitrogenation (de-ni″tro-jĕ-na′shun) removal of the dissolved nitrogen from the body, as a preventive of caisson disease, aeroembolism, etc.

Denman's spontaneous evolution (version, method) (den′manz) [Thomas *Denman,* English obstetrician, 1733–1815] see under *evolution.*

denofungin (de″no-fun′jin) an antibiotic substance produced by a variant of *Streptomyces hygroscopicus,* which has antifungal and antibacterial properties.

Denonvilliers' aponeurosis, fascia, operation (den-aw-vēl-yāz′) [Charles Pierre *Denonvilliers,* surgeon in Paris, 1808–1872] see *septum rectovesicale,* and see under *fascia* and *operation.*

dens (dens), pl. *den′tes* [L.] a tooth or toothlike structure; [NA] a general term for a tooth or the teeth (dentes), the small bonelike structures of the jaws, serving in mastication of food and production of certain sounds in speech. See also *tooth.* **den′tes acus′tici** [NA], elevations along the free surface and margin of the labium limbi vestibulare; called also *auditory teeth of Huschke* and *hair teeth.* **den′tes acu′ti,** the incisor teeth (dentes incisivi [NA]). **d. ax′is** [NA], tooth of axis: the toothlike process that projects from the superior surface of the body of the axis, ascending to articulate with the atlas; called also *d. epistrophei, odontoid bone, odontoid apophysis, odontoid process of axis,* and *tooth of epistropheus.* **den′tes cani′ni** [NA], the canine teeth: the four teeth, one on either side in each jaw, immmediately lateral to the lateral incisors; called also *cuspids* or *cuspid teeth,* and *cynodonts.* **dentes de Chiaie,** mottled enamel. **den′tes decid′ui** [NA], the deciduous teeth: the teeth of the first dentition; see *deciduous tooth,* under *tooth.* **d. epistro′phei,** d. axis. **den′tes incisi′vi** [NA], incisor teeth: the four front teeth of each jaw, called also *dentes acuti* and *primary teeth.* **d. in den′te,** a malformed tooth resulting from invagination of the crown before it is calcified; so named because severe invagination of enamel and dentin gives the appearance of a "tooth within a tooth." Called also *d. invaginatus* and *dilated odontoma.* **d. invagina′tus,** dens in dente. **den′tes mola′res** [NA], molar teeth: the grinders, or double teeth, situated in the back part of either jaw, having the largest and most efficient chewing surfaces. **den′tes permanen′tes** [NA], the teeth of the second dentition; see *permanent teeth,* under *tooth.* **den′tes premola′res** [NA], premolar teeth: the two permanent teeth on either side of each jaw, between the canine teeth and the molars, called also *bicuspids,* or *bicuspid teeth.* **d. sapien′tiae,** d. serotinus. **d. seroti′nus** [NA], the aftermost tooth on each side of each jaw, being the last of the molar teeth to appear; called also *d. sapientiae, molaris tertius, third molar,* and *wisdom tooth.*

densimeter (den-sim′ĕ-ter) [L. *densus* dense + *metron*] densitometer.

densitometer (den″sĭ-tom′ĕ-ter) 1. an apparatus for determining the density of a liquid. Called also *densimeter.* 2. an instrument for determining the degree of darkening of developed photographic or x-ray film by means of a photocell which measures light transmission through a given area of the film. 3. an instrument for determining the density of deposits on electrophoresis strips and chromatographic plates by measuring light absorbancy. **gas d.,** an apparatus for measuring specific gravity of a gas.

densitometry (den″sĭ-tom′ĕ-tre) determination of variations in density by comparison with that of another material, or with a certain standard.

density (den′sĭ-te) [L. *densitas*] 1. the quality of being compact or dense. 2. the quantity of matter in a given space based on the ratio of mass to volume. 3. the quantity of electricity in a given area or in a given volume or in a given time. 4. the degree of darkening of exposed and processed photographic or x-ray film, expressed as the logarithm of the opacity of a given area of the film. 5. density function; see under *function.* **arciform d.,** a trough-shaped body separating the synaptic ribbon and the membrane of the cone pedicle or of the rod spherule in the retina. **background d.,** in radiography, the density of a processed film due to factors other than the radiation exposure received through the recorded objects or structures, e.g., inherent (film) density, scatter radiation, or fogging. **inherent d.,** the density of a processed film due to inherent factors such as the density of the film base, emulsion gelatin, etc. **ionization d.,** the number of ion pairs per unit volume. **optical d. (OD),** absorbance.

dentagra (den-tag′rah, den′tah-grah) [*dent-* + Gr. *agra* seizure] 1. a forceps or key for extracting teeth. 2. toothache.

dental (den′tal) [L. *dentalis*] 1. pertaining to a tooth or teeth. 2. a letter or sound made by or in part by the front teeth.

dentalgia (den-tal′je-ah) [*dent-* + *-algia*] toothache.

dentata (den-ta′tah) the second cervical vertebra or axis, so called from its toothlike process.

dentate (den′tāt) [L. *dentatus*] having teeth or projections like saw teeth on the edges.

dentatothalamic (den-ta″to-thah-lam′ik) pertaining to or connecting the dentate nucleus and the thalamus.

dentatum (den-ta′tum) [L. "toothed"] the nucleus dentatus.

dentes (den′tēz) [L.] plural of *dens.*

denti- see *dent(o)-.*

dentia (den′she-ah) [L.] a condition relating to development or eruption of the teeth. Used also as a combining form, denoting relationship to the teeth. **d. prae′cox,** 1. premature teeth. 2. predeciduous teeth. **d. tar′da,** delayed dentition.

dentibuccal (den-tĭ-buk′al) pertaining to the teeth and cheek.

denticle (den′tĭ-kl) [L. *denticulus* a little tooth] 1. a small toothlike process. 2. a calcified concretion that develops in the dental pulp as part of the aging process; called also *pulp stone.* **adherent d., attached d.,** a calcified formation in a pulp chamber partially fused with the dentin. **embedded d.,** interstitial d. **false d.,** a calcified formation in the pulp chamber of a tooth that does not show the structure of true dentin. **free d.,** a calcified formation in a tooth completely surrounded by the dental pulp. **interstitial d.,** a calcified formation within a tooth, completely surrounded by dentin. **true d.,** a calcified formation in the pulp chamber of a tooth that consists of dentin and shows traces of dentinal tubules and odontoblasts.

denticulated (den-tik′u-lāt″ed) [L. *denticulatus*] having minute teeth.

dentification (den″tĭ-fĭ-ka′shun) dentinogenesis.

dentiform (den′tĭ-form) shaped like a tooth.

dentifrice (den′tĭ-fris) [L. *dentifricium*] a preparation, usually a paste, gel, or powder, used with a toothbrush for cleaning the accessible surfaces of the teeth.

dentigerous (den-tij′er-us) [*denti-* + L. *gerere* to carry] bearing teeth.

dentilabial (den″tĭ-la′be-al) [*denti-* + L. *labium* lip] pertaining to the teeth and lips.

dentilingual (den″tĭ-ling′gwal) [*denti-* + L. *lingua* tongue] pertaining to the teeth and tongue.

dentimeter (den-tim′ĕ-ter) [*denti-* + Gr. *metron* measure] an instrument for measuring teeth.

dentin (den′tin) [L. *dens* tooth] the hard portion of the tooth surrounding the pulp, covered by enamel on the crown and cementum on the root, which is harder and denser than bone but softer than enamel. Called also *dentinum* [NA] and *substantia eburnea dentis.* Sometimes spelled *dentine.* **adventitious d.,** secondary irregular d. **calcified d.,** transparent d. **circumpulpar d.,** the inner portion of the dentin, adjacent to the pulp chamber, consisting of thinner fibrils. See also *predentin.* **cover d.,** mantle d. **functional d.,** secondary regular d. **hereditary opalescent d.,** the brown opalescent-appearing dentin observed in dentinogenesis imperfecta. **interglobular d.,** imperfectly calcified dentinal matrix situated between the calcified globules near the periphery of the dentin. **irregular d.,** secondary irregular d. **mantle d.,** the peripheral portion of the dentin adjacent to the enamel or cementum, consisting mostly of coarse fibers (Korff's fibers). Called also *cover d.* **opalescent d.,** dentin giving an unusual translucent or opalescent appearance to the teeth, as in dentinogenesis imperfecta. **primary d.,** dentin formed subsequently to the time when the tooth takes its anatomic position in the oral cavity; it is separated from secondary dentin by a demarcation line, formed by a change in the directional path of the dentinal tubules. **reparative d.,** secondary irregular d. **sclerotic d.,** transparent d. **secondary d.,** dentin formed and deposited in response to a normal or slightly abnormal stimulus, after the complete formation of the tooth. See *secondary irregular d.* and *secondary regular d.* **secondary irregular d.,** dentin formed in response to stimuli associated with pathologic processes, such as caries or injury, or cavity preparation. Such dentin is usually irregular in nature, being composed of a few tubules that may be tortuous in appearance, and it often demonstrates cellular inclusions. Called also *adventitious d., irregular d., reparative d.,* and *tertiary d.* **secondary regular d.,** dentin formed in response to stimuli associated with normal body processes. Called also *functional d.* **tertiary d.,** secondary irregular d. **transparent d.,** dentin in which some dentinal tubules have become sclerotic or calcified (dental sclerosis), producing the appearance of translucency, usually resulting from injury, abrasion, or normal aging processes. Called also *calcified d.* and *sclerotic d.*

dentinal (den′tĭ-nal) pertaining to dentin.

dentinalgia (den″tĭ-nal′je-ah) (*obs.*) pain in the dentin.

dentine (den′tēn) dentin.

dentinification (den-tin″ĭ-fĭ-ka′shun) (*obs.*) dentinogenesis.

dentinoblast (den′tĭ-no-blast) [*dentin* + *blast*] a cell that forms dentin.

dentinoblastoma (den″tĭ-no-blas-to′mah) dentinoma.

dentinogenesis (den″tĭ-no-jen′ĕ-sis) [*dentin* + *genesis*] the formation of dentin; called also *dentification* and *dentinification.* **d. imperfec′ta,** an autosomal dominant disorder of tooth development characterized by opalescent dentine resulting in discoloration of the teeth, ranging from dusky blue to brownish. The dentine is poorly formed with an abnormally low mineral content; the pulp canal is obliterated, but the enamel is normal. The teeth usually wear down rapidly, leaving short, brown stumps. Called also *odontogenesis imperfecta.*

dentinogenic (den″tĭ-no-jen′ik) forming or producing dentin.

dentinoid (den′tĭ-noid) 1. resembling dentin. 2. (*obs.*) dentinoma. 3. predentin.

dentinoma (den″tĭ-no′mah) a tumor of odontogenic origin, consisting mainly of dentin.

dentinosteoid (den″tin-os′te-oid) a tumor composed of or containing dentin and bone.

dentinum (den-ti′num) [NA] dentin: the chief substance or tissue of the teeth. See *dentin.*

dentiparous (den-tip′ah-rus) bearing teeth.

dentist (den'tist) a person who has received a degree from an accredited school of dentistry and is licensed to practice dentistry by a state board of dental examiners. Called also *odontologist.*

dentistry (den'tis-tre) 1. that department of the healing arts which is concerned with the teeth, oral cavity, and associated structures, including the diagnosis and treatment of their diseases and the restoration of defective and missing tissue. 2. the work done by dentists, such as the creation of restorations, crowns, and bridges, and surgical procedures performed in and about the oral cavity. 3. the practice of the dental profession collectively. Called also *odontoiatria, odontology,* and oral medicine. **cosmetic d., esthetic d.,** that aspect of dental practice concerned with the repair and restoration of carious, broken, or defective teeth in such a manner as to improve their appearance. **forensic d.,** that branch of dentistry that deals with the application of the art and science of dentistry to the purposes of law. *Dental jurisprudence* and *forensic dentistry* are sometimes used synonymously, but some authorities consider dental jurisprudence as a branch of law and forensic dentistry as a branch of dentistry. **geriatric d.,** gerodontics. **legal d.,** forensic d. **operative d.,** that phase of dentistry concerned with restoration of parts of the teeth that are defective through disease, trauma, or abnormal development to a state of normal function, health, and esthetics, including preventive, diagnostic, biological, mechanical, and therapeutic techniques, as well as material and instrument science and application. **pediatric d.,** pedodontics. **preventive d.,** that phase of dentistry concerned with the preservation of healthy teeth and the maintenance of oral structures in a state of optimal health for the longest period of time possible. **prosthetic d.,** prosthodontics. **psychosomatic d.,** that phase of dentistry which considers the mind-body relationship. **restorative d.,** that phase of clinical dentistry concerned with the restoration of existing teeth that are defective through disease, trauma, or abnormal development to the state of normal function, health, and esthetics, including crown and bridgework. See also *restoration.*

dentition (den-tish'un) [L. *dentitio*] the teeth in the dental arch; ordinarily used to designate the natural teeth in position in their alveoli. **artificial d.,** see *denture.* **deciduous d.,** deciduous teeth (dentes decidui [NA]). **delayed d.,** eruption of the first deciduous teeth after the end of the thirteenth month of life or eruption of the first permanent teeth after the seventh year of life. Called also *retarded d., delayed eruption,* and *dentia tarda.* **mixed d.,** the complement of teeth in the jaws after eruption of some of the permanent teeth, before all of the deciduous teeth are shed; called also *transitional d.* **natural d.,** the natural teeth in the dental arch, considered collectively; it may comprise deciduous or permanent teeth, or a mixture of the two, present at one time. **permanent d.,** permanent teeth (dentes permanentes [NA]). **precocious d.,** see *premature teeth,* under tooth. **predeciduous d.,** see under *tooth.* **premature d.,** see under *tooth.* **primary d.,** deciduous teeth (dentes decidui [NA]). **retarded d.,** delayed d. **secondary d.,** permanent teeth (dentes permanentes [NA]). **transitional d.,** mixed d.

dent(o)-, denti- [L. *dens* tooth] a combining form denoting relationship to a tooth or to the teeth. Cf. *odont(o)-.*

dentoalveolar (den″to-al-ve′o-lar) pertaining to a tooth and its alveolus.

dentoalveolitis (den″to-al″ve-o-li′tis) periodontal disease.

dentofacial (den″to-fa′shal) of or pertaining to the teeth and alveolar process and the face.

dentography (den-tog′rah-fe) odontography.

dentoid (den'toid) odontoid.

dentolegal (den″to-le′gal) pertaining to dental jurisprudence.

dentoliva (den″to-li′vah) [*dento-* + L. *oliva* olive] (*obs.*) the olivary nucleus.

dentoma (den-to′mah) dentinoma.

dentomechanical (den″to-mě-kan′i-k'l) pertaining to the mechanics or to the biomechanics of dentistry.

dentonomy (den-ton′o-me) [*dent-* + Gr. *onoma* name] odontonomy.

dentosurgical (den″to-sur′jĭ-k'l) pertaining to or used in dentistry and oral surgery.

dentotropic (den″to-trop′ik) turning toward or having an affinity for tissues composing the teeth.

dentulous (den′tu-lus) possessing natural teeth.

denture (den′chur) [Fr., from L. *dens* tooth] a set of teeth; ordinarily used to designate an artificial or prosthetic replacement for missing natural teeth and adjacent tissues. See also *bridge, dental prosthesis,* under *prosthesis,* and *restoration.* **clasp d.,** a partial denture retained with a clasp. See also *clasp* and *retainer.* **complete d.,** a dental prosthesis replacing all natural teeth and associated mandibular and maxillary structures; it is completely supported by the tissues. Called also *full d.* **conditioning d.,** a temporary denture used to condition the patient to wearing a denture. See also *interim d.* **full d.,** complete d. **immediate d., immediate-insertion d.,** a complete or removable denture made before all teeth are extracted, so constructed that it may be inserted immediately following the removal of the natural teeth. **implant d.,** an artificial denture retained and stabilized through the use of a subperiosteal, intraperiosteal, or intraosseus implant, consisting of the framework (substructure) implanted in contact with the bone, and the overlying structure (superstructure). **interim d.,** a denture to be used for a short interval of time for reasons of esthetics, mastication, occlusal support, convenience, or to condition the patient to the acceptance of an artificial substitute for missing natural teeth until more definite prosthetic dental treatment can be provided. Called also *provisional d.* See also *conditioning d.* and *transitional d.* **overlay d.,** a removable tooth-supported partial or complete denture whose built-in secondary copings overlay or telescope over the primary copings that fit over the prepared natural crowns, posts, or studs. Called *overdenture* and *telescopic d.* **partial d.,** a prosthetic appliance replacing one or more missing teeth in one jaw, and receiving its support and retention from the underlying tissues and/or some or all of the remaining teeth; it may be fixed or removable. See also *bridge,* def. 2. **partial d., distal extension,** a removable partial denture that is retained by natural teeth only at the anterior end of the base segments. A portion of the functional load is carried by the residual ridge. **partial d., fixed,** a dental restoration of one or more missing teeth, which is attached to the prepared natural teeth, roots, or implants by means of cementation. Called also *fixed bridge* and *stationary bridge.* **partial d., removable,** a denture replacing one or more, but less than all, natural teeth, so constructed that it may be readily removed from the mouth; it may be entirely supported by the residual teeth, or it may be supported by both the teeth and the tissue of the residual area. Called also *removable bridge* and *removable bridgework.* **partial d., unilateral,** a partial denture designed to restore the missing teeth on one side of the dental arch. **provisional d.,** interim d. **telescopic d.,** overlay d. **temporary d.,** an artificial denture intended to serve a very short time in a temporary or emergency situation. See *conditioning d., interim d., transitional d.,* and *trial d.* **transitional d.,** a partial denture which is to serve as a temporary prosthesis and to which teeth will be added as more teeth are lost and which will be replaced after postextraction tissue changes have occurred; it may become an interim denture when all of the teeth have been removed from the dental arch. **trial d.,** a denture fabricated for placement in the patient's mouth for verification of its esthetic qualities, the making of records, or other procedures before the final denture is completed.

denturism (den′chur-ism) the practice of fabrication and fitting of dentures by dental technologists without benefit of a dentist's expertise.

denturist (den′chur-ist) a dental technologist who fabricates and fits dentures for patients without benefit of a dentist's expertise. Denturists practice in parts of Canada and the United States but in many states denturism is illegal.

Denucé's ligament (den-u-sāz′) [Jean Henri Maurice *Denucé,* French surgeon, 1859–1924] see under *ligament.*

denucleated (de-nu′kle-āt″ed) deprived of the nucleus; called also *anucleated.*

denudation (den″u-da′shun) [L. *denudare* to make bare] the act of laying bare; removal of the epithelial covering from any surface, by surgery, trauma, or pathologic change.

denutrition (de″nu-trish′un) a withdrawal or failure of the nutritive processes, with consequent atrophy and degeneration.

deodorant (de-o′der-ant) [L. *de* from + *odorare* to perfume] 1. removing undesirable or offensive odors. 2. a substance that masks offensive odors. Called also *antibromic*.

deodorize (de-o′der-īz) [L. *de* from + *odor* odor] to neutralize or absorb odor.

deodorizer (de-o′der-īz-er) a deodorizing agent.

deontology (de″on-tol′o-je) [Gr. *deonta* things that ought to be done + *-logy*] the science of professional duties and etiquette.

deoppilant (de-op′ĭ-lant) removing obstructions.

deoppilation (de-op″ĭ-la′shun) [L. *de* away + *oppilatio* obstruction] the removal of obstructions.

deorsumduction (de-or″sum-duk′shun) infraduction.

deorsumvergence (de-or″sum-ver′jens) infravergence.

deorsumversion (de-or″sum-ver′zhun) infraversion (def. 3).

deossification (de-os″ĭ-fi-ka′shun) [L. *de* from + *os* bone + *facere* to make] loss of or removal of the mineral elements of bone.

deoxidation (de-ok″sĭ-da′shun) [L. *de* from + *oxygen*] the removal of oxygen from a chemical compound.

deoxidize (de-ok′sĭ-dīz) to deprive of chemically combined oxygen.

deoxy- (de-ok′se) a prefix used in naming chemical compounds, to designate a compound containing one less atom of oxygen than the reference substance. For words beginning thus see also those beginning *desoxy-*.

deoxyadenosine (de-ok″se-ah-den′o-sēn) a nucleoside, adenine β-D-deoxyribofuranoside. Symbol dA. **d. diphosphate (dADP),** a nucleotide, deoxyadenosine 5′-pyrophosphate. **d. monophosphate (dAMP),** a nucleotide, deoxyadenosine 5′-phosphate. **d. triphosphate (dATP),** a nucleotide, deoxyadenosine triphosphate, required for DNA synthesis.

5′-deoxyadenosyl transferase cob(1)alamin adenosyltransferase.

deoxyadenylate (de-ok″se-ah-den′ĭ-lāt) a dissociated form of deoxyadenylic acid.

deoxyadenylic acid (de-ok″se-ad″ĕ-nil′ik) deoxyadenosine monophosphate.

deoxyadenylyl (de-ok″se-ad-ĕ-nil′il) the radical formed by removal of OH from the phosphate group of deoxyadenosine monophosphate.

deoxycholaneresis (de-ok″se-ko″lan-er′ĕ-sis) increase in the output of deoxycholic acid in the bile.

deoxycholate (de-ok″se-ko′lāt) the dissociated form of deoxycholic acid.

deoxycholic acid (de-ok″se-ko′lik) a secondary bile acid, 3α, 12α-dihydroxy-5β-cholanic acid.

deoxycholylglycine (de-ok″se-ko″lil-gli′sēn) a bile salt, the glycine conjugate of deoxycholic acid.

deoxycholyltaurine (de-ok″se-ko″lil-taw′rēn) a bile salt, the taurine conjugate of deoxycholic acid.

11-deoxycorticosterone (DOC) (de-ok″se-kor″tĭ-kos′ter-ōn; -kor″tĭ-ko-ster′ōn) 21-hydroxy-4-ene-3,20-dione, a mineralocorticoid produced in small quantities by the human adrenal cortex, having about 3 per cent of the sodium-retaining activity of aldosterone; it has little physiological significance except in rare cases of hypersecretion associated with hypertension but was formerly used medically (called also *desoxycorticosterone*) for mineralocorticoid replacement therapy in patients with Addison's disease.

deoxycytidine (de-ok″se-si′tĭ-dēn) a nucleoside, cytosine β-D-deoxyribofuranoside. Symbol dC. **d. diphosphate (dCDP),** a nucleotide, deoxycytidine 5′-pyrophosphate. **d. monophosphate (dCMP),** a nucleotide, deoxycytidine 5′-phosphate. **d. triphosphate (dCTP),** a nucleotide, deoxycytidine 5′-triphosphate, required for DNA synthesis.

deoxycytidylate (de-ok″se-si-tĭ-dil′āt) a dissociated form of deoxycytidylic acid.

deoxycytidylic acid (de-ok″se-si″tĭ-dil′ik) deoxycytidine monophosphate.

deoxycytidylyl (de-ok″se-si″tĭ-dil′il) the radical formed by removal of OH from the phosphate group of deoxycytidine monophosphate.

deoxygenation (de-ok″sĭ-jen-a′shun) the act of depriving of oxygen.

2-deoxy-D-glucose (de-ok″se-gloo′kōs) an antimetabolite of glucose that has antiviral properties by virtue of its inhibition of the glycosylation of glycoproteins and glycolipids; radioactive 2-deoxyglucose is also used to determine the rate of energy metabolism in cells, since cells (e.g., neurons) adjust their rate of glucose (or 2-deoxyglucose) uptake to fill their metabolic needs.

deoxyguanosine (de-ok″se-gwan′o-sēn) a nucleoside, guanine β-D-deoxyribofuranoside. Symbol dG. **d. diphosphate (dGDP),** a nucleotide, deoxyguanosine 5′-pyrophosphate. **d. monophosphate (dGMP),** a nucleotide, deoxyguanosine 5′-phosphate. **d. triphosphate (dGTP),** a nucleotide, deoxyguanosine 5′-triphosphate.

deoxyguanylate (de-ok″se-gwan′il-āt) a dissociated form of deoxyguanylic acid.

deoxyguanylic acid (de-ok″se-gwah-nil′ik) deoxyguanosine monophosphate.

deoxyguanylyl (de-ok″se-gwah-nil′il) the radical formed by removal of OH from the phosphate group of deoxyguanosine monophosphate.

deoxyhemoglobin (de-ok″se-he″mo-glo′bin) hemoglobin not combined with oxygen, formed when oxyhemoglobin releases its oxygen; called also *deoxygenated* or *reduced hemoglobin*.

deoxynucleotidyl transferase (terminal) DNA nucleotidylexotransferase.

deoxypentosenucleic acid (de-ok″se-pen″tōs-noo-kle′ik) deoxyribonucleic acid.

deoxyribonuclease (de-ok″se-ri′bo-nu′kle-ās) an enzyme of the hydrolase class that catalyzes the hydrolytic cleavage of deoxyribonucleic acid. It may produce a single nucleotide residue by cleavage at the end of the chain (*exodeoxyribonuclease*, EC 3.1.11) or a polynucleotide by cleavage at a position within the chain (*endodeoxyribonuclease*, EC 3.1.21–25). Called also *DNase*. **d. I** [EC 3.1.21.1], an endonuclease that produces 5′-phospho-dinucleotide and 5′-phospho-olingonucleotide as end products. The enzyme occurs in the pancreas and thymus. **d. II** [EC 3.1.22.1], an endonuclease that produces 3′-phospho-mononucleotide and 3′-phospho-oligonucleotide as end products. The enzyme occurs in the pancreas, liver, thymus, and gastric mucosa.

deoxyribonucleic acid (de-ok″se-ri′bo-nu-kle′ik) DNA; a nucleic acid that constitutes the genetic material of all cellular organisms and the DNA viruses. Single-stranded DNA is a linear polymer of deoxyribonucleotides in which the β-D-deoxyribofuranose residues are connected by 5′ 3′ phosphate linkages to form the backbone of the molecule, and the purine bases, adenine (A) and guanine (G), and the pyrimidine bases, cytosine (C) and thymine (T), are attached as side chains, one to each deoxyribose residue. Adenine forms two hydrogen bonds with thymine, and cytosine forms three with guanine; these bonding pairs are referred to as complementary bases. In double-stranded DNA (see illustration) each base in one strand is hydrogen bonded to its complementary base in the other strand, and the strands are twisted to form a double helix. The strands are antiparallel; the 5′ 3′ linkages run in opposite directions. The genetic material is duplicated before cell division by DNA replication, in which the two strands are separated and each serves as a template for the synthesis of a new complementary strand. The genetic information is used in the synthesis of RNAs from DNA templates (transcription) and synthesis of proteins from mRNA templates (translation). **complementary DNA, copy DNA (cDNA),** single-stranded DNA transcribed from an RNA by the enzyme reverse transcriptase; radiolabeled cDNA is used as a "probe" that hybridizes with genes for the RNA or with hnRNA precursors of the RNA.

deoxyribonucleoprotein (de-ok″se-ri″bo-nu″kle-o-pro′te-in) a nucleoprotein in which the nucleic acid sugar is D-2-deoxyribose.

deoxyribonucleoside (de-ok″se-ri″bo-nu′kle-o-sīd) a nucleoside having a purine or pyrimidine base bonded to deoxyribose.

deoxyribonucleotide (de-ok″se-ri″bo-nu′kle-o-tīd) a nucleotide consisting of a purine or a pyrimidine base bonded to deoxyribose, which in turn is bound to a phosphate group.

deoxyribose (de-ok″se-ri′bōs) an aldopentose, CH₂·OH··(CHOH)₂·CH₂·CHO, found in deoxyribonucleic acids (DNA), deoxyribonucleotides, and deoxyribonucleosides.

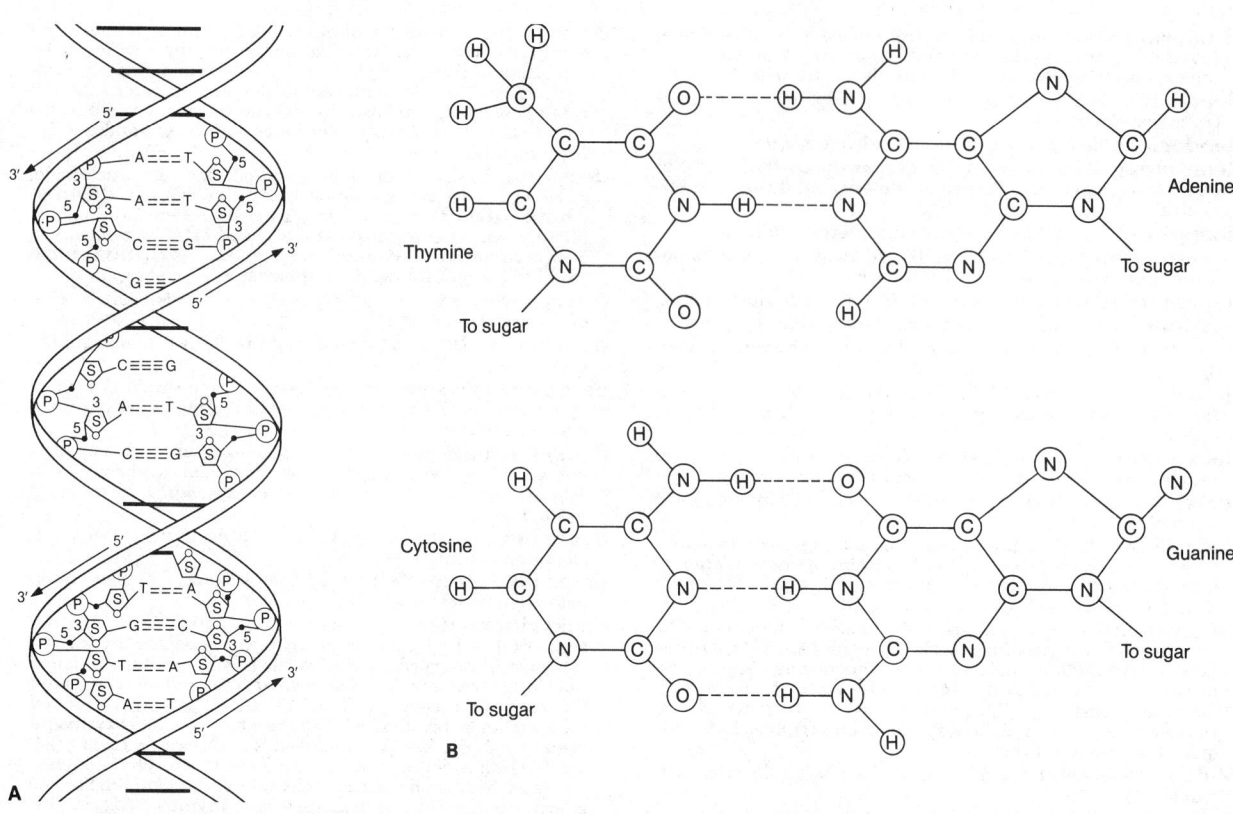

A, The DNA double helix. The base pairs are perpendicular to the long axis and lie stacked on one another. A=adenine, G=guanine, C=cytosine, T=thymine. *B,* The two base pairs of DNA. There are two hydrogen bonds between adenine and thymine, and three hydrogen bonds between cytosine and guanine.

deoxythymidine (de-ok″se-thi′mĭ-dēn) a nucleoside thymine β-D-deoxyribofuranoside; symbol dT. Called also *thymidine* (see note at thymidine). **d. diphosphate (dTDP),** a nucleotide, deoxythymidine 5′-pyrophosphate. **d. monophosphate (dTMP),** a nucleotide, deoxythymidine 5′-phosphate. **d. triphosphate (dTTP),** a nucleotide, deoxythymidine 5′-triphosphate, required for DNA synthesis.

deoxythymidylate (de-ok″se-thi″mĭ-dil′āt) a dissociated form of deoxythymidylic acid.

deoxythymidylic acid (de-ok″se-thi″mĭ-dil′ik) deoxythymidine monophosphate.

deoxythymidylyl (de-ok″se-thi″mĭ-dil′il) the radical formed by removal of OH from the phosphate group of deoxythymidine monophosphate.

Dep. abbreviation for L. *depura′tus,* purified.

Depakene (dep′ah-kēn) trademark for preparations of valproic acid.

dependence (de-pen′dens) a state in which there is a compulsion to take a drug, either continuously or periodically, in order to experience its psychic effects or to avoid the discomfort of its absence; this state can be further classified as *habituation* or *emotional* or *psychological dependence,* use to obtain relief from tension and emotional discomfort, and *physical* or *physiological dependence,* use to prevent withdrawal symptoms. Some use dependence more narrowly to refer only to physiological dependence, and in this sense it may be considered to be a phenomenon distinct from tolerance, a need to increase the dose to maintain the effect, or it may be considered to be a state characterized by either tolerance or withdrawal. **psychoactive substance d.** [DSM III-R], psychoactive substance abuse (q.v.) in which either tolerance or withdrawal is present. DSM III-R includes specific substance dependence disorders for alcohol, amphetamines or similarly acting sympathomimetics, cannabis, cocaine, hallucinogens, inhalants, nicotine, opioids, phencyclidines or similarly acting arylcyclohexylamines, and sedatives, hypnotics, and anxiolytics. **substance d.,** see *psychoactive substance d.*

dependency (de-pen′den-se) a state of relying on another for love, affection, mothering, comfort, security, food, warmth, shelter, protection, and the like—the so-called dependency needs.

dependent (de-pen′dent) 1. exhibiting dependence or dependency. 2. hanging down.

depepsinized (de-pep′sin-īzd) deprived of pepsin; peptically inactivated: said of gastric juice.

depersonalization (de-per″sun-al-ĭ-za′shun) alteration in the perception of the self so that the usual sense of one's own reality is lost, manifested in a sense of unreality or self-estrangement, in changes of body image, or in a feeling that one does not control his own actions and speech; seen in depersonalization disorder, schizophrenic disorders, and schizotypal personality disorder. Some do not draw a distinction between depersonalization and derealization, using depersonalization to include both.

dephosphorylation (de-fos″for-i-la′shun) [*de-* + *phosphorylation*] removal of a phosphate group from an organic molecule.

depigmentation (de″pig-men-ta′shun) [*de-* + *pigmentation*] removal or loss of pigment, especially melanin. Cf. *amelanosis, hypomelanosis,* and *hypopigmentation.*

depilate (dep′ĭ-lāt) [L. *de* away + *pilus* hair] to remove the hair from.

depilation (dep″ĭ-la′shun) epilation.

depilatory (de-pil′ah-to-re) [L. *de* from + *pilus* hair] 1. having the power to remove the hair. 2. an agent for removing or destroying the hair.

deplasmolysis (de″plaz-mol′ĭ-sis) return to the initial volume, after plasmolysis, of the protoplasm of a cell in hypertonic solution.

deplasmolyze (de-plaz′mo-līz) to undergo deplasmolysis.

deplete (de-plēt′) [L. *deplere* to empty] to empty; to unload; to cause depletion.

depletion (de-ple′shun) [L. *deplere* to empty] 1. the act or process of emptying; removal of a fluid, as the blood. 2. exhausted state which results from excessive loss of blood. **plasma d.,** plasmapheresis.

depolarization (de-po″lar-i-za′shun) the process or act of neutralizing polarity. In neurophysiology, the reversal of the resting potential in excitable cell membranes when stimulated, i.e., the tendency of the cell membrane potential to become positive with respect to the potential outside the cell.

depolarize (de-po′lar-īz) [L. *de* from + *polus* pole] to reduce toward a nonpolarized condition; to deprive of polarity. See *depolarization.*

depolarizer (de-po′lar-īz″er) 1. a chemical agent placed in a galvanic cell for preventing the accumulation of gas upon either of the plates. 2. a substance that reduces the voltage across a biological membrane. 3. a muscle relaxant that produces striated muscle paralysis by altering the electrical state of the muscle receptor, thus blocking muscle response to nerve impulse.

depolymerization (de-pol″ĕ-mer-i-za′shun) the conversion of a compound into one of smaller molecular weight and different physical properties without changing the percentage relationships of the elements composing it.

depolymerize (de-pol′ĕ-mer-īz) to cause to undergo depolymerization.

Depo-Provera (dep″o-pro-ver′ah) trademark for a preparation of medroxyprogesterone acetate for intramuscular injection.

deposit (de-poz′it) [L. *de* down + *ponere* to place] 1. sediment or dregs. 2. extraneous inorganic matter collected in the tissues or in a viscus or cavity. 3. tooth d. **tooth d.,** a hard or soft material deposited on a tooth surface, such as dental calculus or plaque and materia alba.

depot (de′po, dep′o) [Fr. *dépôt* from L. *depositum*] a body area in which a substance, e.g., a drug, can be accumulated, deposited, or stored and from which it can be distributed. **fat d.,** a site in the body in which large quantities of fat are stored, as in adipose tissue.

Depo-Testosterone (de″po-tes-tos′ter-ōn) trademark for a sustained-action preparation of testosterone.

depravation (dep″rah-va′shun) [L. *depravare* to vitiate; *de* down + *pravus* bad] deterioration; a change for the worse.

depraved (de-prāvd′) vitiated or perverted.

depressant (de-pres′ant) 1. diminishing functional activity. 2. an agent that reduces functional activity and the vital energies in general by producing muscular relaxation and diaphoresis. **cardiac d.,** an agent that depresses the rate or force of contraction of the heart.

depressed (de-prest′) carried below the normal level; associated with depression.

depression (de-presh′un) [L. *depremere* to press down] 1. a hollow or depressed area; downward or inward displacement. 2. a lowering or decrease of functional activity. 3. a mental state of depressed mood characterized by feelings of sadness, despair, and discouragement. Depression ranges from normal feelings of "the blues" through dysthymia to major depression. It in many ways resembles the grief and mourning that follow bereavement; there are often feelings of low self-esteem, guilt, and self-reproach, withdrawal from interpersonal contact, and somatic symptoms such as eating and sleep disturbances. **agitated d.,** major depression with psychomotor agitation. **anaclitic d.,** impairment of an infant's physical, social, and intellectual development resulting from absence of mothering. **atrial d.** (*obs.*), great lowering in the sphygmographic tracing of the venous pulse, representing the diastole of the right atrium. **congenital chondrosternal d.,** a congenital, deep, funnel-shaped depression in the anterior chest wall. **endogenous d.,** any depression that is not a reactive depression (q.v.); the term implies that some intrinsic biological process rather than environmental influences is the cause. Endogenous depression has been identified with a specific symptom complex—psychomotor retardation, early morning awakening, weight loss, excessive guilt, and lack of reactivity to the environment—that is roughly equivalent to major depression or major depression with melancholia, although there is not much correlation between this symptom complex and the presence or absence of precipitating life events. **freezing point d.,** the depression of the freezing point of a solution below that of the pure solvent; it is proportional to the osmolality. For water the proportionality constant is 1.86°C/(Osm/kg). **involutional d.,** see under *melancholia.*

major d. [DSM III-R], a mental disorder characterized by the occurrence of one or more major depressive episodes (q.v.) and the absence of any history of manic or hypomanic episodes. **neurotic d.,** depressive neurosis; any depression that is not a psychotic depression (q.v.), which means, depending upon which sense of psychotic depression is intended, either any depression without psychotic features (which includes the large majority of major depressions) or only the milder type of depression that would be diagnosed as dysthymia or adjustment disorder with depressed mood by DSM III-R criteria or as reactive (rather than endogenous) depression. **otic d.,** auditory pit. **pacchionian d's,** granular foveolae. **precordial d.,** epigastric fossa, def. 1. **psychotic d.,** in the strict sense, a major depression with psychotic features, such as hallucinations, delusions, mutism, or stupor. However, this term is commonly used in a broader sense to cover all severe depressions causing gross impairment of social or occupational functioning, i.e., as a rough equivalent of major depression or endogenous depression. Cf. *neurotic d.* **pterygoid d.,** pterygoid fovea. **radial d.,** radial fossa of humerus. **reactive d.,** a depression that is precipitated by a stressful life event; as commonly used the term is an equivalent to neurotic depression, depressive neurosis, or dysthymic disorder. See *endogenous d.* **retarded d.,** major depression with psychomotor retardation; melancholia. **situational d.,** reactive d. **supratrochlear d.,** a slight depression on the anterior surface of the femur, above the trochlea. **systolic d.** (*obs.*), a falling of the precordial region of the chest observed during the systole. **tooth d.,** intrusion. **ventricular d.,** that part of the venous pulse tracing which lies between the ventricular and atrial waves.

depressive (de-pres′iv) causing depression.

depressomotor (de-pres″o-mo′tor) [L. *deprimere* to press down + *motor* mover] 1. retarding or abating motion. 2. an agent which lessens or depresses motor activity.

depressor (de-pres′or) [L.] that which depresses, as a muscle, agent, instrument, or apparatus which depresses, or an afferent nerve whose stimulation causes a fall of blood pressure. **d. an′guli o′ris,** see *Table of Musculi.* **d. epiglot′tidis,** a portion of the thyroepiglottic muscle which depresses the epiglottis. **d. la′bii inferio′ris,** see *Table of Musculi.* **tongue d.,** an instrument for pressing the tongue against the floor of the mouth.

deprimens oculi (dep′re-menz ok′u-le) [L.] musculus rectus inferior bulbi.

deprivation (dep-ri-va′shun) [L. *de* from + *privare* to remove] loss or absence of parts, organs, powers, or things that are needed. **emotional d.,** deprivation of adequate and appropriate interpersonal and environmental experience in the early development years. **maternal d.,** the result of premature loss or absence of the mother or of lack of proper mothering; see *maternal deprivation syndrome,* under *syndrome.* **sensory d.,** deprivation of visual, auditory, and tactile stimuli. Experimental total sensory deprivation can produce anxiety, loss of ability to concentrate and organize thoughts, increased suggestibility, and unpleasant vivid hallucinations. Similar symptoms can be produced by solitary confinement, loss of sight or hearing, paralysis, and even by ordinary hospital bed rest. **thought d.,** blocking (def. 2).

deprostil (dĕ-pros′til) chemical name: 15-hydroxy-15-methyl-9-oxoprostan-1-oic acid; a prostaglandin that inhibits gastric secretion, $C_{21}H_{38}O_4$.

deproteinization (de-pro″te-in-i-za′shun) removal of protein.

depside (dep′sīd) one of a class of compounds which are products of the condensation of two or more molecules of the hydroxyacids of benzene, e.g., tannic acid.

depth (depth) an expression of the distance separating the upper and lower surfaces of an object. **focal d., d. of focus,** the measure of the power of a lens to yield clear images of objects at different distances from it.

depula (dep′u-lah) [L., from Gr. *depas* goblet] in zoology, the developing egg in the stage succeeding the blastula and preceding the gastrula.

depurant (dep′u-rant) 1. cleansing or purifying. 2. an agent that cleanses or purifies.

depurate (dep′u-rāt) [L. *depurare* to purify] to cleanse, refine, or purify.

depuration (dep″u-ra′shun) cleansing, purification; especially placement of shellfish in clean water to allow them to cleanse themselves of bacteria.

depurative (dep′u-ra″tiv) tending to purify or cleanse; called also *pellant.*

depurator (dep′u-ra″tor) 1. an agent that cleanses or purifies. 2. (*obs.*) a vacuum-producing apparatus for stimulating the excretory function of the skin.

deradelphus (der″ah-del′fus) [*der-* + Gr. *adelphos* brother] a monster made up of twins fused at or near the navel, and having only one head.

deranencephalia (der-an″en-sĕ-fa′le-ah) [*der-* + *an* neg. + Gr. *enkephalos* brain] monstrosity marked by defect of the brain and upper part of the spinal cord.

derangement (de-rānj′ment) 1. mental disorder. 2. disarrangement of a part or organ. **Hey's internal d.,** partial dislocation of the knee, marked by great pain and spasm of the muscles.

Dercum's disease (der′kumz) [Francis Xavier *Dercum,* American physician, 1856–1931] adiposis dolorosa.

derealization (de-re″al-ĭ-za′shun) a loss of the sensation of the reality of one's surroundings; the feeling that something has happened, that the world has been changed and altered, that one is detached from one's environment. It is seen most frequently in schizophrenic disorders.

dereism (de′re-izm) [L. *de* away + *res* thing] thinking not in accordance with the facts of reality and experience and following illogical, idiosyncratic reasoning. Used interchangeably with *autism,* although not an exact synonym: dereism emphasizes disconnection from reality and autism preoccupation with inner experience. Called also *dereistic thinking.*

dereistic (de″re-is′tik) pertaining to or characterized by dereism.

derencephalocele (der″en-sĕ-fal′o-sēl) [*der-* + Gr. *enkephalos* brain + *kēlē* hernia] protrusion of the brain substance through a slit in one or more of the cervical vertebrae.

derencephalus (der″en-sef′ah-lus) [*der-* + Gr. *enkephalos* brain] a monster with rudimentary skull bones and bifid cervical vertebrae, the brain resting in the bifurcation.

derepression (de″re-presh′un) [*de-* + *repression*] 1. elevation of the level of an enzyme above the normal, either by lowering of the corepressor concentration or by a mutation that decreases the formation of aporepressor or the response to the complete repressor. 2. in genetic theory, the inhibition of the repressor substance produced by the regulator genes with the result that the operator gene is free to initiate the process of polypeptide formation; called also *gene d.* Cf. repression, def. 3. **gene d.,** derepression, def. 2.

dericin (der′ĭ-sin) a light-colored oil derived from castor oil and used as a vehicle for menthol; called also *florizine.*

derivant (der′ĭ-vant) derivative.

derivation (der″ĭ-va′shun) [L. *derivatio,* from *derivare* to draw off] 1. the origin or source of a substance. 2. a lead in electrocardiography.

derivative (de-riv′ah-tiv) 1. producing or causing a derivation. 2. a chemical substance derived from another substance either directly or by modification or partial substitution. 3. an agent which withdraws blood from the seat of a disease. **hematoporphyrin d.,** a material prepared by an acetic acid—sulfuric acid treatment of hematoporphyrin that concentrates selectively in metabolically active tumor tissue; used in photodynamic therapy.

-derm [Gr. *derma* skin] a word termination denoting skin, or a germ layer.

derma (der′mah) [Gr.] the skin, usually with special reference to the dermis.

derma- see *dermat*(o)-.

dermabrader (der-mah-brād′er) any device used for dermabrasion.

dermabrasion (der-mah-bra′shun) planing of the skin done by mechanical means, as by fine sandpaper or wire brushes. See *planing.*

Dermacentor (der″mah-sen′tor) [*derma-* + Gr. *kentein* to prick, stab] a genus of ticks which are important as transmitters of disease. **D. albipic′tus,** a species of brown ticks widely distributed in the United States, parasitic on cattle, horses, deer, elk, and moose. Called also *winter tick.*

D. anderso′ni, a reddish brown tick which is responsible for transmitting Rocky Mountain spotted fever, Colorado tick fever, and tularemia to man and for causing tick paralysis. Its hosts include deer, elk, antelope, grizzly bear, porcupine, prairie dog, and various species of rabbits. Called also *D. venustus, Rocky Mountain wood tick,* and *mountain wood tick.* **D. hal′li,** a yellow-brown tick found on peccaries in Texas. **D. hun′teri,** a brown tick found on Rocky Mountain sheep in the southwestern United States, particularly in southwestern Arizona. **D. margina′tus,** a species that is the vector of a type of tick-borne hemorrhagic fever in Siberia. **D. ni′tens,** *Anocentor nitans.* **D. nuttal′lii,** a tick which transmits Siberian tick typhus. **D. occidenta′lis,** a brown tick found widely distributed along the west coast of the United States, from southwestern Oregon to southern California, the principal hosts being the cow, horse, deer, dog, and man; called also *Pacific coast dog tick.* **D. parumaper′tus,** a reddish brown tick which is found widely distributed in the southwestern United States, found on deer and coyotes, and abundant on various species of rabbits. **D. reticula′tus,** a tick which attacks sheep and oxen, occurring in Europe, Asia, and America; a vector of canine babesiosis in southern Europe. **D. sylva′rum,** a tick which transmits Siberian tick typhus. **D. varia′bilis,** a dark brown tick found along the California coast and widely distributed east of the Rocky Mountains, the dog being the principal host of the adults, which are found also on cattle, horses, rabbits, and man; it is the principal vector of Rocky Mountain spotted fever in the central and eastern United States. Called also *American dog tick* and *dog tick.* **D. venus′tus,** *D. andersoni.*

Dermacentroxenus (der″mah-sen″trok-se′nus) [*Dermacentor* + Gr. *xenos* a guest-friend] a genus name formerly given microorganisms parasitic in ticks, now included in the genus *Rickettsia.* **D. rickett′si,** *Rickettsia rickettsii.* **D. ty′phi,** *Rickettsia typhi (mooseri).*

dermad (der′mad) toward the integument.

dermal (der′mal) 1. pertaining to the dermis. 2. pertaining to the skin; cutaneous; dermic.

dermamyiasis (der″mah-mi-i′ah-sis) [*derma-* + *myiasis*] see *larva migrans.*

Dermanyssidae (der″mah-nis′ĭ-de) a family of mites (order Acarina) parasitizing mammals, reptiles, and birds, whose bite may cause a painful dermatitis in man; *Dermanyssus* is the type genus.

Dermanyssus (der″mah-nis′sus) [*derma-* + Gr. *nyssein* to prick] a genus of mites of the family Dermanyssidae. **D. galli′nae,** the bird mite, poultry (chicken or fowl) mite, or chicken louse, which sometimes infests man.

dermaskeleton (der″mah-skel′ĕ-ton) exoskeleton.

dermatan sulfate (der′mah-tan) a glycosaminoglycan found mostly in the skin but also in blood vessels, tendons, heart valves, and pulmonary connective tissues. It is a stereoisomer of chondroitin 4-sulfate in which most of the β-D-glucuronic acid residues are epimerized at C-5 converting them to α-L-iduronic acid.

dermatitides (der″mah-tit′ĭ-dēz) plural of *dermatitis.*

dermatitis (der″mah-ti′tis), pl. *dermatit′ides* [*dermato-* + *-itis*] inflammation of the skin. **actinic d.,** dermatitis resulting from exposure to actinic radiation, such as that from the sun, ultraviolet waves, or x or gamma radiation. **allergic d.,** 1. atopic d. 2. allergic contact d. **allergic contact d.,** contact dermatitis due to allergic sensitization to various substances that produce inflammatory reactions in the skin of those who have acquired hypersensitivity to the allergen as a result of previous exposure to it. Called also *allergic d., contact d.,* and *d. venenata.* Cf. *irritant d.* **ammonia d.,** a form of diaper dermatitis that has been attributed to irritation of the skin due to the ammonia decomposition products of urine. **d. artefac′ta,** factitial d. **ashy d.,** erythema dyschromicum perstans. **atopic d.,** a chronic inflammatory skin disorder seen in individuals with a hereditary predisposition to a lowered cutaneous threshold to pruritus, often accompanied by allergic rhinitis, hay fever, and asthma, and principally characterized by extreme itching, leading to scratching and rubbing that in turn results in the typical lesions of eczema. In infants (*infantile eczema*), there is a predilection for occurrence of the cheeks, which may extend to other areas of the body; in children, adolescents, and adults, it is found chiefly on the flexural surfaces (*flexural eczema*), especially on the antecubital and popliteal areas, and on the neck, eyelids, and wrists and behind the ears. Called also *allergic dermatitis, allergic* or *atopic eczema, Besnier's prurigo, disseminated neurodermatitis,* and *prurigo of Besnier*. **berlock d., berloque d.,** phytophotodermatitis due to sequential exposure to cologne, perfume, or other toilet articles containing bergamot oil and then to sunlight. In women, the lesions usually present as lavaliere-shaped brown pigmented patches, most often on the sides of the neck and retroauricular areas and sometimes on the face, breasts, shoulders, and elsewhere. Aftershave lotion containing bergamot oil or related substance may cause a similar type of dermatitis on the bearded region in men. Called also *perfume d*. **brown-tail moth d.,** a cutaneous irritation produced by the hairs of the brown-tail moth, *Euproctis chrysorrhoea;* called also *brown-tail rash*. **d. bullo′sa stria′ta praten′sis,** phytophotodermatitis manifested as a bizarrely arranged linear or streaky eruption of vesicles and bullae that heal with intense residual melanoderma, caused by contact with meadow grass, usually *Agrimonia eupatoria,* and then exposure to sunlight. Called also *grass d., meadow d., meadow grass d.,* and *d. striata pratensis bullosa.* **d. calor′ica,** inflammation of the skin due to heat or cold. Cf. *erythema abigne* and *cold erythema*. **caterpillar d.,** see *insect d*. **cercarial d.,** a severely pruritic papular eruption due to hypersensitivity to the cercariae of nonhuman schistosomes that die after penetrating the skin of those who bathe, swim, or wade in fresh or salt water infested with the organisms without gaining access to the circulation and deeper tissues, evoking an inflammatory reaction. Called also *clam digger's itch, cutaneous schistosomiasis, schistosome d.,* and *swimmers′ d.* or *itch*. **contact d.,** 1. acute or chronic dermatitis caused by materials or substances coming in contact with the skin, which may involve either allergic or nonallergic mechanisms. See *allergic contact d.* and *irritant d.* 2. allergic contact d. **contagious pustular d.,** 1. contagious acne of horses. 2. contagious ecthyma. **cosmetic d.,** allergic contact dermatitis caused by some ingredient in a cosmetic preparation. **dhobie mark d.,** dhobie itch. **diaper d.,** a type of irritant dermatitis localized to the area in contact with the diaper in infants, often sparing the skin of the genitocrural folds, occurring as a reaction to prolonged contact with urine and feces, retained soaps and topical preparations, and friction and maceration, and commonly associated with secondary bacterial and yeast infections, especially *Candida albicans* infections. Some consider irritation of the skin by the ammoniac decomposition products of urine to be a contributing etiologic factor. Called also *ammonia d., diaper rash, Jacquet's d., Jacquet's erythema,* and *napkin d.* **eczematous d.,** eczema. **d. exfoliati′va,** exfoliative d. **d. exfoliati′va neonato′rum,** staphylococcal scalded skin syndrome. **exfoliative d.,** widespread involvement of the skin by a scaly erythematous dermatitis occurring as a secondary or reactive process to an underlying cutaneous disorder (e.g., atopic dermatitis, psoriasis, scabies, lichen planus) or as a primary or idiopathic disorder, and often associated with loss of hair and nails, hyperkeratosis of the palms and soles, pruritus, and sometimes severe and debilitating secondary physiological effects. Called also *d. exfoliativa, erythroderma,* and *pityriasis rubra* (Hebra). **exudative discoid and lichenoid d.,** a form of neurodermatitis occurring predominantly in middle-aged or older men of Jewish extraction, characterized by intense pruritus with exudative, weeping discoid and oval patches scattered irregularly over most of the body, many of which are of the eczematous type and undergo lichenification, or they may resemble lesions seen in various other cutaneous disorders such as mycosis fungoides or lichen planus. Called also *oid-oid disease* and *Sulzberger-Garbe syndrome*. **factitial d.,** various types of self-inflicted lesions, usually produced by mechanical means, burning, or application of chemical irritants or caustics. Called also *d. artefacta*. **d. gangreno′sa infan′tum,** a gangrenous disease occurring as a primary condition or secondarily to varicella or another exanthematous disease, chiefly in children under the age of 3, in which multiple small erosive and pustular lesions coalesce to form extensive sloughs, usually over the lower back and buttocks. **grass d.,** d. bullosa striata pratensis. **d. herpetifor′mis,** a chronic, relapsing multisystem disease in which the primary clinical manifestations are cutaneous, presenting as an extremely pruritic eruption consisting of various combinations of grouped, erythematous, symmetrical, papular, papulovesicular, vesicular, eczematous, and

bullous lesions, which frequently heal with hyperpigmentation or occasionally hypopigmentation and sometimes scarring. It usually occurs in association with an asymptomatic gluten-sensitive enteropathy. The cause is unknown, but immunogenetic factors are thought to play a role. Called also *Duhring's disease*. **d. hiema′lis,** dermatitis coming on with cold weather; cf. *winter itch*. **industrial d.,** occupational d. **infectious eczematous d.,** a condition arising from a primary lesion that is the source of an infectious exudate (e.g., a boil, surgical wound, draining ear or nose), spreads by autoinoculation, and has a tendency to the formation of circumscribed eczematous plaques that enlarge gradually, and in which vesicles and pustules may occur. **insect d.,** a transient localized or widespread dermatitis caused by the toxin-containing irritant hairs of certain insects, especially moths and their caterpillars, which may be associated with severe conjunctivitis, pruritus, a burning sensation, and pain; clinical manifestations vary according to the species involved and the intensity of exposure. **irritant d.,** a nonallergic type of contact dermatitis due to exposure to a substance that damages the skin. Called also *primary irritant d.* Cf. *allergic contact d.* **Jacquet's d.,** diaper d. **livedoid d.,** a condition due to temporary or prolonged local ischemia resulting from vasculitis or accidental arterial obliteration from intragluteal administration of medications, marked by severe local pain, swelling, livedoid changes, and local increase in temperature; fever, tachycardia, dyspnea, and albuminuria also occur, and gangrene may supervene. **marine d.,** swimmer's itch occurring in persons wading or swimming in salt water; called also *seabather's eruption*. **meadow d., meadow-grass d.,** d. bullosa striata pratensis. **d. medicamento′sa,** drug eruption. **moth d.,** insect d. **napkin d.,** diaper d. **nummular eczematous d.,** see under *eczema*. **occupational d.,** contact dermatitis caused by primary or allergic contactants found in the work place. Called also *industrial d.* and *industrial dermatosis*. **onion mite d.,** dermatitis affecting handlers of decaying onions, caused by the onion mite, *Acarus rhyzoglypticus hyacinthi*. **d. papilla′ris capilli′tii,** a rare disease seen most commonly in black males, characterized by the development of persistent hard follicular plaques along the posterior hairline of the scalp that fuse to form a thick, sclerotic, hypertrophic, pseudokeloidal band extending across the occiput. Called also *acne keloid, folliculitis keloidalis, keloidal folliculitis,* and *sycosis nuchae*. **perfume d.,** berlock d. **periocular d.,** see *perioral d.* **perioral d.,** a papular eruption of unknown etiology that progresses to residual papular erythema and scaling usually confined to the area about the mouth, and almost exclusively occurring in young women; it may also be localized or extend to involve the eyelids and adjacent glabella area of the forehead (*periocular d.*). **photoallergic contact d.,** the cutaneous manifestations of photoallergy, consisting of a papulovesicular, eczematous, or exudative dermatitis, and occurring chiefly on the light-exposed areas of the skin. Called also *photocontact d.* **photocontact d.,** photoallergic contact d. **phototoxic d.,** an exaggerated sunburn-like reaction, sometimes with vesiculation, resulting in hyperpigmentation and desquamation, which occurs on the light-exposed areas of the skin as the cutaneous manifestation of phototoxicity. **phytophototoxic d.,** phytophotodermatitis. **pigmented purpuric lichenoid d.,** a purpuric cutaneous eruption usually seen in men 40–60 years of age, occurring chiefly on the legs, thighs, and lower trunk, and characterized by the presence of minute, rust-colored, lichenoid papules that tend to fuse into plaques, which may contain variously pigmented papules. Called also *Gougerot-Blum syndrome*. **poison ivy d., poison oak d., poison sumac d.,** see *rhus d.* **precancerous d.,** Bowen's disease. **primary irritant d.,** irritant d. **radiation d.,** radiodermatitis. **rat-mite d.,** dermatitis resulting from the bite of *Ornithonyssus bacoti*. **d. re′pens,** acrodermatitis continua. **rhus d.,** allergic contact dermatitis due to exposure to plants of the genus *Rhus* (*Toxicodendron*) (poison ivy, poison oak, poison sumac), which contain urushiol, a potent skin-sensitizing agent. **roentgen-ray d.,** radiodermatitis. **sabra d.,** a dermatitis somewhat resembling scabies, affecting those who handle the fruit of cacti (sabra or prickly pear) and Indian figs in Israel; thought to be due to the penetration of minute thorns or hairs into the skin. **schistosome d.,** cercarial d. **seborrheic d., d. seborrheica,** a chronic inflammatory disease of the skin of unknown etiology, characterized by moderate erythema, dry, moist, or greasy scaling, and yellow crusted patches on various areas, including the mid-parts of the face, ears, supraorbital regions, umbilicus, genitalia, and especially the scalp, where it is manifested by small patches of scales that progress to involve the entire scalp, with exfoliation of an excessive amount of dry scales (dandruff). The condition is usually accompanied by itching. Called also *seborrheic eczema* and *seborrhea*. **stasis d.,** an often chronic, usually eczematous dermatitis, which initially involves the inner aspect of the lower leg just above the internal malleolus and which later may involve the entire lower leg or portions thereof, characterized by edema, pigmentation, and commonly ulceration; it is due to venous insufficiency. **d. stria′ta praten′sis bullo′sa,** d. bullosa striata pratensis. **swimmer's d.,** cercarial d. **uncinarial d.,** ground itch. **d. veg′etans,** a cutaneous reaction to secondary infection with an eczematous lesion, especially in moist areas of the body such as axillae, groin, genitalia, and lips, which is characterized by the development of exuberant hypertrophic granulation tissue that may erode to form ulcers. A variant involving the oral mucosa and associated with ulcerative colitis or other gastrointestinal disturbance is known as pyostomatitis vegetans. Called also *pemphigus vegetans, Hallopeau type.* **d. venena′ta,** 1. allergic contact d. 2. former name for contact dermatitis due to exposure to sensitizing agents in plants. **verminous d.,** stephanofilariasis. **vesicular d.,** a sometimes fatal disease, believed to be eczematous in nature, affecting young poultry that range over unbroken prairie sod, marked by the formation of blisters and scabs on the feet and legs; called also *sod disease.* **x-ray d.,** radiodermatitis.

dermat(o)-, derma- derm(o)- [Gr. *derma,* gen. *dermatos* skin] combining forms denoting relationship to the skin.

dermatoarthritis (der″mah-to-ar-thri′tis) skin disease associated with arthritis. **lipid d., lipoid d.,** multicentric reticulohistiocytosis.

dermatoautoplasty (der″mah-to-aw′to-plas″-te) [*dermato-* + Gr. *autos* self + *plassein* to mold] the grafting on denuded areas of skin taken from some other portion of the patient's own body.

Dermatobia (der″mah-to′be-ah) [*dermato-* + Gr. *bios* life] a genus of botflies of the family Oestridae. **D. hom′inis,** the human botfly of South America whose larvae (called ver macaque or ver moyocuil) are parasitic in the skin of man, mammals and birds; the eggs are deposited by the female on the bodies of mosquitoes, flies or ticks and by them transported to the host.

dermatobiasis (der″mah-to-bi′ah-sis) the presence of *Dermatobia* in the body.

dermatochalasis, dermatochalazia (der″mah-to-kal′ah-sis; der″mah-to-kal-ah′zi-ah) [*dermato-* + Gr. *chalasthai* to become slack] cutis laxa.

dermatoconjunctivitis (der″mah-to-kon-junk″tĭ-vi′tis) inflammation of the conjunctiva and of the skin around the eyes.

dermatodysplasia (der″mah-to-dis-pla′ze-ah) [*dermato-* + *dysplasia*] abnormal development of the skin.

dermatofibroma (der″mah-to-fi-bro′mah) a fibrous tumor-like nodule of the dermis. **d. protu′berans,** a large-sized molluscum growth that tends to recur after incision; called also *dermatofibrosarcoma protuberans.*

dermatofibrosarcoma (der″mah-to-fi″bro-sar-ko′mah) a fibrosarcoma of the skin. **d. protu′berans,** dermatofibroma protuberans.

dermatofibrosis (der″mah-to-fi-bro′sis) a condition characterized by fibrotic changes in the skin. **d. lenticula′ris dissemina′ta,** an autosomal dominant syndrome, present at birth or appearing before puberty, characterized by the development of connective tissue nevi of the elastic type in association with osteopoikilosis; the skin lesions are manifested as small, firm, yellowish or skin-colored papules or plaques distributed symmetrically, primarily on the lower trunk and extremities. Called also *Buschke-Ollendorff syndrome.*

dermatoglyphics (der″mah-to-glif′iks) [*dermato-* + Gr. *glyphein* to carve] the study of the patterns of ridges of the skin of the fingers, palms, toes, and soles; of interest in anthropology and law enforcement as a means of establishing identity and in medicine, both clinically and as a genetic indicator, particularly of chromosomal abnormalities.

dermatographic (der″mah-to-graf′ik) pertaining to or characterized by dermatographism.

dermatographism (der″mah-tog′rah-fizm) urticaria due to physical allergy, in which moderately firm stroking or scratching of the skin with a dull instrument produces a pale, raised welt or wheal, with a red flare on each side; see also *white d.* and *black d.* **black d.,** black or greenish streaking of the skin caused by deposit of fine metallic particles abraded from jewelry by various dusting powders. **white d.,** linear blanching of (usually erythematous) skin of persons with atopic dermatitis in response to firm stroking with a blunt instrument.

dermatoheteroplasty (der″mah-to-het′er-o-plas″te) [*dermato-* + Gr. *heteros* other + *plassein* to form] the grafting of skin derived from a member of another species.

dermatologic, dermatological (der″mah-to-loj′ik, der″-mah-to-loj′ĭ-kal) pertaining to dermatology; of or affecting the skin.

dermatologist (der″mah-tol′o-jist) a physician who limits his practice to the diagnosis and treatment of skin disorders.

dermatology (der″mah-tol′o-je) the medical specialty concerned with the diagnosis and treatment of diseases of the skin.

dermatolysis (der″mah-tol′ĭ-sis) [*dermato-* + Gr. *lysis* loosening] cutis laxa. **d. palpebra′rum,** blepharochalasis.

dermatome (der′mah-tōm) [*derma-* + Gr. *temnein* to cut] 1. an instrument for cutting thin skin slices for skin grafts. 2. the area of skin supplied with afferent nerve fibers by a single posterior spinal root; called also *dermatomic area.* 3. the lateral portion of a mesodermal somite; the cutis plate. **Brown d.,** an electric dermatome, the first to be developed, for cutting split-thickness skin grafts; it enables the surgeon to rapidly remove long strips of skin. **Castroviejo d.,** an electric dermatome used for cutting mucous membrane grafts for the treatment of eyelid and socket deformities and as an adjunct in the removal of tattoos after the initial excision has been done using either the Brown or Padgett dermatomes. It has a tiny cutting head with special blades and skims to control the thickness of the cut. **Padgett d.,** an instrument for rapid cutting of split-thickness skin grafts of any desired thickness. **Reese d.,** an instrument for cutting split-thickness skin grafts that permits careful calibration of the thickness of the graft.

dermatomegaly (der″mah-to-meg′ah-le) cutis laxa.

dermatomere (der′mah-to-mēr″) [*dermato-* + Gr. *meros* part] any segment or metamere of the embryonic integument.

dermatomic (der″mah-tom′ik) pertaining to a dermatome, def. 2.

dermatomyces (der″mah-to-mi′sēz) dermatophyte.

dermatomycosis (der″mah-to-mi-ko′sis) [*dermato-* + Gr. *mykes* fungus] a superficial infection of the skin or its appendages by fungi. The term includes dermatophytosis and the various clinical forms of tinea, as well as deep fungous infections. Called also *epidermomycosis.*

dermatomyiasis (der″mah-to-mi-i′ah-sis) [*dermato-* + *myiasis*] see *larva migrans.*

dermatomyoma (der″mah-to-mi-o′mah) [*dermato-* + *myoma*] a dermal leiomyoma.

dermatomyositis (der″mah-to-mi″o-si′tis) [*dermato-* + *myositis*] polymyositis occurring in association with characteristic inflammatory skin changes, including Gottron's sign (flat-topped violaceous papules over the dorsal aspects of the knuckles), which is pathognomonic; a violaceous or heliotrope rash on the upper eyelids accompanied by edema of the eyelids and periorbital tissue; and an erythematous rash on the forehead, neck, shoulders, trunk, and arms.

dermatoneurology (der″mah-to-nu-rol′o-je) [*dermato-* + Gr. *neuron* nerve + *-logy*] the study of the nerves of the skin in health and disease.

dermato-ophthalmitis (der″mah-to-of″thal-mi′tis) inflammation of the skin and of the eye, including the conjunctiva, cornea, etc.

dermatopathic (der″mah-to-path′ik) pertaining or attributable to disease of the skin, as dermatopathic lymphadenopathy. Called also *dermopathic.*

dermatopathology (der″mah-to-pah-thol′o-je) microscopic anatomic pathology of the skin.

dermatopathy (der″mah-top′ah-the) [dermato- + Gr. *pathos* disease] dermopathy.

Dermatophagoides (der″mah-tof″ah-goi′dēs) a genus of sarcoptiform mites, usually found on the skin of chickens. **D. pteronyssi′nus,** the house dust mite, which acts as an antigen and produces an allergic asthmatic reaction in atopic persons. **D. scheremetew′skyi,** a species that attacks man and causes a mange-like inflammation.

dermatopharmacology (der″mah-to-fahr″mah-kol′o-je) pharmacology as applied to dermatologic disorders.

Dermatophilaceae (der″mah-to-fi-la′se-e) a family of bacteria of the order Actinomycetales, consisting of gram-positive aerobic microorganisms characterized by mycelial filaments or muriform thalli that divide transversely and in at least two longitudinal planes to form masses of coccoid or cuboid motile cells. It includes genera *Dermatophilus* and *Geodermatophilus.*

dermatophiliasis (der″mah-to-fĭ-li′ah-sis) 1. tungiasis. 2. dermatophilosis.

dermatophilosis (der″mah-to-fi-lo′sis) an actinomycotic disease caused by *Dermatophilus congolense,* affecting cattle, sheep, horses, goats, deer, and sometimes man. In man, it is characterized by nonpainful pustules on the hands and arms; the lesions break down and form shallow red ulcers which regress spontaneously, leaving some scarring. In sheep, it is characterized by exudative red scaling lesions that form pyramidal masses and is known as *lumpy wool, strawberry rot foot,* and formerly *streptotrichosis.* Called also *dermatophiliasis.*

Dermatophilus (der″mah-tof′ĭ-lus) [dermato- + Gr. *philos* loving] 1. a genus of bacteria of the family Dermatophilaceae, order Actinomycetales, consisting of aerobic or facultatively anaerobic, gram-positive, nonacid-fast organisms. The organisms form mycelia containing filaments that segment transversely and longitudinally to produce coccoid cells in packets, which become motile spores. They are pathogenic for mammals, involving the uncornified epidermis. 2. *Tunga.* **D. congolen′sis,** the etiologic agent of dermatophilosis; called also *Streptothrix bovis.* **D. pen′-etrans,** *Tunga penetrans,* or chigoe.

dermatophyte (der′mah-to-fīt″) [dermato- + Gr. *phyton* plant] a fungus parasitic upon the skin; the term embraces the imperfect fungi of the genera *Microsporum, Epidermophyton,* and *Trichophyton.* Called also *cutaneous fungus* and *dermatomyces.*

dermatophytid (der″mah-tof′ĭ-tid) [dermatophyte + -id] an id reaction associated with a dermatophytosis, which may be associated with various types of lesions but with the most common being vesicles occurring on the hands, wrists, and sides of the fingers in association with tinea pedis. Called also *epidermophytid* and *mycid.*

dermatophytosis (der″mah-to-fi-to′sis) [dermatophyte + -osis] any superficial fungal infection caused by a dermatophyte and involving the stratum corneum of the skin, hair, and nails. The term broadly comprises onychophytosis and the various form of tinea (ringworm), sometimes being used specifically to designate tinea pedis (athlete's foot). Called also *epidermomycosis.*

dermatoplastic (der″mah-to-plas′tik) pertaining to dermatoplasty.

dermatoplasty (der′mah-to-plas″te) [dermato- + Gr. *plassein* to form] a plastic operation on the skin; operative replacement of destroyed or lost skin.

dermatopolyneuritis (der″mah-to-pol″e-nu-ri′tis) acrodynia.

dermatorrhagia (der″mah-to-ra′je-ah) discharge of blood into or from the skin. **d. parasit′ica,** a disease of the skin of horses, asses, and mules in Europe and Asia, marked by hard elevations formed by accumulations of blood between the layers of the skin, and caused by the presence of a parasitic filarial worm, *Parafilaria multipapillosa.* Called also *summer bleeding.*

dermatorrhexis (der″mah-to-rek′sis) [dermato- + Gr. *rhēxis* a breaking] rupture of the skin capillaries, as in Ehlers-Danlos syndrome.

dermatosclerosis (der″mah-to-skle-ro′sis) [dermato- + Gr. *sklērōsis* hardening] scleroderma.

dermatosis (der″mah-to′sis), pl. *dermato′ses* [dermat- + -osis] any skin disease, especially one not characterized by inflammation. **acute febrile neutrophilic d.,** a condition usually seen on the upper body of middle-aged women, characterized by the presence of one or more large, rapidly extending, erythematous, tender or painful plaques, and occurring in association with fever and dense infiltration of neutrophilic leukocytes in the upper and mid dermis. Called also *Sweet's syndrome.* **ashy d. of Ramirez,** erythema dyschromicum perstans. **Bowen's precancerous d.,** Bowen's disease. **chick nutritional d.,** a disease of chicks due to a deficiency of pantothenic acid, marked by eruptions on the head and feet. **d. cinecien′ta,** erythema dyschromicum perstans. **dermatolytic bullous d.,** epidermolysis bullosa dystrophica. **industrial d.,** occupational dermatitis. **lichenoid d.,** any skin disorder characterized by lichenification. **d. papulo′sa ni′gra,** a variant of seborrheic keratosis seen almost exclusively in blacks, characterized by the development of small, pedunculated, pigmented papules on the malar regions, upper cheeks, or lateral orbital areas. **precancerous d.,** any skin condition having a tendency to malignant change. **progressive pigmentary d.,** Schamberg's disease. **Schamberg's d.,** Schamberg's progressive pigmented purpuric d., see under *disease.* **subcorneal pustular d.,** a chronic, superficial, pustular disorder with a chronic relapsing course, resembling dermatitis herpetiformis, and chiefly affecting women in middle life, with sterile pustular blebs beneath the horny layer of the epidermis on the trunk and in the major skin folds. Called also *Sneddon-Wilkinson disease.* **transient acantholytic d.,** a self-limited papulovesicular disease occurring in middle-aged individuals and having a predilection for the trunk, in which the histologic changes are suggestive of keratosis follicularis or benign familial pemphigus. It may be an epidermal reaction to actinic injury. **d. veg′etans,** a hereditary disease of young pigs characterized by raised skin lesions, abnormalities of the hooves, and pneumonia.

dermatosome (der′mah-to-sōm″) [dermato- + Gr. *sōma* body] a thickening on each spindle fiber in the equatorial region during mitosis.

dermatosparaxis (der″mah-to-spah-rak′sis) [dermato- + Gr. *sparaxis, sparagmos* a tearing] a disease of cattle and sheep in which the skin is fragile and very easily torn; it is related to the Ehlers-Danlos syndrome of humans, and evidence indicates that the defect may reside in an abnormally low activity of the enzyme procollagen peptidase.

dermatotherapy (der″mah-to-ther′ah-pe) [dermato- + Gr. *therapeia* treatment] treatment of the skin and its diseases.

dermatotropic (der″mah-to-trop′ik) [dermato + Gr. *tropos,* turning toward or affecting] preferentially infecting, infesting, or affecting the skin; said of certain microorganisms. Called also *dermotropic.*

dermatozoiasis (der″mah-to-zo-i′ah-sis) dermatozoonosis.

dermatozoon (der″mah-to-zo′on) [dermato- + Gr. *zōon* animal] any animal parasite of the skin; an ectoparasite.

dermatozoonosis (der″mah-to-zo″o-no′sis) [dermato- + Gr. *zōon* animal + *nosos* disease] a skin disease caused by a dermatozoon; called also *dermatozoiasis.*

dermenchysis (der-men′kĭ-sis) [derma- + Gr. *enchysis* pouring in] the hypodermic administration of medicines.

dermic (der′mik) dermal; cutaneous.

dermis (der′mis) [Gr. *derma* skin, hide] [NA] the layer of the skin deep to the epidermis, consisting of a dense bed of vascular connective tissue; called also *corium* [NA alternative].

derm(o)- see *dermato-.*

dermoblast (der′mo-blast) [dermo- + Gr. *blastos* germ] that part of the mesoblast which develops into the true skin or corium.

dermocyma (der″mo-si′mah) [dermo- + Gr. *kyma* fetus] a monstrosity in which one fetus is inclosed within another.

dermocymus (der″mo-si′mus) dermocyma.

dermohygrometer (der″mo-hi-grom′ĕ-ter) an instrument for measuring skin resistance without inducing a constant current into the skin.

dermoid (der′moid) [derm- + -oid] 1. resembling skin. 2. dermoid cyst. **corneal d.,** a tumorous growth upon the cornea of animals; its surface contains hairs.

dermoidectomy (der″moid-ek′to-me) [dermoid + Gr. *ektomē* excision] excision of a dermoid cyst.

dermolipectomy (der″mo-lĭ-pek′to-me) [dermo + lipectomy] resection of excess skin and fat, usually from the abdomen.

dermolipoma (der″mo-lĭ-po′mah) a congenital yellow fatty growth beneath the bulbar conjunctiva.

dermolysin (der-mol′ĭ-sin) a substance, circulating in the blood, capable of dissolving the skin.

dermometer (der-mom′ĕ-ter) the instrument used in dermometry.

dermometry (der-mom′ĕ-tre) [dermo- + Gr. metron measure] the measurement of areas of skin resistance to a passage of direct electric current; these areas will correspond to the areas of sensory loss.

dermomyotome (der″mo-mi′o-tōm) [dermo- + myo- + -tome] all but the sclerotome of a mesodermal somite; the primordium of skeletal muscle and, perhaps, of corium.

dermoneurotropic (der″mo-nu″ro-trop′ik) having an affinity for the skin and nervous tissue.

dermopathic (der″mo-path′ik) dermatopathic; pertaining to dermopathy.

dermopathy (der-mop′ah-the) [dermo- + -pathy] dermatopathy; any skin disorder. **diabetic d.,** any of several cutaneous manifestations of diabetes mellitus marked by papular, erosive, ulcerated, pigmented, macular, or cicatricial lesions of the shins (shin spots), apparently occurring as a result of a specific angiitis of small cutaneous blood vessels. The lesions are not specific for diabetes and may be seen after trauma in nondiabetic patients. The term is sometimes broadened to include bullae in diabetic patients, especially bullae of the toes, feet, and ankles, and necrobiosis lipoidica diabeticorum. Called also diabetid. **infiltrative d.,** pretibial myxedema.

dermophyte (der′mo-fīt) dermatophyte.

dermoplasty (der′mo-plas″te) dermatoplasty.

dermoreaction (der″mo-re-ak′shun) cutaneous reaction.

dermoskeleton (der″mo-skel′ĕ-ton) exoskeleton.

dermosynovitis (der″mo-sin-o-vi′tis) [dermo- + synovitis] inflammation of skin overlying an inflamed bursa or tendon sheath.

dermotoxin (der″mo-tok′sin) a toxin produced by certain bacteria, especially staphylococci, which causes necrosis and other pathologic changes of the skin.

dermotropic (der″mo-trop′ik) dermatotropic.

dermovascular (der″mo-vas′ku-lar) [dermo- + vas vessel] pertaining to the blood vessels of the skin.

der(o)- [Gr. derē neck] a combining form denoting relationship to the neck.

derodidymus (der″o-did′ĭ-mus) dicephalus.

derrengadera (der″ en-gah-da′ rah) [Sp. "crookedness"] surra.

derriengue (der″e-eng′geh) [Sp.] rabies, usually of the paralytic form, transmitted by vampire bats in Mexico, South and Central America, and Trinidad. It is usually seen in cattle, but infected bats may attack other domestic animals and even humans.

derris (der′is) a plant of the South Sea Islands; extracts of the leaves and dried root are used as insecticides. Cf. rotenone.

Derxia (derk′se-ah) [H. G. Derx, Dutch microbiologist 1894–1953] a genus of gram-negative, aerobic, rod-shaped bacteria of uncertain affiliation, found in tropical soils and water, made up of slime-producing cells that fix nitrogen. The type species is D. gummo′sa.

DES diethylstilbestrol.

desalination (de″sal-ĭ-na′shun) [L. de from + sal salt] the removal of salt from a substance.

desalivation (de″sal-ĭ-va′shun) the depriving of saliva.

De Sanctis-Cacchione syndrome (dah sank′tis kak″e-o′ne) [Carlo De Sanctis, Italian psychiatrist, born 1888; Aldo Cacchione, Italian physician, 20th century] see under syndrome.

desaturation (de-sach″er-a′shun) the process of introducing a double bond between carbon atoms of a fatty acid.

Desault's bandage (apparatus), sign (dĕ-sōz′) [Pierre Joseph Desault, French surgeon, 1744–1795] see under bandage and sign.

Descemet's membrane (des-ĕ-māz′) [Jean Descemet, French anatomist, 1732–1810] lamina limitans posterior corneae.

descemetitis (des″ĕ-mĕ-ti′tis) inflammation of Descemet's membrane.

descemetocele (des″ĕ-met′o-sēl) [Descemet's membrane + Gr. dēlē hernia] herniation of Descemet's membrane.

descendens (de-sen′denz) [L.] [NA] a general term denoting a descending structure or part. **d. cervica′lis, d. cer′vicis,** the inferior root of the ansa cervicalis.

descending (de-send′ing) [L. descendere to go down] extending downward.

descensus (de-sen′sus), pl. descen′sus [L.] the process of descending or falling. **d. tes′tis** [NA], the descent of the testis from its fetal position in the abdominal cavity to the scrotum; it normally occurs during the last three months of fetal life and is essential to spermatogenesis. **d. u′teri,** prolapse of the uterus. **d. ventric′uli,** gastroptosis.

Deschamps' compressor, needle (da-shawz′) [Joseph François Louis Deschamps, French surgeon, 1740–1824] see under compressor and needle.

descinolone acetonide (des-in′o-lōn) chemical name: 9-fluoro-11β-hydroxy-16α,17-[(1-methylethylidene)bis(oxy)]-pregna-1,4-diene-3,20-dione; a glucocorticoid, $C_{24}H_{31}FO_5$.

desensitization (de-sen″sĭ-ti-za′shun) 1. the prevention or reduction of immediate hypersensitivity reactions by administration of graded doses of allergen; called also hyposensitization and immunotherapy. 2. in behavior therapy, the treatment of phobias and related disorders by intentionally exposing the patient, in imagination or in real life, to emotionally distressing stimuli. Common forms of desensitization include flooding (q.v.), implosion (q.v.), and systematic desensitization (q.v.). **systematic d.,** a form of desensitization therapy in which the patient is taught to relax and is then exposed, in imagination, to the mildest or least anxiety-provoking stimuli first; as treatment progresses he is exposed progressively to stronger anxiety-provoking stimuli until he can tolerate the most extreme stimuli.

desensitize (de-sen′sĭ-tīz) 1. to deprive of sensation; paralysis of a sensory nerve by section or blocking. 2. to carry out desensitization.

desequestration (de″se-kwes-tra′shun) (obs.) the release of sequestered material, such as release into the general circulation of blood formerly withheld from it, by either physiological or mechanical means.

deserpidine (de-ser′pĭ-dēn) chemical name: 17α-methoxy -18β - [(3,4,5 - trimethoxybenzoyl)oxy] - 3β -20α-yohimban-16β-carboxylic acid methyl ester. An alkaloid of Rauwolfia canescens, $C_{32}H_{38}N_2O_8$, occurring as a white to light yellow, crystalline powder; used as an antihypertensive and tranquilizer, administered orally.

desexualize (de-seks′u-al-iz″) to deprive of sexual characters; to castrate.

Desferal (des′fer-al) trademark for a preparation of deferoxamine mesylate.

desferrioxamine (des-fer′e-oks′ah-mēn) deferoxamine.

deshydremia (des″hi-dre′me-ah) [L. de from + Gr. hydōr water + haima blood + -ia] deficiency of the watery element of the blood.

desiccant (des′ĭ-kant) 1. promoting dryness; causing to dry up. 2. an agent that promotes dryness. Called also exsiccant.

desiccate (des′ĭ-kāt) [L. desiccare to dry up] to render thoroughly dry.

desiccation (des″ĭ-ka′shun) the act of drying up. **electric d.,** the treatment of a tumor or other disease by drying up the part by the application of a monopolar electric current (short spark) of high frequency and high tension.

desiccative (des′ĭ-ka″tiv) causing to dry up.

desiccator (des′ĭ-ka″tor) a closed vessel for containing apparatus or chemicals that are to be kept free from moisture.

desipramine hydrochloride (des-ip′rah-mēn) [USP] chemical name: 10,11-dihydro-N-methyl-5H-dibenz[b,f]azepine-5-propanamine monohydrochloride. A metabolite of imipramine, $C_{18}H_{22}N_2 \cdot HCl$, occurring as a white to off-white, crystalline powder; used as an antidepressant, administered orally.

-desis [Gr. desis "a binding together"] a word termination denoting a binding or fusion.

Desjardins' point (da″zhar-danz′) [Abel Desjardins, French surgeon, 20th century] see under point.

deslanoside (des-lan′o-sīd) [USP] a digitalis glycoside, $C_{47}H_{74}O_{19}$, occurring as white crystals or as a white crystalline powder; used as a cardiotonic where digitalis is recommended, administered intramuscularly or intravenously. Called also *deacetyllanatoside C.*

desmalgia (des-mal′je-ah) [*desmo-* + *-algia*] pain in a ligament; called also *desmodynia.*

Desmanthos (des-man′thos) [*desmo-* + Gr. *anthos* flower] a genus of gliding bacteria of the provisional family Pelonemataceae, found in mud, made up of colorless cells in filaments attached in bundles to a substrate. The type species is *D. thiocrenoph'ilum.*

desmectasis (des-mek′tah-sis) [*desmo-* + Gr. *ektasis* stretching] the stretching of a ligament.

desmepithelium (des″mep-ĭ-the′le-um) [*desmo-* + *epithelium*] the endothelial lining of blood vessels, lymphatics, and synovial membranes.

desmid (des′mid) unicellular, free-floating, aquatic algae characterized by symmetrical, curved, spiny or lacey bodies with a median constriction dividing the cell into two equal halves.

desmiognathus (des″me-o-nath′us) [Gr. *desmios* binding + *gnathos* jaw] a monster with a parasitic head attached to the jaw or neck; called also *dicephalus parasiticus.*

desmitis (des-mi′tis) [*desmo-* + *-itis*] inflammation of a ligament.

desm(o)- [Gr. *desmos* band, ligament] a combining form denoting relationship to a band, bond, or ligament.

desmocranium (des″mo-kra′ne-um) [*desmo-* + *cranium*] the mass of mesoderm at the cranial end of the notochord in the early embryo, forming the earliest stage of the skull.

desmocyte (des′mo-sīt) [*desmo-* + Gr. *kytos* hollow vessel] fibroblast.

desmocytoma (des″mo-si-to′mah) fibroma.

desmodontium (des″mo-don′she-um) [*desmo-* + Gr. *odous* tooth] [NA] periodontal ligament.

desmodynia (des″mo-din′e-ah) [*desmo-* + Gr. *odynē* pain] desmalgia.

desmogenous (des-moj′ĕ-nus) [*desmo-* + Gr. *gennan* to produce] of ligamentous origin.

desmography (des-mog′rah-fe) [*desmo-* + Gr. *graphein* to write] a description of the ligaments.

desmohemoblast (des″mo-hem′o-blast) [*desmo-* + Gr. *haima* blood + *blastos* germ] mesenchyme.

desmoid (des′moid) [*desmo-* + Gr. *eidos* form] 1. a fibromatous tumor arising in the muscle sheath, usually of the abdominal wall, and closely resembling fibrosarcoma; desmoids are not encapsulated, are locally invasive, and rarely metastasize. Called also *desmoid tumor.* 2. fibrous or fibroid.

desmolase (des′mo-lās) a nonspecific term for an enzyme that catalyzes the cleavage of a carbon-carbon bond in a substrate with formation of two products by a process other than hydrolysis, i.e., an oxidoreductase, a lyase; or a transferase. Used especially for enzymes involved in synthesis of steroid hormones. **17,20-d.,** 17α-hydroxyprogesterone aldolase. **20,22-d.,** cholesterol monooxygenase (side-chain-cleaving).

desmology (des-mol′o-je) [*desmo-* + *-logy*] 1. the study of ligaments, their structure and function. 2. the art of bandaging.

desmoma (des-mo′mah) [*desmo-* + *-oma*] desmoid tumor.

desmon (des′mon) [Gr. *desmos* band] see *amboceptor.*

desmoneoplasm (des″mo-ne′o-plazm) [*desmo-* + *neoplasm*] a connective tissue tumor (q.v.).

desmopathy (des-mop′ah-the) [*desmo-* + Gr. *pathos* disease] any disease of the ligaments.

desmoplasia (des″mo-pla′ze-ah) the formation and development of fibrous tissue.

desmoplastic (des″mo-plas′tik) [*desmo-* + Gr. *plassein* to form] characterized by or causing the growth of fibrous tissue; producing or forming adhesions.

desmopressin (des″mo-pres′in) chemical name: 1-(3-mercaptopropionic acid)-8-*D*-argininevasopressin; a potent synthetic analogue of vasopressin used as an antidiuretic in diabetes insipidus and to increase Factor VIII activity before surgical procedures in patients with hemophilia and von Willebrand's disease.

desmorrhexis (des″mo-rek′sis) [*desmo-* + Gr. *rhēxis* rupture] rupture of a ligament.

desmose (des′mōs) [Gr. *desmos* band, ligament] a filament, fibril, or strand connecting intranuclear (*centrodesmose*) or extranuclear (*paradesmose*) basal bodies during mitosis; seen especially in certain protozoa (e.g., *Dientamoeba fragilis*). The terms *desmose*, *centrodesmose*, and *paradesmose* have been used synonymously by some authorities.

desmosine (des′mo-sin) one of two unusual amino acids found in elastin, the other being isodesmosine.

desmosis (des-mo′sis) [*desmo-* + *-osis*] a disease of the connective tissue.

desmosome (des′mo-sōm) [*desmo-* + Gr. *sōma* body] a small, discrete, circular, dense body that forms the site of attachment between certain epithelial cells, especially those of stratified epithelium of the epidermis. It consists of local differentiations of the apposing cell membranes, with a dense cytoplasmic plaque underlying each membrane, toward which numerous tonofilaments converge; a dense lamina may occur within the intercellular gap. Called also *macula adherens.* See also *intercellular bridge*, under *bridge.* **half d.,** hemidesmosome.

desmosterol (des-mos′ter-ol) the immediate precursor of cholesterol in the biosynthetic pathway, 24-dehydrocholesterol; normally not present in the blood in amounts that can be detected by ordinary means.

Desmothoracida (des″mo-tho-ras′ĭ-dah) [*desmo-* + Gr. *thōrax* chest] an order of protozoa (class Heliozoa, superclass Actinopoda), most species of which are enclosed in a usually spherical, latticed organic, stalked capsule. There is no centroplast, but microtubular stiffening elements, not discernible as axonemes, are present in axopodia of some species.

desmotomy (des-mot′o-me) [*desmo-* + Gr. *tomē* a cutting] the cutting or division of ligaments.

desmotropism (des-mot′ro-pizm) tautomerism.

desoleolecithin (des-o″le-o-les′ĭ-thin) one of the components, the other being oleic acid, into which lecithin is split by the action of cobra venom.

desomorphine (des″o-mor′fin) chemical name: 4,5a-epoxy-17-methylmorphinan-3-ol; a narcotic analgesic, $C_{17}H_{21}NO_2$.

desonide (des′o-nīd) chemical name: 11β,21-dihydroxy-16α,17-[(1-methylethylidene)bis(oxy)]pregna-1,4-diene-3,20-dione. A synthetic corticosteroid, $C_{24}H_{36}O_6$, used as an anti-inflammatory in the treatment of steroid-responsive dermatoses, applied topically.

desorb (de-sorb) to remove a substance from the state of absorption or adsorption.

desorption (de-sorp′shun) the process or state of being desorbed.

desoximetasone (des-ok″se-met′a-sōn) [USP] chemical name: 9-fluoro-11β-21-dihydroxy-16α-methylpregna-1,4-diene-3,20-dione. A corticosteroid, $C_{22}H_{29}FO_4$, having anti-inflammatory, antipruritic, and vasoconstrictive actions; applied topically for the relief of inflammatory manifestations of corticosteroid-responsive dermatoses.

desoxy- a prefix used in names of chemical compounds. See also words beginning *deoxy-*.

desoxycorticosterone (des-ok″se-kor″tĭ-kos′ter-ōn) see *II-desoxycorticosterone* and *desoxycortone.* **d. acetate** [USP] an ester of desoxycorticosterone, $C_{23}H_{32}O_4$, occurring as a white or creamy white, crystalline powder; used for replacement therapy in adrenocortical insufficiency in Addison's disease and in the treatment of salt-losing adrenogenital syndrome, administered by intramuscular injection or by implantation of pellets subcutaneously. Called also *cortexone* and *desoxycortone acetate.* **d. pivalate** [USP], an ester of desoxycorticosterone, $C_{26}H_{38}O_4$, occurring as a white to creamy white, crystalline powder; used the same as the acetate ester, administered in a repository type of intramuscular injection. **d. trimethylacetate,** d. pivalate.

desoxycortone (des″ok-se-kōr′tōn) desoxycorticosterone. **d. acetate,** desoxycorticosterone acetate.

desoxyephedrine (des″ok-se-ef′ĕ-drin) methamphetamine.

desoxymorphine (des″ok-se-mor′fin) a product of the reduction of morphine.

Desoxyn (des-ok′sin) trademark for preparations of methamphetamine hydrochloride.

desoxyphenobarbital (des-ok″se-fe″no-bar′bǐ-tal) primidone.

desoxyribonuclease (des-ok″se-ri″bo-nu′kle-ās) deoxyribonuclease.

desoxyribonucleic acid, desoxyribose nucleic acid (des-ok″se-ri″bo-noo-kle′ik, des-ok″se-ri′bōs noo-kle′ik) deoxyribonucleic acid.

desoxyribose (des″ok-se-ri′bōs) deoxyribose.

desoxy-sugar (des-ok′se-shoog″ar) a sugar having one oxygen atom less than the parent monosaccharide.

despeciate (de-spe′se-āt) to undergo despeciation; to subject to (as by chemical treatment), or to undergo, loss of species antigenic characteristics.

despeciation (de-spe″se-a′shun) deviation from or loss of species characteristics.

despecification (de-spes″ǐ-fǐ-ka′shun) the process of reducing the antigenicity of heterologous antisera used therapeutically, by treating them with enzymes such as pepsin to remove the antigenic Fc regions of the immunoglobulin molecules. This leaves F(ab′)₂ fragments which contain both antigen binding regions of each immunoglobulin molecule.

d'Espine's sign (des-pēnz′) [Jean Henri Adolphe d'Espine, French physician, 1846–1930] see under sign.

despumation (des″pu-ma′shun) [L. de away + spuma froth] the removal of froth or scum from the surface of a liquid.

desquamation (des″kwah-ma′shun) [L. de from + squama scale] the shedding of epithelial elements, chiefly of the skin, in scales or small sheets; exfoliation. **furfuraceous d.,** desquamation in branlike scales. **lamellar d. of the newborn,** see collodion baby, under baby.

desquamative (des-kwam′ah-tiv) pertaining to or characterized by desquamation.

desquamatory (des-kwam′ah-to-re) desquamative.

dest. abbreviation for L. destil′la distil, and destilla′tus, distilled.

desthiobiotin (des″thi-o-bi′o-tin) biotin in which the sulfur has been replaced by two atoms of hydrogen. It is an analogue, CH₂·CH·NH·CO·NH·CH·CH₂·(CH₂)₄·COOH, of ascorbic acid which competitively inhibits the activity of the latter.

destil. abbreviation for L. destil′la, distil.

destructive (de-struk′tiv) characterized by or causing destruction.

desulfhydrase (de″sulf-hi′drās) one of a group of enzymes of the lyase class, a carbon-sulfur lyase (EC 4.4), that catalyzes the removal of hydrogen sulfide or substituted hydrogen sulfide from a compound.

Desulfobacter (de-sul″fo-bak′ter) [de- + sulfo- + Gr. baktron a rod] a genus of gram-negative, anaerobic, rod-shaped to ellipsoidal bacteria that reduce sulfate compounds to hydrogen sulfide, found in the anaerobic sediments from brackish waters. The type species is D. postga′tei.

Desulfobulbus (de-sul″fo-bul′bus) [de- + sulfo- + L. bulbus onion] a genus of anaerobic, ellipsoidal to onion-shaped nonspore-forming bacteria that reduce sulfate compounds to hydrogen sulfide, found in anaerobic sediments from fresh or brackish waters, in bovine rumen fluid, and in animal feces. The type species is D. propion′icus.

Desulfococcus (de-sul″fo-kok′us) [de- + sulfo- + coccus] a genus of anaerobic, gram-negative, nonspore-forming, spherical bacteria that reduce sulfate compounds to hydrogen sulfide, found in anaerobic sediments from fresh and marine waters and in sewage sludge. The type species is D. multivo′rans.

Desulfomonas (de-sul″fo-mo′nas) [de- + sulfo- + Gr. monas unit, from monos single] a genus of bacteria made up of gram-negative, nonspore-forming, anaerobic bacilli that reduce sulfate to hydrogen sulfide. They are part of the normal flora of the oral cavity and the respiratory, intestinal, and urogenital tracts of humans and other animals. The type species is D. pi′gra.

Desulfosarcina (de-sul″fo-sar-si′nah) [de- + sulfo- + sarcina] a genus of gram-negative, anaerobic, irregularly shaped bacteria occurring in packets of eight or more, consisting of organisms that reduce sulfate compounds to

hydrogen sulfide. They are found in the anaerobic sediments of marine waters. The type species is D. variabi′lis.

Desulfotomaculum (de-sul″fo-to-mak′u-lum) [de- + sulfo- + L. tomaculum sausage] a genus of endospore-forming, rod-shaped bacteria of the family Bacillaceae, made up of anaerobic, gram-negative cells that reduce sulfates, sulfites, and other sulfur compounds. They are found in soil, water, and geothermal regions, and in the intestines of insects, and in the contents of animal rumens. The type species is D. nigri′ficans.

Desulfovibrio (de-sul″fo-vib′re-o) [de- + sulfo- + vibrio] a genus of gram-negative, nonspore-forming, anaerobic bacteria, consisting of actively motile curved rods that reduce sulfur compounds to hydrogen sulfide, found in animal intestines and feces, fresh and salt water, soil, and mud. The type species is D. desulfur′icans.

desulfurase (de-sul′fu-rās) desulfhydrase.

Desulfuromonas (de-sul″fer-o-mo′nas) [de- + sulfo- + Gr. monas unit, from monos single] a genus of sulfur-reducing bacteria, consisting of straight or slightly curved rods that are motile with flagella. The organisms occur in anaerobic sediments of salt and fresh waters. The type species is D. acetox′idans.

Det. abbreviation for L. de′tur, let it be given.

detachment (de-tach′ment) [Fr. détacher to unfasten; to separate] the condition of being unfastened, disconnected, or separated. **d. of retina, retinal d.,** see under retina.

detector (de-tek′tor) a device by which the presence of something, or the existence of a certain condition, is discovered. **lie d.,** polygraph. **radiation d.,** any device for converting radiant energy to a form more readily observable.

deterenol hydrochloride (dě-ter′ě-nōl) chemical name: (+)-4-hydroxy-α-[[(1-methylethyl)amino]methyl]benzenemethanol hydrochloride; an adrenergic, $C_{11}H_{17}NO_2\cdot HCl$, used in ophthalmology.

detergent (de-ter′jent) [L. detergere to cleanse] 1. purifying, cleansing. 2. an agent which purifies or cleanses.

determinant (de-ter′mǐ-nant) [L. determinare to bound, limit, or fix] a factor that establishes the nature of an entity or event. **antigenic d.,** a site on the surface of an antigen molecule to which a single antibody molecule binds; generally an antigen has several or many different antigenic determinants and reacts with antibodies of many different specificities. Called also epitope. **hidden d.,** an antigenic determinant located in an unexposed region of a molecule so that it is prevented from interacting with receptors on lymphocytes, or with antibody molecules, and is unable to induce an immune response unless exposed by conformational change or stereochemical alteration of the molecule. Such hidden determinants may appear following stereochemical alterations of molecular structure. **immunogenic d.,** the part of an immunogenic molecule that interacts with a helper T cell in triggering antibody production, as opposed to the antigenic determinant or hapten, which interacts with B cells. **sequential d.,** a polymeric antigenic determinant with antigenic specificity determined by monomer sequence rather than monomer composition.

determination (de-ter″mǐ-na′shun) establishment of the exact nature of an entity or event. **embryonic d.,** the loss of pluripotency in any part of an embryo and its start on the way toward an unalterable fate. **sex d.,** the process by which the sex of an organism is fixed, associated, in man, with the presence or absence of the Y chromosome.

determiner (de-ter′min-er) determinant.

determinism (de-ter′min-izm) the theory that all phenomena are the result of antecedent conditions and that nothing occurs by chance. **psychic d.,** the concept, originated by Freud, that mental events do not occur by chance but have their antecedent mental causes, that even accidents, slips of the tongue, or whims commonly felt to be inexplicable result from unconscious mental processes.

dethyroidize (de-thi′roid-īz) to deprive of the function of the thyroid gland by chemical or surgical means.

Det. in dup., Det. in 2 plo. abbreviations for L. de′tur in du′plo, let twice as much be given.

detonation (de″to-na′shun) [L. de intensive + tonare to thunder] loudly explosive combustion.

detorsion (de-tor′shun) 1. the correction of a twisting or deformity, as the reduction of torsion of the testis. 2. a deficiency in a normal twisting as may occur in the early development of the heart.

detoxicate (de-tok′sĭ-kāt)   detoxify.

detoxication (de-tok″sĭ-ka′shun)   detoxification.

detoxification (de-tok″sĭ-fi-ka′shun)   1. reduction of the toxic properties of poisons.   2. treatment designed to free an addict from his drug habit.   **metabolic d.,** reduction of the toxic properties of a substance by chemical changes induced in the body, producing a compound which is less poisonous or is more readily eliminated.

detoxify (de-tok′sĭ-fi)   to remove the toxic quality of a substance.

detrition (de-trish′un)   [L. *de* away + *terere* to wear]   a wearing away, as of the teeth, by friction. See also *abrasion.*

detritivorous (de″trĭ-tiv′o-rus)   subsisting on particulate matter (detritus), a mode of existence important in certain, such as aquatic, ecosystems.

detritus (de-tri′tus)   [L., from *deterere* to rub away]   particulate matter produced by or remaining after the wearing away or disintegration of a substance or tissue; designated as organic or nonorganic, depending on the nature of the original material. See also *biodetritus.*

detruncation (de″trun-ka′shun)   [L. *de* off + *truncus* trunk]   decapitation, chiefly of a dead fetus.

detrusor (de-troo′sor)   [L., from *detrudere* to push down]   [NA] a general term for any body part that pushes down.   **d. uri′nae,** musculus detrusor vesicae.

D. et s.   abbreviation for L. *de′tur et signe′tur,* let it be given and labeled.

detubation (de″tu-ba′shun)   removal or withdrawal of a tube.

detumescence (de″tu-mes′ens)   [L. *de* down + *tumescere* to swell]   the subsidence of swelling, or turgor.

deutan (doo′tan)   1. pertaining to deuteranomaly or deuteranopia.   2. a person with deuteranomaly or deuteranopia.

deutencephalon (doo″ten-sef′ah-lon)   [Gr. *deuteros* second + *enkephalos* brain]   (*obs.*) diencephalon.

deuteranomal (doo″ter-ah-nom′al)   a person with deuteranomaly.

deuteranomalous (doo″ter-ah-nom′ah-lus)   pertaining to or characterized by deuteranomaly.

deuteranomaly (doo″ter-ah-nom′ah-le)   [*deuter-* + *anomaly*]   a type of anomalous trichromacy in which the second, green-sensitive, cones have decreased sensitivity; therefore a greater than normal proportion of thallium green light to lithium red light is required to match a fixed sodium yellow light. Deuteranomaly is an X-linked trait, affects about 5 per cent of white males and 0.25 per cent of females, and is the most common color vision deficiency.

deuteranope (doo′ter-ah-nōp″)   an individual exhibiting deuteranopia.

deuteranopia (doo″ter-ah-no′pe-ah)   [*deuter-* + *an-* neg. + *-opia*]   a dichromasy characterized by retention of the sensory mechanism for two hues only (blue and yellow) of the normal 4-primary quota, and lacking that for red and green and their derivatives, without loss of luminance or shift or shortening of the spectrum. It is an X-linked trait occurring in about 1 per cent of males, but only rarely in females.

deuteranopic (doo″ter-ah-nop′ik)   pertaining to or characterized by deuteranopia.

deuteranopsia (doo″ter-ah-nop′se-ah)   deuteranopia.

deuterate (du′ter-āt)   to treat (combine) with deuterium.

deuterion (doo-te′re-on)   deuteron.

deuterium (du-te′re-um)   [Gr. *deuteros* second]   the mass two isotope of hydrogen, symbol ^{2}H, or D. It is available as a gas or as heavy water and is used as a tracer or indicator in studying fat and amino acid metabolism; called also *heavy hydrogen* (see *hydrogen*). Cf. *protium* and *tritium.*   **d. oxide,** heavy water; see under *water.*

deuter(o)-, deut(o)-   [Gr. *deuteros* second]   a combining form meaning second.

deuteroconidium (doo″ter-o-ko-nid′e-um)   [*deutero-* + *conidium*]   a reproductive element derived from a hemispore.

deuterofat (doo′ter-o-fat)   a fat containing deuterium.

deuterohemin (du″ter-o-hem′in)   a derivative of hemin, $C_{30}H_{28}O_4N_4FeCl$.

deuterohemophilia (doo″ter-o-he″mo-fil′e-ah)   a group of hemorrhagic disorders resembling classical hemophilia, due to coagulation factor deficiency or to the action of certain anticoagulants. See individual coagulation factors, under *factor.*

Deuteromyces (doo″ter-o-mi′zēz)   Deuteromycetes.

Deuteromycetae (doo″ter-o-mi-se′te)   Deuteromycetes.

deuteromycete (doo″ter-o-mi′sēt)   any individual fungus of the Deuteromycetes; an imperfect fungus.

Deuteromycetes (doo″ter-o-mi-se′tēz)   [*deutero-* + Gr. *mykēs* fungus]   a class of the Eumycetes in which the perfect (sexual) stage is unknown; the Fungi Imperfecti. Called also *Deuteromyces* and *Deuteromycetae.*

deuteron (doo′ter-on)   the nucleus of deuterium, or heavy hydrogen; deuterons are used as bombing particles for nuclear disintegration.

deuteropathic (doo″ter-o-path′ik)   occurring secondarily to some other disease.

deuteropathy (doo″ter-op′ah-the)   [*deutero-* + Gr. *pathos* disease]   a disease that is secondary to another disease.

deuteropine (doo″ter-o′pin)   an alkaloid, $C_{20}H_{21}O_3N$, from opium.

deuteroplasm (doo″ter-o-plazm″)   [*deutero-* + Gr. *plasma* something formed]   the passive or inactive materials in protoplasm, especially reserve foodstuffs, such as yolk. Cf. *energid.*

deuteroporphyrin (doo″ter-o-por′fĭ-rin)   a porphyrin (q.v.) in which two pyrrole rings each have one ethyl and one propionate side chain and the other two pyrrole rings have a single methyl side chain.

deuterosome (doo″ter-o-sōm″)   [*deutero-* + Gr. *sōma* body]   a cytoplasmic organelle of ciliating epithelial cells that plays a role in the formation of ciliary basal bodies, being the precursor of the procentriole.

deuterostome (doo″ter-o-stōm″)   an animal belonging to the Deuterostomia.

Deuterostomia (doo″ter-o-sto′mĭ-ah)   [*deutero-* + Gr. *stoma* mouth + *-ia*]   a series of the Eucoelomata, including the echinoderms, hemichordates, and chordates, in all of which the site of the blastopore is posterior—far from the mouth, which forms a new structure unrelated to the blastopore. Cf. *Protostomia.*

deuterotocia (doo″ter-o-to′se-ah)   [*deutero-* + Gr. *tokos* birth]   asexual reproduction in which the female produces offspring of both sexes.

deuterotoky (doo″ter-ot′o-ke)   deuterotocia.

deuthyalosome (doo″thi-al′o-sōm)   [Gr. *deuteros* second + *hyalos* glass + *sōma* body]   the matured nucleus of an ovum.

deut(o)-   see *deuter(o)-.*

deutomerite (doo″to-me′rīt)   [*deuto-* + Gr. *meros* portion]   the larger posterior, nucleus-containing portion of the body of certain gregarine protozoa, separated from the anterior portion (protomerite) by an ectoplasmic septum.

deuton (doo′ton)   deuteron.

deutonephron (doo″to-nef′ron)   [*deuto-* + Gr. *nephros* kidney]   mesonephros.

deutoplasm (doo′to-plazm)   deuteroplasm.

deutoplasmolysis (doo″to-plaz-mol′ĭ-sis)   destruction or disintegration of deutoplasm.

Deutschländer's disease (doich′len-derz)   [Karl Ernst Wilhelm *Deutschländer,* surgeon in Hamburg, 1872–1942]   1. see under *disease.*   2. march foot.

DEV   duck embryo rabies vaccine.

devasation (de″vas-a′shun)   [L. *de* away + *vas* vessel]   (*obs.*) devascularization.   **senile cortical d.,** interruption of the circulation to the cerebral cortex as a result of arteriosclerosis of the blood vessels.

devascularization (de-vas″ku-lar-i-za′shun)   interruption of the circulation of blood to a part caused by obstruction or destruction of the blood vessels supplying it.

Devegan (dev′e-gan)   trademark for a preparation of acetarsone.

development (de-vel′op-ment)   the process of growth and differentiation.   **arrested d.,** cessation of the development process at some stage prior to its normal completion.   **cognitive d.,** the development of intelligence, conscious thought, and problem solving ability that begins in infancy. **mosaic d.,** the development of an embryo in a fixed, unalterable way, local regions being independent portions of a mosaic whole. **postnatal d.,** that which occurs after birth. **prenatal d.,** that which occurs before birth. **psychosexual d.,** 1. a general term for the developing sexuality of the individual as affected by biological, cultural, and emotional influences from prenatal life onward through the life cycle. 2. in psychoanalysis, libidinal maturation from infancy through adulthood (including the oral, anal, and genital stages). **psychosocial d.,** the development of the personality, including the acquisition of social attitudes and skills, from infancy through maturity. **regulative d.,** the development of an embryo, the determination of the various organs and parts being gradually attained through the action of inductors.

developmental (de-vel″op-men′tal) pertaining to development.

Deventer's diameter (de-ven′terz) [Hendrik van *Deventer*, Dutch obstetrician, 1651–1724] see *diameter obliqua pelvis.*

deviant (de′ve-ant) [L. *deviare* to turn aside] 1. varying from a determinable standard. 2. an individual with characteristics varying from what is considered normal, or standard. **sexual d.,** an individual exhibiting paraphilia (sexual deviation).

deviation (de″ve-a′shun) [L. *deviare* to turn aside] 1. a turning away from the regular standard or course. 2. in ophthalmology, strabismus. 3. in statistics, the difference between a sample datum and some central point, such as the sample mean. **animal d.,** the attracting of zoophilous mosquitos from human beings by the proximity of animals preferred by the insects. **axis d.,** the direction of the mean QRS complex in the electrocardiogram; changes may be due to alteration in the anatomical position of the heart or to intraventricular conduction (ventricular preponderance). **complement d.,** inhibition of complement-mediated immune hemolysis in the presence of excess antibody. Called also *Neisser-Wechsberg phenomenon.* **conjugate d.,** the deflection of two similar parts, as the eyes, in the same direction at the same time. **Hering-Hellebrand d.,** the amount of deviation between any point on the Vieth-Müller horopter and the frontoparallel plane passing through the point of fixation. **immune d.,** modification of the immune response to an antigen by previous inoculation of the same antigen. **latent d.,** heterophoria. **manifest d.,** strabismus. **minimum d.,** the smallest deflection of a ray of light that can be produced by a given prism. **primary d.,** deviation of the visual axis of the squinting eye in strabismus when the sound eye fixates. **sample standard d.,** an estimate of the population standard deviation, usually calculated (from a sample of size n) by dividing the sum of the squared deviations from the sample mean by $n-1$ and taking the square root; $n-1$ is used (rather than n) in order to obtain an unbiased estimate of the population variance. Symbol s. **secondary d.,** deviation of the visual axis of the sound eye in strabismus when the squinting eye fixates. **sexual d.,** paraphilia. **skew d.,** downward and inward rotation of the eye on the side of the cerebellar lesion and upward and outward deviation on the opposite side. Called also *Hertwig-Magendie phenomenon, Magendie's sign,* and *Magendie-Hertwig sign.* **squint d.,** squint angle; see under *angle.* **standard d.,** in statistics an approximate average of the amount by which each value deviates from the mean; equal to the square root of the variance, i.e., the square root of the average of the squared deviations from the mean. It is the most commonly used measure of dispersion of statistical data. Symbol σ. See *sample standard d.* **strabismic d.,** deviation of the visual axis of an eye in strabismus. **d. to the left,** shift to the left. **d. to the right,** shift to the right.

device (de̅-vīs′) something contrived for a specific purpose. **central-bearing d.,** a device that provides a central point of bearing, or support, between upper and lower occlusion rims, consisting of a contacting point attached to one occlusion rim and a plate that provides the surface on which the bearing point rests or moves. **central-bearing tracing d.,** one for determining the central bearing or support between maxillary and mandibular occlusion rims or dentures. **contraceptive d.,** one used to prevent conception, as a diaphragm or condom to prevent entrance of spermatozoa into the uterine cervix, or one inserted into the

uterus (intrauterine contraceptive device) to prevent implantation of a fertilized ovum. **intrauterine d. (IUD),** a coil, loop, T, or triangle of plastic or metallic substance inserted into the uterus to prevent conception. **left ventricular assist d.,** a circulatory support device consisting of a pump with afferent and efferent conduits attached to the left atrium or left ventricular apex and the ascending aorta, respectively; the pump rests on the external chest wall or is implanted into the thorax or abdomen and is connected to an external pneumatic power source and control circuit. Its effect is to augment left ventricular function.

deviometer (de″ve-om′ĕ-ter) strabismometer.

devisceration (de-vis″er-a′shun) [L. *de* away + *viscus* viscus] removal of viscera.

devitalization (de-vi″tal-i-za′shun) the deprivation of vitality or life, as of a tissue. **pulp d.,** the destruction of vitality of the pulp of a tooth.

devitalize (de-vi′tal-īz) [L. *de* from + *vita* life] to deprive of vitality or of life.

devolution (dev″o-lu′shun) [L. *de* down + *volvere* to roll] 1. the reverse of evolution. 2. catabolic change.

devorative (dev′o-ra″tiv) [L. *devorare* to devour] (*obs.*) intended to be swallowed without chewing.

De Vries' theory (de-vrēz′) [Hugo *de Vries,* botanist in Amsterdam, 1848–1935] see *theory of mutations.*

dewatered (de-wah′terd) having the water removed; a term applied to sludge from which the water has been removed by drying or pressing.

dewclaw (doo′klaw) a vestigial digit or claw in an animal.

dewlap (du′lap) a heavy fold of skin on the ventral aspect of the neck in animals.

deworming (de-werm′ing) the destruction and removal of worms from an infected individual.

dexamethasone (dek″sah-meth′ah-sōn) [USP] a synthetic glucocorticoid 25 times as potent as cortisol; used in the diagnosis of Cushing's syndrome (see *dexamethasone suppression test,* under *test*) for replacement therapy in adrenal insufficiency and as an anti-inflammatory agent. Also available as *dexamethasone acetate* [USP] and *dexamethasone sodium phosphate* [USP]. **d. acetate** [USP], an ester of dexamethasone, $C_{24}H_{31}FO_6 \cdot H_2O$, occurring as a clear, white to off-white, odorless powder, having actions and uses similar to those of the base. **d. sodium phosphate** [USP], an ester of dexamethasone, $C_{22}H_{28}FNa_2O_8P$, occurring as a white or slightly yellow, crystalline powder, having actions and uses similar to those of the base; administered by intra-articular, soft tissue, intravenous or intramuscular injection, by inhalation, or applied topically to the skin and conjunctiva.

dexamisole (deks-am′ĭ-sōl) chemical name: (R)-2,3,5,6,-tetrahydro-6-phenyl-imidazo[2,1-b]thiazole; an antidepressant, $C_{11}H_{12}N_2S$.

dexbrompheniramine (deks″brōm-fen-ir′ah-mēn) chemical name: γ-(4-bromophenyl)-N,N-dimethyl-2-pyridine-propanamine. The bromine analogue of dexchlorpheniramine, $C_{16}H_{19}BrN_2$, an antihistaminic drug. **d. maleate** [USP], the maleate salt of dexbrompheniramine, $C_{16}H_{19}Br-N_2 \cdot C_4H_4O_4$, occurring as a white, crystalline powder; administered orally for therapy and prophylaxis of conditions in which antihistamines may be effective.

dexchlorpheniramine (deks″klōr-fen-ir′ah-mēn) chemical name: γ-(4-chlorophenyl)-N,N-dimethyl-2-pyridine-propanamine. The dextrorotatory isomer of chlorpheniramine, $C_{16}H_{19}ClN_2$, an antihistaminic drug. **d. maleate** [USP], the maleate salt of dexchlorpheniramine, $C_{16}H_{19}Cl-N_2 \cdot C_4H_4O_4$, occurring as a white, crystalline powder; administered orally for therapy and prophylaxis of conditions in which antihistamines may be effective.

dexclamol hydrochloride (deks′klah-mōl) chemical name (+)-2,3α,4,4aα,8,9,13bβ,14-octahydro-3-(1-methylethyl)-1H-benzo[6,7]cyclohepta[1,2,3-de]pyrido[2,1-a]iso-quino-line-3-ol hydrochloride; a sedative, $C_{24}H_{29}NO \cdot HCl$.

Dexedrine (dek′sĕ-drēn) trademark for preparations of dextroamphetamine sulfate.

dexetimide (dek-set′ĭ-mīd) chemical name: (S)-3-phenyl-1′-(phenylmethyl)-[3,4′-biperidine]-2,6-dione. An anticholinergic, $C_{23}H_{26}N_2O_2$, which has been tried as an antiparkinsonian agent.

deximafen (dek-sim′ah-fen) chemical name: (+)-2,3,5,6-

tetrahydro-5-phenyl-1*H*-imidazo[1,2-*a*]imidazol; an antidepressant, $C_{11}H_{13}N_3$.

dexiocardia (dek″se-o-kar′de-ah)   dextrocardia.

dexiotropic (dek″se-o-trop′ik) [Gr. *dexios* on the right + *tropos* a turning]   wound in a spiral from left to right, as a shell.

dexivacaine (dek-siv′ah-kān)   chemical name: (*S*)-*N*-(2,6-dimethylphenyl)-1-methyl-2-piperidinecarboxamide; an anesthetic, $C_{15}H_{22}N_2O$.

Dexon (dek′son)   trademark for a synthetic suture material, polyglycolic acid, a polymer that is completely absorbable and nonirritating.

Dexoval (dek′so-val)   trademark for a preparation of methamphetamine hydrochloride.

dexpanthenol (deks-pan′thĕ-nōl)   chemical name: (*R*)-2,4-dihydroxy-*N*-(3-hydroxypropyl)-3,3-dimethylbutamide.   The D(+) form of *panthenol* (pantothenyl alcohol), $C_9H_{19}NO_4$, the alcoholic analogue of pantothenic acid. It is claimed to be a precursor of coenzyme A, and is administered intravenously or intramuscularly to increase peristalsis in atony and paralysis of the lower intestine and orally to help relieve gas retention and abdominal distention in certain conditions. It is also applied topically to the skin to stimulate healing of the lesions of various dermatologic lesions such as burns, infected wounds, eczema, diaper rash, etc.

dexpropranolol hydrochloride (deks″-pro-pran′o-lōl)   chemical name: 1-[(1-methylethyl)amino]-3-(1-naphthalenyl- oxy)-2-propanol hydrochloride. The dextrorotatory isomer of propranolol, $C_{16}H_{21}NO_2 \cdot HCl$, having cardiac depressant properties similar to those of the parent compound; used as an antiarrhythmic.

dexter (dek′ster) [L.]   right; [NA] a term denoting the right-hand one of two similar structures, or the one situated on the right side of the body.

dextrad (deks′trad)   toward the right side.

dextral (deks′tral)   1. right as opposed to left; right-handed. 2. a right-handed person.

dextrality (deks-tral′ĭ-te) [L. *dexter* right]   the preferential use, in voluntary motor acts, of the right member of the major paired organs of the body, as the right ear, eye, hand, or foot.

dextran (dek′stran)   a high-molecular-weight polymer of D-glucose, produced by enzymes (glycosyltransferases) on the cell surface of certain lactic acid bacteria. Dextrans, formed from sucrose by bacteria in the mouth, adhere to the tooth surfaces and produce dental plaque, a major cause of dental caries. Uniform molecular weight dextrans from *Leuconostoc mesenteroides* preparations are used as plasma volume expanders. Specific preparations are designated, according to their average molecular weight in thousands, as *dextran 40, dextran 70*, and so on. Commercial preparations in bead form are also used in gel-filtration chromatography.

dextranomer (deks-tran′o-mer)   a preparation of highly hydrophilic dextran polymers occurring as small beads, used in débridement of secreting wounds, such as venous stasis ulcers; the sterilized beads are poured over secreting wounds to absorb wound exudates and prevent crust formation.

dextrates (deks′trāts)   a tablet binder and diluent, composed of a mixture of sugars (approximately 92 per cent dextrose monohydrate and 8 per cent high saccharides; dextrose equivalent is 95 to 97 per cent) resulting from the controlled enzymatic hydrolysis of starch.

dextraural (deks-traw′ral) [L. *dexter* right + *auris* ear]   hearing better with the right ear than with the left.

dextriferron (deks″trĭ-fer′on) [NF]   a complex of ferric hydroxide and partially hydrolyzed dextrin used in the treatment of iron-deficiency anemia.

dextrin (deks′trin) [L. *dexter* right]   any one, or the mixture, of the intermediate products $(C_6H_{10}O_5)_n$, formed during the hydrolysis of starch, which are dextrorotatory, soluble in water, and precipitable by alcohol. Commercial dextrin or starch sugar is a white or yellowish powder, in aqueous solution forming mucilage. See *erythrodextrin*.

dextrinase (deks′trin-ās)   any enzyme that catalyzes the hydrolysis of dextrins.

α-dextrinase (deks′trin-ās) [EC 3.2.1.10]   an enzyme that catalyzes the hydrolysis of both α-1,6 and α-1,4 bonds in linear and branched oligoglucosides and maltase and isomaltase. It occurs on the brush border of the intestinal mucosa, completes the digestion of starch or glycogen to glucose, and

is present as a complex with sucrase. The formal EC name is *oligo-1,6-α-glucosidase*.

dextrinate, dextrinize (deks′trin-āt; deks′trin-īz)   to convert into dextrin.

dextrin-1,6-glucosidase (deks″trin-glu-ko′sĭ-dās)   amylo-1,6-glucosidase.

dextrinose (deks′trin-ōs)   isomaltose.

dextrinosis (deks″trĭ-no′sis)   accumulation in the tissues of an abnormal polysaccharide.   **limit d.,** glycogen storage disease, type III; see under *disease*.

dextrinuria (deks″trin-u′re-ah) [*dextrin* + Gr. *ouron* urine + *-ia*]   the presence of dextrin in the urine.

dextr(o)- [L. *dexter* right]   1. a combining form denoting relationship to the right. 2. chemical prefix used to designate the dextrorotatory enantiomorph of a substance; opposed to *levo-*. Symbol (+)- (formerly *d-*; sometimes Δ).

dextroamphetamine (deks″stro-am-fet′ah-mēn)   chemical name: (*S*)-α-methylbenzeneethanamine. The dextrorotatory isomer of amphetamine, which has substantially more central nervous system stimulating effect than the levorotatory form (levamphetamine) or racemic forms of amphetamine. Abuse of this drug may lead to dependence; see *amphetamine*, def. 1.   **d. phosphate** [USP], a white, crystalline powder, $C_9H_{13}N \cdot H_3PO_4$, having the same actions as the base, used chiefly for its central stimulant effects in the treatment of mental depression, psychopathic states, narcolepsy, hyperkinetic behavior disorders in children, and exogenous obesity; administered orally.   **d. sulfate** [USP], a white, crystalline powder, $(C_9H_{13}N)_2 \cdot H_2SO_4$, having the same actions and uses as the phosphate salt; administered orally.

dextrocardia (deks″tro-kar′de-ah)   location of the heart in the right hemithorax, with the apex pointing to the right, occurring with transposition (situs inversus) of the abdominal viscera, or without such transposition (*isolated d.*).   **mirror-image d.,** location of the heart in the right side of the chest, the atria being transposed and the right ventricle lying anteriorly and to the left of the left ventricle, usually associated with complete situs inversus.   **secondary d.,** displacement of the heart to the right as a result of disease of the pleura, diaphragm, or lungs.

dextrocardiogram (deks″tro-kar′de-o-gram) [L. *dexter* right + *cardiogram*]   that part of the normal cardiogram which represents the action of the right side of the heart.

dextrocerebral (deks″tro-ser′e-bral) [L. *dexter* right + *cerebrum*]   having the right hemisphere of the brain more active than the left.

dextroclination (deks″tro-klĭ-na′shun) [*dextro-* + L. *clinatus* leaning]   rotation of the upper poles of the vertical meridians of the two eyes to the right; called also *dextrocycloduction* and *dextrotorsion*. Cf. *levoclination*.

dextrocompound (deks″tro-kom′pound)   a dextrorotatory compound.

dextrocular (deks-trok′u-lar)   right eyed; affected with dextrocularity.

dextrocularity (deks″trok-u-lar′ĭ-te) [L. *dexter* right + *oculus* eye]   the condition of having greater visual power in the right eye and, therefore, using it more than the left.

dextrocycloduction (deks″tro-si″klo-duk′shun)   dextroclination.

dextroduction (deks″tro-duk′shun) [*dextro-* + *duction*]   movement of either eye to the right.

dextrogastria (deks″tro-gas′tre-ah) [L. *dexter* right + Gr. *gastēr* stomach]   displacement of the stomach to the right, being simple displacement or situs inversus.

dextroglucose (deks″tro-glu′kōs)   dextrose.

dextrogram (deks′tro-gram) [*dextro-* + Gr. *graphein* to record]   an electrocardiographic tracing showing right axis deviation, indicative of right ventricular hypertrophy.

dextrogyral (deks″tro-ji′ral) [L. *dexter* right + *gyrare* to turn]   dextrorotatory.

dextrogyration (deks″tro-ji-ra′shun) [*dextro-* + *gyration*]   a turning to the right or motion to the right; said of movements of the eye and of the plane of polarization.

dextromanual (deks″tro-man′u-al) [L. *dextro-* + *manus* hand]   right-handed.

dextromenthol (deks″tro-men′thol)   an oxidation product of menthol.

dextromethorphan hydrobromide (dek″stro-meth′or-fan) [USP] chemical name: 3-methoxy-17-methyl-9α,13α,14α-morphinan hydrobromide monohydrate. An antitussive, $C_{18}H_{25}NO \cdot HBr \cdot H_2O$, occurring as practically white crystals or as a crystalline powder; administered orally.

dextropedal (deks-trop′ĕ-dal) [L. dextro- + pes foot] using the right foot in preference to the left.

dextroposition (deks″tro-po-zish′un) displacement to the right.

dextropropoxyphene (dek″stro-pro-pok′se-fēn) propoxyphene.

dextrorotary (deks″tro-ro′tah-re) dextrorotatory.

dextrorotatory (deks″tro-ro′tah-to-re) [L. dexter right + rotare to turn] turning the plane of polarization, or rays of light, to the right; called also dextrogyral.

dextrose (deks′trōs) chemical name: D-glucose monohydrate. A monosaccharide, $C_6H_{12}O_6H_2O$, known as glucose (q.v.) in biochemistry and physiology. The official preparation [USP] is usually obtained by the hydrolysis of starch, and occurs as colorless crystals or as a white, crystalline or granular powder; it is used chiefly as a fluid and nutrient replenisher, usually administered by intravenous infusion. It is also used as a diuretic and alone or in combination with other agents for various other clinical purposes.

dextrosinistral (deks″tro-sin′is-tral) [L. dextro- + sinister left] extending from right to left. The term is also applied to a person naturally left-handed but trained to use the right hand in certain performances.

dextrosozone (deks″tro-so′zōn) glucosazone.

Dextrostix (dek′stro-stiks) trademark for a reagent strip designed for determination of blood-glucose levels with the use of fingertip venous blood.

dextrosuria (deks″tro-su′re-ah) [dextrose + Gr. ouron urine + -ia] the presence of dextrose (D-glucose) in the urine; called also glucosuria.

dextrothyroxine sodium (deks″tro-thi-rok′sin) [USP] chemical name: O-(4-hydroxy-3,5-diiodophenyl)-3,5-diiodo-D-tyrosine monosodium salt hydrate. The sodium salt of the dextrorotatory isomer of thyroxine, $C_{15}H_{10}I_4NNaO_4 \cdot xH_2O$, occurring as a light yellow to buff-colored powder; used as an oral anticholesteremic, mainly to treat hypercholesteremia in euthyroid patients.

dextrotorsion (deks″tro-tor′shun) dextroclination.

dextrotropic (deks″tro-trop′ik) [L. dexter right + Gr. tropos a turning] turning to the right; see also dexiotropic.

dextroversion (deks″tro-ver′shun) [dextro- + version] 1. version to the right side; especially movement of the eyes to the right. 2. location of the heart in the right hemithorax, the left ventricle remaining on the left as in the normal position, but lying anterior to the right ventricle.

dextroverted (deks″tro-vert′ed) turned to the right.

dezocine (dez′o-sēn) chemical name: (−)-13S*-amino-5,6,7,8,9,10,11α,12-octahydro-5α-methyl-5,11-methanobenzocyclodecen-3-ol; an analgesic, $C_{16}H_{23}NO$.

DFDT a powerful insecticide, difluoro-diphenyl-trichloroethane; called also GIX.

DFP diisopropyl flurophosphate.

DF-2 see under bacillus.

dG deoxyguanosine.

dg decigram.

dGDP deoxyguanosine diphosphate.

dGMP deoxyguanosine monophosphate.

dGTP deoxyguanosine triphosphate.

DH delayed hypersensitivity.

DHEA dehydroepiandrosterone.

D.H.E. 45 trademark for dihydroergotamine.

d'Herelle phenomenon (dĕ-rel′) [Félix Hubert d'Herelle of the Pasteur Institute, Paris, 1873–1949] see Twort-d'Herelle phenomenon, under phenomenon.

D.Hg., D.Hy. Doctor of Hygiene.

DHT dihydrotestosterone.

dhurrin (du′rin) a cyanogenetic glycoside, $C_{14}H_{17}NO_7$, from sorghum which hydrolyzes into parahydroxy benzaldehyde, glucose, and hydrocyanic acid.

di- [Gr. dis twice] a prefix meaning twice. In chemical nomenclature, the use of di- is preferred to the use of bi- (q.v.).

dia- [Gr. dia through] a prefix meaning through, between, apart, across, or completely.

diabetes (di″ah-be′tēz) [Gr. diabētēs a syphon, from dia through + bainein to go] a general term referring to disorders characterized by excessive urine excretion (polyuria), as in diabetes mellitus and diabetes insipidus. When used alone, the term refers to diabetes mellitus. **adult-onset d.,** non–insulin-dependent d. **alloxan d.,** an animal model for diabetes mellitus; administration of alloxan produces selective destruction of the beta cells of the pancreatic islets, thereby causing hyperglycemia and ketoacidosis. **brittle d.,** formerly used term for insulin-dependent diabetes, especially that characterized by wide, unpredictable fluctuation of blood glucose values and therefore difficult to control. **bronze d., bronzed d.,** hemochromatosis. **chemical d.,** see impaired glucose tolerance, under tolerance. **gestational d.,** glucose intolerance with onset during pregnancy; this category does not include diabetics who become pregnant or women who become lactosuric; after the pregnancy the woman is reclassified as having diabetes mellitus (DM) or previous abnormality of glucose tolerance (prev AGT) depending upon whether or not the glucose intolerance persists. **growth-onset d.,** insulin-dependent d. **d. insip′idus,** a metabolic disorder due to injury of the neurohypophyseal system, which results in a deficient quantity of antidiuretic hormone being released or produced, and thus in failure of tubular reabsorption of water in the kidney. As a result, a large amount of urine of low specific gravity is excreted, followed by dehydration and great thirst; it is often attended by voracious appetite, loss of strength, and emaciation. It may be inherited, acquired, or idiopathic. Another form occurs (nephrogenic diabetes insipidus) in which the renal tubules are refractory to the antidiuretic effect of vasopressin. **d. insip′idus, nephrogenic,** a rare congenital and familial form of diabetes insipidus, resulting from failure of the renal tubules to reabsorb water; there is excessive production of antidiuretic hormone but the tubules fail to respond to it. **insulin-dependent d. (IDD),** type I diabetes mellitus, characterized by abrupt onset of symptoms, insulinopenia, dependence on exogenous insulin to sustain life, and a tendency to develop ketoacidosis. The peak age of onset is 12 years, but onset can occur at any age. The disorder is due to lack of insulin production by the beta cells of the pancreatic islets. The beta cell injury is associated with viral infection and autoimmune reactions and probably with genetic factors; islet cell antibodies are detectable in most patients at diagnosis. In undiagnosed or inadequately controlled IDD, lack of insulin causes hyperglycemia, protein wasting, and production of ketone bodies as a result of increased fat metabolism. Hyperglycemia leads to overflow glycosuria and osmotic diuresis, resulting in hyperosmolarity and dehydration, followed by diabetic ketoacidosis, hyperosmolar coma, or both. Accompanying symptoms are polyuria, polydipsia, polyphagia, weight loss, lassitude, paresthesias, blurred vision, and irritability; if untreated, diabetic ketoacidosis progresses to nausea and vomiting, stupor, coma, and death. For late complications see d. mellitus. Formerly called juvenile-onset d. and brittle d. **juvenile d., juvenile-onset d.,** insulin-dependent d. **ketosis-prone d.,** insulin-dependent d. **ketosis-resistant d.,** non-insulin-dependent d. **latent d.,** see impaired glucose tolerance, under tolerance. **lipoatrophic d.,** total lipodystrophy. **maturity-onset d.,** non-insulin-dependent d. **maturity-onset d. of youth (MODY),** a subtype of non–insulin-dependent diabetes characterized by autosomal dominant inheritance and onset in late adolescence or early adulthood. **d. melli′tus (DM),** a chronic syndrome of impaired carbohydrate, protein, and fat metabolism secondary to insufficient secretion of insulin or to target tissue insulin resistance. It occurs in two major forms: insulin-dependent diabetes mellitus (type I) and non–insulin-dependent diabetes mellitus (type II), which differ in etiology, pathology, genetics, age of onset, and treatment. Type I diabetes tends to a higher incidence of microangiopathy (affecting the retinas, kidneys, and basement membrane of arterioles throughout the body) than type II; type II diabetes is classically accompanied by macroangiopathy: premature atherosclerosis (myocardial infarction), cerebrovascular accident. Both types are associated with disease of small and large blood vessels. **non–insulin-dependent d. (NIDD),** type II diabetes mellitus, usually characterized by a gradual onset with minimal or no symptoms of metabolic disturbance (glycosuria and its consequences) and no requirement for exogenous insulin to prevent ketonuria and ketoacidosis; dietary control with or without oral hypoglycemics is usually effective. The peak age of onset is 50 to 60 years. Obesity and possibly a genetic factor are usually present. Diagnosis is based on laboratory tests indicating glucose intolerance. Basal insulin secretion is maintained at normal or reduced levels, but insulin release in response to a glucose load is delayed or reduced. Defective glucose receptors on the beta cells of the pancreatic islets may be involved. For late complications see *d. mellitus.* Formerly called *adult-onset d.* and *maturity-onset d.* **phosphate d.,** vitamin D–resistant rickets. **preclinical d.,** see *impaired glucose tolerance,* under *tolerance.* **puncture d.,** a form produced by puncturing the floor of the fourth ventricle in the medulla oblongata; called also *piqûre d.* **renal d.,** renal glycosuria. **steroid d., steroidogenic d.,** glucose intolerance or overt hyperglycemia induced by glucocorticoids or estrogens; it is due in part to target tissue insulin resistance and is characterized by a relatively low incidence of microvascular sequelae. **subclinical d.,** impaired glucose tolerance or previous abnormality of glucose tolerance; see under *tolerance.* **thiazide d.,** glucose intolerance or overt hyperglycemia induced by thiazide diuretics, which inhibit insulin secretion, possibly through thiazide-induced hypokalemia.

diabetic (di″ah-bet′ik) 1. pertaining to or affected with diabetes. 2. a person with diabetes. See under *diabetes* for specific forms.

diabetid (di″ah-be′tid) diabetic dermopathy.

diabetogenic (di″ah-bet″o-jen′ik) [*diabetes* + Gr. *gennan* to produce] producing diabetes.

diabetogenous (di″ah-be-toj′ĕ-nus) produced by diabetes.

diabetograph (di″ah-be′to-graf) [*diabetes* + Gr. *graphein* to write] an instrument used in urinalysis, with a graduated scale to show the proportion of glucose present.

diabetometer (di″ah-be-tom′ĕ-ter) [*diabetes* + Gr. *metron* measure] a polariscope for use in estimating the percentage of sugar in the urine.

Diabinese (di-ab′ĭ-nēs) trademark for chlorpropamide.

diabrosis (di″ah-bro′sis) [*dia-* + Gr. *brōsis* eating] perforation resulting from a corrosive process; perforating ulceration.

diabrotic (di″ah-brot′ik) [Gr. *diabrōtikos*] 1. ulcerative; caustic. 2. a corrosive or escharotic agent.

diacele (di′ah-sēl) (*obs.*) the third ventricle of the cerebrum (ventriculus tertius cerebri [NA]).

diacetate (di-as′ĕ-tāt) any salt of acetoacetic acid.

diacetemia (di″as-ĕ-te′me-ah) [*diacetic acid* + Gr. *haima* blood + *-ia*] the presence of acetoacetic acid (diacetic acid) in the blood.

diacetic acid (di-ah-se′tik, -set′ik) acetoacetic acid

diaceticaciduria (di″ah-set″ik-as″ĭ-du′re-ah) diaceturia.

diacetonuria (di-as″ĕ-to-nu′re-ah) diaceturia.

diaceturia (di″as-ĕ-tu′re-ah) [*diacetic acid* + Gr. *ouron* urine + *-ia*] the excretion of acetoacetic acid (diacetic acid) in the urine; called also *acetoacetic aciduria.*

diacetyl (di-as′ĕ-til) a yellow liquid, 2,3-butane-dione, CH_3-$COCOCH_3$, having the odor of butter. **d. peroxide,** a compound, $CH_3CO\cdot O\cdot O\cdot CO\cdot CH_3$, used in solution as an antiseptic.

diacetylmorphine (di″ah-se″til-mor′fēn) heroin; a white, bitterish, crystalline powder, $C_{17}H_{17}(O\cdot OC\cdot CH_3)_2\cdot NO$, the diacetic acid ester of morphine, formerly used as an analgesic and narcotic. Because it is highly addictive, the importation of heroin and its salts into the United States, as well as its use in medicine, is illegal. Called also *acetomorphine* and *diamorphine.* **d. hydrochloride,** a white, crystalline powder, $C_{17}H_{17}(O\cdot CO\cdot CH_3)_2ON\cdot HCl\cdot H_2O$. See *diacetylmorphine.*

diacetyltannic acid (di″ah-se″til-tan′ik) acetyltannic acid.

Diachlorus (di-ah-klo′rus) a genus of tabanid flies of South America.

diachorema (di″ah-ko-re′mah) [Gr. *diachōrēma*] excrement; feces.

diachoresis (di-ah-ko-re′sis) defecation.

diacid (di-as′id) [Gr. *dis* twice + *acid*] having two replaceable hydrogen atoms; a dibasic acid, having the acid activity of two molecules of a monobasic acid.

diaclasis (di-ak′lah-sis) [*dia-* + Gr. *klasis* fracture] osteoclasis.

diacrinous (di-ak′rĭ-nus) [Gr. *diakrinein* to separate] giving off secretion directly, as from a filter; said of gland cells, as those of the kidney. Opposed to *ptyocrinous.*

diacrisis (di-ak′rĭ-sis) [Gr. *diakrisis* separation] 1. diagnosis. 2. a disease marked by a morbid state of the secretions. 3. a critical discharge or excretion.

diacritic (di-ah-krit′ik) [*dia-* + Gr. *krinein* to judge] distinguishing; diagnostic.

diactinic (di″ak-tin′ik) transmitting chemically active rays.

diactinism (di-ak′tin-izm) [*dia-* + Gr. *aktis* ray] the property of transmitting chemically active rays.

diadochocinesia (di-ad″ŏ-ko-si-ne′se-ah) diadochokinesia.

diadochocinetic (di-ad″ŏ-ko-si-net′ik) diadochokinetic.

diadochokinesia (di-ad″ŏ-ko-ki-ne′se-ah) [Gr. *diadochos* succeeding + *kinēsis* motion] the function of arresting one motor impulse and substituting for it one that is diametrically opposite, to permit sequential alternating movements, as pronation and supination of the arm.

diadochokinesis (di-ad″ŏ-ko-ki-ne′sis) diadochokinesia.

diadochokinetic (di-ad″ŏ-ko-ki-net′ik) pertaining to diadochokinesia.

Diadol (di′ah-dol) trademark for a preparation of allobarbital.

Diafen (di′ah-fen) trademark for a preparation of diphenylpyraline hydrochloride.

diagnose (di′ag-nōs) to make a diagnosis of; to recognize the nature of an attack of disease.

diagnosis (di″ag-no′sis) [*dia-* + Gr. *gnōsis* knowledge] 1. the art of distinguishing one disease from another. 2. the determination of the nature of a case of disease. **biological d.,** diagnosis by tests performed on animals, as by the Aschheim-Zondek test. **clinical d.,** diagnosis based on signs, symptoms, and laboratory findings during life. **cytohistologic d.,** cytologic diagnosis. **cytologic d.,** the diagnosis of disease, both benign and malignant, by study of exfoliated cells; called also *cytohistologic d.* **differential d.,** the determination of which one of two or more diseases or conditions a patient is suffering from, by systematically comparing and contrasting their clinical findings. **direct d.,** pathologic diagnosis by observing structural lesions or pathognomonic symptoms. **d. by exclusion,** recognition of a disease by excluding all other known diseases. **d. ex juvan′tibus,** diagnosis based on the results of treatment. **laboratory d.,** diagnosis based on the findings of various laboratory examinations or measurements. **niveau d.** [Fr. "level diagnosis"], localization of the exact level of a lesion; as, for instance, of an intervertebral tumor. **pathologic d.,** diagnosis by observing the structural lesions present. **physical d.,** determination of disease by inspection, palpation, percussion, and auscultation. **provocative d.,** the induction of a condition for the purpose of diagnosis, as the induction of a fit in a doubtful case of epilepsy. **roentgen d.,** diagnosis made by means of roentgen rays. **serum d.,** diagnosis by means of the analysis of serums; immunodiagnosis.

diagnostic (di″ag-nos′tik) pertaining to or subserving diagnosis; distinctive of or serving as a criterion of a disease, as signs and symptoms.

diagnosticate (di″ag-nos′te-kāt) diagnose.

diagnostician (di″ag-nos-tish′an) an expert in diagnosis.

diagnostics (di″ag-nos′tiks) the science and practice of diagnosis of disease.

diagnosticum (di″ag-nos′te-kum) (*obs.*) a preparation used in tests and experiments.

diagram (di′ah-gram) a graphic representation, in simplest form, of an object or concept, made up of lines and lacking entirely any pictorial elements. **scatter d.,** scatterplot. **vector d.,** a diagram representing the direction and magnitude of electromotive forces of the heart for one entire cycle, based on analysis of the scalar electrocardiogram.

diagrammatic (di″ah-grah-mat′ik) pertaining to or of the nature of a diagram.

diagraph (di′ah-graf) [*dia-* + Gr. *graphein* to write] an instrument for recording outlines; used in craniometry, etc.

diakinesis (di″ah-ki-ne′sis) [*dia-* + Gr. *kinēsis* motion] the stage of first meiotic prophase in which the nucleolus and nuclear envelope disappear and the spindle fibers form.

Dial (di′al) trademark for a preparation of allobarbital.

dial (di′al) [L. *dialis* daily, from *dies* day] a circular area with graduations around the circumference and a centrally fixed pointer for indicating values of time, pressure, etc. **astigmatic d.,** a diagram arranged like the face of a watch used to determine the presence and axis of astigmatism.

Dialister (di″ah-lis′ter) a genus of bacteria the organisms of which have been assigned to the genus *Bacteroides*. **D. pneumosin′tes,** *Bacteroides pneumosintes*.

diallyl (di-al′il) 1. any compound containing two allyl molecules. 2. a liquid unsaturated hydrocarbon, CH₂:CH·-CH₂·CH₂·CH:CH₂, having the odor of radishes.

diallylbisnortoxiferin dichloride (di-al″il-bis-nor-tok′si-fer-in) alcuronium chloride.

Dialog (di′ah-log) trademark for a preparation of allobarbital and acetaminophen.

Dialume (di′ah-loom) trademark for a preparation of dried aluminum hydroxide gel.

dialurate (di-al′u-rāt) a salt of dialuric acid.

dialysance (di″ah-li′sans) [*dialysis* + *-ance* suffix denoting action or process] the minute rate of net exchange of a substance between blood and bath fluid, per unit blood-bath concentration gradient; a parameter in artificial kidney kinetics (nonfiltration) functionally equivalent to the clearance of the natural kidney.

dialysate (di-al′ĭ-sāt) the material that passes through the membrane in dialysis.

dialysis (di-al′ĭ-sis) [*dia-* + Gr. *lysis* dissolution] the process of separating crystalloids and colloids in solution by the difference in their rates of diffusion through a semipermeable membrane: crystalloids pass through readily, colloids very slowly or not at all. See also *hemodialysis*. **cross d.,** dialytic parabiosis. **equilibrium d.,** a technique used to measure antibody-hapten affinities: solutions of pure antibody and hapten are placed in two cells separated by a semipermeable membrane and the hapten diffuses across until the free hapten concentration is the same on both sides. From the known total amounts of antibody and hapten and the measured free hapten concentration, the concentrations of free antibody and antibody-hapten complex and the dissociation constant are calculated. **lymph d.,** removal of urea and other elements from lymph collected from the thoracic duct, treated outside the body, and later reinfused. **peritoneal d.,** dialysis through the peritoneum, the dialyzing solution being introduced into and removed from the peritoneal cavity as either a continuous or an intermittent procedure. **d. re′tinae,** a tear in the retina at the ora serrata.

dialyzable (di-ah-līz′ah-b'l) capable of dialysis or of passing through a membrane.

dialyzed (di′ah-līzd) separated or prepared by dialysis.

dialyzer (di′ah-līz″er) an apparatus for effecting dialysis; see *hemodialyzer*.

Diamanus (di″ah-ma′nus) a genus of fleas. **D. monta′nus,** a flea of rodents in the western United States which has been implicated in the transmission of sylvatic plague; formerly called *Ceratophyllus acustus, C. montanus,* and *Oropsylla montana*.

diameter (di-am′e-ter) the length of a straight line passing through the center of a circle and connecting opposite points on its circumference; hence the distance between two specified opposite points on the periphery of a structure such as the cranium or pelvis. **anteroposterior d.,** the distance between two points located on the anterior and posterior aspects, respectively, of the structure being measured; such as the true conjugate diameter of the pelvis, or the occipitofrontal diameter of the skull. **anterotransverse d.** (of the cranium), temporal d. **Baudelocque's d.,** external conjugate diameter. **biischial d.,** transverse diameter of pelvic outlet. **biparietal d.,** the distance between the two parietal eminences. **bisacromial d.,** the distance between the outermost points of the shoulder. **bisiliac d.,** the distance between the two most remote points of the iliac crests. **bispinous d.,** the dis-

tance between the opposite spines of the ischia. **bitemporal d.,** the distance between the two extremities of the coronal suture. **buccolingual d.,** the distance from the buccal to the lingual surface of a tooth crown at its widest point or greatest curvature. **cervicobregmatic d.,** the distance between the center of the anterior fontanel and the junction of the neck with the floor of the mouth. **coccygeopubic d.,** the distance from the tip of the coccyx to the under margin of the symphysis pubis. **d. conjuga′ta pel′vis** [NA], conjugate diameter of pelvis: the anteroposterior diameter of the superior aperture of the minor pelvis (pelvic inlet), measured from the superior margin of the symphysis pubis to the sacrovertebral angle; called also *conjugata, conjugate,* or *conjugate d., conjugata anatomica, conjugata vera, anatomic, internal,* or *true conjugate,* and *anatomic conjugate d.* **conjugate d.,** 1. the distance between two specified opposite points on the periphery of the pelvic inlet. 2. d. conjugata pelvis. **conjugate d., anatomic,** d. conjugata pelvis. **conjugate d., diagonal,** a diameter of the pelvic inlet: the distance from the posterior surface of the pubis to the tip of the sacral promontory; called also *conjugata diagonalis* and *diagonal conjugate.* **conjugate d., external,** the distance from the depression under the last lumbar spine to the upper margin of the pubis; called also *external conjugate* and *Baudelocque's d.* or *line.* **conjugate d., internal,** true conjugate d. **conjugate d., obstetric,** the shortest anteroposterior diameter of the pelvic inlet; the distance from a point 1 cm. below the top of the pubis to the tip of the sacral promontory, measuring 11 to 13 cm. in the normal pelvis. So called because it is intimately concerned in the process of labor. Called also *obstetric conjugate* and *conjugata vera obstetrica.* **conjugate d. of pelvis,** 1. d. conjugata pelvis. 2. conjugate d. **conjugate d., true,** d. conjugata pelvis. **cranial d's,** distances measured between certain landmarks of the skull, such as the *biparietal d., bitemporal d., cervicobregmatic d., frontomental d., occipitofrontal d., occipitomental d.,* and *suboccipitobregmatic d.* **craniometric d.,** any line connecting two craniometric points of the same name. **frontomental d.,** the distance from the forehead to the chin. **fronto-occipital d.,** occipitofrontal d. **intercristal d.,** the distance between the middle points of the iliac crests. **intertuberal d.,** the distance between the sciatic notches. **longitudinal d., inferior,** the distance from the foramen cecum to the internal occipital protuberance. **mento-occipital d.,** occipitomental d. **mentoparietal d.,** the distance from the chin to the vertex of the skull. **d. obli′qua pel′vis** [NA], **oblique diameter of pelvis,** the oblique diameter of the superior aperture of the minor pelvis, measured from one sacroiliac articulation to the iliopubic eminence of the other side. Designated right or left depending on the sacroiliac joint used for reference; the left is uniformly 0.5 cm. shorter than the right. **occipitofrontal d.,** the distance from the external occipital protuberance to the most prominent midpoint of the frontal bone; called also *fronto-occipital d.* **occipitomental d.,** the distance from the external occipital protuberance to the most prominent midpoint of the chin; called also *mento-occipital d.* **parietal d.,** the distance between tuberosities of parietal bones; called also *posterotransverse d.* **pelvic d.,** any diameter of the pelvis. **posterotransverse d.,** parietal d.

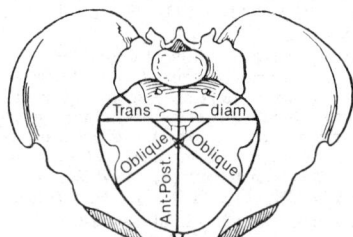

Diameters of pelvic inlet (see also pelvic planes).

pubosacral d., true conjugate d. **pubotuberous d.,** the distance from the tuberosity of the ischium to a point on the superior ramus of the pubis which is located directly perpendicular to the tuberosity. **sacropubic d.,** the distance from the tip of the sacrum or coccyx to the lower margin of the symphysis pubis. **sagittal d.,** the distance from the glabella to the external occipital protuberance. **suboccipitobregmatic d.,** the distance from the lowest posterior point of the occiput to the center of the anterior fontanel. **temporal d.,** the distance between the tips of the alae magnae; called also *anterotransverse d.* **d. transver'sa pel'vis** [NA], transverse diameter of pelvis: the greatest distance from side to side of the superior aperture of the minor pelvis. **transverse d.,** the distance between two points located on the opposite sides of the body part being measured, such as the biparietal diameter of the head. **transverse d. of pelvis,** d. transversa pelvis. **transverse d. of pelvic outlet,** the distance between the medial surfaces of the ischial tuberosities (average length 11 cm.); called also *biischial d.* **vertebromammary d.,** the anteroposterior diameter of the chest. **vertical d.,** the distance between two points situated on the upper and lower aspects of the structure being measured, such as the distance between the occipital foramen and the vertex of the skull.

diamide (di-am'id) [L. *di* two + *amide*] 1. a compound which contains two amido groups. 2. hydrazine.

diamidine (di-am'ĭ-dēn) a compound that contains two amidine groups.

diamido- a prefix indicating the possession of two amido groups.

diamine (di'ah-mēn'; di''ah-min') [L. *di* two + *amine*] 1. a compound which contains two amino groups. 2. hydrazine sulfate, $N_2H_5HSO_4$, used as a germicide.

diamine oxidase (di'ah-mēn ok'sĭ-dās) amine oxidase (copper containing).

diaminoacridine (di-am''ĭ-no-ak'rĭ-din) proflavine.

diaminodiphenylsulfone (di-am''ĭ-no-di-fen''il-sul'fōn) dapsone. **diacetyl d.,** acedapsone.

diaminodiphosphatide (di-am''ĭ-no-di-fos'fah-tīd'') a phosphatide containing two atoms of nitrogen and two of phosphorus to the molecule.

diaminomonophosphatide (di-am''ĭ-no-mon''o-fos'fah-tīd'') a phosphatide containing two atoms of nitrogen and one of phosphorus to the molecule.

diaminuria (di-am''ĭ-nu're-ah) the presence of diamines in the urine.

diamniotic (di''am-ne-ot'ik) having or developing within separate amniotic cavities, as diamniotic twins.

diamocaine cyclamate (di-ah'mo-kān) chemical name: 1-(2-anilinoethyl)-4-[2-(diethylamino)ethoxy]-4-phenylpiperidine; a local anesthetic, $C_{37}H_{63}N_5O_7S_2$.

Diamond-Blackfan syndrome (di'ah-mond-blak'fan) [Louis Klein Diamond, U.S. pediatrician, born 1902; Kenneth D. Blackfan, U.S. pediatrician, 1883–1941] see *congenital hypoplastic anemia,* under *anemia.*

diamonds (di'ah-munz) an urticarial form of swine erysipelas characterized by well-defined quadrangular or rhombic patches on the skin.

diamorphine (di''ah-mor'fēn) diacetylmorphine.

diamorphosis (di''ah-mor-fo'sis) (*obs.*) growth into normal shape.

Diamox (di'ah-moks) trademark for preparations of acetazolamide.

diamthazole dihydrochloride (di-am'thah-zōl) chemical name: 6-(2-diethylaminoethoxy)-2-dimethylaminobenzothiazole dihydrochloride. An antifungal agent, $C_{15}H_{25}Cl_2N_3$-OS, effective against species of *Trichophyton* and *Microsporum* and *Candida albicans;* it has been used in the treatment of various forms of tinea, applied topically.

diamylene (di-am'ĭ-lēn) dipentene.

Dianabol (di-an'ah-bol) trademark for methandrostenolone.

dianhydroantiarigenin (di''an-hi''dro-an''te-ar'ĭ- jen''in) an aglycone, $C_{23}H_{28}O_5$, from antiarin.

dianoetic (di''ah-no-et'ik) [*dia-* + Gr. *nous* mind] pertaining to the intellectual functions, especially to reasoning.

diantebrachia (di''an-te-bra'ke-ah) a developmental anomaly characterized by duplication of a forearm.

diapamide (di-ap'ah-mīd) chemical name: 4-chloro-*N*-methyl-3-(methylsulfamoyl)benzamide; a diuretic and antihypertensive, $C_9H_{11}ClN_2O_3S$.

Diaparene (di-ap'ah-rēn) trademark for preparations of methylbenzethonium chloride.

diapause (di'a-pawz) [*dia-* + Gr. *pausis* pause] a state of inactivity and arrested development accompanied by greatly decreased metabolism, as in many eggs, insect pupae, and plant seeds; it is a mechanism for surviving adverse winter conditions.

diapedesis (di''ah-pĕ-de'sis) [*dia-* + Gr. *pēdan* to leap] the outward passage through intact vessel walls of corpuscular elements of the blood; called also *diapiresis* and *emigration.*

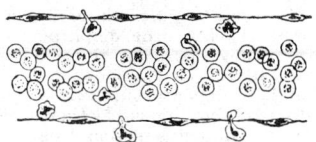

Diapedesis of leukocytes.

diapedetic (di''ah-pĕ-det'ik) pertaining to or characterized by diapedesis.

diaphane (di'ah-fān) [Gr. *diaphanēs* transparent] a minute electric lamp for use in transillumination.

diaphaneity (di''ah-fah-ne'ĭ-te) transparency.

diaphanography (di-af''ah-nog'rah-fe) transillumination of the breast, with photography of the transilluminated light on infrared-sensitive film.

diaphanometer (di-af''ah-nom'ĕ-ter) [Gr. *diaphanēs* transparent + Gr. *metron* measure] an instrument for testing milk, urine, and other fluids by means of transmitted light.

diaphanometry (di-af''ah-nom'ĕ-tre) the measurement of the transparency of a fluid.

diaphanoscope (di-af''ah-no-skōp'') [Gr. *diaphanēs* transparent + *skopein* to examine] an instrument for transilluminating a body cavity; called also *electrodiaphane* and *electrodiaphanoscope.*

diaphanoscopy (di-af''ah-nos'ko-pe) examination with the diaphanoscope; transillumination; called also *electrodiaphanoscopy.*

diaphemetric (di''ah-fĕ-met'rik) [*dia-* + Gr. *haphē* touch + *metron* measure] pertaining to the measurement of tactile sensibility.

diaphorase (di-af'o-rās) 1. any flavoprotein catalyzing the oxidation of reduced nicotinamide-adenine dinucleotide or reduced nicotinamide-adenine dinucleotide phosphate using a nonphysiological compound such as methylene blue as electron acceptor, but not oxygen or cytochromes. The reaction is an artifact arising from removal of the enzyme from the complexes in which it occurs naturally. 2. dihydrolipoamide dehydrogenase.

diaphoresis (di''ah-fo-re'sis) [Gr. *diaphorēsis*] perspiration, especially profuse perspiration. Called also sudoresis.

diaphoretic (di''ah-fo-ret'ik) [Gr. *diaphorētikos*] 1. pertaining to, characterized by, or promoting diaphoresis. 2. an agent that promotes diaphoresis.

diaphragm (di'ah-fram) 1. the musculomembranous partition separating the abdominal and thoracic cavities, and serving as a major inspiratory muscle; called also *diaphragma* [NA], *midriff,* and *diaphragmatic muscle.* 2. any separating membrane or structure. 3. a disk with one or more openings in it, or with an adjustable opening, mounted in relation to a lens or source of radiation by which part of the light or radiation may be excluded from the area. 4. a contraceptive device of molded rubber or other soft plastic material with a metal spring rim that is coated with a spermicidal agent; it is fitted over the cervix uteri prior to intercourse to prevent the entrance of spermatozoa by both mechanical and chemical means. Called also *contraceptive d.* and *vaginal d.* **accessory d.,** diaphragma urogenitale. **Akerlund d.,** a spiral type of diaphragm used in roentgenography. **Bucky d., Bucky-Potter d.,** a grid that is an integral part of the x-ray table, located below the table top and above a cassette tray. It decreases the amount of secondary radiation reaching the film, thus increasing detail and contrast, and moves during exposure so that no grid lines appear in the radiograph. **contraceptive d.,** see diaphragm, def. 4. **epithelial d.,** an epithelial structure, evolving from the root sheath (sheath of Hertwig), that narrows the opening into the pulp chamber, diminishing its caliber. It is in close contact with the bone forming the fundus of the developing alveolus, from which it is separated by the dental sac. **d. of mouth** musculus mylohyoideus. **oral d.,** musculus mylohyoideus. **pelvic d., d. of pelvis,** diaphragma pelvis. **polyarcuate d.,** one showing abnormal scalloping of margins on radiographic visualization. **Potter-Bucky d.,** Bucky d. **secondary d.,** diaphragma urogenitale. **d. of sella turcica,** diaphragma sellae. **urogenital d.,** diaphragma urogenitale. **vaginal d.,** see *diaphragm* (def. 4).

diaphragma (di″ah-frag′mah), pl. *diaphragmata* [Gr. "a partition-wall, barrier"] [NA] the diaphragm: the musculomembranous partition separating the abdominal and thoracic cavities, and serving as a major thoracic muscle. Called also *midriff* and *diaphragmatic muscle.* Also used in anatomical nomenclature in the names of other separating structures. **d. o′ris,** musculus mylohyoideus. **d. pel′vis** [NA], pelvic diaphragm: the portion of the floor of the pelvis formed by the coccygei and levatores ani muscles and their fasciae. **d. sel′lae** [NA], diaphragm of sella turcica: a ring-shaped fold of dura mater covering the sella turcica, and containing an aperture for passage of the infundibulum of the hypophysis. **d. urogenita′le,** urogenital diaphragm: traditional but no longer valid concept that superior and inferior fascial layers enclose the sphincter urethrae and deep transverse perineal muscles and together form a musculomembranous sheet that extends between the ischiopubic rami. Called also *accessory* or *secondary diaphragm, Camper's ligament, deep fascia of perineum* or *deep perineal fascia,* and *fascia of urogenital trigone.* See also *membrana perinei.*

diaphragmalgia (di″ah-frag-mal′je-ah) [*diaphragm* + Gr. *algos* pain + *-ia*] pain in the diaphragm.

diaphragmata (di″ah-frag′mah-tah) [Gr.] plural of *diaphragma.*

diaphragmatic (di″ah-frag-mat′ik) pertaining to or of the nature of a diaphragm.

diaphragmatitis (di″ah-frag″mah-ti′tis) diaphragmitis.

diaphragmatocele (di″ah-frag-mat′o-sēl) [*diaphragm* + Gr. *kēlē* hernia] diaphragmatic hernia.

diaphragmitis (di″ah-frag-mi′tis) inflammation of the diaphragm.

diaphragmodynia (di″ah-frag″mo-din′e-ah) [*diaphragm* + Gr. *odynē* pain] diaphragmalgia.

diaphysary (di-af′ĭ-zār-e) diaphyseal.

diaphyseal (di″ah-fiz′e-al) pertaining to or affecting the shaft of a long bone (diaphysis).

diaphysectomy (di″ah-fiz-ek′to-me) [*diaphysis* + Gr. *ektomē* excision] excision of a portion of the shaft of a long bone.

diaphyses (di-af′ĭ-sēz) [Gr.] plural of *diaphysis.*

diaphysial (di″ah-fiz′e-al) diaphyseal.

diaphysis (di-af′ĭ-sis), pl. *diaph′yses* [Gr. "the point of separation between stalk and branch"] 1. [NA] the elongated cylindrical portion (the shaft) of a long bone, between the ends or extremities (the epiphyses), which are usually articular and wider than the shaft; it consists of a tube of compact bone, enclosing the medullary (marrow) cavity. Called also *shaft.* 2. the portion of a long bone formed from a primary center of ossification.

diaphysitis (di″ah-fiz-i′tis) inflammation of a diaphysis. **tuberculous d.,** inflammation involving intermediate segments of the shafts of long bones, caused by the tubercle bacillus.

Diapid (di′ah-pid) trademark for a preparation of lypressin.

diapiresis (di″ah-pi-re′sis) [Gr. *diapeirein* to drive through] diapedesis.

diaplacental (di″ah-plah-sen′tal) through the placenta.

diapophysis (di-ah-pof′ĭ-sis) [*dia-* + Gr. *apophysis* outgrowth] the superior or articular part of a transverse process of a vertebra.

Diaptomus (di-ap′to-mus) a genus of copepod crustaceans, species of which act as hosts of the larvae of *Diphyllobothrium latum.*

diapyesis (di″ah-pi-e′sis) suppuration.

diapyetic (di″ah-pi-et′ik) promoting suppuration.

diarrhea (di″ah-re′ah) [*dia-* + Gr. *rhein* to flow] abnormal frequency and liquidity of fecal discharges. **bovine virus d.,** an infectious disease of cattle caused by a togavirus (genus *Pestivirus*) marked by ulceration and hemorrhage of the alimentary tract with diarrhea and dehydration. **cachectic d.,** diarrhea associated with cachexia; it may be due to malabsorption, or both the diarrhea and the cachexia may be manifestations of an underlying disease, e.g., neoplasm. **choleraic d.,** acute diarrhea with serous stools, accompanied by circulatory collapse, thus resembling cholera. **chronic bacillary d.,** Johne's disease. **d. chylo′sa,** diarrhea in which the discharge consists of a yellowish white, mucopurulent substance that resembles chyle in gross appearance. **Cochin-China d.,** 1. sprue (def. 1). 2. strongyloidiasis. **colliquative d.,** profuse diarrhea, producing a state of dehydration, sometimes seen in the late stages of pulmonary tuberculosis. **congenital chloride d.,** familial chloride d. **crapulous d.,** that due to excess in eating or drinking. **critical d.,** diarrhea occurring at the crisis of a disease or producing a crisis. **dientameba d.,** a mild though chronic diarrhea caused by infection with *Dientamoeba fragilis.* **dysenteric d.,** diarrhea with mucous and bloody stools. **enteral d.,** diarrhea due to infection within the gastrointestinal tract. **epidemic d. of newborn,** a contagious diarrhea occurring in epidemics among newborn infants in hospitals; called also *neonatal d.* **familial chloride d.,** severe watery diarrhea with an excess of chloride in the stool, beginning in early infancy and marked by distended abdomen, lethargy, and retarded growth and mental development. It is accompanied by alkalosis and hypokalemia, and maternal hydramnios is often associated. The disorder is due to impairment of chloride-bicarbonate exchange in the lower bowel. Called also *congenital chloride d.* and *familial chloridorrhea.* **fermental d., fermentative d.,** diarrhea caused by fermentation due to microorganisms. **flagellate d.,** diarrhea marked by the presence of flagellate organisms (*Giardia*) in the stools. **gastrogenic d.,** diarrhea due to gastric disorder. **hill d.,** a chronic diarrhea peculiar to hot climates and occurring only at elevations of several thousand feet; named from the hill districts of India; it is considered by some to be identical with sprue. **infantile d.,** summer diarrhea. **inflammatory d.,** diarrhea in which there is an inflammation of the intestine due to bacterial action. **irritative d.,** diarrhea due to irritation of the intestine by improper food, poisons, purgatives, etc. **lienteric d.,** diarrhea with fluid stools containing undigested food. **mechanical d.,** diarrhea due to mechanical obstruction to the portal circulation, producing gastrointestinal hyperemia. **morning d.,** a condition marked by diarrhea in the morning only. **mucous d.,** a kind characterized by the presence of mucus in stools. **neonatal d.,** epidemic diarrhea of the newborn. **osmotic d.,** diarrhea resulting from the presence of osmotically active nonabsorbable solutes, e.g., magnesium sulfate, in the intestine. **d. pancreat′ica,** the diarrhea that accompanies parenchymatous degeneration or cystic disease of the pancreas. **pancreatogenous fatty d.,** a diarrhea in which the stools contain an excessive amount of fat owing to dysfunction of the pancreas. **paradoxical d.,** stercoral d. **parenteral d.,** diarrhea due to infections outside the gastrointestinal tract, such as tuberculosis, syphilis, etc. **putrefactive d.,** diarrhea due to putrefaction of the intestinal contents. **serous d.,** discharge of feces softened by copious serous fluid; called also *watery d.* **stercoral d.,** diarrhea accompanied by colic and following two or three days of constipation; called also *paradoxical d.* **summer d.,** acute diarrhea in children during great heat of summer; called also *infantile d.* **traveler's d.,** diarrhea occurring among travelers, particularly in those visiting tropical or subtropical areas where sanitation is suboptimal; it is caused by many different infectious agents, the most common being enterotoxigenic *Escherichia coli.* In Mexico, it is also called *turista.* **trench d.,** a form of diarrhea and dysentery that occurred in troops in the trenches. **tropical d.,** see *sprue*; def. 1. **tubercular d.,** a variety of diarrhea peculiar to cases of tuberculosis. **virus d.,** a specific infectious condition manifested by diarrhea in infants and by stomatitis and diarrhea in older children. **watery d.,** serous d. **white d.,** an infectious disease of young chickens marked by loss of appetite, dullness, and diarrhea, the discharges of which leave white lumps around the cloaca; it is caused by *Salmonella pullorum.* Called also *pullorum disease.*

diarrheal (di″ah-re′al) pertaining to or marked by diarrhea.

diarrheic (di″ah-re′ik) diarrheal.

diarrheogenic (di″ah-re″o-jen′ik) [*diarrhea* + Gr. *gennan* to produce] giving rise to diarrhea.

diarthric (di-ar′thrik) [*di-* + Gr. *arthron* a joint] pertaining to or affecting two different joints.

diarthrodial (di″ar-thro′di-al) of the nature of a diarthrosis.

diarthroses (di″ar-thro′sēz) plural of *diarthrosis*.

diarthrosis (di″ar-thro′sis), pl. *diarthroses* [Gr. *diarthrōsis* a movable articulation] a specialized articulation permitting more or less free movement; a synovial joint. See *articulationes synoviales* [NA]. **d. rotato′ria,** a joint characterized by mobility in a rotary direction.

diarticular (di″ar-tik′u-lar) diarthric.

diaschisis (di-as′kĭ-sis) [*dia-* + Gr. *schizein* to split] the loss of function and electrical activity caused by cerebral lesions in areas which are remote from the lesion but which are neuronally connected to it; called also *Monakow's theory.*

diascope (di′ah-skōp) [*dia-* + Gr. *skopein* to examine] a glass or clear plastic plate, usually a flat blade or microscope slide, pressed against the skin to permit observation of changes produced in the underlying skin after the blood vessels are emptied and the skin is blanched.

diascopy (di-as′ko-pe) 1. examination with the diascope. 2. transillumination.

Diasone (di′ah-sōn) trademark for a preparation of sulfoxone sodium.

diasostic (di″ah-sos′tik) hygienic.

diaspironecrobiosis (di-as″pi-ro-nek″ro-bi-o′sis) [*dia-* + Gr. *speirein* to sow + *necrobiosis*] disseminated necrobiosis.

diaspironecrosis (di-as″pi-ro-ne-kro′sis) disseminated necrosis.

diastalsis (di″ah-stal′sis) [*dia-* + Gr. *stalsis* contraction] (*obs.*) a downward moving wave of contraction with a preceding wave of inhibition occurring in the digestive tube.

diastaltic (di″ah-stal′tik) (*obs.*) 1. pertaining to diastalsis. 2. performed reflexly; reflex.

diastase (di′ah-stās) 1. a mixture of amylolytic enzymes from malt, used to convert starch into simple sugars. 2. (*obs.*) α- or β-amalase.

diastasic (di″as-ta′sik) diastatic.

diastasis (di-as′tah-sis) [Gr.] 1. a form of dislocation in which there is separation of two bones normally attached to each other without the existence of a true joint; as in separation of the pubic symphysis. Also, separation beyond the normal between associated bones, as between the ribs, or the ulna and radius. 2. diastasis cordis. Called also *divarication.* **d. cor′dis,** the rest period of the cardiac cycle, which occurs just before systole. **iris d.,** iridodiastasis. **d. rec′ti abdom′inis,** separation of the rectus muscles of the abdominal wall, sometimes occurring during pregnancy.

diastasuria (di″ah-stās-u′re-ah) the presence of diastase in the urine.

diastatic (di″ah-stat′ik) 1. pertaining to diastase. 2. pertaining to diastasis.

diastem (di′ah-stem) diastema.

diastema (di″ah-ste′mah), pl. *diaste′mata* [Gr. *diastēma* an interval] 1. a space or cleft. 2. [NA] a space between two adjacent teeth in the same dental arch. 3. a narrow zone in the equatorial plane through which the cytosome divides in mitosis. **anterior d.,** a space between the incisor teeth, generally one between the maxillary central incisors.

diastemata (di″ah-stem′ah-tah) [Gr.] pl. of *diastema.*

diastematocrania (di″ah-stem″ah-to-kra′ne-ah) [Gr. *diastēma* an interval + *kranion* cranium] congenital longitudinal fissure of the cranium.

diastematomyelia (di″ah-stem″ah-to-mi-e′le-ah) [Gr. *diastēma* an interval + *myelos* marrow] a congenital defect, often associated with spina bifida, in which the spinal cord is split into halves by a bony spicule or fibrous band, each half being surrounded by a dural sac.

diastematopyelia (di″ah-stem″ah-to-pi-e′le-ah) [Gr.

diastēma an interval + *pyelos* pelvis] congenital median fissure of the pelvis.

diaster (di′as-ter) [*di-* two + Gr. *astēr* star] amphiaster.

diastereoisomer (di″ah-ster″e-o-i′so-mer) diastereomer.

diastereoisomeric (di″ah-ster″e-o-i″so-mer′ik) exhibiting diastereoisomerism.

diastereoisomerism (di″ah-ster″e-o″i-som′er-izm) the relationship between two or more stereoisomers whose molecules are not mirror images of each other, e.g., glucose and galactose or *cis* and *trans* isomers.

diastereomer (di″ah-ster′e-o-mer) one of a group of compounds having a disastereoisomeric relationship.

Diastix (di′ah-stiks) trademark for a reagent strip designed for the quantitative determination of glucose in urine.

diastole (di-as′to-le) [Gr. *diastolē* a drawing asunder; expansion] the dilatation, or period of dilatation, of the heart, especially of the ventricles; it coincides with the interval between the second and the first heart sound.

diastolic (di″ah-stol′ik) of or pertaining to the diastole.

diastomyelia (di-as″to-mi-e′le-ah) diastematomyelia.

diastrophic (di″-ah-strof′ik) [Gr. *diastrephein* distortion] bent or curved; said of structures, such as bones, deformed in such manner.

diataxia (di″ah-tak′se-ah) [*di-* two + *ataxia*] ataxia affecting both sides of the body. **cerebral d., d. cerebra′lis infanti′lis,** infantile cerebral ataxic paralysis.

diathermal (di″ah-ther′mal) pertaining to diathermy; heated by high-frequency electromagnetic radiation.

diathermic (di″ah-ther′mik) pertaining to diathermy; permeable to high-frequency electromagnetic radiation.

diathermy (di′ah-ther″me) [*dia-* + Gr. *thermē* heat] heating of the body tissues due to their resistance to the passage of high-frequency electromagnetic radiation, electric currents, or ultrasonic waves. In *medical d.* (thermopenetration) the tissues are warmed but not damaged; in *surgical d.* (electrocoagulation) tissue is destroyed. **short wave d.,** the therapeutic heating of the body tissues by means of an oscillating electromagnetic field of high frequency; the frequency varies from 10 million to 100 million cycles per second and the wavelength from 30 to 3 meters. **ultrashort wave d.,** diathermy in which the wavelength used is less than 10 meters.

diathesis (di-ath′ĕ-sis) [Gr. "arrangement, disposition"] a constitution or condition of the body which makes the tissues react in special ways to certain extrinsic stimuli and thus tends to make the person more than usually susceptible to certain diseases. Cf. *constitution* (def. 1) and *type.* **gouty d.,** predisposition to gout; status arthriticus. **hemorrhagic d.,** a predisposition to abnormal hemostasis.

diathetic (di″ah-thet′ik) of or pertaining to a diathesis.

diatom (di′ah-tom) any unicellular microscopical form of alga having a wall of silica and belonging to the family Diatomaceae. Several species are toxic, causing the "red blooms" or "red tides." The skeletal siliceous remains of many others are mined from deposits and used as filtering and abrasive agents; see *infusorial earth,* under *earth.*

diatomaceous (di″ah-to-ma′shus) composed of diatoms; said of earth composed of the siliceous skeletons of diatoms. See *infusorial earth,* under *earth.*

diatomic (di″ah-tom′ik) [*di-* + *atom*] 1. made up of two atoms. 2. dibasic. 3. diatomaceous.

diatrizoate (di″ah-tri-zo′āt) the most commonly used water-soluble, iodinated, radiopaque x-ray contrast medium; used as *diatrizoate meglumine* [USP] and *diatrizoate sodium* [USP] for all types of angiography; for splenoportography, hysterosalpingography, and arthrography; for cystography and intravenous and retrograde urography; for intravenous, operative, T-tube, and percutaneous transhepatic cholangiography; and for gastrointestinal tract studies. **d. meglumine** [USP], a radiopaque medium, ($C_7H_{17}NO_5 \cdot C_{11}H_9I_3 N_2O_4$), available in solution, consisting of diatrizoate meglumine in water for injection or of diatrizoic acid in water for injection, prepared with the aid of meglumine; used intra-arterially in angiocardiography, aortography, cerebral angiography, and peripheral arteriography, intravenously in angiocardiography, excretory urography, and venography, and unilaterally in retrograde pyelography. **d. sodium** [USP], a radiopaque medium, $C_{11}H_8I_3N_2NaO_4$, available in solution, consisting of diatrizoate sodium in water for injection or of diatrizoic acid in water for injection, prepared with the aid of sodium hydroxide; used in cholangiography, intravenously in excretory urography, hysterosalpingography, and unilaterally in retrograde pyelography.

diatrizoic acid (di″ah-tri-zo′ik) [USP] chemical name: 3,5-bis(acetylamino)-2,4,6-triiodobenzoic acid. A white powder, $C_{11}H_9I_3N_2O_4$, used in the preparation of certain radiopaque media (see *diatrizoate meglumine* and *diatrizoate sodium*).

diauchenos (di-awk′ĕ-nos) a dicephalic monster with two necks.

diauxic (di-awk′sik) pertaining to or characterized by diauxie; implying two periods of growth separated by a lag period.

diauxie (di-awk′se) [*di-* + Gr. *auxein* to increase in size] a phenomenon of bacterial growth in which an organism given a mixture of organic compounds first grows exclusively on one until that compound is exhausted, and then, after a lag during which it forms induced enzymes for utilizing the second compound, resumes growth on the latter.

diaveridine (di″ah-ver′ĭ-dēn) chemical name: 5-[(3,4-dimethoxyphenyl)methyl]-2,4-pyrimidinediamine. An antiprotozoal and antibacterial, $C_{16}H_{19}ClN_2O$; used as a coccidiostat in poultry.

diaxon (di-ak′son) [*di-* + *axon*] a nerve cell having two axons or axis-cylinder processes.

diaxone (di-ak′sōn) diaxon.

diazepam (di-az′ĕ-pam) [USP] chemical name: 7-chloro-1,3-dihydro-1-methyl-5-phenyl-2*H*-1,4-benzodiazepin-2-one. One of the benzodiazepine tranquilizers, $C_{16}H_{13}ClN_2O$, occurring as an off-white to yellow, crystalline powder. It is administered orally, intravenously, or intramuscularly as a sedative, and is also used as a skeletal muscle relaxant, to produce anesthesia, as an anticonvulsant, and in the management of alcohol withdrawal symptoms and delirium tremens.

diazine (di-az′in) any compound containing a ring of four carbon and two nitrogen atoms.

diazo- (di-az′o) a prefix indicating possession of the group —N═N—.

diazobenzene (di-az″o-ben′zēn) a univalent organic radical, $C_6H_5N_2$.

diazobenzenesulfonic acid (di-az″o-ben″zēn-sul-fon′ik) chemical name: *p*-sulfobenzenediazonium hydroxide inner salt. White or slightly red crystals, $C_6H_4N_2O_3S$, prepared by the diazotization of sulfanilic acid and used in Ehrlich's diazo reaction.

diazoma (di″ah-zo′mah) [Gr. *diazōma* that which is put round] the diaphragm.

diazomethane (di-az″o-meth′ān) an extremely poisonous yellow gas, N_2CH_2, used in organic synthesis.

diazonal (di″ah-zo′nal) 1. situated across or bridging two zones. 2. pertaining to a diazone.

diazone (di′ah-zōn) one of the dark bands that alternate with light bands (parazones) to form the lines of Schreger, which are seen under reflected light in a ground section of a tooth; believed to be an area in which the enamel prisms have been cut in cross section.

diazosulfobenzol (di-az″o-sul′fo-ben′zol) a substance which acts upon certain principles in the urine to form aniline colors.

diazotization (di-az″o-ti-za′shun) conversion into a diazo compound.

diazotize (di-az′o-tīz) to introduce the diazo group into a compound.

diazoxide (di-az-ok′sīd) [USP] chemical name: 7-chloro-3-methyl-2*H*-1,2,4-benzothiadiazine. An antihypertensive, $C_8H_7ClN_2O_2S$, structurally related to chlorothiazide but having no diuretic properties, occurring as white or cream-colored crystals or crystalline powder; administered intravenously. Because it inhibits release of insulin, it is also administered orally in the treatment of hypoglycemia due to hyperinsulinism.

dibasic (di-bā′sik) [*di-* + Gr. *basis* base] containing two hydrogen atoms replaceable by bases, and thus yielding two series of salts, as H_2SO_4.

Dibenamine (di-ben′ah-mēn) trademark for a preparation of dibenzylchlorethamine.

dibenzanthracene (di-benz-an′thrah-sēn) an aromatic polycyclic hydrocarbon, $C_{22}H_{14}$, capable, when injected into the body, of producing epithelial tumors. Abbreviated DBA.

dibenz-dibutyl anthraquinol (di-benz″di-bu′til an″-thrah-kwin′ol) a carcinogenic and estrogenic substance, 1,2,5,6,-dibenz-9,10,di-n-butyl anthraquinol.

dibenzepin hydrochloride (di-benz′ĕ-pin) chemical name: 10-[2-(dimethylamino)ethyl]-5,10-dihydro-5-methyl-11*H*-dibenzo[*b*,*e*][1,4]diazepin-11-one monohydrochloride; a tricyclic antidepressant, $C_{18}H_{21}N_3O·HCl$.

dibenzothiazine (di-ben″zo-thi′ah-zēn) phenothiazine.

dibenzoxazepine (di-benz″oks-az′ĕ-pēn) any of a class of structurally related drugs containing the antipsychotic agent loxapine and the antidepressant amoxapine.

dibenzylchlorethamine (di″ben-zil-klōr-eth′ah-mēn) chemical name: N-(2-chloroethyl)dibenzylamine. An alpha-adrenergic blocking agent, $C_{16}H_{18}ClN$, which has been used in the treatment of peripheral vascular disorders and in the diagnosis of pheochromocytoma.

Dibenzyline (di-ben′zĭ-lēn) trademark for a preparation of phenoxybenzamine hydrochloride.

diblastula (di-blas′tu-lah) [*di-* + *blastula*] a blastula in which the ectoderm and entoderm are both present.

dibothriocephaliasis (di-both″re-o-sef″ah-li′ah-sis) diphyllobothriasis.

Dibothriocephalus (di-both″re-o-sef′ah-lus) [*di-* + Gr. *bothrion* pit + *kephalē* head] *Diphyllobothrium*.

dibrachia (di-bra′ke-ah) [*di-* + Gr. *brachion* arm] a developmental anomaly characterized by duplication of an arm.

dibrachius (di-bra′ke-us) a twin monster having only two arms.

dibromide (di-bro′mīd) any bromide which combines two atoms of bromine with one of another element or radical.

dibromoketone (di-bro″mo-ke′tōn) methyl dibromoethyl ketone, $CH_3COCHBrCH_2Br$, a war gas.

dibromsalan (di-brom′sah-lan) chemical name: 5-bromo-N-(4-bromophenyl)-2-hydroxybenzamide. A disinfectant with antibacterial and antifungal activities, $C_{13}H_9Br_2NO_2$, used mainly in medicated soaps.

dibucaine (di′bu-kān) [USP] chemical name: 2-butoxy-N-[2-(diethylamino)ethyl]-4-quinolinecarboxamide. A potent local anesthetic, $C_{20}H_{29}N_3O_2$, occurring as a white to off-white powder; applied topically to the skin and mucous membranes. **d. hydrochloride** [USP], the monohydrochloride salt of dibucaine, $C_{20}H_{29}N_2O_2·HCl$, occurring as colorless or white to off-white crystals or as a white to off-white, crystalline powder, having the same actions as the base; administered in the form of an aerosol spray to produce anesthesia of the skin and mucous membranes or injected into the subarachnoid space to produce spinal anesthesia.

Dibuline (di′bu-lēn) trademark for a preparation of dibutoline sulfate.

dibutoline sulfate (di-bu′to-lēn) chemical name: bis[ethyl(2-hydroxyethyl)dimethylammonium]sulfate bis(dibutylcarbamate). A quaternary ammonium anticholinergic, $C_{30}H_{66}N_4O_8S$, used as a cycloplegic and gastrointestinal antispasmodic, administered intramuscularly or subcutaneously.

dibutyl (di-būt′il) a hydrocarbon, C_8H_{18}, occurring in mineral oil.

DIC abbreviation for disseminated intravascular coagulation.

dicacodyl (di-kak′o-dīl) cacodyl.

dicalcic (di-kal′sik) having in each molecule two atoms of calcium.

dicalcium phosphate (di-kal′se-um fos′fāt) dibasic calcium phosphate; see under *calcium*.

dicamphendion (di″kam-fen′de-on) a substance, $(C_{10}H_{14}O)_2$, obtained by the action of metallic sodium upon bromocamphor, dicamphor being produced at the same time.

dicamphor (di-kam′for) a principle in colorless needles, $(C_{10}H_{15}O)_2$, produced at the same time and from the same materials as dicamphendion.

dicarbonate (di-kar′bon-āt) bicarbonate.

dicelous (di-se′lus) [*di-* + Gr. *koilos* hollow] 1. hollowed on both sides. 2. having two cavities. 3. amphicelous.

dicentric (di-sen′trik) [*di-* + *center*] in genetics, a structurally abnormal chromosome with two centromeres.

dicephalous (di-sef'ah-lus) having two heads.

dicephalus (di-sef'ah-lus) [*di-* + Gr. *kephalē* head] a monster with two heads. **d. di'pus dibra'chius,** a monster with two heads but only two feet and two arms. **d. di'pus tetrabra'chius,** a monster with only two legs, but with varying degrees of fusion of the upper trunk, each component having a head and pair of arms. **d. di'pus tribra'chius,** a monster with two heads, two feet, but with a median third arm or arm rudiment. **d. dipy'gus,** anakatadidymus. **d. parasit'icus,** desmiognathus. **d. tri'pus tribra'chius,** a monster with a common trunk, but with two heads, three arms, and three legs, the third limbs being either rudimentary or complete.

dicephaly (di-sef'ah-le) a developmental anomaly characterized by the presence of two heads.

dicheilia (di-ki'le-ah) the appearance of a double lip, owing to folding of the oral mucosa.

dicheiria (di-ki're-ah) [*di-* + Gr. *cheir* hand] a developmental anomaly characterized by duplication of a hand.

dicheirus (di-ki'rus) an individual exhibiting dicheiria.

dichlordioxydiamidoarsenobenzol (di-klor''di-ok''se-di-am''ĭ-do-ar''sĕ-no-ben'zol) arsphenamine.

dichlorhydrin (di''klor-hi'drin) a colorless fluid, CH_2Cl·$CHOH$·CH_2Cl, used as a solvent for resins and prepared by heating anhydrous glycerin with sulfur monochloride.

dichloride (di-klo'rīd) a combination of a base or a metal with two atoms of chlorine.

dichlorisone (di-klōr'ĭ-sōn) chemical name: 9,11β-dichloro-17,21-dihydroxy pregna-1,4-diene-3,20-dione. A glucocorticoid, $C_{21}H_{26}Cl_2O_4$, used in the treatment of steroid-responsive pruritic or allergic inflammations, applied topically.

dichlorodiethyl sulfide (di-klo''ro-di-eth'il) chemical name: 1,1'-thiobis[2-chloroethane]. Mustard gas, $(CH_2Cl$-$CH_2)_2S$, a vesicant gas once employed in war. It produces blistering and subsequent sloughing of the skin with involvement of the eyes and respiratory tract. Death results from bronchopneumonia. Called also *yellow cross* and *yperite*.

dichlorodifluoromethane (di-klo''ro-di-floor''o-meth'ān) [NF] a clear, colorless gas with a faint, ethereal odor, CCl_2F_2, used as an aerosol propellant, and also as a refrigerant.

dichloroformoxime (di-klo''ro-for-mok'sim) a suffocating war gas, CCl_2:N·OH; called also *phosgene oxime*.

dichloroisoproterenol (di-klo''ro-i''so-pro-ter'ĕ-nol) chemical name: 3,4-dichloro-α-(isopropylaminomethyl)benzyl alcohol. A beta-adrenergic blocking agent, $C_{11}H_{15}Cl_2NO$, used in the treatment of various cardiac disorders.

dichlorophen (di-klor'o-fen) an anthelmintic effective against the large tapeworms of cats and dogs (*Taenia saginata* and *T. solium*).

2,4-dichlorophenoxyacetic acid (di-klor''o-fen-ok''se-ah-se'tik) 2,4-D.

dichlorotetrafluoroethane (di-klo''ro-tet''rah-floor''o-eth'ān) [NF] chemical name: 1,2-dichlorotetrafluoroethane. A clear, colorless gas with a faint ethereal odor, $CClF_2$-$CClF_2$, used as an aerosol propellant.

dichlorphenamide (di''klōr-fen'ah-mīd) [USP], a carbonic anhydrase inhibitor; used in the treatment of glaucoma.

dichlorvos (di-klor'vos) chemical name: phosphoric acid 2,2-dichloroethenyl dimethyl ester; an organophorous insecticide and anthelmintic, $C_4H_7Cl_2O_4P$.

dichogeny (di-koj'ĕ-ne) [Gr. *dicha* in two + *gennan* to produce] development of tissues in different ways in accordance with changes in conditions affecting them.

dichorial (di-ko're-al) dichorionic.

dichorionic (di''ko-re-on'ik) having two distinct chorions; said of dizygotic twins.

dichotomization (di-kot''ŏ-mi-za'shun) dichotomy.

dichotomy (di-kot'o-me) [Gr. *dicha* in two + *tomē* a cutting] the process or result of division into two parts.

dichroic (di-kro'ik) exhibiting dichroism.

dichroine (di-kro'ēn) an alkaloid from Ch'ang Shan, the root of the shrub *Dichroa febrifuga* Lour. (Saxifragaceae), having three isomeric forms α-, β-, and γ-dichroine.

dichroism (di'kro-izm) [*di-* + Gr. *chroa* color] the quality or condition of presenting one color in reflected and another in transmitted light.

dichromasy (di-kro'mah-se) [*di-* + Gr. *chrōma* color] a defect in color vision in which one of the three cone pigments is missing altogether. The most common forms are protanopia and deuteranopia, each of which is transmitted by X-linked inheritance and affects about 1 per cent of white males. The third form, tritanopia, is very rare; and a fourth, tetartanopia, is of doubtful existence.

dichromat (di'kro-mat) a person with dichromasy.

dichromate (di-kro'māt) any salt containing the bivalent Cr_2O_7 radical.

dichromatic (di''kro-mat'ik) pertaining to or characterized by dichromasy.

dichromatism (di-kro'mah-tism) 1. the quality of existing in or exhibiting two different colors. 2. dichromasy.

dichromatopsia (di''kro-mah-top'se-ah) dichromasy.

dichromic (di-kro'mik) pertaining to two colors.

dichromophil (di-kro'mo-fil) amphophilic; also, an amphophilic element.

dichromophilism (di''kro-mof'ĭ-lizm) capacity for double staining, that is, with both acid and basic dyes.

dick (dik) a vesicant war gas, ethyldichlorarsine, C_2H_5·As-Cl_2, causing sneezing and pulmonary edema.

Dick test (reaction), toxin (dik) [George Frederick *Dick*, 1881–1967, and Gladys Rowena Henry *Dick*, 1881–1963, American physicians] see *tests*, and see *erythrogenic toxin*, under *toxin*.

dicliditis (dik''lĭ-di'tis) [Gr. *diklis* double door + *-itis*] (*obs.*) inflammation of a valve, especially one of the heart valves.

diclidostosis (dik''lid-os-to'sis) [Gr. *diklis* double door + *osteon* bone + *-osis*] ossification of the valves of the veins.

diclofenac sodium (di-klo'fen-ak) chemical name: 2-[(2,6-dichlorophenyl)amino]benzeneacetic acid monosodium salt. An analgesic, antipyretic, and anti-inflammatory, $C_{14}H_{10}Cl_2NNaO_2$, used in the treatment of rheumatic and other inflammatory disorders.

dicloralurea (di''klor-al'u-re'ah) chemical name: *N,N'*-bis(2,2,2-trichloro-1-hydroxyethyl)urea; a food additive for animal feed, $C_5H_6Cl_6N_2O_3$.

dicloxacillin sodium (di-kloks''ah-sil'in) [USP] chemical name: [2S-(2α,5α,6β)]-6[[[3-(2,6-dichlorophenyl)-5-methyl-4-isoxazolyl]carbonyl]amino]-3,3-dimethyl-7-oxo-4-thia-1-azabicyclo[3.2.0]heptane-2-carboxylic acid monosodium salt monohydrate. A semisynthetic penicillinase-resistant penicillin, $C_{19}H_{16}Cl_2N_3NaO_5S$·$H_2O$, occurring as a white to off-white, crystalline powder; used primarily in the treatment of infections due to penicillinase-resistant staphylococci, administered orally. It is also available as *sterile dicloxacillin sodium* [USP].

Dicodid (di-ko'did) trademark for preparations of hydrocodone bitartrate.

dicoelous (di-se'lus) [*di-* + Gr. *koilos* hollow] 1. hollowed on each of two sides. 2. having two cavities.

dicotyledon (di-kot''ĭ-le'don) [Gr. *dis* twice + *kotylēdon* a cup-shaped hollow] a flowering plant with embryos having two seed leaves, or cotyledons.

dicoumarin (di-koo'mah-rin) dicumarol.

dicroceliasis (dik''ro-se-li'ah-sis) infection with *Dicrocoelium*.

Dicrocoelium (dik''ro-se'le-um) [Gr. *dikroos* forked + *koilia* bowel] a genus of trematodes. **D. dendrit'icum,** a lancet-shaped fluke infesting the liver of cattle and sheep in Europe, North and South America, and northern Africa; it has been found in the human bilary passages. **D. hos'pes,** a species found in the gallbladder of cattle in the Sudan. **D. lanceola'tum,** *D. dendriticum.* **D. macrosto'mum,** a species found in the gallbladder of guinea fowl in Egypt.

dicrotic (di-krot'ik) [Gr. *dikrotos* double beating] pertaining to or characterized by dicrotism, as the dicrotic notch.

dicrotism (di'krŏ-tizm) the quality of having two sphygmographic waves or elevations to one beat of the pulse.

dicty(o)- [Gr. *diktyon* net] a combining form denoting a relationship to a net or to a netlike structure.

Dictyocaulus (dik″te-o-kaw′lus) [dictyo- + Gr. kaulos stalk] a genus of nematode parasites of the bronchial tree of horses, sheep, goats, deer, and cattle. **D. fila′ria,** a species that infects the bronchial tree of sheep, goats, and cattle, and causes hoose; called also *Strongylus filaria.* **D. vivipa′-rus,** a species that infects the bronchial tree of cattle and deer, and causes hoose; called also *Strongylus micrurus.*

Dictyocha (dik″te-o′kah) a genus of plantlike, flagellate marine protozoa (order Silicoflagellida, class Phytomastigophorea) having one flagellum, golden-brown or green-brown chloroplasts, and a star-shaped siliceous skeleton.

dictyokinesis (dik″te-o-ki-ne′sis) [dictyo- + kinesis] the migration and distribution of the dictyosomes to the daughter cells in mitosis.

dictyoma (dik″te-o′mah) [dicty- + -oma] diktyoma.

dictyosome (dik′te-o-sōm) [dictyo- + Gr. soma body] a stack of membranous lamellae or cisternae with attached tubules and vesicles in the cytoplasm of various cells; see also *Golgi complex,* under complex.

Dictyosteliia (dik″te-o-stĕ-li′e-ah) [dictyo- + Gr. stechelo stem] a subclass of protozoa (class Eumycetozoea, superclass Rhizopoda) that feed on bacteria, characterized by the formation of a multicellular pseudoplasmodium by aggregation of myxamebae that gives rise to a multispored fruiting body with a stalk tube. It includes one order: Dictyosteliida.

Dictyosteliida (dik″te-o-stĕ-li′ĭ-dah) an order of ameboid protozoa with characters of the subclass (subclass Dictyosteliia, class Eumycetozoea).

dictyotene (dik′te-o-tēn) [dictyo- + -tene] the protracted stage resembling suspended prophase in which the primary oocyte persists from late fetal life until discharged from the ovary at or after puberty.

dicumarol (di-koo′mah-rol) [USP] chemical name: 3,3′-methylenebis[4-hydroxy-2H-1-benzopyran-2-one]. One of the coumarin anticoagulants, $C_{19}H_{12}O_6$, occurring as a white or creamy white, crystalline powder, originally isolated from spoiled sweet clover but now produced synthetically; it acts by inhibiting the hepatic synthesis of vitamin K–dependent coagulation factors (prothrombin, Factors II, VII, IX, and X); administered orally. It is the etiologic agent of the hemorrhagic disease in animals known as *sweet clover disease.* Called also *bishydroxycoumarin* and *dicoumarin.*

Dicurin (di-kur′in) trademark for a preparation of merethoxylline.

dicyclic (di-si′klik) pertaining to or having two cycles; in chemistry, having a molecular structure containing two rings.

dicyclomine hydrochloride (di-si′klo-mēn) [USP] chemical name: [bicyclohexyl]-1-carboxylic acid 2-(diethylamino)ethyl ester. An anticholinergic, $C_{19}H_{35}NO_2 \cdot HCl$, occurring as a fine, white, crystalline powder; used as an antispasmodic in the treatment of functional gastrointestinal disorders, administered orally or intramuscularly.

dicysteine (di″sis-te′in) cystine.

didactic (di-dak′tik) [Gr. didaktikos] conveying instruction by lectures and books rather than by practice.

didactylism (di-dak′til-izm) [di- + Gr. daktylos finger] the condition of having only two digits on a hand or foot.

didactylous (di-dak′tĭ-lus) having only two digits on a hand or foot.

didelphia (di-del′fe-ah) [di- + Gr. delphys uterus] the condition characterized by presence of a double uterus.

didelphic (di-del′fik) pertaining to or possessing a double uterus.

Didelphis (di-del′fis) [di- + Gr. delphys uterus] a genus of marsupials, the opossums, species of which are reservoirs of *Trypanosoma cruzi* in South America.

didermoma (di″der-mo′mah) bidermoma.

Didrex (di′dreks) trademark for a preparation of benzphetamine hydrochloride.

Didronel (di-dro′nel) trademark for preparations of etidronate disodium.

didymalgia (did″ĭ-mal′je-ah) orchialgia.

didymitis (did″ĭ-mi′tis) orchitis.

didymodynia (did″ĭ-mo-din′e-ah) orchialgia.

didymous (did′ĭ-mus) occurring in pairs.

didymus (did′ĭ-mus) [Gr. didymos double, twofold, twain] a testis. Sometimes used as a word termination to designate a

fetus with a duplication of parts or one consisting of conjoined symmetrical twins. See also *-pagus.*

die (di) 1. a form to be used in the construction of something. 2. a positive reproduction of the form of a prepared tooth in a suitable hard substance, such as a metal or a specially prepared artificial stone. **amalgam d.,** a model of a tooth made of amalgam; used in making dental prostheses. **electroformed d.,** a die formed by electroplating an impression, forming a metallic positive reproduction of a prepared tooth. Often called incorrectly *electroplated d.* or *plated d.* **electroplated d.,** electroformed d. **plated d.,** electroformed d. **waxing d.,** a die or model to which wax is adapted for the fabrication of a wax pattern.

Dieb. alt. abbreviation for L. *die′bus alter′nis,* on alternate days.

Dieb. tert. abbreviation for L. *die′bus ter′tiis,* every third day.

diechoscope (di-ek′o-skōp) [di- + Gr. ēchō echo + skopein to examine] an instrument for the simultaneous perception of two different sounds in auscultation.

diecious (di-e′shus) [di- + Gr. oikos house] sexually distinct; denoting species in which male and female genitals do not occur in the same individual. In botany, having staminate and pistillate flowers on separate plants.

Dieffenbach's operation (de′fen-bahks) [Johann Friedrich *Dieffenbach,* Prussian surgeon, 1792–1847] see under *operation.*

dieldrin (di-el′drin) chemical name: 3,4,5,6,9,9-hexachloro-1a,2,2a,3,6,6a,7,7a-octahydro-2,7:3,6-dimethanonaphth[2,3-b]oxirene. A chlorinated insecticide, $C_{12}H_8Cl_6O$, of particular value against the sheep tick *Melophagus ovinus,* and also used to control vectors of insect-borne diseases, especially mosquitoes. Inhalation, ingestion, or skin contact with dieldrin may cause poisoning.

dielectric (di″ĕ-lek′trik) 1. transmitting electric effects by induction, but not by conduction. The term is applied to an insulating substance through or across which electric force is acting or may act, by induction without conduction. 2. a dielectric substance.

dielectrolysis (di″e-lek-trol′ĭ-sis) [Gr. dia through + electrolysis] electrolysis of a drug, the current being passed through a diseased portion of the body, so that the drug passes through the part.

diembryony (di-em′bre-on″e) [di- + embryon embryo] the production of two embryos from a single egg.

diencephalic (di″en-se-fal′ik) pertaining to the diencephalon.

diencephalohypophysial (di″en-sef″ah-lo-hi″po-fiz′-e-al) pertaining to the diencephalon and the pituitary gland.

diencephalon (di″en-sef′ah-lon) [dia- + Gr. enkephalos brain] 1. [NA] the caudal part of the prosencephalon, which largely bounds the third ventricle and connects the mesencephalon to the cerebral hemispheres; each lateral half is divided by the hypothalamic sulcus into a dorsal part, comprising the epithalamus, dorsal thalamus, and metathalamus and a ventral part, comprising the ventral thalamus (subthalamus) and hypothalamus. Called also *betweenbrain, interbrain* and *'tween brain.* See Plate accompanying *brain.* See also *brain stem,* under B. 2. the posterior of the two brain vesicles formed by specialization of the prosencephalon in the developing embryo.

-diene a suffix used in chemistry to denote an unsaturated hydrocarbon containing two double bonds.

diener (de′ner) [Ger. "man-servant"] a man-of-all-work in a laboratory.

dienestrol (di″ēn-es′trol) [USP] chemical name: 4,4′-(1,2-diethylidene-1,2-ethanediyl)bisphenol. A synthetic estrogen, $C_{18}H_{18}O_2$, occurring as colorless, white, or practically white, needle-like crystals or as a white or practically white, crystalline powder; administered orally in the management of menopausal symptoms, in the treatment of functional uterine bleeding, as a postpartum antigalactagogue, for palliative therapy in certain female breast cancers, and in the management of prostatic carcinoma, and applied locally in the treatment of postmenopausal and senile vulvovaginitis, atrophic vaginitis, pruritus vulvae due to atrophic changes in the vulval epithelium, dyspareunia associated with atrophic vaginal epithelium, and prior to plastic pelvic surgery in menopausal patients.

Dientamoeba (di″ent-ah-me′bah) [di-(1) + ent- + ameba] a genus of small highly active, usually nonpathogenic or mildly pathogenic ameboid protozoa (superorder Parabasalidea, order Trichomonadida) parasitic in the large intestine of humans and certain monkeys, and typically characterized by the presence of two nuclei connected by a desmose and an endosome formed by four to eight chromatin granules. D. fragilis has been associated with human infection, which is manifested chiefly by diarrhea, abdominal pain, bloody, mucoid, or loose stools, and flatulence.

dieresis (di-er′ĕ-sis) [Gr. diairesis a taking] 1. the division or separation of parts normally united. 2. in surgery, the operative separation of parts by incision, electrosurgery, or cautery.

diesophagus (di-e-sof′ah-gus) doubling of the esophagus.

diestrum (di-es′trum) diestrus.

diestrus (di-es′trus) a short period of sexual quiescence occurring between metestrus and proestrus in female mammals. **gestational d.,** the period of sexual inactivity occurring during gestation in female mammals. **lactational d.,** the period of sexual inactivity occurring during lactation in female mammals.

diet (di′et) [Gr. diaita way of living] the customary allowance of food and drink taken by any person from day to day, particularly one especially planned to meet specific requirements of the individual, and including or excluding certain items of food. **absolute d.,** fasting. **acid-ash d.,** a diet to produce acidification of the urine, consisting of meat, fish, eggs and cereals, with little fruit and vegetables and no cheese or milk; used in prophylaxis of some types of urolithiasis. **adequate d.,** one that enables an animal to grow, mature, and reproduce in a normal manner. Cf. optimal d. **alkali-ash d.,** a diet of fruit, vegetables, and milk with as little as possible of meat, fish, eggs, and cereals. **balanced d.,** one containing all the nutritive factors in proper proportion for adequate nutrition. **basal d.,** one which is just sufficient to meet the caloric requirements of basal metabolism. **basic d.,** a diet which contains a preponderant proportion of alkaline ash; used for some types of urinary calculus. **bland d.,** one that is free from any irritating or stimulating foods. **diabetic d.,** a diet prescribed in the treatment of diabetes mellitus, usually limited in the amount of sugar or readily available carbohydrate. **elemental d.,** one consisting of a well-balanced, residue-free mixture of all essential and nonessential amino acids combined with simple sugars, electrolytes, trace elements, and vitamins. **elimination d.,** a procedure to identify food allergy in which foods are sequentially omitted in order to detect the one or ones responsible for symptoms. **Feingold d.,** a diet proposed for hyperactive children which excludes artificial colors, artificial flavors, preservatives, and salicylates. **Giordano-Giovannetti d.,** a low protein diet given to alleviate gastrointestinal symptoms of chronic renal failure. **gluten-free d.,** a diet deficient in the cereal protein gluten; used as a specific treatment for celiac disease (gluten enteropathy). **gouty d.,** one for mitigation of gout, restricting nitrogenous, especially high-purine foods, and substituting dairy products, with prohibition of wines and liquors. **high calorie d.,** one that furnishes more calories than needed for the maintenance of weight, often more than 3500–4000 calories per day. **high fat d.,** ketogenic d. **high fiber d.,** one relatively high in dietary fibers, which decreases bowel transit time and relieves constipation. **high protein d.,** one containing large amounts of protein, consisting largely of meats, fish, milk, legumes, and nuts. **Karell d.,** a diet for nephritis and cardiac conditions, consists of 800 ml. of milk per day; the milk diet, running from six days to a week, is amplified gradually by the use of eggs, dry toast, meat, rice, and vegetables. **Keith's low ionic d.,** a diet for chronic nephritis based on decrease in the water content, reduction of the amount of sodium, and the minimum water content kept constant from day to day. **Kempner's d.,** a diet consisting of only rice, fruit juices, and sugar, supplemented with vitamins and iron; for hypertension and chronic renal disease. **ketogenic d.,** one containing a large amount of fat with minimal amounts of protein and carbohydrate, the object of such a diet being to produce ketosis; called also high fat d. **light d.,** a simple mixed diet suitable for convalescents. **low calorie d.,** one containing fewer calories than needed for the maintenance of weight, e.g., less than 1200 calories per day for an adult. **low fat d.,** one containing limited amounts of fat.

low oxalate d., one with no potatoes, beans, or fiber vegetables, and no sweet fruit, tea, chocolate, or sweets; used for the prevention of oxalate stones in the urinary tract. **low purine d.,** one for mitigation of gout, omitting meat, fowl, and fish and substituting milk, eggs, cheese, and vegetable protein. **low residue d.,** a diet which gives the least possible fecal residue: such as gelatin, sucrose, dextrose, broth, hard-boiled egg, meat, liver, rice, and cottage cheese. **low salt d.,** a diet which contains very little sodium chloride; prescribed by some for hypertension and for edematous states. **Meulengracht d.,** a full-feeding diet for peptic ulcer. **Minot-Murphy d.,** see under treatment. **Moro-Heisler d.,** a diet of grated raw apple for diarrheal conditions in infants. **optimal d.,** a diet that produces the most desirable growth, the most successful reproduction, and the maintenance of the best possible health; Cf. adequate d. **Petrén's d.,** a diet once given to diabetics, consisting of extremely small amounts of protein and carbohydrate and very large amounts of fat, chiefly butter. **protein-sparing d.,** one consisting only of liquid proteins or liquid mixtures of proteins, vitamins, and minerals, and containing no more than 600 calories; it is designed to maintain a favorable nitrogen balance. **provocative d.,** a diet designed to include the most common allergenic foods, from which they are eliminated one by one, as a means of determining the offending substances in cases of food allergy. **purine-free d.,** see low-purine d. **rachitic d.,** an inadequate diet which will bring about rickets in an experimental animal. The animal is kept in a room from which all daylight is excluded and the diet consists of whole wheat flour, 33 per cent; yellow maize, 33 per cent; wheat gluten, 15 per cent; gelatin powder, 15 per cent; calcium carbonate, 3 per cent; sodium chloride, 1 per cent; and tap water, ad libitum. **rice d.,** Kempner's d. **salt-free d.,** see low-salt d. **Schemm d.,** a low-sodium, neutral and acid-ash diet for patients with congestive heart failure. **Schmidt d.,** a daily diet consisting of 1.5 liters of milk, 100 gm. of zwieback, 2 eggs, 50 gm. of butter, 125 gm. of beef, 190 gm. of boiled potato, and gruel made from 80 gm. of oatmeal. It contains 102 gm. of protein, 111 gm. of fat, and 191 gm. of carbohydrate, giving 2234 calories. It is used to facilitate examination of the stools in diarrhea of various causation. **Schmidt-Strassburger d.,** Schmidt d. **Sippy d.,** a diet for peptic ulcer and for conditions in which the patient is unable to take bulky foods. It consists of nothing but milk and cream for the first few days, with the addition of crackers, cereals, and eggs on the third day; the amounts increasing gradually until during the later days of the diet puréed vegetables are included. On the twenty-eighth day the patient is placed on the regular ward diet. **smooth d.,** one which avoids the use of foods containing roughage. **subsistence d.,** a diet on which one can just live. **Taylor's d.,** a preparation of white of egg, olive oil, and sugar, given when the urine is to be tested for chlorides. **Wilder's d.,** a low-potassium diet formerly used in Addison's disease.

dietary (di′ĕ-ta″re) a regular or systematic scheme of diet.

dietetic (di″ĕ-tet′ik) [Gr. diaitētikos] pertaining to diet or proper food.

dietetics (di″ĕ-tet′iks) the science or study and regulation of the diet.

diethazine hydrochloride (di-eth′ah-zēn) chemical name: N,N-diethyl-10H-phenothiazine-10-ethanamine hydrochloride. An anticholinergic, $C_{18}H_{23}ClN_2S$, which has been used as an antiparkinsonian agent.

diethylamine (di″eth-il-am′in) a nonpoisonous liquid ptomaine, $NH(C_2H_5)_2$, from decaying fish and putrid sausages.

diethylcarbamazine (di-eth″il-kar-bam′ah-zēn) an antifilarial agent effective against microfilariae of Wuchereria bancrofti, W. malayi, and Loa loa, causing their disappearance from the blood due to phagocytosis by macrophages of the reticuloendothelial system; used as diethylcarbamazine citrate.

diethylenediamine (di-eth″il-ēn-di′ah-mēn) piperazine.

diethyl ether (di-eth′il e′ther) ethyl ether, ether [USP], a colorless, volatile, flammable liquid, $C_2H_5OC_2H_5$, with a characteristic odor; the first inhalational anesthetic used for surgical anesthesia (1846), now little used because of its flammability.

diethylmalonylurea (di-eth″il-mal″o-nil-u-re′ah) (obs.) barbital.

diethylpropion hydrochloride (di-eth′il-pro′pe-on) [USP] chemical name: 2-(diethylamino)-1-phenyl-1-propanone hydrochloride. An adrenergic, $C_{13}H_{19}NO \cdot HCl$, structurally related to amphetamine, methamphetamine, and ephedrine, occurring as a white to off-white, fine crystalline powder; used as an anorexic, administered orally.

diethylstilbestrol (di-eth″il-stil-bes′trol) [USP] chemical name: (E)-4,4′-(1,2-diethyl-1,2-ethenediyl)bis-phenol. A synthetic nonsteroidal estrogen, $C_{18}H_{20}O_2$, occurring as a white, crystalline powder, having estrogenic activity similar to but greater than that of estrone. It is used for many purposes, e.g., to relieve menopausal symptoms, to suppress lactation, in amenorrhea, dysmenorrhea, senile vaginitis, and pruritus vulvae, in the palliative treatment of female breast carcinoma, and to relieve the symptoms of prostatic carcinoma; administered orally, intravaginally, or intramuscularly. Formerly used to prevent threatened or habitual abortion and premature labor. Women who have been exposed *in utero* to diethylstilbestrol show characteristic changes in the cervix and vagina and are subject to an increased risk of vaginal or cervical carcinoma. Called also *estrostilben* and *stilbestrol*. **d. diphosphate** [USP], an ester of diethylstilbestrol, $C_{18}H_{22}O_8P_2$, occurring as an off-white, crystalline powder, having the same actions as the base; used in the treatment of prostatic carcinoma, administered intravenously. **d. dipropionate,** an ester of diethylstilbestrol, $C_{24}H_{28}O_4$, occurring as a white, crystalline powder, having actions and uses similar to those of the base; administered orally, intravaginally, or intramuscularly.

diethyltoluamide (di-eth″il-tol-u′ah-mīd) [USP] chemical name: N,N-diethyl-3-methylbenzamide. An arthropod repellent, $C_{12}H_{17}NO$, occurring as a colorless liquid; applied topically to the skin and to the clothing.

diethyltryptamine (di-eth″il-trip′tah-min) chemical name: N_2N-diethyltryptamine. A hallucinogenic substance closely related to dimethyltryptamine, but prepared synthetically. Abbreviated DET.

dietitian (di-ĕ-tish′an) a person trained in the scientific use of diet in health and disease.

Dietl's crisis (de′tlz) [Józef *Dietl,* physician in Cracow, 1804–1878] see under *crisis.*

dietotherapy (di″ĕ-to-ther′ah-pe) dietetic treatment.

dietotoxic (di″ĕ-to-tok′sik) having the quality of dietotoxicity.

dietotoxicity (di″ĕ-to-tok-sis′ĭ-te) a quality in certain food substances which renders them toxic when used in an unbalanced diet.

Dieulafoy's theory, triad (dyuh-lah-fwahz′) [Georges *Dieulafoy,* physician in Paris, 1839–1911] see under *theory* and *triad.*

difenoxamide hydrochloride (di″fen-oks′ah-mīd) chemical name: 4-[[(2,5-dioxo-1-pyrrolidinyl)oxy]carbonyl]-α,α,4-triphenyl- 1-piperidinebutanenitrile monohydrochloride; an antiperistalic, $C_{32}H_{31}N_3O_4 \cdot HCl$.

difenoxin (di″fen-oks′in) chemical name: 1-(3-cyano-3,3-diphenylpropyl-4-piperidinecarboxylic acid; an antiperistaltic, $C_{28}H_{28}N_2O_2$.

differential (dif″er-en′shal) [L. *differre* to carry apart] pertaining to a difference or differences.

differentiate (dif″er-en′she-āt) 1. to distinguish, on the basis of differences. 2. to develop specialized form, character, or function differing from that of surrounding cytoplasm, cells, or tissue or from the original type.

differentiation (dif″er-en″she-a′shun) 1. the distinguishing of one thing or disease from another. 2. the act or process of acquiring completely individual characters, as occurs in the progressive diversification of cells and tissues of the embryo. 3. increase in morphological or chemical heterogeneity. **correlative d.,** differentiation caused by factors outside the tissue itself, as by an inductor; called also *dependent* d. **dependent d.,** correlative d. **functional d.,** differentiation which results from the functioning of the tissue of a part. **invisible d.,** the development toward a fixed fate, through chemodifferentiation, by cells that show no visible signs of this determination. **regional d.,** the appearance of regional differences within a field of development. **self d.,** differentiation produced by factors solely within the tissue or part.

diffluence (dif′loo-ens) the act of becoming fluid or of flowing readily.

diffluent (dif′loo-ent) [L. *diffluere* to flow off] easily flowing away or dissolving; deliquescent; temporary.

Difflugia (dĭ-floo′je-ah) [L. *diffluere* to flow away or apart, dissolve] a genus of ameboid protozoa (order Arcellinida, subclass Testacealobosia) characterized by the presence of cylindrical pseudopodia with rounded or pointed ends and a test composed of grains of sand, diatoms, and other foreign bodies.

diffraction (dĭ-frak′shun) [L. *dis-* apart + *frangere* to break] the bending or breaking up into its component parts of a ray of light. **d. grating,** a strip of glass ruled closely with fine lines for use in the spectroscope. **x-ray d.,** a technique for studying the cell based on the diffraction of radiations when they encounter small obstacles; used especially in the study of inorganic and organic crystals, in which it is possible to determine the precise spatial relationships between the constituent atoms.

diffusate (dĭ-fu′zāt) material that has passed through a membrane.

diffuse (dĭ-fūs′) [L. *dis-* apart + *fundere* to pour] 1. not definitely limited or localized; widely distributed. 2. (dĭ-fūz′) to pass through or to spread widely through a tissue or structure.

diffusible (dĭ-fūz′ĭ-b′l) susceptible of becoming widely spread.

diffusiometer (dĭ-fu″ze-om′ĕ-ter) an apparatus for measuring the speed of diffusion.

diffusion (dĭ-fu′zhun) 1. the process of becoming diffused, or widely spread; the spontaneous movement of molecules or other particles in solution, owing to their random thermal motion, to reach a uniform concentration throughout the solvent, a process requiring no addition of energy to the system. 2. dialysis. 3. immunodiffusion. **double d.,** immunodiffusion in which both the antigen and antibody diffuse through the medium toward each other. **double d. in one dimension,** antiserum is placed in a test tube and overlaid with agar, which is allowed to solidify, and antigen is layered over the agar. Precipitin lines form where the concentrations of each antigen and antibody are equivalent. Called also *Oakley-Fulthorpe technique.* **double d. in two dimensions,** double diffusion in which antigen and antiserum are placed in wells cut in an agar plate; antigen solutions to be compared are placed in wells equidistant from the antiserum well. Three principal types of reaction may occur, *reaction of identity, reaction of nonidentity,* and *reaction of partial identity* (see under *reaction*), each identified by a characteristic pattern of precipitin lines, indicating the extent to which the antigen samples a share antigenic determinants. Called also *Ouchterlony technique.* **exchange d.,** the process in which diffusion of a molecule across a membrane in one direction brings about diffusion of another molecule in the opposite direction. **facilitated d.,** diffusion across a cell membrane or other biological membrane in which the molecules to be transported form complexes with specific carriers in the membrane, are shuttled across the membrane by the complex, and then released on the other side. **free d.,** diffusion in which there is no obstacle such as a membrane. **gel d.,** immunodiffusion. **impeded d.,** diffusion in which the rate is slowed down by the difficulty of passing through a membrane. **single d.,** immunodiffusion in which either the antibody or antigen remains fixed and the other reactant diffuses through it. **single radial d.,** a quantitative immunodiffusion technique in which the antigen solutions are placed in wells cut in an agar plate containing antiserum; the area or diameter of the precipitin ring around an unknown solution is compared with the rings of a serial dilution of a standard antigen solution to determine the amount of antigen present in the unknown. Called also *radial immunodiffusion (RID).*

diflorasone diacetate (di-flor′ah-sōn) chemical name: 17,21-*bis*(acetyloxy)-6α,9-difluoro-11β-hydroxy-16β- methyl-pregna-1,4-diene-3,20-dione; a topical corticosteroid, $C_{26}H_{32}F_2O_7$, used as a cream or ointment in treatment of certain dermatoses.

difluanine hydrochloride (di-floo′ah-nēn) chemical name: 4-[4,4-bis(4-fluorophenyl)butyl]-N-phenyl-1-piperazineethanamine trihydrochloride; a central nervous system stimulant, $C_{28}H_{33}F_2N_3 \cdot HCl$.

diflucortolone (di″floo-kor′to-lōn) chemical name: 6,9-difluoro-11,21-dihydroxy-16-methyl-pregna-1, 4-diene-3, 20-dione; a glucocorticoid, $C_{22}H_{28}F_2O_4$. **d. pivalate,** the pivalate salt of diflucortolone, $C_{27}H_{36}F_2O_5$; a glucocorticoid.

diflumidone sodium (di-floo′mĭ-dōn) chemical name: *N*-(3-benzoylphenyl)-1,1-difluoromethanesulfonamide: an anti-inflammatory, $C_{14}H_{10}F_2NNaO_3S$.

diflunisal (di-floo′nĭ-sal) a diflurophenyl derivative of salicylic acid; used for relief of mild to moderate pain.

difluprednate (di′′floo-pred′nāt) chemical name: 21-(acetyloxy)-6α,9-difluoro-11β-hydroxy-17-(1-oxobutoxy)-pregna-1,4-diene-3,20-dione; an anti-inflammatory agent, $C_{27}H_{34}F_2$-O_7.

diftalone (dif′tah-lōn) chemical name: phthalazino[2,3-*b*]-phthalazine-5,12-(7*H*,14*H*)-dione; an anti-inflammatory, C_{16}-$H_{12}N_2O_2$.

Dig. abbreviation for L. *digera′tur*, let it be digested.

digallic acid (di-gal′ik) an incorrect term for tannic acid.

digametic (di′′gah-met′ik) 1. pertaining to or producing gametes or sex cells of two different types, female (ova) and male (spermatozoa). 2. heterogametic.

digastric (di-gas′trik) [*di-* + Gr. *gastēr* belly] 1. having two bellies. 2. musculus digastricus.

digenesis (di-jen′ĕ-sis) alternation of generation.

digenetic (di′′jĕ-net′ik) [*di-* + Gr. *genesis* generation] having two stages of multiplication, one sexual in the mature forms, the other asexual in the larval stages; said of flukes and many other parasites.

DiGeorge′s syndrome (dĭ-jor′jez) [Angelo M. *DiGeorge,* American pediatrician, born 1921] see under *syndrome.*

digestant (di-jes′tant) 1. assisting or stimulating digestion. 2. an agent that assists or stimulates digestion.

digestion (di-jest′yun) [L. *digestio,* from *dis-* apart + *gerere* to carry] 1. the process or act of converting food into chemical substances that can be absorbed and assimilated. 2. the subjection of a body to prolonged heat and moisture, so as to disintegrate and soften it. **artificial d.,** that which is performed outside the body. **biliary d.,** the digestive effect of the bile upon food. **gastric d.,** that which is carried on in the stomach by aid of the gastric juice; called also *peptic d.* and *chymification.* **gastrointestinal d.,** the gastric and intestinal digestions together; called also *primary d.* **intercellular d.,** digestion carried on within an organ by secretions from the cells of the organ. **intestinal d.,** that which is carried on in the intestine. **intracellular d.,** digestion carried on within a single cell. **lipolytic d.,** the splitting of fat into fatty acid and glycerol. **pancreatic d.,** that which is performed by the pancreatic secretion. **parenteral d.,** digestion taking place somewhere else in the body than in the alimentary canal, as in the blood or under the skin. **peptic d.,** gastric d. **primary d.,** gastrointestinal d. **salivary d.,** the change of starch into maltose by the saliva. **sludge d.,** the biochemical process by which organic matter in sludge is gasified, liquefied, mineralized, or converted into more stable organic matter.

digestive (di-jes′tiv) 1. pertaining to digestion. 2. digestant.

digit (dij′it) [L. *digitus*] a finger or toe. See also *ossa digitorum manus,* under *os².*

digital (dij′ĭ-tal) 1. of, pertaining to, or performed with, a finger. 2. resembling the imprint of a finger. 3. pertaining to numerical methods or discrete variables.

digitalin (dij′′ĭ-tal′in) 1. true digitalin; a cardiac glycoside, $C_{36}H_{56}O_{14}$, from the seeds of *Digitalis purpurea.* 2. any of several mixtures of digitalis glycosides extracted from the leaves or seeds.

Digitaline Nativelle (dij′′ĭ-tal′ēn na′′tĭ-vel′) trademark for a preparation of digitoxin.

Digitalis (dij′′ĭ-ta′lis) [L. from *digitus* finger, because of the finger-like leaves of the corolla of its flowers] a genus of herbs. *D. purpu′rea* is the purple foxglove whose leaves furnish digitalis. *D. lana′ta* is a Balkan species which yields digoxin and lanatoside.

digitalis (dij′′ĭ-tal′is) 1. [USP] the dried leaf of *Digitalis purpurea,* the purple foxglove, the main systemic effects of which are manifested by an increase in the strength of the heart beat while decreasing its rate. When digitalis is prescribed *powdered digitalis* (see below) is to be dispensed. Called also *d. leaf.* 2. [NA] a general term for any finger-like structure. **d. leaf,** digitalis (def. 1). **powdered**

d. [USP], **prepared d.,** the standardized preparation to be dispensed when digitalis is prescribed; principally used in the treatment of congestive heart failure but also used in other cardiac disorders, administered orally.

digitalization (dij′′ĭ-tal-i-za′shun) the administration of digitalis in a dosage schedule designed to produce and then maintain optimal therapeutic concentrations of its cardiotonic glycosides.

digitaloid (dij′ĭ-tal-oid) resembling or related to digitalis.

digitalose (dij′ĭ-tal-ōs) a hexose sugar, 6-desoxy-*d*-allose, $CH_3(CHOH_3)CH(O\cdot CH_3)\cdot CHO$, from digitalin.

digitate (dij′ĭ-tāt) having several finger-like processes.

digitatio (dij′′ĭ-ta′she-o), pl. *digitatio′nes* [L.] a finger-like process. **digitatio′nes hippocam′pi,** see *pes hippocampi.*

digitation (dij′′ĭ-ta′shun) 1. a finger-like process. 2. surgical creation of a functioning digit.

digitationes (dij′′ĭ-ta′′she-o′nez) [L.] plural of *digitatio.*

digiti (dij′ĭ-ti) [L.] genitive and plural of *digitus.*

digitiform (dij′′ĭ-tĭ-form) resembling a finger; finger-like.

digitigrade (dij′ĭ-tĭ-grād′′) [L. *digitus* finger or toe + *gradi* to walk] characterized by standing or walking on the toes (but not the toe tips as do unguiligrade animals); applied to certain quadrupeds (e.g., cats, dogs) whose digits alone touch the ground, the posterior part of the foot being more or less raised. Cf. *plantigrade.*

digitogenin (dij′′ĭ-toj′ĕ-nin) a sapogenin, $C_{27}H_{44}O_5$, from digitonin.

digitonin (dij′′ĭ-to′nin) [USP] a saponin, $C_{55}H_{90}O_{29}$, from *Digitalis purpurea,* which possesses no cardiotonic action; used as a reagent to precipitate free cholesterol.

digitoplantar (dij′′ĭ-to-plan′tar) [L. *digitus* finger or toe + *planta* sole] pertaining to the toes and the sole of the foot.

digitoxin (dij′′ĭ-tok′sin) [USP] chemical name: 3β-[(*O*-2,6-dideoxy-β-D-*ribo*-hexopyranosyl-(1→4)-*O*-2,6-dideoxy-β-D-*ribo*-hexopyranosyl-(1→4)-2,6-dideoxy-β-D-*ribo*-hexopyranosyl)-oxy]-14-hydroxy-card-5β-20(22)-enolide. A cardiac glycoside, $C_{41}H_{64}O_{13}$, obtained from *Digitalis purpurea, D. lanata,* and other *Digitalis* species, occurring as a white or pale buff, microcrystalline powder. It has actions and uses similar to those of digitalis, administered orally, intramuscularly, or intravenously.

digitoxose (dij′′ĭ-tok′sōs) a hexose sugar, $CH_3(CHOH)_3$-$CH_2\cdot CHO$, derived from several of the digitalis glycosides.

digitus (dij′ĭ-tus), pl. *dig′iti* [L.] digit: a finger or a toe. See also *ossa digitorum manus,* under *os².* **d. annula′ris** [NA], the fourth digit, or ring finger, of the hand. Called also *d. quartus (IV) manus* [NA alternative]. **d. hippocrat′icus,** clubbed finger. **d. mal′leus,** mallet finger. **dig′iti ma′nus** [NA], the digits of the hand; the fingers. **d. me′dius** [NA], the middle, or third, digit of the hand; called also *d. tertius (III) manus* [NA alternative]. **d. min′imus ma′nus** [NA], the fifth digit of the hand; called also *d. quintus (V) manus* [NA alternative]. **d. min′imus pe′dis** [NA], the fifth digit of the foot; called also *d. quintus (V) pedis* [NA alternative]. **d. mor′tuus** [L. "dead finger"], a numb, mottled finger, as seen in acrocyanosis; called also *waxy* or *white finger.* **dig′iti pe′dis** [NA], the digits of the foot; the toes. **d. postmin′imus,** an appendage ranging from a small round mass of fat and connective tissue to a longer mass containing bones and with a nail at its distal end, attached by a small pedicle to the soft tissue covering the lateral surface of the little finger or toe. **d. pri′mus (I) ma′nus,** NA alternative for *pollex* (thumb). **d. pri′mus (I) pedis** NA alternative for *hallux* (great toe). **d. quar′tus (IV) ma′nus,** NA alternative for *d. annularis.* **d. quar′tus (IV) pe′dis** [NA], the fourth digit of the foot. **d. quin′tus (V) ma′nus** NA alternative for *d. minimus manus.* **d. quin′tus (V) pe′dis,** NA alternative for *d. minimus pedis.* **d. recel′lens** (obs.), trigger finger. **d. secun′dus (II) ma′nus,** NA alternative for *index* (finger). **d. secun′dus (II) pe′dis** [NA], the second digit of the foot. **d. ter′tius (III) ma′nus** NA alternative for *d. medius.* **d. ter′tius (III) pe′dis** [NA], the third digit of the foot. **d. V,** the fifth digit of the hand or foot; NA alternative for *d. minimus.* **d. val′gus,** deviation of a digit in the radial direction, or toward the digit of next higher number. **d. va′rus,** deviation of a digit in the ulnar direction, or toward the digit of next lower number.

diglossia (di-glos′e-ah) [*di-* + Gr. *glōssa* tongue] bifid tongue.

diglyceride (di-glis′er-id) a glyceride containing two fatty acid molecules in ester linkage.

dignathus (dig-na′thus) [*di-* + Gr. *gnathos* jaw] a monster with two lower jaws.

digoxin (di-goks′in) [USP] chemical name: 3β-[(O-2,6-dideoxy-β-D-*ribo*-hexopyranosyl-(1→4)-O-2,6-dideoxy-β-D-*ribo*-hexopyranosyl-(1→4)-2, 6-dideoxy-β-*ribo*-hexopyranosyl)oxy] -12 β,14-dihydroxy-card-5β-20(22)-enolide. A cardiotonic glycoside, $C_{41}H_{64}O_{14}$, obtained from the leaves of *Digitalis lanata*, occurring as clear to white crystals or white crystalline powder. It may be used for the same purposes as digitalis, administered orally, intramuscularly, or intravenously.

Digramma brauni (di-gram′ah braw′ni) a larval tapeworm belonging to the family Diphyllobothriidae, reported from man in Roumania; formerly called *Diplogonoporus brauni.*

diheterozygote (di-het″er-o-zi′gōt) [*di-* + *heterozygote*] an individual heterozygous for two pairs of genes; called also *dihybrid.*

dihexyverine hydrochloride (di″heks-ĭ-ver′ēn) chemical name: 2-piperidinoethyl ester of bicyclohexyl-1-carboxylic acid hydrochloride; an anticholinergic, $C_{20}H_{35}NO_2 \cdot HCl$, which has been used as an antispasmodic in uterine hypermotility and intestinal muscle spasm.

dihomocinchonine (di-ho″mo-sin′ko-nin) an alkaloid, $C_{38}H_{44}O_2N_4$, from cinchona.

dihybrid (di-hi′brid) diheterozygous.

dihydrate (di-hi′drāt) [*di-* + Gr. *hydōr* water] 1. any compound containing two hydroxyl groups. 2. any compound containing two molecules of water.

dihydrated (di-hi′drāt-ed) compounded with two molecules of water.

dihydric (di-hi′drik) having two hydrogen atoms in each molecule.

dihydrobiopterin synthetase deficiency (di-hi″dro-bi-op′ter-in sin′thĕ-tās) hyperphenylalaninemia, type V.

dihydrocholesterol (di-hi″dro-ko-les′ter-ol) cholestanol.

dihydrocodeine (di-hi″dro-ko′dēn) chemical name: 4,5α-epoxy-3-methoxy-17-methylmorphinan-6α-ol: a narcotic analgesic and antitussive, $C_{18}H_{23}NO_3$; called also *drocode.*

dihydrocodeinone bitartrate (di-hi″dro-ko′de-ĭ-nōn) hydrocodone bitartrate.

dihydrocollidine (di-hi″dro-kol′ĭ-din) an oily base, $C_8H_{11}NH_2$, from decaying flesh and fish; regarded as a ptomaine.

dihydrodiethylstilbestrol (di-hi″dro-di-eth″il-stil-bes′trol) hexestrol.

dihydroergocornine (di-hi″dro-er″go-kor′nin) an ergot derivative that has sympatholytic and adrenolytic properties.

dihydroergocristine (di-hi″dro-er″go-kris′tin) an ergot derivative that has sympatholytic and adrenolytic properties.

dihydroergocryptine (di-hi″dro-er″go-krip′tin) an ergot derivative that has sympatholytic and adrenolytic properties.

dihydroergotamine mesylate (di-hi″dro-er-got′ah-mēn) [USP] chemical name: 9-10-dihydro-12′-hydroxy-2′-methyl-5′α-(phenylmethyl)-ergotaman-3′,6′,18-trione monomethanesulfonate. An antiadrenergic, $C_{34}H_{41}N_5O_8S$, produced by the catalytic hydrogenation of ergotamine; used as a vasoconstrictor in the treatment of migraine.

dihydrofolate reductase (di-hi″dro-fo′lāt re-duk′tās) [EC 1.5.1.3] an enzyme of the oxidoreductase class that catalyzes the reaction 7,8-dihydrofolate + NADPH = 5,6,7,8-tetrahydrofolate + NADP$^+$, producing reduced folate for amino acid metabolism, purine ring synthesis, and the formation of deoxythymidine monophosphate. Methotrexate and other folic acid antagonists used as chemotherapeutic drugs act by inhibiting this enzyme.

dihydrofolate reductase (DHFR) deficiency a genetic aminoacidopathy of defective folate metabolism; decreased conversion of folate to tetrahydrofolate may cause, depending on the degree of deficiency, spontaneous abortion, stillbirth, or, in surviving infants, failure to thrive and severe megaloblastic anemia. Therapy with folinic acid (leucovorin) is curative.

dihydroindolone (di-hi″dro-in′do-lōn) any of a class of structurally related antipsychotic agents; the prototype is molindone.

dihydrol (di-hi′drol) the associated water molecule,$(H_2O)_2$.

dihydrolipoamide acetyltransferase (di-hi′dro-lip″o-am″īd as″ĕ-til-trans′fer-ās) [EC 2.3.1.12] an enzyme of the transferase class that catalyzes the reaction S-acetyldihydrolipoamide + CoA = dihydrolipoamide + acetyl-CoA. The enzyme is a lipoyl protein and part of the multienzyme pyruvate dehydrogenase complex. Called also *dihydrolipoyltransacetylase.*

dihydrolipoamide dehydrogenase (di-hi″dro-lip″o-am″īd de-hi′dro-jen″ās) [EC 1.8.1.4] an enzyme of the oxidoreductase class that catalyzes the reaction NAD$^+$ + dihydrolipoamide = NADH + lipoamide. The enzyme contains FAD$^+$ and is a component of the oxidative decarboxylation enzyme complexes branched chain α-ketoacid dehydrogenase, α-ketoglutarate dehydrogenase, and pyruvate dehydrogenase (lipoamide).

dihydrolipoamide succinyltransferase (di-hi″dro-lip″o-am″īd suk″sĭ-nil-trans′fer-ās) [EC 2.3.1.61] an enzyme of the transferase class that catalyzes the reaction succinyl-CoA + dihydrolipoamide = CoA + S-succinyldihydrolipoamide. The enzyme is a lipoyl-protein and is a component of the α-ketoglutarate dehydrogenase complex. Called also *transsuccinylase.*

dihydrolipoyltransacetylase dihydrolipoamide acetyltransferase.

dihydrolutidine (di-hi″dro-lu′tĭ-din) an oily, poisonous, caustic base, $C_7H_{11}N$, from rancid cod liver oil.

dihydromorphinone (di-hi″dro-mor′fĭ-nōn) hydromorphone hydrochloride.

dihydroorotase (di-hi″dro-or′o-tās) [E.C. 3.5.2.3] An enzyme of the hydrolase class that catalyzes the reaction: (S)- dihydroorotate + H_2O = N-carbamoyl-L-aspartate. The reverse reaction occurs during pyrimidine biosynthesis.

dihydropteridine reductase (di-hi″dro-ter′ĭ-dēn re-duk′tās) [EC 1.6.99.7] an enzyme of the oxidoreductase class that catalyzes the reaction NADPH + 6, 7-dihydropteridine = NADP$^+$ + 5,6,7,8-tetrahydropteridine. The enzyme regenerates the reduced coenzyme, tetrahydropteridine, which is essential for the conversion of phenylalanine to tyrosine or dopamine and epinephrine, and for the conversion of tryptophan to serotonin. A genetic defect of the enzyme causes hyperphenylalaninemia, type IV.

dihydropteridine reductase (DHPR) deficiency hyperphenylalaninemia, type IV.

dihydrostreptomycin (di-hi″dro-strep″to-mi′sin) an antibiotic substance, $C_{21}H_{41}N_7O_{12}$, produced by the hydrogenation of streptomycin; no longer used in medicine because of its toxicity.

dihydrotachysterol (di-hi″dro-tak-is′tĕ-rol) [USP] chemical name: 9,10-secoergosta-5,7,22-trien-3β-ol. A synthetic reduction product of tachysterol, $C_{28}H_{46}O$, occurring as colorless or white crystals, or white, crystalline powder; used as an antihypocalcemic agent in the treatment of hypocalcemic tetany, administered orally. Called also *A.T. 10.*

dihydrotestosterone (di-hi″dro-tes-tos′ter-ōn) 7β-hydroxy-5α-androstan-3-one (DHT), a powerful androgenic hormone, $C_{19}H_{30}O_2$, formed in peripheral tissue by the action on testosterone of the enzyme 5α-reductase; it is thought to be the essential androgen responsible for somatic virilization during embryogenesis, for development of most male secondary characteristics at puberty, and for adult male sexual function. A semisynthetic preparation is called *stanolone* (q.v.).

dihydroxyacetone (di″hi-drok″se-as′ĕ-tōn) one of the trioses, the ketotriose $CH_2OH \cdot CO \cdot CH_2OH$; formed by the oxidation of glycerin with nitric acid; used as a humectant.

dihydroxyacetone phosphate (di-hi-drok″se-as′ĕ-tōn fos′fāt) the most widely used term for glycerone phosphate.

dihydroxyaluminum (di″hi-drok″se-ah-lu′mĭ-num) an aluminum compound having two hydroxyl groups in the molecule. **d. aminoacetate** [USP], chemical name: (glycinato-N,O)dihydroxyaluminum. A basic aluminum salt of aminoacetic acid, $C_2H_6AlNO_4 \cdot xH_2O$, occurring as a white powder; used as a gastric antacid. Available in tablets and as a magma. Called also *aluminum aminoacetate.* **d. sodium carbonate** [USP], chemical name: [carbonato(2–)-

O,O']dihydroxy-aluminate(1–)sodium hydrate. An aluminum salt of sodium carbonate, $CH_2AlNaO_5 \cdot xH_2O$, occurring as a fine, white powder; used as a gastric antacid in tablet form.

dihydroxycholecalciferol (di″hi-drok″se-ko″le-kal-sif′ĕ-rol) a group of active metabolites of cholecalciferol (vitamin D_3) numbered according to the carbon atom(s) on which a hydroxyl group is substituted. 1,25-Dihydroxycholecalciferol, synthesized in the kidney from 25-hydroxycholecalciferol, is the most active derivative; it increases intestinal absorption of calcium and phosphate, enhances bone resorption, and prevents rickets and, because of these activities at sites distant from the site of its synthesis, is considered to be a hormone. Called also *1,25-dihydroxyvitamin D_3*. Another form, *24,25-dihydroxycholecalciferol*, is almost inert.

dihydroxyfluorane (di″hi-drok″se-floo′o-rān) fluorescein.

3,4-dihydroxyphenylalanine (di-hi-drok″se-fen″il-al′ah-nēn) dopa.

dihydroxyvitamin D_3 (di″hi-drok″se-vi′tah-min) see *dihydroxycholecalciferol.*

dihysteria (di″his-te′re-ah) [*di-* + Gr. *hystera* uterus + *-ia*] the condition of having a double uterus.

diiodide (di-i′o-dīd) a combination of a base or a metal with two atoms of iodine.

diiodohydroxyquin (di″i-o″do-hi-drok′se-kwin) iodoquinol.

3,5-diiodothyronine (di″i-o″do-thi′ro-nēn) chemical name: 3-[4-(*p*-hydroxyphenoxy)-3,5-diiodophenyl] alanine. An organic iodine-containing compound, $C_{15}H_{13}I_2NO_4$, used in the manufacture of thyroxine.

diiodotyrosine (di″i-o″do-ti′ro-sēn) chemical name: 2-amino-3-(3,5-diiodo-4-hydroxyphenol)-propionic acid. A precursor of the thyroid hormone thyroxine: an organic iodine-containing compound liberated from thyroglobulin by hydrolysis, and thought to be formed by the iodination of monoiodotyrosine. Called also *iodogorgoric acid.*

diisopropyl fluorophosphate (di-i″so-pro′pil floo″ro-fos′fāt) DFP; a potent irreversible acetylcholinesterase inhibitor, widely used in biochemistry in the study of serine proteases; radiolabeled $DF^{32}P$ has been used to label red and white blood cells in kinetics studies. DFP is also used (see *isoflurophate*) as an ophthalmic cholinergic agent.

dikaryon (di-ka′re-on) [*di-* + Gr. *karyon* kernel] a growth stage in the mycelium of fungi, especially Basidiomycetes, in which each cell has two haploid nuclei.

dikaryote (di-kar′e-ōt) a cell having two haploid nuclei.

dikaryotic (di″kar-e-ot′ik) pertaining to the dikaryon or to a dikaryote.

diketone (di-ke′tōn) a ketone containing two carbonyl groups.

diketopiperazine (di-ke″to-pi-per′ah-zin) a closed-ring compound produced by the condensation of two amino acids, the carboxyl group of each combining with the amino group of the other.

diktyoma (dik″te-o′mah) [*dicty-* + *-oma*] a benign or malignant tumor of the ciliary epithelium with characteristics resembling those of embryonic retinal tissue.

dikwakwadi (dik″wak-wad′e) witkop.

dil. abbreviation for L. *dil′ue*, dilute or dissolve.

dilaceration (di-las″er-a′shun) [L. *dilaceratio*] 1. a tearing apart, as of a cataract; see *discission*. 2. in dentistry, a condition due to injury to a tooth during its developmental period and characterized by a crease or band at the junction of the crown and root, or by tortuous roots with abnormal curvatures.

Dilantin (di-lan′tin) trademark for preparations of phenytoin.

dilatancy (di-la′tan-se) an unusual behavior observed in cytoplasm (and in some physical systems) during which its viscosity and applied force both increase.

dilatant (di-la′tant) exhibiting dilatancy.

dilatation (dil-ah-ta′shun) 1. the condition, as of an orifice or tubular structure, of being dilated or stretched beyond the normal dimensions. 2. the act of dilating or stretching. **digital d.**, digital dilation. **gastric d.**, d. of the stomach. **d. of the heart,** enlargement of the cavities of the heart, with thinning of its walls. **idiopathic d.,** dilatation of a vessel or other channel, especially of the pulmonary

artery, not associated with any other abnormality. **post-stenotic d.,** dilatation of a vessel distal to a stenosed segment or valve, often seen in the pulmonary artery distal to valvular pulmonary stenosis. **prognathic d., prognathion d.,** dilatation of the pyloric end of the stomach greater than that of the fundus, giving a protruding appearance in the roentgen-ray picture. **d. of the stomach,** distention of the stomach with retained secretions, food, and/or gas due to obstruction, ileus, or denervation; called also *gastric d.*

dilatator (dil″ah-ta′tor) [L.] that which dilates, as a muscle.

dilation (di-la′shun) 1. the act of dilating or stretching. 2. dilatation. **digital d.,** the expansion or stretching of a cavity or orifice by means of a finger.

dilator (di-la′tor) 1. [NA] a general term for a structure (muscle) that dilates. 2. an instrument used in enlarging an orifice or canal by stretching. **anal d.,** an instrument for dilating or stretching the anal sphincter. **Barnes's d.,** see under *bag*. **Einhorn's d.,** a metal dilator used to stretch the cardioesophageal region in cardiospasm. **Hegar's d's,** a series of bougies of varying sizes for dilating the ostium uteri. **Kollmann's d.,** a metallic, expandable urethral dilator. **laryngeal d.,** a bougie-like instrument which is used for distending a stenosed larynx. **d. na′ris,** the alar part of the nasal muscle; see *partes transversa et alaris musculi nasalis*. **Starck d.,** an expandable rubber-covered metal frame used to dilate the cardioesophageal region.

Dilaudid (di-law′did) trademark for preparations of hydromorphone hydrochloride.

dilecanus (di″lě-ka′nus) [*di-* + Gr. *lekanē* a dish] dipygus.

Dilepididae (dil″ě-pid′ĭ-de) a family of medium-sized or small tapeworms of the order Cyclophyllidea, subclass Cestoda, which parasitize mammals, birds, and snakes. The genus *Dipylidium* is of medical importance.

diltiazem hydrochloride (dil-ti′ah-zem) chemical name: (+)-*cis*-3-(acetyloxy)-5-[2-(dimethylamino)ethyl]-2,3-dihydro-2-(4-methoxyphenyl)-1,5-benzothiazepin-4(5*H*)one monohydrochloride. A coronary vasodilator, $C_{22}N_2O_4S \cdot HCl$, used in the symptomatic treatment of angina of effort.

Diluc. abbreviation for L. *dilu′culo*, at daybreak.

diluent (dil′u-ent) [L. *diluere* to wash] 1. diluting. 2. an agent that dilutes or renders less potent or irritant.

dilut. abbreviation for L. *dilu′tus*, diluted.

dilution (di-lu′shun) 1. the act or process of diluting or the state of being diluted. 2. a diluted or attenuated medicine. 3. in homeopathy, the diffusion of a given quantity of a medicinal agent in ten or one hundred times the same quantity of water. **doubling d.,** a serial dilution in which the dilution in each tube is double that of the preceding tube. **nitrogen d.,** the addition of nitrogen to inspired air to lower its oxygen tension, producing an alveolar oxygen tension equal to a desired oxygen pressure. **serial d.,** a set of dilutions in a mathematical sequence. In microbiological technique, serial dilutions are used to obtain a culture plate that yields a countable number of separate colonies. From this, a calculation of viable cells in the original suspension can be made, as a colony picked for pure culture.

dim. abbreviation for L. *dimid′ius*, one half.

dimargarin (di-mar′gar-in) a glyceride having two molecules of margaric acid combined with a molecule of glycerin.

Dimastigamoeba (di-mas″tig-ah-me′bah) *Naegleria*.

dimefadane (di-mef′ah-dān) chemical name: *N,N*-dimethyl-3-phenyl-1-indanamine; an analgesic, $C_{17}H_{19}N$.

dimefilcon A (di″mě-fil′kon) a contact lens material (hydrophilic).

dimefline hydrochloride (di-mef′lēn) chemical name: 8-[(dimethylamino)methyl]-7-methoxy-3-[methyl-2-phenyl-4-*H*-1-benzopyran-4-one] hydrochloride; a respiratory stimulant, $C_{20}H_{21}NO_3 \cdot HCl$.

dimelia (di-me′le-ah) [*di-* + Gr. *melos* limb] a developmental anomaly characterized by duplication of a limb.

dimelus (di-me′lus) a fetus exhibiting dimelia.

dimenhydrinate (di″men-hi′drĭ-nāt) [USP] chemical name: 8-chloro-3,7-dihydro-1,3-dimethyl-1*H*-purine-2,6-dione compound with 2-(diphenylmethoxy)-*N,N*-dimethylethanamine. An antiemetic, $C_{17}H_{21}NO \cdot C_7H_7ClN_4O_2$, occurring as a white, crystalline powder; used in the treatment of motion sickness and in other conditions in which nausea may be a feature, administered orally.

dimension (dĭ-men′shun) a numerical expression, in appropriate units, of a linear measurement of an object, such as an organ or body part. **vertical d.,** the distance between two points, measured perpendicular to the horizontal. In prosthodontics, the length of the face determined by the distance of separation of the jaws. See *contact vertical d., postural vertical d.,* and *vertical d.* **vertical d., contact, vertical d., occlusal,** the lower face height with the teeth in centric occlusion. **vertical d., postural,** the vertical face height when the mandible is suspended in the postural resting position. **vertical d., rest,** the lower face height measured from a chin point just below the nose, with the mandible in the rest position.

dimensionless (dĭ-men′shun-les) denoting a numerical constant or variable that has no units of measurement.

dimer (di′mer) 1. a compound formed by combination of two identical simpler molecules. 2. a capsomer having two structural subunits. **thymine d.,** two adjacent thymine residues linked together by a covalent bond along a single polynucleotide of DNA, which may lead to inactivation of the DNA molecule. It results from exposure to ultraviolet radiation and may be reversed by photoreactivation.

dimercaprol (di″mer-kap′rol) [USP] chemical name: 2,3-dimercaptopropanol. A metal complexing agent, $C_3H_8OS_2$, occurring as a colorless or almost colorless liquid; used as an antidote to poisoning by arsenic, gold, and mercury, and sometimes other metals, administered intramuscularly. It has also been used in the treatment of hepatolenticular degeneration.

dimeric (di′mer-ik) exhibiting the characteristics of a dimer.

dimerous (dim′er-us) [di- + Gr. *meros* part] made up of two parts.

dimetallic (di″mĕ-tal′ik) containing two atoms or equivalents of a metallic element in the molecule.

Dimetane (di′mĕ-tān) trademark for preparations of brompheniramine maleate.

dimethicone (di-meth′ĭ-kōn) 1. a silicone oil consisting of dimethylsiloxane polymers with viscosities from 0.65 to 3,000,000 centistokes at 25° C. The term is used with a numeric suffix which indicates the approximate viscosity of the various grades in centistokes, e.g., the viscosity of dimethicone 200 in centistokes is 190 to 210. Dimethicones are used as ingredients of ointments and other preparations for topical application to protect the skin against water-soluble irritants. 2. simethicone. **activated d.,** simethicone. **d. 350,** a grade of dimethicone having a viscosity of approximately 350 in centistokes at 25° C; a prosthetic aid for soft tissues.

dimethindene maleate (di″meth-in′dēn) [USP] chemical name: N,N-dimethyl-3-[1-(2-pyridinyl)ethyl]-1H-indene-2-ethanamine (Z)-2-butenedioate. An antihistaminic, $C_{20}H_{24}N_2 \cdot C_4H_4O_4$, occurring as a white to off-white, crystalline powder; administered orally.

dimethisoquin hydrochloride (di″mĕ-thi′so-kwin) [USP] chemical name: 2-[(3-butyl-1-isoquinolinyl)oxy]-N,N-dimethylethanamine monohydrochloride. A local anesthetic, $C_{17}H_{24}N_2O \cdot HCl$, occurring as a white to off-white, crystalline powder; applied topically to relieve pain, itching, and burning of the skin.

dimethisterone (di″meth-is′ter-ōn) chemical name: 17-hydroxy-6-methyl-17-(1-propynyl)androst-4-en-3-one monohydrate. An orally effective progestin, $C_{23}H_{32}O_2 \cdot H_2O$, occurring as a white, crystalline powder, having actions and uses similar to those of progesterone; used alone or as the progestin component in combination with ethinyl estradiol as an oral contraceptive.

dimethoxanate hydrochloride (di″mĕ-thok′sĭ-nāt) chemical name: 10H-phenothiazine-10-carboxylic acid 2-[2-(dimethylamino)ethoxy]ethyl ester hydrochloride; an antitussive, $C_{19}H_{22}N_2O_3S \cdot HCl$.

2,5-dimethoxy-4-methylamphetamine (di″mĕ-thok″se-meth′il-am-fet′ah-mēn) a hallucinogenic compound derived from amphetamine; abbreviated DOM and popularly called STP.

3,4-dimethoxyphenylethylamine (di-mĕ-thok″se-fen″il-eth″il-am′in) a substance characteristically found in the urine of schizophrenics; abbreviated DMPE.

dimethylacetal (di″meth-il-as′ĕ-tal) a colorless, volatile liquid, ethylidene dimethyl ether, $CH_3 \cdot CH(OCH_3)_2$, formerly used as an inhalation anesthetic.

dimethylamine (di-meth″il-am′in) a gaseous and liquid ptomaine, $(CH_3)_2NH$, from decaying gelatin, decomposing yeast, rotten fish, etc.

p-dimethylaminoazobenzene (di-meth″il-am″ĭ-no-az″o-ben′zēn) a carcinogenic dye, $C_6H_5N_2C_6H_4 \cdot N(CH_3)_2$; used as an indicator in Töpfer's test for free hydrochloric acid in gastric juice. It has a pH range of 2.9 to 4, being red at 2.9 and yellow at 4. Called also *butter yellow.*

Dimethylane (di-meth′ĭ-lān) trademark for a preparation of promoxolane.

dimethylarsine (di-meth″il-ar′sin) cacodyl hydride.

dimethylarsinic acid (di-meth″il-ar-sin′ik) cacodylic acid.

7,12-dimethylbenz[a]anthracene (di-meth″il-benz-an′-thrah-sēn) 9,10-dimethyl-1,2-benzanthracene; a highly carcinogenic polycyclic aromatic hydrocarbon produced during incomplete combustion of carbonaceous materials. It is a procarcinogen that requires metabolic activation to an epoxide intermediate to exert a mutagenic effect; it is widely used in research on chemical carcinogenesis. Abbreviated DMBA.

dimethylbenzene (di-meth″il-ben′zēn) xylene.

dimethyl carbate (di-meth′il kar′bāt) chemical name: (endo,endo)-bicyclo-[2.2.1]hept-5-ene-2,3-dicarboxylic acid dimethyl ester; an insect repellent, $C_{11}H_{14}O_4$.

dimethylcarbinol (di-meth″il-kar″bĭ-nol) isopropyl alcohol.

dimethylethylpyrrole (di-meth″il-eth″il-pir′ol) a substituted pyrrole obtained from bilirubin.

dimethylguanidine (di-meth″il-guan″ĭ-din) a ptomaine, $CH_3 \cdot NH \cdot C(:NH) \cdot NH \cdot CH_3$, found in small amounts in the urine.

dimethylketone (di-meth″il-ke′ton) acetone.

dimethylphenanthrene (di-meth″il-fe-nan′thrēn) a carcinogenic and weakly estrogenic hydrocarbon.

dimethyl phthalate (di-meth″il-thal′āt) chemical name: 1,2-benzenedicarboxylic acid dimethyl ester. A clear, colorless, oily liquid, $C_6H_4(COO \cdot CH_3)_2$, the normal methyl ester of phthalic acid; used as an insect repellent.

dimethyl sulfate (di-meth″il sul′fāt) an industrial poison and war gas, $(CH_3)_2SO_4$, causing nystagmus, convulsions, and death from pulmonary complications.

dimethyl sulfoxide (di-meth′il sul-fok′sīd) chemical name: sulfinylbis[methane]: an alkyl sulfoxide, C_2H_6OS, practically odorless in its purified form. As a highly polar organic liquid, it is a powerful solvent, dissolving most aromatic and unsaturated hydrocarbons, organic compounds, and many other substances. Its biologic activities include the ability to penetrate plant and animal tissues and to preserve living cells during freezing. It has been used investigationally as a topical analgesic and anti-inflammatory agent and as an agent to increase the penetrability of other substances. It is available as a 50 per cent solution for direct instillation into the bladder for treatment of interstitial cystitis. Abbreviated DMSO.

dimethyltryptamine (di-meth″il-trip′tah-mēn) chemical name: N,N,dimethyltryptamine. A hallucinogenic substance, $C_{12}H_{16}N_2$, derived from the apocynaceous plant *Prestonia amazonica* (Benth.) Macbride (*Haemadictyon amazonicum* Spruce and Benth.) which is native to parts of South America and the West Indies. Abbreviated DMT.

dimetria (di-me′tre-ah) [di- + Gr. *mētra* womb] uterus duplex.

diminution (dim″ĭ-nu′shun) reduction or decrease in size or substance.

Dimmer's keratitis (dim″erz) [Friedrich *Dimmer*, Austrian ophthalmologist, 1855–1926] keratitis nummularis.

Dimocillin (di-mo-sil′in) trademark for preparations of sodium methicillin.

dimorphic (di-mor′fik) dimorphous.

dimorphism (di-mor′fizm) [di- + Gr. *morphē* form] the property of having or existing in two forms, as fungi that can grow as molds or yeasts. See also *dysmorphism,* def. 2. **physical d.,** the property of certain solids of existing in two crystalline or allotropic forms. **sexual d.,** 1. physical or behavioral differences associated with sex. 2. the condition of having some of the properties of both sexes, as in the early embryo and in some hermaphrodites.

dimorphobiotic (di-mor″fo-bi-ot′ik) [di- + Gr. *morphē* form + *biōsis* life] showing alternation of generations and having a parasitic and a nonparasitic stage in the complete life history.

dimorphous (di-mor′fus) [di- + Gr. *morphē* form] occurring in two distinct forms; having the property of dimorphism.

dimoxamine hydrochloride (di-mok′sah-mēn) chemical name: (R)-α-ethyl-2,5-dimethoxy-4-methylbenzene ethanamine hydrochloride; a memory adjuvant, $C_{13}H_{21}NO_2 \cdot HCl$.

dimoxyline phosphate (di-mok′-sĭ-lēn) dioxyline phosphate.

dimple (dim′pl) a slight depression, as in the flesh of the cheek, chin, or sacral region. **Fuchs's d's,** dellen. **postanal d.,** coccygeal foveola.

dimpling (dim′pling) the formation of slight depressions or dimples.

dineric (di-ner′ik) [di- + Gr. *nēros* liquid] denoting a solution made up of two immiscible solvents with a single solute soluble in each.

dineuric (di-nu′rik) having two neurons or axons; said of nerve cells.

dinitrate (di-ni′trāt) a compound of a base or a metal with two nitrate groups, as in lead dinitrate, $Pb(NO_3)_2$.

dinitrated (di-ni′trāt-ed) compounded with or containing two nitrate (NO_3) or nitro (NO_2) groups.

dinitroaminophenol (di-ni″tro-am″ĭ-no-fe′nol) a phenol, $C_6H_2(NO_2)_2 \cdot OH$, found in the blood after poisoning with trinitrophenol, forming red granules, free or in the leukocytes. Called also *aminodinitrophenol* and *picramic acid.*

dinitrobenzene (di-ni″tro-ben′zēn) a poisonous substance, $C_6H_4(NO_2)_2$, whose fumes may cause breathlessness and final asphyxia.

dinitrocellulose (di-ni″tro-sel′u-lōs) pyroxylin.

dinitrochlorobenzene (di-ni″tro-klor″o-ben′zēn) a substance that produces a delayed-type hypersensitivity response (contact dermatitis) in sensitized individuals when applied to the skin; it is a commonly used sensitizing agent in laboratory immunology and has been used to test cellular immune function in evaluation of suspected immunodeficiency. Abbreviated DNCB.

dinitrocresol (di-ni″tro-kre′sol) a poisonous cresol compound, $CH_3C_6H_2(NO_2)_2OH$, used as an insecticide. Dinitro-*o*-cresol has an effect similar to that of α-dinitrophenol.

dinitrofluorobenzene (di-ni″tro-floo″o-ro-ben′zēn) a substance that induces a delayed-type hypersensitivity reaction (contact dermatitis) in sensitized individuals when applied to the skin; a commonly used sensitizing agent and hapten in laboratory immunology. Abbreviated DNFB.

dinitrogen (di-ni′tro-gen) containing two nitrogen atoms. **d. monoxide,** nitrous oxide.

dinitrophenol (di-ni″tro-fe′nol) any one of six isomeric compounds, $C_6H_3(OH)(NO_2)_2$, used in making dyes. 2,4-Dinitrophenol was formerly suggested for administration in the treatment of myxedema and obesity, but it has been reported as a cause of agranulocytosis and cataracts, and is now used only as a reagent and indicator and frequently as a hapten.

dinitroresorcinol (di-ni″tro-re-sor′sin-ol) a green coal tar derivative, $C_6H_2(NO_2)_2(OH)_2$, used in preparing degenerated nerve tissue for study.

Dinobdella (di″nob-del′ah) a genus of leeches of the family Gnathobdellidae, species of which attack the larynx of cattle in India when swallowed in drinking water.

Dinoflagellata (di″no-flaj″ĕ-la′tah) [Gr. *dinos* whirl + *flagellum* whip] Dinoflagellida.

dinoflagellate (di″no-flaj′ĕ-lāt) a protozoan of the order Dinoflagellida.

Dinoflagellida (di″no-flah-jel″lĭ-dah) [Gr. *dinos* + L. *flagellum* whip] an order of minute, plantlike, chiefly marine protozoa (class Phytomastigophorea, subphylum Mastigophora) having two or more flagella in grooves, transverse and longitudinal, which cause the organism to rotate as it advances. Dinoflagellates generally have a cellulose covering and numerous green, yellow, or brown chromatophores. They may be present in sea water in vast numbers, causing a

discoloration known as red tide or red water, which may result in the death of various marine animals and fish by exhaustion of their oxygen supply. Dinoflagellates are an important component of plankton. Some species secrete a powerful neurotoxin that can cause a severe toxic reaction in humans who ingest shellfish that feed on the toxin-producing organisms. Representative genera include *Ceratium, Gonyaulax, Gymnodinium,* and *Prorocentrum.* Called also *Dinoflagellata.*

dinogunellin (di″no-gun′el-lin) the toxic lipoprotein found in the roe of the Japanese blenny *Stichaeus (Dinogunellus) grigorjewi.*

dinoprost (di′no-prōst) prostaglandin $F_{2\alpha}(PGF_{2\alpha})$, used as an oxytocic for induction of abortion, to evacuate the uterus in the management of missed abortion, and in the treatment of hydatidiform mole. Available as *dinoprost tromethamine.* **d. trometanol,** d. tromethamine. **d. tromethamine,** the tromethamine salt of dinoprost, $C_{20}H_{34}O_5 \cdot C_4H_{11}NO_3$, having the same actions as the base; used as an oxytocic for induction of labor, termination of pregnancy, missed abortion, fetal death, and hydatidiform mole. It is administered intravenously, extra-amniotically, or intra-amniotically. Called also *d. trometanol* and *prostaglandin $F_{2\alpha}$.*

dinoprostone (di″no-prōst′ōn) prostaglandin $E_2(PGE_2)$, used as an oxytocic for induction of abortion, to evacuate the uterus in the management of missed abortion, and in the treatment of hydatidiform mole.

D. in p. aeq. abbreviation for L. *div′ide in par′tes aequa′les,* divide into equal parts.

dinsed (din′sed) chemical name: *N-N ′*-ethylenebis[3-nitrobenzenesulfonamide]. A coccidiostat for use in poultry, $C_{14}H_{14}N_4O_8S_2$.

dinucleotide (di-nu′kle-o-tīd) one of the cleavage products into which a polynucleotide may be split; a dinucleotide itself may be split into two mononucleotides.

Diocles (di′ŏ-klēz) **of Carystus** (4th century B.C.) Greek physician and anatomist, a contemporary and student of Aristotle. Diocles was a founder of the Dogmatist school; he studied embryology, gynecology, and obstetrics, and he also performed animal dissections (e.g., on the womb of a mule). See also *Hippocrates* and *Praxagoras.*

diocoele (di′o-sēl) [di- + Gr. *koilos* hollow] (*obs.*) the cavity of the diencephalon; the third ventricle of the cerebrum.

Dioctophyma (di-ok″to-fi′mah) a genus of nematodes of the superfamily Dioctophymoidea. **D. rena′le,** the kidney worm, the largest nematode known, found commonly in dogs, cattle, horses, and other animals, but rarely in man; red in color and 35 cm. (males) to 103 cm. (females) in length, they are found usually in the pelvis of the kidney or free in the peritoneal cavity. The parasite is highly destructive to kidney tissue and may cause death. Called also *Eustrongylus gigas.*

Dioctophymoidea (di-ok″to-fi″moi′de-ah) a superfamily of aphasmids, including the genus *Dioctophyma.*

dioctyl calcium sulfosuccinate (di′ok′til) docusate calcium.

dioctyl sodium sulfosuccinate (di-ok′til) docusate sodium.

Diodon (di′o-don) a genus of tetraodontiform fishes of the family Diodontidae; some species are poisonous when ingested.

Diodoquin (di′o-do′kwin) trademark for a preparation of iodoquinol.

Diodrast (di′o-drast) trademark for a preparation of iodopyracet for injection.

dioecious (di-e′shus) diecious.

diogenism (di-oj′ĕ-nizm) [from *Diogenes,* a Greek philosopher of the 5th century B.C. noted for his contempt of the common aims and conditions of life] an effort or tendency to get rid of the refinements of civilization and to lead a life closer to nature.

diolamine (di-ol′ah-mēn) USAN contraction for diethanolamine.

Dioloxol (di″o-lok′sol) trademark for a preparation of mephenesin.

Dionosil (di-on′o-sil) trademark for preparations of propyliodone.

diopsimeter (di″op-sim′ĕ-ter) [dia- Gr. *opsis* sight + -*meter*] a device for measuring the field of vision.

diopter (di-op′ter) [Gr. *dioptra* optical instrument for measuring angles] a unit of refractive power of lenses: the reciprocal of the focal length in meters is the refractive power in diopters. Symbol D. **prism d.,** a unit of prismatic deviation; deflection of one centimeter at a distance of one meter.

dioptometer (di″op-tom′ĕ-ter) [*dioptric* + -*meter*] an instrument for use in testing ocular refraction.

dioptometry (di″op-tom′ĕ-tre) the measurement of refraction and accommodation of the eye.

dioptoscopy (di″op-tos′ko-pe) [*dioptric* + -*scopy*] measurement of ocular refraction by means of the ophthalmoscope.

dioptre (di-op′ter) diopter.

dioptric (di-op′trik) pertaining to refraction or to transmitted and refracted light; refracting.

dioptrics (di-op′triks) the science of refracted light.

dioptrometer (di″op-trom′ĕ-ter) dioptometer.

dioptrometry (di″op-trom′ĕ-tre) dioptometry.

dioptroscopy (di″op-tros′ko-pe) dioptoscopy.

dioptry (di′op-tre) diopter.

Dioscorea (di″os-ko′re-ah) a genus of plants, the Mexican yams, family Dioscoreaceae. The dried rhizome of *D. villosa* L., which contains saponin and acrid resins, was once used for its diaphoretic, expectorant, and diuretic properties. Several species of *Dioscorea*, e.g., *D. villosa, D. floribunda,* and *D. tokoro,* are used as sources of diosgenin, an important saponin precursor in the synthesis of several medically important steroids, e.g., pregnenolone and progesterone. **D. mexica′na,** the source of botogenin.

Dioscorides (di″ŏ-skōr′ĭ-dēz) **of Anazarbos** (1st century A.D.) a noted botanist and pharmacologist whose encyclopedia of materia medica was widely used for centuries after his death.

diose (di′ōs) the simplest sugar, a monosaccharide containing two carbon atoms in the molecule: $CH_2OH—CHO$. Called also *glycolic aldehyde.*

diosgenin (di-os′jen-in) an aglycone of the saponin dioscin, Δ^5-$20\beta_F,22\alpha$-$F,25\alpha_F$-spirosten-3-β-ol; $C_{27}H_{42}O_3$. Obtained from several species of *Dioscorea,* it is a precursor in the synthesis of pregnenolone, progesterone, and other medically useful steroids.

diospyrobezoar (di″os-pi′ro-be′zŏr) a bezoar made up of persimmon fibers.

diovulatory (di-ov′u-lah-to″re) ordinarily discharging two ova in one ovarian cycle.

dioxane (di-ok′sān) diethylene dioxide, a clear fluid, used for dehydrating and clearing tissues preparatory to paraffin embedding; it is an industrial poison.

dioxide (di-ok′sīd) 1. a binary compound containing two oxide ions, such as silicon dioxide, SiO_2. 2. an oxide of a non-metal with a valence of four, such as sulfur dioxide, SO_2.

dioxin (di-ok′sin) any of the heterocyclic hydrocarbons present as a trace contaminant in herbicides, especially the chlorinated dioxin 2,3,7,8-tetrachlorodibenzo-para-dioxin, thought to have oncogenic and teratogenic properties.

dioxybenzone (di-oks″ĭ-ben′zōn) [USP] chemical name: (2-hydroxy-4-methoxyphenyl) (2-hydroxyphenyl)methanone. A sunscreening agent, $C_{14}H_{12}O_4$, occurring as an off-white to yellow powder; applied topically to the skin.

dioxygen (di″ok′sĭ-gen) molecular oxygen, O_2.

dioxygenase (di-ok′sĭ-jĕ-nās) one of a sub-subclass of enzymes of the oxidoreductase class (EC 1.13.11), which catalyze the incorporation of both atoms of oxygen from O_2 into a single substrate, frequently cleaving a C=C bond. Most of these enzymes require either iron or copper for activity.

dioxyline phosphate (di-ok′sĭ-lēn) chemical name: 1-(4-ethoxy-3-methoxybenzyl)-6,7-dimethoxy-3-methylisoquinoline. A synthetic analogue of papaverine, $C_{22}H_{25}NO_4$, occurring as a white, crystalline powder; used as a vasodilator, mainly in the treatment of vascular spasm associated with acute myocardial infarction, angina of effort, peripheral vascular disease in which there is a vasospastic element, and peripheral and pulmonary embolism, administered orally. Called also *dimoxyline phosphate.*

Dipaxin (di-pak′sin) trademark for a preparation of diphenadione.

dipentene (di-pen′tēn) any terpene found in volatile oils; called also *diamylene.*

dipeptidase (di-pep′tĭ-dās) a peptidase which catalyzes the hydrolysis of the peptide linkage in a dipeptide.

dipeptide (di-pep′tīd) a peptide which, on hydrolysis, yields two amino acids.

dipeptidyl I carboxypeptidase (di-pep″ti-dil karbok″sĕ-pep′tĭ-dās) [EC 3.4.15.1] an enzyme of the hydrolase class that catalyzes the reaction polypeptidyl-dipeptide + H_2O = polypeptide + dipeptide. The reaction cleaves a dipeptide from the C-terminal end of oligopeptides. It also catalyzes the reaction angiotensin I + H_2O = angiotensin II + histidine-leucine, and acts on bradykinin. The enzyme is a zinc-protein, found on the luminal surface of vascular endothelial cells in the lungs and other tissues. Called also *angiotensin converting enzyme.*

dipeptidyl peptidase I (di-pep″tĭ-dil pep′tĭdās) [EC 3.4.14.1] an enzyme of the hydrolase class that catalyzes the reaction dipeptidyl-polypeptide + H_2O = dipeptide + polypeptide. Called also *cathepsin C.*

diperodon (di-per′o-don) [USP] chemical name: 3-(1-piperidinyl)-1,2-propanediolbis(phenylcarbamate)(ester) monohydrate. A local anesthetic, $C_{22}H_{27}N_3O_4 \cdot H_2O$, occurring as a white to cream-colored powder; applied topically to the skin for abrasions, irritations, and pruritus and intrarectally for relief of discomfort associated with hemorrhoids. **d. hydrochloride,** the monohydrochloride salt of diperodon, $C_{22}H_{27}N_3O_4 \cdot HCl$, having the same actions and uses as the base.

Dipetalonema (di-pet″ah-lo-ne′mah) a genus of nematodes of the superfamily Filarioidea. **D. per′stans,** *Mansonella perstans.* **D. recondi′tum,** a species found in the perirenal fat pad of dogs; called also *Filaria recondita.* **D. streptocer′ca,** *Mansonella streptocerca.*

dipetalonemiasis (di-pet″ah-lo-ne-mi′ah-sis) mansonellosis.

diphallia (di-fal′e-ah) [*di-* + Gr. *phallos* penis] duplication of the penis.

diphallus (di′fal-lus) a double penis.

diphasic (di-fa′zik) [*di-* + Gr. *phasis* phase] occurring in two phases or stages. Cf. *monophasic* and *triphasic.*

diphebuzol (di-feb′u-zol) phenylbutazone.

diphemanil methylsulfate (di-fe′mah-nil) [USP] chemical name: 4-(diphenylmethylene)-1,1-dimethylpiperidinium methyl sulfate. A quaternary ammonium anticholinergic, $C_{21}H_{27}NO_4S$, occurring as a white or nearly white, crystalline powder; used in the treatment of peptic ulcer, gastric hyperacidity, and hypermotility in gastritis and pylorospasm, and in the treatment of hyperhidrosis, administered orally.

diphenadione (di-fen-di′ōn) [USP] chemical name: 2-(diphenylacetyl)-1*H*-indene-1,3-(2*H*)-dione. One of the indanedione anticoagulants, $C_{23}H_{16}O_3$, occurring as yellow crystals or as a yellow, crystalline powder; administered orally.

diphenhydramine hydrochloride (di″fen-hi″drah-mēn) [USP] chemical name: 2-(diphenylmethoxy)-*N,N*-dimethylethanamine hydrochloride. An antihistaminic, $C_{17}H_{21}NO \cdot HCl$, occurring as a white, crystalline powder; used in the symptomatic management of allergic symptoms and also for its sedative, antiemetic, antitussive, local anesthetic, and anticholinergic (antispasmodic) effects, administered orally, intramuscularly, and intravenously.

diphenidol (di-fen′ĭ-dōl) chemical name: α,α-diphenyl-1-piperidinebutanol. An antiemetic, $C_{21}H_{27}NO$, used for the treatment of vertigo and to control nausea and vomiting; administered rectally. **d. hydrochloride,** the hydrochloride salt of diphenidol, $C_{21}H_{27}NO \cdot HCl$, having the same actions and uses as the base; administered orally or intramuscularly. **d. pamoate,** the pamoate salt of diphenidol, $(C_{21}H_{27}NO)_2 \cdot C_{23}H_{16}O_6$, having the same actions as the base.

diphenoxylate hydrochloride (di″fen-ok′sĭ-lāt) [USP] chemical name: 1-(3-cyano-3,3-diphenylpropyl)-4-phenyl-4-piperidinecarboxylic acid ethyl ester monohydrochloride. An antiperistaltic derived from meperidine, $C_{30}H_{32}N_2O_2 \cdot HCl$; used as an antidiarrheal, administered orally.

diphenyl (di-fe′nil) a colorless compound, $C_6H_5C_6H_5$, found in coal tar and used as fungistat in containers for shipping oranges. Called also *biphenyl.*

diphenylamine (di-fen″il-am′in) chemical name: *N*-phenylbenzeneamine. A compound, $(C_6H_5)_2NH$, used as a test for oxidizing agents, such as nitric acid and chlorine, and, in veterinary medicine, in the prevention and treatment of screw-worm infestation.

diphenylaminearsine chloride (di-fen″il-am″in-ar′sin klo′rīd) a toxic smoke for war use, $NH(C_6H_4)_2AsCl$; called also *adamsite*.

diphenylamino-azo-benzene (di-fen″il-am″ĭ-no-az″o-ben′zēn) an indicator with a pH range of 1.2 to 2.1.

diphenylbutylpiperidine (di-fen″il-bu″til-pi-per′ĭ-dēn) any of a class of structurally related antipsychotic agents that includes penfluridol and pimozide.

diphenylchlorarsine (di-fen″il-klor-ar′sin) sneezing gas, $(C_6H_5)_2AsCl$, a toxic smoke once used in war, causing sneezing, coughing, headache, salivation, and vomiting; called also *Clark I* and *DA*.

diphenylcyanarsine (di-fen″il-si″an-ar′sin) a lethal war gas, $(C_6H_5)_2AsCN$; called also *Clark II*.

diphenylhydantoin (di-fen″il-hi-dan′to-in) phenytoin.

diphenylpyraline hydrochloride (di-fen″il-pi′rah-lēn) [USP] chemical name: 4-(diphenylmethoxy)-1-methyl-piperidine hydrochloride. An antihistaminic, $C_{19}H_{23}NO$·HCl, occurring as a white powder; used to relieve the symptoms of allergic reactions, administered orally.

diphonia (di-fo′ne-ah) [di- + Gr. *phōnē* voice] a condition in which two different tones are produced in speaking; double voice.

diphosgene (di-fos′jēn) a gas, $ClCOOCCl_3$, which is intensely irritating to the lungs, producing pulmonary edema.

2,3-diphosphoglycerate (di-fos′fo-glis′er-āt) 2,3-bis-phosphoglycerate.

diphosphoglycerate mutase (di-fos″fo-glis′er-āt mu′tās) bisphosphoglycerate mutase.

diphosphoglycerate phosphatase (di-fos″fo-glis′er-āt fos′fah-tās) bisphosphoglycerate phosphatase.

diphosphopyridine nucleotide (di-fos′fo-pir′ĭ-dēn) DPN; former name of nicotinamide-adenine dinucleotide (NAD).

diphosphothiamin (di-fos″fo-thi′ah-min) thiamine diphosphate.

diphosphotransferase (di″fos-fo-trans′fer-ās) a sub-sub-class of enzymes [EC 2.7.6] of the transferase class that catalyze the transfer of diphosphate groups from one molecule to another. Called also *pyrophosphokinase* and *pyrophosphotransferase*.

diphtheria (dif-the′re-ah) [Gr. *diphthera* leather + -*ia*] an acute infectious disease caused by toxigenic strains of *Corynebacterium diphtheriae*, acquired by contact with an infected person or a carrier of the disease, which is usually confined to the upper respiratory tract, and characterized by the formation of a tough membrane (false membrane or pseudo-membrane) attached firmly to the underlying tissue that will bleed if forcibly removed. In the most serious infections the membrane begins in the tonsillar (faucial) area on one tonsil and may spread to involve the other tonsil, uvula, soft palate, and pharyngeal wall, from where it may extend to the larynx, trachea, and bronchial tree, and may cause bronchial obstruction and death by hypoxia. Diphtheria also occurs in a cutaneous form and may rarely involve the eyes, middle ear, buccal mucosa, genitalia and umbilical stump, usually secondarily. Systemic effects, chiefly myocarditis and peripheral neuritis, are caused by the exotoxin produced by *C. diphtheriae*. Called also *Bretonneau's angina* or *disease*. **avian d.,** fowlpox. **Bretonneau's d.,** diphtheria. **calf d.,** a contagious disease of young calves in which grayish patches form in the mouth and throat, caused by *Fusobacterium necrophorum*. Called also *necrotic laryngitis*. **cutaneous d.,** a form of diphtheria involving the skin, occurring as a primary infection, usually seen in warm climates, characterized by a nonhealing, punched-out ulcer with a rolled border, surrounded by a zone of erythema, and sometimes covered by a hard, adherent membrane; or as a secondary infection of a preexisting lesion (burn, abrasion, cut, insect bite, etc.); or as a superinfection of various eczematous lesions. **faucial d.,** see diphtheria. **fowl d.,** fowlpox. **laryngeal d., laryngeotracheal d.,** see diphtheria. **malignant d.,** severe pharyngeal diphtheria characterized by massive cervical lymphadenopathy associated with marked edema on the anterior neck and submandibular region (bull neck appearance). **nasal d.,** diphtheria usually localized to the nasal mucosa, most often seen in the anterior nasal septum of infants, characterized by a serosanguineous discharge, uni-

lateral or bilateral, that becomes mucopurulent and causes skin erosion around the nostrils and upper lip and by the presence of a whitish membrane; constitutional symptoms may be absent or slight. **nasopharyngeal d.,** see diphtheria. **pharyngeal d.,** see diphtheria. **umbilical d.,** see diphtheria.

diphtherial (dif-the′re-al) diphtheritic.

diphtheric (dif-the′rik) diphtheritic.

diphtherin (dif′the-rin) 1. (*obs.*) diphtheria toxin. 2. a polyvalent diphtheritic antigen for use in anaphylactic skin test.

diphtheritic (dif″the-rit′ik) pertaining to, caused by, or resembling diphtheria (with particular reference to the membrane characteristic of diphtheria); diphtherial; diphtheric.

diphtheroid (dif′ther-oid) 1. resembling diphtheria or the diphtheria bacillus. 2. any member of *Corynebacterium* other than *C. diphtheriae*. 3. pseudodiphtheria. 4. former name for organisms now in the genus *Propionibacterium*.

diphtherotoxin (dif″thĕ-ro-tok′sin) see *diphtheria toxin*, under *toxin*.

diphthongia (dif-thon′je-ah) [di- + Gr. *phthongos* sound] the production of double vocal sounds; called also *diplophonia*.

Diphylets (di′fĭ-lets) trademark for a preparation dextroamphetamine sulfate.

diphyllobothriasis (di-fil″o-both-ri′ah-sis) the state of being infected with tapeworms of the genus *Diphyllobothrium*; formerly called *dibothriocephaliosis*.

Diphyllobothriidae (di-fil″o-both-re′ĭ-de) a family of tapeworms of the order Pseudophyllidea, subclass Cestoda, which are parasitic in man and other fish-eating vertebrates. The genera *Diphyllobothrium*, *Diplogonoporus*, and *Spirometra* are of medical importance.

Diphyllobothrium (di-fil″o-both′re-um) [di- + Gr. *phyllon* leaf + *bothrion* pit] a genus of large tapeworms of the family Diphyllobothriidae, order Pseudophyllidea; formerly called *Bothriocephalus* and *Dibothriocephalus*. **D. corda′tum,** the heart-headed tapeworm; a small species found in dogs and in seals in Greenland and very rarely in man. **D. erina′cei,** a species found in the adult form in the dog and other carnivores; formerly called *D. mansoni*. **D. la′tum,** the broad tapeworm or fish tapeworm; a very large tapeworm found in the intestines of man and (somewhat smaller) in cats, dogs, mink, bears, and other fish-eating mammals. It may be $\frac{3}{4}$ inch wide and 30 feet long. The head is marked with two grooves or suckers (bothria). It has two intermediate hosts: the first a crustacean, the second a fish. Infection in man, acquired by eating inadequately cooked fish, may result in a clinical picture resembling that of pernicious anemia. Formerly called *D. taenioides*. Called also *Dibothriocephalus latus*. See accompanying illustration. **D. manso′ni,** *D. erinacei*. **D. mansonoi′des,** a species whose migrating larvae (sparganoa) are one of the causes of sparganosis. **D. par′vum,** a species found in man in Tasmania, Japan, Rumania, Iran, and Minnesota; possibly identical with *D. latum*. **D. taenioi′des,** *D. latum*.

diphyodont (dif′ĭ-o-dont″) [di- + Gr. *phyein* to produce + *odous* tooth] having two dentitions, a deciduous and a permanent, as in humans. Cf. monophyodont and polyphyodont.

dipipanone hydrochloride (di-pip′ah-nōn) chemical name: *dl*-4,4-diphenyl-6-piperidinoheptan-3-one hydrochloride. An analogue of methadone, $C_{24}H_{31}NO$·HCl, occurring as a white, crystalline powder; used as an analgesic, administered subcutaneously, intramuscularly, and intravenously.

dipivefrin (dĭ-piv′ĕ-frin) chemical name: (+)-4-[1-hydroxy-2-(methylamino)ethyl]-1,2-phenylene ester 2,2-dimethylpropanoic acid; an ophthalmic adrenergic, $C_{19}H_{29}NO_5$.

diplacusia (dip″lah-ku′ze-ah) diplacusis.

diplacusis (dip″lah-ku′sis) [Gr. *diplous* double + *akousis* hearing] the perception of a single auditory stimulus as two sounds, as a result of a pathologic condition involving the cochlea; called also *double disharmonic hearing*. **binaural d.,** different perception of a single auditory stimulus by the two ears; the difference may be in tone (disharmonic d.) or in timing (echo d.). **d. binaura′lis dysharmon′ica,** disharmonic d. **d. binaura′lis echo′ica,** echo d. **disharmonic d.,** a form of diplacusis in which a given pure tone is heard differently in the two ears. **echo d.,** a form in which a sound of brief duration is heard in the one ear a

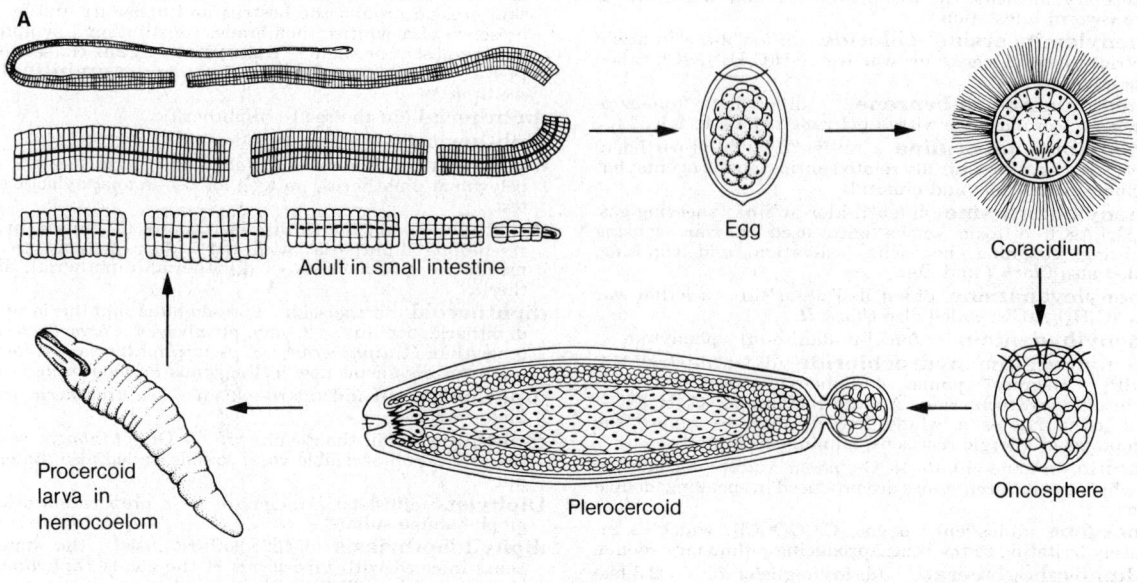

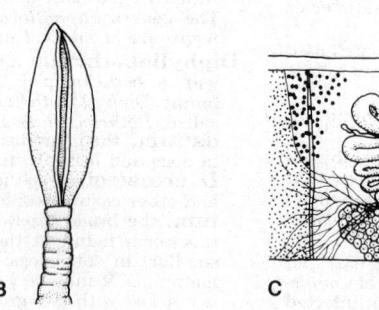

A, Life cycle of *Diphyllobothrium latum. B,* Scolex. *C,* Gravid proglottid.

fraction of a second later than in the other ear. **monaural d., d. monaura′lis,** a form in which a pure tone is heard in the same ear as a split tone of two frequencies.

diplasmatic (di″plaz-mat′ik) [*di-* + Gr. *plasma* something formed] containing substances besides protoplasm; said of cells.

diplegia (di-ple′je-ah) [*di-* + Gr. *plēgē* stroke] paralysis affecting like parts on both sides of the body; bilateral paralysis. **atonic-astatic d.,** diplegia characterized by hypotonia instead of spasticity. **facial d.,** paralysis affecting both sides of the face. **facial d., congenital,** Möbius syndrome. **infantile d.,** birth palsy. **masticatory d.,** paralysis of all the muscles which take part in mastication. **spastic d.,** Little's disease.

diplegic (di-ple′jik) pertaining to or marked by diplegia.

dipl(o)- (dip′lo) [Gr. *diploos* double] a combining form meaning double, twin, twofold, or twice.

diploalbuminuria (dip″lo-al-bu″mĭ-nu′re-ah) [*diplo-* + *albuminuria*] the presence of both physiologic and pathologic albuminuria.

diplobacilli (dip″lo-bah-sil′i) [L.] plural of *diplobacillus.*

diplobacillus (dip″lo-bah-sil′us), pl. *diplobacil′li* [*diplo-* + *bacillus*] a short, rod-shaped bacterium occurring in pairs, joined end to end; diplobacterium. **Morax-Axenfeld d.,** *Moraxella lacunata.*

diplobacteria (dip″lo-bak-te′re-ah) [L.] plural of *diplobacterium.*

diplobacterium (dip″lo-bak-te′re-um), pl. *diplobacteria* [*diplo-* + *bacterium*] a bacterial cell occurring as one of a pair of linked cells.

diploblastic (dip″lo-blas′tik) [*diplo-* + Gr. *blastos* germ] made up of two germ layers.

diplocardia (dip″lo-kar′de-ah) [*diplo-* + Gr. *kardia* heart] a condition in which the right and left heart are somewhat separated by a fissure.

diplocephalus (dip″lo-sef′ah-lus) dicephalus.

diplocephaly (dip″lo-sef′ah-le) dicephaly.

diplococcal (dip″lo-kok′al) pertaining to or caused by diplococci.

diplococci (dip″lo-kok′si) plural of *diplococcus.*

diplococcoid (dip″lo-kok′oid) 1. resembling diplococci. 2. an organism that resembles a diplococcus.

Diplococcus (dip″lo-kok′us) [*diplo-* + *coccus*] in former systems of classification, a genus of bacteria made up of organisms now assigned to various other genera. **D. constella′tus,** *Peptococcus constellatus.* **D. mag′nus,** *Peptococcus anaerobius.* **D. muco′sus,** *Neisseria mucosa.* **D. pneumo′niae,** *Streptococcus pneumoniae.*

diplococcus (dip″lo-kok′us), pl. *diplococ′ci.* 1. a spherical bacterium occurring predominantly in pairs as a consequence of incomplete separation following cell division in a single plane. 2. an organism of the genus *Diplococcus.* **d. of Morax-Axenfeld,** *Moraxella (Moraxella) lacunata.* **d. of Neisser,** *Neisseria gonorrhoeae.*

Diplodia (dĭ-plo′de-ah) a genus of imperfect fungi producing the dry-rot or corn-stalk disease of corn.

diplodiatoxicosis (dip″lo-dĭ″ah-tok″sĭ-ko′sis) a form of mycotoxicosis caused by fungi of the genus *Diplodia*.

diploë (dip′lo-e) [Gr. *diploë* fold] [NA] the loose osseous tissue between the two tables of the cranial bones.

diploetic (dip″lo-et′ik) of or pertaining to the diploë.

Diplogaster (dip″lo-gas″ter) [*diplo-* + Gr. *gastēr* stomach] a genus of free-living coprozoic nematodes which may, in fecal examination, be confused with hookworms or *Strongyloides*.

diplogenesis (dip″lo-jen′ĕ-sis) [*diplo-* + Gr. *genesis* production] the production of a double monster.

Diplogonoporus (dip″lo-go-nop′o-rus) [*diplo-* + Gr. *gonos* seed + *poros* passage] a genus of tapeworms of the family Diphyllobothriidae, characterized by the possession of two sets of reproductive organs in each segment. **D. brau′ni,** former name for *Digramma brauni*. **D. gran′dis,** a common parasite of whales that has been found in man in Japan; it may be up to 10 meters long, and may cause diarrhea or constipation, and secondary anemia.

diplogram (dip′lo-gram) [*diplo-* + Gr. *gramma* a writing] a roentgenogram containing two exposures.

diploic (dip-lo′ik) 1. double. 2. diploetic.

diploid (dip′loid) [Gr. *diploos* twofold] 1. having two sets of chromosomes, as normally found in the somatic cells of higher organisms. Cf. *haploid* (def. 1). 2. an individual or cell having two full sets of homologous chromosomes. Symbol, 2n.

diploidy (dip′loi-de) the state of having two full sets of homologous chromosomes.

diplomate (dip′lo-māt) a person who has received a diploma or certificate. In medicine the term refers particularly to a holder of a certificate of the National Board of Medical Examiners or of one of the American Boards in the Specialties.

diplomonad (dip″lo-mo′nad) [*diplo-* + Gr. *monas* unit, from *monos*, single] 1. pertaining to or caused by protozoa of the order Diplomonadida. 2. a protozoan of the order Diplomonadida.

Diplomonadida (dip″lo-mo-nad′ĭ-dah) [*diplo-* + Gr. *monas* unit, from *monos* single] an order of mostly parasitic, bilaterally symmetrical protozoa (class Zoomastigophorea, subphylum Mastigophora) having one or two karyomastigonts, each with one to four flagella. It includes two suborders: Diplomonadina and Enteromonadina.

Diplomonadina (dip″lo-mo″nah-di′nah) a suborder of mostly parasitic protozoa (order Diplomonadida, class Zoomastigophorea) having two karyomastigonts, each containing four flagella. Representative genera include *Giardia*, *Hexamita*, and *Trepomonas*.

diplomyelia (dip″lo-mi-e′le-ah) [*diplo-* + Gr. *myelos* marrow + *-ia*] lengthwise fissure and seeming doubleness of spinal cord.

diplon (dip′lon) [Gr. *diploos* double] deuteron.

diploneural (dip″lo-nu′ral) [*diplo-* + Gr. *neuron* nerve] (*obs.*) having a double nerve supply.

diplopagus (dip-lop′ah-gus) [Gr. *diploos* double + *pagos* a thing fixed] a double monster in which the component parts are equal to and the symmetrical equivalents of one another; called also *duplicitas symmetros*.

diplophase (dip′lo-fāz) that phase in the life history of certain organisms in which the nuclei are diploid.

diplophonia (dip″lo-fo′ne-ah) [*diplo-* + Gr. *phōnē* voice] diphthongia.

diplopia (dĭ-plo′pe-ah) [*diplo-* + *-opia*] the perception of two images of a single object; called also *ambiopia*, *double vision*, and *binocular polyopia*. **binocular d.,** double vision in which the images of an object are formed on noncorresponding points of the retinas. **crossed d.,** double vision in which the image belonging to the right eye is displaced to the left of the image belonging to the left eye, as occurs in exotropia (divergent squint). Called also *heteronymous d.* **direct d.,** double vision in which the image belonging to the right eye appears to the right of the image belonging to the left eye, as occurs in esotropia (convergent squint). Called also *homonymous d.* and *uncrossed d.* **heteronymous d.,** crossed d. **homonymous d.,** direct d. **horizontal d.,** diplopia in which the images lie in the same horizontal plane, being either crossed or direct. **monocular d.,** the perception by the same eye of two images of a single object, due to double pupil, early cataract, irregular astigmatism, or displacement of the lens. **paradoxical d.,** crossed d. **physiological d.,** diplopia in normal binocular vision; all objects not on the horopter of the fixated object are doubled through stimulation of disparate points of the retinae outside the corresponding retinal areas. For nearer objects, the diplopia is crossed; for farther objects, uncrossed. Called also *stereoscopic d.* **stereoscopic d.,** physiological d. **torsional d.,** double vision in which the upper pole of the vertical axis of one image is inclined toward or away from that of the other. **uncrossed d.,** direct d. **vertical d.,** double vision in which one image appears to be above the other.

diplopiometer (dĭ-plo″pe-om′ĕ-ter) [*diplopia* + *-meter*] an instrument for measuring diplopia.

Diplopoda (di-plop′o-dah) [*diplo-* + Gr. *pous* foot] a class of arthropods of the superclass Myriapoda, which comprises the millipedes.

Diplopylidium (dip″lo-pi-lid′e-um) a genus of small tapeworms of the family *Dilepididae*, species of which are parasites of birds and mammals.

diploscope (dip′lo-skōp) [*diplo-* + *-scope*] an apparatus for the study of binocular vision.

diplosomia (dip″lo-so′me-ah) diplosomatia.

diplosomatia (dip″lo-so-ma′she-ah) [*diplo-* + Gr. *sōma* body] a condition in which complete twins are joined at some part of their bodies.

diplosome (dip′lo-sōm) [*diplo-* + Gr. *sōma* body] the two centrioles of mammalian cells; called also *paired allosomes*.

diplotene (dip′lo-tēn) the stage of the first meiotic prophase, following the pachytene, in which the two chromosomes in each bivalent begin to repel one another and a split occurs between the chromosomes, which are then held together by regions where exchanges have taken place (chiasmata) during crossing over. See also *leptotene*, *pachytene* and *zygotene*.

diploteratology (dip″lo-ter″ah-tol′o-je) [*diplo-* + *teratology*] the sum of what is known regarding joined twin monstrosities.

Dipluridae (dip-lu′rĭ-de) a family of spiders (suborder Orthognatha); two genera, *Atrax* and *Trechona*, have been shown to be harmful to man.

dipodia (di-po′de-ah) [*di-* + Gr. *pous* foot] a developmental anomaly characterized by duplication of a foot.

dipole (di′pōl) 1. a molecule having charges of equal and opposite signs but in which the center of the positive charge does not coincide with that of the negative charge, a property which enables the molecule to be bound electrostatically by both positively and negatively charged groups. See *polar compounds*, under *compound*. 2. a pair of electric charges or magnetic poles separated by a short distance.

dipotassium phosphate (di″po-tas′e-um fos′fāt) potassium phosphate.

dipping (dip′ing) palpation of the liver by a quick depressing movement of the fingers with the hand flat across the abdomen.

Diprosone (di-pro′sōn) trademark for preparations of betamethasone dipropionate.

diprosopus (di-pros′o-pus) [*di-* + Gr. *prosōpon* face] a monster with a single trunk and normal limbs, but with varying degrees of duplication of the face. **d. tetrophthal′mus,** a monster having two fused faces, the median eye of each being fused into a common orbit.

diprotrizoate (di″pro-tri′zo-āt) chemical name: 3,5-dipropionamido-2,4,6-triiodobenzoate; used as a contrast medium in roentgenography of the urinary tract.

dipsesis (dip-se′sis) [Gr. *dipsēsis* a thirst, longing] thirst.

dipsetic (dip-set′ik) [Gr. *dipsētikos* thirsty; provoking thirst] pertaining to, characterized by, or producing dipsesis.

dipsia (dip′se-ah) [Gr. *dipsa* thirst + *-ia*] thirst; often used as a word termination, denoting a condition relative to thirst, or the physiological state of the body leading to the ingestion of fluids.

dipsogen (dip′so-jen) [Gr. *dipsa* thirst + *gennan* to produce] an agent or measure that induces thirst and promotes the ingestion of fluids.

dipsogenic (dip-so-jen′ik) engendering thirst.

dipsomania (dip″so-ma′ne-ah) [Gr. *dipsa* thirst + *mania* madness] (*obs.*) alcoholism.

dipsosis (dip-so′sis) [Gr. *dipsa* thirst + *-osis*] extreme thirst or a craving for unusual things to drink. Cf. *polydipsia.*

dipsotherapy (dip″so-ther′ah-pe) [Gr. *dipsa* thirst + *therapeia* treatment] treatment by strict limitation of the amount of water to be ingested.

dipstick (dip′stik) a strip of cellulose chemically impregnated to render it sensitive to protein, glucose, or other substances in the urine.

Diptera (dip′ter-ah) [Gr. *dipteros* two winged] an order of insects including the flies, gnats, and mosquitoes.

Dipterocarpus (dip″ter-o-kar′pus) [Gr. *dipteros* two winged + *karpos* fruit] a genus of trees from southern Asia, affording gurjun balsam.

dipterous (dip′ter-us) 1. having two wings. 2. pertaining to insects of the order Diptera.

dipus (di′pus) [di- + Gr. *pous* foot] a conjoined twin monster with only two feet.

dipygus (di-pi′gus) [di- + Gr. *pygē* rump] a monster with double pelvis. **d. parasit′icus,** gastrothoracopagus dipygus.

dipylidiasis (dip″ĭ-lĭ-di′ah-sis) infection with *Dipylidium caninum.*

Dipylidium (dip″ĭ-lid′e-um) [Gr. *dipylos* having two entrances] a genus of tapeworms of the family Dilepididae, found in cats and other small carnivores. **D. cani′num,** a common tapeworm of dogs and cats, the larval stage living in fleas (*Ctenocephalides canis*) and lice (*Trichodectes canis*) of dogs, as well as in *Pulex irritans*, which thus act as vectors; it has been found in man. Called also *Taenia elliptica.*

dipyridamole (di″pi-rid′ah-mōl) chemical name: 2,2′,2″,2‴-(4,8-dipiperidinopyrimido[5,4-*d*]pyrimidine-2,6-diyldinitrilo)tetraethanol. A coronary vasodilator, $C_{24}H_{40}N_8O_4$, occurring as a yellow, crystalline powder; administered orally.

dipyrithione (di″pēr-ĭ-thi-ōn) chemical name: 2,2′-dithiobispyridine 1,1′-dioxide; an antibacterial and antifungal, $C_{10}H_8N_2O_2S_2$.

dipyrone (di′pi-rōn) a pyrazolone analgesic and antipyretic; now seldom used because it can cause agranulocytosis.

direct (di-rekt′) [L. *directus*] 1. straight; in a straight line. 2. performed immediately and without the intervention of subsidiary means.

director (di-rek′tor) [L. *dirigere* to direct] any person, thing, or device that guides or directs. **grooved d.,** a grooved instrument used to guide the direction and depth of a surgical incision.

dirhinic (di-ri′nik) pertaining to both nasal cavities.

dirigomotor (dir″ĭ-go-mo′tor) [L. *dirigere* to direct + *motor* mover] controlling muscular activity.

Dirofilaria (di″ro-fĭ-la′re-ah) a genus of filarial nematodes with very long filiform bodies and a striated cuticle. **D. immit′is,** the heartworm, an important pathogen of dogs and other canids, which is of worldwide distribution in tropical and subtropical areas. Mosquitoes, fleas, and gnats transmit the larvae, and adult worms are found in and may occlude the vessels of the heart, primarily the right ventricle and pulmonary artery, of affected animals. **D. magalhae′si,** a species found in the heart of a child in Brazil; it is probably identical with *D. immitis.* **D. re′pens,** a species found in the subcutaneous connective tissues of dogs and occasionally of man.

dirofilariasis (di″ro-fil″ah-ri′ah-sis) infection with a parasite of the genus *Dirofilaria.*

Dir. prop. abbreviation for L. *directio′ne pro′pria*, with proper direction.

dis- a prefix denoting (1) reversal or separation [L. *dis* apart], or (2) duplication [Gr. *dis* twice].

disability (dis″ah-bil′ĭ-te) 1. a lack of the ability to function normally, physically or mentally; incapacity. 2. anything that causes disability. 3. as defined by the federal government: "inability to engage in any substantial gainful activity by reason of any medically determinable physical or mental impairment which can be expected to last or has lasted for a continuous period of not less than 12 months." **developmental d.,** a substantial handicap having its on-

set before the age of 18 years and of indefinite duration, and attributable to mental retardation, autism (when found to be closely related to and requiring treatments similar to that of mental retardation), cerebral palsy, epilepsy, or other neuropathy.

disaccharidase (di-sak′ah-rĭ-dās″) an enzyme that hydrolyzes disaccharides. **intestinal d. deficiency,** disaccharide intolerance. **small-intestinal d's,** disaccharide intolerance.

disaccharide (di-sak′ah-rīd) any of a class of sugars that yield two monosaccharides on hydrolysis and have the general formula $C_n(H_2O)_{n-1}$ or $C_{12}H_{22}O_{11}$. They include sucrose, lactose, and maltose. Formerly called *biose*, *disaccharose*, and *hexabiose.* **reducing d's,** disaccharides that can reduce Fehling's solution or other reagents, owing to the presence of a functional aldehyde group.

disacchariduria (di-sak″ah-ri-du′re-ah) presence of a disaccharide (lactose or sucrose) in the urine.

disaccharose (di-sak′ah-rōs) disaccharide.

disacidify (dis″ah-sid′ĭ-fi) to remove an acid from, or to neutralize an acid in, a mixture.

Disalcid (di-sal′sid) trademark for preparations of salsalate.

disarticulation (dis″ar-tik″u-la′shun) [L. *dis-* apart + *articulus* joint] amputation or separation at a joint.

disassimilate (dis″ah-sim′ĭ-lāt) dissimilate.

disassimilation (dis″ah-sim″ĭ-la′shun) [*dis-* + *assimilation*] dissimilation.

disazo (dis-az′o) diazo-.

disc (disk) [L. *discus*] disk.

discectomy (dis-kek′to-me) diskectomy.

discharge (dis-charj′) 1. a setting free, or liberation. 2. matter or force set free. 3. an excretion or substance evacuated. **brush d.,** in electrotherapeutics, the spark discharge from a static machine or an induction coil; because of its slight ability to penetrate solid matter it was confused with x-rays by early investigators. Called also *spark x-rays.* **disruptive d.,** the passing of a current through an insulating medium due to the breakdown of the medium under the electrostatic stress. **epileptic d.,** the pathophysiological events underlying epilepsy. **nervous d., neural d.,** the propagated excitation produced by stimulation of a center in the nervous system. **systolic d.,** see *stroke volume*, under *volume.*

disci (dis′i) [L.] genitive and plural of *discus.*

disciform (dis′ĭ-form) [L. *discus* disk + *forma* shape] in the form of a disk.

discission (dis-sizh′un) [L. *discissio; dis-* apart + *scindere* to cut] incision, or cutting into, as of a soft cataract. **d. of cataract,** the surgical rupturing of the capsule so that the aqueous humor may gain access to the lens of the eye. **d. of cervix uteri,** incisions on each side of the cervix uteri, formerly done for the relief of stenosis of the cervix. **posterior d.,** incision of the capsule of a cataract from behind.

discitis (dis-ki′tis) diskitis.

disclination (dis″klĭ-na′shun) extorsion.

disc(o)- [L. *discus,* q.v.] a combining form denoting relationship to a disk, or disk-shaped. See also words beginning *disko-.*

discoblastic (dis″ko-blas′tik) [*disco-* + Gr. *blastos* germ] pertaining to a discoblastula or to discoidal cleavage.

discoblastula (dis″ko-blas′tu-lah) the specialized blastula formed by cleavage of a fertilized telolecithal ovum, consisting of a cellular cap—the germinal disk, or blastoderm—separated by the blastocoele from a floor of uncleaved yolk.

discogastrula (dis″ko-gas′troo-lah) a modified, flattened gastrula formed by discoidal cleavage of a highly telolecithal ovum.

discogenetic (dis″ko-jĕ-net′ik) discogenic.

discogenic (dis″ko-jen′ik) [*disco-* + Gr. *gennan* to produce] caused by derangement of an intervertebral disk.

discogram (dis′ko-gram) diskogram.

discography (dis-kog′rah-fe) diskography.

discoid (dis′koid) [Gr. *diskos* disk + *-oid*] 1. shaped like a disk. 2. a disklike medicated tablet. 3. a dental instrument with a circular blade around the entire periphery except where it meets the shank; used to carve dental restorations. 4. a disk-shaped dental excavator designed to remove the carious dentin of a decayed tooth.

discoidectomy (dis″koid-ek′to-me) diskectomy.

Discomyces (dis″ko-mi′sēz) [*disco-* + Gr. *mykēs* fungus] in former systems of classification, a genus of bacteria made up of organisms now assigned to the genera *Actinomyces*, *Nocardia*, and *Streptomyces*.

Discomycetes (dis″ko-mi-se′tēz) [*disco-* + Gr. *mykēs* fungus] a series of ascomycetous fungi of the subclass Euascomycetidae, including the order Pezizales; their fruiting body is an apothecium.

discopathy (dis-kop′ah-the) [*disco-* + Gr. *pathos* disease] disease of an intervertebral cartilage (disk). **traumatic d.**, rupture of an intervertebral disk due to physical trauma.

discophorous (dis-kof′o-rus) [*disco-* + Gr. *phoros* bearing] possessing a disklike organ or part.

discoplacenta (dis″ko-plah-sen′tah) a discoid placenta.

discord (dis′kord) [L. *discordia*] a simultaneous assemblage of two or more inharmonious sounds.

discordance (dis-kor′dans) in genetics, the occurrence of a given trait in only one member of a twin pair, as opposed to *concordance*.

discordant (dis-kor′dant) exhibiting discordance.

discoria (dis-ko′re-ah) dyscoria.

discrepancy (dis-krep′an-se) disagreement or inconsistency. **tooth size d.**, lack of harmony of size of individual or groups of teeth when related to those within the same arch or the opposing arch.

discrete (dis-krēt′) [L. *discretus; discernere* to separate] made up of separated parts or characterized by lesions which do not become blended.

discus (dis′kus), pl. *dis′ci* [L.; Gr. *diskos*] a circular or rounded flat plate; used as a general term in anatomical nomenclature to designate such a structure. Called also *disc* or *disk*. **d. articula′ris** [NA], the articular disk: a pad composed of fibrocartilage or dense fibrous tissue found in some synovial joints; it extends into the joint from a marginal attachment at the articular capsule and in some cases completely divides the joint cavity into two separate compartments. Called also *interarticular disk*. **d. articula′ris articulatio′nis acromioclavicula′ris** [NA], articular disk of acromioclavicular articulation: a pad of fibrocartilage, sometimes present, commonly imperfect, within the articular cavity of the acromioclavicular joint. Called also *Weitbrecht's cartilage* and *meniscus of acromioclavicular joint*. **d. articula′ris articulatio′nis mandibula′ris**, discus articularis articulationis temporomandibularis. **d. articula′ris articulatio′nis radioulna′ris dista′lis** [NA], articular disk of distal radioulnar articulation: a triangular pad of fibrocartilage, attached at its base to the radius and at its apex to the base of the styloid process of the ulna; it usually separates the articular cavity of the distal radioulnar joint from that of the radiocarpal joint. Called also *cartilago triqueta, meniscus of inferior radioulnar joint*, and *triquetrous* or *triquetral cartilage*. **d. articula′ris articulatio′nis sternoclavicula′ris** [NA], articular disk of sternoclavicular articulation: a pad of fibrocartilage, the circumference of which is connected to the articular capsule of the sternoclavicular joint; it is attached superiorly to the clavicle and inferiorly to the first costal cartilage near its union with the sternum, and divides the joint cavity into two parts. Called also *meniscus of sternoclavicular joint*. **d. articula′ris articulatio′nis temporomandibula′ris** [NA], articular disk of temporomandibular joint: a plate of fibrocartilage or fibrous tissue that divides the temporomandibular joint into two separate cavities; its circumference is connected to the articular capsule. Called also *d. articularis articulationis mandibularis* and *meniscus of temporomandibular joint*. **d. interpu′bicus** [NA], interpubic disk: a midline plate of fibrocartilage interposed between the symphysial surfaces of the pubic bones, these surfaces being covered by a thin layer of hyaline cartilage; called also *lamina fibrocartilaginea interpubica*. **dis′ci intervertebra′les** [NA], intervertebral disks: the 23 plates of fibrocartilage found, from the axis to the sacrum, between the bodies of adjacent vertebrae, each consisting of a fibrous ring (annulus fibrosus) enclosing a pulpy center (nucleus pulposus); called also *fibrocartilagines intervertebrales*, and *intervertebral cartilages, fibrocartilage*, or *ligaments*. **d.**

lentifor′mis (obs.), subthalamic nucleus. **d. ner′vi op′tici** [NA], the optic disk: the intraocular portion of the optic nerve formed by fibers converging from the retina and appearing as a pink to white disk; there are no sensory receptors in this region and hence no response to stimuli restricted to it. Called also *blind spot, optic papilla*, and *papilla nervi optici*. **d. ooph′orus**, cumulus oophorus. **d. op′ticus**, d. nervi optici. **d. ovig′erus, d. prolig′erus**, cumulus oophorus.

discussive (dis-kus′iv) discutient.

discutient (dis-ku′she-ent) [L. *discutere* to dissipate] 1. scattering; causing a disappearance. 2. a remedy which so acts. Called also *discussive*.

disdiaclast (dis-di′ah-klast) [Gr. *dis* twice + *diaklan* to break through] any of the doubly refracting elements of the contractile substance of muscle.

disdiadochokinesia (dis-di-ad″o-ko-ki-ne′se-ah) dysdiadochokinesia.

disease (dĭ-zēz′) [Fr. *dès* from + *aise* ease] any deviation from or interruption of the normal structure or function of any part, organ, or system (or combination thereof) of the body that is manifested by a characteristic set of symptoms and signs and whose etiology, pathology, and prognosis may be known or unknown. **accumulation d.**, thesaurismosis. **Acosta's d.**, acute mountain sickness. **Adams′ d., Adams-Stokes d.**, a condition caused by heart block and characterized by sudden attacks of unconsciousness, with or without convulsions; called also *Adams-Stokes syndrome* or *syncope, Stokes-Adams d., syndrome*, or *syncope, Morgagni-Adams-Stokes syndrome*, and *Stokes' syndrome*. See also *heart block*. **d's of adaptation**, a concept introduced by Hans Selye that certain diseases are by-products of physiologic adaptations to chronic stress; he included in this category rheumatoid arthritis, peptic ulcer, essential hypertension, and possibly atherosclerosis. **Addison's d.**, a disease characterized by hypotension, weight loss, anorexia, weakness, and sometimes a bronzelike melanotic hyperpigmentation of the skin; it is due to tuberculosis- or autoimmune-induced disease (hypofunction) of the adrenal glands that results in deficiency of aldosterone and cortisol and, in the absence of replacement therapy, is usually fatal. **adult celiac d.**, the adult form of celiac disease, or nontropical sprue. **airsac d.**, infectious sinusitis of turkeys. **akamushi d.**, scrub typhus. **Akureyri d.**, epidemic neuromyasthenia; named for a town in northern Iceland where more than 1000 cases occurred in 1948. **Åland eye d.**, Forsius-Eriksson syndrome. **Albers-Schönberg d.**, osteopetrosis. **Aleutian mink d.**, a chronic, progressive disease of mink, perhaps of viral origin, marked by inappetance, weight loss, lethargy, polydipsia, and hemorrhages. **Alexander's d.**, an infantile form of leukodystrophy, characterized histologically by the presence of eosinophilic material at the surface of the brain and around its blood vessels, resulting in brain enlargement. **alkali d.**, 1. botulism in ducks. 2. a disease of livestock; see *selenium poisoning*, under *poisoning*. **allogeneic d.**, graft-versus-host reaction occurring in immunosuppressed animals receiving injections of allogeneic lymphocytes. **Almeida's d.**, paracoccidioidomycosis. **Alpers' d.**, poliodystrophia cerebri. **alpha chain d.**, the most common heavy chain disease, occurring predominantly in young adults in the Mediterranean area, and characterized by plasma cell infiltration of the lamina propria of the small intestine resulting in malabsorption with diarrhea, abdominal pain, and weight loss, or, exceedingly rarely, by pulmonary involvement. The gastrointestinal form is called also *immunoproliferative small intestine disease*. **altitude d.**, high-altitude sickness. **Alzheimer's d.**, a progressive degenerative disease of the brain of unknown etiology characterized by diffuse atrophy throughout the cerebral cortex with distinctive histopathologic changes termed "senile plaques" (microscopic lesions composed of fragmented axon terminals and dendrites surrounding a core of amyloid) and "neurofibrillary tangles" (intracellular knots or clumps of neurofibrils). There is a loss of choline acetyltransferase activity in the cortex, and it appears that many of the degenerating neurons are cholinergic neurons projecting from the substantia innominata to the cortex. The first signs of the disease are slight memory disturbance or subtle changes in personality; there is progressive deterioration resulting in profound dementia over a course of 5 to 10 years.

Onset may occur at any age; the disease was originally described as presenile dementia, occurring in persons under 65, as opposed to senile dementia, which was supposed to be a consequence of the aging process, but there is no clinical or pathophysiological distinction between the two classes of patients. Women are affected twice as frequently as men. **Anders' d.,** adiposis tuberosa simplex. **Andersen's d.,** glycogen storage d. (type IV). **Andes d.,** chronic mountain sickness. **anti–glomerular basement membrane (anti-GBM) antibody d.,** glomerulonephritis, usually of a generalized proliferative crescent-forming histologic type with a rapidly progressive course, marked by circulating anti-GBM antibodies and linear deposits of immunoglobulin and complement along the glomerular basement membrane. When associated with pulmonary hemorrhage the condition is called *Goodpasture's syndrome.* **Apert's d.,** acrocephalosyndactyly. **Apert-Crouzon d.,** an autosomal dominant disorder, consisting of the hand and foot malformations associated with Apert's syndrome (see *acrocephalosyndactyly*) together with the facial characteristics of Crouzon's disease (see *craniofacial dysostosis,* under *dysostosis*). Called also *acrocephalosyndactyly type I* and *Vogt's cephalodactyly.* **Aran-Duchenne d.,** spinal muscular atrophy. **arc-welders' d.,** siderosis (def. 1). **Armstrong's d.,** lymphocytic choriomeningitis. **atopic d.,** atopy. **Aujeszky's d.,** pseudorabies. **Australian X d.,** an acute epidemic encephalitis of viral origin observed in Australia during the summer months between 1917 and 1926, which resembled Japanese B encephalitis both symptomatically and pathologically; the virus appeared to be a variant of Japanese B encephalitis virus, but the culture was lost before it could be identified. See also *Murray Valley encephalitis,* under *encephalitis.* **autoimmune d.,** a disorder caused by an immune response directed against self antigens. Ideally there should be not only demonstrable circulating autoantibodies or cell-mediated immunity against autoantigens in conjunction with inflammatory lesions caused by immunologically competent cells or immune complexes in tissues containing the autoantigens but also clinical or experimental evidence that the autoimmune process is pathogenic not secondary to other tissue damage. In practice many diseases, such as systemic lupus erythematosus (SLE) and rheumatoid arthritis are often classified as autoimmune diseases although their pathogenesis is unclear. **aviators' d.,** high-altitude sickness **Ayerza's d.,** a form of polycythemia vera marked by chronic cyanosis, chronic dyspnea, chronic bronchitis, bronchiectasis, enlargement of liver and spleen, hyperplasia of bone marrow, and associated with sclerosis of the pulmonary artery. **Azorean d.,** a progressive degenerative disease of the central nervous system occurring in families of Portuguese-Azorean descent, having a variety of forms and inherited as an autosomal dominant trait. There are four major types: *Type I,* with pyramidal and extrapyramidal deficits; *Type II,* with cerebellar, pyramidal, and extrapyramidal deficits; *Type III,* with cerebellar deficits and distal sensorimotor neuropathy; *Type IV,* with parkinsonism and distal sensory neuropathy. Called also *Joseph's d., Machado-Joseph d.,* and *Portuguese-Azorean d.* **Azorean d. of nervous system,** Machado-Joseph d. **Baastrup's d.,** kissing spine. **Baelz's d.,** see *cheilitis glandularis.* **Baló's d.,** an atypical form of Schilder's disease in which the demyelination is arranged in concentric rings around a central circle; called also *encephalitis periaxialis concentrica* and *leukoencephalitis periaxialis concentrica.* **Bamberger's d.,** 1. saltatory spasm or tic of the lower extremities. 2. Concato's d. **Bamberger-Marie d.,** hypertrophic pulmonary osteoarthropathy. **Bang's d.,** infectious abortion in cattle caused by *Brucella abortus.* **Bannister's d.,** angioedema. **Banti's d.,** originally described as a primary disease of the spleen associated with splenomegaly and pancytopenia, but later considered secondary to portal hypertension; called also *congestive splenomegaly, Klemperer's d.,* and *splenic anemia.* **Barcoo d.,** desert sore. **Barlow's d.,** infantile scurvy. **barometer-maker's d.,** chronic mercurial poisoning in makers of barometers, due to the inhalation of the fumes of mercury. **Barraquer's d.,** partial lipodystrophy. **Basedow's d.,** Graves' d. **Batten d.,** see *amaurotic idiocy,* under *idiocy.* **bauxite workers' d.,** bauxite pneumoconiosis. **Bayle's d.,** general paresis. **Bazin's d.,** see *erythema induratum.* **Beard's d.,** neurasthenia. **Beau's d.,** cardiac insufficiency. **Beauvais' d.,** rheumatoid arthritis. **Beck's d.,** a disease affecting

young people in Siberia and marked by fatigue and swelling of the phalanges; later all the joints of the body become enlarged and normal growth is retarded. **Béguez César d.,** Chédiak-Higashi syndrome. **Behçet's d.,** see under *syndrome.* **Behr's d.,** degeneration of the macula retinae in adult life. **Beigel's d.,** piedra. **Bekhterev's d.,** rheumatoid spondylitis. **Benson's d.,** asteroid hyalosis. **Berger's d.,** IgA glomerulonephritis. **Bergeron's d.,** see under *chorea.* **Berlin's d.,** commotio retinae. **Bernard-Soulier d.,** an autosomal recessive disorder characterized by platelets with a wide range in size and morphology. The platelet membranes lack glycoprotein Ib, the probable receptor for plasma von Willebrand Factor (vWF); this deficiency keeps the platelets from binding the vWF necessary for their adhesion to the subendothelial surfaces of blood vessels. The clinical signs are variable and include mucocutaneous and visceral hemorrhaging, purpura, and prolonged bleeding time. See also *thrombasthenia* and *von Willebrand disease,* under *disease.* Called also *Bernard-Soulier syndrome* and *giant platelet d.* or *syndrome.* **Bernhardt's d., Bernhardt-Roth d.,** meralgia paraesthetica. **Besnier-Boeck d.,** sarcoidosis. **Best's d.,** congenital macular degeneration. **Bettlach May d.,** a fatal disease affecting adult honeybees, principally in Switzerland, marked by paralysis with inability to fly, caused by ingestion of the pollen of certain buttercups, which contains a poisonous substance. **Biedl's d.,** see *Bardet-Biedel syndrome,* under *syndrome.* **Bielschowsky-Jansky d.,** Jansky-Bielschowsky d. **Biermer's d.,** pernicious anemia. **Bilderbeck's d.,** acrodynia. **Billroth's d.,** 1. meningocele due to skull fracture and tearing of the arachnoid; called also *cephalhydrocele traumatica* and *spurious meningocele.* 2. lymphoma. **Binswanger's d.,** see under *dementia.* **black d.,** infectious necrotic hepatitis of sheep: a fatal disease of sheep, and occasionally of man, in the United States (in Montana) and in Australia (in New South Wales, Victoria, Tasmania), marked by necrotic areas in the liver; it is caused by *Clostridium novyi.* **blinding filarial d.,** blindness caused by onchocerciasis. **Blocq's d.,** astasia-abasia. **Bloodgood's d.,** cystic d. of breast. **Blount d.,** tibia vara. **blue d.,** 1. an old term for congenital heart disease; see *morbus caeruleus.* 2. Rocky Mountain spotted fever. **blue nose d.,** a disease of horses, apparently due to photosensitization following the ingestion of certain meadow plants, in which there is usually a blue discoloration of muzzle, sloughing of nonpigmented skin, and frequently intense excitement. **Boeck's d.,** sarcoidosis. **border d. of sheep,** a disease of unknown etiology and very high mortality that affects sheep on the English-Welsh border; it is manifested by an increase in the amount of hair in the fleece, slow growth, diminished stature, slight abnormality of head shape, and a slightly swaying gait. **Borna d.,** a fatal enzootic encephalitis of horses, cattle, and sheep, caused by a virus; called also *enzootic encephalitis of horses, equine encephalitis,* and *crazy d.* **Bornholm d.,** epidemic pleurodynia. **Bostock's d.,** hay fever. **bottom d.,** crotalism. **Bouchard's d.,** dilatation of the stomach from inefficiency of the gastric muscles. **Bouchet-Gsell d.,** swineherd's d. **Bouillaud's d.,** rheumatic endocarditis. **Bourneville's d.,** tuberous sclerosis. **Bouveret's d.,** paroxysmal tachycardia. **Bowen's d.,** intraepidermal squamous cell carcinoma, often occurring in multiple primary sites; called also *Bowen's precancerous dermatosis* and *precancerous dermatitis.* **Bradley's d.,** epidemic nausea and vomiting. **brancher glycogen storage d.,** glycogen storage d. (type IV). **Breda's d.,** yaws. **Breisky's d.,** kraurosis vulvae. **Bretonneau's d.,** diphtheria. **Bright's d.,** a broad descriptive term once used for kidney disease with proteinuria, usually glomerulonephritis. **Brill's d.,** Brill-Zinsser d. **Brill-Symmers d.,** nodular lymphoma. **Brill-Zinsser d.,** a recrudescence of epidemic typhus occurring years after the initial infection, in which the etiologic agent, *Rickettsia prowazekii,* persists in the body tissue in an inactive state (perhaps as long as 70 years), with humans as the reservoir. Compared with epidemic typhus, it is milder, the fever is not as high and is of shorter duration, the rash is less intense and is often absent, and the fatality rate is much lower. Called also *Brill's d.* and *latent* or *recrudescent typhus.* **Brinton's d.,** linitis plastica. **Brion-Kayser d.,** paratyphoid fever. **brisket d.,** a disease resembling mountain sickness in man, affecting young cattle living at altitudes above 7600 feet; it is sometimes seen in sheep and has been produced experimentally in pigs. **broad-beta d.,** familial hyperlipoproteinemia (type III); so called because on electrophoresis the lipoproteins show a broad band of beta lipoproteins. **Brodie's d.,** 1. chronic synovitis, especially of the knee, with a pulpy degeneration of the parts affected. 2. hysterical pseudofracture of the spine. **bronzed d.,** Addison's d. **Brooke's d.,** 1. keratosis follicularis contagiosa. 2. trichoepithelioma papillosum multiplex. **Brown-Séquard d.,** see under *syndrome.* **Brown-Symmers d.,** fatal acute serous encephalitis in children. **Bruck's d.,** a condition marked by deformity of bones, multiple fractures, ankylosis of joints, and atrophy of muscles. **Brushfield-Wyatt d.,** see under *syndrome.* **Bruton's d.,** X-linked infantile agammaglobulinemia. **Budd's d.** (*obs.*), Budd's cirrhosis. **Budd-Chiari d.,** see under *syndrome.* **Buerger's d.,** thromboangiitis obliterans. **Buerger-Grütz d.,** idiopathic hyperlipemia. **buffalo d.,** buffalo encephalitis. **Buhl's d.,** an acute sepsis affecting newborn infants, marked by hemorrhages into the skin, mucous membranes, and navel attended with cyanosis and jaundice; there are also hemorrhages in the intestinal organs. **Buschke's d.,** cryptococcosis. **bush d.,** a disease of sheep and cattle in certain parts of New Zealand, marked by progressive anemia; it is due to an iron or an iron and copper deficiency. **Busquet's d.,** exostoses on the dorsum of the foot due to osteoperiostitis of the metatarsal bones. **Buss d.,** a viral encephalomyelitis with pleuritis affecting cattle in the United States and Japan, marked by dullness, labored breathing, cough, diarrhea, staggering gait, and, sometimes, drooling of saliva and a discharge from the nose; called also *sporadic bovine encephalomyelitis.* **Busse-Buschke d.,** cryptococcosis. **Cacchi-Ricci d.,** sponge kidney. **Caffey's d.,** infantile cortical hyperostosis. **caisson d.,** decompression sickness. **California d.,** coccidioidomycosis. **caloric d.,** any disease due to exposure to high temperature. **Calvé-Perthes d.,** osteochondrosis of the capitular epiphysis of the femur. **Camurati-Engelmann d.,** diaphyseal dysplasia. **Canavan's d., Canavan-van Bogaert-Bertrand d.,** spongy degeneration of the central nervous system; see under *degeneration.* **canine parvovirus d.,** an acute, often fatal gastroenteritis of dogs caused by a parvovirus related to the virus of feline panleukopenia or of mink enteritis. **Caroli's d.,** congenital dilatation of the intrahepatic bile ducts. **Carrión's d.,** bartonellosis. **Castellani's d.,** bronchospirochetosis. **cat-scratch d.,** a usually benign, self-limited infectious disease of the regional lymph nodes, chiefly characterized by subacute painful regional lymphadenitis and mild fever of short duration. It is most often associated with close contact with a cat, the primary symptom being an isolated papule or pustule at the site of a cat scratch. Various organisms, including viruses, rickettsiae, and chlamydiae, have been suspected as etiologic agents. Although the disease has traditionally been considered to be nonbacterial in origin (being called also *nonbacterial regional lymphadenitis*), evidence has implicated a gram-negative, silver-staining bacillus as the causative agent. Called also *benign lymphoreticulosis, cat-scratch fever,* and *regional lymphadenitis.* **Cavare's d.,** familial periodic paralysis. **celiac d.,** a malabsorption syndrome affecting both children and adults, precipitated by the ingestion of gluten-containing foods; its etiology is unknown but a hereditary factor has been implicated. Pathologically, the proximal intestinal mucosa loses its villous structure, surface epithelial cells exhibit degenerative changes, and the absorptive function of these cells is severely impaired. It is characterized by diarrhea in which the stools are bulky, frothy, fatty (steatorrhea), and fetid (occasionally, malabsorption may be associated with the passage of a single bulky stool without diarrhea); abdominal distention; flatulence; weight loss; asthenia; deficiency of vitamins B, D, and K; and electrolyte depletion. Called also *gluten enteropathy* and *nontropical sprue.* In the *infantile form* the onset is insidious, and is marked by irritability, loss of appetite, weakness, extreme wasting, growth retardation, and celiac crisis. The *adult form* is marked by extreme lassitude, fatigue, difficulty in breathing, clubbing of the fingers, bone pain, cramping of the muscles, tetany, abdominal distention during the day, megacolon, tympanitis, and skin pigmentation. Until recently it was thought that the infantile form and the adult form were different entities, but it is now believed that they are the same. **central core d. of muscle,** a rare hereditary disease, transmitted as an autosomal dominant trait, in which severe hypotonia arrests motor development in infancy, but the course is benign and by school age affected children can walk; histologically, the diagnostic feature is a central core in each muscle fiber. **Chabert's d.,** blackleg. **Chagas' d., Chagas-Cruz d.,** an acute, subacute, or chronic form of trypanosomiasis occurring widely in Central and South America, caused by *Trypanosoma cruzi,* and transmitted by the bites of reduviid bugs of the genera *Triatoma, Panstrongylus,* and *Rhodnius,* with various domestic and wild animals, including cats, dogs, rodents, armadillos, bats, foxes, and other mammals, serving as reservoir hosts. The acute form (prevalent in children) is marked initially by an erythematous nodule (chagoma) at the site of inoculation; high fever; unilateral swelling of the face with edema of the eyelid (Romaña's sign); regional lymphadenopathy; hepatosplenomegaly; and meningoencephalic irritation. If death does not occur, the disease may resolve completely, or the subacute or chronic form may follow. Subacute Chagas' disease, which may last for several months or years, is characterized by mild fever, severe asthenia, and generalized lymphadenopathy. The chronic form, which may or may not be preceded by an acute episode, is characterized principally by cardiac manifestations (*chagasic myocarditis*) and gastrointestinal manifestations associated with megaesophagus and megacolon. Called also *Cruz-Chagas d., American, Cruz,* or *South American trypanosomiasis,* and *schizotrypanosomiasis.* **Charcot's d.,** neuropathic arthropathy. **Charcot-Marie-Tooth d.,** progressive neuropathic (peroneal) muscular atrophy. **Charlouis' d.,** yaws. **Chédiak-Higashi d.,** see under *syndrome.* **Cherchevski's (Cherchewski's) d.,** ileus of nervous origin. **Chester's d.,** xanthomatosis of the long bones with spontaneous fractures. **Chiari's d.,** Budd-Chiari syndrome. **Chiari-Frommel d.,** see under *syndrome.* **Chicago d.,** North American blastomycosis. **cholesteryl ester storage d. (CESD),** a relatively mild lysosomal storage disease due to acid lipase deficiency; hepatomegaly may be the only clinical abnormality; hyperbetalipoproteinemia is common, and there is often severe premature atherosclerosis; patients may survive past 40. **Christian's d.,** Hand-Schüller-Christian d. **Christian-Weber d.,** nodular nonsuppurative panniculitis. **Christmas d.,** Factor IX deficiency; see *coagulation factors,* under *factor.* **chronic granulomatous d. (CGD), chronic granulomatous d. of childhood,** a group of immunodeficiencies of X-linked or autosomal recessive inheritance, caused by the failure of the respiratory or metabolic burst, which results in deficient microbicidal ability. Clinically, the picture resembles glucose-6-phosphate dehydrogenase deficiency anemia, and patients usually suffer frequent, severe, and prolonged bacterial and fungal infections affecting the skin, oral and intestinal mucosa, reticuloendothelial system, bones, lungs, and genitourinary tract. The course of the disease varies: symptoms may appear at one week of age, with death during the first decade, or patients may survive well into middle age with no medical intervention. There appear to be no physiologic differences between the X-linked and the autosomal recessive types. Therapy includes antibiotic prophylaxis and supportive treatment against infection. **chronic obstructive pulmonary d. (COPD),** any disorder, e.g., asthma, chronic bronchitis, and pulmonary emphysema, marked by persistent obstruction of bronchial air flow. **chronic respiratory d. of poultry,** a common respiratory disease of chickens caused by mycoplasma, and marked by distressed breathing, swelling of the face, and discharge from the nostrils; abbreviated C.R.D. **chylopoietic d.** (*obs.*), one which affects the digestive organs. **circling d.,** listeriosis. **climatic d.,** any disease thought to be produced by a change of climate. **coast d.,** a disease of domestic animals similar to enzootic marasmus (q.v.), occurring in Tasmania. **Coats' d.,** chronic progressive exudative retinopathy usually occurring in male children and young adults. **Cogan's d.,** see under *syndrome.* **cold agglutinin d.,** see under *syndrome.* **collagen d.,** any of a group of diseases that, although clinically distinct and not necessarily related etiologically, have in common widespread pathologic changes in the connective tissue; they include lupus erythematosus, dermatomyositis, scleroderma, polyarteritis nodosa, thrombotic purpura, rheumatic fever, and rheumatoid arthritis. Collagen disease is not to be confused with collagen disorder (q.v.). **comb d.,** favus of fowl. **combined immunodeficiency d.,** see *immunodeficiency.* **combined system d.,** subacute combined degeneration of the spinal cord; see under *degener-*

ation. **communicable d.,** an infectious disease transmitted from one individual to another, either by direct contact or indirectly by means of a vector or fomites; the terms *communicable disease* and *contagious disease* are used synonymously. Cf. *infectious d.* **complicating d.,** one which occurs in the course of some other disease as a complication. **compressed-air d.,** decompression sickness. **Concato's d.,** progressive malignant polyserositis with large effusions into the pericardium, pleura, and peritoneum. **Conor and Bruch's d.,** boutonneuse fever. **Conradi's d.,** chondrodysplasia punctata. **constitutional d.,** one that involves a system of organs or one characterized by widespread symptoms. **contagious d.,** communicable disease transmitted by contact; the terms *contagious disease* and *communicable disease* are used synonymously. Cf. *infectious d.* **Cooley's d.,** see *β-thalassemia.* **Cooper's d.** (*obs.*), chronic cystic disease of the breast. **Corbus' d.,** gangrenous balanitis. **Cori's d.,** glycogen storage d. (type III). **cornstalk d.,** toxic encephalomalacia of dietary origin affecting horses. **corridor d.,** a tick-borne protozoal disease resembling East Coast fever, due to *Theileria lawrencei,* first reported in the Corridor, a region in South Africa. It is highly pathogenic for cattle, with buffalo serving as a reservoir of infection. **Corrigan's d.,** aortic insufficiency; see also *aortic regurgitation,* under *regurgitation.* **Corvisart's d.,** 1. chronic hypertrophic myocarditis. 2. tetralogy of Fallot associated with right aortic arch. **Cotugno's d.,** sciatica. **covering d.,** dourine. **Cowden's d.,** an autosomal dominant disorder comprising a combination of ectodermal, mesodermal, and endodermal anomalies, characterized by the development of a wide variety of multiple hamartomatous lesions, especially in the skin, oral mucosa, breast, thyroid, colon, and intestines, and associated with a high incidence of malignancies in the organs involved. Called also *Cowden's syndrome* and *multiple hamartoma syndrome.* **crazy d.,** Borna disease. **crazy chick d.,** 1. avian encephalomalacia. 2. avian encephalomyelitis. **creeping d.,** a condition marked by cutaneous lesions similar to those seen in larva migrans, but produced by nematodes of the genus *Gnathostoma.* **Creutzfeldt-Jakob d.,** a rare, usually fatal, transmissible spongiform encephalopathy, occurring in middle life, in which there is partial degeneration of the pyramidal and extrapyramidal systems accompanied by progressive dementia and sometimes wasting of the muscles, tremor, athetosis, and spastic dysarthria. Called also *Creutzfeldt-Jakob syndrome, Jakob's disease, Jakob-Creutzfeldt disease,* and *spastic pseudoparalysis.* **Crigler-Najjar d.,** see under *syndrome.* **Crocq's d.** (*obs.*), acrocyanosis. **Crohn's d.,** a chronic granulomatous inflammatory disease of unknown etiology, involving any part of the gastrointestinal tract from mouth to anus, but commonly involving the terminal ileum with scarring and thickening of the bowel wall; it frequently leads to intestinal obstruction and fistula and abscess formation and has a high rate of recurrence after treatment. Called also *regional enteritis* or *ileitis.* **Crouzon's d.,** craniofacial dysostosis. **Cruveilhier's d.,** 1. spinal muscular atrophy. 2. Cruveilhier's ulcer. **Cruz-Chagas d.,** Chagas' d. **Csillag's d.** (*obs.*), lichen sclerosus et atrophicus. **Curschmann's d.** (*obs.*), perihepatitis chronica plastica. **Cushing's d.,** Cushing's syndrome in which the hyperadrenocorticism is secondary to excessive anterior pituitary secretion of adrenocorticotropic hormone, with or without a pituitary adenoma. **cystic d. of breast,** a form of mammary dysplasia with formation of cysts of various size containing a semitransparent, turbid fluid that imparts a brown to blue color (blue dome cyst) to the unopened cysts; considered to be due to abnormal hyperplasia of the ductal epithelium and dilatation of the ducts of the mammary gland, occurring as a result of an exaggeration and distortion of the cyclic breast changes that normally occur in the menstrual cycle. Called also *chronic cystic mastitis, fibrocystic disease, fibrocystic disease of breast,* and *Schimmelbusch's disease.* **cystic d. of lung,** a condition in which there are abnormally large air spaces in the lung parenchyma; the term is sometimes applied to cystic emphysema. Called also *pseudocysts of lung* and *pulmonary pseudocysts.* **cysticercus d.,** infection with larval forms (*Cysticercus cellulosae*) of *Taenia solium* (the pork tapeworm). **cystine d., cystine storage d.,** cystinosis. **cytomegalic inclusion d.,** any of a group of diseases caused by cytomegalovirus infection marked by characteristic inclusion bodies in enlarged infected cells. The classic disease is congenital, being

acquired in utero from the mother; infection can also be transmitted from mother to infant in passage through the birth canal or from ingestion of the virus present in the mother's milk. Most infected infants are asymptomatic, but in some hepatosplenomegaly, jaundice, chorioretinitis, purpura, microcephaly, cerebral calcifications, and severe central nervous system sequelae resulting in blindness, deafness, quadriplegia, and mental retardation may occur. Acquired disease is transmitted via respiratory droplets or tissue or blood donation, or it may be sexually transmitted. The group also includes an infectious mononucleosis–like syndrome in previously well individuals and in those receiving multiple blood transfusions and a fatal disseminated infection in patients immunosuppressed or otherwise immunocompromised. See also *cytomegalovirus mononucleosis,* under *mononucleosis,* and *postperfusion syndrome,* under *syndrome.* **Czerny's d.,** periodic hydrarthrosis of the knee. **Daae's d.,** epidemic pleurodynia. **Dalrymple's d.,** cyclokeratitis. **Danlos' d.,** *Ehlers-Danlos syndrome.* **Darier's d.,** keratosis follicularis. **Darling's d.,** histoplasmosis. **David's d.,** tuberculosis of the spine. **debrancher glycogen storage d.,** glycogen storage d. (type III). **deficiency d.,** a condition produced by dietary or metabolic deficiency; the term includes all diseases—e.g., kwashiorkor, beriberi, scurvy, pellagra, calcium deficiency, etc.—caused by an insufficient supply of the essential nutrients, i.e., protein (or amino acids), vitamins, and minerals. **degenerative joint d.,** osteoarthritis. **Degos' d.,** malignant papulosis. **Dejerine's d., Dejerine-Sottas d.,** progressive hypertrophic interstitial neuropathy. **demyelinating d.,** any condition characterized by destruction of myelin. **dense deposit d.,** type II membranoproliferative glomerulonephritis. **deprivation d.,** deficiency d. **de Quervain's d.,** painful tenosynovitis due to relative narrowness of the common tendon sheath of the abductor pollicis longus and the extensor pollicis brevis. **Dercum's d.,** adiposis dolorosa. **dermopathic herpesvirus d.,** a herpesvirus disease of cattle, characterized by ulcerative lesions in the skin. It resembles lumpy skin disease (q.v.), a poxvirus disease indigenous to African cattle. **Deutschländer's d.,** 1. tumor of the metatarsal bones. 2. march foot (fracture). **Devic's d.,** neuromyelitis optica. **diamond-skin d.,** the urticarial and mildest form of swine erysipelas. **Di Guglielmo d.,** erythremic myelosis. **diverticular d.,** a general term embracing the prediverticular state, diverticulosis, and diverticulitis. **Döhle d.,** syphilitic aortitis. **Down's d.,** see under *syndrome.* **drug d.,** 1. a morbid condition due to long-continued use of a drug. 2. in homeopathy, the group of symptoms seen after the administration of a drug for the purpose of proving. **Dubin-Sprinz d.,** Dubin-Johnson syndrome. **Dubini's d.,** see under *chorea.* **Dubois' d.,** see under *abscess.* **Duchenne's d.,** 1. spinal muscular atrophy. 2. bulbar paralysis. 3. tabes dorsalis. **Duchenne-Aran d.,** spinal muscular atrophy. **Duchenne-Griesinger d.,** pseudohypertrophic muscular dystrophy. **Duhring's d.,** dermatitis herpetiformis. **Dukes' d.,** a mild febrile disease of childhood characterized by a bright rosy red, generalized exanthematous eruption, probably a viral exanthem of the Coxsackie-ECHO group; it was given the ordinal designation *fourth disease* to differentiate it from other exanthems (see *exanthem,* def. 2). Called also *Filatov-Dukes d.* and *scarlatinella.* **Duncan's d.,** X-linked lymphoproliferative syndrome. **Duplay's d.** (*obs.*), subacromial or subdeltoid bursitis; see *calcific tendinitis,* under *tendinitis.* **Dupré's d.,** meningism, def. 1. **Durand-Nicolas-Favre d.,** lymphogranuloma venereum. **Durante's d.,** osteogenesis imperfecta. **Duroziez's d.,** congenital mitral stenosis. **Eales d.,** a condition marked by recurrent hemorrhages into the retina and vitreous, affecting mainly males in the second and third decades of life. **Ebola virus d.,** a highly fatal, acute hemorrhagic fever, clinically very similar to Marburg virus disease, caused by the Ebola virus, which is morphologically but not antigenically similar to Marburg virus, and occurring in the Sudan and adjacent areas in northwestern Zaire; the natural reservoir and mode of transmission of the virus are unknown, but secondary infection is by direct contact with infected blood and other body secretions and by airborne particles. **Ebstein's d.,** 1. hyaline degeneration and necrosis of the epithelial cells of the renal tubules; seen in diabetes. 2. see under *anomaly.* **echinococcus d.,** hydatid d. **Economo's d.,** lethargic encephalitis. **Eddowes' d.,** see under *syndrome.* **Edsall's d.,** heat cramp. **Ehlers-Danlos d.,** see under *syndrome*. **elevator d.,** respiratory distress affecting persons who work in grain elevators. **endemic d.,** one present or usually prevalent in a population or geographical area at all times; such diseases are usually of low morbidity. Called also *endemia*. See also *holoendemic d.* and *hyperendemic d.* Cf. *epidemic d.* **Engelmann's d.,** diaphyseal dysplasia. **Engel-Recklinghausen d.,** osteitis fibrosa cystica. **English d.,** rickets. **English sweating d.,** anglicus sudor. **enzootic d.,** a disease which is at all times present in a small number of animals in a particular region. **eosinophilic endomyocardial d.,** Löffler's endocarditis. **epidemic d.,** an infectious or other disease that suddenly affects individuals in a population or geographical area clearly in excess of the number of cases normally expected. Cf. *endemic d.* **epizootic d.,** a disease which affects a large number of animals in some particular region within a short period of time. **Epstein's d.,** pseudodiphtheria. **Erb's d.,** progressive muscular dystrophy. **Erb-Charcot d.,** Erb's spastic paraplegia. **Erb-Goldflam d.,** myasthenia gravis. **Erb-Landouzy d.,** muscular dystrophy. **Eulenburg's d.,** paramyotonia congenita. **extensor process d.,** buttress foot. **extrapyramidal d.,** any of a group of clinical disorders marked by abnormal involuntary movements, alterations in muscle tone, and postural disturbances and involving lesions of the extrapyramidal tract; it includes parkinsonism, chorea, athetosis, etc. **Fabry's d.,** an X-linked lysosomal storage disease of glycosphingolipid catabolism, resulting from deficient α-galactosidase A and leading to accumulation of globotriaosylceramide in the cardiovascular and renal systems. Clinical manifestations include telangiectases in the "bathing suit area," corneal opacities, burning pain in the palms, soles, and abdomen, chronic paresthesias of the hands and feet, cardiopulmonary involvement, edema of the legs, osteoporosis, retarded growth, and delayed puberty. Patients usually die of renal failure or cardiac or cerebrovascular disease. Detection of female heterozygotes and prenatal testing (amniocentesis) are available. Called also *angiokeratoma corporis diffusum, diffuse angiokeratoma, α-galactosidase A deficiency,* and *ceramide trihexosidase deficiency.* **Fahr-Volhard d.,** malignant nephrosclerosis. **Fallot's d.,** tetralogy of Fallot. **Fanconi's d.,** see under *syndrome*. **Farber d.,** a lysosomal storage disease of ceramide metabolism due to defective ceramidase and marked by hoarseness, aphonia, and a brownish desquamating dermatitis beginning at about three months of age, followed by foam cell infiltration of bones and joints, resulting in deformations; granulomatous reaction in lymph nodes, heart, lungs, and kidneys, and psychomotor retardation. Called also *Farber lipogranulomatosis,* and *ceramidase deficiency.* **fat-deficiency d.,** a condition characterized by cessation of growth and skin lesions that result when essential fatty acids (arachidonic and linoleic acid) are absent from the diet. **Fauchard d.,** marginal periodontitis. **Favre-Durand-Nicholas d.,** lymphogranuloma venereum. **Feer's d.,** acrodynia. **Fenwick's d.,** idiopathic atrophic gastritis, first described by Fenwick in a patient with pernicious anemia. **fibrocystic d., fibrocystic d. of breast,** cystic d. of breast. **fibrocystic d. of the pancreas,** cystic fibrosis. **Fiedler's d.,** Weil's syndrome. **fifth d.,** erythema infectiosum. **fifth venereal d.,** lymphogranuloma venereum. **Filatov's d.,** infectious mononucleosis. **Filatov-Dukes d.,** Dukes' d. **file-cutters' d.,** lead poisoning from inhaling particles of lead which arise from the bed of lead used in file cutting. **finger and toe d.,** a disease of cabbage and other cruciferous plants due to the protozoan *Plasmodiophora brassicae*, and characterized by knotty enlargement of the affected plant's roots. Called also *clubroot.* **fish-slime d.,** septicemia following a puncture wound made by the spine of a fish. **Flajani's d.,** Graves' d. **Flatau-Schilder d.,** Schilder's d. **flax-dresser's d.,** a pulmonary disorder seen in flax-dressers, and caused by inhaling particles of flax. **Flegel's d.,** hyperkeratosis lenticularis perstans. **Fleischner's d.,** osteochondritis affecting the middle phalanges of the hand. **flint d.,** chalicosis. **floating-beta d.,** broad-beta d. **fluke d.,** infection with flukes; see *Trematoda*. **focal d.,** one which is localized at one or more foci. **Følling's d.,** phenylketonuria. **foot-and-mouth d.,** an acute, naturally occurring, extremely contagious viral disease of wild and domestic animals, chiefly cattle, pigs, sheep, goats, and other ruminants, and very rarely of man. It is marked by an

eruption of vesicles on the lips, buccal cavity, pharynx, legs, and feet; sometimes the skin of the udder or teats is involved. Called also *hoof-and-mouth d.; aftosa; contagious, epizootic,* or *malignant aphthae; aphthous fever;* and *aphthobullous, epidemic,* or *epizootic stomatitis.* **Forbes' d.,** glycogen storage d. (type III). **Fordyce's d.,** 1. see under *granule*. 2. Fox-Fordyce d. **Forestier d.,** hyperostosis of the anterolateral vertebral column, especially in the thoracic region. **Förster's d.,** see under *choroiditis*. **Fothergill's d.,** 1. scarlatina anginosa. 2. trigeminal neuralgia. **Fournier's d.,** see under *gangrene*. **fourth d.,** Dukes' d. **fourth venereal d.,** 1. specific gangrenous and ulcerative balanoposthitis; see under *balanoposthitis*. 2. granuloma inguinale. **Fox-Fordyce d.,** a chronic, usually pruritic disease chiefly seen in women, characterized by the development of small follicular papular eruptions of apocrine gland–bearing areas, especially the axillae and pubes, and caused by obstruction and rupture of the intraepidermal portion of the ducts of affected apocrine glands, resulting in alteration of the regional ductal epidermis, apocrine secretory tubule, and adjacent dermis. Called also *apocrine miliaria.* **Francis' d.,** tularemia. **Frankl-Hochwart's d.,** polyneuritis cerebralis menieriformis. **Frei's d.,** lymphogranuloma venereum. **Freiberg's d.,** osteochondrosis of the head of the second metatarsal. **Friedländer's d.,** endarteritis obliterans. **Friedreich's d.,** 1. paramyoclonus multiplex. 2. Friedreich's ataxia. **fright d.,** canine hysteria; psychic disturbance in dogs marked by symptoms of fright and by hysterical barking and running. **Frommel's d.,** Chiari-Frommel syndrome. **functional d.,** a disease involving functions without tissue damage. **functional cardiovascular d.,** neurocirculatory asthenia. **Fürstner's d.,** pseudospastic paralysis with tremor. **Gaisböck's d.,** stress polycythemia. **gamma chain d.,** a heavy chain disease occurring usually in elderly persons that clinically resembles a malignant lymphoma, with symptoms of lymphadenopathy, hepatosplenomegaly, and recurrent infections. **Gamna's d.,** a form of splenomegaly, with thickening of the splenic capsule and the presence of small brownish areas (Gamna nodules) which are usually surrounded by a hematogenous zone; ferruginous pigment is deposited in the splenic pulp. **Gamstorp's d.,** adynamia episodica hereditaria. **Gandy-Nanta d.,** siderotic splenomegaly. **gannister d.,** pneumoconiosis due to the inhalation of dust by workers in the manufacture of refractory brick or fire clay. **Garré's d.,** sclerosing nonsuppurative osteomyelitis. **Gaucher's d.,** a lipidosis caused by deficient glucocerebrosidase (glucosylceramidase), with glucocerebroside (glucosylceramide) accumulation in storage cells (Gaucher cells) in the liver, spleen, lymph nodes, alveolar capillaries, and bone marrow. There are three clinical types: *type 1* (chronic non-neuronopathic or "adult") may appear at any age and is associated with hypersplenism, thrombocytopenia, anemia, jaundice, and bone lesions; *type 2* (acute neuronopathic or "infantile") is associated with onset in infancy, hepatosplenomegaly, severe CNS impairment, and death usually within the first year; *type 3* (subacute neuronopathic or "juvenile") is the most varied, having the same clinical features as types 1 and 2 but a longer course. Called also *glucosylceramide lipidosis.* **Gee's d., Gee-Herter d., Gee-Herter-Heubner d.,** the infantile form of celiac disease or nontropical sprue. **Gee-Thaysen d.,** adult celiac disease; the adult form of nontropical sprue. **genetic d.,** a general term for any disorder caused by a genetic mechanism, comprising chromosome aberrations or anomalies, mendelian or monogenic or single-gene disorders, and multifactorial disorders. **Gerhardt's d.,** erythromelalgia. **Gerlier's d.,** a disease of the nerves and nerve centers attacking farm laborers and stablemen, and characterized by pain, paresis, vertigo, ptosis, and muscular contractions; called also *endemic paralytic vertigo, paralyzing vertigo,* and *Gerlier's syndrome.* **giant platelet d.,** Bernard-Soulier d. **Gibney's d.,** see under *perispondylitis*. **Gierke's d.,** see *glycogen storage d. (type I).* **Gilbert's d.,** see under *syndrome*. **Gilchrist's d.,** North American blastomycosis. **Gilles de la Tourette's d.,** see under *syndrome*. **Glanzmann's d.,** see *thrombasthenia*. **Glasser's d.,** a disease mainly affecting pigs 5 to 14 weeks old, in which swelling of the hocks or knee joints, or both, is accompanied by fever, lameness, and a disinclination to move: if untreated, death usually results. It is caused by a strain of *Haemophilus influenzae.* **Glénard's d.** (obs.), splanchnoptosis. **Glisson's d.,** rickets. **glucose-6-**

phosphate dehydrogenase (G6PD) d., the most common inborn error of metabolism, affecting over 100 million people with varying degrees of hemolytic anemia. The G6PD locus, Xq28, is very closely linked to the genes for deutanomaly, protanomaly, hemophilia A, and adrenoleukodystrophy, and closely linked to the genes (on Xq27) for the fragile X syndrome and HPRT deficiency (the Lesch-Nyhan syndrome). (G6PD deficiency provides heterozygote advantage against falciparum malaria.) The G6PD gene is highly polymorphous, with over 300 variants known. See also *glucose-6-phosphate dehydrogenase deficiency anemia.* **glycogen storage d.,** any of at least 14 types or subtypes of rare inborn errors of metabolism due to a defect in a specific enzyme involved in glycogen catabolism. In *type I,* defective glucose-6-phosphatase affects liver and kidneys, causing hepatomegaly, hypoglycemia, hyperuricemia, xanthomas, bleeding, and adiposity; patients may live well into adulthood. Called also *Gierke (von Gierke) d., hepatorenal glycogenosis, hepatorenal glycogen storage d.,* and *glucose-6-phosphatase deficiency.* In *type II,* defective α-1,4-glucosidase (acid maltase) causes generalized glycogen accumulation with CNS involvement and psychomotor retardation, with cardiomegaly and cardiorespiratory failure; most infants die by one year of age. Called also *Pompe d., α-1,4-glucosidase deficiency, acid-maltase deficiency,* and *generalized glycogenosis.* In *type III,* a defect in the debranching enzyme amylo-1,6 glucosidase affects the heart and liver; signs include stunted growth, hepatomegaly, hypoglycemia, and acidosis. Six different subgroups (IIIA through IIIF) are known. Called also *debrancher deficiency, Cori d., Forbes d., limit dextrinosis, amylo-1,6 glucosidase deficiency,* and *debrancher glycogen storage d.* In *type IV,* a defect in the branching enzyme amylo-1:4,1:6-transglucosidase causes early cirrhosis with liver failure and hepatosplenomegaly; the child dies usually in his second year. Called also *amylopectinosis, Andersen d., brancher deficiency, brancher deficiency glycogenosis, brancher glycogen storage d., amylo-1:4,1:6-transglucosidase deficiency,* and *α-1,4 glucan: α-1,4 glucan 5-glucosyl-transferase deficiency.* In *type V,* a deficiency of muscle phosphorylase affects the skeletal muscles, causing muscle cramps and a depressed blood lactate level during exercise. Called also *McArdle d., McArdle syndrome, myophosphorylase deficiency glycogenosis,* and *muscle phosphorylase deficiency.* In *type VI,* a deficiency of liver phosphorylase is manifested in the liver and leukocytes, with hepatomegaly, moderate hypoglycemia, mild acidosis, and growth retardation. Called also *Hers d., hepatic phosphorylase deficiency,* and *hepatophosphorylase deficiency glycogenosis.* In *type VII,* a deficiency in phosphofructokinase affects muscle and erythrocytes, with temporary weakness and skeletal muscle cramping after exercise. Called also *muscle phosphofructokinase deficiency* and *Tarui d.* In *type VIII,* an X-linked disorder, a defect in hepatic phosphorylase kinase reduces liver and leukocyte phosphorylase and causes hepatomegaly and increased concentrations of liver glycogen; patients are otherwise asymptomatic. Called also *hepatic phosphorylase kinase deficiency.* **Goldflam's d.,** Goldflam-Erb d., myasthenia gravis. **Goldstein's d.,** hereditary hemorrhagic telangiectasia. **graft-versus-host (GVH) d.,** disease caused by the immune response of histoincompatible, immunocompetent donor cells against the tissues of immunoincompetent host, which can occur as a complication of bone marrow transplantation or as a result of maternal-fetal blood transfusion or therapeutic blood transfusion in which the recipient has a cellular immunodeficiency disease. Clinical manifestations include skin disease ranging from a maculopapular eruption to epidermal necrosis, intestinal disease marked by diarrhea, malabsorption, and abdominal pain, and liver dysfunction caused by cholestatic hepatitis or veno-occulsive disease and marked by serum enzyme abnormalities. Called also *graft-versus-host reaction.* **grass d.,** a usually fatal disease of horses occurring after they have been put to graze on grass, usually between May and July; first seen in Scotland, it has spread to Wales, England, and Sweden. It is marked by dysphagia, severe diarrhea, dehydration, interrupted peristalsis, and priapism. Called also *grass sickness.* **Graves' d.,** a disorder of the thyroid of unknown but probably autoimmune etiology, occurring most often in women, characterized by thyrotoxicosis with diffuse goiter, exophthalmos, or pretibial myxedema, or any combination of the three. Signs and symptoms include fatigability, nervousness, emotional lability and irritability, heat intolerance and increased sweating,

weight loss, palpitation, and tremor of the hands and tongue. Some patients have varying degrees of exophthalmos. Most patients have circulating thyroid-stimulating immunoglobulins (TSI) that cause excessive secretion of thyroid hormones by binding to TSH receptors on thyroid cells. Called *Basedow's d.* in continental Europe. Called also *cachexia exophthalmica, diffuse toxic goiter, exophthalmic goiter, Flajani's d., Parry's d.,* and *tachycardia strumosa exophthalmica.* **greasy pig d.,** seborrhea of piglets, which is thought to be associated with a vitamin B deficiency. **Greenfield's d.,** see *metachromatic leukodystrophy,* under *leukodystrophy.* **Griesinger's d.** (*obs.*), hookworm d. **grinder's d.,** pneumoconiosis of grinders. **Gross d.,** encysted rectum; saccular dilatation of anal wall with retained inspissated feces. **guinea worm d.,** dracunculiasis. **Guinon's d.,** Gilles de la Tourette's syndrome. **Gull's d.,** atrophy of the thyroid with myxedema. **Gumboro d.,** infectious bursal d. **Günther's d.,** congenital erythropoietic porphyria. **H d.,** Hartnup d. **Habermann's d.,** acute lichenoid pityriasis. **Haff d.,** a condition affecting fishermen of the Königsberg (Frisches) Haff, a lagoon joining the Baltic Sea. The men are suddenly seized with severe pain in the limbs, great weariness, and myoglobinuria. The disease is said to be the result of poisoning by arsine introduced into the Haff through the waste water of cellulose factories. Several epidemics occurred prior to World War II. **Haglund's d.,** bursitis in the region of the Achilles tendon. **Hagner's d.,** an obscure bone disease somewhat resembling acromegaly (Pierre Marie described this obscure bone disease in the two Hagner brothers). **Hailey-Hailey d.,** benign familial pemphigus. **Hallervorden-Spatz d.,** see under *syndrome.* **Hamman's d.,** pneumomediastinum. **Hammond's d.,** athetosis. **Hand's d.,** Hand-Schüller-Christian d. **hand-foot-and-mouth d.,** a usually mild and self-limited exanthematous eruption most often caused by coxsackievirus A16, primarily seen in preschool children, and characterized by vesicles on the buccal mucosa, tongue, soft palate, gingivae, and hands and feet, including the palms and soles. Called also *hand-foot-and-mouth syndrome.* **Hand-Schüller-Christian d.,** a chronic idiopathic form of histiocytosis, sometimes with accumulation of cholesterol, characterized classically by the triad of: defects in the membranous bones, exophthalmos, and diabetes insipidus. In most cases this triad is not seen, but there is multiple-system, soft tissue, and bone involvement. Called also *chronic idiopathic xanthomatosis* and *cholesterol thesaurismosis.* **Hanot's d.,** 1. primary biliary cirrhosis. 2. secondary biliary cirrhosis. **Hansen's d.,** leprosy. **d. of the Hapsburgs,** hemophilia. **Harada's d.,** see under *syndrome.* **hard pad d.,** hyperkeratosis of the footpads of young dogs, occurring in canine distemper. **Hartnup d.,** an inborn error of metabolism characterized by cerebellar ataxia, a pellagra-like condition of the skin, and massive aminoaciduria involving a group of neutral monoaminomonocarboxylic amino acids sharing a common renal reabsorption mechanism; patients respond well to prolonged oral administration of nicotinamide. **Hashimoto's d.,** a progressive autoimmune disease of the thyroid gland, with lymphocytic infiltration of the gland and circulating antithyroid antibodies. Women are most commonly affected, and there is a familial predisposition to the disease. It sometimes occurs after the subsidence of Graves' disease. Patients have goiter and gradually develop hypothyroidism. Called also *autoimmune* and *Hashimoto's thyroiditis* and *struma lymphomatosa.* **heart d.,** any organic, mechanical, or functional abnormality of the heart; it may be valvular, myocardial, or neurogenic. **heartwater d.,** see *heartwater.* **heavy-chain d's,** a group of rare malignant neoplasms of lymphoplasmacytic cells that secrete an M component consisting of monoclonal immunoglobulin heavy chains or heavy chain fragments; they are classified according to heavy chain type. See also *alpha chain d., gamma chain d.,* and *mu chain d.* **Heberden's d.,** 1. rheumatism of the smaller joints, accompanied by nodules in or about the distal interphalangeal joints. 2. angina pectoris. **Hebra's d.,** erythema multiforme minor. **Heerfordt's d.,** see under *syndrome.* **Heine-Medin d.,** the major form of poliomyelitis, with involvement of the central nervous system and perhaps paralysis; see *poliomyelitis.* **Heller-Döhle d.,** syphilitic aortitis. **helminthic d.,** a disease caused by worms. **hemoglobin d.,** any of a group of heredity molecular diseases, characterized by the presence of various abnormal hemoglobins, e.g., hemoglobin C, D, E, H, or S, in the red blood cells, in which the homozygous form is manifested by hemolytic anemia. See also *sickle cell anemia*, under *anemia*, and see individual hemoglobins, under *hemoglobin*. **hemoglobin C–thalassemia d.,** a hereditary disorder involving simultaneous heterozygosity for hemoglobin C and thalassemia, manifested by mild hemolytic anemia and persistent splenomegaly; called also *hemoglobin C–thalassemia*. **hemoglobin E–thalassemia d.,** a hereditary condition involving simultaneous heterozygosity for hemoglobin E and thalassemia, manifested by mild hemolytic anemia and persistent splenomegaly; called also *hemoglobin E–thalassemia*. **hemolytic d. of newborn,** erythroblastosis fetalis. **hemorrhagic d. of the newborn,** a self-limited hemorrhagic disorder of the first days of life, caused by a deficiency of the vitamin K–dependent blood coagulation factors II, VII, IX, and X. **Henderson-Jones d.,** osteochondromatosis characterized by the presence of numerous cartilaginous foreign bodies in the joint cavity or in the bursa of a tendon sheath. **hepatolenticular d.,** Wilson's d. **hepatorenal glycogen storage d.,** glycogen storage d. (type I). **hereditary d.,** one that is transmitted genetically from parents to children. **heredoconstitutional d.,** an inherited pathologic condition which does not progress. **heredodegenerative d.,** any disease of the central nervous system characterized by specific loss of neural tissue due to hereditary influence. **Herlitz's d.,** junctional epidermolysis bullosa. **Hers' d.,** glycogen storage d. (type VI). **Herter's d.,** Herter-Heubner d., the infantile form of nontropical sprue. **Heubner's d.,** syphilitic endarteritis of the cerebral vessels; called also *Heubner's specific endarteritis*. **hip-joint d.,** tuberculosis of the hip joint. **Hippel's d.,** see *von Hippel's d.* **Hippel-Lindau d.,** see *von Hippel-Lindau d.* **Hirschsprung's d.,** congenital megacolon. **His d., His-Werner d.,** trench fever. **hock d.,** perosis. **Hodgkin's d.,** a form of malignant lymphoma characterized by painless, progressive enlargement of the lymph nodes, spleen, and general lymphoid tissue; other symptoms may include anorexia, lassitude, weight loss, fever, pruritus, night sweats, and anemia. The characteristic histologic feature is presence of Reed-Sternberg cells. Hodgkin's disease is usually classified as: (1) diffuse, according to the number of lymphocyte and histiocytes (lymphocytes predominant; mixed cellularity; lymphocytes depleted) and (2) nodular sclerosing (marked by birefringent bands of collagen and the presence of the lacunar cells). The condition, which affects twice as many males as females and usually occurs between the ages of 15 and 34 or after 50, is considered by many to be neoplastic in origin, but neither an infectious origin nor an immune response to the development of Reed-Sternberg cells has been excluded. Called also *Hodgkin's lymphoma*. Cf. *non-Hodgkin's lymphoma*. **Hodgson's d.,** an aneurysmal dilatation of the proximal part of the aorta, often accompanied by dilatation or hypertrophy of the heart. **Hoffa's d.,** traumatic proliferation of fatty tissue (solitary lipoma) in the knee joint (Albert Hoffa, 1904). **holoendemic d.,** a disease endemic in most of the children in a population, with the adults in the same population being less often affected. Cf. *hyperendemic d.* **hoof-and-mouth d.,** foot-and-mouth d. **hookworm d.,** a condition due to infection with *Ancylostoma duodenale* or *Necator americanus*, nematode worms that closely resemble each other. (In dogs, the disease is usually caused by *Ancylostoma caninum*.) The disease occurs in practically all tropical and subtropical countries, including the southern United States and the West Indies. In temperate regions, it may occur in mines and tunnels, where conditions of temperature and moisture resemble the tropics. The larvae of the parasite live in soil and gain entrance to the digestive tract indirectly by way of the skin of the feet or legs or directly with contaminated food or water. The percutaneous infection is followed by a transitory eruption known as "ground itch." From here the parasites are carried by the blood to the lungs, ascend the trachea, are swallowed, and settle in the small intestine, where they attach to the intestinal mucosa and ingest blood. Symptoms, which vary with diet and with severity of infection, may include abdominal pain, diarrhea, and colic or nausea. Anemia is seen only in moderate to severe infections or when other adverse nutritional factors operate in conjuction with the parasite-induced blood loss. **Horton's d.,** 1. migrainous neuralgia. 2. temporal arteritis. **Huchard's d.,** continued arterial hypertension, thought to be a cause of arteriosclerosis. **hunger d., hungry d.,** excessive hunger accompa-

nied by weakness and nervousness caused by the hypoglycemia of hyperinsulinism. **Hunt's d.,** 1. dyssynergia cerebellaris myoclonica. 2. Ramsay Hunt syndrome, def. 1. **Huntington's d.,** see under *chorea*. **Hurler's d.,** see under *syndrome*. **Hutchinson's d.,** 1. prurigo estivalis. 2. angioma serpiginosum. 3. Tay's choroiditis. **Hutchinson-Gilford d.,** progeria. **Hutinel's d.,** tuberculous pericarditis with cirrhosis of the liver in children. **hyaline membrane d.,** a disorder affecting newborn infants (usually premature) characterized pathologically by the development of a hyaline-like membrane lining the terminal respiratory passages. Extensive atelectasis is attributed to lack of surfactant. See *respiratory distress syndrome of newborn*, under *syndrome*. **hydatid d.,** an infection, usually of the liver, caused by larval forms (hydatid cysts) of tapeworms of the genus *Echinococcus*, and characterized by the development of expanding cysts. See *hydatid d., alveolar*, and *hydatid d., unilocular*. Called also *hydatidosis, echinococcus d.,* and *echinococcosis*. **hydatid d., alveolar,** infection with larval forms (hydatid cysts) of *Echinococcus multilocularis*, characterized by invasion and destruction of the host's tissues as the cysts undergo endogenous budding to form an aggregate of innumerable small cysts which honeycomb the affected organ (the liver in over 90 per cent of cases) and may metastasize. **hydatid d., unilocular,** infection with the larval forms (hydatid cysts) of *Echinococcus granulosis*, characterized by the formation of single or multiple expanding cysts which are unilocular in nature; as the cysts expand they may give rise to symptoms of related space-occupying lesions in the tissues or organs affected. **hydrocephaloid d.,** a condition similar to hydrocephalus, but marked by depression of the fontanels, due to diarrhea or some other wasting disease with dehydration. **hyperendemic d.,** a disease equally endemic in all age groups of a population. Cf. *holoendemic d.* **hypopigmentation-immunodeficiency d.,** Griscelli syndrome. **Iceland d., Icelandic d.,** epidemic neuromyasthenia. **I-cell d.,** mucolipidosis II. **idiopathic d.,** one not consequent upon any other disease, and of which the cause is unknown. **immune-complex d's,** diseases caused by the formation of immune complexes in tissues or by the deposition of circulating immune complexes in tissues resulting in acute or chronic inflammation. Deposition of circulating immune complexes is generally associated with glomerulonephritis, vasculitis, synovitis, endocarditis, neuritis, and dermatitis. Locally formed complexes are involved in the pathogenesis of some autoimmune diseases. Circulating complexes may result from administration of heterologous antigens (as in serum sickness) or from the immune response to microbial antigens or tumor antigens. **immunodeficiency d.,** any of a group of disorders resulting from the functional impairment of components of the immune system, which may include deficiency or malfunction of a cell population (e.g., phagocytic cells, subpopulations of T lymphocytes), lack of an antibody response, or complement abnormality. Called also *immunodeficiency disorder* or *syndrome*. See also table accompanying *immunodeficiency*. **immunoproliferative small intestine d.,** a condition characterized by diarrhea, malabsorption, abdominal pain, clubbing, plasma cell infiltration of the lamina propria of the small bowel, and presence of an abnormal alpha heavy chain fragment in the serum, occurring predominantly in young adults living around the Mediterranean Sea; it frequently evolves into primary malignant lymphoma. Called also *alpha-chain d.* **inborn lysosomal d's,** lysosomal storage d. **inclusion d.,** any disease in which cell inclusions are found. **infantile celiac d.,** the infantile form of celiac disease, or nontropical sprue. **infectious d.,** a disease caused by a pathogenic microorganism; the etiologic agent may be a bacterium, virus, fungus, or animal parasite, and may be transmitted from another host or arise from the host's own indigenous microflora. See also *infection*. Cf. *communicable d.* and *contagious d.* **infectious bursal d.,** a highly contagious acute disease of chickens, caused by virus provisionally classified as an orbivirus, characterized by a propensity of infected birds to pick at their own vents (cloacal apertures), edema and swelling of the cloacal bursa, soiled wet feathers, whitish watery diarrhea, listlessness, trembling, extreme kidney damage, damage of the bursa of Fabricius, and death. Called also *Gumboro disease* and *avian nephrosis*. **inflammatory bowel d.,** a general term for those inflammatory diseases of the bowel of unknown etiology, including Crohn's disease and ulcerative colitis. **inherited d.,** one transmitted genetically, from parents to offspring. **intercurrent d.,** a disease occurring during the course of another disease with which it has no connection. **interstitial d.,** one in which the stroma of an organ is mainly affected. **interstitial lung d.,** a heterogeneous group of noninfectious, nonmalignant disorders of the lower respiratory tract, affecting primarily the alveolar wall structures but also often involving the small airways and blood vessels of the lung parenchyma; slowly progressive loss of alveolar-capillary units may lead to respiratory insufficiency and death. **iron storage d.,** hemochromatosis. **Isambert's d.,** acute miliary tuberculosis of the larynx and pharynx. **island d.,** scrub typhus. **Isle of Wight d.,** paralysis of the muscles of flight in honey bees caused by the presence of the mite *Acarapis woodi* in the tracheae of the bees. **itch d.,** a dermatomycosis of horses probably caused by the mold *Microsporum canis.* **Jaffe-Lichtenstein d.,** cystic osteofibromatosis; a form of polyostotic fibrous dysplasia characterized by an enlarged medullary cavity with a thin cortex, which is filled with fibrous tissue (fibroma). **Jakob's d., Jakob-Creutzfeldt d.,** Creutzfeldt-Jakob disease. **Jaksch's d.,** anemia pseudoleukemica infantum. **Janet's d.,** psychasthenia. **Jansen's d.,** metaphyseal dysostosis. **Jansky-Bielschowsky d.,** see *amaurotic idiocy,* under *idiocy.* **Jensen's d.,** retinochoroiditis juxtapapillaris. **Johne's d.,** a usually fatal form of chronic enteritis due to *Mycobacterium paratuberculosis,* chiefly affecting cattle but also sheep, goats, and deer. It remotely resembles a tuberculous infection, and is marked by intermittent or persistent diarrhea, progressive emaciation, anemia, and extreme weakness. Called also *chronic dysentery of cattle, bovine leprosy,* and *paratuberculosis.* **Johnson-Stevens d.,** see *Stevens-Johnson syndrome.* **Joseph d.,** Azorean d. **jumping d.,** Gilles de la Tourette's syndrome. **juvenile Paget d.,** hyperostosis corticalis deformans juvenilis. **Kahler's d.,** multiple myeloma. **Kaiserstuhl d.,** a form of chronic arsenic poisoning that occurred in the Kaiserstuhl wine district of Germany. **Kaschin-Beck d.,** Kashin-Beck d. **Kashin-Beck d.,** a slowly progressive, chronic, disabling, degenerative disease of the peripheral joints and spine, which principally occurs in children and is endemic in eastern Siberia, northern China, and Korea. It is believed to be caused by the ingestion of cereal grains infected with *Fusarium sporotrichiella.* Called also *osteoarthritis deformans endemica.* **Katayama d.,** see under *fever.* **Kawasaki d.,** mucocutaneous lymph node syndrome. **Keshan d.,** a fatal, congestive cardiomyopathy first observed in children in the Keshan province of China. It is caused by deficiency of selenium in the diet and occurs in areas with low selenium content in the soil, especially China, New Zealand, and Finland. **Kienböck's d.,** 1. slowly progressive osteochondrosis of the semilunar (carpal lunate) bone; it may affect other bones of the wrist. Called also *lunatomalacia.* 2. traumatic cavity formation in the spinal cord; called also *traumatic syringomyelia.* **Kimberley horse d.,** a disease of horses in the Kimberley district of northeastern Western Australia occurring during the wet season (January to April), due to grazing on *Crotolaria* spp. It is marked by cirrhosis of the liver, dullness, wasting, irritability, biting of other horses, gnawing fence posts, constant yawning, and muscular spasms leading to uncontrollable galloping, which gradually merges into aimless walking with a slow staggering gait and low stiff carriage of the head. Called also *walk-about d.* **Kimura's d.,** angiolymphoid hyperplasia. **kinky hair d.,** Menkes' syndrome. **Kinnier Wilson d.,** hepatolenticular degeneration. **Kirkland's d.,** an acute infection of the throat with regional lymphadenitis. **kissing d.,** popular term for infectious mononucleosis. **Klebs' d.,** glomerulonephritis. **Klemperer's d.,** Banti's d. **Klippel's d.,** arthritic general pseudoparalysis; see under *pseudoparalysis.* **knight's d.,** infection of the perianal region following a minute abrasion of the skin, so called historically because of the frequency of its occurrence in horsemen. **Köhler's bone d.,** 1. osteochondrosis of the tarsal navicular bone in children; called also *tarsal scaphoiditis, epiphysitis juvenilis, osteoarthrosis juvenilis,* and *os naviculare pedis retardatum.* 2. a disease of the second metatarsal bone, with thickening of its shaft and changes about its articular head, characterized by pain in the second metatarsophalangeal joint on walking or standing. Called also *Köhler's second d.,* and *juvenile deforming metatarsophalangeal osteochondritis.* See also *osteochondrosis.* **Köhler's second d.,** Köhler's

bone d., def. 2. **Köhler-Pellegrini-Stieda d.,** Pellegrini's d. **Koshevnikoff's (Koschewnikow's, Kozhevnikov's) d.,** epilepsia partialis continua. **Krabbe's d.,** a lysosomal storage disease due to deficient galactosylceramidase. It begins in infancy with irritability, fretfulness, and rigidity, followed by tonic seizures, convulsions, quadriplegia, blindness, deafness, dysphagia, and progressive mental deterioration. Pathologically, there is rapidly progressive cerebral demyelination and large globoid bodies in the white substance. Called also *galactosylceramide lipidosis, galactosylceramide β-galactosidase deficiency, globoid, globoid cell,* and *Krabbe leukodystrophy.* **Krishaber's d.,** a neurosis characterized by tachycardia, insomnia, lightheadedness or vertigo, and hyperesthesia; called also *cerebrocardiac syndrome.* **Kufs' d.,** see *amaurotic idiocy,* under *idiocy.* **Kugelberg-Welander d.,** a hereditary juvenile form of muscular atrophy, usually transmitted as an autosomal recessive trait, due to lesions of the anterior horns of the spinal cord. It is marked by onset in the first or second decade, principally between two and seventeen years, and atrophy and weakness of the proximal muscles of the lower extremities and pelvic girdle, followed by involvement of the distal muscles and muscular twitchings. Cf. *Werdnig-Hoffman paralysis.* **Kuhnt-Junius d.,** disciform macular degeneration. **Kümmell's d.,** compression fracture of vertebra; a complex of symptoms coming on in a few weeks after spinal injury, and consisting of pain in the spine, intercostal neuralgia, motor disturbances of the legs, and a gibbus of the spine which is painful on pressure and easily reduced by extension; post-traumatic spondylitis. Called also *Kümmell-Verneuil d.,* Kümmell's d. **Kümmell-Verneuil d.,** Kümmell's d. **Kussmaul's d., Kussmaul-Maier d.,** periarteritis nodosa, def. 1. **Kyasanur Forest d.,** a severe hemorrhagic fever marked by fever, hemorrhagic manifestations, and rash, occurring in the Mysore State of India, first found in an epidemic among forest workers and monkeys in the Kyasanur Forest, caused by a flavivirus and transmitted to humans from monkey and vole reservoirs by ticks of the genus *Haemophysalis,* especially *H. spinigera.* **Kyrle's d.,** a rare chronic disorder of keratinization characterized by a papular eruption and the development of hyperkeratotic cone-shaped plugs in the hair follicles and eccrine ducts, which project through the epidermis into the dermis, producing a foreign body giant cell reaction and pain. The usually discrete lesions leave a crateriform depression on removal; they may coalesce to form circinate patches, and coalescing plaques are often seen. Called also *hyperkeratosis follicularis et parafollicularis in cutem penetrans, hyperkeratosis follicularis in cutem penetrans,* and *hyperkeratosis penetrans.* **Laënnec's d.,** 1. see under *cirrhosis.* 2. dissecting aneurysm. **Lafora's d.,** myoclonus epilepsy. **Lancereaux-Mathieu d.,** Weil's syndrome. **Landouzy's d.,** Weil's syndrome. **Landry's d.,** acute febrile polyneuritis. **Lane's d.,** chronic intestinal stasis; small bowel obstruction in chronic constipation. **Larsen's d., Larsen-Johansson d.,** a disease of the patella in which the x-ray shows an accessory center of ossification in the lower pole of the patella. **Lauber's d.,** fundus albipunctatus. **laughing d.,** kuru. **leaf-curl d.,** a viral disease of plants characterized by curling or crinkling of the leaves. **Leber's d.,** 1. Leber's optic atrophy; see under *atrophy.* 2. Leber's congenital amaurosis; see under *amaurosis.* **Legal's d.,** a disease affecting the pharyngotympanic region, and marked by headache and local inflammatory changes; called also *pharyngotympanic cephalalgia.* **Legg's d., Legg-Calvé d., Legg-Calvé-Perthes d., Legg-Calvé-Waldenström d.,** osteochondrosis of the capitular epiphysis of the femur; see *osteochondrosis.* **legionnaires' d.,** a highly fatal disease caused by a gram-negative bacillus (*Legionella pneumophila*), which is not spread by person-to-person contact and is characterized by high fever, gastrointestinal pain, headache, and pneumonia; there may also be involvement of the kidneys, liver, and nervous system. The etiologic agent was identified after an outbreak occurred in the summer of 1976 at an American Legion convention in Philadelphia, Pennsylvania. **Leigh d.,** subacute necrotizing encephalomyelopathy. **Leiner's d.,** a disorder of infancy characterized principally by generalized seborrheic-like dermatitis and erythroderma, intractable, severe diarrhea, recurrent infections, and failure to thrive. The cause is unclear, but familial cases associated with a dysfunction of the C5 component of complement, which results in decreased phagocytosis of the patient's serum (opsonic activity), have been reported. Called also *erythroderma desquamativum*. **Lenegre's d.,** acquired complete heart block due to primary degeneration of the conduction system. **Leriche's d.,** post-traumatic osteoporosis. **Letterer-Siwe d.,** a nonlipid, autosomal recessive reticuloendotheliosis of early childhood, characterized by a hemorrhagic tendency, eczematoid skin eruption, hepatosplenomegaly with lymph node enlargement, and progressive anemia. Called also *L-S d.* and *acute disseminated histiocytosis X*. **Lev's d.,** acquired complete heart block due to sclerosis of the cardiac skeleton. **Lewandowsky-Lutz d.,** epidermodysplasia verruciformis. **Leyden's d.,** a form of periodic vomiting. **Libman-Sacks d.,** atypical verrucous endocarditis. **Lichtheim's d.,** subacute combined degeneration of the spinal cord; see under *degeneration*. **Lignac's d., Lignac-Fanconi d.,** Fanconi syndrome, def. 2. **Lindau's d., Lindau-von Hippel d.,** von Hippel-Lindau d. **lipid storage d.,** lipidosis. **Lipschütz's d.,** ulcus vulvae acutum. **Little's d.,** congenital spastic stiffness of the limbs, a form of cerebral spastic paralysis dating from birth and due to lack of development of the pyramidal tracts; it may be associated with various disorders, including birth trauma, fetal anoxia, or illness of the mother during pregnancy. Clinically, it is characterized by muscular weakness, walking difficulties, and, usually, by convulsions, bilateral athetosis, and mental deficiency. Called also *spastic diplegia*. **Lobo's d.,** keloidal blastomycosis. **Lobstein's d.,** osteogenesis imperfecta, type I. **local d.,** a condition which originates in and remains confined to one part. **loco d.,** locoism. **Lorain's d.,** hyphophysial infantilism. **Lowe's d.,** oculocerebrorenal syndrome. **L-S d.,** Letterer-Siwe d. **Luft's d.,** a hypermetabolic disorder of striated muscle caused by an abnormal quantity and type of mitochondria producing excessive cellular respiration; it is characterized by profuse perspiration, asthenia, progressive weakness, and an abnormally increased basal metabolic rate. **lumpy skin d.,** a highly infectious poxvirus disease indigenous to African cattle, which may result in permanent sterility or death, marked by the formation of nodules in the skin and sometimes in the mucous membranes. It resembles dermopathic herpesvirus disease (q.v.). **lung fluke d.,** parasitic hemoptysis. **lunger d.,** pulmonary adenomatosis, def. 2. **Lutembacher's d.,** see under *syndrome*. **Lutz-Splendore-Almeida d.,** paracoccidoidomycosis. **Lyell's d.,** toxic epidermal necrolysis. **Lyme d.,** a recurrent multisystemic disorder first reported in Old Lyme, Connecticut, beginning with the lesions of erythema chronicum migrans and followed by arthritis of the large joints, myalgia, malaise, and neurologic and cardiac manifestations. It is caused by the spirochete *Borrelia burgdorferi*, with the vector being the tick *Ixodes dammini*. Called also *Lyme arthritis*. **lymphocystic d. of fish,** a disease of fish marked by the formation on the skin of spherical nodules caused by a virus. **lymphoproliferative d's,** see *lymphoproliferative*. **lymphoreticular d's,** see *lymphoreticular*. **lysosomal storage d.,** any inborn error of metabolism having four characteristics: (1) a defect in a specific lysosomal hydrolase; (2) intracellular accumulation of the unmetabolized substrate, (3) clinical progression affecting multiple tissues and organs; (4) considerable phenotypic variation within a disease. All but two of the lysosomal storage disorders are of autosomal recessive inheritance. The term comprises the *mucolipidoses, mucopolysaccharidoses, glycoprotein storage diseases*, and *lipase deficiencies, ceramidase deficiency (Farber lipogranulomatosis), α-galactosidase A deficiency (Fabry disease), lipidoses*, and *gangliosidoses*. See also *inborn errors of metabolism*, under *metabolism*. Called also *lysosomal enzymopathy* and *inborn lysosomal d*. **McArdle's d.,** glycogen storage d. (type V). **Machado-Joseph d.,** Azorean d. **Mackenzie's d.,** x disease, def. 1. **MacLean-Maxwell d.,** a chronic condition of the calcaneus marked by enlargement of its posterior third and attended by pain on pressure. **Madelung's d.,** 1. see under *deformity*. 2. see under *neck*. **Maher's d.,** paracolpitis. **Majocchi's d.,** purpura anularis telangiectodes. **Malassez's d.,** cyst of the testis. **Malibu d.,** surfers' nodules. **Manson's d.,** see under *schistosomiasis*. **maple bark d.,** a granulomatous interstitial pneumonitis caused by inhalation of spores from *Coniosporium corticale*, a mold found beneath the bark of maple logs. **maple syrup urine d., (MSUD),** a genetic aminoacidopathy due to an enzyme deficiency in the second step in branched-chain amino acid (BCAA) catabolism; the

BCAAs and their analogues accumulate in the blood and urine, causing severe ketoacidosis soon after birth, death in about half the newborns, seizures, coma, physical and mental retardation, and a characteristic smell of maple syrup or curry in the urine and on the body. There are five clinical phenotypes of MSUD: classic, intermittent, intermediate, thiamine-responsive, and dihydrolipoyl dehydrogenase (E_3) deficiency. Called also *keto acid decarboxylase deficiency* and *branched-chain ketoaciduria* or *ketoaminoacidemia*. See also *branched-chain α-keto acid dehydrogenase*. **Marburg d., Marburg virus d.,** a severe, acute, often fatal viral hemorrhagic fever, characterized by fever, prostration, hemorrhagic manifestations, pancreatitis, and hepatitis, the first reported primary cases of which were in Marburg and Frankfurt, Germany, and Belgrade, Yugoslavia, in laboratory workers handling infected African green monkeys or their organs; secondary infection is acquired through direct physical contact with infected patients. It has been reported as occurring in Kenya, Zimbabwe, and South Africa. **March's d.,** Graves' d. **Marchiafava-Bignami d.,** progressive degeneration of the corpus callosum characterized by progressive intellectual deterioration, emotional disturbances, confusion, hallucinations, tremor, rigidity, and convulsions. It is a very rare disorder affecting chiefly middle-aged male alcoholics, especially those who consume excessive amounts of crude red wine. **Marchiafava-Micheli d.,** paroxysmal nocturnal hemoglobinuria; see under *hemoglobinuria*. **Marek's d.,** a lymphoproliferative disease of chickens caused by a herpesvirus. Lymphoid cell infiltrations are most common in the peripheral nerves and gonads, but widespread infiltrations may also be found in any of the visceral organs, skin, muscle, and the iris of the eye. Perivascular cuffing of blood vessels in the brain and spinal cord frequently occurs. The location of the lesions dictates the clinical signs, such as paralysis, general depression, and blindness. It was once included in the avian leukosis complex. Called also, according to the symptoms manifested, *acute leukosis, fowl paralysis, ocular lymphomatosis, neural lymphomatosis, neurolymphomatosis gallinarum, range paralysis*, and *skin leukosis*. **margarine d.,** erythema multiforme due to an emulsifier in oleomargarine; it occurred as an explosive epidemic outbreak in Germany and Holland, thought at the time to be infectious in origin. **Marie's d.,** 1. acromegaly. 2. hypertrophic pulmonary osteoarthropathy. **Marie-Bamberger d.,** hypertrophic pulmonary osteoarthropathy. **Marie-Strümpell d.,** rheumatoid spondylitis. **Marie-Tooth d.,** progressive neuropathic (peroneal) muscular atrophy. **Marion's d.,** congenital obstruction of the posterior urethra due to muscular hypertrophy of the bladder neck or absence of the plexiform dilator fibers in the urinary tract. **Marsh's d.,** Graves' d. **Martin's d.,** periosteoarthritis of the foot from excessive walking. **Medin's d.,** see *poliomyelitis*. **Mediterranean d.,** see *β-thalassemia*. **medullary cystic d.,** familial juvenile nephronophthisis. **Meige's d.,** Milroy's d. **Meleda d.,** mal de Meleda. **Ménétrier's d.,** giant hypertrophic gastritis. **Meniere's d.,** hearing loss, tinnitus, and vertigo resulting from nonsuppurative disease of the labyrinth with the histopathologic feature of endolymphatic hydrops (distention of the membranous labyrinth). **Menkes' d.,** see under *syndrome*. **mental d.,** see under *disorder*. **Merzbacher-Pelizaeus d.,** Pelizaeus-Merzbacher d. **metabolic d.,** general term for diseases caused by disruption of a normal metabolic pathway because of a genetically determined enzyme defect. **metazoan d.,** a disease caused by metazoan parasites, such as nematodes, cestodes, trematodes, and arthropods. **Meyer's d.,** adenoid vegetations of the pharynx. **Meyer-Betz d.,** a rare familial disease of unknown etiology, marked by attacks of myoglobinuria, which may be precipitated by strenuous exertion or possibly by an infection, and which results in tenderness, swelling, and weakness of muscles of varying intensity. It may occur with or without diffuse chronic myopathy or dystrophy. Called also *idiopathic, spontaneous*, or *familial myoglobinuria*. **microdrepanocytic d.,** sickle cell–thalassemia d. **Mikulicz's d.,** originally, a chronic, benign, and usually painless inflammatory swelling of the lacrimal and salivary glands; some authorities have broadened the entity to include lacrimal and salivary gland enlargement associated with other diseases, such as Sjögren's syndrome, sarcoidosis, lupus erythematosus, leukemia, lymphoma, and tuberculosis, which they designate *Mukulicz's syndrome* (see under *syndrome*). **milky d., milky-**

white d., a fatal infection of beetle larvae due to *Bacillus papilliae* or *B. lentimorbus,* in which the "blood" of the larvae appears milky white as a result of the profuse multiplication and sporulation of the bacilli. The infection may be produced deliberately in Japanese beetles to control their population. **Miller's d.,** osteomalacia. **Mills' d.,** ascending hemiplegia that eventually develops into quadriplegia; its etiology is unknown. **Milroy's d.,** congenital hereditary lymphedema of the legs caused by chronic lymphatic obstruction; other areas, including the arms, trunk, and face may be involved. Called also *Meige's d., Milroy's edema, Nonne-Milroy-Meige syndrome,* and *congenital lymphedema.* **Milton's d.,** angioedema. **Minamata d.,** a severe neurologic disorder caused by alkyl mercury poisoning, usually characterized by peripheral and circumoral paresthesia, ataxia, dysarthria, and loss of peripheral vision, and leading to severe permanent neurologic and mental disabilities or death. It was prevalent between 1953 and 1958 among those who ate sea food from Minamata Bay, Japan, which contained an excess of alkyl mercury compounds. **Minor's d.,** hematomyelia involving the central parts of the spinal cord. **Mitchell's d.,** erythromelalgia. **mixed connective tissue d.,** a disorder combining features of scleroderma, myositis, systemic lupus erythematosus, and rheumatoid arthritis, and marked serologically by the presence of antibody against extractable nuclear antigen. **Möbius' d.,** periodic migraine with paralysis of the oculomotor muscles. **Moeller-Barlow d.,** subperiosteal hematoma in rickets. **molecular d.,** any disease in which the pathogenesis can be traced to a single molecule, usually a protein, which is either abnormal in structure or present in reduced amounts; the classical example is abnormal hemoglobin in sickle cell anemia. **Molten's d.,** Pictou d. **Mondor's d.,** phlebitis affecting the large subcutaneous veins normally crossing the lateral chest region and breast from the epigastric or hypochondriac region to the axilla, occurring in both males and females. **Monge's d.,** chronic mountain sickness. **Morgagni's d.,** hyperostosis frontalis interna. **Morquio's d.,** see under *syndrome.* **Morquio-Ullrich d.,** Morquio's syndrome. **Morton's d.,** see under *toe.* **Morvan's d.,** 1. syringomyelia. 2. see under *syndrome,* def. 2. **mosaic d's,** infectious diseases of plants caused by viruses and characterized by mottling of the foliage. **Moschcowitz's d.,** thrombotic thrombocytopenic purpura. **motor neuron d.,** any disease of a motor neuron, including spinal muscular atrophy, progressive bulbar paralysis, amyotrophic lateral sclerosis, and lateral sclerosis. **mountain d.,** see under *sickness.* **moyamoya d.** [Jap. *moyamoya* puff of smoke, from the angiographic appearance] cerebral ischemia due to occlusion and small hemorrhages from rupture of an abnormal network of vessels at the base of the brain, causing progressive neurologic disability; it occurs predominantly in the Japanese. **Mozer's d.,** myelosclerosis in adults. **mu chain d.,** the rarest heavy chain disease, found in patients with chronic lymphocytic leukemia, with symptoms of hepatomegaly and splenomegaly. **Mucha's d., Mucha-Habermann d.,** acute lichenoid pityriasis. **mucosal d.,** a disease of cattle, due to the virus of bovine virus diarrhea; ulcerations in the mouth may be the only sign, but often there is fever, diarrhea, loss of appetite, and a drop in milk yield. **mule spinner's d.,** warts or ulcers of the skin, especially of the scrotum, which tend to become malignant; so called because they were found chiefly among the operators of spinning mules in cotton mills. **Münchmeyer's d.,** a diffuse progressive ossifying polymyositis. **Murray Valley d.,** see under *encephalitis.* **mushroom picker's d., mushroom worker's d.,** an allergic respiratory disease closely resembling farmer's lung, developing in persons working with moldy compost prepared for growing mushrooms in closed areas, especially in those handling the dried material after harvesting. **mushy chick d.,** omphalitis of birds; see under *omphalitis.* **Nairobi d.,** an infectious disease of sheep and goats in Africa, especially in the region around Nairobi, marked by acute hemorrhagic gastroenteritis, green, watery diarrhea, mucopurulent nasal discharge, and breathing difficulty; it is caused by a virus transmitted by the ticks *Rhipicephalus appendiculatus* and *Amblyomma variegatum.* **nanukayami d.,** nanukayami. **navicular d.,** necrotic inflammation of the navicular bone in horses, causing intermittent lameness; called also *grog.* **Newcastle d.,** an influenza-like viral disease of birds, including domestic fowl, characterized by respiratory and gastrointesti-

nal or pneumonic and encephalitic symptoms. First seen near Newcastle, England, the infection is also transmissible to man by contact with infected birds. Called also *avian influenza.* **new duck d.,** infectious avian serositis in ducklings. **Nicolas-Favre d.,** lymphogranuloma venereum. **Niemann d., Niemann-Pick d.,** sphingolipidosis due to sphingomyelinase deficiency with sphingomyelin accumulation in the reticuloendothelial system. There are five types distinguished by age of onset and by the amount of CNS involvement and of sphingomyelinase activity. *Type A* (acute neuronopathic) in the classic type, accounting for 85 per cent of the patients: onset is in early infancy; CNS damage is severe; death occurs by 4 years. *Type B* (chronic non-neuronopathic) has onset in early infancy but does not affect the CNS or intelligence; normal life-span is possible. *Type C* (chronic neuronopathic) has variable ages of onset (at 2 years or older) and of death (from age 5 to adulthood) and variable CNS involvement. *Type D* (the Nova Scotia variant) resembles type C; *type E* (the adult, non-neuronopathic form) may be a late-onset variant of type C. Called also *sphingolipidosis, sphingomyelin lipidosis,* and *sphingomyelinase deficiency.* **nodule d., nodular worm d.,** a disease of sheep and cattle, caused by a minute worm, *Oesophagostomum columbianum,* which infests the intestines, becoming embedded in the mucous membrane, where it causes the formation of nodules of varying size. **Norrie's d.,** a congenital, X-linked disorder consisting of bilateral blindness from retinal malformation with possible mental retardation and deafness developing later; called also *atrophia bulborum hereditaria.* **Norum-Gjone d.,** familial lecithin-cholesterol acyltransferase deficiency. **nosema d.,** a disease of bees caused by *Nosema apis,* characterized by dysentery and paralysis. Cf. *pébrine.* **notifiable d.,** one required to be reported to federal, state, or local health officials when diagnosed, because of infectiousness, severity, or frequency of occurrence; called also *reportable d.* **Novy's rat d.,** a viral disease discovered by Novy in his stock of experimental rats. **oasthouse urine d.,** methionine malabsorption syndrome. **occupational d.,** one due to factors involved in one's employment, e.g., various forms of pneumoconiosis or dermatitis. **Oguchi's d.,** a form of congenital night blindness occurring in Japan. **Ohara's d.,** in Japan, tularemia. **oid-oid d.** [from disc*oid* and lichen*oid*], exudative discoid and lichenoid dermatitis. **Ollier's d.,** enchondromatosis. **Ondiri d.,** bovine infectious petechial fever. **Opitz's d.,** thrombophlebitic splenomegaly: enlargement of the spleen due to thrombosis of the splenic vein. **Oppenheim's d.,** amyotonia congenita. **organic d.,** one associated with demonstrable change in a bodily organ or tissue. **Oriental lung fluke d.,** parasitic hemoptysis. **Ormond's d.,** retroperitoneal fibrosis. **Osgood-Schlatter d.,** osteochondrosis of the tuberosity of the tibia; called also *apophysitis tibialis adolescentium, Schlatter's d.,* and *Schlatter-Osgood d.* See also *osteochondrosis.* **Osler's d.,** 1. polycythemia vera. 2. hereditary hemorrhagic telangiectasia. **Osler-Vaquez d.,** polycythemia vera. **Osler-Weber-Rendu d.,** hereditary hemorrhagic telangiectasia. **Otto's d.,** osteoarthritic protrusion of the acetabulum; arthrokatadysis. **overeating d.,** pulpy kidney d. **Owren's d.,** Factor V deficiency; see *coagulation factors,* under *factor.* **ox-warble d.,** see *larva migrans.* **Paas's d.,** a familial disorder marked by skeletal deformities such as coxa valga, shortening of phalanges, scoliosis, spondylitis, etc. **Paget d.,** 1. intraductal carcinoma of the breast extending to involve the nipple and areola, characterized clinically by eczema-like inflammatory skin changes, and histologically by infiltration of the epidermis by malignant cells (*Paget's cells*). 2. a neoplasm of the vulva and sometimes the perianal region histologically and clinically quite similar to Paget's disease of the breast, but having less of a tendency to be associated with underlying invasive carcinoma. 3. osteitis deformans. **Paget's d., extramammary,** Paget d., def. 2. **Panner's d.,** osteochondrosis of the capitellum of the humerus. **parenchymatous d.,** one which attacks the parenchyma of an organ. **Parkinson's d.,** paralysis agitans. **parrot d.,** psittacosis. **Parrot's d.,** see under *pseudoparalysis.* **Parry's d.,** toxic nodular goiter. **Patella's d.,** pyloric stenosis in tuberculous patients following fibrous stenosis. **Pavy's d.,** cyclic proteinuria. **Payr's d.,** constipation with left upper quadrant pain attributed to kinking of an adhesion between the transverse and descending colon with obstruction; probably a manifestation of the irritable colon syndrome rather than an organic lesion. Called also *splenic flexure syndrome.* **pearl d.,** tuberculosis of the peritoneum and mesentery of cattle. **pearl-worker's d.,** recurrent inflammation of bone with hypertrophy, seen in persons who work in pearl dust. **Pel-Ebstein d.,** Hodgkin's d. **Pelizaeus-Merzbacher d.,** a familial form of leukoencephalopathy (q.v.) occurring in early life and running a slowly progressive course into adolescence or adulthood. It is marked by nystagmus, ataxia, tremor, choreoathetotic movements, parkinsonian facies, dysarthria, and mental deterioration. Pathologically, there is diffuse demyelination in the white substance of the brain, which may involve the brain stem, cerebellum, and spinal cord. **Pellegrini's d., Pellegrini-Stieda d.,** a condition characterized by a semilunar bony formation in the upper portion of the medial lateral ligament of the knee, due to traumatism; called also *Köhler-Pellegrini-Stieda d.* and *Stieda's d.* **pelvic inflammatory d.,** any ascending pelvic infection involving the upper female genital tract beyond the cervix. **periodic d.,** a condition characterized by regularly recurring and intermittent episodes of fever, edema, arthralgia, or gastric pain and vomiting, continuing for years without further development in otherwise healthy individuals. **periodontal d.,** any of a group of pathological conditions that affect the surrounding and supporting tissues of the teeth, generally classified as inflammatory (gingivitis and periodontitis), dystrophic (periodontal trauma and periodontosis), and anomalies. Called also *dentoalveolitis.* **Perrin-Ferraton d.,** snapping hip. **Perthes' d.,** osteochondrosis of the capital femoral epiphysis; see *osteochondrosis.* **Peyronie's d.,** induration of the corpora cavernosa of the penis, producing a fibrous chordee; called also *fibrous cavernitis, penis plastica,* and *penile induration.* **Pfeiffer's d.,** infectious mononucleosis. **Phocas' d.,** chronic glandular mastitis with the formation of numerous small nodules. **phytanic acid storage d.,** Refsum d. **Pick's d.,** 1. [Arnold Pick] a rare progressive degenerative disease of the brain very similar in clinical manifestations and course to Alzheimer's disease but having a distinctive histopathology; cortical atrophy is confined to the frontal and temporal lobes; degenerating neurons contain globular intracytoplasmic filamentous inclusions (Pick bodies). Called also *circumscribed cerebral atrophy.* 2. [Friedel Pick] (obs.) pericardial pseudocirrhosis of the liver; congestive cirrhosis resulting from constrictive pericarditis. 3. [Ludwig Pick] Niemann-Pick d. **Pictou d.,** cirrhosis of the liver in horses and cattle in Nova Scotia due to ingestion of *Senecio jacobeus,* the ragwort; called also *Molten's d.* and *Winton d.* **pink d.,** acrodynia. **plaster-of-Paris d.,** atrophy of a limb which has been enclosed in a plaster-of-Paris splint. **Plummer's d.,** toxic nodular goiter. **pneumatic hammer d.,** vasospastic disease in the hands resulting from use of a pneumatic hammer. **policeman's d.,** tarsalgia. **polycystic d. of kidneys,** a heritable disorder marked by cysts scattered throughout both kidneys. It occurs in two unrelated forms: The *infantile* form, transmitted as an autosomal recessive trait, may be congenital or appear at any time during childhood. There is a high perinatal mortality rate, and almost all cases lead to hypertension. In older children cystic and fibrotic disease of the liver may be associated. The *adult* form, transmitted as an autosomal dominant trait, is marked by progressive deterioration of renal function. Called also *polycystic kidneys* and *polycystic renal d.* **polycystic ovary d.,** Stein-Leventhal syndrome. **polycystic renal d.,** polycystic kidney d. **polyendocrine autoimmune d.,** the combination of endocrine and nonendocrine autoimmune diseases. In type I, which occurs in infants and children, candidiasis, hypoparathyroidism, and adrenal insufficiency are associated, and pernicious anemia, vitiligo, gonadal failure, alopecia, insulin-dependent diabetes, and thyroid autoimmune disease may also occur; called also *autoimmune polyendocrine-candidiasis syndrome.* Type II is known as *Schmidt's syndrome* (q.v.). **polyhedral d's,** infectious diseases of insects, especially caterpillars, caused by viruses. **Pompe's d.,** glycogen storage d. (type II). **Poncet's d.,** tuberculous rheumatism. **Portuguese-Azorean d.,** Azorean d. **Posada-Wernicke d.,** coccidioidomycosis. **Pott's d.,** tuberculosis of the spine. **pregnancy d.,** pregnancy toxemia in ewes. **Preiser's d.,** osteoporosis and atrophy of the carpal scaphoid due to trauma or a fracture which has not been kept immobilized. **Pringle's d.,** adenoma sebaceum. **Profichet's d.,** see under *syndrome.* **pullet d.,** pyelonephritis of young hens of unknown etiology, character-

ized by loss of appetite, diarrhea with watery or whitish evacuations, and sometimes darkening of the comb; affected birds appear drowsy. **pullorum d.,** see *white diarrhea* (def. 2), under *diarrhea.* **pulpy kidney d.,** a fatal enterotoxemia usually seen in young animals, chiefly lambs, but which may affect sheep, goats, and cattle of any age; it is caused by *Clostridium perfringens* type D. Pathologically, the kidneys are mottled and soft in consistency and the cortex is jelly-like or almost semifluid; the liver is severely congested with small hemorrhages diffusely scattered over its surface. **pulseless d.,** progressive obliteration of the brachiocephalic trunk and the left subclavian and left common carotid arteries above their origin in the aortic arch, leading to loss of pulse in both arms and carotids and to symptoms associated with ischemia of the brain (syncope, transient hemiplegia, etc.), eyes (transient blindness, retinal atrophy, etc.), face (muscular atrophy, etc.), and arms (claudication, etc.). Called also *arteritis brachiocephalica* or *brachiocephalic arteritis, Martorell's syndrome, reversed coarctation,* and *Takayasu's disease* or *syndrome.* **Purtscher's d.,** traumatic angiopathy of the retina with edema, hemorrhage, and exudation, usually following crush injuries of the chest; called also *Purtscher's angiopathic retinopathy.* **Pyle's d.,** metaphyseal dysplasia. **pyramidal d.,** buttress foot. **Quervain's d.** see *de Quervain's d.* **Quincke's d.,** angioedema. **ragpicker's d., ragsorter's d.,** inhalational anthrax. **railroad d.,** transit tetany. **Ramsay Hunt d.,** see under *syndrome,* def. 1. **rat-bite d.,** see under *fever.* **Raynaud's d.,** 1. a primary or idiopathic vascular disorder characterized by bilateral attacks of Raynaud's phenomenon. The disease affects females more frequently than males. Called also *Raynaud's gangrene.* See *Raynaud's phenomenon,* under *phenomenon.* 2. paralysis of the throat muscles following parotiditis; called also *local asphyxia.* **Recklinghausen's d.,** neurofibromatosis. **Recklinghausen's d. of bone,** osteitis fibrosa cystica. **Recklinghausen-Applebaum d.,** hemochromatosis. **Reclus' d.,** 1. a painless cystic enlargement of the mammae, marked by multiple dilatations of the acini and ducts. 2. cellulitis with induration. **redwater d.,** bacillary hemoglobinuria. **Reed-Hodgkin d.,** Hodgkin's d. **Refsum d.,** an inborn error of metabolism caused by accumulation of phytanic acid, and manifested chiefly by chronic polyneuritis, retinitis pigmentosa, cerebellar ataxia, and persistent elevation of protein in cerebrospinal fluid; there may also be ichthyosis, nerve deafness, and electrocardiographic abnormalities. Called also *phytanic acid storage d., heredopathia atactica polyneuritiformis,* and *Refsum syndrome.* **Reichmann's d.** (obs.), gastrosuccorrhea. **Reiter's d.,** see under *syndrome.* **Rendu-Osler-Weber d.,** hereditary hemorrhagic telangiectasia. **Renikhet d.** (obs.), Newcastle d. in chickens. **reportable d.,** notifiable d. **rheumatic heart d.,** the most important manifestation of and sequel to rheumatic fever (q.v.), consisting chiefly of valvular deformities. **rheumatoid d.,** a systemic condition best known by its articular involvement (rheumatoid arthritis) but emphasizing nonarticular changes, e.g., pulmonary interstitial fibrosis, pleural effusion, and lung nodules. **Ribas-Torres d.,** variola minor. **rice d.,** beriberi. **Riedel's d.,** see under *thyroiditis.* **Riga-Fede d.,** a small sublingual ulceration in infants with natal or neonatal teeth due to rubbing the lower central incisors; most often observed in whooping cough. **Riggs' d.,** marginal periodontitis. **Ritter's d.,** staphylococcal scalded skin syndrome. **Robles' d.,** name for onchocerciasis in Central America. **Roger's d.,** a ventricular septal defect; the term is usually restricted to small, asymptomatic defects. **Rokitansky's d.,** (obs.), massive hepatic necrosis. **rolling d.,** a disease of laboratory mice characterized by lateral rolling movements, by neurolysis and by a polymorphonuclear leukocytic reaction in the brain; it is caused by a potent neurolytic exotoxin produced by *Mycoplasma neurolyticum.* **Romberg's d.,** facial hemiatrophy. **rose d.,** the urticarial form of swine erysipelas. **Rossbach's d.,** hyperchlorhydria. **Rot's d., Rot-Bernhardt d.,** meralgia paresthetica. **Roth's d.,** meralgia paraesthetica. **Roth-Bernhardt d.,** meralgia paraesthetica. **Rougnon-Heberden d.,** angina pectoris. **round heart d.,** a disease of unknown etiology which causes sudden death in apparently healthy poultry; a greatly enlarged heart is seen post mortem. **Roussy-Lévy's d.,** see under *syndrome.* **Rubarth's d.,** hepatitis contagiosa canis. **runt d.,** graft-versus-host disease produced by injection of allogenic lymphocytes into immunologically immature experimental animals. **Rust's d.,** tuberculous spondylitis of the cervical vertebrae. **Ruysch's d.,** Hirschsprung's d. **saccharine d.,** a term proposed for any disease resulting from the overconsumption of refined carbohydrate foods in combination with the removal of dietary fiber and protein, including diabetes, cardiovascular disease, constipation, obesity, peptic ulcer, etc. **Sachs' d.,** Tay-Sachs d. **sacroiliac d.,** chronic tuberculous inflammation of the sacroiliac joint. **salivary gland d.,** cytomegalic inclusion d. **Sanders' d.,** epidemic keratoconjunctivitis. **Sandhoff d.,** a type of GM₂ gangliosidosis with clinical features similar to Tay-Sachs disease although it has been observed only among non-Jews. The underlying defect is deficiency of both hexosaminidase A and hexosaminidase B. **sandworm d.,** larva migrans. **San Joaquin Valley d.,** coccidioidomycosis. **Saunders' d.,** a dangerous condition seen in infants having digestive disturbances to whom is given a large percentage of carbohydrates; it is marked by vomiting, cerebral symptoms, and depression of circulation. **Schamberg's d.,** a chronic, asymptomatic dermatosis occurring in adolescent and young adult males, localized to the shin, ankles, and dorsa of the feet and toes, and characterized by an eruption of orange- to fawn-colored macules with red puncta (cayenne pepper spots) within or on their border. Called also *progressive pigmentary dermatosis, Schamberg's dermatosis,* and *Schamberg's progressive pigmented purpuric dermatosis.* **Schanz's d.,** traumatic inflammation of the tendo Achillis. **Schaumann's d.,** sarcoidosis. **Scheuermann's d.,** osteochondrosis of vertebral epiphyses in juveniles; see *osteochondrosis.* **Schilder's d.,** a subacute or chronic form of leukoencephalopathy of children and adolescents. Clinical symptoms include blindness, deafness, bilateral spasticity, and progressive mental deterioration. There is massive destruction of the white substance of the cerebral hemispheres, cavity formation, and glial scarring. The disease usually occurs sporadically, but a familial form has been reported. Called also *encephalitis peri- axialis diffusa, Flatau-Schilder disease,* and *Schilder's encephalitis.* **Schimmelbusch's d.,** cystic d. of breast. **Schlatter's d., Schlatter-Osgood d.,** Osgood-Schlatter d. **Schmorl's d.,** 1. herniation of the nucleus pulposus into an adjacent ventral body. 2. necrobacillosis of wild and domestic rabbits, rats, and other wild animals, due to infection with *Fusobacterium necrophorum* (Schmorl's bacillus); it is characterized by abscesses on various parts of the body, or by areas of necrosis around the mouth, nose, eyelids, throat, and chest. **Scholz's d.,** metachromatic leukodystrophy (juvenile form). **Schönlein's d.,** see under *purpura.* **Schönlein-Henoch d.,** see under *purpura.* **Schottmüller's d.,** paratyphoid fever. **Schroeder's d.,** a condition characterized by hypertrophic endometrium and excessive uterine bleeding, probably due to deficiency of the gonadotropic hormone. **Schüller's d.,** 1. Hand-Schüller-Christian disease. 2. osteoporosis circumscripta cranii. **Schüller-Christian d.,** Hand-Schüller-Christian d. **Schultz's d.,** agranulocytosis. **Schwediauer's d.,** see *Swediaur's d.* **secondary d.,** 1. a morbid condition occurring subsequent to or as a consequence of another disease. 2. one due to introduction of incompatible immunologically competent cells into a host rendered incapable of rejecting them by heavy exposure to ionizing radiation. **Seitelberger's d.,** infantile neuroaxonal dystrophy. **self-limited d.,** one which by its very nature runs a limited and definite course. **Selter's d.,** acrodynia. **senecio d.,** cirrhosis of the liver occurring as the result of poisoning by the plant *Senecio.* **septic d.,** one which arises from the development of pyogenic or putrefactive organisms. **serum d.,** see under *sickness.* **Sever's d.,** epiphysitis of the calcaneus. **severe combined immunodeficiency d. (SCID),** see under *immunodeficiency.* **sexually transmitted d.,** any of a diverse group of infections caused by biologically dissimilar pathogens and transmitted by sexual contact, which includes both heterosexual and homosexual behavior; sexual transmission is the only important mode of spread of some of the diseases in the group (e.g., the classic venereal diseases), while others (e.g., hepatitis viruses, shigellosis, amebiasis, giardiasis) can also be acquired by nonsexual means. See also *venereal d.* **Shaver's d.,** bauxite pneumoconiosis. **shimamushi d.,** scrub typhus. **shuttlemaker's d.,** a condition in shuttlemakers, marked by faintness, shortness of breath, headache, nausea, etc., attributed to inhaling the dust of poisonous wood from which

the shuttles (devices used in weaving) are made. **sickle-cell d.,** any of the diseases associated with the presence of hemoglobin S, including sickle cell anemia, sickle cell–hemoglobin C or D disease, and sickle cell–thalassemia disease. **sickle cell–hemoglobin C d.,** a genetically determined anemia in which the red cells contain both hemoglobin S and hemoglobin C. **sickle cell–hemoglobin D d.,** a genetically determined anemia characterized by the presence of both hemoglobin S and hemoglobin D in red blood cells. **sickle cell–thalassemia d.,** a hereditary anemia involving simultaneous heterozygosity for hemoglobin S and thalassemia. Called also *microdrepanocytosis, microdrepanocytic d., hemoglobin S–thalassemia, sickle cell–thalassemia,* and *thalassemia–sickle cell disease.* **silo-filler's d.,** pulmonary inflammation, often with acute pulmonary edema, caused by inhalation of the irritant gases (especially oxides of nitrogen) which collect in recently filled silos. **Simmonds' d.,** panhypopituitarism. **Simons' d.,** partial lipodystrophy. **sixth d.,** exanthema subitum. **sixth venereal d.,** lymphogranuloma venereum. **Sjögren's d.,** see under *syndrome.* **Skevas-Zerfus d.,** sponge-diver's d. **sleeping d.,** narcolepsy. **sleepy foal d.,** a form of equulosis affecting foals within the first three days of life, due to infection with *Actinobacillus equuli,* characterized by sudden onset, extreme prostration, and death usually within 12 hours. **Smith-Strang d.,** methionine malabsorption syndrome. **Sneddon-Wilkinson d.,** subcorneal pustular dermatosis. **sod d.,** vesicular dermatitis. **specific d.,** any disease, such as syphilis, due to a characteristic morbific agency. **Spencer's d.,** a form (probably viral) of epidemic gastroenteritis. **Spielmeyer-Vogt d.,** see *amaurotic idiocy,* under *idiocy.* **sponge-diver's d.,** a condition encountered by divers in the Mediterranean who come in contact with the stinging tentacles of sea anemones of the genera *Sagartia* and *Actinia,* which are frequently attached to the base of sponges; it is marked by burning, itching, erythema, necrosis, and ulceration. Called also *Skevas-Zerfus d.* **Stargardt's d.,** hereditary degeneration of the macula lutea occurring between the ages of six and twenty, marked by rapid loss of visual acuity and by abnormal appearance and pigmentation of the macular area. **Steinert's d.,** myotonic dystrophy. **sterility d.,** a deficiency disease observed in experimental animals and due to a lack of vitamin E in the diet. **Sternberg's d.,** Hodgkin's d. **Sticker's d.,** erythema infectiosum. **Stieda's d.,** Pellegrini's d. **stiff lamb d.,** polyarthritis of lambs caused by a chlamydial organism, with stiffness of the legs, reluctance to move, and recumbency. **Still's d.,** a variety of chronic polyarthritis affecting children and marked by enlargement of lymph nodes, generally of the spleen, and irregular fever; called also *juvenile rheumatoid arthritis.* **Stokes-Adams d.,** Adams-Stokes d. **storage d.,** a metabolic disorder in which some substance accumulates or is stored in certain cells in unusually large amounts; the stored substances may be lipids, proteins, carbohydrates, or other substances. See, for example, *glycogen storage d., mucopolysaccharidosis,* and *proteinosis.* Formerly called *thesaurismosis.* **storage pool d,** a blood coagulation disorder due to failure of the platelets to release ADP in response to aggregating agents (collagen, epinephrine, exogenous ADP, thrombin, etc.). It is characterized by mild bleeding episodes, prolonged bleeding time, and reduced aggregation response to collagen or thrombin. **structural d.,** any disease in which there are microscopic changes. **Strümpell's d.,** 1. a hereditary form of lateral sclerosis (q.v. under *sclerosis*) in which the spasticity is principally limited to the legs; called also *Strümpell type.* 2. polioencephalomyelitis. **Strümpell-Leichtenstern d.,** hemorrhagic encephalitis. **Strümpell-Marie d.,** rheumatoid spondylitis. **Sturge's d.,** Sturge-Weber syndrome. **Stuttgart d.,** a nonjaundiced type of canine leptospirosis caused by *Leptospira interrogans* serogroup *canicola;* called also *canine typhus.* **Sudeck's d.,** post-traumatic osteoporosis. **Sutton's d.,** 1. [R. L. Sutton, Sr.] (a) halo nevus; (b) periadenitis mucosa necrotica recurrens. 2. [R. L. Sutton, Jr.] granuloma fissuratum. **Sutton and Gull's d.** (*obs.*), arteriocapillary fibrosis. **Swediaur's (Schwediauer's) d.,** inflammation of the calcaneal bursa. **sweet clover d.,** a hemorrhagic disease of animals, especially cattle, caused by ingestion of spoiled sweet clover, which contains the anticoagulant dicumarol. **Swift's d.,** acrodynia. **Swift-Feer d.,** acrodynia. **swineherd's d.,** leptospirosis, manifested as a benign meningitis, caused by *Leptospira interrogans* serogroups *hyos* or *pomona*, and affecting those who work with swine or pork or come in contact with the urine of carriers. **Sylvest's d.,** epidemic pleurodynia. **Symmers' d.,** nodular lymphoma. **systemic d.,** one affecting a number of organs and tissues. **Takahara's d.,** acatalasia. **Takayasu's d.,** pulseless d. **Talfan d.,** infectious porcine encephalomyelitis. **Talma's d.,** myotonia acquisita. **Tangier d.,** see *familial lipoprotein deficiency,* under *lipoprotein.* **tartaric d.,** gout and calculus (Paracelsus). **Tarui d.,** glycogen storage d. (type VII). **Tay's d.,** see under *choroiditis.* **Tay-Sachs d. (TSD),** the most common ganglioside storage disease, occurring almost exclusively among northeast European Jews. TSD is a GM₂ gangliosidosis specifically characterized by infantile onset (3-6 months), doll-like facies, cherry-red macular spot (90+ per cent of the infants), early blindness, hyperacusis, macrocephaly, seizures, and hypotonia; the children die between 2 and 5 years of age. See also *gangliosidosis; Sandhoff disease,* under *disease;* and *amaurotic familial idiocy,* under *idiocy.* **teart d. in cattle,** a diarrhea that affects cattle that graze on certain pastures in England, due to the presence of molybdenum in the herbage. **Teschen d.,** infectious porcine encephalomyelitis. **thalassemia–sickle cell d.,** sickle cell–thalassemia d. **Thaysen's d.,** nontropical sprue, or celiac disease. **Theiler's d.,** spontaneous encephalomyelitis of mice, caused by invasion of the nervous system by a common viral infection of the intestinal tract; called also *Theiler's mouse encephalomyelitis* and *murine encephalomyelitis.* **Thiemann's d.,** familial avascular necrosis of the phalangeal epiphysis, beginning in childhood or adolescence and resulting in deformity of the interphalangeal joints; called also *familial osteoarthropathy of the fingers.* Similar lesions may occur in the great toes and first tarsometatarsal joints, in which case it is known as *osteochondritis ossis metacarpi et metatarsi.* **Thomsen's d.,** myotonia congenita. **Thomson's d.,** an autosomal recessive skin disorder similar to Rothmund-Thomson syndrome except that saddle nose and cataract are not manifestations. **thyrocardiac d.,** thyrotoxic heart d. **thyrotoxic heart d.,** heart disease associated with hyperthyroidism, marked by atrial fibrillation, cardiac enlargement, and congestive heart failure; called also *thyrocardiac d.* **Tietze's d.,** see under *syndrome.* **Tillaux's d.,** mastitis with the formation of multiple tumors in the breast. **Tommaselli's d.,** pyrexia and hematuria due to excessive use of quinine. **Tooth d.,** progressive neuropathic (peroneal) muscular atrophy. **Tornwaldt's (Thornwaldt's) d.,** see under *bursitis.* **Tourette's d.,** Gilles de la Tourette's syndrome. **Traum's d.,** infectious abortion (brucellosis) in swine. **Trevor's d.,** dysplasia epiphysealis hemimelica. **trophoblastic d.,** a group of disorders that have their origin in the placenta, including hydatidiform mole, chorioadenoma destruens, and gestational choriocarcinoma. **tsutsugamushi d.,** scrub typhus. **tunnel d.,** 1. (*obs.*) hookworm d. 2. decompression sickness. **twin-lamb d.,** pregnancy toxemia in ewes. **twist d.,** whirling d. **Tyzzer's d.,** a disease caused by *Bacillus piliformis* and characterized by necrotic lesions of the liver and intestine; originally described in Japanese waltzing mice; it also affects rats, rabbits, gerbils, dogs, and man. **Tzaneen d.,** a tick-borne protozoal disease, reported in Tzaneen, South Africa, due to *Theileria mutans,* and occurring in cattle and water buffalo, which may manifest as a mild febrile disease or may be severe and fatal. **Underwood's d.,** sclerema. **Unna-Thost d.,** diffuse palmoplantar keratoderma. **Unverricht's d.,** myoclonus epilepsy. **Urbach-Wiethe d.,** lipoid proteinosis. **vagabonds' d.,** **vagrants' d.,** discoloration of the skin in persons subjected to louse (*Pediculus humanus corporis*) bites over long periods; called also *parasitic melanoderma.* **van Buren's d.,** Peyronie's disease. **Vaquez' d., Vaquez-Osler d.,** polycythemia vera. **veld d., veldt d.,** heartwater. **venereal d.,** classically, five infectious diseases (gonorrhea, syphilis, chancroid, lymphogranuloma venereum, granuloma inguinale) that were known to be transmitted by sexual contact, principally sexual intercourse. Infections caused by *Chlamydia trachomatis* are now also included. See *sexually transmitted d.* **veno-occlusive d. of the liver,** symptomatic occlusion of the small hepatic venules, first seen in children in Jamaica where it resulted from ingestion of Senecio tea, also caused by other hepatotoxins and by radiation. Many patients recover after withdrawal of the

offending toxin; some progress to portal hypertension and liver failure, as in Budd-Chiari syndrome. **vent d.,** rabbit syphilis. **Verneuil's d.,** syphilitic disease of the bursae. **Verse's d.,** calcinosis intervertebralis. **vibration d.,** blanching and diminished flexion of the fingers with loss of perception of cold, heat, and pain and osteoarthritic changes in joints of the arm, due to continuous use of vibrating tools. **Vogt's d.,** see under *syndrome.* **Vogt-Spielmeyer d.,** see *amaurotic idiocy,* under *idiocy.* **Volkmann's d.,** a congenital deformity of the foot due to a tibiotarsal dislocation; called also *Volkmann's deformity.* **Voltolini's d.,** an acute purulent inflammation of the internal ear with violent pain, followed by involvement of the meninges with subsequent fever, delirium, and unconsciousness. **von Economo's d.,** lethargic encephalitis. **von Gierke's d.,** glycogen storage d. (type I). **von Hippel's d.,** angiomatosis confined principally to the retina; when associated with hemangioblastoma of the cerebellum, it is known as *von Hippel-Lindau d.* **von Hippel-Lindau d.,** hereditary phakomatosis characterized by congenital angiomatosis of the retina and cerebellum; there may also be similar lesions of the spinal cord and cysts of the pancreas, kidneys, and other viscera. Neurologic symptoms, including seizures and mental retardation, may be present. Called also *cerebroretinal* or *retinocerebral angiomatosis,* and *Lindau-von Hippel d.* **von Jaksch's d.,** anemia pseudoleukemica infantum. **von Recklinghausen's d.,** see *Recklinghausen's d.* **von Willebrand's d.,** a congenital hemorrhagic diathesis, inherited as an autosomal dominant trait, characterized by prolonged bleeding time, deficiency of coagulation Factor VIII, and often impairment of adhesion of platelets on glass beads, associated with epistaxis and increased bleeding after trauma or surgery, menorrhagia, and postpartum bleeding. Called also *angiohemophilia, Minot-von Willebrand syndrome, pseudohemophilia, vascular hemophilia,* and *Willebrand's syndrome.* **Vrolik's d.,** osteogenesis imperfecta congenita. **Waldenström's d.,** osteochondrosis of the capital femoral epiphysis; see *osteochondrosis.* **walkabout d.,** Kimberley horse d. **Wartenberg's d.,** 1. cheiralgia paresthetica. 2. brachialgia statica paresthetica. 3. partial thenar atrophy. **wasting d.** any disease marked especially by progressive emaciation and weakness. **Weber's d.,** Sturge-Weber syndrome. **Weber-Christian d.,** relapsing febrile nodular nonsuppurative panniculitis. **Wegner's d.,** osteochondritic separation of the epiphyses in hereditary syphilis. **Weil's d.,** see under *syndrome.* **Weir Mitchell's d.,** erythromelalgia. **Wenckebach's d.** (*obs.*), cardioptosis. **Werdnig-Hoffmann d.,** Werdnig-Hoffmann spinal muscular atrophy. **Werlhof's d.,** idiopathic thrombocytopenic purpura. **Werner-His d.,** trench fever. **Werner-Schultz d.,** agranulocytosis. **Wernicke's d.,** see under *encephalopathy.* **Wesselsbron d.,** a mosquito-borne viral disease causing death of lambs and abortion and death in ewes in Africa; it is communicable to man, in whom it causes a mild febrile illness. **Westphal-Strümpell d.,** Wilson's d. **Whipple's d.,** a malabsorption syndrome characterized by diarrhea, steatorrhea, skin pigmentation, arthralgia and arthritis, lymphadenopathy, and central nervous system lesions. The intestinal mucosa is infiltrated with macrophages containing PAS-positive material (the remnants of bacillary microorganisms which invade the lamina propria). **whirling d.,** a highly fatal protozoal disease of young salmonid fish caused by *Myxosoma cerebralis,* characterized chiefly by cartilaginous damage in the axial skeleton and granuloma formation involving the auditory-equilibrium apparatus of the fish, causing it to swim rapidly in a circular pattern. Called also *twist d.* **white heifer d.,** a condition reputed to most commonly occur in white heifers, usually of the Shorthorn breed, in which there is a rubber-like sheet of fibrous tissue and membrane stretching across the posterior part of the vagina; the converage may be partial or complete. Called also *persistent hymen.* **white muscle d.,** skeletal muscle degeneration in animals, produced by calcification or muscle fibers, the result of deficiency of selenium in the diet. **white-spot d.,** 1. lichen sclerosus et atrophicus. 2. guttate morphea. 3. a pustular eruption involving the skin, gills, and eyes of marine and freshwater fishes both in the wild and in aquaria, caused by the protozoan *Ichthyophthirius multifiliis,* and often leading to death, and sometimes to great economic loss. Called also *ich, ichthyophthiriasis,* and *ick.* **Whitmore's d.,** melioidosis. **Whytt's d.,** tuberculous meningitis causing acute hydrocephalus. **Wilson's d.,** a rare progressive disease, inherited as an autosomal recessive trait and due to a defect in the metabolism of copper, with accumulation of copper in the liver, brain, kidney, cornea, and other tissues. The disease is characterized by cirrhosis of the liver and degenerative changes in the brain, particularly the basal ganglia. Liver disease is the most likely presenting manifestation in children; neurologic disease is most common in young adults. The characteristic ophthalmic feature is a pigmented ring (Kayser-Fleischer ring) at the outer margin of the cornea. Called also *hepatolenticular degeneration* or *disease, familial hepatitis,* and *Westphal-Strümpell disease* or *pseudosclerosis.* **Winckel's d.,** a fatal disease of newborn infants characterized by jaundice, hemoglobinuria, hemorrhage, bloody urine, cyanosis, polyuria, collapse, and convulsions. **Winiwarter-Buerger d.,** thromboangiitis obliterans. **Winkler's d.,** chondrodermatitis nodularis chronica helicis. **Winton d.,** Pictou d. **Witkop's d.,** Witkop-Von Sallman d. **Wolman d.,** a lysosomal storage disease due to acid lipase deficiency, with onset in early infancy and death before one year of age. Clinical features include hepatosplenomegaly, steatorrhea, abdominal distension, anemia, inanition, and adrenal calcification. Called also *primary familial* and *Wolman xanthomatosis.* **woolsorters' d.,** inhalational anthrax. **Woringer-Kolopp d.,** pagetoid reticulosis. **x d.,** 1. hyperkeratosis (def. 3). 2. aflatoxicosis. **X-linked lymphoproliferative d.,** see under *syndrome.* **Zahorsky's d.,** exanthema subitum. **Ziehen-Oppenheim d.,** dystonia musculorum deformans.

disengagement (dis″en-gāj′ment) liberation of the fetus, or parts thereof, from the vaginal canal.

disequilibrium (dis-e″kwĭ-lib′re-um) a disturbed state of equilibrium, either physical or mental. **linkage d.,** see *linkage.*

disesthesia (dis″es-the′ze-ah) dysesthesia.

disgerminoma (dis-jer″mĭ-no′mah) dysgerminoma.

dish (dish) a shallow vessel of glass or other material for laboratory work. **culture d.,** a shallow glass vessel for making bacterial cultures. **dappen d.,** a small, heavy, solid glass, octagonal dish with a shallow depression to hold a few drops of medicaments or filling material. **evaporating d.,** a laboratory vessel, usually wide and shallow, in which material is evaporated by exposure to heat. **Petri d.,** a round, shallow, flat-bottomed transparent glass or plastic dish with vertical sides and a similar but slightly larger dish that forms a cover; used for the culture of microorganisms on solid media and for tissue cell cultures. **Stender d.,** a vessel of various forms and sizes, used in preparing and staining histologic specimens.

disharmony (dis-har′mo-ne) lacking harmony; discordant. **occlusal d.,** a condition in which (*a*) contacts of opposing occlusal surfaces of teeth are not in harmony with other tooth contacts and with the anatomic and physiologic control of the mandible, or (*b*) occlusions do not coincide with their respective jaw relations.

disinfect (dis″in-fekt′) [*dis-* + L. *inficere* to corrupt] to free from pathogenic organisms, or to render them inert, especially as applied to the treatment of inanimate materials to reduce or eliminate infectious organisms.

disinfectant (dis″in-fek′tant) 1. freeing from infection. 2. an agent that disinfects; applied particularly to agents used on inanimate objects. Cf. *antiseptic.* **coal-tar d.,** creosote.

disinfection (dis″in-fek′shun) the act of disinfecting. **concomitant d., concurrent d.,** immediate disinfection and disposal of discharges and infective matter all through the course of a disease. **terminal d.,** disinfection of a sick room and its contents at the termination of a disease.

disinfestation (dis″in-fes-ta′shun) the extermination or destruction of insects, rodents, or other animal forms which might transmit infection and which are present on the person or clothing of an individual or in his surroundings; defaunation.

disinhibition (dis″in-hĭ-bish′un) 1. removal of inhibitions, as reduction of the inhibitory function of the cerebral cortex by drugs such as ethyl alcohol or reduction in the severity of superego controls in psychotherapy. 2. in experimental psychology, the revival of an extinguished conditioned response by exposure to an unconditioned stimulus.

disinomenine (di″sĭ-nom′ĕ-nin) an alkaloid, $C_{19}H_{25}O_4N$, formed by the oxidation of sinomenine.

disinsected (dis″in-sekt′ed) freed from insects or vermin.

disinsection (dis″in-sek′shun) disinsectization.

disinsectization (dis″in-sek″ti-za′shun) removal of insects from; extermination of insects or vermin.

disinsector (dis″in-sek′tor) an apparatus for the removal of insects or vermin from patients or their clothing.

disinsertion (dis″in-ser′shun) 1. rupture of a tendon from its insertion into a bone. 2. detachment of the retina at its periphery; retinodialysis.

disintegrant (dis-in′tĕ-grant) disintegrator; an agent used in the pharmaceutical preparation of tablets, which causes them to disintegrate and release their medicinal substances on contact with moisture.

disintegration (dis″in-tĕ-gra′shun) [*dis-* + L. *integer* entire] 1. the process of breaking up or decomposing. 2. disruption of integrative functions of personality in mental illness. **radioactive d.,** see under *decay.*

Disipal (dis′ĭ-pal) trademark for a preparation of orphenadrine hydrochloride.

disjoint (dis-joint′) to disarticulate.

disjunction (dis-junk′shun) the act or state of being disjoined. In genetics, the moving apart of bivalent chromosomes at first anaphase of meiosis. **craniofacial d.,** Le Fort III fracture; see under *fracture.*

disk (disk) [L. *discus;* Gr. *diskos*] a circular or rounded flat plate; also *disc.* **A d.,** A band; see under *band.* **abrasive d.,** a thin, flat, oval, or concave circular plate with abrasive materials bonded to its surface or edge; used to polish and finish cavity preparations and for cutting or polishing dental restorations. See *dental d.* **Amici's d.,** Z band; see under *band.* **anangioid d.,** a retinal disk without blood vessels. **anisotropic d., anisotropous d.,** A band; see under *band.* **articular d.,** 1. a pad of fibrocartilage or dense fibrous tissue found in some synovial joints; see *discus articularis,* and for names of articular disks of particular joints, see entries beginning *discus articularis,* under *discus.* 2. meniscus articularis. **Bardeen's primitive d.,** the embryonic structure which develops into the intervertebral ligament. **Blake's d.,** a disk-shaped paper patch for a perforated tympanic membrane. **blastodermic d.,** the early germinal disk during the period of cleavage. **blood d.,** see *platelet.* **Bowman's d's,** flat, disklike plates which make up striated muscle fibers. **Carborundum d.,** a dental disk with Carborundum as the abrasive material. **choked d.,** papilledema. **ciliary d.,** orbiculus ciliaris. **cloth d.,** rag wheel. **cupped d.,** a pathologically depressed and enlarged optic disk, frequently seen in advanced glaucoma. **cutting d.,** a dental disk with abrasive material attached to its surfaces or edge, used for grinding or reducing teeth. **cuttlefish d.,** a dental disk with powdered cuttlefish bone bonded to its surface and edge. **dental d.,** a disk with abrasive material bonded to its surface, used in dentistry for cutting, smoothing, or polishing; an abrasive disk. **diamond d.,** a steel dental disk with diamond chips bonded to its surface or edge. **ectodermal d.,** an elongated plate of epithelial cells developed from the inner cell mass in the human conceptus about a week after fertilization. **embryonic d.,** a flattish area in a cleaved ovum in which the first traces of the embryo are seen; called also *germinal d.* and *gastrodisk.* **emery d.,** a paper or resin dental disk with emery powder attached to its surface. **Engelmann's d.,** H band; see under *band.* **epiphyseal d.,** cartilago epiphysialis. **gelatin d.,** a disk or lamella of gelatin, variously medicated; used chiefly in eye diseases. **germinal d.,** embryonic d. **Hensen's d.,** H band; see under *band.* **I d.,** the light disk or band of a striated muscle fiber; called also *isotropic disk* or *J disk.* **interarticular d.,** articular d., def. 1. **intercalated d.,** dense bands that extend in a serrated fashion transversely across cardiac muscle fibers, separating one fiber from another but containing contact specializations, including desmosomes and gap junctions. **intermediate d.,** Z band; see under *band.* **interpubic d.,** discus interpubicus. **intervertebral d's,** disci intervertebrales. **intra-articular d.,** fibrous structures within the capsules of diarthrodial joints. **isotropic d., J d.,** I band; see under *band.* **M d.,** M band; see under *band.* **Merkel's d's,** menisci tactus. **micrometer d.,** a glass disk, engraved with a scale, used in an ocular in making microscopi-

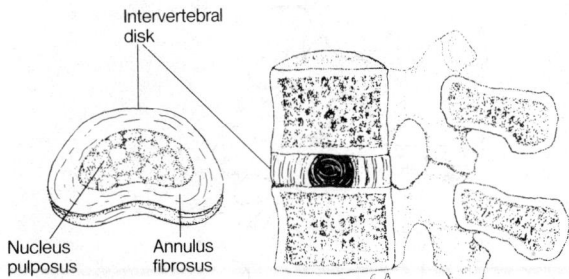

Intervertebral disk

Nucleus pulposus   Annulus fibrosus

cal measurements. **Newton's d.,** a disk which is divided into seven sectors that are colored the seven primary colors of the spectrum and which, when rotated rapidly, appears to be white. **optic d.,** discus nervi optici. **Placido's d.,** a keratoscope. **polishing d.,** a dental disk with a very fine abrasive material, used for finishing and polishing of surfaces. **proligerous d.,** cumulus oophorus. **Q d.,** A band; see under *band*. **Ranvier's tactile d's,** terminations of nerve fibers in cup-shaped bodies in the transparent substance between Grandry's corpuscles. **Rekoss d.,** the rotating device for quickly changing the lenses in the ophthalmoscope. **sandpaper d.,** a dental disk with pulverized silica as the abrasive material. **Schiefferdecker's d's,** a substance in neurons staining black with silver nitrate, assumed to occupy the space in Ranvier's nodes between Schwann's sheath and the axon. **slipped d.,** popular name for herniation of an intervertebral disk. **stenopeic d.,** an opaque disk having a narrow slit; used for testing for astigmatism. **stroboscopic d.,** a revolving disk with alternate open and closed sections that gives successive views of a moving object. **tactile d's,** see under *meniscus*. **thin d.,** Z band; see under *band*. **transverse d.,** A band; see under *band*. **Z d.,** Z band; see under *band*.

diskectomy (dis-kek′to-me) excision of an intervertebral disk.

diskiform (dis′kĭ-form) in the shape of a disk.

diskitis (dis-ki′tis) inflammation of a disk, particularly of an interarticular disk.

disk(o)- [Gr. *diskos* disk] a combining form denoting relationship to a disk, or disk-shaped. See also words beginning *disc(o)-*.

diskogram (dis′ko-gram) a roentgenogram of an intervertebral disk.

diskography (dis-kog′rah-fe) roentgenography of the spine for visualization of an intervertebral disk, after injection into the disk itself of an absorbable contrast medium.

dislocatio (dis″lo-ka′she-o) [L.] dislocation. **d. erec′ta,** subglenoid dislocation of the shoulder with the arm in a vertical position and the hand on top of the head.

dislocation (dis″lo-ka′shun) [*dis-* + L. *locare* to place] the displacement of any part, more especially of a bone; see Plate. Called also *luxation*. **Bell-Dally d.,** nontraumatic dislocation of the atlas. **closed d.,** simple d. **complete d.,** one which completely separates the surfaces of a joint. **complicated d.,** one which is associated with other important injuries. **compound d.,** one in which the joint communicates with the external air. **congenital d.,** one which exists from or before birth. **consecutive d.,** one in which the luxated bone has changed its position since its first displacement. **divergent d.,** one in which the ulna and radius are dislocated separately. **fracture d.,** dislocation complicated by fracture of, or adjacent to, a joint. **habitual d.,** one which often recurs after replacement. **incomplete d.,** a subluxation; a slight displacement. Called also *partial d.* **intrauterine d.,** one which occurs to the fetus in utero. **Kienböck's d.,** isolated dislocation of the semilunar bone. **d. of the lens,** displacement of the crystalline lens of the eye. **Lisfranc's d.,** dislocation of the forefoot at the tarsometatarsal joints. **Monteggia's d.,** dislocation of the hip joint in which the head of the femur is near the anterosuperior spine of the ilium. **Nélaton's d.,** dislocation of the ankle in which the talus is forced up between the end of the tibia and the fibula. **old d.,** a dislocation in which inflammatory or fibrotic changes have occurred. **open d.,** compound d. **partial d.,** incom-

plete d. **pathologic d.,** one which results from paralysis, synovitis, infection, or other disease. **primitive d.,** one in which the bones remain as originally displaced. **recent d.,** one in which there is no complicating inflammation. **simple d.,** one in which the joint is not penetrated by a wound. **Smith's d.,** upward and backward dislocation of the metatarsals and the medial cuneiform bone. **subastragalar d.,** separation of the calcaneus and the navicular bone from the talus. **subspinous d.,** dislocation of the head of the humerus into the space below the spine of the scapula. **traumatic d.,** one due to an injury or to violence.

dismemberment (dis-mem′ber-ment) amputation of a limb or a portion of it.

dismutation (dis″mu-ta′shun) a reaction or reactions involving two identical molecules in which one gains what the other loses. For example, one may be oxidized and the other reduced, or one may be phosphorylated and the other dephosphorylated.

disocclude (dis″ŏ-klood′) to cause loss of contact between opposing teeth as a result of tooth guidance, occlusal interferences, or occlusal adjustment.

disodium (di-so′de-um) having two atoms of sodium in each molecule.

Disomer (di′so-mer) trademark for preparations of dexbrompheniramine maleate.

disomus (di-so′mus) [*di-* + Gr. *sōma* body] a double-bodied monster.

disopyramide (di-so-pēr′ah-mīd) [USP] chemical name: α-[2-[bis(1-methylethyl)amino]ethyl]-α-phenyl-2-pyridineacetamide. A cardiac depressant with anticholinergic properties, $C_{21}H_{29}N_3O$, used as an antiarrhythmic. **d. phosphate,** the phosphate salt of disopyramide, $C_{21}H_{29}N_3O\cdot H_3PO_4$, having the same actions and uses as the base, administered orally.

disorder (dis-or′der) a derangement or abnormality of function; a morbid physical or mental state. **adjustment d.** [DSM III-R], a maladaptive reaction to identifiable stressful life events, such as divorce, loss of job, physical illness, or natural disaster; this diagnosis assumes that the condition will remit when the stress ceases or when the patient adapts to the situation. **affective d's,** mood d's. **amnestic d.** [DSM III-R], either of two DSM III-R diagnostic categories: alcohol amnestic disorder (amnestic syndrome due to prolonged alcohol use, Korsakoff's syndrome) and sedative, hypnotic, or anxiolytic amnestic disorder (a transient amnestic syndrome due to prolonged use of a sedative, hypnotic, or anxiolytic. **anxiety d's** [DSM III-R], a group of mental disorders in which anxiety and avoidance behavior predominate. Included are panic disorder with and without agoraphobia, agoraphobia without history of panic disorders, social phobia, simple phobia, obsessive compulsive disorder, post-traumatic stress disorder, and generalized anxiety disorder. **anxiety d's of childhood or adolescence** [DSM III-R], a group of mental disorders of children and adolescents in which the predominant clinical feature is anxiety, either focused on specific situations (separation anxiety disorder, avoidant disorder of childhood or adolescence) or generalized (overanxious disorder). **attention-deficit hyperactivity d.** [DSM III-R], a controversial childhood mental disorder with onset before age seven characterized by fidgeting and squirming, difficulty in remaining seated, easy distractability, difficulty awaiting one's turn and refraining from blurting out answers to questions before they have been completed, and inability to follow instructions, excessive talking, and other disruptive behavior. Called also minimal brain dysfunction (based on the unproven assumption that brain damage causes the syndrome and the neurological abnormalities) and *hyperkinetic reaction* or *syndrome* and *hyperactive child syndrome*. **autistic d.** [DSM III-R], a severe mental disorder with onset in infancy characterized by qualitative impairment in reciprocal social interaction (e.g., lack of awareness of the existence of feelings of others, failure to seek comfort at times of distress, lack of imitation) and in verbal and nonverbal communication and restricted repertoire of activities and interests. It differs from childhood schizophrenia in its early onset and in the lack of delusions, hallucinations, incoherence, or loosening of associations and from mental retardation in the presence of intelligent, responsive facies and in that the full syndrome of infantile autism is not produced by

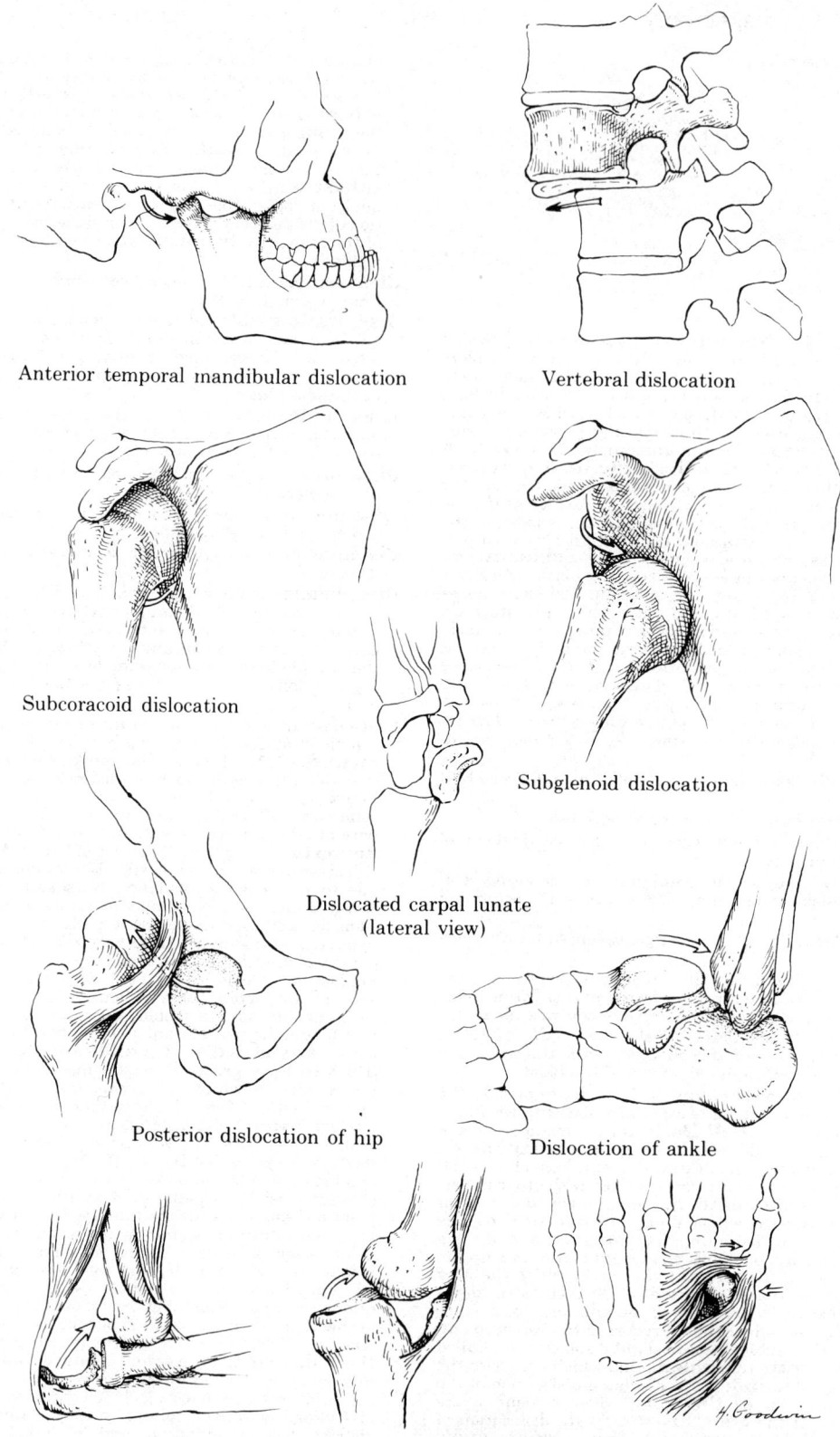

Anterior temporal mandibular dislocation

Vertebral dislocation

Subcoracoid dislocation

Subglenoid dislocation

Dislocated carpal lunate
(lateral view)

Posterior dislocation of hip

Dislocation of ankle

Posterior dislocation of elbow   Posterior dislocation of knee   Dislocation of thumb

PLATE 14 —VARIOUS TYPES OF DISLOCATION

mental retardation. Called also *infantile a.* and *Kanner's syndrome*. **avoidant d. of childhood or adolescence** [DSM III-R], persistent and excessive shrinking from contact with strangers. **behavior d.,** 1. conduct d. 2. (*obs.*) mental disorder characterized by socially unacceptable behavior. **bipolar d.,** 1. [DSM III-R] a mood disorder characterized by the occurrence of one or more manic episodes (q.v.); in almost all cases one or more major depressive episodes (q.v.) will eventually occur. Bipolar disorder is further classified as *mixed* if manic and depressive episodes alternate every few days and otherwise as *manic* or *depressed* according to the type of the most recent episode. Called also *manic-depressive disorder, illness,* or *psychosis*. 2. (pl.) bipolar disorder and cyclothymia. Cf. *unipolar d's*. **body dysmorphic d.** [DSM III-R], a mental disorder characterized by preoccupation with some imagined defect in appearance of a normal-appearing person. **character d.,** see *personality disorder,* under *personality*. See also *character*. **collagen d.,** any inborn error of metabolism involving abnormal structure or metabolism of collagen; the term includes the Ehlers-Danlos syndrome, the Marfan syndrome, cutis laxa, osteogenesis imperfecta, and epidermolysis bullosa. *Collagen disorder* is not to be confused with *collagen disease*. **conduct d.** [DSM III-R], mental disorders of childhood and adolescence characterized by a persistent pattern of conduct in which rights of others and age-appropriate societal norms or rules are violated; classified as *group type, solitary aggressive type,* and *undifferentiated type*. **conversion d.** [DSM III-R], a mental disorder characterized by conversion symptoms (loss or alteration of physical function suggesting physical illness, usually of the sensorimotor system, such as seizures, paralysis, dyskinesia, anesthesia, blindness, or aphonia) having no demonstrable physiological basis and whose psychological basis is suggested by (1) exacerbation of symptoms at times of psychological stress, (2) relief from tension or inner conflicts (primary gain) provided by the symptoms, or (3) secondary gains (support, attention, avoidance of unpleasant responsibilities) provided by the symptoms. Many patients exhibit "la belle indifférence," a lack of concern about the impairment caused by the symptoms; histrionic (hysterical) personality traits are also common. This diagnosis excludes patients whose symptoms are under voluntary control (as in factitious disorder with physical symptoms or malingering), patients with the full syndrome of somatization disorder (q.v.), and patients whose predominant complaint is pain (as in psychogenic pain disorder). Called also *conversion hysteria* and *hysterical neurosis, conversion type*. **cyclothymic d.,** see *cyclothymia*. **delusional (paranoid) d.** [DSM III-R], see *paranoia*. **depersonalization d.** [DSM III-R], a dissociative disorder characterized by one or more episodes of depersonalization (feelings of unreality and strangeness in one's perception of the self or one's body image) not due to another mental disorder, such as schizophrenia. Episodes of depersonalization are usually accompanied by dizziness, anxiety, fears of going insane, and derealization. Called also *depersonalization neurosis* or *syndrome*. **dissociative d's** [DSM III-R], hysterical neuroses, dissociative type; mental disorders characterized by sudden, temporary alterations in identity, memory, or consciousness, segregating normally integrated memories or parts of the personality from the dominant identity of the individual. This category includes *multiple personality disorder, psychogenic fugue, psychogenic amnesia,* and *depersonalization disorder* (depersonalization neurosis). **dysthymic d.,** see *dysthymia*. **emotional d.,** see under *illness*. **factitious d.** [DSM III-R], a mental disorder characterized by repeated, knowing simulation of physical and psychological symptoms for no apparent purpose other than obtaining treatment. It differs from malingering in that there is no recognizable motive for feigning illness. DSM III distinguishes two main types: chronic factitious disorder with physical symptoms (called also Munchausen syndrome) and factitious disorder with psychological symptoms (called also Ganser syndrome). **functional d.,** a disorder of function having no known organic basis. In psychiatry, the term is roughly equivalent to "psychogenic disorder"; in other branches of medicine, to "idiopathic disorder." **generalized anxiety d.** [DSM III-R], a neurotic mental disorder characterized by the presence of unrealistic or excessive anxiety and worry about two or more life circumstances, for six months or longer. **genetic d.,** see under *disease*. **identity d.** [DSM III-R], severe subjective distress, lasting 3 months or longer, about inability to reconcile aspects of the

self into a relatively coherent whole and acceptable sense of self, with uncertainty about career choice, sexual orientation and behavior, moral values, and the like, occurring most commonly in late adolescence. **immunodeficiency d.,** see under *disease*. **induced psychotic d.** [DSM III-R], a delusional system that develops in a second person as a result of a close relationship with another person who already has a psychotic disorder with prominent delusions. Called also *folie à deux*. **intermittent explosive d.** [DSM III-R], a functional mental disorder characterized by multiple discrete episodes of loss of control of aggressive impulses resulting in serious assault or destruction of property that are out of keeping with the individual's normal personality. Formerly called *explosive personality* and *epileptoid personality disorder*, which are misnomers since intermittent behavior is not a personality trait. **isolated explosive d.** [DSM III], a functional mental disorder characterized by a single violent catastrophic act performed for no apparent reason and not attributable to an underlying psychotic or organic mental disorder; classified in DSM III-R as impulse control disorder not otherwise specified. **LDL-receptor d.,** familial hyperlipoproteinemia, type IIa. **major mood d's** [DSM III-R], bipolar disorder and major depression. **manic-depressive d.,** bipolar d. **mendelian d.,** a genetic disease, showing a mendelian pattern of inheritance, and caused by a single mutation in the structure of DNA, which causes a single basic defect that has some pathological consequence or consequences. Called also *monogenic* or *single-gene d*. See also *inborn error of metabolism,* under *metabolism*. **mental d.,** any clinically significant behavioral or psychological syndrome characterized by the presence of distressing symptoms or significant impairment of functioning. Mental disorders are assumed to result from some psychological or organic dysfunction of the individual; the concept does not include disturbances that are essentially conflicts between the individual and society (social deviance). **monogenic d.,** mendelian d. **mood d's** [DSM III-R], mental disorders whose essential feature is a disturbance of mood manifested as a full or partial manic or depressive syndrome. Functional mood disorders are subclassified as *bipolar disorders*, including bipolar disorder and cyclothymia, and *depressive disorders*, including major depression and dysthymia. For organic mood disorders, see *organic mood syndrome,* under *syndrome*. **multifactorial d.,** a disorder caused by interaction of genetic factors and perhaps also nongenetic, environmental factors, e.g. some forms of birth defects and diabetes mellitus. See also *genetic disease*. **multiple personality d.** [DSM III-R], see *multiple personality,* under *personality*. **organic mental d's,** a particular organic brain syndrome (q.v.) in which the etiology is known or presumed, such as delirium tremens or Alzheimer's disease. **overanxious d.** [DSM III-R], an anxiety disorder of childhood or adolescence characterized by excessive worrying and fearful behavior not related to a specific situation or due to recent stress. **panic d.** [DSM III-R], a neurotic mental disorder characterized by recurrent panic (anxiety) attacks, episodes of intense apprehension, fear, or terror associated with somatic symptoms such as dyspnea, palpitations, dizziness, vertigo, faintness, or shakiness and with psychological symptoms such as feelings of unreality (depersonalization or derealization) or fears of dying, going crazy, or losing control; there is usually chronic nervousness and tension between attacks. It may be associated with agoraphobia. This disorder does not include panic attacks that may occur in phobias when the patient is exposed to the phobic stimulus. **paranoid d's,** see *paranoia*. **personality d.** [DSM III], see *personality* and specific personality disorders, under *personality,* and see *organic personality syndrome,* under *syndrome*. **pervasive developmental d's** [DSM III-R], a subclass of disorders in which there is impairment in development of reciprocal social interaction and of verbal and nonverbal communication skills and in imaginative activity; included is autistic disorder. **posttraumatic stress d.** [DSM III-R], a mental disorder caused by a traumatic event outside the range of normal human experience, such as rape or assault, military combat or bombing of civilians, natural disasters or terrible accidents, torture, or death camps, and characterized by reexperiencing the traumatic event in recurrent intrusive recollections, nightmares, or flashbacks, by "psychic numbness" or "emotional anesthesia," by hyperalertness and difficulty in sleeping, remembering, or concentrating, and by guilt about surviving when others have not or about things that had to

be done in order to survive; classified as acute, chronic, or delayed depending on the duration of symptoms and on whether there is a latent period, which may be months or years, between the trauma and the onset of symptoms. Terms formerly used for disorders of this type include *traumatic neurosis, gross stress reaction,* and *combat* (or battle or war) *exhaustion, fatigue,* or *neurosis.* **psychoactive substance-induced organic mental d's** [DSM III-R], organic brain syndromes associated with use of psychoactive substances; DSM III includes ten specific syndromes, *intoxication, withdrawal, delirium, dementia, amnestic disorder, delusional disorder, hallucinosis, mood disorder, perception disorder,* and *personality disorder.* When the causative substance is known, it is specified, e.g., "alcohol intoxication." **psychoactive substance use d's** [DSM III-R], mental disorders involving maladaptive behavior associated with regular use of mood- or behavior-altering substances. See *psychoactive substance abuse,* under *abuse,* and *psychoactive substance dependence,* under *dependence.* **psychogenic pain d.,** see *somatoform pain d.* **psychophysiologic d.,** psychosomatic d. **psychosomatic d.,** a disorder in which the physical symptoms are caused or exacerbated by psychological factors, such as migraine headache, lower back pain, gastric ulcer, or irritable bowel syndrome. The term *psychophysiologic disorders* used in previous official nomenclatures and defined as "physical disorders of presumably psychogenic origin" has been replaced in DSM III-R by the more neutral phrase *psychological factors affecting physical condition,* which may be applied to "any physical condition to which psychological factors are judged to be contributory," and reflects the existing lack of certainty about the actual etiological role of psychological factors in these conditions. **schizoaffective d.** [DSM III-R], a diagnostic category for mental disorders that have features of both schizophrenia and mood disorders (mania or depression). **schizophreniform d.** [DSM III-R], a mental disorder with the signs and symptoms of schizophrenia but duration of less than 6 months. Formerly called *acute schizophrenia.* **seasonal mood d.,** depression with increased need for sleep and increased carbohydrate intake occurring during winter months. **separation anxiety d.** [DSM III-R], distress and apprehension in a child on being removed from parents, home, or familiar surroundings. **shared paranoid d.,** induced psychotic d. **single-gene d.,** mendelian d. **sleep terror d.** [DSM III-R], repeated episodes of awakening shortly after sleep onset with intense anxiety, autonomic symptoms, and unresponsiveness to comforting efforts. Called also *pavor nocturnus.* **sleepwalking d.** [DSM III-R], repeated episodes of somnambulism. **somatization d.** [DSM III-R], classic hysteria (Briquet's syndrome); a mental disorder characterized by multiple somatic complaints that are not caused by a real physical illness; the complaints may involve a general complaint of being sickly or specific conversion (pseudoneurological) symptoms, gastrointestinal symptoms, female reproductive symptoms, psychosexual symptoms, cardiopulmonary symptoms, or pain. Complaints are often presented in a dramatic, vague, or exaggerated way; many physicians become involved in the medical care; and numerous diagnostic evaluations and unnecessary medical treatment or surgery may be performed. Most patients have symptoms of anxiety and depression and a wide range of interpersonal difficulties; many have histrionic (hysterical) personality traits. **somatoform d's** [DSM III-R], mental disorders characterized by symptoms suggesting a physical disorder that are of psychogenic origin but not under voluntary control; this category includes body dysmorphic disorder, conversion disorder (hysterical neurosis, conversion type), hypochondriasis (hypochondriacal neurosis), somatization disorder, and somatoform pain disorder. **somatoform pain d.** [DSM III-R], a mental disorder characterized by a chief complaint of severe chronic pain and that meets the criteria of conversion disorder (the pain is inconsistent with neuroanatomy and known pathophysiological mechanisms or far exceeds what would be expected from what organic pathologic change is present, and there are signs indicating the psychological origin of the symptoms). **substance use d's,** see *psychoactive substance use d's.* **Tourette's d.,** Gilles de la Tourette's syndrome. **unipolar d's,** major depression and dysthymic disorder (depressive neurosis). Cf. *bipolar d's.*
disorganization (dis-or″gan-i-za′shun) the process of destruction of any organic tissue; any profound change in the

tissues of an organ or structure which causes the loss of most or all of its proper characters.
disorientation (dis-o″re-en-ta′shun) the loss of proper bearings, or a state of mental confusion as to time, place, or identity. **spatial d.,** a condition in which a pilot or other air crew member is unable to determine accurately his spatial attitude in relation to the surface of the earth; it occurs only in conditions of poor visibility or when vision is otherwise restricted and results from vestibular illusions. Called also *pilot's vertigo.*
disoxidation (dis″ok-se-da′shun) deoxidation.
dispar (dis′par) [L.] unequal.
disparasitized (dis-par′ah-si-tīzd) freed from parasites.
disparate (dis′pah-rat) [L. *disparatus, dispar* unequal] not situated alike; not exactly paired; dissimilar in kind.
dispensary (dis-pen′sah-re) [L. *dispensarium,* from *dispensare* to dispense] 1. a place where medical or dental skill, treatment, and remedies are provided for the indigent ambulant sick at little or no cost to them. 2. any place where drugs and medicines are actually dispensed.
dispensatory (dis-pen′sah-to-re) [L. *dispensatorium*] a treatise on the qualities and composition of medicines. **D. of the United States of America,** a collection of monographs on unofficial drugs and drugs recognized by the United States Pharmacopoeia, the British Pharmacopoeia, and the National Formulary, and on general tests, processes, reagents, and solutions of the U.S.P. and N.F., as well as drugs used in veterinary medicine.
dispense (dis-pens′) [L. *dispensare, dis-* out + *pensare* to weigh] to prepare and distribute medicines to those who are to use them.
dispermy (di′sper-me) the penetration of two spermatozoa into one ovum.
dispersate (dis′pur-sāt) a suspension of finely divided particles of a substance.
disperse (dis-pers′) [L. *dis-* apart + *spargere* to scatter] to scatter the component parts, as of a tumor or the fine particles in a colloid system; also the particles so dispersed.
dispersible (dis-per′sĭ-b′l) capable of being dispersed.
dispersion (dis-per′shun) [L. *dispersio*] 1. the act of scattering or separating; the condition of being scattered. 2. the incorporation of the particles of one substance into the body of another, comprising solutions, suspensions, and colloid solutions. 3. a colloid solution. **colloid d.,** a colloid solution. **molecular d.,** solution, def. 1.
dispersity (dis-per′sĭ-te) the degree of dispersion of a colloid, i.e., the degree to which the dimensions of the disperse particles have been reduced.
dispersoid (dis-per′soid) a colloid in which the dispersity is relatively great.
dispert (dis′pert) a medicinal preparation obtained from a vegetable drug or endocrine gland by extracting its therapeutical constituents in the cold and then reducing the product to a dry concentrated form.
Dispholidus (dis-fol′ĭ-dus) a genus of venomous colubrid snakes. *D. ty′pus* is the boomslang of South Africa. See table accompanying *snake.*
dispira (di-spi′rah) [*di-* + Gr. *speira* coil] dispireme.
dispireme (di-spi′rem, di-spi′rēm) [*di-* + Gr. *speirēma* coil] the stage of cell division which follows the diaster; so called because the cytoplasm is divided into two parts, in each of which the chromatin appears to assume the form of a coil. See *mitosis.*
displaceability (dis-plās″ah-bil′ĭ-te) the quality of being susceptible to movement from an initial position, or the degree to which such movement is possible.
displacement (dis-plās′ment) 1. removal from the normal position or place; ectopia. 2. percolation. 3. in psychology, a defense mechanism in which emotions, ideas, wishes, or impulses are unconsciously shifted from their original object to a more acceptable substitute. 4. in dentistry, the malposition of the crown and root of one or more teeth from the normal line of occlusion; also the deflection of the mandible from its normal path of closure, i.e., posterior displacement. 5. in chemistry, the replacement, in a chemical reaction, of one atom or group of atoms in a molecule by another. **character d.,** the adaptive characters that evolve and enable one species to exclude another from its ecological niche. See also *competitive exclusion,* under *exclusion.* **condy-**

lar d., an abnormal position of the head of the mandibular condyle in the fossa due to a deviation or shift of the mandible, which is often the result of malocclusion. **fetal d.,** a group of cells which, during fetal development, has become displaced from its normal relations. **fish-hook d.,** a form of displacement of the stomach in which the orifice of the pylorus faces directly upward, and the duodenum runs upward and to the right to join the pylorus at an angle, producing a constricting cause; there is no evidence that such displacement causes symptoms. **gallbladder d.,** wandering gallbladder. **tissue d.,** change in the position of tissues as the result of pressure or other force.

dispore (di′spōr) one of two spores, as the basidia of higher fungi; opposed to tetraspore (four-spored basidium).

disporous (di′spo-rus) having two spores, as the basidia of the higher fungi.

disposition (dis″po-zish′un) a tendency either physical or mental toward certain diseases.

disproportion (dis″pro-por′shun) a lack of the proper relationship between two elements or factors. **cephalopelvic d.,** a condition in which the head of the fetus is too large for the pelvis of the mother.

disruption (dis-rup′shun) [L. *diruptio* a bursting apart] a morphologic defect resulting from the extrinsic breakdown of, or interference with, an originally normal developmental process.

disruptive (dis-rup′tiv) bursting apart; rending.

Disse's spaces (dis′ēz) [Joseph *Disse*, German anatomist, 1852–1912] see under *space*.

dissect (dĭ-sekt′, di-sekt′) [L. *dissecare* to cut up] to cut apart, or separate; applied especially to the exposure of structures of a cadaver, for anatomical study.

dissection (dĭ-sek′shun) [L. *dissectio*] 1. the act of dissecting. 2. a part or whole of an organism prepared by dissecting. **aortic d.,** dissecting aneurysm. **blunt d.,** dissection accomplished by separating tissues along natural cleavage lines, without cutting. **sharp d.,** dissection accomplished by incising tissues with a sharp edge.

dissector (dĭ-sek′tor) 1. one who dissects. 2. a handbook used as a guide for the act of dissecting.

disseminated (dis-sem′ĭ-nāt″ed) [L. *dis-* apart + *seminare* to sow] scattered; distributed over a considerable area.

dissepiment (dis-sep′ĭ-ment) partition; separation.

dissimilate (dis-sim′ĭ-lāt) [L. *dis-* neg. + *similare* to make alike] to decompose a substance into simpler compounds, for the production of energy or of materials that can be eliminated.

dissimilation (dis″sim-ĭ-la′shun) the act or process of dissimilating (see *dissimilate*); the reverse of assimilation.

dissociable (dis-so′shĕ-b'l) easily separable into component parts; separable from associations.

dissociation (dis-so″she-a′shun) [L. *dis-* neg. + *sociatio* union] 1. the act of separating or state of being separated. 2. the separation of a molecule into two or more fragments (atoms, molecules, ions, or free radicals) produced by the absorption of light or thermal energy or by solvation. 3. in psychology, a defense mechanism in which a group of mental processes are segregated from the rest of a person's mental activity in order to avoid emotional distress, as in the dissociative disorders (q.v.), or in which an idea or object is segregated from its emotional significance; in the first sense it is roughly equivalent to *splitting,* in the second, to *isolation.* 4. a defect of mental integration in which one or more groups of mental processes become separated off from normal consciousness and, thus separated, function as a unitary whole. Cf. *unconscious.* **albuminocytologic d.,** increase of protein with normal cell count in the spinal fluid. **atrial d.,** independent beating of the left and right atria, each with normal rhythm or with various combinations of normal rhythm, atrial flutter, or atrial fibrillation. **atrioventricular d.,** control of the atria by one pacemaker and of the ventricles by another, independent pacemaker; when the ventricular rate is more rapid than the atrial rate, ventriculoatrial (retrograde) block is present but atrioventricular conduction (anterograde) usually is not impaired. **auriculoventricular d.,** atrioventricular d. **bacterial d.,** the change, due to mutation and selection, in colonial morphology (usually from mucoid or smooth to rough) of bacteria in culture on laboratory media; called also *microbic d.* See also *smooth-rough variation,* under *variation.* **in-**

terference d., **d. by interference,** control of the atria by the sinoatrial node or other atrial pacemaker and of the ventricles by a lower pacemaker (atrioventricular dissociation) with a phasic rhythm related to capture of the ventricle (anterograde) or atrium (retrograde) by conduction from the pacemaker in the other chamber; called also *atrioventricular interference d.* **microbic d.,** bacterial d. **peripheral d.,** sensory disturbance in which touch, superficial pain, and temperature sensibility are diminished in the hands and feet; seen in polyneuritis. **syringomyelic d.,** loss of pain and temperature sense due to a lesion in the region of the central canal of the spinal cord implicating the spinothalamic fibers with preservation of other sensory modalities. **tabetic d.,** disturbance of the vibratory and muscle-tendon sensibility due to lesion of the dorsal columns.

dissogeny (dĭ-soj′ĕ-ne) [Gr. *dissos* twofold + *gennan* to produce] the state of having sexual maturity in both a larval and an adult stage.

dissolution (dis″so-lu′shun) [L. *dissolutio, dissolvere* to dissolve] 1. the process in which one substance is dissolved in another. 2. separation of a compound into its components by chemical action. 3. liquefaction. 4. the process of loosening, or of relaxing. 5. death.

dissolve (diz-zolv′) 1. to cause a substance to pass into solution. 2. to pass into solution.

dissolvent (diz-zol′vent) 1. a solvent medium. 2. a medicine capable of dissolving concretions within the body. 3. solvent; capable of dissolving substances.

dissonance (dis′so-nans) discord or disagreement. **cognitive d.,** the unpleasant feeling that arises when there is a lack of agreement among a person's ideas, beliefs, attitudes, and experiences.

Dist. abbreviation for L. *distil′la,* distil.

distad (dis′tad) in a distal direction.

distal (dis′tal) [L. *distans* distant] remote; farther from any point of reference; opposed to proximal. In dentistry, used to designate a position on the dental arch farther from the median line of the jaw.

distalis (dis-ta′lis) distal; [NA] a term denoting remoteness from the point of origin or attachment of an organ or part.

distally (dis′tal-le) in a distal direction.

distance (dis′tans) the measure of space intervening between two objects or two points of reference. **angular d.,** the aperture of the angle made at the eye by lines drawn from the eye to two objects. **focal d.,** the distance from the focal point to the optical center of a lens or the surface of a concave mirror. **infinite d.,** in ophthalmology, a distance of 20 feet or more: so called because rays entering the eye from an object at that distance are practically as parallel as if they came from a point at an infinite distance. **interarch d.,** 1. the vertical distance between the maxillary and mandibular arches (alveolar or residual) under certain conditions of vertical dimension that must be specified. 2. the vertical distance between the maxillary and mandibular ridges; called also *interridge d.* **interocclusal d.,** the distance between the occluding surfaces of the maxillary and mandibular teeth when the mandible is in physiologic rest position; called also *freeway space* and *interocclusal clearance, gap,* and *space.* **interocular d.,** the distance between the two eyes, usually used in reference to the interpupillary distance. **interpediculate d.,** the distance between the vertebral pedicles as measured on the roentgenogram. **interpupillary d.,** the distance between the centers of the pupils of the two eyes when the visual axes are parallel; in practice usually measured from the lateral margin of one pupil to the medial margin of the other. **interridge d.,** interarch d. **map d.,** the distance between two genetic loci on a linkage map, measured in centimorgans. **working d.,** the distance between the front lens of a microscope and the object when the instrument is correctly focused.

distemper (dis-tem′per) a name for several infectious diseases of animals, especially canine distemper. **canine d.,** a specific infectious respiratory and sometimes gastrointestinal disease of dogs characterized by fever, dullness, loss of appetite, and a discharge from the eyes and nose. It is caused by a virus and is also infectious for foxes and ferrets. **cat d.,** panleukopenia. **colt d.,** strangles, def. 1.

distemperoid (dis-tem′per-oid) an attenuated canine distemper virus that has been subjected to several passages in ferrets; called also *Green's distemperoid.*

distensibility (dis-ten″sĭ-bil′ĭ-te) capability of being distended.

distention (dis-ten′shun) the state of being distended or enlarged; the act of distending.

distichia (dis-tik′e-ah) distichiasis.

distichiasis (dis″tĭ-ki′ah-sis) [Gr. *distichia* a double line] the presence of a double row of eyelashes on an eyelid, one or both of which are turned in against the eyeball.

distichous (dis′tĭ-kus) arranged in two vertical rows; said of the arrangement of leaves where the leaf at one node is opposite to those just above and below it.

distil, distill (dis-til′) [L. *destillare; de* from + *stillare* to drop] to volatilize by heat and then cool and condense the evaporated matter, as to purify a substance or to separate a volatile substance from other less volatile substances.

distillate (dis′til-lāt) material that has been obtained by distillation.

distillation (dis-til-la′shun) vaporization; the process of vaporizing and condensing a substance to purify the substance or to separate a volatile substance from less volatile substances. **destructive d., dry d.,** decomposition of a solid by heating in the absence of air, which results in volatile liquid products. **fractional d.,** that which is attended by the successive separation of volatilizable substances in the order of their respective volatility. **molecular d.,** a process of purification applied to drugs and pharmaceuticals during which the crude material is evaporated under high vacuum of about one millionth of an atmosphere, and the condensate is caught on a cooled surface held close in front of the evaporating layer. The process is applied currently to vitamins A, D, and E, to animal and vegetable sterols and hormones, and to drugs and intermediates. **vacuum d.,** distillation under reduced pressure to avoid the decomposition which might occur at atmospheric pressure.

distoaxiogingival (dis″to-ak″se-o-jin′jĭ-val) 1. pertaining to the line angle formed by the axial and gingival walls of a cavity preparation on the distal aspect of a tooth. 2. axiodistogingival.

distoaxioincisal (dis″to-ak″se-o-in-si′zal) pertaining to or formed by the distal, axial, and incisal walls of a tooth cavity preparation.

distoaxio-occlusal (dis″to-ak″se-o-ŏ-kloo′zal) pertaining to or formed by the distal, axial, and occlusal walls of a tooth cavity preparation.

distobuccal (dis″to-buk′al) pertaining to or formed by the distal and buccal surfaces of a tooth, or by the distal and buccal walls of a tooth cavity preparation. Called also *buccodistal.*

distobucco-occlusal (dis″to-buk″o-ŏ-kloo′zal) pertaining to or formed by the distal, buccal, and occlusal surfaces of a tooth.

distobuccopulpal (dis″to-buk″o-pul′pal) pertaining to or formed by the distal, buccal, and pulpal walls of a tooth cavity preparation.

distocervical (dis″to-ser′vĭ-kal) 1. pertaining to the distal surface of the neck of a tooth. 2. distogingival.

distoclination (dis″to-kli-na′shun) deviation of a tooth from the vertical, in the direction of the tooth next distal (posterior) to it in the dental arch.

distoclusal (dis″to-kloo′zal) disto-occlusal.

distoclusion (dis″to-kloo′zhun) malocclusion in which the mandibular arch is in a posterior (distal) position in relation to the maxillary arch. Generally considered as identical with Class II in Angle's classification of malocclusion (see *malocclusion*). Called also *disto-occlusion, posterior occlusion, posteroclusion,* and *retrusive occlusion.*

distogingival (dis″to-jin′jĭ-val) pertaining to or formed by the distal and gingival walls of a tooth cavity preparation; called also *distocervical.*

distolabial (dis″to-la′be-al) pertaining to or formed by the distal and labial surfaces of a tooth, or the distal and labial walls of a tooth cavity preparation.

distolabioincisal (dis″to-la″be-o-in-si′zal) pertaining to or formed by the distal, labial, and incisal surfaces of a tooth.

distolingual (dis″to-ling′gwal) pertaining to or formed by

the distal and lingual surfaces of a tooth, or the distal and lingual walls of a tooth cavity preparation.

distolinguoincisal (dis″to-ling″gwo-in-si′zal) pertaining to or formed by the distal, lingual, and incisal surfaces of a tooth.

distolinguo-occlusal (dis″to-ling″gwo-ŏ-kloo′zal) pertaining to or formed by the distal, lingual, and occlusal surfaces of a tooth.

distolinguopulpal (dis″to-ling″gwo-pul′pal) pertaining to or formed by the distal, lingual, and pulpal walls of a tooth cavity preparation.

Distoma (dis′to-mah) [*di-* + Gr. *stoma* mouth] former name of a genus of trematode worms; as now used, a general term including various genera of trematodes or flukes, such as *Paragonimus, Fasciola,* etc. **D. bus′ki,** *Fasciolopsis buski.* **D. conjunc′tum,** *Amphimerus noverca.* **D. feli′neum,** *Opisthorchis felineus.* **D. haemato′bium,** *Schistosoma haematobium.* **D. hepat′icum,** *Fasciola hepatica.* **D. heteroph′yes,** *Heterophyes heterophyes.* **D. rin′geri,** *Paragonimus westermani.* **D. sinen′sis,** *Opisthorchis sinensis.* **D. westerman′i,** *Paragonimus westermani.*

distomatosis (dis″to-mah-to′sis) distomiasis.

distomia (di-sto′me-ah) the presence of two mouths.

distomiasis (dis″to-mi′ah-sis) infection by trematodes or flukes. **hemic d.,** schistosomiasis. **hepatic d.,** infection by *Opisthorchis, Dicrocoelium, Fasciola hepatica,* or *Fasciola gigantica.* **intestinal d.,** infection by *Fasciolopsis* or other intestinal flukes. **pulmonary d.,** parasitic hemoptysis.

distomolar (dis″to-mo′lar) a supernumerary molar; any tooth found distal to a third molar.

Distomum (dis′to-mum) distoma.

distomus (di-sto′mus) [*di-* + Gr. *stoma* mouth] a fetus having a double mouth.

disto-occlusal (dis″to-ŏ-kloo′zal) pertaining to or formed by the distal and occlusal surfaces of a tooth, or the distal and occlusal walls of a tooth cavity preparation; called also distoclusal.

disto-occlusion (dis″to-ŏ-kloo′zhun) distoclusion.

distoplacement (dis-to-plās′ment) displacement of a tooth distally.

distopulpal (dis″to-pul′pal) pertaining to or formed by the distal and pulpal walls of a tooth cavity preparation.

distopulpolabial (dis″to-pul″po-la′be-al) pertaining to or formed by the distal, pulpal, and labial walls of a tooth cavity preparation.

distopulpolingual (dis″to-pul″po-ling′gwal) pertaining to or formed by the distal, pulpal, and lingual walls of a tooth cavity preparation.

distortion (dis-tor′shun) [L. *dis-* apart + *torsio* a twisting] 1. the state of being twisted out of a natural or normal shape or position. 2. in psychology, the process of altering or disguising unconscious ideas or impulses so that they become acceptable to the conscious mind. 3. in optics or radiology, deviation of an image from the true outline or shape of an object or structure. **parataxic d.,** Harry Stack Sullivan's term for distortions in judgment and perception, particularly in interpersonal relations, based upon the need to perceive objects and relationships in accord with a pattern from earlier experience.

distortor (dis-tor′tor) [L.] that which distorts. **d. o′ris,** musculus zygomaticus minor; see *Table of Musculi.*

distoversion (dis″to-ver′zhun) the position of a tooth which is farther than normal from the median line of the face along the dental arch.

distractibility (dis-trak″tĭ-bil′ĭ-te) inability to focus one's attention on the task at hand; the attention is too frequently drawn to irrelevant and unimportant environmental stimuli.

distraction (dĭ-strak′shun) [L. *distrahere* to draw apart] 1. a state in which the attention is diverted from the main portion of an experience or is divided among various portions of it. 2. a form of dislocation in which the joint surfaces have been separated without rupture of their binding ligaments and without displacement. 3. excessive space between fracture fragments due to interposed tissue or too forceful traction. 4. surgical separation of the two parts of a bone after the bone is transected. 5. unusual width of the dental arch; placement of the teeth or other maxillary or mandibular structures farther than normal from the median plane. See also *contraction*, def. 3.

distress (dĭ-stres′) [L. *distringere* to draw apart] physical or mental anguish or suffering. **idiopathic respiratory d. of newborn,** see *respiratory distress syndrome of newborn,* under *syndrome.*

distribution (dis″trĭ-bu′shun) [L. *distributio*] 1. the specific location or arrangement of continuing or successive objects or events in space or time. 2. the extent of a ramifying structure such as an artery or nerve and its branches. 3. the geographical range of an organism or disease. 4. probability d. **Bernouilli d.,** a mathematical formula for calculating the theoretical distribution of male and female children to be born to any given set of parents. **chi-squared d.,** a theoretical probability distribution of the sum of the squares of a number (k) of normally distributed variables whose mean is 0 and standard deviation is 1; the parameter k is the number of degrees of freedom. Cf. *chi-squared test,* under *test.* **density d.,** probability density function. **dose d.,** in radiology, a representation of the variation of dose with position in any region of an irradiated object. **F-d.,** the exact sampling distribution of the sample variances from two independent normal distributions. **frequency d.,** probability density function. **gaussian d.,** normal d. **normal d.,** a symmetric, bell-shaped probability distribution having the density function

$$f(x) = \frac{1}{\sqrt{2\pi}\sigma} e^{-(x-\mu)^2/2\sigma^2}$$

where x is the abscissa, $f(x)$ is the ordinate, e is the base of natural logarithms (2.718) μ is the mean, and δ is the standard deviation. The normal distribution is entirely dependent on μ and δ; it is symmetric about the mean, with both tails extending to infinity; and the mean, the median and the mode are identical. Roughly speaking, the normal distribution characterizes a random variable that is the sum of a large number of independent random effects. More precisely, it is the limiting distribution of the sum of an infinite series of random variables with finite variance, each making a negligible contribution to the total variance (a fact known as the central limit theorem, q.v.). For this reason it is common statistical practice to assume that random sampling distributions of statistical measures are "approximately normal" and apply tests (*t*-tests, analysis of variance) based on the normal distribution. See illustration. Called also *gaussian d.* **Poisson d.,** the probability distribution that describes counts of events randomly distributed in time or space where now-events cannot be counted, such as radioactive decay or blood cell counts. The probability of counting exactly k events in a fixed time period or region is

$$f_\kappa = \frac{\lambda^\kappa e^\lambda}{\kappa!}$$

where λ is average density of events in a period or region of that size and e is the base of natural logarithms (2.718). The mean and variance of the distribution are both equal to λ, thus the coefficient of variation is $1/\sqrt{\lambda}$ (the variability of the count is inversely proportional to the square root of the average count). **probability d.,** a mathematical function that assigns to each measurable event in a sample space the probability that the event will occur; usually a distribution function or a probability density function. **standard normal d.,** the normal distribution with mean 0 and standard deviation 1. **t-d.,** the probability distribution of the statistic $t = (\overline{X}-\mu)/(s/\sqrt{n})$, where $\overline{X}$ is the mean of a sample with a normal distribution of size n and standard deviation s taken from a population of mean μ; used in the *t*-test (q.v.). It is symmetric about zero and approaches the normal distribution as the sample size increases.

districhiasis (dis″trĭ-ki′ah-sis) [Gr. *dis* double + Gr. *thrix* hair + *-iasis*] a condition in which two hairs grow from a single follicle.

distrix (dis′triks) [Gr. *dis* double + Gr. *thrix* hair] the splitting of hairs at their distal ends.

disturbance (dis-tur′bans) a departure or divergence from that which is considered normal. **emotional d.,** see under *illness.* **sexual orientation d.,** ego-dystonic homosexuality. **transient situational d.,** acute stress reaction.

disubstituted (di-sub′stĭ-tūt-ed) having two atoms in each molecule replaced by other atoms or radicals.

disulfate (di-sul′fāt) a compound containing two sulfate ions or radicals, as in titanium disulfate, $Ti(SO_4)_2$ (not to be confused with bisulfate).

disulfide (di-sul′fīd) a compound of a base with two atoms of sulfur; see also under *bond.*

disulfiram (di-sul′fi-ram) [USP] chemical name: tetraethylthioperoxydicarbonic diamide $[(H_2N)C(S)]_2S_2$. An antioxidant, $C_{10}H_{20}N_2S_4$, occurring as a white to off-white, crystalline powder, which inhibits the oxidation of the acetaldehyde metabolized from alcohol, resulting in high concentrations of acetaldehyde in the body. Extremely uncomfortable symptoms occur when alcohol is ingested subsequent to the oral administration of disulfiram (see *mal rouge*); used to produce an aversion to alcohol in the treatment of chronic alcoholism. Called also *tetraethylthiuram disulfide.*

dithiazanine iodide (di″thi-az′ah-nēn) chemical name: 3-ethyl-2-[5-(3-ethyl-2-(3H)-benzothiazolinylidene)-1,3-pentadienyl]benzothiazolium iodide. A dark green crystalline powder, $C_{23}H_{23}IN_2S_2$, used as an anthelminthic against strongylids and whipworms.

dithio (di-thi′o) the chemical group —S_2—.

dithiol (di-thi′ol) a chemical compound containing two sulfhydryl (thiol) radicals.

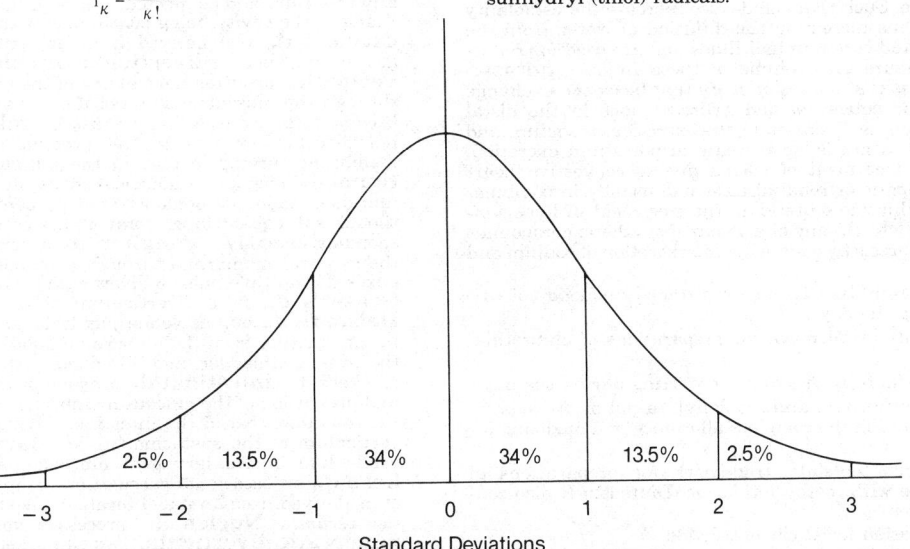

Normal distribution. The approximate percentage of the area (or frequency) lying under the curve between standard deviations is indicated.

dithranol (dith′rah-nōl) anthralin.

dithymol diiodide (di-thi″mol di-i′o-dīd) thymol iodide.

Ditropan (di′tro-pan) trademark for a preparation of oxybutynin hydrochloride.

Ditropenotus aureoviridis (di″tro-pĕ-no′tus aw″re-o-vir′ĭ-dis) former name for *Pyemotes ventricosus.*

Dittel's operation (dit′elz) [Leopold Ritter von *Dittel*, Vienna urologist, 1815–1898] see under *operation.*

Dittrich's plugs (dit′riks) [Franz *Dittrich*, German pathologist, 1815–1859] see under *plug.*

Ditylenchus (dit-ĕ-len′kus) a genus of small nematodes. **D. dip′saci,** the stem and bulb eelworm, a parasite of various grains, grasses, and bulbs, such as lilies, hyacinths, gladioli, narcissi, and onions; when ingested with the latter, it may be found as a pseudoparasite in the feces. Called also *Anguillulina putrifaciens.*

Diucardin (di″u-kar′din) trademark for preparations of hydroflumethiazide.

Diulo (di′u-lo) trademark for preparations of metolazone.

Diupres (di′u-pres) trademark for preparations of chlorothiazide and reserpine.

diurea (di-u-re′ah) a crystalline substance, $C_2H_4N_4O_2$, 1,2,4,5-tetrazine-3,6-dione, derivable from two molecules of urea, slightly soluble in ethanol or water. Called also *p-urazine* or *urazin.*

diureide (di-u′re-id) see *ureide.*

diurese (di″u-rēs′) the act of effecting diuresis.

diureses (di″u-re′sēz) plural of *diuresis.*

diuresis (di″u-re′sis), pl. *diure′ses* [Gr. *diourein* to urinate, to pass in urine] increased excretion of urine. **tubular d.,** diuresis resulting from the presence of nonabsorbable or poorly absorbable, osmotically active substances (mannitol, urea, glucose, etc.) in the renal tubules.

diuretic (di″u-ret′ik) [Gr. *diourētikos* promoting urine] 1. increasing the excretion of urine. 2. an agent that promotes the excretion of urine. **high-ceiling d's,** chemically unrelated compounds that increase the renal excretion of sodium, chloride, potassium, magnesium, and calcium and produce a high level of diuresis whose effect is not altered by acid-base imbalances or hypoalbuminemia; used in the treatment of edema associated with congestive heart failure or hepatic or renal disease and, alone or in combination with other drugs, in the treatment of hypertension. Called also *loop d's,* high-ceiling d's. **loop d.,** high-ceiling d's. **mercurial d's,** a group of organometallic compounds, now rarely used, that inhibit tubular reabsorption of sodium and chloride. **osmotic d.,** a substance, e.g., mannitol, that is filtered at the glomerulus and reabsorbed in the renal tubule only to a limited extent; it thus increases the amount of osmotically active solute in the urine and a corresponding increase in urine volume. Such compounds also increase the osmolality of plasma, thus increasing the diffusion of water from the intraocular and cerebrospinal fluids and are used for reducing the pressure and volume of these fluids. **potassium-sparing d's,** a class of drugs that block the exchange of sodium for potassium and hydrogen ions in the distal tubule, causing an increase in the excretion of sodium and chloride with a negligible increase in potassium excretion; used in the treatment of edema due to congestive heart failure or hepatic or renal disease and, usually in combination with a thiazide diuretic, in the treatment of hypertension. **thiazide d.,** any of a group of synthetic compounds that effect diuresis by enhancing the excretion of sodium and chloride.

diuria (di-u′re-ah) [L. *dies* day + *urine*] frequency of urination during the day.

Diuril (di′u-ril) trademark for preparations of chlorothiazide.

diurnal (di-er′nal) [L. *dies* day] occurring during the day.

diurnule (di-ern′ūl) [L. *diurnus* daily] a pill or other preparation containing the complete allowance of a medicine for one day.

Diutensin (di″u-ten′sin) trademark for preparations of cryptenamine with methyclothiazide (Diutensin-R also contains reserpine).

Div. abbreviation for L. *div′ide,* divide.

divagation (di″vah-ga′shun) rambling, incoherent speech and thought.

divalent (di-va-lent) [Gr. *dis* twice + *valent*] having a valence of two. Called also *bivalent.*

divarication (di-var″ĭ-ka′shun) separation; divergence; diastasis.

divergence (di-ver′jens) a spreading or tending apart; in ophthalmology, the simultaneous abduction of both eyes. **negative vertical d.** (−V.D.), the condition in which the visual line of the left eye deviates upward or the visual line of the right eye deviates downward. **positive vertical d.** (+V.D.), the condition in which the visual line of the right eye deviates upward, or the visual line of the left eye deviates downward.

divergent (di-ver′jent) [L. *divergens; dis-* apart + *vergere* to tend] tending apart; deviating or radiating away from a common point.

diversine (di-ver′sin) an amorphous sinomenine alkaloid, $C_{20}H_{27}O_5N$.

diversion (di-ver′zhun) a turning aside. **antigenic d.,** the change in the antigenic structure of tumor cells or tissue to that normally found in different cells or tissue.

diverticula (di″ver-tik′u-lah) [L.] plural of *diverticulum.*

diverticular (di″ver-tik′u-lar) pertaining to or resembling a diverticulum.

diverticularization (di″ver-tik″u-lar-i-za′shun) the act of forming diverticula, pockets, etc.

diverticulectomy (di″ver-tik″u-lek′to-me) [*diverticulum* + Gr. *ektomē* excision] excision of a diverticulum.

diverticulitis (di″ver-tik-u-li′tis) inflammation of a diverticulum, especially inflammation related to colonic diverticula, which may undergo perforation with abscess formation. Sometimes called *left-sided* or *L-sided appendicitis.*

diverticulogram (di″ver-tik′u-lo-gram) [*diverticulum* + Gr. *gramma* mark] a roentgenogram of a diverticulum.

diverticulopexy (di″ver-tik″u-lo-pek′se) surgical fixation of a diverticulum in a new position following its separation from the initial adjacent or adherent structures.

diverticulosis (di″ver-tik″u-lo′sis) the presence of diverticula, particularly of colonic diverticula, in the absence of inflammation. Cf. *diverticulitis.*

diverticulum (di″ver-tik′u-lum), pl. *divertic′ula* [L. *divertere* to turn aside] a circumscribed pouch or sac of variable size occurring normally or created by herniation of the lining mucous membrane through a defect in the muscular coat of a tubular organ. **acquired d.,** any diverticulum produced secondarily, mechanically, or by disease. **allantoic d.,** the entodermal sacculation that becomes the allantois; called also *allantoic vesicle.* **divertic′ula ampul′lae duc′tus deferen′tis** [NA], sacculations in the wall of the ampulla of the ductus deferens. **caliceal d., calyceal d.,** an epithelial-lined cavity in the kidney, situated peripherally to a calix and connected to it by a narrow isthmus, the lining of the cavity being continuous with that of the calix. **cervical d.,** one derived from an embryonic branchial groove or pouch. **diverticula of colon, colonic diverticula,** acquired herniations of the mucosa of the colon through the muscular layers of the bowel wall, which may become inflamed (see *diverticulitis*). **false d.,** an intestinal diverticulum due to the protrusion of the mucous membrane through a tear in the muscular coat. **functional d.,** a benign radiological entity, in which a diverticulum-like shadow is demonstrated by contrast medium, although subsequent laparotomy shows no sign of any corresponding anomaly. **ganglion d.,** a hernial protrusion of the synovial membrane through a tendon sheath. **Ganser's d.,** multiple pulsion diverticula of the sigmoid flexure. **Graser's d.,** false diverticulum of the sigmoid flexure. **Heister's d.,** bulbus venae jugularis superior. **hepatic d.,** one arising from the embryonic duodenum and forming the liver, gallbladder, and bile ducts. **d. il′ei ve′rum,** Meckel's d. **intestinal d.,** a pouch or sac formed by hernial protrusion of the mucous membrane through a defect in the muscular coat of the intestine. **Kirchner's d.,** a diverticulum of the eustachian tube. **laryngeal d.,** a diverticulum of the laryngeal mucous membrane. **Meckel's d.,** an occasional sacculation or appendage of the ileum, derived from an unobliterated yolk stalk; called also *d. ilei verum.* **Nuck's d.,** processus vaginalis peritonei. **pancreatic diverticula,** two outpocketings from the embryonic duodenum, later forming the pancreas and its ducts. **Pertik's d.,** an unusually deep recessus pharyngeus.

pharyngoesophageal d., a diverticulum at the junction of the pharynx and esophagus; called also *Zenker's d.* **pituitary d.,** Rathke's pouch. **pressure d., pulsion d.,** a sac or pouch formed by hernial protrusion of the mucous membrane through the muscular coat (as of the colon or esophagus) as a result of pressure from within. **Rokitansky's d.,** a traction diverticulum of the esophagus. **supradiaphragmatic d.,** a diverticulum of the esophagus situated just above the diaphragm. **synovial d.,** a hernial protrusion of the synovial membrane of a joint or a tendon sheath. **thyroid d.,** an outpouching of the ventral floor of the embryonic pharynx that becomes the thyroid gland. **diverticula of trachea, tracheal diverticula,** pouches projecting from the trachea. **traction d.,** a localized distortion, angulation, or funnel-shaped bulging of the full thickness of the wall of the esophagus, caused by adhesions resulting from some external lesion. **vesical d.,** diverticulum of the bladder. **Zenker's d.,** pharyngoesophageal d.

divi-divi (div″e-div′e) the leguminous pods of *Caesalpinia coriaria* (Jacq.) Willd., plants of South America; the seeds contain tannin and gallic acid and have been used as an astringent and in tanning.

divinyl (di-vi′nil) a gaseous hydrocarbon, vinyl ethylene, CH_2:CH·CH:CH_2. **d. oxide,** vinyl ether.

divisio (di-viz′e-o), pl. *divisiónes* [L.] 1. the act or process of separating or sectioning into two or more parts. 2. a section or part of a larger structure. **divisio′nes anteri-o′res trunco′rum plex′us brachia′les,** NA alternative for *divisiones ventrales trunco′rum plexus brachialis.* **divisio′nes dorsa′les trunco′rum plex′us brachia′lis** [NA], the dorsal, or posterior, divisions into which each of the three trunks (superior, medial, and inferior) of the brachial plexus splits; all three dorsal divisions unite to form the posterior fasciculus of the plexus. Called also *divisiones posteriores truncorum plexus brachialis* [NA alternative]. **divisio′nes posterio′res trunco′rum plex′us brachia′lis,** NA alternative for *divisiones dorsales truncorum plexus brachialis.* **divisio′nes ventra′les trunco′rum plex′us brachia′lis** [NA], the ventral, or anterior, divisions into which each of the three (superior, medial, inferior) nerve trunks of the brachial plexus splits; the ventral divisions of the superior and medial trunks unite to form the lateral fasciculus and that of the inferior trunk forms the medial fasciculus of the plexus. Called also *divisiones anteriores truncorum plexus brachialis* [NA alternative].

division (dĭ-vizh′un) [L. *divisio*] 1. the act or process of separation or sectioning into two or more parts. 2. a section or part of a larger structure. **cell d.,** the fission of a cell. **cell d., direct,** see *amitosis.* **cell d., indirect,** see *meiosis* and *mitosis.* **craniosacral d.,** see *pars parasympathica systematis nervosi autonomici.* **equational d.,** the second meiotic division, essentially mitotic in type, characterized by the separation of sister chromatids. The latter are genetically identical except where recombination with the homologous chromosome has occurred in the first meiotic division. **maturation d.,** meiosis. **reduction d.,** the first meiotic division, so called because at this stage the chromosome number per cell is reduced from diploid to haploid. **thoracicolumbar d., thoracolumbar d.,** see *pars sympathica systematis nervosi autonomici.* **d's of trunks of brachial plexus,** see *divisiones dorsales truncorum plexus brachialis* and *divisiones ventrales truncorum plexus brachialis.*

divisiones (dĭ-viz″e-o′nēz) [L.] plural of *divisio.*

divulse (dĭ-vuls′) to pull apart forcibly.

divulsion (dĭ-vul′shun) [L. *dis-* apart + *vellere* to pluck] the act of forcibly separating or pulling apart.

divulsor (dĭ-vul′sor) an instrument for dilating the urethra.

Dixon Mann see *Mann.*

dizygotic (di″zi-got′ik) pertaining to or derived from two separate zygotes, as dizygotic (fraternal) twins.

dizygous (di-zi′gus) dizygotic.

dizziness (diz′ĭ-nes) a disturbed sense of relationship to space; a sensation of unsteadiness with a feeling of movement within the head; giddiness; lightheadedness; dysequilibrium. Cf. *vertigo.*

djenkolic acid (jen-kol′ik) an amino acid, S,S′-meth-

ylenebiscysteine, $CH_2SCH_2CH(NH_2)COOH_2$, found in the djenkol bean.

DL a regimen of doxorubicin and lomustine, used in cancer chemotherapy.

DL- (de-el) chemical prefix (small capital D and L) used with the D and L convention to indicate a racemic mixture of enantiomers.

dl- (de-el) chemical prefix used with the *d* and *l* convention to indicate a racemic mixture of enantiomers; the prefix (±)- is used with the same meaning.

DLE discoid lupus erythematosus.

DM diabetes mellitus.

D.M. see *diphenylamine-arsine chloride.*

DMBA 7,12-dimethylbenz[a]anthracene.

D.M.D. Doctor of Dental Medicine.

DMF see under *rate.*

DMPE 3,4-dimethoxyphenylethylamine.

D.M.R.D. Diploma in Medical Radio-Diagnosis (British).

D.M.R.T. Diploma in Medical Radio-Therapy (British).

DMSO dimethyl sulfoxide.

DMT dimethyltryptamine.

DN dibucaine number.

Dn. dekanem.

dn. decinem.

DNA deoxyribonucleic acid. **DNA library,** see *library.* **recombinant DNA,** DNA artificially constructed by insertion of foreign DNA into the DNA of an appropriate organism (usually a bacterial plasmid or bacteriophage) so that the foreign DNA is replicated along with the host DNA.

DNA-directed DNA polymerase [EC 2.7.7.7] an enzyme of the transferase class that catalyzes the reaction n deoxynucleoside triphosphate = n pyrophosphate + DNA_n. A DNA chain acts as a template. The reaction is important in the replication and repair of deoxyribonucleic acids. Called also *DNA nucleotidyltransferase* and *DNA polymerase.*

DNA-directed RNA polymerase [EC 2.7.7.6] an enzyme of the transferase class that catalyzes the reaction n nucleoside triphosphate = n pyrophosphate + RNA_n. A DNA chain acts as a template. The reaction forms ribonucleic acids by step-wise linkages of individual nucleoside triphosphates. Called also *RNA polymerase.*

DNA ligase polydeoxyribonucleotide synthase (ATP).

DNA nucleotidylexotransferase (nu″kle-o-tīd′il-ek″so-trans′fer-ās) [EC 2.7.7.31] an enzyme of the transferase class that catalyzes the reaction n-deoxynucleoside triphosphate + (deoxynucleotide)$_m$=n pyrophosphate + (deoxynucleotide)$_{m+n}$. The enzyme is a polymerase that forms larger nucleotides by the addition of single terminal nucleotide residues. Determination of the enzyme is used clinically in the diagnosis of leukemias.

DNA nucleotidyltransferase (nu″kle-o-tīd′il-trans′fer-ās) DNA-directed DNA polymerase.

DNA polymerase (pol-im′er-ās) see DNA-directed DNA polymerase and RNA directed DNA polymerase.

DNase deoxyribonuclease.

D.N.B. dinitrobenzene; Diplomate of the National Board (of Medical Examiners).

DNCB dinitrochlorobenzene.

DNFB dinitrofluorobenzene.

DNR do not resuscitate.

D.O. Doctor of Osteopathy.

D_2O the symbol for heavy water.

D.O.A. dead on arrival.

Dobie's globule, layer (line) (do′bēz) [William Murray Dobie, English physician, 1828–1915] see under *globule,* and see *Z band,* under *band.*

dobutamine (do-bu′tah-mēn) chemical name: (+)-[2- [[3-(4-hydroxyphenyl)-1-methylpropyl]amino]ethyl]-1,2-benzenediol. A synthetic catecholamine, $C_{18}H_{23}NO_3$, used as an adrenergic with cardiotonic actions. **d. hydrochloride,** the hydrochloride salt of dobutamine, $C_{18}H_{23} NO_3$·HCl, having the same actions as the base.

DOC 11-deoxycorticosterone.

Doca (do′kah) trademark for desoxycorticosterone acetate.

Dochmius duodenalis (dok'me-us du"o-dě-na'lis) former name for *Ancylostoma duodenale.*

Docibin (do'si-bin) trademark for a crystalline preparation of vitamin B_{12}; see *cyanocobalamin.*

docimasia (do"se-ma'ze-ah) [Gr. *dokimazein* to examine] an assay or examination; an official test. **auricular d.,** Wreden's sign. **hepatic d.,** the search for glycogen or glucose in the liver. **pulmonary d.,** determination as to whether air has entered the lungs of a dead infant, as an indication whether it was born dead or alive.

docimastic (do"se-mas'tik) pertaining to docimasia; of the nature of an assay or test.

dock (dok) to remove part or all of the tail of an animal.

doconazole (do-ko'nah-zōl) chemical name: cis-1-[[4-[([1,1'-biphenyl]-4-yloxy)methyl]-2-(2,4-dichlorophenyl)-1,3-dioxolan-2-yl]methyl]1H-imidazole; an antifungal, $C_{26}H_{22}Cl_2N_2O_3$.

doctor (dok'tor) [L. "teacher"] 1. a practitioner of the healing arts, one who has received a degree from a college of medicine, osteopathy, chiropractic, optometry, podiatry, pharmacy, dentistry, or veterinary medicine, licensed to practice by a state. 2. a holder of a diploma of the highest degree from a university, qualified as a specialist in a particular field of learning.

doctrine (dok'trin) a theory supported by authorities and having general acceptance. **Arrhenius' d.,** see under *theory.* **Monro-Kellie d.,** the quantity of blood within the cranium must be approximately constant at all times, in health or disease; the doctrine refers to quantity of blood, not to blood flow. **neuron d.,** the doctrine that the nervous system is entirely cellular, that its cells are distinctive as to morphological type and functional characteristics, and that its cells are not in protoplasmic continuity but are juxtaposed without a significant amount of intervening extracellular substance.

docusate calcium (dok'u-sāt) [USP] chemical name: sulfobutanedioic acid 1,4-bis(2-ethylhexyl) ester calcium salt. An ionic surfactant, $C_{40}H_{74}CaO_{14}S_2$, occurring as a white, amorphous powder; used as a fecal softener, administered orally. Called also *dioctyl calcium sulfosuccinate.*

docusate sodium (dok'u-sāt) [USP] chemical name: sulfobutanedioic acid 1,4-bis(2-ethylhexyl)ester sodium salt. An anionic surfactant, $C_{20}H_{37}NaO_7S$, with wetting, detergent, emulsifying, and dispersing properties, occurring as a white, waxlike plastic solid; used as a fecal softener, administered orally or rectally, and for its solubilizing action as a tablet disintegrant. It has also been used for its dispersing and emulsifying properties in dermatological preparations. Called also *dioctyl sodium sulfosuccinate.*

dodecadactylitis (do"dek-ah-dak"tǐ-li'tis) [*dōdecadactylon* + *-itis*] duodenitis.

dodecadactylon (do"dek-ah-dak'tǐ-lon) [Gr. *dōdeka* twelve + *daktylos* finger, from its length] the duodenum.

Döderlein's bacillus (ded'er-līnz) [Albert Siegmund Gustav *Döderlein,* German obstetrician and gynecologist, 1860–1941] see under *bacillus.*

Dogiel's corpuscles (do-zhe-elz') [Jean von *Dogiel,* Russian physiologist, 1830–1916] see under *corpuscle.*

dögling (deg'ling) [Danish and German] the northern bottle-nosed whale (*Hyperoodon ampullatus*).

dogma (dog'mah) a belief or an opinion, or a system of beliefs or opinions, formally stated, defined, and held to be true.

Dogmatist (dog'mah-tist) a school of medicine formed by Diocles of Carystus. The school put Aristotelian language, system, and speculation into Hippocratic medicine to discover the hidden causes of the constitution of man and of disease: such knowledge, they thought, was necessary for the practice of medicine. See also *Empiric* and *Praxagoras.*

Döhle's disease, inclusion bodies (de'lēz) [Paul *Döhle,* German pathologist, 1855–1928] see *syphilitic aortitis,* under *aortitis,* and see under *body.*

Döhle-Heller aortitis (de'lě-hel'er) [K.G.P. *Döhle;* Arnold Ludwig Gotthilf *Heller,* Kiel pathologist, 1840–1913] syphilitic aortitis.

doigt (dwa) [Fr.] finger or toe. **d. mort** [Fr.], dead finger.

Doisy (doi'se), Edward Adelbert. An American biochemist, born 1893; co-winner, with Carl Peter Henrik Dam, of the Nobel prize for medicine and physiology in 1943, for the isolation and synthesis of vitamin K.

dol (dōl) [L. *do'lor* pain] a unit of pain intensity.

dolabrate (do-lab'rāt) [L. *dolabra* ax] ax-shaped.

dolabriform (do-lab'rǐ-form) dolabrate.

Doléris' operation (dol-a-rēz') [Jacques Amédée *Doléris,* French gynecologist, 1852–1938] see under *operation.*

dolich(o)- [Gr. *dolichos* long] a combining form meaning long.

dolichocephalia (dol"ǐ-ko-sě-fa'le-ah) dolichocephaly.

dolichocephalic, dolichocephalous (dol"ǐ-ko-se-fal'ik; dol"ǐ-ko-sef'ah-lus) [*dolicho-* + Gr. *kephalē* head] long headed; having a cephalic index of 75.9 or less. Called also *mecocephalic.*

dolichocephalism (dol"ǐ-ko-sef'ah-lizm) dolichocephaly.

dolichocephaly (dol"ǐ-ko-sef'ah-le) the quality of being dolichocephalic.

dolichocolon (dol"ǐ-ko-ko'lon) [*dolicho-* + *colon*] an abnormally long colon.

dolichocranial (dol"ǐ-ko-kra'ne-al) having a cranial index of 74.9 or less.

dolichoderus (dol"ǐ-ko-dēr'us) [*dolicho-* + Gr. *dere* neck] an individual with a long neck.

dolichofacial (dol"ǐ-ko-fa'shal) having a long face.

dolichohieric (dol"ǐ-ko-hi-er'ik) having a sacral index below 100.

dolichokerkic (dol"ǐ-ko-ker'kik) having a radiohumeral index above 80.

dolichoknemic (dol"ǐ-ko-ne'mik) having a tibiofemoral index of 83 or above.

dolichomorphic (dol"ǐ-ko-mor'fik) [*dolicho-* + Gr. *morphē* form] built along lines that tend toward the slender or longer type.

dolichopellic, dolichopelvic (dol"ǐ-ko-pel'ik; dol"ǐ-ko-pel'vik) [*dolicho-* + Gr. *pella* bowl] having a pelvic index of 95 or above.

dolichoprosopic (dol"ǐ-ko-pro-sop'ik) dolichofacial.

dolichosigmoid (dol"ǐ-ko-sig'moid) [*dolicho-* + *sigmoid*] (*obs.*) an abnormally long sigmoid flexure.

dolichostenomelia (dol"ǐ-ko-ste"no-me'le-ah) [*dolicho-* + Gr. *stenos* narrow + *melos* limb] arachnodactyly.

Döllinger's tendinous ring (del'ing-erz) [Johann Ignaz Josef *Döllinger,* German physiologist, 1770–1841] see under *ring.*

Dolobid (do'lo-bid) trademark for a preparation of diflunisal.

Dolophine (do'lo-fēn) trademark for preparations of methadone hydrochloride.

dolor (do'lor), pl. *dolo'res* [L.] pain; one of the cardinal signs of inflammation. **d. cap'itis,** headache. **d. cox'ae,** coxalgia, def. 2. **dolo'res praesagien'tes,** false pains late in pregnancy, similar to those experienced during menstruation, indicating that labor is imminent. **d. va'gus,** wandering pain.

dolores (do-lo'rēz) [L.] plural of *dolor.*

dolorific (do"lor-if'ik) producing or causing pain.

dolorimeter (do"lor-im'ě-ter) an instrument for measuring pain in dols.

dolorimetry (do"lor-im'ě-tre) [L. *dolor* pain + Gr. *metrein* to measure] the measurement of pain.

dolorogenic (do-lor"o-jen'ik) dolorific.

DOM 2,5-dimethoxy-4-methylamphetamine.

Domagk (do'mahk), Gerhard Johannes Paul. German physician and biochemist, 1895–1964; winner of the Nobel prize for medicine or physiology in 1939 for his discovery of the effectiveness of Prontosil, the predecessor of sulfa drugs, in treating streptococcal infections.

domain (do-mān') a compact globular structure composed of one section of a polypeptide chain that constitutes a recognizable unit of the tertiary structure of a protein. Domains may fold up independently and maintain their native conformation when the connecting sections of the chain are broken. **immunoglobulin d's.,** see *homology regions* under *region.*

domazoline fumarate (do"mah-zo'lēn) chemical name: 2-[(3,6-dimethoxy-2,4-dimethylphenyl)methyl]-4,5-dihydro-1*H*-imidazole (*E*)-2-butenedioate (1:1); an anticholinergic, $C_{14}H_{20}N_2O_2 \cdot C_4H_4O_4$.

Domeboro (dōm′bor-o) trademark for preparations of aluminum subacetate.

domiciliary (dom″ĭ-sil′e-ār″e) [L. *domus* house] pertaining to or carried on in the house or place of permanent residence, as domiciliary treatment.

dominance (dom′ĭ-nans) [L. *dominari* to govern] in genetics, the full phenotypic expression of a gene in both heterozygotes and homozygotes; see also *Mendel's law*, under *law*. See also *codominant gene*, under *gene*, and also *quasidominance*. **cerebral d.**, the dominance of one cerebral hemisphere over the other, in cerebral functions, demonstrated by laterality in voluntary motor acts. **incomplete d.**, failure of one gene to be competely dominant, the heterozygotes showing a phenotype intermediate between the two parents; called also *partial d.* and *semidominance*. **lateral d.**, the preferential use, in voluntary motor acts, of ipsilateral members of the major paired organs of the body (arm, ear, eye, and leg). **ocular d.**, the preferential use of one eye over the other in vision. **one-sided d.**, lateral d.

dominant (dom′ĭ-nant) 1. exerting a ruling or controlling influence; in genetics, capable of expression when carried by only one of a pair of homologous chromosomes. 2. a dominant allele or trait.

domiphen bromide (do′mĭ-fen) chemical name: *N,N*-dimethyl-*N*-(2-phenoxyethyl)-1-dodecanaminium bromide. A quaternary ammonium compound, $C_{22}H_{40}BrNO$, occurring as colorless to faintly yellow, crystalline flakes, effective against a wide range of gram-negative and gram-positive bacteria and against certain fungi; used as a topical anti-infective and to disinfect instruments and utensils.

domperidone (dom-per′ĭ-dōn) chemical name: 5-chloro-1-[1-[3-(2,3-dihydro-2-oxo-1*H*-benzimidazol-1-yl)propyl]-4-piperidinyl]-1,3-dihydro-2*H*-benzimidazol-2-one; an antiemetic, $C_{22}H_{24}ClN_5O_2$.

Donath-Landsteiner test (do′nath-land′sti-ner) [Julius *Donath,* German immunologist, 1870–1950; Karl *Landsteiner,* Austrian physician in New York, 1868–1943] see under *test.*

donaxine (do-nak′sēn) gramine.

Donders' glaucoma, law (don′derz) [Franciscus Cornelius *Donders,* Dutch physician and ophthalmologist, 1818–1889] see *glaucoma simplex,* and see under *law.*

Donec alv. sol. fuerit abbreviation for L. *do′nec al′vus solu′ta fu′erit,* until the bowels are opened (i.e., until a bowel movement occurs).

donee (do-ne′) recipient; host (def. 2).

Don Juan (don hwan) [after *Don Juan,* legendary Spanish nobleman and libertine] a man who is sexually promiscuous.

Don Juanism (don-hwan′izm) hypersexuality in a man.

Donnan's equilibrium (don′anz) [Frederick George *Donnan,* English chemist, 1870–1956] see under *equilibrium.*

donor (do′nor) 1. an individual organism that supplies living tissue to be used in another body, as a person who furnishes blood for transfusion, or an organ for transplantation in a histocompatible recipient. 2. in chemistry, a substance or compound which contributes part of itself, as an atom or radical, to another substance (acceptor). **F d.**, in bacterial genetics, a cell that donates the F plasmid by means of bacterial conjugation. **general d.**, universal d. **hydrogen d.**, a substance or compound that gives up hydrogen to another substance (the hydrogen acceptor). **universal d.**, a person with group O blood (International Classification); such blood (blood cells preferred, rather than whole blood) is sometimes used in emergency transfusion.

Donovan bodies (don′o-van) [Charles *Donovan,* Irish physician, formerly in Sanitary Service in India, 1863–1951] 1. *Calymmatobacterium granulomatis.* 2. Leishman-Donovan bodies.

Donovania granulomatis (don″o-va′ne-ah gran″u-lo′mah-tis) [Charles *Donovan*] *Calymmatobacterium granulomatis.*

donovanosis (don″o-vah-no′sis) granuloma inguinale.

dopa (do′pah) an amino acid, 3,4-dihydroxyphenylalanine, produced by oxidation of tyrosine by tyrosinase; it is the precursor of dopamine and an intermediate product in the biosynthesis of norepinephrine, epinephrine, and melanin.

L-dopa (*levodopa* [USP]), the naturally occurring form, is used in the treatment of parkinsonism.

dopamantine (do″pah-man′tēn) chemical name: *N*-[2-(3,4-dihydroxyphenyl)ethyl]tricyclo[3,3,1,1^{3,7}]decane-1-carboxamide; an antiparkinsonian agent, $C_{19}H_{25}NO_3$.

dopamine (do′pah-mēn) chemical name: 4-(2-aminoethyl)-1,2-benzenediol. A monoamine, $C_8H_{11}NO_2$, formed in the body by the decarboxylation of dopa; it is an intermediate product in the synthesis of norepinephrine, and acts as a neurotransmitter in the central nervous system. **d. hydrochloride,** the hydrochloride salt of dopamine, $C_8H_{11}NO_2 \cdot HCl$, used to correct hemodynamic balance in the treatment of shock syndrome; administered intravenously.

dopamine β-hydroxylase (do″pah-mēn hi-drok′sĭ-lās) dopamine β-monooxygenase.

dopamine β-monooxygenase (do″pah-mēn mon-o-oks″ĭ-jen-ās) [EC 1.14.17.1] an enzyme of the oxidoreductase class that catalyzes the reaction 3,4-dihydroxyphenylethylamine + ascorbate + O_2 = norepinephrine + dehydroascorbate + H_2O. It is a copper-protein occurring in nervous tissue and the adrenal medulla. Called also *dopamine β-hydroxylase.*

dopaminergic (do″pah-mēn-er′jik) activated or transmitted by dopamine; pertaining to tissues or organs affected by dopamine.

dopa-oxidase (do″pah-ok′sĭ-dās) monophenol monooxygenase.

Dopar (do′par) trademark for a preparation of levodopa.

dopase (do′pās) monophenol monooxygenase.

Doppler effect (phenomenon, principle) (dop′ler) [Christian Johann *Doppler,* Austrian physicist and mathematician, 1803–1853] see under *effect.*

Dopram (do′pram) trademark for a preparation of doxapram hydrochloride.

dorastine hydrochloride (dor′as-tēn) chemical name: 8-chloro-2,3,4,5-tetrahydro-2-methyl-5-[2-(6-methyl-3-pyridyl)ethyl]-1*H*-pyrido[4,3-*b*]indole dihydrochloride; an antihistaminic, $C_{20}H_{22}ClN_3 \cdot 2HCl$.

Dorbane (dor′bān) trademark for a preparation of danthron.

Dorendorf's sign (dor′en-dorfs) [Hans *Dorendorf,* German physician, born 1866] see under *sign.*

Doriden (dor′ĭ-den) trademark for preparations of glutethimide.

dormancy (dor′man-se) [L. *dormire* to sleep] 1. the state of being dormant. 2. in bacteriology, the property exhibited by some bacteria, and especially by bacterial spores, of remaining viable for an extended time with minimal physical or chemical change, often in response to unfavorable growth conditions.

dormant (dor′mant) [L. *dormire* to sleep] sleeping, inactive, quiescent.

dormifacient (dor″mĭ-fa′shent) [L. *dormire* to sleep + *facere* to make] producing sleep; counteracting the conditions which tend to prevent sleep.

Dornavac (dor′nah-vak) trademark for a preparation of pancreatic dornase.

Dorno's rays (dor′no) [Carl Wilhelm *Dorno,* Swiss climatologist, 1865–1942] see under *ray.*

Dorn-Sugarman test [John H. *Dorn,* American obstetrician; Edward J. *Sugarman,* American chemist] see under *tests.*

dorsa (dor′sah) [L.] plural of *dorsum.*

Dorsacaine (dor′sah-kān) trademark for a preparation of benoxinate hydrochloride.

dorsad (dor′sad) toward the back or dorsal aspect.

dorsal (dor′sal) [L. *dorsalis;* from *dorsum* back] 1. pertaining to the back or to any dorsum. 2. denoting a position more toward the back surface than some other object of reference; same as posterior in human anatomy; superior in the anatomy of quadrupeds.

dorsalgia (dor-sal′je-ah) [*dorsum* + *-algia*] pain in the back.

dorsalis (dor-sa′lis) [L.] dorsal; [NA] a term denoting a position closer to the back surface. Cf. *posterior.*

dorsi- see *dors(o)-.*

dorsiduct (dor′sĭ-dukt) [*dorsi* + L. *ducere* to draw] to draw toward the back or dorsum.

dorsiflexion (dor″sĭ-flek′shun) [*dorsi-* + *flexion*] flexion or bending toward the extensor aspect of a limb, as of the hand or foot.

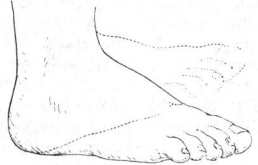

Dorsiflexion of foot.

dorsimesal (dor″sĭ-mes′al) dorsomesial.

dorsispinal (dor″sĭ-spi′nal) pertaining to the back and vertebral column.

dors(o)-, dorsi- [L. *dorsum* back] combining form denoting relationship to a dorsum or to the back (posterior) aspect of the body.

dorsoanterior (dor″so-an-te′re-or) having the back of the fetus toward the front of the mother.

dorsocephalad (dor″so-sef′ah-lad) [*dorso-* + Gr. *kephalē* head] directed toward the back of the head.

dorsodynia (dor″so-din′e-ah) dorsalgia.

dorsointercostal (dor″so-in″ter-kos′tal) situated in the back and between the ribs.

dorsolateral (dor″so-lat′er-al) pertaining to the back and the side.

dorsolumbar (dor″so-lum′bar) pertaining to the back and the loins.

dorsomedian (dor″so-me′de-an) the median line of the back.

dorsomesial (dor″so-me′se-al) pertaining to the median line of the back.

dorsonasal (dor″so-na′sal) pertaining to the bridge of the nose.

dorsonuchal (dor″so-nu′kal) pertaining to the back of the neck.

dorsoposterior (dor″so-pos-te′re-or) having the back of the fetus directed toward the mother's back.

dorsoradial (dor″so-ra′de-al) pertaining to the radial or outer side of the back of the forearm or hand.

dorsoscapular (dor″so-skap′u-lar) pertaining to the posterior surface of the scapula.

dorsoventrad (dor″so-ven′trad) [*dorso-* + *venter* belly] directed from the dorsal toward the ventral aspect.

dorsoventral (dor″so-ven′tral) 1. pertaining to the back and belly surfaces of the body. 2. passing from the back to the belly surface.

dorsum (dor′sum), pl. *dor′sa* [L.] [NA] 1. the back. 2. the aspect of an anatomical part or structure corresponding in position to the back; posterior, in the human. **d. of foot,** d. pedis. **d. of hand,** d. manus. **d. lin′guae** [NA], the superior surface of the tongue. **d. ma′nus** [NA], the back of the hand; the surface opposite the palm. **d. na′si** [NA], **d. of nose,** that part of the external surface of the nose formed by junction of the lateral surfaces. **d. pe′dis** [NA], the upper surface of the foot; the surface opposite the sole. Called also *regio dorsalis pedis* [NA alternative]. **d. pe′nis** [NA], **d. of penis,** the anterior, more extensive surface of the dependent penis, opposite the urethral surface. **d. of scapula,** facies posterior scapulae. **d. sca′pulae,** NA alternative for *facies posterior scapulae.* **d. sel′lae** [NA], the quadrilateral plate on the sphenoid bone that forms the posterior boundary of the sella turcica; the posterior clinoid processes project from its superior extremity, and it is continuous inferiorly with the clivus. **d. of testis,** margo posterior testis. **d. of tongue,** d. linguae.

dosage (do′sij) the determination and regulation of the size, frequency, and number of doses.

dose (dōs) [Gr. *dosis* a giving] 1. a quantity to be administered at one time, such as a specified amount of medication. 2. in radiology, the amount of energy absorbed per unit mass of tissue at a given site. **absorbed d.,** the amount of energy from ionizing radiations absorbed per unit mass of

matter, expressed in rads. **air d.,** air exposure. **average d.,** the quantity of an agent which will usually produce the therapeutic effect for which it is administered. **booster d.,** a dose of an active immunizing agent, usually smaller than the initial dose, given to maintain immunity. **cumulative d., cumulative radiation d.,** the total dose resulting from repeated exposures to radiation. **curative d.,** a dose that is sufficient to restore normal health. **curative d., median,** a dose that abolishes symptoms in 50 per cent of the test subjects. Abbreviated C.D.$_{50}$. **daily d.,** the total amount of a drug administered in a 24-hour period. **depth d.,** the intensity of radiation at a given depth in an irradiated body, expressed as a percentage of that at the surface of the body nearest the portal of entry. **divided d.,** a fraction of the total quantity of the drug prescribed, to be given at intervals, usually during a twenty-four hour period. **doubling d.,** in radiation biology, the dose of ionizing radiation which will result in a doubling of the current rate of spontaneous biological changes, such as mutations or cancers of various kinds, in a population. **effective d.,** that quantity of a drug which will produce the effects for which it is administered; abbreviated E.D. **effective d., median,** a dose that produces the desired effect in 50 per cent of a population. Abbreviation ED$_{50}$. **epilating d.,** the amount of radiation necessary to cause temporary or permanent loss of hair. **erythema d.,** the amount of radiation which, when applied to the skin, causes temporary reddening of the skin. **exit d.,** the intensity of radiation emerging from the body at the surface opposite the portal of entry. **exposure d.,** see *exposure,* def. 3. **fatal d.,** lethal d. **fractional d's,** amounts of an agent less than that usually administered, given at shorter intervals than usual. **infective d.,** that amount of pathogenic microorganisms that will cause infection in susceptible subjects. Abbreviated I.D. **infective d., median,** the amount of pathogenic microorganisms that will produce demonstrable infection in 50 per cent of the test subjects. Abbreviated I.D.$_{50}$. **integral absorbed d.,** in radiation biology, the total energy absorbed by an individual or other biological object during exposure to radiation, expressed in gram-rads (100 ergs). **L + d., L$_{+}$d.,** the limes tod (death) d., the smallest amount of diphtheria toxin that will kill a 250-gm. guinea pig within four days when mixed with one unit of diphtheria antitoxin before being injected subcutaneously. **L0 d., L$_0$d., limes nul d., limes zero d.,** the largest amount of diphtheria toxin that when mixed with one standard unit of antitoxin produces no perceptible reaction when injected subcutaneously into a guinea pig. **lethal d.,** the amount of an agent, such as radiation, which will or may be sufficient to cause death. Called also *fatal d.* **lethal d., median,** the amount of pathogenic bacteria, bacterial toxin, or other poisonous substance, required to kill 50 per cent of uniformly susceptible animals inoculated with it. In radiology, the amount of ionizing radiation that will kill, within a specified period, 50 per cent of individuals in a large group or population. Abbreviated L.D.$_{50}$. **lethal d., minimum (M.L.D.),** 1. the smallest amount of a toxic substance that can cause the death of a laboratory animal. 2. the smallest quantity of diphtheria toxin that will kill a guinea pig of 250-gm. weight in four to five days when injected subcutaneously. **Lf d.,** the limes flocculating d., the amount of diphtheria toxin that in the shortest time produces precipitation when mixed with one standard unit of antitoxin. **Lr d.,** the limes reacting d., the amount of diphtheria toxin that, when mixed with one standard unit of antitoxin, will produce a minimal skin reaction in a guinea pig. **maintenance d.,** a dose (often a daily dose or dosage regimen) sufficient to maintain at the desired level the influence of a drug achieved by earlier administration of larger amounts. **maximum d.,** the largest quantity of an agent that may be safely administered to the average patient. **maximum permissible d.,** the largest amount of ionizing radiation that a person may receive according to recommended limits in current radiation protection guides; abbreviated M.P.D. **median tissue culture infective d.,** that quantity of a cytopathogenic agent (virus) that will produce a cytopathic effect in 50 per cent of the cultures inoculated. Abbreviated TCID$_{50}$. **minimal d., minimum d.,** the smallest quantity of an agent that is likely to produce an appreciable effect. **optimal d., optimum d.,** the quantity of an agent which will produce the effect desired without unfavorable effects. **organ tolerance d.,** in radiology, that amount of radiation which can be administered without appreciable damage to a normal organ; abbreviated OTD. **permissible d.,** that amount of ionizing radiation that, in the light of current knowledge, is not expected to lead to appreciable bodily injury and is allowable according to current radiation protection guides; see also *maximum permissible d.* **priming d.,** a quantity several times larger than the maintenance dose, used at the initiation of therapy to rapidly establish the desired blood and tissue levels of the drug. **radiation absorbed d.,** see *absorbed d.* and *rad,* def. 1. **reacting d.,** the second dose of sensitizing antigen administered to an animal; it is followed by an immediate hypersensitive (e.g., anaphylactic or allergic) response. Cf. *sensitizing d.* **sensitizing d.,** the first dose of sensitizing antigen (e.g., protein) administered to an animal in the induction of a hypersensitivity (e.g., anaphylactic or allergic) response; cf. *reacting d.* **skin d.,** 1. the air dose of radiation at the skin surface, comprising primary radiation plus backscatter. 2. the absorbed dose in the skin. **therapeutic d.,** a quantity several times larger than the maintenance dose, used in vitamin therapy when a marked deficiency exists. **threshold d.,** the minimum dose of ionizing radiation that will produce a detectable degree of any given effect. **threshold erythema d.,** the single skin dose that will produce in 80 per cent of those tested, a faint but definite erythema within 30 days, and in the other 20 per cent, no visible reaction. Abbreviated T.E.D. **tissue d.,** the absorbed dose of radiation in a tissue or organ, expressed in rads. **tolerance d.,** the largest quantity of an agent, such as x-ray energy, that may be administered without harm. **toxic d.,** the amount of an agent which will cause toxic symptoms. **volume d.,** integral d.

dosimeter (do-sim′ĕ-ter) in radiology, an instrument used to detect and measure exposure to radiation, commonly a pencil-sized ionization chamber with a built-in electrometer used in monitoring exposure of personnel. Called also *dosage meter.*

dosimetric (do″se-met′rik) of or pertaining to dosimetry.

dosimetrist (do-sim-ĕ′trist) one who plans an optimum radiation treatment technical dosage pattern or establishes a summation isodose pattern for the radiation treatment by means of isodose curves or other data supplied by a radiation physicist.

dosimetry (do-sim′ĕ-tre) [Gr. *dosis* dose + *metron* measure] the determination by scientific methods of the amount, rate, and distribution of radiation emitted from a source of ionizing radiation.

dosis (do′sis) [L., Gr. "a giving"] dose. **d. curati′va,** the minimum amount of a therapeutic agent that will effect a cure. **d. ef′ficax,** d. curativa. **d. refrac′ta,** fractional dose. **d. tolera′ta,** the largest amount of a therapeutic agent that can be given with safety.

dossier (dos′e-a) [Fr.] the accumulated records of a patient's case history.

dot (dot) a small spot or speck. **Gunn's d's,** white dots seen about the macula lutea on oblique illumination. **Marcus Gunn's d's,** Gunn's d's. **Maurer's d's,** irregular dots, staining red with Leishman's stain, seen in erythrocytes infected with *Plasmodium falciparum;* called also *Maurer's clefts.* **Mittendorf's d.,** a congenital anomaly manifested as a small gray or white opacity just inferior and nasal to the posterior pole of the lens, representing the remains of the lenticular attachment of the hyaloid artery; it does not affect vision. **Schüffner's d's,** minute granules observed in erythrocytes infected with *Plasmodium vivax* when stained by certain methods, such as Romanowsky's or Wright's stain; called also *Schüffner's granules* or *punctuation.* **Trantas' d's,** small, white calcareous looking dots in the limbus of the conjunctiva in vernal conjunctivitis.

dotage (do′tij) senile dementia.

dothiepin hydrochloride (do-thi′ĕ-pin) chemical name: 3-dibenzo [*b,e*] thiepin-11 (6*H*) -ylidene-*N,N* -dimethyl-1-propanamine; a tricyclic antidepressant, $C_{19}H_{21}NS \cdot HCl$.

double-blind (dub″l-blīnd′) pertaining to a clinical trial or other experiment in which neither the subject nor the person administering treatment knows which treatment any particular subject is receiving.

doublet (dub′let) [Middle English, from Old Fr. *double*] a fixed combination of two lenses, as in a telescope or microscope, for reducing aberration and increasing power.

Wollaston's d., a microscopical lens consisting of a combination of two planoconvex lenses for correcting chromatic aberration.

douche (doōsh) [Fr.] a stream of water directed against a part of the body or into a cavity. **air d.,** a current of air blown into a cavity, particularly into the tympanum, for opening the eustachian tube. **alternating d.,** transition douche. **fan d.,** water applied to the body in a fan-shaped spray. **jet d.,** water applied to the body in a single stream. **Scotch d.,** a jet douche of alternating hot and cold water. **Tivoli d.,** a reclining bath in which a hot douche is employed over the patient's abdomen. **transition d.,** a douche of alternating hot and cold water; called also *alternating d.*

Douglas's cul-de-sac, etc. (dug′las) [James *Douglas,* Scottish anatomist in London, 1675–1742] see under *cul-de-sac, fold, ligament, line, pouch, septum,* and *space.*

douglascele (dug′lah-sēl) posterior vaginal hernia.

douglasitis (dug-lah-si′tis) inflammation of Douglas' pouch (excavatio rectouterina).

dourine (doo-rēn′) venereal typanosomiasis affecting horses and asses in Africa, Asia, and certain regions of North and South America, caused by *Trypanosoma equiperdum,* transmitted by coitus, and characterized by edematous swelling of the external genitalia and a mucopurulent discharge from the urethra or vagina, cutaneous plaques, and progressive emaciation and weakness. Called also *covering disease.*

Dover's powder (do′verz) [Thomas *Dover,* English physician, 1660–1742] ipecac and opium powder.

dowel (dow′l) a post or a pin, usually metal, fitted into a prepared posthole within the root canal and cemented in place, serving to retain a dental restoration, such as a crown. Called also *post.*

down (down) lanugo.

Downs' analysis, Y axis (downz) [W.B. *Downs,* American orthodontist] see under *analysis* and see *Y axis,* under *axis.*

Down's syndrome (disease) (downz) [John Langdon Haydon *Down,* English physician, 1828–1896] see under *syndrome.*

doxapram hydrochloride (dok′sah-pram) [USP] chemical name: 1-ethyl-4-[2-(4-morpholinyl)ethyl]-3,3-diphenyl-2-pyrrolidinone monohydrochloride monohydrate. A respiratory stimulant, $C_{24}H_{30}N_2O_2 \cdot HCl \cdot H_2O$, occurring as a white to off-white, crystalline powder; used in the treatment of postanesthetic respiratory depression, administered intravenously.

doxaprost (doks′ah-prost) chemical name: (13*E*)-15-hydroxy-15-methyl-9-oxoprost-13-en-1-oic acid; a bronchodilator, $C_{21}H_{36}O_4$.

doxepin hydrochloride (dok′sĕ-pin) [USP] chemical name: 3-dibenz[*b,e*]oxepin-11(6*H*)ylidene-*N,N*-dimethyl-1-propanamine hydrochloride. A tricyclic compound, $C_{19}H_{21}$-NO·HCl, occurring as a white crystalline powder, having marked antianxiety and significant antidepressant activity; administered orally. It is also used as an antipruritic in veterinary medicine.

Doxinate (dok′sĭ-nāt) trademark for a preparation of dioctyl sulfosuccinate sodium.

doxorubicin (dok″so-roo′bĭ-sin) an anthracycline (q.v.) antibiotic having one of the widest spectrums of antitumor activity of any antineoplastic agent; used for treatment of acute granulocytic and lymphocytic leukemias; Hodgkin's disease and non-Hodgkin's lymphomas; rhabdomyosarcoma and osteogenic, Ewing's and soft-tissue sarcomas; carcinomas of the breast, bladder, endometrium, prostate, testes, and thyroid; small-cell carcinoma of the lung, bronchogenic carcinoma, and squamous cell carcinoma of the head and neck; hepatoma, neuroblastoma, and Wilms' tumor. Available as *doxorubicin hydrochloride* [USP]. **d. hydrochloride** [USP], the hydrochloride salt of doxorubicin, $C_{27}H_{30}Cl$-NO_4, having the same actions, uses, and route of administration as the base.

doxycycline (dok″se-si′klēn) [USP] chemical name: 4αS-(dimethylamino)-1,4,4aα,5,5aα,6,11,12a-octahydro -3,5α,10,1-2aα-pentahydroxy-6α-methyl - 1,11-dioxo-2-naphthacenecarboxamide monohydrate. A semisynthetic broad-spectrum antibacterial of the tetracycline (q.v.) group, $C_{22}H_{24}N_2O_8$-H_2O, derived from methacycline, it occurs as a yellow crystalline powder; administered orally. **d. calcium,** a complex prepared from doxycycline hyclate and calcium chloride, having the same actions and uses as the hyclate salt; administered orally. **d. hyclate [USP], d. hydrochloride,** a salt, $(C_{22}H_{24}N_2O_8 \cdot HCl)_2 \cdot C_2H_{60} \cdot H_2O$, occurring as a yellow crystalline powder, having the antibacterial effects of other tetracyclines; administered orally.

Doxy-II (dok′se) trademark for a preparation of doxycycline.

doxylamine succinate (dok-sil′ah-mēn) [USP] chemical name: *N,N*-dimethyl-2-[1-phenyl-1-(2-pyridinyl)ethoxy] ethanamine butanedioate (1:1). An antihistaminic, $C_{17}H_{22}N_2$-$O \cdot C_4H_6O_4$, occurring as a white or creamy white powder; administered orally.

Doyen's clamp (dwah-yahz′) [Eugène Louis *Doyen*, surgeon in Paris, 1859–1916] see under *clamp.*

Doyère's eminence (hillock) (dwa-yārz′) [Louis Michel François *Doyère*, French physiologist, 1811–1863] see under *eminence.*

Doyne's familial honeycombed choroiditis (doinz) [Robert Walter *Doyne,* Oxford ophthalmologist, 1857–1916] see under *choroiditis.*

D.P. abbreviation for L. *directio′ne prop′ria,* "with proper direction"; Doctor of Pharmacy; Doctor of Podiatry.

D.P.H. Diploma in Public Health.

D.P.M. Diploma in Psychological Medicine; Doctor of Podiatric Medicine.

DPN diphosphopyridine nucleotide; former name for *nicotinamide adenine dinucleotide* (NAD).

DPN kinase (ki′nās) NAD$^+$ kinase.

DPT diphtheria-pertussis-tetanus (vaccine).

DR reaction of degeneration; see under *reaction.*

dr. dram.

drachm (dram) [Gr. *drachmē*] dram.

dracontiasis (drak″on-ti′ah-sis) [Gr. *drakontion* (little dragon) tapeworm] dracunculiasis.

dracuncular (drah-kung′ku-lar) pertaining to or caused by nematodes of the genus *Dracunculus.*

dracunculiasis (drah-kung″ku-li′ah-sis) the state of being infected with nematodes of the genus *Dracunculus;* called also *guinea worm disease.*

Dracunculoidea (drah″kung-ku-loi′de-ah) a superfamily of phasmid nematodes including the genus *Dracunculus.*

dracunculosis (drah-kung″ku-lo′sis) dracunculiasis.

Dracunculus (drah-kung′ku-lus) [L. "little dragon"] a genus of nematode parasites of the superfamily Dracunculoidea. **D. medinen′sis,** the guinea worm or Medina worm, a threadlike worm, 30 to 120 cm. long, which inhabits the subcutaneous and intermuscular tissues of man and several domestic animals in India, Africa, and Arabia. Its embryos are discharged through an opening in the skin upon contact with water, in which they enter the bodies of a small crustacean, *Cyclops,* where they undergo larval development. Called also *dragon* or *serpent worm;* formerly called *Filaria medinensis.*

draft (draft) a potion; dose. **black d.,** the compound infusion of senna. **effervescing d.,** one which contains an acid and sodium or potassium bicarbonate. **mustard d.,** a mild rubefacient paste of mustard and flour. **Riverius' d.,** Rivière's potion.

drag (drag) the lower or cast side of a denture flask to which the cope is fitted.

dragée (drah-zha′) [Fr. "sugar-plum"] a sugar-coated pill, or medicated confection.

drain (drān) any device by which a channel or open area may be established for the exit of fluids or purulent material from any cavity, wound, or infected area. **cigarette d.,** a drain made by drawing a strip of gauze or surgical sponge into the lumen of a rubber tube. **controlled d.,** a drain made by pressing a square of gauze into the wound and then packing with gauze strips, the ends of which, together with the corners of the square, are left projecting from the wound. **Mikulicz's d.,** a drain formed by pushing a single layer of gauze into a wound or cavity, then packing with several thick wicks of gauze as the original layer is forced farther and farther into the defect. **Penrose d.,** a thin rubber tube, usually 0.5 to 1 inch in diameter. **stab wound d.,** drainage accomplished by bringing out the drain through a

small separate wound adjacent to the major operative incision. **sump d.,** a double-lumen drain that allows air to enter the drained area through the smaller lumen and displace fluid into the larger lumen. **sump-Penrose d.** a triple-lumen drain formed by placing a double-lumen tube within a Penrose drain.

drainage (drān′ij) the systematic withdrawal of fluids and discharges from a wound, sore, or cavity. **basal d.,** withdrawal of the cerebrospinal fluid from the basal subarachnoid space for the relief of intracranial pressure. **button d.,** drainage of a peritoneal transudate by means of a special button affixed to all layers of the abdominal wall. **capillary d.,** drainage effected by strands of hair, catgut, spun glass, or other material of tiny diameter which induces capillary attraction. **closed d.,** airtight drainage of a cavity carried out so that the entrance of air or contaminants is prevented. **continuous suction d.,** see *Wangensteen d.* **open d.,** drainage of a cavity through an opening into which one or more rubber drainage tubes are inserted, the opening not being sealed against the entrance of outside air. **postural d.,** removal of secretions in bronchiectasis and lung abscess by changes in the patient's position with accompanying repetitive striking of the chest. **suction d.,** closed drainage of a cavity, with a suction apparatus attached to the drainage tube. **through d.,** drainage achieved by passing a perforated tube or other type of drain through a cavity, so that irrigation may be effected by injecting fluid into one aperture and letting it escape through another. **tidal d.,** drainage of the urinary bladder by an apparatus which alternately fills the bladder to a predetermined extent and then empties it by a combination of siphonage and gravity flow. **Wangensteen d.,** continuous drainage by suction through an indwelling gastric or duodenal tube; for treatment of intestinal obstruction, paralytic ileus, etc.

dram (dram) a unit of weight which, in the apothecaries' system, equals 60 grains, or $\frac{1}{8}$ ounce; in the avoirdupois system it equals 27.34 grains, or $\frac{1}{16}$ ounce. Symbol ℨ; abbreviated dr. Called also *drachm.* **fluid d.,** a unit of capacity (liquid measure) of the apothecaries' system, being 60 minims, or the equivalent of 3.697 ml. Abbreviated fl.dr.

Dramamine (dram′ah-mēn) trademark for preparations of dimenhydrinate.

drastic (dras′tik) [Gr. *drastikos* effective] 1. acting powerfully or thoroughly. 2. a violent purgative.

draught (draft) draft.

dream (drēm) a mental phenomenon occurring during sleep in which images, emotions, and thoughts are experienced with a sense of reality. Dreaming occurs during REM sleep; typically there are four or five such periods a night having a total duration of about 90 minutes. Freud originated psychological interpretation of dreams, theorizing that dreams are the conscious expression of repressed unconscious impulses and wishes. **day d.,** wishful, purposeless reveries, without regard to reality. **wet d.,** a slang term for nocturnal emission.

drench (drench) a draft of medicine given to an animal by pouring it into its mouth.

Drepanidotaenia (drep″ah-nid-o-te′ne-ah) a genus of tapeworms parasitic in birds. *D. lanceola′ta* (*Hymenolepis lanceolata*) is a tapeworm of ducks and geese once reported from man.

drepanocyte (drep′ah-no-sīt″) [Gr. *drepanē* sickle + *kytos* cell] a sickle cell.

drepanocytemia (drep″ah-no-si-te′me-ah) sickle cell anemia.

drepanocytic (drep″ah-no-si′tik) pertaining to drepanocytes (sickle cells); having sickle-shaped cells.

drepanocytosis (drep″ah-no-si-to′sis) an occurrence of drepanocytes in the blood.

Drepanospira (drep″ah-no-spi′rah) [Gr. *drepanē* sickle + *speira* coil] a genus of Spirillaceae parasitic on protozoa.

Dresbach's anemia (syndrome) (dres′bahks) [Melvin *Dresbach,* American physician, 1874–1946] elliptocytosis.

dresser (dres′er) a surgical assistant who dresses wounds, etc.

dressing (dres′ing) any of various materials utilized for covering and protecting a wound. See also *bandage.* **adhesive absorbent d.,** a sterile individual dressing consisting of a plain absorbent compress affixed to a film or fabric coated with a pressure-sensitive adhesive substance. **antiseptic d.**, a dressing of gauze impregnated with an antiseptic material. **bolus d.**, tie-over d. **cocoon d.**, a dressing of gauze affixed to the surrounding skin by collodion or other liquid adhesive in such fashion that its elevated appearance resembles a cocoon. **cross d.**, transvestism. **dry d.**, dry gauze or absorbent cotton applied to a wound. **fixed d.**, a dressing impregnated with plaster of Paris, starch, or silicate of soda, utilized to secure fixation of the part when the material dries. **occlusive d.**, one which seals a wound from contact with air or bacteria. **pressure d.**, one by which pressure is exerted on the area covered to prevent the collection of fluids in the underlying tissues; most commonly used after skin grafting and in the treatment of burns. **protective d.**, a light dressing to prevent exposure to injury or infection. **stent d.**, a dressing in which is incorporated a mold or stent, to maintain position of a graft. **tie-over d.**, a dressing placed over a skin graft or other sutured wound, and tied on by the sutures which have been made of sufficient length for that purpose; called also *bolus d.*

Dressler's syndrome (dres′lerz) [William *Dressler*, Polish-born American physician, born 1890] postmyocardial infarction syndrome.

Dreyer and Bennett hypothesis (dri′er; ben′et) see *recombinational germline theory*, under *theory.*

DRG diagnosis-related group.

drift (drift) [A.S. *drifan* to drive] a chance variation, as in gene frequency between populations; the smaller the population, the greater the chance random variations. Called also *genetic d.* or *random genetic d.* **antigenic d.**, relatively minor changes in the antigenic structure of a virus strain, probably resulting from natural selection of virus variants circulating among an immune or partially immune population. **genetic d.**, see *drift.* **physiologic d.**, physiologic tooth migration. **random genetic d.**, see *drift.*

drill (dril) a rotating cutting instrument for making holes in hard substances, such as bones or teeth; a bur. **cannulated d.**, a drill with a hole through the center of its long axis, to be used over a guide wire.

drilling (dril′ing) the act or process of boring holes with a rotary instrument; the term is sometimes used in connection with cavity preparation.

Drinalfa (drin-al′fah) trademark for preparations of methamphetamine hydrochloride.

drinidene (dri′nĭ-dēn) chemical name: 2-(aminomethylene)-2,3-dihydro-1*H*-inden-1-one; an analgesic, $C_{10}H_9NO$.

drink (drink) a quantity of liquid taken in one or a series of successive swallows; to take a drink. **sham d.**, a drink, as by an esophagostomized dog, in which swallowed water fails to be ingested or retained in the stomach.

Drinker respirator (drink′er) [Philip *Drinker*, American public health engineer, 1894–1972] see under *respirator.*

drip (drip) the slow, drop by drop, infusion of a liquid. **alkalinized milk d. of Winkelstein,** a method of treating certain cases of ulcers, in which a mixture of 5 gm. of sodium bicarbonate in 1 quart of whole milk is allowed to drip into the stomach through a small nasal or oral tube at the rate of 30 drops per minute, producing constant achlorhydria. **intravenous d.**, continuous intravenous instillation, drop by drop, of saline or other solution. **Murphy d.**, see *Murphy method,* 2d def., under *method.* **nasal d.**, a method of giving fluid slowly to dehydrated infants through a catheter inserted into the nose and pushed down into the esophagus. **postnasal d.**, the dripping of discharges from the postnasal region into the pharynx due to hypersecretion of mucus in the nasal or nasopharyngeal mucosa or to chronic sinusitis.

Drisdol (driz′dol) trademark for preparations of ergocalciferol.

drive (drīv) the force which activates human impulses. **aggressive d.**, death instinct. **sexual d.**, life instinct.

drobuline (dro′bu-lēn) chemical name: (±)-α-[[(1-methylethyl)amino]methyl]-γ-phenylbenzenepropanol; a cardiac depressant with antiarrhythmic action, $C_{19}H_{25}NO.$

drocarbil (dro-kar′bil) chemical name: 1,2,5,6-tetrahydro-1-methylnicotinic acid methyl ester, compound with *N*-acetyl-4-hydroxy-*m*-arsanilic acid; a veterinary anthelmintic, $C_{16}H_{23}AsN_2O_7.$

drocinonide (dro-sin′o-nīd) chemical name: 9-fluoro-11β,21-dihydroxy-16α-17-[(1-methylethylidene)bis(oxy)]-5α-pregnane-3,20-dione; an anti-inflammatory, $C_{24}H_{35}FO_6.$

drocode (dro′kod) dihydrocodeine.

Drolban (drol′ban) trademark for a preparation of dromostanolone propionate.

drom(o)- [Gr. *dromos* a course, race] a combining form denoting relationship to conduction, to running, or to speed.

dromograph (drom′o-graf) [*dromo-* + Gr. *graphein* to record] an instrument for recording conduction or flow.

dromostanolone propionate (dro″mo-stan′o-lōn) [USP] chemical name: 2α-methyl-17β-(1-oxopropoxy)-5α-androstan-3-one. An androgenic, anabolic steroid, $C_{23}H_{36}O_3$, occurring as a white to creamy white, crystalline powder; used as an antineoplastic agent in the palliative treatment of advanced metastatic, inoperable breast cancer in certain postmenopausal women, administered intramuscularly.

dromotropic (drom″o-trop′ik) affecting the conductivity of a nerve fiber.

dromotropism (dro-mot′ro-pizm) [Gr. *dromos* a course + *tropē* a turn, turning] the quality or property of affecting the conductivity of a nerve fiber. **negative d.**, the property of diminishing the conductivity of a nerve. **positive d.**, the property of increasing the conductivity of a nerve.

Droncit (dron′cit) trademark for preparations of praziquantel.

drop (drop) [L. *gutta*] a minute sphere of liquid as it hangs or falls. **ear d's,** medicated oil or water to be dropped into the external auditory meatus. **enamel d.**, enameloma. **eye d's,** a medicated solution to be dropped into the conjunctival sac. **foot d.**, footdrop. **Hoffmann's d's,** ether spirit. **nose d's,** a medicated solution to be dropped into the nose. **d. phalangette,** a condition in which the terminal phalanx of a finger or toe is permanently flexed, as in baseball finger or mallet finger. **wrist d.**, wristdrop.

dropacism (drop′ah-sizm) [Gr. *drōpax* plaster] the removal of hairs by means of a plaster or wax.

droperidol (dro-per′ĭ-dol) [USP] chemical name: 1-[1-[4 -(4 -fluorophenyl) -4-oxobutyl] -1,2,3,6 -tetrahydro -4-pyridinyl]-1,3-dihydro-2*H*-benzimidazol-2-one. A drug of the butyrophenone series, $C_{22}H_{22}FN_3O_2$, occurring as a white to light tan, amorphous or microcrystalline powder; used for its antianxiety, sedative, and antiemetic effects as a premedication prior to surgery and during induction and maintenance of anesthesia, administered intravenously or intramuscularly. A combination of droperidol and fentanyl citrate (known as *Innovar*) is administered intramuscularly to produce neuroleptanalgesia.

droplet (drop′let) a diminutive drop, such as the particles of moisture expelled from the mouth in coughing, sneezing, or speaking, which may carry infection to others through the air. See also under *nucleus.*

dropper (drop′er) a pipet or tube for dispensing liquid in drops.

dropping (drop′ing) the limping gait of a horse, which is due to a neurologic disorder affecting the extensors of the limb.

dropsical (drop′sĭ-kal) affected with or pertaining to dropsy.

dropsy (drop′se) [L. *hydrops,* from Gr. *hydōr* water] the abnormal accumulation of serous fluid in the cellular tissue or in a body cavity; see also *hydrops.* **abdominal d.**, ascites. **d. of amnion,** hydramnios. **articular d.**, hydrarthrosis. **d. of belly,** ascites. **d. of brain,** hydrocephalus. **cardiac d.**, gross edema related to heart failure. **d. of chest,** hydrothorax. **cutaneous d.**, edema. **epidemic d.**, a sometimes fatal condition occurring in epidemics in India, Fiji, South Africa, and elsewhere, characterized by edema of the extremities; dilatation of the vessels of the skin, subcutaneous tissues, and uveal tract, resulting in glaucoma; cardiac insufficiency; and liver abnormalities. It is caused by contamination of mustard oil used for cooking by oil from the seeds of the prickly poppy (*Argemona mexicana*), which contains the glycoside sanguinarine, which causes dilatation and increased permeability of capillaries and interferes with pyruvic acid oxidation. **famine d.**, nutritional edema. **d. of head,** hydrocephalus. **hepatic d.**, that which is due to disease of the liver. **nutritional d.**, nutritional edema. **d. of pericar-**

dium (*obs.*), hydropericardium. **peritoneal d.,** ascites. **renal d.,** anasarca due to kidney disease. **salpingian d.,** hydrosalpinx. **war d.,** nutritional edema. **wet d.,** beriberi.

Drosophila (dro-sof′ĭ-lah) [Gr. *drosos* dew + *philein* to love] a genus of flies; the pomace flies (often erroneously called fruit flies). **D. melanogas′ter,** a small fly often seen about decaying fruit; used extensively in experimental genetics.

drosopterin (dro-sop′ter-in) any of a group of bright red pteridine pigments of the eye of *Drosophila* which are readily decomposed by light.

drowning (drown′ing) suffocation and death resulting from filling of the lungs with water or other substance or fluid, so that gas exchange becomes impossible. **secondary d.,** delayed death from drowning, due to such complications as pulmonary alveolar inflammation.

droxacin sodium (droks′ah-sin) chemical name: 5-ethyl-2,3,5,8-tetrahydro-8-oxo-furo[2,3-*g*]quinoline-7-carboxylic acid sodium salt; an antibacterial, $C_{14}H_{12}NNaO_4$.

droxifilcon A (droks″ĭ-fil′kon) a hydrophilic contact lens material.

Dr.P.H. Doctor of Public Health.

drug (drug) 1. any chemical compound that may be used on or administered to humans or animals as an aid in the diagnosis, treatment, or prevention of disease or other abnormal condition, for the relief of pain or suffering, or to control or improve any physiologic or pathologic condition. 2. a narcotic. **antagonistic d.,** one that tends to counteract or neutralize the effect of another. **crude d.,** the whole drug with all its ingredients.

drug-fast (drug′fast) drug-resistant.

druggist (drug′ist) pharmacist.

drug-resistant (drug′re-zis″tant) resistant to the action of drugs; said of microorganisms. Called also *drug-fast*.

drum (drum) 1. loosely, the tympanic membrane (*membrana tympani* [NA]). 2. the tympanic cavity (*cavitas tympanica* [NA]).

drumhead (drum′hed) the tympanic membrane (membrana tympani [NA]).

Drummond's sign (drum′unds) [Sir David *Drummond*, English physician, 1852–1932] see under *sign*.

drumstick (drum′stik) a nuclear lobule attached by a slender strand to the nucleus of a small proportion of polymorphonuclear leukocytes of normal females but not of normal males.

drupe (droop) [L. *drupa* an overripe olive] stone fruits in which the outer part of the ovary wall forms a skin, the middle part becomes fleshy and juicy, and the inner part forms a hard pit or stone around the seed; e.g., peaches, plums, apricots.

drusen (droo′zen) [Ger. "bumps"] 1. hyaline excrescences in Bruch's membrane (lamina basalis choroideae); they usually result from aging, but sometimes occur with pathologic conditions. 2. rosettes of granules occurring in the lesions of actinomycosis.

Drysdale's corpuscles (drīz′dālz) [Thomas Murray *Drysdale*, American gynecologist, 1831–1904] see under *corpuscle*.

D.S.C. Doctor of Surgical Chiropody.

dsDNA double-stranded DNA.

dsRNA double-stranded RNA.

DT diphtheria and tetanus toxoids for pediatric use.

dT deoxythymidine.

D.T.D. abbreviation for L. *da′tur ta′lis do′sis*, give of such a dose.

dTDP deoxythymidine diphosphate.

DTH delayed type hypersensitivity.

DTIC dacarbazine.

DTIC-Dome (dōm) trademark for a preparation of dacarbazine.

dTMP deoxythymidine monophosphate.

DTP diphtheria and tetanus toxoids and pertussis vaccine.

dTTP deoxythymidine triphosphate.

dualism (du′al-izm) [L. *duo* two] 1. the theory that there are two distinct stem cells for blood cell formation: one for the lymphatic cells and the other for the myeloid cells. 2. the

theory that human beings are made up of two independent systems, mind and body, and that psychic and physical phenomena are fundamentally independent and different in nature.

Duane's syndrome (du-ānz′) [Alexander *Duane*, ophthalmologist in New York, 1858–1926] see under *syndrome*.

duazomycin (du-az″o-mi′sin) an antibiotic substance with antineoplastic properties, produced by *Streptomyces ambofaciens;* formerly called *duazomycin A.* **d. A,** former name for duazomycin. **d. B,** former name for azotomycin. **d. C,** former name for ambomycin.

Dubini's chorea (disease) (du-be′nēz) [Angelo *Dubini*, Italian physician, 1813–1902] see under *chorea.*

Dubois' abscess (disease) (du-bwahz′) [Paul *Dubois*, French obstetrician, 1795–1871] see under *abscess.*

DuBois-Reymond's law (dŭ-bwah″ri-maw′) [Emil Heinrich *DuBois-Reymond*, German physiologist, 1818–1896] see under *law.*

Duboisia (du-boi′se-ah) a genus of solanaceous plants; *D. myoporoides* yields hyoscyamine and scopolamine.

Dubos enzyme (crude crystals, lysin) (doo-bos′) [René Jules *Dubos*, French biochemist in America, 1901–1982] see *tyrothricin.*

Duboscq colorimeter (du-bosk′) [Louis Jules *Duboscq*, French optician, 1817–1886] see under *colorimeter.*

Duchenne's disease, etc. (du-shenz′) [Guillaume Benjamin Amand *Duchenne*, French neurologist, 1806– 1875] see under *disease, dystrophy, paralysis,* and *type.*

Duchenne-Aran muscular atrophy (disease, type) (du-shen′ar-an′) [G. B. A. *Duchenne;* F. A. *Aran*] spinal muscular atrophy; see under *atrophy.*

Duchenne-Erb paralysis, syndrome (du-shen′airb) [G. B. A. *Duchenne;* Wilhelm Heinrich *Erb*, German internist, 1840–1921] Erb-Duchenne paralysis.

Duchenne-Landouzy dystrophy (type) [G. B. A. *Duchenne;* L. T. J. *Landouzy*] facioscapulohumeral muscular dystrophy; see under *dystrophy.*

Duckworth's phenomenon (sign) (duk′worths) [Sir Dyce *Duckworth*, British physician, 1840–1928] see under *phenomenon.*

Ducobee (doo′ko-be) trademark for preparations of vitamin B₁₂; see *cyanocobalamin.*

Ducrey's bacillus (doo-krāz′) [Augusto *Ducrey*, Italian dermatologist, 1860–1940] *Haemophilus ducreyi.*

duct (dukt) [L. *ductus,* from *ducere* to draw or lead] a passage with well-defined walls, especially a tube for the passage of excretions or secretions; called also *ductus* [NA]. **aberrant d.,** any duct that is not usually present or that takes an unusual course or direction, such as the ductulus aberrans superior. **acoustic d.,** meatus acusticus externus. **adipose d.,** an elongated sac in the cellular tissue filled with fat. **alimentary d.,** thoracic d. **allantoic d.,** allantoic stalk. **alveolar d's,** ductuli alveolares. **d. of Arantius,** ductus venosus. **archinephric d.,** pronephric d. **arterial d.,** ductus arteriosus. **Bartholin's d.,** ductus sublingualis major. **Bellini's d's,** tubuli renales recti. **Bernard's d.,** ductus pancreaticus accessorius. **bile d.,** any of the ducts that convey bile in and from the liver; called also *biliary d.* and *gall d.* See *ductus choledochus, ductus cysticus, ductus hepaticus dexter,* and *ductus hepaticus sinister.* **bile d., common,** ductus choledochus. **bile d's, interlobular,** ductuli interlobulares. **biliary d.,** 1. bile d. 2. ductus choledochus. **Blasius' d.,** ductus parotideus. **Bochdalek's d.,** ductus thyroglossalis. **d. of Botallo,** ductus arteriosus. **branchial d's,** drawn-out branchial grooves 2, 3, and 4, which open into the temporary cervical sinus of the embryo. **canalicular d's,** ductus lactiferi. **cervical d.,** the opening from the exterior into the temporary cervical sinus of the embryo. **choledochous d.,** ductus choledochus. **chyliferous d.,** thoracic d. **cloacal d.,** Reichel's cloacal d. **cochlear d.,** 1. a spirally arranged membranous tube in the bony canal of the cochlea; see *ductus cochlearis* [NA]. 2. canalis spiralis cochleae. **common bile d.,** the duct formed by union of the cystic duct and the hepatic duct; called also *ductus choledochus* [NA]. **Coschwitz' d.,** a supposed salivary duct forming an arch over the dorsum of the tongue, proved by von Haller to be a vein. **cowperian d.,** ductus glandulae bulbourethralis. **craniopharyngeal d.,** hypophyseal d. **d's of Cuvier,** common cardinal veins: two short venous trunks in the fetus opening into the atrium of the heart; the right one becomes the superior vena cava; called also *Cuvier's sinuses* and *ductus cuvieri*. **cystic d.,** ductus cysticus. **deferent d.,** ductus deferens. **efferent d.,** a duct that gives outlet to a glandular secretion. **ejaculatory d.,** ductus ejaculatorius. **endolymphatic d.,** ductus endolymphaticus. **d. of epididymis,** ductus epididymidis. **d. of epoöphoron, d. of epoöphoron, longitudinal,** ductus epoöphorontis longitudinalis. **excretory d.,** one that is merely conductive and not secretory. **excretory d. of seminal vesicle,** ductus excretorius vesiculae seminalis. **excretory d. of testis,** ductus deferens. **frontonasal d.,** nasofrontal d. **galactophorous d's,** ductus lactiferi. **gall d.,** bile d. **d. of gallbladder,** ductus cysticus. **Gartner's d.,** ductus epoöphorontis longitudinalis. **gasserian d.,** ductus paramesonephricus. **genital d.,** genital canal. **gutteral d.,** auditory tube. **Haller's aberrant d.,** a small coiled tube extending from the lower part of the canal of the epididymis; called also *ductus aberrans halleri.* **Hensen's d.,** ductus reuniens. **hepatic d., common,** ductus hepaticus communis. **hepatic d., left,** ductus hepaticus sinister. **hepatic d., right,** ductus hepaticus dexter. **hepaticopancreatic d.,** ductus pancreaticus. **hepatocystic d.,** ductus choledochus. **d. of His,** ductus thyroglossalis. **hypophyseal d.,** an embryonic structure composed of the elongated Rathke's pouch joining the infundibulum of the embryonic hypophysis; called also *craniopharyngeal duct.* **incisive d., incisor d.,** ductus incisivus. **intercalated d.,** a slender initial portion of the duct system interposed between an acinus of a gland and a secretory duct. **interlobular d's,** channels located between different lobules of a gland; see *ductuli interlobulares.* **lacrimal d.,** canaliculus lacrimalis. **lacrimonasal d.,** ductus nasolacrimalis. **lactiferous d's,** ductus lactiferi. **Leydig's d.,** d. mesonephricus. **lingual d.,** a depression on the dorsum of the tongue at the apex of the terminal sulcus. **Luschka's d's,** tubular structures in the wall of the gallbladder, some connected with bile ducts but none connected with the lumen of the gallbladder; they may be aberrant bile ducts. **lymphatic d's,** channels for conducting lymph. **lymphatic d., left,** thoracic d. **lymphatic d., right,** ductus lymphaticus dexter. **mammary d's, mammillary d's,** ductus lactiferi. **mesonephric d.,** ductus mesonephricus. **metanephric d.,** ureter. **milk d's,** ductus lactiferi. **d. of Müller, müllerian d.,** ductus paramesonephricus. **nasal d.,** ductus nasolacrimalis. **nasofrontal d.,** a duct in the lateral wall of the nasal cavity extending from the infundibulum of the ethmoid bone to the frontal sinus; called also *frontonasal d.* **nasolacrimal d.,** ductus nasolacrimalis. **nasopharyngeal d.,** the lumen of the nasopharynx. **nephric d.,** ureter. **omphalomesenteric d.,** the narrow tube connecting the umbilical vesicle (yolk sac) with the midgut of the embryo; called also *omphalomesenteric canal, umbilical duct, vitelline duct, vitellointestinal duct,* and *yolk stalk.* **ovarian d.,** tuba uterina. **pancreatic d.,** ductus pancreaticus. **pancreatic d., accessory,** **pancreatic d., minor,** ductus pancreaticus accessorius. **papillary d's,** tubuli renales recti. **paramesonephric d's of female urethra,** ductus paramesonephricus. **paraurethral d's of female urethra,** ductus paraurethrales urethrae femininae. **paraurethral d's of male urethra,** ductus paraurethrales urethrae masculinae. **parotid d.,** ductus parotideus. **d. of Pecquet,** thoracic d. **perilymphatic d's,** aqueductus cochleae. **primordial d.,** ductus paramesonephricus. **pronephric d.,** the duct of the pronephros, which later serves as the mesonephric duct (ductus mesonephricus); called also *archinephric d.* or *canal.* **d's of prostate gland, prostatic d's,** ductuli prostatici. **Rathke's d.,** that part of the ductus paramesonephricus lying between its main part and the sinus pocularis. **Reichel's cloacal d.,** the cleft between Douglas' septum and the cloaca in the embryo. **renal d.,** ureter. **d's of Rivinus,** ductus sublinguales minores. **Rokitansky-Aschoff d's,** see under *sinus.* **sacculoutricular d.,** ductus utriculosaccularis. **salivary d's,** the ducts that convey the saliva: they are the ductus parotideus, ductus submandibularis, ductus sublingualis major, and ductus sublinguales minores. **d. of Santorini,** ductus pancreaticus accessorius. **Schüller's d's,** ductus paraurethrales urethrae femininae. **secretory d.,** a smaller duct that is tributary to an excretory duct of a gland and that also has a secretory function.

semicircular d's, the long ducts of the membranous labyrinth of the ear; called also *ductus semicirculares* [NA]. **semicircular d., anterior,** ductus semicircularis anterior. **semicircular d., lateral,** ductus semicircularis lateralis. **semicircular d., posterior,** ductus semicircularis posterior. **semicircular d., superior,** ductus semicircularis anterior. **seminal d's,** passages for the conveyance of spermatozoa and semen, including the ductus deferens, ductus excretorius vesiculae seminalis, and ductus ejaculatorius. **d. of seminal vesicle,** ductus excretorius vesiculae seminalis. **Skene's d's,** ductus paraurethrales urethrae femininae. **spermatic d.,** ductus deferens. **d. of Steno, Stensen's d.,** ductus parotideus. **sublingual d's,** the ducts of the sublingual salivary glands, including the ductus sublingualis major and ductus sublinguales minores. **sublingual d., major,** ductus sublingualis major. **sublingual d's, minor,** ductus sublinguales minores. **submandibular d., submaxillary d. of Wharton,** ductus submandibularis. **sudoriferous d., sweat d.,** ductus sudoriferus. **tear d's,** the ducts conveying the secretion of the lacrimal glands. **testicular d.,** ductus deferens. **thoracic d.,** the canal that ascends from the cisterna chyli to the junction of the left subclavian and left internal jugular vein; called also *ductus thoracicus* [NA], *alimentary d., chyliferous d., d. of Pecquet, left lymphatic d.,* and *Van Hoorne's canal.* **thoracic d., right,** see *ductus lymphaticus dexter.* **thyroglossal d., thyrolingual d.,** ductus thyroglossalis. **umbilical d.,** yolk stalk. **urogenital d's,** the ductus paramesonephricus and ductus mesonephricus. **utriculosaccular d.,** ductus utriculosaccularis. **d. of Vater,** ductus thyroglossalis. **vitelline d., vitellointestinal d.,** yolk stalk. **Walther's d's,** ductus sublinguales minores. **Wharton's d.,** ductus submandibularis. **d. of Wirsung,** ductus pancreaticus. **d. of Wolff, wolffian d.,** ductus mesonephricus.

ductal (duk'tal) pertaining to a duct.

ductile (duk'til) [L. *ductilis,* from *ducere* to draw, to lead] susceptible of being drawn out, as into a wire.

duction (duk'shun) [L. *ductio,* from *ducere* to lead] in ophthalmology, the rotation of an eye by the extraocular muscles around its horizontal, vertical, or anteroposterior axis, the direction of the movement of the eye being indicated by prefixes. See *infraduction, supraduction, abduction, adduction,* and *cycloduction,* and see also *vergence* (def. 2) and *version* (def. 5).

ductless (dukt'les) having no excretory duct.

ductule (dukt'ūl) a minute duct, especially that part or branch of a duct which is nearest the alveolus of a gland; called also *ductulus* [NA]. **aberrant d's,** ductules that are not usually present, or that follow an unusual course or direction; see *ductuli aberrantes* [NA]. **aberrant d., inferior,** ductulus aberrans inferior. **aberrant d., superior,** ductulus aberrans superior. **alveolar d's,** ductuli alveolares. **bile d's, biliary d's,** 1. ductuli biliferi [NA]. 2. cholangioles. **efferent d's of testis,** ductuli efferentes testis. **excretory d's of lacrimal gland,** ductuli excretorii glandulae lacrimalis. **interlobular d's,** ductuli interlobulares. **d's of prostate,** ductuli prostatici. **transverse d's of epoöphoron,** ductuli transversi epoöphorontis.

ductuli (duk'tu-li) [L.] genitive and plural of *ductulus.*

ductulus (duk'tu-lus), pl. *duc'tuli* [L.] [NA] ductule: a general term for a minute duct; applied especially to branches of ducts nearest to the alveoli of a gland, or the smallest beginnings of the duct system of an organ. **d. aber'rans infe'rior** [NA], inferior aberrant ductule: a narrow, coiled tube often connected with the first part of the ductus deferens, or with the lower part of the duct of the epididymis. **d. aber'rans supe'rior** [NA], superior aberrant ductule: a narrow tube of variable length that lies in the epididymis and is connected with the rete testis; called also *ductus aberrans.* **duc'tuli aberran'tes** [NA], aberrant ductules: blind vestiges of mesonephric tubules standing in relation to the epididymis. **duc'tuli alveola'res** [NA], alveolar ductules: small passages connecting the respiratory bronchioles and the alveolar sacs; see Plate 46 accompanying *system.* Called also *alveolar ducts.* **duc'tuli bilif'eri** [NA], biliary ductules: the small channels that connect the interlobular ductules with the right and left hepatic ducts; called also *bile ductule* and *ductus biliferi.*

duc′tuli efferen′tes tes′tis [NA], efferent ductules of testis: ductules entering the head of the epididymis from the rete testis. **duc′tuli excreto′rii glan′dulae lacrima′lis** [NA], excretory ductules of lacrimal gland: numerous ductules that traverse the palpebral part of the lacrimal gland and open into the superior fornix of the conjunctiva. **duc′tuli interlobula′res** [NA], interlobular ductules: small channels between the hepatic lobules, draining into the bile ductules; called also *ductus interlobulares,* and *interlobular biliary canals* or *bile ducts.* **duc′tuli prostat′ici** [NA], ductules of prostate gland: minute ducts from the prostate gland that open on either side into or near the prostatic sinuses on the posterior wall of the urethra: called also *ductus prostatici, ducts of prostate gland,* and *prostatic ducts.* **duc′tuli transver′si epooph′ori,** NA alternative for *ductuli transversi epoöphorontis.* **duc′tuli transver′si epoöphoron′tis** [NA], transverse ductules of epoöphoron: the vestigial remains of the mesonephric ducts, which open into the longitudinal duct of the epoöphoron. Called also *ductuli transversi epoöphori.*

ductus (duk′tus), pl. *duc′tus* [L.] [NA] a duct: a general term for a passage with well-defined walls, especially such a channel for the passage of excretions or secretions. **d. aber′rans,** ductulus aberrans superior. **d. aber′rans hal′leri,** Haller's aberrant duct. **d. Aran′tii,** d. venosus. **d. arterio′sus** [NA], arterial duct: a fetal blood vessel connecting the pulmonary artery directly to the descending aorta; called also *arterial canal, Botallo's duct,* and *pulmoaortic canal.* **d. arteriosus, patent,** abnormal persistence of an open lumen in the ductus arteriosus after birth, the direction of flow being from the aorta to the pulmonary artery, resulting in recirculation of arterial blood through the lungs. **d. arteriosus, reversed,** abnormal persistence of an open lumen in the ductus arteriosus after birth with obstruction of the small vessels of the lungs, the direction of flow being from the pulmonary artery to the aorta, resulting in the return of venous blood to the systemic circulation (the reverse of the normal post-fetal circulation); characterized clinically by cyanosis, especially of the feet. **d. bilia′ris,** NA alternative for *d. choledochus.* **d. bilif′eri,** ductuli biliferi. **d. choled′ochus** [NA], choledochous duct: the duct formed by union of the common hepatic and the cystic ducts which empties into the duodenum at the major duodenal papilla, along with the pancreatic duct; called also *biliary duct, common bile duct, d. biliaris* [NA alternative], *hepatic funiculus,* and *hepatocystic duct.* **d. cochlea′ris** [NA], cochlear duct: a spirally arranged membranous tube in the bony canal of the cochlea along its outer wall, lying between the scala tympani below and the scala vestibuli above; called also *cochlear canal, membranous cochlea, scala media,* and *scala of Löwenberg.* **d. cuvi′eri,** ducts of Cuvier. **d. cys′ticus** [NA], cystic duct: the passage connecting the neck of the gallbladder and the common bile duct; called also *duct of gallbladder.* **d. def′erens** [NA], deferent duct: the excretory duct of the testis, which unites with the excretory duct of the seminal vesicle to form the ejaculatory duct; called also *vas deferens, excretory duct of testis, spermatic duct,* and *testicular duct.* **d. de′ferens vestigia′lis** [NA], the vestigial remnants of the mesonephric duct in the female. **d. ejaculato′rius** [NA], ejaculatory duct: the canal formed by union of the ductus deferens and the excretory duct of the seminal vesicle. It enters the prostatic part of the urethra on the colliculus seminalis. **d. endolymphat′icus** [NA], endolymphatic duct: a canal connecting the utriculosaccular duct with the endolymphatic sac; called also *aqueduct of vestibule, aqueductus vestibuli,* and *aqueductus endolymphaticus.* **d. epididym′idis** [NA], duct of epididymus: the single tube into which the coiled ends of the efferent ductules of the testis open, the convolutions of which make up the greater part of the epididymis; called also *canal of epididymis.* **d. epoöph′ori longitudina′lis,** d. epoöphorontis longitudinalis. **d. epoöphoron′tis longitudina′lis** [NA], longitudinal duct of epoöphoron: a closed rudimentary duct lying parallel to the uterine tube into which the transverse ducts of the epoöphoron open, it is a remnant of the part of the mesonephros that participates in formation of the reproductive organs. Called also *duct of epoöphoron, d. epoöphori longitudinalis,* and *Gartner's canal* or *duct.* **d. excreto′rius vesic′ulae semina′lis** [NA], excretory duct of seminal vesicle: the duct that drains the seminal vesicle and unites with the ductus deferens to form the ejaculatory duct. **d. glan′dulae bulbourethra′lis** [NA], duct of bulbourethral gland: a duct passing from the bulbourethral gland through the urogenital diaphragm into the bulb of the penis and entering the spongy part of the urethra; called also *cowperian duct.* **d. hepat′icus commu′nis** [NA], common hepatic duct: the duct which is formed by union of the right and left hepatic ducts, and in turn joins the cystic duct to form the common bile duct. **d. hepat′icus dex′ter** [NA], right hepatic duct: the duct that drains the right lobe and part of the caudate lobe of the liver. **d. hepat′icus sin′ister** [NA], left hepatic duct: the duct that drains the left and the quadrate lobe and part of the caudate lobe of the liver. **d. inci′sivus** [NA], incisive duct: a passage sometimes found in the incisive canal that interconnects the nasal and oral cavities during embryonic development; it occasionally fails to close. Called also *incisor canaliculis* and *incisor duct.* **d. interlobula′res,** ductuli interlobulares. **d. lacrima′les,** canaliculus lacrimalis. **d. lactif′eri** [NA], lactiferous ducts: channels conveying the milk secreted by the lobes of the breast to and through the nipples; called also *galactophorous tubules, lactiferous tubules,* and *mammary ducts.* **d. lingua′lis,** a depression on the dorsum of the tongue, at the apex of the terminal sulcus. **d. lo′bi cauda′ti dex′ter** [NA], the right duct of the caudate lobe of the liver. **d. lo′bi cauda′ti sinis′ter** [NA], the left duct of the caudate lobe of the liver. **d. lymphat′ici** [NA], lymphatic ducts: the main lymph channels, the right lymphatic duct, thoracic duct, and cisterna chyli (when present), into which the converging lymph vessels drain, which in turn empty into the blood stream. **d. lymphat′icus dex′ter** [NA], right lymphatic duct: a vessel draining the lymph from the upper right side of the body, typically formed by the right jugular, subclavian, and bronchomediastinal lymphatic trunks, any one of which may, however, end separately in the right brachiocephalic vein; when all three lymphatic vessels unite, a right lymphatic duct (called also *d. thoracicus dexter* and *right thoracic duct*) is formed, which empties directly into the junction of the internal jugular and subclavian veins. **d. mesoneph′ricus** [NA], mesonephric duct: an embryonic duct which initiated in association with rudiments of the pronephric kidney, is taken over as an excretory duct by the mesonephros, and develops into the epididymis, the ductus deferens and its ampulla, the seminal vesicles, and the ejaculatory duct in the male and into vestigial structures in the female. Called also *d. Wolffi, wolffian duct, duct of Wolff, Leydig's duct,* and *canal of Oken.* **d. Muel′leri,** ductus paramesonephricus. **d. nasolacrima′lis** [NA], nasolacrimal duct: the passage that conveys the tears from the lacrimal sac into the interior nasal meatus; called also *lacrimonasal* or *nasal duct.* **d. pancrea′ticus** [NA], pancreatic duct: the main excretory duct of the pancreas, which usually unites with the common bile duct before entering the duodenum at the major duodenal papilla; called also *duct* or *canal of Wirsung,* and *hepatopancreatic duct.* **d. pancrea′ticus accesso′rius** [NA], accessory pancreatic duct: a small inconstant duct draining a part of the head of the pancreas into the minor duodenal papilla; called also *minor pancreatic duct,* and *duct of Santorini* or *Bernard.* **d. paramesoneph′ricus** [NA], paramesonephric duct: either of the paired embryonic ducts arising as a peritoneal pocket, extending caudally to join the urogenital sinus, and developing into uterine tubes, uterus, and vagina in the female and into a vestigial structure (appendix testis) in the male. Called also *d. Muelleri, duct of Müller* or *müllerian duct,* and *gasserian* or *primordial duct.* **d. paraurethra′les ure′thrae femini′nae** [NA], paraurethral ducts of female urethra: inconstantly present ducts in the female, which drain a group of the urethral glands into the vestibule; called also *Guérin's ducts, Schüller's ducts* or *glands, Skene's ducts, glands,* or *tubules,* and *paraurethral glands of female urethra.* **d. paraurethra′les ure′thrae masculi′nae** [NA], paraurethral ducts of male urethra: the ducts of the urethral glands situated in the spongy portion of the male urethra; called also *canales paraurethrales urethrae masculinae* [NA alternative] and *paraurethral canals of male urethra.* **d. paroti′deus** [NA], parotid duct: the duct that drains the parotid gland and empties into the oral cavity opposite the second superior molar; called also *Blasius' duct, Stensen's canal* or *duct,* and *duct* or *canal of Steno.* **patent d. arteriosus,** see *d. arteriosus, patent.* **d. perilymphat′ici, d. perilymphaticus,** aqueductus cochleae. **d. prostat′ici,** ductuli prostatici. **d. reu′niens** [NA], a small canal leading from the saccule to the cochlear duct; called also *canalis reuniens, Hensen's canal* or *duct,* and *Reichert's canal.* **reversed d. arteriosus,** see *d. arteriosus, reversed.* **d. semicircula'res** [NA], semicircular ducts: the long ducts of the membranous labyrinth of the ear, corresponding to the semicircular canals of the bony labyrinth and designated anterior, posterior, and lateral, according to the canal they occupy. Their diameter is only one-fourth that of the bony canals containing them, and each is affixed by one wall to the endosteal lining of the canal. They give information about angular acceleration and deceleration. Called also *membranous semicircular canal.* **d. semicircula'ris ante'rior** [NA], anterior semicircular duct: the semicircular duct occupying the anterior semicircular canal; called also *d. semicircularis superior,* or *superior semicircular duct.* See *ductus semicirculares.* **d. semicircula'ris latera'lis** [NA], lateral semicircular duct: the semicircular duct occupying the lateral semicircular canal; see *ductus semicirculares.* **d. semicircula'ris poste'rior** [NA], posterior semicircular duct: the semicircular duct occupying the posterior semicircular canal; see *ductus semicirculares.* **d. semicircula'ris supe'rior,** d. semicircularis anterior. **d. spermat'icus,** d. deferens. **d. sublingua'lis ma'jor** [NA], major sublingual duct: the duct that drains the sublingual gland and opens alongside the submandibular duct on the sublingual caruncle; called also *Bartholin's duct.* **d. sublingua'les mino'res** [NA], minor sublingual ducts: the ducts that drain the sublingual gland and open along the crest of the sublingual fold; called also *canals* or *ducts of Rivinus,* and *Walther's ducts.* **d. submandibula'ris** [NA], **d. submaxilla'ris** [**Wharto'ni**], submandibular duct: the duct that drains the submandibular gland and opens at the sublingual caruncle; called also *submaxillary duct of Wharton,* and *Wharton's duct.* **d. sudorif'erus** [NA], sudoriferous duct: the duct that leads from the body of a sweat gland to the surface of the skin; called also *sweat duct.* **d. thora'cicus** [NA], thoracic duct: the largest lymph channel in the body, which collects lymph from the portions of the body below the diaphragm and from the left side of the body above the diaphragm; it begins in the abdomen (*pars abdominalis*) at the junction of the intestinal, lumbar, and descending intercostal trunks (which consists of a plexus or the *cisterna chyli*) at about the level of the second lumbar vertebra, enters the thorax through the aortic hiatus of the diaphragm (*pars thoracica*), ascends to cross the posterior mediastinum, and enters the neck (*pars cervicalis*), where it forms a downward arch (*arcus ductus thoracici*) across the subclavian artery, and ends at the junction of the subclavian and internal jugular veins. **d. thora'cicus dex'ter,** see *d. lymphaticus dexter.* **d. thyroglossa'lis** [NA], thyroglossal duct: a duct in the embryo extending between the thyroid primordium and the posterior part of the tongue, which opens as the foramen caecum; the distal part usually differentiates to form the pyramidal lobe the thyroid and the remainder becomes obliterated, but occasionally persists into adult life, giving rise to cysts, fistulas, or sinuses. Called also *duct of His* or *Vater, Bochdalek's duct, His' canal,* and *thyrolingual duct.* **d. utriculosaccula'ris** [NA], utriculosaccular duct: a narrow duct uniting the utricle and saccule of the membranous labyrinth; called also *sacculoutricular duct* or *canal* and *utriculosaccular canal.* **d. veno'sus** [NA], a major blood channel that develops through the embryonic liver from the left umbilical vein to the inferior vena cava; called also *canal* or *duct of Arantius, canal of Cuvier,* and *ductus Arantii.* **d. Wol'fii,** ductus mesonephricus.

Duddell's membrane (dud'elz) [Benedict *Duddell,* English physician of the 18th century] lamina limitans posterior corneae.

Dugas' test (sign) (doo'gahz) [Louis Alexander *Dugas,* American physician, 1806–1884] see under *tests.*

Duhot's line (dŭ-hōz') [Robert *Duhot,* urologist and dermatologist in Brussels, born 1867] see under *line.*

Duhring's disease (du'rings) [Louis Adolphus *Duhring,* dermatologist in Philadelphia, 1845–1913] dermatitis herpetiformis.

Dührssen's incisions, operation (dēr'senz) [Alfred *Dührssen,* German gynecologist, 1862–1933] see under *incision* and *operation.*

Duke's method, test (dūks) [William Waddell *Duke,* pathologist in Kansas City, Missouri, 1883–1945] see *bleeding time,* under *time,* and see under *tests.*

Dukes' disease (dūks) [Clement *Dukes,* English physician, 1845–1925] see under *disease.*

Dulbecco (dool-bak'ko) Renato. Italian-born American biologist, born 1914; co-winner, with David Baltimore and Howard Temin, of the Nobel prize for medicine or physiology for 1975, for discoveries concerning the interaction between tumor viruses and the genetic material of host cells and the role of reverse transcriptase.

dulcite, dulcitol (dul'sīt, dul'sĭ-tol) [L. *dulcis* sweet] a polyhydric alcohol, $CH_2OH(CHOH)_4CH_2OH$, occurring in various plants.

dulcose (dul'kōs) dulcite.

dull (dul) not resonant on percussion.

dullness, dulness (dul'nes) diminished resonance on percussion; also a peculiar percussion sound which lacks the normal resonance. **Gerhardt's d.,** see under *triangle.* **Grocco's triangular d.,** Grocco's sign, def. 1. **postcardial d.** (obs.), dullness on percussion on the back over the site of the heart. **shifting d.,** dullness on abdominal percussion, the level of which shifts as the patient is rolled from side to side; indicative of free fluid in the abdominal cavity. **tympanitic d.,** resonance of a dull and diminished quality.

dulse (duls) a coarse red seaweed used as a food in Scotland and other northern countries.

dumb (dum) unable to speak; mute.

dumbbell (dum'bel) a dumbbell-shaped body; a mass consisting of two spherical portions connected by a narrow isthmus. **d's of Schäfer,** microscopic bodies found in striated muscular tissue.

dumbness (dum'nes) [L. *surditas*] mutism, or aphasia.

dummy (dum'e) 1. pontic. 2. placebo.

dumping (dump'ing) see under *syndrome.*

Duncan disease, syndrome (dun'kan) [*Duncan,* the original kindred in which the disease was described] see *X-linked lymphoproliferative syndrome,* under *syndrome.*

Duncan's folds, position, ventricle (dun'kanz) [James Matthews *Duncan,* British gynecologist, 1826–1890] see under *fold* and *position,* and see *cavitas septi pellucidi.*

Dunfermline scale (dun-ferm'lin) [*Dunfermline,* a city in Scotland where the scheme was devised] see under *scale.*

Dunham's fans (cones, triangles) (dun'amz) [Henry Kennon *Dunham,* American physician, 1872–1944] see under *fan.*

duodenal (du''o-de'nal) of, pertaining to, or situated in, the duodenum.

duodenectomy (du''o-dĕ-nek'to-me) [*duodenum* + Gr. *ektomē* excision] excision of the duodenum, total or partial.

duodenitis (du''od-ĕ-ni'tis) inflammation of the duodenal mucosa.

duoden(o)- [L. *duodenum,* q.v.] a combining form denoting relationship to the duodenum.

duodenocholangeitis (du''o-de''no-ko-lan''je-i'tis) inflammation of the duodenum and common bile duct.

duodenocholecystostomy (du''o-de''no-ko''le-sis-tos'to-me) surgical creation of a communication between the gallbladder and the duodenum.

duodenocholedochotomy (du''o-de''no-ko''led-o-kot'o-me) surgical incision of the duodenum and common bile duct.

duodenocolic (du''o-de''no-kol'ik) pertaining to the duodenum and colon.

duodenocystostomy (du''o-de''no-sis-tos'to-me) [*duodeno-* + Gr. *kystis* bladder + *stomoun* to provide with an opening or mouth] surgical formation of a communication between the duodenum and the gallbladder.

duodenoduodenostomy (du''o-de''no-du''o-de-nos'to-me) anastomosis of the two portions of a divided duodenum.

duodenoenterostomy (du''o-de''no-en''ter-os'to-me) surgical formation of a communication from the duodenum to another part of the small intestine.

duodenogram (du-od'ĕ-no-gram'') a roentgenogram of the duodenum.

duodenohepatic (du-od''ĕ-no''hĕ-pat'ik) pertaining to the duodenum and the liver.

duodenoileostomy (du''o-de''no-il''e-os'to-me) surgical formation of a communication between the duodenum and the ileum.

duodenojejunostomy (du″o-de″no-jĕ-joo-nos′to-me) surgical formation of a communication between the duodenum and the jejunum.

duodenolysis (du″o-dĕ-nol′ĭ-sis) the operation of loosening the duodenum from adhesions.

duodenopancreatectomy (du″o-de″no-pan″kre-ah-tek′to-me) pancreatoduodenectomy.

duodenorrhaphy (du″o-dĕ-nor′ah-fe) [*duodeno-* + Gr. *rhaphē* suture] the operation of suturing the duodenum.

duodenoscope (du″o-de″no-skōp) a fiberoptic endoscope inserted via the mouth for examining the duodenum.

duodenoscopy (du″od-ĕ-nos′ko-pe) [*duodeno-* + Gr. *skopein* to examine] endoscopic examination of the duodenum.

duodenostomy (du″od-ĕ-nos′to-me) [*duodeno-* + Gr. *stomoun* to provide with an opening or mouth] surgical formation of a permanent orifice into the duodenum.

duodenotomy (du″od-ĕ-not′o-me) [*duodeno-* + Gr. *tomē* a cutting] incision of the duodenum.

duodenum (du″o-de′num, du-od′ĕ-num) [L. *duode′ni* twelve at a time] [NA] the first or proximal portion of the small intestine, extending from the pylorus to the jejunum; so called because it is about 12 fingerbreadths in length.

duoparental (du″o-pah-ren′tal) [L. *duo* two + *parens* parent] pertaining to or derived from two parents or sexual elements.

Duphalac (du′fah-lak) trademark for a preparation of lactulose.

Duphaston (du-fas′ton) trademark for a preparation of dydrogesterone.

Duplay's bursitis (disease, syndrome), operation (doo-plāz′) [Simon Emanuel *Duplay*, French surgeon, 1836–1924] see under *bursitis* and *operation*.

duplication (doo″plĭ-ka′shun) [L. *duplicatio* doubling] in genetics, the presence in the genome of additional genetic material (a chromosome or segment thereof, a gene or part thereof). **incomplete d. of spinal cord,** diastematomyelia.

duplicitas (du-plis′ĭ-tas) [L.] a doubling, or duplication. **d. ante′rior,** katadidymus. **d. asym′metros,** heteropagus. **d. comple′ta,** a double monster in which each component is completely or almost completely developed. **d. crucia′ta,** conjoined twins with fused heads, each face being a joint product whose midplane forms a right angle with that of the body. **d. incomple′ta,** a double monster in which the two components are not completely developed. **d. infe′rior,** anadidymus. **d. me′dia,** a double monster in which the duplication is restricted to the middle region of the body. **d. paralle′la,** a double monster consisting of two components united in the sagittal plane. **d. poste′rior,** anadidymus. **d. supe′rior,** katadidymus. **d. sym′metros,** diplopagus.

dupp (dup) a syllable used to represent the second sound of the heart in auscultation; it is shorter and higher pitched than the first sound. See *lubb* and *lubb-dupp*.

Dupré's disease, syndrome (du-prāz′) [Ernest Pierre *Dupré*, French physician, 1862–1921] meningism, def. 1.

Dupuy-Dutemps' operation (du-pue′-du-tahm′) [Louis *Dupuy-Dutemps*, Paris ophthalmologist, 1871–1946] see under *operation*.

Dupuytren's contracture, etc. (du-pwe-trahnz′) [Baron Guillaume *Dupuytren*, a celebrated French surgeon, 1777–1835] see under *amputation, contracture, fracture, hydrocele,* and *sign*.

dura (du′rah) [L. "hard"] dura mater.

Durabolin (du-rab′o-lin) trademark for a preparation of nandrolone phenpropionate.

Duracillin (du″rah-sil′in) trademark for preparations of penicillin G procaine.

dural (du′ral) pertaining to the dura mater.

dura mater (du′rah ma′ter) [L. "hard mother"] the outermost, toughest, and most fibrous of the three membranes (meninges) covering the brain and spinal cord; called also *pachymeninx*. **d. m. of brain, d. m. enceph′ali** [NA], the dura mater covering the brain, composed of two mostly fused layers: an endosteal outer layer (endocranium) adherent to the inner aspect of the cranial bones, and an inner, meningeal layer. Venous sinuses and the trigeminal ganglion are located between the layers. **d. m. of spinal cord, d. m. spina′lis** [NA], the dura mater covering the spinal

cord; it is separated from the periosteum of the enclosing vertebrae by an epidural space containing blood vessels and fibrous and areolar tissue.

duramatral (du-rah-ma′tral) (*obs.*) dural.

Duran-Reynals' permeability factor [Francisco *Duran-Reynals*, American bacteriologist, 1899–1958] hyaluronidase.

Durand's disease (du-ranz′) [Paul *Durand*, French physician, born 1895] see under *disease.*

Durand-Nicolas-Favre disease [J. *Durand*, French physician of the 20th century; Joseph *Nicolas*, French physician, born 1868; Maurice Jules *Favre*, French physician, 1876–1954] lymphogranuloma venereum.

Duranest (du′rah-nest) trademark for a preparation of etidocaine hydrochloride.

duraplasty (du′rah-plas-te) [*dura mater* + Gr. *plassein* to form] a plastic operation on the dura mater; graft of the dura.

Dürck's granuloma, nodes (derks) [Hermann *Dürck*, Munich pathologist, 1869–1941] see under *granuloma* and *node.*

Dur. dolor. abbreviation for L. *duran′te dolo′re*, while the pain lasts.

Duret's lesion (du-rāz′) [Henri *Duret*, French neurological surgeon, 1849–1921] see under *lesion.*

Durham rule (dur′um) see under *rule.*

Durham's tube (dur′umz) [1. Arthur Edward *Durham*, English surgeon, 1834–1895. 2. Herbert Edward *Durham*, English bacteriologist, 1866–1945] see under *tube.*

duroarachnitis (du″ro-ar″ak-ni′tis) inflammation of the dura mater and arachnoid.

Duroziez' disease, murmur (sign) (du-ro″ze-ez′) [Paul Louis *Duroziez*, French physician, 1826–1897] see under *disease* and *murmur.*

dust (dust) fine, dry particles of earth or any other substance small enough to be blown by the wind. **blood d. (of Müller),** hemoconia. **chromatin d.,** small red granules, smaller than Howell's bodies, sometimes seen at the periphery of stained erythrocytes. **ear d.,** statoconia.

dust-borne (dust′born) spread through the air in dust particles, as an infectious disease; see under *infection.*

Dutcher body (duch′er) [Thomas F. *Dutcher*, American pathologist, born 1923] see under *body.*

Dutton's relapsing fever, spirochete (dut′unz) [Joseph Everett *Dutton*, English physician, 1877–1905] see under *fever,* and see *Borrelia duttonii.*

Duttonella (dut″o-nel′ah) [J. Everett *Dutton*] in some systems of classification a subgenus of salivarian trypanosomes including *Trypanosoma uniforme* and *T. vivax.*

Duval's nucleus (du-valz′) [Mathias Marie *Duval*, French anatomist, 1844–1907] see under *nucleus.*

Duve (dōōv) Christian René de. British-born Belgian cytologist, born 1917; co-winner, with Albert Claude and George E. Palade, of Nobel prize for medicine or physiology for 1974, for their discoveries concerning the structural and functional organization of the cell.

Duverney's foramen, gland (du-ver-nāz′) [Joseph Guichard *Duverney*, French anatomist, 1648–1730] see *foramen epiploicum* and *glandula bulbourethralis.*

Duvoid (doo′void) trademark for preparations of bethanechol chloride.

d.v. double vibrations (a unit for the measurement of the frequency of sound waves).

D.V.M. Doctor of Veterinary Medicine. Also abbreviated V.M.D.

dwale (dwāl) belladonna leaf.

dwarf (dwarf) an abnormally undersized person. **achondroplastic d.,** a type of dwarf, having a relatively large head with saddle nose and brachycephaly, short extremities, and usually lordosis; see also *achondroplasia.* **Amsterdam d.,** a dwarf affected with de Lange's syndrome. **asexual d.,** an adult dwarf with deficient sexual development. **ateliotic d.,** a dwarf whose skeleton is infantile with persistent nonunion between epiphyses and diaphyses. **bird-headed d., bird-headed d. of Seckel,** a dwarf with a proportionately small head, a narrow birdlike face with a beaklike protrusion of the nose, large eyes, antimongoloid slant of the palpebral fissures, and receding lower jaw; called also *nanocephalic d.* **Brissaud's d.,** one with infantile myxedema. **cretin d.,** a thyroid-deficient dwarf; see *cretinism.* Called also *hypothyroid d.* **diastrophic d.,** a dwarf with progressive structural deformities of the bones and joints, including scoliosis, bilateral clubfoot, deformity of the thumb, micromelia, joint contractures and subluxations, malformation of the pinna with calcification of the cartilage, premature calcification of the costal cartilages, and cleft palate. **geleophysic d.,** a dwarf with a peculiar but pleasant facial appearance and bone dysplasia, especially of the hands and feet. **hypophysial d.,** pituitary d. **hypothyroid d.,** cretin d. **infantile d.,** a person with marked retardation of mental and physical development. **Levi-Lorain d.,** pituitary d. **micromelic d.,** a dwarf with very small limbs. **nanocephalic d.,** bird-headed d. **normal d.,** a person who is abnormally undersized, but is perfectly formed. **phocomelic d.,** a dwarf in whom the diaphyses of the long bones are abnormally short. **physiologic d.,** normal d. **pituitary d.,** a dwarf whose retarded development is due to hypofunction of the anterior pituitary; called also *hypophysial d.* and *Levi-Lorain d.* **primordial d., pure d.,** normal d. **rachitic d.,** a person dwarfed by rickets, having a high forehead with prominent bosses, bent long bones, and Harrison's sulcus or groove. **renal d.,** a dwarf whose failure to achieve normal bone maturation is due to renal failure. **rhizomelic d.,** one with an autosomal recessive form of chondrodysplasia punctata, characterized by symmetric shortening of the extremities, cataracts, optic atrophy, mental retardation, fibrous joint contractures, and ichthyosis; it is lethal in early childhood. **Russell d.,** Silver's syndrome. **sexual d.,** a dwarf with normal sexual development. **Silver d.,** see under *syndrome.* **thanatophoric d.,** a micromelic dwarf having very short ribs and bones of the extremities, and vertebral bodies that are greatly reduced in height with wide intervertebral spaces; death usually occurs in the first few hours of life. **true d.,** normal d.

dwarfism (dwarf′izm) the state of being a dwarf; underdevelopment of the body; nanosomia. See various forms under *dwarf.* **deprivation d.,** maternal deprivation syndrome. **Robinow d.,** see under *syndrome.* **Walt Disney d.,** geroderma osteodysplastica.

Dy chemical symbol for *dysprosium.*

dyad (di′ad) [Gr. *dyas* the number two, from *dyo* two] a double chromosome resulting from the halving of a tetrad in the first meiotic division.

dyaster (di′as-ter) amphiaster.

Dyazide (di′ah-zīd) trademark for preparations of triamterene with hydrochlorothiazide.

Dyclone (di′klōn) trademark for preparations of dyclonine hydrochloride.

dyclonine hydrochloride (di′klo-nēn) [USP] chemical name: 1-(4-butoxyphenyl)-3-(1-piperidinyl)-1-propanone. A local anesthetic having significant bactericidal and fungicidal activity, $C_{18}H_{27}NO_2 \cdot HCl$, occurring as a white, crystalline powder or as white crystals; applied topically to the skin and mucous membranes.

dydrogesterone (di″dro-jes′ter-ōn) an orally effective, synthetic progestin occurring as a white to pale yellow, crystalline powder; used mainly in the diagnosis and treatment of primary amenorrhea and severe dysmenorrhea, and in combination with estrogen in dysfunctional menorrhagia.

dye (di) any of various colored substances that contain auxochromes and thus are capable of coloring substances to which they are applied; used for staining and coloring, as test reagents, and as therapeutic agents in medicine. **acid d., acidic d.,** one which is acidic in reaction and usually unites with positively charged ions of the material acted upon; called also *anionic d.* **amphoteric d.,** one containing both reactive basic and reactive acidic groups, and staining both acidic and basic elements. **anionic d.,** acid d. **basic d.,** one which is basic in reaction and unites with negatively charged ions of material acted upon; called also *cationic d.* **cationic d.,** basic d. **metachromatic d.,** a dye that stains tissues two or more colors. **orthochromatic d.,** a dye that stains tissues a single color. **vital d.,** one that penetrates living cells and colors certain structures, without serious injury to the cells.

Dymelor (di′mĕ-lor) trademark for a preparation of acetohexamide.

dynamic (di-nam′ik) [Gr. *dynamis* power] pertaining to or manifesting force.

dynamics (di-nam′iks) that phase of mechanics which deals with the motions of material bodies taking place under different specific conditions.

dynamization (di″nam-i-za′shun) (*obs.*) the hypothetical increase of medicinal effectiveness by dilution and trituration.

dynam(o)- [Gr. *dynamis* power] a combining form denoting relationship to power or strength.

dynamogenesis (di″nah-mo-jen′ĕ-sis) [*dynamo-* + Gr. *genesis* production] the development of energy or force, as in muscle or nerves.

dynamogenic (di″nah-mo-jen′ik) [*dynamo-* + Gr. *gennan* to produce] producing or favoring the development of power; pertaining to the development of power, as in muscle or nerves.

dynamogeny (di-nah-moj′ĕ-ne) dynamogenesis.

dynamograph (di-nam′o-graf) [*dynamo-* + Gr. *graphein* to write] a self-registering dynamometer.

dynamometer (di″nah-mom′ĕ-ter) [*dynamo-* + Gr. *metron* measure] an instrument for measuring the force of muscular contraction. **squeeze d.,** one by which the grip of the hand is measured.

dynamoneure (di-nam′o-nūr) [*dynamo-* + Gr. *neuron* nerve] a spinal neuron connected with the muscles; a spinal motoneuron.

dynamopathic (di-nam″o-path′ik) [*dynamo-* + Gr. *pathos* disease] affecting function; functional.

dynamophore (di-nam′o-fōr) [*dynamo-* + Gr. *phoros* carrying] food or any substance that supplies energy to the body.

dynamoscope (di-nam′o-skop) [*dynamo-* + Gr. *skopein* to examine] a device for performing dynamoscopy.

dynamoscopy (di″nah-mos′ko-pe) the observation of the performance of function by an organ or structure, as of muscle action or of kidney function by ureteral catheterization.

Dynapen (di′nah-pen) trademark for a preparation of dicloxacillin sodium.

dyne (dīn) the C.G.S. unit of force, being that amount of force which, when acting continuously upon a mass of 1 gram, will impart to it an acceleration of 1 cm. per second per second.

dynein (di′ne-in) a protein from the microtubules of cilia and flagella which functions as an ATP-splitting enzyme and is essential to the motility of cilia and flagella.

dyphylline (di-fil′in) chemical name: 7-(2,3-dihydroxypropyl)-3,7-dihydro-1,3-dimethyl-1*H*-purine-2,6-dione. A theophylline derivative, $C_{10}H_{14}N_4O_4$, occurring as a white, amorphous powder, having the peripheral vasodilator, bronchodilator, diuretic, and myocardial stimulant effects of the parent compound; used chiefly in the treatment of acute bronchial asthma and reversible bronchospasm associated with chronic bronchitis and emphysema; administered orally or intramuscularly. Called also *glyphylline* and *hyphylline.*

Dyrenium (di-ren′i-um) trademark for a preparation of triamterene.

dys- [Gr. *dys-*] a combining form signifying difficult, painful, bad, disordered, abnormal; the opposite of *eu-*.

dysacousia (dis″ah-koo′ze-ah) [*dys-* + Gr. *akousis* hearing + *-ia*] dysacusis.

dysacousis (dis″ah-koo′sis) dysacusis.

dysacousma (dis″ah-koōs′mah) dysacusis.

dysacusis (dis″ah-koo′sis) [*dys-* + Gr. *akousis* hearing] 1. a hearing impairment in which there is distortion of frequency or intensity. 2. a condition in which certain sounds produce discomfort; called also *auditory dysesthesia.*

dysadaptation (dis″ad-ap-ta′shun) dysaptation.

dysadrenalism (dis″ad-re′nal-izm) any disorder of adrenal function, whether of decreased function (hypoadrenalism, hypoadrenocorticism) or heightened function (hyperadrenalism, hyperadrenocorticism).

dysallilognathia (dis-al″il-lo-na′the-ah) a condition characterized by disproportion of the maxilla and mandible.

dysanagnosia (dis″an-ag-no′se-ah) a form of dyslexia in which certain words cannot be recognized.

dysantigraphia (dis″an-te-gra′fe-ah) loss of power to copy writing; it is due to a lesion of the association path between the word-seeing center and the word-writing center.

dysaphia (dis-a′fe-ah) [*dys-* + Gr. *haphē* touch] impairment of the sense of touch.

dysaptation (dis″ap-ta′shun) defective power of accommodation of the iris and retina to light variations.

dysarteriotony (dis″ar-te″re-ot′o-ne) [*dys-* + Gr. *artēria* artery + *tonos* tension] abnormality of blood pressure.

dysarthria (dis-ar′thre-ah) [*dys-* + Gr. *arthroun* to utter distinctly + *-ia*] imperfect articulation of speech due to disturbances of muscular control which result from damage to the central or peripheral nervous system. Cf. *anarthria.* **d. litera′lis,** stuttering. **d. syllaba′ris spasmod′ica,** stuttering.

dysarthric (dis-ar′thrik) characterized by or pertaining to dysarthria.

dysarthrosis (dis″ar-thro′sis) [*dys-* + Gr. *arthrōsis* joint] 1. deformity or malformation of a joint. 2. dysarthria.

dysautonomia (dis″aw-to-no′me-ah) [*dys-* + Gr. *autonomia* autonomy] an autosomal recessive disease of childhood characterized by defective lacrimation, skin blotching, emotional instability, motor incoordination, total absence of pain sensation, and hyporeflexia; seen exclusively in Jews. Called also *familial autonomic dysfunction* and *Riley-Day syndrome.*

dysbarism (dis′bar-izm) a general term applied to any clinical syndrome caused by difference between the surrounding atmospheric pressure and the total gas pressure in the various tissues, fluids, and cavities of the body, including such conditions as barotitis media, barosinusitis, or expansion of gases in the hollow viscera.

dysbasia (dis-ba′ze-ah) [*dys-* + Gr. *basis* step] difficulty in walking, especially that due to a nervous lesion. **d. angiosclerot′ica, d. angiospas′tica, d. intermit′tens angiosclerot′ica** (*obs.*), intermittent claudication. **d. lordot′ica progressi′va,** dystonia musculorium deformans.

dysbetalipoproteinemia (dis-ba″tah-lip″o-pro″te-in-e′me-ah) familial hyperlipoproteinemia, type III. **familial d.,** familial hyperlipoproteinemia, type III.

dysbolism (dis′bo-lizm) [*dys-* + *metabolism*] a condition arising from an error in metabolism not necessarily of a disease nature, as in incomplete oxidation of tyrosine, giving a reddish color to the urine.

dyscalculia (dis″kal-ku′le-ah) impairment of the ability to do mathematical problems because of brain injury or disease.

dyscephaly (dis-sef′ah-le) malformation of the cranium and bones of the face. **mandibulo-oculofacial d.,** oculomandibulofacial syndrome.

dyschesia (dis-ke′se-ah) dyschezia.

dyschezia (dis-ke′ze-ah) [*dys-* + Gr. *chezein* to go to stool + *-ia*] difficult or painful evacuation of feces from the rectum.

dyschiasia (dis-ki-a′se-ah) any disorder of sense localization.

dyschiria (dis-ki′re-ah) [*dys-* + Gr. *cheir* hand + *-ia*] derangement of the power to tell which side of the body has been touched; see *achiria, allochiria,* and *synchiria.*

dyscholia (dis-ko′le-ah) [*dys-* + Gr. *cholē* bile + *-ia*] a disordered condition of the bile.

dyschondroplasia (dis″kon-dro-pla′ze-ah) [*dys-* + Gr. *chondros* cartilage + *plassein* to form + *-ia*] enchondromatosis.

dyschondrosteosis (dis″kon-dros″te-o′sis) a form of dyschondroplasia that may produce micromelia.

dyschromasia (dis″kro-ma′ze-ah) dyschromatopsia.

dyschromatopsia (dis″kro-mah-top′se-ah) [*dys-* + Gr. *chrōma* color + *-opsia*] disorder of color vision.

dyschromia (dis-kro′me-ah) [*dys-* + Gr. *chrōma* color] any disorder of pigmentation of the skin or hair.

dyschronism (dis-kro′nizm) separate in time; disturbance of any time relation.

dyschylia (dis-ki′le-ah) disorder of the chyle.

dyscinesia (dis-si-ne′se-ah) dyskinesia.

dyscoimesis (dis″koi-me′sis) dyskoimesis.

dyscoria (dis-ko′re-ah) [*dys-* + Gr. *korē* pupil] abnormality of the form or shape of the pupil or in the reaction of the two pupils.

dyscorticism (dis-kor′tĭ-sizm) disordered functioning of the adrenal cortex.

dyscrasia (dis-kra′ze-ah) [Gr. *dyskrasia* bad temperament] a term formerly used to indicate an abnormal mixture of the four humors; in surviving usages it now is roughly synonymous with "disease" or "pathologic condition." **blood d.,** a pathologic condition of the blood, usually referring to disorders of the cellular elements of the blood. **plasma cell d's,** a diverse group of neoplastic diseases involving proliferation of a single clone of cells producing a serum M component (a monoclonal immunoglobulin or immunoglobulin fragment); the cells usually have plasma cell morphology, but may have lymphocytic or lymphoplasmacytic morphology; this group includes multiple myeloma, Waldenström's macroglobulinemia, the heavy chain diseases, benign monoclonal gammopathy, and immunocytic amyloidosis. Called also *monoclonal gammopathies* or *immunoglobulinopathies* and *paraproteinemias.*

dyscrasic (dis-kra′sik) dyscratic.

dyscratic (dis-krat′ik) [Gr. *dyskratos*] pertaining to or characterized by dyscrasia.

dysdiadochocinesia (dis″di-ad″ŏ-ko″si-ne′se-ah) dysdiadochokinesia.

dysdiadochocinetic (dis″di-ad″ŏ-ko-si-net′ik) dysdiadochokinetic.

dysdiadochokinesia (dis″di-ad″ŏ-ko-ki-ne′se-ah) impairment of the ability to perform rapid alternating movements, as sequential pronation and supination of the arm.

dysdiadochokinetic (dis″di-ad″ŏ-ko-ki-net′ik) pertaining to or characterized by dysdiadochokinesia.

dysdipsia (dis-dip′se-ah) [*dys-* + Gr. *dipsa* thirst] difficulty in drinking.

dysecoia (dis″ĕ-koi′ah) dysacusis.

dysembryoma (dis-em″bre-o′mah) teratoma.

dysembryoplasia (dis-em″bre-o-pla′se-ah) [*dys-* + Gr. *embryon* embryo + *plasis* formation + *-ia*] malformation occurring during embryonic life.

dysemia (dis-e′me-ah) [*dys-* + Gr. *haima* blood + *-ia*] (*obs.*) disorder of the blood.

dysencephalia splanchnocystica (dis-en″sĕ-fa′le-ah splank″no-sis′tĭ-kah) Meckel's syndrome.

dysenteric (dis″en-ter′ik) pertaining to or of the nature of dysentery.

dysenteriform (dis″en-ter′ĭ-form) resembling dysentery.

dysentery (dis′en-ter″e) [L. *dysenteria,* from Gr. *dys-* + *enteron* intestine] any of various disorders marked by inflammation of the intestines, especially of the colon, and attended by pain in the abdomen, tenesmus, and frequent stools containing blood and mucus. Causes include chemical irritants, bacteria, protozoa, or parasitic worms. **amebic d.,** dysentery due to ulceration of the bowel caused by severe amebiasis; it may be associated with spread of the infection to the liver and other distant sites. Called also *amebic colitis* and *intestinal amebiasis.* **bacillary d.,** an infectious disease caused by bacteria of the genus *Shigella,* and marked by intestinal pain, tenesmus, diarrhea with mucus and blood in the stools, and more or less toxemia; it is especially prevalent in tropical countries, but it frequently occurs elsewhere. Called also *Flexner's d.* and *Japanese d.* **balantidial d.,** dysentery caused by *Balantidium coli.* **bilharzial d.,** dysentery caused by the parasitic worm *Schistosoma haematobium* (*Bilharzia haematobia*). **catarrhal d.,** sprue, def. 1. **chronic d. of cattle,** Johne's disease. **ciliary d., ciliate d.,** dysentery due to ciliate organisms, such as *Balantidium coli.* **epidemic d.,** a variety that becomes epidemic and is often fatal. **flagellate d.,** dysentery due to a flagellate organism, such as *Giardia lamblia* or *Trichomonas.* **Flexner's d.,** bacillary d. **fulminant d.,** bacillary dysentery marked by collapse and toxemia and followed by death. **institutional d.,** bacillary dysentery affecting patients in an institution, especially in mental hospitals. **Japanese d.,** bacillary d. **lamb d.,** a highly fatal form of enterotoxemia affecting young lambs, caused by *Clostridium perfringens* type B, and marked by ulcerative inflammation of the intestine and fetid diarrhea, sometimes tinged with blood; it is also frequently seen in young foals and calves. **malarial d.,** that which is complicated with intermittent febrile attacks. **malignant d.,** a form in which the symptoms are all very intense and progress rapidly to a fatal ending. **protozoal d.,** amebic and balantidial dysentery. **schistosomal d.,** dysentery accompanying intestinal schistosomiasis. **scorbutic d.,** that which is an accompaniment of scurvy. **Sonne d.,** bacillary dysentery occurring in temperate regions, caused by group D dysentery bacillus, *Shigella sonnei.* **spirillar d.,** dysentery caused by spirilla in the intestines. **sporadic d.,** dysentery occurring in scattered cases that have apparently no connection. **swine d.,** a contagious form of enteritis due to *Vibrio coli*, marked by grayish feces. **viral d.,** a virus-caused dysentery occurring in epidemics and marked by acute watery diarrhea. **winter d.,** see under *scours.*

dysequilibrium (dis″e-kwĭ-lib′re-um) any derangement of proper balance.

dyserethesia (dis″er-e-the′ze-ah) [*dys-* + Gr. *erethizein* to irritate] impairment of sensibility to stimuli.

dyserethism (dis-er′e-thizm) dyserethesia.

dysergia (dis-er′je-ah) [*dys-* + Gr. *ergon* work] motor incoordination due to defect of efferent nerve impulse.

dysesthesia (dis″es-the′ze-ah) [*dys-* + Gr. *aisthēsis* perception] 1. impairment of any sense, especially of that of touch. 2. an unpleasant abnormal sensation produced by normal stimuli. **auditory d.,** dysacusis (def. 2).

dysesthetic (dis″es-thet′ik) pertaining to or characterized by dysesthesia.

dysfunction (dis-funk′shun) disturbance, impairment, or abnormality of the functioning of an organ. **constitutional hepatic d.,** Gilbert syndrome. **minimal brain d.,** attention-deficit hyperactivity disorder. **myofascial pain d.,** temporomandibular joint syndrome. **d. of uterus,** inertia uteri.

dysgalactia (dis″gah-lak′te-ah) [*dys-* + Gr. *gala* milk] disordered milk secretion.

dysgammaglobulinemia (dis-gam″mah-glob″u-lĭ-ne′me-ah) an immunological deficiency state characterized by selective deficiencies of one or more, but not all, classes of immunoglobulins.

dysgenesia (dis″jě-ne′ze-ah) [*dys-* + Gr. *gennan* to generate + *-ia*] impairment of the powers of procreation.

dysgenesis (dis-jen′ě-sis) defective development. **epiphyseal d.,** a condition in which epiphyseal centers may be irregularly formed or appear to be fragmented or stippled. **gonadal d.,** Turner's syndrome and its variants. **mixed gonadal d.,** a condition in which there is a testis on one side and a streak gonad on the other; those affected typically show some degree of virilization and ambiguous genitalia, and a uterus, vagina, and at least one fallopian tube are usually present. The most common karyotype is a mosaic, 45,XO/46,XY. **pure gonadal d.,** the gonadal lesions of Turner's syndrome occurring without the somatic features. **reticular d.,** see *severe combined immunodeficiency*, under *immunodeficiency.* **seminiferous tubule d.,** Klinefelter's syndrome.

dysgenic (dis-jen′ik) detrimental to the race or tending to counteract race improvement.

dysgenics (dis-jen′iks) [*dys-* + Gr. *gennan* to produce] the study of racial deterioration. Cf. *eugenics.*

dysgenitalism (dis-jen′ĭ-tal-izm) any abnormality of genital development, as eunuchism.

dysgenopathy (dis″jen-op′ah-the) [*dys-* + Gr. *gennan* to produce + *pathos* disease] a disorder of bodily development.

dysgerminoma (dis″jer-mĭ-no′mah) [*dys-* + *germ* + *-oma*] a malignant ovarian neoplasm, thought to be derived from primordial germ cells of the sexually undifferentiated embryonic gonad; it is the counterpart of the classical seminoma (q.v.) of the testis, to which it is both grossly and histologically identical. Called also *ovarian seminoma.*

dysgeusia (dis-gu′ze-ah) [*dys-* + Gr. *geusis* taste] distortion of the sense of taste.

dysglobulinemia (dis-glob″u-lin-e′me-ah) [*dys-* + *globulin* + Gr. *haima* blood + *-ia*] any disorder of the blood globulins.

dysglycemia (dis″gli-se′me-ah) [*dys-* + Gr. *glykys* sweet + *haima* blood + *-ia*] any derangement of the sugar content of the blood.

dysgnathia (dis-na′the-ah) [*dys-* + *gnath-* + *-ia*] an ab-

normality of the oral cavity and teeth that also involves the jaws. Cf. *eugnathia.*

dysgnathic (dis-nath′ik) [*dys-* + Gr. *gnathos* jaw] pertaining to or characterized by dysgnathia.

dysgnosia (dis-no′se-ah) [Gr. *dysgnōsia* difficulty of knowing] any disorder of intellectual function.

dysgonesis (dis″go-ne′sis) [*dys-* + Gr. *gonē* seed] a functional disorder of the genital organs.

dysgonic (dis-gon′ik) [*dys-* + Gr. *gonē* seed] seeding poorly; said of bacterial cultures, especially of species of *Mycobacterium*, that grow sparsely on culture media. Cf. *eugonic.*

dysgrammatism (dis-gram′ah-tizm) partial impairment of the ability to speak grammatically because of brain injury or disease.

dysgraphia (dis-gra′fe-ah) [*dys-* + Gr. *graphein* to write] inability to write properly; it may be part of a language disorder caused by a disturbance of the parietal lobe or of the motor system. Called also *status dysgraphicus.*

dyshematopoiesis (dis-hem″ah-to″poi-e′sis) defective blood formation.

dyshematopoietic (dis-hem″ah-to-poi-et′ik) pertaining to or characterized by dyshematopoiesis.

dyshemopoiesis (dis-he″mo-poi-e′sis) dyshematopoiesis.

dyshemopoietic (dis-he″mo-poi-et′ik) dyshematopoietic.

dyshepatia (dis-hĕ-pa′she-ah) [*dys-* + Gr. *hēpar* liver] disordered liver function. **lipogenic d.,** a liver disorder of children due to excessive fats in the diet.

dyshesion (dis-he′shun) [*dys-* + L. *haesio*, from *haerere* to stick] 1. disordered cell adherence. 2. loss of intercellular cohesion, a characteristic of malignancy, as determined by aspiration biopsy cytology.

dyshidrosis (dis-hid-ro′sis) [*dys-* + Gr. *hidrōsis* a sweating] 1. pompholyx; so called because it was formerly thought that the condition was a sweat retention disorder. 2. any disorder of the eccrine sweat glands. Spelled also *dyshydrosis.*

dyshydrosis (dis-hid-ro′sis) dyshidrosis.

dysidrosis (dis-id-ro′sis) dyshidrosis.

dysjunction (dis-junk′shun) see *disjunction.*

dyskaryosis (dis-kar″e-o′sis) abnormal changes in cell nuclei, such as those observed in epithelial cells of the cervix during pregnancy.

dyskaryotic (dis″kar-e-ot′ik) [*dys-* + Gr. *karyon* nucleus] pertaining to, characterized by, or promoting dyskaryosis.

dyskeratoma (dis″ker-ah-to′mah) a dyskeratotic tumor. **warty d.,** a benign, usually solitary, typically flesh-colored to brown elevated papule with a depressed and crusted center containing a keratotic plug, occurring in association with the pilosebaceous unit, especially on the scalp, face, neck, and axilla, and principally seen in older men. Histologically, it resembles the individual lesion of keratosis follicularis. Called also *isolated dyskeratosis follicularis.*

dyskeratosis (dis″ker-ah-to′sis) abnormal, premature, or imperfect keratinization of the keratinocytes. **d. conge′nita, congenital d.,** an X-linked syndrome with onset in childhood, and characterized by nail dystrophy, reticular cutaneous hyperpigmentation, mucosal leukokeratosis, and pancytopenia resembling that of Fanconi. Called also *Zinsser-Cole-Engman syndrome.* **hereditary benign intraepithelial d.,** a congenital hereditary disease, transmitted as an autosomal dominant trait, characterized by foamy gelatinous plaques on the conjunctiva and white thickenings resembling leukoplakia on the oral mucosa; photophobia is common in children, and blindness may occur. Called also *Witkop's* or *Witkop-Von Sallmann disease.* **isolated d. follicularis,** warty dyskeratoma.

dyskeratotic (dis″ker-ah-tot′ik) of, relating to, or affected by dyskeratosis.

dyskinesia (dis″ki-ne′ze-ah) [Gr. *dyskinēsia* difficulty of moving] impairment of the power of voluntary movement, resulting in fragmentary or incomplete movements. **biliary d.,** derangement of the filling and emptying mechanism of the gallbladder. **d. intermit′tens,** disability of the limbs, coming on intermittently, and due to impairment of the circulation. **tardive d.,** an iatrogenic extrapyramidal disorder produced by long-term administration of antipsychotic drugs; it is characterized by oral-lingual-buccal dyskinesias that usually resemble continual chewing motions with intermittent darting movements of the tongue; there may also be choreoathetoid movements of the extremities. The disorder is more common in women than in men and in the elderly than in the young, and incidence is related to drug dosage and duration of treatment. In some patients symptoms disappear within several months after antipsychotic drugs are withdrawn; in others symptoms may persist indefinitely. There are two minor variants: *withdrawal-emergent dyskinesia*, in which the symptoms appear when the drug is withdrawn abruptly, and *tardive dystonia*, in which there are dystonic rather than choreic movements.

dyskinetic (dis″ki-net′ik)   pertaining to or characterized by dyskinesia.

dyskoimesis (dis″koi-me′sis) [*dys-* + Gr. *koimēsis* sleeping] difficulty in getting to sleep.

dyslalia (dis-la′le-ah) [*dys-* + Gr. *lalein* to talk + *-ia*] impairment of utterance with abnormality of the external speech organs.

dyslexia (dis-lek′se-ah) [*dys-* + Gr. *lexis* diction]   inability to read, spell, and write words, despite the ability to see and recognize letters; a familial disorder with autosomal dominant inheritance that occurs more frequently in males.

dyslipidoses (dis″lip-ĭ-do′sēz)   plural of *dyslipidosis*.

dyslipidosis (dis″lip-ĭ-do′sis), pl. *dyslipido′ses*.   A general designation applied to a localized or systemic disturbance of fat metabolism.

dyslipoidosis (dis-lip″oi-do′sis), pl. *dyslipoido′ses*.   Dyslipidosis.

dyslipoproteinemia (dis-lip″o-pro″te-in-e′me-ah)   the presence of abnormal lipoproteins in the blood.

dyslochia (dis-lo′ke-ah) [*dys-* + Gr. *lochia* lochia]   disordered lochial discharge.

dyslogia (dis-lo′je-ah) [*dys-* + Gr. *logos* understanding]   impairment of the reasoning power; also impairment of the speech, due to mental disorders.

dysmaturity (dis-mah-tūr′ĭ-te)   placental dysfunction. **pulmonary d.,** Wilson-Mikity syndrome.

dysmegalopsia (dis″meg-ah-lop′se-ah) [*dys-* + Gr. *megas* big + *-opsia*]   a disturbance of the visual appreciation of the size of objects, in which they appear larger than they are.

dysmelia (dis-me′le-ah) [*dys-* + Gr. *melos* limb + *-ia*]   malformation of a limb or limbs as a result of a disturbance in embryonic development; the term includes defects of excessive development as well as reduction deformities. See also *amelia* and *phocomelia*.

dysmenorrhea (dis″men-o-re′ah) [*dys-* + Gr. *mēn* month + *rhein* to flow]   painful menstruation. **acquired d.,** secondary d. **congestive d.,** that which is accompanied by great congestion of the uterus. **essential d.,** painful menstruation for which there is no demonstrable cause; called also *primary d.* **inflammatory d.,** that which comes from or is due to inflammation. **d. intermenstrua′lis,** intermenstrual pain. **mechanical d.,** that which is believed to be due to mechanical interference with the flow, as from clots or flexion of the uterus. **membranous d.,** that which is characterized by membranous exfoliations derived from the uterus. **obstructive d.,** that which is due to mechanical obstruction to the discharge of the menstrual fluid. **ovarian d.,** neuralgic pain which is due to ovarian disease. **primary d.,** essential d. **psychogenic d.,** dysmenorrhea due to disturbance of psychic control. **secondary d.,** dysmenorrhea due to a definite pelvic lesion. **spasmodic d.,** that which is due to spasmodic uterine contractions. **tubal d.,** that which is due to disease of the oviduct, such as chronic salpingitis. **uterine d.,** that which arises from a uterine lesion.

dysmetabolism (dis″mě-tab′o-lizm)   defective metabolism.

dysmetria (dis-me′tre-ah) [*dys-* + Gr. *metron* measure]   a condition in which there is improper measuring of distance in muscular acts; disturbance of the power to control the range of movement in muscular action. In *hypermetria*, voluntary muscular movement overreaches the intended goal, and in *hypometria*, voluntary muscular movement falls short of reaching the intended goal.

dysmetropsia (dis″mě-trop′se-ah) [*dys-* + Gr. *metron* measure + *-opsia*]   defect in the visual appreciation of the measure or size of objects.

dysmimia (dis-mim′e-ah) [*dys-* + Gr. *mimia* imitation]   impairment of the power of expressing thought by gestures.

dysmnesia (dis-ne′se-ah) [*dys-* + Gr. *mnēmē* memory]   impaired memory.

dysmnesic (dis-ne′zik)   characterized by impairment or disorder of memory.

dysmorphic (dis-mor′fik)   pertaining to dysmorphology.

dysmorphism (dis-mor′fizm) [*dys-* + Gr. *morphē* form]   1. allomorphism.   2. the condition of appearing under different morphologic forms; for example, some fungi grow differently under parasitic and under saprophytic conditions.   3. an abnormality in morphological development, as a congenital malformation.

dysmorphologist (dis″mor-fol′o-jist)   a specialist in dysmorphology.

dysmorphology (dis″mor-fol′o-je) [*dys-* + *morpho-* + *-logy*]   a branch of clinical genetics concerned with the diagnosis and interpretation of patterns of the three types of structural defects—malformation, disruption, and deformation (q.q.v.).

dysmorphophobia (dis-mor″fo-fo′be-ah) [Gr. *dysmorphos* deformed + *phobia*]   irrational fear of deformity or of becoming deformed; a delusional belief that one is deformed.

dysmorphopsia (dis″mor-fop′se-ah) [Gr. *dysmorphos* deformed + *-opsia*]   defective vision, with distortion of the shape of objects perceived.

dysmorphosis (dis″mor-fo′sis) [Gr. *dysmorphos* deformed]   malformation.

dysmyotonia (dis″mi-o-to′ne-ah) [*dys-* + Gr. *mys* muscle + *tonos* tension]   muscular dystonia; abnormal tonicity of muscle.

dysnomia (dis-no′me-ah) [*dys-* + Gr. *onoma* name]   partial nominal aphasia; cf. *anomia.*

dysodontiasis (dis″o-don-ti′ah-sis) [*dys-* + *odonto-* + *-iasis*]   imperfect or defective dentition; defective, delayed, or difficult eruption of the teeth.

dysoemia (dis-e′me-ah) [*dys-* + Gr. *oimos* road, path]   a medicolegal term for death from obscure causes, traceable to chronic mineral poisoning.

dysontogenesis (dis″on-to-jen′ĕ-sis) [*dys-* + *ontogenesis*]   defective embryonic development.

dysontogenetic (dis″on-to-jě-net′ik)   pertaining to or characterized by dysontogenesis.

dysopia (dis-o′pe-ah) [*dys-* + *-opia*]   defective vision. **d. al′gera,** disturbances of vision due to pains in the eyes and head on looking at objects.

dysopsia (dis-op′se-ah)   dysopia.

dysorexia (dis″o-rek′se-ah) [*dys-* + Gr. *orexis* appetite]   impaired or deranged appetite.

dysorganoplasia (dis-or″gan-o-pla′se-ah) [*dys-* + Gr. *organon* organ + *plasis* formation]   disordered development of an organ.

dysoria (dis-or′e-ah) [*dys-* + Gr. *oros* serum]   any abnormality of vascular permeability.

dysoric (dis-or′ik)   pertaining to or affected with dysoria.

dysosmia (dis-oz′me-ah) [*dys-* + Gr. *osmē* smell]   distortion of the sense of smell.

dysosteogenesis (dis-os″te-o-jen′ĕ-sis)   defective bone formation; dysostosis.

dysostosis (dis″os-to′sis) [*dys-* + Gr. *osteon* bone]   defective ossification; defect in the normal ossification of fetal cartilages. **cleidocranial d.,** a rare autosomal dominant condition in which there is defective ossification of the cranial bones, with large fontanels and delayed closing of the sutures; complete or partial absence of the clavicles, so that the shoulders may be brought together, or nearly together, in front; wide pubic symphysis; short middle phalanges of the fifth fingers; and dental and vertebral anomalies. Called also *cleidocranial dysplasia.* **craniofacial d.,** an autosomal dominant disorder characterized by acrocephaly, exophthalmos, hypertelorism, strabismus, parrot-beaked nose, and hypoplastic maxilla with relative mandibular prognathism. Called also *Crouzon's disease.* **d. enchondra′lis epiphysa′ria,** dysplasia epiphysealis multiplex. **mandibulofacial d.,** a hereditary disorder occurring in two forms: the complete form (Franceschetti's syndrome) is characterized by antimongoloid slant of the palpebral fissures, coloboma of the lower lid, micrognathia and hypoplasia of the zygomatic arches, and microtia. It is transmitted as an autosomal dominant trait. The incomplete form (Treacher Collins syndrome) is characterized by the same anomalies in

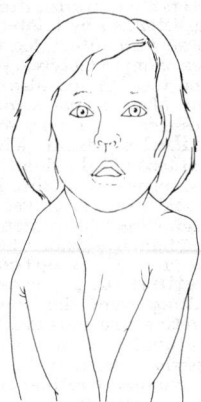

Cleidocranial dysostosis.

less pronounced degree. It occurs sporadically, but an autosomal dominant mode of transmission is suspected. **mandibulofacial d. with epibulbar dermoids,** oculoauriculovertebral dysplasia. **metaphyseal d.,** a skeletal abnormality in which the epiphyses are normal, or nearly so, and the metaphyseal tissues are replaced by masses of cartilage, producing interference with enchondral bone formation, and expansion and thinning of the metaphyseal cortices. Called also *Jansen's disease* and *metaphyseal chondrodysplasia*. **d. mul'tiplex,** a term for the widespread skeletal manifestations typical of the mucopolysaccharidoses. **Nager's acrofacial d.,** a congenital condition in which mandibulofacial dysostosis is associated with limb deformities consisting of absence of the radius, radioulnar synostosis, and hypoplasia or absence of the thumbs. **orodigitofacial d.,** oral-facial-digital syndrome.

dysoxidative (dis-ok′sĭ-da″tiv) due to deficient oxidation.

dysoxidizable (dis-ok′sĭ-diz″ah-b'l) [*dys-* + *oxidizable*] not easily oxidizable.

dyspareunia (dis″pah-roo′ne-ah) [Gr. *dyspareunos* badly mated] difficult or painful coitus.

dyspepsia (dis-pep′se-ah) [*dys-* + Gr. *peptein* to digest] impairment of the power or function of digestion; usually applied to epigastric discomfort following meals. **acid d.,** a variety associated with excessive acidity of the stomach. **appendicular d., appendix d.,** dyspeptic symptoms occurring in chronic appendicitis. **atonic d.** (obs.), a form ascribed to a lack of tone in the digestive organs; a nonspecific symptom of gastrointestinal dysfunction. **catarrhal d.,** a variety accompanied by gastric inflammation. **chichiko d.,** a condition of farinaceous malnutrition found in badly nourished infants who are fed mostly on solutions of polished rice powder. **cholelithic d.,** the sudden dyspeptic attacks characteristic of gallbladder disturbance. **colon d.,** functional disturbance of the large intestine, giving rise to the symptoms of dyspepsia. **fermentative d.,** that characterized by the fermentation of ingested food. **flatulent d.,** that which is associated with the formation of gas in the stomach, especially upper abdominal discomfort accompanied by frequent belching. **functional d.,** that which is either atonic or of reflex or nervous origin. **gastric d.,** that which originates within the stomach. **intestinal d.,** that which arises in the intestines. **nervous d.,** dyspepsia which is functional in origin. **ovarian d.,** a form of reflex indigestion due to ovarian disease. **reflex d.,** that which is due to reflex influence from some disease of an organ not directly concerned in digestion. **salivary d.** (obs.), dyspepsia due to defective or deficient saliva.

dyspeptic (dis-pep′tik) pertaining to or affected with dyspepsia.

dysperistalsis (dis″per-ĭ-stal′sis) [*dys-* + *peristalsis*] painful or abnormal peristalsis.

dysphagia (dis-fa′je-ah) [*dys-* + Gr. *phagein* to eat] difficulty in swallowing. **contractile ring d.,** dysphagia due to an overactive interior esophageal sphincteric mechanism which gives rise to painful sticking sensations under the lower sternum. **d. inflammato′ria,** dysphagia due to

inflammation of the pharynx or esophagus. **d. luso′ria,** dysphagia resulting from compression of the esophagus caused by an anomalous right subclavian artery that arises from the descending aorta and passes behind the esophagus. **d. nervo′sa,** esophagospasm. **d. paralyt′ica,** dysphagia due to paralysis of the pharyngeal or esophageal muscles. **sideropenic d.,** Plummer-Vinson syndrome. **d. spas′tica,** esophagospasm. **vallecular d.,** dysphagia caused by the lodgment of food in the valleculae. **d. valsalvia′na,** dysphagia due to subluxation of the major cornu of the hyoid bone.

dysphagy (dis′fah-je) dysphagia.

dysphasia (dis-fa′ze-ah) [*dys-* + Gr. *phasis* speech] impairment of speech, consisting in lack of coordination and failure to arrange words in their proper order, due to a central lesion.

dysphemia (dis-fe′me-ah) [*dys-* + Gr. *phēmē* speech + *-ia*] stuttering or other speech disorder of psychogenic origin.

dysphonia (dis-fo′ne-ah) [*dys-* + Gr. *phōnē* voice] any impairment of voice; a difficulty in speaking. **d. clerico′rum,** any impairment of voice; a difficulty in speaking, such as that which may be experienced by those who speak at length, e.g., clergymen. **dysplatic d.,** chronic hoarseness due to malformation of the larynx. **d. pli′cae ventricula′ris,** a condition in which phonation is performed with the false vocal cords (ventricular bands). **d. pu′berum,** the harsh, irregular utterance of puberty, and of the change of voice in youth. **spasmodic d., spastic d., d. spas′tica,** difficulty in speaking due to excessively vigorous adduction or, more rarely, abduction, of the vocal cords against each other, so that the voice is hoarse, soft, and strained.

dysphonic (dis-fon′ik) pertaining to or characterized by dysphonia.

dysphoretic (dis″fo-ret′ik) 1. dysphoric. 2. dysphoriant.

dysphoria (dis-fo′re-ah) [Gr. "excessive pain, anguish, agitation"] disquiet; restlessness; malaise.

dysphoriant (dis-fo′re-ant) 1. producing a condition of dysphoria. 2. an agent that produces dysphoria.

dysphoric (dis-for′ik) pertaining to or characterized by dysphoria.

dysphrasia (dis-fra′ze-ah) [*dys-* + Gr. *phrasis* speech + *-ia*] imperfection of utterance due to a central or cerebral defect.

dysphylaxia (dis″fi-lak′se-ah) [*dys-* + Gr. *phylaxis* watching] a condition marked by too early waking.

dyspigmentation (dis″pig-men-ta′shun) a disorder of pigmentation of the skin or hair.

dysplasia (dis-pla′se-ah) [*dys-* + Gr. *plassein* to form] abnormality of development; in pathology, alteration in size, shape, and organization of adult cells. **anhidrotic ectodermal d.,** congenital ectodermal defect. **anteroposterior facial d.,** defective development resulting in abnormal anteroposterior relationship of the maxilla and mandible to each other or to the cranial base with secondary malocclusion. **bronchopulmonary d.,** a chronic lung disease of infants, possibly related to oxygen toxicity or barotrauma, characterized by bronchiolar metaplasia and interstitial fibrosis. **d. of cervix,** cellular deviations from the normal in the epithelium of the uterine cervix, which may begin as basal cell hyperplasia and progress to anaplasia; its relationship to cervical carcinoma has not been established. **chondroectodermal d.,** achondroplasia occurring in association with defective development of skin, hair, and teeth, polydactyly, and defect of the cardiac septum; called also *Ellis-van Creveld syndrome*. **cleidocranial d.,** see under *dysostosis*. **congenital alveolar d.,** respiratory distress syndrome of newborn; see under *syndrome*. **craniocarpotarsal d.,** see under *dystrophy*. **craniodiaphyseal d.,** a hereditary condition transmitted as an autosomal recessive trait, in which progressive cranial and facial hyperostosis results in striking distortion. **craniometaphyseal d.,** metaphyseal dysplasia associated with overgrowth of the head bones, leontiasis ossea, and hypertelorism. **cretinoid d.,** abnormality of development characteristic of cretinism, consisting of dwarfism, retarded ossification, and smallness of the internal and sex organs. **dental d.,** dentoalveolar dysplasia. **dentinal d.,** an apparently hereditary disorder of dentin formation, marked by a normal appearance of coronal dentin associated with pulpal obliteration, faulty root formation, and a tendency for peripheral lesions without obvious cause. The teeth become loose and are exfoliated prematurely, probably because of the short pointed roots and periapical granulomas and cysts that are a common complication. Called also *rootless teeth.* **dentoalveolar d.,** abnormal development of two or more teeth within one or both jaws, producing disharmonious relationships between the teeth and their immediate supporting bone and periodontal structures, and resulting in malocclusion. Called also *dental d.* **diaphyseal d.,** a condition characterized by thickening of the cortex of the mid-shaft area of the long bones, progressing toward the epiphyses, the thickening sometimes occurring also in the flat bones; excessive growth in length of bones of the extremities usually results in abnormal stature. Called also *diaphyseal sclerosis* and *Engelmann's disease.* **ectodermal d's,** a group of hereditary disorders involving tissues and structures derived from the embryonic ectoderm; ectodermal dysplasia is a component of various syndromes, including anhidrotic and hidrotic ectodermal dysplasia and the EEC syndrome. **ectodermal d., anhidrotic,** an X-linked disorder or, rarely, an autosomal recessive disorder with full expression in both sexes, characterized by ectodermal dysplasia associated with aplasia or hypoplasia of the sweat glands, hypothermia, alopecia, anodontia, conical teeth, and typical facies with frontal bossing, midfacial hypoplasia, saddle nose, large chin, and thick lips. Called also *Christ-Siemens-Touraine syndrome, congenital ectodermal defect,* and *hypohidrotic ectodermal d.* **ectodermal d., hidrotic,** an autosomal dominant disorder characterized by ectodermal dysplasia associated with dystrophic, hypoplastic, or absent teeth, hypotrichosis, hyperpigmentation of the skin over the joints, hyperkeratosis of the palms and soles, and occasionally small teeth with extensive decay. Called also *Clouston's syndrome.* **ectodermal d., hypohidrotic,** anhidrotic ectodermal d. **encephaloophthalmic d.,** Krause syndrome. **epiphyseal d.,** faulty growth and ossification of the epiphyses, with roentgenographically apparent stippling and decreased stature, not associated with thyroid disease. See *d. epiphysealis hemimelica, d. epiphysealis multiplex,* and *chondrodysplasia punctata.* **d. epiphysea'lis hemimel'ica,** a rare condition characterized by swellings in the extremities, usually on the inner and outer aspects of the ankles and knees, made up of bone covered with epiphyseal cartilage, and leading to limitation of motion of the joints. Called also *tarsoepiphyseal aclasis* and *Trevor's disease.* **d. epiphysea'lis mul'tiplex,** a developmental abnormality of various epiphyses, which appear late and are mottled, flattened, fragmented, and usually hypoplastic; the digits are short and thick, with blunt ends, and stature may be diminished owing to flattening deformities at the hips, knees, and ankles. Called also *dysostosis enchondralis epiphysaria.* **d. epiphysea'lis puncta'ta,** chondrodysplasia punctata. **faciogenital d.,** Aarskog's syndrome. **familial white folded mucosal d.,** white sponge nevus. **fibrous d. (of bone),** a disease of bone marked by thinning of the cortex and replacement of bone marrow by gritty fibrous tissue containing bony spicules, producing pain, disability, and gradually increasing deformity. Only one bone may be involved (*monostotic fibrous d.*), with the process later affecting several or many bones (*polyostotic fibrous d.*). When associated with melanotic pigmentation of the skin and endocrine disorders, it is known as *Albright's syndrome.* **fibrous d. of jaw,** cherubism. **hereditary bone d.,** a heterogeneous group of more than 80 distinct skeletal disorders associated with abnormalities in the size, shape, and proportions of the limbs, trunk, and skull, often resulting in short, disproportionate stature. **d. linguofacia'lis,** oral-facial-digital syndrome. **metaphyseal d.,** a disturbance in enchondral bone growth, failure of modeling causing the ends of the shafts to remain larger than normal in circumference; called also *Pyle's disease.* See also *craniometaphyseal d.* **multiple epiphyseal d.,** d. epiphysealis multiplex. **oculoauricular d., oculoauriculovertebral (OAV) d.,** a congenital condition in which colobomas of the upper eyelid, epibulbar dermoids, bilateral accessory auricular appendages anterior to the ears, and vertebral anomalies are frequently associated with characteristic facies, consisting of asymmetry of the skull, prominent frontal bossing, low hairline, mandibular hypoplasia, low-set ears, and, sometimes, hemifacial microstomia. Called also *Goldenhar's syndrome, mandibulofacial dysostosis with epibulbar dermoids,* and *OAV syndrome.* **oculodentodigital (ODD) d., oculodentoosseous d. (ODOD),**

a rare hereditary condition transmitted as an autosomal dominant trait, characterized by bilateral microphthalmos, abnormally small nose with anteverted nostrils, hypotrichosis, dental anomalies, camptodactyly, syndactyly, and missing phalanges of the toes. Called also *dysplasia oculodentodigitalis syndrome, Meyer-Schwickerath and Weyers syndrome, oculodento-osseous syndrome,* and *ODD syndrome.* **ophthalmomandibulomelic d.,** a hereditary syndrome transmitted as an autosomal dominant trait, consisting of blindness caused by corneal opacities, temperomandibular fusion, absent coronoid process, obtuse mandibular angle, radiohumeral and radioulnar dislocations, and aplasia of the lateral condyle of the humerus, radial head, and distal ulna. Called also *OMM syndrome.* **progressive diaphyseal d.,** diaphyseal d. **retinal d.,** 1. a general term for a congenital defect resulting from the abnormal growth and differentiation of a retina that fails to develop into functioning tissue and forms tubular, acinic rosettes. Further ocular defects, e.g. microphthalmos, may be present; syndromic abnormalities may accompany retinal changes. 2. amaurosis congenita. 3. a synonym for, or a conspicuous feature of, Krause syndrome and Patau syndrome. **spondyloepiphyseal d.,** a hereditary dysplasia of the vertebrae and extremities resulting in dwarfism of the short-trunk type, often with shortened limbs due to epiphyseal abnormalities. In the delayed onset form, the principal feature is precocious osteoarthritis. There are several forms, including autosomal dominant, autosomal recessive, and X-linked forms, the dominant form often being associated with such ocular anomalies as myopia and detached retina. **Streeter's d.,** congenital ringlike concentric bands on the limbs or trunk. **thymic d.,** any of a group of hereditary disorders, some transmitted as an autosomal recessive trait and others as an X-linked recessive trait, characterized by faulty development of the thymus, which may be associated with (*a*) normal serum immunoglobulin levels and impaired cell-mediated immunity (Nezelof's syndrome), (*b*) Swiss type agammaglobulinemia and impairment of both cell-mediated and humoral immunity, or (*c*) variable deficiencies of immunoglobulins, the severity being dependent on the degree of the deficiency. **ureteral neuromuscular d.,** megaloureter.

dysplastic (dis-plas'tik)   marked by dysplasia.

dyspnea (disp'ne-ah) [Gr. *dyspnoia* difficulty of breathing] difficult or labored breathing. **cardiac d.,** distressful breathing caused by heart disease. **exertional d.,** dyspnea provoked by physical effort or exertion. **expiratory d.,** difficulty in breathing caused by hindrance to the free egress of air from the lungs. **functional d.,** respiratory distress not caused by organic disease and unrelated to exertion but associated with anxiety states; see also *sighing d.* **inspiratory d.,** difficulty in breathing caused by hindrance to the free ingress of air into the lungs. **nocturnal d.,** respiratory distress that is minimal in the morning, and may gradually progress until it becomes quite disturbing at night. **nonexpansional d.,** difficulty in breathing caused by inadequate expansion of the chest. **orthostatic d.,** difficulty in breathing experienced when in the erect position. **paroxysmal nocturnal d.,** a form of respiratory distress related to posture (especially reclining at night) and usually attributed to congestive heart failure with pulmonary edema. **renal d.,** difficulty in breathing attributable to kidney disease. **sighing d.,** a syndrome characterized by intermittent deep sighing respirations, the depth of inspiration being greatly increased, without significant alteration in the respiratory rate and without wheezing; it is associated with functional or emotional rather than organic disorders, and is characteristic of functional dyspnea.

dyspneic (disp-ne'ik)   pertaining to or characterized by dyspnea.

dyspoiesis (dis''poi-e'sis)   a disorder of formation, as of blood cells.

dysponderal (dis-pon'der-al) [*dys-* + L. *pondus* weight] pertaining to disorder of weight, either obesity or underweight.

dysponesis (dis''po-ne'sis) [*dys-* + Gr. *ponēsis* toil, exertion] a reversible physiopathologic state consisting of unnoticed, misdirected neurophysiologic reactions to various agents (environmental events, bodily sensations, emotions, and thoughts) and the repercussions of these reactions throughout the organism. These errors in energy expenditure, which are capable of producing functional disorders, consist mainly of covert errors in action-potential output from the motor and premotor areas of the cortex and the consequences of that output.

dyspragia (dis-pra'je-ah) [Gr. *dyspragia* ill success] painful performance of any function. **d. intermit'tens angiosclerot'ica intestina'lis,** intestinal (abdominal) angina.

dyspraxia (dis-prak'se-ah) [Gr. *dyspraxia* ill success] partial loss of ability to perform coordinated acts.

dysprosium (dis-pro'se-um) one of the rare earth elements, atomic number 66, atomic weight 162.50, symbol Dy.

dysprosody (dis-pros'o-de) disturbance of stress, pitch, and rhythm of speech.

dysproteinemia (dis-pro"te-in-e'me-ah) [*dys-* + *protein* + Gr. *haima* blood + *-ia*] derangement of the protein content of the blood.

dysraphia, dysraphism (dis-ra'fe-ah; dis'rah-fizm) [*dys-* + Gr. *raphē* seam] incomplete closure of a raphe; defective fusion, e.g., of the neural tube.

dysreflexia (dis"re-fleks'e-ah) a condition of disordered response to stimuli. **autonomic d.,** a syndrome affecting persons with lesions of the spinal cord above the mid-thoracic level, characterized by paroxysmal hypertension, bradycardia, excessive sweating, facial flushing, nasal congestion, pilomotor responses, and headache. It is due to an exaggerated autonomic response to such stimuli as distention of the bladder or rectum.

dysrhaphia, dysrhaphism (dis-ra'fe-ah; dis'rah-fizm) dysraphia.

dysrhythmia (dis-rith'me-ah) [*dys-* + Gr. *rhythmos* any regularly recurring motion + *-ia*] disturbance of rhythm, as abnormality of rhythm in speech: *d. pneumophra'sia* is defective breath grouping; *d. proso'dia* is defective placement of stress; *d. to'nia* is defective inflection. **cerebral d.,** disturbance or irregularity in the rhythm of the brain waves as recorded by electroencephalography; called also *electroencephalographic d.* **electroencephalographic d.,** cerebral d. **esophageal d.,** diffuse esophageal spasm.

dyssebacea (dis"se-ba'she-ah) dyssebacia.

dyssebacia (dis"se-ba'she-ah) [*dys-* + *sebum*] a condition clinically indistinguishable from seborrheic dermatitis due to alteration of the pattern of sebaceous gland retention, usually occurring as a manifestation of ariboflavinosis, and characterized by greasy scaling lesions involving the alae nasi, malar areas, canthi of the eyes, and earlobes and sometimes the scrotum or vulva.

dyssocial (dis-so'shal) (*obs.*) denoting antisocial or criminal behavior not associated with the personality traits of antisocial personality disorder and thus not attributable to mental disorder.

dyssomnia (dis-som'ne-ah) [*dys-* + L. *somnus* sleep] any disorder of sleep.

dysspermia (dis-sper'me-ah) [*dys-* + Gr. *sperma* seed + *-ia*] impairment of the spermatozoa, or of the semen.

dysstasia (dis-sta'se-ah) [*dys-* + Gr. *stasis* standing] difficulty in standing; dystasia.

dysstatic (dis-stat'ik) pertaining to or characterized by dysstasia.

dyssymbolia (dis"sim-bo'le-ah) failure of conceptual thinking so that thoughts cannot be intelligently formulated in language.

dyssymboly (dis-sim'bo-le) dyssymbolia.

dyssymmetry (dis-sim'ĕ-tre) a condition characterized by absence of symmetry.

dyssynergia (dis"sin-er'je-ah) [*dys-* + Gr. *synergia* cooperation] disturbance of muscular coordination. **biliary d.,** failure of coordinated action of the different parts of the biliary system. **d. cerebella'ris myoclon'ica,** dyssynergia cerebellaris progressiva associated with myoclonus epilepsy; called also *Hunt's disease.* **d. cerebella'ris progressi'va,** a condition marked by generalized intention tremors associated with disturbance of muscle tone and of muscular coordination; due to disorder of cerebellar function. Called also *Ramsay Hunt syndrome.*

dyssystole (dis-sis'to-le) [*dys-* + *systole*] (*obs.*) abnormal cardiac systole, especially asystole.

dystasia (dis ta'she-ah) [*dys-* + (s)*tasis*] difficulty in standing; dysstasia. **hereditary ataxic d., Roussy-Lévy hereditary ataxic d.,** Roussy-Lévy syndrome.

dystaxia (dis-tak'se-ah) [*dys-* + Gr. *taxis* arrangement] difficulty in controlling voluntary movements; partial ataxia.

dystectia (dis-tek'she-ah) [*dys-* + L. *tectum* roof] defective closure of the neural tube, resulting in such malformations as anencephaly, porencephaly, meningocele, spina bifida, etc.

dysteleology (dis"te-le-ol'o-je) 1. the study of apparently useless organs or parts. 2. lack of purposefulness, or of contribution to the final result.

Dysteriina (dis"ter-i'ĭ-nah) a suborder of mainly marine, free-living or commensal ciliate protozoa (order Cyrtophorida, superorder Phyllopharyngidea), generally having reduced ciliature and a relatively narrow body, a well-developed adhesive organelle (often with a protruding mobile appendix), and a heteromerous macronucleus; the nematodesmata of the cyrtos may be few in number, sometimes with prominent teethlike capitula.

dysthymia (dis-thi'me-ah) [*dys-* + Gr. *thymos* mind] [DSM III-R] a mood disorder characterized by depressed feeling (sad, blue, low, down in the dumps) and loss of interest or pleasure in one's usual activities and in which the associated symptoms have persisted for more than two years but are not severe enough to meet the criteria for major depression. Called also *depressive neurosis.*

dysthymic (dis-thi'mik) depressed.

dysthyreosis (dis"thi-re-o'sis) dysthyroidism.

dysthyroid, dysthyroidal (dis-thi'roid; dis"thi-roid'al) denoting defective functioning of the thyroid gland.

dysthyroidism (dis-thi'roid-izm) imperfect development and function of the thyroid gland.

dystimbria (dis-tim'bre-ah) defect in quality or resonance of the voice.

dystithia (dis-tith'e-ah) [*dys-* + Gr. *tithēnē* a nurse + *-ia*] difficulty in breast feeding.

dystocia (dis-to'se-ah) [*dys-* + Gr. *tokos* birth] abnormal labor or childbirth. **cervical d.,** dystocia caused by mechanical obstruction at the ostium uteri. **constriction ring d., contraction ring d.,** difficult labor caused by contraction of an area of circular muscle fibers, which may occur at various levels of the parturient uterus. **fetal d.,** that which is due to the shape, size, or position of the fetus. **maternal d.,** that which is due to some condition inherent in the mother. **placental d.,** difficulty in delivering the placenta.

dystonia (dis-to'ne-ah) [*dys-* + Gr. *tonos*] disordered tonicity of muscle. **d. defor'mans progressi'va,** d. musculorum deformans. **d. lenticula'ris,** dystonia due to a lesion of the lenticular nucleus. **d. musculo'rum defor'mans,** a rare, chronic, genetic disease marked by involuntary, irregular, clonic contortions of the muscles of the trunk and extremities. The symptoms appear chiefly on walking, at which time the contortions twist the body forward and sideways in a grotesque fashion (tortipelvis). An autosomal recessive form occurs before puberty, principally among Jews; the autosomal dominant form has a later onset and is not as consistent in severity. Called also *Ziehen-Oppenheim disease, dystonia deformans progressiva, dysbasia lordotica progressiva,* and *torsion dystonia* or *neurosis.* **tardive d.,** a variant of tardive dyskinesia in which there are dystonic movements. **torsion d.,** d. musculorum deformans.

dystonic (dis-ton'ik) pertaining to or characterized by dystonia.

dystopia (dis-to'pĕ-ah) [*dys-* + Gr. *topos* place] malposition; faulty placement of an organ.

dystopic (dis-top'ik) misplaced; out of its normal place.

dystopy (dis'to-pe) dystopia.

dystrophia (dis-tro'fe-ah) [L.] dystrophy. **d. adipo'sa cor'neae,** primary fatty degeneration of the cornea; called also *xanthomatosis corneae.* **d. adiposogenita'lis,** adiposogenital dystrophy. **d. brevicol'lis,** a condition of dwarfism characterized especially by shortness of the neck. **d. endothelia'lis cor'neae,** cornea guttata. **d. epithelia'lis cor'neae,** dystrophy of the epithelium of the cornea marked by erosions; called also *Fuchs' dystrophy.* **d. media'na canalifor'mis,** d. unguis mediana canaliformis. **d. mesoderma'lis conge'nita hyperplas'tica,** Weill-Marchesani syndrome. **d. myoto'nica** myotonic dystrophy; see under *dystrophy.* **d. un'guium,** dystrophy of the nails; changes in the color, texture, and structure of the nails. Called also *onychodystrophy.* **d.**

un'guis media'na canalifor'mis, a deep longitudinal split or canal in the nail plate, sometimes showing lateral branches. Called also *d. mediana canaliformis* and *solenonychia.*

dystrophic (dis-trof'ik) pertaining to or characterized by dystrophy.

dystrophodextrin (dis"trof-o-deks'trin) [*dys-* + Gr. *trophē* nutrition + *dextrin*] a starchlike material said to exist in normal blood.

dystrophoneurosis (dis-trof"o-nu-ro'sis) [*dys-* + Gr. *trophē* nutrition + *neurosis*] 1. any nervous disorder due to poor nutrition. 2. impairment of nutrition which is caused by nervous disorder.

dystrophy (dis'tro-fe) [L. *dystrophia*, from *dys-* + Gr. *trephein* to nourish] any disorder arising from defective or faulty nutrition, especially the muscular dystrophies. **adiposogenital d.,** a condition characterized by adiposity of the feminine type and genital hypoplasia associated with lesions of the hypothalamus. Called also *Fröhlich's syndrome.* **Albright's d.,** see under *syndrome.* **asphyxiating thoracic d. (ATD),** a congenital hereditary syndrome transmitted as an autosomal recessive trait, in which chondrodystrophy of the rib cage, usually causing asphyxia early in the newborn period, occurs in association with defects of the phalanges and pelvis; called also *Jeune's syndrome* and *thoracic-pelvic-phalangeal dystrophy.* **Becker's d., Becker's muscular d.,** a form closely resembling pseudohypertrophic muscular dystrophy but having a late onset and slowly progressive course; it is transmitted as an X-linked recessive trait. **Best's macular d.,** a form of early macular degeneration. **Biber-Haab-Dimmer d.,** lattice d. **corneal d.,** see *granular corneal d., lattice d., macular corneal d., Salzmann's nodular corneal d., cornea guttata, dystrophia epithelialis corneae,* and *dystrophia adiposa corneae.* **craniocarpotarsal d.,** a congenital anomaly transmitted as an autosomal dominant trait, consisting of characteristic flattened, masklike facies; microstomia, the lips protruding as in whistling; deep-set eyes with hypertelorism; camptodactyly with ulnar deviation of the fingers; and talipes equinovarus. Called also *Freeman-Sheldon syndrome, whistling face syndrome,* and *whistling face–windmill vane hand syndrome.* **Dejerine-Landouzy d.,** Landouzy-Dejerine d. **distal muscular d.,** late distal hereditary myopathy. **Duchenne type muscular d.,** pseudohypertrophic muscular d. **Duchenne-Landouzy d.,** Landouzy-Dejerine d. **Erb's d.,** pseudohypertrophic muscular d. **facioscapulohumeral muscular d.,** Landouzy-Dejerine d. **familial osseous d.,** Morquio's syndrome. **Fuchs' d.,** dystrophia epithelialis corneae. **Gowers type muscular d.,** late distal hereditary myopathy. **granular corneal d. (Groenouw's type I),** a dominantly transmitted form of corneal dystrophy occurring during the first decade and characterized by the presence of small opacities in the superficial layers of the cornea, which form a granular disk. **hereditary vitelliform d.,** congenital macular degeneration. **infantile neuroaxonal d.,** progressive hereditary degenerative encephalopathy transmitted as an autosomal recessive trait, beginning in infancy with muscular hypotonia and arrest of development in late infancy, followed by dementia, blindness, spasticity, and ataxia. Pathologically it is characterized by widespread focal swellings and degeneration of the axons with scattered spheroids in the brain. Called also *Seitelberger's disease* and *spastic amaurotic axonal idiocy.* **Landouzy's d.,** Landouzy-Dejerine d. **Landouzy d., Landouzy-Dejerine d.,** a relatively benign autosomal dominant form of muscular dystrophy in which there is marked atrophy of the muscles of the face, shoulder girdle, and arm, producing a facial expression called myopathic face. Most patients enjoy a normal life-span.

Called also *facioscapulohumeral muscular d.* or *atrophy.* **lattice d. (of cornea),** hereditary dystrophy of the cornea marked clinically by linear lesions having a filamentous interwoven appearance and histologically by fusiform areas of hyaline degeneration and dense deposits of hyalin between the epithelium and Bowman's membrane; called also *Biber-Haab-Dimmer d.* **Leyden-Möbius d.,** limb-girdle muscular d. **limb-girdle muscular d.,** a slowly progressive form of muscular dystrophy affecting either sex and usually beginning in childhood, sometimes in maturity or later; it is characterized by weakness and wasting in the shoulder or pelvic girdle. Called also *Leyden-Möbius d.* or *type.* **macular corneal d. (Groenouw's type II),** a recessively transmitted form of corneal dystrophy occurring during the first or second decade and characterized by the presence of macular opacities with indistinct irregular borders, between which the stroma is cloudy. **muscular d.,** a group of genetic degenerative myopathies characterized by weakness and atrophy of muscle without involvement of the nervous system. There are three main types: pseudohypertrophic muscular dystrophy, facioscapulohumeral dystrophy, and limb-girdle muscular dystrophy. Other forms include distal muscular dystrophy, ocular myopathy, and myotonic dystrophy. **myotonic d.,** a rare, slowly progressive, hereditary disease transmitted as an autosomal dominant trait, characterized by myotonia followed by atrophy of the muscles (especially those of the face and neck), cataracts, hypogonadism, frontal balding, and cardiac abnormalities; called also *dystrophia myotonica, myotonia atrophica,* and *Steinert's disease.* **oculocerebrorenal d.,** see under *syndrome.* **progressive muscular d.,** muscular d. **progressive tapetochoroidal d.,** choroideremia. **pseudohypertrophic muscular d.,** a chronic progressive disease affecting the shoulder and pelvic girdles, commencing in early childhood. It is characterized by increasing weakness, pseudohypertrophy of the muscles followed by atrophy, lordosis, and a peculiar swaying gait with the legs kept wide apart. The disorder is transmitted as an X-linked trait, and affected individuals, predominantly males, rarely survive to maturity; death is usually due to respiratory weakness or heart failure. Called also *Duchenne muscular d.* or *type, Erb's d.* or *paralysis, pseudohypertrophic muscular atrophy* or *paralysis,* and *Zimmerlin's d.* or *type.* **reflex sympathetic d.,** a disturbance of the sympathetic nervous system marked by pallor or rubor, pain, sweating, edema, or skin atrophy following sprain, fracture or injury to nerves or blood vessels. **Salzmann's nodular corneal d.,** a progressive hypertrophic degeneration of the epithelial layer of the cornea, Bowman's membrane, and the outer portion of the corneal stroma. **Simmerlin's d.,** limb-girdle muscular d. **tapetochoroidal d.,** choroideremia. **thoracic-pelvic-phalangeal d.,** asphyxiating thoracic d. **thyroneural d.,** a condition marked by chorea, athetosis, rigidity, ataxia, and other indications of disturbed function of the autonomic nervous system with mental and thyroid defects. **wound d.,** a syndrome of defective protein metabolism (hypoproteinemia) that sometimes develops after severe injury.

dystrypsia (dis-trip'se-ah) [*dys-* + *trypsin* + *-ia*] derangement of intestinal or pancreatic digestion due to lack of trypsin.

dysuresia (dis-u-re'se-ah) dysuria.

dysuria (dis-u're-ah) [*dys-* + Gr. *ouron* urine + *-ia*] painful or difficult urination. **spastic d.,** difficult urination due to spasm of the bladder.

dysuriac (dis-u're-ak) an individual exhibiting dysuria.

dysuric (dis-u'rik) pertaining to dysuria.

dysvitaminosis (dis"vi-tah-min-o'sis) a disorder due to an excess or deficiency of a vitamin.

dyszoospermia (dis-zo-o-sper'me-ah) [*dys-* + *zoospermia*] a disorder of spermatozoon formation.

E symbol for *exa-*.

E symbol for *elastance, electromotive force* (voltage, redox potential), *energy*, and *expectation* (in probability and statistics).

E- [Ger. *entgegen* opposite] a stereodescriptor used to specify the absolute configuration of compounds having double bonds. The substituents attached to the double-bonded carbons are ranked according to the sequence rules described below; then if the higher priority substituents are on the same side of the double bond the configuration is *Z*, otherwise *E*. In the simple case when both carbons have the same pair of substituents, *Z* is equivalent to *cis-*, *E-* to *trans*. Substituent atoms or groups have higher priority if the atom to which the bond is attached has a higher atomic number (higher mass number for isotopes); e.g., —OH > —NH₂ > —CH₃. In case of ties the ranking is based on the priority of the atoms attached to the first atoms; e.g., —CH₂OH > —CH(CH₃)₂ > —CH₂CH₃ because (O,H,H,) > (C,C,H) > (C,H,H). Double (triple) bonds are treated as if they were two (three) single bonds to identical copies of the multiply bonded substituent; e.g., —CHO > —CH₂OH because (O,O,H) > (O,H,H,). If the secondary atoms are tied, the decision is based on tertiary atoms bonded to the secondary atoms, and so forth; e.g., —CH₂CH₂-CH₃ > —CH₂CH₃.

E° symbol for *standard electrode potential* (*standard reduction potential*).

E₁ estrone.

E₂ estradiol.

E₃ estriol.

E₄ estetrol.

ε epsilon, the fifth letter of the Greek alphabet; symbol for *molar absorptivity*, the heavy chain of IgE, and the ε chain of hemoglobin.

η eta, the seventh letter of the Greek alphabet; symbol for viscosity.

e symbol for base of natural logarithms (approximately 2.7182818285).

e⁺ symbol for *positron*.

e⁻ symbol for *electron*.

EAC symbol for *erythrocyte, antibody,* and *complement,* sometimes used to denote complement complexes, e.g., EAC1 4b2a.

EACA epsilon-aminocaproic acid; see *ε-aminocaproic acid*.

ead. abbreviation for L. *ea'dem,* the same.

EAE experimental allergic encephalomyelitis.

EAHF *e*czema, *a*sthma, *h*ay fever; see *EAHF complex,* under *complex*.

Eales' disease (ēlz) [Henry *Eales,* British physician, 1852–1913] see under *disease*.

EAP epiallopregnanolone.

Ea. R. abbreviation for Ger. *Entartungs-Reaktion,* reaction of degeneration.

ear (ēr) [L. *auris;* Gr. *ous*] the organ of hearing and of equilibrium, consisting of the external ear, the middle ear, and the internal ear; called also *auris* [NA]. See Plate 15.] **acute e.,** acute middle ear catarrh, otitis media catarrhalis acuta. **aviator's e.,** barotitis media. **Aztec e.,** an ear in which the lobule is wanting, the whole ear looking as if it were pushed forward and downward. **bat e.,** lop e. **beach e.,** maceration and inflammation of the auditory canal as a result of ocean bathing. **Blainville e's,** asymmetry of the two ears. **Cagot e.,** an ear in which the lobule is wanting. **cat's e.,** an ear that is folded over on itself. **cauliflower e.,** a partially deformed auricle caused by injury and subsequent perichondritis. **cup e.,** a protruding ear which in its milder form presents a poorly developed or unformed antihelical crus with deficient or faulty development of the superior helix, and exaggerated overdevelopment of its deep "cup-shaped," concave concha. In the severe forms, the ear is smaller than normal and the helical rim is shortened to such an extent that the helix margin, or fold, cups forward and over the scapha as a hood. **Darwin's e.,** an ear having an eminence on the edge of the helix. **diabetic e.,** mastoiditis complicating diabetes. **external e.,** the pinna and external meatus together (auris externa [NA]). **glue e.,** a chronic condition marked by a collection of fluid of high viscosity in the middle ear, due to obstruction of the eustachian tube. **hairy e's,** hypertrichosis pinnae auris. **Hong Kong e.,** otomycosis. **hot weather e.,** an otitis externa, especially of the meatus, which is rather common in the hot and humid tropics and is often caused by *Pseudomonas aeruginosa.* **inner e., internal e.,** the labyrinth, comprising the vestibule, cochlea, and semicircular canals (auris interna [NA]). **insane e.** (*obs.*), hematoma of the ear. **lop e.,** deformity of the external ear in which the conchal portion grows at a right angle to the head; called also *bat e.* **middle e.,** the space in the temporal bone comprising the tympanic cavity, mastoid appendages, and auditory tube; called also *auris media.* [NA]. Formerly, the terms *middle ear* and *tympanic cavity* were regarded as being synonymous. **Morel e.,** a deformed ear marked by abnormal development of the helix, anthelix, and scaphoid fossa, so that the folds of the ear seem obliterated, and the ear is smooth, large, and often prominent, with a thin edge. **Mozart e.,** congenital fusion of the crura of the anthelix and the helix. **outer e.,** external e. **prizefighter e.,** cauliflower e. **satyr e.,** one with a pointed pinna. **scroll e.,** one in which the pinna is rolled up. **Singapore e.,** otomycosis. **swimmer's e.,** otitis externa. **tank e.,** a condition like beach ear from bathing in swimming pools. **tropical e.,** a local infection of the external auditory meatus prevalent in tropical and semitropical countries. **Wildermuth's e.,** a deformed ear with prominent anthelix and poorly developed helix.

earache (ēr'āk) pain in the ear; otalgia.

eardrum (ēr'drum) 1. loosely, tympanic membrane (*membrana tympani* [NA]). 2. the tympanic cavity (*cavitas tympanica* [NA]).

ear-minded (ēr'mīnd-ed) audile.

earth (erth) 1. the soil and other pulverulent substances forming the ground. 2. any amorphous, easily pulverizable mineral. **alkaline e.,** any oxide of the alkaline earth metals. **diatomaceous e.,** infusorial earth. **fuller's e.,** an impure aluminum silicate having decolorizing and purifying properties. **infusorial e.,** a silicious earth composed mostly of the frustules and fragments of diatoms. By boiling with dilute hydrochloric acid, washing, and calcining, it can be so purified as to be a very pure form of silica, SiO_2 (terra silicea purificata). It is often mixed with clay and used in various industries. Called also *diatomaceous e.* **silicious e., purified** [NF], a form of silica (*infusorial e.*), SiO_2, purified by boiling with acid, washing, and calcining; used as a pharmaceutical filtering agent.

earwax (ēr'waks) cerumen.

Eaton-Lambert syndrome (e't'n lam'bert) [L.M. *Eaton,* American neurologist, 1905–1958; Edward H. *Lambert,* American physiologist, born 1915] see under *syndrome*.

E.B. elementary body.

Eberth's lines (ā'berts) [Karl Joseph *Eberth,* pathologist in Halle, 1835–1926] see under *line*.

Eberthella (e″ber-thel'ah) [K. J. *Eberth,* German pathologist, 1835–1926] a genus of bacteria of the family Enterobacteriaceae, made up of organisms now classified in various other genera.

Ebner's fibrils, etc. (eb'nerz) [Victor *Ebner* von Rofenstein, histologist in Vienna, 1842–1925] see under *fibril, gland, line,* and *reticulum*.

ebonation (e″bo-na'shun) [L. *e* out + *bone*] the removal of bone fragments from a wound.

ébranlement (a-brahnl-maw') [Fr.] removal of a polyp by twisting the pedicle of the tumor.

ebriety (e-bri'ĕ-te) drunkenness; inebriety.

Ebstein's angle, anomaly, disease (eb'stīnz) [Wilhelm *Ebstein,* physician in Göttingen, 1836–1912] see *cardiohepatic angle,* under *angle,* and see under *anomaly* and *disease*.

ebullition (eb-u-lish'un) [L. *ebullire* to boil] 1. the process or condition of boiling. 2. the motion of a boiling liquid.

ebur (e'bur) [L.] ivory. **e. den'tis,** dentin.

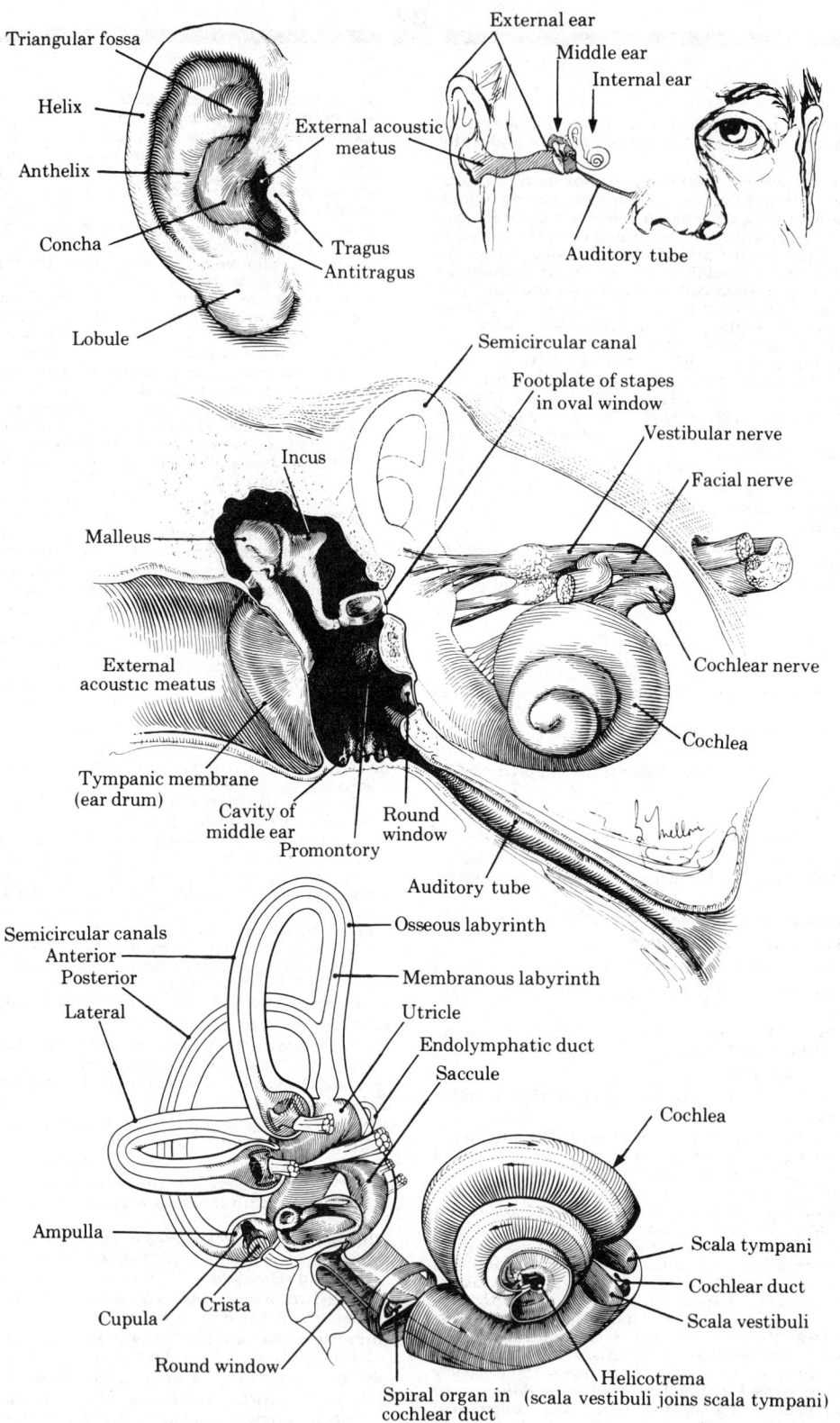

Triangular fossa

Helix

Anthelix

Concha

Lobule

External acoustic meatus

Tragus
Antitragus

External ear
Middle ear
Internal ear

Auditory tube

Semicircular canal

Footplate of stapes in oval window

Vestibular nerve

Facial nerve

Incus

Malleus

External acoustic meatus

Cochlear nerve

Cochlea

Tympanic membrane (ear drum)

Cavity of middle ear
Promontory

Round window

Auditory tube

Semicircular canals
Anterior
Posterior
Lateral

Osseous labyrinth

Membranous labyrinth

Utricle

Endolymphatic duct

Saccule

Cochlea

Ampulla

Cupula   Crista

Round window

Spiral organ in cochlear duct

Scala tympani

Cochlear duct

Scala vestibuli

Helicotrema
(scala vestibuli joins scala tympani)

PLATE 15—EXTERNAL AND INTERNAL STRUCTURES OF THE EAR

eburnation (e''bur-na'shun) [L. *ebur* ivory] 1. the conversion of a bone into an ivory-like mass. In osteoarthritis, the thinning of the articular cartilage due to disorganization and fragmentation of the superficial tissue and extension of degenerative changes to the deeper part of the cartilage, resulting in exposure of the subchondral bone, which becomes denser and the surface of which becomes worn and polished. 2. e. of dentin. **e. of dentin,** a condition observed in arrested dental caries, characterized by a large open cavity, usually on the occlusal surface of the deciduous and permanent teeth, in which decalcified dentin is burnished and takes a brown-stained, polished appearance.

eburneous (e-bur'ne-us) resembling ivory.

eburnitis (e''ber-ni'tis) [L. *eburnus* of ivory + *-itis*] increased hardness and density of dentin, generally occurring in exposed dentin, which may also undergo gradual discoloration, to yellow, to brown, and eventually to black.

EBV Epstein-Barr virus.

EC abbreviation for *Enzyme Commission.*

écarteur (ā-kar-ter') [Fr.] a retractor.

ecaudate (e-kaw'dāt) [L. *e* without + *cauda* tail] without a tail.

ecbolic (ek-bol'ik) [Gr. *ekbolikos* throwing out] oxytocic.

ecbovirus (ek''bo-vi'rus) [from *e*nteric *c*ytopathic *b*ovine *o*rphan + *virus*] an enteric orphan virus isolated from cattle; also written *ECBO virus.*

eccentric (ek-sen'trik) 1. situated or occurring away from a center. 2. proceeding from a center.

eccentrochondroplasia (ek-sen''tro-kon''dro-pla'se-ah) Morquio's syndrome.

eccentro-osteochondrodysplasia (ek-sen''tro-os''te-o-kon''dro-dis-pla'se-ah) [Gr. *ekkentros* from the center + *osteon* bone + *chondros* cartilage + *dys-* + *plassein* to form] Morquio's syndrome.

ecchondroma (ek''kon-dro'mah) [Gr. *ek* out + *chondros* cartilage + *-oma*] a hyperplastic growth of cartilage tissue developing on the surface of a cartilage or projecting under the periosteum of a bone; called also *ecchondrosis.*

ecchondrosis (ek''kon-dro'sis) ecchondroma.

ecchondrotome (ek-kon'dro-tōm) [Gr. *ek* out + *chondros* cartilage + *tomē* a cutting] a knife for excising cartilaginous tissue.

ecchordosis physaliphora (ek''kor-do'sis fis''ah-lif'o-rah) gelatinous nodules of heterotopic notochordal tissue projecting from the clivus or dorsum sellae. True tumors (chordomas) may arise from these or from intraosseous remnants of the notochord.

ecchymoma (ek-ĭ-mo'mah) a swelling due to a bruise and formed by subcutaneous extravasation of blood.

ecchymosed (ek'ĭ-mōsd) characterized by ecchymosis.

ecchymoses (ek''ĭ-mo'sēz) [Gr.] plural of *ecchymosis.*

ecchymosis (ek''ĭ-mo'sis), pl. *ecchymo'ses* [Gr. *ekchymōsis*] a small hemorrhagic spot, larger than a petechia, in the skin or mucous membrane forming a nonelevated, rounded or irregular, blue or purplish patch. **cadaveric e's,** stains seen on the more dependent portions of the body after death, giving the appearance of bruises.

ecchymotic (ek-ĭ-mot'ik) pertaining to or of the nature of an ecchymosis.

Eccles (ek''lz), Sir John Carew. Australian physiologist, born 1903; co-winner, with Alan Lloyd Hodgkin and Andrew Fielding Huxley, of the Nobel prize in medicine or physiology for 1963, for discoveries concerning the ionic mechanisms involved in excitation and inhibition in the peripheral and central portions of the nerve cell membrane.

eccoprotic (ek''o-prot'ik) [Gr. *ek* out + *kopros* dung] cathartic.

eccrine (ek'rin) exocrine, with special reference to ordinary sweat glands.

eccrisis (ek'rĭ-sis) [Gr. *ek* out + *krisis* separation] the excretion or expulsion of waste products.

eccritic (ek-krit'ik) [Gr. *ekkritikos*] 1. promoting excretion. 2. an agent that promotes excretion.

eccyesis (ek''si-e'sis) [Gr. *ek* out + *kyēsis* pregnancy] ectopic pregnancy.

ecdemic (ek-dem'ik) [Gr. *ekdēmos* gone on a journey] neither endemic nor epidemic; said of an infectious disease

introduced into a population or geographical area from without.

ecdovirus (ek''do-vi'rus) [from *e*nteric *c*ytopathic *d*og orphan + *virus*] an enteric orphan virus isolated from dogs; also written *ECDO virus.*

ecdysiasm (ek-di'sĭ-azm) [Gr. *ekdyein* to strip off one's clothes] an abnormal tendency to take off one's clothes.

ecdysis (ek'dĭ-sis) [Gr. *ekdysis* a getting out] desquamation or sloughing; especially the shedding of an outer covering and the development of a new one such as occurs in certain arthropods, crustaceans, lizards, and snakes. Called also *molting.*

ecdysone (ek-di'son) [Gr. *edkysis* a getting out] the hormone produced in the prothoracic glands of arthropods that induces molting (ecdysis) and metamorphosis.

ECF extracellular fluid; eosinophil chemotactic factor.

ECF-A eosinophil chemotactic factor of anaphylaxis; see under *factor.*

ECG electrocardiogram.

ecgonine (ek'go-nin) chemical name: 3β-hydroxy-2β-tropanecarboxylic acid. The final basic product, $C_9H_{15}NO_3$, obtained by hydrolysis of cocaine and several related alkaloids.

echidnase (e-kid'nās) [Gr. *echidna* viper + *-ase*] an enzyme found in the venom of vipers.

echidnin (e-kid'nin) [Gr. *echidna* viper] serpent venom, or a nitrogenous poisonous principle from it.

Echidnophaga (ek''id-nof'ah-gah) a genus of fleas. **E. gallina'cea,** the sticktight flea, which collects in dense masses on the heads of chickens, in the ears of other animals, and which may also parasitize man.

echidnotoxin (e-kid''no-tok'sin) a poisonous principle in the venom of vipers.

echidnovaccine (e-kid''no-vak'sēn) [Gr. *echidna* viper + *vaccine*] viper venom that has been deprived of its poisonous power by heating; it is used as a vaccine against venom.

Echinacea (ek''ĭ-na'se-ah) [Gr. *echinos* hedgehog] a genus of composite plants, the cone flowers. The dried rhizome and roots of *E. angustifo'lia* and *E. purpu'rea* have tonic properties.

echinate (ek'ĭ-nāt) echinulate.

echinenone (e-kin'ĕ-nōn) a carotenoid provitamin prepared from the sex glands of sea urchins and which in the body becomes vitamin A.

echin(o)- [Gr. *echinos* hedgehog] a combining form denoting relationship to spines, or spiny.

Echinochasmus (e-ki''no-kaz'mus) [*echino-* + Gr. *chasma* open mouth] a genus of parasitic intestinal flukes. **E. perfolia'tus,** the causative agent of echinostomiasis in Japan.

echinochrome (e-ki'no-krōm) a brown respiratory pigment found in sea urchins.

echinococciasis (e-ki''no-kok-ki'ah-sis) hydatid disease.

echinococcosis (e-ki''no-kok-o'sis) hydatid disease.

echinococcotomy (e-ki''no-kok-kot'o-me) [*echinococcus* + Gr. *tomē* a cutting] evacuation of an echinococcus (hydatid) cyst.

Echinococcus (e-ki''no-kok'us) [*echino-* + Gr. *kokkos* berry] a genus of small tapeworms of the family Taeniidae. **E. alveola'ris,** *E. multilocularis.* **E. granulo'sus,** a small tapeworm parasitic in dogs and wolves and occasionally in cats. Its larva, known as the hydatid, may develop in nearly all mammals, forming hydatid tumors or cysts in the liver, lungs, kidneys, and other organs. See *hydatid disease, unilocular,* under *disease.* **E. multilocula'ris,** a species whose adults usually parasitize the fox and wild rodents, although man is sporadically infected. It resembles *E. granulosis,* but the larvae form alveolar or multilocular cysts rather than unilocular cysts. See *hydatid disease, alveolar,* under *disease.*

echinocyte (e-ki'no-sīt) [*echino-* + Gr. *kytos* hollow vessel] a burr cell.

echinoderm (e-kin'o-derm) one of the Echinodermata.

Echinodermata (e-ki''no-der'mah-tah) [*echino-* + Gr. *derma* skin] a phylum of the animal kingdom, including starfishes, sea urchins, etc.

Echinolaelaps (e-ki''no-le'laps) a genus of mites found on rats and in stable litter; its bite causes intense itching. Called also *Laelaps* or *Lelaps*. **E. echidni′nus,** a mite that acts as an intermediate host of *Hepatozoon muris* and *H. perniciosum.*

echinophthalmia (e-kin″of-thal′me-ah) [*echino-* + *ophthalmia*] inflammation of the eyelids marked by projection of the lashes.

Echinorhynchus (e-ki″no-ring′kus) [*echino-* + Gr. *rhynchos* beak] a former genus of parasitic worms. **E. gi′gas, E. hom′inis,** *Macracanthorhynchus hirudinaceus.* **E. monilifor′mis,** *Moniliformis moniliformis.*

echinosis (ek″ĭ-no′sis) [Gr. *echinos* hedgehog + *-osis*] irregularity in the form of an erythrocyte, giving it a spiny appearance. Cf. *crenation.*

Echinosteliida (e-ki″no-stĕ-li′ĭ-dah) [*echino-* + Gr. *stechlo* stalk] an order of protozoa (subclass Myxogastria, class Eumycetozoa), characterized by the presence of minute stalked sporangia and a nonreticulate small plasmodium.

Echinostoma (ek″ĭ-nos′to-mah) [*echino-* + Gr. *stoma* mouth] a genus of parasitic flukes. *E. revolu′tum* is found in the intestines of ducks and geese and has been reported in man in Taiwan and Indonesia. *E. iloca′num* has been found in the feces of natives of Java and the Philippine Islands. *E. lindoen′sis* occurs in Celebes; *E. perfolia′tum* in Japan.

echinostomiasis (e-kin″o-sto-mi′ah-sis) infection by flukes of the genus *Echinostoma* or of related genera of the family Echinostomatidae.

echinulate (e-kin′u-lāt) [L. *echinus* hedgehog] having small prickles or spines; applied in bacteriology to cultures showing toothed or pointed outgrowths.

Echis (e′kis) a genus of small venomous vipers ranging from India to North Africa.

echo (ek′o) [Gr. *ēchō* a returned sound] repetition of a sound as a result of reverberation of sound waves; also the reflection of ultrasonic, radio, and radar waves. Sometimes used to refer to repetition of movement. **amphoric e.,** resonant repetition of a sound heard on auscultation of the chest, occurring at an appreciable interval after the vocal sound. **metallic e.,** a peculiar ringing repetition of the heart sounds sometimes heard in patients with pneumopericardium and pneumothorax.

echoacousia (ek″o-ah-koo′ze-ah) [*echo* + Gr. *akousis* hearing + *-ia*] the subjective experience of hearing echoes after normally heard sounds.

echocardiogram (ek″o-kar′de-o-gram″) the record produced by echocardiography.

echocardiography (ek″o-kar″de-og′rah-fe) a method of graphically recording the position and motion of the heart walls or the internal structures of the heart and neighboring tissue by the echo obtained from beams of ultrasonic waves directed through the chest wall. Called also *ultrasonic cardiography.*

echoencephalogram (ek″o-en-sef′ah-lo-gram″) the record produced by echoencephalography.

echoencephalograph (ek″o-en-sef′ah-lo-graf) the instrument used in echoencephalography.

echoencephalography (ek″o-en-sef″ah-log′rah-fe) a diagnostic technique in which pulses of ultrasonic waves are beamed through the head from both sides, and echoes from the midline structures of the brain are recorded as graphic tracings; shifts from the midline may indicate a centrally placed mass.

echogenic (ek″o-jen′ik) in ultrasonography, giving rise to reflections (echoes) of ultrasound waves.

echogram (ek′o-gram) the record made by echography.

echographia (ek-o-gra′fe-ah) [*echo* + Gr. *graphein* to write + *-ia*] an aphasic condition in which the patient can copy writing, but cannot write to express ideas.

echography (ĕ-kog′rah-fe) ultrasonography; the use of ultrasound as a diagnostic aid. Ultrasound waves are directed at the tissues, and a record is made, as on an oscilloscope, of the waves reflected back through the tissues, which indicate interfaces of different acoustic densities and thus differentiate between solid and cystic structures.

echokinesis (ek″o-ki-ne′sis) [*echo* + Gr. *kinesis* motion] echopraxia.

echolalia (ek″o-la′le-ah) [*echo* + Gr. *lalia* speech, babble] stereotyped repetition of another person's words or phrases,

seen in some cases of schizophrenia, particularly in catatonic schizophrenia; called also *echophrasia.*

echolucent (ek″o-loo′sent) permitting the passage of ultrasonic waves without giving rise to echoes, the representative areas appearing black on the sonogram.

echomatism (ĕ-ko′mah-tizm) [*echo* + Gr. *matizein* to strive to do] echopraxia.

echomimia (ek″o-mim′e-ah) [*echo* + Gr. *mimia* imitation] echopraxia.

echomotism (ek″o-mo′tizm) [*echo* + L. *motio* movement] echopraxia.

echopathy (ĕ-kop′ah-the) [*echo* + Gr. *pathos* disease] stereotyped repetition of the words or actions of others; echolalia or echopraxia.

echophonocardiography (ek″o-fo″no-kar″de-og′rah-fe) the combined use of echocardiography and phonocardiography.

echophony (ek-of′o-ne) [*echo* + Gr. *phōne* voice] an echo-like sound heard immediately after a vocal sound on auscultation of the chest.

echophotony (ek″o-fot′o-ne) [*echo* + Gr. *phōs* light + *tonos* tone] the association of certain colors with certain sounds.

echophrasia (ek″o-fra′se-ah) echolalia.

echopraxia (ek″o-prak′se-ah) [*echo* + Gr. *praxia* action, from *prassein* to perform] stereotyped imitation of the movements of another person; seen in some cases of catatonic schizophrenia.

echopraxis (ek″o-prak′sis) echopraxia.

echo-ranging (ek″o-rānj′ing) in ultrasonography, the determining of the position or depth of a body structure on the basis of the time interval between the moment an ultrasonic pulse is transmitted and the moment its echo is received.

echothiophate (ek″o-thi′o-fāt) an anticholinesterase agent applied topically to produce miosis, decrease intraocular pressure, and potentiate accommodation in treatment of open-angle glaucoma and accommodative convergent strabismus. Available as *echothiophate iodide* [USP].

echovirus (ek″o-vi′rus) [enteric cytopathic *h*uman *o*rphan + *virus*] an enteric orphan RNA virus isolated from man, separable into many serotypes, certain of which are associated with human disease, especially aseptic meningitis; also written *ECHO virus.* **e. 28,** a serotype isolated from patients with mild respiratory disease, pathogenic for man but not for conventional laboratory animals, including the suckling mouse and monkey, by the intracerebral route; also written *ECHO 28 virus.*

Eck's fistula (eks) [Nicolai Vladimirovich *Eck,* Russian physiologist, 1847–1908] see under *fistula.*

Ecker's fissure (ek′erz) [Alexander *Ecker,* German anatomist, 1816–1887] see under *convolution* and *fissure.*

Ecker's fluid (ek′erz) [Enrique E. *Ecker,* American bacteriologist, 1887–1966] Rees and Ecker diluting fluid; see under *fluid.*

Eclabron (ek′lah-bron) trademark for preparations of guaithylline.

eclampsia (ĕ-klamp′se-ah) [Gr. *eklampein* to shine forth] convulsions and coma occurring in a pregnant or puerperal woman, associated with preeclampsia, i.e., with hypertension, edema, and/or proteinuria. **puerperal e.,** that occurring after childbirth. **uremic e.,** eclampsia due to uremia.

eclampsism (ĕ-klamp′sizm) preeclampsia.

eclamptic (ĕ-klamp′tik) pertaining to or of the nature of eclampsia.

eclamptism (ĕ-klamp′tizm) the condition due to the autointoxication incident to pregnancy, and marked by headache, visual impairment, and sometimes by convulsions.

eclamptogenic (ĕ-klamp″to-jen′ik) causing convulsions.

eclectic (ĕ-klek′tik) [Gr. *eklektikos* selecting] designating a sect or school which professes to select what is best from all other systems of medicine. See *eclecticism.*

eclecticism (ĕ-klek′tĭ-sizm) [Gr. *eklegein* to pick out] a nineteenth-century medicinal cult popular in America which treats diseases by the application of single remedies to known pathologic conditions, without reference to nosology, special attention being given to developing indigenous plant remedies.

eclipse (e-klips′) in virology, that period of the infective cycle during which infected bacterial cells contain no detectable infective bacteriophage.

eclysis (ek′lĭ-sis) mild syncope.

ecmnesia (ek-ne′ze-ah) [Gr. *ek* out of + *mnēmē* memory] forgetfulness of recent events with normal memory for more remote ones.

ecmovirus (ek″mo-vi′rus) [from *enteric cytopathic monkey orphan* + *virus*] an enteric orphan virus isolated from monkeys; also written *ECMO virus*.

ecogenetics (ek″o-jĕ-net′iks) the study of the relationship between genetic factors and the nature of response to an environmental agent.

ecologist (e-kol′o-jist) an individual skilled in ecology.

ecology (e-kol′o-je) [Gr. *oikos* house + *-logy*] the science of organisms as affected by the factors of their environments; study of the environment and life history of organisms. **human e.,** application of the ecologic approach to the study of human societies.

ecomania (e″ko-ma′ne-ah) [Gr. *oikos* house + *mania* madness] (*obs.*) an attitude of mind that is dominating toward members of the family but humble toward those in authority.

econazole nitrate (ĕ-kon′ah-zōl) chemical name: 1-[2-[(4-chlorophenyl) methoxy] - 2 - (2,4 - dichlorophenyl) ethyl]- 1*H*-imidazole. A broad-spectrum antifungal with some antibacterial activity, $C_{18}H_{15}Cl_3N_2O \cdot HNO_3$; used topically in the treatment of infections due to susceptible organisms, including dermatophytes, and in vaginal candidiasis.

Economo's disease (encephalitis) (a-kon′o-mōz) [Constantin von *Economo*, Austrian neurologist, 1876–1931] encephalitis lethargica.

economy (e-kon′o-me) [Gr. *oikos* house + *nomos* law] the management of domestic affairs. **animal e.,** the system of operation of the bodily processes in organic bodies; also the body as an organized whole. **token e.,** a program of treatment in behavior therapy, usually conducted in a hospital setting, in which the patient may earn tokens by engaging in appropriate personal and social behavior, or lose tokens by inappropriate or antisocial behavior; tokens may be exchanged for tangible rewards (food snacks, clothing, etc.) or for special privileges (watching television, passes to leave the hospital, etc.).

ecoparasite (e″ko-par′ah-sīt) ecosite.

écorché (a″kor-sha′) [Fr.] a painting or sculpture of a man or other animal exhibited as deprived of its skin, so that the muscles are exposed for study.

ecostate (e-kos′tāt) [L. *e* without + *costa* rib] ribless; without ribs.

ecosystem (ek″o-sis′tem) the fundamental unit in ecology, comprising the living organisms and the nonliving elements interacting in a certain defined area.

ecotaxis (ek′o-tak″sis) [Gr. *oikos* house + *taxis* arrangement] the "homing" of recirculating lymphocytes to specific compartments of peripheral lymphoid tissues—B cells to B-dependent areas and T cells to T-dependent areas.

ecotone (ek′o tōn) a transition region where adjacent biomes blend, containing some organisms from each of the adjacent biomes plus some that are characteristic of, and perhaps restricted to, the ecotone; this region tends to have more species and to be more densely populated than either adjacent biome.

Ecotrin (ek′o-trin) trademark for a preparation of aspirin.

écouvillon (a-koo″ve-yaw′) [Fr.] a stiff brush or swab used for swabbing cavities and inflammatory lesions.

écouvillonage (a-koo″ve-yŏ-nahzh′) [Fr.] the scrubbing of a cavity or an infected area.

ecphyaditis (ek″fi-ah-di′tis) [Gr. *ekphyas* appendix + *-itis*] appendicitis.

écrasement (a-krahz-maw′) [Fr.] removal by means of the écraseur.

écraseur (e-krah-zer′) [Fr. "crusher"] an instrument containing a chain or cord to be looped about a part and then tightened in order to transect the portion enclosed within the loop.

ecsomatics (ek″so-mat′iks) [Gr. *ek* out + *sōma* body] the study by laboratory methods of the materials removed from the body.

ecsovirus (ek″so-vi′rus) [from *enteric cytopathic swine or-*

phan + *virus*] an enteric orphan virus isolated from swine; also written *ECSO virus*.

ecstasy (ek′stah-se) [Gr. *ekstasis*] a state of rapture and trancelike elation.

ecstatic (ek-stat′ik) pertaining to or characterized by ecstasy.

ecstrophy (ek′stro-fe) [Gr. *ekstrephein* to turn inside out] exstrophy.

ECT electroconvulsive therapy.

ectacolia (ek″tah-ko′le-ah) ectasia of a portion of the colon.

ectad (ek′tad) [Gr. *ektos* without] outward; the reverse of inward.

ectal (ek′tal) [Gr. *ektos* without] superficial or external.

ectasia (ek-ta′ze-ah) [Gr. *ektasis* + *-ia*] dilatation, expansion, or distention. **alveolar e.,** overdistention of the pulmonary alveoli. **annuloaortic e.,** dilatation of the proximal aorta and the fibrous ring of the heart at the aortic orifice, marked by aortic regurgitation and, when severe, by dissecting aneurysm; it is often associated with Marfan's syndrome. **corneal e.,** keratectasia. **diffuse arterial e.,** racemose aneurysm. **hypostatic e.,** dilatation of a blood vessel from the effect of gravity on the blood. **mammary duct e.,** a condition characterized chiefly by dilatation of the collecting ducts of the mammary gland, inspissation of breast secretion, intraductal inflammation, and marked periductal and interstitial chronic inflammatory reaction in which plasma cells are prominent; a benign process associated with atrophy of the duct epithelium, it generally occurs during or after the menopause. **papillary e.,** a circumscribed dilatation of the capillaries, forming a red spot on the skin. **scleral e.,** see under *staphyloma*. **tubular e.,** a congenital, usually bilateral and diffuse condition of the renal medulla characterized by dilated collecting tubules and medullary cysts.

ectasis (ek′tah-sis) ectasia.

ectasy (ek′tah-se) ectasia.

ectatic (ek-tat′ik) distended or stretched; distensible.

ectental (ek-ten′tal) [Gr. *ektos* without + *entos* within] pertaining to the ectoderm and entoderm, and to their line of junction.

ecterograph (ek′ter-o-graf) [Gr. *ektos* outside + *graphein* to write] an apparatus for recording graphically the movements of the intestines.

ectethmoid (ek-teth′moid) [Gr. *ektos* without + *ethmoid*] one of the paired lateral masses of the ethmoid bone.

ecthyma (ek-thi′mah) [Gr. *ekthyma*] an ulcerative pyoderma usually caused by group A beta-hemolytic streptococcal infection at the site of minor trauma, predominantly involving the shins and dorsal feet, and generally healing with variable scar formation. **contagious e.,** an endemic infectious disease of sheep and goats caused by a poxvirus, characterized by the development on non-wool-bearing areas, especially the lips and oral mucosa, of an erythematous vesiculopustular eruption, the lesions of which may coalesce and crust over, forming large scabs that fall off, which is followed by healing of the tissues without scarring. In humans, who usually acquire the disease by direct contact with infected animals, it is usually manifested by the presence of a single painless pustule (up to 10 lesions may appear) on a finger; when lesions are disseminated systemic symptoms such as lymphadenitis and fever may occur. Called also *contagious pustular dermatitis, orf, sore mouth,* and *ulcerative stomatitis of sheep.* **e. gangreno′sum,** a condition most often seen in debilitated patients in association wiith septicemia caused by gram negative organisms (e.g., gonococcus, meningococcus, *Escherichia coli, Klebsiella, Pseudomonas*), characterized by lesions that begin as vesicles that rapidly progress to pustulation and gangrenous ulcers with undermined purpuric edges.

ecthymiform (ek-thi′mĭ-form) resembling ecthyma.

ect(o)- [Gr. *ektos* outside] a prefix meaning outside, or situated on the outside.

ectoantigen (ek″to-an′te-jen) an antigen which seems to be loosely attached to the outside of bacteria so that it can be readily removed by shaking them in physiologic sodium chloride solution; also an antigen formed in the ectoplasm of a bacterium.

ectobiology (ek″to-bi-ol′o-je) the study of the properties and biochemical constitution of the cell surface and the specific enzymes at the surface.

ectoblast (ek'to-blast) [ecto- + Gr. *blastos* germ] 1. the ectoderm. 2. an external membrane; a cell wall.

ectocardia (ek-to-kar'de-ah) [ecto- + Gr. *kardia* heart] congenital displacement of the heart, either inside or outside the thorax.

ectocervical (ek″to-ser'vĭ-kal) of or pertaining to the ectocervix.

ectocervix (ek″to-ser'viks) the portio vaginalis cervicis, the part of the uterine cervix lined with stratified squamous epithelium; called also *exocervix*.

ectocinerea (ek″to-sĭ-ne're-ah) [ecto- + *cinerea*] (*obs.*) the cortical gray matter of the brain.

ectocinereal (ek″to-sĭ-ne're-al) (*obs.*) relating to the ectocinerea.

ectocolon (ek″to-ko'lon) [Gr. *ektasis* dilatation + *kolon* colon] dilatation of the colon.

ectocommensal (ek″to-kom-men'sal) a commensal organism that lives outside the body of its symbiotic companion, but cannot be separated from it.

ectocondyle (ek″to-kon'dīl) the external condyle of a bone.

ectocuneiform (ek″to-ku-ne'ĭ-form) the lateral cuneiform bone.

ectocytic (ek″to-si'tik) [ecto- + Gr. *kytos* hollow vessel] outside the cell.

ectoderm (ek'to-derm) [ecto- + Gr. *derma* skin] the outermost of the three primary germ layers of the embryo. From it are developed the epidermis and the epidermal tissues, such as the nails, hair, and glands of the skin, the nervous system, the external sense organs, as the ear, eye, etc., and the mucous membrane of the mouth and anus. Cf. *entoderm* and *mesoderm*. **amniotic e.,** the inner layer of the amnion (and covering of the umbilical cord) that is continuous with body ectoderm. **basal e.,** trophoblast covering the eroded uterine tissue that faces the placental sinuses. **blastodermic e.,** the external layer of a blastula or blastodisk; called also *primitive e.* **chorionic e.,** the trophoblast. **extraembryonic e.,** a derivative of epiblast or ectoderm located outside the body of the embryo. **neural e.,** the region of the ectoderm destined to become the neural tube; neuroderm. **primitive e.,** blastodermic e.

ectodermal (ek″to-der'mal) [ecto- + Gr. *derma* skin] pertaining to or derived from the ectoderm.

ectodermatosis (ek″to-der″mah-to'sis) ectodermosis.

ectodermic (ek″to-der'mik) ectodermal.

ectodermoidal (ek″to-der-moid'al) of the nature of or resembling the ectoderm.

ectodermosis (ek″to-der-mo'sis) a disorder based on congenital maldevelopment of the organs of ectodermal derivation, i.e., nervous system, retina, eyeball, and skin. Called also *ectodermatosis*. See also *phakomatosis*. **e. erosi'va pluriorificia'lis,** Stevens-Johnson syndrome.

ectoentad (ek″to-en'tad) from without inward.

ectoenzyme (ek″to-en'zīm) an enzyme secreted from a cell into the surrounding medium; an extracellular enzyme. Cf. *endoenzyme*.

ectogenic (ek″to-jen'ik) ectogenous.

ectogenous (ek-toj'ĕ-nus) [ecto- + Gr. *gennan* to produce] introduced from without; arising from causes outside the organism, as an infectious disease.

ectoglia (ek-tog'le-ah) [ecto- + Gr. *glia* glue] the thin, external marginal layer of the early medullary tube of the embryo.

ectoglobular (ek″to-glob'u-lar) [ecto- + *globule*] (*obs.*) formed outside the blood cells.

ectogony (ek-tog'o-ne) the influence exerted on the mother by the developing embryo. Improperly called *metaxenia*.

ectohormone (ek″to-hor'mōn) a hormone secreted to the outside of the body, as a pheromone.

ectolecithal (ek″to-les'ĭ-thal) [ecto- + Gr. *lekithos* yolk] having the yolk situated peripherally; see under *ovum*.

ectolysis (ek-tol'ĭ-sis) [*ectoplasm* + *lysis*] lysis of the ectoplasm.

ectomere (ek'to-mēr) [ecto- + Gr. *meros* part] any of the blastomeres which share in the formation of the ectoderm.

ectomesoblast (ek″to-mes'o-blast) the layer of cells which has not yet become differentiated into ectoblast and mesoblast.

-ectomize [*ectomy*, q.v.] a word termination meaning to deprive by excision, as in *thyroidectomize, adrenalectomize;* the structure or organ exised is indicated by the root to which the suffix is attached. By extension, used in terms to designate destruction or deprivation by other methods as well.

ectomorph (ek'to-morf) an individual having a type of body build in which tissues derived from the ectoderm predominate: there is a preponderance of linearity and fragility, with large surface area, thin muscles and subcutaneous tissue, and slightly developed digestive viscera, as contrasted with endomorph and mesomorph.

ectomorphic (ek″to-mor'fik) pertaining to or characteristic of an ectomorph.

ectomorphy (ek″to-mor'fe) [*ectoderm* + Gr. *morphē* form] the condition of being an ectomorph.

ectomy (ek'to-me) [Gr. *ektomē*] excision of an organ or part. Used as a word termination to indicate excision of the structure or organ designated by the root to which it is affixed, as *appendectomy, tonsillectomy*. By extension, used in terms to designate destruction or deprivation by other methods as well.

ectonuclear (ek″to-nu'kle-ar) outside the nucleus of a cell.

ectopagus (ek-top'ah-gus) [ecto- + Gr. *pagos* something fixed] a double monster connected along the side of the body, so that the components are definitely right and left, the inner arms and/or legs being represented by a bilateral median limb.

ectoparasite (ek″to-par'ah-sīt) [ecto- + *parasite*] a parasite that lives on the outside of the body of the host.

ectopectoralis (ek″to-pek″to-ra'lis) musculus pectoralis major.

ectoperitoneal (ek″to-per″ĭ-to-ne'al) relating to the external or abdominal surface of the peritoneum.

ectoperitonitis (ek″to-per″ĭ-to-ni'tis) [ecto- + *peritonitis*] inflammation of the external or abdominal side of the peritoneum.

ectophyte (ek'to-fīt) [ecto- + Gr. *phyton* plant] a vegetable parasite or species living on the outside of the body of its host.

ectopia (ek-to'pe-ah) [Gr. *ektopos* displaced + *-ia*] displacement or malposition, especially if congenital. **e. cloa'cae,** exstrophy of cloaca. **e. cor'dis,** congenital displacement of the heart outside the thoracic cavity. **e. cor'dis, pectoral,** location of the heart outside the chest wall, through a fissure in the lower sternum. **e. cor'dis abdomina'lis,** location of the heart in the abdominal cavity. **crossed renal e.,** a condition in which the two kidneys are on the same side of the body, one ureter crossing the midline. **e. len'tis,** displacement of the crystalline lens of the eye. **e. pupil'lae conge'nita,** congenital displacement of the pupil. **renal e., e. re'nis,** displacement of the kidney. **e. tes'tis,** dislocation of the testicle. **e. vesi'cae,** exstrophy of the bladder.

ectopic (ek-top'ik) 1. pertaining to or characterized by ectopia. 2. located away from normal position, as in ectopic pregnancy. 3. arising from an abnormal site or tissue.

ectoplacenta (ek-to-plah-sen'tah) [ecto- + Gr. *placenta* cake] the actively growing trophoblast that becomes the placenta in rodents.

ectoplasm (ek'to-plazm) [ecto- + Gr. *plasma* a thing formed] plasma membrane.

ectoplasmatic (ek″to-plaz-mat'ik) pertaining to ectoplasm.

ectoplast (ek'to-plast) cell membrane.

ectoplastic (ek″to-plas'tik) [ecto- + Gr. *plassein* to shape] having a formative power on the surface, as *ectoplastic* cells.

ectopterygoid (ek″to-ter'ĭ-goid) musculus pterygoideus lateralis.

ectopy (ek'to-pe) ectopia.

ectoscopy (ek-tos'ko-pe) [ecto- + Gr. *skopein* to examine] a diagnostic method based on observation of chest and abdominal movements, and said to be capable of determining the outlines of the lungs and of localized internal conditions.

ectosite (ek'to-sīt) (*obs.*) ectoparasite.

ectoskeleton (ek″to-skel′ĕ-ton) exoskeleton.

ectosphere (ek″to-sfēr) the outer zone of the centrosome.

ectosteal (ek-tos′te-al) pertaining to or situated on the outside of a bone.

ectostosis (ek″to-sto′sis) [ecto- + Gr. *osteon* bone] ossification beneath the perichondrium of a cartilage or the periosteum of a bone.

ectosymbiont (ek″to-sim′be-ont) a symbiont that lives outside the body of the organism with which it is biologically related.

ectotherm (ek′to-therm) [ecto- + Gr. *thermē* heat] 1. an animal that exhibits ectothermy. 2. poikilotherm.

ectothermic (ek″to-therm′ik) 1. pertaining to or characterized by ectothermy. 2. poikilothermic.

ectothermy (ek″to-ther′me) 1. the regulation of body temperature by the external environment rather than by internal metabolism, with thermoregulation being accomplished by behavioral means; i.e., the animal seeks an appropriate environmental temperature. Cf. *endothermy* (def. 2). 2. poikilothermy.

Ectothiorhodospira (ek″to-thi″o-rho-dos′pĭ-rah) [ecto- + Gr. *theion* sulfur + *rhodon* rose + Gr. *speira* coil] a genus of aquatic phototrophic bacteria of the family Chromatiaceae, order Rhodospirillales, consisting of spiral to rod-shaped motile cells that do not contain gas vacuoles. The organisms fix carbon dioxide in the presence of hydrogen sulfide. Cell suspensions are brown to red. The type species is *E. mo′bilis*.

ectothrix (ek′to-thriks) [ecto- + Gr. *thrix* hair] a fungus which grows inside the hair shaft but also produces a sheath of arthrospores on the outside of the hair. Such fungi include *Trichophyton verrucosum* (*large-spored e.*) and *T. mentagrophytes*, *Microsporum audouinii*, *M. canis*, and *M. gypseum* (*small-spored e.'s*).

ectotoxin (ek″to-tok′sin) (*obs.*) exotoxin.

Ectotrichophyton (ek″to-tri-kof′ĭ-ton) [ecto- + Gr. *thrix* hair + *phyton* plant] former name for a genus of fungi, now included in the genus *Trichophyton*.

ectozoa (ek″to-zo′ah) [Gr.] plural of *ectozoon*.

ectozoal (ek″to-zo′al) pertaining to or caused by ectozoa.

ectozoon (ek″to-zo′on), pl. *ectozo′a* [ecto- + Gr. *zōon* animal] ectoparasite.

ectr(o)- [Gr. *ektrōsis* miscarriage] a combining form denoting congenital absence of a part.

ectrodactylia (ek″tro-dak-til′e-ah) ectrodactyly.

ectrodactylism (ek″tro-dak′tĭ-lism) ectrodactyly.

ectrodactyly (ek″tro-dak′tĭ-le) [ectro- + *daktylos* finger] congenital absence of all or of only part of a digit (*partial e.*).

ectrogenic (ek″tro-jen′ik) pertaining to or characterized by ectrogeny.

ectrogeny (ek-troj′ĕ-ne) [ectro- + *gennan* to produce] congenital absence or defect of a part.

ectromelia (ek″tro-me′le-ah) [ectro- + Gr. *melos* limb + -ia] gross hypoplasia or aplasia of one or more long bones of one or more limbs; the term includes amelia, hemimelia, and phocomelia. **infectious e.**, a disease of mice caused by a poxvirus and characterized by gangrene and often loss of one or more of the feet and sometimes of other external parts, and by necrotic areas in the liver, spleen, and other organs; called also *mousepox*.

ectromelic (ek″tro-mel′ik) pertaining to or characterized by ectromelia.

ectromelus (ek-trom′ĕ-lus) [ectros- + *melos* limb] an individual exhibiting ectromelia.

ectrometacarpia (ek″tro-met″ah-kar′pe-ah) [ectro- + *metacarpus* + -ia] congenital absence of a metacarpal bone.

ectrometatarsia (ek″tro-met″ah-tar′se-ah) [ectro- + *metatarsus* + -ia] congenital absence of a metatarsal bone.

ectrophalangia (ek″tro-fah-lan′je-ah) congenital absence of one or more phalanges of a digit.

ectropion (ek-tro′pe-on) [Gr. "an everted eyelid"; *ektropē* a turning aside] the turning outward (eversion) of an edge or margin, as of the eyelid, resulting in exposure of the palpebral conjunctiva. **atonic e.**, eversion due to loss of skin tone or of muscle tone, especially of the orbicularis oculi muscle. **cervical e.**, eversion of uterine cervix. **cicatricial e.**, eversion of the margin of an eyelid caused by contraction of scar tissue in the lid or by contraction of the

skin. **flaccid e.**, ectropion of the lower lid resulting from reduced tone of the orbicularis oculi muscle. **e. luxu′rians**, e. sarcomatosum. **paralytic e.**, eversion of the margin of the lower eyelid as a result of paralysis of the facial nerve, and loss of contractile power of the orbicularis oculi muscle. **e. of pigment layer**, proliferation of the cells in the posteriorly situated pigment layer of the iris, leading to their migration around the pupillary margin to encroach upon the anterior surface of the iris. **e. sarcomato′sum**, eversion of an eyelid resulting from chronic thickening of the palpebral conjunctiva; called also *e. luxurians*. **senile e.**, eversion of the lower eyelid associated with relaxation of the fibers of the palpebral portion of the orbicularis oculi muscle as a concomitant of age, or occurring as a result of atrophic changes in the skin. **spastic e.**, ectropion caused by tonic spasm of the orbicularis oculi muscle. **e. u′veae**, eversion of the margin of the pupil, often congenital (*e. u′veae conge′nitum*), and frequently due to the presence of a newly formed membrane on the anterior layer of the iris, or to the formation of connective tissue in the stroma, particularly in diabetes. Called also *iridectropium*.

ectropionize (ek-tro′pe-ŏ-nīz″) to put into a state of eversion.

ectropium (ek-tro′pe-um) ectropion.

ectrosis (ek-tro′sis) [Gr. *ektrōsis*] 1. abortion. 2. treatment that arrests the development of disease.

ectrosyndactylia (ek″tro-sin″dak-til′e-ah) ectrosyndactyly.

ectrosyndactyly (ek″tro-sin-dak′tĭ-le) [ectro- + *syn* together + *daktylos* finger] a condition in which some of the digits are missing and those that remain are webbed, so that they are more or less attached.

ectrotic (ek-trot′ik) 1. pertaining to or producing abortion. 2. arresting the development of a disease.

ectylurea (ek″til-u-re′ah) chemical name: cis-(2-ethylcrotonyl)urea. A white crystalline powder, $C_7H_{12}N_2O_2$, used as a sedative.

ectyonin (ek″tĭ-on′in) an antimicrobial substance obtained from the sponge *Microciona prolifera*.

eczema (ek′zĕ-mah) [Gr. *ekzein* to boil out] a pruritic papulovesicular dermatitis occurring as a reaction to many endogenous and exogenous agents, characterized in the acute stage by erythema, edema associated with a serous exudate between the cells of the epidermis (spongiosis) and an inflammatory infiltrate in the dermis, oozing and vesiculation, and crusting and scaling; and in the more chronic stages by lichenification or thickening or both, signs of excoriations, and hyperpigmentation or hypopigmentation or both. Atopic dermatitis is the most common type of dermatitis. Called also *eczematous dermatitis*. **allergic e.**, **atopic e.**, atopic dermatitis. **asteatotic e.**, xerotic e. **e. craquelé** (krah-kĕ-lá) [Fr. "marred with cracks"], xerotic e. **dyshidrotic e.**, pompholyx. **facial e. of ruminants**, a photosensitive disease of ruminants, particularly in New Zealand, due to ingestion of the spores of the mold *Pithomyces chartarum* (class Deuteromycetes), which contain sporidesmin. **flexural e.**, see *atopic dermatitis*, under *dermatitis*. **e. herpet′icum**, Kaposi's varicelliform eruption due to infection with the herpes simplex virus superimposed on a preexisting skin condition, usually atopic dermatitis. Cf. *e. vaccinatum*. **infantile e.**, see *atopic dermatitis*, under *dermatitis*. **e. intertri′go**, intertrigo. **nummular e.**, eczema presenting in discrete coin-shaped, ringed, or annular lesions that may coalesce to form extensive patches, which may ooze and crust over, typically distributed on the extensor surfaces of the extremities, lower legs, chest, back, and buttocks, and tending to occur in older men and young women. Called also *exudative* or *nummular neurodermatitis* and *nummular eczematous dermatitis*. **seborrheic e.**, see under *dermatitis*. **e. vaccina′tum**, Kaposi's varicelliform eruption due to infection with the vaccinia virus superimposed upon a preexisting skin condition, usually atopic dermatitis. Cf. *e. herpeticum*. **xerotic e.**, a dehydrated condition of the skin characterized by erythema, dry scaling, fine cracking, and pruritus, which occurs chiefly during the winter when low humidity in heated rooms causes excessive water loss from the stratum corneum. Called also *asteatosis*, *asteatotic eczema*, *eczema craquelé*, *pruritus hiemalis*, *winter itch*, and *xerosis cutis*.

eczematization (ek-zem″ah-ti-za′shun) persistent eczema-like lesions of the skin, usually due to the continued trauma of scratching.

eczematogenic (ek-zem″ah-to-jen′ik) causing eczema.

eczematoid (ek-zem′ah-toid) resembling eczema.

eczematous (ek-zem′ah-tus) affected with or of the nature of eczema.

E.D. erythema dose; effective dose.

ED₅₀ median effective dose; a dose that produces the desired effect in 50 per cent of a population.

edathamil (ĕ-dath′ah-mil) edetate. **calcium disodium e.,** edetate calcium disodium. **e. disodium,** edetate disodium.

Eddowes' syndrome (disease) (ed′ōz) [Alfred *Eddowes,* British physician, 1850–1946] see under *syndrome.*

Edebohls' position (ed′e-bōlz) [George Michael *Edebohls,* New York surgeon, 1853–1908] see under *position.*

Edecrin (ĕ-dek′krin) trademark for preparations of ethacrynic acid.

Edelman (a′d'l-man), Gerald Maurice. American biochemist, born 1929; co-winner, with Rodney Porter, of the Nobel prize for medicine or physiology in 1972 for his work in separating and identifying the heavy and light chains in the antibody molecule.

Edelmann's anemia, cell (a′del-manz) [Adolf *Edelmann,* physician in Vienna, 1885–1939] see under *anemia,* and see *kinetocyte.*

edema (ĕ-de′mah) [Gr. *oidēma* swelling] the presence of abnormally large amounts of fluid in the intercellular tissue spaces of the body; usually applied to demonstrable accumulation of excessive fluid in the subcutaneous tissues. Edema may be localized, due to venous or lymphatic obstruction or to increased vascular permeability, or it may be systemic due to heart failure or renal disease. Collections of edema fluid are designated according to the site, e.g., ascites (peritoneal cavity), hydrothorax (pleural cavity), and hydropericardium (pericardial sac). Massive generalized edema is called *anasarca.* **alimentary e.,** nutritional edema. **ambulant e.** (*obs.*), Calabar swelling; see under *swelling.* **angioneurotic e.,** angioedema. **Berlin's e.,** commotio retinae. **brain e.,** an excessive accumulation of fluid in the brain substance (*wet brain*); it may be due to various causes, including trauma, tumor, and increased permeability of the capillaries occurring as a result of anoxia or exposure to toxic substances. **brown e.,** hardening and infiltration of the lung with a brownish fluid. **e. bullo′sum vesi′cae,** a condition of the mucous lining of the bladder marked by the formation of clear vesicles with small white particles floating between them. **Calabar e.,** Calabar swellings. **e. cal′idum,** inflammatory e. **cardiac e.,** a manifestation of congestive heart failure, caused by increased venous and capillary pressures and often associated with the retention of sodium by the kidneys. **circumscribed e.,** angioedema. **dependent e.,** edema affecting most seriously the lowermost or dependent parts of the body. **famine e.,** nutritional e. **fingerprint e.,** edema in which the whorls of the fingerprint are clearly visible after circumferential manipulation of a pressure point on the forehead or sternum, considered indicative of intracellular fluid excess. **e. frig′idum,** noninflammatory e. **e. fu′gax,** transient accumulation of fluid in a specific region. **gaseous e.,** edema accompanied with gas formation, as in gas bacillus infection and subcutaneous emphysema. **giant e.,** angioedema. **hepatic e.,** edema due to faulty functioning of the liver. **hereditary angioneurotic e. (HANE),** hereditary angioedema. **high-altitude pulmonary e.,** pulmonary edema caused by hypoxia that develops as a result of prolonged exertion after ascending quickly to high altitudes without the benefit of acclimatization; seen especially in mountain climbers. **Huguenin's e.,** acute congestive edema of the brain. **hunger e.,** nutritional e. **hydremic e.,** edema in conditions marked by hydremia. **idiopathic e.,** edema of unknown cause affecting women, occurring intermittently over a period of years and usually worse during the premenstrual phase; it is associated with increased aldosterone secretion. **inflammatory e.,** a form due to inflammation, and attended with redness and pain. **insulin e.,** edema which sometimes follows the injection of insulin. **invisible e.,** the accumulation of a considerable amount of fluid in the subcutaneous tissues before it becomes demonstrable. **e. of lung,** pulmonary e. **lymphatic**

e., edema associated with obstruction of the lymph vessels. **malignant e.,** 1. a form of cutaneous anthrax (q.v.) in which massive spreading edema develops around a necrotic eschar. 2. inflammatory edema in gas gangrene. **Milroy's e.,** see under *disease.* **Milton's e.,** angioedema. **mucous e.,** myxedema. **e. neonato′rum,** a disease of premature and feeble infants that resembles sclerema and is marked by spreading edema with cold, livid skin. **nephrotic e.,** edema occurring in nephrosis and in the intermediate stage of diffuse nephritis. **noninflammatory e.,** edema without redness and pain, occurring from passive congestion or from lowered serum osmolarity. **nonpitting e.,** edema in which the tissues cannot be pitted by pressure. **nutritional e.,** a disorder of nutrition due to long-continued diet deficiency of protein and/or calories, and marked by anasarca and edema; called also *alimentary e., famine e., war e., hunger e.,* and *nutritional, famine,* or *war dropsy.* **paroxysmal pulmonary e.,** pulmonary edema marked by nocturnal attacks of difficult respiration, audible rales, wheezes, and cough, caused by acute left ventricular failure, usually associated with hypertensive heart disease. **passive e.,** edema occurring because of obstruction to vascular or lymphatic drainage from the area. **periodic e.,** angioedema. **periretinal e.,** central serous retinopathy. **pitting e.,** edema in which the tissues show prolonged existence of the pits produced by pressure. **placental e.,** the presence of fluid in the villi of the placenta, the villi being club-shaped and irregularly swollen. **prehepatic e.,** edema occurring in prehepatic hypoproteinemia. **pulmonary e.,** abnormal, diffuse, extravascular accumulation of fluid in the pulmonary tissues and air spaces due to changes in hydrostatic forces in the capillaries or to increased capillary permeability; it is characterized clinically by intense dyspnea and, in the intra-alveolar form, by voluminous expectoration of frothy pink serous fluid and, if severe, by cyanosis. **purulent e.,** a swelling due to the effusion of a purulent fluid. **Quincke's e.,** angioedema. **renal e.,** edema due to nephritis and the consequent hypoproteinemia. **rheumatismal e.,** painful red edematous swellings on the limbs in rheumatism, due to subcutaneous exudation. **salt e.,** edema produced by an increase of sodium chloride in the diet. **solid e.,** myxedema. **solid e. of lungs,** a rubbery consistency and gelatinous appearance of the lungs sometimes associated with hypertensive left ventricular failure and uremia. **terminal e.,** pulmonary edema which frequently develops as an agonal event from circulatory failure. **toxic e.,** edema caused by a poison. **vasogenic e.,** edema characterized by increased permeability of capillary endothelial cells; the most common form of brain edema. **venous e.,** edema in which the effused liquid comes from the blood. **vernal e. of lung,** edema of the lung occurring in spring and considered to be allergic. **war e.,** nutritional e.

edemagen (ĕ-de′mah-jen) an irritant that elicits edema by causing capillary damage but not the cellular response of true inflammation. Cf. *inflammagen.*

edematigenous (ĕ-dem″ah-tij′ĕ-nus) edematogenic.

edematization (ĕ-dem″ah-ti-za′shun) the process of becoming or of making edematous.

edematogenic (ĕ-dem″ah-to-jen′ik) producing or causing edema.

edematous (ĕ-dem′ah-tus) pertaining to or affected by edema.

Edentata (e″den-ta′tah) an order of mammals including armadillos, tree sloths, and anteaters.

edentate (e-den′tāt) edentulous.

edentia (e-den′she-ah) [L. *e* without + *dens* tooth] a condition in which some or all of the teeth are absent from the dental arch; anodontia. See also *Kennedy classification* and *Skinner classification,* under *classification.*

edentulate (e-den′tu-lāt) edentulous.

edentulous (e-den′tu-lus) without teeth; having lost some or all natural teeth. Called also *edentate* and *edentulate.*

edetate (ed′ĕ-tāt) nonproprietary drug name for salts of EDTA (ethylenediamine tetraacetic acid), a chelating agent used as *edetate calcium disodium* [USP], *edetate disodium* [USP], *edetate sodium,* and *edetate trisodium* in the diagnosis and treatment of lead poisoning and for emergency treatment of hypercalcemia. Formerly called *edathamil.* **e. calcium disodium** [USP], **calcium disodium e.,** chemical name: disodium [[*N,N*′-1,2-ethanediylbis[*N*-(carboxymethyl)glycinato]](4–)-*N,N′, O,O′,O*^N*,O*^{N′}calciate (2–). A metal complexing agent, $C_{10}H_{12}CaN_2NaO_8 \cdot xH_2O$, consisting of a mixture of the dihydrate and tetrahydrate calcium disodium salt of edetic acid, used intramuscularly or intravenously in the diagnosis and treatment of lead poisoning. Called also *calcium disodium edathamil, calcium EDTA, sodium calciumedetate,* and *sodium calcium edetate.* **e. disodium** [USP], **disodium e.,** chemical name: *N,N′*-1,2-ethanediylbis[*N*-(carboxymethyl)glycine] disodium salt. A metal complexing agent, $C_{10}H_{14}N_2Na_2O_8 \cdot 2H_2O$, used as a chelating pharmaceutic aid. It is also used in poisoning with lead and other heavy metals and, because of its affinity for calcium, in the treatment of hypercalcemia. Called also *edathamil disodium.* **e. sodium,** the tetrasodium salt of edetic acid, $C_{10}H_{12}N_2NaO_8$, used as a chelating agent. **e. trisodium,** the trisodium salt of edetic acid, $C_{10}H_{13}N_2NaO_8$, sometimes used similarly to edetate disodium.

edetic acid (ĕ-det′ik) EDTA; the free acid of edetate.

edge (ej) a thin side or border. **cutting e.,** the angle formed by the merging of two flat surfaces, by which something may be cut, such as the blade of a knife, or the incisal surface of an anterior tooth. **denture e.,** see under *border.* **incisal e.,** the junction of the labial surface of an anterior tooth with a flattened linguoincisal surface created by occlusal wear.

edge-strength (ej′ strength) the ability of fine edges to resist fracture or abrasion; applied especially to such resistance in dental restorations.

Edinger's law, nucleus (ed′ing-gerz) [Ludwig *Edinger,* German neurologist, 1855–1918] see under *law* and see *nucleus oculomotorius accessorius.*

Edinger-Westphal nucleus (ed′ing-ger vest′fahl) [L. *Edinger;* Carl Friedrich Otto *Westphal,* German neurologist, 1833–1890] nucleus oculomotorius accessorius.

edipism (ed′ĭ-pizm) [from *Oedipus,* King of Thebes. See *Oedipus complex*] intentional injury of one's own eyes.

edisylate (ĕ-dis′ĭ-lāt) USAN contraction for 1,2-ethanedisulfonate.

EDR effective direct radiation; electrodermal response.

edrophonium (ed″ro-fo′ne-um) an anticholinesterase agent with a duration of action of approximately 10 minutes; used for differential diagnosis and evaluation of treatment requirements in myasthenia gravis and as an antagonist to nondepolarizing neuromuscular blocking agents (e.g., tubocurarine). Available as *edrophonium chloride* [USP].

Edsall's disease (ed′salz) [David Linn *Edsall,* American physician, 1869–1945] heat cramp.

EDTA ethylenediaminetetraacetic acid.

educable (edj′u-kah-b′l) capable of being educated; used to describe persons with mild mental retardation (IQ 50–70) who in their late teens can learn academic skills up to about the sixth grade level and can usually achieve social and vocational skills adequate for minimal self-support. Cf. *trainable.*

eduction (e-duk′shun) [L. *e* (*ex*) from + *ducere* to lead] the process of leading out from or the dissipation of a former state, as the restoration to normal physiological state of an anesthetized patient.

edulcorant (e-dul′ko-rant) sweetening.

edulcorate (e-dul′ko-rāt) to sweeten.

Edwardsiella (ed-ward″se-el′ah) [Philip R. *Edwards,* American bacteriologist, 1901–1966] a genus of gram-negative, facultatively anaerobic bacteria of the family Enterobacteriaceae, made up of small rods that are mostly motile with peritrichous flagella. The organisms are pathogenic for aquatic animals and an occasional opportunistic pathogen for humans. **E. hoshi′nae,** a motile species that, isolated from animals and humans, does not produce indole. **E. ic′taluri,** a nonmotile species that does not produce indole, occurring as a pathogen of catfish. **E. tar′da,** an indole-producing species found in the intestinal tract of snakes, and occasionally isolated from the urine, blood, and feces of humans. It can cause acute gastroenteritis and serious septic infections.

Edwardsielleae (ed-ward″se-el′e-e) in some systems of classification, a tribe of gram-negative, facultatively anaerobic, rod-shaped bacteria of the family Enterobacteriaceae, made up of the genus *Edwardsiella.*

EEE eastern equine encephalomyelitis.

EEG electroencephalogram.

eelworm (ēl′wurm) any roundworm, such as ascaris.

E.E.N.T. eye-ear-nose-throat.

EFA essential fatty acids.

E-Ferol (e-fer′ol) trademark for a preparation of an intravenous vitamin E supplement.

effacement (ĕ-fās′ment) the obliteration of the cervix in labor when it is so changed that only the thin external os remains.

effect (ĕ-fekt′) the result produced by an action. **additive e.,** the combined effect produced by the action of two or more agents, being equal to the sum of their separate effects. **anachoretic e.,** see *anachoresis.* **Anrep e.,** augmented resistance to outflow in the heart. **Blinks e's,** brief enhancement in photosynthesis which follows shifts from a long wavelength to a shorter wavelength. **Bohr e.,** displacement of the oxyhemoglobin dissociation curve by a change in partial pressure of carbon dioxide or in pH. **Bruce e.,** the blocking of pregnancy in a newly impregnated female mouse by a pheromone (the odor of a strange male). **clasp-knife e.,** a sudden complete flexion of the limb in the lengthening reaction. **Compton e.,** the change in the wavelength of roentgen or gamma rays due to interaction of an incident photon with an orbital electron of an atom, which produces a recoil electron and a scattered photon of reduced energy. **contrary e.,** Hata's phenomenon. **Crabtree e.,** the inhibition of oxygen consumption on the addition of glucose to tissues or microorganisms having a high rate of aerobic glycolysis; the converse of the Pasteur effect. **Danysz e.,** see under *phenomenon.* **Deelman e.,** scarification of the skin in artificial carcinogenesis tends to localize the subsequent carcinomata at the scarified area. **Doppler e.,** the relationship of the apparent frequency of waves, as of sound, light, and radio waves, to the relative motion of the source of the waves and the observer, the frequency increasing as the two approach each other and decreasing as they move apart. **Emerson e.,** the photosynthetic efficiency of a long wavelength of light is enhanced by simultaneous exposure of plant cells to shorter wavelengths of light. **experimenter e's,** see *demand characteristics,* under *characteristic.* **Fahraeus-Lindqvist e.,** blood viscosity is lower in small vessels (diameter less than 1.5 mm) than in large vessels, the viscosity in capillaries being less than half that in large vessels; the effect is due to red cells moving together in single file through the small vessels. **Hallberg e.,** the crests and troughs of ultrashort standing-wave field have opposite electrical signs. **Hallwachs e.,** photoelectrical e. **heel e.,** in radiology, variation in intensity through the cross section of the useful beam due to differential attenuation of roentgen rays emerging at varying angles from beneath the focal spot; the intensity is greater on the cathode side. **interpolar e.,** the effect of an electric current throughout the whole region of the body between the two electrodes or poles, as contrasted with polar effects. **isomorphic e.,** Koebner phenomenon. **Mierzejewski e.,** the disharmonious development of gray and white matter of the brain, the gray being in excess. **Nagler e.,** gas-filled tubes, placed in high frequency fields, will act as rectifiers, causing a unidirectional current. **Orbeli e.,** see under *phenomenon.* **Pasteur e.,** the decrease in the rate of glucose utilization (glycolysis) and the suppression of lactate accumulation by tissues or microorganisms in the presence of oxygen. Cf. *Crabtree e.* **photechic e.,** Russell e. **photoelectrical e.,** the ejection of electrons from matter when light of short wavelengths falls upon it; called also *Hallwachs e.* **placebo e.,** the sum total of all nonspecific effects, both good and adverse, of medical treatment, primarily psychological and psychophysiological effects associated with the physician-patient relationship and the patient's expectations and apprehensions concerning the treatment. **polar e.,** the effect of the electric current which is manifested at one of the poles. **position e.,** in genetics, the changed effect produced by alteration of the relative positions of various genes on the chromosomes. **pressure e.,** the sum of the changes that are due to obstruction of tissue drainage by pressure. **Purkinje e.,** see under *phenomenon.* **Raman e.,** when a substance is irradiated with monochromatic light, the spectrum which the substance scatters contains, in addition to a line of the same wavelength as the incident radiation, lines which are satellites of the primary line moving with it when the wavelength of the primary radiation is altered.

Russell e., the rendering of a photographic plate developable by agents other than light; called also *photechic effect.* **side e.,** see under S. **Somogyi e.,** see under *phenomenon.* **Soret e.,** when a solution is maintained for some time in a temperature gradient, a difference in concentration develops along the temperature gradient. **specific dynamic e.,** see under *action.* **Staub-Traugott e.,** a second dose of dextrose by mouth to a normal person one hour after a first dose does not elevate the blood sugar level. **Tyndall e.,** see under *phenomenon.* **Whitten e.,** initiation and synchronization of the estrous cycles and reduction of the frequency of reproductive abnormalities in female mice by the odor (pheromone) of a male mouse placed among them; when more than four female mice are placed together in a cage their estrous cycles become very erratic. **Wolff-Chaikoff e.,** inhibition of the synthesis of thyroid hormone after administration of large doses of iodide. **Zeeman e.,** separation of a single line in the spectrum by suitable magnetic fields.

effectiveness (ĕ-fek′tiv-nes) the ability to produce a specific result or to exert a specific measurable influence. **relative biological e.,** an expression of the effectiveness of other types of radiation in comparison with that of gamma or roentgen rays. Abbreviated RBE.

effector (ef-fek′tor) 1. an agent that mediates a specific effect, e.g., an allosteric effector or an effector cell. 2. an organ that produces an effect, e.g., contraction or secretion, in response to nerve stimulation. Cf. *receptor.* **allosteric e.,** an enzyme inhibitor or activator that has its effect at a site other than the catalytic site of the enzyme; see also under *site,* and see *allosterism.*

effemination (ĕ-fem″ĭ-na′shun) feminization.

efferent (ef′er-ent) [L. *ex* out + *ferre* to bear] centrifugal; conveying away from a center, as an efferent nerve.

efferential (ef″er-en′shal) efferent.

effervescent (ef-er-ves′ent) [L. *effervescens*] bubbling; sparkling; giving off gas bubbles.

effleurage (ef-loo-rahzh′) [Fr.] stroking movement in massage; frottage.

efflorescence (ef″lo-res′ens) [L. *efflorescentia*] a rash or eruption; any skin lesions, especially numerous and conspicuous lesions.

efflorescent (ef″lo-res′ent) [L. *efflorescere* to bloom] becoming powdery in consequence of losing water of crystallization.

effluve (ef-loōv′) a conductive discharge of a high voltage current through a dielectric.

effluvia (ef-floo′ve-ah) [L.] plural of *effluvium.*

effluvium (ef-floo′ve-um), pl. *efflu′via* [L. "a flowing out"] 1. an outflowing, or shedding, especially of the hair. 2. an exhalation or emanation, applied especially to one of noxious character. **anagen e.,** abnormal loss of hair during the anagen phase, which may occur following administration of certain cancer chemotherapeutic agents or exposure to certain chemicals, or in association with various other factors and diseases. **telluric e.,** an emanation arising from the earth; see *miasma* and *tellurium.* **telogen e.,** the early, excessive, temporary loss of normal club hairs from normal resting follicles in the scalp as a result of traumatization by some stimulus (e.g., surgery, starvation diet, parturition, drugs, traction, high fever, certain diseases, or psychogenic stress) that prematurely precipitates the anagen phase into catagen and telogen phases, altering the normal hair cycle.

effraction (ef-frak′shun) a breaking open; a weakening.

effumability (ef″u-mah-bil′ĭ-te) [L. *ex* out + *fumus* smoke] the property of being easily volatilized.

effuse [L. *effusus,* from *ex* out + *fundere* to pour] 1. (ĕ-fūs′) spread out, profuse; said of bacterial growth that is thin, veily, and unusually widely spread. 2. (ĕ-fūz′) to pour out and spread widely.

effusion (ĕ-fu′zhun) [L. *effusio* a pouring out] 1. the escape of fluid into a part or tissue, as an exudation or a transudation. 2. an effused material, which may be classified according to protein content as an exudate or transudate. **hemorrhagic e.,** an effusion of bloody liquid. **pleural e.,** the presence of fluid in the pleural space.

Efudex (ef′u-deks) trademark for a preparation of fluorouracil for topical application.

egagropilus (e″gah-grop′ĭ-lus) [Gr. *aigagros* wild goat + *pilos* felt] trichobezoar.

egersimeter (e″ger-sim′ĕ-ter) an instrument for testing the electric excitability of nerves and muscles and for measuring chronaxia.

egersis (e-ger′sis) [Gr.] (*obs.*) extreme wakefulness.

egesta (e-jes′tah) [L. *e* out + *gerere* to bear] undigested material thrown out from the body.

egestion (e-jes′chun) the casting out of material which is indigestible.

egg (eg) [L. *ovum*] 1. an ovum; a female gamete. 2. an oocyte. 3. a female reproductive cell at any stage before fertilization and its derivatives after fertilization and even after some development.

Eggleston's method (eg′el-stunz) [Cary *Eggleston,* New York physician, 1884–1966] see under *method.*

egilops (e′jĭ-lops) [Gr. *aix* goat + *ōps* eye] perforating abscess at the inner canthus of the eye.

eglandulous (e-gland′u-lus) [L. *e* without + *glandula* glandule] having no glands.

ego (e′go) [L. "I"] in modern psychoanalytic theory, the psychologic segment of the personality, dominated by the reality principle, comprising integrative and executive aspects that function to adapt the forces and pressures exerted by the impulses of the id, the demands of the superego, and the requirements of external reality through conscious perception, thought, reasoning, learning, and all other activities necessary to interact effectively with the world. Cf. *id* (def. 1) and *superego.*

ego-alien (e″go-āl′yen) ego-dystonic.

egobronchophony (e″go-bron-kof′o-ne) [Gr. *aix* goat + *bronchophony*] increased vocal resonance with high-pitched bleating quality of the transmitted voice, detected by auscultation of the lungs, especially over lung tissue compressed by pleural effusion.

egocentric (e″go-sen′trik) [L. *ego* I + *centric*] self-centered, conceited, egotistical; preoccupied with one's own interests and needs; lacking concern for others.

ego-dystonic (e″go-dis-ton′ik) denoting aspects of a person's thoughts, impulses, attitudes, and behavior that are felt to be repugnant, distressing, unacceptable, or inconsistent with the rest of his personality. Cf. *ego-syntonic.*

ego-ideal (e′go-i′de-al) see under *ideal.*

egoism (e′go-izm) 1. a healthy awareness and advancement of one's own interests. 2. the philosophical doctrine that self-interest is the proper basis of all human conduct. 3. self-centeredness, egotism.

egomania (e″go-ma′ne-ah) [Gr. *egō* I + *mania* madness] extreme self-centeredness; extreme egotism.

egophony (e-gof′o-ne) [Gr. *aix* goat + *phōnē* voice] egobronchophony.

ego-syntonic (e″go-sin-ton′ik) denoting aspects of a person's thoughts, impulses, attitudes, and behavior that are felt to be acceptable and consistent with the rest of his personality. Cf. *ego-dystonic.*

egotism (e′go-tizm) conceit, selfishness, self-centeredness; an inflated sense of one's importance.

egotropic (e″go-trop′ik) [Gr. *egō* I + *tropos* a turning] egocentric.

E_h symbol for *redox potential.*

EHBF estimated hepatic blood flow.

EHDP ethane-1-hydroxy-1,1-diphosphonate; see *etidronate.*

Ehlers-Danlos syndrome (disease) (a′lerz-dan′los) [Edvard *Ehlers,* Danish dermatologist, 1863–1937; Henri Alexandre *Danlos*] see under *syndrome.*

Ehrenritter's ganglion (er′en-rit″erz) [Johann *Ehrenritter,* Austrian anatomist, died 1790] ganglion superius nervi glossopharyngei.

Ehrlich (ār′lik) Paul. German physician and bacteriologist, 1854–1915; co-winner, with Elie Metchnikoff, of the Nobel prize for medicine or physiology in 1908 for developing the side chain theory.

Ehrlich's reaction, etc. (ār′lik) [Paul *Ehrlich*] see under *body, granule, reaction, stain, test,* and *theory,* and see *arsphenamine.*

Ehrlich-Hata preparation, remedy, treatment [Paul

Ehrlich; Sahachiro *Hata,* Japanese physician, 1872–1938] arsphenamine.

Ehrlich-Heinz granules (ār′lik hĭnts) [Paul *Ehrlich;* Robert *Heinz,* German pathologist, 1865–1924]   Ehrlich's granules.

Ehrlichia (ār-lik′e-ah) [Paul *Ehrlich*]   a genus of bacteria of the tribe Ehrichieae, family Rickettsiaceae, order Rickettsiales that produce disease in dogs, cattle, sheep, and humans. **E. ca′nis,** a species causing disease in dogs, transmitted by the tick *Rhipicephalus sanguineus.* Called also *Rickettsia canis.*

Ehrlichieae (ār″lĭ-ki′e-e)   a tribe of bacteria of the family Rickettsiaceae, order Rickettsiales, made up of rickettsia-like organisms adapted to existence in invertebrates, chiefly arthropods, and pathogenic for certain mammals, including humans. It includes the genera *Cowdria, Ehrlichia,* and *Neorickettsia.*

EIA   enzyme immunoassay.

Eichhorst's atrophy (type), corpuscles (ik′horsts) [Hermann Ludwig *Eichhorst,* Swiss physician, 1849–1921]   see under *atrophy* and *corpuscle.*

Eicken's method (i′kenz) [Carl von *Eicken,* German laryngologist and otologist, 1873–1960]   see under *method.*

eiconometer (i″ko-nom′ĕ-ter)   eikonometer.

eicosanoate (i-ko″sah-no′āt)   systematic name for arachidate, denoting that it has twenty (*eicosa* twenty) carbon atoms in a straight chain.

eicosanoic acid (i″ko-sah-no′ik)   arachidic acid.

eicosanoid (i-ko″sah-noid) [*eicosane* + *-oid*]   any of the biologically active substances derived from arachidonic acid, including the prostaglandins and leukotrienes.

eidetic (i-det′ik) [Gr. *eidos* that which is seen; form or shape]   pertaining to or characterized by exact visualization of events or of objects previously seen. By extension, sometimes used to designate an individual possessing such an ability.

eidogen (i′do-jen) [Gr. *eidos* form + *genesthai* produced]   a substance elaborated by a second grade inductor, which is capable of modifying the form of an embryonic organ already in the process of formation.

eidoptometry (i″dop-tom′ĕ-tre) [Gr. *eidos* form + *opto-* + *-metry*]   measurement of the acuteness of vision for the perception of form.

Eijkman (ik′man)   Christiaan. Dutch physiologist, 1858–1930; co-winner, with Sir Frederick Gowland Hopkins, of the Nobel prize for medicine or physiology in 1929 for his discovery of the antineuritic vitamin, B₁ thiamine.

Eijkman's test (ik′manz) [Christiaan *Eijkman*]   see under *tests.*

Eikenella (i″ken-el′ah) [M. *Eiken*]   a genus of gram-negative, facultatively anaerobic, rod-shaped bacteria. The organisms are part of the normal flora of the human oral cavity and upper respiratory tract but may cause infections of the head, neck, and abdominal area and general systemic disease. The single species is *E. corrodens.*

eikonometer (i″ko-nom′ĕ-ter) [Gr. *eikōn* image + *-metry*]   an instrument used in making an examination for aniseikonia.

eiloid (i′loid) [Gr. *eilein* to roll up + *eidos* form]   having a coiled appearance.

Eimeria (i-me′re-ah) [Gustav Heinrich Theodor *Eimer,* German zoologist, 1843–1898]   a genus of homoxenous coccidian protozoa (suborder Eimeriina, order Eucoccidiida) found principally as parasites of the gastrointestinal tract of birds and herbivorous mammals, characterized by the presence of four spores in each oocyst and two sporozoites in each spore, the oocysts being passed in the feces. It comprises numerous species, many of which are of economic importance. Some of the common pathogenic species found in domestic animals are *E. bovis, E. ellipsoidalis,* and *E. zuernii* in cattle; *E. arloingi* A (*ovina*), *E. weybridgensis* (*E. arloingi* B), *E. crandallis, E. ahsata, E. ovinoidalis,* and *E. gilruthi* in sheep; *E. debliecki, E. scabra,* and *E. perminuta* in swine; *E. leukarti* in horses and donkeys; *E. arloingi, E. faurei, E. caprina,* and *E. ninakohlyakimovae* in goats; *E. magna, E. stieda, E. sciurorum,* and *E. perforans* in rabbits; and *E. acervulina, E. maxima, E. meleagridis, E. necatrix,* and *E. tenella* in poultry. See also *coccidiosis.*

Eimeriina (i″me-ri′ĭ-nah)   a suborder of homoxenous or heteroxenous protozoa (order Eucoccidiida, subclass Coccidia), usually parasitizing the gut epithelium of the host, in which the macrogamete and microgametocyte develop independently, syzygy does not occur, the microgametocyte gives rise to numerous biflagellated microgametes, the zygont is not mobile, and the sporozoites are typically enclosed in an oocyst. Representative genera include *Aggregata, Besnoitia, Cryptosporidium, Eimeria, Isospora, Sarcocystis, Toxoplasma,* and *Tyzzeria.*

Einhorn's saccharimeter, string test (in′hornz) [Max *Einhorn,* physician in New York, 1862–1953]   see under *saccharimeter* and *string test.*

einsteinium (in-sti′ne-um) [Albert *Einstein,* theoretical physicist, born in Germany, became a naturalized citizen of Switzerland, then of the United States, 1879–1955; winner of Nobel prize for physics in 1921]   the chemical element of atomic number 99, atomic weight 254, symbol Es, originally discovered in debris from a thermonuclear explosion in 1952.

Einthoven (in′to-ven)   Willem. Dutch physiologist, 1860–1927; winner of the Nobel prize for medicine or physiology in 1924 for his invention of a string galvanometer to produce the electrocardiogram.

Einthoven's formula, galvanometer, triangle (in′to-venz) [Willem *Einthoven*]   see under *formula, galvanometer,* and *triangle.*

eisanthema (is-an′the-mah) [Gr. *eis* into + *anthein* to bloom]   an eruption on a mucous membrane.

Eisenia (i-se′ne-ah)   a genus of chaelopod worms. *E. fo-e′tida,* a species reportedly found in the urine of man.

Eisenmenger's complex (i′sen-meng″erz) [Victor *Eisenmenger,* German physician, 1864–1932]   see under *complex.*

eisodic (i-sod′ik) [Gr. *eis* into + *hodos* way]   afferent or centripetal.

EIT   erythrocyte iron turnover.

Eitelberg's test (i′tel-bergz) [Abraham *Eitelberg,* Austrian physician, born 1847]   see under *tests.*

eiweissmilch (i′vis-milkh) [Ger.]   albumin milk; see under *milk.*

ejaculate (e-jak′u-lāt)   1. to expel suddenly, especially semen.   2. the semen expelled in a single ejaculation; ejaculum.

ejaculatio (e-jak″u-la′she-o) [L.]   ejaculation.   **e. defi′ciens,** defective ejaculation.   **e. prae′cox,** ejaculation of the semen immediately after the beginning of the sexual act.   **e. retarda′ta,** unduly delayed ejaculation.

ejaculation (e-jak″u-la′shun) [L. *ejaculatio*]   a sudden act of expulsion, as of the semen.   **premature e.,** ejaculatio praecox.

ejaculator (e-jak″u-la′tor) [L.]   that which or one who ejaculates.   **e. sem′inis,** musculus bulbospongiosus.

ejaculatory (e-jak′u-lah-to″re) [L. *ejaculatorius*]   pertaining to ejaculation.

ejaculum (e-jak′u-lum)   the semen discharged in a single ejaculation in the male, consisting of the secretions of Cowper's gland, epididymis, ductus deferens, seminal vesicles, and prostate, and containing the spermatozoa. Called also *ejaculate.*

ejecta (e-jek′tah) [L. pl.; from *e* out + *jacere* to cast]   materials which have been cast out from the body. Excrementitious material; refuse.

ejection (e-jek′shun)   1. the act of ejecting or the state of being ejected.   2. something ejected.   **milk e.,** let-down reflex.

Ejusd.   abbreviation for L. *ejus′dem,* of the same.

eka- (e′kah) [Sanscrit, "one" or "first"]   a prefix added to the name of a known chemical element as a provisional designation of the unknown element which should occur next in the same group in the periodic system.

eka-iodine (e′kah i′o-dīn)   the name formerly used to designate element 85, now officially known as astatine.

EKG   electrocardiogram.

ekiri (ĕ-ke′re)   an acute cerebral and cardiovascular disorder occurring in children with shigellosis in Japan.

EKY   electrokymogram.

elaborate (e-lab′o-rāt) [L. *elabora′re* to work out]   to produce complex substances out of simpler materials.

elaboration (e-lab″o-ra′shun)   1. the process of producing complex substances out of simpler materials.   2. in psychiatry, an unconscious mental process of expansion and embellishment of detail, especially of a symbol or representation in a dream; called also *secondary e.*

elacin (el′ah-sin)　degenerated elastic tissue.

elae(o)-, elai(o)-　for words beginning thus, see those beginning *ele(o)-*.

elaidic acid (el″ah-id′ik)　the *trans* isomer of oleic acid.

elaioma (e-le-o′mah)　eleoma.

elaiometer (e″la-om′ĕ-ter)　eleometer.

elaiopathia (e″la-o-path′e-ah)　elaiopathy.

elaiopathy (e″la-op′ah-the) [Gr. *elaion* oil + *pathos* disease] a diffuse fatty edema, usually attacking the joints of the lower extremities, the effect of contusions or distortions incurred in war, and attributed to the formation of an irritating oily substance and its action upon the subcutaneous cellular tissue (C. Blondi, 1917).　**pathomimic e.,** the simulation of disease produced by the injection of liquid petrolatum subcutaneously.

elaioplast (e-la′o-plast) [Gr. *elaion* oil + *plassein* to form] a fat-producing plastid.

elantrine (el′an-trēn)　chemical name: 3-(5,6-dihydro-5-methyl)-11*H*-dibenz[*b,e*]azepin-11-ylidine-*N*, *N*-dimethyl-1-propanamine. An anticholinergic, $C_{20}H_{24}N_2$, which has been used in the treatment of drug-induced extrapyramidal syndrome.

elapid (el′ah-pid)　1. any snake of the family Elapidae. 2. of or pertaining to the family Elapidae.

Elapidae (e-lap′ĭ-de)　a family of usually terrestrial, venomous snakes, which have cylindrical tails and front fangs that are short, stout, immovable, and grooved. It includes cobras, kraits, coral snakes, Australian copperheads, Australian blacksnakes, brown snakes, tiger snakes, death adders, and mambas.

Elaps (e′laps)　*Micruris.*

elasmobranch (e-las′mo-brank) [Gr. *elasmos* plate + L. *branchia* gill]　1. any cartilaginous fish having platelike gills, each gill slit opening independently on the body surface, such as sharks, skates, rays, and sawfish. 2. of or pertaining to elasmobranchs.

elassosis (el″ah-so′sis) [Gr. *elassōn* smaller, less]　a diminutive type of mitosis characteristic of the small cells of the thymus.

elastance (e-las′tans)　the quality of recoiling on removal of pressure without disruption, or an expression of the measure of the ability to do so, as an expression of the recoil of an air- or fluid-filled organ, e.g., the lung or urinary bladder, in terms of unit of pressure change per unit of volume change. It is the reciprocal of compliance.

elastase (pancreatic) (e-las′tās)　[EC 3.4.21.36] an enzyme of the hydrolase class that catalyzes the hydrolysis of peptide bonds containing the carboxyl groups of alanine, glycine, isoleucine, leucine, or valine, so named because it was once thought to attack elastin preferentially. It is a serine proteinase secreted by the pancreas as the zymogen proelastase, and is involved in the intestinal digestion of proteins.

elastic (e-las′tik) [L. *elasticus*]　1. susceptible of resisting and recovering from stretching, compression, or distortion applied by a force. Cf. *resiliency.* 2. an elastic band, usually of rubber, used in orthodontic therapy.　**intermaxillary e.,** an elastic band used to produce traction between the upper and lower teeth in orthodontic therapy.　**intramaxillary e.,** an elastic band applied within the same dental arch to achieve space closure.　**vertical e.,** an elastic band applied in a direction perpendicular to the occlusal plane, connecting one arch wire to the other, usually for approximating teeth to improve intercuspation.

elastica (e-las′tĭ-kah) [L.]　1. gum elastic or caoutchouc. 2. a general term for elastic tissue of the body, such as that found in the tunica media of blood vessels. 3. tunica media.

elasticin (e-las′tĭ-sin)　elastin.

elasticity (e″las-tis′ĭ-te)　the quality or condition of being elastic.　**physical e. of muscle,** the physical quality of muscle of being elastic, of yielding to passive physical stretch.　**physiologic e. of muscle,** the biologic quality, unique to muscle, of being able to change and resume size under neuromuscular control.　**total e. of muscle,** the combined effect of physical and physiologic elasticity of muscle.

elastin (e-las′tin)　a yellow scleroprotein, the essential constituent of yellow elastic connective tissue: it is brittle when dry, but when moist is flexible and elastic.

elastinase (e-las′tin-ās)　elastase.

elastofibroma (e-las″to-fi-bro′mah)　a tumor consisting of both elastin and fibrous elements.　**e. dor′si,** a tumor-like nodule of subscapular soft tissue, occurring in old age, consisting of an elastin-filled central core and a surrounding elastase-resistant matrix impregnated with elastin.

elastogel (e-las′to-jel)　a gel which possesses great elasticity.

elastoid (e-las′toid)　a substance formed by the hyaline degeneration of the internal elastic lamina of blood vessels; seen in the vessels of the uterus after delivery.

elastoidosis, (e-las″toi-do′sis)　changes in the skin resembling elastosis.　**nodular e.,** see under *elastosis.*

elastolysis (e″las-tol′ĭ-sis) [*elasto-* + *lysis*]　a defect in the elastic tissue, resulting in atrophy and laxity of the skin. See *anetoderma, atrophoderma,* and *cutis laxa.*　**generalized e.,** cutis laxa.　**perifollicular e.,** see under *anetoderma.*　**postinflammatory e.,** see under *anetoderma.*

elastolytic (e-las″to-lit′ik)　capable of catalyzing the digestion of elastic tissue.

elastoma (e″las-to′mah)　a tumor or focal excess of elastic tissue fibers or abnormal collagen fibers of the skin.　**juvenile e.,** connective tissue nevus.

elastomer (ĕ-las′to-mer)　a synthetic rubber; any of various soft, elastic, rubber-like polymers; used in dentistry as an impression material.

elastometer (e″las-tom′ĕ-ter)　an instrument for determining the elasticity of tissues, and thus measuring the degree of edema.

elastometry (e″las-tom′ĕ-tre)　the measurement of elasticity.

elastomucin (e-las″to-mu′sin)　a polysaccharide component of elastic tissue.

elastopathy (e″las-top′ah-the)　deficiency of elastic tissue.

Elastoplast (e-las′to-plast)　trademark for an elastic bandage.

elastorrhexis (e-las″to-rek′sis)　rupture of fibers composing elastic tissue.

elastose (e-las′tōs)　an albumose formed by treating elastin with ferments, acids, or alkalis.

elastosis (e″las-to′sis)　1. degeneration of elastic tissue. 2. degenerative changes in the dermal connective tissue with increased amounts of elastotic material having the staining properties of elastin. 3. any disturbance of the dermal connective tissue.　**actinic e.,** premature aging of the skin due to solar damage caused by prolonged exposure to sunlight, occurring especially in light-skinned individuals, and chiefly characterized by inelasticity, thinning or sometimes thickening (see *cutis rhomboidalis nuchae,* and *nodular elastosis,* under *elastosis*), wrinkling, dryness with fine scaling, and variable hyperpigmentation of the skin, often associated with the development of cherry angiomas, telangiectasis, senile lentigines, ecchymosis, milea, and senile keratosis. Called also *farmers'* or *sailors' skin, senile e.,* and *solar e.*　**nodular e. of Favre-Racouchot,** actinic elastosis occurring chiefly in elderly men, in which giant comedones, pilosebaceous cysts, and large folds of furrowed and yellowish skin are seen in the periorbital region. Called also *Favre-Racouchot syndrome* and *nodular elastoidosis.*　**e. per′forans serpigino′sa, perforating e.,** a chronic disorder of the dermal connective tissue, usually occurring in males below 30 years of age, alone or in association with more widespread disease, typically characterized by the development of a skin-colored keratopapular eruption consisting of clustered arciform serpiginous lesions that gradually form a circular or horseshoe-shaped pattern, especially on the sides and nape of the neck but sometimes also on the upper arms, face, trunk, and other areas of the body. Elongated tortuous channels in the epidermis into which abnormal elastic tissue perforates and is extruded into the dermis are the most significant histopathologic features.　**senile e.,** 1. senile atrophy of skin. 2. actinic e.　**solar e.,** actinic e.

elastotic (e″las-tot′ik)　1. pertaining to or characterized by elastosis. 2. resembling elastic tissue; having the staining properties of elastin.

elater (el′ah-ter) a specialized structure of certain plants, such as liverworts and slime molds, which aids in the distribution of spores.

elation (e-la′shun) emotional excitement marked by speeding up of mental and bodily activity.

Elavil (el′ah-vil) trademark for preparation of amitriptyline hydrochloride.

elbow (el′bo) [L. *cubitus*] 1. the joint that connects the arm and forearm; called also *cubitus* [NA]. 2. any angular bend. **baseball pitchers' e.,** a disorder of the elbow in baseball pitchers due to a piece of cartilage or bone torn from the head of the radius. **capped e.,** hygroma of the elbow; a swelling of the bursa or a hard, fibrous mass on the point of the elbow in horses or cattle. Called also *shoe boil.* **dropped e.,** radial paralysis (def. 2). **golfer's e.,** pain due to medial epicondylitis, the lesion being in the origin of the flexor muscles. **little leaguer's e.,** medial epicondylitis of the elbow due to repeated stress on the flexor muscles of the forearm, a frequent problem of adolescent ballplayers. **miners' e.,** enlargement of the bursa over the point of the elbow (olecranon bursitis) caused by resting the weight of the body on the elbow as in mining. **nursemaids' e.,** pulled e. **pulled e.,** subluxation of the head of the radius distally under the annular ligament, produced by sudden traction on the hand with the elbow extended and the forearm pronated; called also *nursemaid's e., Goyrand's injury,* and *Malgaigne's luxation.* **tennis e.,** a painful condition localized to the outer aspect of the elbow, due to inflammation or irritation of the extensor tendon attachment to the lateral humeral condyle; called also *external humeral epicondylitis,* and *radiohumeral bursitis* or *epicondylitis.*

elcosis (el-ko′sis) helcosis.

Eldadryl (el′dah-dril) trademark for a preparation of diphenhydramine hydrochloride.

Eldecort (el′dĕ-kort) trademark for preparations of hydrocortisone.

elder (el′der) the plants, *Sambucus nigra,* L., of Europe, S. *canadensis,* L. (Caprifoliaceae), of America, and other congeneric species; the flowers, which contain a volatile oil, have been used in dressing wounds, burns, ulcers, etc., and as a diaphoretic, laxative and diuretic.

Eldodram (el′do-dram) trademark for a preparation of dimenhydrinate.

Eldopaque (el′do-pāk) trademark for preparations of hydroquinone.

Eldoquin (el′do-kwin) trademark for a preparation of hydroquinone.

eldrin (el′drin) rutin.

elective (e-lek′tiv) 1. tending to combine with or act on one substance rather than another. 2. subject to the choice or decision of the patient or physician; applied to procedures that are advantageous to the patient but not urgent.

Electra complex (e-lek-trah) see under *complex.*

electro- [Gr. *ēlektron* amber, because an electric charge can be produced in amber by rubbing] a combining form denoting relationship to electricity.

electroacupuncture (e-lek″tro-ak″u-pung′-cher) acupuncture in which the needles are stimulated electrically.

electroaffinity (e-lek″tro-ah-fin′ĭ-te) electronegativity.

electroanalgesia (e-lek″tro-an″al-je′ze-ah) the reduction of pain by electrical stimulation of a peripheral nerve or the dorsal column of the spinal cord.

electroanalysis (e-lek″tro-ah-nal′ĭ-sis) chemical analysis performed by the aid of the electric current.

electroanesthesia (e-lek″tro-an″es-the′ze-ah) anesthesia, either local or general, induced by electricity.

electroaugmentation (e-lek″tro-awg″men-ta′shun) electrical pacing of the heart.

electrobasograph (e-lek″tro-ba′so-graf) [*electro-* + Gr. *basis* step + *graphein* to record] an apparatus for recording the duration of weight bearing on the respective part while walking, i.e., a record of the gait.

electrobiology (e-lek″tro-bi-ol′o-je) [*electro-* + *biology*] the study of electric phenomena in living tissue.

electrobioscopy (e-lek″tro-bi-os′ko-pe) [*electro-* + Gr. *bios* life + *skopein* to examine] the determination of the presence or absence of life by means of an electric current.

electrocardiogram (e-lek″tro-kar′de-o-gram″) [*electro-* +

Gr. *kardia* heart + *gramma* mark] a graphic tracing of the variations in electrical potential caused by the excitation of the heart muscle and detected at the body surface. The normal electrocardiogram shows deflections resulting from atrial and ventricular activity. The first deflection, P, is due to excitation of the atria. The QRS deflections are due to excitation (depolarization) of the ventricles. The T wave is due to recovery of the ventricles (repolarization). The U wave is a potential undulation of unknown origin immediately following the T wave, seen in normal electrocardiograms and accentuated in hypokalemia. Abbreviated ECG or EKG. See also *lead*[2]. **scalar e.,** a conventional tracing showing

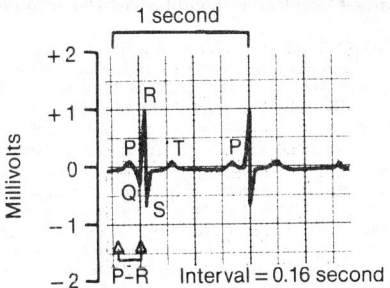

Normal electrocardiogram.

only changes in magnitude of voltage and polarity (positive and negative) with time.

electrocardiograph (e-lek″tro-kar′de-o-graf″) an instrument for performing electrocardiography, i.e., for making electrocardiograms.

electrocardiography (e-lek″tro-kar″de-og′rah-fe) the making of graphic records of the variations in electrical potential caused by electrical activity of the heart muscle and detected at the body surface, as a method for studying the action of the heart muscle; see *electrocardiogram.* **intracardiac e.,** that performed by introducing an electrode through a cardiac catheter. **precordial e.,** an electrocardiographic technique in which potentials over the chest wall near the surface of the heart are recorded; see *precordial leads,* under *lead*[2].

electrocardiophonogram (e-lek″tro-kar″de-o-fo′no-gram) (*obs.*) a record of the heart sounds made by an electrocardiophonograph.

electrocardiophonograph (e-lek″tro-kar″de-o-fo′no-graf) (*obs.*) an apparatus for recording electrically the heart sounds.

electrocardioscopy (e-lek″tro-kar-de-os′ko-pe) [*electro-* + Gr. *kardia* heart + *skopein* to examine] (*obs.*) electrocardiography by means of a cathode-ray oscillograph which throws a record on a luminous screen.

electrocatalysis (e-lek″tro-kah-tal′ĭ-sis) the catalytic effect produced by electricity on the bodily processes.

electrocautery (e-lek″tro-kaw′ter-e) an apparatus for cauterizing tissue, consisting of a platinum wire in a holder which is heated to a red or white heat when the instrument is activated by an electric current.

electrochemistry (e-lek″tro-kem′is-tre) study of chemical changes produced by electric action.

electrochromatography (e-lek″tro-kro″mah-tog′rah-fe) electrophoresis.

electrocoagulation (e-lek″tro-ko-ag″u-la′shun) coagulation of tissue usually accomplished by means of a biterminal high frequency electric current.

electrocochleogram (e-lek″tro-kok′le-o-gram) the record obtained by electrocochleography.

electrocochleograph (e-lek″tro-kok′le-o-graf″) the instrument used in electrocochleography.

electrocochleographic (e-lek″tro-kok′le-o-graf′ik) pertaining to or accomplished by electrocochleography.

electrocochleography (e-lek″tro-kok′le-og′rah-fe) measurement of electrical potentials (cochlear microphonics and action potentials of the eighth cranial nerve) in response to acoustic stimuli applied by an electrode to the external acoustic canal or to the promontory or the round window through the tympanic membrane.

electrocontractility (e-lek″tro-kon-trak-til′ĭ-te) contractility in response to electric stimulation.

electroconvulsive (e-lek″tro-con-vul′siv) inducing convulsions by means of electric shock; see under *therapy*.

electrocorticogram (e-lek″tro-kor′tĭ-ko-gram″) the record obtained by electrocorticography.

electrocorticography (e-lek″tro-kor′tĭ-kog′rah-fe) electroencephalography with the electrodes applied directly to the cortex of the brain.

electrocution (e-lek″tro-ku′shun) the taking of life by passage of electric current through the body.

electrocystography (e-lek″tro-sis-tog′rah-fe) the recording of changes of electric potential in the human urinary bladder.

electrode (e-lek′trōd) [Gr. *ēlektron* amber + *hodos* way] a medium used between an electric conductor and the object to which the current is to be applied. In electrotherapy, an instrument with a point or surface from which to transmit an electric current to the body of a patient or to another instrument. **active e.,** one smaller in size than an indifferent electrode, and producing electrical stimulation in a concentrated area. **calomel e.,** an electrode capable of both collecting and giving up chloride ions in neutral or acidic aqueous media, consisting of mercury in contact with mercurous chloride; used as a reference electrode in pH measurements. **depolarizing e.,** one which has a resistance greater than that of the portion of the body inclosed in the circuit. **dispersing e.,** indifferent e. **exciting e.,** active e. **impregnated e.,** one with an absorbent tip impregnated with prescribed medicament. **indifferent e.,** one larger in size than an active electrode, and dispersing electrical stimulation over a larger area. **localizing e.,** active e. **multiple point e.,** an electrode possessing multiple contact points. **point e.,** an electrode with a metallic point for use in applying an electric current to a small area. **silent e.,** indifferent e. **therapeutic e.,** active e.

electrodermal (e-lek″tro-der′mal) pertaining to the electrical properties of the skin, especially to changes in its resistance.

electrodermatome (e-lek″tro-der′mah-tōm) an electrical dermatome for cutting off even layers of large areas of skin in a short time; used in skin grafting, shaving scars, etc.

electrodesiccation (e-lek″tro-des″ĭ-ka′shun) dehydration of tissue by the use of a high frequency electric current; see *fulguration*.

electrodiagnosis (e-lek″tro-di″ag-no′sis) the use of electrical devices in the diagnosis of pathologic conditions.

electrodiagnostics (e-lek″tro-di″ag-nos′tiks) the science and practice of electrodiagnosis.

electrodialysis (e-lek″tro-di-al′ĭ-sis) dialysis under the influence of an electric field.

electrodialyzer (e-lek″tro-di″ah-li′zer) a blood dialyzer utilizing an applied electric field and semipermeable membranes for separating the colloids from the solution.

electrodiaphake (e-lek″tro-di-af′ah-ke) [*electro-* + *dia-* + Gr. *phakos* lentil] an instrument for removing the lens by diathermy.

electrodiaphane (e-lek″tro-di′ah-fān) [*electro-* + Gr. *diaphainein* to show through] diaphanoscope.

electrodiaphanoscope (e-lek″tro-di-af′ah-no-skōp″) diaphanoscope.

electrodiaphanoscopy (e-lek″tro-di-af″ah-nos′ko-pe) diaphanoscopy.

electroencephalogram (e-lek″tro-en-sef′ah-lo-gram″) a recording of the potentials on the skull generated by currents emanating spontaneously from nerve cells in the brain. The dominant frequency of these potentials is about 8 to 10 cycles per second and the amplitude about 10 to 100 microvolts. Variations in wave characteristics correlate well with neurological conditions and so have been useful as diagnostic criteria. Abbreviated EEG. **flat e., isoelectric e.,** one in which no brain waves are recorded, indicating a complete lack of brain activity.

electroencephalograph (e-lek″tro-en-sef′ah-lo-graf″) an instrument for performing electroencephalography.

electroencephalography (e-lek″tro-en-sef″ah-log′rah-fe) the recording of the electric currents developed in the brain, by means of electrodes applied to the scalp, to the surface of

Excited

Relaxed

Drowsy

Asleep

Deep Sleep

1 second   50 μV

Electroencephalogram. Recordings made while the subject was excited, relaxed, and in various stages of sleep. During excitement the brain waves are rapid and of small amplitude, whereas in sleep they are much slower and of greater amplitude.

the brain (*intracranial e.*), or placed within the substance of the brain (*depth e.*). See *electroencephalogram*.

electroencephaloscope (e-lek″tro-en-sef′ah-lo-skōp) an instrument for detecting brain potentials at many different sections of the brain and displaying them on a cathode-ray tube.

electroendosmosis (e-lek″tro-en″dos-mo′sis) endosmosis under the influence of an electric field.

electroexcision (e-lek″tro-ek-siz′zhun) excision performed by electrosurgical means.

electrofluoroscopy (e-lek″tro-floo″o-ros′ko-pe) (*obs.*) fluoroscopic electrocardiography.

electrofocusing (e-lek″tro-fo′kus-ing) isoelectric focusing.

electrogastrogram (e-lek″tro-gas′tro-gram) the graphic record obtained by electrogastrography.

electrogastrograph (e-lek″tro-gas′tro-graf) an instrument for recording the electrical activity of the stomach by means of swallowed gastric electrodes.

electrogastrography (e-lek″tro-gas-trog′rah-fe) the recording of the electrical activity of the stomach as measured between its lumen and the surface of the body.

electrogoniometer (e-lek″tro-go″ne-om′ĕ-ter) an instrument for measuring angular positions, as of a finger, arm, limb.

electrogram (e-lek′tro-gram) any record produced by changes in electric potential. **His bundle e.,** an intracardiac electrocardiogram of potentials in the bundle of His, done through a cardiac catheter.

electrograph (e-lek′tro-graf) electrogram.

electrography (e″lek-trog′rah-fe) [*electro-* + Gr. *graphein* to record] the graphic recording of changes in electric potential, as in electrocardiography, electroencephalography, etc.

electrogustometry (e-lek″tro-gus-tom′ĕ-tre) the testing of the sense of taste by application of galvanic stimuli to the tongue.

electrohemostasis (e-lek″tro-he-mos′tah-sis) [*electro-* + *hemostasis*] the arrest of hemorrhage by the application of a high frequency current to coagulate the bleeding point or surface.

electrohysterogram (e-lek″tro-his′ter-o-gram) the graphic record obtained by electrohysterography.

electrohysterography (e-lek″tro-his″ter-og′rah-fe) the recording of the changes in electric potential associated with contractions of the uterine muscle.

electroimmunodiffusion (e-lek″tro-im″u-no-dif-u′zhun) the combination of immunodiffusion with electrophoresis, using an applied electric field to speed up the migration of antigen and antibody. Two such techniques have achieved widespread use: *counterimmunoelectrophoresis* (one-dimensional double electroimmunodiffusion) and *Laurell's rocket immunoelectrophoresis* (one-dimensional single electroimmunodiffusion).

electrokinetic (e-lek″tro-ki-net′ik) pertaining to motion produced by an electric current.

electrokymogram (e-lek″tro-ki′mo-gram) the graphic record produced by electrokymography; abbreviated EKY.

electrokymograph (e-lek″tro-ki′mo-graf) an instrument for graphically recording motion of or changes in density of organs by recording variations in intensity of a small beam of roentgen rays; it consists of three essential parts—a fluoroscope, a pick-up unit, and a recording instrument; used especially for showing motion of the cardiac silhouette.

electrokymography (e-lek″tro-ki-mog′rah-fe) the photography on x-ray film of the motion of the heart or of other moving structures which can be visualized radiologically. See *electrokymograph.*

electrolepsy (e-lek′tro-lep″se) electric chorea.

electrolithotrity (e-lek″tro-lĭ-thot′rĭ-te) the disintegration of calculi by the application of electric current.

electrolysis (e″lek-trol′ĭ-sis) [*electro-* + Gr. *lysis* dissolution] destruction by passage of a galvanic electric current, as in disintegration of a chemical compound in solution or removal of excessive hair from the body.

electrolyte (e-lek′tro-līt) [*electro-* + Gr. *lytos* that may be dissolved] a substance that dissociates into ions when fused or in solution, and thus becomes capable of conducting electricity; an ionic solute. **amphoteric e.,** a compound which dissociates into both hydrogen (H^+) and hydroxyl (OH^-) ions; called also *ampholyte.* **colloidal e.,** an electrolyte in which one or more of the ionic components is of macromolecular dimensions.

electrolytic (e-lek′tro-lit′ik) pertaining to or characterized by electrolysis.

electrolyzable (e-lek′tro-līz″ah-bl) susceptible of being decomposed by electric current.

electromagnet (e-lek″tro-mag′net) a temporary magnet made by passing an electric current through a coil of wire surrounding a core of soft iron.

electromagnetism (e-lek″tro-mag′net-izm) magnetism produced by an electric current.

electromanometer (e-lek″tro-man-om′ĕ-ter) an instrument for measuring the pressure of gases or liquids by electronic methods.

electrometer (e″lek-trom′ĕ-ter) [*electro-* + Gr. *metron* measure] an electrostatic instrument for measuring the difference in potential between two points. In radiology, it is used to measure changes in the potential of charged electrodes due to ionization occasioned by radiation.

electrometrogram (e-lek″tro-met′ro-gram) [*electro-* + Gr. *mētra* uterus + *gramma* mark] an apparatus for recording changes in electric potential associated with contraction of the uterine muscle.

electromigratory (e-lek″tro-mi′grah-to″re) moving under the influence of electric current.

electromotive (e-lek″tro-mo′tiv) causing electric activity to be propagated along a conductor.

electromyogram (e-lek″tro-mi′o-gram) the record obtained by electromyography.

electromyograph (e-lek″tro-mi′o-graf) the instrument used in electromyography.

electromyography (e-lek″tro-mi-og′rah-fe) [*electro-* + *myography*] the recording and study of the intrinsic electrical properties of skeletal muscle (1) by means of surface or needle electrodes to determine merely whether the muscle is contracting or not (useful in kinesiology); or (2) by insertion of a needle electrode into the muscle and observing by cathode-ray oscilloscope and loud-speaker the action potentials spontaneously present in a muscle (abnormal) or induced by voluntary contractions, as a means of detecting the nature and location of motor unit lesions; or (3) by recording the electrical activity evoked in a muscle by electrical stimulation of its nerve (called also *electroneuromyography*), a procedure useful for study of several aspects of neuromuscular function, neuromuscular conduction, extent of nerve lesion, reflex responses, etc. Abbreviated EMG. **ureteral e.,** recording of the action potentials produced by peristalsis of the ureter.

electron (e-lek′tron) the unit or "atom" of negative electricity. It is equivalent to 4.77×10^{-10} absolute electrostatic units or 1.59×10^{-20} absolute electromagnetic units, and its mass when moving at moderate speed is $\frac{1}{1845}$ that of a hydrogen atom or 9×10^{-28} grams. Electrons flowing in a conductor constitute an electric current; when ejected from a radioactive substance, the beta rays; and when revolving about the nucleus of an atom they determine all of its physical and chemical properties except mass and radioactivity. Cf. *atom.* **emission e.,** one of the electrons which give radioactivity to the atom. **free e.,** an electron which is not bound to the nucleus of an atom but may move from one atom nucleus to another. **valence e.,** any electron able to participate in the formation of chemical bonds, the electrons in the outermost shell of an atom.

electronarcosis (e-lek″tro-nar-ko′sis) anesthesia produced by passing an electric current through the brain by electrodes placed on the temples; used in treating a wide variety of psychiatric disorders in the U.S.S.R. It differs from electroconvulsive therapy in not producing convulsions.

electron-dense (e-lek′tron-dens″) in electron microscopy, having a density that prevents electrons from penetrating.

electronegative (e-lek″tro-neg′ah-tiv) bearing a negative electric charge.

electronegativity (e-lek″tro-neg″ah-tiv′ĭ-te) the relative power of an atom to attract electrons.

electroneurography (e-lek″tro-nu-rog′rah-fe) the measurement of the conduction velocity and latency of peripheral nerves.

electroneurolysis (e-lek″tro-nu-rol′ĭ-sis) neurolysis by means of the electric needle.

electroneuromyography (e-lek″tro-nu″ro-mi-og′rah-fe) electromyography in which the nerve of the muscle under study is stimulated by application of an electric current.

electronic (e″lek-tron′ik) pertaining to or carrying electrons.

electronics (e″lek-tron′iks) the science which treats of the conduction of electricity through gases, solids, or a vacuum.

electron-microscopic (e-lek′tron-mi-kro-skop′ik) visible under the electron microscope.

electron-microscopical (e-lek′tron-mi″kro-skop′ĭ-kal) observable with the aid of an electron microscope; of such size as to be so observed.

electronograph (e″lek-tron′o-graf) electron micrograph.

electronystagmogram (e-lek″tro-nis-tag′mo-gram) the record obtained by electronystagmography.

electronystagmograph (e-lek″tro-nis-tag′mo-graf) an instrument for recording eye movements induced by electrical stimulation; abbreviated ENG.

electronystagmography (e-lek″tro-nis″tag-mog′rah-fe) the recording of changes in the corneoretinal potential due to eye movements that provide objective documentation of induced and spontaneous nystagmus.

electro-oculogram (e-lek″tro-ok′u-lo-gram″) the electroencephalographic tracings made by moving the eyes a constant distance between two fixation points, inducing a deflection of fairly constant amplitude; abbreviated EOG.

electro-oculography (e-lek″tro-ok″u-log′rah-fe) the production and interpretation of electro-oculograms.

electro-olfactogram (e-lek″tro-ol-fak′to-gram) a recording of electrical potential changes detected by an electrode placed on the surface of the olfactory mucosa as the mucosa is subjected to an odorous stimulus. Abbreviated EOG.

electro-osmosis (e-lek″tro-oz-mo′sis) the movement of a solution past a stationary colloid material when an electric potential is applied; see also *iontophoresis.*

electroparacentesis (e-lek″tro-par″ah-sen-te′sis) puncture of the eyeball with a needle, using galvanic current and holding the needle in position until bubbles of hydrogen appear in the aqueous humor.

electropathology (e-lek″tro-pah-thol′o-je) [*electro-* + Gr. *pathos* disease + *-logy*] the study of pathologic conditions of the body as revealed by electricity.

electropherogram (e-lek″tro-fer′o-gram) electrophoretogram.

electrophile (e-lek′tro-fil) an electron acceptor that is covalently bonded to a nucleophile.

electrophilic (e-lek″tro-fil′ik) having an affinity for electrons; serving as an electrophile.

electrophoregram (e-lek″tro-fo′rĕ-gram) electrophoretogram.

electrophoresis (e-lek″tro-fo-re′sis) [*electro-* + Gr. *phoros* bearing + *-esis* process] a technique using separate mixtures of ionic solutes by differences in their rates of migration in an applied electric field. The original method, in which the movement of the solvent is unrestricted is termed *moving boundary electrophoresis*, because all of the particles of a single species move at the same rate, maintaining a sharp boundary. Widely used methods involve a support medium, such as paper, cellulose acetate, agarose gel, starch gel, or polyacrylamide gel, which prevents convective motion of the solvent; this is termed *zone electrophoresis*. The particular methods are usually designated by reference to the support, e.g., cellulose acetate electrophoresis. **counter e.,** counterimmunoelectrophoresis. **disc e.,** a method of polyacrylamide gel electrophoresis involving discontinuous (hence the name) gel layers. The sample starts in a large-pore "spacer" gel and rapidly moves to and is concentrated at the interface with a small-pore "separation" gel; then it separates into components as it slowly moves through the separation gel. **lipoprotein e.,** electrophoretic separation and quantitation of serum lipoproteins, most commonly by paper or agarose gel electrophoresis at pH 8.6. **protein e.,** electrophoretic separation and quantitation of serum, urine, or cerebrospinal fluid proteins, most commonly by cellulose acetate electrophoresis at pH 8.6. Proteins are separated into seven bands: in order of electrophoretic mobility, prealbumin, albumin, α_1, α_2, β_1, β_2, and γ globulins. **pulsed field gradient e.,** a technique permitting the study of chromosomal regions several hundreds or thousands of kb long rather than 100-150 kb as with older methods.

electrophoretic (e-lek″tro-fo-ret′ik) pertaining to electrophoresis.

electrophoretogram (e-lek″tro-fo-ret′o-gram) the record produced on or in a supporting medium by bands of material which have been separated by the process of electrophoresis. Called also *electropherogram* and *electrophoregram*.

electrophorus (e-lek-trof′o-rus) [*electro-* + Gr. *phoros* bearing] an instrument for obtaining static electricity by means of induction.

electrophotometer (e-lek″tro-fo-tom′ĕ-ter) an instrument equipped with a photoelectric sensor for colorimetric determinations.

electrophysiologic (e-lek″tro-fis″ĭ-o-loj′ik) pertaining to electrophysiology.

electrophysiology (e-lek″tro-fiz″e-ol′o-je) the science of physiology in its relations to electricity; the study of the mechanisms of the production of electrical phenomena, and their consequences, in the living organism; the electrical phenomena involved in physiological processes.

electroplating (ĕ-lek″tro-plāt′ing) plating or coating of an object with a layer of metal through the use of electrolytic processes. See also *electroplated die*, under *die*.

electroplax (e-lek′tro-plaks) the electric units of the specialized organs in the muscle fibers of electric fish.

electroplexy (e-lek′tro-plek″se) [*electro-* + Gr. *plēgē* stroke] electric shock.

electropositive (e-lek″tro-poz′ĭ-tiv) [*electro-* + *positive*] bearing a positive electric charge.

electroradiometer (e-lek″tro-ra-de-om′ĕ-ter) an electroscope for measuring radiant energy.

electroresection (e-lek″tro-re-sek′shun) excision by electrosurgical means.

electroretinogram (e-lek″tro-ret′ĭ-no-gram) the record obtained by electroretinography; abbreviated ERG.

electroretinograph (e-lek″tro-ret″in-o-graf) an instrument for measuring the electrical response of the retina to light stimulation; abbreviated ERG.

electroretinography (e-lek″tro-ret″ĭ-nog′rah-fe) the recording of the changes in electric potential in the retina after stimulation by light.

electrosalivogram (e-lek″tro-sah-li′vo-gram) [*electro-* + *saliva* + *-gram*] a graphic record or curve showing the action potential of the salivary glands, obtained with an electrically operated instrument.

electroscission (e-lek″tro-sizh′un) cutting tissue by use of the electrocautery.

electroscope (e-lek′tro-skōp) [*electro-* + Gr. *skopein* to examine] an instrument for measuring the intensity of radia-

tion by detecting the motion imparted to charged strips suspended from a conductor.

electrosection (e-lek″tro-sek′shun) an incision made by electrosurgical means.

electroselenium (e-lek″tro-sĕ-le′ne-um) a form of colloidal selenium.

electroshock (e-lek′tro-shok) shock produced by application of electric current to the brain; see *electroconvulsive therapy*, under *therapy*.

electrosleep (e-lek′tro-slēp) see *cerebral electrotherapy* under *electrotherapy*.

electrosol (e-lek′tro-sol) a colloidal solution of a metal obtained by passing electric sparks through distilled water between poles formed of the metal.

electrosome (e-lek′tro-sōm) (*obs.*) a chrondriosome considered as a center of chemical activity.

electrospectrogram (e-lek″tro-spek′tro-gram) a record produced in electrospectrography.

electrospectrography (e-lek″tro-spek-trog′rah-fe) the isolation and recording of the constituent wave systems that are merged in an electroencephalogram.

electrospinogram (e-lek″tro-spi′no-gram) a tracing of the action potential of the spinal cord.

electrostatic (e-lek″tro-stat′ik) pertaining to static electricity.

electrostenolysis (e-lek″tro-stĕ-nol′ĭ-sis) the oxidation and reduction which occur on opposite surfaces of a high resistance membrane in a solution when there is a steep electric potential gradient across the membrane, reduction occurring on the surface facing the anode.

electrostethograph (e-lek″tro-steth′o-graf) (*obs.*) an apparatus for recording the amplified heart sounds over the chest.

electrostimulation (e-lek″tro-stim″u-la′shun) electrical stimulation of tissues, as for therapeutic or experimental purposes.

electrostriatogram (e-lek″tro-stri-āt′o-gram) a record of waves derived by the bipolar technique from the several structures of the corpus striatum.

electrosurgery (e-lek″tro-sur′jer-e) surgery performed by electrical methods.

electrosynthesis (e-lek″tro-sin′thĕ-sis) chemical reactions effected by means of electricity.

electrotaxis (e-lek″tro-tak′sis) [*electro-* + Gr. *taxis* arrangement] the movement of organisms or cells under the influence of electric currents.

electrothanasia (e-lek″tro-thah-na′ze-ah) [*electro-* + Gr. *thanotos* death] death by electricity; electrocution.

electrotherapeutics (e-lek″tro-ther-ah-pu′tiks) treatment of disease by means of electricity.

electrotherapeutist (e-lek″tro-ther-ah-pu′tist) a physician who specializes in the therapeutic use of electricity.

electrotherapist (e-lek″tro-ther′ah-pist) a person trained in using electricity for therapeutic purposes.

electrotherapy (e-lek″tro-ther′ah-pe) electrotherapeutics. **cerebral e. (CET),** the use of low intensity electricity, usually employing positive pulses or direct current, in the treatment of insomnia, anxiety, and neurotic depression. It has been called *electrosleep*, a misleading term because the treatment does not induce sleep.

electrotherm (e-lek′tro-therm) [*electro-* + Gr. *thermē* heat] an electrosurgical appliance used for cutting.

electrotome (e-lek′tro-tōm) [*electro-* + Gr. *tomē* a cut] an electric surgical cutting instrument.

electrotomy (e-lek-trot′o-me) electroexcision with low current, high voltage, and high frequency; a procedure in which the tissues are not coagulated.

electrotonic (e-lek″tro-ton′ik) 1. pertaining to electrotonus. 2. denoting the direct spread of current in tissues by electrical conduction, without the generation of new current by action potentials.

electrotonus (e-lek-trot′o-nus) the altered electrical state of a nerve or muscle cell when a constant electric current is passed through it.

electrotropism (e″lek-trot′ro-pizm) [*electro-* + Gr. *tropos* a turning, change] the tendency of a cell or organism to react in a definite manner in response to an electric stimulus.

negative e., the tendency of a cell to be repelled by an electric stimulus. **positive e.,** the tendency of a cell to be attracted by an electric stimulus.

electroultrafiltration (e-lek″tro-ul″trah-fil-tra′shun) ultrafiltration in an electric field.

electroureterogram (e-lek″tro-u-re″ter-o-gram) the record obtained by electroureterography.

electroureterography (e-lek″tro-u-re″ter-og′rah-fe) electromyography in which the action potientials produced by peristalsis of the ureter are recorded.

electrovagogram (e-lek″tro-va′go-gram) vagogram.

electrovalence (e-lek″tro-va′lens) 1. the number of charges an atom acquires by the gain or loss of electrons in forming an ionic bond. 2. the bonding resulting from such a transfer of electrons.

electrovalent (e-lek″tro-va′lent) pertaining to electrovalence or to an electrovalent (ionic) bond.

electroversion (e-lek″tro-ver′zhun) the act of electrically terminating a cardiac dysrhythmia.

electrovert (e-lek′tro-vert) to apply electricity to the heart or precordium to depolarize the heart and terminate a cardiac dysrhythmia.

electuary (e-lek′tu-a-re) [L. *electuarium*, from *e* out + *legere* to select] a medicinal preparation consisting of a powdered drug made into a paste with honey or syrup; a confection. Called also *lincture* and *linctus*. **e. of senna,** a mixture of senna, syrup, and tamarind pulp.

eledoisin (el-ĕ-doi′sin) chemical name: L-pyroglutamyl-L-prolyl-L-seryl-L-lysyl-L-aspartyl-alanyl-phenylalanyl-L-isoleucyl-glycyl-L-leucyl-L-methioninamide. An endecapeptide, $C_{54}H_{85}N_{13}O_{15}S$, from the posterior salivary gland of a species of small octopus (*Eledone*), which is a precursor of a large group of biologically active peptides. It has vasodilator, hypotensive, and extravascular smooth muscle stimulant properties.

eleidin (el-e′ĭ-din) a substance of peculiar nature, allied to keratin and protoplasm, found in the cells of the stratum lucidum of the skin.

element (el′ĕ-ment) [L. *elementum*] 1. any of the primary parts or constituents of a thing. 2. in chemistry, a simple substance which cannot be decomposed by chemical means and which is made up of atoms which are alike in their peripheral electronic configurations and so in their chemical properties, and also in the number of protons in their nuclei, but which may differ in the number of neutrons in their nuclei and so in their atomic weight and in their radioactive properties. [See accompanying *Table of Elements*.] **anatomic e.,** morphological e. **appendicular e's,** a set of cartilaginous rods attached to the chondral skull of the embryo; from them are developed the ear bones, the hyoid, and the styloid process. **electronegative e.,** any chemical element that adds electrons (or tends to add electrons)

TABLE OF ELEMENTS

NAME	SYMBOL	AT. NO.	AT. WT.*	NAME	SYMBOL	AT. NO.	AT. WT.*
Actinium	Ac	89	227.028	Mendelevium	Md	101	(258)
Aluminum	Al	13	26.982	Mercury	Hg	80	200.59
Americium	Am	95	(243)	Molybdenum	Mo	42	95.94
Antimony	Sb	51	121.75	Neodymium	Nd	60	144.24
Argon	Ar	18	39.948	Neon	Ne	10	20.179
Arsenic	As	33	74.922	Neptunium	Np	93	237.0482
Astatine	At	85	(210)	Nickel	Ni	28	58.69
Barium	Ba	56	137.33	Niobium	Nb	41	92.906
Berkelium	Bk	97	(247)	Nitrogen	N	7	14.007
Beryllium	Be	4	9.012	Nobelium	No	102	259
Bismuth	Bi	83	208.980	Osmium	Os	76	190.2
Boron	B	5	10.811	Oxygen	O	8	15.999
Bromine	Br	35	79.904	Palladium	Pd	46	106.42
Cadmium	Cd	48	112.41	Phosphorus	P	15	30.974
Calcium	Ca	20	40.08	Platinum	Pt	78	195.08
Californium	Cf	98	(251)	Plutonium	Pu	94	(244)
Carbon	C	6	12.011	Polonium	Po	84	(209)
Cerium	Ce	58	140.12	Potassium	K	19	39.098
Cesium	Cs	55	132.905	Praseodymium	Pr	59	140.908
Chlorine	Cl	17	35.453	Promethium	Pm	61	(145)
Chromium	Cr	24	51.996	Protactinium	Pa	91	231.036
Cobalt	Co	27	58.933	Radium	Ra	88	226.025
Copper	Cu	29	63.546	Radon	Rn	86	(222)
Curium	Cm	96	(247)	Rhenium	Re	75	186.207
Dysprosium	Dy	66	162.50	Rhodium	Rh	45	102.906
Einsteinium	Es	99	(252)	Rubidium	Rb	37	85.468
Element 106		106	(263)	Ruthenium	Ru	44	101.07
Erbium	Er	68	167.26	Rutherfordium	Rf	104	(261)
Europium	Eu	63	151.96	Samarium	Sm	62	150.36
Fermium	Fm	100	(257)	Scandium	Sc	21	44.956
Fluorine	F	9	18.998	Selenium	Se	34	78.96
Francium	Fr	87	(223)	Silicon	Si	14	28.086
Gadolinium	Gd	64	157.25	Silver	Ag	47	107.868
Gallium	Ga	31	69.72	Sodium	Na	11	22.990
Germanium	Ge	32	72.59	Strontium	Sr	38	87.62
Gold	Au	79	196.967	Sulfur	S	16	32.064
Hafnium	Hf	72	178.49	Tantalum	Ta	73	180.948
Hahnium	Ha	105	(261)	Technetium	Tc	43	(98)
Helium	He	2	4.003	Tellurium	Te	52	127.60
Holmium	Ho	67	164.930	Terbium	Tb	65	158.925
Hydrogen	H	1	1.008	Thallium	Tl	81	204.383
Indium	In	49	114.82	Thorium	Th	90	232.038
Iodine	I	53	126.905	Thulium	Tm	69	168.934
Iridium	Ir	77	192.22	Tin	Sn	50	118.69
Iron	Fe	26	55.847	Titanium	Ti	22	47.88
Krypton	Kr	36	83.80	Tungsten	W	74	183.85
Lanthanum	La	57	138.906	Uranium	U	92	238.029
Lawrencium	Lw	103	(260)	Vanadium	V	23	50.942
Lead	Pb	82	207.2	Xenon	Xe	54	131.29
Lithium	Li	3	6.941	Ytterbium	Yb	70	173.04
Lutetium	Lu	71	174.967	Yttrium	Y	39	88.906
Magnesium	Mg	12	24.312	Zinc	Zn	30	65.38
Manganese	Mn	25	54.938	Zirconium	Zr	40	91.22

*Atomic weights are corrected to conform with the 1979 values of the International Union of Pure and Applied Chemistry, expressed to the fourth decimal point, rounded off to the nearest thousandth. The numbers in parentheses are the mass numbers of the most stable or most common isotope.

during chemical combination. **electropositive e.,** a chemical element that loses electrons (or tends to lose electrons) during chemical combination. **F e.,** see under *factor*. **formed e's (of the blood),** erythrocytes, leukocytes, and platelets. **labile e.,** tissue cells which continue to multiply during the life of the individual. **morphological e.,** any cell, fiber, or other of the ultimate structures which go to make up tissues and organs. **radioactive e.,** a chemical element which spontaneously transmutes into another element with emission of corpuscular or electromagnetic radiations. The natural radioactive elements are all those with atomic number above 83, and some other elements, such as potassium (at. no. 19) and rubidium (at. no. 37), which are very weakly radioactive. **rare earth e's,** elements of the lanthanum series, comprising elements with atomic numbers 57 to 71. **sarcous e.,** any of the elementary granules into which the primitive fibril of an elementary muscle fiber is divisible. **stable e.,** 1. a chemical element which does not spontaneously transmute into another element with emission of corpuscular or electromagnetic radiations; the stable elements are those with atomic number below 84, except for a few, such as potassium and rubidium, which are weakly radioactive. 2. a tissue cell of mature tissues which does not alter by mitosis. **tissue e.,** morphological e. **trace e's,** chemical elements that are distributed throughout the tissues in very small amounts and are either essential in nutrition, such as cobalt, copper, magnesium, manganese, and zinc, or may be harmful, such as selenium. **tracer e's,** see *radioactive tracer*, under *tracer*. **transcalifornium e's,** the elements with atomic numbers higher than that of californium, and discovered subsequent to its discovery in 1950. They are einsteinium 99, fermium 100, mendelevium 101, nobelium 102, and lawrencium 103. **transuranic e's, transuranium e's,** the elements with atomic numbers higher than that of uranium. Applied originally to neptunium 93, plutonium 94, americium 95, curium 96, berkelium 97, and californium 98, the term now, by definition, includes the transcalifornium elements as well.

elementary (el″ĕ-men′tah-re) not resolvable or divisible into simpler parts or components; see also under *particle*.

elemi (el″ĕ-me) [Turkish *eleme* hand picked] a resinous substance, of extremely various origin, the best coming from *Canarium commune*, of the Philippine Islands. It furnishes a volatile oil, and was formerly used externally, generally in an ointment, for ulcers and sores.

ele(o)- [Gr. *elaion* oil] combining form denoting relationship to oil.

eleoma (el″e-o′mah) [*eleo-* + *-oma*] a tumor or swelling caused by the injection of oil into the tissues.

eleometer (el″e-om′ĕ-ter) [*eleo-* + Gr. *metron* measure] an instrument for determining percentage of oil in a mixture, also specific gravity of oils.

eleopathy (el″e-op′ah-the) elaiopathy.

eleoplast (el-e′o-plast) [*eleo-* + Gr. *plastos* formed] a globular body made up of granular protoplasm and containing drops of oil.

eleopten (el″e-op′ten) [*eleo-* + Gr. *ptēnos* volatile] the more volatile constituent of a volatile oil, as distinguished from its stearopten.

eleosaccharum (el″e-o-sak′ah-rum), pl. *eleosacch′ara* [Gr. *elaion* oil + *sakcharon* sugar] a mixture of sugar with a volatile oil; an oil sugar. Called also *oleosaccharum*.

eleotherapy (el″e-o-ther′ah-pe) [*eleo-* + *therapy*] oleotherapy.

elephantiasic (el″ĕ-fan′te-as′ik) pertaining to elephantiasis.

elephantiasis (el″ĕ-fan-ti′ah-sis) [Gr. *elephas* elephant + *-iasis*] 1. a chronic filarial disease most commonly occurring in the tropics due to infection of the lymphatic channels with the nematode *Wuchereria bancrofti* or *Brugia malayi*, and characterized by inflammation and obstruction of the lymphatics and hypertrophy of the skin and subcutaneous tissues (pachyderma). The legs and external genitals are principally affected, the disease beginning in attacks of dermatitis, with enlargement of the part, attended by chills and fever (elephantoid fever) and followed by the formation of ulcers and tubercles, with thickening, discoloration, and fissuring of the skin. Called also *Barbados leg, chyloderma, elephant leg, mal de Cayenne,* and *pes febricitans*. 2. hypertrophy and thickening of the tissues from any cause. **e.**

chirur′gica, Halsted's name for massive edema of the arm after mastectomy. **congenital e.,** Milroy's disease. **e. gingi′vae,** fibromatosis gingivae. **lymphangiectatic e.,** elephantiasis of a part due to lymphangiectasis. **e. neuromato′sa,** neurofibroma. **nevoid e.,** a variety marked by great dilatation of the lymph vessels. **e. nos′tras,** that due to either chronic recurrent streptococcal erysipelas or chronic recurrent cellulitis. **e. oc′uli,** thickening and protrusion of the eyelids. **e. scro′ti,** that in which the scrotum is the principal seat of the disease; called also *parasitic chylocele,* and *lymph scrotum*.

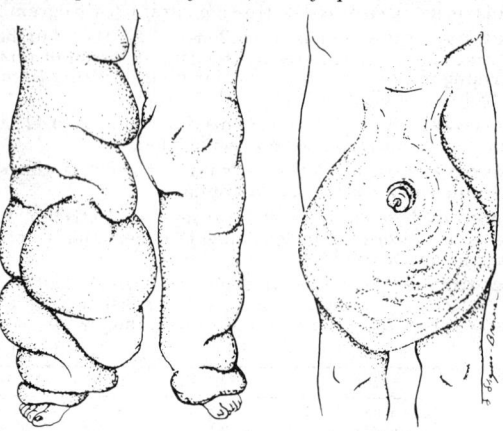

Elephantiasis of the legs and of the scrotum.

elephantoid (el″ĕ-fan′toid) relating to or resembling elephantiasis.

Elettaria cardamomum (L.) Maton (Zingiberaceae) (el″ĕ-ta′re-ah kar″dah-mo′mum) a species of plants of tropical areas of the Old World, which afford cardamom and grains of paradise.

elevation (el″ĕ-va′shun) a raised area, or point of greater height. **boiling point e.,** elevation of the boiling point of a solution above that of the pure solvent; it is proportional to the osmolality. For water the proportionality constant is 0.512° C/(Osm/kg). **tactile e's,** toruli tactiles.

elevator (el′ĕ-va″tor) [L. *elevare* to lift] an instrument for elevating tissues or for removing osseous fragments or roots of teeth. **angular e.,** one in which the blade angles from the shank to the right or to the left. **apical e.,** an instrument for removing fractured root tips retained in the apex of the tooth socket following tooth extraction; its shank has an angle to provide access within the socket and its tip has a barb for reaching a fractured root tip. Called also *apical pick* and *root pick.* **cross bar e.,** one in which the handle is at a right angle to the shank. Called also T-*bar e.* **Cryer e.,** a dental instrument for removing the roots of molar teeth; furnished in pairs, one for mesial and one for distal roots, which are reversed for use on opposite sides of the jaw. **dental e.,** an instrument having a blade that engages the teeth or their roots and extracts teeth by elevating them from their alveoli through leverage applied to the handle. **malar e.,** an instrument used to elevate or reposition the zygomatic bone and/or arch. **periosteum e.,** a flat steel bar for separating the attachments of the periosteum to bone. **root e.,** a dental elevator for extracting a fractured root of a tooth; they may be designed in pairs, a right and a left, and as single, straight, mitered, or double ended. **screw e.,** a dental instrument designed to be screwed into a root canal for subsequent removal of the root, usually of the apical third. **straight e.,** one in which the shank continues in a straight line with the handle. **T-bar e.,** cross bar e. **wedge e.,** one used as a lever in tooth extraction, being placed in a hole drilled into the root of the tooth below the investing bony tissue to rework a tooth.

elfazepam (el-faz′ĕ-pam) chemical name: 7-chloro-1-[2-(ethylsulfonyl)ethyl]-5-(2-fluorophenyl)-1,3-dihydro-2*H*-1,4-benzodiazepin-2-one; a veterinary appetite stimulant, $C_{19}H_{18}ClFN_2O_3S$.

eliminant (e-lim′ĭ-nant) 1. causing an evacuation. 2. an agent that promotes evacuation.

elimination (e-lim″ĭ-na′shun) [L. *eliminatio*, from *e* out + *limen* threshold] 1. the act of expulsion or of extrusion, especially of expulsion from the body. 2. omission or exclusion, as in an elimination diet. Cf. *excretion*. **immune e.**, the period of accelerated degradation of antigen (e.g., foreign gamma globulin) as a result of its removal and destruction by antibodies. Also, a technique for determining antibody response by measuring the rate of removal of labeled antigen from the circulation of an immunized animal. Called also *immune clearance*.

elinin (el′ĭ-nin) a lipoprotein fraction of red cells containing the Rh and A and B factors.

Elipten (e-lip′ten) trademark for a preparation of aminoglutethimide.

ELISA (e-li′sah) [*Enzyme-Linked ImmunoSorbent Assay*] any enzyme immunoassay utilizing an enzyme-labeled immunoreactant (antigen or antibody) and an immunosorbent (antigen or antibody bound to a solid support). A variety of methods (e.g., competitive binding between the labeled reactant and unlabeled unknown (e.g., a sandwich technique in which the unknown (an antigen) binds both the immunosorbent and labeled antibody) may be used to measure the unknown concentration.

elixir (e-lik′ser) [L., from Arabic] a clear, sweetened, usually hydroalcoholic liquid containing flavoring substances and sometimes active medicinal agents, used orally as a vehicle or for the effect of the medicinal agent contained. **acetaminophen e.** [USP], an elixir containing not less than 95 per cent and not more than 105 per cent of the labeled amount of acetaminophen, $C_8H_9NO_2$; used as an analgesic and antipyretic. **amobarbital e.** [USP], an elixir containing not less than 95.0 per cent and not more than 105.0 per cent of the labeled amount of amobarbital; used as a sedative and hypnotic. **aprobarbital e.**, an elixir containing not less than 92.5 per cent and not more than 107.5 per cent of aprobarbital; used as a sedative. **aromatic e.** [NF], a preparation containing orange, lemon, coriander, and anise oils, syrup, talc, and alcohol in purified water; used as a flavored vehicle for pharmaceutical preparations. **aromatic e., red,** aromatic elixir colored by addition of amaranth solution. **benzaldehyde e., compound,** a preparation of benzaldehyde, vanillin, orange flower water, alcohol, simple syrup, and water; used as a vehicle for pharmaceutical preparations. **bromodiphenhydramine hydrochloride e.** [USP], an elixir containing not less than 93 per cent and not more than 107 per cent of the labeled amount of bromodiphenhydramine hydrochloride; used as an antihistaminic. **brompheniramine maleate e.** [USP], an elixir containing not less than 95 per cent and not more than 105 per cent of the labeled amount of brompheniramine maleate; used as an antihistaminic. **butabarbital sodium e.** [USP], an elixir containing not less than 95 per cent and not more than 105 per cent of the labeled amount of sodium butabarbital; used as a sedative. **carbinoxamine maleate e.** [USP], an elixir containing not less than 95 per cent and not more than 105 per cent of the labeled amount of carbinoxamine maleate; used as an antihistaminic. **chlorpheniramine maleate e.,** see under *syrup*. **dexamethasone e.** [USP], an elixir containing not less than 90 per cent and not more than 110 per cent of the labeled amount of dexamethasone; used as a glucocorticoid. **dextroamphetamine sulfate e.** [USP], a preparation containing, in each 100 ml., between 90 and 110 mg. of dextroamphetamine sulfate; used as a central nervous system stimulant in the treatment of mental depression, psychopathic states, narcolepsy, hyperkinetic behavior disorders in children, and exogenous obesity. **digoxin e.** [USP], an elixir containing, in each 100 ml., not less than 4.60 mg. and not more than 5.40 mg. of digoxin; used as a cardiotonic. **diphenhydramine hydrochloride e.** [USP], a preparation containing 94 to 106 per cent of the labeled amount of diphenhydramine hydrochloride; used as an antihistaminic, antiemetic, antitussive, and antispasmodic. **fluphenazine hydrochloride e.** [USP], a preparation containing 95 to 105 per cent of the labeled amount of fluphenazine hydrochloride; used as a tranquilizer in the treatment of the manifestations of psychotic disorders and as an antiemetic. **gentian e., glycerinated,** a preparation of gentian and taraxacum fluidextracts, compound cardamon tincture, raspberry syrup, sweet orange peel tincture, phosphoric acid, ethyl acetate, glycerin, sucrose, and alcohol, in purified water; used as a flavored vehicle for drugs.

high-alcoholic e., see *iso-alcoholic e.* **homatropine methylbromide e.,** a preparation containing 90 to 110 per cent of the labeled amount of homatropine methylbromide; used as an anticholinergic to reduce spasms and inhibit secretions, especially in gastrointestinal disorders. **e. I. Q. & S., iron, quinine, and strychnine e.,** a preparation of iron, quinine, and strychnine, with compound orange spirit, alcohol, glycerin, and purified water; used as a bitter tonic. **iso-alcoholic e.** [NF], a mixture of low-alcoholic elixir and high-alcoholic elixir to produce a solution whose strength is suitable for the medicament for which it serves as a vehicle. *Low-alcoholic e.*: compound orange spirit 10 ml., alcohol 100 ml., glycerin 200 ml., sucrose 320 gm., and sufficient purified water to make a total of 1000 ml. *High-alcoholic e.*: compound orange spirit 4 ml., saccharin 3 gm., glycerin 200 ml., and sufficient alcohol to make a total of 1000 ml. **low-alcoholic e.,** see *iso-alcoholic e.* **methenamine e.** [USP] an elixir containing 90 to 110 per cent of the labeled amount of methenamine; used as a urinary antibacterial. **oxtriphylline e.** [USP], an elixir containing between 90 and 110 per cent of the labeled amount of oxtriphylline; used as a bronchodilator. **pentobarbital e.** [USP], an elixir containing between 92.5 and 107.5 per cent of the labeled amount of pentobarbital; used as a sedative and hypnotic. **pentobarbital sodium e.** [USP], pentobarbital sodium 4.0 gm., glycerin 450.0 ml., alcohol 150.0 ml., orange oil 0.75 ml., caramel 2 gm., syrup 150.0 ml., diluted hydrochloric acid 6.0 ml., and sufficient purified water to make a total of 1000 ml.; used as a sedative and hypnotic. **pepsin e., lactated,** a water preparation containing a proteolytic enzyme from the glandular layer of the fresh stomach of the hog, with lactic acid, glycerin, alcohol, orange oil, and amaranth solution. **phenobarbital e.** [USP], an elixir containing between 92.5 and 107.5 per cent of the labeled amount of phenobarbital; used as a sedative, hypnotic, and anticonvulsant. **potassium chloride e.** [USP], an elixir containing between 90 and 110 per cent of the labeled amount of potassium chloride, KCl; used as an electrolyte replenisher. **potassium gluconate e.** [USP], an elixir containing 97 to 103 per cent of the labeled amount of potassium gluconate; used as an electrolyte replenisher in the prophylaxis and treatment of hypokalemia. **reserpine e.,** [USP], an elixir containing between 90 and 110 per cent of the labeled amount of reserpine; used as an antihypertensive agent. **secobarbital e.** [USP], an elixir containing, in each 100 ml., not less than 417 mg. and not more than 461 mg. of secobarbital in a suitable, flavored vehicle; used as a hypnotic. **terpin hydrate e.** [USP], terpin hydrate 17 gm., sweet orange peel tincture 20 ml., benzaldehyde 50μl., glycerin 400 ml., alcohol 430 ml., syrup 100 ml., and sufficient purified water to make 1000 ml.; used as an expectorant. **terpin hydrate and codeine e.** [USP], 2 gm. of codeine dissolved in a sufficient quantity of terpin hydrate elixir to make 1000 ml.; used as an expectorant and antitussive. **terpin hydrate and dextromethorphan hydrobromide e.** [USP], 2 gm. of dextromethorphan hydrobromide dissolved in a sufficient quantity of terpin hydrate elixir to make 1000 ml.; used as an expectorant and antitussive. **theophylline sodium glycinate e.** [USP], an elixir containing an amount of theophylline between 47 and 54 per cent of the labeled amount of theophylline sodium glycinate; used as a bronchodilator and smooth muscle relaxant. **three bromides e.,** a mixture of ammonium, potassium, and sodium bromides, amaranth solution, and compound benzaldehyde elixir, occasionally used as a sedative in grand mal seizures. See also *bromide*. **trihexyphenidyl hydrochloride e.** [USP], an elixir containing, in each 100 ml., not less than 37.2 mg. and not more than 42.8 mg. of trihexyphenidyl hydrochloride; used as an antiparkinsonian agent. **tripelennamine citrate e.** [USP], an elixir containing, in each 100 ml., not less than 705 mg. and not more than 795 mg. of tripelennamine citrate; used as an antihistaminic in the symptomatic treatment of allergic disorders.

Elixophyllin (e-lik″so-fil′in) trademark for preparations of theophylline.

Elkosin (el′ko-sin) trademark for preparations of sulfisomidine.

elkosis (el′ko-sis) helcosis.

Elliot's operation (el′ĭ-ots) [Col. Robert Henry *Elliot*, of the Indian Medical Service, 1864–1936] see under *operation*.

Elliot's position [John Wheelock *Elliot*, American surgeon, 1852–1925] see under *position.*

Elliot's sign [George T. *Elliot*, American dermatologist, 1851–1935] see under *sign.*

ellipsin (e-lip′sin) the insoluble constituents of cells which remain after the removal of the soluble proteins.

ellipsoid (e-lip′soid) [Gr. *ellipēs* (*kyklos*), defective (circle) + *-oid*] 1. any structure shaped like a spindle or an ellipse. 2. any of the spindle-shaped masses of cells surrounding the second portion of the arterioles of the spleen; see *sheathed artery*, under *artery.* 3. in ophthalmology, the acidophilic outer region of the inner segment of the dendritic process of a retinal rod or cone, lying between the cilium and the myoid, and containing some glycogen and many mitochondria; called also *visual cell e.*

elliptocytary (e-lip″to-si′tah-re) pertaining to elliptocytes.

elliptocyte (e-lip′to-sīt) an elliptical erythrocyte.

elliptocytosis (e-lip″to-si-to′sis) a hereditary disorder in which the greater proportion of erythrocytes are elliptical in shape, and which is characterized by varying degrees of increased red cell destruction and anemia.

elliptocytotic (e-lip″to-si-tot′ik) pertaining to or characterized by elliptocytosis.

Ellis's line (curve), sign (el′ĭ-sez) [Calvin *Ellis*, Boston physician, 1826–1883] see under *line* and *sign.*

Ellis-Garland line (el′is-gar′land) [Calvin *Ellis*; George Minot *Garland*, American physician, 1849–1926] Ellis' line.

Eloesser flap (el-es′er) [Leo *Eloesser*, San Francisco surgeon, born 1881] see under *flap.*

elongation (e″long-ga′shun) 1. the act, process or condition of increasing in length. 2. pathologic migration of a tooth in the occlusal or incisal direction. 3. radiographic distortion in which the image is proportionally longer than that which is being x-rayed.

Elorine (el′o-rēn) trademark for a preparation of tricyclamol chloride.

Elsberg's test (els′bergz) [Charles Albert *Elsberg*, New York surgeon, 1871–1948] see under *solution* and *test.*

Elschnig's bodies (pearls) (elsh′nig) [Anton *Elschnig*, German ophthalmologist, 1863–1939] see under *body.*

Elsner's asthma (els′nerz) [Christoph Friedrich *Elsner*, German physician, 1749–1820] angina pectoris.

Elspar (el′spar) trademark for a preparation of L-asparaginase.

eluate (el′u-āt) the substance separated out by, or the product of, elution or elutriation.

elucaine (ĕ-lu′kān) chemical name: α-(diethylamino)-methyl] benzenemethanol benzoate (ester); an anticholinergic (gastric), $C_{19}H_{23}NO_2$.

eluent (e-lu′ent) a solution used in elution.

elution (e-lu′shun) [L. *e* out + *luere* to wash] in chemistry, the separation of material by washing, as in the freeing of an enzyme from its absorbent. **membrane e.,** a method of selecting cells in which a culture of cells is collected on a membrane filter, over which a fresh warm culture fluid is then slowly passed, washing off excess cells and leaving only adsorbed cells at a particular developmental stage.

elutriation (e-lu″tre-a′shun) [L. *elutriare* to wash out] the operation of pulverizing substances and mixing them with water in order to separate the heavier constituents, which settle out in solution, from the lighter constituents.

Ely's test (sign) (e′lēz) [Leonard Wheeler *Ely*, American orthopedic surgeon, 1868–1944] see under *test.*

elytr(o)- [Gr. *elytron* a covering, sheath] a combining form denoting relationship to the vagina or to a sheath; for words beginning thus, see those beginning *colp(o)-.*

Em. *emmetropia.*

emaciation (e-ma″se-a′shun) [L. *emaciare* to make lean] excessive leanness; a wasted condition of the body.

eman (em′an) a unit for expressing the concentration of radium emanation in solution: it is the concentration present when one tenth of a millimicrocurie of radium emanation is dissolved in 1 liter of air or water, or 10^{-10} curie.

emanation (em-ah-na′shun) [L. *e* out + *manare* to flow] that which is given off, such as a gaseous disintegration product given off from radioactive substances or an efflu-

vium. **actinium e.,** one member of the radioactive series derived from actinium. It is produced from actinium X, has an atomic weight of 218, its atomic number is 86, and by the loss of alpha particles it becomes actinium A. Called also *actinon.* **radium e.,** radon. **thorium e.,** one member of the radioactive series derived from thorium. It is produced from thorium X, has an atomic weight of 220, its atomic number is 86, and by the loss of alpha particles it changes into thorium A. Called also *thoron.*

emancipation (e-man″sĭ-pa′shun) [L. *emancipare* to release, give up] the establishment of local autonomy within restricted fields of a developing embryo.

emasculation (e-mas″ku-la′shun) [L. *emasculare* to castrate] castration; removal of the testes or of the testes and penis.

embalming (em-bahm′ing) the treatment of the dead body with antiseptics and preservatives, to prevent putrefaction.

embarrass (em-bar′as) to impede the function of; to obstruct.

Embden ester (em′den) [Gustav *Embden*, German biochemist, 1874–1933] see under *ester.*

Embden-Meyerhof-Parnas pathway (em′den mi′er-hof par′nas) [Gustav Embden; Otto Fritz *Meyerhof*; Jakub Karol *Parnas*, Polish biochemist, 1884–1949] see *Embden-Meyerhof pathway*, under *pathway.*

Embden-Meyerhof pathway (em′den mi′er-hof) [Gustav *Embden*; Otto Fritz *Meyerhof*, German physiologist, 1884–1951] see under *pathway.*

embedding (em-bed′ing) the fixation of a tissue specimen in a firm medium, in order to keep it intact during the cutting of thin sections.

Embelia (em-be′le-ah) a genus of myrtaceous East Indian climbing plants. **E. ri′bes, E. robus′ta,** species whose fruit has been used for its anthelminthic and cathartic principles.

embelin (em′bĕ-lin) chemical name: 2,5-dihydroxy-3-undecyl-*p*-benzoquinone. An active principle, $CH_3(CH_2)_{10} \cdot C_6 HO_2(OH)_2$, from *Embelia ribes*, formerly used as a teniacide.

emboitement (ahm-bwat′maw) [Fr. "encasement"] the supposed encasement of miniature individuals within the germ cells of predecessors, advanced as one theory of preformation.

embolalia (em″bo-la′le-ah) embololalia.

embole (em′bo-le) [Gr. *embolē* a throwing in] 1. the reducing of a dislocated limb. 2. emboly.

embolectomy (em″bo-lek′to-me) [*embolus* + Gr. *ektomē* excision] surgical removal of an embolus from a blood vessel.

emboli (em′bo-li) [L.] plural of *embolus.*

embolia (em-bo′le-ah) embole.

embolic (em-bol′ik) pertaining to an embolus or to embolism.

emboliform (em-bol′ĭ-form) 1. shaped like a wedge. 2. resembling an embolus.

embolism (em′bo-lizm) [L. *embolismus*, from Gr. *en* in + *ballein* to throw] the sudden blocking of an artery by a clot or foreign material which has been brought to its site of lodgment by the blood current. **air e.,** that due to air bubbles entering the veins after trauma or surgical procedures. **amniotic fluid e.,** embolism due to amniotic fluid forced into the maternal circulation near the end of normal pregnancy by strong uterine contractions. **bacillary e.,** obstruction of a vessel by an aggregation of bacilli. **bland e.,** that in which the thrombotic plug is composed of nonseptic material. **bone marrow e.,** embolism caused by material from a fractured long bone. **capillary e.,** blocking of the capillaries with bacteria. **cerebral e.,** embolism of a cerebral artery. **coronary e.,** embolism of one of the coronary arteries. **crossed e.,** paradoxical e. **direct e.,** embolism occurring in the direction of the blood stream. **fat e.,** embolism of fat that has entered the circulation, especially after fractures of large bones, or after corticosteroid administration. **infective e.,** embolism in which the embolus is infective. **lymph e., lymphogenous e.,** embolism of a lymph vessel. **miliary e.,** that which affects at the same time many small blood vessels. **multiple e.,** embolism by a number of small emboli. **oil e.,** fat e. **pantaloon e.,** saddle e. **paradoxical e.,** blockage of a systemic artery by a thrombus originating in a systemic vein, which has passed through a defect that permits direct communication between the right and the left side of the heart, notably an open foramen ovale; called also *crossed e.* **plasmodium e.,** the occlusion of a coronary artery by *Plasmodium falciparum.* **pulmonary e.,** the closure of the pulmonary artery or one of its branches by an embolus, sometimes associated with infarction of the lung. **pyemic e.** (*obs.*), infective e. **retinal e.,** embolism of the central artery of the retina. **saddle e.,** an embolism lodging at the bifurcation of the aorta, causing sudden severe pain of the legs, abdomen, and back, with numbing and coldness. Called also *pantaloon e.* **spinal e.,** embolism of an artery in the spinal cord. **trichinous e.,** embolism due to trichinae. **tumor e.,** embolism due to tumor fragments, especially from cancer of the stomach. **venous e.,** embolism in which the clot or plug originates in the veins.

embolization (em″bo-li-za′shun) 1. the process or condition of becoming an embolus. 2. therapeutic introduction of a substance into a vessel in order to occlude it. **poppet e.,** the embolization of the ball of a poppet valve used as a heart valve prosthesis.

embololalia (em″bŏ-lo-la′le-ah) [Gr. *emballein* to insert + *lalia* babble] the interpolation of meaningless words or phrases into the speech; called also *embolophrasia.*

embolomycotic (em″bŏ-lo-mi-kot′ik) pertaining to or marked by an infectious embolus.

embolophrasia (em″bŏ-lo-fra′ze-ah) [Gr. *emballein* to insert + *phrasis* utterance] embololalia.

embolus (em′bo-lus), pl. em′boli [Gr. *embolos* plug] 1. a clot or other plug brought by the blood from another vessel and forced into a smaller one, thus obstructing the circulation. See accompanying illustration. 2. the emboliform nucleus of the cerebellum. **air e.,** a bubble of air obstructing a

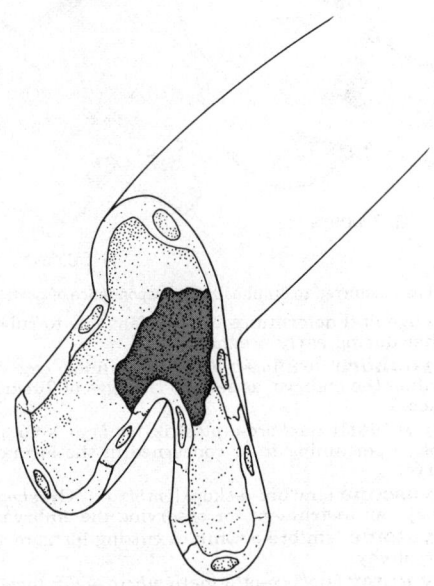

Embolus impacted at site of branching of an artery.

blood vessel. **cancer e.,** a small mass of cells detached from a cancer and carried by the blood stream to lodge in a distant location. **cellular e.,** one consisting of tissue cells of various kinds. **fat e.,** one composed of oil or fat. **foam e.,** one formed by a mixture of a gas and blood. **obturating e.,** one completely blocking a vessel. **riding e., saddle e., straddling e.,** one at the bifurcation of an artery, blocking both branches.

emboly (em′bo-le) [Gr. *embolē* a throwing in] the invagination of the blastula by which the gastrula is formed.

embouchement (aw-boosh-maw′) [Fr.] the opening of one vessel into another.

embrasure (em-bra′zhur) a space continuous with an interproximal space, produced by curvatures of teeth in contact in the same arch, that provides a channel or passage through

which food escapes from the occlusal surfaces of the teeth during mastication. Called also *spillway.* **buccal e.,** the embrasure opening out toward the cheek between molar and premolar teeth. **incisal e.,** occlusal e. **interdental e.,** the space formed by the interproximal contours of adjoining teeth, beginning at the contact area and extending lingually, facially, occlusally, and apically. **labial e.,** the embrasure that widens out from the area of contact toward the lips between the canine and incisor teeth. **lingual e.,** the embrasure that widens out from the area of contact toward the lingual sides of the teeth. **occlusal e.,** the space bounded by the marginal ridges as they join the cusps and incisal ridges. Called also *incisal e.*

embrocation (em-bro-ka′shun) [L. *embrocatio*] 1. the application of a liquid medicament to the surface of the body. 2. a liquid medicine for external use.

embryectomy (em″bre-ek′to-me) [*embryo* + Gr. *ektomē* excision] excision of the embryo in extrauterine pregnancy.

embryo (em′bre-o) [Gr. *embryon*] 1. in plants, the element of the seed that develops into a new individual. 2. in animals, those derivatives of the fertilized ovum that eventually become the offspring, during their period of most rapid development, i.e., after the long axis appears until all major structures are represented. In man, the developing organism is an embryo from about two weeks after fertilization to the end of seventh or eighth week. **hexacanth e.,** the six-hooked embryo, or onchosphere, characteristic of most tapeworms of man and domestic animals. **Janošik's e.,** a human embryo having three aortic arches and two gill pouches. **presomite e.,** the embryo at any stage prior to the appearance of the first somite. **previllous e.,** the conceptus before the chorionic villi develop. **somite e.,** the embryo at any stage between the appearances of the first and the last somites. **Spee's e.,** a 1.5 mm. human embryo, horizon IX, about 20 days old as described by Spee.

embryoblast (em′bre-o-blast″) [*embryo-* + Gr. *blastos* germ] inner cell mass.

embryocardia (em″bre-o-kar′de-ah) [*embryo* + Gr. *kardia* heart] a symptom in which the sounds of the heart resemble those of fetal life, there being very little difference in the quality of the first and second sounds.

embryoctony (em″bre-ok′tŏ-ne) [*embryo* + Gr. *kteinein* to kill] the artificial destruction of the living embryo, or fetus.

embryogenesis (em″bre-o-jen′ĕ-sis) [*embryo* + *genesis*] the development of a new individual by means of sexual reproduction, that is, from a fertilized ovum; the process of embryo formation.

embryogenetic (em″bre-o-jĕ-net′ik) embryogenic.

embryogenic (em″bre-o-jen′ik) 1. pertaining to the development of the embryo. 2. producing an embryo.

embryogeny (em″bre-oj′ĕ-ne) [*embryo* + Gr. *gennan* to produce] the production or origin of the embryo.

embryograph (em′bre-o-graf) [*embryo* + Gr. *graphein* to write] a combination of a microscope and a camera lucida; used in drawing figures of the embryo.

embryography (em″bre-og′rah-fe) [*embryo* + Gr. *graphein* to write] 1. a treatise or description of the embryo. 2. the drawing of an embryo by means of the embryograph.

embryoid (em′bre-oid) [*embryo* + Gr. *eidos* form] resembling an embryo.

embryoism (em′bre-o-izm) the condition of being an embryo.

embryologist (em″bre-ol′o-jist) an expert in embryology.

embryology (em″bre-ol′o-je) [*embryo* + *-logy*] the science of the development of the individual during the embryonic stage and, by extension, in several or even all preceding and subsequent stages of the life cycle. **causal e.,** experimental e. **comparative e.,** embryology applied with a comparative view to various species studied with reference to their taxonomy and the principle that ontogeny recapitulates phylogeny. **descriptive e.,** the study of embryos and fetuses and their components with reference to anatomical and chronological sequence so as to define stages and report the course of development. **experimental e.,** analysis of the factors and relations in development, obtained by subjecting embryos to experimental procedures; called also *causal embryology.*

embryoma (em″bre-o′mah) 1. a general term applied to

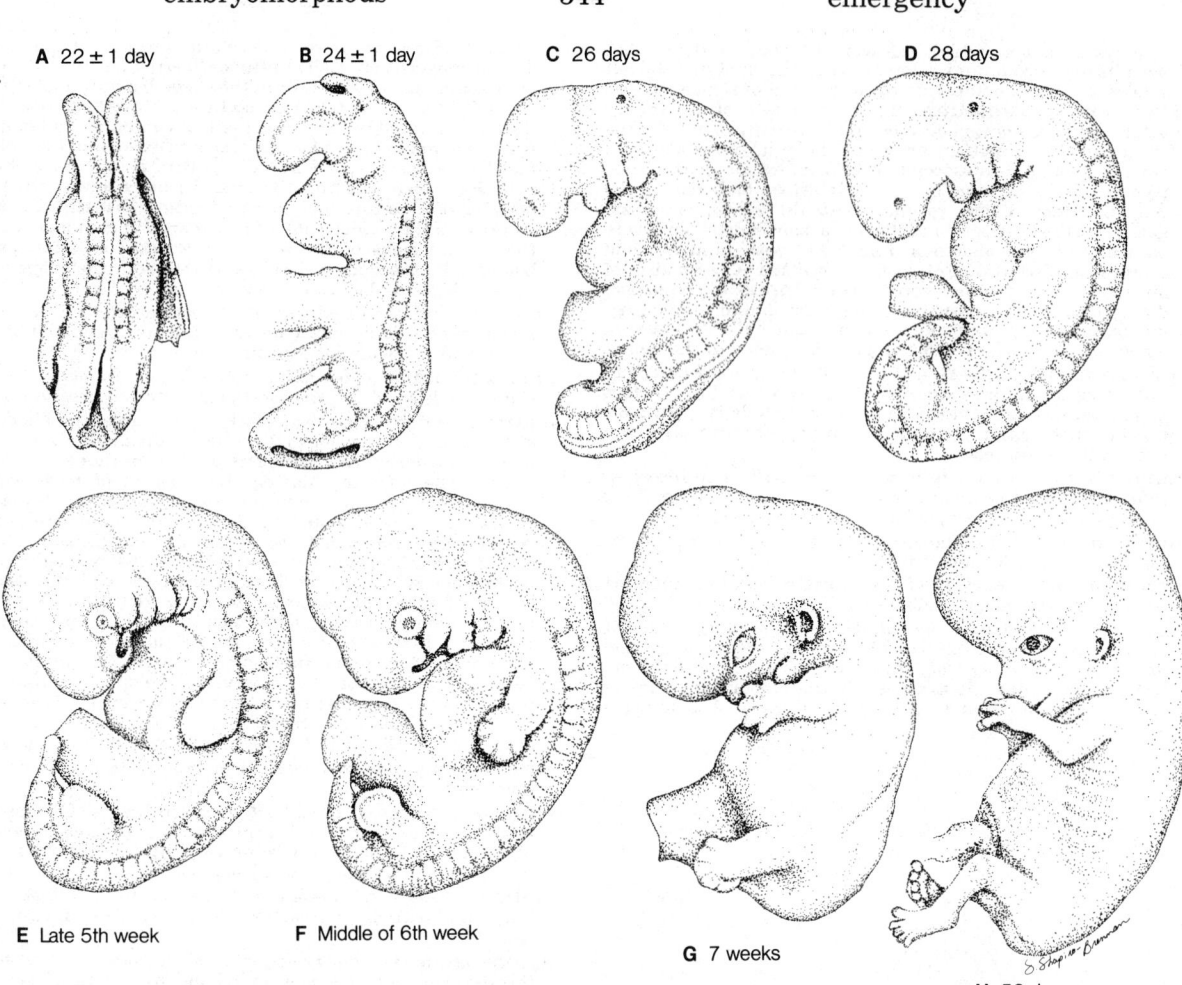

A 22 ± 1 day   **B** 24 ± 1 day   **C** 26 days   **D** 28 days

E Late 5th week   **F** Middle of 6th week   **G** 7 weeks   **H** 56 days

Human embryo at various stages of development. The relative size has been distorted to emphasize correspondence of parts.

neoplasms thought to be derived from embryonic cells or tissues, including dermoid cysts, teratomas, embryonal carcinomas and sarcomas, nephroblastomas, hepatoblastomas, etc. 2. a former term for neoplasms once thought to be derived from cells of a blighted ovum. **e. of kidney,** Wilms' tumor.

embryomorphous (em″bre-o-mor′fus) [*embryo* + Gr. *morphē form*] having a form suggestive of an embryo; said of certain abnormal tissue elements supposed to be relics of a conceptus.

embryonal (em′bre-o-nal) pertaining to the embryo.

embryonate (em′bre-o-nāt) 1. pertaining to or resembling an embryo. 2. containing an embryo. 3. impregnated; fecundated.

embryonic (em″bre-on′ik) of or pertaining to the embryo.

embryoniform (em″bre-on′ĭ-form) resembling an embryo.

embryonism (em′bre-o-nizm) embryoism.

embryonization (em″bre-o-ni-za′shun) reversion to the embryonic form on the part of a tissue or cell.

embryonoid (em′bre-o-noid″) resembling an embryo.

embryony (em′bre-o-ne) the production of an embryo.

embryopathia (em″bre-o-path′e-ah) embryopathy. **e. rubeola′ris,** developmental anomalies observed in infants of mothers who had rubeola during pregnancy.

embryopathology (em″bre-o-pah-thol′o-je) the study of abnormal embryos or of defective development.

embryopathy (em″bre-op′ah-the) [*embryo-* + Gr. *pathos* disease] a morbid condition of the embryo or a disorder resulting from abnormal embryonic development. **rubella**

e., congenital deformities in an infant due to rubella in the mother during early pregnancy.

embryophore (em′bre-o-fōr) the inner egg shell surrounding the embryo, as seen in the eggs of *Taenia* found in the feces.

embryoplastic (em″bre-o-plas′tik) [*embryo* + Gr. *plassein* to shape.] pertaining to or concerned in the formation of an embryo.

embryoscope (em″bre-o-skōp) [*embryo* + Gr. *skopein* to examine] an instrument for observing the embryo.

embryotome (em′bre-o-tōm) a cutting instrument used in embryotomy.

embryotomy (em″bre-ot′o-me) [*embryo* + Gr. *tomē* a cutting] 1. the dismemberment of a fetus in the uterus or vagina to facilitate delivery. 2. the dissection of embryos and fetuses.

embryotoxon (em″bre-o-tok′son) arcus corneae; see under *arcus*. **anterior e.,** arcus corneae. **posterior e.,** Axenfeld's anomaly.

embryotroph (em′bre-o-trōf″) [*embryo* + Gr. *trophē* nourishment] the total nutriment (histotroph and hemotroph) made available to the embryo.

embryotrophy (em″bre-ot′ro-fe) [*embryo* + Gr. *trophē* nourishment] the nutrition of the embryo.

EMC encephalomyocarditis (virus).

Emcyt (em′sīt) trademark for a preparation of estramustine.

emedullate (e-med′u-lāt) [L. *e* out + *medulla* marrow] to extract bone marrow.

emeiocytosis (e″me-o-si-to′sis) emiocytosis.

emergency (e-mer′jen-se) [L. *emergere* to raise up] an unlooked for or sudden occasion; an accident; an urgent or pressing need.

emergent (e-mer'jent) 1. pertaining to an emergency. 2. coming into being through consecutive stages of development, as in emergent evolution.

emery (em'er-e) impure crystalline corundum mixed with iron oxide; used as an abrasive.

emesia (ĕ-me'ze-ah) emesis.

emesis (em'ĕ-sis) [Gr. *emein* to vomit] vomiting; an act of vomiting. Also used as a word termination, as in *hematemesis*. **e. gravida'rum**, the vomiting of pregnancy.

emetatrophia (em''ĕ-tah-tro'fe-ah) [Gr. *emetos* vomiting + *atrophia* atrophy] atrophy or wasting due to persistent vomiting.

emetic (ĕ-met'ik) [Gr. *emetikos*; L. *emeticus*] 1. bringing on or causing the act of vomiting. 2. an agent that causes vomiting. **central e.**, one carried by the blood stream to the vomiting center, upon which it acts; called also *indirect e.* and *systemic e.* **direct e.**, one that acts directly on the stomach; called also *mechanical e.* **indirect e.**, central e. **mechanical e.**, direct e. **systemic e.**, central e. **tartar e.**, antimony potassium tartrate.

emeticology (ĕ-met''ĭ-kol'o-je) the sum of knowledge regarding emetics.

emetine (em'ĕ-tin) chemical name: 6',7',10-11-tetramethoxyemetan; an alkaloid, $C_{29}H_{40}N_2O_4$, obtained from ipecac or prepared by methylation of cephaeline. **e. and bismuth iodide**, a complex iodide of emetine and bismuth, occurring as a reddish-orange powder; used as an antiamebic in amebic dysentery, administered orally. **e. hydrochloride** [USP], the dihydrochloride salt of emetine, $C_{29}H_{40}N_2O_4 \cdot HCl$, occurring as a white or very slightly yellowish crystalline powder; used as an antiamebic, administered subcutaneously or intramuscularly.

emetocathartic (em''ĕ-to-kah-thar'tik) 1. both emetic and cathartic. 2. an agent that is both emetic and cathartic.

emetology (em''ĕ-tol'o-je) emeticology.

E.M.F. electromotive force; erythrocyte maturation factor.

EMG *electromyogram.*

-emia [Gr. *haima* blood + *-ia*] a word termination denoting the presence of a substance in the blood.

emigration (em''ĭ-gra'shun) [L. *e* out + *migrare* to wander] the escape of leukocytes through the walls of small blood vessels; diapedesis.

emilium tosylate (ĕ-mil'e-um) chemical name: *N*-ethyl-3-methoxy-*N,N*-dimethylbenzenemethanaminium salt with 4-methylbenzenesulfonic acid (1:1); a cardiac depressant with antiarrhythmic action, $C_{19}H_{27}NO_4S$.

eminence (em'ĭ-nens) a prominence or projection, especially one upon the surface of a bone; called also *eminentia* [NA]. **antithenar e.**, hypothenar (def. 1). **arcuate e.**, eminentia arcuata. **articular e. of temporal bone**, tuberculum articulare ossis temporalis. **bicipital e.**, tuberositas radii. **canine e.**, a prominent bony ridge overlying the root of either canine tooth on the labial surface of both the maxilla and the mandible. **capitate e.**, capitulum humeri. **e. of cartilage of Santorini**, tuberculum corniculatum. **caudate e. of liver**, processus caudatus hepatis. **coccygeal e.**, cornu sacrale. **cochlear e. of sacral bone**, promontorium ossis sacri. **collateral e. of lateral ventricle**, eminentia collateralis ventriculi lateralis. **e. of concha**, eminentia conchae. **cruciate e., cruciform e. of occipital bone**, eminentia cruciformis. **cuneiform e. of head of rib**, crista capitis costae. **deltoid e.**, tuberositas deltoidea humeri. **Doyère's e.**, the papilla marking the entrance of a nerve filament into a muscle fiber; called also *Doyère's hillock.* **facial e. of eminentia teres**, colliculus facialis. **frontal e.**, tuber frontale. **genital e.**, genital tubercle. **gluteal e. of femur**, tuberositas glutea femoris. **hypobranchial e.**, copula linguae. **hypothenar e.**, hypothenar (def. 1). **e. of humerus**, capitulum humeri. **iliopectineal e., iliopubic e.**, eminentia iliopubica. **intercondylar e., intercondyloid e., intermediate e.**, eminentia intercondylaris. **jugular e.**, tuberculum jugulare ossis occipitalis. **mamillary e.**, corpus mamillare. **e. of maxilla**, tuber maxillae. **medial e. of rhomboid fossa**, eminentia medialis fossae rhomboideae. **median e.**, the raised area on the infundibulum hypothalami at the floor of the third ventricle of the brain. Continuous

below with the infundibular stem or stalk of the pituitary gland, it contains the primary capillary network of the hypophysial portal system. In some anatomical classification systems it is included as part of the neurohypophysis and in others as part of the tuber cinereum. **nasal e.**, the prominence above the root of the nose. **oblique e. of cuboid bone**, tuberositas ossis cuboidei. **occipital e.**, a ridge on the lateral ventricle of the embryonic brain, corresponding to the occipital fissure in the adult. **olivary e. of sphenoid bone**, tuberculum sellae turcicae. **orbital e. of zygomatic bone**, eminentia orbitalis ossis zygomatici. **parietal e.**, tuber parietale. **postchiasmatic e.**, an inconstant protuberance on the floor of the third ventricle posterior to the optic chiasm; called also *postfundibular e.* **postfundibular e.**, postchiasmatic e. **pyramidal e.**, eminentia pyramidalis. **radial e. of wrist**, eminentia carpi radialis. **e. of scapha**, eminentia scaphae. **e. of superior semicircular canal**, eminentia arcuata. **terete e.**, eminentia medialis fossae rhomboideae. **thenar e.**, thenar (def. 1). **thyroid e.**, prominentia laryngea. **triangular e., e. of triangular fossa of auricle**, eminentia fossa triangularis auriculae. **e. of triquetral fossa**, eminentia fossae triangularis auriculae. **trochlear e.**, trochlea humeri. **ulnar e. of wrist**, eminentia carpi ulnaris. **vagal e.**, trigonum nervi vagi.

eminentia (em''ĭ-nen'she-ah), pl. *eminen'tiae* [L.] [NA] an eminence: a general term for a prominence or projection, especially one on the surface of a bone. **e. abducen'tis** (*obs.*), colliculus facialis. **e. arcua'ta** [NA], arcuate eminence: an arched prominence on the internal surface of the petrous part of the temporal bone in the floor of the middle cranial fossa, marking the position of the superior semicircular canal. It is particularly prominent in young skulls. Called also *eminence of superior semicircular canal.* **e. articula'ris os'sis tempora'lis**, tuberculum articulare ossis temporalis. **e. capita'ta**, capitulum humeri. **e. car'pi radia'lis**, an eminence on the palmar surface of the radial side of the wrist, formed by the tubercles on the scaphoid and trapezium bones; called also *radial eminence of wrist.* **e. car'pi ulna'ris**, an eminence on the palmar surface of the ulnar side of the wrist, formed by the pisiform bone and the hook of the hamate bone; called also *ulnar eminence of wrist.* **e. ciner'ea cuneifor'mis**, trigonum nervi vagi. **e. collatera'lis ventric'uli latera'lis** [NA], collateral eminence of lateral ventricle: an elevation in the floor of the temporal horn of the lateral ventricle, produced by the collateral sulcus. **e. con'chae** [NA], eminence of concha: the projection on the medial surface of the auricle that corresponds to the concha on the lateral surface. **e. crucia'ta**, e. cruciformis. **e. crucifor'mis** [NA], cruciform eminence of occipital bone: the cross-shaped bony prominence on the internal surface of the squama of the occipital bone, at the intersection of the ridges associated with the sulci of the superior sagittal sinus and the transverse sinuses. Called also *e. cruciata, internal occipital crest,* and *cruciate line.* **e. facia'lis**, colliculus facialis. **e. fallo'pii**, a ridge on the inner wall of the tympanum, showing the position of the facial nerve. **e. fos'sae triangula'ris auric'ulae** [NA], eminence of triangular fossa of auricle: the protuberance on the medial surface of the auricle of the ear that corresponds to the triangular fossa on the lateral surface. Called also *agger perpendicularis, e. triangularis, eminence of triquetral fossa,* and *triangular eminence.* **e. fronta'le**, NA alternative for *tuber frontale.* **e. grac'ilis**, fasciculus gracilis medullae oblongatae. **e. hypoglos'si**, trigonum nervi hypoglossi. **e. hypothena'ris**, NA alternative for *hypothenar* (def. 1). **e. iliopectin'ea**, e. iliopubica. **e. iliopu'bica** [NA], iliopubic eminence: a diffuse enlargement just anterior to the acetabulum, marking the junction of the ilium with the superior ramus of the pubis; called also *e. iliopectinea, iliopectineal eminence, iliopubic tuber* or *tubercle,* and *iliopectineal tubercle* or *crest of pubis.* **e. intercondyla'ris** [NA], **e. intercondyloi'dea, e. interme'dia**, intercondylar eminence: an eminence on the proximal extremity of the tibia, surmounted on either side by a prominent tubercle, on to the sides of which the articular facets are prolonged; called also *intermediate eminence* and *tuberculum intercondyloideum.* **e. jugula'ris**, tuberculum jugulare ossis occipitalis. **e. latera'lis cartilag'inis crico'deae**, facies articularis thyroidea. **e. maxillae**, tuber maxillae. **e. media'lis fos'sae rhomboi'deae** [NA], medial eminence of rhomboid fossa: an eminence in the medial part of the floor of the fourth ventricle, bounded laterally by the sulcus limitans and produced by the facial colliculus and the trigone of the hypoglossal nerve. Called also *e. teres* and *terete eminence.* **e. orbita′lis os′sis zygomat′ici** [NA], orbital eminence of zygomatic bone: a small tubercle that is usually present on the orbital surface of the frontal process of the zygomatic bone, within the orbital opening below the frontozygomatic suture. **e. papilla′ris,** e. pyramidalis. **e. pyramida′- lis** [NA], pyramidal eminence: the hollow elevation in the posterior wall of the middle ear, which contains the stapedius muscle; called also *e. papillaris.* **e. sca′phae** [NA], eminence of scapha: the prominence on the medial side of the auricle of the external ear that corresponds to the scapha on the lateral side. **e. styloi′dea,** prominentia styloidea. **e. sym′physis,** the prominent lower border of the middle of the chin. **e. te′res,** e. medialis fossae rhomboideae. **e. thena′ris,** NA alternative for *thenar* (def. 1). **e. triangula′ris,** e. fossae triangularis auriculae. **e. tri- gem′ina, e. trigem′ini,** tuberculum trigeminale. **e. va′gi,** trigonum nervi vagi.

emiocytosis (e″me-o-si-to′sis) the ejection of material from a cell. Cf. *exocytosis* (def. 1).

emissaria (em″ĭ-sa′re-ah) [L.] plural of *emissarium.*

emissarium (em″ĭ-sa′re-um), pl. *emissa′ria* [L.] an emissary vein; see *venae emissariae.* **e. condyloi′deum,** vena emissaria condyloidea. **e. mastoi′deum,** vena emissaria mastoidea. **e. occipita′le,** vena emissaria occipitalis. **e. parieta′le,** vena emissaria parietalis.

emissary (em′ĭ-sa″re) [L. *emissarium* drain] affording an outlet, referring especially to the venous outlets from the dural sinuses through the skull.

emission (e-mish′un) [L. *emissio,* a sending out] a discharge; specifically an involuntary discharge of semen. **nocturnal e.,** reflex emission of the semen during sleep. **thermionic e.,** the emission of electrons and ions by incandescent bodies.

emissivity (e″mis-siv′ĭ-te) the ratio of emissive power (of radiant energy) of a surface to that of a black surface having the same temperature.

EMIT (e-mit′) [*Enzyme-Multiplied Immunoassay Technique*] trademark for a homogeneous (single phase) enzyme immunoassay which utilizes the change in enzyme activity of an enzyme-labeled hapten that occurs on binding with antibody to determine the amount of unlabeled hapten (the unknown) present in a biologic specimen.

emmenagogic (ĕ-men″ah-goj′ik) inducing menstruation.

emmenagogue (ĕ-men′ah-gog) [Gr. *emmēna* menses + *agōgos* leading] an agent or measure that induces menstruation. **direct e.,** an agent that induces menstruation by acting directly upon the reproductive organs. **indirect e.,** an agent or measure that acts to induce menstruation by relieving another condition of which amenorrhea is a secondary result.

emmenia (ĕ-me′ne-ah) [Gr. *emmēna*] the menses.

emmenic (ĕ-men′ik) pertaining to the menses; menstrual.

emmeniopathy (ĕ-me″ne-op′ah-the) [Gr. *emmēnios* menses + *pathos* disease] any disorder of menstruation.

emmenology (em″ĕ-nol′o-je) [Gr. *emmēna* menses + *-logy*] the sum of knowledge regarding menstruation and its disorders.

Emmet's operation, retractor (em′ets) [Thomas Addis *Emmet,* gynecologist in New York, 1818–1919] see under *operation* and *retractor.*

emmetrope (em′ĕ-trōp) an individual who has no refractive error of vision.

emmetropia (em-ĕ-tro′pe-ah) [Gr. *emmetros* in proper measure + *-opia*] a state of proper correlation between the refractive system of the eye and the axial length of the eyeball, rays of light entering the eye parallel to the optic axis being brought to a focus exactly on the retina.

emmetropic (em″ĕ-trop′ik) pertaining to or characterized by emmetropia.

Emmonsia (ĕ-mon′se-ah) a genus of imperfect, saprophytic, soil fungi of the order Moniliales, family Moniliaceae. Two species, *E. cres′cens* and *E. par′va,* cause adiospiromycosis in rodents and man. Called also *Haplosporangium.*

emodin (em′o-din) [from *Rheum emodi,* a Himalayan rhubarb] a purgative compound, trihydroxymethyl anthraquinone, from rhubarb, aloes, senna, and cascara sagrada.

emollient (e-mol′e-ent) [L. *emolliens* softening, from *e* out + *mollis* soft] 1. softening or soothing; called also *malactic.* 2. an agent which softens or soothes the skin, or soothes an irritated internal surface; called also *malagma.*

emotion (e-mo′tion) [L. *emovere* to disturb] any strong feeling state, such as excitement, distress, happiness, sadness, love, hate, fear, or anger. The external manifestation of emotion is called *affect;* a pervasive and sustained emotional state, *mood.*

emotional (e-mo′shun-al) pertaining to the emotions.

Emp. abbreviation for L. *emplas′trum,* a plaster.

empacho (em-pah′cho) a Mexican term for chronic indigestion in children with diarrhea.

empasma (em-paz′mah) [Gr. *en* in + *passein* to sprinkle] a powder for external use.

empathic (em-path′ik) pertaining to or characterized by empathy.

empathize (em′pah-thīz) to experience or feel empathy.

empathy (em′pah-the) [Gr. *en* into + *pathos* feeling] intellectual and emotional awareness and understanding of another person's thoughts, feelings, and behavior, even those that are distressing and disturbing. *Empathy* emphasizes understanding, *sympathy* emphasizes sharing, of another person's feelings and experiences.

Empedocles (em-ped′o-klēz) (c. 493 to c. 433 B.C.) a Greek philosopher born in Acragas, Sicily. He accepted and combined pneumatism with his own theories of the four "roots" (earth, air, fire, and water) and of the two opposite, complementary forces (love and strife), which unite and reunite or separate and disintegrate the four roots in diverse proportions to form or destroy matter; thus health is a balance, disease an imbalance, of the roots by the forces. See also *Alcmaeon* and *humoralism.*

emphraxis (em-frak′sis) [Gr.] a stoppage or obstruction.

emphysema (em″fĭ-se′mah, em″fĭ-ze′mah) [Gr. "an inflation"] a pathological accumulation of air in tissues or organs; applied especially to such a condition of the lungs (see *pulmonary e.*). **alveolar e.,** overdistention of the alveolar spaces in the lungs. **alveolar duct e.,** distention of the alveolar ducts as seen in elderly individuals, often producing little or no functional disturbance. **atrophic e.,** overdistention and stretching of lung tissues due to atrophic changes, especially loss of elastic tissue. **bullous e.,** single or multiple large cystic alveolar dilatations of lung tissue; see also *paraseptal e.* **centriacinar e., centrilobular e.,** focal dilatations of air spaces distributed throughout the lung in the midst of grossly normal lung tissue; the dilatations affect respiratory bronchioles rather than alveoli. **chronic hypertrophic e.,** panacinar e. **compensating e., compensatory e.,** overdistention of lung tissue which fills a void produced by contraction, atelectasis, surgical resection, fibrosis, or otherwise reduced volume of another part of the lung. **cutaneous e.,** subcutaneous e. **cystic e.,** dilatations of lung tissue characterized by multiple alveolar cysts. **diffuse e.,** panacinar e. **ectatic e.,** vesicular e. **false e.,** deformity of the thoracic cage which simulates the form associated with pulmonary emphysema (increased anterior-posterior diameter, elevated rib angle, etc.); the lungs may or may not be normal. Called also *skeletal e.* **focal-dust e.,** a form of pulmonary emphysema associated with inhalation of environmental dusts, producing dilatation of the terminal and respiratory bronchioles. **gangrenous e.,** a malignant emphysema of microbic origin. **generalized e.,** pulmonary emphysema affecting all portions of both lungs in a similar manner. **glass blower's e.,** emphysema of the lungs attributed to overstrain in glass blowers. **hypertrophic e.,** a discarded term for chronic obstructive pulmonary edema (atrophy rather than hypertrophy is involved). **hypoplastic e.,** pulmonary emphysema due to a developmental abnormality resulting in reduced number of alveoli, which are abnormally large; it may affect a pulmonary segment, lobe, or an entire lung. **idiopathic unilobar e.,** a syndrome characterized by emphysematous expansion of one lobe of the lung, with the production of dyspnea and cyanosis. **interlobular e.,** accumulation of air in interlobar spaces, between the lobes of lungs. **interstitial e.,** the escape of air into the connective tissue of the lung, mediastinum (see *pneumomediastinum*), or subcutaneous tissue (see *subcutaneous e.*) resulting from a tear or rupture of the respiratory passages or alveoli, which may occur in association with bronchiolar obstruction or be caused by a penetrating wound of the chest wall of the lung. **intestinal e.,** a condition marked by accumulation of gas under the serous tunic of the intestine. **lobar e.,** emphysema involving fewer than all the lobes of the affected lung. **lobar e., infantile,** a condition characterized by overinflation, commonly affecting one of the upper lobes and causing respiratory distress in early life; called also *congenital lobar e.* **e. of lungs,** pulmonary e. **mediastinal e.,** pneumomediastinum. **obstructive e.,** overinflation of the lungs associated with partial bronchial obstruction which interferes with exhalation. **obstructive e., localized,** overinflation of a lobe or segment of lung, often due to partial bronchial obstruction; called also *obstructive pulmonary overinflation.* **panacinar e., panlobular e.,** generalized obstructive emphysema affecting all lung segments, with atrophy and dilatation of the alveoli and destruction of the vascular bed. **paracicatricial e.,** alveolar distention occurring in the vicinity of pulmonary scars. **paraseptal e.,** alveolar distention localized to the lung periphery, including the interlobar septa; a form of bullous emphysema. **pulmonary e.,** a condition of the lung characterized by increase beyond normal in the size of air spaces distal to the terminal bronchioles, either from dilatation of the alveoli (*panacinar e.*), or from destruction (*interstitial e.*) of their walls. **pulmonary e. of cattle, acute,** fog fever. **senile e.,** pulmonary emphysema due to dilatation of the alveoli occurring with age. **skeletal e.,** false e. **small-lunged e.,** atrophic e. **subcutaneous e.,** interstitial emphysema characterized by the presence of air in the subcutaneous tissue, usually caused by intrathoracic injury, and in most instances associated with pneumothorax and pneumomediastinum. Called also *cutaneous e.* and *pneumoderma.* **surgical e.,** subcutaneous emphysema following surgical operation. **traumatic e.,** subcutaneous, interstitial, or mediastinal emphysema due to trauma. **unilateral e.,** emphysema affecting only one lung, frequently due to congenital defects in circulation; called also *hyperlucent lung.* **vesicular e.,** panlobular e.

emphysematous (em″fi-sem′ah-tus) of the nature of or affected with emphysema.

Empiric (em-pir′ik) [Gr. *empeirikos* experienced] the second of the post-hippocratic schools of medicine, which arose in the second century, B.C., under the leadership of Philinos of Cos and Serapion of Alexandria. As opposed to the Dogmatists, the Empirics declared that the search for the ultimate causes of phenomena was vain, but they were active in endeavoring to discover the immediate causes. They paid particular attention to the totality of symptoms. In their search for a line of treatment to benefit a particular set of symptoms they employed the "tripod of the Empirics": (1) their own chance observations—their own experience; (2) learning obtained from contemporaries and predecessors —the experience of others; and (3), in cases of new diseases, the formation of conclusions from other diseases which they resembled—analogy. The Empirics paid great attention to clinical observation, and were guided in their methods of treatment almost entirely by experience.

empiric (em-pir′ik) 1. empirical. 2. a practitioner whose skill is based on experience.

empirical (em-pir′e-kal) based on experience.

empiricism (em-pir′ĭ-sizm) [Gr. *empeirikos,* experienced] 1. the method of the Empiric school of medicine; opposed to rational medicine. 2. reliance on mere experience; empirical practice. 3. quackery.

Empirin (em′pĭ-rin) trademark for tablets containing acetylsalicylic acid, phenacetin, and caffeine.

emplastic (em-plas′tik) [Gr. *emplastikos* stopping up] 1. adhesive or glutinous. 2. a constipating medicine.

emplastrum (em-plas′trum) [L.; Gr. *emplastron*] plaster (def. 2).

emporiatrics (em-po″re-at′riks) [Gr. *emporos* one who goes on shipboard as a passenger + *iatrike* medicine] that branch of medicine which treats of the health problems of travelers about the world.

emprosthotonos (em″pros-thot′o-nos) [Gr. *emprosthen* forward + *tonos* tension] a form of tetanic spasm in which the head and feet are brought forward and the body is rendered tense; called also *episthotonos.*

emprosthotonus (em″pros-thot′o-nus) emprosthotonos.

emptysis (emp′tĭ-sis) [Gr.] expectoration, especially of blood.

Empusa (em-pu′sah) former name for *Entomophora.*

empyema (em″pi-e′mah) [Gr. *empyema*] accumulation of pus in a cavity of the body; when used without a descriptive qualifier, it refers to thoracic empyema (q.v.). **e. artic′uli,** acute suppurative synovitis. **e. benig′num,** thoracic empyema in which fever is absent and there is a fair condition of general health. **e. of the chest,** thoracic e. **e. of gallbladder,** cholecystitis in which the contents of the acutely inflamed gallbladder are turbid or appear to be frankly purulent. **interlobar e.,** empyema situated between two lobes of the lung. **latent e.,** empyema unaccompanied by any symptoms. **loculated e.,** pus in a group of loculi. **mastoid e.,** suppurative inflammation of the mucous lining of the cavities of the mastoid process. **metapneumonic e.,** empyema developing some time after the subsidence of the pneumonia; cf. *synpneumonic e.* **e. necessita′tis,** empyema in which the pus can make a spontaneous escape toward the chest wall. **e. of pericardium,** purulent pericarditis. **pneumococcal e.,** that which is due to the pneumococcus, *Streptococcus pneumoniae.* **pulsating e.,** thoracic empyema in which the movements of the heart produce a visible vibration of the chest wall. **putrid e.,** empyema in which the pus has become more or less decomposed. **streptococcal e.,** a form due to *Streptococcus pyogenes.* **synpneumonic e.,** empyema which arises during the course of pulmonary inflammation. Cf. *metapneumonic e.* **thoracic e.,** suppurative inflammation of the pleural space; called also *pyothorax.* **tuberculous e.,** a form of empyema due to *Mycobacterium tuberculosis.*

empyemic (em″pi-e′mik) pertaining to or of the nature of empyema.

empyesis (em″pi-e′sis) [Gr. *empyēsis* suppuration] 1. a pustular eruption. 2. any disease characterized by phlegmonous vesicles becoming filled with purulent fluid.

empyocele (em′pi-o-sēl) [Gr. *empyein* to suppurate + *kēlē* tumor] a collection of pus at the umbilicus.

empyreuma (em″pi-roo′mah) [Gr. *empyreuma* a live coal] the peculiar odor of animal or vegetable matter when charred in a closed vessel.

empyreumatic (em″pi-roo-mat′ik) pertaining to empyreuma; pertaining to or produced by destructive distillation of organic matter.

E.M.S. Emergency Medical Service (British).

emul. abbreviation for L. *emul′sum* emulsion.

emulgent (e-mul′jent) [L. *emulgere* to milk or drain out] 1. effecting a straining or purifying process. 2. a renal artery or vein. 3. a medicine that stimulates the flow of bile or urine.

emulsifier (e-mul″si-fi′er) an agent used to produce an emulsion.

emulsify (e-mul′sĭ-fi) to convert or to be converted into an emulsion.

emulsion (e-mul′shun) [L. *emulsio, emulsum*] a preparation of one liquid distributed in small globules throughout the body of a second liquid. The dispersed liquid is the discontinuous phase, and the dispersion medium is the continuous phase. When oil is the dispersed liquid and an aqueous solution is the continuous phase, it is known as an oil-in-water emulsion, whereas when water or aqueous solution is the dispersed phase and oil or oleaginous substance is the continuous phase, it is known as a water-in-oil emulsion. Pharamaceutical emulsions for which official standards have been promulgated include cod liver oil emulsion, cod liver oil emulsion with malt, liquid petrolatum emulsion, and phenolphthalein in liquid petrolatum emulsion. **hexachlorophene cleansing e.** [USP], an emulsion containing between 90 and 110 per cent of the labeled amount of hexachlorophene in a suitable aqueous vehicle; used as a topical anti-infective and detergent. **kerosene e.,** an emulsion of kerosene in soap solution, used as an insecticide. **liquid petrolatum e.,** mineral oil e. **mineral oil e.** [USP], an emulsion of mineral oil, acacia, syrup, vanillin, and alcohol in purified water, used as a cathartic; called also *liquid petrolatum e.* **photographic e.,** a light- and radiation-sensitive gelatinous coating incorporating silver halide which is applied to film. **Pusey's e.,** a preparation of powdered tragacanth, glycerin, phenol, oil of bergamot, and olive oil in water, used in infantile eczema.

emulsive (e-mul′siv) 1. capable of emulsifying a substance. 2. susceptible of being emulsified. 3. affording an oil on pressure.

emulsoid (e-mul′soid) an emulsion colloid.

emulsum (e-mul′sum), pl. *emul′sa* [L.] an emulsion.

emunctory (e-munk′to-re) [L. *emungere* to cleanse] 1. excretory or depurant. 2. any excretory organ or duct.

E-Mycin (e-mi′sin) trademark for a preparation of erythromycin.

emylcamate (e-mil′kah-māt) chemical name: 3-methyl-3-pentanol carbamate. A white crystalline powder, C_7H_{15}-NO_2, freely soluble in alcohol, used as a tranquilizer.

ENA extractable nuclear antigens.

enalapril (e-nal′ah-pril) a converting enzyme inhibitor used as an antihypertensive.

enamel (en-am′el) [O.F. *esmail*] 1. the glazed surface of baked porcelain, metal, or pottery. 2. any hard, smooth, glossy coating or enamel-like surface. 3. dental e. **curled e.,** dental enamel in which the columns are bent and are wavy and intertwined with one another. Called also *gnarled e.* Cf. *straight e.* **dental e.,** a hard, thin, translucent layer of calcified substance that envelops and protects the dentin of the crown of the tooth; it is the hardest substance in the body and is almost entirely composed of calcium salts. Called also *adamantine layer, enamel, enamelum* [NA], and *substantia adamantina dentis.* **dwarfed e.,** nanoid e. **gnarled e.,** curled e. **hereditary brown e.,** amelogenesis imperfecta. **hypoplastic e.,** enamel hypoplasia. **mottled e.,** a chronic endemic form of hypoplasia of the dental enamel caused by drinking water with a high fluorine content during the time of tooth formation, and characterized by defective calcification that gives a white chalky appearance to the enamel, which gradually undergoes brown discoloration. Called also *dental fluorosis, dentes de Chiaie,* and *mottled teeth.* **nanoid e.,** imperfectly formed dental enamel that is thinner than normal. Called also *dwarfed e.* **straight e.,** dental enamel in which the rods are straight. Cf. *curled e.*

enameloblast (en-am′el-o-blast) ameloblast.

enameloblastoma (en-am″el-o-blas-to′mah) ameloblastoma.

enameloma (en-am″el-o′mah) [*enamel* + *-oma*] a non-neoplastic excrescence sometimes found at the bifurcation of a multirooted tooth, at the end of an enamel spur, or on the root surface, which may be composed only of enamel, contain a small dentin nucleus, or contain a minute strand of dentin and pulp. Called also *enamel drop* and *enamel pearl.*

enamelum (e-nam′el-um) [NA] dental enamel.

enanthate (en-an′thāt) USAN contraction for heptanoate, the anionic form of enanthic acid.

enanthem (en-an′them) enanthema.

enanthema (en″an-the′ma), pl. *enanthe′mas, enanthem′ata* [Gr. *en* in + *anthema* a blossoming] an eruption upon a mucous surface.

enanthematous (en″an-them′ah-tus) pertaining to or of the nature of an enanthema.

enanthic acid (ĕ-nan′thik) trivial name for heptanoic acid.

enanthrope (en-an′thrōp) [Gr. *en* in + *anthrōpos* man] any source of disease situated within the human body.

enantiobiosis (en-an″te-o-bi-o′sis) [Gr. *enantios* opposite + *bios* life] the condition in which organisms living together antagonize one another's development. Cf. *symbiosis,* def. 1.

enantiomer (en-an′te-o-mer) one of a pair of compounds having a mirror image relationship. Called also *enantiomorph.*

enantiomerism (en-an″te-om′er-izm) [Gr. *emantios* opposite + *meros* part] the relationship between two stereoisomers having molecules that are mirror images of each other. Enantiomers have identical chemical and physical properties in an achiral environment. However, they form different products when reacted with other chiral molecules, and they exhibit optical activity. The enantiomer that rotates the plane of polarization of a beam of polarized light in the clockwise direction is indicated by the prefix (+) –, formerly *d*- or dextro-. The other enantiomer rotates the plane of

polarization an equal amount in the counterclockwise direction and is indicated by the prefix (–), formerly *l*- or levo-. Two conventions are used to designate the actual configurations of enantiomers. The D, L system (see D-) is used to denote the configuration of carbohydrates relative to D-(+)-glyceraldehyde and of amino acids relative to L-(–)-serine. The *R,S* system (see *R*-) is a more general system used to specify the absolute configuration at every asymmetric carbon atom. An equimolar mixture of enantiomers (a racemic form or racemic modification) is optically inactive and is designated by the prefixes (±)-, DL-, or *dl*-.

enantiomorph (en-an′te-o-morf″) enantiomer.

enantiomorphic (en-an″te-o-mor′fik) pertaining to or exhibiting enantiomerism.

enantiomorphism (en-an″te-o-mor′fizm) enantiomerism.

Enantiothamnus (en-an″te-o-tham′nus) a former genus of yeastlike imperfect fungi.

enarkyochrome (en-ar′ke-o-krōm″) [Gr. *en* in + *arkys* network + *chrōma* color] an arkyochrome nerve cell containing a single network of chromatin substance.

enarthritis (en″ar-thri′tis) inflammation of an enarthrosis.

enarthrodial (en″ar-thro′de-al) of or pertaining to an enarthrosis.

enarthrosis (en″ar-thro′sis) [Gr. *en* in + *arthrosis* joint] a joint in which the globular head of one bone is received into a socket in another, as in the hip joint.

en bloc (aw blok′) [Fr.] in a lump; as a whole.

encanthis (en-kan′this) [Gr. *en* in + *kanthos* the angle of the eye] a small red excrescence on the semilunar fold of the conjunctiva and inner lacrimal caruncle.

encapsulated (en-kap′su-lāt-ed) [Gr. *en* in + L. *capsula* a little box] enclosed within a capsule.

encapsulation (en-kap″su-la′shun) 1. any act of inclosing in a capsule. 2. a physiologic process of inclosure in a sheath made up of a substance not normal to the part.

encapsuled (en-kap′sūld) encapsulated.

encarditis (en″kar-di′tis) endocarditis.

encatarrhaphy (en″kah-tar′ah-fe) [Gr. *enkatarrhaptein* to sew in] the operation of burying a structure by suturing together the sides of the tissues adjacent to it.

enceinte (aw-sawt′) [Fr.] pregnant; with child.

encelialgia (en″se-le-al′je-ah) [Gr. *en* in + *koilia* belly + *-algia* pain] pain in an abdominal viscus.

enceliitis (en-se″le-i′tis) [Gr. *en* in + *koilia* belly + *-itis*] inflammation of an intra-abdominal organ.

encelitis (en″se-li′tis) enceliitis.

encephalalgia (en-sef″ah-lal′je-ah) [*encephalo-* + *-algia*] pain within the head.

encephalatrophy (en-sef″ah-lat′ro-fe) [*encephalo-* + *atrophy*] atrophy of the brain.

encephalauxe (en″sef-ah-lawk′se) [*encephalo-* + Gr. *auxē* increase] hypertrophy of the brain.

encephalemia (en-sef″ah-le′me-ah) [*encephalo-* + Gr. *haima* blood + *-ia*] congestion of the brain.

encephalic (en″se-fal′ik) 1. pertaining to the encephalon. 2. within the skull.

encephalitic (en″sef-ah-lit′ik) pertaining to or affected with encephalitis.

encephalitides (en″sef-ah-lit′ĭ-dēz) [Gr.] plural of *encephalitis.*

encephalitis (en″sef-ah-li′tis), pl. *encephalit′ides* [*encephalo-* + *-itis*] inflammation of the brain. **e. A,** lethargic e. **acute disseminated e.,** see under *encephalomyelitis.* **acute necrotizing e.,** morphological term for encephalitis characterized by a particularly destructive reaction in the brain. **Australian X e.,** see under *disease.* **e. B,** Japanese B e. **benign myalgic e.,** epidemic neuromyasthenia. **Binswanger's e.,** see under *dementia.* **bovine e.,** encephalitis of cows caused by microorganisms of the psittacosis-lymphogranuloma venereum group (*Chlamydia*). **buffalo e.,** a viral encephalitis of the Asiatic water buffalo. **e. C,** St. Louis e. **California e.,** an acute viral encephalitis caused by an arbovirus, primarily a disease of children. **Central European e.,** Russian spring-summer e. **chronic subcortical e.,** Binswanger's dementia. **cortical e., e. cortica′lis,** encephalitis affecting the cortex of the brain only. **Dawson's e.,** subacute sclerosing panencephalitis. **eastern equine e.,** see under *encephalomyelitis.* **Economo's e.,** lethargic e. **enzootic e. of horses,** Borna disease. **epidemic e., e. epidem′ica,** a viral encephalitis occurring epidemically in several types (see *influenzal e., Japanese B e., lethargic e., Russian spring-summer e.,* and *St. Louis e.*). **equine e.,** see *equine encephalomyelitis,* under *encephalomyelitis,* and *Borna disease,* under *disease.* **forest-spring e.,** Russian spring-summer e. **fox e.,** a viral disease of foxes, raccoons, and coyotes. **Hayem's e.,** e. hyperplastica. **hemorrhagic e.,** herpes encephalitis in which there is inflammation of the brain with hemorrhagic foci and perivascular exudate; called also *Strümpell-Leichtenstern type of encephalitis.* **hemorrhagic arsphenamine e.,** a rapidly progressive form which sometimes follows the administration of arsphenamine. **herpes e., herpes simplex e., herpetic e.,** a disease caused by herpesvirus, resembling equine encephalomyelitis. See *hemorrhagic e.* **e. hyperplas′tica,** an acute nonsuppurating form of encephalitis; called also *Hayem's encephalitis.* **Ilhe′us e.,** a viral encephalitis transmitted by mosquitoes in Brazil. See also under *virus.* **infantile e.,** inflammation of the brain in children from infectious disease. **influenzal e.,** encephalitis occurring as a complication of influenza. **Japanese B e.,** a form of epidemic encephalitis occurring in Japan and other Pacific islands, China, Manchuria, U.S.S.R., and probably much of the Far East; it may occur as a symptomless, subclinical infection, or an acute meningoencephalomyelitis with cortical damage and cord lesions resembling those of poliomyelitis. Called also *e. B.* and *Russian autumnal e.* See also under *virus.* **lead e.,** encephalitis with marked cerebral edema, caused by lead poisoning. **Leichtenstern's e.,** hemorrhagic e. **lethargic e., e. lethar′gica,** a form of epidemic encephalitis, the original type described by von Economo, characterized by increasing languor, apathy, and drowsiness, passing into lethargy; observed in various parts of the world between 1915 and 1926. Called also *e. A, Economo's e.* or *disease,* and *Vienna e.* **Murray Valley e.,** a viral encephalitis that occurred epidemically in 1950 and 1951 in the Murray Valley, Victoria, Australia, believed to be a recrudescence of Australian X disease; a few cases occurred in 1956, and it has been reported in New Guinea. **e. neonato′rum,** encephalitis in the newborn. **e. periaxia′lis concen′trica,** Baló's disease. **e. periaxia′lis diffu′sa,** Schilder's disease. **postinfectious e., postvaccinal e.,** acute disseminated encephalomyelitis. **Powassan e.,** a form reported from Canada, caused by a tickborne virus and closely resembling Russian spring-summer encephalitis. **purulent e., pyogenic e.,** suppurative e. **Russian autumnal e.,** Japanese B e. **Russian endemic e., Russian forest-spring e.,** Russian spring-summer e. **Russian spring-summer e.,** a form of epidemic encephalitis which is acquired in forests from infected ticks (*Ixodes persulcatus*), but is also transmitted in other ways, as by ingestion of the flesh of infected mammals and birds, or milk of infected goats. It ranges in severity from mild to fatal cases, with degenerative changes in organs other than those of the nervous system. See also under *virus.* **Russian tick-borne e., Russian vernal e.,** Russian spring-summer e. **St. Louis e.,** a viral disease first observed in Illinois in 1932, closely similar to western equine encephalomyelitis clinically, occurring in late summer and early fall and transmitted usually by mosquitoes of the genus *Culex;* it ranges from an abortive type of infection to severe disease. Called also *e. C.* See also under *virus.* **Schilder's e.,** see under *disease.* **Semliki Forest e.,** a form due to a virus transmitted by mosquitoes in the Semliki Forest of western Uganda. See also under *virus.* **e. sid′erans,** a form of epidemic encephalitis terminating fatally in a few hours. **subacute inclusion body e.,** subacute sclerosing panencephalitis. **e. subcortica′lis chron′ica,** Binswanger's dementia. **summer e.,** Japanese B e. **suppurative e.,** encephalitis accompanied by suppuration and abscess formation; called also *purulent e.* and *pyogenic e.* **toxoplasmic e.,** encephalitis due to infection with *Toxoplasma.* **van Bogaert e.,** subacute sclerosing panencephalitis. **Venezuelan equine e.,** see under *encephalomyelitis.* **vernal e.,** Russian spring-summer e. **vernoestival e.,** Russian spring-summer e. **Vienna e.,** lethargic e. **von Economo's e.,** lethargic e. **western equine e.,** see under *encephalomyelitis.* **West Nile e.,** a mild, febrile, sporadic disease of viral origin, probably transmitted by the mosquito *Culex univittatus,* occurring chiefly in the summer; frequently, infection does not lead to encephalitis. It may be of sudden onset, and symptoms may include drowsiness, severe frontal headache, maculopapular rash, abdominal pain, loss of appetite, nausea, and generalized lymphadenopathy. It was first reported in Uganda, but is widespread in Africa and has been reported in Israel. See also under *virus.* **woodcutter's e.,** Russian spring-summer e.

encephalitogen (en-sef″ah-lit′o-jen) any agent that causes encephalitis.

encephalitogenic (en-sef″ah-lit-o-jen′ik) [*encephalitis* + Gr. *gennan* to produce] causing encephalitis.

Encephalitozoon (en″sĕ-fal″ĭ-to-zo′on) [*encephal-* + Gr. *zōon* animal] a genus of parasitic protozoa (suborder Apansporoblastina, order Microsporida), formerly thought to be identical with *Nosema,* first reported in the brains of rabbits. Called also *Nosema.* **E. cunic′uli,** a species causing encephalitozoonosis in various domestic mammals, including rabbits, mice, rats, guinea pigs, dogs, and cats, involving chiefly the brain and kidney but also such other organs as the liver and spleen. Called also *Nosema cuniculi.*

encephalitozoonosis (en″sĕ-fal″ĭ-to-zo″o-no′sis) [*encephal-* + *zoonosis*] infection with protozoa of the genus *Encephalitozoon,* especially *E. cuniculi.* Called also *nosematosis.*

encephalization (en-sef″ah-li-za′shun) the developmental process by which the cerebral cortex has taken over the functions of the lower (spinal) centers.

encephal(o)- [L. *encephalon,* q.v.] a combining form denoting relationship to the brain.

encephalo-arteriography (en-sef″ah-lo-ar-te″re-og′rah-fe) a combination of encephalography and arteriography for examining the blood supply of the brain.

encephalocele (en-sef′ah-lo-sēl″) [*encephalo-* + Gr. *kēlē* hernia] hernia of the brain, manifested by protrusion of brain substance through a congenital or traumatic opening of the skull.

encephaloclastic (en-sef″ah-lo-klas′tik) [*encephalo-* + Gr. *klastōs* broken] exhibiting the residues of a destructive lesion in the brain; see under *porencephaly,* def. 2.

encephalocoele (en-sef″ah-lo-se′le) [*encephalo-* + Gr. *koilos* hollow] 1. the entire cavity of the cranium. 2. the ventricles and other spaces of the brain.

encephalocystocele (en-sef″ah-lo-sis″to-sēl) [*encephalo-* + Gr. *kystis* sac, bladder + *kēlē* hernia] hernia of the brain, the protrusion being distended by a collection of fluid communicating with the ventricle; called also *hydrencephalocele.*

encephalodialysis (en-sef″ah-lo-di-al′ĭ-sis) [*encephalo-* + Gr. *dialysis* loosening] softening of the brain.

encephalodysplasia (en-sef″ah-lo-dis-pla′se-ah) any congenital anomaly of the brain.

encephalogram (en-sef′ah-lo-gram″) the film made by encephalography.

encephalography (en-sef″ah-log′rah-fe) [*encephalo-* + Gr. *graphein* to write] roentgenography demonstrating the intracranial fluid-containing spaces after the withdrawal of cerebrospinal fluid and introduction of air or other gas; it includes pneumoencephalography and ventriculography.

encephaloid (en-sef′ah-loid) [*encephalo-* + Gr. *eidos* form] 1. resembling the brain or brain substance. 2. medullary carcinoma.

encephalolith (en-sef′ah-lo-lith″) [*encephalo-* + Gr. *lithos* stone] a brain calculus.

encephalology (en″sef-ah-lol′o-je) [*encephalo-* + *-logy*] the sum of knowledge regarding the brain, its functions, and its diseases.

encephaloma (en″sef-ah-lo′mah) 1. any swelling or tumor of the brain. 2. medullary carcinoma.

encephalomalacia (en-sef″ah-lo-mah-la′she-ah) [*encephalo-* + Gr. *malakia* softness] softening of the brain. **avian e.,** a disease of young chickens due to vitamin E deficiency, in which there is ataxia, incoordination, paralysis, and severe encephalomalacia in several areas of the brain, especially the cerebellum. It must be differentiated from avian encephalomyelitis. Called also *crazy chick disease.*

encephalomeningitis (en-sef″ah-lo-men″in-ji′tis) [*encephalo-* + *meningitis*] meningoencephalitis.

encephalomeningocele (en-sef″ah-lo-me-ning′go-sēl) [*encephalo-* + Gr. *mēninx* membrane + *kēlē* hernia] meningoencephalocele.

encephalomeningopathy (en-sef″ah-lo-men″in-gop′ah-the) meningoencephalopathy.

encephalomere (en-sef′ah-lo-mēr″) [*encephalo-* + Gr. *meros* part] any one of the succession of segments which make up the embryonic brain.

encephalometer (en-sef″ah-lom′ĕ-ter) [*encephalo-* + Gr. *metron* measure] an instrument used in locating certain of the regions of the brain.

encephalomyelitis (en-sef″ah-lo-mi″ĕ-li′tis) inflammation involving both the brain and the spinal cord. **acute disseminated e.,** an acute or subacute encephalomyelitis or myelitis characterized by perivascular lymphocyte and mononuclear cell infiltration and demyelination; it occurs most commonly following an acute viral infection, especially measles, but may occur without a recognizable antecedent, and formerly occurred as a complication of rabies vaccination before the introduction of duck embryo and human diploid vaccines and of smallpox vaccination. Clinical manifestations include fever, headache, vomiting, and drowsiness progressing to lethargy and coma; tremor, seizures, and paralysis may also occur; mortality ranges from 5 to 20 per cent; many survivors have residual neurologic deficits. Called also *acute perivascular myelinoclasis, postinfectious e., postvaccinal e.,* and *acute disseminated, postinfectious,* or *postvaccinal encephalitis.* **avian e.,** a viral disease of chickens under six weeks old, marked by weakness of the legs followed by partial or complete paralysis of the legs, trembling of the head and neck, and degeneration of the neurons in the pons, medulla, and anterior horns of the spinal cord. Clinically, it resembles avian encephalomalacia and must be differentiated from that condition. Called also *crazy chick disease* and *epidemic tremor.* **benign myalgic e.,** epidemic neuromyasthenia. **equine e.,** a viral disease of horses and mules, communicable to man, occurring as summer epizootics in the Western Hemisphere. Three forms are recognized: *eastern equine e., western equine e.,* and *Venezuelan equine e.* Called also *equine encephalitis.* See also under *virus.* **equine e., eastern,** a viral disease similar to western equine encephalomyelitis, but occurring in the United States in a region extending from New Hampshire to Texas and as far west as Wisconsin, and in Canada, Mexico, the Carribean, and parts of Central and South America. Abbreviated EEE. **equine e., Venezuelan,** a viral disease of horses and mules first observed in Colombia in 1935, the causative agent being isolated in Venezuela in 1938. It has since been reported in other South American countries and in Mexico, Texas, and Florida. The infection in man resembles influenza, with little or no indication of central nervous system involvement. Abbreviated VEE. **equine e., western,** a viral disease of horses and mules, communicable to man, occurring chiefly as a meningoencephalitis, with little involvement of the medulla or spinal cord; observed west of the Mississippi River in the United States, but present also along the Gulf and Atlantic coasts. Abbreviated WEE. **experimental allergic e. (EAE),** an animal model for acute disseminated encephalomyelitis in which the characteristic pathophysiology and clinical signs of this disease are produced by immunization of an animal with extracts of brain tissue or with myelin basic protein together with Freund's complete adjuvant; it is transferable by adoptive transfer of lymphocytes but not by serum. **granulomatous e.,** a disease marked by granulomas and necrosis of the walls of the cerebral and spinal ventricles. **infectious porcine e.,** a highly fatal encephalomyelitis of swine, caused by a picornavirus, and characterized by a flaccid ascending paralysis, similar in character to the paralysis of human poliomyelitis. First reported in the Teschen district of Czechoslovakia, it occurs throughout Europe. Called also *porcine encephalomyelitis, porcine poliomyelitis, Talfan disease,* and *Teschen disease.* **Mengo e.,** a form of encephalomyelitis the virus of which was first isolated from animals in the Mengo region of Uganda. See also under *virus.* **mouse e., murine e.,** Theiler's disease. **porcine e.,** infectious porcine e. **postinfectious e., postvaccinal e.,** acute disseminated e. **sporadic bovine e.,** Buss disease. **Theiler's mouse e.,** Theiler's disease. **toxoplasmic e.,** encephalomyelitis due to infection with *Toxoplasma.* **viral e., virus e.,** encephalomyelitis caused by a virus. See *equine e.*

encephalomyelocele (en-sef″ah-lo-mi-el′o-sēl) [*encephalo-*

+ Gr. *myelon* spinal cord + *kēlē* hernia] abnormality of the foramen magnum and absence of the laminae and spinal processes of the cervical vertebrae, with herniation of meninges, brain substance, and spinal cord.

encephalomyeloneuropathy (en-sef″ah-lo-mi″ĕ-lo-nurop′ah-the) disease involving the brain, spinal cord, and peripheral nerves.

encephalomyelopathy (en-sef″ah-lo-mi″ĕ-lop′ah-the) [*encephalo-* + Gr. *myelos* marrow + *pathos* disease] any disease or diseased condition of the brain and spinal cord. **postinfection e.,** demyelination secondary to common viral diseases such as measles, varicella, rubella, mumps, and influenza. **postvaccinial e.,** demyelination complicating the reaction to vaccination against smallpox. **subacute necrotizing e.,** an encephalopathy of unclear clinical and pathological criteria, causing neuropathologic and brain stem damage like that from the Wernicke-Korsakoff syndrome. It occurs in two forms: In the *infantile,* which may be the same as pyruvate carboxylase deficiency, the chief pathological finding is degeneration of the gray matter with foci of necrosis and capillary proliferation in the brain stem, and the chief biochemical findings are high lactate and pyruvate in the blood and low glucose in the blood and CSF. There is a wide variety of manifestation, including anorexia and vomiting, slow or arrested development, hypotonia, seizures, abnormal movements, ocular and respiratory disorders, and dementia, with death usually occurring before age 3. In the *adult* form, the first manifestation is bilateral optic atrophy with central scotoma and colorblindness, which is followed by a quiescent period of up to 30 years, after which ataxia, spastic paresis, clonic jerks, grand mal seizures, psychic lability, and mild dementia, appear. Called also *subacute necrotizing encephalopathy* and *Leigh disease* or *syndrome.*

encephalomyeloradiculitis (en-sef″ah-lo-mi″ĕ-lo-rahdik″u-li′tis) inflammation of the brain, spinal cord, and spinal nerve roots.

encephalomyeloradiculoneuritis (en-sef″ah-lo-mi″ĕ-lo-rah-dik″u-lo-nu-ri′tis) acute febrile polyneuritis.

encephalomyeloradiculopathy (en-sef″ah-lo-mi″ĕ-lo-rah-dik″u-lop′ah-the) disease involving the brain, spinal cord, and spinal nerve roots.

encephalomyocarditis (en-sef″ah-lo-mi″o-kar-di′tis) a viral disease characterized by degenerative and inflammatory changes in skeletal and cardiac muscle, and lesions of the central nervous system resembling those of poliomyelitis.

encephalon (en-sef′ah-lon) [L., from Gr. *enkephalos,* from *en-* in + *kephalē* head] [NA] the brain: that part of the central nervous system contained within the cranium, comprising the prosencephalon, mesencephalon, and rhombencephalon; it is derived (developed) from the anterior part of the embryonic neural tube. See illustration accompanying *brain.* See also *cerebrum.*

encephalonarcosis (en-sef″ah-lo-nar-ko′sis) [*encephalo-* + Gr. *narkē* stupor] stupor due to brain disease.

encephalopathia (en-sef″ah-lo-path′e-ah) encephalopathy. **e. alcohol′ica,** polioencephalitis haemorrhagica superior.

encephalopathic (en-sef″ah-lo-path′ik) pertaining to encephalopathy.

encephalopathy (en-sef″ah-lop′ah-the) [*encephalo-* + Gr. *pathos* illness] any degenerative disease of the brain. **biliary e.,** kernicterus. **bilirubin e.,** kernicterus. **boxer's e.,** traumatic e. **demyelinating e.,** a degenerative disease of the brain characterized by demyelination; see *Schilder's disease,* under *disease.* **dialysis e.,** a degenerative disease of the brain associated with long-term use of hemodialysis, marked by speech disorders and constant myoclonic jerks, progressing to global dementia, with associated psychological changes; it is often accompanied by osteomalacia and is due to high levels of aluminum in the water used in the dialysis fluid or to aluminum-containing compounds given to control phosphorus levels. Called also *progressive dialysis e.* **hepatic e.,** a condition usually occurring secondarily to advanced disease of the liver but also seen in the course of any severe disease or in patients with portacaval shunts. It is marked by disturbances of consciousness which may progress to deep coma (hepatic coma), psychiatric changes of varying degree, flapping tremor, and fetor hepaticus. Called also *portal-systemic encephalopathy.* **hypernatremic e.,** a severe hemorrhagic encephalopathy induced by the hyperosmolarity accompanying hypernatremia and dehydration. **hypertensive e.,** a complex of cerebral phenomena (headache, convulsions, coma, etc.) occurring in the course of malignant hypertension. **hypoglycemic e.,** metabolic encephalopathy induced by severe hypoglycemia, as in glycogen storage disease, oversecretion or overdose of insulin, etc. **lead e.,** brain disorder caused by lead poisoning; called also *saturnine e.* **metabolic e.,** neuropsychiatric disturbances due to metabolic brain disease. It may occur primarily as a result of hypoxia, ischemia, or hypoglycemia, or secondarily to disease of other organs, such as the kidney, lung, or liver. **mink e.,** a progressive viral disease of the central nervous system of mink, characterized by locomotor incoordination, progressing to semicoma and death within three to eight weeks. **myoclonic e. of childhood,** a neurologic disorder of unknown etiology with onset between ages one and three, characterized by myoclonus of trunk and limbs and by opsoclonus, with ataxia of gait and intention tremor; some cases have been associated with occult neuroblastoma. Called also *Kinsbourne syndrome.* **portal-systemic e., portasystemic e.,** hepatic e. **progressive dialysis e.,** dialysis e. **progressive subcortical e.,** Schilder's disease; see under *disease.* **punch-drunk e.,** a state of forgetfulness, slowness in thinking, dysarthric speech, and slow, uncertain movements, especially of the legs, the cumulative effects of repeated cerebral injuries in boxers; called also *dementia pugilistica* and *punchdrunk.* **saturnine e.,** lead e. **spongiform e.,** encephalopathy involving extensive vacuolization of the cerebral cortex; the term embraces Creutzfeldt-Jakob syndrome, kuru, scrapie of sheep, and mink encephalopathy. Called also *status spongiosus.* **subacute necrotizing e.,** see under *encephalomyelopathy.* **subacute spongiform e.,** transmissible spongiform e. **subcortical arteriosclerotic e.,** Binswanger's dementia. **transmissible spongiform e., transmissible spongiform virus e.,** any of a group of transmissible infections of the nervous system caused by a slow virus, including Creutzfeldt-Jakob syndrome, kuru, scrapie, and mink encephalopathy, characterized pathologically by neuronal loss, astrogliosis, and extensive vacuolization of the cerebral cortex. Called also *subacute spongiform e.* **traumatic e.,** a syndrome due to cumulative punishment absorbed in the boxing ring, characterized by the general slowing of mental functions, occasional bouts of confusion, and scattered memory loss. **Wernicke's e.,** a neurological disorder characterized by confusion, apathy, drowsiness, ataxia of gait, nystagmus, and ophthalmoplegia. It was described as "acute superior hemorrhagic polioencephalitis" by Wernicke in 1881, because he observed hemorrhagic lesions of the gray matter around the third and fourth ventricles and aqueduct of Sylvius and supposed an inflammatory process was involved. The disease is now known to be due to thiamine deficiency. It most commonly results from chronic alcohol abuse and is almost invariably accompanied by or followed by Korsakoff's syndrome (organic amnesia) and frequently accompanied by other nutritional polyneuropathies. Called also *Wernicke's disease* or *syndrome.* See also *Wernicke-Korsakoff syndrome,* under *syndrome.*

encephalopuncture (en-sef″ah-lo-punk′tūr) surgical puncture of the brain.

encephalopyosis (en-sef″ah-lo-pi-o′sis) [*encephalo-* + Gr. *pyōsis* suppuration] suppuration or abscess of the brain.

encephalorachidian (en-sef″ah-lo-rah-kid′e-an) [*encephalo-* + Gr. *rhachis* spine] cerebrospinal.

encephaloradiculitis (en-sef″ah-lo-rah-dik′u-li″tis) inflammation of the roots of spinal nerves and of the brain.

encephalorrhagia (en-sef″ah-lo-ra′je-ah) [*encephalo-* + Gr. *rhēgnynai* to burst out] hemorrhage within the brain or from the brain, especially cerebral pericapillary hemorrhage.

encephalosclerosis (en-sef″ah-lo-skle-ro′sis) [*encephalo-* + Gr. *sklērōsis* hardness] hardening of the brain.

encephaloscope (en-sef′ah-lo-skōp) an instrument for examining a cavity (such as an abscess cavity) in the brain.

encephaloscopy (en-sef″ah-los′ko-pe) [*encephalo-* + Gr. *skopein* to examine] inspection or examination of the brain.

encephalosepsis (en-sef″ah-lo-sep′sis) [*encephalo-* + Gr. *sēpsis* decay] gangrene of brain tissue.

encephalosis (en-sef″ah-lo′sis) [*encephalo-* + *-osis*] any organic brain disease; as used by Winkelman, the term

indicates a degenerative process as distinguished from true encephalitis.

encephalospinal (en-sef″ah-lo-spi′nal) pertaining to the brain and spinal column.

encephalothlipsis (en-sef″ah-lo-thlip′sis) [*encephalo-* + Gr. *thlipsis* pressure] compression of the brain.

encephalotome (en-sef′ah-lo-tōm) an instrument for performing encephalotomy.

encephalotomy (en-sef″ah-lot′o-me) [*encephalo-* + Gr. *tomē* a cutting] 1. the destruction of the head of a fetus in order to facilitate delivery. 2. incision of the brain.

enchondral (en-kon′dral) endochondral.

enchondroma (en″kon-dro′mah) [Gr. *en* in + *chondros* cartilage + *-oma*] a benign growth of cartilage arising in the metaphysis of a bone; called also *true chondroma* and *enchondrosis.* When multiple bones are involved, the condition is called *enchondromatosis.* **multiple congenital e.,** enchondromatosis.

enchondromatosis (en-kon″dro-mah-to′sis) a condition characterized by hamartomatous proliferation of cartilage cells within the metaphysis of several bones, causing thinning of the overlying cortex and distortion of the growth in length; called also *multiple* or *skeletal e., dyschondroplasia,* and *Ollier's disease.* In combination with multiple cutaneous or visceral hemangiomas, the disorder is known as *Maffucci's syndrome.* **multiple e., skeletal e.,** enchondromatosis.

enchondromatous (en″kon-dro′mah-tus) of the nature of or pertaining to enchondroma.

enchondrosarcoma (en-kon″dro-sar-ko′mah) central chondrosarcoma.

enchondrosis (en″kon-dro′sis) 1. an outgrowth from cartilage. 2. an enchondroma.

enchylema (en″ki-le′mah) [Gr. *en* in + *chylos* juice] hyaloplasm, def. 1.

enchyma (en′ki-mah) [Gr. *en* in + *chymos* juice] the substance elaborated from absorbed nutritive materials; the formative juice of the tissues.

enclave (en′klāv, aw-klahv′) [Fr.] a tissue detached from its normal connection and enclosed within another organ or tissue.

enclitic (en-klit′ik) [Gr. *enklinein* to incline] having the planes of the fetal head inclined to those of the maternal pelvis; not synclitic.

enclomiphene (en-klo′mi-fēn) chemical name: (*E*)-2-[4-(2-chloro-1,2-diphenylethenyl)phenoxy]-*N,N*-diethylethanamine; the *cis*-isomer of the gonad-stimulating principle clomiphene citrate (q.v.), $C_{26}H_{28}ClNO$. Called also *cisclomiphene.* Cf. *zuclomiphene.*

encolpism (en-kol′pizm) [Gr. *en* in + *kolpos* vagina] medication administered via the vagina.

encopresis (en-ko-pre′sis) incontinence of feces not due to organic defect or illness.

encranius (en-kra′ne-us) [Gr. *en* in + *kranion* skull] a teratoid parasitic twin located within the cranium of the autosite.

encyesis (en″si-e′sis) [Gr. *en* in + *kyēsis* pregnancy] normal uterine pregnancy.

encyopyelitis (en-si″o-pi″ĕ-li′tis) [*encyesis* + *pyelitis*] dilatation of the ureters and/or renal pelvis during normal pregnancy with associated edema, but seldom with all the classical signs of inflammation.

encysted (en-sist′ed) [Gr. *en* in + *kystis* sac, bladder] enclosed in a sac, bladder, or cyst.

encystment (en-sist′ment) the process or condition of being or becoming encysted.

endadelphos (end″ah-del′fos) [*end-* + Gr. *adelphos* brother] a monster in which a parasitic twin is inclosed within the body of the autosite, or within a tumor upon the larger twin.

endangiitis (en″dan-je-i′tis) inflammation of the endangium; intimitis.

endangium (en″dan′je-um) [*end-* + Gr. *angeion* vessel] the innermost coat of a blood vessel (tunica intima vasorum [NA]).

endaortic (en″da-or′tik) pertaining to the interior of the aorta.

endaortitis (end″a-or-ti′tis) inflammation of the lining membrane of the aorta. **bacterial e.,** the formation of bacterial vegetations on the endothelial surface of the aorta.

endarterectomy (end″ar-ter-ek′to-me) excision of the thickened, atheromatous tunica intima of an artery. **gas e.,** endarterectomy performed by utilizing high-pressure carbon dioxide to remove plaque deposits from the coronary blood vessels in the treatment of atherosclerosis.

endarterial (end″ar-te′re-al) within an artery.

endarteritis (end″ar-ter-i′tis) [end- + Gr. *artēria* artery + *-itis*] inflammation of the tunica intima of an artery; intimitis. Cf. *arteritis* and *periarteritis*. **e. defor′mans** (*obs.*), chronic endarteritis characterized by fatty degeneration of the arterial tissues, with the formation of deposits of lime salts. **Heubner's specific e.,** see under *disease*. **e. oblit′erans,** endarteritis in which the lumina of the smaller vessels become narrowed or obliterated as a result of proliferation of the tissue of the intimal layer; called also *arteritis obliterans* and *Friedländer's disease*. **e. prolif′-erans,** overgrowth of fibrous tissue in the internal layers of the aorta.

endarterium (end″ar-te′re-um) [end- + Gr. *artēria* artery] the tunica intima of an artery.

endarteropathy (end″ar-ter-op′ah-the) disorder of the innermost coat (tunica intima) of an artery. **digital e.,** disorder of the tunica intima of the arteries of the digits, associated with Raynaud's phenomenon and nutritional lesions of the pulp of the fingers.

end-artery (end′ar-ter-e) an artery that does not anastomose with other arteries.

endaural (end-aw′ral) within the ear.

endbrain (end′brān) telencephalon.

end-brush (end′brush) the brushlike or tufted arrangement sometimes forming the termination of the process of a nerve cell.

end-bud (end′bud) see under *bud*.

end-bulb (end′bulb) see under *bulb*.

endchondral (end-kon′dral) endochondral.

endeictic (en-dīk′tik) [Gr. *endeixis* a pointing out] symptomatic.

endemia (en-de′me-ah) any endemic disease.

endemial (en-de′me-al) endemic.

endemic (en-dem′ik) [Gr. *endēmos* dwelling in a place] present or usually prevalent in a population or geographical area at all times; said of a disease or agent. Called also *endemial*. See also *holoendemic* and *hyperendemic*. Cf. *epidemic*.

endemoepidemic (en″dĕ-mo-ep″ĭ-dem′ik) endemic, but occasionally becoming epidemic.

endepidermis (end″ep-ĭ-der′mis) the epithelium or internal epidermis.

endergic (end-er′jik) [end- + Gr. *ergon* work] taking in work: a term applied to chemical reactions in which the products have a higher free energy than the reactants.

endergonic (end″er-gon′ik) [end(o)- + Gr. *ergon* work] characterized by or accompanied by the absorption of energy; said of chemical reactions that require energy in order to proceed, so that the products have a higher free energy than the reactants. Opposed to *exergonic*.

enderon (en′der-on) [Gr. *en* in + *deros* skin] the deeper part of the skin or mucous membrane, as distinguished from the epithelium or epidermis.

enderonic (en″der-on′ik) pertaining to the enderon or derived from it.

Enders (en′derz), John Franklin. American microbiologist, 1897–1985; co-winner with Thomas Huckle Weller and Frederick Chapman Robbins, of the Nobel prize in medicine or physiology for 1954, for the discovery that many viruses (specifically, poliomyelitis viruses) can be grown in tissue culture and thereby studied and isolated, making possible the production of vaccines.

end-feet (end′feet) button-like or knoblike terminal enlargements of naked nerve fibers which end in relation to the dendrite of another cell; called also *terminal buttons*, *boutons terminaux*, and *synaptic knobs*. **e. of Held,** end-feet.

end-flake (end′flāk) end-plate.

ending (end′ing) a termination or finish, especially the peripheral termination of a nerve or nerve fiber. **annulo-spiral e's,** wide, ribbon-like sensory nerve endings which are wrapped around the fibers of a muscle spindle. **club**

e. of Bartelmez, a type of nerve fiber ending in the vertebrate central nervous system, terminating abruptly on the dendrite of another neuron. **encapsulated nerve e's,** corpuscula nervosa terminalia. **epilemmal e's,** sensory nerve endings in striated muscle in which the nerve endings are in close contact with the muscle fibers but do not penetrate the sarcolemma. **flower-spray e's,** branched, slender sensory nerve endings on the sarcolemma of muscle spindles. **free nerve e's,** terminationes nervorum liberae. **grape e's,** sensory nerve endings in muscle which have the form of terminal swellings. **nerve e's,** the fine branchlike terminations of axons.

end-nuclei (end-nu′kle-i) terminal nuclei; see under *nucleus*.

end(o)- [Gr. *endon* within] prefix denoting an inward situation, within.

endoabdominal (en″do-ab-dom′ĭ-nal) pertaining to the interior of the abdomen.

endo-amylase (en″do-am′ĭ-las) α-amylase.

endoaneurysmorrhaphy (en″do-an″u-riz-mor′ah-fe) [*endo-* + Gr. *aneurysma* aneurysm + *rhaphē* suture] Matas' operation for aneurysm by opening the aneurysmal sac and narrowing the internal lumen by suture; of historical interest.

endoangiitis (en″do-an-je-i′tis) endangiitis.

endoantitoxin (en″do-an-te-tok′sin) (*obs.*) an antitoxin contained within the elaborating cell.

endoaortitis (en″do-a″or-ti′tis) endaortitis.

endoappendicitis (en″do-ah-pen″dĭ-si′tis) inflammation of the mucous membrane lining the vermiform appendix.

endoarteritis (en″do-ar″ter-i′tis) endarteritis.

endoauscultation (en″do-aws″kul-ta′shun) auscultation of the stomach and thoracic organs by means of a tube passed into the stomach.

endobacillary (en″do-bas′ĭ-lār-e) contained within a bacillus.

endobiotic (en″do-bi-ot′ik) [*endo-* + Gr. *biōsis* living] living parasitically within the tissues of the host.

endoblast (en′do-blast) [*endo-* + Gr. *blastos* germ] entoderm.

endoblastic (en″do-blas′tik) entodermic.

endobronchitis (en″do-brong-ki′tis) inflammation of the epithelial lining of the bronchi.

endocardial (en″do-kar′de-al) [*endo-* + Gr. *kardia* heart] 1. situated or occurring within the heart. 2. pertaining to the endocardium.

endocardiopathy (en″do-kar″de-op′ah-the) any noninflammatory disease of the endocardium.

endocarditic (en″do-kar-dit′ik) pertaining to endocarditis.

endocarditis (en″do-kar-di′tis) exudative and proliferative inflammatory alterations of the endocardium, characterized by the presence of vegetations on the surface of the endocardium or in the endocardium itself, and most commonly involving a heart valve, but sometimes affecting the inner lining of the cardiac chambers or the endocardium elsewhere. It may occur as a primary disorder or as a complication of or in association with another disease. **atypical verrucous e.,** nonbacterial endocarditis found in association with systemic lupus erythematosus, in which the vegetations consist of necrotic debris, fibrinoid material, and trapped, disintegrating, fibroblastic and inflammatory cells. Called also *Libman-Sacks e.* or *disease*, *e. benigna*, and *nonbacterial verrucous e.* **bacterial e.,** infectious endocarditis (q.v.), acute or subacute, caused by various bacteria, including streptococci, staphylococci, enterococci, gonococci, gram-negative bacilli, etc. **e. benig′na,** atypical verrucous e. **e. chorda′lis,** endocarditis affecting particularly the chordae tendineae. **chronic e.,** chronic deforming disease of the heart valves. **constrictive e.,** Löffler's e. **fungal e.,** mycotic e. **infectious e., infective e.,** endocarditis caused by infection with microorganisms, especially bacteria and fungi, and sometimes other organisms, such as spirochetes, rickettsiae, and the etiologic agent of psittacosis. It has been classified according to course as acute and subacute. The *acute* form, which may be due to staphylococci, pneumococci, gonococci, streptococci, and other bacteria and other microorganisms, usually involves a normal heart valve, has a high mortality rate with or without treatment, and causes rapid destruction and metastases; the *subacute* form, which may be caused by viridans streptococci, fungi, or other organisms, usually affects a previously damaged heart valve, produces additional damage slowly, and responds well to therapy. **e. len'ta,** the subacute form of infectious endocarditis. **Libman-Sacks e.,** atypical verrucous e. **Löffler's e., Löffler's parietal fibroplastic e.,** endocarditis associated with eosinophilia, marked by fibroplastic thickening of the endocardium, and resulting in congestive heart failure, persistent tachycardia, hepatomegaly, splenomegaly, serous effusions into the pleural cavity, edema of the legs, and edema and ascites of the arms; called also *constrictive e.* and *eosinophilic endomyocardial disease.* **malignant e.,** a term sometimes applied to a rapidly fatal form of acute infectious endocarditis marked by ulcerated valvular lesions (*ulcerative e.*); called also *septic e.* **marantic e.,** nonbacterial thrombotic e. **mural e.,** a form affecting the lining of the walls of the heart chambers, as distinguished from *valvular e.;* called also *parietal e.* **mycotic e.,** infectious endocarditis (q.v.), usually subacute, due to various fungi, most commonly *Candida* (especially *C. albicans*), *Aspergillus,* and *Histoplasma.* Called also *fungal e.* **nonbacterial thrombotic e.,** endocarditis in which the vegetations, single or multiple, consist of fibrin and other blood elements. **nonbacterial verrucous e.,** atypical verrucous e., mural e. **parietal e.,** mural e. **prosthetic valve e.,** infective endocarditis as a complication of implantation of a prosthetic valve in the heart; the vegetations usually occur along the line of suture. **pulmonic e.,** endocarditis involving the pulmonic valve. **rheumatic e.,** endocarditis associated with rheumatic fever; called also *Bouillaud's disease.* **rickettsial e.,** endocarditis caused by invasion of the heart valves with *Coxiella burnetii;* it is a sequela of Q fever, usually occurring in persons who have had rheumatic fever. **right-side e.,** primary acute endocarditis of the right side of the heart. **septic e.,** malignant e. **syphilitic e.,** endocarditis resulting from extension of syphilitic infection from the aorta. **tuberculous e.,** a rare form of endocarditis in which the endocardium is involved by extension of a tuberculous perimyocarditis or of miliary tuberculosis. **ulcerative e.,** see *malignant e.* **valvular e.,** endocarditis affecting the membrane over the valves of the heart only, as distinguished from *mural e.* **vegetative e., verrucous e.,** endocarditis, infectious or noninfectious, the characteristic lesions of which are vegetations or verrucae on the endocardium. **viridans e.,** the subacute form of infectious endocarditis due to infection with viridans streptococci.

endocardium (en″do-kar′de-um) [*endo-* + Gr. *kardia* heart] [NA] the endothelial lining membrane of the cavities of the heart and the connective tissue bed on which it lies.

endoceliac (en″do-se′le-ak) [*endo-* + Gr. *koilia* cavity] inside one of the body cavities.

endocellular (en″do-sel′u-lar) within a cell.

endocervical (en″do-ser′vĭ-kal) pertaining to the interior of the cervix uteri.

endocervicitis (en″do-ser″vĭ-si′tis) [*endo-* + L. *cervix* neck] inflammation of the mucous membrane of the cervix uteri; called also *endotrachelitis.*

endocervix (en″do-ser′viks) 1. the mucous membrane lining the canal of the cervix uteri. 2. the region of the opening of the uterine cervix into the uterine cavity.

endochondral (en″do-kon′dral) situated, formed, or occurring within cartilage.

endochorion (en″do-ko′re-on) [*endo-* + Gr. *chorion* chorion] the inner chorionic layer.

endochrome (en′do-krōm) [*endo-* + Gr. *chrōma* color] the coloring matter within a cell.

endocolitis (en″do-ko-li′tis) inflammation of the mucous membrane of the colon.

endocommensal (en″do-kom-men′sal) a commensal organism which lives inside the body of its symbiotic companion.

endoconidiotoxicosis (en″do-ko-nĭd″e-o-tok″sĭ-ko′sis) a form of mycotoxicosis caused by a fungus of the genus *Endoconidium.*

endocorpuscular (en″do-kor-pus′ku-lar) situated within a corpuscle.

endocranial (en″do-kra′ne-al) situated within the cranium.

endocraniosis (en″do-kra″ne-o′sis) intracranial hyperostosis described by Morgagni.

endocranitis (en″do-kra-ni′tis) inflammation of the endocranium.

endocranium (en″do-kra′ne-um) [*endo-* + Gr. *kranion* skull] the endosteal outer layer of the dura mater of the brain.

endocrine (en′do-krīn, en′do-krin) [*endo-* + Gr. *krinein* to separate] 1. secreting internally; applied to organs and structures whose function is to secrete into the blood or lymph a substance (hormone) that has a specific effect on another organ or part. See also under *system.* 2. pertaining to internal secretions; hormonal. Cf. *exocrine.*

endocrinic (en″do-krin′ik) endocrinous.

endocrinism (en-dok′rĭ-nism) endocrinopathy.

endocrinium (en″do-krin′e-um) the endocrine system.

endocrinologist (en″do-krĭ-nol′o-jist) an individual skilled in endocrinology, and in the diagnosis and treatment of disorders of the glands of internal secretion, i.e., the endocrine glands.

endocrinology (en″do-krĭ-nol′o-je) [*endocrine* + *-logy*] the study of the endocrine system and its role in the physiology of the body.

endocrinopathic (en″do-krin″o-path′ik) pertaining to or characterized by endocrinopathy.

endocrinopathy (en″do-krĭ-nop′ah-the) [*endocrine* + Gr. *pathos* disease] any disease due to disorder of the endocrine system; hormonal imbalance.

endocrinosis (en″do-krĭ-no′sis) a disordered condition due to dysfunction of the endocrine system.

endocrinotherapy (en″do-kri″no-ther′ah-pe) treatment of disease by the administration of endocrine preparations; hormonotherapy.

endocrinotropic (en″do-kri″no-trop′ik) having an endocrine tendency.

endocuticle (en″do-ku′tĭ-kl) [*endo-* + L. *cuticula*] the inner layer of the procuticle in certain crustaceans and arthropods, which is almost entirely composed of protein and chitin.

endocyclic (en″do-sik′lik) a term applied to cyclic compounds in which the bond occurs in the ring.

endocyst (en′do-sist) the inner, germinative, or embryonic membrane of the hydatid cyst.

endocystitis (en″do-sis-ti′tis) inflammation of the lining membrane of the bladder.

endocyte (en′do-sīt) [*endo-* + Gr. *kytos* hollow vessel] any cell inclusion.

endocytosis (en″do-si-to′sis) [*endo-* + Gr. *kytos* a hollow vessel] the uptake by a cell of material from the environment by invagination of its plasma membrane; it includes both phagocytosis and pinocytosis.

endodeoxyribonuclease (en″do-de-ok″se-ri″bo-nu′kle-ās) [EC 3.1.21–25] one of several sub-sub classes of enzymes of the hydrolase class that catalyze the hydrolysis of interior bonds of deoxyribonucleotides, producing oligonucleotides or polynucleotides.

endoderm (en′do-derm) [*endo-* + Gr. *derma* skin] entoderm.

endodermal (en″do-der′mal) entodermal.

Endodermophyton (en″do-der-mof′ĭ-ton) [*endo-* + Gr. *derma* skin + *phyton* a growth] the former name of a genus of fungi, now called *Trichophyton.*

endodiascope (en″do-di′ah-skōp) a roentgen-ray tube which may be placed inside a body cavity for roentgenography and radiotherapy.

endodiascopy (en″do-di-as′ko-pe) [*endo-* + Gr. *dia* through + *skopein* to examine] roentgenoscopic examination of a body cavity by means of an endodiascope.

endodontia (en″do-don′she-ah) (*obs.*) endodontics.

endodontics (en″do-don′tiks) [*end-* + *odont-* + *-ics*] that branch of dentistry concerned with the etiology, prevention, diagnosis, and treatment of diseases and injuries affecting the dental pulp, tooth root, and periapical tissue. In current terminology, the term *endodontics* is used in a more restrictive sense than the term *endodontology,* which comprises the scientific study of the dental pulp and associated processes in health and disease. Sometimes the terms are used interchangeably.

endodontist (en″do-don′tist)   a dentist who specializes in endodontics; called also *endodontologist.*

endodontium (en″do-don′she-um)   the dental pulp (pulpa dentis [NA]).

endodontologist (en″do-don-tol′o-jist)   endodontist.

endodontology (en″do-don-tol′o-je) [*end-* + *odont-* + *-logy*] the scientific study of the dental pulp and associated processes in health and disease. In current terminology, the term *endodontology* is used in a broader sense than the term *endodontics,* which is restricted to the etiology, prevention, diagnosis, and treatment of disease and injuries of the dental pulp and associated processes. Sometimes the terms are used interchangeably.

endodyogeny (en″do-di-oj′ĕ-ne)   reproduction by the formation of two daughter cells within the wall of the mother cell (internal budding, the progeny being released by rupture of the mother cell, as in the protozoan *Toxoplasma.*

endoectothrix (en″do-ek′to-thriks)   a ringworm fungus which produces spores both on the interior and exterior of the hairs.

endoenteritis (en″do-en″ter-i′tis)   inflammation of the mucous membrane of the intestine.

endoenzyme (en″do-en′zīm)   an intracellular enzyme; an enzyme that is retained in a cell and does not normally diffuse out of the cell into the surrounding medium. Cf. *ectoenzyme.*

endoepidermal (en″do-ep″ĭ-der′mal)   within the epidermis.

endoepithelial (en″do-ep″ĭ-the′le-al)   within the epithelium.

endoergic (en″do-er′jik)   characterized by or accompanied by the absorption of free energy; requiring energy for its completion, as a chemical reaction to which energy must be supplied if it is to proceed. Cf. *exoergic* and *exothermic.*

endoesophagitis (en″do-e-sof″ah-ji′tis)   inflammation of the lining membrane of the esophagus.

endoexoteric (en″do-ek″so-ter′ik) [*endo-* + Gr. *exōterikos* pertaining to the outside]   resulting from certain causes internal to the body, and from others of external origin.

endofaradism (en″do-far′ah-dizm)   the application of alternating current to an internal organ, as to the stomach.

endogalvanism (en″do-gal′vah-nizm)   the application of direct current to an internal organ, as to the stomach.

endogamous (en-dog′ah-mus)   characterized by endogamy.

endogamy (en-dog′ah-me) [*endo-* + Gr. *gamos* marriage] 1. fertilization by the union of separate cells having the same genetic ancestry; called also *pedogamy.* Cf. *autogamy* (def. 1) and *exogamy* (def. 1).   2. restricting marriage to persons within the community; inbreeding.

endogastric (en″do-gas′trik)   pertaining to the interior of the stomach.

endogastritis (en″do-gas-tri′tis)   inflammation of the mucous membrane of the stomach.

endogenetic (en″do-jĕ-net′ik)   endogenous.

endogenic (en″do-jen′ik)   endogenous.

Endogenina (en″do-jĕ-ni′nah) [*endo-* + Gr. *gennan* to produce]   a suborder of ciliate protozoa (order Suctorida, subclass Suctoria) found in various habitats with some species being endocommensal in various hosts. Some species are stalkless, several have atypically huge ramified bodies, and bundles of tentacles, sometimes branched, are characteristic. They reproduce by endogenous budding, with the small, motile larvae occurring free in a cortical pouch before emergence.

endogenote (en″do-je′nōt)   in bacterial genetics, the recipient cell's own complement of genetic information, as opposed to the exogenote introduced by transduction.

endogenous (en-doj′ĕ-nus) [*endo-* + Gr. *gennan* to produce]   1. growing from within.   2. developing or originating within the organism, or arising from causes within the organism.

endoglobar (en″do-glo′bar)   endoglobular.

endoglobular (en″do-glob′u-lar)   situated or occurring within the blood corpuscles.

endognathion (en″do-na′the-on) [*endo-* + Gr. *gnathos* jaw]   the inner segment of the incisive bone.

endogonidium (en″do-go-nid′e-um)   a gonidium developed within a cell, especially in the algal component of a lichen.

endoherniorrhaphy (en″do-her″ne-or′ah-fe)   surgical repair of a hernia by suture of the interior of its sac.

endointoxication (en″do-in-tok″sĭ-ka′shun)   poisoning caused by an endogenous toxin.

endolabyrinthitis (en″do-lab″ĭ-rin-thi′tis)   inflammation of the membranous labyrinth.

endolaryngeal (en″do-lah-rin′je-al) [*endo-* + Gr. *larynx*]   situated on or occurring within the larynx.

endolarynx (en′do-lar″inks)   the interior or cavity of the larynx.

endolymph (en′do-limf) [*endo-* + *lymph*]   the fluid contained in the membranous labyrinth of the ear; it is entirely separate from the perilymph. Called also *endolympha* [NA], *liquor scarpae, liquor of Scarpa,* and *Scarpa's fluid.*

endolympha (en″do-lim′fah) [NA]   the endolymph.

endolymphatic (en″do-lim-fat′ik)   pertaining to the endolymph.

endolysin (en-dol′ĭ-sin) [*endo-* + *lysin*]   a bactericidal substance existing in cells, acting directly on bacteria, e.g., leukin.

endolysis (en-dol′ĭ-sis) [*endo-* + Gr. *lysis* dissolution]   dissolution or breaking up of the cytoplasm of a cell.

endomastoiditis (en″do-mas″toi-di′tis)   inflammation within the mastoid cavity and cells.

endomesoderm (en″do-mes′o-derm) [*endo-* + Gr. *mesos* middle + *derma* skin]   mesoderm originating from the entoderm of the two-layered blastodisk.

endometria (en″do-me′tre-ah) [Gr.]   plural of *endometrium.*

endometrial (en″do-me′tre-al)   pertaining to the endometrium.

endometrioid (en″do-me′tre-oid)   resembling endometrium.

endometrioma (en″do-me″tre-o′mah)   a solitary, non-neoplastic mass containing endometrial tissue.

endometriosis (en″do-me″tre-o′sis) [*endometrium* + *-osis*]   a condition in which tissue more or less perfectly resembling the uterine mucous membrane (the endometrium) and containing typical endometrial granular and stromal elements occurs aberrantly in various locations in the pelvic cavity; called also *adenomyosis externa* and *endometriosis externa.* **e. exter′na,** endometriosis.   **e. inter′na,** adenomyosis. **ovarian e., e. ova′rii,** occurrence in the ovary of tissue resembling the uterine mucous membrane, either in the form of small superficial islands or in the form of endometrial ("chocolate") cysts of various sizes; called also *adenoma endometrioides ovarii.*   **stromal e.,** adenomyosis in which all or nearly all of the tissue infiltrating the myometrium consists of stroma.   **e. uteri′na,** adenomyosis.   **e. ves′icae,** endometriosis involving the bladder.

endometriotic (en″do-me″tre-ot′ik)   pertaining to or characterized by endometriosis.

endometritis (en″do-mĕ-tri′tis) [*endometrium* + *-itis*]   inflammation of the endometrium.   **bacteriotoxic e.,** endometritis caused by the toxins of bacteria, as distinguished from that caused by the presence of the organisms themselves.   **decidual e.,** inflammation of the decidua of pregnancy.   **exfoliative e.,** endometritis with the casting off of portions of the membrane.   **glandular e.,** endometritis of the uterine glands.   **membranous e.,** endometritis with an exudate which forms a false membrane.   **puerperal e.,** endometritis following childbirth.   **syncytial e.,** a benign tumor-like lesion with infiltration of the uterine wall by large syncytial trophoblastic cells; called also *syncytioma.*   **tuberculous e.,** inflammation of the endometrium due to infection by *Mycobacterium tuberculosis,* with the presence of tubercles; usually the uterine tubes are also involved.   **e. tubero′sa papulo′sa,** a cast of the uterine cavity expelled at abortion.

endometrium (en-do-me′tre-um), pl. *endome′tria* [*endo-* + Gr. *metra* uterus]   the inner mucous membrane of the uterus, the thickness and structure of which vary with the phase of the menstrual cycle. It is functionally divisible into three layers: the stratum basale, stratum spongiosum, and stratum compactum; the latter two layers together form the *stratum functionale.* Accepted by NA as an alternative term for *tunica mucosa uteri.*   **Swiss-cheese e.,** hyperplasia of the endometrium, under the influence of progesterone, in which the glands vary in size and shape, producing an appearance like that of Swiss cheese, with its large and small holes.

endometry (en-dom′ĕ-tre) [*endo-* + Gr. *metron* measure] the measurement of the capacity of a cavity.

endomitosis (en″do-mi-to′sis) reproduction of nuclear elements not followed by chromosome movements and cytoplasmic division; called also *endopolyploidy.*

endomitotic (en″do-mi-tot′ik) pertaining to or characterized by endomitosis.

endomorph (en′do-morf) an individual having a body build in which tissues derived from the endoderm predominate: there is relative preponderance of soft roundness throughout the body, with large digestive viscera and accumulations of fat, and with large trunk and thighs and tapering extremities, as contrasted with ectomorph and mesomorph (def. 1).

endomorphic (en″do-mor′fik) pertaining to or characteristic of an endomorph.

endomorphy (en′do-mor″fe) [*endoderm* + Gr. *morphē* form] the condition of being an endomorph.

Endomyces (en″do-mi′sēz) [*endo-* + Gr. *mykēs* fungus] a genus of ascomycetous fungi of the order Endomycetales, which includes a number of yeasts from soil, nectar, and decaying fruit. **E. al′bicans,** former name for *Candida albicans.* **E. capsula′tus, E. epidermat′idis, E. epider′midis,** former name for *Blastomyces dermatitidis.*

Endomycetales (en″do-mi″sĕ-ta′lēz) an order of mostly saprophytic ascomycetous fungi of the subclass Hemiascomycetidae in which the zygote results from fusion of two cells and immediately forms an ascus; it includes the family Saccharomycetaceae.

endomyocarditis (en″do-mi″o-kar-di′tis) [*endo-* + Gr. *mys* muscle + *kardia* heart] inflammation of the endocardium and myocardium.

endomysium (en″do-mis′e-um) [*endo-* + Gr. *mys* muscle] the sheath of delicate reticular fibrils which surrounds each muscle fiber.

endonasal (en″do-na′zal) within the nose.

endoneural (en″do-nu′ral) pertaining to or situated within a nerve.

endoneurial (en″do-nu′re-al) pertaining to the endoneurium.

endoneuritis (en″do-nu-ri′tis) inflammation of the endoneurium.

endoneurium (en″do-nu′re-um) [*endo-* + Gr. *neuron* nerve] [NA] the interstitial connective tissue in a peripheral nerve, separating the individual nerve fibers; called also *epilemma.*

endoneurolysis (en″do-nu-rol′ĭ-sis) [*endo-* + Gr. *neuron* nerve + *lysis* dissolution] hersage.

endonuclear (en″do-nu′kle-ar) within a cell nucleus.

endonuclease (en″do-nu′kle-ās) [EC 3.1.21–31] any of the enzymes of the hydrolase class that catalyze the hydrolysis of interior bonds of ribonucleotide or deoxyribonucleotide chains, producing poly- or oligonucleotides. Cf. *exonuclease.* **restriction e.,** an endonuclease that hydrolyzes any deoxyribonucleic acid molecule not having the specific base pattern peculiar to the cell producing the endonuclease, thus destroying foreign deoxyribonucleic acid. Cleavage is highly specific for an individual site in a specific sequence. Restriction endonucleases isolated from bacterial sources have been used extensively for sequencing of deoxyribonucleic acid and recombinant technology.

endonucleolus (en″do-nu-kle′o-lus) a nonstaining spot near the center of the nucleolus of a cell.

endoparasite (en″do-par′ah-sīt) [*endo-* + *parasite*] a parasite that lives within the body of its host.

endopelvic (en″do-pel′vik) within the pelvis.

endopeptidase (en″do-pep′tĭ-dās) [EC 3.4.21–24] any of several sub-subclasses of enzymes of the hydrolase class that catalyze the hydrolysis of peptide bonds in the interior of the peptide chain. Called also *protease.*

endoperiarteritis (en″do-per″ĭ-ar″ter-i′tis) (*obs.*) inflammation involving both the internal and the external coat of an artery.

endopericardial (en″do-per″ĭ-kar′de-al) pertaining to the endocardium and pericardium.

endopericarditis (en″do-per″ĭ-kar-di′tis) inflammation involving both the endocardium and pericardium.

endoperimyocarditis (en″do-per″ĭ-mi″o-kar-di′tis) inflammation of the endocardium, pericardium, and myocardium.

endoperineuritis (en″do-per″ĭ-nu-ri′tis) inflammation of the endoneurium and perineurium.

endoperitoneal (en″do-per″ĭ-to-ne′al) within the peritoneum.

endoperitonitis (en″do-per″ĭ-to-ni′tis) inflammation of the serous lining of the peritoneal cavity.

endophlebitis (en″do-fle-bi′tis) [*endo-* + Gr. *phleps* vein + *-itis*] inflammation of the intima of a vein. **e. hepat′ica oblit′erans,** Budd-Chiari syndrome. **proliferative e.,** phlebosclerosis.

endophthalmitis (en″dof-thal-mi′tis) [*end-* + *ophthalmitis*] inflammation involving the ocular cavities and their adjacent structures; called also *entophthalmia.* **phacoanaphylactic e.,** phacoantigenic uveitis.

endophylaxination (en″do-fi-lak″si-na′shun) resistance to infection developed entirely within the body of the animal possessing it.

endophyte (en′do-fīt) [*endo-* + Gr. *phyton* plant] a parasitic plant organism living within the body of its host.

endophytic (en″do-fit′ik) [*endo-* + Gr. *phyein* to grow] 1. pertaining to an endophyte. 2. growing inward; proliferating on the interior or inside of an organ or other structure, as a tumor.

endoplasm (en′do-plazm) [*endo-* + Gr. *plasma* something formed] the central portion of the cytoplasm of a cell. Cf. *ectoplasm.*

endoplasmic (en″do-plas′mik) composed of or pertaining to endoplasm; see under *reticulum.*

endoplast (en′do-plast) [*endo-* + Gr. *plassein* to form] the nucleus of a cell; see *nucleus,* def. 1.

endoplastic (en″do-plas′tik) entoplastic.

endopolyploid (en″do-pol′e-ploid) having reduplicated chromatin within an intact nucleus, with or without an increase in the number of chromosomes (applied only to cells and tissues); see also *endomitosis.*

endopolyploidy (en″do-pol′e-ploi″de) [*endo-* + *polyploidy*] 1. endomitosis. 2. polysomaty. 3. autopolyploidy resulting from a previous endomitotic cycle. See also *polysomaty.*

endopredator (en″do-pred′ah-tor) an individual or species that lives within the body of an organism of another species which it feeds upon and destroys.

endoradiography (en″do-ra″de-og′rah-fe) the radiographic demonstration of the condition of internal organs and cavities by means of radiopaque materials.

endoradiosonde (en″do-ra″de-o-sond′) a small radio transmitter inserted within a body cavity or tube, as within the intestinal lumen to measure the pressure.

endoreduplication (en″do-re-du″plĭ-ka′shun) replication of the chromosomes without subsequent cell division.

end-organ (end′or-gan) one of the larger, encapsulated endings of the sensory nerves; for names of specific types, see under *corpuscle.*

endorhinitis (en″do-ri-ni′tis) [*endo-* + Gr. *rhis* nose] inflammation of the lining membrane of the nasal passages.

endoribonuclease (en″do-ri″bo-nu′kle-as) [EC 3.1.26–27] one of two sub-subclasses of enzymes of the hydrolase class that catalyze the hydrolysis of interior bonds of ribonucleotides, producing oligonucleotides or polynucleotides.

endorphin (en-dor′fin, en′dor-fin) [*endo*genous + *morphine*] any of three neuropeptides: β-endorphin, the C-terminal 30 amino acid residues of β-lipotropin, and α- and γ-endorphin, the N-terminal 16 and 17 residues, respectively, of β-endorphin, all of which bind to opioid receptors in the brain and have potent analgesic activity; β-endorphin is found in the adenohypophysis, hypothalamus, and other sites in the brain; one function appears to be mediation of pain perception.

endosalpingitis (en″do-sal″pin-ji′tis) [*endosalpinx* + *-itis*] inflammation of the endosalpinx.

endosalpingoma (en″do-sal″pin-go′mah) adenomyoma of the uterine tube.

endosalpingosis (en″do-sal″pin-go′sis) 1. endometriosis of the uterine tube. 2. ovarian endometriosis in which the abnormal mucosa resembles tubal mucosa rather than endometrial mucosa.

endosalpinx (en″do-sal′pinks) [endo- + Gr. *salpinx* tube] the mucous membrane lining the uterine tube, arranged in longitudinal rugae, or folds, and continuous with the mucous lining of the uterus (tunica mucosa tubae uterinae [NA]).

endosarc (en′do-sark) endoplasm.

endoscope (en′do-skōp) [endo- + Gr. *skopein* to examine] an instrument for the examination of the interior of a hollow viscus, such as the bladder.

endoscopic (en″do-skop′ik) performed by means of an endoscope; pertaining to endoscopy.

endoscopy (en-dos′ko-pe) visual inspection of any cavity of the body by means of an endoscope. **peroral e.,** examination of organs accessible to observation through an endoscope passed through the mouth. **transcolonic e.,** examination of the lumen of the colon by means of an endoscope inserted through an incision in its wall.

endosecretory (en-do-se′kre-to-re) [endo- + secretory] pertaining to the internal secretions; secreting internally; endocrine.

endosepsis (en″do-sep′sis) septicemia originating within the organism.

endosite (en′do-sīt) (obs.) an endoparasite.

endoskeleton (en″do-skel′ĕ-ton) [endo- + Gr. *skeleton*] the bony and cartilaginous skeleton of the body, exclusive of that part of the skeleton which is of dermal origin; called also *neuroskeleton.*

endosmometer (en″dos-mom′ĕ-ter) [endosmosis + Gr. *metron* measure] an instrument for determining the rate and extent of endosmosis.

endosmosis (en″dos-mo′sis) [endo- + Gr. *ōsmos* impulsion] a movement in liquids separated by a membranous or porous septum, by which one fluid passes through the septum into the cavity which contains another fluid of a different density. Cf. *exosmosis.*

endosmotic (en″dos-mot′ik) of the nature of endosmosis.

endosome (en′do-sōm) [endo- + Gr. *soma* body] a nucleolus-like, intranuclear, RNA-containing organelle of certain flagellate protozoa that persists during mitosis.

endosperm (en′do-sperm) a substance containing reserve food materials, formed within the embryo sac of plants.

endospore (en′do-spōr) [endo- + Gr. *sporos* seed] 1. a thick-walled body formed within the vegetative cells of certain bacteria (e.g., *Bacillus, Clostridium, Sarcina*) that is able to withstand adverse environmental conditions for prolonged periods; under favorable conditions it will germinate to form a vegetative bacterium. See also *spore.* 2. a fungal spore produced within the hyphae or cell, as in a spherule of *Coccidioides immitis.*

endosporium (en″do-spōr′e-um) the inner layer of the envelope of a spore.

endosteal (en-dos′te-al) pertaining to the endosteum; occurring or located within a bone.

endosteitis (en-dos″te-i′tis) inflammation of the endosteum.

endosteoma (en-dos″te-o′mah) [endo- + Gr. *osteon* bone + -oma] a tumor in the medullary cavity of a bone.

endostethoscope (en″do-steth′o-skōp) a stethoscope passed into the esophagus for auscultating the heart.

endosteum (en-dos′te-um) [endo- + Gr. *osteon* bone] [NA] the tissue lining the medullary cavity of a bone.

endostitis (en″dos-ti′tis) endosteitis.

endostoma (en″dos-to′mah) endosteoma.

endosymbiont (en″do-sim′be-ont) [endo- + symbiont] a symbiont which lives within the cells of its partner.

endosymbiosis (en″do-sim″bi-o′sis) the state achieved between a virus and its host cell in which cellular division is inhibited but the cell is not immediately destroyed.

endotendineum (en″do-ten-din′e-um) [endo- + L. *tendo, tendines,* after Gr. *tenōn*] the delicate connective tissue separating the secondary bundles (fascicles) of a tendon.

endotenon (en″do-ten′on) [endo- + Gr. *tenōn* tendon] endotendineum.

endothelia (en″do-the′le-ah) [Gr.] plural of *endothelium.*

endothelial (en″do-the′le-al) pertaining to or made up of endothelium.

endothelialization (en″do-the″le-al-ĭ-za′shun) the healing of the inner surfaces of vessels or grafts by endothelial cells.

endotheliitis (en″do-the-le-i′tis) inflammation of the endothelium.

endothelioblastoma (en″do-the″le-o-blas-to′mah) [endothelium + Gr. *blastos* germ + -oma] a tumor derived from primitive vasoformative tissue with formation of usually small and slitlike vascular spaces lined by prominent endothelial cells; the term, which now includes hemangioendothelioma, angiosarcoma, lymphangioendothelioma, and lymphangiosarcoma, was applied formerly to such tumors arising from mesothelial tissue as well.

endotheliochorial (en″do-the″le-o-ko′re-al) [endothelium + chorion] denoting a type of placenta in which syncytial trophoblast embeds maternal vessels bared to their endothelial lining.

endotheliocyte (en″do-the′le-o-sīt″) [endothelia + Gr. *kytos* hollow vessel] a term formerly applied to certain macrophages and monocytes reflecting the erroneous theory that they were derived from vascular endothelium.

endotheliocytosis (en-do-the″le-o-si-to′sis) an abnormal increase in the number of endotheliocytes.

endothelioid (en″do-the′le-oid) resembling endothelium.

endotheliolysin (en″do-the″le-ol′ĭ-sin) a cytolysin capable of lysing epithelial cells.

endotheliolytic (en″do-the″le-o-lit′ik) capable of destroying endothelial tissue.

endothelioma (en″do-the″le-o′mah) [endothelium + -oma] a tumor which originates from the endothelial linings of blood vessels (*hemangioendothelioma*), lymphatics (*lymphangioendothelioma*), or serous cavities (*mesothelioma*). **e. angiomato′sum,** angioma. **e. cap′itis,** a large multiple hemangioma on the scalp. **e. cu′tis,** endothelioma of the skin, manifested as violaceous papules. **diffuse e.,** Ewing sarcoma. **dural e.,** meningioma. **perithelial e.,** hemangiopericytoma.

endotheliomatosis (en″do-the″le-o-mah-to′sis) the formation of multiple and diffuse endotheliomas in a tissue.

endotheliomyoma (en″do-the″le-o-mi-o′mah) (obs.) a vascular leiomyoma.

endotheliosarcoma (en″do-the″le-o-sar-ko′mah) Kaposi's sarcoma.

endotheliosis (en″do-the″le-o′sis) proliferation of endothelium.

endotheliotoxin (en″do-the″le-o-tok′sin) a specific toxin which acts on the endothelium of capillaries and small veins, producing hemorrhage. Cf. *hemorrhagin.*

endothelium (en″do-the′le-um), pl. *endothe′lia* [endo- + Gr. *thēlē* nipple] [NA] the layer of epithelial cells that lines the cavities of the heart and of the blood and lymph vessels, and the serous cavities of the body, originating from the mesoderm. **e. ca′merae anterio′ris bul′bi,** epithelium posterius corneae. **corneal e., e. cornea′le,** epithelium posterius corneae. **extraembryonic e.,** endothelium which arises outside of the body of the embryo, such as that lining the vitelline vessels.

endotherm (en′do-therm″) [endo- + Gr. *thermē* heat] 1. an animal that exhibits endothermy (def. 2). 2. homeothermic.

endothermal (en″do-ther′mal) endothermic.

endothermic (en″do-ther′mik) 1. characterized by or accompanied by the absorption of heat, as a chemical reaction accompanied by absorption of heat and to which heat must be supplied if it is to proceed: storing up heat or energy in a potential form. Cf. *endoergic* and *exothermic.* 2. pertaining to or characterized by endothermy (def. 2). 3. homeothermic.

endothermy (en′do-ther″me) [endo- + Gr. *thermē* heat] 1. diathermy. 2. thermoregulation accomplished by internal heat production. Cf. *ectothermy* (def. 1). 3. homeothermy.

endothoracic (en″do-tho-ras′ik) within the thorax; situated internal to the ribs.

endothrix (en′do-thriks) [endo- + Gr. *thrix* hair] a dermatophyte whose growth and spore production are confined chiefly within the shaft of the hair, without formation of conspicuous external spores; such fungi include *Trichophyton tonsurans* and *T. violaceum.*

endotoxemia (en″do-toks-e′me-ah) the presence of endotoxins in the blood, which may result in shock.

endotoxicosis (en″do-tok″sĭ-ko′sis) (obs.) poisoning caused by an endotoxin.

endotoxin (en″do-tok′sin) [endo- + L. toxicum poison] a heat-stable toxin associated with the outer membranes of certain gram-negative bacteria, including the brucellae, the enterobacteria, neisseriae, and vibrios. Endotoxins are not secreted and are released only when the cells are disrupted. They are less potent and less specific than the exotoxins, and do not form toxoids. They are composed of complex lipopolysaccharide molecules. The polysaccharide unit (somatic O antigen) is responsible for antigenicity, occurring in hundreds of variations; the phospholipid moiety (lipid A) is the source of toxicity. When injected in large quantities the endotoxins produce hemorrhagic shock and severe diarrhea; smaller amounts cause fever, altered resistance to bacterial infection, leukopenia followed by leukocytosis, and numerous other biologic effects. Called also bacterial pyrogen. See also toxin.

endotracheal (en″do-tra′ke-al) [endo- + trachea] 1. within or through the trachea. 2. performed by passage through the lumen of the trachea.

endotracheitis (en″do-tra-ke-i′tis) inflammation of the mucosa of the trachea.

endotrachelitis (en″do-tra-kel-i′tis) [endo- + Gr. trachēlos neck] endocervicitis.

endourethral (en″do-u-re′thral) within the urethra.

endouterine (en″do-u′ter-in) within the uterus.

endovaccination (en″do-vak″sĭ-na′shun) [endo- + vaccination] the administration of vaccines by the mouth.

endovasculitis (en″do-vas″ku-li′tis) [endo- + L. vasculum vessel] endangiitis.

endovenitis (en″do-ve-ni′tis) endophlebitis.

endovenous (en″do-ve′nus) intravenous.

Endoxan (en-dok′san) trademark for a preparation of cyclophosphamide.

endozoite (en″do-zo′ĭt) tachyzoite.

end plate, end-plate (end plāt) a flat termination. **motor e.p.,** the discoid expansion of a terminal branch of the axon of a motor nerve fiber, which apposes the sole plate of a skeletal muscle fiber forming the neuromuscular junction (q.v.).

end-pleasure (end′plezh-er) the pleasure produced by the sexual orgasm, as contrasted with the fore-pleasure which precedes it.

end point (end′ point) in titration, the highest dilution of a substance that produces a reaction with a given volume of another substance.

end product (end prod′ukt) the chemical compound resulting from the completion of a sequence of metabolic reactions.

Endrate (en′drāt) trademark for preparations of edetate disodium.

endrin (en′drin) chemical name: 1,2,3,4,10,10-hexachloro-6,7-epoxy-1,4,4a,5,6,7,8,8a-octahydro-1,4,5,8-endo-endo-dimethanonaphthalene; a highly toxic insecticide of the chlorinated hydrocarbon group.

endrysone (en′drĭ-sōn) chemical name: 11β-hydroxy-6α-methylpregna-1,4-diene-3,20-dione; a topical anti-inflammatory for use in ophthalmology, $C_{22}H_{30}O_3$.

Enduron (en′du-ron) trademark for a preparation of methyclothiazide.

Enduronyl (en-dūr′o-nil) trademark for preparations of methyclothiazide with reserpine.

endyma (en′dĭ-mah) ependyma.

-ene a suffix used in chemistry to indicate an unsaturated hydrocarbon containing one double bond.

enema (en′ĕ-mah), pl. enemas or enem′ata [Gr.] a clyster or injection; a liquid injected or to be injected into the rectum. **analeptic e.,** an enema consisting of a pint of tepid water containing ¼ teaspoonful of salt; called also thirst e. **barium e.,** a suspension of barium administered as a clyster and retained in the intestines during roentgenologic examination, the presence of deformities of the intestine, produced by neoplasm or other abnormality, being demonstrated by filling defects revealed by the column of radiopaque barium. Called also contrast e. **blind e.,** the insertion of a soft-rubber tube into the rectum to aid in the expulsion of flatus. **contrast e.,** barium e. **double contrast e.,** injection and evacuation of a suspension of barium, followed by inflation of the intestines with air under light pressure; used in mucosal relief roentgenography. **flatus e.,** an enema made of ½ oz. of magnesium sulfate, 1 oz. of glycerin, and 4 oz. of warm water. **Fleet e.,** trademark for an enema containing, in each 100 ml., 16 gm. sodium biphosphate and 6 gm. sodium phosphate, packaged in a plastic squeeze bottle fitted with a 2-inch, prelubricated rectal tube. **hydrocortisone e.** [USP], a suspension containing 100 mg. of hydroxycortisone per 60 ml.; used in the treatment of various conditions responsive to the anti-inflammatory action of glucocorticoids. **nutrient e., nutritive e.,** an enema of predigested nutrient matter. **pancreatic e.,** an enema containing pancreatin. **small bowel e.,** enteroclysis, def. 2. **soapsuds e.,** an enema made by dissolving 2 oz. of soap in a pint of warm water. **sodium phosphate and biphosphate e., sodium phosphate e.** [USP], a solution of sodium phosphate and sodium biphosphate, or sodium phosphate and phosphoric acid in purified water, containing in each 100 ml., 5.7 to 6.3 gm. of sodium phosphate and 15.2 to 16.8 gm. of sodium biphosphate; used as a cathartic. **theophylline olamine e.** [USP], an enema containing an amount of anhydrous theophylline equivalent to 72 to 78 per cent of the labeled amount of theophylline olamine and an amount of monethanolamine equivalent to 22 to 28 per cent of the labeled amount of theophylline olamine. **thirst e.,** analeptic enema. **turpentine e.,** an enema of 1 pint of soapsuds containing 2 oz. olive oil and 1 oz. turpentine.

enemator (en′ĕ-ma″tor) an apparatus for giving enemas.

energetics (en″er-jet′iks) the study of energy; the science of energy.

energid (en′er-jid) living, active protoplasm, as distinguished from deuteroplasm.

energizer (en′er-jīz″er) that which gives energy to, activates, or charges. **psychic e.,** (colloq.) any drug that produces mood elevation, such as a sympathomimetic amine or an antidepressant.

energometer (en″er-gom′ĕ-ter) an apparatus for studying the pulse.

energy (en′er-je) [Gr. energeia] the capacity to operate or work; power to produce motion, to overcome resistance, and to effect physical changes. **activation e.,** in a chemical reaction, the energy that must be supplied to the reactants in order to form an activated complex or transition state, which then breaks down to form the products. **atomic e.,** energy that can be liberated by changes in the nucleus of an atom (as by fission of a heavy nucleus or fusion of light nuclei into heavier ones with accompanying loss of mass). **binding e.,** energy equal to the difference between the weight of the nucleus of an atom and the sum of the weights of its constituent particles. **chemical e.,** energy which shows itself in chemical transformations. **free e., Gibbs free e.** (G), the thermodynamic function $G=H-TS$, where H is enthalpy, T absolute temperature, and S entropy. For chemical reactions occurring at a constant temperature, the free energy change $\Delta G=\Delta H - T\Delta S$ determines the direction in which a reaction proceeds; ΔG is negative for a spontaneous (exergonic) reaction; ΔG is positive for a nonspontaneous (endergonic) reaction. The free energy change can be determined from the equation $\Delta G=\Delta G^\circ + RT \ln Q$, where R is the gas constant, Q is the reaction quotient (q.v.), and ΔG° is the standard free energy change (the free energy change when all products and reactants are in their standard states; solids and liquids are pure substances; gases are at 1 atm pressure; the temperature is specified, usually 0° C or 25° C; and all solutions have a concentration of 1M). ΔG° is by adding the tabulated values for the products and subtracting the tabulated values for the reactants. For a reaction at equilibrium, $\Delta G=0$; thus $\Delta G^\circ=-RT \ln K$, where K is the equilibrium constant. **free e.,** the energy equal to the maximum amount of work that can be obtained from a process occurring under conditions of fixed temperature and pressure. **kinetic e.,** energy of motion; equal to one-half the mass of a body times the square of its velocity. **nuclear e.,** atomic e. **potential e.,** the energy that a body has due to its position, equal to the work required to move the body to that position from some reference position; e.g., a body has a gravitational potential energy equal to its mass times the acceleration due to gravity times its height above the reference position. **radiant e.,** the energy of electromagnetic waves, such as radio waves, visible light, x-rays, and gamma rays.

enervation (en″er-va′shun) [L. *enervatio*] 1. lack of nervous energy; languor. 2. removal of a nerve or a section of a nerve.

enflagellation (en″flaj-el-la′shun) the formation of flagella.

enflurane (en′floo-rān) [USP] chemical name: 2-chloro-1,1,2-trifluroethyl difluromethyl ether, a potent inhalational anesthetic agent, widely used for induction and maintenance of general anesthesia; it is nonflammable, induction and recovery are smooth and rapid, and the depth of anesthesia is rapidly altered; the incidence of arrhythmias and postoperative nausea and vomiting are somewhat less than with halothane or methoxyflurane.

ENG electronystagmography.

engagement (en-gāj′ment) in obstetrics, the entrance of the fetal head, or presenting part, into the superior pelvic strait and beginning descent through the pelvic canal.

engastrius (en-gas′tre-us) [Gr. *en* in + *gastēr* belly] a monster in which a parasitic twin is contained within the abdomen of the autosite.

Engel's alkalimetry (eng′elz) [Rodolphe Charles *Engel,* Alsatian chemist, 1850–1916] see under *alkalimetry.*

Engelmann's disease (eng′el-mahnz) [Guido *Engelmann,* German surgeon, born 1876] diaphyseal dysplasia.

Engelmann's disk (eng′el-mahnz) [Theodor Wilhelm *Engelmann,* a German physiologist, 1843–1909] H band; see under *band.*

engine (en′jin) a machine by which energy is converted into mechanical motion. **dental e.,** a machine operated by electricity, water, or compressed air that provides power for rotary dental instruments.

englobe (en-glōb′) phagocytize; to absorb within the substance of a globe.

Engman's disease (eng′manz) [Martin Feeney *Engman,* American dermatologist in St. Louis, 1869–1953] dermatitis infectiosa eczematoides.

engorged (en-gorjd′) distended or swollen with fluids.

engorgement (en-gorj′ment) hyperemia; local congestion; excessive fullness of any organ, vessel, or tissue due to accumulation of fluids, especially that due to accumulation of blood.

engram (en′gram) [Gr. *en* in + *gramma* mark] a lasting mark or trace. The term is applied to the definite and permanent trace left by a stimulus in nerve tissue. See *engraphia.* In psychology it is the lasting trace left in the psyche by anything that has been experienced psychically; a latent memory picture.

engraphia (en-graf′e-ah) the process hypothesized in the theory that stimuli leave definite traces (engrams) on the protoplasm which, when regularly repeated, induce a habit that persists after the stimuli cease.

enhancement (en-hans′ment) immunologic enhancement; prolonged survival of tumor cells in animals previously immunized with antigens of the tumor owing to the presence of "enhancing" or "facilitating" antibodies that prevent an immune response against these antigens.

enhexymal (en-hek′sĭ-mal) hexobarbital.

Enhydrina (en″hi-dri′nah) a genus of sea snakes. **E. schisto′sa,** a venomous sea snake commonly found in Indo-Pacific waters.

enkatarrhaphy (en″kah-tar′ah-fe) encatarrhaphy.

enkephalin (en-kef′ah-lin) either of two simple pentapeptides having the formula H_2N-Tyr-Gly-Gly-Phe-X, where X is leucine or methionine, referred to as leu-enkephalin and met-enkephalin. Although met-enkephalin is the N-terminal 5 residues of the endorphins and both enkephalins and endorphins bind to opioid receptors, the two groups derive from functionally and anatomically distinct groups of neurons. The enkephalins function as neurotransmitters or neuromodulators at many locations in the brain and spinal cord and play a part in pain perception, movement, mood, behavior, and neuroendocrine regulation; they are also found in nerve plexuses and exocrine glands of the gastrointestinal tract.

enkephalinergic (en-kef″ah-lin-er′jik) denoting synaptic transmission by enkephalin neurotransmitters.

enlargement (en-larj′ment) 1. an increase in the size of an organ or part; see *hypertrophy* and *hyperplasia.* 2. in anatomy, a prominence or swelling; an intumescence. **cardiac e.,** dilatation or hypertrophy of the heart, due to compensatory mechanisms or secondary to disease. **cervical e.,** intumescentia cervicalis. **gingival e.,** hyperplastic enlargement of the gingival tissue. It may occur as a result of inflammatory or fibrous lesions resulting from irritation or injury brought about by mechanical or chemical factors or systemic or localized pathologic processes. See also *fibromatosis gingivae* and *gingival hyperplasia.* **e. of heart,** cardiac e. **lumbar e., lumbosacral e.,** intumescentia lumbosacralis. **tympanic e.,** intumescentia tympanica.

enniatin (en-e-a′tin) a cyclic polypeptide antibiotic with a ring of 18 atoms, produced by a fungus of the genus *Fusarium.* It is active against certain gram-positive bacteria, functioning as an ionophore and altering membrane permeability.

enol (e′nol) a compound with a hydroxy group attached to a double-bonded carbon. See *enol-keto tautomerism* under *tautomerism.*

R.CH   R.CH₂
‖ |
R.C.OH   R.C:O
Enol form   Keto form

enolase (e′no-lās) [EC 4.2.1.11] an enzyme of the lyase class that catalyzes the reaction 2-phospho-D-glycerate = phosphoenolpyruvate + H_2O, a part of the Embden-Meyerhof pathway of glucose metabolism.

enology (e-nol′o-je) [Gr. *oinos* wine + *-logy*] the scientific study of the production and composition of wine.

enophthalmos (en-of-thal′mos) [Gr. *en* in + *ophthalmos* eye] a backward displacement of the eyeball into the orbit.

enophthalmus (en″of-thal′mus) enophthalmos.

enorganic (en-or-gan′ik) existing as a permanent quality of the organism.

enostosis (en″os-to′sis) [Gr. *en* in + *osteon* bone] a morbid bony growth developed within the cavity of a bone or on the internal surface of the bone cortex.

Enovid (en-o′vid) trademark for preparations of mestranol and norethynodrel.

enoxidase (e-nok′sĭ-dās) [Gr. *oinos* wine + *oxidase*] an oxidizing ferment found in spoiled wines.

en plaque (ahn-plak′) [Fr.] in the form of a plaque or plate.

enpromate (en′pro-māt) chemical name: 1,1-diphenyl-2-propynyl cyclohexanecarbamate; an antineoplastic agent, $C_{22}H_{23}NO_2$.

enrichment (en-rich′ment) the addition of nutrients, as to culture media; the medium resulting from such addition.

ens (enz) [L. "being"] an abstract or existent being. **e. mor′bi,** the nature or essential principle of a disease considered apart from its causation; the pathology of a disease as distinguished from its etiology.

ensiform (en′sĭ-form) [L. *ensis* sword + *forma* form] shaped like a sword; xiphoid.

ensisternum (en″sis-ter′num) [L. *ensis* sword + *sternum*] xiphoid process (processus xiphoideus [NA]).

ensomphalus (en-som′fah-lus) [Gr. *en* in + *sōma* a body + *omphalos* navel] a double monster with blended bodies, two separate navels, and two umbilical cords.

enstrophe (en′stro-fe) entropion.

E.N.T. ear, nose, and throat.

entad (en′tad) toward the center; inwardly.

ental (en′tal) [Gr. *entos* within] inner; central.

entamebiasis (en″tah-me-bi′ah-sis) infection with *Entamoeba.*

Entamoeba (en″tah-me′bah) [*ent-* + *ameba*] a genus of naked ameboid protozoa (suborder Tubulina, order Amoebida) parasitic in invertebrates and vertebrates, including humans, and characterized by the presence of a vesicular nucleus with a comparatively small central karyosome with a number of peripheral chromatin granules attached to the nuclear membrane. **E. bucca′lis,** *E. gingivalis.* **E.**

co′li, a very common nonpathogenic species found in the human intestinal tract. **E. gingiva′lis,** a species often found in the mouth of humans with periodontal disease; it has not been shown to be pathogenic. Called also *E. buccalis.* **E. hartman′ni,** a nonpathogenic species found in the human intestinal tract that is almost indistinguishable from but smaller than *E. histolytica;* it was formerly designated "small race" *E. histolytica.* **E. histolyt′ica,** the only species of parasitic protozoa with the potential for producing human amebiasis, transmitted through ingestion of cysts in contaminated food and water. Trophozoites may invade the tissue of the large intestine and may be spread to extraintestinal sites such as the liver, spleen, brain, lungs, and pericardium. **E. inva′dens,** the only pathogenic species of the genus *Entamoeba* other than *E. histolytica,* producing lesions of the stomach, colon, duodenum, ileum, colon, and liver in reptiles. **E. polec′ki,** an intestinal parasite of hogs, sheep, monkeys, and cattle; it has rarely been found in man.

entasia (en-ta′ze-ah) [Gr. *entasis*] a constrictive spasm; spasmodic muscular action.

entasis (en′tah-sis) entasia.

entelechy (en-tel′ĕ-ke) [Gr. *entelecheia* actuality] 1. completion; full development or realization; the complete expression of some function. 2. a supposed vital principle operating in living creatures as a directive spirit.

entepicondyle (en-tep″ĭ-kon′dīl) the internal epicondyle of the humerus.

enteque (en-ta′ka) chronic hemorrhagic septicemia of unknown etiology affecting chiefly cattle and sometimes horses and sheep in the Argentine. It occurs in two forms: the *intestinal* form, marked by wasting, diarrhea, and death within three to four months, and a *wasting* form, (*e. seca*), marked by progressive emaciation, anemia, inflammation of the joints, and calcification of the lungs.

enteraden (en-ter′ad-en) [*enter-* + Gr. *adēn* gland] any intestinal gland.

enteradenitis (en″ter-ad″ĕ-ni′tis) [*enteraden* + *-itis*] inflammation of the intestinal glands.

enteral (en′ter-al) [Gr. *enteron* intestine] within, by way of, or pertaining to the small intestine.

enteralgia (en″ter-al′je-ah) [*enter-* + *-algia*] pain or neuralgia of the intestine.

enteramine (en″ter-am′in) serotonin.

enterauxe (en″ter-awk′se) [*enter-* + Gr. *auxē* increase] (*obs.*) hypertrophy of the intestinal wall.

enterectasis (en″ter-ek′tah-sis) [*enter-* + Gr. *ektasis* extension] distention of the intestines.

enterectomy (en″ter-ek′to-me) [*enter-* + Gr. *ektomē* excision] excision of a part of the intestine; resection of the intestine.

enterepiplocele (en″ter-e-pip′lo-sēl) enteroepiplocele.

enteric (en-ter′ik) [Gr. *enterikos* intestinal] pertaining to the small intestine.

enteric-coated (en-ter″ik-kōt′ed) a term designating a special coating applied to tablets or capsules which prevents release and absorption of their contents until they reach the intestines.

entericoid (en-ter′ĭ-koid) resembling enteric or typhoid fever.

enteritis (en″ter-i′tis) [*enter-* + *-itis*] inflammation of the intestine, applied chiefly to inflammation of the small intestine; see also *enterocolitis.* **cat e.,** panleukopenia. **choleriform e.,** an acute, cholera-like diarrheal disease with a high case fatality rate, prevalent in epidemic and endemic form in the Western Pacific area since 1938, caused by the El Tor or Celebes vibrio, immunologically identical with the cholera vibrio. **chronic cicatrizing e.,** Crohn's disease. **e. cys′tica chron′ica,** a form marked by cystic dilatation of the intestinal glands, due to closure of the openings of their ducts. **diphtheritic e.,** enteritis characterized by the presence of a false membrane and severe ulceration of the mucosa beneath the membrane. **duck virus e.,** duck plague. **feline e.,** panleukopenia. **e. gra′vis,** an often fatal disease characterized by acute onset of severe abdominal pain, nausea, vomiting, and bloody diarrhea, with mucosal necrosis and hemorrhage and edema of the submucosa, most prominent in the jejunum and proximal ileum. **infectious feline e.,** panleukopenia. **mink viral e.,** a highly contagious viral disease of mink resembling feline panleukopenia and caused by a similar, but

not identical, virus. **mucous e.,** former term for irritable bowel syndrome. **e. necrot′icans,** an inflammation of the intestines in man, caused by *Clostridium perfringens* type F, and characterized by necrosis. **e. nodula′ris,** enteritis with enlargement of the lymph nodes. **phlegmonous e.,** a condition with symptoms resembling those of peritonitis; it may be secondary to other intestinal diseases, as chronic obstruction, strangulated hernia, carcinoma, etc. **e. polypo′sa,** enteritis marked by polypoid growths in the intestine, due to proliferation of the connective tissue. **protozoan e.,** enteritis in which the intestine is infested with protozoan organisms of various species. **pseudomembranous e.,** pseudomembranous enterocolitis. **regional e., segmental e.,** Crohn's disease. **specific feline e.,** panleukopenia. **streptococcus e.,** primary phlegmonous enteritis, due to *Streptococcus pyogenes.* **terminal e.,** Crohn's disease. **tuberculous e.,** enteritis secondary to advanced pulmonary tuberculosis, believed to be caused by the swallowing of large amounts of positive sputum; now rare due to antibiotic tuberculosis therapy.

enter(o)- [Gr. *enteron* intestine] a combining form denoting relationship to the intestines.

enteroanastomosis (en″ter-o-ah-nas″to-mo′sis) the surgical formation of an anastomosis between two portions of the intestine.

enteroanthelone (en″ter-o-ant-he′lōn) enterogastrone.

Enterobacter (en″ter-o-bak′ter) [*entero-* + Gr. *baktron* a rod] a genus of gram-negative, facultatively anaerobic rod-shaped bacteria of the family Enterobacteriaceae, made up of motile, peritrichously flagellated cells, some being encapsulated. The organisms, widely distributed in nature, occur in the intestinal tract of humans and animals. They are frequently a cause of nosocomial infections, arising from contaminated medical devices and personnel. **E. aerog′enes,** a species isolated from feces, sewage, soil, and dairy products. Called also *Aerobacter aerogenes* and *Bacterium aerogenes.* **E. agglo′merans,** a species found on plants, in water, and in the human intestinal tract. It is a potential pathogen, causing a variety of infections, including those of nosocomial origin. Called also *Erwinia herbicola.* **E. amni′genus,** a species found in natural waters but not identified as a pathogen of humans. **E. cloa′cae,** the most commonly occurring species, found in feces, soil, and water and, less commonly, in urine, pus, and pathological material. Called also *Aerobacter cloacae* and *Bacterium cloacae.* **E. gergo′viae,** a species that is lysine decarboxylase positive, a cause of human urinary, pulmonary, and bloodstream infections. **E. haf′nia,** *Hafnia alvei.* **E. interme′dium,** a species isolated from natural sources, but not found in human clinical specimens. **E. sakaza′kii,** a species that produces a yellow pigment at 25°C, found in environment and foods, but rarely in human clinical specimens.

Enterobacteriaceae (en″ter-o-bak-te″re-a′se-e) a family of gram-negative, facultatively anaerobic, rod-shaped bacteria, usually motile with peritrichous flagella, made up of saprophytes and plant and animal parasites of worldwide distribution, found in soil, water, and plants and in animals from insects to humans. Many species are important economically, causing disease in agricultural, fish, cattle, and poultry industries. In humans, disease is produced by both invasive action and production of toxin. Species not normally associated with disease are often opportunistic pathogens. Enterobacteriaceae have been responsible for as many as half of the nosocomial infections reported annually in the United States, most frequently by species of *Escherichia, Klebsiella, Enterobacter, Proteus, Providencia,* and *Serratia.* The family includes the following genera: *Buttiauxella, Cedecea, Citrobacter, Edwardsiella, Enterobacter, Erwinia, Escherichia, Hafnia, Klebsiella, Kluyvera, Morganella, Obesumbacterium, Proteus, Providencia, Rahnella, Salmonella, Serratia, Shigella, Tatumella, Xenorhabdus,* and *Yersinia;* two additional genera are proposed: *Ewingella* and *Levinea.*

enterobiasis (en″ter-o-bi′ah-sis) infection with nematode worms of the genus *Enterobius,* especially *E. vermicularis.*

enterobiliary (en″ter-o-bil′e-er-e) pertaining to the small intestine and the bile passages.

Enterobius (en″ter-o′be-us) [*entero-* + Gr. *bios* life] a genus of intestinal nematode worms of the superfamily Oxyuroidea. **E. vermicula′ris,** the seatworm, threadworm, or pinworm, a small white worm parasitic in the upper part of the large intestine, and occasionally in the female genitals and bladder. Infection is frequent in children, sometimes causing itching. Formerly called *Ascaris vermicularis* or *Oxyuris vermicularis*.

enterocele (en″ter-o-sēl″) [*entero-* + Gr. *kēlē* hernia] 1. a hernia containing intestine. 2. posterior vaginal hernia.

enterocentesis (en″ter-o-sen-te′sis) [*entero-* + Gr. *kentēsis* puncture] surgical puncture of the intestine.

enterocholecystostomy (en″ter-o-ko″le-sis-tos′to-me) [*entero-* + Gr. *cholē* bile + *kystis* bladder + *stoma* mouth] formation of an opening from the gallbladder into the small intestine; it may be created surgically or occur spontaneously by rupture due to an impacted stone.

enterocholecystotomy (en″ter-o-ko″lo-sis-tot′o-me) [*entero-* + *cholecystotomy*] incision into the gallbladder and the intestine.

enterocinesia (en″ter-o-si-ne′ze-ah) [*entero-* + Gr. *kinēsis* motion] peristalsis.

enterocinetic (en″ter-o-si-net′ik) pertaining to or stimulating peristalsis.

enterocleisis (en″ter-o-kli′sis) [*entero-* + Gr. *kleisis* closure] 1. closure of a wound in the intestine. 2. occlusion of the lumen of the intestine. **omental e.,** closure of an intestinal perforation by suturing the omentum over the defect.

enteroclysis (en″ter-ok′lĭ-sis) [*entero-* + Gr. *klysis* a drenching] 1. the injection of a nutrient or medicinal liquid into the bowel. 2. the introduction of barium directly into the small bowel through a nasogastric tube whose end is positioned beyond the duodenojejunal junction; used in radiographic examination of the small bowel. Called also *small bowel enema*.

enterococcemia (en″ter-o-kok-se′me-ah) [*enterococcus* + Gr. *haima* blood + *-ia*] the presence of enterococci in the blood.

enterococci (en″ter-o-kok′si) [L.] plural of *enterococcus*.

enterococcus (en″ter-o-kok′us), pl. *enterococ′ci* [*entero-* + *coccus*] any streptococcus of the human intestine; the enterococcus group includes *Streptococcus durans, S. faecalis,* and *S. faecium.*

enterocoel (en″ter-o-sēl) enterocoele.

enterocoele (en″ter-o-se′le) [*entero-* + Gr. *koilia* belly] the body cavity formed by the outpouchings from the archenteron, typically found in echinoderms and chordates. Cf. *schizocoele.*

enterocoelom (en″ter-o-se′lom) enterocoele.

enterocoelomate (en″ter-o-sēl′o-māt) 1. having an enterocoele. 2. any of a group of animals, such as echinoderms and chordates, having a body cavity (enterocoele) derived from the archenteron.

enterocolectomy (en″ter-o-ko-lek′to-me) resection of the intestines, including the ileum, cecum, and ascending colon.

enterocolitis (en″ter-o-ko-li′tis) [*entero-* + *colitis*] inflammation involving both the small intestine and the colon; see also *enteritis.* **antibiotic-associated e.,** that in which treatment with antibiotics alters the bowel flora and results in diarrhea and pseudomembranous enterocolitis. Called also *antibiotic-associated colitis.* **hemorrhagic e.,** an inflammation of the small intestine and colon, characterized by hemorrhagic breakdown of the intestinal mucosa with inflammatory-cell infiltration. **necrotizing e.,** pseudomembranous e. **pseudomembranous e.,** an acute inflammation of the bowel mucosa with the formation of pseudomembranous plaques overlying an area of superficial ulceration, and the passage of the pseudomembranous material in the feces; it may result from shock and ischemia or be associated with antibiotic therapy. Called also *necrotizing e.* and *pseudomembranous colitis* or *enteritis.* **regional e.,** Crohn's disease.

enterocolostomy (en″ter-o-ko-los′to-me) [*entero-* + Gr. *kolon* colon + *stomoun* to provide with an opening, or mouth] the surgical formation of a communication between the small intestine and the colon; also, the opening so constructed.

enterocrinin (en″ter-ok′rĭ-nin) an extract of the mucosa of the small intestine, said to be a physiological hormone, which stimulates the intestine to secretory activity.

enterocutaneous (en″ter-o-ku-ta′ne-us) pertaining to or communicating with the intestine and the cutaneous surface of the body, as an enterocutaneous fistula.

enterocyst (en′ter-o-sist″) [*entero-* + *cyst*] enteric cyst.

enterocystocele (en″ter-o-sis′to-sēl) [*entero-* + Gr. *kystis* bladder + *kēlē* hernia] hernia of the bladder and intestine.

enterocystoma (en″ter-o-sis-to′mah) [*entero-* + *cyst* + *-oma*] enteric cyst.

enterocyte (en′ter-o-sīt″) an intestinal epithelial cell.

enterodynia (en″ter-o-din′e-ah) [*entero-* + Gr. *odynē* pain] pain in the intestine.

enteroenterostomy (en″ter-o-en″ter-os′to-me) surgical anastomosis between two segments of the intestine.

enteroepiplocele (en″ter-o-e-pip′lo-sēl) [*entero-* + Gr. *epiploon* omentum + *kēlē* hernia] hernia of the small intestine and omentum.

enterogastric (en″ter-o-gas′trik) of or pertaining to the intestine and stomach.

enterogastritis (en″ter-o-gas-tri′tis) [*entero-* + Gr. *gastēr* stomach + *-itis*] gastroenteritis.

enterogastrone (en″ter-o-gas′trōn) [*entero-* + *gastro-* + *chalone*] a hormone of the duodenum that mediates the humoral inhibition of gastric secretion and motility produced by the ingestion of fat; called also *enteroanthelone.*

enterogenous (en″ter-oj′ĕ-nus) [*entero-* + Gr. *gennan* to produce] 1. arising from the primitive foregut. 2. originating within the small intestine.

enteroglucagon (en″ter-o-gloo′kah-gon) [*entero-* + *glucagon*] a glucagon-like hyperglycemic peptide released by special cells of the mucosa of the upper intestine in response to the ingestion of glucose. It is immunologically distinct from pancreatic glucagon but has similar activities. Called also *intestinal glucagon.*

enterogram (en′ter-o-gram″) a tracing made by an instrument of the movements of the intestine.

enterograph (en′ter-o-graf) [*entero-* + Gr. *graphein* to write] an instrument for recording the intestinal movements.

enterography (en″ter-og′rah-fe) 1. recording of the intestinal movements by means of an enterograph. 2. a description of the intestines.

enterohepatitis (en″ter-o-hep-ah-ti′tis) [*entero-* + Gr. *hēpar* liver + *-itis*] 1. inflammation of the bowel and liver. 2. histomoniasis of turkeys.

enterohepatocele (en″ter-o-hep′ah-to-sēl″) an infantile umbilical hernia which contains intestines and liver.

enterohydrocele (en″ter-o-hi′dro-sēl) [*entero-* + *hydrocele*] hernia with hydrocele.

enteroidea (en″ter-oi′de-ah) the intestinal fevers; the fevers caused by intestinal bacteria, including typhoid fever, paratyphoid fever, etc.

enterointestinal (en″ter-o-in-tes′tĭ-nal) [*entero-* + *intestine*] intestino-intestinal.

enterokinase (en″ter-o-ki′nās) enteropeptidase.

enterokinesia (en″ter-o-ki′ne-se-ah) peristalsis.

enterokinetic (en″ter-o-ki-net′ik) pertaining to or stimulating peristalsis.

enterokinin (en″ter-o-ki′nin) an extract of the mucosa of the small intestine, said to be a physiological hormone, which stimulates intestinal motility.

enterolith (en′ter-o-lith″) [*entero-* + Gr. *lithos* stone] an intestinal calculus; any concretion found in the intestine.

enterolithiasis (en″ter-o-lĭ-thi′ah-sis) [*entero-* + *lithiasis*] a condition characterized by the presence of intestinal calculi.

enterology (en″ter-ol′o-je) [*entero-* + *-logy*] the sum of what is known regarding the intestines.

enterolysis (en″ter-ol′ĭ-sis) [*entero-* + Gr. *lysis* dissolution] the operative division of adhesions between loops of intestine or between the intestine and abdominal wall.

enteromegalia (en″ter-o-mĕ-ga′le-ah) enteromegaly.

enteromegaly (en″ter-o-meg′ah-le) [*entero-* + Gr. *megaleia* bigness] enlargement of the intestine.

enteromere (en′ter-o-mēr″) [*entero-* + Gr. *meros* part] any segment of the embryonic alimentary tract.

enteromerocele (en″ter-o-me′ro-sēl) [*entero-* + Gr. *mēros* thigh + *kēlē* hernia] femoral hernia.

Enteromonadina (en″ter-o-mo″nah-di′nah) a suborder of parasitic protozoa (order Diplomonadida, class Zoomastigophorea) having one karyomastigont containing one to four flagella. *Enteromonas* is a representative genus.

Enteromonas (en″ter-o-mo′nas) [*entero-* + Gr. *monas* unit, from *monos* single] a genus of nonpathogenic parasitic intestinal protozoa (suborder Enteromonadina, order Diplomonadida) having four anterior flagella, one of which passes along the body and emerges and extends posteriorly.

enteromycodermitis (en″ter-o-mi″ko-der-mi′tis) [*entero-* + Gr. *myxa* mucus + *derma* skin] endoenteritis.

enteromycosis (en″ter-o-mi-ko′sis) [*entero-* + Gr. *mykēs* fungus + *-osis*] disease of the intestine due to bacteria or fungi. **e. bacteria′cea,** a general name for certain infections of the intestine due to nonspecific bacteria.

enteromyiasis (en″ter-o-mi-i′ah-sis) [*entero-* + Gr. *myia* fly] presence of larvae of flies in the intestine.

enteron (en′ter-on) [Gr.] the gut or alimentary canal; usually used in medicine with specific reference to the small intestine.

enteroneuritis (en″ter-o-nu-ri′tis) inflammation of the nerves of the intestine.

enteronitis (en″ter-o-ni′tis) enteritis.

entero-oxyntin (en″ter-o-oks′in-tin) a polypeptide postulated to be secreted by the small intestine and to stimulate secretion of hydrochloric acid by parietal (oxyntic) cells when protein is introduced into the small intestine.

enteroparesis (en″ter-o-par′e-sis) [*entero-* + Gr. *paresis* relaxation] relaxation of the intestine resulting in dilatation.

enteropathogen (en″ter-o-path′o-jen) a microorganism which causes a disease of the intestines.

enteropathogenesis (en″ter-o-path″o-jen′ĕ-sis) the production of disease or disorder of the intestines.

enteropathogenic (en″ter-o-path″o-jen′ik) pertaining to or effective in production of disease of the intestines.

enteropathy (en″ter-op′ah-the) [*entero-* + Gr. *pathos* illness] any disease of the intestine. **gluten e.,** nontropical sprue. **protein-losing e.,** a nonspecific term referring to conditions associated with excessive enteric loss of plasma protein. It occurs in extensive ulceration (e.g., inflammatory bowel disease), diffuse mucosal disease (e.g., adult celiac disease) in which there is more rapid desquamation of mucosal epithelial cells, and in intestinal lymphatic obstruction (intestinal lymphangiectasia).

enteropeptidase (en″ter-o-pep′tĭ-dās) [EC 3.4.21.9] an enzyme of the hydrolase class that catalyzes the cleavage of the Lys^6 - Ile^7 bond in trypsinogen, thus converting it to trypsin. It is secreted by the small intestine. Called also *enterokinase*.

enteropexy (en′ter-o-pek″se) [*entero-* + Gr. *pēxis* fixation] surgical fixation of the intestine to the anterior or posterior abdominal wall, or occasionally of one segment to another.

enteroplasty (en′ter-o-plas″te) [*entero-* + Gr. *plassein* to mold] plastic surgery of the intestine, especially to enlarge the caliber of a constricted segment or area of bowel.

enteroplegia (en″ter-o-ple′je-ah) [*entero-* + Gr. *plēgē* stroke] adynamic ileus.

enteroptosia (en″ter-op-to′se-ah) enteroptosis.

enteroptosis (en″ter-op-to′sis) [*entero-* + Gr. *ptōsis* fall] descent or downward displacement of the intestine in the abdominal cavity; a term based on the outmoded concept that variations of position of abdominal organs are pathological.

enteroptotic (en″ter-op-tot′ik) pertaining to or characterized by enteroptosis.

enteroptychia, enteroptychy (en″ter-o-ti′ke-ah; en″ter-o-ti′ke) [*entero-* + Gr. *ptychē* a fold] plication of the intestine, an operation for the prevention of intestinal adhesions.

enterorenal (en″ter-o-re′nal) pertaining to the intestine and the kidney.

enterorrhagia (en″ter-o-ra′je-ah) [*entero-* + Gr. *rhēgnynai* to burst forth] hemorrhage from the intestine.

enterorrhaphy (en″ter-or′ah-fe) [*entero-* + Gr. *rhaphē* suture] repair or suture of the intestine. **circular e.,** the suturing of two completely divided portions of intestine after invaginating one segment over the other so that they are joined end to end.

enterorrhea (en″ter-o-re′ah) diarrhea.

enterorrhexis (en″ter-o-rek′sis) [*entero-* + Gr. *rhēxis* rupture] rupture of the intestine.

enteroscope (en′ter-o-skōp″) [*entero-* + Gr. *skopein* to examine] an endoscope for examining the lumen of the intestine.

enterosepsis (en″ter-o-sep′sis) [*entero-* + Gr. *sēpsis* putrefaction] intestinal sepsis due to putrefaction of the contents of the intestines.

enterosorption (en″ter-o-sorp′shun) accumulation of a substance in the bowel by virtue of its passage from the circulating blood; occurring when its exsorption exceeds its insorption.

enterospasm (en′ter-o-spazm″) [*entero-* + Gr. *spasmos* spasm] a spasm of the intestine.

enterostasis (en″ter-o-sta′sis) [*entero-* + Gr. *stasis* stoppage] intestinal stasis.

enterostaxis (en″ter-o-stak′sis) [*entero-* + Gr. *staxis* dripping] slow hemorrhage through the intestinal mucous membrane.

enterostenosis (en″ter-o-stĕ-no′sis) [*entero-* + Gr. *stenōsis* contraction] narrowing or stricture of the intestine.

enterostomal (en″ter-o-sto′mal) relating to or having undergone enterostomy.

enterostomy (en″ter-os′to-me) [*entero-* + Gr. *stomoun* to provide with an opening, or mouth] the formation of a permanent opening into the intestine through the abdominal wall, usually by surgical means; also, the opening so created. **gun-barrel e.,** enterostomy in which the two segments of the divided intestine are parallel to one another as they emerge through the abdominal wall, like the tubes of a double-barreled shotgun.

enterotome (en′ter-o-tōm″) [*entero-* + Gr. *tomē* a cutting] an instrument for cutting the intestine.

enterotomy (en″ter-ot′o-me) [*entero-* + Gr. *tomē* a cutting] incision into the intestine.

enterotoxemia (en″ter-o-tok-se′me-ah) a condition characterized by presence in the blood of toxins produced in the intestines. **hemorrhagic e.,** struck. **infectious e. of sheep,** pulpy kidney disease (q.v., under *disease*) of sheep.

enterotoxication (en″ter-o-tok″sĭ-ka′shun) enterotoxism.

enterotoxigenic (en″ter-o-tok″sĭ-jen′ik) producing or containing a toxin specific for the cells of the intestinal mucosa.

enterotoxin (en″ter-o-tok′sin) [*entero-* + L. *toxicum* poison] a toxin specifically affecting cells of the intestinal mucosa, causing vomiting and diarrhea, e.g., those elaborated by species of *Bacillus, Clostridium, Escherichia, Staphylococcus,* and *Vibrio.* See also *toxin.* **cholera e.,** choleragen.

enterotoxism (en″ter-o-tok′sizm) Autointoxication of enteric origin.

enterotropic (en″ter-o-trop′ik) [*entero-* + Gr. *tropos* a turning] having a special affinity for or exerting its principal effect upon the intestines.

enterovaginal (en″ter-o-vaj′ĭ-nal) pertaining to or communicating with the intestine and the vagina, as an enterovaginal fistula.

enterovenous (en″ter-o-ve′nus) communicating between the intestinal lumen and the lumen of a vein.

enterovesical (en″ter-o-ves′ĭ-kal) pertaining to or communicating with the intestine and urinary bladder, as an enterovesical fistula.

Entero-Vioform (en″ter-o-vi′o-form) trademark for a preparation of iodochlorhydroxyquin.

enteroviral (en″ter-o-vi′ral) pertaining to or caused by enteroviruses.

enterovirus (en″ter-o-vi′rus) one of a subgroup of the picornaviruses infecting the gastrointestinal tract and discharged in the excreta, including poliovirus, the coxsackieviruses, and the echoviruses.

enterozoic (en″ter-o-zo′ik) relating to or caused by an enterozoon.

enterozoon (en″ter-o-zo′on), pl. *enterozo′a* [*entero-* + Gr. *zōon* animal] an animal parasite or species inhabiting or infecting the intestinal canal.

enteruria (en″ter-u′re-ah) [*entero-* + Gr. *ouron* urine + *-ia*] the presence of fecal constituents in the urine.

enthalpy (en′thal-pe) [Gr. *en* within + *thalpein* to warm] the heat content or chemical energy of a physical system; it is a thermodynamic function equal to the internal energy plus the product of the pressure and volume.

enthesis (en′the-sis) [Gr. "a putting in; insertion"] 1. the use of artificial material in the repair of a defect or deformity of the body. 2. the site of attachment of a muscle or ligament to bone.

enthesitis (en-thĕ-si′tis) inflammation of the muscular or tendinous attachment to bone.

enthesopathy (en-thĕ-sop′ah-the) disorder of the muscular or tendinous attachment to bone.

enthetic (en-thet′ik) [Gr. *enthetikos* fit for implanting] 1. pertaining to enthesis. 2. introduced from without.

enthetobiosis (en-thet″o-bi-o′sis) [Gr. *enthesis* a putting in + *biōsis* way of life] dependency on a mechanical implant, as on an artificial cardiac pacemaker.

enthlasis (en′thlah-sis) [Gr. "a dent caused by pressure"] comminuted fracture of the skull, with depression of the bony fragments.

entire (en-tīr′) smooth and continuous with no projections or indentations; used to describe the border of a bacterial colony.

entiris (en-ti′ris) [ent- + *iris*] the posterior pigment layer of the iris.

entity (en′tĭ-te) [L. *ens* being] an independently existing thing; a reality.

ent(o)- [Gr. *entos* inside] a prefix signifying within, or inner.

entoblast (en′to-blast) [*ento-* + Gr. *blastos* germ] 1. entoderm. 2. a cell nucleolus.

entochondrostosis (en″to-kon″dros-to′sis) [*ento-* + Gr. *chondros* cartilage + *osteon* bone] the development of bone taking place within cartilage.

entochoroidea (en″to-ko-roid′e-ah) lamina choroidocapillaris.

entocnemial (en″tok-ne′me-al) on the inner side of the tibia.

entocornea (en″to-kor′ne-ah) [*ento-* + *cornea*] lamina limitans posterior cornea.

entocranial (en″to-kra′ne-al) endocranial.

entocuneiform (en″to-ku′ne-ĭ-form) os cuneiform mediale.

entocyte (en′to-sīt) [*ento-* + Gr. *kytos* hollow vessel] the cell contents.

entoderm (en′to-derm) [*ento-* + Gr. *derma* skin] the innermost of the three primary germ layers of the embryo; from it are derived the epithelium of the pharynx, respiratory tract (except the nose), the digestive tract, bladder and urethra. Called also *endoderm*, *endoblast*, *entoblast*, and *hypoblast*. Cf. *ectoderm* and *mesoderm*. **primitive e.,** the primary internal layer of the gastrula that becomes both gut and yolk sac. **yolk-sac e.,** the epithelial lining of the yolk sac.

entodermal (en″to-der′mal) pertaining to or derived from the entoderm.

entodermic (en″to-der′mik) entodermal.

Entodiniomorphida (en″to-di″ne-o-mor′fĭ-dah) [*ento-* + Gr. *dinos* a whirling + *morphē* form] an order of ciliate protozoa (subclass Vestibuliferia, class Kinetofragminophorea) found as commensals in mammalian herbivores, including anthropoid apes. The somatic ciliature is reduced to unique tufts or bands and the oral ciliature is conspicuous, with the adoral zone being composed of membranelles that spiral toward the cytostome; the oral area is sometimes retractable, the pellicle is generally firm and may be drawn out into processes, and skeletal plates are present in many species.

entoectad (en″to-ek′tad) [*ento-* + Gr. *ektos* without] directed or proceeding from within outward.

entomere (en′to-mēr) [*ento-* + Gr. *meros* part] a blastomere destined to become entoderm.

entomesoderm (en″to-mes′o-derm) endomesoderm.

entomion (en-to′me-on) [Gr. *entomē* notch] the point at the tip of the mastoid angle of the parietal bone in the parietal notch of the temporal bone.

entom(o)- [Gr. *entomon* insect] a combining form denoting relationship to an insect, or to insects.

Entomobrya (en″to-mo-bri′ah) a genus of insects, the spring tails, of the order Collembola, Australian species of which cause irritation by their bite.

entomogenous (en″to-moj′ĕ-nus) [*entomo-* + Gr. *gennan* to produce] 1. derived from insects, their bites, emanations, etc. 2. growing in the body of an insect.

entomologist (en″to-mol′o-jist) an expert in entomology.

entomology (en″to-mol′o-je) [*entomo-* + *-logy*] that branch of zoology which deals with the study of insects. **medical e.,** that concerned with insects that cause disease or serve as vectors of microorganisms that cause disease in man.

entomophilous (en″to-mof′ĭ-lus) [*entomo-* + Gr. *philein* to love] fertilized by insect-borne pollen; said of certain flowers.

Entomophthora (en″to-mof′thor-ah) [*entomo-* + Gr. *phthora* destruction, death] a genus of phycomycetous fungi of the order Entomophthorales, which comprises pathogens of insects and spiders. Formerly called *Empusa*. **E. corona′ta,** a parasite of spiders, termites, and other insects, which causes a subcutaneous infection of the nose (rhinoentomophthoromycosis) in man, and has been isolated from nasal polyps in horses. **E. mus′cae,** a species developing in the bodies of flies, thus destroying them.

Entomophthoraceae (en″to-mof″tho-ra′se-e) a family of fungi of the order Entomophthorales, subclass Zygomycetes, found as parasites on man, horses, and insects; it includes the genera *Basidiobolus* and *Entomophthora*.

Entomophthorales (en″to-mof″tho-ra′lēz) an order of phycomycetous fungi of the subclass Zygomycetes, which are typically parasites of insects, but may cause entomophthoromycosis in man; it includes the family Entomophthoraceae.

entomophthoromycosis (en″to-mof″tho-ro-mi-ko′sis) any disease caused by phycomycetous fungi of the order Entomophthorales, such as rhinoentomophthoromycosis and subcutaneous phycomycosis.

entophthalmia (en″tof-thal′me-ah) endophthalmitis.

entophyte (en′to-fīt) [*ento-* + Gr. *phyton* plant] endophyte.

entopic (en-top′ik) [Gr. *en* in + *topos* place] occurring in the proper place, as opposed to ectopic.

entoplasm (en′to-plazm) [*ento-* + Gr. *plasma* something formed] 1. endoplasm. 2. (*obs.*) the blue-staining, or nonchromatinic, portion of certain bacteria.

entoplastic (en″to-plas′ik) [*ento-* + Gr. *plastikos* formative] having a formative power lodged within.

entoptic (en-top′tik) [*ent-* + *optic*] denoting visual phenomena which have their seat within the eye.

entoptoscope (en-top′to-skōp) an instrument for examining the media of the eye, to ascertain their transparency.

entoptoscopy (en″top-tos′ko-pe) [*ent-* + *opto-* + *-scopy*] the observation of the interior of the eye and its light and shadows.

entoretina (en″to-ret′ĭ-nah) [*ento-* + *retina*] the internal or nervous portion of the retina, disposed in five layers, which are named respectively outer molecular, inner nuclear, inner molecular, ganglion, and nerve fiber layers.

entorganism (ent-or′gan-izm) [*ento-* + *organism*] endoparasite.

entosarc (en′to-sark) [*ento-* + Gr. *sarx* flesh] endoplasm.

entosthoblast (en-tos′tho-blast) [Gr. *entosthen* from within + *blastos* germ] the hypothetical nucleus of the nucleolus.

entostosis (ent″os-to′sis) [*ento-* + Gr. *osteon* bone] enostosis.

entotympanic (en″to-tim-pan′ik) within the tympanum of the ear.

entozoa (en″to-zo′ah) [Gr.] plural of *entozoon*.

entozoal (en″to-zo′al) pertaining to or caused by entozoa.

entozoon (en″to-zo′on), pl. *entozo′a* [*ento-* + Gr. *zōon* animal] a parasitic animal organism living within the body of its host.

entripsis (en-trip′sis) [Gr. *en* in + *tripsis* rubbing] inunction.

entropion (en-tro′pe-on) [Gr. *en* in + *tropein* to turn] the turning inward (inversion) of an edge or margin, as of the margin of the eyelid, with the tarsal cartilage turned inward toward the eyeball; called also *blepharelosis*, *enstrophe*, and *trichoma*. **cicatricial e.,** inversion of the margin of an eyelid caused by contraction of scar tissue in the palpebral conjunctiva or underlying tarsus. **spastic e.,** inversion of the eyelid caused by tonic spasm of the orbicularis oculi muscle. **e. u′veae,** inversion of the margin of the pupil, usually the result of an iritis attended with exudate, and occurring rarely as a congenital condition.

entropionize (en-tro′pe-o-nīz″) to put into a state of entropion or inversion; to turn inward.

entropium (en-tro′pe-um) entropion.

entropy (en′tro-pe) [Gr. *entropē* a turning inward] 1. the measure of that part of the heat or energy of a system which is not available to perform work; entropy increases in all natural (spontaneous and irreversible) processes. 2. diminished capacity for spontaneous change, as occurs in aging.

entsulfon sodium (ent′sul-fon) chemical name: 2-[2-[2-[4-(1,1,3,3-tetramethylbutyl) phenoxy]ethoxy]ethoxy]ethonesulfonic acid sodium salt; a detergent, $C_{20}H_{33}NaO_6S$.

entwicklungsmechanik (ent″wik-lungs″mĕ-kan′ik) [Ger. "developmental mechanics"] mechanisms of embryological development, as revealed by experimental study.

entypy (en′ti-pe) [Gr. *entypē* pattern] a method of gastrulation in which the entoderm lies external to the amniotic ectoderm.

enucleate (e-nu′kle-āt) [L. *enucleare*] to remove whole and clean, as a tumor from its envelope or the eyeball; see *enucleation*.

enucleated (e-nu′kle-āt″ed) removed; said of an organ, tumor, or cell nucleus.

enucleation (e-nu″kle-a′shun) [L. *e* out + *nucleus* kernel] the removal of an organ, of a tumor, or of another body in such a way that it comes out clean and whole, like a nut from its shell. Used in connection with the eye, it denotes removal of the eyeball after the eye muscles and optic nerve have been severed.

enuresis (en″u-re′sis) [Gr. *enourein* to void urine] involuntary discharge of urine after the age at which urinary control should have been achieved; often used alone with specific reference to involuntary discharge of urine occurring during sleep at night (*bed-wetting; nocturnal enuresis*).

enuretic (en″u-ret′ik) 1. pertaining to enuresis. 2. an agent which causes enuresis. 3. a person who exhibits enuresis.

envelope (en′vĕ-lōp) an encompassing structure or membrane. In virology, a coat surrounding the capsid and usually furnished at least partially by the host cell. In bacteriology, the cell wall and the plasma membrane considered together. **cell e.**, the plasma membrane and the cell wall considered together. **egg e.**, egg membrane; see under *membrane*. **nuclear e.**, the condensed double layer of lipids and proteins enclosing the cell nucleus and separating it from the cytoplasm; its two concentric membranes, inner and outer, are separated by a perinuclear space. Called also *nuclear membrane*.

envenomation (en-ven″o-ma′shun) the poisonous effects caused by the bites, stings, or effluvia of insects and other arthropods, or the bites of snakes.

environment (en-vi′ron-ment) [Fr. *environner* to surround, to encircle] the sum total of all the conditions and elements which make up the surroundings and influence the development and actions of an individual.

envy (en′ve) a desire to have another's possessions or qualities for oneself. **penis e.**, Freud's concept that the little girl envies the little boy his possession of a penis; also, a woman's generalized envy of men.

Enzactin (en-zak′tin) trademark for preparations of triacetin.

enzootic (en″zo-ot′ik) [Gr. *en* in + *zōon* animal] 1. present in an animal community at all times, but occurring in only small numbers of cases. 2. a disease of low morbidity which is constantly present in an animal community. Cf. *epizootic*.

Enzopride (en′zo-prīd) trademark for a preparation of nadide.

enzygotic (en″zi-got′ik) developed from the same fertilized ovum.

enzymatic (en″zi-mat′ik) relating to, caused by, or of the nature of an enzyme.

enzyme (en′zīm) [Gr. *en* in + *zymē* leaven] a protein molecule that catalyzes chemical reactions of other substances without itself being destroyed or altered upon completion of the reactions. Enzymes are classified according to the recommendations of the Nomenclature Committee of the International Union of Biochemistry. Each enzyme is assigned a recommended name and an Enzyme Commission (EC) number. They are divided into six main groups: oxidoreductases, transferases, hydrolases, lyases, isomerases, and ligases. For individual enzymes, see under the specific name, e.g., *glucose-6-phosphate dehydrogenase*. **adaptive e.**, induced e. **allosteric e.**, one containing an allosteric site; see under *site*. See also *allosterism*. **angiotensin converting e.**, dipeptidyl carboxypeptidase I. **brancher e., branching e.**, 1,4-α-glucan branching enzyme. **catheptic e.**, cathepsin. **clotting e., coagulating e.**, an enzyme, such as thrombin, that catalyzes the conversion of soluble into insoluble proteins. **constitutive e.**, one produced by a microorganism regardless of the presence or absence of the specific substrate. Cf. *induced e.* **cryptic e.**, in bacteriology, an enzyme that can attack added substrate in a cell lysate but not in intact cells, owing to selective action of a permeability barrier. **debrancher e., debranching e.**, amylo-1-6-glucosidase. See also *isoamylase*. **extracellular e.**, exoenzyme. **fat-splitting e.**, lipase. **glycolytic e.**, one that catalyzes the conversion of sugar to pyruvic acid. **hydrolytic e.**, hydrolase. **induced e.**, one whose production has been or may be stimulated by another compound, often a substrate or a structurally related compound (inducer). The inducers studied first were substrates whose utilization thus became possible; hence these enzymes were known earlier as *adaptive enzymes*. Cf. *constitutive e.* **inducible e.**, induced e. **intracellular e.**, endoenzyme. **old yellow e.**, NADPH dehydrogenase. **proteolytic e.**, protease. **Q e.**, 1,4-α-glucan branching enzyme (amylopectin producing). **receptor-destroying e.**, one that renders red cells insusceptible to viral hemolysis by destroying its receptors. **redox e.**, oxidoreductase. **repressible e.**, one whose rate of formation is decreased by an increased concentration of one or more endproducts. The process serves as a control mechanism in certain bacterial and mammalian metabolic systems. **respiratory e.**, an enzyme in an oxidative system that transfers electrons from a substrate to molecular oxygen. **restriction e.**, restriction endonuclease. **Schardinger's e.**, xanthine oxidase. **terminal addition e.**, DNA nucleotidylexotransferase. **transferring e.**, transferase. **yellow e's**, any of a number of enzymes having a flavin as a prosthetic group. Historically, NADPH dehydrogenase was called the *old yellow enzyme* to distinguish it from D-amino acid oxidase, known as the *new yellow enzyme*. See also *flavoprotein*.

Enzyme Commission (EC) the International Commission on Enzymes, a committee established in 1956 by the International Union of Biochemistry to standardize enzyme classification and nomenclature.

enzymic (en-zim′ik) enzymatic.

enzymology (en″zi-mol′o-je) the study of enzymes and enzymatic action.

enzymolysis (en″zi-mol′ĭ-sis) [*enzyme* + Gr. *lysis* dissolution] cleavage of a substance by enzymatic action.

enzymopathy (en″zi-mop′ah-the) an inborn error of metabolism consisting of defective or absent enzymes, as in the glycogen storage diseases or the mucopolysaccharidoses. **lysosomal e.**, lysosomal storage disease.

enzymosis (en″zi-mo′sis) [*enzyme* + *-osis*] (*obs.*) fermentation induced by an enzyme.

EOG electro-olfactogram.

eonism (e′o-nizm) [Chevalier *d'Eon*, French political adventurer, 1728–1810; having adopted woman's dress when sent on a secret mission to Russia in 1755, he was later forced by decree of Louis XVI to wear such apparel to the end of his life] (*obs.*) transvestism.

eosin (e′o-sin) [Gr. *ēōs* dawn] a rose-colored stain or dye: typically the sodium salt of tetrabromfluorescein, $C_{20}H_6Br_4$-Na_2O_5, C.I. 45380. Commercially, several other red coal tar dyes are called eosin. All the eosins are bromine derivatives of fluorescin. Eosin is an important plasma stain, used especially with hematoxylin, methylene blue, and methyl green. **e. B, e. I bluish**, dibromodinitrofluorescein, a dye having staining properties similar to eosin, but of a distinctly bluer shade. **ethyl e.**, the ethyl ester of eosin. **water-soluble e., e. W or W S, yellowish e., e. Y**, eosin.

eosinocyte (e″o-sin′o-sīt) eosinophil.

eosinopenia (e″o-sin-o-pe′ne-ah) [*eosinophil* + Gr. *penia* poverty] abnormal deficiency of eosinophilic leukocytes in the blood.

eosinophil (e″o-sin′o-fil) [*eosin* + Gr. *philein* to love] a structure, cell, or histologic element readily stained by eosin, especially a granular leukocyte with a nucleus that usually has two lobes connected by a slender thread of chromatin, and cytoplasm containing coarse, round granules that are uniform in size; called also *acidocyte, eosinocyte, eosinophilic leukocyte,* and *Rindfleisch's cell.*

eosinophile (e″o-sin′o-fīl) 1. eosinophil. 2. eosinophilic.

eosinophilia (e″o-sin″o-fil′e-ah) [*eosin* + Gr. *philein* to love] 1. the formation and accumulation of an abnormally large number of eosinophils in the blood. 2. the condition of being readily stained with eosin. **Löffler's e.,** see under *syndrome.* **pulmonary infiltration e.,** infiltration of the pulmonary parenchyma by eosinophils, as in Löffler's syndrome. **tropical e., tropical pulmonary e.,** a subacute or chronic form of occult filariasis, usually involving *Brugia malayi* or *Wuchereria bancrofti,* occurring in the tropics, and chiefly affecting Asiatic Indians, in whom it may represent a genetic predisposition. It is characterized by episodic nocturnal wheezing and coughing, strikingly elevated eosinophilia, and diffuse reticulonodular infiltrations of the lung. Microfilariae are seldom detected in peripheral blood films since the parasites are confined primarily to the lungs. Called also *eosinophilic lung, filarial hypereosinophilia,* and *Weingarten's syndrome.*

eosinophilic (e″o-sin″o-fil′ik) readily stainable with eosin; pertaining to eosinophils or to eosinophilia.

eosinophilopoietin (e″o-sin″o-fil″o-poi′ĕ-tin) a peptide of low molecular weight that induces production of eosinophils.

eosinophilosis (e″o-sin″o-fĭ-lo′sis) eosinophilia, def. 1.

eosinophilotactic (e″o-sin″o-fil″o-tak′tik) having the power of attracting eosinophils; chemotactic for eosinophils.

eosinophilous (e″o-sin-of′ĭ-lus) eosinophilic.

eosinophiluria (e″o-sin″o-fil-u′re-ah) the presence of eosinophils in the urine.

eosinotactic (e″o-sin″o-tak′tik) [*eosinophil* + Gr. *taktikos* regulating] exhibiting an influence on eosinophilic cells, either repelling them (*negatively e.*) or attracting them (*positively e.*).

eosolate (e-o′so-lāt) acetyl guaiacol trisulfonate; the silver salt is used as an antiseptic.

ep- see *epi-.*

epacmastic (ep″ak-mas′tik) pertaining to the epacme.

epacme (ep-ak′me) [Gr. *epakmazein* to come to its height] in evolution, the stage or period of development.

epactal (e-pak′tal) [Gr. *epaktos* brought in] 1. supernumerary. 2. a wormian bone; see *ossa suturalium.*

epallobiosis (ep-al″lo-bi-o′sis) [*epi-* + Gr. *allo-* other + *biōsis* way of life] dependency on an external life-support system, as on a heart-lung machine or hemodialyzer.

eparsalgia (ep″ar-sal′je-ah) [Gr. *epairein* to lift + *-algia*] any painful disorder due to overstrain of a part, including dilatation of the heart, hernia, enteroptosis, coughing, etc.

eparterial (ep″ar-te′re-al) [Gr. *epi* upon + *artēria* artery] over an artery; applied especially to the first branch of the right primary bronchus which is so situated.

epaxial (ep-ak′se-al) [Gr. *epi* upon + *axis*] situated upon or above an axis.

epencephal (ep″en-sef′al) epencephalon.

epencephalic (ep″en-se-fal′ik) pertaining to the epencephalon.

epencephalon (ep″en-sef′ah-lon) [Gr. *epi* upon + *enkephalos* brain] 1. cerebellum. 2. metencephalon.

ependopathy (ep″en-dop′ah-the) ependymopathy.

ependyma (ĕ-pen′dĭ-mah) [Gr. *ependyma* upper garment] [NA] the lining membrane of the ventricles of the brain and of the central canal of the spinal cord.

ependymal (ĕ-pen′dĭ-mal) pertaining to or composed of ependyma.

ependymitis (ĕ-pen″dĭ-mi′tis) inflammation of the ependyma.

ependymoblast (ĕ-pen′dĭ-mo-blast) an embryonic ependymal cell; an ependymal spongioblast.

ependymoblastoma (ĕ-pen″dĭ-mo-blas-to′mah) a malignant tumor composed of primitive ependymal cells; some neuropathologists classify such tumors as malignant ependymoma.

ependymocyte (ĕ-pen′dĭ-mo-sīt″) [*ependyma* + Gr. *kytos* hollow vessel] an ependymal cell.

ependymocytoma (ĕ-pen″dĭ-mo-si-to′mah) ependymoma.

ependymoma (ĕ-pen″dĭ-mo′mah) a neoplasm composed of differentiated ependymal cells; most ependymomas are slow growing and benign, but malignant varieties occur.

ependymopathy (ĕ-pen″dĭ-mop′ah-the) disease of the ependyma.

Eperythrozoon (ep″ĕ-rith″ro-zo′on) [*epi-* + *erythros-* + Gr. *zoon* animal] a genus of parasitic bacteria of the family Anaplasmataceae, order Rickettsiales, sometimes causing disease in rodents, cattle, sheep, and swine. The type species is *E. coccoi′des.*

eperythrozoonosis (ep″ĕ-rith″ro-zo″o-no′sis) infection with organisms of the genus *Eperythrozoon.*

ephapse (e-faps′) [Gr. *ephapsis* a touching] a point of lateral contact (other than a synapse) between nerve fibers across which impulses are conducted directly through the nerve membranes from one fiber to the other. Cf. *synapse.*

ephaptic (e-fap′tik) denoting the conduction of a nerve impulse across an ephapse, as opposed to synaptic conduction.

epharmony (ep-har′mo-ne) development in complete harmony with environment; harmonic relation between structure and environment.

ephebiatrics (ĕ-fe″be-at′riks) [Gr. *ephēbos* one arrived at puberty + *iatrikē* surgery, medicine] that department of medicine which deals especially with the diagnosis and treatment of the diseases of youth (18–25 years).

ephebic (ĕ-feb′ik) [Gr. *ephēbikos* pertaining to puberty] pertaining to youth or the period of puberty and adolescence.

ephebogenesis (ef″ĕ-bo-jen′ĕ-sis) [Gr. *ephēbos* one arrived at puberty + *genesis*] the bodily changes occurring at puberty.

ephebogenic (ef″e-bo-jen′ik) pertaining to or caused by ephebogenesis.

ephebology (ef″ĕ-bol′o-je) [Gr. *ephēbos* one arrived at puberty + *-logy*] the study of puberty.

Ephedra (e-fed′rah) [Gr. *epi* upon + *hedra* seat] a genus of low, branching, gnetaceous shrubs indigenous to China and India. *E. equisetina, E. sinica, E. vulgaris,* and other species, known as *ma huang* in China, furnish ephedrine.

ephedrine (ĕ-fed′rin, ef′ĕ-drin) [USP] chemical name: $[R-(R^*, S^*)]-\alpha$-[1-(methylamino)ethyl]benzenemethanol. An adrenergic, $C_{10}H_{15}NO$, obtained from *Ephedra* species or prepared synthetically, occurring as an unctuous, almost colorless solid or white crystals or granules. Its principal uses, in the form of the hydrochloride or sulfate salt, are: to decongest the nasal mucosa in allergic states and to relax bronchiolar muscles in bronchial asthma; to stimulate the central nervous system in narcolepsy and in poisoning by central nervous system depressants; to prevent hypotension during spinal and infiltration anesthesia; and as a mydriatic. **e. hydrochloride** [USP], the hydrochloride salt of ephedrine, $C_{10}H_{15}NO\cdot HCl$, occurring as fine, white crystals or as a powder, having the same actions, uses, and routes of administration as the sulfate salt. **e. sulfate** [USP], the sulfate salt of ephedrine, $(C_{10}H_{15}NO)_2H_2SO_4$, occurring as fine, white crystals or powder, having the same actions as the base; administered orally, parenterally, or intranasally.

ephelides (ĕ-fel′ĭ-dēz) [Gr.] plural of *ephelis.*

ephelis (ĕ-fe′lis), pl. *ephel′ides* [Gr. *ephēlis*] a freckle.

ephemera (ĕ-fem′er-ah) [Gr. *ephēmeros* short-lived] a transitory condition or thing.

ephemeral (ĕ-fem′er-al) short-lived; transient.

Ephemerida (e″fĕ-mer′ĭ-dah) a family of flies (class Insecta), the exuviae of which may cause sensitization and severe asthmatic paroxysms when inhaled.

ephippium (ep-hip′e-um) [Gr. *epi* upon + *hippos* horse] (obs.) sella turcica.

Ephynal (ef′ĭ-nal) trademark for a preparation of vitamin E; see *tocopherol.*

epi- ep- [Gr. *epi* on] a prefix meaning upon, above, or beside. In chemistry, it denotes a chemical compound or group that is related to another chemical compound or group.

epiallopregnanolone (ep″ĭ-al″o-preg-nan′o-lōn) a 21 corticoid hormone present in pregnancy urine, thought to arise from the fetal adrenal cortex; probably a precursor of C19 androgens. Abbreviated EAP.

epiandrosterone (ep″ĭ-an-dros′ter-ōn)   chemical name: 3β-hydroxy-17-androstan-17-one. An androgenic steroid, one of the urinary 17-ketosteroids, less active than androsterone and excreted in small amounts in normal human urine. Called also *isoandrosterone*.

epiblast (ep′ĭ-blast) [*epi-* + Gr. *blastos* germ] 1. ectoderm. 2. ectoderm, except for the neural plate.

epiblastic (ep″ĭ-blas′tik) pertaining to or arising from the epiblast; ectodermal.

epiblepharon (ep″ĭ-blef′ah-ron) [*epi-* + Gr. *blepharon* eyelid] a developmental anomaly in which a horizontal fold of skin stretches across the border of the eyelid, pressing the eyelashes inward against the eyelid.

epibole (e-pib′o-le) epiboly.

epiboly (e-pib′o-le) [Gr. *epibolē* cover] a method of gastrulation by which the smaller blastomeres at the animal pole of the fertilized ovum grow over and enclose the cells of the vegetal hemisphere.

epibulbar (ep″ĭ-bul′bar) upon the eyeball.

epicanthal, epicanthic (ep″ĭ-kan′thal; ep″ĭ-kan′thik) 1. pertaining to the epicanthus. 2. overlying the canthus.

epicanthine (ep″ĭ-kan′thīn) epicanthal.

epicanthus (ep″ĭ-kan′thus) [*epi-* + *canthus*] a vertical fold of skin on either side of the nose, sometimes covering the inner canthus. It is present as a normal characteristic in persons of certain races and sometimes occurs as a congenital anomaly in others. Called also *epicanthic fold, palpebronasal fold*, and *plica palpebronasalis* [NA].

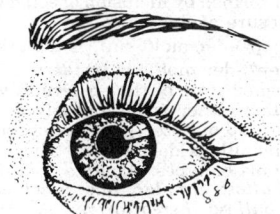

Epicanthus.

epicarcinogen (ep″ĭ-kar-sin′o-jen) an agent that increases the effect of a carcinogen.

epicardia (ep″ĭ-kar′de-ah) the lower portion of the esophagus, extending from the hiatus esophagi to the cardia.

epicardial (ep″ĭ-kar′de-al) pertaining to the epicardium or to the epicardia.

epicardiectomy (ep″ĭ-kar″de-ek′to-me) surgical removal of the epicardium, usually performed in constrictive pericarditis to permit greater diastolic filling of the heart.

epicardium (ep″ĭ-kar′de-um) [*epi-* + Gr. *kardia* heart] NA alternative for *lamina visceralis pericardii*, the layer of serous pericardium on the surface of the heart.

epicauma (ep″ĭ-kaw′mah) [*epi-* + Gr. *kauma* a burn] a superficial burn or ulcer on the eye.

Epicauta (ep″ĭ-kaw′tah) a genus of blister beetles that secrete cantharidin, which if rubbed into the skin, causes severe vesicular dermatitis. *E. pennsylva′nica* and *E. vitta′ta* are found in the eastern United States, *E. cine′rea* in the southwestern United States, and *E. tormento′sa* and *E. sapphiri′na* in Africa.

epicele (ep′ĭ-sēl) (*obs.*) epicoele.

epicentral (ep″ĭ-sen′tral) attached to the centrum of a vertebra.

epichitosamine (ep″ĭ-ke-to′sah-min) D-2-aminomannose: a hexosamine homologous with glucosamine, but containing mannose instead of D-glucose.

epichordal (ep″ĭ-kor′dal) situated dorsad of the notochord.

epichorion (ep″ĭ-ko′re-on) [*epi-* + *chorion*] that part of the uterine mucosa which encloses the implanted conceptus.

epicillin (ep-ĭ-sil′in) chemical name: [2S-[2α,5α,6β(S*)]]-6-[(amino-1,4-cyclohexadien-1-ylacetyl)amino]-3,3-dimethyl-7-oxo-4-thia-1-azabicyclo[3.2.0] heptane-2-carboxylic acid. An antibacterial, $C_{16}H_{21}N_3O_4S$, effective against various gram-negative and gram-positive organisms.

epicoele (ep′ĭ-sēl) [*epi-* + Gr. *koilia* hollow] (*obs.*) the cavity of the myelencephalon.

epicoeloma (ep″ĭ-se-lo′mah) the portion of the coeloma nearest the notochord.

epicomus (e-pik′o-mus) [*epi-* + Gr. *komē* hair] a monster with a parasitic twin joined at the summit of the head.

epicondylalgia (ep″ĭ-kon-dĭ-lal′je-ah) [*epicondyle* + *-algia*] pain in the muscles or tendons attached to the epicondyle of the humerus; see also *tennis elbow*, under *elbow*.

epicondyle (ep″ĭ-kon′dĭl) [*epi-* + Gr. *kondylos* condyle] an eminence upon a bone, above its condyle; called also *epicondylus* [NA]. **external e. of femur,** epicondylus lateralis femoris. **external e. of humerus,** epicondylus lateralis humeri. **internal e. of femur,** epicondylus medialis femoris. **internal e. of humerus,** epicondylus medialis humeri. **lateral e. of femur,** epicondylus lateralis femoris. **lateral e. of humerus,** epicondylus lateralis humeri. **medial e. of femur,** epicondylus medialis femoris. **medial e. of humerus,** epicondylus medialis humeri.

epicondyli (ep″ĭ-kon′dĭ-li) [L.] plural of *epicondylus*.

epicondylian, epicondylic (ep″ĭ-kon-di′le-an; ep″ĭ-kon-dil′ik) pertaining to an epicondyle.

epicondylitis (ep″ĭ-kon″dĭ-li′tis) inflammation of the epicondyle or of the tissues adjoining the epicondyle of the humerus. **external humeral e., radiohumeral e.,** tennis elbow.

epicondylus (ep″ĭ-kon′dĭ-lus), pl. *epicon′dyli* [L.] [NA] epicondyle: a general term for an eminence upon a bone, above its condyle. **e. latera′lis fem′oris** [NA], lateral epicondyle of femur: a projection from the distal end of the femur, above the lateral condyle, for the attachment of collateral ligaments of the knee. Called also *external epicondyle of femur*. **e. latera′lis hu′meri** [NA], lateral epicondyle of humerus: a projection from the distal end of the humerus, giving attachment to a common tendon of origin of the extensor carpi radialis brevis, extensor digitorum communis, extensor digiti quinti proprius, extensor carpi ulnaris, and supinator muscles. Called also *external epicondyle of humerus, external, extensor, lateral,* or *radial condyle of humerus,* and *condylus lateralis humeri*. **e. media′lis fem′oris** [NA], medial epicondyle of femur: a projection from the distal end of the femur, above the medial condyle, for the attachment of collateral ligaments of the knee; called also *internal epicondyle of femur*. **e. media′lis hu′meri** [NA], medial epicondyle of humerus: a projection from the distal end of the humerus, giving attachment to the pronator teres above; a common tendon of origin of the flexor carpi radialis, palmaris longus, flexor digitorum sublimis, and flexor carpi ulnaris muscles in the middle, and the ulnar collateral ligament below. Called also *condylus medialis humeri, internal epicondyle of humerus,* and *flexor, internal, medial,* or *ulnar condyle of humerus*.

epicoracoid (ep″ĭ-kor′ah-koid) situated above the coracoid process.

epicorneascleritis (ep″ĭ-kor″ne-ah-skle-ri′tis) a chronic inflammatory condition affecting the cornea and sclera.

epicostal (ep″ĭ-kos′tal) [*epi-* + L. *costa* rib] situated upon a rib.

epicotyl (ep″i-kot′il) the part of the stem of a plant embryo or seedling above the cotyledons and below the leaves.

epicranium (ep″ĭ-kra′ne-um) [*epi-* + Gr. *kranion* skull] the integument, aponeurosis, and muscular expansions of the scalp.

epicrisis (ep″ĭ-kri′sis) [*epi-* + *crisis*] 1. a second or supplementary crisis. 2. a critical analysis or discussion of a case of disease after its termination.

epicritic (ep″ĭ-krit′ik) [Gr. *epikrisis* determination] relating to or serving the purpose of accurate determination; applied to cutaneous nerve fibers that serve the purpose of perceiving fine variations of touch or temperature. See under *sensibility*.

epicuticle (ep″ĭ-ku′tĭ-kl) [*epi-* + L. *cuticula*] the thin, flexible, colorless, outermost layer of the exoskeleton of certain crustaceans and arthropods, composed of wax and cuticulin.

epicystitis (ep″ĭ-sis-ti′tis) [*epi-* + Gr. *kystis* bladder] inflammation of the structures above the bladder.

epicystotomy (ep″ĭ-sis-tot′o-me) [*epi-* + Gr. *kystis* bladder + *tomē* a cutting] suprapubic cystotomy.

epicyte (ep′ĭ-sīt) [epi- + cyte]   the cell membrane covering gregarine trophozoites.

epidemic (ep′′ĭ-dem′ik) [Gr. epidēmios prevalent]   occurring suddenly in numbers clearly in excess of normal expectancy; said especially of infectious diseases but applied also to any disease, injury, or other health-related event occurring in such outbreaks. Cf. endemic and sporadic.

epidemicity (ep′′ĭ-dĕ-mis′ĭ-te)   the state or quality of being epidemic.

epidemiography (ep′′ĭ-de′′me-og′rah-fe) [epidemic + Gr. graphein to write]   a treatise upon or an account of epidemics.

epidemiologist (ep′′ĭ-de′′me-ol′o-jist)   one who specializes in epidemiology.

epidemiology (ep′′ĭ-de′′me-ol′o-je) [epidemic + -logy]   the science concerned with the study of the factors determining and influencing the frequency and distribution of disease, injury, and other health-related events and their causes in a defined human population for the purpose of establishing programs to prevent and control their development and spread. Also, the sum of knowledge gained in such a study.

epiderm (ep′ĭ-derm)   epidermis.

epidermal (ep′ĭ-der′mal)   1. pertaining to or resembling epidermis. Called also epidermic.   2. epidermoid, def. 1.

epidermatitis (ep′′ĭ-der-mah-ti′tis)   a term sometimes used to denote an inflammation restricted to the epidermis; in actuality the inflammation also invariably affects the dermis. Called also epidermitis.

epidermatoplasty (ep′′ĭ-dₑr-mat′o-plas′′te) [epidermis + Gr. plassein to form]   skin grafting done by transplanting pieces of epidermis to denuded areas.

epidermic (ep′ĭ-der′mik)   epidermal, def. 1.

epidermicula (ep′′ĭ-der-mik′u-lah)   a very thin membrane or cuticula, such as that covering a hair.

epidermidalization (ep′′ĭ-der′′mid-ah-li-za′shun)   development of epidermic cells (stratified epithelium) from mucous cells (columnar epithelium).

epidermides (ep′′ĭ-der′mĭ-dēz) [Gr.]   plural of epidermis.

epidermis (ep′′ĭ-der′mis), pl. epider′mides [epi- + Gr. derma skin] [NA]   the outermost and nonvascular layer of the skin, derived from the embryonic ectoderm, varying in thickness from 0.07 to 0.12 mm., except on the palms and soles where it may be 0.8 and 1.4 mm., respectively. On the palmar and plantar sufaces, it exhibits maximal cellular differentiation and layering, and comprises, from within outward, five layers: (1) a basal layer (stratum basale epidermidis), composed of columnar cells arranged perpendicularly; (2) a prickle-cell or spinous layer (stratum spinosum epidermidis), composed of polyhedral cells with short processes or spines; (3) a granular layer (stratum granulosum epidermidis), composed of flattened granular cells; (4) a clear layer (stratum lucidum epidermidis), composed of several layers of clear, transparent cells in which the nuclei are indistinct or absent; and (5) a horny layer (stratum corneum epidermidis), composed of flattened, cornified, non-nucleated cells. In the thinner epidermis of the general body surface, the basal, prickle-cell, and horny layers are constantly present and the granular layer is usually identifiable, but the clear layer is usually absent. Called also cuticle.

epidermitis (ep′′ĭ-der-mi′tis)   epidermatitis.

epidermization (ep′′ĭ-der′′mi-za′shun)   1. the process of covering or of becoming covered with epidermis.   2. skin grafting.

epidermodysplasia (ep′′ĭ-der′′mo-dis-pla′se-ah)   faulty development of the epidermis.   **e. verrucifor′mis,** the widespread and persistent, sometimes for decades, dissemination of verruca plana associated with a tendency to malignant degeneration. It typically begins in early childhood with the development of flat-topped papules, varying in color from pink and flesh to gray or brown, which increase in number and coalesce to form large plaques, especially on the knees, elbows, and trunk. Familial occurrence, parental consanguinity, and mental retardation are often associated with the disorder. Called also Lewandowsky-Lutz disease.

epidermoid (ep′′ĭ-der′moid)   1. resembling the epidermis. Called also epidermal.   2. epidermal, def. 1.   3. any tumor occurring in a noncutaneous site (such as the skull, brain, or meninges) and formed by inclusion of epidermal elements, e.g., an intracranial cholesteatoma.

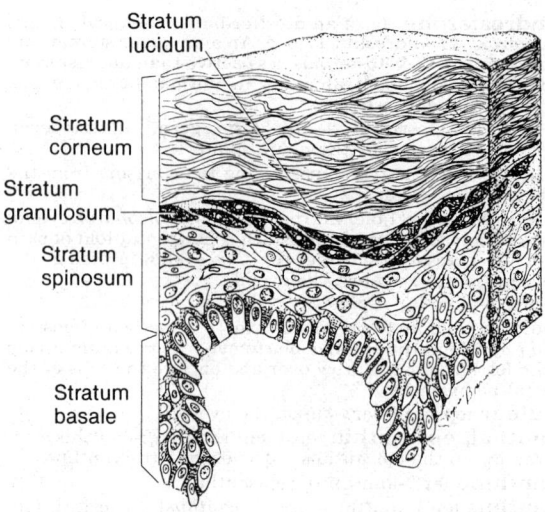

Section of epidermis.

epidermoidoma (ep′′ĭ-der′′moi-do′mah)   a cerebral or meningeal tumor formed by inclusion of ectodermal elements at the time of closure of the neural groove.

epidermolysin (ep′′ĭ-der-mol′ĭ-sin)   exfoliatin.

epidermolysis (ep′′ĭ-der-mol′ĭ-sis) [epidermis + Gr. lysis dissolution]   a loosened state of the epidermis, with formation of blebs and bullae either spontaneously or after trauma.   **e. bullo′sa,** a group of heterogeneous, chronic, mostly hereditary, mechanobullous dermatoses. The group has been classified in four major types: acquired e. bullosa, e. bullosa dystrophica, e. bullosa simplex, and junctional e. bullosa. Called also e. bullosa hereditaria.   **e. bullo′sa, acquired, e. bullo′sa acquisi′ta,** a form of epidermolysis bullosa presenting in adulthood with evidence of genetic transmission, and occurring in association with such diseases as diabetes mellitus, tuberculosis, amyloidosis, colitis, and multiple myeloma and with penicillamine therapy. The blisters, which occur most often on the pressure areas of the hands and feet but can occur anywhere on the body, heal leaving atrophic scars and milia; nail dystrophy and lesions of the oral mucosa are often seen. There is evidence of deposition of immunoglobulin on the dermal side of the dermal-epidermal basement membrane.   **e. bullo′sa dystroph′ica,** a generalized form of epidermolysis bullosa often present at birth or in early infancy, and marked by atrophy of previously blistered areas, severe scarring after healing, and dystrophy or absence of the nails. It occurs in autosomal dominant and recessive forms. Called also dermatolytic bullous dermatosis.   **e. bullo′sa dystroph′ica, albopapuloid,** the Pasini variant of epidermolysis bullosa dystrophica.   **e. bullo′sa dystroph′ica, dominant,** the relatively mild autosomal dominant form of epidermolysis dystrophica, occurring in two main variants: The Pasini (albopapuloid) variant, which is the more severe of the two, is usually present at birth or in infancy, and is characterized by extensive blistering that heals with atrophic scarring, primarily confined to skin over the joints and extremities but sometimes generalized; spontaneous flesh-colored, scarlike (albopapuloid) lesions on the trunk, usually appearing during adolescence; and frequent involvement of the mucous membranes, including the oral, esophageal, and pharyngeal mucosa. The Cockayne-Touraine (dysplastic or hyperplastic) variant usually occurs in infancy or early childhood, and is characterized by keratotic lesions that may show ichthyotic changes, generally confined to the extremities, which may heal with hypertrophic rather than atrophic scars. See also Bart's syndrome, under syndrome.   **e. bullo′sa dystroph′ica, dysplastic,** the Cockayne-Touraine variant of dominant epidermolysis bullosa dystrophica.   **e. bullo′sa dystroph′ica, hyperplastic,** the Cockayne-Touraine variant of dominant epidermolysis bullosa dystrophica.   **e. bullo′sa dystroph′ica, polydysplastic,** recessive e. bullosa dystrophica.   **e.**

bullo'sa dystroph'ica, recessive, the autosomal recessive form of epidermolysis bullosa dystrophica, tending to be more severe than the dominant disorder, characterized by the presence of extensive denuded hemorrhagic erosions and blisters on all body surfaces at birth or in early infancy, including mucous membranes, the subsequent healing of which produces esophageal strictures that may impair feeding and atrophic scars that may restrict mobility owing to fusion of the digits, mitten-like deformity of the hands and feet, and flexion contractures of joints. Called also *polydysplastic e. bullosa dystrophica.* **e. bullo'sa heredita'ria,** e. bullosa. **e. bullo'sa, junctional,** an autosomal recessive disorder having onset at birth or during the neonatal period, characterized clinically by severe generalized blistering, particularly on the perioral area, scalp, legs, diaper area, and trunk, and extensive denudation that may be associated with secondary infection and death from septicemia, nail dystrophy, and dental dysplasia; growth retardation and refractory anemia are frequent findings in those who survive. On electron microscopy, a cleavage plane between the plasma membranes of the basal cells and the basement membrane is seen. Called also *e. bullosa letalis* and *Herlitz disease.* **e. bullo'sa leta'lis,** junctional e. bullosa. **e. bullo'sa sim'plex,** a dominantly inherited, relatively benign, nonscarring form of epidermolysis bullosa, most often involving the extremities, and usually presenting during the first few years of life; blistering may cease in adulthood. It occurs in two forms: generalized and localized. **bullo'sa sim'plex, generalized,** a form of epidermolysis bullosa simplex present at birth or occurring in early infancy, in which the lesions, consisting of vesicles, bullae, and milia, are usually located on areas subjected to repeated minor trauma, such as the elbows, knees, hands, and feet. **e. bullo'sa sim'plex, localized,** a form of epidermolysis bullosa primarily confined to the hands and feet, especially the palms and soles, appearing in infancy or later life, and often associated with hyperhidrosis. It may be exacerbated by unusual trauma such as prolonged walking. Called also *Weber-Cockayne syndrome.* **toxic bullous e.,** toxic epidermal necrolysis.

epidermolytic (ep″ĭ-der-mo-lit′ik) pertaining to or characterized by epidermolysis.

epidermomycosis (ep″ĭ-der″mo-mi-ko′sis) dermatophytosis.

epidermophytid (ep″ĭ-der-mof′ĭ-tid) dermatophytid.

Epidermophyton (ep″ĭ-der-mof′ĭ-ton) [*epidermis* + Gr. *phyton* plant] a monotypic genus of imperfect fungi (dermatophytes) of the order Moniliales, family Moniliaceae. **E. flocco'sum,** a species that attacks both skin and nails but not hair, and one of the causative organisms of tinea cruris, tinea pedis (athlete's foot), and onychomycosis; formerly called *Acrothesium floccosum.*

epidermophytosis (ep″ĭ-der″mo-fi-to′sis) infection by fungi, especially of the genus *Epidermophyton*; dermatophytosis.

epididymal (ep″ĭ-did′ĭ-mal) pertaining to the epididymis.

epididymectomy (ep″ĭ-did″ĭ-mek′to-me) [*epididymis* + Gr. *ektomē* excision] surgical removal of the epididymis.

epididymis (ep″ĭ-did′ĭ-mis), pl. *epididym'ides* [*epi-* + Gr. *didymos* testis] [NA] the elongated cordlike structure along the posterior border of the testis, whose elongated coiled duct provides for storage, transit, and maturation of spermatozoa and is continuous with the ductus deferens. It consists of a head (caput epididymis), body (corpus epididymis), and tail (cauda epididymis). Called also *parorchis.*

epididymitis (ep″ĭ-did″ĭ-mi′tis) inflammation of the epididymis. **spermatogenic e.,** an inflammatory reaction to spermatozoa that have escaped from the lumen of the epididymal tubules into the tissues of the epididymis.

epididymodeferentectomy (ep″ĭ-did″ĭ-mo-def″er-entek′to-me) epididymovasectomy.

epididymodeferential (ep″ĭ-did″ĭ-mo-def″er-en′shal) pertaining to the epididymis and ductus deferens.

epididymo-orchitis (ep″ĭ-did″ĭ-mo-or-ki′tis) inflammation of the epididymis and testis.

epididymotomy (ep″ĭ-did″ĭ-mot′o-me) [*epididymis* + Gr. *tomē* a cut] incision of the epididymis.

epididymovasectomy (ep″ĭ-did″ĭ-mo-vaz-ek′to-me) excision of the epididymis and a large portion of the ductus deferens.

epididymovasostomy (ep-e-did″e-mo-vaz-os′to-me) [*epididymo-* + *vas* vessel + Gr. *stomoun* to provide with an opening, or mouth] surgical creation of a new communication between the epididymis and a formerly distal portion of the vas (ductus) deferens.

epidural (ep″ĭ-du′ral) situated upon or outside the dura mater.

epidurography (ep″ĭ-du-rog′rah-fe) radiography of the spine after a radiopaque medium has been injected into the epidural space.

epiestriol (ep″ĭ-es′tre-ol) any epimer of estriol found in the urine of pregnant women and originating in the fetoplacental unit.

epifascial (ep″ĭ-fash′e-al) upon a fascia.

epigamous (ĕ-pig′ah-mus) [*epi-* + Gr. *gamos* marriage] occurring after fertilization; a term descriptive of the erroneous theory that the sex of an embryo is determined by external factors acting on the embryo during its development.

epigaster (ep″ĭ-gas′ter) [*epi-* + Gr. *gastēr* belly] the hindgut: the embryonic structure from which the large intestine is formed.

epigastralgia (ep″ĭ-gas-tral′je-ah) [*epigastrium* + *-algia*] pain in the epigastrium.

epigastric (ep″ĭ-gas′trik) [*epi-* + Gr. *gastēr* belly] pertaining to the epigastrium.

epigastrium (ep″ĭ-gas′tre-um) [Gr. *epigastrion*] NA alternative for *regio epigastrica.*

epigastrius (ep″ĭ-gas′tre-us) [*epi-* + Gr. *gastēr* belly] a double monster in which the parasite is small and forms a tumor upon the epigastrium of the autosite.

epigastrocele (ep″ĭ-gas′tro-sēl) [*epigastrium* + Gr. *kēlē* hernia] hernia in the epigastric region.

epigenesis (ep″ĭ-jen′ĕ-sis) [*epi-* + *genesis*] the development of an organism from an undifferentiated cell, consisting in the successive formation and development of organs and parts that do not preexist in the fertilized egg; opposed to the erroneous theory of preformation.

epigenetic (ep″ĭ-jĕ-net′ik) pertaining to epigenesis.

epigenetics (ep″ĭ-jĕ-net′iks) the science concerned with the analysis of development.

epiglottectomy (ep″ĭ-glot-tek′to-me) epiglottidectomy.

epiglottic (ep″ĭ-glot′ik) pertaining to the epiglottis.

epiglottidean (ep″ĭ-glo-tid′e-an) pertaining to the epiglottis.

epiglottidectomy (ep″ĭ-glot″ĭ-dek′to-me) [*epiglottis* + Gr. *ektomē* excision] excision of the epiglottis.

epiglottiditis (ep″ĭ-glot″ĭ-di′tis) inflammation of the epiglottis.

epiglottis (ep″ĭ-glot′is) [*epi-* + Gr. *glōttis* glottis] [NA] the lidlike cartilaginous structure overhanging the entrance to the larynx and serving to prevent food from entering the larynx and trachea while swallowing.

epiglottitis (ep″ĭ-glot-ti′tis) epiglottiditis.

epignathous (ĕ-pig′nah-thus) of the nature of an epignathus.

epignathus (ĕ-pig′nah-thus) [*epi-* + Gr. *gnathos* jaw] a fetal tumor arising from the soft or hard palate in the region of Rathke's pouch, filling the buccal cavity and protruding from the mouth. Because the tumor sometimes shows a certain degree of organization, it has been considered a parasitic fetus.

epigonal (ĕ-pig′o-nal) [*epi-* + Gr. *gonē* seed] situated on an embryonic gonad.

epiguanine (ep″ĭ-gwan′in) one of the purine bodies found in the urine after the ingestion of theobromine (cocoa). It is 7-methyl-2-amino-6-oxypurine, $C_6H_7N_5O$.

epihydrinaldehyde (ep″ĭ-hi″drin-al′dĕ-hīd) a chemical compound, one of the substances that give rancid fats their disagreeable odor.

epihyoid (ep″ĭ-hi′oid) situated upon the hyoid bone.

epilamellar (ep″ĭ-lah-mel′ar) situated upon the basement membrane.

epilate (ep′ĭ-lāt) to remove hair by the roots.

epilation (ep″ĭ-la′shun) [L. *e* out + *pilus* hair] the removal of hair by the roots.

epilemma (ep″ĭ-lem′ah) [*epi-* + Gr. *lemma* scale] the endoneurium.

epilemmal (ep″ĭ-lem′al) pertaining to the epilemma (endoneurium).

epilepsia (ep″ĭ-lep′se-ah) [L.; Gr. *epilēpsia*] epilepsy. **e. cursi′va,** cursive epilepsy. **e. gra′vior, e. major,** grand mal epilepsy. **e. minor, e. mit′ior,** minor epilepsy. **e. nu′tans,** head nodding attacks in children, a minor form of astatic seizure. **e. partia′lis contin′ua,** continuous clonic movements of a limited part of the body, due to an abnormal neuronal discharge. **e. procursi′va,** cursive epilepsy. **e. rotato′ria,** an epileptic seizure in which the body rotates. **e. tar′da,** epilepsy beginning in middle age or later.

epilepsy (ep′ĭ-lep′se) [Gr. *epilēpsia* seizure] paroxysmal transient disturbances of brain function that may be manifested as episodic impairment or loss of consciousness, abnormal motor phenomena, psychic or sensory disturbances, or perturbation of the autonomic nervous system. Symptoms are due to paroxysmal disturbance of the electrical activity of the brain. On the basis of origin, epilepsy is idiopathic (cryptogenic, essential, genetic) or symptomatic (acquired, organic). On the basis of clinical and electroencephalographic phenomenon, four subdivisions are recognized: (1) *grand mal e.* (major e., haut mal e.)—subgroups: generalized, focal (localized), jacksonian (rolandic), (2) *petit mal e.*, (3) *psychomotor e.* (temporal lobe e., psychic, psychic equivalent, or variant)—subgroups: psychomotor proper (tonic with adversive or torsion movements or masticatory phenomena), automatic (with amnesia), and sensory (hallucinations, or dream states or déjà vu), (4) *autonomic e.* (diencephalic), with flushing, pallor, tachycardia, hypertension, perspiration, or other visceral symptoms. Called also *epilepsia*. **abdominal e.,** paroxysmal abdominal pain, the expression of an abnormal neuronal discharge from the brain. **acquired e.,** epilepsy due to cerebral disease acquired after birth; see *symptomatic e.* **activated e.,** epileptic seizures induced by electrical or drug stimulation for the purpose of observing the pattern of clinical and electroencephalographic response. **automatic e.,** automatisms, often ambulatory with quasipurposive acts, but with amnesia for the events. **Bravais-jacksonian e.,** jacksonian e. **cortical e.,** seizure phenomena originating in the cerebral cortex. **cryptogenic e.,** idiopathic e. **cursive e.,** psychomotor epilepsy manifested by running. **diurnal e.,** epileptic attacks occurring in the daytime or when the patient is awake. **essential e.,** idiopathic e. **focal e.,** minor epileptic seizures in which the seizures are predominantly one-sided or local, or present localized features. **focal e., chronic,** epilepsia partialis continua. **focal e., minor,** an epileptic attack consisting of the aura without convulsions; called also *paraepilepsy.* **gelastic e.,** epilepsy in which there are episodes of uncontrollable mirthless laughter. **generalized e.,** epilepsy in which the seizures are generalized; they may have a focal onset or be generalized from the beginning. **generalized flexion e.,** hypsarrhythmia. **grand mal e.,** epilepsy, frequently preceded by an aura, in which a sudden loss of consciousness is immediately followed by generalized convulsions; called also *grand mal, major e.,* and *haut mal e.* Cf. *petit mal e.* **haut mal e.,** grand mal e. **hysterical e.,** seizures associated with hysteria, which may mimic epilepsy. **idiopathic e.,** epilepsy of unknown origin, possibly associated with some inherited predisposition for seizures; called also *cryptogenic e., essential e.,* and *genetic e.* **jacksonian e.,** epilepsy characterized by unilateral clonic movements that start in one group of muscles and spread systematically to adjacent groups, reflecting the march of the epileptic activity through the motor cortex. The seizures are due to a discharging focus in the contralateral motor cortex; called also *Bravais-jacksonian e.* and *rolandic e.* **Koshevnikoff's (Koschewnikow's, Kozhevnikov's) e.,** epilepsia partialis continua. **larval e.,** unerupted epileptic seizures, represented only by characteristic waves in the electroencephalogram; called also *latent e.* **laryngeal e.,** tussive syncope. **latent e.,** larval e. **localized e.,** focal e. **major e.,** grand mal e. **matutinal e.,** epileptic seizures occurring in the morning on awakening. **menstrual e.,** epileptic seizures associated with menstruation. **minor e.,** slight epileptic attacks consisting of brief impairment or loss of consciousness, or localized motor or sensory symptoms, as in petit mal epilepsy and psychomotor epilepsy. Called also *epilepsia minor* or *epilepsia mitior.* **musicogenic e.,** reflex epilepsy occurring in response to a musical stimulus. **myoc-**

lonus e., a slowly progressive autosomal recessive form of epilepsy beginning in childhood and characterized by attacks of intermittent or continuous clonus of muscle groups, resulting in difficulties in voluntary movement; there is mental deterioration, sometimes progressing to complete dementia, and the presence of Lafora bodies in various cells, including those of the nervous system, retina, heart, muscle, and liver. Called also *Lafora's disease, progressive familial myoclonic e., Unverricht's disease* or *syndrome,* and *myoclonia epileptica.* **nocturnal e.,** epileptic attacks occurring at night or while the patient is asleep. **organic e.,** symptomatic e. **petit mal e.,** epilepsy in which there is sudden momentary loss of consciousness with only minor myoclonic jerks, seen especially in children, and accompanied by 3-c.p.s. spike and wave discharges on the electroencephalogram; called also *petit mal* and *absence seizure.* Cf. *grand mal e.* **photogenic e.,** epilepsy in which seizures are induced by a flickering light. **physiologic e.,** biologic or electrobiologic seizures based on physiologic and not on organic or structural abnormalities of the brain. **post-traumatic e.,** recurring convulsions due to head injury. **procursive e.,** cursive e. **progressive familial myoclonic e.,** myoclonus e. **psychic e.,** a seizure manifested by a predominance of psychic or psychotic features; called also *psychic equivalent.* **psychomotor e.,** epileptic seizures associated with disease of the temporal lobe and characterized by variable degrees of impairment of consciousness, the patient performing a series of coordinated acts which are out of place, bizarre, and serve no useful purpose and for which he is amnesic. **reflex e.,** an epileptic seizure occurring in response to a sensory (tactile, visual, auditory, or musical) stimulus. **rolandic e.,** see *jacksonian e.* **sensory e.,** seizures manifested by hallucinations of sight, smell, or taste. **serial e.,** seizures occurring in series, with return of consciousness between the individual attacks. **spinal e.,** a succession of clonic and tonic spasms in spastic paraplegia. **symptomatic e.,** acquired epileptic seizures caused by disease of the central nervous system itself, a generalized systemic disorder, such as hypoglycemia or uremia, or poisoning, as with lead or pentylenetetrazol; called also *organic e.* **tardy e.,** epilepsia tarda. **temporal lobe e.,** psychomotor e. **thalamic e.,** epilepsy ascribed to disease of the thalamus. **tonic e.,** a seizure characterized by generalized rigidity. **traumatic e.,** epileptic seizures occurring as the result of trauma (gunshot wound or other injury) to the brain. **uncinate e.,** epileptic seizures originating in the uncinate region of the temporal lobe, associated with hallucinations of smell and taste.

epileptic (ep″ĭ-lep′tik) [Gr. *epilēptikos*] 1. pertaining to or affected with epilepsy. 2. a person affected with epilepsy.

epileptiform (ep″ĭ-lep′tĭ-form) [Gr. *epilēptikos* + [L.] *forma* shape] 1. resembling epilepsy or its manifestations. 2. occurring in severe or sudden paroxysms.

epileptogenic (ep″ĭ-lep-to-jen′ik) [*epilepsy* + Gr. *gennan* to produce] producing epileptic attacks.

epileptogenous (ep″ĭ-lep-toj′ĕ-nus) epileptogenic.

epileptoid (ep″ĭ-lep′toid) epileptiform.

epileptologist (ep″ĭ-lep-tol′o-jist) a practitioner who makes a special study of epilepsy.

epileptology (ep″ĭ-lep-tol′o-je) the study of epilepsy.

epiloia (ep″ĭ-loi′ah) tuberous sclerosis.

epimandibular (ep″ĭ-man-dib′u-lar) [*epi-* + L. *mandibulum* jaw] situated upon the lower jaw.

epimastigote (ep″ĭ-mas′tĭ-gōt) [*epi-* + Gr. *mastix* whip] any of the bodies representing the morphologic (crithidial) stage in the life cycle of certain trypanosomatid protozoa resembling the typical adult form of members of the genus *Crithidia,* in which the kinetoplast and basal body are located anterior to the central vesicular nucleus of the slender elongate cell and the flagellum is attached to the body up to the anterior end by a short undulating membrane before becoming free-flowing. Cf. *amastigote, choanomastigote, opisthomastigote, promastigote,* and *trypomastigote.*

epimenorrhagia (ep″ĭ-men″o-ra′je-ah) too frequent and too excessive menstruation.

epimenorrhea (ep″ĭ-men″o-re′ah) abnormally frequent menstruation; menstrual irregularity in which the patient has a menstrual cycle less than the normal twenty-eight days.

epimer (ep′ĭ-mer) either of two diastereomers that differ in the configuration around one asymmetric carbon atom.

epimerase (ĕ-pim′er-ās) [EC 5.1] any of a subclass of enzymes of the isomerase class that catalyze inversion of the configuration about an asymmetric carbon atom in a substrate (epimer) having more than one center of asymmetry. Cf. *racemase.*

epimere (ep′ĭ-mēr) [epi- + Gr. *meros* a part] the dorsal portion of a somite, from which is formed muscles innervated by the dorsal ramus of a spinal nerve.

epimerite (ep″ĭ-mer′ĭt) [epi- + Gr. *meros* part] a modification of the protomerite of certain gregarine protozoa that serves to anchor the organism to the host's tissues, remaining attached after the parasite has matured and become detached. Cf. *mucron.*

epimerization (ĕ-pim″er-i-za′shun) the changing of one epimeric form of a compound into another, as by enzymatic action.

epimestrol (ep″ĭ-mes′trōl) chemical name: 3-methoxyestra-1,3,5(10)-triene-16α,17α-diol; an anterior pituitary activator, $C_{19}H_{26}O_3$.

epimicroscope (ep″ĭ-mī′kro-skōp) (*obs.*) a microscope in which the specimen is illuminated by light passing though a condenser built around the objective.

epimorphic (ep″ĭ-mor′fik) pertaining to or characterized by epimorphosis.

epimorphosis (ep″ĭ-mor-fo′sis) [epi- + Gr. *morphē* form] the regeneration of a part of an organism by proliferation at the cut surface.

Epimys (ep′ĭ-mis) [epi- + Gr. *mys* mouse] *Rattus.*

epimysium (ep″ĭ-mis′e-um) [epi- + Gr. *mys* muscle] [NA] the fibrous sheath about an entire muscle; called also *perimysium externum* or *external perimysium.*

Epinal (ep′ĭ-nal) trademark for a preparation of epinephryl borate.

epinephrine (ep′ĭ-nef′rin) chemical name: 4-[1-hydroxy-2-(methylamino)ethyl]-1,2-benzenediol. A hormone, C_9H_{13}-NO_3, secreted by the adrenal medulla in response to splanchnic stimulation, and stored in the chromaffin granules; it is released also in response to hypoglycemia. It is a potent stimulator of the sympathetic nervous system (adrenergic receptors), and a powerful vasopressor, increasing blood pressure, stimulating the heart muscle, accelerating the heart rate, and increasing cardiac output. It also increases such metabolic activities as glycogenolysis and glucose release. The official preparation [USP], produced synthetically as the levorotatory form (*l*-form), occurs as white to nearly white, microcrystalline powder or granules and is used chiefly as a topical vasoconstrictor, cardiac stimulant, and bronchodilator; administered intranasally, orally, and parenterally, or by inhalation. Called also *adrenaline.* **e. bitartrate** [USP], the bitartrate salt of epinephrine, $C_9H_{13}NO_3$·$C_4H_6O_6$, occurring as a white, or grayish white or light brownish gray, crystalline powder, having the same actions as the base; applied topically to the conjunctiva to reduce intraocular pressure in the management of chronic simple (open-angle) glaucoma and administered by inhalation as a bronchodilator.

epinephrinemia (ep″ĭ-nef″rĭ-ne′me-ah) the presence of epinephrine in the blood.

epinephroma (ep″ĭ-nĕ-fro′mah) (*obs.*) renal cell carcinoma.

epinephros (ep″ĭ-nef′ros) [epi- + Gr. *nephros* kidney] an adrenal gland (glandula suprarenalis [NA]).

epinephryl borate (ep-ĭ-nef′ril) chemical name: (S)-2-hydroxy-α-[(methylamino)methyl]-1,3,2-benzodioxaborole-5-methanol. A compound containing epinephrine as a borate complex, $C_9H_{12}BNO_4$; used as an adrenergic in ophthalmology.

epineural (ep″ĭ-nu′ral) situated upon a neural arch.

epineurial (ep″ĭ-nu′re-al) pertaining to the epineurium.

epineurium (ep″ĭ-nu′re-um) [epi- + Gr. *neuron* nerve] [NA] the connective tissue covering of a peripheral nerve.

epiorchium (ep″e-or′ke-um) lamina visceralis tunicae vaginalis testis.

epiotic (ep″e-ot′ik) [epi- + Gr. *ous* ear] situated on or above the ear.

epipastic (ep″ĭ-pas′tik) [epi- + Gr. *passein* to sprinkle] 1.

suitable for use as a dusting powder. 2. a powder to be sprinkled upon the surface of the body.

epipharyngeal (ep″ĭ-fah-rin′je-al) nasopharyngeal.

epipharyngitis (ep″ĭ-far″in-ji′tis) nasopharyngitis.

epipharynx (ep′ĭ-far′inks) nasopharynx.

epiphenomenon (ep″ĭ-fĕ-nom′ĕ-non) [epi- + Gr. *phainomenon* phenomenon] an accessory, exceptional, or accidental occurrence in the course of an attack of any disease.

epiphora (ĕ-pif′o-rah) [Gr. *epiphora* sudden burst] an abnormal overflow of tears down the cheek, mainly due to stricture of the lacrimal passages; called also *illacrimation.*

epiphyseal (ep″ĭ-fiz′e-al) pertaining to or of the nature of an epiphysis.

epiphyseodesis (ep″ĭ-fiz″e-od′ĕ-sis) epiphysiodesis.

epiphyses (ĕ-pif′ĭ-sēz) [Gr.] plural of *epiphysis.*

epiphysial (ep″ĭ-fiz′e-al) epiphyseal.

epiphysiodesis (ep″ĭ-fiz″e-od′ĕ-sis) [epiphysis + Gr. *desis* a binding] the operation of premature fusion of an epiphysis to arrest growth.

epiphysioid (ep″ĭ-fiz′e-oid) resembling epiphyses; a term applied to carpal and tarsal bones which develop like epiphyses from centers of ossification.

epiphysiolysis (ep″ĭ-fiz″e-ol′ĭ-sis) [epiphysis + Gr. *lysis* loosening] separation of an epiphysis from its bone; especially slipping of the upper femoral epiphysis.

epiphysiometer (ep″ĭ-fiz″e-om′ĕ-ter) an instrument for measuring the epiphyses, used in the diagnosis of rickets.

epiphysiopathy (ep″ĭ-fiz″e-op′ah-the) [epiphysis + Gr. *pathos* disease] 1. any disease of the pineal body. 2. any disease of an epiphysis of a bone.

epiphysis (ĕ-pif′ĭ-sis), pl. *epiph′yses* [Gr. "an ongrowth; excrescence"] [NA] the expanded articular end of a long bone, developed from a secondary ossification center, during which the period of growth is either entirely cartilaginous or is separated from the shaft by the epiphyseal cartilage. Called also *apophysis ossium.* **capital e.,** the epiphysis at the head of a long bone. **e. cer′ebri,** pineal body. **slipped e.,** dislocation of the epiphysis of a bone, as of the epiphysis of the head of the femur. **stippled epiphyses,** chondrodysplasia punctata.

epiphysitis (ĕ-pif″ĭ-si′tis) inflammation of an epiphysis or of the cartilage that separates it from the main bone. **vertebral e.,** osteochondrosis (q.v.) of the vertebra.

epiphyte (ep′ĭ-fīt) [epi- + Gr. *phyton* plant] 1. a plant organism growing upon another plant. 2. a plant organism parasitic upon the exterior of the human or an animal body.

epiphytic (ep″ĭ-fit′ik) 1. pertaining to or caused by epiphytes. 2. a widely diffused outbreak of an infectious disease in plants.

epipial (ep″ĭ-pi′al) situated on the pia mater.

epipleural (ep″ĭ-ploo′ral) situated on a pleural element, or pleurapophysis.

epipl(o)- [Gr. *epiploon* omentum] a combining form denoting relationship to the epiploon (omentum).

epiplocele (ĕ-pip′lo-sēl) [epiplo- + Gr. *kēlē* hernia] a hernia that contains omentum.

epiploectomy (ep″ĭ-plo-ek′to-me) [epiplo- + Gr. *ektomē* excision] omentectomy; excision of the omentum.

epiploenterocele (ĕ-pip″lo-en′ter-o-sēl) [epiplo- + Gr. *enteron* intestine + *kēlē* hernia] hernia containing intestine and omentum.

epiploic (ep″ĭ-plo′ik) omental.

epiploitis (ĕ-pip″lo-i′tis) omentitis.

epiplomerocele (ĕ-pip″lo-me′ro-sēl) [epiplo- + Gr. *mēros* thigh + *kēlē* hernia] femoral hernia containing omentum.

epiplomphalocele (ep″ĭ-plom-fal′o-sēl″) [epiplo- + Gr. *omphalos* navel + *kēlē* hernia] umbilical hernia containing omentum.

epiploon (ĕ-pip′lo-on) [Gr.] the omentum. **great e.,** omentum majus. **lesser e.,** omentum minus.

epiplopexy (ĕ-pip′lo-pek″se) [epiplo- + Gr. *pēxis* fixation] omentopexy.

epiploplasty (ĕ-pip′lo-plas″te) [epiplo- + Gr. *plassein* to form] omentoplasty.

epiplorrhaphy (e″pip-lor′ah-fe) [epiplo- + Gr. *rhaphē* suture] omentorrhaphy.

epiploscheocele (e″pip-los′ke-o-sēl″) [*epiplo-* + Gr. *oscheon* scrotum + *kēlē* hernia] scrotal hernia containing omentum.

epipygus (ep″ĭ-pi′gus) pygomelus.

epipyramis (ep″ĭ-pir′ah-mis) a small supernumerary carpal bone sometimes found between the triquetrum, lunate, hamate, and capitate bones; called also *epitriquetrum*.

epirizole (ĕ-pēr′ĭ-zōl) chemical name: 4-methoxy-2-(5-methoxy-3-methyl-1*H*-pyrazol-1-yl)-6-methylpyrimidine; an analgesic and anti-inflammatory, $C_{11}H_{14}N_4O_2$.

epirotulian (ep″ĭ-ro-tu′le-an) [*epi-* + L. *rotula* patella] upon the patella.

episarkin (ep″ĭ-sar′kin) one of the alloxur bases, $C_4H_6N_3O$, occurring in the normal urine and in excess in the urine of leukemia.

episclera (ep″ĭ-skle′rah) the loose connective tissue forming the external surface of the sclera.

episcleral (ep″ĭ-skle′ral) 1. overlying the sclera. 2. of or pertaining to the episclera.

episcleritis (ep″ĭ-skle-ri′tis) inflammation of tissues overlying the sclera; also inflammation of the outermost layers of the sclera. **e. partia′lis fu′gax,** sudden hyperemia of the sclera and overlying conjunctiva, lasting a short time.

episclerotitis (ep″ĭ-skle″ro-ti′tis) episcleritis.

episi(o)- [Gr. *epision* pubic region] a combining form denoting relationship to the vulva.

episioperineoplasty (ĕ-piz″e-o-per″ĭ-ne′o-plas″te) [*episio-* + *perineum* + Gr. *plassein* to form] plastic repair of the vulva and perineum.

episioperineorrhaphy (ĕ-piz″e-o-per″ĭ-ne-or′ah-fe) the suturing of the vulva and perineum for the support of a prolapsed uterus.

episioplasty (ĕ-piz′e-o-plas″te) [*episio-* + Gr. *plassein* to shape] plastic repair of the vulva.

episiorrhaphy (ĕ-piz″e-or′ah-fe) [*episio-* + Gr. *rhaphē* suture] 1. the suturing of the labia majora. 2. suture repair of an episiotomy.

episiostenosis (ĕ-piz″e-o-stĕ-no′sis) [*episio-* + Gr. *stenōsis* contraction] the narrowing of the vulvar orifice.

episiotomy (ĕ-piz″e-ot′o-me) [*episio-* + Gr. *tomē* a cutting] surgical incision into the perineum and vagina to prevent traumatic tearing during delivery.

episode (ep′ĭ-sōd) a noteworthy happening or series of happenings occurring in the course of continuous events, as an episode of illness; a separate but not unrelated incident. **acute schizophrenic e.,** acute schizophrenia. **hypomanic e.,** a pathological disturbance of mood similar to a manic episode but not as severe. **major depressive e.** [DSM III-R], a period of depressed mood with loss of interest or pleasure in one's usual activities. Associated symptoms of the depressive syndrome are appetite or sleep disturbance, change in weight, psychomotor agitation or retardation, difficulty in thinking and concentration, lack of energy and fatigue, feelings of worthlessness, self-reproach, or inappropriate guilt, and recurrent thoughts of death or suicide. **manic e.** [DSM III-R], a period of predominantly elevated, expansive, or irritable mood accompanied by some of the associated symptoms of the manic syndrome: inflated self-esteem or grandiosity, decreased need for sleep, talkativeness, flight of ideas, distractability, hyperactivity or psychomotor agitation, hypersexuality, and reckless behavior. **psycholeptic e.,** a sudden and vivid psychic experience to which a patient attributes the beginning of his mental illness, and which so possesses his mind that he is unable to shake it off.

episome (ep′ĭ-sōm) in bacterial genetics, any accessory extrachromosomal replicating genetic element that can exist either autonomously or integrated with the chromosome, e.g., the F factor, colicinogens, and (drug) resistance transfer factor. See also *plasmid*.

epispadia (ep″ĭ-spa′de-ah) epispadias.

epispadiac (ep″ĭ-spa′de-ak) pertaining to or exhibiting epispadias; by extension, sometimes used to designate an individual exhibiting epispadias.

epispadial (ep″ĭ-spa′de-al) pertaining to epispadias.

epispadias (ep″ĭ-spa′de-as) [*epi-* + Gr. *spadōn* a rent] congenital absence of the upper wall of the urethra, occurring in various degrees of severity in both sexes, but affecting males

more commonly, the urethral opening being anywhere on the dorsum of the penis, and manifested as a groove or cleft without a covering. **balanic e., balanitic e.,** incom-

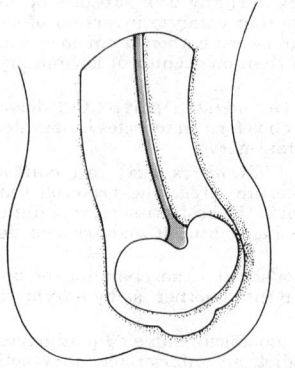

Epispadias.

plete epispadias in which the urethral opening is above and behind the glans, the dorsum of the penis usually being indented to its tip, but the opening may end at the corona or proximal to it. Called also *glandular e.* **clitoric e.,** incomplete epispadias in which the urethra opens cephalad to the clitoris or into it. **complete e.,** epispadias in which the urethra is entirely open to the bladder neck in males, and there may be complete failure of fusion of the anterior urethral wall in the female; it is frequently associated with exstrophy of the bladder. **glandular e.,** balanic e. **incomplete e.,** epispadias in which the bladder does not entirely open to the outside; designated according to the location of urethral opening in the male as *balanic* and *penile*, and in the female as *clitoric* and *subsymphyseal*. **penile e.,** incomplete epispadias in which the urethral orifice is somewhere between the postglandular sulcus and the suspensory ligament, but is usually at the base of the penis. **penopubic e.,** complete epispadias in which the urethral opening is at the junction of the penis and pubis; unless associated with exstrophy of the bladder, the urethral passage emerges between the corpora cavernosa under the pubic symphysis. **subsymphyseal e.,** incomplete epispadias in which the urethral opening is beneath the symphysis.

epispinal (ep″ĭ-spi′nal) situated upon the spinal cord or the spinal column.

episplenitis (ep″ĭ-splĕ-ni′tis) [*epi-* + Gr. *splēn* spleen + *-itis*] inflammation of the capsule of the spleen.

epistasis (ĕ-pis′tah-sis) [*epi-* + Gr. *stasis* a standing] 1. suppression of a secretion or excretion, as of blood, menses, or lochia. 2. a scum or pellicle on the surface of urine. 3. the interaction between genes at different loci, as a result of which one hereditary character is unexpressed, or is masked by the superimposition of another upon it. Cf. *dominance*.

epistasy (e-pis′tah-se) epistasis.

epistatic (ep″ĭ-stat′ik) 1. pertaining to or characterized by epistasis. 2. superimposed.

epistaxis (ep″ĭ-stak′sis) [Gr.] nosebleed; hemorrhage from the nose. **Gull's renal e.,** essential hematuria.

epistemology (ep″ĭ-stĕ-mol′o-je) [Gr. *epistēmē* knowledge + *-logy*] the science of the methods and validity of knowledge.

episternal (ep″ĭ-ster′nal) 1. situated on or over the sternum. 2. pertaining to the episternum.

episternum (ep″ĭ-ster′num) [*epi-* + Gr. *sternon* sternum] a bone present in reptiles and monotremes that may be represented as part of the manubrium, or first piece of the sternum.

episthotonos (e″pis-thot′o-nos) emprosthotonos.

epistropheus (ep″ĭ-stro′fe-us) [Gr. "the pivot"] the second cervical vertebra (axis [NA]).

epitarsus (ep″ĭ-tar′sus) [*epi-* + *tarsus*] a congenital anomaly of the eye consisting of a fold of conjunctiva passing from the fornix to near the lid border; called also congenital *pterygium*.

epitaxy (ep″ĭ-tak′se) the oriented growth and binding of a crystalline substance on a substrate of another crystalline compound, as in the embryonic formation of bone.

epitela (ep″ĭ-te′lah) [*epi-* + L. *tela* web] the delicate tissue of Vieussen's valve (velum medullare superius).

epitendineum (ep″ĭ-ten-din′e-um) the fibrous sheath covering a tendon.

epitenon (ep″ĭ-te′non) [*epi-* + Gr. *tenōn* tendon] the connective tissue covering a tendon within its sheath.

epithalamic (ep″ĭ-thah-lam′ik) 1. overlying the thalamus. 2. pertaining to the epithalamus.

epithalamus (ep″ĭ-thal′ah-mus) [NA] the caudal part of the roof and the adjoining lateral walls of the third ventricle of the diencephalon, comprising the habenular nuclei and their commissure, pituitary body, and commissure of the epithalamus.

epithalaxia (ep″ĭ-thah-lak′se-ah) [*epithelium* + Gr. *allaxis* exchange] desquamation of the epithelium, especially of the intestinal mucosa.

epithelia (ep″ĭ-the′le-ah) plural of *epithelium*.

epithelial (ep″ĭ-the′le-al) pertaining to or composed of epithelium.

epithelialization (ep″ĭ-the″le-al-i-za′shun) healing by the growth of epithelium over a denuded surface.

epithelialize (ep″ĭ-the′le-al-iz″) to cover with epithelium.

epitheliitis (ep″ĭ-the″le-i′tis) inflammation of epithelium.

epitheli(o)- [L. *epithelium*, q.v.] a combining form denoting relationship to the epithelium.

epithelioblastoma (ep″ĭ-the″le-o-blas-to′mah) [*epithelio-* + Gr. *blastos* cell + *-oma*] (obs.) an undifferentiated carcinoma.

epithelioceptor (ep″ĭ-the″le-o-sep′tor) the region in a gland cell which receives a nerve stimulus from the end-organ of the nerve fibril.

epitheliochorial (ep″ĭ-the″le-o-ko′re-al) [*epithelium* + *chorion*] denoting a type of placenta in which the chorion is apposed to the uterine epithelium but does not erode it.

epitheliofibril (ep″ĭ-the′le-o-fi″bril) one of the fibrils which run through the cytoplasm of epithelial cells.

epitheliogenetic (ep″ĭ-the″le-o-jĕ-net′ik) [*epithelio-* + Gr. *gennan* to produce] due to epithelial proliferation.

epitheliogenic (ep″ĭ-the″le-o-jen′ik) tending to produce epithelium.

epithelioglandular (ep″ĭ-the″le-o-glan′du-lar) pertaining to the epithelial cells of a gland.

epithelioid (ep″ĭ-the′le-oid) resembling epithelium.

epitheliolysin (ep″ĭ-the-le-ol′ĭ-sin) a cytolysin formed in the serum of an animal when epithelial cells from an animal of a different species are injected. The epitheliolysin has the power of destroying epithelial cells of an animal of the same species as that from which the epithelial cells were originally taken.

epitheliolysis (ep″ĭ-the″le-ol′ĭ-sis) [*epithelio-* + Gr. *lysis* dissolution] destruction of epithelial cells.

epitheliolytic (ep″ĭ-the″le-o-lit′ik) pertaining to, characterized by, or causing epitheliolysis.

epithelioma (ep″ĭ-the″le-o′mah) [*epithelium* + *-oma*] 1. a neoplasm of epithelial origin, ranging from benign (adenoma and papilloma) to malignant (carcinoma). 2. loosely and incorrectly, a carcinoma. **e. adamanti′num,** ameloblastoma. **e. adenoi′des cys′ticum,** trichoepithelioma. **basal cell e.,** basal cell carcinoma. **benign calcifying e.,** pilomatricoma. **calcified e., calcifying e., calcifying e. of Malherbe,** pilomatricoma. **chorionic e.,** choriocarcinoma. **columnar e., cylindrical e.,** one composed of columnar cells arranged in glandlike tubules; when benign, it is *adenoma,* and when malignant, *adenocarcinoma.* **e. contagio′sum,** fowlpox. **diffuse e.,** infiltrating carcinoma. **glandular e.,** a variety consisting of gland cells and affecting mucous surfaces; when benign, it is *adenoma,* and when malignant, *adenocarcinoma.* **Malherbe's calcifying e.,** pilomatricoma. **malignant e.,** carcinoma. **multiple self-healing squamous e.,** 1. self-healing squamous e. 2. multiple keratoacanthoma. **self-healing squamous e.,** a hereditary type of generalized multiple keratoacanthoma, transmitted as an autosomal dominant trait, and associated with extreme pruritus. Called also *multiple self-healing squamous e.* **suprarenal e.** (obs.), renal cell carcinoma.

epitheliomatosis (ep″ĭ-the″le-o-mah-to′sis) the state of being subject to or afflicted with epitheliomas.

epitheliomatous (ep″ĭ-the″le-o′mah-tus) pertaining to or of the nature of epithelioma.

epitheliomuscular (ep″ĭ-the″le-o-mus′ku-lar) composed of epithelium and muscle.

epitheliosis (ep″ĭ-the″le-o′sis) a disease caused by a virus exhibiting a special affinity for the epithelial structures of the body, including variola, vaccinia, sheeppox, molluscum contagiosum, and contagious epithelioma of birds.

epitheliotoxin (ep″ĭ-the″le-o-tok′sin) a cytotoxin which destroys epithelial cells.

epithelite (ep″ĭ-the′līt) a lesion produced as a reaction to irradiation, in which the epithelium is replaced by a fibrous exudate.

epithelium (ep″ĭ-the′le-um), pl. *epithe′lia* [*epi-* + Gr. *thēlē* nipple] [NA] the covering of internal and external surfaces of the body, including the lining of vessels and other small cavities. It consists of cells joined by small amounts of cementing substances. Epithelium is classified into types on the basis of the number of layers deep and the shape of the superficial cells. **e. ante′rius cor′neae** [NA], ante-

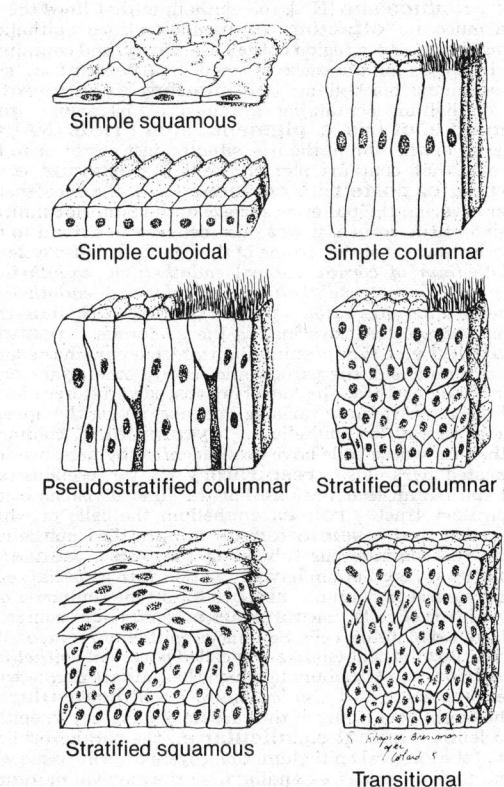

Simple squamous

Simple cuboidal

Simple columnar

Pseudostratified columnar

Stratified columnar

Stratified squamous

Transitional

Epithelium of different types.

rior **e. of cornea,** the outer epithelial layer of the cornea, consisting of stratified squamous epithelium continuous with that of the conjunctiva; called also *e. corneae* or *corneal e.* **Barrett's e.,** the columnar epithelium of the esophagus seen in Barrett's syndrome. **capsular e.,** the outer, or parietal, layer of the renal glomerular capsule, composed of simple squamous epithelium, and separated from the inner, or visceral, layer by the capsular (Bowman's) space. Cf. *glomerular e.* **ciliated e.,** any type bearing vibratile cilia on the free surface. **columnar e.,** a type composed of tall prismatic cells. **e. cor′neae, corneal e.,** e. anterius corneae. **cubical e., cuboidal e.,** a type composed of cells which have a cubical shape. **e. duc′tus semicircula′ris,** the inner, simple, low epithelium lining the semicircular ducts. **enamel e.,** in the developing tooth, the inner or internal layer of cells (ameloblasts) of the enamel organ that deposit the organic matrix of enamel, plus the outer or external layer of cuboidal cells. The reduced enamel epithelium is the remains of both layers after enamel formation is complete. **false e.,** the lining of joint cavities. **germinal e.,** thickened peritoneal epithelium covering the gonad from earliest development; formerly thought to give rise to the germ cells, hence the name. **gingival e.,** the stratified squamous epithelial covering of the gingival tissues, varying in architecture according to location, functional demands, and adaptation. **glandular e.,** epithelium made up of glandular or secreting cells. **glomerular e.,** the inner, or visceral, layer of the renal glomerular capsule, overlying the capillaries, composed of podocytes, and separated from the outer, or parietal, layer by the capsular (Bowman's) space. Cf. *capsular e.* **junctional e.,** a collarlike band of stratified squamous epithelium adhering on one side to the free gingiva and on the other to the crown of a tooth. **laminated e.,** stratified e. **e. of lens, e. len′tis** [NA], the cuboidal epithelium on the front of the lens; called also *subcapsular e.* **mesenchymal e.,** the epithelium which lines the subdural and subarachnoid spaces, the perilymphatic spaces in the inner ear, and the chamber of the eye. **e. muco′sae** [NA], the epithelium that lines the tunica mucosa. **olfactory e.,** pseudostratified epithelium lining the olfactory region of the nasal cavity, and containing the receptors for the sense of smell. **pavement e.,** simple squamous epithelium. **pigmentary e., pigmented e.,** epithelium containing granules of pigment. **pigmented e. of iris, e. pigmento′sum i′ridis** [NA], the anterior epithelium of the iris, situated just posterior to the stroma, that contains pigment cells. **posterior e. of cornea, e. poste′rius cor′neae** [NA], the mesothelial layer covering the posterior surface of the posterior limiting lamina of the cornea; it was once believed to extend to the anterior surface of the stroma of the iris. Called also *anterior endothelium of cornea, corneal endothelium, endothelium anterius corneae, endothelium corneale,* and *endothelium camerae anterioris bulbi.* **protective e.,** epithelium that forms a protective covering, as the epidermis. **pseudostratified e.,** a type of epithelium which occurs in the large excretory ducts of the parotid and several other glands and in the male urethra. The nuclei are spaced at different levels and the cells are quite variable in shape, giving the appearance of a stratified epithelium. **pyramidal e.,** columnar epithelium whose cells have been modified by pressure into truncated pyramids. **respiratory e.,** the pseudostratified epithelium that lines all but the finer divisions of the respiratory tract. **rod e.,** epithelium the cells of which are rod-shaped. **seminiferous e.,** stratified epithelium lining the seminiferous tubules of the testis. **sense e., sensory e.,** epithelium having relation with a special sense organ; neuroepithelium. **simple e.,** a type composed of a single layer of cells. **squamous e.,** epithelium composed of flattened platelike cells. Squamous epithelium composed of a single layer of cells (*simple e.*) is called *pavement epithelium.* **stratified e.,** epithelium in which the cells are arranged in several layers; called also *laminated e.* **subcapsular e.,** 1. the epithelioid lining of the capsule of ganglia. 2. epithelium lentis. **sulcal e., sulcular e.,** the parakeratinized part of the gingival epithelium that covers the soft tissue wall of the gingival sulcus, extending from the gingival margin to the line of attachment of the epithelium to the tooth surface. **tessellated e.,** simple squamous epithelium. **transitional e.,** epithelium that was originally thought to represent a transitional form between stratified squamous and columnar epithelium, found characteristically in the mucous membrane of the excretory passages of the urinary system; in the contracted condition it consists of many cell layers, whereas in the stretched condition usually only two layers can be distinguished.

epithelization (ep″ĭ-the″li-za′shun) epithelialization.

epithelize (ep″ĭ-the′līz) epithelialize.

epithesis (ĕ-pith′ĕ-sis) [Gr. "a laying on"] 1. the surgical correction of deformity or of crooked limbs. 2. a splint or other appliance to be worn.

epithiazide (ep″ĭ-thi′ah-zīd) chemical name: 6-chloro-3,4-dihydro-3-[[(2,2,2-trifluoroethyl)thio]-methyl]-2*H*,1,2,4-benzothiadiazine-7-sulfonamide 1,1-dioxide; an antihypertensive and diuretic, $C_{10}H_{11}ClF_3N_3O_4S_3$.

epitonic (ep″ĭ-ton′ik) [Gr. *epitonos* strained] abnormally tense or tonic; exhibiting an abnormal degree of tension or of tone.

epitope (ep′ĭ-tōp) antigenic determinant.

epitoxoid (ep″ĭ-tok′soid) (*obs.*) any toxoid that has less affinity for an antitoxin than does the corresponding toxin.

Epitrate (ep′ĭ-trāt) trademark for a preparation of epinephrine bitartrate.

epitrichium (ep″ĭ-trik′e-um) [epi- + Gr. *trichion* hair] periderm, def. 1.

epitriquetrum (ep″ĭ-tri-kwe′trum) epipyramis.

epitrochlea (ep″ĭ-trok′le-ah) [epi- + Gr. *trochilia*, L. *trochlea* pulley] the inner condyle of the humerus.

epituberculosis (ep″ĭ-tu-ber″ku-lo′sis) a form of primary tuberculosis in children, producing mild symptoms despite large, usually lobar, consolidations as seen roentgenographically; probably due to bronchial compression by enlarged hilar lymph nodes, with atelectasis.

epiturbinate (ep″ĭ-ter″bĭ-nāt) the soft tissue covering a nasal concha (turbinate bone).

epitympanic (ep″ĭ-tim-pan′ik) 1. situated upon or over the tympanum. 2. pertaining to the epitympanum (recessus epitympanicus [NA]).

epitympanum (ep″ĭ-tim′pah-num) recessus epitympanicus.

epitype (ep′ĭ-tīp) a group of related epitopes.

epityphlitis (ep″ĭ-tif-li′tis) [epi- + Gr. *typhlon* cecum + -*itis*] 1. appendicitis. 2. paratyphlitis.

epityphlon (ep″ĭ-ti′flon) [epi- + Gr. *typhlon* cecum] the vermiform appendix.

epivaginitis (ep″ĭ-vaj″ĭ-ni′tis) a venereal disease of cattle, probably of viral origin, in Kenya, southern Africa, and the United States, marked in cows by vaginal inflammation and discharge and by sterility. In bulls it is marked by epididymitis.

epizoa (ep″ĭ-zo′ah) [Gr.] plural of *epizoon.*

epizoic (ep″ĭ-zo′ik) pertaining to or caused by epizoa.

epizoicide (ep″ĭ-zo′ĭ-sīd) [epizoon + L. *caedere* to kill] an agent that destroys epizoa.

epizoon (ep″ĭ-zo′on), pl. *epizo′a* [epi- + Gr. *zōon* animal] an animal parasite living upon the exterior of the body of the host.

epizootic (ep″ĭ-zo-ot′ik) 1. attacking many animals in any region at the same time; widely diffused and rapidly spreading. 2. a disease of high morbidity which is only occasionally present in an animal community. Cf. *enzootic.*

epizootiology (ep″ĭ-zo-ot″e-ol′o-je) the study of epizootics; the field of science dealing with the relationships of the various factors which determine the frequencies and distributions of infectious diseases among animals.

épluchage (a″ploo-shahzh′) [Fr. "cleaning," "picking"] removal of the contused and contaminated tissues of a wound. Cf. *débridement.*

epontic (ĕ-pon′tik) growing on any surface, plant, animal, or mineral.

eponychium (ep″o-nik′e-um) [epi- + Gr. *onyx* nail] 1. [NA] the narrow band of epidermis that extends from the nail wall onto the nail surface; commonly called *cuticle.* 2. the horny fetal epidermis at the site of the future nail.

eponym (ep′o-nim) [Gr. *epōnymos* named after] a name or phrase formed from or including the name of a person, as Hodgkin's disease.

eponymic, eponymous (ep″o-nim′ik; ĕ-pon′ĭ-mus) named for some person; pertaining to an eponym.

epoophorectomy (ep″o-of″o-rek′to-me) [epi- + Gr. *ōophoron* ovary + *ektomē* excision] surgical removal of the epoophoron.

epoöphoron (ep″o-of′o-ron) [epi- + Gr. *ōophoron* ovary] [NA] a vestigial structure associated with the ovary, consisting of a more cranial group of mesonephric tubules and a corresponding portion of the mesonephric duct; called also *corpus pampiniforme, pampiniform body, parovarium,* and *Rosenmüller's body* or *organ.*

epoprostenol (ep″o-pro′sten-ol) prostacyclin.

epornithology (ep-or″nĭ-thol′o-je) the scientific study of diseases of high morbidity which are only occasionally present in a bird community.

epornitic (ep″or-nit′ik) [epi- + Gr. *ornis* bird] 1. attacking many birds in any region at the same time. 2. a disease of high morbidity which is only occasionally present in a bird population.

epoxide (ĕ-pox′sīd) an organic compound containing a reactive group resulting from the union of an oxygen atom with two other atoms, usually carbon. Commonly referred to as *epoxy*. See also *epoxy resin*, under *resin*.

epoxy (ĕ-pok′se) 1. epoxide. 2. see under *resin*.

epoxytropine tropate (e-pok″se-tro′pēn tro′pāt) methscopolamine.

Eppy (ep′e) trademark for a preparation of epinephryl borate.

EPR electrophrenic respiration.

Eprolin (ep′ro-lin) trademark for a preparation of vitamin E, consisting of a concentrate of distilled natural tocopherols.

epsilon (ep′si-lon) [E,ϵ] the fifth letter of the Greek alphabet.

EPSP excitatory postsynaptic potential.

Epstein's disease, pearls (ep′stīnz) [Alois *Epstein*, a pediatrician in Prague, 1849–1918] see *pseudodiphtheria*, and see under *pearl*.

Epstein's nephrosis, syndrome (ep′stīnz) [Albert Arthur *Epstein*, New York physician, 1880–1965] see under *nephrosis*, and see *nephrotic syndrome*, under *syndrome*.

Epstein-Barr virus (ep′stīn-bar′) [Michael Anthony Epstein, English physician, born 1921; Y. M. Barr, English virologist of the 20th century] see under *virus*.

eptatretin (ep″tah-tre′tin) a potent cardiostimulant obtained from the branchial heart of the Pacific hagfish *Eptatretus stouti* and reported to be a highly unstable aromatic amine. Its chemical structure has not been fully defined, but it is not a catecholamine or other commonly occurring biochemical.

epulides (ĕ-pu′lĭ-dēz) [Gr.] plural of *epulis*.

epulis (ĕ-pu′lis), pl. *epu′lides* [Gr. *epoulis* gumboil] 1. a nonspecific term applied to tumors and tumor-like masses of the gingiva. 2. peripheral ossifying fibroma. **congenital e.,** a benign, nonencapsulated soft, pedunculated tumor of the mucosa of the jaws, usually the maxilla, of newborn infants. It is often found in the incisor region, arising on the crest of the alveolar ridge or process. Microscopically, it resembles granular cell tumor. Called also *e. of newborn*. **e. fibromato′sa,** a fibroma arising from the alveolar periosteum and the periodontal ligament. **e. fissura′ta,** fibrous inflammatory hyperplasia. **giant cell e., e. gigantocellula′ris,** a sessile or pedunculated lesion of the gingiva, or less often the mucous membrane covering edentulous ridges, which represents inflammatory reactions to injury or hemorrhage, and is not considered a true neoplasm. Histologically, it is composed of a spindle cell stroma punctuated by multinucleate giant cells. Called also *peripheral giant cell granuloma*. **e. granulomato′sa,** a pyogenic granuloma on the gingiva resulting from mechanical or other irritation. **e. of newborn,** congenital e.

epulofibroma (ep″u-lo″fi-bro′mah) a fibroma of the gingiva.

epuloid (ep′u-loid) resembling an epulis.

epulosis (ep″u-lo′sis) [Gr. *epoulōsis*] cicatrization.

epulotic (ep″u-lot′ik) [Gr. *epoulōtikos*] pertaining to, characterized by, or promoting cicatrization.

Equanil (ek′wah-nil) trademark for preparations of meprobamate.

equate (e-kwāt′) to make equal or equivalent. In color vision, the physiologic faculty of combining two colors to match a third, as to combine red and green to make a homogeneous yellow.

equation (e-kwa′zhun) [L. *aequatio*, from *aequare* to make equal] an expression made up of two members connected by the sign of equality, =. **Arrhenius′ e.,** an equation describing the temperature dependence of a reaction rate constant, $k = A^e - \Delta E_a/RT$, where k is the rate constant, ΔE_a the activation energy, R the gas constant, T the absolute temperature, and A is a constant called the frequency factor. **Ayala's e.,** see under *quotient*. **chemical e.,** an equation that expresses a chemical reaction, the symbols on the left of the equation denoting the substances before, and those on the right those after, the reaction. **Harden and Young e.,** an equation showing the chemical reaction in the fermentation of glucose to carbon dioxide, alcohol, and hexose diphosphate. **Henderson-Hasselbalch e.,** an equation giving the pH of a buffer system:

$$pH = pKa + \log \frac{[A^-]}{[HA]}$$

where [HA] is the concentration of the free acid, $[A^-]$ is the concentration of the ionized form, and pK_a is the negative logarithm of the dissociation constant (K_a) of the acid. **Lineweaver-Burk e.,** a rearrangement of the Michaelis-Menten equation of enzyme kinetics to give $1/v = (K_m/V_{max})(1/[S]) + 1/V_{max}$, where v is the reaction velocity, [S] is the substrate concentration, V_{max} is the maximum velocity, and K_m is the Michaelis constant. If an enzyme reaction follows Michaelis-Menten kinetics, a plot of $1/v$ against $1/[S]$ results in a straight line (Lineweaver-Burk plot). **Michaelis-Menten e.,** a fundamental equation of enzyme kinetics:

$$v = \frac{V_{max}[S]}{k_m + [S]}$$

where v is the "initial velocity" of an enzyme-catalyzed reaction (the velocity when the product concentration is near zero); [S] is the substrate concentration; and V_{max} and K_m are two constants that characterize a specific enzyme: V_{max}, the maximum velocity, is the initial velocity seen when the enzyme is completely saturated with substrate, and K_m, the Michaelis constant, is the *apparent* affinity constant of the enzyme for the substrate. K_m is defined operationally as the substrate concentration at which $v = V_{max}/2$. The Michaelis-Menten equation does not apply to allosteric enzymes for which the binding of the substrate at the active site is altered by binding of the substrate at a second (allosteric) site. See also *Lineweaver-Burk e.* **Nernst e.,** an equation for the voltage produced by an electrochemical reaction:

$$E = E° - \frac{RT}{zF} \ln Q$$

where E is the voltage produced, E is the standard reduction potential for the reaction, R is the gas constant, T the absolute temperature, z the number of electrons transferred in the reaction, F Faraday's constant, Q the reaction quotient (q.v.), and ln the natural logarithm. The same formula gives the membrane potential produced by a concentration of a diffusible ion across a membrane; in this case E is zero, z is the ionic charge, and Q is the ratio of the concentrations on the two sides of the membrane. **Poiseuille e., (Hagenbach extension)** an equation for the volume flow (V) of a fluid through a capillary tube in terms of the pressure drop P, the radius R, and the length L of the system, and the viscosity η, of the fluid:

$$V = \frac{P\pi R^4}{8\eta L}$$

Ussing e., a method for determining active transport across a biologic membrane, by considering the unidirectional fluxes.

equator (e-kwa′tor) [L. *aequator* equalizer] an imaginary line encircling a globe, equidistant from the poles. Used in anatomical nomenclature to designate such a line on a spherical organ, dividing the surface into two approximately equal parts. Called also *aequator*. **e. bul′bi o′culi** [NA], an imaginary line encircling the eyeball equidistant from the anterior and the posterior poles, dividing the eye into anterior and posterior halves. Called also *e. of eyeball*. **e. of cell,** the boundary of the plane of separation of a dividing cell. **e. of crystalline lens,** e. lentis. **e. of eyeball,** e. bulbi oculi. **e. of lens, e. len′tis** [NA], the rounded peripheral margin of the lens at which the anterior and posterior surfaces meet.

equatorial (e″kwah-to′re-al) pertaining to an equator; occurring at the same distance from each extremity of an axis.

equiaxial (e″kwe-ak′se-al) having axes of the same length.

equicaloric (e″kwi-kah-lōr′ik) isocaloric.

Equidae (ek′wĭ-de) [L. *equus* horse] a family of perissodactyl mammals containing a single living genus, *Equus*, which includes horses, asses, zebras, and onagers.

equilateral (e″kwĭ-lat′er-al) having sides that are equal or identical; called also *isolateral*.

equilibration (e″kwĭ-lĭ-bra′shun) the achievement of a balance between opposing elements or forces. **mandibular e.,** 1. the act or acts performed to place the mandible in equilibrium. 2. a condition in which all of the forces acting upon the mandible are neutralized. 3. a term applied to adjustive grinding of an interfering tooth structure during the functional stroke. **occlusal e.,** see under *adjustment.*

equilibrator (e″kwĭ-lĭ-bra′tor) an apparatus used to produce or maintain a state of balance between opposing forces.

equilibrium (e″kwĭ-lib′re-um) [L. *aequus* equal + *libra* balance] a state of balance or equipoise; a condition in which opposing forces exactly counteract each other. **acid-base e.,** see under *balance.* **body e.,** the condition in which the materials taken into the body are balanced by corresponding excretions. **carbon e.,** the condition in which the total carbon of the excreta is balanced by the carbon of the food. **Donnan's e.,** the conditions which exist at equilibrium when two solutions are separated by a membrane which is permeable to some of the ions of the solutions, but not to all of them. There is a complex distribution of the ions between the two solutions, an electrical potential develops between the two sides of the membrane and the two solutions vary in osmotic pressure. Called also *Gibbs-Donnan e.* **dynamic e.,** the condition of balance between varying, shifting, and opposing forces which is characteristic of living processes. **fluid e.,** see under *balance.* **genetic e.,** the condition that exists when the gene pool in a population is constant in successive generations (unless altered by selection or mutation); i.e., the frequency of each allele in the population remains unchanged in successive generations. **Gibbs-Donnan e.,** Donnan e. **Hardy-Weinberg e.,** see *genetic e.* **linkage e.,** in genetics, the situation in which the coupling and repulsion phases for two linked loci are equally frequent, so that the frequency of each combination of alleles is equal to the product of their individual frequencies. **nitrogen e., nitrogenous e.,** the condition in which the body is metabolizing and excreting as much nitrogen as it is receiving in the food; called also *protein e.* **nutritive e.,** physiologic e. **physiologic e.,** the condition in which the amount of material taken into the body exactly equals the amount discharged. **protein e.,** nitrogen e. **radioactive e.,** the fixed ratio between a radioactive element and one of its disintegration products that results after the lapse of a suitable time, owing to their half value periods. That of uranium and radium is as 2,380,000 to 1. **water e.,** fluid balance.

equilin (ek′wil-in) chemical name: 3-hydroxyestra-1,3,5(10),7-tetraen-17-one. A conjugated estrogen, $C_{18}H_{20}O_2$, with both rings A and B aromatized, isolated from urine of pregnant horses.

equimolar (e″kwĭ-mo′lar) containing the same number of moles, or having the same molarity.

equimolecular (e″kwĭ-mo-lek′u-lar) containing the same number of molecules; said of solutions.

equine (e′kwīn) [L. *equus* a horse] pertaining to, characteristic of, or derived from the horse.

equinophobia (e-kwi″no-fo′be-ah) [L. *equinus* relating to horses + *phobia*] irrational fear of horses.

equinovalgus (e-kwi″no-val′gus) talipes equinovalgus.

equinovarus (e-kwi″no-va′rus) talipes equinovarus.

equinus (e-kwi′nus) talipes equinus.

equipotential (e″kwĭ-po-ten′shal) [L. *aequus* equal + *potentia* ability, power] possessed of similar and equal power; capable of developing in the same way and to the same extent.

equipotentiality (e″kwe-po-ten″she-al′ĭ-te) the quality or state of having similar and equal power; the capacity for developing in the same way and to the same extent.

equisetosis (ek″wĭ-sĕ-to′sis) poisoning of horses from eating equisetum.

equisetum (ek″wĭ-se′tum) a common weed, *E. arvense,* horsetail or jointed rush, that causes a form of poisoning in horses that eat it with hay. It is used as a diuretic drug in eclectic practice.

equivalence (e-kwiv′ah-lens) 1. the condition of being equivalent; having equal valence. 2. in immunology, the ratio of antigen to antibody concentration at which maximal antigen-antibody combination takes place, yielding a precipitate or aggregate; see also *precipitin reaction,* under *reaction.*

equivalent (e-kwiv′ah-lent) [L. *aequivalens,* from *aequus* equal + *valere* to be worth] 1. having the same value; neutralizing or counterbalancing each other. 2. chemical equivalent. 3. in medicine, a symptom that replaces one that is usual in a given disease. **aluminum e.,** the thickness of pure aluminum affording the same radiation attenuation, under specified conditions, as the material or

materials being considered. **combustion e.,** the heat value of a gram of fat or carbohydrate burned outside the body. It measures the amount of potential energy of the substance available, in the form of food, for the production of heat or the supply of energy. **concrete e.,** the thickness of concrete having a density of 2.35 gm./cm.^{3} which would afford the same radiation attenuation, under specified conditions, as the material or materials being considered. **dose e.,** in radiation biology, the product of absorbed dose in rads and the modifying factors, namely the quality factor (QF), distribution factor (DF), and any other necessary factors. The unit of dose equivalent is the rem. **endosmotic e.,** the number which represents the quantity of water that will pass through a diaphragm by endosmosis in the same time that a unit of any other given substance will pass in the other direction by exosmosis. **epileptic e.,** a disturbance, mental or bodily, that may take the place of an epileptic attack. **gold e.,** the amount of protective colloid, expressed in milligrams, which is just enough to prevent the precipitation of 10 ml. of a 0.0055 per cent gold solution by 1 ml. of a 10 per cent sodium chloride solution. **gram e.,** chemical e. **isodynamic e.,** the ratio, from a food-energy standpoint, between carbohydrate and fat. It is 9.3 to 4.1, or 2.3 to 1; that is, one part of fat is equivalent to 2.3 parts of sugar or starch. **lead e.,** the thickness of pure lead which would afford the same radiation attenuation, under specified conditions, as the material or materials under consideration. **lethal e.,** a gene carried in the heterozygous state which, if homozygous, would be lethal, or any combination of genes which would be lethal to 100 percent of homozygotes; for example, a combination of two genes in the heterozygous state either of which in the homozygous state would have 50 per cent lethality. **neutralization e.,** the equivalent weight of an acid as determined by neutralization with a base regarded as a primary standard. **protein e.,** the protein content of a food plus the nonprotein content that can be converted into protein in the animal body. **psychic e.,** psychic epilepsy. **starch e.,** a number (nearly 2.4) expressing the amount of oxygen which a given weight of fat will require for its complete combustion as compared with the amount required by the same weight of starch. **toxic e.,** the amount of poison per kilogram of body weight necessary to kill an animal. **ventilation e.,** 1. the ratio of the total volume of ventilation to the volume of expired carbon dioxide per unit of time. 2. the ratio of the total volume of ventilation to the volume of oxygen absorbed by the lungs per unit of time. **water e.,** the product of the weight of an animal by its specific heat, it being also the number which represents the specific thermal capacity of an equal weight of water.

equulosis (ek″kwoo-lo′sis) [L. *equulus* a foal + *-osis*] a purulent arthritis, synovitis, and enteritis, often with formation of kidney abscesses, affecting primarily young foals but occasionally mature horses and caused by *Actinobacillus equuli.* When manifested as extreme prostration, it is known as *sleepy foal disease* (q.v.).

Equus (ek′wus) the single living genus of the family Equidae, including horses, asses, and zebras.

Er chemical symbol for *erbium.*

erabutoxin (ĕ-rab″u-tok′sin) the active toxic principle of the venom of the sea snake *Laticauda semifasciata.*

erasion (e-ra′zhun) [L. *erasio*] removal by scraping, or curettage.

Erasistratus (er″ah-sis′trah-tus) (c. 300 to c. 250 B.C.) a Greek physician born on Ceos, who studied at Alexandria and was a contemporary of Herophilus. Though believing bodily functions to be mechanical, Erasistratus adopted pneumatism to explain physiology, and rejected humoralism; he also invoked an external force, Nature, as shaper of the ends to which the body works. Erasistratus reputedly performed human vivisection and post mortems; he inferred that the greater number and complexity of convolutions in the human brain than in the animal implied greater intelligence (opposing Aristotle); and he distinguished the cerebrum from the cerebellum and the sensory from the motor nerves. Erasistratus ascribed disease to plethora, hyperemia from indigested food, yet he opposed phlebotomy and purgation (and other violent remedies) and advocated Hippocratic-like diet, exercise, and steam baths. See also *Alcmaeon of Crotona* and *Democritus.*

Eratyrus (er″ah-ti′rus) a genus of reduviid bugs that transmit Chagas' disease.

Erb (erb), Wilhelm Heinrich. A celebrated German internist (1840–1921). See *progressive muscular dystrophy* and *pseudohypertrophic muscular dystrophy*, under *dystrophy*, *Erb's spastic paraplegia*, under *paraplegia*, *Erb-Duchenne paralysis*, under *paralysis*, and see under *point, sclerosis, sign*, and *syndrome*.

Erb-Charcot disease (erb′shar-ko′) [W. H. *Erb*; Jean Martin *Charcot*, French neurologist, 1825–1893] Erb's spastic paraplegia.

Erb-Duchenne paralysis (erb′du-shen′) [Willhelm Heinrick *Erb*; Guillaume Benjamin Amand *Duchenne*, French neurologist, 1806–1875] see under *paralysis*.

Erb-Goldflam disease (erb′golt′flahm) [W. H. *Erb*; Samuel V. *Goldflam*, Polish neurologist, 1825–1932] myasthenia gravis.

Erben's reflex (phenomenon, sign) (er′benz) [Siegmund *Erben*, neurologist in Vienna, born 1863] see under *reflex*.

ERBF effective renal blood flow.

erbium (er′be-um) a rare metallic element: symbol, Er; atomic number, 68; atomic weight, 167.26.

ERCP endoscopic retrograde cholangiopancreatography.

erectile (ĕ-rek′tĭl) capable of erection; see under *tissue*.

erection (ĕ-rek′shun) [L. *erectio*] the condition of being made rigid and elevated; as erectile tissue when filled with blood.

erector (ĕ-rek′tor) [L.] [NA] a general term for a structure that erects, as a muscle which raises or holds up a part.

eremacausis (er″ĕ-mah-kaw′sis) [Gr. *ērema* gently + *kausis* burning] the slow oxidation, combustion, or decay of organic matter.

eremophobia (er″ĕ-mo-fo′be-ah) [Gr. *erēmos* solitary + *phobia*] irrational fear of being alone.

erethism (er′ĕ-thizm) [Gr. *erethisma* stimulation] (*obs.*) excessive irritability, excitability, or sensitivity to stimulation. **sexual e.**, (*obs.*), hypersexuality, nymphomania, and satyriasis.

erethismic (er″ĕ-thiz′mik) erethistic.

erethistic (er″ĕ-this′tik) [Gr. *erethistikos*] pertaining to, characterized by, or producing erethism.

erethitic (er″ĕ-thit′ik) erethistic.

Erethmapodites (ĕ-reth″mah-pod′ĭ-tēz) a genus of mosquitoes, species of which transmit Rift Valley fever.

ereuth(o)- [Gr. *ereuthos* redness] for words beginning thus, see those beginning *eryth-*.

ERG electroretinogram.

erg (erg) [Gr. *ergon* work] a unit of work or energy, being the work performed when a force of 1 dyne moves its point of operation through a distance of 1 centimeter; equivalent to 2.4×10^{-8} gram calories, or to 0.624×10^{12} electron volts.

ergasia (er-ga′se-ah) [Gr. "work"] Adolf Meyer's term for the total activity or functioning of a person, encompassing both behavior and mental activity.

ergasiophobia (er-ga″se-o-fo′be-ah) [*ergasia* + Gr. *phobein* to be affrighted by + *ia*] (*obs.*) pathological aversion to work.

ergasthenia (er″gas-the′ne-ah) [Gr. *ergon* work + *astheneia* weakness] (*obs.*) a condition of debility from overwork.

ergastoplasm (er-gas′to-plazm) [*ergasia* + *plasm*] 1. granular endoplasmic reticulum. 2. (*obs.*) Garnier's concept of cytoplasm, the fibrillar or flocculent masses found in many gland cells and elsewhere.

erg(o)- [Gr. *ergon* work] a combining form denoting relationship to work.

ergobasine (er″go-ba′sin) ergonovine.

ergocalciferol (er″go-kal-sif′er-ol) [USP] chemical name: 9,10-secoergosta-5,7,10(19),22-tetraen-3β-ol. An activation product, $C_{28}H_{44}O$, of ergosterol, produced by ultraviolet irradiation or electronic bombardment, occurring in white odorless crystals, insoluble in water but soluble in alcohol, chloroform, ether, and fatty oils; used chiefly as an oral antirachitic vitamin. Called also *calciferol, activated ergosterol, viosterol*, and *vitamin D₂*.

ergocardiogram (er″go-kar′de-o-gram) the graphic record obtained by ergocardiography.

ergocardiography (er″go-kar″de-og′rah-fe) the recording of moment-to-moment electromotive forces of the heart while the subject is engaging in muscular activity.

ergocornine (er″go-kor′nēn) an alkaloid, $C_{31}H_{39}N_5O_5$, from ergot, once used in peripheral vascular disorders.

ergocristine (er″go-kris′tēn) an alkaloid, $C_{35}H_{39}N_5O_5$, from ergot, once used in peripheral vascular disorders.

ergocryptine (er″go-krip′tēn) an alkaloid, $C_{32}H_{41}N_5O_5$, from ergot, once used in peripheral vascular disorders.

ergodynamograph (er″go-di-nam′o-graf) [*ergo-* + Gr. *dynamis* force + *graphein* to record] an apparatus for recording the force exhibited and the work done in muscular contraction.

ergoesthesiograph (er″go-es-the′ze-o-graf) [*ergo-* + Gr. *aisthēsis* sensation + *graphein* to record] an apparatus for recording graphically muscular reactions to various stimuli.

ergogenic (er″go-jen′ik) [*ergo-* + Gr. *gennan* to produce] tending to increase work output.

ergogram (er′go-gram) [*ergo-* + Gr. *gramma* a mark] a tracing made by an ergograph.

ergograph (er′go-graf) [*ergo-* + Gr. *graphein* to record] an instrument for recording work done in muscular exertion. **Mosso's e.** (1890), an apparatus for recording the force and frequency of flexion of the fingers.

ergographic (er″go-graf′ik) pertaining to the ergograph.

Ergomar (er′go-mar) trademark for a preparation of ergotamine tartrate.

ergometer (er-gom′ĕ-ter) [*ergo-* + Gr. *metron* measure] a dynamometer. **bicycle e.**, an apparatus for measuring the muscular, metabolic, and respiratory effects of exercise.

ergometrine (er″go-met′rin) ergonovine.

ergon (er′gon) a unit representing the stability of a particular gene throughout a lifetime; it is a function of the ratio of the adenine-thymine to guanine-cytosine content of the gene and is reflected in the persistence of the resultant phenotypical trait. Cf. *chronon*.

ergonomics (er″go-nom′iks) [*ergo-* + Gr. *nomos* law] the science relating to man and his work, embodying the anatomic, physiologic, psychologic, and mechanical principles affecting the efficient use of human energy.

ergonovine (er″go-no′vin) chemical name: D-lysergic acid 1-hydroxy-methylethylamide. A water-soluble alkaloid, $C_{19}H_{23}N_3O_2$, from ergot or produced synthetically; used as an oxytocic and to relieve migraine headache. Called also *ergobasine, ergometrine, ergostetrine*, and *ergotocine*. **e. maleate** [USP], the bimaleate salt of ergonovine, $C_{19}H_{23}N_3O_2 \cdot C_4H_4O_4$, occurring as a grayish white to faintly yellow odorless powder; used as an oxytocic, administered orally, intramuscularly, or intravenously. It is also used in the treatment of migraine and as a provocative test in detection of variant angina due to coronary artery spasm.

ergoplasm (er′go-plazm) ergastoplasm.

ergosome (er′go-sōm) polyribosome.

ergostat (er′go-stat) a machine to be worked for muscular exercise.

ergosterol (er-gos′tĕ-rol) a sterol, $C_{28}H_{43} \cdot OH$, occurring in animal and plant tissues which, on irradiation with ultraviolet rays, becomes a potent antirachitic substance, ergocalciferol (vitamin D₂). The substance was originally isolated by Tanret from ergot and named accordingly. **activated e., irradiated e.**, ergocalciferol.

ergostetrine (er″go-stet′rin) ergonovine.

ergot (er′got) [Fr.; L. *ergota*] 1. the dried sclerotium of *Claviceps purpurea*, which is developed on rye plants (*Secale cereale*); ergot alkaloids are used as oxytocics and in the treatment of migraine. 2. (*obs.*) calcar avis. 3. a small mass of horn in the tuft of hair at the flexion surface of the fetlock in horses.

ergotamine (er-got′ah-min) an alkaloid derived from ergot, consisting of lysergic acid, ammonia, proline, phenylalanine, and pyruvic acid combined in amide linkages; used in the treatment of migraine. **e. tartrate** [USP], the tartrate salt of ergotamine, $(C_{33}H_{35}H_5O_5)_2 \cdot C_4H_6O_6$, occurring as colorless crystals or as a yellowish crystalline powder; used as an analgesic in the treatment of migraine.

ergotaminine (er″go-tam′ĭ-nēn) an isomer, $C_{33}H_{35}N_5O_5$, of ergotamine.

ergotherapy (er″go-ther′ah-pe) [*ergo-* + Gr. *therapeia* treatment] treatment of disease by physical effort.

ergothioneine (er″go-thi″o-ne′in) the trimethylbetaine of thiolhistidine, $C_3HN_2(SH) \cdot CH_2 \cdot CH \cdot CO \cdot ON(CH_3)_3 \cdot 2H_2O$, found in ergot and in the blood and in abnormal amounts in the urine of cancer patients; called also *thioneine* and *erythrothioneine*.

ergotism (er′got-izm)   chronic poisoning from excessive or misdirected use of ergot as a medicine, or from eating ergotized grain; it is marked by cerebrospinal symptoms, spasms, and cramps, or by a kind of dry gangrene. Called also *St. Anthony's fire*.

ergotized (er′got-īzd)   diseased or otherwise affected by ergot.

ergotocine (er″go-to′sēn)   ergonovine.

ergotoxicosis (er″go-tok″si-ko′sis)   a form of mycotoxicosis caused by one of the ergot (*Claviceps*) species.

ergotoxine (er″go-tok′sēn)   a toxic crystalline alkaloid originally isolated from ergot (*Claviceps purpurea*), consisting of a mixture of ergocornine, ergocristine, and ergocryptine, which exert both oxytocic and adrenergic blocking effects. Because of the variability of these effects, neither ergotoxine nor its constituents are currently used in medicine.

Ergotrate (er′go-trāt)   trademark for preparations of ergonovine maleate.

ergusia (er-ju′se-ah)   a hypothetical lipoid substance which, liberated from a cell, reduces surface tension and enables the cell to migrate.

Erichsen's ligature, sign (test) (er′ik-senz) [Sir John Eric *Erichsen*, English surgeon, 1818–1896]   see under *ligature* and *spine*.

Eriodictyon (er″e-o-dik′te-on) [Gr. *erion* wool + *diktyon* net]   a genus of hydrophyllaceous plants. *E. califor′nicum* H. & A. Greene (*E. glutino′sum*), also known as yerba santa or mountain balm, was once used in bronchitis. See *eriodictyon*.

eriodictyon (er″e-o-dik′te-on) [NF]   the dried leaf of *Eriodictyon californicum*; its fluidextract is used as a flavor and its aromatic syrup as a vehicle for dispensing drugs.

erisiphake (er-is′ī-fāk)   erysiphake.

Eristalis (er-is′tah-lis)   a genus of flies, the hover flies, of the family Syrphidae. **E. te′nax,** the "drone fly," the "rat-tail" maggots (larvae), which occasionally cause intestinal and nasal myiasis.

Erlenmeyer flask (ār′len-mi″er) [Emil Richard August Carl *Erlenmeyer*, German chemist, 1825–1909]   see under *flask*.

Erni's sign (er′nēz) [H. *Erni*, Swiss physician, 1859–1937]   see under *sign*.

erode (e-rōd′)   to wear away.

erogenous (ĕ-roj′ĕ-nus)   erotogenic; arousing erotic feelings.

erose (e-rōs′) [L. *erodere* to eat away]   having an irregularly toothed edge.

erosio (e-ro′se-o) [L., from *erodere* to eat away]   erosion. **e. interdigita′lis blastomyce′tica,** candidal intertrigo manifested by an area of macerated white skin in the interdigital webs between and extending onto the sides of the fingers, and particularly involving the webs between the third and fourth fingers of those whose hands are frequently or continually immersed in water such as domestic, laundry, and cannery workers, bartenders, and dishwashers.

erosion (e-ro′zhun) [L. *erosio*, from *erodere* to eat out]   1. an eating away; destruction of the surface of a tissue, material, or structure. 2. progressive loss of the hard substance of a tooth by chemical processes that do not involve bacterial action. See also *abrasion* and *attrition*. 3. a gradual breakdown or very shallow ulceration of the skin which involves only the epidermis and heals without scarring. **cervical e.,** a condition caused by irritation and characterized by destruction of the squamous epithelium of the vaginal portion of the cervix; the eroded area is covered by columnar epithelium.

erosive (e-ro′siv)   1. causing, characterized by, or producing erosion. 2. an agent that produces erosion.

erotic (ĕ-rot′ik) [Gr. *erōtikos*]   charged with sexual feeling; pertaining to sexual desire.

eroticism (e-rot′ĭ-sizm)   erotism.

eroticize (ĕ-rot′ĭ-sīz)   erotize.

eroticomania (ĕ-rot″ĭ-ko-ma′ne-ah)   erotomania.

erotism (er′o-tizm)   a sexual instinct or desire; the expression of one's instinctual energy or drive, especially the sex drive. **anal e.,** fixation of libido at (or regression to) the anal phase of infantile development, said in psychoanalytic

theory to produce egotistic, dogmatic, stubborn, miserly character. **oral e.,** 1. fixation of libido at (or regression to) the oral phase of infantile development, said in psychoanalytic theory to produce passive, insecure, sensitive character. 2. the pleasure derived from the use of the mouth for other than nutritional satisfactions.

erotize (er′o-tīz)   to endow with erotic or libidinous instinct or energy.

erot(o)- [Gr. *erōs* sexual desire]   a combining form denoting relationship to sexual desire.

erotogenesis (ĕ-ro″to-jen′ĕ-sis)   the formation or production of erotic feeling.

erotogenic (ĕ-ro″to-jen′ik) [*eroto-* + Gr. *gennan* to produce]   producing erotic feelings; erogenous.

erotomania (ĕ-rot″to-ma′ne-ah) [*eroto-* + Gr. *mania* madness]   pathologic preoccupation with sexual fantasies or activities.

erotopathy (er″o-top′ah-the) [*eroto-* + Gr. *pathos* disease]   (*obs.*) disorder of the sexual impulse.

erotophobia (ĕ-ro″to-fo′be-ah) [*eroto-* + *phobia*]   fear of love, especially of sexual feelings and activity.

ERPF   effective renal plasma flow; see under *flow*.

erratic (ĕ-rat′ik) [L. *errare* to wander]   1. roving or wandering. 2. eccentric; deviating from an accepted course of thought or conduct.

errhine (er′īn) [Gr. *en* in + *rhis* nose]   1. promoting a nasal discharge. 2. a medicine that promotes nasal discharge or secretion.

error (er′or)   a defect in structure or function; a deviation. **inborn e. of metabolism,** see under *metabolism*. **random e.,** error in a measurement process that varies randomly from measurement to measurement; it is measurable by statistical methods. **systematic e.,** error in a measurement process that is in the same direction in all measurements; it may not be detectable by statistical methods. Called also *bias*. **Type I e.,** in a hypothesis test, the rejection of the null hypothesis when it is true; the probability of a Type I error (the significance level) is denoted by α. **Type II e.,** in a hypothesis test, accepting the null hypothesis when it is false; the probability of a Type II error is denoted by β.

Ertron (er′tron)   trademark for preparations of ergocalciferol (vitamin D_2).

erucic acid (ĕ-roo′sik)   an unsaturated fatty acid, *cis*-13-docosenoic acid, found in rape seed and mustard oils.

eructation (ĕ-ruk-ta′shun) [L. *eructatio*]   the act of belching, or of casting up wind from the stomach through the mouth.

eruption (e-rup′shun) [L. *eruptio* a breaking out]   1. the act of breaking out, appearing, or becoming visible, as eruption of the teeth (see *tooth e.*). 2. visible efflorescent lesions of the skin due to disease, especially an exanthematous disease, and marked by redness and prominence; a rash. See also *exanthem*. **active e.,** the continued eruption of the teeth after complete formation of their dentinal roots, consisting of movement of the teeth in the direction of the occlusal plane, and being coordinated with attrition. **continuous e.,** a concept that tooth eruption continues throughout life and does not cease when teeth meet their functional antagonists. See also *active e.* and *passive e.* **creeping e.,** 1. cutaneous larva migrans. 2. a term used to describe the development of migratory lesions corresponding to the movements of various parasites beneath the skin, such as occurs in cutaneous larva migrans and cutaneous migratory myiasis. **delayed e.,** see under *dentition*. **drug e.,** an adverse cutaneous reaction produced by ingestion, parenteral use, or local application of a drug, which may produce various morphologic patterns and types of lesions. Called also *dermatitis medicamentosa* and *drug rash*. **fixed e.,** a circumscribed inflammatory skin lesion(s) that recurs at the same site(s) over a period of months or years; each attack lasts only a few days but leaves residual pigmentation which is cumulative. **fixed drug e.,** a drug eruption that recurs at the same site; see *fixed e.* **Kaposi's varicelliform e.,** a generalized and serious vesiculopustular, umbilicated eruption of viral origin, superimposed upon a preexisting atopic dermatitis; it may be caused by the virus of herpes simplex (eczema herpeticum) or vaccinia (eczema vaccinatum). Called also *pustulosis vacciniformis* (or *varioliformis*) *acuta*. **passive e.,** the apparent eruption of a tooth that is actually the exposure of the crown of the tooth by separation of the epithelial attachment from the enamel and migration to the cementoenamel junction. **polymorphous light e.,** a cutaneous eruption occurring after exposure to sunlight without evidence of any other precipitating factor, which may consist of papular, papulovesicular, nodular, eczematoid, or plaquelike lesions. **seabather's e.,** marine dermatitis. **serum e.,** an eruption or exanthem accompanying serum sickness. **surgical e.,** surgical removal of tissue blocking an unerupted tooth to permit eruption. **tooth e.,** the final stage of odontogenesis, in which a tooth breaks out from its crypt through surrounding tissue.

eruptive (e-rup′tiv) pertaining to or characterized by eruption.

ERV expiratory reserve volume; see under *volume*.

Erwinia (er-win′e-ah) [*Erwin F. Smith*, American bacteriologist, 1854–1927] a genus of gram-negative, facultatively anaerobic, rod-shaped bacteria of the family Enterobacteriaceae, made up of plant pathogens, epiphytes, and saprophytes. The genus includes organisms formerly classified as *Pectobacterium*. **E. amylo′vora,** a species that causes fire blight of apples and pears, rarely isolated from humans. **E. caroto′vora,** a species that causes soft spots in carrots, potatoes, and other plants; not found in clinical specimens. **E. herbic′ola,** a species found on plant surfaces, and occasionally isolated from human clinical specimens. It has been associated with nosocomial septicemia. Called also *Enterobacter agglomerans*.

Erwinieae (er″wĭ-ni′e-e) in some systems of classification, a tribe of gram-negative, facultatively anaerobic, rod-shaped bacteria of the family Enterobacteriaceae, made up of the genera *Erwinia* and *Pectobacterium*.

erysipelas (er″ĭ-sip′ĕ-las) [Gr. *erythros* red + *pella* skin] an acute superficial form of cellulitis involving the dermal lymphatics, usually caused by infection with group A streptococci, and chiefly characterized by a peripherally spreading hot, bright red, edematous, brawny, infiltrated, and sharply circumscribed plaque with a raised indurated border. Formerly called *St. Anthony's fire.* Cf. *cellulitis* and *phlegmon*, def. 1. **coast e.** (Sp. *erisipela de la costa*), a cutaneous manifestation of onchocerciasis seen in Central America, so called because of its resemblance to streptococcal erysipelas, characterized by an erythematous macular rash and edema of the face; in chronic cases the skin loses its elasticity, atrophies, becomes wrinkled, and causes leonine facies. **gangrenous e.,** necrotizing fasciitis. **e. gra′ve inter′num,** erysipelas in the vagina, uterus, and peritoneum; a form of puerperal fever. **malignant e.,** one of the forms of puerperal fever. **necrotizing e.,** see under *fasciitis*. **swine e.,** a contagious disease of swine of worldwide distribution, caused by *Erysipelothrix rhusiopathiae* (*E. insidiosa*). Of great economic importance, it occurs in four clinical forms: An *acute septicemic form*, marked by high fever, lesions of the internal organs and viscera, and a high mortality rate. An *urticarial form*, marked by sudden onset, high fever, general debility, formation of reddish or purplish quadrangular or rhomboid blotches on the neck and body and sometimes by involvement of the viscera; this is the mildest form and is rarely fatal. Called also *diamonds, diamond skin disease, rose disease,* and *rouget du porc.* A *chronic form*, marked by difficulty in breathing, vegetative endocarditis, and ultimately death. An *arthritic form*, marked by stunting of growth; this form may occur alone or may complicate other forms of the disease, and is not usually fatal.

erysipelatous (er″ĭ-sĭ-pel′ah-tus) pertaining to or of the nature of erysipelas.

erysipeloid (er″ĭ-sip′ĕ-loid) [*erysipelas* + *-oid*] 1. bacterial cellulitis due to infection with *Erysipelothrix rhusiopathiae*, usually occurring as an occupational disease associated with the handling of infected fish, shellfish, meat, or poultry. It presents in three forms: in a usually self-limited, mild localized form manifested by an erythematous and painful swelling at the site of inoculation, which spreads peripherally with central clearing; in a generalized or diffuse form, which may be accompanied by fever and arthritis symptoms, and resolves spontaneously; and in a rare and sometimes fatal systemic form associated with endocarditis. 2. loosely, erysipelas-like.

Erysipelothrix (er″ĭ-sip′ĕ-lo-thriks″) [*erysipelas* + Gr. *thrix* hair] a genus of bacteria of uncertain affiliation, consisting of gram-positive, asporogenous, rod-shaped organisms

that form long filaments. They occur as parasites in mammals, birds, and fish. **E. insidio′sa,** *E. rhusiopathiae*. **E. rhusiopath′iae,** a species widely distributed in nature, the cause of swine erysipelas. It is the etiologic agent of an erysipeloid disease in humans following contact with injected fish, meats, hides, or bones (see *erysipeloid*). Called also *E. insidiosa* and *swine rotlauf bacillus*.

erysipelotoxin (er″ĭ-sip″ĕ-lo-tok′sin) the toxin produced by certain strains of *Streptococcus pyogenes* in bacterial erysipelas.

Erysiphaceae (er-is″ĭ-fa′se-e) a family of fungi of the order Erysiphales, series Pyrenomycetes, which are plant pathogens and include the genus *Erysiphe*.

erysiphake (er-is′ĭ-fāk) [Gr. *erysis* a drawing + *phakos* lentil] an instrument for removing the lens in cataract by suction. Cf. *phacoerysis*.

Erysiphales (er-is″ĭ-fa′lēz) the powdery mildews, an order of ascomycetous fungi of the series Pyrenomycetes, subclass Euascomycetidae, which are parasitic on higher plants and usually have closed ascocarps and large spherical stalked asci; it includes the family Erysiphaceae.

Erysiphe (er-is′ĭ-fe) a genus of ascomycetous fungi of the family Erysiphaceae, order Erysiphales, including *E. polygoni*, the powdery mildews; its imperfect (sexual) stage is *Oidium*.

erythema (er″ĭ-the′mah) [Gr. *erythēma* flush upon the skin] a name applied to redness of the skin produced by congestion of the capillaries, which may result from a variety of causes, the etiology or a specific type of lesion often being indicated by a modifying term. **e. ab ig′ne,** permanent erythema or a brown to red reticulated residual pigmentation produced by prolonged exposure to excessive nonburning heat. It is seen most often on the legs of women, but under appropriate environmental circumstances, it can occur anywhere on the body in either sex. **e. annula′re,** 1. gyrate erythema in which the lesions are ring shaped. 2. e. marginatum rheumaticum. **e. annula′re centrif′ugum,** an often mild but chronic and recurrent form of gyrate erythema characterized by the occurrence of crops of annular wheal-like lesions with edematous, sometimes vesicular, borders and commonly a yellowish central region that exhibits a fine branny scaling, which may coalesce. Called also *e. figuratum perstans* and *e. gyratum perstans*. **e. annula′re rheumat′icum,** e. marginatum rheumaticum. **e. arthrit′icum epidem′icum,** Haverhill fever. **e. calor′icum,** that caused by exposure to heat or cold. See *e. ab igne* and *cold e.* **e. chro′micum figura′tum melanoder′micum,** e. dyschromicum perstans. **e. chron′icum mi′grans,** a deep form of gyrate erythema characterized by the development at the site of a bite by an ixodid tick of a red papule that expands slowly, producing an annular lesion with central clearing, and often associated with systemic symptoms, including chills, fever, headache, malaise, vomiting, backache, and stiff neck; a similar clinical presentation has been seen in association with a mosquito bite or with no history of a preceding bite. See also *Lyme arthritis*, under *arthritis*. **e. circina′tum, e. circina′tum rheumat′icum,** e. marginatum rheumaticum. **cold e.,** a congenital hypersensitivity to cold seen in children, characterized by localized pain, widespread erythema, occasional muscle spasms, and vascular collapse on exposure to cold, and vomiting after drinking cold liquids. **diaper e.,** see under *dermatitis*. **e. dyschro′micum per′stans,** an idiopathic dermatosis occurring predominantly in dark-skinned individuals, particularly in Latin Americans, characterized by the presence of single or multiple sharply demarcated ashen macules of variable size and shape, which in their acute phase have a fine erythematous border. Called also *ashy dermatitis, ashy dermatosis of Ramirez, dermatosis cinecienta,* and *e. chromicum figuratum melanodermicum*. **e. eleva′tum diu′tinum,** a benign cutaneous, small vessel vasculitis of unknown etiology characterized by the development of red, brown, purple, and orange-yellow nodules and plaques, usually on the acral extremities and buttocks, which are sometimes associated with erosions, ulcers, and vesiculopustules. The lesions exhibit polymorphonuclear neutrophils and nuclear fragments infiltrating vessel walls in association with fibrinoid material, and lymphocytes, plasma cells, and eosinophils can be seen in perivascular and stromal locations. Intracellular and extracellular lipid deposits, chiefly cholesterol esters, occur in chronic lesions. See also *extracellular cholesterosis*, under *cholesterosis*. **epidemic**

e., acrodynia. **epidemic arthritic e.,** Haverhill fever. **figurate e., e. figura'tum,** gyrate e. **e. figura'tum per'stans,** e. annulare centrifugum. **e. fu'gax,** redness of the skin that comes and goes quickly. **gyrate e., e. gyra'tum,** erythema multiforme characterized by the development of gyrate, figurate, circinate, annular, arcuate, polycyclic, serpiginous, or reticulate lesions that tend to migrate and spread peripherally with central clearing. There are three basic types: *erythema annulare centrifugum, erythema chronicum migrans,* and *erythema gyratum repens.* Called also *figurate e.* and *e. figuratum.* **e. gyra'tum per'stans,** e. annulare centrifugum. **e. gyra'tum re'pens,** a superficial form of gyrate erythema almost always associated with internal malignancy, which is characterized by the presence of migratory wavy bands of slightly elevated erythema with a scaly collarette over the entire body, and sometimes accompanied by pruritus. **e. indura'tum,** a type of panniculitis characterized histologically by the presence of granulomas, vasculitis, and caseation necrosis, traditionally considered to be the tuberculous counterpart of nodular vasculitis, but now known often to occur without tuberculous causation, although of uncertain etiology. It is seen most commonly in adolescent and menopausal women, is initiated or exacerbated by cold weather, and typically presents as one or more recurrent erythrocyanotic nodules or plaques on the calves, which may progress to form deep-seated indurations, ulcerations, and scars. Those cases of tuberculous origin are called also *Bazin's disease, tuberculosis cutis indurativa,* and *tuberculosis indurativa.* **e. infectio'sum,** a moderately contagious, benign epidemic disease seen mainly in children, probably of viral etiology, and characterized by the abrupt onset of a rash, which occurs in three stages: livid erythema appears on the cheeks, giving them the appearance of having been slapped; an erythematous maculopapular rash then involves the trunk and extremities; the rash fades with central clearing, leaving a lacelike pattern. Called also *fifth disease,* and *Sticker's disease.* **e. i'ris,** the characteristic bull's eye or targetlike lesion of erythema multiforme. **Jacquet's e.,** diaper dermatitis. **e. margina'tum,** e. marginatum rheumaticum. **e. margina'tum rheumat'icum,** a superficial, often asymptomatic, form of gyrate erythema associated with some cases of rheumatic fever, which is characterized by the presence on the trunk and extensor surfaces of the extremities of a transient eruption of flat to slightly indurated, nonscaling, and usually multiple lesions. Called also *e. annulare, e. annulare rheumaticum, e. circinatum, e. circinatum rheumaticum,* and *e. marginatum.* **e. mi'grans,** benign migratory glossitis. **Milian's e.,** a scarlatiniform eruption with malaise and fever, occurring seven to nine days after injection of arsphenamine, or as a toxic reaction to other drugs; called also *ninth-day e.* **e. multifor'me,** a symptom complex representing a reaction pattern of the skin and mucous membranes secondary to various known, suspected, and unknown factors, including infections, ingestants, physical agents, malignancy, and pregnancy. The conditions in the complex are characterized by the sudden onset of an erythematous macular, bullous, papular, nodose, or vesicular eruption, the characteristic lesion being the iris, bull's eye, or target lesion, which consists of a central papule with two or more concentric rings. The complex comprises a mild self-limited mucocutaneous form (*e. multiforme minor*) and a severe, sometimes fatal, multisystem form (*Stevens-Johnson syndrome*). **e. multifor'me ma'jor,** Stevens-Johnson syndrome. **e. multifor'me mi'nor,** a mild self-limited mucocutaneous form of erythema multiforme that may have a prodrome of fever, cough, and pharyngitis. In addition to the characteristic iris lesions, erythematous macules and papules, purpura, and occasional vesiculobullous lesions may be present, which are usually asymptomatic, but may burn or itch slightly. Called also *Hebra's disease.* **necrolytic migratory e.,** a generalized symmetrical scaling eczematous dermatitis, followed by migratory necrolysis of the upper epidermis, liquefaction of the granular layer, and subcorneal clefting, flaccid bulla formation, erosions, crusts, and postinflammatory hyperpigmentation, which is seen on the central third of the face, lower abdomen, perineum, groin, buttocks, thighs, and distal extremities. It usually occurs in association with a glucagon-secreting tumor of the alpha cells of the pancreas. See also *glucagonoma syndrome,* under *syndrome.* **e. necrot'icans,** Lucio's phenomenon. **ninth-day e.,** Milian's e. **e. nodo'sum,** a type of panniculitis occurring usually as a hypersensitivity reaction to multiple provoking agents, including various infections, especially beta-hemolytic streptococcal infections and tuberculosis; drugs, especially oral contraceptives and sulfonamides; sarcoidosis; and certain enteropathies. It may also be of idiopathic origin. It most often affects young women and is characterized by the development of crops of transient, inflammatory, nonulcerating nodules that are usually tender, multiple, and bilateral, and most commonly located on the shins; the lesions involute slowly, leaving bruiselike patches without scarring. The acute disease is often associated with mild constitutional symptoms, including fever, malaise, and arthralgias. A chronic variant sometimes occurs without any serious associated systemic disease. See also *e. nodosum migrans.* **e. nodo'sum lepro'sum,** a recurrent Arthus-like lepra reaction occurring during the course of chemotherapy in lepromatous leprosy, sometimes in the borderline form, and occasionally spontaneously, usually characterized histologically by vasculitis and clinically by the appearance of crops of small erythematous, tender cutaneous nodules or plaques, which are widely distributed, especially on the extremities and face; it may be associated with severe systemic symptoms and visceral manifestations. Cf. *Lucio's phenomenon.* **e. nodo'sum mi'grans,** a variant of erythema nodosum in which the lesions are asymmetrical, often unilateral, usually less acute and less numerous than those in the classic disorder, and characterized by the coalescence and clearing of older central nodules and formation of new lesions nearby, which gives the appearance of migration. *Subacute nodular migratory panniculitis* may be the same variant. **palmar e., e palma're,** persistent redness of the palms, which may be seen in pregnancy, liver disease, rheumatoid arthritis, regional ileitis, and certain skin diseases, e.g., psoriasis, pityriasis rubra pilaris, and genodermatoses, and rarely as an autosomal dominant condition. **e. per'nio,** chilblain. **e. streptog'enes,** pityriasis alba. **toxic e., e. tox'icum,** a generalized, diffuse erythematous eruption or a widespread erythematomacular eruption occurring as a result of hypersensitivity to certain foods or drugs, or caused by bacterial or other toxins, or associated with various systemic diseases. **e. tox'icum neonato'rum,** a benign, idiopathic, very common, generalized, transient eruption occurring in infants during the first week of life, usually consisting of small papules or pustules that become sterile, yellow-white, firm vesicles surrounded by an erythematous halo and some edema.

erythematous (er″ĭ-them′ah-tus) characterized by erythema.

erythemogenic (er″ĭ-the″mo-jen′ik) causing erythema.

Erythraea (er″ĭ-thre′ah) [Gr. *erythraios* red] a genus of red-flowered gentianaceous plants. *E. centau′rium,* the lesser centaury, and various other species are tonic and stomachic.

erythralgia (er″ĭ-thral′je-ah) [*erythro-* + *-algia*] erythromelalgia.

erythrasma (er″ĭ-thraz′mah) a chronic, superficial bacterial infection of the skin involving the body folds and toe webs, sometimes becoming generalized, caused by *Corynebacterium minutissimum,* and characterized by the presence of sharply demarcated, dry, brown, slightly scaly, and slowly spreading patches.

erythredema polyneuropathy (ĕ-rith″rĕ-de′mah pol″e-nu-rop′ah-the) [*erythro-* + Gr. *oidēma* swelling] acrodynia.

erythremia (er″ĭ-thre′me-ah) [*erythro-* + Gr. *haima* blood] polycythemia vera.

erythremomelalgia (er-ith″rĕ-mo-mel-al′je-ah) [Gr. *erythrēma* redness + *melos* limb + *-algia*] erythromelalgia.

Erythrina (er″ĭ-thri′nah) a genus of tropical shrubs and trees of the legume family, long used in native medicines. Several species yield the alkaloids α-erythroidine and β-erythroidine.

erythrism (ĕ-rith′rizm) redness of the hair and beard with a ruddy complexion.

erythristic (er″ĭ-thris′tik) characterized by erythrism. Called also *rufous.*

erythritol (ĕ-rith′rĭ-tol) chemical name: tetrahydroxybutane. A polyhydric alcohol, $CH_2OH(CHOH)_2CH_2OH$, occurring in algae, lichens, grasses, and several fungi; it is about twice as sweet as sucrose. Called also *erythrol.* See also *erythrityl.*

erythrityl (ĕ-rith′rĭ-til) the univalent radical C_4H_9 from erythritol. **e. tetranitrate,** chemical name: erythritol tetranitrate. A synthetic compound, $C_4H_6(NO_3)_4$, with actions similar to those of nitroglycerin. Percussion or excessive heat can cause undiluted erythrityl tetranitrate to explode. The official pharmaceutical preparations, prepared in accordance with USP standards, are used as a coronary vasodilator in the prophylaxis of angina pectoris and in long-term treatment of coronary insufficiency, administered orally or sublingually.

erythr(o)- [Gr. *erythros* red] a combining form meaning red, or denoting a relationship to red or to erythrocytes.

erythroblast (ĕ-rith′ro-blast) [*erythro-* + Gr. *blastos* germ] a term used by Ehrlich to indicate any type of nucleated erythrocyte, but now more generally, and somewhat inaccurately, used to designate an immature cell from which a red corpuscle develops. The precise position assigned to it in the red cell lineage varies with the specific theory of blood maturation being propounded. **acidophilic e.,** orthochromatic normoblast. **basophilic e.,** basophilic normoblast. **early e.,** basophilic normoblast. **eosinophilic e.,** orthochromatic normoblast. **intermediate e.,** polychromatic normoblast. **definitive e′s,** basophil cells in the primordium of the liver that give rise to the mature non-nucleated erythrocytes; cf. *primitive e′s.* **late e.,** orthochromatic normoblast. **orthochromatic e.,** orthochromatic normoblast. **oxyphilic e.,** orthochromatic normoblast. **polychromatic e.,** polychromatic normoblast. **primitive e′s,** cells arising from the blood islands of the yolk sac which are the precursors of the nucleated erythrocytes characteristic of the early embryo; cf. *definitive e′s.*

erythroblastemia (ĕ-rith″ro-blas-te′me-ah) the presence in the peripheral blood of abnormally large numbers of nucleated red cells; erythroblastosis.

erythroblastic (ĕ-rith″ro-blas′tik) of, or relating to, erythroblasts.

erythroblastoma (ĕ-rith″ro-blas-to′mah) a tumor-like mass composed of nucleated red blood corpuscles.

erythroblastomatosis (ĕ-rith″ro-blas″to-mah-to′sis) a condition marked by the formation of erythroblastomas.

erythroblastopenia (ĕ-rith″ro-blas″to-pe′ne-ah) abnormal deficiency of the erythroblasts; see *aplastic crisis,* under *crisis.*

erythroblastosis (ĕ-rith″ro-blas-to′sis) 1. the presence of erythroblasts in the circulating blood; erythroblastemia. 2. a disease of fowl classified in the avian leukosis complex, marked by an increase in the number of immature red blood cells in the circulating blood; called also *erythroleukosis.* **e. feta′lis, e. neonato′rum,** hemolytic anemia of the fetus or newborn infant, caused by the transplacental transmission of maternally formed antibody, usually secondary to an incompatibility between the blood group of the mother and that of her offspring, characterized by accelerated destruction of erythrocytes and consequent jaundice and by increased red cell regeneration (nucleated red cells in the blood) and hepatosplenomegaly. In infants with severe jaundice, kernicterus may result. The most severe form is *hydrops fetalis.* Called also *hemolytic disease of newborn.*

erythroblastotic (ĕ-rith″ro-blas-tot′ik) pertaining to or characterized by erythroblastosis.

erythrocatalysis (ĕ-rith″ro-kah-tal′ĭ-sis) erythrokatalysis.

erythrochromia (ĕ-rith″ro-kro′me-ah) [*erythro-* + Gr. *chrōma,* color] hemorrhagic pigmentation of the spinal fluid, giving it a red color.

Erythrocin (ĕ-rith′ro-sin) trademark for a preparation of erythromycin.

erythroclasis (er″ĕ-throk′lah-sis) [*erythro-* + Gr. *klasis* a breaking] fragmentation or splitting up of red blood cells.

erythroclast (ĕ-rith′ro-klast) [*erythro-* + Gr. *klastos* broken] a degenerating or fragmented erythrocyte with no hemoglobin; called also *ghost cell* (def. 2) and *shadow cell.*

erythroclastic (ĕ-rith″ro-klas′tik) pertaining to, characterized by, or producing erythroclasis.

erythrocruorin (ĕ-rith″ro-kroo′o-rin) a respiratory protein from the blood of the marine worm, *Spirographis spallanzanii,* and certain other worms.

erythrocuprein (ĕ-rith″ro-koo′prin) superoxide dismutase.

erythrocyanosis (ĕ-rith″ro-si″ah-no′sis) [*erythro-* + *cyano-*

sis] a condition seen in young girls and women following prolonged exposure to cold, characterized by the presence of a slight swelling and a bluish pink tint of the skin of the legs and thighs.

erythrocytapheresis (ĕ-rith″ro-si″tah-fĕ-re′-sis) [*erythrocyte* + Gr. *aphairesis* removal] the withdrawal of blood, separation and retention of red blood cells, and retransfusion of the remainder into the donor.

erythrocyte (ĕ-rith′ro-sīt) [*erythro-* + Gr. *kytos* hollow vessel] one of the elements found in peripheral blood; called also *red blood cell* or *corpuscle.* Normally, in the human, the mature form is a non-nucleated, yellowish, biconcave disk, adapted, by virtue of its configuration and its hemoglobin content, to transport oxygen. For immature forms in the erythrocytic series, see *normoblast.* **achromic e.,** a colorless erythrocyte; see *achromocyte.* **basophilic e.,** one that takes the basic stain; see *basophilia* (def. 1). **burr e.,** burr cell. **crenated e.,** an erythrocyte that shows a scalloped border. **hypochromic e.,** one that contains less than the normal concentration of hemoglobin and as a result appears paler than normal; it is usually also microcytic. Cf. *normochromic e.* **immature e.,** any erythrocyte prior to achievement of its complete development; see *normoblast* and *rubicyte.* **"Mexican hat" e.,** target cell. **normochromic e.,** one of normal color with a normal concentration of hemoglobin; cf. *hypochromic e.* **nucleated e.,** any of the immature forms of an erythrocyte, e.g., a normoblast. **orthochromatic e.,** one that takes only the acid stain. **polychromatic e., polychromatophilic e.,** an erythrocyte that, on staining, shows various shades of blue, combined with tinges of pink. **target e.,** see under *cell.*

erythrocythemia (ĕ-rith″ro-si-the′me-ah) an increase in the number of erythrocytes in the blood, as in erythrocytosis and polycythemia vera.

erythrocytic (ĕ-rith″ro-sit′ik) 1. pertaining to, characterized by, or of the nature of erythrocytes. 2. pertaining to the erythrocytic series; see under *series.*

erythrocytoblast (ĕ-rith″ro-si′to-blast) erythroblast.

erythrocytolysin (ĕ-rith″ro-si-tol′ĭ-sin) a substance that causes dissolution of erythrocytes and escape of hemoglobin.

erythrocytolysis (ĕ-rith″ro-si-tol′ĭ-sis) [*erythrocyte* + Gr. *lysis* dissolution] dissolution of erythrocytes and escape of the hemoglobin.

erythrocytometer (ĕ-rith″ro-si-tom′ĕ-ter) [*erythrocyte* + Gr. *metron* measure] a device for measuring or counting erythrocytes.

erythrocytometry (ĕ-rith″ro-si-tom′ĕ-tre) the measurement or counting of erythrocytes.

erythrocyto-opsonin (ĕ-rith″ro-si″to-op-so′nin) [*erythrocyte* + *opsonin*] hemopsonin.

erythrocytopenia (ĕ-rith″ro-si″to-pe′ne-ah) erythropenia.

erythrocytophagous (ĕ-rith″ro-si-to-tof′ah-gus) pertaining to or characterized by erythrocytophagy.

erythrocytophagy (ĕ-rith″ro-si-tof′ah-je) [*erythrocyte* + Gr. *phagein* to devour] the engulfment or consumption of erythrocytes by other cells, such as the histiocytes of the reticuloendothelial system.

erythrocytopoiesis (ĕ-rith″ro-si″to-poi-e′sis) erythropoiesis.

erythrocytorrhexis (ĕ-rith″ro-si″to-rek′sis) [*erythrocyte* + Gr. *rhēxis* rending] a morphological change in erythrocytes, consisting in the escape from the cells of round, shiny granules and the splitting off of particles.

erythrocytoschisis (ĕ-rith″ro-si-tos′kĭ-sis) [*erythrocyte* + Gr. *schisis* division] a morphological change in erythrocytes, consisting in the degeneration of the cells into disklike bodies similar to the blood platelets.

erythrocytosis (ĕ-rith″ro-si-to′sis) any absolute increase in the total red cell mass secondary to any of a number of nonhematopoietic systemic disorders in response to a known stimulus (*secondary polycythemia* [q.v.]), in contrast to erythremic or primary polycythemia (polycythemia vera). **leukemic e., e. megalosplen′ica,** polycythemia vera. **stress e.,** see under *polycythemia.*

erythrocyturia (ĕ-rith″ro-si-tu′re-ah) hematuria.

erythrodegenerative (ĕ-rith″ro-de-jen′er-a″tiv) characterized by degeneration of erythrocytes.

erythroderma (ĕ-rith″ro-der′mah) [*erythro-* + Gr. *derma* skin] 1. abnormal redness of the skin, usually applied to a condition of abnormal redness over widespread areas of the body. 2. exfoliative dermatitis. Called also *erythrodermia*. **congenital ichthyosiform e., bullous,** epidermolytic hyperkeratosis. **congenital ichthyosiform e., nonbullous,** former name for *lamellar ichthyosis*. **e. desquamati'vum,** Leiner's disease. **e. psoriat'icum,** erythrodermic psoriasis. **Sézary e.,** see under *syndrome*.

erythrodermia (ĕ-rith″ro-der′me-ah) erythroderma.

erythrodextrin (ĕ-rith″ro-dek′strin) a dextrin, *e-dextrin*, which is turned red by iodine and changed by various digestive enzymes into maltose.

erythrodontia (ĕ-rith″ro-don′she-ah) [*erythro-* + Gr. *odous* tooth] reddish brown pigmentation of the teeth.

erythrogen (ĕ-rith′ro-jen) a fatty, crystalline compound from diseased bile.

erythrogenesis (ĕ-rith″ro-jen′ĕ-sis) the production of erythrocytes. **e. imperfec'ta,** congenital hypoplastic anemia, def. 1.

erythrogenic (ĕ-rith″ro-jen′ik) [*erythro-* + Gr. *gennan* to produce] 1. producing erythrocytes. 2. producing a sensation of red. 3. producing or causing erythema.

erythrogone (ĕ-rith′ro-gōn) promegaloblast.

erythrogonium (ĕ-rith″ro-go′ne-um) [*erythro*cyte + Gr. *gonē* seed] promegaloblast.

erythrogranulose (ĕ-rith″ro-gran′u-lōs) an amylodextrin colored red by iodine.

erythroid (er″ĭ-throid) 1. of a red color; reddish. 2. pertaining to the developmental series of cells ending in erythrocytes.

β-erythroidine (ĕ-rith′roi-din) an alkaloid, $C_{16}H_{19}NO_3$ from *Erythrina americana*: it has a curare-like action.

erythrokatalysis (ĕ-rith″ro-kah-tal′ĭ-sis) [*erythro-* + Gr. *katalysis* dissolution] the dissolution of erythrocytes; erythrocytolysis.

erythrokeratodermia (ĕ-rith″ro-ker″ah-to-der′me-ah) a reddening and hyperkeratosis of the skin. **e. varia'bilis,** a very rare autosomal dominant form of ichthyosis characterized by the presence at birth of two types of lesions: transient, migratory areas of discrete macular erythroderma with angular, arcuate, gyrate, and circinate configurations as well as fixed hyperkeratotic plaques.

erythrokinetics (ĕ-rith″ro-ki-net′iks) [*erythro*cyte + Gr. *kinētikos* of or for putting in motion] the kinetics of erythrocytes, described by laboratory measurements of total red cell volume, rate of red cell production, and red cell life-span (rate of destruction).

erythrol (er′ith-rol) erythritol. **e. tetranitrate,** erythrityl tetranitrate.

erythrolabe (ĕ-rith′ro-lāb) [*erythro-* + Gr. *lambanein* to take] name proposed for the pigment in retinal cones that is more sensitive to the red range of the spectrum than are the other pigments (chlorolabe and cyanolabe).

erythrolein (er″ĭ-thro′le-in) the ether-soluble fraction of the acid-precipitable part of the water-soluble pigments of litmus, occurring as a red oily substance.

erythroleukemia (ĕ-rith″ro-lu-ke′me-ah) a malignant blood dyscrasia, one of the myeloproliferative disorders, characterized by neoplastic proliferation of erythroblastic and myeloblastic elements, with atypical erythroblasts and myeloblasts in the peripheral blood, and showing a variable (acute or chronic) clinical course. Called also *di Guglielmo's disease* or *syndrome*. Cf. *erythremic myelosis*.

erythroleukoblastosis (ĕ-rith″ro-lu″ko-blas-to′sis) icterus gravis neonatorum.

erythroleukosis (ĕ-rith″ro-lu-ko′sis) 1. a condition seen in malaria in which the erythrocytes are changed into brassy bodies. 2. erythroblastosis, def. 2.

erythroleukothrombocythemia (ĕ-rith″ro-lu″ko-throm″bo-si-the′me-ah) di Guglielmo's term for hyperplasia of the erythroblastic, leukoblastic, and megakaryocytic tissue, with the appearance of immature cells in the blood.

erythrolitmin (e-rith″ro-lit′min) the alcohol-soluble fraction of the acid-precipitable part of the water-soluble pigments of litmus, occurring as a bright red powder.

erythrolysin (er″ĭ-throl′ĭ-sin) erythrocytolysin.

erythrolysis (er″ĭ-throl′ĭ-sis) erythrocytolysis.

erythromelalgia (ĕ-rith″ro-mel-al′je-ah) [*erythro-* + Gr. *me-*

los limb + *-algia*] a disease affecting chiefly the extremities of the body, the feet more often than the hands, and marked by paroxysmal, bilateral vasodilatation, particularly of the extremities, with burning pain, and increased skin temperature and redness; called also *erythremomel, acromelalgia*, and *Gerhardt's, Mitchell's*, or *Weir Mitchell's disease*. **e. of the head,** a severe recurring headache caused by vascular dilatation, both induced by and cured by doses of histamine.

erythrometer (er″ĭ-throm′ĕ-ter) [*erythro-* + *-meter*] 1. an instrument or color scale for measuring degrees of redness. 2. erythrocytometer.

erythrometry (er″ĭ-throm′ĕ-tre) 1. the measurement of the degree of redness. 2. erythrocytometry.

erythromycin (ĕ-rith″ro-mi′sin) [USP] an intermediate spectrum macrolide antibiotic, $C_{37}H_{67}NO_{13}$, produced by *Streptomyces erythreus*, occurring as a slightly yellow, crystalline powder, effective against most gram-positive and certain gram-negative bacteria, such as *Neisseria* and *Haemophilus influenzae*, and against spirochetes, some rickettsias, and *Entamoeba*, and highly effective against *Mycoplasma pneumoniae*; used in the treatment of infections due to susceptible organisms, especially in patients allergic to penicillin, in penicillin-resistant infections, and in legionnaire's disease, administered orally or topically. **e. B,** berythromycin. **e. estolate** [USP], the lauryl sulfate ester of propionyl erythromycin, $C_{40}H_{71}NO_{14}·C_{12}H_{26}O_4S$, occurring as a white, crystalline powder, having the same actions and uses as the base; administered orally. **e. ethylcarbonate,** a salt of erythromycin, $C_{40}H_{71}NO_{15}$, used for oral administration. **e. ethylsuccinate** [USP], a salt of erythromycin, $C_{43}H_{75}NO_{16}$, occurring as a white or slightly yellow crystalline powder, having the same actions and uses as the base; administered orally or intramuscularly. **e. gluceptate** [USP], a salt of erythromycin, $C_{37}H_{67}NO_{13}·C_7H_{14}O_8$, occurring as a white powder, having the same actions and uses as the base; administered by intravenous infusion. **e. lactobionate** [USP], a salt of erythromycin, $C_{37}H_{67}NO_{13}·C_{12}H_{22}O_{12}$, occurring as white or slightly yellow crystals or powder, having the same actions and uses as the base; administered by intravenous infusion. **e. propionate,** a salt of erythromycin, $C_{40}H_{71}NO_{14}$, suitable for oral use. **e. propionate lauryl sulfate,** former name for *e. estolate*. **e. stearate** [USP], a salt of erythromycin, $C_{37}H_{67}NO_{13}·C_{18}H_{36}O_2$, suitable for oral use.

erythromyeloblastosis (ĕ-rith″ro-mi″ĕ-lo-blas-to′sis) a neoplastic disease of chickens caused by a fowl tumor virus.

erythron (er′ĭ-thron) [Gr. *erythros* red] the circulating erythrocytes in the blood, their precursors, and all the elements of the body concerned in their production; it is the counterpart of the leukon and thrombon.

erythroneocytosis (ĕ-rith″ro-ne″o-si-to′sis) [*erythro-* + Gr. *neos* new + *kytos* hollow vessel] the presence of immature erythrocytes in the blood.

erythronoclastic (ĕ-rith″ro-no-klas′tik) causing lysis or destruction of erythron.

erythroparasite (ĕ-rith″ro-par′ah-sīt) a parasite of erythrocytes.

erythropathy (er″ĭ-throp′ah-the) [*erythro-* + Gr. *pathos* disease] an archaic term for any disorder of the erythrocytes.

erythropenia (ĕ-rith″ro-pe′ne-ah) [*erythro-* + Gr. *penia* poverty] deficiency in the number of erythrocytes; called also *erythrocytopenia*.

erythrophage (ĕ-rith′ro-fāj) [*erythro-* + Gr. *phagein* to eat] a phagocyte that takes up erythrocytes and blood pigments.

erythrophagia (ĕ-rith″ro-fa′je-ah) erythrocytophagy.

erythrophagocytosis (ĕ-rith″ro-fag″o-si-to′sis) erythrocytophagy.

erythrophagous (er″ĭ-throf′ah-gus) erythrocytophagous.

erythrophil (ĕ-rith′ro-fil) [*erythro-* + Gr. *philein* to love] 1. a cell or other element that is easily stained red. 2. erythrophilous.

erythrophilous (er″ĭ-throf′ĭ-lus) easily stained with red.

Erythrophloeum (ĕ-rith″ro-fle′um) [*erythro-* + Gr. *phloios* bark] a genus of leguminous trees. *E. guineen'se* affords casca or Mancona bark, an African ordeal poison.

erythrophobia (ĕ-rith″ro-fo′be-ah) [*erythro-* + *phobia*] 1. irrational fear of the color red, often accompanied by fear of blood (hematophobia).　2. fear of blushing; a distressing tendency to blush frequently.

erythrophobic (ĕ-rith″ro-fo′bik)　having no affinity for red dye (acid fuchsin).

erythrophore (ĕ-rith′ro-fōr) [*erythro-* + Gr. *phoros* bearing] a chromatophore containing granules of a red or brown alcohol-resistant pigment; called also *allophore.*

erythrophose (ĕ-rith′ro-fōz) [*erythro-* + Gr. *phōs* light] any red phose.

erythrophyll (ĕ-rith′ro-fil) [*erythro-* + Gr. *phyllon* leaf] a red coloring matter occurring in plants.

erythropia (er″ĕ-thro′pe-ah)　erythropsia.

erythroplakia (ĕ-rith″ro-pla′ke-ah) [*erythro-* + Gr. *plax* plate + *-ia*]　erythroplasia of Queyrat involving the oral mucosa.　**speckled e.,** see *e. of Queyrat.*

erythroplasia (ĕ-rith″ro-pla′ze-ah)　a condition of the mucous membrane characterized by erythematous papular lesions.　**e. of Queyrat,** a form of epithelial dysplasia, which may range in severity from mild disorientation of epithelial cells with variable cellular pleomorphism to changes of carcinoma in situ and even invasive carcinoma, usually found on the glans penis and prepuce, although it rarely involves the lips, oral mucosa, tongue, vulva, and glabrous skin. It is typically characterized by the development of a slowly growing, circumscribed, erythematous, usually moist, velvety, and shiny patch. Lesions in the oral cavity may be interspersed with patches of leukoplakia, giving the affected area a "speckled" appearance; this form is called also *erythroplakia.*　**Zoon's e.,** balanitis circumscripta plasmacellularis.

erythroplastid (ĕ-rith″ro-plas′tid)　a red blood cell of mammalian animals, characterized by having no nucleus.

erythropoiesis (ĕ-rith″ro-poi-e′sis) [*erythro-* + Gr. *poiēsis* making]　the production of erythrocytes.

erythropoietic (ĕ-rith″ro-poi-et′ik)　pertaining to, characterized by, or promoting erythropoiesis.

erythropoietin (ĕ-rith″ro-poi′ĕ-tin)　a glycoprotein hormone secreted chiefly by the kidney in the adult and by the liver in the fetus, which acts on stem cells of the bone marrow to stimulate red blood cell production (erythropoiesis).

erythroprosopalgia (ĕ-rith″ro-pros″o-pal′je-ah) [*erythro-* + Gr. *prosōpon* face + *-algia*]　a nervous disorder, analogous to erythromelalgia, marked by redness and pain in the face.

erythropsia (er″ĭ-throp′se-ah) [*erythro-* + *-opsia*]　a chromatopsia in which all objects appear to have a red tinge, a symptom of aphakia.

erythropsin (er″ĕ-throp′sin) [*erythro-* + Gr. *opsis* vision] rhodopsin.

erythropyknosis (ĕ-rith″ro-pik-no′sis) [*erythro-* + *pyknosis*] pyknosis.

erythrorrhexis (ĕ-rith″ro-rek′sis) [*erythro-* + Gr. *rhēxis* rupture]　erythrocytorrhexis.

erythrose (er″ĭ-thrōs)　one of the aldotetroses.　**e. péribuccale pigmentaire of Brocq,** a patchy facial melanoderma seen chiefly in women that may involve an inflammatory photosensitivity, perhaps phototoxic, reaction, and characterized by the presence of a combination of erythema and a diffuse brownish red pigmentation of the perioral region.

erythrosedimentation (ĕ-rith″ro-sed″ĭ-men-ta′shun)　the sedimentation of erythrocytes; see *erythrocyte sedimentation rate,* under *rate.*

erythrosin (ĕ-rith′ro-sin)　a red compound, $C_{13}H_{18}O_6N_2$, used as a histologic stain.

erythrosine sodium (ĕ-rith′ro-sēn) [USP]　chemical name: 3′,6′-dihydroxy-2′,4′,5′,7′-tetraiodospiro[isobenzofuran-1(3*H*),9′-[9*H*]xanthen]-3-one disodium salt monohydrate. A coloring agent, $C_{20}H_6I_4Na_2O_5 \cdot H_2O$, occurring as a red or brownish red powder; used to disclose plaque on teeth; applied topically in solution, or tablets containing erythrosine sodium are chewed, after which the mouth is rinsed with water.

erythrosis (er″ĭ-thro′sis)　1. a reddish or purplish discoloration of the skin and mucous membranes seen in polycythemia vera.　2. hyperplasia of the hematopoietic tissue.

erythrostasis (ĕ-rith″ro-sta′sis)　the stoppage of erythrocytes in the capillaries, as in sickle cell anemia.

erythrothioneine (ĕ-rith″ro-thi″o-ne′in)　ergothioneine.

erythrulose (ĕ-rith′roo-lōs)　a ketose sugar, $C_4H_8O_4$, formed by the oxidation of erythrol.

erythruria (er″ĭ-throo′re-ah) [*erythro-* + Gr. *ouron* urine + *-ia*]　the passing of red urine.

Es　chemical symbol for *einsteinium.*

escape (es-kāp′)　the act of becoming free.　**aldosterone e.,** limitation to a finite period of time of the usual renal sodium-retaining effects of mineralocorticoid hormones when aldosterone is administered exogenously, after which sodium balance of natriuresis supervenes.　**nodal e.,** extrasystole in which the atrioventricular node is the pacemaker.　**vagal e.,** the exhaustion of or adaptation to neural chemical mediators in the regulation of systemic arterial pressure.　**ventricular e.,** extrasystole in which a ventricular pacemaker becomes effective before the sinoatrial pacemaker; it usually occurs with slow sinus rates and often, but not necessarily, with increased vagal tone.

eschar (es′kar) [Gr. *eschara* scab]　1. a slough produced by a thermal burn, by a corrosive application, or by gangrene.　2. the lesion seen in certain rickettsioses; see *tache noire.*

escharotic (es-kah-rot′ik) [Gr. *escharōtikos*]　1. corrosive; capable of producing an eschar.　2. a corrosive or caustic agent.

escharotomy (es″kah-rot′o-me)　surgical incision of the constricting eschar of a circumferentially burned limb in order to permit the cut edges to separate and restore blood flow to unburned tissue distal to the eschar.

Escherich's bacillus, sign (reflex) (esh′er-iks) [Theodor *Escherich,* German physician, 1857–1911]　see *Escherichia coli,* and under *sign.*

Escherichia (esh″er-i′ke-ah) [T. *Escherich,* German physician, 1857–1911]　a genus of gram-negative, facultatively anaerobic, rod-shaped bacteria of the tribe Escherichieae, family Enterobacteriaceae, found in the large intestine of warm-blooded animals. The organisms are nonpathogenic or opportunistic pathogens. They are members of the "coliform" group of bacteria, their presence in water supplies being used as an indicator of fecal contamination.　**E. aures′cens,** a variant of *E. coli,* characterized by the production of yellow-orange carotenoid pigments.　**E. blat′tae,** a species isolated from cockroaches.　**E. co′li,** the principal species of the genus and the predominant facultative organism of the intestine of humans and animals. The organisms are characteristically positive to indole and methyl red and negative to the Voges-Proskauer and citrate tests; serotypes are based on the distribution of heat-stable O antigens, envelope K antigens of varying heat stability, and flagellar H antigens that are heat labile. They are usually nonpathogenic, but pathogenic strains producing pyogenic infections and diarrhea are common. The pyogenic strains are found in infections in the urinary tract, abscesses, conjunctivitis, and occasionally septicemia, such as the hemorrhagic septicemia in newborn infants known as *Winckel's disease.* The enteropathogenic strains (EPEC) produce intestinal disease, especially in hospitalized infants. The enterotoxicogenic species (ETEC) cause diarrhea in piglets and calves and a cholera-like disease in human infants and adults. Enteroinvasive serogroups (EIEC) related to *Shigella* invade the epithelial cells of the human colon, causing dysentery, sometimes associated with food poisoning. They often become the predominant bacteria in the flora of the mouth and throat during antibiotic therapy. Enterohemorrhagic groups (EHEC) cause acute bloody diarrhea. See Plate 8, accompanying *bacterium.* Called also *Bacterium coli, Bacterium colicommune, colibacillus* or *colon bacillus* and *Escherich's bacillus, Shigella alkalescens, Shigella dispar,* and *Shigella madampensis.*　**E. ferguso′nii,** a species (enteric group 10) found in human clinical specimens.　**E. freun′dii,** *Citrobacter freundii.*　**E. herma′nii,** a species that produces a yellow pigment, found in human clinical specimens.　**E. interme′dia,** *Citrobacter intermedius.*　**E. vul′neris,** a species found in human clinical specimens.

Escherichieae (esh″ĕ-rik′e-e)　in some systems of classification, a tribe of gram-negative, facultatively anaerobic, rod-shaped bacteria of the family Enterobacteriaceae, made up of the genera *Escherichia* and *Shigella.*

Eschscholtzia (esh-skōlt′ze-ah)　a genus of papaveraceous plants. *E. califor′nica* Cham. (California poppy) is a hypnotic and anodyne.

escin (es′kin)　a strongly hemolytic saponin derived from horse-chestnut.

escorcin (es-kor′sin) a brown powder, $C_9H_8O_4$, prepared from a substance extracted from the horse chestnut; used in detecting corneal and conjunctival lesions.

esculapian (es″ku-la′pe-an) aesculapian.

esculent (es′ku-lent) edible; fit for eating.

esculin (es′ku-lin) [L. *aesculus* horse-chestnut] a coumarin glycoside, $C_9H_{11}O_5O \cdot C_9H_4O(O:) \cdot OH$, from *Aesculus hippocastanum* L. (Hippocastanaceae) (horse-chestnut) bark, having febrifuge properties.

escutcheon (es-kuch′an) [L. *scutum* a shield] the pattern of distribution of the pubic hair.

eseptate (e-sep′tāt) having no septa.

eserine (es′er-in) [*esere*, an African name of the Calabar bean] physostigmine.

E.S.F. erythropoietic stimulating factor.

Esidrix (es′ĭ-driks) trademark for a preparation of hydrochlorothiazide.

Esimil (es′ĭ-mil) trademark for preparations of guanethidine monosulfate with hydrochlorothiazide.

-esis [Gr.] a word termination denoting action, process, or condition; see also *-sis*.

Eskabarb (es′kah-barb) trademark for a preparation of phenobarbital.

Eskadiazine (es″kah-di′ah-zēn) trademark for a preparation of sulfadiazine.

Eskalith (es′kah-lith) trademark for a preparation of lithium carbonate.

esmarch (es′mark) an Esmarch bandage.

Esmarch's bandage, tourniquet, tube (es′marks) [Johann Friedrich August von *Esmarch*, German surgeon, 1823–1908] see under *bandage, tourniquet,* and *tube*.

eso- [Gr. *esō* inward] a combining form meaning within.

esocataphoria (es″o-kat-ah-fo′re-ah) [*eso-* + *cataphoria*] a phoria in which the visual axes turn downward and inward.

esocine (es′o-sin) a protamine from the sperm of the pike, *Esox lucius.*

esodeviation (e″so-de″ve-a′shun) 1. esophoria. 2. esotropia.

esodic (es-sod′ik) [Gr. *es* toward + *hodos* way] (*obs.*) afferent, as esodic nerves.

esoethmoiditis (es″o-eth″moi-di′tis) [*eso-* + *ethmoiditis*] inflammation within the sinuses of the ethmoid bone.

esogastritis (es″o-gas-tri′tis) [*eso-* + *gastritis*] inflammation of the mucous membrane of the stomach.

esophagalgia (ĕ-sof″ah-gal′je-ah) [*esophagus* + *-algia*] pain in the esophagus.

esophageal (ĕ-sof″ah-je′al, ĕ-so-fa′je-al) pertaining to or belonging to the esophagus.

esophagectasia (ĕ-sof″ah-jek-ta′se-ah) [*esophagus* + Gr. *ektasis* distention + *-ia*] dilatation of the esophagus.

esophagectasis (ĕ-sof″ah-jek′tah-sis) esophagectasia.

esophagectomy (ĕ-sof″ah-jek′to-me) [*esophagus* + Gr. *ektomē* excision] excision of part (*partial*) or all (*total*) of the esophagus.

esophagism (ĕ-sof′ah-jism) esophagospasm. **hiatal e.,** cardiospasm.

esophagismus (ĕ-sof″ah-jiz′mus) esophagospasm.

esophagitis (ĕ-sof″ah-ji′tis) [*esophagus* + *-itis*] inflammation of the esophagus. **chronic peptic e.,** reflux e. **e. dis′secans superficia′lis,** infection of the esophagus, with sloughing of the squamous epithelial lining in the form of a tubular cast. **reflux e.,** a chronic, pathologic, potentially life-threatening disease manifested by the various sequelae associated with reflux of the stomach and duodenal contents into the esophagus (*gastroesophageal reflux*), which is principally characterized by heartburn and regurgitation. It may occur as a primary condition or be associated with other diseases such as hiatal hernia. Called also *chronic peptic e.*

esophagobronchial (ĕ-sof″ah-go-brong′ke-al) pertaining to or communicating with the esophagus and a bronchus.

esophagocardiomyotomy (ĕ-sof″ah-go-kar″de-o-mi-ot′o-me) incision through the muscular coats of the esophagus and cardiac part of the stomach, the incision extending equal distances above and below the esophagogastric junction; done in achalasia of the esophagus. Called also *cardiomyotomy.*

esophagocele (ĕ-sof″ah-go-sēl″) [*esophagus* + Gr. *kēlē* hernia] abnormal distention of the esophagus; hernia of the esophagus: protrusion of the mucous and submucous coats of the esophagus through a rupture in the muscular coat, producing a pouch or diverticulum.

esophagocologastrostomy (ĕ-sof″ah-go-ko″lo-gas-tros′to-me) surgical creation of a new connection between the esophagus and stomach, by interposition of a segment of colon.

esophagocoloplasty (ĕ-sof″ah-go-ko′lo-plas″te) excision of a portion of the esophagus and its replacement by a segment of the colon.

esophagoduodenostomy (ĕ-sof″ah-go-du″o-de-nos′to-me) surgical anastomosis between the esophagus and the duodenum.

esophagodynia (ĕ-sof″ah-go-din′e-ah) [*esophagus* + Gr. *odynē* pain] pain in the esophagus.

esophagoenterostomy (ĕ-sof″ah-go-en″ter-os′to-me) [*esophagus* + Gr. *enteron* intestine + *stomoun* to provide with an opening, or mouth] surgical formation of an anastomosis between the esophagus and small intestine after total gastrectomy.

esophagoesophagostomy (ĕ-sof″ah-go-ĕ-sof″ah-gos′to-me) anastomosis between two parts of the esophagus.

esophagofundopexy (ĕ-sof″ah-go-fun″do-pek′se) surgical fixation of the fundus of the stomach to the esophagus.

esophagogastrectomy (ĕ-sof″ah-go-gas-trek′to-me) excision of the esophagus and stomach, usually the distal portion of the esophagus and the proximal stomach.

esophagogastric (ĕ-sof″ah-go-gas′trik) pertaining to the esophagus and the stomach.

esophagogastroanastomosis (ĕ-sof″ah-go-gas″tro-ah-nas″to-mo′sis) surgical formation of an anastomosis between the esophagus and the stomach.

esophagogastromyotomy (ĕ-sof″ah-go-gas″tro-mi-ot′o-me) esophagocardiomyotomy.

esophagogastroplasty (ĕ-sof″ah-go-gas′tro-plas″te) plastic repair of the esophagus and stomach; cardioplasty.

esophagogastroscopy (ĕ-sof″ah-go-gas-tros′ko-pe) [*esophagus* + Gr. *gastēr* stomach + *skopein* to examine] endoscopic examination of the esophagus and the stomach.

esophagogastrostomy (ĕ-sof″ah-go-gas-tros′to-me) [*esophagus* + Gr. *gastēr* stomach + *stomoun* to provide with an opening, or mouth] surgical creation of a communication between the stomach and esophagus.

esophagogram (ĕ-sof′ah-go-gram) a roentgenogram of the esophagus.

esophagography (ĕ-sof″ah-gog′rah-fe) roentgenography of the esophagus.

esophagojejunogastrostomosis (ĕ-sof″ah-go-je″ju-no-gas″tros-to-mo′sus) esophagojejunogastrostomy.

esophagojejunogastrostomy (ĕ-sof″ah-go-je-ju″no-gas-tros′to-me) the operation of mobilizing an isolated segment of jejunum and anastomosing its proximal end to the esophagus and its distal end to the stomach.

esophagojejunoplasty (ĕ-sof″ah-go-jĕ-joo′no-plas″te) replacement of the esophagus with a segment of jejunum.

esophagojejunostomy (ĕ-sof″ah-go-je-ju-nos′to-me) surgical anastomosis between the esophagus and the jejunum.

esophagolaryngectomy (ĕ-sof″ah-go-lar″in-jek′to-me) en bloc excision of the upper cervical esophagus and larynx.

esophagology (ĕ-sof″ah-gol′o-je) the study and treatment of diseases of the esophagus.

esophagomalacia (ĕ-sof″ah-go-mah-la′she-ah) [*esophagus* + Gr. *malakia* softness] softening of the walls of the esophagus.

esophagomycosis (ĕ-sof″ah-go-mi-ko′sis) [*esophagus* + Gr. *mykēs* fungus] any disease of the esophagus caused by fungi.

esophagomyotomy (ĕ-sof″ah-go-mi-ot′o-me) incision through the muscular coat of the esophagus, the term usually referring to incision through the muscular coat of the distal part of the esophagus.

esophagopharynx (ĕ-sof″ah-go-făr′inks) the distal portion of the pharynx where the fibers of the inferior constrictor are arranged in circular form.

esophagoplasty (ĕ-sof′ah-go-plas″te) [esophagus + Gr. plassein to form] a plastic operation on the esophagus.

esophagoplication (ĕ-sof″ah-go-pli-ka′shun) the operation of narrowing the esophagus by folding in its wall.

esophagoptosis (ĕ-sof″ah-gop-to′sis) [esophagus + Gr. ptōsis falling] prolapse of the esophagus.

esophagorespiratory (ĕ-sof″ah-go-rĕ-spir′ah-to″re) pertaining to or communicating with the esophagus and respiratory tract (the trachea or a bronchus).

esophagoscope (ĕ-sof′ah-go-skōp) [esophagus + Gr. skopein to examine] a flexible or rigid instrument for inspecting the lumen of the esophagus and carrying out diagnostic and therapeutic maneuvers such as taking biopsy specimens and removing foreign bodies.

esophagoscopy (ĕ-sof″ah-gos′ko-pe) endoscopic examination of the esophagus.

esophagospasm (ĕ-sof′ah-go-spazm″) [esophagus + spasm] spasm of the esophagus.

esophagostenosis (ĕ-sof″ah-go-stĕ-no′sis) [esophagus + Gr. stenōsis constriction] stricture or constriction of the esophagus.

esophagostoma (e″sof-ah-gos′to-mah) [esophagus + Gr. stoma mouth] the external opening of an artificial opening leading into the esophagus.

esophagostomiasis (ĕ-sof″ah-go-sto-mi′ah-sis) infestation with nematodes of the genus Oesophagostomum.

esophagostomy (ĕ-sof″ah-gos′to-me) [esophagus + Gr. stomoun to provide with an opening, or mouth] the creation of an opening into the esophagus.

esophagotome (e″so-fag′o-tōm) a cutting instrument for use in esophagotomy.

esophagotomy (ĕ-sof″ah-got′o-me) [esophagus + Gr. tomē a cutting] incision of the esophagus.

esophagotracheal (ĕ-sof″ah-go-tra′ke-al) pertaining to or communicating with esophagus and trachea.

esophagram (ĕ-sof′ah-gram) esophagogram.

esophagus (ĕ-sof′ah-gus) [Gr. oisophagos, from oisein to carry + phagēma food] [NA] the musculomembranous passage extending from the pharynx to the stomach. Called also gullet. Written also oesophagus [NA]. **Barrett's e.,** see under syndrome. **nutcracker e.,** a motility disorder characterized by high-amplitude peristaltic contractions, often of prolonged duration, arising from the distal esophagus.

esophoria (es″o-fo′re-ah) [eso- + phoria] a form of heterophoria in which there is a deviation of the visual axis of an eye toward that of the other eye after the visual fusional stimuli have been eliminated; called also esodeviation.

esophoric (es″o-for′ik) pertaining to or characterized by esophoria.

esosphenoiditis (es″o-sfe″noi-di′tis) [eso- + sphenoid + -itis] osteomyelitis of the sphenoid bone.

esotropia (es″o-tro′pe-ah) [eso- + tropia] strabismus in which there is manifest deviation of the visual axis of an eye toward that of the other eye, resulting in diplopia. Called also cross-eye and convergent or internal strabismus.

esotropic (es″o-trop′ik) pertaining to or characterized by esotropia.

ESP extrasensory perception.

espnoic (esp-no′ik) [Gr. es into + pnoē vapor, blast] pertaining to the injection of vapors or gases.

esponja (es-pong′ah) cutaneous habronemiasis.

esproquin hydrochloride (es′pro-kwin) chemical name: 2-[3-(ethylsulfinyl)propyl]-1,2,3,4-tetrahydroisoquinoline hydrochloride; an adrenergic, $C_{14}H_{21}NOS$·HCl.

espundia (es-poon′de-ah) mucocutaneous leishmaniasis.

esquillectomy (es″kwil-lek′to-me) [Fr. esquille fragment + Gr. ektomē excision] excision of fragments of bone following fractures caused by projectiles.

ESR erythrocyte sedimentation rate.

essence (es′ens) [L. essentia quality or being] 1. that which is or necessarily exists as the cause of the properties of a body. 2. a solution of a volatile oil in alcohol. **e. of peppermint,** peppermint spirit; see under spirit.

essentia (ĕ-sen′she-ah) [L.] essence.

essential (ĕ-sen′shal) [L. essentialis] 1. constituting the

necessary or inherent part of a thing; giving a substance its peculiar and necessary qualities. 2. idiopathic; self-existing; having no obvious external exciting cause; said of a disease. 3. indispensable; required in the diet, as essential fatty acids.

Esser's graft, operation (es′erz) [Johannes Fredericus Samuel Esser, Holland surgeon, 1878–1946] see under graft, and see epithelial inlay, under inlay.

EST electric shock therapy; electroshock therapy.

ester (es′ter) a compound formed by removal of water from an acid and an alcohol, e.g., carboxylic acid esters, R—O—CO—R′, and phosphoric acid esters (organic phosphates), R-PO₄²⁻; esters are named as if they were salts of the parent acid, e.g., methyl acetate, glucose 6-phosphate. **Cori e.,** glucose 1-phosphate. **Embden e.,** an equilibrium mixture of 75-80 per cent glucose 6-phosphate and 20-25 per cent fructose 6-phosphate. **Harden-Young e.,** fructose 1,6-bisphosphate. **Neuberg e.,** fructose 6-phosphate. **Robison e.,** glucose 6-phosphate.

esterapenia (es″ter-ah-pe′ne-ah) [esterase + Gr. penia poverty] deficiency in the cholinesterase content of the blood.

esterase (es′ter-ās) any of a subclass of enzymes [EC 3.1] of the hydrolase class that catalyze the hydrolysis of ester bonds, yielding an alcohol or phenol and an acid anion. **C1 e.,** C1s; see under complement.

esterification (es-ter″ĭ-fi-ka′shun) the process of converting an acid into an ester.

esterify (es-ter′ĭ-fi) to combine with an alcohol with elimination of a molecule of water, forming an ester.

esterize (es′ter-īz) to convert, or be converted, into an ester.

esterolysis (es″ter-ol′ĭ-sis) [ester + Gr. lysis dissolution] the hydrolysis of an ester into its alcohol and acid.

esterolytic (es″ter-o-lit′ik) effecting or pertaining to esterolysis.

Estes' operation (es′tēz) [William Lawrence Estes, Jr., American surgeon, 1885–1940] see under operation.

estetrol (es′tĕ-trol) 15α, 16α, 17β-estetrol, an estrogen produced in the fetoplacental unit by 15α-hydroxylation of estriol or estrogen precursors and found in the maternal serum, amniotic fluid, and urine.

esthematology (es″them-ah-tol′o-je) [Gr. aisthēma sensation + -logy] the science of the senses and sense organs.

esthesia (es-the′ze-ah) [Gr. aisthēsis perception] perception, feeling, or sensation.

esthesic (es-the′sik) [Gr. aisthēsis perception] pertaining to the mental perception of sensations.

esthesi(o)- [Gr. aisthēsis perception, sensation] a combining form denoting relationship to feeling or to perception. Spelled also aesthesi(o)-.

esthesioblast (es-the′ze-o-blast″) [esthesio- + Gr. blastos germ] a ganglioblast; an embryonic cell of the spinal ganglia.

esthesiodic (es-the″ze-od′ik) esthesodic.

esthesiogenic (es-the″ze-o-jen′ik) producing sensation.

esthesiology (es-the″ze-ol′o-je) [esthesio- + -logy] the science of sensation and the senses.

esthesiometer (es-the″ze-om′ĕ-ter) [esthesio- + Gr. metron measure] an instrument for measuring tactile sensibility; tactometer.

esthesioneure (es-the′ze-o-nūr) [esthesio- + Gr. neuron nerve] a sensory neuron.

esthesioneuroblastoma (es-the″ze-o-nu″ro-blas-to′mah) a radiosensitive glioma occurring in the nasal cavity.

esthesioneurosis (es-the″ze-o-nu-ro′sis) [esthesio- + neurosis] any disorder of the sensory nerves.

esthesionosus (es-the″ze-on′o-sus) [esthesio- + Gr. nosos disease] esthesioneurosis.

esthesiophysiology (es-the″ze-o-fiz″e-ol′o-je) the physiology of sensation and the sense organs.

esthesodic (es″thĕ-zod′ik) [esthesio- + Gr. hodos path] conducting or pertaining to the conduction of sensory impulses.

esthetic (es-thet′ik) [Gr. aisthēsis sensation] 1. pertaining to sensation. 2. pertaining to beauty, or the improvement of appearance. Also spelled aesthetic.

esthetics (es-thet′iks) the branch of philosophy dealing with beauty. In dentistry, a philosophy concerned especially with the appearance of a dental restoration, as achieved through its color and/or form. Also spelled *aesthetics.*

estimate (es′tĭ-mit) [L. *aestimare* to value, to estimate] 1. a rough calculation or one based on incomplete data. 2. a statistic used to characterize the value of a population parameter. Called also *estimator.* 3. (es′tĭ-māt) to produce or use such a calculation or statistic. **biased e.,** a point estimate that is not unbiased. **consistent e.,** a statistic that converges to the parameter being estimated as the sample size increases; i.e., the sampling error can be made as small as desired by taking a large enough sample. **interval e.,** a statistical estimate that states with a specified degree of confidence that the parameter lies within a specified interval. Cf. *point e.* **point e.,** a statistical estimate that specifies a value for the parameter. Cf. *interval e.* **product-limit e.,** Kaplan-Meier survival curve. **unbiased e.,** a point estimate having a sampling distribution with a mean equal to the parameter being estimated; for example, the sample mean and variance, if calculated appropriately, are unbiased estimates of the population mean and variance.

estimator (es′tĭ-ma″tor) estimate (def. 2).

Estinyl (es′tĭ-nil) trademark for a preparation of ethinyl estradiol.

estival (es′tĭ-val, ĕ-sti′val) [L. *aestivus,* from *aestas* summer] pertaining to or occurring in summer.

estivation (es″tĭ-va′shun) [L. *aestivus,* from *aestas* summer] the dormant state of decreased metabolism in which certain animal species, as some tropical amphibians, survive a hot, dry summer; summer dormancy. Cf. *hibernation.*

estivoautumnal (es″tĭ-vo-aw-tum′nal) pertaining to the summer and autumn; formerly applied, in the United States, to a form of malaria; see *falciparum malaria,* under *malaria.*

Estlander's operation (est′land-erz) [Jakob August *Estlander,* Finnish surgeon, 1831–1881] see under *operation.*

estolate (es′to-lāt) USAN contraction for propionate lauryl sulfate.

eston (es′ton) aluminum acetate.

Estrace (es′trās) trademark for a preparation of estradiol.

estradiol (es″trah-di′ol, es-tra′de-ol) chemical name: estra-1,3,5(10)-triene-3,17β-diol. The most potent naturally occurring ovarian and placental estrogen in human subjects, $C_{18}H_{24}O_2$, the chief functions of which are to prepare the uterus for implantation of the fertilized ovum and to induce and maintain the female secondary sex characteristics; it has also been isolated from hog ovaries and the urine of pregnant mares and has been produced semisynthetically. Estradiol exists in two isomeric forms: the most active isomer is *estradiol-17β* (formerly called β-estradiol), and the much less active *estradiol-17α* (formerly called α-estradiol). The official preparation [NF], occurring as white or creamy white, small crystals or crystalline powder, is administered by intramuscular injection or implanted subcutaneously in pellets. For functions and uses, see *estrogen.* Called also (rarely) *dihydroxyestrin, dihydrofolliculin,* and *dihydrotheelin.* **e. benzoate** [USP], an ester of estradiol, $C_{25}H_{28}O_3$, occurring as a white to creamy white, crystalline powder; injected intramuscularly in oil solution. **e. cypionate** [USP], an ester of estradiol, $C_{26}H_{36}O_3$, occurring as a white to practically white, crystalline powder, injected intramuscularly in oil solution. **e. dipropionate,** an ester of estradiol, $C_{24}H_{32}O_4$, occurring as small, white or slightly off-white crystals or as a crystalline powder; injected intramuscularly in oil solution. **e. enanthate,** an ester of estradiol, $C_{25}H_{36}O_3$, injected intramuscularly in oil solution. **ethinyl e.** [USP], chemical name: 19-norpregna-1,3,5(10)-trien-20-yne-3,17α-diol. An orally effective semisynthetic derivative of estradiol, $C_{20}H_{24}O_2$, occurring as a white to creamy white, crystalline powder, which is one of the most potent estrogens. It is also used as the estrogen component in combination with progestins in many oral contraceptives. **e. undecylate,** an ester of estradiol, $C_{29}H_{44}O_3$, injected intramuscularly in oil solution. **e. valerate** [USP], an ester of estradiol, $C_{23}H_{32}O_3$, occurring as a white, crystalline powder; injected intramuscularly in oil solution.

estradiol 6β-hydroxylase (es″trah-di′ol hi′drok′sĭ-lās) estradiol 6β-monooxygenase.

estradiol 6β-monooxygenase (es″trah-di′ol mon″o-ok′sĭ-jen-ās) [EC 1.14.99.11] an enzyme of the oxidoreduc-

tase class that catalyzes the reaction estradiol-17β + hydrogen donor (reduced) + O_2 = 6β-hydroxy-estradiol + donor + H_2O. The reaction, occurring in the liver, inactivates estrogen.

estramustine (es″trah-mus′tēn) chemical name: 3-[bis(2-chlorothyl)carbamate]estra-1,3,5(10)-triene-3,17β-diol; an antineoplastic, $C_{23}H_{31}Cl_2NO_3$.

estrane (es′trān) the organic chemist's name for the parent hydrocarbon, $C_{18}H_{30}$, of the estrogenic steroids.

estrapentaene (es″trah-pen′tah-ēn) a steroid nucleus with five double bonds and one methyl group, $C_{18}H_{20}$.

estratetraene (es″trah-tet′rah-ēn) a steroid nucleus with four double bonds and one methyl group, $C_{18}H_{22}$.

estratriene (es″trah-tri′ēn) a steroid nucleus with three double bonds and one methyl group, $C_{18}H_{24}$.

Estraval (es-trah-val) trademark for preparations of estradiol valerate.

estrazinol hydrobromide (es-trah′zĭ-nōl) chemical name: (+)-3-methoxy-8-aza-19-nor-17α-1,3,5(10)-trien-20-yn-17-ol hydrobromide; an estrogen, $C_{20}H_{25}NO_2 \cdot HBr$.

estrenol (es′trĕ-nol) a crystalline estrogenic steroid, $C_{18}H_{24}O$, 1,3,5(10)estratriene-3-ol.

estriasis (es-tri′ah-sis) oestriasis.

Estridae (es′trĭ-de) Oestridae.

estrin (es′trin) estrogen.

estrinization (es″trin-ĭ-za′shun) production of the cellular changes in the vaginal epithelium characteristic of estrus.

estriol (es′tre-ol) chemical name: estra-1,3,5(10)-triene-3β, 16α,17β-triol. A reduction product of estradiol and estrone, $C_{18}H_{24}O_3$, having relatively weak estrogenic activity and detectable in high concentrations in the urine, especially human pregnancy urine. The official preparation [USP], rarely used clinically, is a white, microcrystalline powder, to be administered orally. For uses, see *estrogen.* Called also *trihydroxyestrin.*

estrofurate (es-tro-fūr′āt) chemical name: 21,23-epoxy-19, 24-dinorchola-1, 3, 5 (10),7,20, 22-hexaene -3,17α-diol 3-acetate; an estrogen, $C_{24}H_{26}O_4$.

estrogen (es′tro-jen) a generic term for estrus-producing steroid compounds; the female sex hormones. In humans, estrogen is formed in the ovary, possibly the adrenal cortex, the testis, and the fetoplacental unit; it has various functions in both sexes. It is responsible for the development of the female secondary sex characteristics, and during the menstrual cycle it acts on the female genitalia to produce an environment suitable for the fertilization, implantation, and nutrition of the early embryo. Estrogen is used in oral contraceptives and as a palliative in cancer of the breast after menopause and cancer of the prostate; other uses include the relief of the discomforts of menopause, inhibition of lactation, and treatment of osteoporosis, threatened abortion, and various functional ovarian disorders. See also *estradiol, estrone,* and *estriol.* **conjugated e's** [USP], a mixture of the sodium salts of the sulfate esters of estrogenic substances, principally estrone and equilin, that are of the type excreted by pregnant mares, occurring as a buff-colored, amorphous powder; the actions and uses are those of estrogens (q.v.), administered orally. **esterified e's** [USP], a mixture of the sodium salts of esters of estrogenic substances, principally estrone, that are of the type excreted by pregnant mares, occurring as a white or buff-colored, amorphous powder; the actions and uses are those of estrogens (q.v.), administered orally.

estrogenic (es-tro-jen′ik) producing estrus; of, pertaining to, having the properties of, or similar to an estrogen.

estrogenicity (es″tro-jĕ-nis′ĭ-te) the quality of exerting or the ability to exert an estrus-producing or an estrogenic effect.

estrogenous (es-troj′ĕ-nus) estrogenic; arising from estrogens or their effects.

estrone (es′trōn) chemical name: 3-hydroxyestra-1,3,5(10)-triene-17-one. An oxidation product of estradiol, $C_{18}H_{22}O_2$, the first of the estrogens isolated in pure form, found in human pregnancy urine, male human urine, human plasma, mare pregnancy urine, stallion urine, human ovarian follicular fluid and placenta, and palm kernel oil; also produced synthetically. Less potent than estradiol but more so than estriol, it is secreted by the ovary but circulating estrone is for the most part derived from peripheral metabolism of estradiol and especially androstenedione. Pharmaceutical preparations are made in conformance with USP standards; see under *estrogen* for uses. Called also *folliculin*, *ketohydroxyestrin*, and *thelykinin*.

estrophilin (es″tro-fil′in) a cell protein that acts as a receptor for estrogen, found in estrogenic target tissue and in estrogen-dependent tumors and metastases.

estropipate (es′tro-pĭ-pāt) [USP] a compound of estrone sulfate with piperazine, used as estrone; formerly called *piperazine estrone sulfate.*

estrostilben (es″tro-stil′ben) diethylstilbestrol.

estrous (es′trus) pertaining to estrus.

estrual (es′troo-al) pertaining to estrus.

estruation (es″troo-a′shun) estrus.

Estrugenone (es″troo-jen′on) trademark for a preparation of estrone.

estrum (es′trum) estrus.

estrus (es′trus) [L. *oestrus* gadfly; Gr. *oistros* anything that drives mad, any vehement desire] the recurrent, restricted period of sexual receptivity in female mammals other than human females, marked by intense sexual urge. See also *estrous cycle*, under *cycle.*

estuarium (es″tu-a′re-um) [L.] a vapor bath.

e.s.u. electrostatic unit.

esylate (es′ĭ-lāt) USAN contraction for ethanesulfonate.

Et ethyl group.

eta (a′tah) [H, η] the seventh letter of the Greek alphabet.

etafedrine hydrochloride (et-ah-fed′rin) chemical name: α-[1-(ethylmethylamino)ethyl]benzylmethanol hydrochloride; an adrenergic, $C_{12}H_{19}NO \cdot HCl$, administered orally in the treatment of bronchial asthma.

etafilcon A (et″ah-fil′kon) a hydrophilic contact lens material.

Etamon (et′ah-mon) trademark for a preparation of tetraethylammonium chloride.

état (a-tah′) [Fr.] state, condition. **é. criblé** (a-tah′krēb-la′), 1. a condition in which the necrotic Peyer's patches in typhoid fever are riddled with small, irregular perforations. 2. status cribralis. **é. lacunaire** (a-tah′lah-ku-nār′), status lacunaris. **é. mammelonné** (a-tah′mah-mel-un-a′), hyperplasia of the mucous membrane of the stomach in chronic gastritis, resulting in the formation of small elevations. **é. marbré** (a-tah′ mar-bra′), status marmoratus. **é. vermoulu** (a-tah′ vār-moo-lu′) ["worm-eaten state"], an irregularly ulcerated condition of the surface of the brain, sometimes seen in advanced arteriosclerosis.

etazolate hydrochloride (ĕ-taz′o-lāt) chemical name: 1-ethyl-4-[(1-methylethylidene)hydrazino]-1*H*-pyrazolo[3,4-*b*]pyridine-5-carboxylic acid ethyl ester monohydrochloride; a tranquilizer, $C_{14}H_{19}N_5O_2 \cdot HCl$.

Eternod's sinus (a-ter-nōz′) [Auguste François Charles *Eternod*, Swiss histologist, 1854–1932] see under *sinus.*

eterobarb (ĕ-tēr′o-barb) chemical name: 5-ethyl-1,3-bis-(methoxymethyl)-5-phenyl-2,4,6(1*H*, 3*H*, 5*H*)-pyrimedine-trione; a barbiturate with anticonvulsant properties, $C_{16}H_{20}N_2O_5$.

ethacrynate (eth″ah-krin′āt) the conjugate base of ethacrynic acid, used as *ethacrynate sodium* [USP].

ethacrynic acid (eth-ah-krin′ik) [USP] a powerful, rapid-acting diuretic of short duration used orally or, in the form of a sodium salt, intravenously.

ethal (eth′al) cetyl alcohol.

ethambutol hydrochloride (ĕ-tham′bu-tōl) [USP] chemical name: [*R*-(*R* *,R* *)*]-2,2′-(1,2-ethanediyldiimino)-bis-1-butanol dihydrochloride. An antibacterial, $C_{10}H_{24}N_2O_2 \cdot 2HCl$, occurring as a white crystalline powder, specifically effective against *Mycobacterium*, including *M. tuberculosis*; used in conjunction with one or more other antituberculous drugs in the treatment of pulmonary tuberculosis, administered orally.

ethamivan (eth-am′ĭ-van″) [USP] chemical name: *N,N*-diethyl-4-hydroxy-3-methoxybenzamide. A central nervous system stimulant and analeptic, $C_{12}H_{17}NO_3$, occurring as a white or practically white, crystalline powder; used as a respiratory stimulant, administered intravenously.

ethamsylate (ĕ-tham′sĭ-lāt) chemical name: 2,5-dihy-

droxybenzenesulfonic acid compound with *N*-ethylethanamine; a hemostatic agent, $C_6H_6O_5S \cdot C_4H_{11}N$.

ethanal (eth′ah-nal) acetaldehyde.

ethane (eth′ān) a hydrocarbon of the methane series, C_2H_6, forming a constituent of natural gas, which occurs as a colorless, odorless, flammable gas.

ethanedial (eth-ān-di′al) glyoxal.

ethanoic acid (eth″ah-no′ik) systematic name for acetic acid.

ethanol (eth′ah-nol) alcohol.

ethanolamine (eth″ah-nol′ah-mēn) monoethanolamine.

ethanolism (eth′ah-nol″izm) ethanol-induced hypoglycemia.

ethaverine hydrochloride (eth″ah-ver′ēn) chemical name: 1-[(3,4-diethoxyphenyl)methyl]-6,7-diethoxyisoquinoline. The tetrahydroxy analogue of papaverine, $C_{24}H_{29}NO_4 \cdot HCl$, used as an antispasmodic in peripheral and vascular insufficiency associated with arterial spasm and as a smooth muscle relaxant in spasticity of the gastrointestinal and genitourinary tracts; administered orally.

ethchlorvynol (eth-klōr′vĭ-nol) [USP] chemical name: 1-chloro-3-ethyl-1-penten-4-yn-3-ol. A nonbarbiturate sedative and hypnotic, C_7H_9ClO, occurring as a colorless to yellow, slightly viscous liquid; administered orally.

ethene (eth-ēn′) ethylene.

ethenoid (eth′ĕ-noid) containing an ethylene linkage.

ether (e′ther) [L. *aether*, Gr. *aithēr* "the upper and purer air"] 1. an organic compound having an oxygen atom bonded to two carbon atoms; general formula, R–O–R′. 2. [USP] diethyl ether. **anesthetic e.,** diethyl ether; also any other ether inhalational anesthetic, e.g., vinyl ether. **petroleum e.,** petroleum benzin. **thio e.,** an ether in which sulfur replaces oxygen.

ethereal (e-the′re-al) 1. pertaining to, prepared with, containing, or resembling ether. 2. evanescent; delicate.

etherification (e″ther-ĭ-fi-ka′shun) the formation of an ether from alcohol.

etherion (e-the′re-on) (*obs.*) 1. a gas said to have been discovered in 1898 in the atmosphere; said to be about $\frac{1}{1000}$ part as dense as hydrogen, and to exist in less than $\frac{1}{1,000,000}$ part of its proportion in the air. 2. Mathews' name for one of the minute spheres once believed to make up the ether.

etherization (e″ther-i-za′shun) the administration of ether by inhalation, and the consequent production of anesthesia.

etherize (e′ther-iz) to put under the anesthetic influence of ether.

etherometer (e″ther-om′ĕ-ter) [*ether* + Gr. *metron* measure] a device for administering ether by which the number of drops per minute can be accurately controlled.

ethical (eth′ĭ-kal) in accordance with the principles which govern right conduct.

ethics (eth′iks) [Gr. *ēthos* the manner and habits of man or of animals] the rules or principles which govern right conduct. **medical e.,** the values and guidelines that should govern decisions in medicine.

ethidene (eth′ĭ-dēn) ethylidene. **e. chloride,** ethylene dichloride. **e. diamine,** a harmful ptomaine, $C_2H_8N_2$, from fish.

ethidium (ĕ-thid′e-um) homidium.

ethinamate (ĕ-thin′ah-māt) [USP] chemical name: 1-ethynylcyclohexanol carbamate. A short-acting nonbarbiturate sedative, $C_9H_{13}NO_2$, occurring as a white powder; used as a hypnotic, administered orally.

ethinyl (eth′ĭ-nil) ethynyl. **e. estradiol,** see under *estradiol.*

Ethiodol (ĕ-thi′o-dol) trademark for a preparation of ethiodized oil, used as a contrast medium.

ethionamide (ĕ-thi″on-am′īd) [USP] chemical name: 2-ethyl-4-pyridine-carbothioamide. An antibacterial, $C_8H_{10}N_2S$, occurring as a bright yellow powder, effective against *Myobacterium tuberculosis;* used in conjunction with one or more other antituberculous drugs in the treatment of pulmonary tuberculosis, administered orally.

ethionine (ĕ-thi′o-nin) the ethyl homologue of methionine.

ethisterone (ĕ-this′ter-ōn) chemical name: 17α-hydroxy-pregn-4-en-20-yn-3-one; a semisynthetic progestin, $C_{21}H_{28}O_2$, which may be considered a derivative of both progesterone and of testosterone. Called also *anhydrohydroxyprogesterone*, *pregneninolone*, and *ethinyl testosterone*.

ethmocarditis (eth″mo-kar-di′tis) [Gr. *ēthmos* sieve + *kardia* heart + *-itis*] inflammation of the connective tissue of the heart.

ethmocephalus (eth″mo-sef′ah-lus) [Gr. *ēthmos* sieve + *kephalē* head] a monster with an imperfect head, more or less union of the eyes, and a rudimentary nose, which may often be displaced upward.

ethmofrontal (eth″mo-fron′tal) pertaining to the ethmoid and frontal bones.

ethmoid (eth′moid) [Gr. *ēthmos* sieve + *eidos* form] cribriform; sievelike.

ethmoidal (eth-moi′dal) of or pertaining to the ethmoid bone.

ethmoidectomy (eth″moi-dek′to-me) [ethmoid + Gr. *ektomē* excision] excision of the ethmoid cells or of a portion of the ethmoid bone.

ethmoiditis (eth″moi-di′tis) inflammation of the ethmoid bone.

ethmoidotomy (eth″moi-dot′o-me) surgical incision into the ethmoid sinus.

ethmolacrimal (eth″mo-lak′rĭ-mal) pertaining to the ethmoid and the lacrimal bones.

ethmomaxillary (eth″mo-mak′sĭ-lār-e) pertaining to the ethmoid and maxillary bones.

ethmonasal (eth″mo-na′zal) pertaining to the ethmoid and nasal bones.

ethmopalatal (eth″mo-pal′ah-tal) pertaining to the ethmoid and palatine bones.

ethmosphenoid (eth″mo-sfe′noid) pertaining to the ethmoid and sphenoid bones.

ethmoturbinal (eth″mo-tur′bĭ-nal) pertaining to the superior and middle nasal conchae.

ethmovomerine (eth″mo-vo′mer-in) pertaining to the ethmoid bone and the vomer.

ethnic (eth′nik) [Gr. *ethnikos* of a nation; national] pertaining to a social group who share cultural bonds (religious, national, etc.) or physical (racial) characteristics.

ethnics (eth′niks) [Gr. *ethnikos* of a nation; national] ethnology.

ethnobiology (eth″no-bi-ol′o-je) the scientific study of physical characteristics of different races of mankind.

ethnography (eth-nog′rah-fe) [Gr. *ethnos* race + *graphein* to write] a description of the races of man. Cf. *anthropography*.

ethnology (eth-nol′o-je) [Gr. *ethnos* race + *-logy*] the science which deals with the races of man, their descent, relationship, etc.

ethobrom (eth′o-brōm) tribromoethanol.

ethocaine (eth′o-kān) procaine hydrochloride.

ethoglucid (eth″o-glu′sid) chemical name: triethylene glycol diglycidyl ether. A clear colorless viscous liquid, $C_{12}H_{22}O_6$, with antineoplastic properties.

ethoheptazine citrate (eth″o-hep′tah-zēn) chemical name: ethylhexahydro-1-methyl-4-phenyl-1*H*-azepine-4-carboxylate dihydrogen citrate. An analgesic, $C_{16}H_{23}NO_2 \cdot C_6H_8O_7$, used to control mild or moderate pain; administered orally.

ethohexadiol (eth″o-heks-a′de-ol) chemical name: 2-ethyl-1,3-hexamediol. An arthropod repellant, $C_8H_{18}O_2$, applied topically to the skin and clothing.

ethological (eth″o-loj′ĭ-kal) pertaining to ethology.

ethologist (e-thol′o-jist) an individual skilled in ethology.

ethology (e-thol′o-je) [Gr. *ēthos* the manners and habits of man, or of animals + *-logy*] The scientific study of animal behavior, particularly in the natural state, the evolution of behavior, and its biologic significance.

ethomoxane hydrochloride (eth″o-moks′ān) chemical name: *N*-butyl-8-ethoxy-2,3-dihydro-1,4-benzodioxin-2-methanamine hydrochloride; a tranquilizer, $C_{15}H_{23}NO_3 \cdot HCl$.

ethonam nitrate (eth′o-nam) chemical name: 1-(1,2,3,4-tetrahydro-1-naphthalenyl)-1*H*-imidazole-5-carboxylic acid ethyl ester mononitrate; an antifungal agent, $C_{16}H_{18}N_2O_2 \cdot HNO_3$.

ethopropazine hydrochloride (eth″o-pro′pah-zēn) [USP] chemical name: *N,N*-diethyl-α-methyl-10*H*-phenothiazine-10-ethanamine monohydrochloride. A phenothiazine derivative, $C_{19}H_{24}N_2S \cdot HCl$, occurring as a white to slightly off-white, crystalline powder, having anticholinergic, antihistaminic, adrenergic-blocking, ganglion-blocking, local anesthetic, and central nervous system depressant effects; used as an antiparkinsonian agent, administered orally. Called also *isothiazine hydrochloride* and *phenopropazine hydrochloride*.

ethosuximide (eth″o-suk′sĭ-mīd) [USP] chemical name: 3-ethyl-3-methyl-2,5-pyrrolidinedione. An anticonvulsant, $C_7H_{11}NO_2$, occurring as a white to off-white crystalline powder or waxy solid; used in the treatment of petit mal epilepsy, administered orally.

ethotoin (ĕ-tho′to-in) chemical name: 3-ethyl-5-phenyl-2,4-imidazolidinedione. An anticonvulsant, $C_{11}H_{12}N_2O_2$, occurring as a white, crystalline powder; used in the treatment of grand mal epilepsy and psychomotor seizures, administered orally. Called also *ethylphenylhydantoin*.

ethoxazene hydrochloride (ĕ-thok′sah-zēn) chemical name: 4-[(4-ethoxyphenyl)azo]-1,3-benzenediamine hydrochloride. A local analgesic, $C_{14}H_{16}N_4O \cdot HCl$, occurring as a reddish powder; used to relieve pain associated with urinary tract infections, administered orally.

ethoxzolamide (eth″oks-zōl′ah-mīd) [USP] a carbonic anhydrase inhibitor, used in the treatment of glaucoma and edema.

Ethrane (eth′rān) trademark for a preparation of enflurane.

Ethril (eth′ril) trademark for preparations of erythromycin stearate.

ethybenztropine (eth″ĭ-benz-tro′pēn) chemical name: *endo*-3-(diphenylmethoxy)-8-ethyl-8-azabicyclo[3.2.1]octane. An anticholinergic with high antihistaminic action, $C_{22}H_{27}NO$, which has been used as an antiparkinsonian agent and in the treatment of drug-induced extrapyramidal syndrome.

ethyl (eth′il) [*ether* + Gr. *hylē* matter] the univalent alcohol radical, $CH_3 \cdot CH_2$. Symbol Et. **e. acetate** [NF], a transparent, colorless liquid, $CH_3COOC_2H_5$, used as a flavoring agent in pharmaceutical preparations. Called also *acetic ether*, *naphtha aceti*, and *vinegar naphtha*. **e. aminobenzoate**, benzocaine. **e. biscoumacetate**, chemical name: 4-hydroxy-α-(4-hydroxy-2-oxo-2*H*-1-benzopyran-3-yl)-2-oxo-2*H*-1-benzopyran-3-acetic acid ethyl ester. One of the synthetic, orally effective coumarin anticoagulants, $C_{22}H_{16}O_8$. **e. butyrate**, the butyric acid ester of ethyl alcohol, $C_3H_7 \cdot CO \cdot O \cdot C_2H_5$, with the odor of pineapple. **e. carbamate**, urethan. **e. carbinol**, propyl alcohol. **e. chloride** [USP], a colorless, extremely volatile, flammable liquid, C_2H_5Cl, sprayed on skin to produce local anesthesia by superficial freezing caused by its rapid evaporation; formerly used as an inhalational anesthetic. **e. cyanide**, a colorless liquid, C_2H_5CN; called also *propionitril*. **e. diacetate**, a substance which has been used in urinary tests. **e. dibunate**, chemical name: 3,6-*bis*(1,1-dimethylethyl)-naphthalenesulfonic acid ethyl ester; an antitussive, $C_{20}H_{28}O_3S$. **e. ether**, see *diethyl ether*. **e. linoleate**, ethyl, (9,12)-cis, cis-octadecadienoate: a lipid occurring on the skin of warm-blooded animals and responsible for its passive water-holding capacity; also prepared synthetically. **e. mercaptan**, a thioalcohol, C_2H_5SH, which has a revolting odor and contributes to the odor of feces. **e. nitrate**, a compound, $CH_3 \cdot CH_2 \cdot NO_3$, formerly used as a vasodilator. **e. nitrite**, $C_2H_5NO_2$, a liquid which is mixed with alcohol to form ethyl nitrite spirit. Called also *nitrous ether*. **e. oleate** [NF], chemical name: (Z)-9-octadecenoic acid ethyl ester. A mobile, practically colorless liquid, $C_{20}H_{38}O_2$, consisting of esters of ethyl alcohol and high-molecular-weight fatty acids; used as a vehicle for pharmaceutical preparations. **e. orange**, a dye, the sodium salt of diethylaniline-azo-benzene-sulfonic acid, $C_6H_4 \cdot N(C_2H_5)_2 \cdot N_2 \cdot C_6H_4 \cdot SO_2 \cdot ONa$; used as an indicator, being turned red by acids and yellow by alkalis. **e. pelargonate**, the pelargonic acid ester of ethyl alcohol, $C_8H_{17} \cdot CO \cdot O \cdot C_2H_5$. **e. phenylcinchoninate**, a yellowish powder once used in gout. **e. phenylephrine**, see *ethylphenylephrine*. **e. salicylate**, the salicylic acid ester of ethyl alcohol, $CH_3 \cdot CH_2 \cdot O \cdot CO \cdot C_6H_4 \cdot OH$, formerly used internally for rheumatism and as a counterirritant. **e. urethan**, a compound which inhibits cellular respiration and interferes with a large number of enzymes in the cell.

ethylaldehyde (eth″il-al′dĕ-hīd) acetaldehyde.

ethylamine (eth″il-am′in) a liquid ptomaine, CH_3CH_2-NH_2, from decaying plant tissue, possessing many of the properties of ammonia.

ethylate (eth′il-āt) any compound of ethyl alcohol in which the hydrogen of the hydroxyl is replaced by a base.

ethylation (eth″il-a′shun) the act of combining or causing to combine with the ethyl radical.

ethylcellulose (eth″il-sel′u-lōs) [NF] chemical name: cellulose ethyl ester. A free-flowing, white to light tan powder, used as a tablet binder in pharmaceutical preparations.

ethylene (eth″ĭ-lēn) ethene, $CH_2{=}CH_2$, a colorless, flammable gas with a sweet taste and odor, formerly used as an inhalational anesthetic. **e. dichloride,** a colorless heavy liquid, $C_2H_4Cl_2$, with a pungent odor, used as a solvent; called also *ethidine chloride*. **e. oxide,** a bactericidal agent, occurring as a colorless gas with a pleasant ethereal odor; used as a disinfectant, especially for disposable equipment.

ethylenediamine (eth″ĭ-lēn-di′ah-mēn) [USP] chemical name: 1,2-ethanediamine. A clear, colorless or slightly yellow liquid, $C_2H_8N_2$, having an ammonia-like odor and a strong alkaline reaction; used as a component of aminophylline injection.

ethylenediaminetetraacetate (eth″ĭ-lēn-di″ah-mēn-tet-ras′ĕ-tāt) a salt of ethylenediaminetetraacetic acid (EDTA). Called also *edetate*.

ethylenediaminetetraacetic acid (eth″il-ēn-di′ah-mēn-tet″rah-ah-se′tik) EDTA; a chelating agent that binds calcium and heavy metal ions; used as an anticoagulant for blood specimens and also (see *edetate*) for treatment of lead poisoning and hypercalcemia.

ethylenimine (eth″il-en′ĭ-mēn) a group of cytotoxic alkylating agents that includes triethylenemelamine (TEM) and thiotepa (triethylenethiophosphoramide).

ethylestrenol (eth″il-es′trĕ-nōl) chemical name: 19-nor-17α-pregn-4-en-17β-ol; an anabolic-androgenic steroid, C_{20}-$H_{32}O$.

ethylic (e-thil′ik) pertaining to or derived from ethyl.

ethylidene (eth′il-ĭ-dēn) the bivalent radical, $CH_3 \cdot CH$; called also *ethidene*.

ethylism (eth′il-izm) poisoning or intoxication by ethyl alcohol.

ethylmorphine hydrochloride (eth″il-mor′-fen) chemical name: 7,8-didehydro-4,5α-epoxy-3-ethoxy-17-methylmorphinan-6α-ol hydrochloride. The chloride salt of the ethyl ester of morphine, $C_{10}H_{15}NO_3 \cdot HCl$, having some of the actions of morphine and codeine; used as a chemotic in the treatment of glaucoma, iritis, and corneal ulcers, applied topically to the conjunctiva. It has also been used as an antitussive.

ethylnoradrenaline (eth″il-nor-ah-dren″ah-lin) ethylnorepinephrine.

ethylnorepinephrine hydrochloride (eth″ĭl-nor-ep″ĭ-nef′rin) [USP] chemical name: 4-(2-amino-1-hydroxybutyl)-1,2-benzendiol hydrochloride. A synthetic adrenergic, $C_{10}H_{15}NO_3 \cdot HCl$, used for the relief of bronchospasm in bronchial asthma; administered intramuscularly or subcutaneously.

ethylnorsuprarenin (eth″il-nor-su″prah-ren′in) ethylnorepinephrine.

ethylparaben (eth″il-par′ah-ben) [NF] chemical name: 4-hydroxybenzoic acid ethyl ester. An antifungal agent, $C_9H_{10}O_3$, occurring as small, colorless crystals or white powder; used as a preservative in pharmaceutical preparations.

ethylphenylhydantoin (eth″il-fen″il-hi-dan′to-in) ethotoin.

ethylstibamine (eth″il-sti′bah-mēn) neostibosan.

ethynodiol diacetate (ĕ-thi″no-di′ōl) [USP] chemical name: 19-norpregn-4-en-20-yne-3β,17α-diol diacetate. A progestin, $C_{24}H_{32}O_4$, occurring as a white, crystalline powder; used in combination with an estrogen as an oral contraceptive.

ethynyl (eth″ĭ-nil) the radical —C≡CH, when it occurs in organic compounds; called also *ethinyl*.

etidocaine hydrochloride (ĕ-te′do-kān) chemical name: (±) N-(2,6-dimethylphenyl)-2-(ethylpropylamino)-butanamide hydrochloride. A local anesthetic of the amide type, $C_{17}H_{28}N_2O \cdot HCl$, used for percutaneous infiltration anesthesia, peripheral nerve blocks, and caudal and epidural blocks.

etidronate (ĕ-tĭ-drō′nāt) a diphosphonate compound, ethane-1-hydroxy-1,1-diphosphonate (EHDP), that inhibits the resorption and deposition of hydroxyapatite crystals in bone and is used for treatment of Paget's disease of bone. It is also used in bone scanning (see *technetium Tc 99m etidronate*).

etidronic acid (e-ti-dro′nik) an acid used as a bone calcium regulator.

etiocholanolone (e″te-o-ko-lan′o-lōn) 3α-hydroxy-5β-androstan-17-one, a reduced form of testosterone, androstenedione, and dehydroepiandrosterone excreted in the urine.

etiogenic (e″te-o-jen′ik) [Gr. *aitia* cause + *gennan* to produce] causative.

etiolation (e″te-o-la′shun) [Fr. *étioler* to blanch] 1. a blanching or paleness of color in a plant due to lack of chlorophyll when grown in the dark. 2. the process by which the skin becomes pale when deprived of sunlight.

etiologic, etiological (e″te-o-loj′ik; e″te-o-loj′e-kal) pertaining to etiology, or to the causes of disease.

etiology (e″te-ol′o-je) [Gr. *aitia* cause + *-logy*] the study or theory of the factors that cause disease and the method of their introduction to the host; the cause(s) or origin of a disease or disorder. Cf. *pathogenesis*.

etiopathology (e″te-o-pah-thol′o-je) pathogenesis.

etioporphyrin (e″te-o-por′fīr-in) a porphyrin (q.v.) in which each pyrrole ring has one methyl and one ethyl side chain.

etiotropic (e″te-o-trop′ik) [Gr. *aitia* cause + *tropos* turning] directed against the cause of a disease.

etodolic acid (e-to-do′lik) an acid with anti-inflammatory and analgesic properties.

etofenamate (ĕ-to-fen′ah-māt) a nonsteroidal anti-inflammatory agent of the fenamate class.

etoformin hydrochloride (et″o-for′min) chemical name: N-butyl-N″-ethylimidodicarbonimidic diamide monohydrochloride; an antidiabetic, $C_8H_{19}N_5 \cdot HCl$.

etomidate (ĕ-tom′ĭ-dāt) chemical name: (+)-1-(1-phenylethyl)-1H-imidazole-5-carboxylic acid ethyl ester; a sedative–hypnotic, $C_{14}H_{16}N_2O_2$; administered intravenously for the induction and maintenance of anesthesia and as a sedative for critically ill patients.

etoposide (e-to-po′sīd) a semisynthetic derivative of podophyllotoxin used as an antineoplastic; administered intravenously.

etoprine (et′o-prēn) chemical name: 5-(3,4-dichlorophenyl)-6-ethyl-2,4-pyrimidinediamine; an antineoplastic, $C_{12}H_{12}Cl_2N_4$.

etoxadrol hydrochloride (ĕ-toks′ah-drōl) chemical name: (+)-2-(2-ethyl-2-phenyl-1,3-dioxolan-4-yl) piperidine hydrochloride; an anesthetic, $C_{16}H_{23}NO_2 \cdot HCl$.

etozolin (et″o-zo′lin) chemical name: [3-methyl-4-oxo-5-(1-piperidinyl)-2-thiazolidinylidene]acetic acid ethyl ester; a diuretic, $C_{13}H_{20}N_2O_3S$.

etryptamine acetate (e-trip′tah-min) chemical name: 3-(2-aminobutyl) indole acetate. A compound, $C_{12}H_{16}N_2 \cdot C_2$-$H_4O_2$, formerly used as a central stimulant, now removed from the market because of serious toxic reactions.

Eu chemical symbol for *europium*.

eu- (u) [Gr. *eu* well] a combining form meaning well, easily, or good; the opposite of *dys-*.

euadrenocorticism (u″ah-dre″no-kōr′tĭ-sizm) the normal state of adrenal cortical secretion, as distinguished from hypo- or hyperadrenocorticism.

euangiotic (u″an-je-ot′ik) [*eu-* + Gr. *angeion* vessel] well supplied with blood vessels.

Euascomycetidae (u-as″ko-mi-se′tĭ-de) a subclass of ascomycetous fungi in which the asci most commonly develop from hyphae, and functional sex organs are usually present; it includes the series Plectomycetes, Pyrenomycetes, and Discomycetes.

eubacteria (u″bak-te′re-ah) 1. bacteria of the genus *Eubacterium*. 2. formerly, bacteria of the order Eubacteriales.

Eubacteriales (u″bak-te″re-a′lēz) in former systems of classification, an order of the class Schizomycetes, made up of the so-called true bacteria, i.e., bacteria that possess peritrichous flagella; cf. *Pseudomonodales.*

Eubacterium (u″bak-te′re-um) [*eu-* + Gr. *baktērion* small rod] a genus of bacteria of the family Propionibacteriaceae, consisting of nonsporulating, gram-positive, anaerobic rod-shaped organisms found as saprophytes in soil and water. They are normal inhabitants of the skin and cavities of humans and other mammals, occasionally causing infections of soft tissues. **E. alactoly′ticum,** a species isolated from dental tartar, various infections, and abscesses. **E. len′tum,** a species isolated from various infections, including infected postoperative wounds and abscesses, and from human blood and feces. Called also *Bifidobacterium cornutum, Corynebacterium diphtheroides,* and group 3 *corynebacterium.* **E. limo′sum,** a species that synthesizes vitamin B₁₂. It has been isolated from the feces of humans and other animals, from human infections, and from mud.

eubacterium (u″bak-te′re-um), pl. *eubacte′ria.* 1. an organism of the genus *Eubacterium.* 2. an organism of the order Eubacteriales.

eubiotics (u″bi-ot′iks) [*eu-* + Gr. *bios* life] the science of healthy living.

eucaine (u′kān) chemical name: 2,2,6-trimethyl-4-piperidinol benzoate ester. A substance, $C_{15}H_{21}NO_2$, closely resembling cocaine in action and composition, but less depressant to the heart; formerly used as a local anesthetic. In veterinary medicine, the hydrochloride is used as a substitute for cocaine. Called also *benzamine.*

eucalyptol (u″kah-lip′tol) a colorless liquid with a characteristic aromatic, camphoraceous odor, and a cooling, pungent, spicy taste, obtained from eucalyptus oil and other sources, used as a flavoring agent, expectorant, and local antiseptic, and formerly as a vermifuge. Used in veterinary medicine as an inhalant in bronchitis and as an expectorant.

Eucalyptus (u″kah-lip′tus) [*eu-* + Gr. *kalyptos* covered] a genus of myrtaceous trees and shrubs, chiefly Australian, of many species; on distillation, the leaves yield eucalyptus oil, the major constituent of which is eucalyptol. Called also *blue gum.*

eucapnia (u-kap′ne-ah) [*eu-* + Gr. *kapnos* smoke] the condition in which the carbon dioxide tension of the blood is normal.

eucaryon (u-kar′e-on) eukaryon.

eucaryosis (u″kar-e-o′sis) eukaryosis.

Eucaryotae (u-kar″e-o′te) [*eu-* + Gr. *karyon* nucleus] in some systems of classification, a kingdom of organisms that includes higher plants and animals, fungi, protozoa, and most algae (except blue-green algae), which are made up of eukaryotic cells, i.e., which have a true nucleus. Also written *Eukaryotae.* Cf. *Prokaryotae.*

eucaryote (u-kar′e-ōt) eukaryote.

eucaryotic (u″kar-e-ot′ik) eukaryotic.

eucatropine hydrochloride (u-kat′ro-pēn) [USP] chemical name: α-hydroxybenzeneacetic acid 1,2,2,6-tetramethyl-4-piperidinyl ester hydrochloride. An anticholinergic, $C_{17}H_{25}NO_3 \cdot HCl$, occurring as a white, granular powder; used as a mydriatic, applied topically to the eye.

Eucestoda (u-ses-to′dah) Cestoda.

euchlorhydria (u″klōr-hi′dre-ah) [*eu-* + *chlorhydric acid*] the presence of the normal proportion of free hydrochloric acid in the gastric juice.

eucholia (u-ko′le-ah) [*eu-* + Gr. *cholē* bile] normal condition of the bile.

euchromatic (u-kro-mat′ic) of or relating to euchromatin.

euchromatin (u-kro′mah-tin) [*eu-* + *chromatin*] the condensed state of chromatin in which it stains lightly, is genetically active, and is partially or fully uncoiled, being the interphase form of the chromosome.

euchromatopsy (u-kro′mah-top″se) [*eu-* + *chromat-* + *opsio*] normal color vision.

euchylia (u-kil′e-ah) [*eu-* + Gr. *chylos* chyle] a normal condition of the chyle.

Eucoccidia (u″kok-sid′e-ah) [*eu-* + Gr. *kokkos* berry] an order of parasitic protozoa (subclass Coccidia, class Sporozoea) found in the blood and epithelial cells of invertebrates, and having a life cycle involving merogony. It includes three suborders: Adeleina, Eimeriina, and Haemosporina.

eucoelom (u-se′lom) [*eu-* + *coelom*] coelom.

Eucoelomata (u″se-lo-ma′tah) the major division of the higher invertebrates, the coelomates, including mollusks, annelids, arthropods, echinoderms, and chordates, which all have a separate mouth and anus, a true coelom, and a well-developed circulatory system. It is divided into two series, the Deuterostomia and the Protostomia.

eucoelomate (u-sēl′o-māt″) any member of the Eucoelomata; a coelomate.

eucolloid (u-kol′oid) a colloid in which each dispersed particle consists of a single large molecule.

eucrasia (u-kra′se-ah) [*eu-* + Gr. *krasis* mixture] 1. a state of health; proper balance of different factors constituting a healthy state. 2. a state in which there is a decreased bodily reaction to ingested or injected drugs, proteins, etc.

eudiemorrhysis (u″di-ĕ-mor′ĭ-sis) [*eu-* + Gr. *dia* through + *haima* blood + *rhysis* flow] the normal flow of blood through the capillaries.

eudiometer (u″de-om′ĕ-ter) [Gr. *eudia* fine weather + *metron* measure] an instrument used in testing the purity of the air.

eudipsia (u-dip′se-ah) [*eu-* + Gr. *dipsa* thirst + *-ia*] ordinary, mild thirst.

euesthesia (u″es-the′ze-ah) [*eu-* + Gr. *aisthēsis* perception] a normal state of the senses.

Euflagellata (u-flaj″ĕ-la′tah) [*eu-* + L. *flagellum whip*] former name for Mastigophora.

euflavine (u-fla′vin) acriflavine.

eugamy (u′gah-me) [Gr. *eu* well + *gamos* marriage] the union of gametes, each of which contains the proper (haploid) complement of chromosomes.

Eugenia (u-je′ne-ah) an extensive genus of myrtaceous trees and shrubs. *E. caryophyllata* Thunb. furnishes clove, clove oil.

eugenic acid (u-jen′ik) eugenol.

eugenicist (u-jen′ĭ-sist) a person who is versed in eugenics.

eugenics (u-jen′iks) [*eu-* + Gr. *gennan* to generate] the improvement of a population by selection of its best specimens for breeding; called also *orthogenics.* Cf. *dysgenics.* **negative e.,** that concerned with prevention of reproduction (procreation) by individuals possessing inferior or undesirable traits. **positive e.,** that concerned with promotion of optimal reproduction of individuals possessing superior or desirable traits.

eugenism (u′jen-izm) that condition of heredity and environment which tends to produce healthy and happy existence.

eugenist (u-jen′ist) eugenicist.

eugenol (u′jen-ol) [USP] chemical name: 2-methoxy-4-(2-propenyl)phenol. A dental analgesic, $C_{10}H_{12}O_2$, occurring as a colorless or pale yellow liquid, obtained from clove oil or other natural sources; applied topically to dental cavities and also used as a component of dental protectives. Called also *allylguaiacol* and *eugenic acid.*

Euglena (u-gle′nah) [*eu-* + Gr. *glēnē* pupil of the eye] a genus of green, plantlike, flagellate protozoa (suborder Euglenina, order Euglenida) commonly found in great abundance in stagnant water. They have a pellicle usually marked by spiral or longitudinal striations; those with a thin pellicle are very plastic. *E. viridis* and *E. gracilis* are common species.

Euglenamorpha (u-glen″nah-mor′fah) [*eu-* + Gr. *glēnē* pupil of the eye + *morphē* form, shape] a genus of plantlike, flagellate protozoa, (suborder Euglenamorphina, order Euglenida) resembling *Euglena* but having three flagella. It comprises a single species, *E. hegneri,* which is found in the gut of tadpoles.

Euglenamorphina (eu-gle″nah-mor-fi′nah) a suborder of plantlike, flagellate protozoa (order Euglenida, class Phytomastigophorea) having three or more flagella. *Euglenamorpha* is a representative genus.

euglenid (u-gle′nid) a protozoan of the order Euglenida; euglenoid.

Euglenida (u-gle′nĭ-dah) an order of plantlike, flagellate protozoa (class Phytomastigophora, subphylum Mastigophora) having green chromatophores when present; one or two, rarely more, flagella protruding from an anterior invagination; and a small stigma located anteriorly in colored forms.

The organisms are usually found in freshwater, although some inhabit salt or brackish water, and a few are parasitic. The order comprises six suborders: Eutriptiina, Euglenina, Rhabdomonadina, Sphenomonadina, Heteronematina, and Euglenamorphina. Called also *Euglenoidina.* See also *euglenoid movement,* under *movement.*

Euglenina (u″glĕ-ni′nah) a suborder of plantlike, biflagellate protozoa (order Euglenida, class Phytomastigophorea), having one highly mobile flagellum emergent from an anterior recess and the other short and nonemergent. *Euglena* is a representative genus.

euglenoid (u-gle′noid) 1. pertaining to the order Euglenoid; see also under movement. 2. a protozoa of the order Euglenoida, euglinid.

Euglenoidina (u-gle″noi-di′nah) Euglenida.

euglobulin (u-glob′u-lin) one of a class of globulins characterized by being insoluble in water but soluble in saline solutions; see also under *globulin.*

euglycemia (u″gli-se′me-ah) a normal level of glucose in the blood.

euglycemic (u″gli-se′mik) pertaining to, characterized by, or conducive to euglycemia.

Euglypha (u-glif′ah) [*eu-* + Gr. *glyphē* carving] a genus of freshwater ameboid protozoa (order Gromiida, class Filosea), having a scaly test and dichotomously branching filopodia.

eugnathia (u-na′the-ah) [*eu-* + *gnath-* + *-ia*] an abnormality of the oral cavity, which is limited to the teeth and their immediate alveolar supports, and does not include the jaws. Cf. *eugnathism.*

eugnathic (u-nath′ik) [*eu-* + Gr. *gnathos* jaw] pertaining to or characterized by eugnathia.

eugnosia (u-no′se-ah) [*eu-* + Gr. *gnōsis* perception] ability to recognize and synthesize sensory stimuli into a normal perception.

eugnostic (u-nos′tik) pertaining to eugnosia.

eugonic (u-gon′ik) [*eu-* + Gr. *gonē* seed] growing luxuriantly; said of bacterial cultures, especially of species of *Mycobacterium,* that produce heavy growth on culture media. Cf. *dysgonic.*

Eugregarinida (u″greg-ah-ri′nĭ-dah) [*eu-* + L. *gregarius* crowding together] an order of parasitic protozoa (subclass Gregarinia, class Sporozoea) typically found in annelids and arthropods and occasionally other invertebrates. Their life cycle includes gametogony and sporogony but not merogony; schizogony does not occur, and syzygy is usually seen. They move progressively by gliding or undulation of longitudinal ridges. The order comprises three suborders: Blastogregarinina, Aseptatina, and Septatina.

euhydration (u-hi-dra′shun) a normal state of body water content; absence of absolute or relative hydration or of dehydration.

eukaryon (u-kar′e-on) [*eu-* + Gr. *karyon* nucleus] 1. a highly organized nucleus bounded by a nuclear membrane, a characteristic of cells of higher organisms. Cf. *prokaryon.* 2. eukaryote.

eukaryosis (u″kar-e-o′sis) [*eu-* + Gr. *karyon* nucleus + *-osis*] the state of having a true nucleus, the nuclear material being surrounded by a membrane and the cytoplasm containing organelles; generally a characteristic of all cell types except bacteria. Cf. *prokaryosis.*

Eukaryotae (u-kar″e-o′te) Eucaryotae.

eukaryote (u-kar′e-ōt) [*eu-* + Gr. *karyon* nucleus] an organism whose cells have a true nucleus, i.e., one bounded by a nuclear membrane, within which lie the chromosomes combined with proteins, and that exhibit mitosis; eukaryotic cells also contain many membrane-bound compartments (organelles) in which cellular functions are performed. The cells of higher plants and animals, fungi, protozoa, and most algae are eukaryotic. See also *Eucaryotae.* Cf. *prokaryote.*

eukaryotic (u″kar-e-ot′ik) pertaining to a eukaryon or a eukaryote or to eukaryosis.

eukeratin (u-ker′ah-tin) a true keratin found in hair, nails, feathers, and horns.

eukinesia (u″ki-ne′se-ah) [Gr. *eu* well + *kinēsis* movement + *-ia*] the state of possessing normal or proper motor function or activity; normal or proper mobility.

eukinesis (u″ki-ne′sis) eukinesia.

eukinetic (u″ki-net′ik) pertaining to or characterized by eukinesia.

eulachon (u′lah-kon) the candle-fish, *Thaleichthys pacificus;* its oil is used like cod liver oil.

eulaminate (u-lam′ĭ-nāt) having the normal number of lamina, as certain areas of the cerebral cortex.

Eulenburg's disease (oil′en-burgz) [Albert *Eulenburg,* German neurologist, 1840–1917] paramyotonia congenita.

Euler (oi′ler) Ulf Svante von. Swedish physiologist, born 1905; co-winner, with Julius Axelrod and Sir Bernard Katz, of the Nobel prize for medicine or physiology in 1970 for his discovery of noradrenalin, showing that it is a chemical intermediary for neurotransmission in the sympathetic nervous system.

eumenorrhea (u″men-o-re′ah) [*eu-* + Gr. *mēn* menses + *rhoia* flow] normal menstruation.

Eumetazoa (u-met″ah-zo′ah) in some classifications, a subdivision of the Metazoa comprising all multicellular animals with organ systems, a mouth, and a digestive cavity. Cf. *Parazoa.*

eumetria (u-me′tre-ah) [Gr. "good measure," "good proportion"] a normal condition of nerve impulse, so that a voluntary movement just reaches the intended goal; the proper range of movement.

eumorphism (u-mor′fizm) [*eu-* + Gr. *morphē* form] retention of the normal form of a cell.

Eumycetes (u″mi-se′tēz) a taxonomic division comprising the true or proper fungi. It includes three classes of perfect fungi (Ascomycetes, Phycomycetes, and Basidiomycetes) and all the imperfect fungi (Deuteromycetes, or Fungi Imperfecti). Called also *Eumycophyta.*

eumycetoma (u″mi-se-to′mah) [*eu-* + *mycetoma*] eumycotic mycetoma.

Eumycetozoea (u″mi-se″to-zo′e-ah) [*eu-* + *myceto-* + Gr. *zōon* animal] a class of protozoa (superclass Rhizopoda, subphylum Sarcodina) consisting of myxamebae with filiform subpseudopodia and flagella that when present usually occur in unequal apical pairs, and producing aerial fruiting bodies; in some species, a stalk tube is present in the fruiting body. It comprises three subclasses: Dictyosteliia, Myxogastria, and Protosteliia. See also *Mycetozoida.*

Eumycophyta (u-mi″ko-fi′tah) Eumycetes.

eunoia (u-noi′ah) [*eu-* + Gr. *nous* mind] (*obs.*) normality or soundness of mind or will.

eunuch (u′nuk) [Gr. *eunouchos* a castrated person, employed in Asia, and later in Greece, to take charge of the women and act as a chamberlain] a man or boy deprived of the testes or the external genital organs, especially one castrated before puberty (so that male secondary sex characteristics fail to develop).

eunuchism (u′nuk-izm) [Gr. *eunouchismos* castration] the condition of being a eunuch or of undeveloped sexual organs in which testicular hormones are not produced. **pituitary e.,** that due to deficiency of pituitary hormones.

eunuchoid (u′nŭ-koid) [Gr. *eunouchoeidēs*] 1. resembling a eunuch; having the characteristics of a eunuch. 2. a hypogonadal male with defective masculinity of appearance, causing him to resemble a eunuch.

eunuchoidism (u′nŭ-koi″dizm) a deficiency of the testes or of the testicular secretion, with impaired sexual power and eunuch-like symptoms. **female e.,** hypogonadism in which the ovaries fail to function at puberty, resulting in infertility, absence of development of secondary sex characteristics, infantile sexual organs, and excessive growth of the long bones. **hypergonadotropic e.,** that associated with high levels of gonadotropins, as in Klinefelter's syndrome. **hypogonadotropic e.,** that due to lack of gonadotropin secretion; either luteinizing hormone or follicle-stimulating hormone or both may be deficient, and anosmia or hyposmia may be associated. Called also *Kallmann's syndrome.*

euosmia (u-os′me-ah) [*eu-* + Gr. *osmē* smell] 1. normal state of the sense of smell. 2. a pleasant odor.

eupancreatism (u-pan′kre-ah-tizm″) a normal condition of the pancreatic function.

eupatorin (u″pah-to′rin) 3′,5-dihydroxy-4′,6,7-trimethoxyflavone; an active (emetic) principle from *Eupatorium perfoliatum.*

Eupatorium (u″pah-to′re-um) a genus of composite-flowered plants. The leaves and tops of *E. perfoliatum*, boneset or thoroughwort, are tonic, diuretic, diaphoretic, and stomachic. The ingestion of *E. rugosum* (*E. urticaefolium*), the white snakeroot, which contains the toxic principle tremetol, causes a disease known as trembles in cattle and sheep.

eupepsia (u-pep′se-ah) [*eu-* + Gr. *pepsis* digestion + -*ia*] good digestion; particularly the presence of a normal amount of pepsin in the gastric juice. Cf. *dyspepsia*.

eupepsy (u′pep-se) eupepsia.

eupeptic (u-pep′tik) pertaining to, characterized by, or promoting eupepsia. Cf. *dyspeptic*.

euperistalsis (u-per″ĭ-stal′sis) normal or painless peristalsis.

Euphorbia (u-for′be-ah) an extensive genus of euphorbiaceous trees, shrubs, and herbs, the spurges, which are actively poisonous, emetic, and cathartic. including *E. antisyphilitica* Zucca., the source of candelilla wax.

euphoretic (u″fo-ret′ik) 1. pertaining to, characterized by, or producing a condition of euphoria. 2. an agent that produces euphoria.

euphoria (u-fo′re-ah) [Gr. "the power of bearing easily"] an exaggerated feeling of physical and mental well-being, especially when not justified by external reality. Euphoria may be induced by drugs such as opioids, amphetamines, and alcohol and is also a feature of mania.

euphoriant (u-fo′re-ant) euphoretic.

euphoric (u-fo′rik) characterized by euphoria.

euphorigenic (u-fōr″ĭ-jen′ik) tending to produce euphoria.

euphoristic (u″fo-ris′tik) causing euphoria.

euplastic (u-plas′tik) [*eu-* + Gr. *plastikos* plastic] readily becoming organized; adapted to the formation of tissue, as in embryonic development or wound healing.

euploid (u′ploid) [*eu-* + -*ploid*] 1. having a balanced set or sets of chromosomes, in any number. 2. an individual or cell having a balanced set or sets of chromosomes, in any number, that is an exact multiple of the haploid number.

euploidy (u-ploi′de) the state of being euploid.

eupnea (ūp-ne′ah) [*eu-* + Gr. *pnein* to breathe] easy or normal respiration.

eupneic (ūp-ne′ik) pertaining to or characterized by eupnea.

eupractic (u-prak′tic) [*eu-* + Gr. *praktikos* active, able, effective] pertaining to, characterized by, or promoting eupraxia.

eupraxia (u-prak′se-ah) [Gr. "good conduct"] intactness of reproduction of coordinated movements.

eupraxic (u-prak′sik) 1. concerned in the proper performance of a function. 2. eupractic.

euprocin hydrochloride (u′pro-sin) chemical name: (8α,9*R*)-10,11-dihydro-6′-(3-methylbutoxy) cinchonan-9-ol dihydrochloride; a topical anesthetic, $C_{24}H_{34}N_2O_2 \cdot 2HCl$.

Euproctis (u-prok′tis) a genus of moths. **E. chrysorrhoe′a (phaeorrhoe′a),** the brown-tail moth, which is the cause of brown-tail rash.

eupyrene (u-pi′rēn) having a normal nucleus or chromatic material; said of certain spermatozoa.

eupyrexia (u″pi-rek′se-ah) a slight fever in the early stage of an infection, regarded as an attempt on the part of the individual to combat the infection.

eupyrous (u′pi-rus) eupyrene.

Eurax (u′raks) trademark for preparations of crotamiton.

Euresol (u′rĕ-sol) trademark for a preparation of resorcinol monoacetate.

eurhythmia (u-rith′me-ah) [Gr. "harmony"] 1. harmonious relationships in body or organ development. 2. regularity of the pulse.

europium (u-ro′pe-um) a rare element, atomic number 63, atomic weight 151.96, symbol Eu.

Eurotiaceae (u-ro″she-a′se-e) a family of ascomycetous fungi of the order Eurotiales, series Plectomycetes, containing the perfect, or sexual, stages of certain species of *Aspergillus* and *Penicillium*, and also the genus *Allescheria*.

Eurotiales (u-ro″she-a′lēz) an order of ascomycetous fungi (series Plectomycetes, subclass Euascomycetidae), in which the asci are irregularly arranged within the primitive cleistothecium.

Eurotium (u-ro′she-um) [Gr. *eurōs* mold] a genus of ascomycetous fungi or molds of the family Eurotiaceae, order Eurotiales. The imperfect (sexual) stage of these fungi includes some of the aspergilli. **E. malig′num,** former name for *Aspergillus fumigatus*. **E. re′pens,** a species sometimes seen on bread and on preserved fruits, and rarely found in human pulmonary infections. Its imperfect stage is *Aspergillus repens*.

eury- [Gr. *eurys* wide] a combining form meaning wide or broad.

eurycephalic (u″re-sĕ-fal′ik) [*eury-* + Gr. *kephalē* head] brachycephalic.

eurycranial (u″re-kra′ne-al) [*eury-* + Gr. *kranian* upper part of the head] brachycranic.

eurygnathic (u″rig-nath′ik) pertaining to or characterized by eurygnathism.

eurygnathism (u-rig′nah-thizm) [*eury-* + Gr. *gnathos* jaw] the state of having a wide jaw.

euryon (u′re-on) [Gr. *eurys* wide] the point on the right and left parietal bones marking the greatest transverse diameter of the skull or head.

euryopia (u″re-o′pe-ah) [*eury-* + -*opia*] abnormally wide opening of the eyes.

Eurypelma (u″re-pel′mah) a genus of tarantulas. **E. hent′zii,** an American tarantula.

Eurysporina (u″re-spo-ri′nah) [*eury-* + *spore*] a suborder of parasitic protozoa (order Bivalvulida, class Myxosporea) having two to four polar capsules at one pole of the spore in a plane perpendicular to the sutural plane. *Ceratomyxa* is a representative genus.

eurythermal (u″re-ther′mal) [*eury-* + Gr. *thermē* heat] able to grow in a wide range of temperature, said of bacteria capable of good growth from 28° C. to 50° C. and above.

eurythermic (u″re-ther′mik) [*eury-* + Gr. *thermē* heat] eurythermal.

Euscorpius (u-skor′pe-us) a genus of scorpions. **E. ital′icus,** the black scorpion of Europe and North Africa.

Eusimulium (u″sĭ-mu′le-um) a genus of flies of the family Simuliidae, various species of which are common hosts of *Onchocerca volvulus*, a filarial worm parasitic in man.

eusitia (u-sit′e-ah) [*eu-* + Gr. *sitos* food] normal appetite.

eusplanchnia (u-splank′ne-ah) [Gr. *eu* well + *splanchna* viscera + -*ia*] a normal condition of the internal organs.

eusplenia (u-sple′ne-ah) normal splenic function.

eustachian (u-sta′ke-an) [named after Bartolommeo *Eustachio* (L. *Eustachius*), an Italian anatomist, 1524–1574] see under *canal, cartilage, tube,* and *valve*.

eustachitis (u″sta-ki′tis) inflammation of the eustachian tube.

eustachium (u-sta′ke-um) the eustachian tube (tuba auditiva [NA]).

eusthenia (u-sthen′e-ah) [*eu-* + Gr. *sthenos* strength] a condition of normal strength and activity.

eusthenuria (u″sthen-u′re-ah) [*eu* + G. *sthenos* strength + *ouron* urine + -*ia*] a normal state of the urine as regards osmolality.

Eustrongylus (u-stron′jĭ-lus) genus of nematode parasites of aquatic birds. **E. gi′gas,** *Dioctophyma renale*.

eusystole (u-sis′to-le) [*eu-* + *systole*] a normal state of the systole of the heart.

eusystolic (u″sis-tol′ik) pertaining to or characterized by eusystole.

Eutamias (u-tam′e-as) the western chipmunk, which harbors the plague-infected flea, *Monopsyllus eumolpi*, and has been found infected with plague.

eutectic (u-tek′tik) [Gr. *eutēktos* easily melted or dissolved] melting readily; said of a mixture that melts at a lower temperature than any of its ingredients.

eutelolecithal (u-tel″o-les′ĭ-thal) [*eu-* + *telolecithal*] having deutoplasm greatly in excess of the cell protoplasm; said of the ova of birds and many reptiles. Cf. *oligolecithal* and *telolecithal*.

euthanasia (u″thah-na′zhe-ah) [*eu-* + Gr. *thanatos* death] 1. an easy or painless death. 2. mercy killing; the deliberate ending of the life of a person suffering from an incurable and painful disease.

euthenic (u-then′ik) conducive to race improvement through environment.

euthenics (u-then′iks) [Gr. *euthēnia* well-being] the science of race improvement through the regulation of environment. Cf. *eugenics*.

eutherapeutic (u-ther″ah-pu′tik) [*eu-* + *therapeutic*] having good therapeutic properties.

Eutheria (u-the′rĭ-ah) [*eu-* + Gr. *thērion* beast, animal] in some systems of classification, a subclass of the Mammalia and in others an infraclass of the subclass Theria, including all the true placental mammals, and excluding the monotremes and marsupials.

eutherian (u-the′rĭ-an) any member of the Eutheria.

euthermic (u-ther′mik) [Gr. *euthermos* very warm] characterized by the proper temperature; promoting warmth.

Euthroid (u′throid) trademark for a preparation of liothrix.

euthymism (u-thi′mizm) a normal condition of thymus activity.

Euthyneura (u″thĕ-nu′rah) a subclass of hermaphroditic mollusks (class Gastropoda) found chiefly in fresh-water or terrestrial habitats; many species are primary or intermediate hosts of various pathogens.

euthyroid (u-thi′roid) having a normally functioning thyroid gland.

euthyroidism (u-thi′roid-ism) a condition of normal thyroid function.

eutocia (u-to′se-ah) [Gr. *eutokia*] normal labor, or childbirth.

Eutonyl (u′to-nil) trademark for a preparation of pargyline hydrochloride.

eutopic (u-top′ik) [*eu-* + Gr. *topos* place] situated normally; arising from the normal site or tissue. Cf. *ectopic*.

Eutreptiina (u-trep″tĭ-i′nah) a suborder of plantlike, flagellate protozoa (order Euglenida, class Phytomastigophorea) having two highly emergent flagella, one directed anteriorly and the other laterally.

Eutriatoma (u″trĭ-at′o-mah) a genus of reduviid bugs, species of which transmit Chagas' disease.

Eutrombicula (u″trom-bik′u-lah) a subgenus of *Trombicula*; see *chigger*. **E. alfredugé′si,** the common chigger of the United States; called also *Trombicula irritans*. **E. splen′dens,** a troublesome species found in southeastern localities.

Eutron (u′tron) trademark for preparations of pargyline hydrochloride and methyclothiazide.

eutrophia (u-tro′fe-ah) [*eu-* + Gr. *trophē* nourishment + *-ia*] a state of normal (good) nutrition.

eutrophic (u-trof′ik) pertaining to, characterized by, or conducive to good nutrition.

eutrophication (u″tro-fĭ-ka′shun) the promotion of excessive growth of an organism to the disadvantage of other organisms in the same ecosystem by oversupplying the former with nutrients; e.g., the stimulation of excessive growth of plants and algae in natural waters by an oversupply of inorganic nitrogen and phosphate compounds found in fertilizers.

euvolia (u-vo′le-ah) normal water content or volume of a given body compartment, e.g., extracellular euvolia.

euxanthon (u-zan′thon) chemical name: 1,7-dihydroxyxanthon. A ketone, dioxydiphenylene ketone oxide, $CO(C_6H_3-OH)_2O$, obtained from Indian yellow.

eV, ev electron volt.

evacuant (e-vak′u-ant) [L. *evacuans* making empty] 1. emptying; serving to clear the bowels. 2. a remedy which empties any organ; a cathartic, emetic, or diuretic.

evacuation (e-vak″u-a′shun) [L. *evacuatio*, from *e* out + *vacuus* empty] 1. an emptying, as of the bowels. 2. a dejection or stool; material discharged from the bowels.

evacuator (e-vak′u-a-tor) an instrument for removing fluid or small particles from a body cavity or container; formerly applied to one for compelling evacuation of the bowels or bladder.

evagination (e-vaj″ĭ-na′shun) an outpouching of a layer or part. **optic e.,** optic vesicle (vesicula ophthalmica [NA]).

Evaginogenina (e-vaj″ĭ-no-jĕ-ni′nah) [*evagination* + Gr. *gennan* to produce] a suborder of ciliate protozoa (suborder Suctorida, subclass Suctoria) found on marine and freshwater organisms with some species being endoparasites, characterized by a large, single, flattened larva with distinct patterns of ventral ciliature; some adults have branched bundles of tentacles. They reproduce by budding that involves evagination of the entire cortical pouch with the bud still attached.

evanescent (ev″ah-nes′ent) [L. *evanescere* to vanish away] vanishing; passing away quickly; unstable; unfixed.

evaporation (e-vap″o-ra′shun) [L. *e* out + *vaporare* to steam] conversion of a liquid or solid into vapor.

evasion (e-va′zhun) in psychiatry, suppression of an idea that comes next in a thought sequence and substitution of a closely related idea; called also *paralogia*.

Eve's method (ēvz) [Frank Cecil *Eve*, English physician, 1871–1952] a method of artificial respiration; see under *respiration, artificial*.

eventration (e″ven-tra′shun) [L. *eventratio* disembowelment, from *e* out + *venter* belly] 1. protrusion of the bowels from the abdomen. 2. removal of the abdominal viscera. **diaphragmatic e.,** elevation of the dome of the diaphragm, usually the result of paralysis of a phrenic nerve. **umbilical e.,** omphalocele.

Eversbusch's operation (a′vārz-boosh″ez) [Oskar *Eversbusch*, German ophthalmologist, 1853–1912] see under *operation*.

eversion (e-ver′zhun) [L. *eversio*] a turning inside out; a turning outward, as of the foot.

evert (e-vert′) [L. *e* out + *vertere* to turn] to turn inside out; to turn outward.

evertor (e-ver′tor) a muscle that turns a part outward.

Evex (e′veks) trademark for a preparation of esterified estrogens.

évidement (a-vēd-maw′) [Fr.] the operation of scooping out a cavity or diseased portion of an organ.

évideur (a-ve-dur′) [Fr.] an instrument for performing évidement.

evil (e′vil) an illness or disease. **poll e.,** an abscess behind the ears of a horse, caused by a dual infection of the supra-atlantal bursa by *Brucella* and *Actinomyces*. **quarter e.,** blackleg.

Evipal (ev′ĭ-pal) trademark for a preparation of hexobarbital.

eviration (e″vi-ra′shun) [L. *e* out + *vir* man] 1. castration, emasculation, effemination, feminization. 2. delusional belief of a man that he has become a woman.

evisceration (e-vis″er-a′shun) [*ex-* + *viscus*] 1. extrusion of viscera outside the body, especially through a surgical incision. 2. removal of viscera; disembowelment. 3. in ophthalmology the removal of the contents of the eyeball, with the sclera being left intact.

evocation (ev″o-ka′shun) [L. *e* out + *vocare* to call] the calling forth of morphogenetic potentialities through contact with organizer material.

evocator (ev′o-ka″ter) a chemical substance emitted by an organizer region of an embryo that evokes a specific morphogenetic response from competent embryonic tissue in contact with it.

evolution (ev″o-lu′shun) [L. *evolutio*, from *e* out + *volvere* to roll] 1. an unrolling. 2. a process of development in which an organ or organism becomes more and more complex by the differentiation of its parts; a continuous and progressive change according to certain laws and by means of resident forces. 3. preformation. Cf. *devolution*. **bathmic e.,** evolution due to something in the organism itself independent of environment; called also *orthogenic e.* **convergent e.,** the appearance of similar forms and/or functions in two or more lines not sufficiently related phylogenetically to account for the similarity. **Denman's spontaneous e.,** a mechanism of spontaneous version in shoulder presentations in which the head rotates behind, and as the breech descends the shoulder ascends in the pelvis, the breech finally coming down and emerging. Called also *Denman's spontaneous version.* **determinate e.,** orthogenesis, def. 2. **Douglas' spontaneous e.,** a mechanism of spontaneous evolution of the fetus in the back anterior position with prolapse of the arm: the head, arrested above the inlet, rotates to the pubis; the neck is applied to the pelvic brim; the chest, abdomen, and breech roll alongside the shoulder; the legs drop out, followed by the other arm and the head. **emergent e.,** the assumption that each step in evolution produces something new and something that could not be predicted from its antecedents. **organic e.,** the origin and development of species; the theory that existing organisms are the result of descent with modification from those of past times. **orthogenic e.,** bathmic e. **parallel e.,** the independent evolution of similar structures in two or more rather closely related organisms. **Roederer's spontaneous e.,** a mechanism of spontaneous evolution in which the fetus is folded like the letter V: the shoulder and back advance and the head is pressed deep into the chest and abdomen. **saltatory e.,** evolution showing sudden changes; mutation or saltation. **spontaneous e.,** the unaided expulsion of a transversely placed fetus without the process of version or turning.

evulsio (e-vul′se-o) [L., from *evellere* to pull out] evulsion.

evulsion (e-vul′shun) [L. *evulsio*] forcible extraction; see *avulsion.*

Ewart's sign (u′arts) [William *Ewart,* English physician, 1848–1929] see under *sign.*

Ewingella (u″ing-el′ah) [W. H. *Ewing,* American bacteriologist] a proposed genus of gram-negative, facultatively anaerobic, rod-shaped bacteria of the family Enterobacteriaceae. The organisms belong to enteric group 40. The type species is *E. americana.*

Ewing's tumor (sarcoma) (u′ingz) [James *Ewing,* New York pathologist, 1866–1943] see under *tumor.*

ex- [L. *ex* out of, away from] a prefix meaning away from, without, or outside; it is sometimes used to denote completely, as in *exacerbation.*

exa- a combining form used in naming units of measurement to indicate a quantity one quintillion (10^{18}) times the unit designated by the root with which it is combined. Symbol, E.

exacerbation (eg-zas″er-ba′shun) [*ex-* + L. *acerbus* harsh] increase in the severity of a disease or any of its symptoms.

exairesis (eks-er′ĕ-sis) [Gr. "a taking out"] exeresis.

exaltation (eg″zawl-ta′shun) a feeling of extreme elation, often associated with delusions of grandeur.

examination (eg-zam″ĭ-na′tion) [L. *examinare*] inspection or investigation, especially as a means of diagnosing disease, qualified according to the methods employed, as physical examination, roentgen examination, cystoscopic examination, etc. **double-contrast e.,** radiologic examination of the stomach using first a high concentration of contrast medium and then (after the stomach empties) a lower concentration of contrast material. The lower concentration is sometimes used first.

exangia (eks-an′je-ah) [*ex-* + Gr. *angeion* vessel] (*obs.*) dilatation of a blood vessel.

exania (ek-sa′ne-ah) [*ex-* + L. *anus*] prolapse of the rectum.

exanimation (eg-zan″ĭ-ma′shun) unconsciousness; coma.

exanthem (eg-zan′them) [Gr. *exanthēma*] 1. a skin eruption or rash. 2. a disease in which skin eruptions or rashes are a prominent manifestation. Classically, six exanthems, or exanthematous diseases, were described that had somewhat similar rashes and were numbered in the order in which they were reported: first (*measles*), second (*scarlet fever*), third (*rubella*), fourth (*Dukes' disease*), fifth (*erythema infectiosum*), and sixth (*exanthema subitum*); only the latter three ordinal designations are sometimes used as synonyms in current terminology. **Boston e.,** a mild febrile exanthematous illness caused by echovirus 16, an epidemic of which occurred in Boston, Massachusetts. **e. subi′tum,** exanthema subitum. **vesicular e.,** a viral disease of swine marked by the formation of vesicles on the snout, lips, tongue, feet, and teats. A local eruption may be produced experimentally in horses by injection into the tongue.

exanthema (eg″zan-the′mah), pl. *exanthe′mas, exanthem′ata* [Gr. *exanthēma*] exanthem. **e. subitum,** an acute, short-lived, probably viral, disease of infants and young children in which after a high fever of 3 to 4 days' duration the temperature suddenly drops to normal and a macular or maculopapular rash appears on the trunk and spreads to

other areas shortly before, simultaneously with, or shortly after the subsidence of the fever; it was given the ordinal designation *sixth disease* to differentiate it from other exanthems (see *exanthem,* def. 2.). Called also *exanthem subitum, roseola,* and *roseola infantum.*

exanthemata (eg″zan″-them′ah-tah) [Gr.] plural of *exanthema.*

exanthematous (eg″zan-them′ah-tus) pertaining to, characterized by, or of the nature of an exanthem.

exanthrope (ek′zan-thrōp) [*ex-* + Gr. *anthrōpos* man] any source of disease not situated within the human body.

exanthropic (ek″zan-throp′ik) of the nature of an exanthrope; not situated within the human body.

exarteritis (eks″ar-tĕ-ri′tis) [*ex-* + *arteritis*] (*obs.*) inflammation of the outer arterial coat.

exarticulation (eks″ar-tik-u-la′shun) [*ex-* + L. *articulus* joint] amputation at a joint; removal of a portion of a joint.

excalation (eks″kah-la′shun) absence or exclusion of one member of a normal series, such as a vertebra.

excarnation (eks″kar-na′shun) [*ex-* + L. *caro, carnis* flesh] removal of superfluous fleshy tissue from a preparation.

excavatio (eks″kah-va′she-o), pl. *excavatio′nes* [L., from *ex* out + *cavus* hollow] excavation: [NA] a general term for a hollowed-out space, or pouchlike cavity. **e. dis′ci** [NA], a depression in the center of the optic disk; called also *optic* or *physiological cup* and *e. papillae nervi optici.* **e. papill′-lae ner′vi op′tici,** e. disci. **e. rectouteri′na** [NA], rectouterine excavation: a sac or recess formed by a fold of the peritoneum dipping down between the rectum and the uterus; called also *cul-de-sac of Douglas, pouch of Douglas, Douglas' space,* and *rectouterine, rectovaginal, uterovesical,* or *vesicouterine pouch.* **e. rectovesica′lis** [NA], rectovesical excavation: the space between the rectum and the bladder in the peritoneal cavity of the male; called also *rectovesical pouch.* **e. vesicouteri′na** [NA], vesicouterine excavation: the space between the bladder and the uterus in the peritoneal cavity; called also *uterovesical* or *vesicouterine pouch.*

excavation (eks″kah-va′shun) [L. *excavatio*] 1. the act of hollowing out. 2. a hollowed-out space, or pouchlike cavity. **atrophic e.,** the cupping of the optic disk, caused by atrophy of the optic nerve fibers. **dental e.,** removal of carious material from a tooth in preparation for restoration. See also *cavity preparation,* under *preparation,* and *prepared cavity,* under *cavity.* **glaucomatous e.,** see under *cup.* **ischiorectal e.,** fossa ischiorectalis. **e. of optic disk, physiologic e.,** excavatio disci. **rectoischiadic e.,** fossa ischiorectalis. **rectouterine e.,** excavatio rectouterina. **rectovesical e.,** excavatio rectovesicalis. **vesicouterine e.,** excavatio vesicouterina.

excavationes (eks″kah-va″she-o′nēz) [L.] plural of *excavatio.*

excavator (eks′kah-va″tor) 1. an instrument for hollowing out something by removing the outer or inner part, or for making a hole or cavity. 2. a scoop or gouge for surgical use. **dental e.,** a handcutting instrument designed for removing the carious dentin of a decayed tooth. See also *discoid,* def. 4. **hatchet e.,** hatchet. **spoon e.,** a dental excavator having a spoonlike blade with the entire margin tapered and sharpened to cut carious dentin out of tooth cavities. Called also *spoon.*

excelsin (ek-sel′sin) a crystalline globulin from the Brazil nut.

excerebration (ek″ser-ĕ-bra′shun) [*ex-* + L. *cerebrum* brain] the removal of the brain, chiefly that of the fetus in embryotomy.

excernent (ek-ser′nent) [L. *excernere* to sift, to separate] causing an evacuation or discharge.

excess (ek-ses′, ek′ses) the state of exceeding that which is normal, sufficient, or needed; superfluous. **antibody e.,** see *prozone.* **antigen e.,** see *precipitin reaction,* under *reaction.*

exchange (eks-chānj) 1. the substitution of one thing for another. 2. to substitute one thing for another. **plasma e.,** the removal of plasma from withdrawn blood, usually to a greater extent than in plasmapheresis, with retransfusion of the formed elements into the donor; done for removal of circulating antibodies or abnormal plasma constituents. The plasma removed is replaced by type-specific frozen plasma or albumin. **sister chromatid e.,** the exchange of segments of DNA between sister chromatids, which occurs very often in patients with Bloom syndrome.

exchanger (eks-chānj'er) an apparatus by which something may be exchanged. **heat e.,** a device which is placed in the circuit of extracorporeal circulation to induce rapid cooling and rewarming of blood.

excipient (ek-sip'e-ent) [L. *excipiens*, from *ex* out + *capere* to take] any more or less inert substance added to a prescription in order to confer a suitable consistency or form to the drug; a vehicle.

excise (ek-sīz') to cut out or off.

excision (ek-sizh'un) [L. *excisio*, from *ex* out + *caedere* to cut] removal, as of an organ, by cutting.

excitability (ek-sīt"ah-bil'ĭ-te) readiness to respond to a stimulus; irritability.

excitable (ek-sīt'ah-b'l) [L. *excitabilis*] susceptible of stimulation; responding to a stimulus.

excitant (ek-sīt'ant) any agent that produces excitation of the vital functions, or of those of the brain.

excitation (ek"si-ta'shun) [L. *excitatio*, from *ex* out + *citare* to call] an act of irritation or stimulation or of responding to a stimulus; the addition of energy, as the excitation of a molecule by absorption of photons. **anomalous atrioventricular e.,** Wolff-Parkinson-White syndrome. **direct e.,** electrostimulation of a muscle by placing the electrode on the muscle itself. **indirect e.,** electrostimulation of a muscle by placing the electrode on its nerve.

excitatory (ek-si'tah-to"re) 1. tending to excitation or stimulation. 2. tending to disassimilation.

excitoanabolic (ek-si"to-an"ah-bol'ik) stimulating anabolism.

excitocatabolic (ek-si"to-kat"ah-bol'ik) stimulating catabolism.

excitoglandular (ek-si"to-glan'du-lar) causing glands to secrete.

excitometabolic (ek-si"to-met"ah-bol'ik) producing metabolic changes.

excitomotor (ek-si"to-mo'tor) 1. tending to produce motion or motor function. 2. an agent that induces motion or functional activity.

excitomotory (ek-si"to-mo'to-re) excitomotor.

excitomuscular (ek-si"to-mus'ku-lar) stimulating muscular activity.

excitonutrient (ek-si"to-nu'tre-ent) exciting or stimulating nutrition.

excitor (ek-si'tor) a nerve, the stimulation of which excites greater action in the part which it supplies.

excitosecretory (ek-si"to-se-kre'to-re) producing increased secretion.

excitovascular (ek-si"to-vas'ku-lar) causing vascular changes.

exclave (eks'klāv) [*ex-* + L. *clavis* key, by analogy with *enclave*] a detached part of an organ, as of the pancreas or of some other gland.

exclusion (eks-kloo'zhun) [L. *exclusio*, from *ex* out + *claudere* to shut] elimination, rejection, or extrusion. Specifically, an operation in which a portion of an organ is separated from the remainder but is not removed from the body. **allelic e.,** the phenomenon in which only a single immunoglobulin is produced by any one B cell or plasma cell. Although the cell possesses two (maternal and paternal) heavy chain genes and four (two κ and two λ) light chain genes, at most one heavy or light chain gene undergoes successful DNA rearrangement and is expressed. **competitive e.,** the tendency for the better adapted species to exclude another related species from its particular ecological niche. See also *character displacement*, under *displacement*.

excochleation (eks-kok"le-a'shun) [*ex-* + L. *cochlea* spoon] the operation of curetting or scooping out a cavity.

exconjugant (eks-kon'joo-gant) [*ex-* + L. *conjugare* to join] either member of a pair of ciliate protozoa or bacteria (conjugants) after separation following conjugation.

excoriation (eks-ko"re-a'shun) [L. *excoriare* to flay, from *ex* out + *corium* skin] a scratch or abrasion of the skin. **neurotic e.,** a self-induced skin lesion, inflicted by the fingernails or other physical means.

excrement (eks'krĕ-ment) [L. *excrementum*, from *ex* out + *cernere* to sift, to separate] fecal matter; matter cast out as waste from the body; called also *ordure.*

excrementitious (eks"krĕ-men-tish'us) pertaining to or of the nature of excrement; fecal.

excrescence (eks-kres'ens) [*ex-* + L. *crescere* to grow] any abnormal outgrowth; a projection of morbid origin. **fungating e., fungous e.,** a fungous growth in the umbilicus after separation of the umbilical cord; granuloma of the umbilicus. **Lambl's e's,** small papillary projections on the cardiac valves seen post mortem on many adult hearts.

excrescent (eks-kres'ent) resembling or of the nature of an excrescence.

excreta (eks-kre'tah) [L., pl.] excretion products; waste materials excreted by the body.

excrete (eks-krēt') [L. *excernere*] to throw off or eliminate, as waste matter, by a normal discharge.

excretin (eks'kre-tin) a crystalline compound, $C_{20}H_{36}O$, derivable from human feces.

excretion (eks-kre'shun) [L. *excretio*] 1. the act, process, or function of excreting. 2. material which is excreted. Cf. *elimination.* **pseudouridine e.,** increased excretion of pseudouridine in the urine of gouty patients, the significance of which remains to be established; a greater turnover of some forms of RNA has been suggested, possibly adding to the hyperuricemia of gout.

excretory (eks'kre-to-re) of, pertaining to, or subserving excretion.

excurrent (eks-kur'ent) excretory; efferent.

excursion (eks-kur'zhun) [L. *excurrere* to run out from] movements occurring from a normal, or rest, position of a movable part in performance of a function, as those of the mandible to attain functional contact between the cusps of the mandibular and maxillary teeth in mastication, or of the chest wall in respiration. Called also *excursive movements.* **lateral e.,** sideward movement of the mandible between the position of closure and that in which the tips of the cusps of opposing teeth are in vertical proximity. **protrusive e.,** movement of the mandible between the position of closure and that in which the incisal edges of the anterior teeth are in vertical approximation. **retrusive e.,** the slight backward and return movement of the mandible between the position of closure and one slightly posterior, more often present with mandibular overclosure.

excursive (eks-kur'sive) pertaining to or characterized by excursion.

excyclophoria (ek"si-klo-fo're-ah) [*ex-* + *cyclophoria*] cyclophoria in which the upper pole of the vertical axis of the eye deviates away from the midline of the face and toward the temple; called also *positive* (or *plus*) *cyclophoria.* Cf. *incyclophoria.*

excyclotropia (ek"si-klo-tro'pe-ah) [*ex-* + *cyclotropia*] cyclotropia in which the upper pole of the vertical axis of the eye deviates away from the midline of the face, and toward the temple; called also *positive* (or *plus*) *cyclotropia.*

excystation (ek"sis-ta'shun) escape from a cyst or envelope; especially a stage in the life cycle of parasites occurring after the cystic form has been swallowed by the host.

exelcin (ek-sel'sin) a substance extracted from Brazil nut.

exemia (ek-se'me-ah) [*ex-* + Gr. *haima* blood + *-ia*] loss of fluid from the blood vessels, the red cells being left behind. Cf. *hemoconcentration.*

exencephalia (eks"en-sĕ-fa'le-ah) exencephaly.

exencephalon (eks"en-sef'ah-lon) exencephalus.

exencephalous (eks"en-sef'ah-lus) characterized by exencephaly.

exencephalus (eks"en-sef'ah-lus) [*ex-* + Gr. *enkephalos* brain] a monster exhibiting exencephaly.

exencephaly (eks"en-sef'ah-le) [*ex-* + Gr. *enkephalos* brain] a developmental anomaly characterized by an imperfect cranium, the brain lying outside of the skull.

exenteration (eks-en"ter-a'shun) [*ex-* + Gr. *enteron* bowel] surgical removal of the inner organs; commonly used to indicate radical excision of the contents of a body cavity, as of the pelvis. Used in connection with the eye, it denotes removal of the entire contents of the orbit. **pelvic e.,** excision of the organs and adjacent structures of the pelvis. **pelvic e., anterior,** excision en masse of the bladder, lower ureters, vagina, adnexa, pelvic lymph nodes, and pelvic peritoneum, with implantation of the ureters into the intact pelvic colon or an ileal conduit. **pelvic e., posterior,** excision en masse of the pelvic colon, uterus, vagina, and adnexa, with or without pelvic lymph node excision, the lower urinary tract being undisturbed. **pelvic e., total,** excision en masse of the bladder, lower ureters, vagina, uterus, adnexa, and the pelvic and lower sigmoid colon, with excision of the pelvic lymph nodes, removal of all the pelvic peritoneum, and replantation of the ureters into an isolated ileal segment.

exenterative (eks-en'ter-ah-tiv) pertaining to or requiring exenteration, as exenterative surgery.

exenteritis (eks-en'ter-i'tis) inflammation of the peritoneal covering of the intestine; visceral peritonitis.

exercise (ek'ser-sīz) the performance of physical exertion for improvement of health or the correction of physical deformity. **active e.,** motion imparted to a part by voluntary contraction and relaxation of the muscles controlling the part. **active assisted e.,** motion imparted to a part of the body by voluntary contraction of muscles controlling the part, assisted by a therapist or by some other means. **active resistive e.,** that performed voluntarily by the patient against resistance. **corrective e.,** the scientific use of bodily movement to maintain or restore normal function in diseased or injured tissues. **free e.,** active exercise in which no aid is derived from external forces. **isokinetic e.,** dynamic muscle activity performed at a constant angular velocity. **isometric e.,** active exercise performed against stable resistance, without change in the length of the muscle. **isotonic e.,** active exercise without appreciable change in the force of muscular contraction, with shortening of the muscle. **muscle-setting e.,** voluntary contraction and relaxation of skeletal muscles without movement of the associated part of the body; called also *static e.* **passive e.,** motion imparted to a segment of the body by another individual, machine, or other outside force, or produced by voluntary effort of another segment of the patient's own body. **static e.,** muscle-setting e. **therapeutic e.,** corrective e. **underwater e.,** exercise performed in a pool or a large tub. Cf. *Hubbard tank.*

exeresis (eks-er'ĕ-sis) [Gr. *exairesis* a taking out] surgical removal or excision.

exergic (ek-ser'jik) [*ex-* + Gr. *ergon* work] giving out work; a term applied to chemical reactions which occur with a decrease in free energy. Cf. *endergic.*

exergonic (ek"ser-gon'ik) [*ex*(o)- + Gr. *ergon* work] characterized or accompanied by the release of energy; said of chemical reactions that release free energy, so that the products have a lower free energy than the reactants. Opposed to *endergonic.*

exesion (eg-ze'zhun) [L. *exedere* to eat out] the gradual destruction of superficial parts of a tissue.

exfetation (eks"fe-ta'shun) [*ex-* + L. *fetus*] ectopic or extrauterine pregnancy.

exflagellation (eks"flaj-ĕ-la'shun) [*ex-* + L. *flagellum*] the rapid formation in the gut of the insect vector of microgametes from the microgamont in *Plasmodium* and certain other sporozoan protozoa.

exfoliatin (eks-fō"le-a'tin) [*ex-* + L. *folium* leaf] an erythrogenic, epidermolytic, heat-stabile, acid-labile exotoxin produced by certain strains of *Staphylococcus aureus* (phage group II), which causes intraepidermal separation by disturbing the adhesive forces between cells in the stratum granulosum to give rise to the clinical manifestations of the scalded skin syndrome. Called also *epidermolysin.*

exfoliatio (eks"fo-le-a'she-o) [L., from *ex* away from + *folium* leaf] exfoliation. **e. area'ta lin'guae,** benign migratory glossitis.

exfoliation (eks"fo-le-a'shun) [L. *exfoliatio*] a falling off in scales or layers. **lamellar e. of newborn,** see *collodion baby,* under *baby.*

exfoliative (eks-fo'le-a"tiv) characterized by exfoliation.

exhalation (eks"hah-la'shun) [L. *exhalatio,* from *ex* out + *halare* to breathe] 1. the giving off of watery or other vapor, or of an effluvium. 2. a vapor or other substance exhaled or given off. 3. the act of breathing out.

exhale (eks-hāl') [*ex-* + L. *halare* to breathe] 1. to expel from the lungs by breathing. 2. to give off a watery or other vapor.

exhaustion (eg-zaws'chun) [*ex-* + L. *haurire* to drain] 1. a state of extreme mental or physical fatigue. 2. the state of being drained, emptied, consumed, or used up. **combat e.,** a general term applicable to any psychiatric combat casualty. See *combat fatigue,* under *fatigue,* and *combat neurosis,* under *neurosis.* **heat e.,** an effect of excessive exposure to heat occurring commonly among workers in furnace rooms, foundries, etc., although it may occur from exposure to the sun's heat. It is marked by subnormal temperature, with dizziness, headache, nausea, and sometimes delirium and/or collapse. Distinguished from heat stroke, in which the body temperature may be dangerously elevated. Called also *heat prostration.* Cf. *sunstroke.* **nervous e.,** neurasthenia.

Exhib. abbreviation for L. *exhibea'tur,* let it be given.

exhibition (ek"sĭ-bish'un) administration of a drug.

exhibitionism (ek"sĭ-bish'ŭ-nizm") [DSM III-R] a paraphilia characterized by recurrent intense sexual urges and sexually arousing fantasies of exposing the genitals to an unsuspecting stranger. Exhibitionism occurs almost exclusively in males.

exhibitionist (ek"sĭ-bish'ŭ-nist) a person affected with exhibitionism.

exhilarant (eg-zil'ar-ant) [L. *exhilarare* to gladden] (*obs.*) 1. causing elevation or gladness. 2. an enlivening or elating agent.

exhumation (eks"hu-ma'shun) [*ex-* + L. *humus* earth] disinterment; removal of the dead body from the earth after burial.

exitus (ek'sĭ-tus), pl. *exitus* [L. "a going out"] 1. death. 2. an exit or outlet. **e. pel'vis,** apertura pelvis inferior.

Exna (eks'nah) trademark for a preparation of benzthiazide.

Exner's plexus (eks'nerz) [Siegmund *Exner,* Austrian physiologist, 1846–1926] see under *plexus.*

exo- [Gr. *exō* outside] a prefix meaning outside, or outward.

exo-amylase (ek"so-am'ĭ-lās) β-amylase.

exoantigen (ek"so-an'te-jen) ectoantigen.

exobiology (ek"so-bi-ol'o-je) the science concerned with the study of life on planets other than the earth.

exocardia (ek"so-kar'de-ah) ectocardia.

exocardial (ek"so-kar'de-al) situated, occurring, or developed outside the heart.

exocarp (ek'so-karp) the outer layer of the pericarp of a flower.

exocataphoria (ek"so-kat"ah-fo're-ah) [*exo-* + *cataphoria*] a phoria in which the visual axes turn downward and outward.

exocele (ek'so-sēl) extraembryonic coelom.

exocellular (eks"o-sel'u-lar) external to the cell membrane, yet still attached, e.g., flagella, capsule.

exocervix (ek"so-ser'viks) ectocervix.

exochorion (ek"so-ko're-on) that part of the chorion which is derived from the ectoderm, as in those species in which extraembryonic membranes form by folding.

exocoelom (ek"so-se'lom) [*exo-* + *coelom*] extraembryonic coelom.

exocoeloma (ek"so-se-lo'mah) extraembryonic coelom.

exocolitis (ek"so-ko-li'tis) [*exo-* + *colitis*] inflammation of the outer coat of the colon.

exocrine (ek'so-krin) [*exo-* + Gr. *krinein* to separate] 1. secreting outwardly, via a duct; Cf. *endocrine.* 2. denoting such a gland or its secretion. See also under *gland.*

exocrinology (ek"so-krī-nol'o-je) the study of substances secreted externally by individual organisms which effect integration of a group of organisms.

exocrinosity (ek"so-krī-nos'ĭ-te) the quality or state of secreting externally.

exocuticle (ek"so-ku'tĭ-kl) [*exo-* + L. *cuticula*] the outer layer of the procuticle of certain crustaceans and arthropods, which contains cuticulin, chitin, and phenolic substances that are oxidized to produce the dark pigment of the cuticle.

exocyclic (ek-so-si'klik) a term applied to cyclic chemical compounds having their double bond in the side chain.

exocytosis (ek"so-si-to'sis) 1. the discharge from a cell of particles that are too large to diffuse through the wall; the opposite of endocytosis. 2. the aggregation of migrating leukocytes in the epidermis as part of the inflammatory response.

exodeoxyribonuclease (ek″so-de-ok″se-ri″bo-nu′kle-ās) [EC 3.1.11] any of a sub-sub class of enzymes of the hydrolase class that catalyze the hydrolysis of terminal bonds of deoxyribonucleotides, releasing mononucleotides.

exodeviation (ek″so-de″ve-a′shun) 1. exophoria. 2. exotropia.

exodic (ek-sod′ik) [ex- + Gr. hodos way] centrifugal or efferent.

exodontia (ek″so-don′she-ah) exodontics.

exodontics (ek″so-don′tiks) that branch of dentistry dealing with extraction of the teeth. Called also exodontia.

exodontist (ek″so-don′tist) a dentist who practices exodontics.

exoenzyme (ek″so-en′zīm) an extracellular enzyme; an enzyme that acts outside of the cells in which it originates.

exoergic (ek″so-er′jik) characterized by or accompanied by loss of free energy; releasing energy, as in a chemical reaction during and by which energy is released; energy releasing. Cf. endoergic and endothermic.

exoerythrocytic (ek″so-ĕ-rith″ro-si′tik) outside the erythrocyte, a term applied to stages in the development of malarial parasites which takes place in tissue cells instead of in erythrocytes.

exogamy (ek-sog′ah-me) [exo- + Gr. gamos marriage] protozoan fertilization by the union of elements that are not derived from the same cell. Cf. autogamy (def. 1) and endogamy (def. 1).

exogastric (ek″so-gas′trik) pertaining to the external surface of the stomach.

exogastritis (ek″so-gas-tri′tis) inflammation of the external coat of the stomach.

exogastrula (ek″so-gas′troo-lah) [exo- + gastrula] a gastrula in which invagination is hindered and the mesentoderm bulges outward.

exogastrulation (eks″o-gas″troo-la′shun) the evagination to the exterior (or turning inside out) of the gut due to an interference with the normal processes of gastrulation, which can occur if the morula is cut transversely below the equator. It is usually followed by a migration of mesenchyme cells into the interior.

Exogemmina (ek″so-jem′ĭ-nah) [exo- + gemmare to bud] a suborder of endocommensal ciliate, mostly stalked protozoa (order Chonotrichida, superorder Phyllopharyngidea) found in fresh and brackish waters. They reproduce by external budding and have a relatively large, long cylindrical body with a well-developed collar.

exogenetic (ek″so-jĕ-net′ik) [exo- + Gr. gennan to produce] exogenous.

exogenic (ek″so-jen′ik) exogenous.

Exogenina (ek″so-jĕ-ni′ah) [exo- + Gr. gennan to produce] a suborder of ciliate protozoa (order Suctorida, subclass Suctoria), most species of which are large and either solitary and marine, free-living, or endocommensal organisms, and some species have both prehensile and suctorial tentacles; the larvae of some species are long, vermiform, nonmotile, and practically naked. The organisms reproduce by exogenous budding without invagination of the parental cortex.

exogenote (eks″o-je′nōt) in bacterial genetics, the extra piece of genetic information introduced by transduction into the recipient cell by the donor cell. Cf. endogenote.

exogenous (eks-oj′ĕ-nus) [exo- + Gr. gennan to produce] 1. developed or originating outside the organism, as exogenous disease. 2. growing by additions to the outside.

exognathia (ek″sog-na′the-ah) prognathism.

exognathion (ek″sog-na′the-on) [exo- + Gr. gnathos jaw] the maxilla exclusive of the premaxilla.

exomphalos (eks-om′fah-los) [ex- + Gr. omphalos navel] congenital umbilical hernia.

exomysium (eks″o-mis′e-um) perimysium.

exon (eks′on) a coding sequence in a gene; see intron.

exonuclease (ek″so-nu′kle-ās) [EC 3.1.11,16] any of the enzymes of the hydrolase class that catalyze the hydrolysis of terminal bonds of deoxyribonucleotide or ribonucleotide chains, releasing mononucleotides. Cf. endonuclease.

exopathic (ek″so-path′ik) of the nature of an exopathy; originating outside the body.

exopathy (eks-op′ah-the) [exo- + Gr. pathos disease] a disease originating in some cause lying outside the organism; exogenous disease.

exopeptidase (ek″so-pep′tĭ-dās) any enzyme of the hydrolase class that catalyzes the hydrolysis of a terminal peptide bond, releasing a single amino acid from that chain.

exophoria (ek-so-fo′re-ah) [exo- + phoria] a form of heterophoria in which there is deviation of the visual axis of one eye away from that of the other eye in the absence of visual fusional stimuli. Called also exodeviation.

exophoric (ek″so-for′ik) pertaining to or characterized by exophoria.

exophthalmic (ek″sof-thal′mik) of or pertaining to or characterized by exophthalmos.

exophthalmogenic (ek″sof-thal″mo-jen′ik) causing or producing exophthalmos.

exophthalmometer (ek″sof-thal-mom′ĕ-ter) an instrument for measuring the amount of exophthalmos; called also ophthalmostatometer, orthometer, proptometer, protometer, and statometer.

exophthalmometric (ek″sof-thal″mo-met′rik) pertaining to exophthalmometry.

exophthalmometry (ek″sof-thal-mom′ĕ-tre) [exophthalmos + -metry] measurement of the extent of protrusion of the eyeball in exophthalmos.

exophthalmos (ek″sof-thal′mos) [ex- + Gr. ophthalmos eye] abnormal protrusion of the eyeball; called also proptosis. **endocrine e.,** exophthalmos associated with disorder of an endocrine gland, commonly thyrotoxicosis. **malignant e.,** the severe exophthalmos of Graves' disease in which there is marked edema and infiltration of the orbital tissues and extraocular muscles, proptosis, and stare. It was formerly attributed to overactivity of thyrotropin, and so was formerly called thyrotropic e. **pulsating e.,** exophthalmos with pulsation and bruit, often due to aneurysm pushing the eye forward. **thyrotoxic e.,** a mild form due to thyrotoxicosis. **thyrotropic e.,** malignant e.

exophthalmus (ek″sof-thal′mus) exophthalmos.

exophytic (ek″so-fit′ik) [exo- + Gr. phyein to grow] growing outward; in oncology, proliferating on the exterior or surface epithelium of an organ or other structure, in which the growth originated.

exoplasm (ek′so-plazm) plasma membrane.

exorbitism (ek-sor′bĭ-tizm) exophthalmos.

exoribonuclease (ek″so-ri″bo-nu′kle-ās) [EC 3.1.13–14] any enzyme of two sub-subclasses of the hydrolase class that catalyzes the hydrolysis of terminal bonds of ribonucleotides, producing mononucleotides.

exosepsis (ek″so-sep′sis) [ex- + Gr. sēpsis decay] septic poisoning which does not originate within the organism.

exoserosis (ek″so-se-ro′sis) an oozing of serum or exudate, as in moist skin diseases and edema.

exoskeleton (ek″so-skel′ĕ-ton) [exo- + skeleton] a hard structure developed on the outside of the body, as the shell of a crustacean. In vertebrates the term is applied to structures produced by the epidermis, as hair, nails, hoofs, teeth, etc.

exosmose (ek′sos-mōs) to diffuse from within outward.

exosmosis (ek″sos-mo′sis) [ex- + Gr. ōsmos impulsion] diffusion or osmosis from within outward; movement outward through a diaphragm or through vessel walls. Cf. endosmosis.

exospore (ek′so-spōr) conidium.

exosporium (ek″so-spo′re-um) the external layer of the envelope of a spore.

exostosectomy (ek-sos″to-sek′to-me) excision of an exostosis.

exostosis (ek″sos-to′sis) [ex- + Gr. osteon bone] a benign bony growth projecting outward from the surface of a bone, characteristically capped by cartilage. **e. bursa′ta,** an exostosis from the epiphyseal portion of a bone, consisting of bone and cartilaginous tissue covered by a connective-tissue capsule. **e. cartilagin′ea,** a variety of osteoma consisting of a layer of cartilage developing beneath the periosteum of a bone. **hereditary multiple exostoses,** multiple e. **ivory e.,** a bony growth of great density. **multiple exostoses,** a hereditary disorder characterized by exostoses near the extremities of diaphyses of long bones, which may be cartilaginous or osteocartilaginous growths. Transmitted as an autosomal dominant, it is generally benign, although sarcomatous changes have occurred. Called also *diaphyseal aclasis* and *multiple cartilaginous exostoses*. **multiple cartilaginous exostoses,** multiple exostoses. **osteocartilaginous e.,** osteochondroma.

exostotic (ek″sos-tot′ik) pertaining to or of the nature of exostosis.

exoteric (ek″so-ter′ik) [Gr. *exōterikos* outer] generated or developed outside the organism; exogenous.

exothelioma (ek″so-the″le-o′mah) meningioma.

exothermal (ek″so-ther′mal) exothermic.

exothermic (ek″so-ther′mik) [*exo-* + Gr. *thermē* heat] characterized or accompanied by the evolution of heat, as in a chemical reaction during and by which heat is released; liberating heat or energy from its potential forms. Cf. *endothermic* and *exoergic*.

exotic (eg-zot′ik) of foreign origin; not native.

exotoxic (ek″so-tok′sik) [*exo-* + *toxic*] pertaining to or produced by an exotoxin.

exotoxin (ek″so-tok′sin) [*exo-* + *toxin*] a toxic substance formed by species of certain bacteria (e.g., *Bacillus*, *Bordetella*, *Clostridium*, *Corynebacterium*, *Escherichia*, *Pseudomonas*, *Staphylococcus*, *Streptococcus*, *Vibrio*, *Salmonella*, *Shigella*, *Yersinia*) that is found outside the bacterial cell, or free in the culture medium. Exotoxins are heat-labile and protein in nature. They are detoxified with retention of antigenicity by treatment with formaldehyde (formol toxoid), and are the most poisonous substances known to man; the LD_{50} of crystalline botulinum type A toxin for the mouse is 4.5×10^{-9} mg.

exotropia (ek″so-tro′pe-ah) [*exo-* + *tropia*] strabismus in which there is permanent deviation of the visual axis of one eye away from that of the other, resulting in diplopia; called also *divergent* or *external strabismus*, and *walleye*.

exotropic (ek″so-tro′pik) pertaining to or characterized by exotropia.

expander (ek-span′der) [L. *expandere* to spread out] extender. **plasma volume e.,** artificial plasma extender.

expansion (ek-span′shun) [L. *expandere* to spread out] 1. the process or state of being increased in extent, surface, or bulk. 2. a region or area of increased bulk or surface. **e. of the arch,** maxillary e. **clonal e.,** an immunological response in which lymphocytes stimulated by antigen proliferate and amplify the population of relevant cells. **cubical e.,** increase in volume by an increase in all dimensions. **hygroscopic e.,** an increase in dimensions of a body or substance as a result of absorption of moisture. **maxillary e.,** an orthodontic method of correcting narrow or collapsed maxillary arches and functional posterior crossbite, whereby increased maxillary arch width is obtained with the use of various appliances that provide laterally expansive force resulting in orthopedic and orthodontic movements. Called also *e. of the arch*. **setting e.,** the increase in dimensions of a material, such as plaster of Paris, which occurs concurrently with its hardening. **thermal e.,** an increase in dimensions of a body or substance as a result of an increase in its temperature. **wax e.,** an increase, ordinarily thermally induced, in the dimensions of a wax pattern for a dental restoration to compensate for shrinkage of the gold during the casting process.

expansiveness (ek-span′siv-nes) behavior marked by euphoria, loquacity, and grandiosity.

expectancy (ek-spek′tan-se) the probability of occurrence of a specific event. **life e.,** the number of years, based on statistical averages, that a given person of a specific age or class may reasonably expect to continue living.

expectorant (ek-spek′to-rant) [*ex-* + L. *pectus* breast] 1. promoting the ejection, by spitting, of mucus or other fluids from the lungs and trachea. 2. an agent that promotes the ejection of mucus or exudate from the lungs, bronchi, and trachea; sometimes extended to all remedies that quiet cough (antitussives). **liquefying e.,** an expectorant that promotes the ejection of mucus from the respiratory tract by decreasing its viscosity. **stimulant e.,** an expectorant that stimulates secretion of mucus by the respiratory tract mucosa. **Stokes's e.,** expectorant mixture.

expectoration (ek-spek″to-ra′shun) 1. the act of coughing up and spitting out materials from the lungs, bronchi, and trachea. 2. sputum.

experiment (ek-sper′ĭ-ment) [L. *experimentum* "proof from experience"] a procedure done in order to discover or to demonstrate some fact or general truth. **bulbocapnine e.,** the experimental injection of the alkaloid bulbocapnine into animals, which produces in them the motor phenomena typical of catatonia. **check e.,** crucial e. **control e.,** an experiment that is made under standard conditions, to test the correctness of other observations; see also *control*. **crucial e.,** an experiment so designed and so prepared for by previous work that it will definitely settle some point. **Cyon's e.,** the application of a stimulus to an intact anterior spinal nerve root, which induces a stronger contraction of muscle than the same stimulus to the peripheral end of a divided nerve root. **defect e.,** observation of an embryo, after destruction of a region or part, to ascertain the effect on development. **Goltz's e.,** the striking of a frog on the abdomen, which produces stoppage of the heart's action. **Küss's e.,** injection of a solution of opium or belladonna into the bladder, which produces no symptoms of poisoning and thus proves the impermeability of the bladder epithelium to these substances. **Mariotte's e.,** (to demonstrate the blind spot of the eye), the eye is fixed on the center of a cross marked on a card on which is also marked a large spot; the card is moved to or from the face, and at a certain distance the image of the spot will disappear. **Müller's e.,** the converse of Valsalva's maneuver, i.e., making a forced inspiratory effort with the glottis closed. **Nussbaum's e.,** ligation of the renal arteries of an animal in order to isolate the glomeruli of the kidneys from the circulation. **Scheiner's e.,** an experiment in accommodation: one looks at an object through two pinholes closer together than pupil diameter in a card. If the object is in focus, only one image is observed; if it is not, two or more images are seen. **Stensen's e.,** the experiment of cutting off the blood supply from the lumbar region of the spinal cord of an animal by compressing the abdominal aorta; it produces paralysis of the posterior parts of the body. **Toynbee's e.,** the experiment of partially exhausting the air in the tympanic cavity by swallowing while the nose and mouth are closed. **Valsalva's e.,** see under *maneuver*.

expirate (eks′pĭ-rāt) expired gas (or air); the gas expired in one expiration is called *single expirate*.

expiration (eks″pĭ-ra′shun) [*ex-* + L. *spirare* to breathe] 1. the act of breathing out, or expelling air from the lungs. 2. termination, or death.

expiratory (eks-pi′rah-to″re) subserving or pertaining to expiration.

expire (ek-spīr′) 1. to breathe out. 2. to die, or terminate.

expirium (eks-pi′re-um) (*obs.*) an expiration.

expiscation (eks″pis-ka′shun) (*obs.*) the long-continued study of symptoms for diagnostic purposes.

explant 1. (eks-plant′) to take from the body and place in an artificial medium for growth. 2. (eks′plant) tissue taken from its original site and transferred to an artificial medium for growth.

explode (eks-plōd′) [L. *explodere*, from *ex* out + *plaudere* to clap the hands] 1. to undergo sudden and violent decomposition or combustion. 2. to burst; to spread rapidly, as an epidemic.

exploration (eks″plo-ra′shun) [L. *exploratio*, from *ex* out + *plorare* to cry out] investigation or examination for diagnostic purposes.

exploratory (eks-plo′rah-to″re) [L. *exploratorius*] pertaining to exploration or investigation.

explorer (eks-plōr′er) 1. an instrument for use in exploration, particularly for foreign bodies. 2. an instrument with a flexible, sharp point, used to examine the crown of a tooth for defects or caries.

explosion (eks-plo′zhun) [L. *explosio*] 1. the act of exploding. 2. a sudden and violent outbreak, as of emotion. 3. the discharge of a neural cell.

explosive (eks-plo′siv) characterized by explosions, or by sudden and violent outbreaks.

exponent (ek-spo′nent, eks′po-nent) a number or symbol placed above and to the right of another number or symbol indicating the number of times that that value is to be multiplied by itself; a negative exponent indicates the reciprocal of the quantity arrived at by multiplication. For example, $3^3 = 3 \times 3 \times 3 = 27$, and $x^{-2} = \frac{1}{x \times x}$.

exponential (eks″po-nen′shul) denoting a mathematical

function in which the variable or variables appear in exponents, e.g., $y = a^x$, where a is a constant and x is a variable.

exposure (eks-po′zhur) [L. *exponere* to put out]　1. the act of laying open, as surgical exposure. 2. the condition of being subjected to something, as to infectious agents, extremes of weather or radiation, which may have a harmful effect. 3. in radiology, a measure of the roentgen ray or gamma radiation at a certain place based on its ability to cause ionization. The unit of exposure is the roentgen. Symbol X. Called also *exposure dose*. 4. in radiology, the product of the intensity of roentgen rays and the time the film is exposed.　**acute e.,** radiation exposure of short duration, usually referring to a heavy dose. See also *acute radiation syndrome*, under *syndrome*.　**air e.,** radiation exposure measured in a small mass of air, excluding backscatter from irradiated objects; called also *air dose*.　**chronic e.,** a long-term radiation exposure, either continuous (*protraction exposure*) or intermittent (*fractionation exposure*), usually referring to exposure to low-intensity radiation; effects may include accelerated aging, neoplastic disease, and genetic damage.

expressate (eks-pres′āt)　the material forced out by expression.

expression (eks-presh′un) [L. *expressio*]　1. the aspect or appearance of the face as determined by the physical or emotional state.　2. the act of squeezing or evacuating by pressure; a term used in pharmacy, surgery, and obstetrics. **Kristeller e.,** see under *method*.

expressivity (eks″pres-iv′ĭ-te)　in genetics, the extent to which a genetic defect is expressed. It there is variable expressivity, the trait may vary in expression from mild to severe but is never completely unexpressed in those who have the corresponding genotype.

expulsive (ek-spul′siv) [*ex-* + L. *pellere* to drive]　driving or forcing out; tending to expel.

exsanguinate (eks-sang′gwĭ-nāt) [*ex-* + L. *sanguis* blood]　1. to deprive of blood. 2. bloodless; anemic.

exsanguination (eks-sang″wĭ-na′shun)　extensive loss of blood due to internal or external hemorrhage.

exsanguine (eks-sang′win)　bloodless.

exsanguinotransfusion (eks-sang″gwĭ-no-trans-fu′zhun)　exchange transfusion.

exsect (ek-sekt′)　to excise; to cut out.

exsection (ek-sek′shun)　excision.

exsector (ek-sek′tor)　a cutting instrument for use in performing exsections (excisions).

exsiccant (ek-sik′ant)　desiccant.

exsiccate (ek′sĭ-kāt) [L. *exsiccare*, from *ex* out + *siccus* dry]　desiccate.

exsiccation (ek″sĭ-ka′shun)　the act of drying; in chemistry, the deprival of a crystalline substance of its water of crystallization.

exsorption (ek-sorp′shun)　the movement of substances out of cells, especially the movement of substances out of the blood, through the intestinal epithelial cells, and into the intestinal lumen.

exstrophy (ek′stro-fe) [*ex-* + Gr. *strephein* to turn oneself]　the congenital eversion or turning inside out of an organ, as the bladder.　**e. of the bladder,** a developmental anomaly marked by absence of a portion of the lower abdominal wall and the anterior vesical (urinary bladder) wall, with eversion of the posterior vesical wall through the deficit and with an open pubic arch and widely separated ischia connected by a fibrous band. Called also *ectopia vesicae*.　**e. of cloaca, cloacal e.,** a developmental anomaly in which two segments of bladder (hemibladders) are separated by an area of intestine with a mucosal surface, which appears as a large red tumor in the midline of the lower abdomen. Called also *ectopia cloacae*.

exsufflation (ek″suf-fla′shun) [*ex-* + L. *sufflatio* a blowing up]　the act of exhausting the air content of a cavity by artificial or mechanical means, especially such action upon the lungs by means of an exsufflator.

exsufflator (ek″suf-fla′tor)　an apparatus which, by the sudden production of negative pressure, can reproduce in the bronchial tree the effects of a natural, vigorous cough.

ext.　extract.

extender (ek-sten′der) [*ex-* + L. *tendere* to stretch]　something which enlarges or prolongs.　**artificial plasma e.,** a substance which can be transfused, to maintain fluid volume of the blood in event of great necessity, supplemental to the use of whole blood and plasma.

extension (ek-sten′shun) [L. *extensio*]　1. the movement by which the two elements of any jointed part are drawn away from each other.　2. a movement which brings the members of a limb into or toward a straight relation.　**Buck's e.,** the extension of a fractured leg by weights, the foot of the bed being raised so that the body makes counterextension.　**nail e.,** extension exerted on the distal fragment of a fractured bone by means of a nail or pin driven into the fragment.　**e. per contiguita′tem,** the spreading of a morbid process through one tissue or part into one adjacent to it.　**e. per continuita′tem,** the spreading of a morbid process throughout a single tissue or part.　**e. per sal′tam,** the spreading of a morbid condition from one part to a part or tissue distant from it, with normal tissues intervening; metastasis.　**ridge e.,** an intraoral surgical operation for deepening the vestibular and oral sulci so as to increase the relative intraoral height of the alveolar ridge to facilitate denture retention.

extensometer (eks″ten-som′ĕ-ter) [L. *extensus* extension + Gr. *metron* measure]　an instrument for measuring distortion of specimens under test.

extensor (eks-ten′sor) [L.]　[NA] a general term for any muscle that extends a joint.

exterior (eks-te′re-or) [L.]　situated on or near the outside; outer.

exteriorize (eks-te′re-or-īz)　1. to form a correct mental reference of the image of an object seen.　2. in psychiatry, to turn one's interest outward.　3. to transpose an internal organ to the exterior of the body.

extern (eks′tern)　a medical student or graduate in medicine who assists in the care of patients in a hospital but does not reside in the hospital.

external (eks-ter′nal) [L. *externus* outside]　situated or occurring on the outside; many anatomical structures formerly called external are now more correctly termed lateral.

externalia (eks″ter-na′le-ah)　the external genitals.

externalization (eks-ter″nal-ĭ-za′shun)　the tendency to perceive in the external world and external objects components of one's own personality, including instinctual impulses, conflicts, moods, attitudes, and ways of thinking.

externe (eks′tern)　extern.

externus (eks-ter′nus)　external; [NA] a term denoting a structure or an aspect farther from the center of a part or cavity.

exteroceptive (eks″ter-o-sep′tiv)　Sherrington's term for the external surface field of distribution of receptor organs; see *interoceptive, proprioceptive,* and *receptor* (def. 3).

exteroceptor (eks″ter-o-sep′tor)　a sensory nerve terminal which is stimulated by the immediate external environment, such as those in the skin and mucous membranes; cf. *interoceptor, proprioceptor,* and *receptor* (def. 3).

exterofection (eks″ter-o-fek′shun)　the response of the body made to changes in external environment, effected by the cerebrospinal system.

exterofective (eks″ter-o-fek′tiv)　responding to external stimuli; a term applied by Cannon to the cerebrospinal nervous system.

exterogestate (eks″ter-o-jes′tāt)　1. developing outside the uterus, but still requiring complete care to meet all physical needs.　2. an infant during the period of exterior gestation.

extima (eks′tĭ-mah) [L.]　outermost.

extinction (eks-ting′shun)　in psychology, the disappearance of a conditioned response as a result of nonreinforcement; also, the process by which the disappearance is accomplished.

extinguish (eks-ting′gwish) [L. *extinguere*]　to render extinct.

extirpation (ek″ster-pa′shun) [L. *extirpare* to root out, from *ex* out + *stirps* root]　complete removal or eradication of an organ or tissue.　**dental pulp e.,** pulpectomy.

extorsion (eks-tor′shun) [*ex-* + *torsion*]　outward rotation of the upper pole of the vertical meridian of each eye; called also *obtorsion* and *disclination*. Cf. *intorsion*.

extra- [L. *extra* outside] a prefix meaning outside of, beyond, or in addition.

extra-adrenal (eks″trah-ah-dre′nal) situated or occurring outside the adrenal gland.

extra-anthropic (eks″trah-an-throp′ik) exanthropic.

extra-articular (eks″trah-ar-tik′u-lar) [*extra-* + L. *articulus* joint] situated or occurring outside a joint.

extrabronchial (eks″trah-brong′ke-al) outside or independent of the bronchial tubes; usually used in contrast to intrabronchial.

extrabuccal (eks″trah-buk′al) outside the mouth or cheek.

extrabulbar (eks″trah-bul′bar) outside or away from a bulb, as the medulla oblongata or the urethral bulb.

extracapsular (eks″trah-kap′su-lar) situated or occurring outside a capsule.

extracardial (eks″trah-kar′de-al) outside the heart.

extracarpal (eks″trah-kar′pal) just outside the region of the wrist.

extracellular (eks″trah-sel′u-lar) outside a cell or cells.

extracerebral (eks″trah-ser′ĕ-bral) situated or having its origin outside the cerebrum.

extracorporal (eks″trah-kor′po-ral) extracorporeal.

extracorporeal (eks″trah-kor-po′re-al) [*extra-* + L. *corpus* body] situated or occurring outside the body.

extracorpuscular (eks″trah-kor-pus′ku-lar) outside the corpuscles.

extracorticospinal (eks″trah-kor″tĭ-ko-spi′nal) outside the corticospinal tract; see under *tract*.

extracranial (eks″trah-kra′ne-al) outside the cranium.

extract (eks′trakt) [L. *extractum*] a concentrated preparation of a vegetable or animal drug obtained by removing the active constituents therefrom with a suitable menstruum, evaporating all or nearly all the solvent, and adjusting the residual mass or powder to a prescribed standard. Extracts are prepared in three forms: semiliquid or of syrupy consistency, pilular or solid, and as dry powder. **allergenic e.,** an extract of allergenic components from a crude preparation of an allergen, e.g., weed, grass, or tree pollen, molds, house dust, or animal dander, used for diagnostic skin testing or for immunotherapy (hyposensitization) of allergy. **animal e.,** one prepared from material of animal origin. **beef e.,** a concentrate from beef broth, used in compounding certain prescriptions; called also *extractum carnis*. **belladonna e.** [USP], a preparation, available in pilular and powdered form, containing in each 100 grams, 1.15–1.35 gm. of the alkaloids of belladonna leaf; used as an anticholinergic for the same purposes as atropine and hyoscyamine. **cascara sagrada e.** [USP], a powdered preparation of cascara sagrada, each gram of which represents 3 gm. of cascara sagrada; a cathartic. Called also *Rhamnus purshiana e.* **cell-free e.,** the solution obtained by rupturing cells and removing all particulate matter. **chondodendron tomentosum e.,** an alcoholic extract of a desiccated substance (curare) obtained from the bark and stem of *Chondodendron tomentosum;* used in producing relaxation of skeletal muscle. **chondrus e.,** a tan powder prepared from chondrus, used as a protective; called also *Irish moss e.* **colocynth e.,** a powdered preparation each gram of which represents 4 gm. of colocynth; formerly used as a cathartic. **colocynth e., compound,** a preparation of colocynth extract with finely powdered ipomea, aloe, and cardamon seed; formerly used as a cathartic. **compound e.,** one prepared from more than one drug. **dry e.,** powdered e. **glycyrrhiza e.,** a brown powder prepared from the rhizome and roots of species of *Glycyrrhiza*, used as a flavoring agent; called also *licorice root e.* **glycyrrhiza e., pure** [NF], preparation of the dried rhizome and roots of varieties of *Glycyrrhiza glabra*, used in the compounding of aromatic cascara sagrada fluidextract; called also *pure licorice root e.* **Goulard's e.,** lead subacetate solution. **henbane e.,** hyoscyamus e. **hyoscyamus e.,** a preparation of hyoscyamus, formerly used as an anticholinergic for the same purposes as atropine. **Irish moss e.,** chondrus e. **licorice root e.,** glycyrrhiza e. **licorice root e., pure,** glycyrrhiza e., pure. **liver e.,** a brownish, somewhat hygroscopic powder prepared from mammalian livers; used as a hematopoietic. **liver e., liquid,** liver solution. **e. of male fern,** aspidium oleoresin; see under *oleoresin*.

malt e., a product containing dextrin, maltose, a small amount of glucose, and amylolytic enzymes, obtained by extracting the partially and artificially germinated grain of one or more varieties of *Hordeum vulgare* (barley); used as a nutritive and emulsifying agent. **nux vomica e.,** a powder prepared from nux vomica, each 100 gm. of which contains 7–7.75 gm. of strychnine. **ox bile e.,** a brownish to greenish yellow powder or granules, with a characteristic odor and bitter taste, prepared from the fresh bile of the ox and containing not less than 45 per cent of cholic acid; used as a choleretic. **oxgall e., powdered,** ox bile e. **parathyroid e.,** parathyroid injection. **pilular e.,** an extract prepared as a plastic mass, with liquid glucose, malt extract, or glycerin being used as a diluent. **poison ivy e.,** an extract of the fresh leaves of poison ivy, *Rhus (Toxicodendron), radicans*, L., used in desensitization for prevention of rhus dermatitis due to poison ivy. **poison ivy e., alum precipitated,** a repository form of a pyridine extract of poison ivy, *Rhus (Toxicodendron) radicans*, L., used to counteract rhus dermatitis due to poison ivy. **poison oak e.,** an extract of the fresh leaves of poison oak, *Rhus (Toxicodendron) diversiloba*, L., used for desensitization in prevention of rhus dermatitis due to poison oak. **pollen e.,** a preparation of the pollen of certain plants, such as ragweed, used in the diagnosis and treatment of inhalant allergy. **powdered e.,** an extract prepared in a dry powdered form, with starch, sucrose, lactose, powdered glycyrrhiza, magnesium carbonate, magnesium oxide, or calcium phosphate being used as a diluent. Called also *dry e.* **Rhamnus purshiana e.,** cascara sagrada e. **rice polishings e.,** a preparation of rice polishings, used as a source of vitamin B_1, or thiamine. **semiliquid e.,** one evaporated to a syrupy consistency. **solid e.,** pilular e. **tikitiki e.,** rice polishings e. **trichinella e.,** an aqueous extract of specially treated larvae of *Trichinella spiralis*, usually obtained from inoculated rodents; used as a skin test for trichinella infection. **yeast e.,** a powder prepared from a water-soluble, peptone-like derivative of yeast cells (*Saccharomyces*).

extraction (eks-trak′shun) [L. *ex* out + *trahere* to draw] 1. the process or act of pulling or drawing out. 2. the preparation of an extract. **breech e.,** extraction of the infant from the uterus in breech presentation, i.e., when the buttocks of the fetus are presented in labor. **breech e., partial,** extraction of the remainder of the infant's body after it has been extruded from the uterus by natural forces as far as the umbilicus. **breech e., total,** extraction of the entire body of the infant from the uterus in cases of breech presentation. **cataract e.,** the surgical removal of a cataractous lens. **cataract e., extracapsular,** the surgical removal of the anterior capsule of a cataractous lens and of the lens contents (cortex and nucleus). **cataract e., intracapsular,** the surgical removal of a cataractous lens and its capsule. **flap e.,** extraction of cataract by an incision which makes a flap of cornea. **serial e.,** the selective extraction of deciduous teeth during the stage of mixed dentition in accordance with the shedding and eruption of the teeth; it is done over an extended period to allow autonomous adjustment to relieve crowding of the dental arches during the eruption of the lateral incisors, canines, and premolars, eventually involving the extraction of the first premolar teeth. Called also *selected e.* and *progressive e.* **tooth e.,** the surgical removal of a tooth; odontectomy.

extractive (eks-trak′tiv) any substance present in an organized tissue, or in a mixture in a small quantity, and requiring to be extracted by a special method.

extractor (eks-trak′tor) an instrument used for removing a calculus or foreign body. **vacuum e.,** a device to assist delivery consisting of a metal traction cup that is attached to the fetus' head; negative pressure is applied and traction is made on a chain passed through the suction tube.

extractum (eks-trak′tum), gen. *extrac′ti*, pl. *extrac′ta* [L., from *ex* out + *trahere* to draw] an extract. **e. car′nis,** beef extract. **e. fel′lis bo′vis,** ox bile extract. **e. hep′a-tis,** liver extract. **e. nu′cis vom′icae,** nux vomica extract. **e. perpolitio′num ory′zae,** rice polishings extract.

extracystic (eks″trah-sis′tik) outside a cyst or the bladder.

extradural (eks″trah-du′ral) situated or occurring outside the dura mater.

extraembryonic (eks″trah-em″bre-on′ik) external to the

embryo proper, as the extraembryonic coelom or extraembryonic membranes.

extraepiphyseal (eks″trah-ep″ĭ-fiz′e-al) away from, or unconnected with, an epiphysis.

extragenital (eks″trah-jen′ĭ-tal) unrelated to, not originating in, or remote from the genital organs.

extrahepatic (eks″trah-hĕ-pat′ik) situated or occurring outside the liver.

extraligamentous (eks″trah-lig″ah-men′tus) occurring outside a ligament.

extramalleolus (eks″trah-mal-le′o-lus) the outer malleolus of the ankle joint.

extramastoiditis (eks″trah-mas″toi-di′tis) inflammation of the outer surface of the mastoid process and of the superincumbent tissues.

extramedullary (eks″trah-med′u-la″re) situated or occurring outside any medulla, especially the medulla oblongata.

extrameningeal (eks″trah-mĕ-nin′je-al) occurring outside the meninges.

extramural (eks″trah-mu′ral) [L. *extra* + *murus* wall] situated or occurring outside the wall of an organ or structure.

extraneous (eks-tra′ne-us) [L. *extraneus* external] existing or belonging outside the organism.

extranuclear (eks″trah-nu′kle-ar) situated or occurring outside a cell nucleus.

extraocular (eks″trah-ok′u-lar) situated outside the eye.

extraosseous (eks″trah-os′e-us) occurring outside a bone or bones.

extraparenchymal (eks″trah-par-en′kĭ-mal) occurring or formed outside the parenchyma.

extrapelvic (eks″trah-pel′vik) unconnected with the pelvis.

extrapericardial (eks″trah-per″ĭ-kar′de-al) outside the pericardium.

extraperineal (eks″trah-per″ĭ-ne′al) away from the perineum.

extraperiosteal (eks″trah-per″e-os′te-al) outside or independent of the periosteum.

extraperitoneal (eks″trah-per″ĭ-to-ne′al) situated or occurring outside the peritoneal cavity.

extraplacental (eks″trah-plah-sen′tal) outside of or independent of the placenta.

extraplantar (eks″trah-plan′tar) on the outside of the sole of the foot.

extrapleural (eks″trah-ploo′ral) outside the pleural cavity.

extrapolation (eks″trap-o-la′shun) inference of a value(s) on the basis of that which is known or has been observed.

extraprostatic (eks″trah-pros-tat′ik) not connected with the prostate gland.

extraprostatitis (eks″trah-pros″tah-ti′tis) paraprostatitis.

extrapsychic (eks″trah-si′kik) occurring outside the mind; taking place between the mind and the external environment.

extrapulmonary (eks″trah-pul′mo-na″re) not connected with the lungs.

extrapyramidal (eks″trah-pi-ram′ĭ-dal) outside of the pyramidal tracts; see under *system*.

extrarectus (eks″trah-rek′tus) musculus rectus lateralis bulbi.

extraserous (eks″trah-se′rus) outside a serous cavity.

extrasomatic (eks″trah-so-mat′ik) unconnected with the body.

extrasuprarenal (eks″trah-su″prah-re′nal) extra-adrenal.

extrasystole (eks″trah-sis′to-le) a premature contraction of the heart that is independent of the normal rhythm and arises in response to an impulse in some part of the heart other than the sinoatrial node; called also *premature beat*. **atrial e.,** an extrasystole in which the stimulus is thought to arise in the atrium elsewhere than at the sinus. **auriclar e.,** former name for *atrial e.* **atrioventricular e.,** one in which the stimulus is supposed to arise in the atrioventricular node; called also *nodal e.* **auriculoventricular e.,** former name for *atrioventricular e.* **infranodal e.,** ventricular e. **interpolated e.,** a contraction

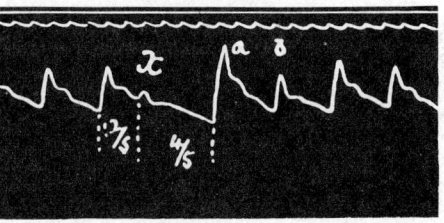

Extrasystole. In this tracing of the radial pulse, the extrasystole occurs at *x*. A compensatory pause of four fifths of a second follows, ending in a large pulse wave.

taking place between two normal heart beats. **nodal e.,** atrioventricular e. **retrograde e.,** a premature ventricular contraction followed by a premature atrial contraction, due to transmission of the stimulus backward, usually over the bundle of His. **ventricular e.,** one in which either a pacemaker or re-entry site is in the ventricular structure.

extrathoracic (eks″trah-tho-ras′ik) outside the thorax.

extratracheal (eks″trah-tra′ke-al) situated or occurring outside the trachea.

extratubal (eks″trah-tu′bal) outside a tube.

extratympanic (eks″trah-tim-pan′ik) outside the tympanum of the ear.

extrauterine (eks″trah-u′ter-in) situated or occurring outside the uterus.

extravaginal (eks″trah-vaj′ĭ-nal) outside the vagina.

extravasation (eks-trav″ah-sa′shun) [*extra-* + L. *vas* vessel] 1. a discharge or escape, as of blood, from a vessel into the tissues. 2. the process of being extravasated. 3. blood or other substance which has been extravasated. **punctiform e.,** extravasation which causes a tissue to be covered with minute bloody points.

extravascular (eks″trah-vas′ku-lar) situated or occurring outside a vessel or the vessels.

extraventricular (eks″trah-ven-trik′u-lar) situated or occurring outside a ventricle.

extraversion (eks″trah-ver′zhun) 1. in orthodontics, malocclusion in which the teeth or other maxillary structures are further from the median plane than normal, resulting in a wide dental arch; Cf. *intraversion*. Called also *extroversion*. 2. extroversion.

extravert (eks′trah-vert) extrovert.

extremital (eks-trem′ĭ-tal) pertaining to or situated at an extremity.

extremitas (eks-trem′ĭ-tas), pl. *extremita′tes* [L.] 1. [NA] a general term denoting the distal or terminal portion of elongated or pointed structures. 2. the arm or leg (membrum [NA]). Called also *extremity* and *limb*. **e. acromia′lis clavic′ulae** [NA], acromial extremity of clavicle: the lateral end of the clavicle, which articulates with the acromion of the scapula; called also *external* or *scapular extremity of clavicle*. **e. ante′rior lie′nis,** NA alternative for *e. anterior splenis.* **e. ante′rior sple′nis** [NA], anterior extremity of spleen: the lower pole of the spleen, which is situated anterior to the upper pole; called also *e. anterior lienis* [NA alternative] and *e. inferior lienis.* **e. infe′rior,** membrum inferius. **e. infe′rior lie′nis,** e. anterior splenis. **e. infe′rior re′nis** [NA], inferior extremity of kidney: the lower, smaller pole of the kidney; called also *caput lienis* and *head of spleen.* **e. infe′rior tes′tis** [NA], inferior extremity of testis: the lower end of the testis, which is attached to the tail of the epididymis. **e. poste′rior lie′nis,** NA alternative for *e. posterior splenis.* **e. poste′rior sple′nis** [NA], posterior extremity of spleen: the uppermost pole of the spleen, situated somewhat posterior to the lower pole; called also *e. posterior lienis* [NA alternative] and *e. superior lienis.* **e. sterna′lis clavic′ulae** [NA], sternal extremity of clavicle: the medial end of the clavicle, which articulates with the sternum; called also *internal extremity of clavicle.* **e. supe′rior,** membrum superius. **e. supe′rior lie′nis,** e. posterior splenis. **e. supe′rior re′nis** [NA], superior extremity of kidney: the upper, larger pole of the kidney. **e. supe′rior tes′tis** [NA], superior extremity of testis: the upper end of the testis, which is attached to the head of the epididymis. **e. tuba′le ova′rii,** e. tubaria ovarii. **e. tuba′ria ova′rii** [NA], tubal extremity of ovary: the upper end of the ovary, related to the free end of the uterine tube; called also *e. tubale ovarii.* **e. uteri′na ova′rii** [NA], uterine extremity of ovary: the lower end of the ovary, directed toward the uterus; called also *pelvic extremity.*

extremitates (eks-trem″ĭ-ta′tēz) [L.] plural of *extremitas.*

extremity (eks-trem′ĭ-te) 1. a distal or terminal portion; for names of specific anatomical structures, see official terms under *extremitas.* 2. a limb; an arm or leg (membrum [NA]); sometimes applied specifically to a hand or foot. **cartilaginous e. of rib,** cartilago costalis. **external e. of clavicle,** extremitas acromialis claviculae. **fimbriated e. of fallopian tube,** fimbria ovarica. **internal e. of clavicle,** extremitas sternalis claviculae. **lower e.,** membrum inferius. **pelvic e. of ovary,** extremitas uterina ovarii. **proximal e. of phalanx of finger,** basis phalangis digitorum manus. **proximal e. of phalanx of toe,** basis phalangis digitorum pedis. **scapular e. of clavicle,** extremitas acromialis claviculae. **upper e.,** membrum superius. **uterine e. of ovary,** extremitas uterina ovarii.

extrinsic (eks-trin′sik) [L. *extrinsecus* situated on the outside] coming from or originating outside; having relation to parts outside the organ or limb in which found.

extro- [L. *extra* outside] a prefix meaning outward, outside.

extrogastrulation (eks″tro-gas″troo-la′shun) the formation of an embryonic monster by gastrular evagination instead of invagination.

extrophia (eks-tro′fe-ah) exstrophy.

extroversion (eks″tro-ver′zhun) [L. *extroversio,* from *extra* outside + *vertere* to turn] 1. a turning inside out; exstrophy. 2. the turning outward to the external world of one's interest; cf. *introversion.* Called also *extraversion.* 3. extraversion.

extrovert (eks′tro-vert) a person whose interest is turned outward to the external world.

extrude (eks-trood′) 1. to force, thrust, or press out. 2. to force out, or to occupy a position mesial, distal, labial or buccal, or lingual or palatal to that normally occupied. 3. to occupy a position occlusal to that normally occupied, said of an overerupted tooth.

extrusion (eks-troo′zhun) 1. thrusting or pushing out; expulsion by force. 2. the overeruption or movement of a tooth beyond its normal occlusal plane in the absence of opposing occlusal force. 3. an orthodontic technique for the elongation or elevation of a tooth. Cf. *intrusion.*

extubate (eks-tu′bāt) [*ex-* + L. *tuba* tube] to remove a tube from.

extubation (eks″tu-ba′shun) the removal of a previously inserted tube.

exuberant (eg-zu′ber-ant) [L. *exuberare* to be very fruitful] copious or excessive in production; showing excessive proliferation.

exudate (eks′u-dāt) [L. *exsudare* to sweat out] material, such as fluid, cells, or cellular debris, which has escaped from blood vessels and has been deposited in tissues or on tissue surfaces, usually as a result of inflammation. An exudate, in contrast to a transudate, is characterized by a high content of protein, cells, or solid materials derived from cells. **cotton-wool e's,** see under *spot.*

exudation (eks″u-da′shun) 1. the escape of fluid, cells, and cellular debris from blood vessels and their deposition in or on the tissues, usually as the result of inflammation. 2. an exudate.

exudative (eks-oo′dah-tiv) of or pertaining to a process of exudation.

exulcerans (eks-ul′ser-anz) [L.] ulcerating.

exulceratio (eks-ul″ser-a′she-o) [L.] ulceration. **e. sim′plex,** superficial ulceration.

exumbilication (eks″um-bil″ĭ-ka′shun) [*ex-* + *umbilicus*] 1. marked protrusion of the navel. 2. umbilical hernia.

exuviation (eks-u″ve-a′shun) [L. *exuere* to divest oneself of] the shedding of any epithelial structure, as of the deciduous teeth.

ex vivo (eks″ve′vo) outside the living body; denoting removal of an organ (e.g., the kidney) for reparative surgery, after which it is returned to the original site.

eye (i) [L. *oculus;* Gr. *ophthalmos*] the organ of vision. Called also *oculus* [NA]. In shape the eyeball (bulbus oculi [NA]) is of a large sphere, with the segment of a smaller sphere, the cornea, in front. It is composed of three coats—the *sclera* and *cornea,* the *choroid,* and the *retina*—each coat being divided into several layers. Within the three coats are the refracting media—namely, the *aqueous humor,* the *crystalline lens,* and the *vitreous humor.* The sclerotic, or external coat, is white and fibrous. Posteriorly the fibers of the optic nerve enter through small perforations in the *lamina cribrosa.* The inner surface is attached to the choroid by delicate connective tissue, the *lamina fusca.* The *cornea* is composed of five layers, the internal layer being a serous membrane, sometimes called *Descemet's membrane.* The *uvea,* or middle coat, is chiefly composed of blood vessels and pigment. Anteriorly, it terminates near the periphery of the lens in folds called the *ciliary processes.* The *retina,* or internal coat, is chiefly composed of nerve tissue, and is made up of three principal layers. The external layer, or Jacob's membrane, is composed of terminal nerve cells, which, from their shape, are called the *rods* and *cones.* The *iris* is a curtain with a central perforation, the *pupil,* and is composed of smooth muscular fibers arranged both in a circular and in a radiating manner. It varies in color, and is suspended in the aqueous humor in front of the lens. The *ciliary ligament* is a ring of connective tissue fibers surrounding the iris. The *ciliary muscle* surrounds the periphery of the iris and controls the convexity of the lens during accommodation. The *aqueous humor* fills the cavity between the cornea in front and the lens behind. The *vitreous humor* fills the space behind the lens and is a clear, jelly-like substance containing mucin. It is surrounded by the *hyaloid membrane.* The *lens,* or *crystalline humor,* is a double convex transparent body between the vitreous and aqueous humors, and is held in place by an elastic *capsule* and *suspensory* ligament. The arteries of the eye are the short ciliary, the long ciliary, the anterior ciliary, and the central artery of the retina. The nerves are the optic and the long and short ciliary nerves. **aphakic e.,** an eye lacking the crystalline lens; see also *aphakia.* **artificial e.,** a ready-made (stock) or custom-made prosthesis of glass or plastic shaped and colored to resemble the anterior portion of a normal eye and inserted for cosmetic reasons in the socket of an enucleated or eviscerated eye. **black e.,** ecchymosis of the eyelids and surrounding area. **blear e.,** blepharitis ciliaris. **cinema e.,** Klieg e. **compound e.,** the multifaceted eye of arthropods composed of units (ommatidia), each of which contains all of the structural and functional elements of the eye (including lens, retina, and photoreceptor cells). **crossed e's,** esotropia. **cystic e.,** a malformed eye consisting of a cystic structure. **dark-adapted e.,** an eye that has undergone the changes produced by adequate exposure to darkness; it is more sensitive to very weak light. **deviating e.,** in strabismus, the nonfixating eye; called also *following e.* **epiphyseal e.,** a modification of the parapineal organ of certain lower vertebrates to form an eyelike structure lying subepidermally on the median dorsal aspect of the head; it is a photoreceptor rather than an image forming eye, enabling the organism to respond to darkness or to light. Called also *parietal e., parietal body,* and *pineal e.* **exciting e.,** the eye that is primarily injured and from which the influences start which involve the other eye in sympathetic ophthalmia; called also *primary e.* **fixating e.,** in strabismus, the eye directed toward the object of vision. **following e.,** deviating e. **hare's e.** (*obs.*), lagophthalmos. **hop e.,** conjunctivitis in hop pickers caused by irritation from the spinelike hairs of the hop plant. **Klieg e.,** a condition marked by conjunctivitis, edema of the eyelids, lacrimation, and photophobia due to exposure to intense lights (Klieg lights); called also *cinema e.* **light-adapted e.,** an eye that has undergone the changes produced by adequate exposure to rather strong light; it is less sensitive to weak light. **median e.,** an organ on the top of the head of many reptiles; it plays an important role in the response to light. **monochromatic e.,** an eye that can perceive only one color. **parietal e.,** epiphyseal e. **pineal e.,** epiphyseal e. **pink e.,** acute contagious conjunctivitis. **primary e.,** exciting e. **pseudophakic e.,** an eye with an intraocular lens implant. **reduced e.,** a mathematical model of the eye in which the optical systems are diagrammatically reduced to one refracting unit. **schematic e.,** 1. a diagrammatic illustration of the ideal normal eye, with constants for curvature, indices of refraction, and

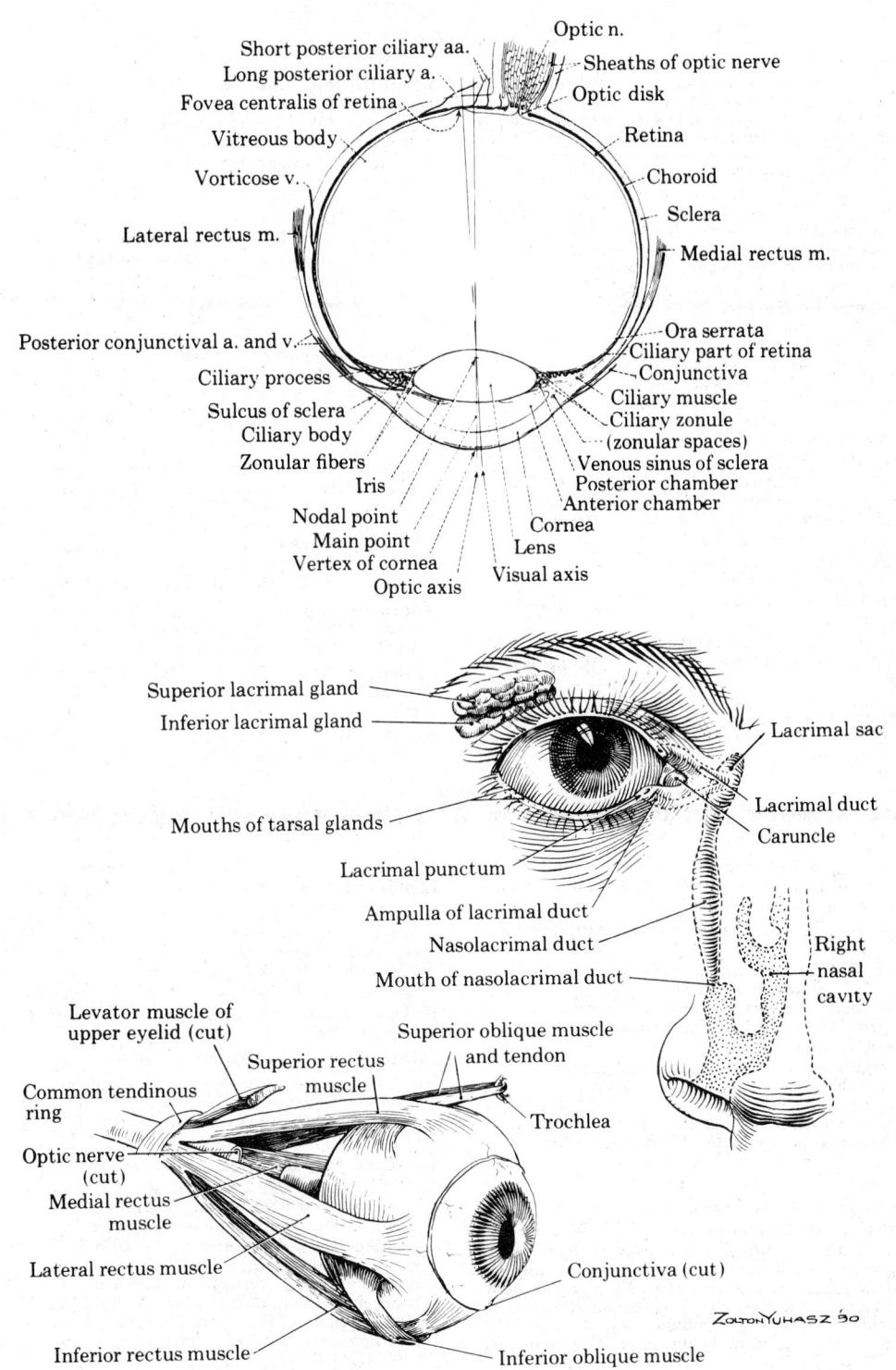

Short posterior ciliary aa.
Long posterior ciliary a.
Fovea centralis of retina
Vitreous body
Vorticose v.
Lateral rectus m.
Posterior conjunctival a. and v.
Ciliary process
Sulcus of sclera
Ciliary body
Zonular fibers
Iris
Nodal point
Main point
Vertex of cornea
Optic axis

Optic n.
Sheaths of optic nerve
Optic disk
Retina
Choroid
Sclera
Medial rectus m.
Ora serrata
Ciliary part of retina
Conjunctiva
Ciliary muscle
Ciliary zonule (zonular spaces)
Venous sinus of sclera
Posterior chamber
Anterior chamber
Cornea
Lens
Visual axis

Superior lacrimal gland
Inferior lacrimal gland
Mouths of tarsal glands
Lacrimal punctum
Ampulla of lacrimal duct
Nasolacrimal duct
Mouth of nasolacrimal duct
Lacrimal sac
Lacrimal duct
Caruncle
Right nasal cavity

Levator muscle of upper eyelid (cut)
Common tendinous ring
Optic nerve (cut)
Medial rectus muscle
Lateral rectus muscle
Superior rectus muscle
Superior oblique muscle and tendon
Trochlea
Conjunctiva (cut)
Inferior rectus muscle
Inferior oblique muscle

ZoltonYuhasz '80

PLATE 16—THE EYE AND RELATED STRUCTURES

601

distances between the optical elements. 2. a model of the eye, usually simplified and enlarged, showing its anatomical and mechanical features. **secondary e.**, sympathizing e. **shipyard e.**, epidemic keratoconjunctivitis. **Snellen's reform e.**, an artificial eye composed of two concavoconvex plates with an empty space between. **squinting e.**, in strabismus, the eye the visual axis of which deviates from the object of vision while the sound eye fixates. **sympathizing e.**, the uninjured eye which becomes secondarily involved in sympathetic ophthalmia; called also *secondary e.* **wall e.**, 1. leukoma of the cornea. 2. exotropia.

eyeball (i′bawl)　the globe or ball of the eye; called also *bulbus oculi* [NA] and *orb*. See *eye*.

eyebrow (i′brow)　1. the transverse elevation at the junction of the forehead and the upper eyelid, consisting of five layers: skin, subcutaneous tissue, a layer of interwoven fibers of the orbicularis oculi and occipitofrontalis muscles, a submuscular areolar layer, and pericranium; called also *supercilium* [NA]. 2. the hairs growing on the transverse elevation at the junction of the forehead and the upper eyelid; called also *supercilia* [NA].

eyecup (i′kup)　1. a small vessel for the application of cleansing or medicated solution to the exposed area of the eyeball. 2. physiologic cup. 3. caliculus ophthalmicus.

eyeglass (i′glas)　a lens for aiding the sight.

eyeground (i′ground)　the fundus of the eye as revealed by ophthalmoscopical examination.

eyelash (i′lash)　one of the hairs growing at the edge of an eyelid; collectively called *cilia* [NA].

eyelet (i′let)　an orthodontic attachment, usually used with an edgewise appliance, welded or soldered for better rotational control.

eyelid (i′lid)　either of the two movable folds (upper and lower) that protect the anterior surface of the eyeball; called also *palpebra* [NA]. **third e.**, the nictitating membrane; see under *membrane*.

eye-minded (i′mīnd-ed)　visile.

eyepiece (i′pēs)　the lens or system of lenses in a microscope (or telescope) that is nearest to the eye of the user and that serves to further magnify the image produced by the objective. **comparison e.**, an eyepiece which presents, as though in juxtaposition, the images of separate objects being transmitted through two different objectives. **compensating e.**, an eyepiece especially designed to correct chromatic and spherical aberrations of the light rays produced by the objective. **demonstration e.**, a device consisting of two eyepieces which may be affixed to the eyepiece tube of a microscope, permitting two observers to see the same field simultaneously. **high-eyepoint e.**, one with an eyepoint higher than usual, which may be used by viewers wearing eyeglasses. **huygenian e.**, a negative eyepiece consisting of two planoconvex lenses, the convexities being directed toward the objective. **negative e.**, a combination of two lenses, one of which is below the plane in which the real image from the objective is formed. **positive e.**, a single lens combination, consisting of two planoconvex lenses or of an achromatic doublet or triplet, the combination being above the plane in which the real image from the objective is formed. **Ramsden's e.**, a positive eyepiece consisting of two planoconvex lenses with the convexities turned toward each other. **widefield e.**, a positive eyepiece consisting of a doublet and a single element, giving a wider field of view than that afforded by other eyepieces.

eyepoint (i′point)　the point above a microscope eyepiece where the image is focused and where the eye should be positioned for viewing.

eyespot (i′spot)　1. the light-sensitive pigmented spot of certain invertebrates. 2. stigma, def. 5. 3. eye spot; see under *spot*.

eyestrain (i′strān)　fatigue of the eye from overuse or from uncorrected defect in focus of the eye.

F

F　chemical symbol for *fluorine*; symbol for *Faraday's constant, force, gilbert*; in bacterial genetics, symbol for *fertility*.

°F　symbol for degree Fahrenheit.

F.　Fahrenheit; fiat; field of vision; French (catheter size); formula.

F₁　1. the "first filial generation," produced by crossing two individuals. 2. a fluorescent substance found in small amounts in normal urine, and in larger quantities in the urine of pellagrins; said to be present in larger amounts after the ingestion of thiamine.

F₂　1. the "second filial generation," produced by mating two members of the F₁ generation. 2. a substance in urine which develops fluorescence after alkali is added; it may appear in small amounts in normal urine or in large amounts in the urine of normal persons after the ingestion of nicotinic acid.

f　symbol for *femto-*.

FA　fatty acid; fluorescent antibody.

F and R　force and rhythm (of pulse).

Fab [*fragment, antigen-binding*]　originally, either of two identical fragments, each containing an antigen combining site, obtained by papain cleavage of the IgG molecule; now generally used as an adjective, e.g., Fab region, segment, to refer to an "arm" of any immunoglobulin monomer, i.e., one light chain and the adjoining heavy chain V_H and C_H1 domains. Cf. *Fc*.

F(ab′)₂　the fragment, containing both Fab regions and the hinge region connecting them by interchain disulfide bonds, obtained by pepsin cleavage of the IgG molecule; called also F(ab′)₂ fragment.

fabella (fah-bel′ah), pl. *fabel′lae* [L. "little bean"]　a sesamoid fibrocartilage occasionally found on the gastrocnemius muscle; it is visible roentgenographically as a small bony shadow behind the knee joint.

fabellae (fah-bel′e) [L.]　plural of *fabella*.

Faber's anemia, syndrome (fah′berz) [Knud Helge *Faber*, Danish physician, 1862–1956]　see *achylanemia*, and see *hypochromic anemia*, under *anemia*.

fabism (fa′bizm) [L. *faba* bean]　favism.

fabrication (fab″rĭ-ka′shun)　confabulation.

Fabricius (fah-bris′e-us)　**(ab Aquapendente),** Hieronymus [It. Girolamo *Fabrizio*] (1537–1619)　an Italian anatomist and surgeon who was the pupil and successor (at Padua) of Gabriele Falloppio. He was the teacher of William Harvey, and the first demonstrator of the valves of the veins.

Fabry's disease (fah′brez) [Johannes *Fabry*, German dermatologist, 1860–1930]　see under *disease*.

fabulation (fab″u-la′shun)　confabulation.

Facb [*fragment, antigen-and-complement-binding*]　the fragment, containing both light chains and the V_H, C_H2 domains of both heavy chains, obtained by plasmin cleavage of an IgG molecule.

F.A.C.D.　Fellow of the American College of Dentists.

face (fās) [L. *facies*]　1. the anterior, or ventral, aspect of the head from the forehead to the chin, inclusive. 2. any presenting aspect, or surface. See also *facies*. **adenoid f.**, adenoid facies. **bovine f.**, facies bovina. **cleft f.**, macrostomia. **cow f.**, facies bovina. **dish f., dished f.**, a facial deformity characterized by a prominence of the forehead, a recession of the midface and lower half of the nose, a lengthening of the upper lip, and a prognathic chin; called also *facies scaphoidea*. **frog f.**, flatness of the face due to intranasal disease. **hippocratic f.**, facies hippocratica. **moon f., moon-shaped f.**, the peculiar rounded face observed in various conditions, such as Cushing's syndrome, or following administration of adrenal corticoids.

face-bow (fās′bo)　a caliperlike device used in dentistry to record the positional relationship of the maxillary arch to the temporomandibular joints (or opening axis of the jaw) and to orient dental casts in this same relationship to the opening axis of the articulator. **adjustable axis f.-b.**, a facebow with caliper ends (condyl ends) that can be adjusted in such a way as to permit location of the hinge axis of rotation of the mandible. Called also *hinge-bow* and *kinematic f.-b*. **kinematic f.-b.**, adjustable axis f.-b.

faceometer (fās-om'ĕ-ter) an instrument for measuring the dimensions of the face.

facet (fas'et) [Fr. *facette*] a small plane surface on a hard body, as on a bone; see also *fovea*. **articular f.,** a small plane surface on a bone at the site where it articulates with another structure; see terms beginning *facies articularis*, under *facies*. **articular f. of atlas, circular,** fovea dentis atlantis. **articular f. of atlas, inferior,** fovea articularis inferior atlantis. **articular f. of atlas, superior,** fovea articularis superior atlantis. **articular f. of axis, anterior,** facies articularis anterior axis. **articular f's for rib cartilages,** incisurae costales sterni. **f. of calcaneus, posterior, medial,** facies articularis talaris media calcanei. **clavicular f.,** incisura clavicularis sterni. **costal f., anterior, costal f., inferior,** facies articularis tuberculi costae. **costal f., posterior, costal f., superior,** facies articularis capitis costae. **costal f. of sternum,** incisurae costales sterni. **costal f. of vertebra, superior,** fovea costalis superior. **lateral f's of sternum,** incisurae costales sterni. **locked f's of spine,** dislocation of articular processes of the spine. **malleolar f. of tibia, internal,** facies articularis malleolaris tibiae. **squatting f.,** a smooth area observed on the anterior surface of the lower end of the tibia in races whose members habitually sit in the squatting position. **f. for tubercle of rib,** fovea costalis transversalis.

facetectomy (fas"ĕ-tek'to-me) [*facet* + Gr. *ektomē* excision] excision of the articular facet of a vertebra.

facette (fah-set') [Fr.] facet.

facial (fa'shal) [L. *facialis*, from *facies* face] 1. of or pertaining to the face. 2. see *facies vestibularis dentis*.

-facient [L. *faciens*, present participle of *facere* to do, to make] a word termination meaning making or causing to become.

facies (fa'she-ēz), pl. **fa'cies** [L.] 1. a term used in anatomical nomenclature to designate (*a*) the anterior, or ventral, aspect of the head, from forehead to chin, inclusive, and (*b*) a specific surface of a body structure, part, or organ. 2. the expression or appearance of the face. **f. abdomina'lis,** the expression of the face characteristic of abdominal disease: it is pinched, anxious, and furrowed, with the nose and upper lip drawn up. **adenoid f.,** the dull expression, with open mouth, sometimes seen in children with adenoid growths. **antebrachial f., anterior,** regio antebrachialis anterior. **antebrachial f., posterior,** regio antebrachialis posterior. **f. antebrachia'lis ante'rior,** NA alternative for regio antebrachialis anterior. **f. antebrachia'lis poste'rior,** NA alternative for *regio antebrachialis posterior*. **f. ante'rior cor'dis,** f. sternocostalis cordis. **f. ante'rior cor'neae** [NA], the anterior surface of the cornea. **f. ante'rior den'tium premola'rium et mola'rium,** the contact surface of the premolar and molar teeth that is directed toward the midline of the dental arch. **f. ante'rior glan'dulae suprarena'lis** [NA], the anterior, or front, surface of the adrenal gland. **f. ante'rior i'ridis** [NA], the anterior surface of the iris, directed toward the anterior chamber of the eye. **f. ante'rior latera'lis hu'meri** [NA], the anterolateral surface of the humerus, which provides attachment to the deltoid muscle and lateral part of the brachialis muscle. Called also *f. anterolateralis humeri* [NA alternative]. **f. ante'rior len'tis** [NA], the surface of the lens directed toward the anterior surface of the eye. **f. ante'rior maxil'lae** [NA], the surface of the body of the maxilla that is directed forward and somewhat laterally; it is bounded roughly by the infraorbital margin, root of the frontal process, nasal notch, alveolar process, and zygomatic process. **f. ante'rior media'lis hu'meri** [NA], the anteromedial surface of the humerus, which begins above at the intertubercular groove and spreads out inferiorly to form the wide smooth area for origin of the brachialis muscle. Called also *f. anteromedialis humeri* [NA alternative]. **f. ante'rior palpebra'rum** [NA], the anterior, or external, surface of the eyelids. **f. ante'rior pancre'atis** [NA], the front, or anterior, surface of the pancreas, directed toward the ventral surface of the body. **f. ante'rior par'tis petro'sae os'sis tempora'lis** [NA], the surface of the petrous part of the temporal bone that forms the posterior portion of the floor of the middle cranial fossa; called also *f. anterior pyramidis ossis temporalis*. **f. ante'rior patel'lae** [NA], the slightly convex, longitudinally striated anterior, or front, surface of the patella, which is perforated by small openings for the

nutrient vessels. **f. ante'rior prosta'tae** [NA], the anterior, or ventral, surface of the prostate, separated from the pubic symphysis by the pudendal venous plexus. **f. ante'rior pyram'idis os'sis tempora'lis,** f. anterior partis petrosae ossis temporalis. **f. ante'rior ra'dii** [NA], the anterior, or volar, surface of the radius, which gives attachment to the flexor pollicis longus and pronator quadratus muscles; called also *f. volaris radii.* **f. ante'rior re'nis** [NA], the anterior, peritoneum-covered surface of the kidney which is directed toward the viscera. **f. ante'rior scap'ulae,** NA alternative for *f. costalis scapulae*. **f. ante'rior ul'nae** [NA], the front, or anterior, surface of the ulna; called also *f. volaris ulnae.* **f. anterolatera'lis cartilag'inis arytenoi'deae** [NA], the external surface of the arytenoid cartilage, which bears the triangular pit, the oblong pit, and the arcuate crest. **f. anterolatera'lis hu'meri,** NA alternative for *f. anterior lateralis humeri.* **f. anteromedia'lis hu'meri,** NA alternative for *f. anterior medialis humeri.* **f. articula'res inferio'res atlan'tis,** see *fovea articularis inferior atlantis.* **f. articula'res inferio'res vertebra'rum,** the surfaces on the inferior articular processes of the vertebrae. **f. articula'ris acromia'lis clavic'ulae** [NA], the smooth area on the lateral end of the clavicle for articulation with the acromion of the scapula. **f. articula'ris acromia'lis scap'ulae,** f. articularis acromii scapulae. **f. articula'ris acro'mii scap'ulae** [NA], a small variable area on the acromion of the scapula, for articulation with the acromial end of the clavicle; called also *f. articularis acromialis.* **f. articula'ris ante'rior ax'is** [NA], anterior articular facet of axis: an oval facet on the ventral surface of the odontoid process of the axis, articulating with the fovea dentis of the atlas; called also *f. articularis anterior epistrophei.* **f. articula'ris ante'rior calca'nei,** f. articularis talaris anterior calcanei. **f. articula'ris ante'rior epistro'phei,** f. articularis anterior axis. **f. articula'ris arytenoi'dea cartila'geinis cricoi'deae** [NA], the surface of the cricoid cartilage that articulates with the arytenoid cartilage. **f. articula'ris calca'nea ante'rior ta'li** [NA], the small surface on the head of the talus that rests upon the anterior articular surface of the calcaneus. **f. articula'ris calca'nea me'dia ta'li** [NA], the convex part of the head of the talus that articulates with the sustentaculum tali of the calcaneus. **f. articula'ris calca'nea poste'rior ta'li** [NA], a transverse concavity on the inferior surface of the talus, articulating with the calcaneus. **f. articula'ris cap'itis cos'tae** [NA], the surface on the head of a rib where it articulates with the body of a vertebra. Typically it is divided into two facets by a transverse crest, the lower facet articulating with the corresponding vertebra, and the upper facet with the suprajacent vertebra. The articular surfaces of the heads of the first, tenth, eleventh, and twelfth ribs generally consist of only one facet. Called also *f. articularis capituli costae*, and *posterior* or *superior costal facet.* **f. articula'ris cap'itis fib'ulae** [NA], the medial surface of the head of the fibula, which articulates with the lateral condyle of the tibia; called also *f. articularis capituli fibulae.* **f. articula'ris capit'uli cos'tae,** f. articularis capitis costae. **f. articula'ris capit'uli fib'ulae,** f. articularis capitis fibulae. **f. articula'ris carpa'lis ra'dii,** NA alternative for *f. articularis carpi radii.* **f. articula'ris car'pea ra'dii,** f. articularis carpi radii. **f. articula'ris car'pi ra'dii** [NA], the convex surface of the distal end of the radius, which articulates with the lunate and scaphoid carpal bones. Called also *f. articularis carpalis radii* [NA alternative]. **f. articula'ris cartilag'inis arytenoi'dea** [NA], the surface of the arytenoid cartilage that articulates with the cricoid cartilage. **f. articula'ris cuboi'dea calca'nei,** [NA], the saddle-shaped area on the anterior surface of the calcaneus where it articulates with the cuboid bone; called also *cuboid articular surface of calcaneus.* **f. articula'ris fibula'ris tib'iae** [NA], the articular surface on the posteroinferior aspect of the lateral condyle of the tibia, which articulates with the head of the fibula. **f. articula'ris fos'sae mandibula'ris,** f. articularis ossis temporalis. **f. articula'ris infe'rior tib'iae** [NA], the surface on the distal end of the tibia where it articulates with the talus. **f. articula'ris malleola'ris tib'iae** [NA], the lateral aspect of the medial malleolus, which articulates with the talus; called also *fovea of lateral malleolus* and *internal malleolar facet of tibia.* **f. articula'ris malle'oli fib'ulae** [NA], the anterosuperior surface of the lateral malleolus, which articulates with the lateral side of the talus; called also *lateral malleolar fovea of fibula.* **f. articula′- ris me′dia calca′nei,** f. articularis talaris media calcanei. **f. articula′ris navicula′ris ta′li** [NA], the surface of the head of the talus that articulates with the navicular bone. **f. articula′ris os′sis tempora′lis** [NA], the articular surface found in the deep part of the mandibular fossa of the temporal bone; called also *f. articularis fossae mandibularis.* **f. articula′ris os′sium** [NA], the surface by which a bone articulates with another; called also *articular surface.* **f. articula′ris patel′lae** [NA], the posterior, or back, surface of the patella, which is largely covered by a thick cartilaginous layer. **f. articula′ris poste′rior ax′is** [NA], a smooth groove on the dorsal surface of the odontoid process of the axis, which lodges the transverse ligament of the atlas. **f. articula′ris sterna′lis clavic′ulae** [NA], a triangular surface on the medial end of the clavicle for articulation with the sternum. **f. articula′ris supe′rior tib′iae** [NA], the surface on the proximal end of the tibia that articulates with the condyles of the femur; called also *condyloid surface of tibia.* **f. articula′ris tala′ris ante′rior calca′nei** [NA], the small area on the superior surface of the calcaneus just anterior to the middle articular surface, which articulates with the talus; called also *f. articularis anterior calcanei.* **f. articula′ris tala′ris me′dia calca′nei** [NA], the area on the superior surface of the calcaneus just in front of the calcaneal sulcus, which articulates with the talus; called also *f. articularis media calcanei* and *medial posterior facet of calcaneus.* **f. articula′ris tala′ris poste′rior calca′nei** [NA], the area on the superior surface of the calcaneus just posterolateral to the calcaneal sulcus, which articulates with the talus. **f. articula′ris thyroi′dea cartilag′inis cricoi′deae** [NA], the surface of the cricoid cartilage that articulates with the thyroid cartilage; called also *eminentia lateralis cartilaginis cricoideae.* **f. articula′ris tuber′culi cos′tae** [NA], the convex facet on the costal tubercle that articulates with the transverse process of a vertebra; called also *anterior* or *inferior costal facet.* **f. auricula′ris os′sis il′ium,** [NA], **f. auricula′ris os′sis il′ii,** a somewhat ear-shaped area on the sacropelvic surface of the ilium, which articulates with the auricular surface of the sacrum to form the sacroiliac joint. **f. auricula′ris os′sis sa′cri** [NA], the broad irregular surface on the superior half of the lateral aspect of the sacrum, which articulates with the ilium; called also *auricular surface of sacrum.* **f. bovi′na** [L. "cow face"], a term sometimes applied to the appearance of the face in craniofacial dysostosis; called also *bovine* or *cow face.* **brachial f., anterior,** regio brachialis anterior. **brachial f., posterior,** regio brachialis posterior. **f. brachia′lis ante′rior,** NA alternative for *regio brachialis anterior.* **f. brachia′lis poste′rior,** NA alternative for *regio brachialis posterior.* **f. bucca′lis den′tis,** buccal surface. **f. cerebra′lis a′lae mag′nae, f. cerebra′lis a′lae majo′ris** [NA], the smooth, concave part of the great wing of the sphenoid bone that forms the anterior part of the floor of the middle cranial fossa, lying in front of the petrous and squamous parts of the temporal bone. **f. cerebra′lis os′sis fronta′lis,** f. interna ossis frontalis. **f. cerebra′lis os′sis parieta′lis,** f. interna ossis parietalis. **f. cerebra′lis squa′mae tempora′lis, f. cerebra′lis par′tis squamo′sae os′sis tempora′lis** [NA], the inner surface of the squamous part of the temporal bone, forming the lateral wall of the middle cranial fossa. **f. co′lica lie′nis,** NA alternative for *f. colica splenis.* **f. co′lica sple′nis** [NA], the surface of the spleen in contact with the colon; called also *f. colica lienis* [NA alternative]. **f. contac′tus den′tis** [NA], contact surface: the area where the mesial and distal surfaces of the teeth touch each other; called also *centric stop* and *contact area.* **f. convex′a cer′ebri,** f. superolateralis hemispherii cerebri. **f. costa′lis pulmo′nis** [NA], the convex surface of each lung in close adaptation to the curvatures of the ribs and the costal cartilages, which joins the mediastinal surface at the anterior and posterior borders and the diaphragmatic surface at the inferior border. It is related behind to the sides of the vertebral bodies (*pars vertebralis faciei costalis*). **f. costa′lis scap′ulae** [NA], the anteromedially facing, concave surface of the scapula; called also *anterior, costal,* or *ventral surface of scapula,* f. anterior scapulae [NA alternative], and *f. ventralis scapulae.* **f. crura′lis ante′rior,** NA alternative for *regio cruralis anterior.* **f. crura′lis poste′rior,** NA alternative for *regio cruralis posterior.* **cubi-**

tal f., anterior, regio cubitalis anterior. **cubital f., posterior,** regio cubitalis posterior. **f. cubita′lis ante′rior,** NA alternative for *regio cubitalis anterior.* **f. cubita′lis poste′rior,** NA alternative for *regio cubitalis posterior.* **f. dex′tra cor′dis,** margo dexter cordis. **f. diaphragmat′ica cor′dis** [NA], the surface of the heart (within the pericardium) that rests on the diaphragm and is directed inferiorly and somewhat posteriorly; it is formed by the two ventricles, the left ventricle contributing a little more than the right; called also *f. inferior cordis.* **f. diaphragmat′ica hep′atis** [NA], the surface of the liver that lies in contact with the diaphragm, being composed of the superior, anterior, right, and posterior aspects. **f. diaphragmat′ica lie′nis,** NA alternative for *f. diaphragmatica splenis.* **f. diaphragmat′ica pulmo′nis** [NA], the surface area of each lung that is adjacent to the diaphragm. **f. diaphragmat′ica sple′nis** [NA], the convex posterolateral surface of the spleen which is directed toward the diaphragm; called also *f. diaphragmatica lienis* [NA alternative]. **f. digita′les,** the digital surfaces of the hand (*f. digitales manus*), or of the foot (*f. digitales pedis*). **f. digita′les dorsa′les ma′nus** [NA], the posterior or back (dorsal) surfaces of the fingers. **f. digita′les dorsa′les pe′dis,** the superior or upper (dorsal) surfaces of the toes. **f. digita′les fibula′res pe′dis,** f. digitales laterales pedis. **f. digita′les latera′les ma′nus,** the lateral surfaces of the fingers; called also *f. digitales radiales manus.* **f. digita′les latera′les pe′dis,** the lateral surfaces of the toes; called also *f. digitales fibulares pedis.* **f. digita′les media′les ma′nus,** the medial surfaces of the fingers; called also *f. digitales ulnares manus.* **f. digitales media′les pe′dis,** the medial surfaces of the toes; called also *f. digitales tibiales pedis.* **f. digita′les palma′res ma′nus,** NA alternative for *f. digitales ventrales manus.* **f. digita′les planta′res pe′dis,** f. digitales ventrales pedis. **f. digita′les radia′les ma′nus,** f. digitales laterales manus. **f. digita′les tibia′les pe′dis,** f. digitales mediales pedis. **f. digita′les ulna′res ma′nus,** f. digitales mediales manus. **f. digita′les ventra′les ma′nus** [NA], the anterior or palmar (ventral) surfaces of the fingers; called also *f. digitales palmares manus* [NA alternative], *f. palmares digitorum manus,* and *f. volares digitorum manus.* **f. digita′les ventra′les pe′dis,** the inferior or plantar (ventral) surfaces of the toes; called also *f. digitales plantares pedis.* **f. dista′lis den′tis** [NA], distal surface: the proximal or contact surface of a tooth that is farthest from the midline of the dental arch. **f. doloro′sa,** the facial expression of a patient experiencing pain or severe sickness. **f. dorsa′lis os′sis sac′ri** [NA], the markedly convex and rough posterior, or dorsal, surface of the sacrum, which gives origin to the sacrospinalis and multifidus muscles; called also *posterior surface of sacral bone.* **f. dorsa′lis ra′dii,** f. posterior radii. **f. dorsa′lis scap′ulae** f. posterior scapulae. **f. dorsa′lis ul′nae,** f. posterior ulnae. **f. exter′na os′sis fronta′lis** [NA], the external surface of the squama of the frontal bone; called also *f. frontalis ossis frontalis.* **f. exter′na os′sis parieta′lis** [NA], the externally directed surface of the parietal bone; called also *f. parietalis ossis parietalis.* **f. facia′lis den′tis,** NA alternative for *f. vestibularis dentis.* **f. femora′lis anterior,** NA alternative for *regio femoralis anterior.* **f. femora′lis poste′rior,** NA alternative for *regio femoralis anterior.* **f. fronta′lis os′sis fronta′lis,** f. externa ossis frontalis. **f. gas′trica lie′nis,** NA alternative for *f. gastrica splenis.* **f. gas′trica sple′nis** [NA], the surface of the spleen in contact with the stomach; called also *f. gastrica lienis* [NA alternative]. **f. glu′tea os′sis il′ii** [NA], the large external, or dorsal, surface of the ala of the ilium, on which are located the three gluteal lines; called also *gluteal surface of ilium.* **f. hepat′ica,** a thin face with sunken eyeballs, sallow complexion, and yellow conjunctivae, characteristic of certain chronic disorders of the liver. **f. hippocrat′ica,** a drawn, pinched, and pale appearance of the face, indicative of approaching death. **Hutchinson's f.,** a peculiar appearance in ophthalmoplegia externa, the eyeballs being fixed, the eyebrows raised, and the lids drooping. **f. infe′rior cer′ebri,** the lower, or inferior, surface of the cerebrum; called also *basis cerebri* and *basis encephali.* **f. infe′rior cor′dis,** f. diaphragmatica cordis. **f. infe′rior hemisphe′rii cerebel′li** [NA], the inferior surface of the cerebellar hemisphere, formed by the inferior semilunar lobule, the biventral lobule, the tonsilla, and the flocculus. **f. infe′rior hemisphe′rii cer′ebri** [NA], the part of the cerebral hemisphere that rests on the tentorium and in the anterior and middle cranial fossae. **f. infe′rior hep′atis,** f. visceralis hepatis. **f. infe′rior lin′guae** [NA], the under surface of the body of the tongue. **f. infe′rior pancre′atis** [NA], the inferior surface of the pancreas. **f. infe′rior par′tis petro′sae os′sis tempora′lis** [NA], **f. infe′rior pyram′idis os′sis tempora′lis,** that surface of the petrous part of the temporal bone which appears on the external surface of the base of the cranium. **f. inferolatera′lis prosta′tae** [NA], the convex inferolateral surface of the prostate, separated from the superior fascia of the pelvic diaphragm by a venous plexus. **f. infratempora′lis maxil′lae** [NA], the posterior convex surface of the body of the maxilla, bounded roughly by the inferior orbital fissure, the zygomatic process and associated ridge, maxillary tuberosity, and posterior margin of the nasal surface. **f. interloba′res pulmo′nis** [NA], the surface area of each lung lying within the oblique and horizontal fissures. **f. inter′na os′sis fronta′lis** [NA], the vertically situated, concave cerebral surface of the frontal bone; in its midline the sagittal sulcus is seen superiorly and the frontal crest inferiorly. Called also *f. cerebralis ossis frontalis.* **f. inter′na os′sis parieta′lis** [NA], the internal, or cerebral, surface of the parietal bone; called also *f. cerebralis ossis parietalis.* **f. intestina′lis u′teri** [NA], the convex posterior surface of the uterus, adjacent to the intestine. **f. labia′lis den′tis,** labial surface. **f. latera′lis cor′dis,** f. pulmonalis cordis. **f. latera′lis den′tium incisivo′rum et canino′rum,** the contact surface of the incisor and canine teeth that is directed away from the midline of the dental arch. **f. latera′lis fib′ulae** [NA], the area between the anterior and posterior borders of the body of the fibula. **f. latera′lis os′sis zygomat′ici** [NA], the anterior convex surface of the zygomatic bone; called also *f. malaris ossis zygomatici.* **f. latera′lis ova′rii** [NA], the surface of the ovary in contact with the lateral pelvic wall. **f. latera′lis ra′dii** [NA], the surface of the radius that gives attachment to the supinator and pronator teres muscles proximally, and underlies the tendons of the extensor carpi radialis longus and brevis muscles distally. **f. latera′lis tes′tis** [NA], the surface of the testis that is directed away from its fellow of the opposite side. **f. latera′lis tib′iae** [NA], the surface of the body of the tibia between the interosseous and anterior borders; called also *external border of tibia.* **leonine f.,** f. **leonti′na** [L. "lion's face"], a peculiar, deeply furrowed, lion-like appearance of the face, seen in certain cases of advanced lepromatous leprosy (see *leontiasis*) and in other diseases associated with facial edema such as coast erysipelas, a cutaneous manifestation of onchocerciasis seen in Central America. **f. lingua′lis den′tis** [NA], lingual surface: the surface of a tooth that faces inward toward the tongue (oral cavity), and opposite the vestibular (or facial) surface. Called also *oral surface.* **f. luna′ta acetab′uli** [NA], the articular portion of the acetabulum. **f. mala′ris os′sis zygomat′ici,** f. lateralis ossis zygomatici. **f. malleola′ris latera′lis ta′li** [NA], the large triangular facet on the talus that articulates with the lateral malleolus. **f. malleola′ris media′lis ta′li** [NA], the narrow facet on the talus continuous with the superior surface; it articulates with the medial malleolus. **Marshall Hall's f.,** the facies of hydrocephalus: a triangular face with a broad forehead and prominent frontal bones. **f. masticato′ria den′tis,** 1. f. occlusalis dentis. 2. working occlusal surface. **f. maxilla′ris a′lae majo′ris** [NA], a small surface on the inferior part of the great wing of the sphenoid bone above the pterygoid processes; it is perforated by the foramen rotundum. Called also *f. sphenomaxillaris alae magnae.* **f. maxilla′ris lam′inae perpendicula′ris os′sis palati′ni** [NA], **f. maxilla′ris par′tis perpendicula′ris os′sis palati′ni,** the lateral surface of the perpendicular plate of the palatine bone, which is in relation to the maxilla. Posteriorly and inferiorly it contains the greater palatine sulcus, which forms the greater palatine canal with a corresponding groove on the maxilla. **f. media′lis cartilag′inis arytenoi′deae** [NA], the surface of the arytenoid cartilage that faces medially, toward the opposite arytenoid cartilage. **f. media′lis cer′ebri** [NA], the surface of the cerebrum parallel to and facing the median plane. **f. media′lis den′tium incisivo′rum et canino′rum,** the contact surface of the incisor and canine teeth that is directed toward the midline of the dental

arch. **f. media′lis fib′ulae** [NA], the narrow area on the body of the fibula between the interosseous and anterior borders. **f. media′lis hemisphe′rii cer′ebri** [NA], the surface of the cerebral hemisphere parallel to and facing both the median plane and the corresponding surface of the opposite hemisphere. **f. media′lis ova′rii** [NA], the side of the ovary in contact with the fimbriated end of the uterine tube and the intestine. **f. media′lis pulmo′nis,** f. mediastinalis pulmonis. **f. media′lis tes′tis** [NA], the surface of the testis that is directed toward its fellow of the opposite side. **f. media′lis tib′iae** [NA], the slightly convex surface of the body of the tibia between the anterior and medial borders. **f. media′lis ul′nae** [NA], the smooth, rounded, internal surface of the ulna. **f. mediastina′lis pulmo′nis** [NA], the surface of each lung lying medially to the vertebral column and mediastinum; it contains the cardiac impression. Called also *f. medialis pulmonis.* **f. mesia′lis den′tis** [NA], mesial surface: the contact or proximal surface of the incisor or canine tooth that is closest to the midline of the dental arch. **mitral f., mitrotricuspid f.,** the appearance of the face of some patients with mitral disease of long duration, marked by rosy, flushed cheeks and dilated capillaries. **moon f.,** see under *face.* **myasthenic f.,** the characteristic facial expression in myasthenia gravis, caused by ptosis and weakness of the facial muscles. **myopathic f.,** the peculiar facial expression produced by relaxation of the facial muscles, as in Landouzy-Dejerine dystrophy. **f. nasa′lis lam′inae horizonta′lis os′sis palati′ni** [NA], the superior surface of the horizontal part of the palatine bone; it forms the posterior part of the floor of the nasal cavity. Called also *f. nasalis partis horizontalis ossis palatini.* **f. nasa′lis lam′inae perpendicula′ris os′sis palati′ni** [NA], the medial surface of the perpendicular plate of the palatine bone; it articulates with the middle and inferior nasal conchae. Called also *f. nasalis partis perpendicularis ossis palatini.* **f. nasa′lis maxil′lae** [NA], the surface of the body of the maxilla that helps form the lateral wall of the nasal cavity; it is bounded roughly by the following: medial margin of the orbital surface, medial margin of the infratemporal surface, the palatine process, and the nasal notch. **f. nasa′lis par′tis horizonta′lis os′sis palati′ni,** f. nasalis laminae horizontalis ossis palatini. **f. nasa′lis par′tis perpendicula′ris os′sis palati′ni,** f. nasalis laminae perpendicularis ossis palatini. **f. occlusa′lis den′tis** [NA], occlusal surface of teeth: the surface of the posterior or artificial teeth coming in contact with those of the opposite jaw during the act of occlusion. In natural teeth, restricted to the anatomic tooth surfaces of the posterior teeth limited mesially and distally by the marginal ridges and buccally and lingually by the buccal and lingual boundaries of the cusp eminences. By extension, the term *occlusal surface* is used to designate the incisal surface of the anterior teeth. Called also *f. masticatoria dentis* and *masticatory surface.* See also *incisal s.* and *occlusal s., working.* **f. orbita′lis a′lae mag′nae, f. orbita′lis a′lae majo′ris** [NA], the quadrilateral surface on the great wing of the sphenoid bone that forms the major part of the lateral wall of the orbit; called also *orbital border* or *surface of sphenoid bone.* **f. orbita′lis maxil′lae** [NA], a triangular surface on the body of the maxilla that forms the greater part of the floor of the orbit. **f. orbita′lis os′sis fronta′lis** [NA], the triangularly shaped plates of the frontal bone that form most of the roof of each orbit and the floor of the anterior cranial fossa; they are separated by the ethmoidal notch. **f. orbita′lis os′sis zygomat′ici** [NA], the part of the zygomatic bone that helps form the lateral wall of the orbit. **f. [os′sea] cra′nii,** the bony skeleton of the face. **f. palati′na lam′inae horizonta′lis os′sis palati′ni** [NA], **f. palati′na par′tis horizonta′lis os′sis palati′ni,** the inferior surface of the horizontal part of the palatine bone; it forms the posterior part of the hard palate. **f. parieta′lis os′sis parieta′lis,** f. externa ossis parietalis. **Parkinson's f., parkinsonian f.,** a stolid masklike expression of the face, with infrequent blinking, pathognomonic of parkinsonism; see also *parkinsonian syndrome,* under *syndrome,* and see *paralysis agitans.* **f. patella′ris fem′oris,** the smooth anterior continuation of the condyles that forms the surface of the femur articulating with the patella; called also *anterior intercondylar fossa of femur,* and *patellar fossa of femur.* **f. pel′vica os′sis sa′cri** [NA], **f. pelvi′na os′sis sac′ri,** the smooth, concave, ventrocaudally directed surface of the sacrum that helps form the posterior wall of the pelvis; called also *anterior surface of sacral bone.* **f. poplit'ea fem'oris** [NA], the triangular lower third of the posterior surface of the femur, between the medial and lateral supracondylar lines, which forms the superior part of the floor of the popliteal fossa; called also *planum popliteum femoris.* **f. poste'rior cartilag'inis arytenoi'deae** [NA], the concave dorsal surface of the arytenoid cartilage, to which various laryngeal muscles are attached. **f. poste'rior cor'neae** [NA], the posterior surface of the cornea, which forms the anterior boundary of the anterior chamber. **f. poste'rior den'tium premola'rium et mola'rium,** posterior surface of premolar and molar teeth: the contact surface of the premolar and the molar teeth that is directed away from the midline of the dental arch. **f. poste'rior fib'ulae** [NA], the large area between the posterior and interosseous borders of the body of the fibula, presenting the medial crest. **f. poste'rior glan'dulae suprarena'lis** [NA], the portion of the adrenal gland that is directed toward the posterior body wall. **f. poste'rior hep'atis,** pars posterior faciei diaphragmaticae hepatis. **f. poste'rior hu'meri** [NA], the surface of the humerus that is subdivided obliquely by the radial groove to give attachment to the lateral and medial heads of the triceps muscle. **f. poste'rior i'ridis** [NA], the posterior surface of the iris, directed toward the posterior chamber of the eye. **f. poste'rior len'tis** [NA], the posterior surface of the lens, directed toward the vitreous body of the eye. **f. poste'rior palpebra'rum** [NA], the internal surface of the eyelids in contact with the eyeball and covered by the conjunctiva. **f. poste'rior pancre'atis** [NA], the posterior surface of the pancreas. **f. poste'rior par'tis petro'sae os'sis tempora'lis** [NA], the surface of the petrous part of the temporal bone that forms part of the anterior portion of the floor of the posterior cranial fossa; called also *f. posterior pyramidis ossis temporalis.* **f. poste'rior prosta'tae** [NA], the dorsal surface of the prostate, separated by fascia from the anterior wall of the rectum. **f. poste'rior pyram'idis os'sis tempora'lis,** f. posterior partis petrosae ossis temporalis. **f. poste'rior ra'dii** [NA], the posterior surface of the radius, which gives attachment to the supinator, abductor pollicis longus, and extensor pollicis brevis muscles; called also *f. dorsalis radii.* **f. poste'rior re'nis** [NA], the dorsal surface of the kidney, directed toward the posterior body wall, and not covered by peritoneum. **f. poste'rior scap'ulae** [NA], the convex posterior surface of the scapula, which is divided into two unequal parts by the spine of the scapula. Called also *dorsal* or *posterior surface of scapula, dorsum of scapula, dorsum scapulae* [NA alternative], and *f. dorsalis scapulae.* **f. poste'rior tib'iae** [NA], the surface of the body of the tibia between the medial and interosseous borders; in the proximal third presenting the soleal line. **f. poste'rior ul'nae** [NA], the posterolaterally directed surface of the ulna; called also *f. dorsalis ulnae.* **Potter f.,** the facial appearance characteristic of bilateral renal agenesis: flattened nose, receding chin, wide interpupillary space, and large, low-set ears. **f. pulmona'lis cor'dis** [NA], the surface of the heart that faces the lung; called also *f. lateralis cordis* and *left surface of heart.* **f. rena'lis glan'dulae suprarena'lis** [NA], the surface of the adrenal gland that is directed toward the kidney, being separated from it by a layer of fat; called also *basis glandulae suprarenalis* and *inferior margin of suprarenal gland.* **f. rena'lis lie'nis,** NA alternative for *f. renalis splenis.* **f. rena'lis sple'nis** [NA], the surface of the spleen in contact with the left kidney; called also *f. renalis lienis* [NA alternative]. **f. sacropelvi'na os'sis il'ii** [NA], an irregular area on the inner surface of the ala of the ilium, posterior to the iliac fossa; it contains the iliac tuberosity and the auricular surface. Called also *sacropelvic surface of the ilium.* **f. scaphoi'dea,** dish face. **f. sphenomaxilla'ris a'lae mag'nae,** f. maxillaris alae majoris. **f. sternocosta'lis cor'dis** [NA], the convex surface of the heart, which in general is directed anteriorly and somewhat superiorly, being formed mainly by the right ventricle and, to a lesser degree, by the left ventricle and the atria; called also *f. anterior cordis.* **f. supe'rior hemisphe'rii cerebel'li,** the superior surface of the cerebellar hemisphere, consisting of the ala of the lobulus centralis, the lobulus quadrangularis, the lobulus simplex, and the superior semilunar lobule. **f. supe'rior hep'atis,** pars superior faciei diaphragmaticae hepatis. **f. supe'rior troch'leae ta'li** [NA], the broad, smooth surface of the talus that articulates with the tibia. **f. superolatera'lis cer'ebri, f. superolatera'lis hemisphe'rii cer'ebri** [NA], the convex outer surface of the cerebrum, which faces the calvaria; called also *f. convexa cerebri.* **f. symphys'eos os'sis pu'bis, f. symphysia'lis** [NA], the rough, ovoid, medial surface of the body of the pubic bone, by which it articulates at the pubic symphysis with its fellow of the opposite side. **f. tempora'lis a'lae mag'nae, f. tempora'lis a'lae majo'ris** [NA], the lateral and inferior surface of the great wing of the sphenoid bone, divided by the infratemporal crest into a superior part that forms a portion of the wall of the temporal fossa, and an inferior part that forms part of the wall of the infratemporal fossa. **f. tempora'lis os'sis fronta'lis** [NA], the slightly concave surface of the frontal bone that forms the upper part of the wall of the temporal fossa and gives attachment to the anterosuperior part of the temporalis muscle. **f. tempora'lis os'sis zygomat'ici** [NA], the internal, concave surface of the zygomatic bone, facing the temporal and infratemporal fossae. **f. tempora'lis par'tis squamo'sae** [NA], **f. tempora'lis squa'mae tempora'lis,** the external surface of the squamous part of the temporal bone, the anterior part of which forms a portion of the temporal fossa. **f. urethra'lis pe'nis** [NA], the surface of the penis overlying the urethra, and opposite the dorsum penis. **f. ventra'lis scap'ulae,** f. costalis scapulae. **f. vesica'lis u'teri** [NA], the flat anterior surface of the uterus, adjacent to the urinary bladder. **f. vestibula'ris den'tis** [NA], vestibular surface: the surface of a tooth that is directed outward toward the vestibule of the mouth, including the buccal and labial surfaces, and opposite the lingual (or oral) surface. Called also *f. facialis dentis* [NA alternative] and *facial surface.* **f. viscera'lis hep'atis** [NA], the posteroinferior surface of the liver, which is in contact with various abdominal viscera; called also *f. inferior hepatis.* **f. viscera'lis lie'nis,** NA alternative for *f. visceralis splenis.* **f. viscera'lis sple'nis** [NA], the surface of the spleen which comes in contact with various other viscera, including the colon (facies colica), kidney (facies renalis), and stomach (facies gastrica); called also *f. visceralis lienis* [NA alternative]. **f. vola'ris ra'dii,** f. anterior radii. **f. vola'ris ul'nae,** f. anterior ulnae.

facilitation (fah-sil″ĭ-ta'shun) [L. *facilis* easy] the promotion or hastening of any natural process; the reverse of inhibition; specifically, the effect of a nerve impulse acting across a synapse, and resulting in an increase in the efficacy of subsequent impulses in that nerve fiber, or impulses in other convergent nerve fibers, in exciting the postsynaptic element. See *law of facilitation.* **Wedensky f.,** facilitation across a block; when there is a complete block to nerve conduction the threshold of the nerve below the block to electric stimulation is lowered.

facilitative (fah-sil'ĭ-ta″tiv) in pharmacology, denoting a reaction arising as an indirect result of drug action, as development of an infection after the normal microflora has been altered by an antibiotic.

facilitory (fah-sil'ĭ-tōr-e) making easier; promoting or hastening a natural process; acting so as to render a neural element more easily excitable.

facing (fās'ing) a porcelain reproduction of the labial or buccal surface of a tooth; it may be constructed with or without pins and is soldered or cemented to a metal backing.

faci(o)- [L. *facies* face] a combining form denoting relationship to the face.

faciobrachial (fa″she-o-bra'ke-al) [*facio-* + Gr. *brachiōn* arm] pertaining to the face and arm.

faciocephalalgia (fa″she-o-sef″ah-lal'je-ah) [*facio-* + Gr. *kephalē* head + *-algia*] neuralgic pain in the face and neck attributed to disorders of the autonomic (vegetative) nervous system.

faciocervical (fa″she-o-ser'vĕ-kal) [*facio-* + L. *cervix* neck] pertaining to or affecting the face and neck.

faciolingual (fa″she-o-ling'gwal) [*facio-* + L. *lingua* tongue] pertaining to the face and tongue.

facioplasty (fa″she-o-plas'te) [*facio-* + Gr. *plassein* to form] plastic surgery of the face.

facioplegia (fa″she-o-ple'je-ah) [*facio-* + Gr. *plēgē* stroke] facial paralysis.

facioscapulohumeral (fa″she-o-skap″u-lo-hu'mer-al) pertaining to the face, scapula, and arm.

faciostenosis (fa″she-o-stĕ-no′sis) failure of the midface to grow.

F.A.C.O.G. Fellow of the American College of Obstetricians and Gynecologists.

F.A.C.P. Fellow of the American College of Physicians.

FACS fluorescence-activated cell sorter.

F.A.C.S. Fellow of the American College of Surgeons.

F.A.C.S.M. Fellow of the American College of Sports Medicine.

F-actin see *actin.*

factitial (fak-tish′al) produced by artificial means; unintentionally produced.

factitious (fak-tish′us) [L. *factitiosus*] artificial; not natural.

factor (fak′tor) [L. "maker"] 1. any of several substances or activities that are necessary to produce a result, e.g., a coagulation factor. Often, use of the term "factor" indicates that the chemical nature of the substance or its mechanism of action is unknown, as in endocrinology, where "factors" are renamed as "hormones" when their chemical nature is determined. 2. any of the numbers of algebraic symbols multiplied together to form a product. 3. a coefficient or conversion factor, a number by which a quantity is multiplied to produce a change of units of measurement. 4. a gene (hereditary factor). **f. A,** C3 (in the alternative complement pathway); see *complement.* **accelerator f.,** see *Factor V,* under *coagulation f's.* **activation f.,** see *Factor XII,* under *coagulation f's.* **adrenocorticotropic releasing f. (ACTH-RF),** corticotropin releasing f. **angiogenesis f.,** a substance that causes the growth of new blood vessels, found in tissues with high metabolic requirements such as cancers and the retina. It is also released by hypoxic macrophages at the edges or outer surface of a wound and initiates revascularization in wound healing. **animal protein f.,** an element in animal proteins found to be essential to maximal growth of animals; vitamin B_{12}. Abbreviated APF. **antiachromotrichia f.,** pantothenic acid. **antiacrodynia f.,** pyridoxine. **antialopecia f.,** inositol. **antianemia f.,** cyanocobalamin. **antianemia f. for chicks,** a vitamin, folic acid, in spinach and other green leaves, which prevents anemia in chicks. **antiblack tongue f.,** niacin. **anticanities f., antidermatitis f. of chicks,** pantothenic acid. **antidermatitis f. of rats,** pyridoxine. **anti-egg white f.,** biotin. **antigen-specific T-cell helper f.,** a soluble factor produced by helper T cells that activates other lymphocytes that are specific for the stimulating antigen; it may itself bind antigen. **antigen-specific T-cell suppressor f.,** a soluble factor produced by suppressor T cells following immunization; it produces antigen-specific suppression of the immune response and may itself bind antigen. **antigray hair f.,** pantothenic acid. **antihemophilic f.,** 1. see *Factor VIII,* under *coagulation f's.* Abbreviated AHF. 2. [USP] a sterile freeze-dried powder containing the Factor VIII fraction obtained from suitable whole-blood donors. **antihemophilic f., cryoprecipitated** [USP], a sterile, frozen concentrate of human antihemophilic factor prepared from the Factor VIII–rich cryoprotein fraction of human venous plasma obtained from suitable whole-blood donors from a single unit of plasma derived from whole blood or by plasmapheresis, collected and processed in a closed system. Called also *human antihemophilic f.* **antihemophilic f., human,** antihemophilic f., def. 2. **antihemophilic f. A,** see *Factor VIII,* under *coagulation f's.* **antihemophilic f. B,** see *Factor IX,* under *coagulation f's.* **antihemophilic f. C,** see *Factor XI,* under *coagulation f's.* **antihemorrhagic f.,** vitamin K. **antineuritic f.,** thiamine. **antinuclear f. (ANF),** see under *antibody.* **antipellagra f.,** niacin. **anti-pernicious anemia f.,** cyanocobalamin. **antirachitic f.,** vitamin D. **antiscorbutic f.,** ascorbic acid. **antisterility f.,** vitamin E. **antixerophthalmia f., antixerotic f.,** vitamin A. **atrial natriuretic f. (ANF),** a peptide secreted by specific endocrine cells in the right atrium of the mammalian heart that, in response to atrial dilatation or increased intravascular fluid volume, exerts a natriuretic effect on the kidney. **f. B,** a complement component C3 proactivator which participates in the alternative pathway of complement activation. The factor B-C3b complex is split by factor D, which leads to formation of C3 convertase, which in turn acts in the alternative pathway. **basophil chemotactic f.**

(BCF), a lymphokine produced by activated lymphocytes that is chemotactic for basophils, possibly responsible for the influx of basophils into sites of inflammation (Jones-Mote reaction). **B cell differentiation f's (BCDF),** factors derived from T cells that stimulate B cells to differentiate into antibody-secreting cells. Cf. *B lymphocyte stimulatory f's.* **B cell growth f's (BCGF),** factors derived from T cells that stimulate B cells to proliferate in vitro but (unlike B cell differentiation factors) do not stimulate antibody secretion. Cf. *B lymphocyte stimulatory f's.* **B-lymphocyte stimulatory f's (BSF),** a system of nomenclature for factors that stimulate B cells, replacing individual factor names (e.g., B cell differentiation factors). Each factor is designated by BSF and a number, BSF1, BSF2, etc., with the letter p prefixed to the number for factors that have not been purified or whose structure has not been identified, e.g., BSF-p1. **Bittner milk f.,** mouse mammary tumor virus. **blastogenic f. (BF),** lymphocyte mitogenic f. **bone f.,** in periodontal disease, the systemic influence on alveolar bone loss in response to local inflammatory processes. **Bx f.,** aminobenzoic acid. **C f.,** a factor found in the soluble part of cytoplasm which promotes the contraction of mitochondria. **C3 nephritic f. (C3 NeF),** an autoantibody specific for the alternative complement pathway C3 convertase C3b,Bb found in the serum of many patients with type II membranoproliferative glomerulonephritis. It stabilizes the C3b,Bb complex and prevents its inactivation by factor H, resulting in chronic fluid phase alternative pathway activation. **CAMP f.,** see under *tests.* **Castle's f.,** intrinsic factor. **chemotactic f.,** a substance that induces chemotaxis. Called also *chemoattractant* and *chemotactin.* **chick antidermatitis f.,** pantothenic acid. **chick antipellagra f.,** pantothenic acid. **chick growth f. S,** streptogenin. **Christmas f.,** see *Factor IX,* under *coagulation f's.* **chromotrichial f.,** aminobenzoic acid. **citrovorum f.,** folinic acid. **clonal inhibitory f., cloning inhibitory f. (CIF),** see *growth inhibitory f's.* **coagulation f's,** substances in the blood that are essential to the clotting process and hence, to the maintenance of normal hemostasis. They are designated by Roman numerals, to which the notation "a" is added to indicate the activated state. Platelet factors, designated by Arabic numerals, also play a role in coagulation. *Factor I,* fibrinogen: a high-molecular-weight plasma protein which is converted to fibrin through the action of thrombin. Deficiency of this factor results in afibrinogenemia or hypofibrinogenemia. Several molecular forms of this factor have been recognized. *Factor II,* prothrombin: a protein present in the plasma that, in theoretical hematology, is converted to thrombin by extrinsic prothrombin converting principle. More than one molecular form has been detected. Deficiency of this factor leads to hypoprothrombinemia. *Factor III,* tissue thromboplastin: a material derived from several sources in the body (brain, lung, etc.) and important in the formation of extrinsic prothrombin converting principle in the extrinsic pathway of blood coagulation. Called also *tissue factor. Factor IV,* calcium: a factor required in many phases of blood coagulation. *Factor V,* proaccelerin: a heat- and storage-labile material, present in plasma but not in serum, functioning in both the intrinsic and extrinsic pathways of blood coagulation. Deficiency of this factor, an autosomal recessive trait, leads to a rare hemorrhagic tendency, known as Owren's disease or parahemophilia, which varies greatly in severity. Called also *accelerator globulin (AcG)* and *labile factor. Factor VI,* a factor (accelerin) previously thought to be an activated form of Factor V. It is no longer is considered in the scheme of hemostasis, and hence it is assigned neither a name nor a function at this time. *Factor VII,* proconvertin: a heat- and storage-stable factor participating only in the extrinsic pathway of blood coagulation. Deficiency of this factor, which deficiency may be hereditary (autosomal recessive) or acquired (associated with vitamin K deficiency), results in a hemorrhagic tendency. Called also *prothromboki-nase, autoprothrombin I, serum prothrombin conversion accelerator (SPCA),* and *stable factor. Factor VIII,* antihemophilic factor (AHF): a relatively storage-labile factor participating only in the intrinsic pathway of blood coagulation. Deficiency of this factor, when transmitted as a sex-linked recessive trait, causes classical hemophilia (hemophilia A). More than one molecular form of this factor has been discovered. Called also *antihemophilic globulin (AHG)* and *antihemophilic factor A. Factor IX,* plasma thromboplastin component (PTC): a relatively storage-stable substance involved only in the intrinsic pathway of blood coagulation. Deficiency of this factor results in a hemorrhagic syndrome called hemophilia B or Christmas disease, which is similar to classical hemophilia (hemophilia A). More than one molecular form has been discovered. A transient form, known as *hemophilia B Leyden*, is clinically indistinguishable from ordinary hemophilia, but the bleeding tendency abates after puberty. Called also *autoprothrombin II, Christmas factor*, and *antihemophilic factor B*. **Factor X**, Stuart factor: a storage-stable factor that participates in both the intrinsic and extrinsic pathways of blood coagulation. Deficiency of this factor may cause a systemic coagulation disorder (Factor X deficiency). Called also *autoprothrombin C, Prower factor, Stuart-Prower factor*, and *thrombokinase*. **Factor XI**, plasma thromboplastin antecedent (PTA): a stable factor involved in the intrinsic pathway of blood coagulation. Deficiency of this factor results in a systemic blood-clotting defect called hemophilia C or Rosenthal's syndrome, that may resemble classical hemophilia. Called also *antihemophilic factor C*. **Factor XII**, Hageman factor: a stable factor activated by contact with glass or other foreign surfaces, which initiates the intrinsic process of blood coagulation *in vitro*. Deficiency of this factor results in prolonged *in vitro* blood clotting but overt clinical bleeding is rare. Called also *glass, contact*, or *activation factor*. **Factor XIII**, fibrin stabilizing factor (FSF): a factor that polymerizes fibrin monomers so that they become stable and insoluble in urea, thus enabling fibrin to form a firm blood clot. Deficiency of this factor produces a clinical hemorrhagic diathesis. Called also *fibrinase* and *Laki-Lorand factor (LLF)*. The inactive form is also known as *protransglutaminase*, and the active form as *transglutaminase*. *platelet factor 1*, adsorbed Factor V from the plasma. *platelet factor 2*, an accelerator of the thrombin-fibrinogen reaction, attached to platelets. *platelet factor 3*, a substance, probably a lipoprotein, extracted from platelets, which contributes to the interaction of plasma coagulation proteins in the generation of intrinsic prothrombin converting principle. *platelet factor 4*, an intracellular protein component of blood platelets, capable of neutralizing the antithrombic activity of heparin in the fibrinogen-fibrin reaction and the inhibitory effect of heparin in the thromboplastin generation test. **colony-stimulating f. (CSF)**, a glycoprotein lymphokine produced by blood monocytes, tissue macrophages, and stimulated lymphocytes required for differentiation of stem cells into granulocyte and monocyte cell colonies, and which may be required in granulopoiesis. It has been used as an experimental cancer agent. **conglutinogen activating f. (KAF)**, factor I. **contact f.**, see *Factor XII*, under *coagulation f's*. **cord f.**, a mycoside produced by those strains of *Mycobacterium tuberculosis* that characteristically grow in long serpentine cords. **corticotropin releasing f. (CRF)**, a factor or hormone (43 amino acids) elaborated by the hypothalamus at the median eminence, which stimulates the release of corticotropin by the anterior pituitary gland. Called also *corticotropin releasing hormone*. **crystal-induced chemotactic f. (CCF)**, a glycoprotein, mol. wt. 8400, produced by neutrophils upon ingestion of monosodium urate or calcium pyrophosphate crystals that is directly chemotactic for neutrophils and is thought to be involved in the inflammatory process in gouty arthritis. **Curling f.**, griseofulvin. **f. D**, a protein of the alternate complement pathway; see *complement*. **Day's f.**, folic acid. **decay-activating f. (DAF)**, an intrinsic red blood cell protein that prevents the assembly of convertase on the cell surface, thus protecting it from injury by autologous complement. **diabetogenic f.**, a substance of unknown constitution associated with extracts of growth hormone from the anterior pituitary which, when injected into normal dogs, causes them to become diabetic. **diffusion f.**, hyaluronidase. **Duran-Reynals f.**, hyaluronidase. **elongation f.**, one of two soluble proteins (EF-1 and EF-2) involved in the addition of each amino acid to the growing polypeptide chain in protein synthesis (see *translation*). **eluate f.**, pyridoxine. **eosinophil chemotactic f. (ECF)**, 1. eosinophil chemotactic f. of anaphylaxis. 2. a lymphokine produced by activated lymphocytes that is chemotactic for eosinophils. **eosinophil chemotactic f. of anaphylaxis (ECF-A)**, eosinophil chemoattractants released by basophils and mast cells in immediate hypersensitivity reactions. ECF-A activity is associated with two acidic tetrapeptides (Ala-Gly-Ser-Glu and Val-Gly-Ser-Glu) and with less well characterized larger peptides, which are chemotactic for eosinophils and, to a lesser degree, for neutrophils. Some ECF-A activity is due to arachidonic acid metabolites (leukotriene B, 12-HETE, and 12-HHT). Called also *eosinophil chemotactic f. (ECF)*. **epidermal growth f.**, a protein extractable from the submaxillary glands of male mice that stimulates proliferation of cells of ectodermal and mesodermal origin and inhibits gastric secretion; it is very similar or identical to urogastrone. **erythrocyte maturation f. (E.M.F.)**, a former name for vitamin B_{12} (cyanocobalamin). **erythropoietic stimulating f. (E.S.F.)**, a name given a factor in the body which stimulates the production of erythrocytes; probably identical with erythropoietin. **extrinsic f.**, vitamin B_{12} (cyanocobalamin). **F (fertility) f.**, F plasmid. **fermentation Lactobacillus casei f.**, pteropterin. **fibrin stabilizing f.**, see *Factor XIII*, under *coagulation f's*. **filtrate f.**, **filtrate f. II**, pantothenic acid. **follicle stimulating hormone releasing f. (FRF, FSH-RF)**, gonadotropin releasing hormone. **galactopoietic f.**, prolactin. **gastric anti-pernicious anemia f., gastric intrinsic f.**, intrinsic f. **glass f.**, see *Factor XII*, under *coagulation f's*. **glucose tolerance f.**, a biologically active complex of chromium and nicotinic acid that facilitates the reaction of insulin with receptor sites on tissues. **gonadotropin releasing f. (GnRF)**, see under hormone. **growth hormone releasing f. (GRF, GH-RF)**, a peptide hormone elaborated by the median eminence of the hypothalamus, which stimulates the release of growth hormone from the anterior pituitary gland. Called also *growth hormone releasing hormone (GH-RH)* and *somatotropin releasing hormone (SRF)*. **growth inhibitory f's**, two lymphokines, clonal inhibitory factor (CIF) and proliferation inhibitory factor (PIF) that inhibit the growth of certain target cells, permanently at higher concentrations and temporarily at lower concentrations. Both inhibitory factors and lymphotoxin (q.v.) may be activities of the same substance. **f. H**, a glycoprotein that binds to C3b (see *complement*) and acts as an alternative pathway complement inhibitor by interfering with the binding of factor B to C3b; it also acts as a cofactor in the conversion of C36 to C3bi by factor I. **Hageman f. (HF)**, see *Factor XII*, under *coagulation f's*. **high-molecular-weight neutrophil chemotactic f. (HMW-NCF)**, neutrophil chemotactic f. **histamine releasing f.**, a lymphokine that produces basophil degranulation. **hydrazine-sensitive f. (HSF)**, C3 (in the alternative complement pathway); see *complement*. **hyperglycemic-glycogenolytic f.**, see *glucagon*. **f. I**, a plasma enzyme that inactivates C3b (see *complement*) by cleaving it to form C3bi; factor H is required as a cofactor for its activity. **f. II**, 1. see under *coagulation f's*. 2. pantothenic acid. **f. III**, see under *coagulation f's*. **immunoglobulin-binding f. (IBF)**, a lymphokine having the ability to bind IgG complexed with antigen and prevent complement activation, possibly Fc receptors shed from T cells. **inhibiting f's**, factors elaborated by one structure (as by the hypothalamus) that inhibit the release of hormones by another structure (as by the anterior pituitary gland), including melanocyte-stimulating hormone inhibiting factor and prolactin inhibiting factor (presumably peptides). The term is applied to substances of unknown chemical structure, while substances of established chemical identity are called *inhibiting hormones* (see under *hormone*). **initiation f.**, one of three soluble proteins (IF-1, IF-2, and IF-3) involved in the binding of mRNA and the first aminoacyl-tRNA to the small ribosomal subunit and the attachment of the small subunit to the large subunit at the beginning of protein synthesis (see *translation*). **insulin-like growth f's (IGF)**, insulin-like substances in serum that do not react with insulin antibodies; they are growth hormone–dependent and possess all the growth-promoting properties of the somatomedins. Called also *nonsuppressible insulin-like activity*. **intermediate lobe inhibiting f.**, melanocyte-stimulating hormone inhibiting f. **intrinsic f.**, a glycoprotein secreted by the parietal cells of the gastric glands, necessary for the absorption of vitamin B_{12} (cyanocobalamin, extrinsic factor). Lack of intrinsic factor, with consequent deficiency of vitamin B_{12}, results in pernicious anemia. **f. IV**, see under *coagulation f's*. **f. IX**, see under *coagulation f's*. **labile f.**, see *Factor V*, under *coagulation f's*. **Lactobacillus casei f.**, folic acid. **Lactobacillus lactis Dorner f.**, cyanocobalamin. **lactogenic f.**, prolactin. **Laki-Lorand f.**, see *Factor XIII*, under *coagulation f's*. **LE f.**, an antibody having a sedimentation rate of 7S that reacts with leukocyte nuclei in the LE cell test, now referred to as antinuclear antibody (q.v.). **leukocyte inhibitory f. (LIF),** a lymphokine that inhibits the migration of polymorphonuclear leukocytes but not macrophages. **liver filtrate f.,** pantothenic acid. **liver Lactobacillus casei f.,** folic acid. **LLD f.,** cyanocobalamin. **luteinizing hormone releasing f. (LRF, LH-RF),** a factor elaborated by the hypothalamus at the median eminence, which stimulates the release of luteinizing hormone by the anterior pituitary gland. **lymph node permeability f. (LNPF),** a vasoactive factor, distinct from histamine, serotonin, bradykinin, and kallikrein, that is released without immunologic stimulus from many tissues, including lymph nodes, spleen, kidney, liver, and muscle. **lymphocyte activating f.,** interleukin 1. **lymphocyte blastogenic f. (BF),** lymphocyte mitogenic f. **lymphocyte mitogenic f. (LMF),** a nondialyzable heat-stable macromolecule, mol. wt. approximately 20,000–30,000, released by lymphocytes stimulated by specific antigen, that causes nonstimulated lymphocytes to undergo blast transformation and cell division. Called also *lymphocyte blastogenic f. (BF)* and *lymphocyte transforming f. (LTF).* **lymphocyte transforming f. (LTF),** lymphocyte mitogenic f. **lysogenic f.,** bacteriophage. **macrophage-activating f. (MAF),** a lymphokine that, after a 72-hour incubation period, induces or increases macrophage adherence, phagocytosis, oxygen consumption, and bactericidal and tumoricidal activity. MAF and MIF (macrophage inhibitory factor) appear to be activities of the same macromolecule. **macrophage chemotactic f. (MCF),** a lymphokine produced by activated lymphocytes that is chemotactic for macrophages. **macrophage-derived growth f.,** a substance released by macrophages below the surface of a wound that induces the proliferation of fibroblasts, with consequent deposition of collagen, fibronectin, and glycosaminoglycan. **macrophage growth f. (MGF),** glycoproteins that permit macrophages harvested from peritoneal exudates to proliferate in liquid-suspension cultures and form colonies consisting solely of mononuclear phagocytes. **macrophage inhibitory f., migration inhibiting f. (MIF),** a lymphokine that causes temporary inhibition of macrophage migration, lasting about 24 hours. **melanocyte stimulating hormone inhibiting f. (MIF),** a tripeptide, Pro-Leu-Gly-NH$_2$, formed in the hypothalamus by enzymatic cleavage of oxytocin that inhibits the release of MSH by the intermediate lobe of the pituitary gland in fish and amphibians. **melanocyte stimulating hormone releasing f. (MRF, MSH-RF),** a hypothalamic factor or factors of undetermined chemical nature reported to cause release of MSH from the pituitary gland in lower animals. **milk f.,** mouse mammary tumor virus. **mitogenic f.,** lymphocyte mitogenic f. **mouse antialopecia f.,** inositol. **mouse mammary tumor f.,** see under *virus.* **MSH inhibiting f.,** melanocyte-stimulating hormone inhibiting f. **müllerian regression f., müllerian duct inhibitory f.,** a factor postulated to be present in the male embryo which inhibits development of the wolffian ducts. **multiple f's,** in heredity, two or more genes or environmental variants that act in combination to produce a certain trait. **myocardial depressant f. (MDF),** a peptide formed in response to a fall in systemic blood pressure that has a negatively inotropic effect on myocardial muscle fibers. **N f.,** a factor occurring in yeast, meat, liver, and wheat germ, the absence of which from an otherwise complete diet causes rats to voluntarily consume more alcohol than they do when factor N is present in the diet. **necrotizing f.,** necrotoxin. **nerve growth f.,** a protein consisting of two identical polypeptide chains associated with two gamma subunits (enzymes) and two alpha subunits; first isolated from mouse sarcoma and later from snake venom and mouse salivary glands, it stimulates the growth of sensory and sympathetic nerve cells and of the adrenal medulla and has been found to be secreted by a variety of normal and neoplastic cells, including those of man. Abbreviated NGF. **neutrophil chemotactic f. (NCF),** 1. a poorly characterized chemotactic factor, mol. wt. approximately 750,000, that attracts neutrophils but not eosinophils or monocytes and is released by basophils or mast cells in immediate hypersensitivity reactions. Called also *high-molecular-weight neutrophil chemotactic f. (HMW-NCF).* 2. a lymphokine produced by activated lymphocytes that is chemotactic for neutrophils. **osteoclast activating f. (OAF),** a lymphokine that stimulates bone resorption; it is a small protein unrelated to parathyroid hormone and may be involved in the bone resorption associated with multiple myeloma and other hematologic neoplasms or inflammatory disorders such as rheumatoid arthritis and periodontal disease. **f. P,** properdin; a nonimmunoglobulin gamma globulin component of the alternative pathway; it complexes with C3b and stabilizes alternative pathway C3 convertase. **pellagra-preventive f.,** niacin. **platelet f's,** factors important in hemostasis which are contained in or attached to the platelets. See *platelet factors 1, 2, 3,* and *4,* under *coagulation f's.* See also *platelet cofactors,* under *cofactor.* **platelet activating f. (PAF),** a substance released by basophils and mast cells in immediate hypersensitivity reactions and macrophages and neutrophils in other inflammatory reactions that is an extremely potent mediator of bronchoconstriction and of the platelet aggregation and release reactions. It differs from other known biochemical mediators in being a phospholipid. Called also *PAF-acether* or *AGEPC* (acetyl glyceryl ether phosphoryl choline). **platelet-derived growth f.,** a substance contained in the alpha granules of platelets and capable of inducing proliferation of vascular endothelial cells, vascular smooth muscle cells, fibroblasts, and glia cells; its action contributes to the repair of damaged vascular walls. **P.-P. f.,** niacin. **prolactin inhibiting f. (PIF),** a factor elaborated by the hypothalamus at the median eminence, which inhibits the secretion of prolactin by the anterior pituitary gland. **prolactin releasing f. (PRF),** a factor(s) elaborated by the hypothalamus at the median eminence, which stimulates the release of prolactin by the anterior pituitary gland. In human subjects, thyrotropin releasing hormone can also act as prolactin releasing factor(s). **proliferation inhibitory f. (PIF),** see *growth inhibitory f's.* **Prower f.,** see *Factor X,* under *coagulation f's.* **R f.,** R plasmid. **rat acrodynia f.,** pyridoxine. **recruitment f.,** lymphocyte mitogenic f. **releasing f.,** one of two soluble proteins (RF-1 and RF-2) involved in the release of the completed polypeptide chain from the ribosome when a termination codon is encountered during protein synthesis (see translation; RF-1 recognizes the termination codons UAA or UAG and RF-2 recognizes UAA or UGA. **releasing f's,** factors elaborated in one structure (as in the hypothalamus) that effect the release of hormones from another structure (as from the anterior pituitary gland), including corticotropin releasing factor, melanocyte stimulating hormone releasing factor, and prolactin releasing factor. The term is applied to substances of unknown chemical structure, while substances of established chemical identity are called *releasing hormones* (see under *hormone*). **resistance-inducing f.,** see *Rubin's test* (def. 2), under *tests.* **resistance transfer f.,** the portion of an R plasmid in a bacterial cell that contains the genes for conjugation and replication. **Rh f., Rhesus f.,** antigens (agglutinogens) present on the membrane of red blood cells; see *blood group.* **rheumatoid f., (RF),** antibodies directed against antigenic determinants, i.e., Gm, in the Fc region of IgG, found in the serum of about 80 per cent of patients with classical or definite rheumatoid arthritis; but in only about 20 per cent of patients with juvenile rheumatoid arthritis; rheumatoid factors may be IgM, IgG, or IgA antibodies, although serologic tests measure only IgM. Rheumatoid factors also occur in other connective tissue diseases and infectious diseases (Sjögren's syndrome, systemic lupus erythematosus, sarcoidosis, subacute bacterial endocarditis, infectious hepatitis, leprosy). **risk f.,** a clearly defined occurrence or characteristic that has been associated with the increased rate of a subsequently occurring disease. **f. S,** biotin. **separation f.,** the ratio of the relative concentration of two isotopes after processing, to their relative concentration before processing. **sex f.,** F plasmid. **Simon's septic f.,** decrease of eosinophils and increase of neutrophils in the blood in pyogenic infections. **skin reactive f. (SRF),** a lymphokine derived from antigen-stimulated lymphocytes that augments the delayed hypersensitivity skin reaction, increasing capillary permeability and infiltration of monocytes, perhaps a mixture of other lymphokines. **somatotropin releasing f. (SRF),** growth hormone releasing f. **specific macrophage arming f. (SMAF),** a lymphokine reported to be a nonimmunoglobulin factor produced by activated T cells that is capable of activating macrophages so that they are capable of specifically recognizing and killing tumor cells. **spreading f.,** hyaluronidase. **stable f.,** see *Factor VII,* under *coagulation f's.* **Stuart f., Stuart-Prower f.,** see *Factor X,* under *coagulation f's.* **sulfation f.,** a formerly used term for somatomedin. **T-cell**

growth f., interleukin 2. **thyrotropin releasing f. (TRF),** see under *hormone.* **transfer f. (TF),** a dialyzable extract obtained from lysates of peripheral blood lymphocytes that is capable of transferring antigen-specific cell-mediated immunity (delayed type hypersensitivity) from donor to recipient and also has nonspecific immunostimulatory activity; it appears to contain both protein and RNA but not DNA and consist of small molecules (mol. wt. less than 10,000). TF is nonantigenic and does not transfer humoral immunity. Clinical trials have shown promising results in treatment of immunodeficiency diseases, including Wiskott-Aldrich syndrome, severe combined immunodeficiency disease, and ataxia-telangiectasia, and in fungal infections refractory to chemotherapy, including disseminated mucocutaneous candidiasis and disseminated coccidioidomycosis; the use of TF in viral infections, parasitic diseases, and cancer is also under investigation. **Trapp's f.,** the last two figures expressive of the specific gravity of urine; when multiplied by 2 they give the number of parts of solids per 1000. **tumor-angiogenesis f.,** a factor produced by cancer cells of solid tumors that stimulates the growth of blood vessels into the tumor. **tumor necrosis f. (TNF),** a lymphokine produced by macrophages capable of causing in vivo hemorrhagic necrosis of certain tumor cells, but not affecting normal cells. It is the same substance as cachectin. It has been used as an experimental anticancer agent. **V f.,** an accessory substance required for the growth of certain species of *Haemophilus,* replaceable by nicotinamide-adenine dinucleotide (NAD) or nicotinamide-adenine dinucleotide phosphate (NADP) and present in red blood cells. Cf. *X f.* **f. V,** see under *coagulation f's.* **f. VI,** see under *coagulation f's.* **f. VII,** see under *coagulation f's.* **f. VIII,** see under *coagulation f's.* **von Willebrand's f.,** the attribute of Factor VIII (see under *coagulation f's*) necessary for the adhesion of platelets to vascular elements. Deficiency of this factor results in the prolonged bleeding time seen in von Willebrand's disease. Called also *Factor VIII$_{VWF}$.* **f. W,** biotin. **Wills f.,** folic acid. **f. X,** see under *coagulation f's.* **X f.,** an accessory substance required for the aerobic growth of certain species of *Haemophilus* replaceable by hemin or other iron porphyrin compounds, and present in red blood cells. It is heat stable and not destroyed by autoclaving. Cf. *V f.* **f. XI,** see under *coagulation f's.* **f. XII,** see under *coagulation f's.* **f. XIII,** see under *coagulation f's.* **yeast eluate f.,** pyridoxine. **yeast filtrate f.,** pantothenic acid.

facultative (fak'ul-ta''tiv) 1. not obligatory; capable of adaptation to different conditions. 2. in bacteriology, a bacterium that can grow either aerobically or anaerobically.

faculty (fak'ul-te) [L. *facultas*] 1. any normal power or function, especially a mental one. 2. the corps of professors and instructors of a college or university. **fusion f.,** the power of blending into one the two images viewed by the two eyes.

FAD flavin adenine dinucleotide.

fading (fād'ing) an illness of puppies marked by progressive weakness which makes suckling impossible, a falling body temperature, and paddling movements; it usually results in death within a few days of birth.

fae- for words beginning thus, see those beginning *fe-.*

fagopyrism (fag-op'ĭ-rizm) [L. *fagopyrum* buckwheat] poisoning by buckwheat.

Fahrenheit scale, thermometer (far'en-hīt) [Gabriel Daniel *Fahrenheit,* German physicist, 1686–1736] see under *scale* and *thermometer.*

failure (fāl'yer) inability to perform. **heart f.,** see under *H.* **kidney f.,** renal f. **renal f.,** the inability of a kidney to excrete metabolites at normal plasma levels under conditions of normal loading, or the inability to retain electrolytes under conditions of normal intake. In the acute form, it is marked by uremia and usually by oliguria or anuria, with hyperkalemia and pulmonary edema. **respiratory f.,** a persistent condition of abnormally low arterial oxygen tension (PaO$_2$) or abnormally high carbon dioxide tension (PaCO$_2$).

faint (fānt) syncope.

falcadina (fal''kah-de'nah) a disease of Istria, a peninsula in northwestern Yugoslavia, characterized by the formation of papillomas.

falcate (fal'kāt) falciform.

falces (fal'sēz) [L.] plural of *falx.*

falcial (fal'shal) pertaining to a falx.

falciform (fal'sĭ-form) [L. *falx* sickle + *forma* form] shaped like a sickle.

falcular (fal'ku-lar) [L. *falx* sickle] sickle-shaped.

fallopian aqueduct (arch), artery, ligament, tube (fal-lo'pe-an) [Gabriele *Falloppio* (L. *Fallopius*), 1523–1562; an important Italian anatomist, pupil of Vesalius, and later professor at Padua] see *canalis facialis, arteria uterina, ligamentum inguinale,* and *tuba uterina.*

Fallot's tetralogy (disease, syndrome, tetrad), trilogy (fal-ōz') [Étienne-Louis Arthur *Fallot,* French physician, 1850–1911] see *tetralogy of Fallot* and *trilogy of Fallot.*

fallout (fawl'out) the settling to the earth's surface of radioactive fission products that have been projected into the atmosphere by the explosion of a nuclear device.

false (fawls) [L. *falsus*] not true; not genuine; apparent, but not real.

false-negative (fawls'neg'ah-tiv) 1. denoting a test result that wrongly excludes an individual from a diagnostic or other category. 2. an individual so excluded. 3. an instance of a false-negative result.

false-positive (fawls'pos'ĭ-tiv) 1. denoting a test result that wrongly assigns an individual to a diagnostic or other category. 2. an individual so categorized. 3. an instance of a false-positive result. **biologic f. (BFP),** a positive result on a serologic test for syphilis (STS), such as the VDRL test, when syphilis is not present. Acute BFP is associated with infectious disease, e.g., bacterial and mycoplasma pneumonias, subacute bacterial endocarditis, varicella, infectious mononucleosis, and scarlet fever. Chronic BFP is associated with immune complex diseases, systemic lupus erythematosus, and leprosy.

falsification (fawl''sĭ-fĭ-ka'shun) a deliberate misstatement or misrepresentation. **retrospective f.,** unconscious distortion of memories of past experiences to conform to present emotional needs.

Falta's coefficient, triad (fahl'taz) [Wilhelm *Falta,* Vienna physician, born 1875] see under *coefficient* and *triad.*

falx (falks), pl. *fal'ces* [L. "sickle"] a sickle-shaped organ or structure; used as a general term in anatomical nomenclature to designate such a structure. **aponeurotic f., f. aponeurot'ica,** f. inguinalis. **f. cerebel'li** [NA], **f. of cerebellum,** the small fold of dura mater in the midline of the posterior cranial fossa, projecting forward toward the vermis of the cerebellum. **f. cer'ebri** [NA], **f. of cerebrum,** the sickle-shaped fold of dura mater that extends downward in the longitudinal cerebral fissure and separates the two cerebral hemispheres. **inguinal f., f. inguina'lis** [NA], the united tendons of the transverse and internal oblique muscles going to the linea alba and pectineal line of the pubic bone; called also *Henle's ligament* and *tendo conjunctivus.* **ligamento'sa, f. ligamento'sa,** processus falciformis ligamenti sacrotuberosi. **f. sep'ti,** NA alternative for *valvula foraminis ovalis.*

fames (fa'mēz) [L.] hunger.

familial (fah-mil'e-al) [L. *familia* family] occurring in or affecting more members of a family than would be expected by chance.

family (fam'ĭ-le) 1. a group of individuals descended from a common ancestor. 2. a taxonomic subdivision subordinate to an order (or suborder) and superior to a tribe (or subfamily). **systematic f.,** see *family* (def. 2).

famotine hydrochloride (fam'o-tēn) chemical name: 1-[(4 - chlorophenoxy)methyl]-3,4-dihydroisoquinoline hydrochloride; an antiviral agent, C$_{16}$H$_{14}$ClNO·HCl.

fan (fan) an area, figure, or structure resembling an open fan. **Dunham's f's,** formations seen in the roentgenogram of the lung in silicosis, made up of nodules connected by fine lines in a pyramidal arrangement; called also *Dunham's cones* or *triangles.*

F and R force and rhythm (of pulse).

fang (fang) 1. the root of a tooth. 2. a carnassial tooth of a carnivore or the envenomed tooth of a serpent.

fango (fan'go) volcanic mud.

fangotherapy (fan''go-ther'ah-pe) the therapeutic use of fango in packs or baths.

Fannia (fan'e-ah) a genus of flies (family Muscidae), the larvae of which have caused both intestinal and urinary myiasis in man. In some systems of classification, it is included in the family Anthomyiidae. **F. canicula′ris,** the lesser house fly: a species of small grayish flies, visibly different from the housefly; they lay their eggs on decaying vegetable matter or animal manure, from which the eggs or larvae may gain access to human hosts. **F. scala′ris,** a species of flies, the latrine flies, similar to but larger than *F. canicularis,* and commonly depositing its eggs on excrement, rather than on vegetable matter.

fantasy (fan′tah-se) [Gr. *phantasia* imagination; the power by which an object is made apparent to the mind] a daydream; an imagined situation or sequence of events. Fantasy can serve as a realistic rehearsal of future events; it may also serve as an unconscious defense mechanism providing wish-fulfillment, gratification of repressed impulses, and resolution of unconscious conflicts.

fantridone hydrochloride (fan′trĭ-dōn) chemical name: 5-[3-(dimethylamino)propyl]-6(5*H*)-phenanthridinone monohydrochloride monohydrate; an antidepressant, $C_{18}H_{20}N_2O\cdot$-$HCl\cdot H_2O$.

F.A.P.H.A. Fellow of the American Public Health Association.

Farabeuf's amputation, triangle (far″ah-bufs′) [Louis Hubert *Farabeuf,* French surgeon, 1841–1910] see under *amputation* and *triangle.*

farad (far′ad) [Michael *Faraday*] the International System (SI) unit of electrical capacitance. The capacitance of a condenser which, charged with 1 coulomb, gives a difference of potential of 1 volt. Symbol, F. This unit is so large that one-millionth part of it has been adopted as a practical unit called a microfarad.

faraday (far′ah-da) the quantity of electrical charge associated with one gram equivalent of an electrochemical reaction, equal to about 96,510 coulombs.

Faraday's constant, law, dark space (far′ah-dāz) [Michael *Faraday,* English physicist, 1791–1867] see under *constant, law,* and *space.*

faradic (fah-rad′ik) pertaining to faradism.

faradimeter (far″ah-dim′ĕ-ter) [*farad* + Gr. *metron* measure] an instrument for measuring faradic electricity.

faradism (far′ah-dizm) 1. induced current. 2. induced current in a rapidly alternating current. 3. faradization. **surging f.,** a faradic current of gradually increasing and decreasing amplitude; obtained by introducing a rhythmically varying series resistance into the circuit.

faradization (far″ah-di-za′shun) the therapeutic use of an interrupted current; principally for the stimulation of muscles and nerves. Such a current is derived from an induction coil.

faradocontractility (far″ah-do-kon″trak-til′ĭ-te) contractility in response to faradic stimulus.

faradomuscular (far″ah-do-mus′cu-lar) pertaining to the reaction of a muscle when a faradic current is applied to it.

faradopalpation (far″ah-do-pal-pa′shun) galvanopalpation.

faradotherapy (far′ah-do-ther″ah-pe) faradization.

farcy (far′se) cutaneous glanders, the more chronic and constitutional lymphatic form of glanders, marked by thickening of the superficial lymph vessels; see *glanders.* **button f.,** farcy characterized by the formation of small tubercular nodules in the skin of the limbs, thorax, and abdomen. **cattle f.,** a disease of cattle caused by infection with *Nocardia farcinica,* and characterized by the formation of cheesy nodules in the subcutaneous tissue and the organs. **cryptococcus f.,** lymphangitis epizootica. **Japanese f., Neapolitan f.,** lymphangitis epizootica. **f. pipes,** acute farcy along the lymphatic vessels. **water f.,** inflammation of the lymphatics of a horse's leg.

fardel-bound (far′del-bownd) having an inflamed abomasum and distended omasum, so that chewing of the cud is impossible; a condition affecting cattle and sheep.

farina (fah-re′nah) [L., from *far* spelt (a kind of grain)] 1. meal or flour. 2. a starchy food prepared from cereal grains, usually from wheat. **f. ave′na,** oatmeal. **f. trit′ici,** wheaten flour.

farinaceous (far″ĭ-na′shus) [L. *farinaceus*] 1. of the nature of flour or meal. 2. starchy; containing starch.

farinometer (far″ĭ-nom′ĕ-ter) an instrument for determining the percentage of gluten in flour.

farnoquinone (far-no-kwin′ōn) menaquinone.

Farr's law (farz) [William *Farr,* English medical statistician, 1807–1883] see under *law.*

Farre's tubercles (farz) [John Richard *Farre,* an English physician, 1775–1862] see under *tubercle.*

Farre's white line (farz) [Arthur *Farre,* British obstetrician, 1811–1887] see under *line.*

farsighted (far-sīt′ed) hyperopic.

farsightedness (far-sīt′ed-nes) hyperopia.

fasc. abbreviation for L. *fascic′ulus,* bundle.

fascia (fash′e-ah), pl. *fas′ciae* [L. "band"] [NA] a sheet or band of fibrous tissue such as lies deep to the skin or forms an investment for muscles and various other organs of the body. **abdominal f., internal,** f. transversalis. **Abernethy's f.,** f. iliaca. **f. adher′ens,** that portion of the junctional complex of the cells of an intercalated disk which is the counterpart of the zonula adherens of epithelial cells, but instead of being beltlike it has multiple, moderately extensive but discontinuous areas with irregular and variable outlines. **anal f.,** f. diaphragmatis pelvis inferior. **anoscrotal f.,** f. perinei superficialis. **antebrachial f., f. antebra′chii** [NA], the investing fascia of the forearm; called also (*deep*) *f. of forearm.* **aponeurotic f.,** f. profunda. **f. of arm,** f. brachii. **f. axilla′ris** [NA], **axillary f.,** the investing fascia of the armpit which passes between the lateral borders of the pectoralis major and latissimus dorsi muscles. **bicipital f.,** aponeurosis musculi bicipitis brachii. **brachial f.,** f. brachii. **f. brachia′lis,** NA alternative for *f. brachii.* **f. bra′chii** [NA], the investing fascia of the arm. **buccinator f., f. buccopharyn′gea** [NA], **buccopharyngeal f., f. buccopharyngea′lis** [NA], a fibrous membrane forming the external covering of the constrictor muscles of the pharynx, and passing forward superiorly to the surface of the buccinator muscle. **Buck's f.,** the deep fascia of the penis, being continuous with Colles' fascia of the perineum and with Scarpa's fascia of the abdominal wall. **bulbar f., f. bul′bi** [Teno′ni], vagina bulbi. **f. of Camper,** the superficial layer of the superficial fascia of the abdomen. **cervical f.,** f. cervicalis. **cervical f., deep,** f. nuchae. **f. cervica′lis** [NA], the fascia of the neck, comprising a superficial layer deep to the skin, a pretracheal layer anterior to the trachea, and a prevertebral layer anterior to the vertebrae; it also forms a sheath enclosing the carotid vessels and vagus nerve. Called also *f. colli, cervical f.,* and *f. of neck.* **f. cine′rea** (*obs.*), gyrus fasciolaris. **clavipectoral f., f. clavipectora′lis** [NA], a fascial sheet investing the subclavius muscle, attached to the clavicle above and continuing to the pectoralis minor muscle below; called also *f. coracoclavicularis* and *coracoclavicular f.* **f. clitor′idis** [NA], **f. of clitoris,** the dense fibrous tissue that encloses the two corpora cavernosa of the clitoris. **Cloquet's f.,** the condensation of extraperitoneal tissue closing the femoral ring (septum femorale). **Colles' f.,** f. diaphragmatis urogenitalis inferior. **f. col′li,** f. cervicalis. **fasciae of colon,** teniae coli. **Cooper's f.,** 1. fascia cremasterica. 2. see *fibrae intercrurales.* **coracoclavicular f., f. coracoclavicula′ris, coracocostal f.,** f. clavipectoralis. **cremasteric f., f. cremaster′ica** [NA], the thin covering of the spermatic cord formed by the investing fascia of the cremasteric muscle; it is adjacent to the external surface of the internal spermatic fascia. Called also *Cooper's f.* and *intercolumnar f.* **cribriform f.,** 1. fascia cribrosa. 2. septum femorale. **f. cribro′sa** [NA], cribriform fascia: the part of the superficial fascia of the thigh that covers the saphenous opening. **crural f., f. cru′ris** [NA], the investing fascia of the leg; called also *crural aponeurosis.* **Cruveilhier's f.,** f. perinei superficialis. **dartos f. of scrotum,** tunica dartos. **deep f.,** f. profunda. **deep f. of arm,** f. brachii. **deep f. of back,** f. thoracolumbalis. **deep f. of forearm,** f. antebrachii. **deep f. of perineum,** diaphragma urogenitale. **deep f. of thigh,** f. lata femoris. **deltoid f., f. deltoi′dea** [NA], the deep fascia covering the deltoid muscle of the shoulder. **Denonvilliers' f.,** septum rectovesicale. **f. denta′ta hippocam′pi, dentate f.,** gyrus dentatus. **f. diaphrag′matis pel′vis infe′rior** [NA], the fascia that covers the lower surface of the coccygeus and levator ani muscles, forming the medial wall of the ischiorectal fossa;

called also *ischiorectal f.* and *ischiorectal aponeurosis*. **f. diaphrag′matis pel′vis supe′rior** [NA], the fascia on the upper surface of the levator ani and coccygeus muscles. **f. diaphrag′matis urogenita′lis infe′rior,** membrana perinei. **f. diaphrag′matis urogenita′lis supe′rior,** see *diaphragma urogenitale*. **dorsal f., deep,** f. thoracolumbalis. **dorsal f. of foot,** f. dorsalis pedis. **dorsal f. of hand, f. dorsa′lis ma′nus** [NA], the investing fascia of the back of the hand. **f. dorsa′lis pe′dis** [NA], the investing fascia on the dorsum of the foot. **endoabdominal f.,** f. transversalis. **endopelvic f., endopelvi′na,** a name given to fascia forming part of the general layer lining the pelvic walls and serving as a packing for the pelvic organs, as well as ensheathing the blood vessels, various specific parts of which have been known by various names. **endothoracic f., f. endothora′cica** [NA], the fascial sheet beneath the serous lining of the thoracic cavity. **external intercostal f.,** f. thoracica. **extraperitoneal f., f. extraperitonea′lis** [NA], the thin layer of areolar connective tissue separating the parietal peritoneum from the abdominal walls; called also *extraperitoneal tissue, subperitoneal f.,* and *f. subperitonealis*. **extrapleural f.,** a prolongation of the endothoracic fascia sometimes found at the root of the neck, which is important as possibly modifying the auscultatory sounds at the apex of the lung. **femoral f.,** f. lata femoris. **fibroareolar f.,** f. superficialis. **f. of forearm,** f. antebrachii. **fusion f.,** a double connective tissue band derived from the fusion of closely apposed surfaces of peritoneum as a result of degeneration of the lubricating serous layer between them; such fasciae are seen in the pelvic and abdominal cavities where crowding of organs occurs. **f. of Gerota, Gerota's f.,** f. renalis. **hypogastric f.,** f. pelvis. **iliac f.,** 1. fascia iliaca. 2. arcus iliopectineus. **f. ili′aca** [NA], a strong fascia covering the inner surface of the iliac and psoas muscles. **f. iliopectin′ea, iliopectineal f.,** arcus iliopectineus. **infundibuliform f.,** f. spermatica interna. **intercolumnar f.,** 1. fascia cremasterica. 2. see *fibrae intercrurales*. **f. la′ta fem′oris** [NA], the external investing fascia of the thigh. **f. of leg,** f. cruris. **longitudinal f., anterior,** ligamentum longitudinale anterius. **longitudinal f., posterior,** ligamentum longitudinale posterius. **lumbodorsal f., f. lumbodorsa′lis,** f. thoracolumbalis. **masseteric f., f. masseter′ica** [NA], a layer of fascia covering the masseter muscle. **muscular fasciae of eye, fas′ciae muscula′res bul′bi** [NA], **fas′cial muscula′res oc′uli,** the sheets of fascia investing the extraocular muscles, continuous with the vagina bulbi. **f. of nape,** f. nuchae. **f. of neck,** f. cervicalis. **f. nu′chae** [NA], **nuchal f.,** the fascia on the muscles in the dorsal region of the neck. Called also *f. nuchalis* [NA alternative]. **f. nucha′lis,** NA alternative for *f. nuchae*. **obturator f., f. obturato′ria** [NA], the part of the parietal fascia of the pelvis covering the internal obturator muscle. **orbital fasciae, fas′ciae orbita′les** [NA], fibrous tissue surrounding the posterior part of the eyeball, supporting and binding together the structures within the orbit. **palmar f.,** aponeurosis palmaris. **palpebral f., f. palpebra′lis,** septum orbitale. **parietal f. of pelvis,** f. pelvis parietalis. **parotid f., f. parotide′a** [NA], a layer of cervical fascia enclosing the parotid gland. **f. parotideomasseter′ica,** the fascia enclosing the parotid gland and masseter muscle; separately called *f. parotidea* and *f. masseterica* [NA]. **f. pectin′ea, pectineal f.,** the pubic portion of the fascia lata; called also *Cowper's ligament*. **pectoral f., f. pectora′lis** [NA], the sheet of fascia investing the pectoralis major muscle. **pelvic f.,** f. pelvis. **pelvic f., parietal,** f. pelvis parietalis. **pelvic f., visceral,** f. pelvis visceralis. **f. pel′vica parieta′lis,** NA alternative for *f. pelvis parietalis*. **pelviprostatic f.,** f. prostatae. **f. pel′vis** [NA], pelvic fascia: an inclusive term for the fascia that forms part of the general layer lining the walls of the pelvis and invests the pelvic organs; called also *hypogastric f.* **f. pel′vis parieta′lis** [NA], the fascia on the wall of the pelvis that covers the muscles which pass from the interior of the pelvis to the thigh. Called also *f. pelvica parietalis* [NA alternative]. **f. pel′vis viscera′lis** [NA], visceral fascia of pelvis: the fascia that covers the organs and vessels of the pelvis. **f. pe′nis profun′da** [NA], the firm inner fascial layer that surrounds the corpora cavernosa and the corpus spongiosum collectively. **f. pe′nis superficia′lis** [NA], the loose external layer of fascial tissue of the penis, continuous with the tunica dartos and with the superficial perineal fascia. **perineal f., deep,** diaphragma urogenitale. **perineal f., middle,** f. diaphragmatis urogenitalis superior. **perineal f., superficial,** f. perinei superficialis. **f. perine′i superficia′lis** [NA], superficial fascia of perineum: the subcutaneous tissue of the urogenital region, comprising a superficial fatty and a deep membranous layer; called also *Cruveilhier's f.* **peritoneoperineal f., f. peritoneoperinea′lis** [NA], the fusion fascia that passes from the front of the rectum to form the floor of the rectovesical or rectovaginal pouch, contributing to the rectovesical or rectovaginal septum. **pharyngobasilar f., f. pharyngobasila′ris** [NA], a strong fibrous membrane in the wall of the pharynx, lined internally with mucous membrane and incompletely covered on its outer surface by the overlapping constrictor muscles of the pharynx. It blends with the periosteum at the base of the skull. Called also *pharyngeal* or *pharyngobasilar aponeurosis*, and *aponeurosis pharyngis* or *pharyngobasilaris*. **phrenicopleural f., f. phrenicopleura′lis** [NA], the fascial layer on the upper surface of the diaphragm, beneath the pleura. **plantar f.,** aponeurosis plantaris. **prevertebral f., f. prevertebra′lis,** lamina prevertebralis. **f. profun′da** [NA], deep fascia: a dense, firm, fibrous membrane investing the trunk and limbs, and giving off sheaths to the various muscles; called also *aponeurotic f.* **proper f. of neck, f. pro′pria col′li,** f. cervicalis. **f. pro′pria coo′peri,** fascia spermatica interna. **f. prosta′tae** [NA], **f. of prostate,** the reflection of the superior fascia of the pelvic diaphragm onto the prostate. **rectal f.,** f. diaphragmatis pelvis superior. **rectoabdominal f.,** vagina musculi recti abdominis. **rectovesical f.,** f. diaphragmatis pelvis superior. **renal f., f. rena′lis** [NA], a thin membranous sheath that encloses the kidney, formed by condensation of the fibroareolar tissue surrounding the kidney and the perirenal fat; called also *f. of Gerota, Gerota's f.,* and *Gerota's capsule*. **Richet's f.,** a fold of extraperitoneal fascia enveloping the obliterated umbilical vein. **scalene f.,** membrana suprapleuralis. **Scarpa's f.,** 1. the deep, membranous layer of subcutaneous abdominal fascia. 2. see *fibrae intercrurales*. **semilunar f.,** aponeurosis musculi bicipitis brachii. **Sibson's f.,** membrana suprapleuralis. **spermatic f., external,** f. spermatica externa. **spermatic f., internal,** f. spermatica interna. **f. spermat′ica exter′na** [NA], external spermatic fascia: the thin outer covering of the spermatic cord, which is continuous with the investing fascia of the external oblique muscle. **f. spermat′ica inter′na** [NA], internal spermatic fascia: the thin innermost covering of the spermatic cord, derived from the transversalis fascia of the abdominal wall. **subperitoneal f., f. subperitonea′lis** f. extraperitonealis. **superficial f.,** 1. f. superficialis. 2. subcutaneous tissue (tela subcutanea [NA]). **superficial f. of perineum,** f. perinei superficialis. **f. superficia′lis,** [NA], a fascial sheet lying directly beneath the skin. **f. superficia′lis perine′i,** f. perinei superficialis. **f. of Tarin, f. tari′ni,** gyrus dentatus, def. 1. **temporal f., f. tempora′lis [lam′ina profun′da et lam′ina superficia′lis]** [NA], a strong fibrous sheet covering the temporal muscle; it has a deep and a superficial part which attach inferiorly to the zygomatic arch. Called also *temporal aponeurosis*. **f. of Tenon,** vagina bulbi. **f. of thigh,** f. lata femoris. **thoracic f., f. thora′cica** [NA], the deep fascia that covers the outside of the thoracic cavity; called also *external intercostal fascia*. **f. thoracolumba′lis** [NA], **thoracolumbar f.,** the fascia of the back that attaches medially to the spinous processes of the vertebral column for its entire length and blends laterally with the aponeurosis of the transversus abdominis muscle; inferiorly it attaches to the iliac crest and the sacrum. Called also *f. lumbodorsalis* and *lumbodorsal f.* **thyrolaryngeal f.,** fascia investing the thyroid body and attaching to the cricoid cartilage. **f. transversa′lis** [NA], **transverse f.,** part of the inner investing layer of the abdominal wall, continuous with the fascia of the other side behind the rectus abdominis and the rectus sheath, and continuous also with the diaphragmatic fascia, iliac fascia, and the parietal pelvic fascia. **triangular f. of abdomen,** ligamentum inguinale reflexum. **triangular f. of Macalister,** musculus pyramidalis. **triangular f. of Quain,** ligamentum inguinale reflexum. **Tyrrell's f.,** septum rectovesicale. **f. of urogenital diaphragm, inferior,** f. diaphragmatis urogenitalis inferior. **f. of urogenital diaphragm, superior,** see *diaphragma urogenitale*.

f. of urogenital trigone, diaphragma urogenitale. **visceral f. of pelvis,** f. pelvis visceralis. **volar f.,** aponeurosis palmaris.

fasciae (fash′e-e) [L.] genitive and plural of *fascia*.

fasciagram (fash′e-ah-gram) a roentgenogram obtained by fasciagraphy.

fasciagraphy (fash″e-ag′rah-fe) roentgenography of fasciae after the injection of air into them.

fascial (fash′e-al) pertaining to or of the nature of a fascia.

fasciaplasty (fash′e-ah-plas″te) [*fascia* + Gr. *plassein* to form] a plastic operation on fascia.

fascicle (fas′ĭ-k′l) a small bundle or cluster, especially of nerve or muscle fibers; see also *fasciculus*. **longitudinal f's of cruciform ligament,** fasciculi longitudinales ligamenti cruciformis atlantis.

fascicular (fah-sik′u-lar) 1. pertaining to a fascicle. 2. fasciculated.

fasciculated (fah-sik′u-lāt-ed) clustered together or occurring in bundles.

fasciculation (fah-sik″u-la′shun) 1. the formation of fasciculi. 2. a small local contraction of muscles, visible through the skin, representing a spontaneous discharge of a number of fibers innervated by a single motor nerve filament.

fasciculi (fah-sik′u-li) [L.] genitive and plural of *fasciculus*.

fasciculus (fah-sik′u-lus), pl. *fascic′uli* [L. dim. of *fascis* bundle] 1. a fascicle: a small bundle or cluster; [NA] a general term for a small bundle of nerve, muscle, or tendon fibers. 2. a tract, bundle, or group of nerve fibers that are more or less associated functionally; see also *tractus*. **f. aberrans of Monakow,** tractus rubrospinalis. **f. acus′ticus** (obs.), striae medullares ventriculi quarti. **f. ante′rior pro′prius,** see *fasciculi proprii medullae spinalis*. **f. arcua′tus,** f. longitudinalis superior cerebri. **f. atrioventricula′ris** [NA], a small band of atypical cardiac muscle fibers originating in the atrioventricular node; see *bundle of His*. **f. of Burdach,** 1. f. longitudinalis superior cerebri. 2. pars temporalis radiationis corporis callosi. **cuneate f. of Burdach,** f. cuneatus medullae spinalis. **cuneate f. of medulla oblongata,** f. cuneatus medullae oblongatae. **cuneate f. of spinal cord,** f. cuneatus medullae spinalis. **f. cunea′tus medul′lae oblonga′tae** [NA], cuneate fasciculus of medulla oblongata: the continuation into the medulla oblongata of the fasciculus cuneatus of the spinal cord; called also *funiculus cuneatus medullae oblongatae*. **f. cunea′tus medul′lae spina′lis** [NA], the lateral portion of the dorsal funiculus of the spinal cord, composed of ascending fibers that terminate in the nucleus cuneatus of the medulla oblongata; called also *cuneate f. of spinal cord* or *of Burdach*. **dorsolateral f., f. dorsolatera′lis,** tractus dorsolateralis. **f. exi′lis,** a cluster of muscle fibers connecting the flexor pollicis longus with the medial condyle of the humerus, or with the coronoid process of the ulna. **extrapyramidal motor f.,** rubrospinal tract. **fibrous f. of biceps muscle,** aponeurosis musculi bicipitis brachii. **Flechsig's f.,** fasciculus proprii medullae spinalis. **f. of Foville,** a term that has been applied to the tractus spinocerebellaris posterior, but which more properly relates to the stria terminalis. **f. of Goll,** f. gracilis medullae spinalis. **Gowers' f.,** tractus spinocerebellaris ventralis. **f. gra′cilis medul′lae oblonga′tae** [NA], the continuation into the medulla oblongata of the fasciculus gracilis of the spinal cord; called also *posteromedian column of medulla oblongata*. **f. gra′cilis medul′lae spina′lis** [NA], the median portion of the dorsal funiculus of the spinal cord, composed of ascending fibers that terminate in the nucleus gracilis of the medulla oblongata; called also *column of Goll*. **interfascicular f., f. interfascicula′ris** [NA], a collection of fibers situated between the fasciculus gracilis and the fasciculus cuneatus, containing some of the descending branches of the fibers of the medial division of the dorsal roots of the spinal nerves; called also *comma tract of Schultze, f. semilunaris* [NA alternative], *Schultze's bundle* or *tract,* and *semilunar f. or tract*. **intersegmental fasciculi of spinal cord,** fasciculi proprii medullae spinalis. **intersegmental fasciculi of spinal cord, anterior,** fasciculi proprii ventrales medullae spinalis. **intersegmental fasciculi of spinal cord, dorsal,** fasciculi proprii dorsales medullae spinalis. **intersegmental fasciculi of spinal cord, lateral,** fasciculi proprii laterales medullae spinalis. **intersegmental fasciculi of spinal cord, posterior,**

fasciculi proprii dorsales medullae spinalis. **intersegmental fasciculi of spinal cord, ventral,** fasciculi proprii ventrales medullae spinalis. **f. latera′lis plex′us brachia′lis** [NA], the lateral cord of the brachial plexus, formed by the union of the anterior divisions of the superior and middle trunks, C5 through C7, and from which arise the lateral pectoral and musculocutaneous nerves and the lateral root of the median and the ulnar nerves. **f. latera′lis pro′prius,** see *fasciculi proprii medullae spinalis*. **lenticular f., f. lenticula′ris,** a bundle of pallidofugal nerve fibers that arise from the dorsal surface of the globus pallidus, pass through the internal capsule, traverse field H₂ of Forel, join and mingle with the fibers of the ansa lenticularis, and continue to the nuclei of the ventral thalamus. In official anatomical nomenclature [NA], the fasciculus lenticularis and the ansa lenticularis are considered together, and are designated *ansa et fasciculus lenticulares*. **longitudinal f., dorsal,** f. longitudinalis dorsalis. **longitudinal f., medial,** f. longitudinalis medialis. **longitudinal f. of cerebrum, inferior,** f. longitudinalis inferior cerebri. **longitudinal f. of cerebrum, superior,** f. longitudinalis superior cerebri. **longitudinal fasciculi of colon,** see *teniae coli*. **longitudinal fasciculi of cruciform ligament,** fasciculi longitudinales ligamenti cruciformis atlantis. **longitudinal f. of medulla oblongata, posterior,** f. longitudinalis medialis. **f. longitudina′lis dorsa′lis** [NA], dorsal longitudinal fasciculus: a lightly myelinated fiber bundle that runs in the periventricular gray substance throughout the extent of the mesencephalon, near the medial longitudinal fasciculus; called also *Schutz's bundle*. **f. longitudina′lis infe′rior cer′ebri** [NA], inferior longitudinal f. of cerebrum: a bundle of association fibers interconnecting the cortex of the occipital and temporal lobes, extending through the occipital and temporal lobes of the cerebrum, and consisting chiefly of geniculocalcarine projection fibers. **fascic′uli longitudina′les ligamen′ti crucifor′mis atlan′tis** [NA], longitudinal fasciculi of cruciform ligament: vertical midline longitudinal fibers that, together with the transverse ligament of the atlas, form the cruciform ligament of the atlas. The fibers arise in two groups from the root of the dens—one group extending cranially to the anterior margin of the foramen magnum, the other caudally to the body of the axis. **f. longitudina′lis media′lis** [NA], medial longitudinal fasciculus: a fiber tract extending between the mesencephalon and the upper part of the spinal cord; it lies close to the median plane, just ventral to the central gray matter, and interconnects the vestibular nuclei with motor nuclei, chiefly those of the third, fourth, sixth, and eleventh cranial nerves. **f. longitudina′lis media′lis medul′lae oblonga′tae,** the portion of the fasciculus longitudinalis medialis within the medulla oblongata. **f. longitudina′lis media′lis pon′tis,** the portion of the fasciculus longitudinalis medialis within the pons. **fascic′uli longitudina′les pon′tis** [NA], **fascic′uli longitudina′les [pyramida′les] pon′tis,** a former term for the corticopontine fibers (corticopontine tract), together with the corticonuclear and corticopontine fibers of the pyramidal tract in the pars ventralis pontis. **f. longitudina′lis supe′rior cer′ebri** [NA], superior longitudinal fasciculus of cerebrum: a bundle of association fibers in the cerebrum, extending from the frontal lobe to the posterior end of the lateral sulcus, and interrelating the cortex of the frontal, temporal, parietal, and occipital lobes; called also *f. arcuatus*. **macrary f.,** a system of nerve fibers originating in the macula lutea; some are uncrossed (on the temporal side) and others are crossed fibers (on the nasal side of the retina). **mamillotegmental f., f. mamillotegmenta′lis** [NA], a bundle of fibers from the mamillary body to the tegmental nuclei of the reticular formation of the mesencephalon; called also *mamillotegmental tract*. **mamillothalamic f., f. mamillothalam′icus** [NA], a stout bundle of fibers from the mamillary body to the anterior nucleus of the thalamus; called also *bundle of Vicq d'Azyr, mamillothalamic tract, thalamomamillary bundle,* and *thalamomamillary f.* **f. margina′lis ventra′lis** (obs.), a fasciculus made up of the tectospinal tract and the vestibulospinal tract. **medial prosencephalic f.,** f. prosencephalicus medialis. **medial telencephalic f.,** f. prosencephalicus medialis. **f. media′lis plex′us brachia′lis** [NA], the medial cord of the brachial plexus, formed by the anterior division of the inferior trunk, C8 through T1, and from which arise the medial pectoral, medial brachial cutaneous, and medial antebrachial cutaneous nerves, and the medial root of the ulnar and the median nerves. **Meynert's f.,** tractus habenulo-interpeduncularis. **Monakow's f.,** tractus rubrospinalis. **f. occipitofronta'lis infe'rior,** a collection of association fibers in the inferior part of the extreme capsule near the uncinate fasciculus, connecting various inferior gyri of the temporal and frontal lobes. **f. occipitofronta'lis supe'rior,** f. subcallosus. **olivochlear f.,** tractus olivocochlearis. **oval f.,** an area of descending fibers in the posterior funiculus of the spinal cord near the posterior septum; called also *median root zone.* **f. parieto-occipitoponti'nus** [NA], a bundle of nerve fibers that arise in the parietal and occipital lobes and pass through the retrolenticular part of the posterior limb of the internal capsule to end in the pontine nuclei. **f. poste'rior plex'us brachia'lis** [NA], the posterior cord of the brachial plexus, formed by the union of the posterior divisions of the superior, middle, and inferior trunks, C5 through C8 and sometimes T1, and from which arise the subscapular, thoracodorsal, radial, and axillary nerves. **proper fasciculi of spinal cord,** fasciculi proprii medullae spinalis. **proper fasciculi of spinal cord, ventral,** fasciculi proprii ventrales medullae spinalis. **fascic'uli pro'prii dorsa'les medul'lae spina'lis** [NA], the bundles of white substance in the deepest part of the dorsal funiculus of the spinal cord, consisting chiefly of intersegmental fibers derived from the cells of the dorsal gray column, which divide into ascending and descending association fibers that reenter the gray substance and ramify in it; called also *dorsal* or *posterior intersegmental fasciculi* or *tracts of the spinal cord* and *fasciculi proprii posteriores medullae spinalis* [NA alternative]. **fascic'uli pro'prii latera'les** [NA], the bundles of white substance in the lateral funiculus of the spinal cord, consisting of intersegmental fibers, some of which have passed from the contralateral side, and probably reticulospinal and autonomic fibers; called also *lateral intersegmental fasciculi* or *tracts of spinal cord.* **fascic'uli pro'prii medul'lae spina'lis,** proper fasciculi of spinal cord: a term formerly used to refer to the bundles of fibers in the white substance of the spinal cord surrounding the gray substance, consisting of short ascending and descending association fibers, and including those of the anterior or ventral, funiculus (f. anterior pro'prius) and the lateral funiculus (f. lateralis proprius); see *fasciculi proprii dorsales, fasciculi proprii laterales,* and *fasciculi proprii ventrales.* Called also *Flechsig's fasciculi, intersegmental fasciculi* or *tracts of spinal cord,* and *fundamental* or *ground bundles of spinal cord.* **fascic'uli pro'prii posterio'res medul'lae spina'lis,** NA alternative for *fasciculi proprii dorsales medullae spinalis.* **fascic'uli pro'prii ventra'les medul'lae spina'lis** [NA], the bundles of white substance in the ventral funiculus of the spinal cord, consisting of intersegmental fibers, some of which pass from the contralateral side, and, probably, reticulospinal and descending autonomic fibers; called also *anterior* or *ventral intersegmental fasciculi* or *tracts of spinal cord* and *fasciculi proprii anteriores medullae spinalis* [NA alternative]. **f. prosencephal'icus media'lis** [NA] prosencephalic fasciculus: a fiber system that is the main pathway for longitudinal connection in the hypothalamus; it runs through the lateral hypothalamic region, connecting the tegmentum of the mesencephalon and elements of the limbic system. Called also *f. telencephalicus medialis, medial forebrain bundle,* and *medial telencephalic fasciculus.* **pyramidal f. of medulla oblongata,** f. pyramidalis medullae oblongatae. **f. pyramida'lis medul'lae oblonga'tae** [NA], pyramidal fasciculus of medulla oblongata: the corticonuclear and corticospinal fibers considered collectively; see *pyramidal tract,* under *tract.* **f. retroflex'us,** tractus habenulo-interpeduncularis. **f. rotun'dus** (*obs.*), tractus solitarius medullae oblongatae. **semilunar f., f. semiluna'ris,** NA alternative for *f. interfascicularis.* **septomarginal f., f. septomargina'lis** [NA], a bundle of nerve fibers situated along the dorsal periphery of the dorsal funiculus of the spinal cord in the thoracic region and bordering the dorsal median septum in the lumbar region; called also *septomarginal tract.* **solitary f.,** tractus solitarius medullae oblongatae. **subcallosal f.,** f. subcallosus. **f. subcallo'sus** [NA], subcallosal fasciculus: a collection of association fibers lying just internal to the intersection of the internal capsule and corpus callosum, interconnecting the cortex of the occipital and temporal lobes with that of the insula and frontal lobe, and

probably comprising a significant part of the tapetum. Called also *f. occipitofrontalis superior.* **subthalamic f., f. subthalam'icus** [NA], a bundle of fibers passing through the internal capsule and connecting the subthalamic nucleus with the globus pallidus and putamen. **sulcomarginal f., f. sulcomargina'lis,** [NA], a layer of descending branches from the midbrain tectum situated in the ventral funiculus of the spinal cord, along the border of the ventral median fissure. **f. telencephal'icus media'lis,** f. prosencephalicus medialis. **f. te'res** (*obs.*), f. longitudinalis medialis pontis. **thalamamillary f.,** f. mamillothalamicus. **thalamic f., f. thalam'icus** [NA], a bundle of nerve fibers ascending through field H of Forel to pass dorsal to and partly through the zona incerta to reach some of the ventral nuclei of the thalamus; it contains continuations of the ansa lenticularis and the fasciculus lenticularis and dentatothalamic, rubrothalamic, and thalamostriate fibers. See also *fields of Forel,* under *field.* **fascic'uli transver'si aponeuro'sis palma'ris** [NA], transverse fasciculi of palmar aponeurosis: the transverse fascial bands that support the webs between the fingers. **fascic'uli transver'si aponeuro'sis planta'ris** [NA], transverse fasciculi of plantar aponeurosis: transverse bundles in the plantar aponeurosis near the toes. **f. of Türck,** tractus pyramidalis anterior. **unciform f., uncinate f., f. uncina'tus** [NA], a collection of association fibers which interconnect the cortex of the orbital surface of the frontal lobe with the parahippocampal gyrus and perhaps with the amygdala; other temporofrontal connections probably also exist. **f. of Vicq d'Azyr,** f. mamillothalamicus.

fasciectomy (fas"e-ek'to-me) [*fascia* + Gr. *ektomē* excision] excision of fascia.

fasciitis (fas"e-i'tis) inflammation of fascia. **exudative calcifying f.,** calcinosis. **necrotizing f.,** a fulminating group A streptococcal infection beginning with severe or extensive cellulitis that spreads to involve the superficial and deep fascia, producing thrombosis of the subcutaneous vessels and gangrene of the underlying tissues. A cutaneous lesion usually serves as a portal of entry for the infection, but sometimes no such lesion is found. Called also *gangrenous* or *necrotizing erysipelas.* **nodular f.,** proliferative f. **perirenal f.,** retroperitoneal fibrosis. **proliferative f.,** a benign reactive proliferation of fibroblasts with a distinct microscopic pattern superficially resembling that of sarcoma; the lesions are located in the subcutaneous tissues and commonly associated with the deep fascia. **pseudosarcomatous f.,** a benign soft-tissue tumor occurring subcutaneously and sometimes arising from deep muscle and fascia, and histologically resembling a malignant sarcoma.

fasciodesis (fas"e-od'ĕ-sis) [L. *fascia* + Gr. *desis* binding] the operation of suturing a fascia to skeletal attachment.

Fasciola (fah-si'o-lah) [L. *fasciola* a band] a genus of flukes. **F. cer'vi,** former name for *Paramphistomum cervi.* **F. gigan'tica,** the giant liver fluke of Africa, Asia, and Hawaii, which occasionally infects man. **F. hepat'ica,** the common liver fluke of sheep, oxen, goats, horses, and other herbivorous animals. It is occasionally found in the human liver, where it may cause dangerous symptoms by obstructing the biliary passages and by invasion of the liver parenchyma. Several snails of the genus *Lymnaea* act as invertebrate hosts. Called also *Distoma hepaticum.* **F. heteroph'yes,** *Heterophyes heterophyes.* **F. mag'na,** *Fascioloides magna.*

fasciola (fah-se'o-lah, fah-si'o-lah), pl. *fasci'olae* [L., dim. of *fascia*] 1. a small band or striplike structure. 2. a small bandage. **f. cine'rea, f. cine'rea cin'guli,** gyrus fasciolaris. **f. denta'ta** (*obs.*), gyrus dentatus.

fasciolae (fah-se'o-le, fah-si'o-le) [L.] genitive and plural of *fasciola.*

fasciolar (fah-se'o-lar, fah-si'o-lar) pertaining to a fasciola.

Fascioletta (fas"e-o-let'tah) a genus of parasitic flukes. **F. ilioca'na,** *Echinostoma ilocanum.*

fascioliasis (fas"e-o-li'ah-sis) infection with *Fasciola hepatica* or *F. gigantea.*

Fascioloides (fas"e-o-loi'dēz) a genus of flukes. **F. mag'na,** the large American liver fluke, a trematode found in the liver and lungs of herbivorous animals in North America; formerly called *Fasciola magna.*

fasciolopsiasis (fas"e-o-lop-si'ah-sis) the state of being infected with flukes of the genus *Fasciolopsis.*

Fasciolopsis (fas''e-o-lop'sis) [*fasciola* + Gr. *opsis* appearance] a genus of trematode worms. **F. bus'ki,** a trematode worm found in the small intestine of residents in many parts of Asia. It is the largest of the intestinal flukes, and may cause nausea, diarrhea, and a malabsorption syndrome if present in large numbers. The intermediate hosts are the snails *Planorbis coenosus* and various species of *Segmentina*. Other names given this species are *F. fuelleborni* from Calcutta and Egypt, *F. goddardi* and *F. spinifera* from China, and *F. rathouisi* from Asia. Formerly called *Distoma buski*.

fascioplasty (fash'e-o-plas''te) plastic operation on fascia.

fasciorrhaphy (fash''e-or'ah-fe) [*fascia* + Gr. *rhaphē* suture] suture of lacerated fascia.

fasciotomy (fash''e-ot'o-me) [*fascia* + Gr. *temnein* to cut] surgical incision or transection of fascia.

fascitis (fah-si'tis) fasciitis.

fast (fast) [A.S. faest firm; *faestan* to abstain from food] 1. immovable, or unchangeable; resistant to the action of a specific drug, stain, or destaining agent, as in acid-fast. 2. abstention from food.

fastidious (fas-tid'e-us) in bacteriology, a microorganism having complex nutritional or cultural requirements for growth.

fastidium (fas-tid'e-um) [L.] loathing, disgust. **f. ci'bi,** loathing of food. **f. po'tus,** loathing of drink.

fastigatum (fas''tĭ-ga'tum) [L.] pointed; sharpened to a point.

fastigial (fas-tij'e-al) of or pertaining to the fastigium.

fastigium (fas-tij'e-um) [L. "gable end"] 1. the highest point in the roof of the fourth ventricle of the brain, at the junction between the superior medullary velum and the nodulus. 2. the acme, or highest point, as of a fever.

fastness (fast'nes) the quality, in bacteria, of being resistant to the action of specific stains or inhibitors.

fat (fat) 1. adipose tissue; a white or yellowish tissue which forms soft pads between various organs of the body, serves to smooth and round out bodily contours, and furnishes a reserve supply of energy. 2. an ester of glycerol with fatty acids, usually oleic acid, palmitic acid, or stearic acid; tri-acyl glycerol; neutral fat. **bound f.,** masked f. **brown f.,** brown adipose tissue. **chyle f.,** fat in the form of an extremely fine emulsion taken into the chyle by the lymphatics of the intestine. **corpse f.,** adipocere. **fetal f.,** a term sometimes used in pathology to refer to brown adipose tissue. **grave f.,** adipocere. **masked f.,** fat that can be detected in a cell or tissue by chemical methods but is not revealed by staining methods; called also *bound f.* **milk f.,** the suspension in milk which tends to separate out as cream. **molecular f.,** fat occurring in fine specks within the cells. **moruloid f., mulberry f.,** brown adipose tissue. **neutral f.,** see *fat* (def. 2). **paranephric f., pararenal f.,** corpus adiposum pararenale. **perinephric f., perirenal f.,** capsula adiposa renis. **polyunsaturated f.,** a fat containing fatty acid that has more than one double bond in its carbon chain. **saturated f.,** one containing fatty acid that has only single bonds in its carbon chain. **unsaturated f.,** a fat containing fatty acid that has one or more double bonds in its carbon chain. **wool f.,** anhydrous lanolin. **wool f., hydrous,** lanolin. **wool f., refined,** anhydrous lanolin.

fatal (fa'tal) causing death; deadly; mortal; lethal.

fate (fāt) [L. *fatum* what is ordained by the gods] the ultimate disposition or decreed outcome. In pharmacology, the intermediate and ultimate disposition of a drug in the body. **prospective f.,** the development normally achieved by any region of the egg or early embryo when there is no interference.

fatigability (fat''ĭ-gah-bil'ĭ-te) easy susceptibility to fatigue.

fatigue (fah-tēg') [Fr.; L. *fatigatio*] a state of increased discomfort and decreased efficiency resulting from prolonged or excessive exertion; loss of power or capacity to respond to stimulation. **battle f.,** combat f. **combat f.,** a term applied to psychiatric combat casualties, especially to those with healthy premorbid personalities who have been overwhelmed by combat stress; the applicable DSM III diagnosis would in most cases be post-traumatic stress disorder. Cf. *combat neurosis*. **pseudocombat f.,** a term applied to psychiatric combat casualties whose functional impairment is attributed to preexisting personality disorder rather than to reaction to combat stress. **stimulation f.,** an increase in the threshold of a neural element due to repeated stimulation.

fatty (fat'e) pertaining to or characterized by fat.

fatty acid (fah'te) any straight-chain monocarboxylic acid, especially those naturally occurring in fats; generally classified as *saturated fatty acids*, those with no double bonds, *monounsaturated fatty acids*, those with one double bond, and *polyunsaturated fatty acids*, those with multiple double bonds. Those that cannot be synthesized by the human body and must be obtained from dietary sources, e.g., linoleic acid, linolenic acid, and arachidonic acid, are termed *essential fatty acids*. Consumption of less saturated fats and more polyunsaturated fats lowers the serum LDL (low density lipoprotein) and cholesterol levels, and some evidence suggests that it may reduce the incidence of coronary heart disease. **free f. a's (FFA),** nonesterified fatty acids. **nonesterified f. a's (NEFA),** the fraction of plasma fatty acids that are not in the form of glycerol esters. Called also *free fatty a's* (a misnomer because they are transported complexed with albumin). **polyunsaturated f. a's** acids with abundant unsaturated bonds; in large amounts in diets, they tend to lower plasma cholesterol levels.

fatty acid synthase [EC 2.3.1.85] an enzyme complex catalyzing the synthesis of long chain fatty acids: acetyl CoA + n malonyl CoA + $2n$ NADPH→long chain fatty acid anion + n CO_2 + $2n$ NADPH + (NH). CoA palmitate is the preferred product with the mammalian liver enzyme complex. The complex includes catalytic sites for seven reactions.

fauces (faw'sēz) [L., pl. of *faux* "a gorge, narrow pass"] [NA] the passage from the mouth to the pharynx, including both the lumen and its boundaries; the throat.

Fauchard's disease (fo-sharz') [Pierre *Fauchard*, French dentist, 1678–1761] marginal periodontitis.

faucial (faw'shal) pertaining to the fauces.

faucitis (faw-si'tis) inflammation of the fauces.

Faught's sphygmomanometer (fawtz) [Francis Ashley *Faught*, American chemist, born 1881] see under *sphygmomanometer*.

fauna (faw'nah) [L. *Faunus* mythical deity of herdsmen] the animal life present in or characteristic of a given region or locality. It may be discernible with the unaided eye (macrofauna), or only with the aid of a microscope (microfauna).

Fauvel's granules (fo-velz') [Sulpice Antoine *Fauvel*, French physician, 1813–1884] see under *granule*.

fava (fa'vah) *Vicia faba* L. (Leguminosae).

faveolar (fa-ve'o-lar) pertaining to the faveolus (foveola).

faveolate (fa-ve'o-lāt) [L. *faveolus*, from *fa'vus* honeycomb] honeycombed; alveolate.

faveoli (fa-ve'o-li) [L.] genitive and plural of *faveolus*.

faveolus (fa-ve'o-lus), pl. *fave'oli* [L.] foveola.

favid (fa'vid) a secondary skin eruption due to allergy in favus.

favism (fa'vism) [Italian *fava* bean] an acute hemolytic anemia caused by ingestion of fava beans or inhalation of the pollen of the plant *Vicia faba* (*fava*), occurring in certain individuals, usually as a result of a hereditary deficiency of glucose-6-phosphate dehydrogenase in erythrocytes. See *glucose-6-phosphate dehydrogenase anemia*, under *anemia*.

favus (fa'vus) [L. "honeycomb"] a distinctive type of ringworm usually caused by *Trichophyton schoenleini*, most often involving the scalp but may also affect glabrous skin, and characterized by the formation of perifollicular yellow, cup-shaped crusts (scutula) composed of dense mats of mycelia and epithelial debris and having a cheesy or mousy odor; scutula may enlarge and coalesce to form prominent honeycomb-like masses that may be associated with hair loss and cutaneous atrophy and scarring. Called also *honeycomb ringworm* and *tinea favosa*. **f. of fowl,** a chronic dermatomycosis affecting the comb of fowl, caused by *Trichophyton gallinae*; called also *comb disease*, usually in male birds. **f. herpetifor'mis,** mouse favus. **mouse f.,** a disease of mice, caused by the fungus *Trichophyton mentagrophytes* var. *quinkeanum*; it may be transmitted to man. **f. mu'rium,** mouse f.

Fc [*f*ragment, *c*rystallizable] originally, the fragment, not containing antigen combining sites, obtained by papain cleavage of the IgG molecule; now generally used as an adjective, e.g., Fc region, segment, to refer to the part of any immunoglobulin monomer comprising the hinge region and C_H2, C_H3, and C_H4 domains of both heavy chains. The Fc region contains the allotypic markers and mediates all biologic activities including complement activation, binding to cell-surface receptors (Fc receptors, IgE receptors), and transplacental transport of IgG. Cf. *Fab.*

Fc′   a fragment produced in minute quantities by papain digestion of IgG molecules, a noncovalently bonded dimer containing most of the C_H3 domains of both heavy chains.

fCi   femtocurie.

Fd   the heavy chain portion of an Fab fragment.

FDA   Food and Drug Administration, a division of the Department of Health and Human Services.

F.D.A.   fronto-dextra anterior (right frontoanterior, a position of the fetus); Food and Drug Administration.

F.D.I.   abbreviation for *Fédération Dentaire Internationale* [Fr. International Dental Association].

F.D.P.   fronto-dextra posterior (right frontoposterior, a position of the fetus).

F.D.T.   fronto-dextra transversa (right frontotransverse, a position of the fetus).

F-duction (ef-duk′shun)   in bacterial genetics, the process whereby part of the bacterial chromosome is attached to the autonomous F factor (fertility factor) and thus is transferred with high frequency from the donor (male) bacterium to the recipient (female) bacterium. Called also *sexduction.*

Fe   chemical symbol for *iron* (L. *ferrum*).

FE$_{Na}$ excreted fraction of filtered sodium; see under *test.*

fear (fēr)   the unpleasant emotional state consisting of psychological and psychophysiological responses to a real external threat or danger. Cf. *anxiety.*

febantel (feb′an-tel)   chemical name: [[2-[(methoxyacetyl) amino] -4- (phenylthio) phenyl] carbonimidoyl]biscarbamic acid dimethyl ester; a veterinary antihelmintic, $C_{20}H_{22}N_4$-O_6S.

Feb. dur.   abbreviation for L. *feb′re duran′te,* while the fever lasts.

febricant (feb′rĭ-kant)   causing fever.

febricide (feb′rĭ-sīd) [*febris* + L. *caedere* to kill]   1. lowering body temperature in fever. 2. an agent that reduces fever.

febricity (fe-bris′ĭ-te)   feverishness; the quality of being febrile.

febricula (fe-brik′u-lah) [L.]   a slight or temporary attack of fever of indefinite origin or pathology.

febrifacient (feb″rĭ-fa′shent) [*febris* + L. *facere* to make]   producing fever.

febrific (fĕ-brif′ik)   producing fever.

febrifugal (fĕ-brif′ŭ-gal) [*febris* + L. *fugare* to put to flight]   dispelling or relieving fever.

febrifuge (feb′rĭ-fūj)   an agent that reduces body temperature in fever; antipyretic.

febrifugine (feb-rif′u-jin)   an antimalarial alkaloid, C_{16}-$H_{19}O_3N_3$, from Ch'ang Shan.

febrile (feb′ril) [L. *febrilis*]   pertaining to or characterized by fever.

febris (fe′bris) [L.]   fever. **f. meliten′sis,** brucellosis. **f. un′dulans,** brucellosis.

fecal (fe′kal)   pertaining to or of the nature of feces.

fecalith (fe′kah-lith) [*feces* + Gr. *lithos* stone]   an intestinal concretion formed around a center of fecal matter.

fecaloid (fe′kal-oid)   resembling fecal matter.

fecaloma (fe″kah-lo′mah) [*feces* + *-oma*]   stercoroma.

fecaluria (fe″kah-lu′re-ah) [*feces* + Gr. *ouron* urine + *-ia*]   the presence of fecal matter in the urine.

feces (fe′sēz) [L. *faeces,* pl. of *faex* refuse]   the excrement discharged from the intestines, consisting of bacteria, cells exfoliated from the intestines, secretions, chiefly of the liver, and a small amount of food residue.

Fechner's law (fek′nerz) [Gustav Theodor *Fechner,* Prussian natural philosopher, 1801–1887]   see under *law.*

FeCO$_3$ ferrous carbonate.

fecula (fek′u-lah) [L. *faecula* lees, dregs]   1. lees or sediment. 2. starch; also the starchy part of a seed.

feculent (fek′u-lent) [L. *faeculentus*]   1. having dregs or a sediment. 2. excrementitious.

fecundate (fe′kun-dāt) [L. *fecundare* to fertilize]   to impregnate or fertilize.

fecundatio (fe″kun-da′she-o) [L., from *fecundare* to fertilize]   fecundation. **f. ab ex′tra,** impregnation occurring without entrance of the penis into the vagina.

fecundation (fe″kun-da′shun) [L. *fecundatio*]   impregnation or fertilization. **artificial f.,** artificial insemination.

fecundity (fĕ-kun′dĭ-te) [L. *fecunditas*]   ability to produce offspring rapidly and in large numbers. In demography, the physiological ability to reproduce, as opposed to fertility.

Federici's sign (fe-de-re′chēz) [Cesare *Federici,* an Italian physician, 1838–1892]   see under *sign.*

feeblemindedness (fe″b'l-mīnd′ed-nes)   former name for mental retardation. The feebleminded were divided into three grades: idiots, with a mental age below two years; imbeciles, with a mental age between two and seven years; and morons, with a mental age between seven and twelve years.

feedback (fēd′bak)   the return of some of the output of a system as input so as to exert some control in the process; see also *endproduct inhibition,* under *inhibition.* **alpha f.,** see under *biofeedback.* **negative f.,** the condition of maintaining a constant output of a system by exertion of an inhibitory control on a key step in the system by a product of that system. **positive f.,** a condition causing the output of a system to increase continually by exertion of a stimulatory effect on a key step in the system by a product of that system.

feed-forward (fēd-for′ward)   the anticipatory effect that one intermediate in a metabolic or endocrine control system exerts on another intermediate further along in the pathway; such effect may be stimulatory (positive f.) or inhibitory (negative f.).

feeding (fēd′ing)   the taking or giving of food. **artificial f.,** feeding of a baby with food other than mother's milk. **breast f.,** breast-feeding. **extrabuccal f.,** the administration of nutriment other than by mouth. **Finkelstein's f.,** feeding of infants based upon decrease in the milk sugar of the food. **forced f., forcible f.,** the administration of food by force to those who cannot or will not receive it. **sham f.,** feeding in which the food is chewed and swallowed but does not enter the stomach, because of diversion to the exterior by an esophageal fistula or other device.

Feer's disease (fairz) [Emil *Feer,* Swiss pediatrician, 1864–1955]   acrodynia.

fee-splitting (fe-split′ing)   the division of moneys received by a specialist, such as a surgeon, between himself and the physician who referred the patient to him.

feet (fēt)   see *foot.*

Fehleisen's streptococcus (fa′līs-enz) [Friedrich *Fehleisen,* German (later American) physician, 1854–1924]   *Streptococcus pyogenes.*

Fehling's solution, test (fa′lingz) [Hermann Christian von *Fehling,* German chemist, 1812–1885]   see under *solution* and *tests.*

fel (fel), gen. *fel′lis* [L. "bile"]   the bile. **f. bo′vis,** ox bile. **f. bo′vis purifica′tum, f. tau′ri purifica′tum,** ox bile extract.

Feldene (fel′dēn)   trademark for preparations of piroxicam.

Felderstruktur (fel″der-shtrook′tur) [Ger.]   the term used to describe the pattern of organization of the myofilaments in cardiac and red skeletal muscles, in which the myofilaments are not associated in discrete myofibrils, but instead form a continuous field interrupted by mitochondria. Cf. *Fibrillenstruktur.*

Feleky's instrument (fa-la′kēz) [Hugó von *Feleky,* Budapest urologist, 1860–1932]   see under *instrument.*

Felicola (fel-ĭ-ko′lah)   a genus of parasitic insects of the order Mallophaga, the biting lice. It includes *F. subrostratus,* a parasite of cats.

feline (fe′līn) [L. *feles* cat]   pertaining to, characteristic of, or derived from a cat.

Felix-Weil reaction (fa′liks-vīl) [Arthur *Felix,* Prague bacteriologist, 1887–1956; Edmund *Weil,* German physician in Prague, 1880–1922]   Weil-Felix reaction.

fellatio (fĕ-la′she-o) [L. *fellare* to suck] oral stimulation or manipulation of the penis.

felon (fel′on) an extremely painful abscess on the palmar aspect of the fingertips, occurring as the result of infection in the closed space of the terminal phalanx, usually following inoculation into the skin of a pathogenic microorganism. Called also *whitlow*.

Felsules (fel′sulz) trademark for a preparation of chloral hydrate.

Felton's phenomenon (fel′tunz) [Lloyd D. *Felton*, Boston physician, 1885–1953] see under *phenomenon*.

feltwork (felt′werk) a complex of closely interwoven fibers, as of nerve fibrils. **Kaes' f.**, a dense network of nerve fibers in the cerebral cortex.

Felty's syndrome (fel′tēz) [Augustus Roi *Felty*, American physician, born 1895] see under *syndrome*.

female (fe′māl) [L. *femella* young woman] 1. an individual organism of the sex that bears young or that produces ova or eggs. 2. feminine.

feminine (fem′ĭ-nin) pertaining to the female sex, or possessing qualities normally characteristic of the female.

femininity (fem″ĭ-nin′ĭ-te) womanhood; the possession of normal female qualities by a woman.

feminism (fem′ĭ-nizm) the appearance or existence of female secondary sex characters in the male. **mammary f.**, gynecomastia.

feminization (fem″ĭ-ni-za′shun) 1. the normal induction or development of female sex characters. 2. the induction or development of female secondary sex characters in the male. **testicular f.**, a condition, due to lack of cellular receptors for testosterone and dihydrotestosterone, in which the subject is phenotypically female but lacks nuclear sex chromatin and is of XY chromosomal sex; the uterus and tubes are absent or rudimentary, and the gonads are typically testes and may be abdominal or inguinal in position. The *incomplete* form is marked by partial fusion of the labioscrotal folds and clitoromegaly, and at puberty, variable feminization and partial virilization may both take place.

Feminone (fem′ĭ-nōn) trademark for a preparation of ethinyl estradiol.

feminonucleus (fem″ĭ-no-nu′kle-us) the female pronucleus.

Fem. intern. abbreviation for L. *femor′ibus inter′nus*, at the inner side of the thighs.

femme (fahm) [Fr.] woman. **sage f.** (sahzh-fahm′) [Fr. "wise woman"], a midwife.

Femogen (fem′o-gen) trademark for preparations of esterified estrogens.

femora (fem′o-rah) [L.] plural of *femur*.

femoral (fem′or-al) [L. *femoralis*] pertaining to the femur, or to the thigh.

femorocele (fem′o-ro-sēl″) [L. *femur* thigh + Gr. *kēlē* hernia] femoral hernia.

femoroiliac (fem″o-ro-il′e-ak) pertaining to the femur and the ilium.

femorotibial (fem″o-ro-tib′e-al) pertaining to the femur and the tibia.

femto- [Danish *femten* fifteen] a combining form used in naming units of measurement to indicate one-quadrillionth (10^{-15}) of the unit designated by the root with which it is combined. Symbol, f.

femtocurie (fem″to-cu′rie) a unit of radioactivity, being one-quadrillionth (10^{-15}) curie, or the quantity of radioactive material in which the number of nuclear disintegrations is 3.7×10^{-5} per second. Abbreviated fCi.

femur (fe′mur), pl. *fem′ora* [L.] 1. [NA] the bone that extends from the pelvis to the knee, being the longest and largest bone in the body; its head articulates with the acetabulum of the hip bone, and distally the femur, along with the patella and tibia, forms the knee joint. Called also *femoral bone, os femorale* [NA alternative] and *thigh bone*. See also illustration accompanying *skeleton*. 2. the thigh.

fenalamide (fen-al′ah-mīd) chemical name α-[[[2-(diethylamino)ethyl]amino]carbonyl]-α-ethylbenzeneacetic acid ethyl ester; a smooth muscle relaxant, $C_{19}H_{30}N_2O_3$.

fenamate (fen′ah-māt) any of a class of analgesic and anti-inflammatory agents derived from *N*-phenylanthranilic acid.

fenbendazole (fen-ben′dah-zōl) chemical name: [5-(phenylthio)-1*H*-benzimidazol-2-yl] carbamic acid methyl ester; an anthelmintic, $C_{15}H_{13}N_3O_2S$.

fenbufen (fen-bu′fen) chemical name: γ-oxo-[1,1′-biphenyl]-4-butanoic acid; an anti-inflammatory, $C_{16}H_{14}O_3$.

fenclofenac (fen-klo′fen-ak) chemical name: 2-(2,4-dichlorophenoxy)benzeneacetic acid; an anti-inflammatory, $C_{14}H_{10}Cl_2O_3$.

fenclonine (fen′klo-nēn) chemical name: DL-3-(4-chlorophenyl)alanine; a serotonin inhibitor, $C_9H_{10}ClNO_2$.

fenclorac (fen-klor′ak) chemical name: α,3-dichloro-4-cyclohexylbenzeneacetic acid; an anti-inflammatory, $C_{14}H_{16}Cl_2O_2$.

fendosal (fen′do-sal) chemical name: 5-(4,5-dihydro-2-phenyl-3*H*-benz[*e*]indol-3-yl)-2-hydroxy-5-benzoic acid; an anti-inflammatory, $C_{25}H_{19}NO_3$.

fenestra (fĕ-nes′trah), pl. *fenes′trae* [L. "window"] a window-like opening; [NA] a general term for an opening or open area. Also, an opening in a bandage or cast, or in the blade of a forceps. **f. of cochlea, f. coch′leae** [NA], a round opening in the inner wall of the middle ear inferior to and a little posterior to the fenestra vestibuli; it is covered by the secondary tympanic membrane. Called also *round window*. **f. nov-ova′lis**, a surgically created oval window in the lateral semicircular canal in Lempert's fenestration operation. **f. ova′lis**, f. vestibuli. **f. rotun′da**, f. cochleae. **f. vestib′uli** [NA], an oval opening in the inner ear, which is closed by the base of the stapes; called also *f. ovalis* and *oval window*.

fenestrae (fĕ-nes′tre) [L.] genetive and plural of *fenestra*.

fenestrate (fen′es-trāt) to pierce with one or more openings.

fenestrated (fen′es-trāt″ed) [L. *fenestratus*] pierced with one or more openings.

fenestration (fen″es-tra′shun) [L. *fenestratus* furnished with windows] 1. the act of perforating, or the condition of being perforated. 2. the surgical creation of a new opening in the labyrinth of the ear for the restoration of hearing in cases of otosclerosis. **alveolar plate f.**, apical f. **aortopulmonary f.**, aortic septal defect. **apical f.**, perforation of the cortical plate of bone overlying a portion of a pulpless primary tooth with round or oval openings, which may involve all the primary teeth but most often affect the plate overlying the upper primary incisors. Called also *alveolar plate fenestration*.

fenestrel (fen-es′trel) chemical name: 5-ethyl-6-methyl-4-phenyl-3-cyclohexene-1-carboxylic acid; an estrogen, $C_{16}H_{20}O_2$.

fenethylline hydrochloride (fen-eth′ĭ-lin) chemical name: 3,7-dihydro-1,3-dimethyl-7-[2-[(1-methyl-2-phenylethyl)amino]ethyl]-1*H*-purine-2,6-dione monohydrochloride; a central nervous system stimulant, $C_{18}H_{23}N_5O_1 \cdot HCl$.

fenfluramine hydrochloride (fen-floor′ah-mēn) chemical name: *N*-ethyl-α-methyl-3-(trifluoromethyl)benzeneethanamine hydrochloride. An adrenergic, $C_{12}H_{16}F_3N \cdot HCl$, used as an anorexic in the short-term treatment of exogenous obesity; administered orally.

fenisorex (fen-i′so-reks) chemical name: *cis*-7-fluoro-3,4-dihydro-1-phenyl-1*H*-2-benzopyran-3-methanamine; an anorexic, $C_{16}H_{16}FNO$.

fenmetozole hydrochloride (fen-met′o-zōl) chemical name: 2-[(3,4-dichlorophenoxy)methyl]-4,5-dihydro-1*H*-imidazole monohydrochloride; an antidepressant and narcotic antagonist, $C_{10}H_{10}Cl_2N_2O \cdot HCl$.

fenobam (fen′o-bam) chemical name: *N*-(3-chlorophenyl)-*N*′-(4,5-dihydro-1-methyl-4-oxo-1*H*-imidazol-2-yl)urea; a tranquilizer, $C_{11}H_{11}ClN_4O_2$.

fenoprofen (fen″o-pro′fen) a nonsteroidal anti-inflammatory agent that is a propionic acid derivative; used as fenoprofen calcium [USP] for the treatment of rheumatoid arthritis and osteoarthritis.

fenoterol (fen″o-ter′ōl) chemical name: 3,5-dihydroxy-α-[[(*p*-hydroxy-α-methylphenethyl)amino]methyl]benzyl alcohol; a bronchodilator, $C_{17}H_{21}NO_4$.

fenpipalone (fen-pip′ah-lōn) chemical name: 5-[-2-(3,6-dihydro-4-phenyl-1(2*H*)-pyridinyl)ethyl]-3-methyl-2-oxazolidinone; an anti-inflammatory, $C_{17}H_{22}N_2O_2$.

fenspiride hydrochloride (fen-spēr′īd) 8-(2-phenethyl)-1-oxa-3,8-diazaspiro[4.5]decan-2-one monohydrochloride. An antiadrenergic compound, $C_{15}H_{20}N_2O_2 \cdot HCl$, used as a bronchodilator.

fentanyl citrate (fen′tah-nil) [USP] chemical name: N-phenyl-N-[1-(2-phenylethyl)-4-piperidineyl] propanamide 2-hydroxy-1,2,3-propanetricarboxylate (1:1). A narcotic analgesic, $C_{22}H_{28}N_2O \cdot C_6H_8O_7$, derivative of piperidine, occurring as a white, crystalline powder or white, glistening crystals; used mainly preoperatively, postoperatively, and during surgery, administered intravenously or intramuscularly. A combination of fentanyl citrate and droperidol (known as *Innovar*) is administered intramuscularly to produce neuroleptanalgesia.

fenticlor (fen′tĭ-klor) chemical name: 2,2′-thiobis[4-chlorophenol]. A topical anti-infective, $C_{12}H_8Cl_2O_2S$, which has been used in candidial and dermatophytic infections of the skin and mucous membranes.

fenugreek (fen′u-grēk) [L. *faenum graecum* Greek hay] the leguminous annual herb, *Trigonella foenumgraecum* L., grown in Southern Europe, India, and Northern Africa for its oily seeds, which are used in making curry. The seeds are used in veterinary medicine in poultices, ointments, and plasters, and to flavor medicinal powders that are mixed with the food of livestock. See also *trigonelline*.

Fenwick's disease (fen′wiks) [Samuel *Fenwick*, English physician, 1821–1902] see under *disease*.

Fe₂O₃ ferric oxide.

Fe(OH)₃ ferric hydroxide.

Feosol (fe′o-sol) trademark for preparations of ferrous sulfate.

feral (fe′ral) [L. *feralis*] savage; wild; deadly; living in the wild state, especially after having been domesticated.

fer-de-lance (făr-dĕ-lahs′) [Fr. "lance head"] a large venomous snake, *Bothrops atrox*, of South and Central America, Mexico and the West Indies; see table accompanying *snake*.

Fergon (fer′gon) trademark for preparations of ferrous gluconate.

Fergusson's incision (operation), speculum (fer′-gus-unz) [Sir William *Fergusson*, British surgeon, 1808–1877] see under *incision* and *speculum*.

Fer-In-Sol (fer′in-sōl) trademark for a preparation of ferrous sulfate.

ferment [L. *fermentum* leaven] 1. (fer-ment′) to undergo fermentation; the term is applied to decomposition of carbohydrates. 2. (fer′ment) (*obs.*) enzyme.

fermentation (fer″men-ta′shun) [L. *fermentatio*] the anaerobic enzymatic conversion of organic compounds, especially carbohydrates, to simpler compounds, especially to ethyl alcohol, resulting in energy in the form of adenosine triphosphate (ATP); the process is used in the production of alcohol, bread, vinegar, and other food or industrial products. It differs from respiration in that organic substances rather than molecular oxygen are used as electron acceptors. Fermentation occurs widely in bacteria and yeasts, the process usually being identified by the product formed; e.g., acetic, alcoholic, butyric, and lactic fermentation are those that result in the formation of acetic acid, alcohol, butyric acid, and lactic acid, respectively. **heterolactic f.,** one that produces lactic acid and one or more additional products, such as ethanol, acetic acid, and carbon dioxide. **homolactic f.,** one that produces only lactic acid as a product. **mixed acid f.,** one that forms more than one acid (e.g., acetic, lactic, succinic, and formic) as a product. **stormy f.,** the rapid fermentation of milk produced by *Clostridium perfringens*, marked by rupture of the clotted milk by the pressure of the gas which develops.

fermentemia (fer″men-te′me-ah) [*ferment* + Gr. *haima* blood + *-ia*] the presence of a ferment in the blood.

fermentum (fer-men′tum) [L. "ferment"] yeast.

fermium (fer′me-um) [Enrico *Fermi*, Italian physicist, 1901–1954; winner of the Nobel prize for physics in 1938] the chemical element number 100, atomic weight 253, symbol Fm, originally discovered in debris from a thermonuclear explosion in 1952.

ferning (fern′ing) the appearance of a fernlike pattern in a dried specimen of cervical mucus, an indication of the presence of estrogen; called also *fern phenomenon*.

-ferous [L. *ferre* to bear] a word termination meaning bearing or producing.

Ferrata's cell (fer-at′az) [Adolfo *Ferrata*, Italian physician, 1880–1946] hemohistioblast.

ferrated (fer-āt′ed) charged with iron.

ferredoxin (fer″ĕ-dok′sin) a nonheme iron-containing protein, also having a high sulfide content and a very low redox potential; the ferredoxins participate in electron transport in photosynthesis, nitrogen fixation, and various other biological processes.

Ferrein's canal, etc. (fer′inz) [Antoine *Ferrein*, French physician, 1693–1769] see under *canal, foramen, ligament, pyramid, tube,* and *tubule*.

ferri (fer′e) [L., gen. of *ferrum*] see *iron*.

ferri-albuminic (fer″e-al-bu-min′ik) containing iron and albumin.

Ferribacterium (fer″re-bak-te′re-um) [*ferri* + Gr. *baktērion* little rod] a genus of gram-negative chemolithotrophic bacteria of uncertain status, affiliated with the family Siderocapsaceae.

ferric (fer′ik) [L. *ferrum*] containing iron in its plus-three oxidation state, Fe(III) (sometimes designated Fe^{3+}). For ferric compounds see under the salt, e.g., arsenate and citrate. **f. fructose,** an oral iron preparation used in the treatment of iron deficiency. **f. oxide, red** [NF], a red pigment used as a pharmaceutic aid in preparations for application to the skin. **f. oxide, yellow** [NF], a yellow pigment used as a pharmaceutic aid in preparations for application to the skin.

ferritin (fer′ĭ-tin) the iron-apoferritin complex, which is one of the chief forms in which iron is stored in the body; it occurs at least in the gastrointestinal mucosa, liver, spleen, bone marrow, and reticuloendothelial cells generally. See also *immunoferritin*.

Ferrobacillus (fer″o-bah-sil′us) *Thiobacillus*.

ferrochelatase (fer″o-ke′la-tās) [EC 4.99.1.1] an enzyme of the lyase class that catalyzes the reaction protoporphyrin + Fe^{2+} = protoheme + 2 H^+. The reaction incorporates ferrous iron into protoporphyrin and is the final step in biosynthesis of heme. Inhibition of the enzyme in lead poisoning results in accumulation of protoporphyrin IX. Deficiency of the enzyme, an autosomal dominant trait, results in protoporphyria and is associated with variegate porphyria.

ferrocholinate (fer″o-ko′lin-āt) a chelate prepared by reacting equimolar quantities of freshly precipitated ferric chloride with choline dihydrogen citrate, the metallic ion being sequestered and firmly bound into a ring within the molecule; used in the treatment of iron-deficiency anemias. Called also *iron choline citrate*.

ferroflocculation (fer″o-flok″u-la′shun) a flocculation test for malaria, performed with a fine-grained iron antigen; see *Henry's test*, under *tests*.

ferrokinetic (fer″ro-kĭ-net′ik) pertaining to ferrokinetics.

ferrokinetics (fer″ro-kĭ-net′iks) the movement of iron in the body from plasma transferrin to red cell precursors in the bone marrow to circulating red cells to macrophages in the reticuloendothelial system and back to plasma transferrin. Ferrokinetic studies, using the radioisotope iron-59 as a tracer, measure kinetic parameters (*plasma iron clearance half-time, plasma iron turnover, red cell utilization,* and *erythrocyte iron turnover*) helpful in evaluating certain anemias and detect abnormal iron storage or extramedullary hematopoiesis by external counting over the liver, spleen, and bone marrow.

Ferrolip (fer′o-lip) trademark for preparations of ferrocholinate.

ferroprotein (fer″o-pro′te-in) a protein combined with an iron-containing radical; the ferroproteins are respiratory carriers. Cf. *Warburg's enzyme*, under *enzyme*, and *cytochrome* (def. 1.).

ferrosilicon (fer″o-sil′ĭ-kon) an alloy of iron and silicon made by electrothermal reduction, and used for the deoxidation of steel.

ferrosoferric (fer-o″so-fer′ik) combining a ferrous with a ferric compound; containing iron in two different oxidation states, as in the oxide Fe_3O_4.

ferrotherapy (fer″o-ther′ah-pe) [*ferrum* + *therapy*] therapeutic use of iron and iron compounds.

ferrous (fer′us) containing iron in its plus-two oxidation state, Fe(II) (sometimes designated Fe^{2+}). For ferrous compounds see under the salt, e.g., arsenate and sulfate. **f. fumarate** [USP], an oral iron preparation used in the treatment of iron deficiency. **f. gluconate** [USP], an oral iron preparation used in the treatment of iron deficiency. **f. lactate,** a salt formerly used as a hematinic (iron supplement). **f. sulfate** [USP], an oral iron preparation used in the treatment of iron deficiency.

ferroxidase (fer-ok′sĭ-dās) [EC 1.16.3.1] an enzyme of the oxidoreductase class that catalyzes the reaction 4 Fe(II) + O_2 = 4 Fe(III) + 2 H_2O. The enzyme, a deep blue α-globulin of blood plasma, contains eight atoms of copper per molecule. It oxidizes iron to Fe(III) for transport in the blood by transferrins. It is also a principal means of transport and maintenance of tissue levels of copper. Ferroxidase activity in plasma is increased in stress, infectious disease, and pregnancy, and during oral contraceptive use; it is decreased in Wilson's disease. Called also *ceruloplasmin.*

ferruginous (fer-u′jĭ-nus) [L. *ferruginosus; ferrugo* iron rust] 1. containing iron or iron rust; chalybeate. 2. of the color of iron rust.

ferrum (fer′um) [L.] iron.

Ferry-Porter law (fer′re-por′ter) [Erwin Sidney *Ferry,* American scientist, 1890–1933; T.C. *Porter,* English scientist] see under *law.*

fertile (fer′til) [L. *fertilis*] fruitful; susceptible of being developed into a new individual (of ova); not sterile or barren.

fertility (fer-til′ĭ-te) 1. the capacity to conceive or induce conception. 2. the ratio of the number of births per year to the number of women of child-bearing age; see *birth rate,* under *rate.*

fertilization (fer′tĭ-lĭ-za′shun) the act of rendering gametes fertile or capable of further development; fecundation. Fertilization begins with contact between spermatozoon and ovum, leading to their fusion, which stimulates the completion of ovum maturation with release of the second polar body. Male and female pronuclei then form and perhaps merge; synapsis follows, which restores the diploid number of chromosomes and results in biparental inheritance and the determination of sex. The process of fertilization leads to the formation of a zygote and ends with the initiation of its cleavage. **cross f.,** the fertilization of one flower by the pollen of another; allogamy. **external f.,** union of the gametes outside the bodies of the originating organisms, as in most fish. **internal f.,** union of the gametes inside the body of the female, the sperm having been transferred from the body of the male by an accessory sex organ or other means. **in vitro f.,** removal of an ovum, fertilization in a culture medium in the laboratory, and placement of the fertilized ovum into the uterus.

fertilizin (fer″tĭ-li′zin) a substance of the plasma membrane and gelatinous coat of the ovum of some species. It is considered to possess the specific receptor groups that bind the spermatozoon to the ovum. In sea-urchins, it has been characterized chemically as a glycoprotein of about 300,000 molecular weight.

Ferv. abbreviation for L. *fer′vens,* boiling.

fervescence (fer-ves′ens) [L. *fervescere* to become hot] development of an increased body temperature, or fever.

fescue (fes′ku) 1. any of the grasses belonging to the genus *Festuca.* 2. a condition resembling ergotism, affecting cattle and sometimes sheep, in New Zealand, Australia, and the United States, grazing on tall fescue (*Festuca aruncinea*) contaminated by a fungus which contains a toxic principle similar to ergot; it is characterized by lameness of the hind feet, which may progress to necrosis of the affected extremities, sometimes involving the ears or tail. Called also *fescue foot.*

Fesotyme (fe′so-tīm) trademark for a preparation of ferrous sulfate.

fester (fes′ter) to suppurate superficially.

festinant (fes′tĭ-nant) accelerating.

festination (fes″tĭ-na′shun) [L. *festinatio*] an involuntary tendency to take short accelerating steps in walking (festinating gait), as in paralysis agitans and other neurologic diseases.

festoon (fes-toon′) a carving in the base material of a denture that simulates the contours of the natural tissues being replaced by the denture. **gingival f.,** the contour of the gingiva and oral mucosa over the roots of teeth with a thin alveolar process. **McCall's f.,** a lifesaverlike enlarge-

ment of the marginal gingiva occurring on the vestibular surface, most commonly in the canine and premolar areas.

festschrift (fest′shrift) [Ger.] a memorial volume; a book made up of articles contributed by pupils or associates and friends of a scientist or leader, published usually to honor some special occasion, such as a birthday or other anniversary.

fetal (fe′tal) of or pertaining to a fetus; pertaining to *in utero* development after the embryonic period.

fetalism (fe′tal-izm) fetalization.

fetalization (fe″tal-i-za′shun) the retention, into adult life, of bodily characters which at some earlier stage of evolutionary history were actually only infantile and were rapidly lost as the organism attained maturity.

fetation (fe-ta′shun) 1. the development of a fetus within the uterus. 2. pregnancy.

feticide (fe′tĭ-sid) [*fetus* + L. *caedere* to kill] the destruction of the fetus.

fetid (fe′tid) [L. *foetidus*] having a rank or disagreeable smell.

fetish (fet′ish, fe′tish) [Fr. *fétiche,* from Port. *feitico* charm, sorcery] 1. a material object, such as an idol, charm, or talisman, believed by primitive people to have supernatural powers. 2. an inanimate object used to obtain sexual gratification.

fetishism (fet′ish-izm, fe′tish-izm) 1. a primitive religion marked by belief in fetishes. 2. [DSM III-R] a paraphilia characterized by recurrent, intense sexual urges and sexually arousing fantasies of the use of inanimate objects (fetishes), most commonly articles of clothing, such as shoes, gloves, female undergarments, or hose as a preferred or necessary adjunct to sexual arousal or orgasm. The fetish is often associated with a childhood caretaker. This disorder arbitrarily excludes fetishistic cross-dressing (transvestism). **transvestic f.** [DSM III-R], recurrent, intense sexual urges and sexually arousing fantasies involving cross-dressing.

fetishist (fet′ish-ist, fe′tish-ist) a person who obtains sexual gratification from a fetish.

fetlock (fet′lok) the metacarpophalangeal and metatarsophalangeal regions in the horse.

fetography (fe-tog′rah-fe) [*fetus* + Gr. *graphein* to write] roentgenography of the fetus in utero.

fetology (fe-tol′o-je) that branch of medicine dealing with the fetus *in utero.*

fetometry (fe-tom′ĕ-tre) [*fetus* + Gr. *metron* measure] the measurement of the fetus, especially of the diameters of its head. **roentgen f.,** measurement of the fetal head in the uterus by means of the roentgen ray.

fetoplacental (fe″to-plah-sen′tal) pertaining to the fetus and placenta.

α-fetoprotein (fe″to-pro′te-in) see *alpha-fetoprotein.*

fetor (fe′tor) [L.] stench, or offensive odor. **f. ex o′re,** halitosis. **f. hepat′icus,** the peculiar odor of the breath characteristic of hepatic disease; liver breath. **f. o′ris,** halitosis.

fetoscope (fe′to-skōp) 1. a specially designed stethoscope for listening to the fetal heart beat. 2. an endoscope for viewing the fetus *in utero.*

fetoscopic (fe″to-skop′ik) pertaining to or accomplished by fetoscopy.

fetoscopy (fe-tos′ko-pe) viewing of the fetus *in utero* by means of the fetoscope.

fetoxylate hydrochloride (fĕ-toks′ĭ-lāt) chemical name: 1-(3-cyano-3,3-diphenylpropyl)-4-phenyl-4-piperidinecarboxylic acid 2-phenoxyethyl ester monohydrochloride; a smooth muscle relaxant, $C_{36}H_{36}N_2O_3 \cdot HCl$.

fetuin (fe′tu-in) a low-molecular-weight globulin which constitutes nearly the total globulin in the blood of the fetus and newborn of ungulates.

fetus (fe′tus) [L.] the unborn offspring of any viviparous animal; specifically, the unborn offspring in the postembryonic period, after major structures have been outlined, in man from seven or eight weeks after fertilization until birth. **f. acardi′acus,** acardius. **f. amor′phus,** holoacardius amorphus. **calcified f.,** lithopedion. **f. compres′sus,** f. papyraceus. **harlequin f.,** a fetus covered with thick, horny armorlike plates as a result of an autosomal recessive keratinizing disorder; it may also be a severe form of collodion baby or it may represent the extreme form of lamellar ichthyosis. Those affected are usually stillborn or die shortly after birth. **f. in fe′tu,** a small, imperfect fetus, incapable of independent life, contained within the body of another fetus, the autosite. **mummified f.,** a shriveled and dried-up fetus. **paper-doll f., papyraceous f.,** f. papyraceus. **f. papyra′ceus,** a dead fetus pressed flat by the growth of a living twin. **parasitic f.,** an incomplete minor fetus attached to a larger, more completely developed fetus, or autosite. **f. sanguinolen′tis,** a dead fetus which has undergone maceration. **sireniform f.,** a sirenomelus, or sympus apus.

Feulgen test (reaction) (foil′gen) [Robert *Feulgen*, German physiologic chemist, 1884–1955] see under *test.*

fever (fe′ver) [L. *febris*] 1. elevation of body temperature above the normal; pyrexia. It may be due to such physiological stress as ovulation, excess thyroid hormone secretions, vigorous exercise, central nervous system lesions, or to infection by microorganisms, or to a host of noninfectious processes, as that accompanying inflammation or resulting from release of pyrogenic materials, as in leukemia. 2. any disease characterized by fever. **Aden f.,** dengue. **adynamic f.,** asthenic f. **African coast f.,** East Coast f. **African tick f.,** relapsing fever caused by *Borrelia duttonii.* **aphthous f.,** foot-and-mouth disease. **Argentine hemorrhagic f., Argentinian hemorrhagic f.,** a hemorrhagic fever primarily affecting agricultural field hands in northern Argentina, and caused by the Junin virus, transmitted by contact with the excreta of infected rodents, especially of the genus *Calomys.* It is characterized chiefly by high fever, leukopenia, thrombocytopenia, generalized myalgia, hemorrhagic manifestations, exanthema, renal involvement, and shock. Called also *Junin f.* **artificial f.,** elevation of bodily temperature produced by artificial means, as by external heat or the injection of typhoid vaccine or malarial parasites. **aseptic f.,** fever associated with aseptic wounds, presumably due to the disintegration of leukocytes or to the absorption of avascular or traumatized but uninfected tissue. **asthenic f.,** a fever with nervous depression, feeble pulse, and a cool, moist skin. **Australian Q f.,** Q fever. **autumn f.,** 1. nanukaymi. 2. mud f. **biliary f. of dogs,** canine babesiosis. **biliary f. of horses,** equine babesiosis. **bilious f. of cattle,** gallsickness. **black f.,** 1. Rocky Mountain spotted f. 2. the classic form of visceral leishmaniasis. **blackwater f.,** a severe complication of malaria characterized by intravascular hemolysis, hemoglobinuria, renal failure, and passage of dark brown or red urine, seen in association with intermittent quinine therapy, with *Plasmodium falciparum* infection in the nonimmune, or with interrupted exposure in the partially immune. Called also *hemolytic malaria, malarial hemoglobinuria,* and *West African f.* **blue f.,** Rocky Mountain spotted f. **Bolivian hemorrhagic f.,** a hemorrhagic fever occurring in rural areas of northeastern Bolivia, caused by the Machupo virus, the clinical manifestations and epidemiology of which are almost identical with those of Argentine hemorrhagic fever (q.v.). **boutonneuse f.,** an acute febrile disease caused by *Rickettsia conorii,* transmitted by the bites of various ixodid ticks, with dogs and rodents being the chief hosts, and characterized by a primary lesion (tache noire) at the site of the tick bite, maculopapular or petechial skin rash, headache, arthralgia, myalgia, chills, fever, and photophobia; there are usually no sequelae. The disease is widely distributed along the Mediterranean, Black Sea, and Caspian Sea littorals, and apparent variant forms of the infection occur in Africa and on the Indian subcontinent. Called also *boutonneuse, Conor and Bruch's disease,* and *fièvre boutonneuse,* and known also by various names according to geographical area, e.g., *Marseilles f., South African tickbite f.,* and *Indian* or *Kenya tick typhus.* **bovine epizootic f.,** ephemeral f. of cattle. **bovine infectious petechial f.,** a disease of cattle in Kenya, characterized by hemorrhages of the visible mucous membranes, fever, and diarrhea; there may be severe conjunctivitis and protrusion of the eyeball, and death within one to three days is not uncommon. The cause is believed to be a rickettsial-like organism, *Cytoectes ondiri,* spread by a biting insect. Called also *Ondiri disease.* **brain f.,** inflammation of the brain or meninges, or both together. **brassfounder's f.,** metal fume fever (q.v.) caused by fumes of any of several metals, most commonly zinc, copper, or magnesium; called also *brass* or *brazier's chill.* **Brazilian purpuric f.,** an

acute illness in children characterized by fever, abdominal pain, vomiting, petechiae, purpura, and a recent history of conjunctivitis. **Brazilian spotted f.,** Rocky Mountain spotted f. **breakbone f.,** dengue. **Bullis f.,** a febrile, probably rickettsial, disease transmitted by the tick *Amblyomma americanum,* observed in soldiers who had been at Camp Bullis, Texas, in 1942, marked by very low leukocyte count with neutropenia, headache, and constant lymphadenitis. Called also *Lone Star f.* and *Texas tick f.* **Bwamba f.,** a mild, mosquito-borne, febrile viral infection occurring in eastern, central, western, and parts of southern Africa. **cachectic f., cachexial f.,** the classic form of visceral leishmaniasis. **camp f.,** epidemic typhus. **cane-field f.,** mild leptospirosis caused by *Leptospira interrogans* serogroup *australis,* which is transmitted by rodents. **canicola f.,** Stuttgart disease. **carbuncular f.,** a variety of anthrax affecting cattle and horses, marked by the formation of circumscribed swellings in the skin, which at first are hard, hot, and painful, but later become gangrenous. **catscratch f.,** see under *disease.* **central f.,** sustained fever resulting from damage to the thermoregulatory centers of the hypothalamus. **cerebrospinal f.,** epidemic cerebrospinal meningitis. **Charcot's f.,** intermittent hepatic f. **childbed f.,** puerperal f. **Choix f.,** a disease observed in northern Mexico, identical with Rocky Mountain spotted fever. **Colombian tick f.,** a variety of spotted fever occurring in Colombia, identical with Rocky Mountain spotted fever. **Colorado tick f.,** an acute, benign febrile infection caused by an orbivirus, transmitted by the bite of the wood tick, *Dermacentor andersoni,* occurring in areas in which the tick is distributed, i.e., the Rocky Mountain area and Pacific slope of the United States and Canada, and characterized chiefly by a biphasic course and leukopenia. Called also *mountain tick f.* **Congolian red f.,** murine typhus. **continued f.,** one which does not vary more than 1.0° to 1.5° F. in twenty-four hours. **continuous f.,** persistently elevated body temperature, showing no or little variation and never falling to normal during any 24-hour period. **cotton-mill f.,** byssinosis. **Crimean hemorrhagic f.,** Congo-Crimean hemorrhagic f. by the tick *Hyalomma marginatum,* occurring in the Crimea and the Lower Don and Volga River Valleys of the U.S.S.R. **dandy f.,** dengue. **deer fly f.,** tularemia. **dehydration f.,** 1. inanition f. 2. fever due to loss of body water or inadequate fluid intake, sometimes occurring as a postoperative complication. **dengue f.,** dengue. **dengue hemorrhagic f.,** hemorrhagic dengue. **desert f.,** the primary stage of coccidioidomycosis. **digestive f.,** a slight rise of temperature during the process of digestion. **drug f.,** a febrile reaction marked by prolonged temperature elevation during the course of administration of a drug, such as an antibiotic, antineoplastic, vaccine, etc.; it may be associated with vasculitis affecting small vessels, and usually disappears rapidly on discontinuance of the drug. **Dumdum f.,** [*Dum Dum,* India] the classic form of visceral leishmaniasis. **Dutton's relapsing f.,** the central African form of relapsing fever caused by *Borrelia duttonii.* **East Coast f.,** a highly fatal form of theileriasis in African cattle, caused by *Theileria parva,* transmitted by ticks of *Rhipicephalus* and *Hyalomma* spp., and characterized by high fever, dyspnea, emaciation, lymphadenopathy, and tarry feces. Called also *African Coast f., bovine theileriasis, Rhodesian f., Rhodesian redwater f.,* and *Rhodesian tick f.* **elephantoid f.,** a recurrent acute febrile condition occurring with filariasis; it may be associated with elephantiasis or lymphangitis. **enteric f.,** any of a group of various febrile illnesses associated with enteric symptoms caused by salmonellae, especially *typhoid fever,* the prototype of the severe enteric salmonellal infections, produced by *Salmonella typhi;* and *paratyphoid fever,* which is clinically indistinguishable from typhoid fever but milder in its symptomatology and caused by *Salmonella* serotypes other than *S. typhi.* Cf. *salmonellosis.* **entericoid f.,** any fever which resembles typhoid fever in its clinical manifestations. **ephemeral f.,** a slight fever persisting or lasting only a day or two. **ephemeral f. of cattle,** stiff sickness; three-day sickness: an acute infectious disease symptomatically resembling a benign form of African horse sickness, which affects cattle in South Africa. It is characterized by high fever, stiffness, and lameness, and is thought to be of viral origin. **epidemic hemorrhagic f.,** an acute, febrile viral disease occurring in epidemics in northeastern Asia, including Korea, Japan, and Manchuria, and in a milder form in the U.S.S.R., Eastern Europe, and

Scandinavia, characterized by fever, prostration, vomiting, hemorrhagic phenomena, shock, and renal failure. It is caused by the Hantaan (Hataan) virus, which is believed to be transmitted to humans by contact, direct or indirect, with saliva and excreta of infected rodents such as the field mouse and ground vole. Called also *Far Eastern* or *Korean hemorrhagic f., hemorrhagic* or *Korean hemorrhagic nephrosonephritis, hemorrhagic f. with renal syndrome, Korin f., nephropathia epidemic,* and *nephrosonephritis.* **equine biliary f.,** equine babesiosis. **eruptive f.,** any fever accompanied by an eruption on the skin. **essential f.,** fever for which no cause has been found. **exanthematous f.,** eruptive f. **familial Mediterranean f.,** a hereditary disease transmitted in an autosomal recessive manner, usually occurring in Armenians and Sephardic Jews, and characterized by short recurrent attacks of fever with pain in the abdomen, chest, or joints and erythema resembling that seen in erysipelas; it is sometimes complicated by amyloidosis, in which the deposits of fibrillar protein are of the AA type. Called also *benign paroxysmal peritonitis, periodic peritonitis, familial recurrent polyserositis,* and *periodic* or *recurrent polyserositis.* **Far East hemorrhagic f.,** epidemic hemorrhagic f. **fatigue f.,** a febrile attack due to overexercise and the absorption of waste products. **field f.,** 1. harvest f. 2. mud f. See also *cane-field f.* and *rice-field f.* **five-day f.,** trench f. **fog f.,** a highly fatal, acute adenomatoid reaction in the lungs of cattle, believed to be a response to chemicals generated in the rumen by cattle grazing on "fog" (second growth pasture grasses). **food f.,** sudden fever with digestive disturbance lasting from a few days to some weeks; once attributed to intestinal autointoxication, these symptoms may be due to viral gastroenteritis. **Fort Bragg f.,** pretibial f. **foundryman's f.,** metal fume f. **glandular f.,** infectious mononucleosis. **Hankow f.,** schistosomiasis japonica. **harvest f.,** a form of spirochetosis affecting harvest workers; it is marked by fever, conjunctivitis, stupor, diarrhea, vomiting, and abdominal pains, and is caused by *Leptospira interrogans* serogroup *grippotyphosa;* called also *field f.* **Hasami f.,** mild leptospirosis caused by *Leptospira interrogana* serogroup *autumnalis* in Japan. **Haverhill f.,** the bacillary form of rat-bite fever (q.v.), caused by *Streptobacillus moniliformis,* and transmitted through contaminated raw milk and its products. It was first reported in an epidemic in Haverhill, Massachusetts in 1925. Called also *epidemic arthritic erythema* and *erythema arthriticum epidemicum.* **hay f.,** a seasonal variety of allergic rhinitis, marked by acute conjunctivitis with lacrimation and itching, swelling of the nasal mucosa, nasal catarrh, sudden attacks of sneezing, and often with asthmatic symptoms. It is regarded as an anaphylactic or allergic condition excited by a specific allergen (e.g., a pollen) to which the individual is sensitized. Known by various names, including *allergic conjuctivitis* and *pollenosis.* Cf. *nonseasonal allergic rhinitis.* **hay f., nonseasonal, hay f., perennial,** nonseasonal allergic rhinitis. **hectic f.,** a daily recurring fever with profound sweating, chills, and flushed countenance. **hemoglobinuric f.,** malaria attended with hemoglobinuria; see *blackwater f.* **hemorrhagic f's,** a group of diverse, severe epidemic viral infections of worldwide distribution, but occurring mainly in tropical climates, usually transmitted to humans by arthropod bites or contact with virus-infected rodents, and sharing certain common clinicopathological features, including fever, hemorrhagic manifestations, thrombocytopenia, shock, and neurologic disturbances. The group comprises Argentine hemorrhagic fever, Bolivian hemorrhagic fever, chikungunya, Congo-Crimean hemorrhagic fever, dengue hemorrhagic fever, Ebola virus disease, epidemic hemorrhagic fever, Kyasanur Forest disease, Lassa fever, Marburg virus disease, Omsk hemorrhagic fever, Rift Valley fever, and yellow fever. Called also *viral hemorrhagic f's.* **hemorrhagic f. with renal syndrome,** epidemic hemorrhagic f. **herpetic f.,** primary infection with herpes simplex virus, with diffuse involvement of mucous membranes of the mouth and lips and the surrounding skin; fever and sometimes chills occur. **inanition f.,** a transitory fever that frequently occurs in infants during the first few days of life; it is believed to be due to dehydration and is also called *dehydration f.* **intermenstrual f.,** fever sometimes seen in women between menstrual periods. **intermittent f.,** an attack of malaria or other fever characterized by recurring paroxysms of elevated temperature separated by intervals during which the temperature is normal. **intermittent**

hepatic f., a fever occurring intermittently as the result of intermittent impaction of stone in the common duct and inflammation of the bile ducts; called also *Charcot fever* and *Charcot syndrome.* **inundation f.,** scrub typhus. **island f.,** scrub typhus. **Jaccoud's dissociated f.,** fever with slow and irregular pulse in tuberculosis meningitis of adults. **jail f.,** epidemic typhus. **Japanese flood f., Japanese river f.,** scrub typhus. **jungle f.,** malaria. **jungle yellow f.,** a form of yellow fever endemic in parts of Africa and South America; it occurs in or near uncut forest or jungle. **Junin f.,** Argentine hemorrhagic f. **Katayama f.,** acute systemic schistosomiasis causing a distinct serum sickness–like syndrome, usually associated with heavy infection by *Schistosoma japonicum,* characterized by fever, chills, nausea and vomiting, cough, headache, urticaria, hepatosplenomegaly, lymphadenopathy, marked eosinophilia, and usually increased levels of IgE and IgG. It was first reported from the Katayama River Valley in Japan. **Kedani f.,** scrub typhus. **Kew Gardens spotted f.,** rickettsialpox. **Kinkiang f.,** schistosomiasis japanica. **Korean hemorrhagic f.,** epidemic hemorrhagic f. **Korin f.,** epidemic hemorrhagic f. **land f.,** a set of symptoms resembling seasickness sometimes experienced when, after an ocean voyage, the ship enters a relatively landlocked body of water. **Lassa f.,** an acute, highly fatal infectious disease caused by an arenavirus occurring epidemically in Nigeria, Sierra Leone, and Liberia, although serological evidence suggests the presence of the virus in Central and West African countries, and transmitted by contact with the multimammate rat (*Mastomys natalensis*), which sheds the virus in its urine, or spread by interpersonal contact. Chief symptoms include fever, prostration, severe pharyngitis, vomiting, abdominal pain, and dyspnea, which may be followed by serous effusions, generalized hemorrhages, and fatal shock. **lechuguilla f.,** a disease of sheep and goats in western Texas, marked by toxic encephalitis, nephritis, photosensitization, listlessness, icterus, and a yellow discharge from the eyes and nostrils; it is caused by eating the plant *Agave lechuguilla.* Commonly called *swellhead.* **Lone Star f.,** Bullis f. **lung f.,** lobar or other pneumonia. **malarial f.,** malaria. **Malta f.,** brucellosis. **Marseilles f.,** boutonneuse f. **marsh f.,** 1. mud f. 2. malaria. **Mediterranean f.,** 1. brucellosis. 2. boutonneuse f. **Mediterranean Coast f.,** tropical theileriasis. **metal fume f.,** an occupational disorder occurring in those engaged in welding and other metallic operations and due to inhalation of volatilized metals; it is characterized by sudden onset of thirst and a metallic taste in the mouth, followed by high fever, muscular aches and pains, shaking chills, headache, weakness, diaphoresis, and leukocytosis. The symptoms usually subside within 24 to 48 hours, but repeated attacks are common. The disorder includes *brassfounder's f.* (*brass chill, brazier's chill, brassfounders's ague*) and *spelter's f.* (*spelter's chill, zinc chill, zinc fume f.*). Cf. *polymer fume f.* **Meuse f.,** trench f. **milk f.,** 1. a fever said to attend the establishment of lactation after delivery. 2. an endemic fever said to be caused by the use of unwholesome cow's milk. 3. a form of paralysis affecting cows near delivery; usually accompanied by hypocalcemia, it is due to a metabolic disorder. Called also *parturient apoplexy, parturient fever,* and *parturient paralysis.* **Mossman f.,** scrub typhus. **mountain tick f.,** Colorado tick f. **mud f.,** leptospirosis occurring in the summer and late autumn in Bavaria, Silesia, and the Volga region, usually caused by *Leptospira interroganis* serogroup *grippotyphosa,* transmitted by a field mouse, *Microtus arvalis,* and affecting workers in flooded fields or in swamps. Called also *autumn f., marsh f., slime f.,* and *swamp f.* **Murchison-Pel-Ebstein f.,** Pel-Ebstein f. **nanukayami f.,** nanukayami. **nine-mile f.,** Q f. **Omsk hemorrhagic f.,** a hemorrhagic fever similar in its clinical manifestations to Kyasanur Forest disease, endemic in a forested region of western Siberia, and caused by a flavivirus, transmitted to humans by the bites of infected ticks of the genus *Dermacentor* or by direct contact with infected muskrats, as by fur trappers. **O'nyong-nyong f.,** O'nyong-nyong. **Oroya f.,** see *bartonellosis.* **Pahvant Valley f.,** tularemia. **pappataci f.,** phlebotomus f. **paratyphoid f.,** a prolonged febrile illness clinically indistinguishable from but usually less severe than typhoid fever, caused by *Salmonella* serotypes other than *S. typhi,* especially *S. enteritidis* serotypes *paratyphi A* and *B* and *S. cholerae-suis;* occasionally, the symptoms of paratyphoid fever may occur following an attack of salmonella food poisoning. Called also *Brion-Kayser disease, paratyphoid,* and *Schöttmuller's disease.* **parenteric f.,** a disease clinically resembling typhoid fever and paratyphoid fever, but not caused by *Salmonella.* **parrot f.,** psittacosis. **parturient f.,** milk f., def. 3 **Pel-Ebstein f.,** a cyclic fever occasionally seen in Hodgkin's disease and also associated with other diseases, characterized by irregular episodes of pyrexia of several days duration, with intervening afebrile periods lasting for days or weeks. Called also *Murchison-Pel-Ebstein f., Pel-Ebstein pyrexia,* and *Pel-Ebstein symptom.* **periodic f.,** a hereditary condition characterized by repetitive febrile episodes and autonomic disturbances, occurring in precise or irregular cycles of days, weeks, or months. Transmitted as an autosomal dominant trait, it may begin at any time of life and may last for decades with temporary remissions, or may cease. See also *etiocholanolone f.* and *familial Mediterranean f.* **petechial f.,** cerebrospinal meningitis. **Pfeiffer's glandular f.,** infectious mononucleosis. **pharyngoconjunctival f.,** a febrile disease caused by an adenovirus, occurring in epidemic form, largely in school children, and characterized by fever, pharyngitis, rhinitis, conjunctivitis, and enlarged cervical lymph nodes. **Philippine hemorrhagic f.,** hemorrhagic dengue. **phlebotomus f.,** an acute, self-limited, influenza-like febrile viral disease occurring chiefly during the warm months in parts of the Mediterranean littoral, central Asia, the Middle East, and Central and South America. It is caused by at least five immunologically distinct arboviruses (family Bunyaviridae), especially the Naples and Sicilian serogroups, and transmitted by the urban sandfly *Phlebotomus papatasii,* except in tropical America, where the vectors are sylvan sandflies of the genus *Lutzomyia.* Called also *pappataci f., sandfly f.,* and *three-day f.* **pinta f.,** a disease observed in northern Mexico, identical with Rocky Mountain spotted fever. **pneumonic f.,** pneumonia. **polymer fume f.,** an occupational disorder due to exposure to the products of combustion of polymers, chiefly polytef (also known as Teflon or paratetrafluoroethylene), the manifestations of which are quite similar to those of metal fume fever (q.v.). Called also *Teflon shakes.* **Pomona f.,** leptospirosis caused by *Leptospira interrogans* serogroup *pomona.* **Pontiac f.,** a self-limited disease first noted in an outbreak in 1968 in a single building in Pontiac, Michigan, marked by fever, cough, muscle aches, chills, headache, chest pain, confusion, and pleuritis; it is now known to be caused by a strain of *Legionella pneumophila.* **pretibial f.,** leptospirosis marked by a rash on the pretibial region accompanied by lumbar and postorbital pain, malaise, coryza, and fever; it is caused by *Leptospira interrogans* serogroup *autumnalis.* Called also *Fort Bragg f.* **prison f.,** epidemic typhus. **protein f.,** heightened temperature produced by the injection of protein material into the body. **puerperal f.,** septicemia accompanied by fever, in which the focus of infection is a lesion of the mucous membrane of the parturient canal due to trauma during childbirth; the etiologic agent is usually a streptococcus. Called also *childbed f.,* and *puerperal sepsis* or *septicemia.* **pulmonary f.,** pneumonia. **Q f.** [Q for *query;* so-called because the etiologic agent was unknown when it was first reported in Queensland, Australia, in 1935], an acute, generally self-limited rickettsial infection caused by *Coxiella burnettii,* characterized by fever, chills, headache, myalgia, malaise, and very rarely rash, and sometimes complicated by pneumonitis, hepatitis, and endocarditis. In humans, it is usually acquired by inhalation of airborne organisms in infected dust or aerosols derived from infected domestic animals, with no vector being involved in transmission as in other rickettsial diseases. Called also *Australian Q f.* and *nine-mile f.* **quartan f.,** a fever that occurs every fourth day; see under *malaria.* **quintan f.,** trench f. **quotidian f.,** a fever that recurs every day; see under *malaria.* **rabbit f.,** tularemia. **rat-bite f.,** either of two clinically similar but etiologically distinct, acute infectious diseases, usually transmitted through the bite of a rat, and occurring in a bacillary form caused by *Streptobacillus moniliformis,* and in a spirillary form caused by *Spirillum minus.* In the bacillary form, there is a latent period of a week to ten days, during which time the initial wound heals promptly without inflammation, but then the bite site becomes inflamed, painful, and indurated, followed by adenitis, chills, vomiting, headache, high fever, morbilliform eruption, especially on the hands and feet, and polyarthritis that is often severe. This form also may be associated with ingestion of contaminated raw milk or its products (*Haverhill*

fever), in which case there is no initial wound, the first symptoms being systemic. In the spirillary form (*sodoku*), the latent period is most commonly greater than ten days, inflammation recurs at the primary wound site, the rash is less evident than in the bacillary form, arthritis is rare, and the fever is commonly of the relapsing type. **recurrent f.,** 1. relapsing f. 2. recurrent paroxysmal fever occurring in various diseases, including tularemia, meningococcemia, malaria, and rat-bite fever. **red-water f.,** bovine babesiosis. **relapsing f.,** an acute infectious, systemic, usually self-limited disease of worldwide distribution, caused by various species of the genus *Borrelia,* which is endemic or occurs epidemically, and is transmitted by the bites of either the body louse (*Pediculus humanus humanus*), for which man is the reservoir, or by soft ticks of the genus *Ornithodor,* for which rodents and other animals are the principal reservoirs. It is characterized by one or more episodes of fever and spirochetemia alternating with afebrile periods without spirochetemia, each lasting for several days. During the febrile period symptoms include chills, headache, fatigue, myalgia, arthralgia, anorexia, cough, abdominal pain, and sometimes coagulation disturbance, hepatosplenomegaly, psychic disturbances, petechial rash, and vomiting; treatment may be complicated by severe Jarisch-Herxheimer reaction. Both epidemiological forms of the disease are known by various descriptive and local names, including *famine, recurrent,* or *spirillum f.* See also *recurrent f.,* def. 2. **remittent f.,** a fever in which the diurnal variation is 2° F. or more, but in which the temperature never falls to a normal level; see *malaria.* **rheumatic f.,** a febrile disease occurring as a delayed sequela of infections with group A hemolytic streptococci and characterized by multiple focal inflammatory lesions of the connective tissue structures, especially of the heart, blood vessels, and joints (polyarthritis), and by the presence of Aschoff bodies in the myocardium and skin. Typically, the onset is signalled by the sudden occurrence of fever and joint pain, followed by manifestations of heart and pericardial disease, abdominal pain, skin changes, and chorea. Atypical manifestations, particularly in adults, are not uncommon. Called also *acute articular rheumatism, acute rheumatic fever* or *arthritis,* and *polyarthritis rheumatica acuta.* **Rhodesian f., Rhodesian redwater f., Rhodesian tick f.,** East Coast f. **rice-field f.,** leptospirosis caused by *Leptospira interrogans* serogroup *bataviae.* **Rift Valley f.,** an acute febrile infection of domestic animals (e.g., sheep, cattle) and humans caused by a bunyavirus, transmitted by moquitoes of the genera *Aedes, Culex,* and *Erethmapodites* and also by contact with tissues and secretions of diseased animals. In humans, it may be manifested by nonspecific influenza-like symptoms, or in severe cases, it may be associated with encephalitis, retinitis, or hemorrhagic fever. In animals, it is characterized by fever, listlessness, hepatitis, melena, blood-stained nasal discharge, and abortion in pregnant animals. First observed in the Rift Valley of Kenya, it is now seen throughout southern and eastern Africa to Egypt. **Rocky Mountain spotted f.,** an acute infectious sometimes fatal disease caused by *Rickettsia rickettsii,* usually transmitted by the bites of several species of infected ixodid ticks, the two most important vectors being *Dermacentor andersoni* (wood tick) and *D. variablis* (dog tick), and occurring only in North and South America. It is characterized by sudden onset, with chills; fever lasting about 2 to 3 weeks; cutaneous rash that generally appears between the second and sixth day of illness, at first involving the wrists, ankles, palms, soles, and forearms and spreading to the proximal extremities, trunk, and face; myalgias; severe headache; and prostration. Called also *black, blue, chroix, mountain,* or *pinta fever, blue disease,* and tickborne typhus. It is also known by many local names including *Brazilian spotted, Colombian tick,* or *Tobia fever, exanthematic typhus of Sao Paulo,* and *Sao Paulo typhus.* **Salinem f.,** see under *infection.* **salt f.,** fever associated with excess of salt in the body, due to the retention by the salt of the water normally eliminated in perspiration. **sandfly f.,** phlebotomus f. **San Joaquin f.,** the primary stage of coccidioidomycosis. **scarlet f.,** infection with group A β-hemolytic streptococci of varying severity, although it usually has a milder course than in the past when septic complications such as otitis media, mastoiditis, and suppurative lymphadenitis were not rare. It is characterized by pharyngitis and tonsillitis concurrent with a typical erythematous rash, produced by an erythrogenic toxin elaborated by the streptococci, progressing from the trunk and neck to the extremities (except the palms and soles), forehead, and face, with flushed face and circumoral pallor, red or white strawberry tongue, and lines of hyperpigmentation (Pastia's sign) in the body creases; the rash disappears and is followed by desquamation of the skin. Similar clinical manifestations, but usually with involvement of the pharynx and tonsils, may follow infection of wounds, burns, or the skin with group A β-hemolytic streptococci, or with any strain of streptococci that elaborates an erythrogenic toxin. Called also *scarlatina*. **Schottmüller's f.,** paratyphoid f. **septic f.,** fever due to septicemia. **seven-day f.,** 1. a fever affecting Europeans in India, and marked by symptoms similar to those of dengue. 2. benign leptospirosis. 3. nanukayami. 4. sakushu f. **sheep f.,** heartwater. **shin bone f.,** trench f. **ship f.,** epidemic typhus. **shipping f.,** a disease of cattle caused by *Pasteurella haemolytica* in association with a virus; infection occurs when the resistance of the animal is lowered by stress. **shoddy f.,** a febrile disease, with cough, dyspnea, and headache, caused by dust in shoddy factories. **Sinbis f.,** an epidemic-endemic febrile disease caused by an alphavirus, transmitted by mosquitoes of the genus *Culex*, and occurring in southern and eastern Africa, Egypt, Israel, India, the Philippines, and eastern Australia; symptoms include macular rash and arthritis. **slime f.,** mud f. **Songo f.,** epidemic hemorrhagic f. **South African tick-bite f.,** see *boutonneuse f.* **spelter's f.,** metal fume fever caused by fumes in zinc smelters; called also *spelter's chill, zinc chill,* and *zinc fume f.* **spirillum f.,** sodoku or rat-bite fever due to *Spirillum minus.* **splenic f.,** anthrax. **spotted f.,** a febrile disease typically characterized by a skin eruption, such as Rocky Mountain spotted fever, boutonneuse fever, and other infections caused by tick-borne rickettsiae, and typhus and epidemic cerebrospinal meningitis. **sthenic f.,** fever characterized by a full, strong pulse, hot and dry skin, high temperature, thirst, and active delirium. **stiff-neck f.,** epidemic cerebrospinal meningitis. **stockyards f.,** a complex of bacterial and viral diseases of the respiratory system of cattle. **swamp f.,** 1. mud f. 2. equine infectious anemia. 3. malaria. **swine f.,** hog cholera. **swine f., African,** a viral disease similar to but more severe than hog cholera, and caused by an immunologically distinct agent; recognized first in Africa and found also in western Europe, Cuba, the Dominican Republic, and Haiti. **tertian f.,** a fever that occurs every third day; see under *malaria.* **tetanoid f.,** cerebrospinal meningitis. **Texas f., Texas cattle f.,** bovine babesiosis. **Texas tick f.,** Bullis f. **Thai hemorrhagic f.,** hemorrhagic dengue. **therapeutic f.,** pyretotherapy, def. 1. **thermic f.,** sunstroke. **three-day f.,** phlebotomus f. **threshing f.,** irritation of the respiratory tract, headache, and fever, occurring in workers at threshing grain. **tick f.,** any infectious disease transmitted by the bite of a tick; the causative parasite may be a rickettsia, as in Rocky Mountain spotted fever; a *Babesia*, as in Texas fever; a *Borrelia*, as in relapsing fever; or a virus, as in Colorado tick fever. **Tobia f.,** Rocky Mountain spotted f. **trench f.,** a self-limited louse-borne rickettsial disease due to *Rochalimaea quintana*, transmitted by the body louse, *Pediculus humanus*, and characterized by intermittent fever, generalized aches and pains, particularly severe in the shins, chills, sweating, vertigo, malaise, typhus-like rash, and multiple relapses. It was first recognized during the trench warfare of World War I and also was a major problem among military personnel in Europe in World War II, and is endemic in Mexico, North Africa, eastern Europe, and parts of Asia. Called also *five-day f., Meuse f., quintan f., shin bone f., Wolhynia f., His' disease, His-Werner disease,* and *Werner-His disease.* **tsutsugamushi f.,** scrub typhus. **typhoid f.,** an acute generalized, systemic febrile illness caused by *Salmonella typhi*, usually spread by ingestion of contaminated food and water, and characterized by sustained bacteremia and invasion by the pathogen and multiplication within the mononuclear phagocytic cells of the liver, spleen, lymph nodes, and Peyer's patches of the ileum, associated with prolonged hectic fever, malaise, transient characteristic skin rash (rose spots), abdominal pain, splenomegaly, bradycardia, delirium, and leukopenia; significant intestinal hemorrhages and frank perforation may be late complications. Called also *typhoid.* See also *paratyphoid f.* **typhomalarial f.,** a fever showing typhoid symptoms, but believed to be malarial in origin. **typhus f.,** see *typhus.* **undulant f.,** brucellosis. **urethral f., urinary f.,** fever following the use of the urethral bougie, catheter, or sound. **uveoparotid f.,**

Heerfordt's syndrome. **vaccinal f.,** the slight fever that sometimes follows vaccination. **valley f.,** the primary stage of coccidioidomycosis. **viral hemorrhagic f's,** hemorrhagic f's. **war f.,** epidemic typhus. **West African f.,** blackwater f. **West Nile f.,** see under *encephalitis.* **Whitmore's f.,** melioidosis. **Wolhynia f.,** trench f. **wound f.,** traumatic f. **Yangtze Valley f.,** schistosomiasis japonica. **yellow f.,** an acute infectious disease caused by a flavivirus, transmitted to man by mosquitoes which acquire the infection either from man (urban type) or from animals (jungle type). In its severe form it is marked by fever, jaundice, hemorrhage, and renal damage, the jaundice resulting from necrosis of the liver; it may also occur as a mild febrile illness, with inapparent infections being frequent. Yellow fever occurs endemically and epidemically in tropical regions of the Americas and Africa. *Urban yellow fever* affects chiefly persons living in close contact with one another, and is transmitted by *Aedes aegypti*, which usually breeds near human habitations. *Jungle (or sylvan) yellow fever* most often affects those working in or living near forests; it has a variety of mosquito vectors, including several species of *Haemagogus* in South America, and *Aedes africanus* and *A. simpsoni* in Central Africa. **zinc fume f.,** spelter's f.

Fèvre-Languepin syndrome (fevr lan'gĕ-pah) [Marcel *Fèvre;* Anne *Languepin*] see under *syndrome.*

FFA free fatty acids.

F.F.T. flicker fusion threshold.

F.h. abbreviation for L. *fi'at haus'tus,* let a draught be made.

FIA fluoroimmunoassay.

fiat (fi'at), pl. *fi'ant* [L.] let there be made.

fiber (fi'ber) 1. an elongated, threadlike structure; see also *fibra* [NA]. 2. in nutrition, the sum of the constituents of the diet that are not digested by gastrointestinal enzymes; see *dietary f.* **A f's,** myelinated fibers of the somatic nervous system having a diameter of 1μ to 22μ and a conduction velocity of 5 to 120 meters per second; they include the alpha, beta, delta, and gamma fibers. **accelerating f's, accelerator f's,** adrenergic fibers that transmit the impulses that accelerate the heart beat; called also *augmentor f's* and *cardiac accelerator f's.* **accessory f's,** those fibers of the zonule of Zinn running perpendicularly to the chief fibers and not reaching the lens of the eye; supporting the fibers running from the ciliary body to the chief fibers and bracing them, including the interciliary fibers and the orbiculociliary fibers. Called also *auxiliary fibers.* **adrenergic f's,** nerve fibers that liberate epinephrine-like substances at the time of passage of nerve impulses across a synapse. **afferent f's, afferent nerve f's,** nerve fibers that convey sensory impulses from the periphery to the central nervous system; classified according to function as somatic afferent and visceral afferent fibers. Called also *afferent neurofibers* and *neurofibrae afferentes* [NA]. **alpha f's,** motor and proprioceptive fibers of the A type having conduction velocities of 70 to 120 meters per second and ranging from 13μ to 22μ in diameter. **alveolar f's,** fibers of the periodontal ligament extending from the cementum of the tooth root to the walls of the alveolus, distinguished as alveolar crest, horizontal, oblique, and apical fibers. Called also *cementoalveolar f's.* **alveolar crest f's,** fibers of the periodontal ligament extending from the cementum of the tooth root to the alveolar crest. **anastomosing f's, anastomotic f's,** fibers extending from one muscle bundle or nerve trunk to another. **apical f's,** fibers of the periodontal ligament extending from the cementum to the fundus of the alveolus. **archiform f's,** fibrae intercrurales. **arcuate f's, anterior external,** fibrae arcuatae externae ventrales. **arcuate f's, dorsal external,** fibrae arcuatae externae dorsales. **arcuate f's, ventral external,** fibrae arcuatae externae ventrales. **arcuate f's, internal,** fibrae arcuatae internae. **arcuate f's of cerebrum,** fibrae arcuatae cerebri. **arcuate f's, posterior external,** fibrae arcuatae externae dorsales. **argentaffin f's, argentophil f's, argentophilic f's,** reticular f's. **asbestos f's,** fibers formed in degenerating hyaline cartilage by ossification of the collagen fibers. **association f's, association nerve f's,** nerve fibers that interconnect portions of the cerebral cortex within a hemisphere. Short association fibers interconnect neighboring gyri; long fibers interconnect more widely separated gyri and are arranged into bundles or fasciculi. Called also *association neurofibers* and *neurofibrae associationes* [NA]. **astral f.,** see under *ray.* **augmentor f's,** accelerating f's. **auxiliary f's,** accessory f's. **axial f.,** the axon of a nerve fiber. **B f's,** myelinated preganglionic autonomic axons having a fiber diameter $\leq 3\mu$ and a conduction velocity of 3 to 15 meters per second. **basilar f's,** fibers that form the middle layer of the zona arcuata and the zona pectinata of the basilar membrane in the inner ear; called also *auditory strings.* **Bergmann's f's,** processes which radiate from the molecular layer of the cerebellum and enter the pia. **Bernheimer's f's,** a tract of nerve fibers connecting the optic tract to Luys' body. **beta f's,** touch and temperature fibers of the A type having conduction velocities of 30 to 70 meters per second and ranging from 8μ to 13μ in diameter. **bone f's,** Sharpey's f's. (def. 1). **Brücke's f's,** fibrae meridionales musculi ciliaris. **bulbospiral f's,** spiral muscular fibers forming a portion of the musculature of the atria and ventricles of the heart. **Burdach's f's,** nerve fibers connected with Burdach's nucleus (nucleus cuneatus). **C f's,** unmyelinated postganglionic fibers of the autonomic nervous system, also the unmyelinated fibers found at the dorsal roots, and at free nerve endings, which have a conduction velocity of 0.6 to 2.3 meters per second and a diameter of 0.3μ to 1.3μ. **capsular f's,** the nerve fibers within the internal capsule of the brain. **cardiac accelerator f's,** accelerating f's. **cardiac depressor f's,** vagal fibers to the heart which when activated cause a decrease in cardiac output. **cardiac pressor f's,** sympathetic nerve fibers to the heart which when activated cause an increase in cardiac output. **cemental f's,** the fibers of the periodontal ligament extending from the cementum to the zone of the intermediate plexus, where their terminations are interspersed with the terminations of the alveolar group of periodontal fibers. **cementoalveolar f's,** alveolar f's. **cerebrospinal f's,** the fibers in the internal capsule of the brain which run from the motor region of the cortex to the pyramids of the medulla oblongata. **chief f's,** those fibers of the zonule of Zinn which run from the ciliary body to the lens, including the orbiculoposterocapsular, the orbiculoanterocapsular, the cilioposterocapsular, and cilioequatorial fibers; called also *main* or *principal f's.* **cholinergic f's,** nerve fibers that liberate acetylcholine at the synapse. **chromatic f.,** the long fiber of chromatin into which the nucleus is resolved during the early stages of karyokinesis and which afterward separates into the chromosomes. **chromosomal f.,** traction f. **cilioequatorial f's,** those chief fibers which pass from the summits of the ciliary processes to the equator of the lens. **cilioposterocapsular f's,** the most numerous of the chief zonular fibers, arising from the tips and sides of the ciliary processes, passing posteriorly and crossing the anteriorly directed fibers, to insert into the posterior capsule anterior to the insertion of the orbiculoposterocapsular fibers. **circular f's,** gingival fibers that pass through the connective tissue of the marginal and interdental gingivae and encircle the tooth in ringlike fashion. **circular f's of ciliary muscle,** fibrae circulares musculi ciliaris. **circular f's of eardrum,** see *stratum circulare membranae tympani.* **climbing f's, clinging f's,** afferent fibers arising in part from the middle cerebellar peduncle and passing through the granular layer of the cerebellar cortex to terminate on Purkinje cell dendrites. Called also *tendril f's.* Cf. *mossy f's.* **collagen f's, collagenic f's,** collagenous f's. **collagenous f's,** the soft, flexible, white fibers which are the most characteristic constituent of all types of connective tissue, consisting of the protein collagen, and composed of bundles of fibrils that are in turn made up of smaller units (microfibrils) which show a characteristic crossbanding with a major periodicity of 65 nm. See also *fibrous long-spacing collagen* and *segment long-spacing collagen,* under *collagen,* and see also *tropocollagen.* **collateral f's of Winslow,** fibrae intercrurales. **commissural f's, commissural nerve f's,** the nerve fibers which pass between the cortex of opposite hemispheres of the brain, or between two sides of the brain stem or spinal cord. Called also *commissural neurofibers* and *neurofibrae commissurales* [NA]. **cone f.,** a fiber-like extension of a retinal cone, running from the inner segment of the dendrite to the nucleus to the pedicle. **continuous f's,** the spindle fibers in mitosis which extend from pole to pole. **Corti's f's,** rods of Corti. **corticobulbar f's, corticonuclear f's,** fibrae corticonucleares. **corticopontine f's,** fibrae corticopontinae. **corticoreticular f's,** fibrae corticoreticulares. **corticorubral f's,** fibrae

corticorubrales. **corticospinal f's,** fibrae corticospinales. **corticotectal f's,** fibrae corticotectales. **corticothalamic f's,** fibrae corticothalamicae. **dark f's,** muscle fibers rich in sarcoplasm and having a dark appearance. **Darkshevich's f's,** nervous fibers of the cerebrum running from the optic tract to the habenular ganglion. **decussating f's,** any set of interconnecting fibers. **dendritic f's,** fibers which pass in a treelike form from the cortex to the white substance of the brain. **dentatorubral f's,** fibrae dentatorubrales. **dentatothalamic f's,** nerve fibers in the cranial cerebellar peduncle that make up the dentatothalamic tract. **dentinal f.,** process of odontoblast. **dentinogenic f's,** Korff's f's. **depressor f's,** 1. nerve fibers which, when stimulated reflexly, cause a diminished vasomotor tone and thereby a decrease in arterial pressure. 2. cardiac depressor f's. **dietary f.,** that part of whole grains, vegetables, fruits, and nuts that resists digestion in the gastrointestinal tract; it consists of carbohydrate (cellulose, etc.) and lignin. **Edinger's f's,** fibers in the cerebrum of amphibia, forming part of the visual paths. **efferent f's, efferent nerve f's,** nerve fibers that convey motor impulses away from the central nervous system toward the periphery; classified according to function as somatic efferent and visceral efferent fibers. Called also *efferent neurofibers* and *neurofibrae efferentes* [NA]. **elastic f's,** yellowish fibers of elastic quality traversing the intercellular substance of connective tissue; called also *yellow f's.* **endogenous f's,** nerve fibers of the spinal cord which arise from cells the bodies of which are situated inside the cord. **exogenous f's,** fibers of the spinal cord which arise from cells the bodies of which are situated outside the cord. **extraciliary f's,** see *fleece.* **extrafusal f's,** ordinary muscle fibers, as opposed to the intrafusal fibers of the muscle spindle. **forklike f's,** branching fibers in the tunica media of arteries. **frontopontine f's,** fibrae frontopontinae. **gamma f's,** A fibers that conduct touch and pressure impulses and innervate the intrafusal fibers of the muscle spindle; they conduct at velocities of 15 to 40 meters per second and range from 3μ to 7μ in diameter. **Gerdy's f's,** the fibers of the superficial ligament connecting the clefts of the palmar surfaces of the fingers. **gingival f's,** the collagen fibers which make up the gingival corium and support the gingiva. They are attached and adapted to the tooth surface and act as a barrier to the apical migration of the epithelial attachment. **gingivodental f's,** gingival fibers of the vestibular, oral, and interproximal surfaces, embedded in the cementum just beneath the epithelium at the base of the gingival crevice. **Goll's f's,** fibers extending from Goll's nucleus (nucleus gracilis) to the vermis of the cerebellum. **Gottstein's f's,** the external hair cells, and nerve fibers associated with them, forming a part of the expansion of the auditory nerve in the cochlea. **Gratiolet's radiating f's,** radiatio optica. **gray f's,** unmyelinated nerve fibers, found largely, but not exclusively, in the sympathetic nerves; called also *f's of Remak.* **hair f.,** any one of the horny fibers, each containing relics of a nucleus, which make up the main substance of a hair. **half-spindle f's,** spindle fibers in mitosis which extend from one pole to the chromosomes. **Henle's f's,** the fibers of the fenestrated membrane which exists in certain arteries between the external and middle coats; some are elastic, others nucleated. **Herxheimer's f's,** minute spiral fibers in the stratum mucosum of the skin; called also *Herxheimer's spirals.* **heterodesmotic f's,** white fibers connecting dissimilar gray structures of the nervous system. **homodesmotic f's,** white fibers connecting similar gray structures of the central nervous system. **horizontal f's,** fibers of the periodontal ligament extending horizontally from the cementum of the tooth root to the walls of the alveolus. **impulse-conducting f's,** Purkinje's f's. **interciliary f's,** those accessory fibers running between the ciliary processes. **intercolumnar f's,** fibrae intercrurales. **intercrural f's,** fibrae intercrurales. **internuncial f's,** fibers connecting nerve cells. **interzonal f's,** the delicate fibers of achromatin forming the central spindle during karyokinesis. **intrafusal f's,** modified muscle fibers which, surrounded by fluid and enclosed in a connective tissue envelope, compose the muscle spindle. **James f.,** junctional tissue or a tract which bypasses the atrioventricular node, thus permitting ventricular preexcitation. **Korff f's,** collagen fibrils extending from fibroblasts (preodontoblasts), which project their processes toward the inner enamel epithelium (preameloblasts), whence they reach the area of aperiodic fibrils and basal lamina, where they form bundles and make up the matrix for dentin, particularly the mantle dentin. **lattice f's,** reticular f's. **f's of lens,** fibrae lentis. **light f's,** muscle fibers poor in sarcoplasm and therefore more transparent than dark fibers. **longitudinal f's of ciliary muscle,** fibrae meridionales musculi ciliaris. **longitudinal f's of pons,** fibrae longitudinales pontis. **Luschka's f's,** fibers of the levator ani muscle that meet between the anus and the vagina in the perineal body. **Mahaim f's,** fibers arising from the proximal main atrioventricular bundle, which allow early excitation of the base of the ventricular septum. **main f's,** chief f's. **mantle f.,** any one of the cytoplasmic filaments which assist in drawing the daughter chromosomes toward the poles of the central spindles. **Mauthner's f.,** an axon that extends from the metencephalon to the caudal end of the spinal cord of fishes and amphibians, and provides the final common path for impulses to the tail. **medullated f's,** myelinated f's. **meridional f's of ciliary muscle,** fibrae meridionales musculi ciliaris. **moss f's, mossy f's,** thick afferent nerve fibers arising from the inferior cerebellar peduncle and passing into the cerebellar cortex to terminate in numerous branches or mosslike appendages around the cells of the granular layer. Cf. *climbing f's.* **motor f.,** a fiber in a mixed nerve which transmits impulses to a muscle fiber. **Müller's f's,** elongated neuroglial cells traversing all the layers of the retina and forming its most important supporting element; called also *sustentacular f's, cells of Müller, radial cells of Müller,* and *retinal gliocytes.* **muscle f.,** any of the cells of skeletal or cardiac muscle tissue. Skeletal muscle fibers are cylindrical multinucleate cells containing contracting myofibrils, across which run transverse striations, enclosed in a sarcolemma. Cardiac muscle fibers contain one or sometimes two nuclei and myofibrils and are separated from one another by an intercalated disk; although striated, cardiac muscle fibers branch to form an interlacing network. See also *muscle cell,* under *cell.* **muscle f's, intermediate,** muscle fibers having characteristics intermediate between red and white muscle fibers. **muscle f's, red,** the small dark fibers that predominate in red muscle (q.v.). **muscle f's, white,** the large pale fibers that predominate in white muscle (q.v.). **myelinated f's, myelinated nerve f's,** grayish white nerve fibers whose axons are encased in a myelin sheath, which may in turn be enclosed by a neurilemma; called also *medullated f's* and *medullated nerve f's.* Cf. *unmyelinated f's.* **nerve f.,** a slender process of a neuron, especially the prolonged axon which conducts nerve impulses away from the cell. Nerve fibers are classified on the basis of the presence or absence of a myelin sheath as myelinated or unmyelinated. Called also *neurofibra* [NA] and *neurofiber.* **nerve f's, afferent,** afferent f's. **nerve f's, association,** association f's. **nerve f's, commissural,** commissural f's. **nerve f's, efferent,** efferent f's. **nerve f's, postganglionic,** postganglionic f's. **nerve f's, preganglionic,** preganglionic f's. **nerve f's, projection,** projection nerve f's. **nerve f's, somatic,** somatic f's. **nerve f's, tangential,** tangential nerve f's. **nerve f's, visceral,** visceral f's. **neuroglial f.,** one of the fibrillar structures embedded in the cytoplasm and expansions of neuroglial cells. **nonmedullated f's, nonmedullated nerve f's,** unmyelinated f's. **oblique f's,** the largest fibers of the periodontal ligament, extending from the cementum in a coronal direction obliquely to the apical two thirds of the alveolus; they suspend and anchor the tooth in its socket and resist surface tooth pressures. **oblique f's of ciliary muscle,** fibrae radiales musculi ciliaris. **oblique f's of stomach, oblique gastric f's,** fibrae obliquae gastricae. **odontogenic f's,** fibers of connective tissue (periodontium and pulp) contributing to the matrix of dentin and cementum. **olivocerebellar f's,** see *tractus olivocerebellaris.* **orbiculoanterocapsular f's,** those chief fibers which have the most posterior and internal position, lying in close relation to the anterior boundary of the vitreous. **orbiculociliary f's,** those accessory fibers which pass from the pars orbicularis to the ciliary processes. **orbiculoposterocapsular f's,** those chief fibers which spring from the prolongation of the hyaloid membrane investing the ciliary ring. **osteocollagenous f's,** fibers gathered together into bundles and united by a special binding substance in the interstitial substance of bone. **osteogenetic f's,** osteogenic f's. **osteogenic f's,** pre-

collagenous fibers formed by osteoclasts and becoming the fibrous component of bone matrix. **oxytalan f.,** a connective tissue fiber, resistant to acid hydrolysis, found in structures subjected to mechanical stress, such as tendons, ligaments, adventitia, and connective tissue sheaths that surround the skin appendages. **paraventriculoventricular f's,** fibrae paraventriculares. **parietotemporoporopontine f's,** fibrae parietotemporoporopontinae. **periventricular f's,** Sharpey's f's (def. 2). **periventricular f's,** fibrae periventriculares. **pilomotor f's,** unmyelinated nerve fibers going to the small muscles of the hair follicles. **pontocerebellar f's,** fibrae pontocerebellares. **postcommissural f's,** the fibers of the posterior commissure lying just behind the pineal body. **postganglionic f's, postganglionic nerve f's,** the axons of postganglionic neurons; called also *neurofibrae postganglionares* [NA] and postganglionic *neurofibers.* **precollagenous f's,** a name given reticular fibers on the supposition that they are immature collagenous fibers. **preganglionic f's, preganglionic nerve f's,** the axons of preganglionic neurons; called also *neurofibrae preganglionares* [NA] and *preganglionic neurofibers.* **pressor f's,** 1. nerve fibers which, when stimulated reflexly, cause or increase vasomotor tone. 2. cardiac pressor f's. **principal f's,** 1. chief f's. 2. fibers of the periodontal ligament, which are collagen fibers arranged in bundles along the length of the root of a tooth that suspend and anchor the tooth to the alveolus. They include the transseptal, alveolar crest, horizontal, oblique, and apical fibers. **projection f's, projection nerve f's,** nerve fibers that connect the cerebral cortex with the subcortical centers, the brain stem, and the spinal cord; called also *projection neurofibers* and *neurofibrae projectiones* [NA]. **Prussak's f's,** two short fibers from the end of the short process of the malleus to the notch of Rivinus. **Purkinje f's,** modified cardiac fibers in the subendocardial tissue that constitute the terminal ramifications of the conducting system of the heart. The term is sometimes used loosely to denote the entire system of conducting fibers. See also *rami subendocardiales* and *systema conducens cordis.* **radial f's of ciliary muscle,** fibrae radiales musculi ciliaris. **radiating f's of anterior chondrosternal ligaments,** ligamenta sternocostalia radiata. **radiating f's of eardrum,** see *stratum radiatum membranae tympani.* **radicular f's,** fibers in the roots of the spinal nerves. **Rasmussen's nerve f's,** efferent fibers in both the vestibular and cochlear divisions of the eighth cranial nerve, which originate bilaterally from the vicinity of the superior olive. **Reissner's f.,** a highly refractive longitudinal fiber in the central canal of the spinal cord. **f's of Remak,** gray f's. **reticular f's,** immature connective tissue fibers, staining with silver, forming the reticular framework of lymphoid and myeloid tissue and occurring also in the interstitial tissue of glandular organs, the papillary layer of the skin, and elsewhere; called also *argentaffin f's, argentophilic f's, lattice f's,* and *Gitterfasern.* **Retzius' f's,** the stiff filaments of Deiters' cells in the organ of Corti. **Ritter's f.,** a fiber in the axis of a retinal rod, probably a nerve fiber. **rod f.,** a fiber-like extension of a retinal rod, running from the inner segment of the dendrite to the nucleus to the spherule. **Sappey's f's,** smooth muscle fibers in the check ligaments of the eye near their orbital attachments. **Sharpey's f's,** 1. collagenous fibers that pass from the periosteum and are embedded in the outer circumferential and interstitial lamellae of bone; called also *bone f's.* 2. terminal portions of principal fibers that insert into the cementum of a tooth. Called also *perforating f's.* **short association f's,** fibers in the cerebrum that connect adjacent gyri. **sinospiral f's,** spiral muscular fibers forming a portion of the musculature of the atria and ventricles of the heart. **somatic f's, somatic nerve f's,** nerve fibers, afferent or efferent, that stimulate or activate skeletal muscle and somatic tissues; called also *neurofibrae somaticae* [NA] and *somatic neurofibers.* **sphincter f's of ciliary muscle,** fibrae circulares musculi ciliaris. **spindle f's,** the microtubules radiating from the centrioles during mitosis and forming a spindle-shaped configuration. See *spindle.* **Stilling's f's,** a term applied, probably incorrectly, to association fibers of the cerebellum; more correctly refers to the reticular formation of the medulla oblongata. **f's of stria terminalis,** fibrae striae terminalis. **sudomotor f's,** unmyelinated nerve fibers going to the sweat glands. **supraoptic f's,** fibrae supraopticae. **sustentacular f's,** Müller's f's. **T f.,** a nerve fiber that branches at right angles from the axon of a nerve cell. **tangential f's, tangential nerve f's,** tangentially oriented nerve fibers arranged in striae in the superficial layers of the hippocampus and cerebral cortex; called also *tangential neurofibers* and *neurofibrae tangentiales* [NA]. **temporopontine f's,** fibrae temporopontinae. **tendril f's,** climbing f's. **thalamocortical f's,** sensory nerve fibers that connect the dorsal thalamus to the cerebral cortex, which together form the peduncles of the thalamus; called also *thalamic radiations, radiations of thalamus,* and *thalamocortical projections.* **thalamoparietal f's,** fibrae thalamoparietales. **Tomes f.,** process of odontoblast. **traction f's,** the fibers of the spindle in mitosis along which the daughter chromosomes move apart; called also *chromosomal f's.* **transilient f's,** short association fibers, especially those that pass from one gyrus to another not next to it. **transseptal f's,** fibers of the periodontal ligament extending interproximally over the alveolar crest and embedding in the cementum of adjacent teeth; they support the interproximal gingiva and secure the adjacent tooth. **transverse f's of pons,** fibrae pontis transversae. **ultraterminal f.,** a thin unmyelinated twig given off from the ramifications of the axon in the motor plate. **unmyelinated f's, unmyelinated nerve f's,** nerve fibers (axons) that lack the myelin sheath but may be enclosed by a neurilemma. Called also *nonmedullated f's* and *nonmedullated nerve f's.* Cf. *myelinated f's.* **varicose f's,** certain myelinated fibers which have no neurilemma; after death a fluid accumulates between the myelin and the axon, giving the fibers a varicose appearance. **vasomotor f's,** unmyelinated nerve fibers going chiefly to arteriolar muscles. **visceral f's, visceral nerve f's,** nerve fibers, afferent or efferent, that stimulate or activate smooth muscle and glandular tissues; called also *neurofibrae viscerales* [NA] and *visceral neurofibers.* **von Monakow's f's,** ansa lenticularis. **Weissmann's f's,** fibers within the muscle spindle. **white f's,** collagenous f's. **yellow f's,** elastic f's. **zonular f's,** fibrae zonulares.

fibercolonoscope (fi″ber-ko-lōn′-o-skōp) a fiberoptic instrument for viewing the colon.

fibergastroscope (fi″ber-gas′tro-skōp) a fiberoptic instrument for viewing the stomach.

fiber-illuminated (fi′ber-ĭ-loo′mĭ-na″ted) transmitting light by means of bundles of glass or plastic fibers, utilizing a lens system to transmit the image; said of endoscopes of such design.

fiberoptic (fi″ber-op′tik) pertaining to fiberoptics; coated with glass or plastic fibers having special optical properties.

fiberoptics (fi″ber-op′tiks) 1. the transmission of an image along flexible bundles of coated parallel glass or plastic fibers that propagate light by internal reflections. 2. the branch of optics dealing with such transmission.

fiberscope (fi′ber-skōp) a flexible endoscope whose lumen is coated with glass or plastic fibers having special optical properties; see *fiberoptics.*

Fibiger (fe′bĕ-ger) Johannes Andreas Grib, Danish pathologist, 1867–1928; winner of the Nobel prize in medicine or physiology for 1926 for his discovery of the Spiroptera carcinoma and thus of a method for the experimental induction of cancer.

fibra (fi′brah), pl. *fi′brae* [L.] [NA] a fiber: a general term designating an elongated, threadlike structure. **fi′brae annula′res,** see *pars anularis vaginae fibrosae digitorum manus* and *pars anularis vaginae fibrosae digitorum pedis.* **fi′brae arcua′tae cer′ebri** [NA], arcuate fibers of cerebrum: short association fibers within the cerebral cortex, connecting adjacent gyri; called also *fibrae propriae.* **fi′brae arcua′tae exter′nae anterio′res,** NA alternative for *fibrae arcuatae externae ventrales.* **fi′brae arcua′tae exter′nae dorsa′les** [NA], dorsal external arcuate fibers: fibers that arise from the accessory cuneate nucleus and enter the cerebellum by way of the ipsilateral caudal (inferior) cerebellar peduncle; called also *fibrae arcuatae externae posteriores* [NA alternative] and *posterior external arcuate fibers.* **fi′brae arcua′tae exter′nae posterio′res,** NA alternative for *fibrae arcuatae externae dorsales.* **fi′brae arcua′tae exter′nae ventra′les** [NA], ventral external arcuate fibers: fibers that arise from the arcuate nuclei, emerging from the ventral median fissure, they run laterally, backward, and upward over the medulla oblongata to reach the cerebellum by way of the caudal

inferior cerebellar peduncle; called also *anterior external arcuate fibers* and *fibrae arcuatae externae anteriores* [NA alternative]. **fi′brae arcua′tae inter′nae** [NA], internal arcuate fibers: fibers that arise from the nucleus cuneatus and nucleus gracilis and pass ventromedially around the central gray substance of the medulla oblongata to form the decussation of the medial lemnisci. **fi′brae circula′res mus′culi cilia′ris** [NA], circular fibers of ciliary muscle: the most internal fibers of the ciliary muscle that form a discrete portion of the ciliary muscle and extending around the apex of the ciliary body close to the root of the iris. Called also *Müller fibers* or *muscle* and *sphincteric fibers of ciliary muscle.* **fi′brae corticonuclea′res** [NA], corticonuclear fibers: longitudinal fibers of the pyramidal tract (q.v.) that arise in the cerebral cortex, descend in the internal capsule, and synapse in the various motor nuclei of the mesencephalon, pons, and medulla oblongata. Together they form the corticonuclear tract. Called also *corticobulbar fibers.* **fi′brae corticoponti′nae** [NA], corticopontine fibers: nerve fibers that arise in the cerebral cortex of the frontal, temporal, parietal, and occipital lobes, descend in the internal capsule and cerebral peduncle, and terminate at different levels in the pontine nuclei where they are relayed chiefly to the opposite cerebellar hemisphere. Formerly collectively called *corticopontine tract* and *tractus corticopontinus.* **fi′brae corticoreticula′res** [NA], corticoreticular fibers: nerve fibers that arise chiefly in the sensorimotor areas of the cerebral cortex, descend with corticospinal fibers, and synapse with cells of the reticular formation, especially in the pons and medulla oblongata. **fi′brae corticorubra′les** [NA], corticorubral fibers: nerve fibers that descend from the cortex of the frontal lobe through the posterior limb of the internal capsule to terminate in the red nucleus. **fi′brae corticospina′les** [NA], corticospinal fibers: longitudinal fibers that arise in the cerebral cortex, descend in the internal capsule, mesencephalon, pons, and pyramids of the medulla oblongata and which form, upon reaching the spinal cord, the lateral and ventral corticospinal tracts; see also *pyramidal tract,* under *tract.* **fi′brae corticothala′micae** [NA], corticothalamic fibers: nerve fibers that project from the cerebral cortex through the posterior limb of the internal capsule to terminate in the thalamus. **fi′brae dentatorubra′les** [NA], dentatorubral fibers: afferent nerve fibers received by the red nucleus from the contralateral dentate nucleus; called also *fibrae dentatae rubrales* and *red dentate fibers.* **fi′brae frontoponti′nae** [NA], frontopontine fibers: nerve fibers that arise in the frontal lobe of the cerebral hemisphere and traverse the internal capsule and end in the pontine nuclei. Together they form the frontopontine tract. **fi′brae intercrura′les** [NA], intercrural fibers: fibers joining the medial and lateral crura of the superficial inguinal ring; called also *Cooper's* or *Scarpa's fascia, Todd's process,* and *collateral fibers of Winslow.* **fi′brae len′tis** [NA], fibers of lens: long bands, derived from the epithelium, that make up the substance of the lens; called also *cellulae lentis.* **fi′brae longitudina′les mus′culi cilia′ris,** fibrae meridionales musculi ciliaris. **fi′brae meridiona′les mus′culi cilia′ris** [NA], meridional fibers of ciliary muscle: the most external fibers of the ciliary muscle that run meridionally or longitudinally from the reticulum trabeculae toward the ciliary processes. Called also *Brücke's fibers* and *longitudinal fibers of ciliary muscle.* **fi′brae obli′quae gas′tricae** [NA], oblique gastric fibers: the inner obliquely coursing fibers of the muscular coat of the stomach; called also *fibrae obliquae ventriculi* [NA alternative] and *oblique fibers of stomach.* **fi′brae obli′quae ventric′uli,** NA alternative for *fibrae obliquae gastricae.* **fi′brae paraventricula′res** [NA], paraventricular fibers: the efferent fiber components of the hypothalamicohypysial tract that arise in the paraventricular nucleus and form the paraventriculohypophysial tract. **fi′brae parietotemporoponti′nae** [NA], parietotemporopontine fibers: nerve fibers that arise in the cerebral cortex of the parietal and temporal lobes, descend in the sublentiform part of the posterior limb of the internal capsule to become constituent fibers of the basis pedunculi cerebri of the ventral part of the cerebral peduncle, and end in the pontine nuclei. Formerly divided into the *tractus parietopontinus (parietopontine tract)* and *tractus temporopontinus (temporopontine tract).* **fi′brae periventricula′res** [NA], periventricular fibers: fibers that arise from the hypothalamus, then descend in the central gray matter through the tegmentum of the mesencephalon and the reticular formation of the pons and medulla oblongata; some are found in the dorsal longitudinal fasciculus. **fi′brae pon′tis longitudina′les** [NA], longitudinal fibers of pons: a group of longitudinal nerve fibers that arise in the crus cerebri and run to the ventral part of the pons, where they become dispersed into smaller bundles, separated by the nuclei of the pons and the transverse fibers of the pons. The group includes the corticospinal, corticonuclear, corticoreticular, corticopontine, transverse, and pontocerebellar fibers. **fi′brae pon′tis profun′dae,** the more deeply situated of the fibrae pontis transversae. **fi′brae pon′tis superficia′les,** the more superficial of the fibrae pontis transversae. **fi′brae pon′tis transver′sae** [NA], transverse fibers of pons: fibers within the ventral part of the pons which arise from the pontine nuclei and run laterally to form the middle cerebellar peduncles. Most of these fibers cross the midline. **fi′brae pontocerebella′res** [NA], pontocerebellar fibers: longitudinal fibers in the ventral part of the pons that terminate in the vermis of the cerebellum. **fi′brae pro′priae,** fibrae arcuatae cerebri. **fi′brae radia′les mus′culi cilia′ris** [NA], radial fibers of ciliary muscle: the fibers of the ciliary muscle lying between the meridional (external) fibers and the circular (internal) fibers; they run in a radial or oblique direction from one to another and may form a fibrous network. Called also *oblique fibers of ciliary muscle.* **fi′brae stri′ae termina′lis** [NA], fibers of stria terminalis: the myelinated nerve fibers that make up the stria terminalis. **fi′brae supraop′tica** [NA], supraoptic fibers: the efferent fiber components of the hypothalamicohypophysial tract that arise in supraoptic nucleus and form the supraopticohypophysial tract. **fi′brae temporoponti′nae** [NA], temporopontine fibers: nerve fibers that arise in the temporal lobe and pass through the posterior limb of the internal capsule to end in the pontine nuclei. **fi′brae thalamoparieta′les** [NA], thalamoparietal fibers: nerve fibers that project from the parietal lobe through the posterior limb of the internal capsule to end in the thalamus. **fi′brae zonula′res** [NA], zonular fibers: the fibers that anchor the lens capsule to the ciliary body and the retina; called also *aponeurosis of Zinn.*

fibrae (fi′bre) [L.]   genitive and plural of *fibra.*

fibre (fi′ber)   fiber.

fibrescope (fi′ber-skōp)   fiberscope.

fibril (fi′bril) [L. *fibrilla*]   a minute fiber or filament; often a component of a compound fiber. **border f's,** myoglia. **collagen f's,** delicate fibrils of collagen in connective tissue, usually cemented together in wavy bundles; they are composed of molecules of tropocollagen. Cf. *fibroblast.* **dentinal f's,** component fibrils of the dentinal matrix. **Dirck's f's,** fibrils of elastic tissue binding together the layers of elastic fibers of the tunica media of an artery. **Ebner f's,** (*obs.*) threadlike fibrils in the dentin and in the cementum of a tooth. **fibroglia f's,** see *fibroglia.* **muscle f., muscular f.,** myofibril. **nerve f.,** an axon. **side f. of Golgi,** a delicate twig given off at right angles from a neuraxon near its junction with the ganglion cells. **Tomes f.,** process of odontoblast.

fibrilla (fi-bril′ah), gen. and pl. *fibril′lae* [L., dim. of *fibra*] a fibril.

fibrillae (fi-bril′e) [L.]   genitive and plural of *fibrilla.*

fibrillar, fibrillary (fi′brĭ-lar, fi′brĭ-lār-e)   pertaining to a fibril or to fibrils.

fibrillated (fi′brĭ-lāt-ed)   made up of fibrils.

fibrillation (fi-brĭ-la′shun)   1. the quality of being fibrillar. 2. a small, local, involuntary contraction of muscle, invisible under the skin, resulting from spontaneous activation of single muscle cells or muscle fibers. 3. the initial degenerative changes in osteoarthritis, characterized by softening of the articular cartilage and development of vertical clefts between groups of cartilage cells. **atrial f.,** atrial arrhythmia characterized by rapid randomized contractions of the atrial myocardium, causing a totally irregular, often rapid ventricular rate. **auricular f.,** atrial f. **ventricular f.,** arrhythmia characterized by fibrillary contractions of the ventricular muscle due to rapid repetitive excitation of myocardial fibers without coordinated contraction of the ventricle, an expression of randomized circus movement or of an ectopic focus with a very rapid cycle.

Fibrillenstruktur (fib″ril-len-shtrook′tur) [Ger.]   the

term used to describe the pattern of separate myofibrils that is typical of white skeletal muscles. Cf. *Felderstruktur.*

fibrilloblast (fi-bril′o-blast) [*fibril* + Gr. *blastos* germ] odontoblast.

fibrillogenesis (fi-bril″o-jen′ĕ-sis)   the formation of fibrils.

fibrillolysis (fi″brĭ-lol′ĭ-sis)   the destruction or dissolution of fibrils or fibrillae.

fibrillolytic (fi″bril-o-lit′ik)   destroying or dissolving fibrillae.

fibrin (fi′brin)   the insoluble protein formed from fibrinogen by the proteolytic action of thrombin during normal clotting of blood. Fibrin forms the essential portion of the blood clot. **gluten f.,** a form of fibrin from the seeds of various plants. **Henle's f.,** fibrin formed by precipitating semen with water. **myosin f.,** an insoluble variety of myosin, probably actomyosin. **stroma f.,** fibrin obtained from the stroma of blood corpuscles. **vegetable f.,** gluten f.

fibrinase (fi′brin-ās)   Factor XIII; see *coagulation factors,* under *factor.*

fibrinocellular (fi″brĭ-no-sel′u-lar)   made up of fibrin and cells.

fibrinogen (fi-brin′o-jen) [*fibrin* + Gr. *gennan* to produce] 1. Factor I; see *coagulation factors,* under *factor.* 2. human fibrinogen: a sterile fraction of normal human plasma, dried from the frozen state, which in solution has the property of being converted into soluble fibrin when thrombin is added; administered by intravenous infusion to increase the coagulability of the blood.

fibrinogenase (fi″brin-oj′ĕ-nās)   [*fibrinogen* + *-ase*] thrombin.

fibrinogenemia (fi-brin″o-jĕ-ne′me-ah)   hyperfibrinogenemia.

fibrinogenesis (fi″brĭ-no-jen′ĕ-sis)   the production or formation of fibrin.

fibrinogenic (fi″brĭ-no-jen′ik)   producing or causing the formation of fibrin.

fibrinogenolysis (fi″brĭ-no-jĕ-nol′ĭ-sis) [*fibrinogen* + Gr. *lysis* dissolution]   the dissolution or inactivation of fibrinogen in the blood.

fibrinogenolytic (fi″brĭ-no-jen″o-lit′ik)   pertaining to or inducing fibrinogenolysis.

fibrinogenopenia (fi-brin″o-jen″o-pe′ne-ah)   deficiency of fibrinogen in the blood.

fibrinogenopenic (fi″brin-o-jen″o-pe′nik)   pertaining to or caused by fibrinogenopenia.

fibrinogenous (fi″brĭ-noj′ĕ-nus)   caused by fibrin, or resulting from the formation of fibrin.

fibrinoid (fi′brĭ-noid) [*fibrin* + Gr. *eidos* form]   1. resembling fibrin. 2. a homogeneous, eosinophilic, refractile, relatively acellular material with some of the tinctorial properties of fibrin.

fibrinokinase (fi″brĭ-no-ki′nās)   a name proposed for a plasminogen factor derived from animal tissues.

fibrinolysin (fi″brĭ-nol′ĭ-sin)   plasmin.

fibrinolysis (fi″brĭ-nol′ĭ-sis) [*fibrin* + Gr. *lysis* dissolution] the dissolution of fibrin by enzymatic action.

fibrinolytic (fi″brĭ-no-lit′ik)   pertaining to, characterized by, or causing fibrinolysis.

fibrinopenia (fi″brĭ-no-pe′ne-ah) [*fibrin* + Gr. *penia* poverty]   deficiency of fibrinogen in the blood.

fibrinopeptide (fi″brĭ-no-pep′tid)   a substance split off from fibrinogen, during coagulation, by the action of thrombin.

fibrinoplastin (fi″brĭ-no-plas′tin)   paraglobulin.

fibrinoplatelet (fi″brin-o-plāt′let)   composed of fibrin and platelets, as a blood clot.

fibrinopurulent (fi″brĭ-no-pu′roo-lent)   characterized by the presence of both fibrin and pus.

fibrinorrhea (fi″brĭ-no-re′ah)   a profuse discharge containing fibrin.

fibrinoscopy (fi-brĭ-nos′ko-pe) [*fibrin* + Gr. *skopein* to examine]   inoscopy.

fibrinous (fi′brĭ-nus)   pertaining to or of the nature of fibrin.

fibrinuria (fi″brin-u′re-ah)   the presence of fibrin in the urine.

fibr(o)- [L. *fibra* fiber] a combining form denoting relationship to fibers.

fibroadenia (fi″bro-ah-de′ne-ah) [*fibro-* + Gr. *adēn* gland] fibroid degeneration of gland tissue, especially the reduction in lymphocytes and increase in stroma in the malpighian bodies in Banti's disease.

fibroadenoma (fi″bro-ad″ĕ-no′mah) adenoma containing fibrous tissue. **giant f. of the breast,** a fibroadenoma of large size that may involve much of the mammary gland.

fibroadenosis (fi″bro-ad″ĕ-no′sis) a nodular condition of the breast not due to neoplasm.

fibroadipose (fi″bro-ad′ĭ-pōs) both fibrous and fatty.

fibroangioma (fi″bro-an″je-o′mah) an angioma containing much fibrous tissue. **nasopharyngeal f.,** see under *angiofibroma*.

fibroareolar (fi″bro-ah-re′o-lar) [*fibro-* + L. *areola*] both fibrous and areolar.

fibroatrophy (fi″bro-at′ro-fe) a combination of fibrosis and atrophy.

fibroblast (fi′bro-blast) [*fibro-* + Gr. *blastos* germ] 1. a connective tissue cell; a flat elongated cell with cytoplasmic processes at each end, having a flat, oval, vesicular nucleus. Fibroblasts, which differentiate into chondroblasts, collagenoblasts, and osteoblasts, form the fibrous tissues in the body, tendons, aponeuroses, supporting and binding tissues of all sorts. Called also *fibrocyte* and *desmocyte*. 2. collagenoblast; the collagen-producing cell. Such cells also proliferate at the site of chronic inflammation. **pericryptal f's,** flattened fibroblasts forming a sheath around the intestinal glands of the colon.

fibroblastic (fi″bro-blas′tik) 1. pertaining to fibroblasts. 2. fibroplastic.

fibroblastoma (fi″bro-blas-to′mah) a tumor arising from a fibroblast; such tumors are now differentiated as fibromas or fibrosarcomas. **perineural f.,** a tumor arising from the connective tissue sheath of a neuron, as an acoustic neuroma.

fibrobronchitis (fi″bro-brong-ki′tis) croupous bronchitis.

fibrocalcific (fi″bro-kal-sif′ik) pertaining to or characterized by partially calcified fibrous tissue.

fibrocarcinoma (fi″bro-kar″sĭ-no′mah) scirrhous carcinoma.

fibrocartilage (fi″bro-kar′tĭ-lij) a type of cartilage made up of typical cartilage cells (chondrocytes), with parallel thick, compact collagenous bundles forming the interstitial substances, separated by narrow clefts enclosing the encapsulated cells; called also *stratified cartilage*. For names of specific structures composed of such tissue, see under *fibrocartilago*. **basal f.,** fibrocartilago basalis. **basilar f.,** synchondrosis sphenooccipitalis. **circumferential f.,** fibrocartilage that forms a rim about a joint cavity. **connecting f.,** a disk of fibrocartilage that attaches opposing bones to each other by synchondrosis; called also *spongy f.* **cotyloid f.,** labrum acetabulare. **elastic f.,** fibrocartilage containing elastic fibers. **interarticular f.,** an articular disk (def. 1); see terms beginning *discus articularis*, under *discus*. **intervertebral f's,** disci intervertebrales. **semilunar f's,** crescent-shaped structures resting on the articulating surfaces of the upper end of the tibia, increasing the concavity of the tibial condyles and acting as cushions or shock absorbers; the lateral and medial menisci. **spongy f.,** connecting f. **stratiform f.,** cartilage such as that lining the bony grooves lodging certain tendons. **white f.,** fibrocartilage in which strong bundles of white fibrous tissue predominate. **yellow f.,** fibrocartilage containing bundles of yellow elastic fibers but with little or no white fibrous tissue.

fibrocartilagines (fi″bro-kar″tĭ-laj′ĭ-nēz) [L.] plural of *fibrocartilago*.

fibrocartilaginous (fi″bro-kar″tĭ-laj′ĭ-nus) pertaining to or composed of fibrocartilage.

fibrocartilago (fi″bro-kar″tĭ-lah′go), pl. *fibrocartilag′ines* [L.] [NA] fibrocartilage: a general term for an anatomical structure composed of cartilage the matrix of which contains a considerable amount of fibrous tissue; called also *stratified cartilage*. **f. basa′lis,** basal fibrocartilage: the cartilage that fills the foramen lacerum of the skull. **f. basila′ris,** synchondrosis sphenooccipitalis. **fibrocartilag′ines intervertebra′les,** disci intervertebrales. **f. navicula′-**

ris, a fibrocartilaginous facet on the dorsal surface of the plantar calcaneonavicular ligament that helps form the articular cavity for the head of the talus.

fibrocaseous (fi″bro-ka′se-us) both fibrous and caseous.

fibrocellular (fi″bro-sel′u-lar) partly fibrous and partly cellular.

fibrochondritis (fi″bro-kon-dri′tis) [*fibro-* + *chondritis*] inflammation of a fibrocartilage.

fibrochondroma (fi″bro-kon-dro′mah) [*fibro-* + *chondroma*] chondroma that contains areas of fibrosis.

fibrocollagenous (fi″bro-kol-laj′ĕ-nus) both fibrous and collagenous; pertaining to or composed of fibrous tissue mainly composed of collagen.

fibrocyst (fi′bro-sist) [*fibro-* + Gr. *kystis* sac, bladder] cystic fibroma.

fibrocystic (fi″bro-sis′tik) characterized by the development of cystic spaces, especially in relation to some duct or gland, accompanied by an overgrowth of fibrous tissue.

fibrocystoma (fi″bro-sis-to′mah) cystic fibroma.

fibrocyte (fi′bro-sīt) [*fibro-* + Gr. *kytos* hollow vessel] fibroblast.

fibrocytogenesis (fi″bro-si″to-jen′ĕ-sis) [*fibrocyte* + Gr. *genesis* production] the development of connective tissue fibrils.

fibrodysplasia (fi″bro-dis-pla′se-ah) fibrous dysplasia.

fibroelastic (fi″bro-e-las′tik) composed of fibrous and elastic tissue.

fibroelastosis (fi″bro-e″las-to′sis) overgrowth of fibroelastic elements. **endocardial f.,** a condition characterized by hypertrophy of the wall of the left ventricle and conversion of the endocardium into a thick fibroelastic coat, with the capacity of the ventricle sometimes reduced, but often increased.

fibroenchondroma (fi″bro-en″kon-dro′mah) enchondroma containing fibrous elements.

fibroepithelioma (fi″bro-ep″ĭ-the″le-o′mah) a tumor composed of fibrous and epithelial elements. **premalignant f.,** an uncommon variant of basal cell carcinoma presenting as a firm sessile to pedunculated papule that may have a smooth or nodular surface and variable coloration, usually located on the lower trunk or lumbosacral area in middle-aged or older adults. Histologically, there are interlacing ribbons of cells that extend downward from the surface to form an epithelial meshwork upon a hyperplastic mesodermal stroma. Although the tumor is typically indolent, it may occasionally evolve into a true basal cell carcinoma. Called also *premalignant epithelial tumor*.

fibrofascitis (fi″bro-fah-si′tis) fibrositis.

fibrofatty (fi″bro-fat′e) both fibrous and fatty.

fibrofibrous (fi″bro-fi′brus) joining or connecting fibers.

fibrogenesis (fi″bro-jen′ĕ-sis) [*fibro-* + *genesis*] the development of fibers. **f. imperfec′ta os′sium,** a rare collagen disorder causing osteomalacia, with progressive skeletal pain and tenderness.

fibrogenic (fi″bro-jen′ik) conducive to the development of fibers.

fibroglia (fi-brog′le-ah) [*fibro-* + Gr. *glia* glue] border fibrils in close relation to the surface of fibroblasts, and thought by some to be transformations of the ectoplasm.

fibroglioma (fi″bro-gli-o′mah) a glioma containing an excessive amount of fibrous tissue.

fibrohemorrhagic (fi″bro-hem″o-raj′ik) attended with hemorrhage and fibrin formation.

fibrohistiocytic (fi″bro-his″te-o-sit′ik) having fibrous and histiocytic elements.

fibroid (fi′broid) [*fibro-* + Gr. *eidos* form] 1. having a fibrous structure; resembling a fibroma. 2. a fibroma. 3. leiomyoma; *fibroids* is a colloquial clinical term for leiomyoma uteri.

fibroidectomy (fi″broid-ek′to-me) [*fibroid* + Gr. *ektomē* excision] excision of a fibroma of the uterus.

fibroin (fi-bro′in) a white albuminoid, $C_{15}H_{23}N_3O_6$, from spiders' webs and the cocoons of insects.

fibrolipoma (fi″bro-lĭ-po′mah) [*fibro-* + Gr. *lipos* fat + *-oma*] lipoma containing an excess of fibrous tissue.

fibrolipomatous (fi″bro-lĭ-po′mah-tus) pertaining to fibrolipoma.

fibroma (fi-bro'mah) a tumor composed mainly of fibrous or fully developed connective tissue; called also *fibroid*. **ameloblastic f.,** an odontogenic tumor characterized by the simultaneous proliferation of both epithelial and mesenchymal tissue, without the formation of enamel or dentin. **f. caverno'sum,** a cavernous hemangioma containing an excess of fibrous tissue. **cementifying f.,** cementoblastoma; a tumor usually occurring in the mandible of older persons and consisting of fibroblastic tissue containing masses of cementum-like tissue. **chondromyxoid f.,** a rare, benign, slowly growing tumor of bone of chondroblastic origin, usually affecting the large long bones of the lower extremity; it has distinct histological characteristics and is sometimes mistaken for chondrosarcoma. **concentric f.,** a uterine fibroma surrounding the uterine cavity. **f. cu'tis,** fibroma of the skin. **cystic f.,** a fibroma that has undergone cystic degeneration. **f. du'rum,** hard f. **hard f.,** one composed of fibrous tissue with few cells; called also *f. durum.* **intracanalicular f.,** fibroadenoma of the breast. **juvenile nasopharyngeal f.,** nasopharyngeal angiofibroma. **f. mucino'sum,** a fibroma affected with mucoid degeneration. **f. myxomato'des,** a myxofibroma. **nonosteogenic f.,** a common degenerative and proliferative lesion of the medullary and cortical tissues of bone, occurring most commonly near the ends of the diaphyses of the large long bones, particularly of the lower extremities, often causing no symptoms and discovered only incidentally in roentgenograms of the skeleton made for other reasons. **odontogenic f.,** a rare benign central tumor of the jaw, usually the mandible, originating from the embryonic structures of the tooth germ, dental papilla, or dental follicle. **ossifying f., ossifying f. of bone,** a benign, relatively slow-growing, central bone tumor, usually of the jaws, especially the mandible, which is composed of fibrous connective tissue within which bone is formed. **ossifying f., peripheral,** a fibroma, usually of the gingiva, showing areas of calcification or ossification. Called also *epulis.* **osteogenic f.,** osteoblastoma. **parasitic f.,** a pedunculated, subperitoneal fibroid of the uterus which obtains part or all of its blood supply from the omentum. **f. pen'dulum,** soft f. **rabbit f.,** a naturally occurring benign viral disease of the wild cottontail rabbit, which is transmissible to laboratory rabbits, and marked by the development of fibromas that regress; called also *Shope f.* **recurrent digital f. of childhood,** digital fibromatosis. **f. sarcomato'sum,** fibrosarcoma. **Shope f.,** rabbit f. **soft f.,** a large pedunculated acrochordon. Called also *f. pendulum.* **telangiectatic f.,** angiofibroma. **f. thecocellula're xanthomato'des,** theca cell tumor. **f. xantho'ma,** fibroxanthoma.

fibromatogenic (fi-bro"mah-to-jen'ik) producing or causing the formation of fibroma.

fibromatoid (fi-bro'mah-toid) [*fibroma* + Gr. *eidos* form] resembling fibroma; fibroma-like.

fibromatosis (fi"bro-mah-to'sis) the formation of a fibrous, tumor-like nodule arising from the deep fascia with a tendency to local recurrence, as in desmoid tumor. **f. col'li,** a firm, fusiform, fibrous mass in the midportion of the sternocleidomastoid muscle, usually occurring between two weeks and two months of age, and commonly disappearing in four to eight months; in some instances, torticollis may develop. It is believed by some to be a small hematoma due to injury to the muscle at birth. **congenital generalized f.,** a condition in which multiple small, firm, spherical or ovoid fibromas of the subcutaneous and muscle tissues, the viscera, and osseous systems are characteristically present at birth. Visceral involvement may be responsible for various symptoms, such as intestinal obstruction, diarrhea due to diffuse involvement of the intestines, and respiratory disturbances. Death frequently occurs during the neonatal period or early infancy. **f. gingi'vae, gingival f.,** generalized or localized diffuse fibrous overgrowth of the gingival tissue, usually transmitted as an autosomal dominant trait, but some cases are idiopathic and others produced by drugs (see *Dilantin gingivitis,* under *gingivitis*). The enlarged gingiva is pink, firm, and has a leather-like consistency with a minutely pebbled surface and in severe cases the teeth are almost completely covered and the enlargement projects into the oral vestibule. Called also *elephantiasis gingivae, keloid of gums,* and *macrogingivae.* **infantile digital f.,** a rare, often recurrent, condition, usually occurring in infants less than a year old, in which one or more small, smooth,

dome-shaped, skin-colored to slightly red nodules occur on the lateral or dorsal aspects of the fingers and toes; histologically, the lesions are composed of fibrous connective tissue and abundant collagen, and contain characteristic virus-like, black intracellular inclusions. Called also *recurring digital fibrous tumors of childhood.* **palmar f.,** fibromatosis involving the palmar fascia, and resulting in Dupuytren's contracture. **plantar f.,** fibromatosis involving the plantar fascia, manifested as single or multiple nodular swellings, sometimes accompanied by pain but usually unassociated with contractures. **subcutaneous pseudosarcomatous f.,** proliferative fasciitis. **f. ventric'uli,** linitis plastica.

fibromatous (fi-bro'mah-tus) pertaining to or of the nature of fibroma.

fibromectomy (fi"bro-mek'to-me) [*fibroma* + Gr. *ektomē* excision] excision of a fibroma.

fibromembranous (fi"bro-mem'brah-nus) composed of membrane containing much fibrous tissue.

fibromuscular (fi"bro-mus'ku-lar) composed of fibrous and muscular tissue.

fibromyitis (fi"bro-mi-i'tis) [*fibro-* + Gr. *mys* muscle + *-itis*] inflammation and fibrous degeneration of a muscle.

fibromyoma (fi"bro-mi-o'mah) [*fibro* + Gr. *mys* muscle + *-oma*] leiomyoma. **f. u'teri,** leiomyoma uteri.

fibromyomectomy (fi"bro-mi"o-mek'to-me) excision of a fibromyoma (leiomyoma).

fibromyositis (fi"bro-mi"o-si'tis) [*fibro-* + Gr. *mys* muscle + *-itis*] inflammation of fibromuscular tissue. **nodular f.,** a disease marked by inflammation and the formation of nodules in the muscles.

fibromyxoma (fi"bro-mik-so'mah) myxofibroma.

fibromyxosarcoma (fi"bro-mik"so-sar-ko'mah) myxosarcoma or myxoid liposarcoma that is undergoing fibrosis.

fibronectin (fi"bro-nek'tin) [*fibro-* + L. *nexus* a connecting] an adhesive glycoprotein: one form circulates in plasma, acting as an opsonin; another is a cell-surface protein which mediates cellular adhesive interactions. Fibronectins are important in connective tissue, where they cross-link to collagen, and they are also involved in aggregation of platelets.

fibroneuroma (fi"bro-nu-ro'mah) neurofibroma.

fibronuclear (fi"bro-nu'kle-ar) made up of nucleated fibers.

fibro-osteoma (fi"bro-os"te-o'mah) an ossifying fibroma.

fibropapilloma (fi"bro-pap"ĭ-lo'mah) a papilloma containing much fibrous tissue; called also *fibroepithelial papilloma.*

fibropituicyte (fi"bro-pĭ-tu"ĭ-sīt) see *pituicyte.*

fibroplasia (fi"bro-pla'se-ah) the formation of fibrous tissue, as occurs normally in the healing of wounds and abnormally in some tissues. **retrolental f.,** a bilateral retinopathy occurring in premature infants treated with excessively high concentrations of oxygen, characterized by vascular dilatation, proliferation, and tortuosity, edema, and retinal detachment, with ultimate conversion of the retina into a fibrous mass that can be seen as a dense retrolental membrane; usually, growth of the eye is arrested and may result in microophthalmia, and blindness may occur. Called also *retinopathy of prematurity, RLF,* and *Terry's syndrome.*

fibroplastic (fi"bro-plas'tik) [*fibro-* + Gr. *plassein* to form] giving origin to fibrous tissue.

fibroplate (fi'bro-plāt) an interarticular fibrocartilage.

fibropolypus (fi"bro-pol'ĭ-pus) a polyp containing fibrous elements.

fibropurulent (fi-bro-pu'roo-lent) characterized by the presence of both fibers and pus.

fibroreticulate (fi"bro-re-tik'u-lāt) composed of a network of fibers.

fibrosarcoma (fi"bro-sar-ko'mah) a sarcoma derived from fibroblasts that produce collagen. **odontogenic f.,** a malignant tumor of the jaws, originating from one of the mesenchymal components of the tooth or tooth germ, and histologically identical with other fibrosarcomas; the malignant counterpart of odontogenic fibroma.

fibrosclerosis (fi"bro-skle-ro'sis) fibrosis associated with sclerosis. **multifocal f.,** any of a group of disorders of unknown etiology characterized by fibrosis, including mediastinal, hilar, and retroperitoneal fibrosis, Reidel's struma, and sclerosing cholangitis.

fibrose (fi′brōs) 1. to form fibrous tissue. 2. fibrous.

fibroserous (fi″bro-se′rus) composed of both fibrous and serous elements.

fibrosis (fi-bro′sis) the formation of fibrous tissue; fibroid or fibrous degeneration. **African endomyocardial f.,** endomyocardial f. **congenital hepatic f.,** a developmental disorder of the liver marked by formation of irregular broad bands of fibrous tissue containing multiple cysts formed by disordered terminal bile ducts, chiefly in the portal areas, resulting in vascular constriction, which leads to portal hypertension. It may be associated with polycystic renal disease. **cystic f., cystic f. of the pancreas,** a generalized, autosomal recessive disorder of infants, children, and young adults, in which there is widespread dysfunction of the exocrine glands; characterized by signs of chronic pulmonary disease (due to excess mucus production in the respiratory tract), pancreatic deficiency, abnormally high levels of electrolytes in the sweat, and occasionally by biliary cirrhosis. Pathologically, the pancreas shows obstruction of the pancreatic ducts by amorphous eosinophilic concretions, with consequent deficiency of pancreatic enzymes, resulting in steatorrhea and azotorrhea. The degree of involvement of organs and glandular systems may vary greatly, with consequent variations in the clinical picture. Called also *fibrocystic disease of the pancreas* and *mucoviscidosis.* **diatomite f.,** a form of silicosis caused by inhalation of diatomaceous earth (silicon dioxide). **diffuse interstitial pulmonary f.,** idiopathic pulmonary f. **endomyocardial f.,** idiopathic myocardiopathy occurring endemically in various regions of Africa and rarely in other areas, characterized by cardiomegaly, marked thickening of the endocardium with dense, white fibrous tissue that frequently extends to involve the inner third or half of the myocardium, and congestive heart failure. Called also *African endomyocardial f.* **graphite f.,** a form of silicosis caused by the inhalation of graphite, which may contain as much as 10 per cent silicon dioxide. **idiopathic pulmonary f.,** chronic inflammation and progressive fibrosis of the pulmonary alveolar walls, with steadily progressive dyspnea, resulting finally in death from oxygen lack or right heart failure. Called also *diffuse interstitial pulmonary f.* The acute, rapidly fatal form is often called *Hamman-Rich syndrome.* **idiopathic retroperitoneal f.,** retroperitoneal f. **mediastinal f.,** development of whitish, hard fibrous tissue in the upper mediastinum, causing compression, distortion, or obliteration of the superior vena cava, and sometimes constriction of the bronchi and large pulmonary vessels. **neoplastic f.,** proliferative f. **nodular subepidermal f.,** the formation, beneath the epidermis, of multiple fibrous nodules as the result of productive inflammation. **panmural f. of the bladder,** chronic interstitial cystitis. **periureteric f.,** progressive development of fibrous tissue, spreading laterally from the great midline vessels, gradually engulfing, distorting, and finally causing strangulation of one or both ureters. **postfibrinous f.,** fibrosis occurring in tissues in which fibrin has been deposited. **proliferative f.,** fibrosis in which the fibrous elements continue to proliferate after the original causative factor has ceased to operate; called also *neoplastic f.* **pulmonary f.,** see *idiopathic pulmonary f.* **replacement f.,** the development of fibrous tissues to replace tissue that has been damaged. **retroperitoneal f.,** deposition of fibrous tissue in the retroperitoneal space, producing vague abdominal discomfort, and often causing blockage of the ureters, with resultant hydronephrosis and impaired renal function, which may result in renal failure. **root sleeve f.,** fibrosis and thickening of the dura mater resulting from prolonged nerve root pressure. **f. u′teri,** a morbid condition characterized by overgrowth of the smooth muscle and increase in the collagenous fibrous tissue, producing a thickened, coarse, tough myometrium.

fibrositis (fi″bro-si′tis) [*fibrous* tissue + *-itis*] inflammatory hyperplasia of the white fibrous tissue of the body, especially of the muscle sheaths and fascial layers of the locomotor system; it is marked by pain and stiffness. Called also *fibrofascitis* and *muscular rheumatism.*

fibrothorax (fi″bro-tho′raks) a condition characterized by adhesion of the two layers of pleura, the lung being covered by a thick layer of nonexpansible fibrous tissue; often a consequence of traumatic hemothorax or of effusion.

fibrotic (fi-brot′ik) pertaining to or characterized by fibrosis.

fibrous (fi′brus) composed of or containing fibers.

fibrovascular (fi″bro-vas′ku-lar) both fibrous and vascular.

fibroxanthoma (fi″bro-zan-tho′mah) a type of xanthoma containing fibromatous elements.

fibula (fib′u-lah) [L. "buckle"] [NA] the outer and smaller of the two bones of the leg, which articulates proximally with the tibia and distally is joined to the tibia in a syndesmosis. See Plate accompanying *skeleton.*

fibular (fib′u-lar) pertaining to the fibula; peroneal.

fibularis (fib″u-la′ris) fibular; [NA] a term designating relationship to the fibula.

fibulocalcaneal (fib″u-lo-kal-ka′ne-al) pertaining to the fibula and calcaneus.

F.I.C.D. Fellow of the International College of Dentists.

ficin (fi′sin) [EC 3.4.22.3] an enzyme of the hydrolase class that catalyzes the hydrolysis of proteins preferentially at lysine, alanine, tyrosine, glycine, asparagine, leucine, and valine bonds. It is a cysteine proteinase derived from the sap of fig trees. It is used as a protein digestant, as a veterinary anthelmintic, and to enhance the agglutination of red blood cells with IgG antibodies such as Rh antibodies.

Fick principle (formula, method) (fik) [Adolph Eugen *Fick,* German physiologist, 1829–1901] see under *principle.*

Ficker's diagnosticum (fik′erz) [Philipp Martin *Ficker,* German bacteriologist, 1868–1950] see under *diagnosticum.*

F.I.C.S. Fellow of the International College of Surgeons.

fidicinales (fi-dis″ĭ-na′lez) [pl., from L. *fidicen, fidicinis,* a player on the harp] musculi lumbricales manus.

fieber (fe′ber) [Ger.] fever.

Fiedler's disease, myocarditis (fēd′lerz) [Carl Ludwig Alfred *Fiedler,* German physician, 1835–1921] see *Weil's syndrome,* under *syndrome,* and see *acute isolated myocarditis,* under *myocarditis.*

field (fēld) 1. an area or open space, as an operative field or visual field. 2. a range of specialization in knowledge, study, or occupation. 3. in embryology, the developing region within a range of modifying factors. **absolute f.,** that area of the cerebral cortex in which injury always causes paralysis or spasm. **auditory f.,** the space or range within which stimuli may be perceived as sound. **Cohnheim's f's,** see under *area.* **dark-f.,** see under *microscope,* and see *ultramicroscope.* **f. of fixation,** the region bounded by the utmost limits of central or clear vision, the eye being allowed to move, but the head being fixed. **Flechsig's f.,** the myelinogenetic field. **f's of Forel, Forel's f's,** three areas in the ventral thalamus that are rich in nerve fibers and associated with cell groups. They are designated: *Field H,* lying medial to the subthalamic nucleus, immediately rostral to the red nucleus, is a large area in which pallidofugal, dentatothalamic, and rubrothalamic fibers and associated nuclei merge, uniting fields H_1 and H_2; called also *f. H. of Forel, prerubral f.,* and *tegmental f. Field H_1* is the area occupied by the thalamic fasciculus, although the term is sometimes used synonymously with thalamic fasciculus; called also *f. H_1 of Forel. Field H_2* is the area along the course of the lenticular fasciculus where the fibers of the fasciculus merge with the dorsal aspect of the subthalamic nucleus and the ventral aspect of the zona incerta; called also *f. H_2 of Forel.* Called also *areas of Forel.* **gamma f.,** any area subjected to radiation from an unshielded or slightly shielded gamma radiation source. **f. H, f. H of forel,** see under *f's of Forel.* **f. H_1, f. H_1 of Forel,** see under *f's of Forel.* **f. H_2, f. H_2 of Forel,** see under *f's of Forel.* **high-power f.,** the area of a slide visible under the high magnification system of a microscope. **individuation f.,** a region in which an organizer influences adjacent tissue to become a part of a total embryo. **Krönig's f.** (obs.), the area of resonance on the chest due to the apices of the lungs. **low-power f.,** the area of a slide visible under the low magnification system of a microscope. **magnetic f.,** that portion of space about a magnet in which its action is perceptible. **f. of a microscope,** the area that can be seen through a microscope at one time. The *high-power field* is that area which is visible under the high-power objective; the *low-power field* is that which is visible under low power.

morphogenetic f., an embryonic region, larger than its main derivatives, out of which definite structures normally develop. **myelinogenetic f.,** a collection of fibers in the neuraxis which at a definite stage of development receive myelin sheaths; called also *Flechsig's field*. **penumbra f.,** the region of free space which is irradiated by primary photons coming from only part of the radiation source. **prerubral f.,** see *f. H,* under *f's of Forel.* **primary nail f.,** a flat area on the terminal phalanx in the embryo where the nail is to develop. **relative f.,** an area of the cerebral cortex in which a lesion may or may not cause paralysis. **surplus f.,** the portion of the field of vision in partial hemianopia which passes beyond the point of fixation. **tegmental f.,** see *f. H,* under *f's of Forel.* **f. of vision,** visual f. **f. of vision, cribriform,** a field of vision over which a number of isolated scotomas lie dispersed. **visual f.,** the area within which stimuli will produce the sensation of sight when the eye in a straight-ahead position; also called *field of vision.* **Wernicke's f.,** see under *area.*

Fielding's membrane (fēld'ingz) [George Hunsley *Fielding,* English anatomist, 1801–1871] the tapetum, def. 2.

fièvre (fe-evr') [Fr.] fever. **f. boutonneuse** (fe-evr' boo-ton-uz'), boutonneuse fever.

FIGLU formiminoglutamic acid.

figuratum (fig"u-ra'tum) [L.] figured; a term used to describe skin lesions that have a geometric, usually circular or annular, pattern.

figure (fig'ūr) [L. *figura,* from *fingere* to shape or form] 1. an object of a particular form. 2. a number, or numeral. **fortification f's,** a form of migraine aura characterized by scintillating, colored lights or zigzag luminous bands suggestive of the walls of a turret. **Minkowski's f.,** a numerical expression of the relation between dextrose and nitrogen in the urine on a pure meat diet, and when fasting. It is 2.8:1. **mitotic f's,** stages of chromosome aggregation exhibiting a pattern characteristic of mitosis. **Purkinje's f's,** patterns of shadows of retinal blood vessels cast onto the retina by obliquely projected light; called also *Purkinje's shadows.* **Stifel's f.,** a black disk having a white spot in the center, used for locating and measuring the blind spot in the eye. **Zöllner's f's,** see under *line.*

fila (fi'lah) [L.] plural of *filum.*

filaceous (fi-la'shus) made up of filaments.

filament (fil'ah-ment) [L. *filamentum,* from *filum* thread] a delicate fiber or thread. **acrosomal f.,** a long, thin, rigid filament projecting from the head of a spermatozoon; it is formed by elongation of the central part of the acrosome in preparation for the fertilization process, and is used to make contact with and to penetrate the cell membrane of the ovum. **axial f.,** axoneme. **linin f.,** a network of linin spread throughout the cell nucleus. **lymphatic anchoring f's,** filaments that attach the endothelial cells of lymphatic capillaries to the connective tissue between surrounding tissue cells. **meningeal f., f. of meninges,** filum terminale. **polar f.,** a hollow, extensible, filamentous tubular organelle found coiled in the polar capsule of spores of certain protozoa that serves to anchor the parasite to the host's tissues. Called also *polar tube.* 2. see under *tube,* def. 1. **root f's of spinal nerves,** fila radicularia nervorum spinalium. **spermatic f.,** end piece, def. 2. **spinal f.,** filum terminale. **terminal f.,** 1. filum terminale. 2. end piece (def. 2). **terminal f., dural, terminal f., external,** filum terminale externum. **terminal f., internal, terminal f., pial,** filum terminale internum. **terminal f. of spinal dura mater,** filum terminale externum.

filamenta (fil"ah-men'tah) [L.] plural of *filamentum.*

filamentous (fil-ah-men'tus) composed of long, threadlike structures; said of bacterial colonies.

filamentum (fil"ah-men'tum), pl. *filamen'ta* [L.] a filament.

filar (fi'lar) [L. *filum* thread] threadlike; filamentous.

Filaria (fi-la're-ah) [L. *filum* thread] a former loosely applied generic name for members of the superfamily Filarioidea. **F. bancrof'ti,** *Wuchereria bancrofti.* **F. conjuncti'vae,** a species, possibly identical with *Dirofilaris conjunctivae,* found in the eye of horses and asses, and sometimes in man; called also *F. palpebralis.* **F. demarquay'i,** *Mansonella ozzardi.* **F. diur'na,** *Loa loa.* The name was actually applied to the microfilaria (*microfilaria diurna*). **F. equi'na,** *Setaria equina.* **F. immit'is,**

Dirofilaria immitis. **F. jun'cea,** *Mansonella ozzardi.* **F. lo'a,** *Loa loa.* **F. medinen'sis,** *Dracunculus medinensis.* **F. noctur'na,** *Wuchereria bancrofti.* **F. oz-zar'di,** *Mansonella ozzardi.* **F. palpebra'lis,** *F. conjunctivae.* **F. per'stans,** *Mansonella perstans.* **F. recon'dita,** *Dipetalonema reconditum.* **F. san'guin-is-hom'inis,** *Wuchereria bancrofti.* **F. vol'vulus,** *Onchocerca volvulus.*

filaria (fi-la're-ah), pl. *fila'riae* [L. *filum* thread] a nematode worm of the superfamily Filarioidea. **Bancroft's f.,** *Wuchereria bancrofti.* **Brug's f.,** *Brugia malayi.*

filariae (fi-la're-e) [L.] plural of *filaria.*

filarial (fi-la're-al) pertaining to, caused by, or denoting filariae.

filariasis (fil"ah-ri'ah-sis) a diseased state due to the presence of filariae within the body. **Bancroft's f., f. bancrof'ti, bancroftian f.,** infection with the filarial worm *Wuchereria bancrofti,* the adults of which reside in the lymphatic system, producing recurrent lymphangitis with fibrosis and obstruction. In extensive obstruction, chronic edema may result, progressing to elephantiasis. The disease is transmitted by mosquitoes, which harbor the larval forms (microfilariae). **Brug's f., Malayan f., ma'layi,** infection with the filarial worm *Brugia malayi,* the adult forms of which reside in the lymphatics, lymph nodes, and connective tissue; symptoms range from asymptomatic adenitis, to periodic attacks of fever and lymphangitis, to elephantiasis, especially of the legs and feet. The disease is transmitted by mosquitoes. **occult f.,** a condition in which microfilariae are present in the tissues but not in the blood; see *tropical eosinophilia,* under *eosinophilia.* **Ozzard's f.,** infection with *Mansonella ozzardi.*

filaricidal (fi-lār"i-sīd'al) [*filaria* + L. *caedere* to kill] destructive to filariae.

filaricide (fi-lār'i-sīd) an agent that is destructive to filariae.

filariform (fi-lār'i-form) threadlike; resembling filariae; denoting that developmental stage in the life cycle of certain nematodes which is characterized by the possession of an esophagus of uniform diameter and which is often, as in hookworms, the infective stage.

Filarioidea (fi-lār"e-oi'de-ah) a superfamily or order of nematode parasites, the adults being threadlike worms which invade the tissues and body cavities where the female deposits embryonated eggs (prelarvae) known as microfilariae. These microfilariae are ingested by blood-sucking insects in whom they pass their developmental stage and are returned to man by the bites of such insects. The filariae of man belong to the genera *Wuchereria, Onchocerca, Loa, Dipetalonema, Mansonella, Dirofilaria,* and *Brugia.*

Filatov's (Filatow's) disease (fi-lat'ofs) [Nils Fédorovich *Filatov,* pediatrician in Moscow, 1847–1902] infectious mononucleosis.

Filatov-Dukes disease (fi-lat'of-dūks) [Nils Fédorovich *Filatov;* Clement *Dukes,* English physician, 1845–1925] Dukes' disease.

Fildes enrichment agar (fil'dez) [Paul Gordon *Fildes,* English bacteriologist, born 1882] see *Table of Culture Media,* under *culture medium.*

file (fīl) a surgical or a dental instrument with a finely serrated surface, for reducing surplus hard substance such as bone or materials used in dental restorations, or for smoothing roughened surfaces. **endodontic f.,** root canal f. **root canal f.,** an endodontic instrument for cleaning and shaping the root canals of a tooth. Called also *endodontic f.*

filicic acid (fi-lis'ik) an acid from filix mas (male fern); it has limited use in veterinary medicine as an anthelmintic for cattle, sheep, and goats. Called also *filixic acid.*

filicin (fil'i-cin) a compound found in aspidium.

filiform (fil'i-form, fi'li-form) [L. *filum* thread + *forma* form] 1. thread shaped. 2. an extremely slender bougie.

filioparental (fil"e-o-pah-ren'tal) pertaining to the relationships between children and their parents.

filipin (fi'li-pin) chemical name: 4,6,8,10,12,14,16,27-octahydroxy-3-(1-hydroxyethyl)-17,28-dimethyloxacyclooctacosa-17,19,21,23,25-pentaen-2-one; an antifungal antibiotic, $C_{35}H_{58}O_{11}$. Called also *filipin III.*

Filipovitch's (Filipowicz's) sign (fi-le'po-vich"ez) [Casimir *Filipovitch*, Polish physician of the 19th century] see under *sign*.

filix (fi'liks), pl. *fil'ices* [L.] a fern. **f. mas,** male fern; see *aspidium*.

filixic acid (fĭ-lik'sik) filicic acid.

fillet (fil'et) 1. a loop, as of cord or tape, for making traction on the fetus. 2. in the nervous system, a long band of nerve fibers, such as the medial lemniscus.

filling (fil'ing) 1. the material inserted into a prepared tooth cavity, usually gold, amalgam, cement, or a synthetic resin. 2. the process of inserting, condensing, shaping, and finishing a filling in a prepared tooth cavity or root canal. Called also *restoration*. **complex f.,** a filling for a complex cavity. **composite f.,** a filling that consists of a composite resin. **compound f.,** a filling for a cavity that involves two surfaces of a tooth. **direct f.,** one that is formed and completed directly in the prepared tooth cavity. **direct resin f.,** a direct filling made from a synthetic resin. **ditched f.,** the marginal failure of an amalgam restoration due to fracture of either the material or the tooth structure itself in the affected area. **indirect f.,** one that is constructed on a die that has been made from an accurate impression of the tooth and that is then inserted into the tooth cavity. **permanent f.,** a filling intended to provide complete function while the tooth remains in the oral cavity. **retrograde f.,** an amalgam or other restoration placed in the apical portion of a tooth to seal the root canal following surgical removal of a periapical lesion, which is performed through the apex of a tooth, approached through the alveolar bone. Called also *retrograde amalgam*. **reverse f.,** retrofilling. **root canal f.,** 1. material(s) placed inside a root canal for the purpose of obturating or sealing it. 2. canal obturation. **root-end f.,** retrofilling. **temporary f.,** a filling placed in a tooth cavity with the intention of removing it within a short period of time. **treatment f.,** a filling used to allay sensitive dentin prior to final preparation of the cavity.

film (film) 1. a thin layer or coating. 2. a thin transparent sheet of cellulose acetate or similar material coated on one or both sides with an emulsion that is sensitive to light or radiation. **bite-wing f.,** one with a central protruding tab or wing to be held between the upper and lower teeth; used in dental radiography. **fixed blood f.,** a thin film of blood spread on a slide, dried quickly, and fixed. **gelatin f., absorbable** [USP] a sterile, nonantigenic, absorbable, water-insoluble gelatin film, used as a local hemostatic. **lateral jaw f.,** a radiograph showing either the ramus or the body of the mandible. **occlusal f.,** a radiograph showing topographic and cross-sectional views of the maxillary or mandibular dental structure and adjacent tissue. **periapical f.,** one used in radiography of the root apex of a tooth and the surrounding structures. **plain f.,** a radiograph made without the use of a contrast medium. **spot f.,** a radiograph of a small anatomic area obtained (*a*) by rapid exposure during fluoroscopy to provide a permanent record of a transiently observed abnormality, or (*b*) by limitation of radiation passing through the area to improve definition and detail of the image produced. **sulfa f.,** a film made from an emulsion of sulfadiazine, sulfanilamide, and methyl cellulose; used as a dressing for burns, cuts, and skin grafts. **x-ray f.,** a film specially prepared for use in roentgenograph; also, a roentgenogram.

film badge (film baj) a pack of radiographic film or films, used for the detection and approximate measurement of radiation exposure of personnel.

filopodia (fi''lo-po'de-ah) [L.] plural of *filopodium*.

filopodium (fi''lo-po'de-um), pl. *filopo'dia* [L. *filum* thread + Gr. *pous* foot] a slender filamentous pseudopodium with a pointed end, branched or unbranched, consisting mostly of ectoplasm. Cf. *axopodium, lobopodium,* and *reticulopodium*.

filopressure (fi'lo-presh''ūr) [L. *filum* thread + *pressura* pressure] the compression of a blood vessel by a thread.

Filosea (fi-lo'se-ah) [L. *filum* thread] a class of ameboid protozoa (superclass Rhizopoda, subphylum Sarcodina) characterized by the presence of hyaline filiform pseudopodia that often branch and sometimes anastomose. It includes two orders: Aconchulinida and Gromida.

filovaricosis (fi'lo-var''ĭ-ko'sis) the development of varicosities on the axon of a nerve fiber.

filter (fil'ter) [L. *filtrum*] 1. a device for the straining of wa-

ter or other liquid. 2. in radiology, a solid screen usually of varying thickness of metal (aluminum, copper, tin, lead, etc.) which when placed in the pathway of the radiation beam prevents transmission of beta particles and photons of longer wavelengths. **Berkefeld f.,** a bacterial filter made of diatomaceous earth, available in three porosities: V (*viel*, or coarse), N (normal), and W (*wenig*, or fine). Most bacteria are removed by the V filter; all are usually removed by the N; and the W is used for exceedingly small organisms. **Chamberland f.,** a bacterial filter made of unglazed porcelain, available in several graded porosities. **collodion f.,** a synthetic cellulose nitrate membrane with uniform pore sizes, used as a microbiological filter and for estimating the size of viral particles. **Hemming f.,** a bacterial filter that uses centrifugal force to move liquid through a filter pad into a receiving vessel. **intermittent sand f.,** a sand filter to which sewage is applied for only a short time and then is allowed to drain away so that aeration and oxidation may take place. **Kimray-Greenfield f.,** an umbrella filter consisting of six stainless-steel struts; small hooks on the ends of the struts anchor the filter in the vena cava when it is opened. **mechanical f.,** a filter of sand or other porous material through which water is forced rapidly to remove gross particles; these particles may be the precipitate caused by the addition of some coagulant. **membrane f.,** a filter made up of a thin film of collodion, cellulose acetate, or other material, available in a wide range of defined pore sizes, the smaller ones being capable of retaining all the known viruses. **Millipore f.,** trademark for a cellulose acetate filter used to sterilize heat-labile solutions, e.g., intravenous solutions. **Mobin-Uddin f.,** an umbrella filter consisting of six stainless-steel spokes connected to a hub and covered by a perforated, heparin-impregnated Silastic membrane. **percolating f.,** trickling f. **roughing f., scrubbing f.,** a coarse-grained filter through which turbid water is passed to remove the larger particles and thus protect the sand filter from clogging. **Seitz f.,** a bacterial filter in which the filtering element is an asbestos or asbestos and cellulose pad, fitted between sample and receiving vessels. **sintered glass f.,** a filter of sintered glass, available in various porosities, sometimes designed C (coarse), M (medium), F (fine), and UF (ultrafine); only the ultrafine is bacteria-proof. **slow sand f.,** a filter made of sand and gravel through which water passes slowly and is purified largely by the action of the microorganisms growing on the surface of the grains of sand near the top of the filter. **sprinkling f.,** a trickling filter in which the sewage is applied by spray. **trickling f.,** beds of porous material on which sewage is distributed and allowed to percolate through to drains laid on a tight floor; the purpose is to so oxidize the organic material as to make it nonputrescible. Called also *percolating f*. **umbrella f.,** a filter used in transvenous interruption of the inferior vena cava for the prevention of pulmonary embolism; it is inserted in a folded position and springs open like an umbrella to engage the caval wall. **Wood's f.,** see under *light*.

filterable (fil'ter-ah-b'l) capable of passing through the pores of a filter; usually referring to living infectious agents (i.e., viruses) able to pass through a filter that retains the usual pathogenic bacteria.

filtrable (fil'trah-b'l) filterable.

filtrate (fil'trāt) a liquid that has passed through a filter. **glomerular f.,** the ultrafiltrate of plasma that passes across the membranes of the malpighian corpuscles of the kidney to the lumen of Bowman's capsule.

filtration (fil-tra'shun) 1. the passage of a liquid through a filter, accomplished by gravity, pressure, or vacuum (suction). 2. in radiology, the use of a solid screen usually made of metal (aluminum, copper, tin, lead, etc.) to absorb beta particles and photons of longer wavelengths. **gel f.,** column chromatography in which high molecular weight substances are separated according to molecular size.

fil'trum ventric'uli [L.] a depression between the two projections formed in the lateral wall of the vestibule of the larynx by the arytenoid and cuneiform cartilages; called also *Merkel's filtrum*.

filum (fi'lum), pl. *fi'la* [L.] [NA] a threadlike structure or part. **fi'la anastomot'ica ner'vi acus'tici,** an anastomotic filament between the vestibulocochlear and facial nerves in the internal acoustic meatus. **f. du'rae ma'tris spina'le** [NA], f. terminale externum. **f. menin'gea'le, f. menin'geum,** f. terminale. **fi'la olfac-**

to′ria, nervi olfactorii. fi′la radicula′ria nervo′rum spina′lium [NA], the threadlike filaments by which the dorsal and ventral roots of each spinal nerve are attached to the spinal cord; called also *root filaments of spinal nerves.* f. spina′le, f. terminale. f. termina′le [NA], terminal filament: a slender threadlike filament of connective tissue that descends from the conus medullaris to the base of the coccyx. Called also *f. meningeale, f. meningeum, f. spinale, meningeal filament, filament of meningeum,* and *spinal filament.* See also *f. terminale externum* and *f. terminale internum.* f. termina′le dura′le, NA alternative for *f. terminale externum.* f. termina′le exter′num [NA], external terminal filament: the downward prolongation of the spinal dura mater from the lower border of the second sacral vertebra to the first coccygeal vertebral segment. Called also *dural terminal filament, f. durae matris spinale, f. terminale durale* [NA alternative], and *terminal filament of spinal dura mater.* f. termina′le inter′num [NA], internal terminal filament: the prolongation of the spinal pia mater, surrounded by extensions of the dural and arachnoid meninges, from the conus medullaris to the lower border of the second sacral vertebra. Called also *f. terminale pialis* [NA alternative] and *pial terminal filament.* f. termina′le pia′lis, NA alternative for *f. terminale internum.*

fimbria (fim′bre-ah) [L. *fimbriae* (pl.) a fringe] 1. a fringe, border, or edge; [NA] a general term for such a structure. 2. pilus (def. 2). f. hippocam′pi [NA], the band of white matter along the medial edge of the ventricular surface of the hippocampus; called also *corpus fimbriatum hippocampi.* ovarian f., f. ova′rica [NA], the longest of the processes that make up the fimbriae tubae uterinae, extending along the free border of the mesosalpinx; called also *fimbriated extremity.* fim′briae of tongue, plica fimbriata. fim′briae tu′bae uteri′nae [NA], fimbriae of uterine tube, the numerous divergent fringelike processes on the distal part of the infundibulum of the uterine tube.

Fimbriaria (fim″bre-a′re-ah) a genus of tapeworms of the family Hymenolepididae, which are parasites of anseriform birds. F. fascio·la′ris, a tapeworm infecting wild and domestic fowl.

fimbriated (fim′bre-āt-ed) [L. *fimbriatus*] fringed.

fimbriation (fim″bre-a′shun) the formation of or the possession of fimbriae.

fimbriatum (fim″bre-a′tum) [L.] fringed.

fimbriocele (fim′bre-o-sēl″) [*fimbria* + Gr. *kēlē* hernia] hernia containing fimbriae of the uterine tube.

finder (fīnd′er) a device on a microscope to facilitate the finding of some object in the field.

finding (fīnd′ing) an observation; a condition discovered.

finger (fing′ger) any of the five digits of the hand. **baseball f.,** partial permanent flexion of the terminal phalanx of a finger caused by a ball or other object striking the end or back of the finger, resulting in rupture of the attachment of the extensor tendon; called also *mallet f.* **blubber f.,** seal f. **bolster f's,** the swollen fingers that result from a *Candida* infection in workers who handle sugar. **clubbed f.,** a deformity produced by proliferation of the soft tissues about the terminal phalanx, with no constant osseous changes; seen in various cases of chronic disease of the thoracic organs. **dead f.,** a numb, mottled finger, as one seen in acrocyanosis. **drop f.,** mallet f. **drumstick f.,** clubbed f. **first f.,** the thumb (*pollex* [NA]). **giant f.,** macrodactyly. **hammer f.,** mallet f. **hippocratic f's,** enlargement of the terminal phalanges, with coarse nails curving over the ends of the fingers (hippocratic nails); see *hypertrophic pulmonary osteoarthropathy,* under *osteoarthropathy.* **index f.,** the second digit of the hand, the thumb being considered the first; the forefinger. **lock f.,** one that is fixed in a flexed position, owing to the presence of a small fibrous growth in the sheath of the flexor tendon. **Madonna f's,** the thin, delicate fingers seen in acromicria. **mallet f.,** permanent flexion of the distal phalanx; called also *drop* or *hammer f.* See also *baseball f.* **ring f.,** the fourth finger of the hand (*digitus annularis* [NA]). **seal f.,** a disease caused by *Erysipelothrix rhusiopathiae,* clinically resembling erysipeloid, occurring in handlers of seals and seal skins; called also *blubber f.* **snapping f.,** trigger f. **spider f.,** arachnodactyly. **spring f.,** a condition in which flexion and extension of the finger beyond certain points are difficult. **trigger f.,** a finger liable to be af-

fected with a momentary spasmodic arrest of flexion or extension, followed by a snapping into place; it is due to stenosing tendovaginitis, or a nodule in the flexor tendon (see *lock f.*). **tulip f's,** dermitis of the fingers caused by handling tulip bulbs. **waxy f.,** dead f. **webbed f's,** fingers united to a greater or less extent by a fold of skin; syndactyly. **white f.,** dead f.

fingeragnosia (fing″ger-ag-no′se-ah) [*finger + agnosia*] inability to recognize, indicate on command, name, or choose the individual fingers of one's own hand or of the hands of others.

fingernail (fing′er-nāl) the nail of a finger; see *unguis* [NA].

fingerprint (fing′ger-print) 1. an impression of the cutaneous ridges of the fleshy distal portion of a finger, made by applying ink and pressing the finger on paper; such records (as well as prints of hand or foot) are used as means of establishing identification. 2. in biochemistry, a photomicrograph obtained by fingerprinting; also, the characteristic positioning of the peptide fragments of a protein subjected to fingerprinting.

fingerprinting (fing″ger-print′ing) a technique for determining the structure of a protein in which the protein is split into peptides by digestion with protease and the fragments are separated in one direction by electrophoresis and at right angles by chromatography. After staining, the peptide fragments are seen to be in characteristic locations.

Finkelstein's albumin milk, feeding [Heinrich *Finkelstein,* German pediatrician, 1865–1942] see *albumin milk,* under *milk,* and see under *feeding.*

Finkler-Prior spirillium (fink′ler-pri′or) [Dittmar *Finkler,* German bacteriologist, 1852–1912; J. *Prior,* German bacteriologist, 19th century] *Vibrio proteus.*

Finney's pyloroplasty (operation) (fin′ez) [John M. T. *Finney,* Baltimore surgeon, 1863–1942] see under *pyloroplasty.*

Finochietto's stirrup (fe-no″ke-at′ōz) [Enrique *Finochietto,* surgeon in Buenos Aires, 1880–1948] see under *stirrup.*

Finsen (fin′sen) Niels Ryberg. Danish physician, 1860–1904; winner of the Nobel prize for medicine or physiology in 1903 for his discovery of the curative effects of ultraviolet rays, especially for lupus vulgaris.

Finsen bath, lamp (apparatus), light (rays) (fin′sen) [Niels Ryberg *Finsen*] see under *bath, lamp,* and *light.*

fire (fīr) fever; inflammation. **St. Anthony's f.,** 1. former name for *ergotism.* 2. former name for *erysipelas.*

firing (fīr′ing) the fusing of a mixture of a powder containing feldspar, kaolin, and other substances with distilled water in the process of producing porcelain.

Firmacutes (fer-mak′u-tēz; fer″mah-ku′tēz) Firmicutes.

Firmibacteria (fer″mĭ-bak-te′re-ah) [L. *firmus* strong + *bacteria*] a class of bacteria of the division Firmicutes, consisting of simple, gram-positive, asporogenous and sporogenous rods and cocci, including the medically important families: Micrococcaceae, Streptococcacea, Peptococcaceae, Bacillaceae, and Lactobacillaceae.

Firmicutes (fer-mik′u-tēz; fer″mĭ-ku′tēz) [L. *firmus* strong + *cutis* skin] a division of bacteria of the kingdom Procaryotae made up of organisms with a gram-positive type of cell wall that consists of a thick layer of peptidoglycan containing muramic acid. The division includes simple asporogenous and sporogenous rods and cocci (Firmibacteria) as well as the actinomycetes and related organisms (Thallobacteria). Called also *Firmacutes.*

firpene (fir′pēn) pinene.

first aid (ferst ād) emergency care and treatment of an injured or ill person before definitive medical and surgical management can be secured.

Fischer's sign (fish′erz) [Louis *Fischer,* pediatrician in New York, 1864–1945] see under *sign.*

Fishberg concentration test (fish′berg) [Arthur Maurice *Fishberg,* American physician, born 1898] see under *tests.*

Fisher's exact test (fish′erz) [Ronald Aylmer *Fisher,* British statistician, 1890–1962] see under *tests.*

fishpox (fish′poks) a hyperplastic epidermal disease of viral origin occurring in fresh-water and marine fish.

fissile (fis′il) capable of being split; fissionable.

fission (fish′un) [L. *fissio*] 1. the act of splitting. 2. a form of asexual reproduction in which the cell divides into two or more daughter parts of equal size, each of which becomes a new, independent organism; it is seen chiefly in unicellular organisms, such as bacteria. See also *binary f.* and *multiple f.*   **binary f.,** fission of a cell in which the cell divides into two approximately equal daughter parts.   **cellular f.,** see *fission,* 2nd def.   **multiple f.,** fission of a cell in which the cell divides into a number of daughter cells.   **nuclear f.,** the splitting of the nucleus of an atom, releasing a great quantity of kinetic energy.

fissionable (fish'un-ah-b'l)   capable of undergoing fission.

fissiparous (fi-sip'ah-rus) [L. *fissus* cleft + *parere* to produce] propagated by fission.

fissula (fis'u-lah) [L., dim. of *fissura*]   a little cleft.   **f. an'te fenes'tram,** an irregular ribbon of connective tissue that extends through the bony otic capsule from the vestibule just anterior to the oval window, to the tympanic cavity near the processus cochleariformis.

fissura (fis-su'rah), pl. *fissu'rae* [L., from *findere* to split] [NA] fissure: a general term for a cleft or groove, especially a deep fold in the cerebral cortex that involves its entire thickness.   **f. in a'no,** anal fissure.   **f. antitragohelici'na,** antitragohelicine fissure: a fissure in the auricular cartilage between the cauda helicis and the antitragus; called also *posterior fissure of auricle.*   **f. au'ris congen'ita,** preauricular fistula; see under *fistula.*   **f. calcari'na,** sulcus calcarinus.   **fissu'rae cerebel'li** [NA], fissure of the cerebellum: any of the numerous shallow grooves in the cortex of the cerebellum, on the surface and within the deep fissures, which divide the cortex into folia.   **f. choroi'dea** [NA], choroid fissure: the line in the lateral ventricle along which the choroid plexus invaginates.   **f. collatera'lis,** sulcus collateralis.   **f. dorsolatera'lis cerebel'li** [NA], dorsolateral fissure of cerebellum: the fissure separating the nodulus from the uvula of the vermis and the flocculus from the tonsilla of the cerebellar hemisphere; called also *f. posterolateralis cerebelli* [NA alternative] and *posterolateral fissure of cerebellum.*   **f. hippocam'pi,** sulcus hippocampi.   **f. horizonta'lis cerebel'li** [NA], horizontal fissure of cerebellum: the fissure that separates the cranial from the caudal semilunar lobule of the cerebellum. Called also *sulcus horizontalis cerebelli* and *great horizontal fissure.*   **f. horizonta'lis pulmo'nis dex'tri** [NA], horizontal fissure of right lung: the cleft that extends forward from the oblique fissure in the right lung, separating the upper and middle lobes.   **f. ligamen'ti te'retis** [NA], fissure for ligamentum teres: the fossa on the visceral surface of the liver lodging the ligamentum teres in the adult, and helping separate the right and left lobes of the liver; called also *fossa venae umbilicalis, fissure of round ligament,* and *umbilical fissure.*   **f. ligamen'ti veno'si** [NA], fissure for ligamentum venosum: a fossa on the posterior part of the diaphragmatic surface of the liver lodging the ligamentum venosum in the adult.   **f. longitudina'lis cer'ebri** [NA], longitudinal fissure of cerebrum: the deep fissure between the cerebral hemispheres extending inferiorly to the corpus callosum.   **f. media'na ante'rior medul'lae oblonga'tae,** NA alternative for *f. mediana ventralis medullae oblongatae.*   **f. media'na ante'rior medul'lae spina'lis,** NA alternative for *f. mediana ventralis medullae spinalis.*   **f. media'na poste'rior medul'lae oblonga'tae,** sulcus medianus dorsalis medullae oblongatae.   **f. media'na ventra'lis medul'lae oblonga'tae,** ventral median fissure of medulla oblongata: the longitudinal fissure in the median plane of the ventral aspect of the medulla oblongata, continuous with the ventral median fissure of the spinal cord; it separates the pyramids and is partially obliterated below by their decussation. Called also *anterior median fissure of medulla oblongata, anteromedian groove of medulla oblongata,* and *f. mediana anterior medullae oblongatae* [NA alternative].   **f. media'na ventra'lis medul'lae spina'lis** [NA], ventral median fissure of spinal cord: the deep longitudinal fissure in the median plane of the ventral aspect of the spinal cord; it contains the anterior spinal artery ensheathed in the linea splendens. Called also *anterior median fissure of spinal cord, anteromedian groove of spinal cord, fissura mediana anterior medullae spinalis* [NA alternative], *Haller's line,* and *sulcus ventralis medullae spinalis.*   **f. obli'qua pulmo'nis** [NA], oblique fissure of lung: 1. the cleft that separates the lower from the middle lobe in the right lung. 2. the cleft that separates the upper from

the lower lobe in the left lung.   **f. orbita'lis infe'rior** [NA], inferior orbital fissure: a cleft in the inferolateral wall of the orbit bounded by the great wing of the sphenoid and the orbital process of the maxilla; it transmits the infraorbital and zygomatic nerves and the infraorbital vessels. Called also *inferior sphenoidal fissure* and *sphenomaxillary fissure.*   **f. orbita'lis supe'rior** [NA], superior orbital fissure: an elongated cleft between the small and great wings of the sphenoid bone, which transmits various nerves and vessels; called also (*superior) sphenoidal fissure.*   **f. parietooc-cipita'lis,** sulcus parietooccipitalis.   **f. petro-oc-cipita'lis** [NA], petro-occipital fissure: a fissure extending backward from the foramen lacerum to the jugular foramen, between the basioccipital and the posterior and inner border of the petrous portion of the temporal bone; called also *petrobasilar fissure.*   **f. petrosquamo'sa** [NA], petro-squamous fissure: a slight fissure of varying distinctness in the floor of the middle cranial fossa, marking the line of fusion between the squamous and petrous portions of the temporal bone.   **f. petrotympan'ica** [NA], petrotympanic fissure: a narrow transversely running slit just posterior to the articular surface of the mandibular fossa of the temporal bone; an arteriole and the chorda tympani nerve pass through it, and it lodges a portion of the malleus. Called also *glaserian, tympanic,* or *tympanosquamous fissure.*   **f. posterolatera'lis cerebel'li,** NA alternative for *f. dorsolateralis cerebelli.*   **f. pri'ma cerebel'li** [NA], primary fissure: the fissure that separates the cranial from the caudal lobe in the cerebellum; it lies between the culmen and declive of the vermis, and between the quadrangular lobule and the lobulus simplex in the hemisphere of the cerebellum.   **f. pterygoi'dea,** pterygoid fissure: a fissure on the inferior portion of each pterygoid process where the pyramidal process of the palatine bone is inserted between the diverging medial and lateral pterygoid plates; called also *palatine* or *pterygoid notch,* and *palatine* or *pterygoid incisure.*   **f. pterygomaxilla'ris** [NA], pterygomaxillary fissure: a cleft just behind the inferior orbital fissure between the lateral pterygoid plate and the maxilla; called also *pterygo-palatine fissure.*   **f. secun'da cerebel'li** [NA], secondary fissure: a fissure that lies between the uvula of the cerebellum and the pyramid; called also *postpyramidal fissure.*   **f. sphenooccipita'lis,** sphenooccipital fissure: the fissure between the basilar part of the occipital bone and the body of the sphenoid bone; called also *basilar* or *occipito-sphenoidal fissure.*   **f. sphenopetro'sa** [NA], sphenope-trosal fissure: a fissure in the floor of the middle cranial fossa between the posterior edge of the great wing of the sphenoid bone and the petrous part of the temporal bone; called also *angular* or *petrosphenoidal fissure.*   **f. transver'sa cer'ebri** [NA], transverse fissure of cerebrum: the fissure between the dorsal surface of the diencephalon and the ventral surface of the cerebral hemispheres, produced by the folding back of the hemispheres during their development; called also *great (transverse) fissure of cerebrum* and *fissure of Bichat.*   **f. tympanomastoi'dea** [NA], tympanomastoid fissure: an external fissure on the inferior and lateral aspect of the skull between the tympanic portion and the mastoid process of the temporal bone; the auricular branch of the vagus nerve often passes through it. Called also *petromastoid fissure.*   **f. tympanosquamo'sa** [NA], tympanosqua-mous fissure: a line seen on the posterior wall of the external acoustic meatus at the junction between the tympanic and squamous parts of the temporal bone.

fissurae (fĭ-su're) [L.]   genitive and plural of *fissura.*

fissural (fish'u-ral)   pertaining to a fissure.

fissure (fish'ūr) [L. *fissura*]   1. any cleft or groove, normal or otherwise; especially a deep fold in the cerebral cortex which involves the entire thickness of the brain wall. See *fissura.* Cf. *sulcus.* 2. a deep ditch or cleft in the tooth surface, which is usually due to imperfect fusion of the enamel of the adjoining dental lobes. To be distinguished from a groove or sulcus. Considered as belonging to Class I in Black's classification of dental caries (see table accompanying *caries*). Called also *enamel f.* See also *pit,* def. 3.   **abdominal f.,** a congenital cleft in the abdominal wall.   **adoccipital f.,** an inconstant sulcus which crosses the caudal part of the precuneus and joins the occipital fissure.   **Ammon's f.,** a pear-shaped aperture in the sclera at an early fetal period.   **amygdaline f.,** a slight groove inconstantly present near the extremity of the temporal lobe.   **anal f., f. in a'no,** a painful linear ulcer at the margin of the anus.   **angular**

f., fissura sphenopetrosa. **antitragohelicine f.**, fissura antitragohelicina. **f. of aqueduct of vestibule,** apertura externa aqueductus vestibuli. **f. of auricle, posterior,** fissura antitragohelicina. **auricular f. of temporal bone,** fissura tympanomastoidea. **basilar f.**, fissura spheno-occipitalis. **basisylvian f.**, the part of the lateral sulcus between the temporal lobe and the orbital surface of the frontal bone. **f. of Bichat,** fissura transversa cerebri. **branchial f's,** see under *cleft.* **Broca's f.**, a term loosely applied to the anterior and ascending rami of the cerebral lateral sulcus which invade the left inferior frontal gyrus. **Burdach's f.**, the groove between the lateral surface of the insula and the inner surface of the operculum. **calcarine f.**, sulcus calcarinus. **callosal f.**, sulcus corporis callosi. **callosomarginal f.**, sulcus cinguli. **central f.**, sulcus centralis cerebri. **cerebral f's, f's of cerebrum,** sulci cerebri. **cerebral f., lateral,** sulcus lateralis cerebri. **choroid f.** 1. a ventral fissure formed by invagination of the optic vesicle and its stalk in the embryo, permitting the ingrowth of the mesoblast for the formation of the vitreous humor, etc. 2. fissura choroidea. **collateral f.**, sulcus collateralis. **corneal f.**, the cleft or groove in the scleral margin into which the limbus corneae fits; called also *rima cornealis* and *corneal cleft.* **craniofacial f.**, a vertical fissure separating the mesethmoid into two parts. **dentate f.**, sulcus hippocampi. **dorsolateral f. of cerebellum,** fissura dorsolateralis cerebelli. **f. of ductus venosus,** fossa ductus venosi. **Ecker's f.**, sulcus occipitalis transversus. **enamel f.**, a fault in the enamel surface of a tooth; see *fissure* (def. 2). **entorbital f.**, a sulcus occasionally seen between the orbital and olfactory sulci. **ethmoid f.**, meatus nasi superior. **glaserian f.**, fissura petrotympanica. **f. of glottis,** rima glottidis. **great f. of cerebrum,** fissura transversa cerebri. **great horizontal f.**, fissura horizontalis cerebelli. **Henle's f's,** spaces filled with connective tissue between the muscular fibers of the heart. **hippocampal f., f. of hippocampus,** sulcus hippocampi. **horizontal f. of cerebellum,** fissura horizontalis cerebelli. **horizontal f. of right lung,** fissura horizontalis pulmonis dextri. **inferofrontal f.**, sulcus frontalis inferior. **interparietal f.**, sulcus intraparietalis. **intratonsillar f.**, fossa supratonsillaris. **lacrimal f.**, sulcus lacrimalis ossis lacrimalis. **lateral f. of cerebrum,** sulcus lateralis cerebri. **f. for ligamentum teres,** fissura ligamenti teretis. **f. for ligamentum venosum,** fissura ligamenti venosi. **longitudinal f.** 1. fissura longitudinalis cerebri. 2. tenia omentalis. **longitudinal f. of cerebellum,** vallecula cerebelli. **longitudinal f. of cerebrum,** fissura longitudinalis cerebri. **mandibular f's,** the two lowest facial fissures of the embryo. **maxillary f.**, a groove on the maxilla for the maxillary process of the palatal bone. **median f. of medulla oblongata, anterior,** fissura mediana ventralis medullae oblongatae. **median f. of medulla oblongata, dorsal,** sulcus medianus dorsalis medullae oblongatae. **median f. of medulla oblongata, posterior,** sulcus medianus dorsalis medullae oblongatae. **median f. of medulla oblongata, ventral,** fissura mediana ventralis medullae oblongatae. **median f. of spinal cord, anterior,** fissura mediana ventralis medullae spinalis. **median f. of spinal cord, dorsal,** sulcus medianus dorsalis medullae spinalis. **median f. of spinal cord, posterior,** sulcus medianus dorsalis medullae spinalis. **median f. of spinal cord, ventral,** fissura mediana ventralis medullae spinalis. **f. of Monro,** sulcus hypothalamicus. **oblique f. of lung,** fissura obliqua pulmonis. **occipital f.**, sulcus parietooccipitalis. **occipitosphenoidal f.**, fissura spheno-occipitalis. **oral f.**, rima oris. **orbital f., inferior,** fissura orbitalis inferior. **orbital f., superior,** fissura orbitalis superior. **f. of palpebrae, palpebral f.**, rima palpebrarum. **Pansch's f.**, sulcus interparietalis. **paracentral f., anterior** (*obs.*), sulcus precentralis. **parietooccipital f.**, sulcus parietooccipitalis. **parietosphenoid f.**, incisura parietalis ossis temporalis. **paroccipital f.** (*obs.*), the posterior portion of the sulcus intraparietalis. **petrobasilar f.**, fissura petro-occipitalis. **petromastoid f.**, fissura tympanomastoidea. **petro-occipital f.**, fissura petro-occipitalis. **petrosal f., superficial,** hiatus canalis nervi petrosi majoris. **petrosphenoidal f.**, fissura sphenopetrosa. **petrosquamosal f., petrosquamous f.**, fissura petrosquamosa. **petrotympanic f.**, fissura petrotympanica.

portal f., porta hepatis. **postcentral f.**, sulcus postcentralis. **posterolateral f. of cerebellum,** fissura dorsolateralis cerebelli. **postpyramidal f.**, fissura secunda cerebelli. **precentral f.**, sulcus precentralis. **precuneal f.**, a sulcus in the precuneus. **prepyramidal f.**, a fissure between the pyramis vermis and the uvula vermis. **presylvian f.**, the anterior branch of the lateral cerebral sulcus. **primary f.**, fissura prima cerebelli. **pterygoid f.**, fissura pterygoidea. **pterygomaxillary f.**, fissura pterygomaxillaris. **pterygopalatine f.**, fissura pterygomaxillaris. **pterygopalatine f. of palatine bone,** sulcus palatinus major ossis palatini. **pterygotympanic f.**, fissura petrotympanica. **pudendal f., f. of pudendum,** rima pudendi. **retrocuticular f.**, a fissure in the oral epithelium made by a tooth at the time of eruption. **f. of Rolando,** sulcus centralis cerebri. **f. of round ligament,** fissura ligamenti teretis. **sagittal f. of liver,** fossa sagittalis sinistra hepatis. **Santorini's f's,** incisurae cartilaginis meatus acustici. **Schwalbe's f.**, fissura choroidea. **secondary f.**, fissura secunda cerebelli. **sphenoidal f.**, fissura orbitalis superior. **sphenoidal f., inferior,** fissura orbitalis inferior. **sphenoidal f., superior,** fissura orbitalis superior. **sphenomaxillary f.** 1. fissura orbitalis inferior. 2. fossa pterygopalatina. **sphenooccipital f.**, fissura spheno-occipitalis. **sphenopetrosal f.**, fissura sphenopetrosa. **squamotympanic f.**, fissura petrotympanica. **subfrontal f.**, sulcus frontalis inferior. **subsylvian f.** (*obs.*), 1. an occasional fissure on the ventral surface of the frontal lobe of the brain. 2. ramus posterior sulci lateralis cerebri. **subtemporal f.**, an occasional fissure in the inferior and middle temporal convolutions. **superfrontal f.**, sulcus frontalis superior. **supertemporal f.**, sulcus temporalis superior. **sylvian f., f. of Sylvius,** sulcus lateralis cerebri. **tentorial f.** (*obs.*), sulcus collateralis. **transtemporal f.**, an occasional short fissure on the lateral surface of the temporal lobe. **transverse f.**, porta hepatis. **transverse f. of cerebrum,** fissura transversa cerebri. **transverse f. of cerebrum, great,** fissura transversa cerebri. **transverse occipital f.**, sulcus occipitalis transversus. **tympanic f.**, fissura petrotympanica. **tympanomastoid f.**, fissura tympanomastoidea. **tympanosquamous f.**, 1. fissura tympanosquamosa. 2. fissura petrotympanica. **umbilical f.**, fissura ligamenti teretis. **f. of the venous ligament,** fossa ductus venosi. **f. of the vestibule,** rima vestibuli. **zygal f.**, a fissure that consists of two portions united by a third portion. **zygomaticosphenoid f.**, a fissure between the orbital surface of the great wing of the sphenoid bone and the zygomatic bone.

fistula (fis′tu-lah), pl. *fistulas* or *fis′tulae* [L. "pipe"] an abnormal passage or communication, usually between two internal organs, or leading from an internal organ to the surface of the body; frequently designated according to the organs or parts with which it communicates, as anovaginal, bronchocutaneous, hepatopleural, pulmonoperitoneal, rectovaginal, urethrovaginal, and the like (see illustrations). Such passages are frequently created experimentally for the purpose of obtaining body secretions for physiologic study. **abdominal f.**, an abnormal passage leading from one of the hollow abdominal viscera to the surface of the abdomen. **amphibolic f.**, an opening made into the gallbladder of an animal in order to obtain bile for study, with the common bile duct left intact so that the bile may flow through it when the fistula is closed. **anal f., f. in a′no,** one opening on the cutaneous surface near the anus, which may or may not communicate with the rectum. **arteriovenous f.**, an abnormal communication between an artery and a vein; it may result from injury (*traumatic arteriovenous f.*), or occur as a congenital abnormality (*congenital arteriovenous fistula*). **f. au′ris congen′ita,** preauricular f., congenital. **biliary f.**, an abnormal passage communicating with the biliary tract. **f. bimuco′sa,** a complete fistula of the anus, both ends of which open on the mucous surface of the anal canal. **blind f.**, a fistula that is open at one end only; it may open only upon the cutaneous surface of the body (*external blind f.*), or on an internal mucous surface (*internal blind f.*). Called also *incomplete f.* **branchial f.**, an abnormal passage resulting from failure of closure of a branchial cleft; called also *cervical f.* **cervical f.** 1. branchial f. 2. an abnormal passage communicating with the canal of the cervix uteri. **f. cervicovagina′lis laqueat′ica,** a fistula in the vaginal portion of the cervix

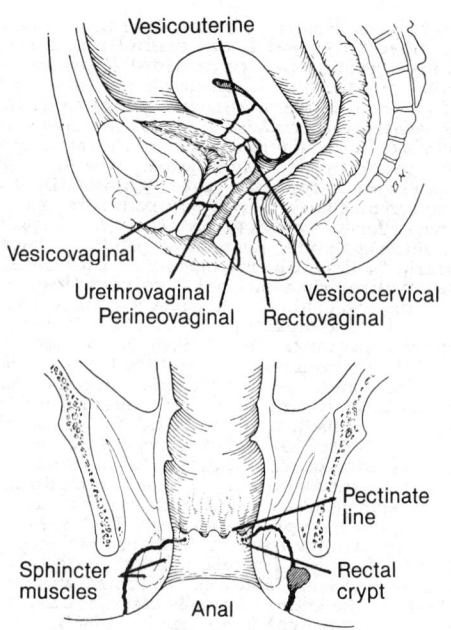

Various types of fistulae, designated according to site or to the organs with which they communicate.

uteri, communicating with the cervical canal and the vagina. **f. ciba′lis,** the esophagus. **f. col′li congen′ita,** a congenital fistula in the neck, opening into the pharynx. **colonic f.,** an abnormal passage communicating with the colon and the cutaneous surface of the body (*external colonic f.*), or with the colon and another hollow organ (*internal colonic f.*). **complete f.,** an abnormal passage in the body, each end of which opens on a mucous surface or on the cutaneous surface of the body. **f. cor′neae,** an orifice remaining after failure of a corneal ulcer to heal. **coronary arteriovenous f.,** a congenital condition in which there is an abnormal communication between a coronary artery and vein. **coronary artery f.,** a congenital condition in which there is an abnormal communication between a coronary artery and the right heart, or with the pulmonary or bronchial arteries. **craniosinus f.,** a fistula between the intracranial space and one of the paranasal sinuses, permitting the escape of cerebrospinal fluid into the nose. **Eck′s f.,** an artificial communication made between the portal vein and the vena cava; used in animal experiments. **Eck′s f. in reverse,** an artificial communication created to route all the blood from the posterior (lower) part of the body through the portal vein and liver; used in animal experiments. **external f.,** an abnormal communication between a hollow organ and the external surface of the body. **fecal f.,** a colonic fistula opening on the external surface of the body and discharging feces. **gastric f.,** an abnormal passage communicating with the stomach; often applied to an artificially created opening through the abdominal wall into the stomach (gastrostoma). **hepatic f.,** an abnormal communication between the liver and another body part or organ. **horseshoe f.,** a semicircular fistulous tract near the anus, both openings being on the cutaneous surface. **incomplete f.,** blind f. **internal f.,** an abnormal communication between two internal organs. **intestinal f.,** an abnormal passage communicating with the intestine, often designating an artificially created opening through the abdominal wall into the intestine. **lacrimal f.,** an abnormal passage communicating with the lacrimal sac or duct. **lacteal f.,** an abnormal passage communicating with a lacteal duct. **lymphatic f., f. lymphat′ica,** an abnormal passage communicating with a lymphatic vessel. **Mann-Bollman f.,** an artificial opening into an isolated segment of intestine, the proximal end of which is sutured to the abdominal wall and the distal end attached by end-to-side anastomosis to the duodenum or other part of the small

intestine; used in animal experiments. **parietal f.,** an abnormal passage in the body wall, ending blindly or communicating with an internal organ or body cavity. **pharyngeal f.,** an abnormal passage communicating with the pharynx. **pilonidal f.,** pilonidal sinus. **preauricular f., congenital,** an epidermis-lined tract communicating with a pitlike depression just in front of the helix and above the tragus (ear pit), resulting from imperfect fusion of the first and second branchial arches in formation of the auricle; called also *f. auris congenita.* **pulmonary f.,** an abnormal passage communicating with the lung. **pulmonary arteriovenous f., congenital,** a congenital anomaly characterized by existence of a direct communication between the pulmonary arterial and venous systems, allowing unoxygenated blood to enter the systemic circulation. **rectovaginal f.,** one between the rectum and vagina. **rectovesical f.,** one between the rectum and urinary bladder. **salivary f.,** one between a salivary duct or gland and the cutaneous surface, or into the oral cavity through other than a normal pathway. **spermatic f.,** an abnormal passage communicating with the seminal ducts. **stercoral f.,** fecal f. **submental f.,** a salivary fistula opening below the chin. **Thiry′s f.,** an artificial opening into an isolated segment of intestine, the proximal end of which is sutured to the abdominal wall and the distal end is closed; used in animal experiments. **Thiry-Vella f.,** an artificial opening into an internal closed loop of intestine, which communicates with the abdominal wall through an intestinal segment interposed between the surface and the loop; used in animal experiments. **thoracic f.,** an abnormal passage communicating with the thoracic cavity. **tracheal f.,** an abnormal passage communicating with the trachea. **umbilical f.,** an abnormal passage communicating with the gut or with the urachus at the umbilicus. **urachal f.,** an abnormal passage communicating with the urachus. **urinary f.,** an abnormal passage communicating with the urinary tract. **Vella′s f.,** an artificial opening into an isolated segment of intestine, both open ends of which are sutured to the abdominal wall; used in animal experiments. **vesical f.,** an abnormal passage communicating with the urinary bladder. **vesicovaginal f.,** one from the bladder to the vagina.

fistulae (fis′tu-le) [L.]   genitive and plural of *fistula.*

fistulatome (fis′tu-lah-tōm″) [*fistula* + Gr. *temnein* to cut] an instrument for incising a fistula; syringotome.

fistulectomy (fis″tu-lek′to-me) [*fistula* + Gr. *ektomē* excision]   excision of a fistulous tract.

fistulization (fis″tu-li-za′shun)   1. the process of becoming fistulous. 2. the surgical creation of an opening into a hollow organ, cavity, or abscess; the creation of a communication between two structures which were not previously connected.

fistuloenterostomy (fis″tu-lo-en″ter-os′to-me)   the operation of making a fistula empty permanently into the intestine.

fistulotomy (fis″tu-lot′o-me)   incision of a fistula.

fistulous (fis′tu-lus) [L. *fistulosus*]   pertaining to or of the nature of a fistula.

fit (fit)   1. an episode characterized by inappropriate and involuntary motor or psychic activity. See also *epilepsy.* 2. the adaptation of one structure into another, as the adaptation of any dental restoration to its site in the mouth. **running f.,** 1. fright disease. 2. cursive epilepsy.

FITC   fluorescein isothiocyanate.

fitness (fit′nes)   in genetics, the probability of transmitting one's genes to the next generation and having them survive in that generation and be passed on to the next, relative to the average probability for the population.

Fitz Gerald method, treatment [William Henry Hope *Fitz Gerald,* American physician, 1872–1939]   zone therapy.

fix (fiks)   to fasten or hold firm; see *fixation.*

fixation (fik-sa′shun) [L. *fixatio*]   1. the act or operation of holding, suturing, or fastening in a fixed position. 2. the condition of being held in a fixed position. 3. in psychiatry, a term with two related but distinct meanings: (1) arrest of development at a particular stage, which like regression (return to an earlier stage), if temporary is a normal reaction to setbacks and difficulties but if protracted or frequent is a cause of developmental failures and emotional problems, and (2) a close and suffocating attachment to another person, especially a childhood figure, such as one's mother or father. Both meanings are derived from psychoanalytic theory and refer to "fixation" of libidinal energy either in a specific erogenous zone, hence fixation at the oral, anal, or phallic stage, or in a specific object, hence mother or father fixation. 4. the use of a fixative (q.v.) to preserve histological or cytological specimens. 5. in chemistry, the process whereby a substance is removed from the gaseous or solution phase and localized, as in carbon dioxide fixation or nitrogen fixation. 6. in ophthalmology, direction of the gaze so that the visual image of the object falls on the fovea centralis. 7. in film processing, the chemical removal of all undeveloped salts of the film emulsion, leaving only the developed silver to form a permanent image. **autotrophic f.,** the cyclic mechanism whereby carbon dioxide is fixed into organic linkage by autotrophic organisms, e.g., plants and autotrophic bacteria. **bifoveal f., binocular f.,** training both eyes on the same object as in ordinary vision. **Bovin f.,** an acetic fixation which destroys the mitochrondria of the cell. **carbon dioxide f.,** conversion of atmospheric carbon dioxide to organic carbon compounds, as in photosynthesis. **complement f., f. of complement,** the consumption of complement upon reaction with immune complexes containing complement-fixing antibodies, the basis of *complement fixation tests,* widely used procedures for the detection of antigens or antibodies. These are two-stage procedures in which heat-inactivated antiserum (or antigen) is reacted with the test material in the presence of a known amount of complement. If the homologous antigen (or antibody) is present in the test material, complement is fixed. Then sheep red blood cells and antisheep erythrocyte antibody are added; lack of hemolysis indicates complement fixation, i.e., a positive best result. Quantitive results are obtained by determining the highest dilution of antiserum or test material that gives a positive reaction. Called also *Bordet-Gengou phenomenon* or *reaction.* **elastic band f.,** the stabilization of fractured segments of the jaws by means of intermaxillary elastic bands applied to splints or appliances. **external pin f.,** in oral surgery, a method for stabilizing fractures by means of pins drilled into the bony parts through the overlying skin and connected by metal bars. **external pin f., biphase,** external pin fixation in which the rigid metal bar connector is replaced with an acrylic bar adapted at the time of the reduction. **internal f., intraosseous f.,** the open reduction and stabilization of fractured bony parts by direct fixation to one another with surgical wires, screws, pins, and plates. **maxillomandibular f.,** the fixation of fractures of the maxilla or mandible in a functional relationship with the opposing dental arch, through the use of elastics, wire ligatures, arch bars, or other splints. **nasomandibular f.,** mandibular immobilization, especially for edentulous jaws, using maxillomandibular splints; a circummandibular wire is connected with an intraoral interosseous wire passed through a hole drilled into the anterior nasal spine of the maxilla. **nitrogen f.,** the union of the free atmospheric nitrogen with other elements to form chemical compounds, such as ammonia and nitrates or amino groups. This occurs primarily through the action of soil bacteria of the genus *Rhizobium* in symbiosis with leguminous plants. Organisms capable of nitrogen fixation are also found in the genera *Azotobacter, Beijerinckia, Bacillus, Cyanobacteria, Clostridium,* and *Rhodospirillum.* Nonbiological nitrogen fixation processes include electrical methods and chemical catalysis (Haber process). **skeletal f.,** immobilization of the ends of a fractured bone by metal wires or plates applied directly to the bone (*internal skeletal fixation*) or on the body surface (*external skeletal fixation*).

fixative (fik′sah-tiv) a fluid, often a mixture of several reactive chemicals, into which histological or cytological specimens are placed so that, by processes such as denaturation and cross-linking of proteins, autolysis is prevented, the specimen is hardened to withstand further processing, and the specimen is preserved in a close facsimile of the living state in regard to both cellular morphology and the location of subcellular constituents. A standard fixative for routine use is buffered neutral formalin. A wide variety of fixatives, containing ingredients such as formalin, glutaraldehyde, and other aldehydes, ethanol, methanol, and other alcohols, acetone, acetic acid, chromates, mercuric salts, and picric acid, are used for special purposes. Osmium tetroxide and glutaraldehyde are standard fixatives for processing specimens for electron microscopy. **glutaraldehyde f.,** a fixative used in specimen preparation for electron microscopy

that does not simultaneously stain the tissue. **Kaiserling's f.,** see under *solution.* **Maximow's f.,** a solution composed of Zenker's fixative, formol, and osmic acid, used in preserving vertebrate cells for study with the visible light microscope. **Zenker's f.,** a fixative solution containing corrosive mercuric chloride, potassium bichromate, sodium sulfate, glacial acetic acid, and water; the sodium sulfate is frequently omitted. The most widely used variations of this fixative are the modifications by Maximow, by Helly, and by Custer, in which formalin replaces the acetic acid. **Zenker-formol f.,** a solution composed of Zenker's fixative with added formalin; see *Helly's fluid,* under *fluid.*

Fl. fluid.

F.L.A. fronto-laeva anterior (left frontoanterior—a position of the fetus).

F.l.a. abbreviation for L. *fi'at le'ge ar'tis,* let it be done according to rule.

Flabellina (flab″ĕ-li′nah) [L. *flabellum* fan] a suborder of ameboid protozoa (order Amoebida, class Lobosea) having a flattened, broad, sometimes discoid body with an extensive hyaline zone but no obvious pellicle-like layer.

flaccid (flak′sid) [L. *flaccidus*] weak, lax, and soft.

flacherie (flash-er-e′) [Fr.] a fatal disease of silkworms occurring in two forms: an infectious form due to a small nonoccluded virus and a noninfectious form due to environmental changes, such as a sudden increase in temperature and humidity. It is marked by diarrhea, weakness, flaccidity, and death, after which the body quickly turns dark and the tissues liquefy. See also *gattine.*

Flack's node, test (flaks) [Martin William Flack, physiologist in London, 1882–1931] see *Keith-Flack's node,* under *node,* and see under *tests.*

flagella (flah-jel′ah) [L.] plural of *flagellum.*

flagellantism (flaj′ĕ-lan-tizm) flagellation.

flagellar (flah-jel′ar) of or relating to a flagellum.

Flagellata (flaj″ĕ-la′tah) former name for Mastigophora.

flagellate (flaj′ĕ-lāt) 1. any microorganism having flagella as organs of locomotion. 2. any protozoon of the subphylum Mastigophora. 3. having flagella. 4. to practice flagellation. **animal-like f.,** any protozoan of the class Phytomastigophorea. **plantlike f.,** any protozoan of the class Phytomastigophorea.

flagellation (flaj″ĕ-la′shun) 1. a form of massage by tapping a part with the fingers. 2. sexual sadism or masochism in which whipping or being whipped produces sexual arousal and gratification. Called also *flagellantism.* 3. the protrusion of flagella; exflagellation.

flagelliform (flah-jel′i-form) [L. *flagellum* whip + *forma* shape] shaped like a flagellum, or lash.

flagellin (flaj′ĕ-lin) a protein (mol. wt. approximately 40,000) occurring in the flagella of bacteria, which is composed of subunits arranged in several-stranded helix formation somewhat resembling myosin in structure, and sometimes containing ∊-N-methyl lysine. Its composition varies with the species; thus flagellin antibodies are species specific.

flagellosis (flaj″ĕ-lo′sis) infection with a flagellate protozoon.

flagellospore (flah-jel′o-spōr) zoospore.

flagellula (flah-jel′u-lah) zoospore.

flagellum (flah-jel′um), pl. *flagel′la* [L. "whip"] a long, mobile, whiplike projection from the free surface of a cell, serving as a locomotor organelle; it is composed of nine pairs of microtubules arrayed around a central pair. Arising from basal bodies, flagella are common to all mastigophoran protozoa and occur in such specialized cells as spermatozoa. Bacterial flagella are thinner and simpler, being composed of strands of flagellin tightly woven in a helical filament, attached to a basal body in the cell wall. Bacteria having a single flagellum are *monotrichous,* those with two or more at one end are *lophotrichous,* those with one flagellum at each end are *amphitrichous,* and those with flagella around the entire surface are *peritrichous.* Cf. *cilium,* def. 3.

Flagyl (flag″l) trademark for a preparation of metronidazole.

flail (flāl) exhibiting abnormal or paradoxical mobility, as flail joint, flail chest, or flail valve.

Flajani's disease (flah-jan′ēz) [Giuseppe *Flajani,* Italian surgeon, 1741–1808] Graves' disease.

flame (flām) 1. the luminous, irregular appearance usually accompanying combustion caused by the light emitted from energetically excited chemical species, or an appearance resembling it. 2. to render an object sterile by exposure to a flame. **manometric f.,** a gas flame in an enclosed box arranged so that it pulsates with the vibration of air caused by sound; such pulsations may be seen on a mirror or recorded photographically (flame picture).

flange (flanj) 1. a projecting rim, collar, or ring on a shaft, pipe, or machine housing. 2. that part of the denture base which extends from the cervical ends of the teeth to the border of the denture. Called also *denture f.* **buccal f.,** the portion of the flange of a denture that occupies the buccal vestibule of the mouth and extends distally from the buccal notch. **denture f.,** flange, def. 2. **labial f.,** the portion of the flange of a denture that occupies the labial vestibule of the mouth. **lingual f.,** the portion of the flange of a mandibular denture which occupies the space adjacent to the residual ridge and next to the tongue.

flank (flank) the part of the body below the ribs and above the ilium.

flap (flap) 1. a mass of tissue for grafting, usually including skin, only partially removed from one part of the body so that it retains its own blood supply during its transfer to a new location; used to repair defects in an adjacent or distant part of the body. 2. an uncontrolled movement. **Abbe f.,** a triangular, full-thickness flap from the median portion of the lower lip used to fill a defect in the upper lip. **advancement f.,** a flap carried to its new position by a sliding technique of surgical advancement; called also *sliding f.* **bilobed f.,** a surgical flap consisting of a large lobe, which is transposed into the primary defect, and a smaller second lobe, which is transposed to fill the secondary defect produced by mobilization of the large lobe. **bipedicle f.,** a pedicle flap with two vascular attachments. **cross-arm f.,** a surgical flap cut from one arm and attached to the other to repair a defect. **cross-leg f.,** a surgical flap cut from one leg and attached to the other to repair a defect. **delayed transfer f.,** a surgical flap that is partially raised from its donor bed and then replaced; done to permit development of collateral circulation through the pedicle. **direct transfer f.,** immediate transfer f. **distant f.,** a pedicle flap brought from a distant area and transplanted by bringing the donor area and the recipient site into close approximation; called also *Italian f.* **double pedicle f.,** bipedicle f. **Eloesser f.,** a flap of skin created over the ribs for open drainage of chronic empyema. **envelope f.,** a mucoperiosteal flap retracted from a horizontal linear incision (as along the free gingival margin) with no vertical component of that incision. **Estlander f.,** a triangular flap from the side of the lower lip used to fill a defect in the lateral upper lip. **free f.,** an island flap detached from the body and reattached at the distant recipient site by microvascular anastomosis. **French f.,** advancement f. **gauntlet f.,** pedicle f. **Gillies' f.,** tube f. **immediate transfer f.,** a surgical flap that is applied to the recipient site immediately after it is elevated from its bed; called also *direct transfer f.* **Indian f.,** interpolated f. **interpolated f.,** a pedicle flap that is twisted or rotated on its base and placed into a contiguous area; called also *Indian f.* **island f.,** a skin flap consisting of the skin and subcutaneous tissue with a pedicle made up of only the nutrient vessels. **Italian f.,** distant f. **jump f.,** a flap cut from the abdomen and attached to the forearm; the flap is transferred later to some other part of the body to fill a defect there. **Langenbeck's pedicle mucoperiosteal f.,** von Langenbeck's bipedicle mucoperiosteal f. **lingual tongue f.,** a combination flap used to repair fistulae of the hard palate: a palatal flap forms the floor of the nose, and a flap taken from the back or edge of the tongue forms the palatal surface. **local f.,** a surgical flap cut from the tissue neighboring the defect. **mucoperiosteal f.,** a flap of mucosal tissue, including the periosteum, reflected from bone. **liver f.,** asterixis. **musculocutaneous f., mycocutaneous f.,** a compound flap of skin and muscle with adequate vascularity to permit sufficient tissue to be transferred to the recipient site. **pedicle f.,** a flap consisting of the full thickness of the skin and the subcutaneous tissue, attached by tissue through which it receives its blood supply. **rope f.,** tube f. **rotation f.,** a pedicle flap whose width is increased by transforming the edge of the flap distal to the defect into a curved line; the flap is then rotated and a counterincision is

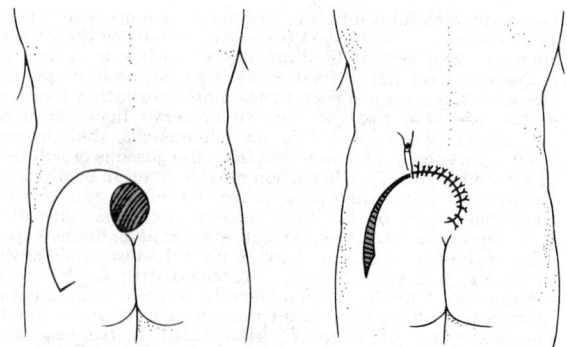

Rotation flap.

made at the base of the curved line, which increases the mobility of the flap. **skin f.,** a full-thickness mass or flap of tissue containing epidermis, dermis, and subcutaneous tissue. **sliding f.,** advancement f. **tube f., tubed pedicle f.,** a bipedicle flap made by elevating a long strip of tissue from its bed except at the two ends, the cut edges then being sutured together to form a tube; called also *rope* or *tunnel f.* and *Gillies' f.* **tunnel f.,** tube f. **von Langenbeck's bipedicle mucoperiosteal f.,** a bipedicle flap of the conjoined mucoperiosteal tissues, used for closure of a cleft palate. **V-Y f.,** a flap in which the incision is made in the shape of a V and is sutured in the shape of a Y so as to lengthen an area of tissue; or conversely the incision is Y-shaped and the closure V-shaped to shorten an area of tissue. **Widman f., modified,** see *surgical curettage,* under *curettage.* **Z-f.,** a flap in which the incision is made in the shape of a Z so as to distribute contraction in more than one direction; often used to correct scars. **Zimany's bilobed f.,** bilobed f.

flaps (flaps) severe swelling of the lips in horses.

flare (flār) 1. the red outermost zone of the "triple response" (Sir Thomas Lewis) urticarial wheal reaction, a manifestation of immediate, as opposed to delayed, allergy or hypersensitivity. 2. a spreading flush or area of redness on the skin, spreading out around an infective lesion or extending beyond the main point of reaction to an irritant. 3. sudden exacerbation of a disease.

flash (flash) excess material extruded from a mold, as in the packing of a denture by the compression technique.

flask (flask) 1. a container, such as a narrow-necked vessel of glass for containing liquid. 2. a metal case in which the materials used in the creation of artificial dentures are placed for processing. 3. to place a denture in a flask for processing. **casting f.,** refractory f. **crown f.,** denture f. **denture f.,** a sectional, boxlike metal, ceramic, or polymer case that can be tightly closed, and with which sectional molds of plaster of Paris or dental stone are used to compress and form a resinous denture base or crown material during curing. Called also *crown f.* **Erlenmeyer f.,** a glass flask with a conical body, broad base, and narrow neck. **refractory f.,** a metal tube in which a refractory mold is made for casting metal dental restorations or appliances; called also *cast f.* and *cast r.* **volumetric f.,** a narrow-necked vessel of glass calibrated to contain or deliver an exact volume at a given temperature.

flasking (flask'ing) 1. the act of investing in a flask. 2. the process of investing the cast and a wax denture in a flask preparatory to molding the denture base material into the form of the denture.

flat (flat) 1. lying in one plane; having an even surface. 2. having little or no resonance. 3. slightly below the normal pitch of a musical tone. **optical f.,** a glass plate so perfectly flat that only an interferometer can measure its unevenness.

Flatau's law (flat-owz') [Edward *Flatau,* Polish neurologist, 1869–1932] see under *law.*

flatfoot (flat'foot) a condition in which one or more of the arches of the foot have flattened out; called also *pes planovalgus, pes planus,* and *pes valgus.* **rocker-bottom f.,** see under *foot.* **spastic f.,** a painful form of flatfoot due to spasm of the peroneal muscles.

flatness (flat'nes) a peculiar sound lacking resonance, heard on percussing a part that is abnormally solid.

flatulence (flat′u-lens) [L. *flatulentia*] the presence of excessive amounts of air or gases in the stomach or intestine, leading to distention of the organs.

flatulent (flat′u-lent) [L. *flatulentus*] pertaining to or characterized by flatulence; distended with gas.

flatus (fla′tus) [L. "a blowing"] 1. gas or air in the gastrointestinal tract. 2. gas or air expelled through the anus. **f. vagina′lis**, noisy expulsion of gas from the vagina.

flatworm (flat′werm) any worm belonging to the phylum Platyhelminthes.

flavanoid (fla′vah-noid) flavonoid.

flavanone (fla′vah-nōn) colorless, flavonoid compounds formed by reduction of the 2:3 double bond of a flavone; they occur in free form or as glycosides. A subgroup, the *flavanonols*, have a 3-hydroxy group and seldom occur as glycosides.

flavanonol (fla′vah-non-ol) a subgroup of flavanone (q.v.).

flavectomy (fla-vek′to-me) [L. *flavus* yellow + Gr. *ektomē* excision] excision of the ligamentum flavum.

flavescent (flah-ves′ent) [L. *flavescere* to become gold colored] yellowish.

flavin (fla′vin) [L. *flavus* yellow] any one of a group of compounds containing the isoalloxazine nucleus, especially riboflavin. Flavin compounds are characterized by a yellow color and intense green fluorescence in the oxidized form; the reduced form is colorless. **f.-adenine dinucleotide (FAD)**, a coenzyme composed of riboflavin 5′-phosphate (FMN) and adenosine 5′-phosphate linked by a pyrophosphate bond; it forms the prosthetic group of many flavoprotein enzymes, including D-amino acid oxidase and xanthine oxidase, and is important in electron transport in mitochondria and the endoplasmic reticulum. **f. mononucleotide (FMN)**, riboflavin 5′-phosphate; it acts as a coenzyme for a number of oxidative enzymes including NADH dehydrogenase. **f. monooxygenase**, monooxygenase (unspecific).

flavine (fla′vīn) acriflavine hydrochloride.

flavivirus (fla″ve-vi′rus) a subcategory of togaviruses; the type species is the yellow fever virus.

flav(o)- [L. *flavus* yellow] a combining form meaning yellow.

Flavobacterium (fla″vo-bak-te′re-um) [L. *flavus* yellow + Gr. *baktērion* little rod] a genus of gram-negative, aerobic or facultatively anaerobic, rod-shaped bacteria of uncertain affiliation, characterized by production of a yellow pigment. The organisms occur widely in soil and water, and are opportunistic pathogens in humans. **F. bre′ve**, a species of uncertain pathogenicity, occasionally recovered from clinical specimens. **F. meningosep′ticum**, a pathogenic species that is a major cause of nosocomial infections, producing meningitis and septicemia with a high fatality rate in premature and newborn infants. In adults, it causes a milder bacteremia. **F. odora′tum**, a pathogenic species usually producing yellow pigment and a fruity odor, recovered from infections of wounds and the urinary tract.

flavoenzyme (fla″vo-en′zīm) any enzyme that is a flavoprotein.

flavone (fla′vōn) a colorless crystalline substance, the 4-keto series of flavonoids, able to reverse increased capillary fragility. Numerous yellow dyestuffs having similar properties are derived from it.

flavonoid (fla′vo-noid) a generic term for a group of aromatic oxygen heterocyclic compounds derived from 2-phenylbenzopyran or its 2,3-dehydro derivative. They are widely distributed in higher plants, one subgroup, the anthocyanins, accounting for the majority of yellow, red, and blue pigmentation. Another subgroup, varying somewhat in structure, has physiologic properties formerly referred to as "vitamin P" activity, now called *bioflavonoids*, e.g., citrin, rutin, etc. The flavonoids are grouped in order of increasing oxidation state: catechins; leucoanthocyanidins and flavanones, flavanols, flavones, and anthocyanidins; and flavonols.

flavonol (fla′vo-nol) a yellow crystalline flavonoid, formed by introduction of an OH group at C-3 of a flavone; it is grouped with the flavones and isoflavones.

flavoprotein (fla″vo-pro′tēn) a protein containing a flavin nucleotide (FAD or FMN) as a prosthetic group. Most flavoproteins are enzymes; many are found in complexes containing metal ions and an iron-sulfur complex or a heme. They catalyze a wide variety of oxidation-reduction reactions.

flavor (fla′vor) 1. that quality of any substance which affects the taste. 2. a pharmaceutical or other preparation for improving the taste of a food or medicine.

flavoxanthin (fla″vo-zan′thin) a minor, yellow, carotenoid pigment, $C_{40}H_{56}O_3$, from the petals of ranunculaceous plants, structurally related to vitamin A but having no vitamin A activity.

flavoxate hydrochloride (fla-voks′āt) chemical name: 3-methyl-4-oxo-2-phenyl-4*H*-1-benzopyran-8-carboxylic acid 2-(1- piperidinyl)ethyl ester hydrochloride. A smooth muscle relaxant, $C_{24}H_{25}NO_4 \cdot HCl$, occurring as an off-white, crystalline powder; used as an antispasmodic for the urinary system, administered orally.

Flaxedil (flaks′e-dil) trademark for a preparation of gallamine triethiodide.

flaxseed (flaks′sēd) linseed.

flazalone (fla′ză-lōn) chemical name: [(4-fluorophenyl)[4-(4-fluorophenyl)-4-hydroxy-1-methyl-3-piperidinyl]methanone]; an anti-inflammatory agent, $C_{19}H_{19}F_2NO_2$.

fld. fluid.

fl.dr. fluid dram.

flea (fle) any insect of the order *Siphonaptera*; many are parasitic and may act as carriers of disease. The genera of medical importance are: *Cediopsylla*, *Ceratophyllus*, *Ctenocephalides*, *Ctenophthalmus*, *Leptopsylla*, *Diamanus*, *Echidnophaga*, *Hoplopsyllus*, *Monopsyllus*, *Neopsylla*, *Nosopsyllus*, *Oropsylla*, *Pulex*, *Rhopalopsyllus*, *Tunga*, *Xenopsylla*. **Asiatic rat f.**, *Xenopsylla cheopis*. **burrowing f.**, *Tunga penetrans*. **cat f.**, *Ctenocephalides felis*. **cavy f.**, *Rhopalopsyllus cavicola*. **chigoe f.**, *Tunga penetrans*. **common f.**, *Pulex irritans*. **common rat f.**, *Nosopsyllus fasciatus*. **dog f.**, *Ctenocephalides canis*. **European mouse f.**, *Ctenophthalmus agrytes*. **European rat f.**, *Nosopsyllus fasciatus*. **human f.**, *Pulex irritans*. **Indian rat f.**, *Xenopsylla astia*. **jigger f.**, *Tunga penetrans*. **mouse f.**, *Leptopsylla segnis*. **sand f.**, *Tunga penetrans*. **squirrel f.**, *Hoplopsyllus anomalus*. **sticktight f.**, *Echidnophaga gallinacea*. **suslik f.**, any of several species of fleas which infest Russian ground squirrels. **tropical rat f.**, *Xenopsylla cheopis*.

flecainide (fle-ka′nīd) a fluorinated benzamide derivative, $C_{17}H_{20}F_6N_2O_3$, administered orally for treatment of ventricular arrhythmias. Available as *flecainide acetate*.

Flechsig's area, etc. (flek′sigz) [Paul Emil *Flechsig*, neurologist in Leipzig, 1847–1929] see under *area*, *cuticulum*, *fasciculus*, *field*, and *law*.

fleck (flek) a flake, particle, speckle, or spot. **tobacco f's**, Gamna-Gandy nodules.

fleckfieber (flek-fe′ber) [Ger.] epidemic typhus; see under *typhus*.

fleckmilz (flek′milts) [Ger.] a condition of the spleen in malignant nephrosclerosis in which necrotic follicles appear as translucent areas.

flection (flek′shun) flexion.

Flectobacillus (flek″to-bah-sil′lus) [L. *flecto* curve + *bacillus*] a genus of nonmotile, gram-negative, straight to curved, rod-shaped bacteria of the family Spirosomaceae, usually occurring as C-shaped or ring-shaped cells; they are found in fresh and marine water. The type species is *F. májor*.

fleece (flēs) a network of interlacing fibers. **f. of Stilling**, the lacework of white fibers surrounding the dentate nucleus.

Fleming (flem′ing), Sir Alexander. Scottish bacteriologist, 1881–1955; co-winner, with Ernst Boris Chain and Sir Howard Walter Florey, of the Nobel prize for medicine or physiology for 1945 for the discovery of penicillin.

flemingen (flĕ-min′jin) any of several chalcone dyes from waras; a natural dyestuff (C.I. natural yellow 22) from shrubs of the genus *Flemingia*.

Flemming's center, solution (fixing fluid) [Walther *Flemming*, German anatomist, 1843–1905] see *germinal center*, under *center*, and see under *solution*.

flesh (flesh) the soft, muscular tissue of the animal body. **goose f.**, cutis anserina. **proud f.**, exuberant amounts of soft, edematous, granulation tissue that may develop during the healing of large surface wounds.

fletazepam (flĕ-taz′e-pam) chemical name: 7-chloro-5-(2-fluorophenyl)-2,3-dihydro-1-(2,2,2-trifluoroethyl)-1*H*-1,4-benzodiazepine; a skeletal muscle relaxant, $C_{17}H_{13}ClF_4N_2$.

fletcherism (flech′er-izm) [Horace *Fletcher*, American dietitian, 1849–1919] the thorough mastication of solid food and the taking of liquids by sips.

flex (fleks) [L. *flexus* bent] to bend or put in a state of flexion.

Flexibacter (flek″sĭ-bak′ter) [L. *flexus* flexible + Gr. *baktron* a rod] a genus of gliding bacteria of the family Cytophagaceae, found in soil and water, made up of flexible, rod-shaped, single or filamentous cells. The type species is *F. flex′ilis.*

flexibilitas (flek-sĭ-bil′ĭ-tas) [L.] flexibility. **f. ce′rea,** cerea flexibilitas.

flexibility (flek″sĭ-bil′ĭ-te) [L. *flexibilitas*] the quality of being flexible. **waxy f.,** cerea flexibilitas.

flexible (flek′sĭ-bl) [L. *flexibilis, flexilis*] readily bent without tendency to break.

flexile (fleks′īl) flexible.

fleximeter (fleks-im′ĕ-ter) an instrument for measuring the amount of flexion of a joint.

flexion (flek′shun) [L. *flexio*] 1. the act of bending or condition of being bent. 2. in gynecology, a displacement of the uterus in which the organ is bent so far forward or backward that an acute angle forms between the fundus and the cervix. See *version* (def. 3). 3. in obstetrics, the normal bending forward of the head of the fetus in the uterus or the birth canal.

Flexithrix (flek′sĭ-thriks) [L. *flexus* flexible + Gr. *thrix* hair] a genus of gliding bacteria of the family Cryptophagaceae, found in sea water, made up of rod-shaped cells usually in sheathed filaments. The type species is *F. dorothe′ae.*

Flexner's bacillus, dysentery (fleks′nerz) [Simon *Flexner*, American pathologist, 1863–1946] see *Shigella flexneri,* and see *bacillary dysentery,* under *dysentery.*

flexor (flek′sor) [L.] any muscle that flexes a joint; see *Table of Musculi.* **f. retinac′ulum,** see *retinaculum flexorum manus* and *retinaculum musculorum flexorum pedis.*

flexorplasty (flek′sor-plas″te) plastic surgery of flexor muscles.

flexuose (fleks′u-ōs) winding or wavy.

flexura (flek-shoo′rah), pl. *flexu′rae* [L.] flexure: a bending; [NA] a general term for a bent portion of a structure or organ. **f. co′li dex′tra** [NA], right flexure of colon: the bend in the large intestine at which the ascending colon becomes the transverse colon; called also *f. hepatica coli* and *hepatic flexure of colon.* **f. co′li sinis′tra** [NA], left flexure of colon: the bend in the large intestine at which the transverse colon becomes the descending colon; called also *f. lienalis coli* and *splenic flexure of colon.* **f. duode′ni infe′rior** [NA], inferior flexure of duodenum: the bend in the duodenum at which the descending duodenum becomes horizontal or transverse. Called also *inferior angle of duodenum.* **f. duode′ni supe′rior** [NA], superior flexure of duodenum: the bend in the first or superior part of the duodenum; called also *superior angle of duodenum.* **f. duodenojejuna′lis** [NA], duodenal flexure: the bend in the small intestine at the junction between the duodenum and jejunum; the suspensory muscle of the duodenum attaches to this point. **f. hepat′ica co′li,** f. coli dextra. **f. liena′lis co′li,** f. coli sinistra. **f. perinea′lis rec′ti** [NA], perineal flexure of rectum: the dorsal and caudal bend at the caudal end of the rectum. **f. sacra′lis rec′ti** [NA], sacral flexure of rectum: the dorsal first bend in the rectum.

flexurae (flek-shoo′re) [L.] plural of *flexura.*

flexural (flek′shur-al) pertaining to or affecting a flexure.

flexure (flek′sher) a bending; a bent portion of a structure or organ; see *flexura.* **basicranial f.,** pontine f. **caudal f.,** the bend at the aboral end of the embryo; called also *sacral f.* **cephalic f.,** the curve in the midbrain of the embryo; called also *cranial f.* **cerebral f.,** one of the bends in the embryonic brain; called also *nuchal f.* **cervical f.,** a bend in the neural tube of the embryo at the junction of the brain and spinal cord. **cranial f.,** cephalic f. **dorsal f.,** one of the flexures of the embryo in the mid-dorsal region. **duodenojejunal f.,** flexura duodenojejunalis. **hepatic f. of colon,** flexura coli dextra. **inferior f. of duodenum,** flexura duodeni inferior. **left f. of colon,** flexura coli sinistra. **lumbar f.,** the ventral curvature of the back in the lumbar region. **mesencephalic f.,** a flexure in the neural tube of the vertebrate embryo at the level of the mesencephalon. **nuchal f.,** cervical f. **peri-**

neal f. of rectum, flexura perinealis recti. **pontine f.,** a flexure in the hindbrain of the embryo; called also *basicranial f.* **right f. of colon,** flexura coli dextra. **sacral f.,** caudal f. **sacral f. of rectum,** flexura sacralis recti. **sigmoid f.,** sigmoid colon. **splenic f. of colon,** flexura coli sinistra. **superior f. of duodenum,** flexura duodeni superior.

flicker (flik′er) [A.S. *flicorian* to flutter] the visual sensation produced by regular flashes of light. The flashes may appear to flutter or to be steady according to the rate of interruption (*flicker phenomenon*). The number of flashes per second at which the light just appears to be continuous is known as the *flicker fusion threshold (fusion frequency; critical fusion frequency)*. The *flicker test,* an application of the flicker fusion threshold, has been used to diagnose hypertension and angina pectoris, to determine vessel spasm, or to indicate conditions of fatigue or anoxemia. A low threshold indicates disease.

Fliess treatment (therapy) (flēs) [Wilhelm *Fliess*, Berlin physician, 1858–1928] see under *treatment.*

flight of ideas a nearly continuous flow of rapid speech that jumps from topic to topic, usually based on discernible associations, distractions, or plays on words, but in severe cases wholly disorganized and incoherent. It is most commonly seen in manic episodes but may also occur in psychotic disorders and organic mental disorders.

Flint's arcade, law (flints) [Austin *Flint*, American physiologist, 1836–1915] see under *arcade* and *law.*

Flint's murmur (flints) [Austin *Flint*, American physician, 1812–1886] see under *murmur.*

floaters (flo′ters) "spots before the eyes"; deposits in the vitreous of the eye, usually moving about and probably representing fine aggregates of vitreous protein occurring as a benign degenerative change. Called also *vitreous f's* and *muscae volitantes.*

floccilegium (flok″sĭ-le′je-um) floccillation.

floccillation (flok″sĭ-la′shun) [L. *floccilatio*] the picking at bedclothes by a delirious patient.

floccose (flok′ōs) [L. *floccosus* full of flocks of wool] woolly; said of a bacterial growth which is composed of short, curved chains variously oriented.

floccular (flok′u-lar) pertaining to the flocculus.

flocculation (flok″u-la′shun) 1. a colloid phenomenon in which the disperse phase separates in discrete, usually visible, particles rather than in a continuous mass, as in coagulation. 2. in immunology, the formation of downy masses of precipitate in a precipitin test or of agglutinated bacteria in an agglutination test for the H antigens of *Salmonella* species.

floccule (flok′ūl) flocculus. **toxoid-antitoxin f.,** a suspension of the precipitate formed when toxoid and antitoxin are mixed.

flocculent (flok′u-lent) containing downy or flaky masses.

flocculi (flok′u-li) [L.] genitive and plural of *flocculus.*

flocculus (flok′u-lus), pl. *floc′culi* [L. "tuft"] 1. a small tuft, as of wool or similar material, or a small mass of other fibrous material such as one of the flakes of a flocculent solution. 2. [NA] one of the small paired, partially detached lateral lobules continuous with the nodulus of the cerebellum, separated from each cerebellar hemisphere by the dorsolateral fissure, and forming part of the flocculonodular lobe. **accessory f.,** paraflocculus.

floctafenine (flok″tah-fen′ēn) chemical name: 2-[[8-(trifluoromethyl)-4-quinolinyl]amino]benzoic acid; an analgesic, $C_{20}H_{17}F_3N_2O_4.$

Flood's ligament (fludz) [Valentine *Flood*, Irish surgeon, 1800–1847] see under *ligament.*

flooding (flud′ing) in behavior therapy, a form of desensitization (q.v.) for the treatment of phobias and related disorders in which the patient is repeatedly exposed, in imagination or real life, to emotionally distressing stimuli of high intensity. Cf. *implosion* and *systematic densensitization.*

Flor. abbreviation for L. *flo′res,* flowers.

flora (flo′rah) [L. *Flora,* the goddess of flowers] the plant life present in or characteristic of a special location; it may be discernible with the unaided eye (macroflora), or only with the aid of a microscope (microflora). **intestinal f.,** the bacteria normally residing within the lumen of the intestine.

florantyrone (flo-ran'tĭ-rōn) chemical name: γ-oxo-8-fluoranthenebutyric acid. A hydrocholeretic agent, $C_{20}H_{14}O_3$, occurring as yellow, crystalline platelets; administered orally in the treatment of chronic cholecystitis, cholangitis, and biliary dyskinesia, and in the prevention of cholelithiasis.

Floraquin (flor'ah-kwin) trademark for a preparation of iodoquinol.

florentium (flo-ren'she-um) former name for promethium.

flores (flo'rēz) [L., pl. of *flos* flower] 1. the blossoms or flowers of a plant. 2. a drug after sublimation. **f. benzoi'ni,** benzoic acid. **f. sul'furis,** sublimed sulfur.

Florey (flor'e) Sir Howard Walter. Australian-born British pathologist, 1898–1968; co-winner, with Ernst Boris Chain and Sir Alexander Fleming, of the Nobel prize for medicine or physiology in 1945 for the discovery of penicillin.

Florey unit (flor'ē) [Sir Howard W. *Florey*, English pathologist, 1898–1968; co-winner, with Ernst Boris Chain and Sir Alexander Fleming, of the Nobel prize for medicine in 1945 for the discovery of penicillin] see *Oxford unit,* under *unit.*

florid (flor'id) [L. *floridus* blossoming] 1. in full bloom; occurring in fully developed form. 2. having a bright red color.

Floridin (flor'ĭ-din) trademark for a preparation of fuller's earth.

florigen (flor'ĭ-jen) a hypothetical flower-producing hormone of unknown chemical composition, believed to be produced in the leaves and transported in the phloem to the buds.

Florinef (flor'ĭ-nef) trademark for preparations of fludrocortisone acetate.

florizine (flor'ĭ-zēn) dericin.

Floropryl (flor'o-pril) trademark for preparations of isoflurophate.

Florschütz formula (flor'shitz) [Georg *Florschütz*, German physician, born 1859] see under *formula.*

flow (flo) the amount of a fluid that flows through an organ or part in a specified time. **effective renal blood f.,** that portion of the total renal blood flow that perfuses functional renal tissue, e.g., the glomeruli; abbreviated ERBF. **effective renal plasma f., (ERPF),** the amount of plasma that perfuses the renal tubules per unit time, generally measured by the *p*-aminohippurate clearance. **gene f.,** the movement of genes between populations due to migration and interbreeding. **renal plasma f. (RPF),** the amount of plasma that perfuses the kidneys per unit time, approximately 10 per cent greater than the effective renal plasma flow.

Flower's index (flow'erz) [Sir William Henry *Flower*, British physician, 1831–1899] dental index; see under *index.*

flowers (flow'erz) 1. the blossoms of a plant. 2. a sublimed drug, as sulfur or benzoin. **f. of arsenic,** arsenic trioxide. **f. of benzoin,** benzoic acid. **f. of camphor,** powdered camphor prepared by sublimation. **pyrethrum f's,** the dried powdered flowers of the perennial herbs *Chrysanthemum (Pyrethrum) cinerariaefolium* (Trév.) Vis., indigenous to Dalmatia and Montenegro, and *C. coccineum* and *C. marschalli,* indigenous to western Asia; they are used in the preparation of insecticides, and have been used as a scabicide. Called also *Dalmatian,* or *Persian, insect powder.* **f. of sulfur,** sublimed sulfur.

flowmeter (flo'me-ter) an apparatus for measuring the rate of flow of liquids or gases. **blood f.,** an instrument for determining the rate of blood flow in the arteries or veins.

flow tract (flo'trakt) the path of the blood within the chambers of the heart. In the *left flow tract,* blood enters the left atrium through the pulmonary veins, flows through the mitral valve into the left ventricle, and passes through the aortic valve and on into the aorta and systemic circulation. In the *right flow tract,* blood enters the right atrium through the venae cavae, flows through the tricuspid valve into the right ventricle, and passes through the pulmonary valve and on into the pulmonary artery and the pulmonary circulation.

floxacillin (floks"ah-sil'in) chemical name: 6-[3-(2-chloro-6-fluorophenyl)-5-methyl-4-isoxazolecarboxamido]-3,3-dimethyl-7-oxo-4-thia-1-azabicyclo[3.2.0]heptane-2-carboxylic acid. A penicillinase-resistant, semisynthetic penicillin, C_{19}-$H_{17}ClFN_3O_5S$, which has been used primarily in the treat-

ment of infections due to benzylpenicillin-resistant staphylococci. Called also *flucloxacillin.*

floxuridine (floks-ur'ĭ-dēn) [USP] 5-fluorodeoxyuridine, 5-fluorouracil deoxyribonucleoside (FUDR, FUdR); a deoxyuridine analogue, which is metabolically activated to the monophosphate nucleotide (F-dUMP), the metabolite of 5-fluorouracil (q.v.) that blocks DNA synthesis; FUDR is also metabolized to 5-fluorouracil; it is used as an antineoplastic by intra-arterial administration for treatment of liver metastases from gastrointestinal malignancies.

fl.oz. fluidounce; see under *ounce.*

F.L.P. fronto-laeva posterior (left frontoposterior—a position of the fetus).

F.L.T. fronto-laeva transversa (left frontotransverse—a position of the fetus).

flu (floo) popular name for *influenza.*

fluazacort (floo-az'ah-kort) chemical name: 21-(acetyloxy)-9-fluoro-11β,21-hydroxy-2'-methyl-5'βH-pregna-1,4-dieno[17,16-d]oxazole-3,20-dione; an anti-inflammatory, $C_{25}H_{30}$-FNO_6.

flubendazole (floo-ben'dah-zōl) chemical name: [5-(4-fluorobenzoyl)-1H-benzimidazol-2-yl]carbamic acid methyl ester; an antiprotozoal, $C_{16}H_{12}FN_3O_3$.

flucindole (floo-sin'dōl) chemical name: 6,8-difluoro-2,3,4,9-tetrahydro-N,N-dimethyl-1H-carbazol-3-amine; a tranquilizer, $C_{14}H_{16}F_2N_2$.

flucloronide (floo-klor'o-nīd) chemical name: 9,11β-dichloro-6α-fluoro-21-hydroxy-16α,17-[(1-methylethylidene)bis(oxy)]-pregna-1,4-diene-3,20-dione. A synthetic glucocorticoid, $C_{24}H_{29}Cl_2FO_5$, used in the treatment of steroid-responsive dermatoses.

flucloxacillin (floo"kloks-ah-sil'in) floxacillin.

Flucort (floo'kort) trademark for a preparation of flumethasone.

flucrylate (floo'krĭ-lāt) chemical name: 2,2,2-trifluoro-1-methylethyl 2-cyanoacrylate; a tissue adhesive, $C_7H_6F_3NO_2$.

fluctuant (fluk'tu-ant) 1. showing varying levels. 2. conveying the sensation of or exhibiting wavelike motion on palpation, owing to a liquid content.

fluctuation (fluk"tu-a'shun) [L. *fluctuatio*] 1. a variation, as about a fixed value or mass. 2. a wavelike motion, as of a fluid in a cavity of the body after succussion.

flucytosine (flu-si'to-sēn") [USP] chemical name: 5-fluorocytosine. An antifungal, $C_4H_4FN_3O$, occurring as a white to off-white, crystalline powder; used in the treatment of serious infections, such as septicemia, endocarditis, and urinary tract infections, due to *Candida* and/or *Cryptococcus* species, administered orally.

fludalanine (floo-dal'ah-nēn) chemical name: 3-fluoro-d-alanine-2-d; an antibacterial, $C_3H_5DFNO_2$.

fludazonium chloride (floo"dah-zo'ne-um) chemical name: 1-[2-(2,4-dichlorophenyl)-2-[(2,4-dichlorophenyl)methoxy]ethyl]-3-[2-(4-fluorophenyl)-2-oxoethyl]-1H-imidazolium chloride; a topical anti-infective, $C_{26}H_{20}Cl_5FN_2O_2$.

fludorex (floo'do-reks) chemical name: β-methoxy-3-[(trifluoromethyl)benzeneethanamine]; an anorexic and antiemetic, $C_{11}H_{14}F_3NO$.

fludrocortisone (floo"dro-kor'tĭ-sōn) a synthetic steroid with potent mineralocorticoid and high glucocorticoid activity, used as *fludrocortisone acetate* [USP] in replacement therapy for primary or secondary adrenocortical insufficiency in Addison's disease and for the treatment of salt-losing adrenogenital syndrome.

flufenamic acid (floo-fen-am'ik) an anthranilic acid derivative with analgesic, anti-inflammatory, and antipyretic properties.

flufenisal (floo-fen'ĭ-sal) chemical name: [4-(acetyloxy)-4'-fluoro-[1,1'-biphenyl]-3-carboxylic acid]; an analgesic, C_{15}-$H_{11}FO_4$.

flügelplatte (fle"gel-plah'teh) [Ger.] lamina alaris.

fluid (floo'id) [L. *fluidus*] 1. a liquid or a gas. 2. composed of elements or particles which freely change their relative positions without their separating. See also *liquid, liquor,* and *solution.* **allantoic f.,** the fluid contained in the allantois. **Altmann's f.,** a histologic fixing fluid composed of equal parts of 2 per cent osmic acid solution and a 5 per cent potassium dichromate solution. **amniotic f.,** fluid within the amniotic cavity produced by the amnion at the very earliest period of fetation and later by lungs and kidneys; at first crystal clear, it later becomes cloudy. The amount at term normally varies from 500 to 2000 ml. Called also *aqua* or *liquor amnii*, and, popularly, *waters*. **ascitic f.**, the serous fluid which accumulates in the peritoneal cavity in ascites. **Bamberger's f.**, an albuminous mercuric solution for use in the treatment of syphilis. **bleaching f.**, a fluid prepared by passing chlorine gas into an emulsion of calcium hydrate. **Bouin's f.**, a histologic fixing fluid consisting of formaldehyde solution, glacial acetic acid, and saturated solution of trinitrophenol (picric acid). **Burnett's disinfecting f.**, a strong aqueous solution of zinc chloride. **Callison's f.**, a solution of distilled water, Löffler's aniline methylene blue, solution of formaldehyde, glycerin, ammonium oxalate, and sodium chloride; used as a diluent in counting red blood corpuscles. **Carrel-Dakin f.**, diluted sodium hypochlorite solution. **cerebrospinal f. (C.S.F.)**, the fluid contained within the four ventricles of the brain, the subarachnoid space, and the central canal of the spinal cord; it is formed by the choroid plexus and brain parenchyma, is circulated through the ventricles into the subarachnoid space, and is absorbed into the venous system. Called also *liquor cerebrospinalis* [NA]. **chlorpalladium f.**, a decalcifying fluid for anatomical and other specimens, containing palladium chloride and hydrochloric acid; called also *Waldeyer's f.* **Condy's f.**, a disinfecting solution of sodium and potassium permanganates. **Dakin's f.**, sodium hypochlorite solution, diluted. **decalcifying f.**, a solution of formic acid and formalin. **Delafield's f.**, a fixing fluid for delicate histologic tissues, containing osmic acid, chromic acid, acetic acid, and alcohol. **Ecker's f.**, Rees and Ecker diluting f. **extracellular f.**, a general term for all the body fluids outside the cells, including the interstitial fluid, plasma, lymph, cerebrospinal fluid, etc. Extracellular fluid consists of ultrafiltrates of the blood plasma and transcellular fluid, i.e., fluid produced by active cellular secretion. It provides a constant external environment for the cells. **Flemming's fixing f.**, Flemming's solution. **follicular f.**, liquor folliculi. **formol-Müller f.**, Müller's fluid to which formaldehyde has been added. **Helly's f.**, a histologic fixative consisting of Zenker's fluid in which the glacial acetic acid is replaced by formalin; the most widely used formula consists of 9 parts Zenker stock solution and 1 part neutral formalin (Zenker-Helly-Maximow) and is usually called *Zenker-formol fixative*. **interstitial f.**, the extracellular fluid that bathes the cells of most tissues but which is not within the confines of the blood or lymph vessels and is not a transcellular fluid; it is formed by filtration through the blood capillaries and is drained away as lymph. It is the extracellular fluid volume minus the lymph volume, the plasma volume, and the transcellular fluid volume. **intracellular f.**, the portion of the total body water with its dissolved solutes which are within the cell membranes. **Kaiserling's f.**, see under *solution*. **labyrinthine f.**, perilymph. **Lang's f.**, a hardening fluid containing corrosive mercuric chloride, sodium chloride, and acetic acid, in water. **Locke's f.**, see under *solution*. **Morton's f.**, a mixture of iodine, potassium iodide, and glycerin; formerly used by injection in spinal meningocele. **Müller's f.**, a hardening solution consisting of potassium dichromate, sodium sulfate, and water. **Parker's f.**, a hardening fluid composed of formaldehyde and alcohol. **pericardial f.**, liquor pericardii. **Piazza's f.**, a blood-coagulating fluid composed of sodium chloride and ferric chloride in water. **Pitfield's f.**, a diluting fluid for counting leukocytes, made by dissolving acacia gum in distilled water and adding glacial acetic acid and gentian violet. **Rees and Ecker diluting f.**, a solution of sodium citrate, formaldehyde solution, brilliant cresyl blue, and distilled water, used as a diluting fluid for blood platelets. **Scarpa's f.**, endolymph (of the ear). **Schaudinn's f.**, a hardening fluid consisting of mercury bichloride, alcohol, and distilled water. **seminal f.**, semen, def. 2. **serous f.**, normal lymph of a serous cavity. **synovial f.**, synovia. **Tellyesniczky's f.**, a fixing solution consisting of potassium dichromate, water, and glacial acetic acid. **Thoma's f.**, a decalcifying fluid for histologic work, consisting of alcohol and pure nitric acid. **tissue f.**, interstitial f. **Toison's f.**, see under *solution*. **transcellular f.**, that portion of the extracellular fluid produced by active cellular secretion. **ventricular f.**, that portion of the cerebrospinal fluid contained in the cerebral ventricles. **Waldeyer's f.**, chlorpalladium f. **Wickersheimer's f.**, a fluid

composed of arsenic trioxide, sodium chloride, and the sulfate, carbonate, and nitrate of potassium in a mixture of water, alcohol, and glycerin; used for preserving anatomical specimens. **Zenker's f.**, see under *fixative*.

fluidextract (floo″id-ek′strakt) a liquid preparation of a vegetable drug containing alcohol as a solvent or as a preservative, or both, of such strength that each milliliter contains the extraction of 1 gm. of the standard drug which it represents. The official preparations are *aromatic cascara f.* [USP], *cascara sagrada f.* [USP], *glycyrrhiza f.* [NF], and *senna f.* [USP], all of which are used as cathartics, and *eriodictyon f.* [NF], used as a flavoring agent for pharmaceutical preparations.

fluidextractum (floo″id-eks-trak′tum), gen. *fluidextrac′ti*, pl. *fluidextrac′ta* [L.] fluidextract.

fluidism (floo′id-izm) humoralism.

fluidounce (floo-id-ouns′) fluid ounce; see under *ounce*.

fluidrachm (floo″id-ram′) fluid dram; see under *dram*.

fluidram (floo″id-ram′) fluid dram; see under *dram*.

fluke (flook) any trematode worm; see *Trematoda*. **blood f.**, Schistosoma. **intestinal f's**, see *Echinostoma, Fasciolopsis, Gastrodiscoides, Heterophyes, Metagonimus*, and *Watsonius*. **liver f's**, see *Clonorchis, Dicrocoelium, Fasciola*, and *Opisthorchis*. **lung f.**, see *Paragonimus*.

flumen (floo′men), pl. *flu′mina* [L.] a stream. **flu′mina pilo′rum** [NA], hair streams: continuous lines formed by the pattern of hair growth on various parts of the body, the hairs lying in the same direction.

flumequine (floo′mě-kwin) chemical name: 9-fluoro-6,7-dihydro-5-methyl-1-oxo-1H,5H-benzo[ij]quinolizine-2-carboxylic acid; an antibacterial, $C_{14}H_{12}FNO_3$.

flumethasone pivalate (floo-meth′ah-sōn) [USP] chemical name: 21-(2,2-dimethyl-1-oxopropoxy)-6α,9-difluoro-6,9-difluoro-11β,17-dihydroxy-16α-methylpregna-1,4-diene-3,2-0-dione. A synthetic glucocorticoid, $C_{27}H_{36}F_2O_6$, occurring as a white to off-white, crystalline powder; used as a topical anti-inflammatory in steroid-responsive dermatoses.

flumethiazide (floo″mě-thi′ah-zīd) chemical name: 6-trifluoromethyl-2H-1,2,4-benzothiadiazine-7-sulfonamide-1,1--dioxide; a thiazide diuretic, $C_8H_6F_3N_3O_4S_2$.

flumina (floo′mi-nah) [L.] plural of *flumen*.

flumizole (floo′mi-zōl) chemical name: 4,5-bis(4-methoxyphenyl)-2-(trifluoromethyl)-1H-imidazole; an anti-inflammatory, $C_{18}H_{15}F_3N_2O_2$.

flumoxonide (floo-mok′so-nīd) chemical name: 6α,9-difluoro- 11β-hydroxy-21,21-dimethoxy-16α,17-[(1-methylethylidene)bis(oxy)]pregna-1,4-diene-3,20-dione; an adrenocortical steroid, $C_{26}H_{34}F_2O_7$.

flunarizine hydrochloride (floo-nar′i-zēn) chemical name: 1-[bis-(4-fluorophenyl)methyl]-4-(3-phenyl-2-propenyl)piperazine dihydrochloride; a vasodilator, $C_{26}H_{26}F_2$-$N_2 \cdot 2HCl$.

flunidazole (floo-ni′dah-zōl) chemical name: 2-(4-fluorophenyl)-5-1H-imidazole-1-ethanol; an antiprotozoal agent, $C_{11}H_{10}$ FN_3O_3.

flunisolide (floo-nis′o-līd) chemical name: 6α-fluoro-11β,21-dihydroxy-16α,17-[(1-methylethylidine)bis(oxy)]pregna-1,4-diene-3,20-dione; a glucocorticoid, $C_{24}H_{31}FO_6$. **f. acetate**, the 21-acetate ester of flunisolide, $C_{26}H_{33}FO_7$; an anti-inflammatory.

flunitrazepam (floo″ni-trāz′ě-pam) chemical name: 5-(2-fluorophenyl)-1,3-dihydro-1-methyl-7-nitro-2H-1,4-benzodiazepin-2- one; a hypnotic and induction agent in anesthesia, $C_{16}H_{12}FN_3O_3$.

flunixin (floo-nik′sin) chemical name: 2-[[2-methyl-3-(trifluoromethyl)phenyl]amino]-3-pyridinecarboxylic acid; an anti-inflammatory and analgesic, $C_{14}H_{11}F_3N_2O_2$. **f. meglumine**, the meglumine salt of flunixin, $C_{14}H_{11}F_3N_2O_2 \cdot C_7$-$H_{17}NO_5$; an anti-inflammatory and analgesic.

fluocinolone acetonide (floo″o-sin′o-lon) [USP] chemical name: 6α,9-difluoro-11β,21-dihydroxy-16α,17-[(1-methylethylidene)bis(oxy)]pregna-1,4-diene,3,20-dione. A synthetic glucocorticoid, $C_{24}H_{30}F_2O_6$, occurring as a white or practically white, crystalline powder; used as a topical anti-inflammatory in steroid-responsive dermatoses.

fluocinonide (floo″o-sin′o-nīd) [USP] The 21-acetate ester of fluocinolone acetonide, occurring as a white to cream-colored, crystalline powder, which has anti-inflammatory, antipruritic, and vasoconstrictive properties; used topically in the treatment of certain dermatoses.

fluocortin butyl (floo″o-kor′tin) chemical name: 6α-fluoro-11β-hydroxy-16α-methyl-3,20-dioxopregna-1,4-dien-21-oic acid butyl ester; an anti-inflammatory, $C_{26}H_{35}FO_5$.

Fluogen (floo′o-jen) trademark for a preparation of influenza virus vaccine.

Fluonid (floo′o-nid) trademark for preparations of fluocinolone acetonide.

fluor (floo′or) [L. "a flow"] a discharge. **f. al′bus,** leukorrhea.

fluorane (floo′or-ān) the parent compound of fluorescein and related dyes; 9-hydroxy-9-xanthene-o-benzoic acid lactone.

fluorescein (floo″o-res′e-in) chemical name: resorcinolphthalein. The simplest of the fluorane dyes and the parent compound of eosin; used intravenously in tests to assess by its fluorescence the adequacy of the circulation, and combined with radioactive iodine in localization of brain tumors, etc. Called also *dihydroxyfluorane.* **f. isothiocyanate (FITC),** a form capable of being conjugated to protein and hence used as a label in fluorescent antibody staining procedures. **sodium f. [USP], soluble f.,** chemical name: resorcinolphthalein sodium. An odorless, water-soluble, orange-red powder, $C_{20}H_{10}Na_2O_5$, used in dilute solution to reveal corneal lesions and as a test of circulation in the extremities and retina. Called also *uranin.*

fluoresceinuria (floo″o-res″e-in-u′re-ah) the presence of fluorescein in the urine.

fluorescence (floo″o-res′ens) [first observed in *fluor spar*] the property of emitting light while exposed to light, the wavelength of the emitted light being only slightly longer than that of the light absorbed. Cf. *phosphorescence.* **secondary f.** fluorescence in tissues which is induced by staining with fluorescent dyes (*fluorochromes*). Cf. *autofluorescence.*

fluorescent (floo″o-res′ent) exhibiting fluorescence.

fluorescin (floo″o-res′in) a reduced form of fluorescein used to detect oxidative activity. As the sodium salt, it may be used for the same purposes as sodium fluorescein.

fluoridation (floo″or-ĭ-da′shun) treatment with fluorides; specifically, the addition of fluoride to the public water supply as part of the public health program to prevent or reduce the incidence of dental caries.

fluoride (floo′o-rīd) a binary compound of fluorine (q.v.). **stannous f. [USP],** a compound, SnF_2, containing not less than 71.2 per cent stannous tin and between 22.3 and 25.5 per cent fluoride; applied topically to the teeth as a dental caries prophylactic.

fluorimeter (floo″o-rim′ĕ-ter) fluorometer.

fluorimetry (floo″o-rim′ĕ-tre) fluorometry.

fluorine (floo′ŏ-rēn) [from *fluor spar*, from which it is derived] a nonmetallic, gaseous element, belonging to the halogen group; symbol, F; atomic number, 9; atomic weight, 18.998. Fluorine, in the form of fluoride, is incorporated into the structure of bone and teeth and provides protection against dental caries; an excess of fluorine may result in fluorosis.

fluoroacetate (floo″or-o-ah′sĕ-tāt) a salt of fluoroacetic acid.

fluorochrome (floo′or-o-krōm) any fluorescent dye used as a stain or label, e.g., fluorescein isothiocyanate attached to an antibody.

fluorocyte (floo′or-o-sīt) a reticulocyte showing red fluorescence.

fluorography (floo″or-og′rah-fe) photofluorography.

fluoroimmunoassay (flōōr′o-im″u-no-as″a) any immunoassay using fluorochrome-labeled antibody or antigen; classified as heterogeneous assays requiring separation of the bound label (antigen-antibody complex) from the free labeled immunoreactant by physicochemical methods and homogeneous (single-phase) assays utilizing a change in fluorescence (e.g., quenching, increased polarization) accompanying antigen-antibody binding to measure the amount of bound label without separation. Abbreviated FIA.

Fluoromar (floor′o-mar) trademark for a preparation of fluroxene.

fluorometer (floo″or-om′ĕ-ter) 1. an apparatus for measuring the quantity of rays given out by a roentgen-ray tube.

2. an attachment to the fluoroscope, enabling the operator to secure a correct and undistorted shadow of the object and to locate exactly the position of the object. 3. the instrument used in fluorimetry, consisting of an energy source (e.g., a mercury arc lamp or xenon lamp) to induce fluorescence, monochromators for selection of the wavelength, and a detector; called also *fluorimeter.*

fluorometholone (floor″o-meth′o-lōn) [USP] chemical name: 9-fluoro-11β,17-dihydroxy-6α-methylpregna-1,4-diene-3,20-dione. A synthetic glucocorticoid, $C_{22}H_{29}FO_4$, occurring as a white to yellowish white, crystalline powder; used as a topical anti-inflammatory in steroid-responsive dermatoses.

fluorometry (floo″o-rom′ĕ-tre) an analytical technique for identifying minute amounts of a substance by detection and measurement of the characteristic wavelength of the light it emits during fluorescence. Called also *fluorimetry.*

fluoronephelometer (floo″o-ro-nef″ĕ-lom′ĕ-ter) an instrument for analysis of a solution by measuring the light scattered or emitted by it. Called also *nefluorophotometer.*

p-**fluorophenylalanine** (floo″o-ro-fen″il-al′ĭ-nīn) a modified molecule of phenylalanine that binds to enzymes but is incapable of performing the functions of the natural molecule and thus acts as an antagonist.

fluorophosphate (floo″or-o-fos′fāt) an organic compound containing fluorine and phosphorus. **diisopropyl f.,** isoflurophate.

fluorophotometry (floo″o-ro-fo-tom′ĕ-tre) the measurement of light given off by fluorescent substances. **vitreous f.,** the measurement of light given off by intravenously injected fluorescein that has leaked through the retinal vessels into the vitreous; done to detect the breakdown of the blood-retinal barrier, an early ocular change in diabetes mellitus.

Fluoroplex (floo′oro-pleks) trademark for a preparation of fluorouracil for topical application.

fluororoentgenography (floo″o-ro-rent″gen-og′rah-fe) photofluorography.

fluoroscope (floo′ŏ-ro-skōp) [*fluorescence* + Gr. *skopein* to examine] a device used for examining deep structures by means of roentgen rays; it consists of a screen (*fluorescent screen*) covered with crystals of calcium tungstate on which are projected the shadows of x-rays passing through the body placed between the screen and the source of irradiation. **biplane f.,** a fluoroscope by which examinations can be made in two planes, horizontal and vertical.

fluoroscopical (floo″o-ro-skop′ĭ-kal) pertaining to fluoroscopy.

fluoroscopy (floo″or-os′ko-pe) examination by means of the fluoroscope.

fluorosilicate (floo″o-ro-sil′ĭ-kāt) a compound of silicon and some other base with fluorine, such as sodium silicofluoride; fluorosilicates are sometimes used as insecticides, and are very toxic when ingested. Called also *silicofluoride.*

fluorosis (floo″o-ro′sis) a condition due to exposure to excessive amounts of fluorine or its compounds. Fluoride intoxication may occur as a result of such factors as accidental ingestion of fluoride-containing insecticides and rodenticides, chronic inhalation of industrial dusts or gases containing fluorides, or prolonged ingestion of water containing large amounts of fluorides; it is characterized by skeletal changes, consisting of combined osteosclerosis and osteomalacia (osteofluorosis) and by mottled enamel (q.v.) of the teeth when exposure occurs during enamel formation. A similar condition is seen in cattle, sheep, and other livestock, and is due to the same factors that cause intoxication in humans and also to ingestion of animal feed containing toxic levels of fluorides and grazing on pastures contaminated with fluorides in industrial dusts or gases. Called also *chronic endemic f.* and *chronic fluoride,* or *fluorine, poisoning.* **dental f.,** mottled enamel. **endemic f., chronic,** fluorosis.

5-fluorouracil (flōōr″o-ur′ah-sil) 5-FU; a uracil analog metabolically activated like uracil; used as an antineoplastic for palliative treatment of carcinomas of the breast and gastrointestinal tract and also as a component of combination chemotherapy regimens. Major side effects are nausea and vomiting, ulceration of the oral and gastrointestinal mucosa, and bone marrow depression; 5-FU is also used topically, without these systemic side effects, for treatment of actinic keratoses and superficial basal cell and squamous cell skin carcinoma. Available as *fluorouracil* [USP].

Fluosol (floo′o-sol) a frozen perfluorochemical blood substitute that, when administered with oxygen, fulfills the functions of hemoglobin but lacks clotting factors and other properties of blood.

Fluothane (floo′o-thān) trademark for a preparation of halothane.

fluotracen hydrochloride (floo″o-tra′sen) chemical name: *cis*-(±)-9,10-dihydro-N,N,10-trimethyl-2-(trifluoromethyl)-9-anthracenepropanamine hydrochloride; a tranquilizer and antidepressant, $C_{21}H_{24}F_3N \cdot HCl$.

fluoxetine (floo-ok′sĕ-tēn) chemical name: (±)-N-methyl-γ-[4-(trifluoromethyl)phenoxy]benzenepropanamine; an antidepressant, $C_{17}H_{18}F_3NO$.

fluoxymesterone (floo-ok″se-mes′ter-ōn) [USP] chemical name: 9-fluoro-11β,17β-dihydroxy-17-methylandrost-4-en-3-one. An androgen, $C_{20}H_{29}FO_3$, occurring as a white or practically white, crystalline powder; used in the treatment of male hypogonadism and in the palliative therapy of inoperable female breast cancer in selected patients, administered orally.

fluperamide (floo-per′ah-mīd) chemical name: 4-[4-chloro-3-(trifluoromethyl)phenyl]-4-hydroxy-N,N-dimethyl-α,α-diphenyl-1-piperidinebutamide; an antiperistaltic, $C_{30}H_{32}ClF_3N_2O_2$.

fluphenazine (floo-fen′ah-zēn) chemical name: 4-[3-[2-(trifluoromethyl)-10H-phenothiazin-10-yl]-propyl]-1-piperazineethanol. The 2-trifluromethyl derivative of perphenazine, $C_{22}H_{26}F_3N_3OS$, the most potent of the phenothiazine tranquilizers. **f. enanthate** [USP], the enanthate ester of fluphenazine, $C_{22}H_{38}F_3N_3O_2S$, occurring as pale yellow to yellow-orange, clear to slightly turbid, viscous liquid, having the same uses as those of the hydrochloride salt, but of longer duration; administered intramuscularly and subcutaneously. **f. hydrochloride** [USP], the dihydrochloride salt of fluphenazine, $C_{22}H_{26}F_3N_3OS \cdot 2HCl$, occurring as a white or nearly white, crystalline powder; used as a tranquilizer in the treatment of manifestations of psychotic disorders, and as an antiemetic, administered orally and intramuscularly.

fluprednisolone (floo″pred-nis′o-lōn) chemical name: 6α-fluoro-11β17,21-trihydroxypregna-1,4-diene-3,20-dione. A synthetic glucocorticoid, $C_{21}H_{27}FO_5$, occurring as a white to off-white, crystalline powder; used in the treatment of various conditions responsive to the anti-inflammatory actions of glucocorticoids, administered orally. **f. valerate**, an ester of fluprednisolone, $C_{26}H_{35}FO_6$, with actions similar to those of the base.

fluprostenol sodium (floo-pros′tĕ-nōl) chemical name: [1α(Z), 2β(1E,3R*), 3α,5α]-7-[3,5-dihydroxy-2-[3-hydroxy-4-[3-(trifluoromethyl)phenoxy]-1-butenyl]cyclopentyl]-5-heptenoic acid sodium salt; a prostaglandin of the F series, $C_{23}H_{28}F_3NaO_6$, used in the treatment of infertility.

fluquazone (floo′kwah-zōn) chemical name: 6-chloro-4-phenyl-1-(2,2,2-trifluoroethyl-2(1H)-quinazolinone; an anti-inflammatory, $C_{16}H_{10}ClF_3N_2O$.

flurandrenolide (floor″an-dren′o-līd) [USP] chemical name: 6α-fluoro-11β,21-dihydroxy-16α,17-[(1-methylethylidine)bis(oxy)]pregn-4-ene-3,20-dione. A glucocorticoid, $C_{24}H_{33}FO_6$, occurring as a white to off-white, fluffy, crystalline powder; used as an anti-inflammatory in the treatment of steroid-responsive dermatoses, applied topically. Called also *flurandrenolone*.

flurandrenolone (floor″an-dren′o-lōn) flurandrenolide.

flurazepam hydrochloride (floor-az′ĕ-pam) [USP] chemical name: 7-chloro-1-[2-(diethylamino)ethyl]-5-(2-fluorophenyl)-1,3-dihydro-2H-1,4-benzodiazepin-2-one dihydrochloride. A hypnotic, $C_{21}H_{23}ClFN_3O \cdot 2HCl$, occurring as an off-white to yellow, crystalline powder; administered orally.

flurbiprofen (floor-bip′ro-fen) a nonsteroidal anti-inflammatory agent that is a propionic acid derivative.

Flurobate (floor′o-bāt) trademark for preparations of betamethasone benzoate.

flurocitabine (floo″ro-si′tah-bēn) chemical name: [(2R-(2α,3β,3aβ,9aβ)]-7-fluoro-2,3,3a,9a-tetrahydro-3-hydroxy-6-imino-6H-furo[2′,3′:4,5]oxazolo(3,2-a)pyrimidine-2-methanol; an antineoplastic, $C_9H_{10}FN_3O_4$.

flurogestone acetate (floor″o-jes′tōn) chemical name:

17-(acetyloxy-9-9-fluoro-11β,17-hydroxypregn-4-ene-3,20-dione; a progestin, $C_{23}H_{31}FO_5$.

flurothyl (floor′o-thil) [USP] an inhalant convulsive agent, hexafluorodiethyl ether; see *convulsive therapy*, under *therapy*.

flush (flush) transient, episodic redness of the face and neck caused by certain diseases, ingestion of certain drugs or other substances, heat, emotional factors, or physical exertion. **atropine f.,** flushing and dryness of the skin of the face and neck from overdosage with atropine. **breast f.,** a condition sometimes occurring in the early puerperium consisting of a tense and flushed state of the breasts with prominent veins. **carcinoid f.,** extensive blotchy red or bluish flushing on the face or trunk, often associated with diarrhea and abdominal pain and sometimes bronchospasm; it is possibly due to vasoactive kinins or other peptides associated with carcinoid tumor. **hectic f.,** a persistent or chronic flush associated with chronic debilitating disease, usually febrile, such as pulmonary tuberculosis. **histamine f.,** sudden symmetric erythema of the face and upper trunk, usually associated with throbbing headache and bounding pulse, and histaminuria; seen in urticaria pigmentosa, it may also occur a few minutes after eating fish of the scombroid family (red snapper or mahimahi) contaminated by *Proteus* during cold storage prior to cooking. **mahogany f.,** a deep red or mahogany-colored, circumscribed spot seen on one cheek in some cases of lobar pneumonia. **malar f.,** hectic flush at the malar eminence.

fluspiperone (floo-spip′er-ōn) chemical name: 1-(4-fluorophenyl)-8-[4-(4-fluorophenyl)-4-oxobutyl]-1,3,8-triazaspiro[4.5]decan-4-one; a tranquilizer, $C_{23}H_{25}F_2N_3O_2$.

fluspirilene (floo-spēr′ĭ-lēn) chemical name: 8-[4,4-bis(4-fluorophenyl) butyl] -1-phenyl-1, 3, 8-triazaspiro-[4.5]decan-4-one; a tranquilizer, $C_{29}H_{31}F_2N_3O$.

flutamide (floo′tah-mīd) chemical name: 2-methyl-N-[4-nitro-3-(trifluormethyl)phenyl]propanamide. A nonsteroidal antiandrogen, $C_{11}H_{11}F_3N_2O_3$; used to increase the flow of urine in benign hypertrophy of the prostate.

flutiazin (floo-ti′ah-zin) chemical name: 8-(trifluoromethyl)-10H-phenothiazine-1-carboxylic acid; an anti-inflammatory agent for veterinary use, $C_{14}H_8F_3NO_2S$.

flutter (flut′er) a rapid vibration or pulsation. **atrial f.,** a condition of cardiac arrhythmia in which the atrial contractions are rapid (200 to 320 per minute), but regular. In many instances, a circus pathway is probably present. The ventricles are unable to respond to each atrial impulse, so that a partial block usually is present. Formerly called *auricular f.* **auricular f.,** atrial f. **diaphragmatic f.,** peculiar, wavelike fibrillations of the diaphragm of unknown cause; the condition may be paroxysmal or persist indefinitely. **impure f.,** atrial flutter in which the atrial rhythm is irregular. **mediastinal f.,** a condition of abnormal motility of the mediastinum during respiratory movements. **pure f.,** atrial flutter in which the atrial rhythm is regular. **ventricular f.,** a possible transition stage between ventricular tachycardia and ventricular fibrillation, the electrocardiogram showing rapid, uniform, and virtually regular oscillations, 250 or more per minute.

flutter-fibrillation (flut′er-fi-brĭ-la′shun) impure flutters that vary from moment to moment in their resemblance to flutter or fibrillation, respectively.

flux (fluks) [L. *fluxus*] 1. an excessive flow or discharge. 2. a borax-containing substance that maintains the cleanliness of metals to be united and facilitates the easy flow and attachment of solder. **celiac f.,** diarrhea accompanied by the discharge of undigested food. **hepatic f.,** bilious f. **ionic f.,** the number of mols per second passing through an area of 1 cm. oriented perpendicularly to the direction of flow of the substance. **menstrual f.,** the menses. **neutral f.,** a fusible material, usually an inorganic salt, which does not unite with the combined oxygen in the metal but merely dissolves the metal oxide (barium chloride, sodium chloride). **oxidizing f.,** a material which, when heated, gives up oxygen that may unite with base metals and form oxides (as potassium nitrate, potassium chlorate). **reducing f.,** a flux which unites with the oxygen of metallic oxides and frees the metal from such combinations.

fluxion (fluk′shun) a flowing; especially an abnormal or excessive flow of fluid to a part.

fly (fli) a dipterous, or two-winged, insect. Called also *musca*. **black f.,** a name given various individuals of the family Simuliidae. **blackbottle f.,** see *Phormia*. **bloodsucking f's,** see *Chrysops* and *Tabanus*. **blow f., bluebottle f.,** see *Calliphora*. **bot f.,** see *botfly*. **caddis f.,** a fly of the order Trichoptera; hairs and scales from these flies are a cause of allergic symptoms in susceptible persons. **cheese f.,** see *Piophila*. **deer f.,** *Chrysops discalis*. **drone f.,** *Eristalis tenax*. **dung f.,** *Sepsis violacea*. **eye f.,** any fly which attacks the eye; see *Hippelates* and *Siphunculina funicola*. **face f.,** *Musca autumnalis*. **filth f.,** *Musca domestica*. **flesh f.,** see *Sarcophaga* and *Wohlfahrtia*. **fruit f.,** see *Drosophila*. **gad f.,** see *Tabanus*. **gold f.,** *Lucilia caesar*. **green-bottle f.,** see *Lucilia* and *Phaenicia*. **heel f.,** see *Hypoderma*. **horn f.,** see *Haematobia*. **horse f.,** see *Tabanus*. **house f.,** *Musca domestica*. **hover f's,** flies, such as *Helophilus* and *Eristalis*, of the family Syrphidae. **lake f.,** see *Hexagenia bilineata*. **latrine f.,** *Fannia scalaris*. **mango f., mangrove f.,** *Chrysops dimidiata*. **moth f.,** a fly of the family Psychodidae. **motuca f.,** *Lepidoselaga lepidota*. **nose f., nostril f.,** *Oestrus ovis*. **owl f.,** a name given individuals of the family Psychodidae. **ox-warble f.,** see *Hypoderma*. **phlebotomus f.,** see *Phlebotomus*. **Russian f.,** *Lytta*. **sand f.,** see *sandfly*. **screw-worm f.,** *Cochliomyia hominivorax*. **Seroot f.,** *Tabanus gratus*. **snipe f.,** see *Rhagionidae*. **soldier f.,** *Hermetia illucens*, the larvae of which sometimes cause intestinal myiasis in man. **Spanish f.,** *Lytta vesicatoria*. **stable f.,** see *Stomoxys calcitrans*. **tick f.,** see *Hippobosca*. **tsetse f.,** see *Glossina*. **tumbu f.,** *Cordylobia anthropophaga*. **typhoid f.** (obs.), *Musca domestica*. **vinegar f.,** see *Drosophila*. **warble f.,** *Hypoderma*.

Fm chemical symbol for *fermium*.

F.M. abbreviation for L. *fi'at mistu'ra*, make a mixture.

FMN flavin mononucleotide (riboflavin 5'-phosphate).

FNTC fine needle transhepatic cholangiography.

focal (fo'kal) pertaining to or occupying a focus.

foci (fo'si) [L.] genitive and plural of *focus*.

focil, focile (fo'sil, fo'sĭ-le) [L. *fusillus*, a little spindle] one of the bones of the forearm or leg.

focimeter (fo-sim'ĕ-ter) [*focus* + *-meter*] an apparatus for finding the focus of a lens.

focus (fo'kus), pl. *fo'ci* [L. "fire-place"] 1. the point of convergence of light rays or of the waves of sound. 2. the chief center of a morbid process. **aplanatic f.,** that focus or point from which diverging rays pass the lens without spherical aberration. **Assmann f.,** the early exudative lesion of pulmonary tuberculosis, occurring most frequently in the subapical region; called also *Assmann's tuberculous infiltrate*. **conjugate f.,** the point at which rays that come from some definite point are brought together. **epileptogenic f.,** the area of the cerebral cortex responsible for causing epileptic seizures, as revealed in the encephalogram. **Ghon f.,** the primary parenchymal lesion of primary pulmonary tuberculosis in children; when associated with a corresponding lymph node focus, it is known as the *primary*, or *Ghon, complex*. Called also *Ghon's primary lesion* and *Ghon tubercle*. **principal foci,** points of convergence of rays parallel with the principal axis of a lens, or system: in the *eye* (approx.) 18 mm. from the anterior nodal point, and 24 mm. from the posterior nodal point, and holding the ratio of the indices of air and vitreum. **real f.,** the point at which convergent rays intersect. **Simon's foci,** hematogenous areas in the apices of the lungs of children regarded as precursors of apical tuberculosis in later life. **virtual f.,** the point at which divergent rays would intersect if prolonged backward.

focusing (fo'kus-ing) the act of converging at a point. **isoelectric f.,** electrophoresis in which the protein mixture is subjected to an electric field in a gel medium in which a pH gradient has been established; each protein then migrates until it reaches the site (or focus) at which the pH is equal to its isoelectric point. Called also *electrofocusing*.

foe- for words beginning thus, see those beginning *fe-*.

Foerster see *Förster*.

fog (fog) a colloid system in which the dispersion medium is a gas and the disperse particles are liquid, e.g., a cloudlike mass of water droplets dispersed in air.

fogging (fog'ing) in ophthalmology, a method employed in determining the refractive error, the patient being first made artificially myopic by means of plus spheres, in order to relax all accommodation before using cylinders.

fogo (fo'go) [Port. "fire"] a name given to a skin condition in Brazil. **f. selva'gem** [Port. "wild fire"] a progressive and sometimes fatal variant of pemphigus foliaceous endemic in certain areas of Brazil, most often affecting children, and characterized by flaccid blisters that rupture easily, forming erosions with peripheral rolls of epidermis, associated with a burning sensation. Called also *Brazilian, South American,* or *wildfire pemphigus*.

foil (foil) metal in the form of an extremely thin, pliable sheet. **gold f.,** pure gold beaten and/or rolled into thin sheets, used as a direct filling material in dental restorations; gold foil used in direct restorations has a thickness of 0.5 μm or less. Occasionally used loosely to refer to mat gold and powdered gold. **gold f., cohesive,** gold foil that has been rendered cohesive by the process of annealing or degassing; two pieces of gold foil are welded together into a single sheet that can be hammered, rolled, or otherwise fashioned into a desired shape or thinness. Called also *cohesive gold*. **mat f.,** foil produced by sandwiching mat gold between two sheets of cohesive gold foil; used as a direct filling dental material. **platinum f.,** a very thin foil of pure platinum with a high fusing point, thus being suitable for use as a matrix for soldering procedures. Also used to provide internal forms for porcelain restorations during their fabrication. **tin f.,** a thin sheet rolled from tin or an alloy of tin and lead, used as a protective wrapping; also used as a separating material between the cast and denture base material during flasking and curing. Written also *tinfoil*.

Fol. abbreviation for L. *fo'lia*, leaves.

folacin (fōl'ah-sin) folic acid.

folate (fo'lāt) the anionic form of folic acid.

fold (fōld) a thin, recurved margin, or doubling; called also *plica*. **alar f's,** plicae alares. **amniotic f.,** the folded edge of the amniotic membrane where it rises over and finally encloses the embryo. **aryepiglottic f.,** plica aryepiglottica. **aryepiglottic f. of Collier,** plica triangularis. **axillary f.,** the fold of skin and muscle bounding the armpit, formed by the anterior and posterior axillary folds. **axillary f., anterior,** plica axillaris anterior. **axillary f., posterior,** plica axillaris posterior. **Brachet's mesolateral f.,** mesolateral f. **bulboventricular f.,** a fold between the bulbus cordis and the ventricle that disappears as the bulbus cordis is absorbed into the right ventricle. **caval f.,** a ridge that contains the superior segment of the embryonic inferior vena cava. **cecal f's,** plicae caecales. **cholecystoduodenocolic f.,** an occasionally present fold of peritoneum sometimes uniting the colon, duodenum, and gallbladder. **ciliary f's,** plicae ciliares. **circular f's, circular f's of Kerckring,** plicae circulares. **conjunctival f.,** the cul-de-sac formed where the conjunctiva is reflected from the eyeball to the upper or lower eyelid; called also *palpebral f.* and *retrotarsal f.* **costocolic f.,** ligamentum phrenicolicum. **Douglas' f.,** 1. plica rectouterina. 2. linea arcuata vaginae musculi recti abdominis. **Duncan's f's,** the loose folds of peritoneum which cover the uterus immediately following delivery. **duodenojejunal f.,** plica duodenalis superior. **duodenomesocolic f.,** plica duodenalis inferior. **epicanthal f., epicanthine f.,** epicanthus (plica palpebronasalis [NA]). **epigastric f.,** plica umbilicalis lateralis, def. 1. **falciform f. of fascia lata,** margo falciformis hiatus saphenus. **fimbriated f.,** plica fimbriata. **gastric f's,** plicae gastricae. **gastropancreatic f., left,** plica gastropancreatica. **gastropancreatic f., right,** plica hepatopancreatica. **genital f.,** genital ridge. **glossoepiglottic f's,** folds of mucous membrane extending from the base of the tongue to the epiglottis. **glossoepiglottic f., median,** plica glossoepiglottica mediana. **gluteal f.,** sulcus glutealis. **Guérin's f.,** a fold of mucous membrane occasionally seen in the fossa navicularis of the urethra. **Hasner's f.,** plica lacrimalis. **head f.,** a crescentic, ventral fold of the blastoderm at the future head end of the embryo. **Heister's f.,** plica spiralis. **Hensing's f.,** see under *ligament*. **hepatopancreatic f.,** plica hepatopancreatica. **horizontal f's of rectum,** plicae transversales recti. **ileocecal f.,** plica ileocaecalis. **ileocolic f.,** a crescentic fold of peritoneum forming a part of the mesentery, mesocecum, and mesocolon. **incudal f.,** plica incudis. **inferior duodenal f.,** plica duodenalis inferior. **interarticular f. of hip,** ligamentum capitis femoris. **inter-**

arytenoid f., plica interarytenoidea. **interdigital f.,** the free border of the web connecting the bases of adjoining digits. **interureteric f.,** plica interureterica. **iridial f's,** plicae iridis. **Jonnesco's f., Juvara's f.,** parietoperitoneal f. **Kerckring's f's (of small intestine),** plicae circulares. **Kohlrausch's f's,** plicae transversales recti. **lacrimal f.,** plica lacrimalis. **f's of large intestine,** plicae semilunares coli. **longitudinal f. of duodenum,** plica longitudinalis duodeni. **mallear f. of mucous coat of tympanic cavity, anterior,** plica mallearis anterior tunicae mucosae cavitatis tympanicae. **mallear f. of mucous coat of tympanic cavity, posterior,** plica mallearis posterior tunicae mucosae cavitatis tympanicae. **mallear f. of tympanic membrane, anterior,** plica mallearis anterior membranae tympani. **mallear f. of tympanic membrane, posterior,** plica mallearis posterior membranae tympani. **mammary f.,** the primordium of the mammary gland in the early embryo; it extends from the root of the upper extremity to the inguinal fold. **Marshall's f.,** plica venae cavae sinistrae. **medullary f.,** neural f. **mesolateral f.,** the right lamella of the primitive mesentery running to the right lobe of the liver; called also *Brachet's mesolateral f.* **mesonephric f.,** mesonephric ridge. **mesouterine f.,** a fold of peritoneum supporting the uterus. **mucobuccal f.,** the cul-de-sac formed where the mucous membrane is reflected from the upper or lower jaw to the cheek. **mucolabial f.,** the line of flexure of the oral mucous membrane as it passes from the mandible or maxilla to the lip. **mucosal f.,** a fold of mucous membrane; called also *mucous f.* **mucosobuccal f.,** mucobuccal f. **mucous f.,** mucosal f. **mucous f's of rectum,** columnae anales. **nail f.,** the fold of palmar skin around the base and sides of the nail. **nasopharyngeal f.,** plica salpingopalatina. **Nélaton's f.,** a transverse fold of mucous membrane in the rectum, marking the junction of its lower and middle thirds. **neural f.,** one of the paired folds, lying one on either side of the neural plate, that form the neural tube; called also *medullary f.* **opercular f.,** a fold of tissue constituting an adhesion between the tonsil and the anterior pillar of the fauces. **palatine f's, palatine f's, transverse,** plicae palatinae transversae. **palmate f's,** plicae palmatae. **palpebral f.,** conjunctival f. **palpebronasal f.,** epicanthus (plica palpebronasalis [NA]). **pancreaticogastric f., left,** plica gastropancreatica. **paraduodenal f.,** plica paraduodenalis. **parietocolic f.,** Hensing's ligament. **parietoperitoneal f.,** a fold of peritoneum in the fetus, arising at the left side of the ascending colon and attached to the parietal peritoneum at the right of the ascending colon; called also *Jonnesco's f.* and *Juvara's f.* **pharyngoepiglottic f.,** a fold of mucous membrane running backward from the epiglottis. **pituitary f's** (*obs.*), diaphragma sellae. **primitive f.,** one of the two ridges flanking the primitive groove, one on either side. **Rathke's f's,** two fetal folds of mesoderm which unite at the median line to form Douglas' septum and to render the rectum a complete canal. **rectal f's,** plicae transversales recti. **rectouterine f.,** plica rectouterina. **rectovaginal f.,** a fold of peritoneum interposed between the rectum and vagina. **rectovesical f.,** plica rectouterina. **retrotarsal f.,** conjunctival f. **Rindfleisch's f's,** folds in the serous surface of the pericardium around the beginning of the aorta. **sacrogenital f.,** plica rectouterina. **salpingopalatine f.,** plica salpingopalatina. **salpingopharyngeal f.,** plica salpingopharyngea. **Schultze's f.,** a sickle-shaped fold of the amnion extending from the point of insertion of the cord into the placenta to the remains of the umbilical vesicle. **semilunar f.,** plica semilunaris. **semilunar f's of colon,** plicae semilunares coli. **semilunar f. of conjunctiva,** plica semilunaris conjunctivae. **semilunar f. of transversalis fascia,** ligamentum interfoveolare. **serosal f., serous f.,** a fold of serous membrane. **sigmoid f's of colon,** plicae semilunares coli. **spiral f.,** plica spiralis. **spiral f. of cystic duct,** plica spiralis. **stapedial f.,** plica stapedis. **sublingual f.,** plica sublingualis. **superior duodenal f.,** plica duodenalis superior. **synovial f.,** plica synovialis. **synovial f., infrapatellar, synovial f., patellar,** plica synovialis infrapatellaris. **synovial f. of hip,** ligamentum capitis femoris. **tail f.,** a crescentic, ventral fold of the blastoderm, at the future caudal end of the embryo. **transverse f's of rectum,** plicae transversales recti. **Treves' f.,** plica ileocecalis. **triangular f.,** plica trian-

gularis. **tubal f's of uterine tube,** plicae tubariae tubae uterinae. **umbilical f., lateral,** plica umbilicalis lateralis, def. 1. **umbilical f., medial,** plica umbilicalis medialis. **umbilical f., median, umbilical f., middle,** plica umbilicalis mediana. **urogenital f.,** urogenital ridge. **vaginal f's,** rugae vaginales. **vascular cecal f.,** plica cecalis vascularis. **ventricular f.,** plica vestibularis. **vesical f., transverse,** plica vesicalis transversa. **vestibular f.,** false vocal cord (plica vestibularis [NA]). **vestigial f. of Marshall,** plica venae cavae sinistrae. **villous f's of stomach,** plicae villosae gastris. **vocal f.,** true vocal cord (plica vocalis [NA]). **vocal f., false,** plica vestibularis.

Foley catheter (fo'le) [Frederic Eugene Basil *Foley*, American urologist, 1891–1966] see under *catheter.*

folia (fo'le-ah) plural of *folium.*

foliaceous (fo''le-a'shus) [L. *folia* leaves] having, pertaining to, or resembling leaves.

folian (fo'le-an) pertaining to Folius' process; see *processus anterior mallei.*

folic acid (fo'lik) [USP] pteroylglutamic acid, a vitamin of the B complex, which serves as a carrier of one-carbon groups in many metabolic reactions. After absorption, dietary folate is reduced to dihydrofolate and then tetrahydrofolate, the active form of the coenzyme; usually several additional glutamate residues are added to form tetrahydropteroyl polyglutamates, which cannot diffuse out of cells. Tetrahydrofolate is required for the synthesis and catabolism of several amino acids, the formation of creatine and choline, the methylation of RNAs, the synthesis of purines, and the synthesis of deoxythymidine monophosphate (dTMP), a DNA precursor. Deficiency of folic acid causes megaloblastic anemia. Called also *Lactobacillus casei factor, liver Lactobacillus casei factor, vitamin B$_c$* and *vitamin M.*

folie (fo-le') [Fr.] psychosis; insanity. **f. à deux** (ah-duh') mental disorder affecting two persons who share the same delusions; classified as induced psychotic disorder by DSM III-R. **f. circulaire** (seer-ku-lair') (*obs.*), circular psychosis. **f. du doute** (du-doot'), pathologic inability to make even the most trifling decisions, an extreme obsessive-compulsive reaction. **f. du pourquoi** (du-poor-kwah'), psychopathologic constant questioning. **f. gémellaire** (zha''mě-lār'), psychosis occurring simultaneously in twins. **f. raisonnante** (rez-un-ahnt'), the delusional form of any psychosis.

folinic acid (fo-lin'ik) a derivative of folic acid necessary for the growth of *Leuconostoc citrovorum;* the calcium salt (*leucovorin calcium* [USP]) is used as an antidote for folic acid antagonists when there is need to reverse the toxic effects of the latter and in the treatment of megaloblastic anemias due to folic acid deficiency. Called also *citrovorum factor* and *leucovorin.*

folium (fo'le-um), pl. *fo'lia* [L. "leaf"] [NA] a general term for a leaflike structure, especially one of the leaflike subdivisions of the cerebellar cortex. **f. cacu'minis** (*obs.*), f. vermis. **fo'lia cerebel'li** [NA], **folia of cerebellum,** the numerous long narrow folds of the cerebellar cortex, separated by sulci and supported by white laminae; they are aggregated into the various subdivisions of the cerebellum. Called also *gyri cerebelli.* **lingual f.,** a foliate papilla of the tongue. **f. ver'mis** [NA], the part of the vermis of the cerebellum between the declive and the tuber vermis.

Folius' muscle, process (fo'le-us) [Caecilius *Folius,* anatomist of Venice, 1615–1660] see *ligamentum mallei laterale* and *processus anterior mallei.*

follicle (fol'lĭ-k'l) 1. a sac or pouchlike depression or cavity; see also *folliculus.* 2. a former name for a lymph nodule. **aggregated f's,** folliculi lymphatici aggregati. **aggregated f's of vermiform appendix,** folliculi lymphatici aggregati appendicis vermiformis. **antral f's,** folliculi ovarici vesiculosi. **atretic f.,** an ovarian follicle which has involuted. **dental f.,** tooth f. **Fleischmann's f.,** an occasional follicle in the mucosa of the floor of the mouth, near the anterior border of the genioglossus muscle. **gastric f's,** 1. glandulae gastricae [propriae]. 2. folliculi lymphatici gastrici. **graafian f's,** folliculi ovarici vesiculosi. **hair f.,** folliculus pili. **intestinal f's,** the intestinal glands; see *glandulae intestinales.* **lenticular f's,** folliculi lymphatici gastrici. **Lieberkühn's f's,** the intestinal glands; see *glandulae intestinales.* **lingual f's,** folliculi linguales. **lymph f., lymphatic f.,** nodulus lymphaticus. **lymph f's of stomach,** folliculi lymphatici gastrici. **lymphatic f's, aggregated, of Peyer,** folliculi lymphatici aggregati. **lymphatic f's, laryngeal,** folliculi lymphatici laryngei. **lymphatic f's of large intestine, solitary,** folliculi lymphatici solitarii intestini crassi. **lymphatic f's of tongue,** folliculi linguales. **Montgomery's f's,** Naboth's f's. **mucous f's, nasal,** glandulae nasales. **Naboth's f's, nabothian f's,** cystlike formations caused by occlusion of the lumina of glands in the mucosa of the uterine cervix, causing them to be distended with retained secretion; called also *Montgomery's f's, Naboth's cysts, glands,* or *ovules,* and *ovula nabothi.* **ovarian f.,** the egg and its encasing cells, at any stage of its development. **ovarian f's, primary,** folliculi ovarici primarii. **ovarian f's, vesicular,** folliculi ovarici vesiculosi. **primordial f.,** an ovarian follicle consisting of an egg enclosed by a single layer of cells. **sebaceous f.,** a hair follicle supplied with a relatively large sebaceous gland, and producing a relatively insignificant hair. **secondary f's,** folliculi ovarici vesiculosi. **solitary f's,** see *folliculi lymphatici solitarii intestini crassi* and *folliculi lymphatici solitarii intestini tenuis.* **f. of Stannius,** a lymphoid unit in chicks, resembling the thymus and developing from nodules formed by proliferation of points of the epithelium of the bursa of Fabricius. **thyroid f's, f's of thyroid gland,** folliculi glandulae thyroideae. **f's of tongue,** folliculi linguales. **tooth f.,** the structure within the developing alveolar bone of the jaws enclosing the tooth germ. Called also *dental f.* **unilaminar f.,** primordial f.

folliclis (fol′ĭ-klis) a term applied to a superficial form of papulonecrotic tuberculid with a predilection for the dorsa of the hands, feet, forearms, and legs.

follicular (fo-lik′u-lar) [L. *follicularis*] of or pertaining to a follicle or follicles.

folliculi (fo-lik′u-li) [L.] genitive and plural of *folliculus.*

folliculin (fŏ-lik′u-lin) an obsolete name for estrone.

folliculitis (fŏ-lik″u-li′tis) inflammation of a follicle or follicles; used ordinarily in reference to hair follicles, but sometimes in relation to follicles of other kinds. **f. abscē′dens et suffo′diens,** perifolliculitis capitis abscedens et suffodiens. **agminate f.,** inflammation of a number of follicles in one area. **f. bar′bae,** sycosis barbae. **f. decal′vans,** a rare, localized, spreading, suppurative folliculitis of unknown cause, leading to scarring, with permanent hair loss. **f. gonorrhoe′ica,** littritis caused by gonococci. **gram-negative f.,** a superinfection complicating long-term systemic antibiotic treatment of acne vulgaris, particularly tetracyclines, usually caused by species of *Enterobacter, Klebsiella,* or *Proteus.* Infection with the first two species is manifested by a superficial pustular eruption, often occurring around the nares; deep nodular cysts, usually on the back, are associated with *Proteus* infections. **keloidal f., f. keloida′lis,** dermatitis papillaris capillitii. **f. na′res per′forans,** inflammation of a hair follicle in the nose, with pustulation and destruction of the follicle, leading to extension of the process through the tissues to the external surface. **f. ulerythemato′sa reticula′ta,** atrophodermia vermiculata usually confined to the cheek but sometimes spreading to involve the ears, forehead, and scalp. Called also *atrophoderma reticulatum symmetricum faciei.* See also *ulerythema ophryogenes.* **f. variolifor′mis,** see under *acne.*

folliculoma (fo-lik″u-lo′mah) granulosa–theca cell tumor; see under *tumor.* **f. lipidique,** a granulosa– theca cell tumor in which streamers or trabeculae of tall, columnar, lipid-laden cells are interspersed among the more characteristic collections of granulosa cells.

folliculosis (fo-lik″u-lo′sis) a disease characterized by excessive development of lymph follicles.

folliculus (fo-lik′u-lus), pl. *follic′uli* [L., dim. of *follis* a leather bag] [NA] a follicle; [NA] a general term for a very small excretory or secretory sac or gland. **follic′uli glan′dulae thyroi′deae,** follicles of thyroid gland: discrete, cystlike units of the thyroid gland that are lined with cuboidal epithelium and are filled with a colloid substance; there are about 30 to each lobule. Called also *thyroid follicles.* **follic′uli lingua′les** [NA], lingual follicles: projections on the mucosa of the root of the tongue, caused by underlying nodular masses of lymphoid tissue, making up the lingual tonsil. **f. lymphat′icus,** NA alternative for *nodulus lymphaticus.* **follic′uli lymphat′ici aggrega′ti** [NA],

oval elevated areas of lymphoid tissue on the mucosa of the small intestine, composed of many lymphoid follicles closely packed together; called also *noduli lymphatici aggregati* [*Peyeri*] and *Peyer's patches.* **follic′uli lymphat′ici aggrega′ti appen′dicis vermifor′mis** [NA], aggregated follicles of vermiform appendix: oval elevated areas of lymphoid tissue occupying the greater part of the submucosa of the vermiform appendix; called also *noduli aggregati processus vermiformis.* **follic′uli lymphat′ici gas′trici** [NA], lymph follicles of stomach: small lymphocytic aggregates in the interstitial tissue of the lamina propria of the stomach, especially in the pyloric region; called also *lenticular glands of stomach, lymphatic nodules of stomach,* and *noduli lymphatici gastrici.* **follic′uli lymphat′ici laryn′gei** [NA], laryngeal lymphatic follicles: lymphatic aggregations in the mucosa of the ventricle of the larynx and on the posterior surface of the epiglottis; called also *noduli lymphatici laryngei.* **follic′uli lymphat′ici liena′les,** folliculi lymphatici splenici. **follic′uli lymphat′ici rec′ti** [NA], concentrations of lymphoid tissue in the tunica mucosa of the rectum; called also *noduli lymphatici recti.* **follic′uli lymphat′ici solita′rii intesti′ni cras′si** [NA], solitary lymphatic follicles of large intestine: the areas of concentrated lymphatic tissue in the tunica mucosa of the colon; called also *noduli lymphatici solitarii intestini crassi.* **follic′uli lymphat′ici solita′rii intesti′ni ten′uis** [NA], small lymph follicles scattered throughout the mucosa and submucosa of the small intestine; called also *noduli lymphatici solitarii intestini tenuis, solitary glands of small intestine,* and *solitary lymphatic nodules of small intestine.* **follic′uli lymphat′ici sple′nici** [NA], aggregations of lymphatic tissue that ensheath the arteries in the spleen. Called also *f. lymphatici lienalis, lymphonoduli splenici* [NA alternative], *malpighian bodies* or *corpuscles (of spleen),* and *white pulp.* **follic′uli ooph′ori prima′rii,** folliculi ovarici primarii. **follic′uli ooph′ori vesiculo′si** [Graaf′i], folliculi ovarici vesiculosi. **follic′uli ovar′ici prima′rii** [NA], primary ovarian follicles: immature ovarian follicles, each comprising an immature ovum and the specialized epithelial cells (follicle cells) that surround it; called also *folliculi oophori primarii.* **follic′uli ovar′ici vesiculo′si** [NA], vesicular ovarian follicles: maturing ovarian follicles among whose cells fluid has begun to accumulate, leading to the formation of a single cavity or antrum and leaving the ovum eccentrically located in a hillock of follicle cells, the cumulus oophorus; called also *folliculi oophori vesiculosi [Graafi],* and *graafian follicles* or *vesicles.* **f. pi′li** [NA], hair follicle: one of the tubular invaginations of the epidermis that enclose the hairs, and from which the hairs grow.

Follutein (fol-lu′te-in) trademark for a preparation of chorionic gonadotropin.

Foltz's valve (fōlts′ez) [Jean Charles Eugène *Foltz,* French ophthalmologist, 1822–1876] see under *valve.*

Folvite (fōl′vīt) trademark for preparations of folic acid.

fomentation (fo″men-ta′shun) [L. *fomentatio; fomentum,* a poultice] treatment by warm and moist applications; also the substance thus applied.

fomes (fo′mēz), pl. *fo′mites* [L. "tinder"] fomite.

fomite (fo′mīt) an object, such as a book, wooden object, or an article of clothing, that is not in itself harmful, but is able to harbor pathogenic microorganisms and thus may serve as an agent of transmission of an infection. Called also *fomes.*

fomites (fo′mĭ-tēz) plural of *fomes.*

fonazine mesylate (fo′nah-zēn) chemical name: 10-[2-(dimethylamino)propyl]-*N,N*-dimethyl-10*H* phenothiazine-2-sulfonamide monomethanesulfonate; a serotonin inhibitor, $C_{20}H_{29}N_3O_5S_3$.

Fonsecaea (fon-se-se′ah) a genus of dematiacious Fungi Imperfecti, some species of which were formerly included in the genera *Hormodendrum* and *Cladosporium. F. pedrosoi* and *F. compactum* are etiologic agents of chromomycosis.

fontactoscope (fon-tak′to-skōp) an instrument for measuring the radioactivity of water and gas.

Fontana's markings, spaces (fon-tah′nahz) [Felice *Fontana,* Italian naturalist and physiologist, 1720–1805] see under *marking* and *space,* and see *spatia anguli iridocornealis.*

fontanel (fon″tah-nel) fontanelle.

fontanelle (fon″tah-nel′) [Fr., dim. of *fontaine* spring, filter] a soft spot, such as one of the membrane-covered spaces (*fonticuli cranii* [NA]) remaining in the incompletely ossified skull of a fetus or infant. See also *fonticulus.* **anterior f.,** fonticulus anterior. **anterolateral f.,** fonticulus sphenoidalis. **bregmatic f.,** fonticulus anterior. **Casser's f., casserian f., Casserio's f.,** fonticulus mastoideus. **cranial f's,** fonticuli cranii. **frontal f.,** fonticulus anterior. **Gerdy's f.,** a fontanelle occasionally occurring in the sagittal suture; called also *sagittal f.* **mastoid f.,** fonticulus mastoideus. **occipital f., posterior f.,** fonticulus posterior. **posterolateral f., posterotemporal f.,** fonticulus mastoideus. **quadrangular f.,** fonticulus anterior. **sagittal f.,** Gerdy's f. **sphenoidal f.,** fonticulus sphenoidalis. **triangular f.,** fonticulus posterior.

fonticuli (fon-tik′u-li) [L.] genitive and plural of *fonticulus.*

fonticulus (fon-tik′u-lus), pl. *fontic′uli* [L., dim. of *fons* fountain] [NA] fontanelle; a soft spot; one of the membrane-covered spaces remaining in the incompletely ossified skull of the fetus or infant. **f. ante′rior** [NA], anterior fontanelle: the unossified area of the skull situated at the junction of the frontal, coronal, and sagittal sutures; called also *f. frontalis* [*major*], and *frontal fontanelle.* **f. anterolatera′lis,** NA alternative for *f. sphenoidalis.* **fontic′uli cra′nii** [NA], the membrane-covered spaces, or soft spots, remaining at the incomplete angles of the parietal and adjacent bones, until ossification of the skull is completed; called also *fontanelles.* **f. fronta′lis [major],** f. anterior. **f. guttu′ris,** fossa jugularis. **f. ma′jor,** f. anterior. **f. mastoi′deus** [NA], mastoid fontanelle: the unossified area of the skull at the junction of the lambdoidal, parietomastoid, and occipitomastoid sutures. Called also *posterolateral fontanelle, f. posterolateralis* [NA alternative], and *posterotemporal fontanelle.* **f. mi′nor,** f. posterior. **f. occipita′lis, f. poste′rior** [NA], posterior fontanelle: the unossified area of the skull at the junction of the sagittal and lambdoidal sutures; called also *f. minor,* and *occipital* or *triangular fontanelle.* **f. posterolatera′lis,** NA alternative for *f. mastoideus.* **f. sphenoida′lis** [NA], sphenoidal fontanelle: the unossified area at the junction of the parietal and frontal bones, the greater wing of the sphenoidal, and the squamous part of the temporal bones. Called also *anterolateral fontanelle* and *f. anterolateralis* [NA alternative].

food (fōōd) anything which, when taken into the body, serves to nourish or build up the tissues or to supply body heat; aliment; nutriment. **isodynamic f's,** foods which generate equal amounts of energy in heat units.

foot (foot) [L. *pes*] 1. the distal portion of the primate leg, upon which an individual stands and walks. It consists, in man, of the tarsus, metatarsus, and phalanges and the tissues encompassing them. See also *pes* and *talipes.* 2. a unit of linear measure, 1/3 yard, or 12 inches, being the equivalent of 30.48 cm. **athlete's f.,** tinea pedis. **broad f.,** metatarsus latus. **burning feet,** a deficiency disease, possibly pantothenic acid deficiency, occurring among the poor in South India and West Africa. It is marked by burning sensations in the soles and palms. **buttress f.,** a condition of periostitis or ostitis in the region of the pyramidal process of the os pedis of the horse, with fracture of the process, deformity of the hoof, and alteration of the normal angle of the joint. Called also *extensor process disease, pyramidal disease,* and *low ring-bone.* **Charcot's f.,** the deformed foot seen in tabetic arthropathy. **cleft f.,** a deformed foot in which the division between the third and fourth toes extends into the metatarsal region. **club f.,** see *talipes.* **contracted f.,** see *hoof-bound.* **crooked f.,** a condition of the horse's hoof in which one wall is concave and the opposite wall convex, giving the hoof a bent appearance; it is due to improper trimming and shoeing. **dangle f., drop f.,** a condition in which the foot hangs in a plantar-flexed position, due to lesion of the peroneal nerve. **end f.,** see *end-feet.* **fescue f.,** fescue (def. 2). **flat f.,** flatfoot. **forced f.,** a painful swelling of the feet of soldiers after forced marches, due to fracture of a metatarsal bone. **Friedreich's f.,** pes cavus, with hyperextension of the toes; seen in hereditary ataxia. **Hong Kong f.,** an infectious mycotic disease (dermatophytosis) of the foot occurring in China. **immersion f.,** a condition resembling trench foot occurring in persons who have spent long periods in water. **immersion f., tropical,** maceration, blanching, and wrinkling of the skin of the feet and swelling of the soles with ridging of the surface, caused by prolonged immersion of the feet in warm water. **Madura f.,** myce-

toma. **march f.,** painful swelling of the forefoot, often associated with fracture of one of the metatarsal bones, following excessive foot strain. **Morand's f.,** a foot having eight toes. **Morton's f.,** see under *toe.* **mossy f.,** chromomycosis involving the foot. **perivascular feet,** terminal expansions of the cytoplasmic processes of some astrocytes by which they are attached to blood vessels. **pricked f.,** a condition in the horse in which the sole or the frog has been punctured either in the forge or by the animal treading on a nail or some other object. **red f.,** redfoot. **reel f.,** clubfoot; see *talipes.* **rocker-bottom f.,** 1. congenital convex pes valgus, due to primary dislocation of the talonavicular joint; it may occur as an isolated primary deformity or be associated with autosomal trisomy, including trisomy 13–15 and trisomy 18; called also *rocker-bottom flatfoot.* 2. talipes equinovarus in which the foot is shaped like a rocker of a rocking-chair, occurring as a result of a transverse break in the midtarsal area; called also *rocker-bottom deformity.* **sag f.,** sagging of the arch of the foot. **spatula f.,** a foot in which several toes are fused together. **spread f.,** metatarsus latus. **strawberry rot f.,** dermatophilus of sheep involving the legs and feet. **sucker f.,** a pyramidal expansion of a process of an astrocyte by which the latter is attached to a small blood vessel; called also *sucker apparatus* or *process, podium,* and *vascular foot plate.* **tabetic f.,** the flat, distorted foot seen in tabes, and due to disease of the tarsus. **taut f.,** a shortening and contraction of the calf muscles and plantar flexors of the foot, due to high-heeled shoes. **trench f.,** a condition of the feet resembling frostbite. It is due to the prolonged action of water on the skin combined with circulatory disturbance due to cold and inaction. Called also *water-bite.* **weak f.,** an early stage of flatfoot.

foot-candle (foot kan′d′l) a unit of illumination being 1 lumen per square foot or equivalent to 1.0764 milliphots. Cf. *lux.*

footdrop (foot′drop) dropping of the foot from paralysis of the anterior muscles of the leg.

foot lambert (foot lam′bert) see *lambert.*

footplate (foot′plāt) the flat portion of the stapes, which is set into the oval window on the medial wall of the middle ear. Called also *base of stapes.*

foot-pound (foot-pownd′) the work done in raising a mass of one pound the distance of one foot against gravity. Abbreviated f.p.

foram (for′am) foraminiferan.

foramen (fo-ra′men), pl. *foram′ina* [L.] a natural opening or passage; [NA] a general term for such a passage, especially one into or through a bone. **accessory f.,** a lateral or accessory orifice, other than the main apical foramen, opening into the root canal of a tooth; called also *lateral f.* **alveolar foramina of maxilla, foram′ina alveola′ria maxil′lae** [NA], the openings of the alveolar canals at the deepest portion of the tooth sockets in the maxilla. **aortic f.,** hiatus aorticus. **apical f. of tooth, f. a′picis den′tis** [NA], a minute aperture usually at or near the apex of a root of a tooth but on occasion located on a side of a root, which gives passage to the vascular, lymphatic, and neural structures supplying the pulp; the main foramen sometimes branches near the apex to form two or more apical ramifications. Called also *f. radicis dentis, pulpal f.,* and *root f.* **auditory f., external,** meatus acusticus externus. **auditory f., internal,** porus acusticus internus. **Bartholin's f.** (*obs.*), f. obturatum. **Bichat's f.,** cisterna venae magnae cerebri. **f. of Bochdalek,** hiatus pleuroperitonealis. **Botallo's f.,** f. ovale cordis. **Bozzi's f.** (*obs.*), macula retinae. **f. cae′cum lin′guae,** [NA], foramen cecum of tongue: a depression on the dorsum of the tongue at the end of the median sulcus, representing the remains of the upper end of the thyroglossal duct of the embryo; called also *f. cecum linguae* [NA alternative]. **f. cae′cum medul′lae oblonga′tae,** a small triangular expansion at the lower border of the pons, formed by the termination of the anterior median fissure of the medulla oblongata; called also *f. caecum posterius, Schwalbe's f.,* and *f. of Vicq d'Azyr.* **f. cae′cum os′sis fronta′lis** [NA], foramen cecum of frontal bone: a blind opening formed between the frontal crest and the crista galli, which sometimes transmits a vein from the nasal cavity to the superior sagittal sinus; called also *cecal f.* and *f. cecum ossis frontalis* [NA alternative]. **f. cae′cum poste′rius, f. caecum of Vicq d'Azyr,** f.

caecum medullae oblongatae. **caroticotympanic fo-ramina,** canaliculi caroticotympanici. **carotid f.,** the inferior aperture of the carotid canal, giving passage to the carotid vessels. **cecal f., f. cecum of frontal bone,** f. caecum ossis frontalis. **f. ce′cum lin′guae,** NA alternative for *f. caecum linguae.* **f. ce′cum os′sis fronta′lis,** NA alternative for *f. caecum ossis frontalis.* **f. cecum of tongue,** f. cecum linguae. **condyloid f., anterior,** canalis hypoglossalis. **condyloid f., posterior,** canalis condylaris. **conjugate f.,** a foramen formed by a notch in each of two opposed bones. **f. costotransver-sa′rium** [NA], **costotransverse f.,** the narrow space be-tween the dorsal surface of the neck of a rib and the ventral surface of the transverse process of the corresponding verte-bra. **cotyloid f.,** a passage between the margin of the ac-etabulum and the transverse ligament. **cribroethmoid f.,** f. ethmoidale anterius. **foram′ina cribro′sa os′sis ethmoida′lis,** the openings in the cribriform plate of the ethmoid bone for passage of the olfactory nerves. In official anatomical nomenclature [NA], the cribriform plate and the foramina of the ethmoid bone are considered together, and are designated *lamina et foramina cribrosa ossis ethmoidalis.* **dental foramina,** see *foramina alveolaria maxillae* and *foramina mandibulae.* **f. diaphrag′matis [sel′lae],** the opening in the center of the diaphragm of the sella through which the infundibulum passes. **Duverney's f.,** f. epiploicum. **emissary f.,** any foramen in a cranial bone that gives passage to an emissary vein. **epiploic f., f. epiplo′icum,** NA alternative for *f. omentale.* **esoph-ageal f.,** hiatus esophageus. **ethmoidal f., anterior,** f. ethmoidale anterius. **ethmoidal f., posterior,** f. eth-moidale posterius. **ethmoidal foramina,** foramina ethmoidalia. **foram′ina ethmoida′lia** [NA], ethmoidal foramina: small openings in the ethmoid bone at the junction of the medial wall with the roof of the orbit, the anterior (*f. ethmoidale anterius*) transmitting the nasal branch of the ophthalmic nerve and the anterior ethmoid vessels, the posterior (*f. ethmoidale posterius*) transmitting the posterior ethmoid vessels. Called also *orbital canals.* **f. of Fallo-pio,** hiatus canalis nervi petrosi majoris. **Ferrein's f.,** hiatus canalis nervi petrosi majoris. **frontal f., f. fron-ta′le** [NA], see *incisura frontalis.* **frontoethmoidal f.,** a foramen lying on the line of the frontoethmoidal suture. **Galen's f.,** the opening of an anterior cardiac vein into the right atrium. **glandular foramina of Littre,** lacu-nae urethrales. **glandular f. of Morgagni, glandu-lar f. of tongue,** f. cecum linguae. **great f.,** f. mag-num. **Hartigan's f.,** a foramen said to exist in the base of the transverse process of a lumbar vertebra but seldom persisting to adult life. **Huschke's f.,** a perforation found near the inner extremity of the tympanic plate between the tympanum and the jugular fossa caused by arrest of development. **incisive f., f. incisi′vum** [NA], one of the openings in the incisive fossa of the hard palate that transmit the nasopalatine nerves. **incisor f., me-dian,** Scarpa's f. **infraorbital f., f. infraorbita′le** [NA], the opening of the infraorbital canal on the anterior surface of the maxilla giving passage to the infraorbital nerve and vessels; called also *suborbital f.* **infrapiriform f.,** an opening below the piriformis muscle through which the inferior gluteal vessels and nerve pass out of the pelvis. **innominate f.,** an occasional opening in the temporal bone for passage of the small superficial petrosal nerve. **inter-sacral foramina,** foramina intervertebralia ossis sacri. **interventricular f., f. interventricula′re** [NA], a pas-sage through which the lateral and third ventricles commu-nicate. **intervertebral f., f. intervertebra′le** [NA], the passage formed by the inferior and superior notches on the pedicles of adjacent vertebrae; it transmits a spinal nerve and vessels. **intervertebral foramina of sacrum,** foramina intervertebralia ossis sacri. **intervertebral foramina of sacrum, foram′ina intervertebra′lia os′sis sa′cri** [NA], the four short, forked tunnels in each lateral wall of the sacral canal, connecting it with the pelvic and dorsal sacral foramina; called also *intersacral canals* or *foramina.* **ischiadic f., greater,** f. ischiadicum majus. **ischiadic f., lesser** f. ischiadicum minus. **f. is-chia′dicum ma′jus** [NA], greater ischiadic foramen: a hole converted from the major sciatic notch by the sacrotu-beral and sacrospinal ligaments; called also *f. sciaticum majus* [NA alternative], *greater sciatic f.,* and *great ischiac-atic f.* **f. ischia′dicum mi′nus** [NA], lesser ischiadic foramen: a hole converted from the minor sciatic notch by the

sacrotuberal and sacrospinal ligaments; called also *f. sciati-cum minus* [NA alternative], *lesser sciatic f.,* and *small sacrosciatic f.* **ischiopubic f.,** f. obturatum. **jugular f., f. jugula′re** [NA], the opening formed by the jugular notches on the temporal and occipital bones, for the transmis-sion of various veins, arteries, and nerves. **f. of Key and Retzius,** apertura lateralis ventriculi quarti. **lacerate f., anterior,** fissura orbitalis superior. **lacerate f., middle,** f. lacerum. **lacerate f., posterior,** f. jugulare. **f. lac′erum** [NA], an irregular gap formed at the junction of the base of the great wing of the sphenoid bone, the tip of the petrous part of the temporal bone, and the basilar part of the occipital bone; in life, it does not exist, being occupied by an unossified part of the petrous part of the temporal bone. **f. lac′erum ante′rius,** fissura orbitalis superior. **f. lac′erum me′dium,** f. lacerum. **f. lac′erum post-e′rius,** f. jugulare. **lateral f.,** accessory f. **left f., in-ferior,** hiatus aorticus. **left f., superior,** hiatus esoph-ageus. **f. of Luschka,** apertura lateralis ventriculi quarti. **f. of Magendie,** apertura mediana ventriculi quarti. **f. mag′num** [NA], great foramen: the large opening in the anterior and inferior part of the occipital bone, interconnecting the vertebral canal and the cranial cavity; called also *f. occipitale magnum* and *great occipital f.* **ma-lar f.,** f. zygomaticofaciale. **f. mandib′ulae** [NA], **f. mandibula′re,** the opening on the medial surface of the ramus of the mandible, leading into the mandibular canal. **mastoid f., f. mastoi′deum** [NA], a prominent opening in the temporal bone posterior to the mastoid process and near its occipital articulation; an artery and vein usually pass through it. **maxillary f.,** hiatus maxillaris. **maxil-lary f., anterior,** f. mentale. **maxillary f., inferior,** f. ovale basis cranii. **maxillary f., internal, maxil-lary f., posterior,** f. mandibulae. **maxillary f., su-perior,** f. rotundum ossis sphenoidalis. **medullary f., f. vertebrale. meibomian f.,** f. cecum linguae. **mental f., f. menta′le** [NA], an opening on the lateral part of the body of the mandible, opposite the second biscuspid tooth, for passage of the mental nerve and vessels. **f. of Monro,** f. interventriculare. **Morand's f.,** f. cecum linguae. **Morgagni's f., morgagnian f.,** 1. a small gap on either side, between the sternal and costal portions of the dia-phragm, for the passage of the superior epigastric blood vessels and a few lymphatic vessels; called also *pleuroperito-neal f.* 2. foramen cecum linguae. 3. foramen singulare. **nasal foramina, foram′ina nasa′lia,** openings in the outer surface of each nasal bone for the transmission of blood vessels. **foram′ina nervo′sa lam′inae spira′lis,** fo-ramina nervosa limbus laminae spiralis. **foram′ina nervo′sa lim′bus lam′inae spira′lis** [NA], numerous small openings in the labium limbi tympanicum for the passage of the cochlear nerves; called also *foramina nervosa laminae spiralis* and *habenulae perforatae.* **f. nu-tric′ium** [NA], **f. nu′triens, nutrient f.,** any one of the passages that admit the nutrient vessels to the medullary cavity of a bone. **obturator f., f. obtura′tum** [NA], the large opening between the os pubis and the ischium. Called also *f. obturatorium* [NA alternative]. **f. ob-turato′rium,** NA alternative for *f. obturatum.* **occipi-tal f., great, occipital f., inferior,** f. magnum. **f. oc-cipita′le mag′num,** f. magnum. **olfactory f.,** any one of the many openings of the cribriform plate of the ethmoidal bone. **omental f., f. omenta′le** [NA], the opening connecting the greater and the lesser peritoneal sacs, situated below and behind the porta hepatis; called also *epiploic f.* and *f. epiploicum* [NA alternative]. **optic f. of sclera,** lamina cribrosa sclerae. **optic f. of sphenoid bone, f. op′ticum os′sis sphenoida′lis,** canalis opti-cus. **orbitomalar f.,** f. zygomatico-orbitale. **oval f. of fetus,** fossa ovalis cordis. **oval f. of hip bone,** f. ob-turatum. **oval f. of sphenoid bone,** f. ovale basis cra-nii. **f. ova′le ba′sis cra′nii** [NA], an opening in the posterior part of the medial portion of the great wing of the sphenoid bone; it transmits the mandibular branch of the trigeminal nerve and some vessels. Called also *f. ovale ossis sphenoidalis* and *oval f. of sphenoid bone.* **f. ova′le cor′-dis** [NA], the aperture in the septum secundum of the fetal heart that provides a communication between the atria; called also *Botallo's f.* and *oval f. of fetus.* **f. ova′le os′-sis sphenoida′lis,** f. ovale basis cranii. **f. of Pacchi-oni, pacchionian f.,** f. diaphragmatis [sellae]. **pala-tine foramina, accessory,** foramina palatina minora. **palatine f., anterior,** f. incisivum. **palatine f.,**

greater, f. palatinum majus. **palatine foramina, lesser,** foramina palatina minora. **palatine f., posterior,** f. palatinum majus. **foramina of palatine tonsil,** fossulae tonsillares tonsillae palatinae. **f. palati′num ma′jus** [NA], greater palatine foramen: the inferior opening of the great palatine canal, found laterally on the horizontal plate of each palatine bone opposite the root of each third molar tooth; it transmits a palatine nerve and artery. Called also *posterior palatine f., pterygopalatine f.,* and *sphenopalatine f.* **foram′ina palati′na mino′ra** [NA], lesser palatine foramina: the openings of the palatine canals behind the palatine crest and the greater palatine foramina; called also *accessory palatine foramina.* **foram′ina papilla′ria re′nis** [NA], **papillary foramina of kidney,** minute openings in the summit of each renal papilla, the orifices of the collecting tubules; called also *foveolae papillae.* **parietal f., f. parieta′le** [NA], an opening on the posterior part of the superior portion of the parietal bone near the sagittal suture, for the passage of a vein and arteriole. **f. petro′sum** [NA], petrosal foramen: a small opening sometimes present behind the oval foramen for transmission of the lesser petrosal nerve; called also *canaliculus innominatus of Arnold* and *innominate canaliculus.* **pleuroperitoneal f.,** 1. hiatus pleuroperitonealis. 2. Morgagni's f. (def. 1). **f. proces′sus transver′si** [NA], foramen of transverse process: the passage in either transverse process of a cervical vertebra that, in the upper six vertebrae, transmits the vertebral vessels; it is small or may be absent in the seventh. Called also *f. transversarium, f. vertebroarteriale* [NA alternative], *transverse f.,* and *vertebroarterial f.* **pterygopalatine f.,** f. palatinum majus. **pulpal f.,** f. apicis dentis. **quadrate f.,** f. venae cavae. **f. rad′icis den′tis,** f. apicis dentis. **Retzius' f.,** apertura lateralis ventriculi quarti. **right f.,** f. venae cavae. **rivinian f., Rivinus' f.,** incisura tympanica. **root f.,** f. apicis dentis. **f. rotun′dum os′sis sphenoida′lis** [NA], a round opening in the medial part of the great wing of the sphenoid bone that transmits the maxillary branch of the trigeminal nerve; called also *superior maxillary f.* or *canal.* **sacral foramina, anterior,** foramina sacralia anteriora. **sacral foramina, dorsal,** foramina sacralia posteriora. **sacral foramina, internal,** foramina sacralia anteriora. **sacral foramina, posterior,** foramina sacralia dorsalia. **sacral foramina, ventral,** foramina sacralia anteriora. **f. of sacral canal,** hiatus sacralis. **foram′ina sacra′lia anterio′ra,** [NA], anterior sacral foramina: the eight openings (four on each side) on the pelvic surface of the sacral bone for the ventral rami of the sacral nerves. Called also *internal* or *ventral sacral foramina, foramina sacralia pelvica* [NA alternative], *foramina sacralia pelvina,* and *foramina sacralia ventralia.* **foram′ina sacra′lia dorsa′lia** [NA], foramina sacralia posteriora. **foram′ina sacra′lia pel′vica,** NA alternative for *foramina sacralia anteriora.* **foram′ina sacra′lia pelvi′na,** foramina sacralia anteriora. **foram′ina sacra′lia posterio′ra,** [NA], posterior sacral foramina: the eight openings (four on each side) on the dorsal surface of the sacral bone for the dorsal rami of the sacral nerves. Called also *dorsal sacral foramina* and *foramina sacralia dorsalia.* **foram′ina sacra′lia ventra′lia,** foramina sacralia anteriora. **sacrosciatic f., great,** f. ischiadicum majus. **sacrosciatic f., small,** f. ischiadicum minus. **f. of saphenous vein,** hiatus saphenus. **Scarpa's f.,** one of the two foramina, one behind either upper medial incisor, for transmission of the nasopalatine nerves; called also *median incisor f.* **Schwalbe's f.,** f. caecum medullae oblongatae. **sciatic f., greater,** f. ischiadicum majus. **sciatic f., lesser,** f. ischiadicum minus. **f. scia′ticum ma′jus,** NA alternative for *f. ischiadicum majus.* **f. scia′ticum mi′nus,** NA alternative for *f. ischiadicum minus.* **f. singula′re** [NA], the opening in the inferior vestibular area of the fundus of the internal acoustic meatus that gives passage to the nerves of the ampulla of the posterior semicircular duct; called also *Morgagni's* or *morgagnian f.* **foramina of smallest veins of heart,** foramina venarum minimarum cordis. **Soemmering's f.** (*obs.*), fovea centralis retinae. **sphenopalatine f.,** 1. foramen sphenopalatinum. 2. foramen palatinum majus. **f. sphenopalati′num** [NA], sphenopalatine foramen: an opening on the medial wall of the pterygopalatine fossa, interconnecting this fossa with the nasal cavity, and transmitting the sphenopalatine artery and nasal nerves. **sphenotic f.,** f. lacerum. **spinal f., f. of**

spinal cord, f. vertebrale. **f. spino′sum** [NA], **spinous f.,** an opening in the great wing of the sphenoid bone, near its posterior angle, for the middle meningeal artery. **Spöndel's f.,** a small transient foramen in the cartilaginous base of the developing skull between the ethmoid bone and the lower wings of the sphenoid. **f. of Stensen,** 1. foramen incisivum. 2. canalis incisivus. **stylomastoid f., f. stylomastoi′deum** [NA], a foramen on the inferior part of the temporal bone between the styloid and mastoid processes, for the facial nerve and the stylomastoid artery. **suborbital f.,** f. infraorbitale. **supraorbital f., f. supraorbita′le** [NA], **f. supraorbita′lis,** an opening in the frontal bone in the supraorbital margin, giving passage to the supraorbital artery and nerve; it is often present as a notch (*incisura supraorbitalis*) bridged only by fibrous tissue. **suprapiriform f.,** an opening above the piriformis muscle through which the gluteal vessels and superior gluteal nerve pass out of the pelvis. **f. of Tarin** (*obs.*), hiatus canalis nervi petrosi majoris. **temporomalar f.,** f. zygomatico-temporale. **thebesian foramina, foram′ina thebes′-ii,** foramina venarum minimarum cordis. **thyroid f.,** 1. f. thyroideum. 2. obturator f. **f. thyroi′deum** [NA], thyroid foramen: an inconstantly present opening in the upper part of the lamina of the thyroid cartilage, resulting from incomplete union of the fourth and fifth branchial cartilages. **tonsillar foramina,** see *fossulae tonsillares tonsillae palatinae* and *pharyngeae.* **f. transversa′rium** [NA], **transverse f.,** f. processus transversi. **vena caval f., f. ve′nae ca′vae** [NA], the opening in the respiratory diaphragm that transmits the inferior vena cava and some branches of the right vagus nerve; called also *venal caval hiatus* and *venous f.* **foram′ina vena′rum minima′rum cor′dis** [NA], foramina of smallest veins of heart: minute openings in the walls of the right atrium of the heart, through which small veins, the venae cordis minimae, empty their blood directly into the heart; called also *Vieussen's foramina* and *thebesian foramina.* **f. veno′sum** [NA], venous foramen: an opening occasionally found medial to the foramen ovale of the sphenoid, for the passage of a vein from the cavernous sinus; called also *f. of Vesalius* and *f. Vesalii.* **venous f.,** 1. f. venae cavae. 2. f. venosum. **vertebral f.,** foramen vertebrale. **f. vertebra′le** [NA], vertebral foramen: the large opening in a vertebra formed by its body and arch; called also *medullary f.,* and *spinal f.* or *aperture.* **vertebroarterial f.,** f. processus transversi. **f. vertebroarteria′le,** NA alternative for *f. processus transversi.* **f. Vesa′lii, f. of Vesalius,** f. venosum. **f. of Vicq d'Azyr,** f. caecum medullae oblongatae. **Vieussen's foramina,** foramina venarum minimarum cordis. **Weitbrecht's f.,** an opening in the capsule of the shoulder joint through which passes the synovial membrane to the bursa that lines the under surface of the subscapularis muscle. **f. of Winslow,** f. epiploicum. **zygomatic f., anterior, zygomatic f., external, zygomatic f., facial,** f. zygomaticofaciale. **zygomatic f., inferior, zygomatic f., internal, of Arnold,** f. zygomatico-orbitale. **zygomatic f., internal, of Meckel,** f. zygomaticotemporale. **zygomatic f., orbital,** f. zygomatico-orbitale. **zygomatic f., posterior,** f. zygomaticotemporale. **zygomatic f., superior,** f. zygomatico-orbitale. **zygomatic f., temporal,** f. zygomaticotemporale. **zygomaticofacial f., f. zygomaticofacia′le** [NA], the opening on the anterior surface of the zygomatic bone for the zygomaticofacial nerves and vessels. **zygomatico-orbital f., f. zygomatico-orbita′le** [NA], either of the two openings on the orbital surface of each zygomatic bone, which transmit branches of the zygomatic branch of the trigeminal nerve and branches of the lacrimal artery. **zygomaticotemporal f., f. zygomaticotempora′le** [NA], the opening on the temporal surface of the zygomatic bone for passage of the zygomaticotemporal nerve.

foramina (fo-ram′ĭ-nah) [L.] plural of *foramen.*

foraminifer (for″ah-min′ĭ-fer) foraminiferan.

foraminiferal (fo-ra″mi-nif′er-al) foraminiferous, def. 2.

foraminiferan (fo-ra″mĭ-nif′er-an) a protozoan of the order Foraminiferida. Called also *foram* and *foraminifer.*

Foraminiferida (fo-ram″ĭ-nĭ-fer′ĭ-dah) [*foramen* + L. *ferre* to bear] an order of large, uninucleate or multinucleate, chiefly benthic marine protozoa (class Granuloreticulosea, subphylum Sarcodina), found chiefly as components of the ocean bottom and characterized by the presence of a calcareous, sometimes silaceous test, usually consisting of many successively formed chambers with minute perforations and pseudopodia protruding from an aperture in the last-formed chamber or through the wall perforations or both to form an adhesive net for food gathering and locomotion. It includes five suborders: Allogromiina, Fusulinina, Miliolina, Rotaliina, and Textulariina, many of which are known only as fossils.

foraminiferous (for″am-ĭ-nif′er-us) [foramen + L. ferre to bear] 1. having foramina. 2. pertaining or relating to protozoa of the order Foraminiferida; foraminiferal.

foraminotomy (for″am-ĭ-not′o-me) [foramina + Gr. tomē a cutting] the operation of removing the roof of intervertebral foramina, done for the relief of nerve root compression.

foraminulum (for″ah-min′u-lum), pl. foramin′ula [L.] a minute foramen.

Forane (for′ān) trademark for preparations of isoflurane.

force (fōrs) [L. fortis strong] energy, or power; that which originates or arrests motion. **catabolic f.**, energy derived from the metabolism of food. **chewing f.**, masticatory f. **electromotive f.**, the force which, by reason of differences in potential, causes a flow of electricity from one place to another, giving rise to an electric current; it is measured in volts. **extraoral f.**, force applied by orthodontic anchorage units (calvarial, occipital, or cervical) outside the oral cavity. **field f's**, hypothetical forces which have a part in the individuation processes of the early embryo. **masticatory f.**, the degree of force applied against the occlusal surfaces of the teeth by the muscles of mastication during the chewing of food. Called also chewing f. **occlusal f.**, the force exerted on opposing teeth when the jaws are brought into approximation. **reciprocal f.**, a force applied by an orthodontic anchorage in which the

resistance of one or more dental units is utilized to move one or more opposing dental units. Cf. reciprocal anchorage. **reserve f.**, energy above that required for normal functioning; in the heart it is the power which will take care of the additional circulatory burden imposed by bodily exertion. **rest f.**, the power of the heart necessary to maintain the circulation when the patient is at rest. **Van der Waals f's**, the relatively weak, short-range forces of attraction existing between atoms and molecules, which results in the attraction of nonpolar organic compounds to each other (hydrophobic bonding). **vital f.**, the energy which characterizes a living organism.

forceps (fōr′seps) [L.] 1. an instrument with two blades and a handle for compressing or grasping tissues in surgical operations, and for handling sterile dressings and other surgical supplies. 2. any forcipate organ or part, particularly the terminal fibers of the corpus callosum. **alligator f.**, a long, sharply angled forceps with a jawlike mechanism at the tip. **Allis f.**, one with opposing serrated edges with short teeth, used for grasping fascia. **f. anterior**, f. occipitalis. **artery f.**, forceps for grasping and compressing an artery. **Asch f.**, forceps used for reduction and fixation of nasal fractures. **axis-traction f.**, specially jointed obstetrical forceps so constructed that traction may be applied in the line of the pelvic axis. **Bailey-Williamson f.**, a special obstetrical forceps used in mid- and high-forceps delivery and in breech presentations with aftercoming head. **Barton f.**, an obstetrical forceps with a hinge in one blade, which can be applied correctly to the fetal head without disturbing its relationship to the pelvic axis. **bayonet f.**, a forceps whose blades are offset from the axis of the handle. **Brenner f.**, a special obstetrical

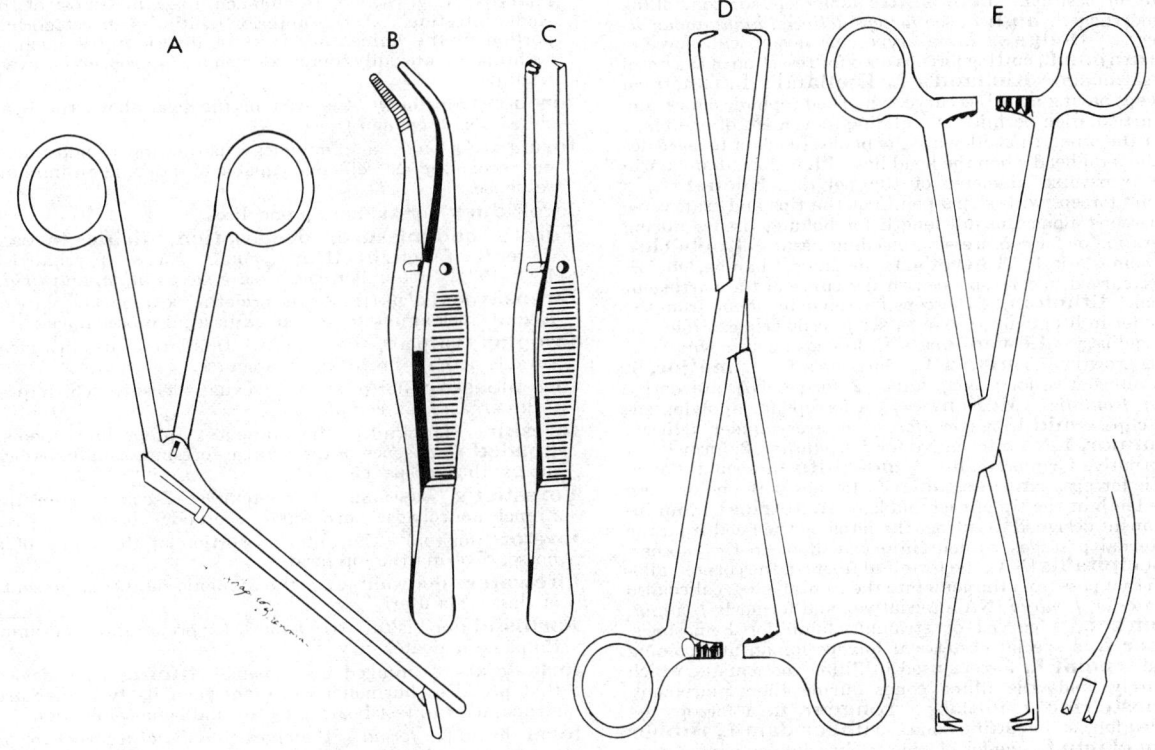

Some types of forceps: A, Struycken ear forceps; B, serrated forceps; C, Iris forceps, fine mouse tooth; D, Schroeder tenaculum forceps; E, Schroeder vulsellum forceps (with side view of blade).

forceps used in breech presentations. **bulldog f.,** spring forceps for seizing an artery to arrest or prevent hemorrhage; the jaws are usually covered with rubber tubing to prevent injury to the vascular wall. **bullet f.,** a forceps for extracting bullets. **capsule f.,** forceps for removing the lens capsule in membranous cataract. **chalazion f.,** a thumb forceps with a flattened plate at the end of one arm and a matching ring on the other; it is an ophthalmologic instrument, also used for isolation of lip and cheek lesions to facilitate removal. **Chamberlen f.,** the original form of obstetrical forceps, invented by Peter Chamberlen (1560–1631), and disclosed by Hugh Chamberlen (1664–1728). **clamp f.,** 1. a forceps with an automatic lock, used for compressing arteries, the pedicle of a tumor, etc.; called also *pedicle clamp.* 2. rubber dam f. **clip f.,** a double-action forceps for applying wound clips; also used to designate a McKenzie forceps for applying brain clips. **Cornet's f.,** a forceps for holding a coverglass. **DeLee f.,** a modified Simpson forceps. **dental f.,** forceps for the extraction of teeth. Called also *extracting f.* **disk f.,** a forceps for grasping the scleral disk in trephining the eyeball. **dressing f.,** forceps with scissor-like handles for grasping lint, drainage tubes, etc., in dressing wounds. **ear f.,** delicate forceps for extracting foreign bodies from the auditory canal. **Elliot f.,** a special obstetrical forceps used in low-forceps delivery and frank breech presentations. **epilating f.,** forceps for use in plucking out hairs. **extracting f.,** dental f. **fixation f.,** forceps for holding a part during an operation. **f. fronta′lis** [NA], the terminal fibers of the corpus callosum that pass from the splenium into the occipital lobes; called also *f. minor* [NA alternative], *f. posterior,* and formerly *f. major.* **galea f.,** Willett f. **Garrison's f.,** an obstetrical forceps with unfenestrated blades; called also *Luikart's f.* **Good f.,** a special obstetrical forceps used in midforceps delivery in the anterior position. **Haig Ferguson f.,** a special obstetrical forceps used in low-forceps delivery. **Hawks-Dennen f.,** a special obstetrical forceps used in midforceps delivery in the anterior position. **hemostatic f.,** forceps for controlling hemorrhage. **high f.,** see *forceps delivery, high,* under *delivery.* **Hodge's f.,** a type of obstetrical forceps. **Kazanjian f.,** cutting forceps used for resection of the nasal dorsal hump. **Kielland's f., Kjelland's f.,** obstetrical forceps having no pelvic curve, a marked cephalic curve, and an articulation permitting a gliding movement of one blade over the other, thus allowing the blades to adapt to the sides of the fetal head when the head lies with its long diameter in the transverse diameter of the pelvis. **Kocher f.,** a strong forceps with sharp points at the tips and transverse serrations along the full length for holding tissues during operation or for compressing bleeding tissue. **Koeberlé's f.,** hemostatic f. **Levret's f.,** modified Chamberlen forceps, curved to correspond with the curve of the parturient canal. **lithotomy f.,** forceps for removing stone from the bladder in lithotomy. **low f.,** see *forceps delivery, low,* under *delivery.* **Löwenberg's f.,** forceps for removing adenoid growths. **Luikart f.,** Garrison's f. **f. ma′jor,** 1. NA alternative for *f. occipitalis.* 2. former NA alternative for *f. frontalis.* **McKenzie f.,** a forceps for applying silver clips. **mid f.,** see *midforceps delivery,* under *delivery.* **f. mi′nor,** 1. NA alternative for *f. frontalis.* 2. former NA alternative for *f. occipitalis.* **mosquito f.,** a small hemostatic forceps. **mouse-tooth f.,** forceps with one or more fine teeth at the tip of each blade. **obstetrical f.,** an instrument designed to extract the fetus by the head from the maternal passages without injury to it or to the mother. **f. occipita′lis** [NA], the terminal fibers of the corpus callosum that pass from the genu into the frontal lobes; called also *f. anterior, f. major* [NA alternative], and formerly *f. minor.* **Péan's f.,** a curved or straight clamp for hemostasis. **Piper f.,** a special obstetrical forceps for an aftercoming head. **point f.,** forceps used in filling root canals, which securely holds the filling cones during their placement. **f. poste′rior,** f. frontalis. **rongeur f.,** a forceps designed for use in cutting bone. **rubber dam f., rubber dam clamp f.,** one for placing rubber dam clamps in position. Called also *clamp f.* **sequestrum f.,** forceps with small but strong serrated jaws for removing the portions of bone forming a sequestrum. **Simpson's f.,** a form of obstetrical forceps. **speculum f.,** long slender forceps for use through a speculum. **suture f.,** forceps used to hold the needle in passing a suture; a needle holder. **Tarni-**

er's f., a form of axis-traction forceps. **tenaculum f.,** forceps having a sharp hook at the end of each jaw. **thumb f.,** tissue f. **tissue f.,** forceps with one or more fine teeth at the tip of each blade, designed for handling tissues with minimal trauma during surgery; called also *thumb f.* **torsion f.,** forceps for making torsion on an artery to arrest hemorrhage. **Tucker-McLean f.,** a long obstetrical forceps with a solid blade. **volsella f., vulsellum f.,** a forceps with teeth for grasping tissues and applying traction. **Walsham f's,** forceps used for reduction and fixation of nasal fractures. **Willett f.,** a vulsellum for applying scalp traction in the control of hemorrhage from placenta previa; called also *galea f.* and *Willett clamp.*

forcipate (for′sĭ-pāt) shaped like forceps.

Forcipomyia (for″po-mi′yah) a genus of midges, family Chironomidae. *F. townsen′di* and *F. u′tae* were once thought to transmit mucocutaneous leishmaniasis.

forcipressure (for′sĭ-presh″ur) pressure with forceps, chiefly for the arrest of hemorrhage.

Fordyce's disease, granule (spot) (for′dīs-es) [John Addison *Fordyce,* New York dermatologist, 1858–1925] see *Fox-Fordyce disease,* under *disease,* and see under *granule.*

forearm (fōr′arm) the part of the upper limb of the body between the elbow and the wrist; called also *antebrachium* [NA].

forebrain (fōr′brān) prosencephalon.

foreconscious (fōr-kon′shus) that part of the mind which contains memory impressions which may be brought into consciousness under certain conditions.

forefinger (fōr-fing′ger) the index finger.

forefoot (fōr′foot) 1. one of the front feet of a quadruped. 2. the fore part of the foot.

foregilding (fōr′gild-ing) the treatment of fresh nerve tissue with salts in histologic technique.

foregut (fōr′gut) 1. the endodermal canal of the embryo cephalic to the junction of the yolk stalk; it gives rise to the pharynx, lung, esophagus, stomach, liver, and most of the small intestine. 2. the anterior, chitin-lined, ectodermal portion of the alimentary tract of invertebrates, such as arthropods; it usually comprises a pharynx, crop, and proventriculus.

forehead (fōr′hed) the part of the face above the eyes; called also *brow* and *frons* [NA].

foreign (for′en) in immunology, pertaining to substances not recognized as "self" and capable of inducing an immune response.

forekidney (fōr-kid′ne) pronephros.

Forel's commissure, decussation, fields (areas) (fo-relz′) [Auguste Henri *Forel,* Swiss psychiatrist, 1848–1931] see under *commissure, decussation,* and *field.*

forensic (fo-ren′zik) [L. *forēnsis* relating to a market place or forum] pertaining to or applied in legal proceedings.

foreplay (fōr′pla) the sexually stimulating, usually pleasurable activity preceding intercourse.

fore-pleasure (fōr′plezh-er) sexual pleasure which precedes orgasm. Cf. *end-pleasure.*

foreskin (fōr′skin) the prepuce (preputium penis). **hooded f.,** absence of the ventral foreskin, usually associated with hypospadias.

Forestier's disease (fo″res-tě-āz′) [Jacques *Forestier,* French neurologist, born 1890] see under *disease.*

foretop (fōr′top) the anterior portion of the mane of a horse, covering the forehead.

forewaters (fōr′waht-erz) the amniotic fluid that presents at the cervix uteri.

Forhistal (for-his′tal) trademark for preparations of dimethindene maleate.

fork (fork) a pronged instrument. **tuning f.,** a device that produces harmonic vibration when its two tines are struck; used to test hearing by air and bone conduction.

form (form) [L. *forma*] the characteristic of a structure or entity generally determined by its shape and size, or other external or visible feature. **accolé f.** (ak″o-la′), appliqué f. **appliqué f.** (ap″le-ka′), a term used to describe the early trophozoite of *Plasmodium falciparum* that does not assume a ring form but lies spread out along the periphery of the infected cell where it appears to have been "applied." Called also *accolé f.* **arch f.,** the shape and contour of a dental arch. **band f's,** band cell; see under *cell.* **involution f's,** an abnormally shaped bacterial cell that occurs in an old culture or one that has been exposed to unfavorable conditions. **juvenile f.,** metamyelocyte. **L-f.,** L-phase variant; see under *variant.* **racemic f.,** see *racemate.* **retention f.,** adaptation of the form of a tooth cavity in such a way as to help maintain the filling material in the cavity. **ring f.,** the early trophozoite in the erythrocytic stage of the life cycle of hemosporian protozoa, which after Romanovsky staining has blue cytoplasm surrounding a clear zone with a red nucleus at one side, giving the cell the appearance of a signet ring. Called also *ring stage* and *signet ring.* **spherical f. of occlusion,** an arrangement of teeth which places their occlusal surfaces on the surface of an imaginary sphere (usually 8 inches in diameter) with its center above the level of the teeth. **tooth f.,** the characteristic contour of a tooth, with its curves, lines, and angles, which permits the tooth to be differentiated from other teeth and its identity to be established. **young f.,** metamyelocyte.

Formad's kidney (fōr′madz) [Henry F. *Formad,* American physician, 1847–1892] see under *kidney.*

formaldehyde (fōr-mal′dĕ-hīd) a powerful disinfectant gas, HCHO, formerly used as a disinfectant for rooms, clothing, etc. A 37 per cent solution of formaldehyde gas in water (formalin) is widely used as a fixing fluid for pathologic specimens or as a preservative, and dilutions have also been used as a surgical and general antiseptic and as an astringent.

formaldehyde dehydrogenase (for-mal′dĕ-hīd de-hi′-dro-jen-ās) [EC 1.2.1.46] an enzyme of the oxidoreductase class that catalyzes the reaction formaldehyde + NAD$^+$ + H$_2$O = formate + NADH. The reaction occurs in mitochondria and is a major source of formate in the cell.

formaldehydogenic (for-mal″dĕ-hīd″o-jen′ik) [*formaldehyde* + *-genic*] producing formaldehyde; pertaining to the production of formaldehyde by certain compounds when subjected to chemical reactions (i.e., steroids with α-ketol grouping in the C-17 position which on treatment with periodic acid liberate formaldehyde).

formalin (fōr′mah-lin) see *formaldehyde.*

formalinize (fōr′mah-lin-īz) to treat with formaldehyde.

formamidase (for-mam′ĭ-dās) 1. [EC 3.5.1.49] an enzyme of the hydrolase class that catalyzes the reaction formamide + H$_2$O = formate + NH$_3$. The enzyme also acts on acetamide, propanamide, and butanamide. 2. arylformamidase.

formant (fōr′mant) a combination of tones produced in the articulation of a vowel phoneme (speech sound).

formate (fōr′māt) any salt of formic acid.

formate dehydrogenase (fōr′māt de-hi′dro-jen-ās) [EC 1.2.1.2] an enzyme of the oxidoreductase class that catalyzes the reaction formate + NAD$^+$ = CO$_2$ + NADH. The reaction occurs in bacteria but not in mammals. The fact that bacteria containing the enzyme (e.g., *Escherichia coli*) produce gas in mixed acid fermentations, and those that do not form the enzyme (e.g., *Shigella*) produce acid but no gas, is the basis for a test for the identification of Enterobacteriaceae. Called also *formate hydrogenlyase.*

formate hydrogenlyase (fōr′māt hi″dro-jen-li′ās) formate dehydrogenase.

formatio (for-ma′she-o), pl. *formatio′nes* [L.] [NA] formation: a general term designating a structure of definite shape. **f. reticula′ris medul′lae oblonga′tae** [NA], reticular formation of medulla oblongata: the phylogenetically old part of the medulla oblongata which has a reticular structure, i.e., which is structurally comprised of diffuse aggregations of nerve cells in the midst of a wealth of nerve fibers and, with certain exceptions, lacks circumscribed cell groups; it fills the spaces between the major nuclei and fiber tracts. Called also *reticular substance of medulla oblongata* and *substantia reticularis medullae oblongatae* [NA alternative]. **f. reticula′ris medul′lae spina′lis** [NA], reticular formation of spinal cord: numerous small islets of gray matter and intersecting white fibers which together constitute part of the intermediate gray substance of the spinal cord; in the thoracic cord, the formation occurs immediately dorsal to the lateral horn. **f. reticula′ris mesenceph′ali** [NA], **f. reticula′ris pedun′culi cer′ebri,** reticular formation of mesencephalon: the part of the mesencephalon that has a reticular structure like that of the medulla oblongata; it lies

between the substantia nigra and the central gray matter. **f. reticula′ris pon′tis** [NA], reticular formation of pons: the part of the pars dorsalis pontis, anterior to the central gray matter, that has a structure similar to that of the reticular formation of the medulla oblongata.

formation (fōr-ma′shun) 1. the process of giving shape or form; the creation of an entity, or of a structure of definite shape. 2. a structure of definite shape; see *formatio.* **coffin f.,** the surrounding of dead nerve cells by satellite cells in neuronophagia. **compromise f.,** in psychoanalysis, a disguised idea or act representing and permitting partial expression of a repressed conflict. **Gothic arch f.,** Henning's sign. **gray reticular f.,** substantia reticularis grisea medullae oblongatae. **palisade f.,** an arrangement in cells of a glioma, the fusiform cells being arranged in compact manner pointing radially from a central area comparatively free of vessels. **reaction f.,** a defense mechanism in which a person adopts conscious attitudes, interests, or feelings that are the opposites of his unconscious feelings, impulses, or wishes, e.g., excessive moralistic zeal may defend against an unconscious wish to do the very behavior that one castigates, or conscious revulsion or repugnance may defend against an unconscious desire or attraction. **reticular f. of medulla oblongata,** formatio reticularis medullae oblongatae. **reticular f. of mesencephalon,** formatio reticularis mesencephali. **reticular f. of pons,** formatio reticularis pontis. **reticular f. of spinal cord,** formatio reticularis medullae spinalis. **rouleaux f.,** the aggregation of erythrocytes in structures resembling piles of coins, caused by adhesion of their flat surfaces. **white reticular f.,** substantia reticularis alba medullae oblongatae.

formationes (for-ma-she-o′nēz) [L.] plural of *formatio.*

formative (fōr′mah-tiv) concerned in the origination and development of an organism, part, or tissue.

formboard (fōrm′bōrd) a board containing variously shaped cutouts into which blocks corresponding to the cutouts are to be fitted; used as a test in mental retardation.

form-class (form-klas) an artificial taxonomic category comparable to a class, to which organisms are provisionally assigned, as are imperfect fungi until their perfect (sexual) stages are identified. Form-classes are subdivided into form-orders, form-families, and so on.

forme (fōrm), pl. *formes* [Fr.] form. **f. fruste** (fōrm froost), pl. *formes frustes* [Fr. "defaced"], an atypical, especially a mild or incomplete, form, as of a disease or anomaly. **f. tardive** (fōrm tahr-dēv′) [Fr. "late"], a late-occurring form of a disease that usually makes its appearance at an earlier age.

form-family (form-fam′ĭ-le) see *form-class.*

formic acid (for′mik) an acid from the distillation of ants and derivable from oxalic acid, glycerine, and the oxidation of formaldehyde. Formic acid resembles acetic acid in its actions but is far more irritating and pungent and is dangerously caustic to skin. The acid and its sodium and calcium salts are used as food preservatives.

formication (fōr″mĭ-ka′shun) [L. *formica* ant] a tactile hallucination in which there is a sensation of tiny insects crawling over the skin; most commonly seen in cocaine or amphetamine intoxication.

formiciasis (for″mĭ-si′ah-sis) [L. *formica* ant] a condition produced by poisoning resulting from ant bites.

Formicoidea (for″mĭ-koi-de′ah) a superfamily of ants (order Hymenoptera), some members of which may inflict painful stings.

formimino (for-mim′ĭ-no) the group —CH=NH.

formiminoglutamate (for- mim″ĭ- no-gloo′tah- māt) NH= CH—NH-CH(COO⁻)CH$_2$CH$_2$COO⁻, the anionic form of formiminoglutamic acid and an intermediate in the degradation of histidine to glutamate. It may be excreted in the urine in genetic deficiency of glutamate formiminotransferase, in vitamin B$_{12}$ or folic acid deficiency and in liver disease.

formiminotransferase (for-mim″ĭ-no-trans′fer-ās) glutamate formiminotransferase.

Formin (fōr′min) trademark for preparations of methenamine.

formocortal (for-mo-kor′tal) chemical name: 21-(acetyloxy)-3-(2-chloroethoxy)-9-fluoro-11β-hydroxy-16α,17[(1-methylethylidene)bis(oxy)]-20-oxo-pregna-3,5-diene-6-carboxaldehyde,cyclic 16,17-acetal with acetone, 21-acetate; a gluco-corticoid, $C_{29}H_{38}ClFO_8$.

formol (fŏr′mol)   see *formaldehyde solution,* under *solution.*

form-order (form-or′der)   see *form-class.*

formula (fŏr′mu-lah), pl. *formulas* or *formulae* [L., dim. of *forma* form] a specific statement, using numerals and other symbols, of the composition of, or of the directions for preparing, a compound, such as a medicine, or of a procedure to follow for obtaining a desired value or result; a simplified statement, using numerals and symbols, of a single concept. See also *chemical f.* **acoustic f.,** Brenner's f. in which *Ur* represents the proportion of urea in the blood; *D,* the total urea for twenty-four hours in grams; *P,* the body weight of the patient in kilograms; *C,* the proportion of urea in the urine. **Arneth's f.,** see under *count.* **Arrhenius′ f.,** log x = θc, in which *x* is the viscosity of the solution relative to that of the medium of suspension, *c* the percentage of volume occupied by the suspended particles, and θ a constant. **Beckmann's f.,** a formula used in cryoscopy, ΔT = Km, in which ΔT is the difference in freezing points of the pure solvent and the solution containing a solute at molality *m,* and *K* is a constant characteristic of the particular solvent. For water, K = 1.860 deg(KgH₂O) per mole solute. **Bernhardt's f.,** the ideal weight of an adult in kilograms equals height in centimeters multiplied by chest circumference in centimeters divided by 240. **Bird's f.,** the last two figures expressive of the specific gravity of urine closely represent the number of grains of solids in each ounce. **Black's f.,** F = (W + C) − H. *W* represents the weight in pounds; *C,* the chest measurement in inches at full inspiration; and *H,* the height in inches. When *F* is over 120 a man is classed as very strong; between 110 and 120, strong; between 100 and 110, good; between 90 and 100, fair; between 80 and 90, weak; under 80, very weak. Cf. *Pignet's f.* **Brenner's f.** (*obs.*), with the cathode in the external meatus of the ear, a loud sound is heard on closing the circuit, intensity is diminished during closure, and the sound ceases when the circuit is broken. With the anode in the meatus, no sound is heard on closing or during closure; a weak sound is heard at the break. **Broca's f.,** the ideal weight of a full-grown man in kilograms equals the number of centimeters by which his height exceeds 1 meter. **chemical f.,** a combination of symbols used to express the chemical constitution of a substance; in practice, different types of formulas, of varying complexity, are employed. See *empirical f., molecular f., spatial f., structural f.* **Christison's f.,** Trapp's f. **configurational f.,** spatial f. **constitutional f.,** structural f. **Demoivre's f.,** the expectation of life is equal to two thirds of the difference between the age of the person and eighty. **dental f.,** an expression in symbols of the number and arrangement of teeth in the jaws. Letters represent the various types of teeth: I, *incisor;* C, *canine;* P, *premolar;* M, *molar.* Each letter is followed by a horizontal line. Numbers above the line represent maxillary teeth; those below, mandibular teeth. The human dental formula is $I\frac{2}{2}C\frac{1}{1}M\frac{2}{2} = 10$ (one side only) for deciduous teeth, and $I\frac{2}{2}C\frac{1}{1}P\frac{2}{2}M\frac{3}{3} = 16$ (one side only) for permanent teeth. **digital f.,** a formula expressing the relative lengths of the digits, usually 3 > 4 > 2 > 5 > 1, or 3 > 2 > 4 > 5 > 1, for the fingers, and 1 > 2 > 3 > 4 > 5, or 2 > 1 > 3 > 4 > 5, for the toes. **Dreser's f.,** a formula comparing the molecular concentration of the urine with that of the blood, to show the work done by the kidney. **Einthoven's f.,** e¹ + e³ × e². See *Einthoven's triangle,* under *triangle.* **empirical f.,** a chemical formula which expresses the proportions of the elements present in a substance. For substances composed of discrete molecules, it expresses the relative numbers of atoms present in a molecule of the substance in the smallest whole numbers. For example, the *empirical formula* for ethane is written CH₃, whereas its actual *molecular formula* is C_2H_6. **Fick f.,** see under *principle.* **Florschütz's f.,** L : (2B − L), in which *L* represents body length, and *B,* circumference of abdomen. An index of 5 is normal; an index below 5 indicates the degree of overweight. **Gale's f.,** pulse rate − pulse pressure − 111 closely represents the basal metabolic rate. **Gompertz f.,** see under *law.* **graphic f.,** a term occasionally used to describe a "complete" structural formula, i.e., one in which every individual atom and bond is represented in the formula. The distinction is made because structural formulas are frequently written in a simplified or shortened form. See *structural f.* **Guthrie's f.,** the ideal weight of an adult in pounds equals 110 + (5.5 × number of inches

body height exceeds 5 feet). **Haines′ f.,** the product obtained by multiplying by 1.1 (Haines' coefficient) the last two digits of the number expressing the specific gravity of urine; the result closely represents the number of grains of solids in one fluid ounce of urine. **Hamilton-Stewart f.,** a formula for measuring cardiac output following the rapid intravenous injection of an indicator dye: F = i/ct, in which *F* represents the blood flow in liters per minute; *i,* the injected substance in milligrams; *c,* the average dye concentration of the primary curve; and *t,* the duration of the primary curve in seconds, i.e., the time from appearance to disappearance of the dye at a fixed site if there were no recirculation of the dye. **Häser's f.,** the product obtained by multiplying by 2.33 (Häser's coefficient) the last two digits of the number expressing the specific gravity of urine; the result closely represents the number of grains of solids in one liter of urine. **Loebisch's f.,** the product obtained by multiplying by 2.2 (Loebisch's coefficient) the last two digits of the number expressing the specific gravity of urine; the result closely represents the number of grains of solids in one liter of urine. **Long's f.,** the product obtained by multiplying by 2.6 (Long's coefficient) the last two digits of the number expressing the specific gravity of urine; the result closely represents the number of grains of solids in one liter of urine. **Mall's f.,** the age (in days) of a human embryo is equal to the square root of its length (in millimeters) from vertex to breech multiplied by 100. **Meeh's f.,** the surface area, *O,* is equal to K √P², in which *K* is a constant (12.3), and *P* is the weight of the body. **molecular f.,** a chemical formula giving the number of atoms of each element present in a molecule of a substance, without indicating how they are linked. **official f.,** one officially established by a pharmacopeia or other recognized authority. **paretic f.,** the findings in the cerebrospinal fluid characteristic of dementia paralytica: normal or slightly increased pressure, moderate pleocytosis, moderate increase in protein, change in the colloidal gold test, and positive cerebrospinal fluid Wassermann test. **Pignet's f.,** F = H − (C + W). *H* represents the height in centimeters; *C,* the chest measurement in centimeters at greatest expiration; and *W,* the weight in kilograms. When *F* is less than 10 a person is classed as very strong; between 10 and 15, strong; between 15 and 20, good; between 20 and 25, medium; between 25 and 30, weak; above 30, very weak. Cf. *Black's f.* **projection f.,** a planar, and therefore simplified, representation of a spatial formula. **Ranke's f.,** the number expressive of the specific gravity − 1000 × 0.52 − 5.406 closely represents the amount in grams of the albumin per liter of a serous fluid. **rational f.,** structural f. **Read's f.,** 0.75 × pulse rate + 0.75 × pulse pressure − 72 closely represents the basal metabolic rate. **Reuss′ f.,** $\frac{3}{8}$(S − 1000) − 2.8, in which *S* is the specific gravity, closely represents the percentage of albumin present in a pathologic fluid exudate or transudate. **Runeberg's f.,** a modification of Reuss' formula in which 2.8 is replaced by 2.73 in the case of a transudate and by 2.88 in the case of an inflammatory exudate. **spatial f.,** a chemical formula giving the numbers of atoms of each element present in a molecule of a substance, which atom is linked to which, the types of linkages involved, and the relative positions of the atoms in space. **stereochemical f.,** spatial f. **structural f.,** a chemical formula tell-

$$H-\underset{\underset{H}{|}}{\overset{\overset{H}{|}}{C}}-\underset{\underset{H}{|}}{\overset{\overset{H}{|}}{C}}-O-H \qquad\qquad C_2H_5OH$$

Complete   Abbreviated

Structural formulas for ethyl alcohol.

ing how many atoms of each element are present in a molecule of a substance, which atom is linked to which, and the type of linkages involved; for convenience, abbreviated structural formulas are sometimes used. Called also *constitutional f., graphic f.,* and *rational f.* **Trapp's f.,** the product obtained by multiplying the last two digits of the number expressing its specific gravity by 2 (Trapp's coefficient) closely represents the number of grains of solids in one liter of urine. **Van Slyke's f.,** the urinary coefficient of various substances is equal to D/(Bl × √Wt × V), in which *D* is the daily output in grams of the substance in the urine; *Bl,* the grams of the same substance per liter of blood; *Wt,* the weight of the patient in kilograms; and *V,* the total volume of urine in twenty-four hours. **vertebral f.,** an expression in symbols of the number of vertebrae in each region of the spinal column; for man it is $C_7T_{12}L_5S_5Cd_4 = 33$.

formulary (fōr′mu-lār″e) a collection of recipes, formulas, and prescriptions. **National F.,** see under *N*.

formulate (fōr′mu-lāt) 1. to state in the form of a formula. 2. to prepare in accordance with a prescribed or specified method.

formulation (fōr″mu-la′shun) the act or product of formulating. **American Law Institute f.,** a section of the American Law Institute Model Penal Code: "A person is not responsible for criminal conduct if at the time of such conduct as a result of mental disease or defect he lacks substantial capacity either to appreciate the criminality [wrongfulness] of his conduct or to conform his conduct to the requirements of the law ... the terms 'mental disease or defect' do not include an abnormality manifested only by repeated criminal or otherwise anti-social conduct [antisocial personality]." This test of criminal responsibility or closely related rules have been adopted by many state and federal jurisdictions.

formyl (fōr′mil) [L. *formic* + Gr. *hylē* matter] the radical, HCO or H·C:O—, of formic acid. **f. phenetidin,** colorless crystals, para-ethoxyformanilid, $C_2H_5O·C_6H_4·NH··COH$; formerly used as an antiseptic and analgesic.

formylase (form′ĭ-lās) axylformamidase.

formylkynurenine hydrolase (for″mil-ki″nu-re′nin hi′dro-lās) arylformamidase.

formyltransferase (for″mil-trans′fer-ās) an enzyme of the transferase class [EC 2.1.2] that catalyzes the transfer of a formyl group from a donor to an acceptor compound.

fornicate (fōr′nĭ-kāt) 1. [L. *fornicatus* arched] shaped like an arch. 2. [L. *fornix*, a brothel] to engage in illicit sexual intercourse.

fornix (fōr′niks), pl. *for′nices* [L. "arch"] 1. a general term for an archlike structure or the vaultlike space created by such a structure. 2. fornix cerebri. **anterior f.,** see *f. vaginae*. **f. cer′ebri** [NA], **f. of cerebrum,** the efferent pathway of the hippocampus, projecting chiefly to the mamillary bodies and habenular nuclei; each fornix of the pathway is an arched tract that is united under the corpus callosum with the other fornix, so that together they comprise two columns, a body, and two crura. **f. conjuncti′vae infe′rior** [NA], inferior conjunctival fornix: the inferior line of reflection of the conjunctiva from the eyelid to the eyeball. **f. conjuncti′vae supe′rior** [NA], superior conjunctival fornix: the superior line of reflection of the conjunctiva from the eyelid to the eyeball; it receives the openings of the lacrimal duct. **gastric f.,** f. gastricus. **f. gas′tricus** [NA], gastric fornix: a term used in radiographic anatomy to refer to the arch of the fundus of the stomach. Called also *f. of stomach*, *f. ventricularis* [NA alternative], and *f. ventriculi*. **lateral f.,** see *f. vaginae*. **f. pharyn′gis** [NA], **f. of pharynx,** the vault of the pharynx. **posterior f.,** see *f. vaginae*. **f. sac′ci lacrima′lis** [NA], fornix of lacrimal sac: the upper, blind extremity of the lacrimal sac. **f. of stomach,** f. gastricus. **f. vagi′nae** [NA], the recess formed between the vaginal wall and the vaginal part of the cervix; sometimes subdivided to *pars anterior, pars posterior,* and *pars lateralis,* depending on its relation to the wall of the vagina; called also *fundus vaginae* or *fundus of vagina.* **f. ventricula′ris,** NA alternative for *f. gastricus.* **f. ventric′uli,** f. gastricus.

Foroblique (fōr″ob-lek′) trademark for an obliquely forward visual telescopic system used in panendoscopes.

Forssell's sinus (fōr′selz) [Gösta *Forssell*, Swedish radiologist, 1876–1950] see under *sinus*.

Forssman's antigen (fōrs′manz) [John *Forssman*, Swedish pathologist, 1868–1947] see under *antigen*.

Forssmann (fors′man), Werner Theodor Otto. German surgeon, 1904–1979; co-winner, with André Frédéric Cournand and Dickinson Woodruff Richards, Jr., of the Nobel prize for medicine or physiology in 1956 for developing cardiac catheterization.

Förster's choroiditis (disease), photometer (fers′terz) [Carl Friedrich Richard *Förster*, German ophthalmologist, 1825–1902] see under *choroiditis*, and see *photoptometer*.

Fortaz (for′taz) trademark for a preparation of ceftazidime.

Forthane (for′thān) trademark for a preparation of methylhexaneamine.

fortuitous (fōr-tu′ĭ-tus) pertaining to or occurring by chance.

fosazepam (fos-az′ĕ-pam) chemical name: 7-chloro-1-[(dimethylphosphenyl)methyl]-1,3-dihydro-5-phenyl-2*H*-1,4-benzodiazepin-2-one. A benzodiazepine derivative, $C_{18}H_{18}ClN_2O_2P$, which has been used as a hypnotic.

fosfomycin (fos-fo-mi′sin) chemical name: (–)-(1*R*,2*S*)-(1,2-epoxypropyl)phosphonic acid; an antibiotic, $C_3H_7O_4P$, produced by *Streptomyces fradiae*.

fosfonet sodium (fos′fo-net) chemical name: phosphonoacetic acid monosodium salt monohydrate; an antiviral agent, $C_2H_3Na_2O_5P·H_2O$.

Foshay's test [Lee *Foshay*, American bacteriologist, 1896–1961] see under *tests*.

fospirate (fos′pĭ-rāt) chemical name: dimethyl 3,5,6-trichloro-2-pyridinyl ester; an anthelmintic for veterinary use, $C_7H_7Cl_3NO_4P$.

fossa (fos′ah), pl. *fos′sae* [L.] a trench or channel; [NA] a general term for a hollow or depressed area. **acetabular f., f. acetab′uli** [NA], a rough nonarticular area in the floor of the acetabulum above the acetabular notch. **adipose fossae,** spaces in the female breast, just beneath the skin, which contain fat. **Allen's f.** (*obs.*), a fossa on the neck of the femur. **anconal f., anconeal f.,** f. olecrani. **antecubital f.,** f. cubitalis. **f. anthel′icis** [NA], **f. of anthelix,** the depression on the medial surface of the auricle of the ear that corresponds to the anthelix on the lateral surface. **articular f. of atlas, inferior,** fovea articularis inferior atlantis. **articular f. of atlas, superior,** fovea articularis superior atlantis. **articular f. of mandible,** f. mandibularis. **articular f. for odontoid process of axis,** fovea dentis atlantis. **articular f. of temporal bone,** f. mandibularis. **f. axilla′ris** [NA], **axillary f.,** the small hollow, underneath the arm, where it joins the body at the shoulder, which contains axillary vessels, the brachial plexus of nerves, many lymph nodes and vessels, and loose areolar tissue; called also *armpit, axilla,* and *axillary space.* **Biesiadecki's f.,** f. iliacosubfascialis. **Broesike's f.,** parajejunal f. **f. caeca′lis,** a peritoneal recess at the beginning medial to and behind the cecum; it is formed by the cecal folds. **f. cani′na** [NA], **canine f.,** a wide depression on the external surface of the maxilla superolateral to the canine tooth socket; the levator anguli oris muscle arises from it. Called also *maxillary f.* **f. capitel′li,** the depression for the head of the malleus. **f. cap′itis fem′oris,** fovea capitis femoris. **f. carot′ica,** trigonum caroticum. **cerebellar f.** (*obs.*), f. cranii posterior. **cerebral f.,** any one of the depressions on the floor of the cranial cavity; see *f. cranii anterior, f. cranii media,* and *f. cranii posterior.* **f. cer′ebri latera′lis** [Syl′vii], f. lateralis cerebri. **f. chor′dae duc′tus veno′si,** f. ductus venosi. **cochleariform f.,** semicanalis musculi tensoris tympani. **condylar f., f. condyla′ris** [NA], **condyloid f.,** either of two pits situated on the lateral portions of the occipital bone, one on either side of the foramen magnum, posterior to the occipital condyle; called also *f. condyloidea, postcondyloid f.,* and *posterior condyloid f.* **condyloid f., posterior,** f. condylaris. **condyloid f. of atlas,** fovea articularis superior atlantis. **condyloid f. of mandible,** f. mandibularis. **condyloid f. of temporal bone,** f. mandibularis. **f. condyloi′dea,** f. condylaris. **coronoid f. of humerus, f. coronoi′dea hu′meri** [NA], the cavity in the humerus that receives the coronoid process of the ulnar when the elbow is flexed. **f. of coronoid process,** f. coronoidea humeri. **costal f., inferior,** fovea costalis inferior. **costal f., superior,** fovea costalis superior. **costal f. of transverse process,** fovea costalis processus transversus. **cranial f., anterior,** f. cranii anterior. **cranial f., middle,** f. cranii media. **cranial f., posterior,** f. cranii posterior. **f. crania′lis ante′rior,** f. cranii anterior. **f. crania′lis me′dia,** f. cranii media. **f. crania′lis posterior,** f. cranii posterior. **f. cra′nii ante′rior** [NA], anterior cranial fossa: the anterior subdivision of the floor of the cranial cavity, supporting the frontal lobes of the brain, and composed of portions of three bones: the ethmoid, frontal, and sphenoid. Called also *f. cranialis anterior.* **f. cra′nii me′dia** [NA], middle cranial fossa: the middle subdivision of the floor of the cranial cavity, supporting the temporal lobes of the brain and the pituitary gland; it is composed of the body and greater wings of the sphenoid bone and the squamous and petrous portions of the temporal bone. Called also *f. cranialis media.* **f. cra′nii poste′rior** [NA], posterior cranial fossa: the posterior subdivision of the floor of the cranial cavity, lodging the cerebellum, pons, and medulla oblongata; it is formed by portions of the sphenoid, temporal, parietal, and occipital bones. Called also *f. cranialis posterior.* **crural f.,** annulus femoralis. **cubital f.,** 1. fossa cubitalis. 2. fossa coronoidea humeri. **f. cubita′lis** [NA], cubital fossa: the depression in the anterior region of the elbow. **f. cys′tidis fel′leae,** f. vesicae felleae. **digastric f.,** 1. fossa digastrica. 2. incisura mastoidea ossis temporalis. **f. digas′trica** [NA], digastric fossa: a depression on the internal surface of the body of the mandible on each side of the symphysis to which is attached the anterior belly of the digastric muscle; called also *f. musculi biventeris,* and *digastric fovea* or *impression.* **digital f. of femur,** f. trochanterica. **digital f., inferior,** annulus femoralis. **digital f., superior,** f. inguinalis lateralis. **f. duc′tus veno′si** [NA], f. of ductus venosus, an impression on the posterior part of the diaphragmatic surface of the liver in the fetus, lodging the ductus venosus. **duodenal f., inferior,** recessus duodenalis inferior. **duodenal f., superior,** recessus duodenalis superior. **duodenojejunal f.,** recessus duodenalis superior. **epigastric f.,** 1. fossa epigastrica. 2. the urachal fossa. **f. epigas′trica** [NA], epigastric fossa: a fossa in the epigastric region; called also *scrobiculus cordis* and *fovea cardiaca.* **ethmoid f.,** a groove situated in the cribriform plate of the ethmoid bone; it lodges the olfactory bulb of the brain. Called also *olfactory f.* or *groove.* **f. of eustachian tube,** f. scaphoidea ossis sphenoidalis. **femoral f.,** annulus femoralis. **floccular f.,** f. subarcuata ossis temporalis. **f. of gallbladder,** f. vesicae felleae. **f. of gasserian ganglion,** impressio trigemini ossis temporalis. **Gerdy′s hyoid f.,** superior carotid triangle. **f. glan′dulae lacrima′lis** [NA], fossa of lacrimal gland: a shallow depression in the lateral part of the roof of the orbit, lodging the lacrimal gland; called also *lacrimal f.* **glandular f. of frontal bone,** f. glandulae lacrimalis. **glenoid f.,** f. mandibularis. **glenoid f. of scapula,** cavitas glenoidalis. **glenoid f. of temporal bone,** f. mandibularis. **greater f. of Scarpa,** trigonum femorale. **Gruber′s f.,** a diverticulum of the suprasternal space alongside of the inner end of the clavicle. **Gruber-Landzert f.,** a recess in the peritoneum in the same situation as the superior duodenal recess, but extending downward behind the duodenojejunal angle. **harderian f.,** the depression in which the harderian glands are lodged. **f. of head of femur,** fovea capitis femoris. **f. hel′icis,** scapha. **f. hemiellip′tica,** recessus ellipticus vestibuli. **f. hemisphe′rica,** recessus sphericus vestibuli. **hyaloid f., f. hyaloi′dea** [NA], a depression on the anterior surface of the vitreous body, in which the lens is lodged; called also *lenticular f. of vitreous body* and *patellar f.* **hypogastric f.,** f. inguinalis medialis. **hypophyseal f., f. hypophys′eos, f. hypophysia′lis** [NA], a deep depression in the middle of the sella turcica of the sphenoid bone, lodging the hypophysis cerebri; called also *pituitary f.* and *sellar f.* **ileocecal f., inferior,** recessus ileocecalis inferior. **ileocecal f., superior,** recessus ileocecalis superior. **ileocolic f.,** recessus ileocecalis superior. **iliac f., f. ili′aca** [NA], a large, smooth concave area occupying much of the inner surface of the ala of the ilium, especially anteriorly; from it arises the iliacus muscle. **iliacosubfascial f., f. iliacosubfascia′lis,** an inconstant depression on the inner surface of the abdomen between the psoas muscle and the crest of the ilium; called also *Biesiadecki′s f.* **f. iliopecti′nea, iliopectineal f.,** a depression between the iliopsoas and pectineus muscles in the center of the femoral triangle; called also *lesser f. of Scarpa.* **implantation f.,** a shallow depression at the site where the tail of a spermatozoon attaches to the head. **incisive f. of maxilla,** a slight depression on the anterior surface of the maxilla above the incisor teeth; called also *myrtiform f., f. praenasalis,* and *prenasal f.* **incudal f., incu′dis** [NA], f. of incus, a groove in the posterior wall of the tympanic cavity, lodging the short limb of the incus. **infraclavicular f., f. infraclavicula′ris** [NA], the triangular region of the chest just below the clavicle, between the deltoid and pectoralis major muscles; called also *infraclavicular region* or *triangle, Mohrenheim′s f.* or *triangle, regio infraclavicularis,* and

trigonum deltoideopectorale. **infraduodenal f.,** a recess in the peritoneum below the third portion of the duodenum. **f. infraspina′ta** [NA], **infraspinous f.,** the large, slightly concave area below the spinous process on the dorsal surface of the scapula; it is the site of origin of the infraspinatus muscle. **infratemporal f., f. infratempora′lis** [NA], the area on the side of the cranium limited superiorly by the infratemporal crest, posteriorly by the mandibular fossa, anteriorly by the infratemporal surface of the maxilla, and laterally by the zygomatic arch and part of the ramus of the mandible; called also *zygomatic f., infratemporal region,* and *regio infratemporalis.* **inguinal f., external,** f. inguinalis lateralis. **inguinal f., internal,** f. inguinalis medialis. **inguinal f., lateral,** f. inguinalis lateralis. **inguinal f., medial, inguinal f., middle,** f. inguinalis medialis. **f. inguina′lis latera′lis** [NA], lateral inguinal fossa: the depression on the inside of the anterior abdominal wall lateral to the lateral umbilical fold; called also *fovea inguinalis lateralis* and *lateral inguinal fovea.* **f. inguina′lis media′lis** [NA], medial inguinal fossa: the depression on the inside of the anterior abdominal wall between the medial and lateral umbilical folds; called also *fovea inguinalis medialis.* **innominate f. of auricle,** cavitas conchae. **intercondylar f. of femur,** f. intercondylaris femoris. **intercondylar f. of femur, anterior,** facies patellaris femoris. **intercondylar f. of tibia, anterior,** area intercondylaris anterior tibiae. **intercondylar f. of tibia, posterior,** area intercondylaris posterior tibiae. **f. intercondyla′ris fem′oris** [NA], intercondylar fossa of femur: the posterior depression between the condyles of the femur; called also *f. intercondyloidea femoris.* **f. intercondyl′ica,** f. intercondylaris femoris. **intercondyloid f.,** see *f. intercondylaris femoris, area intercondylaris anterior tibiae,* and *area intercondylaris posterior tibiae.* **f. intercondyloi′dea ante′rior tib′iae,** area intercondylaris anterior tibiae. **f. intercondyloi′dea fem′oris,** f. intercondylaris femoris. **f. intercondyloi′dea poste′rior tib′iae,** area intercondylaris posterior tibiae. **f. intercrura′lis,** f. interpedunuclaris. **f. intermesocol′ica transver′sa,** a recess of the peritoneum in the same situation as the recessus duodenalis superior, but extending transversely. **interpeduncular f., f. interpeduncula′ris** [NA], a depression between the two cerebral peduncles, the floor of which is the posterior perforated substance; called also *Tarin′s f.* **intersigmoid f.,** recessus intersigmoideus. **ischiorectal f., f. ischiorecta′lis** [NA], the potential space between the pelvic diaphragm and the skin below it; an anterior recess extends a variable distance between the pelvic and urogenital diaphragms, sometimes reaching the retropubic space. **Jobert′s f.,** the fossa in the popliteal region bounded above by the adductor magnus and below by the gracilis and sartorius, best seen when the knee is bent and the thigh strongly rotated outward. **f. of Jonnesco,** the duodenojejunal fossa between the superior and inferior duodenal folds. **jugular f., f. jugula′ris,** 1. the depression at the base of the neck just above the sternum; called also *suprasternal space.* 2. jugular f. of temporal bone. **jugular f. of temporal bone, f. jugula′ris os′sis tempora′lis** [NA], a prominent depression on the inferior surface of the petrous part of the temporal bone, forming the major part of the jugular notch; it forms the anterior and lateral wall of the jugular foramen and lodges the superior bulb of the internal jugular vein. **lacrimal f.,** 1. fossa glandulae lacrimalis. 2. sulcus lacrimalis ossis lacrimalis. **f. of lacrimal gland,** f. glandulae lacrimalis. **f. of lacrimal sac,** f. sacci lacrimalis. **Landzert′s f.,** recessus paraduodenalis. **lateral f. of cerebrum,** f. lateralis cerebri. **f. of lateral malleolus,** f. malleoli lateralis. **f. latera′lis cer′ebri** [NA], lateral fossa of cerebrum: a depression, in fetal life, on the lateral surface of each cerebral hemisphere at the bottom of which lies the insula; later it is closed over by the operculum, the edges of which form the lateral sulcus. Called also *f. cerebri lateralis* [Sylvii] and *f. of Sylvius.* **lenticular f., lenticular f. of vitreous body,** f. hyaloidea. **lesser f. of Scarpa,** f. iliopectinea. **f. for ligamentum teres,** fissura ligamenti teretis. **f. of little head of radius,** fovea capituli radii. **longitudinal fossae of liver, right,** fossae sagittales dextrae hepatis. **f. longitudina′lis hep′atis,** f. sagittalis sinistra hepatis. **Luschka′s f.,** recessus ileocecalis superior. **Malgaigne′s f.,** see *carotid triangle, superior,* under *triangle.* **f. malle′oli latera′lis** [NA], fossa of lateral malleolus: a depression on the medial aspect of the lateral malleolus behind its articular surface. **mandibular f., f. mandibula'ris** [NA], a prominent depression in the inferior surface of the squamous part of the temporal bone at the base of the zygomatic process, in which the condyloid process of the mandible rests. **mastoid f.,** 1. mastoid f. of temporal bone. 2. foveola suprameatica. **mastoid f. of temporal bone,** a small triangular area between the posterior wall of the external acoustic meatus and the posterior root of the zygomatic process of the temporal bone; called also mastoid f., *Macewen's triangle,* and *suprameatal triangle.* **maxillary f.,** f. canina. **mesentericoparietal f.,** parajejunal f. **mesocranial f.** (*obs.*), f. cranii media. **mesogastric f.,** recessus duodenalis superior. **middle cranial f.,** f. cranii media. **Mohrenheim's f.,** f. infraclavicularis. **f. of Morgagni,** f. navicularis urethrae. **f. mus'culi biven'teris,** f. digastrica. **mylohyoid f. of mandible,** fovea sublingualis. **myrtiform f.,** incisive f. of maxilla. **nasal f.,** the portion of the nasal cavity anterior to the middle meatus. **navicular f. of Cruveilhier,** f. scaphoidea ossis sphenoidalis. **navicular f. of male urethra,** f. navicularis urethrae. **navicular f. of sphenoid bone,** f. scaphoidea ossis sphenoidalis. **f. navicula'ris ure'thrae** [NA], **f. navicula'ris ure'thrae [Morgag'nii],** the lateral expansion of the urethra in the glans penis. **f. navicula'ris [vestib'uli vagi'nae],** f. vestibuli vaginae. **f. occipita'lis cerebra'lis** (*obs.*), f. lateralis cerebri. **f. olec'rani** [NA], **olecranon f.,** a depression on the posterior surface of the humerus, above the trochlea, for lodging the olecranon of the ulna when the elbow is extended. **olfactory f.,** ethmoid f. **f. of omental sac, inferior,** recessus inferior omentalis. **f. of omental sac, superior,** recessus superior omentalis. **oral f.,** stomodeum. **oval f. of heart,** f. ovalis cordis. **oval f. of thigh,** hiatus saphenus. **f. ova'lis cor'dis** [NA], oval f. of heart: a depression on the right side of the interatrial septum of the heart, representing the remains of the fetal foramen ovale. **f. ova'lis fem'oris,** hiatus saphenus. **ovarian f., f. ova'rica,** [NA], a shallow pouch on the posterior surface of the broad ligament, in which the ovary is located. **paraduodenal f.,** recessus duodenalis superior. **parajejunal f.,** a pouch of peritoneum below the lower end of the first part of the jejunum. **paravesical f., f. paravesica'lis** [NA], the fossa formed by the peritoneum on each side of the urinary bladder. **parietal f.,** the deepest portion of the inner surface of the parietal bone. **patellar f.,** f. hyaloidea. **patellar f. of femur,** facies patellaris femoris. **patellar f. of tibia,** area intercondylaris anterior tibiae. **perineal f.,** f. ischiorectalis. **petrosal f., f. for petrosal ganglion,** fossula petrosa. **piriform f.,** recessus piriformis. **pituitary f.,** f. hypophysialis. **f. poplit'ea** [NA], **popliteal f.,** the depression in the posterior region of the knee; called also *popliteal cavity.* **popliteal f. of femur,** f. intercondylaris femoris. **popliteal f. of tibia,** area intercondylaris posterior tibiae. **postcondyloid f.,** f. condylaris. **posterior f. of humerus,** f. olecrani. **f. praenasa'lis, prenasal f.,** incisive f. of maxilla. **prescapular f., prespinous f.,** a depression in the anterior surface of the spine of the scapula. **pterygoid f. of inferior maxillary bone,** fovea pterygoidea mandibulae. **pterygoid f. of sphenoid bone, f. pterygoi'dea os'sis sphenoida'lis** [NA], the posteriorly facing fossa which is formed by the divergence of the medial and lateral pterygoid plates of the sphenoid bone, and lodges the origins of the internal pterygoid muscle and tensor veli palatini muscle. **pterygomaxillary f.,** f. pterygopalatina. **f. pterygopalati'na** [NA], **pterygopalatine f.,** a small space between the front of the root of the pterygoid process of the sphenoid bone and the back of the maxilla. **radial f. of humerus, f. radia'lis hu'meri** [NA], a depression on the anterior surface of the humerus just above the capitulum. **retrocecal f.,** recessus retrocecalis. **retroduodenal f.,** a pouch of peritoneum below and behind the third portion of the duodenum. **retromandibular f., f. retromandibula'ris,** the depression posterior to the angle of the jaw, on either side, inferior to the auricle. **rhomboid f., f. rhomboi'dea** [NA], the floor of the fourth ventricle of the brain, made up of the dorsal surfaces of the medulla oblongata and pons. **Rosenmüller's f.,** recessus pharyngeus. **f. sac'ci lacrima'lis** [NA], the fossa that lodges the lacrimal sac, formed by the lacrimal sulcus of the lacrimal bone and the frontal process of the

maxilla; called also *lacrimal groove.* **fossae sagitta'les dex'trae hep'atis,** a longitudinal fissure in the right lobe of the liver. **fossae sagitta'les hep'atis,** f. sagittalis sinistra hepatis. **f. sagitta'lis sinis'tra hep'atis,** a longitudinal fissure in the left lobe of the liver, composed of the fossa venae umbilicalis in front and the fossa ductus venosi dorsally. **scaphoid f.,** 1. f. scaphoidea ossis sphenoidalis. 2. scapha. **scaphoid f. of sphenoid bone, f. scaphoi'dea os'sis sphenoida'lis** [NA], a depression on the superior part of the posterior portion of the medial plate of the pterygoid process of the sphenoid bone, giving attachment to the tensor veli palatini muscle. Called also *f. of Eustachian tube, navicular f. of Cruveilher, navicular f. of sphenoid bone,* and *scaphoid f.* **f. scar'pae ma'jor,** trigonum femorale. **sellar f.,** f. hypophysialis. **semilunar f. of ulna,** incisura trochlearis ulnae. **sigmoid f.,** sulcus sinus transversi. **sigmoid f. of temporal bone,** sulcus sinus sigmoidei ossis temporalis. **sigmoid f. of ulna,** incisura trochlearis ulnae. **sigmoid f. of ulna, lesser,** incisura radialis ulnae. **sphenomaxillary f.,** f. pterygopalatina. **splenic f. of omental sac,** recessus lienalis. **f. subarcua'ta os'sis tempora'lis** [NA], **subarcuate f. of temporal bone,** a small fossa on the internal surface of the petrous part of the temporal bone just below the arcuate eminence, most prominent in the fetus. In the adult it lodges a piece of dura and transmits a small vein. **subcecal f.,** recessus ileocecalis inferior. **sublingual f.,** fovea sublingualis. **submandibular f.,** fovea submandibularis. **submaxillary f.,** fovea submandibularis. **subpyramidal f.,** a fossa on the inferior wall of the middle ear, inferior to the round window and posterior to the pyramid. **subscapular f., f. subscapula'ris** [NA], the concave ventral surface of the body of the scapula. **subsigmoid f.,** a fossa between the mesentery of the sigmoid flexure and that of the descending colon. **supraclavicular f., greater,** f. supraclavicularis major. **supraclavicular f., lesser,** f. supraclavicularis minor. **f. supraclavicula'ris ma'jor** [NA], greater supraclavicular fossa: a depression on the surface of the body, located above and behind the clavicle, lateral to the tendon of the sternocleidomastoid muscle. See also *trigonum omoclaviculare.* **f. supraclavicula'ris mi'nor** [NA], lesser supraclavicular fossa: the region of the neck in the depression behind the clavicle, about the interval between the two tendons of the sternocleidomastoid muscle; called also *Zang's space.* **supracondyloid f.,** a depression on the femur between the internal tuberosity and the internal supracondyloid tubercle. **supramastoid f.,** foveola suprameatica. **suprasphenoidal f.,** f. hypophysialis. **f. supraspina'ta** [NA], **supraspinous f.,** the deeply concave area above the spinous process on the dorsal surface of the scapula from which the supraspinous muscle takes origin. **supratonsillar f., f. supratonsilla'ris** [NA], the space between the palatoglossal and palatopharyngeal arches superior to the tonsil. **supratrochlear f., posterior,** f. olecrani. **supravesical f., f. supravesica'lis** [NA], the depression on the inside of the anterior abdominal wall between the median and the medial umbilical fold; called also *fovea supravesicalis peritonaei.* **sylvian f., f. of Sylvius,** 1. fossa lateralis cerebri. 2. sulcus lateralis cerebri. **Tarin's f.,** f. interpeduncularis. **temporal f.,** 1. fossa temporalis. 2. fossa cranii media. **f. tempora'lis** [NA], temporal fossa: the area on the side of the cranium outlined posteriorly and superiorly by the temporal lines, anteriorly by the frontal and zygomatic bones, laterally by the zygomatic arch, and inferiorly by the infratemporal crest. **terminal f.,** f. navicularis urethrae. **tibiofemoral f.,** a palpable space between the articular surfaces of the tibia and femur mesial (internal tibiofemoral f.) or lateral (external tibiofemoral f.) to the inferior pole of the patella. **tonsillar f., f. tonsilla'ris** [NA], the depression between the palatoglossal and palatopharyngeal arches in which the palatine tonsil is located; called also *sinus tonsillaris* and *tonsillar sinus.* **f. transversa'lis hep'atis,** porta hepatis. **f. of Treitz,** recessus duodenalis superior. **triangular f. of auricle, f. triangular'is auric'ulae** [NA], the cavity just above the concha of the ear between the crura of the anthelix. **trochanteric f., f. trochanter'ica** [NA], a deep depression on the medial surface of the greater trochanter that receives the insertion of the tendon of the obturator externus muscle. **trochlear f., f. trochlea'ris,** fovea trochlearis. **ulnar f.,** f. coronoidea humeri. **umbilical f., medial,** f. inguinalis medialis.

f. umbilica'lis hep'atis, fissura ligamenti teretis. **urachal f.,** a depression on the inner surface of the anterior abdominal wall, between the urachus and the hypogastric artery; called also *epigastric f.* **f. ve'nae ca'vae,** sulcus venae cavae. **f. ve'nae umbilica'lis,** fissura ligamenti teretis. **f. vesi'cae fel'leae** [NA], the fossa on the posteroinferior surface of the liver that lodges the gallbladder; it helps separate the left and right lobes. Called also *f. of gallbladder.* **vestibular f., f. of vestibule of vagina, f. vestib'uli vagi'nae** [NA], the part of the vestibule between the orifice of the vagina and the frenulum of the pudendal labia; called also *f. navicularis* [*vestibuli vaginae*]. **Waldeyer's f.,** the recessus duodenalis inferior and recessus duodenalis superior considered as one space. **zygomatic f.,** f. infratemporalis.

fossae (fos'e) [L.] genitive and plural of *fossa.*

fossette (fos-et') [Fr.] 1. a small depression. 2. a small and deep corneal ulcer.

fossil (fos'il) [L. *fossilis* to dig] any remains of an organism that have been preserved in the earth's crust.

fossula (fos'u-lah), pl. *fos'sulae* [L., dim. of *fossa*] a small fossa; [NA] a general term for a slight depression in the surface of a structure or organ. **f. of cochlear window,** f. fenestrae cochleae. **costal f., inferior,** fovea costalis inferior. **costal f., superior,** fovea costalis superior. **f. fenes'trae coch'leae** [NA], fenestra of cochlea: a depression on the medial wall of the tympanic cavity, at the bottom of which is the fenestra cochleae; called also *f. of round window.* **f. fenes'trae vestib'uli** [NA], fenestra of vestibule: a depression on the medial wall of the tympanic cavity, at the bottom of which is the fenestra vestibuli; called also *f. of oval window* and *niche of round window.* **f. of oval window,** f. fenestrae vestibuli. **f. petro'sa** [NA], **petrosal f., f. of petrous ganglion,** a small depression on the under surface of the petrous portion of the temporal bone, on a small ridge separating the jugular fossa from the external carotid foramen. **f. post fenes'tram,** a connective tissue tract just behind the oval window, resembling the fissula ante fenestram, but smaller and less constant. **f. of round window,** f. fenestrae cochleae. **tonsillar fossulae of palatine tonsil,** fossulae tonsillares tonsillae palatinae. **tonsillar fossulae of pharyngeal tonsil,** fossulae tonsillares tonsillae pharyngeae. **fos'sulae tonsilla'res tonsil'lae palati'nae** [NA], tonsillar fossulae of palatine tonsil: the mouths of the tonsillar crypts of the palatine tonsils. **fos'sulae tonsilla'res tonsil'lae pharyn'geae** [NA], tonsillar fossulae of pharyngeal tonsil: the mouths of the tonsillar crypts of the pharyngeal tonsil.

fossulae (fos'u-le) [L.] genitive and plural of *fossula.*

fossulate (fos'u-lāt) marked by a small fossa; hollowed or grooved.

Foster Kennedy see *Kennedy.*

Fothergill's disease (sore throat), neuralgia, pill (foth'er-gilz) [John *Fothergill*, English physician, 1712–1780] see *scarlatina anginosa* and *trigeminal neuralgia,* under *neuralgia,* and see under *pill.*

Fothergill's operation (foth'er-gilz) [William Edward *Fothergill,* Manchester gynecologist, 1865–1926] see *Manchester operation,* under *operation.*

Fouchet's test (foo-shāz') [André *Fouchet,* French chemist, born 1894] see under *tests.*

foudroyant (foo''drah-yaw') [Fr.] fulminant.

foulage (foo-lahzh') [Fr. "treading, pressing of grapes"] massage in which the muscles are kneaded and pressed; called also *pétrissage.*

foulbrood (fowl'brood) a contagious disease of honeybees caused by *Bacillus larvae* (American f.) or *Bacillus alvei* (European f.).

foundation (fown-da'shun) the structure or basis on which something is built. **denture f.,** denture-bearing area.

founder (fown'der) the crippled condition of a horse afflicted with laminitis. **chest f.,** founder accompanied by atrophy of the chest muscles. **grain f.,** a condition of indigestion or overloaded stomach in the horse due to overeating.

fourchette (foor-shet') [Fr. "a fork-shaped object"] frenulum labiorum pudendi.

Fourneau 309 (fur'no) trademark for a preparation of suramin sodium.

Fournier's gangrene (disease), etc. (foor-ne-āz') [Jean Alfred *Fournier,* dermatologist in Paris, 1832–1914] see under *gangrene, sign,* and *tests.*

fovea (fo've-ah), pl. *fo'veae* [L.] a pit or depression; [NA] a general term for a small pit in the surface of a structure or organ. Often used alone to indicate the central fovea of the retina. **anterior f. of humerus, greater,** fossa coronoidea humeri. **anterior f. of humerus, lesser,** fossa radialis humeri. **articular foveae for rib cartilages,** incisurae costales sterni. **articular f. of temporal bone,** fossa mandibularis. **f. articula'ris cap'itis ra'dii** [NA], a depression on the proximal surface of the head of the radius for articulation with the capitulum of the humerus. **f. articula'ris infe'rior atlan'tis** [NA], inferior articular fovea of atlas: either of the two inferior articular surfaces (facies articulares inferiores atlantis) found on the lateral masses of the atlas; called also *inferior articular facet* or *fossa of atlas.* **f. articula'ris supe'rior atlan'tis** [NA], either of the two superior articular surfaces (facies articulares superiores atlantis) found on the lateral masses of the atlas; called also *superior articular surface, facet,* or *fossa of atlas,* and *condyloid fossa of atlas.* **calcaneal f.,** sulcus calcanei. **f. cap'itis fem'oris** [NA], fovea of head of femur: a depression in the head of the femur where the ligamentum teres is attached; called also *fossa capitis femoris* and *fossa of head of femur.* **f. capit'uli ra'dii,** a shallow cup on the upper surface of the head of the radius for articulation with the capitulum of the humerus. **f. cardi'aca,** fossa epigastrica. **caudal f., f. cauda'lis** [NA], a slight depression in the inferior part of the floor of the fourth ventricle, at the upper end of the vagal triangle, marking the end of the sulcus limitans; called also *inferior f.* and *f. inferior* [NA alternative]. **central f. of retina, f. centra'lis ret'inae** [NA], a tiny pit, about 1 degree wide, in the center of the macula lutea, which in turn presents an extremely small depression (foveola) containing rodlike elongated cones; it is the area of clearest vision, because here the layers of the retina are spread aside, permitting light to fall directly on the cones. Called also *Soemmering's foramen.* **f. of condyloid process,** f. pterygoidea mandibulae. **f. of coronoid process,** fossa coronoidea humeri. **costal f., inferior,** f. costalis inferior. **costal f., superior,** f. costalis superior. **costal f., transverse,** f. costalis transversalis. **costal foveae of sternum,** incisurae costales sterni. **f. costa'lis infe'rior** [NA], inferior costal fovea: a small facet on the lower edge of the body of a vertebra articulating with the head of a rib; called also *inferior costal fossa* or *fossula.* **f. costa'lis supe'rior** [NA], superior costal fovea: a small facet on the upper edge of the body of a vertebra articulating with the head of a rib; called also *superior costal facet, fossa,* or *fossula.* **f. costa'lis proces'sus transver'sus,** [NA], transverse costal fovea: a facet on the transverse process of a vertebra for articulation with the tubercle of a rib; called also *costal fossa of transverse process.* **cranial f., f. crania'lis** [NA], an angular depression in the floor of the fourth ventricle produced by widening of the sulcus limitans at the level of the facial colliculus; called also *superior f.* and *f. superior* [NA alternative]. **crural f.,** annulus femoralis. **dental f. of atlas, f. den'tis atlan'tis** [NA], the facet on the inner surface of the anterior arch of the atlas for the articulation of the dens of the axis. **digastric f.,** fossa digastrica. **femoral f.,** annulus femoralis. **f. of fourth ventricle,** see *f. cranialis* and *f. caudalis.* **glandular foveae of Luschka,** foveolae granulares. **f. of head of femur,** f. capitis femoris. **f. for head of radius,** fossa radialis humeri. **f. hemiellip'tica,** recessus ellipticus vestibuli. **f. hemisphe'rica,** recessus sphericus vestibuli. **inferior f., f. caudalis.** **f. infe'rior,** NA alternative for *f. caudalis.* **inferior articular f. of atlas,** f. articularis inferior atlantis. **inguinal f., external,** fossa inguinalis lateralis. **inguinal f., internal,** fossa inguinalis medialis. **inguinal f., lateral,** fossa inguinalis lateralis. **inguinal f., medial,** fossa inguinalis medialis. **inguinal f., middle,** fossa inguinalis medialis. **f. ingui'nalis latera'lis,** fossa inguinalis lateralis. **f. ingui'nalis media'lis,** fossa inguinalis medialis. **interligamentous f. of peritoneum,** fossa supravesicalis. **f. of lateral malleolus,** facies articularis malleolaris tibiae. **f. lim'bica,**

a sulcus marking the lateral border of the lateral area olfactoria and gyrus hippocampi in lower mammals. **f. of little head of radius,** f. capituli radii. **malleolar f., lateral, of fibula,** facies articularis malleoli fibulae. **f. of Morgagni,** fossa navicularis urethrae. **oblong f. of arytenoid cartilage,** f. oblonga cartilaginis arytenoideae. **f. oblon′ga cartilag′inis arytenoi′deae** [NA], oblong fovea of arytenoid cartilage: a depression on the anterolateral surface of the arytenoid cartilage, separated from the triangular pit above by the arcuate crest; called also *oblong pit of arytenoid cartilage.* **pterygoid f., f. pterygoi′dea mandib′ulae** [NA], **f. pterygoi′dea proces′sus condyloi′dei,** a depression on the inner side of the neck of the condyloid process of the mandible, for attachment of the external pterygoid muscle; called also *fovea of condyloid process,* and *pterygoid depression* or *pit.* **sublingual f., f. sublingua′lis** [NA], a depression on the inner surface of the body of the mandible, lodging a portion of the sublingual gland. **submandibular f., f. submandibula′ris** [NA], **f. submaxilla′ris,** a depression on the medial aspect of the body of the mandible, lodging a small portion of the submandibular gland; called also *submandibular* or *submaxillary fossa.* **f. supe′rior,** NA alternative for *f. cranialis.* **superior f.,** f. cranialis. **supratrochlear f., anterior,** fossa coronoidea humeri. **supratrochlear f. of humerus,** fossa coronoidea humeri. **f. supravesica′lis peritonae′i,** fossa supravesicalis. **f. of talus,** sulcus tali. **f. of tooth of atlas,** f. dentis atlantis. **f. triangula′ris cartilag′inis arytenoi′deae** [NA], a depression on the anterolateral surface of the arytenoid cartilage, separated from the oblong pit below by the arcuate crest; called also *triangular pit of arytenoid cartilage.* **trochlear f., f. trochlea′ris** [NA], a depression on the anteromedial part of the orbital surface of the frontal bone for the attachment of the trochlea of the superior oblique muscle; it is often replaced by the trochlear spine. Called also *trochlear fossa* and *fossa trochlearis.*

foveate (fo′ve-āt) [L. *foveatus*] pitted.

foveation (fo″ve-a′shun) a pitted condition.

foveola (fo-ve′o-lah), pl. *fove′olae* [L., dim. of *fovea*] a small pit; [NA] a general term for an extremely small depression. **f. coccyg′ea** [NA], **coccygeal f.,** a dermal pit near the tip of the coccyx, indicative of the site of attachment of the embryonic neural tube to the skin; called also *postanal dimple* or *pit.* **fove′olae gas′tricae** [NA], the numerous pits in the gastric mucosa marking the openings of the gastric glands; called also *gastric pits.* **granular foveolae, fove′olae granula′res** [NA], **fove′olae granula′res [Pacchio′ni],** small pits on the internal surface of the cranial bones on either side of the sagittal sulcus; they are occupied by the arachnoidal granulations. **fove′olae papil′lae,** foramina papillaria renis. **f. re′tinae** [NA], foveola of retina: an extremely small depression in the floor of the fovea centralis, which is devoid of rod cells but contains rodlike elongated cones. **f. suprameata′lis,** NA alternative for *f. suprameatica.* **f. supramea′tica** [NA], suprameatal pit: a small depression at the junction of the posterior and superior borders of the external acoustic meatus, posterior to the suprameatal spine; called also *f. suprameatalis* [NA alternative], *mastoid fossa,* and *suprameatal fossa.*

foveolae (fo-ve′o-le) [L.] genitive and plural of *foveola.*

foveolate (fo-ve′o-lāt) pitted.

Foville's syndrome (fo-vēlz′) [Achille Louis François *Foville,* French psychiatrist, 1831–1887] see under *syndrome.*

Fowler's position (fow′lerz) [George Ryerson *Fowler,* American surgeon, 1848–1906] see under *position.*

Fowler's solution (fow′lerz) [Thomas *Fowler,* English physician, 1736–1801] potassium arsenite solution.

Fowler-Murphy treatment [G. R. *Fowler;* John Benjamin *Murphy,* Chicago surgeon, 1857–1916] Murphy's treatment (def. 2).

fowlpox (fowl′poks) a contagious disease of domestic poultry and birds, due to a poxvirus, and marked by epithelial nodules on the unfeathered parts of the skin, especially the wattles, comb, and legs, and sometimes by membranous lesions in the respiratory passages; called also *epithelioma contagiosum.*

Fox's disease (foks′ez) [G. H. *Fox;* New York dermatologist, 1846–1937] Fox-Fordyce disease.

Fox-Fordyce disease (foks-for′dīs) [G. H. *Fox;* John Addison *Fordyce,* New York dermatologist, 1858–1925] see under *disease.*

foxglove (foks′glov) see *digitalis.* **purple f.,** digitalis.

F.p. abbreviation for L. *fi′at po′tio,* let a potion be made; freezing point.

f.p. foot-pound.

F.pil. abbreviation for L. *fi′ant pil′ulae,* let pills be made.

Fr chemical symbol for *francium.*

Fracastorius (frah″kahs-to′re-us) [It. Girolamo *Fracastoro*] an Italian physician, born in Verona (1483–1553), a poet and geologist, who published in 1530 a medical poem, *Syphilis sive morbus gallicus,* in which the name syphilis was first given to the disease.

Fract. dos. abbreviation for L. *frac′ta do′si,* in divided doses.

fraction (frak′shun) in chemistry, one of the separable constituents of a substance. **ejection f.,** a measure of ventricular contractility, equal to

$$\frac{\text{end diastolic volume} - \text{end systolic volume}}{\text{end diastolic volume}} \times 100,$$

normally 65 + 8 per cent; lower values indicate ventricular dysfunction. **filtration f.,** the portion of the plasma that is filtered through the renal glomerular membranes, calculated as the ratio of the plasma flow through both kidneys to the glomerular filtration rate per minute. **human plasma protein f.,** plasma protein f. **mol f.,** the ratio of the number of moles of a solute to total number of moles in the solution. **plasma f's,** the various components separated from the blood plasma by electrophoresis or by other means. **plasma protein f.** [USP], a sterile preparation of serum albumin and globulin obtained by fractionating material (source blood, plasma, or serum) from healthy human donors and tested for the absence of hepatitis B surface antigen; used as a blood volume supporter.

fractional (frak′shun-al) [L. *fractio* a breaking] accomplished by repeated divisions; see under *dose.*

fractionation (frak″shun-a′shun) 1. in radiology, division of the total dose of radiation into small doses administered at intervals; radiation given in this manner usually causes less biological damage than the same total dose given at one time; called also *dose fractionation.* 2. in chemistry, separation of a substance into components, as by distillation or crystallization. 3. in histology, isolation of components of living cells by differential centrifugation. **dose f.,** see *fractionation* (def. 1).

fractography (frak-tog′rah-fe) [L. *fractus* broken + Gr. *graphein* to record] a technique of photography which permits observation of jagged surfaces at high magnification.

fracture (frak′chur) [L. *fractura,* from *frangere* to break] 1. the breaking of a part, especially a bone. 2. a break or rupture in a bone. **agenetic f.,** spontaneous fracture due to imperfect osteogenesis. **apophyseal f.,** one in which a small smear fragment or a bony prominence is torn from the bone. **articular f.,** a fracture of the joint surface of a bone; called also *joint f.* **atrophic f.,** a spontaneous fracture resulting from atrophy of the bone. **avulsion f.,** an indirect fracture caused by avulsion or pull of a ligament. **Barton's f.,** fracture of the distal end of the radius into the wrist joint. **basal neck f.,** fracture of the neck of the femur at its junction with the trochanteric region. **bending f.,** an indirect fracture caused by bending of the limb. **Bennett's f.,** a fracture of the base of the first metacarpal bone running into the carpometacarpal joint and complicated by subluxation. **blow-out f.,** fracture of the orbital floor caused by a sudden increase of intraorbital pressure due to traumatic force; the orbital contents herniate into the maxillary sinus so that the inferior rectus or inferior oblique muscle may become incarcerated in the fracture site, producing diplopia on looking up. In the pure type there is disruption of the orbital floor without involvement of the orbital rim; the impure type involves the rim, i.e., there is concomitant midfacial fracture. **boxer's f.,** fracture of the metacarpal neck with volar displacement of the metacarpal head. **bucket-handle f.,** a tear in the semilunar cartilage, along the middle portion, leaving a loop of cartilage lying in the intercondylar notch. **bumper f.,** fracture of one or both legs immediately below the knee caused by an automobile bumper, often involving the tibial plateau.

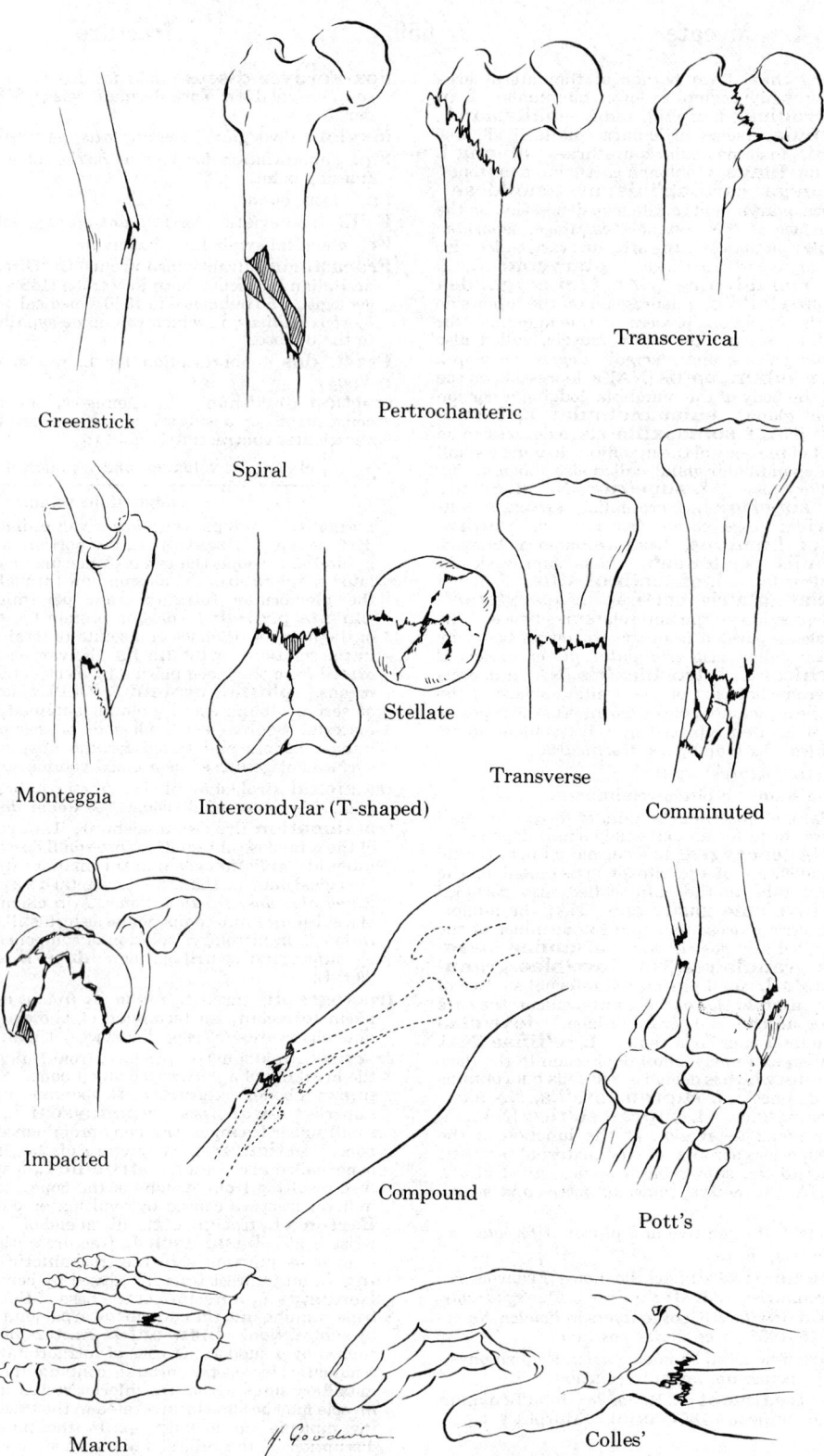

Greenstick

Spiral

Pertrochanteric

Transcervical

Monteggia

Intercondylar (T-shaped)

Stellate

Transverse

Comminuted

Impacted

Compound

Pott's

March

Colles'

H. Goodwin

PLATE 17 —VARIOUS TYPES OF FRACTURES

bursting f., a comminuted fracture of the distal phalanx; called also *tuft f.* **butterfly f.,** a comminuted fracture in which there are two fragments on each side of a main fragment, somewhat resembling the wings of a butterfly. **buttonhole f.,** fracture in which the bone is perforated by a missile; called also *perforating f.* **capillary f.,** a fracture that appears in the roentgenogram as a fine hairlike line, the segments of bone not being separated; sometimes seen in fractures of the skull. **cemental f., cementum f.,** see under *tear.* **chisel f.,** oblique detachment of a piece from the head of the radius. **cleavage f.,** shelling off of cartilage with a small fragment of bone from the upper surface of the capitellum humeri (Kocher). **closed f.,** a fracture which does not produce an open wound in the skin; called also *simple f.* **Colles' f.,** fracture of the lower end of the radius in which the lower fragment is displaced posteriorly (see illustration). If the lower fragment is displaced anteriorly, it is a *reverse Colles' fracture* (Smith's fracture). **comminuted f.,** one in which the bone is splintered or crushed (see illustration). **complete f.,** one in which the bone is entirely broken across. **complicated f.,** fracture with injury of the adjacent parts. **compound f.,** open f. **compression f.,** one produced by compression; e.g., vertebral fracture. **condylar f.,** fracture of the humerus in which a small fragment including the condyle is separated from the inner or outer aspect of the bone. **congenital f.,** intrauterine f. **f. by contrecoup,** a fracture of the skull opposite to the site of impact. **deferred f.,** in the horse, one that does not separate at the time of injury because of the presence of powerful muscles or a strong covering of periosteum, but does separate when extra strain is put upon the injured part. **depressed f.,** a fracture of the skull in which a fragment is depressed. **diacondylar f.,** transcondylar f. **direct f.,** a fracture at the point of injury. **dislocation f.,** fracture of a bone near an articulation with concomitant dislocation of that joint. **double f.,** fracture of a bone in two places; called also *segmental f.* **Dupuytren's f.,** 1. Pott's fracture. 2. (of forearm) Galeazzi's fracture. **Duverney's f.,** fracture of the ilium just below the anterior superior spine. **dyscrasic f.,** fracture due to weakening of the bone from debilitating disease. **f. en coin** (ah kwahn), a V-shaped fracture. **f. en rave** (ah rahv), a fracture in which the break is transverse at the surface, but not within. **endocrine f.,** fracture of a bone weakened by endocrine disorder, such as hyperparathyroidism. **epiphyseal f.,** fracture at the point of union of an epiphysis with the shaft of a bone. **extracapsular f.,** a fracture of the humerus or femur outside of the capsule. **fatigue f.,** a fracture attributed to the strain of prolonged walking or exercise; see *march f.* **fissure f., fissured f.,** a crack extending from a surface into, but not through, a long bone. **Galeazzi's f.,** fracture of the radius above the wrist combined with dislocation of the distal end of the ulna; called also *Dupuytren's f.* **Gosselin's f.,** a V-shaped fracture of the distal end of the tibia, extending into the ankle joint. **greenstick f.,** fracture in which one side of a bone is broken, the other being bent (see illustration); an infraction; called also *hickory-stick* or *willow f.* **grenade-thrower's f.,** fracture of the humerus caused by muscular contraction in throwing a grenade. **Guérin's f.,** Le Fort I f. **gutter f.,** a fracture of the skull in which the depression is elliptic in form. **hangman's f.,** fracture through the pedicles of the axis (C2) with or without subluxation of the second cervical vertebra on the third. **hickory-stick f.,** greenstick f. **horizontal maxillary f.,** Le Fort I f. **impacted f.,** fracture in which one fragment is firmly driven into the other. **incomplete f.,** one which does not entirely destroy the continuity of the bone. **indirect f.,** a fracture at a point distant from the site of injury. **inflammatory f.,** fracture of a bone weakened by inflammatory disease. **interperiosteal f.,** incomplete or greenstick fracture. **intra-articular f.,** a fracture of the articular surface of a bone. **intracapsular f.,** one within the capsule of a joint. **intraperiosteal f.,** a fracture without rupture of the periosteum. **intrauterine f.,** fracture of a fetal bone occurring in utero; called also *congenital f.* **Jefferson f.,** fracture of the atlas (first cervical vertebra). **joint f.,** articular fracture. **Jones f.,** diaphyseal fracture of the fifth metatarsal. **lead pipe f.,** fracture in which the cortex of the bone is slightly compressed and bulged on one side with a slight crack on the opposite side of the bone. **Le Fort's f.,** bilateral horizontal fracture of the maxilla. Le Fort frac-

tures are classified as follows: *Le Fort I f.,* a horizontal segmented fracture of the alveolar process of the maxilla, in which the teeth are usually contained in the detached portion of the bone; called also *Guérin's f.* and *horizontal maxillary f. Le Fort II f.,* unilateral or bilateral fracture of the maxilla, in which the body of the maxilla is separated from the facial skeleton and the separated portion is pyramidal in shape; the fracture may extend through the body of the maxilla down the midline of the hard palate, through the floor of the orbit, and into the nasal cavity. Called also *pyramidal f. Le Fort III f.,* a fracture in which the entire maxilla and one or more facial bones are completely separated from the craniofacial skeleton; such fractures are almost always accompanied by multiple fractures of the facial bones. Called also *craniofacial disjunction* and *transverse facial f.* **linear f.,** a fracture extending lengthwise of the bone. **longitudinal f.,** a break in a bone extending in a longitudinal direction. **loose f.,** a fracture in which the bone is completely broken so that the broken ends have free play. **march f.,** fracture of a bone of the lower extremity, developing after repeated stresses, as seen in soldiers; called also *fatigue f.* Cf. *march foot.* **Montegia's f.,** fracture in the proximal half of the shaft of the ulna, with dislocation of the head of the radius. Sometimes called parry fracture because it is often caused by attempts to fend off blows with the forearm. **Moore's f.,** fracture of the lower end of the radius with dislocation of the head of the ulna and imprisonment of the styloid process beneath the annular ligaments. **multiple f.,** a variety in which there are two or more lines of fracture of the same bone not communicating with each other. **neoplastic f.,** fracture due to weakening of the bone as a result of a malignant process. **neurogenic f.,** fracture due to weakening of the bone as a result of tabes, paresis, etc. **oblique f.,** fracture in which the break extends in an oblique direction. **open f.,** one in which there is an external wound leading to the break of the bone; called also *compound f.* **paratrooper f.,** fracture of the posterior articular margin of the tibia and/or of the internal or external malleolus. **parry f.,** Montegia f. **pathologic f.,** one due to weakening of the bone structure by pathologic processes, such as neoplasia, osteomalacia, osteomyelitis, and other diseases. Called also *secondary f.* and *spontaneous f.* **perforating f.,** buttonhole f. **periarticular f.,** a fracture extending close to, but not into, a joint. **pertrochanteric f.,** fracture of the femur passing through the great trochanter. **pillion f.,** a fracture of the lower end of the femur occurring when the knee of a person riding pillion on a motorcycle is struck in a collision; it is a T-shaped fracture with displacement of the condyles behind the femoral shaft. **ping-pong f.,** an indented fracture of the skull, resembling the indentation that can be produced with the finger in a ping-pong ball; when elevated it resumes and retains its normal position. **pond f.,** fracture of the skull in which a fissure circumscribes the radiating lines, giving the depressed area a circular form. **Pott's f.,** fracture of the lower part of the fibula, with serious injury of the lower tibial articulation, usually a chipping off of a portion of the medial malleolus, or rupture of the medial ligament; called also *Dupuytren's f.* **pressure f.,** one caused by pressure on the bone from an adjoining tumor. **pyramidal f. (of maxilla),** Le Fort II f. **Quervain's f.,** fracture of the navicular bone together with a volar luxation of the os lunatum. **resecting f.,** a fracture in which a piece of the bone is removed by violence, as by a bullet. **secondary f.,** pathologic f. **segmental f.,** double f. **Shepherd's f.,** fracture of the astragalus, with detachment of the outer protecting edge. **silver-fork f.,** fracture of the lower ends of the radius (*Colles' f.*); so called because of the shape of the deformity that it causes. **simple f.,** closed f. **simple f., complex,** a closed fracture in which there is considerable injury to adjacent soft tissues. **Skillern's f.,** complete fracture of the lower third of the radius with greenstick fracture of the lower third of the ulna. **Smith's f.,** a fracture of the lower end of the radius near its articular surface with forward displacement of the lower fragment; sometimes called *reverse Colles' fracture.* **spiral f.,** one in which the bone has been twisted apart; called also *torsion f.* **splintered f.,** a comminuted fracture in which the bone is splintered into thin, sharp fragments. **spontaneous f.,** one occurring as a result of disease of a bone or from some undiscoverable cause, and not due to trauma; called also *pathologic f.* **sprain f.,** the separation of a tendon or ligament from its insertion, taking with it a piece of bone. **sprinter's f.,** fracture of the anterior superior or of the anterior inferior spine of the ilium, a fragment of the bone being pulled off by muscular violence, as at the start of a sprint. **stellate f.,** a fracture with a central point of injury, from which radiate numerous fissures. **Stieda's f.,** fracture of the internal condyle of the femur. **subcapital f.,** fracture of a bone just below its head; especially an intracapsular fracture of the neck of the femur at the junction of the head and neck. **subcutaneous f.,** closed f. **subperiosteal f.,** a crack through a bone without alteration in its alignment or contour, the supposition being that the periosteum is not broken. **supracondylar f.,** fracture of the humerus in which the line of fracture is through the lower end of the shaft of the humerus. **torsion f.,** spiral f. **torus f.,** a fracture in which there is a localized expansion or torus of the cortex, with little or no displacement of the lower end of the bone. **transcervical f.,** fracture through the neck of the femur. **transcondylar f.,** fracture of the humerus in which the line of fracture is at the level of the condyles, traverses the fossae, and is in part within the capsule of the joint; called also *diacondylar f.* **transverse f.,** a fracture at right angles to the axis of the bone. **transverse facial f.,** Le Fort III f. **transverse maxillary f.,** a term sometimes used for horizontal maxillary fracture (Le Fort I f.). **trimalleolar f.,** fracture of the medial and lateral malleoli and the posterior tip of the tibia. **trophic f.,** one due to a trophic (nutritional) disturbance. **tuft f.,** bursting f. **Wagstaffe's f.,** separation of the internal malleolus. **willow f.,** greenstick f.

fracture-dislocation (frak′chur dis″lo-ka′shun) a fracture of a bone near a joint, also involving dislocation.

Fraenkel (freng′kel) see *Fränkel.*

fragiform (fraj′ĭ-form) [L. *fraga* strawberry + *forma* shaped] shaped like a strawberry.

fragilitas (frah-jil′ĭ-tas) [L., from *frangere* to break] fragility. **f. crin′ium,** a brittle condition of the hair. **f. os′sium,** abnormal brittleness of the bones; see *osteogenesis imperfecta.* **f. un′guium** [L. "fragility of the nails"], abnormal brittleness of the nails.

fragility (frah-jil′ĭ-te) susceptibility, or lack of resistance, to factors capable of causing disruption of continuity or integrity. **f. of blood,** erythrocyte f. **capillary f.,** susceptibility, or lack of resistance, of capillaries to disruption under conditions of increased stress. **erythrocyte f.,** the susceptibility, or lack of resistance, of erythrocytes to hemolysis when exposed to increasingly hypotonic saline solutions (*osmotic f.*) or when subjected to mechanical trauma (*mechanical f.*). **hereditary f. of bone,** osteogenesis imperfecta. **mechanical f.,** see *erythrocyte f.* **osmotic f.,** see *erythrocyte f.*

fragilocyte (frah-jil′o-sīt) an erythrocyte which is less than normally resistant to hypotonic saline solution.

fragilocytosis (frah-jil″o-si-to′sis) the presence of fragilocytes in the blood.

fragment (frag′ment) one of the small pieces into which a larger entity has been broken. **Fab f.,** see *Fab.* **F (ab′)₂ f.,** see F (ab′)₂. **Fc f.,** see *Fc.* **restriction f.,** a DNA fragment produced by a restriction endonuclease. **Spengler's f's,** small round bodies seen in tuberculous sputum.

fragmentation (frag″men-ta′shun) 1. a division into fragments. 2. a form of reproduction seen in certain organisms, such as flatworms, in which the body of the parent may break into several pieces, each piece then regenerating the missing parts and developing into a whole animal. **f. of myocardium,** transverse rupture of the muscle fibers of the heart.

fragmentography, mass (frag″men-tog′rah-fe) combined gas chromatography and mass spectrometry in which quantitative analysis of the substance in question (e.g., a steroid) is based on a determination of the abundance of certain fragments characteristic of that substance.

fraise (frāz) [Fr. "strawberry"] a conical or hemispherical burr for cutting osteoplastic flaps or enlarging trephine openings.

frambesia (fram-be′ze-ah) [Fr. *framboise* raspberry] yaws. **f. trop′ica,** yaws.

frambesioma (fram-be″ze-o′mah) mother yaw; see under *yaw.*

framboesia (fram-be′ze-ah) yaws.

framboesioma (fram-be″ze-o′mah) mother yaw; see under *yaw.*

frame (frām) a structure, usually rigid, designed for giving support to or for immobilizing a part. **Balkan f.,** a rectangular frame attached to and overhanging a bed; particularly useful in allowing bedridden patients to move more effectively and for attachment of splints. Called also *Balkan splint.* **Bradford f.,** a rectangular frame of pipe to which is attached a sheet of heavy canvas; used as a bed frame for patients who must remain immobile. **Deiters' terminal f.,** plates in the lamina reticularis uniting Deiters' phalanges with the cells of Hensen. **Foster f.,** one similar to the Stryker frame. **occluding f.,** a dental articulator. **quadriplegic standing f.,** a device for supporting in the upright position a patient whose four limbs are paralyzed. **reading f.,** one of the three possible ways of reading a nucleotide sequence as a series of triplets. An open reading frame contains no termination codons and is thus potentially translatable into protein. **Stryker f.,** one consisting of canvas stretched on anterior and posterior frames, on which the patient can be rotated around his longitudinal axis. **trial f.,** a frame specially devised to permit easy insertion of different lenses used in correcting refractive errors of vision. **Whitman's f.,** a frame similar to the Bradford frame except that it is curved.

framework (frām′werk) 1. the basic structure about which something is formulated or built. 2. the metallic skeletal portion of a prosthesis to which are attached the resin flange and base components of the partial denture and the artificial teeth. **implant f.,** see under *substructure.* **scleral f.,** the larger and coarser part of the angle of the iris which is adjacent to the sclera. **uveal f.,** ligamentum pectinatum anguli iridocornealis.

Franceschetti's syndrome (frahn″cha-skāt′tēz) [Adolphe *Franceschetti,* Swiss ophthalmologist, born 1896] mandibulofacial dysostosis.

Franceschetti-Jadassohn syndrome (frahn″cha-skāt′te-yah′das-ōn) [Adolphe *Franceschetti;* Josef *Jadassohn,* German dermatologist, 1863–1936] see under *syndrome.*

Francis' disease (fran′siz) [Edward *Francis,* American physician, 1872–1957] tularemia.

Francisella (fran-sĭ-sel′ah) [Edward *Francis*] a genus of gram-negative, aerobic, coccoid or rod-shaped bacteria of uncertain affiliation, made up of very small, nonmotile organisms that are human pathogens, found in rabbits, voles, muskrats, beavers, squirrels, and sheep, and in waters frequented by these animals. **F. novi′cida,** the etiologic agent of a disease resembling tularemia in guinea pigs, hamsters, and white mice; not known to infect man. Formerly called *Pasteurella novicida.* **F. tularen′sis,** the etiologic agent of tularemia in man. It is transmitted from wild animals, usually rabbits, to man by contact with infected tissue, from the bites of blood-sucking insects, by inhalation, and by ingestion. It is also the cause of a severe form of conjunctivitis (oculoglandular tularemia). Called also *Brucella tularensis* and *Pasteurella tularensis.*

francium (fran′se-um) the chemical element of atomic number 87, atomic weight 223, symbol Fr, all isotopes of which are radioactive; formerly called *virginium.*

Franco's operation (frah′ko) [Pierre *Franco,* French surgeon, 1500–1561] suprapubic cystotomy.

frange (franzh) [Fr. "brush"] a fringe or band of cilia in the oral area of certain ciliate protozoa, made up of kinetofragments. Called also *hypostomial frange.* Cf. *pseudomembranelle.*

Franke's operation (frang′kez) [Felix *Franke,* German surgeon, born 1858] see under *operation.*

Fränkel's sign (freng′kelz) [Albert *Fränkel,* German physician, 1848–1916] see under *sign.*

Fränkel's speculum, test (freng′kelz) [Bernhard *Fränkel,* German laryngologist, 1836–1911] see under *speculum* and *tests.*

Fränkel's treatment (freng′kelz) [Albert *Fränkel,* Heidelberg physician, 1864–1938] see under *treatment.*

Frankenhäuser's ganglion (frang′ken-hoy″zerz) [Ferdinand *Frankenhäuser,* German gynecologist, 1832–1894] see under *ganglion.*

Frankia (frank′e-ah) [B. *Frank,* Swiss microbiologist] a genus of bacteria of the family Frankiaceae, consisting of actinomycete organisms that occur free in the soil or in symbiotic nodules on nitrogen-fixing plants. The type species is *F. al'ni.*

Frankiaceae (frank"e-a'se-e) a family of bacteria of the order Actinomycetales, consisting of gram-positive aerobic organisms that produce a true mycelium. They occur as soil saprophytes and symbionts in nitrogen-fixing plant nodules. The single genus is *Frankia.*

Frankl-Hochwart's disease (frank'l-hoch'warts) [Lothar von *Frankl-Hochwart,* Vienna neurologist, 1862–1914] polyneuritis cerebralis menieriformis.

Franklin glasses (frangk'lin) [Benjamin *Franklin,* American patriot, 1706–1790] bifocal glasses.

franklinism (frangk'lin-izm) [Benjamin *Franklin*] 1. static or frictional electricity. 2. franklinization.

franklinization (frangk"lin-i-za'shun) the therapeutic use of static electricity.

Frasera (fra'zer-ah) [after John *Fraser,* 1750–1817] a genus of gentianaceous plants.

Frateuria (frah-ter'e-a) [Joseph *Frateur,* Belgian microbiologist, 1903–1974] a genus of gram-negative, aerobic, rod-shaped bacteria of the family Pseudomonadaceae, consisting of organisms that are nonmotile or motile by polar flagella, and are found in plants. The type species is *F. auran'tia.*

Fraunhofer's lines (frown'hof-erz) [Joseph von *Fraunhofer,* German optician, 1787–1826] see under *line.*

Frazier-Spiller operation (fra'zher-spil'er) [Charles Harrison *Frazier,* American surgeon, 1870–1936; William Gibson *Spiller,* American neurologist, 1863–1940] see under *operation.*

FRC functional residual capacity.

F.R.C.P. Fellow of the Royal College of Physicians.

F.R.C.P.(C.) Fellow of the Royal College of Physicians of Canada.

F.R.C.P.E. Fellow of the Royal College of Physicians of Edinburgh.

F.R.C.P.(Glasg.) Fellow of the Royal College of Physicians and Surgeons of Glasgow *qua* Physician.

F.R.C.P.I. Fellow of the Royal College of Physicians in Ireland.

F.R.C.S. Fellow of the Royal College of Surgeons.

F.R.C.S.(C.) Fellow of the Royal College of Surgeons of Canada.

F.R.C.S.E. Fellow of the Royal College of Surgeons of Edinburgh.

F.R.C.S.(Glasg.) Fellow of the Royal College of Physicians and Surgeons of Glasgow *qua* Surgeon.

F.R.C.S.I. Fellow of the Royal College of Surgeons in Ireland.

F.R.C.V.S. Fellow of the Royal College of Veterinary Surgeons.

FreAmine II (fre-am'ēn) trademark for a crystalline amino acid solution for intravenous administration, containing a mixture of essential and nonessential amino acids but no peptides.

freckle (frek'l) a benign, small, tan to brown macule occurring on sun-exposed skin, especially in children and tending to fade in adult life. Freckles resemble lentigines, but they darken after exposure to sunlight, whereas lentigines do not; and in freckles, the number of melanocytes is not increased. Called also *ephelis.* **melanotic f. of Hutchinson,** see *lentigo maligna melanoma,* under *melanoma.*

Fredet-Ramstedt operation (frĕ-da' rahm'stet) [Pierre *Fredet,* French surgeon, 1870–1946; Conrad *Ramstedt,* German surgeon, born 1867] see under *operation.*

freemartin (fre'mar-tin) a sexually maldeveloped female calf born as a twin to a normal male calf; it is commonly sterile and intersexual as the result of male hormone reaching it through anastomosed placental vessels.

freeze-cleaving (frēz-clēv'ing) freeze-etching.

freeze-drying (frēz-dri'ing) a method of tissue preparation in which the tissue specimen is frozen and then dehydrated at low temperature in a high vacuum.

freeze-etching (frēz-ech'ing) a method used to study unfixed cells by electron microscopy, in which the object to be

studied is placed in 20 per cent glycerol, frozen at –100° C., and then mounted on a chilled holder.

freeze-fracturing (frēz-frak'chur-ing) a method of preparing cells for electron-microscopical examination: a tissue specimen is frozen at –150 °C., inserted into a vacuum chamber, and fractured by a microtome; a platinum carbon replica of the exposed surfaces is made, freed of the underlying specimen, and then examined.

freeze-substitution (frēz-sub-stĭ-tu'shun) a modification of freeze-drying in which the ice within the frozen tissue is replaced by alcohol or other solvents at a very low temperature.

Frei's antigen, disease, test (frīz) [Wilhelm Siegmund *Frei,* German dermatologist, 1885–1943] see *lymphogranuloma venereum,* and see under *antigen* and *tests.*

Freiberg's infraction (fri'bergz) [Albert Henry *Freiberg,* American surgeon, 1868–1940] see under *infraction.*

fremitus (frem'ĭ-tus) [L.] a vibration perceptible on palpation. **bronchial f.,** rhonchal f. **friction f.,** the vibration caused by the rubbing together of two dry body surfaces; called also *friction rub.* **hydatid f.,** see under *thrill.* **pectoral f.,** vocal f. **pericardial f.,** a thrill of the chest wall due to the friction of the surfaces of the pericardium over each other. **pleural f.,** a palpable vibration of the wall of the thorax due to friction of the opposing surfaces of the pleura over each other. **rhonchal f.,** palpable vibrations produced by the passage of air through a large bronchial tube filled with mucus; called also *bronchial f.* **subjective f.,** a thrill felt by the patient on humming with his mouth closed. **tactile f.,** a thrill, as in the chest wall, which may be felt by a hand applied to the thorax while the patient is speaking. **tussive f.,** a thrill felt on the chest when the patient coughs. **vocal f.,** a thrill caused by speaking, perceived by the ear of the auscultator applied to the chest; called also *pectoral f.*

frena (fre'nah) [L.] plural of *frenum.*

frenal (fre'nal) pertaining to a frenum.

French (french') see *French scale,* under *scale.*

frenectomy (fre-nek'to-me) [*frenum* + Gr. *ektomē* excision] excision of the frenum (frenulum).

Frenkel's movements (treatment) (freng-kelz') [Heinrich S. *Frenkel,* Berlin neurologist, 1860–1931] see under *movement.*

frenoplasty (fre"no-plas'te) the correction of an abnormally attached frenum by surgically repositioning it.

frenotomy (fre-not'o-me) [L. *frenum* + Gr. *tomē* a cutting] cutting the frenum (frenulum), especially for release of ankyloglossia (tongue-tie). **lingual f.,** incision of the lingual frenum; ankylotomy.

frenula (fren'u-lah) [L.] plural of *frenulum.*

frenulum (fren'u-lum), pl. *fren'ula* [L., dim. of *frenum*] a small bridle; [NA] a general term for a small fold of integument or mucous membrane that checks, curbs, or limits the movements of an organ or part; see also *frenum.* **f. clito'ridis** [NA], the tissue fold on the under surface of the clitoris formed by union of the two medial parts of the labia minora; called also *crus glandis clitoridis.* **f. of ileocecal valve,** f. valvae ileocaecalis. **f. of inferior lip, f. la'bii inferio'ris** [NA], the fold of mucous membrane on the inside of the middle of the lower lip, connecting the lip with the gums. **f. la'bii superio'ris** [NA], frenulum of superior lip; the fold of mucous membrane on the inside of the middle of the upper lip, connecting the lip with the gums. **f. labio'rum puden'di** [NA], frenulum of pudendal labia: the posterior union of the labia minora, anterior to the posterior commissure; called also *f. pudendi, fourchette,* and *frenum of labia.* **f. lin'guae** [NA], frenulum of tongue: the vertical fold of mucous membrane under the tongue, attaching it to the floor of the mouth; called also frenum of tongue. **f. lin'guae cerebel'li,** vincula lingulae cerebelli. **f. of prepuce of penis, f. prepu'tii pe'nis** [NA], the fold on the lower surface of the glans penis that connects it with the prepuce. **f. of pudendal labia, f. puden'di,** f. labiorum pudendi. **f. of rostral medullary velum,** f. veli medullaris rostralis. **f. of superior lip,** f. labii superioris. **f. of superior medullary velum,** f. veli medullaris rostralis. **f. of tongue,** f. linguae. **f. val'vae ilea'lis,** frenulum of ileal valve: a narrow ridge formed by the coalescence of the flaps of the ileocecal valve at the ends of the ileocecal orifice; called also *f. valvae ileocecalis* and *frenum of Morgagni.* **f. val'vae**

ileocaeca′lis [NA], frenulum of iliocecal valve: a fold formed by the joined extremities of the ileocecal valve, extending partly around the lumen of the colon; called also *frenum of Morgagni*. **f. ve′li medulla′ris crania′lis,** f. veli medullaris rostralis. **f. ve′li medulla′ris rostra′lis** [NA], frenulum of rostral medullary velum: a median ridge that descends upon the rostral medullary velum from between the caudal colliculi; called also *f. of cranial medullary velum, f. of superior medullary velum, f. veli medullaris cranialis,* and *f. veli medullaris superius* [NA alternative]. **f. ve′li medulla′ris supe′rius,** NA alternative for *f. veli medullaris rostralis.*

frenum (fre′num), pl. *fre′na* [L. "bridle "] a restraining structure or part; see *frenulum*. **f. of labia,** frenulum labiorum pudendi. **lingual f.,** frenulum linguae. **Macdowel's f.,** a group of fibers attached to the tendon of the pectoralis muscle and strengthening the intermuscular septum. **f. of Morgagni,** frenulum valvae ileocaecalis. **f. of tongue,** frenulum linguae.

frenzy (fren′ze) [Gr. *phrenitizein* to be delirious or frantic] (*obs.*) extreme agitation or excitement; mania.

frequency (fre′kwen-se) 1. the number of occurrences of a periodic or recurrent process per unit time, e.g., the number of vibrations of a particle per second or the number of repetitions of a complete wave form (cycles) per second. 2. the number of occurrences of a particular event or the number of members of a population or statistical sample falling in a particular class. 3. relative frequency; the average number of occurrences of a particular event in a large number of repeated trials. **audio f.,** any frequency corresponding to a normally audible sound wave. **fusion f.,** see under *flicker*. **gene f.,** the proportion of loci at which a given allele is found in a given population. **high f.,** the rate of oscillation in an alternating current exceeding the rate at which muscular contraction ceases—approximately 10,000 per second. **infrasonic f.,** any frequency below the audio frequency range. **low f.,** an alternating current where frequency in cycles per second is low in reference to a certain standard, such as the pitch frequency of middle C. **recombination f.,** the frequency with which new combinations of linked genes are formed because of crossing over occurring between their loci, i.e., the number of recombinants divided by the total number of progeny. Because an even number of crossovers does not result in recognizable recombination, the recombination frequency underestimates the crossover frequency unless the loci are very closely linked. **subsonic f.,** infrasonic f. **supersonic f.,** ultrasonic f. **ultrasonic f.,** any frequency above the audio frequency range; see *ultrasonics*. **urinary f.,** urination at short intervals without increase in daily volume of urinary output, due to reduced bladder capacity.

Frerichs' theory (fra′riks) [Friedrich Theodor *Frerichs*, Berlin physician, 1819–1885] see under *theory*.

fressreflex (fres′re-fleks) [Ger. "eating reflex"] rhythmic sucking, chewing, and swallowing movements elicited by stroking of the lips and cheeks.

freta (fre′tah) [L.] plural of *fretum*.

fretum (fre′tum), pl. *fre′ta* [L.] a constriction, or strait. **f. hal′leri,** a constriction between the atria and ventricles of the fetal heart; called also *Haller's isthmus*.

Freud (froid) Sigmund. Austrian psychiatrist, 1856–1939; the founder of psychoanalysis. He developed such fundamental concepts as the unconscious, infantile sexuality, repression, sublimation, and superego, ego, and id formation and their applications to all human behavior.

freudian (froid′e-an) 1. pertaining to Sigmund Freud or his psychological theories and method of psychotherapy (psychoanalytic theory and technique). 2. an adherent or user of freudian theory or methods.

Freund adjuvant (froind) [Jules Thomas *Freund*, Hungarian-born bacteriologist in the United States, 1891–1960] see under *adjuvant*.

Freund's anomaly, operation (froindz) [Wilhelm Alexander *Freund*, German surgeon, 1833–1918] see under *anomaly* and *operation*.

Frey's hairs (frīz) [Max von *Frey*, German physiologist, 1852–1932] see under *hair*.

Frey's syndrome (frīz) [Lucie *Frey*, Polish physician, 1852–1932] auriculotemporal syndrome; see under *syndrome*.

Freyer's operation (fri′erz) [Sir Peter Johnston *Freyer*, British surgeon, 1857–1921] see under *operation*.

FRF follicle-stimulating hormone releasing factor; see gonadotropin releasing hormone, under *hormone*.

F.R.F.P.S.G. Fellow of the Royal Faculty of Physicians and Surgeons of Glasgow.

friable (fri′ah-b'l) [L. *friabilis*] easily pulverized or crumbled.

fricative (frik′ah-tiv) a speech sound produced by forcing an air stream through a narrow opening and resulting in audible high-frequency vibrations, such as *f* or *s*.

Fricke's bandage (frik′ez) [Johann Karl Georg *Fricke*, German surgeon, 1790–1841] see under *bandage*.

friction (frik′shun) [L. *frictio*] the act of rubbing; attrition.

Friderichsen-Waterhouse syndrome (frid″er-ik′sen-wah″ter-hows) [Carl *Friderichsen*, Danish physician, born 1886; Rupert *Waterhouse*, British physician, 1873–1958] Waterhouse-Friderichsen syndrome.

Fridericia's method (frid″er-ĭ-che-ahz) [Louis Sigurd *Fridericia*, Danish hygienist, born 1881] see under *method*.

Friedländer's bacillus, disease, pneumobacillus, pneumonia (frēd′len-derz) [Karl *Friedländer*, German pathologist, 1847–1887] see *Klebsiella pneumoniae* (for bacillus and pneumobacillus); see *endarteritis obliterans* (for disease); and see under *pneumonia*.

Friedman's test (frēd′manz) [Maurice Harold *Friedman*, American physician, born 1903] see under *test*.

Friedmann's vasomotor syndrome (complex) (frēd′manz) [Max *Friedmann*, German neurologist, 1858–1925] see under *syndrome*.

Friedreich's ataxia (tabes), disease, foot, sign (frēd′rīks) [Nikolaus *Friedreich*, Heidelberg physician, 1825–1882] see under *ataxia, foot,* and *sign,* and see *paramyoclonus multiplex*.

frigidity (frĭ-jid′ĭ-te) coldness; especially, lack of sexual response in the female.

frigolabile (frig″o-la′bĭl) [L. *frigor* cold + *labilis* unstable] easily affected or destroyed by cold.

frigorific (frig″o-rif′ik) [L. *frigorificus*] producing coldness.

frigostabile (frig″o-sta′bĭl) frigostable.

frigostable (frig″o-sta′bl) [L. *frigor* cold + *stabilis* firm] resistant to cold or low temperature.

frigotherapy (frig′o-ther′ah-pe) cryotherapy.

Frisch (frish) Karl Ritter von. Austrian zoologist, born 1886; co-winner, with Konrad Loren and Nikolaas Tinbergen, of the Nobel prize for medicine or physiology in 1973 for his work on the behavior of bees.

frit (frit) a fused mass produced by firing a mixture of quartz, kaolin, pigments, opacifiers, a suitable flux, and other substances, which is ground to form a fine powder for use in fabricating dental porcelain restorations and artificial teeth.

Fritsch's catheter (frich′es) [Heinrich *Fritsch*, German gynecologist, 1844–1914] Bozeman's catheter; see under *catheter*.

froe- for words beginning thus, see those beginning *fre-*.

frog (frog) 1. a tailless, leaping amphibian with a smooth skin and fully webbed feet, commonly used as a laboratory animal. 2. the band of horny substance in the middle of the sole of a horse's foot, dividing into two branches and running toward the heel in the form of a fork.

frog stay (frog sta) see *spine* (def. 3).

Fröhlich's syndrome (fra′liks) [Alfred *Fröhlich*, Vienna neurologist, 1871–1953] adiposogenital dystrophy.

Frohn's test (reagent) (frohnz) [Damianus *Frohn*, German physician, born 1843] see under *tests*.

Froin's syndrome (frow-anz′) [Georges *Froin*, French physician, born 1874] see under *syndrome*.

frolement (frōl-maw′) [Fr.] 1. a rustling sound often heard in auscultation in disease of the pericardium. 2. a massage movement consisting of light brushing with the palm of the hand.

Froment's paper sign (fro-mahz′) [Jules *Froment*, French physician, 1878–1946] see under *sign*.

Frommann's lines (from′anz) [Carl *Frommann*, anatomist in Heidelberg, 1831–1892] see under *line*.

Frommel's disease (from'elz) [Richard Julius Ernst *Frommel*, German gynecologist, 1854–1912] see *Chiari-Frommel syndrome*, under *syndrome*.

Frommel-Chiari syndrome (from'el-ke-ar'e) [Richard Julius Ernst *Frommel*; Johann Baptist *Chiari*, German obstetrician 1817–1854] Chiari-Frommel syndrome.

frondose (fron'dōs) [L. *frondosus* leafy] bearing fronds, or villi, as the chorion frondosum.

frons (fronz) [L. "the front, forepart"] [NA] the forehead; the region of the face above the eyes.

frontad (frun'tad) toward a frontal aspect.

frontal (frun'tal) [L. *frontalis*] 1. pertaining to the forehead. 2. denoting a longitudinal plane of the body at right angles to the sagittal plane; see under *plane*.

frontalis (frun-ta'lis) [L.] frontal; in official anatomical nomenclature, the term designates a relationship to the frontal or coronal plane.

frontipetal (frun-tip'ĕ-tal) [L. *frontalis* in front + *petere* to seek] directed to the front; moving in a frontal direction.

frontomalar (frun″to-ma'lar) pertaining to the frontal and malar bones.

frontomaxillary (frun″to-mak'sĭ-lār″e) pertaining to the frontal bone and the upper jaw.

frontonasal (frun″to-na'zal) pertaining to the frontal sinus and the nose.

fronto-occipital (frun″to-ok-sip'ĭ-tal) pertaining to the forehead and the occiput.

frontoparietal (frun″to-pah-ri'e-tal) pertaining to the frontal and parietal bones.

frontotemporal (frun″to-tem'po-ral) pertaining to the frontal and temporal bones.

Froriep's ganglion (fro'rēps) [August von *Froriep*, German anatomist, 1849–1917] see under *ganglion*.

Froriep's induration (fro'rēps) [Robert *Froriep*, Berlin surgeon, 1804–1861] myositis fibrosa.

frost (frost) a deposit resembling that of frozen dew or vapor. **urea f.,** urhidrosis crystallina.

frostbite (frost'bīt) damage to tissues as the result of exposure to low environmental temperatures; called also *congelation*. **deep f.,** damage resulting from exposure to extremely low temperatures, involving not only the skin and subcutaneous tissue but also deeper tissues, sometimes leading to gangrene and loss of affected parts; it is marked by persistent ischemia, secondary thrombosis, and livid cyanosis. **superficial f.,** damage resulting from exposure to low temperatures, involving only the skin or extending to the tissue immediately beneath it; it may be manifested as simple erythema, transient anesthesia, and superficial bullae.

frottage (frŏ-tahzh') [Fr. "rubbing"] 1. a rubbing movement in massage; effleurage. 2. a paraphilia in which sexual arousal or orgasm is achieved by rubbing up against another person, who is unaware of the activity, as when pressed close to others in a crowd, usually without specific genital contact. Called also *frotteurism*.

frotteur (frŏ-tur') an individual who achieves sexual gratification by practicing frottage.

F.R.S. Fellow of the Royal Society.

fructification (fruk″tĭ-fĭ-ka'shun) 1. the production of fruit. 2. a fruiting body. 3. a spore-bearing structure.

fructivorous (fruk-tiv'o-rus) subsisting on or eating fruits.

fructofuranose (fruk″to-fu'rah-nōs) the combining form and the more reactive form of fructose.

$$CH_2OH \cdot CH \cdot (CHOH)_2 \cdot CHO \cdot CH_2OH$$
$$\underline{\hspace{1.2cm} O \hspace{1.2cm}}$$

fructokinase (frook″to-ki'nās) 1. [EC 2.7.1.3] an enzyme of the transferase class that catalyzes the reaction ATP + D-fructose = ADP + D-fructose-1-phosphate. The enzyme is present in the liver, intestine, and kidney cortex. A deficiency of the enzyme, inherited as an autosomal recessive trait, is the cause of essential fructosuria.

fructopyranose (fruk″to-pi'rah-nōs) fructose.

fructosamine (fruk″to-sa'min) an amino sugar formed by the reduction of the osazone of glucosamine.

fructosan (fruk'to-san) a hexosan, $C_6H_{10}O_5$, an anhydride of fructose; called also *levulan*.

fructosazone (fruk″to-sa'zōn) a phenyl-osazone of fructose identical with glucosazone; called also *levulosazone*.

fructose (fruk'tōs) [L. *fructus* fruit] chemical name: D-fructose. A ketohexose, $C_6H_{12}O_6$, occurring in honey and many sweet fruits and a component of many di- and polysaccharides; it is obtainable by inversion of aqueous solutions of sucrose and subsequent separation of fructose from glucose. The official preparation [USP], occurring as colorless crystals or as a white, crystalline powder, is administered intravenously as a fluid and nutrient replenisher. Called also *fructopyranose, fruit sugar,* and *levulose.* **f. 1,6-bisphosphate, f. 1,6-diphosphate,** an intermediate in the Embden-Meyerhof pathway (q.v.) of glucose metabolism. **f. 6-phosphate,** an intermediate in the Embden-Meyerhof pathway (q.v.) of glucose metabolism.

fructose-1,6-bisphosphatase (frook'tōs bis-fos'fah-tās″) [EC 3.1.3.11] an enzyme of the hydrolase class that catalyzes the reaction D-fructose-1,6-bisphosphate + H_2O = D-fructose-6-phosphate + orthophosphate. The reaction is part of the route of gluconeogenesis in the liver and kidneys. Deficiency of the enzyme, an autosomal recessive trait, results in infant hypoglycemia. Formerly called *fructose-1,6-diphosphatase.*

fructose-2,6-bisphosphatase (frook'tōs bis-fos'fah-tās) [EC 3.1.3.46] An enzyme of the hydrolase class that catalyzes the reaction: fructose 2,6-bisphosphate + H_2O = fructose 6-phosphate + orthophosphate. The enzyme occurs in liver as part of a mechanism for regulating carbohydrate metabolism; it is phosphorylated by the CAMP-dependent protein kinase. Phosphorylation activates the enzyme, thus increasing the removal of fructose 2,6-bisphosphate when glucagon or catecholamines are secreted.

fructose 1,6-bisphosphate (frook'tōs bis-fos'fāt) a key intermediate in the Embden-Meyerhof pathway and in gluconeogenesis.

fructose 2,6-bisphosphate (frook'tōs bis-fos'fāt) an effector synthesized in small amounts in the liver to activate phosphofructokinase and inhibit fructose 1,6 bisphosphatase. Its formation is inhibited by catecholamines or glucagon, which thereby promote gluconeogenesis and diminish conversion of glucose to fatty acids.

fructose bisphosphate aldolase (frook'tōs bis-fos'fāt al'do-lās) [EC 4.1.2.13] an enzyme of the lyase class that catalyzes the reaction D-fructose-1,6-bisphosphate = glycerone phosphate (dihydroxyacetone phosphate) + D-glyceraldehyde-3-phosphate, a reaction that is part of the Embden-Meyerhof pathway. The enzyme also catalyzes the conversion of fructose-1-phosphate to glycerone phosphate (dihydroxyacetone phosphate) and D-glyceraldehyde. Three isozymes are recognized: A (occurring primarily in skeletal muscle), B (in liver, kidney, small intestine, and leukocytes), and C (brain). Isozyme B, often referred to as fructose-1-phosphate aldolase, has greater affinity for fructose-1-phosphate. Deficiency of this latter activity, an autosomal recessive trait, results in hereditary fructose intolerance. Called also *aldolase* and *fructose-1-phosphate aldolase.*

fructose-1,6-diphosphatase (frook'tos di-fos'fah-tās″) fructose bisphosphatase.

fructose-1,6-diphosphatase (FDP) deficiency, hereditary, an autosomal recessive disorder marked by apnea, hyperventilation, hypoglycemia, ketosis, and lactic acidosis resulting from impaired gluconeogenesis due to deficient hepatic fructose-1,6-diphosphatase; it may be fatal to newborns, but patients past early childhood develop normally.

fructose-6-phosphate (frook'tōs fos'fāt) an intermediate in carbohydrate metabolism,

$$CH_2OH \cdot CHO \cdot (CHOH)_2 CH \cdot CH_2O \cdot PO(OH)_2$$
$$\underline{\hspace{1.2cm} O \hspace{1.2cm}}$$

See also *Embden-Meyerhof pathway,* under *pathway.* Called also *Neuberg ester.*

fructose-1-phosphate aldolase (frook'tōs fos'fāt al'do-lās) fructose bisphosphate aldolase isozyme B.

fructosemia (fruk″to-se'me-ah) the presence of fructose in the blood; seen in fructose intolerance. Called also *levulosemia.*

fructosidase (fruk-to-si'dās) β-fructofuranosidase.

fructoside (fruk-to'sīd) a compound that bears the same relation to fructose as a glucoside does to glucose.

fructosuria (fruk″to-su′re-ah) [*fructose* + Gr. *ouron* urine + *-ia*] the presence of fructose in the urine; seen in fructose intolerance. Called also *levulosuria*. **essential f.,** a benign, asymptomatic hereditary disorder of carbohydrate metabolism, transmitted as an autosomal recessive trait, caused by a defect in the hepatic enzyme fructokinase, and in which the only manifestations are fructosemia and fructosuria. See also *hereditary fructose intolerance,* under *intolerance.*

fructosyl (fruk′to-sil) a radical of fructose.

fructosyltransferase (frook″to-sil-trans′fer-ās) [EC 2.4.1] any of several enzymes of the transferase class that catalyze the transfer of a fructose group from a donor to an acceptor compound.

fructovegetative (fruk″to-vej′ĕ-ta″tiv) composed of or pertaining to fruits and vegetables.

frugivorous (froo-jiv′o-rus) [L. *frux* fruit + *vorare* to eat] fructivorous; eating or subsisting on fruit.

fruit (froot) [L. *fructus*] the developed ovary of a plant, including the seed and its envelopes.

fruitarian (froo-ta′re-an) a person whose diet consists chiefly of fruits.

fruitarianism (froo-ta′re-an-izm) the use of an exclusively fruit diet.

frusemide (frus′ĕ-mīd) BAN for furosemide.

Frust. abbreviation for L. *frustilla′tim,* in small pieces.

frustration (frus-tra′shun) 1. the blocking or thwarting of purposes, desires, actions, or impulses. 2. a feeling of tension arising when such thwarting occurs.

F.s.a. abbreviation for L. *fi′at secun′dum ar′tem,* let it be made skillfully.

FSH follicle-stimulating hormone.

FSH/LH-RH follicle-stimulating hormone and luteinizing hormone releasing hormone; see *gonadotropin releasing hormone,* under *hormone.*

FSH-RF follicle-stimulating hormone releasing factor; see *gonadotropin releasing hormone,* under *hormone.*

FSH-RH follicle stimulating hormone releasing hormone; see *gonadotropin releasing hormone,* under *hormone.*

ft. abbreviation for L. *fi′at* or *fi′ant,* let there be made, and for *foot* and *feet.*

Ft. mas. div. in pil. abbreviation for L. *fi′at mas′sa dividen′da in pil′ulae,* let a mass be made and divided into pills.

Ftorafur (ftor′ah-fur) trademark for preparations of tegafur.

Ft. pulv. abbreviation for L. *fi′at pul′vis,* let a powder be made.

5-FU fluorouracil.

Fuadin (fu′ah-din) trademark for a preparation of stibophen.

Fuchs' coloboma, etc. (fooks) [Ernst *Fuchs,* German ophthalmologist, 1851–1930] see under *coloboma, dimple, dystrophy,* and *syndrome.*

fuchsin (fook′sin) [from the pink, red, or purple flower *fuchsia,* after Leonard *Fuchs,* German botanist, 1501–1566] any of several red to purple triaminotriphenylmethane dyes. **acid f.,** a mixture of sulfonated fuchsins used in Andrade's indicator and in various complex stains; called also *acid magenta.* **basic f.** [USP], a triphenylmethane dye, a mixture of rosanilin and pararosanilin hydrochlorides and magenta II, used in the form of carbolfuchsin in the Gram and Ziehl-Neelsen stains, as an antifungal agent in Castellani's paint, as a germicide, and as a histologic stain. Called also *basic magenta.* **new f.,** a basic dye with staining properties much like those of basic fuchsin; it is triaminotritolylmethane chloride, or trimethyl fuchsin, [CH₃(NH₂)·C₆H₃]₂C·C₆H₃(CH₃)·NH₄Cl.

fuchsinophil (fook-sin′o-fil) [*fuchsin* + Gr. *philein* to love] 1. any cell or other element readily stained with fuchsin. 2. fuchsinophilic.

fuchsinophilia (fook″sin-o-fil′e-ah) the property of staining readily with fuchsin dyes; especially the affinity of infarcted areas of the heart for acid fuchsin, which is an aid in determining diagnosis in cases of unexplained death.

fuchsinophilic (fook″sin-o-fil′ik) readily stained by fuchsin; pertaining to or characterized by fuchsinophilia.

fuchsinophilous (fook″sin-of′ĭ-lus) fuchsinophilic.

fucosan (fu′ko-san) a methylpentosan that is a constituent of the cell wall of many seaweeds, and is derived from L-fucose, or 6-deoxygalactose.

fucose (fu′kōs) an unusual monosaccharide occurring as L-fucose (6-deoxy-L-galactose) in a number of mucopolysaccharides and mucoproteins, including the blood group polysaccharides.

α-L-fucosidase (fu-ko′sĭ-dās″, fu′ko-sīd-ās″) [EC 3.2.1.51] an enzyme of the hydrolase class that catalyzes the reaction α-L-fucoside + H₂O = alcohol + L-fucose. The enzyme is important in the metabolism of mucopolysaccharide lipids. Genetic deficiency of the enzyme, transmitted as an autosomal recessive trait, results in fucosidosis.

fucoside (fu′ko-sīd) an acetal derivative of fucose.

fucosidosis (fu″ko-si-do′sis) a lysosomal storage disease caused by defective α-L-fucosidase and accumulation of fucose. Clinical symptoms include psychomotor deterioration, growth retardation, hepatosplenomegaly, cardiomegaly, and seizures. There are two clinical types based on age of onset: *Type I,* the fatal infantile type, has age of onset by 18 months and causes death before six years of age. Marked increase of sodium chloride in sweat is an additional feature. *Type II,* the juvenile form, has age of onset by four years of age and slower psychomotor and neurologic deterioration; patients survive to their twenties.

fucoxanthin (fu″ko-zan′thin) [L. *fucus* rock lichen + Gr. *xanthos* yellow] the brown carotenoid found in diatoms, brown algae, and dinoflagellates.

FUDR, FUdR 5-fluorouracil deoxyribonucleoside; see *floxuridine.*

Fuerbringer (fer′bring-er) see *Fürbringer.*

fugacity (fu-gas′ĭ-te) [L. *fugacitas,* from *fugere* to flee] a measure of the escaping tendency of a substance from one phase to another phase, or from one part of a phase to another part of the same phase. The logarithm of the fugacity is proportional to the chemical potential.

-fugal (fu′gal) 1. [L., *fugare* to put to flight] a word termination implying banishing, or driving away, affixed to a stem designating the object of banishment, as *culicifugal,* driving away mosquitoes and gnats (*Culex*), or *febrifugal,* relieving or dispelling fever. 2. [L., *fugere* to flee from] a word termination implying traveling away from, affixed to a stem designating the object from which flight is made, as *centrifugal* traveling away from a center, or *corticifugal,* directed away from the cortex.

-fuge [L. *fugare* to put to flight] a word termination denoting an agent that drives away or banishes, as *febrifuge,* that which drives away fever.

fugitive (fu′jĭ-tiv) [L. *fugitivus*] 1. wandering. 2. transient.

Fugu (fu′gu) [Jap.] a genus of Japanese puffer fish that contain a potent neurotoxin (tetrodotoxin) concentrated in the gonads and viscera, which when eaten without special cooking preparation causes generalized paralysis and in severe cases unconsciousness and death.

fugue (fūg) [L. *fuga* a flight] a pathological state of altered consciousness in which an individual may act and wander around as though conscious but his behavior is not directed by his complete normal personality and is not remembered after the fugue ends. **epileptic f.,** a fuguelike state of running or wandering that occasionally occurs as an ictal or postictal phenomenon in psychomotor (temporal lobe) epilepsy.

fuguism (foo′goo-izm) [Jap. *fugu* the tetraodon fish + *-ism*] tetrodotoxism.

fuguismus (foo″goo-iz′mus) [see *fuguism*] tetrodotoxism.

fugutoxin (foo-goo-tok′sin) tetrodotoxin.

Fukala's operation (foo-kah′lahz) [Vincenz *Fukala,* Vienna ophthalmologist, 1847–1911] see under *operation.*

fulgurant (ful′gu-rant) [L. *fulgurans,* from *fulgur* lightning] coming and going like a flash of lightning.

fulgurate (ful′gu-rāt) 1. to come and go like a flash of lightning. 2. to destroy by contact with electric sparks generated by a high frequency current; see *fulguration.*

fulguration (ful″gu-ra′shun) [L. *fulgur* lightning] destruction of living tissue by electric sparks generated by a high frequency current. This may be direct or indirect. *Direct:* An insulated fulguration electrode with a metal point is connected to the uniterminal of the high frequency apparatus and a spark of electricity is allowed to impinge on the area to be treated. *Indirect:* In this procedure the patient is connected directly by a metal handle to the uniterminal and the operator utilizes an active electrode to complete an arc from the patient.

fuliginous (fu-lij′ĭ-nus) [L. *fuligo* soot]   sooty in color or appearance.

Fülleborn's method (fēl′ĕ-bornz) [Friedrich *Fülleborn*, German parasitologist, 1866–1933]   see under *method*.

Fuller's operation [Eugene *Fuller*, New York urologist, 1858–1930]   see under *operation*.

füllkörper (fēl′ker-per) [Ger., pl., "fill-bodies"]   glia cells which have become degenerated; called also *filling cells*.

fulminant (ful′mĭ-nant) [L. *fulminare* to flare up]   sudden, severe; occurring suddenly and with great intensity.

fulminate (ful′mĭ-nāt)   to occur suddenly with great intensity.

Fulvicin (ful′vĭ-sin)   trademark for a preparation of griseofulvin.

fumagillin (fu″mah-jil′in)   chemical name: 2,4,6,8-decatetraenedioic acid mono[5-methoxy-4-[2-methyl-3-(3-methyl-2-butenyl)oxiranyl]-1-oxaspiro[2.5]oct-6-yl]ester. An antibiotic, $C_{26}H_{34}O_7$, produced by *Aspergillus fumigatus*.

fumarase (fu′mah-rās)   fumarate hydratase.

fumarate (fu′mar-āt)   a salt or anionic form of fumaric acid.

fumarate hydratase (fu′mah-rāt hi′drah-tās) [EC 4.2.1.2]   an enzyme of the lyase class that catalyzes the reaction (S)-malate = fumarate + H_2O. The reaction is a part of the citric (tricarboxylic) acid cycle of carbohydrate oxidation. Called also *fumarase*.

fumaric acid (fu-mar′ik)   *trans*-butanedioic acid, the trans isomer of maleic acid, an intermediate in the tricarboxylic acid cycle (q.v.).

fumaroylacetoacetate hydrolase (fu-mar″o-il-ah-se″to-as′ĕ-tat hi′dro-lās)   fumarylacetoacetase.

fumarylacetoacetase (fu″mar-il-ah-se″to-as′ĕ-tās) [EC 3.7.1.2]   an enzyme of the hydrolase class that catalyzes the reaction 4-fumarylacetoacetate + H_2O = acetoacetate + fumarate. The reaction is part of the tyrosine catabolic pathway. Deficiency of the enzyme results in a form of tyrosinemia characterized by progressive hepatic and renal damage.

fumigant (fu′mĭ-gant)   a substance used in fumigation.

fumigation (fu″mĭ-ga′shun) [L. *fumus* smoke, steam, vapor]   exposure of an area or object to disinfecting fumes.

fuming (fūm′ing) [L. *fumus* smoke]   smoking; emitting a visible vapor.

Fumiron (fūm′i-ron)   trademark for a preparation of ferrous fumarate.

functio (funk′she-o) [L.]   function.   **f. lae′sa,** loss of function, one of the cardinal signs of inflammation.

function (funk′shun) [L. *functio*, from *fungi* to do]   1. the special, normal, or proper physiologic activity of an organ or part.   2. to perform such activity.   3. in chemistry, a characteristic behavior of a chemical compound due to the presence of a specific functional group (q.v.)   4. in mathematics, a rule that assigns to each member of one set (the domain) a value in another set (the range).   **cumulative distribution f. (cdf),** distribution f.   **distribution f.,** a mathematical function that defines the probability distribution of a random variable by giving for each *x* the probability of observing a value less than or equal to *x*. Called also *cumulative distribution f.*   **frequency f.,** density f.   **probability density f.,** in statistics, a mathematical function that describes the distribution of measurements on a scale for a specific population; a curve that describes a population. The probability that an individual measurement will fall between two numbers *a* and *b* is equal to the proportion of the area under the curve between points *a* and *b*. Called also *frequency distribution* and *frequency f.*

functional (funk′shun-al)   1. of or pertaining to a function.   2. affecting the function but not the structure; said of disturbances with no detectable organic cause; idiopathic.

functionalis (funk″she-o-na′lis) [L.]   1. functional.   2. stratum functionale.

functionating (funk′shun-āt-ing)   in a condition of performing the proper function.

fundal (fun′dal)   pertaining to a fundus.

fundament (fun′dah-ment) [L. *fundamentum*]   1. a base or foundation, such as the breech or rump.   2. the anus and parts adjacent to it.

fundamental (fun″dah-men′tal)   pertaining to a base or foundation.

fundectomy (fun-dek′to-me)   fundusectomy.

fundi (fun′di) [L.]   genitive and plural of *fundus*.

fundic (fun′dik)   pertaining to a fundus.

fundiform (fun′dĭ-form) [L. *funda* sling + *forma* form]   shaped like a sling.

fundoplication (fun″do-pli-ka′shun)   mobilization of the lower end of the esophagus and plication of the fundus of the stomach around it (fundic wrapping), in the treatment of reflux esophagitis that may be associated with various disorders, such as hiatal hernia. Called also *Nissen f.* or *Nissen operation*.

Fundulus (fun′du-lus)   a genus of killifish of the order Cyprinodontidae; the common or green killifish, *F. heteroclitus*, is much used in biological research.

fundus (fun′dus), pl. *fun′di* [L.]   the bottom or base of anything; [NA] a general term for the bottom or base of an organ, or the part of a hollow organ farthest from its mouth.   **albinotic f.,** a fundus of the eye which permits clear visualization of the choroidal vasculature, owing to lack of pigment in the pigment epithelium and choroid.   **f. albipuncta′tus,** a disorder in which gray or white mottling of the fundus of the eye is associated with night blindness; called also *Lauber's disease*.   **f. of bladder,**   1. fundus vesicae urinariae.   2. apex vesicae urinariae.   **f. diabe′ticus,** an ocular fundus with dilated veins, a prodrome of diabetic retinopathy.   **f. of eye,** f. oculi.   **f. flavimacula′tus,** a condition characterized by the presence of yellow to white atrophic lesions in the midperiphery or perimacular region of the fundus of the eye.   **f. of gallbladder,** f. vesicae biliaris.   **gastric f.,** f. gastricus.   **f. gas′tricus** [NA], gastric fundus: that part of the stomach to the left and above the level of the entrance of the esophagus; called also *f. of stomach, f. ventricularis* [NA alternative], and *f. ventriculi*. See also *fornix gastricus*.   **f. of internal acoustic meatus, f. mea′tus acus′tici inter′ni** [NA], the laterally placed end or bottom of the internal acoustic meatus.   **leopard f.,** the mottled ocular fundus of tapetoretinal degeneration; called also *leopard retina*.   **f. o′culi,** fundus of the eye: the back portion of the interior of the eyeball, as seen by means of the ophthalmoscope.   **salt and pepper f.,** an ocular fundus dusted with fine blue pigmented and orange depigmented spots, characteristic of hereditary syphilis; also seen in other disorders, e.g., rubella.   **f. of stomach,** f. gastricus.   **tessellated f., t. tigr′e, tigroid f.,** a normal, nonpathological fundus of the eye with marked exposure of the choroidal vessels due to scanty pigmentation; called also *tessellated* or *tigroid retina*.   **f. tym′pani,** paries jugularis cavi tympani.   **f. of urinary bladder,**   1. fundus vesicae urinariae.   2. apex vesicae urinariae.   **f. u′teri** [NA], **f. of uterus,** the part of the uterus above the orifices of the uterine tubes.   **f. of vagina, f. vagi′nae,** fornix vaginae.   **f. ventricula′ris,** NA alternative for *f. gastricus*.   **f. ventric′uli,** f. gastricus.   **f. vesi′cae bilia′ris** [NA], fundus of gallbladder: the inferior dilated portion of the gallbladder; called also *f. vesicae felleae* [NA alternative].   **f. vesi′cae fel′leae,** NA alternative for *f. vesicae biliaris*.   **f. ves′icae urina′riae** [NA], fundus of urinary bladder: the base or posterior surface of the bladder; called also *f. of bladder* and *infundibulum of urinary bladder*.

funduscope (fun′dus-skōp)   ophthalmoscope.

funduscopy (fun-dus′ko-pe)   ophthalmoscopy.

fundusectomy (fun″dŭ-sek′to-me) [*fundus* + Gr. *ektomē* excision]   excision of the fundus of an organ as of the fundus of the stomach or uterus.

fungal (fung′gal)   pertaining to or caused by a fungus.

fungate (fung′gāt)   to produce fungus-like growths; to grow rapidly, like a fungus.

fungemia (fun-je′me-ah)   the presence of fungi in the blood stream.

fungi (fun′ji) [L.]   plural of *fungus*.

Fungi Imperfecti (fun′ji im″per-fek′ti) [L., pl. "imperfect fungi"]   a large heterogeneous group of fungi which have septate mycelium and in which the perfect (sexual) stage is unknown. This group includes many of the fungi that are pathogenic for animals including man and plants, among them *Candida*, *Cryptococcus*, *Histoplasma* and *Pityrosporon*. Imperfect fungi are classified in form-classes, form-orders, and so on, until their perfect stages are identified. Called also *Deuteromycetes*.

fungicidal (fun″jĭ-si′dal) [*fungus* + L. *caedere* to kill] destroying fungi.

fungicide (fun′jĭ-sīd) an agent that destroys fungi.

fungicidin (fun″jĭ-si′din) nystatin.

fungiform (fun′jĭ-form) shaped like a fungus or mushroom.

fungistasis (fun-jĭ-sta′sis) [*fungus* + Gr. *stasis* a stopping] inhibition of growth of fungi.

fungistat (fun′jĭ-stat) a substance that inhibits the growth of fungi.

fungistatic (fun″jĭ-stat′ik) inhibiting the growth of fungi.

fungisterol (fun-jis′ter-ol) a sterol, $C_{25}H_{44}O$, found in ergot and other fungi.

fungitoxic (fun″jĭ-tok′sik) exerting a toxic effect upon fungi.

fungitoxicity (fun″jĭ-tok-sis′ĭ-te) the quality of exerting a toxic effect upon fungi.

Fungizone (fun′jĭ-zōn) trademark for a preparation of amphotericin B.

fungoid (fung′goid) [*fungus* + Gr. *eidos* form] resembling a fungus, or mushroom.

fungosity (fun-gos′ĭ-te) a fungoid growth or excrescence.

fungous (fung′gus) [L. *fungosus*] of the nature of, caused by, or resembling a fungus.

fungus (fung′gus), pl. *fun′gi* [L.] a general term used to denote a group of eukaryotic protists, including mushrooms, yeasts, rusts, molds, smuts, etc., which are characterized by the absence of chlorophyll and by the presence of a rigid cell wall composed of chitin, mannans, and sometimes cellulose. They are usually of simple morphological form or show some reversible cellular specialization, such as the formation of pseudoparenchymatous tissue in the fruiting body of a mushroom. The dimorphic fungi grow, according to environmental conditions, as molds or yeasts. **algae-like f.,** Phycomycetes. **alpha f.** (*obs.*), the fungus *Trichophyton menlagrophytes* var. *quinckeanum*. **beta f.** (*obs.*), the fungus *Trichophyton schoenleinii*. **f. of the brain,** hernia cerebri. **cerebral f., f. cere′bri,** hernia cerebri. **club f.,** Basidiomycetes. **fission f.,** a bacterium. **foot f.,** a fungus, such as *Madurella mycetomi*, which produces maduromycosis, or other foot infection. **gamma f.,** a strain of the fungus *Trichophyton schoenleinii*. **f. haemato′des** (*obs.*), a soft, bleeding, malignant tumor. **imperfect f.,** a fungus whose perfect (sexual) stage is unknown; Fungi Imperfecti (Deuteromycetes). **kefir fungi,** a mixture of bacteria and yeasts capable of causing lactic acid fermentation of milk of the kefir type. **mold f.,** mycelial f. **mosaic f.,** a mycelium-like intercellular deposit of cholesterol sometimes seen in scrapings from lesions thought to be fungal in origin. **mycelial f.,** any fungus that forms mycelia, in contrast to a yeast fungus; called also *mold f.* and *thread f.* **perfect f.,** a fungus for which both sexual and asexual types of spore formation are known; see *Ascomycetes*, *Phycomycetes*, and *Basidiomycetes*. **proper f.,** Eumycetes. **ray f.,** *Actinomyces*. **sac f.,** Ascomycetes. **slime f.,** see *Mycetozoida*. **f. tes′tis,** protrusion from a scrotal sinus of a mass of granulation tissue in tuberculous epididymitis. **thread f.,** mycelial f. **true f.,** Eumycetes. **yeast f.,** any single-celled budding form of a fungus, in contrast to a mold fungus. **yeastlike f.,** single-celled budding fungi, such as yeasts.

funic (fu′nik) pertaining to the funis.

funicle (fu′nĭ-kl) funiculus.

funicular (fu-nik′u-lar) pertaining to a funiculus.

funiculi (fu-nik′u-li) genitive and plural of *funiculus*.

funiculitis (fu-nik″u-li′tis) 1. inflammation of the spermatic cord. 2. inflammation of that portion of a spinal nerve root which lies within the intervertebral canal. **endemic f.,** a disease of unknown etiology occurring chiefly in Ceylon and southern India, marked by painful swelling of the spermatic cord, chills, nausea, and vomiting. The disease also occurs sporadically in temperate climates. **filarial f.,**

secondary involvement of the spermatic cord in lymphatic filariasis.

funiculoepididymitis (fu-nik″u-lo-ep″ĭ-did″ĭ-mi′tis) inflammation of the spermatic cord and the epididymis.

funiculopexy (fu-nik′u-lo-pek″se) [L. *funiculus* cord + Gr. *pēxis* fixation] surgical fixation of the spermatic cord to the surrounding tissues in the correction of undescended testes.

funiculus (fu-nik′u-lus), pl. *funic′uli* [L.] a cord; [NA] a general term for a cordlike structure or part. **f. am′nii,** a cord of tissue by which the amnion and chorion are temporarily united in certain ruminant animals. **f. ante′rior medul′lae spina′lis,** NA alternative for *f. ventralis medullae spinalis*. **anterior f. of spinal cord,** f. ventralis medullae spinalis. **cuneate f., f. cunea′tus [Burdachi],** fasciculus cuneatus medullae spinalis. **f. cunea′tus latera′lis,** a longitudinal ridge on the oblongata between the line of roots of the spinal accessory nerve and the fasciculus cuneatus. **f. cunea′tus medul′lae oblonga′tae,** fasciculus cuneatus medullae oblongatae. **f. dorsal′is medul′lae spina′lis** [NA], the white substance of the spinal cord lying on either side between the dorsal median sulcus and the dorsal roots of the spinal nerves; called also *posterior f. of spinal cord* and *f. posterior medullae spinalis* [NA alternative]. **dorsal f. of spinal cord,** f. dorsalis medullae spinalis. **f. gra′cilis** (*obs.*), fasciculus gracilis medullae spinalis. **f. grac′ilis medul′lae oblonga′tae** (*obs.*), fasciculus gracilis medullae oblongatae. **hepatic f.,** ductus choledochus. **lateral f. of medulla oblongata, f. latera′lis medul′lae oblonga′tae** [NA], the continuation into the medulla oblongata of all the fiber tracts of the lateral funiculus of the spinal cord, with the exception of the lateral pyramidal tract. **f. latera′lis medul′lae spina′lis** [NA], lateral funiculus of spinal cord: the white substance of the spinal cord that lies on either side between the dorsal and ventral roots of the spinal nerves; called also *anterolateral column* and *lateral white commissure of spinal cord*. **ligamentous f.,** ligamentum collaterale carpi ulnare. **funic′uli medul′lae spina′lis** [NA], funiculi of spinal cord: the large bundles of fiber tracts that make up the white substance of the spinal cord. **f. poste′rior medul′lae spina′lis,** NA alternative for *f. dorsalis medullae spinalis*. **posterior f. of spinal cord,** f. dorsalis medullae spinalis. **f. se′parans,** a narrow translucent ridge of thickened ependyma in the floor of the fourth ventricle that runs across the lower part of the trigone of the vagus nerve and separates it from the area postrema; the blood-brain barrier may be modified in this area. **f. solita′rius** (*obs.*), tractus solitarius medullae oblongatae. **f. spermat′icus** [NA], the structure that extends from the abdominal inguinal ring to the testis; called also *chorda spermatica*. See *spermatic cord*, under *cord*. **funiculi of spinal cord,** funiculi medullae spinalis. **f. of spinal cord, anterior,** f. ventralis medullae spinalis. **f. of spinal cord, lateral,** f. lateralis medullae spinalis. **f. of spinal cord, posterior,** f. dorsalis medullae spinalis. **f. umbilica′lis** [NA], the flexible structure connecting the umbilicus with the placenta and giving passage to the umbilical arteries and vein; called also *chorda umbilicalis* and *funis*. See *umbilical cord*, under *cord*. **ventral f. of spinal cord, f. ventra′lis medul′lae spina′lis** [NA], the white substance of the spinal cord lying on either side between the ventral median fissure and the ventral roots of the spinal nerves; called also *anterior f. of spinal cord* and *f. anterior medullae spinalis* [NA alternative].

funiform (fu′nĭ-form) [L. *funis* rope + *forma* shape] resembling a rope or cord.

funis (fu′nis) [L. "cord"] any cordlike structure; particularly the umbilical cord. **f. bra′chii,** the median cephalic vein of the arm (vena mediana cephalica). **f. hippoc′ratis,** tendo calcaneus.

funnel (fun′el) a conic, hollow structure with a narrow opening at the apex, such as the vessels used in chemistry and pharmacy in filtering and for other purposes. **accessory müllerian f.,** a rudiment similar to the primordial uterine tube. **mitral f.,** the cone-shaped mitral valve seen in mitral stenosis, the orifice being at the apex of the cone. **muscular f.,** the funnel-shaped space bounded by the four rectus muscles of the eye. **pial f.,** a sheath of adventitia, extended from the pia mater, loosely surrounding the blood vessels of the substance of the brain or cord. **vascular f.,**

the light colored depression at the center of the disk of the retina.

F.U.O. fever of undetermined origin.

Furacin (fu′rah-sin) trademark for preparations of nitrofurazone.

Furadantin (fur″ah-dan′tin) trademark for preparations of nitrofurantoin.

furan, furane (fu′ran) a colorless liquid,

$$CH{:}CH{\cdot}CH{:}CH,$$
$$\underbrace{\qquad\qquad}_{O}$$

from wood tar.

furanose (fu′rah-nōs) a sugar in which the oxygen ring bridges carbon atoms 1 and 4 in the aldoses or carbon atoms 2 and 5 in the ketoses.

Furaspor (fur′ah-spōr) trademark for a preparation of nitrofurfuryl methyl ether; see under *ether*.

furazolidone (fu″rah-zol′ĭ-dōn) chemical name: 3-[[(5-nitro-2-furanyl)methylene]amino]-2-oxazolidinone. An antibacterial and antiprotozoal, $C_8H_7N_3O_5$, occurring as a white to slightly yellow, crystalline powder, effective against many gram-negative enteric organisms; used in the treatment of diarrhea and enteritis due to susceptible organisms, administered orally, and (combined with nifuroxime) in bacterial, candidal, and trichomonal vaginitis, administered intravaginally.

furazolium (fūr″ah-zo′le-um) chemical name: 6,7-dihydro-3-(5-nitro-2-furyl)-5*H*-imidazo [2,1-*b*] thiazolium; an antibacterial. **f. chloride,** the chloride salt of furazolium, $C_9H_8ClN_3O_3S$; an antibacterial. **f. tartrate,** the tartrate salt of furazolium, $C_{13}H_{13}N_3O_9S$; an antibacterial.

Fürbringer's sign, test (fer′bring-erz) [Paul *Fürbringer*, Berlin physician, 1849–1930] see under *sign* and *tests*.

furca (fer′kah), gen. and pl., *fur′cae* [L. "fork"] furcation.

furcal (fur′kal) [L. *furca* fork] shaped like a fork; forked.

furcation (fur-ka′shun) the anatomical area of a multirooted tooth where the roots divide.

furcocercous (fur″ko-ser′kus) [L. *furca* fork + Gr. *kerkos* tail] having a forked tail.

furcula (fur′ku-la) [L. "little fork"] a horseshoe-shaped ridge in the embryonic larynx, bounding the pharyngeal aperture in front and laterally.

furfuraceous (fur″fu-ra′shus) [L. *furfur* bran] fine and loose; said of scales resembling bran or dandruff.

furfural (fur′fu-ral) furfurol.

furfuran (fur′fu-ran) furan.

furfurol (fur′fu-rol) [L. *furfur* bran] an aromatic compound,

$$CH{:}CH{\cdot}CH{:}C{\cdot}CHO$$
$$\underbrace{\qquad\qquad}_{O}$$

from the distillation of bran, sawdust, etc. It causes convulsions in animals.

furobufen (fur″o-bu′fen) chemical name: γ-oxo-2-dibenzofuranbutanoic acid; an anti-inflammatory, $C_{16}H_{12}O_4$.

furocoumarin (fu″ro-koo′mah-rin) any of a group of antifungal dyestuffs produced by certain species of plants (e.g., parsley and figs) which, on contact with skin, cause photosensitization.

furodazole (fur-o′dah-zōl) chemical name: 2-(2-furanyl)-7-methyl-1*H*-imidazol hydrate; an anthelmintic, $C_{15}H_{11}N_3O_2 \cdot xH_2O$.

furor (fu′ror) [L.] fury; rage. **f. epilep′ticus,** an attack of intense anger occurring in epilepsy.

furosemide (fu-ro′sĕ-mīd) [USP] a high-ceiling diuretic; used in the treatment of hypertension and edema. Called also *frusemide* (BAN).

Furoxone (fur-ok′sōn) trademark for preparations of furazolidone.

furrow (fur′o) a groove or trench. **atrioventricular f.,** the transverse groove marking off the atria of the heart from the ventricles. **digital f.,** any one of the transverse folds across the joints on the palmar surface of a finger. **genital f.,** a groove that appears on the genital tubercle of the fetus at the end of the second month. **gluteal f.,** sulcus glutealis. **Jadelot's f's,** see under *line*. **Liebermeister's f's,** depressions sometimes seen on the upper surface of the liver from pressure of the ribs, generally caused by tight garments or tight lacing of a girdle or corset. **mentola-**

bial f., see under *sulcus*. **nympholabial f.,** a groove separating the labium majus and labium minus on either side. **primitive f.,** primitive groove. **scleral f.,** sulcus sclerae. **Sibson's f.,** the lower border of the pectoralis major muscle. **skin f's,** sulci cutis.

fursalan (fur′sah-lan) chemical name: 3,5-dibromo-2-hydroxy-*N*-[(tetrahydro-2-furanyl)methyl]benzamide; a disinfectant, $C_{12}H_{13}Br_2NO_3$.

Fürstner's disease (ferst′nerz) [Carl *Fürstner*, German psychiatrist, 1848–1906] see under *disease*.

furuncle (fu′rung-k'l) [L. *furunculus*] a painful nodule formed in the skin by circumscribed inflammation of the corium and subcutaneous tissue, enclosing a central slough or "core." It is caused by staphylococci, which enter through the hair follicles, and its formation is favored by constitutional or digestive derangement and local irritation. Called also *boil* and *furunculus*.

furuncular (fu-rung′ku-lar) pertaining to or of the nature of a furuncle or boil.

furunculoid (fu-rung′ku-loid) resembling a furuncle or boil.

furunculosis (fu-rung″ku-lo′sis) 1. the persistent sequential occurrence of furuncles over a period of weeks or months. 2. the simultaneous occurrence of a number of furuncles. **f. blastomycet′ica, f. cryptococ′cica,** any systemic fungous infection in which the lesions resemble furuncles.

furunculus (fu-rung′ku-lus), pl. *furun′culi* [L.] furuncle.

fusaridiosis (fu″sah-rid″e-o′sis) a dermatomycosis of horses thought to be caused by the mold *Fusarium equinum* (a species now considered to be identical with *Microsporum canis*).

fusariotoxicosis (fu-sar″ĭ-o-tok″sĭ-ko′sis) a form of mycotoxicosis caused by fungi of the genus *Fusarium*.

Fusarium (fu-sa′re-um) a genus of Fungi Imperfecti of the order Moniales, family Tuberculariaceae, the perfect stages of many species are included in the class Ascomycetes, order Hypocreales. Some are important pathogens of plants, and some are opportunistic infectious agents of man and animals. They have been isolated from otomycosis externa and mycotic keratitis. *F. oxysporum* and *F. solani* are frequently associated with mycotic keratitis, often destroying the eye. The *F. equinum* reported to cause a dermatomycosis of horses is probably *Microsporum canis*. **F. oxyspor′um,** a species causing banana wilt. **F. sol′anae,** a species causing potato wilt and, occasionally, mycotic keratitis of man. **F. sporotri′chiella,** a species believed to be the etiologic agent of Kashin-Beck disease.

fuscin (fu′sin) [L. *fuscus* brown] a brown pigment of the retinal epithelium.

fuse (fūz) 1. a bar, strip, or wire of easily fusible metal inserted for safety in an electric circuit; when the current increases beyond a safe strength the metal melts, thus breaking the circuit and thereby saving an apparatus from overload. 2. to join together, as the abnormal coherence of adjacent body structures.

fuseau (fĕ-zō′), pl. *fuseaux* [Fr.] a macroaleuriospore or macrocondium.

fusi (fu′si) [L.] plural of *fusus*.

fusible (fu′zĭ-b'l) susceptible of being melted or fused.

fusicellular (fu″sĭ-sel′u-lar) fusocellular.

fusidate (fu′si-dāt) a salt of fusidic acid.

fusidic acid (fu-si′dik) a fermentation product of *Fusidium coccineum* used as an antibiotic.

fusiform (fu′zĭ-form) [L. *fusus* spindle + *forma* form] spindle shaped.

Fusiformis (fu″sĭ-for′mis) a name formerly given to the genus *Fusobacterium*. **F. necroph′orus,** *Fusobacterium necrophorum*.

fusimotor (fu″sĭ-mo′tor) denoting motor nerve fibers (of gamma motoneurons) that innervate intrafusal fibers of the muscle spindle.

fusion (fu′zhun) [L. *fusio*] 1. the act, process, or result of melting. 2. the merging or coherence of adjacent parts or bodies. 3. the coordination of the separate images of the same object in the two eyes into one. 4. the operative formation of an ankylosis or arthrodesis (*f. of joint*). **binocular f.,** see *fusion*, def. 3. **centric f.,** Robertsonian translocation. **diaphyseal-epiphyseal f.,** operative establishment of bony union between the diaphysis and epiphysis, to arrest growth in length of a bone. **nuclear f.,** the fusion of two atomic nuclei to form a single heavier nucleus, resulting in the release of large amounts of energy. **spinal f.,** operative immobilization or ankylosis of two or more vertebrae; called also spondylosyndesis.

fusional (fu′zhun-al) marked by fusion.

Fusobacterium (fu″zo-bak-te′re-um) [L. *fusus* spindle + *bacteria*] a genus of gram-negative, anaerobic, nonsporulating bacteria of the family Bacteroidaceae, consisting of slender cells with tapered ends that are normal inhabitants of the cavities of humans and animals. Some species are pathogenic, causing purulent or gangrenous infections. Formerly called *Fusiformis*. **F. gonidiafor′mans,** a species isolated from human infections of the respiratory, urogenital, and gastrointestinal tracts. Called also *Actinomyces gonidiaformis*. **F. mortif′erum,** a species isolated from normal sources and from abscesses, septicemia, pleurisy, and urinary tract infections. **F. navifor′me,** a species isolated from human abscesses and other clinical specimens, and from the intestines of rats. **F. necroph′-orum,** a pleomorphic species found in normal body cavities, which is also the cause of virulent disseminated infection involving necrotic lesions, abscesses, and bacteremia. Called also *Actinomyces necrophorus, Actinomyces pseudonecrophorus, Bacteroides fundiliformis, Fusiformis necrophorus, Schmorl's bacillus,* and *Sphaerophorus necrophorus*. See also *foot rot of cattle* and *foot rot of sheep* under *rot; necrobacillosis; calf diphtheria,* under *diphtheria,* and *Schmorl's disease,* under *disease*. **F. nuclea′tum,** a species isolated from the normal mouth, the upper respiratory, genital, and gastrointestinal tracts, and infections of the mouth, lungs, and brain. It is the organism most commonly found, in association with spirochetes (*Treponema vincentii*), in acute necrotizing gingivitis. Called also *Bacillus fusiformis*. **F.**

plau′ti-vincen′ti, *Leptotrichia buccalis*. **F. rus′sii,** a species isolated from perianal abscesses, and from human and animal feces. **F. va′rium,** a species isolated from the intestinal cavities of humans and animals, and from human purulent infections.

fusobacterium (fu″zo-bak-te′re-um), pl. *fusobacte′ria*. 1. a rod-shaped bacterium in which the cell is thicker in the center and tapers toward the ends. 2. an organism of the genus *Fusobacterium*.

fusocellular (fu″so-sel′u-lar) [L. *fu′sus* spindle + *cellular*] having spindle-shaped cells.

fusospirillary (fu″so-spi′rĭ-lār″e) pertaining to or caused by fusiform bacilli and spirilla, as in acute necrotizing ulcerative gingivitis.

fusospirillosis (fu″so-spi″rĭ-lo′sis) acute necrotizing ulcerative gingivitis.

fusospirochetal (fu″so-spi″ro-ke′tal) pertaining to or caused by fusobacteria and spirochetes.

fusospirochetosis (fu″so-spi″ro-ke-to′sis) infection with fusobacteria and streptococci.

fustic (fus′tik) a yellow dye wood from a South American tree, *Chlorophora tinctoria*.

fustigation (fus″tĭ-ga′shun) [L. *fustigatio*] flagellation (def. 2).

fusus (fu′sus), pl. *fu′si* [L.] a spindle-like object; applied especially to minute air vesicles in a hair shaft. **cortical fusi,** the delicate air spaces appearing among the cells of the cortex as a hair grows out, produced by drying out of the fluid which fills the spaces in the living portion of the hair root. **fracture fusi,** minute rifts or ruptures observed between the keratinized cells of the cortex of a mature hair shaft which has been subjected to pressure sufficient to dissociate the cells of the particular region.

F. vs. abbreviation for L. *fi′at venaesec′tio,* let the patient be bled.

G

G 1. symbol for *conductance, gauss, Gibbs free energy, giga-,* and *gravitational constant*. 2. glycine, glucose, and guanidine or guanosine.

g 1. symbol for gram. 2. symbol for standard gravity (9.80665 m/s²).

g. gram (or grams).

Γ the Greek capital letter gamma.

γ gamma, the third letter of the Greek alphabet; symbol for *photon* (gamma ray), the heavy chain of IgG, and the γ chains of fetal hemoglobin ($^{A}\gamma$ and $^{G}\gamma$, produced by two different genetic loci and differing in the amino acid [alanine or glycine] at position 136); former symbol for microgram (now μg).

γ- a prefix designating (1) a plasma protein migrating with the γ band in protein electrophoresis (a gamma globulin) and (2) the third carbon atom from the one attached to the principal functional group, e.g., γ-aminobutyric acid.

Ga chemical symbol for *gallium*.

GABA γ-aminobutyric acid.

G-actin see *actin*.

gadfly (gad′fli) see *Tabanus*.

gadoleic acid (gad″o-le′ik) 9-eicosenoic acid; an unsaturated fatty acid from cod liver oil.

gadolinium (gad″o-lin′e-um) a rare element of atomic number 64, atomic weight 157.25, symbol Gd.

gaduhiston (gad″u-his′ton) [L. *gadus* cod + *histon*] a histone occurring in the spermatozoa of the codfish.

Gadus (ga′dus) [L.; Gr. *gados*] a genus of fishes. **G. mor′rhua,** the codfish; from its liver, cod liver oil is prepared.

Gaenslen's sign (test) (genz′lenz) [Frederick Julius *Gaenslen,* Milwaukee surgeon, 1877–1937] see under *sign*.

Gaertner see *Gärtner*.

Gaffky scale (table) (gaf′ke) [Georg Theodor August *Gaffky,* German bacteriologist, 1850–1918] see under *scale*.

Gaffkya (gaf′ke-ah) [G. T. A. *Gaffky*] in former systems of classification, a genus of bacteria species of which are now included in the genus *Aerococcus*.

GAG glycosaminoglycan.

gag (gag) 1. a surgical device for holding the mouth open. 2. to retch, or strive to vomit.

gage (gāj) gauge.

Gaillard-Arlt suture (ga-yahr′arlt) [François Lucien *Gaillard,* French physician, 1805–1869; Carl Ferdinand Ritter von *Arlt,* ophthalmologist in Vienna, 1812–1887] see under *suture*.

gain (gān) 1. an increase in amount or value; a benefit or advantage; the increase achieved by amplification of a signal. 2. to acquire, obtain, or increase. **antigen g.,** the acquisition by cells of new antigenic determinants not normally present or not normally accessible in the parent tissue. **primary g.,** the direct alleviation of anxiety by a defense mechanism; the relief from emotional conflict or tension provided by neurotic symptoms or illness. **secondary g.,** the external and incidental advantage derived from an illness such as personal attention, release from responsibility, and disability benefits.

Gairdner's test (gārd′nerz) [Sir William Tennant *Gairdner,* Scotch physician, 1824–1907] coin test; see under *tests*.

Gaisböck's disease, syndrome (gīs′bekz) [Felix *Gaisböck,* German physician, 1868–1955] stress polycythemia.

gait (gāt) the manner or style of walking. **antalgic g.,** a limp adopted so as to avoid pain on weight-bearing structures (as in hip injuries), characterized by a very short stance phase. **ataxic g.,** an unsteady, uncoordinated walk, with a wide base and the feet thrown out, coming down first on the heel and then on the toes with a double tap. **calcaneous g.,** the gait resulting when the gastrocnemius-soleus muscles are paralyzed, with lack of push-off and shift of the tibia posteriorly over the talus at the end of the stance phase. **cerebellar g.,** a staggering gait indicative of cerebellar disease. **Charcot's g.,** the peculair gait seen in Friedreich's ataxia. **double step g.,** a gait in which the length and/or timing of alternate steps is noticeably differ-

ent. drag-to g., a gait in which the feet are dragged (rather than lifted) toward the crutches. **drop-foot g.,** steppage g. **dystrophic g.,** exaggerated alternation of lateral trunk movements with an exaggerated elevation of the hip, suggesting the gait of a duck or penguin; characteristic of progressive muscular dystrophy. **equine g.,** a walk accomplished mainly by flexing the hip joint; seen in crossed-leg palsy. **festinating g.,** a gait in which the patient involuntarily moves with short, accelerating steps, often on tiptoe, as seen in paralysis agitans and other nervous disorders; festination. **four-point g.,** a gait in forward motion is as follows: first one crutch and then the opposite leg, followed by the other crutch and then the other leg, and so on. **gluteal g.,** the gait characteristic of paralysis of the gluteus medius muscle, marked by a listing of the trunk toward the affected side at each step; called also *Trendelenburg g.* **heel-toe g.,** a gait in which the heel touches down first and the toes last. **helicopod g.,** a gait in which the feet describe half-circles, as in some cases of hysterical disorder. **hemiplegic g.,** a gait involving flexion of the hip because of drop-foot and circumduction of the leg. **intermittent double-step g.,** a hemiplegic gait in which there is a pause after the short step of the normal foot, or in some cases after the step of the affected foot. **Oppenheim's g.,** a gait marked by irregular oscillation of the head, limbs, and body; seen in some cases of multiple sclerosis. **scissor g.,** a gait in which one foot is passed in front of the other, producing a cross-legged progression. **spastic g.,** a walk in which the legs are held together and move in a stiff manner, the toes seeming to drag and catch. **staggering g.,** a reeling, tottering, and tipping gait in which the individual appears as if he may fall backward or lose his balance; it is associated with alcoholic and barbiturate intoxication. **steppage g.,** the gait in drop foot in which the advancing leg is lifted high in order that the toes may clear the ground. It is due to paralysis of the anterior tibial and peroneal muscles and is seen in lesions of the lower motor neuron, such as multiple neuritis, lesions of the anterior motor horn cells, and lesions of the cauda equina. **swaying g.,** cerebellar g. **swing-through g.,** a gait in which the crutches are advanced and then the legs are swung past them. **swing-to g.,** a gait in which the crutches are advanced and the legs are swung to the same point. **tabetic g.,** ataxic g. **three-point g.,** a gait in which both crutches and the affected leg are advanced together and then the normal leg is moved forward. **Trendelenburg g.,** gluteal g. **two-point g.,** a gait in which the right foot and left crutch (or cane) are advanced together, and then the left foot and right crutch. **waddling g.,** dystrophic g.

Gajdusek (gi'doo-shek) Daniel Carleton. American pediatrician, born 1923; co-winner, with Baruch Samuel Blumberg, of the Nobel prize for medicine or physiology in 1976 for their discoveries of new mechanisms for the origin and dissemination of infectious diseases.

galactacrasia (gal"ak-tah-kra'se-ah) [galact- + a neg. + Gr. krasis mixture + -ia] abnormal condition of the breast milk.

galactagogin (gah-lak"tah-gog'in) human placental lactogen.

galactagogue (gah-lak'tah-gog) [galact- + Gr. agōgos leading] 1. promoting the flow of milk. 2. an agent that promotes the flow of milk.

galactan (gah-lak'tan) a hemicellulose carbohydrate that yields galactose upon hydrolysis; agar is a well-known example.

galactemia (gal"ak-te'me-ah) [galact- + Gr. haima blood + -ia] the presence of milk in the blood.

galactic (gah-lak'tik) 1. pertaining to milk. 2. galactagogue.

galactin (gah-lak'tin) an obsolete term for prolactin.

galactischia (gal"ak-tisk'e-ah) [galact- + Gr. ischein to suppress] suppression of the secretion of milk.

galactitol (gah-lak'tĭ-tol) dulcitol.

galact(o)- [Gr. gala, gen. galaktos milk] a combining form denoting relationship to milk.

galactoblast (gah-lak'to-blast) [galacto- + Gr. blastos germ] a colostrum corpuscle found in the acini of the mammary gland.

galactobolic (gah-lak"to-bol'ik) of or relating to the action of neurohypophyseal peptides which contract the mammary myoepithelium and cause ejection of milk.

galactocele (gah-lak'to-sēl) [galacto- + Gr. kēlē tumor] 1. a cystic enlargement of the mammary gland containing milk. 2. a hydrocele filled with a milky fluid. Called also galactoma.

galactocerebroside (gah-lak"to-ser'ĕ-bro-sīd) cerebroside.

galactocerebroside β-galactosidase (gah-lak"to-ser'ĕ-bro-sīd gah-lak"to-si'dās) galactosylceramidase.

galactochloral (gah-lak-to-klo'ral) a derivative, $C_8H_4Cl_3O_6$, of chloral and galactose in glossy scales; it is used as a hypnotic.

galactogen (gah-lak'to-jen) a polysaccharide in the eggs of snails which yields galactose on hydrolysis.

galactogenous (gal"ak-toj'ĕ-nus) [galacto- + Gr. gennan to produce] favoring the production of milk.

galactogogue (gah-lak"to-gog) galactagogue.

galactography (gal"ak-tog'rah-fe) [galacto- + -graphy] radiography of the mammary ducts after injection of a radiopaque substance into the duct system.

galactokinase (gah-lak"to-ki'nās) [EC 2.7.1.6] an enzyme of the transferase class that catalyzes the reaction ATP + D-galactose = ADP + α-D-galactose 1-phosphate. The reaction is the initial step of galactose utilization. Deficiency of the enzyme, an autosomal recessive trait, results in accumulation of galactitol in the lens of the eye and causes cataracts in infants.

galactolipid (gah-lak"to-lip'id) galactolipin.

galactolipin, galactolipine (gah-lak"to-li'pin) a cerebroside which yields galactose on hydrolysis; found abundantly in nervous tissue, usually as structural material. See cerebroside.

galactoma (gal"ak-to'mah) [galact- + -oma] galactocele.

galactometastasis (gah-lak"to-mĕ-tas'tah-sis) galactoplania.

galactometer (gal"ak-tom'ĕ-ter) [galacto- + Gr. metron measure] an instrument for measuring the specific gravity of milk.

galactopexic (gah-lak"to-pek'sik) fixing or holding galactose.

galactopexy (gah-lak'to-pek"se) the fixation of galactose by the liver.

galactophagous (gal"ak-tof'ah-gus) [galacto- + Gr. phagein to eat] feeding upon milk.

galactophlebitis (gah-lak"to-fle-bi'tis) [galacto- + phlebitis] phlegmasia alba dolens.

galactophlysis (gal"ak-tof'lĭ-sis) [galacto- + Gr. phlysis eruption] a vesicular eruption containing a milky fluid.

galactophore (gah-lak'to-for) 1. galactophorous. 2. a milk duct.

galactophoritis (gah-lak"to-fo-ri'tis) [galacto- + Gr. pherein to carry + -itis] inflammation of the milk ducts.

galactophorous (gal"ak-tof'o-rus) [galacto- + Gr. pherein to bear] conveying milk.

galactophygous (gal-ak-tof'ĭ-gus) [galacto- + Gr. phygē flight] arresting the milk secretion.

galactoplania (gah-lak"to-pla'ne-ah) [galacto- + Gr. planē wandering] the secretion of milk in some abnormal part; the metastasis of milk. Called also galactometastasis.

galactopoiesis (gah-lak"to-poi-e'sis) the production of milk by the mammary glands; lactogenesis.

galactopoietic (gah-lak"to-poi-et'ik) [galacto- + Gr. poiein to make] 1. pertaining to, characterized by, or promoting the production of milk. 2. an agent that promotes the secretion of milk.

galactopyra (gah-lak"to-pi'rah) [galacto- + Gr. pyr fire] milk fever.

galactopyranose (gah-lak"to-pi'rah-nōs) the pyranose form of galactose, $CH_2OH \cdot CH \cdot CH \cdot (CHOH)_3 \cdot CHOH$.

galactorrhea (gah-lak"to-re'ah) [galacto- + Gr. rhoia flow] excessive or spontaneous flow of milk; persistent secretion of milk irrespective of nursing.

galactosamine (gah-lak"to-sam'in) an amino sugar, $NH_2 \cdot CH_2 \cdot C(CHOH)_4CHOH$.

galactosamine-6-sulfate sulfatase (gah-lak″to-sam′in sul′fāt sul′fah-tās) N-acetylgalactosamine-6-sulfatase.

galactosan (gah-lak′to-san) a polysaccharide occurring in plants, yielding galactose on hydrolysis.

galactosazone (gah-lak″to-sa′zōn) the phenylosazone of galactose, CHOH(CHOH)$_3$C(:N·NH·C$_6$H$_5$)·CH·N·NH·C$_6$H$_5$. It is a yellow, crystalline substance formed by treating galactose with phenylhydrazine and acetic acid. The crystals melt at 193° C. and may be used in identifying galactose.

galactoschesis (gal″ak-tos′kĕ-sis) [galacto- + Gr. schesis suppression] galactischia.

galactoscope (gah-lak′to-skōp) [galacto- + Gr. skopein to examine] a device for showing the proportion of cream in the milk.

galactose (gah-lak′tōs) an aldohexose, CH$_2$OH(CHOH)$_4$-CHO, obtained from lactose or milk sugar by enzymatic action or by boiling with a mineral acid. It is a white crystalline substance, resembles glucose in most of its properties, but is less soluble, less sweet, and forms mucic acid when oxidized with nitric acid. D-Galactose is found in milk sugar, in the cerebrosides of the brain, in the raffinose of the sugar beet, and in many gums and seaweeds; L-galactose, in flaxseed mucilage.

galactose epimerase (gah-lak′tōs ĕ-pim′er-ās″) UDP-glucose 4-epimerase.

galactosemia (gah-lak″to-se′me-ah) [galactose + -emia] any of three genetic disorders resulting from defective galactose metabolism. *Classic galactosemia* occurs in 1 of 60,000 births, is often fatal to neonates, is caused by deficient galactose-1-phosphate uridyl transferase, and is marked by accumulation of galactose-1-phosphate and galactose, cirrhosis of the liver, hepatomegaly, cataracts, and mental retardation in survivors, with vomiting, diarrhea, jaundice, poor weight gain, and malnutrition in early infancy. *Galactokinase deficiency* occurs in 1 of 500,000 births and results in accumulation of galactose in blood and tissues and formation of cataracts. *Galactose epimerase deficiency* is of unknown prevalence, is caused by defective uridine diphosphogalactose-4-epimerase, results in accumulation of galactose-1-phosphate in the red blood cells, and is nearly always benign. See *disorder of carbohydrate metabolism,* under *metabolism.*

galactose-1-phosphate uridyltransferase (gah-lak′tōs fos′fāt u″rĭ-dil-trans′fer-ās) UDPglucose-hexose-1-phosphate uridyltransferase.

α-D-galactosidase (gah-lak″to-si′dās) [EC 3.2.1.22] an enzyme of the hydrolase class that catalyzes the hydrolysis of terminal, nonreducing α-D-galactose residues in α-D-galactosides. **α-D-g. A**, the heat labile, lysosomal enzyme that catalyzes the reaction ceramide-glucose-galactose-galactose + H$_2$O = ceramide-glucose-galactose + galactose. Deficiency of the enzyme, an X-linked trait, leads to the accumulation of ceramide trihexoside in plasma and tissues, a condition known as diffuse angiokeratoma (see *Fabry's disease,* under *disease*). Called also *ceramide trihexosidase.* **α-D-g. B**, α-N-acetylgalactosaminidase.

α-D-galactosidase A deficiency Fabry disease.

β-galactosidase (gah-lak″to-si′dās) [EC 3.2.1.23] an enzyme of the hydrolase class that catalyzes the hydrolysis of terminal nonreducing residues in β-D-galactosides with release of D-galactose. The enzyme in the brush border membrane of the intestinal mucosa (lactase) catalyzes the hydrolysis of lactose to galactose and glucose and the hydrolysis of β-D-galactosides in gangliosides and keratan. Genetic deficiency of one variant in cell lysosomes (β-galactosidase A), an autosomal recessive trait, causes generalized gangliosidosis. Deficiency of another variant causes Morquio syndrome type B (mucopolysaccharidosis IVB). Called also *lactosyl ceramidase II.* See also *galactosylceramidase.* **neutral β-g.**, lactosylceramidase. **neutral β-g. deficiency**, lactosylceramidosis.

galactoside (gah-lak′to-sīd) a glycoside containing galactose.

galactosis (gal″ak-to′sis) the formation of milk by the lacteal glands.

galactostasia (gah-lak″to-sta′se-ah) galactostasis.

galactostasis (gal″ak-tos′tah-sis) [galacto- + Gr. stasis halt]

1. cessation of the milk secretion. 2. an abnormal collection of milk in the mammary glands.

galactosuria (gah-lak″to-su′re-ah) [galactose + Gr. ouron urine + -ia] presence of galactose in the urine.

galactosylceramidase (gah-lak″to-sil-ser-am′ĭ-dās) [EC 3.2.1.46] an enzyme of the hydrolase class that catalyzes the reaction D-galactosyl-N-acylsphingosine + H$_2$O = D-galactose + N-acylsphingosine. The enzyme is a β-galactosidase, specific for ceramide galactosides. Genetic deficiency of the enzyme, inherited as an autosomal recessive trait, causes Krabbe's disease.

galactosylceramide β-galactosidase (gah-lak″to-sil-ser′ah-mīd gah-lak″to-si′dās) galactosylceramidase.

galactosylceramide β-galactosidase deficiency Krabbe disease.

galactosylceramide β-galactosyl-hydrolase (gah-lak″to-sil-ser′ah-mīd gah-lak″to-sil hi′dro-lās) galactosylceramidase.

galactotherapy (gah-lak″to-ther′ah-pe) [galacto- + Gr. therapeia treatment] 1. the treatment of suckling children by giving remedies to the mother or wet nurse. 2. milk cure. 3. lactotherapy.

galactotoxin (gah-lak″to-tok′sin) [galacto- + Gr. toxikon poison] a basic substance formed in milk.

galactotoxism (gah-lak″to-tok′sizm) poisoning by milk.

galactotrophy (gal″ak-tot′ro-fe) [galacto- + Gr. trophē nutrition] feeding with milk.

galactowaldenase (gah-lak″to-wal′den-ās) UDP glucose 4-epimerase.

galactoxism (gal″ak-tok′sizm) galactotoxism.

galactoxismus (gah-lak″tok-siz′mus) galactotoxism.

galacturia (gal″ak-tu′re-ah) [galact- + Gr. ouron urine + -ia] the discharge of milklike urine; chyluria.

galacturonic acid (gah-lak″tu-ron′ik) the uronic acid formed by the oxidation of C-6 of galactose to a carboxy group; it occurs in pectins.

galantamine hydrobromide (gah-lan′tah-mēn) galanthamine hydrobromide.

galanthamine hydrobromide (gah-lan′thah-mēn) the hydrobromide salt of an alkaloid, C$_{17}$H$_{21}$NO$_3$·HBr, obtained in the U.S.S.R. from the Caucasian snowdrop *Galanthus woronowii* and closely related species. It is a cholinesterase inhibitor and is used in the U.S.S.R. in the treatment of myasthenia, myopathy, and sensory and motor dysfunction associated with disorders of the central nervous system and may be used as an antidote to nonpolarizing muscle relaxants. Called also *galantamine hydrobromide.*

galea (ga′le-ah) [L.] a helmet; [NA] a general term for a helmetlike structure. **g. aponeurot′ica** [NA], the aponeurotic structure of the scalp, connecting the frontal and occipital bellies of the occipitofrontalis muscle.

Galeati's glands (gal″e-ah′tēz) [Domenico Maria *Galeati,* Italian physician, 1686–1775] glandulae duodenales.

galeatus (gal″e-a′tus) [L. *galea* helmet] born with a caul.

Galeazzi's fracture, sign (gal″e-at′zēz) [Riccardo *Galeazzi,* Italian orthopedic surgeon, 1866–1952] see under the nouns.

Galen (ga′len) (c. 129 to c. 200) a Greek physician and teacher, born in Pergamum (Asia Minor), author of 500 books on philosophy, philology, and medicine (83 medical books survive). Galen was also court physician to Marcus Aurelius, a former surgeon to gladiators, and a practicing anatomist (he performed vivisections and post mortems on the Barbary ape [*Macaca sylvana*], but not on humans). Galen was an eclectic Dogmatist; he worshipped Hippocrates and Plato and respected Aristotle, but he also freely advanced his own findings and opinions. Galen was the great compiler and systemizer of Greco-Roman medicine, physiology, and anatomy. He accepted Aristotelian teleology and the theories of humoralism, the four qualities, and pneumatism, and he promulgated that of the four temperaments (cf. *temperament*). Galen's piety, half-Stoic, half-Christian, appealed strongly to late antiquity and the Middle Ages. By experiment he showed that arteries carried blood, believed the brain to be the seat of intelligence, and understood the diagnostic value of the pulse. His work was superseded by Vesalius in anatomy and by Harvey in physiology. See also under *anastomosis* and *foramen,* and see *venae cerebri internae,* and *magna,* and *ventriculus laryngis.*

galenic (gah-len′ik) pertaining to the ancient system of medicine taught and practiced by Galenus, or Galen.

galenica (gah-len′ĭ-kah) galenicals.

galenicals (gah-len′ĭ-kalz) medicines prepared according to the formulas of Galen; the term is now used to denote standard preparations containing one or several organic ingredients, as contrasted with pure chemical substances.

galenics (gah-len′iks) galenicals.

Galeodes araneoides (gal″e-o′dēz ah-ra″ne-oi′dēz) a spider-like arachnid of the Old World, with a venomous bite.

galeophobia (gal″e-o-fo′be-ah) (obs.) ailurophobia.

galeropia, galeropsia (gal″er-o′pe-ah, gal″er-op′se-ah) [Gr. galeros cheerful + -opia, -opsia] abnormal clearness of vision due to a pathological condition.

gall (gawl) [L. galla] 1. the bile. 2. nutgall. **Aleppo g.,** nutgall. **ox g.,** see ox bile extract, under extract. **Smyrna g.,** nutgall. **wind g.,** windgall.

Gall's craniology (gawlz) [Franz Joseph Gall, anatomist in Vienna and Paris, 1758–1828] phrenology.

gallacetophenone (gal-as″e-to-fe′non) chemical name: 2′,3′,4′-trihydroxyacetophenone. A yellowish powder, CH_3·CO·$C_6H_2(OH)_3$, used as an antiseptic.

gallamine triethiodide (gal′ah-mĭn tri″ĕ-thi′o-dīd) [USP] chemical name: 2,2′,2″-[1,2,3,-benzenetriyltris(oxy)]tris[N,N,N-triethyl]ethanaminium triiodide. A quaternary ammonium compound, $C_{30}H_{60}I_3N_3O_3$, occurring as a white, amorphous powder; used to induce skeletal muscle relaxation during surgery and other procedures, such as endoscopy or intubation, administered intravenously. Called also benzurine iodide.

gallate (gal′āt) any salt of gallic acid.

gallbladder (gawl′blad-der) the pear-shaped reservoir for the bile on the posteroinferior surface of the liver, between the right and the quadrate lobe; from its neck, the cystic duct projects to join the common bile duct. Called also cholecyst, vesica biliaris [NA], and vesica fellea [NA alternative]. **Courvoisier's g.,** a distended gallbladder resulting from biliary tract obstruction. **fish-scale g.,** a gallbladder with a fish-scale-like appearance due to multiple small cysts of the mucosa. **floating g.,** wandering g. **folded fundus g.,** phrygian cap. **hourglass g.,** a gallbladder in which there is an annular constriction dividing it into a wide upper and a narrower lower compartment; the anomaly may be congenital or acquired. **mobile g.,** wandering g. **sandpaper g.,** a rough state of the mucous membrane of the gallbladder caused by the presence of the cholesterin crystals. **stasis g.,** a gallbladder that contracts sluggishly in response to a fatty meal. **strawberry g.,** a gallbladder with a strawberry-like appearance, due to fine grains of cholesterin-fat material embedded in the mucosa as a result of chronic catarrhal inflammation. **wandering g.,** abnormal mobility of the fundus and body of the gallbladder.

gallein (gal′e-in) dioxyfluorescein, an aniline dye indicator which is changed in color by an alkali to red and by an acid to yellow.

gallic acid (gal′ik) 3,4,5-trihydroxybenzoic acid, obtained from nutgalls and formerly used as an astringent.

Gallie transplant (gal′e) [William Edward Gallie, Toronto surgeon, 1882–1959] see under transplant.

Galli Mainini test (gal′e mi-ne′ne) [Carlos Galli Mainini, Argentinian physician, 1879–1943] see under test.

Gallionella (gal″le-o-nel′ah) [Benjamin Gallion, French zoologist, 1782–1839] a genus of appendaged bacteria found in iron-containing waters and soils, made up of kidney-shaped or rounded cells that produce long, twisted stalks and reproduce by fission. The type species is G. ferrugin′ea.

gallipot (gal′ĭ-pot) a small pot for ointments or confections.

gallisin (gal′ĭ-sin) a substance analogous to dextrin.

gallium (gal′e-um) [L., from Gallia Gaul] a rare metal liquid at room temperature; atomic number, 31, atomic weight, 69.72; symbol, Ga: some of its compounds are poisonous.

gallnut (gawl′nut) nutgall.

gallon (gal′on) [L. congius] a measure of volume, four quarts (3785 ml.); in the United States, 231 cubic inches.

gallop (gal′op) a disordered rhythm of the heart; see under rhythm.

gallotannic acid (gal-o-tan′ik) tannic acid.

gallsickness (gawl-sik′nes) anaplasmosis.

gallstone (gawl′stōn) a concretion, usually of cholesterol, formed in the gallbladder or bile duct.

GALT gut-associated lymphoid tissue; see under tissue.

Galton's law of regression (gawl′tonz) [Sir Francis Galton, English scientist, 1822–1911] see under law.

Galv. galvanic.

galvanic (gal-van′ik) 1. named for or discovered by Luigi Galvani, Italian physician and physiologist, 1737–1798. 2. pertaining to galvanism.

galvanism (gal′vah-nizm) [Luigi Galvani] 1. galvanic electricity: unidirectional electric current derived from a chemical battery. 2. the therapeutic use of direct current. **dental g.,** production of galvanic current in the oral cavity due to the presence of two or more dissimilar metals in dental restorations that are bathed in saliva, or a single metal restoration and two electrolytes, saliva and pulp tissue fluid, thus producing an electrolytic cell and an electric current. When such restorations touch each other, the current may be high enough to irritate the dental pulp and cause sharp pain. The anodic restoration or areas of a restoration are subject to electrolytic corrosion.

galvanization (gal″vah-ni-za′shun) treatment by galvanic electricity.

galvanocautery (gal″vah-no-kaw′ter-e) cautery accomplished by application of a wire heated with a galvanic current.

galvanochemical (gal″vah-no-kem′e-kal) pertaining to the chemical action of the galvanic current.

galvanocontractility (gal″vah-no-kon″trak-til′ĭ-te) contractility in response to a galvanic stimulus.

galvanogustometer (gal″vah-no-gus-tom′ĕ-ter) an apparatus for the clinical determination of taste thresholds by the use of a galvanic current.

galvanoionization (gal″vah-no-i″on-i-za′shun) (obs.) iontophoresis.

galvanolysis (gal″vah-nol′ĭ-sis) [galvanism + Gr. lysis dissolution] electrolysis.

galvanometer (gal″vah-nom′ĕ-ter) [galvanism + -meter] an instrument for measuring current by electromagnetic action. **Einthoven's g., string g., thread g.** (obs.), a forerunner of the electrocardiograph, consisting of a delicate thread of silvered quartz or platinum stretched between the poles of a strong magnet; the thread is displaced by an electric current flowing through it in proportion to the strength of the current.

galvanonervous (gal″vah-no-ner′vus) produced by application of the galvanic current to a nerve trunk.

galvanopalpation (gal″vah-no-pal-pa′shun) a method of testing the sensory and vasomotor nerves of the skin by applying a sharp-pointed anode electrode to the part of the skin to be tested, the cathode being applied to some other part of the body.

galvanosurgery (gal″vah-no-sur′jer-e) the employment of galvanic cautery in surgery.

galvanotaxis (gal″vah-no-tak′sis) the tendency of an organism to arrange itself in a medium so that its axis bears a certain relation to the direction of the current in the medium.

galvanotherapeutics, galvanotherapy (gal-vah-no-ther″ah-pu′tiks, gal″vah-no-ther′ah-pe) the therapeutic use of galvanic current.

galvanotropism (gal″vah-not′ro-pizm) [galvanism + Gr. tropos a turn] the tendency of an organism to turn or move under the action of an electric current.

galziekte (gahl-zēk′te) [Dutch gal gall + ziekte sickness] South African name for gallsickness.

gamasid (gam′ah-sid) a mite of the Gamasides group.

Gamasidae (gah-mas′ĭ-de) former name for a family of mites of the order Acarina, the spider mites or beetle mites; they are parasitic on birds and animals. See Gamasides group; under group.

Gamasides (gah-mas′ĭ-dēz) see under group.

gamasoidosis (gam″ah-soi-do′sis) infestation by mites of the Gamasides group, such as the dermatitis caused by the fowl mite, Dermanyssus.

Gamastan (gam′ah-stan″) trademark for a preparation of immune human serum globulin.

Gambian horse disease, sickness (gam′be-an) [*Gambia*, a country on the west coast of Africa] see under *disease* and *sickness*.

gambir (gam′bēr) the dried aqueous, astringent extract from the leaves and twigs of *Uncaria gambier*, a rubiaceous climbing shrub of southeastern Asia, the chief constituents of which are catechin, catechutannic acid, and quercetin; formerly used as an antidiarrheal and as a gargle for sore throat. Called also *catechu* or *pale catechu*.

gamboge (gam-bōj′, gam-booj′) the yellow gum-resin from *Garcinia hanburyi* Hook. f., and other guttiferous plants of Cambodia and the East Indies; used as a drastic hydragogue cathartic. Abbreviated G.G.G. Called also *cambogia* and *gutti*.

Gambusia (gam-bu′se-ah) a genus of fish effective in destroying mosquito larvae. **G. affin′is,** a top minnow which has been introduced into every major malarious region in the world; it feeds upon the larvae of *Anopheles* mosquitoes along the surface of the water.

gamefar (gah′mĕ-fahr) pamaquine.

gametangia (gam-ĕ-tan′je-ah) [L.] plural of *gametangium*.

gametangium (gam-ĕ-tan′je-um), pl. *gametan′gia* [*gamete* + Gr. *angeion* vessel] the structure in which zygospores are developed. See *spore*.

gamete (gam′ēt) [Gr. *gametē* wife, *gametēs* husband] 1. a haploid reproductive cell (ovum or spermatozoon), whose union is necessary in sexual reproduction to initiate the development of a new individual. 2. the malarial parasite in its sexual form in the gut of the mosquito vector, either male (*microgamete*) or female (*macrogamete*); the latter fertilizes the former to develop into an ookinete.

gametic (gah-met′ik) pertaining to gametes or the primitive sexual elements.

gamet(o)- [Gr. *gametē* wife, *gametēs* husband] a combining form denoting relationship to a gamete.

gametocidal (gah-me″to-si′dal) capable of destroying gametes or gametocytes.

gametocide (gah-me′to-sīd) [*gameto-* + L. *caedere* to kill] an agent that destroys gametes or gametocytes.

gametocyst (gah-me′to-sist) [*gameto-* + *cyst*] a cyst containing two gregarine protozoa (macrogamete and microgamete) enclosed in a protective wall, within which the gametes are formed.

gametocyte (gah-me′to-sīt) [*gameto-* + *cyte*] 1. a cell that produces gametes; an oocyte or spermatocyte. 2. gamont.

gametocytemia (gah-me″to-si-te′me-ah) the presence of malarial gametocytes in the blood.

gametogenesis (gam″e-to-jen′ĕ-sis) [*gameto-* + Gr. *genesis* production] the development of the male and female sex cells, or gametes.

gametogenic (gam″e-to-jen′ik) producing or favoring the production of germ cells.

gametogony (gam″e-tog′o-ne) 1. the development of merozoites of malarial plasmodia and other sporozoa into male and female gametes, which later fuse to form a zygote; called also *gamogony*. 2. reproduction by means of gametes.

gametoid (gam′ĕ-toid) resembling gametes or reproductive cells.

gametokinetic (gam″ĕ-to-ki-net′ik) [*gameto-* + Gr. *kinein* to move] stimulating gamete action.

gametophagia (gam″ĕ-to-fa′je-ah) gamophagia.

gametophyte (gam′ĕ-to-fīt) [*gameto-* + Gr. *phyton* plant] the haploid or sexual stage in organisms having alternation of generations (metagenesis); it may be female (megagametophyte) or male (microgametophyte).

Gamgee tissue (gam′je) [Joseph Sampson *Gamgee*, British surgeon, 1828–1886] see under *tissue*.

gamic (gam′ik) sexual; applied to eggs which develop only after fertilization.

gamma (gam′ah) [Γ, γ] 1. the third letter of the Greek alphabet. 2. an obsolete equivalent for microgram.

gamma-aminobutyric acid (ah-me″no-bu-tir′ik) γ-aminobutyric acid; see under *A*.

gamma benzene hexachloride (gam′ah ben′zēn hek″sah-klōr′īd) lindane.

gammacism (gam′ah-sizm) [Gr. *gamma* the letter G] the

imperfect utterance of velar consonants, especially *g* and *k* sounds.

gamma globulin see under *globulin*.

gammaglobulinopathy (gam″ah-glob″u-lin-op′ah-the) any gammopathy.

gammagram (gam′ah-gram) a graphic record of the gamma rays emitted by an object or substance.

gammagraphic (gam″ah-graf′ik) pertaining to the recording of gamma rays in the study of organs after the administration of radioactive isotopes.

gamma-lactone (gam″ah-lak′tōn) a compound having a five-membered ring structure formed by internal reaction of a carboxylic acid group with a hydroxyl group on the gamma carbon of a carbon chain.

gamma-pipradol (gam″ah-pip′rah-dol) azacyclonol.

gammopathy (gam-op′ah-the) [*gamma* globulin + *pathy*] a condition marked by disturbed immunoglobulin synthesis. **benign monoclonal g.,** the presence of a serum M component without signs or symptoms of multiple myeloma, Waldenström's macroglobulinemia, or other plasma cell neoplasms; it occurs in about 3 per cent of the population over age 70. A few patients eventually develop a malignant plasma cell dyscrasia, most do not. **monoclonal g.,** plasma cell dyscrasia.

gam(o)- [Gr. *gamos* marriage] a combining form denoting relationship to marriage or sexual union.

gamobium (gah-mo′be-um) [*gamo-* + Gr. *bios* life] in biology, the sexually reproducing generation in cases of metagenesis (alternation of generations). Cf. *agamobium*.

gamogenesis (gam″o-jen′ĕ-sis) [*gamo-* + Gr. *genesis* production] sexual reproduction.

gamogenetic (gam″o-jĕ-net′ik) pertaining to or exhibiting sexual reproduction.

gamogony (gam-og′o-ne) gametogony.

gamone (gam′ōn) a hypothetical substance supposed to be released by the ovum (gynogamone) and spermatozoa (androgamone) to facilitate their fusion.

gamont (gam′ont) [*gam-* + Gr. *ōn* being] 1. the sexual (gametic) stage in the sporozoan life cycle, produced by gamogony from a trophozoite or a merozoite. Called also *gametocyte*. 2. either of the conjugating individuals in ciliate reproduction; see also *syzygy*.

gamophagia (gam″o-fa′je-ah) [*gamo-* + Gr. *phagein* to eat] the disappearance of the male or female element in the conjugation of unicellular organisms.

gampsodactyly (gamp″so-dak′tĭ-le) [Gr. *gampsos* crooked + *daktylos* digit] deformity of the toes marked by hyperextension of the first phalanx on the metatarsal and flexion of the other two phalanges; called also *clawfoot*.

Gamulin Rh (gam′u-lin) trademark for a preparation of Rh₀(D) immune serum globulin.

ganglia (gang′gle-ah) [Gr.] plural of *ganglion*.

ganglial (gang′gle-al) pertaining to a ganglion.

gangliated (gang′gle-āt″ed) ganglionated.

gangliectomy (gang″gle-ek′to-me) ganglionectomy.

gangliform (gang′glĭ-form) having the form of a ganglion.

gangliitis (gang″gle-i′tis) ganglionitis.

gangli(o)- [Gr. *ganglion*, q.v.] a combining form denoting relationship to a ganglion.

ganglioblast (gang′gle-o-blast″) [*ganglio-* + Gr. *blastos* germ] an embryonic cell of the cerebrospinal ganglia.

gangliocyte (gang′gle-o-sīt″) [*ganglio-* + Gr. *kytos* hollow vessel] a ganglion cell.

gangliocytoma (gang″gle-o-si-to′mah) ganglioneuroma.

ganglioform (gang′gle-o-form″) gangliform.

ganglioglioma (gang″gle-o-gli-o′mah) a glioma rich in mature neurons or ganglion cells.

ganglioglioneuroma (gang″gle-o-gli″o-nu-ro′mah) ganglioneuroma.

gangliolytic (gang″gle-o-lyt′ik) ganglioplegic.

ganglioma (gang″gle-o′mah) [*ganglio-* + -*oma*] ganglioneuroma.

ganglion (gang′gle-on), pl. *ganglia* or *ganglions* [Gr. "knot"] 1. a knot, or knotlike mass. 2. [NA] a general term for a group of nerve cell bodies located outside the central nervous system; occasionally applied to certain nuclear groups within

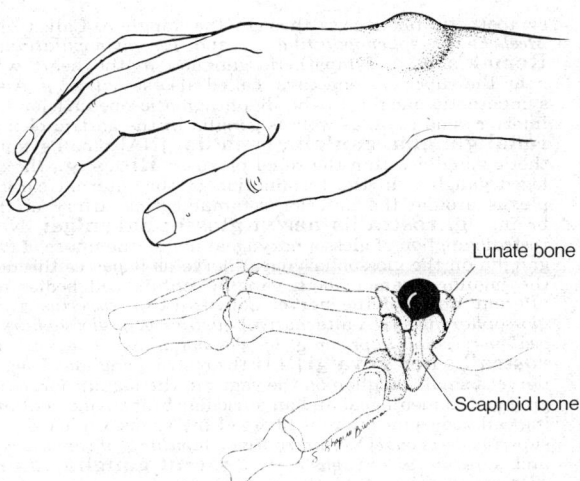

Lunate bone

Scaphoid bone

Ganglion of wrist arising from a tendon.

the brain or spinal cord, e.g., basal ganglia. 3. a benign cystic tumor occurring on an aponeurosis or tendon, as in the wrist or dorsum of the foot; it consists of a thin fibrous capsule enclosing a clear mucinous fluid. **accessory ganglia,** ganglia intermedia. **acousticofacial g.,** a ganglion of early embryonic life, a portion of which persists as the geniculate ganglion. **Acrel's g.,** a cystic tumor on an extensor tendon of the wrist. **Andersch's g.,** g. inferius nervi glossopharyngei. **aorticorenal g., ganglia aorticorena'lia** [NA], a more or less detached inferolateral extension of the celiac ganglion. **auditory g.,** see *nuclei cochlearis, ventralis et dorsalis.* **Auerbach's g.,** any of the small ganglia of Auerbach's plexus. **autonomic ganglia, gan'glia autonom'ica** [NA], the ganglia found along the sympathetic trunks, on the peripheral plexuses, and within the walls of organs supplied by the autonomic nervous system; they are divided into two structurally similar groups, the sympathetic ganglia and the parasympathetic ganglia. Called also *visceral ganglia* and *ganglia visceralia* [NA alternative]. **ganglia of autonomic plexuses,** ganglia plexuum autonomicorum. **azygous g.,** glomus coccygeum. **basal ganglia,** see under *nucleus.* **Bezold's g.,** a series of ganglion cells in the interatrial septum. **Bidder's ganglia,** ganglia on the cardiac nerves, situated at the lower end of the atrial septum. **Blandin's g.,** g. submandibulare. **Bochdalek's g., g. Bochdalek'ii,** plexus dentalis superior. **Bock's g.,** carotid g. **cardiac ganglia, gan'glia cardi'aca** [NA], ganglia of the cardiac plexus near the arterial ligament; called also *Wrisberg's g.* and *g. wrisbergi.* **carotid g.,** a ganglion of the internal carotid plexus in the cavernous sinus; called also *Bock's g.* **carotid g., inferior,** a ganglion of the internal carotid plexus in the lower part of the carotid canal; called also *Laumonier's g.* and *Schmiedel's g.* **carotid g., superior,** a ganglion of the internal carotid plexus in the upper part of the carotid canal. **g. cauda'lis ner'vi glossopharyn'gei** [NA], caudal ganglion of glossopharyngeal nerve: the lower of two ganglia on the glossopharyngeal nerve as it passes through the jugular foramen; both contain cell bodies for the afferent fibers of the nerve. Called also *g. inferius nervi glossopharyngei* [NA alternative], *inferior g. of glossopharyngeal nerve, inferior petrosal g.,* and *petrosal* or *petrous g.* **g. cauda'lis ner'vi va'gi** [NA], caudal ganglion of vagus: a ganglion of the vagus nerve located just below the jugular foramen, in front of the transverse processes of the first and second cervical vertebrae; it contains cell bodies for afferent fibers of the vagus. Called also *g. inferius nervi vagi* [NA alternative], *inferior g. of vagus nerve, nodose g.,* and *g. nodosum.* **celiac ganglia, ganglia celi'aca,** ganglia coeliaca. **cephalic g.,** parasympathetic ganglia in the head, consisting of the ciliary, otic, pterygopalatine, and submandibular ganglia. **cerebrospinal ganglia,** the ganglia associated with the cranial and spinal nerves. **cervical g., inferior,** a portion of the ganglion cervicothoracicum. **cervical g., middle,** g. cervicale medium. **cervical g.,**

superior, g. cervicale superius. **cervical g. of uterus,** a ganglion situated near the cervix uteri; called also *Lee's g.* and *Frankenhäuser's g.* **g. cervica'le infe'rius,** a portion of the ganglion cervicothoracicum. **g. cervica'le me'dium** [NA], middle cervical ganglion: a variable ganglion, often fused with the vertebral ganglion, on the sympathetic trunk at about the level of the cricoid cartilage; its postganglionic fibers are distributed mainly to the heart, cervical region, and upper limb. Formerly called *inferior* or *superior thyroid g.* **g. cervica'le supe'rius** [NA], superior cervical ganglion: the uppermost ganglion on the sympathetic trunk, lying behind the internal carotid artery and in front of the second and third cervical vertebrae; it gives rise to postganglionic fibers to the heart via cervical cardiac nerves, to the pharyngeal plexus and thence to the larynx and pharynx and to the head via the external and internal carotid plexuses. **cervicothoracic g., g. cervicothora'cicum** [NA], a ganglion on the sympathetic trunk at the level of the 7th cervical and 1st thoracic vertebrae, anterior to the 8th cervical and 1st thoracic nerves; it has two components, the inferior cervical and first thoracic ganglia, which are usually fused, partially or completely. Its postganglionic fibers are distributed to the head and neck, heart, and upper limb. Called also *stellate g.* and *g. stellatum* [NA alternative]. **cervicouterine g.,** cervical g. of uterus. **g. cilia're** [NA], **ciliary g.,** a parasympathetic ganglion in the posterior part of the orbit; it receives preganglionic fibers from the oculomotor nerve, and its postganglionic fibers supply the ciliary muscle and the sphincter pupillae. Sensory and postganglionic sympathetic fibers pass through the ganglion. **Cloquet's g.,** an enlargement of the nasopalatine nerve in the anterior palatine canal. **cochlear g., g. cochlea're** [NA], the sensory ganglion located within the spiral canal of the modiolus. It consists of bipolar cells that send fibers peripherally through the foramina nervosa to the spiral organ and centrally through the internal acoustic meatus to the cochlear nuclei of the brain stem. Called also *Corti's g., g. spirale cochleare* [NA alternative], *spiral g.,* and *spiral g. of cochlea.* **g. coelia'ca** [NA], two irregularly shaped ganglia, one on each crus of the diaphragm, within the celiac plexus; each contains sympathetic nerve cells and preganglionic sympathetic fibers from the greater and lesser splanchnic nerves; preganglionic parasympathetic and sensory fibers pass through the ganglion. Called also *celiac g.* and *g. celiaca.* **collateral ganglia,** prevertebral ganglia. **compound g.,** a cystic tumor of a tendon sheath that has been compressed into two parts by a ligament. **Corti's g.,** g. cochleare. **craniospinal ganglia, gan'glia craniospina'lia** [NA], collections of sensory neurons that form nodular enlargements on the dorsal roots of the spinal nerves (ganglia spinalia) and on the sensory roots of cranial nerves (ganglia sensorialia nervorum cranialium). Called also *encephalospinal ganglia, ganglia encephalospinalia* [NA alternative], *ganglia sensorialia* or *sensoria,* and *sensory ganglia.* **diffuse g.,** a swelling of several adjoining tendon sheaths due to inflammatory effusion. **dorsal root g.,** spinal g. **Ehrenritter's g.,** g. superius nervi glossopharyngei. **encephalospinal ganglia,** ganglia craniospinalia. **gan'glia encephalospina'lia,** NA alternative for *ganglia craniospinalia.* **false g.,** an enlargement on a nerve that does not have a true ganglionic structure. **Frankenhäuser's g.,** cervical g. of uterus. **Froriep's g.,** the ganglion of the lowest occipital segment in the human embryo. **ganglia of autonomic plexuses,** ganglia plexuum autonomicrorum. **Ganser's g.,** nucleus interpeduncularis. **Gasser's g., gasserian g.,** g. trigeminale. **geniculate g., g. genic'uli ner'vi facia'lis** [NA], the sensory ganglion of the facial nerve, situated on the geniculum nervi fascialis. Called also *g. geniculatum nervi facialis* [NA alternative]. **g. genicula'tum ner'vi facia'lis,** NA alternative for *g. geniculi nervi facialis.* **g. of glossopharyngeal nerve, caudal, g. of glossopharyngeal nerve, inferior,** g. caudalis nervi glossopharyngei. **g. of glossopharyngeal nerve, rostral, g. of glossopharyngeal nerve, superior,** g. rostralis nervi glossopharyngei. **hepatic g.,** a ganglion situated near the hepatic artery. **hypogastric g.,** either of two ganglia on each side of the cervix uteri, connected with the sacral and hypogastric plexuses. **hypoglossal g.,** a ganglion of the hypoglossal nerve; rarely found in man, except in the embryo. **g. im'par** [NA], the ganglion commonly found in front of the coccyx, where the sympathetic trunks of the two sides unite.

g. infe′rius ner′vi glossopharyn′gei, NA alternative for *g. caudalis nervi pharyngei.* **g. infe′rius ner′vi va′gi** NA alternative for *g. caudalis nervi vagi.* **inhibitory g.,** any ganglion performing an inhibitory function. **gan′glia interme′dia** [NA], **intermediate ganglia,** small groups of sympathetic nerve cells present on spinal nerves and on rami communicantes, especially in the cervical, lower thoracic, and upper lumbar regions; called also *accessory ganglia.* **g. intermédiaire,** g. vertebrale. **jugular g. of glossopharyngeal nerve,** g. rostralis glossopharyngei. **jugular g. of vagus nerve, g. jugula′re ner′vi va′gi,** g. rostralis nervi vagi. **Küttner′s g.,** nodus lymphaticus jugulodigastricus. **Langley′s g.,** a collection of nerve cells in the hilus of the submaxillary gland in some animals. **Laumonier′s g.,** 1. carotid g. 2. inferior carotid g. **Lee′s g.,** cervical g. of the uterus. **lesser g. of Meckel,** g. submandibulare. **Lobstein′s g.,** a ganglion on the greater splanchnic nerve above the diaphragm; probably the same as the splanchnic ganglion. **lower g. of glossopharyngeal nerve,** g. inferius nervi glossopharyngei. **lower g. of vagus nerve,** g. inferius nervi vagi. **Ludwig′s g.,** a ganglion connected with the cardiac plexus and situated near the right atrium of the heart. **gan′glia lumba′lia** [NA], **lumbar ganglia,** the ganglia on the lumbar part of the sympathetic trunk, usually four or five on either side. Called also *ganglia lumbaria* [NA alternative]. **gan′glia lumba′ria,** NA alternative for *ganglia lumbalia.* **Luschka′s g.,** glomus coccygeum. **gan′glia lymphat′ica,** lymph nodes; see *nodus lymphaticus.* **Meckel′s g.,** g. pterygopalatinum. **Meissner′s g.,** one of the small groups of nerve cells in the submucosal (Meissner′s) plexus. **mesenteric g., inferior,** g. mesentericum inferius. **mesenteric g., superior,** g. mesentericum superius. **g. mesenter′icum infe′rius** [NA], inferior mesenteric ganglion: a sympathetic ganglion in the inferior mesenteric plexus near the beginning of the inferior mesenteric artery. **g. mesenter′icum supe′rius** [NA], superior mesenteric ganglion: one or more sympathetic ganglia at the sides of, or just below, the superior mesenteric artery; commonly fused with the celiac ganglia. **g. of Müller,** g. superius nervi glossopharyngei. **nerve g., neural g.,** ganglion, def. 2. **g. ner′vi splanch′nici,** g. splanchnicum. **nodose g., g. nodo′sum,** g. caudalis nervi vagi. **olfactory g.,** a mass of tissue in the embryo which develops into the olfactory nerves. **otic g., g. o′ticum** [NA], a parasympathetic ganglion in the infratemporal fossa, medial to the mandibular nerve and just inferior to the foramen ovale: its preganglionic fibers are derived from the glossopharyngeal nerve via the lesser petrosal nerve, and its postganglionic fibers supply the parotid gland. Sensory and postganglionic sympathetic fibers pass through the ganglion. **parasympathetic g., g. parasympathet′icum,** NA alternative for *g. parasympathicum.* **g. parasympath′icum** [NA], one of the aggregations of cell bodies of primarily cholinergic neurons of the parasympathetic nervous system, which are located near to or within the wall of the organs being innervated; called also *g. parasympatheticum* [NA alternative] and *parasympathetic g.* See also *cholinergic.* **pelvic ganglia, gan′glia pelvi′na** [NA], small sympathetic and parasympathetic ganglia located within the pelvic plexus. **periosteal g.,** periostitis albuminosa. **petrosal g., petrosal g., inferior, petrous g.,** g. caudalis nervi glossopharyngei. **phrenic g., gan′glia phren′ica** [NA], a small sympathetic ganglion often found within the phrenic plexus at its junction with the celiac plexus. **gan′glia plex′uum autonomico′rum** [NA], **gan′glia plex′uum sympathico′rum,** ganglia of autonomic plexuses: groups of nerve cell bodies found in the autonomic plexuses, composed primarily of sympathetic postganglionic neurons; called also *ganglia of sympathetic* or *visceral plexuses* and *ganglia plexuum visceralium* [NA alternative]. **gan′glia plex′uum viscera′lium,** NA alternative for *g. plexuum autonomicorum.* **prevertebral ganglia,** sympathetic ganglia (other than those of the sympathetic trunk) in the prevertebral plexuses of the thorax and abdomen. **primary g.,** a ganglion on a tendon or aponeurosis that does not follow a local inflammation. **pterygopalatine g., g. pterygopalati′num** [NA], a parasympathetic ganglion in the pterygopalatine fossa; its preganglionic fibers are derived from the facial nerve via the greater petrosal nerve and the nerve of the pterygopalatine canal. Its postganglionic fibers supply the lacrimal, nasal, and palatine glands; sensory and

sympathetic fibers pass through the ganglion. Called also *Meckel′s g., sphenopalatine g.,* and *g. sphenopalatinum.* **Remak′s g.,** a sympathetic ganglion in the heart wall near the superior vena cava; called also *sinoatrial g.* Also, sympathetic ganglia in the diaphragmatic opening for the inferior vena cava, as well as ganglia in the gastric plexus. **renal ganglia, gan′glia rena′lia** [NA], small sympathetic ganglia within the renal plexus. **Ribes′ g.,** the alleged ganglion in the termination of the internal carotid plexus around the anterior communicating artery of the brain. **g. rostra′lis ner′vi glossopharyn′gei** [NA], rostral ganglion of glossopharyngeal nerve: the upper of two ganglia on the glossopharyngeal nerve as it passes through the jugular foramen; both ganglia contain cell bodies of afferent fibers of the nerve. Called also *g. superius nervi glossopharyngei* [NA alternative], *jugular g. of glossopharyngeal nerve,* and *superior g. of glossopharyngeal nerve.* **g. rostra′lis ner′vi va′gi** [NA], the rostral ganglion of vagus nerve: a small ganglion on the vagus in the jugular foramen, giving off a meningeal and an auricular branch and containing cell bodies for afferent fibers of the vagus. Called also *g. superius nervi vagi* [NA alternative], *jugular g. of vagus nerve,* and *superior g. of vagus nerve.* **sacral ganglia, gan′glia sacra′lia** [NA], the ganglia of the sacral part of the sympathetic trunk, usually three or four on either side. **Scarpa′s g.,** g. vestibulare. **Schacher′s g.,** g. ciliare. **Schmiedel′s g.,** 1. carotid g. 2. inferior carotid g. **semilunar g.,** 1. ganglion trigeminale. 2. [pl.] ganglia celiaca. **g. semiluna′re [Gas′seri],** g. trigeminale. **gan′glia senso′ria, sensory ganglia,** 1. ganglia craniospinalia. 2. ganglia spinalia. **g. sensoria′le,** NA alternative for *g. spinale.* **gan′glia sensoria′lia,** 1. ganglia craniospinalia. 2. ganglia spinalia. **gan′glia senso′ria nervo′rum crania′lium** [NA], sensory ganglia of cranial nerves: the ganglia on the roots of the cranial nerves that contain the cell bodies of afferent (sensory) neurons; called also *ganglia sensorialia nervorum encephalici* [NA alternative], *sensory ganglia of cranial nerves,* and *sensory ganglia of encephalic nerves.* **gan′glia senso′ria′lia ner′vi encepha′lici,** NA alternative for *ganglia sensorialia nervi cranialium.* **g. senso′rius, sensory g.,** g. spinale. **sensory ganglia of cranial nerves, sensory ganglia of encephalic nerves,** ganglia sensorialia nervi cranialium. **simple g.,** a cystic tumor in a tendon sheath. **sinoatrial g.,** Remak′s g. **sinus g.,** a group of nerve cells around the junction of the coronary sinus and the right atrium of the heart. **sphenomaxillary g., sphenopalatine g., g. sphenopalati′num,** g. pterygopalatinum. **spinal ganglia, gan′glia spina′lia** [NA], the craniospinal ganglia on the dorsal roots of the spinal nerves; called also *ganglia sensorialia* [NA alternative], *ganglia sensoria,* and *sensory ganglia.* See also *ganglion spinale.* **spinal g., g. spina′le** [NA], the ganglion found on the dorsal root of each spinal nerve, composed of the unipolar nerve cell bodies of the sensory neurons of the nerve. Called also *g. sensorius* [NA alternative], *sensory g.,* and *g. sensoriale.* See also *ganglia spinalia.* **spiral g., spiral g. of cochlea,** g. cochleae. **spiral g. of cochlear nerve,** g. spirale partis cochlearis nervi octavi. **g. spira′le coch′leae,** NA alternative for *g. cochleare.* **splanchnic g., splanchnic thoracic g., g. splanch′nicum,** g. thoracicus splanchnicum. **stellate g.,** g. cervicothoracicum. **g. stella′tum,** NA alternative for *g. cervicothoracicum.* **sublingual g., g. sublingua′le** [NA], a ganglion of nerve cells sometimes found on the fibers passing distally from the submandibular ganglion to the lingual nerve. **submandibular g., g. submandibula′re** [NA], **g. submaxilla′re, submaxillary g.,** a parasympathetic ganglion located superior to the deep part of the submandibular gland, on the lateral surface of the hyoglossus muscle; its preganglionic fibers are derived from the facial nerve by way of the chorda tympani and lingual nerve, and its postganglionic fibers supply the submandibular and sublingual glands; sensory and postganglionic sympathetic fibers pass through the ganglion. **g. supe′rius ner′vi glossopharyn′gei,** NA alternative for *g. rostralis nervi glossopharyngei.* **g. supe′rius ner′vi va′gi,** NA alternative for *g. rostralis nervi vagi.* **suprarenal g.,** a small sympathetic ganglion in the suprarenal plexus. **sympathetic ganglia,** aggregations of cell bodies of primarily adrenergic neurons of the sympathetic nervous system; these ganglia are arranged in chainlike fashion on either side of the spinal cord. See also *adrenergic.*

ganglia of sympathetic plexuses, ganglia plexuum autonomicorum. **ganglia of sympathetic trunk,** ganglia trunci sympathici. **g. sympathet'icum,** NA alternative for *g. sympathicum.* **g. sympath'icum** [NA], any of the aggregations of cell bodies of primarily adrenergic neurons of the sympathetic nervous system, which are arranged in a chainlike fashion on either side of the spinal cord or in a collateral (paravertebral or prevertebral) position; called also *g. sympatheticum* [NA alternative] and *sympathetic g.* See also *adrenergic.* **synovial g.,** a myxoid cyst. **terminal g., g. termina'le** [NA], a group of nerve cells found along the terminal nerves, medial to the olfactory bulb. **gan'glia thoraca'lia, thoracic ganglia, gan'glia thora'cica** [NA], the ganglia on the thoracic portion of the sympathetic trunk, usually about eleven or twelve on either side. **g. thora'cicum pri'mum,** a portion of ganglion cervicothoracicum; it is present sometimes as a separate ganglion. **g. thora'cicum splanch'nicum** [NA], splanchnic thoracic ganglion: a small ganglion formed on the greater thoracic splanchnic nerve near the twelfth thoracic vertebra; called also *ganglion splanchnicum* and *splanchnic g.* **trigeminal g., g. of trigeminal nerve, g. trigemina'le** [NA], a ganglion on the sensory root of the fifth cranial nerve, situated in a cleft within the dura mater (trigeminal cave) on the anterior surface of the petrous portion of the temporal bone, and giving off the ophthalmic and maxillary and part of the mandibular nerve; it contains the cells of origin of most of the sensory fibers of the trigeminal nerve. Called also *semilunar g.,* and *g. semilunare* [Gasseri]. **Troisier's g.,** an enlarged lymph node sometimes seen above the clavicle in cases of retrosternal tumor. **gan'glia trun'ci sympath'ici** [NA], ganglia of sympathetic trunk: groups of nerve cell bodies found along each sympathetic trunk, about twenty to twenty-three on either side. **tympanic g.,** intumescentia tympanica. **tympanic g. of Valentin,** 1. a ganglion on a superior dental nerve. 2. intumescentia tympanica. **g. tympan'icum,** intumescentia tympanica. **upper g.,** g. superius nervi glossopharyngei. **vagal g., inferior,** g. inferius nervi vagi. **vagal g., superior,** g. superius nervi vagi. **g. of vagus nerve, caudal, g. of vagus nerve, inferior,** g. caudalis nervi vagi. **g. of vagus nerve, rostral, g. of vagus nerve, superior,** g. rostralis nervi vagi. **Valentin's g.,** 1. intumescentia tympanica. 2. a ganglion on a superior dental nerve. **ventricular g.,** Bidder's g. **vertebral g., g. vertebra'le** [NA], a small ganglion almost always present between the middle and inferior sympathetic ganglion, usually anterior to the vertebral artery; it contributes to the ansa subclavia and sends postganglionic fibers to the vertebral nerve and plexus and to the brachial plexus. Called also *g. intermediaire.* **vestibular g., g. vestibula're** [NA], the sensory ganglion located in the upper part of the lateral end of the internal acoustic meatus; the bipolar nerve cells of which give rise to the fibers of the vestibular nerve. **gan'glia viscera'lia,** NA alternative for *ganglia autonomica.* **ganglia of visceral plexuses,** ganglia plexuum autonomicorum. **Wrisberg's g., g. Wrisbergi,** see *ganglia cardiaca.* **wrist g.,** cystic enlargement of a tendon sheath on the back of the wrist.

ganglionated (gang'gle-o-nāt-ed) provided with ganglia.

ganglionectomy (gang''gle-o-nek'to-me) [*ganglio-* + Gr. *ektomē* excision] excision of a ganglion.

ganglioneure (gang'gle-o-nūr'') [*ganglio-* + Gr. *neuron* nerve] any cell of a nervous ganglion.

ganglioneuroblastoma (gang''gle-o-nu''ro-blas-to'mah) a tumor composed of ganglioneuromatous and neuroblastomatous elements.

ganglioneurofibroma (gang''gle-o-nu''ro-fi-bro'mah) ganglioneuroma.

ganglioneuroma (gang''gle-o-nu-ro'mah) a benign neoplasm composed of nerve fibers and mature ganglion cells; regarded by many as a fully differentiated neuroblastoma.

ganglionic (gang''gle-on'ik) pertaining to a ganglion.

ganglionitis (gang''gle-on-i'tis) inflammation of a ganglion. **acute posterior g.,** herpes zoster. **gasserian g.,** herpes zoster ophthalmicus.

ganglionoplegic (gang''gle-on''o-ple'jik) ganglioplegic.

ganglionostomy (gang''gle-o-nos'to-me) [*ganglio-* + Gr. *stomoun* to provide with an opening, or mouth] surgical creation of an opening into a cystic tumor on a tendon sheath or aponeurosis.

ganglioplegic (gang''gle-o-ple'jik) [*ganglio-* + Gr. *plēgē* stroke] 1. blocking transmission of impulses through the sympathetic and parasympathetic ganglia. 2. an agent that blocks the transmission of impulses through the sympathetic and parasympathetic ganglia.

ganglioside (gang'gle-o-sīd) a general designation for a member of a class of galactose-containing cerebrosides found in the tissues of the central nervous system. Gangliosides are glycolipids of the basic composition ceramide-glucose-galactose-N-acetyl neuraminic acid. **g. GM₁,** a ganglioside with the addition of an N-acetyl galactosamine and a galactose group; it accumulates in tissues in generalized gangliosidosis. **g. GM₂,** a ganglioside with the addition of N-acetyl galactosamine at the terminal; it accumulates in tissues in Tay-Sachs disease.

gangliosidosis (gang''gle-o-si-do'sis), pl. *gangliosidoses.* a group of lysosomal storage diseases of which most are generally characterized by a defective glycohydrolase, by storage of GM_1 or GM_2 ganglioside and related glycolipids or oligosaccharides, and by progressive psychomotor deterioration usually beginning in infancy or childhood and usually fatal. There are two subgroups of gangliosidosis. *GM_1 gangliosidosis* is caused by a defect in acid β-galactosidase, is characterized by defective bones, foam cells in the bone marrow, vacuolated lymphocytes, visceral histiocytosis, and dysarthria; it occurs in three main types: *infantile* or *type 1* or *generalized; juvenile* or *type 2;* and *adult* or *type 3.* Gm_2 *gangliosidosis* occurs in four main types: *Tay-Sachs disease,* caused by a severe deficiency of hexosaminidase A; *Sandhoff disease,* caused by a severe deficiency of hexosaminidase A and B; and *juvenile GM_2 gangliosidosis* and *adult (chronic) GM_2 gangliosidosis,* both caused by a deficiency of hexosaminidase A. See *amaurotic familial idiocy,* under *idiocy.* **generalized g.,** the severest type of GM_1 gangliosidosis, characterized by onset at birth, coarse facies, edema, hepatosplenomegaly, cherry-red macular spot (in 50 per cent of the infants), early blindness, hyperacusis, macroglossia, seizures, glomerular epithelial ballooning, and hypotonia; mucopolysacchariduria may be present; the children die by the age of 2. **GM₁ g.,** generalized g. **GM₁ g., adult,** the least severe type of GM_1 gangliosidosis, characterized by onset in the teens, spasticity, and ataxia; patients survive to over 20 years of age. **GM₁ g., infantile,** generalized g. **GM₁ g., juvenile,** a less severe type of GM_1 gangliosidosis, characterized by onset between 6 and 20 months, seizures, late blindness, glomerular epithelial ballooning, spasticity, and ataxia; mucopolysacchariduria may be present; the children survive to between 3 and 10 years of age. **GM₂ g.,** Tay-Sachs disease. **GM₂ g., adult,** the least severe type of GM_2 gangliosidosis, characterized by onset in the teens, dysarthria, spasticity, and ataxia; psychomotor deterioration and retinitis pigmentosa are sometimes present; patients survive to over 20 years of age. **GM₂ g., juvenile,** a less severe type of GM_2 gangliosidosis, characterized by onset between 2 and 6 years of age, hyperacusis, seizures, late blindness, dysarthria, spasticity, and ataxia; patients survive to between 5 and 15 years of age.

gangliospore (gang'gle-o-spōr) a fungal spore developed from the swollen tip of a hypha.

gangliosympathectomy (gang''gle-o-sim''pah-thek'to-me) excision of a sympathetic ganglion.

gangosa (gang-go'sah) [Sp. "muffled voice"] a late sequel of yaws, leprosy, leishmaniasi and endemic syphilis manifested by a massive and grossly mutilating ulcerative destruction of the nose, soft and hard palates, and pharynx. Called also *rhinopharyngitis mutilans.*

gangrene (gang'grēn) [L. *gangraena;* Gr. *gangraina* an eating sore, which ends in mortification] death of tissue, usually in considerable mass and generally associated with loss of vascular (nutritive) supply and followed by bacterial invasion and putrefaction. Cf. *necrosis* and *necrobiosis.* **angiosclerotic g.,** dry gangrene caused by vascular sclerosis. **circumscribed g.,** gangrene that is clearly separated from normal tissue by a zone of inflammatory reaction. **cold g.,** gangrene that is not preceded by inflammation. **diabetic g.,** moist gangrene occurring in a person with diabetes; called also *glycemic g.* **dry g.,** necrosis occurring without subsequent bacterial decomposition, the tissues becoming dry and shriveled. **embolic g.,** that which follows the blocking of the blood supply by an embolism. **emphysematous g.,** gas g. **epidemic g.,** ergotism. **Fournier's g.,** an acute gangrenous infection of the scrotum, penis, or perineum involving gram-positive organisms, enteric bacilli, and anaerobes, which occurs following local trauma, operative procedures, an underlying urinary tract disease, or a distant acute inflammatory process. Called also *Fournier's disease.* **gas g., gaseous g.,** an acute, severe, and painful condition often resulting from dirty, lacerated wounds in which the muscles and subcutaneous tissues become filled with gas and a serosanguineous exudate. The condition is due to histotoxic infection by anaerobic bacteria, among which are *Clostridium perfringens, C. novyi, C. septicum* (*vibrion septique*), *C. sporogenes,* and other species of *Clostridium.* Called also *clostridial myonecrosis.* **glycemic g., glykemic g.,** diabetic g. **hot g.,** gangrene which follows an inflammation. **humid g.,** moist g. **inflammatory g.,** gangrene due to acute inflammation. **Meleney's g.,** see under *ulcer.* **Meleney's synergistic g.,** progressive synergistic g. **mephitic g.,** gas g. **moist g.,** necrosis of tissues, with proteolytic decomposition resulting from bacterial action. **pressure g.,** gangrene due to pressure, as in decubitus ulcer. **primary g.,** gangrene occurring without preceding inflammation of the part. **progressive g.,** gangrene in which an effective limiting zone of inflammatory reaction does not form. **progressive bacterial synergistic g.,** progressive synergistic g. **progressive synergistic g., progressive synergistic bacterial g.,** gangrene of the skin due to a mixed infection caused by the synergistic action of aerobic hemolytic *Staphylococcus aureus* and a microaerophilic nonhemolytic streptococcus as well as gram-negative rods, which may occur as a complication of abdominal or thoracic surgery or after any type of traumatic wound. The characteristic lesion presents as a wide area of pale red cellulitis that subsequently ulcerates and gradually enlarges to form a large ulcerative plaque, typically with a central area of granulation tissue encircled by gangrenous skin that is in turn surrounded by a markedly undermined and rolled, bluish purple border. Called also *burrowing phagedenic ulcer, Meleney's ulcer, Meleney's chronic undermining ulcer, Meleney's synergistic g., progressive bacterial synergistic g.,* and *undermining burrowing ulcer.* See also *Meleney's ulcer* (def. 1), under *ulcer.* **Raynaud's g.,** Raynaud's disease, def. 1. **secondary g.,** a form which follows a local inflammation. **senile g.,** dry gangrene affecting the extremities of the aged. **static g.,** gangrene that results from stasis of blood in a part. **symmetric g.,** gangrene of corresponding digits on both sides, due to vasomotor disturbances. **sympathetic g.,** gangrene which results from some primary condition. **thrombotic g.,** gangrene from thrombosis of an artery. **traumatic g.,** gangrene which occurs as a consequence of accidental injury. **trophic g.,** gangrene due to lesion of the trophic nerve supply of a part. **venous g.,** static g.

gangrenosis (gang″grĕ-no′sis) the development of gangrene.

gangrenous (gang′grĕ-nus) pertaining to, characterized by, or of the nature of gangrene.

ganja (gan′jah) an Asian Indian preparation of *Cannabis sativa* in which an infusion is made from the mature female plant tops of very carefully selected, cultivated varieties. It may also be smoked and, when incorporated into sweet-meats, is known as majoon.

ganoblast (gan′o-blast) ameloblast.

Ganser's commissure, ganglion, symptom, syndrome (gan′serz) [Sigbert Joseph Maria *Ganser,* psychiatrist in Dresden, 1853–1931] see under *symptom* and *syndrome,* and see *nucleus interpeduncularis* and *supraoptic commissure,* under *commissure.*

Gant's clamp (gants) [Samuel Goodwin *Gant,* New York proctologist, 1870–1944] see under *clamp.*

Gantanol (gan′tah-nol) trademark for preparations of sulfamethoxazole.

Gantrisin (gan′trĭ-sin) trademark for preparations of sulfisoxazole.

gap (gap) an unoccupied interval in time; an opening or hiatus. **air-bone g.,** the lag between the audiographic curves for air- and bone-conducted stimuli, as an indication of a conductive hearing loss. **auscultatory g.,** time in which sound is not heard in the auscultatory method of sphygmomanometry, occurring particularly in hypertension

and in aortic stenosis. **Bochdalek's g.,** hiatus pleuroperitonealis. **chromatid g.,** a nonstaining region in a chromatid, the portions of the chromatid immediately proximal and distal to the site remaining in alignment. **interocclusal g.,** see under *distance.* **isochromatid g.,** a nonstaining region of the same level in two sister chromatids, the distal segments remaining in alignment with the proximal portions. **silent g.,** auscultatory g.

GAPD glyceraldehyde-3-phosphate dehydrogenase.

gapes (gāps) a disease of young fowls and turkeys caused by the gapeworm *Syngamus trachea* and marked by gasping and choking.

Garamycin (gar-ah-mi′sin) trademark for a preparation of gentamicin sulfate.

Garcinia (gar-sin′e-ah) a genus of guttiferous fruit trees widely cultivated in the tropics. *G. hanburyi* Hook. f. is the source of gamboge, *G. mangostana* L. of mangosteen, a delicious berry.

Gardiner-Brown's test [Alfred *Gardiner-Brown,* English otologist] see under *tests.*

Gardner's syndrome (gard′nerz) [Eldon J. *Gardner,* American geneticist, born 1909] see under *syndrome.*

Gardnerella (gard″ner-el′ah) [H. L. *Gardner,* American bacteriologist] a genus of small, pleomorphic, gram-negative, rod-shaped bacteria found in the normal female genital tract and also as a major cause of bacterial vaginitis. It comprises a single species, *G. vagina′lis.* Formerly called *Haemophilus vaginalis.*

Garel's sign (gar-elz′) [Jean *Garel,* French physician, 1852–1931] see under *sign.*

Garg. abbreviation for L. *gargaris′mus,* gargle.

gargalanesthesia (gar″g′l-an″es-the′ze-ah) absence of the tickle sense.

gargalesthesia (gar″g′l-es-the′ze-ah) the sense which perceives tickling sensations.

gargalesthetic (gar″g′l-es-thet′ik) pertaining to the tickle sense.

garget (gar′get) mastitis in the cow.

gargle (gar′g′l) [L. *gargarisma*] 1. to agitate a solution in the throat by forcing air through it so as to rinse or medicate the mucous membranes. 2. a solution used for rinsing or medicating the mouth and throat.

gargoylism (gar′goil-izm) Hurler's syndrome.

Garland's curve, triangle (gar′landz) [George Minot *Garland,* American physician, 1848–1926] see *Ellis' line,* under *line,* and see under *triangle.*

garment (gar′ment) an article of clothing. **pneumatic antishock g.,** an inflatable garment used to combat shock, stabilize fractures, promote hemostasis, increase peripheral vascular resistance, and permit autotransfusion of small amounts of blood.

garnet (gar′net) a silicate of any combination of aluminum, cobalt, magnesium, iron, and manganese. Garnet particles are one of the abrasives commonly used on dental disks.

Garré's osteomyelitis (disease, osteitis) (gar-āz′) [Carl *Garré,* Swiss surgeon, 1858–1928] sclerosing nonsuppurative osteomyelitis; see under *osteomyelitis.*

Gärtner's bacillus (gairt′nerz) [August *Gärtner,* German bacteriologist, 1848–1934] *Salmonella enteritidis.*

Gartner's cyst, duct (canal) (gart′nerz) [Hermann Treschow *Gartner,* Danish surgeon and anatomist, 1785–1827] see under *cyst,* and see *ductus epoöphorontis longitudinales.*

Gärtner's phenomenon, tonometer (gairt′nerz) [Gustav *Gärtner,* Austrian pathologist, 1855–1937] see under *phenomenon* and *tonometer.*

Garymicin (gar″ĭ-mi′sin) trademark for a preparation of gentamicin.

gas (gas) any elastic aeriform fluid in which the molecules are separated from one another and so have free paths. **alveolar g.,** the gas in the alveoli of the lungs, where gaseous exchange with the capillary blood takes place; called also *alveolar air.* **coal g.,** a gas produced by the destructive distillation of coal and much used for domestic cooking; it is poisonous because it contains carbon monoxide. **ethyl g.,** tetraethyl lead. **expired g.,** gas expired from the lungs, especially a mixture of gas from the dead space and alveolar gas. **hemolytic g.,** arsine. **inert g.,** a gas that does not react chemically with the other constituents of a system, especially in reference to the noble gases, such as helium and argon. **lacrimator g.,** tear g. **laughing g.,** nitrous oxide. **marsh g.,** methane. **mustard g.,** dichlorodiethyl sulfide. **noble g.,** the gas elements of group VIII of the periodic table, i.e., helium, neon, argon, krypton, xenon, and radon. **sewer g.,** the mixture of gases and vapors from a sewer; often dangerous from the contained materials resulting from the decay of organic matter. **sneezing g.,** diphenylchlorarsine. **suffocating g.,** any of several war gases, e.g., phosgene or dephosgene oxychlor carbon, that causes intense irritation of the bronchial tubes and lungs, resulting in pulmonary edema. **sweet g.,** carbon monoxide. **tear g.,** a gas which produces severe lacrimation by irritating the conjunctivae. **vesicating g.,** dichlorodiethyl sulfide. **war g.,** any noxious gas manufactured for possible use in warfare.

gaseous (gas′e-us, gash′us) of the nature of a gas.

gasiform (gas′ĭ-form) gaseous.

Gaskell's bridge (gas′kelz) [Walter Holbrook *Gaskell*, English physiologist, 1847–1914] bundle of His.

gaskin (gas′kin) the thigh of a horse.

gasogenic (gas-o-jen′ik) producing gas.

gasometer (gas-om′ĕ-ter) a calibrated container for measuring the volume of gases.

gasometric (gas″o-met′rik) pertaining to gasometry.

gasometry (gas-om′ĕ-tre) [*gas* + Gr. *metron* measure] the chemical determination of the amount of gas present in a mixture.

Gasser (gas′er), Herbert Spencer. American physiologist, 1888–1963, noted for his work on the nervous system; co-winner, with E. Joseph Erlanger, of the Nobel prize for medicine or physiology in 1944.

Gasser's ganglion (gas′erz) [Johann Laurentius *Gasser*, professor in Vienna from 1757 to 1765] ganglion trigeminale.

Gasser's syndrome (gas′erz) [Konrad Joseph *Gasser*, Swiss pediatrician, born 1912] see *hemolytic-uremic syndrome,* under *syndrome.*

gasserian (gas-se′re-an) named for Johann Laurentius *Gasser,* as gasserian (trigeminal) ganglion.

gaster (gas′ter) [Gr. *gastēr* the stomach] [NA] the stomach: the musculomembranous expansion of the alimentary tract between the esophagus and the duodenum. Called also *ventriculus* [NA alternative]. The proximal portion is the cardiac part; the portion above the entrance of the esophagus is the fundus; the distal portion is the pyloric part; and the body is between the fundus and the pyloric part. The upper concave surface or edge is the *lesser* curvature; the lower convex edge is the *greater* curvature. The coats of the stomach are four; an outer, peritoneal, or *serous* coat; a *muscular* coat, made up of longitudinal, oblique, and circular fibers; a *submucous* coat; and the *mucous* coat or membrane forming the inner lining. Gastric glands, which are in the mucous coat, secrete gastric juice containing hydrochloric acid, pepsin, and various other digestive enzymes into the cavity of the stomach. Food mixed with this secretion forms a semifluid substance (chyme) suitable for further digestion by the intestine.

gasteralgia (gas-ter-al′je-ah) (*obs.*) gastric colic.

gasterangiemphraxis (gas″ter-an″je-em-frak′sis) [*gaster* + Gr. *angeion* vessel + *emphraxis* obstruction] (*obs.*) obstruction of the blood vessels of the stomach.

gasteremphraxis (gas″ter-em-frak′sis) (*obs.*) 1. gasterangiemphraxis. 2. distention of the stomach.

Gasteromycetes (gas″ter-o-mi-se′tēz) a series of basidiomycetous fungi of the subclass Homobasidiomycetidae, including the puffballs and stinkhorns, in which the spores are arranged around a columella; it includes the genera *Lycoperdon, Calvatia, Geaster,* and *Phallus.*

Gasterophilus (gas″ter-of′i-lus) [*gaster* + Gr. *philein* to love] a genus of dipterous insects of the family Oestridae. *G. intestinalis* is the botfly whose larva infests horses. Migration of the larva beneath the skin of their occasional human hosts may give rise to a form of creeping eruption (larva migrans). *G. hemorrhoidalis,* the nose botfly, which has orange-red terminal segments, sometimes infests man.

gastradenitis (gas″trad-ĕ-ni′tis) [*gastr-* + Gr. *adēn* gland + *-itis*] inflammation of the stomach glands.

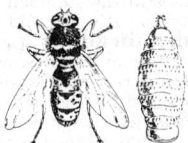

Gasterophilus and larva.

gastralgia (gas-tral′je-ah) [*gastr-* + *-algia*] gastric colic.

gastralgokenosis (gas-tral″go-ke-no′sis) [*gastr-* + Gr. *algos* pain + *kenōsis* emptiness] paroxysmal gastric pain when the stomach is empty, which is easily relieved by taking food.

gastramine hydrochloride (gas′trah-min) betazole hydrochloride.

gastratrophia (gas″trah-tro′fe-ah) [*gastr-* + Gr. *atrophia* atrophy] atrophic gastritis.

gastrectasia, gastrectasis (gas-trek-ta′ze-ah; gas-trek′tah-sis) [*gastr-* + Gr. *ektasis* stretching] (*obs.*) dilatation of the stomach.

gastrectomy (gas-trek′to-me) [*gastr-* + Gr. *ektomē* excision] excision of the whole (total g.) or part (subtotal g., partial g., gastric resection) of the stomach.

gastric (gas′trik) [L. *gastricus;* Gr. *gastēr* stomach] pertaining to, affecting, or originating in the stomach.

gastricsin (gas-trik′sin) pepsin C.

gastrin (gas′trin) a polypeptide hormone released from peptidergic fibers in the vagus nerve and from G cells in the pyloric glands in the gastric antrum. It occurs in several molecular sizes, among them little gastrin (G_{17}), with a chain length of 17 amino acids, big gastrin (G_{34}), minigastrin (G_{14}), big big gastrin, and component I. Gastrin stimulates secretion of gastric acid (causing contraction of the lower esophageal sphincter and modifying gastric and esophageal motility) and pepsin, increases growth of acid-secreting mucosa, and weakly stimulates secretion of pancreatic enzymes and gallbladder contraction.

gastrinoma (gas″trin-o′mah) a gastrin-secreting non–beta islet cell tumor associated with Zollinger-Ellison syndrome, usually found within the substance of the pancreas but also occurring at other sites, as in the antrum of the stomach, hilus of the spleen, and regional lymph nodes.

gastritic (gas-trit′ik) pertaining to or affected with gastritis.

gastritis (gas-tri′tis) [*gastr-* + *-itis*] inflammation of the stomach. **antral g., antrum g.,** inflammation affecting the antrum of the stomach. **atrophic g.,** chronic gastritis with atrophy of the mucous membrane and glands. **atrophic-hyperplastic g.,** a variant of atrophic gastritis in which the mucosa is of normal or even increased thickness. **catarrhal g.,** inflammation of the mucous membrane of the stomach, with hypertrophy of the membrane, secretion of an excessive quantity of mucus, and alteration of the gastric juice. The condition is marked by loss of appetite, nausea, pain, vomiting, and tympanitic distention of the stomach. **chemical g.,** inflammation caused by the ingestion of corrosive substances, with complete mucosal destruction in fatal cases; called also *corrosive g.* **chronic cystic g.,** gastritis in which the gastric and pyloric glands are dilated and lined by flattened epithelium, suggestive of a degenerative rather than an inflammatory condition. **chronic follicular g.,** an atrophic gastritis in which the size and number of lymphoid follicles in the mucosa and submucosa are greatly increased, with heavy infiltration of the entire mucosa by lymphocytes. **cirrhotic g.,** linitis plastica. **corrosive g.,** chemical g. **eosinophilic g.,** gastritis in which there is considerable edema and a heavy infiltration of all coats of the wall of the pyloric antrum by eosinophils. **erosive g.,** gastritis in which the surface epithelium is eroded, manifesting as a patchy or a diffuse lesion; exfoliative g. **exfoliative g.,** chronic gastritis in which bits of the surface of the mucous membrane are shed; erosive g. **follicular g.,** inflammation of the glands of the stomach. **giant hypertrophic g.,** excessive proliferation of the gastric mucosa, producing diffuse thickening of the stomach wall; inflammatory changes may be associated. Called also *Ménétrier's disease.* **hemorrhagic g.,** erosive gastritis with bleeding. **hypertrophic g.,** gastritis with infiltration and enlargement of the glands. **phlegmonous g.,**

a variety with abscesses in the stomach walls. **polypous g.,** hypertrophic gastritis with polypoid projections into the stomach. **pseudomembranous g.,** a variety in which a false membrane occurs in patches within the stomach. **radiation g.,** gastritis resulting from radiation injury. **toxic g.,** gastritis caused by the action of a poison or a corrosive agent. **zonal g.,** gastritis occurring in the vicinity of a gastric lesion, as that associated with peptic ulcer and gastric carcinoma.

gastr(o)- [Gr. *gastēr* stomach]   a combining form denoting relationship to the stomach.

gastroacephalus (gas″tro-a-sef′ah-lus) [*gastro-* + *a* neg. + Gr. *kephalē* head]   a twin monster, the autosite bearing a headless parasite on its abdomen.

gastroadenitis (gas″tro-ad″ĕ-ni′tis)   gastradenitis.

gastroadynamic (gas″tro-a″di-nam′ik)   marked by an adynamic condition of the stomach.

gastroamorphus (gas″tro-a-mor′fus) [*gastro-* + Gr. *a* neg. + *morphē* form]   a presumptive twin monster in which the parasite consists of fetal parts concealed within the abdomen of the autosite.

gastroanastomosis (gas″tro-ah-nas″to-mo′sis)   gastrogastrostomy.

gastroatonia (gas″tro-ah-to′ne-ah)   (obs.) atony of the stomach.

gastrocamera (gas″tro-kam′er-ah)   a small camera which can be swallowed or passed down the esophagus on an appropriate instrument to photograph the inside of the stomach; it is attached to an external control box by a hollow flexible tube, and fitted with a flash lamp and inflation bulb. After the camera is inserted into the stomach, the bulb is inflated and pictures are taken as the flash lamp is triggered.

gastrocardiac (gas″tro-kar′de-ak)   pertaining to the stomach and the heart.

gastrocele (gas′tro-sēl) [*gastro-* + Gr. *kēlē* hernia]   hernial protrusion of the stomach or of a gastric pouch.

gastrocnemius (gas″trok-ne′me-us) [*gastro-* + Gr. *knēmē* leg]   see Table of *Musculi*.

gastrocoele (gas′tro-sēl) [*gastro-* + Gr. *koilos* hollow]   the archenteron.

gastrocolic (gas″tro-kol′ik)   pertaining to or communicating with the stomach and colon, as a gastrocolic fistula.

gastrocolitis (gas″tro-ko-li′tis) [*gastro-* + Gr. *kolon* colon + *-itis*]   inflammation of the stomach and colon.

gastrocolostomy (gas″tro-ko-los′to-me) [*gastro-* + Gr. *kolon* colon + *stomoun* to provide with an opening, or mouth]   the creation of an artificial opening between the stomach and the colon; also, the opening so established.

gastrocolotomy (gas″tro-ko-lot′o-me) [*gastro-* + Gr. *kolon* colon + *tomē* a cutting]   incision into the stomach and colon.

gastrocutaneous (gas″tro-ku-ta′ne-us)   pertaining to the stomach and skin, or communicating with the stomach and the cutaneous surface of the body, as a gastrocutaneous fistula.

gastrodermis (gas″tro-der′mis) [*gastro-* + Gr. *derma* skin]   the tissue lining the gut cavity of an invertebrate, which is responsible for digestion and absorption.

gastrodiaphane (gas″tro-di′ah-fān) [*gastro-* + Gr. *dia* through + *phainein* to show]   a small electric lamp introduced into the stomach in gastrodiaphany.

gastrodiaphanoscopy (gas″tro-di-af″ah-nos′ko-pe) [*gastro-* + Gr. *dia* through + *phainein* to show + *skopein* to examine]   gastrodiaphany.

gastrodiaphany (gas″tro-di-af′ah-ne) [*gastro-* + Gr. *dia* through + *phainein* to show]   the exploration of the stomach by means of an electric lamp passed down the esophagus.

gastrodidymus (gas″tro-did′ĭ-mus) [*gastro-* + Gr. *didymos* twin]   symmetrical conjoined twins joined in the abdominal region.

gastrodisciasis (gas″tro-dis-ki′ah-sis)   infection caused by *Gastrodiscoides hominis.*

Gastrodiscoides (gas″tro-dis-koi′dēz) [*gastro-* + Gr. *diskos* disk + *eidos* form]   a genus of trematodes parasitic in the intestinal tract; called also *Gastrodiscus.* **G. hom′inis,** a species common in the cecum and large intestine of pigs and occasionally in man, in Indochina, India, and Malaysia. Called also *Amphistomum hominis.*

Gastrodiscus (gas″tro-dis′kus)   *Gastrodiscoides.*

gastrodisk (gas′tro-disk)   the embryonic disk.

gastroduodenal (gas″tro-du″o-de′nal)   pertaining to or communicating with the stomach and duodenum, as a gastroduodenal fistula.

gastroduodenectomy (gas″tro-du″o-dĕ-nek′to-me)   excision of stomach and duodenum.

gastroduodenitis (gas″tro-du-od″ĕ-ni′tis) [*gastro-* + *duodenitis*]   an inflammation of the stomach and duodenum.

gastroduodenoscopy (gas″tro-du″o-dĕ-nos′ko-pe) [*gastro-* + *duodenum* + Gr. *skopein* to examine]   examination of the stomach and duodenum, the gastroscope usually being passed through the mouth and esophagus; occasionally performed through incisions in the abdominal and gastric walls during laparotomy.

gastroduodenostomy (gas″tro-du″o-dĕ-nos′to-me) [*gastro-* + *duodenum* + Gr. *stomoun* to provide with an opening, or mouth]   surgical creation of an anastomosis between the stomach and the duodenum.

gastrodynia (gas″tro-din′e-ah) [*gastro-* + Gr. *odynē* pain]   pain in the stomach.

gastroenteralgia (gas″tro-en″ter-al′je-ah) [*gastro-* + Gr. *enteron* intestine + *-algia*]   pain in the stomach and intestines.

gastroenteric (gas″tro-en-ter′ik) [*gastro-* + Gr. *enteron* intestine]   pertaining to the stomach and intestines.

gastroenteritis (gas″tro-en-ter-i′tis) [*gastro-* + *enteritis*]   an acute inflammation of the lining of the stomach and intestines, characterized by anorexia, nausea, diarrhea, abdominal pain, and weakness, which has various causes, including food poisoning due to infection with such organisms as *Escherichia coli, Staphylococcus aureus,* and *Salmonella* species; consumption of irritating food or drink; or psychological factors such as anger, stress, and fear. Called also *enterogastritis.* **acute infectious g.,** gastritis with acute onset, caused by various bacteria and viruses. **eosinophilic g.,** a disorder marked by infiltration of the mucosa of the small intestine by eosinophils, with edema but without vasculitis, and by eosinophilia of the peripheral blood. Symptoms, including abdominal pain, diarrhea, nausea, fever, and malabsorption, depend on the site and extent of the disorder. The stomach is also frequently involved. The disorder is commonly associated with intolerance to specific foods. See also *eosinophilic granuloma* (def. 2), under *granuloma.* **Norwalk g.,** gastroenteritis caused by the Norwalk virus. **transmissible g. (T.G.E.) of swine,** a viral disease of swine occurring chiefly during the winter and characterized by severe diarrhea and acute inflammation of the gastric mucosa which may lead to ulceration and hemorrhage. The mortality rate among piglets is very high.

gastroenteroanastomosis (gas″tro-en″ter-o-ah-nas″to-mo′sis)   anastomosis between the stomach and small intestine in gastroenterostomy.

gastroenterocolitis (gas″tro-en″ter-o-ko-li′tis)   inflammation of the stomach, small intestine, and colon.

gastroenterocolostomy (gas″tro-en″ter-o-ko-los′to-me) [*gastro-* + Gr. *enteron* intestine + *kolon* colon + *stomoun* to provide with an opening, or mouth]   surgical creation of an opening between the stomach, intestine, and colon; also, the opening so established.

gastroenterologist (gas″tro-en″ter-ol′o-jist)   a practitioner who specializes in diseases of the digestive tract.

gastroenterology (gas″tro-en″ter-ol′o-je) [*gastro-* + Gr. *enteron* intestine + *-logy*]   the study of the stomach and intestines and their diseases.

gastroenteropathy (gas″tro-en″ter-op′ah-the)   any disease of the stomach and intestines.

gastroenteroplasty (gas″tro-en″ter-o-plas′te)   a plastic operation on the stomach and small intestine.

gastroenteroptosis (gas″tro-en″ter-op-to′sis) [*gastro-* + Gr. *enteron* intestine + *ptōsis* falling]   downward displacement, or prolapse, of the stomach and intestines; a term based on the concept that variations in the positions of organs cause disease.

gastroenterostomy (gas″tro-en-ter-os′to-me) [*gastro-* + Gr. *enteron* intestine + *stomoun* to provide with an opening, or mouth]   surgical creation of an artificial passage (anastomosis) between the stomach and intestines (usually the jejunum); see illustration.

gastroenterotomy (gas″tro-en″ter-ot′o-me) [*gastro-* + Gr. *enteron* intestine + *temnein* to cut] surgical incision into the stomach and intestine.

gastroepiploic (gas″tro-ep″ĭ-plo′ik) [*gastro-* + Gr. *epiploon* caul] pertaining to the stomach and epiploon (omentum).

gastroesophageal (gas″tro-ĕ-sof″ah-je′al) pertaining to the stomach and esophagus, as the gastroesophageal junction.

gastroesophagitis (gas″tro-ĕ-sof″ah-ji′tis) inflammation of the stomach and esophagus.

gastroesophagostomy (gas″tro-ĕ-sof″ah-gos′to-me) surgical creation of an anastomosis between the stomach and the esophagus; done for stricture of the lower end of the esophagus.

gastrofiberscope (gas″tro-fi′ber-skōp) a fiberoptic instrument for viewing the stomach.

gastrogastrostomy (gas″tro-gas-tros′to-me) [*gastro-* + *gastro-* + Gr. *stomoun* to provide with an opening, or mouth] surgical creation of an anastomosis between the pyloric and cardiac ends of the stomach, usually performed because of hourglass contraction of the middle third of the stomach; also, the anastomosis so established.

gastrogavage (gas″tro-gah-vazh′) [*gastro-* + Fr. *gavage* cramming] the introduction of nutriment into the stomach by means of a tube passed through the esophagus.

gastrogenic (gas″tro-jen′ik) formed or originating in the stomach.

Gastrografin (gas″tro-graf′in) trademark for a preparation of meglumine diatrizoate.

gastrograph (gas′tro-graf) [*gastro-* + Gr. *graphein* to record] an apparatus for recording the motions of the stomach.

gastrohepatic (gas″tro-hĕ-pat′ik) [*gastro-* + Gr. *hēpar* liver] pertaining to the stomach and liver.

gastrohepatitis (gas″tro-hep-ah-ti′tis) inflammation of the stomach and liver.

gastrohypertonic (gas″tro-hi″per-ton′ik) marked by excessive tonicity of the stomach.

gastroileac (gas″tro-il′e-ak) pertaining to stomach and ileum.

gastroileitis (gas″tro-il-e-i′tis) inflammation of the stomach and ileum.

gastroileostomy (gas″tro-il-e-os′to-me) surgical creation of an anastomosis between the stomach and ileum; also, the anastomosis so established.

gastrointestinal (gas″tro-in-tes′tĭ-nal) [*gastro-* + *intestinal*] pertaining to or communicating with the stomach and intestine, as a gastrointestinal fistula.

gastrojejunocolic (gas″tro-jĕ-ju″no-kol′ik) pertaining to or communicating with the stomach, jejunum, and colon, as a gastrojejunocolic fistula.

gastrojejunoesophagostomy (gas″tro-jĕ-ju″no-ĕ-sof″ah-gos′to-me) esophagojejunogastrostomy.

gastrojejunostomy (gas″tro-jĕ-ju-nos′to-me) [*gastro-* + *jejunostomy*] surgical creation of an anastomosis between the stomach and jejunum; also, the anastomosis so established.

gastrokinesograph (gas″tro-ki-nes′o-graf) [*gastro-* + Gr. *kinēsis* motion + *graphein* to record] a device for recording the mechanical motions of the stomach.

gastrolienal (gas″tro-li′en-al) [*gastro-* + L. *lien* spleen] pertaining to the stomach and spleen.

gastrolith (gas′tro-lith) [*gastro-* + Gr. *lithos* stone] a calcareous or other concretion formed in the stomach; called also *gastric* or *stomachic calculus.*

gastrolithiasis (gas″tro-lĭ-thi′ah-sis) [*gastro-* + Gr. *lithos* stone + *-iasis*] the presence or formation of gastroliths.

gastrologist (gas-trol′o-jist) a specialist in diseases of the stomach.

gastrology (gas-trol′o-je) [*gastro-* + *-logy*] the sum of knowledge regarding the stomach.

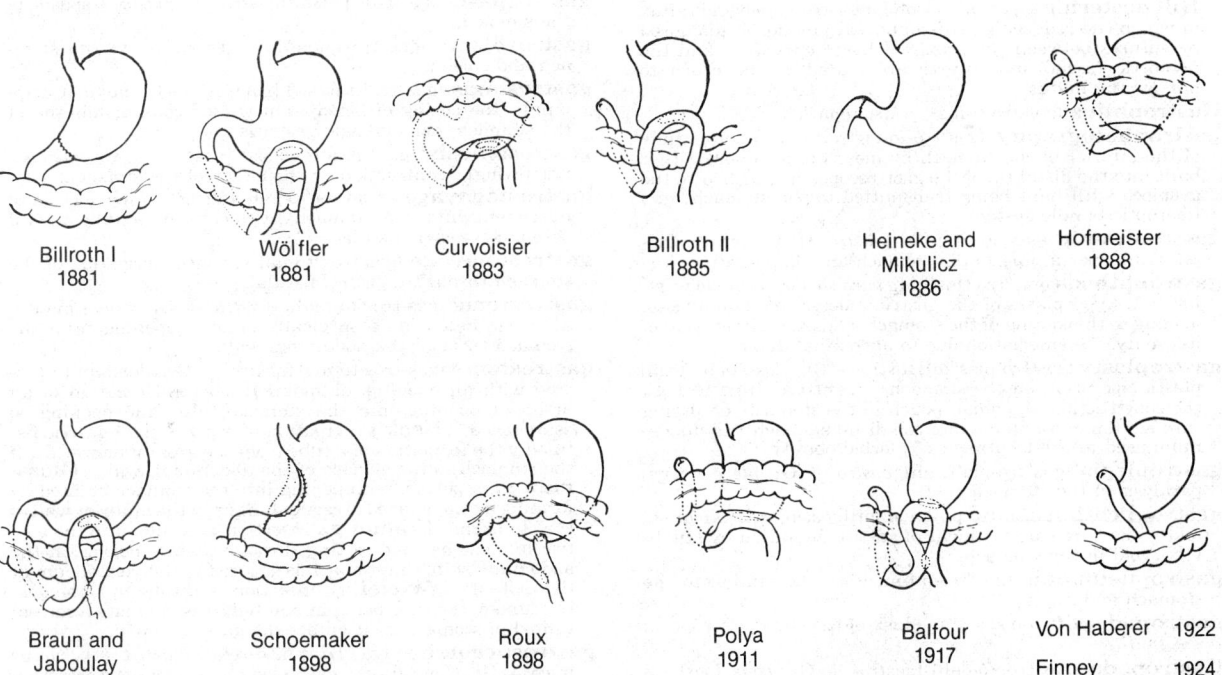

Billroth I 1881   Wölfler 1881   Curvoisier 1883   Billroth II 1885   Heineke and Mikulicz 1886   Hofmeister 1888

Braun and Jaboulay 1892   Schoemaker 1898   Roux 1898   Polya 1911   Balfour 1917   Von Haberer 1922   Finney 1924

Types of gastroenterostomy.

gastrolysis (gas-trol′ĭ-sis) [*gastro-* + Gr. *lysis* loosening] surgical division of perigastric adhesions in order to mobilize the stomach.

gastromalacia (gas″tro-mah-la′she-ah) [*gastro-* + Gr. *malakia* softening] an abnormal softening or softness of the wall of the stomach; see *softening of the stomach.*

gastromegaly (gas″tro-meg′ah-le) [*gastro-* + Gr. *megas* large] enlargement of the stomach.

gastromelus (gas-trom′ĕ-lus) [*gastro-* + Gr. *melos* limb] a monster with a supernumerary leg attached to the abdomen.

gastromycosis (gas″tro-mi-ko′sis) [*gastro-* + Gr. *mykēs* fungus] a disease of the stomach caused by fungi.

gastromyotomy (gas″tro-mi-ot′o-me) [*gastro-* + Gr. *mys* muscle + *temnein* to cut] incision through the muscular coats of the stomach down to the mucosa.

gastromyxorrhea (gas″tro-mik″so-re′ah) [*gastro-* + Gr. *myxa* mucus + *rhoia* flow] excessive secretion of mucus by the stomach.

gastrone (gas′trōn) a reputed hormonal inhibitor of gastric acid secretion, extracted from gastric mucus.

gastropancreatitis (gas″tro-pan″kre-ah-ti′tis) inflammation of the stomach and pancreas.

gastroparalysis (gas″tro-pah-ral′ĭ-sis) paralysis of the stomach; gastric atony; gastroparesis.

gastroparesis (gas″tro-par′ĕ-sis) [*gastro-* + Gr. *paresis* paralysis] paralysis of the stomach.

gastroparietal (gas″tro-pah-ri′ĕ-tal) pertaining to the stomach and the body wall.

gastropathic (gas″tro-path′ik) pertaining to disease of the stomach.

gastropathy (gas-trop′ah-the) [*gastro-* + Gr. *pathos* disease] any disease of the stomach.

gastroperiodynia (gas″tro-per″e-o-din′e-ah) [*gastro-* + Gr. *periodos* period + *odynē* pain] periodic attacks of pain in the stomach.

gastroperitonitis (gas″tro-per″ĭ-to-ni′tis) inflammation of the stomach and peritoneum.

gastropexy (gas′tro-pek″se) [*gastro-* + Gr. *pēxis* fixation] surgical fixation of the stomach to prevent displacement. **Hill posterior g.,** an operation for gastroesophageal reflux in which the reduced gastroesophageal junction is anchored by sutures between the proximal lesser curvature and the preaortic fascia, and sutures are placed in the crura to narrow the hiatus.

Gastrophilus (gas-trof′ĭ-lus) *Gasterophilus.*

gastrophotography (gas″tro-fo-tog′rah-fe) photography of the interior of the stomach by means of a camera either built into the distal tip of the gastroscope, or attached to the eyepiece with light being transmitted to the stomach by a fiberoptic bundle system.

gastrophrenic (gas″tro-fren′ik) [*gastro-* + Gr. *phrēn* diaphragm] pertaining to the stomach and diaphragm.

gastrophthisis (gas″tro-this′is) [*gastro-* + Gr. *phthisis* wasting] 1. hyperplasia of the gastric mucosa and submucosa, leading to thickening of the stomach walls and diminution of its cavity. 2. emaciation due to abdominal disease.

gastroplasty (gas′tro-plas″te) [*gastro-* + Gr. *plassein* to form] plastic operation on the stomach. **vertical banded g.,** the construction of a small pouch in the stomach, emptying through a narrow stoma into the distal stomach and duodenum; used in the treatment of morbid obesity.

gastroplegia (gas″tro-ple′je-ah) [*gastro-* + Gr. *plēgē* stroke] paralysis of the stomach.

gastroplication (gas″tro-pli-ka′shun) [*gastro-* + L. *plicare* to fold] the surgical treatment of gastric dilatation by stitching a fold in the stomach.

gastropneumonic (gas″tro-nu-mon′ik) pertaining to the stomach and lungs.

gastropod (gas′tro-pod) a mollusk of the class Gastropoda; see *snail.*

Gastropoda (gas-trop′ŏ-dah) [*gastro-* + Gr. *pous* foot] a class of mollusks embracing the snails, slugs, whelks, abalones, etc., including many species that serve as primary and intermediate hosts of pathogens.

gastroptosis (gas″tro-to′sis) [*gastro-* + Gr. *ptosis* falling] downward displacement of the stomach; a term based on the outmoded concept that variation in position of abdominal organs is pathological.

gastropulmonary (gas″tro-pul′mo-nar-e) [*gastro-* + L. *pulmo* lung] pertaining to the stomach and lungs.

gastropylorectomy (gas″tro-pi″lo-rek′to-me) [*gastro-* + Gr. *pylōros* pylorus + *ektomē* excision] excision of the pyloric portion of the stomach.

gastropyloric (gas″tro-pi-lor′ik) pertaining to the stomach in its entirety and to the pylorus.

gastroradiculitis (gas″tro-rah-dik″u-li′tis) [*gastro-* + L. *radix* root + *-itis*] inflammation of the posterior roots of spinal nerves involving irritation of the sensory fibers in them which are connected with the stomach.

gastrorrhagia (gas″tro-ra′je-ah) [*gastro-* + Gr. *rhēgnynai* to break forth] hemorrhage from the stomach.

gastrorrhaphy (gas-tror′ah-fe) [*gastro-* + Gr. *rhaphē* suture] suture of a wound of the stomach.

gastrorrhea (gas″tro-re′ah) [*gastro-* + Gr. *rhoia* flow] excessive secretion of mucus or gastric juice in the stomach; gastric hypersecretion.

gastrorrhexis (gas″tro-rek′sis) [*gastro-* + Gr. *rhēxis* rupture] rupture of the stomach.

gastroschisis (gas-tros′kĭ-sis) [*gastro-* + Gr. *schisis* cleft] a congenital fissure of the abdominal wall not involving the site of insertion of the umbilical cord, and usually accompanied by protrusion of the small and part of the large intestine.

gastroscope (gas′tro-skōp) [*gastro-* + Gr. *skopein* to examine] an endoscope for inspecting the interior of the stomach. **fiberoptic g.,** a fiberscope for examining the stomach.

gastroscopic (gas″tro-skop′ik) pertaining to gastroscopy or the gastroscope.

gastroscopy (gas-tros′ko-pe) [*gastro-* + Gr. *skopein* to examine] inspection of the interior of the stomach by means of the gastroscope.

gastroselective (gas″tro-sĕ-lek′tiv) having an affinity for receptors involved in regulation of gastric activities.

gastrosia (gas-tro′se-ah) a disease of the stomach. **g. fungo′sa,** a disease of the stomach caused by fungi or molds.

gastrosis (gas-tro′sis) any disease of the stomach.

gastrospasm (gas′tro-spazm) [*gastro-* + *spasm*] spasm of the stomach.

gastrosplenic (gas″tro-splen′ik) pertaining to the stomach and spleen.

gastrostaxis (gas″tro-stak′sis) [*gastro-* + Gr. *staxis* a dripping] the oozing of blood from the mucous membrane of the stomach; hemorrhagic gastritis.

gastrostenosis (gas″tro-stĕ-no′sis) [*gastro-* + Gr. *stenōsis* narrowing] contraction or shrinkage of the stomach.

gastrostogavage (gas-tros″to-gah-vahzh′) introduction of nutriment into the stomach by means of a tube passed through a gastric fistula.

gastrostolavage (gas-tros″to-lah-vahzh′) irrigation of the stomach through a gastric fistula.

gastrostoma (gas-tros′to-mah) [*gastro-* + Gr. *stoma* mouth] a gastric fistula or a surgically created opening from the stomach through the abdominal wall.

gastrostomy (gas-tros′to-me) [*gastro-* + Gr. *stomoun* to provide with an opening, or mouth] surgical creation of an artificial opening into the stomach; also, the opening so established. **Beck g.,** creation of a permanent gastric fistula by the formation of a tube from the greater curvature of the stomach to the surface of the abdominal wall. **Glassman g.,** a permanent opening into the stomach created by forming a cone-shaped diverticulum from the anterior wall of the stomach. **Stamm g.,** insertion of a tube into the gastric lumen, the tube exiting through a stab incision in the abdominal skin; the stomach is sutured to the peritoneum at the exit site. **Witzel g.,** insertion of a tube into the gastric lumen, the tube being implanted so as to create a serosal tunnel of stomach as it enters the gastric lumen.

gastrosuccorrhea (gas″tro-suk″o-re′ah) [*gastro-* + L. *succus* juice + Gr. *rhoia* flow] excessive and continuous secretion of gastric juice. **digestive g.,** a condition in which there is excessive secretion of gastric juice during digestion only.

gastrothoracopagus (gas″tro-tho″rah-kop′ah-gus) [*gastro-* + Gr. *thōrax* chest + *pagos* thing fixed] a double monster joined at the abdomen and thorax. **g. dipy′gus,** a double monster in which there is attached to the abdomen of the autosite a parasite consisting of the pelvis and lower extremities only; called also *dipygus parasiticus*.

gastrotome (gas′tro-tōm) a cutting instrument used in gastrotomy.

gastrotomy (gas-trot′o-me) [*gastro-* + Gr. *temnein* to cut] incision into the stomach.

gastrotonometer (gas″tro-to-nom′ĕ-ter) [*gastro-* + Gr. *tonos* tension + *metron* measure] an instrument for measuring intragastric pressure.

gastrotonometry (gas″tro-tro-nom′ĕ-tre) the measurement of intragastric pressure.

gastrotoxin (gas″tro-tok′sin) a substance that exerts a toxic effect on the stomach.

Gastrotricha (gas″tro-trik′ah) [*gastro-* + Gr. *trichos* hair] a class of very small aquatic animals of the phylum Aschelminthes, which have cilia on the ventral surface and a triradiate esophagus. In some systems of classification, they are considered to be a separate phylum.

gastrotropic (gas″tro-trop′ik) [*gastro-* + Gr. *tropos* a turning] having an affinity for or exerting a special effect upon the stomach.

gastrotympanites (gas″tro-tim″pah-ni′tēz) [*gastro-* + *tympanites*] tympanitic distention of the stomach.

gastrula (gas′troo-lah) that early embryonic stage which follows the blastula. The simplest type consists of two layers, the ectoderm and the mesentoderm, and of two cavities, one lying between the ectoderm and the entoderm; the other (the archenteron) formed by invagination so as to lie within the entoderm and having an opening (the blastopore).

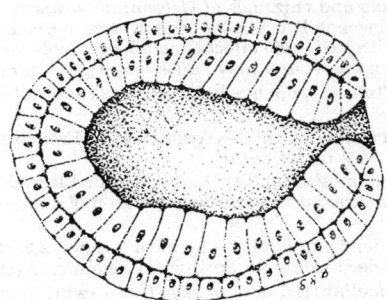

Section of a gastrula.

gastrulation (gas″troo-la′shun) the process by which a blastula becomes a gastrula or, in forms without a true blastula, the process by which three germ cell layers are acquired.

Gatch bed (gach) [Willis Dew *Gatch*, American surgeon, 1878–1954] see under *bed*.

gate (gāt) an electronic circuit that passes a pulse only when a signal (the gate pulse) is present at a second input; called also *gate circuit*.

gating (gāt′ing) the selection of electrical signals by a gate, which passes signals only when a control signal, the gate pulse, is present, or which passes only signals with certain characteristics, such as a pulse height.

gatism (ga′tizm) [Fr. *gâter* to spoil] rectal, vesical, or rectovesical incontinence.

gatophobia (gat″o-fo′be-ah) (*obs.*) ailurophobia.

gattine (gat′ēn) a form of flacherie (a disease of silkworm larvae) in which the cephalic end of affected larvae may become swollen and almost translucent; thought to be caused by a mixed infection with an unidentified virus and an enterococcus closely related to *Streptococcus faecalis*.

Gaucher's cells, disease (splenomegaly) (go-shāz′) [Phillippe Charles Ernest *Gaucher*, French physician, 1854–1918] see under *cell* and *disease*.

gauge (gāj) an instrument for determining physical properties of anything, including caliber, dimensions, or pressure. **Boley g.,** a watchmaker's gauge used in dentistry for accurate measurement of arch, tooth, and facial dimensions.

catheter g., a plate with graduated perforations for measuring the outside diameter of catheters.

Gaultheria (gawl-the′re-ah) [Jean François *Gaultier*, Quebec physician and botanist, 1708–1756] a genus of ericaceous plants; the leaves of *G. procumbens*, of North America, afford a fragrant volatile oil rich in methyl salicylate.

gauntlet (gawnt′let) [Fr. *gant* glove] a bandage which covers the hand and fingers like a glove.

gauss (gows) [Johann Karl F. *Gauss*, German physicist, 1777–1855] the cgs unit of magnetic flux density, equal to one maxwell per square centimeter or 10^{-4} tesla. Symbol, G.

gaussian curve (gow′shun) [J. K. F. *Gauss*] see under *curve*.

Gauvain's fluid (go-vānz′) [Ernest Almore *Gauvain*, American dermatologist, born 1893] see under *fluid*.

gauze (gawz) a light, open-meshed fabric of muslin or similar material used in bandages, dressings, and surgical sponges. Before use in surgery, it is usually sterilized and frequently impregnated with various antiseptics. **absorbable g.,** gauze made from oxidized cellulose. **absorbent g.** [USP], a well-bleached cotton cloth of plain weave, of various thread counts (20–44 per inch warp, 12–36 filling) and various weights (17.2–44.5 gm. per yard). **absorbent g., sterile,** absorbent gauze which has been sterilized and subsequently protected from contamination. **petrolatum g.** [USP], absorbent gauze saturated with white petrolatum; used as a protective covering for wounds. **zinc gelatin impregnated g.** [USP], absorbent gauze impregnated with zinc gelatin that may contain a small amount of ferric oxide.

gavage (gah-vahzh′) [Fr. "cramming"] 1. forced feeding, especially through a tube passed into the stomach. 2. the therapeutic use of a very full diet; superalimentation.

Gavard's muscle (gah-vahrz′) [Hyacinthe *Gavard*, French anatomist, 1753–1802] see under *muscle*.

Gay's glands (gāz) [Alexander H. *Gay*, Russian anatomist, 1880–1930] glandulae circumanales.

Gay-Lussac's law (ga″lū-sahks′) [Joseph Louis *Gay-Lussac*, French naturalist, 1778–1850] Charles' law; see under *law*.

gaze (gāz) [Middle English *gazen*] to look steadily in one direction.

GBG glycine-rich β glycoprotein; see *complement*.

GBGase glycine-rich β glycoproteinase; see *complement*.

GBM glomerular basement membrane.

GC gas chromatography.

g-cal. gram calorie; see *small calorie*, under *calorie*.

Gd chemical symbol for *gadolinium*.

GDP guanosine diphosphate.

Ge chemical symbol for *germanium*.

gear (gēr) equipment. **cervical g.,** an extraoral appliance by means of which the back of the neck is used for anchorage or as a base of traction in effecting tooth movement. **head g.,** headgear.

Geaster (je-as′ter) a genus of basidiomycetous fungi of the order Lycoperdales, series Gasteromycetes, including the star fungi.

Gee's disease (gēz) [Samuel Jones *Gee*, London physician, 1839–1911] the infantile form of nontropical sprue.

Gee-Herter disease (ge′her′ter) [S. J. *Gee*; Christian Archibald *Herter*, American physician, 1865–1910] the infantile form of nontropical sprue.

Gee-Herter-Heubner disease, syndrome (ge′her′ter-hoib′ner) [S. J. *Gee*; C. A. *Herter*; Johann Otto L. *Heubner*, pediatrician in Berlin, 1843–1926] the infantile form of nontropical sprue.

Gee-Thaysen disease (ge′thi′sen) [S. J. *Gee*; Thorwald Einar Hess *Thaysen*, Copenhagen physician, 1883–1936] the adult form of nontropical sprue.

geeldikkop (gēl-dik′kop) [Dutch "yellow, thick head"] tribulosis.

Gegenbaur's cell (ga′gen-bow″erz) [Carl *Gegenbaur*, German anatomist, 1826–1903] osteoblast.

gegenhalten (ga″gen-halt′en) [Ger.] an involuntary resistance to passive movement, as may occur in cerebral cortical disorders.

Geigel's reflex (gi′gelz) [Richard *Geigel*, German physician, 1859–1930] see under *reflex*.

Geiger counter, Geiger-Müller counter (gi′ger, gi′ger-mil′er) [Hans *Geiger*, German physicist in England, 1882–1945] see under *counter*.

Geissler's tube (gīs′lerz) [Heinrich *Geissler*, German inventor, 1814–1879] see under *tube*.

gel (jel) a colloid which is firm in consistency, although containing much liquid, a colloid in a gelatinous form. See *sol*. **aluminum hydroxide g.** [USP], a suspension of 3.6 to 4.4 per cent of aluminum oxide (Al₂O₃), in the form of aluminum hydroxide and hydrated oxide, used as a gastric antacid, especially in the treatment of peptic ulcer. Called also *colloidal aluminum hydroxide gel*. **aluminum hydroxide g., dried** [USP], a white, amorphous powder suitable for preparing tablets and capsules, obtained by drying aluminum hydroxide gel, and containing not less than 50 per cent aluminum oxide; used as an antacid. **aluminum carbonate g., basic,** an aqueous suspension containing the equivalent of 4.9 to 5.3 per cent aluminum oxide and not less than 2.4 per cent carbon dioxide; used as an antacid. **aluminum phosphate g.** [USP], a water suspension of aluminum phosphate and some flavoring agents; it contains 4 to 5 per cent aluminum phosphate (AlPO₄) and is used as a gastric antacid, especially in the treatment of gastric ulcer. **betamethasone benzoate g.** [USP], a gel containing 90 to 110 per cent of the labeled amount of betamethasone benzoate; used as a topical glucocorticoid. **corticotropin g.,** repository corticotropin injection [USP]. **fluocinonide g.** [USP], a gel containing 90 to 110 per cent of the labeled amount of fluocinonide; used as a topical glucocorticoid. **silica g.** [NF], a gel obtained by the reaction of sodium silicate with hydrochloric or sulfuric acid, and containing not less than 99 per cent of silica; used as a dispersing and suspending agent. **sodium fluoride and orthophosphoric acid g., sodium fluoride and phosphoric acid g.** [USP], a preparation containing 90 to 110 per cent of the labeled amount of fluoride ion, in an aqueous medium containing a suitable viscosity-inducing agent; used as a dental caries prophylactic, applied topically to the teeth. **tolnaftate g.** [USP], a gel containing 90 to 110 per cent of the labeled amount of tolnaftate; used as an antifungal agent. **tretinoin g.** [USP], a gel containing 90 to 130 per cent of the labeled amount of tretinoin; used as a topical keratolytic.

Gel. quav. abbreviation for L. *gelati′na qua′vis*, in any kind of jelly.

gelasmus (jĕ-las′mus) [G. *gelasma* a laugh] hysterical laughter.

gelastic (jĕ-las′tik) [Gr. *gelastos* laughable] pertaining to laughter.

gelate (jel′āt) to form a gel.

gelatification (jĕ-lat″ĭ-fi-ka′shun) conversion into gelatin.

gelatigenous (jel″ah-tij′ĕ-nus) producing or forming gelatin.

gelatin (jel′ah-tin) [L. *gelatina*, from *gelare* to congeal] [USP] a product obtained by partial hydrolysis of collagen derived from the skin, white connective tissue, and bones of animals; used as a suspending agent. It is also used pharmaceutically in the manufacture of capsules and suppositories, and has been suggested for intravenous use as a plasma substitute, and has been used as an adjuvant protein food. **glycerinated g.,** a preparation of gelatin and glycerin. **medicated g.,** gelatin mixed with medicated substances for local application. **silk g.,** sericin. **g. of Wharton,** Wharton's jelly. **zinc g.** [USP], a preparation of zinc oxide, gelatin, glycerin, and purified water, applied topically as a protective.

gelatinase (jĕ-lat′ĭ-nās) a nonspecific extracellular proteolytic enzyme, produced by certain microorganisms, that hydrolyzes gelatin.

gelatiniferous (jel″ah-tĭ-nif′er-us) [L. *gelatina* gelatin + *ferre* to bear] producing gelatin.

gelatinize (jĕ-lat′ĭ-nīz) 1. to convert into gelatin. 2. to become converted into gelatin.

gelatinoid (jĕ-lat′ĭ-noid) resembling gelatin.

gelatinolytic (jel″ah-tĭ-no-lit′ik) [*gelatin* + Gr. *lysis* dissolution] dissolving or splitting up gelatin.

gelatinosa (jel″ah-tĭ-no′sah) [L.] gelatinous; see entries beginning *substantia gelatinosa*, under *substantia*.

gelatinous (jĕ-lat′ĭ-nus) [L. *gelatinosus*] like jelly or softened gelatin.

gelatinum (jel-ah-ti′num) [L., from *gelare* to congeal] gelatin. **g. glycerina′tum,** glycerinated gelatin.

gelation (jĕ-la′shun) the conversion of a sol into a gel.

gelatose (jel′ah-tōs) an albumose formed by hydrolyzing gelatin by acid, alkalis, or an enzyme.

gelatum (jĕ-la′tum) [L., from *gelare* to congeal] jelly, or gel.

geld (geld) to remove the testes, especially of the horse.

gelding (gel′ding) a castrated male animal, especially a horse.

Gelfilm (jel′film) trademark for absorbable gelatin film (q.v., under *film*).

Gelfoam (jel′fōm) trademark for an absorbable gelatin sponge (q.v., under *sponge*).

gelidusi (ga″le-doo′se) pelidisi.

Gélineau's syndrome (zha-lĭ-no′) [Jean Baptiste Edouard *Gélineau*, French neurologist, born 1859] narcolepsy.

Gellé's test (zhel-āz′) [Marie Ernest *Gellé*, French otologist, 1834–1923] see under *tests*.

gelometer (jel-om′ĕ-ter) a device for determining the time required for a solution to gel.

gelose (jel′ōs) agar.

gelosis (jĕ-lo′sis), pl. *gelo′ses* [L. *gelare* to freeze] a hard lump in a tissue, especially such a lump in a muscle.

gelotripsy (jel′o-trip″se) [*gelosis* + Gr. *tripsis* a rubbing] the breaking up of geloses in muscle by massage.

gelsemine (jel′sĕ-mēn) an alkaloid, C₂₀H₂₂N₂O₂, obtained from the roots and rhizomes of *Gelsemium sempervirens* (L.) Ait., (Loganiaceae). It acts as a mild central nervous system stimulant with toxic side effects, including double vision and muscular weakness, and may cause respiratory arrest.

Geltabs (jel′tabz) trademark for a preparation of ergocalciferol.

Gély's suture (zha-lēz′) [Jules Aristide *Gély*, French surgeon, 1806–1861] see under *suture*.

gemästete (gĕ-mes′tĕ-tĕ) [Ger.] swollen or bloated: a term applied to enlarged astrocytes in the region of a degenerated area.

gemcadiol (jem″kah-di′ōl) chemical name: 2,2,9,9-tetramethyl-1,10-decanediol; an antihyperlipidemic, C₁₄H₃₀O₂.

Gemella (jĕ-mel′ah) [L., dim. of *gemellus* a twin] a genus of aerobic or facultatively anaerobic cocci of the family Streptococcaceae, occurring singly or in pairs with adjacent sides flattened; they are found as parasites of mammals. **G. haemoly′sans,** a species found in bronchial secretions and slime from the repiratory tract.

gemellary (jem′ĕ-lār″e) pertaining to twins.

gemellipara (jem″el-lip′ah-rah) [L. *gemelli* twins + *parere* to produce] a woman who has given birth to twins.

gemellology (jem″el-ol′o-je) [L. *gemellus* twin + *-logy*] the scientific study of twins and twinning.

gemfibrozil (gem-fib′ro-zil) a hypolipidemic drug chemically and pharmacologically related to clofibrate that lowers elevated serum lipids by decreasing triglyceride levels; administered orally in the treatment of very high serum triglyceride levels that are not responsive to diet.

geminate (jem′ĭ-nāt) [L. *geminatus*] paired; occurring in pairs.

gemination (jem-ĭ-na′shun) a doubling; a form of fusion of two teeth which results in the formation of two teeth or of a double crown formed on a single root with a single pulp canal. The term is usually applied to fusion of two supernumerary teeth or union of one supernumerary with a regular tooth.

gemini (jem′ĭ-ni) [L.] plural of *geminus*.

geminous (jem′ĭ-nus) geminate.

geminus (jem′ĭ-nus), pl. *gem′ini* [L.] a twin. **gem′ini aequa′les,** monozygotic twins.

gemistocyte (jem-is′to-sīt) [Gr. *gemistos* laden, full + *cyte*] an astrocyte in which the cell body swells considerably, the nucleus assumes an eccentric position, and the cytoplasm is clearly visible. Called also *gemistocytic astrocyte*.

gemistocytic (jem-is″to-si′tik) composed of large round

cells (gemistocytes); a term applied to astrocytomas composed of such cells.

gemma (jem′ah) [L. "bud"] a budlike body or structure.

gemmangioma (jem″an-je-o′mah) hemangioendothelioma.

gemmation (jĕ-ma′shun) [L. *gemmare* to bud] reproduction by budding, a kind of reproduction in cells in which a portion of the cell body is thrust out and then becomes separated, forming a new individual; used particularly to describe the formation of chlamydospores in fungi. See *budding*, def. 1.

Gemminges (jĕ-min′jēz) a genus of bacteria made up of gram-positive anaerobic cocci, occasionally isolated from human specimens.

gemmule (jem′ūl) [L. *gemmula*, dim. of *gemma* bud] 1. a reproductive bud; the immediate product of gemmation. 2. any one of the many little excrescences upon the dendrites of a nerve cell; called also *dendritic spine*. 3. hypothetical units assumed to be thrown off by the somatic cells, to be stored in the germ cells, and to determine the development of certain characters.

Gemonil (jem′o-nil) trademark for a preparation of metharbital.

-gen [Gr. *-genēs* born, with an alteration in meaning to "producing"] a word termination denoting an agent productive of the object or state indicated by the word stem to which it is affixed, as allergen (allergy), cryogen (cold), and pathogen (disease).

genal (je′nal) [L. *gena* cheek] pertaining to the cheek; buccal.

gender (jen′der) sex; the category to which an individual is assigned on the basis of sex.

gene (jēn) [Gr. *gennan* to produce] a segment of a DNA molecule that contains all the information required for synthesis of a product (polypeptide chain or RNA molecule), including both coding and non-coding sequences. It is the biological unit of heredity, self-reproducing, and transmitted from parent to progeny. Each gene has a specific position (locus) on the chromosome map. From the standpoint of function, genes are conceived of as structural, operator, and regulatory genes (see subentries). **allelic g's,** alleles. **autosomal g.,** a gene located on any chromosome that is not a sex chromosome. **cell interaction (CI) g's,** genes of the major histocompatibility complex that control cell-cell interactions between B cells, T cells, and macrophages and between cytotoxic T cells and target cells. **CI g's,** cell interaction g's. **codominant g's,** alleles that are both fully expressed in the heterozygote; called also *codominance*. **complementary g's,** two independent pairs of nonallelic genes, neither of which will produce its effect in the absence of the other; called also *reciprocal g's*. **g. complex,** a DNA segment containing a number of genes coding for products with related functions, e.g. the human major histocompatibility complex (MHC). **cumulative g's,** polygenes. **derepressed g.,** in genetic theory, one that in response to an environmental demand for a particular enzyme functions to increase production of that enzyme; cf. *repressed g.* **dominant g.,** one that is phenotypically expressed when present either in homozygous or heterozygous form. See *recessive g.* **H g., histocompatibility g.,** a gene that determines a histocompatibility antigen. **holandric g's,** genes in the nonhomologous region of the Y chromosome. **immune response (Ir) g's,** genes that govern the immune response to certain antigens. Animals carrying the gene are responders; those lacking the gene are nonresponders. In all species studied they are autosomal dominant genes that map with the genes for class II MHC antigens; thus the HLA-D/DR genes are probably immune response genes in humans. **immune suppressor (Is) g's,** genes governing the ability of suppressor T cells to respond to certain antigens. **immunoglobulin g's,** the genes coding for immunoglobulin heavy and light chains, which are organized in three loci coding for κ light chains, λ light chains, and heavy chains found on human chromosomes 2, 22, and 14, respectively. These genes undergo several DNA rearrangements during the differentiation of stem cells into B cells and plasma cells, permitting synthesis of the various immunoglobulin classes. **Ir g's,** immune response g's. **Is g's,** immune suppressor g's. **leaky g.,** one in which a switch in the sequence of bases in a nucleotide results in the production of a mutant protein that, because of a single

amino acid replacement, has only partial enzymatic activity; a hypomorph. **lethal g.,** a gene the presence of which brings about the death of the organism, or permits its survival only under certain conditions; see also *lethal equivalent.* **major g.,** a gene whose effect on the phenotype is always evident, regardless of how this effect is modified by other genes. **mutant g.,** a gene in which the loss, gain, or exchange of material has resulted in a permanent transmissible change in function. Such a gene may have become practically inactive (*amorph*), may act to antagonize or inhibit normal activity (*antimorph*), may act to increase normal activity (*hypermorph*), or may show only a slight reduction in its effectiveness (*leaky gene* or *hypomorph*). **nonstructural g's,** the operator and regulator genes, i.e., those not concerned in the formation of templates for messenger RNA. **operator g.,** a gene that serves as a starting point for reading the genetic code and controls the activity of the structured genes by interacting with a repressor. Called also *operator* and *operator locus.* **pleiotropic g.,** one producing many effects in the phenotype. **recessive g.,** one that is phenotypically expressed only when homozygous. See *dominant g.* **reciprocal g's,** complementary g's. **regulator g., regulatory g.,** in genetic theory, a gene that synthesizes repressor, a substance which, through interaction with the operator gene, switches off the activity of the structural genes associated with it in the operon. More generally, a gene whose product affects the activity of other genes. **repressed g.,** in genetic theory, one that under normal conditions does not always function to produce the maximum number of enzymes; cf. *derepressed g.* **repressor g.,** regulator g. **sex-conditioned g., sex-influenced g.,** a gene that is fully expressed in one sex only, e.g. human baldness. **sex-limited g.,** a sex-linked or autosomal gene that will produce an effect in one sex only. **sex-linked g.,** a gene carried on a sex chromosome (X or Y); only X linkage has clinical significance, and sex linkage has become synonymous with X linkage. **silent g.,** a mutant gene having no detectable phenotypic effect. **structural g.,** a gene that specifies the amino acid sequence of a polypeptide chain. Messenger RNA is its primary product. **sublethal g.,** a gene the presence of which handicaps or impairs the function of the organism. **supplementary g's,** two independent pairs of genes which interact in such a way that one dominant will produce its effect even in the absence of the other, but the second requires the presence of the first to be effective. **suppressor g.,** see under *mutation.* **syntenic g's,** genes located on the same chromosome. **wild-type g.,** the normal allele of a rare mutant gene, sometimes symbolized by +. **X-linked g.,** a gene carried on the X chromosome; the corresponding trait, whether dominant or recessive, is always expressed in males, who have only one X chromosome. X linkage is used synonymously with sex linkage since no genetic disorders have as yet been associated with genes on the Y chromosome. **Y-linked g.,** a gene located on the Y chromosome; the trait determined by it is therefore exhibited only by males and is transmitted by a father to all of his sons. Other than the genes that determine maleness, no clinically significant Y-linked genes have been identified in human beings.

genera (jen′er-ah) [L.] plural of *genus.*

general (jen′er-al) [L. *generalis*] affecting many parts or all parts of the organism; not local.

generalization (jen″er-al-i-za′shun) 1. act or process of generalizing. 2. a general principle or idea. **stimulus g.,** exhibition of a conditioned response to stimuli similar but not identical to the conditioned stimulus.

generalize (jen′er-al-īz) 1. to spread throughout the body, as when local disease becomes systemic. 2. to form a general principle; to reason inductively.

generation (jen″ĕ-ra′shun) [L. *generatio*] 1. the act or process of reproduction. 2. a class composed of all individuals removed by the same number of successive ancestors from a common predecessor, or occupying positions on the same level in a genealogical chart. **alternate g.,** the alternate reproduction by asexual and sexual means in an animal or plant species. **asexual g.,** production of a new organism by budding, fission, or any method not requiring the union of sexual elements. **direct g.,** asexual g. **filial g., first,** all of the offspring produced by the mating of two individuals, as in a hybrid cross; symbol F_1. **filial g., second,** all of the offspring produced by the mating of two individuals of the first filial generation; symbol F_2. **nonsexual g.,** asexual

g. **parental g.,** the generation with which a particular genetic study is begun; symbol P₁. **sexual g.,** production of a new individual (organism) by the union of male and female elements (gametes). **spontaneous g.,** abiogenesis; the discredited concept of the development of living organisms from nonliving matter.

generative (jen′ĕ-ra″tiv) pertaining to the reproduction of the species.

generator (jen′er-a″tor) something that produces or causes to exist; a machine that converts mechanical to electrical energy. **pulse g.,** the power source for a cardiac pacemaker system, usually fueled by lithium or plutonium-238, supplying impulses to the implanted electrodes, either at a fixed rate or in some programmed pattern.

generic (jĕ-ner′ik) [L. *genus, generis* kind] 1. pertaining to a genus. 2. nonproprietary; denoting a drug name not protected by a trademark, usually descriptive of its chemical structure; sometimes called *public name.*

genesial, genesic (jĕ-ne′ze-al; jĕ-nes′ik) pertaining to generation or to origin.

genesiology (jĕ-ne″ze-ol′o-je) [*genesis* + *-logy*] the sum of what is known concerning reproduction.

genesis (jen′ĕ-sis) [Gr. "production," "generation"] the coming into being of anything; the process of originating. Often used as a word termination to denote the production, formation, or development of the object or state indicated by the word stem to which it is affixed, as biogenesis, gametogenesis, and pathogenesis.

genesistasis (jen″ĕ-sis′tah-sis) [*genesis* + Gr. *stasis* a stopping] interruption of the reproduction of organisms by chemotherapy so as to permit the body cells or fluids to dispose of them.

genestatic (gen″ĕ-stat′ik) tending to prevent sporulation.

genetic (jĕ-net′ik) 1. pertaining to reproduction, or to birth or origin. 2. determined by genes.

geneticist (jĕ-net′ĭ-sist) a specialist in genetics.

genetics (jĕ-net′iks) [Gr. *gennan* to produce] the study of genes and their heredity. **bacterial g.,** the study of mechanisms of heredity in bacteria. **biochemical g.,** the science concerned with the chemical and physical nature of genes and the mechanism by which they control the development and maintenance of the organism. **clinical g.,** the study of the possible genetic factors influencing the occurrence of clinical disorders. **mathematical g.,** the statistical analysis of probabilities of genetic transmission, genes in populations, and hypothesis testing. **molecular g.,** that branch of genetics concerned with the molecular structure and activities of the genetic material, including the replication of DNA, its transcription into RNA, and the translation of RNA to form proteins. **population g.,** the study of the distribution of genes in populations and of how genes and genotype frequencies are maintained or changed. See also *Hardy-Weinberg law,* under *Law.* **reverse g.,** the indirect exploration of a genetic disease by learning the location of the responsible gene, isolating and cloning its DNA, and translating the DNA to determine the protein product. By comparing this product with the product of the normal allele, one can also analyze the nature of the normal protein altered by the mutation.

genetotrophic (jĕ-net″o-trōf′ik) pertaining to genetics and nutrition; relating to problems of nutrition which are hereditary in nature, or transmitted through the genes.

genetous (jĕ-net′us) dating from fetal life.

Geneva Convention an international agreement of 1864 whereby, among other pledges, the signatory nations pledged themselves to treat the wounded and the army medical and nursing staffs as neutrals on the field of battle.

Gengou phenomenon (zhaw-goo′) [Octave *Gengou,* French bacteriologist, 1875–1957] complement fixation.

genial, genian (jĕ-ni′al; jĕ-ni′an) [Gr. *geneion* chin] pertaining to the chin.

genic (jen′ik) pertaining to or caused by genes.

-genic [Gr. *gennan* to produce] a word termination meaning producing, or productive of.

genicula (jĕ-nik′u-lah) [L.] plural of *geniculum.*

genicular (jĕ-nik′u-lar) pertaining to the knee.

geniculate (jĕ-nik′u-lāt) [L. *geniculatus*] bent, like a knee.

geniculum (jĕ-nik′u-lum), pl. *genic′ula* [L., dim. of *genu*] a

little knee; [NA] a general term designating a sharp, kneelike bend in a small structure or organ, such as a nerve. **g. cana′lis facia′lis** [NA], **g. of facial canal,** the bend in the facial canal which lodges the geniculum nervi facialis; called also *genu of facial canal* and *knee of aquaeductus fallopii.* **g. of facial nerve, g. ner′vi facia′lis** [NA], the part of the facial nerve at the lateral end of the internal acoustic meatus, where the fibers turn sharply posteroinferiorly, and where the geniculate ganglion is found; called also *external genu of facial nerve.*

genin (jen′in) aglycon.

geni(o)- [Gr. *geneion* chin] a combining form denoting relationship to the chin. See also words beginning *mento-.*

geniocheiloplasty (je″ne-o-ki′lo-plas″te) [*genio-* + Gr. *cheilos* lip + *plassein* to form] plastic surgery of the chin and lip.

genioglossus (je″ne-o-glos′us) see *Table of Musculi.*

geniohyoglossus (je″ne-o-hi″o-glos′us) musculus genioglossus.

geniohyoid (je″ne-o-hi′oid) pertaining to the chin and hyoid bone.

geniohyoideus (je″ne-o-hi-oi′de-us) see *Table of Musculi.*

genioplasty (jĕ-ni′o-plas″te) [*genio-* + Gr. *plassein* to shape] plastic surgery of the chin.

genital (jen′ĭ-tal) [L. *genitalis* belonging to birth] 1. pertaining to reproduction or generation. 2. pertaining to the genitalia.

genitalia (jen″ĭ-ta′le-ah) [L., pl.] the various external and internal organs concerned with reproduction; see *organa genitalia.* **external g.,** see *organa genitalia feminina externa* and *organa genitalia masculina externa.* **indiffer-**

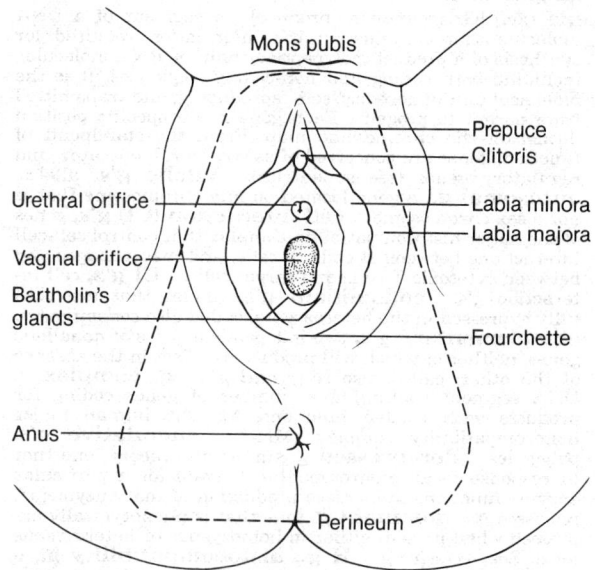

Female external genitalia.

ent g., the reproductive organs of the embryo prior to the establishment of definitive sex. **internal g.,** see *organa genitalia feminina interna* and *organa genitalia masculina interna.*

genitaloid (jen′ĭ-tal-oid) [*genitalia* + Gr. *eidos* form] pertaining to the primordial sex cells, before future sexuality is distinguishable.

genit(o)- [*genital,* q.v.] a combining form denoting relationship to the organs of reproduction.

genitocrural (jen″ĭ-to-kroo′ral) [*genital* + *crural*] pertaining to the genitalia and the leg.

genitofemoral (jen″ĭ-to-fem′or-al) genitocrural.

genitography (jen″ĭ-tog′rah-fe) radiography of the urogenital sinus and internal duct structures after injection of a contrast medium through the opening of the sinus.

genitoplasty (jen′ĭ-to-plas″te) [*genital* + Gr. *plassein* to mold] plastic surgery on the genital organs.

genitourinary (jen″ĭ-to-u′rĭ-nar-e) pertaining to the genital and urinary organs; urogenital; urinosexual.

genius (jēn′yus) 1. distinctive character or peculiar nature. 2. superlative aptitude or ability. 3. a person with superlative aptitude or ability. **g. epidem′icus** (obs.), Sydenham's theory of "epidemic constitutions," that contagious diseases are influenced by cosmic or atmospheric conditions which may change the character of and produce variations in these diseases.

Gennari's line (band, stria, stripe) (jen-nah′rēz) [Francisco Gennari, Italian anatomist of the 18th century] see under line.

gen(o)- [Gr. genos offspring, race, kind] a combining form denoting relationship to (1) reproduction, (2) sex, (3) race or kind, or (4) a gene or genes.

genoblast (jen′o-blast) [geno- + Gr. blastos germ] 1. the nucleus of the fertilized ovum. 2. a mature germ cell.

genocopy (jen′o-kop″e) a genetic trait that is a phenotypic copy of another trait but caused by a different mechanism. See also phenocopy.

genodermatology (jen″o-der″mah-tol′o-je) that branch of dermatology which treats hereditary skin diseases.

genodermatosis (jen″o-der-mah-to′sis) [geno- + dermatosis] a genetically determined disorder of the skin, usually generalized; if circumscribed, it is usually called nevus.

genome (je′nōm) [gene + chromosome] 1. the complete gene complement of an organism, contained in a set of chromosomes in eukaryotes, a single chromosome in bacteria, or a DNA or RNA molecule in viruses. 2. the full set of genes in an individual, either haploid (the set derived from one parent) or diploid (the double set, derived from both parents). In a human being the haploid set contains about 3 billion base pairs of DNA and 50,000–100,000 genes.

genomic (je-nom′ik) pertaining to the genome.

genotoxic (je″no-tok′sic) damaging to DNA: pertaining to agents (radiation or chemical substances) known to damage DNA, thereby causing mutations or cancer.

genotype (jen′o-tīp) [geno- + Gr. typos type] 1. the entire genetic constitution of an individual. 2. the alleles present at one or more specific loci. 3. the type species of a genus.

genotypic (jen″o-ti′pik) pertaining to or expressive of the genotype.

-genous [Gr. -genēs born] a word termination with two opposite meanings: (1) arising or resulting from, or produced by (endogenous, pyogenous); (2) producing (androgenous).

gentamicin (jen″tah-mi′sin) an antibiotic complex isolated from the actinomycetes Micromonospora purpurea and M. echinospora, consisting of components designated A, B, C, etc. The form in medicinal use is a mixture of three fractions of the C component (C₁, C₁ₐ, C₂); it is bactericidal for a wide range of pathogens, being highly effective against many gram-negative bacteria, especially Pseudomonas species, as well as some gram-positive species, especially Staphylococcus aureus. **g. sulfate** [USP], the sulfate salt of the antibiotic substances isolated from Micromonospora purpurea. It is used as an antibacterial in the treatment of infections caused by susceptible organisms involving almost all body organs and systems, especially in gram-negative bacillary infections of the urinary tract, in burns contaminated by Pseudomomas, sepsis, and toxemias. It is administered intramuscularly, intravenously, or applied topically to the skin, and is also applied topically to the conjunctiva in eye infections due to responsive bacteria.

gentamycin (jen″tah-mi′sin) gentamicin.

gentian (jen″shun) the dried rhizome and roots of Gentiana lutea L. (Gentianaceae); it has been used as a bitter tonic. It contains gentiin, gentiamarin, gentisin, gentisic acid, gentiopicrin, gentianose, and pectin. Also known as yellow or pale gentian. **g. violet** [USP], chemical name: N-[4-[bis [4-(dimethylamino)phenyl]methylene]-2,5-cyclohexadiene-1-ylidene]-N-methylmethanaminium chloride. A dye occurring as a dark green powder or greenish glistening pieces having a metallic luster, with antibacterial, antifungal, and anthelmintic properties, applied topically in the treatment of infections of the skin and mucous membranes associated with gram-positive bacteria and molds, and administered orally in pinworm and liver fluke infections. It has been given in strongyloidosis.

gentianophil (jen′shan-o-fil) 1. an element staining readily with gentian violet. 2. gentianophilic.

gentianophilic (jen″shan-o-fil′ik) [gentian + Gr. philein to love] staining readily with gentian violet.

gentianophilous (jen″shan-of′ĭ-lus) gentianophilic.

gentianophobic (jen″shan-o-fo′bik) not staining readily with gentian violet.

gentianophobous (jen″shan-of′o-bus) gentianophobic.

gentianose (jen′shen-ōs) a trisaccharide, $C_{18}H_{32}O_{16}$, occurring in the rhizomes of gentian.

gentiavern (jen′shah-vern) gentian violet.

gentiopicrin (jen″she-o-pik′rin) [gentian + Gr. pikros bitter] a bitter, crystalline glycoside, $C_{16}H_{20}O_9$, from gentian root.

gentisate (jen′tĭ-sāt) a salt of gentisic acid.

gentisic acid (jen-tis′ik) trivial name for 2,5-dihydroxybenzoic acid.

Gentran (jen′tran) trademark for a preparation of dextran 70.

gentrogenin (jen″tro-jen′in) botogenin.

genu (je′nu), gen. ge′nus, pl. gen′ua [L.] [NA] 1. the knee; the site of articulation between the thigh (femur) and leg. 2. a general term used to designate any anatomical structure bent like the knee. **g. cap′sulae inter′nae** [NA], genu of internal capsule: the blunt angle formed by the union of the two limbs of the internal capsule, situated posterior to the caudate nucleus, anterior to the thalamus, and medial to the lentiform nucleus; called also knee of internal capsule. **g. cor′poris callo′si** [NA], **g. of corpus callosum**, the sharp ventral curve at the anterior end of the trunk of the corpus callosum. **g. extror′sum**, g. varum. **g. of facial canal**, geniculum canalis facialis. **g. of facial nerve**, properly genu nervi facialis (internal g.), but also applied to geniculum nervi facialis (external g.). **g. of facial nerve, external**, geniculum nervi facialis. **g. of facial nerve, internal**, g. nervi facialis. **g. impres′sum**, a flattening and bending of the knee joint to one side, with consequent displacement of the patella up and to the same side. **g. of internal capsule**, g. capsulae internae. **g. [inter′num] ra′dicis ner′vi facia′lis**, g. nervi facialis. **g. intror′sum**, g. valgum. **g. ner′vi facia′lis** [NA], genu of facial nerve: the bend in the fibers arising from the nucleus of the facial nerve, which produces the facial colliculus in the floor of the fourth ventricle; it is at this point that the fibers loop around the abducens nucleus. **g. recurva′tum**, hyperextension of the knee; called also back knee. **g. val′gum**, a deformity in which the knees are abnormally close together and the space between the ankles is increased; known also as knock knee. **g. va′rum**, a deformity in which the knees are abnormally separated and the lower extremities are bowed inwardly; the deformity may be in the thigh or leg, or both. Known also as bowleg.

genua (jen′u-ah) [L.] plural of genu.

genual (jen′u-al) relating to or resembling a genu.

genucubital (jen″u-ku′bĭ-tal) [L. genu knee + cubitus elbow] pertaining to the knees and elbows; see under position.

genufacial (jen″u-fa′shal) [L. genu knee + facies face] pertaining to the knees and face; see under position.

genupectoral (jen″u-pek′tor-al) [L. genu knee + pectus breast] pertaining to the knees and chest; see under position.

genus (je′nus), pl. gen′era [L.] a taxonomic category subordinate to a tribe (or subtribe) and superior to a species (or subgenus).

-geny [Gr. -geneia, from -genēs born] a combining form meaning generation or origin.

ge(o)- [Gr. gē earth] a combining form denoting relationship to the earth, or to soil.

geobiology (je″o-bi-ol′o-je) [geo- + biology] the biology of terrestrial life.

geochemistry (je″o-kem′is-tre) [geo- + chemistry] the science concerned with study of the elements in the earth's crust and the chemical changes that occur therein.

Geocillin (je″o-sil′in) trademark for a preparation of carbenicillin indanyl sodium.

geode (je′ōd) [Gr. geōdes earthlike: so called from a fancied resemblance to a mineral geode] a dilated lymph space.

Geodermatophilus (je″o-der″mah-tof′ĭ-lus) [geo- + Gr.

derma skin + *philus* loving] a genus of nonpathogenic soil bacteria of the family Dermatophilaceae, order Actinomycetales, occurring as aerobic, gram-positive organisms that produce a tuber-shaped, nonencapsulated thallus containing cuboid and coccoid nonmotile cells, some of which develop into motile zoospores.

geogen (je′o-jen) an aspect of the geography or geochemistry of an area that affects organisms in it, particularly with reference to disease.

geomedicine (je″o-med′ĭ-sin) [*geo-* + *medicine*] the branch of medicine dealing with the influence of geographic factors, such as climate and environmental conditions, on health and disease. Called also *nosochthonography* and *nosogeography*. See also *geographic pathology*, under *pathology*.

geopathology (je″o-pah-thol′o-je) [*geo-* + *pathology*] the study of the peculiarities of disease in relation to topography, climate, food habits, etc., of various regions of the earth.

Geopen (je′o-pen) trademark for a preparation of carbenicillin disodium.

geophagia (je-o-fa′je-ah) [*geo-* + Gr. *phagein* to eat] the habit of eating clay or earth.

geophagism (je-of′ah-jizm) geophagia.

geophagy (je-of′ah-je) geophagia.

geophilic (je″o-fil′ik) [Gr. *ge* earth + *philein* to love] characterized by an affinity for soil.

geotactic (je″o-tak′tik) pertaining to geotaxis.

geotaxis (je″o-tak′sis) [*geo-* + *taxis*] taxis of an animal in response to gravitational force.

geotrichosis (je″o-tri-ko′sis) infection by *Geotrichum candidum*, which may attack the bronchi, lungs, mouth, or intestinal tract; its manifestations resemble those of candidiasis.

Geotrichum (je-ot′rĭ-kum) a genus of yeastlike imperfect fungi of the family Cryptococcaceae, order Moniliales. *G. candidum*, found in the feces and in dairy products, is the etiologic agent of geotrichosis.

geotropic (je″o-trop′ik) influenced by gravity; pertaining to geotropism.

geotropism (je-ot′ro-pizm) [*geo-* + *tropism*] tropism in an organism in response to gravitational force, as the downward growth of the roots of a plant (*positive g.*), while the stem grows upward (*negative g.*).

geraniol (jĕ-ra′ne-ol) 1. a 10-carbon branched-chain alcohol, 2,6-dimethyl-2,6-octadien-8-ol, occurring widely in essential oils of plants. 2. a pheromone of certain species of bees, being secreted by worker bees to signal the location of food.

geratic (jĕ-rat′ik) [Gr. *gēras* old age] pertaining to old age.

geratology (jer″ah-tol′o-je) gereology.

gerbil (jer′bil) a small burrowing rodent of the genus *Gerbillus*, which is native to the more arid parts of Africa and southwestern Asia, and is capable of serving as an agent for the transmission of plague.

Gerdy's fibers, etc. (zher-dēz′) [Pierre Nicholas *Gerdy*, French physician, 1797–1856] see under *fiber*, *fontanelle*, *fossa*, *loop*, and *ligament*.

gereology (jer″e-ol′o-je) [Gr. *gēras* old age + *-logy*] the science which deals with old age and its phenomena.

Gerhardt's disease, sign (phenomenon), test (reaction) (ger′harts) [Carl Adolf Christian Jacob *Gerhardt*, German physician, 1833–1902] see *erythromelalgia*, and see under *sign* and *tests*.

Gerhardt's test (zher-harts′) [Charles Frédéric *Gerhardt*, French chemist, 1816–1856] see under *tests*.

Gerhardt-Semon law [Carl Adolf Christian Jacob *Gerhardt*; Sir Felix *Semon*, German laryngologist in London, 1849–1921] see under *law*.

geriatric (jer″e-at′rik) pertaining to the treatment of the aged.

geriatrician (jer″e-ah-trish′an) a specialist in geriatrics.

geriatrics (jer″e-at′riks) [Gr. *gēras* old age + *iatrikē* surgery, medicine] that branch of medicine which treats all problems peculiar to old age and the aging, including the clinical problems of senescence and senility. **dental g.**, gerodontics.

geriodontics (jer″e-o-don′tiks) gerodontics.

geriodontist (jer″e-o-don′tist) gerodontist.

Gerlach's network, valve (ger′laks) [Joseph von *Gerlach*, German anatomist, 1820–1896] see under *network*, and see *valvula processus vermiformis*.

Gerlier's disease (zher-le-āz′) [Felix *Gerlier*, French physician, 1840–1914] see under *disease*.

germ (jerm) [L. *germen*] 1. a pathogenic microorganism. 2. living substance capable of developing into an organ, part, or organism as a whole; a primordium. **dental g.**, tooth g. **enamel g.**, the epithelial rudiment of the enamel organ. **hair g.**, see *hair matrix*, under *matrix*. **tooth g.**, a budlike thickening of the dental lamina that is the primordium of a tooth, and in which the enamel knot develops; the collective structures from which a tooth is formed, including the dental follicle, enamel organ, and dental papilla. Called also *dental g.* See also *tooth bud*, under *bud*. **wheat g.**, the embryo of wheat, which contains tocopherol, thiamine, riboflavin, and other vitamins.

germanin (jer′mah-nin) suramin sodium.

germanium (jer-ma′ne-um) a rare element, having the appearance of a bluish gray metalloid, atomic number 32, atomic weight 72.59; symbol, Ge.

germerine (jer′mer-ēn) a crystalline alkaloid, $C_{36}H_{57}O_{11}N$, from *Veratrum senecio*.

germicidal (jer″mĭ-si′dal) [L. *germen* germ + *caedere* to kill] lethal to pathogenic microorganisms.

germicide (jer′mĭ-sīd) an agent that kills pathogenic microorganisms.

germinal (jer′mĭ-nal) [L. *germinalis*] pertaining to or of the nature of a germ cell or the primitive stage of development.

germination (jer″mĭ-na′shun) [L. *germinatio*] the sprouting of a seed or spore or of a plant embryo.

germinative (jer′mĭ-na″tiv) [L. *germinativus*] pertaining to or causing germination.

germinoma (jer″mĭ-no′mah) a neoplasm of germ tissue (testis or ovum), e.g., a seminoma.

germitrine (jer′mĭ-trēn) an antihypertensive alkaloid isolated from green hellebore (*Veratrum viride* Ait. [Liliaceae]).

germline, germ line (jerm′līn) the sequence of cells in the line of direct descent from zygote to gamete, as opposed to somatic cells (all other body cells). Mutations in germline cells are transmitted to progeny; those in somatic cells are not.

germogen (jer′mo-jen) [*germ* + Gr. *gennan* to produce] a mass of protoplasm from which reproductive cells arise.

ger(o)- (jer′o, jer-on′to) [Gr. *gēras* old age] combining form denoting relationship to old age or to the aged.

gerocomia (jer″o-ko′me-ah) [*gero-* + Gr. *komein* to care for] the care of old men; the hygiene of old age.

gerocomy (jer′o-ko″me) gerocomia.

geroderma, gerodermia (jer-o-der′mah, jer-o-der′me-ah) [*gero-* + *derma*] dystrophy of the skin and genitals, producing the appearance of old age. **g. osteodysplas′tica**, a condition believed to be transmitted as an autosomal recessive trait, in which geroderma is associated with osseous changes, including osteoporosis and lines in the bones somewhat resembling growth rings of a tree. Called also *Walt Disney dwarfism*.

gerodontia (jer-o-don′she-ah) gerodontics.

gerodontic (jer″o-don′tik) [*gero-* + Gr. *odous* tooth] 1. pertaining to changes in the dental tissues with age. 2. pertaining to the practice of gerodontics.

gerodontics (jer″o-don′tiks) [Gr. *gēras* old age + *odous* tooth] the delivery of dental care to aging persons; the diagnosis, prevention, and treatment of problems peculiar to advanced age. Called also *dental geriatrics* and *gerodontia*.

gerodontist (jer″o-don′tist) a dentist who practices gerodontics.

gerodontology (jer″o-don-tol′o-je) the study of the dentition and dental problems in the aged or aging.

gerokomy (jer′o-ko″me) gerocomia.

geromarasmus (jer″o-mah-raz′mus) [*gero-* + Gr. *marasmos* a wasting] the emaciation sometimes characteristic of old age.

geromorphism (jer″o-mor′fizm) [*gero-* + Gr. *morphē* form] premature senility. **cutaneous g.,** a condition in which the skin shows at a very early age the characteristics of old age.

gerontal (jer-on′tal) pertaining to an old man or old age; senile.

gerontin (jer-on′tin) a base from the nuclei of the cells of a dog's liver, identical with spermin.

geront(o)- [Gr. *gerōn,* gen. *gerontos* old man] combining from denoting relationship to old age or to the aged.

gerontologist (jer″on-tol′o-jist) a specialist in gerontology.

gerontology (jer″on-tol′o-je) [*geronto-* + *-logy*] the scientific study of the problems of aging in all their aspects—clinical, biological, historical, and sociological.

gerontophilia (jer″on-to-fil′e-ah) [*geronto-* + Gr. *philein* to love] special fondness for old people.

gerontopia (jer″on-to′pe-ah) [*geronto-* + *-opsia*] senopia.

gerontotherapeutics (jer-on″to-ther″ah-pu′-tiks) [*geronto-* + *therapeutics*] therapeutic management of aging persons designed to retard and prevent the development of many of the aspects of senescence.

gerontotherapy (jer-on″to-ther′ah-pe) gerontotherapeutics.

gerontotoxon, gerontoxon (jer-on″to-tok′son, jer-on-tok′-son) arcus corneae; see under *arcus.* **g. len′tis,** equatorial couching of the lens in the aged; no longer done.

geropsychiatry (jer″o-si-ki′ah-tre) a subspecialty of psychiatry dealing with mental illness in the elderly.

Gerota's capsule, method (ga-ro′tahz) [Dimitru *Gerota,* anatomist in Bucharest, 1867–1939] see under *capsule* and *method.*

Gerovital H3 (jer″o-vi′tal) trademark for a preparation of 2 per cent procaine hydrochloride solution with small amounts of benzoic acid, potassium metabisulfite, and disodium phosphate; it is purported to increase longevity, retard the aging process, rejuvenate the senile, and prevent or relieve various disorders, such as arthritis, arteriosclerosis, angina pectoris, etc.

Gerson-Herrmannsdorfer diet (gār′son-Har′mans-dor-fer) [Max Bernhard *Gerson,* Austrian-born American physician, born 1881; Adolph H. *Herrmannsdorfer,* German surgeon, born 1889] Gerson diet.

Gerstmann's syndrome (garst′manz) [Josef *Gerstmann,* Vienna neurologist, 1887–1969] see under *syndrome.*

gerüstmark (gĕ-rist′mark) [Ger. *Gerüst* scaffolding + *Mark* marrow] a unique, collagen-poor zone of connective tissue lying across the bone marrow adjoining the growing ends of bones; observed in scurvy.

Gesell developmental schedule (geh-zel′) [A. *Gesell,* American pediatrician and psychologist, 1880–1961] see under *schedule.*

gestaclone (jes′tah-klōn) chemical name: 17β-acetyl-6-chloro-1β,1a,2β,8β,9α,10,11,12,13,14α,15,16,β-17-tetradeca-hydro-10β,13β-dimethyl-3H-dicyclopropa[1,2:16,17]cyclopenta[a]-phenanthren-3-one; a progestin, $C_{23}H_{27}ClO_2$.

gestagen (jes′tah-jen) any hormone with progestational activity, progesterone being the most important.

gestalt (gĕ-stawlt′, gĕ-shtawlt) [Ger.] form, shape; a whole perceptual configuration. See *gestaltism.*

gestaltism (gĕ-stawl′tizm, gĕ-shtawl′tizm) [Ger. *Gestalt* form] that theory in psychology which claims that the objects of mind, as immediately presented to direct experience, come as complete, unanalyzable wholes or forms (Gestalten) which cannot be split up into parts; called also *gestalt theory.*

gestation (jes-ta′shun) [L. *gestatio,* from *gestare* to bear] the period of development of the young in viviparous animals, from the time of fertilization of the ovum until birth; see also *pregnancy.* **exterior g.,** the development of an infant after emergence from the uterus, until the time of quadrupedal locomotion, or about the age of nine months, during the period when it is in need of maternal care and might still be regarded by some as a fetus. **interior g.,** development of a fetus before birth; a term used only in contradistinction to external gestation.

gestodene (jes′to-dēn) chemical name: 13-ethyl-17α-hydroxy-18,19-dinorpregna-4,15-diene-20-yn-3-one; a progestin, $C_{21}H_{26}O_2$.

gestosis (jes-to′sis), pl. *gesto′ses* [L. *gestare* to bear] any toxemic manifestation of pregnancy.

gestrinone (jes′trĭ-nōn) chemical name: 13-ethyl-17-hydroxy-18,19-dinor-17α-pregna-4,9-11-trien-20-yn-3-one; a progestin, $C_{21}H_{24}O_2$.

GeV, Gev giga electron volt.

GFR glomerular filtration rate.

G.G.G. abbreviation for L. *gum′mi gut′tae gam′biae;* see *gamboge.*

GH growth hormone.

Ghilarducci's reaction (ge″lar-doot′shēz) [Francesco *Ghilarducci,* Italian physician, 1857–1924] see under *reaction.*

Ghon-Sachs bacillus (gahn saks) [Anton *Ghon,* Prague pathologist, 1866–1936; Anton *Sachs,* Czech physician, 19th century] *Clostridium septicum.*

Ghon-Sachs complex, focus (primary lesion, tubercle) [Anton *Ghon;* Anton *Sachs*] see *primary complex,* under *complex,* and see under *focus.*

ghost (gōst) a faint or shadowy figure, lacking the customary substance of reality. **red cell g.,** an erythrocyte membrane that remains intact after hemolysis.

GH-RH growth hormone releasing hormone.

G.I. gastrointestinal.

Giacomini's band (jah-ko-me′nēz) [Carlo *Giacomini,* Italian anatomist, 1841–1898] see under *band.*

Giannuzzi's crescents, (bodies, cells, demilunes) (jah-noot′zēz) [Guiseppe *Giannuzzi,* Italian anatomist, 1839–1876] see under *crescent.*

Gianotti-Crosti syndrome (jah-not′e-kraw′ste) [Fernando *Gianotti,* Italian dermatologist, born 1920; Agostino *Crosti,* Italian dermatologist, born 1896] see under *syndrome.*

giant (ji′ant) [Gr. *gigas*] a person or organism of very great size; see *gigantism.*

giantism (ji′ant-izm) 1. gigantism. 2. excessive size, as of cells or nuclei.

Giardia (je-ar′de-ah) [Alfred *Giard,* biologist in Paris, 1846–1908] a genus of usually nonpathogenic, flagellate intestinal protozoa (suborder Diplomonadina, order Diplomonadida) parasitic in various vertebrates, including humans, characterized by the presence of a large sucking disk on the ventral body surface, by means of which the organism adheres to the microvilli of the host's intestinal epithelium; two anterior nuclei; and eight flagella in four pairs. **G. intestina′lis,** *G. lamblia.* **G. lamb′lia,** a species that may cause giardiasis in humans. Called also *G. intestinalis* and *Lamblia intestinalis.*

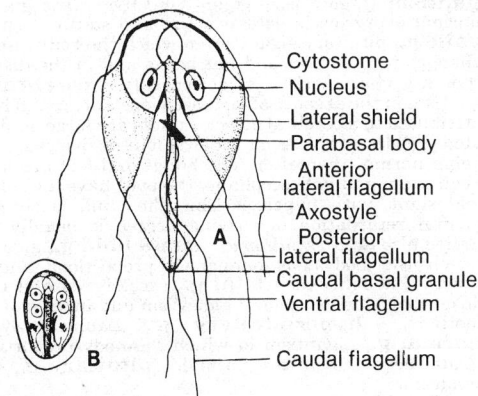

Giardia lamblia: A, trophozoite; B, cyst.

giardiasis (je″ar-di′ah-sis) a common infection of the lumen of the small intestine with the flagellate protozoan *Giardia lamblia,* and spread via contaminated food and water and by direct person-to-person contact. Most of those infected are asymptomatic, but a small percentage of cases present a wide range of symptoms, including nonspecific gastrointestinal discomfort, mild to profuse diarrhea, nausea, lassitude, anorexia, and weight loss. Called also *lambliasis* and *lambliosis*.

gibberellin (gib-ber-el'in) any of a class of phytohormones whose most striking activity is the promotion of lateral bud development in decapitated plant stems; first isolated from fungi of the genus *Gibberella*.

Gibbon-Landis test (gib'on-lan'dis) [John Heysham *Gibbon*, Jr., American physician, 1903–1973; Eugene Markley *Landis*, American physician, born 1901] see under *tests*.

gibbosity (gǐ-bos'ǐ-te) [L. *gibbosus* crooked] the condition of being humped; kyphosis.

gibbous (gib'us) [L. *gibbosus*] convex; humped; protuberant; humpbacked.

Gibbs' free energy theory (gibz) [Josiah Willard *Gibbs*, American physicist, 1839–1903] see under *energy* and *theorem*.

Gibbs-Donnan equilibrium (gibz-don'an) [J. W. *Gibbs*; Frederick George *Donnan*, English chemist, 1870–1956] see under *equilibrium*.

gibbus (gib'us) [L.] a hump.

Gibney's bandage (strapping), perispondylitis (disease) (gib'nēz) [Virgil Pendleton *Gibney*, New York surgeon, 1847–1927] see under *bandage* and *perispondylitis*.

Gibson's murmur, rule (gib'sunz) [George Alexander *Gibson*, Edinburgh physician, 1854–1913] see under *murmur* and *rule*.

gid (gid) a functional and organic disease of the brain and spinal cord of domestic animals, especially a disease of sheep caused by the presence of *Coenurus cerebralis* (the larva of the dog tapeworm, *Multiceps multiceps*), and marked by unsteadiness of gait. Called also *coenurosis*, *staggers*, and *sturdy*.

giddiness (gid'e-nes) dizziness.

Giemsa stain (gēm'sah) [Gustav *Giemsa*, chemist and bacteriologist in Hamburg, 1867–1948] see *Table of Stains and Staining Methods*.

Gierke's corpuscles (gēr'kez) [Hans Paul Bernhard *Gierke*, German anatomist, 1847–1886] see under *corpuscle*.

Gierke's disease (gēr'kez) [Edgar Otto Konrad von *Gierke*, German pathologist, 1877–1945] glycogen storage disease, type I; see under *disease*.

Gieson (ge'son) see *van Gieson*.

Gifford's operation, reflex, sign (gif'ordz) [Harold *Gifford*, American oculist, 1858–1929] see under *operation* and *sign*, and see *orbicularis pupillary reflex*, under *reflex*.

giga- [Gr. *gigas* mighty] a combining form designating gigantic size; used in naming units of measurement to indicate a quantity one billion (10⁹) times the unit designated by the root with which it is combined. Symbol, G.

gigantism (ji-gan'tizm) (jī'gan-tizm) [Gr. *gigas* giant] abnormal overgrowth; excessive size and stature. **acromegalic g.,** pituitary gigantism in which the body also has the changes in the short and flat bones and in the distal parts that are characteristic of acromegaly. **cerebral g.,** gigantism in the absence of increased levels of growth hormone, attributed to a cerebral defect; infants are large, and accelerated growth continues for the first four or five years, the rate being normal thereafter. The hands and feet are large, the head large and dolicocephalic, the eyes have an antimongoloid slant, with hypertelorism. The child is clumsy, and mental retardation of varying degree is usually present. Called also *Sotos' syndrome*. **eunuchoid g.,** gigantism in which the body has eunuchoid proportions and sexual function is deficient. **fetal g.,** excessive size of the fetus or newborn, as in cerebral gigantism and infants of diabetic mothers. **hyperpituitary g.,** Launois' syndrome. **normal g.,** gigantism in which the body proportions and sexual development are normal. **pituitary g.,** Launois' syndrome.

gigant(o)- [Gr. *gigas*, gen. *gigantos* huge] a combining form meaning huge.

gigantomastia (ji-gan″to-mas'te-ah) extreme hypertrophy of the breast.

gigantosoma (ji-gan″to-so'mah) [*giganto-* + Gr. *sōma* body] gigantism, or great size and stature.

Gigli's operation, wire saw (jēl'yēz) [Leonardo *Gigli*, gynecologist in Florence, 1866–1908] see under *operation* and *saw*.

gikiyami (ge″ke-yam'e) nanukayami.

gilbert (gil'bert) [W. *Gilbert*, English physicist, 1544–1603] the unit of magnetomotive force; symbol, F.

Gilbert's disease (cholemia, syndrome), sign (zhēl-bārz') [Nicolas Augustin *Gilbert*, French physician, 1858–1927] see under *disease* and *sign*.

Gilchrist's disease, mycosis (gil'krists) [Thomas Caspar *Gilchrist*, American dermatologist, 1862–1927] North American blastomycosis.

gildable (gil'dah-b'l) susceptible of being colored with gold stains.

gill (gil) 1. the respiratory organ of aquatic animals, such as fish, mollusks, and many arthropods, usually a thin-walled projection from the body surface or from some part of the digestive tract whose surface is increased by filaments, lamellae, or other folds. 2. one of the thin perpendicular plates found on the underside of a mushroom cap and along which the basidia are produced.

Gillenia (jil-le'ne-ah) [L.; after Arnold *Gill*] a genus of rosaceous plants; the root of *G. trifoliata* and *G. stipulacea*, of North America, is mildly emetic and aperient.

Gilles de la Tourette's syndrome (disease) [Georges *Gilles de la Tourette*, French physician, 1857–1904] see under *syndrome*.

Gilliam's operation (gil'ĭ-amz) [David Tod *Gilliam*, Columbus gynecologist, 1844–1923] see under *operation*.

Gillies' flap, operation (gil'ēz) [Sir Harold Delf *Gillies*, British plastic surgeon, 1882–1960] see *tube flap*, under *flap*, and see under *operation*.

Gilmer's splint (gil'merz) [Thomas Lewis *Gilmer*, American oral surgeon, 1849–1931] see under *splint*.

Gimbernat's ligament, reflex ligament (him-ber-nats') [Antonio de *Gimbernat*, Spanish surgeon and anatomist, 1734–1816] see *ligamenta lacunare* and *ligamentum inguinale reflexum*.

ginger (jin'jer) [L. *zingiber*; Gr. *zingiberis*] the dried rhizome of the tropical plant *Zingiber officinale*, used as a flavoring agent. It has been used in the treatment of flatulence and colic, and is used in veterinary medicine as a stimulant and carminative in atonic indigestion of horses and cattle, and in the treatment of spasmodic colic in horses.

gingiva (jin-ji'vah, jin'jĭ-vah), pl. *gingi'vae* [L. "gum of the mouth"] that part of the oral mucosa overlying the crowns of unerupted teeth and encircling the necks of those that have erupted, serving as the supporting structure for subadjacent tissues. It is formed by pale pink tissue immovably attached to the bone and the teeth, which joins the alveolar mucosa at the mucogingival junction. See also *gingivae* [NA]. **alveolar g.,** that part of the nonkeratinized oral mucosa which overlies the alveolar process. **areolar g.,** the oral mucous membrane lying beyond the keratinized mucosa over the alveolar process, being continuous with the buccal and labial mucosa. **attached g.,** that portion of the gingiva which is firm and resilient and is bound to the underlying cementum and the alveolar bone, thus being immovable. Called also *periodontium protectoris* [NA]. **buccal g.,** that portion of the gingiva located on the buccal aspect of the teeth. **cemental g.,** that portion of the attached gingiva adherent to the cementum. **free g.,** the unattached portion of the gingiva forming the wall of the gingival crevice. Called also *unattached g.* and *free gum*, and *periodontium insertionis*. See also *margo gingivalis*, under *margo*. **interdental g., interproximal g.,** the portion of the gingiva occupying the interproximal space beneath the area of tooth contact, consisting of two papillae and a depression (col) that connects the papillae and conforms to the shape of the interproximal contact area; called also *papillary g.* and *septal g.* **labial g.,** that portion of the gingiva found on the labial aspect of the teeth. **lingual g.,** that portion of the gingiva found on the lingual aspect of the teeth. **marginal g.,** margo gingivalis [NA]. **papillary g.,** interdental g. **septal g.,** interdental g. **unattached g.,** free g.

gingivae (jin-ji've, jin'jĭ-ve) [L., plural of *gingiva*] [NA] the gums: the mucous membrane, with the supporting fibrous tissue, which overlies the crowns of unerupted teeth and encircles the necks of those that have erupted. See also under *gingiva*.

gingival (jin'jĭ-val, jin-ji'val) pertaining to the gingivae.

gingivalgia (jin″jĭ-val'je-ah) [*gingivo-* + *-algia*] pain in the gingivae.

gingivally (jin′jĭ-val″le) toward the gingivae.

gingivectomy (jin″jĭ-vek′to-me) [*gingiv-* + *ectomy*] surgical excision of the gingiva at the level of its attachment, thus creating new marginal gingiva; used to eliminate gingival or periodontal pockets or to provide an approach for extensive surgical interventions, and to gain access necessary to remove calculus within the pocket.

gingivitis (jin″jĭ-vi′tis) [*gingiv-* + *-itis*] inflammation of the gingivae. Gingivitis associated with bony changes is referred to as *periodontitis.* Called also *oulitis* and *ulitis.* **acute necrotizing ulcerative g. (ANUG),** a progressive painful infection, also occurring in subacute and recurrent forms, marked by crateriform lesions of the interdental papillae that are covered by pseudomembranous slough and circumscribed by linear erythema. Fetid breath, increased salivation, and spontaneous gingival hemorrhage are additional features. The etiology is uncertain, but fusiform bacilli and spirochetes, together with other microorganisms, are present in the lesions; many authorities believe that the disease is caused by a bacterial complex in the presence of predisposing factors such as pre-existing gingival disease and nutritional deficiency. Although the disease often occurs in an epidemic pattern, it has not been shown to be contagious. Called also *acute ulcerative g., acute ulceromembranous g., fusospirillary g., fusospirillosis, fusospirochetal g., necrotizing ulcerative g., phagedenic g., trench mouth,* and *Vincent's g., infection,* or *stomatitis.* When the condition extends to other parts of the oral mucosa, with lesions involving the palate or pharynx, it is called *necrotizing ulcerative gingivostomatitis* (q.v.) and *Vincent's angina* (q.v.). **acute ulcerative g., acute ulceromembranous g.,** acute necrotizing ulcerative g. **atrophic senile g.,** inflammation of the gingiva and oral mucosa in menopausal and postmenopausal women, characterized microscopically by atrophy of the germinal and prickle cell layers of the gingival epithelium and sometimes by areas of ulceration; considered to be caused by altered estrogen metabolism. **bismuth g.,** see under *stomatitis.* **catarrhal g.,** transitory gingivitis, sometimes associated with stomatitis, accompanied by erythema, swelling, and occasionally epithelial desquamation; believed to be caused by the oral bacterial flora. **cotton-roll g.,** secondary infection of denuded areas of gingivae caused by adherence of epithelium to cotton rolls placed in the mouth during dental procedures. **desquamative g.,** an inflammatory condition characterized by tendency of the surface epithelium of the gingivae to desquamate. Chronic desquamative gingivitis is called also *gingivosis.* **Dilantin g.,** generalized hyperplasia of the gingivae, which may also rarely involve other areas of the oral mucosa, resulting from overgrowth of the fibrous tissue following anticonvulsant therapy with Dilantin (phenytoin). Called also *Dilantin hyperplasia.* **eruptive g.,** gingivitis occurring at the time of tooth eruption, particularly the permanent teeth; food impaction and debris accumulation may be associated. **fusospirochetal g.,** acute necrotizing ulcerative g. **g. gravida′rum,** pregnancy g. **hemorrhagic g.,** gingivitis characterized by profuse bleeding, as in ascorbic acid deficiency. **herpetic g.,** that due to herpesvirus infection. See also under *gingivostomatitis.* **hormonal g.,** that associated with endocrine imbalance. **hyperplastic g.,** that associated with proliferation of the gingival cells. See *gingival enlargement,* under *enlargement,* and *gingival hyperplasia,* under *hyperplasia.* **marginal g.,** inflammation of the marginal gingivae. **marginal g., generalized,** inflammation of the marginal gingivae in all the teeth, frequently extending to the interdental papillae. **marginal g., simple,** hyperemia of the gingivae with edema of the margins and gingival papillae, resulting from slight trauma or neglected dental hygiene. **marginal g., suppurative, g. margina′lis suppurati′va,** inflammation of the gingival margins, with formation of a purulent discharge. **necrotizing ulcerative g.,** acute necrotizing ulcerative g. **papillary g.,** inflammation of the interdental papillae. **phagedenic g.,** acute necrotizing ulcerative g. **pregnancy g.,** any of various gingival changes during pregnancy, ranging from gingivitis to the so-called pregnancy tumor; called also *g. gravidarum.* **scorbutic g.,** gingivitis associated with vitamin C deficiency (scurvy). **streptococcal g.,** inflammation of the gingival margins caused by streptococcal infection. **tuberculous g.,** tuberculous infection of the gingiva, characterized by diffuse, hyperemic, nodular or papillary proliferation of the gingival tissue. See also *oral tuberculosis,* under

tuberculosis. **Vincent's g.,** acute necrotizing ulcerative g.

gingiv(o)- [L. *gingiva* gum] a combining form denoting relationship to the gingivae.

gingivobuccoaxial (jin″jĭ-vo-buk″o-ak′se-al) pertaining to or formed by the gingival, buccal, and axial walls of a tooth cavity preparation.

gingivoglossitis (jin″jĭ-vo-glos-si′tis) [*gingivo-* + *gloss-* + *-itis*] inflammation of gingivae and tongue.

gingivolabial (jin″jĭ-vo-la′be-al) pertaining to the gingivae and lips.

gingivolinguoaxial (jin″jĭ-vo-ling″gwo-ak′se-al) pertaining to or formed by the gingival, lingual, and axial walls of a tooth cavity preparation.

gingivoperiodontitis (jin″jĭ-vo-per″e-o-don-ti′tis) inflammation involving the gingivae and periodontium. **necrotizing ulcerative g.,** a severe form of periodontitis occurring after prolonged repeated bouts of acute necrotizing ulcerative gingivitis, manifested by generalized or localized destruction of interdental bone, and characterized by periods of exacerbation in which a gray pseudomembrane may be present in affected areas and by necrotic odor.

gingivoplasty (jin′jĭ-vo-plas″te) [*gingivo-* + *-plasty*] surgical reshaping of the gingivae and papillae for correction of deformities (particularly enlargements) and to provide the gingivae with a normal and functional form, the incision creating an external bevel.

gingivosis (jin″jĭ-vo′sis) [*gingiv-* + *-osis*] chronic desquamative gingivitis.

gingivostomatitis (jin″jĭ-vo-sto″mah-ti′tis) inflammation involving both the gingivae and the oral mucosa. **herpetic g.,** an infection of the oral mucosa (including the gingivae) by the herpes simplex virus, characterized by redness of oral tissues, formation of multiple vesicles and painful ulcers, and fever. **necrotizing ulcerative g.,** that caused by extension to the oral mucosa of necrotizing ulcerative gingivitis, characterized by ulceration, pseudomembrane, and odor, with lesions involving the palate or pharynx as well as the oral mucosa. Called also *fusospirochetal stomatitis, Plaut's angina,* and *pseudomembranous angina.*

ginglyform (jin′glĭ-form) ginglymoid.

ginglymoarthrodial (jin″glĭ-mo-ar-thro′de-al) partly ginglymoid and partly arthrodial.

ginglymoid (jin′glĭ-moid) [*ginglymus* + Gr. *eidos* form] resembling a ginglymus.

ginglymus (jin′glĭ-mus) [L.; Gr. *ginglymos* hinge] [NA] a type of synovial joint that allows movement in but one plane, forward and backward, as the hinge of a door; called also *ginglymoid* or *hinge joint.*

ginseng (jin′seng) [Chinese *jin-tsan* life of man] 1. any herb of the genus *Panax,* especially *P. schinseng* (Chinese ginseng) and *P. quinquefolius* (American ginseng), whose roots are used by the Chinese as a tonic, stimulant, and aphrodisiac. 2. the root of Chinese or American ginseng.

Giordano's sphincter (jor-dan′oz) [Davide *Giordano,* Italian surgeon, 1864–1954] musculus sphincter ductus choledochi.

GIP gastric inhibitory polypeptide.

Giraldés' organ (he-ral′dās) [Joachim Albin Cardozo Cazado *Giraldés,* Portuguese surgeon in Paris, 1808–1875] paradidymis.

Girard's treatment (method) (jir-ardz′) [Brig. Gen. Alfred C. *Girard,* Swiss surgeon, 1850–1916] see under *treatment.*

Girardinus (jĭ-rar′dĭ-nus) *Poecilia.* **G. poeciloi′des,** *Poecilia reticulata.*

girdle (ger′d'l) an encircling structure, or part; anything that encircles a body. Called also *cingulum* [NA]. Cf. *belt.* **Hitzig's g.,** an encircling zone of analgesia at the level of the breasts, in the area supplied by the third and sixth dorsal nerves, seen in the early stages of tabes dorsalis. **g. of inferior member,** cingulum membri inferioris. **limbus g.,** a corneal degeneration in the form of an opaque line concentric with the limbus; called also *white limbal g. of Vogt.* **pectoral g.,** cingulum membri superioris. **pelvic g.,** cingulum membri inferioris. **shoulder g.,** cingulum membri superioris. **g. of superior member,** thoracic g., cingulum membri superioris. **Venus' g.,** mercurial plaster spread on leather or linen, once used in the

treatment of syphilis; called also *balteum venereum*.
white limbal g. of Vogt, limbus g.

Girdner's probe (gerd″nerz) [John Harvey *Girdner*, physician in New York, 1856–1933] an electric probe; see under *probe*.

gitaligenin (jĭ-tal′ĭ-jen″in) the aglycone of gitalin.

Gitaligin (jĭ-tal′ĭ-jin) trademark for a preparation of gitalin (def. 2).

gitalin (jit′ah-lin) 1. a crystalline cardiac glycoside, $C_{35}H_{56}O_{12}$, from the leaves of *Digitalis purpurea*. 2. a mixture of the digitalis glycosides gitoxin, gitaloxin, and digitoxin, having the same actions as digitalis and used like digitalis in the treatment of congestive heart failure and other cardiac disorders; administered orally. Called also *amorphous g.*

gitaloxin (jit″ah-loks′in) a cardiac glycoside from *Digitalis purpurea*.

githagism (gith′ah-jizm) poisoning by the seeds of *Agrostemma githago*, or corn cockle.

gitogenin (jit-oj′ĕ-nin) a sapogenin, $C_{27}H_{44}O_4$, from gitonin.

gitonin (jit′o-nin) a neutral saponin, $C_{50}H_{82}O_{23}$, from digitalis seed.

gitoxigenin (jĭ-tok′sĭ-jen-in) an aglycone of gitoxin, $C_{23}H_{35}O_5$.

gitoxin (jĭ-tok′sin) a cardiac glycoside, $C_{41}H_{64}O_{14}$, principally from *Digitalis purpurea* but also a constituent of *D. lanata*.

Gitterfasern (git′er-fas″ern) [Ger.] the reticular lattice fibers of the corium.

Giuffrida-Ruggieri stigma (joof-re″dah-roo″je-er′e) [Vincenzo *Giuffrida-Ruggieri*, Italian anthropologist, 1872–1922] see under *stigma*.

Givens' method (giv′enz) [Maurice Hope *Givens*, American biochemist, born 1888] see under *method*.

GIX an insecticidal compound, DFDT.

gizzard (giz′ard) [L. *gigeria* cooked entrails of poultry] a portion of the digestive tract specialized for the mechanical breakdown of food before digestion begins. In birds, it is the highly modified posterior portion of the stomach, characterized by muscular walls and glands that secrete a horny lining, in which food passed from the proventriculus is ground with the aid of gravel swallowed by the bird. A similar gizzard-like organ is seen in the alimentary tract of certain invertebrates, such as insects.

GL abbreviation for *greatest length*, an axis of measurement or dimension used for small flexed embryos.

Gl chemical symbol for *glucinium* (beryllium).

gl. abbreviation for L. *glan′dula* and *glan′dulae* (gland, glands).

GL 54 athomin.

glabella (glah-bel′ah) [L. *glaber* smooth] 1. the smooth area on the frontal bone between the superciliary arches. 2. [NA] the most prominent point in the midsagittal plane between the eyebrows; used as an anthropometric landmark.

glabellad (glah-bel′ad) toward the glabella.

glabellum (glah-bel′um) glabella.

glabrificin (glah-brif′ĭ-sin) [L. *glaber* smooth + *facere* to make] (*obs.*) an antibody; so called because of its property of rendering bacteria smooth or glabrous.

glabrous (gla′brus) [L. *glaber* smooth] smooth and bare.

glacial (gla′shal) [L. *glacialis*] 1. resembling ice; vitreous; solid. 2. designating a highly pure state of certain acids, e.g., acetic or phosphoric acid, so called because the freezing point is only slightly below room temperature.

gladiate (gla′de-āt) [L. *gladius* sword] sword-shaped.

gladiolus (glah-di′o-lus) [L., dim. of *gladius* sword] corpus sterni.

gladiomanubrial (glad″e-o-mah-nu′bre-al) pertaining to gladiolus (corpus sterni) and manubrium.

glairin (glār′in) [L. *clarus* clear] a gelatinous substance of bacterial origin found on the surface of certain thermal and sulfur waters.

glairy (glār′e) resembling the white of an egg.

gland (gland) [L. *glans* acorn] an aggregation of cells, specialized to secrete or excrete materials not related to their ordinary metabolic needs; called also *glandula* [NA]. **absorbent g.,** lymph node. **accessory g.,** a minor mass

of glandular tissue situated near or at some distance from a gland of similar structure. **acid g's,** glandulae gastricae [propriae]. **acinar g.,** acinous g. **acinotubular g.,** tuboloacinar g. **acinous g.,** a gland made up of one or more acini. **admaxillary g.,** glandula parotis accessoria. **adrenal g.,** a flattened body situated in the retroperitoneal tissues at the cranial pole of each kidney. In man, the adrenal gland is the result of fusion of two organs of different embryologic origin, recognizable as cortex and medulla. The adrenal cortex, under control of the pituitary hormone corticotropin, elaborates steroid hormones—glucocorticoids, mineralocorticoids, androgens, and progestins. The adrenal medulla elaborates the catecholamines epinephrine and norepinephrine. Called also *glandula suprarenalis* [NA] and *suprarenal g.* **adrenal g's, accessory,** accessory adrenal glandular tissue found near the adrenals or in the abdomen or pelvis. Such tissue is usually either cortical or medullary. Called also *glandulae suprarenales accessoriae* [NA] and *accessory suprarenal glands.* **aggregate g's, agminated g's,** folliculi lymphatici aggregati. **Albarrán's g.,** that part of the median lobe of the prostate underneath the uvula vesicae. **alveolar g.,** acinous g. **anal g's,** circumanal g's. **anteprostatic g.,** bulbourethral g. **apical g's of tongue,** glandulae linguales anteriores. **apocrine g.,** one the discharged secretion of which contains part of the secreting cells; see *glandulae sudoriferae.* **aporic g.,** endocrine g's. **areolar g's,** glandulae areolares. **arterial g.,** any knot of small arteries, or mass of vascular tissue, such as the glomus coccygeum. **arteriococcygeal g.,** glomus coccygeum. **arytenoid g's,** glandulae laryngeae posteriores. **Aselli's g's,** see under *pancreas.* **Avicenna's g.,** an encapsulated tumor. **axillary g's,** nodi lymphatici axillares. **Bartholin's g.,** one of the two small bodies on either side of the vaginal orifice, homologues of the bulbourethral glands in the male; called also *glandula vestibularis major* [NA]. **Bauhin's g's,** glandulae linguales anteriores. **g's of biliary mucosa,** glandulae mucosae biliosae. **Blandin's g's, Blandin and Nuhn's g's,** glandulae linguales anteriores. **blood g's, blood vessel g's,** endocrine g's. **Bonnot's g.,** brown adipose tissue. **Bowman's g's,** glandulae olfactoriae. **brachial g's,** nodi lymphatici cubitales. **bronchial g's,** glandulae bronchiales. **Bruch's g's,** the lymph follicles of the conjunctiva of the lower lid. **Brunner's g's,** glandulae duodenales. **buccal g's,** glandulae buccales. **bulbocavernous g.,** bulbourethral g. **bulbourethral g.,** one of two glands embedded in the substance of the sphincter of the urethra, just posterior to the membranous part of the urethra; called also *Cowper's g.* and *glandula bulbourethralis* [NA]. **cardiac g's,** mucin-secreting glands at the cardiac end of the stomach surrounding the entrance of the esophagus into the stomach. **carotid g.,** glomus caroticum. **celiac g's,** lymph nodes anterior to the abdominal aorta. **ceruminous g's,** the glands in the skin of the external auditory canal that secrete the cerumen; called also *glandulae ceruminosae* [NA]. **cervical g's of uterus,** glandulae cervicales uteri. **cheek g's,** glandulae buccales. **choroid g.** (*obs.*), the choroid plexus, regarded as one of the sites of formation of the cerebrospinal fluid. **Ciaccio's g's,** glandulae lacrimales accessoriae. **ciliary g's, ciliary g's of conjunctiva,** glandulae ciliares conjunctivales. **circumanal g's,** specialized sweat and sebaceous glands situated around the anus; called also *anal g's* and *glandulae circumanales* [NA]. **Cloquet's g.,** see under *node.* **closed g's,** endocrine g's. **Cobelli's g's,** mucous glands in the mucosa of the esophagus just above the cardia. **coccygeal g.,** glomus coccygeum. **coil g.,** eccrine g. **compound g.,** one made up of a number of smaller units whose excretory ducts combine to form ducts of progressively higher order. **conglobate g.,** a lymph node. **conjunctival g's,** glandulae conjunctivales. **Cowper's g.,** bulbourethral g. **cutaneous g's,** glandulae cutis. **cytogenic g.,** a term applied to the testis and the ovary because they form free living cells. **ductless g.,** one without a duct; a gland of internal secretion. See *endocrine g's.* **duodenal g's,** glandulae duodenales. **Duverney's g.,** bulbourethral g. **Ebner's g's,** serous secreting glands in the posterior part of the tongue near the vallate papillae; called also *gustatory g's.* **eccrine g.,** one of the ordinary, or simple, sweat glands of the body, which is of the merocrine type; see *glandulae sudoriferae.* **Eglis' g's,** glandulae mucosae ureteris. **endocrine g's,** ductless organs that secrete specific sub-

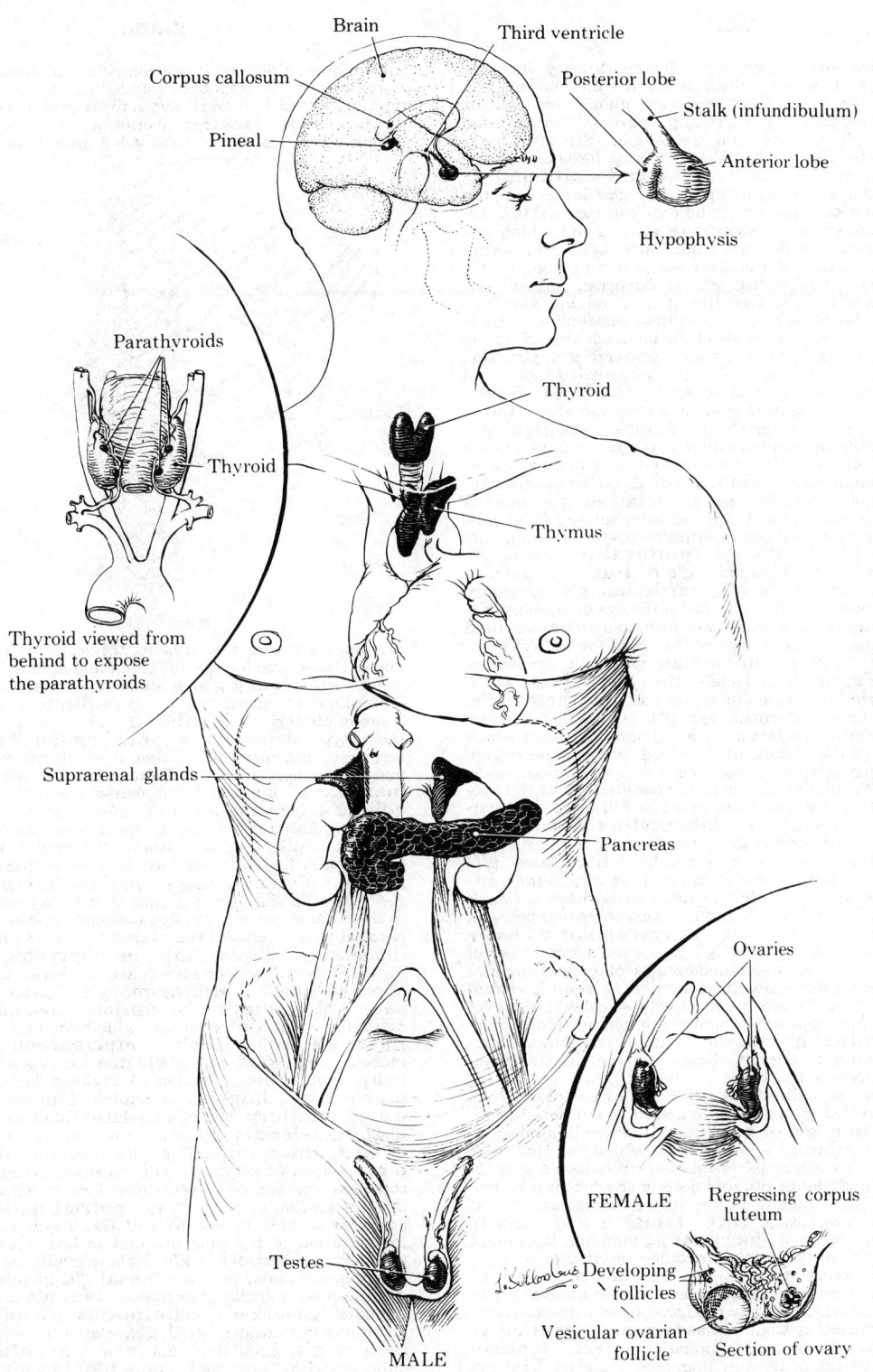

Brain

Third ventricle

Corpus callosum

Posterior lobe

Stalk (infundibulum)

Pineal

Anterior lobe

Hypophysis

Parathyroids

Thyroid

Thyroid

Thymus

Thyroid viewed from
behind to expose
the parathyroids

Suprarenal glands

Pancreas

Ovaries

FEMALE

Regressing corpus
luteum

Testes

Developing
follicles

Vesicular ovarian
follicle

Section of ovary

MALE

PLATE 18 —THE ENDOCRINE GLANDS

stances (hormones) which are released directly into the circulatory system and which influence metabolism and other body processes. The endocrine glands include the hypothalamus, pituitary, thyroid, parathyroid, and adrenal glands, the pineal body, and the gonads. See also under *system*, and see Plate XIX. Called also *glandulae endocrinae* [NA] and *glandulae sine ductibus*. **endoepithelial g.**, intraepithelial g. **esophageal g's**, glandulae oesophageae. **excretory g.**, any gland that excretes waste products from the system. **exocrine g.**, a gland which discharges its secretion through a duct opening on an internal or external surface of the body, as a lacrimal gland. Cf. *endocrine g's*. **follicular g's of tongue**, folliculi linguales. **fundic g's, fundus g's**, glandulae gastricae [propriae]. **Galeati's g's**, glandulae duodenales. **gastric g's**, the secreting glands of the stomach, including the fundic, cardiac, and pyloric glands. **gastric g's, proper**, glandulae gastricae [propriae]. **gastroepiploic g's**, nodi lymphatici gastrici [dextri et sinistri]. **Gay's g's**, glandulae circumanales. **genal g's**, glandulae buccales. **genital g.**, 1. ovary (ovarium [NA]). 2. testis. **gingival g's**, glandlike infoldings of epithelium at the junction of gingiva and tooth. **Gley's g's**, glandulae parathyroideae. **globate g.**, lymph node. **glomiform g.**, anastomosis arteriovenosa glomeriformis. **glossopalatine g's**, mucous glands at the posterior end of the smaller sublingual glands. **Guérin's g's**, ductus paraurethrales urethrae femininae. **gustatory g's**, Ebner's g's. **guttural g.**, one of the mucous glands of the pharynx. **g's of Haller**, glandulae preputiales. **Harder's g's, harderian g's**, accessory lacrimal glands at the inner corner of the eye in animals that possess nictitating membranes and excrete an unctuous fluid that facilitates the movement of the third eyelid. They are rudimentary in man. **haversian g's**, villi synoviales. **hedonic g's**, glands in some of the lower animals which function during the season of sexual activity. **hemal g's**, see under *node*. **hemal lymph g's**, hemal nodes. **hematopoietic g's** (*obs.*), certain glandlike bodies which take a part in the making of the blood, such as the spleen. **hemolymph g's**, 1. hemal nodes. 2. see under *node*. **Henle's g's**, tubular glands in the conjunctiva of the eyelids. **hepatic g's**, glandulae mucosae biliosae. **heterocrine g's**, seromucous g's. **hibernating g.**, brown adipose tissue. **holocrine g.**, a gland whose discharged secretion contains entire secreting cells. **incretory g's**, endocrine g's. **intercarotid g.**, glomus caroticum. **intermediate g's**, according to some authorities, a fourth type of gastric gland (q.v.) found in a narrow region between the fundic and pyloric glands. **interscapular g.**, brown adipose tissue. **interstitial g.**, 1. (pl.) the aggregations of Leydig cells of the testis; so called because of their occurrence in clusters and their endocrine function. 2. the interstitial cells (see def. 2) of the ovary, collectively; so called because of their epithelioid appearance and presumed secretory function. **intestinal g's**, straight tubular glands in the mucous membrane of the intestines, opening, in the small intestine, between the bases of the villi, and containing argentaffin cells; called also *glandulae intestinalis* [NA]. **intraepithelial g.**, a gland situated in an epithelial layer. **intramuscular g's of tongue**, glandulae linguales anteriores. **jugular g.**, a lymph node behind the clavicular insertion of the sternomastoid muscle. **Krause's g's**, accessory lacrimal glands situated deep in the subconjunctival connective tissue, mainly in the upper fornix; called also *glandulae conjunctivales* [NA]. **labial g's of mouth**, glandulae labiales oris. **lacrimal g.**, glandula lacrimalis. **lacrimal g's, accessory**, glandulae lacrimales accessoriae. **lactiferous g.**, mammary g's. **g's of large intestine**, see *glandulae intestinales*. **large sweat g.**, an apocrine gland which usually produces an odoriferous secretion. **laryngeal g's**, glandulae laryngeae. **lenticular g's of stomach**, folliculi lymphatici gastrici. **lenticular g's of tongue**, folliculi linguales. **g's of Lieberkühn**, glandulae intestinales. **lingual g's**, glandulae linguales. **lingual g's, anterior (of Blandin and Nuhn)**, glandulae linguales anteriores. **Littre's g's**, 1. glandulae preputiales. 2. glandulae urethrales urethrae masculinae. **Luschka's g.**, glomus coccygeum. **lymph g., lymphatic g.**, lymph node. **lymph g's, extraparotid**, lymph nodes overlying the parotid gland, between the superficial and deep fasciae. **malar g's**, glandulae buccales. **mammary g.**, the specialized accessory gland of the skin of female mammals that secretes milk.

In the human female, it is a compound tubuloalveolar gland composed of 15 to 25 lobes arranged radially about the nipple and separated by connective and adipose tissue, each lobe having its own excretory (lactiferous) duct opening on the nipple. The lobes are subdivided into lobules, with the

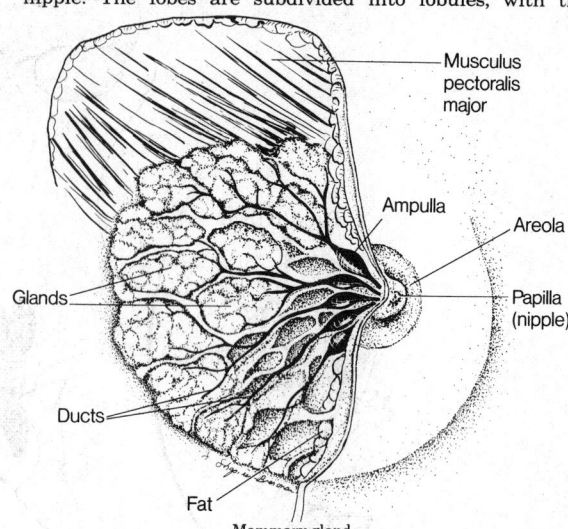

Musculus pectoralis major

Ampulla

Areola

Papilla (nipple)

Glands

Ducts

Fat

Mammary gland.

alveolar ducts and alveoli being the secretory portion of the gland. Called also *lactiferous gland* and *glandula mammaria* [NA]. **mammary g's, accessory**, mammae accessoriae [femininae et masculinae]. **mandibular g.**, glandula submandibularis. **Mehlis' g.**, gland cells surrounding the ootype of trematodes. **meibomian g's**, glandulae tarsales. **merocrine g.**, one in which the secretory cells maintain their integrity throughout the secretory cycle. **mesenteric g's**, nodi lymphatici mesenterici. **mesocolic g's**, lymph nodes in the mesentery of the colon; see *nodi lymphatici colici dextri, medii*, and *sinistri, nodi lymphatici ileocolici*, and *nodi lymphatici mesenterici inferiores*. **mixed g's**, 1. glands that have both endocrine and exocrine portions. 2. seromucous g's. **molar g's**, glandulae molares. **Moll's g's**, sweat glands that have become arrested in their development, situated obliquely in contact with and parallel to the bulbs of the eyelashes. Called also *glandulae ciliares conjunctivales* [NA]. **monoptychic g.**, a gland in which the tubules or alveoli are lined with a single layer of secreting cells. **Montgomery's g's**, glandulae areolares. **Morgagni's g's**, glandulae urethrales urethrae masculinae. **g's of mouth**, glandulae oris. **mucilaginous g's**, villi synoviales. **muciparous g.**, glandula mucosa. **mucous g.**, a gland that secretes a slimy, chemically inert material; called also *glandula mucosa* [NA]. **mucous g's, lingual**, glandulae linguales. **mucous g's of auditory tube**, glandulae tubariae. **mucous g's of duodenum**, glandulae duodenales. **mucous g's of eustachian tube**, glandulae tubariae. **multicellular g.**, one in which many cells cooperate to produce a gland complex, represented in its simplest form by a secretory sheet (q.v.) of epithelial cells. **myometrial g.**, a tissue supposed to develop in the wall of the uterus at the site of implantation of the placenta and to last until the end of pregnancy. **Naboth's g's**, Naboth's follicles. **nabothian g's**, see under *follicle*. **nasal g's**, glandulae nasales. **g. of neck**, tonsilla pharyngea. **Nuhn's g's**, glandulae linguales anteriores. **odoriferous g's of prepuce**, glandulae preputiales. **oil g's**, glandulae sebaceae. **olfactory g's**, glandulae olfactoriae. **oxyntic g's**, glandulae gastricae [propriae]. **pacchionian g's** (*obs.*), granulationes arachnoideales. **palatine g's**, glandulae palatinae. **palpebral g's**, glandulae tarsales. **pancreaticosplenic g's**, nodi lymphatici pancreaticolienales. **parafrenal g's**, glands opening near the frenum of the prepuce. **parathyroid g's**, small bodies apposed to the posterior surface of the thyroid gland, developed from the entoderm of the branchial clefts, occurring in a variable number of pairs, commonly two (*glandula parathyroidea inferior* and *glandula parathyroidea superior* [NA]) (see inset on accompanying Plate). The parenchyma consists of masses and cords of epithelial cells, which have been divided into two main types: chief cells and oxyphil cells, but intermediate forms exist. The parathyroid glands secrete parathyroid hormone and are concerned chiefly with the metabolism of calcium and phosphorus. Called also *epithelial* or *parathyroid bodies.* **paraurethral g's,** see *ductus paraurethrales urethrae femininae* and *ductus paraurethrales urethrae masculinae.* **parotid g.,** the largest of the three chief, paired salivary glands; see *glandula parotidea* [NA]. **parotid g., accessory,** glandula parotidea accessoria. **pectoral g's,** see *nodi lymphatici axillares.* **peptic g's,** glandulae gastricae [propriae]. **perspiratory g's** (*obs.*), glandula sudoriferae. **Peyer's g's,** folliculi lymphatici aggregati. **pharyngeal g's,** glandulae pharyngeae. **Philip's g's,** enlarged glands above the clavicle, seen in children with tuberculosis. **pineal g.,** see under *body,* def. 1. **pituitary g.,** the epithelial body of dual origin located at the base of the brain in the sella turcica. It is attached by a stalk to the hypothalamus, from which it receives an important neural and vascular outflow. The pituitary gland (or *hypophysis* [NA]) is composed of two main lobes: the *adenohypophysis* [NA] (anterior lobe, lobus anterior, anterior pituitary), which arises from the buccal epithelium in the embryo, and the *neurohypophysis* [NA] (posterior lobe, lobus posterior, posterior pituitary), which originates in the embryo as an evagination from the floor of the diencephalon. The adenohypophysis comprises the *pars tuberalis* (or pars infundibularis), a thin cloak of cells on the anterior and lateral surfaces of the infundibulum; the *pars distalis,* the main body of the adenohypophysis; and the *pars intermedia,* an ill-defined region between the two lobes (assigned in some systems of nomenclature to the neurohypophysis). The neurohypophysis comprises the *infundibulum* (neural stalk), which is continuous with the hypothalamus, and the *neural lobe* (infundibular process, pars nervosa), which is the main body of the neurohypophysis. The median eminence is also often classified (in nonofficial anatomical nomenclature) as part of the neurohypophysis. The adenohypophysis secretes several important hormones (growth hormone, ACTH, β-lipotropin, TSH, FSH, LH, and prolactin) which are released or inhibited by the actions on the pituitary by hypophysiotropic factors secreted by the hypothalamus, and which regulate the proper functioning of the thyroid, gonads, adrenal cortex, and other endocrine organs. As a consequence, the hypothalamo-pituitary unit is of vital importance to the growth, maturation, and reproduction of the individual. The neurohypophysis, formerly thought to be the source of hypothalamic neurohormones having antidiuretic and oxytocic action, is now known to serve only as a reservoir for them, releasing them as needed. Called also *glandula pituitaria* [NA alternative], *hypophysis cerebri* [NA], and *pituitary body.* **Poirier's g's,** lymph nodes on the conoid ligament at the upper border of the isthmus of the thyroid. **polyptychic g.,** a gland in which the tubules or alveoli are lined with more than one layer of secreting cells. **preen g.,** a large, compound alveolar structure present on the back of birds, above the base of the tail, which secretes an oily "water-proofing" material that the bird applies to its feathers and skin by preening. **pregnancy g's,** the glands containing female genital hormone, that is, the ovarian follicle, corpus luteum, and placenta. **prehyoid g's,** glandulae thyroidea accessoriae. **preputial g's,** glandulae preputiales. **prostate g.,** prostate. **pyloric g's,** glandulae pyloricae. **racemose g's,** glands composed of acini arranged like grapes on a stem. **retrolingual g.,** a rather large gland in some animals situated near the mandibular gland. **retromolar g's,** glandulae molares. **Rivinus g.,** glandula sublingualis. **Rosenmüller's g.,** 1. pars palpebralis glandulae lacrimalis. 2. [pl.] nodi lymphatici inguinalis profundi. **saccular g.,** a gland consisting of a sac or sacs, lined with glandular epithelium. **salivary g's,** the glands of the oral cavity whose combined secretion constitutes the saliva; they include the parotid, sublingual, and submandibular glands, as well as numerous small glands in the tongue, lips, cheeks, and palate. See *glandulae salivariae majores* and *glandulae salivariae minores.* **salivary g., abdominal,** the pancreas. **salivary g., external,** glandula parotidea. **salivary g., internal,** see *glandula sublingualis* and *glandula submandibularis.* **salivary g's, major,** glandulae salivariae majores. **salivary g's, minor,** glandulae salivariae minores. **Sandström's g's,** glandulae thyroideae accessoriae. **Schüller's g's,** ductus paraurethrales urethrae femininae. **sebaceous**

g's, glandulae sebaceae. **sebaceous g's of conjunctiva,** glandulae sebaceae conjunctivales. **seminal g.,** vesicula seminalis. **sentinel g.,** an enlarged lymph node, considered to be pathognomonic of some pathological condition elsewhere. **seromucous g.,** one that contains both serous and mucous secreting cells; called also *glandula seromucosa* [NA]. **serous g.,** a gland that secretes a watery albuminous material commonly but not always containing enzymes; called also *glandula serosa* [NA]. **Serres' g's,** pearly masses of epithelial cells near the surface of the gum of the infant. **sexual g.,** see *testis* and *ovary.* **Sigmund's g's,** the epitrochlear lymph nodes. **simple g.,** one with a nonbranching duct. **Skene's g's,** ductus paraurethrales urethrae femininae. **g's of small intestine,** see *glandulae intestinales.* **solitary g's of large intestine,** folliculi lymphatici solitarii intestini crassi. **solitary g's of small intestine,** folliculi lymphatici solitarii intestini tenuis. **splenoid g.,** an apparently compensatory new growth that sometimes follows extirpation of the spleen. **Stahr's g.,** a lymph node situated on the facial artery. **staphyline g's,** glandulae palatinae. **subauricular g's,** nodi lymphatici retroauriculares. **sublingual g.,** the smallest of the three chief, paired salivary glands; see *glandula sublingualis* [NA]. **submandibular g., submaxillary g.,** one of the three chief, paired salivary glands; see *glandula submandibularis* [NA]. **sudoriferous g's, sudoriparous g's,** glandulae sudoriferae. **suprarenal g.,** adrenal g. **suprarenal g's, accessory,** adrenal g's, accessory. **Suzanne's g.,** a mucous gland of the mouth, beneath the alveololingual groove. **sweat g's,** glandulae sudoriferae. **synovial g's,** villi synoviales. **target g.,** a gland specifically affected by a pituitary hormone; such glands include the thyroid, adrenal cortex, and gonads. **tarsal g's, tarsoconjunctival g's,** glandulae tarsales. **Theile's g's,** glandlike formations in the walls of the cystic duct and in the pelvis of the gallbladder. **thymus g.,** thymus. **thyroid g.,** one of the endocrine glands, normally situated in the lower part of the front of the neck and consisting of two lobes, one on either side of the trachea and joined in front by a narrow isthmus. It secretes, stores, and liberates as neccessary the thyroid hormones (thyroxine and triiodothyronine), which require iodine for their elaboration and which play the major endocrine role in regulating the metabolic rate. It also secretes thyrocalcitonin. Called also *glandula thyroidea* [NA] and *thyroid body.* See also *thyroid.* **thyroid g's, accessory,** glandulae thyroideae accessoriae. **g's of tongue,** glandulae linguales. **tracheal g's,** glandulae tracheales. **trachoma g's,** lymphoid follicles of the conjunctiva, found chiefly near the inner canthus of the eye. **tubular g.,** any gland made up of or containing a tubule or a number of tubules. **tubuloacinar g.,** one that is both tubular and acinous. **tympanic g's,** glandulae tympanicae. **g's of Tyson,** glandulae preputiales. **ultimobranchial g's,** see under *body.* **unicellular g.,** a single cell that functions as a gland, e.g., a goblet cell. **urethral g's,** see entries beginning *glandulae urethrales,* under *glandula.* **urethral g's of female urethra,** glandulae urethrales urethrae femininae. **uropygial g.,** preen g. **uterine g's,** glandulae uterinae. **utricular g's,** glandulae uterinae. **vaginal g.,** any gland occurring exceptionally in the vaginal mucous membrane. **vascular g.,** 1. glomus. 2. a hemal node. **vestibular g., greater,** glandula vestibularis major [NA]. **vestibular g's, lesser,** glandulae vestibulares minores. **Virchow's g.,** signal node. **vitelline g.,** see *vitellarium.* **vulvovaginal g.,** glandula vestibularis major. **Waldeyer's g's,** acinotubular glands in the inner skin of the attached edge of the eyelid. **Weber's g's,** the tubular mucous glands of the tongue. **g's of Wolfring,** small tubuloalveolar glands in the subconjunctival tissue above the upper border of the tarsal plate, their ducts opening on the conjunctival surface. **g's of Zeis,** modified rudimentary sebaceous glands attached directly to the follicles of the eyelashes; called also *glandulae sebaceae conjunctivales* [NA]. **Zuckerkandl's g.,** corpora paraaortica.

glanderous (glan′der-us) of the nature of or affected with glanders.

glanders (glan′derz) [L. *malleus*] a contagious disease of horses, communicable to man, and caused by the glanders bacillus, *Pseudomonas mallei.* It is marked by a purulent inflammation of mucous membranes and an eruption of nodules on the skin which coalesce and break down, forming deep ulcers, which may end in necrosis of cartilages and bones. Called also *maliasmus* and *malleus;* the more chronic and constitutional lymphatic form is known as *farcy.* **African g., Japanese g.,** lymphangitis epizootica.

glandes (glan′dēz) [L.] plural of *glans.*

glandilemma (glan″dĭ-lem′ah) [*gland* + Gr. *lemma* sheath] the capsule or outer envelope of a gland.

glandula (glan′du-lah), pl. *glan′dulae* [L.] [NA] a gland: an aggregation of cells, specialized to secrete or excrete materials not related to their ordinary metabolic needs. **g. adrena′lis,** NA alternative for *g. suprarenalis.* **glan′dulae areola′res** [NA], **glan′dulae areola′res [Montgomer′ii],** areolar glands: sebaceous glands of the mammary areola; called also *Montgomery's glands.* **glan′dulae bronchia′les** [NA], bronchial glands: seromucous glands in the mucosa and submucosa of the bronchial walls. **glan′dulae bucca′les** [NA], buccal glands: the serous and mucous glands on the inner surface of the cheeks. **g. bulbourethra′lis** [NA], **g. bulbourethra′lis [Cow′peri],** bulbourethral gland: either of two glands embedded in the substance of the sphincter of the male urethra, just posterior to the membranous part of the urethra; they are homologues of the greater vestibular glands in the female. Called also *Cowper's gland.* **glan′dulae cerumino′sae** [NA], ceruminous glands: the glands in the skin of the external auditory canal that secrete the cerumen. **glan′dulae cervica′les u′teri** [NA], cervical glands of uterus: compound clefts in the wall of the uterine cervix. **glan′dulae cilia′res conjunctiva′les** [NA], **glan′dulae cilia′res [Mol′li],** ciliary glands of conjunctiva: sweat glands that have become arrested in their development, situated obliquely in contact with and parallel to the bulbs of the eyelashes; called also *Moll's glands.* **glan′dulae circumana′les** [NA], circumanal glands: specialized sweat and sebaceous glands situated in an annular zone around the anus; called also *anal glands* and *Gay's glands.* **gland′dulae conjunctiva′les** [NA], conjunctival glands: accessory lacrimal glands situated deep in the subconjunctival connective tissue, mainly in the upper fornix; called also *glandulae mucosae conjunctivae [Krausei]* and *Krause's glands.* **glan′dulae cu′tis** [NA], cutaneous glands: the glands of the skin, including the sweat glands (glandulae sudoriferae), sebaceous glands (glandulae sebaceae), and the modified sweat glands that secrete cerumen (glandulae ceruminosae). **glan′dulae duodena′les** [NA], **glan′dulae duodena′les [Brun′neri],** duodenal glands: tubuloalveolar glands in the submucous layer of the duodenum which open into the crypts of Lieberkühn; they secrete urogastrone. Called also *Brunner's glands.* **glan′dulae endocri′nae** [NA], the endocrine glands (q.v.), including the thyroid, parathyroid, pituitary, and adrenal glands, and the gonads; called also *glandulae sine ductibus.* **glan′dulae esopha′geae,** NA alternative for *glandulae oesophageae.* **glan′dulae gas′tricae [pro′priae]** [NA], gastric glands proper: very numerous, nearly straight tubular glands located in the mucosa of the fundus and body of the stomach; they contain the cells that produce acid and pepsin. Called also *fundic glands.* **g. glomifor′mis,** anastomosis arteriovenosa glomeriformis. **glan′dulae hepat′icae,** glandulae mucosae biliosae. **g. incisi′va,** a small intraoral gland in the median line of the upper jaw near the incisors. **glan′dulae intestina′les** [NA], intestinal glands: simple tubular glands in the mucous membrane of the small intestine (*intestinales intestini tenuis*), opening between the bases of the villi and containing argentaffin cells; of the large intestine (*g. intestinales intestini crassi*); and of the rectum (*g. intestinales intestini recti*). Called also *crypts, glands,* or *follicles of Lieberkühn,* and *intestinal follicles.* **glan′dulae labia′les o′ris** [NA], labial glands of the mouth: the serous and mucous glands on the inner part of the lips. **g. lacrima′lis** [NA], lacrimal gland: one of the glands that lie at the upper outer angle of the orbit and secrete the tears; they are divided into two portions, the orbital and palpebral, by the orbital fascia. **glan′dulae lacrima′les accesso′riae** [NA], accessory lacrimal glands: portions of the lacrimal gland sometimes found near the superior fornix of the conjunctiva. **g. lacrima′lis infe′rior,** pars palpebralis glandulae lacrimalis. **g. lacrima′lis supe′rior,** pars orbitalis glandulae lacrimalis. **glan′dulae laryn′geae** [NA], laryngeal glands: the mucous glands in the mucosa of the larynx. **glan′dulae laryn′geae anterio′res,** mucous glands in the anterior of the larynx. **glan′dulae laryn′geae me′diae,** mucous glands located in the aryteno-epiglottic fold. **glan′dulae laryn′geae posteri-o′res,** mucous glands in the posterior wall of the larynx; called also *arytenoid glands.* **glan′dulae lingua′les** [NA], lingual glands: the mucous and serous glands on the surface of the tongue. **glan′dulae lingua′les anteri-o′res** [NA], anterior lingual glands: deeply placed mucoserous glands near the apex of the tongue. **g. mamma′ria** [NA], mammary gland: the collective glandular elements of the mamma, or breast, which secrete milk for nourishment of the young; see *mammary gland,* under *gland.* **glan′dulae mola′res** [NA], molar glands: the glands on the external aspect of the buccinator muscle, their ducts piercing it to open on the internal aspect of the cheek; called also *retromolar glands.* **g. muco′sa** [NA], mucous gland: a gland that secretes a slimy, chemically inert material. **g. muco′sae tu′bae auditi′vae,** g. tubariae. **glan′dulae muco′sae bilio′sae** [NA], glands of biliary mucosa: tubuloalveolar glands in the mucosa of the bile ducts and the neck of the gallbladder; called also *hepatic glands* and *glandulae hepaticae.* **glan′dulae muco′sae conjuncti′vae [Kraus′ei],** glandulae conjunctivales. **glan′dulae muco′sae ure′teris,** mucous glands of the ureter. **glan′dulae nasa′les** [NA], nasal glands: numerous large mucous and serous glands in the respiratory part of the nasal cavity. **glan′dulae oesopha′geae** [NA], esophageal glands: the mucous glands in the submucosa of the esophagus. Written also *glandulae esophageae* [NA alternative]. **glan′dulae olfacto′riae** [NA], olfactory glands: small mucous glands in the olfactory mucosa; called also *Bowman's glands.* **glan′dulae o′ris** [NA], the glands of the mouth. **glan′dulae palati′nae** [NA], palatine glands: the mucous glands on the soft palate and the posteromedial part of the hard palate; called also *staphyline glands.* **glan′dulae parathyroi′deae** [NA], small bodies in the region of the thyroid gland occurring in a variable number of pairs, commonly two, named *glandula parathyroidea superior* and *glandula parathyroidea inferior,* according to their position; see *parathyroid glands,* under *gland.* **g. parotid′ea** [NA], parotid gland: the largest of the three chief, paired glands which, together with numerous small glands in the mouth, constitute the salivary glands; it is located below the zygomatic arch, below and in front of the external acoustic meatus. **g. parotid′ea accesso′ria** [NA], accessory parotid gland: a more or less detached portion of the parotid gland that is frequently present. **glan′dulae pel′vis rena′lis,** mucous glands in the wall of the kidney pelvis. **glan′dulae pharyn′geae** [NA], pharyngeal glands: mucous glands beneath the tunica mucosa of the pharynx. Called also *glandulae pharyngeales* [NA alternative]. **glan′dulae pharyngea′les,** NA alternative for *glandulae pharyngeae.* **g. pinea′lis,** NA alternative for *corpus pineale.* **g. pituita′ria** [NA alternative], pituitary gland; see under *gland.* **glan′dulae preputia′les** [NA], preputial glands: small sebaceous glands of the corona of the penis and the inner surface of the prepuce, which secrete smegma; called also *Littre's crypts* or *glands.* **g. prosta′ta, g. prostat′ica,** prostate. **glan′dulae pylo′ricae** [NA], pyloric glands: the mucin-secreting glands of the pyloric part of the stomach. **glan′dulae saliva′riae majo′res** [NA], major salivary glands: the larger exocrine glands of the oral cavity, which together with the smaller salivary glands (*glandulae salivariae minores*) secrete saliva; the group includes the sublingual, submandibular, and parotid glands. **glan′dulae saliva′riae mino′res** [NA], minor salivary glands: the smaller exocrine glands of the oral cavity, which together with the larger salivary glands (*glandulae salivariae majores*) secrete saliva; the group includes the labial, buccal, molar, palatine, and lingual glands, and the anterior lingual gland. **glan′dulae seba′ceae** [NA], sebaceous glands: holocrine glands of the skin, secreting an oily substance, sebum, and situated in the corium. Called also *oil glands.* **glan′dulae seba′ceae conjunctiva′les** [NA], sebaceous glands of conjunctivae: modified rudimentary sebaceous glands attached directly to the follicles of the eyelashes; called also *glands of Zeis.* **glan′dulae seba′ceae la′bii majo′ris pudenda′lis,** sebaceous glands in the skin of the labia majora. **glan′dulae seba′ceae mam′mae,** glandulae areolares. **g. semina′lis,** NA alternative for *vesicula seminalis.* **g. seromuco′sa** [NA], seromucous gland: a gland composed of both mucous and serous secreting cells, such as the labial glands. **g. sero′sa** [NA], serous gland: a gland that secretes a watery albuminous material, commonly but not always containing enzymes. **glan′dulae si′ne duc′tibus** [L. "glands without ducts"] glandulae endocrinae. **g. sublingua′lis** [NA], sublingual gland: the smallest of the three chief, paired salivary glands, predominantly mucous in type, and draining into the oral cavity through 10 to 30 sublingual ducts; called also *Rivinus gland.* **g. submandibula′ris** [NA], **g. submaxilla′ris,** submandibular gland: one of the three chief, paired salivary glands, predominantly serous, lying partly above and partly below the posterior half of the base of the mandible. **glan′dulae sudorif′erae** [NA], sudoriferous or sweat glands: the glands that secrete sweat, situated in the corium or subcutaneous tissue, and opening by a duct on the surface of the body. They are of two types: The ordinary or *eccrine sweat glands* are unbranched, coiled, tubular glands that are distributed over almost all of the body surface, and promote cooling by evaporation of their secretion. The *apocrine sweat glands* are large, branched, specialized glands that empty into the upper portion of a hair follicle instead of directly onto the skin surface, and are found only on certain areas of the body, such as around the anus and in the axilla. Called also *sudoriparous glands.* **g. suprarena′lis** [NA], a flattened body situated in the retroperitoneal tissues at the superior pole of each kidney; called also *g. adrenalis* [NA alternative]. See *adrenal gland,* under *gland.* **glan′dulae suprarena′les accesso′riae** [NA], accessory suprarenal glands: accessory adrenal glandular tissue found in the abdomen or pelvis. See *adrenal g's, accessory,* under *gland.* **glan′dulae tarsa′les** [NA], **glan′dulae tarsa′les [Meibo′mi],** tarsal glands: sebaceous follicles between the tarsi and the conjunctiva of the eyelids; called also *palpebral* or *meibomian glands.* **g. thyroi′dea** [NA], thyroid gland (see under *gland*), one of the endocrine glands, normally situated in the front of the lower part of the neck and consisting of two lobes, one on each side of the trachea and joined in front by a narrow isthmus. **glan′dulae thyroi′deae accesso′riae** [NA], accessory thyroid glands: small exclaves of the thyroid gland that may be found any place along the course of the thyroglossal duct, as well as in the thorax. **glan′dula thyroi′dea accesso′ria suprahyoi′dea,** accessory thyroid tissue found above the hyoid bone. **glan′dulae trachea′les** [NA], tracheal glands: mucous glands in the elastic submucous coat between the cartilaginous rings and on the posterior wall of the trachea. **glan′dulae tuba′riae** [NA], mucous glands within the mucosa of the auditory tube, especially near its nasopharyngeal end; called also *glandulae mucosae tubae auditivae* and *mucous glands of auditory* or *eustachian tube.* **g. tympan′icae,** tympanic gland: a small mass situated on Jacobson's nerve in the tympanic canal. **glan′dulae urethra′les [Lit′trei],** glandulae urethrales urethrae masculinae. **glan′dulae urethra′les ure′thrae femini′nae** [NA], urethral glands of female urethra: numerous small mucous glands in the mucosa of the female urethra, some of which on either side are drained by the inconstant paraurethral duct opening into the vestibule. **glan′dulae urethra′les ure′thrae masculi′nae** [NA], mucous glands in the wall of the male urethra; called also *Littre's glands.* **glan′dulae urethra′les ure′thrae mulie′bris,** glandulae urethrales urethrae femininae. **g. uropygia′lis,** preen gland. **glan′dulae uteri′nae** [NA], uterine glands: simple tubular glands throughout the entire thickness and extent of the endometrium, which become enlarged during the premenstrual period. **glan′dulae vesica′les ves′icae urina′riae,** mucous glands in the wall of the urinary bladder. **g. vestibula′ris ma′jor** [NA], either of two small reddish yellow bodies in the vestibular bulbs, one on each side of the vaginal orifice; they are homologues of the bulbourethral glands in the male. Called also *Bartholin's gland* and *greater vestibular gland.* **glan′dulae vestibula′res mino′res** [NA], small mucous glands opening upon the vestibular mucous membrane between the urethral and the vaginal orifice; called also *lesser vestibular glands.*

glandulae (glan′du-le) [L.] genitive and plural of *glandula.*

glandular (glan′du-lar) 1. pertaining to or of the nature of a gland. 2. pertaining to the glans penis or glans clitoridis.

glandule (glan′dūl) [L. *glandula*] a small gland.

glandulous (glan′du-lus) [L. *glandulosus*] abounding in kernels or small glands.

glans (glanz), pl. *glan′des* [L. "acorn"] [NA] a general term for a small rounded mass, or glandlike body. **g. clitor′idis** [NA], **g. of clitoris,** erectile tissue at the end of the clitoris, which is continuous with the intermediate part of the vestibular bulbs. **g. pe′nis** [NA], the cap-shaped expansion of the corpus spongiosum at the end of the penis; called also *balanus.*

glanular (glan′u-lar) pertaining to the glans penis or glans clitoris.

Glanzmann's thrombasthenia (disease) (glahnz′manz) [Edward *Glanzmann,* Swiss pediatrician, 1887–1959] see *thrombasthenia.*

glare (glār) [Middle English *glaren*] a condition of discomfort in the eye and of depression of central vision produced when a bright light enters the field of vision, especially when the eye is adapted to dark. The amount of glare is directly proportional to the candle power of the light and inversely proportional to the square of the distance of the light from the eye and to its angular distance from the visual axis. *Direct g.,* when the image of the light falls on the fovea; *peripheral g.,* when it falls outside of the fovea.

glarometer (glār-om′ĕ-ter) [*glare* + *-meter*] an instrument for measuring a person's resistance to glare from the lights of an approaching automobile.

glaserian fissure, etc. (gla-se′re-an) [named for or described by Johann Heinrich *Glaser* (Glaserius), Swiss anatomist, 1629–1675] fissura petrotympanica.

Glasgow's sign (glas′gōz) [William Carr *Glasgow,* American physician, 1845–1907] see under *sign.*

glass (glas) [L. *vit′rum*] 1. a hard, brittle, and often transparent material, usually consisting of the fused amorphous silicates of potassium or sodium, and of calcium, with silica in excess. 2. a container, usually cylindrical, made from glass. 3. (pl.) lenses worn to aid or improve vision; see *glasses, lens,* and *spectacles.* **cover g.,** a thin glass plate used to cover an object for microscopical examination. Spelled also *coverglass.* **crown g.,** a glass of low refractive index (achieved by incorporating a considerable percentage of phosphorus pentoxide); used in combination with flint glass in multielement lenses. **cupping g.,** a vessel of glass from which the air has been or can be exhausted, applied to the body for the purpose of drawing blood to the surface; no longer used. **flint g.,** a highly refractive glass in which calcium has been replaced in large part by lead; used for lenses and prisms and in the manufacture of cut glass. **lithium g.,** glass containing lithium, used in grenz ray x-ray tubes. **object g.,** see *objective.* **optical g.,** glass of high quality and controlled composition, used for lenses. **quartz g.,** pure fused silica, SiO_2; used for prisms, lenses, and chemical vessels (1) because its index of thermal expansion is so small that it does not crack when heated or cooled, and (2) because it transmits more ultraviolet radiation than does ordinary glass. **test g.,** a small glass vessel, resembling a beaker, used in a chemical laboratory. **Wood's g.,** see under *light.*

glasses (glas′ez) spectacles; a pair of lenses arranged in a frame holding them in the proper position before the eyes, as an aid to vision. See also *lens* and *spectacles.* **bifocal g.,** lenses which have two different refracting powers, one for distant and one for near vision. **contact g.,** see *contact lens.* **crutch g.,** glasses which will elevate and support the upper lid of patients with ptosis. **Hallauer's g.,** glasses with grayish-green lenses which prevent the passage of blue and ultraviolet rays. **safety g.,** see under *lens.* **trifocal g.,** glasses with lenses which have three different refracting powers, one for distant, one for intermediate, and one for near vision.

glassy (glas′e) like glass; hyaline or vitreous.

Glauber's salt (glow′berz) [Johann Rudolf *Glauber,* German physician and chemist, 1604–1688] sodium sulfate.

glaucarubin (glaw″kah-ru′bin) a crystalline glycoside obtained from the fruit of *Simaruba glauca* D.C. (Simarubaceae); formerly used as an amebicide.

glaucoma (glaw-ko′mah) [Gr. *glaukōma* opacity of the crystalline lens (from the dull gray gleam of the affected eye)] a group of eye diseases characterized by an increase in intraocular pressure which causes pathological changes in the optic disk and typical defects in the field of vision.

absolute g., the final stage of glaucoma characterized by pain in the eye and blindness. **acute congestive g.,** narrow-angle g. **air-block g.,** a form of postoperative glaucoma, resulting from blockage of the flow of aqueous by air injected inadvertently behind the iris either through the pupillary opening or through a peripheral iridectomy. **angle-closure g.,** glaucoma caused by closure of the anterior angle by contact between the iris and the inner surface of the trabecular meshwork; called also *closed-angle g., narrow-angle g.,* and *pupillary block g.* **angle-closure g., acute,** the third phase of angle-closure glaucoma and a grave medical emergency. Initially the symptoms resemble intermittent angle-closure glaucoma. Then, as the intraocular pressure continues increasing, the cornea becomes swollen and steamy; the iris fixes in mid-dilation; there is excruciating ocular pain radiating to the other areas of the trigeminal distribution, and there may be nausea and vomiting. Finally the eye may become red and congested; visual acuity fails rapidly as the cornea keeps swelling, and severe visual field loss or even blindness may result if the intraocular pressure is not lowered. **angle-closure g., chronic,** the fourth, last stage of angle-closure glaucoma, it is an irreversible increase of intraocular pressure resulting from progressive damage to the angle structures and from permanent, at least partial closure of the anterior angle by synechiae. **angle-closure g., intermittent,** the second phase of angle-closure glaucoma, usually lasting for several months, and characterized by intermittent, transient attacks of glaucoma with rapidly rising intraocular pressure, edematous cornea, and dull or throbbing pain in or around the eye. **angle-closure g., latent,** the first phase of angle-closure glaucoma; patients may be free of symptoms or have minor attacks of varying severity, duration, and frequency for months or years before a crisis. Gonioscopy reveals narrow angles capable of closure. Called also *prodromal g.* **angle-recession g.,** glaucoma secondary to contusion injury of the eye, in which the anterior chamber is deep and the angle recedes, with exposure of the ciliary body, as seen gonioscopically, with blocking of the trabecular spaces; called also *contusion g.* **aphakic g.,** a general term referring to glaucoma in an eye from which the lens has been removed; the glaucoma may be related to the cataract extraction or to its sequelae, or it may have existed prior to the cataract extraction. **apoplectic g.,** hemorrhagic g. **auricular g.,** that associated with increased intralabyrinthine pressure. **capsular g., g. capsulare,** an open-angle glaucoma associated with the exfoliation syndrome, and with particles of iris pigment scattered in the anterior angle. **chronic narrow-angle g.,** a form of narrow angle glaucoma without a severe congestive episode. **chronic g.,** open-angle g. **chymotrypsin-induced g.,** enzyme g. **closed-angle g.,** angle-closure g. **congenital g.,** infantile g. **congestive g.,** narrow-angle g. **g. consumma'tum,** absolute g. **contusion g.,** angle-recession g. **Donders' g.,** advanced open-angle g. **enzyme g.,** a transient glaucoma developing postoperatively in patients in whom trypsin has been used in the lysis of the zonule during cataract surgery; it is usually self-limited, with no permanent damage. **ghost cell g.,** an open-angle glaucoma caused by rigid erythroclasts obstructing aqueous outflow, occurring after vitreous hemorrhage caused by trauma or by retinal neovascularization or by cataract extraction. **hemolytic g.,** an open-angle glaucoma caused by blood clots filling the anterior angle or by erythrocytes infiltrating the trabecular network. **hemorrhagic g.,** that which is caused by pressure from retinal hemorrhage. **infantile g.,** a form of congenital glaucoma that may be fully developed at birth, with characteristic signs (enlargement and hazing of the corneas), or it may develop at any time up to two or three years of age; these signs result from inability of the cornea and sclera to withstand the increased intraocular pressure. Called also *buphthalmos.* Cf. *juvenile g.* **inflammatory g.,** a form attended with ciliary congestion, corneal opacity, and blindness, recurring in paroxysmal attacks. **juvenile g.,** glaucoma differing from infantile glaucoma in that it occurs in older children and young adults up to 30 years of age, and there is no gross enlargement of the eyeball. **lenticular g.,** glaucoma occurring in association with congenital or traumatic dislocation of the lens, or with swelling of the lens, usually due to mechanical obstruction at the peripheral angle of the anterior chamber. **low-tension g.,** open-angle glaucoma without increased intraocular pressure. **malignant g.,** glaucoma that grows rapidly worse

in spite of iridectomy. **melanomalytic g.,** glaucoma caused by mechanical blockage of the angle by macrophages in the eye with necrotic malignant melanoma. **narrow-angle g.,** angle-closure g. **neovascular g.,** a form of secondary glaucoma; glaucoma caused by neovascularization in the chamber angle. **noncongestive g.,** open-angle g. **obstructive g.,** narrow-angle g. **open-angle g.,** any glaucoma in which the angle of the anterior chamber remains open, but filtration is gradually diminished because of the tissues of the angle; called also *chronic simple g., simple g.,* and *wide-angle g.* **phacogenic g., phacolytic g.,** an open-angle glaucoma secondary to leakage of lens protein into the aqueous from a mature or hypermature cataract with subsequent ingestion of the protein by macrophages, which swell and block the trabecular spaces. **pigmentary g.,** a form of open-angle glaucoma associated with an abnormal amount of pigment dispersion in the anterior segment of the eye. **primary g.,** increased intraocular pressure occurring in an eye without previous disease; see *angle-closure g.* and *open-angle g.* **prodromal g.,** latent angle-closure g. **pupillary block g.,** angle-closure g. **secondary g.,** increased intraocular pressure resulting from a preexisting disease or injury. **simple g.,** primary open-angle g. **steroid g.,** a secondary open-angle glaucoma due to chronic use of topical or systemic corticosteroids. **traumatic g.,** an increase in intraocular pressure due to a nonperforating injury of the globe, resulting in vascular congestion. **vitreous-block g.,** postoperative glaucoma in which vitreous plugs the pupil, so that the aqueous, which is unable to move to the anterior chamber, forces the vitreous and iris forward, producing occlusion of the chamber angle and eventually peripheral anterior synechiae. **wide-angle g.,** open-angle g.

glaucomatous (glaw-ko'mah-tus)   pertaining to or of the nature of glaucoma.

glaucosis (glaw-ko'sis)   blindness caused by glaucoma.

glaucosuria (glaw″ko-su're-ah) [Gr. *glaukos* silvery + *ouron* urine + *-ia*]   indicanuria.

glaukomflecken (glou′kōm-flek′n) [Ger. "glaucoma spots"]   glaucomatous cataract.

glaze (glāz)   1. to cover with a glossy, smooth surface or coating. 2. a ceramic veneer added to a dental porcelain restoration after it has been fired, to give a completely nonporous, glossy or semiglossy surface. 3. the critical stage in the final firing of dental porcelain when complete fusion takes place, with the formation of a thin, vitreous, glossy surface.

GLC   gas-liquid chromatography.

gleet (glēt)   1. a chronic form of gonorrheal urethritis. 2. a urethral discharge, especially one that is mucous or purulent. **vent g.,** cloacitis.

gleety (glēt′e)   pertaining to or of the nature of gleet.

Glénard's disease (gla-narz′) [Frantz *Glénard,* French physician, 1848–1920]   see *splanchnoptosis.*

Glenn operation (procedure, shunt) (glen) [William W. L. *Glenn,* American surgeon, born 1914]   see under *operation.*

glenohumeral (gle″no-hu′mer-al)   pertaining to the glenoid cavity and to the humerus.

glenoid (gle′noid) [Gr. *glēnē* socket + *eidos* form]   resembling a pit or socket; see *cavitas glenoidalis.*

Glenosporella (gle″no-spo-rel′ah)   former name for the genus *Chrysosporium.*

Gley's cells, glands (glāz) [Marcel Eugène Émile *Gley,* French physiologist, 1857–1930]   see under *cell* and see *glandulae thyroidea accessoriae.*

GLI   glucagon-like immunoreactivity; see *enteroglucagon.*

glia (gli′ah) [Gr. "glue"]   the neuroglia. **ameboid g.,** degenerated neuroglial cells which are rich in pale protoplasm, possess few processes, and have densely staining nuclei. **cytoplasmic g.,** enlarged neuroglial cells, rich in cytoplasm, containing vacuoles and supplied with fibrils; seen in degeneration of the spinal cord. **g. of Fañana,** a form of neuroglial cell occurring in the molecular layer of the cerebellar cortex. **fibrillary g.,** degenerated neuroglial cells containing an abundance of fibrils.

-glia [Gr. *glia* glue]   a word termination denoting neuroglia.

gliacyte (gli′ah-sīt) [*glia* + Gr. *kytos* hollow vessel]   a neuroglia cell.

gliadin (gli′ah-din) [Gr. *glia* glue] an alcohol-soluble protein present in wheat and occurring in various forms (α-, β-, γ-, and W-gliadins); it contains the toxic factor associated with celiac disease.

glial (gli′al) of or pertaining to the neuroglia or glia.

gliamilide (gli-am′ĭ-lid) chemical name: *endo*-N-[2-[1-[[[[(bicyclo[2.2.1]hept-5-en-2-ylmethyl)amino]carbonyl]amino]sulfonyl]-4-piperidinyl]ethyl]-2-methoxy-3-pyridinecarboxamide; an oral hypoglycemic, $C_{23}H_{33}N_5O_5S$.

gliarase (gli′ah-rās) an aggregation of astrocytes whose cytoplasm has undergone incomplete fission.

glibenclamide (gli-ben′klah-mīd) glyburide.

glibornuride (gli-born′ūr-īd) chemical name: *N*-[[(3-hydroxy-4,7,7-trimethylbicyclo[2.2.1]hept-2-yl)amino]carbonyl]-4-methylbenzenesulfonamide; an orally effective hypoglycemic agent of the sulfonylurea group, $C_{18}H_{26}N_2O_4S$.

glicentin (gli-sen′tin) enteroglucagon.

glicetanile sodium (glĭ-set′ah-nīl) chemical name: *N*-(5-chloro-2-methoxyphenyl)-4-[[[5-(2-methyl propyl)-2-pyrimidinyl]amino]sulfonyl]benzeneacetamide monosodium salt; an oral hypoglycemic, $C_{23}H_{24}ClN_4NaO_4S$. Called also *glydanile sodium*.

glide (glīd) a smooth continuous movement. **mandibular g.,** the side-to-side, protrusive, and intermediate movement of the mandible occurring when the teeth or other occluding surfaces are in contact. **occlusal g.,** the movement induced by deflective tooth contact that diverts the mandible from a normal path of closure to a centric jaw relation.

gliflumide (glĭ-floo′mīd) chemical name: (−)-(S)-*N*-[1-(5-fluoro-2-methoxyphenyl)ethyl]-4-[[[5-(2-methylpropyl)-2-pyrimidinyl]amino]sulfonyl]benzeneacetamide; an oral hypoglycemic, $C_{25}H_{29}FN_4O_4S$.

gli(o)- [Gr. *glia* glue] a combining form denoting relationship to a gluey substance or, specifically, to the neuroglia.

gliobacteria (gli″o-bak-te′re-ah) [*glio-* + *bacteria*] bacteria that are surrounded by a gelatinous matrix.

glioblast (gli′o-blast) spongioblast.

glioblastoma (gli″o-blas-to′mah) [*glio-* + Gr. *blastos* germ + *-oma*] a general term for malignant forms of astrocytoma. **g. multifor′me,** an astrocytoma of Grade III or IV; it is a rapidly growing tumor, usually confined to the cerebral hemispheres and composed of a mixture of spongioblasts, astroblasts, and astrocytes. Called also *spongioblastoma multiforme* and *anaplastic astrocytoma*.

gliococcus (gli″o-kok′us) [*glio-* + Gr. *kokkos* berry] a micrococcus that forms gelatinous matter.

gliocyte (gli′o-sīt) gliacyte. **retinal g's,** Müller's fibers.

gliocytoma (gli″o-si-to′mah) glioma.

gliofibrillary (gli″o-fi′brĭ-lār-e) pertaining to fibrils of the neuroglia.

gliogenous (gli-oj′ĕ-nus) [*glio-* + Gr. *gennan* to produce] produced or formed by glial (neuroglial) cells.

glioma (gli-o′mah) [*glio-* + *-oma*] a tumor composed of tissue which represents neuroglia in any one of its stages of development. The term is sometimes extended to include all the primary intrinsic neoplasms of the brain and spinal cord, including astrocytomas, ependymomas, neurocytomas, etc. **astrocytic g.,** astrocytoma. **g. endo′phytum,** retinoblastoma beginning in the inner layers of the retina and spreading toward the center of the globe. **ependymal g.,** a bulky, solid, rather firm but vascular tumor of the fourth ventricle. **g. exoph′ytum,** retinoblastoma beginning in the outer layers of the retina and spreading away from the center of the globe. **ganglionic g.,** a glioma that contains also ganglion cells of nearly adult type; see *neuroblastoma*. **mixed g.,** a glioma in which the cytological components are of more than one cell type, the commonest form consisting of oligodendrogliomatous foci in an otherwise typical astrocytoma. **nasal g.,** a tumor-like mass composed of ectopic neural tissue in the nasal cavity. **optic g.,** a slow-growing glioma of the optic nerve or optic chiasm heralded by visual loss, often with secondary strabismus, followed by proptosis and loss of ocular movement. **peripheral g.,** schwannoma. **g. ret′inae,** retinoblastoma. **g. sarcomato′sum,** a gliosarcoma. **telangiectatic g.,** glioma containing blood vessels.

gliomatosis (gli″o-mah-to′sis) excessive development of

the neuroglia, especially of the spinal cord, in certain cases of syringomyelia.

gliomatous (gli-o′mah-tus) affected with or of the nature of glioma.

glioneuroma (gli″o-nu-ro′mah) a tumor containing both gliomatous and neuromatous elements.

gliophagia (gli″o-fa′je-ah) [*glio-* + Gr. *phagein* to eat] phagocytosis of neuroglial cells.

gliopil (gli′o-pil) [*glio-* + Gr. *pilos* felt] a dense feltwork of glial processes, as in the subependymal matrix of the ventricular system.

gliosa (gli-o′sah) (obs.) the gray matter of the spinal cord which covers the head of the dorsal horn and surrounds the central canal.

gliosarcoma (gli″o-sar-ko′mah) [*glio-* + *sarcoma*] a spindle cell glioma; see also *spongioblastoma*. **g. ret′inae,** retinoblastoma.

gliosis (gli-o′sis) an excess of astroglia in damaged areas of the central nervous system. **basilar g.,** gliosis affecting the brain stem, thalamus, and corpus striatum. **cerebellar g.,** gliosis affecting the cerebellum. **diffuse g.,** gliosis affecting the whole of the cerebral tissue, or widely scattered through it. **g. endome′trii,** g. uteri. **hemispheric g.,** gliosis affecting one of the cerebral hemispheres. **hypertrophic nodular g.,** a form of gliosis in which the brain is symmetrically enlarged because of hyperplasia of the neuroglial tissue. **isomorphic g.,** gliosis in which there is a regular and parallel arrangement of glial fibers. **lobar g.,** gliosis affecting a single lobe of the brain. **perivascular g.,** a form of arteriosclerosis of the cerebral vessels, marked by increase of the neuroglia about the vessels. **spinal g.,** gliosis of the spinal cord. **unilateral g.,** hemispheric gliosis. **g. u′teri,** proliferation of fetal neural tissue in the endometrium or endocervix.

gliosome (gli′o-sōm) [*glio-* + Gr. *sōma* body] one of the small cytoplasmic granules seen in neuroglial cells.

gliotoxin (gli″o-tok′sin) an antibiotic substance, $C_{13}H_{14}N_2O_4S_2$, obtained from several unrelated species of fungi, including species of *Trichoderma*, *Aspergillus*, and *Penicillium*; it is a neutral, nitrogen- and sulfur-containing compound first isolated from culture filtrates of *Gliocladium* (*Trichoderma*).

glipizide (glip′ah-zīd) chemical name: *N*-[2-[4-[[[(cyclohexylamino)carbonyl]amino]sulfonyl]phenyl]ethyl]-5-methylpyrazine carboxamide. An orally effective hypoglycemic, $C_{21}H_{27}N_5O_4S$, used in the treatment of diabetes mellitus in certain patients.

Gliricola (gli-rik′o-lah) a genus of biting lice. **G. porcel′li,** a biting louse found on guinea pigs.

glischrin (glis′krin) [Gr. *glischros* gluey] a mucin produced in urine by bacterial activity.

glischruria (glis-kroo′re-ah) [Gr. *glischros* gluey + *ouron* urine + *-ia*] the presence of glischrin in the urine.

glissade (glis-ād′) [Fr. "sliding"] a gliding involuntary movement of the eye in changing the point of fixation; it is a slower, smoother movement than is a saccade.

glissadic (glis-sad′ik) pertaining to a glissade.

Glisson's capsule, disease, sling (glis′unz) [Francis *Glisson*, English physician and anatomist, 1597–1677, one of the founders of the Royal Society] see *capsula fibrosa perivascularis*, and *rickets*, and see under *sling*.

glissonitis (glis″o-ni′tis) inflammation of Glisson's capsule (capsula fibrosa perivascularis [NA]).

globi (glo′bi) [L.]. 1. genitive and plural of *globus*. 2. encapsulated globular masses containing bacilli, seen in smears of lepromatous leprosy lesions.

globidiosis (glob-bid″i′o-sis) former name for besnoitiosis.

Globidium (glo-bid′e-um) former name for *Besnoitia*.

globin (glo′bin) the protein constituent of hemoglobin; also any member of a group of proteins similar to the typical globin. **g. zinc insulin injection,** see under *injection*.

globinometer (glo″bĭ-nom′ĕ-ter) an instrument used in determining the proportion of oxyhemoglobin in the blood.

globoid (glo′boid) globe-shaped; spheroid.

globose (glo′bōs) [L. *globus* a ball] globe-shaped, spherical.

globoside (glob′o-sīd) a sphingoglycolipid containing acetylated aminosugars and simple hexoses of the general composition: ceramide-(glucose)$_m$-(galactose)$_n$-(*N*-acetylhexosamine)$_p$. It occurs in human serum, spleen, liver, and erythrocytes, accumulates in tissues in Sandhoff's disease, and is probably a precursor of glucocerebroside and ceramide trihexoside.

globular (glob′u-lar) 1. like a globe or globule. 2. composed of globules.

Globularia (glob″u-la′re-ah) a European shrub; *G. alypum* L. (Globulariaceae), a perennial herb indigenous to the Mediterranean region, is used as a purgative and for intermittent fevers.

globulariacitrin (glob″u-la″re-ah-sit′rin) rutin.

globule (glob′ūl) [L. *globulus* a globule] 1. a small spherical mass or body. 2. a small spherical drop of fluid or semifluid substance, e.g., a fat droplet in milk or a drop of water. 3. a little globe or pellet, as of medicine. **dentin g's,** small spherical bodies in the peripheral dentin, created by beginning calcification of the matrix about discrete foci. **Dobie's g.,** a minute stainable mass in the middle of the transparent disk of a muscle fibril. **Marchi's g's,** fragments and particles of broken-up myelin which stain by Marchi's method, seen in degeneration of the spinal cord. **milk g's,** the small round masses of fat in milk which tend to separate out as cream. **Morgagni's g's,** round fragments of cells in the cortex of the lens; they are a sign of mature cataract. **myelin g's,** colorless globules resembling fat droplets and sometimes spirally marked, seen in some sputa. **polar g's,** polar bodies.

globuli (glob′u-li) [L.] genitive and plural of *globulus*.

globulin (glob′u-lin) [L. *globulus* globule] a class of proteins characterized by being insoluble in water, but soluble in saline solutions (euglobulins), or water soluble proteins (pseudoglobulins) whose other physical properties closely resemble true globulins. See *serum g.* **AC g., accelerator g.,** Factor V; see *coagulation factors,* under *factor.* **alpha g's,** serum globulins having α electrophoretic mobility. **antihemophilic g. (AHG),** Factor VIII; see *coagulation factors,* under *factor.* **anti–human g. serum** [USP], monospecific or broad spectrum antiserum produced by immunizing a rabbit or other animal with human plasma proteins; used in the antiglobulin test (Coombs' test) and immunoelectrophoresis. **antilymphocyte g. (ALG),** the gamma globulin fraction of antilymphocyte serum (q.v.). **antithymocyte g. (ATG),** the gamma globulin fraction of equine antiserum against human thymocytes, an immunosuppressive agent that causes specific destruction of T lymphocytes, used experimentally in treatment of renal allograft rejection and graft-versus-host (GVH) disease. **beta g's,** globulins of plasma which have an electrophoretic mobility in neutral or alkaline solutions intermediate between that of the alpha and the gamma globulins. **corticosteroid-binding g., cortisol-binding g. (CBG),** transcortin. **gamma g's,** serum globulins having γ electrophoretic mobility. Since the gamma globulin fraction is composed almost entirely of immunoglobulins, gamma globulin came to be used as a synonym of "immunoglobulin" or "immune globulin." This usage is imprecise, because some immunoglobulins have α or β electrophoretic mobility, and is in decline. **hepatitis B immune g.** [USP], a specific immune globulin derived from plasma of human donors with high titers of antibodies against hepatitis B surface antigen (HB$_s$Ag); used for postexposure prophylaxis following contact with HB$_s$Ag-positive materials, also administered to infants of HB$_s$Ag-positive mothers. **immune g.** [USP], a concentrated preparation containing gamma globulins, predominantly IgG, from a large pool of human donors; used for prophylaxis of measles or hepatitis A and for treatment of hypogammaglobulinemia in immunodeficient patients. Formerly called *immune human serum g.* Called also *gamma g.* **immune human serum g.,** immune g. **pertussis immune g.** [USP], a specific immune globulin derived from human donors immunized with pertussis vaccine; used for prophylaxis and treatment of pertussis. Formerly called *pertussis immune human g.* **rabies immune g.** [USP], a specific immune globulin derived from plasma of human donors hyperimmunized with rabies vaccine; administered in conjunction with rabies vaccine in cases of bite or scratch exposure to animals known or suspected to be rabid. **Rh$_o$(D) immune g.** [USP], a specific immune globulin derived from plasma of human donors immunized to produce high levels of antibodies against the Rh$_o$ antigen (D antigen); used to prevent Rh-sensitization of Rh-negative females and thus prevent erythroblastosis fetalis in subsequent pregnancies; administered within 72 hours after exposure to Rh-positive blood resulting from delivery of an Rh-positive child, abortion, or miscarriage of an Rh-positive fetus, or transfusion of Rh-positive blood. Formerly called *Rh$_o$(D) immune human g.* **testosterone-estradiol–binding g. (TEBG),** a plasma protein that transports testosterone in the blood. **tetanus immune g.** [USP], a specific immune globulin derived from blood of human donors hyperimmunized with tetanus toxoid; used for prophylaxis and treatment of tetanus. Formerly called *tetanus immune human g.* **thyroxine-binding g.,** a plasma carrier inter-α-globulin that transports thyroxine in the blood. **vaccinia immune g. (VIG)** [USP], a specific immune globulin derived from blood of human donors immunized with vaccinia virus smallpox vaccine; used for prophylaxis and treatment of vaccinia or smallpox. Formerly called *vaccinia immune human g.* **varicella-zoster immune g. (VZIG),** a specific immune globulin derived from plasma of human donors with high titers of varicella-zoster antibodies; used for prevention or amelioration of varicella in immunodeficient or immunosuppressed patients exposed to the disease and in neonates whose mothers develop varicella in the perinatal period. **g. X,** a globulin occurring in the intracellular spaces of muscle.

globulinuria (glob″u-lin-u′re-ah) [*globulin* + Gr. *ouron* urine + *-ia*] the presence of globulin in the urine.

globulose (glob′u-lōs) a proteose produced by action of pepsin on the globulins; several varieties have been described.

globulus (glob′u-lus), pl. *glob′uli* [L.] 1. the globose nucleus. 2. a pill, bolus, or spherical suppository. **glob′uli os′sei,** globules of bone tissue contained within lacunae of the calcified cartilage matrix in intrachondrial bone.

globus (glo′bus), pl. *glo′bi* [L.] 1. a sphere or ball; [NA] a general term denoting a spherical structure. 2. see *globi,* def. 2. **g. of the heel,** that portion of the wall of a horse's hoof where it curves around the heel to form the bar. **g. hyster′icus,** the disturbing subjective sensation of a lump in the throat; seen in hysteria. **g. ma′jor epididym′idis,** caput epididymidis. **g. mi′nor epididym′idis,** cauda epididymidis. **g. pal′lidus,** the smaller and more medial part of the lentiform nucleus of the brain, separated from the putamen by the lateral medullary lamina. In official anatomical nomenclature, it is divided by the medial medullary lamina into two parts, lateral and medial (see *g. pallidus lateralis* and *g. pallidus medialis*), both of which have extensive connections with the corpus striatum, thalamus, and mesencephalon. Called also *pallidum.* See also *paleostriatum.* **g. pal′lidus latera′lis** [NA], the larger, lateral part of the globus pallidus, separated from the putamen by the lateral medullary lamina and from the smaller, medial part of the globus pallidus by the medial medullary lamina; called also *pallidum I.* See also *globus pallidus.* **g. pal′lidus media′lis** [NA], the smaller, medial part of the globus pallidus, separated from the larger, lateral part by the medial medullary lamina; called also *pallidum II.* See also *globus pallidus.*

glomangioma (glo-man″je-o′mah) [*glomus* + Gr. *angeion* vessel + *-oma*] glomus tumor.

glomectomy (glo-mek′to-me) excision of a glomus, especially of the glomus caroticum.

glomera (glom′er-ah) [L.] plural of *glomus.*

glomerate (glom′er-āt) [L. *glomeratus* wound into a ball] crowded together into a ball.

glomerular (glo-mer′u-lar) pertaining to or of the nature of a glomerulus, especially a renal glomerulus.

glomeruli (glo-mer′u-li) [L.] genitive and plural of *glomerulus.*

glomerulitis (glo-mer″u-li′tis) inflammation of the glomeruli of the kidney, with proliferative or necrotizing changes of the endothelial or epithelial cells or thickening of the basement membrane.

glomerul(o)- [L. *glomerulus,* q.v.] combining form denoting relationship to the renal glomeruli.

glomerulonephritis (glo-mer″u-lo-ně-fri′tis) [*glomerulus* + *nephritis*] a variety of nephritis characterized by inflammation of the capillary loops in the glomeruli of the kidney. It occurs in acute, subacute, and chronic forms and may be secondary to hemolytic streptococcal infection. Evidence also supports possible immune or autoimmune mechanisms.

acute g., glomerulonephritis, typically preceded by tonsillitis or febrile pharyngitis, and characterized by proteinuria, edema, hematuria, renal failure, and hypertension. **chronic g.,** a slowly progressive glomerulonephritis generally leading to irreversible renal failure; it may be a primary disease, follow acute glomerulonephritis, or be secondary to systemic disease. Symptoms and course vary widely. **chronic hypocomplementemic g.,** membranoproliferative g. **focal g.,** a condition in which only some glomeruli show inflammatory changes, others appearing normal. **focal embolic g.,** focal glomerulonephritis associated with bacterial endocarditis; see *Löhlein-Baehr lesion,* under *lesion.* **IgA g.,** a chronic form marked by hematuria and proteinuria and by deposits of IgA immunoglobulin in the mesangial areas of the renal glomeruli, with subsequent reactive hyperplasia of mesangial cells; called also *Berger's disease* and *IgA nephropathy.* **immune complex g.,** see *immune complex disease,* under *disease.* **lobular g.,** membranoproliferative g. **lobulonodular g.,** membranoproliferative g. **malignant g.,** rapidly progressive g. **membranoproliferative g.,** a chronic glomerulonephritis characterized by mesangial cell proliferation and irregular thickening of the glomerular capillary wall. There are two subtypes: *Type I* marked by subendothelial electron-dense deposits and classic complement pathway activation and *Type II* marked by heavy electron-dense deposits in the glomerular basement membrane and alternative complement pathway activation involving C3 nephritic factor. It occurs in older children and young adults and follows a slowly progressing course with irregular remissions ultimately resulting in renal failure. Called also *chronic hypocomplementemic g., lobular g., mesangiocapillary g.,* and (type II only) *dense deposit disease.* **membranous g.,** a form characterized histologically by proteinaceous deposits on the glomerular capillary basement membrane or by thickening of the membrane. The clinical features are those of chronic glomerulonephritis, occasionally with transient nephrotic syndrome. **mesangiocapillary g.,** membranoproliferative g. **nodular g.,** membranoproliferative g. **rapidly progressive g.,** acute glomerulonephritis marked by a rapid progression to end-stage renal failure and, histologically, by profuse epithelial proliferation; principal signs are anuria, proteinuria, hematuria, and anemia. **segmental g.,** focal glomerulonephritis in which only limited segments of affected glomeruli are diseased. **subacute g.,** persistence of acute glomerulonephritis, with or without periods of remission, which may develop into the lobular or malignant forms.

glomerulonephropathy (glo-mer″u-lo-ně-frop′ah-the) any noninflammatory disease of the renal glomeruli.

glomerulopathy (glo-mer″u-lop′ah-the) any disease of the renal glomeruli. **diabetic g.,** intercapillary glomerulosclerosis.

glomerulosclerosis (glo-mer″u-lo-skle-ro′sis) fibrosis and scarring which result in senescence of the renal glomeruli. **diabetic g.,** intercapillary g. **focal segmental g.,** focal glomerular sclerosis. **intercapillary g.,** a degenerative complication of diabetes, manifested as albuminuria, nephrotic edema, hypertension, renal insufficiency, and retinopathy.

glomerulose (glo-mer′u-lōs) glomerular.

glomerulotropin (glo-mer″u-lo-tro′pin) a substance, probably secreted by the diencephalon, capable of stimulating the zona glomerulosa of the adrenals to produce aldosterone; its rate of secretion is increased by lowered plasma sodium concentration.

glomerulus (glo-mer′u-lus), pl. *glomer′uli* [L., dim. of *glomus* ball] a tuft or cluster; used in anatomical nomenclature as a general term to designate such a structure, as one composed of blood vessels or nerve fibers. Often used alone to designate one of the glomeruli of the kidney (glomeruli renis [NA]). **glomer′uli arterio′si coch′leae** [NA], an arterial network surrounding the cochlea. **glomeruli of kidney, malpighian glomeruli,** glomeruli renis. **nonencapsulated nerve g.,** a nerve ending in the connective tissue of various organs in which the terminal branches of the nerve form spherical or elongated structures resembling glomeruli. **olfactory g.,** one of the small globular masses of dense neuropil in the olfactory bulb containing the first synapse in the olfactory pathway. **renal glomeruli, glomer′uli re′nis** [NA], globular tufts of capillaries, one projecting into the expanded end or capsule of each of the

uriniferous tubules, which together with its surrounding capsule (*glomerular capsule*) constitute the renal corpuscle. Called also *glomeruli of kidney,* and *malpighian glomeruli.* See also plate accompanying *kidney.* **Ruysch's glomeruli,** glomeruli renis.

glomic (glo′mik) pertaining to or affecting a glomus.

glomoid (glo′moid) resembling a glomus.

glomus (glo′mus), pl. *glom′era* [L. "a ball"] 1. [NA] a small, histologically recognizable body, composed of fine arterioles connecting directly with veins, and possessing a rich nerve supply. 2. anastomosis arteriovenosa glomeriformis. **glom′era aor′tica,** NA alternative for corpora para-aortica. **carotid g., g. carot′icum** [NA], carotid body: a small neurovascular structure lying in the bifurcation of the right and left carotid arteries, made up of richly innervated epithelioid glomus cells (type I) surrounded by type II cells. It functions as an arterial chemoreceptor (although which component is responsible is uncertain), with stimulation by hypoxia, hypercapnia, or elevated hydrogen ion concentration resulting in an increase in blood pressure, cardiac rate, and respiratory movements. Another function may be as an endocrine gland. **choroid g., g. choroi′deum** [NA], an enlargement of the choroid plexus of the lateral ventricle where the inferior horn joins the central part. **coccygeal g., g. coccyg′eum** [NA], an oval structure consisting of irregular masses of spherical or polyhedral epithelioid cells grouped around a dilated, sinusoidal capillary vessel, occurring anterior to, or immediately inferior to, the apex of the coccyx, at the termination of the median sacral vessels. Called also *coccygeal body, corpus coccygeum,* and *Luschka's body, ganglion,* or *gland.*

glossa (glos′ah) [Gr. *glōssa*] the tongue (lingua [NA]).

glossagra (glos-sa′grah, glos′ag-rah) [*gloss-* + Gr. *agra* seizure] gouty pain of the tongue.

glossal (glos′al) pertaining to the tongue; lingual.

glossalgia (glos-sal′je-ah) [*gloss-* + *-algia*] pain in the tongue, glossodynia. See also *glossopyrosis.*

glossanthrax (glos-san′thraks) [*gloss-* + *anthrax*] carbuncle of the tongue.

glossectomy (glos-sek′to-me) [*gloss-* + Gr. *ektomē* excision] partial or total surgical excision of the tongue.

Glossina (glos-si′nah) a genus of biting flies of the family Muscidae; the tsetse flies. **G. mor′sitans,** a fly of South Africa which transmits by its bite *Trypanosoma brucei,* the cause of nagana in horses; it also transmits *T. rhodesiense,* the cause of Rhodesia trypanosomiasis. **G. pallid′ipes,** a fly which transmits *Trypanosoma brucei.* **G. palpa′lis,** a species of Central Africa which transmits by its bite *Trypanosoma gambiense,* the organism causing African trypanosomiasis. Other species which probably transmit trypanosomes to animals and to man are: *G. brevipalpis, G. fusca, G. longipalpis, G. longipennis, G. morsitans, G. pallicera, G. pallidipes, G. swynnertoni, G. tachinoides.*

glossitis (glos-si′tis) [*gloss-* + *-itis*] inflammation of the tongue. **g. area′ta exfoliati′va,** benign migratory g. **atrophic g.,** Hunter's g. **benign migratory g.,** an inflammatory disease of the tongue of unknown etiology, characterized by multiple annular areas of desquamation of the filiform papillae on the dorsal surface of the tongue, usually presenting pinkish-red central lesions outlined by thin, yellowish lines or bands that change patterns and shift from one area to another every few days. Called also *g. areata exfoliativa, g. migrans, erythema migrans, exfolatio areata linguae, geographic tongue, lingua geographica, mappy tongue, pityriasis linguae,* and *wandering rash.* **Hunter's g.,** a chronic condition of the tongue seen in pernicious anemia, characterized by glossitis, glossodynia, glossopyrosis, and altered sense of taste; the pain and burning sensation are usually confined to the tongue but may also extend to other parts of the oral mucosa. Ultimately, the tongue becomes atrophic and assumes a beefy red color and a smooth shiny appearance, sometimes with small ulcers spreading over its surface. Called also *atrophic g.* **idiopathic g.,** inflammation of the substance of the tongue and its mucous membrane. **median rhomboid g.,** a congenital disorder of noninflammatory origin, characterized by a somewhat rhomboid reddish, smooth, and shiny lesion with some opalescent spots, occurring at about the middle third of the dorsal surface of the tongue, immediately anterior to the circumvallate papillae. **g. mi'grans,** benign migratory g. **Moeller's g.,** a chronic condition of the tongue characterized by superficial excoriation, principally of the tip and edges. The lesions are beefy red, well-defined, irregular patches, in which the filiform papillae are thinned or absent and the fungiform papillae are swollen. Called also *bald tongue* and *glossodynia exfoliativa*. **psychogenic g.,** glossopyrosis. **g. rhomboi'dea media'na,** median rhomboid g.

gloss(o)- [Gr. *glōssa* tongue] a combining form denoting relationship to the tongue.

glossocele (glos'o-sēl) [*glosso-* + Gr. *kēlē* tumor] swelling and protrusion of the tongue.

glossocinesthetic (glos"o-sin-es-thet'ik) glossokinesthetic.

glossocoma (glŏ-sok'o-mah) retraction of the tongue.

glossodynamometer (glos"o-di"nah-mom'ĕ-ter) [*glosso-* + *dynamometer*] an instrument for recording the power of the tongue to resist pressure.

glossodynia (glos"o-din'e-ah) [*glosso-* + Gr. *odynē* pain] pain in the tongue; glossalgia. See also *glossopyrosis*. **g. exfoliati'va,** Moeller's glossitis.

glossoepiglottic (glos"o-ep-ĭ-glot'ik) glossoepiglottidean.

glossoepiglottidean (glos"o-ep-ĭ-glo-tid'e-an) pertaining to the tongue and epiglottis.

glossograph (glos'o-graf) [*glosso-* + Gr. *graphein* to record] an apparatus for recording the tongue movements in speech.

glossohyal (glos"o-hi'al) [*glosso-* + *hyoid*] pertaining to the tongue and hyoid bone.

glossokinesthetic (glos"o-kin"es-thet'ik) [*glosso-* + *kinesthetic*] pertaining to the subjective perception of the movements of the tongue in speech.

glossolalia (glos"o-la'le-ah) [*glosso-* + Gr. *lalein* to babble] speech in unknown or imaginary language; gibberish.

glossology (glŏ-sol'o-je) [*glosso-* + *-logy*] 1. the sum of knowledge regarding the tongue. 2. a treatise on nomenclature.

glossomantia (glos"o-man-ti'ah) [*glosso-* + Gr. *manteia* divination] prognosis based on the appearance of the tongue.

glossoncus (glŏ-song'kus) [*glosso-* + Gr. *onkos* mass] a swelling of the tongue.

glossopalatinus (glos"o-pal"ah-ti'nus) musculus palatoglossus.

glossopathy (glŏ-sop'ah-the) [*glosso-* + Gr. *pathos* disease] any disease of the tongue.

glossopexy (glos'o-pek'se) lip-tongue adhesion.

glossopharyngeal (glos"o-fah-rin'je-al) [*glosso-* + *pharynx*] pertaining to the tongue and pharynx.

glossopharyngeum (gos"o-fah-rin'je-um) [*glosso-* + *pharynx*] the tongue and pharynx together.

glossopharyngeus (glos"o-fah-rin'je-us) see *pars glossopharyngea musculi constrictoris pharyngis superioris*.

glossophobia (glos"o-fo'be-ah) lalophobia.

glossophytia (glos"o-fit'e-ah) [*glosso-* + Gr. *phyton* plant] black tongue.

glossoplasty (glos"o-plas"te) [*glosso-* + Gr. *plassein* to mold] plastic surgery of the tongue.

glossoptosis (glos"op-to'sis) [*glosso-* + Gr. *ptōsis* fall] downward displacement or retraction of the tongue.

glossopyrosis (glos"o-pi-ro'sis) [*glosso-* + Gr. *pyrōsis* burning] a form of paresthesia characterized by pain, burning, itching, and stinging of the mucous membranes of the tongue without apparent lesions of the affected areas. Called also *burning t.*

glossorrhaphy (glŏ-sor'ah-fe) [*glosso-* + Gr. *rhaphē* suture] suture of the tongue.

glossoscopy (glŏ-sos'ko-pe) [*glosso-* + Gr. *skopein* to examine] examination of the tongue.

glossospasm (glos'o-spazm) [*glosso-* + Gr. *spasmos* spasm] spasm of the tongue muscles.

glossosteresis (glos"o-ster-e'sis) glossectomy.

glossotilt (glos'o-tilt) [*glosso-* + Gr. *tillein* to pull] a lever which holds the tongue during one of the processes for artificial respiration.

glossotomy (glŏ-sot'o-me) [*glosso-* + Gr. *temnein* to cut] incision of the tongue.

glossotrichia (glos"o-trik'e-ah) [*glosso-* + Gr. *thrix* hair] hairy tongue.

glottal (glot'al) pertaining to the glottis.

glottic (glot'ik) 1. pertaining to the glottis. 2. pertaining to the tongue.

glottides (glot'ĭ-dēz) [Gr.] plural of *glottis*.

glottis (glot'is), pl. *glot'tides* [Gr. *glōttis*] [NA] the vocal apparatus of the larynx, consisting of the true vocal cords (plica vocalis) and the opening between them (rima glottidis). **false g.,** rima vestibuli. **intercartilaginous g., respiratory g.,** pars intercartilaginea rimae glottidis. **true g.,** rima glottidis.

glottology (glŏ-tol'o-je) glossology.

glou-glou (gloo'gloo) [Fr.] a gurgling sound produced in the stomach by various causes, such as the pressure of a girdle.

glow (glo) incandescence; also brightness or warmth of color.

gloxazone (gloks'ah-zōn) chemical name: 2,2'-[1-(1-ethoxyethyl)-1,2-ethanediylidene]bishydrazine carbothioamide; a compound, $C_8H_{16}N_6OS_2$, used in *Anaplasma* infections in cattle.

Glu glutamic acid.

glucagon (gloo'kah-gon) 1. a polypeptide hormone secreted by the alpha cells of the islets of Langerhans in response to hypoglycemia or to stimulation by the growth hormone of the anterior pituitary; it stimulates glycogenolysis in the liver by inducing activation of liver phosphorylase. Called also *hyperglycemic-glycogenolytic factor (HGF)*. 2. [USP] the polypeptide occurring in the pancreas of those domestic mammals used for food by man, $C_{153}H_{225}N_{43}O_{49}S$, which has the property of increasing the blood glucose concentration, occurring as a fine, white or faintly colored crystalline powder; used in the form of the hydrochloride salt as an antihypoglycemic, administered parenterally. **gut g.,** enteroglucagon.

glucagonoma (glu"kah-gon-o'mah) a glucagon-secreting, usually malignant tumor of the alpha cells of the pancreatic islets. See under *syndrome*.

glucal (gloo'kal) an aldehyde derivative, $C_6H_{10}O_4$, of glucose.

glucan (gloo'kan) any polysaccharide (e.g., glycogen, starch, and cellulose) composed only of recurring units of glucose; a homopolymer of glucose.

1,4-α-glucan branching enzyme (gloo'kan bran'ching en'zīm) [EC 2.4.1.18] an enzyme of the transferase class that catalyzes the transfer of a segment of a 1,4-α-D-glucan chain to a primary hydroxyl group in a similar glucan chain, resulting in a new branch in a glycogen molecule (glycogen branching enzyme) or an amylopectin molecule (amylopectin branching enzyme in plants). Genetic deficiency, transmitted as an autosomal recessive trait, occurs in type IV glycogen storage disease. Called also *brancher* or *branching enzyme*.

α-glucan–branching glycosyltransferase (gloo'kan bran'ching gli"ko-sil-trans'fer-ās) 1,4-α-glucan branching enzyme.

α-1,4-glucan:α-1,4-glucan 6-glucosyl-transferase deficiency glycogen storage disease.

glucan-1,4-α-glucosidase (gloo'kan gloo-ko'sĭ-dās) [EC 3.2.1.3] an enzyme of the hydrolase class that catalyzes the hydrolysis of terminal 1,4-linked α-D-glucose residues from nonreducing ends of the chains with release of β-D-glucose. Genetic defect in the enzyme, an autosomal recessive trait, results in glycogen storage disease, type II (Pompe disease). Called also *lysosomal α-glucosidase*.

α-glucan glycosyl 4:6-transferase (gloo'kan gli"ko-sil trans'fer-ās) 1,4-α-glucan branching enzyme.

glucaric acid (gloo-kar'ik) the saccharic acid produced by oxidation of C-1 and C-6 of glucose to carboxyl groups.

glucatonia (gloo-kah-to'ne-ah) reduction of blood sugar to a point where pathologic symptoms are produced.

glucemia (gloo-se'me-ah) glycemia.

gluceptate (glu-sep'tāt) USAN contraction for glucoheptonate.

glucide (gloo'sīd) an organic substance consisting in whole or in part of carbohydrates; a general term, embracing the carbohydrates and glycosides.

glucidtemns (gloo'sid-tems) a collective name for the

products produced by the digestion of starch, namely, dextrin, maltose, and glucose.

glucinium (gloo-sin′e-um) beryllium.

gluciphore (gloo′sĭ-fōr) glucophore.

gluc(o)- [Gr. *glykys* sweet] a combining form denoting relationship to sweetness, or to glucose. Cf. *glyc(o)-*.

glucoascorbic acid (gloo″ko-ah-skor′bik) a seven-carbon homologue of ascorbic acid having no vitamin C activity.

glucocerebrosidase (gloo″ko-ser″ĕ-bro-si′dās) glucosylceramidase.

glucocerebroside (gloo″ko-ser′ĕ-bro-sīd″) a cerebroside with a glucose sugar; it accumulates in the tissues in Gaucher's disease.

glucocinin (gloo″ko-sin′in) glucokinin.

glucocorticoid (gloo″ko-kor′tĭ-koid) 1. any of the group of C21 corticosteroids predominantly affecting carbohydrate metabolism (promotion of gluconeogenesis and liver glycogen deposition and elevation of blood glucose levels). They also influence fat and protein metabolism and have many other activities; e.g., they affect muscle tone and the excitation of nerve tissue and the microcirculation, participate in the maintenance of arterial blood pressure, increase gastric secretion, alter connective tissue response to injury, impede cartilage production, inhibit inflammatory, allergic, and immunological responses, suppress pituitary release of corticotropin and hence production of adrenocortical steroids, induce shrinkage of lymphatic tissue, reduce the number of circulating lymphocytes, and affect the functions of the central nervous system. Some also exhibit varying degrees of mineralocorticoid activity. In man, the most important glucocorticoid is cortisol (hydrocortisone). Cf. *mineralocorticoid*. 2. of, pertaining to, having the properties or effects of, or resembling a glucocorticoid.

Gluco-Ferrum (gloo″ko-fer′rum) trademark for preparations of ferrous gluconate.

glucofuranose (gloo″ko-fu′rah-nōs) a form of glucose in which carbon atoms 1 and 4 are bridged by an oxygen atom.

glucogenesis (gloo″ko-jen′ĕ-sis) the formation of glucose by the breakdown of glycogen.

glucogenic (gloo″ko-jen′ik) giving rise to or producing glucose.

glucohemia (gloo″ko-he′me-ah) glycemia.

glucokinase (gloo″ko-ki′nās) 1. [EC 2.7.1.2] an enzyme of the transferase class that catalyzes the reaction ATP + D-glucose = ADP + D-glucose-6-phosphate. The enzyme is found in invertebrates and microorganisms and is highly specific for glucose. 2. hexokinase [EC 2.7.1.1] type IV.

glucokinetic (gloo″ko-ki-net′ik) activating sugar so as to maintain the sugar level of the blood.

glucokinin (gloo″ko-kin′in) [*gluco-* + Gr. *kinein* to move] a hormone-like substance obtained from vegetable tissues and yeast, subcutaneous injection of which produces hypoglycemia in animals and acts on depancreatized dogs in a manner similar to insulin.

glucolactone (gloo″ko-lak′tōn) a lactone from gluconic acid.

glucolysis (gloo-kol′ĭ-sis) glycolysis.

glucolytic (gloo″ko-lit′ik) glycolytic.

gluconate (gloo′ko-nāt) a salt, ester, or anionic form of gluconic acid.

gluconeogenesis (gloo″ko-ne″o-jen′ĕ-sis) the formation of glucose from molecules that are not themselves carbohydrates, as from amino acids, lactate, and the glycerol portion of fats. Called also *glyconeogenesis*.

gluconeogenetic (gloo″ko-ne″o-jĕ-net′ik) pertaining to or involved in gluconeogenesis.

gluconic acid (gloo-kon′ik) the hexonic acid derived from glucose by oxidation of the aldehyde group at C-1 to a carboxy group.

Gluconobacter (gloo″ko-no-bak′ter) [*gluconic acid* + Gr. *baktron* a rod] a genus of gram-negative, aerobic, rod-shaped bacteria of the family Acetobacteraceae. The organisms produce acetic acid from ethanol, and are found in soil, plants, fruits, and vegetables. The type species is *G. ox′ydans*.

glucopenia (gloo-ko-pe′ne-ah) glycopenia.

glucophenetidin (gloo″ko-fĕ-net′ĭ-din) a derivative from paraphenetidin and dextrose, in silky white needles.

glucophore (gloo′ko-fōr) [*gluco-* + Gr. *phoros* bearing] the group of atoms in a molecule of a compound which is responsible for its sweet taste.

glucoprotein (gloo″ko-pro′te-in) glycoprotein.

glucopyranose (gloo″ko-pi′rah-nōs) a form of glucose in which carbon atoms 1 and 5 are bridged by an oxygen atom.

glucoregulation (gloo″ko-reg″u-la′shun) regulation of glucose metabolism.

glucosamine (gloo-kōs′ah-mēn) chemical name: 2-amino-2-deoxy-D-glucose. An amino acid derivative of glucose, $C_6H_{13}NO_5$, obtained from mucin and chitin by hydrolysis and occurring in many polysaccharides of vertebrate tissue; called also *glycosamine*. **acetyl g.,** the structural unit of chitin.

α-glucosaminide-N-acetyltransferase (gloo″kōs-am′ĭ-nīd as″ĕ-til-trans′fer-ās) heparan-α-glucosaminide acetyltransferase.

glucosan (gloo′ko-san) an anhydro-polymer which on hydrolysis yields a hexose.

glucosazone (gloo″ko-sa′zōn) a yellow crystalline substance, $CH_2OH(CHOH)_3C{:}N{\cdot}NH{\cdot}C_6H_5{\cdot}CH{:}N{\cdot}NH{\cdot}C_6H_5$, produced by treating dextrose with phenylhydrazine and acetic acid; the crystals melt at 205° C. and may be used in the identification of glucose.

glucose (gloo′kōs) [Gr. *gleukos* sweetness; *glykys* sweet] 1. D-glucose, a monosaccharide (hexose), $C_6H_{12}O_6$, also known as *dextrose* (q.v.), found in certain foodstuffs, especially fruits, and in the normal blood of all animals. It is the end product of carbohydrate metabolism and is the chief source of energy for living organisms, its utilization being controlled by insulin. Excess glucose is converted to glycogen and stored in the liver and muscles for use as needed and, beyond that, is converted to fat and stored as adipose tissue. Glucose appears in the urine in diabetes mellitus. 2. liquid g. **Brun's g.,** a histologic clearing solution composed of glucose, distilled water, camphor, and glycerin. **gamma g.,** a very reactive form of glucose that can be isolated only as a derivative. **liquid g.** [NF], an odorless, colorless or yellowish, thick syrupy liquid, with a sweet taste, consisting chiefly of dextrose, with dextrins, maltose, and water, and obtained by the incomplete hydrolysis of starch; used as a flavoring agent, tablet binder, and coating agent in pharmaceutical preparations. It may be used as a food, often administered rectally, and has been used in the treatment of dehydration. Sometimes simply called *glucose*. **g. 1-phosphate,** an intermediate in carbohydrate metabolism,

$$CH_2OH{\cdot}CH(CHOH)_3CH{\cdot}O{\cdot}PO{\cdot}(OH)_2$$
$$\underset{O}{\rule{1.8cm}{0.4pt}}$$

See also *Embden-Meyerhof pathway*, under *pathway*. Called also *Cori ester*. **g. 6-phosphate,** an intermediate in carbohydrate metabolism,

$$CHOH(CHOH)_3{\cdot}CH{\cdot}CHO_2{\cdot}PO(OH)_2$$
$$\underset{O}{\rule{1.8cm}{0.4pt}}$$

See also *Embden-Meyerhof pathway*, under *pathway*. Called also *Robison ester*.

glucose oxidase (gloo′kōs ok′sĭ-dās) [EC 1.1.3.4] an enzyme of the oxidoreductase class that catalyzes the reaction β-D-glucose + O_2 = D-glucono-1,5-lactone + H_2O_2. It is a flavoprotein, highly specific for β-D-glucose. The enzyme is produced by *Penicillium notatum* and other fungi and has antibacterial activity in the presence of glucose and oxygen. It is used to estimate glucose concentration in blood or urine samples through the formation of colored dyes by the hydrogen peroxide produced in the reaction.

glucose-6-phosphatase (gloo′kōs fos″fah-tās″) [EC 3.1.3.9.] an enzyme of the hydrolase class that catalyzes the reaction D-glucose-6-phosphate + H_2O = D-glucose + orthophosphate. The enzyme also catalyzes transphosphorylation and pyrophosphate hydrolytic reactions of uncharacterized physiological significance. It occurs in the endoplasmic reticulum of liver, kidney, and intestinal mucosa, but not of muscle, and its reaction is the principal route for hepatic glucogenesis. Deficiency in the enzyme, an autosomal recessive trait, results in glycogen storage disease, type I (von Gierke disease).

glucose-6-phosphatase deficiency glycogen storage disease, type I.

glucose-6-phosphate dehydrogenase (G6PD) (gloo′kōs fos′fāt de-hi′dro-jen-ās) [EC 1.1.1.49] an enzyme of the oxidoreductase class that catalyzes the reaction D-glucose-6-phosphate + NADP⁺ = D-glucono-1,5-lactone 6-phosphate + NADPH. The reaction is the first step in the pentosephosphate pathway of glucose metabolism. Genetic deficiency of the enzyme causes severe hemolytic crises in affected individuals. See also *glucose-6-phosphate dehydrogenase deficiency.*

glucose-6-phosphate dehydrogenase (G6PD) deficiency the most common inborn error of metabolism, affecting over 100 million people with varying degrees of hemolytic anemia. The G6PD locus, Xq28, is very closely linked to the genes for deutanomaly, protanomaly, hemophilia A, and adrenoleukodystrophy, and closely linked to the genes (on Xq27) for the fragile X syndrome and HPRT deficiency (the Lesch-Nyhan syndrome). (G6PD deficiency provides heterozygote advantage against falciparum malaria.) The G6PD gene is highly polymorphic, with over 300 variants known. See also *glucose-6-phosphate dehydrogenase deficiency anemia,* under *anemia.*

glucose-6-phosphate isomerase (gloo′kōs fos′fāt i-som′er-ās) [EC 5.3.1.9] an enzyme of the isomerase class that catalyzes the reaction D-glucose-6-phosphate = D-fructose-6-phosphate. The reaction is the first step in the conversion of glucose-6-phosphate to triose phosphates in the Embden-Meyerhof pathway. Deficiency of the enzyme, an autosomal recessive trait, results in hemolytic anemia.

α-glucosidase (gloo-ko′sĭ-dās) [EC 3.2.1.3, 3.2.1.20] an enzyme of the hydrolase class that catalyzes the hydrolysis of terminal, nonreducing 1,4-linked α-D-glucose residues, primarily in oligosaccharides but also in polysaccharides, with release of α-D-glucose. Deficiency in the lysosomal (acid) α-glucosidase, an autosomal recessive trait, results in glycogen storage disease, type II (Pompe disease). **lysosomal α-g.,** glucan-1,4-α-glucosidase.

α-1,4-glucosidase (gloo-ko′sĭ-dās) α-D-glucosidase.

α-1,4-glucosidase deficiency glycogen storage disease, type II.

glucoside (gloo′ko-sīd) a glycoside in which the sugar constituent is glucose; originally the term glucoside was given to any of a variety of natural plant products containing a sugar, but it is now generally restricted to those in which the sugar is glucose. See *glycoside.*

glucosidolytic (gloo″ko-si″do-lit′ik) causing the splitting up of glucosides.

glucosin (gloo′ko-sin) any one of a group of bases derived from glucose by the action of ammonia; some are highly toxic.

glucosulfone sodium (gloo″ko-sul′fōn) chemical name: 1,1′-[sulfonylbis(4,1-phenyleneimino)]bis[1-deoxy-1-sulfo-D-glucitol]disodium salt. An antibacterial derivative of dapsone, C₂₄H₃₄N₂Na₂O₁₈S₃, having actions similar to those of the parent compound, occurring as white to faintly yellow, amorphous solid; used primarily as a leprostatic in the treatment of lepromatous and tuberculoid leprosy, administered intravenously.

glucosum (gloo-ko′sum) glucose.

glucosuria (gloo″ko-su′re-ah) [*glucose* + Gr. *ouron* urine + *-ia*] 1. the presence of glucose in the urine. 2. dextrosuria.

glucosyl (gloo′ko-sil) a glucose radical.

glucosylceramidase (gloo″ko-sil-ser-am′ĭ-dās) [EC 3.2.1.45] an enzyme of the hydrolase class that catalyzes the reaction D-glucosyl-*N*-acylsphingosine + H₂O = D-glucose + *N*-acylsphingosine. The reaction occurs in the lysosomal degradation of sphingolipids. Defect in the enzyme, an autosomal recessive trait, results in Gaucher disease. Called also *cerebroside β-glucosidase* and *glucocerebrosidase.*

glucosyltransferase (gloo″ko-sil-trans′fer-ās) [EC 2.4.1] an enzyme that catalyzes the transfer of a glucosyl group from a donor to an acceptor compound. Called also *glucosyltransferase* and *transglucosylase.*

glucoxylose (gloo″ko-zi′lōs) a disaccharide, C₁₁H₂₀O₁₀, occurring in the leaves and branches of *Daviesia latifolia.*

glucurolactone (gloo″ku-ro-lak′tōn) chemical name: γ-lactone of D-glucofuranuronic acid; formerly used in treatment of arthritis, neuritis, and fibrositis.

glucuronate (gloo-ku′ro-nāt) a salt, ester, or anionic form of glucuronic acid.

glucuronic acid (gloo″ku-ron′ik) a constituent of glycosaminoglycans (mucopolysaccharides), conjugated by hepatic microsomal enzymes and forming soluble glucuronides that are then excreted in the bile and urine. This is the primary pathway of biotransformation for many drugs and poisons.

β-glucuronidase (gloo″ku-ron′ĭ-dās) [EC 3.2.1.31] an enzyme of the hydrolase class that catalyzes the reaction β-D-glucuronide + H₂O = alcohol + D-glucuronate. The enzyme occurs in the lysosomes of many types of cells. It hydrolyzes various β-glucuronides, including breakdown products of proteoglycans. Deficiency of the enzyme, an autosomal recessive trait, results in mucopolysaccharidosis VII (Sly syndrome).

β-glucuronidase (GUSB) deficiency Sly syndrome.

glucuronide (gloo″ku-ron′īd) common term for glucuronoside.

glucuronide transferase (gloo-ku′ron-īd trans′fer-ās) glucuronosyltransferase.

glucuronolactone (gloo″ku-ro″no-lak′tōn) glucurolactone.

glucuronoside (gloo″ku-ron′o-sīd) a compound in which glucuronic acid, combined as a sugar (hexose), not as an acid, is linked by a glycosidic bond to a hydroxyl or carboxyl group on another compound. Less accurately called *glucuronide.*

glucuronosyltransferase (gloo″ku-ron″o-sil-trans′fer-ās) [EC 2.4.1.17] an enzyme of the transferase class that catalyzes the reaction UDPglucuronate + acceptor = UDP + acceptor β-D-glucuronoside. The reaction occurs with a wide range of substrates. It is important in the conversion of bilirubin to the more soluble glucuronide, which is then secreted into the bile. Deficiency of the enzyme, an autosomal recessive trait, results in Crigler-Najjar syndrome.

glucuronyl transferase (gloo-ku′ron-il trans′fer-ās) a less accurate term for glucuronosyltransferase.

glue (gloo) an adhesive preparation in the form of impure gelatin derived from boiling certain animal substances, such as hoofs, in water.

Gluge's corpuscles (gloo′gez) [Gottlieb *Gluge,* German pathologist, 1812–1898] see under *corpuscle.*

Glugea (gloo′je-ah) a genus of intracellular protozoa (suborder Apansporoblastina, order Microsporida) parasitic in fishes.

glutamate (gloo′tah-māt) a salt, ester, or anionic form of glutamic acid.

glutamic acid hydrochloride (gloo-tam′ik as′id hi″dro-klo′rīd) a white crystalline powder, C₅H₉NO₄·HCl, used as gastric acidifier; formerly used in the treatment of achlorhydria and hypochlorhydria, and as an antiepileptic.

glutamate decarboxylase (gloo′tah-māt de″kar-bok′sĭ-lās) [EC 4.1.1.15] an enzyme of the lyase class that catalyzes the reaction L-glutamate = 4-aminobutyrate + CO₂. The enzyme is a pyridoxal phosphate protein. The reaction provides an important neurotransmitter and is a step in the metabolism of glutamate in brain tissue. Defect in the enzyme, an autosomal recessive trait, is the cause of pyridoxine-dependent infantile convulsions.

glutamate dehydrogenase (gloo′tah-māt de-hi′dro-jen-ās) [EC 1.4.1.2-4] an enzyme of the oxidoreductase class that catalyzes the reaction L-glutamate + H₂O + NAD⁺ (or NADP⁺) = 2-ketoglutarate + NH₃ + NADH (or NADPH). The reaction operates in either direction, having a major function in both the synthesis and degradation of glutamic acid and other amino acids.

glutamate formiminotransferase (gloo′tah-māt for-mim″ĭ-no-trans′fer-ās) [EC 2.1.2.5] an enzyme of the transferase class that catalyzes the reaction tetrahydrofolate + *N*-formimino-L-glutamate = 5-formiminotetrahydrofolate + L-glutamate. The reaction is a step in the degradation of histidine. Urinary excretion of formiminoglutamate and mental retardation have been associated with decreased enzyme activity, resulting from either a genetic disorder or a deficiency of tetrahydrofolate. The enzyme also has catalytic sites with formiminoglutamate deaminase activity.

glutamic acid (gloo-tam′ik) a nonessential amino acid (q.v.) occurring in proteins. It also serves as an excitatory neurotransmitter in all regions of the central nervous system. Symbols Glu and E. **g.a. hydrochloride,** a compound used as a gastric acidifier in replacement therapy for achlorhydria and hypochlorhydria.

glutamic-oxaloacetic transaminase (GOT) (gloo′-tam-ik oks″al-o-ah-se′tik trans-am′ĭ-nās) aspartate aminotransferase.

glutamic-pyruvic transaminase (GPT) (gloo′tam-ik pi-roo′vik trans-am′ĭ-nās) alanine aminotransferase.

glutaminase (gloo-tam′ĭ-nās) [EC 3.5.1.2] an enzyme of the hydrolase class that catalyzes the reaction L-glutamine + H_2O = L-glutamate + NH_3. The enzyme occurs in the small intestine and kidneys. The ammonia formed is converted to urea by way of the urea cycle in the liver or excreted in acidic urines.

glutamine (gloo′tah-min) the monoamide of glutamic acid, $C_5H_{10}N_2O_3$, occurring in the juices of many plants and in some animal tissues; it is an important carrier of urinary ammonia and is broken down in the kidney by the enzyme glutaminase.

glutaminyl (gloo-tam′ĭ-nil) the acyl radical of glutamine.

glutaminyl-peptide-γ-glutamyltransferase (gloo-tam′ĭ-nil pep′tĭd gloo″tah-mil-trans′fer-ās) protein-glutamine γ-glutamyltransferase.

glutamyl (gloo′tah-mil) the acyl radical of glutamic acid.

γ-glutamylcyclotransferase (gloo′tah-mil-si-klo-trans′fer-ās) [E.C. 2.3.2.4] an enzyme catalyzing the reaction: (5-L-glutamyl)-L-amino acid = 5-oxoproline + L-amino acid. It is part of a mechanism for transporting amino acids across the plasma membrane.

γ-glutamylcysteine synthetase deficiency (gloo″-tah-mil-sis-te′in sin′thĕ-tās) a genetic aminoacidopathy of glutathione synthesis, consisting of hemolytic anemia, spinocerebellar degeneration, peripheral neuropathy, myopathy, and aminoaciduria.

γ-glutamyltransferase (GGT) (gloo″tah-mil-trans′fer-as) [EC 2.3.2.2] an enzyme of the transferase class that catalyzes the reaction (5-L-glutamyl)-peptide + amino acid = peptide + 5-L-glutamyl-amino acid. The enzyme occurs in all cells, primarily in the plasma membrane. It is involved in the transfer of amino acids across the cell membrane in kidney, small bowel, brain, and red blood cells. Deficiency of the enzyme, an autosomal recessive trait, results in glutathionemia and glutathionuria.

glutamyl transpeptidase (gloo′tah-mil trans-pep′tĭ-dās) γ-glutamyltransferase.

γ-glutamyl transpeptidase deficiency a genetic aminoacidopathy of glutathione synthesis, marked by mental retardation, behavioral disorders, glutathionemia, and urinary excretion of glutathione, γ-glutamyl cysteine, and cysteine. Called also *glutathionuria.*

glutaral (gloo′tah-ral) glutaraldehyde. **g. concentrate** [USP], a solution of glutaraldehyde in purified water, containing not less than 49 per cent and not more than 51 per cent by weight of glutaraldehyde; used as a disinfectant.

glutaraldehyde (gloo′tah-ral′dĕ-hīd) chemical name: pentanedial. A disinfectant, $C_5H_8O_2$, effective against vegetative gram-positive, gram-negative, and acid-fast bacteria, bacterial spores, some fungi, and viruses; used in an aqueous solution for sterilization of endoscopic equipment, thermometers, and plastic, rubber, or other non-heat-resistant equipment. It is also used topically as an anhidrotic and may be used in the treatment of warts. Glutaraldehyde is also used as a tissue fixative for light and electron microscopy because of its preservation of fine structural detail and localization of enzyme activity. Called also *glutaral.*

glutargin (gloo′tar-jin) arginine glutamate.

glutaric acid (gloo-tar′ik) pentanedioic acid, an intermediate in the metabolism of tryptophan and lysine.

glutathione (gloo″tah-thi′ōn) a tripeptide, γ-glutamyl-cysteinyl-glycine, $^-OOC \cdot CH(NH_3{}^+) \cdot \cdot CH_2 \cdot CH_2 \cdot CO \cdot NH \cdot CH(CH_2 \cdot SH) \cdot CO \cdot NH \cdot CH_2 \cdot COO^-$, composed of glutamate, cysteine, and glycine. It is widely distributed in animal and plant tissues. It exists in reduced (GSH) and oxidized (GSSG) forms, and it functions in various redox reactions: (1) in the

destruction of peroxides and free radicals, (2) as a cofactor for enzymes, and (3) in the detoxification of harmful compounds. In erythrocytes, these reactions prevent oxidative damage by reduction of methemoglobin and peroxides. Glutathione is also involved in the maintenance of SH bonds in proteins and in membrane amino acid transport.

glutathione peroxidase (gloo″tah-thi′ōn pĕ-rok′sĭ-dās) [EC 1.11.1.9] an enzyme of the oxidoreductase class that catalyzes the reaction 2 glutathione + H_2O_2 = oxidized glutathione + $2H_2O$. The reaction reduces toxic hydrogen peroxide formed within the cell. The enzyme is a selenium protein. Deficiency of the enzyme causes jaundice in newborn infants.

glutathione reductase (NAD(P)H) (gloo″tah-thi′ōn re-duk′tās) [EC 1.6.4.2] an enzyme of the oxidoreductase class that catalyzes the reaction NAD(P)H + oxidized glutathione = NAD(P)$^+$ + 2 glutathione. It is a flavoprotein, occurring in erythrocytes, and is involved in many redox reactions. A deficiency of the enzyme, possibly a genetic trait, has been associated with damage to neutrophils, causing a weakened immune response, and with fava bean–induced hemolytic anemia.

glutathione synthetase (gloo″tah-thiōn′ sin′thĕ-tās) [EC 6.3.2.3] an enzyme of the ligase class that catalyzes the reaction ATP + γ-L-glutamyl-L-cysteine + glycine = ADP + orthophosphate + glutathione. The reaction is a step in the pathway of glutathione synthesis. Congenital glutathione synthetase deficiency, inherited as an autosomal recessive trait, gives rise to hemolytic anemia and severe acidosis associated with oxoprolinemia.

glutathione (GSH) synthetase deficiency a genetic aminoacidopathy due to decreased GSH synthesis, occurring in two types: type one shows a low GSH level in erythrocytes but only a slightly reduced GSH level in leukocytes and causes a well-compensated hemolytic anemia; type two shows a low GSH level in leukocytes and very high 5-oxoproline levels in plasma and urine, resulting in severe metabolic acidosis.

glutathionemia (gloo″tah-thi″o-ne′me-ah) the presence of glutathione in the blood.

glutathionuria (gloo″tah-thi″o-nu′re-ah) [*glutathione* + *-uria*] 1. the excretion of excessive amounts of glutathione in the urine. 2. γ-glutamyl transpeptidase deficiency.

gluteal (gloo′te-al) [Gr. *gloutos* buttock] pertaining to the buttocks.

glutelin (gloo′tĕ-lin) a simple protein, insoluble in all neutral solvents, but readily soluble in very dilute acids and alkalis and coagulable by heat; it occurs in seeds of cereals.

gluten (gloo′ten) [L. "glue"] the protein of wheat and other grains which gives to the dough its tough elastic character.

glutenin (gloo′tĕ-nin) the glutelin of wheat.

gluteofemoral (gloo″te-o-fem′or-al) [*gluteal* + *femoral*] pertaining to the buttock and thigh.

gluteoinguinal (gloo″te-o-in′gwĭ-nal) pertaining to the buttock and groin.

glutethimide (gloo-teth′ĭ-mīd) [USP] chemical name: 3-ethyl-3-phenyl-2,6-piperidinedione. A nonbarbiturate structurally related to phenobarbital, $C_{13}H_{15}NO_2$, occurring as a white, crystalline powder; used as a sedative and hypnotic, administered orally.

glutinous (gloo′tĭ-nus) [L. *glutinosus*] sticky; adhesive; gluey; viscid.

glutitis (gloo-ti′tis) [Gr. *gloutos* buttock + *-itis*] inflammation of the buttock.

glutose (gloo′tōs) an artificial glucoside that resembles glucose in many of its chemical reactions, but which seems to be inert in the body.

Gluzinski's test (gloo-zin′skēz) [Wladyslaw Antoni *Gluzinski,* a physician in Lemberg, 1856–1935] see under *tests.*

Gly glycine.

glyburide (gli′būr-īd) chemical name: 5-chloro-N-[2-[4-[[[(cyclohexylamino)carbonyl]amino]sulfonyl]phenyl]ethyl]-2-methoxybenzamide; an orally effective hypoglycemic agent of the sulfonylurea group, $C_{23}H_{28}ClN_3O_5S$. Called also *glibenclamide.*

glycal (gli′kal) an unsaturated sugar, —CH=CH—.

glycan (gli′kan) polysaccharide.

glycemia (gli-se′me-ah) [Gr. *glykys* sweet + Gr. *haima* blood + *-ia*] the presence of glucose in the blood.

glycemin (gli′sĕ-min) a substance, secreted by the liver, in the blood of diabetics which has an antagonistic action toward insulin by inhibition to fixation of dextrose by erythrocytes.

glycentin (gli-sen′tin) enteroglucagon.

glyceraldehyde (glis″er-al′de-hīd) a compound, glyceric aldehyde, $CH_2OHCHOHCHO$, formed by the oxidation of glycerol. **g. phosphate,** a triosephosphate which results from the decomposition of hexosephosphate in the chemistry of muscle contraction.

glyceraldehyde-3-phosphate dehydrogenase (GAPD) (glis″er-al′dĕ-hīd fos′fāt de-hi′dro-jen-ās) [EC 1.2.1.12] an enzyme of the oxidoreductase class that catalyzes the reaction D-glyceraldehyde 3-phosphate + orthophosphate + NAD^+ = 3-phospho-D-glyceroyl phosphate + NADH. The reaction is one of two by which high-energy phosphate is generated in the Embden-Meyerhof pathway.

glycerate (glis′er-āt) a salt or ester of glyceric acid.

glyceric acid (glĭ-sēr′ik) trivial name for 2,3-dihydroxypropanoic acid formed by oxidation of glycerol.

glyceridase (glis′er-ĭ-dās) lipase.

glyceride (glis′er-īd) an organic acid ester of glycerol; the natural fats are glycerides of the higher fatty acids.

glycerin (glis′er-in) [L. *glycerinum*] [USP] chemical name: 1,2,3-propanetriol. A clear, colorless, syrupy liquid, $C_3H_8O_3$, obtained as a by-product of soap, by carbohydrate fermentation, and by propylene synthesis; administered rectally as a cathartic and orally as a diuretic to reduce intraocular pressure. It is also used as a solvent, humectant, and vehicle in various pharmaceutical preparations. See also *glycerol*.

glycerinated (glis′er-in-āt-ed) treated with or preserved in glycerin.

glycerinum (glis″er-i′num) [L.] glycerin.

glycerite (glis′er-īt) [L. *glyceritum*] a solution or mixture of a medicinal substance in glycerin; the glycerites for which official standards have been promulgated are boroglycerin, starch, and tannic acid glycerites. **boroglycerin g.,** see under *boroglycerin*. **starch g.** [NF], a preparation of starch, benzoic acid, glycerin, and purified water; used topically as an emollient; called also *glyceritum amyli*. **tannic acid g.,** a preparation of tannic acid, sodium citrate, exsiccated sodium sulfite, and glycerin, containing about 20 per cent of tannic acid; used as an astringent. Called also *glyceritum acidi tannici*.

glyceritum (glis″er-i′tum), gen. *glyceri′ti*, pl. *glyceri′ta* [L.] glycerite. **g. ac′idi tan′nici,** tannic acid glycerite. **g. am′yli,** starch glycerite. **g. boroglyceri′ni,** boro-glycerin glycerite.

glycerogel (glis′er-o-jel) a gel in which glycerin is the dispersed medium.

glycerogelatin (glis″er-o-jel′ah-tin) glycerin jelly.

glycerol (glis′er-ol) a trihydric sugar alcohol, $CH_2OH\cdot CHOH\cdot CH_2OH$, being the alcoholic component of the fats; it is soluble in water and alcohol. Glycerol is an intermediate in the metabolism of fatty acids and serves as a phosphate acceptor. Pharmaceutical preparations are called glycerin (q.v.). **g. boroglycerite,** boroglycerin glycerite. **iodinated g.,** chemical name: 2-(1-iodoethyl)-1,3-dioxolane-4-methanol; an isomeric mixture of the iodinated dimers of glycerol, $C_6H_{11}IO_3$, used as an expectorant. **g. phosphate,** an intermediate in glycolysis and alcoholic fermentation, $CH_2OH\cdot CHOH\cdot CH_2\cdot O\cdot PO(OH)_2$.

glycerolize (glis′er-o-līz) to treat with or preserve in glycerol, as in the exposure of red blood cells to glycerol solution so that glycerol diffuses into the cells before they are frozen for preservation.

glycerol kinase (glis′er-ol ki′nās) [EC 2.7.1.30] an enzyme of the transferase class that catalyzes the reaction ATP + glycerol = ADP + *sn*-glycerol 3-phosphate.

glycerol-3-phosphate dehydrogenase (glis′er-ol fos′fāt de-hi′dro-jĕ-nās) [EC 1.1.99.5] an enzyme of the oxidoreductase class that catalyzes the reaction *sn*-glycerol 3-phosphate + acceptor = glycerone phosphate (dihydroxyacetone phosphate) + reduced acceptor. In mitochondria of striated muscle and of nervous tissue, the enzyme contains iron and the acceptor is flavin-adenine-dinucleotide. The glycerone phosphate (dihydroxyacetone phosphate) formed can cross

into the cytosol, where glycerol 3-phosphate is regenerated by glycerol-3-phosphate dehydrogenase (NAD^+). See also *glycerol phosphate shuttle*, under *shuttle*.

glycerol-3-phosphate dehydrogenase (NAD^+) (glis′er-ol fos′fāt de-hi′dro-jĕ-nās) [EC 1.1.1.8] an enzyme of the oxidoreductase class that catalyzes the reaction *sn*-glycerol 3-phosphate + NAD^+ = glycerone phosphate + NADH. The enzyme is found in the cytosol; NADH formed from NAD^+ by other reactions displaces its equilibrium to produce glycerol 3-phosphate and NAD^+, thus regenerating the oxidized nucleotide. The glycerol phosphate produced can cross into the mitochondria, where it is reoxidized by glycerol-3-phosphate dehydrogenase. See also *glycerol phosphate shuttle*, under *shuttle*.

glycerone phosphate (glis′er-ōn fos′fāt) *dihydroxyacetone phosphate*, the ketone formally derived from glycerol.

glycerophilic (glis″er-o-fil′ik) having a special affinity for glycerol.

glycerophosphatase (glis″er-o-fos′fah-tās) see *acid phosphatase* and *alkaline phosphatase*.

glycerose (glis′er-ōs) a sugar formed by oxidizing glycerol; there are two glyceroses, glyceraldehyde and dihydroxyacetone.

glyceryl (glis′er-il) the mono-, di-, or trivalent radical formed by removal of a hydrogen from one, two, or three of the hydroxy groups of glycerol. **g. guaiacolate,** guaifenesin. **g. monostearate** [NF], a compound prepared from glycerin and stearic acid, occurring as a white, waxlike solid, or white, waxlike beads or flakes with a slight, pleasant, fatty odor and taste; used as an emulsifying agent. **g. triacetate,** triacetin. **g. trinitrate,** nitroglycerin.

glycide (gli′sid) glycidol.

glycidol (glis′id-ol) the oxide of hydroxypropene, isomeric with lactic aldehyde and acetol.

glycinate (gli′sin-āt) any salt of glycine (aminoacetic acid).

glycine (gli′sēn) chemical name: aminoacetic acid. A nonessential amino acid (q.v. under *amino acid*), H_2NCH_2COOH, occurring as a constituent of many proteins. It has been synthesized and is used as a gastric antacid and dietary supplement; it has also been used in the treatment of various myopathies. Glycine has also been postulated to be a neurotransmitter, inhibiting neural excitation in the central nervous system.

glycinemia (gli″sĭ-ne′me-ah) hyperglycinemia.

glycinin (glis″i-nin) a globulin which constitutes 90 to 95 per cent of the protein content of soy bean.

Glyciphagus (gli-sif′ah-gus) *Glycyphagus*. **G. domes′ticus (G. pruno′rum),** *Glycyphagus domesticus*.

glyc(o)- [Gr. *glykys* sweet] a combining form denoting relationship to (*a*) sweetness, (*b*) sugar, sometimes specifically glucose, (*c*) glycerine, or (*d*) glycogen. Cf. *gluc(o)-*.

glycobiarsol (gli″ko-bi-ar′sol) [USP] chemical name: [[4-(hydroxyacetyl)amino]phenyl]arsonato(1−) oxobismuth. An arsenic- and bismuth-containing compound, $C_8H_9AsBiNO_6$, occurring as a yellowish white to beige-pink, amorphous powder; used as an intestinal antiamebic, administered orally. It is also effective in trichomonal and candidal vaginitis and other nongonococcal vaginal infections, administered intravaginally.

glycocalix, glycocalyx (gli″ko-kal′iks) the glycoprotein and polysaccharide covering that surrounds many cells; in bacterial cells the glycocalyx forms masses of fibers which extend from the cell and by means of which the cell adheres to surfaces.

glycochenodeoxycholate (gli″ko-ke″no-de-ok-se′ko-lāt) chenodeoxycholylglycine.

glycochenodeoxycholic acid (gli″ko-ke″no-de-ok″se-ko′-lik) chenodeoxycholylglycine.

glycocholate (gli″ko-ko′lāt) cholylglycine.

glycocholic acid (gli″ko-ko′lik) cholylglycine.

glycocine (gli′ko-sin) aminoacetic acid.

glycoclastic (gli″ko-klas′tik) [*glyco-* + Gr. *klan* to break] glycolytic.

glycocoll (gli′ko-kol) [*glyco-* + Gr. *kolla* glue] glycine.

glycocyamine (gli″ko-si′ah-min) guanidinoacetic acid.

glycogelatin (gli″ko-jel′ah-tin) an ointment base containing glycerin and gelatin.

glycogen (gli′ko-jen) [*glyco-* + Gr. *gennan* to produce] a polysaccharide, $(C_6H_{10}O_5)_x$, the chief carbohydrate storage material in animals. It is a long-chain polymer of glucose, formed in and largely stored in the liver and to a lesser extent in muscles, being depolymerized to glucose and liberated as needed. Called also *animal starch, tissue dextrin,* and *hepatin.* **hepatic g.,** glycogen stored in the liver. **tissue g.,** glycogen stored in tissues other than the liver, especially in muscle.

glycogenase (gli′ko-jĕ-nās″) α-amylase.

glycogenesis (gli″ko-jen′ĕ-sis) [*glyco-* + *genesis*] 1. the formation or synthesis of glycogen. 2. the production of sugar.

glycogenetic (gli″ko-jĕ-net′ik) glycogenic.

glycogenic (gli″ko-jen′ik) pertaining to, characterized by, or promoting glycogenesis; pertaining to glycogen.

glycogenolysis (gli″ko-jĕ-nol′ĭ-sis) [*glycogen* + Gr. *lysis* dissolution] the breakdown of glycogen to glucose by hydrolysis (as in digestion or within lysosomes) or phosphorolysis (as in mobilization of glycogen as a fuel).

glycogenolytic (gli″ko-jen′o-lit″ik) pertaining to, characterized by, or promoting glycogenolysis.

glycogenosis (gli″ko-jĕ-no′sis) glycogen storage disease; see under *disease.* **brancher deficiency g.,** glycogen storage disease, type IV. **generalized g.,** glycogen storage disease, type II; see under *disease.* **hepatophosphorylase deficiency g.,** glycogen storage disease, type VI. **hepatorenal g.,** glycogen storage disease, type I; see under *disease.* **myophosphorylase deficiency g.,** glycogen storage disease, type V; see under *disease.*

glycogenous (gli-koj′ĕ-nus) glycogenetic.

glycogen phosphorylase (gli′ko-jen fos-for′ĭ-lās) [EC 2.4.1.1] an enzyme of the transferase class that catalyzes the reaction $(1,4-α-D-glucosyl)_n$ + orthophosphate = $(1,4-α-D-glucosyl)_{n-1}$ + α-D-glucose 1-phosphate. The reaction in liver enables replenishment of blood glucose; the reaction in muscle mobilizes glycogen as a fuel. The enzyme exists in two forms: the inactive form (phosphorylase *b*, phosphorylase H) is converted to the active form (phosphorylase *a*, phosphorylase P) by phosphorylase kinase. Phosphorylase *b* can also be activated by 5′-AMP without being phosphorylated. Deficiency of glycogen phosphorylase, an autosomal recessive trait, causes glycogenosis. The muscle enzyme is absent in glycogen storage disease, type V (McArdle's disease); the liver enzyme is deficient in type VI (Hers' disease).

glycogen phosphorylase kinase (gli′ko-jen fos-for′ĭ-lās ki′nās) phosphorylase kinase.

glycogen synthase (gli′ko-jen sin′thās) [EC 2.4.1.11] an enzyme of the transferase class that catalyzes the reaction UDPglucose + $(1,4-α-D-glucosyl)_n$ = UDP + $1,4-α-D-glucosyl)_{n+1}$. The reaction is highly regulated by allosteric effectors, by phosphorylation reactions, and by insulin. Glycogen synthase *a* (active) is not phosphorylated; it was formerly called the I (independent) form. The phosphorylated form is glycogen synthase *b* (inactive unless glucose 6-phosphate is present); it was formerly called the D (dependent) form. Insulin secretion causes an increase in enzyme activity.

glycogen synthetase (gli′ko-jen sin′thĕ-tās) glycogen synthase.

glycogeusia (gli′ko-ju′se-ah) [*glyco-* + Gr. *geusis* taste] a condition in which there is a sweet taste in the mouth.

glycohemia (gli′ko-he′me-ah) [*glyco-* + Gr. *haima* blood + *-ia*] glycemia.

glycohemoglobin (gli″ko-he″mo-glo′bin) a glycosylated hemoglobin; see hemoglobin A_{1c}.

glycohistechia (gli″ko-his-tek′e-ah) [*glyco-* + Gr. *histos* tissue + *echein* to hold] the presence of an abnormally large amount of sugar in a tissue (Urbach).

glycol (gli′kol) any of a group of aliphatic dihydric alcohols, having marked hygroscopic properties and useful as solvents and plasticizers. *Diethylene glycol* should not be used for oral administration. **polyethylene g.,** see under P.

glycolate (gli′ko-lāt) a salt or ester of glycolic acid.

glycolic acid (gli-kol′ik) trivial name for hydroxyacetic acid, an intermediate in the conversion of serine to glycine.

glycolipid (gli″ko-lip′id) a lipid containing carbohydrate groups, usually galactose but also glucose, inositol, or others. Phosphate may or may not be present, and glycerol or sphingosine may occur. The simplest are the glycodiacylglycerols. The glycolipids include the cerebrosides.

glycoluric acid (gli″kōl-ūr′ik) a crystalline acid, a ureide of glycolic acid, $NH_2 \cdot CO \cdot NH \cdot CH_2$, formed by heating urea with aminoacetic acid. Called also *hydantoic a.* and *uraminoacetic a.*

glycolyl (gli′ko-lil) the radical $HOCH_2CO—$ of glycolic acid, $HO \cdot CH_2 \cdot COOH$.

glycolysis (gli-kol′ĭ-sis) [*glyco-* + Gr. *lysis* solution] the anaerobic enzymatic conversion of glucose to the simpler compounds lactate or pyruvate, resulting in energy stored in the form of adenosine triphosphate (ATP), as occurs in muscle; it differs from respiration in that organic substances, rather than molecular oxygen, are used as electron acceptors. See *Embden-Meyerhof pathway,* under *pathway.*

glycolytic (gli″ko-lit′ik) pertaining to, characterized by, or promoting glycolysis.

glycometabolic (gli″ko-met-ah-bol′ik) pertaining to the metabolism of sugar.

glycometabolism (gli″ko-mĕ-tab′o-lizm) the metabolism of sugar.

glycone (gli′kōn) a glycerin suppository.

glyconeogenesis (gli″ko-ne″o-jen′ĕ-sis) [*glyco-* + Gr. *neos* new + *gennan* to produce] gluconeogenesis.

glyconucleoprotein (gli″ko-nu″kle-o-pro′te-in) a nucleoprotein bearing carbohydrate groups.

glycopenia (gli″ko-pe′ne-ah) [*glyco-* + Gr. *penia* poverty] a deficiency of sugar in the tissues.

glycopeptide (gli″ko-pep′tid) any of a class of peptides that contain carbohydrates, including those that contain amino sugars.

glycopexic (gli″ko-pek′sik) pertaining to, characterized by, or promoting glycopexis.

glycopexis (gli″ko-pek′sis) [*glyco-* + Gr. *pēxis* fixation] the fixation or storing of sugar or glycogen.

Glycophagus (gli-kof′ah-gus) *Glycyphagus.*

glycophenol (gli″ko-fe′nol) glucide.

glycophilia (gli″ko-fil′e-ah) [*glyco-* + Gr. *philein* to love] a condition in which a very small amount of dextrose produces hyperglycemia.

glycophorin (gli″ko-for′in) a protein that projects through the thickness of the cell membrane of erythrocytes; it is attached to oligosaccharides at the outer cell membrane surface and to contractile proteins (spectrin and actin) at the cytoplasmic surface.

glycopolyuria (gli″ko-pol″e-u′re-ah) [*glyco-* + Gr. *polys* much + *ouron* urine + *-ia*] polyuria due to glucosuria.

glycoprival (gli″ko-pri′val) [*glyco-* + L. *privus* deprived of] pertaining to or characterized by deprivation of carbohydrates.

glycoprotein (gli″ko-pro′te-in) any of a class of conjugated proteins consisting of a compound of protein with a carbohydrate group. They are distinguished by yielding in decomposition a product frequently capable of reducing alkaline solutions of cupric oxide. The glycoproteins include the mucins, the mucoids, and the chondroproteins. Glycoproteins having a very high content of polysaccharides are called *proteoglycans.* **glycine-rich β g. (GBG),** factor B.

glycoptyalism (gli″ko-ti′al-izm) [*glyco-* + Gr. *ptyalon* saliva] glycosialia.

glycopyrrolate (gli″ko-pir′ro-lāt) [USP] chemical name: 3-[(cyclopentylhydroxyphenylacetyl)oxy]-1,1-dimethyl pyrrolidinium bromide. A synthetic quaternary anticholinergic, $C_{19}H_{28}BrNO_3$, occurring as a white, crystalline powder; used in the treatment of peptic ulcer and other gastrointestinal disturbances in which hyperacidity, hypermotility, and/or spasm occur, administered orally, subcutaneously, intramuscularly, or intravenously. Called also *glycopyrronium bromide.*

glycopyrronium bromide (gli″ko-pir-ro′ne-um) glycopyrrolate.

glycoregulation (gli″ko-reg″u-la′shun) the control of sugar metabolism.

glycoregulatory (gli″ko-reg′u-lah-to″re) pertaining to the control of sugar metabolism.

glycorrhachia (gli″ko-ra′ke-ah) [*glyco-* + Gr. *rhachis* spine + *-ia*] presence of glucose in the cerebrospinal fluid.

glycorrhea (gli″ko-re′ah) [*glyco-* + Gr. *rhoia* flow] any sugary discharge, as of urine.

glycosamine (gli″ko-sam′in) an amino sugar.

glycosaminoglycan (gli″kōs-ah-me″no-gli′kan) any of several high molecular weight linear heteropolysaccharides having disaccharide repeating units containing an *N*-acetylhexosamine and a hexose or hexuronic acid; either or both residues may be sulfated. This class of compounds includes the chondroitin sulfates, dermatan sulfates, heparan sulfate and heparin, keratan sulfates, and hyaluronic acid. All except heparin occur in proteoglycans. Inborn errors of glycosaminoglycan-degrading lysosomal enzymes, which cause the lysosomal accumulation and urinary excretion of glycosaminoglycans, are called mucopolysaccharidoses. Abbreviated GAG.

glycosaminolipid (gli″kos-am″ĭ-no-lip′id) any of a class of lipids that contain amino sugars.

glycosecretory (gli″ko-se-kre′to-re) causing or concerned in the deposition of glycogen.

glycosemia (gli-ko-se′me-ah) glycemia.

glycosene (gli′ko-sēn) an anhydrosugar in which there is a double bond between two adjacent carbon atoms having hydroxyl groups in the *trans* position.

glycosialia (gli″ko-si-a′le-ah) [*glyco-* + Gr. *sialon* saliva + *-ia*] presence of glucose in the saliva.

glycosialorrhea (gli″ko-si″ah-lo-re′ah) [*glyco-* + Gr. *sialon* saliva + *rhoia* flow] excessive flow of saliva containing glucose.

glycosidase (gli-ko′sĭ-dās) [EC 3.2] any of a large group of enzymes of the hydrolase class that break the hemiacetal bonds of glycosides. See also *glucosidase*.

glycoside (gli′ko-sīd) any compound that contains a carbohydrate molecule (sugar), particularly any such natural product in plants, convertible, by hydrolytic cleavage, into sugar and a nonsugar component (aglycone), and named specifically for the sugar contained, as glucoside (glucose), pentoside (pentose), fructoside (fructose), etc. **cardiac g.,** any one of a group of glycosides occurring in certain plants (*Digitalis, Strophanthus, Urginea,* and others), which have a characteristic action on the contractile force of cardiac muscle. **cyanophoric g.,** a glycoside which on hydrolysis yields hydrocyanic acid. **sterol g.,** phytosterolin.

glycosometer (gli″ko-som′ĕ-ter) [*glyco-* + Gr. *metron* measure] an instrument used in determining the proportion of glucose in the urine.

glycosphingolipid (gli″ko-sfing″o-lip′id) a sphingolipid containing the sugar glucose or galactose.

glycosphingolipidosis (gli″ko-sfing″o-lip″ĭ-do′sis) [*glycosphingolipid* + *-osis*] Fabry's disease.

glycostatic (gli″ko-stat′ik) tending to maintain a constant sugar level.

glycosuria (gli″ko-su′re-ah) [*glyco-* + Gr. *ouron* urine + *-ia*] the presence of glucose in the urine; especially the excretion of an abnormally large amount of sugar (glucose) in the urine, i.e., more than 1 gm. in 24 hours. **alimentary g.,** digestive g. **benign g.,** renal g. **digestive g.,** normal glycosuria following the ingestion of sugar. **emotional g.,** glycosuria induced by violent emotion. **epinephrine g.,** glycosuria following the injection of epinephrine. **hyperglycemic g.,** glycosuria associated with hyperglycemia. **magnesium g.,** glycosuria due to high concentration of magnesium in the blood. **nervous g.,** glycosuria produced by puncture of the fourth ventricle of the brain or by stimulation of the great splanchnic nerve. **nondiabetic g., nonhyperglycemic g., normoglycemic g., orthoglycemic g.,** renal g. **pathologic g.,** a condition in which large amounts of sugar appear in the urine for a considerable period of time. **phloridzin g., phlorhizin g.,** glycosuria following the administration of phlorhizin. **renal g.,** glycosuria occurring when there is only the normal amount of sugar in the blood, due to inherited inability of the renal tubules to reabsorb glucose completely. **toxic g.,** glycosuria produced by poisons.

glycosuric acid (gli″ko-su′rik) homogentisic acid.

glycosyl (gli′ko-sil) a radical derived from a carbohydrate.

glycosylated (gli-ko′sĭ-lāt″ed) having formed a linkage with a glycosyl group.

glycosylation (gli″ko-sĭ-la′shun) the formation of linkages with glycosyl groups.

glycosyltransferase (gli″ko-sil-trans′fer-ās) [EC 2.4] any enzyme that catalyzes the transfer of glycosyl groups from one molecule to another; the glycosyltransferases include the hexosyltransferases (EC 2.4.1), the pentosyltransferases (EC 2.4.2), and those transferring other glycosyl groups (EC 2.4.99). Called also *transglycosylase*.

glycotaxis (gli″ko-tak′sis) [*glyco-* + Gr. *taxis* arrangement] the metabolic distribution of glucose to the body tissues.

glycotropic (gli″ko-trop′ik) [*glyco-* + Gr. *tropos* a turning] having an affinity for or attracting sugar; mediated by sugar; causing hyperglycemia.

glycuresis (gli″ku-re′sis) the normal increase in the glucose content of the urine which follows an ordinary carbohydrate meal.

glycuronic acid (gli″ku-ron′ik) any uronic acid.

glycuronide (gli-ku′ro-nīd) a compound formed by the union of glycuronic acid and some other substance, frequently an aromatic body.

glycuronuria (gli-ku″ro-nu′re-ah) the presence of glucuronic acid in the urine.

glycyl (glis′il) the acyl radical of glycine.

glycylglycine (glis″il-glis′in) the simplest dipeptide, $CH_2(NH_2) \cdot CO \cdot NH \cdot CH_2 \cdot CO_2 \cdot H$.

glycyltryptophan (glis″il-trip′to-fan) a dipeptide consisting of glycine and tryptophan radicals; used as a test for cancer of stomach. See under *tests*.

Glycyphagus (gli-sif′ah-gus) [Gr. *glykys* sweet + *phagein* to eat] a genus of mites. **G. domes′ticus,** the food mite; the causative agent of grocers' itch.

Glycyrrhiza (glis″ĭ-ri′zah) [Gr. *glykys* sweet + *rhiza* root] a genus of leguminous plants.

glycyrrhiza (glis″ir-ri′zah) [NF] the dried rhizome and roots of *Glycyrrhiza glabra* (Spanish licorice) or its variety *glandulifera* (Russian licorice), or of other varieties; used as a pharmaceutic necessity for the preparation of pure glycyrrhiza extract; see under *extract*. Called also *licorice, licorice root,* and *liquorid*.

glycyrrhizic acid (glis″ĭ-ri′zik) glycyrrhizin.

glycyrrhizin (glis″ĭ-ri′zin) [L. *glycyrrhizinum*] a very sweet substance, $C_{42}H_{62}O_{16}$, from glycyrrhiza; has been used in the treatment of Addison's disease.

glydanile sodium (gli′dah-nīl) glicetanile sodium.

glykemia (gli-ke′me-ah) glycemia.

glymidine sodium (gli′mĭ-dēn) chemical name: *N*-[5-(2-methoxyethoxy)-2-pyrimidinyl] benzene sulfonamide sodium salt; an oral hypoglycemic, $C_{13}H_{14}N_3NaO_4S$.

glyoxal (gli-ok′sal) a yellow crystalline compound, $O{:}HC \cdot CH{:}O$, prepared by the oxidation of acetaldehyde; called also *biformyl, ethanedial,* and *oxalaldehyde*.

glyoxalase (gli-ok′sah-lās) (obs) a term used to describe the enzyme activity that converts methylglyoxal to lactic acid. It is composed of two enzymes: lactoylglutathione lyase (glyoxalase I) and hydroxyacylglutathione hydrolase (glyoxalase II).

glyoxalin (gli-ok′sah-lin) iminazole.

glyoxisome (gli-ok′sĭ-sōm) glyoxosome.

glyoxosome (gli-ok′so-sōm) any of the microbodies present in certain plants and microorganisms, resembling the peroxisomes of vertebrate animal cells, but having, in addition to catalase and oxidase enzymes, the enzymes of the glyoxylate cycle, a metabolic pathway involved in the conversion of fat to carbohydrate. Glyoxosomes, in association with chloroplasts, also participate in the process of photorespiration. Called also *glyoxisome*. See also *microbody* and *peroxisome,* def. 1.

glyoxylate (gli-ok′sĭ lăt) a salt of ester of glyoxylic acid.

glyoxylic acid (gli-ok-sil′ik) a crystalline acid, dihydroxyacetic acid, $O{:}HC \cdot COOH)_2$, used in Hopkins-Cole test for protein; called also *ethanal a*. See also *glyoxylate cycle*.

glyphylline (gli-fil′lin) dyphylline.

Glyptocranium (glip″to-kra′ne-um) *Mastophora*. **G. gasteracanthoi′des,** *Mastophora gasteracanthoides*.

Glytheonate (gli-the′o-nāt) trademark for a preparation of theophylline sodium glycinate.

Gm See under *allotype*.

gm *gram*.

G.M.C. General Medical Council (British).

Gmelin's test (ma′linz) [Leopold *Gmelin*, German physiologist, 1788–1853] see under *tests*.

GMK a preparation of green monkey kidney cells used as culture system for growing viruses, e.g., for recovering the rubella virus.

GMP guanosine monophosphate. **cGMP,** cyclic GMP. **3′,5′-GMP,** cyclic GMP.

gnat (nat) a small dipterous insect. In England the term is applied to mosquitoes; in America to insects smaller than mosquitoes. See *Chironomidae.* **buffalo g.,** a name given various individuals of the family Simuliidae. **eye g.,** *Hippelates pusio.* **fungus g.,** a gnat whose larvae feed on fungi; see *Bradysia* and *Sciaria.* **turkey g.,** a name given various individuals of the family Simuliidae.

gnathalgia (nath-al′je-ah) [*gnath-* + *-algia*] pain in the jaw.

gnathic (nath′ik) pertaining to the jaw or cheek.

gnathion (nath′e-on) [NA] an anthropometric landmark indicating the lowest point on the median line of the mandible.

gnathitis (nath-i′tis) [*gnath-* + *-itis*] inflammation of the jaw.

gnath(o)- [Gr. *gnathos* jaw] a combining form denoting relationship to the jaw.

Gnathobdellidae (nath″ob-del′ĭ-de) a family of the Hirudinea, which includes leeches of the genera *Hirudo, Limnatis, Haemadipsa, Macrobdella, Theromyzon, Haemopis, Dinobdella,* and *Hirudinaria.*

gnathocephalus (nath″o-sef′ah-lus) [*gnatho-* + Gr. *kephalē* head] a monster with no head except the jaws.

gnathodynamics (nath″o-di-nam′iks) [*gnatho-* + Gr. *dynamis* power] the study of the physical forces used in mastication.

gnathodynamometer (nath″o-di″nah-mom′ĕ-ter) [*gnatho-* + *dynamometer*] an instrument for measuring the force exerted in closing the jaws; called also *occlusometer.* **bimeter g.,** a gnathodynamometer equipped with a central-bearing point of adjustable height.

gnathodynia (nath″o-din′e-ah) [*gnatho-* + *odynē* pain] gnathalgia.

gnathography (nath-og′rah-fe) [*gnatho-* + *-graphy*] the recording of the strength of a patient's bite by a tracing of the changes in the flow of an electric current through a bite gauge.

gnathologic (nath″o-loj′ik) relating to gnathology.

gnathology (nath-ol′o-je) [*gnatho-* + *-logy*] the science that deals with the anatomy, histology, physiology, and pathology of the jaws and the masticatory system as a whole, including the applicable diagnostic, therapeutic, and rehabilitative procedures.

gnathoplasty (nath′o-plas″te) [*gnatho-* + Gr. *plassein* to mold] plastic surgery of the jaw.

gnathoschisis (nath-os′kĭ-sis) [*gnatho-* + Gr. *schisis* splitting] cleft jaw.

gnathosoma (nath″o-so′mah) [*gnatho-* + Gr. *soma* body] the capitulum of an acarine.

gnathostat (nath′o-stat) a jaw-positioning device used in dental radiology, facial photography, cephalometry, and other procedures requiring exact positioning of the jaws. See also *cephalostat.*

gnathostatics (nath″o-stat′iks) [*gnatho-* + Gr. *statikē* the art of weighing] a method of prosthodontic and orthodontic diagnosis based on determination of the basal and osteometric relationships between the teeth and their supporting structures.

Gnathostoma (nath-os′to-mah) [*gnatho-* + Gr. *stoma* mouth] a genus of nematode worms of the superfamily Spiruroidea, which are parasitic in cats, swine, cattle, and sometimes in man. **G. spinig′erum,** a nematode parasitic in the stomach of cats and dogs that ingest fish which contain the larvae; man acquires the larvae when he eats undercooked fish. See *gnathostomiasis.*

gnathostomiasis (nath″o-sto-mi′ah-sis) infection with the nematode *Gnathostoma spinigerum,* acquired when undercooked fish harboring the larvae are eaten. The larvae migrate, often in the subcutaneous tissue, causing a creeping eruption associated with intense eosinophilia. Occasionally they migrate to deeper tissues and cause abscesses or to the central nervous system, causing eosinophilic myeloencephalitis (q.v.).

Gnathostomum (nath-os′to-mum) *Gnathostoma.*

gnosia (no′se-ah) the faculty of perceiving and recognizing.

gnosis (no′sis) [Gr. *gnōsis* knowledge] Edinger's term for the arousal of associative mnemonic complexes by sensory pallial impulses; one of the functions of the cerebral cortex. Cf. *praxis.*

gnotobiology (no″to-bi-ol′o-je) gnotobiotics.

gnotobiota (no″to-bi-o′tah) the specifically and entirely known microfauna and microflora of a specially reared laboratory animal.

gnotobiote (no′to-bi-ōt) a specially reared laboratory animal the microfauna and microflora of which are specifically known in their entirety.

gnotobiotic (no′to-bi-ot′ik) pertaining to a gnotobiote or to gnotobiotics. Cf. *axenic.*

gnotobiotics (no″to-bi-ot′iks) [Gr. *gnotos* known + *biota* the fauna and flora of a region] the science of rearing laboratory animals the microfauna and microflora of which are specifically known in their entirety.

gnotophoresis (no″to-for′ĕ-sis) [Gr. *gnotos* known + *phōresis* a being borne] the state of existence of an organism bearing one or more known species in intimate contact with it and no other demonstrable viable microorganisms.

gnotophoric (no″to-for′ik) pertaining to gnotophoresis.

Gn-RH gonadotropin-releasing hormone; see under *hormone.*

Goa powder (go′ah) [*Goa* a city of India] see under *powder.*

goatpox (gōt′poks) an acute, highly infectious disease of goats marked by a vesicular eruption with catarrh of the respiratory mucous membranes and caused by a poxvirus. It is less severe than sheep-pox. Called also *variola caprina.*

Godélier's law (go-da-lyāz′) [Charles Pierre *Godélier,* French physician, 1813–1877] see under *law.*

goiter (goi′ter) an enlargement of the thyroid gland, causing a swelling in the front part of the neck. **aberrant g.,** enlargement of an ectopic or supernumerary thyroid gland. **adenomatous g.,** enlargement of the thyroid gland caused by adenomas of the gland, or by multiple colloid nodules. **Basedow's g.,** a colloid goiter which has become hyperfunctioning after administration of iodine. **colloid g.,** a large and soft form of goiter in which the follicles of the gland are greatly distended with colloid. **congenital g.,** enlargement of the thyroid gland which is present at birth, or which results from a congenital absence of enzymes leading to inadequate production of thyroxine, with consequent overstimulation of the thyroid by thyrotropin. **cystic g.,** an enlarged thyroid gland containing cysts formed by mucoid or colloid degeneration. **diffuse g.,** a thyroid gland which is diffusely enlarged, as in Graves' disease. **diving g.,** a movable goiter located sometimes above and sometimes below the sternal notch. **endemic g.,** enlargement of the thyroid gland occurring in certain districts, particularly in the mountain regions of the Alps, Pyrenees, Carpathians, Andes, and Himalayas, and other areas where the iodine content of the normal diet is low. **exophthalmic g.,** enlargement of the thyroid gland with protrusion of the eyeballs; see *Graves' disease,* under *disease.* **fibrous g.,** enlargement of the thyroid gland caused by hyperplasia of

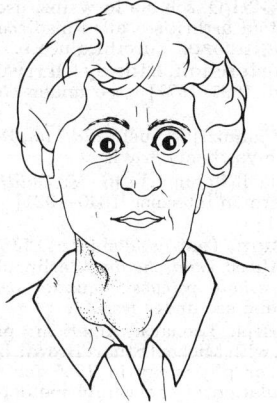

Exophthalmic goiter.

the capsule and stroma. **follicular g.**, parenchymatous g. **intrathoracic g.**, goiter in which a portion of the enlarged thyroid is situated in the thoracic cavity. **iodide g.**, that occurring in reaction to exogenous iodides at high concentrations, due to inhibition of iodide organification (Wolff-Chaikoff effect). **lingual g.**, an enlargement of the upper end of the original thyroglossal duct, forming a tumor at the posterior part of the dorsum of the tongue. **lymphadenoid g.**, Hashimoto's disease. **multinodular g.**, an enlarged thyroid gland containing circumscribed nodules within its substance. **nontoxic g.**, that occurring sporadically and not associated with hyperthyroidism; such goiters may be either diffuse or nodular. **parenchymatous g.**, goiter marked by increase in the follicles and proliferation of the epithelium. **perivascular g.**, one which surrounds a large blood vessel. **plunging g.**, diving g. **retrovascular g.**, goiter with a process or processes behind an important blood vessel. **simple g.**, simple hyperplasia of the thyroid gland. **substernal g.**, goiter in which a portion of the enlarged gland is situated beneath the sternum. **suffocative g.**, one which causes dyspnea by pressure on the trachea. **toxic g., diffuse** Graves' disease. **toxic multinodular g.**, hyperthyroidism arising in a multinodular goiter, usually of long standing. Called also *Parry's disease* and *Plummer's disease.* **vascular g.**, enlargement of the thyroid gland due chiefly to dilatation of the blood vessels. **wandering g.**, diving g.

goitre (goi′ter) [Fr.] goiter.

goitrin (goi′trin) a goitrogenic substance isolated from rutabagas and turnips.

goitrogen (goi′tro-jen) a goiter-producing compound.

goitrogenic (goi-tro-jen′ik) producing goiter.

goitrogenicity (goi″tro-jĕ-nis′ĭ-te) the tendency to produce goiter.

goitrogenous (goi-troj′ĕ-nus) producing goiter.

goitrous (goi′trus) pertaining to or of the nature of goiter.

gold (gōld) a yellow metallic element occurring in masses or veins in rocks or in grains in the sand of rivers. Its symbol is Au (L. *au′rum*); atomic number, 79; atomic weight, 196.967; specific gravity, 19.32. When alloyed, in carats, pure gold has 24 parts (or carats). Gold compounds are used in medicine, chiefly in arthritis, and all the compounds are poisonous. **g. aurothiosulfate**, g. sodium thiosulfate. **cohesive g.**, cohesive gold foil. **colloidal g.**, a purplish suspension of minute particles of metallic gold, made by reducing a solution of bromauric acid or other acid or salt of gold, used in medicine since alchemical times. The radioactive form, made by exposure to neutrons, is used as a suspension in the pleural cavity to treat lung cancer. **Dutch g.**, an alloy of copper and zinc. **mat g.**, spongy strips of pure gold produced by the process of electroplating, which can be formed into ropes and cylinders and used in the base of dental restorations and as a direct filling material. See also under *foil.* **radioactive g.**, radiogold. **g. sodium thiomalate** [USP], a monovalent gold salt used in the treatment of early active rheumatoid arthritis not controlled by nonsteroidal anti-inflammatory agents, rest, and physical therapy. Called also *sodium aurothiomalate* [INN]. **g. sodium thiosulfate**, white, needle-like or prismatic small glistening crystals, $Na_3Au(S_2O_3)_2 \cdot 2H_2O$, soluble in water; used in the treatment of rheumatoid arthritis. Called also *sodium aurothiosulfate.* **g. thioglucose**, aurothioglucose.

Goldblatt's clamp, hypertension, kidney [Harry Goldblatt, Cleveland physician, 1891–1977] see under *clamp, hypertension*, and *kidney.*

Goldflam's disease (gōlt′flahmz) [Samuel *Goldflam*, Polish neurologist, 1852–1932] myasthenia gravis.

Goldflam-Erb disease (gōlt′flahm-ērb) [S. V. *Goldflam;* Wilhelm Heinrich *Erb*, German internist, 1840–1921] myasthenia gravis.

Goldscheider's percussion, test (gōld′shi-derz) [Johannes Karl August Eugen Alfred *Goldscheider*, Berlin physician, 1858–1935] see *threshold percussion*, under *percussion*, see *orthopercussion;* and see under *tests.*

Goldstein (gōld′stīn) Joseph Leonard. American physician, born 1940; co-winner, with Michael Stuart Brown, of the Nobel prize for medicine or physiology in 1985 for their discoveries about the regulation of cholesterol metabolism

and the treatment of diseases caused by abnormally high levels of cholesterol in the blood.

Goldstein's disease, etc. (gōld′stīnz) [Hyman Isaac *Goldstein*, American physician, 1887–1954] see under *disease, hematemesis, hemoptysis*, and *sign.*

Goldstein rays (gōld′stīn) [Eugene *Goldstein*, German physicist, 1850–1930] see under *ray.*

Goldthwait's brace, sign (symptom) (gōld′thwāts) [Joel Ernest *Goldthwait*, American orthopedic surgeon, 1866–1971] see under *brace* and *sign.*

Golgi (gol′je) Camillo. Italian neurologist and histologist, 1843–1926; co-winner, with Santiago Ramón y Cajal, of the Nobel prize for medicine or physiology in 1906 for their work on the structure of the nervous system.

Golgi's complex, etc. (gol′jēz) [Camillo *Golgi*] see under *complex, corpuscle, law, neuron, organ, Table of Stains*, and *theory.*

golgiosome (gol′je-o-sōm) mitochondrion-sized, platelike structures which make up the Golgi complex of the cell; the platelike structure consists of stacks of flattened vessels (cisternae) more commonly known as dictyosomes.

Goll's column, fasciculus (column, tract), fibers, nucleus (golz) [Friedrich *Goll*, Swiss anatomist, 1829–1903] see *fasciculus gracilis medullae spinalis*, and *nucleus gracilis*, and see under *fiber.*

Goltz's experiment, theory (gōlts′ez) [Friedrich Leopold *Goltz*, German physician, 1834–1902] see under *experiment* and *theory.*

Gombault's degeneration, neuritis (gom-bōz′) [François Alexis Albert *Gombault*, French neurologist, 1844–1904] progressive hypertrophic interstitial neuropathy.

Gombault-Philippe triangle (gom-bo′fe-lēp′) [F. A. A. *Gombault;* Claudius *Philippe*, French pathologist, 1866–1903] see under *triangle.*

gomitoli (go-mit′o-li) a network of capillaries in the upper infundibular stem (of the hypothalamus) that surround terminal arterioles of the superior hypophyseal arteries and that lead into portal veins to the adenohypophysis.

Gomori methods, stains [George *Gomori*, Hungarian histochemist in Chicago, 1904–1957] see *Table of Stains and Staining Methods*, under *stain.*

Gompertz formula, law (gom′pertz) [Benjamin *Gompertz*, British actuary, 1779–1865] see under *law.*

gomphosis (gom-fo′sis) [Gr. *gomphōsis* a bolting together] [NA] a type of fibrous joint in which a conical process is inserted into a socket-like portion, such as the styloid process in the temporal bone, or the teeth in the dental alveoli. Called also *articulatio dentoalveolaris* and *dentoalveolar articulation.*

gon- 1. see *gon(o)-.* 2. [Gr. *gony* knee] a combining form denoting relationship to the knee. Cf. *gony-.*

gonacratia (gon″ah-kra′she-ah) [*gon-(1)* + Gr. *akrateia* incontinence] spermatorrhea.

gonad (go′nad, gon′ad) [L. *gonas*, from Gr. *gonē* seed] a gamete-producing gland; an ovary or testis. **indifferent g.**, the sexually undifferentiated gonad of the early embryo. **streak g's**, undeveloped gonadal structures found in the broad ligament below the fallopian tube and composed of whorled connective-tissue stroma with no germinal or secretory cells; seen most often in Turner's syndrome.

gonadal (go′nad-al) pertaining to a gonad.

gonadectomize (go″nah-dek′to-mīz) to deprive of the gonads by surgical excision.

gonadectomy (go″nah-dek′to-me) [*gonad* + Gr. *ektomē* excision] removal of an ovary or testis.

gonadial (go-nad′e-al) pertaining to a gonad.

gonadoblastoma (gon″ah-do-blas-to′mah) a dysgerminoma that contains all gonadal elements—germ cells, sex cord derivatives, and stromal derivatives; occurring almost exclusively in abnormal gonads, most often associated with some form of gonadal dysgenesis, frequently associated with abnormal chromosomal karyotype.

gonadogenesis (gon″ah-do-jen′ĕ-sis) [*gonado-* + Gr. *genesis* production] the development of the gonads in the embryo, especially the development of gonads typical of one or the other sex.

gonadoinhibitory (gon″ah-do-in-hib′ĭ-to-re) inhibiting or preventing gonadal activity.

gonadokinetic (gon″ah-do-ki-net′ik) [*gonad* + Gr. *kinēsis* motion] stimulating gonadal activity.

gonadopathy (gon″ah-dop′ah-the) [*gonad* + Gr. *pathos* disease] any disease of the gonads.

gonadopause (go-nad′o-paws) the loss of gonadal activity which accompanies the aging process.

gonadorelin (go″nad-o-rel′in) synthetic gonadotropin releasing hormone.

gonadotrope (go-nad′o-trōp) 1. gonadotroph. 2. a gonadotropic substance.

gonadotroph (go-nad′o-trōf) 1. any of the basophils (beta cells) of the adenohypophysis, the granules of which secrete follicle-stimulating hormone and luteinizing hormone. A single cell type probably secretes both hormones; called also *delta basophil* and *delta cell*. 2. a gonadotropic substance.

gonadotrophic (gon″ah-do-tro′fik) gonadotropic.

gonadotrophin (gon″ah-do-tro′fin) gonadotropin.

gonadotropic (gon″ah-do-trōp′ik) [*gonad* + Gr. *tropos* a turning] stimulating the gonads; applied to hormones of the anterior pituitary which influence the gonads.

gonadotropin (gon″ah-do-tro′pin) any hormone having a stimulating effect on the gonads. Two such hormones are secreted by the anterior pituitary: follicle-stimulating hormone and luteinizing hormone, both of which are active, but with differing effects, in the two sexes. See also *chorionic g.* **chorionic g.,** 1. a glycopeptide hormone produced by the syncytiotrophoblasts of the fetal placenta that is thought to maintain the function of the corpus luteum during the first few weeks of pregnancy, to promote steroidogenesis in the fetoplacental unit, and to stimulate fetal testicular secretion of testosterone. It can be detected by immunoassay in the maternal urine within days after fertilization and thus provides the basis of the most commonly used pregnancy test. 2. [USP] the same principle obtained from the urine of pregnant women, occurring as a white or practically white amorphous powder; used in the treatment of certain cases of cryptorchidism and male hypogonadism, and to induce ovulation and pregnancy in certain infertile, anovulatory women, administered intramuscularly. **equine g.,** pregnant mare serum g. **human chorionic g. (hCG),** see *chorionic g.* **human menopausal g. (hMG),** menotropins. **pregnant mare serum g.,** a preparation of the follicle-stimulating substance obtained from the blood serum of pregnant mares; it has been used in the treatment of cryptorchidism, sterility, pituitary dwarfism, and other conditions in both men and women. Called also *equine g.* Abbreviated PMSG.

gonaduct (gon′ah-dukt) the duct of a gonad; an oviduct or seminal duct.

gonagra (gon-ag′rah) [*gon-*(2) + Gr. *agra* seizure] gout in the knee.

gonalgia (go-nal′je-ah) [*gon-*(2) + *-algia*] pain in the knee.

gonarthritis (gon″ar-thri′tis) [*gon-*(2) + Gr. *arthron* joint + *-itis*] inflammation of a knee or knee joint.

gonarthrocace (gon″ar-throk′a-se) [*gon-*(2) + Gr. *arthron* joint + *kakē* evil] white swelling of the knee, produced by tuberculous arthritis.

gonarthromeningitis (gon-ar″thro-men″in-ji′tis) [*gon-*(2) + Gr. *arthron* joint + *mēninx* membrane] inflammation of the synovial membrane of the knee joint.

gonarthrosis (gon″ar-thro′sis) arthritic affection of the knee joint, due to degeneration or trauma.

gonarthrotomy (gon″ar-throt′o-me) [*gon-*(2) + Gr. *arthron* joint + *temnein* to cut] surgical incision of the knee joint.

gonatocele (go-nat′o-sēl) [*gon-*(2) + Gr. *kēlē* tumor] tumor of the knee.

gonecyst, gonecystis (gon′ĕ-sist, gon″ĕ-sis′tis) [Gr. *gonē* seed + *kystis* bladder] vesicula seminalis.

gonecystitis (gon″ĕ-sis-ti′tis) inflammation of a seminal vesicle.

gonecystolith (gon″ĕ-sis′to-lith) [*gonecyst* + Gr. *lithos* stone] a concretion in a seminal vesicle.

gonecystopyosis (gon″ĕ-sis″to-pi-o′sis) [*gonecyst* + Gr. *pyōsis* suppuration] suppuration in a seminal vesicle.

goneitis (gon″e-i′tis) [*gon-*(2) + *-itis*] inflammation of the knee.

gonepoiesis (gon″e-poi-e′sis) [Gr. *gonē* seed + *poiein* to make] the secretion or formation of the semen.

gonepoietic (gon″e-poi-et′ik) pertaining to, characterized by, or promoting gonepoiesis.

Gongylonema (gon″jĭ-lo-ne′mah) [Gr. *gongylos* round + *nēma* thread] a genus of nematodes of the superfamily Spiruroidea. **G. ingluvic′ola,** a species found in chickens. **G. neoplas′ticum,** a species occurring in the anterior portion of the digestive tract of rats. **G. pul′chrum,** a common parasite in the esophageal mucosa of sheep, goats, cattle, and pigs in the United States; it has been found in the mucosa and submucosa of the lips and mouth of man. **G. scuta′tum,** G. pulchrum.

gongylonemiasis (gon″jĭ-lo-ne-mi′ah-sis) infection with Gongylonema.

gonia (go′ne-ah) [Gr.] plural of *gonion*.

gonial (go′ne-al) pertaining to the gonion.

gonidangium (gon″id-an′je-um) a cell within which gonidia are formed.

gonidia (go-nid′e-ah) [L.] plural of *gonidium*.

gonidiospore (go-nid′e-o-spōr) 1. a general term for a sexual spore of fungi, as one produced from an antherium. 2. a spore produced from the algal part of a lichen. See *spore*.

gonidium (go-nid′e-um), pl. *gonid′ia* [Gr. *gonē* seed] 1. the algal cell part of the thallus of a lichen. 2. a motile reproductive unit of the nitrogen-fixing bacteria *Azotobacter* and *Rhizobium*.

Gonin's operation (go-nāz′) [Jules *Gonin*, Swiss ophthalmic surgeon, 1870–1935] see under *operation*.

goni(o)- [Gr. *gōnia* angle] a combining form denoting relationship to an angle.

Goniobasis (go″ne-o-ba′sis) a genus of small fresh-water snails. **G. sili′cula,** the host of *Troglotrema salmincola* in northwestern United States.

gonioma (gon″e-o′ma) [*gon-*(1) + *-oma*] a term formerly applied to testicular tumors thought to be derived from sexual cells.

goniometer (go″ne-om′ĕ-ter) [*gonio-* + Gr. *metron* measure] 1. an instrument for measuring angles. 2. a plank, one end of which may be tilted to any height, used in testing for labyrinthine disease. **finger g.,** an apparatus for measuring the limits of flexion and extension of the interphalangeal joints of the fingers.

gonion (go′ne-on), pl. *go′nia* [Gr. *gōnia* angle] [NA] an anthropometric landmark located at the most inferior, posterior, and lateral point on the external angle of the mandible, being the apex of the maximum curvature of the mandible, where the ascending ramus becomes confluent with the corpus.

goniophotography (go″ne-o-fo-tog′rah-fe) photography of the angle of the anterior chamber of the eye.

Goniops (gon′e-ops) a genus of tabanid flies.

goniopuncture (go″ne-o-punk′tūr) [*gonio-* + *puncture*] a rarely used filtering operation for glaucoma, done by inserting a knife blade through clear cornea just within the limbus, across the anterior chamber, and through the opposite corneoscleral wall.

gonioscope (go′ne-o-skōp″) [*gonio-* + *-scope*] an optical instrument for examining the angle of the anterior chamber and for demonstrating ocular motility and rotation.

gonioscopy (go″ne-os′ko-pe) examination of the angle of the anterior chamber of the eye with the gonioscope.

goniosynechia (go′ne-o-sĭ-nek′e-ah) adhesion of the iris to the cornea at the angle of the anterior chamber of the eye.

goniotomy (go″ne-ot′o-me) [*gonio-* + *-tomy*] an operation for glaucoma characterized by an open angle and normal depth of the anterior chamber; it consists of the opening of Schlemm's canal under direct vision secured by a contact glass.

gonitis (go-ni′tis) [*gon-*(2) + *-itis*] inflammation of the knee. **fungous g.,** inflammation of the knee joint in which the capsule is diffusely thickened. **g. tuberculo′sa,** tuberculosis of the knee joint.

gon(o)- [Gr. *gonē* offspring, seed, genitalia] a combining form meaning sexual or generative, or denoting relationship to semen or seed, or to the reproductive organs.

gonoblennorrhea (gon″o-blen″o-re′ah) gonococcal conjunctivitis.

gonocampsis (gon″o-kamp′sis) permanent flexion of the knee.

gonocele (gon′o-sēl) spermatocele.

gonochorism (gon-ok′o-rizm) [*gono-* + Gr. *chōrizein* to separate] differentiation of the gonads with normal development of the reproductive organs appropriate to the sex; the opposite of hermaphroditism.

gonococcal (gon″o-kok′al) pertaining to gonococci.

gonococcemia (gon″o-kok-se′me-ah) [L. *gonococci* + Gr. *haima* blood + *-ia*] the presence of gonococci in the blood.

gonococci (gon″o-kok′si) [L.] plural of *gonococcus*.

gonococcic (gon″o-kok′sik) gonococcal.

gonococcide (gon″o-kok′sīd) [*gonococcus* + L. *caedere* to kill] an agent that kills gonococci.

gonococcocide (gon″o-kok′o-sīd) [*gonococcus* + L. *caedere* to kill] gonococcide.

gonococcus (gon″o-kok′us), pl. *gonococ′ci* [*gono-* + *coccus*] an individual microorganism of the species *Neisseria gonorrhoeae*, the organism causing gonorrhea.

gonocyte (gon′o-sīt) [*gono-* + Gr. *kytos* hollow vessel] 1. the primitive reproductive cell of the embryo. 2. a secondary gamete-producing cell.

gonomery (gon-om′er-e) [*gono-* + Gr. *meros* part] the condition in which the paternal and the maternal chromosomes remain in separate groups and do not completely fuse, as occurs in certain hybrids.

gononephrotome (gon″o-nef′ro-tōm) [*gono-* + Gr. *nephros* kidney + *tomē* a section] that part of the mesoderm which develops into the reproductive and excretory organs of the embryo.

gonophage (gon′o-fāj) a bacteriophage having the gonococcus as its natural host.

gonophore (gon′o-fōr) [*gono-* + Gr. *phoros* bearing] an accessory generative organ, such as the uterine tube and uterus in the female, or spermiduct and seminal vesicle in the male.

gonorrhea (gon″o-re′ah) [*gono-* + Gr. *rhein* to flow] infection due to *Neisseria gonorrhoeae* transmitted sexually in most cases, but also by contact with infected exudates in neonatal children at birth, or by infants in households with infected inhabitants. It is marked in males by urethritis with pain and purulent discharge, but is commonly asymptomatic in females, although it may extend to produce suppurative salpingitis, oophoritis, tubo-ovarian abscess, and peritonitis. Bacteremia occurs in both sexes, resulting in cutaneous lesions, arthritis, and rarely meningitis or endocarditis. Formerly called *blennorrhagia* and *blennorrhea*.

gonorrheal (gon″o-re′al) of or pertaining to gonorrhea.

gonotokont (gon″o-to′kont) auxocyte.

gonotome (gon′o-tōm) [*gono-* + Gr. *tomē* a section] that part of the mesoderm which develops into the reproductive organs of the embryo.

gony- [Gr. *gony* knee] a combining form denoting relationship to the knee.

Gonyaulax (gon″e-aw′laks) [*gony-* + Gr. *aulakos* a furrow] a genus of plantlike marine protozoa (order Dinoflagellida, class Phytomastigophorea) having mainly brown to yellow chromatophores. Like other dinoflagellates, they produce discoloration of the water (red tide) when present in vast numbers, and certain species have been associated with a form of shellfish poisoning (q.v.). Representative species include *G. acatenella, G. catenella, G. polyedra,* and *G. tamarensis*.

gonycampsis (gon″ĭ-kamp′sis) [*gony-* + Gr. *kampsis* bending] abnormal curvature of the knee.

gonycrotesis (gon″e-kro-te′sis) [*gony-* + Gr. *krotēsis* striking] genu valgum.

gonyectyposis (gon″e-ek″tĭ-po′sis) [*gony-* + Gr. *ektypōsis* a modelling in relief] genu varum.

gonyocele (gon′e-o-sēl″) [*gony-* + Gr. *kēlē* tumor] synovitis or tuberculous arthritis of the knee.

gonyoncus (gon″e-ong′kus) [*gony-* + Gr. *onkos* bulk] tumor of the knee.

Good's syndrome (goodz) [R. A. *Good,* American pediatrician, born 1922] immunodeficiency with thymoma.

Goodell's sign (law) (good′elz) [William *Goodell,* American gynecologist, 1829–1894] see under *sign*.

Goodpasture's stain, syndrome (good-pas′churs) [Ernest William *Goodpasture,* American pathologist, 1886–1960]

see *Table of Stains and Staining Methods,* under *stain,* and see under *syndrome*.

Goormaghtigh's apparatus (cells) [Norbert *Goormaghtigh,* Belgian physician, 1890–1960] juxtaglomerular cells.

Gordiacea (gor″de-a′se-ah) Nematomorpha.

Gordius (gor′de-us) [Gordian knot] a genus of the Gordiacea, the hair snakes or horsehair worms. **G. aquat′icus,** a species occasionally found as a pseudoparasite of the intestinal tract of man; its presence is the result of the accidental ingestion of infected insects. **G. medinen′sis,** *Dracunculus medinensis*. **G. robus′tus,** a species that is generally a pseudoparasite of the intestinal tract (see *G. aquaticus*), but has also been reported as invading the periorbital tissues of man.

Gordon (gor′don), Alexander (1752–1799). Scottish obstetrician who, in his *Treatise on the Epidemic Puerperal Fever of Aberdeen* (1795), first demonstrated the contagiousness of this disease.

Gordon's bodies, test (gor′donz) [Mervyn Henry *Gordon,* English physician, 1872–1953] see under *body* and *tests*.

Gordon's reflex, sign (gor′donz) [Alfred *Gordon,* American neurologist, 1874–1953] see *flexor reflex, paradoxical,* under *reflex,* and *finger phenomenon* (def. 1), under *phenomenon*.

gorget (gor′jet) a wide-grooved lithotome director.

Gorlin's syndrome (gor′linz) [Robert James *Gorlin,* American physician, born 1923] see *basal cell nevus syndrome,* and *Gorlin-Chaudhry-Moss syndrome,* under *syndrome*.

Gorlin-Chaudhry-Moss syndrome (gor′lin chaw′dre maws) [Robert James *Gorlin;* Anand P. *Chaudhry,* Indian-born American oral pathologist, born 1922; Melvin Lionel *Moss,* American anatomist] see under *syndrome*.

Gorlin-Goltz syndrome (gor′lin gōltz) [Robert James *Gorlin;* Robert William *Goltz,* American physician, born 1923] basal cell nevus syndrome.

Gorlin-Psaume syndrome (gor′lin sōm) [Robert James *Gorlin;* Jean *Psaume,* French stomatologist, 20th century] orofaciodigital syndrome.

gorondou (go-ron′doo) goundou.

Goslee tooth (goz′le) [Hart J. *Goslee,* American dentist, 1871–1930] see under *tooth*.

Gosselin's fracture (gos-laz′) [Léon Athanase *Gosselin,* French surgeon, 1815–1887] see under *fracture*.

Gossypium (gŏ-sip′e-um) [L.] a genus of tropical and subtropical malvaceous plants found in both hemispheres, including ten species, three of which (*G. barbadense, G. herbaceum,* and *G. hirsutum*) yield most of the world's cotton. The dried bark of the root of various species (cotton root bark) was formerly used as an oxytocic. See *cotton,* and see *cottonseed oil,* under *oil*.

gossypium (gŏ-sip′e-um), gen. *gossyp′ii* [L.] cotton. **g. asep′ticum, g. depura′tum, g. purifica′tum,** purified cotton.

gossypol (gos′ĭ-pol) chemical name: 2,2′-bis[8-formyl-1,6,7-trihydroxy-5-isopropyl-3-methylnaphthyl]. A poisonous yellow pigment, $C_{30}H_{30}O_8$, found in cottonseed (and named for *Gossypium*), which is detoxified by heating. Gossypol has male antifertility properties, apparently having its effects in the seminiferous tubules, where spermatozoa are produced.

GOT glutamine-oxaloacetic transaminase, now known as aspartate aminotransferase.

Göthlin's test (index) (get′linz) [Gustaf Fredrik *Göthlin,* Swedish physiologist, 1874–1949] see under *tests*.

Gottlieb's epithelial attachment (got′lēbz) [Bernhard *Gottlieb,* Vienna dentist, 1885–1950] see under *attachment*.

Gottron's papules, sign (got′ronz) [Heinrich Adolf *Gottron,* German dermatologist, born 1890] see under *papule* and *sign*.

Gottstein's fibers, process (got′stīnz) [Jacob *Gottstein,* otologist in Breslau, 1832–1895] see under *fiber* and *process*.

gouge (gowj) a hollow chisel used in cutting and removing bone. **Kelley g.,** an instrument for removing cartilage grafts.

Gougerot-Blum syndrome (goo-zher-o′ blum) [Henri *Gougerot,* French physician, 1881–1955; Paul *Blum,* French physician, 1878–1933]   pigmented purpuric lichenoid dermatitis.

Gougerot-Carteaud syndrome (goo-zher-o′ kar-to′) [Henri *Gougerot;* Alexandre *Carteaud,* French physician, born 1897]   confluent and reticulated papillomatosis.

Goulard's extract, lotion, water (goo-larz′) [Thomas *Goulard,* French surgeon, 1720–1790]   see *lead subacetate solution* and *diluted lead subacetate solution.*

Gouley's catheter (goo′lēz) [John Williams Severin *Gouley,* American surgeon, 1832–1920]   see under *catheter.*

goundou (goon′doo) [West African]   a late sequel of yaws and endemic syphilis manifested by massive periostitis of the nasal processes of the maxillae, characterized by the formation of bony hornlike exostoses at the sides of the nose, leading to distortion of the facial features and destruction of the nose and orbit. Called also *anakhré, gorondou,* and *henpuye.*

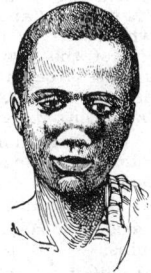

Goundou.

gousiekte (goo-sek′te) [Dutch "rapid disease"]   a condition in sheep marked by myocarditis, dilatation, and heart failure, caused by eating the poisonous plant *Vangueria pygmora.*

gout (gowt) [L. *gutta* a drop, because of the ancient belief that the disease was due to a "noxa" falling drop by drop into the joint]   a group of disorders of purine and pyrimidine metabolism. Fully developed gout is manifested by various combinations of (1) hyperuricemia; (2) recurrent, characteristic acute inflammatory arthritis induced by crystals of monosodium urate monohydrate and normally responsive to colchicine; (3) tophaceous deposits of these crystals in and around the joints of the extremities, which may lead to joint destruction and severe crippling; and (4) uric acid urolithiasis. All forms of gout are characterized by inflammatory arthritis and tophi. **abarticular g.,** that which does not affect the joints. **articular g.,** gout affecting the joints. **calcium g.,** calcinosis. **chalky g.,** tophaceous g. **idiopathic g.,** a gout of uncertain classification; primary or secondary gout. **irregular g.,** abarticular g. **latent g., masked g.,** lithemia without the typical features of gout. **lead g.,** gout ascribed to lead poisoning. **misplaced g.,** gout in which the arthritic symptoms have disappeared and are followed by severe constitutional disturbances. **oxalic g.,** oxalism. **polyarticular g.,** an atypical form of gout which attacks many joints and which resembles rheumatic fever in that an attack may last for weeks. **poor man's g.,** gout ascribed to hard work, exposure, ill feeding, and excess in the use of malt liquors. **primary g.,** a gout that seems to be innate, not a consequence of an acquired disorder (e.g., from using diuretics of the thiazide group or from chronic hemolysis) and not a later, secondary manifestation of some other unlike inborn error of metabolism (e.g., glycogen storage disease, type I); it afflicts chiefly men (about 95 per cent of the cases) and postmenopausal women; peak of incidence is relatively early (thirties through fifties). **regular g.,** articular g. **rheumatic g.,** rheumatoid arthritis. **saturnine g.,** lead g. **secondary g.,** that resulting from an acquired disorder (e.g., polycythemia vera or chronic myelogenous leukemia) or from some other unlike inborn error of metabolism (e.g., the Lesch-Nyhan syndrome); mean age of onset is relatively late (59 years); a greater percentage of women are afflicted (14 per cent of the cases). **tophaceous g.,** gout in which there are tophi or chalky deposits of sodium urate. **visceral g.,** a disease of birds characterized by the deposition of sodium urates on the viscera.

gouty (gow′te)   affected with or of the nature of gout.

Gowers' column, etc. (gow′erz) [Sir William Richard *Gowers,* celebrated English neurologist, 1845–1915]   see under *column, fasciculus, sign, solution,* and *tract,* and see *vasovagal attack,* under *attack.*

G.P.   general practitioner; general paresis (see *dementia paralytica*).

G6PD   glucose-6-phosphate dehydrogenase.

G.P.I.   general paralysis of the insane.

GPT   glutamic-pyruvic transaminase.

gr.   grain.

graafian follicle, vesicle (graf′e-an) [Reijnier (Regner) de *Graaf,* a celebrated Dutch physician and anatomist, 1641–1673]   see *folliculi ovarici vesiculosi.*

gracile (gras′il) [L. *gracilis*]   slender or delicate.

Gracilicutes (gras″ĭ-lik′u-tēz; grah-sil′ĭ-ku″tēz) [L. *gracilis* thin + *cutis* skin]   a division of the kingdom Procaryotae comprising bacteria with a gram-negative type of cell wall consisting of an outer membrane and a thin inner peptidoglycan layer containing muramic acid. It contains three classes: Scotobacteria, Anoxyphotobacteria, and Oxyphotobacteria.

Grad.   abbreviation for L. *grada′tim,* by degrees.

gradatim (gra-da′tim) [L.]   gradually; by degrees.

Gradenigo's syndrome (grah-dě-ne′gōz) [Giuseppe *Gradenigo,* Italian physician, 1859–1926]   see under *syndrome.*

gradient (gra′dē-ent)   the rate of increase or decrease of a variable magnitude; also the curve which represents it. **density g.,** the continuous variation in density (concentration) of a solute along the height or width of a confined solution. **mitral g.,** the difference in pressure in the left atrium and the left ventricle in diastole. **systolic g.,** the difference in pressure between the left atrium and left ventricle in systole. **ventricular g.,** the net differences in ventricular electrical activity of varying duration, as determined by the algebraic sum of the electrocardiographic vectors representing the QRS and T-wave areas.

graduate (grad′u-āt) [L. *graduatus*]   1. a person who has received a degree from a university or college. 2. a measuring vessel marked by a series of lines.

graduated (grad′u-āt-ed) [L. *gradus* step]   marked by a succession of lines, steps, or degrees.

Graefe's knife, operation, sign (gra′fēz) [Albrecht von *Graefe,* German ophthalmologist, 1828–1870]   see under *knife, operation,* and *sign.*

Gräfenberg's ring (graf′en-burg) [Ernest *Grafenberg,* German gynecologist in United States, 1881–1957]   see under *ring.*

graft (graft)   1. any tissue or organ for implantation or transplantation. 2. to implant or transplant such tissues. See also *flap.* **accordion g.,** mesh g. **activated g.,** a graft in which the nerves and blood supply have grown to nourish it, after a period of denervation and tenuous vascularity. **allogeneic g.,** allograft. **autochthonous g.,** autograft. **autodermic g., autoepidermic g.,** a skin graft taken from the patient's own body. **autogenous g., autologous g., autoplastic g.,** autograft. **avascular g.,** a graft of tissue in which not even transient vascularization is achieved. **Blair-Brown g.,** a split-thickness skin graft of intermediate depth. **bone g.,** bone transplanted from one site to another. **brephoplastic g.,** the transplantation of tissue from an embryo or newborn to an adult animal. **cable g.,** a nerve graft made up of several sections of nerve in the manner of a cable. **chorioallantoic g.,** the placing of cells, tissues, or parts on the chorioallantoic membrane of the embryonic chick. **cutis g.,** dermal g. **Davis g.,** pinch g. **delayed g.,** a skin graft which is sutured back into its bed and subsequently shifted to a new recipient bed. **dermal g., dermic g.,** skin from which epidermis and subcutaneous fat have been removed; used instead of fascia in various plastic procedures. Called also *cutis g.* **diced cartilage g's,** numerous small segments of cartilage that can be packed or molded into any desired contour like wet grains of sand; used to repair faulty cartilage or bone structure. **epidermic g.,** a piece of epidermis implanted upon a raw surface; called also *Reverdin g.* **Esser g.,** inlay g. **fascia g.,** a graft taken from the fascia lata or from the lumbar fascia. **fascicular g.,** a nerve graft in which the bundles of nerve fibers are approximated and sutured separately. **fat g.,** a graft of fat completely freed from its bed; used in filling depressions.

filler g., one used for the filling of defects, as the filling of depressions with fatty tissue or of a bony cyst cavity with bone chips or dried cartilage. **free g.,** a graft of tissue completely freed from its bed, in contrast to a flap. **full-thickness g.,** a skin graft consisting of the epidermis and the full depth of the dermis. **heterodermic g.,** a skin graft taken from a donor of another species. **heterologous g., heteroplastic g.,** xenograft. **homologous g.,** allograft. **homoplastic g.,** allograft. **hyperplastic g.,** a skin graft that is in a state of active repair. **inlay g.,** a skin or mucosal graft applied by spreading the graft over a stent and suturing the graft and mold into a prepared pocket; called also *Esser g.* and *Stent g.* **island g.,** see under *flap.* **isogeneic g., isologous g., isoplastic g.,** syngraft. **jump g.,** see under *flap.* **Krause-Wolfe g.,** a graft of full thickness of the skin. **lamellar g.,** replacement of the superficial layers of an opaque cornea by a thin layer of clear cornea from a donor eye. **mesh g.,** a thin split-thickness skin graft in which many tiny splits have been made to allow the graft to expand and be stretched to cover a large area. **mucosal g.,** a graft of mucosal tissue, usually comprising the entire mucosal thickness. **nerve g.,** replacement of an area of defective nerve with a segment from a sound one. **Ollier-Thiersch g.,** a very thin skin graft consisting of epidermis and a thin layer of dermis, often cut in long, broad strips. **omental g's,** free or attached segments of omentum used to cover suture lines following gastrointestinal or colonic surgery. **onlay bone g.,** bone used as a graft that is laid on or over cortical bone of the recipient site(s). **osseous g.,** bone g. **outlay g.,** a modification of an inlay graft, used in ectropion of the eyelid. **patch g.,** a graft of living tissue or prosthetic material used to repair a vascular incision in order to enlarge the lumen of the vessel. **pedicle g.,** see under *flap.* **penetrating g.,** a full-thickness corneal transplant. **periosteal g.,** a piece of periosteum applied to a denuded area of a bone. **Phemister g.,** a bone graft of cortical bone with cancellous bone chips to enhance callus formation. **pinch g.,** a small split-thickness skin graft. **Reverdin g.,** epidermic g. **sieve g.,** a skin graft from which very small circular islands of skin are removed so that a larger denuded area can be covered, the sievelike portion being placed over one area, and the individual islands over surrounding or other denuded areas. **skin g.,** skin transplanted to replace a lost portion of the body skin surface; it may be a full-thickness or split-thickness graft. **sleeve g.,** a graft for repairing traumatic gaps in nerves by a sleevelike extension from the distal stump which is sutured to the central stump. **split-skin g.,** a skin graft consisting of the epidermis and about one third of the dermis. **split-thickness g.,** a skin graft consisting of the epidermis and a portion of dermis. **Stent g.,** inlay g. **syngeneic g.,** syngraft. **thick-split g.,** a skin graft consisting of the epidermis and about two thirds of the dermis. **Thiersch's g.,** Ollier-Thiersch g. **thin-split g.,** Ollier-Thiersch g. **tube g., tunnel g.,** tube flap. **white g.,** avascular g. **Wolfe's g., Wolfe-Krause g.,** Krause-Wolfe g.

grafting (graft′ing) the implanting or transplanting of any tissue or organ. **skin g.,** implantation of patches of healthy skin on a denuded area to provide epithelial covering.

Graham's law (gra′amz) [Thomas *Graham*, English chemist, 1805–1869] see under *law.*

Graham's test (gra′amz) [Evarts Ambrose *Graham*, American surgeon, 1883–1957] see under *test.*

Graham Little syndrome (gra′am-lit′el) [Sir Ernest Gordon *Graham Little*, English physician, 1867–1950] see under *syndrome.*

Graham Steell murmur (gra′am stēl) [Graham *Steell*, English physician, 1851–1942] see under *murmur.*

Grahamella (gra″am-el′lah) [G. S. *Graham* Smith] a genus of bacteria of the family Bartonellaceae, order Rickettsiales, made up of Bartonella-like microorganisms occurring as parasites in erythrocytes of mammals other than humans. It occurs as two species, *G. peromys′ci* and *G. tal′pae,* infecting deer mice and moles, respectively.

grahamellosis (gra″am-el-o′sis) infection with organisms of the genus *Grahamella.*

grain (grān) [L. *gra′num*] 1. a seed, especially of a cereal plant. 2. the twentieth part of a scruple: 0.065 gram. Ab-

breviated gr. **cayenne pepper g's,** brown crystals of uric acid in the urine.

grainage (grān′ij) weight in grains or parts of a grain.

gram (gram) [Fr. *gramme*] the basic unit of mass (weight) of the metric system, being the equivalent of 15.432 grains, or 0.035 ounces avoirdupois. Abbreviated gm.

-gram [Gr. *gramma* something drawn or written] a word termination meaning that which is drawn, written, or recorded.

Gram's method, stain, solution (gramz) [Hans Christian Joachim *Gram,* Danish physician, 1853–1938] see *Table of Stains and Staining Methods,* under *stain,* and see *gram-negative* and *gram-positive.*

gram-equivalent (gram″e-kwiv′ah-lent) see under *equivalent.*

gramicidin (gram″ĭ-si′din) [USP] an antibiotic produced by *Bacillus brevis,* consisting of linear polypeptides with formyl groups at the N-terminal and ethanolamine residues at the C-terminal, which acts by damaging bacterial cell membranes. It is one of the two major components of tyrothricin, the other being tyrocidine. Gramicidin is applied topically in pyodermic, ocular, and other localized infections due to susceptible gram-positive organisms.

gramine (gram′in) chemical name: 3-(dimethylaminomethyl) indole. A crystalline indole alkaloid, $C_{11}H_{14}N_2$, from barley; called also *donaxine.*

graminin (gram′ĭ-nin) a fructosan from rye flour.

graminivorous (gram″ĕ-niv′o-rus) feeding or subsisting on grass or cereal grains.

gram-ion (gram-i′on) that quantity of an ion whose weight in grams is numerically equal to the atomic weight of the ion.

grammeter (gram′me-ter) a unit of work, representing the energy expended in raising 1 gm. of weight 1 meter vertically against gravitational force. It is one thousandth of a kilogrammeter, or about 98,000 ergs.

grammole (gram′mol) gram-molecule.

gram-molecule (gram-mol′ĕ-kūl) as many grams of a substance as are numerically equal to its molecular weight. See *mole,* def. 3.

gram-negative (gram-neg′ah-tiv) losing the stain or decolorized by alcohol in Gram's method of staining, a primary characteristic of bacteria having a cell wall composed of a thin layer of peptidoglycan covered by an outer membrane of lipoprotein and lipopolysaccharide. Cf. *gram-positive.*

gram-positive (gram-poz′ĭ-tiv) retaining the stain or resisting decolorization by alcohol in Gram's method of staining, a primary characteristic of bacteria whose cell wall is composed of a thick layer of peptidologlycan with attached teichoic acids. Cf. *gram-negative.*

grana (gra′nah) [pl. of L. *granum* grain] dense green, chlorophyll-containing bodies in chloroplasts consisting of numerous, closely-packed lamellae which make them appear to be suspended in a matrix.

granatum (grah-na′tum), gen. *grana′ti* [L.] pomegranate.

Grancher's system (grahn-shāz) [Jacques Joseph *Grancher,* French physician, 1843–1907] see *splenopneumonia,* and see under *system.*

grandiose (gran′dĭ-ōs) in psychiatry, pertaining to exaggerated belief or claims of one's importance or identity, often manifested by delusions of great wealth, power, or fame.

grandiosity (gran″de-os′ĭ-te) the condition of being grandiose; an exaggerated belief of one's importance or identity.

grand mal (grahn mahl) see under *epilepsy.*

Grandry's corpuscles (grahn′drēz) [M. *Grandry,* Belgian physician of the 19th century] menisci tactus.

Granger line, sign (grān′jer) [Amedee *Granger,* New Orleans radiologist, 1879–1939] see under *line* and *sign.*

Granit (grahn′it) Ragnar Arthur. Finnish-born Swedish physiologist, born 1900; co-winner, with Haldan Keffer Hartline and George Wald, of the Nobel prize for medicine or physiology in 1967 for discoveries on the chemical and physiological visual processes in the eye.

granoplasm (gran′o-plazm) granular protoplasm.

granula (gran′u-lah), pl. *gran′ulae* [L.] granule, def. 2. **g. irid′ica,** a black or brown outgrowth from the edge of the iris in horses; called also *nigroid body.*

granular (gran′u-lar) [L. *granularis*] made up of or marked by presence of granules or grains.

granulatio (gran″u-la′she-o), pl. *granulatio′nes* [L.] [NA] a general term denoting a granule, or granular mass. **granulatio′nes arachnoidea′les** [NA], **granulatio′nes arachnoidea′les** [Pacchio′ni], arachnoidal granulations: small elevations, visible to the naked eye, thought by some to be enlargements of arachnoid villi, which project into the superior sagittal sinus and associated venous lacunae and create slight depressions on the inner surface of the cranium; these granulations are the structures through which cerebrospinal fluid is reabsorbed into the blood in the venous system. Called also *arachnoid villi*, and *pacchionian bodies* or *granulations*. **granulatio′nes cerebra′les**, **granulatio′nes pacchio′ni**, granulationes arachnoideales.

granulation (gran″u-la′shun) [L. *granulatio*] 1. the process of forming granulation tissue. 2. the process of forming cytoplasmic granules. 3. granule, def. 1. 4. any granular material on the surface of a tissue, membrane, or organ. 5. the rendering of hard or metallic substances into granules or grains. **arachnoidal g′s**, granulationes arachnoideales. **Bayle's g′s**, gray tubercular nodules of the lung that have undergone fibroid degeneration. **Bright's g′s**, the granulations seen in chronic interstitial nephritis. **cell g′s**, small masses seen in the cytoplasm of certain cells that give the latter a characteristic appearance when stained; see the various granules, under *granule*. **exuberant g′s**, excessive proliferation of granulation tissue in healing wounds. **pacchionian g′s**, granulationes arachnoideales. **pyroninophilic g′s**, structures seen in liver and other cells, which stain red with methyl green–pyronine by Pappenheim's stain; they are one of the early effects of carbon tetrachloride poisoning. **Reilly g′s**, large azurophilic granules in the cytoplasm of polymorphonuclear leukocytes and lymphocytes, occurring in gargoylism. **Virchow's g′s**, granulations containing ependymal and glia fibers, found in the walls of the cerebral ventricles in general paralysis.

granulationes (gran″u-la″she-o′nēz) [L.] plural of *granulatio*.

granule (gran′ūl) [L. *granulum*] 1. a small particle or grain, as the small beadlike masses of tissue formed on the surface of wounds, or the insoluble nonmembranous particles found in cytoplasm. 2. a small pill made from sucrose. **acidophil g′s**, granules staining with acid dyes, such as those of the alpha cells of the adenohypophysis; see also *carminophil* (def. 3) and *orangeophil* (def. 3). **acrosomal g.**, a large globule formed by the coalescence of proacrosomal granules, contained within a membrane-bounded *acrosomal vesicle*, which enlarges further to become the core of the acrosome of a spermatozoon. **albuminous g′s**, granules seen in the cytoplasm of many normal cells; they optically disappear on the addition of acetic acid, but are not affected by ether or chloroform; called also *cytoplasmic g′s*. **aleuronoid g′s**, colorless myeloid colloidal bodies found in the base of pigment cells. **alpha g′s**, 1. oval granules found in blood platelets; their membrane structure and the contained acid phosphatase suggest that they are lysosomes. 2. large granules in the alpha cells of the islets of Langerhans, which are insoluble in alcohol and secrete glucagon. 3. the acidophilic granules in the alpha cells of the adenohypophysis; see also *carminophil* and *orangeophil*. **Altmann's g′s**, mitochondria. **amphophil g′s**, granules that stain with either acid or basic dyes. **argentaffine g′s**, granules which stain with silver. **atrial g′s**, membrane-bound, spherical, electron-dense granules in the cytoplasm of the cells of the cardiac atrium, located in the Golgi region; they contain the polypeptide hormones cardionatrin and cardilatin, and are involved in the control of sodium excretion and blood pressure, respectively. **azur g.**, **azurophil g.**, a granule which stains easily with azure dyes; they are coarse reddish granules seen in many lymphocytes. **Babès-Ernst g.**, metachromatic g. **basal g.**, basal body. **basophil g′s**, granules staining with basic dyes, such as those of the beta cells of the adenohypophysis; see also *gonadotrope* (def. 3) and *thyrotrope* (def. 2). **beta g′s**, 1. the granules in the beta cells of the islets of Langerhans, which secrete insulin and are soluble in alcohol. 2. basophilic granules in the beta cells of the adenohypophysis; see also *gonadotrope* (def. 3) and *thyrotrope* (def. 2). **Birbeck g′s**, peculiar membrane-bound, rod- or tennis racquet–shaped inclusions

with a central linear, longitudinally striated nucleus, found in the cytoplasm of the Langerhans cells of the epidermis. Called also *Langerhans' g′s* and *vermiform g′s*. **Bollinger's g′s**, 1. Bollinger's bodies. 2. small, yellowish white granules in mulberry-like masses, containing micrococci, seen in the granulation tissue of botryomycosis. **Bütschli's g′s**, swellings on the bipolar rays of the amphiaster in the ovum. **carbohydrate g′s**, particles of carbohydrate matter in the body fluids in the course of being assimilated. **chromatic g′s, chromophilic g′s**, Nissl's bodies; see under *body*. **cone g′s**, the nuclei of the visual cells of the retina in its outer nuclear layer which are connected with the cones. **cortical g′s**, special structures in the cortex of the ovum of many animals, which break up during fertilization and supply the material for the development of the fertilization membrane. **cytoplasmic g′s**, albuminous g′s. **delta g′s**, fine basophilic granules occurring in the lymphocytes. **Ehrlich's g′s, Ehrlich-Heinz g′s**, cell granules which stain with Ehrlich's triacid stain. **elementary g′s**, hemoconia. **eosinophil g′s**, granules staining with eosin; an eosinophil. **Fauvel's g′s**, peribronchitic abscesses. **fuchsinophil g′s**, granules staining with fuchsin. **Fordyce g′s**, ectopic sebaceous glands found on the lips and gums and in the mucosa of the cheeks, which present as yellowish white milia. Called also *Fordyce's disease* and *Fordyce's spots*. **gamma g′s**, a name applied to basophilic granules found in the blood, marrow, and in the tissues. **Heinz g′s**, Heinz-Ehrlich bodies. **hyperchromatin g.**, azur g. **iodophil g′s**, granules staining brown with iodine, seen in polymorphonuclear leukocytes in various acute infectious diseases. **juxtaglomerular g′s**, stainable osmophilic secretory granules present in the juxtaglomerular cells, closely resembling zymogen granules. **kappa g.**, azur g. **keratohyalin g′s**, irregularly shaped granules, representing deposits of keratohyalin on tonofibrils in the stratum granulosum epidermidis. They stain with some acid dyes and with certain basic dyes. See also *keratohyalin*, def. 1. **Kölliker's interstitial g′s**, various sized granules seen in the sarcoplasm of muscle fibers. **Kretz's g′s**, granules found in the liver in cirrhosis. **Langerhans' g′s**, Birbeck's g′s. **Langley's g′s**, granules seen in secreting serous glands. **membrane-coating g′s**, keratinosome. **meningeal g′s**, granulationes arachnoideales. **metachromatic g.**, a granular cell inclusion that stains a color different from that of the dye used. In certain bacteria, yeasts, yeastlike fungi, and protozoa, metachromatic granules appear red when stained with a blue dye. They are composed of complex polyorthophosphate, lipid, and nucleoprotein molecules (volutin) and serve as an intracellular phosphate reserve. Called also *Babès-Ernst bodies* or *granule*. **Mezei g′s** (*obs.*), spherical brownish granules seen in smears from the lesions of cutaneous actinomycosis. **Much's g′s**, gram-positive, nonacid-fast granules and rods found in tuberculous sputum and thought to be modified tubercle bacilli. **Neusser's g′s** (*obs.*), basophil granules seen about the nuclei of leukocytes. **Nissl's g′s**, Nissl's bodies. **oxyphil g′s**, acidophil g′s. **Paschen's g′s**, see under *body*. **perichromatin g′s**, granules believed to contain nucleic acid, found near the masses of nuclear chromatin in the hepatic parenchymal cells. **pigment g′s**, small masses of coloring matter occurring in pigment cells. **polar g′s**, polar bodies. **proacrosomal g.**, any of the small, dense bodies found inside one of the vacuoles of the Golgi body, which fuse to form an acrosomal granule. **protein g′s**, microscopically observable particles of various proteins, some anabolic and others catabolic. **rod g′s**, the nuclei of rod visual cells in the outer nuclear layer of the retina which are connected with the rods. **Schrön's g.**, a small body, of doubtful origin, seen in the germinal spot of the ovum. **Schrön-Much g′s**, Much's g′s. **Schüffner's g′s**, see under *dot*. **secretory g′s**, granules in secretory cells which apparently represent material that helps to form the secretion. **seminal g′s**, the small granular bodies seen in the spermatic fluid. **specific atrial g′s**, membrane-bound spherical granules with a dense homogeneous interior concentrated in the core of sarcoplasm of the atrial cardiac muscle, extending in either direction from the poles of the nucleus, usually near the Golgi complex; they also may be found in limited numbers in other regions of the cell. **sphere g.**, a large granular cell or corpuscle seen in serous exudation. **sulfur g′s**, peculiar granular bodies of a yellow color found in actinomycotic lesions and discharges.

thread g's, mitochondria.   **toxic g's,** dark-staining basophilic granules observed in neutrophils in infections and other toxic states; they are probably phagosomes or autophagic vacuoles.   **trichohyalin g's,** see *trichohyalin.*   **vermiform g's,** Birbeck's g's.   **volutin g's,** see *volutin.*   **zymogen g's,** secretory granules in certain cells, containing the precursors of enzymes that become active after they have left the cell.

granuliform (gran′u-lĭ-form)   in the form of, or resembling, small grains.

granuloadipose (gran″u-lo-ad′ĭ-pōs)   showing fatty degeneration which contains granules of fat.

granuloblast (gran′u-lo-blast)   myeloblast.

granuloblastosis (gran″u-lo-blas-to′sis)   a form of avian leukosis marked by an increase in the circulating blood of immature blood cells of the granular series; there may be infiltration of the liver or spleen.

granulocorpuscle (gran″u-lo-kor′pus′l)   a small corpuscle observed in infected tissue in lymphogranuloma venereum.

granulocyte (gran′u-lo-sīt″) [*granular* + Gr. *kytos* hollow vessel]   any cell containing granules, especially a leukocyte containing neutrophil, basophil, or eosinophil granules in its cytoplasm. See also *granular leukocytes,* under *leukocyte,* and *granular series,* under *series.*   **band-form g.,** band cell.   **segmented g.,** see under *cell.*

granulocytic (gran″u-lo-sit′ik)   1. pertaining to, characterized by, or of the nature of granulocytes. 2. pertaining to the granulocytic series; see under *series.*

granulocytopathy (gran″u-lo-si-top′ah-the)   any disorder of the granular leukocytes (granulocytes).

granulocytopenia (gran″u-lo-si″to-pe′ne-ah) [*granulocyte* + Gr. *penia* poverty]   agranulocytosis.

granulocytopoiesis (gran″u-lo-si″to-poi-e′sis)   the production of granulocytes.

granulocytopoietic (gran″u-lo-si″to-poi-et′ik)   pertaining to, characterized by, or stimulating granulocytopoiesis.

granulocytosis (gran″u-lo-si-to′sis)   an abnormally large number of granulocytes in the blood.

granulofatty (gran″u-lo-fat′e)   granuloadipose.

granuloma (gran″u-lo′mah), pl. *granulomas* or *granulo′mata* [*granulo-* + *-oma*]   an imprecise term applied to (1) any small nodular delimited aggregation of mononuclear inflammatory cells, or (2) such a collection of modified macrophages resembling epithelial cells (*epithelioid cells*), usually surrounded by a rim of lymphocytes, often with multinucleated giant cells. Some granulomas contain eosinophils and plasma cells, and fibrosis is commonly seen around the lesion. Granuloma formation represents a chronic inflammatory response initiated by various infectious and noninfectious agents. See also *granulomatosis.*   **amebic g.,** granulomatous lesions of the colon sometimes seen in amebiasis.   **g. annula′re,** a benign, usually self-limited granulomatous disease of unknown etiology, chiefly involving the dermis, clinically characterized by annularly grouped, localized or disseminated, perforating papules or subcutaneous nodules, which predominantly affects female children. Histopathologic findings include the presence of palisading histiocytes surrounding foci of altered collagen (necrobiosis) in the mid and upper dermis.   **apical g.,** a slowly expanding, spherical, granulomatous lesion adjacent to the root apex of a tooth, usually occurring as a complication of pulpitis, which consists of a proliferating mass of chronic inflammatory tissue enclosed within a fibrous capsule that is an extension of the periodontal ligament. Mild pain on biting and sensitivity to percussion are the chief symptoms, but many cases are asymptomatic. Called also *dental g.*   **benign g. of thyroid,** a chronic inflammation of the thyroid gland which changes it into a bulky tumor which later becomes extremely hard.   **beryllium g.,** a chronic, local, noncaseating, sarcoid-like granulomatous reaction to the presence of beryllium in the tissues, which often progresses to fibrosis and hyalinization. See also *berylliosis.*   **candida g., candidal g.,** a rare response to invasive candidiasis of the skin occurring in children who may have defects of the immune system causing them to be predisposed to the condition, characterized by the presence of granulomatous lesions manifested by primary vascularized papules covered with thick, adherent, yellow-brown crusts, which may develop into horns or protrusions, located on the face, scalp, fingernails, trunk, legs, and pharynx. Called also *monilial g.*   **cholesterol g.,** a gran-

ulomatous lesion in which crystals of cholesterol esters are surrounded by foreign-body giant cells in a mass of fibrotic granulation tissue.   **coccidioidal g.,** coccidioidomycosis.   **dental g.,** apical g.   **eosinophilic g.,** 1. Langerhans cell granulomatosis. 2. a disorder similar to eosinophilic gastroenteritis and characterized by localized nodular or pedunculated lesions of the gastric submucosa and muscle walls, especially of the pyloric area of the stomach, caused by infiltration of eosinophils, but without peripheral eosinophilia and allergic symptoms. It may also affect the small intestine. 3. anisakiasis.   **g. fissura′tum,** a circumscribed, firm, reddish, fissured, fibrotic granuloma of the gum and buccal mucosa, occurring on an edentulous alveolar ridge and in the fold between the ridge and cheek; it is caused by an ill-fitting denture.   **foreign-body g.,** a localized histiocytic skin reaction to a foreign body in the tissue, such as starch, talc, or oil.   **g. fungoi′des,** mycosis fungoides.   **g. gangraenes′cens,** a condition beginning with the formation of proliferating granulations in the nasal mucous membrane which invade the adjacent tissues and soon become gangrenous.   **giant cell reparative g., central,** a lesion of the jaws considered by some authorities to be a giant cell tumor occurring in both benign and malignant forms, and by others as a form of osteogenic sarcoma, varying in degree of malignancy. Most consider it to be a central lesion of the bone of the jaws, presenting an inflammatory reaction of injury or hemorrhage, which is not regarded as a true neoplasm. It is composed of a spindle cell stroma punctuated by multinucleate giant cells.   **giant cell reparative g., peripheral,** giant cell epulis.   **g. glutea′le infan′tum,** a dermatosis occurring in the diaper area or buttocks of infants, characterized clinically by the development of oval, hemangioma-like or hematoma-like nodules, and histologically by hyperkeratosis and acanthosis, associated with a polymorphonuclear infiltrate mixed with plasma cells, histiocytes, and macrophages throughout the dermis. Spontaneous recovery usually occurs.   **Hodgkin's g.,** see under *disease.*   **infectious g.,** a granulomatous lesion due to an infectious agent, such as a bacterium or fungus.   **infective g.,** one due to the presence in the tissues of living agents.   **g. inguina′le,** a chronic, slowly progressive, ulcerative granulomatous disease, assumed to be sexually transmitted, caused by *Calymmatobacterium granulomatis,* and primarily involving the skin and lymphatics of the anogenital region but sometimes spreading to the perineum and perianal area or the inguinal region; it occurs principally in the tropics and is usually seen in dark-skinned people even in temperate areas, where it is rare. Called also *donovanosis, fourth venereal disease, g. pudendi, g. venereum,* and *pudendal ulcer.*   **laryngeal g.,** a firm nodule on the larynx due to trauma, particularly from endotracheal intubation or from excessive use of the voice.   **lethal midline g.,** a progressive, localized, destructive process occurring chiefly in males, predominantly involving the nose, paranasal sinuses, and palate, with erosion through contiguous structures such as the orbit and face and destruction of soft tissue, bone, and cartilage, and associated with nonspecific acute and chronic inflammation and necrosis with or without granuloma formation. Called also *midline g.*   **lipoid g.,** a granuloma containing lipoid cells; xanthoma.   **lipophagic g.,** a granuloma attended by the loss of subcutaneous fat.   **Majocchi's g.,** trichophytic g.   **malarial g.,** a granulomatous lesion sometimes seen in the brain in fatal cases of cerebral malaria.   **midline g.,** lethal midline g.   **Mignon's eosinophilic g.,** a solitary destructive lesion affecting the skull and other bones of children and young adults.   **monilial g.,** candidal g.   **g. multifor′me,** a condition seen in Nigerian women, presumed to be an atypical form of granuloma annulare, characterized by the presence of multiple, sometimes very large, papulonodular circinate lesions, accompanied by plaques and nodules, which usually heal spontaneously without residual scarring but often with some hypopigmentation.   **paracoccidioidal g.,** paracoccidioidomycosis.   **plasma cell g.,** granuloma in which other inflammatory cells are very greatly outnumbered by plasma cells.   **pseudopyogenic g.,** a superficial variant of angiolymphoid hyperplasia.   **g. puden′di, g. inguinale.**   **g. pu′dens trop′icum** g. inguinale.   **pyogenic g., g. pyogen′icum,** a usually solitary polypoid capillary hemangioma often associated with trauma or local irritation, representing a vasoproliferative inflammatory response, found on the skin and gingival or oral mucosa, which presents as a small erythematous papule that enlarges and may become pedunculated and may become infected and ulcerate with accompanying purulent exudate. Called also *g. telangiecticum.* See also *pregnancy tumor,* under *tumor.* Cf. *angiogranuloma.* **reticulohistiocytic g.,** 1. reticulohistiocytoma. 2. multicentric reticulohistiocytosis. 3. a solitary reticulohistiocytoma, seen mainly in men, which is not associated with systemic involvement, as in multicentric reticulohistiocytosis. **rheumatic g's,** nodules occurring in various parts of the body in rheumatism. **silicotic g.,** pseudotuberculoma silicoticum. **swimming pool g.,** a chronic granulomatous bacterial infection caused by contamination of an abrasion sustained in a swimming pool by *Mycobacterium marinum,* which histologically and clinically resembles tuberculosis. It is characterized by the development of a reddish papule or pustule at the site of inoculation that enlarges and may break down and become covered by a brownish crust; it tends to heal spontaneously within a few months to 2 years. **g. telangiectat'icum,** pyogenic g. **trichophytic g., g. trichophyt'icum,** a rare form of tinea corporis, occurring chiefly on the lower legs, which is caused by *Trichophyton rubrum* infecting hairs at the site of involvement. It is characterized by the development of elevated, sharply circumscribed, rather boggy granulomas, from rose red to a cyanotic hue, disseminated or arranged in chains; after persisting for three or four months the lesions are slowly absorbed, or undergo necrosis, leaving depressed scars. Called also *Majocchi's g.* and *tinea profunda.* **umbilical g.,** granulation tissue on the stem of the umbilical cord in newborn infants. **g. vene'reum,** g. inguinale. **xanthomatous g.,** eosinophilic g. **zirconium g.,** a papular granulomatous eruption consisting of brownish red, dome-shaped, shiny lesions representing an allergic reaction to the zirconium ion or salts, which may be components of certain antiperspirants and deodorants and lotions used in the treatment of poison ivy.

granulomatosis (gran″u-lo″mah-to′sis) any condition characterized by the formation of multiple granulomas. **allergic g.,** allergic granulomatous angiitis. **g. discifor'mis progressi'va et chron'ica,** a condition clinically resembling necrobiosis lipoidica in nondiabetics (and believed by some authorities to be a variant), characterized by the development on the dorsa of the hands, forearms, shins, and sometimes the face of yellowish red, sharply marginated, smooth, plaquelike granulomas with a tendency to enlarge peripherally. **Langerhans cell g.,** a benign disorder found most frequently in males in childhood or early adulthood, occurring in unifocal and multifocal forms. In the unifocal form a single osteolytic lesion is found, usually in a long or flat bone, that produces bone pain, tenderness, and swelling and sometimes pathologic fractures or is asymptomatic. The multifocal form usually presents with bony lesions, and lung, skin, gingiva, and other sites may also be involved. The Hand-Schüller-Christian syndrome (exophthalmos, diabetes insipidus, and bone destruction) occurs in some cases. **lipophagic intestinal g.,** intestinal lipodystrophy. **lymphomatoid g.,** a multisystem disease involving predominantly the lungs, skin, central nervous system, and kidneys, caused by invasion and destruction of vessels by atypical lymphocytoid and plasmacytoid cells resembling a lymphoma; many affected patients develop frank lymphoma. It usually affects males, and the most frequent presenting symptoms are cough, shortness of breath, and chest pain. Extrapulmonary manifestations are common, with protean skin lesions being present in many cases. **malignant g.,** Hodgkin's disease. **g. siderot'ica,** a condition in which brownish nodules (Gamna nodules) are seen in the enlarged spleen. **Wegener's g.,** a multisystem disease chiefly affecting males, characterized by necrotizing granulomatous vasculitis involving the upper and lower respiratory tracts, glomerulonephritis, and variable degrees of systemic, small vessel vasculitis, which is generally considered to represent an aberrant hypersensitivity reaction to an unknown antigen.

granulomatous (gran″u-lom′ah-tus) composed of granulomas.

granulomere (gran′u-lo-mēr″) the center portion of a platelet in a dry, stained blood smear, apparently filled with fine purplish red granules. Cf. *hyalomere.*

granulopenia (gran″u-lo-pe′ne-ah) agranulocytosis.

granuloplasm (gran′u-lo-plazm) endoplasm.

granuloplastic (gran″u-lo-plas′tik) [*granule* + Gr. *plassein* to form] forming granules.

granulopoiesis (gran″u-lo-poi-e′sis) [*granulocyte* + Gr. *poiein* to make] the formation of granulocytes.

granulopoietic (gran″u-lo-poi-et′ik) pertaining to or concerned in the formation of granulocytes.

granulopoietin (gran″u-lo-poi-e′tin) hypothetical substance(s) believed to serve as the humoral regulator of granulopoiesis; leukopoietin.

granulopotent (gran″u-lo-po′tent) capable of forming granules.

Granuloreticulosea (gran″u-lo-re-tik″u-lo′se-ah) [*granulo-* + *reticular*] a class of ameboid protozoa (superclass Rhizopoda, subphylum Sarcodina), the organisms of which have delicate, finely granular or hyaline reticulopodia or, rarely, finely pointed, granular but nonanastomosing pseudopodia. It includes three orders: Athalamida, Monothalamida, and Foraminiferida.

granulosa (gran″u-lo′sah) cumulus oophorus; see also under *cell.*

granulose (gran′u-lōs) 1. a bacterial polysaccharide resembling amylopectin, occurring as cytoplasmic granules and staining red violet with iodine. 2. having a granular appearance.

granulosis (gran″u-lo′sis) the formation of a mass of granules. **g. ru'bra na'si,** sweating and hyperhidrosis confined to the nose and surrounding area of the face and sometimes the chin, associated with red papules and sometimes many small vesicles; it occurs most often in children, usually clearing up at puberty. There is some evidence that an inheritable trait is involved in the etiology.

granulosity (gran″u-los′ĭ-te) a mass of granulations.

granulovacuolar (gran″u-lo-vak′u-o-lar) characterized by granules and vacuoles.

granum (gra′num), pl. **gra′na** [L.] grain; see *grana.*

grapes (grāps) 1. granulomas formed in severe cases of grease in horses. 2. bovine tuberculosis.

graph (graf) [Gr. *graphein* to write, or record] a diagram or curve representing varying relationships between sets of data. Often used as a word termination denoting an instrument for writing or recording; also, the record made by such an instrument.

graphesthesia (graf″es-the′ze-ah) [Gr. *graphein* to write + *aisthēsis* perception] the sense by which are recognized figures or numbers written on the skin with a dull-pointed object.

graphic (graf′ik) [Gr. *graphein* to write] written or drawn; pertaining to representation by diagrams.

graphite (graf′it) [L. *graphites,* from Gr. *graphis* a style, or writing instrument] plumbago, a form of native mineralized carbon.

graphitosis (graf″ĭ-to′sis) pneumoconiosis due to inhalation of and tissue reaction to graphite dust.

Graphium (graf′e-um) a genus of imperfect fungi which produce several cultural spore types.

graph(o)- [Gr. *graphein* to write] a combining form denoting relationship to writing or to a record.

graphoanalysis (graf″o-ah-nal′ĭ-sis) analysis of personality based on handwriting.

graphokinesthetic (graf″o-kin″es-thet′ik) [*grapho-* + Gr. *kinein* to move + *aisthēsis* perception] pertaining to the sensation aroused by the act of writing.

graphology (graf-ol′o-je) [*grapho-* + *-logy*] the study of handwriting, applied to personal identification or psychological study of the writer.

graphomotor (graf″o-mo′tor) [*grapho-* + *motor*] pertaining to, or affecting, the movements required in writing.

graphorrhea (graf″o-re′ah) [*grapho-* + Gr. *rhoia* flow] the writing of a long succession of meaningless and unconnected words.

graphospasm (graf′o-spazm) [*grapho-* + Gr. *spasmos* spasm] writer's cramp.

-graphy [Gr. *-graphia,* from *graphein* to write] a word termination meaning the process of writing or recording, or a method of recording.

Grashey's aphasia (grash′ēz) [Hubert von *Grashey,* Munich psychologist, 1839–1911] see under *aphasia.*

grass (gras) any plant of the family Gramineae. Some of the grasses which by their pollen are important causes of hay

fever are: Bermuda g., *Cynodon dactylon;* June g., *Poa pratensis;* Johnson g., *Sorghum halepense;* Orchard g., *Dactylis glomerata;* Redtop g., *Agrostis alba;* Sweet vernal g., *Anthoxanthum odoratum;* and Timothy g., *Phleum pratense.*
couch g., *Agropyron repens* (L.) Beauv. (Gramineae).
scurvy g., a cruciferous plant, *Cochlearia officinalis,* once used as a remedy for scurvy.

Grasset's law, phenomenon (sign) (grah-sāz') [Joseph *Grasset,* French physician, 1849–1918] see *Landouzy-Grasset law,* under *law,* and see under *phenomenon.*

Grasset-Gaussel phenomenon (grah-sa'go-sel') [Joseph *Grasset;* Amans *Gaussel,* French physician, 1871–1937] Grasset's phenomenon; see under *phenomenon.*

Grasset-Gaussel-Hoover sign (grah-sa'-go-sel'-hoo'ver) [Joseph *Grasset;* Amans *Gaussel;* Charles Franklin *Hoover,* American physician, 1865–1927] see under *sign.*

Gratiola (grah-ti'o-lah) a genus of plants. **G. officina'-lis,** the hedge hyssop, a scrophulariaceous plant of Europe; it is purgative, emetic, and diuretic.

Gratiolet's radiating fibers, optic radiation (grah-te''o-lāz') [Louis Pierre *Gratiolet,* French anatomist, 1815–1865] see under *fiber,* and see *radiatio optica.*

grattage (grah-tahzh') [Fr.] the removal of granulations (as in trachoma) by scraping or by friction with a stiff brush.

grave (grāv) [L. *gravis*] severe or serious.

gravedo (gra-ve'do) [L.] cold in the head, or nasal catarrh.

gravel (grav'el) a term applied to fairly coarse concretions of mineral salts, as from the kidneys or bladder, of smaller size than the so-called stones.

Graves' disease (grāvz) [Robert James *Graves,* Irish physician, 1796–1853] see under *disease.*

grave-wax (grāv'waks) adipocere.

gravid (grav'id) [L. *gravida* heavy, loaded] pregnant; containing developing young.

gravida (grav'ĭ-dah) a pregnant woman. Called *gravida I* or *primigravida* during the first pregnancy, *gravida II* or *secundigravida* during the second pregnancy, *gravida III* or *tertigravida* during the third pregnancy, and so on. Cf. *Para.*

gravidic (grah-vid'ik) occurring in pregnancy.

gravidism (grav'id-izm) pregnancy, or the sum of symptoms, signs, and conditions associated with it.

graviditas (grah-vid'ĭ-tas) pregnancy. **g. examnia'lis,** pregnancy in which the amnion has burst and is retracted around the insertion of the umbilical cord, but the chorion is intact. **g. exochoria'lis,** pregnancy in which the membranes have burst and shrunk, leaving the fetus in the uterus but outside of the chorion.

gravidity (grah-vid'ĭ-te) [L. *graviditas*] pregnancy; the condition of being pregnant, without regard to the outcome. Cf. *parity.*

gravidocardiac (grav''ĭ-do-kar'de-ak) [L. *gravida* + Gr. *kardia* heart] pertaining to heart disease of pregnancy.

gravidopuerperal (grav''ĭ-do-pu-er'per-al) pertaining to pregnancy and the puerperium.

gravimeter (grah-vim'ĕ-ter) [L. *gravis* heavy + *metrum* measure] an instrument for determining specific gravities.

gravimetric (grav''ĭ-met'rik) pertaining to measurement by weight; performed by weight, as gravimetric method of drug assay.

gravistatic (grav''ĭ-stat'ik) due to gravitation, as *gravistatic* pulmonary congestion.

gravitation (grav''ĭ-ta'shun) the phenomenon of attraction between massive bodies; see *law of gravitation.*

gravitometer (grav''ĭ-tom'ĕ-ter) a balance for measuring specific gravity.

gravity (grav'ĭ-te) [L. *gravitas*] the force of gravitational attraction at the surface of the earth or other body. **specific g.,** the weight of a substance compared with that of an equal volume of another substance taken as a standard. **standard g.,** the acceleration due to gravity at mean sea level, 9.80665 meters per second squared. Symbol, g.

Grawitz's tumor (grah'vits-ez) [Paul Albert *Grawitz,* pathologist in Greifswald, 1850–1932] see under *tumor.*

gray (gra) 1. of a hue between white and black. 2. the gray matter of the nervous system. 3. a unit of absorbed radiation dose equal to 100 rads. Abbreviated Gy. **central g.,** relatively undifferentiated gray matter which re-

tains its primitive position near the ventricles and central canal. **perihypoglossal g.,** see under *complex.* **silver g., steel g.,** nigrosin.

grease (grēs) an inflammatory swelling in a horse's leg in the region of the fetlocks and pasterns, with the formation of cracks in the skin and the excretion of oily matter.

grease-heel (grēs-hēl') grease.

green (grēn) 1. having the color of fresh leaves or of grass. 2. a green coloring matter or dye. **acid g.,** any of several green acid dyes, generally light g. S F. **brilliant g.,** a basic dye having powerful bacteriostatic properties for grampositive organisms; used topically as an anesthetic. **bromocresol g.** [USP] an indicator used in the determination of hydrogen ion concentration, being yellow at pH 4.0 and blue at pH 5.4. **Brunswick g.,** 1. chrome g. 2. copper arsenite. 3. copper subcarbonate. 4. copper oxychloride. **diazin g. S,** Janus g. B. **ethyl g.,** brilliant g. **fast acid g. N,** light g. S F yellowish. **Hoffman g.,** iodine g. **indocyanine g.** [USP], a tricarbocyanine dye, $C_{43}H_{47}N_2$-NaO_6S_2, occurring as an olive-brown, dark green, dark blue, or black powder; used intravenously as a diagnostic aid in the determination of blood volume, cardiac output, and hepatic function. **iodine g.,** a triphenylmethane dye used as a chromatin stain. **Janus g. B,** an azo dye used supravitally for the demonstration of mitochondria. **light g., 2 G or 2 GN,** light g. S F. yellowish. **light g. N,** malachite g. **light g. S F yellowish,** an acid dye used as a plasma stain. **malachite g.,** a triphenylmethane dye used as a stain for bacteria and as an antiseptic for wounds. **malachite g. G,** brilliant g. **methyl g.,** 1. a mixture of hepta and hexa methyl-pararosaniline. 2. ethyl g. **methylene g.,** a mononitromethylene blue, interesting for its dark green metachromasia. **new solid g.,** malachite g. **Paris g.,** a double salt of copper acetate and copper meta- arsenite, $Cu(C_2H_3O_2)_2 \cdot 3Cu(AsO_2)_2$, used as an insecticide. **Schweinfurt g.,** Paris g. **solid g.,** malachite g. **Victoria g.,** malachite g.

Greene's sign (grēnz) [Charles Lyman *Greene,* American physician, 1862–1929] see under *sign.*

gregaloid (greg'ah-loid) [L. *grex* flock + Gr. *eidos* form] see under *colony.*

Gregarina (greg''ah-ri'nah) [L. *gregarius,* crowding together] a genus of parasitic gregarine protozoa (suborder Septatina, subclass Eugregarinida) found in the gut of various arthropods, characterized by the presence of a small, globular, or cylindrical epimerite and dolioform to cylindrical spores.

gregarine (greg'ah-rīn) 1. pertaining or relating to protozoa of the subclass Gregarinia or to the genus *Gregarina.* 2. any protozoan of the subclass Gregarinia or of the genus *Gregarinia.*

Gregarinia (greg''ah-ri'ne-ah) a subclass of generally homoxenous, parasitic protozoa (class Sporozoea, subphylum Apicocomplexa) found in the digestive tract or body cavity of invertebrates, especially insects and annelids, or lower chordates, although the large gamonts occur extracellularly. Some gregarines have compartmentalized bodies (gamonts) that are separated into an anterior uninucleate segment (protomerite) and a larger posterior segment (deutomerite) by an ectoplasmic septum. In some, the conoid is modified into an epimerite or a mucron for attachment to the host's tissues. Their life cycle typically consists of gametogony and sporogony. It comprises three orders: Archigregarinida, Eugregarinida, and Neogregarinida.

Gregory's mixture (greg'o-rēz) [James *Gregory,* Scotch physician, 1753–1821] compound powder of rhubarb; see under *powder.*

GRF growth hormone releasing factor; see under *hormone.*

GRH growth hormone releasing hormone.

grid (grid) 1. an arrangement of thin lead strips separated by a radiolucent material; used to reduce the amount of scattered radiation reaching the x-ray film. 2. a chart with horizontal and perpendicular lines for plotting curves. **baby g.,** a direct reading control chart on infant growth. **crossed g.,** two parallel grids arranged so that the lead strips of one are at right angles to the lead strips of the other. **focused g.,** one in which the lead strips are angled so that they all point toward a focus at a specified distance. **moving g.,** a grid which is moved continuously or oscillated throughout the making of a radiograph; used to eliminate the grid lines that occur with the use of a stationary grid.

parallel g., in radiography, one in which the lead strips are oriented parallel to each other; rather than angled as in a focused grid. **Potter-Bucky g.,** Bucky diaphragm. **stationary g.,** one placed in apposition to a roentgenographic film for its accentuation of detail; the grid lines will be visible on the resultant roentgenograms. **Wetzel g.,** a direct reading chart for evaluating physical fitness in terms of body build, developmental level, and basal metabolism.

grief (grēf) the normal emotional response to an external and consciously recognized loss; it is self-limited, gradually subsiding within a reasonable time. See also *mourning.*

Griesinger's disease, sign (symptom) (gre′zing-erz) [Wilhelm *Griesinger,* German neurologist, 1817–1868] see *hookworm disease,* under *disease,* and see under *sign.*

Grignard's reagent (compound) (grēn-yahrz′) [François Auguste Victor *Grignard,* French chemist, 1871–1935] see under *reagent.*

Grifulvin (grĭ-ful′vin) trademark for a preparation of griseofulvin.

Grindelia (grin-de′le-ah) [H. *Grindel,* 1776–1836] a genus of American composite-flowered plants; the leaves and flowering tops of *G. camporum, G. cuneifolia,* and *G. squarrosa,* of the western United States, are used as a mild expectorant.

grinding (grīnd′ing) 1. rubbing together with force; wearing away or polishing by rubbing. 2. crushing of food by the posterior teeth in mastication, especially by molars. 3. bruxism. 4. shaping of a tooth contour through the use of abrasive tools. See also *occlusal adjustment,* under *adjustment.* **selective g.,** modification of the occlusal forms of teeth by grinding at selected places. **spot g.,** elimination of high places or occlusal interferences on natural dentitions or dentures by grinding.

grinding-in (grīnd′ing-in) the process of correcting errors in the centric and eccentric occlusions of natural or artificial teeth. See also *milling-in.*

grip (grip) 1. [Fr. *grippe*] influenza. 2. a grasping or seizing. **devil's g.,** epidemic pleurodynia. **hook g.,** a functional posture of the hand, as that usually assumed when grasping handles or straps or suspending or pulling upon an object: the fingers are flexed toward the palm, to a degree depending on the size of the grasped object. **power g.,** a functional posture of the hand, as that usually assumed when holding a hammer or piece of rope: the fingers are flexed around an object, with counter pressure from the thumb, which is positioned to bring either its pad or its medial border firmly against the held object. **precision g.,** a functional posture of the hand, as that usually assumed when holding a pen or pencil: the object is grasped between the tips of the thumb and fingers (most often the index, with the middle often involved).

grippal (grip′al) pertaining to grip, or influenza.

grippe (grip) influenza. **g. aurique′,** a polyneuritis sometimes resulting from the therapeutic use of gold salts.

Grisactin (gris-ak′tin) trademark for a preparation of griseofulvin.

griseofulvin (gris″e-o-ful′vin) [USP] chemical name: (1′*S-trans*)-7-chloro-2′,4,6-trimethoxy-6′-methylspiro[benzofuran-2(3*H*),1′-[2]cyclohexene]-3,4′-dione. An antibiotic produced by *Penicillium griseofulvum* or by other means, $C_{17}H_{17}ClO_6$, occurring as a white to creamy white powder; used as an antifungal in the treatment of dermatophytic infections of the hands, feet, nails, and scalp, administered orally. Called also *Curling factor.*

griseomycin (gris″e-o-mi′sin) proactinomycin B.

Grisolle's sign (gre-zolz′) [Augustin *Grisolle,* French physician, 1811–1869] see under *sign.*

Gris-PEG (gris′peg) trademark for a preparation of griseofulvin.

Gritti's amputation (operation) (gre′tēz) [Rocco *Gritti,* surgeon in Milan, 1828–1920] see under *amputation.*

Gritti-Stokes amputation (gre′te-stōks) [Rocco *Gritti;* Sir William *Stokes,* Irish surgeon, 1839–1900] see under *amputation.*

Grocco's sign (triangle, triangular dullness) (grok′ōz) [Pietro *Grocco,* physician in Florence, 1856–1916] see under *sign.*

grog (grog) navicular disease.

groin (groin) [L. *inguen*] the junctional region between the abdomen and thigh; called also *inguen* [NA].

Gromia (grom′e-ah) [L. *groma* pole] a genus of uninucleate or multinucleate ameboid protozoa (order Gromiida, class Filosea) found in salt or fresh water, and having a thin rigid or flexible test with a terminal aperture and many branching and anastomosing filopodia.

Gromiida (gro-mi′ĭ-dah) an order of ameboid protozoa (class Filosea, superclass Rhizopoda), the bodies of which are enclosed by a test or rigid external membrane with a distinct aperture. Representative genera include *Euglypha* and *Gromia.*

Grönblad-Strandberg syndrome (gren′blad- strand′berg) [Ester Elizabeth *Grönblad,* Swedish ophthalmologist, born 1898; James Victor *Strandberg,* Swedish dermatologist, born 1883] see under *syndrome.*

groove (grōōv) a shallow linear depression, especially one appearing during embryonic development or persisting in definitive bone or tooth substance; see also *fissure* and *sulcus.* **alveolingual g.,** the groove between the lower jaw and the tongue. **anal intersphincteric g.,** Hilton's white line. **anterolateral g. of medulla oblongata,** sulcus ventrolateralis anterior medullae oblongatae. **anterolateral g. of spinal cord,** sulcus ventrolateralis anterior medullae spinalis. **anteromedian g. of medulla oblongata,** fissura mediana ventralis medullae oblongatae. **anteromedian g. of spinal cord,** fissura mediana ventralis medullae spinalis. **arterial g's,** sulci arteriosi. **atrioventricular g., auriculoventricular g.,** sulcus coronarius cordis. **basilar g.,** sulcus basilaris pontis. **basilar g. of occipital bone,** clivus ossis occipitalis. **basilar g. of sphenoid bone,** clivus ossis sphenoidalis. **bicipital g. of humerus,** sulcus intertubercularis humeri. **bicipital g., lateral,** sulcus bicipitalis lateralis. **bicipital g., medial,** sulcus bicipitalis medialis. **bicipital g., radial,** sulcus bicipitalis lateralis. **bicipital g., ulnar,** sulcus bicipitalis medialis. **Blessig's g.,** a trace in the eye of the developing embryo corresponding in position with the future ora serrata retinae. **branchial g.,** an external furrow, lined with ectoderm, occurring in the embryo between two branchial arches. **buccal g., buccal developmental g.,** a groove on the buccal surface of a posterior tooth; see also *distobuccal g.* and *mesiobuccal g.* **carotid g. of sphenoid bone, cavernous g. of sphenoid bone,** sulcus caroticus ossis sphenoidalis. **central g., central developmental g.,** a groove in the central part of the occlusal surface of bicuspid and first molar teeth. **costal g.,** sulcus costae. **dental g., primitive,** a groove in the border of the jaws of the embryo. **developmental g's,** fine grooves or lines marking the fusion area between adjacent cusps, named according to the portion of the crown which they connect. Called also *developmental lines* and *segmental lines.* **digastric g.,** incisura mastoidea ossis temporalis. **distobuccal g., distobuccal developmental g.,** the distal of the two buccal grooves ordinarily found on the mandibular first molar. **distolingual g., distolingual developmental g.,** the distal of the lingual grooves of the bicuspid and maxillary molar teeth. **enamel g's,** the grooves bounding the enamel knot. **ethmoidal g.,** ethmoidal sulcus of nasal bone. **g. for eustachian tube,** sulcus tubae auditivae. **genital g.,** urethral g. **gingival g., free,** a shallow groove on the facial surface of the gingiva, running parallel to the margin of the gingiva at a distance of 0.5 to 1.5 mm., and usually at the level of, or somewhat apical to, the bottom of the gingival sulcus. **g. of great superficial petrosal nerve,** sulcus nervi petrosi majoris. **hamular g.,** sulcus hamuli pterygoidei. **Harrison's g.,** a horizontal depression along the lower border of the thorax, corresponding to the costal insertion of the diaphragm; seen in advanced rickets in children. **infraorbital g. of maxilla,** sulcus infraorbitalis maxillae. **interatrial g.,** a slight depression on the external surface of the heart, marking the separation of the atria. **interdental g.,** a linear, vertical depression on the surface of the interdental papillae; it functions as a sluiceway for the egress of food from the interproximal areas. **interosseous g. of calcaneus,** sulcus calcanei. **intertubercular g. of humerus,** sulcus intertubercularis humeri. **interventricular g., anterior,** sulcus interventricularis anterior. **interventricular g. of heart,** see *sulcus interventricularis anterior* and *sulcus interventricularis posterior.* **interventricular g., inferior,** sulcus interventricularis posterior. **interventricular g., posterior,** sulcus interventricularis posterior. **labial g.,** an embryonic groove produced by degeneration of the central cells of the labial lamina, which later becomes the vestibule of the oral cavity. **lacrimal g.,** fossa sacci lacrimalis. **g. of lacrimal bone,** sulcus lacrimalis ossis lacrimalis. **laryngotracheal g.,** a furrow at the caudal end of the embryonic pharynx that develops into the respiratory tract. **lateral g. for lateral sinus of occipital bone,** sulcus sinus transversi. **lateral g. for lateral sinus of parietal bone,** sulcus sinus sigmoidei ossis parietalis. **lateral g. for sigmoidal part of lateral sinus,** sulcus sinus sigmoidei ossis temporalis. **Liebermeister's g's,** developmental grooves on the surface of the liver. **lingual g., lingual developmental g.,** a developmental groove on the lingual surface of a posterior tooth. **medullary g.,** neural g. **mesiobuccal g., mesiobuccal developmental g.,** the mesial of the two buccal grooves ordinarily found on the mandibular first molar. **mesiolingual g., mesiolingual developmental g.,** a groove marking the junction of the fifth cusp with the palatal surface on an upper molar tooth. **g. for middle temporal artery,** sulcus arteriae temporalis mediae. **musculospiral g.,** sulcus nervi radialis. **mylohyoid g. of inferior maxillary bone,** mylohyoid sulcus of mandible; see under *sulcus*. **nail g.,** a pathological linear depression of the nail plate running either lengthwise or, much more often, transversely. **nasal g., g. for nasal nerve,** ethmoidal sulcus of nasal bone. **nasolacrimal g.,** an epithelial ingrowth parallel with but medial to the nasomaxillary groove of the embryo, which marks the site of later development of the nasolacrimal duct. **nasomaxillary g.,** a furrow located between the maxillary and the lateral nasal process of the same side in the embryo. **nasopalatine g.,** a furrow on the lateral surface of the vomer for the nasopalatine nerve and vessels. **nasopharyngeal g.,** a faint line between the nasal cavity and the nasopharynx. **neural g.,** the groove produced by the invagination of the neural plate of the embryo during the process of formation of the neural tube; called also *medullary* g. **obturator g.,** sulcus obturatorius ossis pubis. **occipital g.,** sulcus arteriae occipitalis. **occlusal g.,** one of the developmental grooves on the occlusal surface of a posterior tooth. **olfactory g.,** ethmoid fossa. **optic g.,** sulcus prechiasmaticus. **palatine g's of maxilla,** sulci palatini maxillae. **palatine g. of palatine bone,** sulcus palatinus major ossis palatini. **palatomaxillary g. of palatine bone,** sulcus palatinus major ossis palatini. **paraglenoid g's of hip bone,** sulci paraglenoidales ossis coxae. **paramedian g. of spinal cord, posterior** (*obs.*), sulcus intermedius posterior medullae spinalis. **posterolateral g. of medulla oblongata,** sulcus dorsolateralis medullae oblongatae **posterolateral g. of spinal cord,** sulcus dorsolateralis medullae spinalis. **preauricular g's of ilium,** sulci paraglenoidales ossis coxae. **primitive g.,** a lengthwise furrow on the outer surface of the primitive streak of the embryo. **pterygopalatine g. of pterygoid plate,** sulcus pterygopalatinus processus pterygoidei. **radial g., g. for radial nerve,** sulcus nervi radialis. **sagittal g.,** sulcus sinus sagittalis superioris. **Sibson's g.,** a furrow sometimes seen at the lower border of the pectoralis major muscle. **sigmoid g. of temporal bone,** sulcus sinus sigmoidei ossis temporalis. **g. of small superficial petrosal nerve,** sulcus nervi petrosi minoris. **spiral g.,** sulcus nervi radialis. **subclavian g.,** sulcus musculi subclavi. **subcostal g.,** sulcus costae. **g. for superior longitudinal sinus,** sulcus sagittalis ossis parietalis. **supplemental g's,** grooves on the surface of a tooth which do not mark (as do the developmental grooves) the junction of the primary lobes of the tooth. **supra-acetabular g.,** sulcus supra-acetabularis. **g. for tibialis posticus muscle,** sulcus malleolaris tibiae. **trigeminal g.,** the embryonic structure which develops into the gasserian ganglion. **ulnar g., g. of ulnar nerve,** sulcus nervi ulnaris. **urethral g.,** the embryonic groove that becomes the penile urethra as the genital folds at each side bridge it. **venous g's,** venous sulci. **Verga's lacrimal g.,** a groove running downward from the lower orifice of the nasal duct. **vertebral g.,** the depression on each side of the spine between the spinous processes, laminae, and transverse processes; it lodges the deep back muscles. **vomeral g.,** sulcus vomeris.

gross (grōs) [L. *grossus* rough] coarse or large; visible to the naked eye, as gross pathology; macroscopic; taking no account of minutiae.

Gross's disease (grōs′ez) [Samuel David *Gross*, American surgeon, 1805–1884] see under *disease*.

Gross's method, test (grōs) [Oskar *Gross*, German physician] see under *method* and *tests*.

Grossman's sign (grōs′manz) [Morris *Grossman*, American neurologist, born 1881] see under *sign*.

ground-glass (grownd-glas) having a filmy, hazy appearance, as in radiographs of a lung containing excess fluid.

group (grōōp) 1. an assemblage of objects having certain things in common. 2. a number of atoms forming a recognizable and usually a transferable portion of a molecule. **alcohol g.,** a combination of carbon, hydrogen, and oxygen atoms in a molecule, which is characteristic of a chemical compound known as an alcohol. There are three: $-CH_2OH$, the primary, $=CHOH$, the secondary, and $\equiv COH$, the tertiary alcohol group. **azo g.,** a bivalent chemical group composed of two nitrogen atoms, $-N:N-$. **blood g.,** see *blood group*, under *B*. **CMN g.,** a group of bacteria composed of the genera *Clostridium*, *Mycobacterium*, and *Nocardia*, characterized by common peptidoglycan and mycolic acid constituents in the cell walls. Organisms of this group can be used as adjuvants in experimental immunization. **coli-aerogenes g.,** coliform bacteria. **colon-typhoid-dysentery g.,** a collective term referring to bacteria of the genera *Escherichia*, *Salmonella*, and *Shigella*. **coryneform g.,** see under *bacterium*. **diagnosis-related g's,** groupings of diagnostic categories used as a basis for hospital payment schedules by Medicare and other third-party payment plans. **encounter g.,** a sensitivity group in which the members strive to gain emotional rather than intellectual insight with emphasis on the expression of interpersonal feelings in the group situation. **functional g.,** a part of a molecule that gives it characteristic chemical properties, e.g., an aldehyde, alcohol, amine, carboxylic acid, ester, ether, or ketone group. **glucophore g.,** see *glucophore*. **hemorrhagic-septicemia g.,** a group of bacteria of which *Pasteurella multocida* is the type organism. **methyl g.,** a monovalent chemical group, $-CH_3$. **osmophore g.,** see *osmophore*. **paratyphoid-enteritidis g.,** a group of organisms of the genus *Salmonella*, causing food poisoning in man and various diseases in animals. **peptide g.,** the bivalent radical, $-CO\cdot NH-$, formed by reaction between the NH_2 and $COOH$ groups of adjacent amino acids, and by such linkage building up compounds known as di-, tri-, tetra-[etc.] peptides, depending on the number of amino acids making up the molecule. **prosthetic g.,** a low molecular weight, nonprotein compound that binds with a protein component (apoprotein, specifically apoenzyme) to form a protein (e.g., holoenzyme) with biologic activity. **saccharide g.,** a combination of carbon, hydrogen, and oxygen atoms in a hypothetical molecule, $C_6H_{10}O_5$, the number of which in the compound determines the specific name of the polysaccharide, as di-, tri-, or tetrasaccharide. **sapophore g.,** see *sapophore*. **sensitivity g.,** sensitivity training g. **sensitivity training g.,** a nonclinical group not intended for persons with mental illnesses or substantial emotional problems, which, in an effort to develop the assets of leadership, management, counseling, or other roles, focuses on self-awareness and understanding and on interpersonal interactions. Called also *training* g. (T g. or T-g.). **sulfonic g.,** a monovalent radical, $-SO_2OH$. **T g., T-g.,** sensitivity g. **training g.,** sensitivity g.

grouping (grōōp′ing) the classification of individual entities according to certain common characteristics. **blood g.,** the classification of blood (erythrocytes) according to the type to which it belongs; employed in determination of the suitability of blood for transfusion in a particular recipient, in cases of disputed paternity, and in certain criminal cases. See *blood group*, under *B*. **haptenic g.,** hapten.

group-specific (grōōp″spĕ-sif′ik) specific for a given group; as a blood group or certain microorganisms; said of agglutinins.

group-transfer (grōōp″trans′fer) denoting a chemical reaction, excluding oxidation and reduction, in which molecules exchange functional groups, a process catalyzed by enzymes called transferases.

growth (grōth) 1. a normal process of increase in size of an organism as a result of accretion of tissue similar to that originally present. Cf. *differentiation.* 2. an abnormal formation, such as a tumor. 3. the proliferation of cells, as in a bacterial culture. **absolute g.,** an expression of the actual increase in size of an individual, or of a particular organ or part. **accretionary g.,** increase in size resulting from increase in number of special cells by mitotic division, other more differentiated cells which perform various physiological functions having lost the ability to proliferate. **allometric g.,** the growth of different organs or parts of an organism at different rates. **appositional g.,** growth by addition at the periphery of a particular structure or part. Cf. *interstitial g.* **auxetic g.,** auxesis. **balanced g.,** a steady state condition in which every component of the cell doubles in a cell generation (time between divisions). **condylar g.,** the growth of the condyle of the temporomandibular joint, usually reflected in a downward and forward positioning of the mandible and teeth. **differential g.,** an expression of the comparison of the increases in size of dissimilar organisms, organs, or parts. **heterogonous g.,** growth of such a nature that, when it is plotted logarithmetically, it gives a straight line. **histiotypic g.,** uncontrolled growth of cells as occurs in tissue cultures. **interstitial g.,** growth occurring in the interior of parts or structures already formed. Cf. *appositional g.* **intussusceptive g.,** auxesis. **isometric g.,** the growth of different organs or parts of an organism at the same rate. **multiplicative g.,** increase in the size of an organism, organ, or part, resulting from increase in the number of cells brought about by their mitotic division, the average size of the cells remaining about the same. **new g.,** a neoplasm, or tumor. **organotypic g.,** controlled growth of cells as occurs normally in the production of organs and parts. **relative g.,** an expression of the comparison of the increases in size of similar organisms, organs, or parts.

grübelsucht (grē′bel-sōōkt) [Ger.] the drawing of overly fine distinctions (hair-splitting); worrying over trifles. Seen in obsessive-compulsive personalities.

Gruber's bougies, speculum, test (groo′berz) [Josef *Gruber,* Austrian otologist, 1827–1900] see under *bougie, speculum,* and *tests.*

Gruber's fossa, hernia, suture (groo′berz) [Wenaslaus Leopoldovich *Gruber,* Russian anatomist, 1814–1890] see under *fossa* and *hernia,* and see *fissura petrosphenooccipitalis.*

Gruber's reaction test (groo′berz) [Max von *Gruber,* bacteriologist in Munich, 1853–1927] Widal's test.

Gruber-Widal reaction, test (groo′ber-ve-dahl′) [Max von *Gruber;* Georges Fernand Isidore *Widal,* French physician, 1862–1929] Gruber's reaction.

Grubyella (groo″be-el′ah) former name for the genus *Trichophyton.*

gruel (groo′el) a thin paste or porridge made of cereal grain.

gruffs (grufs) the coarse part of a drug.

grumose, grumous (groo′mōs, groo′mus) [L. *grumus* heap] clotted or lumpy.

Grünbaum-Widal test (grēn′bowm-ve-dahl′) [A. S. *Grünbaum,* English physician, 1869–1921; Georges Fernand Isidore *Widal,* French physician, 1862–1929] Gruber's reaction.

grundplatte (groont-plaht′tĕ) [Ger.] lamina basalis.

Grynfeltt's hernia, triangle (grin′felts) [Joseph Casimir *Grynfeltt,* French surgeon, 1840–1913] see under *hernia,* and see *Lesgaft's space,* under *space.*

Grynfeltt-Lesgaft triangle (grin′feltt-les′gaft) [Joseph Casimir *Grynfeltt;* Peter Frantsevich *Lesgaft,* Russian physician, 1837–1909] Lesgaft's space.

gryochrome (gri′o-krōm) [Gr. *gry* morsel + *chrōma* color] a nerve cell in which the stainable matter of the cell body appears as fine granules; used also adjectively.

gryphosis (gri-fo′sis) abnormal curvature; see *gryposis.*

gryposis (gri-po′sis) [Gr. *grypōsis* a crooking, hooking] abnormal curvature, as of the nails. **g. pe′nis** chordee.

GSC gas-solid chromatography.

GSH reduced glutathione.

GSSG oxidized glutathione.

gt. abbreviation for L. *gut′ta,* drop.

GTH gonadotropic hormone.

GTP guanosine triphosphate.

GTP cyclohydrolase (si′klo-hi′dro-lās) [EC 3.5.4.16] an enzyme of the hydrolase class that catalyzes the reaction: guanosine triphosphate + H_2O = D-erythro-7,8-dihydroneopterin triphosphate. The reaction is a step in the biosynthesis of tetrahydrobiopterin. A deficiency of the enzyme is a rare cause of hyperphenylalanemia.

gtt. abbreviation for L. *gut′tae,* drops.

GU genitourinary.

guaco (gwah′ko) [Spanish American] a name given to many South American plants, and especially to *Mikania guaco* Humb. & Bonpl. (Compositae); used by certain South American natives in asthma, dyspepsia, gout, rheumatism, and skin diseases, and reportedly for snakebite.

guaiac (gwi′ak) a resin from the wood of *Guajacum officinale* L. and *G. sanctum* L. (Zygophyllaceae), trees of Haiti and the Dominican Republic; used as a reagent in tests for occult blood and formerly in the treatment of rheumatism.

guaiacol (gwi′ah-kol) the methyl ether of pyrocatechin, a solid or a colorless oily liquid, $OH \cdot C_6H_4O \cdot CH_3$, derived from beech creosote; formerly used as an expectorant.

guaifenesin (gwi-fen′ĕ-sin) [USP] chemical name: 3-(2-methoxyphenoxy)-1,2-propanediol. The glyceryl ester of guaiacol, $C_{10}H_{14}O_4$, occurring as a white or slightly gray, crystalline powder; used as an expectorant, administered orally. Called also *glyceryl guaiacolate, guaiphenesin,* and *methphenoxydiol.*

guaiphenesin (gwi-fen′ĕ-sin) guaifenesin.

guaithylline (gwi′thĭ-lin) chemical name: theophylline compound with 3-(o-methoxyphenoxy)-1,2-propanediol; a bronchodilator and expectorant, $C_7H_8N_4O_2 \cdot C_{10}H_{14}O_4$.

guanabenz (gwan′ah-benz) chemical name: 2-[(2,6-dichlorophenyl)methylene]hydrazinecarboximidamide; an antihypertensive, $C_8H_8Cl_2N_4$.

guanacline sulfate (gwan′ah-klēn) chemical name: [2-(3,6-dihydro-4-methyl-1(2*H*)-pyridyl)ethyl]guanidine sulfate (1:1) dihydrate; an antihypertensive, $C_9H_{18}N_4 \cdot H_2SO_4 \cdot 2H_2O$.

guanadrel sulfate (gwan′ah-drel) chemical name: (1,4-dioxaspiro[4.5]dec-2-ylmethyl)guanidine sulfate (2:1); an antihypertensive, $(C_{10}H_{19}N_3O_2)_2 \cdot H_2SO_4$.

guanase (gwan′ās) guanine deaminase.

guancydine (gwan′sĭ-dēn) chemical name: N″-cyano-N-(1,1-dimethylpropyl) guanidine; an antihypertensive, $C_7H_{14}N_4$.

guanethidine (gwan-eth′ĭ-dēn) chemical name: [2-(hexahydro-1(2*H*)-azocinyl)ethyl]guanidine; an adrenergic blocking agent, $C_{10}H_{22}N_4$, which has prolonged and marked hypotensive effects. **g. monosulfate,** the monosulfate salt of guanethidine, $C_{10}H_{22}N_4 \cdot H_2SO_4$, used as an antihypertensive. **g. sulfate** [USP], the sulfate salt of guanethidine, $(C_{10}H_{22}N_4)_2 \cdot H_2SO_4$, used as an oral antihypertensive.

guanidase (gwan′ĭ-dās) an enzyme produced by several organisms, including *Aspergillus niger;* it hydrolyzes guanidine into urea and ammonia.

guanidine (gwan′ĭ-din) a poisonous base, the amidine of amino carbamic acid, $NH:C(NH_2)_2$. **g. hydrochloride,** a compound used in the treatment of myasthenia gravis.

guanidine-acetic acid (gwan′ĭ-din-ah-se′tik) guanidinoacetic acid.

guanidinemia (gwan″ĭ-din-e′me-ah) the presence of guanidine in the blood.

guanidinoacetic acid (gwan″ĭ-de″no-ah-se′tik) a nitrogenous compound, $C_3H_7N_3O_2$, formed enzymatically in the liver, pancreas, and kidney by a transamidination reaction between arginine and glycine, and N-methylated in the liver by S-adenosylmethionine to form creatine. Called also *glycocyamine, guanidine-acetic acid,* and *guanido-acetic acid.*

guanido-acetic acid (gwan′ĭ-do-ah-se′tik) guanidinoacetic acid.

guanidylate (gwan″ĭ-dil′āt) a dissociated form of guanidylic acid.

guanine (gwan′in) a white, crystalline base, 2-amino-6-oxypurine, $C_5H_5N_5O$, found in guano, fish scales, leguminous seedlings, and various animal tissues. It is a fundamental constituent of DNA and RNA, and occurs as a white deposit in the tissues of swine affected with a kind of gout. **g. nucleotide,** guanylic acid.

guanine deaminase (gwan′in de-am′ĭ-nās) [EC 3.5.4.3] an enzyme of the hydrolase class that catalyzes the reaction guanine + H_2O = xanthine + NH_3. The reaction is a step in the degradation of guanine to uric acid. The enzyme is present in liver, kidney, spleen, and other tissues. Called also *guanase.*

guanochlor sulfate (gwan′o-klor) chemical name: 2-[2-(2,6-dichlorophenoxy)ethyl]hydrazinecarboximidamide sulfate (2:1); an antihypertensive, $[C_9H_{12}Cl_2N_4O]_2 \cdot H_2SO_4$.

guanophore (gwan′o-for) [*guanine* + Gr. *phoros* bearing] a cell filled with guanine crystals which produce interference in the light and thus give the cell a silvery appearance.

guanosine (gwan′o-sin) a nucleoside, guanine β-D-ribofuranoside, $C_{10}H_{13}O_5N_5$, a major constituent of DNA and RNA; it is extracted from the leaves and unripe berries of the coffee plant and is used in biochemical research. Symbol G. **cyclic g. monophosphate (cyclic GMP, cGMP, 3′,5′-GMP),** a cyclic nucleotide, guanosine 3′,5′-cyclic monophosphate, an intracellular "second messenger" similar in action to cyclic adenosine monophosphate (q.v.); the two cyclic nucleotides activate different protein kinases and usually produce opposite effects on cell function. **g. diphosphate (GDP),** a nucleotide, guanosine 5′-pyrophosphate, which serves as a carrier for mannose residues in glycoprotein synthesis. **g. monophosphate (GMP),** a nucleotide, guanosine 5′-phosphate. Called also *guanylic acid.* **g. triphosphate (GTP),** a nucleotide, guanosine 5′-triphosphate, required for RNA synthesis. It is also involved in energy metabolism, being produced from GDP by substrate level phosphorylation in the tricarboxylic acid (Krebs) cycle and serving as a source of free energy to drive protein synthesis. The ratio of GTP to ATP is maintained by the reversible transfer of phosphate catalysed by GDP kinase.

guanoxabenz (gwahn-oks′ah-benz) chemical name: 2-[(2,6-dichlorophenyl)methylene]-*N*-hydroxyhydrazine carboximidamide; an antihypertensive, $C_8H_8Cl_2N_4O$.

guanoxan sulfate (gwan-oks′an) chemical name: (2,3-dihydro-1,4-benzodioxin-2-ylmethyl)guanidine; an antihypertensive, $[C_{10}H_{13}N_3O_2]_2 \cdot H_2SO_4$.

guanylic acid (gwah-nil′ik) guanosine monophosphate.

guanylyl (gwah-nil′il) the radical formed by removal of OH from the phosphate group of guanosine monophosphate.

guarana (gwah-rah′nah) [Tupi-Guarani] a dried paste prepared from the seeds of *Paullinia cupana*, a tree of Brazil; used as an astringent in diarrhea.

guaranine (gwah-rah′nin) caffeine.

guard (gahrd) a protective device. **bite g.,** occlusal g. **mouth g.,** a removable, soft plastic intraoral appliance that covers all occlusal surfaces and the palate and extends to the border of the attached gingiva on the vestibular surface of the teeth; used to protect the teeth, lips, and cheeks during contact sports. **night g.,** occlusal g. **occlusal g.,** a removable dental appliance, usually constructed of plastic, that covers one or both dental arches, designed to minimize the damaging effect of bruxism and other occlusal habits, being usually worn at night. Called also *bite g.* and *night g.*

Guarnieri's bodies (corpuscles) (gwar″ne-er′ēz) [Giuseppi *Guarnieri*, Italian physician, 1856–1918] see under *body.*

guayule (gwi-oo′la) the Mexican rubber plant, *Parthenium argentatum*, which may produce a severe allergic dermatitis (guayule dermatitis).

gubernacula (gu″ber-nak′u-lah) plural of *gubernaculum.*

gubernacular (gu″ber-nak′u-lar) pertaining to a gubernaculum.

gubernaculum (gu″ber-nak′u-lum), pl. *guberna′cula* [L. "helm, rudder"] a structure that guides. **chorda g.,** a portion of the gubernaculum testis and round ligament that develops in the body wall of the embryo. **Hunter's g.,** g. testis. **g. tes′tis** [NA], the fetal ligament attached to the lower end of the epididymis and testis and, at its other end, to the bottom of the scrotum; it is present during, and is thought to guide, the descent of the testis into the scrotum and then atrophies. Called also *Hunter's g.*

Gubler's hemiplegia, etc. (gōōb′lerz) [Adolphe Marie *Gubler*, French physician, 1821–1879] see under *hemiplegia, line, paralysis, sign,* and *tumor.*

Gubler-Robin typhus [A. M. *Gubler*; Albert Edouard

Charles *Robin*, French physician, 1847–1928] see under *typhus.*

Gudden's commissure, law [Bernhard Alloys von *Gudden*, German neurologist, 1824–1886] see *supraoptic commissures*, under *commissure*, and see under *law.*

Guelpa treatment (gwel′pah) [Guglielmo *Guelpa*, Italian physician in Paris, 1850–1930] see under *treatment.*

Guéneau de Mussy's point (ga-no′dŭ-mis-sĕz′) [Noel François Odon *Guéneau de Mussy*, French physician, 1813–1885] see *de Mussy's point*, under *point.*

Guenz (gints) see *Günz.*

Guenzburg (gints′boorg) see *günzburg.*

Guérin's fold, etc. (ga-ranz′) [Alphonse François Marie *Guérin*, French surgeon, 1816–1895] see under *fold, fracture, gland, sinus,* and *valve.*

guidance (gīd′ans) 1. a guide. 2. an act of guidance. **condylar g.,** the path that the horizontal rotation axis of the condyles travels during normal mandibular opening, measured in degrees as related to the Frankfort Horizontal plane. It also influences mandibular movements from the temporomandibular joint, articular guidance, or condylar elements. Called also *condylar guide.* See also under *inclination.* **incisal g.,** the influence on mandibular movements by the contacting surfaces of the mandibular and maxillary anterior teeth.

guide (gīd) a device by which another object is led in its proper course, such as a grooved sound, or a filiform bougie over which a tunneled sound is passed, as in stricture of the urethra. **adjustable anterior g.,** an anterior guide whose superior surface may be varied to provide desired separation of dental casts in various eccentric relationships. **anterior g.,** that part of a dental articulator on which the anterior guide pin rests to maintain the vertical dimension of occlusion; it influences the degree of separation of the casts in eccentric relationships. **condylar g.,** see under *guidance.* **incisal g.,** that part of a dental articulator which maintains the incisal guide angle.

guideline (gīd′līn) any line used as a marker or indicator. **clasp g.,** survey line, def. 3.

Guidi's canal (gwe′dēz) [Guido *Guidi* (L., *Vidius* (Vidus), Italian physician, 1500–1569] canalis pterygoideus.

Guillain-Barré syndrome (ge-yan′-bar-ra′) [Georges *Guillain*, French neurologist, 1876–1961; Jean Alexander *Barré*, French neurologist, born 1880] acute febrile polyneuritis.

Guillemin (ge-ah-men′) Roger Charles Louis. French-born American physician, born 1924; co-winner, with Andrew Victor Schally and Rosalyn Sussman Yalow, of the Nobel prize for medicine or physiology in 1977 for showing that the hypothalamus secretes hormones that control the pituitary gland and for developing methods for isolating peptide hormones.

guillotine (gil′o-tēn) [Fr.] an instrument for excising a tonsil or the uvula.

Guinard's treatment (method) (ge-narz′) [Aimé *Guinard*, French surgeon, 1856–1911] see under *treatment.*

guinea pig (gin′e pig) a small rodent, *Cavia cobaya*, used extensively for experimental work.

Guinon's disease (ge-nawz′) [Georges *Guinon*, French physician, 1859–1929] Gilles de la Tourette syndrome.

Gull's disease (gulz) [Sir William Withey *Gull*, English physician, 1816–1890] see under *disease.*

gullet (gul′et) the esophagus.

Gullstrand (gul′strand) Allvar. Swedish ophthalmologist, 1862–1930; winner of the Nobel prize for medicine or physiology in 1911 for elucidating the formation of optical images in the eye and incorporating it in the general laws governing optical image formation.

Gullstrand's slit lamp, law (gul′strandz) [Allvar *Gullstrand*] see *slit lamp* under *lamp*, and see under *law.*

gulonic acid (gu-lon′ik) a hexonic acid formed by the reduction of the aldehyde group of glucuronic acid to an alcohol; it is an intermediate in the synthesis of ascorbic acid by many mammals.

L-gulonolactone (gu″lo-no-lak′tōn) the immediate precursor of ascorbic acid in plants and in those animals capable of its biosynthesis; gulonolactone is itself formed from L-gulonic acid.

gulose (gu'lōs)   a hexose, $CH_2OH(CHOH)_4CHO$, isomeric with glucose but nonfermentable.

gum (gum) [L. *gummi*]   1. a mucilaginous excretion from various plants; on hydrolysis gums yield hexoses, pentoses, and uronic acids.   2. see *gingiva* and *gingivae*.   **acaroid g.**, a resin derived from *Xanthorrhoea hastilis* and *X. arborea*, tall liliaceous plants growing in Australia.   **animal g.**, a polysaccharide isolated from various proteins and tissues; possibly an impure chondroitin.   **g. arabic**, acacia.   **Australian g.**, wattle g.   **g. benjamin, g. benzoin**, benzoin, def. 1.   **blackboy g.**, acaroid g.   **blue g.**, 1. eucalyptus.   2. the bluish discoloration of the gums seen in lead poisoning.   **Botany Bay g.**, acaroid gum.   **British g.**, dextrin.   **g. camphor**, camphor.   **cape g.**, a gum from *Acacia horrida*.   **eucalyptus g.**, red g.   **free g.**, see under *gingiva*.   **ghatti g.**, a gum from the dhava tree of India; used like acacia.   **guar g.** [NF], a gum obtained from the ground endosperms of the leguminous tree *Cyamopsis tetragonolobus;* used as a tablet binder and disintegrant in pharmaceutical preparations.   **Indian g.**, karaya g.   **karaya g.**, the dried gummy exudation from *Sterculia urens* or other species of *Sterculia*, which becomes gelatinous when moisture is added; used as a bulk laxative. Because of its adhesive properties, products containing karaya gum are used as dental adhesives and as skin adhesives and protective skin barriers in the fitting and care of colostomy appliances and in other conditions involving an artificial stoma. Called also *sterculia g.*   **Kordofan g.**, the best variety of acacia from Kordofan and adjacent region.   **mesquite g.**, a gum from *Prosopis juliflora*, of Texas; used as a substitute for acacia.   **g. opium**, opium.   **red g.**, an exudation from the bark of *Eucalyptus rostrata* and other species; used as an astringent in throat affections.   **g. senegal**, acacia.   **sterculia g.**, karaya g.   **g. thus**, turpentine.   **g. tragacanth**, tragacanth.   **xanthan g.** [NF], a high molecular weight polysaccharide gum produced by a pure-culture fermentation of a carbohydrate with *Xanthomonas campestris*, then purified by recovery with isopropyl alcohol, dried, and milled; it contains D-glucose and D-mannose as the dominant hexose units, along with D-glucuronic acid, is prepared as the sodium, potassium, or calcium salt, and is used as a suspending agent in pharmaceutical preparations.   **wattle g.**, the gum of several Australian species of *Acacia*, an excellent substitute for acacia.

gumboil (gum'boil)   parulis.

Gumboro disease (gum'bur-o) [*Gumboro*, Delaware]   see *infectious bursal disease*, under *disease*.

gumma (gum'ah), pl. *gummas* or *gum'mata* [L. *gummi* gum]   1. a chronic focal area of inflammatory destruction in tertiary syphilis thought to be due to localization of *Treponema pallidum* in a tissue, manifested by an indolent lesion with a center of rubbery, gray-white coagulation necrosis surrounded by epithelioid and fibroblastic cells and sometimes giant cells. Gummata, which vary in size from microscopic to large tumorous masses of necrotic material, may be single or multiple and may involve any organ or tissue, most commonly the mucocutaneous tissues, liver, bones, and testes. Those found in the skin resemble other chronic granulomatous lesions caused by tuberculosis, sarcoidosis, leprosy, and deep fungal infections. Called also *syphiloma.*   2. late benign syphilis.   **tuberculous g.**, a subcutaneous nodule(s) that becomes fluctuant and drains, with undermined ulceration and sinus formation; caused by hematogenous spread of tubercle bacilli from a primary focus of infection during a period of lowered resistance or immunodeficiency, especially in children. Called also *metastatic tuberculous abscess, tuberculosis colliquativa,* and *tuberculosis colliquativa cutis.* Cf. *scrofuloderma.*

gummata (gum'ah-tah) [L.]   plural of *gumma.*

gummate (gum'āt)   an arabate.

gummatous (gum'ah-tus)   of the nature of gumma.

gummi (gum'i) [L., from Gr. *kommi*]   gum (of plants).

gummy (gum'e)   resembling a gum or a gumma.

gum-resin (gum-rez'in)   a concrete juice exuding from various trees. The gum-resins consist of a principle soluble in water and insoluble in alcohol, combined with a volatile oil or resin soluble in alcohol, but not in water, and include ammoniac, gamboge, myrrh, and scammony.

guncotton (gun-kot'n)   pyroxylin.

Gunn's dots, pupillary phenomenon, syndrome

(phenomenon, sign) (gunz) [Robert Marcus *Gunn*, English ophthalmologist, 1850–1909]   see under *dot*, see *swinging flashlight sign*, under *sign*, and see under *syndrome.*

Gunning's test (reaction) (gun'ingz) [Jan Willem *Gunning*, Dutch chemist, 1827–1901]   see under *test.*

Gunning's splint (gun'ingz) [Thomas Brian *Gunning*, American dentist, 1813–1889]   see under *splint.*

Günz's ligament (gints'ez) [Justus Gottfried *Günz*, German anatomist, 1714–1754]   see under *ligament.*

Günzberg's test (gints'boorgz) [Alfred *Günzberg*, German physician, born 1861]   see under *tests.*

gurgulio (gur-gu'le-o) [L. "gullet"]   uvula palatina.

gurney (ger'ne)   a wheeled cot used in hospitals.

gustation (gus-ta'shun) [L. *gustatio*, from *gustare* to taste]   the act of tasting or the sense of taste.   **colored g.**, the association of colors with tastes.

gustatism (gus'tah-tizm)   a sensation of taste produced indirectly by other than gustatory stimuli.

gustatory (gus'tah-to″re) [L. *gustatorius*]   pertaining to the sense of taste.

gustin (gus'tin)   a polypeptide (molecular weight, 27,000) present in saliva and containing two zinc atoms; it is apparently necessary for normal development of the taste buds.

gustometer (gus-tom'ĕ-ter) [L. *gustare* to taste + Gr. *metron* measure]   an apparatus used in the quantitative determination of taste thresholds.

gustometry (gus-tom'ĕ-tre)   the clinical determination of thresholds of the sense of taste.

gut (gut)   1. the intestine or bowel.   2. the primitive digestive tube, consisting of the fore-, mid-, and hindgut.   3. catgut.   **blind g.**, caecum (def. 2).   **postanal g.**, a temporary extension of the embryonic gut caudal to the cloaca.   **preoral g.**, Seessel's pouch.   **primitive g.**, archenteron.   **ribbon g.**, an absorbable ribbon of the intestinal tissue of animals used for suturing where broad support is to be secured.   **tail g.**, postanal g.

Guthrie's formula (guth'rēz) [Clyde Graeme *Guthrie*, American physician, 1880–1931]   see under *formula.*

Guthrie's muscle (guth'rēz) [George James *Guthrie*, English surgeon, 1785–1856]   musculus sphincter urethrae.

Guthrie test (guth're) [R. *Guthrie*, American pediatrician, born 1916]   see under *tests.*

gutta (gut'ah), pl. *gut'tae* [L.]   a drop.

guttae (gut'e) [L.]   plural of *gutta.*

gutta-percha (gut″ah-per'chah)   [USP] the coagulated, dried, purified latex of trees of the genera *Palaguium* and *Payena*, most commonly *Palaguium gutta;* used in orthopedics for fracture splints, in surgery for temporary sealing of cavities, and in dentistry in the form of cones for filling the root canal and in the form of sticks for sealing cavities over treatment. See also under *baseplate.*

Guttat.   abbreviation for L. *gutta'tim*, drop by drop.

guttate (gut'āt)   characterized by lesions that are drop-shaped.

guttatim (gut-ta'tim) [L.]   drop by drop.

guttation (gut-ta'shun)   the secretion of water by plant cells under humid conditions, an indication that the cells actively transport some materials against a concentration gradient.

gutti (gut'i)   cambogia.

gut-tie (gut'ti)   1. a twisting of the intestine of animals, causing colicky pains.   2. a condition in cattle in which a loop of intestine passes through a tear in the peritoneum and is held there, producing obstruction of the bowels.

Gutt. quibusd.   abbreviation for L. *gut'tis quibus'dam*, with a few drops.

guttur (gut'ur) [L.]   throat.

guttural (gut'ur-al)   pertaining to the throat.

gutturophony (gut″ur-of'o-ne) [*guttur* + Gr. *phōnē* voice]   throaty quality of the voice.

gutturotetany (gut″ur-o-tet'ah-ne) [*guttur* + *tetany*]   a guttural spasm, resulting in a kind of stutter.

Gutzeit's test (goot'zītz) [Max Adolf *Gutzeit*, Leipzig chemist, 1847–1915]   see under *tests.*

Guy de Chauliac   see *Chauliac.*

Guyon's amputation (operation), sign (ge-yonz′) [Felix Jean Casimir *Guyon*, surgeon in Paris, 1831–1920] see under *amputation* and *sign*.

GVH graft-versus-host (disease or reaction).

Gwathmey's oil-ether anesthesia (gwath′mēz) [James Taylor *Gwathmey*, New York surgeon, 1863–1944] see under *anesthesia*.

Gy gray, def. 3.

Gymnamoebia (jim″nah-me′bah) [gymn- + *ameba*] a class of free-living ameboid protozoa (superclass Rhizopoda, subphylum Sarcodina), the organisms of which are "naked"; i.e., they lack a test. It comprises three orders: Amoebida, Schizopyrenida, and Pelobiontida.

gymnastics (jim-nas′tiks) [Gr. *gymnastikos* pertaining to athletics] systematic muscular exercise. **ocular g.,** systematic exercise of the eye muscles in order to secure proper movement, accommodation, or fixation. **Swedish g.,** a system of exercise following a rigid pattern of carefully chosen free, active, deliberate movement, utilizing little equipment and stressing correct bodily posture. **vocal g.,** methodical exercise for the purpose of increasing the lung expansion and strengthening the voice.

Gymnema (jim-ne′mah) a genus of trees. The leaves of *G. sylvestre* R. Bv. (Asclepiadaceae), of Africa, are used to disguise the taste of unpleasant medicines. See also *gymnemic acid*, under *acid*.

gymn(o)- [Gr. *gymnos* naked] a combining form meaning naked or denoting relationship to nakedness.

Gymnoascaceae (jim″no-as-ka′se-e) a family of the ascomycetous fungi, order Eurotiales, series Plectomycetes, in which the reproductive organs are in the form of naked asci. It includes the genera *Ajellomyces*, *Arthroderma*, *Gymnoascus*, and *Nannizzia*.

Gymnoascus (jim″no-as′kus) a genus of keratinophilic fungi of the family Gymnoascaceae, some species of which have been isolated from skin lesions of domestic animals and man.

gymnocarpous (jim″no-kar′pus) [gymno- + Gr. *karpos* fruit] having the hymenium, or fertile layer, exposed during spore formation; said of certain fungi.

gymnocyte (jim′no-sīt) [gymno- + Gr. *kytos* hollow vessel] a cell with no cell wall.

Gymnodinium (jim″no-din′e-um) [gymno- + Gr. *dinein* to whirl] a genus of plantlike marine and freshwater protozoa (order Dinoflagellida, class Phytomastigophorea), most species of which have many colored (yellow, brown, green, or blue) chromatophores. Like other dinoflagellates, they produce discoloration of the water (red tide) when present in vast numbers, and certain species, especially *G. breve*, have been associated with a type of shellfish poisoning (q.v.).

gymnoplast (jim′no-plast) [gymno- + Gr. *plastos* formed] a mass of protoplasm without an enclosing wall.

gymnosperm (jim′no-sperm) [gymno- + Gr. *sperma* seed] a plant in which the seeds are not enclosed in an ovary.

gymnospore (jim′no-spōr) a spore without any protective envelope.

Gymnostomatia (jim″no-sto-ma′she-ah) [gymno- + Gr. *stoma* mouth] a subclass of protozoa (class Kinetofragminophorea, phylum Ciliophora) characterized by the presence of a cytostome at or near the body surface, located apically or laterally; the somatic ciliature is usually uniform, and toxicysts are commonly present. Protostomatida and Pleurostomatida are representative orders.

gymnothecium (jim″no-the′se-um) the fruiting body produced by the sexual (perfect) stage of dermatophytes of the genera *Arthroderma* and *Nannizzia*; it is a loose network of mycelium through which ascospores filter and are released following maturation. Cf. *apothecium*, *cleistothecium*, and *perithecium*.

Gymnothorax (jim″no-tho′raks) [gymno- + Gr. *thōrax* chest] a genus of moray eels whose flesh is sometimes used as food.

gynaec(o)- for words beginning thus, see those beginning *gynec(o)-*.

gynander (ji-nan′der) [gyn- + Gr. *anēr*, *andros* man] 1. a hermaphrodite. 2. a masculine woman.

gynandria (ji-nan′dre-ah) gynandrism.

gynandrism (ji-nan′drizm) [gyn- + *andr-* + *-ism*] 1. hermaphroditism. 2. female pseudohermaphroditism. 3. the state of a virilized woman.

gynandroblastoma (ji-nan″dro-blas-to′mah) [gyn- + andro- + *blastoma*] a rare ovarian tumor containing histological features of both arrhenoblastoma and granulosa cell tumor.

gynandroid (ji-nan′droid) [gyn- + andr- + Gr. *eidos* form] 1. hermaphrodite. 2. female pseudohermaphrodite. 3. like a virilized woman.

gynandromorph (ji-nan′dro-morf) an individual exhibiting gynandromorphism.

gynandromorphism (ji-nan″dro-mor′fizm) [gyn- + andro- + Gr. *morphē* form] the presence of chromosomes of both sexes in different tissues of the body, producing a mosaic of male and female characteristics; a condition common among bees and silkworms. **bilateral g.,** bilateral hermaphroditism.

gynandromorphous (ji-nan″dro-mor′fus) 1. pertaining to or characterized by gynandromorphism. 2. pertaining to a gynandromorph.

gynandry (ji′nan-dre) gynandrism.

gynatresia (jin″ah-tre′ze-ah) [gyn- + *a* neg. + Gr. *trēsis* perforation] occlusion of some part of the female genital tract, especially of the vagina.

gyne- see *gynec(o)-*.

gynecic (ji-nes′ik) pertaining to women.

gynecium (ji-ne′se-um) [gyn- + Gr. *oikos* house] the female part of a flower; called also *pistil*.

gynec(o)-, gynaec(o)-, gyne-, gyn(o)- [Gr. *gynē*, gen. *gynaikos* woman] a combining form meaning female or denoting relationship to women or to the female reproductive organs.

gynecogen (jin′ĕ-ko-jen) any substance (female sex hormones) which produces or stimulates female characteristics.

gynecogenic (jin″ĕ-ko-jen′ik) [gyneco- + Gr. *gennan* to produce] causing or producing female characteristics.

gynecography (jin″e-kog′rah-fe) roentgenography of the female reproductive tract.

gynecoid (jin′ĕ-koid) [gyneco- + Gr. *eidos* form] womanlike; resembling a woman.

gynecologic (gi″nĕ-ko-loj′ik, jin″ĕ-ko-loj′ik) pertaining to or affecting the female reproductive tract.

gynecological (gi″nĕ-ko-loj′ĭ-k'l, jin″ĕ-ko-loj′ĭ-k'l) pertaining to gynecology.

gynecologist (gi″nĕ-kol′o-jist, jin″ĕ-kol′o-jist) a person skilled in gynecology.

gynecology (gi″ne-kol′o-je, jin″ĕ-kol′o-je) [gyneco- + *-logy*] that branch of medicine which treats of diseases of the genital tract in women.

gynecomania (jin″ĕ-ko-ma′ne-ah) [gyneco- + Gr. *mania* madness] satyriasis.

gynecomastia (jin″ĕ-ko-mas′te-ah) [gyneco- + Gr. *mastos* breast] excessive development of the male mammary glands, even to the functional state. **nutritional g.,** refeeding g. **refeeding g.,** transitory enlargement of the male breast developing during rehabilitation and recovery from a state of malnutrition. **rehabilitation g.,** refeeding g.

gynecomastism (jin″ĕ-ko-mas′tizm) gynecomastia.

gynecomasty (jin′ĕ-ko-mas″te) gynecomastia.

gynecomazia (jin″ĕ-ko-ma′ze-ah) gynecomastia.

gynecopathy (jin″ĕ-kop′ah-the) [gyneco- + Gr. *pathos* disease] a disease peculiar to women.

gynecophoral (jin″ĕ-kof′o-ral) see under *canal*.

gyneduct (jin′ĕ-dukt) [gyne- + *duct*] the primitive female duct; ductus paramesonephricus.

gynephobia (jin″ĕ-fo′be-ah) [gyne- + *phobia*] irrational fear of or aversion to women.

gyneplasty (jin′ĕ-plas″te) gynoplasty.

Gynergen (jin′er-jen) trademark for preparations of ergotamine tartrate.

gynesin (jin′ĕ-sin) trigonelline.

gyn(o)- see *gynec(o)-*.

gynogamon (ji-no-gam′ōn) a gamone released by the ovum.

gynogenesis (jin″o-jen′ĕ-sis) [gyno- + Gr. *genesis* production] development of an egg that is stimulated by a sperm in the absence of any participation of the sperm nucleus.

gynomerogon (jin″o-mer′o-gon) an organism developed from a fertilized ovum containing the female pronucleus only, the cells, as a result, containing only the maternal set of chromosomes.

gynomerogone (jin″o-mer′o-gon) gynomerogon.

gynomerogony (jin″o-mĕ-rog′o-ne) [*gyno-* + Gr. *meros* part + *gonos* procreation] development of a portion of a fertilized ovum containing the female pronucleus only. Cf. *andromerogony* and *merogony*.

gynopathic (jin″o-path′ik) [*gyno-* + Gr. *pathos* disease] caused by or pertaining to disease of women.

gynopathy (jin-op′ah-the) any disease of women.

gynophobia (ji″no-fo′be-ah) gynephobia.

gynoplastic (ji″no-plas′tik) pertaining to gynoplastics.

gynoplastics (ji″no-plas′tiks) [*gyno-* + Gr. *plastos* formed] the plastic or reconstructive surgery of the female reproductive organs.

gynoplasty (ji′no-plas″te) plastic or reconstructive surgery of the female reproductive organs.

Gynorest (gi′no-rest) trademark for a preparation of dydrogesterone.

gypsum (jip′sum) [L.; Gr. *gypsos* chalk] native calcium sulfate dihydrate; when calcined, it becomes plaster of Paris, much used in making permanent dressings for fractures and in dentistry for taking dental impressions. See also *calcium sulfate.*

gyrate (ji′rāt) [L. *gyratus* turned round] twisted in a ring or spiral shape.

gyration (ji-ra′shun) revolution in a circle or in circles.

gyre (jīr) gyrus.

gyrectomy (ji-rek′to-me) excision or resection of a cerebral gyrus, or of a portion of the cerebral cortex. **frontal g.,** topectomy.

Gyrencephala (ji″ren-sef′ah-lah) [*gyrus* + Gr. *enkephalos* brain] a group of higher mammals in which the brain is characteristically marked by convolutions. Cf. *Lissencephala.*

gyrencephalic (ji″ren-sĕ-fal′ik) pertaining to the Gyrencephala; having a brain marked by convolutions. Cf. *lissencephalic.*

gyri (ji′ri) [L.] genitive and plural of *gyrus.*

gyr(o)- [Gr. *gyros* circle] a combining form meaning round or denoting relationship to a gyrus.

gyrochrome (ji′ro-krōm) [*gyro-* + Gr. *chrōma* color] a nerve cell in which the Nissl bodies have a ringlike arrangement in the cytoplasm. Cf. *arkyochrome, perichrome,* and *stichochrome.*

gyrometer (ji-rom′ĕ-ter) [*gyro-* + Gr. *metron* measure] an instrument for measuring the cerebral gyri.

Gyropus (ji′ro-pus) a genus of biting lice. **G. ova′lis,** a biting louse found on guinea pigs.

gyrose (ji′rōs) marked by curved lines or circles.

gyrospasm (ji′ro-spazm) [*gyro-* + Gr. *spasmos* spasm] rotatory spasm of the head.

gyrotrope (ji′ro-trōp) rheotrope.

gyrous (ji′rus) gyrose.

gyrus (ji′rus), gen. and pl. **gy′ri** [L., from Gr. *gyros* circle] [NA] one of the tortuous elevations (convolutions) of the surface of the brain caused by infolding of the cortex; see *gyri cerebri.* **angular g., g. angula′ris** [NA], a convolution of the inferior parietal lobule, arching over the posterior end of the superior temporal sulcus and continuous with the middle temporal gyrus. **annectant gyri, gy′ri annecten′tes, gy′ri transitivi cerebri. gy′ri bre′ves in′sulae** [NA], short gyri of insula: the short, rostrally placed gyri on the surface of the insula; called also *preinsular gyri.* **Broca's g.,** see under *convolution.* **callosal g., g. callo′sus,** g. cinguli. **central g., anterior,** g. precentralis. **central g., posterior,** g. postcentralis. **g. centra′lis ante′rior,** g. precentralis. **g. centra′lis poste′rior,** g. postcentralis. **g. cerebel′li,** folia cerebelli. **gy′ri cer′ebri** [NA], **gyri of cerebrum,** the tortuous elevations (convolutions) of the surface of the cerebral hemisphere, caused by infolding of the cortex and separated by the fissures or sulci. Many are constant enough that they have been given special names. **cingulate g.,** g. cinguli. **g. cin-**

gula′tus, NA alternative for *g. cinguli.* **g. cin′guli** [NA], arch-shaped convolution closely related to the surface of the corpus callosum, from which it is separated by the callosal sulcus; called also *callosal g.* or *g. callosus* and *cingulate g.* or *g. cingulatus* [NA alternative]. **dentate g.,** 1. gyrus dentatus (def. 1). 2. gyrus fasciolaris. **g. denta′tus,** 1. [NA], the dentate gyrus: a serrated strip of gray matter under the medial border of the hippocampus and in its depths; it is an archicortex which develops along the edge of the hippocampal fissure and which consists of molecular, granular, and polymorphic layers. Called also *fascia dentata hippocampi.* 2. gyrus fasciolaris. **g. fasciola′ris** [NA], a posterior and upward extension of the dentate gyrus, forming a transitional area between the dentate gyrus and the indusium griseum; called also *fasciola cinerea.* **g. fornica′tus,** the marginal portion of the cerebral cortex on the medial aspect of the hemisphere, including the gyrus cinguli, gyrus parahippocampalis, isthmus, and uncus; it forms a major part of the limbic system. **frontal g., ascending,** g. precentralis. **frontal g., inferior,** g. frontalis inferior. **frontal g., middle,** g. frontalis medius. **frontal g., superior,** g. frontalis superior. **g. fronta′lis infe′rior** [NA], inferior frontal gyrus: a convolution of the frontal lobe below the inferior frontal sulcus; it is divided by the anterior and ascending branches of the lateral sulcus into orbital, triangular, and opercular parts. **g. fronta′lis media′lis** [NA], the medial surface of the frontal lobe, separated from the cingulate gyrus by the cingulate sulcus, and continuous with the superior frontal gyrus above and the gyrus rectus below. **g. fronta′lis me′dius** [NA], middle frontal gyrus: a convolution of the frontal lobe between the superior and inferior frontal sulci, extending anteriorly from the precentral gyrus. **g. fronta′lis supe′rior** [NA], superior frontal gyrus: a convolution of the frontal lobe above the superior frontal sulcus, extending anteriorly from the precentral gyrus. **fusiform g., g. fusifor′mis,** a gyrus of the temporal lobe on the inferior surface of the hemisphere between the inferior temporal gyrus and the parahippocampal gyrus. It consists of a lateral and a medial part, called [NA] *g. occipitotemporalis lateralis* and *g. occipitotemporalis medialis.* **g. genic′uli,** a vestigial gyrus at the anterior end of the corpus callosum. **Heschl's gyri,** gyri temporales transversi. **hippocampal g.,** g. parahippocampalis. **g. hippocam′pi,** NA alternative for *g. parahippocampalis.* **infracalcarine g., g. infracalcari′nus,** g. lingualis. **gy′ri in′sulae** [NA], the gyri that are found on the surface of the insula, including the *gyrus longus insulae* and the *gyri breves insulae.* **g. lim′bicus,** gyrus fornicatus. **lingual g., g. lingua′lis** [NA], a gyrus of the occipital lobe on the inferior surface of the hemisphere, forming the inferior lip of the calcarine sulcus and, with the cuneus, the visual cortex; it is continuous anteriorly with the parahippocampal gyrus. **long g. of insula, g. lon′gus in′sulae** [NA], the long, occipitally directed gyrus on the surface of the insula. **marginal g.,** g. frontalis medialis. **marginal g. of Turner,** g. frontalis medialis. **g. margina′lis,** g. frontalis medialis. **occipital gyri, lateral,** see *occipital g., inferior* and *occipital g., superior.* **occipital g., inferior,** the lower of the two gyri separated by the lateral occipital sulcus on the lateral aspect of the occipital lobe. **occipital g., superior,** the upper of the two gyri separated by the occipital lateral sulcus on the lateral aspect of the occipital lobe. **occipitotemporal g., lateral,** g. occipitotemporalis lateralis. **occipitotemporal g., medial,** g. occipitotemporalis medialis. **g. occipitotempora′lis latera′lis** [NA], lateral occipitotemporal gyrus: the lateral portion of a gyrus (g. fusiformis) on the inferior surface of the cerebral hemisphere, separated from the medial portion by the occipitotemporal sulcus, and continuous laterally with the inferior temporal gyrus. **g. occipitotempora′lis media′lis** [NA], middle occipitotemporal gyrus: the medial portion of a gyrus (g. fusiformis) on the inferior surface of the cerebral hemisphere, separated from the lateral portion by the occipitotemporal sulcus, and from the parahippocampal gyrus by the collateral sulcus. **gy′ri olfacto′rii media′lis et latera′lis** [NA], the layers of gray substance that cover the striae olfactoriae medialis et lateralis. **g. olfacto′rius media′lis,** area subcallosa. **olfactory g., lateral,** see *gyri olfactorii medialis et lateralis.* **olfactory g., medial,** see *gyri olfactorii medialis et lateralis.* **orbital gyri, gy′ri orbita′les** [NA], the various irregular convolutions lateral to the olfactory sulcus on the orbital surface of the frontal lobe. **paracentral g., g. paracentra'lis,** lobulus paracentralis. **parahippocampal g., g. parahippocampa'lis** [NA], a convolution on the inferior surface of each cerebral hemisphere, lying between the hippocampal and collateral sulci; called also *hippocampal g.* or *g. hippocampi* [NA alternative]. **paraterminal g., g. paratermina'lis** [NA], a thin sheet of gray substance in front of and ventral to the genu of the corpus callosum; called also *g. subcallosus* and *subcallosal g.* See also *septum precommissurale.* **parietal g.,** any one of the convolutions into which the surface of the parietal lobe is divided. **parietal g., ascending, postcentral g., g. postcentra'lis** [NA], the convolution of the parietal lobe lying between the central and postcentral sulci; the primary sensory area of the cerebral cortex. Called also *g. centralis posterior* and *posterior central g.* **precentral g., g. precentra'lis** [NA], the convolution of the frontal lobe lying between the precentral and central sulci; the primary motor area of the cerebral cortex. Called also *g. centralis anterior* and *anterior central g.* **preinsular gyri,** gyri breves insulae. **gy'ri profun'di cer'ebri,** the deeply placed cerebral convolutions. **quadrate g.** (*obs.*), precuneus. **g. rec'tus** [NA], a convolution on the orbital surface of the frontal lobe, medial to the olfactory sulcus and continuous with the medial frontal gyrus on the medial surface. **short gyri of insula,** gyri breves insulae. **subcallosal g., g. subcallo'sus,** g. paraterminalis. **subcollateral g.** (*obs.*), the occipitotemporal gyri. **supracallosal g., g. supracallo'sus,** indusium griseum. **supramarginal g., g. supramargina'lis** [NA], the convolution of the inferior parietal lobe that curves around the upper end of the posterior branch of the lateral fissure and is continuous behind it with the superior temporal gyrus. **temporal g.,** any gyrus of the temporal lobe. **temporal g., inferior,** g. temporalis inferior. **temporal g., middle,** g. temporalis medius. **temporal g., superior,** g. temporalis superior. **temporal gyri, transverse,** gyri temporales transversi. **g. tempora'lis infe'rior** [NA], inferior temporal gyrus: the convolution of the temporal lobe lying between the inferior temporal sulcus and the lateral occipitotemporal gyrus, the two gyri being continuous at the inferolateral margin of the temporal lobe. **g. tempora'lis me'dius** [NA], middle temporal gyrus: the convolution of the temporal lobe lying between the superior and the inferior temporal sulci; it is continuous posteriorly with the angular gyrus. **g. tempora'lis supe'rior** [NA], superior temporal gyrus: the convolution of the temporal lobe lying between the superior temporal sulcus and the lateral sulcus, continuous behind with the supramarginal gyrus. **gy'ri tempora'les transver'si** [NA], transverse temporal gyrus: the transverse convolutions marking the posterior extremity of the superior temporal gyrus and lying mostly in the lateral sulcus; the more marked of these, the anterior transverse temporal gyrus (Heschl's convolution), represents the cortical center for hearing. Called also *Heschl's g.* **gy'ri transiti'vi cer'ebri,** various small folds on the cerebral surface that are too inconstant to bear special names; called also *annectant gyri* and *gyri annectentes.* **uncinate g., g. uncina'tus,** uncus.

H

H chemical symbol for *hydrogen;* symbol for *henry* and *Hounsfield unit.*

H symbol for *enthalpy.*

H. abbreviation for [L.] *haustus* (a draft), *horizontal,* [L.] *ho'ra* (hour), *hypermetropia* or *hyperopia* and *Holzknecht unit.*

H⁺ symbol for *hydrogen ion.*

[H⁺] symbol for *hydrogen ion concentration.*

h symbol for *hecto-* or *hour.*

h Planck's constant.

H_0 null hypothesis.

H_1 alternate hypothesis.

H & E hematoxylin and eosin stain; see *Table of Stains and Staining Methods.*

HA hemadsorbent.

Ha symbol for *hahnium.*

HAA hepatitis-associated antigen.

Haab's magnet, reflex (hahbz) [Otto *Haab,* professor of ophthalmology in Zurich, 1850–1931] see under *magnet* and *reflex.*

habena (hah-be'nah), pl. *habe'nae* [L. "rein"] see *habenula* (def. 2).

habenal, habenar (hah-be'nal, hah-be'nar) pertaining to the habena.

habenula (hah-ben'u-lah), gen. and pl. *haben'ulae* [L., dim. of *habena,* q.v.] 1. a frenulum, or reinlike structure, such as one of a set of such structures in the cochlea. 2. [NA] a component of the epithalamus, being the small eminence on the dorsomedial eminence of the thalamus, just in front of the dorsal commissure on the lateral edge of the habenular trigone; called also *pineal peduncle.* **h. arcua'ta,** the inner portion of the basilar membrane of the cochlea. **h. cona'rii,** habenula (def. 2). **Haller's h.,** vestigium processus vaginalis. **h. pectina'ta,** the outer portion of the basilar membrane of the cochlea. **haben'ulae perfora'tae,** foramina nervosa limbus laminae spiralis; see under *foramen.* **h. urethra'lis,** either of two whitish lines extending from the urinary meatus to the clitoris in girls and young women.

habenulae (hah-ben'u-le) [L.] genitive and plural of *habenula.*

habenular (hah-ben'u-lar) pertaining to the habenula.

Habermann's disease (hah'ber-manz) [Rudolf *Habermann,* German dermatologist, 1884–1941] acute lichenoid pityriasis.

habit (hab'it) [L. *habitus,* from *habere* to hold] 1. a fixed or constant practice established by frequent repetition. 2. predisposition or bodily temperament; see under *type.* **clamping h., clenching h.,** centric bruxism. **endothelioid h.,** a condition in which the nucleus of a cell is relatively small as compared with the cytoplasm. **glaucomatous h.,** shallowness of the anterior chamber of the eye with dilated pupil; seen in persons who have a predisposition to glaucoma. **leukocytoid h.,** endothelioid habit. **oral h.,** one that causes changes in occlusal relationships, e.g., finger, thumb, and lip sucking, tongue thrusting, and the like. See also *habit-breaking appliance,* under *appliance.*

habitat (hab'ĭ-tat) the natural abode or home of an animal or plant species.

habituation (hah-bit"u-a'shun) 1. the gradual adaptation to a stimulus or to the environment. 2. the extinction of a conditioned reflex by repetition of the conditioned stimulus. 3. a condition resulting from the repeated consumption of a drug, with a desire to continue its use, but with little or no tendency to increase the dose; there may be psychic, but no physical, dependence on the drug, and detrimental effects, if any, are primarily on the individual.

habitus (hab'ĭ-tus) [L. "habit"] 1. posture or position of the body. 2. physique; body build and constitution. See also under *type.* **Buddha-like h.,** the froglike posture of the fetus due to abdominal enlargement.

Habronema (hab"ro-ne'mah) [Gr. *habros* graceful + *nema* thread] a genus of nematode worms of the superfamily Spiruroidea, which are parasitic in the stomach of horses. The larval forms are taken up from the feces of horses by flies and the flies, swallowed by horses with their feed, transmit the larvae to the horses' stomachs. The larvae may also be transmitted to the skin of horses where they produce a dermatitis and a form of granuloma; in the conjunctiva they produce bungeye. The species are *H. megastoma, H. muscae, H. microstoma,* and *H. zebrae.*

habronemiasis (hab"ro-ne-mi'ah-sis) infection with *Habronema.* **cutaneous h.,** a disease of horses in various parts of the world, including the southern United States, Brazil, India, and the Philippines, caused by infection with larvae of *Habronema,* and characterized by cutaneous granulomas that grow in size until the skin over and around the lesions is destroyed, leaving a large raw surface. Because of the clinical similarity between cutaneous habronemiasis and hyphomycosis destruens equi, the disorders are often confused. Called also *bursautee, esponja,* and *summer sores.*

habu (hah′boo) [native name in Ryukyu Islands]   an extremely venomous pit viper, *Trimeresurus flavorviridis,* inhabiting the warmer parts of East Asia, especially the Ryukyu Islands.

hachement (ash-maw′) [Fr.]   a chopping or hacking stroke in massage.

Hackenbruch's experience (hah′ken-brooks) [Peter Theodor *Hackenbruch,* German surgeon, 1865–1924]   (*obs.*) the rhombic-shaped area of anesthesia produced by the injection of a local anesthetic.

hae-   for words beginning thus, see also those beginning *he-.*

Haeckel's law (hek′elz) [Ernst Heinrich Philipp August *Haeckel,* German naturalist, 1834–1919]   see *recapitulation theory,* under *theory.*

haem (hēm)   heme.

haema (he′mah) [Gr. *haima, haimatos* blood]   [NA] the blood; the fluid that circulates through the heart, arteries, capillaries, and veins, carrying nutriment and oxygen to the cells of the body. Spelled also *hema* [NA alternative], and called also *sanguis.* See *blood.*

haema-   see *hem*(o) -; for words beginning thus, see also those beginning *hema-.*

Haemadipsa (he″mah-dip′sah) [*haema-* + Gr. *dipsa* thirst]   a genus of leeches, the land leeches, of the family Gnathobdellidae.   **H. ceylon′ica,** a species common in Ceylon, which is annoying to man and animals because of its painful bite.   **H. chilia′ni,** a species attacking horses and cattle in South America.   **H. japon′ica,** a species found in Japan.   **H. zeylan′dica,** a species attacking mammals in the tropical jungles of Asia.

Haemagogus (hem″ah-go′gus) [*haem-* + Gr. *agōgos* leading]   a genus of mosquitoes some of which transmit jungle yellow fever in tropical Central and South America.

Haemaphysalis (hem″ah-fis′ah-lis) [Gr. *haima* blood + *physallis* bubble]   a genus of ticks.   **H. concin′na,** one of the vectors of *Rickettsia sibirica,* the etiologic agent of Siberian tick typhus.   **H. humero′sa,** the bandicoot tick, one of the vectors of *Coxiella burneti.*   **H. leach′i,** the common dog tick of South Africa; it transmits canine babesiosis.   **H. leporispalus′tris,** the rabbit tick, one of the vectors of Rocky Mountain spotted fever and tularemia among wild animals.   **H. puncta′ta,** a species of tick which acts as a vector of babesiosis in Southern Europe, and which has been considered the cause of tick paralysis in chickens.   **H. spiniger′a,** a species occurring in the tropical forests of India that is a vector of Kyasanur Forest disease in forest workers.

haemat(o)-   see *hemat*(o)-.

Haematobia (hem″ah-to′be-ah)   a genus of flies of the family Muscidae.   **H. ir′ritans,** a genus of small flies, "horn flies," which are very troublesome to cattle; called also *Lyperosia irritans* and *Siphona irritans.*

Haematopinus (hem″ah-to-pi′nus) [*haemato-* + Gr. *pinein* to drink]   a genus of sucking lice, species of which infest horses, swine, and cattle.

Haematosiphon (hem″ah-to-si′fon)   a genus of insects closely related to the genus *Cimex,* but having longer legs and a very long beak.   **H. in′dorus,** a species of the southwestern United States and Mexico, which may be a serious pest of poultry and sometimes attacks man.

Haematoxylon (he″mah-tok′sĭ-lon) [*haemato-* + Gr. *xylon* wood]   a genus of leguminous trees of Central America and the West Indies; the heart-wood of *H. campechianum* L. (Leguminosae), or logwood, contains tannin, hematoxylin, and resin, and is used mainly as a dye.

Haementeria (hem″en-te′re-ah)   a genus of leeches.   **H. officina′lis,** a species used for medicinal purposes in Mexico and South America.

haem(o)-   see *hem*(o)-.

Haemobartonella (he″mo-bar″to-nel′lah) [*haemo-* + *Bartonella,* from A. L. *Barton,* Peruvian physician]   a genus of bacteria of the family Anaplasmataceae, order Rickettsiales, occurring as parasites in various lower animals.   **H. ca′nis,** a nonpathogenic species found in dogs.   **H. fe′lis,** a species causing severe or fatal anemia in cats, probably transmitted from cat to cat by biting during fights.   **H.**

mu′ris, a common parasite of the laboratory rat, in which the infection is activated by splenectomy.

Haemodipsus (hem″o-dip′sus)   a genus of lice.   **H. ventrico′sus,** the common sucking louse of the rabbit which transmits the infective agent of tularemia from rabbit to rabbit.

Haemogregarina (hem″o-greg″ah-ri′nah) [*hemo-* + L. *gregarius* crowding together]   a genus of coccidian protozoa (suborder Adeleina, order Eucoccidiida) in which the life cycle involves two hosts, the vertebrate circulatory system (e.g., reptiles, amphibians, birds, certain mammals) and the invertebrate digestive system (e.g., blood-sucking invertebrates such as an insect or leech).

Haemonchus (he-mon′kus)   a genus of parasitic nematode worms of the family Trichostrongylidae.   **H. contor′tus,** the wireworm or stomach worm; a small nematode parasite of the abomasum (fourth stomach) of sheep and other ruminants, which produces weakness, wasting, and death of the infected animal; it has also been reported as having been found in man.   **H. pla′cei,** *H. contortus.*

Haemophilus (he-mof′ĭ-lus) [*hemo-* + Gr. *philein* to love]   a genus of gram-negative, aerobic or facultatively anaerobic, rod-shaped or coccobacillary bacteria of the family Pasteurellaceae, made up of cells that sometimes form threads and filaments. The organisms require one or both growth factors (X factor, which can be replaced by hematin, or V factor, which can be replaced by nicotinamide adenine dinucleoside) present in blood. They are normal inhabitants of the upper respiratory tract but may become primary or secondary pathogens. Spelled also *Hemophilus.*   **H. aegyp′tius,** a species similar to *H. influenzae* that produces infectious conjunctivitis in humans, especially in hot climates. Called also *Koch-Weeks bacillus.*   **H. aphroph′ilus,** a species that is part of the normal oral microflora, and occasionally found as a cause of endocarditis.   **H. bronchisep′ticus,** *Bordetella bronchiseptica.*   **H. ducrey′i,** a species that causes soft chancres or chancroids on the genitals of humans. Called also *Ducrey's bacillus.*   **H. du′plex,** *Moraxella (Moraxella) lacunata.*   **H. haemolyt′icus,** a nonpathogenic species found as a normal inhabitant of the upper respiratory tract.   **H. influen′zae,** a species once thought to be the cause of epidemic influenza in humans. Noncapsulated strains are normal inhabitants of the human nasopharynx (biotypes II and III). In children, capsulated strains of biotype I are the major cause of bacterial meningitis, and may also cause potentially fatal acute epiglottitis (obstructive laryngitis). Called also *Pfeiffer's bacillus.*   **H. parainfluen′zae,** a species that is part of the normal oral flora and is occasionally associated with bacterial endocarditis.   **H. paraphroph′ilus,** a species that is part of the normal oral microflora. It has been associated with endocarditis and isolated from clinical specimens of abscessed internal organs.   **H. parasu′is,** a species found as a normal inhabitant of the upper respiratory tract of swine. It is a potential pathogen, causing respiratory tract infections and polyserositis in swine. Called also *H. suis.*   **H. pertus′sis,** *Bordetella pertussis.*   **H. su′is,** *H. parasuis.*   **H. vagina′lis,** *Gardnerella vaginalis.*

Haemophoructus (hem″o-fo-ruk′tus)   a genus of bloodsucking flies of the family Heleidae.

Haemopis (he-mo′pis)   a genus of leeches, the horse leeches, of the family Gnathobdellidae. *H. paludum* is parasitic in the nose and throat in Ceylon. *H. sanguisuga* of Europe and North Africa infests the nasal passages.

Haemoproteus (he″mo-pro′te-us) [*hemo-* + Gr. *prōteus* a many-formed deity]   a genus of coccidian protozoa (suborder Haemosporina, order Eucoccidiida) in which the vectors are blood-sucking insects other than mosquitoes and the vertebrate hosts are mammals, reptiles, and commonly wild birds and domestic ducks, pigeons, and turkeys. In these oganisms merogony takes place not in erythrocytes but in the vascular endothelial cells, and the gametocytes are found only in the circulating erythrocytes.

haemorrhagia (hem″o-ra′je-ah) [L.]   hemorrhage.

Haemosporina (he″mo-spo-ri′nah) [*hemo-* + *spore*]   a suborder of heteroxenous protozoa (subclass Coccidia, class Sporozoea) in which merogony takes place in a vertebrate, usually in the blood, and sporogony in the alimentary canal of a blood-sucking insect. Hemosporians are characterized by the independent development of macrogamete and microgamont; the absence of syzygy; the usual absence of a conoid; the production by the microgamont of eight flagellated microgametes; and the formation of a motile zygote (ookinete). Representative genera include *Haemoproteus*, *Hepatocystis*, *Leucocytozoon*, and *Plasmodium*.

haemozoin (he″mo-zo′in) hemozoin.

Haenel's symptom (ha′nelz) [Hans *Haenel*, German neurologist, 1874–1942] see under *symptom*.

Haeser (ha′ser) see *Häser*.

Haff disease (haf) [named for Königsberg *Haff*, a lagoon connected with the Baltic Sea, where epidemics occurred in 1924–5, 1932–3, and 1940] see under *disease*.

Hafnia (haf′ne-ah) [L. *Hafnia* the old name for Copenhagen] a genus of gram-negative facultatively anaerobic rod-shaped bacteria of the family Enterobacteriaceae, made up of motile, peritrichously flagellated, unencapsulated organisms. **H. al′vei,** a species found in feces, sewage, soil, water, and dairy products. Called also *Enterobacter hafnia*.

hafnium (haf′ne-um) [L. *Hafnia*, Copenhagen] a chemical element of atomic number 72 and atomic weight 178.49; symbol Hf. Discovered in a zircon, in 1923, by Coster and Hevesy of Copenhagen.

Hagedorn needle (hahg′ĕ-dorn) [Werner *Hagedorn*, German surgeon, 1831–1894] see under *needle*.

Haglund's disease (hahg′loondz) [Sims Emil Patrik *Haglund*, Swedish orthopedist, 1870–1937] see under *disease*.

Hagner bag, (hag′nerz) [Francis Randall *Hagner*, American surgeon, 1873–1940] see under *bag*.

hahnemannian (hah″nĕ-man′e-an) pertaining to Christian Friedrich Samuel *Hahnemann* (1755–1843), founder of homeopathy.

hahnemannism (hah′nĕ-man″izm) homeopathy.

hahnium (hah′ne-um) [named for Otto *Hahn*, German physical chemist, 1879–1968] a transuranic element of atomic number 105, atomic weight 260, symbol Ha, produced by an induced nuclear reaction.

HAI hemagglutination inhibition; see under *tests*.

Haidinger's brushes (hi′ding-erz) [Wilhelm von *Haidinger*, Austrian mineralogist, 1795–1871] see under *brush*.

Haines' formula (coefficient), reagent, test (hānz′) [Walter Stanley *Haines*, Chicago chemist, 1850–1923] see under *formula, reagent,* and *tests*.

hair (hār) [L. *pilus;* Gr. *thrix*] a long slender filament. Applied especially to such filamentous appendages of the skin (pili [NA]), consisting of keratin; also the aggregate of such filaments, especially that of the scalp (capilli [NA]). Each hair consists of a cylindrical *shaft* and a root, which is contained in a flasklike depression (*hair follicle*) in the corium and subcutaneous tissue. The base of the root is expanded into the *hair bulb*, which rests upon and encloses the *hair papilla*. **auditory h's,** hairlike attachments of the specialized epithelial cells of the cristae acusticae and the maculae acusticae. **bamboo h.,** trichorrhexis nodosa. **beaded h.,** hair marked with alternate swellings and constrictions, as seen in monilethrix. Called also *moniliform h.* **burrowing h.,** one which does not emerge from the skin but grows horizontally beneath its surface, exciting a foreign body papule, which may become infected. Called also *pilus cuniculatus.* Cf. *ingrown h.* **club h.,** a hair the root of which is surrounded by a bulbous enlargement composed of completely keratinized cells, preliminary to normal loss of the hair from the follicle; see *telogen.* **exclamation point h.,** a hair which, when pulled out, shows atrophy and attenuation of the bulb; it is characteristic of alopecia areata. **h's of eyebrow,** supercilia. **Frey's h's,** stiff hairs mounted in a handle; used for testing the sensitiveness of the pressure points of the skin. **ingrown h.,** one which emerges from the skin but curves and reenters it, exciting a foreign body papule, which may become infected. Called also *pilus incarnatus.* Cf. *burrowing h.* **knotted h.,** trichonodosis. **lanugo h.,** the fine hair growing on the body of the fetus, constituting the lanugo. **moniliform h.,** beaded h. **h's of nose,** vibrissae. **olfactory h's,** modified cilia that are extremely long and nonmotile, which project from the bulblike distal part of an olfactory cell (*olfactory vesicle* [def. 2]), and function as sensory receptors. Called also *olfactory cilia.* **pubic h.,** pubes, def. 1. **resting h.,** see *telogen.* **sensory h's,** hairlike projections on the surface of sensory epithelial cells. **stellate h.,** a hair split at the end in a starlike form. **tactile h's,** hairs which are sensitive to touch, as the vibrissae of certain animals. **taste h's,** short hairlike processes projecting freely into the lumen of the pit of a taste bud from the peripheral ends of the taste cells. **terminal h.,** the coarse hair growing on various areas of the body during adult years. **twisted h.,** a hair which at spaced intervals is twisted through an axis of 180 degrees, being abnormally flattened at the site of twisting. Called also *pilus tortus.* **vellus h.,** the downy hair growing on the body during the prepuberal years, constituting the vellus.

hairball (hār′bawl) trichobezoar.

haircap (hār′kap) *Polytrichum juniperinum.*

haircast (hār′kast) a trichobezoar filling and assuming the shape of the stomach.

halation (hal-a′shun) [Gr. *halōs* halo] indistinctness or blurring of the visual image by strong illumination coming from the same direction as the viewed object.

halazepam (hal-az′e-pam) chemical name: 7-chloro-1,3-dihydro-5-phenyl-1-(2,2,2-trifluoroethyl)-2*H*-1,4-benzodiazepin-2-one; a tranquilizer, $C_{17}H_{12}ClF_3N_2O$.

halazone (hal-ah-zōn) [USP] chemical name: *p*-(dichlorosulfamoyl)benzoic acid. A white, crystalline powder, $C_7H_5Cl_2NO_4S$, having a chlorine-like odor; used as a disinfectant for water supplies.

halcinonide (hal-sin′o-nīd) chemical name: 21-chloro-9-fluoro-11β-hydroxy-16α,17-[(1-methylethylidene)bis(oxy)]-pregn-4-ene-3,20-dione. A synthetic glucocorticoid, $C_{24}H_{32}ClFO_5$; used as a topical anti-inflammatory in the treatment of various steroid-responsive dermatoses.

Haldane chamber (apparatus) (hawl′dān) [John Scott *Haldane*, English physiologist, 1860–1936] see under *chamber.*

Haldol (hal′dol) trademark for a preparation of haloperidol.

Haldrone (hal′drōn) trademark for a preparation of paramethasone acetate.

Hales' piesimeter (hālz) [Stephen *Hales*, English physiologist, 1677–1761] see under *piesimeter.*

half-life (haf′līf) the time required for the decay of half of a sample of particles of a radionuclide or elementary particle, equal to 0.693 divided by the decay constant; symbol $t_{\frac{1}{2}}$ or $T_{\frac{1}{2}}$. **antibody h.,** a measure of the mean survival time of antibody molecules following their formation, usually expressed as the time required to eliminate 50% of a known quantity of immunoglobulin from the animal body. Half-life varies from one immunoglobulin class to another. **biological h.,** the time required for a living tissue, organ, or organism to eliminate one-half of a radioactive substance which has been introduced into it. **effective h.,** the time required for the radioactivity of a radioactive nuclide to be diminished 50 per cent through the combined action of radioactive decay and biological elimination.

half-time (haf′tīm) the time required for one half of a quantity of a substance to be eliminated from a system when the substance is eliminated at a rate proportional to its concentration (i.e., exhibits first-order kinetics); symbol $t_{\frac{1}{2}}$ or $T_{\frac{1}{2}}$. **plasma iron clearance h.,** the time required for half of the iron in the blood plasma at a given time to be removed, determined from the slope of the best-line line to a semilogarithmic plot of the plasma radioactivity after administration of iron-59 bound to the patient's own transferrin.

half-value see under *layer.*

halfway house (haf′wa hous″) a residence for patients, such as mental patients, drug addicts, and alcoholics, who do not require hospitalization but who need an intermediate degree of care until they have again become established in the community.

halide (hal′īd) 1. haloid. 2. a binary compound of one of the halogens (fluorine, chlorine, bromine, or iodine).

hali-ichthyotoxin (hal″ĭ-ik″the-o-tok′sin) a poisonous base of bacterial origin from stale fish.

halisteresis (hah-lis″tĕ-re′sis) [Gr. *hals* salt + *sterēsis* privation] osteomalacia; a loss or lack of the lime salts (calcium) of bone. **h. ce′rea,** waxy softening of the bones.

halisteretic (hah-lis″tĕ-ret′ik) affected with or of the nature of halisteresis.

halitosis (hal-ĭ-to′sis) [L. *halitus* exhalation] offensive breath; bad breath. Called also *fetor ex ore, fetor oris,* and *stomatodysodia.*

halituous (hah-lit′u-us) [L. *halitus* exhalation] covered with moisture or vapor.

halitus (hal′ĭ-tus) [L.] an exhalation or vapor; an expired breath. **h. saturni′nus,** lead breath.

Hall band (hawl) [Herbert H. *Hall,* Bohemian obstetrician and gynecologist in the United States, born 1914] see under *band.*

Hall's method (hawlz) [Marshall *Hall,* English physician, 1790–1857] see *artificial respiration,* under *respiration.*

hallachrome (hal′ah-krōm) a compound formed from dihydroxyphenylalanine by tyrosinase.

Hallauer's glasses (hal′ow-erz) [Otto *Hallauer,* Basel ophthalmologist, born 1866] see under *glasses.*

Hallberg effect (hawl′berg) [Josef Hendrik *Hallberg,* American electrician, born 1874] see under *effect.*

Hallé's point (al-āz′) [Adrien Joseph Marie Noël *Hallé,* French physician, 1859–1947] see under *point.*

Haller's ansa, etc. (hal′erz) [Albrecht von *Haller,* Swiss physiologist, 1708–1777, the master physiologist of his time] see under *arch, circle, cone, crypt, duct, fretum, habenula, layer, line, membrane, plexus, rete,* and *tripod.*

hallex (hal′eks), pl. **hal′lices.** Hallux.

Hallion's test (al-yawz′) [Louis *Hallion,* French physiologist, 1862–1940] Tuffier's test.

Hallopeau's acrodermatitis (al-o-pōz′) [François Henri *Hallopeau,* French dermatologist, 1842–1919] see *acrodermatitis continua.*

hallucal (hal′u-kal) pertaining to the hallux, or great toe.

halluces (hal′ŭ-sēz, hal′lu-sēz) [L.] plural of *hallux.*

hallucination (hah-lu″sĭ-na′shun) [L. *hallucinatio;* Gr. *alyein* to wander in the mind] a sense perception without a source in the external world; a perception of an external stimulus object in the absence of such an object. **auditory h.,** a hallucination involving the sense of hearing. **gustatory h.,** a hallucination involving the sense of taste. **haptic h.,** tactile h. **hypnagogic h.,** a vivid dreamlike hallucination occurring at sleep onset or awakening. **hypnopompic h.,** a vivid dreamlike hallucination occurring on awakening. **kinesthetic h.,** a hallucination involving the sense of bodily movement. **lilliputian h.,** a visual hallucination in which things seem smaller than they actually are; called also *micropsia.* **olfactory h.,** a hallucination involving the sense of smell. **somatic h.,** a hallucination involving the perception of a physical experience occurring with the body. **stump h.,** phantom limb. **tactile h.,** a hallucination involving the sense of touch. **visual h.,** a hallucination involving the sense of sight.

hallucinative, hallucinatory (hah-lu′sĭ-na-tiv; hah-lu′sĭ-nah-to″re) characterized by hallucinations.

hallucinogen (hah-lu′sĭ-no-jen″) [*hallucin*ation + Gr. *gennan* to produce] an agent which induces hallucinations.

hallucinogenesis (hah-lu″sĭ-no-jen′ĕ-sis) the production of hallucinations.

hallucinogenetic (hah-lu″sĭ-no-jĕ-net′ik) hallucinogenic.

hallucinogenic (hah-lu″sĭ-no-jen′ik) producing hallucinations.

hallucinosis (hah-lu″sĭ-no′sis) a state characterized by the presence of hallucinations without other impairment of consciousness. **organic h.** [DSM III-R], an organic brain syndrome characterized by the presence of hallucinations caused by a specific organic factor and not associated with delirium. Causes include hallucinogen use, chronic alcohol abuse, sensory deprivation, and seizure foci.

hallucinotic (hah-lu″sĭ-not′ik) pertaining to or characterized by hallucinosis.

hallux (hal′uks), gen. **hal′lucis,** pl. **hal′luces** [L.] [NA] the great toe, or first digit of the foot; called also *digitus primus (I) pedis* [NA alternative]. **h. doloro′sa,** a painful disease of the great toe usually associated with flatfoot. **h. flex′us,** h. rigidus. **h. mal′leus,** hammer toe of the hallux. **h. rig′idus,** painful flexion deformity of the great toe in which there is limitation of motion at the metatarsophalangeal joint. **h. val′gus,** angulation of the great toe away from the midline of the body, or toward the other toes; the great toe may ride under or over the other toes. **h. va′rus,** angulation of the great toe toward the midline of the body, or away from the other toes.

Hallwachs effect (hal′vaks) [Franz *Hallwachs,* physiologist

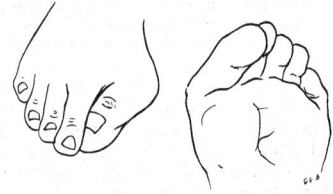

Hallux valgus.

in Dresden, 1859–1922] photoelectrical effect; see under *effect.*

halmatogenesis (hal″mah-to-jen′ĕ-sis) [Gr. *halma* a jump + *genesis*] a sudden alteration of type from one generation to another; called also *saltatory variation.*

halo (ha′lo) [L.; Gr. *halōs*] 1. a luminous or colored circle, such as the colored circle seen around a light in glaucoma. 2. a ring seen around the macula lutea in ophthalmoscopical examination. 3. the imprint of the ciliary processes upon the vitreous body. **Fick's h.,** a colored circle appearing around a light, caused by the wearing of contact lenses; see *Fick's phenomenon.* **h. glaucomato′sus, glaucomatous h.,** peripapillary atrophy seen in severe or chronic glaucoma. **h. saturni′nus,** lead line. **senile h.,** a zone of variable width surrounding the optic papilla, caused by exposure of various elements of the choroid as a result of senile atrophy of the pigmented epithelium.

hal(o)- [Gr. *hals,* gen. *halos* salt] a combining form denoting relationship to a salt.

halobacteria (hal″o-bak-te′re-ah) plural of *halobacterium.*

Halobacteriaceae (hal″o-bak″te-re-a′se-e) a family of aerobic, rod-shaped and coccoid bacteria, made up of chemo-organotrophic organisms that require at least 8 per cent and in most cases 17 to 23 per cent sodium chloride for growth. These extremely halophilic bacteria, which belong to the archaeobacteria group, do not contain peptidoglycan in their cell walls and differ from other bacteria in ribosomal RNA and cell lipid structures. They contain carotenoid pigments, and they are found in pools of evaporating sea water and material preserved with sea salts. The family contains the genera *Halobacterium* and *Halococcus.*

Halobacterium (hal″o-bak-te′re-um) [halo- + Gr. *baktērion* little rod] a genus of gram-negative, aerobic, pleomorphic, rod-shaped bacteria of the family Halobacteriaceae that require a high concentration of sodium chloride (15 per cent or greater) for growth. They contain a red carotenoid pigment (bacterioruferin) and a purple pigment (bacteriorhodopsin), which powers a system of photosynthesis. They are found in evaporating sea water, salt lakes, and heavily salted protein materials. The type species is *H. salina′rium.*

halobacterium (hal″o-bak-te′re-um), pl. *halobacte′ria.* Any member of the genus *Halobacterium.*

Halococcus (hal″o-kok′us) [halo- + Gr. *kokkos* berry] a genus of gram-negative aerobic bacteria of the family Halobacteriaceae, made up of coccoid cells that require a high concentration of sodium chloride (15 per cent or greater) for growth. They contain a red carotenoid pigment and are found in salted meats and fish. The type species is *H. morrhu′ae.*

halodermia (hal″o-der′me-a) any skin eruption caused by a halide.

haloduric (hal″o-du′rik) [Gr. *hals* salt + L. *durare* to endure] capable of existing in a medium containing a high concentration of salt.

halofenate (hal″lo-fen′āt) chemical name: 4-chloro-α-[3-(trifluoromethyl)phenoxy]benzeneacetic acid 2-(acetylamino) ethyl ester; an antihyperlipidemic and uricosuric agent, $C_{19}H_{17}ClF_3NO_4$.

Halog (hal′og) trademark for preparations of halcinonide.

halogen (hal′o-jen, ha′lo-jen) [halo- + Gr. *gennan* to produce] an element of a closely related chemical family, all of which form similar (saltlike) compounds in combination with sodium and most other metals. The halogens are bromine, chlorine, fluorine, iodine, and astatine.

halogeton (hal-o-ge′ton) a small grayish brown plant introduced into the southwestern U.S. that contains soluble oxalates, which can be highly poisonous, causing respiratory difficulty and hemorrhage as well as hypocalcemia. The major species is *Halogeton glomera'tus* (Bieb.) C. A. Mey. (Polygonaceae).

haloid (hal′oid) [halo- + Gr. *eidos* form] saltlike; derived from or resembling a halogen.

halometer (hah-lom′ĕ-ter) [halo + -meter] 1. an instrument for measuring ocular halos. 2. an instrument for estimating the size of red corpuscles by measuring the diffraction halos which they produce.

halometry (hah-lom′ĕ-tre) 1. the measurement of ocular halos. 2. the measurement of the size of red blood corpuscles by utilizing the blood smear as a diffraction grating.

Halomonas (ha″lo-mo′nas) [halo- + Gr. *monas* unit, from *monos* single] a genus of gram-negative, aerobic, rod-shaped bacteria of uncertain affiliation, made up of motile cells capable of growth in high-salt concentrations, occurring in saline waters. The type species is *H. elonga'ta.*

halopemide (hal″o-pem′id) chemical name: *N*-[2-[4-(5-chloro- 2,3-dihydro-2-oxo-1*H*-benzimidazol-1-yl)-1-piperidinyl]ethyl]-4- fluorobenzamide; a tranquilizer, $C_{21}H_{22}ClFN_4O_2$.

haloperidol (hah″lo-per′ĭ-dol) [USP] chemical name: 4-[4-(4-chlorophenyl)-4-hydroxy-1-piperidinyl]-1-butanone. A tranquilizer, $C_{21}H_{23}ClFNO_2$, which also has antiemetic, hypotensive, and hypothermic actions, occurring as a white to faintly yellowish, amorphous or microcrystalline powder; used especially in the management of psychoses and for the control of the vocal utterances and tics of Gilles de la Tourette's syndrome, administered orally and intramuscularly.

halophil (hal′o-fil) a microorganism that requires a high concentration of salt for optimal growth.

halophile (hal′o-fīl) 1. halophil. 2. halophilic.

halophilic (hal″o-fil′ik) [Gr. *hals* salt + *philein* to love] pertaining to or characterized by an affinity for salt; applied to microorganisms which require a high concentration of salt for optimal growth.

halopredone acetate (hal′o-pre″don) chemical name: 17,21- bis(acetyloxy)-2- bromo- 6β, 9- difluoro- 11β- hydroxypregna-1,4-diene-3,20-dione; a topical anti-inflammatory, $C_{25}H_{29}BrF_2O_7$.

haloprogin (hah″lo-pro′jin) chemical name: 1,2,4-trichloro-5-[(3-iodo-2-propynyl)oxy]benzene. A synthetic topical antifungal, $C_9H_4Cl_3IO$, occurring as a pale yellow, crystalline powder; used in the treatment of various forms of tinea.

halosteresis (hah-los″tĕ-re′sis) halisteresis.

Halotestin (hal′o-tes″tin) trademark for a preparation of fluoxymesterone.

Halotex (hal′o-teks) trademark for a preparation of haloprogin.

halothane (hal′o-thān) [USP] chemical name: 2-bromo-2-chloro-1,1,1-trifluoroethane, a potent inhalational anesthetic, widely used for induction and maintenance of general anesthesia; it is nonflammable, induction and recovery are smooth and rapid, and the depth of anesthesia is rapidly altered.

haloxon (hah-loks′on) an organophosphorus compound, $C_{14}H_{14}Cl_3O_6P$, used in veterinary medicine against intestinal nematodes.

halquinol (hal′kwin-ōl) halquinols.

halquinols (hal′kwin-ōls) a topical anti-infective compound, consisting of a mixture of 5,7-dichloro-8-quinolinol, 5-chloro-8-quinolinol, and 7-chloro-8-quinolinol in proportions resulting naturally from chlorination of 8-quinolinol; it has antiamebic, antifungal, and antibacterial actions.

Halsted's operation, suture (hal′stedz) [William Stewart *Halsted*, Baltimore surgeon, 1852–1922] see under *operation* and *suture.*

Haly Abbas see *Ali Abbas.*

halzoun (hal′zun) a pharyngeal form of fascioliasis occurring in the Middle East, caused by eating raw animal livers infected with *Fasciola;* young adult worms attach to the pharyngeal mucosa and produce pain, bleeding, and facial and neck edema.

Ham's test (hamz) [Thomas Hale *Ham*, American physician, born 1905] acidified serum test.

Hamamelis (ham″ah-me′lis) [Gr. *hama* together + *mēlon*

apple] a genus of trees and shrubs. The leaves of *H. virginia′na* L. (Hamamelidaceae), or witch hazel, contain tannin and hamamelose.

hamamelis (ham″ah-me′lis) the dried leaves of *Hamamelis virginiana,* or witch hazel, which have been used as an astringent, and in veterinary medicine in the treatment of anal irritation of dogs.

hamamelose (ham-am′e-lōs) a natural sugar, CH_2OH-$(CHOH)_2\cdot COH(CH_2OH)\cdot COH$, from the bark of *Hamamelis virginiana,* or witch hazel.

hamarthritis (ham″ar-thri′tis) [Gr. *hama* together + *arthritis*] arthritis of all the joints at the same time.

hamartia (ham-ar′she-ah) [Gr. "defect"] a defect in tissue combination during development.

hamartial (ham-ar′she-al) pertaining to or exhibiting a hamartia.

hamart(o)- [Gr. *hamartia* fault] a combining form denoting relationship to a defect or to a hamartoma.

hamartoblastoma (ham-ar″to-blas-to′mah) [hamarto- + Gr. *blastos* germ + -oma] a tumor developing from a hamartoma.

hamartoma (ham″ar-to′mah) [hamarto- + -oma] a benign tumor-like nodule composed of an overgrowth of mature cells and tissues that normally occur in the affected part, but often with one element predominating.

hamartomatosis (ham″ar-to-mah-to′sis) the development of multiple hamartomas.

hamartomatous (ham″ar-to′mah-tus) pertaining to a disturbance in growth of a tissue in which the cells of a circumscribed area outstrip those of the surrounding areas.

hamate (ham′at) hooked, as the hamate bone.

hamatum (hah-ma′tum) [L. "hooked"] the os hamatum, or unciform bone.

Hamberger's schema (ham′ber-gerz) [Georg Erhard *Hamberger,* German physician, 1697–1755] see under *schema.*

Hamburger interchange (ham′boor-ger) [Hartog Jacob *Hamburger,* Dutch physiologist, 1859–1924] the ionic interchange between the corpuscles and plasma of the blood; bicarbonate passes from the erythrocytes into the plasma, and chloride ions pass from the plasma into the erythrocytes. Called also *secondary buffering.*

Hamilton's bandage, test (ham′il-tonz) [Frank Hastings *Hamilton,* American surgeon, 1813–1886] see under *bandage* and *tests.*

Hamman's disease, syndrome, sign (ham′anz) [Louis *Hamman,* American physician, 1877–1946] see *pneumomediastinum,* and see under *sign.*

Hamman-Rich syndrome (ham′an rich) [Louis *Hamman;* Arnold Rice *Rich,* American pathologist, 1893–1968] idiopathic pulmonary fibrosis.

Hammarsten's test (ham′er-stenz) [Olof *Hammarsten,* physiologist in Upsala, 1841–1932] see under *tests.*

hammer (ham′er) 1. an instrument with a head designed for striking blows. 2. the hammer-shaped bone of the middle ear; the malleus. **Neef's h., Wagner's h.,** an instrument for the rapid opening and closing of a galvanic circuit.

Hammerschlag's method (test) (ham′er-shlahgz) [Albert *Hammerschlag,* physician in Vienna, 1863–1935] see under *method.*

Hammond's disease (ham′undz) [William Alexander *Hammond,* American neurologist, 1828–1900] athetosis.

hamster (ham′ster) a ratlike rodent, the most common of which is *Cricetus cricetus* of Europe and Western Asia, bred and used extensively as a laboratory animal. Other species are *Cricetulus larabensis,* the Chinese hamster, and *Mesocretus auratus,* the Syrian hamster.

hamstring (ham′string) one of the tendons that bound the popliteal fossa laterally and medially. **inner h.,** the tendons of the gracilis, sartorius, and two other muscles. **outer h.,** the tendon of the biceps flexor femoris.

hamular (ham′u-lar) shaped like a hook.

hamulus (ham′u-lus), pl. *ham′uli* [L. "little hook"] [NA] a general term denoting a hook-shaped process. **h. coch′leae,** h. laminae spiralis. **h. ethmoid bone,** processus uncinatus ossis ethmoidalis. **frontal h., h. fronta′lis,** ala cristae galli. **h. of hamate bone,** h. ossis hamati. **lacrimal h., h. lacrima′lis** [NA], the hooklike process on the anterior part of the inferolateral border of the lacrimal bone, articulating with the maxilla. **h. lam'i-nae spira'lis** [NA], the hooklike upper end of the osseous spiral lamina. **h. os'sis hama'ti** [NA], hamulus of hamate bone: a hooklike process on the volar surface of the hamate bone, to which numerous structures are attached. **pterygoid h., h. pterygoi'deus** [NA], a hooklike process on the inferior extremity of the medial pterygoid plate of the sphenoid bone, around which the tendon of the tensor veli palatini muscle passes. **trochlear h.**, spina trochlearis.

hamycin (hah-mi'sin) an antibiotic derived from *Streptomyces pimprina*, having antifungal, antitrichomonal, and anti-inflammatory actions; it has been used topically in various fungal infections of the skin.

Hancock's amputation (han'koks) [Henry *Hancock*, English surgeon, 1809–1880] see under *amputation*.

hand (hand) [L. *manus*] the part of the upper limb distal to the forearm: the carpus, metacarpus, and fingers together; called also *manus* [NA]. **accoucheur's h.**, obstetrician's h. **ape h.**, a hand with the thumb permanently extended. **benediction h.**, a hand in which the ring and little fingers are flexed; there is weakness of abduction and adduction of the index and middle fingers but they can be extended normally, and the thumb remains normal; seen in ulnar paralysis and syringomyelia. **claw h.**, see *clawhand*. **cleft h.**, malformation of the hand in which the division between the fingers extends into the metacarpus; also, a hand in which the middle digits are absent, and the remaining fingers are abnormally large; called also *lobster-claw hand* and *main fourché*. **club h.**, clubhand; see *talipomanus*. **dead h.**, an occupational disorder seen sometimes in those who use vibratory tools, and apparently caused by the multitude of concussions. The hands are painful and dark blue in color, but blanch on exposure to cold. **drop h.**, see *wristdrop*. **flat h.**, manus plana. **frozen h.**, stiffness of the hand resulting from edema accompanying trauma. **ghoul h.**, a condition in which the skin of the palm is depigmented and of a dead-white, tallow-yellow color, with blotchy areas of brownish hyperpigmentation, observed in black Africans and associated with late yaws. **lobster-claw h.**, cleft h. **Marinesco's succulent h.**, main succulente. **mirror h's**, a deformity in which there are two crude hands growing from a common wrist. **mitten h.**, a hand in which several fingers are fused together and have a common nail. **monkey h.**, a hand showing atrophy of the thenar muscles; called also *main en singe*. **obstetrician's h.**, the contraction of the hand in tetany; the hand is flexed at the wrist, the fingers at the metacarpophalangeal joints but extended at the interphalangeal joints, the thumb being strongly flexed into the palm; so called because of a dubious resemblance to the position assumed by the hand of the obstetrician when examining the vagina. Called also *accoucheur's h.* and *main d'accoucheur*. **opera-glass h.**, a pawlike hand marked by telescoping of the fingers caused by absorption of the phalanges; occurs in chronic arthritis. **phantom h.**, a paresthetic feeling as if the hand were still present after amputation. **preacher's h.**, benediction h. **skeleton h.**, a hand markedly atrophied and held in a position of extension; seen in progressive muscular atrophy; called also *main en squelette*. **spade h.**, the thick square hand of myxedema and acromegaly. **split h.**, cleft hand. **trench h.**, contracture or other incapacity of the hand from frostbite in the trenches; called also *main de tranchées*. **trident h.**, the characteristic hand of achondroplasia: the fingers are relatively of the same length, and there is a peculiar separation of the second and third fingers at the second phalangeal joint, causing the fingers to spread out. **writing h.**, a peculiar position of the hand in which the hand appears poised for writing; seen in paralysis agitans.

Hand's disease, syndrome (handz) [Alfred *Hand*, Jr., Philadelphia pediatrician, 1868–1949] Hand-Schüller-Christian disease; see under *disease*.

Hand-Schüller-Christian disease (syndrome) (hand-shil'er-kris'chan) [Alfred *Hand*; Artur *Schüller*; Henry A. *Christian*] see under *disease*.

handedness (hand'ed-nes) the preferential use in voluntary motor acts of the hand of one side. **left h.**, the preferential use in voluntary motor acts of the left hand. **right h.**, the preferential use in voluntary motor acts of the right hand.

handicap (han'dǐ-kap) any physical or mental defect or characteristic, congenital or acquired, preventing or restricting a person from participating in normal life or limiting his capacity to work.

handpiece (hand'pēs) a hand-held device that engages rotary instruments used for removing tooth structures, cleaning teeth, and polishing dental restorations, connected to the dental engine by an adjustable arm in the case of a belt-driven instrument or by flexible tubing if air driven.

HANE hereditary angioneurotic edema; see *hereditary angioedema*, under *angioedema*.

Hanger's test (hang'erz) [Franklin M. *Hanger*, Jr., American physician, 1894–1971] see *cephalin-cholesterol flocculation test*, under *tests*.

hangnail (hang'nāl) a shred of eponychium on a proximal or lateral nail fold.

Hannover's canal (han'o-verz) [Adolph *Hannover*, Danish anatomist, 1814–1894] see under *canal*.

Hanot's cirrhosis (disease, syndrome) (an-ōz') [Victor Charles *Hanot*, French physician, 1844–1896] 1. primary biliary cirrhosis. 2. secondary biliary cirrhosis.

Hanot-Chauffard syndrome (an-o'sho-far') [Victor Charles *Hanot*; Anatole Marie Emile *Chauffard*, French physician, 1855–1932] see under *syndrome*.

Hansen's bacillus, disease (han'sunz) [Gerhard Henrik Armauer *Hansen*, Norwegian physician, 1841–1912] see *Mycobacterium leprae* and *leprosy*.

Hansenula (han-sen'u-lah) a genus of ascomycetous yeasts of the order Endomycetales, family Saccharomycetaceae; formerly called *Willia*. **H. anom'ala**, a nonpathogenic species commonly found in soil and in the respiratory and intestinal tracts.

haphalgesia (haf"al-je'ze-ah) [Gr. *haphē* touch + *algēsis* sense of pain + *-ia*] the sensation of pain on touching nonirritating objects or when the skin is lightly touched.

haphephobia (haf"e-fo'be-ah) [Gr. *haphē* touch + *phobia*] irrational fear of being touched.

hapl(o)- [Gr. *haploos* simple, single] a combining form meaning simple or single.

Haplochilus (hap"lo-ki'lus) a genus of fish. **H. pan'chax**, a small fish, called *ikan kapala timah* in Malay, which is placed in fishponds in Indonesia to eat the larvae of *Anopheles* mosquitoes.

haplodiploidy (hap"lo-dip'loi-de) [*hapto-* + *diploidy*] the state in which males develop from unfertilized eggs and are haploid, and females develop from fertilized eggs and are diploid, as in honeybees.

haplodont (hap'lo-dont) [*haplo-* + Gr. *odous* tooth] having molar teeth without cusps or ridges.

haploid (hap'loid) [*hapl-* + *-oid*] 1. having a single set of chromosomes, as normally carried by a gamete, or having one complete set of nonhomologous chromosomes. In man, the haploid number is 23. Symbol, n. Cf. *diploid* (def. 2). 2. an individual or cell having only one member of each pair of homologous chromosomes.

haploidentical (hap"lo-i-den'tǐ-kal) sharing a haplotype; having the same alleles at a set of closely linked genes on one chromosome.

haploidentity (hap"lo-i-den'tǐ-te) the condition of being haploidentical.

haploidy (hap'loi-de) the state of having only one member of each pair of homologous chromosomes.

haplomycosis (hap"lo-mi-ko'sis) adiospiromycosis.

haplont (hap'lont) [Gr. *haploun* to make single] a haploid individual.

Haplopappus (hap-lo-pap'pus) a genus of composite-flowered plants, the ingestion of which causes a disease similar to trembles.

haplopathy (hap-lop'ah-the) [*haplo-* + Gr. *pathos* disease] an uncomplicated disease.

haplophase (hap'lo-fāz) that phase in the life history of germ cells when the nuclei are haploid.

haplopia (hap-lo'pe-ah) [*hapl-* + *-opia*] single vision; the condition in which an object looked at is seen single and not double.

Haplorchis (hap-lor'kis) a genus of minute trematodes found in tropical areas, which are intestinal parasites of dogs, cats, and other vertebrates. **H. tai′chui,** an intestinal parasite of birds and mammals, rarely including man.

haploscope (hap′lo-skōp) [haplo- + -scope] an instrument that presents two separate views to the two eyes so that the views may be seen as one integrated view; it is used to measure, test, or stimulate various binocular functions. **mirror h.,** a haploscope that uses mirrors to separate or displace the fields of vision of the two eyes.

haploscopic (hap-lo-skop′ik) pertaining to a haploscope; stereoscopic.

haplosporangin (hap″lo-spo-ran′jin) an antigen derived from the fungus Emmonsia parva.

Haplosporangium (hap″lo-spo-ran′je-um) Emmonsia.

Haplosporidium (hap″lo-spo-rid′e-um) [haplo- + spore] a genus of parasitic protozoa (order Balanosporida, class Stellatosporea) found in the gut epithelium and connective tissue of annelids and the digestive glands of mollusks.

haplosporosome (hap″lo-spor′o-sōm) [haplo- + sporo- + Gr. soma body] a membrane-bound ultrastructural body found in the sarcoplasm of protozoa of the class Stellalosporea.

haplotype (hap′lo-tīp) [haplo- + type] 1. a set of alleles of a group of closely linked genes, such as the HLA complex, which is usually inherited as a unit. 2. the genetic constitution of an individual at a set of closely linked genes.

Hapsburg jaw, lip [Hapsburg, a German-Austrian royal family, including among its members many rulers of European states, such as Austria (1278–1918) and Spain (1504–1700)] see under jaw and lip; see also hemophilia (disease of the Hapsburgs).

hapten (hap′ten) [Ger., from Gr. haptein to fasten] a small molecule, not antigenic by itself, that can react with antibodies of appropriate specificity and elicit the formation of such antibodies when conjugated to a larger antigenic molecule, usually a protein, called in this context the carrier or schlepper. Antibody production involves activation of B lymphocytes by the hapten and helper T lymphocytes by the carrier.

haptene (hap′tēn) hapten.

haptenic (hap-ten′ik) pertaining to or caused by haptens.

haptephobia (hap″te-fo′be-ah) [Gr. haptein to touch + phobia] haphephobia.

haptic (hap′tik) [Gr. haptikos able to lay hold of] tactile.

haptics (hap′tiks) the science of touch, or the sense of contact.

hapt(o)- [Gr. haptein to fasten, grasp, touch] a combining form denoting relationship to touch or to binding.

haptocyst (hap′to-sist) [hapto- + cyst] one of the minute extensible organelles occurring at the tips of the tentacles of suctorians; believed to contain lytic enzymes and to function in the capture of prey.

haptoglobin (hap″to-glo′bin) a 100,000-dalton plasma glycoprotein with alpha, electrophoretic mobility that irreversibly binds free hemoglobin resulting in prompt removal of the hemoglobin-haptoglobin complex by the liver, preventing loss of free hemoglobin in the urine. Haptoglobin levels are decreased by hemolysis and increased owing to increased synthesis in conditions resulting in extensive tissue damage and necrosis. Haptoglobin has two major genetic variants, designated Hp 1 and Hp 2.

haptometer (hap-tom′ĕ-ter) [hapto- + Gr. metron measure] an instrument for measuring sensitivity to touch.

Haptorina (hap″to-ri′nah) [Gr. haptein touch, seize upon, or hold fast] a suborder of carnivorous ciliate protozoa (order Protostomalida, subclass Gymnostomatina), characterized by the presence of an oval or slitlike apical or subapical cytostome, a cytopharynx, clavate sensory cilia near the anterior end of the body, and toxicysts in the oral or circumoral region or in a proboscis or tentacles.

harara (hah-rar′ah) an allergic skin reaction caused by bites of the sand fly Phlebotomus papatasii. It occurs in the Middle East, and is characterized by urticarial and inflammatory papules and blisters. Immunity usually follows the initial exposure. Called also urticaria multiformis endemica. The term is also a popular name for various types of skin eruptions.

hardening (hard′en-ing) the procedure of rendering tissue firm, so that it may be more readily cut for purposes of microscopic examination.

Harden-Young ester (har′den yung) [Sir Arthur Harden, English biochemist, 1865–1940; William John Young, Australian biochemist, 20th century] see fructose-1,6-diphosphate.

Harder's glands (hard′erz) [Johann Jacob Harder, Swiss anatomist, 1656–1711] see under gland.

harderian (hard′er-e-an) named for Johann Jacob Harder, as harderian fossa or glands.

hardness (hard′nes) 1. a quality of water produced by soluble salts of calcium and magnesium or other substances which form an insoluble curd with soap and thus interfere with its cleansing power. 2. the quality of firmness produced by cohesion of the particles composing a substance, as evidenced by its inflexibility or resistance to indentation or distortion. 3. the quality of x-rays that determines their penetrating power; hardness depends on wavelength: the shorter the wavelength the harder the rays and the greater their penetrating power. 4. the degree of refraction of the residual gas in a glass tube: the higher the vacuum the shorter the wavelength of the resulting roentgen rays. **diamond pyramid h.,** Vickers hardness number. **permanent h.,** hardness of water not removed by boiling; it is usually due to sulfates and chlorides. **temporary h.,** hardness of water removed by boiling; it is due to soluble bicarbonates, which lose CO_2 on boiling and precipitate as normal carbonates.

Hare's syndrome (hārz) [Edward Selleck Hare, British surgeon, 1812–1838] Pancoast's syndrome, def. 1.

harelip (hār′lip) cleft lip.

harlequin (hahr′lĕ-kwin) a venomous snake belonging to the genus Elaps.

Harley's disease (har′lēz) [George Harley, English physician, 1829–1896] intermittent hemoglobinuria.

harmonia (har-mo′ne-ah) [L.] sutura plana.

harmony (har′mo-ne) the state of working together smoothly. **occlusal h.,** proper occlusion of the teeth occurring in various positions of the mandible. **occlusal h., functional,** such occlusion of the teeth in all positions of the mandible during mastication as will provide the greatest masticatory efficiency without imposing undue strain or trauma on the supporting tissues.

Harmonyl (har′mo-nil) trademark for preparations of deserpidine.

Harpirhynchus (har″pe-ring′kus) [Gr. harpē bird of prey + Gr. rhynchos snout] a genus of mites parasitic on birds.

harpoon (har-pōōn′) [Gr. harpazein to seize] an instrument for removing small pieces of living tissue for diagnostic examination.

Harrington instrumentation (har′ing-ton) [Paul R. Harrington, American orthopedic surgeon, born 1911] see under instrumentation.

Harrington's solution (har′ing-tonz) [Charles Harrington, American physician, 1856–1908] see under solution.

Harris' segregator (separator) (har′is) [Malcolm La Salle Harris, Chicago surgeon, 1862–1936] see under segregator.

Harris' staining method (har′is) [Downey Lamar Harris, American pathologist, 1875–1956] see under Table of Stains.

Harris' syndrome (har′is) [Seale Harris, American physician, 1870–1957] see under syndrome.

Harrison's groove (curve, sulcus) (har′ĭ-sunz) [Edward Harrison, London physician, 1766–1838] see under groove.

Hartel's treatment (har′telz) [Fritz Hartel, German surgeon of the 20th century] see under treatment.

Hartley-Krause operation (hart′le-krows) [Frank Hartley, New York surgeon, 1857–1913; Fedor Krause, German surgeon, 1857–1937] see under operation.

Hartline (hart′lin) Haldan Keffer. American physician and physiologist, born 1903; co-winner, with Ragnar Arthur Granit and George Wald, of the Nobel prize for medicine or physiology in 1967 for discoveries regarding the primary chemical and physiological visual processes in the eye.

Hartmann's curet, speculum (hart′manz) [Arthur Hartmann, laryngologist in Berlin, 1849–1931] see under curet and speculum.

Hartmann's point, pouch, procedure (operation, colostomy) (hart′manz) [Henri Hartmann, French surgeon,

1860–1952] See *Sudeck's critical point*, under *point*, and see under *pouch* and *procedure*.

Hartmannella (hart″mah-nel′ah) a genus of free-living protozoa (order Amoebida, class Rhizopoda) found in fresh water and soil, species of which, e.g., *H. hyalina*, are capable of facultative parasitism, causing a primary amebic meningo-encephalitis, especially in the immunocompromised host.

hartmannelliasis (hart″mah-nel-li′ah-sis) infection with *Hartmannella*.

hartshorn (harts′horn) 1. ammonium carbonate. 2. the horn of the stag or hart; cornu cervi.

harveian (har′ve-an) named in honor of William *Harvey*.

harvest (har′vest) to remove tissues or cells from a donor and preserve for transplantation.

Harvey (har′ve), William (1578–1657). English physician, student of Fabricius; he practiced in London and was physician to James I and Charles I. In his *Exercitatio anatomica de motu cordis et sanguinis* (1628), Harvey proved, among other things, that (1) contraction of the heart muscle coincides with the pulse as the ventricles pump blood into the aorta and pulmonary artery; (2) the pulse is produced by the arteries' filling with blood; (3) the septum is impervious; (4) venous and arterial blood are the same; and (5) the blood in the right ventricle goes through the arteries to the lungs and thence through the pulmonary veins to the left ventricle and thence through the arteries to the body venous it returns along the smaller veins to the venae cavae and then into the right ventricle—a complete circulation of the blood. Harvey's work was not fully substantiated until 1827.

Häser's formula (coefficient) (ha′zerz) [Heinrich *Häser*, German physician, 1811–1884] see under *formula*.

Hashimoto's thyroiditis, (disease, struma) (hash″ĭ-mo′tōz) [Hakaru *Hashimoto*, Japanese surgeon, 1881–1934] see under *thyroiditis*.

hashish (hash-ēsh′) [Arabic "herb"] a preparation of the unadulterated resin scraped from the flowering tops of cultivated female hemp plants, *Cannabis sativa* L. (Cannabaceae), which is smoked or chewed for its intoxicating effects. It is far more potent than marihuana. See *cannabis*. Also referred to as *charas* or *churus*.

Hasner's fold, valve (hahs′nerz) [Joseph Ritter von Artha *Hasner*, an ophthalmologist in Prague, 1819–1892] see *plica lacrimalis*.

Hassall's corpuscles (bodies) (has′alz) [Arthur Hill *Hassall*, English chemist and physician, 1817–1894] see under *corpuscle*.

HAT hypoxanthine-aminopterin-thymidine (medium); see under *medium*.

Hata's phenomenon, preparation (hah′tahs) [Sahachiro *Hata*, Japanese physician, 1873–1938] see under *phenomenon* and *preparation*.

hatchet (hach′it) a bibeveled or single beveled cutting dental instrument having its cutting edge in line with the axis of its blade; used for breaking down tooth structure undermined by caries, smoothing cavity walls, and sharpening line and point angles. Called also *hatchet excavator*. **enamel h.**, one in which the broad side of the blade is parallel with the angle of the shank; used with a chipping or a lateral scraping stroke in developing an internal cavity form.

Hauch (howkh) [Ger. "breath"] See *H antigen*, under *antigen*.

Haudek's sign (niche) (haw′deks) [Martin *Haudek*, roentgenologist in Vienna, 1880–1931] see under *sign*.

haunch (hawnch) the hip and buttock.

hauptganglion of Küttner (howpt′gang″gle-on) nodus lymphaticus jugulodigastricus.

Haust. abbreviation for L. *haus′tus*, a draft.

haustellum (haw-stel′lum), pl. *haustel′la* [L. from *haustus* draw up] a mouthpart of certain ectoparasites, such as bedbugs and lice, modified for piercing and sucking, consisting of a hollow tube with an eversible set of five stylets, by which the organism attaches itself to the host and through which the blood is drawn up.

haustorium (haw-stor′ĭ-um), pl. *haus′tra* [L. from *haustus* draw up] a structure of certain parasites adapted specially to penetrate the host's tissues and absorb nutrients and water.

haustra (haws′trah) [L.] plural of *haustrum*.

haustral (hos′tral) pertaining to the haustra of the colon.

haustration (hos-tra′shun) 1. the formation of a haustrum. 2. a haustrum.

haustrum (hows′trum), pl. *haus′tra* [L. *haustor* drawer] [NA] a general term denoting a recess. **haus′tra co′li** [NA], **haustra of colon,** sacculations in the wall of the colon produced by adaptation of its length to that of the tenia coli, or by the arrangement of the circular muscle fibers.

haut-mal (o-mahl′) [Fr.] grand mal; see under *epilepsy*.

HAV hepatitis A virus.

Haverhill fever (ha′ver-il) [*Haverhill*, Mass., where an epidemic occurred in 1925] see under *fever*.

Haverhillia multiformis (ha″ver-il′e-ah mul″tĭ-for′mis) the name given to a slender gram-negative streptobacillus which was found in cases of Haverhill fever; now called *Streptobacillus moniliformis*.

haversian canal (space), glands, lamella, system (ha-ver′shan) [Clopton *Havers*, English physician and anatomist, 1650–1702; known for his researches on the minute structure of bone, which were recorded in his *Osteologia nova* (1691)] see *canalis nutricius ossis* and *villi synoviales*, and see under *lamella* and *system*.

hawkinsin (haw′kin-sin) [2-L-cystein-S-y 1-1,4-dihydroxy-cyclohex-5-en-lyl] acetic acid, a metabolite of tyrosine excreted in the urine in a rare form of tyrosinemia. It is formed from an intermediate of the 4-hydroxyphenylpyruvate dioxygenase reaction combined with glutathione.

hawkinsinuria (haw″kin-sin″u-re′ah) an autosomal dominant form of tyrosinemia associated with a defect of 4-hydroxyphenylpyruvate hydroxylase, manifested by the excretion of hawkinsin in the urine.

Hawley retainer (appliance) (haw′le) [C. A. *Hawley*, American dentist] see under *retainer*.

Hay's test (hāz) [Matthew *Hay*, Scotch physician, 1855–1932] see under *tests*.

Hayem's corpuscles, encephalitis, icterus (jaundice), solution (a-yawz′) [Georges *Hayem*, physician in Paris, 1841– 1933] see *platelet* and *encephalitis hyperplastica*, see *hemolytic anemia*, under *anemia*, and see under *solution*.

Hayem-Widal syndrome (a-yaw-ve′dal) [Georges *Hayem*; Georges Fernand Isidore *Widal*, French physician, 1862–1929] hemolytic anemia.

hay fever (ha fe′ver) see under *fever*.

Haygarth's nodes (nodosities) (ha′garths) [John *Haygarth*, English physician, 1740–1827] see under *node*.

Hazen's theorem (ha′zenz) [Allen *Hazen*, American hydraulic engineer, 1869–1930] see under *theorem*.

HB hepatitis B.

HB_c hepatitis B core (antigen).

HB_e hepatitis B e (antigen).

HB_s hepatitis B surface (antigen).

Hb symbol for *hemoglobin*.

HB_cAg hepatitis B core antigen.

HB_eAg hepatitis B e antigen.

HB_sAg hepatitis B surface (antigen).

HbO₂ oxyhemoglobin.

H₃BO₃ boric acid.

HBr hydrobromic acid.

HBV hepatitis B virus.

H.C. hospital corps.

HCG, hCG human chorionic gonadotropin.

HCHO formaldehyde.

HCl hydrochloric acid.

HCN hydrocyanic acid.

HCO₃ the bicarbonate radical.

H₂CO₃ carbonic acid.

HCT hematocrit.

H.d. abbreviation for L. *ho′ra decu′bitus*, at bedtime.

HDCV human diploid cell rabies vaccine.

HDL high-density lipoprotein.

HDL₁ Lp(a) lipoprotein.

HDL₂ see *high-density lipoprotein*, under *lipoprotein*.

HDL₃ see *high-density lipoprotein*, under *lipoprotein*.

HDN hemolytic disease of the newborn; see *erythroblastosis fetalis*.

H and E hematoxylin and eosin (stain). See *Table of Stains*.

He chemical symbol for *helium*.

he- for words beginning thus, see also those beginning *hae-*.

head (hed) [L. *caput*; Gr. *kephalē*] the upper, anterior, or proximal extremity of a structure or body, especially that part of an organism which contains the brain and the organs of special sense; called also *caput* [NA]. **angular h. of quadratus labii superioris muscle,** musculus levator labii superioris alaeque nasi. **articular h.,** an eminence on a bone by which it articulates with another bone. **h. of astragalus,** caput tali. **big h.,** bighead. **h. of caudate nucleus,** caput nuclei caudati. **h. of condyloid process of mandible,** caput mandibulae. **coronoid h. of pronator teres muscle,** caput ulnare musculi pronatoris teretis. **deep h. of triceps brachii muscle,** caput mediale musculi tricipitis brachii. **deep h. of triceps extensor cubiti muscle,** caput mediale musculi tricipitis brachii. **h. of dorsal horn of spinal cord,** caput cornus dorsalis medullae spinalis. **drum h.,** membrana tympani. **engaged h.,** the position of the fetal head when the biparietal eminences have passed the pelvic inlet. **h. of epididymis,** caput epididymidis. **h. of femur,** caput femoris. **h. of fibula,** caput fibulae. **first h. of triceps brachii muscle,** caput longum musculi tricipitis brachii. **first h. of triceps extensor cubiti muscle,** caput longum musculi tricipitis brachii. **floating h.,** the head of the fetus when it is freely movable above the inlet of the birth canal. **great h. of adductor hallucis muscle,** caput obliquum musculi adductoris hallucis. **great h. of triceps brachii muscle,** caput laterale musculi tricipitis brachii. **great h. of triceps extensor cubiti muscle,** caput laterale musculi tricipitis brachii. **great h. of triceps femoris muscle,** musculus adductor magnus. **hot cross bun h.,** caput natiforme. **hourglass h.,** a head in which the coronal suture is depressed. **humeral h. of flexor carpi ulnaris muscle,** caput humerale musculi flexoris carpi ulnaris. **humeral h. of flexor digitorum sublimis muscle,** caput humero-ulnare musculi flexoris digitorum superficialis. **humeral h. of pronator teres muscle,** caput humerale musculi pronatoris teretis. **humeroulnar h. of flexor digitorum superficialis muscle,** caput humero-ulnare musculi flexoris digitorum superficialis. **h. of humerus,** caput humeri. **infraorbital h. of quadratus labii superioris muscle,** musculus levator labii superioris. **lateral h. of gastrocnemius muscle,** caput laterale musculi gastrocnemii. **lateral h. of triceps brachii muscle,** caput laterale musculi tricipitis brachii. **lateral h. of triceps extensor cubiti muscle,** caput laterale musculi tricipitis brachii. **little h. of humerus,** capitulum humeri. **little h. of mandible,** processus condylaris mandibulae. **long h. of adductor hallucis muscle,** caput obliquum musculi adductoris hallucis. **long h. of adductor triceps muscle,** musculus adductor longus. **long h. of biceps brachii muscle,** caput longum musculi bicipitis brachii. **long h. of biceps femoris muscle,** caput longum musculi bicipitis femoris. **long h. of biceps flexor cruris muscle,** caput longum musculi bicipitis femoris. **long h. of biceps flexor cubiti muscle,** caput longum musculi bicipitis brachii. **long h. of triceps brachii muscle,** caput longum musculi tricipitis brachii. **long h. of triceps extensor cubiti muscle,** caput longum musculi tricipitis brachii. **long h. of triceps femoris muscle,** musculus adductor longus. **h. of malleus,** caput mallei. **h. of mandible,** 1. caput mandibulae. 2. processus condylaris mandibulae. **medial h. of biceps brachii muscle,** caput breve musculi bicipitis brachii. **medial h. of biceps flexor cubiti muscle,** caput breve musculi bicipitis brachii. **medial h. of gastrocnemius muscle,** caput mediale musculi gastrocnemii. **medial h. of triceps brachii muscle,** caput mediale musculi tricipitis brachii. **medial h. of triceps extensor cubiti muscle,** caput mediale musculi tricipitis brachii. **medusa h.,** caput medusae. **h. of metacarpal,** caput metacarpalis. **h. of metatarsal,** caput metatarsalis. **middle h. of triceps brachii muscle,** caput longum musculi tricipitis brachii. **middle h. of triceps extensor cubiti muscle,** caput lon-

gum musculi tricipitis brachii. **h. of muscle,** the end of a muscle at the site of its attachment (origin) to a bone or other fixed structure; called also *caput musculi*. **nasal h. of levator labii superioris alaeque nasi muscle,** musculus levator labii superioris alaeque nasi. **oblique h. of adductor hallucis muscle,** caput obliquum musculus adductoris hallucis. **oblique h. of adductor pollicis muscle,** caput obliquum musculi adductoris pollicis. **overriding h.,** the condition of the fetal head when it overrides the symphysis pubis instead of sinking into the pelvic cavity. **h. of pancreas,** caput pancreatis. **h. of penis,** glans penis. **h. of phalanx of fingers,** caput phalangis digitorum manus. **h. of phalanx of toes,** caput phalangis digitorum pedis. **plantar h. of flexor digitorum pedis longus muscle,** musculus quadratus plantae. **h. of posterior horn of spinal cord,** caput cornus dorsalis medullae spinalis. **quadrate h. of flexor digitorum pedis longus muscle,** musculus quadratus plantae. **radial h. of flexor digitorum sublimis muscle,** caput radiale musculi flexoris digitorum superficialis. **radial h. of flexor digitorum superficialis muscle,** caput radiale musculi flexoris digitorum superficialis. **radial h. of humerus,** capitulum humeri. **h. of radius,** caput radii. **h. of rib,** caput costae. **saddle h.,** a head with a sunken crown. **scapular h. of triceps brachii muscle,** caput longum musculi tricipitis brachii. **scapular h. of triceps extensor cubiti muscle,** caput longum musculi tricipitis brachii. **second h. of triceps brachii muscle,** caput laterale musculi tricipitis brachii. **short h. of biceps brachii muscle,** caput breve musculi bicipitis brachii. **short h. of biceps femoris muscle,** caput breve musculi bicipitis femoris. **short h. of biceps flexor cruris muscle,** caput breve musculi bicipitis femoris. **short h. of biceps flexor cubiti muscle,** caput breve musculi bicipitis brachii. **short h. of coracoradialis muscle,** caput breve musculi bicipitis brachii. **short h. of triceps brachii muscle,** caput mediale musculi tricipitis brachii. **short h. of triceps extensor cubiti muscle,** caput mediale musculi tricipitis brachii. **short h. of triceps femoris muscle,** musculus adductor brevis. **h. of spleen,** extremitas posterior lienis. **h. of stapes,** caput stapedis. **steeple h.,** oxycephaly. **swelled h.,** bighead, def. 2. **h. of talus,** caput tali. **tower h.,** oxycephaly. **transverse h. of adductor hallucis muscle,** caput transversum musculi adductoris hallucis. **transverse h. of adductor pollicis muscle,** caput transversum musculi adductoris pollicis. **h. of ulna,** caput ulnae. **ulnar h. of flexor carpi ulnaris muscle,** caput ulnare musculi flexoris carpi ulnaris. **ulnar h. of pronator teres muscle,** caput ulnare musculi pronatoris teretis. **white h.,** witkop. **zygomatic h. of quadratus labii superioris muscle,** musculus zygomaticus minor.

Head's zones [Sir Henry *Head*, London neurologist, 1861–1940] see under *zone*.

headache (hed'āk) pain in the head; cephalalgia. **anemic h.,** headache ascribed to anemia, local or general. **bilious h.,** headache associated with gastrointestinal symptoms; usually migrainous. See *migraine*. **blind h.,** migraine. **cluster h.,** migrainous neuralgia. **congestive h.,** headache ascribed to congestion or hyperemia. **cough h.,** stabbing pain produced by the traction on pain-sensitive structures resulting from coughing or straining. **dynamite h.,** a severe headache occurring in persons handling high explosives. **functional h.,** headache due to tension or other emotional upset. **helmet h.,** pain involving the upper half of the head. **histamine h.,** Horton's h. **h.,** migrainous neuralgia. **hyperemic h.,** congestive h. **lumbar puncture h.,** headache in the erect position, relieved by recumbency after lumbar puncture, due to lowering of intracranial pressure by leakage of cerebrospinal fluid through the needle tract. **migraine h.,** see *migraine*. **miners' h.,** headache due to the gases produced by exploded nitroglycerin. **Monday morning h.,** a term sometimes applied to cases of malingering or "hangover." **organic h.,** headache due to intracranial disease or other organic disease. **postspinal h.,** lumbar puncture h. **puncture h.,** lumbar puncture h. **pyrexial h.,** that due to fever. **reflex h.,** that associated with disease of some organ, as the stomach, eyes, etc.; called also *symptomatic h.* **rhinogenous h.,** headache due to nasal disease. **sick h.,** migraine. **spinal h.,** lumbar puncture h. **symptomatic h.,** reflex h. **tension h.,** a type due to prolonged overwork or emotional strain, or both, affecting especially the occipital region. **toxic h.,** headache due to systemic poisoning. **vacuum h.,** headache due to obstruction of the outlet of the frontal sinus. **vasomotor h.,** migrainous neuralgia.

headcap (hed′kap) headgear.

headgear (hed′gēr) a harnesslike device fitting over the top and back of the head, serving as a source of resistance for extraoral anchorage for an orthodontic appliance. Called also *headcap.*

headgrit (hed′grit) yellows, def. 2.

headgut (hed′gut) the foregut.

Heaf test [Frederick R. G. *Heaf,* British physician, born 1894] see *tuberculin test, Sterneedle,* under *tests.*

heal (hēl) to restore wounded parts or to make healthy; to become well or healthy.

healing (hēl′ing) a process of cure; the restoration of integrity to injured tissue. **h. by first intention,** healing in which union or restoration of continuity occurs directly without the intervention of granulations. **h. by granulation,** healing by second intention. **h. by second intention,** union by closure of a wound with granulations which form from the base and both sides toward the surface of the wound.

health (helth) a state of optimal physical, mental, and social well-being, and not merely the absence of disease and infirmity. **holistic h.,** a system of preventive medicine that takes into account the whole individual, his own responsibility for his well-being and the total influences—social, psychological, environmental—that affect health, including nutrition, exercise, and mental relaxation. **public h.,** the field of medicine concerned with safeguarding and improving the health of the community as a whole.

health maintenance organization (HMO) a broad term encompassing a variety of health care delivery systems utilizing group practice and providing alternatives to the fee-for-service private practice of medicine and allied health professions. They are essentially prepaid, organized systems for providing comprehensive health care within a geographic area to all persons under contract and they emphasize preventive medicine.

healthy (hel′the) pertaining to, characterized by, or promoting health.

hearing (hēr′ing) [L. *auditus*] the sense by which sounds are perceived; capacity to perceive sound. **color h.,** chromesthesia. **double disharmonic h.,** diplacusis. **monaural h.,** hearing with one ear. **visual h.,** lip reading.

hearing loss (hēr-ing los′) partial or complete loss of hearing; see also *deafness.* **Alexander's h.l.,** congenital deafness due to cochlear aplasia involving chiefly the organ of Corti and adjacent ganglion cells of the basal coil of the cochlea; a high-frequency hearing loss results. Called also *Alexander's deafness.* **conductive h.l.,** hearing loss due to a defect of the sound conducting apparatus, i.e., of the external auditory canal or middle ear. Called also *transmission h.l.* **pagetoid h.l.,** that occurring in osteitis deformans (Paget's disease) of the bones of the skull. **paradoxic h.l.,** hearing loss in which the hearing is better during loud noise. Called also *paracusia willisana.* **sensorineural h.l.,** hearing loss due to a defect in the inner ear or the acoustic nerve. **transmission h.l.,** conductive h.l.

heart (hart) [L. *cor;* Gr. *kardia*] the viscus of cardiac muscle that maintains the circulation of the blood. Called also *cor* [NA]. It is divided into four cavities—two atria and two ventricles. The left atrium receives oxygenated blood from the lungs. From there the blood passes to the left ventricle, which forces it via the aorta through the arteries to supply the tissues of the body. The right atrium receives the blood after it has passed through the tissues and given up much of its oxygen. The blood then passes to the right ventricle, and then to the lungs, to be oxygenated. The major valves are four in number: the *left atrioventricular valve* (bicuspid, or *mitral*), between the left atrium and ventricle; the *right atrioventricular valve* (tricuspid), between the right atrium and ventricle; the *aortic,* at the orifice of the aorta; and the *pulmonary,* at the orifice of the pulmonary trunk. The heart tissue itself is nourished by the blood in the coronary arteries.

abdominal h., a heart displaced into the abdominal cavity. **armored h., armour h.,** a condition marked by calcareous deposits in the pericardium. **artificial h.,** a pumping mechanism that duplicates the output, rate, and blood pressure of the natural heart. It may replace the function of the entire heart or a portion of it, and may be an intracorporeal, extracorporeal, or paracorporeal heart. **athlete's h.,** aortic incompetence due to strain in athletic exercise. **athletic h.,** hypertrophy of the heart with no disease of the valves, sometimes seen in athletes. **beer h.,** hypertrophy and dilatation of the heart attributed to excessive beer drinking; recently cobalt, as an additive in beer, has been implicated in some instances. See also *alcoholic myocardiopathy,* under *myocardiopathy.* **beriberi h.,** heart failure from thiamine deficiency. **boat-shaped h.,** the heart of aortic regurgitation due to dilatation and hypertrophy of the left ventricle. **bony h.,** a heart or pericardium containing calcareous deposits. **booster h.,** auxiliary ventricle. **bovine h.,** cor bovinum, a greatly enlarged heart. **cervical h.,** one situated in the neck. **chaotic h.,** a heart which exhibits frequent premature systoles. **dynamite h.,** a condition occurring in workers exposed to nitroglycerin, in which the blood vessels become dilated during exposure and then, when exposure is discontinued, contract and thus reduce the blood supply to heart. **encased h.,** a heart affected with chronic constrictive pericarditis. **extracorporeal h.,** an artificial heart located outside the body and usually performing a pumping and an oxygenating function. **fat h., fatty h.,** 1. a heart affected with fatty degeneration. Called also *cor adiposum.* 2. a condition in which there is an excessive layer of fat deposited about and in the heart muscle. **fibroid h.,** a heart affected with chronic myocarditis in which fibrous tissue replaces portions of the myocardium. **flask-shaped h.,** the x-ray appearance of the heart in pericarditis with effusion. **frosted h.,** a condition in which the pericardium is thickened, giving the heart the appearance of being frosted like a cake. Cf. *hyaloserositis.* **hairy h.,** cor villosum. **hanging h.,** a condition as seen in the roentgenogram in cardioptosis, in which the heart appears as if hanging straight down from the aorta. **horizontal h.,** a counterclockwise rotation of the electrical axis (deviation to the left) of the heart; a moderate deviation (0° to −20°) is normally observed in asthenic persons with a transversely situated heart, in the obese, and in pregnant women. **hyperthyroid h.,** the heart in thyrotoxic heart disease. **hypoplastic h.,** a heart of small size. **icing h.,** frosted h. **intracorporeal h.,** an artificial heart implanted in the body. **irritable h.,** neurocirculatory asthenia. **left h.,** the left atrium and ventricle; that portion of the heart which propels the blood in systemic circulation. **lymph h.,** an organ in frogs and fishes concerned in the distribution of lymph. **mechanical h.,** artificial h. **myxedema h.,** an enlarged heart associated with hypothyroidism. **ox h.,** cor bovinum. **paracorporeal h.,** an artificial heart worn at the side of the body. **parchment h.,** see *hypoplasia of right ventricle.* **pear-shaped h.,** the x-ray appearance of the heart in combined aortic and mitral disease. **pectoral h.,** a heart situated in the front of the chest where it produces a bulging area. **pulmonary h.,** right heart. **Quain's fatty h.,** a fatty degeneration of the heart muscle. **right h.,** the right atrium and ventricle; that portion of the heart which propels the blood in the pulmonary circulation. **round h.,** the x-ray appearance of the heart in mitral stenosis and regurgitation. **sabot h.,** coeur en sabot. **soldier's h.** neurocirculatory asthenia. **systemic h.,** left heart. **tabby cat h.,** a condition of the heart in which the inner surface of the ventricular wall and the papillary muscles are streaked and spotted; seen in marked cases of fatty degeneration. Called also *thrush breast h., tiger h.,* and *tiger lily h.* **three-chambered h.,** a developmental anomaly in which the heart has a single or common ventricle with two atria emptying into it (absence of the ventricular septum), or a single or common atrium and two normal ventricles (absence of the atrial septum); called also *cor triloculare* or *trilocular h.* **thrush breast h., tiger h., tiger lily h.,** tabby cat h. **tobacco h.,** a heart showing irregularity of action attributed to excessive use of tobacco. **Traube's h.,** heart disease resulting from kidney disorder. **triatrial h.,** cor triatriatum. **trilocular h.,** three-chambered h. **vertical h.,** a clockwise rotation of the electrical axis (deviation to the right) of the heart; a moderate deviation (90° to 100°) is normally observed in asthenic persons with a vertically situated heart

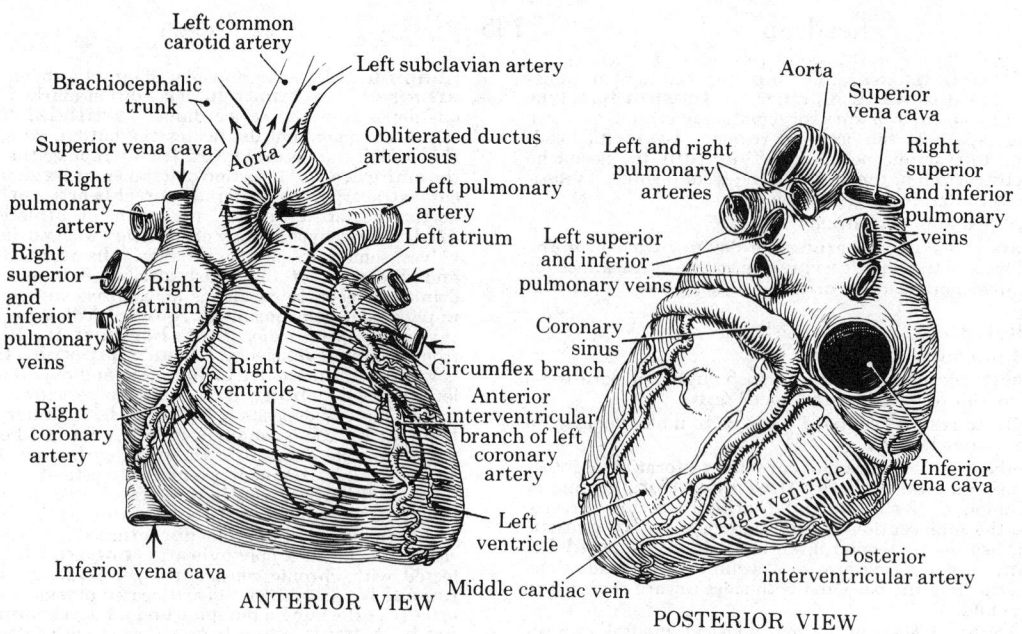

Left common
carotid artery

Brachiocephalic
trunk

Left subclavian artery

Superior vena cava

Right
pulmonary
artery

Right
superior
and
inferior
pulmonary
veins

Obliterated ductus
arteriosus

Left pulmonary
artery

Left atrium

Aorta

Right
atrium

Right
ventricle

Right
coronary
artery

Circumflex branch

Anterior
interventricular
branch of left
coronary
artery

Left
ventricle

Inferior vena cava

Middle cardiac vein

ANTERIOR VIEW

Aorta

Superior
vena cava

Left and right
pulmonary
arteries

Right
superior
and inferior
pulmonary
veins

Left superior
and inferior
pulmonary veins

Coronary
sinus

Right ventricle

Inferior
vena cava

Left ventricle

Posterior
interventricular artery

POSTERIOR VIEW

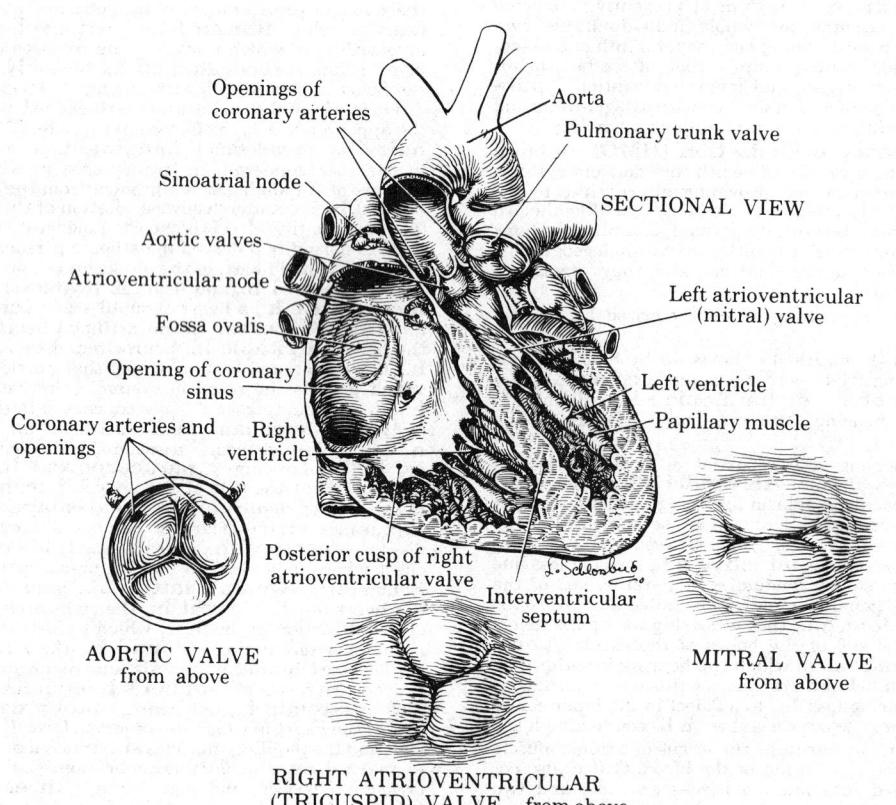

Openings of
coronary arteries

Sinoatrial node

Aortic valves

Atrioventricular node

Fossa ovalis

Opening of coronary
sinus

Coronary arteries and
openings

Right
ventricle

Posterior cusp of right
atrioventricular valve

Interventricular
septum

Aorta

Pulmonary trunk valve

SECTIONAL VIEW

Left atrioventricular
(mitral) valve

Left ventricle

Papillary muscle

L. Schlossberg

AORTIC VALVE
from above

RIGHT ATRIOVENTRICULAR
(TRICUSPID) VALVE   from above

MITRAL VALVE
from above

PLATE 19 — STRUCTURES OF THE HEART

736

and in early infancy. **wandering h.,** an abnormally movable heart. **wooden-shoe h.,** coeur en sabot.

heart block (hart′blok) impairment of conduction in heart excitation; often applied specifically to atrioventricular heart block (q.v.). **arborization h.b.** (*obs.*), an intraventricular conduction defect attributed to loss of function of the distal ramifications of the bundle branches and/or Purkinje tissue. **atrioventricular h.b.,** a form in which the block occurs in the atrioventricular junctional tissue (atrioventricular node, bundle of His, or its branches); it is called *first degree h.b.* when conduction time is prolonged but all atrial beats are followed by ventricular beats; *second degree* (*partial*) *h.b.* when some, but not all, atrial beats are conducted; and *third degree* (*complete*) *h.b.* when no impulses whatsoever are conducted by the junctional tissues, owing to pathologic factors. The condition may be permanent or paroxysmal and if syncopal attacks occur, it is known as *Adams-Stokes disease.* **bundle-branch h.b.,** a form in which one ventricle is excited before the other because of absence of conduction in one of the branches of the bundle of His. **complete h.b.,** loss of conduction through the atrioventricular junctional tissue due to pathologic factors, with atrioventricular dissociation in which a sinus or atrial beat excites the atria while an idioventricular pacemaker below the site of block excites the ventricles; see also *atrioventricular h.b.* **congenital h.b.,** heart block due to defective development of junction conduction tissues of the heart; it may be associated with other cardiac anomalies. **incomplete h.b.,** second degree h.b.; see *atrioventricular h.b.* **interventricular h.b.,** bundle-branch h.b. **intraventricular h.b.,** a general term denoting an abnormal excitation pattern of the ventricles due to absence of conduction in the bundle branches or their ramifications. **Mobitz h.b.,** second degree atrioventricular heart block marked by a periodic dropped beat with a fixed P–R interval. **partial h.b.,** second degree h.b.; see *atrioventricular h.b.* **sinoatrial h.b.,** partial or complete impairment of conduction from the sinoatrial node to the atria, resulting in delay or absence of an atrial beat. **Wenckebach h.b.,** second degree atrioventricular heart block marked by a periodic dropped beat with a varying P–R interval.

heartburn (hart′bern) an esophageal symptom consisting of a retrosternal sensation of warmth or burning occurring in waves and tending to rise upward toward the neck; it may be accompanied by a reflux of fluid into the mouth (water brash). It is often associated with gastroesophageal reflux. Called also *pyrosis.*

heart failure (hart′fāl-yer) a clinical syndrome characterized by distinctive symptoms and signs resulting from disturbances in cardiac output or from increased venous pressure. Most often applied to myocardial failure with increased pressures distending the ventricle (high end-diastolic pressure [EDP]) and a cardiac output inadequate for the body's needs; often subclassified as right- or left-sided heart failure depending on whether the systemic or pulmonary veins are predominantly distended. Cf. *cardiac arrest,* under *arrest.* **acute congestive h.f.,** rapidly occurring deficiency in cardiac output marked by venocapillary congestion and hypertension and edema, usually pulmonary edema. **backward h.f.,** that produced by passive engorgement of the systemic venous system caused by a rise in distending (diastolic) pressures in the right heart. **congestive h.f.,** a clinical syndrome due to heart disease and characterized by breathlessness and abnormal sodium and water retention, resulting in edema. The congestion may occur in the lungs or in the peripheral circulation, or in both, depending on whether the heart failure is right-sided, left-sided, or general. **forward h.f.,** a concept of heart failure that emphasizes the inadequacy of cardiac output relative to body needs; edema is attributed primarily to renal retention of sodium and water, and venous distention is considered a secondary feature. **high output h.f.,** heart failure in which the cardiac output remains high, most often associated with hyperthyroidism. **left-sided h.f., left ventricular h.f.,** failure of adequate output by the left ventricle despite an increase in distending pressure and in end-diastolic volume, with dyspnea, orthopnea, etc.; see *heart failure.* **right-sided h.f., right ventricular h.f.,** failure of proper functioning of the right ventricle, with venous engorgement, hepatic enlargement, and subcutaneous edema; it is often combined with left-sided heart failure.

heartwater (hart-wot′er) a fatal disease of cattle, sheep, and goats, marked by fluid accumulation in the pleura, pericardium, and pleural cavity. It is caused by *Cowdria ruminantium,* which is transmitted by the ticks *Amblyomma hebraeum* and *A. variegata.*

heartworm (hart′werm) *Dirofilaria immitis.*

heat (hēt) [L. *calor;* Gr. *thermē*] 1. the sensation of an increase in temperature. 2. the energy which produces the sensation of heat. It exists in the form of molecular or atomic vibration (thermal agitation) and may be transferred by conduction through a substance, by convection by a substance, and by radiation as electromagnetic waves. 3. energy that is transferred as a consequence of a gradient in temperature. 4. estrus. **atomic h.,** the product of the atomic weight of an element and its specific heat. **conductive h.,** heat transmitted to the body by contact with a heated object, such as a hot water bag. **convective h.,** heat conveyed to the surface of the body from warm currents of water or air. **conversive h.,** heat developed in the tissues by the resistance of the tissues to the passage of high-frequency electromagnetic radiation through them. **dry h.,** heat that is not moist. Heated dry air is used in an apparatus such as a covered "baker," designed for the production of hyperemia. The dry air rapidly absorbs from the skin the moisture of perspiration induced in the apparatus during treatment. **h. of fusion,** the enthalpy change at constant temperature and pressure in converting a unit amount of a substance from the solid to the liquid state, usually specified in cal/g or cal/mol. Called also *latent h. of fusion.* **latent h.,** heat which is absorbed by a body without a rise in temperature. Cf. *sensible h.* **latent h. of fusion,** h. of fusion. **latent h. of sublimation,** h. of sublimation. **latent h. of vaporization,** h. of vaporization. **molecular h.,** the product of the molecular weight of a substance multiplied by its specific heat. **prickly h.,** miliaria rubra. **radiant h.,** heat applied to the surface of the body by rays from a source of infrared radiation, such as a heat lamp. **sensible h.,** (obs.) heat which is absorbed by a body producing a rise in temperature. Cf. *latent h.* **specific h.,** the ratio of amount of heat absorbed in raising a unit mass of a substance one degree Celsius at a specified temperature to the amount of heat absorbed in raising an equal mass of water one degree Celsius at the same temperature. See *specific heat capacity* under *capacity.* **h. of sublimation,** the enthalpy change at constant temperature and pressure in converting a unit amount of a substance from the solid to the gas state, usually specified in cal/g or cal/mol. Called also *latent h. of sublimation.* **h. of vaporization,** the enthalpy change at constant temperature and pressure in converting a unit amount of a substance from the liquid to the gas state, usually specified in cal/g or cal/mol. Called also *latent h. of vaporization.*

Heath's operation (hēths) [Christopher *Heath,* English surgeon, 1835–1905] see under *operation.*

heatstroke (hēt′strōk″) see under *stroke.*

heaves (hēvz) a respiratory disturbance, most common in the Equidae, resulting from reduced elasticity in and rupture of the elastic network of the respiratory bronchioles and pulmonary alveoli and characterized by partly forced expiration.

Hebdom. abbreviation for L. *hebdom′ada,* a week.

hebdomadal (heb-dom′ah-dal) [L. *hebdomada* a week] pertaining to the first week of life.

hebephrenia (heb″ĕ-fre′ne-ah) [Gr. *hebē* youth + *phrēn* mind] (*obs.*) disorganized (hebephrenic) schizophrenia.

hebephrenic (heb′ĕ-fren-ik) 1. pertaining to hebephrenia, disorganized (hebephrenic) schizophrenia. 2. a person affected with disorganized schizophrenia.

Heberden's asthma, disease, nodes (signs), rheumatism (he′ber-denz) [William *Heberden,* English physician, 1710–1801] see *angina pectoris,* and see under *disease, node,* and *rheumatism.*

hebetic (hĕ-bet′ik) [Gr. *hebētikos* youthful] pertaining to or occurring at the time of puberty.

hebetude (heb′ĕ-tūd) [L. *hebetudo*] apathy or dullness from any cause; in psychiatry, emotional dullness, a characteristic of schizophrenia.

hebiatrics (he″be-at′riks) ephebiatrics.

Hebra's disease, prurigo (he′brahs) [Ferdinand von *Hebra,* Austrian dermatologist, 1816–1880, founder of the histologic school of dermatology] see *erythema multiforme minor,* and see under *prurigo.*

hecatomeral (hek″ah-tom′er-al) hecatomeric.

hecatomeric (hek″ah-to-mer′ik) [Gr. *hekateron* each of two + *meros* part] having processes which divide into two, one going to each side of the spinal cord; said of certain neurons.

Hecht's phenomenon (hekts) [Adolf Franz *Hecht,* Vienna pediatrist, born 1876] Rumpel-Leede phenomenon.

hectic (hek′tik) [L. *hecticus;* Gr. *hektikos* consumptive] associated with tuberculosis or with septic poisoning, as hectic fever.

hecto- [Fr., from Gr. *hekaton* one hundred] a combining form designating one hundred; used in naming units of measurement to indicate a quantity 100 (10^2) times the unit designated by the root with which it is combined. Symbol, h.

hectogram (hek′to-gram) a unit of mass of the metric system, being 10^2 grams; the equivalent of 3.527 ounces avoirdupois, or 3.215 ounces apothecaries' weight.

hectoliter (hek′to-le-ter) a unit of capacity of the metric system, being 10^2 liters; the equivalent of 26.4 United States or 22 Imperial gallons.

hectometer (hek-tom′ĕ-ter) a unit of linear measure of the metric system, being 10^2 meters, or the equivalent, roughly, of 328 feet, one inch.

H.E.D. abbreviation for German *Haut-Einheits-Dosis* (unit skin dose), a unit of roentgen-ray dosage established by Seitz and Wintz.

hedonic (he-don′ik) pertaining to pleasure.

hedonism (he′do-nizm) [Gr. *hēdonē* pleasure] pleasure-seeking behavior; the doctrine that regards pleasure and happiness as the highest good.

Hedulin (hed′u-lin) trademark for a preparation of phenindione.

heel (hēl) the hindmost part of the foot; called also *calx* [NA alternative] and *regio calcanea.* **anterior h.,** a triangular-shaped piece of leather fastened obliquely across the ball of the shoe just behind the heads of the metatarsal bones, the object being to support the heads, equalize the pressure, and support the anterior arch. **basketball h.,** black heel (q.v.) in basketball players. **black h.,** a benign condition characterized by the sudden appearance of unilateral or bilateral minute, blood-filled punctate black macules on the bottom of the heel and sometimes the distal toe(s); it is due to the shearing stress of certain athletic activities such as basketball, volleyball, tennis, and lacrosse. Called also *calcaneal petechiae* and *talon noir.* **contracted h.,** hoofbound. **cracked h's,** pitted keratolysis. **gonorrheal h.,** the development of exostoses on the heel, attributed to gonorrheal infection. **painful h.,** a condition in which pain is caused by pressure on the heel. **policeman's h.,** calcanodynia in a policeman. **prominent h.,** a swelling on the back of the heel due to thickening of the periosteum of the os calcis. **Thomas h.,** a shoe correction consisting a heel $\frac{1}{2}$ in. longer and $\frac{1}{8}$-$\frac{1}{6}$ in. higher on the inside, used to bring the heel of the foot into varus and to prevent depression in the region of the head of the talus.

Heerfordt's syndrome (disease) (hār′forts) [Christian Frederik *Heerfordt,* Danish oculist, born 1871] see under *syndrome.*

hefilcon A (hĕ-fil′kon) either of two hydrophilic contact lens materials, designated A or B.

Hegar's dilator, sign (ha′garz) [Alfred *Hegar,* gynecologist in Freiburg, 1830–1914] see under *dilator* and *sign.*

Heiberg-Esmarch maneuver (hi′berg es′mark) [Jacob *Heiberg,* Norwegian surgeon, 1843–1888; Johann Friedrich August von *Esmarch,* German surgeon, 1823–1908] see under *maneuver.*

Heidenhain's cells, law, rods, stain (hi′den-hīnz) [Rudolf Peter *Heidenhain,* German physiologist, 1834–1897] see *chief cells* (def. 1) and *parietal cells,* under *cell,* and see under *law, rod,* and *stain.*

height (hīt) the vertical measurement of an object or body. **apex h.,** the magnitude of the ordinates of the summated twitches of a muscle following application of electric or other stimulation. **h. of contour,** the line encircling a tooth at its greatest bulge with reference to a predetermined path of insertion for a removable partial denture. **h. of contour, surveyed,** a line scribed or marked on a cast that designates the greatest bulge or diameter with respect to a

selected path of denture placement or removal. **cusp h.,** 1. the shortest distance between the tip of a cusp of a tooth and its base plane. 2. the shortest distance between the deepest part of the central fossa of a posterior tooth and a line connecting the points of the cusps of the tooth. **facial h.,** the linear measurement of portions of the face, in the midline, using specific reference points: *anterior facial height* is the distance between the nasion and the menton, gnathion, or pogonion; *posterior facial height* is a measure of a perpendicular line from the sella-nasion plane intersecting the mandibular plane, or the distance from the sella to the gonion; *lower facial height* is the distance from the interdentale inferius to the gnathion, or the distance between the acanthion and the gnathion; *upper facial height* is the distance between the nasion and the interdentale superius, or between the nasion and the anterior nasal spine or the prosthion. **sitting h.,** sitting vertex h. **sitting suprasternal h.,** the distance from the middle of the anterior-superior border of the manubrium sterni to the surface on which the subject is seated. **sitting vertex h.,** the distance from the highest point of the head in the sagittal plane to the surface on which the subject is seated; commonly called *sitting height.* Cf. *crown-rump length.* **standing h.,** the distance from the highest point of the head in the sagittal plane to the surface on which the individual is standing, measured when the subject is not wearing shoes. Cf. *crown-heel length.*

Heilbronner's thigh (sign) (hīl′bron-erz) [Karl *Heilbronner,* Dutch physician, 1869–1914] see under *thigh.*

Heim-Kreysig sign (hīm-kri′sig) [Ernst Ludwig *Heim,* German physician, 1747–1834; Friedrich Ludwig *Kreysig,* German physician, 1770–1839] see under *sign.*

Heimlich maneuver (hīm′lik) [Henry *Heimlich,* American surgeon, born 1920] see under *maneuver.*

Heine's operation (hi′nez) [Leopold *Heine,* German oculist, 1870–1940] see under *operation.*

Heine-Medin disease (hi′nĕ ma′din) [Jacob von *Heine,* German physician, 1806–1879; Karl Oskar *Medin,* Swedish physician, 1847–1927] see *poliomyelitis.*

Heineke-Mikulicz pyloroplasty (operation) (hi′nĕ-kĕ mik′u-lich) [Walter Hermann *Heineke,* German surgeon, 1834– 1901; Johann von *Mikulicz*-Radecki, Polish surgeon, 1850– 1905] see under *pyloroplasty.*

Heinz bodies (granules) (hīnts) [Robert *Heinz,* German pathologist, 1865–1924] Heinz-Ehrlich bodies; see under *body.*

Heinz-Ehrlich bodies (hīnts-ār′lik) [Robert *Heinz;* Paul *Ehrlich,* German bacteriologist, 1854–1915] see under *body.*

Heisrath's operation (hīs′raths) [Friedrich *Heisrath,* German ophthalmologist, 1850–1904] see under *operation.*

Heister's diverticulum, fold, valve (hīs′terz) [Lorenz *Heister,* German anatomist, 1683–1758] for *diverticulum,* see *bulbus superior venae jugularis;* and for *fold* and *valve,* see *plica spiralis.*

HEK human embryo kidney (cell culture).

Hektoen phenomenon (hek′tōn) [Ludvig *Hektoen,* Chicago pathologist, 1863–1951] see under *phenomenon.*

HEL human embryo lung (cell culture).

HeLa cells (he′lah) [from the name of the patient from whose carcinoma of the cervix uteri the parent carcinoma cells were isolated in 1951 at Johns Hopkins Hospital by Dr. George O. Gey] see under *cell.*

helcoid (hel′koid) [Gr. *helkos* ulcer + *eidos* form] resembling an ulcer.

helcology (hel-kol′o-je) [Gr. *helkos* ulcer + *-logy*] the scientific study of ulcers.

helcoma (hel-ko′mah) [Gr.] corneal ulcer.

helcosis (hel-ko′sis) [Gr. *helkōsis*] ulceration; the formation of an ulcer.

Heleidae (hĕ-le′ĭ-de) a family of flies of the suborder Nematocera, order Diptera, containing, among others, the four genera *Culicoides, Haemophoructus, Lasiohelea,* and *Leptoconops,* various species of which suck the blood of man, and may serve as vectors of disease. Called also *Ceratopogonidae.*

helenine (hel′ĕ-nēn) an antiviral substance produced by *Penicillium funiculosum* that is active against nucleic acid synthesis; thought to be a ribonucleoprotein.

helianthin (he-le-an′thin) methyl orange; see under *orange*.

heliation (he″le-a′shun) treatment by exposure to the sun's rays.

helical (hel′ĭ-kal) shaped like a helix.

Helicella (he″lĭ-sel′ah) a genus of snails that serves as a host of *Dicrocoelium dentriticum*.

Helicellidae (he″lĭ-sel′ĭ-de) a family of snails (suborder Stylommatophora, order Pulmonata) that serves as a host of trematodes infecting man.

helicin (hel′ĭ-sin) a glycoside formed by oxidizing salicin, which on hydrolysis yields glucose and salicylic aldehyde.

helicine (hel′ĭ-sīn) 1. of spiral form. 2. of or pertaining to a helix.

helic(o)- [Gr. *helix* coil, gen. *helikos*] a combining form denoting relationship to a coil, or to a snail (*Helix*).

helicoid (hel′ĭ-koid) [*helico-* + Gr. *eidos* form] resembling a coil or helix.

helicopod (hel′ĭ-ko-pod″) denoting a peculiar dragging gait; see under *gait*.

helicopodia (hel″ĭ-ko-po′de-ah) helicopod gait.

helicoprotein (hel″ĭ-ko-pro′te-in) [*helico-* + *protein*] a glucoprotein substance obtained from the snail, *Helix pomata*.

helicotrema (hel″ĭ-ko-tre′mah) [*helico-* + Gr. *trēma* hole] [NA] the passage of the ear that connects the scala tympani and scala vestibuli at the apex of the cochlea; called also *Breschet's* or *Scarpa's hiatus*.

heliencephalitis (he″le-en-sef″ah-li′tis) encephalitis from exposure to the sun (sunstroke).

heli(o)- [Gr. *hēlios* sun] a combining form denoting relationship to the sun.

helioaerotherapy (he″le-o-a″er-o-ther′ah-pe) [*helio-* + Gr. *aēr* air + *therapeia* treatment] treatment by exposure to the sun's rays and to fresh air.

helion (he′le-on) helium.

heliopathia (he″le-o-path′e-ah) [*helio-* + Gr. *pathos* disease] any pathological disturbance caused by sunlight.

heliosin (he″le-o′sin) a compound containing keratin and various inorganic salts.

heliosis (he″le-o′sis) [*helio-* + *-osis*] sunstroke.

heliotaxis (he″le-o-tak′sis) [*helio-* + Gr. *taxis* arrangement] the movement of cells and microorganisms in response to either or both light and heat from the sun. The response may be toward (*positive h.*) or away (*negative h.*) from the source of stimulus. Cf. *heliotropism*, *phototaxis*, and *thermotaxis*.

heliotherapy (he″le-o-ther′ah-pe) [*helio-* + *therapy*] the treatment of disease by exposing the body to the sun's rays; the therapeutic use of the sun bath.

Heliotiales (he″le-o-she-a′lēz) an order of ascomycetes (series Pyrenomycetes, subclass Euascomycetidae), some members of which are saprophytes and others are parasites of plants. It includes the genus *Sclerotinia*.

heliotrope B (he′le-o-trōp″) amethyst violet; see under *violet*.

heliotropism (he″le-ot′ro-pizm) [*helio-* + Gr. *tropē* a turn, turning] the turning of an organism, especially a plant, toward (*positive h.*) or away from (*negative h.*) the sun. Cf. *heliotaxis*.

Heliozoa (he″le-o-zo′ah) [*helio-* + Gr. *zōon* animal] a class of spherical, mostly freshwater protozoa (superclass Actinopoda, subphylum Sarcodina, the bodies of which are free floating or attached to the substratum by a stalk and composed of a uninucleated or multinucleated central cytoplasmic core not enclosed in a capsular membrane and an outer region of highly vacuolated cytoplasm. They have axopodia radiating from all sides of the body, which arise from a centroplast in some species, and contain central cytoplasmic microtubules extending from the central core. Many have a skeleton of a silaceous or organic material. The class comprises four orders: Actinophryida, Centrohelida, Desmothoracida, and Taxopodida.

heliozoa (he″le-o-zo′ah) plural of *heliozoan*.

heliozoan (he″le-o-zo′an), pl. *heliozo′a*. 1. any individual protozoan of the class Heliozoa. 2. heliozoic.

heliozoic (he″le-o-zo′ik) of or pertaining to the Heliozoa; heliozoan.

helium (he′le-um) [Gr. *hēlios* sun] a colorless, odorless, tasteless gas, which is not combustible and does not support combustion. It is one of the inert gaseous elements, which was first detected in the sun and is now obtained from natural gas. Symbol, He; atomic number, 2; atomic weight, 4.003. Used in medicine [USP] as a diluent for other gases, being especially useful with oxygen in the treatment of certain cases of respiratory obstruction, and as a vehicle for general anesthetics.

Helix (he′liks) a genus of gastropods that contains the common garden snails.

helix (he′liks) [Gr. "snail," "coil"] 1. a coiled structure, such as the coil of wire in an electromagnet. 2. [NA] the superior and posterior free margin of the pinna of the ear. **α-h., alpha h.,** a secondary structure occurring in many proteins; it is a right-handed helix with 3.6 amino acid residues per turn stabilized by hydrogen bonds between the imino hydrogen of each peptide bond and the carbonyl oxygen of the peptide bond four residues further along the polypeptide chain. **double h., Watson-Crick h.,** a double helix, each chain of which contains information completely specifying the other chain, representing a structural formulation of the mechanism by which the genetic information in DNA reproduces itself; see at *deoxyribonucleic acid*.

Hellat's sign (hel′ats) [Piotr *Hellat*, Russian otologist, 1857–1912] see under *sign*.

hellebore (hel′ĕ-bōr) [L. *helleborus*; Gr. *helleboros*] a violent gastrointestinal poison, having hydragogue, cathartic, and emmenagogue properties. **American h.,** *Veratrum viride.* **black h.,** the root of *Helleborus niger.* **green h.,** *Veratrum viride.* **white h.,** *Veratrum album.*

Hellendall's sign (hel′en-dahlz) [Hugo *Hellendall*, gynecologist in Düsseldorf, born 1872] Cullen's sign.

Heller's operation (hel′erz) [Ernst *Heller*, Leipzig surgeon, 1877–1964] esophagocardiomyotomy.

Heller's test (hel′erz) [Johann Florian *Heller*, Vienna pathologist, 1813–1871] see under *tests*.

Heller-Döhle disease (hel′er-de′le) [Arnold Ludwig Gotthilf *Heller*, Kiel pathologist, 1840–1913; Karl Gottfried Paul *Döhle*, German pathologist, 1855–1928] syphilitic aortitis.

Hellin's law (hel′inz) [Dyonizy *Hellin*, Polish pathologist, 1867–1935] see under *law*.

Helmholtz's ligament, theory (helm′holtz-ez) [Hermann Ludwig Ferdinand von *Helmholtz*, German physiologist, who in 1851 invented the ophthalmoscope, 1821–1894] see under *ligament* and *theory*.

helminth (hel′minth) [Gr. *helmins* worm] a parasitic worm.

helminthagogue (hel-min′thah-gog) [*helminth* + Gr. *agōgos* leading] anthelmintic.

helminthemesis (hel″min-them′ĕ-sis) [*helminth* + Gr. *emesis* vomiting] the vomiting of worms.

helminthiasis (hel″min-thi′ah-sis) an infection with worms. **h. elas′tica,** the occurrence of elastic tumors in the groin and axilla, probably due to filariae.

helminthic (hel-min′thik) pertaining to or caused by parasitic worms.

helminthicide (hel-min′thĭ-sīd) [*helminth* + L. *caedere* to kill] vermicide.

helminthism (hel′min-thizm) the presence of worms in the body.

helminthoid (hel-min′thoid) [*helminth* + Gr. *eidos* form] wormlike.

helminthology (hel″min-thol′o-je) [*helminth* + *-logy*] the scientific study of parasitic worms.

helminthoma (hel″min-tho′mah) [*helminth* + *-oma*] a tumor caused by a parasitic worm.

helminthous (hel-min′thus) pertaining to or infected with worms.

hel(o)- [Gr. *hēlos* nail, corn, callus] a combining form denoting relationship to a nail, or to a wart or callus.

Heloderma (he″lo-der′mah) [*helo-* + Gr. *derma* skin] a genus of venomous lizards of Arizona and New Mexico. *H. hor′ridum,* the Mexican beaded lizard. *H. suspec′tum,* the Gila monster.

heloma (he-lo′mah) [*helo-* + *-oma*] a corn or callosity on the hand or foot. **h. du′rum,** hard corn, the usual type occurring over joints of the toes. **h. mol′le,** a soft corn.

Helophilus (hĕ-lof′ĭ-lus) a genus of flies, hover flies, of the family Syrphidae, whose "rat-tail" maggots (larvae) may cause nasal and intestinal myiasis.

helosis (he-lo′sis) the condition of having corns.

helotomy (he-lot′o-me) [helo- + Gr. *temnein* to cut] the excision or, more often, the paring of corns or calluses.

Helvella (hel-vel′ah) a genus of fungi of the family Helvellaceae, the saddle fungi, species of which contain a heat-stable hemolysin. Helvellic acid is a constituent of *H. infula.* Other species, including *H. esculenta,* cause a form of mycetismus.

Helvellaceae (hel″vel-a′se-e) a family of ascomycetous fungi of the order Pezizales, series Discomycetes, some species of which are edible; it includes the genus *Helvella.*

Helweg's bundle, tract (hel′vegz) [Hans Kristian Saxtorph *Helweg,* Danish physician, 1847–1901] tractus olivospinalis.

hema (he′mah) [Gr. *haima, haimatos* blood] NA alternative for *haema.*

hema- see hem(o)-.

hemachromatosis (hem″ah-kro″mah-to′sis) hemochromatosis.

hemachrome (hem′ah-krōm) an oxygen-carrying blood pigment, e.g., hemoglobin or hemocyanin.

hemacyte (hem′ah-sīt) hemocyte.

hemacytometer (hem″ah-si-tom′ĕ-ter) hemocytometer.

hemacytometry (hem″ah-si-tom′ĕ-tre) the counting of blood corpuscles by means of a hemacytometer.

hemacytozoon (hem″ah-si″to-zo′on), pl. *hemacytozo′a.* (obs.) hemocytozoon.

hemadostenosis (hem″ad-o-stĕ-no′sis) [Gr. *haimas* blood stream + *stenōsis* narrowing] the narrowing or obliteration of a blood vessel.

hemadsorbent (hem″ad-sor′bent) inducing or characterized by hemadsorption, as hemadsorbent viruses.

hemadsorption (hem″ad-sorp′shun) the adherence of red cells to other cells, particles, or surfaces; see under *tests.*

hemadynamometry (hem″ah-di″nah-mom′ĕ-tre) measurement of blood pressure.

hemafacient (hem″ah-fa′shent) hematopoietic.

hemafecia (hem″ah-fe′se-ah) [hema- + *feces*] blood in the feces.

hemagglutination (hem″ah-gloo″tĭ-na′shun) agglutination of erythrocytes, which may be caused by antibodies (hemagglutinins), by certain viruses (e.g., of influenza and mumps viruses), or by other substances (e.g., lectins). **indirect h., passive h.,** agglutination of erythrocytes due to the reaction of specific antibody with antigen passively adsorbed on the surface or chemically coupled to the cells; the basis of many serologic tests. **viral h.,** the agglutination of erythrocytes by viruses, either by intact virions or by viral products; the basis of hemagglutination or hemagglutination inhibition methods for viral titration.

hemagglutinative (hem″ah-gloo′tĭ-na″tiv) pertaining to, characterized by, or causing agglutination of erythrocytes.

hemagglutinin (hem″ah-gloo′tĭ-nin) [hem- + *agglutinin*] an agglutinin, e.g., an antibody or lectin, that agglutinates erythrocytes. **cold h.,** a cold agglutinin (q.v.) that agglutinates red cells. **warm h.,** a warm agglutinin (q.v.) that agglutinates red cells.

hemal (he′mal) 1. pertaining to the blood or the blood vessels. 2. ventral to the spinal axis, where the heart and great vessels are located, as, e.g., the hemal arches. Cf. *neural.*

hemalum (hem-al′um) a mixture of hematoxylin and alum introduced by Mayer, widely used as a nuclear stain, especially in combination with eosin as a general oversight method. Also, any alum and hematoxylin stain. Called also *alum hematoxylin.*

hemanalysis (hem″ah-nal′ĭ-sis) [hem- + *analysis*] analysis or examination of the blood.

hemangiectasia (hem″an-je-ek-ta′se-ah) angiectasis.

hemangiectasis (hem″an-je-ek′tah-sis) [hem- + Gr. *angeion* vessel + *ektasis* dilatation] angiectasis.

hemangioameloblastoma (hĕ-man″je-o-ah-mel″o-blas-to′mah) a highly vascular ameloblastoma.

hemangioblast (hĕ-man′je-o-blast) a mesodermal cell which gives rise to both vascular endothelium and hemocytoblasts.

hemangioblastoma (hĕ-man″je-o-blas-to′mah) a capillary hemangioma of the brain consisting of proliferated blood vessel cells or angioblasts.

hemangioblastomatosis (hĕ-man″je-o-blas″to-mah-to′sis) multiple or widespread hemangioblastomas.

hemangioendothelioblastoma (hĕ-man″je-o-en″do-the″le-o-blas-to′mah) [hem- + Gr. *angeion* vessel + *endothelium* + Gr. *blastos* germ + *-oma*] a tumor of mesenchymal origin of which the cells tend to form endothelial cells and line blood vessels.

hemangioendothelioma (hĕ-man″je-o-en″do-the″le-o′mah) [hem- + *endothelioma*] a hemangioma in which the endothelial cells are the most prominent component. **benign h.,** a benign neoplasm of blood-vessel endothelium. **malignant h.,** hemangiosarcoma.

hemangioendotheliosarcoma (hĕ-man′je-o-en″do-the″le-o-sar-ko′mah) hemangiosarcoma.

hemangiofibroma (hĕ-man″je-o-fi-bro′mah) a hemangioma containing fibrous tissue.

hemangioma (hĕ-man″je-o′mah) [hem- + *angioma*] an extremely common benign tumor, occurring most commonly in infancy and childhood, made up of newly formed blood vessels, and resulting from malformation of angioblastic tissue of fetal life. There are two main types: capillary and cavernous. Cf. *angioma* and *lymphangioma.* **ameloblastic h.,** a highly vascular ameloblastoma. **capillary h.,** 1. the most common type of hemangioma, characteristically composed of closely packed aggregations of capillaries separated by scant connective stroma, which for the most part conform to the caliber of normal capillaries. According to one classification, strawberry hemangioma, nevus flammeus, cherry angioma, and pyogenic granuloma are all types of capillary hemangiomas. Cf. *cavernous h.* and *vascular nevus.* 2. strawberry h. **cavernous h.,** a vascular tumor proponderantly composed of large dilated blood vessels, often containing large amounts of blood, occurring in the skin, subcutaneously, or both, and also in many viscera, particularly the liver, spleen, pancreas, and sometimes the brain. Most present in early life but are usually not present at birth. The typical superficial lesions are bright to dark red in color; deep lesions have a blue color. Called also *angioma cavernosum* and *strawberry mark* or *nevus.* See also *vascular nevus,* under *nevus.* Cf. *capillary h.* **sclerosing h.,** a sol-

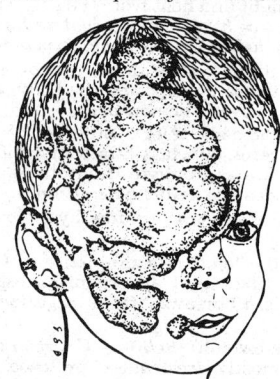

Cavernous hemangioma.

idly cellular lesion (dermatofibroma or histiocytoma) purportedly developing from a hemangioma by proliferation of endothelial cells and connective tissue stroma. **h. sim′plex,** strawberry h. **strawberry h.,** a dull red, firm, dome-shaped hemangioma sharply demarcated from surrounding skin, usually located on the head and neck, which grows rapidly and generally undergoes regression and involution without scarring. It is caused by proliferation of immature capillary vessels in active stroma, and is usually present at birth or occurs within the first 2 or 3 months of life. Called also *h. simplex* and *strawberry mark* or *nevus.* See also *capillary h.* (def. 1), and *vascular nevus,* under *nevus.* 2. vascular n.

hemangiomatosis (hĕ-man″je-o-mah-to′sis) a condition in which multiple hemangiomas are developed.

hemangiopericyte (hĕ-man″je-o-per′ĭ-sīt) pericyte.

hemangiopericytoma (hĕ-man″je-o-per″ĕ-si-to′mah) a tumor composed of spindle cells with a rich vascular network, which apparently arises from pericytes. It is related to a glomus tumor but, unlike the latter, has no nerve elements.

hemangiosarcoma (hĕ-man″je-o-sar-ko′mah) a malignant tumor formed by proliferation of endothelial and fibroblastic tissue.

hemapheic (hem″ah-fe′ik) pertaining to or characterized by hemaphein.

hemaphein (hem″ah-fe′in) [hema- + Gr. phaios dusky, gray] a brown coloring matter of the blood and urine.

hemapheism (hem″ah-fe′izm) the presence of hemaphein in the urine.

hemapheresis (hem″ah-fĕ-re′sis) [hema + Gr. aphairesis removal] any procedure in which blood is withdrawn, a portion (plasma, leukocytes, platelets, etc.) is separated and retained, and the remainder is retransfused into the donor.

hemaphotograph (hem″ah-fo′to-graf) hemophotograph.

hemapoiesis (hem″ah-poi-e′sis) [hema- + Gr. poiēsis formation] hematopoiesis.

hemapoietic (hem″ah-poi-et′ik) hematopoietic.

hemapophysis (hem″ah-pof′ĭ-sis) [hem- + apophysis] a costal cartilage regarded as an apophysis of the hemal spine.

hemarthros (hem-ar′thros) hemarthrosis.

hemarthrosis (hem″ar-thro′sis) [hem- + Gr. arthron joint] extravasation of blood into a joint or its synovial cavity.

hemartoma (hem″ar-to′mah) hemangioma.

hemastrontium (hem″as-tron′she-um) a tissue stain prepared by adding strontium chloride to a solution of hematein and aluminum chloride in alcohol and citric acid.

hematal (hem′ah-tal) pertaining to blood or blood vessels.

hematapostema (hem″at-ah-pos-te′mah) [hemat- + Gr. apostēma abscess] an abscess containing effused blood.

hematein (hem″ah-te′in) [NF] a brownish-red, crystalline substance, $C_{16}H_{12}O_6$, derived from hematoxylin by oxidation; used as an indicator and stain.

hematemesis (hem″ah-tem′ĕ-sis) [hemat- + Gr. emesis vomiting] the vomiting of blood. **Goldstein's h.,** hematemesis due to bleeding telangiectases in the stomach.

hematencephalon (hem″at-en-sef′ah-lon) the effusion of blood into the brain.

hematherapy (hem″ah-ther′ah-pe) hemotherapy.

hemathermal (hem″ah-ther′mal) homoiothermic.

hemathermous (hem″ah-ther′mus) homoiothermic.

hemathorax (hem″ah-tho′raks) hemothorax.

hematic (he-mat′ik) 1. pertaining to or contained in blood. 2. hematinic.

hematidrosis (hem″at-i-dro′sis) [hemat- + Gr. hidrōsis sweating] the excretion of bloody sweat. Called also hematohidrosis and sudor sanguineus.

hematimeter (hem″ah-tim′ĕ-ter) hemocytometer.

hematimetry (hem″ah-tim′ĕ-tre) hemacytometry.

hematin (hem′ah-tin) a porphyrin chelate of iron(III), cf. heme (def. 2). Called also metheme.

hematinemia (hem″ah-tĭ-ne′me-ah) [hematin + Gr. haima blood + -ia] the presence of hematin (heme) in the blood.

hematinic (hem″ah-tin′ik) 1. pertaining to hematin. 2. an agent which improves the quality of the blood, increasing the hemoglobin level and the number of erythrocytes.

hematinometer (hem″ah-tin-om′ĕ-ter) hemoglobinometer.

hematinuria (hem″ah-tin-u′re-ah) [hematin + -uria] the presence of hematin (heme) in the urine.

hemat(o)-, haemat(o)- [Gr. haima, gen. haimatos blood] a combining form denoting relationship to the blood.

hematobilia (hem″ah-to-bil′e-ah) hemobilia.

hematoblast (hem′ah-to-blast″) hemocytoblast.

hematocele (hem′ah-to-sēl″) [hemato- + Gr. kēlē tumor] an effusion of blood into a cavity, especially into the tunica vaginalis testis. **parametric h., pelvic h.,** a tumor formed by effusion of blood into Douglas' pouch. **pudendal h.,** a sanguineous tumor in a labium of the pudenda.

retrouterine h., parametric h. **scrotal h.,** effusion of blood into the tissues of the scrotum. **vaginal h.,** effusion of blood into the tunica vaginalis testis.

hematocelia (hem″ah-to-se′le-ah) hematocoelia.

hematocephalus (hem″ah-to-sef′ah-lus) [hemato- + Gr. kephalē head] a fetus born with its head distended with blood.

hematochezia (hem″ah-to-ke′ze-ah) [hemato- + Gr. chezein to go to stool] the passage of bloody stools.

hematochlorin (hem″ah-to-klo′rin) [hemato- + Gr. chlōros green] a green coloring matter occurring in the placenta and derived from hemoglobin.

hematochromatosis (hem″ah-to-kro″mah-to′sis) [hemato- + Gr. chrōma color] staining of tissues with blood pigment; hemochromatosis.

hematochyluria (hem″ah-to-ki-lu′re-ah) [hemato- + Gr. chylos chyle + -uria] the discharge of blood and chyle with the urine, a symptom of Wuchereria bancrofti infection.

hematocoelia (hem″ah-to-se′le-ah) [hemato- + Gr. koilia cavity] effusion of blood into the peritoneal cavity.

hematocolpometra (hem″ah-to-kol″po-me′trah) [hemato- + Gr. kolpos vagina + mētra uterus] accumulation of menstrual blood in the vagina and uterus.

hematocolpos (hem″ah-to-kol′pos) [hemato- + Gr. kolpos vagina] an accumulation of menstrual blood in the vagina.

hematocrit (he-mat′o-krit) [hemato- + Gr. krinein to separate] 1. a tube with graduated markings used to determine the volume of packed red cells in a blood specimen by centrifugation. 2. by extension, the measurement obtained using this procedure or the corresponding measurements produced by automated blood cell counters. Abbreviated HCT. **large vessel h.,** the ratio of red cell volume to blood volume in large vessels, the hematocrit determined from a venous blood specimen. **Wintrobe h.,** a thick-walled glass tube that has a uniform internal bore and flat bottom and is graduated in millimeters from 0 to 105. **total body h., whole body h.,** the ratio of the total red cell volume to the total blood volume as determined by tracer dilution methods; it is approximately .92 times the large vessel hematocrit.

hematocryal (hem″ah-tok′re-al) [hemato- + Gr. kryos cold] poikilothermic.

hematocyanin (hem″ah-to-si′ah-nin) [hemato- + Gr. kyanos blue] hemocyanin.

hematocyst (hem′ah-to-sist″) [hemato- + Gr. kystis sac, bladder] an effusion of blood into the bladder or into a cyst.

hematocystis (hem″ah-to-sis′tis) hematocyst.

hematocyte (hem′ah-to-sīt) hemocyte.

hematocytoblast (hem″ah-to-si′to-blast) hemocytoblast.

hematocytolysis (hem″ah-to-si-tol′ĭ-sis) hemolysis.

hematocytometer (hem″ah-to-si-tom′ĕ-ter) hemocytometer.

hematocytopenia (hem″ah-to-si″to-pe′ne-ah) [hematocyte + Gr. penia poverty] deficiency in all the cellular elements of the blood.

hematocyturia (hem″ah-to-si-tu′re-ah) [hematocyte + -uria] the presence of red blood cells in the urine.

hematodialysis (hem″ah-to-di-al′ĭ-sis) hemodialysis.

hematoencephalic (hem″ah-to-en″sĕ-fal′ik) [hemato- + Gr. enkephalos brain] pertaining to the blood and the brain.

hematogenesis (hem″ah-to-jen′ĕ-sis) [hemato- + genesis] hematopoiesis.

hematogenic (hem″ah-to-jen′ik) 1. hematopoietic. 2. hematogenous.

hematogenous (hem″ah-toj′ĕ-nus) produced by or derived from the blood; disseminated by the circulation or through the blood stream.

hematoglobin (hem″ah-to-glo′bin) hemoglobin.

hematoglobinuria (hem″ah-to-glo-bin-u′re-ah) hemoglobinuria.

hematoglobulin (hem″ah-to-glob′u-lin) hemoglobin.

hematogone (hem′ah-to-gōn) a name applied to a morphologic type once thought to represent a blood cell precursor.

hematohidrosis (hem″ah-to-hid-ro′sis) hematidrosis.

hematohistioblast (hem″ah-to-his′te-o-blast) hemohistioblast.

hematohyaloid (hem″ah-to-hi′ah-loid) [hemato- + hyaloid] the hyaline matter formed by degeneration of thrombi through conglutination of the red corpuscles or blood platelets.

hematoid (hem′ah-toid) [hemato- + Gr. eidos form] resembling blood.

hematoidin (hem-ah-toid′in) a substance which is apparently chemically identical with bilirubin but which has a different site of origin, being formed locally in the tissues from hemoglobin, particularly under conditions of reduced oxygen tension.

hematokolpos (hem″ah-to-kol′pos) hematocolpos.

hematolith (hem′ah-to-lith) (obs.) hemolith.

hematologist (hem″ah-tol′o-jist) a specialist in the study of the blood.

hematology (hem″ah-tol′o-je) [hemato- + -logy] that branch of medical science which treats of the morphology of the blood and blood-forming tissues.

hematolymphangioma (hem″ah-to-lim″fan-je-o′mah) [hemato- + L. lympha lymph + Gr. angeion vessel + -ome] a tumor composed of blood vessels and lymph vessels. Called also hemolymphangioma.

hematolysis (hem″ah-tol′ĭ-sis) hemolysis.

hematolytic (hem″ah-to-lit′ik) hemolytic.

hematoma (hem″ah-to′mah), pl. hemato′mas [hemato- + -oma] a localized collection of blood, usually clotted, in an organ, space, or tissue, due to a break in the wall of a blood vessel. **aneurysmal h.,** false aneurysm. **h. au′ris,** hematoma of the perichondrium of the ear. **epidural h.,** accumulation of blood in the epidural space, due to damage to the middle meningeal artery and producing compression of the dura mater and thus compression of the brain. Unless evacuated, it may result in herniation through the tentorium, and death. **pelvic h.,** a collection of blood in the pelvic cellular tissue. **perianal h.,** a hematoma under the perianal skin, caused by rupture of a subcutaneous vessel, the blood being kept localized by fibroelastic septa and causing much pain. **retrouterine h.,** an effusion of blood into the retrouterine connective tissue. **subchorionic tuberous h.,** Breus' mole. **subdural h.,** accumulation of blood in the subdural space. In the severe acute form, both blood and cerebrospinal fluid enter the space as a result of laceration of the brain and a tear in the arachnoid, adding subdural compression to the direct injury to the brain. In the chronic form, only blood effuses into the subdural space as a result of rupture of the bridging veins, usually due to closed head injury. The effusion is a gradual process resulting, weeks after the injury, in headache, progressive stupor, and hemiparesis, followed by dilating pupil, a sign of herniation of the tentorium. **subungual h.,** an accumulation of blood under the nail plate.

hematomanometer (hem″ah-to-mah-nom′ĕter) sphygmomanometer.

hematomediastinum (hem″ah-to-me″de-as-ti′num) [hemato- + mediastinum] hemomediastinum.

hematometer (hem″ah-tom′ĕ-ter) [hemato- + Gr. metron measure] a hemoglobinometer.

hematometra (hem″ah-to-me′trah) [hemato- + Gr. mētra uterus] an accumulation of blood in the uterus.

hematometry (hem″ah-tom′ĕ-tre) [hemato- + Gr. metron measure] measurement of the hemoglobin and estimation of the percentage of the various cells in the blood.

hematomole (he-mat′o-mōl) Breus' mole.

hematomycosis (hem″ah-to-mi-ko′sis) (obs.) fungemia.

hematomyelia (hem″ah-to-mi-e′le-ah) [hemato- + Gr. myelos marrow + -ia] hemorrhage into the spinal cord, usually confined to the gray substance, most often due to trauma, and marked by the sudden onset of flaccid paralysis with sensory disturbances.

hematomyelitis (hem″ah-to-mi″ĕ-li′tis) [hemato- + myelitis] acute myelitis with bloody effusion within the spinal cord.

hematomyelopore (hem″ah-to-mi′el-o-pōr″) [hemato- + Gr. myelos marrow + poros opening] a disease marked by the formation of canals in the spinal cord, due to hemorrhage.

hematonephrosis (hem″ah-to-nĕ-fro′sis) presence of blood in the pelvis of the kidney.

hematonic (hem″ah-ton′ik) a blood tonic.

hematopathology (hem″ah-to-pah-thol′o-je) hemopathology.

hematopenia (hem″ah-to-pe′ne-ah) [hemato- + Gr. penia poverty] deficiency of blood.

hematopericardium (hem″ah-to-per″ĭ-kar′de-um) hemopericardium.

hematoperitoneum (hem″ah-to-per″ĭ-to-ne′um) hemoperitoneum.

hematopexis (hem″ah-to-pek′sis) hemopexis.

hematophage (hem′ah-to-fāj) hemophagocyte.

hematophagia (hem″ah-to-fa′je-ah) 1. blood drinking. 2. the act of subsisting on the blood of another animal. 3. hemocytophagia.

hematophagocyte (hem″ah-to-fag′o-sīt) hemophagocyte.

hematophagous (hem″ah-tof′ah-gus) [hemato- + Gr. phagein to eat] pertaining to or characterized by hematophagia.

hematophagy (hem″ah-tof′ah-je) hematophagia.

hematophilia (hem″ah-to-fil′e-ah) hemophilia.

hematophobia (hem″ah-to-fo′be-ah) hemophobia.

hematopiesis (hem″ah-to-pi′ĕ-sis) [hemato- + Gr. piesis pressure] blood pressure.

hematoplastic (hem″ah-to-plas′tik) [hemato- + Gr. plassein to mold] concerned in the elaboration of the blood.

hematopoiesis (hem″ah-to-poi-e′sis) [hemato- + Gr. poiein to make] the formation and development of blood cells. **extramedullary h.,** the formation and development of blood cells outside the bone marrow, as in the spleen, liver, and lymph nodes.

hematopoietic (hem″ah-to-poi-et′ik) [hemato- + Gr. poiein to make] 1. pertaining to or effecting the formation of blood cells. 2. an agent that promotes the formation of blood cells.

hematopoietin (hem″ah-to-poi′e-tin) erythropoietin.

hematoporphyria (hem″ah-to-por-fi′re-ah) porphyria.

hematoporphyrin (hem″ah-to-por′fĭ-rin) a porphyrin (q.v.) in which two pyrrole rings each have one methyl and one propionate side chain and the other two pyrrole rings each have one methyl and one 1-hydroxyethyl side chain.

hematoporphyrinemia (hem″ah-to-por-fĭ-rin-e′me-ah) the presence of hematoporphyrin in the blood.

hematoporphyrinism (hem″ah-to-por′fĭ-rin-izm) a state characterized by hematoporphyrinemia and a sensitiveness to sunlight.

hematoporphyrinuria (hem″ah-to-por′fĭ-rin-u′re-ah) the occurrence of hematoporphyrin in the urine.

Hematopota (hem″ah-top′o-tah) Chrysozona.

hematorrhachis (hem″ah-tor′ah-kis) [hemato- + Gr. rhachis spine] hematomyelia.

hematorrhea (hem″ah-to-re′ah) [hemato- + Gr. rhoia flow] a free or copious hemorrhage.

hematosalpinx (hem″ah-to-sal′pinks) an accumulation of blood in the uterine tube.

hematoscheocele (hem″ah-tos′ke-o-sēl″) [hemato- + Gr. oscheon scrotum + kēlē tumor] a collection of blood within the scrotum.

hematosepsis (hem″ah-to-sep′sis) septicemia.

hematosis (hem″ah-to′sis) (obs.) the formation of the blood.

hematospectrophotometer (hem″ah-to-spek″tro-fo-tom′ĕ-ter) a spectrophotometer for determining the amount of hemoglobin in the blood.

hematospectroscope (hem″ah-to-spek′tro-skōp) [hemato- + spectroscope] a spectroscope for examining thin layers of blood.

hematospectroscopy (hem″ah-to-spek-tros′ko-pe) [hemato- + spectroscopy] the spectroscopic examination of the blood.

hematospermatocele (hem″ah-to-sper-mat′o-sēl) [hemato- + Gr. sperma seed + kēlē tumor] a spermatocele containing blood.

hematospermia (hem″ah-to-sper′me-ah) hemospermia.

hematospherinemia (hem″ah-to-sfēr″ĭ-ne′me-ah) [*hemato-* + Gr. *sphaira* sphere + *haima* blood + *-ia*] hemoglobinemia.

hematostatic (hem″ah-to-stat′ik) [*hemato-* + Gr. *stasis* standing] due to or characterized by stagnation of the blood.

hematosteon (hem″ah-tos′te-on) [*hemat-* + Gr. *osteon* bone] hemorrhage into the medullary cavity of a bone.

hematotherapy (hem″ah-to-ther′ah-pe) hemotherapy.

hematothermal (hem″ah-to-ther′mal) [*hemato-* + Gr. *thermē* heat] homoiothermic.

hematothorax (hem″ah-to-tho″raks) hemothorax.

hematotoxic (hem″ah-to-tok′sik) [*hemato-* + *toxic*] 1. pertaining to hematotoxicosis. 2. poisonous to the blood and hematopoietic system.

hematotoxicosis (hem″ah-to-tok″sĭ-ko′sis) toxic damage to the hematopoietic system.

hematotrachelos (hem″ah-to-trah-ke′los) [*hemato-* + Gr. *trachēlos* neck] distention of the cervix of the uterus with blood, owing to atresia of the external os or of the vagina.

hematotropic (hem″ah-to-trop′ik) [*hemato-* + Gr. *tropos* a turning] having a special affinity for or exerting a specific effect on the blood or blood cells.

hematotympanum (hem″ah-to-tim′pah-num) [*hemato-* + *tympanum*] a hemorrhagic exudation into the midde ear.

hematoxic (hem″ah-tok′sik) hematotoxic.

hematoxylin (hem″ah-tok′sĭ-lin) a colorless crystalline compound, $C_{16}H_{14}O_6 + 3H_2O$, obtained by extracting logwood (*Haematoxylon campechianum*) with ether. It may be used as an indicator with a pH range of 5–6, but is mainly used in oxidized form as a stain in microscopy. See also *Table of Stains and Staining Methods*. **alum h.,** hemalum. **Delafield's h.,** see *Table of Stains and Staining Methods*. **iron h.,** see *iron hematoxylin method, Heidenhain's iron hematoxylin stain,* and *Weigert's hematoxylin stain,* all in the *Table of Stains and Staining Methods*.

Hematoxylon (he″mah-tok′sĭ-lon) *Haematoxylon*.

hematozemia (hem″ah-to-ze′me-ah) [*hemato-* + Gr. *zēmia* loss] a gradual loss of blood.

hematozoa (hem″ah-to-zo′ah) plural of *hematozoon*.

hematozoal (he″mah-to-zo′al) hematozoan, def. 1.

hematozoan (he″ah-to-zo′an) [*hemato-* + Gr. *zōon* animal] 1. pertaining to or caused by animal parasites living in the host's blood. Called also *hematozoal, hematozoic,* and *hemozoic.* 2. any animal parasite living in the host's blood. Called also *hematozoon* and *hemozoon.*

hematozoic (hem″ah-to-zo′ik) hematozoan, def. 1.

hematozoon (hem″ah-to-zo′on), pl. *hematozo′a.* hematozoan, def. 2.

hematuresis (hem″ah-tu-re′sis) hematuria.

hematuria (hem″ah-tu′re-ah) [*hemat-* + Gr. *ouron* urine + *-ia*] blood in the urine. **endemic h.,** urinary schistosomiasis. **enzootic bovine h.,** a disease of cattle marked by passing of blood in the urine, anemia, and debilitation. **essential h.,** hematuria for which no cause has been determined; called also *primary h.* **false h.,** redness of the urine due to food or drugs containing pigment. **microscopic h.,** blood in the urine, the presence of which can be demonstrated only by the microscope. **primary h.,** essential h. **renal h.,** hematuria in which the blood comes from the kidney. **urethral h.,** hematuria in which the blood comes from the urethra. **vesical h.,** hematuria in which the blood comes from the bladder.

heme (hēm) 1. any quadridentate chelate of iron with the four pyrrole groups of a porphyrin, further distinguished as ferroheme or ferriheme referring to the chelates of Fe(II) and Fe(III) respectively. The four porphyrin ligands form a square-planar complex; the fifth and sixth coordination positions of the iron atom are perpendicular to the plane of the porphyrin and both may be occupied by strong field ligands, such as a nitrogen atom of a histidine residue of a protein, as in cytochromes, or only one may be so occupied, as in hemoglobin where the sixth position reversibly binds oxygen. 2. ferroheme, the Fe(II) chelate. Cf. *hematin.* 3. protoheme IX, the heme of hemoglobin.

hemendothelioma (hem″en-do-the″le-o′mah) hemangioendothelioma.

Hementaria (he″men-ta′re-ah) *Haementaria.*

hemeralope (hem′er-al-ōp) a person affected with hemeralopia.

hemeralopia (hem″er-ah-lo′pe-ah) [Gr. *hēmera* day + *alaos* blind + *-opia*] day blindness; defective vision in a bright light.

Hemerocampa (hem″er-o-kam′pah) a genus of moths. **H. leukostig′ma,** the white-marked tussock moth; in the larval stage the smaller white hairs are venomous and may produce severe urticaria.

hemerythrin (hēm″ĕ-rith′rin) [*hem-* + Gr. *erythros* red] the coloring matter of the blood of earthworms which is contained in the plasma.

heme synthetase (hēm sin′thĕ-tās) ferrochelatase.

hemi- [Gr. *hēmi-* half] a prefix meaning one half.

hemiacardius (hem″e-ah-kar′de-us) [*hemi-* + *a* neg. + Gr. *kardia* heart] one of twin fetuses in which only a part of the circulation is accomplished by its own heart.

hemiacephalus (hem″e-ah-sef′ah-lus) [*hemi-* + *a* neg. + Gr. *kephalē* head] a monster whose head lacks a brain and calvarium.

hemiacetal (hem″ĭ-as′ĕ-tal) a derivative formed by a combination of an aldehyde with an alcohol.

hemiachromatopsia (hem″e-ak″ro-mah-top′se-ah) [*hemi-* + *achromatopsia*] color blindness in one half, or in corresponding halves, of the visual field.

hemiacidrin (hem″e-as′ĭ-drin) a solution containing citric and gluconic acids, magnesium hydroxycarbonate, magnesium acid citrate, and calcium carbonate; it is capable of dissolving struvite calculi.

hemiageusia (hem″e-ah-gu′ze-ah) [*hemi-* + *a* neg. + Gr. *geusis* taste + *-ia*] loss or absence of the sense of taste on one side of the tongue.

hemiageustia (hem″e-ah-gūs′te-ah) hemiageusia.

hemialbumin (hem″e-al-bu′min) [*hemi-* + *albumin*] hemialbumose.

hemialbumose (hem″e-al′bu-mōs) a crystallizable product of the digestion of certain proteins; normally found in bone marrow, and occurring in the urine of osteomalacia and diphtheria.

hemialbumosuria (hem″e-al-bu″mo-su′re-ah) [*hemialbumose* + *-uria*] the presence of hemialbumose in the urine.

hemialgia (hem″e-al′je-ah) [*hemi-* + *-algia*] pain affecting one side of the body only.

hemiamblyopia (hem″e-am″ble-o′pe-ah) hemianopia.

hemiamyosthenia (hem″e-ah-mi″os-the′ne-ah) [*hemi-* + *a* neg. + Gr. *mys* muscle + *sthenos* strength + *-ia*] lack of muscular power on one side of the body.

hemianacusia (hem″e-an″ah-ku′ze-ah) [*hemi-* + *an* neg. + Gr. *akousia* hearing] loss of hearing in one ear only.

hemianalgesia (hem″e-an″al-je′ze-ah) [*hemi-* + *analgesia*] analgesia of one side of the body.

hemianencephaly (hem″e-an″en-sef′ah-le) [*hemi-* + Gr. *an* neg. + *enkephalos* brain] congenital absence of one side of the brain.

hemianesthesia (hem″e-an″es-the′ze-ah) anesthesia affecting only one side of the body; called also *unilateral anesthesia.* **alternate h.,** h. cruciata. **cerebral h.,** that which is due to lesion of the internal capsule of the lenticular nucleus. **crossed h.,** h. cruciata. **h. crucia′ta,** loss of sensation on one side of the face with contralateral loss of pain and temperature sense on the body, resulting from a lateral lesion in the pons or medulla, affecting both the sensory root of the trigeminal nerve and the spinothalamic tract. **mesocephalic h., pontile h.,** that which is due to disease of the pons. **spinal h.,** that which is due to a lesion of the spinal cord.

hemianopia (hem″e-ah-no′pe-ah) [*hemi-* + *an.* neg. + *-opia*] defective vision or blindness in half of the visual field of one or both eyes; loosely, scotoma in less than half of the visual field of one or both eyes. **absolute h.,** blindness to light, color, and form, in half of the visual field. **altitudinal h.,** hemianopia in the upper or lower half of the visual field. **bilateral h.,** hemianopia affecting both eyes. **binasal h.,** heteronymous hemianopia in which the defects are in the nasal half of the field of vision in each eye. **binocular h.,** bilateral h. **bitemporal h.,** heteronymous hemianopia in which the defects are in the temporal half of the field of vision in each eye. **complete h.,** hemianopia affecting an entire half of the visual field of each eye. **congruous h.,** homonymous hemianopia in which the defects in the field of vision in each eye are symmetrical in position, shape, size, and degree. **crossed h.,** altitudinal hemianopia affecting the upper field of one eye and the lower field of the other. **heteronymous h.,** hemianopia affecting the nasal or the temporal half of the field of vision of each eye. **homonymous h.,** hemianopia affecting the right halves or the left halves of the visual fields of the two eyes. **horizontal h.,** altitudinal h. **incomplete h.,** hemianopia affecting less than an entire half of the visual field. **incongruous h.,** homonymous hemianopia in which the defects in the field of vision in the two eyes differ in one or more respects, as in extent or intensity. **lateral h.,** homonymous h. **nasal h.,** hemianopia in the nasal halves of the visual fields. **quadrant h., quadrantic h.,** quadrantanopia. **relative h.,** defective vision of or blindness to form or color in half of the visual field, the perception of light being retained. **temporal h.,** hemianopia in the temporal halves of the visual fields. **unilateral h.,** hemianopia in one eye only.

hemianopic (hem″e-ah-no′pik) pertaining to or characterized by hemianopia.

hemianopsia (hem″e-an-op′se-ah) hemianopia.

hemianoptic (hem″e-an-op′tik) hemianopic.

hemianosmia (hem″e-an-oz′me-ah) [hemi- + anosmia] loss of the sense of smell in one of the nostrils.

hemiapraxia (hem″e-ah-prak′se-ah) [hemi- + apraxia] apraxia affecting one side of the body only.

hemiarthrosis (hem″e-ar-thro′sis) [hemi- + arthrosis] a spurious synchondrosis.

Hemiascomycetidae (hem″e-as″ko-mi-se′tĭ-de) a subclass of primitive ascomycetous fungi in which the mycelium is small or lacking and the asci develop without hyphae, including the family Endomycetales.

hemiasynergia (hem″e-ah″sin-er′je-ah) [hemi- + asynergia] asynergia affecting one side of the body only.

hemiataxia (hem″e-ah-tak′se-ah) [hemi- + ataxia] ataxia affecting one side of the body only.

hemiataxy (hem″e-ah-tak′se) hemiataxia.

hemiathetosis (hem″e-ath″ĕ-to′sis) [hemi- + athetosis] athetosis affecting one side of the body only.

hemiatrophy (hem″e-at′ro-fe) [hemi- + atrophy] atrophy of one side of the body or of one half of an organ or part. **facial h.,** atrophy of one half of the face which is sometimes progressive, and is of unknown cause; called also *Romberg's disease*. **progressive lingual h.,** progressive atrophy of one lateral half of the tongue.

hemiaxial (hem″e-aks′e-al) at any oblique angle to the long axis of the body or a part.

hemiballism (hem″e-bal′izm) hemiballismus.

hemiballismus (hem″e-bal-iz′mus) [hemi- + Gr. ballismos jumping] a violent form of motor restlessness involving only one side of the body and being most marked in the upper extremity, resulting from a destructive lesion of the hypothalamic nucleus; called also *body of Luys syndrome*.

hemibladder (hem″ĭ-blad′er) a half bladder; a developmental anomaly in which the bladder is formed as two physically separated parts, each with its own ureter.

hemiblock (hem′ĭ-blok) failure in conduction of the cardiac impulse in either of the two main divisions of the left ventricular conducting system (bundle of His); it is called *left anterior hemiblock* when the anterior-superior division is interrupted and *left posterior hemiblock* when the posterior division is interrupted.

hemic (he′mik, hem′ik) [Gr. haima blood] pertaining to the blood.

hemicanities (hem″e-kah-nish′e-ēz) grayness of the hair on one side of the body.

hemicardia (hem″e-kar′de-ah) [hemi- + Gr. kardia heart] a congenital anomaly characterized by the presence of only half of a four-chambered heart. **h. dex′tra,** hemicardia in which the right side of the heart is present. **h. sinis′tra,** hemicardia in which the left side of the heart is present.

hemicardius (hem″e-kar′de-us) a free twin fetus whose development is greatly reduced but whose body form and various parts are still recognizable.

hemicellulose (hem″e-sel′u-lōs) a general name for a group of high molecular weight carbohydrates that resemble

cellulose but are more soluble and more easily decomposed. They can be extracted by dilute alkali and precipitated with dilute acid, and usually contain a hexose, a pentose, and a uronic acid.

hemicentrum (hem″e-sen′trum) [hemi- + centrum] either lateral half of a vertebral centrum.

hemicephalia (hem″e-sĕ-fa′le-ah) [hemi- + Gr. kephalē head] congenital absence of the cerebrum.

hemicephalus (hem″e-sef′ah-lus) a monster exhibiting hemicephalia.

hemicerebrum (hem″e-ser′ĕ-brum) [hemi- + cerebrum] a cerebral hemisphere.

hemichorea (hem″e-ko-re′ah) [hemi- + chorea] chorea which affects only one side; see *Huntington's chorea,* under *chorea.*

hemichromatopsia (hem″e-kro″mah-top′se-ah) hemiachromatopsia.

hemicolectomy (hem″e-ko-lek′to-me) [hemi- + colectomy] excision of approximately half of the colon. **left h.,** resection of the left half of the colon, from the middle of the transverse segment to the rectum. **right h.,** resection of the right half of the colon, from the ileum to the middle of the transverse segment.

hemicorticectomy (hem″e-kor″tĭ-sek′to-me) excision of a cerebral hemisphere leaving the basal ganglia intact; done in intractable epilepsy.

hemicrania (hem″e-kra′ne-ah) [hemi- + Gr. kranion skull] 1. pain or aching in one side of the head. 2. incomplete anencephaly.

hemicraniectomy (hem″e-kra″ne-ek′to-me) [hemi- + Gr. kranion skull + ektomē excision] exposure of half of the brain by sectioning the vault of the skull from front to back near the median line and forcing the entire side outward.

hemicraniosis (hem″e-kra″ne-o′sis) a condition marked by hyperostosis on one half of the cranium or face, with cerebral involvement. The condition is believed to be due to endothelioma of the dura.

hemicraniotomy (hem″e-kra″ne-ot′o-me) [hemi- + Gr. kranion skull + temnein to cut] hemicraniectomy.

hemidecortication (hem″e-de-kor″tĭ-ka′shun) removal of one half of the cerebral cortex.

hemidesmosome (hem″e-des′mo-sōm) [hemi- + desmosome] a structure similar to a desmosome but representing only half of it, found on the basal surface of some epithelial cells, forming the site of attachment between the basal surface of the cell and the basement membrane. Called also *half desmosome.*

Hemidesmus (hem″e-des′mus) a genus of asclepiadaceous plants. The root of *H. in′dicus* R. Br. has been used as a demulcent, diuretic, and alterative.

hemidiaphoresis (hem″e-di″ah-fo-re′sis) [hemi- + diaphoresis] hemihyperhidrosis.

hemidiaphragm (hem″e-di′ah-fram) one half of the diaphragm.

hemidrosis (hem″ĭ-dro′sis) hemihidrosis.

hemidysergia (hem″e-dis-er′je-ah) dysergia affecting one side of the body.

hemidysesthesia (hem″e-dis″es-the′ze-ah) [hemi- + dys- + aisthēsis feeling] a disorder of sensation affecting one side of the body only.

hemidystrophy (hem″e-dis′tro-fe) unequal development of the two sides of the body.

hemiectromelia (hem″e-ek-tro-me′le-ah) a developmental anomaly characterized by imperfect development of the limbs of one side of the body.

hemielastin (hem″e-e-las′tin) a substance formed by the digestion or hydrolysis of elastin.

hemiencephalus (hem″e-en-sef′ah-lus) [hemi- + Gr. enkephalos brain] a fetus that lacks one cerebral hemisphere.

hemiepilepsy (hem″e-ep′ĭ-lep-se) [hemi- + epilepsy] epilepsy affecting one side of the body only.

hemifacial (hem″e-fa′shal) pertaining to or affecting one half of the face.

hemigastrectomy (hem″e-gas-trek′to-me) excision of half of the stomach.

hemigeusia (hem″e-gu′se-ah) [hemi- + Gr. geusis taste + -ia] presence of taste perception on one side of the tongue only.

hemigigantism (hem″ĭ-ji′gan-tizm) overgrowth of one side of the entire body or of a portion of one side, as of the face.

hemiglossal (hem″e-glos′sal) [*hemi-* + Gr. *glōssa* tongue] affecting one side of the tongue; hemilingual.

hemiglossectomy (hem″e-glos-sek′to-me) [*hemi-* + Gr. *glōssa* tongue + *ektomē* excision] resection of one side of the tongue.

hemiglossitis (hem″e-glos-si′tis) [*hemi-* + Gr. *glōssa* tongue + *-itis*] inflammation involving only one side of the tongue.

hemignathia (hem″e-nath′e-ah) [*hemi-* + Gr. *gnathos* jaw + *-ia*] a developmental anomaly characterized by partial to complete lack of the lower jaw on one side.

hemihepatectomy (hem″e-hep″ah-tek′to-me) excision of half of the liver.

hemihidrosis (hem″e-hĭ-dro′sis) [*hemi-* + Gr. *hidrōs* sweat] sweating on one side of the body only. Called also *hemidrosis.*

hemihypalgesia (hem″e-hi″pal-je′ze-ah) [*hemi* + *hypalgesia*] diminished sensitiveness to pain affecting one side of the body.

hemihyperesthesia (hem″e-hi″per-es-the′ze-ah) [*hemi-* + *hyperesthesia*] abnormally increased acuteness of sensation on one side of the body.

hemihyperidrosis (hem″e-hi″per-ĭ-dro′sis) [*hemi-* + Gr. *hyper* over + *hidrōs* sweat] excessive sweating on one side of the body only; called also *hemidiaphoresis.*

hemihypermetria (hem″e-hi″per-me′tre-ah) hypermetria affecting one side of the body.

hemihyperplasia (hem″e-hi″per-pla′ze-ah) overdevelopment of one side of the body, or of one half of an organ or part, as of the cranium.

hemihypertonia (hem″e-hi″per-to′ne-ah) [*hemi-* + Gr. *hyper* over + *tonos* tension + *-ia*] increased tone of the muscles of one side, which may result in contractures; sometimes seen after a stroke. Called also *hemitonia.*

hemihypertrophy (hem″e-hi-per′tro-fe) [*hemi-* + *hypertrophy*] overgrowth of one half of the body or unilateral hypertrophy of a part. **facial h.,** hypertrophy of half of the face.

hemihypesthesia (hem″e-hi″pes-the′ze-ah) abnormally decreased acuteness of sensation on one side of the body.

hemihypoesthesia (hem″e-hi″po-es-the′ze-ah) hemihypesthesia.

hemihypometria (hem″e-hi″po-me′tre-ah) hypometria affecting one side of the body.

hemihypoplasia (hem″e-hi″po-pla′ze-ah) underdevelopment of one side of the body, or of one half of a part or organ, as of the brain.

hemihypotonia (hem″e-hi″po-to′ne-ah) [*hemi-* + Gr. *hypo* under + *tonos* tension + *-ia*] reduced muscle tone of one side of the body.

hemikaryon (hem″e-kar′e-on) [*hemi-* + Gr. *karyon* nucleus] a cell nucleus which contains the haploid number of chromosomes.

hemiketal (hem″e-ke′tal) a derivative formed by a combination of a ketone group with an alcohol.

hemilaminectomy (hem″e-lam″ĭ-nek′to-me) surgical removal of one side of the vertebral lamina.

hemilaryngectomy (hem″e-lar″in-jek′to-me) excision of one lateral half of the larynx.

hemilateral (hem″e-lat′er-al) affecting one lateral half.

hemilesion (hem″e-le′zhun) a lesion of one side of the spinal cord only.

hemilingual (hem″e-ling′gwal) [*hemi-* + L. *lingua* tongue] affecting one side of the tongue; hemiglossal.

hemimacroglossia (hem″e-mak″ro-glos′e-ah) enlargement of one side of the tongue.

hemimandibulectomy (hem″e-man-dib-u-lek′to-me) surgical excision of half of the mandible.

hemimaxillectomy (hem″ĭ-mak″sĭ-lek′to-me) [*hemi-* + *maxillectomy*] surgical excision of half or part of the maxilla.

hemimelia (hem″e-me′le-ah) [*hemi-* + Gr. *melos* limb + *-ia*] a developmental anomaly characterized by absence of all or part of the distal half of a limb; see illustration under *amelia.* **fibular h.,** hemimelia of the lower limb in which the fibular side is absent. **radial h.,** hemimelia of the upper limb in which the radial side is absent. **tibial h.,** hemimelia of the lower limb, in which the tibial side is absent. **ulnar h.,** hemimelia of the upper limb, in which the ulnar side is absent.

hemimelus (hem-im′ĕ-lus) an individual exhibiting hemimelia.

hemin (he′min) hematin crystallized as the chloride or other salt.

heminephrectomy (hem″e-nĕ-frek′to-me) excision of a portion of a kidney.

heminephroureterectomy (hem″e-nef″ro-u-re″ter-ek′to-me) excision of a portion of a kidney and ureter.

hemineurasthenia (hem″e-nu″ras-the′ne-ah) neurasthenia affecting one side of the body only.

hemiobesity (hem″e-o-bēs′ĭ-te) [*hemi-* + *obesity*] obesity of one side of the body only.

hemiopalgia (hem″e-op-al′je-ah) [*hemi-* + Gr. *ōps* eye + *-algia*] pain in one side of the head and in one eye.

hemiopia (hem″e-o′pe-ah) hemianopia.

hemiopic (hem″e-op′ik) hemianopic.

hemipagus (hem-ip′ah-gus) [*hemi-* + Gr. *pagos* thing fixed] twin fetuses united laterally at the thorax.

hemiparalysis (hem″e-pah-ral′ĭ-sis) hemiplegia.

hemiparanesthesia (hem″e-par″an-es-the′ze-ah) [*hemi-* + Gr. *para* below + *anesthesia*] anesthesia of the lower half of one side of the body.

hemiparaplegia (hem″e-par″ah-ple′je-ah) [*hemi-* + *paraplegia*] paralysis of the lower half of one side of the body.

hemiparesis (hem″e-par′e-sis) [*hemi-* + *paresis*] muscular weakness or partial paralysis affecting one side of the body.

hemiparesthesia (hem″e-par″es-the′ze-ah) [*hemi-* + *paresthesia*] perverted sensation on one side of the body.

hemiparetic (hem″e-pah-ret′ik) 1. pertaining to hemiparesis. 2. one affected with hemiparesis.

hemiparkinsonism (hem″e-par″kin-son-izm) parkinsonism affecting only one side of the body.

hemipelvectomy (hem″e-pel″vek′to-me) amputation of a lower limb through the sacroiliac joint.

hemipeptone (hem″e-pep′tōn) [*hemi-* + *peptone*] one of the intermediate products of pepsin digestion of protein; it is formed along with antipeptone, and differs from the latter in being convertible into amino acids by trypsin.

hemiphalangectomy (hem″e-fal″an-jek′to-me) the excision of part of a digital phalanx.

hemiplacenta (hem″e-plah-sen′tah) [*hemi-* + *placenta*] an organ, composed of the chorion, yolk sac, and, usually, allantois, which puts marsupial embryos into temporary relation with the maternal uterus.

hemiplegia (hem″e-ple′je-ah) [*hemi-* + Gr. *plēgē* stroke] paralysis of one side of the body. **h. al′ternans hypoglos′sica,** hemiplegia due to lesion of the hypoglossal nerve on the side opposite the paralyzed part. **alternate h.,** that which affects a part on one side of the body and another part on the opposite side. **alternating oculomotor h.,** syndrome of Weber. **ascending h.,** ascending paralysis of one lateral half of the body. **capsular h.,** hemiplegia due to lesion of the internal capsule. **cerebral h.,** that which is due to a lesion of the brain. **contralateral h.,** hemiplegia on the side of the body opposite the site of the brain lesion causing it. **crossed h.,** alternate h. **h. crucia′ta,** alternate h. **facial h.,** paralysis of one side of the face, the body being unaffected. **faciobrachial h.,** paralysis of one half of the face and of the arm on the same side. **faciolingual h.,** paralysis of one side of the face and tongue. **flaccid h.,** hemiplegia with loss of tone of the muscles of the paralyzed part and absence of tendon reflexes. Cf. *spastic h.* **Gubler's h.,** Millard-Gubler syndrome. **infantile h.,** hemiplegia due to cerebral thrombosis or hemorrhage at delivery or occurring before birth. **puerperal h.,** hemiplegia of women occurring shortly after childbirth. **spastic h.,** hemiplegia marked by spasticity of the muscles of the paralyzed part and increased tendon reflexes. Cf. *flaccid h.* **spinal h.,** a form due to a lesion of the spinal cord. **Wernicke-Mann h.,** partial hemiplegia of the extremities; called also *Wernicke-Mann type.*

hemiplegic (hem″e-ple′jik) pertaining to or of the nature of hemiplegia.

Hemiptera (he-mip′ter-ah) [*hemi-* + Gr. *pteron* wing] an order of insects which may be winged or wingless, including ordinary bugs and lice, characterized by having the mouth parts adapted to piercing or sucking. The families Cimicidae and Reduviidae (suborder Heteroptera) contain species of considerable medical importance.

hemipterous (he-mip′ter-us) of or pertaining to insects of the order Hemiptera.

hemipylorectomy (hem″e-pi″lor-ek′to-me) excision of half of the pylorus.

hemipyocyanin (hem″e-pi″o-si′ah-nin) an antibiotic produced by the growth of *Pseudomonas aeruginosa* which is active against *Trichophyton schoenleini* and *Candida albicans*.

hemipyonephrosis (hem″e-pi″o-nĕ-fro′sis) a hydronephrotic sac in a portion of the kidney; or pyonephrosis of half of a double kidney.

hemirachischisis (hem″e-rah-kis′kĭ-sis) rachischisis without prolapse of the spinal cord.

hemisacralization (hem″e-sa″kral-i-za′shun) fusion of the fifth lumbar vertebra to the first segment of the sacrum on only one side.

hemiscotosis (hem″e-sko-to′sis) hemianopia.

hemisection (hem″e-sek′shun) division into two equal parts.

hemisectomy (he″me-sek′to-me) [*hemi-* + Gr. *ektomē* excision] amputation of one of two roots of a two-rooted mandibular tooth. Cf. *apicoectomy*.

hemiseptum (hem″e-sep′tum) either half of a septum, especially the lamina of the septum pellucidum of the brain. **h. cer′ebri,** the lateral half of the septum pellucidum of the brain.

hemisomus (hem″e-so′mus) [*hemi-* + Gr. *sōma* body] an imperfectly developed fetus.

hemisotonic (hem″i-so-ton′ik) [Gr. *haima* blood + *isotonic*] having the same osmotic pressure as the blood.

hemispasm (hem″e-spazm) spasm affecting one side only.

hemisphaeria (hem″ĭ-sfe′re-ah) [L.] plural of *hemisphaerium*.

hemisphaerium (hem″ĭ-sfe′re-um), pl. *hemisphae′ria* [L.] Hemisphere; see also *hemispherium*. **hemisphae′ria bul′bi ure′thrae,** the lateral halves of the bulb of the urethra.

hemisphere (hem′ĭ-sfēr) [*hemi-* + Gr. *sphaira* a ball or globe] half of any spherical or roughly spherical structure or organ, as the cerebral hemisphere or the cerebellar hemisphere. **animal h.,** the half of the mass of cells formed by cleavage of a fertilized telolecithal ovum that is nearest the animal pole. **cerebellar h.,** hemispherium cerebelli. **cerebral h.,** hemispherium cerebri. **dominant h.,** that cerebral hemisphere which is more concerned than the other in the integration of sensations and the control of many functions, such as the preferential use of one or the other of paired organs in voluntary movements, e.g., the left cerebral hemisphere in right-handed persons, and vice versa. However, the left hemisphere is usually dominant for speech, regardless of the handedness. **vegetal h.,** the half of the mass of cells formed by cleavage of a fertilized telolecithal ovum that is nearest the vegetal pole.

hemispherectomy (hem″ĭ-sfēr-ek′to-me) [*hemisphere* + Gr. *ektomē* excision] resection of a cerebral hemisphere.

hemispherium (hem″ĭ-sfe′re-um), pl. *hemisphe′ria*. [L.] 1. a general term denoting half of a spherical or spheroid structure. 2. h. cerebri. 3. h. cerebelli. **h. cerebel′li** [NA], cerebellar hemisphere: the part of the cerebellum lateral to the vermis. See also *cerebellum*. **h. cerebra′lis,** NA alternative for *h. cerebri*. **h. cer′ebri** [NA], cerebral hemisphere: either of the pair of structures, formed by evagination of the embryonic telencephalon, lying on either side of the midline, partly separated by the longitudinal cerebral fissure, containing a central cavity, the lateral ventricle, and covered by a layer of gray substance, the cerebral cortex; together they constitute the largest part of the brain in humans. Called also *hemispherium* and *h. cerebralis* [NA alternative].

hemisphygmia (hem″ĭ-sfig′me-ah) [*hemi-* + Gr. *sphygmos* pulse] a condition in which there appears to be twice as many pulse beats as there are heart beats (pulsus bisferiens).

Hemispora stellata (hem-is′po-rah stel-la′tah) a dematiacious imperfect soil fungus reported to have been isolated from cold abscesses, periosteitis, and lesions resembling sporotrichosis.

hemispore (hem′e-spōr) a spore formed by the differentiation and division of the terminal portion of a hypha.

hemisyndrome (hem″e-sin′drōm) a syndrome indicative of a unilateral lesion of the spinal cord.

hemiterata (hem″e-ter′ah-tah) [*hemi-* + Gr. *teras* monster] a group of congenitally deformed individuals who cannot be classed as teratisms or monstrosities.

hemiteratic (hem″e-ter-at′ik) congenitally deformed, but not monstrous.

hemitetany (hem″e-tet′ah-ne) tetany limited to one side of the body.

hemithermoanesthesia (hem″e-ther″mo-an″es-the′ze-ah) absence of temperature sensation on one side of the body.

hemithorax (hem″e-tho′raks) [*hemi-* + *thorax*] one side of the chest.

hemithyroidectomy (hem″e-thi″roi-dek′to-me) excision of one lobe of the thyroid gland.

hemitomias (hem″ĭ-to′me-as) [Gr. *hēmitomias* half a eunuch] a person deprived of one testis.

hemitonia (hem″ĭ-to′ne-ah) [*hemi-* + Gr. *tonos* tension + *-ia*] hemihypertonia.

hemitoxin (hem″ĭ-tok′sin) a toxin the toxicity of which has been reduced by one half.

hemitremor (hem″e-tre′mor) tremor of one side of the body.

hemivagotony (hem″e-va-got′o-ne) hyperexcitability of the vagus nerve on one side.

hemivertebra (hem″e-ver′te-brah) 1. a developmental anomaly characterized by incomplete development of one side of a vertebra. 2. (pl., *hemiver′tebrae*) a vertebra which is incompletely developed on one side.

hemizygosity (hem″e-zi-gos′ĭ-te) [*hemi-* + *zygosity*] possession of only one of a pair of alleles; refers particularly to the state of the male for X-linked genes, and also to abnormal conditions in which a segment of DNA has been deleted from one member of chromosome pair, so that the individual is *hemizygous* for the genes lost with that segment.

hemizygote (hem″e-zi′gōt) an individual or cell exhibiting hemizygosity.

hemizygous (hem″e-zi′gus) possessing only one instead of a pair of genes of a particular kind; see *hemizygosity*.

hemlock (hem′lok) 1. any fir tree of the genus *Tsuga*, especially *T. canadensis* (L.) Carr. (Pinaceae), the source of Canada pitch, of the volatile oil of hemlock, and of an astringent extract. 2. *Conium maculatum* L., or poison hemlock, a large, toxic, umbelliferous herb, which contains the poisonous alkaloid coniine; the dried, fully grown, unripe fruit has sedative, anodyne, and antispasmodic properties. 3. any of the plants of the genera Cicuta and Conium. **poison h.,** see *hemlock*, def. 2. **water h.,** *Cicuta maculata*.

hem(o)-, haem(o)-, hema-, haema- [Gr. *haima* blood] combining form denoting relationship to the blood.

hemoaccess (he″mo-ak′ses) a site of entry into a blood vessel, as one maintained for recurrent hemodialysis.

hemoagglutination (he″mo-ah-gloo″tĭ-na′shun) hemagglutination.

hemoagglutinin (he″mo-ah-gloo″tĭ-nin) hemagglutinin.

hemobilia (he″mo-bil′e-ah) bleeding into the biliary passages.

hemobilinuria (he″mo-bi-lin-u′re-ah) [*hemo-* + *bilin* + Gr. *ouron* urine + *-ia*] the presence of urobilin in the blood and urine.

hemoblast (he′mo-blast) hemocytoblast. **lymphoid h. of Pappenheim,** pronormoblast.

hemoblastosis (he″mo-blas-to′sis) (*obs.*) proliferation of the blood-forming tissues; the term includes leukosis, erythrosis, and reticuloendotheliosis.

hemocatheresis (he″mo-kah-ther′ĕ-sis) [*hemo-* + Gr. *kathairesis* destruction] the destruction of blood, especially of erythrocytes.

hemocatheretic (he″mo-kath″er-et′ik) pertaining to, characterized by, or promoting hemocatheresis.

Hemoccult (he′mo-kult) trademark for a modification of the guaiac test for occult blood, in which guaiac-impregnated filter paper is used; the test is positive if the specimen turns blue.

hemocele (he'mo-sēl) .hemocoelom.

hemocelom (he''mo-se'lom) hemocoelom.

hemocholecyst (he''mo-ko'le-sist) nontraumatic hemorrhage of the gallbladder.

hemocholecystitis (he''mo-ko-le-sis-ti'tis) cholecystitis with hemorrhage into the gallbladder.

hemochorial (he''mo-ko're-al) [*hemo-* + *chorion*] denoting a type of placenta in which maternal blood comes in direct contact with the chorion.

hemochromatosis (he''mo-kro''mah-to'sis) [*hemo-* + *chromatosis*] a disorder due to deposition of hemosiderin in the parenchymal cells, causing tissue damage and dysfunction of the liver, pancreas, heart, and pituitary. Other clinical signs include bronze pigmentation of skin, arthropathy, diabetes, cirrhosis, hepatosplenomegaly, hypogonadism, and loss of body hair. Full development of the disease among women is restricted by menstruation, pregnancy, and lower dietary intake of iron. *Acquired hemochromatosis* may be the result of blood transfusions, excessive dietary iron, or secondary to other disease, e.g., thalassemia or sideroblastic anemia. *Idiopathic* or *genetic hemochromatosis* is an autosomal recessive disorder of metabolism associated with a gene tightly linked to the A locus of the HLA complex on chromosome 6.

hemochromatotic (he''mo-kro''mah-tot'ik) pertaining to or characterized by hemochromatosis.

hemochrome (he'mo-krōm) [*hemo-* + Gr. *chrōma* color] a heme compound in which the fifth and sixth coordination positions of the central iron atom are occupied by strong field ligands, usually nitrogen atoms, as in cytochromes; originally a complex of 2 moles of a nitrogenous base per mole of heme. Called also *hemochromogen*.

hemochromogen (he''mo-kro'mo-jen) [*hemo-* + *chromo-* + *-gen*] hemochrome. **hemoglobin h.,** a hemoglobin in which the globin has been denatured.

hemoclasia (he''mo-kla'se-ah) the occurrence of postalimentary leukopenia; see *hemoclastic crisis,* under *crisis.*

hemoclasis (he-mok'lah-sis) [*hemo-* + Gr. *klasis* a breaking] hemolysis.

hemoclastic (he-mo-klas'tik) pertaining to, characterized by, or causing destruction or dissolution of erythrocytes; see also under *crisis.*

hemoclip (he'mo-klip) a metal clip used to ligate blood vessels.

hemocoagulin (he''mo-ko-ag'u-lin) a constituent of the venom of certain snakes which causes coagulation of the blood.

hemocoelom (he''mo-se'lom) [*hemo-* + *coelom*] 1. the part of the coelom in which the heart is developed. 2. collectively, the spaces between the cells and tissues of many invertebrates, such as most mollusks, arthropods, and tunicates, through which a bloodlike fluid (hemolymph) circulates. Sometimes spelled *hemocele* and *hemocoel.*

hemocoeloma (he''mo-se-lo'mah) [*hemo-* + *coeloma*] hemocoelom.

hemoconcentration (he''mo-kon''sen-tra'shun) decrease of the fluid content of the blood, with resulting increase in its concentration. Cf. *exemia.*

hemoconia (he''mo-ko'ne-ah) [*hemo-* + Gr. *konia* dust] small, round or dumbbell-shaped particles demonstrating brownian movement, observed in blood platelets in a wet film of blood under darkfield microscopy. Called also *blood dust (of Müller)* and *Müller's dust bodies.*

hemoconiosis (he''mo-ko''ne-o'sis) the presence in the blood of abnormal amounts of hemoconia.

hemocryoscopy (he''mo-kri-os''ko-pe) [*hemo-* + *cryoscopy*] cryoscopy of the blood; the ascertaining of the freezing point of the blood.

hemoculture (he'mo-kul'tūr) [*hemo-* + *culture*] a bacteriological culture of the blood.

hemocuprein (he''mo-ku'prein) superoxide dismutase.

hemocyanin (he''mo-si'ah-nin) a nonheme blue respiratory pigment that is found in the blood plasma of many mollusks and arthropods and is composed of monomers each of which contains two atoms of Cu^+ and can bind one molecule of O_2. **keyhole-limpet h. (KLH),** the hemocyanin from the keyhole limpet, a marine gastropod mollusk related to snails and slugs; KLH is a commonly used antigen in laboratory immunology.

hemocyte (he'mo-sīt) [*hemo-* + Gr. *kytos* hollow vessel] any blood corpuscle, or formed element of the blood.

hemocytoblast (he''mo-si'to-blast) [*hemocyte* + Gr. *blastos* germ] the free stem cell from which, according to the monophyletic theory, all blood cells are derived; in modern terminology the totipotent hematopoietic stem cell.

hemocytoblastoma (he''mo-si''to-blas-to'mah) a tumor containing all the cells typical of bone marrow.

hemocytocatheresis (he''mo-si''to-kah-ther'ĕ-sis) [*hemocyte* + Gr. *kathairesis* destruction] the destruction of erythrocytes.

hemocytoma (he'mo-si-to'mah) a tumor containing undifferentiated blood cells.

hemocytometer (he''mo-si-tom'ĕ-ter) a device used in manual blood cell counts consisting of a counting chamber of uniform depth that is covered by a ruled cover glass so that the region under each ruled square contains a known volume of the diluted blood specimen.

hemocytometry (hem''o-si-tom'ĕ-tre) [*hemo-* + Gr. *kytos* hollow vessel + Gr. *metron* measure] the counting of blood cells using a hemocytometer.

hemocytophagia (he''mo-si''to-fa'je-ah) [*hemocyte* + Gr. *phagein* to devour] the ingestion and destruction of blood corpuscles by the histiocytes of the reticuloendothelial system.

hemocytophagic (he''mo-si''to-faj'ik) pertaining to or characterized by hemocytophagia.

hemocytopoiesis (he''mo-si''to-poi-e'sis) hematopoiesis.

hemocytotripsis (he''mo-si''to-trip'sis) [*hemocyte* + Gr. *tribein* to rub] the disintegration of the blood corpuscles by reason of pressure.

hemodiagnosis (he''mo-di''ag-no'sis) [*hemo-* + *diagnosis*] diagnosis by examination of the blood.

hemodialysis (he''mo-di-al'ĭ-sis) the removal of certain elements from the blood by virtue of the difference in the rates of their diffusion through a semipermeable membrane, e.g., by means of a hemodialyzer.

hemodialyzer (he''mo-di'ah-līz''er) an apparatus by which hemodialysis may be performed, blood being separated by a semipermeable membrane from a solution of such composition as to secure diffusion of certain elements out of the blood. Popularly called *artificial kidney.*

hemodiapedesis (he''mo-di''ah-pĕ-de'sis) [*hemo-* + *diapedesis*] the extravasation of blood through the skin.

hemodilution (he''mo-di-lu'shun) increase of the fluid content of the blood with resulting decrease in concentration of its erythrocytes.

hemodynamic (he''mo-di-nam'ik) pertaining to the movements involved in the circulation of the blood.

hemodynamics (he''mo-di-nam'iks) [*hemo-* + Gr. *dynamis* power] the study of the movements of the blood and of the forces concerned therein.

hemodynamometry (he''mo-di''nah-mom'ĕ-tre) measurement of blood pressure.

hemodystrophy (he''mo-dis''tro-fe) [*hemo-* + *dys-* + Gr. *trophē* nutrition] any blood disease due to faulty blood nutrition.

hemoendothelial (he''mo-en-do-the'le-al) [*hemo-* + *endothelium*] denoting a type of placenta in which maternal blood comes in contact with the endothelium of chorionic vessels.

Hemofil (he'mo-fil) trademark for a highly concentrated preparation of antihemophilic factor (coagulation Factor VIII).

hemofilter (he'mo-fil''ter) a filter used in hemofiltration.

hemofiltration (he''mo-fil-tra'shun) the removal of waste products from the blood by passing the blood through extracorporeal filters. **continuous arteriovenous h.,** hemofiltration by means of small-volume, low-resistance hemofilters powered by the patient's arterial pressure, without need for a mechanical pump; used as an alternative to conventional hemodialysis.

hemoflagellate (he''mo-flaj'ĕ-lāt) [*hemo-* + L. *flagellum* whip] any flagellate microorganism parasitic in the blood, especially protozoa of the suborder Trypanosomatina.

hemofuscin (he″mo-fūs′in) [hemo- + L. *fuscus* brown] a brownish-yellow pigment that results from the decomposition of hemoglobin; it gives the urine a deep ruddy color.

hemogenesis (he″mo-jen′ĕ-sis) hematopoiesis.

hemogenic (he″mo-jen′ik) hematogenic.

hemoglobin (he′mo-glo″bin) the oxygen-carrying pigment of the erythrocytes, formed by the developing erythrocyte in bone marrow. It is a conjugated protein containing four heme groups and globin, F having the property of reversible oxygenation. A molecule of hemoglobin contains four globin polypeptide chains. They are designated α, β, γ, δ, in the adult; and each is composed of several hundred amino acids. Different types of hemoglobin are determined by the specific combination of these chains, the number of chains of the different types in the molecule being indicated by subscript numerals. For example, *hemoglobin F* (*fetal h.*), which is the predominant type in the newborn, may be written as $\alpha_2{}^A\gamma_2{}^F$. *Hemoglobin A* (*adult h.*), which is normally predominant in the adult is designated $\alpha_2{}^A\beta_2{}^A$ or $\alpha_2\beta_2$. Another hemoglobin, *hemoglobin A₂* (designated $\alpha_2{}^A\delta_2{}^{A2}$ or $\alpha_2{}^A\delta_2$), is usually present in limited minor concentrations. Many hemoglobins with differing electrophoretic mobilities and characteristics have been reported, for example, S, C, D, E, G, H, I, J, K, L, M, N, Q, Norfolk, Barts, and many others. (See also *hemoglobinopathy.*) Because refined biochemical techniques may lead to the discovery of additional hemoglobins, certain standards for nomenclature have been devised. The hemoglobin electrophoretic mobility is designated by a capital letter; if two or more hemoglobins have the same mobility, the geographic area of discovery is indicated as a subscript, for example, hemoglobin M_S, or $M_{Saskatoon}$, and hemoglobin M_M, or $M_{Milwaukee}$. To restrict the increasing use of capital letters new hemoglobins are named simply for the laboratory, hospital, or town where they were discovered, for example, hemoglobin$_{Norfolk}$. When known, the number of each amino acid substituting in each polypeptide(s) in the molecule should be indicated by the appropriate superscript numeral. Symbol *Hb*. **h. A,** normal adult hemoglobin, composed of two alpha and two beta chains, $\alpha_2{}^A\beta_2{}^A$. **h. A₁c,** a glycosylated hemoglobin A, having a hexose attached to the N-terminal of its β-chain; its levels are increased in poorly controlled diabetics. **h. A₂,** a normal adult hemoglobin, $\alpha_2{}^A\delta_2$, present in small amounts, in which delta chains replace the beta chains. **Bart's h.,** an abnormal hemoglobin composed of four gamma chains having high oxygen affinity. **h. C,** a relatively common, abnormal hemoglobin in which lysine replaces glutamic acid at position six of the beta chains. It was one of the earliest hemoglobins to have its molecular abnormality defined. In the homozygous state, it produces splenomegaly, moderate or mild hemolytic anemia, recurrent jaundice, and an increased number of target cells and reticulocytes in the peripheral blood, while in the heterozygous state (*h. C trait*) anemia or disease is absent, although increased numbers of target cells are seen in the peripheral blood. **h. carbamate,** a compound of hemoglobin and CO_2, important for the transporation of CO_2 in red cells. **h. Chesapeake,** an abnormal hemoglobin in which the amino acid substitution (leucine for arginine in the alpha chain) results in a molecule so structurally abnormal that it has a high oxygen affinity. **h. D,** an abnormal hemoglobin existing in several molecular forms, all characterized by electrophoretic migration on paper or cellulose acetate at a rate identical to that of hemoglobin S, but differentiated on acid agar gel electrophoresis. The homozygous state is manifested by mild hemolytic anemia with numerous target cells in the peripheral blood, while in the heterozygous state no clinical or hematologic abnormality occurs. **deoxygenated h.,** deoxyhemoglobin. **h. E,** an abnormal hemoglobin resulting from a beta chain mutation in the hemoglobin molecule, occurring most commonly in Southeast Asia, especially Thailand. The homozygous state is manifested by mild hemolytic anemia, usually without splenomegaly, and large numbers of normochromic target cells in the peripheral blood, while in the heterozygous state no clinical or hematologic abnormality occurs. **h. F,** fetal h. **"fast" h's,** those with greater mobility on electrophoresis (in an alkaline buffer) than normal adult hemoglobin (h. A), including hemoglobin K, J, and N. **fetal h.,** the form of hemoglobin normally comprising more than half of the hemoglobin in the fetus, composed of two alpha and two gamma polypeptides ($\alpha_2{}^A\gamma_2{}^F$); it is also present in minimal amounts in adulthood and is abnormally elevated in aplastic anemia,

leukemia, and certain types of thalassemia. It has higher affinity for oxygen under physiologic conditions than does hemoglobin A. Called also *h. F*. **glycosylated h.,** hemoglobin A₁c. **Gower h.,** a normal hemoglobin present in two forms, I and II, in early embryonic life, composed either entirely of epsilon chains (ϵ_4) or of two alpha and two epsilon chains ($\alpha_2{}^A\epsilon_2$) and disappearing *in utero*. **h. Gun Hill,** an unstable hemoglobin resulting from a segmental deletion of amino acids in the beta polypeptide of the hemoglobin molecule, resulting in inability to bind heme and leading to mild hemolytic anemia. **h. H,** a rapidly migrating, abnormal hemoglobin composed of four beta chains, having a high oxygen affinity, found in a form of α-thalassemia in various ethnic groups, manifested by chronic hemolytic anemia associated with splenomegaly clinically and hypochromia, anisocytosis, and poikilocytosis of the red blood cells, with inclusion bodies detectable by supravital staining. **h. I,** an abnormal hemoglobin resulting from an amino acid substitution in the alpha chain which causes sickling in an unknown manner. **h. Lepore,** an abnormal hemoglobin having two normal alpha chains associated with two chains resulting from fusion of beta and delta chain segments. Although of considerable theoretical genetic interest, it produces only a mild anemia and, by itself, poses no special clinical problems. **h. M,** any of several hemoglobins having amino acid substitutions either in the alpha or beta chains and all associated with methemoglobinemia. **mean corpuscular h.,** see *MCH*. **muscle h.,** myoglobin. **nitric oxide h.,** a stable compound of nitric oxide and hemoglobin. **oxidized h., oxygenated h.,** oxyhemoglobin. **h. Rainier,** a hemoglobin in which histidine replaces tyrosine at position 145 in the beta chain; it has increased oxygen affinity and is associated with erythrocytosis. **reduced h.,** deoxyhemoglobin. **h. S,** the most common abnormal hemoglobin, in which valine is substituted for glutamic acid at position six of the beta chain; the heterozygous state results in sickle cell trait, the homozygous in sickle cell anemia. The delineation of the basic abnormality in molecular structure is a milestone in biochemical genetics, for it paved the way for further investigation and demonstrated that a single amino acid substitution may produce widespread, untoward clinical effects. **h. Seattle,** an abnormal hemoglobin in which glutamic acid is substituted for alanine at position 76 of the beta chain; it has decreased oxygen affinity. **"slow" h's,** those less mobile on electrophoresis (in an alkaline buffer) than normal adult hemoglobin (h. A), including hemoglobin S and D. **h. Yakima,** an abnormal hemoglobin in which histidine is substituted for aspartic acid at position 99 of the beta chain; it has increased oxygen affinity and is associated with erythrocytosis.

hemoglobinated (he″mo-glo′bin-āt-ed) containing hemoglobin.

hemoglobinemia (he″mo-glo″bĭ-ne′me-ah) [*hemoglobin* + -*emia*] the presence of free hemoglobin in the blood plasma, an indication of significant intravascular hemolysis.

hemoglobinocholia (he″mo-glo″bĭ-no-ko′le-ah) [*hemoglobin* + Gr. *cholē* bile + -*ia*] the occurrence of hemoglobin in the bile.

hemoglobinolysis (he″mo-glo″bĭ-nol′ĭ-sis) [*hemoglobin* + Gr. *lysis* dissolution] splitting up of hemoglobin.

hemoglobinometer (he″mo-glo″bĭ-nom′ĕ-ter) [*hemoglobin* + Gr. *metron* measure] an instrument for measuring the hemoglobin of the blood.

hemoglobinometry (he″mo-glo″bĭ-nom′ĕ-tre) the measurement of the hemoglobin of the blood.

hemoglobinopathy (he″mo-glo″bĭ-nop′ah-the) [*hemoglobin* + Gr. *pathos* disease] a hematologic disorder caused by alteration in the genetically determined molecular structure of hemoglobin, which results in a characteristic complex of clinical and laboratory abnormalities and often, but not always, overt anemia. The specific features of these hemoglobin abnormalities are related to variation of the composite globin polypeptide chains, designated α, β, γ, δ, to changes or substitutions in the sequential arrangement of the amino acids constituting these chains, or to their deletion from their appropriate place in the molecule. When analysis has revealed the site of biochemical aberration, the abnormality of the peptide chain and the number of the altered amino acid and nature of its replacement also should be indicated. For example, hemoglobin S is expressed as $\alpha_2{}^A\beta_2{}^S$, or $\alpha_2{}^A\beta_2{}^{6\,valine}$, and, more completely, hemoglobin G$_{Philadelphia}$ is expressed as $\alpha_2{}^G\beta_2{}^A$, or $\alpha_2{}^{6\,lysine}\beta_2{}^A$. If more than one hemoglobin is present, the phenotype should be designated by listing them in order of decreasing concentrations; for example, the phenotype for sickle cell trait is expressed as AS, for sickle cell anemia as SS, and for sickle cell–hemoglobin C disease as SC.

hemoglobinopepsia (he″mo-glo″bĭ-no-pep′se-ah) [*hemoglobin* + Gr. *pepsis* digestion] hemoglobinolysis.

hemoglobinous (he″mo-glo′bĭ-nus) containing hemoglobin.

hemoglobinuria (he″mo-glo″bĭ-nu′re-ah) [*hemoglobin* + Gr. *ouron* urine + *-ia*] the presence of free hemoglobin in the urine. **bacillary h.,** an infectious toxemic disease caused by *Clostridium haemolyticum*, affecting primarily cattle, occasionally sheep, and rarely dogs. In cattle, it is marked by inappetence, by cessation of rumination, lactation, and defecation, by fever, bloody diarrhea, and dark-red urine, and by anemia and hemoglobinuria. Called also *bovine h.* and *redwater disease.* **bovine h.,** 1. Texas fever. 2. bacillary h. **malarial h.,** blackwater fever. **march h.,** a benign condition in which hemolysis is produced by repeated uncushioned shocks to some body part; seen occasionally in soldiers after long marches, in marathon runners, or in karate experts. **paroxysmal cold h.,** an autoimmune or postviral disease marked by episodes of hemoglobinemia and hemoglobinuria after exposure to cold, caused by complement-dependent hemolysis due to IgG antibody directed against the P blood group antigen; it is detected by the Donath-Landsteiner test. **paroxysmal nocturnal h. (PNH),** a chronic acquired blood cell dysplasia in which there is proliferation of a clone of stem cells producing erythrocytes, platelets, and granulocytes that are abnormally susceptible to lysis by complement; it is marked by episodes of intravascular hemolysis, particularly following infections, and by venous thromboses, particularly of the hepatic veins; diagnosis is based on the acidified serum test (Ham's test) or the sucrose lysis test. Called also *Marchiafava-Micheli disease* or *syndrome.* **toxic h.,** that which is consequent upon the ingestion of various poisons.

hemoglobinuric (he″mo-glo″bĭ-nu′rik) pertaining to or characterized by hemoglobinuria.

hemogram (he′mo-gram) [*hemo-* + Gr. *gramma* a writing] the blood picture; a written record or a graphic representation of the differential blood count.

hemohistioblast (he″mo-his′te-o-blast″) [*hemo-* + Gr. *histos* tissue + *blastos* germ] Ferrata's name for the hypothetical stem cell of all blood cells; in modern terminology, the totipotential hematopoietic stem cell. Called also *Ferrata's cell.*

hemokinesis (he″mo-ki-ne′sis) [*hemo-* + Gr. *kinēsis* movement] the flow of blood in the body.

hemokinetic (he″mo-ki-net′ik) pertaining to or promoting the flow of blood in the body.

hemolith (he′mo-lith) [*hemo-* + Gr. *lithos* stone] (*obs.*) a concretion in the wall of a blood vessel.

hemology (he-mol′o-je) hematology.

hemolymph (he′mo-limf) [*hemo-* + *lymph*] 1. the blood and lymph. 2. the bloodlike fluid moving through the hemocoelom of those invertebrates (e.g., mollusks, arthropods, and tunicates) with open circulatory systems, which combines the properties of blood and lymphlike interstitial fluid.

hemolymphangioma (he″mo-lim-fan″je-o′mah) hematolymphangioma.

hemolysate (he-mol′ĭ-sāt) the product resulting from hemolysis.

hemolysin (he-mol′ĭ-sin) [*hemo-* + Gr. *lysis* dissolution] a substance that causes hemolysis. **alpha h.,** 1. one producing alpha hemolysis. 2. the hemolysin of the alpha toxin of *Staphylococcus aureus*, which hemolyzes rabbit, sheep, cow, and goat but not human erythrocytes. See also *staphylococcal toxin*, under *toxin.* **bacterial h.,** a toxic substance produced by bacteria that lyses erythrocytes. **beta h.,** 1. one producing beta hemolysis. 2. the hemolysin of the beta toxin of *Staphylococcus aureus*. It is a sphingomyelinase that lyses human and sheep erythrocytes in the cold following a warm incubation. See also *staphylococcal toxins*, under *toxin.* **heterophile h.,** a hemolysin which has affinity for the red cells of some animal besides the one for which it is specific. **hot-cold h.,** a hemolytic substance (e.g., *Staphylococcus aureus* beta-hemolysin) that lyses erythrocytes in the cold following preliminary warm incubation. **immune h.,** a hemolysin produced by deliberate immunization of an animal with blood or blood corpuscles foreign to it, as with rabbit anti-sheep red blood cell serum (hemolysin) used in complement fixation tests.

hemolysis (he-mol′ĭ-sis) [*hemo-* + Gr. *lysis* dissolution] disruption of the integrity of the red cell membrane causing release of hemoglobin. Hemolysis may be caused by bacterial hemolysins, by antibodies that cause complement-dependent lysis, by placing red cells in a hyptonic solution, or by defects in the red cell membrane. **alpha h.,** the production of a zone of greenish discoloration surrounding a bacterial colony on blood-agar medium, caused by partial decomposition of hemoglobin and characteristic of pneumococci and certain streptococci. **beta h.,** the production of a clear zone immediately surrounding a bacterial colony on blood-agar medium, which is characteristic of certain pathogenic bacteria. **contact h.,** the hastened hemolysis of blood cells in contact with a surface. **gamma h.,** the absence of hemolysis around a bacterial colony on blood agar, indicating a nonhemolytic organism. **immune h.,** the lysis by complement of erythrocytes sensitized as a consequence of interaction with specific antibody to the erythrocytes. **passive h.,** the lysis of erythrocytes on which antigen has been adsorbed in the presence of complement and antiserum to that antigen. **venom h.,** hemolysis produced by snake venom.

hemolytic (he″mo-lit′ik) pertaining to, characterized by, or producing hemolysis.

hemolyzable (he″mo-liz′ah-b'l) capable of undergoing hemolysis.

hemolyzation (he″mo-li-za′shun) the production of hemolysis.

hemolyze (he′mo-līz) to subject to or to undergo hemolysis.

hemomanometer (he″mo-mah-nom′ĕ-ter) a manometer for determining blood pressure.

hemomediastinum (he″mo-me″de-as-ti′num) an effusion of blood in the mediastinum.

hemometer (he-mom′ĕ-ter) hemoglobinometer.

hemometra (he″mo-me′trah) hematometra.

hemometry (he-mom′ĕ-tre) hematometry.

hemonephrosis (he″mo-nĕ-fro′sis) hematonephrosis.

hemopathic (he″mo-path′ik) pertaining to disease of the blood; due to blood disorder.

hemopathology (he″mo-pah-thol′o-je) [*hemo-* + *pathology*] study of diseases of the blood.

hemopathy (he-mop′ah-the) [*hemo-* + Gr. *pathos* disease] any disease of the blood.

hemopericardium (he″mo-per″ĭ-kar′de-um) [*hemo-* + *pericardium*] an effusion of blood within the pericardium.

hemoperitoneum (he″mo-per″ĭ-to-ne′um) [*hemo-* + *peritoneum*] an effusion of blood in the peritoneal cavity.

hemopexin (he″mo-pek′sin) a plasma glycoprotein, mol. wt. 57,000, in the β_1-globulin band; it is produced by hepatocytes and its function is the binding of free heme in plasma; it has one binding site for hematin forming a tight complex that is taken up and degraded by hepatocytes.

hemophage (he′mo-fāj) hemophagocyte.

hemophagocyte (he″mo-fag′o-sīt) [*hemo-* + *phagocyte*] a phagocyte which destroys blood cells.

hemophagocytosis (he″mo-fag″o-si-to′sis) hemocytophagia.

hemophil (he′mo-fil) [*hemo-* + Gr. *philein* to love] 1. thriving on blood. 2. a microorganism which grows best in media containing hemoglobin.

hemophilia (he″mo-fil′e-ah) [*hemo-* + *-philia*] a hemorrhagic diathesis occurring in two main forms: (1) hemophilia A (classic hemophilia, factor VIII deficiency), an X-linked disorder due to deficiency of coagulation factor VIII; (2) hemophilia B (factor IX deficiency, Christmas disease), also X-linked, due to deficiency of coagulation factor IX. Both forms are determined by a mutant gene near the telomere of the long arm of the X chromosome (Xq), but at different loci, and are characterized by subcutaneous and intramuscular hemorrhages; bleeding from the mouth, gums, lips, and tongue; hematuria; and hemarthroses. **h. A,** hemophilia due to lack of coagulation Factor VIII; see *hemophilia.*

h. B, Factor IX deficiency; see *coagulation factors,* under *factor.*   **h. B, Leyden,** a transient form of Factor IX deficiency; see *coagulation factors,* under *factor.*   **h. C,** Factor XI deficiency; see *coagulation factors,* under *factor.* **classical h.,** hemophilia A.   **h. neonato'rum,** purpura in newborn children.   **vascular h.,** von Willebrand's disease.

hemophiliac (he″mo-fil′e-ak) an individual exhibiting hemophilia.

hemophilic (he-mo-fil′ik) 1. having an affinity for blood; living in blood. In bacteriology, growing especially well in culture media containing blood or having a nutritional affinity for constituents of fresh blood; said of bacteria of the genera *Haemophilus* and *Bordetella.* 2. pertaining to or characterized by hemophilia.

hemophilioid (he″mo-fil′e-oid) [*hemophilia* + Gr. *eidos* form] resembling classical hemophilia clinically. Applied to a number of hereditary or acquired hemorrhagic disorders that are not due solely to a deficiency of blood coagulation Factor VIII. See *coagulation factors,* under *factor.*

Hemophilus (he-mof′ĭ-lus) *Haemophilus.*

hemophilus (he-mof′ĭ-lus) any bacterium of the genus *Haemophilus.*

hemophobia (he″mo-fo′be-ah) irrational fear of blood.

hemophthalmia, hemophthalmos, hemophthalmus (he″mof-thal′me-ah; he″mof-thal′mos; he″mof-thal′mus) [*hemo-* + Gr. *ophthalmos* eye] an extravasation of blood within the eye.

hemophthisis (he-mof′thĭ-sis) [*hemo-* + Gr. *phthisis* wasting] a term once used to indicate anemia due to insufficient nutrition of blood cells.

hemopiezometer (he″mo-pi″e-zom′ĕ-ter) [*hemo-* + Gr. *piesis* pressure + *metron* measure] any apparatus for measuring blood pressure.

hemoplastic (he″mo-plas′tik) hematoplastic.

hemopleura (he″mo-ploo′rah) hemothorax.

hemopneumopericardium (he″mo-nu″mo-per″ĭ-kar′de-um) pneumopericardium with hemorrhagic effusion.

hemopneumothorax (he″mo-nu″mo-tho′raks) pneumothorax with hemorrhagic effusion.

hemopoiesic (he″mo-poi-e′sik) hematopoietic.

hemopoiesis (he″mo-poi-e′sis) hematopoiesis.

hemopoietic (he″mo-poi-et′ik) hematopoietic.

hemopoietin (he″mo-poi-e′tin) [*hemo-* + Gr. *poein* to make] erythropoietin.

hemopoietine (he″mo-poi-e′tin) a name originally given to a substance which stimulated erythropoiesis; probably the same as erythropoietin.

hemoposia (he″mo-po′ze-ah) [*hemo-* + Gr. *posis* drinking + *-ia*] the drinking of blood, as by parasites.

hemoprecipitin (he″mo-pre-sip′ĭ-tin) a precipitin that precipitates leukoantigens.

hemoproctia (he″mo-prok′she-ah) [*hemo-* + Gr. *prōktos* anus] hemorrhage from the rectum.

hemoprotein (he″mo-pro′tēn) a conjugated protein containing heme as the prosthetic group.

hemopsonin (he″mop-so′nin) [*hemo-* + *opsonin*] an opsonin that renders red blood cells more liable to phagocytosis; called also *hemotropin.*

hemoptic, hemoptoic (he-mop′tik; he-mop-to′ik) hemoptysic.

hemoptysic (he″mop-ti′sik) pertaining to or marked by hemoptysis.

hemoptysis (he-mop′tĭ-sis) [*hemo-* + Gr. *ptyein* to spit] the expectoration of blood or of blood-stained sputum. **cardiac h.,** hemoptysis due to heart disease and related pulmonary hypertension, as in mitral stenosis or Eisenmenger's syndrome. **endemic h.,** parasitic h. **Goldstein's h.,** hemoptysis due to bleeding telangiectases in the tracheobronchial tree. **Manson's h.,** hemoptysis due to infection of the lungs with *Paragonimus westermani;* parasitic h. **oriental h.,** parasitic h. **parasitic h.,** a disease caused by infection of the lungs with *Paragonimus westermani* and other lung flukes of the genus *Paragonimus.* It is marked by cough and spitting of blood and by gradual deterioration of health. Called also *endemic h., pulmonary distomiasis,* and *lung fluke disease.* **vicarious h.,** that

which occurs at the time of normal menstruation; see *vicarious menstruation.*

hemopyelectasis (he″mo-pi-ĕ-lek′tah-sis) [*hemo-* + Gr. *pyelos* pelvis + *ektasis* dilatation] dilatation of the renal pelvis with an accumulation of bloody fluid.

hemorrhachis (he-mor′ah-kis) hematomyelia.

hemorrhage (hem′or-ij) [*hemo-* + Gr. *rhēgnynai* to burst forth] the escape of blood from the vessels; bleeding. Small hemorrhages are classified according to size as petechiae (very small), purpura (up to 1 cm.), and ecchymoses (larger). The massive accumulation of blood within a tissue is called a hematoma. **alveolar h.,** hemorrhage from a dental alveolus. **arterial h.,** the escape of blood from an artery, e.g., ruptured aneurysm. **brain h.,** bleeding into the substance of the brain; see *stroke syndrome,* under *syndrome.* **capillary h.,** the oozing of blood from the minute vessels. **capsuloganglionic h.,** hemorrhage into the basal ganglia and internal and external capsule of the brain. **cerebral h.,** a hemorrhage into the cerebrum. See *stroke syndrome,* under *syndrome.* **concealed h.,** internal h. **essential h.,** one not attributable to an established cause. **expulsive h.,** hemorrhage of the eye, breaking through both the choroid and the retina and extruding the ocular contents before it; usually occurring during the course of intraocular surgical procedure. **external h.,** one in which blood escapes from the body. **extradural h.,** intracranial hemorrhage into the epidural space. **fetomaternal h.,** the leakage of fetal red blood cells into the maternal circulation. **fibrinolytic h.,** hemorrhage resulting from abnormalities in the fibrinolytic system. **flame-shaped h's,** large hemorrhagic spots in the eyeground; called also *flame spots.* **gravitating h.,** hemorrhage into the spinal canal, in which the blood settles to the lower part of the canal from the force of gravity. **internal h.,** hemorrhage in which the extravasated blood remains within the body. **intracerebral h.,** hemorrhage within the cerebrum; see *cerebral h.* **intracranial h.,** bleeding within the cranium, which may be extradural, subdural, subarachnoid, or cerebral. See *stroke syndrome,* under *syndrome.* **intramedullary h.,** hematomyelia. **intrapartum h.,** hemorrhage occurring during parturition. **massive h.,** loss of blood so rapid and profuse that shock supervenes unless appropriate replacement is instituted promptly. **nasal h.,** epistaxis. **parenchymatous h.,** capillary hemorrhage into the substance of an organ. **h. per rhexin,** hemorrhage from rupture of a blood vessel. **petechial h.,** hemorrhage that occurs in minute points beneath the skin. **postpartum h.,** that which occurs soon after labor or childbirth. **primary h.,** that which occurs immediately following injury. **pulmonary h.,** hemorrhage from the lungs; pneumorrhagia. **punctate h.,** spots of blood effused into the tissues from capillary hemorrhage. **recurring h.,** intermittent episodes of bleeding. **renal h.,** hemorrhage from the kidney; nephrorrhagia. **secondary h.,** bleeding which follows an accident or injury after a lapse of time. **splinter h's,** linear hemorrhages beneath the nail; when located near the base of the nail they are characteristic of subacute bacterial endocarditis. **spontaneous h.,** bleeding occurring without overt provocation. **subarachnoid h.,** intracranial hemorrhage into the subarachnoid space. **subdural h.,** cerebral hemorrhage into the subdural space; see under *hematoma,* and see *stroke syndrome,* under *syndrome.* **unavoidable h.,** that which results from the detachment of a placenta previa. **uterine h., essential,** a condition marked by hemorrhage from the uterus, and usually showing hypertrophy of the uterine mucosa and cystic disease of the ovary; called also *metropathia hemorrhagica.* **venous h.,** the escape of blood from the venous system; phleborrhagia.

hemorrhagenic (hem″o-rah-jen′ik) [*hemorrhage* + Gr. *gennan* to produce] causing hemorrhage.

hemorrhagic (hem″o-raj′ik) pertaining to or characterized by hemorrhage; descriptive of any tissue into which bleeding has occurred.

hemorrhagin (hem″o-ra′jin) a cytolysin existing in certain venoms and poisons, such as snake venom and ricin, which is destructive to endothelial cells and blood vessels. Cf. *endotheliotoxin.*

hemorrhagiparous (hem″o-rij-ip′ah-rus) [*hemorrhage* + L. *parere* to produce] hemorrhagenic.

hemorrhea (hem-o-re′ah) hematorrhea.

hemorrheology (he″mo-re-ol′o-je) [*hemo-* + Gr. *rhoia* flow

+ *logos* treatise] the scientific study of the deformation and flow properties of cellular and plasmatic components of blood in macroscopic, microscopic, and submicroscopic dimensions, and the rheological properties of vessel structure with which the blood comes in direct contact.

hemorrhoid (hem′o-roid) [Gr. *haimorrhois*] a varicose dilatation of a vein of the superior or inferior hemorrhoidal plexus, resulting from a persistent increase in venous pressure. **combined h.,** mixed h. **external h.,** a varicose

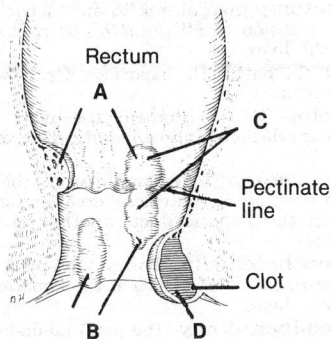

Hemorrhoids: *A*, internal; *B*, external; *C*, combined; *D*, thrombosed.

dilatation of a vein of the inferior hemorrhoidal plexus, situated distal to the pectinate line and covered with modified anal skin. **internal h.,** a varicose dilatation of a vein of the superior hemorrhoidal plexus, originating above the pectinate line, and covered by mucous membrane. **mixed h.,** a varicose dilatation of a vein connecting the superior and inferior hemorrhoidal plexuses, forming an external and an internal hemorrhoid in continuity. **mucocutaneous h.,** mixed h. **prolapsed h.,** an internal hemorrhoid which has descended below the pectinate line and protruded outside the anal sphincter. **strangulated h.,** an internal hemorrhoid which has been prolapsed sufficiently and for long enough time for its blood supply to become occluded by the constricting action of the anal sphincter. **thrombosed h.,** one containing clotted blood.

hemorrhoidal (hem″o-roi′dal) pertaining to, or of the nature of, hemorrhoids.

hemorrhoidectomy (hem″o-roid-ek′to-me) excision of hemorrhoids.

hemosalpinx (he″mo-sal′pinks) [hemo- + Gr. *salpinx* tube] hematosalpinx.

hemosiderin (he″mo-sid′er-in) [hemo- + Gr. *sideros* iron] an intracellular storage form of iron; the granules consist of an ill-defined complex of ferric hydroxides, polysaccharides, and proteins having an iron content of about 33 per cent by weight.

hemosiderinuria (he″mo-sid″er-in-u′re-ah) the presence of hemosiderin in the urine.

hemosiderosis (he″mo-sid″er-o′sis) a focal or general increase in tissue iron stores without associated tissue damage. Cf. *hemochromatosis.* **hepatic h.,** the deposit of an abnormal quantity of hemosiderin in the liver, usually in Kupffer cells; such deposition is not associated with cirrhosis, as is hemochromatosis. **pulmonary h.,** the deposition of abnormal amounts of hemosiderin in the lungs, due to bleeding into the lung interstitium. An idiopathic form, affecting primarily children, is marked by microcytic hypochromic anemia, diffuse pulmonary infiltration, and occasionally hemoptysis; hemosiderin-laden macrophages are abundant in the lungs and may be found in the sputum.

hemosite (he′mo-sīt) (*obs.*) a blood parasite.

hemospermia (he″mo-sper′me-ah) [hemo- + Gr. *sperma* seed + *-ia*] the presence of blood in the semen.

hemosporian (he″mo-spo′re-an) 1. any protozoan of the suborder Haemosporina. 2. pertaining to protozoa of the suborder Haemosporina. Called also *hemosporidian.*

hemosporidian (hem″o-spo-rid′e-an) hemosporian.

hemostasia (he″mo-sta′ze-ah) hemostasis.

hemostasis (he″mo-sta′sis, he-mos′tah-sis) [hemo- + Gr. *stasis* halt] 1. the arrest of bleeding, either by the physiolog-

ical properties of vasoconstriction and coagulation or by surgical means. 2. interruption of the flow of blood through any vessel or to any anatomical area.

hemostat (he′mo-stat) 1. a small surgical clamp for constricting a blood vessel. 2. an agent that checks hemorrhage when properly applied to a bleeding point.

hemostatic (he″mo-stat′ik) [hemo- + Gr. *statikos* standing] 1. checking the flow of blood. 2. an agent that arrests the flow of blood. **capillary h.,** an agent that reduces capillary bleeding time by increasing the contractility and resistance and decreasing the permeability of the capillary wall.

hemostyptic (he″mo-stip′tik) hemostatic.

hemotherapeutics (he″mo-ther″ah-pu′tiks) hemotherapy.

hemotherapy (he″mo-ther′ah-pe) [hemo- + Gr. *therapeia* treatment] treatment of disease by the administration of blood or blood products, such as blood plasma.

hemothorax (he″mo-tho′raks) [hemo- + Gr. *thōrax* chest] a collection of blood in the pleural cavity.

hemotoxic (he″mo-tok′sik) hematotoxic.

hemotoxin (he″mo-tok′sin) an exotoxin characterized by hemolytic activity. **cobra h.,** the constituent of cobra venom which is able to lyse red blood cells of man and of various other animals without the presence of blood serum.

hemotroph (he′mo-trof) [hemo- + Gr. *trophē* nourishment] the sum total of the nutritive substances supplied to the embryo from the maternal blood during gestation. Cf. *histiotroph.*

hemotrophe (he′mo-trof) hemotroph.

hemotrophic (he″mo-trōf-ik) pertaining to or derived through hemotroph.

hemotropic (he″mo-trop′ik) hematotropic.

hemotympanum (he″mo-tim′pah-num) hematotympanum.

hemozoic (he″mo-zo′ik) hematozoan, def. 1.

hemozoin (he″mo-zo′in) [hemo- + Gr. *zōon* animal] a pigment produced by malarial parasites, derived from the hemoglobin in the host's cells, and consisting of insoluble ferriprotoporphyrin polymers that enable the parasites to sequester in benign form. In chronic cases of malaria, hemozoin collects in tissues, e.g., the spleen, giving the organ a grayish to dark brown or black color. Also written *haemozoin.*

hemozoon (he″mo-zo′on) [hemo- + Gr. *zōon* animal] hematozoan, def. 2.

hemuresis (hem″u-re′sis) [hem- + *uresis*] the voiding of bloody urine.

henbane (hen′bān) hyoscyamus.

Hench (hench) Philip Showalter. American physician, 1896–1965; co-winner, with Edward Calvin Kendall and Tadeus Reichstein, of the Nobel prize for medicine or physiology in 1950 for his treatment of rheumatoid arthritis with ACTH and cortisone.

Hench-Aldrich test (index) (hench al′drich) [Philip S. *Hench;* Martha *Aldrich,* American biochemist, born 1897] see under *test.*

Henderson-Hasselbalch equation (hen′der-son-has′el-balk) [Lawrence Joseph *Henderson,* Boston chemist, 1878–1942; Karl A. *Hasselbalch,* Copenhagen scientist, 1874–1962] see under *equation.*

Henderson-Jones disease (hen′der-son-jōnz′) [Melvin Starkey *Henderson,* American orthopedic surgeon, 1883–1954; Hugh T. *Jones,* American orthopedic surgeon, born 1892] see under *disease.*

Henke's space, triangle (trigone) (hen′kēz) [Philipp Jakob Wilhelm *Henke,* German anatomist, 1834–1896] see under *space* and *triangle.*

Henle's loop, etc. (hen′lēz) [Friedrich Gustav Jakob *Henle,* German anatomist, 1809–1885, a celebrated anatomist and histologist] see under *ampulla, ansa, canal, cell, fiber, fissure, gland, layer, ligament, loop, membrane, reaction, sheath, sphincter, spine,* and *tubule.*

Henle-Coenen test (sign) (hen′le-ke′nan) [Adolf Richard *Henle,* German surgeon, born 1864; Hermann *Coenen,* German surgeon, born 1875] see under *tests.*

henna (hen′ah) the dried and powdered leaves of *Lawsonia inermis* L. (Lythraceae) and other species, which have fungicidal properties; it has been used in intestinal candidiasis, and is used as a cosmetic and hair dye.

Hennebert's sign (test) (en-bārz′) [Camille *Hennebert*, Belgian otologist, 1867–1958] see under *sign*.

Henoch's chorea, purpura (disease) (hen′ōks) [Edouard Heinrich *Henoch*, German pediatrist, 1820–1910] see *spasmodic tic*, under *tic*, and under *purpura*.

henogenesis (hen″o-jen′ĕ-sis) [Gr. *hen* one + *genesis* origin] ontogeny.

henpuye (hen-poo′ye) [West African] goundou.

henry (hen′re) [Joseph *Henry*, American physicist, 1797–1878] the unit of electric induction.

Henry's law (hen′rēz) [William *Henry*, English chemist, 1774–1836] see under *law*.

Henry's melanin test (reaction) [Adolf Felix Gerhard *Henry*, Istanbul pathologist, born 1894] see under *tests*.

Hensen's canal, etc. (hen′sen) [Victor *Hensen*, German anatomist and physiologist, 1835–1924] see under *body, canal, cell, disk, duct, knot, line,* and *node*.

Henshaw test (hen′shaw) [Russell *Henshaw*, New York physician] see under *tests*.

Hensing's ligament (fold) (hen′singz) [Frederich Wilhelm *Hensing*, German anatomist, 1719–1745] see under *ligament*.

hepar (he′par) [Gr. *hēpar* liver] 1. [NA] a large gland of a dark red color situated in the upper part of the abdomen on the right side; see *liver*. 2. the liver of certain animals, used in pharmaceutical preparations. 3. a liver-like or liver-colored substance. **h. adipo′sum,** fatty liver. **h. loba′tum,** a liver divided into numerous lobes by deep fissures produced by syphilis. **h. sicca′tum,** the dried and powdered liver of pigs; used as a food and medicine in organic diseases of the liver. **h. sul′furis,** sulfurated potash.

heparan-α-glucosaminide acetyltransferase (hep′-ah-ran gloo″ko-sam′ĭ-nīd as″ĕ-til-trans′fer-ās) [EC 2.3.1.78] an enzyme of the transferase class that catalyzes the reaction acetyl-CoA + heparan α-D-glucosaminide = CoA + heparan N-acetyl-α-D-glucosaminide. The reaction is a step in the degradation of heparan sulfate. A defect in the enzyme, an autosomal recessive trait, results in Sanfilippo syndrome type C.

heparan N-sulfatase (hep′ah-ran sul′fah-tās) an enzyme of the hydrolase class that catalyzes the removal of sulfate from the terminal N- sulfated glucosamine of heparan sulfate chains. A defect in the enzyme, an autosomal recessive trait, is the cause of Sanfilippo syndrome type A.

heparan sulfate (hep′ah-ran) a glycosaminoglycan occurring in the liver, aorta, and lung. It has a structure similar to heparin, but there are more N-acetyl groups and fewer O- and N-sulfate groups. It is an accumulation product in several mucopolysaccharidoses. Called also *heparitin sulfate*.

heparan sulfate sulfamidase (hep′ah-ran sul′fāt sul-fam′ĭ-dās) heparan N-sulfatase.

heparan sulfate sulfatase (hep′ah-ran sul′fāt sul′fah-tās) heparan N-sulfatase.

heparin (hep′ah-rin) an acidic mucopolysaccharide composed of D-glucuronic acid and D-glucosamine, present in many tissues, especially the liver and lungs, and having potent anticoagulant properties. It is believed to act by inhibiting conversion of prothrombin to thrombin, and thus fibrinogen to fibrin. Heparin also has lipotrophic properties, promoting transfer of fat from blood to the fat depots by activation of lipoprotein lipase. **h. sodium** [USP], a mixture of active principles capable of prolonging blood clotting time, usually obtained from the lungs, intestinal mucosa, or other suitable tissues of domestic mammals used for human consumption; used in the prophylaxis and treatment of disorders in which there is excessive or undesirable clotting, such as thrombophlebitis, pulmonary embolism, and certain cardiac conditions, administered intravenously or subcutaneously.

heparinate (hep′ah-rin-āt) any salt of heparin.

heparinemia (hep″ah-rin-e′me-ah) the presence of heparin in the blood.

heparinize (hep′er-ĭ-nīz″) to treat with heparin in order to increase the clotting time of the blood.

heparitin sulfate (hep′ah-rĭ-tin) heparan sulfate.

hepatalgia (hep″ah-tal′je-ah) [*hepat-* + Gr. *algos* pain + *-ia*] pain in the liver.

hepatatrophia (hep″ah-tah-tro′fe-ah) [*hepat-* + Gr. *atrophia* atrophy] atrophy of the liver.

hepatatrophy (hep″ah-tat′ro-fe) hepatatrophia.

hepatauxe (hep″ah-tawk′se) [*hepat-* + Gr. *auxē* increase] (obs.) hepatomegaly.

hepatectomize (hep″ah-tek′to-mīz) to deprive of the liver by surgical removal.

hepatectomy (hep″ah-tek′to-me) [*hepat-* + Gr. *ektomē* excision] excision of all (*total h.*) or part (*partial* or *subtotal h.*) of the liver.

hepatic (hĕ-pat′ik) [L. *hepaticus;* Gr. *hēpatikos*] pertaining to the liver.

hepatic(o)- [Gr. *hēpatikos* of the liver] a combining form denoting relationship to a hepatic duct, or, sometimes, to the liver.

hepaticocholangiojejunostomy (hĕ-pat″ĭ-ko-ko-lan″je-o-je″ju-nos′to-me) surgical creation of a communication between the hepatic duct, another biliary duct, and the jejunum.

hepaticocholedochostomy (hĕ-pat″ĭ-ko-ko-led″o-kos′to-me) surgical anastomosis of the hepatic duct and the common bile duct.

hepaticodochotomy (hĕ-pat″ĭ-ko-do-kot′o-me) surgical incision of the hepatic duct and the common bile duct.

hepaticoduodenostomy (hĕ-pat″ĭ-ko-du″o-de-nos′to-me) surgical creation of a communication between the hepatic duct and the duodenum.

hepaticoenterostomy (hĕ-pat″ĭ-ko-en″ter-os′to-me) [*hepatico-* + Gr. *enteron* intestine + *stomoun* to provide with an opening, or mouth] surgical creation of a communication between the hepatic duct and the intestine.

hepaticogastrostomy (hĕ-pat″ĭ-ko-gas-tros′to-me) [*hepatico-* + Gr. *gastēr* stomach + *stomoun* to provide with an opening, or mouth] surgical creation of a communication between the hepatic duct and the stomach.

hepaticojejunostomy (hĕ-pat″ĭ-ko-je″ju-nos′to-me) [*hepatico-* + *jejunum* + Gr. *stomoun* to provide with an opening, or mouth] surgical creation of a communication between the hepatic duct and the jejunum.

Hepaticola (hep″ah-tik′o-lah) [*hepat-* + *colere* to inhabit] *Capillaria*.

hepaticoliasis (hĕ-pat″ĭ-ko-li′ah-sis) capillariasis.

hepaticolithotomy (hĕ-pat″ĭ-ko-lĭ-thot′o-me) incision of the hepatic duct and removal of one or more calculi.

hepaticolithotripsy (hĕ-pat″ĭ-ko-lith′o-trip-se) the operation of crushing a stone in the hepatic duct.

hepaticopulmonary (hĕ-pat″ĭ-ko-pul′mo-nar″e) pertaining to the liver and the lungs.

hepaticostomy (hĕ-pat″ĭ-kos′to-me) [*hepatico-* + Gr. *stomoun* to provide with an opening, or mouth] surgical creation of an artificial opening into the hepatic duct.

hepaticotomy (hĕ-pat″ĭ-kot′o-me) [*hepatico-* + Gr. *tomē* cutting] incision of the hepatic duct.

hepatin (hep′ah-tin) glycogen.

hepatism (hep′ah-tizm) ill health due to liver disease.

hepatitides (hep″ah-tit′ĭ-dēz) plural of *hepatitis*.

hepatitis (hep″ah-ti′tis), pl. *hepatit′ides* [*hepat-* + *-itis*] inflammation of the liver. **h. A.,** a self-limited viral disease of worldwide distribution caused by the hepatitis A virus, which is more prevalent in areas of poor hygiene and low socioeconomic standards, being transmitted almost exclusively by the fecal-oral route, although parenteral transmission is possible; there is no carrier state. The incubation period is about 30 days, with a range of 15 to 50 days. Most cases are clinically inapparent or have mild flulike symptoms; jaundice, if present, is usually mild. Massive hepatic necrosis (fulminant hepatitis) can occur but much less commonly than with hepatitis B or non-A, non-B hepatitis. Formerly called *epidemic h., jaundice infectious h., MS-1 h.,* and *short-incubation h.* **acute parenchymatous h.,** massive hepatic necrosis. **amebic h.,** invasion of liver parenchyma by trophozoites of *Entamoeba histolytica,* leading to amebic abscess. **anicteric h.,** viral hepatitis without jaundice. **autoimmune h.,** chronic active h. **h. B.,** a viral disease caused by the hepatitis B virus that is endemic worldwide, the areas of highest endemicity being China and

Southeast Asia, sub-Saharan Africa, most Pacific islands, and the Amazon basin. The virus is shed in all body fluids by individuals with acute or chronic infections and by asymptomatic carriers, and is transmitted primarily by parenteral routes, such as by blood transfusion or by sharing of needles among drug users; oral transmission can occur but has low efficiency, and it can be spread by intimate personal contact, especially sexual contact, and by vertical transmission from mother to neonate. The incubation period averages about 90 days, with a range of 40 to 180 days, and the clinical course is more variable than in hepatitis A. In the prodromal phase there may be fever, malaise, anorexia, nausea, and vomiting, which decline with the onset of clinical jaundice, and urticaria, angioedema, arthritis, or, rarely, glomerulonephritis or a serum sickness–like syndrome may occur. Most patients recover completely and become HB$_S$ Ag-negative in 3 to 4 months, but some remain chronic carriers or develop chronic active hepatitis or chronic persistent hepatitis. Massive hepatic necrosis (fulminant hepatitis) is an infrequent complication. In areas of high endemicity a relationship has been shown between hepatitis and virus infection, cirrhosis, and primary hepatocellular carcinoma, with the latter being one of the most common neoplasms. Formerly called *inoculation h.*, *long-incubation h.*, *MS-2 h.*, *serum h.*, and *homologous serum h.* or *jaundice.* See also under *antigen.* **canine virus h.**, h. contagiosa canis. **cholangiolitic h.**, cholestatic h. (def. 1). **cholangitic h.**, cholestatic h. (def. 1). **cholestatic h.**, 1. a rare form of viral hepatitis in which there is cholestasias with obstructive jaundice, pruritus, dark urine, light stools, and elevated alkaline phosphatase and conjugated bilirubin and in which the course is prolonged compared to that of other forms. Called also *cholangitic h.* and *cholangiolitic h.* 2. hepatic inflammation and cholestasis resulting from reaction to drugs such as estrogens, methyltestosterone, and chlorpromazine. **chronic active h.**, a chronic inflammation of the liver occurring as a sequel to hepatitis B or non-A, non-B hepatitis. The same disease may occur in congenital or acquired hypogammaglobulinemia, or in association with the administration of certain drugs. It is characterized by infiltration of portal areas by plasma cells and macrophages, piecemeal necrosis (destruction of hepatocytes in the periphery of lobules), and fibrosis. The course is highly variable; there may be long asymptomatic periods interspersed with periods of symptomatic hepatitis with jaundice, malaise, anorexia, and fever; there may be extrahepatic manifestations, including amenorrhea, arthritis, skin rashes, vasculitis, thyroiditis, glomerulonephritis ulcerative colitis, and Sjögren's syndrome; or the disease may progress to cirrhosis and liver failure. An autoimmune pathogenesis is suspected. Called also *chronic aggressive h.*, *lupoid h.*, *autoimmune h.*, *plasma cell h.*, *subacute h.*, and *acute juvenile cirrhosis.* **chronic aggressive h.**, chronic active h. **chronic interstitial h.**, cirrhosis of the liver. **chronic persisting h.**, a chronic, nonprogressive inflammatory process affecting primarily the portal areas without producing fibrosis, necrosis, or cirrhosis, an uncommon sequel of viral hepatitis; the disease may be asymptomatic or may produce symptoms of mild hepatitis; it does not progress to cirrhosis or liver failure but may persist for years. **h. contagio'sa ca'nis**, an infectious hepatitis of dogs caused by an adenovirus. **delta h.**, infection with hepatitis delta virus, occurring either simultaneously with or as a superinfection in hepatitis B, whose severity it may increase. **duck virus h.**, a highly fatal, rapidly spreading picornavirus disease of waterfowl ducklings, characterized primarily by hepatitis marked by an enlarged, mottled, hemorrhagic liver. **epidemic h.**, h. A. **familial h.**, Wilson's disease. **fulminant h.**, massive hepatic necrosis (q.v.) resulting from viral hepatitis, usually hepatitis B or non-A, non-B hepatitis. **giant cell h.**, neonatal h. **halothane h.**, the extremely rare cases of transient jaundice or massive hepatic necrosis associated with halothane anesthesia. **homologous serum h.**, h. B. **infectious h.**, h. A. **infectious necrotic h. of sheep**, black disease. **inoculation h.**, h. B. **long-incubation h.**, h. B. **lupoid h.**, chronic active hepatitis with autoimmune manifestations. Called also *Bearn-Kunkel-Slater syndrome* and *Kunkel syndrome.* **MS-1 h.**, h. A. **MS-2 h.**, h. B. **neonatal h.**, hepatitis of unknown etiology with onset in the first few weeks of life; some cases are associated with viral or bacterial infection; a few are familial. It is characterized by the transformation of hepatocytes into multinucleated giant cells and by conjugated hyperbilirubi-

nemia with jaundice. Most patients recover completely, some develop chronic disease or fatal cirrhosis. Called also *giant cell h.* **neonatal giant cell h.**, neonatal h. **non-A, non-B h.**, a clinical syndrome of acute viral hepatitis occurring without the serologic markets of hepatitis A or B. It is the major cause of post-transfusion hepatitis, and occurs commonly following parenteral drug abuse. **plasma cell h.**, chronic active h. **post-transfusion h.**, viral hepatitis, now primarily non-A, non-B hepatitis, transmitted via transfusion of blood or blood products, especially multiple pooled donor products such as clotting factor concentrates. Called also *transfusion h.* **serum h.**, h. B. **short-incubation h.**, h. A. **subacute h.**, chronic active h. **toxic h.**, hepatitis produced by hepatotoxins such as *Amanita phalloides toxin*, carbon tetrachloride, yellow phosphorus, and a variety of drugs. Cf. *drug-induced h.* **transfusion h.**, post-transfusion h. **viral h.**, *h. A, h. B, delta h.*, and *non-A, non-B h.*

hepatization (hep″ah-ti-za′shun) transformation into a liver-like mass, as the solidified state of the lung in pneumonia. **gray h.**, hepatization of the lung in which the affected tissue has a gray color. **red h.**, a form in which the affected tissue is red from excess of blood. **yellow h.**, a stage in hepatization in which the exudate is purulent.

hepatized (hep′ah-tīzd) changed into a liver-like substance.

hepat(o)- [Gr. *hēpar*, gen. *hēpatos* liver] combining form denoting relationship to the liver.

hepatobiliary (hep″ah-to-bil′e-ār″e) pertaining to the liver and the bile or the biliary ducts.

hepatoblastoma (hep″ah-to-blas-to′mah) a malignant intrahepatic tumor occurring in infants and young children and consisting chiefly of embryonic hepatic tisssue.

hepatobronchial (hep″ah-to-brong′ke-al) pertaining to or communicating with the liver and a bronchus, as a hepatobronchial fistula.

hepatocarcinogenesis (hep″ah-to-kar″si-no-jen′ĕ-sis) the production of carcinoma of the liver.

hepatocarcinogenic (hep″ah-to-kar″sĭ-no-jen′ik) causing carcinoma of the liver.

hepatocarcinoma (hep″ah-to-kar″sin-o′mah) hepatocellular carcinoma.

hepatocele (he-pat′o-sēl) [*hepato-* + Gr. *kēlē* hernia] hernial protrusion of a part of the liver.

hepatocellular (hep″ah-to-sel′u-lar) pertaining to or affecting liver cells.

hepatocholangeitis (hep″ah-to-ko-lan″je-i′tis) inflammation of the liver and bile ducts.

hepatocholangiocarcinoma (hep″ah-to-ko-lan″je-o-kar″sin-o′mah) cholangiohepatoma.

hepatocholangioduodenostomy (hep″ah-to-ko-lan″je-o-du″o-dĕ-nos′to-me) the operation of establishing drainage of the hepatic duct into the duodenum.

hepatocholangioenterostomy (hep″ah-to-ko-lan″je-o-en″ter-os′to-me) [*hepato-* + Gr. *cholē* bile + *angeion* vessel + *enteron* intestine + *stomoun* to provide with an opening, or mouth] surgical creation of a communication between the hepatic duct and the intestine.

hepatocholangiogastrostomy (hep″ah-to-ko-lan″je-o-gas-tros′to-me) the operation of establishing drainage of the hepatic duct into the stomach.

hepatocholangiostomy (hep″ah-to-ko-lan″je-os′to-me) the operation of establishing drainage of the hepatic duct either through the abdominal wall (*external h.*) or into some part of the gastrointestinal tract (*internal h.*).

hepatocholangitis (hep″ah-to-ko″lan-ji′tis) inflammation of the liver and bile ducts.

hepatocirrhosis (hep″ah-to-sĭ-ro′sis) [*hepato-* + *cirrhosis*] cirrhosis of the liver.

hepatocolic (hep″ah-to-kol′ik) pertaining to the liver and the colon.

hepatocuprein (hep″ah-to-koo′prin) a soluble, bluish-green copper protein present in liver tissue; it contains about 0.34 per cent copper.

hepatocystic (hep″ah-to-sis′tik) pertaining to the liver and gallbladder.

Hepatocystis (hep″ah-to-sis′tis) [*hepato-* + *cyst*] a genus of coccidian protozoa (suborder Haemosporina, subclass

Sporozoea) comprising parasites of Old World lower monkeys, fruit bats, and squirrels, in which merogony takes place in the hepatocytes, resulting in large glistening schizonts (merocysts) on the surface of the liver, from which merozoites are released to invade erythrocytes and develop into gametocytes.

hepatocyte (hep′ah-to-sīt) a hepatic cell.

hepatoduodenostomy (hep″ah-to-du″o-dĕ-nos′to-me) [*hepato-* + *duodenum* + Gr. *stomoun* to provide with an opening, or mouth] the surgical creation of a communication between the liver and the duodenum.

hepatodynia (hep″ah-to-din′e-ah) [*hepato-* + Gr. *odynē* pain] pain in the liver.

hepatodystrophy (hep″ah-to-dis′tro-fe) acute yellow atrophy; see under *atrophy*.

hepatoenteric (hep″ah-to-en-ter′ik) pertaining to the liver and intestine.

hepatoenterostomy (hep″ah-to-en″ter-os′to-me) surgical creation of a communication between the liver and the intestine.

hepatoflavin (hep″ah-to-fla′vin) riboflavin obtained from liver tissue.

hepatofugal (hep″ah-tof′u-gal) [*hepato-* + L. *fugere* to flee from] directed or flowing away from the liver.

hepatogastric (hep″ah-to-gas′trik) pertaining to the liver and stomach.

hepatogenic (hep″ah-to-jen′ik) 1. giving rise to or forming liver tissue. 2. hepatogenous.

hepatogenous (hep″ah-toj′ĕ-nus) 1. produced in or originating in the liver. 2. hepatogenic.

hepatogram (hep′ah-to-gram″) 1. a tracing of the liver pulse in the sphygmogram. 2. a roentgenogram of the liver.

hepatography (hep″ah-tog′rah-fe) [*hepato-* + Gr. *graphein* to record] 1. a treatise on the liver. 2. the recording of a tracing of the liver pulse. 3. the making of a roentgenogram of the liver.

hepatoid (hep″ah-toid) [*hepato-* + Gr. *eidos* form] resembling the liver in structure.

hepatojugular (hep″ah-to-jug′u-lar) pertaining to the liver and jugular vein; see under *reflux*.

hepatolenticular (hep″ah-to-len-tik′u-lar) pertaining to the liver and the lenticular nucleus.

hepatolienal (hep″ah-to-li′e-nal) pertaining to the liver and spleen.

hepatolienography (hep″ah-to-li″ĕ-nog′rah-fe) [*hepato-* + L. *lien* spleen + Gr. *graphein* to record] roentgenography of the liver and spleen after intravenous injection of an opaque medium.

hepatolienomegaly (hep″ah-to-li″ĕ-no-meg′ah-le) hepatosplenomegaly.

hepatolith (hep′ah-to-lith″) [*hepato-* + Gr. *lithos* stone] a gallstone, especially one within the liver.

hepatolithectomy (hep″ah-to-lĭ-thek′to-me) [*hepato-* + Gr. *lithos* stone + *ektomē* excision] removal of a calculus from the liver.

hepatolithiasis (hep″ah-to-lĭ-thi′ah-sis) [*hepato-* + *lithiasis*] the formation or presence of calculi in the intrahepatic biliary ducts.

hepatologist (hep″ah-tol′o-jist) a specialist in hepatology.

hepatology (hep″ah-tol′o-je) [*hepato-* + *-logy*] the study of the liver.

hepatolysin (hep″ah-tol′ĭ-sin) a cytolysin destructive to liver cells.

hepatolysis (hep″ah-tol′ĭ-sis) [*hepato-* + Gr. *lysis* dissolution] destruction of the liver cells.

hepatolytic (hep″ah-to-lit′ik) pertaining to, characterized by, or causing hepatolysis.

hepatoma (hep″ah-to′mah) a tumor of the liver, especially hepatocellular carcinoma. **malignant h.,** hepatocellular carcinoma.

hepatomalacia (hep″ah-to-mah-la′she-ah) [*hepato-* + Gr. *malakia* softening] softening of the liver.

hepatomegalia (hep″ah-to-mĕ-ga′le-ah) [*hepato-* + Gr. *megas* big] hepatomegaly.

hepatomegaly (hep″ah-to-meg′ah-le) enlargement of the liver.

hepatomelanosis (hep″ah-to-mel″ah-no′sis) melanosis of the liver.

hepatometry (hep″ah-tom′ĕ-tre) determination of the size of the liver.

hepatomphalocele (hep″ah-tom′fah-lo-sēl″) omphalocele with the liver also being projected into the membranous sac outside the abdomen.

hepatomphalos (hep″ah-tom′fah-los) [*hepat-* + Gr. *omphalos* navel] projection of the liver through the abdominal wall near the umbilicus.

hepatonephric (hep″ah-to-nef′rik) pertaining to the liver and kidney.

hepatonephritic (hep″ah-to-nĕ-frit′ik) pertaining to or characterized by hepatonephritis.

hepatonephritis (hep″ah-to-nĕ-fri′tis) [*hepato-* + Gr. *nephros* kidney] a form of severe jaundice due to simultaneous inflammation of the liver and kidneys from the same cause, e.g., leptospiral infection.

hepatonephromegaly (hep″ah-to-nef″ro-meg′ah-le) [*hepato-* + Gr. *nephros* kidney + *megas* large] enlargement of the liver and kidney.

hepatopancreas (hep″ah-to-pan′kre-as) any of certain digestive glands of invertebrates, as the so-called liver of certain crustaceans, which secretes a fluid acting on both fats and proteins.

hepatopath (hep′ah-to-path) a person with liver disease.

hepatopathy (hep″ah-top′ah-the) [*hepato-* + Gr. *pathos* disease] any disease of the liver.

hepatoperitonitis (hep″ah-to-per″ĭ-to-ni′tis) [*hepato-* + *peritonitis*] inflammation of the peritoneum covering the liver.

hepatopetal (hep″ah-top′ĕ-tal) [*hepato-* + L. *petere* to seek] directed or flowing toward the liver.

hepatopexy (hep′ah-to-pek″se) [*hepato-* + Gr. *pēxis* fixation] surgical fixation of the displaced liver.

hepatophage (hep′ah-to-fāj) [*hepato-* + Gr. *phagein* to eat] a giant cell supposed to destroy the liver cells.

hepatophlebitis (hep″ah-to-flĕ-bi′tis) inflammation of the veins of the liver.

hepatophlebography (hep″ah-to-fle-bog′rah-fe) radiologic visualization of the outflow of the venous network of the liver performed through retrograde injection of a radiopaque solution.

hepatopleural (hep″ah-to-ploo′ral) pertaining to the liver and the pleura, or communicating with the liver and pleural cavity, as a hepatopleural fistula.

hepatopneumonic (hep″ah-to-nu-mon′ik) [*hepato-* + Gr. *pneumonikos* of the lungs] pertaining to, affecting, or communicating with the liver and lungs; hepatopulmonary.

hepatoportal (hep″ah-to-por′tal) pertaining to the portal system of the liver.

hepatoptosis (hep″ah-to-to′sis) [*hepato-* + Gr. *ptōsis* falling] 1. displacement of the liver because of laxness of suspensory ligaments, diminished tone of abdominal muscles, emphysema, right pleural effusion or empyema, subphrenic abscess, spinal deformity. 2. positioning of the colon between liver and diaphragm on x-ray.

hepatopulmonary (hep″ah-to-pul′mo-nar″e) hepatopneumonic.

hepatorenal (hep″ah-to-re′nal) pertaining to the liver and kidneys.

hepatorrhagia (hep″ah-to-ra′je-ah) [*hepato-* + Gr. *rhēgnynai* to burst forth] hemorrhage from the liver.

hepatorrhaphy (hep″ah-tor′ah-fe) [*hepato-* + Gr. *rhaphē* suture] operative repair of the liver.

hepatorrhea (hep″ah-to-re′ah) [*hepato-* + Gr. *rhoia* flow] a morbidly excessive secretion of bile; any morbid flow from the liver.

hepatorrhexis (hep″ah-to-rek′sis) [*hepato-* + Gr. *rhēxis* rupture] rupture of the liver.

hepatoscan (hep′ah-to-skan) a surface scintiscan of the liver.

hepatoscopy (hep″ah-tos′ko-pe) [*hepato-* + Gr. *skopein* to examine] examination of the liver.

hepatosis (hep″ah-to′sis) any functional disorder of the liver. **serous h.,** veno-occlusive disease of the liver; see under *disease*.

hepatosolenotropic (hep″ah-to-so-le″no-trop′ik) [*hepato-* + Gr. *sōlēn* a channel, gutter, pipe + *tropē* a turn, turning] having an affinity for or exerting a specific effect on the cholangioles and interlobular ducts of the liver.

hepatosplenitis (hep″ah-to-splĕ-ni′tis) inflammation of the liver and spleen.

hepatosplenography (hep″ah-to-splĕ-nog′rah-fe) roentgenography of the liver and spleen.

hepatosplenomegaly (hep″ah-to-sple″no-meg′ah-le) [*hepato-* + Gr. *splēn* spleen + *megas* big] enlargement of the liver and spleen.

hepatosplenometry (hep″ah-to-splĕ-nom′ĕ-tre) determination of the size of the liver and spleen.

hepatosplenopathy (hep″ah-to-splĕ-nop′ah-the) any combined disorder of the liver and spleen.

hepatostomy (hep″ah-tos′to-me) [*hepato-* + Gr. *stoma* mouth] surgical creation of an opening into the liver.

hepatotherapy (hep″ah-to-ther′ah-pe) [*hepato-* + Gr. *therapeia* treatment] treatment of disease by the administration of liver or liver extract.

hepatotomy (hep″ah-tot′o-me) [*hepato-* + Gr. *tomē* a cutting] surgical incision of the liver. **transthoracic h.,** incision of the liver by resecting a rib, opening the pleural sac, and incising the diaphragm; often performed in two or three stages.

hepatotoxemia (hep″ah-to-tok-se′me-ah) [*hepato-* + *toxemia*] blood poisoning originating in the liver.

hepatotoxic (hep″ah-to-tok′sik) toxic to liver cells.

hepatotoxicity (hep″ah-to-tok-sis′ĭ-te) the quality or property of exerting a destructive or poisonous effect upon liver cells.

hepatotoxin (hep″ah-to-tok′sin) [*hepato-* + *toxin*] a toxin that destroys liver cells.

hepatotropic (hep″ah-to-trop′ik) [*hepato-* + Gr. *tropos* a turning] having a special affinity for or exerting a specific effect on the liver.

hepatoxic (hep″ah-tok′sik) hepatotoxic.

Hepatozoon (hep″ah-to-zo′on) [*hepato-* + Gr. *zōon* animal] a genus of coccidian protozoa (suborder Adeleina, order Eucoccidiida) found in the red blood cells of birds and mammals. *H. canis* is transmitted to canines by the tick *Rhipicephalus sanguineus* (see *hepatozoonosis*). *H. muris,* found in the liver cells of rats, and *H. perniciosum,* found in dogs, are transmitted by the mite *Echinolaelaps echidninus.*

hepatozoonosis (hep″ah-to-zo″o-no′sis) an infectious, sometimes fatal disease of dogs caused by *Hepatozoon canis,* and characterized by intermittent fever, emaciation, mild anemia, muscular hyperesthesia, especially affecting the back, purulent ocular and nasal discharge, and sometimes diarrhea.

Hepicebrin (hep′ĭ-se′brin) trademark for a preparation of hexavitamin.

hept-, hepta- [Gr. *hepta* seven] a combining form meaning seven.

heptabarbital (hep″tah-bar′bĭ-tal) chemical name: 5-(1-cyclohepten-1-yl)-5-ethyl-2,4-6(1*H*,3*H*,5*H*)-pyrimidinetrione. A short-acting barbiturate, $C_{13}H_{18}N_2O_3$, occurring as a white, crystalline powder, used as a sedative and hypnotic, administered orally.

heptachromic (hep″tah-kro′mik) [*hepta-* + Gr. *chrōma* color] 1. pertaining to or exhibiting seven colors. 2. able to distinguish all seven colors of the spectrum; possessing full color vision.

heptad (hep′tad) any element having a valency of seven.

heptadactylia (hep″tah-dak-til′e-ah) heptadactyly.

heptadactylism (hep″tah-dak′tĭ-lizm) heptadactyly.

heptadactyly (hep″tah-dak′tĭ-le) [*hepta-* + Gr. *daktylos* finger] the occurrence of seven digits (fingers or toes) on one limb.

heptaene (hep′tah-ēn) a chemical compound in which there are seven conjugated double bonds.

heptanal (hep′tah-nal) oenanthol.

heptapeptide (hep″tah-pep′tīd) a polypeptide containing seven amino acids.

heptatomic (hep″tah-tom′ik) septivalent.

heptavalent (hep-tav′ah-lent) [*hepta-* + L. *valere* to be able] septivalent.

Heptavax-B (hep′tah-vaks) trademark for a preparation of hepatitis B vaccine.

heptoglobin (hep″to-glo′bin) a protein which is one of the fractions of blood plasma; it is said to be increased in infections, malignancy, and certain endocrine disorders.

heptoglobinemia (hep″to-glo-bĭ-ne′me-ah) abnormal increase in heptoglobin in the blood plasma.

heptose (hep′tōs) [*hept-* + *-ose*] a monosaccharide containing seven carbon atoms in a molecule.

heptosuria (hep″to-su′re-ah) presence of a heptose in the urine.

herb (erb, herb) [L. *herba*] any leafy plant without a woody stem, especially one used as a household remedy or as a flavoring. **death's h.,** belladonna leaf. **vulnerary h.,** an herb anciently regarded as healing wounds.

herbaceous (her-ba′shus) having the characters of an herb.

herbal (her′bal) a book on herbs.

herbalist (her′bal-ist) a herb doctor, or one versed in herbal lore.

Herbert's operation, pits (her′berts) [Major Herbert *Herbert,* Indian Medical Service, 1865–1942] see under *operation* and *pit.*

herbicide (her′bĭ-sīd) [L. *herba* herb + *caedere* to kill] an agent that is destructive to weeds or causes an alteration in their normal growth.

herbivore (her′bĭ-vōr) a herbivorous animal.

herbivorous (her-biv′o-rus) [L. *herba* herb + *vorare* to eat] subsisting upon plants.

Herb. recent. abbreviation for L. *herba′rium recen′tium,* of fresh herbs.

Herbst's corpuscles (herbsts) [Ernst Friedrich Gustav *Herbst,* German physician, 1803–1893] see under *corpuscle.*

hereditary (he-red′ĭ-ter-e) [L. *hereditarius*] genetically transmitted from parent to offspring.

heredity (he-red′ĭ-te) [L. *hereditas*] 1. the genetic transmission of a particular quality or trait from parent to offspring. 2. the genetic constitution of an individual. **autosomal h.,** the transmission of a quality or trait by a gene located on an autosome. **sex-linked h.,** the transmission of a quality or trait by a gene located on a sex-chromosome, for practical clinical purposes limited to transmission of a trait by a gene carried on the X chromosome. **X-linked,** sex-linked h.

heredoataxia (her″ĕ-do-ah-tak′se-ah) hereditary ataxia, as in Friedreich's ataxia.

heredodegeneration (her″ĕ-do-de-jen″er-a′shun) hereditary degeneration due to disease or defect of the hyaloplasm; hereditary cerebellar ataxia.

heredodiathesis (her″ĕ-do-di-ath′ĕ-sis) [L. *heres* heir + *diathesis*] hereditary diathesis or predisposition.

heredofamilial (her″ĕ-do-fah-mil′e-al) occurring in certain families under circumstances that implicate a hereditary basis, as heredofamilial disease. The term is being discarded in favor of *familial, hereditary,* or *genetic,* whichever is more appropriate.

heredoinfection (her″ĕ-do-in-fek′shun) germinal infection.

heredolues (her″ĕ-do-lu′ēz) congenital syphilis.

heredoluetic (her″ĕ-do-lu-et′ik) pertaining to congenital syphilis.

heredopathia (her″ĕ-do-path′e-ah) an inherited pathological condition. **h. atac′tica polyneuritifor′mis,** Refsum's disease.

heredoretinopathia congenita (her″ĕ-do-ret″ĭ-no-path′e-ah kon-jen′ĭ-tah) [L] hereditary retinopathy; see *amaurosis congenita,* under *amaurosis.*

heredosyphilis (her″ĕ-do-sif′ĭ-lis) congenital syphilis.

heredosyphilitic (her″ĕ-do-sif″ĭ-lit′ik) a person affected with congenital syphilis.

heredosyphilology (her″ĕ-do-sif″ĭ-lol′o-je) the study of congenital syphilis.

Hérelle see *d'Hérelle.*

Herellea (hĕ-rel′e-ah) in former systems of classification, a genus of bacteria, species of which are now included in the genus *Acinetobacter*. **H. vagini′cola,** *Acinetobacter calcoaceticus.*

Hering's law, etc. (her′ingz) [Carl Ewald Konstantin *Hering,* physiologist in Leipzig, 1834–1918] see under *law, test,* and *theory.*

Hering's nerve, phenomenon (her′ingz) [Heinrich Ewald *Hering,* physiologist in Cologne, 1866–1948] see *ramus sinus carotici nervi glossopharyngei,* and see under *phenomenon.*

heritability (her″ĭ-tah-bil′ĭ-te) 1. the quality of being heritable. 2. a measure of the extent to which a phenotype is influenced by the genotype.

heritable (her′ĭ-tah-b′l) capable of being inherited, as a genetic trait.

Herlitz's disease (her′litz) [Gillis *Herlitz,* Swedish pediatrician, born 1902] junctional epidermolysis bullosa.

Hermann-Perutz reaction, test (her′man-pa′root) [Otto *Hermann,* Vienna physician; Alfred *Perutz,* Austrian dermatologist, born 1885] Perutz's reaction.

Hermansky-Pudlak syndrome (her′mahn-ske-pood′lak) [F. *Hermansky,* Czechoslovakian internist, 20th century; P. *Pudlak,* Czechoslovakian internist, 20th century] see under *syndrome.*

hermaphrodism (her-maf′ro-dizm) hermaphroditism.

hermaphrodite (her-maf′ro-dīt) [Gr. *hermaphroditos*] an individual exhibiting hermaphroditism (q.v.). **pseudo-h.,** see *pseudohermaphrodite.* **true h.,** an individual who has both testicular and ovarian tissue and exhibits ambiguous morphological criteria of sex; called also *true intersex.*

hermaphroditism (her-maf′ro-di-tizm″) [Gr. *hermaphroditos* a person partaking of the attributes of both sexes] originally, a state characterized by the presence of both male and female sex organs. In humans, *true hermaphroditism* is caused by anomalous differentiation of the gonads, with the presence of both ovarian and testicular tissue and of ambiguous morphologic criteria of sex. If only testicular tissue is present, but there are some female morphological criteria of sex, it is known as *male pseudohermaphroditism.* If only ovarian tissue is present, but there are some male morphological criteria of sex, it is known as *female pseudohermaphroditism.* See also *intersex* and *pseudohermaphroditism.* **bilateral h.,** that in which gonadal tissue typical of both sexes occurs on each side of the body. **h. with excess,** a condition characterized by the presence of the normal organs typical of one sex with some that pertain to the opposite sex. **false h.,** pseudohermaphroditism. **lateral h.,** presence of gonadal tissue typical of one sex on one side of the body and tissue typical of the other sex on the opposite side. **spurious h.,** pseudohermaphroditism. **transverse h.,** a condition in which the external genital organs are characteristic of one sex and the gonads are typical of the other. **true h.,** coexistence, in the same individual, of both ovarian and testicular tissue, with somatic characters typical of both sexes; called also *true intersex.* **unilateral h.,** presence of gonadal tissue typical of both sexes on one side and of an ovary or testis on the other.

hermaphroditismus (her-maf″ro-di-tiz′mus) hermaphroditism. **h. ve′rus,** true hermaphroditism. **h. ve′rus bilatera′lis,** bilateral hermaphroditism. **h. ve′rus latera′lis,** lateral hermaphroditism. **h. ve′rus unilatera′lis,** unilateral hermaphroditism.

Hermetia illucens (her-me′she-ah il-lu′senz) the soldier fly, the larvae of which may cause intestinal myiasis or pseudomyiasis in man.

hermetic (her-met′ik) [L. *hermeticus*] impervious to air; airtight.

hermetically (her-met′ĭ-kal-le) in an airtight manner.

hernia (her′ne-ah) [L.] the protrusion of a loop or knuckle of an organ or tissue through an abnormal opening. **abdominal h.,** the protrusion of some internal body structure through the abdominal wall. **acquired h.,** one brought on by lifting or by a strain or other injury. **h. adipo′sa,** fat h. **axial hiatal h.,** sliding hiatal h. **Barth's h.,** hernia of loops of intestine between the serosa of the abdominal wall and that of a persistent vitelline duct. **Béclard's h.,** femoral hernia through the saphenous opening. **Birkett's h.,** synovial h. **Bochdalek's h.,** congenital posterolateral diaphragmatic hernia, with extrusion of bowel and other abdominal viscera into the thorax; it is due to failure of closure of the pleuroperitoneal hiatus (foramen

of Bochdalek). **cecal h.,** one that contains the cecum or a part of it. **h. cere′bri,** protrusion of the brain substance through the skull, usually occurring after a brain tumor operation. **Cloquet's h.,** pectineal h. **complete h.,** one in which the sac and its contents have passed through the orifice. **concealed h.,** hernia not perceptible on palpation. **congenital h.,** that which exists at birth, most commonly scrotal or umbilical. **Cooper's h.,** a femoral hernia with additional tracts into the scrotum, toward the labium majus, and toward the obturator foramen. **crural h.,** femoral h. **diaphragmatic h.,** herniation of the abdominal or retroperitoneal structures into the thorax. **direct h.,** see under *inguinal h.* **diverticular h.,** Littre's h. **dry h.,** a hernia in which the sac and its contents have become intimately adherent to each other. **duodenojejunal h.,** Treitz's h. **encysted h.,** scrotal or oblique inguinal hernia in which the bowel, enveloped in its own proper sac, passes into the tunica vaginalis in such a way that the bowel has three coverings of peritoneum; called also *Hey's h.* **epigastric h.,** a hernia through the linea alba above the navel. **external h.,** see under *inguinal h.* **extrasaccular h.,** sliding h. **fat h.,** hernial protrusion of properitoneal fat through the abdominal wall; called also *h. adiposa.* **femoral h.,** hernia into the femoral canal. **foraminal h.,** hernia through the epiploic foramen. **gastroesophageal h.,** paraesophageal h. **Grynfeltt h.,** hernia through Lesgaft's space (Grynfeltt's triangle). **Hesselbach's h.,** hernia with a diverticulum through the cribriform fascia. **Hey's h.,** encysted h. **hiatal h., hiatus h.,** herniation of an abdominal organ, usually the stomach, through the esophageal hiatus of the diaphragm. It occurs in two major anatomic patterns: the *sliding hiatal hernia* (type I) (q.v.), which is the more common type, and the *paraesophageal hernia* (type II) (q.v.). **Holthouse's h.,** an inguinal hernia which has turned outward into the groin. **incarcerated h.,** hernia that cannot be returned or reduced by manipulation; it may or may not become strangulated. Called also *irreducible h.* **incisional h.,** hernia occurring at the site of a previously made incision in the abdominal wall. **incomplete h.,** one which has not passed quite through the orifice. **indirect h.,** see under *inguinal h.* **infantile h.,** oblique inguinal hernia behind the funicular process of the peritoneum. **inguinal h.,** hernia into the inguinal canal. An *indirect* inguinal hernia (*external* or *oblique* hernia) leaves the abdomen through the deep inguinal ring, and passes down obliquely through the inguinal canal, lateral to the inferior epigastric artery. A *direct* inguinal hernia (*internal* hernia) emerges between the inferior epigastric artery and the edge of the rectus muscle. **inguinocrural h., inguinofemoral h.,** a combined inguinal and femoral hernia. **inguinoproperitoneal h.,** hernia that is partly inguinal and partly properitoneal; called also *Krönlein's h.* **inguinosuperficial h.,** interstitial hernia which passes through the internal inguinal ring, the inguinal canal, and the external inguinal ring, but at this point is deflected upward and outward so as to lie upon the aponeurosis of the external oblique muscle. **intermuscular h., interparietal h.,** an interstitial hernia which lies between one or another of the fascial or muscular planes of the abdomen. **internal h.,** see under *inguinal h.* **intersigmoid h.,** hernia of the intestine through the intersigmoid fossa. **interstitial h.,** a hernia in which a knuckle of intestine lies between two layers of the abdominal wall. **h. of the iris,** protrusion of a part of the iris. **irreducible h.,** incarcerated h. **ischiatic h.,** hernia through the sacrosciatic foramen. **ischiorectal h.,** perineal h. **Krönlein's h.,** inguinoproperitoneal h. **labial h.,** the protrusion of a knuckle of the gut into a labium majus. **labial h., posterior,** vaginolabial h. **Laugier's h.,** a femoral hernia perforating Gimbernat's ligament. **levator h.,** pudendal h. **Littre's h.,** protrusion of a Meckel's diverticulum; called also *diverticular h.* **lumbar h.,** hernia in the lumbar region, through Lesgaft's space (Grynfeltt's triangle) or the trigonum lumbale (Petit's triangle). **mesenteric h.,** the passage of a portion of the gut through an opening in the mesentery. **Morgagni's h.,** congenital retrosternal diaphragmatic hernia, with extrusion of tissue into the thorax through the foramen of Morgagni. **oblique h.,** see under *inguinal h.* **obturator h.,** protrusion through the obturator foramen. **omental h.,** a protrusion of a knuckle of omentum. **ovarian h.,** hernial protrusion of an ovary. **paraesophageal h.,** hiatal hernia in which part or almost all of the stomach protrudes

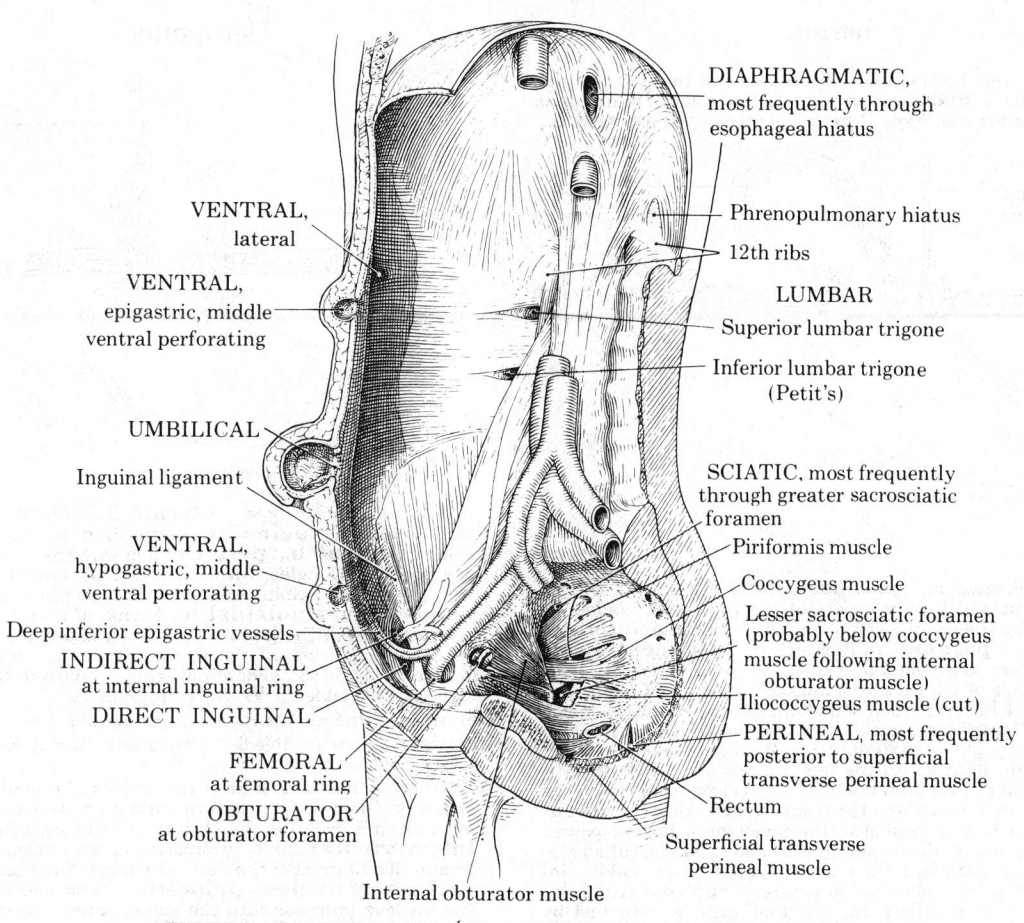

VENTRAL,
lateral

VENTRAL,
epigastric, middle
ventral perforating

UMBILICAL

Inguinal ligament

VENTRAL,
hypogastric, middle
ventral perforating

Deep inferior epigastric vessels

INDIRECT INGUINAL
at internal inguinal ring

DIRECT INGUINAL

FEMORAL
at femoral ring

OBTURATOR
at obturator foramen

Internal obturator muscle

DIAPHRAGMATIC,
most frequently through
esophageal hiatus

Phrenopulmonary hiatus

12th ribs

LUMBAR

Superior lumbar trigone

Inferior lumbar trigone
(Petit's)

SCIATIC, most frequently
through greater sacrosciatic
foramen

Piriformis muscle

Coccygeus muscle

Lesser sacrosciatic foramen
(probably below coccygeus
muscle following internal
obturator muscle)

Iliococcygeus muscle (cut)

PERINEAL, most frequently
posterior to superficial
transverse perineal muscle

Rectum

Superficial transverse
perineal muscle

TYPES OF INTESTINAL HERNIA: ABDOMINAL AND PELVIC OPENINGS

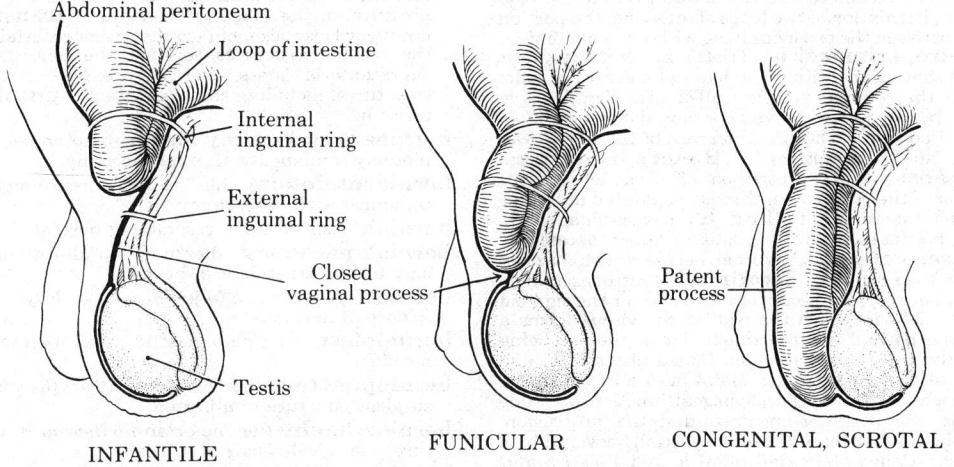

Abdominal peritoneum

Loop of intestine

Internal
inguinal ring

External
inguinal ring

Closed
vaginal process

Testis

Patent
process

INFANTILE   FUNICULAR   CONGENITAL, SCROTAL

TYPES OF INDIRECT INGUINAL HERNIA

PLATE 20 —INTESTINAL AND INGUINAL HERNIAS

through the hiatus into the thorax to the left of the esophagus, with the gastroesophageal junction remaining in place. Called also *Type II hiatal hernia*. **parahiatal h.,**

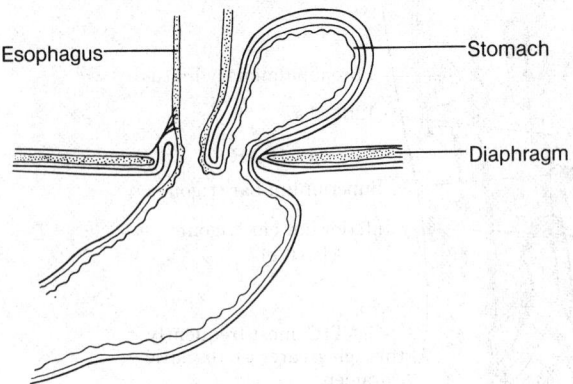

Paraesophageal hernia.

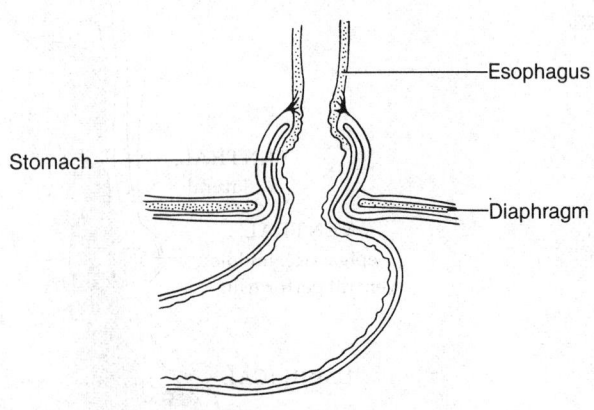

Sliding hiatal hernia.

paraesophageal h. **paraperitoneal h.,** hernia of the bladder in which only a part of the protruded bladder is covered by the peritoneum of the sac. **parasaccular h.,** sliding h. **parietal h.,** Richter's h. **pectineal h.,** one that enters the femoral canal and then perforates the aponeurosis of the pectineus muscle; called also *Cloquet's h.* **perineal h.,** protrusion of abdominal viscera into the perineum. **Petit's h.,** hernia through the trigonum lumbale (Petit's triangle). **prevascular h.,** a hernia in the femoral sheath, anterior to the femoral vessels. **properitoneal h.,** an interstitial hernia which is located between the parietal peritoneum and the transversalis fascia. **pudendal h.,** a hernia located in the pudendum, having passed through a rent in the levator muscle and its fascia; called also *levator h.* **pulsion h.,** a hernia produced by sudden increase of intra-abdominal pressure. **rectovaginal h.,** rectocele. **reducible h.,** one that may be returned by manipulation. **retrocecal h.,** protrusion of the intestine into a pouch behind the cecum; called also *Rieux's h.* **retrograde h.,** herniation of two loops of intestine, the portion of intestine between the two loops lying within the abdominal cavity. **retroperitoneal h.,** Trietz's h. **retrovascular h.,** one that passes within the femoral sheath but exits posterior to the femoral vessels; called also *Serafini's h.* **Richter's h.,** an incarcerated or strangulated hernia in which only a portion of the circumference of the bowel wall is involved; called also *parietal h.* **Rieux's h.,** retrocecal h. **Rokitansky's h.,** protrusion of a sac of mucous membrane or of the peritoneum through separated muscular fibers of the intestine. **rolling h.,** paraesophageal h. **sciatic h.,** hernia through the greater or lesser sacrosciatic foramen. **scrotal h.,** an inguinal hernia which has descended into the scrotum. **Serafini's h.,** retrovascular h. **sliding h.,** hernia of the cecum (on the right) or the sigmoid colon (on the left) in which the wall of the viscus forms a portion of the hernial sac, the remainder of the sac being formed by the parietal peritoneum. Called also *slip h.* and *slipped h.* **sliding hiatal h.,** hiatal hernia in which the upper stomach and the cardioesophageal junction protrude upward into the posterior mediastinum; the protrusion, which may be fixed or intermittent, is partially covered by a peritoneal sac. Called also *axial hiatal h.* and *Type I hiatal h.* **slip h., slipped h.,** sliding h. **spigelian h.,** abdominal hernia through the linea semilunaris. **strangulated h.,** an incarcerated hernia that is so tightly constricted as to compromise the blood supply of the contents of the hernial sac, leading to gangrene. **synovial h.,** protrusion of the inner lining membrane through the stratum fibrosum of a joint capsule; called also *Birkett's h.* **tonsillar h.,** the extrusion of the tonsilla cerebelli through the foramen magnum. **Treitz's h.,** hernia of the intestine through the superior duodenal recess; called also *duodenojejunal h.* and *retroperitoneal h.* **umbilical h.,** protrusion of part of the intestine at the umbilicus, the defect in the abdominal wall and protruding bowel being covered with skin and subcutaneous tissue; called also *exomphalos.* **h. u′teri inguina′le,** see *persistent müllerian duct syn-*

drome, under *syndrome.* **uterine h.,** hernial protrusion of the uterus. **vaginal h.,** hernia into the vagina; colpocele. **vaginal h., posterior,** downward protrusion of the pouch of Douglas, with its intestinal contents, between the posterior vaginal wall and the rectum; called also *enterocele.* **vaginolabial h.,** hernia of a viscus into the posterior end of the labium majus. **Velpeau's h.,** femoral hernia in front of the femoral vessels. **ventral h.,** hernia through the abdominal wall. **vesical h.,** protrusion of the bladder. **W h.,** retrograde h.

hernial (her′ne-al) pertaining to a hernia.

herniated (her′ne-āt″ed) protruding like a hernia; enclosed in a hernia.

herniation (her″ne-a′shun) the abnormal protrusion of an organ or other body structure through a defect or natural opening in a covering membrane, muscle, or bone. **h. of intervertebral disk,** protrusion of the nucleus pulposus or annulus fibrosus of the disk, which may impinge on nerve roots. **h. of nucleus pulposus,** rupture or prolapse of the nucleus pulposus into the spinal canal. **painful fat h.,** piezogenic papules. **tonsillar h.,** protrusion of the cerebellar tonsils through the foramen magnum, exerting pressure on the medulla oblongata. **transtentorial h.,** downward displacement (caudal transtentorial h.; uncal h.) of the medial structures through the tentorial notch by a supratentorial mass, exerting pressure on the underlying structures, including the brain stem. **uncal h.,** transtentorial h.

hernioappendectomy (her″ne-o-ap″en-dek′to-me) herniotomy combined with appendectomy.

hernioenterotomy (her″ne-o-en″ter-ot′o-me) herniotomy conjoined with enterotomy.

hernioid (her′ne-oid) resembling hernia.

herniolaparotomy (her″ne-o-lap″ah-rot′o-me) laparotomy for the treatment of hernia.

herniology (her″ne-ol′o-je) [*hernia* + *-logy*] the study and science of hernias.

hernioplasty (her′ne-o-plas″te) operation for the repair of hernia.

herniopuncture (her″ne-o-pungk′tūr) [*hernia* + *puncture*] surgical puncture of a hernia.

herniorrhaphy (her″ne-or′ah-fe) [*hernia* + Gr. *rhaphē* suture] surgical repair of a hernia.

herniotomy (her″ne-ot′o-me) [*hernia* + Gr. *tomē* a cutting] a surgical operation for the repair of hernia; kelotomy.

heroin (her′o-in) diacetylmorphine.

Herophilus (hě-rof′ĭ-lus) **of Chalcedon** (c. 300 B.C.) a Greek physician at Alexandria, a pupil of Praxagoras and an elder contemporary of Erasistratus. He performed public human post mortems and possibly also vivisection on condemned criminals. In his studies of the brain (for him the seat of intelligence and the organ of the soul) he distinguished the cerebrum from the cerebellum, described and named the meninges, calamus scriptorius, and the torcular Herophili. He studied the vascular and nervous systems and distinguished sensory from motor nerves, tendons from nerves, and veins from arteries. Herophilus recognized that the pulse derives from the heart and is not an innate function of the arteries, and he classified pulses by speed, regularity, etc., and furnished a methematical law of systole and diastole.

herpangina (herp″an-ji′nah) [*herpes* + *angina*] an acute infectious disease caused by either group A or B coxsackievirus or by echoviruses, chiefly affecting young children in the summer, and characterized by vesiculoulcerative lesions on the mucous membranes of the throat, dysphagia, fever, vomiting, and prostration.

herpes (her′pēz) [L.; Gr. *herpēs*, a spreading cutaneous eruption, from *herpein* to creep] any inflammatory skin disease caused by a herpesvirus and characterized by the formation of clusters of small vesicles. When used alone, the term may refer to *herpes simplex* or to *herpes zoster*. **h. cor′neae,** herpetic inflammation involving the cornea. **h. digita′lis,** herpes simplex of the fingers. **h. facia′lis,** herpes simplex of the face. **h. febri′lis,** herpes simplex caused by type 1 virus, and primarily spread by oral secretions, usually occurring as a concomitant of fever, but sometimes also developing in the absence of fever or prior illness, and commonly involving the facial region, especially the vermillion border of the lips (*h. labialis*) and the nares; the vesicular lesions are self-limited. Called also *cold sore* and *fever blister*. **genital h., h. genita′lis,** herpes simplex due to type 2 virus, primarily transmitted sexually via genital secretions, and contact with viroids, and involving the genital region in both sexes; although symptoms in the female are more severe than in the male, the vesicular lesions are self-limited. Genital herpes at term in the pregnant female may lead to infection of the neonate and result in disseminated or localized infection or progress from localized to disseminated disease. Called also *h. progenitalis*. **h. gestatio′nis,** a rare, self-limited blistering cutaneous disorder of unknown origin usually beginning on the abdomen during the second and third trimesters of pregnancy and spreading to other sites, and characterized by the presence of an intensely pruritic polymorphous eruption, which may recur with subsequent pregnancies. **h. gladiato′rum,** see *traumatic h.* **h. labia′lis,** h. febrilis. **ocular h.,** herpes of the eye and its adnexa; see *herpetic keratoconjunctivitis.* **h. ophthal′micus,** h. zoster ophthalmicus. **h. progenita′lis,** genital h. **h. sim′plex,** a group of acute infections caused by herpes simplex virus type 1 or type 2, characterized by the development of one or more small fluid-filled vesicles with a raised erythematous base on the skin or mucous membrane, and occurring as a primary infection or recurring because of reactivation of a latent infection. Type 1 infections usually involve nongenital regions of the body, whereas in type 2 infections the lesions are primarily seen on the genital and surrounding areas. Precipitating factors include fever, exposure to cold temperature or to ultraviolet rays, sunburn, cutaneous or mucosal abrasions, emotional stress, and nerve injury. **traumatic h.,** primary cutaneous herpes simplex acquired by direct exogenous infection of traumatized skin, usually associated with localization of lesions to the area of trauma and regional lymphadenopathy and often by symptoms of systemic illness such as fever and malaise. Such infections have been seen in wrestler's h. (*h. gladiatorum*), and acquired from mats or body contact. **wrestler's h.,** see *traumatic h.* **h. zos′ter,** an acute infectious, usually self-limited, disease believed to represent activation of latent varicella-zoster virus in those who have been rendered partially immune after a previous attack of chickenpox. It involves the sensory ganglia and their areas of innervation, characterized by severe neuralgic pain along the distribution of the affected nerve and crops of clustered vesicles over the area of the corresponding dermatome, and is usually unilateral and confined to a single or adjacent dermatomes. Postherpetic neuralgia may be a complication. Called also *acute posterior ganglionitis, shingles, zona,* and *zoster*. **h. zos′ter auricula′ris,** Ramsay Hunt syndrome, def. 1. **h. zos′ter ophthal′micus,** herpes zoster involving the ophthalmic division of the trigeminal nerve, characterized by a cutaneous vesicular rash on an erythematous base along the nerve path, preceded by lancinating pain, usually accompanied by conjunctivitis and sometimes by keratitis, scleritis, iridocyclitis, extraocular muscle palsies, ptosis, and mydriasis. Called also *gasserian ganglionitis, h. ophthalmicus,* and *ophthalmic zoster*. **h. zos′ter o′ticus,** Ramsay Hunt syndrome, def. 1.

herpesencephalitis (her″pēz-en-sef″ah-li′tis) see under *encephalitis.*

Herpesviridae (her″pēs-vi′rĭ-de) a systematic name for the family of herpesviruses.

Herpesvirus hominis (her″pēz-vi′rus hom′ĭ-nis) the herpesvirus that causes herpes simplex; it occurs in two immunological types: Type 1 infections are primarily nongenital (e.g., herpes labialis and ocular herpes), whereas type II infections are primarily genital (herpes genitalis).

herpesvirus (her″pēz-vi′rus) [*herpes* + *virus*] any of a large group of DNA viruses found in many animal species, with a nucleocapsid about 100 nm in diameter, composed of 162 capsomers, and sometimes enclosed in a loose membrane; the nucleic acid is a single molecule of double-stranded DNA with a molecular weight of about 100 million daltons; the viruses mature in the nucleus of the infected cell, where they induce formation of a characteristic inclusion body; some also induce formation of a cytoplasmic inclusion body. Herpesviruses are causative agents of such conditions as oral herpes simplex, genital herpes simplex, varicella, herpes zoster, cytomegalic inclusion disease in humans, and of pseudorabies and other diseases of animals. See also *herpes.*

herpetic (her-pet′ik) [L. *herpeticus*] pertaining to or of the nature of herpes; relating to or caused by herpesviruses.

herpetiform (her-pet′ĭ-form) [*herpet-*(1) + L. *forma* form] resembling herpes; having grouped vesicles.

herpet(o)- [Gr. *herpeton* creeping thing, crawler, reptile, from *herpein* to creep] a combining form denoting a relationship to (1) herpes or (2) a snake or other reptile.

herpetologist (her″pĕ-tol′o-gist) a specialist in herpetology.

herpetology (her″pĕ-tol′o-ge) [*herpeto-*(2) + *-logy*] the branch of zoology that specializes in the study of reptiles and amphibians.

herpetophobia (her-pet″o-fo′be-ah) irrational fear of reptiles or amphibians.

Herpetosiphon (her″pe-to-si′fon) [Gr. *herpeton* creeper + *siphon* tube] a genus of gliding bacteria of the family Cytophagaceae, found in water, made up of unbranched, flexible, sheathed rods or filaments. Some species attack cellulose. The type species is *H. auranti′acus.*

Herpetosoma (her-pet″o-so′mah) [*herpeto-*(2) + Gr. *soma* body] in some systems of classification, a subgenus of stercorarian trypanosomes, including among others the species *Trypanosoma lewisi, T. duttoni,* and *T. rangeli.*

Herplex (her′pleks) trademark for a preparation of idoxuridine.

Herrick's anemia (her′iks) [James Bryan *Herrick,* Chicago physician, 1861–1954] sickle cell anemia; see under *anemia.*

Herring bodies (her′ing) [Percy Theodore *Herring,* English physiologist, 1872–1967] see under *body.*

Herrmannsdorfer diet (her″mans-dor′fer) [Adolf *Herrmannsdorfer,* Berlin surgeon, born 1889] see *Gerson's diet,* under *diet.*

hersage (ār-sahzh′) [Fr. "combing"] surgical dissociation of the fibers of a peripheral nerve by splitting the sheath and separating the nerve, throughout the diseased area, into a ribbon of fine free fibers.

Hershey (her′she), Alfred Day. American biologist, born 1908; co-winner, with Max Delbruck and Salvador E. Luria, of the Nobel Prize in medicine or physiology for 1969, for research on the mechanism and materials of inheritance of viruses.

Herter's disease (infantilism), test (her′terz) [Christian Archibald *Herter,* American physician, 1865–1910] see *infantile form of nontropical sprue;* under *sprue,* and see under *tests.*

Herter-Heubner disease (her′ter-hoib′ner) [C. A. *Herter;* Johann Otto Leonhard *Heubner,* pediatrician in Berlin, 1843–1926] the infantile form of nontropical sprue, or celiac disease.

Hertig-Rock ova (her′tig rok) [Arthur T. *Hertig,* American pathologist, born 1904; John *Rock,* American gynecologist, born 1890] see under *ovum.*

Hertwig's sheath (hert′vigz) [Richard *Hertwig,* German zoologist, 1850–1937] root sheath, def. 1.

Hertwig-Magendie phenomenon, sign (hert′vig mahjen′de) [Richard *Hertwig;* François *Magendie,* French physiologist, 1783–1855] skew deviation.

hertz (hertz) a unit of frequency equal to one cycle per second; abbreviated Hz.

hertzian waves (rays) (hertz′e-an) [Heinrich Rudolf *Hertz*, German physicist, 1857–1894] see under *wave*.

Herxheimer's fibers (spirals), reaction (herks′-hĭm-erz) [Karl *Herxheimer*, German dermatologist, 1861–1944] see under *fiber*, and see *Jarisch-Herxheimer reaction*, under *reaction*.

Heryng's sign (her′ingz) [Teodor *Heryng*, Polish laryngologist, 1847–1925] see under *sign*.

Heschl's convolution, gyrus (hesh′l′z) [Richard L. *Heschl*, Austrian pathologist, 1824–1881] see *gyri temporales transversi*.

hesperidin (hes-per′ĭ-din) chemical name: 7-[[6-*O*-(6-deoxy-α-L-mannopyranosyl)-β-D-glucopyranosyl]oxy]-2,3-dihydro-5-hydroxy-2-(3-hydroxy-4-methoxyphenyl)-H-benzopyran-4-one. A bioflavonoid, $C_{28}H_{34}O_{15}$, found in certain citrus fruits; it has been reported to reduce capillary fragility.

Hess (hes), Walter Rudolf. Swiss physiologist, 1881–1973; co-winner, with Antonio Egas Moniz, of the Nobel prize for medicine or physiology for 1949, for his discovery of the functional organization of the interbrain as a coordinator of the activities of the internal organs.

Hesselbach's hernia, ligament, triangle (hes′el-bahks) [Franz Kaspar *Hesselbach*, German surgeon, 1759–1816] see under *hernia*, and see *ligamentum interfoveolare* and *trigonum inguinale*.

hetacillin (het″ah-sil′in) [USP] chemical name: 6-(2,2-dimethyl-5-oxo-4-phenyl-1-imidazolidinyl)-3,3-dimethyl-7-oxo-4-thia-1-azabicyclo[3.2.0]heptane-2-carboxylic acid. A semisynthetic penicillin, $C_{19}H_{23}N_3O_4S$, occurring as a white to off-white powder, which itself has no antibacterial activity, but is converted in the body to ampicillin and has actions and uses similar to those of ampicillin (q.v.); administered orally. **h. potassium** [USP], the potassium salt of hetacillin, $C_{19}H_{22}KN_3O_4S$, having antibacterial actions and uses similar to those of ampicillin; administered intravenously and intramuscularly.

hetaflur (het′ah-floor) chemical name: hexadecylamine hydrofluoride; a dental caries prophylactic, $C_{16}H_{35}N·HF$.

hetastarch (het′ah-starch) a starch containing not more than 90 per cent of amylopectin, and that has been etherified so that an average of 7 to 8 of the OH groups in every 10-D-glucopyranose units of starch polymer have been converted into OCH_2CH_2OH groups; used as a plasma volume expander, administered by infusion.

HETE hydroxyeicosatetaraenoic acid.

heteradelphia (het″er-ah-del′fe-ah) [*heter-* + Gr. *adelphos* brother] a joined twin monstrosity in which one fetus is much more fully developed than the other.

heteradelphus (het″er-ah-del′fus) a monster exhibiting heteradelphia.

heteradenia (het″er-ah-de′ne-ah) [*heter-* + Gr. *adēn* gland] any abnormality of the gland tissue.

heteradenic (het″er-ah-den′ik) pertaining to, affected with, or of the nature of heteradenia.

Heterakis (het″er-a′kis) [*heter-* + Gr. *akis* pointed object] a genus of nonpathogenic nematodes parasitic in the ceca of chickens, turkeys, and the like, including *H. gallinae*, a species that serves as a paratenic host for *Histomonas meleagridis*, the etiologic agent of histomoniasis.

heteralius (het″er-a′le-us) [*heter-* + Gr. *halios* fruitless] an extreme example of heteradelphia.

heterauxesis (het″er-awk-ze′sis) [*heter-* + Gr. *auxēsis* growth] disproportionate growth of a part in relation to another part.

heteraxial (het″er-ak′se-al) [*heter-* + *axis*] having axes of unequal length.

heterecious (het″er-e′shus) [*heter-* + Gr. *oikos* house] living upon one host in one stage or generation and upon another in the next.

heterecism (het″er-e′sizm) the state of being heterecious.

heterergic (het″er-er′jik) [*heter-* + Gr. *ergon* work] having different effects; said of two drugs one of which produces a particular effect and the other does not.

heteresthesia (het″er-es-the′ze-ah) [*heter-* + Gr. *aisthēsis* perception] variation in the degree of cutaneous sensibility on adjoining areas of the body surface.

heter(o)- [Gr. *heteros* other, different] a combining form meaning other, different, or abnormal, or denoting relationship to another.

heteroagglutination (het″er-o-ah-gloo″tĭ-na′shun) agglutination of particulate antigens (on cells or adsorbed on inert carrier particles) of one species by agglutinins derived from organisms of another species.

heteroagglutinin (het″er-o-ah-gloo′tĭ-nin) an agglutinin with reactive specificity for particulate antigen(s) in one or more species other than the species in which it originates.

heteroalbumose (het″er-o-al′bu-mōs) a form of hemialbumose that is not soluble in water, but is soluble in hydrochloric acid and sodium chloride solutions.

heteroalbumosuria (het″er-o-al″bu-mo-su′re-ah) [*heteroalbumose* + *-uria*] the presence of heteroalbumose in the urine.

heteroantibody (het″er-o-an′tĭ-bod′e) an antibody specific for antigens originating in a species other than that of the antibody producer.

heteroantigen (het″er-o-an′tĭ-jen) an antigen originating in a species different from, and therefore foreign to, the antibody producer.

heteroatom (het″er-o-at′om) any atom with a ring-shaped chemical nucleus other than the carbon atoms.

heteroauxin (het″er-o-auk′sin) a compound occurring in urine which acts as a plant growth hormone; called also *auxin B*.

Heterobasidiomycetidae (het″er-o-bah-sid″e-o-mi-se′tĭ-de) a subclass of true fungi of the Basidiomycetes, made up of the rusts and smuts, in which the basidiospores germinate by budding, repetition, or by the production of conidia, and the basidium starts as a hyphal cell with two nuclei.

Heterobilharzia (het″er-o-bil-har′ze-ah) a genus of schistosomes that parasitize mammals, including human beings. **H. america′na,** a species whose cercariae may cause a nonpatent visceral schistosomiasis in man.

heteroblastic (het″er-o-blas′tik) [*hetero-* + Gr. *blastos* germ] having origin in different kinds of tissue.

heterocellular (het″er-o-sel′u-lar) composed of cells of different kinds.

heterocentric (het″er-o-sen′trik) [*hetero-* + L. *centrum* center] made up of rays that are neither parallel nor meet in one point; said of a ray of light.

heterocephalus (het″er-o-sef′ah-lus) [*hetero-* + Gr. *kephalē* head] a monster with two unequal heads.

heterochiral (het″er-o-ki′ral) [*hetero-* + Gr. *cheir* hand] reversed as regards right and left, but otherwise the same in form and size, as the hands.

Heterochlorida (het″er-o-klor′ĭ-dah) [*hetero-* + Gr. *chlōros* green] an order of plantlike protozoa (class Phytomastigophorea, subphylum Mastigophorea) having two unequal flagella, yellow-green chloroplasts, and silaceous cyst walls.

heterochromatin (het″er-o-kro′mah-tin) [*hetero-* + *chromatin*] that state of chromatin in which it is dark-staining and tightly coiled, forming irregular clumps (karyosomes) or Barr bodies in the nuclei of cells in interphase, or stains densely in certain areas of mitotic chromosomes. Cf. *euchromatin*. **constitutive h.,** the chromatin in regions of the chromosomes that are invariably heterochromatic, located in secondary constrictions of chromosomes 1, 9, and 16, the distal end of the long arm of the Y chromosome, and centromeric and telomeric regions; it contains highly repetitive sequences of DNA that are genetically inactive, and serves as a structural element of the chromosome. See also *C banding*, under *banding*. **facultative h.,** the chromatin in regions of the chromosomes that become heterochromatic in certain cells and tissues; e.g., it makes up the inactive X chromosome in female somatic cells.

heterochromatinization (het″er-o-kro″mah-tin-i-za′shun) 1. the condensation of euchromatin into heterochromatin. Called also *heterochromatization*. 2. lyonization.

heterochromatization (het″er-o-kro″mah-ti′za-shun) 1. heterochromatinization. 2. lyonization.

heterochromatosis (het″er-o-kro″mah-to′sis) heterochromia.

heterochromia (het″er-o-kro′me-ah) [*hetero-* + Gr. *chrōma* color + *-ia*] diversity of color in a part or parts that should normally be of one color. **h. i′ridis,** difference of color in the two irides, or in different areas of the same iris.

heterochromosome (het″er-o-kro′mo-sōm) [*hetero-* + *chromosome*] a sex chromosome.

heterochromous (het″er-o-kro′mus) marked by diversity of color; exhibiting heterochromia.

heterochron (het″er-o-krōn′) having different or varying chronaxy.

heterochronia (het″er-o-kro′ne-ah) [*hetero-* + Gr. *chronos* time + *-ia*] 1. the formation of parts or tissues, or the occurrence of a phenomenon, at an unusual time. Cf. *synchronia* (def. 2). 2. a difference in the rate or time of occurrence between two processes. 3. difference of more than 100 per cent between the chronaxy of a muscle and that of its nerve.

heterochronic (het″er-o-kron′ik) [*hetero-* + Gr. *chronos* time] 1. pertaining to or characterized by heterochronia. 2. denoting different ages or stages of development, as between the excised organ and the implanted organ in transplantation procedures.

heterochronous (het″er-ok′ro-nus) heterochronic.

heterochthonous (het″er-ok′tho-nus) [*hetero-* + Gr. *chthōn* a particular land or country] originating in a region other than that in which it is found. Cf. *autochthonous.*

heterochylia (het″er-o-ki′le-ah) the sudden varying of the gastric secretion from normal acidity to hyperacidity or anacidity.

heterocladic (het″er-o-klad′ik) [*hetero-* + Gr. *klados* branch] indicating an anastomosis between terminal branches from different arteries.

heterocrine (het′er-o-krin) [*hetero-* + Gr. *krinein* to separate] secreting more than one kind of matter.

heterocrisis (het″er-ok′rĭ-sis) [*hetero-* + Gr. *krisis* division] an abnormal crisis with unusual timing and symptoms.

heterocyclic (het″er-o-sīk′lik) [*hetero-* + Gr. *kyklos* circle] having or pertaining to a closed chain or ring formation which includes atoms of different elements.

heterocytotropic (het″er-o-si″to-trop′ik) [*hetero-* + *cyto-* + Gr. *tropos* a turning] having an affinity for cells of different species; see under *antibody.*

Heterodera radicicola (het″er-od′er-ah rad″ĭ-sik′o-lah) a nematode parasitic on the common root vegetables, such as radishes, carrots, turnips, potatoes, etc., as well as on celery. When infested vegetables are eaten, ova of the parasite may appear in the stools and must be distinguished from those of true parasites.

heterodermic (het″er-o-der′mik) [*hetero-* + Gr. *derma* skin] denoting a skin graft taken from a member of another species. See *dermatoheteroplasty.*

heterodesmotic (het″er-o-des-mot′ik) [*hetero-* + Gr. *desmos* a bond] joining dissimilar parts of the central nervous system; see under *fiber.*

heterodidymus (het″er-o-did′ĭ-mus) heterodymus.

heterodimer (het″er-o-di′mer) [*hetero-* + *dimer*] a dimer consisting of unlike subunits.

heterodont (het′er-o-dont) [*heter-* + Gr. *odous* tooth] having teeth of different types, such as incisors and molars.

Heterodoxus (het″er-o-dok′sus) a genus of insects of the order Mallophaga, the biting lice. *H. longitarsus* is parasitic on kangaroos, wallabies, and sometimes dogs in Australia. *H. spiniger* is parasitic on coyotes and wolves in the New World, and may also infest dogs.

heterodromous (het″er-od′ro-mus) [*hetero-* + Gr. *dromos* running] moving, acting, or arranged in the opposite direction.

heterodymus (het″er-od′ĭ-mus) [*hetero-* + Gr. *didymos* twin] a monster with a second head, neck, and thorax attached to the thorax.

heteroecious (het′er-o-e-shus) requiring two or more hosts to complete the life cycle; said of certain fungi and insects. Cf. *autoecious.*

heteroeroticism (het″er-o-ĕ-rot′ĭ-sizm) sexual feeling directed toward another person; cf. autoeroticism.

heteroerotism (het″er-o-er′o-tizm) heteroeroticism.

heterofermentation (het″er-o-fer″men-ta′shun) fermentation producing more than one major product.

heterofermenter (het″er-o-fer-ment′er) a microorganism that exhibits heterofermentation.

heterogamete (het″er-o-gam′ēt) a gamete of different size and structure than the one with which it unites.

heterogametic (het″er-o-gah-met′ik) pertaining to the sex that produces gametes of different kinds, in terms of their sex chromosomes. In human beings the male, who possesses X-bearing and Y-bearing sperm, is the heterogametic sex.

heterogamety (het″er-o-gam′ĕ-te) the production of unlike gametes by an individual of one sex, as the production of X- and Y-bearing gametes by the human male.

heterogamous (het″er-og′ah-mus) pertaining to heterogamy.

heterogamy (het″er-og′ah-me) [*hetero-* + Gr. *gamos* marriage] reproduction resulting from the union of two cells (gametes) that differ in size and structure; oogamy. See also *homogamy* and *isogamy.*

heteroganglionic (het″er-o-gang″gle-on′ik) [*hetero-* + Gr. *ganglion* ganglion] connecting various ganglia (of the sympathetic nervous system).

heterogeneity (het″er-o-jĕ-ne′ĭ-te) the state or quality of being heterogeneous. In genetics, the production of identical or similar phenotypes by different genetic mechanisms. A phenotype resembling a known phenotype but determined by a different genetic mechanism is called a genocopy or genetic mimic. **genetic h.,** the production of a specific clinical or biochemical phenotype by more than one genetic mechanism.

heterogeneous (het″er-o-je′ne-us) [*hetero-* + Gr. *genos* kind] 1. consisting of or composed of dissimilar elements or ingredients; not having a uniform quality throughout. 2. in genetics, the term denotes a trait that can be produced by different genes or combinations of genes.

heterogenesis (het″er-o-jen′ĕ-sis) [*hetero-* + Gr. *genesis* generation] 1. alternation of generations; reproduction that differs in character in successive generations. 2. asexual generation. 3. (*obs.*) the development of a living thing from some other kind of living thing. 4. spontaneous generation.

heterogenetic (het″er-o-jĕ-net′ik) 1. pertaining to heterogenesis. 2. not arising within the organism.

heterogenic (het″er-o-jen′ik) derived from a different source of species; see *xenograft.*

heterogenicity (het″er-o-jĕ-nis′ĭ-te) heterogeneity.

heterogenote (het″er-o-je″nōt) [*hetero-* + *gene* (analogy with *zygote*)] in bacterial genetics, a merozygote in which the corresponding alleles at a specific locus of the diploid region of the genome are different. See also *homogenote* and *merozygote.*

heterogenous (het″er-oj′ĕ-nus) 1. derived from a different source or species; see *xenograft.* 2. heterogeneous.

heteroglobulose (het″er-o-glob′u-lōs) a heteroalbumose obtained from a globulin.

heterogony (het″er-og′ŏ-ne) [*hetero-* + Gr. *gonos* procreation] heterogenesis.

heterograft (het′er-o-graft) xenograft.

heterography (het″er-og′rah-fe) [*hetero-* + Gr. *graphein* to record] the writing of words other than those intended by the writer.

heterohemagglutination (het″er-o-hem″ah-gloo″tĭ-na′shun) agglutination of erythrocytes of one species by hemagglutinins derived from an individual of a different species.

heterohemagglutinin (het″er-o-hem″ah-gloo′tĭ-nin) a hemagglutinin derived from one species that agglutinates erythrocytes of organisms of one or more other species.

heterohemolysin (het″er-o-he-mol′ĭ-sin) 1. a hemolysin occurring spontaneously in the blood of an untreated animal that will hemolyze the blood cells of an animal of another species. 2. hemolysin established in one species by deliberate immunization with blood cells of an animal of another species.

heterohexosan (het″er-o-hek′so-san) any one of a class of heterosaccharides which contain hexose units; they are lignocellulose, pectocellulose, and lipocellulose.

heteroimmune (het″er-o-im-mūn′) pertaining to or characterized by heteroimmunity.

heteroimmunity (het″er-o-im-mu′nĭ-te) 1. an immune state that results from the immunization of an animal belonging to one species with cells of an animal of a different species. 2. a state in which immunological response by the body to exogenous antigens, which include drugs and infectious agents, results in immunopathological changes.

heterointoxication (het″er-o-in-tok″sĭ-ka′shun) poisoning by material introduced from outside the body.

heterokaryon (het″er-o-kar′e-on) [hetero- + karyon] a cell or hypha containing two or more nuclei of different genetic constitutions.

heterokaryosis (het″er-o-kar″e-o′sis) [heterokaryon + -osis] the formation of, or the state of containing, heterokaryons.

heterokeratoplasty (het″er-o-ker′ah-to-plas″te) [hetero- + keratoplasty] grafting of corneal tissue from an individual of a species other than that of the recipient.

heterokinesis (het″er-o-ki-ne′sis) [hetero- + kinesis] the differential distribution of the sex chromosomes (X and Y in humans) in the developing gametes of a heterogametic organism.

heterolactic (het″er-o-lak′tik) bacterial fermentation which produces large quantities of lactic acid along with acetic acid, ethanol, and CO_2.

heterolalia (het″er-o-la′le-ah) [hetero- + Gr. lalia utterance] heterophasia.

heterolateral (het″er-o-lat′er-al) [hetero- + L. latus side] relating to the opposite side; contralateral.

heteroliteral (het″er-o-lit′er-al) marked by the substitution of one letter for another in pronouncing words.

heterolith (het′er-o-lith) [hetero- + Gr. lithos stone] an intestinal concretion not formed of mineral matter.

heterologous (het″er-ol′o-gus) [hetero- + Gr. logos due relation, proportion] 1. made up of tissue not normal to the part. 2. xenogeneic. 3. pertaining to antigen and antibody that are not homologous, i.e., the antigen is not the one that elicited the production of the antibody.

heterology (het″er-ol′o-je) abnormality in structure, arrangement, or manner of formation. In chemistry, the relationship between substances of partial identity of structure but of different properties.

heterolysin (het″er-ol′ĭ-sin) a lysin that dissolves cells of species other than the one in which it is formed, by leading to interruption of the integrity of the cell membranes; a lysin that is formed on the introduction of antigen from a different species.

heterolysis (het″er-ol′ĭ-sis) [hetero- + Gr. lysis dissolution] lysis of the cells of one species by lysin from a different species.

heterolysosome (het″er-o-li′so-sōm) a vacuole of lysosome containing exogenous substances with digestion in progress.

heterolytic (het″er-o-lit′ik) pertaining to or caused by heterolysis or a heterolysin.

heteromastigote (het″er-o-mas″tĭ-gōt) [hetero- + Gr. mastix lash] having one or more forward flagella together with at least one directed backward.

heteromeral (het″er-om′er-al) heteromeric.

heteromeric (het″er-o-mer′ik) [hetero- + Gr. meros part] sending processes through one of the commissures to the white matter of the other side of the spinal cord; said of nerve cells.

heteromerous (het″er-om′er-us) heteromeric.

heterometaplasia (het″er-o-met″ah-pla′se-ah) [hetero- + metaplasia] development of tissue into a variety foreign to the part where it is produced.

heterometropia (het″er-o-mĕ-tro′pe-ah) [hetero- + Gr. metron measure + -opia] the state in which there are differences in degree of refraction in the two eyes.

heteromorphic (het″er-o-mor′fik) heteromorphous.

heteromorphosis (het″er-o-mor-fo′sis) [hetero- + Gr. morphōsis a forming] the development, in regeneration, of an organ or structure different from the one that was lost.

heteromorphous (het″er-o-mor′fus) [hetero- + -morphous] 1. of abnormal shape or structure; differing from the type. 2. having synaptic chromosome mates which differ in size, form, or structure.

Heteronematina (het″er-o-ne″mah-ti′nah) [hetero- + Gr. nēma thread] a suborder of plantlike biflagellate protozoa (order Euglenida, class Phytomastigophoreae) having one large flagellum directed anteriorly and another smaller one trailing. Peranema is a representative genus.

heteronomous (het″er-on′o-mus) [hetero- + Gr. nomos law] in biology, subject to different laws of growth; specialized along different lines.

heteronymous (het″er-on′ĭ-mus) [heter- + Gr. onyma name] in ophthalmology, pertaining to the noncorresponding vertical halves of the visual fields of both eyes, i.e., the nasal half of the left eye and the nasal of the right, or the temporal half of the left eye and the temporal of the right.

hetero-osteoplasty (het″er-o-os′te-o-plas″te) [hetero- + Gr. osteon bone + plassein to shape] the grafting of bone from an individual of one species to an individual of another.

hetero-ovular (het″er-o-ov′u-lar) pertaining to or derived from different ova; dizygotic.

heteropagus (het″er-o-op′ah-gus) [hetero- + Gr. pagos thing fixed] a twin monster in which one component (the parasite) is much smaller than and dependent on the other (the autosite).

heteropancreatism (het″er-o-pan′kre-ah-tizm) an irregular condition of functioning on the part of the pancreas.

heteropathy (het″er-op′ah-the) [hetero- + Gr. pathos disease] 1. abnormal or morbid sensitiveness to stimuli. 2. allopathy.

heteropentosan (het″er-o-pen′to-san) a heterosaccharide which contains pentose units, such as gums, mucilages, and pectic substances.

heterophagosome (het′er-o-fag′o-sōm) [hetero- + phagosome] an intracytoplasmic vacuole formed by phagocytosis or pinocytosis, which becomes fused with a lysosome, subjecting its contents to enzymatic digestion. Called also heterophagic vacuole.

heterophagy (het″er-of′ah-je) [hetero- + Gr. phagein to eat] the taking into a cell of exogenous material by phagocytosis or pinocytosis and the digestion of the ingested material after fusion of the newly formed vacuole with a lysosome. Cf. autophagy.

heterophany (het″er-of′ah-ne) [hetero- + Gr. phainein to appear] a difference in the manifestations of the same condition.

heterophasia (het″er-o-fa′ze-ah) [hetero- + Gr. phasis speech + -ia] the uttering of words other than those intended by the speaker.

heterophasis (het″er-o-fa′sis) heterophasia.

heterophemia (het″er-o-fe′me-ah) [hetero- + Gr. phēmē word] heterophasia.

heterophil (het′er-o-fil″) 1. a granular leukocyte represented by neutrophils in man but characterized in other mammals by granules which have variable sizes and staining characteristics; called also heterophilic leukocyte. See also neutrophil (def. 2). 2. pertaining to any group of cross-reacting antigens occurring in several species and having a species distribution that does not correspond to phylogenetic relationships or to antibody directed against such antigens.

heterophile (het″er-o-fīl,-fil) heterophil.

heterophilic (het″er-o-fil′ik) [hetero- + Gr. philein to love] 1. heterophil. 2. staining with a type of stain other than the usual one.

heterophoralgia (het″er-o-fo-ral′je-ah) [hetero- + Gr. phoros bearing + -algia] heterophoria associated with pain.

heterophoria (het″er-o-fo′re-ah) [hetero- + Gr. phora movement, range] failure of the visual axes to remain parallel after the visual fusional stimuli have been eliminated. The various forms of heterophoria are called phorias, their direction being indicated by the appropriate prefix. See cyclophoria, esophoria, exophoria, hyperphoria, hypophoria, and latent deviation.

heterophoric (het″er-o-fo′rik) pertaining to or characterized by heterophoria.

heterophthalmia (het″er-of-thal′me-ah) [hetero- + Gr. ophthalmos eye + -ia] difference in the direction of the axes, or in the color, of the two eyes.

heterophthalmos (het″er-of-thal′mos) heterophthalmia.

heterophydiasis (het″er-o-fĭ-di′ah-sis) heterophyiasis.

Heterophyes (het″er-of′ĭ-ēz) [hetero- + Gr. phyē stature] a genus of minute trematode worms found in the middle third of the small intestine of man, dogs, cats, and other fish-eating mammals. H. heterophyes is found in Egypt, Asia, and Asia Minor. H. katsuradai and H. brevicaeca have been reported in man in Japan and the Philippines.

heterophyiasis (het″er-o-fi-i′ah-sis) infection with trematodes of the genus Heterophyes; it is generally asymptomatic.

heteroplasia (het″er-o-pla′ze-ah) [hetero- + Gr. plassein to mold] the replacement of normal by abnormal tissue; malposition of normal cells.

heteroplasm (het′er-o-plazm) any heterologous tissue.

heteroplastic (het″er-o-plas′tik) pertaining to heteroplasia or to heteroplasty.

heteroplastid (het″er-o-plas′tid) a xenograft.

heteroplasty (het′er-o-plas″te) [hetero- + Gr. plassein to mold] heterotransplantation.

heteroploid (het′er-o-ploid″) 1. pertaining to or characterized by heteroploidy. 2. an individual or cell with an abnormal number of chromosomes.

heteroploidy (het′er-o-ploi″de) the state of having an abnormal number of chromosomes.

Heteropoda (het″er-op′o-dah) a genus of large spiders sometimes confused with tarantulas. **H. venato′ria,** a large spider found in shipments of tropical fruit, particularly bananas; its bite is painful, but not serious.

heteropodal (het″er-op′o-dal) [hetero- + Gr. pous foot] having branches or processes of different kinds; said of nerve cells.

heteropolymeric (het″er-o-pol″e-mer′ik) [hetero- + poly- + Gr. meros part] composed of dissimilar constituent building units, as a macromolecule, e.g., a protein.

heteropolysaccharide (het″er-o-pol″e-sak′ah-rīd) any polysaccharide macromolecule containing two or more different sugars, its function varying with the nature of its residues.

heteroprosopus (het″er-o-pro′so-pus) [hetero- + Gr. prosōpon face] janiceps.

heteroproteose (het″er-o-pro′te-ōs) a primary proteose that is insoluble in water, but soluble in dilute salt solution.

heteropsia (het″er-op′se-ah) [hetero- + Gr. opsis vision] unequal vision in the two eyes.

Heteroptera (het″er-op′ter-ah) [hetero- + Gr. pteron wing] a suborder of Hemiptera characterized by the possession of two pairs of wings, one horny, the other membranous; it includes the medically important families Cimicidae and Reduviidae.

heteroptics (het″er-op′tiks) [hetero- + Gr. optikos optic] false or perverted vision; visual perception of objects not in the field of vision or misinterpretation of visual images.

heteropyknosis (het″er-o-pik-no′sis) [hetero- + Gr. pyknōsis condensation] 1. the quality of showing variations in density throughout. 2. a state of differential condensation observed in comparison of different chromosomes, or of different regions of the same chromosome. **negative h.,** attenuation of condensation observed in comparison of different chromosomes, or of different regions of the same chromosome. **positive h.,** accentuation of condensation observed in comparison of different chromosomes, or of different regions of the same chromosome.

heteropyknotic (het″er-o-pik-not′ik) pertaining to or characterized by heteropyknosis. **negatively h.,** showing areas of lesser condensation than normal. **positively h.,** showing areas of greater condensation than normal.

heterosaccharide (het″er-o-sak′ah-rīd) a polysaccharide containing a carbohydrate and a noncarbohydrate unit. Cf. holosaccharide.

heteroscedasticity (het″er-o-skĕ-das-tis′ĭ-te) [hetero- + Gr. skedastikos tending to scatter] the property of having unequal variances.

heteroscope (het′er-o-skōp) [heterophoria + -scope] a pair of fusion tubes so mounted as to subserve the observation of the progress of cases of heterophoria.

heteroscopy (het″er-os′ko-pe) 1. inequality of vision in the two eyes. 2. examination with a heteroscope.

heterosexual (het″er-o-sek′shoo-al) 1. pertaining to the opposite sex; directed toward a person of the opposite sex; opposite of homosexual. 2. one who is sexually attracted to persons of the opposite sex.

heterosexuality (het″er-o-sek″shoo-al′ĭ-te) [hetero- + sexuality] sexual attraction toward those of the opposite sex, as distinguished from homosexuality.

heterosis (het″er-o′sis) [Gr. heterōsis alteration] the condition in which the first generation hybrid shows more vigor as measured by growth, survival, and fertility, than either of the parent strains; it is believed to be caused by the dominance

(or interaction) of favorable alleles not common to both parental populations. Called also hybrid vigor.

heterosmia (het″er-os′me-ah) [hetero- + Gr. osmē smell] a condition in which odors are incorrectly interpreted.

heterosome (het″er-o-sōm) [hetero- + Gr. sōma body] a sex chromosome.

heterospore (het′er-o-spōr) a heterosporous organism.

heterosporous (het″er-os′po-rus) [hetero- + Gr. sporos seed] having spores of two kinds, which reproduce asexually.

heterosuggestion (het″er-o-sug-jes′chun) [hetero- + suggestion] suggestion received from another person; opposed to autosuggestion.

heterotaxia (het″er-o-tak′se-ah) [hetero- + Gr. taxis arrangement] anomalous placement or transposition of viscera or parts.

heterotaxic (het″er-o-tak′sik) affected with heterotaxia.

heterotaxis (het″er-o-tak′sis) heterotaxia.

heterotaxy (het′er-o-tak′se) heterotaxia.

heterothallic (het″er-o-thal′ik) pertaining to or exhibiting heterothallism.

heterothallism (het″er-o-thal′izm) a form of sexual reproduction in which the isogamete must fuse with a gamete formed by a cell of a different mating type, as in various algae and fungi.

heterotherapy (het″er-o-ther′ah-pe) [hetero- + Gr. therapeia treatment] treatment of disease by remedies which are antagonistic to the principal symptoms of the disease; nonspecific therapy.

heterotherm (het′er-o-therm″) an animal which exhibits heterothermy.

heterothermic (het″er-o-ther′mik) pertaining to or characterized by heterothermy.

heterothermy (het′er-o-ther″me) [hetero- + Gr. thermē heat] the exhibition of widely different body temperatures at different times or under different conditions, as certain species of birds, marsupials, or hibernating species.

heterotonia (het″er-o-to′ne-ah) [hetero- + Gr. tonos tension + -ia] a state characterized by variations in tension or tone.

heterotonic (het″er-o-ton′ik) pertaining to or characterized by heterotonia.

heterotopia (het″er-o-to′pe-ah) [hetero- + Gr. topos place + -ia] 1. displacement or misplacement of parts or organs; the presence of a tissue in an abnormal location. 2. a jumbling of sounds in words.

heterotopic (het″er-o-top′ik) occurring at an abnormal place or upon the wrong part of the body.

heterotopy (het″er-ot′o-pe) heterotopia.

heterotransplant (het″er-o-trans′plant) xenograft.

heterotransplantation (het″er-o-trans″plan-ta′shun) the operative replacement of lost or damaged parts or tissues by tissue taken from an individual of a different species (a xenograft).

Heterotrichia (het″er-o-trik′e-ah) [hetero- + Gr. thrix hair] an order of usually large to very large, often highly contractile, sometimes pigmented, parasitic or free-living, ciliate protozoa (subclass Spirotrichia, class Polyhymenophorea), characterized by the presence of a conspicuous adoral zone of membranelles but also commonly bearing holotrichous cilia. It comprises six suborders: Heterotrichina, Clevellandellina, Armophorina, Coliphorina, Plagiotomina, and Licnophorina.

Heterotrichina (het″er-o-trĭ-ki′nah) a suborder of very contractile, ciliate protozoa (order Heterotrichida, subclass Spirotrichia), characterized by the presence of well-developed somatic ciliature, a single, conspicuous vacuole at the posterior end of the body, and peristomial ciliature comprising numerous membranelles and membranes.

heterotrichosis (het″er-o-tri-ko′sis) [hetero- + Gr. trichōsis growth of hair] growth of hair of different colors on the body. **h. supercilio′rum,** difference in color of the hairs of the two eyebrows (von Walther).

heterotroph (het′er-o-trōf″) a heterotrophic organism.

heterotrophia (het″er-o-tro′fe-ah) [hetero- + Gr. trophē nourishment] any disorder or fault of nutrition.

heterotrophic (het″er-o-trōf′ik) [hetero- + Gr. trophē nutrition] not self-sustaining; said of a type of nutrition in which organisms derive energy from the oxidation of organic compounds either by consumption or absorption of other organisms. Called also *organotrophic.* Cf. *autotrophic.*

heterotrophy (het″er-ot′ro-fe) 1. the state of being heterotrophic; heterotrophic nutrition. 2. heterotrophia.

heterotropia (het″er-o-tro′pe-ah) strabismus.

heterotropy (het″er-ot′ro-pe) heterotropia.

heterotypic (het″er-o-tip′ik) pertaining to, characteristic of, or belonging to a different type.

heterotypical (het″er-o-tip′e-k′l) of a type differing from that usually or normally encountered; having characteristics peculiar to a different type; sometimes applied to the first meiotic division of the germ cells.

heterovaccine (het″er-o-vak′sēn) a vaccine made from some microorganism other than the one causing the disease for which the vaccine is used; it is one form of nonspecific therapy.

heteroxenous (het″er-ok′se-nus) [*hetero-* + Gr. *xenos* strange, foreign] requiring more than one host in the life cycle; said of certain parasites.

heterozoic (het″er-o-zo′ik) [*hetero-* + Gr. *zöon* animal] pertaining to another animal or species of animal.

heterozygosis (het″er-o-zi-go′sis) the formation of a zygote by the union of gametes of unlike genetic constitution.

heterozygosity (het″er-o-zi-gos′ĭ-te) [*hetero-* + *zygosity*] the state of possessing different alleles at a given locus in regard to a given character.

heterozygote (het″er-o-zi′gōt) [*hetero-* + *zygote*] an individual possessing different alleles in regard to a given character. **manifesting h.,** a female heterozygous for an X-linked disorder in whom, because of unfavorable X inactivation, the trait is expressed clinically with about the same severity as in hemizygous affected males.

heterozygous (het″er-o-zi′gus) pertaining to heterozygosity. *Doubly heterozygous:* having different alleles at each of two separate loci. See also *homozygous.*

Hetrazan (het′rah-zan) trademark for preparations of diethylcarbamazine citrate.

Heublein method (hoib′lin) [Arthur Carl *Heublein,* radiologist, 1879–1932] see under *method.*

Heubner's disease (endarteritis) (hoib′nerz) [Johann Otto Leonhard *Heubner,* pediatrician in Berlin, 1843–1926] see under *disease.*

Heubner-Herter disease (hoib′ner-her′ter) [J. O. L. *Heubner;* Christian Archibald *Herter,* American physician, 1865–1910] the infantile form of nontropical sprue, or celiac disease.

heuristic (hu-ris′tik) [Gr. *heuriskein* to find out, discover] encouraging or promoting investigation; conducive to discovery.

Heuser's membrane (hoi′zerz) [Chester *Heuser,* American embryologist, 1885–1965] see under *membrane.*

H.E.W. Department of Health, Education, and Welfare; succeeded by the Department of Health and Human Services (H.H.S.).

hex-, hexa- [Gr. *hex* six] a combining form meaning six.

hexabasic (hek″sah-ba′sik) [*hexa-* + *basic*] having six atoms replaceable by a base.

Hexa-Betalin (hek″sah-be′tah-lin) trademark for preparations of pyridoxine hydrochloride.

hexabiose (hek″sah-bi′ōs) disaccharide.

hexachlorobenzene (hek″sah-klor″o-ben′zēn) a compound, C_6Cl_6, used in organic synthesis and as a fungicide.

hexachlorocyclohexane (hek″sah-klo″ro-si″klo-hek′sān) benzene hexachloride.

hexachloroethane (hek″sah-klor″o-eth′ān) a crystal compound, CCl_3CCl_3, used against liver flukes in cattle and sheep.

hexachlorophene (hek″sah-klo′ro-fēn) [USP] chemical name: 2,2′-methylenebis-(3,4,6-trichlorophenol). An antibacterial, $C_{13}H_6Cl_6O_2$, occurring as a white to light tan, crystalline powder, effective against gram-positive organisms; used as a topical anti-infective and detergent, mainly in soaps and dermatological preparations, and in veterinary medicine to combat flukes in ruminants.

hexacosane (heks-ak′o-sān) [*hexa-* + Gr. *eikosi* twenty] an aliphatic hydrocarbon, $C_{26}H_{54}$, extracted from plant waxes; called also *cerane.*

hexad (hek′sad) 1. a group or combination of six similar or related entities. 2. any element having a valency of six.

hexadactylia (hek″sah-dak-til′e-ah) hexadactyly.

hexadactylism (hek″sah-dak′tĭ-lizm) hexadactyly.

hexadactyly (hek″sah-dak′tĭ-le) [*hexa-* + Gr. *daktylos* finger + *-ia*] the occurrence of six digits (fingers or toes) on one limb.

hexadecanoate (hek″sah-dek″ah-no′āt) systematic name for palmitate, denoting that it has sixteen (*hexa* six + *deca* ten) carbon acids in a straight chain.

Hexadrol (hek′sah-drol) trademark for dexamethasone.

hexaene (hek′sah-ēn) a chemical compound in which there are six conjugated double bonds.

hexafluorenium bromide (hek″sah-flūr-en′ĭ-um) [USP] chemical name: N,N'-di-9H-fluoren-9-yl-N,N,N',N'-tetramethyl-1,6-hexanediaminium dibromide. A neuromuscular blocking agent, $C_{36}H_{42}Br_2N_2$, occurring as a white, crystalline powder; used in anesthesiology to prolong and potentiate the skeletal muscle relaxing action of succinylcholine during surgery, administered intravenously.

Hexagenia bilineata (hek″sah-je′ne-ah bi-lin″e-a′tah) a mayfly of the shores of Lake Erie whose cast skins may cause asthma; called also *lake fly.*

hexahydric (hek″sah-hi′drik) containing six atoms of hydrogen.

hexamer (heks′ah-mer) 1. a polymer molecule composed of six monomers. 2. a capsomer having six structural subunits.

hexamethonium (hek″sah-mĕ-tho′ne-um) chemical name: N,N,N,N',N',N'-hexamethyl-1,6-hexanediaminium; a quaternary ammonium ganglion-blocking agent, $C_{10}H_{24}N_2$. **h. bromide,** the dibromide ester of hexamethonium, $C_{12}H_{30}Br_2N_2$, having the same actions as the base; has been used as an antihypertensive but has been largely replaced by more effective drugs. **h. chloride,** the dichloride salt of hexamethonium, $C_{12}H_{30}Cl_2N_2$, having the same actions as the base; used as an antihypertensive, administered orally and parenterally.

hexamethylated (hek″sah-meth′ĭ-lāt-ed) containing six methyl groups.

hexamethylenamine (hek″sah-meth″il-ēn-am′in) methenamine.

hexamethylendiamine (hek″sah-meth″il-ēn-di′am-in) a ptomaine, $NH_2(CH_2)_6NH_2$, from decomposing pancreas and muscle.

hexamethylmelamine (hek″sah-meth″il-mel′ah-mēn) HMM; an investigational antineoplastic agent with potential use for treatment of bronchogenic carcinoma, ovarian carcinoma, and lymphomas. Although structurally related to the alkylating agent triethylenemelamine, HMM does not act as an alkylating agent; its activity is related to the degree to which it is demethylated by the hepatic microsomal enzyme system, but the exact mechanism is unknown.

hexamethylpararosanilin (hek″sah-meth″il-par″ah-ro-san′ĭ-lin) see *gentian violet,* under *violet.*

hexamine (hek′sah-min) methenamine.

Hexamita (heks-am′ĭ-tah) [*hexa-* + Gr. *mitos* thread] a genus of flagellate protozoa (suborder Diplomonadina, order Diplomonadida), characterized by the presence of two anterior nuclei and six anterior and two posterior flagella. It comprises free-living species as well as intestinal parasites. *H. meleagridis* causes severe enteritis in wild and domestic fowl, including turkeys, chickens, quail, and partridges. *H. muris* is found in rats, mice, hamsters, and various wild rodents, *H. salmonis* in trout and salmon, and *H. columbae* in pigeons.

hexamitiasis (heks-am″ĭ-ti′ah-sis) infection with parasites of the genus *Hexamita.*

hexamylose (heks-am′ĭ-lōs) a crystalline amylose, $(C_6H_{10}O_5)_6$.

hexane (hek′sān) *n*-hexane; an aliphatic hydrocarbon of the methane series, C_6H_{14}, obtained by distillation from petroleum, occurring as a colorless, volatile, highly flammable liquid with a characteristic odor; it is a constituent of petroleum benzin, and is used as a solvent and in spectrophotometry.

Hexanicotol (hek″sah-nik′o-tol) trademark for a preparation of inositol niacinate.

Hexapoda (heks-ap′o-dah) [hexa- + Gr. pous foot] insecta.

hexatomic (hek″sah-tom′ik) 1. containing six atoms of an element, or six replaceable univalent atoms.

hexavalent (hek″sah-va′lent) having a valence of six.

Hexavibex (hek″sah-vi′beks) trademark for a preparation of pyridoxine hydrochloride.

hexavitamin (hek″sah-vi′tah-min) [NF] a preparation, in capsule or tablet form, containing vitamin A, vitamin D, ascorbic acid, thiamine hydrochloride, riboflavin, and niacinamide.

hexedine (hek′sĕ-dēn) chemical name: 2,6-bis(2-ethylhexyl)-hexahydro -7a-methyl-1H -imidazo [1,5-c] imidazole; an antibacterial, $C_{22}H_{45}N_3$.

hexenmilch (hek′sen-milkh) [Ger. "witches' milk"] a milklike secretion from the breast of a newborn infant; witch's milk.

hexestrol (hek-ses′trol) chemical name: 4,4′-(1,2-diethyl-1,2-ethanediyl)bisphenol. A diethylstilbestrol derivative, $C_{18}H_{22}O_2$, occurring as a white, crystalline powder, having the uses of estrogen (q.v.); administered orally and parenterally.

hexethal sodium (hek′sĕ-thal) chemical name: 5-ethyl-5-hexyl-2,4,6(1H,3H,5H)-pyrimidinetrione monosodium salt. A short-acting barbiturate, $C_{12}H_{19}N_2NaO_5$, used as a sedative and hypnotic.

hexetidine (heks-et′ĭ-dēn) chemical name: 1,3-bis(2-ethylhexyl)hexahydro-5-methyl-5-pyrimidinamine. An antifungal, antiprotozoal, and antibacterial agent, $C_{21}H_{45}N_3$, used mainly as a topical anti-infective in the treatment of vaginitis.

hexhydric (heks-hi′drik) containing six atoms of replaceable hydrogen.

hexobarbital (hek″so-bar′bĭ-tal) [USP] chemical name: 5-(1-cyclohexen-1-yl)-2,4,6(1H,3H,5H)-pyrimidinetrione. A short-acting barbiturate, $C_{12}H_{16}N_2O_3$, occurring as colorless crystals or white, crystalline powder; used as a sedative, administered orally. **h. sodium,** the sodium salt of hexobarbital, $C_{12}H_{15}N_2NaO_3$, which is a very short-acting barbiturate; used for pre- and postanesthesia sedation and hypnosis, administered orally, and for induction of short anesthesia, administered intravenously.

hexobarbitone (hek″so-bar′bĭ-tōn) hexobarbital.

hexobendine (hek″so-ben′dēn) chemical name: 3,4,5-trimethoxybenzoic acid 1,2-ethanediylbis[(methylimino)-3,1-propanediyl]ester. A vasodilator, $C_{20}H_{44}N_2O_{10}$, which has been used in the treatment of coronary insufficiency and angina of effort.

hexocyclium methylsulfate (hek″so-si′kle-um) chemical name: 4-(2-cyclohexyl-2-hydroxy-2-phenylethyl)-1,1-dimethylpiperazinium methyl sulfate (salt). A quaternary ammonium anticholinergic, $C_{21}H_{36}N_2O_5S$, occurring as a white crystalline powder, which inhibits gastric secretion and gastrointestinal motility; used especially as an adjunct in the treatment of peptic ulcer, administered orally.

hexokinase (hek″so-ki′nās) [EC 2.7.1.1] an enzyme of the transferase class that catalyzes the reaction ATP + D-hexose = ADP + D-hexose 6-phosphate. The reaction is the initial step in the cellular utilization of free hexoses. The enzyme occurs in all tissues and exists as various isoenzymes. Those in brain and muscles are relatively nonspecific; glucose, fructose, and mannose are effective substrates at low concentrations. The liver isoenzyme, often designated type IV, is called also glucokinase because it is more specific to glucose.

hexonate (hek′so-nāt) chemical name: hexamethylene-1,6-bis-(trimethylammonium) nicotinate. A ganglionic blocking agent.

hexone (hek′sōn) see under base.

hexonic acid (heks-on′ik) an aldonic acid formed by oxidation of the aldehyde group of a hexose to a carboxy group, e.g., gluconic acid.

hexosamine (hek′sōs-am″in) a nitrogenous sugar in which an amino group replaces a hydroxyl group.

hexosaminidase (heks″ōs-ah-min′ĭ-dās) any enzyme that cleaves N-acetyl hexosamine residues (glucosamine or galactosamine from glycosphingolipids. The term is usually used specifically to refer to β-N-acetylgalactosaminidase, whose isozymes are known as hexosaminidase A and hexosaminidase B. See also α-N-acetylglucosaminidase.

hexosan (hek′so-san) an anhydride or a polymerized form of a hexose.

hexosazone (hek″so-sa′zōn) an osazone formed from a hexose.

hexose (hek′sōs) a monosaccharide containing six carbon atoms in a molecule. **h. diphosphate,** see Harden-Young ester, under ester. **h. monophosphate,** see hexosephosphate.

hexosediphosphoric acid (hek″sōs-di″fos-for′ik as′id) a normal intermediate of the glycolytic pathway that may accumulate in the products of fermentation of sugars by yeasts in the presence of phosphates.

hexosephosphatase (hek″sōs-fos′fah-tās) an enzyme that catalyzes the removal of a phosphate group from hexose phosphates.

hexosephosphate (hek″sōs-fos′fāt) an ester of glucose with phosphoric acid, e.g., glucose-1-phosphate, glucose-6-phosphate, fructose-6-phosphate, and fructose-1,6-diphosphate.

hexosephosphate isomerase (hek″sōs-fos′fat i-som′er-ās) glucose-6-phosphate isomerase.

hexose-1-phosphate uridylyltransferase (hek′sōs fos′fāt u″ri-dil′il-trans′fer-ās) UDPglucose-hexose-1-phosphate uridylyltransferase.

hexosyltransferase (hek″so-sil-trans′fer-ās) [EC 2.4.1] any of a group of enzymes of the transferase class that catalyze the transfer of a hexose group from one compound to another.

hexuronic acid (heks″u-ron′ik) a uronic acid formed by oxidation of C-6 of a hexose to a carboxy group.

hexyl (hek′sil) [hex- + Gr. hylē matter] a hydrocarbon, C_6H_{13}, in many isomeric forms.

n-hexylamine (hek″sil-ah′mēn) a poisonous ptomaine, $CH_3(CH_2)_5NH_2$, from spoiled yeast and rancid cod liver oil; called also caproylamine.

hexylcaine hydrochloride (hek′sil-kān) [USP] chemical name: 1-cyclohexylamino-2-propanol benzoate (ester) hydrochloride. A local anesthetic, $C_{16}H_{23}NO_2 \cdot HCl$, occurring as a white powder; used for infiltration, block, and topical anesthesia.

hexylresorcinol (hek″sil-rĕ-zor′sĭ-nol) [USP] chemical name: 4-hexyl-1,3-benzenediol. An anthelmintic, $C_{12}H_{18}O_2$, occurring as white, or yellowish white, needle-shaped crystals; used in the treatment of roundworm and trematode infections, administered orally.

Hey's amputation (operation), derangement, hernia, ligament, saw (hāz) [William Hey, English surgeon, 1736– 1819] see under amputation, derangement, and saw; see encysted hernia, under hernia; and see margo falciformis hiatus saphenus.

Heymans (hay′manz), Corneille. Belgian physiologist, 1892–1968; winner of the Nobel prize for medicine or physiology in 1938 for his discovery of the role played by the sinus and aortic mechanisms in the regulation of respiration.

Heynsius' test (hīn′se-oos) [Adrian Heynsius, Dutch physician, 1831–1885] see under tests.

HF Hageman factor (coagulation Factor XII).

Hf chemical symbol of hafnium.

Hfr high frequency of recombination; Hfr cells are the sexual or donor (male) stage of bacteria having the F (fertility) factor in the chromosome, which enables them to transfer chromosomal material to recipient (female) bacteria not having this factor.

Hg chemical symbol for mercury (L. hydrargyrum).

Hgb hemoglobin.

HgCl₂ corrosive mercuric chloride.

Hg₂Cl₂ mild mercurous chloride.

HGF hyperglycemic-glycogenolytic factor (glucagon).

HGG human gamma globulin.

HGH, hGH human (pituitary) growth hormone.

hGHr growth hormone recombinant.

HgI₂ mercuric iodide.

Hg₂I₂ mercurous iodide.

Hg(NO₃)₂ mercuric nitrate.

HgO mercuric oxide.

Hg₂O mercurous oxide.

HGPRT hypoxanthine-guanine phosphoribosyltransferase,

a common name for hypoxanthine phosphoribosyl transferase (HPRT).

H.H.S. Department of Health and Human Services; formerly Department of Health, Education, and Welfare (H.E.W.).

HHT hydroxyheptadecatrienoic acid.

HI hemagglutination inhibition; see under *tests*.

5-HIAA 5-hydroxyindoleacetic acid.

hiatal (hi-a'tal) pertaining to or affecting a hiatus.

hiation (hi-a'shun) the act of yawning.

hiatus (hi-a'tus) [L.] [NA] general term for a gap, cleft, or opening. **adductor h.,** h. tendineus. **h. adducto'rius,** NA alternative for *h. tendineus.* **aortic h., h. aor'ticus** [NA], the opening in the diaphragm through which the aorta and thoracic duct pass. **Breschet's h.,** helicotrema. **h. of canal for greater petrosal nerve,** h. canalis nervi petrosi majoris. **h. of canal for lesser petrosal nerve,** h. canalis nervi petrosi minoris. **h. cana'lis facia'lis, h. cana'lis ner'vi pe-tro'si majo'ris** [NA], hiatus of canal for greater petrosal nerve: an opening in the petrous part of the temporal bone in the floor of the middle cranial fossa that transmits the greater petrosal nerve and a branch of the middle meningeal artery. **h. cana'lis ner'vi petro'si mino'ris** [NA], hiatus of canal for lesser petrosal nerve: the small, laterally placed opening on the anterior surface of the pyramid of the temporal bone that transmits the lesser petrosal nerve. **esophageal h.,** h. oesophageus. **h. esopha'geus,** NA alternative for *h. oesophageus.* **h. of facial canal, h. of fallopian canal, h. fallo'pii, false h. of fallopian canal,** h. canalis nervi petrosi majoris. **h. femora'lis,** annulus femoralis. **h. fina'lis sacra'lis,** a cleft in the lowermost sacral vertebra. **h. for greater superficial petrosal nerve,** h. canalis nervi petrosi majoris. **h. interme'dius lumbosacra'lis,** a cleft in the region of the first sacral vertebra, considered to represent a normally delayed ossification in young subjects. **h. interos'seus,** the opening above the interosseous membrane of the forearm for the passage of the posterior interosseous vessels. **h. leuke'micus,** a condition observed in acute myeloblastic leukemia in which there are numerous myeloblasts and a number of mature neutrophils in the peripheral blood, with few or no intermediate forms; called also *hiatus leukemicus of Naegeli.* **h. lumbosacra'lis,** the gap between the arches of the fifth lumbar and first sacral vertebrae, which is greater than the space between any vertebrae at a higher level. **h. maxilla'ris** [NA], **maxillary h., h. of maxillary sinus,** a very irregular opening on the medial surface of the maxillary sinus, in the articulated skull, being largely filled by parts of several adjoining bones. **neural h.,** an opening in the neural tube during the process of closure. **h. oesophage'us** [NA], esophageal hiatus: the opening in the diaphragm for the passage of the esophagus and the vagus nerves. Called also *h. esophageus* [NA alternative]. **h. pleuroperitonea'lis,** an opening in the fetal diaphragm; its failure to close leaves a congenital defect which may become a site for congenital diaphragmatic hernia. Called also *foramen of Bochdalek.* **sacral h., h. sacra'lis** [NA], the opening at the inferior end of the sacral canal formed by failure of the laminae of the fifth and sometimes the fourth sacral vertebrae to meet in the midline. **saphenous h., h. saphe'nus** [NA], the depression in the fascia lata that is bridged by the cribriform fascia and perforated by the great saphenous vein; called also *fossa ovalis femoris* and *oval fossa of thigh.* **Scarpa's h.,** helicotrema. **semilunar h., h. semiluna'ris** [NA], the deep semilunar groove anterior and inferior to the bulla of the ethmoid bone; the anterior ethmoidal air cells, the maxillary sinus, and sometimes the frontonasal duct drain through it via the ethmoid infundibulum. **subarcuate h.,** fossa subarcuata ossis temporalis. **h. tendin'eus** [NA], the opening between the long tendon of the adductor magnus and the femur, marking the distal end of the adductor canal; called also *h. adductorius.* **tentorial h.,** incisura tentorii cerebelli. **h. tota'lis sacra'lis,** a cleft in all of the sacral vertebrae, sometimes also involving one or several of the contiguous lumbar vertebrae. **vena caval h.,** foramen venae cavae. **h. of Winslow,** foramen epiploicum.

Hibbs' operation (hibz) [Russell Aubra *Hibbs,* New York surgeon, 1869–1932] see under *operation.*

hibernation (hi"ber-na'shun) [L. *hiberna* winter] the dormant state in which certain animal species pass the winter; it is characterized by narcosis and by sharp reduction in body temperature and metabolic activity. Cf. *estivation.* **artificial h.,** a state of reduced metabolism, muscle relaxation, and a twilight sleep resembling narcosis, produced pharmacodynamically by controlled inhibition of the sympathetic nervous system and reducing the level of the homeostatic reactions of the organism.

hibernoma (hi"ber-no'mah) a rare tumor made up of large polyhedral cells with coarsely granular cytoplasm, occurring on the back or around the hips. So called because it is considered by some to be a manifestation of a vestigial fat storage organ and comparable to the dorsal fat pads of hibernating animals. See also *lipoma.*

hiccough (hik'up) hiccup.

hiccup (hik'up) an involuntary spasmodic contraction of the diaphragm, causing a beginning inspiration which is suddenly checked by closure of the glottis, causing the characteristic sound; called also *singultus.* **epidemic h.,** a condition frequently seen in epidemic encephalitis.

Hicks contractions (sign), version (hiks) [John Braxton *Hicks,* English gynecologist, 1823–1897] see *Braxton Hicks contractions,* under *contraction,* and *Braxton Hicks version,* under *version.*

hidebound (hīd'bownd) bound down tightly to the subcutaneous tissues, said of the skin in scleroderma.

hidradenitis (hi"drad-ĕ-ni'tis) [Gr. *hidrōs* sweat + *adēn* gland + *-itis*] inflammation of a sweat gland, usually of the apocrine type. Called also *hidrosadenitis* and *hydradenitis.* **h. axilla'ris,** h. suppurativa. **h. suppurati'va,** a chronic suppurative and cicatricial disease of the apocrine gland–bearing areas, chiefly the axillae (especially in young women) and anogenital region (especially in men), which is caused by poral occlusion with secondary bacterial infection of apocrine sweat glands. It is characterized by the development of one or more tender red abscesses that enlarge and eventually break through the skin, yielding purulent or seropurulent drainage. Healing occurs with fibrosis, and recurrences lead to sinus tract formation and progressive scarring. Called also *apocrinitis* and *hidradenitis axillaris.*

hidradenoid (hi-drad'ĕ-noid) resembling a sweat gland; having components resembling elements of a sweat gland.

hidradenoma (hi"drad-ĕ-no'mah) a general term for tumors of the skin the components of which resemble epithelial elements of sweat glands. Several subtypes are recognized, and these are variously designated according to histologic pattern and specific component of the sweat gland unit from which the particular tumor is thought to be derived. The tumors may be nodular (solid) or papillary. The nodular types show various histologic patterns, each of which has been given a different designation: clear cell hidradenoma, epithelioma, or carcinoma; clear cell myoepithelioma; myoepithelioma; eccrine spiradenoma; eccrine acrospiroma; and mixed tumor of the skin (chondroid syringoma). The papillary hidradenoma (also known as syringocystadenoma papilliferum) is generally found only in the vulvar or perianal region. **h. erupti'vum,** hidradenoma that develops about the time of puberty, in which the lesions appear as small, yellowish papules on the chest, limbs, and lower eyelids.

hidr(o)- [Gr. *hidrōs* sweat] a combining form denoting relationship to sweat or to a sweat gland.

hidroadenoma (hid"ro-ad"ĕ-no'mah) hidradenoma.

hidrocystoma (hid"ro-sis-to'mah) [*hidro-* + *cystoma*] a retention cyst of a sweat gland.

hidropoiesis (hid"ro-poi-e'sis) [*hidro-* + Gr. *poiēsis* formation] the formation and secretion of sweat.

hidropoietic (hid"ro-poi-et'ik) pertaining to, characterized by, or promoting hidropoiesis.

hidrosadenitis (hi"dros-ad"ĕ-ni'tis) [*hidro-* + Gr. *adēn* gland + *-itis*] hidradenitis.

hidroschesis (hid-ros'kĕ-sis) [*hidro-* + Gr. *schesis* holding] anhidrosis.

hidrotic (hi-drot'ik, hi-drot'ik) pertaining to, characterized by, or causing sweating.

hiemal (hi'ĕ-mal) pertaining to or occurring in winter.

hier(o)- [Gr. *hieron* sacred, or *sacrum*] a combining form denoting relationship to the sacrum.

Highmore's antrum, body (hi′mōrz) [Nathaniel *Highmore*, English surgeon, 1613–1685] see *sinus maxillaris* and *mediastinum testis.*

hila (hi′lah) [L.] plural of *hilum.*

hilar (hi′lar) pertaining to a hilus.

Hildebrandt's test (hil′de-brants) [Fritz *Hildebrandt*, German pharmacologist, born 1887] see under *tests.*

hili (hi′li) [L.] plural of *hilus.*

hilitis (hi-li′tis) inflammation of a hilus, especially of the hilus of the lung.

Hill (hil′), Archibald Vivian. English biochemist, 1886–1977; co-winner, with Otto Fritz Meyerhof, of the Nobel prize for medicine or physiology in 1922 for his discovery relating to the production of heat in the muscle.

hillock (hil′ok) a small prominence or elevation. **auricular h's,** embryonic tubercles adjoining the first branchial groove that give rise to the auricle of the ear. **axon h.,** the conical expansion of an axon at its point of attachment to the body of the nerve cell. **Doyère's h.,** see under *eminence.* **germ h., germ-bearing h.,** cumulus oophorus. **seminal h.,** colliculus seminalis.

Hill posterior gastropexy (hil) [Lucius D. *Hill*, American surgeon, born 1921] see under *gastropexy.*

Hilton's law, line, muscle, sac (hil′tunz) [John *Hilton*, English surgeon, 1804–1878] see under *law* and *line;* and see *musculus aryepiglotticus* and *sacculus laryngis.*

hilum (hi′lum), pl. *hi′la* [L. "a small thing," "a trifle"][NA] a general term for a depression or pit at that part of an organ where the vessels and nerves enter. Formerly called *hilus* in NA. **h. of caudal olivary nucleus,** h. nuclei olivaris caudalis. **h. glan′dulae supraren′alis,** hilum of suprarenal gland: the depression on the anterior surface of the suprarenal gland where the suprarenal vein enters the gland. **h. of inferior olivary nucleus,** h. nuclei olivaris caudalis. **h. lie′nis,** NA alternative for *h. splenicum.* **h. nu′clei denta′ti** [NA], hilum of dentate nucleus: the white core of the dentate nucleus of the cerebellum. **h. nu′clei oliva′ris cauda′lis** [NA], hilum of caudal olivary nucleus: the white core of the caudal olivary nucleus of the medulla oblongata, most prominent medially. Called also *inferior h. of caudal olivary nucleus* and *h. nuclei olivaris inferior* [NA alternative]. **h. nu′clei oliva′ris inferio′ris,** NA alternative for *h. nuclei olivaris caudalis.* **h. of spleen,** h. splenicum. **h. sple′nicum** [NA], hilum of spleen: the fissure on gastric surface of the spleen where the vessels and nerves enter; called also *h. lienis* [NA alternative]. **h. of suprarenal g.,** h. glandulae suprarenalis.

hilus (hi′lus), pl. *hi′li.* hilum. **h. hep′atis,** porta hepatis. **h. of kidney,** h. renalis. **h. of lung,** h. pulmonis. **h. of lymph node,** h. nodi lymphatici. **h. lymphoglan′dulae,** h. nodi lymphatici. **h. no′di lymphat′ici** [NA], hilus of lymph node: the indentation on a lymph node where the arteries enter and the veins and efferent lymphatic vessels leave; called also *h. lymphoglandulae.* **h. ova′rii** [NA], **h. of ovary,** the point on the mesovarial border of the ovary where the vessels and nerves enter. **h. pulmo′nis** [NA], hilus of the lung: the depression on the mediastinal surface of the lung where the bronchus and the blood vessels and nerves enter. **h. rena′lis** [NA], hilus of the kidney: the point on the medial margin of the kidney where the vessels, nerves, and ureter enter.

himantosis (hi″man-to′sis) [Gr. *himantōsis,* from *himas* strap] elongation of the uvula.

hinchazon (hinch″ah-zon′) [Cuban] beriberi.

hindbrain (hīnd′brān) rhombencephalon.

Hindenlang's test (hin′den-lahngz) [Karl *Hindenlang,* German physician, 1854–1884] see under *tests.*

hindfoot (hīnd′foot) the posterior portion of the foot, comprising the region of the talus and calcaneus.

hindgut (hīnd′gut) 1. the embryonic structure from which chiefly the colon is formed. 2. the posterior ectodermal portion of the alimentary tract of invertebrates, such as arthropods; it comprises an intestine and rectum.

hind-kidney (hīnd-kid′ne) the metanephros.

Hines-Brown test (hīnz-brown) [Edgar Alphonso *Hines,* Jr., American physician, born 1906; George Elgie *Brown,* American physician, 1885–1935] see under *tests.*

hinge-bow (hinj′bo) adjustable axis face-bow.

Hinton test (hin′ton) [William Augustus *Hinton,* American bacteriologist, 1883–1959] see under *tests.*

HIO₃ iodic acid.

hip (hip) 1. the area of the body lateral to and including the hip joint; called also *coxa* [NA]. 2. loosely, the hip joint. **h. pointer,** contusion of the bone of the iliac crest or avulsion of muscle attachments of the iliac crest. **snapping h.,** a condition marked by a slipping around of the hip joint, sometimes with an audible snap, due to the slipping of a tendinous band over the greater trochanter; called also *Perrin-Ferraton disease.*

hipped (hipt) having a fracture at the point of the hip; said of horses.

Hippel's disease (hip′elz) [Eugen von *Hippel,* German ophthalmologist, 1867–1939] von Hippel's disease; see under *disease.*

Hippelates (hip″ĕ-la′tēz) a genus of insects of the family Chloropidae, order Diptera. **H. fla′vipes,** the probable mechanical vector of yaws in Haiti. **H. pal′lipes,** a species that is thought to be the mechanical vector of yaws in Jamaica; called also *Oscinis pallipes.* **H. pu′sio,** the "eye gnat" of California and Florida and other southern states, which is the mechanical vector of epidemic conjunctivitis, usually of a severe, follicular type.

Hippel-Lindau disease (hip′el-lin′dow) [Eugen von *Hippel;* Arvid *Lindau,* Swedish pathologist, 1892–1958] von Hippel-Lindau disease; see under *disease.*

Hippeutis (hi-pu′tis) a genus of fresh-water snails. **H. canto′ri,** one of the principal intermediate hosts of the trematode *Fasciolopsis buski* in eastern China.

hippo (hip′po) ipecac.

hipp(o)- [Gr. *hippos* horse] a combining form denoting relationship to a horse.

Hippobosca (hip-o-bos′kah) [*hippo-* + Gr. *boskein* to feed] the typical genus of the family Hippoboscidae. They are pupiparous, dipterous, parasitic insects, called winged tick flies. **H. ru′fipes,** a fly of South America whose bite transmits *Trypanosoma theileri.*

Hippoboscidae (hip″o-bos′kĭ-de) a family of parasitic flies found on bird and mammals; some have wings, others are wingless. It includes the genera *Hippobosca, Melaphagus,* and *Pseudolynchia.*

hippocampal (hip″o-kam′pal) pertaining to the hippocampus.

hippocampus (hip″o-kam′pus) [Gr. *hippokampos* sea horse] [NA] a curved elevation of gray matter extending the entire length of the floor of the temporal horn of the lateral ventricle. Starting on its ventricular aspect, the hippocampus is usually considered to comprise seven sublayers: ependyma, alveus, stratum oriens, stratum pyramidale, stratum radiatum, stratum lacunosum, and stratum moleculare. **h. ma′jor,** hippocampus. **h. mi′nor,** calcar avis.

hippocoprosterol (hip″o-ko-pros′ter-ol) [*hippo-* + Gr. *kopros* dung + *sterol*] a sterol found in the feces of herbivorous animals and derived from the phytosterol of grass and other food plants, $C_{27}H_{54}O$; possibly related to coprostanol.

Hippocrates (hip-pok′rah-tēz) **of Cos** (c. 460 to c. 375 B.C.) the Father of Medicine, a student and teacher, not founder, of the medical school on Cos. According to Plato and Aristotle, Hippocrates was a great physician. None of the works in the Hippocratic corpus can be surely ascribed to Hippocrates. His anatomy was vague: he knew only bones in detail, not being sure of the organs, muscles, nerves, tendons, or blood vessels. Hippocrates' physiology was based on humoralism; his diagnosis was directed toward general pathology; his prognosis, to (fore)tell the stages, duration, and end of disease. Hippocrates closely observed fevers, skin, the tongue, eyes, sweat, urine, and feces. Malarial and pulmonary diseases, common in the ancient Mediterranean, provided Hippocrates with ample evidence of humors—hemorrhagic blood, black and yellow bile from fits of vomiting in remittent malaria, and phlegm in mucus and expectoration. Hippocrates' therapy was to restore the humoral equilibrium: rid the excess humors and replace the deficient humors. He relied on the healing power of nature and recommended diet and moderate exercise, but rejected drugs. The Hippocratic Oath is as follows:

"I swear by Apollo the physician, by Æsculapius, Hygeia, and Panacea, and I take to witness all the gods, all the goddesses, to keep according to my ability and my judgment the following Oath:

"To consider dear to me as my parents him who taught me this art; to live in common with him and if necessary to share my goods with him; to look upon his children as my own brothers, to teach them this art if they so desire without fee or written promise; to impart to my sons and the sons of the master who taught me and the disciples who have enrolled themselves and have agreed to the rules of the profession, but to these alone, the precepts and the instruction. I will prescribe regimen for the good of my patients according to my ability and my judgment and never do harm to anyone. To please no one will I prescribe a deadly drug, nor give advice which may cause his death. Nor will I give a woman a pessary to procure abortion. But I will preserve the purity of my life and my art. I will not cut for stone, even for patients in whom the disease is manifest; I will leave this operation to be performed by practitioners (specialists in this art). In every house where I come I will enter only for the good of my patients, keeping myself far from all intentional ill-doing and all seduction, and especially from the pleasures of love with women or with men, be they free or slaves. All that may come to my knowledge in the exercise of my profession or outside of my profession or in daily commerce with men, which ought not to be spread abroad, I will keep secret and will never reveal. If I keep this oath faithfully, may I enjoy my life and practice my art, respected by all men and in all times; but if I swerve from it or violate it, may the reverse be my lot."

hippocratic (hip″o-krat′ik)   pertaining to or described by Hippocrates of Cos, or pertaining to his school of medicine.

hippocratism (hip-pok′rah-tizm)   the system of medicine attributed to Hippocrates and his school, based on imitating the processes of nature, and emphasizing treatment and prognosis.

hippocratist (hip-pok′rah-tist)   a believer in or practitioner of the system of medicine attributed to Hippocrates and his school.

hippolite (hip′o-līt)   hippolith.

hippolith (hip′o-lith) [*hippo-* + Gr. *lithos* stone]   a bezoar, or concretion, from the alimentary tract of the horse.

hippomane (hĭ-pom′ah-ne)   small, rounded, flat, amber bodies found in the allantoic fluid of various animals, especially the ungulates and ruminants.

hippomelanin (hip″o-mel′ah-nin) [*hippo-* + Gr. *melas* black]   a black pigment from tumors and marrow of horses affected with melanosis.

hippostercorin (hip″o-ster′ko-rin)   hippocoprosterol.

hippulin (hip′u-lin)   a crystalline estrogenic steroid, $C_{18}H_{20}O_2$, with four double bonds, obtained from the urine of pregnant mares.

hippurate (hip′u-rāt)   any salt of hippuric acid.

hippuria (hĭ-pu′re-ah) [*hippo-* + *-uria*]   excess of hippuric acid in the urine.

hippuric acid (hip-ūr-ik)   a crystallizable acid, $C_6H_5 \cdot CO \cdot NH \cdot CH_2 \cdot COOH$, from the urine of domestic animals; more rarely found in human urine. Called also *benzoylaminoacetic a.*, *benzoylglycine*, and *urobenzoic a.*

hippuricase (hĭ-pu′ri-kās)   aminoacylase.

hippus (hip′us) [Gr. *hippos*]   abnormally exaggerated rhythmic contraction and dilation of the pupil, independent of changes in illumination or in fixation of the eyes; called also *pupillary athetosis.*

Hiprex (hi′preks)   trademark for a preparation of methenamine hippurate.

hirci (hir′si) [L., plural of *hircus*] [NA]   the hairs growing in the axilla.

hircismus (hir-siz′mus) [L. *hircus* goat]   the strong odor of the axillae caused by bacterial decomposition of apocrine sweat, formed only in that site.

hircus (hir′kus), pl. *hir′ci* [L. "a goat"]   see *hirci.*

Hirschberg's magnet, method (hirsh′bergz) [Julius *Hirschberg*, German ophthalmologist, 1843–1925]   see under *magnet* and *method.*

Hirschfeld's canals (hirsh′feldz) [I. *Hirschfeld*, American dentist 1881–1965]   interdental canals.

Hirschfeld's disease [Felix *Hirschfeld*, German physician, born 1863]   see under *disease.*

Hirschsprung's disease (hirsh′sproongz) [Harald *Hirschsprung*, a Danish physician, 1830–1916]   see under *disease.*

hirsute (her′soot) [L. *hirsutus*]   shaggy; having abundant or excessive hair.

hirsuties (her-soo′she-ēz)   hirsutism.

hirsutism (her′soot-izm)   abnormal hairiness, especially an adult male pattern of hair distribution in women. Cf. *hypertrichosis.*

hirudicidal (hĭ-roo″dĭ-si′dal)   destructive to leeches.

hirudicide (hĭ-roo′dĭ-sīd)   an agent that is destructive to leeches.

hirudin (hĭ-roo′din) [L. *hirudo* leech]   the active principle of the secretion of the buccal glands of leeches; it has the power of preventing coagulation of the blood by acting as an antithrombin.

Hirudinaria (hir″u-dĭ-na′re-ah)   a genus of leeches of the family Gnathobdellidae.

Hirudinea (hir″u-din′e-ah)   a class of the Annelida; the leeches. It includes the genera *Haementeria, Hirudo, Hirudinaria, Haemadipsa, Limnatis, Macrobdella,* and *Haemopis.*

hirudiniasis (hir″u-dĭ-. i′ah-sis)   invasion of the nose, mouth, pharynx, or larynx by leeches; attachment of leeches to the skin.

hirudinization (hĭ-roo″dĭ-ni-za′shun) [L. *hirudo* leech]   1. the process of rendering the blood noncoagulable by the injection of hirudin. 2. the application of leeches; leeching.

hirudinize (hĭ-roo′dĭ-nīz)   to render the blood noncoagulable by the injection of hirudin.

Hirudo (hĭ-roo′do), pl. *hiru′dines* [L. "leech"]   a genus of leeches of the family Gnathobdellidae, class Hirudinea. **H. aegypti′aca,** *Limnatis nilotica.* **H. japon′ica,** the medicinal leech of Japan. **H. javan′ica,** a leech of Java, Batavia, and Burma, reported to produce internal hirudiniasis. **H. medicina′lis,** olive-gray leech formerly used extensively for therapeutic purposes. **H. quinquestria′ta,** a leech occurring in Australia. **H. sanguisor′ba,** *Haemopis sanguisuga.* **H. trocti′na,** the common European leech, which is marked with green, orange, and black somewhat like a trout.

His   histidine.

His' bundle (band), disease, spindle (his′ez) [Wilhelm *His*, Jr., Swiss physician, 1863–1934]   see under *bundle,* and see *trench fever,* under *fever,* and *aortic spindle* under *spindle.*

His' bursa, canal, duct, space, zones [Wilhelm *His,* eminent German anatomist and embryologist, 1831–1904]   see under *bursa, canal, space,* and *zone,* and see *ductus thyroglossalis.*

His-Werner disease (his′ ver′ner) [Wilhelm *His,* Jr.; Heinrich *Werner,* German physician, 1874–1946]   trench fever.

Hispril (his′pril)   trademark for a preparation of diphenylpyraline hydrochloride.

Hiss capsule stain (his) [Philip Hanson *Hiss,* Jr., American bacteriologist, 1869–1913]   see under *Table of Stains.*

Histadyl (his′tah-dil)   trademark for preparations of methapyrilene.

histadyl (his′tah-dil)   the acyl radical of histadine.

Histalog (his′tah-log)   trademark for a preparation of betazole.

histaminase (his-tam′ĭ-nās)   amine oxidase (copper containing).

histamine (his′tah-mēn)   chemical name: 1*H*-imidazole-4-ethanamine. A decarboxylation product of histidine, $C_5H_9N_3$, found in all body tissues, particularly in the mast cells and their related blood basophils, the highest concentration being in the lungs. It is also present in ergot and other plants and may be synthesized outside the body from histidine or citric acid. It has several functions, including (1) dilation of capillaries, which increases capillary permeability and results in a drop of blood pressure, (2) contraction of most smooth muscle tissue, including bronchial smooth muscle of the lung, (3) induction of increased gastric secretion, and (4) acceleration of the heart rate. It is also responsible for the triple response, and is implicated as a mediator of immediate hypersensitivity. On the basis of the antagonistic effects of antihistamines, it is postulated that cellular receptors of histamine are of two types: The H_1 receptors mediate the contraction of smooth muscle and the effects on capillaries; the H_2 receptors mediate the acceleration of heart rate and the promotion of gastric acid secretion. Both H_1 and H_2 receptors mediate the contraction of vascular smooth muscle. Histamine has also been postulated to be a neurotransmitter in the central nervous system.   **h.$_1$,** the cellular receptor site for histamine responsible for the dilation of blood vessels and the contraction of smooth muscle; abbreviated H_1. **h.$_2$,** the cellular receptor site for histamine responsible for the stimulation of heart rate and gastric secretion; abbreviated H_2. **h. hydrochloride,** the dihydrochloride salt of histamine, $C_5H_9N_3 \cdot 2HCl$, having the same actions as the base; used as an active ingredient of several analgesic dermatological preparations. **h. phosphate** [USP], the phosphate salt of histamine, $C_5H_9N_3 \cdot 2H_3PO_4$, occurring as colorless, long prismatic crystals, having the same actions as the base; used as a diagnostic aid in testing gastric secretion, administered subcutaneously. It is also used in the diagnosis of pheochromocytoma and has been used in treating various allergic manifestations, for desensitization in cases of hypersensitivity, and in the treatment of peripheral vascular diseases, Meniere's disease, and headache.

histaminemia (his-tam″ĭ-ne′me-ah) the presence of histamine in the blood.

histaminergic (his″tah-min-er′jik) denoting those responses by histamine receptors to histamine that are blocked by histamine antagonists (e.g., cimetidine).

histanoxia (his″tan-ok′se-ah) [hist- + anoxia] oxygen deprivation of the tissues due to a lessening of the blood supply.

Histaspan (his′tah-span) trademark for preparations of chlorpheniramine maleate.

histic (his′tik) pertaining to or of the nature of tissue.

histidase (his′tĭ-dās) histidine ammonia-lyase.

histidinase (his′tĭ-dĭ-nās) histidine ammonia-lyase.

histidine (his′tĭ-din, dēn) an α-amino acid, beta-4-imidazolyl alanine, $N:CH \cdot NH \cdot CH:C \cdot CH_2CH(NH_2)COOH$, essential for optimal growth in infants; first found as a decomposition product of the protamine of the sturgeon testes (Kossel, 1896), it is obtainable from many proteins by the action of sulfuric acid and water. The decarboxylation of histidine results in the formation of histamine.

histidine ammonia-lyase (his′tĭ-dēn ah-mo′ne-ah li′ās) [EC 4.3.1.3] an enzyme of the lyase class that catalyzes the reaction L-histidine = urocanate + NH_3. The reaction is the initial step of histidine catabolism. Genetic deficiency of the enzyme, transmitted as an autosomal recessive trait, causes histidinemia. Called also histidase. **h. monohydrochloride,** a crystalline substance, $C_6H_9N_3O_2 \cdot HCl$, once believed to be useful in the treatment of peptic ulcer.

histidinemia (his″tĭ-dĭ-ne′me-ah) an inborn aminoacidopathy characterized by excessive amounts of histidine in the blood and urine owing to deficient histidase activity, with consequent failure to metabolize histidine to urocanic acid. Many affected persons suffer modest mental retardation and disordered speech development. It is transmitted as an autosomal recessive trait. Called also ahistidasia.

histidinuria (his″tĭ-dĭ-nu′re-ah) an excess of histidine in the urine; see histidinemia.

histi(o)- [Gr. histion, web] a combining form denoting relationship to tissue.

histioblast (his′te-o-blast″) a local histiocyte (macrophage).

histiocyte (his′te-o-sīt″) [histio- + -cyte] macrophage. **cardiac h.,** Anitschkow's myocyte. **sea-blue h.,** a morphologically distinct, granulated histiocyte, sea-blue in color; see under syndrome. **wandering h's,** an active macrophage.

histiocytic (his″te-o-sit′ik) pertaining to or containing histiocytes.

histiocytoma (his″te-o-si-to′mah) [histiocyte + -oma] a tumor containing histiocytes (macrophages). **fibrous h.,** dermatofibroma. **lipoid h.,** fibroxanthoma.

histiocytomatosis (his″te-o-si-to″mah-to′sis) any generalized disorder of the reticuloendothelial system, such as xanthomatosis, Gaucher's disease, Niemann-Pick disease, lymphogranulomatosis, etc.

histiocytosis (his″te-o-si-to′sis) a condition marked by the abnormal appearance of histiocytes (macrophages) in the blood. **sinus h.,** a disorder of the lymph nodes in which the distended sinuses are completely, or nearly completely, filled by histiocytes, as a result of active multiplication of the littoral cells. **h. X,** a generic term embracing eosinophilic granuloma, Letterer-Siwe disease, and Hand-Schüller-Christian disease, and indicating a shared common origin for the three entities and a common morphologic characteristic: a granulomatous infiltration composed of large histiocytes with pale eosinophilic, foamy cytoplasm and well-delimited nuclei.

histiogenic (his″te-o-jen′ik) histogenous.

histioid (his′te-oid) histoid.

histio-irritative (his″te-o-ir′ĭ-ta″tiv) [histio- + irritative] having an irritative effect on connective tissue.

histioma (his″te-o′mah) histoma.

histionic (his″te-on′ik) pertaining to or derived from a tissue.

hist(o)- [Gr. histos web] a combining form denoting relationship to tissue.

histoblast (his′to-blast) [histo- + Gr. blastos germ] a tissue-forming cell.

histochemical (his″to-kem′ĭ-kal) pertaining to histochemistry or to the chemical components or activities of cells or tissues.

histochemistry (his″to-kem′is-tre) that branch of histology which deals with the identification of chemical components in cells and tissues.

histochemotherapy (his″to-ke″mo-ther′ah-pe) see chemotherapy.

histochromatosis (his″to-kro″mah-to′sis) [histo- + Gr. chrōma color] a general term for affections of the reticuloendothelial system, including xanthochromatosis, Gaucher's disease, and lymphogranulomatosis.

histoclastic (his″to-klas′tik) [histo- + Gr. klastos broken] breaking down tissue; said of certain cells.

histoclinical (his″to-klin′ĭ-kal) combining histological and clinical evaluation.

histocompatibility (his″to-kom-pat″ĭ-bil′ĭ-te) 1. the quality or state of being histocompatible. 2. the degree to which two individuals are histocompatible.

histocompatible (his″to-kom-pat′ĭ-b'l) pertaining to a donor and recipient who share a sufficient number of histocompatibility antigens (q.v.) so that a graft is accepted and remains functional.

histocyte (his′to-sīt) histiocyte.

histodiagnosis (his″to-di″ag-no′sis) [histo- + diagnosis] diagnosis by microscopical examination of the tissues.

histodialysis (his″to-di-al′ĭ-sis) [histo- + dialysis] the disintegration or breaking down of tissues.

histodifferentiation (his″to-dif″er-en″she-a′shun) the acquisition of tissue characteristics by cell groups.

histofluorescence (his″to-floo″o-res′ens) fluorescence produced in the body by exposure to roentgen rays following the administration of a fluorescing drug.

histogenesis (his″to-jen′ĕ-sis) [histo- + Gr. genesis production] the formation or development of tissues from the undifferentiated cells of the germ layers of the embryo.

histogenetic (his″to-jĕ-net′ik) pertaining to histogenesis.

histogenous (his-toj′ĕ-nus) [histo- + Gr. gennan to produce] formed by the tissues.

histogeny (his-toj′ĕ-ne) histogenesis.

histogram (his′to-gram) [Gr. histos mast + -gram] a graph of a frequency distribution in which the class frequencies are represented by vertical bars with bases covering the class intervals on the horizontal axis and heights equal to the class frequencies.

histography (his-tog′rah-fe) [histo- + Gr. graphein to write] description of the tissues.

histohematogenous (his″to-hem″ah-toj′ĕ-nus) [histo- + Gr. haima blood + gennan to produce] formed from both the tissues and the blood.

histohydria (his″to-hi′dre-ah) the presence of an excessive amount of water in body tissue.

histohypoxia (his″to-hi-pok′se-ah) an abnormally diminished concentration of oxygen in the tissues.

histoid (his′toid) [histo- + Gr. eidos form] 1. weblike. 2. developed from but one kind of tissue. 3. like one of the tissues of the body.

histoincompatibility (his″to-in″kom-pat″ĭ-bil′ĭ-te) the quality or state of being histoincompatible.

histoincompatible (his″to-in″kom-pat′ĭ-b'l) pertaining to a donor and recipient who have sufficient differences in histocompatibility antigens to cause rejection of grafts.

histokinesis (his″to-ki-ne′sis) [*histo-* + Gr. *kinēsis* motion] movement in the tissues of the body.

histologic, histological (his″-to-log′-ik; his″to-log′ĭ-kal) pertaining to histology.

histologist (his-tol′o-jist) one who specializes in histology.

histology (his-tol′o-je) [*histo-* + *-logy*] that department of anatomy which deals with the minute structure, composition, and function of the tissues; called also *microscopical anatomy*. **normal h.,** the histology of normal tissues. **pathologic h.,** the histology of diseased tissues; histopathology.

histolysate (his-tol′ĭ-zāt) a substance formed by histolysis.

histolysis (his-tol′ĭ-sis) [*histo-* + Gr. *lyein* to loosen] the dissolution or the breaking down of tissues.

histolytic (his″to-lit′ik) pertaining to, characterized by, or causing histolysis.

histoma (his-to′mah) [*histo-* + *-oma*] any tissue tumor, as a fibroma.

histometaplastic (his″to-met″ah-plas′tik) pertaining to, characterized by, or stimulating metaplasia of tissue.

Histomonas (his″to-mo′nas) [*histo-* + Gr. *monas* unit, from *monos* single] a genus of ameboflagellate protozoa (super-order Parabasalidea, order Trichomonadida) parasitic in the cecum and liver of turkeys, chickens, pheasants, guinea fowl, and other wild and domestic fowl. *H. meleagridis* is the only pathogenic species, being the etiologic agent of histomoniasis, which is especially severe in turkeys. It is usually transmitted in the eggs of the nematode coparasite *Heterakis gallinae*.

histomoniasis (his″to-mo-ni′ah-sis) an infectious proto-zoal disease caused by *Histomonas meleagridis*, which is especially lethal to turkeys although chickens and other fowl may also be affected. It is characterized by ulcerative and necrotic lesions of the cecum and liver, and the head may be cyanotic. Called also *blackhead* and *enterohepatitis*. **h. of turkeys,** an infectious disease of turkeys caused by *Histomonas meleagridis*, with lesions of the intestine and liver and a dark discoloration of the comb; called also *blackhead*, *enterohepatitis*, and *typhlohepatitis*.

histomorphology (his″to-mor-fol′o-je) the morphology of tissues; histology.

histone (his′tōn) a simple protein containing many basic groups, soluble in water and insoluble in dilute ammonia. The globin of hemoglobin is a histone. Combined with nucleic acids they form nucleohistone, and are associated with DNA in chromatin. Some are decidedly poisonous and contain a considerable amount of phosphorus. Blood treated with histone is altered so that it coagulates with difficulty. Histone has been found in the urine in leukemia and febrile conditions. Cf. *protamine*. **h. nucleinate,** a compound of nucleic acid and histone, the characteristic constituent of lymph glands, spleen, and thymus.

histoneurology (his″to-nu-rol′o-je) [*histo-* + *neurology*] the histology of the nervous system; neurohistology.

histonomy (his-ton′o-me) [*histo-* + Gr. *nomos* law] the sci-entific study of tissues based on the translation, into biological terms, of quantitative laws derived from histological measurement.

histonuria (his-tōn-u′re-ah) [*histone* + *-uria*] the presence of histone in the urine.

histopathology (his″to-pah-thol′o-je) [*histo-* + *pathology*] pathologic histology.

histophagous (his-tof′ah-gus) [*histo-* + *phagein* to eat] eating or subsisting on tissues; applied to certain protozoa, especially those ciliates ectoparasitic or endoparasitic in or on nonvital tissues of their hosts.

histophysiology (his″to-fiz″e-ol′o-je) [*histo-* + *physiology*] the correlation of function with the microscopic structure of cells and tissues.

Histoplasma (his″to-plaz′mah) a genus of imperfect fungi of the family Moniliaceae, order Moniliales. **H. cap-sula′tum,** the etiologic agent of classic histoplasmosis, oc-curring as small, oval, yeastlike cells which in tissue seem to be encapsulated but are not. It grows as a mycelial fungus in the soil and as a yeast at 37° C. on agar or in tissue. Formerly called *Cryptococcus capsulatus*. **H. capsula′tum** var. **duboi′sii,** a species larger than *H. capsulatum* and *H. farci-minosus*, that is the cause of the African form of histoplasmo-sis. **H. farcimino′sus,** the etiologic agent of lymphangi-

tis epizootica, differing from *H. capsulatum* and *H. duboisii* in having smooth macroaleuriospores in the saprophytic stage; formerly called *Blastomyces farciminosus*, *Leishmania farciminosa*, and *Zymonema farciminosum*.

histoplasmin (his″to-plaz′min) [USP] a skin test antigen prepared from mycelial phase *Histoplasma capsulatum* or-ganisms. Because positive skin tests are common in endemic areas and indicate only previous exposure, not necessarily active disease, histoplasmin is not useful in diagnosis of histoplasmosis. It is used primarily in epidemiologic surveys and in testing for cutaneous anergy in diagnosis of im-munodeficiency.

histoplasmoma (his″to-plaz-mo′mah) [*Histoplasma* + Gr. *-oma* tumor] a rounded granulomatous density of the lung caused by infection with *Histoplasma capsulatum* and seen radiographically as a coin-shaped lesion.

histoplasmosis (his″to-plaz-mo′sis) infection resulting from inhalation or, infrequently, the ingestion of spores of *Histoplasma capsulatum*. Worldwide in distribution, it is particularly common in the midwestern United States. The infection is asymptomatic in most cases, but in 1–5 per cent, it causes acute pneumonia, or disseminated reticuloendothe-lial hyperplasia with hepatosplenomegaly and anemia, or an influenza-like illness with joint effusion and erythema nodo-sum. Reactivated infection involves the lungs, meninges, heart, peritoneum, and adrenals in that order of frequency. It can be diagnosed by culture, or by demonstration of a rise in complement-fixing antibody titers in serum. **African h.,** a disease differentiated from the classic form of histoplas-mosis by large yeast forms of *Histoplasma capsulatum* var. *duboisii* in the tissues. **ocular h.,** disseminated choroidi-tis resulting in scars in the periphery of the fundus near the optic nerve, and characteristic disciform macular lesions; *Histoplasma capsulatum* is strongly implicated as the causa-tive agent.

historadiography (his″to-ra″de-og′rah-fe) [*histo-* + *radiog-raphy*] roentgenography of microscopic sections of tissue.

historetention (his″to-re-ten′shun) retention of matter by the tissues.

historrhexis (his″to-rek′sis) [*histo-* + Gr. *rhēxis* rupture] breaking up of tissue; Southard's term for focal destruction of nerve tissue of noninfectious nature.

histoteliosis (his″to-tel″e-o′sis) [*histo-* + Gr. *tēle* + *-osis*] the final differentiation of cells whose fate has already been determined irreversibly.

histotherapy (his″to-ther′ah-pe) [*histo-* + *therapy*] the treatment of disease by the administration of animal tissues.

histothrombin (his″to-throm′bin) thrombin from connec-tive tissue.

histotome (his′to-tōm) [*histo-* + Gr. *tomē* a cutting] micro-tome.

histotomy (his-tot′o-me) [*histo-* + Gr. *temnein* to cut] the dissection of the tissues; microtomy.

histotoxic (his″to-tok′sik) [*histo-* + Gr. *toxikon* poison] poisonous to tissue or tissues.

histotroph (his′to-trof) [*histo-* + Gr. *trophē* nourishment] the sum total of nutritive substances supplied to the embryo in viviparous animals from sources other than the mother's blood. Cf. *hemotroph*.

histotrophic (his″to-trof′ik) 1. encouraging the formation of tissue. 2. pertaining to histotroph; with reference to nu-trition through histotroph.

histotropic (his″to-trop′ik) [*histo-* + Gr. *tropos* a turning] having special affinity for tissue cells.

histozoic (his″to-zo′ik) [*histo-* + Gr. *zōē* life] living on or within the tissues; said of parasites.

histrionic (his″tre-on′ik) pertaining to or characterized by histrionism.

histrionism (his′tre-o-nizm″) [L. *histrio* actor] dramatic, attention-seeking, excitable behavior.

Hittorf's number, tube (hit′orf) [Johann Wilhelm *Hittorf*, German physicist, 1824–1914] see under *number*, and see *Crookes' tube*, under *tube*.

Hitzig's girdle, test (hits′igz) [Eduard *Hitzig*, German psy-chiatrist, 1838–1907] see under *girdle* and *tests*.

HIV human immunodeficiency virus.

hive (hīv) wheal.

hives (hīvz) urticaria.

Hl symbol for *latent hyperopia.*

HLA see under *antigen.*

Hm symbol for *manifest hyperopia.*

HMM hexamethylmelamine.

HMO health maintenance organization.

HMW-NCF high-molecular-weight neutrophil chemotactic factor.

HN2 mechlorethamine.

HNO₂ nitrous acid.

HNO₃ nitric acid.

Ho chemical symbol for *holmium.*

H₂O water.

H₂O₂ hydrogen peroxide.

hoarseness (hōrs′nes) a rough or noisy quality of voice.

Hoboken's nodules, valves (ho′bo-kenz) [Nicolas von *Hoboken,* Dutch anatomist and physician, 1632–1678] see under *nodule* and *valve.*

Hoche's bandelette (hōk′ez) [Alfred Erich *Hoche,* German psychiatrist, 1865–1943] a small bundle of nerve fibers forming part of the fasciculi proprii.

Hochenegg's operation (hōk′en-egz) [Julius von *Hochenegg,* Vienna surgeon, 1859–1940] see under *operation.*

Hochsinger's phenomenon, sign (hōk′sing-erz) [Karl *Hochsinger,* Austrian pediatrician, born 1860] see under *phenomenon* and *sign.*

hock (hok) the tarsal joint or region of the tarsus in the hind leg of the horse or ox. **capped h.,** a cyst or a thickening of the skin over the point of the calcaneus in the horse. **curby h.,** a hock affected with curb. **spring h.,** stringhalt.

hodegetics (hod″ĕ-jet′iks) [Gr. *hodēgētikos* fitted for guiding] medical ethics.

Hodge's forceps, pessary, plane, etc. (hoj′ez) [Hugh Lenox *Hodge,* American gynecologist, 1796–1873] see under the nouns.

Hodgen splint (apparatus) (hoj′en) [John Thompson *Hodgen,* American surgeon, 1826–1882] see under *splint.*

Hodgkin (hoj′kin), Alan Lloyd. British physiologist, born 1914; co-winner, with Sir John Carew Eccles and Andrew Fielding Huxley, of the Nobel prize for medicine or physiology for 1963, for discoveries concerning the ionic mechanisms involved in excitation and inhibition in the peripheral and central portions of the nerve cell membrane.

Hodgkin's cells, disease (granuloma), sarcoma (hoj′-kinz) [Thomas *Hodgkin,* English physician, 1798–1866] see *Reed-Sternberg cells,* under *cell,* and see under *disease* and *sarcoma.*

Hodgson's disease (hoj′sonz) [Joseph *Hodgson,* English physician, 1788–1869] see under *disease.*

hodoneuromere (ho″do-nu′ro-mēr) [Gr. *hodos* path + *neuron* nerve + *meros* part] a segment of the embryonic trunk with its pair of nerves and their branches.

hoe (ho) a cutting dental instrument having its cutting edge at a right angle to the axis of its blade and no constriction at the junction of its shank and blade; used for breaking down tooth structure undermined by caries, smoothing cavity walls, and sharpening line and point angles.

Hoehne's sign (ha′nez) [Ottomar *Hoehne,* German gynecologist, 1871–1932] see under *sign.*

hof [Ger. "court"] the area of the cytoplasm of a cell encircled by the concavity of the nucleus.

Hofbauer cells (hof′bow-er) [J. Isfred Isidore *Hofbauer,* American gynecologist, 1878–1961] see under *cell.*

Hoff see *van't Hoff.*

Hoffa's disease, operation (hof′az) [Albert *Hoffa,* German surgeon, 1859–1907] see under *disease,* and see *Lorenz's operation,* under *operation.*

Hoffa-Lorenz operation (hof′ah-lo′rents) [A. *Hoffa;* Adolf *Lorenz,* Austrian surgeon, 1854–1946] Lorenz's operation.

Hoffmann's anodyne, drops (hof′manz) [Friedrich *Hoffmann,* German physician, 1660–1742] see *compound ether spirit* and *ether spirit,* under *spirit.*

Hoffmann's atrophy, sign (phenomenon, reflex) [Johann *Hoffmann,* German neurologist, 1857–1919] see *Werdnig-Hoffman paralysis,* under *paralysis,* and see under *sign.*

Hoffmann's duct [Moritz *Hoffmann,* German anatomist, 1622–1698] ductus pancreaticus.

Hoffmann-Werdnig syndrome (hof′man verd′nig) [Johann *Hoffmann;* Guido *Werdnig,* Austrian neurologist, 1844–1919] Werdnig-Hoffmann paralysis.

Hoffmann's bacillus [Georg von *Hofmann*-Wellenhof, Austrian bacteriologist] *Corynebacterium pseudodiphtheriticum.*

Hofmann's violet [August Wilhelm von *Hofmann,* German chemist, 1818–1892] dahlia.

Hofmeister's test (hōf′mĭs-terz) [Franz *Hofmeister,* German physiologic chemist, 1850–1922] see under *tests.*

Holacanthida (hol″ah-kan′thĭ-dah) [*hol-* + Gr. *akantha* thorn, prickle] an order of marine protozoa (class Acantharea, superclass Actinopoda), characterized by the presence of 10, sometimes 16, diametral spines crossing in the cell center; when present, the capsular membrane is situated far outside the central cell mass.

holagogue (hol′ah-gog) [*hol-* + Gr. *agōgos* leading] a medicine capable of expelling all disease humors; a drastic or radical remedy.

holandric (hol-an′drik) [*hol-* + *aner* man] inherited exclusively through the male descent; transmitted through genes located on the Y chromosome.

holarthritis (hol″ar-thri′tis) hamarthritis.

Holden's line (hōl′denz) [Luther *Holden,* English surgeon, 1815–1905] see under *line.*

holdfast (hōld′fast) a mass of material secreted by a cell or organism by which it is attached to a substrate or surface; called also *holdfast organ* or *organelle.*

holism (hōl′izm) [Gr. *holos* whole] the theory that the determining factors in nature are organisms, which are wholes and not mechanisms and are irreducible, autonomous, and functionally greater than the sums of their parts.

holistic (ho-lis′tik) considering man as a functioning whole, or relating to the conception of man as a functioning whole; see also under *health.*

Holley (hol′e), Robert William. American biochemist, born 1922; co-winner, with Har Gobind Khorana and Marshall Warren Nirenberg, of the Nobel prize for medicine or physiology in 1968 for their interpretation of the genetic code and its function in protein synthesis.

hollow (hol′o) a depressed area or concavity. **Sebileau's h.,** a depressed area beneath the tongue, formed by the oral mucosa and the sublingual glands.

hollow-back (hol′o-bak) see *lordosis.*

Holmes (hōmz), Oliver Wendell (1809–1894). Noted American physician, anatomist, and writer, whose paper *On the Contagiousness of Puerperal Fever* (1843) antedated the work of Semmelweis in its appeal for surgical cleanliness to combat this disease.

Holmes's degeneration phenomenon (sign) (hōmz) [Gordon Morgan *Holmes,* English neurologist, 1876–1965] see under *degeneration,* and see *rebound phenomenon,* under *phenomenon.*

Holmes-Stewart phenomenon (hōmz-stu′art) [Gordon *Holmes;* Purves *Stewart,* London physician, 1869–1949] rebound phenomenon.

Holmgren's test (holm′grenz) [Alarik Fritniof *Holmgren,* Swedish physiologist, 1831–1897] see under *tests.*

holmium (hol′me-um) one of the rare earths; symbol, Ho; atomic number, 67; atomic weight, 164.930.

hol(o)- [Gr. *holos* entire] a combining form meaning entire, or denoting relationship to the whole.

holoacardius (hol″o-ah-kar′de-us) [*holo-* + *a* neg. + Gr. *kardia* heart] a separate, monozygotic twin represented by a more or less shapeless and unidentifiable mass; the vascular systems of the two fetuses are connected, and the circulation is accomplished solely by the heart of the more perfect twin. **h. aceph′alus,** an imperfectly formed free twin fetus lacking the cranial part of the body. **h. acor′mus,** an imperfectly formed free twin fetus lacking the caudal part of the body. **h. amor′phus,** an imperfectly formed free twin fetus entirely without form and recognizable parts.

holoantigen (hol″o-an′tĭ-jen) complete antigen, as opposed to hapten.

holoblastic (hol″o-blas′tik) [*holo-* + Gr. *blastos* germ] undergoing cleavage in which the entire ovum participates; dividing completely.

Holocaine (ho″lo-kān) trademark for a preparation of phenacaine hydrochloride.

holocarboxylase synthetase deficiency (hol″o-kar-bok′sĭ-tās sin′thĕ-tās) multiple carboxylase d.

holocephalic (hol″o-sĕ-fal′ik) [holo- + Gr. kephalē head] having the head entire; said of a monster.

holocrine (ho′lo-krin) [holo- + Gr. krinein to separate] wholly secretory: denoting that type of glandular secretion in which the entire secreting cell, along with its accumulated secretion, forms the secreted matter of the gland, as in the sebaceous glands. Cf. merocrine and apocrine.

holodiastolic (hol″o-di″ah-stol′ik) [holo- + diastole] pertaining to the entire diastole.

holoendemic (hol″o-en-dem′ik) [holo- + Gr. endēmos dwelling in a place] 1. endemic in most of the children in a population, with the adults in the same population being less often affected. Cf. hyperendemic.

holoenzyme (hol″o-en′zīm) the functional compound formed by the combination of an apoenzyme and its appropriate coenzyme.

hologamy (ho-log″ah-me) [holo- + Gr. gamos marriage] the condition in which the gametes are of the same size and structural type as the somatic cells.

hologastroschisis (hol″o-gas-tros′kĭ-sis) [holo- + Gr. gaster belly + schisis cleft] a developmental anomaly characterized by a fissure extending the entire length of the abdomen.

hologenesis (hol″o-jen′ĕ-sis) [holo- + Gr. genesis formation] the theory that man originated everywhere on earth, instead of in certain special region or regions.

hologram (hol′o-gram″) a three-dimensional image produced by holography.

holography (hol-og′raf-e) the recording of images in three-dimensional form on photographic film by exposing it to a laser beam reflected from the object under study. **acoustical h.,** holography in which sound waves reflected from an object under study are converted into light waves, which act on the emulsion of the film. The film is then exposed to a laser beam to give a three-dimensional effect.

holomastigote (hol″o-mas′tĭ-gōt) [holo- + Gr. mastix lash] having numerous flagella scattered over the body.

holomorphosis (hol″o-mor-fo′sis) [holo- + Gr. morphōsis formation] the complete regeneration of a lost part.

holomyarial (hol″o-mi-a′re-al) a type of arrangement of the muscular system in the Nematoda. The muscle cells are small, numerous, close together, and form a band below the cuticle.

holophytic (hol″o-fit′ik) [holo- + Gr. phyton plant] having a type of nutrition or feeding resembling that of a plant; said of certain photosynthesizing protozoa. Cf. holozoic.

holoprosencephaly (hol″o-pros″en-sef′ah-le) [holo- + prosencephalon] failure of cleavage of the prosencephalon with a deficit in midline facial development. Cyclopia occurs in the severe form. In that due to an extra chromosome 13 (trisomy 13, Patau syndrome) there are, characteristically, low-set ears, bilateral cleft lip and palate, microcephaly, ocular anomalies, hypotelorism, mental retardation, deafness, convulsions, and ventricular septal defects. **familial alobar h.,** a form in which the chromosomes are normal but otherwise resembling that due to trisomy 13–15 (see holoprosencephaly).

holorachischisis (hol″o-rah-kis′kĭ-sis) [holo- + Gr. rhachis spinal column + schisis cleft] fissure of the entire spinal cord.

holosaccharide (hol″o-sak′ah-rīd) a polysaccharide composed of sugar units only. Cf. heterosaccharide.

holoschisis (hol″o-ski′sis) [holo- + Gr. schisis cleft] amitosis.

Holospora (hol″o-spo′rah) [holo- + Gr. sporos seed] a genus of bacteria of uncertain affiliation that are parasites of paramecia.

holosystolic (hol″o-sis-tol′ik) [holo- + systole] pertaining to the entire systole.

holothurin (hol″o-thu′rin) a hemotoxic mixture of steroid glycosides obtained from holothurians, or sea cucumbers.

Holothyrus (hol″o-thi′rus) a genus of mites. The toxic secretions of H. coccinella, of Mauritius, may cause the death

of ducks, geese, and chickens after ingestion; in humans it may produce a painful swelling of the tongue and throat.

holotonia (hol″o-to′ne-ah) [holo- + Gr. tonos tension + -ia] muscular spasm of the whole body.

holotonic (hol″o-ton′ik) pertaining to, characterized by, or causing holotonia.

holotopy (ho-lot′o-pe) [holo- + Gr. topos place] the position of an organ in relation to the whole body.

holotrichous (ho-lot′rĭ-kus) [holo- + Gr. thrix hair] covered uniformly with cilia.

holotype (hol′o-tīp) the type culture of a species or subspecies of microoorganisms, either because it was so designated in the original description or because the original description was based on only one strain.

holoxenic (hol″o-zen′ik) [holo- + Gr. xenos a guestfriend, stranger] raised under usual circumstances; said of an animal not raised under special laboratory conditions, as opposed to one raised in a germ-free environment. See also axenic and gnotobiotic.

holozoic (hol″o-zo′ik) [holo- + Gr. zōon animal] having a type of nutrition or feeding resembling that of an animal; i.e., ingestion of whole organisms or relatively large particles. Called also phagotrophic. Cf. holophytic and saprozoic.

Holten's test (hol′tenz) [Cai Holten, Danish physician, born 1894] see under test.

Holth's operation (holths) [Sören Holth, Oslo ophthalmologist, 1863–1937] see under operation.

Holthouse's hernia (holt′howz-es) [Carsten Holthouse, English surgeon, 1810–1901] see under hernia.

Holzknecht's space (holtz′knekts) [Guido Holzknecht, radiologist in Vienna, 1872–1931] see under space.

homalocephalus (hom″ah-lo-sef′ah-lus) [Gr. homalos level + kephalē head] a person with a flat head.

homalography (hom″ah-log′rah-fe) [Gr. homalos level + graphein to write] (obs.) the study of anatomy by means of plane sections of the parts.

homaluria (hom″ah-lu′re-ah) [Gr. homalos level, even + ourein to urinate + -ia] production and excretion of urine at a normal, even rate.

Homans' sign (ho′manz) [John Homans, American physician, 1877–1954] see under sign.

Homapin (ho′mah-pin) trademark for preparations of homatropine methylbromide.

homarine (hom′ah-rin) an organic nitrogen compound which is found in lobster muscle and tissues of other marine animals. It is the methyl betaine of picolinic acid, C_5H_4-$N^+(CH_3)CO_2^-$.

homatropine (ho-mat′ro-pēn) chemical name: endo-α-hydroxybenzeneacetic acid 8-methyl-8-azabicyclo[3.2.1]oct-3-yl. The tropine ester of mandelic acid, $C_{16}H_{21}NO_3$, having anticholinergic effects similar to but weaker than those of atropine. **h. hydrobromide** [USP], the hydrobromide salt of homatropine, $C_{16}H_{21}NO_3 \cdot HBr$, occurring as white crystals or white, crystalline powder; used in ophthalmology as a cycloplegic and mydriatic, applied topically to the conjunctiva. **h. methylbromide** [USP], the 8-methyl derivative of homatropine hydrobromide, $C_{17}H_{24}BrNO_3$, occurring as a white powder; used as an antispasmodic and inhibitor of secretions, especially in gastrointestinal disorders, administered orally.

homaxial (ho-mak′se-al) having axes of the same length.

Homén's syndrome [Ernest Alexander Homén, Finnish physician, 1851–1926] see under syndrome.

home(o)-, homoe(o)-, homoi(o)- [Gr. homoios like, resembling] a combining form denoting sameness or similarity.

homeochrome (ho′me-o-krōm″) [homeo- + Gr. chrōma color] staining with mucin stains after formol-bichromate fixation; applied to certain serous cells of the salivary glands. Cf. tropochrome.

homeokinesis (ho″me-o-ki-ne′sis) [homeo- + Gr. kinēsis motion] the stage of meiosis in which the daughter cells receive equal amounts and kinds of chromatin.

homeomorphous (ho″me-o-mor′fus) [homeo- + Gr. morphē form] of like form and structure.

homeo-osteoplasty (ho″me-o-os″te-o-plas′te) [homeo- + Gr. osteon bone + plassein to mold] the grafting of bone from one individual to another within the same species.

homeopath (ho′me-o-path) homeopathist.

homeopathic (ho″me-o-path′ik) pertaining to homeopathy.

homeopathist (ho″me-op′ah-thist) one who practices homeopathy.

homeopathy (ho″me-op′ah-the) [homeo- + Gr. *pathos* disease] a system of therapeutics founded by Samuel Hahnemann (1755–1843), in which diseases are treated by drugs which are capable of producing in healthy persons symptoms like those of the disease to be treated, the drug being administered in minute doses. Cf. *allopathy*.

homeoplasia (ho″me-o-pla′ze-ah) [homeo- + Gr. *plassein* to form] the formation of new tissue like that adjacent to it and normal to the part.

homeoplastic (ho″me-o-plas′tik) 1. resembling in structure the adjacent parts. 2. pertaining to, characterized by, or stimulating homeoplasia.

homeorrhesis (ho″me-o-re′sis) [homeo- + Gr. *rhein* to flow] the tendency to maintain a biological process, as a growth process, along a particular pathway despite the operation of factors tending to divert it.

homeosis (ho″me-o′sis) [Gr. *homoiōsis* likeness, resemblance] the formation of a body part having the characteristics normally found in a related part at a different body site.

homeostasis (ho″me-o-sta′sis) [homeo- + Gr. *stasis* standing] a tendency to stability in the normal body states (internal environment) of the organism. It is achieved by a system of control mechanisms activated by negative feedback; e.g., a high level of carbon dioxide in extracellular fluid triggers increased pulmonary ventilation, which in turn causes a decrease in carbon dioxide concentration.

homeostatic (ho″me-o-stat′ik) pertaining to homeostasis.

homeotherapy (ho″me-o-ther′ah-pe) [homeo- + Gr. *therapeia* treatment] treatment or prevention of disease with a substance similar to but not the same as the causative agent of the disease.

homeotherm (ho′me-o-therm) [homeo- + Gr. *thermē* heat] 1. an animal that exhibits homoiothermy; a so-called warm-blooded animal, as opposed to a poikilotherm. 2. endotherm.

homeothermal (ho″me-o-ther′mal) [homeo- + Gr. *thermē* heat] homeothermic.

homeothermic (ho″me-o-ther′mik) 1. pertaining to or characterized by homeothermy (def. 1). 2. endothermic (def. 2).

homeothermism (ho″me-o-ther′mizm) homeothermy.

homeothermy (ho″me-o-ther″me) 1. the maintenance of a constant body temperature despite changes in the environmental temperature. Cf. *poikilothermy* (defs. 1 and 2).

homeotypic, homeotypical (ho″me-o-tip′ik; ho″me-o-tip′ĭ-k′l) [homeo- + Gr. *typos* type] resembling the normal or usual type.

homergic (hŏm-er′jik) [hom(o)- + Gr. *ergon* work] having the same effect; said of two drugs each of which produces the same overt effect.

homicide (hom′ĭ-sīd) [L. *homo* man + *caedere* to kill] the taking of the life of another individual.

homidium (ho-mid′e-um) chemical name: 3,8-diamino-5-ethyl-6-phenylphenanthridium, an effective trypanosomicide. Its bromide and chloride are used in the treatment of infections with *Trypanosoma congolense* and *T. vivax* in cattle and horses. Called also *ethidium*.

hominal (hom′ĭ-nal) [L. *homo* man] pertaining to man; pertaining to human beings.

hominid (hom′ĭ-nid) 1. pertaining to the family of humans (Hominidae). 2. a living or extinct human or humanlike type.

Hominidae (ho-min′ĭ-de) [L. *homo* man + Gr. *eidos* resemblance] a family of primates (superfamily Hominoides, suborder Anthropoidea), including both modern man (*Homo sapiens*) and fossil hominids.

homininoxious (hom″in-e-nok′shus) injurious to man.

hominoid (hom′ĭ-noid) 1. pertaining to the Hominoidea. 2. a member of the Hominoidea.

Hominoidea (hom″ĭ-noi′de-ah) [L. *homo* man + Gr. *oeidos* likeness] a superfamily of primates (suborder Anthropoidea), including the families Pongidae (anthropoid apes) and Hominidae (man, both modern and extinct).

homme (um) [Fr.] man. **h. rouge** (um-roozh′) [Fr. "red man"], a stage in mycosis fungoides in which the red plaques become infiltrated and coalesce over a wide area of the body.

Homo (ho′mo) [L. *man*] the genus of primates (family Hominidae, superfamily Hominoides) that includes man (*H. sapiens*) and fossil hominids.

hom(o)- [Gr. *homos* same] 1. a combining form meaning the same. 2. a prefix in chemical names indicating the addition of one CH_2 group to the main compound.

homoarterenol hydrochloride (ho″mo-ar″tĕ-re′nol) nordefrin hydrochloride.

Homobasidiomycetidae (ho″mo-bah-sid″e-o-mi-se′tĭ-de) a subclass of true fungi of the Basidiomycetes, including the series Hymenomycetes and Gasteromycetes.

homobiotin (ho″mo-bi′o-tin) a homologue of biotin having an additional CH_2 group in the side chain and acting as a biotin antagonist.

homobody (ho′mo-bod″e) an antibody with an idiotypic determinant that is stereochemically similar to the epitope on the antigen against which the antibody was originally directed; it is therefore able to mimic the behavior of the antigen.

homocarnosinase (ho″mo-kar′no-sĭ-nās) an uncharacterized enzyme of the hydrolase class that catalyzes the reaction homocarnosine + H_2O = 4-aminobutanoate + L-histidine. Absence of the enzyme, inherited as an autosomal recessive trait, results in homocarnosinosis.

homocarnosine (ho″mo-kar′no-sēn) a dipeptide consisting of γ-aminobutyric acid and histidine that is a normal constituent of the human brain.

homocarnosinosis (ho″mo-kar-no″sin-o′sis) [*homocarnosin* + -*osis*] an inherited aminoacidopathy caused by a deficient homocarnosinase with accumulation of homocarnosine in CSF and the brain, but not in plasma or urine. Clinical features include progressive spastic paraplegia, mental deterioration, and retinal pigmentation.

homocentric (ho″mo-sen′trik) [homo- + Gr. *kentron* center] having the same center or focus.

homochronous (ho-mok′ro-nus) [homo- + Gr. *chronos* time] occurring at the same age in successive generations.

homocinchonine (ho″mo-sin′ko-nin) an alkaloid, $C_{19}H_{22}$-ON_2, from cinchona, isomeric with cinchonine.

homocladic (ho″mo-klad′ik) [homo- + Gr. *klados* branch] formed between small branches of the same artery; said of such an anastomosis.

homocyclic (ho″mo-sik′lik) having or pertaining to a closed chain or ring formation which includes only atoms of the same element.

homocysteine (ho″mo-sis-te′in) a transmethylation product of methionine, $HSCH_2CH_2CHNH_2COOH$; it is an intermediate in the synthesis of cysteine.

homocysteine-tetrahydrofolate methyltransferase (ho″mo-sis-te′in tet″rah-hi″dro-fo′lāt meth″il-trans′fer-ās) 5-methyltetrahydrofolate-homocysteine methyltransferase.

homocystine (ho″mo-sis′tin) a synthetic alpha-alpha′-dithiobis-alpha-aminobutyric acid, $[S \cdot CH_2 \cdot CH_2 \cdot CH(NH_2) \cdot COOH]_2$, which results from the demethylation of methionine. It is homologous with cystine and able to function as a source of sulfur in the body.

homocystinemia (ho″mo-sis″tin-e′me-ah) an excess of homocystine in the blood; see *homocystinuria*.

homocystinuria (ho″mo-sis″tin-u′re-ah) an autosomal recessive aminoacidopathy characterized by excessive homocystine in plasma and urine. Three forms are known. *Homocystinuria I*, the most common, is due to defective cystathione β-synthase; plasma methionine is elevated; patients develop ectopia lentis, mental retardation, hepatomegaly, and cardiovascular and skeletal deformities. *Homocystinuria II* is due to defective 5,10-methylenetetrahydrofolate reductase; plasma levels of methionine are normal; symptoms include seizures, mental retardation, cerebral atrophy, behavioral changes and weakness. *Homocystinuria III* is due to defective methylcobalamin synthesis resulting in decreased activity of 5-methyltetrahydrofolate-homocysteine methyltransferase; plasma methionine is decreased; mental retardation and neurological abnormalities result.

homocytotropic (ho″mo-si″to-trop′ik) [homo- + *cyto-* + Gr. *tropos* a turning] having an affinity for cells from the same species; see under *antibody*.

homodesmotic (ho″mo-des-mot′ik) [*homo-* + Gr. *desmos* bond] joining similar parts of the central nervous system; see under *fiber.*

homodont (ho′mo-dont) [*hom-* + Gr. *odous* tooth] having teeth of only one type.

homodromous (ho-mod′ro-mus) [*homo-* + Gr. *dromos* running] moving or acting in the same direction.

homoe(o)- see *home(o)-.*

homoeosis (ho″me-o′sis) homeosis.

homoerotic (ho″mo-ĕ-rot′ik) pertaining to homoeroticism.

homoeroticism (ho″mo-ĕ-rot′ĭ-sizm) sexual feeling directed toward a person of the same sex.

homoerotism (ho″mo-er′o-tizm) homoeroticism.

homofermentation (ho″mo-fer″men-ta′shun) fermentation that produces one major product, primarily lactic acid, by way of the Embden-Meyerhof-Parnas pathway.

homofermenter (ho″mo-fer-ment′er) a microorganism that exhibits homofermentation.

homogamete (ho″mo-gam′ēt) one of two gametes of the same size and structure, as the X chromosome in the human female.

homogametic (ho″mo-gah-met′ik) pertaining to the sex that produces gametes of only one kind, in terms of their sex chromosomes. In human beings, the female is the homogametic sex.

homogamous (ho-mog′ah-mus) characterized by or pertaining to homogamy.

homogamy (ho-mog′ah-me) [*homo-* + Gr. *gamos* marriage] 1. inbreeding. 2. reproduction resulting from the union of two cells (gametes) that are identical in size and structure. 3. maturation of the male (stamens) and female (pistils) gametes of a flower at the same time. Cf. *heterogamy* and *isogamy.*

homogenate (ho-moj′ĕ-nāt) material subjected to homogenization, as tissue that is finely shredded and mixed.

homogeneity (ho″mo-jĕ-ne′ĭ-te) the state or quality of being homogeneous.

homogeneization (ho″mo-je″nĕ-i-za′shun) homogenization.

homogeneous (ho″mo-je′ne-us) [*homo-* + Gr. *genos* kind] consisting of or composed of similar elements or ingredients; of a uniform quality throughout.

homogenesis (ho″mo-jen′ĕ-sis) [*homo-* + Gr. *genesis* production] the reproduction by the same process in each generation, as contrasted with heterogenesis.

homogenetic (ho″mo-jĕ-net′ik) pertaining to or characterized by homogenesis.

homogenic (ho″mo-jen′ik) homozygous.

homogenicity (ho″mo-jĕ-nis′ĭ-te) homogeneity.

homogenization (ho-moj″ĕ-ni-za′shun) the act or process of rendering homogeneous.

homogenize (ho-moj′ĕ-nīz) to render homogeneous, or of uniform quality or consistency throughout.

homogenote (ho″mo-je′nōt) in bacterial genetics a merozygote in which the corresponding alleles at a specific locus of the diploid region of the genome are identical.

homogenous (ho-moj′ĕ-nus) having a similarity of structure because of descent from a common ancestor.

homogentisate (ho″mo-jen-tis′āt) the anionic form of homogentisic acid.

homogentisate 1,2-dioxygenase (ho″mo-jen″tĭ-sāt di-ok′sĭ-jĕ-nās) [EC 1.13.11.5] an enzyme of the oxidoreductase class that catalyzes the reaction homogentisate + O_2 = 4-maleylacetoacetate. The reaction is a step in the degradation of tyrosine. Genetic deficiency of the enzyme, transmitted as an autosomal recessive trait, causes alkaptonuria. Called also *homogentisate oxidase.*

homogentisate oxidase (ho″mo-jen″tĭ-sāt ok′sĭ-dās) homogentisate 1,2-dioxygenase.

homogentisic acid (ho″mo-jen-tis′ik) 2,5-dihydroxyphenylacetic acid, an intermediate in the catabolism of tyrosine. It is excreted in the urine in homogentisuria (alkaptonuria) an inborn error of metabolism in which there is a deficiency of the enzyme homogentisate oxidase. See also *alkapton bodies* under *body.*

homogentisic acid oxidase deficiency alkaptonuria.

homogentisuria (ho″mo-jen″tĭ-su′re-ah) the excretion of homogentisic acid in the urine, as in spontaneous alkaptonuria.

homogeny (ho-moj′ĕ-ne) homogenesis.

homoglandular (ho″mo-glan′du-lar) pertaining to the same gland.

homograft (ho′mo-graft) allograft.

homoi(o)- see *home(o)-.*

homoiopodal (ho″moi-op′o-dal) [*homoio-* + Gr. *pous* foot] having processes of one kind only; said of nerve cells.

homoiostasis (ho″moi-os′tah-sis) homeostasis.

homoiotoxin (ho″moi′o-tok-sin) a toxin from one individual which is toxic for other individuals of the same species.

homokeratoplasty (ho″mo-ker′ah-to-plas″te) [*homo-* + *keratoplasty*] corneal grafting with tissue derived from another individual of the same species.

homolactic (ho″mo-lak′tik) bacterial fermentation that produces lactic acid by way of the Embden-Meyerhof-Parnas pathway.

homolateral (ho″mo-lat′er-al) situated on, pertaining to, or affecting the same side; ipsilateral.

homologen (ho-mol′o-jen) homologue, def. 2.

homologous (ho-mol′o-gus) [Gr. *homologos* agreeing, correspondent] 1. corresponding in structure, position, origin, etc., as (*a*) the feathers of a bird and the scales of a fish, (*b*) antigen and its specific antibody, (*c*) allelic chromosomes. Cf. *analogous.* 2. allogeneic. 3. pertaining to an antibody and the antigen that elicited its production.

homologue (hom′o-log) 1. any homologous organ or part; an organ similar in structure, position, and origin to another organ, as the front flippers of a seal and human hands. See *analogue.* 2. in chemistry, one of a series of compounds, each of which is formed from the one before it by the addition of a constant element or a constant group of elements, as in the homologous series CH_4, C_2H_6, C_3H_8, etc.; called also *homologen.*

homology (ho-mol′o-je) [Gr. *homologia* agreement] the quality of being homologous; the morphological identity of corresponding parts; structural similarity due to descent from a common form.

homolysin (ho-mol′ĭ-sin) a lysin (e.g., isohemolysin) produced by injection into the body of antigen derived from an individual of the same species.

homolysis (ho-mol′ĭ-sis) [*homo-* + Gr. *lysis* dissolution] lysis of a cell by extracts of the same type of tissue.

homomorphic (ho-mo-mor′fik) [*homo-* + Gr. *morphē* form] having chromosome mates of similar size and form during synapsis of the first meiotic division.

homomorphosis (ho″mo-mor-fo′sis) [*homo-* + Gr. *morphōsis* formation] regenerative replacement of a lost part by a similar part.

homonomous (ho-mon′o-mus) [*homo-* + Gr. *nomos* law] designating homologous serial parts, such as somites.

homonymous (ho-mon′ĭ-mus) [*hom-* + Gr. *onoma* name] in ophthalmology, pertaining to the corresponding vertical halves of the visual fields of both eyes, i.e., the right visual field (the nasal half of the left eye, the temporal of the right) and the left visual field (the temporal half of the left eye, the nasal of the right).

homophil (ho′mo-fil) pertaining to antibody that reacts only with its homologous antigen.

homophilic (ho″mo-fil′ik) [*homo-* + Gr. *philein* to love] having affinity for or reacting with a specific antigen; said of an antibody.

homoplastic (ho″mo-plas′tik) [*homo-* + Gr. *plassein* to form] 1. denoting a transplantation or grafting of tissue taken from another individual of the same species or from a member of another inbred strain of the same species. 2. denoting organs or parts, as the wings of birds and insects, that resemble one another in structure and function but not in origin or development.

homoplasty (ho′mo-plas″te) 1. operative replacement of lost parts or tissues by similar parts from another individual of the same species or from a member of another inbred strain of the same species. 2. similarity between organs or parts not due to common ancestry.

homopolymer (ho″mo-pol′ĭ-mer) [*homo-* + *polymer*] a

polymer containing the same repeating units of one amino acid in a molecule.

homopolysaccharide (ho″mo-pol″e-sak′ah-rīd) a polysaccharide consisting of a single recurring monosaccharide unit, as glycogen is a polymer of glucose.

homorganic (hom″or-gan′ik) [homo- + Gr. organon organ] produced by the same or by homologous organs.

homosalate (ho″mo-sal′āt) chemical name: 2-hydroxybenzoic acid 3,3,5-trimethylcyclohexyl ester; an ultraviolet sunscreen, $C_{16}H_{22}O_3$.

homoscedasticity (ho″mo-skĕ-das-tis′ĭ-te) [homo- + Gr. skedastikos tending to scatter] the property of having equal variances.

homosexual (ho″mo-sek′shoo-al) 1. pertaining to the same sex; directed toward a person of the same sex; the opposite of heterosexual. 2. one who is sexually attracted to persons of the same sex.

homosexuality (ho″mo-sek″shoo-al′ĭ-te) [homo- + sexuality] sexual attraction toward those of the same sex, as distinguished from heterosexuality. **female h.,** that between women; lesbianism.

homospore (ho′mo-spōr) a homosporous organism.

homosporous (ho-mos′po-rus) [homo- + Gr. sporos seed] having spores of only one kind, which reproduce asexually.

homostimulant (ho″mo-stim′u-lant) 1. stimulating the same organ from which it is derived. 2. an extract from an organ which, on injection into the body, stimulates the same organ from which it is derived.

homostimulation (ho″mo-stim″u-la′shun) treatment by a homostimulant.

Homo-Tet (ho-mo-tet′) trademark for a preparation of tetanus immune human globulin.

homothallic (hom″o-thal′ik) pertaining to or exhibiting homothallism.

homothallism (hom″o-thal′izm) a form of sexual reproduction in which the isogamete produced by one cell can fuse with another isogamete produced by the same cell, as in various algae and fungi. Cf. heterothallism.

homotherm (ho′mo-therm) homeotherm.

homothermal (ho″mo-ther′mal) homeothermic.

homothermic (ho″mo-ther′mik) homeothermic.

homotopic (ho″mo-top′ik) [homo- + Gr. topos place] occurring at the same place upon the body.

homotransplant (ho″mo-trans′plant) allograft.

homotropism (ho-mot′ro-pizm) [homo- + Gr. tropos a turning] the property of cells to attract cells of a like order.

homotype (hom′o-tīp) [homo- + Gr. typos type] a part that has a reversed symmetry with its fellow of the opposite side of the body, as the hand.

homotypic (ho″mo-tip′ik) pertaining to or characteristic of a homotype.

homovanillic acid (ho″mo-vah-nil′ik) a product of catecholamine metabolism; elevated urinary levels occur in patients with pheochromocytoma or other catecholamine-secreting tumors. Abbreviated HVA.

homoxenous (ho-mok′sĕ-nus) [homo- + Gr. xenos strange, foreign] requiring only one host in the life cycle; said of certain parasites. Called also monoxenous.

homozoic (ho″mo-zo′ik) [homo- + Gr. zōon animal] pertaining to the same animal or same species.

homozygosis (ho″mo-zi-go′sis) the formation of a zygote by the union of gametes that possess one or more identical alleles.

homozygosity (ho″mo-zi-gos′ĭ-te) [homo- + zygosity] the state of possessing a pair of identical alleles at a given locus.

homozygote (ho″mo-zi′gōt) [homo- + zygote] an individual possessing a pair of identical alleles at a given locus.

homozygous (ho″mo-zi′gus) possessing a pair of identical alleles at a given locus; called also homogenic. See also heterozygous.

homunculus (ho-munk′u-lus) [L. "a little man"] 1. a dwarf without deformity or disproportion of parts. 2. the miniature human form once thought to be preformed in the sperm or ovum.

honey (hon′e) a sweet-tasting substance deposited by the honeybee, which contains between 62 and 83 per cent

dextrose and fructose, and small amounts of sucrose, dextrin, and malic and acetic acids; its pH is 3.8 to 4.3.

hood (hood) a flexible covering. **tooth h.,** dental operculum.

hoof (hoof) [L. ungula] the hard, horny casing of the foot or ends of the digits of many animals which are, because of this feature, designated ungulates. **curved h.,** a condition in which the hoof has the wall of one side concave and the other convex. **dished h.,** a hoof which is concave from the coronet to the plantar surface. **false h.,** the hoof of an unused digit. **ribbed h., ringed h.,** a condition in which the wall of a horse's hoof is marked by ridges running parallel with the coronary margin.

hoof-bound (hoof′bound) dryness and contraction of a horse's hoof, causing lameness; called also contracted foot and contracted heel.

hook (hook) a curved instrument, usually with a sharp point, designed for holding, elevating, or exerting traction on a tissue. **blunt h.,** an instrument for exercising traction on a dead fetus in breech presentation. **Bose's h's,** small hooks used in tracheostomy. **Braun's h.,** a hook for decapitating the fetus. **Loughnane's h.,** a double-pronged hook for removing fragments of the prostate in transurethral prostatectomy. **muscle h.,** a hook for securing and isolating an extraocular muscle; called also squint h. **Pajot's h.,** a hook for decapitating the fetus. **palate h.,** a hook for raising the palate in posterior rhinoscopy. **squint h.,** muscle h. **Tyrrell's h.,** a slender hook used in eye surgery.

hook-up (hook′up) the method of arranging circuits, appliances, and electrodes for a particular diagnostic or therapeutic procedure.

hookworm (hook′werm) a nematode parasitic in the intestine of man and other vertebrates; infection may cause serious illness. See also under disease, and see ground itch, under itch. **American h.,** Necator americanus. **h. of the dog,** Ancylostoma caninum. **European h.,** Ancylostoma duodenale. **New World h.,** Necator americanus. **Old World h.,** Ancylostoma duodenale. **h. of the rat,** Nippostrongylus muris. **h. of ruminants,** Bunostomum.

hoolamite (hoo′lah-mīt) a chemical detector for carbon monoxide, containing fuming sulfuric acid, iodine pentoxide, and powdered pumice; it changes from light gray to green under the influence of carbon monoxide.

hoose (hooz) a disease of sheep, cattle, goats, and swine, caused by the presence of various species of nematodes of the genera Dictyocaulus, Metastrongylus, and Protostrongylus in the bronchial tubes or in the lungs. It is marked by cough, dyspnea, anorexia, and constipation. Called also verminous bronchitis.

Hoover's sign (hoo′verz) [Charles Franklin Hoover, American physician, 1865–1927] see under sign.

HOP 1. high oxygen pressure. 2. a regimen of hydroxydaunomycin (doxorubicin), Oncovin (vincristine), and prednisone, used in cancer chemotherapy.

Hope's sign (hōps) [James Hope, London physician, 1801–1841] see under sign.

Hopkins (hop′kinz), Sir Frederick Gowland. British biologist, 1861–1947; co-winner, with Christiaan Eijkmann, of the Nobel prize for medicine or physiology in 1929 for his discovery of the growth-stimulating vitamins.

Hopkins-Cole test (hop′kinz-kol) [Sir Frederick Gowland Hopkins, English biochemist, 1861–1947; Sidney William Cole, English physiologist, 1877–1952] see under tests.

Hoplopsyllus anomalus (hop″lo-sil′us ah-nom′ah-lus) a species of flea found in the ground squirrels of western United States and transmitting plague.

Hopmann's polyp (papilloma) (hop′manz) [Carl Melchior Hopmann, German rhinologist, 1849–1925] see under polyp.

Hoppe-Seyler's test (hop″ĕ-si′lerz) [Ernst Felix Immanuel Hoppe-Seyler, German physiologic chemist, 1825–1895] see under tests.

hoquizil hydrochloride (ho′kwĭ-zil) chemical name: 2-hydroxy-2-methylpropyl 4-(6,7-dimethoxy-4-quinazolinyl)-1-piperazinecarboxylate monohydrochloride; a bronchodilator, $C_{19}H_{26}N_4O_5 \cdot HCl$.

Hor. decub. abbreviation for L. *ho'ra decu'bitus*, at bedtime.

hordein (hor'de-in) [L. *hordeum*, barley] a simple native protein from barley, a prolamine insoluble in water, but soluble in 80 per cent alcohol.

hordeolum (hor-de'o-lum) [L. "barleycorn"] a localized, purulent, inflammatory staphylococcal infection of one or more sebaceous glands (meibomian or zeisian) of the eyelids; called also *stye*. An *external hordeolum* occurs on the surface of the skin at the edge of the lid. An *internal hordeolum* is marked by swelling on the conjunctival surface of the lid.

horehound (hōr'hound) the labiate plant, *Marrubium vulgare* (Tourn.) L. (Labiatae), also its leaves and tops (L. *marrubium*); used as an expectorant, bitter tonic, vermifuge, and laxative.

Hor. interm. abbreviation for L. *ho'ris interme'diis*, at the intermediate hours.

horizon (hŏ-ri'zon) a numbered stage of human embryonic development defined by anatomical characteristics in order to circumvent individual uncertainties of age and variations of dimension from both natural and technical causes. Streeter outlined 23 horizons, each spanning 2 or 3 days, covering the 7-week period beginning with fertilization. **Streeter's h's,** see *horizon*.

horizontalis (hor''ĭ-zon-ta'lis) horizontal, or parallel to the plane of the horizon; [NA] a term denoting relationship to this orientation when the body is in the anatomical, i.e., the upright, position.

hormesis (hor-me'sis) [Gr. *hormēsis* rapid motion] the stimulating effect of subinhibitory concentrations of any toxic substance on any organism.

hormion (hor'me-on) [Gr. *hormos* a wreath] the median anterior point of the spheno-occipital bones.

Hormocardiol (hor''mo-kar'de-ol) [*hormone* + Gr. *kardia* heart] a commercial preparation of an extract from the sinus of the frog's heart that stimulates the contraction of the frog's ventricle; used as a coronary vasodilator.

Hormodendrum (hor''mo-den'drum) a former genus of Fungi Imperfecti; at present, most saprophytic species are placed in the genus *Cladosporium*, and the human pathogens, e.g., *H. pedrosoi*, in the genus *Fonsecaea*.

hormonagogue (hor-mōn'ah-gog) [*hormone* + Gr. *agōgos* leading] an agent that stimulates the production of hormones.

hormonal (hor'mo-nal) pertaining to or of the nature of a hormone.

hormone (hor'mōn) [Gr. *hormaein* to set in motion, spur on] a chemical substance, produced in the body by an organ or cells of an organ which has a specific regulatory effect on the activity of a certain organ or organs; originally applied to substances secreted by various endocrine glands and transported in the bloodstream to the distant target organ on which their effect was produced, the term was later applied to various substances not produced by special glands but having similar action, both local and anatomically remote. See also *endocrine system*, under *system*. **adaptive h.,** one, such as corticotropin or the corticoids, which is secreted during the organism's adaptation to unusual circumstances. **adenohypophysial h.,** anterior pituitary h. **adipokinetic h.,** 1. a hypothetical lipolytic hormone secreted by the pituitary gland. 2. any lipolytic h. **adrenocortical h.,** any of the corticosteroids elaborated by the adrenal cortex, the major ones being the glucocorticoids and mineralocorticoids, and including some androgens, progesterone, and perhaps estrogens. See also *corticosteroid*. **adrenocorticotropic h.,** corticotropin. **adrenomedullary h's,** substances secreted by the adrenal medulla, including epinephrine and norepinephrine. **androgenic h's,** the masculinizing hormones, including testosterone, androsterone, dehydroepiandrosterone, and others. **anterior pituitary h.,** any of the several protein or polypeptide hormones secreted by the anterior lobe of the pituitary gland, including growth hormone, thyrotropin, prolactin, follicle-stimulating hormone, luteinizing hormone, β-lipotropin, and corticotropin. **antidiuretic h.,** vasopressin. **Aschheim-Zondek h.,** luteinizing h. **chondrotropic h.,** growth h. **chromaffin h.,** epinephrine. **conjugated estrogen h's,** an amorphous preparation of naturally-occurring, water-soluble, conjugated forms of mixed estrogens, chiefly sodium estrone sulfate, extracted from the urine of pregnant mares; used in estrogen hormone therapy. **corpus luteum h.,** progesterone. **cortical h.,** see *adrenocortical h*. **corticotropin releasing hormone (CRH),** corticotropin releasing factor. **diabetogenic h.,** a formerly used term for substance(s) in extracts of the anterior pituitary that tends to elevate the blood sugar by acting as an antagonist to insulin. It is probably not a single entity; its effects are probably related to those of known pituitary hormones, especially human growth hormone. **estrogenic h's,** substances capable of producing certain characteristic biological effects, e.g., the changes that occur in mammals at estrus; the most common naturally occurring estrogenic hormones are β-estradiol, estrone, and estriol. **fat-mobilizing h's,** lipolytic h's. **follicle-stimulating h. (FSH),** one of the gonadotropic hormones of the anterior pituitary, a glycopeptide of 24,000 to 35,000 daltons, which stimulates the growth and maturation of graafian follicles in the ovary, as well as inducing the endometrial changes characteristic of the first portion (proliferative phase) of the mammalian menstrual cycle, and stimulates spermatogenesis in the male. An extract from postmenopausal urine, known as human follicle-stimulating hormone or *menotropins* (q.v.), is used to induce ovulation and to promote spermatogenesis. **follicle-stimulating h., human,** 1. follicle-stimulating h. 2. menotropins. **follicle-stimulating hormone releasing h. (FSH-RH),** gonadotropin releasing h. **galactopoietic h.,** prolactin. **gastrointestinal h's,** hormones that originate in and regulate motor and secretory activity of the digestive system, e.g., gastrin, secretin, and cholecystokinin. **gonadotropic h.,** any hormone that has an influence on the gonads. **gonadotropic h's, pituitary,** gonadotropin. **gonadotropin releasing h. (Gn-RH)** a decapeptide hormone elaborated by the median eminence of the hypothalamus that stimulates the release of follicle-stimulating hormone and luteinizing hormone from the anterior lobe of the pituitary gland. A preparation of the acetate and hydrochloride salts of the same principle obtained from pigs, sheep, or other species is used in the differential diagnosis of hypothalamic, pituitary, and gonadal dysfunction, and in the treatment of certain forms of female and male infertility and hypogonadism. Called also *gonadorelin*. **growth h. (GH),** any substance that stimulates growth, especially one secreted episodically by the anterior pituitary that exerts a direct effect on protein, carbohydrate, and lipid metabolism, and controls the rate of skeletal and visceral growth. Its secretion is in part controlled by the hypothalamus. Human growth hormone (hGH) is composed of a single chain of 191 amino acids (about 21,500 daltons) without carbohydrate substituents. A synthetic preparation, growth hormone recombinant (hGHr), is used to treat growth failure (dwarfism) in children with congenital deficiency of growth hormone. Called also *somatotropin*. **growth hormone release inhibiting h. (GH-RIH),** somatostatin. **growth hormone releasing h. (GH-RH),** see under *factor*. **human (pituitary) growth h. (hGH),** see *growth h*. **hypophysiotropic h.,** any of the hormones of the hypothalamus that stimulate or inhibit the hypophysis, including the releasing factors. **inhibiting h's,** hormones elaborated by one structure (as by the hypothalamus) that inhibit release of hormones from another structure (as from the anterior pituitary gland), e.g., *somatostatin* (growth hormone release inhibiting h.). The term is applied to substances of established clinical identity, whereas substances of unknown chemical structure are called *inhibiting factors* (see under *factor*). **inhibitory h.,** a substance that exerts a depressing influence on any of its target organs, e.g., enterogastrone. **interstitial cell-stimulating h.,** luteinizing h.; so called because it also stimulates the Leydig (interstitial) cells of the testis. Abbreviated ICSH. **juvenile h.,** the secretion of the corpora allata which prevents metamorphosis, keeping the insect in the larval state and ensuring that the larva will molt several times and reach large size before pupating. **ketogenic h's,** lipolytic h's. **lactation h.,** prolactin. **lactogenic h's,** prolactin. **lipolytic h's,** any hormone that serves to mobilize fat, i.e., to induce lipolysis, including the catecholamines, glucagon, tropic hormones of the anterior pituitary (ACTH, TSH, β-lipoprotein, etc.), and growth hormone; called also *fat-mobilizing h's* and *ketogenic h's*. **local h.,** a substance with hormone-like properties, produced from blood or another body fluid, that acts at an anatomically restricted site and usually is rapidly destroyed. **luteal h.,** one secreted by the corpus luteum; see *progester-*

one. **luteinizing h.,** a glycoprotein gonadotropic hormone (28,000 daltons) of the anterior pituitary which acts with the follicle-stimulating hormone to cause ovulation of mature follicles and secretion of estrogen by luteal cells. It instigates and maintains the second (secretory) portion of the mammalian estrus and menstrual cycle. It is also concerned with corpus luteum formation and, in the male, stimulates the development and functional activity of testicular Leydig (interstitial) cells. **luteinizing hormone releasing h. (LH-RH),** gonadotropin releasing h. **luteotropic h.,** luteotropin. **mammotropic h.,** an obsolete name for prolactin. **melanocyte-stimulating h., melanophore-stimulating h. (MSH),** either of two peptide hormones, α-MSH and β-MSH that are released by the intermediate lobe of the pituitary gland in fish and amphibians and cause the dispersion of pigment granules of melanocytes producing a rapid change in skin coloration; α-MSH is identical to the N-terminal 13 residues of ACTH (adrenocorticotropic hormone), and β-MSH to the C-terminal 18 residues of γ-lipotropin (γ-LPH); immunoreactive "β-MSH" in humans consists of β- and γ-LPH. Administration of α-MSH or elevation of ACTH in humans causes a slight increase in melanization. Neither α-MSH nor β-MSH is secreted as a primary pituitary hormone by the human pituitary. **neurohypophysial h's,** posterior pituitary h's. **ovarian h.,** one secreted by the ovary, including the estrogens and progestins. **parathyroid h.,** a polypeptide hormone (84 amino acid residues) secreted by the parathyroid glands, which promotes release of calcium from bone into the extracellular fluid by activating osteoclasts and promotes increased intestinal absorption and renal tubular reabsorption of calcium, as well as increased renal excretion of phosphates; it is the principal regulator of bone metabolism. Secretion of parathyroid hormone is induced by decreased levels of calcium in the extracellular fluid. Its action is opposed by that of calcitonin. Called also *parathormone* and *parathyrin.* **placental h's,** any of the hormones produced by the placenta during pregnancy, including chorionic gonadotropin and other substances having estrogenic, progesteronic, or adrenocorticoid activity. **placental growth h.,** human placental lactogen. **plant h.,** phytohormone. **posterior pituitary h's,** hormones derived from the posterior lobe of the pituitary, including vasopressin (antidiuretic hormone), oxytocin, and neurophysins; now believed to be formed in the neuronal cells of the hypothalamic nuclei and to be stored in nerve cell endings in the posterior pituitary (neurohypophysis) for release in response to appropriate signals. **progestational h.,** 1. progesterone. 2. [pl.] see under *agent.* **proparathyroid h.,** an inactive biosynthetic precursor of parathyroid hormone; it is of larger molecular size than the active hormone. **prothoracicotropic h.,** in the development of insects, the hormone that controls secretion of ecdysone by the prothoracic glands. It is secreted by the intercerebral gland in the brain. **releasing h's,** hormones elaborated in one structure (as in the hypothalamus) that effect the release of hormones from another structure (as from the anterior pituitary gland); they include gonadotropin releasing hormone and thyrotropin releasing hormone. The term is applied to substances of established chemical identity, whereas substances of unknown chemical structure are called *releasing factors* (see under *factor*). **sex h's,** hormones having estrogenic (*female sex h's*) or androgenic (*male sex h's*) activity. **somatotrophic h., somatotropic h.,** growth h. **somatotropin release inhibiting h.,** somatostatin. **somatotropin releasing h. (SRH),** growth hormone releasing f. **steroid h's,** a group of biologically active heterocyclic organic compounds that are secreted by the adrenal cortex, testis, ovary, and placenta and which have in common a cyclopentanoperhydrophenanthrene nucleus; included are estrogens (C18), androgens (C19), mineralocorticoids, progesterones (C21), and glucocorticoids (C21). **testicular h., testis h.,** testosterone. **thyroid h's,** thyroxine, triiodothyronine, "reverse" triiodothyronine, and calcitonin; in the singular, it refers to thyroxine or triiodothyronine or both. **thyroid-stimulating h. (TSH),** thyrotropin. **thyrotropic h.,** thyrotropin. **thyrotropin releasing h. (TRH),** a tripeptide hormone elaborated by the median eminence of the hypothalamus or obtained by synthesis, which stimulates release of thyrotropin from the anterior pituitary gland. In human subjects, it also acts as a prolactin releasing factor. A preparation is used in the diagnosis of mild hyperthyroidism and Graves' disease, and in differentiating among primary, secondary, and tertiary hypothyroidism. Called also *protirelin.*

hormonic (hor-mon′ik) hormonal.

hormonogen (hor′mon-o-jen″) prohormone.

hormonogenesis (hor″mo-no-jen′ĕ-sis) the production of hormones.

hormonogenic (hor″mo-no-jen′ik) pertaining to, characterized by, or stimulating hormonogenesis.

hormonology (hor″mo-nol′o-je) the science of hormones; clinical endocrinology.

hormonopoiesis (hor″mo-no-poi-e′sis) [*hormone* + Gr. *poiesis* a making, creation] hormonogenesis.

hormonopoietic (hor″mo-no-poi-et′ik) hormonogenic.

hormonoprivia (hor-mōn″o-priv′e-ah) [*hormone* + L. *privus* without, deprived of] lack of hormone, or the condition produced by a deficiency of hormone in the body.

hormonosis (hor-mo-no′sis) the condition of having an excess of hormones; exogenous hormonosis is a result of therapeutic administration, as in cortisone therapy.

hormonotherapy (hor″mo-no-ther′ah-pe) treatment by the use of hormones; endocrinotherapy.

horn (horn) [L. *cornu*] a pointed projection such as the paired processes on the head of various animals; any structure resembling a horn in shape. Called also *cornu* [NA]. **h. of Ammon,** hippocampus. **anterior h. of lateral ventricle,** cornu frontale ventriculi lateralis. **anterior h. of spinal cord,** cornu ventrale medullae spinalis. **cicatricial h.,** a hard, dry outgrowth from a cicatrix, commonly scaly and very rarely osseous. **coccygeal h.,** cornu coccygeum. **cutaneous h.,** a horny excrescence of the skin, chiefly seen on the scalp and face; called also *cornu cutaneum.* **dorsal h. of spinal cord,** cornu dorsale medullae spinalis. **frontal h. of lateral ventricle,** cornu frontale ventriculi lateralis. **gray h's of spinal cord,** see *columna griseae.* **greater h. of hyoid bone,** cornu majus ossis hyoidei. **inferior h. of falciform margin,** cornu inferius marginis falciformis. **inferior h. of lateral ventricle,** cornu temporale ventriculi lateralis. **inferior h. of thyroid cartilage,** cornu inferius cartilaginis thyroideae. **lateral h. of hyoid bone,** cornu majus ossis hyoidei. **lateral h. of spinal cord,** cornu laterale medullae spinalis. **lesser h. of hyoid bone,** cornu minus ossis hyoidei. **occipital h. of lateral ventricle,** cornu occipitale ventriculi lateralis. **posterior h. of lateral ventricle,** cornu occipitale ventriculi lateralis. **posterior h. of spinal cord,** cornu dorsale medullae spinalis. **h. of pulp,** an extension of the pulp into an accentuation of the roof of the pulp chamber directly under a cusp or a developmental lobe of the tooth. **sacral h.,** cornu sacrale. **superior h. of falciform margin,** cornu superius marginis falciformis. **superior h. of hyoid bone,** cornu minus ossis hyoidei. **superior h. of thyroid cartilage,** cornu superius cartilaginis thyroideae. **temporal h. of lateral ventricle,** cornu temporale ventriculi lateralis. **h. of uterus, right and left,** cornu uterinum dextrum/sinistrum. **ventral h. of spinal cord,** cornu ventrale medullae spinalis.

Horn's sign (hornz) [C. ten *Horn*, Dutch surgeon] see under *sign.*

Horner's law, syndrome (ptosis) (hor′nerz) [Johann Friedrich *Horner*, Swiss ophthalmologist, 1831–1886] see under *law* and *syndrome.*

Horner's muscle (hor′nerz) [William Edmonds *Horner*, American anatomist, 1793–1853] pars lacrimalis musculi orbicularis oculi.

hornification (hor″nĭ-fi-ka′shun) cornification.

horny (hor′ne) having the nature and appearance of horn.

horopter (ho-rop′ter) [Gr. *horos* limit + *optēr* observer] the sum of all the spatial points whose images at a given distance fall on corresponding points of the retina. If the point of fixation is 2 meters, the horopter is a straight line across the observer's front (the *apparent frontoparallel plane h.*); if the point of fixation is less than 2 meters, the horopter is a curve concave to the observer (*concave h.*); and if the point of fixation is more than 2 meters, the horopter is a curve convex to the observer (*convex h.*). **Vieth-Müller h.,** a circle which joins the fixation point with the nodal points of the two eyes; called also *Vieth-Müller circle.*

horopteric (hor″op-ter′ik)   pertaining to a horopter.

horripilation (hor″ĭ-pi-la′shun) [L. *horrere* to bristle, to stand on end + *pilus* hair]   erection of the fine hairs of the skin, as in cutis anserina.

horror (hor′or) [L.]   dread; terror.   **h. autotox′icus** [L. "fear of self poisoning"], a term coined by Ehrlich and Morgenroth in 1900 to express the refusal of a normal animal to form autoantibodies; it was believed that formation of such antibodies might result in self-destruction of the antibody producer as a result of the reaction between autoantibody and the corresponding antigen present in tissues. Now called *self-tolerance.*

horsepox (hors′poks)   a mild form of poxvirus infection affecting horses, marked by a pustular eruption of the skin and sometimes of the mucosa of the mouth and nose; called also *equine smallpox.*

horse-sickness (hors-sik′nes)   see *African horse sickness* and *Gambian horse sickness,* under *sickness.*

Horsley's operation, test, wax (hors′- lēz) [Sir Victor Alexander Haden *Horsley,* English surgeon, 1857–1916]   see under *operation, tests,* and *wax.*

Hortega cell, method (hor-ta′gah) [Pio del Rio *Hortega,* Spanish histologist in Buenos Aires, 1882–1945]   see *microglia* and under *Table of Stains.*

hortobezoar (hor″to-be-zōr′)   phytobezoar.

Horton's headache, disease (arteritis, syndrome) (hōr′tunz) [Bayard Taylor *Horton,* American physician, born 1895]   see *migrainous neuralgia,* under *neuralgia,* and *temporal arteritis,* under *arteritis.*

Hor. un. spatio   abbreviation for L. *ho′rae uni′us spa′tio,* at the end of one hour.

H₂OsO₄   osmic acid.

hospice (hos′pis)   a facility that provides palliative and supportive care for terminally ill patients and their families, either directly or on a consulting basis.

hospital (hos′pit-′l) [L. *hospitalium; hospes* host, guest]   an institution for the treatment of the sick. "An institution suitably located, constructed, organized, managed and personneled, to supply, scientifically, economically, efficiently and unhindered, all or any recognized part of the complex requirements for the prevention, diagnosis, and treatment of physical, mental, and the medical aspect of social ills; with functioning facilities for training new workers in the many special professional, technical and economic fields essential to the discharge of its proper functions; and with adequate contacts with physicians, other hospitals, medical schools and all accredited health agencies engaged in the better health program."—Council on Medical Education.   **base h.,** a hospital unit within the line of communication of the army, usually in a permanent building, designed for the reception of wounded and other patients received via field hospitals from the front, and for cases originating within the line of communication itself.   **camp h.,** an immobile military unit organized and equipped for the care of the sick and wounded in camp in order to prevent immobilization of field hospitals or other mobile sanitary organizations.   **closed h.,** a hospital in which only members of the staff are permitted to treat patients.   **cottage h.,** a hospital consisting of a number of detached cottages.   **day h.,** see *partial hospitalization,* under *hospitalization.*   **evacuation h.,** a mobile advance hospital unit within the line of communication, designed to take over the functions of field hospitals when they move away with their divisions and to supplement base hospitals in their functions.   **field h.,** a portable military hospital, manned by noncommissioned officers and men, located beyond the zone of conflict, 3–4 miles beyond the dressing stations, designed to shelter and care for wounded brought in by ambulance companies until they can be transported to the line of communications.   **lying-in h.,** an institution for the care of obstetric patients; called also *maternity h.*   **night h.,** see *partial hospitalization,* under *hospitalization.*   **open h.,** 1. a mental hospital, or section of a hospital, without locked doors or other forms of physical restraint. 2. a hospital to which physicians who are not staff members may send their own patients and supervise their treatment.   **teaching h.,** one that allocates a substantial part of its resources to conduct, in its own name or in association with a college or university, formal educational programs or courses of instruction that lead to granting of recognized certificates, diplomas, or degrees, or that are required for professional certification or licensure.   **weekend h.,** see *partial hospitalization,* under *hospitalization.*

hospitalization (hos″pit-′l-i-za′shun)   the confinement of a patient in a hospital, or the period of such confinement.   **partial h.,** a psychiatric treatment program for patients who do not need full-time hospitalization, involving a special facility or an arrangement within a hospital setting to which the patient may come for treatment during the day and return home at night (*day hospital*); or return at night after a day in the community to receive treatment during the evening and to remain all night (*night hospital*); or return at the end of the week to receive treatment and remain all weekend, resuming his normal activities during the week (*weekend hospital*).

hospitalize (hos′pit-′l-īz)   to place a patient in a hospital.

host (hōst) [L. *hospes*]   1. an animal or plant that harbors or nourishes another organism (parasite). 2. the recipient of an organ or other tissue transplanted from another organism (the donor).   **accidental h.,** one that harbors an organism that is not ordinarily parasitic in the particular species.   **definitive h., final h.,** a host in which a parasite attains sexual maturity; called also *primary h.*   **intermediate h.,** a host in which a parasite passes one or more of its asexual stages; usually designated first and second, if there is more than one.   **paratenic h.,** a potential or substitute intermediate host that serves until the appropriate definitive host is reached, and in which no development of the parasite occurs; it may or may not be necessary to the completion of the parasite's life cycle. Called also *transfer h.* and *transport h.*   **h. of predilection,** the host preferred by a parasite.   **primary h.,** definitive h.   **reservoir h.,** reservoir, def. 2.   **secondary h.,** intermediate h.   **transfer h., transport h., h.,** paratenic h.

hot (hot)   1. characterized by high temperature. 2. containing dangerous radioactive material; dangerously radioactive.

hot line (hot līn)   telephone assistance for those in need of crisis intervention (q.v.), as in suicide prevention, usually available 24 hours a day, seven days a week, and staffed by nonprofessionals with mental health professionals serving as advisors or in a back-up capacity.

Hottentot bustle (hot′ten-tot) [*Hottentot,* a people of southern Africa]   steatopygia.

hottentotism (hot′en-tot-izm)   an exaggerated form of stuttering.

hough (hok)   hock.

Hounsfield (hounz′fēld), Sir Godfrey Newbold.   British research scientist, born 1919; co-winner, with Allan MacLeod Cormack, of the Nobel prize for medicine or physiology in 1979 for their development of computerized axial tomography.

Hounsfield unit (howns′fēld) [Godfrey *Hounsfield*]   see under *unit.*

Houssay (ou-si′), Bernardo Alberto.   Argentine physiologist, 1887–1971; co-winner, with Carl Ferdinand Cori and Gerty Theresa Cori, of the Nobel prize for medicine or physiology in 1947 for his demonstrations that a hormone secreted by the pituitary gland prevents metabolism of sugar and that injections of pituitary extract induce diabetes symptoms.

Houssay animal, phenomenon (ou-siz′) [Bernardo Alberto *Houssay*]   see under *animal* and *phenomenon.*

Houston's muscle, valve (hu′stonz) [John *Houston,* Irish surgeon, 1802–1845]   see under *muscle* and *valve.*

hoven (ho′ven)   tympany of the stomach.

Hoverbed (hov′er-bed)   trademark for a bed used for burn victims in which the entire body of the victim is supported on a stream of warm sterile air flowing upward through openings along the length of the bed.

Hovius' canal, circle, membrane, plexus (ho′ve-us) [Jacob *Hovius,* Dutch ophthalmologist, born c. 1675]   see under *canal, circle,* and *plexus,* and see *entochoroidea.*

Howard's method (how′ardz) [Benjamin Douglas *Howard,* American physician, 1840–1900]   see under *respiration, artificial.*

Howel-Evans' syndrome (how′el-ev′anz) [W. *Howel-Evans*]   see under *syndrome.*

Howell's bodies, method, test (how′elz) [William Henry *Howell,* American physiologist, 1860–1945]   see *Howell-Jolly bodies,* under *body,* and see under *method* and *tests.*

Howell-Jolly bodies [W. H. *Howell;* Justin Marie Jules *Jolly,* French histologist, 1870–1953] see under *body.*

Howship's lacuna (how'ships) [John *Howship,* English surgeon, 1781–1841] see *absorption lacuna,* under *lacuna.*

H.P. house physician.

Hp haptoglobin.

HPETE hydroperoxyeicosatetraenoic acid.

HPL, hPL human placental lactogen.

HPLC high-performance liquid chromatography.

HPO₃ metaphosphoric acid.

H₃PO₂ hypophosphorous acid.

H₃PO₃ phosphorous acid.

H₃PO₄ orthophosphoric acid; phosphoric acid.

H₄P₂O₆ hypophosphoric acid.

H₄P₂O₇ pyrophosphoric acid.

HPRT hypoxanthine phosphoribosyltransferase.

HRF histamine releasing factor.

H.S. house surgeon.

h.s. abbreviation for L. *ho'ra som'ni,* at bedtime.

H₂S hydrogen sulfide.

HSA human serum albumin.

HSF hydrazine-sensitive factor; see *complement.*

H₂SiO₃ metasilicic acid.

H₄SiO₄ orthosilicic acid.

H₂SO₃ sulfurous acid.

H₂SO₄ sulfuric acid.

5-HT 5-hydroxytryptamine (serotonin).

Ht symbol for *total hyperopia.*

HTACS human thyroid adenylate cyclase stimulators.

HTC homozygous typing cells.

³H-TdR tritium-labeled thymidine.

HTLV human T-cell leukemia/lymphoma virus.

Hua (hu'ah) a genus of fresh-water snails. **H. ningpoen'sis,** a species of central and southern China that ingests the eggs of *Clonorchis sinensis* and in whose body the eggs hatch. **H. tou'cheana,** a first intermediate host of *Paragonimus westermani.*

Hubel (hu'b'l), David Hunter. Canadian-born American neurobiologist, born 1926; co-winner, with Tolsten Nils Wiesel and Roger Wolcott Sperry, of the Nobel prize for medicine or physiology for 1981 for their research on information processing in the visual system.

Huchard's disease, sign (symptom) (e-sharz') [Henri *Huchard,* physician in Paris, 1844–1910] see under *disease* and *sign.*

Hueck's ligament (heks) [Alexander Friedrich *Hueck,* German anatomist, 1802–1842] reticulum trabeculare anguli iridocornealis.

Huët-Pelger nuclear anomaly (hew'et-pel'ger) [G. J. *Huët,* Dutch physician, born 1879; Karel *Pelger,* Dutch physician, 1885–1931] see *Pelger-Huët nuclear anomaly,* under *anomaly.*

Hueter's line, etc. (he'terz) [Karl *Hueter,* German surgeon, 1838–1882] see under *line, maneuver,* and *sign.*

Huggins (hug'inz), Charles Brenton. Canadian-born American surgeon, born 1901; co-winner, with Francis Peyton Rous, of the Nobel prize for medicine or physiology in 1966 for his discoveries in hormonal treatment of cancer of the prostate.

Huggins operation (hug'inz) [Charles Brenton *Huggins*] see under *operation.*

Hughes' reflex (hūz) [Charles Hamilton *Hughes,* American neurologist, 1839–1916] virile reflex, def. 2.

Huguenin's edema (e-gen-az') [Gustave *Huguenin,* Swiss psychiatrist, 1841–1920] see under *edema.*

Huguier's canal, etc. (e-ge-āz') [Pierre Charles *Huguier,* French surgeon, 1804–1873] see under *canal, circle,* and *sinus.*

Huhner test (hoon'er) [Max *Huhner,* New York urologist, 1873–1947] see under *tests.*

HuIFN human interferon.

hum (hum) an indistinct, low, prolonged sound. **venous h.,** a continuous blowing, singing, or humming murmur heard on auscultation over the right jugular vein in the sitting or erect position; it is an innocent sign that is obliterated on assumption of the recumbent position or on exerting pressure over the vein. Called also *bruit de diable* and *humming-top murmur.*

Human's sign (hu'manz) [J. U. *Human,* London physician] chin-retraction sign.

Humatin (hu'mah-tin) trademark for preparations of paromomycin sulfate.

humectant (hu-mek'tant) [L. *humectus,* from *humectare* to be moist] 1. moistening. 2. a moistening or diluent substance.

humectation (hu″mek-ta'shun) the act of moistening.

humeral (hu'mer-al) [L. *humeralis*] of or pertaining to the humerus.

humeri (hu'mer-i) [L.] genitive and plural of *humerus.*

humeroradial (hu″mer-o-ra'de-al) pertaining to the humerus and the radius.

humeroscapular (hu″mer-o-skap'u-lar) pertaining to the humerus and the scapula.

humeroulnar (hu″mer-o-ul'nar) pertaining to the humerus and the ulna.

humerus (hu'mer-us), gen. and pl. *hu'meri* [L.] [NA] the bone that extends from the shoulder to the elbow articulating proximally with the scapula and distally with the radius and ulna; see Plate accompanying *skeleton.* **h. va'rus,** a bent humerus.

humidifier (hu-mid'ĭ-fi″er) an apparatus for controlling humidity by adding to the content of moisture in the air of a room.

humidity (hu-mid'ĭ-te) [L. *humiditas*] the degree of moisture, especially of that in the air. **absolute h.,** the actual amount of vapor in the atmosphere expressed in grains per cubic foot. **relative h.,** the percentage of moisture in the air as compared to the amount necessary to cause saturation, which is taken as 100.

humor (hu'mor), pl. *humors, humo'res* [L. "a liquid"] a fluid or semifluid substance; used in anatomical nomenclature to designate certain fluid materials in the body. See also *humoralism.* **aqueous h., h. aquo'sus** [NA], the fluid produced in the eye, occupying the anterior and posterior chambers, and diffusing out of the eye into the blood; regarded as the lymph of the eye, its composition varies from that of lymph in the body generally. Called also *aqueous* and *hydatoid.* **h. cristalli'nus, crystalline h.,** 1. the crystalline lens. 2. the vitreous body. **ocular h.,** one of the humors of the eye—the aqueous or vitreous. **plasmoid h.,** aqueous or vitreous humor containing an abnormally high amount of protein; formed after trauma or inflammation, it has a cloudy appearance and the proteins tend to coalesce. **vitreous h.,** 1. corpus vitreum. 2. humor vitreus. **h. vi'treus** [NA], the vitreous humor: the watery substance, resembling aqueous humor, contained within the interstices of the stroma in the vitreous body.

humoral (hu'mor-al) 1. pertaining to the humors of the body. See also under *theory.* 2. pertaining to elements dissolved in the blood or body fluids, e.g., humoral immunity from antibodies in the blood as opposed to cellular immunity.

humoralism (hu'mor-al-izm″) the ancient theory that health and illness result from a balance or imbalance of bodily liquids ("humors"). The theory is especially associated with Hippocratic writers, but it long antedates Hippocrates. Humoralism is a variant of Empedocles' theory of the four "roots" (earth, air, fire, water), the later four "elements," then the four qualities (hot, cold, moist, dry), then the four temperaments (cf. *temperament*). The four humors and the four qualities are (1) phlegm (water, or a watery substance), which is cold and moist; (2) blood, which is hot and moist; (3) black bile or gall, secreted from the kidneys and spleen, cold and dry; and (4) yellow bile or choler, secreted from the liver, hot and dry. Humoralism was decisively displaced only in 1858 by Rudolf Virchow's *Cellularpathologie.*

humorism (hu'mor-izm) humoralism.

Humorsol (hu'mor-sol) trademark for a solution of demecarium bromide.

humpback (hump'bak) kyphosis.

Humphry's ligament (hum'frēz) [Sir George Murray *Humphry,* English anatomist, 1820–1896] ligamenta meniscofemorale anterius.

humus (hu'mus) [L.] a dark mold of decayed vegetable material, used therapeutically in certain forms of the mud bath.

hunchback (hunch′bak) 1. kyphosis. 2. an individual characterized by a rounded deformity of the back, or kyphosis.

hunger (hung′ger) a craving, as for food. **air h.,** a distressing dyspnea occurring in paroxysms; called also *Kussmaul's* or *Kussmaul-Kien respiration*. **calcium h.,** a condition due to calcium defect, marked by severe headache during and after menstruation. **chlorine h.,** a desire for salt due to deficiency of chlorine in the blood.

Hunner's ulcer (hun′erz) [Guy LeRoy *Hunner*, American surgeon, 1868–1957] see under *ulcer*.

Hunt's atrophy, etc. (huntz) [James Ramsay *Hunt*, American neurologist, 1872–1937] see under *atrophy* and *phenomenon;* see *dyssynergia cerebellaris myoclonica;* and see *Ramsay Hunt syndrome,* under *syndrome*.

Hunter's canal, gubernaculum, operation (hunt′erz) [John *Hunter*, Scottish anatomist and surgeon, 1728–1793] see *canalis adductorius* and *gubernaculum testis,* and see under *operation*.

Hunter's glossitis [William *Hunter*, English physician, 1861– 1937] see under *glossitis*.

Hunter's ligament, line [William *Hunter*, Scottish anatomist, 1718–1783, brother of John Hunter] see *ligamentum teres uteri* and *linea alba*.

hunterian (hun-te′re-an) named for or described by John Hunter, as hunterian chancre (hard chancre).

Huntington's chorea (disease) (hunt′ing-tunz) [George *Huntington*, American physician, 1850–1916] see under *chorea*.

Huppert's test (hoōp′erts) [Hugo *Huppert*, Bohemian physician, 1832–1904] see under *tests*.

Hurler's syndrome (disease) (hoor′lerz) [Gertrud *Hurler*, Austrian pediatrician, 20th century] see under *syndrome*.

Hürthle cells, cell tumor (her′tel) [Karl *Hürthle*, German histologist, 1860–1945] see under *cell* and *tumor*.

Hurtley's test (hert′lēz) [William Holdsworth *Hurtley*, English scientist, 1867–1936] see under *tests*.

Huschke's canal, foramen, ligaments, valve (hoosh′kez) [Emil *Huschke*, German anatomist, 1797–1858] see under *canal* and *foramen,* and see *plicae gastropancreaticae* and *plica lacrimalis,* under *plica*.

husk (husk) hoose.

Hutchinson's disease, etc. (huch′in-sunz) [Sir Jonathan *Hutchinson*, English surgeon, 1828–1913] see under *disease, facies, mask, pupil, sign, tooth,* and *triad,* and see *salmon patch,* def. 1, under *patch*.

Hutchinson-Gilford disease, syndrome (huch′in-sun-gil′ford) [Sir Jonathan *Hutchinson*; Hastings *Gilford*, English physician, 1861–1941] progeria.

hutchinsonian (huch″in-so′ne-an) named for or described by Sir Jonathan Hutchinson.

Hutchison type (syndrome) (huch′ĭ-son) [Sir Robert *Hutchison*, English pediatrician, 1871–1960] see under *type*.

Hu-Tet (hu′tet) trademark for a preparation of tetanus immune human globulin.

Hutinel's disease (e-tin-elz′) [Victor Henri *Hutinel*, pediatrician in Paris, 1849–1933] see under *disease*.

Huxley (huks′le), Andrew Fielding. British physiologist, born 1917; co-winner, with Sir John Carew Eccles and Alan Lloyd Hodgkin, of the Nobel prize for medicine or physiology for 1963, for discoveries concerning the ionic mechanism involved in excitation and inhibition in peripheral and central parts of the nerve cell membrane.

Huxley's layer (membrane) (huks′lēz) [Thomas Henry *Huxley*, English physiologist and naturalist, 1825–1895] see under *layer*.

huygenian (hi-jen′e-an) named for Christian *Huygens* (or Huyghens), a Dutch physicist, 1629–1695; see under *eyepiece*.

HVA homovanillic acid.

HVL half-value layer.

hyal (hi′al) hyoid.

hyalin (hi′ah-lin) [Gr. *hyalos* glass] 1. a translucent albuminoid substance, one of the products of amyloid degeneration. 2. a substance composing the walls of hydatid cysts. **hematogenous h.,** hematohyaloid.

hyaline (hi′ah-lin) [Gr. *hyalos* glass] glassy and transparent or nearly so; see also under *membrane*.

hyalinization (hi″ah-lin″i-za′shun) conversion into a substance resembling glass.

hyalinosis (hi″ah-lin-o′sis) hyaline degeneration. **h. cu′tis et muco′sae,** lipoid proteinosis.

hyalinuria (hi″ah-lin-u′re-ah) the discharge of hyalin in the urine, usually in the form of casts composed of protein in an acid pH.

hyalitis (hi″ah-li′tis) [*hyal-* + *-itis*] an inflammation of the hyaloid membrane of the eye or of the vitreous humor. **asteroid h.,** see under *hyalosis*. **h. puncta′ta, punctate h.,** inflammation of the vitreous body marked by the formation of small opacities. **h. suppurati′va, suppurative h.,** a purulent inflammation of the vitreous body.

hyalo-, hyal- [Gr. *hyalos* glass] a combining form denoting a relationship to glass or to the vitreous body or vitreous humor, or denoting a resemblance to glass.

hyalogen (hi-al′o-jen) [*hyalo-* + Gr. *gennan* to produce] an albuminous substance occurring in cartilage, the vitreous body, etc., and convertible into hyalin.

hyaloid (hi′ah-loid) [*hyal-* + Gr. *eidos* form] resembling glass.

hyaloidin (hi″ah-loid′in) a carbohydrate radical from mucoproteins; it resembles chondroitin, but contains no sulfuric acid.

hyaloiditis (hi″ah-loi-di′tis) hyalitis.

hyalomere (hi′ah-lo-mēr″) [*hyalo-* + Gr. *meros* part] a zone of homogeneous or finely fibrillar pale blue cytoplasm surrounding the central granular portion (granulomere) of a platelet in a dry, stained blood smear. Cf. *granulomere*.

hyalomitome (hi″ah-lo-mit′ōm) hyaloplasm, def. 1.

Hyalomma (hi″ah-lom′ah) [*hyal-* + Gr. *omma* eye] a genus of ticks. *H. anatol′icum* is a cattle tick of Africa, India, and southern Europe, which may transmit Uzbekistan hemorrhagic fever and a Near Eastern variety of equine encephalomyelitis. *H. margina′tum* transmits Crimean hemorrhagic fever. *H. mauritan′icum* transmits *Theileria parva,* a protozoan parasite that causes many deaths in cattle in northern Africa.

hyalomucoid (hi″ah-lo-mu′koid) [*hyalo-* + *mucoid* (def. 1)] the mucoid of the vitreous body.

hyalonyxis (hi″ah-lo-nik′sis) [*hyalo-* + Gr. *nyxis* pricking] the surgical puncturing of the vitreous body.

hyalophagia (hi″ah-lo-fa′je-ah) [*hyalo-* + Gr. *phagein* to eat] the eating of glass.

hyalophagy (hi″ah-lof′ah-je) hyalophagia.

hyaloplasm (hi′ah-lo-plazm″) [*hyalo-* + Gr. *plasma* anything formed] 1. the more fluid, finely granular substance of the cytoplasm of cells; called also *paraplasm, interfilar mass, interfilar substance, interfibrillar substance of Flemming, paramitome, enchylema,* and *cytolymph.* 2. axoplasm. **nuclear h.,** karyolymph.

hyaloserositis (hi″ah-lo-se″ro-si′tis) [*hyalo-* + *serum* + *-itis*] a form of inflammation of serous membranes marked by hyalinization of the serous exudate into a pearly investment of the organ concerned. Cf. *frosted heart* and *perihepatitis chronica hyperplastica.* **progressive multiple h.,** Concato's disease.

hyalosis (hi″ah-lo′sis) [*hyal-* + *-osis*] degenerative changes in the vitreous humor. **asteroid h.,** a usually unilateral condition of the eye, most frequently seen in older men, characterized by the presence of spherical or star-shaped, calcium-containing opacities in the vitreous humor, which, when illuminated under an examining light, appear to sparkle; vision is usually unaffected. Called also *asteroid hyalitis* and *Benson's disease*.

hyalosome (hi-al′o-sōm) [*hyalo-* + Gr. *sōma* body] a structure resembling the nucleolus of a cell, but staining only slightly.

hyalotome (hi-al′o-tōm) hyaloplasm.

hyaluronate (hi″ah-lu′ro-nāt) a salt or ester of hyaluronic acid.

hyaluronate lyase (hi″ah-lu′ro-nāt li′as) [EC 4.2.2.1] an enzyme of the lyase class that catalyzes the reaction hyaluronate = *n* 3-(4-deoxy-β-D-gluco-4-enuronosyl)-*N*-acetyl-D-glucosamine. Cf. *hyaluronoglucosaminidase* and *hyaluronoglucuronidase*.

hyaluronic acid (hi″ah-lu-ron′ik)   a glycosaminoglycan found in lubricating proteoglycans of synovial fluid, vitreous humor, cartilage, blood vessels, skin, and the umbilical cord. It is a linear chain of about 2500 repeating disaccharide units, each containing one residue of D-glucuronic acid (GlcUA) and N-acetyl-D-glucosamine (GlcNAc) linked by glycosidic bonds that are alternately 1→3 and 1→4 so that the formula for the repeating unit is (1→3)-β-GlcNAc-(1→4) = β-GlcUA.

hyaluronidase (hi″ah-lu-ron′ĭ-dās)   1. any of three enzymes (hyaluronate lyase, hyaluronoglucosaminidase, and hyaluronoglucuronidase) that catalyze the breakdown of hyaluronic acid. These enzymes are found in mammalian testicular and spleen tissue, in bee and snake venoms, and in certain species of *Clostridium*, *Staphylococcus*, and *Streptococcus*. Called also *Duran-Reynals factor*, *invasion*, and *diffusion* or *spreading factor*. 2. a pharmaceutical preparation suitable for injection [NF], which is a sterile, dry, soluble, enzyme product prepared from mammalian testes and capable of hydrolyzing mucopolysaccharides of the type of hyaluronic acid, used to aid absorption and dispersion of other injected drugs and fluids, for hypodermoclysis, and for improving resorption of radiopaque media.

hyaluronoglucosaminidase (hi″ah-lu-ron″o-gloo″-ko-să-min′ĭ-dās) [EC 3.2.1.35]   an enzyme of the hydrolase class that catalyzes the hydrolysis of 1,4-linkages between N-acetyl-β-D-glucosamine and D-glucuronate residues in hyaluronate to form tetrasaccharide units. It also hydrolyzes chondroitin, chondroitin 4- and 6-sulfates, and dermatan. Cf. *hyaluronate lyase* and *hyaluronoglucuronidase*.

hyaluronoglucuronidase (hi″ah-lu-ron″o-gloo″ku-ron′ĭ-dās) [EC 3.2.1.36]   an enzyme of the hydrolase class that catalyzes the hydrolysis of 1,3-linkages between β-D-glucuronate and N-acetyl-D-glucosamine residues in hyaluronate. Cf. *hyaluronate lyase* and *hyaluronoglucosaminidase*.

Hyazyme (hi′ah-zīm)   trademark for a preparation of hyaluronidase for injection.

hybaroxia (hi″bār-ok′se-ah)   inhalation therapy using hyperbaric oxygen, i.e., oxygen under pressures greater than 1 atmosphere.

hybenzate (hi-ben′zāt)   USAN contraction for *o*-(4-hydroxybenzoyl)benzoate.

hybrid (hi′brid) [L. *hybrida* mongrel]   an animal or plant produced from parents different in kind, such as parents belonging to two different strains, varieties, or species. **false h.,** an individual produced by a form of gynogenesis in which the foreign spermatozoon enters the ovum and activates it to cell division, but does not fuse with the egg nucleus.

hybridism (hi′brid-izm)   1. the state of being a hybrid. 2. the production of hybrids.

hybridity (hi-brid′ĭ-te)   the state of being a hybrid.

hybridization (hi″brid-i-za′shun)   1. the act or process of producing hybrids. In molecular genetics, the creation of RNA-DNA hybrids by annealing a radioactively labeled RNA fraction with denatured DNA, so that the RNA becomes associated with the complementary DNA. 2. the technique of fusing somatic cells of different species or of inserting foreign DNA into a bacterial plastid. 3. in chemistry, a procedure whereby orbitals of intermediate energy and desired directional character are constructed by taking an appropriate linear combination of atomic orbitals, e.g., sp³ hybrid orbitals are formed from one s and three p orbitals.

hybridoma (hi″brĭ-do′mah) [*hybrid* + *-oma*]   a somatic cell hybrid formed by fusion of normal lymphocytes and tumor cells; the resulting hybridoma cells will produce the same secretion as the normal parent cells and proliferate indefinitely in culture like the parent tumor cells. B cell hybridomas are formed by the fusion of antibody-secreting B lymphocytes and nonsecretory myeloma cells and are used in the production of monoclonal antibodies. T cell hybridomas, formed by the fusion of T lymphocytes and myeloma cells, are particularly useful in the production of T lymphocyte–derived lymphokines.

hycanthone (hi-kan′thōn)   a thioxanthone antischistosomal agent effective against *Schistosoma haematobium* and *S. mansoni*; used as *hycanthone mesylate*. **h. mesylate,** the mesylate salt of hycanthone, $C_{20}H_{24}N_2O_2S \cdot CH_3SO_3H$, having the same actions as the base; administered intramuscularly.

hyclate (hi′klāt)   USAN contraction for monohydrochloride hemiethanolate hemihydrate.

Hycodan (hi′ko-dan)   trademark for preparations of hydrocodone bitartrate.

hydantoic acid (hi-dan′to-ik)   glycoluric a.

hydantoin (hi-dan′to-in)   a crystalline base derivable from allantoin, $CO \cdot NH \cdot CH_2 \cdot CO \cdot NH$.

hydantoinate (hi″dan-to′in-āt)   any salt of hydantoin.

hydathode (hi′dah-thōd)   a water-secreting structure found on the edges and tips and leaves of many plants.

hydatid (hi′dah-tid) [L. *hydatis*, a drop of water]   1. a hydatid cyst. 2. any cystlike structure; see under *mole*. **alveolar h's,** see *hydatid disease, alveolar*, under *disease*. **h. of Morgagni**, see *appendix testis* and *appendices vesiculosae epoöphorontis*. **sessile h.**, appendix testis. **Virchow's h.**, alveolar hydatid disease.

hydatidiform (hi″dah-tid′ĭ-form)   resembling a hydatid cyst; see under *mole*.

hydatidosis (hi″dah-tĭ-do′sis)   hydatid disease; infection with *Echinococcus*.

hydatidostomy (hi″dah-tĭ-dos′to-me) [*hydatid* + Gr. *stoma* mouth]   incision and drainage of a hydatid cyst.

hydatiduria (hi″dah-tĭ-du′re-ah)   the excretion of hydatid material in the urine.

Hydatigena (hi″dah-tij′en-ah)   *Taenia*.

hydatism (hi′dah-tizm) [Gr. *hydatis* water]   the sound caused by the presence of fluid in a cavity.

hydatoid (hi′dah-toid) [Gr. *hydōr* water + *-oid*]   1. the aqueous humor. 2. the hyaloid membrane (membrana vitrea [NA]). 3. pertaining to the aqueous humor.

Hydeltra (hi-del′trah)   trademark for preparations of prednisolone.

Hydergine (hi′der-jin)   trademark for a mixture of equal parts of dihydroergocornine, dihydroergocristine, and dihydroergocryptine, in the form of methansulfonate salts, used as a vasodilator for the treatment of peripheral vascular disease.

Hydnocarpus (hid″no-kar′pus)   a genus of Indomalayan trees. *H. wightiana* Blume and *H. anthelmintica* Pierre (Flacourtiaceae) are sources of chaulmoogra oil.

hydracetin (hi-dras′ĕ-tin)   acetylphenylhydrazine.

hydradenitis (hi″drad-ĕ-ni′tis)   hidradenitis.

hydradenoma (hi″drad-ĕ-no′mah)   hidradenoma.

hydraeroperitoneum (hi-dra″ĕ-ro-per″ĭ-to-ne′um) [*hydr-* + Gr. *aēr* air + *peritoneum*]   a collection of watery fluid and gas in the peritoneal cavity.

hydragogue (hi′drah-gog) [*hydr-* + Gr. *agōgos* leading]   1. producing watery discharge, especially from the bowels. 2. a cathartic which causes watery purgation.

hydralazine hydrochloride (hi-dral′ah-zēn) [USP]   chemical name: 1-hydrazinophthalazine hydrochloride. An antihypertensive, $C_8H_8N_4 \cdot HCl$, occurring as a white crystalline powder; administered orally, intramuscularly, or intravenously.

hydramine (hi′drah-min)   an amine derived from a glycol in which one hydroxyl is replaced by an amino group.

hydramnion (hi-dram′ne-on)   hydramnios.

hydramnios (hi-dram′ne-os) [*hydr-* + *amnion*]   excess of amniotic fluid.

hydranencephaly (hi″dran-en-sef′ah-le)   complete or almost complete absence of the cerebral hemispheres, the space they normally occupy being filled with cerebrospinal fluid.

Hydrangea (hi-dran′je-ah)   a genus of saxifragaceous trees and shrubs. A glycoside from the dried rhizome and roots of *H. arborescens* L. (Saxifragaceae) was formerly used as a diuretic. Called also *seven barks*.

hydrargyri (hi-drar′jĭ-ri)   genitive of L. *hydrargyrum*, mercury. **h. bichlo′ridum**, mercury bichloride. **h. chlo′ridum corrosi′vum**, mercury bichloride. **h. iodi′dum fla′vum**, mercurous iodide, yellow. **h. iodi′dum ru′brum**, mercuric iodide, red. **h. ox′idum fla′vum**, mercuric oxide, yellow. **h. sali′cylas**, mercuric salicylate.

hydrargyria, hydrargyrism (hi″drar-jir′e-ah; hi-drar′jĭ-rizm)   mercury poisoning; see under *poisoning*.

hydrargyromania (hi-drar′jĭ-ro-ma′ne-ah)   mental disorder due to mercury poisoning.

hydrargyrorelapsing (hi-drar″jĭ-ro-re-laps′ing) relapsing after apparently successful mercurial treatment.

hydrargyrosis (hi-drar″jĭ-ro′sis) mercury poisoning; see under *poisoning*.

hydrargyrum (hi-drar′jĭ-rum), gen. *hydrar′gyri* [L. "liquid silver"] mercury. **h. ammonia′tum,** ammoniated mercury. **h. chlo′ridum mi′te,** calomel. **h. olea′tum,** mercury oleate.

hydrarthrodial (hi″drar-thro′de-al) pertaining to hydrarthrosis.

hydrarthrosis (hi″drar-thro′sis) [*hydr-* + Gr. *arthron* joint + *-osis*] an accumulation of watery fluid in the cavity of a joint. **intermittent h.,** serous effusion into a joint occurring periodically.

hydrase (hi′drās) hydratase.

hydratase (hi′drah-tās) [EC 4.2.1] any enzyme of the hydro-lyase sub-subclass of lyases that catalyzes the reversible hydration of a double bond. Formerly called *hydrase.*

hydrate (hi′drāt) [L. *hydras*] 1. any compound of a radical with H_2O. 2. any salt or other compound that contains water of crystallization.

hydrated (hi′drāt-ed) [L. *hydratus*] combined with water; forming a hydrate or a hydroxide.

hydration (hi-dra′shun) 1. the act of combining or causing to combine with water. 2. the condition of being combined with water.

hydraulics (hi-draw′liks) [*hydr-* + Gr. *aulos* pipe] the branch of physics which treats of the action of liquids under physical laws.

hydrazine (hi′drah-zin) a colorless, gaseous diamine, H_2-$N \cdot NH_2$; also any member of a group of its substitution derivatives. Called also *diamide.*

hydrazinolysis (hi″drah-zin-ol′ĭ-sis) cleavage of the peptide bonds of a peptide by hydrazine, with the C-terminal residue appearing as a free amino acid.

hydrazone (hi-drah-zōn) a compound formed from an aldehyde or ketone by the action of phenylhydrazine.

Hydrea (hi-dre′ah) trademark for a preparation of hydroxyurea.

hydremia (hi-dre′me-ah) [*hydr-* + Gr. *haima* blood] excess of water in the blood; a condition in which the proportion of the serum in the blood to the corpuscles is excessive.

hydrencephalocele (hi″dren-sef′ah-lo-sēl) [*hydr-* + *encephalocele*] encephalocystocele.

hydrencephalomeningocele (hi″dren-sef″ah-lo-mě-ning′go-sēl) hernial protrusion through a cranial defect of the meninges containing cerebrospinal fluid and brain substance.

hydrencephalus (hi″dren-sef′ah-lus) hydrocephalus.

hydrencephaly (hi″dren-sef′ah-le) hydrocephalus.

hydrepigastrium (hi″drep-ĭ-gas′tre-um) [*hydr-* + *epigastrium*] a collection of watery fluid between the peritoneum and the abdominal wall.

hydriatric (hi″dre-at′rik) [*hydr-* + Gr. *iatikos, iatrikos* healing] pertaining to hydrotherapy.

hydriatrics (hi″dre-at′riks) hydrotherapy.

hydric (hi′drik) pertaining to or combined with hydrogen; containing replaceable hydrogen.

hydride (hi′drīd) [Gr. *hydōr* water] any compound of hydrogen with an element or radical.

hydrindicuria (hi″drin-dĭ-ku′re-ah) the presence in the urine of indoles related to both tryptophan and phenylalanine.

hydriodic acid (hi″dri-o′dik) a term applied to aqueous solutions of hydrogen iodide, HI, a strong mineral acid.

hydrion (hi-dri′on) hydrogen ion.

hydr(o)- [Gr. *hydōr* water] a combining form denoting (*a*) relationship to water, (*b*) the accumulation of fluid in a body part, or (*c*) the presence of hydrogen in a chemical compound.

hydroa (hid-ro′ah) [*hydro-* + Gr. *ōon* egg] a vesicular or bullous eruption. **h. estiva′le,** h. vacciniforme. **h. vaccinifor′me,** a vesicular and bullous eruption, which may be preceded by pruritus and burning sensation, having a tendency to recur each summer during childhood on sun-exposed areas of the skin; the lesions dry up with the formation of brown adherent crusts, and each lesion is surrounded by an erythematous zone, giving the appearance

of a vaccination vesicle. Called also *h. estivale* and *summer prurigo of Hutchinson.*

hydroadipsia (hi″dro-ah-dip′se-ah) [*hydro-* + *a* neg. + Gr. *dipsa* thirst] absence of thirst for water.

hydroappendix (hi″dro-ah-pen′diks) distention of the vermiform appendix with a watery fluid.

Hydrobiidae (hi″dro-be′ĭ-de) a family of snails (order Mesogastropoda) that includes the subfamilies Hydrobiinae and Buliminae, which are intermediate hosts of various species of parasitic flukes.

Hydrobiinae (hi″dro-be′ĭ-ne) a subfamily of snails (family Hydrobiidae, order Mesogastropoda) that includes the genus *Oncomelania,* the intermediate host of *Schistosoma japonicum.*

hydrobilirubin (hi″dro-bil″ĭ-roo′bin) [*hydro-* + *bilirubin*] a brownish-red pigment, $C_{32}H_{40}N_4O_7$, derivable from bilirubin by reduction. It is believed to be identical with stercobilin and urobilin.

hydroblepharon (hi″dro-blef′ah-ron) [*hydro-* + Gr. *blepharon* eyelid] edema of the eyelids.

hydrobromic acid (hi-dro-bro′mik) a term applied to aqueous solutions of hydrogen bromide, HBr, a strong mineral acid.

hydrobromide (hi″dro-bro′mīd) an addition salt of hydrobromic acid. Cf. *hydrochloride.*

Hydrocal (hi′dro-kal) trademark for an artificial stone produced by the calcination of gypsum in an autoclave at a steam pressure sufficient to produce a temperature of 120° to 130°C; used in dentistry.

hydrocalycosis (hi″dro-kal″ĭ-ko′sis) [*hydro-* + *calyx* + *-osis*] a usually asymptomatic cystic dilatation of a major renal calix, lined by transitional epithelium and due to obstruction of the infundibulum.

hydrocalyx (hi″dro-kal′iks) a cyst in the renal cortex caused by obstruction at the infundibulum; the entire calyx dilates to form the cyst wall.

hydrocarbarism (hi″dro-kar′bar-izm) hydrocarbonism.

hydrocarbon (hi″dro-kar′bon) an organic compound that contains carbon and hydrogen only. The hydrocarbons are divided into *alicyclic, aliphatic,* and *aromatic* hydrocarbons, according to the arrangement of the atoms and the chemical properties of the compounds. **alicyclic h.,** a hydrocarbon that has cyclic structure and aliphatic properties. **aliphatic h.,** a hydrocarbon in which no carbon atoms are joined to form a ring. **aromatic h.,** a hydrocarbon that has cyclic structure and a closed conjugated system of double bonds that gives it the characteristic chemical properties of the parent aromatic hydrocarbon, benzene (C_6H_6); other typical aromatic hydrocarbons are toluene (C_7H_8), naphthalene ($C_{10}H_8$), anthracene ($C_{14}H_{10}$), and phenanthrene (C_{14}-H_{10}). **carcinogenic h.,** a condensed nuclear aromatic hydrocarbon that tends to cause cancer when applied to the skin or when otherwise administered. **cyclic h.,** one of a series of hydrocarbons having the general formula C_nH_{2n}, the carbon atoms being thought of as having a closed ring structure. **saturated h.,** a hydrocarbon that has the maximum number of hydrogen atoms for a given carbon structure, such as methane, ethane, propane, cyclopropane, and the butanes. **unsaturated h.,** an aliphatic or alicyclic hydrocarbon that has less than the maximum number of hydrogen atoms for a given carbon structure, such as ethylene, acetylene, propylene, cyclohexene, and the butanes.

hydrocarbonism (hi″dro-kar′bon-izm) poisoning by hydrocarbons.

hydrocardia (hi″dro-kar′de-ah) hydropericardium.

hydrocele (hi′dro-sēl) [*hydro-* + Gr. *kēlē* tumor] a circumscribed collection of fluid, especially a collection of fluid in the tunica vaginalis of the testicle or along the spermatic cord. **cervical h.,** a serous dilatation of a persistent cervical duct, or sometimes of a deep cervical lymph space; called also *h. colli* and *Maunoir's h.* **chylous h.,** a form in which the fluid is milky in appearance. **h. col′li,** cervical h. **communicating h.,** hydrocele in which the processus vaginalis testis is patent. **congenital h.,** hydrocele in the unobliterated canal between the peritoneal cavity and that of the tunica vaginalis. **diffused h.,** a collection of fluid diffused in the loose connective tissue of the spermatic cord. **Dupuytren's h.,** bilocular hydrocele of the tunica vaginalis testis. **encysted h.,** one which occurs in cysts outside the cavity of the tunica vaginalis testis. **h. fem′inae,** an

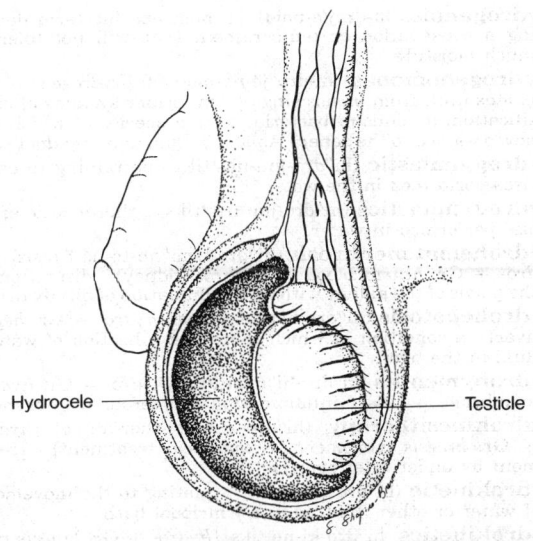

Hydrocele — — Testicle

affection of the round ligament of the female resembling ordinary hydrocele. **funicular h.,** hydrocele of the tunica vaginalis of the spermatic cord in a space closed toward the testis and open toward the peritoneal cavity. **hernial h.,** distention of the hernial sac with a fluid. **Maunoir's h.,** cervical hydrocele. **h. mulie′bris** (obs.), a watery dilatation of the canal of Nuck; called also *Nuck's h.* **h. of neck,** cervical h. **Nuck's h.** (obs.), h. muliebris. **h. rena′lis,** a condition in which the renal capsule forms part of a cyst wall so that the kidney is partially or almost wholly surrounded by the cyst; although often found after trauma in adults, such a cyst is of congenital origin. **scrotal h.,** a circumscribed collection of fluid in the scrotum. **h. spina′lis,** spina bifida.

hydrocelectomy (hi″dro-se-lek′to-me) [*hydrocele* + Gr. *ektomē* excision] excision of a hydrocele.

hydrocephalic (hi″dro-sĕ-fal′ik) pertaining to or affected with hydrocephalus.

hydrocephalocele (hi″dro-sef′ah-lo-sēl″) encephalocystocele.

hydrocephaloid (hi″dro-sef′ah-loid) 1. resembling hydrocephalus. 2. see under *disease.*

hydrocephalus (hi-dro-sef′ah-lus) [*hydro-* + Gr. *kephalē* head] a condition marked by dilatation of the cerebral ventricles, most often occurring secondarily to obstruction of the cerebrospinal fluid pathways (see *ventricular block,* under *block*), and accompanied by an accumulation of cerebrospinal fluid within the skull; the fluid is usually under increased pressure, but occasionally may be normal or nearly so. It is typically characterized by enlargement of the head, prominence of the forehead, brain atrophy, mental deterioration, and convulsions; may be congenital or acquired; and may be of sudden onset (*acute h.*) or be slowly progressive (*chronic* or *primary h.*). **communicating h.,** hydrocephalus in which there is no obstruction in the ventricular system, and cerebrospinal fluid passes readily out of the brain into the spinal canal, but is not absorbed. **h. ex vac′uo,** a compensatory replacement by cerebrospinal fluid of the volume of tissue lost in atrophy of the brain. **noncommunicating h.,** obstructive h. **normal-pressure h., normal-pressure occult h.,** dementia, ataxia, and urinary incontinence with pneumoencephalographic evidence of hydrocephalus, i.e., with enlarged ventricles associated with inadequacy of the subarachnoid spaces, but with normal cerebrospinal fluid pressure; occurring in middle-aged and older persons. Called also *occult normal-pressure h.* **obstructive h.,** hydrocephalus due to ventricular block (q.v.); called also *noncommunicating h.* **occult normal-pressure h.,** normal-pressure h. **otitic h.,** acute hydrocephalus caused by spread of the inflammation of otitis media to the cranial cavity. **secondary h.,** hydrocephalus resulting from meningitis.

hydrocephaly (hi″dro-sef′ah-le) hydrocephalus.

hydrochloric acid (hi″dro-klor′ik) a term applied to aqueous solutions of hydrogen chloride, HCl. It is a highly corrosive strong mineral acid commonly used as a laboratory reagent. HCl is secreted by the gastric parietal cells in response to gastrin, histamine, and vagal stimulation. This normally reduces the pH of the gastric content to below 2.0.

hydrochloride (hi″dro-klo′rīd) a salt formed by addition of hydrochloric acid; chemically it is a chloride salt of the moiety formed by protonation of a neutral organic compound. The term *hydrochloride* is used primarily in drug names.

$$\begin{array}{ccc} & H & \\ H- & N & H \\ H & & Cl \end{array}$$

hydrochlorothiazide (hi″dro-klor″o-thi′ah-zīd) [USP] a thiazide diuretic; used for treatment of hypertension and edema.

hydrocholecystis (hi″dro-ko″le-sis′tis) [*hydro-* + Gr. *cholē* bile + *kystis* bladder] distention of the gallbladder with watery fluid; hydrops of the gallbladder.

hydrocholeresis (hi″dro-ko″lĕ-re′sis) [*hydro-* + Gr. *cholē* bile + *hairesis* a taking] choleresis characterized by increase in water output, or induction of the excretion of bile relatively low in specific gravity, viscosity, and total solid content.

hydrocholeretic (hi″dro-ko″lĕ-ret′ik) pertaining to, characterized by, or producing hydrocholeresis.

hydrocholesterol (hi″dro-ko-les′ter-ol) a reduced form of cholesterol.

hydrocinchonidine (hi″dro-sin-kon′ĭ-din) an alkaloid, $C_{19}H_{24}ON_2$, isomeric with cinchonine.

hydrocirsocele (hi″dro-sir′so-sēl) [*hydro-* + *cirsocele*] hydrocele combined with varicocele.

hydrocodone bitartrate (hi″dro-ko′dōn) [USP] a semisynthetic product of codeine, $C_{18}H_{21}NO_3\cdot C_4H_6O_6\cdot 2\frac{1}{2}H_2O$, occurring as a fine, white, crystalline powder, having narcotic analgesic effects similar to but more active than those of codeine; used as an antitussive, administered orally. Called also *dihydrocodeinone bitartrate.*

hydrocollidine (hi″dro-kol′ĭ-din) [*hydro-* + *collidine*] a poisonous oily ptomaine, $C_8H_{13}N$, from nicotine, decayed flesh, and stale fish.

hydrocolloid (hi″dro-kol′loid) [*hydro-* + *colloid*] a colloid system in which water is the dispersion medium. **irreversible h.,** a hydrocolloid which can be converted from the sol to the gel condition but cannot be reverted to a sol by any simple means. **reversible h.,** a hydrocolloid which can be reverted from the gel to the sol condition by increase in temperature.

hydrocolpos (hi″dro-kol′pos) [*hydro-* + Gr. *kolpos* vagina] a collection of watery fluid in the vagina.

hydroconion (hi″dro-ko′ne-on) [*hydro-* + Gr. *konis* dust] an atomizer or vaporizer for throwing liquids in a fine spray.

hydrocortamate hydrochloride (hi″dro-kor′tah-māt) chemical name: cortisol 21-ester with *N,N*-diethylglycine hydrochloride. A synthetic glucocorticoid, $C_{27}H_{41}NO_6\cdot HCl$, used topically as an anti-inflammatory in the treatment of steroid-responsive dermatoses.

hydrocortisone (hi″dro-kor′tĭ-sōn) chemical name: $11\beta,17\alpha,21$-trihydroxypregn-4-ene-3,20-dione. The major glucocorticoid, $C_{21}H_{30}O_5$, elaborated by the human adrenal cortex (or *cortisol,* as it is usually referred to by biochemists), or the same substance produced synthetically; it has life-maintaining and blood pressure–sustaining properties and also has appreciable mineralocorticoid activity. The official preparation [USP] and its salts are used in the treatment of inflammations, allergies, pruritus, collagen diseases (rheumatoid arthritis, lupus erythematosus, etc.), some neoplasms, acute or chronic adrenocortical deficiency, severe status asthmaticus, and shock. **h. acetate** [USP], an ester of hydrocortisone, $C_{23}H_{32}O_6$, occurring as a white to practically white, crystalline powder, having actions and uses similar to those of the base; administered by intra-articular or soft-tissue injection or applied topically to the skin or conjunctiva. **h. cyclopentylpropionate, h. cypionate** [USP], an ester of hydrocortisone, $C_{29}H_{42}O_6$, occurring as a white to practically white, crystalline powder, having actions and uses similar to those of the base; administered orally. **h. hemisuccinate** [USP], an ester of hydrocortisone, $C_{25}H_{34}O_8$, having actions and uses similar to those of the base. **h. sodium phosphate** [USP], a water-soluble ester of hydrocortisone, $C_{21}H_{29}Na_2O_8P$, occurring as a white to light yellow powder, having actions and uses similar to those of the base; administered intravenously or intramuscularly, especially for adrenocortical insufficiency. **h. sodium succinate** [USP], a water-soluble ester of hydrocortisone, $C_{25}H_{33}NaO_8$, occurring as a white or nearly white crystalline powder, having actions and uses similar to those of the base; administered intravenously or intramuscularly, especially for acute adrenocortical insufficiency. **h. valerate,** an ester of hydrocortisone, $C_{26}H_{38}O_6$, having actions similar to those of the base.

Hydrocortone (hi″dro-kor′tōn)   trademark for preparations of hydrocortisone.

hydrocyanic acid (hi″dro-si-an′ik)   hydrogen cyanide.

hydrocyanism (hi″dro-si′an-izm)   poisoning with hydrocyanic acid.

hydrocyst (hi′dro-sist) [hydro- + Gr. *kystis* sac, bladder] a cyst with watery contents.

hydrocystadenoma (hi″dro-sis″tad-ĕ-no′mah)   papillary hidradenoma; see *hidradenoma.*

hydrodiffusion (hi″dro-dĭ-fu′zhun)   diffusion in an aqueous medium.

hydrodipsia (hi″dro-dip′se-ah)   thirst for water.

hydrodipsomania (hi″dro-dip″so-ma′ne-ah)   an epileptic condition characterized by attacks of insatiable thirst.

hydrodiuresis (hi″dro-di′u-re′sis) [hydro- + *diuresis*] copious secretion of urine of low specific gravity.

HydroDIURIL (hi″dro-di′u-ril)   trademark for a preparation of hydrochlorothiazide.

hydrodynamics (hi″dro-di-nam′iks) [hydro- + *dynamics*] that branch of the science of mechanics which treats of the movement of fluids and of solids contained in fluids.

hydroelectric (hi″dro-e-lek′trik)   pertaining to water and electricity.

hydroencephalocele (hi″dro-en-sef′ah-lo-sēl)   encephalocystocele.

hydroflumethiazide (hi″dro-floo″mĕ-thi′ah-zīd) [USP] a thiazide diuretic; used for treatment of hypertension and edema.

hydrofluoric acid (hi″dro-floor′ik)   a term applied to aqueous solutions of hydrogen fluoride, HF, an extremely poisonous and corrosive acid.

hydrogel (hi′dro-jel)   a gel that has water as its dispersion medium.

hydrogen (hi′dro-jen) [hydro- + Gr. *gennan* to produce] the lightest element, an odorless, tasteless, colorless gas that is inflammable and explosive when mixed with air. It is found in water and in almost all organic compounds. Its ion is the active constituent of all acids in the water system. Its symbol is H; atomic number, 1; atomic weight, 1.00797; specific gravity, 0.069. Hydrogen exists in three isotopes: ordinary, or light, hydrogen is the mass 1 isotope, also called *protium;* heavy hydrogen is the mass 2 isotope, also called *deuterium;* the mass 3 isotope is *tritium.* **arseniuretted h.,** see under *arsine.* **h. cyanide,** an extremely poisonous colorless liquid or gas, HCN; inhalation can cause death within a minute; see *cyanide poisoning* under *poisoning.* Called also *hydrocyanic acid.* **h. disulfide,** an ill-smelling liquid, H_2S_2. **heavy h.,** see *hydrogen.* **light h.,** see *hydrogen.* **h. monoxide,** water, H_2O. **ordinary h.,** see *hydrogen.* **h. peroxide,** a strongly disinfectant cleansing and bleaching liquid, H_2O_2, used in dilute solution in water, mainly as a wash or spray. **h. selenide,** a poisonous gas, H_2Se; its inhalation causes an obstinate coryza and destroys the sense of smell. **h. sulfide,** an offensive and poisonous gas, H_2S, used as a chemical reagent; called also *hydrosulfuric* or *sulfhydric acid.* **sulfuretted h.,** h. sulfide.

hydrogenate (hi′dro-jĕ-nāt″)   to cause to combine with hydrogen; to reduce with hydrogen.

hydrogenize (hi′dro-jen-īz)   hydrogenate.

hydrogenlyase (hi″dro-jen-li′ās)   1. hydrogenase. 2. formerly, an enzyme system in certain bacteria that converts formic acid to carbon dioxide and hydrogen. In *Escherichia coli,* the reaction involves formate dehydrogenase and cytochrome C_3 hydrogenase.

hydrogenoid (hi-droj′ĕ-noid)   a homeopathic term denoting a constitution or temperament that will not tolerate much moisture.

Hydrogenomonas (hi-dro″jĕ-no-mo′nas) [*hydrogen* + Gr. *monas* unit, from *monos* single]   in former systems of classification, a genus of bacteria, certain species of which are now assigned to the genera *Aquaspirillum* and *Pseudomonas.*

hydrogymnastic (hi″dro-jim-nas′tik)   pertaining to exercises performed in the water.

hydrogymnastics (hi″dro-jim-nas′tiks)   therapeutic exercise performed in water.

hydrohematonephrosis (hi″dro-hem″ah-to-nĕ-fro′sis) [*hydro-* + Gr. *haima* blood + *nephros* kidney]   distention of the pelvis of the kidney with an accumulation of bloody urine.

hydrohepatosis (hi″dro-hep″ah-to′sis) [hydro- + Gr. *hēpar* liver]   a condition in which there is a collection of watery fluid in the liver.

hydrohymenitis (hi″dro-hi″men-i′tis) [hydro- + Gr. *hymēn* membrane + *-itis*]   inflammation of a serous membrane.

hydrokinesitherapy (hi″dro-ki-ne″sĭ-ther′ah-pe) [*hydro-* + Gr. *kinēsis* movement + *therapeia* treatment]   treatment by underwater exercise.

hydrokinetic (hi″dro-ki-net′ik)   relating to the movement of water or other fluid, as in a whirlpool bath.

hydrokinetics (hi″dro-ki-net′iks) [*hydro-* + Gr. *kinēsis* motion]   that branch of mechanics which treats of fluids in motion.

hydrokollag (hi″dro-kol′ag)   a suspension of finely particulate graphite, used in experimental study of ciliary action and lymphatic drainage.

hydrol (hi′drol)   a final mother liquor obtained in the manufacture of glucose from cornstarch.

hydrolabile (hi″dro-la′bil)   having a tendency to lose weight under carbohydrate or salt restriction or following infections or gastrointestinal disease. Cf. *hydrostabile.*

hydrolability (hi″dro-lah-bil′ĭ-te) [hydro- + L. *labilis* liable to change]   a condition in which tissue fluids tend to vary in quantity.

hydrolase (hi′dro-lās)   [EC 3] one of the six main classes of enzymes, consisting of those that catalyze the hydrolytic cleavage of a chemical bond with the addition of water, e.g., esterases, glycosidases, lipases, nucleotidases, peptidases, phosphatases, and proteinases.

hydrology (hi-drol′o-je) [*hydro-* + *-logy*]   the sum of knowledge regarding water and its uses.

Hydrolose (hi′dro-lōs)   trademark for a preparation of methylcellulose.

hydro-lyase (hi″dro-li′ās)   [EC 4.2.1] a sub-subclass of enzymes of the lyase class. These enzymes catalyze the removal of water from a substrate by breakage of a carbon-oxygen bond, leading to formation of a double bond. The recommended name is usually dehydratase. The term synthase or hydratase is used when the reverse aspect of the reaction is dominant. Called also *dehydratase* and *hydratase.*

hydrolymph (hi′dro-limf) [*hydro-* + *lymph*]   the thin, watery nutritive fluid of certain of the lower animals.

hydrolysate (hi-drol′ĭ-zāt)   a compound produced by hydrolysis. **protein h.,** a mixture of amino acids prepared by splitting a protein with acid, alkali, or enzyme. Such preparations provide the nutritive equivalent of the original material (casein, lactalbumin, fibrin, etc.) in the form of its constituent amino acids; used in special diets or for patients unable to take the ordinary food proteins.

hydrolysis (hi-drol′ĭ-sis) pl. *hydrol′yses* [*hydro-* + Gr. *lysis* dissolution]   the splitting of a compound into fragments by the addition of water, the hydroxyl group being incorporated in one fragment, and the hydrogen atom in the other.

hydrolyst (hi′dro-list)   an agent that promotes hydrolysis.

hydrolyte (hi′dro-līt)   a substance undergoing hydrolysis.

hydrolytic (hi-dro-lit′ik)   pertaining to, characterized by, or promoting hydrolysis.

hydrolyze (hi′dro-līz)   to subject to hydrolysis.

hydroma (hi-dro′mah)   hygroma.

hydromassage (hi″dro-mah-sahzh′)   massage by means of moving water.

hydromeningitis (hi″dro-men″in-ji′tis) [*hydro-* + *meningitis*]   meningitis with serous effusion.

hydromeningocele (hi″dro-mĕ-ning′go-sēl) [*hydro-* + Gr. *mēninx* membrane + *kēlē* hernia] protrusion of the meninges through a defect in the skull or spine, forming a sac containing cerebrospinal fluid.

hydrometer. (hi-drom′ĕ-ter) [*hydro-* + Gr. *metron* measure] an instrument for determining the specific gravities of a fluid.

hydrometra (hi″dro-me′trah) [*hydro-* + Gr. *mētra* uterus] a collection of watery fluid in the uterus.

hydrometric (hi″dro-met′rik) pertaining to hydrometry.

hydrometrocolpos (hi″dro-me″tro-kol′pos) [*hydro-* + Gr. *mētra* uterus + *kolpos* vagina] a collection of watery fluid in the uterus and vagina

hydrometry (hi-drom′ĕ-tre) the measurement of the specific gravity of a fluid by means of the hydrometer.

hydromicrocephaly (hi″dro-mi″kro-sef′ah-le) microcephaly with an abnormal amount of cerebrospinal fluid.

hydromorphone (hi″dro-mor′fōn) chemical name: 4,5α-epoxy-3-hydroxy-17-methyl-methylmorphinan-6-one. A morphine alkaloid, $C_{17}H_{19}NO_3$, occurring as a fine, white or practically white, crystalline powder, having narcotic analgesic effects similar to but greater and of shorter duration than those of morphine; administered as the sulfate salt by subcutaneous injection. **h. hydrochloride** [USP], the hydrochloride salt of hydromorphone, $C_{17}H_{19}NO_3 \cdot HCl$, having the same actions as the base; administered orally and subcutaneously. Called also *dihydromorphinone hydrochloride*.

Hydromox (hi′dro-moks) trademark for preparations of quinethazone.

hydromphalus (hi-drom′fah-lus) [*hydro-* + Gr. *omphalos* navel] a cystic accumulation of watery fluid at the umbilicus.

hydromyelia (hi″dro-mi-e′le-ah) [*hydro-* + Gr. *myelos* marrow + *-ia*] a pathological condition in which there is dilation of the central canal of the spinal cord with increased fluid accumulation. Cf *syringobulbia* and *syringomyelia*.

hydromyelocele (hi″dro-mi′el-o-sēl) [*hydro-* + *myelocele*] hydromyelomeningocele.

hydromyelomeningocele (hi″dro-mi″ĕ-lo-mĕ-ning′go-sēl) [*hydro-* + Gr. *myelos* marrow + *mēninx* membrane + *kēlē* hernia] a defect of the spine marked by protrusion of the membranes and tissue of the spinal cord, forming a fluid-filled sac.

hydromyoma (hi″dro-mi-o′mah) [*hydro-* + *myoma*] uterine leiomyoma with cystic degeneration.

hydronephrosis (hi″dro-nĕ-fro′sis) [*hydro-* + Gr. *nephros* kidney] distention of the pelvis and calices of the kidney with urine, as a result of obstruction of the ureter, with accompanying atrophy of the parenchyma of the organ. **closed h.,** a permanent condition, resulting from complete obstruction of the ureter. **open h.,** an intermittent condition, resulting from sporadic or incomplete obstruction of the ureter.

hydronephrotic (hi″dro-nĕ-frot′ik) pertaining to or characterized by hydronephrosis.

hydronium (hi-dro′ne-um) the hydrated proton, H_3O^+; it is the form in which the proton (hydrogen ion, H^+) exists in aqueous solution, a combination of H^+ and H_2O.

hydropancreatosis (hi″dro-pan″kre-ah-to′sis) the accumulation of watery fluid in the pancreas.

hydroparotitis (hi″dro-par″o-ti′tis) distention of the parotid gland with watery fluid.

hydropathic (hi″dro-path′ik) pertaining to hydropathy.

hydropathy (hi-drop′ah-the) [*hydro-* + Gr. *pathos* disease] (*obs.*) treatment of disease by the application of water; particularly a system of treatment which professes to cure all diseases by the use of water; water cure.

hydropenia (hi″dro-pe′ne-ah) [*hydro-* + Gr. *penia* poverty] deficiency of water in the body.

hydropenic (hi″dro-pe″nik) relating to hydropenia.

hydropericarditis (hi″dro-per″ĭ-kar-di′tis) pericarditis associated with a watery effusion in the pericardial sac.

hydropericardium (hi″dro-per″ĭ-kar′de-um) [*hydro-* + *pericardium*] abnormal accumulation of serous fluid in the pericardial cavity.

hydroperinephrosis (hi″dro-per″ĭ-nĕ-fro′sis) [*hydro-* + Gr. *peri* around + *nephros* kidney + *-osis*] a collection of fluid in the retroperitoneal connective tissue and opening into the pelvis of the kidney.

hydroperion (hi″dro-per′e-on) [*hydro-* + Gr. *peri* around + *ōon* egg] the fluid between the capsular and parietal decidua.

hydroperitoneum (hi″dro-per″ĭ-to-ne′um) [*hydro-* + *peritoneum*] ascites, or abnormal accumulation of fluid in the peritoneal cavity.

hydroperitonia (hi″dro-per″ĭ-to′ne-ah) ascites.

hydroperoxyeicosatetraenoic acid (hi″dro-per-ok″se-i-ko″sah-tet″rah-e-no′ik) any of several arachidonic acid metabolites produced by lipoxygenases. 5-HPETE (5-hydroperoxy-6,8,11,14-eicosatetraenoic acid) is the precursor of the leukotrienes. 12-HPETE (12-hydroperoxy-5,8,10,14-eicosatetraenoic acid is the precursor of 12-HETE, which is chemotactic for neutrophils and eosinophils.

hydropexia (hi″dro-pek′se-ah) hydropexis.

hydropexic (hi″dro-pek′sik) [*hydro-* + Gr. *pēxis* fixation] fixing or holding water; pertaining to the holding of water.

hydropexis (hi″dro-pek′sis) the fixation or holding of water.

hydrophagocytosis (hi″dro-fag″o-si-to′sis) [*hydro-* + *phagocytosis*] the absorption by macrophages of plasma surrounding them; called also *Lewis' phenomenon*.

hydrophil (hi′dro-fil) hydrophilic.

hydrophilia (hi-dro-fil′e-ah) [*hydro-* + Gr. *philein* to love + *-ia*] the property of absorbing water.

hydrophilic (hi″dro-fil′ik) readily absorbing moisture; hygroscopic; having strongly polar groups that readily interact with water.

hydrophilism (hi-drof′ĭ-lizm) hydrophilia.

hydrophilous (hi-drof′ĭ-lus) hydrophilic.

Hydrophiodae (hi-drof′ĭ-o-de) a family of venomous sea snakes of the Indo-Pacific region, characterized by an oarlike tail and immovable hollow fangs. See table accompanying *snake*.

hydrophobia (hi″dro-fo′be-ah) [*hydro-* + Gr. *phobein* to be affrighted by + *-ia*] 1. choking, gagging, and fear on attempts to drink in the acute neurologic phase of rabies, caused by pain from spasms of the pharynx or larynx. 2. former term for rabies. **paralytic h.,** see under *rabies*.

hydrophobic (hi″dro-fo′bik) 1. pertaining to or affected with hydrophobia (rabies). 2. not readily absorbing water, or being adversely affected by water, as a hydrophobic colloid. 3. lacking polar groups and, therefore, insoluble in water.

hydrophorograph (hi″dro-fo′ro-graf) [*hydro-* + Gr. *phora* a being borne, or carried along + *graphein* to record] an instrument for measuring and recording the pressure and/or flow of a fluid, especially the flow of urine or the pressure of the spinal fluid.

hydrophthalmia (hi″drof-thal′me-ah) hydrophthalmos; buphthalmos.

hydrophthalmos (hi″drof-thal′mos) [*hydro-* + Gr. *ophthalmos* eye] a form of glaucoma characterized by marked enlargement and distention of the fibrous coats of the eye; buphthalmos. **h. ante′rior,** that which affects the anterior portion of the eyeball only. **h. poste′rior,** that affecting the posterior part of the eyeball only. **h. tota′lis,** that which affects the entire eyeball.

hydrophthalmus (hi″drof-thal′mus) hydrophthalmos; buphthalmos.

hydrophysometra (hi″dro-fi″so-me′trah) [*hydro-* + *physometra*] physohydrometra.

hydrophyte (hi′dro-fīt) [Gr. *hydrō* water + *phyton* plant] a plant adapted to grow in a very wet environment, either completely aquatic or rooted in water or mud but with stems and leaves above the water.

hydropic (hi-drop′ik) [L. *hydropicus*; Gr. *hydrōpikos*] pertaining to or affected with dropsy.

hydroplasma (hi″dro-plaz′mah) [*hydro-* + Gr. *plasma* something formed] the watery or liquid part of the protoplasm.

hydropneumatosis (hi″dro-nu″mah-to′sis) [*hydro-* + Gr. *pneumatōsis* inflation] a collection of fluid and gas within the tissues.

hydropneumogony (hi″dro-nu-mo′go-ne) [*hydro-* + Gr. *pneuma* air + *gony* knee] the injection of air into a joint to detect effusion or other abnormality.

hydropneumopericardium (hi″dro-nu″mo-per″ĭ-kar′de-um) [*hydro-* + Gr. *pneuma* air + *pericardium*] a collection of watery fluid and gas within the pericardium.

hydropneumoperitoneum (hi″dro-nu″mo-per″ĭ-to-ne′um) [*hydro-* + Gr. *pneuma* air + *peritoneum*] a collection of watery fluid and gas in the peritoneal cavity.

hydropneumothorax (hi″dro-nu″mo-tho′raks) [*hydro-* + Gr. *pneuma* air + *thōrax* chest] a collection of fluid and gas within the pleural cavity.

hydroponics (hi″dro-pon′iks) the soil-less cultivation of plants on liquid media containing the necessary nutrient.

Hydropres (hi′dro-pres) trademark for preparations of hydrochlorothiazide with reserpine.

hydrops (hi′drops) [L.; Gr. *hydrōps*] the abnormal accumulation of serous fluid in the tissues or in a body cavity; called also *dropsy.* **h. abdom′inis,** ascites. **h. ad mat′-ulam,** polyuria. **h. am′nii,** hydramnios. **h. an′tri,** effusion of serous fluid into the maxillary sinus. **h. ar-tic′uli,** hydrarthrosis. **endolymphatic h.,** an accumulation of endolymph in the inner ear resulting in deafness and tinnitus, and sometimes vertigo (Meniere's disease); called also *labyrinthine h.* **fetal h., h. feta′lis,** gross edema of the entire body, associated with severe anemia, occurring in erythroblastosis fetalis. **h. follic′uli,** accumulation of fluid in the graafian follicle, forming a large solitary follicular cyst. **h. labyrin′thi, labyrinthine h.,** endolymphatic h. **h. pericar′dii,** hydropericardium. **h. spu′rius,** pseudomyxoma peritonaei. **h. tu′bae,** hydrosalpinx. **h. tu′bae prof′luens,** a condition in which the abdominal opening of the uterine tube becomes closed, and the tube may reach enormous proportions as it fills with serum; peristaltic action of the tube causes colicky pain, until the fluid escapes through the uterine opening. Called also *intermittent hydrosalpinx.*

hydropyonephrosis (hi″dro-pi″o-nĕ-fro′sis) [*hydro-* + Gr. *pyon* pus + *nephros* kidney + *-osis*] the accumulation of urine and pus in the pelvis of the kidney.

hydroquinone (hi″dro-kwin′ōn) [USP] chemical name: 1,4-benzenediol. A depigmenting agent, $C_6H_6O_2$, occurring as fine white needles; applied topically to the skin.

hydrorachis (hi-dror′ah-kis) [*hydro-* + Gr. *rhachis* spine] a collection of water in the vertebral canal.

hydrorachitis (hi″dro-rah-ki′tis) [*hydro-* + Gr. *rhachis* spine + *-itis*] inflammation within the vertebral canal, attended with a watery effusion.

hydrorrhea (hi″dro-re′ah) [*hydro-* + Gr. *rhoia* flow] a copious watery discharge. **h. gravida′rum,** a periodic or intermittent discharge of clear, yellowish, or bloody fluid from the uterus, caused by escape of amniotic fluid or resulting from decidual metritis. **nasal h.,** watery discharge from the nose.

hydrosalpinx (hi″dro-sal′pinks) [*hydro-* + Gr. *salpinx* trumpet] a collection of watery fluid in a uterine tube, occurring as the end-stage of pyosalpinx. **h. follicula′ris,** hydrosalpinx in which there is no central cystic cavity, the lumen being broken up into compartments as the result of fusion of the tubal plicae. **intermittent h.,** hydrops tubae profluens. **h. sim′plex,** hydrosalpinx characterized by excessive distention and thinning of the wall of the uterine tube, the plicae being few and widely separated.

hydrosarcocele (hi″dro-sar′ko-sēl) [*hydro-* + *sarcocele*] combined hydrocele and sarcocele.

hydroscope (hi″dro-skōp) [*hydro-* + Gr. *skopein* to examine] an instrument for detecting the presence of water.

hydrosol (hi′dro-sol) a sol in which the dispersion medium is water.

hydrosoluble (hi″dro-sol′u-b'l) soluble in water.

hydrosphygmograph (hi″dro-sfig′mo-graf) [*hydro-* + Gr. *sphygmos* pulse + *graphein* to record] a sphygmograph with water for an index.

hydrospirometer (hi″dro-spi-rom′ĕ-ter) [*hydro-* + L. *spirare* to breathe + Gr. *metron* measure] a spirometer in which a column of water serves as an index.

hydrostabile (hi″dro-sta′bil) preserving a stable weight under diet restrictions or gastrointestinal disease. Cf. *hydrolabile.*

hydrostat (hi′dro-stat) [*hydro-* + Gr. *histanai* to halt] a device by which the height of fluid in a container (column or reservoir) is regulated.

hydrostatic (hi″dro-stat′ik) [*hydro-* + Gr. *statikos* standing] pertaining to a liquid in a state of equilibrium; see under *pressure.*

hydrostatics (hi″dro-stat′iks) the science of liquids in a state of rest or equilibrium and of the pressures they exert.

hydrosynthesis (hi″dro-sin′the-sis) a chemical reaction in which water is formed.

hydrosyringomyelia (hi″dro-sĭ-ring″go-mi-e′le-ah) [*hydro-* + Gr. *syrinx* tube + *myelos* marrow] coexistence of hydromyelia and syringomyelia.

Hydrotaea (hi″dro-te′ah) a genus of flies. **H. meteor′ica,** a species which attacks the eyes and nostrils of man and animals.

hydrotaxis (hi″dro-tak′sis) [*hydro-* + Gr. *taxis* arrangement] an orientation movement of motile organisms or cells in response to stimulation by water or moisture.

hydrotherapeutics (hi″dro-ther″ah-pu′tiks) hydrotherapy.

hydrotherapy (hi″dro-ther′ah-pe) [*hydro-* + Gr. *therapeia* service done to the sick] 1. the application of water in any form, but usually externally, in the treatment of disease. 2. hydropathy.

hydrothermic (hi″dro-ther′mik) relating to the temperature effects of water, as in hot baths.

hydrothionammonemia (hi″dro-thi″o-nam″o-ne′me-ah) [*hydro-* + Gr. *theion* sulfur + *ammonium* + *haima* blood] the occurrence of ammonium hydrosulfide in the blood.

hydrothionemia (hi″dro-thi″o-ne′me-ah) [*hydro-* + Gr. *theion* sulfur + *haima* blood] the presence of hydrogen sulfide in the blood.

hydrothionuria (hi″dro-thi″o-nu′re-ah) [*hydro-* + Gr. *theion* sulfur + *ouron* urine + *-ia*] the presence of hydrogen sulfide in the urine.

hydrothorax (hi″dro-tho′raks) [*hydro-* + Gr. *thorax* chest] a collection of watery fluid in the pleural cavity; pleural effusion with transudate. **chylous h.,** the presence of chyle in the thoracic cavity, due to obstruction of or rupture of the thoracic duct.

hydrotomy (hi-drot′o-me) [*hydro-* + Gr. *tomē* a cutting] the dissection or separation of parts by the forcible injection of water.

hydrotropism (hi-drot′ro-pizm) [*hydro-* + Gr. *tropē* a turn, turning] a growth response of a nonmotile organism elicited by the presence of water or moisture.

hydrotubation (hi″dro-too-ba′shun) introduction of saline solution into the uterine tube; saline solution containing dye may be used in determining patency of the tube, and that containing hydrocortisone followed by chymotrypsin to maintain patency after salpingostomy.

hydroureter (hi″dro-u-re′ter) abnormal distention of the ureter with urine or with a watery fluid, due to obstruction from any cause; cf. *megaloureter.*

hydroureteronephrosis (hi″dro-u-re″ter-o-nĕfro′sis) [*hydro-* + *uretero-* + *nephr-* + *-osis*] distention of both the ureter and the renal pelvis and calices with urine because of obstruction of the ureter.

hydroureterosis (hi″dro-u-re″ter-o′sis) hydroureter.

hydrouria (hi″dro-u′re-ah) [*hydro-* + Gr. *ouron* urine + *-ia*] hydruria.

hydrous (hi′drus) containing water.

hydrovarium (hi″dro-va′re-um) [*hydro-* + L. *ovarium* ovary] a collection of serous fluid in an ovary.

hydroxide (hi-drok′sīd) any compound of hydroxyl radical (OH), or of hydroxide ion, OH⁻, with another radical or atom. **ferric h.,** the hydrated oxide of iron, $Fe(OH)_3$, a reddish brown substance, formerly used as an antidote in arsenic poisoning. Called also *iron hydroxide.*

hydroxocobalamin (hi-drok″so-ko-bal′ah-min) [USP] chemical name: cobinamide dihydroxide, dihydrogen phosphate (ester), mono(inner salt),3′-ester with 5,6-dimethyl-1-α-D-ribofuranosylbenzimidazole. An analogue of cyanocobalamin, $C_{62}H_{89}CoN_{13}O_{15}P$, in which the cyanide ion is replaced with a hydroxyl ion, occurring as dark red crystals or as a red crystalline powder; it possesses exceptionally long-acting hematopoietic activity. Called also *vitamin B₁₂ᵦ.*

hydroxy- (hi-drok′se) a chemical prefix indicating presence of the univalent radical OH.

hydroxyacetanilide (hi-drok″se-as″ĕ-tan′ĭ-lid) acetaminophen.

3-hydroxyacyl-CoA dehydrogenase (hi-drok″se-as′il de-hi′dro-jĕ-nās) [EC 1.1.1.35] an enzyme of the oxidoreductase class that catalyzes the reaction (S)-3-hydroxyacyl-CoA + NAD $^+$ = 3-ketoacyl-CoA + NADH. The reaction is one of the steps in fatty acid oxidation.

hydroxyacylglutathione hydrolase (hi-drok″se-as″il-gloo″ah-thi′ōn hi′dro-lās) [EC 3.1.2.6] an enzyme of the hydrolase class that catalyzes the reaction S-(2-hydroxyacyl) glutathione + H_2O = gluthathione + 2-hydroxy acid anion. The enzyme is found in red cells and other animal tissues. It converts glyoxal into lactic acid and substituted glyoxals to the corresponding hydroxy acid. Formerly called *glyoxalase II*.

hydroxyamphetamine hydrobromide (hi-drok″se-am-fet′ah-mēn) [USP] chemical name: 4-(2-aminopropyl)-phenol hydrobromide. An adrenergic, $C_9H_{13}NO \cdot HBr$, occurring as a white, crystalline powder; used as a mydriatic, applied topically to the conjunctiva. It is also used topically as a nasal decongestant and orally as a pressor agent in the treatment of heart block, carotid sinus syndrome, and postural hypotension.

hydroxyapatite (hi-drok″se-ap′ah-tīt) an inorganic compound, $Ca_{10}(PO_4)_6(OH)_2$, found in the matrix of bone and the teeth, which gives rigidity to these structures.

hydroxybenzene (hi-drok″se-ben′zēn) phenol.

3-hydroxybutyrate dehydrogenase (hi-drok″se-bu′tĭ-rāt de-hi′dro-jĕ-nās) an enzyme of the oxidoreductase class that catalyzes the reaction D-3-hydroxybutyrate + NAD $^+$ = acetoacetate + NADH. The enzyme functions in nervous tissues and muscles, enabling use of circulating hydroxybutyrate as a fuel. Called also *beta-hydroxybutyrate dehydrogenase*.

hydroxybutyric acid (hi-drok″se-bu′tĭ-rik) a poisonous acid, $CH_3CHOHCH_2COOH$, sometimes occurring in the urine in diabetes (ketoacidosis) and sometimes in the blood; it frequently occurs in several isomeric forms. Called also *oxybutyric a.* See also *beta-oxybutyric a.*

β-hydroxybutyric acid (hi-drok″se-bu-ter-ik) 3-hydroxybutanoic acid, $CH_3CHOH CH_2COOH$, one of the ketone bodies (q.v.) produced in diabetic ketoacidosis.

β-hydroxybutyric dehydrogenase (hi-drok″se-bu-tĭ′rik de-hi′dro-jĕ-nās) 3-hydroxybutyrate dehydrogenase.

hydroxychloroquine sulfate (hi-drok″se-klo′ro-kwin) [USP] chemical name: 7-chloro-4-{4-[ethyl(2-hydroxyethyl) amino]-1-methylbutylamino}-quinoline sulfate. A quinoline derivative, $C_{18}H_{26}ClN_3O \cdot H_2SO_4$, occurring as a white or nearly white, crystalline powder; used as an antimalarial and as a lupus erythematosus suppressant, administered orally. It has also been used in the treatment of rheumatoid arthritis and symptomatic cases of giardiasis.

25-hydroxycholecalciferol (hi-drok″se-ko″le-kal-sif′ĕ-rol) a metabolically activated form of vitamin D (cholecalciferol), which is synthesized in the liver. It is the precursor of 1,25-dihydroxycholecalciferol. Called also *calcidiol* and *calcifediole*.

17-hydroxycorticosteroid (hi-drok″se-kor″tĭ-ko-ste′-roid) any adrenocorticosteroid with a dihydroxyacetone side chain, including hydrocortisone (cortisol) and 11-deoxycortisone. Abbreviated 17-OH-CS. Called also *Porter-Silber chromogen*.

17-hydroxycorticosterone (hi-drok″se-kor″tĭ-ko-ster′ōn) hydrocortisone.

hydroxydione sodium succinate (hi-drok″se-di′ōn) chemical name: 21-(3-carboxy-1-oxopropoxy)-5β-pregnane-3,20-dione sodium succinate. A steroid, $C_{25}H_{35}NaO_6$, used as a general anesthetic, administered intravenously.

hydroxyeicosatetraenoic acid (hi-drok″se-i-ko″sah-tet rah-e-no′ik) any of several arachidonic acid metabolites produced by peroxidases from HPETE (hydroperoxyeicosatetraenoic acid). 5-HETE (5-hydroxy-6,8,11,14-eicosatetraenoic acid) is a byproduct of leukotriene metabolism. 12-HETE (12-hydroxy-5,8,10,14-eicosatetraenoic acid) and 5,12-HETE (5,12-dihydroxy-6,8,10,14-eicosatetraenoic acid) are chemotactic for neutrophils and eosinophils.

25-hydroxyergocalciferol (hi″drok-se-er″go-kal-sif′ĕ-rol) an activated form of vitamin D (ergocalciferol) synthesized in the liver.

hydroxyestrin benzoate (hi-drok″se-es′trin) estradiol benzoate.

hydroxyformobenzoylic acid (hi-drok″se-for″mo-ben″zo-il′ik) a crystalline compound, parahydroxyphenyl-glycolic acid, $OH-C_6H_4 \cdot CHOH \cdot COOH$, sometimes occurring in the urine in acute yellow atrophy of the liver; called also *oxyamygdalic a.*, *oxyformobenzoylic a.*, and *oxymandelic a.*

hydroxyheptadecatrienoic acid (hi-drok″se-hep″tah-dek″ah-tri-e-no′ik) HHT, a prostaglandin metabolite (12-L-hydroxy-5,8,10-heptadecatrienoic acid) that is a chemoattractant for neutrophils and eosinophils.

5-hydroxyindoleacetic acid (hi-drok″se-in″dōl-ah-se′tik) a product of serotonin metabolism excreted in large amounts in patients with carcinoid tumors. Abbreviated 5-HIAA.

3-hydroxyisobutyryl-CoA hydrolase (hi-drok″se-i″so-bu′tĭ-ril hi′dro-lās) [EC 3.1.2.4] an enzyme of the hydrolase class that catalyzes the reaction 3-hydroxy-2-methylpropanoyl-CoA + H_2O = CoA + 3-hydroxy-2-methylpropanoate. The reaction is a step in the use of valine as a fuel.

hydroxyl (hi-drok′sil) the univalent radical OH.

hydroxylapatite (hi″drok-sil″ap′ah-tīt) hydroxyapatite.

hydroxylase (hi-drok′sĭ-lās) [EC 1.13 or 1.14] an enzyme of the oxidoreductase class that catalyzes the formation of a hydroxyl group on a substrate by incorporation of oxygen from O_2. Most are monooxygenases incorporating one atom of oxygen; more rarely the term is applied to a dioxygenase hydroxylating two substrates. **11β-h.,** steroid 11β-monooxygenase. **17-h.,** steroid 17α-monooxygenase. **21-h.,** steroid 21-monooxygenase. **24-h.,** 5β-cholestane-3α,7α,-12α,25-24S-hydroxylase.

hydroxylysine (hi″drok-sil′ĭ-sin) one of the alpha amino acids, $NH_2 \cdot CH_2 \cdot CHOH(CH_2)_2 \cdot CH(NH_2) \cdot COOH$.

hydroxymethylglutaryl-CoA lyase (hi-drok″se-meth″-il-gloo″tah-ril li′ās) [EC 4.1.3.4] an enzyme of the lyase class that catalyzes the reaction (S)-3-hydroxy-3-methyl-glutaryl-CoA = acetyl-CoA + acetoacetate. The reaction occurs in the liver or kidneys. It is a step in the ketogenic path of fatty acid oxidation, which is exaggerated in diabetes or starvation and in the use of leucine as a fuel. Genetic deficiency of the enzyme leads to ketoacidosis and hypoglycemia.

3-hydroxy-3-methylglutaryl CoA (HMG CoA) lyase deficiency a genetic aminoacidopathy due to deficient HMG CoA lyase, the last enzyme in the leucine catabolic pathway. Severe hypoglycemia and acidemia result, giving the urine a strong odor of tom cat. The disorder begins a few days after birth and can cause quick death, but it is treatable by dietary restriction of leucine and supplement of glucose against hypoglycemia, with normal development thereafter.

hydroxymethyltransferase (hi-drok″se-meth″il-trans′fer-ās) [EC 2.1.2] an enzyme of the transferase class that catalyzes the transfer of a hydroxymethyl group from one compound to another.

hydroxynervone (hi-drok″se-ner′vōn) a cerebroside occurring in brain tissue.

hydroxyphenamate (hi-drok″se-fen′ah-māt) chemical name: 2-phenyl-1,2-butanediol-1-carbamate; a minor tranquilizer, $C_{11}H_{15}NO_3$, formerly used in the treatment of anxiety and tension.

hydroxyphenylethylamine (hi-drok″se-phen″il- eth″il-am′in) tyramine.

4-hydroxyphenylpyruvate dioxygenase (hi″drok″se-phen″il-pi′roo-vat di-ok′sĭ″jĕ-nās) [EC 1.13.11.27] an enzyme of the oxidoreductase class that catalyzes the reaction 4-hydroxyphenylpyruvate + O_2 = homogentisate + CO_2. The reaction is a step in the use of tyrosine and phenylalanine as fuels. Genetic deficiency of the enzyme has been postulated as the cause of tyrosinosis. Called also *p-hydroxyphenylpyruvate oxidase*.

p-hydroxyphenylpyruvate oxidase (hi-drok″se-phen″-il-pi′roo-vāt ok′sĭ-dās) 4-hydroxyphenylpyruvate dioxygenase.

hydroxyprogesterone caproate (hi-drok″se-pro-jest′-ter-ōn) [USP] chemical name: 17α-[(1-oxohexyl)oxy] pregna-4-ene-3,20-dione. A synthetic progestin, $C_{27}H_{40}O_4$, occurring as a white or creamy white, crystalline powder; used in the treatment of dysfunctional uterine bleeding, abnormalities of the menstrual cycle, endometriosis, and endometrial cancer, administered intramuscularly. Called also *h. hexanoate.*

hydroxyproline (hi-drok″se-pro′lin) an amino acid, gamma-hydroxy-alpha-pyrrolidin-carboxylic acid, produced in the digestion or hydrolytic decomposition of proteins, especially of collagens.

hydroxyprolinemia (hi-drok″se-pro″len-e′me-ah) [*hydroxyproline* + *-emia*] a disorder of amino acid metabolism characterized by an excess of free hydroxyproline in the plasma and urine, due to a defect in the enzyme hydroxyproline oxidase; it may be associated with mental retardation. Called also *4-hydroxy-L-proline oxidase deficiency.*

hydroxyproline oxidase (hi-drok″se-pro′len ok′sĭ-dās) an enzyme of the oxidoreductase class that catalyzes the reaction 4-hydroxy-L-proline + O_2 = Δ'-pyrroline-3-hydroxy-5-carboxylic acid. The reaction occurs in the degradation of free hydroxyproline. Defect of the enzyme, an autosomal recessive trait, results in hyperhydroxyprolinemia.

4-hydroxy-L-proline oxidase deficiency hydroxyprolinemia.

hydroxypropyl methylcellulose (hi-drok″sĭ-pro′pil) chemical name: cellulose 2-hydroxypropyl methyl ether. The propylene glycol ether of methylcellulose, occurring as a white to slightly off-white, fibrous or granular powder, and supplied in differing degrees of viscosity; used as a suspending and viscosity-increasing agent and tablet excipient in pharmaceutical preparations, and applied topically to the conjunctiva to protect the cornea during certain ophthalmic procedures and to lubricate the cornea.

17-hydroxysteroid (hi-drok″se-ste′roid) an excretion product of adrenocorticosteroids; usually used as a synonym for 17-hydroxycorticosteroid.

3β-hydroxy-Δ⁵-steroid dehydrogenase (hi-drok″se-ste′roid de-hi′dro-jĕ-nās) [EC 1.1.1.145] an enzyme of the oxidoreductase class that catalyzes the reaction 3β-hydroxy-Δ^5-steroid + NAD^+ = 3-keto-Δ^5-steroid + NADH. The reaction is a step in the biosynthesis of adrenal corticosteroids. A genetic defect of the enzyme causes accumulation of 17-hydroxypregnenolone in the blood and results in congenital adrenal hyperplasia II.

hydroxystilbamidine isethionate (hi-drok″se-stil-bam′ĭ-dēn) [USP] chemical name: 4-[2-[4-(aminoiminomethyl)phenyl]ethenyl]-3-hydroxybenzenecarboximidamide bis-(2-hydroxyethanesulfonate) (salt). An antifungal and antiprotozoal, $C_{16}H_{16}N_4O \cdot 2C_2H_6O_4S$, occurring as a fine, yellow, crystalline powder; used as an antileishmanial, administered by intramuscular or intravenous infusion. It has also been used in the treatment of some fungal infections, such as North American blastomycosis.

5-hydroxytryptamine (hi-drok″se-trip′tah-mēn) serotonin.

hydroxyurea (hi-drok″se-u-re′ah) [USP] a compound, H_2-$N \cdot CO \cdot NH \cdot OH$, that is an inhibitor of the enzyme ribonucleoside diphosphate reductase, which catalyzes the conversion of ribonucleotides to deoxyribonucleotides, an essential step in DNA synthesis; it is used as an antineoplastic agent primarily for treatment of busulfan-resistant chronic granulocytic leukemia. The major side effect is bone marrow depression.

hydroxyvaline (hi-drok″se-val′in) an amino acid obtained by protein hydrolysis.

hydroxyzine (hi-drok′sĭ-zēn) chemical name: 2-[2-[4-[(4-chlorophenyl)phenylmethyl]- 1- piperazinyl]ethoxy]ethanol. A synthetic drug, $C_{21}H_{27}ClN_2O_2$, with central nervous system depressant, antispasmodic, antihistaminic, and antifibrillatory actions. **h. hydrochloride** [USP], the dihydrochloride salt of hydroxyzine, $C_{21}H_{27}ClN_2O_2 \cdot 2HCl$, occurring as white powder; used in the treatment of anxiety, tension, and agitation in conditions of emotional stress, in acute and chronic urticaria and other manifestations of allergic dermatoses, as an antiemetic, and as pre- and postoperative sedative, administered orally or intramuscularly. **h. pamoate** [USP], the pamoate salt of hydroxyzine, $C_{21}H_{27}Cl$-$N_2O_2 \cdot C_{23}H_{16}O_6$, occurring as light yellow powder, having the actions and uses of the hydrochloride salt; administered orally.

Hydrozoa (hi″dro-zo′ah) [Gr. *Hydra* a mythical nine-headed monster + *zoon* animal] a class of coelenterates that usually possess colonial branching polyps and small medusae, including the genus *Physalia* (Portuguese man-of-war).

hydrozoan (hi″dro-zo′an) an individual of the class Hydrozoa.

hydruria (hi-droo′re-ah) [*hydr-* + Gr. *ouron* urine + *-ia*] excretion of urine of low osmolality or specific gravity.

hydruric (hi-droo′rik) characterized by hydruria.

hyenanchin (hi″ĕ-nan′kin) a poisonous substance, $C_{15}H_{18}$-O_7, from the outer envelopes of the fruit of *Hyaenanche globosa*, of South Africa. It somewhat resembles strychnine in its action.

Hygeia (hi-je′ah) [Gr. *Hygieia*] the goddess of health, one of the daughters of Aesculapius.

hygieist (hi-je′ist) hygienist.

hygiene (hi′jēn) [Gr. *hygieia* health] the science of health and of its preservation. **dental h.,** oral h. **industrial h.,** that branch of preventive medicine which is concerned with the protection of health of the industrial population. **mental h.,** (*obs.*) the science which deals with the development of healthy mental and emotional reactions and habits; psychophylaxis. **mouth h.,** oral h. **oral h.,** the personal maintenance of cleanliness and hygiene of the teeth and oral structures by toothbrushing, tissue stimulation, gum massage, hydrotherapy, and other procedures recommended by the dentist or dental hygienist for the preservation of dental and oral health. Called also *dental h.* and *mouth h.* **radiation h.,** the science of practices involved in human protection from radiation injury.

hygienic (hi″je-en′ik) pertaining to hygiene, or conducive to health.

hygienics (hi″je-en′iks) a system of principles for promoting health; hygiene.

hygienist (hi-je′nist, hi″je-en′ist) a specialist in hygiene. **dental h.,** a dental auxiliary specially trained in dental prophylaxis, who meets certain prescribed standards of education and clinical competence. Dental hygienists work under the direct supervision of the dentist; their functions include scaling and polishing the teeth, dental radiography, and teaching oral hygiene. Some states permit them to apply fluoride solution to the teeth.

hygienization (hi″je-en″i-za′shun) the establishment of hygienic conditions.

hygieology (hi″je-ol′o-je) [Gr. *hygieia* health + *-logy*] the complete science upon which the arts of hygiene and sanitation are based.

hygiogenesis (hi″je-o-jen′ĕ-sis) [Gr. *hygiēs* healthy + *gennan* to produce] the mechanism of the processes which lead to maintenance of health.

hygiology (hi″je-ol′o-je) hygieology.

hygrechema (hi″grĕ-ke′mah) an auscultation sound caused by the presence of water.

hygric (hi′grik) [Gr. *hygros* moist] pertaining or relating to moisture.

hygr(o)- [Gr. *hygros* moist] a combining form meaning moist or denoting relationship to moisture.

hygroblepharic (hi″gro-blĕ-far′ik) [*hygro-* + Gr. *blepharon* eyelid] 1. denoting an excessive watery condition of the eyelids. 2. pertaining to any gland bringing moisture to the eyelids.

hygroma (hi-gro′mah), pl. *hygro′mas* or *hygro′mata* [*hygro-* + *-oma*] a sac, cyst, or bursa distended with a fluid. **h. col′li,** a watery tumor of the neck. **cystic h., h. cys′ticum,** a cystic lymphangioma, often very large, usually occurring in the neck area, and composed of large, multiocular, thin-walled cysts. Called also *cavernous* or *cystic lymphangioma* and *lymphangioma cavernosum* or *cysticum.* **h. praepatella′re,** housemaid's knee. **subdural h.,** a collection of fluid in the subdural space resulting from liquefaction of a subdural hematoma; see under *hematoma.*

hygromatous (hi-gro′mah-tus) pertaining to or of the nature of hygroma.

hygrometer (hi-grom′ĕ-ter) [*hygro-* + Gr. *metron* measure] an instrument for measuring the moisture of the atmosphere. **hair h., Saussure's h.,** a hygrometer whose action is determined by the elongation and contraction of a hair under the influence of moisture.

hygrometric (hi″gro-met′rik) pertaining to hygrometry.

hygrometry (hi-grom′ĕ-tre) [*hygro-* + Gr. *metron* measure] the measurement of the proportion of moisture in the air.

hygromycin (hi″gro-mi′sin) an antibiotic, $C_{23}H_{29}NO_{12}$, produced by *Streptomyces hygroscopicus* and *S. noboritoensis;* called also *hygromycin A.* **h. B,** an anthelmintic, $C_{15}H_{28}$-O_{10}, used in swine.

hygroscopic (hi″gro-skop′ik) taking up and retaining moisture readily.

Hygroton (hi′gro-ton) trademark for a preparation of chlorthalidone.

Hykinone (hi′kin-ōn) trademark for a preparation of menadione sodium bisulfite.

hyla (hi′lah) (*obs.*) a lateral extension of the aqueduct of Sylvius (aqueductus cerebri).

hyle (hi′le) [Gr. *hylē* matter] the theoretical primitive substance from which all matter was once thought to be composed. See *protyl.*

hyle- see *hyl(o)-*.

Hylemyia (hi″lĕ-mi′ah) a genus of flies, the larvae of which infest vegetables and may be swallowed if the latter are eaten raw. *H. anti′qua,* onion root maggot. *H. bras′icae,* the cabbage root maggot.

hylergography (hi″ler-gog′rah-fe) [Gr. *hylē* matter + *ergon* work + *graphein* to write] a recording of the effect of environmental materials on a cell.

hylic (hi′lik) [Gr. *hylē* matter] composed of matter; a term applied by Adami to the pulp tissues of the embryo.

hyl(o)-, hyle- [Gr. *hylē* matter] a combining form denoting relationship to matter, material, or substance.

hylopathism (hi-lop′ah-thizm) [*hylo-* + Gr. *pathos* disease] the obsolete doctrine that disease is due to changes in the constitution of matter.

hylotropic (hi″lo-trop′ik) pertaining to or characterized by hylotropy.

hylotropy (hi-lot′ro-pe) [Gr. *hylē* matter + *tropē* a turn, turning] the ability of a substance to change from one physical form to another (e.g., solid to liquid, liquid to gas) without change in chemical composition; change of phase.

hylozoism (hi-lo′zo-izm) [*hylo-* + Gr. *zōon* animal] the doctrine that all matter in the universe is alive.

hymecromone (hi″mĕ-kro′mōn) chemical name: 7-hydroxy-4-methyl-2*H*-1-benzopyran-2-one; a choleretic and biliary antispasmodic, $C_{10}H_8O_3$.

hymen (hi′men) [Gr. *hymēn* membrane] [NA] the membranous fold which partially or wholly occludes the external orifice of the vagina. **annular h.,** circular g. **h. bifenestra′tus, h. bifo′ris,** a hymen with two openings side by side and a broad septum between them. **circular h.,** a hymen with a circular opening. **cribriform h.,** a hymen pierced by many small perforations. **denticular h.,** a hymen with an opening which has serrate edges. **falciform h.,** a sickle-shaped hymen. **fenestrated h.,** cribriform h. **imperforate h.,** one which completely closes the vaginal orifice. **infundibuliform h.,** a hymen that has a central opening with sloping sides. **lunar h.,** a moon-shaped hymen. **septate h., h. sep′tus,** a hymen in which the opening is divided by a narrow septum. **h. subsep′tus,** a hymen in which the opening is partially filled by a septum growing out of one wall, but not reaching the other.

hymenal (hi′men-al) pertaining to the hymen.

hymenectomy (hi″men-ek′to-me) [*hymeno-* + Gr. *ektomē* excision] excision of the hymen.

hymenitis (hi″men-i′tis) [*hymen-* + *-itis*] inflammation of the hymen.

hymenium (hi-me′ne-um) [dim. of Gr. *hymēn* membrane] the fertile, or spore-forming, surface of a fungus, which is composed of hyphae lining the fruiting body.

hymen(o)- [Gr. *hymēn* membrane] a combining form denoting a relationship to a membrane or a membranous structure, or to the hymen.

hymenolepiasis (hi″mĕ-no-lep-i′ah-sis) infection with *Hymenolepis.*

Hymenolepididae (hi″men-o-lep′ĭ-di-de) a family of small to medium-sized tapeworms of the order Cyclophyllidea, subclass Cestoda, which parasitizes birds and mammals, including man. *Hymenolepis* is the genus of medical importance.

Hymenolepis (hi″mĕ-nol′ĕ-pis) [Gr. *hymēn* membrane + *lepis* rind] a genus of tapeworms of the family Hymenolepididae. **H. diminu′ta,** a tapeworm of rats

and mice, occasionally found in man. **H. frater′na,** the rodent form of *H. nana;* often called *H. nana* var. *fraterna.* **H. lanceola′ta,** *Drepanidotaenia lanceolata.* **H. na′na,** the dwarf tapeworm, a species about 7 to 80 mm. long that is parasitic in rats, mice, and man, especially children. Infected persons are usually asymptomatic, but in massive infection symptoms may include dizziness, abdominal pain, diarrhea, insomnia, convulsions, etc. **H. na′na** var. **frater′na,** *H. fraterna.*

hymenology (hi″men-ol′o-je) [*hymeno-* + *-logy*] the sum of what is known regarding the membranes of the body.

Hymenomycetes (hi″mĕ-no-mi-se′tēz) [*hymeno-* + Gr. *mykēs* fungus] a series of fungi of the subclass Homobasidiomycetes, class Basidiomycetes, including the orders Polyporales and Agaricales.

Hymenoptera (hi″men-op′ter-ah) [*hymeno-* + Gr. *pteron* wing] an order of insects usually having two pairs of well developed membranous wings, as the bees, wasps, ants, etc.

hymenopteran (hi″men-op′ter-an) any insect of the order Hymenoptera.

hymenopterism (hi″men-op′ter-izm) poisoning by the stings or bites of insects of the order Hymenoptera, as of a bee or wasp.

hymenorrhaphy (hi″men-or′ah-fe) [*hymeno-* + Gr. *rhaphē* seam] the closure of the vagina by sutures at the hymen.

Hymenostomatia (hi″mĕ-no-sto-ma′she-ah) [*hymeno-* + Gr. *stoma* mouth] a subclass of chiefly freshwater, ciliate protozoa (class Oligohymenophorea, phylum Ciliophora) with uniform, heavy body ciliature and a ventral buccal cavity when one is present; if kinetodesmata are present, they are usually conspicuous. It comprises three orders: Hymenostomatida, Scuticociliatida, and Astomatida.

Hymenostomatida (hi″mĕ-no-sto-ma′tĭ-dah) an order of ciliate protozoa (subclass Hymenostomatia, class Oligohymenophorea) characterized by the presence of a well-defined buccal cavity containing membranelles or peniculi with infraciliary bases typically three to four rows of kinetosomes wide; and by a ventral oral area, usually in the anterior half of the body. It comprises three suborders: Tetrahymenina, Ophryoglenina, and Peniculina.

hymenotomy (hi″men-ot′o-me) [*hymeno-* + Gr. *temnein* to cut] surgical incision of the hymen.

hyobasioglossus (hi″o-ba″se-o-glos′us) the basal part of the hyoglossus muscle.

hyodeoxycholaneresis (hi″o-de-ok″se-ko″lah-ner′ĕ-sis) [*hyodeoxycholic* acid + Gr. *hairesis* a taking] (*obs.*) increase in the output or elimination of hyodeoxycholic acid in the bile. Cf. *cholaneresis.*

hyodeoxycholic acid (hi″o-de-ok″se-ko′lik) 3,6-dihydroxycholanic acid, a major bile acid of the hog.

hyoepiglottic (hi″o-ep″ĭ-glot′ik) pertaining to the hyoid bone and the epiglottis.

hyoepiglottidean (hi″o-ep″ĭ-glo-tid′e-an) hyoepiglottic.

hyoglossal (hi″o-glos′al) [hyoid bone + Gr. *glōssa* tongue] pertaining to the hyoid bone and the tongue or to the hyoglossal muscle.

hyoid (hi′oid) [Gr. *hyoeides* shaped like the Greek letter upsilon (υ)] 1. shaped like the lower case Greek letter upsilon (υ). Cf. *hypsiloid.* 2. pertaining to the hyoid bone.

hyoscine (hi′o-sin) [L. *hyoscina*] scopolamine.

hyoscyamine (hi″o-si′ah-min) [USP] chemical name: [3(S)-endo]-α-(hydroxymethyl)benzeneacetic acid 8-methyl-8-azabicyclo[3.2.1]oct-3-yl ester. An anticholinergic alkaloid, $C_{17}H_{23}NO_3$, derived from *Hyoscyamus niger, Atropa belladonna,* and other solanaceous plants, occurring as a white, crystalline powder; it is the levorotatory component of racemic atropine with actions and uses similar to those of atropine but with more potent central and peripheral effects. It is administered orally or parenterally. **h. hydrobromide** [USP], a salt of hyoscyamine, $C_{17}H_{23}NO_3HBr$, occurring as white crystals or as a crystalline powder, having actions and uses similar to those of atropine, administered orally or parenterally. **h. sulfate** [USP], a salt of hyoscyamine, $(C_{17}H_{23}NO_3)_2 \cdot H_2SO_4 \cdot 2H_2O$, occurring as white crystals or as a crystalline powder, having actions and uses similar to those of atropine, administered orally or parenterally.

Hyoscyamus (hi″o-si′ah-mus) [L.; Gr. *hys* swine + *kyamos* bean] a genus of annual or biennial solanaceous plants;

the leaves, seeds, flowers, and tops of *H. ni'ger* L. contain the anticholinergic alkaloids hyoscyamine and scopolamine.

hyoscyamus (hi"o-si'ah-mus) the dried leaf of *Hyoscyamus niger* L., with or without its stem and top, which contains the anticholinergic alkaloids hyoscyamine and scopolamine; formerly used as a smooth muscle relaxant and to produce parasympathetic blockade. Called also *henbane* and *black henbane*.

Hyostrongylus rubidus (hi"o-stron'ji-lus roo'bi-dus) a small red nematode worm found in the stomach of pigs.

hyothyroid (hi"o-thi'roid) pertaining to the hyoid bone and the thyroid cartilage.

hypacidemia (hi-pas"i-de'me-ah) [Gr. *hypo* under + *acid* + *haima* blood] deficiency of an acid in the blood.

hypacusia (hi"pah-ku'ze-ah) hypoacusis.

hypacusis (hi"pah-ku'sis) [Gr. *hypo* under + *akousis* hearing] hypoacusis.

hypalbuminemia (hi"pal-bu"mi-ne'me-ah) hypoalbuminemia.

hypalgesia (hi"pal-je'ze-ah) [Gr. *hypo* under + *algēsis* pain] diminished sensitiveness to pain.

hypalgesic (hi"pal-je'sik) pertaining to, characterized by, or producing hypalgesia.

hypalgetic (hi"pal-jet'ik) hypalgesic.

hypalgia (hi-pal'je-ah) hypalgesia.

hypamnion (hi-pam'ne-on) hypamnios.

hypamnios (hi-pam'ne-os) [Gr. *hypo* under + *amnion*] deficiency of the amniotic fluid.

hypanakinesia (hi-pan"ah-ki-ne'ze-ah) [Gr. *hypo* under + *anakinēsis* exercise + *-ia*] hypokinesia.

hypanakinesis (hi-pan"ah-ki-ne'sis) hypokinesia.

hypaphorine (hi-paf'o-rin) a crystalline alkaloid, $C_{14}H_{18}N_2O_2$, obtained from *Erythrina americana* Mill., and other members of the leguminosae; it is a convulsive poisonous alkaloid.

Hypaque (hi'pāk) trademark for preparations of diatrizoate meglumine and diatrizoate sodium.

hyparterial (hi"par-te're-al) [Gr. *hypo* under + *artēria* artery] beneath an artery, applied especially to the bronchi which are so situated.

hypaxial (hi-pak'se-al) ventral to the long axis of the body.

hypazoturia (hi-paz"o-tu're-ah) [Gr. *hypo* under + *azoturia*] excretion of urine of low nitrogen concentration.

hypencephalon (hi"pen-sef'ah-lon) [Gr. *hypo* under + *enkephalos* brain] (*obs.*) the mesencephalon, pons, and medulla.

hypenchyme (hi'pen-kim) the primitive embryonic tissue formed in the cavity of the archenteron.

hyper- [Gr. *hyper* above] a prefix meaning above, beyond, more than normal, or excessive.

hyperabsorption (hi"per-ab-sorp'shun) increased intestinal absorption of a substance.

hyperacanthosis (hi"per-ak"an-tho'sis) [*hyper-* + Gr. *akantha* prickle + *-osis*] acanthosis.

hyperacid (hi"per-as'id) [*hyper-* + L. *acidus* sour] abnormally or excessively acid.

hyperacidaminuria (hi"per-as"id-am"i-nu're-ah) excess of amino acids in the urine.

hyperacidity (hi"per-ah-sid'i-te) an excessive degree of acidity. **gastric h.,** hyperchlorhydria.

hyperacousia (hi"per-ah-koo'ze-ah) hyperacusis.

hyperactive (hi"per-ak'tiv) pertaining to or characterized by hyperactivity; hyperkinetic.

hyperactivity (hi"per-ak-tiv'i-te) excessive or abnormally increased activity; hyperkinesis, hyperkinesia. For hyperactivity in children see *attention-deficit hyperactivity disorder,* under *disorder*.

hyperacusia (hi"per-ah-ku'ze-ah) hyperacusis.

hyperacusis (hi"per-ah-ku'sis) [*hyper-* + Gr. *akousis* hearing] an exceptionally acute sense of hearing, the hearing threshold being unusually low. The term has been used to denote a painful sensitiveness to sounds, but there is no necessary relationship between the threshold of hearing and that of discomfort.

hyperacute (hi"per-ah-kūt') extremely acute.

hyperadenosis (hi"per-ad"ĕ-no'sis) [*hyper-* + Gr. *adēn* gland + *-osis*] a condition characterized by enlargement of the glands.

hyperadiposis (hi"per-ad"i-po'sis) [*hyper-* + *adiposis*] extreme adiposity or fatness.

hyperadiposity (hi"per-ad"i-pos'i-te) hyperadiposis.

hyperadrenalism (hi"per-ah-dre'nal-izm) abnormally increased secretory activity of the adrenal gland.

hyperadrenocorticism (hi"per-ah-dre"no-kor'ti-sizm) a condition characterized by abnormally increased functional activity of the cortex of the adrenal gland. See *Cushing's syndrome* (def. 1), under *syndrome*.

hyperakusis (hi"per-ah-koo'sis) hyperacusis.

hyperalbuminemia (hi"per-al-bu"mi-ne'me-ah) an abnormally high albumin content of the blood.

hyperalbuminosis (hi"per-al-bu"mi-no'sis) a condition characterized by presence of an excess of albuminoids.

hyperaldosteronemia (hi"per-al"do-stēr"ōn-e'me-ah) abnormal increase in the level of aldosterone in the blood.

hyperaldosteronism (hi"per-al"do-ster'ōn-izm) aldosteronism.

hyperaldosteronuria (hi"per-al"do-stēr"ōn-u're-ah) the presence of excessive amounts of aldosterone in the urine.

hyperalgesia (hi"per-al-je'ze-ah) [*hyper-* + Gr. *algēsis* pain] excessive sensitiveness or sensibility to pain. **auditory h.,** the condition in which slight noises cause pain. **muscular h.,** the condition in which slight exertion causes great pain.

hyperalgesic (hi"per-al-je'sik) pertaining to or characterized by hyperalgesia.

hyperalgetic (hi"per-al-jet'ik) hyperalgesic.

hyperalgia (hi-per-al'je-ah) [*hyper-* + *-algia*] hyperalgesia.

hyperalimentation (hi"per-al"i-men-ta'shun) the ingestion or administration of a greater than optimal amount of nutrients. **parenteral h.,** see *total parenteral alimentation,* under *alimentation*.

hyperalimentosis (hi"per-al"i-men-to'sis) disease due to excess in eating.

hyperalkalescence (hi"per-al"kah-les'ens) an excess of alkalinity.

hyperalkalinity (hi"per-al"kah-lin'i-te) excessive alkalinity.

hyperallantoinuria (hi"per-ah-lan"to-in-u're-ah) an excess of allantoin in the urine.

hyperalonemia (hi"per-al"o-ne'me-ah) [*hyper-* + Gr. *hals* salt + *haima* blood] excess of salts in the blood.

hyperalphalipoproteinemia (hi"per-al"fah-lip"o-pro"te-in-e'me-ah) the presence of abnormally high levels of α-lipoproteins in the serum.

hyperaminoacidemia (hi"per-am"i-no-as"i-de'me-ah) presence of amino acids in the blood in excess of the normal amount.

hyperammonemia (hi"per-am"mo-ne'me-ah) [*hyper-* + *-emia*] elevated levels of ammonia or its compounds in the blood. Called also *ammonemia*. **cerebroatrophic h.,** Rett syndrome. **congenital h., type I,** carbamoyl phosphate synthetase deficiency. **congenital h., type II,** ornithine carbamoyl phosphate deficiency.

hyperammoniemia (hi"per-ah-mo"ne-e'me-ah) hyperammonemia.

hyperammonuria (hi"per-am"mo-nu're-ah) increased excretion of ammonia in the urine.

hyperamylasemia (hi"per-am"il-ās-e'me-ah) abnormally high elevation of amylase in the blood serum.

hyperanacinesia (hi"per-an"ah-si-ne'ze-ah) hyperkinesia.

hyperanakinesia (hi"per-an"ah-ki-ne'ze-ah) [*hyper-* + Gr. *anakinēsis* exercise + *-ia*] hyperkinesia.

hyperandrogenism (hi"per-an'dro-jen-izm) a state characterized or caused by an excessive secretion of androgens.

hyperaphia (hi"per-a'fe-ah) [*hyper-* + Gr. *haphē* touch] tactile hyperesthesia.

hyperaphic (hi"per-af'ik) pertaining to or characterized by hyperaphia (tactile hyperesthesia).

hyperargininemia (hi″per-ar″jin-in-e′me-ah) arginase deficiency.

hyperarousal (hi″per-ah-row′sal) a state of increased psychological and physiological tension marked by such effects as reduced tolerance to pain, insomnia, fatigue, accentuation of personality traits, etc.

hyperazotemia (hi″per-az″o-te′me-ah) [hyper- + azotemia] an excess of nitrogenous matter, usually urea, in the blood.

hyperazoturia (hi″per-az″o-tu′re-ah) presence of an excessive amount of nitrogenous matter in the urine.

hyperbaric (hi″per-băr′ik) [hyper- + Gr. baros weight] characterized by greater than normal pressure or weight; applied to gases under greater than atmospheric pressure, as hyperbaric oxygen, or to a solution of greater specific gravity than another taken as a standard of reference.

hyperbarism (hi″per-bar′izm) the condition resulting from exposure to ambient gas pressure or atmospheric pressures that exceed the pressure within body tissues, fluids, and cavities.

hyperbasophilic (hi″per-bas″o-fil′ik) staining intensely with basic dyes.

hyper-beta-alaninemia (hi″per-ba″tah-al″ah-nēn-e′me-ah) a rare disorder of β-alanine metabolism, possibly an autosomal recessive trait, due to deficient aminobutyrate aminotransferase. It is marked by an increased concentration of free β-aminoisobutyric acid and taurine as well as β-alanine in the blood and urine. It is characterized by lethargy, somnolence, and grand mal seizures. Called also β-alaninemia.

hyperbetalipoproteinemia (hi″per-ba″tah-lip″o-pro″te-in-e′me-ah) increased accumulation of β-lipoproteins in the blood. **familial h.,** familial hyperlipoproteinemia, type IIa.

hyperbicarbonatemia (hi″per-bi-kar″bo-nāt-e′me-ah) the presence of an excessive amount of bicarbonate in the blood.

hyperbilirubinemia (hi″per-bil″ĭ-roo″bĭ-ne′me-ah) excessive concentrations of bilirubin in the blood, which may lead to jaundice; the hyperbilirubinemias are classified as conjugated or unconjugated, according to the predominant form of bilirubin in the blood. **congenital h.,** Crigler-Najjar syndrome. **conjugated h.,** that due to defective excretion of conjugated bilirubin by the liver cells or to anatomic obstruction to bile flow within the liver or in the extrahepatic bile duct system, it includes Dubin-Johnson syndrome and Rotor's syndrome. **constitutional h.,** Gilbert syndrome. **h. I,** Gilbert syndrome. **neonatal h.,** a mild, transient, "physiological" hyperbilirubinemia of the unconjugated type occurring in the normal neonate; a transient familial form also occurs, with onset of jaundice within four days after birth, which may lead to kernicterus. **unconjugated h.,** that due to excessive bilirubin production (hemolysis), to defective clearance of bilirubin from the blood by the liver, or to defective conjugation by the liver; it includes hemolytic states, Crigler-Najjar syndrome, Gilbert syndrome, and neonatal hyperbilirubinemia.

hyperblastosis (hi″per-blas-to′sis) [hyper- + Gr. blastos germ] an overgrowth of some specific tissue.

hyperbrachycephalic (hi″per-brak″e-sĕ-fal′ik) having a cephalic index of 85.5 or more.

hyperbrachycephaly (hi″per-brak″e-sef′ah-le) the condition of being hyperbrachycephalic.

hyperbradykininemia (hi″per-brad″ĕ-ki″nin-e′me-ah) elevated levels of bradykinin in the blood, marked by a feeling of warmth, flushing, wheezing, or nausea.

hyperbradykininism (hi″per-brad″ĕ-ki′nin-izm) a syndrome characterized by high plasma levels of bradykinin, in which standing produces a fall in systolic blood pressure, an increase in diastolic pressure and heart rate, and a purplish discoloration and ecchymoses over the legs.

hypercalcemia (hi″per-kal-se′me-ah) [hyper- + calcium + Gr. haima blood] an excess of calcium in the blood; manifestations include fatigability, muscle weakness, depression, anorexia, nausea, and constipation. **familial hypocalciuric h.,** a benign disorder with vague and mild symptoms and few signs that is transmitted as an autosomal dominant trait. **idiopathic h.,** a condition of infants, associated with vitamin D intoxication, and characterized by elevated serum calcium levels and increased density of the skeleton,

with mental deterioration progressing to idiocy, and nephrocalcinosis causing chronic uremia.

hypercalcinemia (hi″per-kal″sĭ-ne′me-ah) hypercalcemia.

hypercalcinuria (hi″per-kal″sĭ-nu′re-ah) hypercalciuria.

hypercalcipexy (hi″per-kal′sĭ-pek″se) excessive fixation of calcium.

hypercalcitoninemia (hi″per-kal″sĭ-to″nĭ-ne′me-ah) an excess of calcitonin in the blood.

hypercalciuria (hi″per-kal″sĭ-u′re-ah) excess of calcium in the urine.

hypercapnia (hi″per-kap′ne-ah) [hyper- + Gr. kapnos smoke] excess of carbon dioxide in the blood.

hypercapnic (hi″per-kap′nik) pertaining to or characterized by hypercapnia.

hypercarbia (hi″per-kar′be-ah) hypercapnia.

hypercarotenemia (hi″per-kar″o-tēn-e′me-ah) an excess of carotene in the blood.

hypercarotinemia (hi″per-kar″o-tĭ-ne′me-ah) hypercarotenemia.

hypercatabolic (hi″per-kat″ah-bol′ik) pertaining to, characterized by, or causing hypercatabolism.

hypercatabolism (hi″per-kah-tab′o-lizm) abnormally increased catabolism.

hypercatharsis (hi″per-kah-thar′sis) [hyper- + Gr. katharsis purge] excessive purgation.

hypercathartic (hi″per-kah-thar′tik) [hyper- + Gr. kathartikos purgative] excessively cathartic.

hypercellular (hi″per-sel′u-lar) pertaining to or characterized by hypercellularity.

hypercellularity (hi″per-sel″u-lār′ĭ-te) a state characterized by an abnormal increase in the number of cells present, as in bone marrow.

hypercementosis (hi″per-se″men-to′sis) a regressive change of teeth characterized by excessive development of secondary cementum on the tooth surface; it may occur on any part of the root, but the apical two-thirds are most commonly affected. Called also cementosis and cementum hyperplasia.

hyperchloremia (hi″per-klo-re′me-ah) an excess of chloride in the blood.

hyperchloremic (hi″per-klo-re′mik) pertaining to or characterized by hyperchloremia.

hyperchlorhydria (hi″per-klōr-hi′dre-ah) excessive secretion of hydrochloric acid by the stomach cells.

hyperchloruration (hi″per-klōr″u-ra′shun) an excess of chlorides in the body.

hyperchloruria (hi″per-klōr-u′re-ah) excess of chlorides in the urine.

hypercholesteremia (hi″per-ko-les″ter-e′me-ah) hypercholesterolemia.

hypercholesteremic (hi″per-ko-les″ter-e′mik) hypercholesterolemic.

hypercholesterinemia (hi″per-ko-les″ter-in-e′me-ah) hypercholesterolemia.

hypercholesterolemia (hi″per-ko-les″ter-ol-e′me-ah) [hyper- + cholesterol + Gr. haima blood + -ia] excess of cholesterol in the blood. **familial h.,** familial hyperlipoproteinemia, type IIa, in which the genetic defect is the mutation of the gene specifying the cellular receptor for plasma low-density lipoprotein.

hypercholesterolemic (hi″per-ko-les″ter-ol-e′mik) pertaining to, characterized by, or tending to produce hypercholesterolemia.

hypercholesterolia (hi″per-ko-les″ter-ol′e-ah) abnormally high cholesterol content of the bile.

hypercholia (hi″per-ko′le-ah) [hyper- + Gr. cholē bile + -ia] excessive secretion of bile.

hyperchondroplasia (hi″per-kon″dro-pla′se-ah) excessive development of cartilage.

hyperchromaffinism (hi″per-kro-maf″ĭ-nizm) a condition caused by excessive secretion of chromaffin in the body, marked by paroxysms of arterial hypertension.

hyperchromasia (hi″per-kro-ma′se-ah) hyperchromatism.

hyperchromatic (hi″per-kro-mat′ik) 1. staining more intensely than is normal. 2. pertaining to or marked by hyperchromatism.

hyperchromatin (hi″per-kro′mah-tin) the part of the chromatin that stains with blue aniline dyes.

hyperchromatism (hi″per-kro′mah-tizm) [hyper- + Gr. *chrōma* color] excessive pigmentation, especially a form of degeneration of a cell nucleus in which it becomes filled with particles of pigment, or chromatin.

hyperchromatosis (hi″per-kro″mah-to′sis) 1. increased staining capacity. 2. hyperchromatism.

hyperchromemia (hi″per-kro-me′me-ah) [hyper- + Gr. *chrōma* color + *haima* blood + *-ia*] a high color index of the blood.

hyperchromia (hi″per-kro′me-ah) hyperchromatism.

hyperchromic (hi″per-kro′mik) highly or excessively stained or colored.

hyperchylia (hi″per-ki′le-ah) excessive secretion of gastric juice.

hyperchylomicronemia (hi″per-ki″lo-mi″kro-ne′me-ah) the presence in the blood of an excessive number of particles of fat (chylomicrons); see *familial hyperlipoproteinemia, type I*, under *hyperlipoproteinemia*. Called also *chylomicronemia*. **familial h.,** familial hyperlipoproteinemia, type I.

hypercinesia (hi″per-si-ne′ze-ah) hyperkinesia.

hypercoagulability (hi″per-ko-ag″u-lah-bil′ĭ-te) the state of being more readily coagulated than normal.

hypercoagulable (hi″per-ko-ag′u-lah-b'l) characterized by abnormally increased coagulability.

hypercoria (hi″per-ko′re-ah) hyperkoria.

hypercorticalism (hi″per-kor″tĭ-kal-izm) hyperadrenocorticism.

hypercorticism (hi″per-kor′tĭ-sizm) hyperadrenocorticism.

hypercortisolism (hi″per-kor′tĭ-sōl″izm) a complex of symptoms and signs due to excessive production or administration of hydrocortisone (cortisone) or its semisynthetic analogues; hyperadrenocorticism.

hypercreatinemia (hi″per-kre″ah-tĭ-ne′me-ah) an abnormality of creatine metabolism in skeletal muscle, a common feature of thyrotoxicosis.

hypercryalgesia (hi″per-kri″al-je′ze-ah) [hyper- + Gr. *kryos* cold + *algēsis* pain] excessive sensitiveness to cold.

hypercryesthesia (hi″per-kri″es-the′ze-ah) [hyper- + Gr. *kryos* cold + *aisthēsis* perception] hypercryalgesia.

hypercupremia (hi″per-ku-pre′me-ah) an excess of copper in the blood.

hypercupriuria (hi″per-ku″pre-u′re-ah) an excess of copper in the urine.

hypercyanotic (hi″per-si″ah-not′ik) extremely cyanotic.

hypercyesis (hi″per-si-e′sis) [hyper- + Gr. *kyēsis* gestation] superfetation.

hypercythemia (hi″per-si-the′me-ah) [hyper- + Gr. *kytos* hollow vessel + *haima* blood + *-ia*] abnormal increase in the number of erythrocytes in the blood.

hypercytochromia (hi″per-si″to-kro′me-ah) [hyper- + Gr. *kytos* hollow vessel + *chrōma* color] increased staining capacity of a blood cell.

hypercytosis (hi″per-si-to′sis) [hyper- + Gr. *kytos* hollow vessel + *-osis*] a condition characterized by an abnormally increased number of cells, especially of leukocytes.

hyperdactylia (hi″per-dak-til′e-ah) hyperdactyly.

hyperdactylism (hi″per-dak′tĭ-lizm) hyperdactyly.

hyperdactyly (hi″per-dak′tĭ-le) [hyper- + Gr. *daktylos* finger] the presence of more than the normal number of fingers or toes.

hyperdicrotic (hi″per-di-krot′ik) [hyper- + *dicrotic*] exhibiting marked dicrotism.

hyperdicrotism (hi″per-dik′ro-tizm) [hyper- + *dicrotism*] the quality of being hyperdicrotic; extreme dicrotism.

hyperdipsia (hi″per-dip′se-ah) [hyper- + Gr. *dipsa* thirst + *-ia*] intense thirst of relatively brief duration.

hyperdistention (hi″per-dis-ten′shun) excessive distention.

hyperdiuresis (hi″per-di″u-re′sis) [hyper- + *diuresis*] excessive excretion of urine.

hyperdontia (hi″per-don′she-ah) [hyper- + *odont-* + *-ia*] an anomaly characterized by the presence of an excessive number of teeth.

hyperdynamia (hi″per-di-na′me-ah) [hyper- + Gr. *dynamis* force] excessive muscular activity. **h. u′teri,** excessive uterine contractions in labor.

hyperdynamic (hi″per-di-nam′ik) pertaining to or characterized by hyperdynamia.

hypereccrisia (hi″per-ek-kris′e-ah) [hyper- + Gr. *ekkrisis* excretion + *-ia*] a state characterized by abnormally increased excretion.

hypereccrisis (hi″per-ek′krĭ-sis) hypereccrisia.

hypereccritic (hi-per-ek-krit′ik) pertaining to or exhibiting hypereccrisia.

hyperechema (hi″per-e-ke′mah) [hyper- + Gr. *ēchēma* sound] exaggeration of auditory sensations.

hyperelectrolytemia (hi-per-e-lek″tro-li-te′me-ah) an abnormally high concentration of electrolytes in the blood.

hyperemesis (hi″per-em′ĕ-sis) [hyper- + Gr. *emesis* vomiting] excessive vomiting. **h. gravida′rum,** pernicious vomiting of pregnancy. **h. lacten′tium,** excessive vomiting of nursing babies.

hyperemetic (hi″per-e-met′ik) characterized by excessive vomiting.

hyperemia (hi″per-e′me-ah) [hyper- + Gr. *haima* blood + *-ia*] an excess of blood in a part; engorgement. **active h.,** excess of blood in a part due to local or general relaxation of the arterioles. **arterial h.,** active h. **collateral h.,** increased flow of blood through collateral vessels when the flow through the main artery is arrested. **fluxionary h.,** active h. **leptomeningeal h.,** congestion of the pia-arachnoid. **passive h.,** an excess of blood in a part resulting from obstruction to its outflow from the area. **reactive h.,** an excess of blood in a part following restoration of its temporarily arrested flow. **venous h.,** passive h.

hyperemic (hi″per-e′mik) marked by hyperemia.

hyperemization (hi″per-e″mi-za′shun) the production of hyperemia, especially when employed for therapeutic purposes.

hyperencephalus (hi″per-en-sef′ah-lus) [hyper- + Gr. *enkephalos* brain] a monster with the cranial vault absent and the brain exposed.

hyperendemic (hi″per-en-dem′ik) [hyper- + Gr. *endēmos* dwelling in a place] equally endemic in all age groups of a population. Cf. *holoendemic*.

hyperenergia (hi″per-en-er′je-ah) excessive energy or activity.

hypereosinophilia (hi″per-e″o-sin-o-fil′e-ah) excessive eosinophilia. **filarial h.,** tropical eosinophilia.

hyperepinephrinemia (hi″per-ep″ĭ-nef″rĭ-ne′me-ah) [hyper- + *epinephrine* + Gr. *haima* blood] an excess of epinephrine in the blood, as in pheochromocytoma.

hyperequilibrium (hi″per-e″kwĭ-lib′re-um) an excessive tendency to vertigo.

hypererethism (hi″per-er′ĕ-thizm) extreme irritability.

hyperergasia (hi″per-er-ga′se-ah) [hyper- + Gr. *ergon* work] abnormally increased functional activity.

hyperergia (hi″per-er′je-ah) 1. hyperergasia. 2. hyperergy.

hypererythrocythemia (hi″per-ĕ-rith″ro-si-the′me-ah) hypercythemia.

hyperesophoria (hi″per-es″o-fo′re-ah) [hyper- + Gr. *esō* inward + *phorein* to bear] a tendency of the visual axis to deviate upward and inward.

hyperesthesia (hi″per-es-the′ze-ah) [hyper- + Gr. *aisthēsis* sensation + *-ia*] increased sensitivity to stimulation. **acoustic h., auditory h.,** hyperacusis. **cerebral h.,** that due to a cerebral lesion. **gustatory h.,** hypergeusia. **muscular h.,** muscular oversensitivity to pain or fatigue. **olfactory h.,** hyperosmia. **oneiric h.,** increase of sensitivity or of pain during sleep and dreams. **optic h.,** abnormal sensitivity of the eye to light. **tactile h.,** excessive tactile sensibility; called also *hyperaphia* and *hyperpselaphesia*.

hyperesthetic (hi″per-es-thet′ik) pertaining to or characterized by hyperesthesia.

hyperestrinemia (hi″per-es-trĭ-ne′me-ah) hyperestrogenemia.

hyperestrinism (hi″per-es′trin-izm) a condition due to excessive secretion of estrogen (estrin) and characterized by functional uterine bleeding (menometrorrhagia).

hyperestrogenemia (hi″per-es″tro-jĕ-ne′me-ah) an excessive amount of estrogens in the blood.

hyperestrogenism (hi″per-es′tro-jen-izm″) a state characterized or caused by excessive secretion of estrogen.

hyperestrogenosis (hi″per-es″tro-jĕ-no′sis) an abnormally elevated level of estrogens in the body.

hypereuryopia (hi″per-u″re-o′pe-ah) euryopia.

hyperevolutism (hi″per-e-vol′u-tizm) a condition characterized by development in excess of the normal.

hyperexcretory (hi″per-eks′kre-to-re) marked by excessive secretion.

hyperexophoria (hi″per-ek″so-fo′re-ah) [hyper- + Gr. exō outward + phorein to bear + -ia] a tendency of the visual axis to deviate upward and outward.

hyperexplexia (hi″per-eks-pleks′e-ah) a congenital condition of exaggerated startle reactions with hypertonia, hypokinesia, and brisk cerebral bulbar reflexes at birth.

hyperextension (hi″per-ek-sten′shun) extreme or excessive extension of a limb or part.

hyperferremia (hi″per-fer-re′me-ah) an excess of iron in the blood.

hyperferremic (hi″per-fer-re′mik) pertaining to or characterized by hyperferremia.

hyperferricemia (hi″per-fer″ĭ-se′me-ah) hyperferremia.

hyperfibrinogenemia (hi″per-fi-brin″o-jĕ-ne′me-ah) an excess of fibrinogen in the blood.

hyperflexion (hi″per-flek′shun) forcible overflexion of a limb or part.

hyperfunctioning (hi″per-funk′shun-ing) excessive functioning of an organ.

hypergalactia (hi″per-gah-lak′she-ah) [hyper- + Gr. gala milk] excessive secretion of milk.

hypergalactosis (hi″per-gal″ak-to′sis) hypergalactia.

hypergalactous (hi″per-gah-lak′tus) pertaining to, characterized by, or causing hypergalactia.

hypergammaglobulinemia (hi″per-gam″ah-glob″u-lĭ-ne′me-ah) an excess of gamma globulins in the blood; it is seen frequently in chronic infectious diseases. **monoclonal h.,** plasma cell dyscrasia.

hypergasia (hip″er-ga′se-ah) hypoergasia.

hypergastrinemia (hi″per-gas″trin-e′me-ah) the presence of an excess of gastrin in the blood.

hypergenesis (hi″per-jen′ĕ-sis) [hyper- + Gr. genesis development] excessive development, hypertrophy, or redundancy.

hypergenetic (hi″per-jĕ-net′ik) pertaining to or characterized by hypergenesis.

hypergenitalism (hi″per-jen′ĭ-tal-izm) hypergonadism.

hypergeusesthesia (hi″per-gūs″es-the′ze-ah) hypergeusia.

hypergeusia (hi″per-gu′se-ah) [hyper- + Gr. geusis taste] increased sensitivity of taste.

hypergia (hi-per′je-ah) 1. hypoergasia. 2. diminished sensitivity in allergy.

hyperglandular (hi″per-glan′du-lar) marked by abnormally increased activity of any gland.

hyperglobulinemia (hi″per-glob″u-lĭ-ne′me-ah) abnormally high globulin content of the blood.

hyperglucagonemia (hi″per-gloo″kah-gŏn-e′me-ah) abnormally high levels of glucagon in the blood.

hyperglycemia (hi″per-gli-se′me-ah) [hyper- + Gr. glykys sweet + haima blood + -ia] abnormally increased content of sugar in the blood.

hyperglycemic (hi″per-gli-se′mik) 1. pertaining to, characterized by, or causing hyperglycemia. 2. an agent that causes an increase in the level of glucose in the blood.

hyperglyceridemia (hi″per-glis″er-ĭ-de′me-ah) an excess of glycerides, usually triglycerides, in the blood.

hyperglyceridemic (hi″per-glis′er-ĭ-de′mik) pertaining to, characterized by, or producing hyperglyceridemia.

hyperglycinemia (hi″per-gli″sĭ-ne′me-ah) [hyper- + glycine + -emia] an aminoacidopathy in which glycine accumulates in body fluids, and occurring in two main forms: ketotic

hyperglycinemia is secondary to several organic acidemias, and is characterized by vomiting, lethargy, dehydration, ketosis, intolerance of dietary protein, hyperglycinuria, hypogammaglobulinemia, neutropenia, increased susceptibility to infection, thrombocytopenia, and periodic purpura. Nonketotic hyperglycinemia, an autosomal recessive aminoacidopathy with excess glycine in body fluids, but no excess organic acids in the blood or urine, is characterized by neonatal onset, no cerebral development, no reflexes, hypotonia, lethargy, weak cry, intolerance of dietary glycine, myoclonic jerks, but no vomiting, ketosis, neutropenia, or thrombocytopenia. Called also glycinemia.

hyperglycinuria (hi″per-gli″sĭ-nu′re-ah) an excess of glycine in the urine; see hyperglycinemia.

hyperglycistia (hi″per-gli-sis′te-ah) [hyper- + Gr. glykys sweet + histos tissue] excess of sugar in the bodily tissues.

hyperglycogenolysis (hi″per-gli″ko-jen-ol′ĭ-sis) excessive splitting up of glycogen, resulting in an excess of dextrose in the body.

hyperglycorrhachia (hi″per-gli″ko-ra′ke-ah) [hyper- + Gr. glykys sweet + rhachis spine] the presence of a greater than normal concentration of glucose in the cerebrospinal fluid.

hyperglycosemia (hi″per-gli″ko-se′me-ah) hyperglycemia.

hyperglycosuria (hi″per-gli″ko-su′re-ah) [hyper- + glycosuria] extreme glycosuria.

hyperglycystia (hi″per-gli-sis′te-ah) hyperglycistia.

hyperglykemia (hi″per-gli-ke′me-ah) hyperglycemia.

hypergnosis (hi″per-no′sis) [hyper- + Gr. gnōsis knowledge] an exaggerated perception, e.g., expansion of an isolated idea into a complex philosophical system; seen in paranoia.

hypergonadism (hi″per-go′nad-izm) a condition resulting from or characterized by abnormally increased functional activity of the gonads, with excessive growth and precocious sexual development.

hypergonadotropic (hi″per-gon″ah-do-trop′ik) relating to or caused by excessive amounts of gonadotropins.

hyperguanidinemia (hi″per-gwan″ĭ-dĭ-ne′me-ah) the presence of an excess of guanidine in the blood.

hyperhedonia (hi″per-hĕ-do′ne-ah) [hyper- + Gr. hēdonē pleasure] pathological increase of the feeling in pleasure in agreeable acts.

hyperhedonism (hi″per-he′do-nizm) hyperhedonia.

hyperhemoglobinemia (hi″per-he″mo-glo″bĭ-ne′me-ah) the presence of an excessive amount of hemoglobin in the blood.

hyperheparinemia (hi″per-hep″ah-rĭ-ne′me-ah) the presence of an excessive amount of heparin in the blood.

hyperhepatia (hi″per-he-pat′e-ah) [hyper- + Gr. hēpar liver] hyperfunction of the liver.

hyperhidrosis (hi″per-hi-dro′sis) [hyper- + Gr. hidrōsis sweating] excessive perspiration. Called also hyperidrosis, polyhidrosis, and polyidrosis. **h. unilatera′lis,** excessive sweating on one side of the body only.

hyperhidrotic (hi″per-hi-drot′ik) pertaining to, characterized by, or causing hyperhidrosis.

hyperhydration (hi″per-hi-dra′shun) a state of excessive water content of the body.

hyperhydrochloria (hi″per-hi-dro-klo′re-ah) hyperchlorhydria.

hyperhydrochloridia (hi″per-hi-dro-klo-rid′e-ah) hyperchlorhydria.

hyperhydroxyprolinemia (hi″per-hi-drok″se-pro″lin-e′me-ah) [hyper- + hydroxyproline oxidase + -emia] a genetic aminoacidopathy resulting from defective hydroxyproline oxidase; collagen metabolism is not affected, and there is no clinical dysfunction.

hyperidrosis (hi″per-i-dro′sis) hyperhidrosis.

hyperimidodipeptiduria (hi″per-im″id-o-di″pep-ti-doo′re-ah) prolidase deficiency.

hyperimmune (hi″per-im-mūn′) possessing very large quantities of specific antibodies in the serum.

hyperimmunity (hi″per-ĭ-mu′nĭ-te) the high levels of specific antibody produced by hyperimmunization.

hyperimmunization (hi″per-im″u-nĭ-za′shun) any process of immunization that produces very high levels of circulating antibodies, especially immunization of an animal or human donor with repeated doses of antigen for the production of therapeutic antisera or immune globulins.

hyperimmunoglobulinemia (hi″per-im″u-no-glob″u-lin-e′me-ah) abnormally high levels of immunoglobulins in the serum. **h. E,** extremely high levels of IgE in the serum, associated with cutaneous anergy and deficient antibody response, as occurs in Job's syndrome.

hyperinflation (hi″per-in-fla′shun) excessive inflation or expansion, as of the lungs; overinflation.

hyperingestion (hi″per-in-jes′chun) ingestion of a greater than optimal amount of nutrients.

hyperinsulinar (hi″per-in′su-lin-ar) pertaining to or characterized by excessive secretion of insulin.

hyperinsulinemia (hi″per-in″su-lĭ-ne′me-ah) the presence of an excessive amount of insulin in the blood.

hyperinsulinism (hi″per-in′su-lin-izm″) 1. excessive secretion of insulin by the pancreas, resulting in hypoglycemia. 2. insulin shock. 3. hyperinsulinemia.

hyperinvolution (hi″per-in″vo-lu′shun) superinvolution.

hyperiodemia (hi″per-i″o-de′me-ah) the presence of an excessive amount of iodine in the blood.

hyperirritability (hi″per-ir″ĭ-tah-bil′ĭ-te) pathological responsiveness to slight stimuli.

hyperisotonia (hi″per-i″so-to′ne-ah) [hyper- + Gr. isos equal + tonos tension] marked equality of tone or of tonicity.

hyperisotonic (hi″per-i″so-ton′ik) [hyper- + Gr. isos equal + tonos tension, or tone] hypertonic.

hyperkalemia (hi″per-kah-le′me-ah) abnormally high potassium concentration in the blood, most often due to defective renal excretion. It is characterized clinically by electrocardiographic abnormalities (elevated T waves and depressed P waves, and eventually by atrial asystole). In severe cases, weakness and flaccid paralysis may occur. Called also *hyperpotassemia.*

hyperkaliemia (hi″per-kal″e-e′me-ah) hyperkalemia.

hyperkeratinization (hi″per-ker″ah-tin″i-za′shun) [hyper- + keratinization] the excessive development or retention of keratin by the epidermis.

hyperkeratosis (hi″per-ker″ah-to′sis) [hyper- + keratosis] 1. hypertrophy of the corneous layer of the skin, or any disease characterized by it. Cf. keratoderma, keratoma (def. 1), keratosis, tyloma, and tylosis. 2. hypertrophy of the cornea. 3. a skin disease of cattle marked by inflammation and thickening of the horny layer, and caused by the ingestion of grease containing high levels of chlorinated hydrocarbons. Once thought to be caused by a virus, it was called x disease. Called also *perkeratosis.* **epidermolytic h.,** a form of ichthyosis present at birth, inherited as an autosomal dominant trait, and characterized by generalized erythroderma and severe hyperkeratosis with small, hard verrucous scales over the entire body, accentuated in flexural areas, which may involve the palms and soles. Recurrent bullae usually localized to the lower limbs are characteristic in infancy and childhood. Formerly called *bullous congenital ichthyosiform erythroderma.* See also *ichthyosis hystrix.* **follicular h.,** a skin condition characterized by hyperkeratosis of hair follicles, resulting in rough, cone-shaped, elevated papules, the openings of which are often closed with a white plug of encrusted sebum. Deficiencies of vitamins A and E, B complex vitamins, and essential fatty acids have all been implicated in the etiology. Called also *phrynoderma* and *toadskin.* **h. follicula′ris in cu′tem pen′etrans, h. follicula′ris et parafollicula′ris in cu′tem pen′etrans,** Kyrle's disease. **h. lacuna′ris,** a condition in which the tonsillar crypts contain hard, firmly attached masses. **h. lenticula′ris per′stans,** an autosomal dominant skin disorder, usually occurring in the third or fourth decade of life, characterized clinically by the presence of pink or reddish or yellowish brown hyperkeratotic scaly papules on the lower leg and dorsum of the foot, sometimes involving the trunk, thigh, arms, and dorsum of the hand, and usually associated with punctate keratoses on the palms and soles; and histologically by a lack of keratinosomes and a reduction of keratohyalin granules in the epidermis underlying the lesions. Called also *Flegel's disease.* **h. of palms and soles,** palmoplantar keratoderma. **h. pen′etrans,** hyperkeratosis follicularis in cutem penetrans. **progressive dystrophic h.,** keratoma

hereditarium mutilans. **h. subungua′lis,** hyperkeratosis affecting the nail beds.

hyperketonemia (hi″per-ke″to-ne′me-ah) an abnormally increased concentration of ketone bodies in the blood.

hyperketonuria (hi″per-ke″to-nu′re-ah) the presence of an excessive quantity of ketone in the urine.

hyperketosis (hi″per-ke-to′sis) the formation of an excess of ketone.

hyperkinemia (hi″per-ki-ne′me-ah) [hyper- + Gr. kinein move + haima blood + -ia] abnormally high cardiac output (blood circulation) when at rest and supine, as in the hyperkinetic syndrome.

hyperkinemic (hi″per-ki-ne′mik) 1. increasing blood flow through a tissue. 2. an agent which increases the flow of blood through a tissue area.

hyperkinesia (hi″per-ki-ne′ze-ah) [hyper- + Gr. kinēsis motion + -ia] abnormally increased motor function or activity; hyperactivity.

hyperkinesis (hi″per-ki-ne′sis) hyperkinesia.

hyperkinetic (hi″per-ki-net′ik) pertaining to or characterized by hyperkinesia.

hyperkoria (hi″per-ko′re-ah) [hyper- + Gr. koros satiety + -ia] an early sense of satiety.

hyperlactacidemia (hi″per-lakt″as-ĭ-de′me-ah) an excessive amount of lactic acid in the blood.

hyperlactation (hi″per-lak-ta′shun) lactation in greater than normal amount or for a longer than usual period.

hyperlecithinemia (hi″per-les″ĭ-thĭ-ne′me-ah) excess of lecithin in the blood.

hyperlethal (hi″per-le′thal) more than sufficient to cause death.

hyperleukocytosis (hi″per-lu″ko-si-to′sis) [hyper- + leukocyte + -osis] an abnormally excessive increase in the number of leukocytes in the blood.

hyperleydigism (hi″per-li′dig-izm) overactivity of Leydig's cells.

hyperlipemia (hi″per-li-pe′me-ah) hyperlipidemia. **carbohydrate-induced h.,** hyperlipoproteinemia, type IV. **combined fat- and carbohydrate-induced h.,** familial hyperprotein lipoproteinemia, type V. **familial h., essential,** familial hyperlipoproteinemia, type I. **fat-induced h., familial,** familial hyperlipoproteinemia, type I. **idiopathic h.,** familial hyperlipoproteinemia, type I. **mixed h.,** familial hyperlipoproteinemia, types IIb and V.

hyperlipidemia (hi″per-lip″ĭ-de′me-ah) [hyper- + lipid + -emia] a general term for elevated concentrations of any or all of the lipids in the plasma, including hyperlipoproteinemia, hypercholesterolemia, etc. **combined h., familial,** familial hyperlipoproteinemia, types II, IIb, and IV. **mixed h.,** familial hyperlipoproteinemia, type IIb. **multiple lipoprotein-type h.,** familial hyperlipoproteinemia, types II and IV.

hyperlipoidemia (hi″per-li″poi-de′me-ah) hyperlipidemia.

hyperlipoproteinemia (hi″per-lip″o-pro″te-in-e′me-ah) [hyper- + lipoprotein + -emia] an excess of lipoproteins in the blood, due to a disorder of lipoprotein metabolism, and occurring as an acquired or familial condition. See also *hyperlipidemia.* **acquired h.,** hyperlipoproteinemia occurring secondarily to some other disorder, such as hypothyroidism, nephrotic syndrome, or hypoadrenocorticism, or as a result of environmental factors, including diet. **broad-beta h., familial,** familial h., type III. **combined h., familial,** familial h., types II and IIb. **familial h.,** a group of genetic disorders of lipoprotein metabolism, classified into five major phenotypes based on clinical features, enzymatic abnormalities, and serum lipoprotein electrophoretic patterns. *Type I,* a recessive trait, due to lipoprotein lipase deficiency, is manifested by abdominal pain and vomiting, acute pancreatitis, xanthomas, hepatosplenomegaly, and lipemia retinalis. Called also *familial lipoprotein lipase (LPL)* or *familial apolipoprotein C-II (apo C-II) deficiency, familial hyperchylomicronemia, essential familial* or *familial fat-induced* or *idiopathic hyperlimpemia,* and *Bürger-Grütz syndrome. Type II,* of unknown biochemistry, a dominant trait with severe homozygous and less severe heterozygous forms, is characterized by xanthomas, xanthelasmas, corneal arcus, and coronary atherosclerosis.

Called also *familial combined h.* or *hyperlipidemia*, and *multiple, lipoprotein-type hyperlipidemia.* Two subtypes of Type II have been described: Type *IIa*, called also *LDL-receptor disorder, familial hypercholesterolemia,* and *familial hyperbetalipoproteinemia;* and Type *IIb*, called also *familial combined h.* or *hyperlipidemia, mixed h.* or *hyperlipidemia,* and *hypertriglyceridemia. Type III*, of unclear inheritance and biochemistry, characterized by accumulation of abnormal β-lipoproteins resembling prebetalipoproteins, is manifested by xanthomas and less often by coronary and peripheral atherosclerosis; called also *broad-beta disease* or *proteinemia, floating-beta disease* or *proteinemia, familial dysbetalipoproteinemia, familial broad-beta h., familial hyperbeta-* and *hyperprebetalipoproteinemia,* and *carbohydrate-induced hyperlipemia* or *hypertriglyceridemia. Type IV,* of unclear inheritance and biochemistry, characterized by elevated serum triglycerides, is manifested by vascular disease, abnormal glucose tolerance, and family history of diabetes mellitus. Called also *familial lipoprotein lipase (LPL)* or *apolipoprotein C-II (apo C-II) deficiency, familial hyperchylomicronemia with hyperprebetalipoproteinemia, combined fat-* and *carbohydrate-induced hyperlipemia,* and *mixed h.* or *hyperlipemia.* **mixed h.,** familial h., types II b and V.

hyperliposis (hi″per-lĭ-po′sis) an excess of fat in the blood serum or tissues.

hyperlithemia (hi″per-lĭ-the′me-ah) presence in the blood of a high concentration of lithium.

hyperlithic (hi″per-lith′ik) pertaining to or characterized by an excess of lithic (uric) acid.

hyperlithuria (hi″per-lith-u′re-ah) excess of lithic (uric) acid in the urine.

hyperlordosis (hi″per-lor-do′sis) extremely marked lordosis.

hyperlucency (hi″per-loo′sen-se) increased radiolucency.

hyperluteinization (hi″per-lu″te-in-i-za′shun) excessive luteinization of the cystic follicles of the ovary.

hyperlysinemia (hi″per-li″sēn-e′me-ah) [*hyper- + lysine + -emia*] a genetic aminoacidopathy due to defective lysine dehydrogenase and occurring in two types: *periodic hyperlysinemia,* associated with hyperammonemia; and *persistent hyperlysinemia,* without hyperammonemia. Called also *1-lysine:nad-oxido-reductase deficiency* and *lysine intolerance.*

hypermagnesemia (hi″per-mag″nĕ-se′me-ah) an abnormally large magnesium content of the blood plasma; manifestations include lethargy, weakness, electrocardiographic abnormalities and, as levels increase, loss of deep tendon reflexes, somnolence, and coma.

hypermania (hi″per-ma′ne-ah) intense mania with overwhelming tensions and marked disorientation.

hypermastia (hi″per-mas′te-ah) [*hyper- + Gr. mastos* breast] 1. the presence of one or more supernumerary mammary glands. 2. hypertrophy of the mammary gland.

Hypermastigida (hi″per-mas-tij′ĭ-dah) [*hyper- + Gr. mastix* whip] an order of mononucleate, parasitic, anaerobic protozoa (superorder Parabasalidea, class Zoomastigophorea), found as symbionts in the gut of wood-eating termites, cockroaches, and woodroaches. Hypermastigotes digest cellulose, and the products of the process are supplied to their insect hosts. They are characterized by the presence of numerous flagella with parabasal bodies arranged anteriorly in a circle, plate(s), or longitudinial or spiral rows. Most species reproduce asexually but sexual reproduction occurs in certain species. The order comprises two suborders: Lophomonadina and Trichonymphina.

hypermastigote (hi″per-mas′tĭgōt) 1. of or pertaining to protozoa of the order Hypermastigida. 2. any protozoan of the order Hypermastigida.

hypermature (hi″per-mah-tūr) past the stage of maturity.

hypermelanotic (hi″per-mel″ah-not′ik) characterized by an excessive deposit of melanin.

hypermenorrhea (hi″per-men″o-re′ah) [*hyper- + Gr. mēn* month + *rhein* to flow] excessive uterine bleeding occurring at regular intervals, the period of flow being of usual duration.

hypermetabolic (hi″per-met″ah-bol′ik) exhibiting an increased metabolic rate.

hypermetabolism (hi″per-mĕ-tab′o-lizm) abnormally increased utilizaton of material by the body; increased metabolism. **extrathyroidal h.,** abnormally elevated basal metabolism unassociated with thyroid disease.

hypermetamorphosis (hi″per-met″ah-mor″fo-sis) too rapid drift of thought activity, leading to mental distraction and confusion, and forming a chief element in mania; excessive attentiveness to visual stimuli, as in the Klüver-Bucy syndrome.

hypermetaplasia (hi″per-met″ah-pla′se-ah) abnormally increased metaplasia.

hypermetria (hi″per-me′tre-ah) [Gr. "a passing all measure, overflow"] a condition in which voluntary muscular movement overreaches the intended goal.

hypermetrope (hi″per-me′trōp) hyperope.

hypermetropia (hi″per-me-tro′pe-ah) hyperopia.

hypermimia (hi″per-mim′e-ah) [*hyper- + Gr. mimia* representation by means of art] excessive use of gestures when speaking.

hypermineralization (hi″per-min″er-al-i-za′shun) the presence of an excess of mineral elements in the body.

hypermnese (hi″perm-ne′ze-ah) [*hyper- + Gr. mnēmē* memory] excessive crowding or unusual clarity of memory images.

hypermnesic (hi″perm-ne′sik) 1. pertaining to or characterized by hypermnesia. 2. marked by excessive mental activity.

hypermodal (hi″per-mo′dal) in statistics, relating to the values or items falling above the mode frequency distribution.

hypermorph (hi′per-morf) [*hyper- + Gr. morphē* form] a mutant gene characterized by an increase in the activity it influences. Cf. *hypomorph.*

hypermotility (hi″per-mo-til′ĭ-te) excessive or abnormally increased motility, as of the gastrointestinal tract.

hypermyotonia (hi″per-mi″o-to′ne-ah) [*hyper- + Gr. mys* muscle + *tonos* tension + *-ia*] excess of muscular tonicity.

hypermyotrophy (hi″per-mi-ot′ro-fe) [*hyper- + Gr. mys* muscle + *trophē* nourishment] excessive development of the muscular tissue.

hypernasality (hi″per-na-zal′ĭ-te) a quality of voice in which the emission of air through the nose is excessive due to velopharyngeal incompetence; it causes deterioration of intelligibility of speech.

hypernatremia (hi″per-nah-tre′me-ah) [*hyper- + L. natron* sodium + *Gr. haima* blood + *-ia*] excessive amount of sodium in the blood. **hypodipsic h.,** an uncommon syndrome of chronic or recurrent episodes of severe hypernatremia with dehydration and lack of thirst, seen in persons with various congenital or acquired diseases of the brain.

hypernatremic (hi″per-na-tre′mik) pertaining to, characterized by, or causing hypernatremia.

hypernatronemia (hi″per-nat″ro-ne′me-ah) hypernatremia.

hyperneocytosis (hi″per-ne″o-si-to′sis) [*hyper- + Gr. neos* new + *kytos* hollow vessel + *-osis*] leukocytosis in which an excessive number of immature forms of leukocytes are present.

hypernephroid (hi″per-nef′roid) resembling the adrenal gland.

hypernephroma (hi″per-nĕ-fro′mah) [*hyper- + Gr. nephros* kidney + *-oma*] renal cell carcinoma whose structure resembles that of the cortical tissue of the adrenal gland. See also *Grawitz's tumor,* under *tumor.*

hypernitremia (hi″per-ni-tre′me-ah) [*hyper- + nitrogen + Gr. haima* blood] excessive nitrogen in the blood.

hypernomic (hi″per-nom′ik) [*hyper- + Gr. nomos* law] above the law; unrestrained; excessive.

hypernormal (hi″per-nor′mal) in excess of what is normal.

hypernutrition (hi″per-nu-trish′un) overfeeding and its ill effects.

hyperonychia (hi″per-o-nik′e-ah) [*hyper- + Gr. onyx* nail + *-ia*] onychauxis.

hyperope (hi″per-ōp) an individual exhibiting hyperopia.

hyperopia (hi″per-o′pe-ah) [*hyper- + -opia*] that error of refraction in which rays of light entering the eye parallel to the optic axis are brought to a focus behind the retina, as a result of the eyeball being too short from front to back. Called also *farsightedness* (because the near point is more distant than it is in emmetropia with an equal amplitude of accommodation) and *hypermetropia*. **absolute h.,** that amount of hyperopia which cannot be corrected by accommodation. **axial h.,** that which is due to shortness of the anteroposterior axis of the eye. **curvature h.,** hyperopia due to insufficient convexity of the refracting surfaces. **facultative h.,** that amount of hyperopia which can be entirely corrected by the ciliary muscle, i.e., by the effort of accomodation. **index h.,** hyperopia caused by deficient refractive power in the media of the eye. **latent h.,** that part of the total hyperopia corrected by the physiologic tone of the ciliary muscle and revealed only when that muscle is paralyzed by the use of a drug, such as atropine. **manifest h.,** that part of the total hyperopia not corrected by the physiologic tone of the ciliary muscle nor revealed with cycloplegic examination. **relative h.,** facultative hyperopia allowing clear vision, but causing excessive convergence or convergent strabismus. **total h.,** the sum of manifest and latent hyperopia; it can be determined only with mydriasis.

hyperopic (hi″per-o′pik) pertaining to or exhibiting hyperopia; farsighted.

hyperorchidism (hi″per-or′kĭ-dizm) [*hyper-* + Gr. *orchis* testicle] abnormally increased functional activity of the testes.

hyperorexia (hi″per-o-rek′se-ah) [*hyper-* + Gr. *orexis* appetite + *-ia*] an abnormally increased appetite.

hyperorthocytosis (hi″per-or″tho-si-to′sis) [*hyper-* + Gr. *orthos* straight + *kytos* hollow vessel + *-osis*] leukocytosis in which the proportion of the various forms of leukocytes is normal.

hyperosmia (hi″per-oz′me-ah) [*hyper-* + Gr. *osmē* smell] increased sensitivity of smell.

hyperosmolality (hi″per-os″mo-lal′ĭ-te) an increase in the osmolality of the body fluids.

hyperosmolarity (hi″per-oz″mo-lar′ĭ-te) abnormally increased osmolar concentration.

hyperosmotic (hi″per-os-mot′ik) 1. producing or caused by abnormally rapid osmosis. 2. containing a higher concentration of osmotically active components than a standard solution.

hyperosphresia (hi″per-os-fre′ze-ah) [*hyper-* + Gr. *osphrēsis* smell + *-ia*] hyperosmia.

hyperosteogeny (hi″per-os″te-oj′ĕ-ne) [*hyper-* + Gr. *osteon* bone + *gennan* to produce] excessive development of bone.

hyperostosis (hi″per-os-to′sis) [*hyper-* + Gr. *osteon* bone + *-osis*] hypertrophy of bone; exostosis. **h. cortica′lis defor′mans juveni′lis,** an autosomal recessive disorder beginning in childhood and marked by multiple fractures and bowing of all extremities, by thickening of the frontal, parietal, and occipital bones, by osteoporosis, and by elevated concentrations of serum alkaline phosphatase and of urinary hydroxyproline. Called also *juvenile Paget disease, chronic congenital idiopathic hyperphosphatasemia,* and *familial osteoectasia.* **h. cortica′lis generalisa′ta,** a hereditary disorder, transmitted as an autosomal recessive trait, characterized principally by osteosclerosis of the skull, mandible, clavicles, ribs, and diaphyses of long bones, associated with elevated blood alkaline phosphatase; beginning during puberty, it sometimes leads to optic atrophy and perceptive deafness due to nerve pressure exerted by thickening of the base of the skull. Called also *hyperphosphatasemia tarda* and *van Buchem's syndrome.* **h. cra′nii,** hyperostosis involving the cranial bones. **flowing h.,** melorheostosis. **h. fronta′lis inter′na,** thickening of the inner table of the frontal bone, which may be associated with hypertrichosis and obesity; it most commonly affects women near menopause. Called also *Morel's syndrome; Morgagni's disease, hyperostosis,* or *syndrome; Morgagni-Stewart-Morel syndrome;* and *Stewart-Morel syndrome.* **infantile cortical h.,** a disease of young infants characterized by soft tissue swellings over the affected bones, fever, and irritability, and marked by periods of remission and exacerbation; called also *Caffey's disease.* **Morgagni's h.,** h. frontalis interna. **senile ankylosing h. of spine,** a disorder of the elderly characterized by large osteophytes that bridge vertebrae and, in association with calcified ligaments, may resemble ankylosing spondylitis.

hyperostotic (hi″per-os-tot′ik) pertaining to or exhibiting hyperostosis.

hyperovarianism (hi″per-o-va′re-an-izm) [*hyper* + L. *ovarium* ovary] sexual precocity in girls due to excessive and untimely ovarian secretion.

hyperovarism (hi″per-o′vah-rizm) hyperovarianism.

hyperoxaluria (hi″per-ok″sah-lu′re-ah) the excretion of an excessive amount of oxalate in the urine; high concentrations of oxalates in the urine may lead to the formation of urinary calculi. Called also *oxaluria.* **enteric h.,** a form occurring after extensive resection or disease of the ileum and resulting from excessive absorption of oxalate from the colon, with formation of calcium oxalate calculi in the urinary tract. **primary h.,** a genetic disorder characterized by urinary excretion of large amounts of oxalate, with nephrolithiasis, nephrocalcinosis, early onset of renal failure, and often a generalized deposit of calcium oxalate (oxalosis), resulting from a defect in glyoxalate metabolism. The disorder occurs in two types: Type 1, hyperoxaluria accompanied by glycolic aciduria, is due to a defect of the enzyme soluble α-ketoglutarate: glyoxylate carboligase. Type 2, hyperoxaluria with D-glyceric aciduria, is due to a defect of the enzyme glyoxalate reductase. Both types are autosomal recessive traits.

hyperoxemia (hi″per-ok-se′me-ah) [*hyper-* + Gr. *oxys* sharp + *haima* blood] excessive acidity of the blood.

hyperoxia (hi″per-ok′se-ah) an excess of oxygen in the system, resulting from exposure to high oxygen concentrations, especially to hyperbaric pressures of oxygen.

hyperoxic (hi″per-ok′sik) pertaining to or characterized by hyperoxia.

hyperoxidation (hi″per-ok″sĭ-da′shun) excessive oxidation.

hyperpallesthesia (hi″per-pal″es-the′ze-ah) [*hyper-* + *pallesthesia*] abnormally increased sensibility to vibrations.

hyperpancreorrhea (hi″per-pan″kre-o-re′ah) excessive secretion from the pancreas.

hyperparasite (hi″per-par′ah-sīt) [*hyper-* + *parasite*] a parasite that preys on a parasite. **second degree h.,** a parasite that preys on a hyperparasite.

hyperparasitic (hi″per-par-ah-sit′ik) living parasitically upon a parasite; biparasitic.

hyperparasitism (hi″per-par′ah-si″tizm) infestation with a hyperparasite.

hyperparathyroidism (hi″per-par″ah-thi′roid-izm) abnormally increased activity of the parathyroid glands, which may be primary or secondary. *Primary hyperparathyroidism* is associated with neoplasia (chiefly benign adenomas) or hyperplasia. The excess of parathyroid hormone leads to alteration in function of cells of bone, renal tubules, and gastrointestinal mucosa. It may result in kidney stones and calcium deposits in the renal tubules; in generalized decalcification of bone (osteoporosis), resulting in pain and tenderness of bones and spontaneous fractures or in localized bone cysts; and in hypercalcemia, leading to muscular weakness, gastrointestinal symptoms such as anorexia, nausea, vomiting, and abdominal pains, and drowsiness or obtundity. *Secondary hyperparathyroidism* occurs when the serum calcium tends to fall below normal, as in chronic renal disease, vitamin D deficiency, etc. *Tertiary hyperparathyroidism* refers to that due to a parathyroid adenoma arising from secondary hyperplasia caused by chronic renal failure.

hyperpathia (hi″per-path′e-ah) abnormally exaggerated subjective response to painful stimuli.

hyperpepsia (hi″per-pep′se-ah) [*hyper-* + Gr. *pepsis* digestion] impairment of digestion, due to hyperchlorhydria.

hyperpepsinemia (hi″per-pep″sĭ-ne′me-ah) an abnormally high level of pepsin in the blood.

hyperpepsinia (hi″per-pep-sin′e-ah) abnormally profuse secretion of pepsin in the stomach.

hyperpepsinuria (hi″per-pep″sĭ-nu′re-ah) an abnormally high level of pepsin in the urine.

hyperperistalsis (hi″per-per″ĭ-stal′sis) excessively active peristalsis.

hyperpermeability (hi″per-per″me-ah-bil′ĭ-te) undue or abnormal permeability, as of a cell membrane or a vessel wall.

hyperpexia (hi″per-pek′se-ah) [*hyper-* + Gr. *pēxis* fixation + *-ia*] fixation of an excessive amount of a substance by a tissue.

hyperpexy (hi″per-pek′se) hyperpexia.

hyperphagia (hi″per-fa′je-ah) [*hyper-* + Gr. *phagein* to eat] ingestion of a greater than optimal quantity of food.

hyperphalangia (hi″per-fah-lan′je-ah) presence of more than the normal number of phalanges in the longitudinal axis of a digit.

hyperphalangism (hi″per-fah-lan′jizm) hyperphalangia.

hyperphenylalaninemia (hi″per-fen″il-al′ah-nĭ-ne′me-ah) a group of genetic aminoacidopathies due to the impaired hydroxylation of phenylalanine to tyrosine by defective phenylalanine hydroxylase; there is an accumulation of phenylalanine with increased shunting of its metabolities. There are eight types of hyperphenylalaninemia based on biochemical defect: *type I* is classic phenylketonuria (q.v.); *type II* or *persistent hyperphenylalaninemia* and *type III* or *transient mild hyperphenylalaninemia* are usually clinically normal; *type IV* or *dihydropteridine reductase deficiency* or *malignant hyperphenylalaninemia* or *phenylketonuria II*, and *type V* or *dihydrobiopterin synthetase deficiency* or *atypical phenylketonuria* or *phenylketonuria III* show clinical manifestations in the first year of life, with severe neurologic damage; *type VI* or *persistent hyperphenylalaninemia and tyrosinemia* shows progressive ataxia and seizures during the second year of life; *type VII* or *neonatal tyrosinemia* (q.v.) is the only X-linked form; and *type VIII* is hereditary tyrosinemia (q.v.). Called also *phenylalaninemia*. **malignant h.**, hyperphenylalaninemia, type IV.

hyperphonesis (hi″per-fo-ne′sis) [*hyper-* + Gr. *phōnēsis* sounding] an increase in intensity of the vocal sound in auscultation, or of the percussion note.

hyperphonia (hi″per-fo′ne-ah) [*hyper-* + Gr. *phōnē* voice] excessively energetic phonation, as in stuttering.

hyperphoria (hi″per-fo′re-ah) [*hyper-* + *phoria*] a form of heterophoria in which there is permanent upward deviation of the visual axis of an eye after the visual fusional stimulus has been eliminated.

hyperphosphatasemia (hi″per-fos″fah-ta-se′me-ah) high levels of alkaline phosphatase in the blood. **chronic congenital idiopathic h.**, hyperostosis corticalis deformans juvenilis. **h. tar′da**, hyperostosis corticalis generalisata.

hyperphosphatasia (hi″per-fos″fah-ta′ze-ah) hyperphosphatasemia.

hyperphosphatemia (hi″per-fos″fah-te′me-ah) an excessive amount of phosphates in the blood; it is usually asymptomatic.

hyperphosphaturia (hi″per-fos″fah-tu′re-ah) an excessive amount of phosphates in the urine.

hyperphosphoremia (hi″per-fos″fo-re′me-ah) an excessive amount of phosphorus compounds in the blood.

hyperphrenia (hi″per-fre′ne-ah) [*hyper-* + Gr. *phrēn* mind] 1. great mental excitement. 2. excessive mental activity.

hyperpigmentation (hi″per-pig″men-ta′shun) abnormally increased pigmentation.

hyperpinealism (hi″per-pi′ne-al-izm) abnormally increased activity of the pineal body.

hyperpituitarism (hi″per-pĭ-tu′ĭ-tah-rizm″) a condition due to pathologically increased secretion of pituitary hormones resulting from functioning adenomas producing growth hormone (resulting in acromegaly, pituitary gigantism), corticotropin (resulting in Cushing's disease), or prolactin (resulting in galactorrhea-amenorrhea syndrome).

hyperplasia (hi″per-pla′ze-ah) [*hyper-* + Gr. *plasis* formation] the abnormal multiplication or increase in the number of normal cells in normal arrangement in a tissue. Cf. *hypertrophy*. **adrenal cortical h.**, hyperplasia of adrenal cortical cells, as in adrenogenital syndrome and Cushing's syndrome. **angiolymphoid h.**, one or more erythematous dermal or subcutaneous nodules occurring primarily on the head and neck of young adults, sometimes associated with lymphadenopathy and peripheral eosinophilia. The more superficial, usually larger, lesions have been called *pseudopyogenic granuloma*. Called also *Kimura disease*. **cementum h.**, hypercementosis. **chronic perforating pulp h.**, internal tooth resorption (def. 1). **congenital adrenal h.**, adrenogenital syndrome. **congenital**

virilizing adrenal h., adrenogenital syndrome. **cutaneous lymphoid h.**, a term for several benign cutaneous disorders with lesions clinically and histologically resembling those of malignant lymphoma. The lesions may be lymphoreticular, granulomatous, and follicular and include lymphocytes, histiocytes, eosinophils, plasma cells, and lymphoid follicles. The disorders may be of unknown etiology or be reactions to insect bites, allergy hyposensitization injections, light, trauma, and tattoo pigment. The term embraces lymphocytoma cutis, lymphadenosis benigna cutis, Spiegler-Frendt sarcoid, lymphocytic infiltration of the skin, and insect bite granuloma. Called also *cutaneous lymphoplasia*. **Dilantin h.**, see under *gingivitis*. **endometrial h., h. endome′trii**, abnormal overgrowth of the endometrium. **fibrous inflammatory h.**, masses of collagenized, fibrous connective tissue along the borders of ill-fitting dentures or in other areas where chronic irritation exists. Called also *epulis fissuratum*. **giant follicular h.**, a disorder of the lymph nodes, generally confined to the cervical lymph nodes, which may simulate follicular lymphoma, but cytologically the follicles contain both macrophages and lymphoblasts. **gingival h.**, noninflammatory enlargement of the gingivae produced by factors other than local irritation. See also under *enlargement*. **inflammatory h.**, hyperplasia brought about by inflammation. **juxtaglomerular cell h.**, a syndrome in which hypertrophy and hyperplasia of juxtaglomerular cells produces hypokalemic alkalosis and hyperaldosteronism; it is characterized by absence of hypertension in the presence of markedly increased plasma renin concentrations, and by insensitivity to the pressor effects of angiotensin. It usually affects children, may be autosomal recessive, and may be associated with other anomalies, such as mental retardation and short stature. Called also *Bartter's syndrome*. **lipoid h.**, increased formation of lipoid-containing cells. **neoplastic h.**, hyperplasia brought about by a new growth. **nodular lymphoid h.**, a proliferation of small nodules of lymphoid tissue, seen in the terminal ileum and colon of children, in the small intestine and sometimes colon and stomach of adults with primary immunodeficiency disease, and, rarely, in the small intestine of adults with malignant lymphoma. **ovarian stromal h.**, thecomatosis. **polar h.**, excessive development at either extremity of the embryo, producing a monster either with two heads or with three or more lower limbs. **pseudoepitheliomatous h.**, a benign proliferative epithelial hyperplasia, the cytoarchitectural features of which are suggestive of squamous cell carcinoma; occurring in certain inflammatory diseases, especially granulomatous reactions and ulcerations. **Swiss-cheese h.**, hyperplasia of a tissue which on section shows openings as in Swiss cheese.

hyperplasmia (hi″per-plaz′me-ah) [*hyper-* + *plasma*] 1. excess in the proportion of blood plasm to corpuscles. 2. abnormally large size of erythrocytes through the absorption of plasma.

hyperplastic (hi″per-plas′tik) pertaining to or characterized by hyperplasia.

hyperploid (hi′per-ploid) [*hyper-* + *-ploid*] 1. having more than the typical number of chromosomes in unbalanced sets, as in Down's syndrome. 2. an individual or cell having more than the typical number of chromosomes in unbalanced sets.

hyperploidy (hi″per-ploi′de) the state of being hyperploid. Cf. *aneuploidy*.

hyperpnea (hi″perp-ne′ah) [*hyper-* + Gr. *pnoia* breath] abnormal increase in the depth and rate of the respiratory movements.

hyperpneic (hi″perp-ne′ik) pertaining to or characterized by hyperpnea.

hyperpolarization (hi″per-po″lar-i-za′shun) any increase in the amount of electrical charge separated by the cell membrane and hence in the strength of the transmembrane potential.

hyperpolypeptidemia (hi″per-pol″e-pep″tĭ-de′me-ah) excess of polypeptides in the blood.

hyperponesis (hi″per-po-ne′sis) [*hyper-* + Gr. *ponesis* toil, exertion] dysponesis in which there is excessive action-potential output from the motor and premotor areas of the cortex.

hyperponetic (hi″per-po-net′ik) pertaining to or characterized by hyperponesis.

hyperposia (hi″per-po′ze-ah) [hyper- + Gr. *posis* drinking + -*ia*] abnormally increased ingestion of fluids for relatively brief periods. Cf. *polyposia*.

hyperpotassemia (hi″per-pot″ah-se′me-ah) excess of potassium in the blood. See *hyperkalemia*.

hyperpragic (hi″per-praj′ik) characterized by excessive mental activity.

hyperpraxia (hi″per-prak′se-ah) [hyper- + Gr. *praxis* exercise] abnormal mental activity.

hyperprebetalipoproteinemia (hi″per-pre-ba″tah-lip″o-pro″- te-in-e′me-ah) an excess of prebetalipoproteins (very low-density lipoproteins) in the blood; see *hyperlipoproteinemia*, type IV. Called also *prebetalipoproteinemia*. **familial h.,** familial hyperlipoproteinemia, type IV.

hyperpresbyopia (hi″per-pres″be-o′pe-ah) excessive presbyopia.

hyperproinsulinemia (hi″per-pro-in″su-lin-e′me-ah) elevated levels of proinsulin or proinsulin-like material in the blood.

hyperprolactinemia (hi″per-pro-lak″tin-e′me-ah) increased levels of prolactin in the blood, which, in women, is associated with amenorrhea and galactorrhea, and, in men, has been reported to cause hypogonadism and impotence; often but not invariably associated with microadenoma of the anterior pituitary.

hyperprolactinemic (hi″per-pro-lak″tĭ-ne′mik) pertaining to, characterized by, or affected by hyperprolactinemia.

hyperprolinemia (hi″per-pro″lĭ-ne′me-ah) a disorder of amino acid metabolism characterized by an excess of proline in the body fluids. It occurs in two types, both of which are probably benign. *Type I* is caused by a defect in the oxidation of proline to pyrroline carboxylate. *Type II* involves a defect in the oxidation of pyrroline carboxylate and is characterized by a greater degree of hyperprolinemia and by urinary excretion of pyrroline carboxylate.

hyperprosexia (hi″per-pro-sek′se-ah) [hyper- + Gr. *prosechein* to heed] a condition in which the mind is occupied by one idea to the exclusion of others.

hyperproteinemia (hi″per-pro″te-in-e′me-ah) [hyper- + protein + Gr. *haima* blood + -*ia*] the presence of an abnormally high amount of protein in the blood; see also *hyperlipoproteinemia*.

hyperproteosis (hi″per-pro″te-o′sis) a condition caused by an excess of protein in the diet.

hyperpselaphesia (hi″perp-sel″ah-fe′ze-ah) [hyper- + Gr. *psēlaphēsis* touch + -*ia*] tactile hyperesthesia.

hyperptyalism (hi″per-ti′al-izm) [hyper- + Gr. *ptyalon* spittle] ptyalism.

hyperpyremia (hi″per-pi-re′me-ah) [hyper- + Gr. *pyreia* fuel + *haima* blood + -*ia*] excess of unoxidized carbonaceous matter in the blood.

hyperpyretic (hi″per-pi-ret′ik) pertaining to, exhibiting, or causing hyperpyrexia.

hyperpyrexia (hi″per-pi-rek′se-ah) [hyper- + Gr. *pyressein* to be feverish] a highly elevated body temperature. **malignant h.,** see under *hyperthermia*.

hyperpyrexial (hi″per-pi-rek′se-al) pertaining to hyperpyrexia.

hyperreactive (hi″per-re-ak′tiv) pertaining to or characterized by a greater than normal response to stimuli.

hyperreflexia (hi″per-re-flek′se-ah) [hyper- + reflex + -*ia*] exaggeration of reflexes. **autonomic h.,** paroxysmal hypertension, bradycardia, sweating of the forehead, severe headache, and gooseflesh due to distention of the bladder and rectum; it is associated with lesions above the outflow of the splanchnic nerves.

hyperreninemia (hi″per-re″nin-e′me-ah) a condition of elevated levels of renin in the blood, which may lead to aldosteronism and hypertension.

hyperreninemic (hi″per-re″nin-e′mik) producing or characterized by hyperreninemia.

hyperresonance (hi″per-rez′o-nans) an exaggerated resonance.

hypersalemia (hi″per-sal-e′me-ah) abnormally increased content of salt in the blood.

hypersaline (hi″per-sa′lin) excessively saline: a term applied to treatment by the administration of large doses of sodium chloride.

hypersalivation (hi″per-sal″ĭ-va′shun) ptyalism.

hypersarcosinemia (hi″per-sar″ko-sēn-e′me-ah) an inborn error of metabolism due to a defect of sarcosine dehydrogenase and marked by elevated levels of sarcosine in the blood.

hypersecretion (hi″per-se-kre′shun) excessive secretion. **gastric h.,** hyperchlorhydria.

hypersegmentation (hi″per-seg″men-ta′shun) the appearance of being divided into multiple segments or lobes. **hereditary h. of neutrophils,** a hereditary condition in which the neutrophils are multilobed; called also *Undritz anomaly.*

hypersensibility (hi″per-sen″sĭ-bil′ĭ-te) excessive sensibility or sensitivity to a substance or stimulus.

hypersensitive (hi″per-sen′sĭ-tiv) 1. exhibiting abnormally increased sensitivity. 2. having the specific or general ability to react with characteristic signs and symptoms to the application or contact with certain substances (allergens) in amounts innocuous to normal (nonsensitized) individuals. See *hypersensitivity*.

hypersensitivity (hi″per-sen′sĭ-tiv″ĭ-te) a state of altered reactivity in which the body reacts with an exaggerated immune response to a foreign substance. Hypersensitivity reactions are classified as immediate or delayed, types I and IV, respectively, in the Gell and Coombs classification (q.v.) of immune responses. **contact h.,** contact dermatitis

MEDIATORS OF IMMEDIATE HYPERSENSITIVITY

MEDIATOR	ACTIONS
Preformed—Released from storage vesicles	
Histamine	Increased vascular permeability Smooth muscle contraction
ECF-A	Chemotactic for eosinophils
Lysosomal enzymes	Tissue damage and repair Activation of kinin system
Heparin	Anticoagulant
NCF	Chemotactic for neutrophils
Serotonin	Increased vascular permeability
Newly formed—Produced upon stimulation	
SRS-A (leukotrienes LTC$_4$, LTD$_4$, LTE$_4$)	Smooth muscle contraction Increased vascular permeability
Prostaglandins (PGD$_2$)	Smooth muscle contraction
HETE, HHT	Chemotactic for eosinophils
PAF	Platelet aggregation Platelet mediator release

ECF-A, eosinophil chemotactic factor of anaphylaxis; *NCF*, neutrophil chemotactic factor; *SRS-A*, slow reacting substance of anaphylaxis; *HETE*, hydroxyeicosatetraenoic acid; *HHT*, hydroxyheptadecatrienoic acid; *PAF*, platelet activating factor.

(def. 1). **cutaneous basophil h.,** Jones-Mote reaction. **delayed h. (DH), delayed-type h. (DTH),** the type of hypersensitivity exemplified by the tuberculin reaction, which (as opposed to immediate hypersensitivity) take 12 to 48 hours to develop and which can be transferred by lymphocytes but not by serum. Delayed hypersensitivity can be induced by most viral infections, many bacterial infections, all mycotic infections, and a few protozoal infections (leishmaniasis and toxoplasmosis). It is produced only by natural infection, by vaccination with live virus vaccines, or by injection of antigen in conjunction with Freund's complete adjuvant. Intradermal injection of antigen (skin test) in sensitized individuals results in the formation of erythema and induration at the injection site characterized histologically by perivascular infiltration of monocytes and lymphocytes and the presence of large numbers of lymphoblasts produced by in situ transformation. Delayed hypersensitivity reactions are mediated by T lymphocytes both through release of lymphokines and through exertion of direct cytotoxicity. The scope of the term is sometimes expanded to cover all aspects of cell-mediated immunity including contact dermatitis, granulomatous reactions, and allograft rejection. Called also *tuberculin-type h.* and *Type IV h.* (Gell and Coombs classification; see under *classification*). **immediate h.,** antibody-mediated hypersensitivity occurring within minutes when a sensitized individual is exposed to antigen; clinical manifestations include systemic anaphylaxis and atopic allergy (allergic rhinitis, asthma, dermatitis, urticaria, and angioedema). The first exposure to the antigen induces the production of IgE antibodies (cytotropic antibodies, reagin) that bind to receptors on mast cells and basophils. Upon subsequent exposure the antigen cross-links receptor-bound IgE molecules, triggering production and release of a diverse array of mediators (see table) that act on other cells, producing symptoms such as bronchospasm, edema, mucous secretion, and inflammation. Called also *Type I h.* (Gell and Coombs classification; see under *classification*). **tuberculin-type h.,** delayed h.

hypersensitization (hi″per-sen″sĭ-ti-za′shun) the process of rendering or the condition of being abnormally sensitive. See *hypersensitivity.*

hyperserotonemia (hi″per-se″ro-to-ne′me-ah) an elevation of the serum serotonin level.

hypersexuality (hi″per-sek″shoo-al′ĭ-te) abnormally increased sexual desire or activity; nymphomania; satyriasis.

hyperskeocytosis (hi″per-ske″o-si-to′sis) [*hyper-* + Gr. *skaios* left + *kytos* hollow vessel + *-osis*] hyperneocytosis.

hypersomatotropism (hi″per-so-mat″ah-trop′izm) increased secretion of growth hormone.

hypersomia (hi″per-so′me-ah) [*hyper-* + Gr. *sōma* body] gigantism.

hypersomnia (hi″per-som′ne-ah) [*hyper-* + L. *somnus* sleep] excessive sleep.

hypersomnolence (hi″per-som′no-lens) a sleep disorder that includes excessive amounts of sleep and excessive daytime sleepiness.

hypersphyxia (hi″per-sfik′se-ah) [*hyper-* + Gr. *sphyxis* pulse + *-ia*] increased activity of the circulation with increased blood pressure.

hypersplenia (hi″per-sple′ne-ah) hypersplenism.

hypersplenism (hi″per-splen′izm) a condition characterized by exaggeration of the suggested inhibitory or destructive functions of the spleen, resulting in deficiency of the peripheral blood elements, singly or in combination, hypercellularity of the bone marrow, and usually, but not always, splenomegaly.

hyperspongiosis (hi-per-spon″je-o′sis) proliferation of the substantia spongiosa ossium.

Hyperstat (hi′per-stat) trademark for a preparation of diazoxide.

hypersteatosis (hi″per-ste-ah-to′sis) [*hyper-* + *steatosis*] increased or excessive sebaceous secretion, as in seborrhea.

hyperstereoroentgenography (hi″per-ste″re-o-rent″-gen-og′rah-fe) stereoroentgenography with great distance between the homologous points.

hyperstereoskiagraphy (hi″per-ste″re-o-ski-ag′rah-fe) hyperstereoroentgenography.

hypersthenia (hi″per-sthe′ne-ah) [*hyper-* + Gr. *sthenos* strength] great strength or tonicity.

hypersthenic (hi″per-sthen′ik) pertaining to or characterized by hypersthenia.

hypersthenuria (hi″per-sthĕ-nu′re-ah) [*hyper-* + Gr. *sthenos* strength + *ouron* urine + *-ia*] increased osmolality of the urine.

hypersuprarenalism (hi″per-su″prah-re′nal-izm) hyperadrenalism.

hypersusceptibility (hi″per-sŭ-sep″tĭ-bil′ĭ-te) a condition of abnormally increased susceptibility to poisons, infective agents, or agents which in the normal individual are entirely innocuous.

hypersympathicotonus (hi″per-sim-path″ĕ-ko-to′nus) an increased tone of the sympathetic nervous system.

hypertarachia (hi″per-tah-rak′e-ah) [*hyper-* + Gr. *tarachē* confusion] extreme irritability of the nervous system.

hypertaurodontism (hi″per-taw″ro-don′tizm) [*hyper-* + Gr. *tauros* bull + *odont-* + *-ism*] taurodontism in which the tooth roots do not branch.

hypertelorism (hi″per-te′lor-izm) [*hyper-* + Gr. *tēlouros* distant] 1. abnormally increased distance between two organs or parts. 2. ocular h. **ocular h., orbital h.,** a condition characterized by abnormal increase in the interorbital distance, often associated with cleidocranial or craniofacial dysostosis, and occasionally accompanied by mental deficiency.

Hypertensin (hi″per-ten′sin) trademark for a preparation of angiotensin amide.

hypertensinogen (hi″per-ten-sin′o-jen) angiotensinogen.

hypertension (hi″per-ten′shun) [*hyper-* + *tension*] persistently high arterial blood pressure. Various criteria for its threshold have been suggested, ranging from 140 mm. Hg systolic and 90 mm. Hg diastolic to as high as 200 mm. Hg systolic and 110 mm. Hg diastolic. Hypertension may have no known cause (*essential* or *idiopathic h.*) or be associated with other primary diseases (*secondary h.*); see also *blood pressure,* under *pressure.* **accelerated h.,** progressive hypertension marked by the funduscopic vascular changes of malignant hypertension but without papilledema. **adrenal h.,** hypertension associated with an adrenal tumor that secretes mineral corticosteroids, e.g., hyperaldosteronism. **benign intracranial h.,** pseudotumor cerebri. **borderline h.,** a condition in which the arterial blood pressure is sometimes within the normotensive range and sometimes within the hypertensive range; called also *labile h.* **essential h.,** hypertension occurring without discoverable organic cause; called also *primary h.* and *idiopathic h.* **Goldblatt h.,** see under *kidney.* **idiopathic h.,** essential h. **intracranial h.,** a syndrome of increased intracranial pressure and papilledema with no focal neurologic signs and with normal-sized cerebral ventricles. **labile h.,** borderline h. **low-renin h.,** essential hypertension associated with low levels of plasma-renin concentration or low renin activity. **malignant h.,** a severe hypertensive state with poor prognosis; it is characterized by papilledema of the ocular fundus with vascular exudative and hemorrhagic lesions, medial thickening of small arteries and arterioles, and left ventricular hypertrophy. Diastolic pressures as high as 130 mm. Hg or more are commonly present. **neuromuscular h.,** a condition of hyperexcitability and hyperirritability of reflex response; called also *anxiety tension state.* **ocular h.,** persistently elevated intraocular pressure in the absence of any other signs of glaucoma; it may or may not progress to chronic simple glaucoma. **pale h.,** malignant h. **portal h.,** abnormally increased blood pressure in the portal venous system, a frequent complication of cirrhosis of the liver. **primary h.,** essential h. **pulmonary h.,** increased pressure (above 30 mm. Hg systolic and 12 mm. Hg diastolic) within the pulmonary circulation. **red h.,** benign h. **renal h.,** hypertension due to or associated with renal disease with a factor of parenchymal ischemia. **renovascular h.,** hypertension due to occlusive disease of the renal arteries. **secondary h.,** hypertension due to or associated with a variety of primary diseases, such as renal disorders, disorders of the central nervous system, endocrine diseases, and vascular diseases. **splenoportal h.,** obstruction of the splenic venous system resulting in enlargement of the liver and manifestation of ascites and other evidence of portal cirrhosis. **symptomatic h.,** secondary h. **systemic venous h.,** elevation of systemic venous pressure, usually detected by inspection of the jugular veins. **vascular h.,** hypertension.

hypertensive (hi″per-ten′siv) 1. characterized by or causing increased tension or pressure, as abnormally high blood pressure. 2. a person with abnormally high blood pressure.

hypertensor (hi″per-ten′sor) a pressor agent.

Hyper-Tet (hi′per-tet″) trademark for a preparation of tetanus immune human globulin.

hyperthecosis (hi″per-the-ko′sis) hyperplasia with excessive luteinization of the cells of the inner stromal layer, the theca interna, of the ovary; it may be associated with hirsutism and amenorrhea.

hyperthelia (hi″per-the′le-ah) [*hyper-* + Gr. *thēlē* nipple] the presence of supernumerary nipples.

hyperthermal (hi″per-ther′mal) marked by abnormally high temperature.

hyperthermalgesia (hi″per-ther″mal-je′ze-ah) [*hyper-* + Gr. *thermē* heat + *algēsis* pain] abnormally increased sensitivity to heat.

hyperthermesthesia (hi″per-ther″mes-the′ze-ah) [*hyper-* + Gr. *thermē* heat + *aisthēsis* perception + *-ia*] increased sensibility for heat.

hyperthermia (hi″per-ther′me-ah) [*hyper-* + Gr. *thermē* heat + *-ia*] abnormally high body temperature, especially that induced for therapeutic purposes. **h. of anesthesia,** malignant h. **malignant h.,** an autosomal dominantly and multifactorially inherited condition, occurring in patients undergoing general anesthesia, and causing a sudden, rapid rise in body temperature, associated with signs of increased muscle metabolism, such as tachycardia, tachypnea, sweating, and cyanosis, and, usually, muscle rigidity. Called also *h. of anesthesia* and *malignant hyperpyrexia*.

hyperthermoesthesia (hi″per-ther″mo-es-the′ze-ah) hyperthermesthesia.

hyperthermy (hi″per-ther′me) hyperthermia.

hyperthrombinemia (hi″per-throm″bĭ-ne′me-ah) abnormally high thrombin content of the blood.

hyperthymia (hi″per-thi′me-ah) [*hyper-* + Gr. *thymos* spirit + *-ia*] excessive emotionalism.

hyperthymic (hi″per-thi′mik) marked by hyperthymia.

hyperthymism (hi″per-thi′mizm) a condition attributed to excessive activity of the thymus gland.

hyperthyrea (hi″per-thi′re-ah) hyperthyroidism.

hyperthyreosis (hi″per-thi″re-o′sis) hyperthyroidism.

hyperthyroid (hi″per-thi′roid) marked by or due to hyperthyroidism.

hyperthyroidism (hi″per-thi′roi-dizm) a condition of excessive functional activity of the thyroid gland and excess secretion of thyroid hormones marked by goiter, tachycardia or atrial fibrillation, widened pulse pressure, palpitations, fatigability, nervousness and tremor, heat intolerance and excessive sweating, warm, smooth, moist skin, weight loss, muscular weakness, hyperdefecation, emotional lability, and ocular signs (stare, lid lag, photophobia, sometimes exophthalmos). **masked h.,** hyperactivity of the thyroid gland in which the classic signs and symptoms are subtle, and predominance of cardiovascular symptoms leads to suspicion of heart disease rather than thyroid disease; it occurs chiefly in middle-aged or elderly persons.

hyperthyroidosis (hi″per-thi″roi-do′sis) hyperthyroidism.

hyperthyroxinemia (hi″per-thi-rok″sĭ-ne′me-ah) excess of thyroxine in the blood. **familial dysalbuminemic h.,** a familial syndrome, with autosomal dominant inheritance, in which total serum thyroxine concentration is elevated, suggesting the presence of hyperthyroidism, but since there is an excess of a T$_4$-binding serum albumin, free thyroxine concentration and triiodothyroxine resin uptake are normal, and the patients are euthyroid by clinical evaluation and other tests.

hypertonia (hi″per-to′ne-ah) [*hyper-* + Gr. *tonos* tension] a condition of excessive tone of the skeletal muscles; increased resistance of muscle to passive stretching. **h. polycythae′mica,** increased blood pressure associated with polycythemia.

hypertonic (hi″per-ton′ik) a biological term denoting a solution which when bathing body cells causes a net flow of water across the semipermeable cell membrane out of the cell. Also, denoting a solution having a greater tonicity than another solution, e.g., the blood, with which it is compared.

hypertonicity (hi″per-to-nis′ĭ-te) the state or quality of being hypertonic.

hypertonus (hi″per-to′nus) hypertonia.

hypertoxic (hi″per-tok′sik) excessively toxic.

hypertoxicity (hi″per-tok-sis′ĭ-te) the state or quality of being excessively toxic.

hypertrichosis (hi″per-tri-ko′sis) [*hyper-* + Gr. *thrix* hair + *-osis*] excessive growth of the hair. Called also *polytrichia* and *polytrichosis*. Cf. *hirsutism*. **h. lanugino′sa,** persistent or acquired production of lanugo. It may be a congenital, autosomal dominant disorder in which there is excessive hair distributed over the entire body throughout life, usually in association with other congenital anomalies, called also *h. universalis*; or it may be acquired, with the degree of hairiness being variable, and usually involving the face, and in most cases associated with internal carcinoma. **h. pin′nae au′ris,** hypertrichosis involving the pinna of the ear; it may be a Y-linked or an autosomal dominant trait. Called also *hairy ears*. **h. universa′lis,** the congenital form of hypertrichosis lanuginosa.

hypertriglyceridemia (hi″per-tri-glis″er-i-de′me-ah) [*hyper-* + *triglyceride* + *-emia*] an excess of triglycerides in the blood; it is an autosomal dominant disorder with the phenotype of hyperlipoproteinemia, type IV. **carbohydrate-induced h.,** familial hyperlipoproteinemia, types III and IV. **familial h.,** familial hyperlipoproteinemia, type IV.

hypertrophia (hi″per-tro′fe-ah) hypertrophy.

hypertrophic (hi″per-trof′ik) pertaining to or marked by hypertrophy.

hypertrophy (hi-per′tro-fe) [*hyper-* + Gr. *trophē* nutrition] the enlargement or overgrowth of an organ or part due to an increase in size of its constituent cells. Cf. *hyperplasia*. **adaptive h.,** increase in size in response to changed conditions, as, for example, increased thickness of the walls of a hollow organ when the outflow is obstructed. **Billroth h.,** idiopathic benign hypertrophy of the pylorus. **compensatory h.,** that which results from an increased workload due to some physical defect, as of the left ventricle of the heart due to hypertension. **complementary h.,** increase in size of the remaining part of an organ to take the place of a portion which has been lost. **concentric h.,** increased thickness of the walls of an organ, with no enlargement and with diminished capacity. **eccentric h.,** hypertrophy of a hollow organ, with dilatation of its cavity. **false h.,** enlargement due to an increase in only one constituent element of an organ or part, commonly the stroma. **functional h.,** hypertrophy of an organ or part caused by its increased activity. **hemifacial h.,** overgrowth of one side of the face. **Marie's h.,** enlargement of the soft parts of the joints resulting from periostitis. **numeric h.,** that which is due to an increased number of structural elements. **physiologic h.,** temporary increase in the size of an organ produced by physiologic activity, as in the female breast during pregnancy and lactation. **pseudomuscular h.,** pseudohypertrophic muscular dystrophy. **quantitative h.,** hyperplasia. **simple h.,** that which is due to a simple increase of the number of structural elements. **true h.,** enlargement due to an increase of all the component elements of an organ or part. **unilateral h.,** overgrowth of one side of the entire body or of a portion of one side, as of the face. **ventricular h.,** hypertrophy of the myocardium of a ventricle. **vicarious h.,** hypertrophy of an organ in consequence of the failure of another organ of allied function.

hypertropia (hi″per-tro′pe-ah) [*hyper-* + Gr. *trepein* to turn] strabismus in which there is permanent upward deviation of the visual axis of an eye.

Hypertussis (hi′per-tus″sis) trademark for a preparation of pertussis immune human globulin.

hyperuresis (hi″per-u-re′sis) polyuria.

hyperuricacidemia (hi″per-u″rik-as″ĭ-de′me-ah) hyperuricemia.

hyperuricaciduria (hi″per-u″rik-as″ĭ-du′re-ah) hyperuricuria.

hyperuricemia (hi″per-u″rĭ-se′me-ah) excess of uric acid or urates in the blood; it is a prerequisite for the development of gout and may lead to renal disease. Called also *uricacidemia* and, formerly, *lithemia*.

hyperuricemic (hi″per-u″rĭ-se′mik) pertaining to or characterized by hyperuricemia.

hyperuricuria (hi″per-u″rik-u′re-ah) excess of uric acid or urates in the urine. Called also *uricaciduria* and, formerly, *lithuria*.

hypervaccination (hi″per-vak″sĭ-na′shun) the subsequent inoculation (one or more times) of a previously immunized animal with enough vaccine to enable it to afford a serum protective to other animals.

hypervalinemia (hi″per-val″ĭ-ne′me-ah) an inborn error of metabolism, possibly due to a defect in valine transamination, characterized by elevated levels of valine in the plasma and urine and by failure to thrive; it may occur alone or with elevated levels of other amino acids, as in maple syrup urine disease. Called also *valinemia*.

hypervascular (hi″per-vas″ku-lar) extremely vascular.

hyperventilation (hi″per-ven″tĭ-la′shun) 1. a state in which there is an increased amount of air entering the pulmonary alveoli (increased alveolar ventilation), resulting in reduction of carbon dioxide tension and eventually leading to alkalosis. 2. abnormally prolonged, rapid, and deep breathing, frequently used as a test procedure in epilepsy and tetany.

hyperviscosity (hi″per-vis-kos′ĭ-te) excessive viscosity, as of the blood; see under *syndrome*.

hypervitaminosis (hi″per-vi″tah-mĭ-no′sis) a condition due to ingestion of an excess of one or more vitamins; called also *supervitaminosis*. **h. A,** a symptom complex resulting from ingestion of excessive amounts of vitamin A, with skin pigmentation, generalized pruritus, changes in the horny structures of the skin, and loss of hair; serum levels of vitamin A usually are elevated to more than 100 mg. per 100 ml. **h. D,** a symptom complex resulting from ingestion of excessive amounts of vitamin D, with weakness, fatigue, loss of weight, and other symptoms.

hypervitaminotic (hi″per-vi″tah-mĭ-not′ik) pertaining to or characterized by hypervitaminosis.

hypervolemia (hi″per-vo-le′me-ah) [*hyper-* + *volume* + Gr. *haima* blood + *-ia*] abnormal increase in the volume of circulating fluid (plasma) in the body.

hypervolemic (hi″per-vo-le′mik) pertaining to or characterized by hypervolemia.

hypervolia (hi″per-vo′le-ah) augmented water content or volume of a given compartment, e.g., as of a cell.

hypesthesia (hĭp″es-the′ze-ah) hypoesthesia.

hypha (hi′fah), pl. *hy′phae* [L., from Gr. *hyphe* web] 1. one of the filaments or threads composing the mycelium of a fungus. 2. branching filamentous outgrowths produced by certain bacteria (e.g., *Actinomyces, Hyphomicrobium*), sometimes forming a mycelium.

hyphae (hi′fe) [L.] plural of *hypha.*

hyphal (hi′ful) pertaining to a hypha.

hyphedonia (hĭp″hĕ-do′ne-ah) [*hypo-* + Gr. *hēdonē* pleasure + *-ia*] pathologic diminution of the feeling of pleasure in acts that normally give pleasure.

hyphema (hi-fe′mah) [Gr. *hyphaimos* suffused with blood, blood-shot; especially of the eyes] hemorrhage within the anterior chamber of the eye. Called also *hyphemia.*

hyphemia (hi-fe′me-ah) 1. (*obs.*) oligemia. 2. hyphema.

hyphidrosis (hĭp″hid-ro′sis) [*hypo-* + Gr. *hidrōs* sweat + *-osis*] hypohidrosis.

Hyphomicrobiaceae (hi″fo-mi-kro″be-a′se-e) in former systems of classification, a family of budding bacteria consisting of the genera *Hyphomicrobium* and *Rhodomicrobium,* which are now classified in separate taxa.

Hyphomicrobiales (hi″fo-mi-kro″be-a′lēz) in former systems of classification, an order of bacteria made up of cells that reproduce by budding or binary fission. They are now classified in the genera *Hyphomicrobium, Pasteuria, Planctomyces,* and *Rhodomicrobium.*

Hyphomicrobium (hi″fo-mi-kro′be-um) [Gr. *hyphe* web + Gr. *mikros* small + *bios* life] a genus of budding bacteria found in soils and sea water, made up of ovoid cells growing in a dense clump from which filaments radiate outward. Multiplication is by budding at the tips of hyphae. The type species is *H. vulga′re.*

Hyphomonas (hi″fo-mo′nas) [Gr. *hyphe-* web + Gr. *monas* a unit, from *monos* single] a genus of budding bacteria made up of oval or pear-shaped cells that produce prosthecae that may be branched. The type species is *H. polymor′pha.*

Hyphomyces (hi-fo-mi′sēz) a genus of phycomycetous fungi the members of which do not sporulate; they appear to be related to the genus *Mortierella* (order Mucorales, family Mucoraceae). **H. des′truens,** the etiologic agent of hyphomycosis destruens equi.

hyphomycete (hi″fo-mi-sēt) any individual organism of the Hyphomycetes, an imperfect mold in contrast to an imperfect yeast.

Hyphomycetes (hi″fo-mi-se′tēz) [pl., Gr. *hyphē* web + Gr. *mykēs* fungus] the mycelial (hyphal) fungi, i.e., molds, of the Fungi Imperfecti (Deuteromycetes).

hyphomycetic (hi″fo-mi-set′ik) (*obs.*) due to the presence of mold, or mycelial, fungi.

hyphomycetoma (hi″fo-mi″se-to′mah) (*obs.*) a tumor caused by hyphomycetes (imperfect fungi).

hyphomycosis (hi″fo-mi-ko′sis) 1. infection with fungi of the genus *Hyphomyces.* 2. (*obs.*) infection with hyphomycetes (imperfect fungi). **h. des′truens e′qui,** a disease of horses and mules in India, Indonesia, Europe, and southern United States, caused by *Hyphomyces destruens;* it is marked by the formation of subcutaneous abscesses that enlarge until the skin over and around the lesions is destroyed, leaving large raw surfaces. Because of the clinical similarity between hyphomycosis destruens equi and cutaneous habronemiasis, the disorders are often confused.

hyphylline (hi-fil′in) dyphylline.

hypisotonic (hīp″i-so-ton′ik) less than isotonic.

hypnagogic (hip″nah-goj′ik) 1. producing sleep. 2. occurring just before sleep; applied to hallucinations occurring at sleep onset.

hypnagogue (hip′nah-gog) [*hypno-* + Gr. *agōgos* leading] 1. hypnotic; pertaining to drowsiness. 2. an agent that induces sleep or drowsiness.

hypnalgia (hip-nal′je-ah) [*hypno-* + Gr. *algos* pain + *-ia*] pain that occurs during sleep.

hypnic (hip′nik) [Gr. *hypnikos*] inducing or pertaining to sleep.

hypn(o)- [Gr. *hypnos* sleep] a combining form denoting relationship to sleep or to hypnosis.

hypnoanalysis (hip″no-ah-nal′ĭ-sis) [*hypno-* + *analysis*] a method of psychotherapy in which psychoanalysis is employed in conjunction with hypnosis.

hypnoanesthesia (hip″no-an″es-the′ze-ah) induction of the anesthetic state by hypnosis.

hypnocinematograph (hip″no-sin″ĕ-mat′o-graf) [*hypno-* + Gr. *kinēma* movement + *graphein* to record] an apparatus for recording the movements made by a sleeping person.

hypnocyst (hip′no-sist) [*hypno-* + *cyst*] a quiescent cyst.

hypnodontia (hip″no-don′she-ah) hypnodontics.

hypnodontics (hip″no-don′tiks) [*hypnosis* + Gr. *odous* tooth] the application of controlled suggestion and hypnosis in the practice of dentistry.

hypnogenetic (hip″no-jĕ-net′ik) hypnogenic.

hypnogenic (hip″no-jen′ik) [*hypno-* + Gr. *gennan* to produce] inducing sleep or a hypnotic state.

hypnogenous (hip-noj′ĕ-nus) hypnogenic.

hypnoid (hip′noid) resembling hypnosis or the hypnotic state.

hypnoidal (hip-noi′dal) pertaining to a state resembling hypnosis.

hypnolepsy (hip′no-lep″se) [*hypno-* + Gr. *lēpsis* seizure] narcolepsy.

hypnology (hip-nol′o-je) [*hypno-* + *-logy*] the sum of what is known regarding sleep or hypnosis.

hypnopedia (hip″no-pe′de-ah) [*hypno-* + *paideia* education] sleep learning; learning during sleep, as by listening to recordings.

hypnopompic (hip″no-pom′pik) [*hypno-* + Gr. *pompē* a sending away, a sending home] persisting after sleep; applied to hallucinations occurring on awakening.

hypnosis (hip-no′sis) a state of altered consciousness, usually artificially induced, characterized by focusing of attention, heightened responsiveness to suggestions and commands, suspension of disbelief with lowering of critical judgment, the potential of alteration in perceptions, motor control, or memory in response to suggestions, and the subjective experience of responding involuntarily.

hypnosophy (hip-nos′o-fe) [*hypno-* + Gr. *sophia* wisdom] the study of sleep and its phenomena.

hypnotherapy (hip″no-ther′ah-pe) [*hypno-* + Gr. *therapeia* treatment] the use of hypnosis in the treatment of disease.

hypnotic (hip-not′ik) [Gr. *hypnōtikos*] 1. inducing sleep. 2. pertaining to or of the nature of hypnotism. 3. a drug that acts to induce sleep.

hypnotism (hip′no-tizm) 1. the method or practice of inducing hypnosis. 2. hypnosis.

hypnotist (hip′no-tist) one who induces hypnosis.

hypnotization (hip″no-ti-za′shun) the induction of hypnosis.

hypnotize (hip′no-tiz) to induce hypnosis.

hypnotoxin (hip″no-tok′sin) a toxic substance derived from the tentacles of *Physalia,* the Portuguese man-of-war, characteristically causing a central nervous system depression, affecting both motor and sensory elements.

hypnozoite (hip″no-zo′ĭt) [*hypno-* + Gr. *zōon* animal] a latent hemosporian sporozoite, i.e., one that does not undergo schizogony but remains capable of doing so; believed to be associated with relapse in malaria.

hypo (hi′po) 1. a popular designation for a hypodermic inoculation or syringe. 2. a contraction for sodium thiosulfate, used as a photographic fixing agent.

hyp(o)- [Gr. *hypo* under] a prefix signifying beneath, under, below normal, or deficient. Cf. *sub-*. In chemistry, it denotes a compound, usually an acid or a salt, containing the lowest proportion of oxygen in a series of similar compounds, e.g., hypochlorous acid (HClO) or sodium hypochlorite (NaClO).

hypoacidity (hi″po-ah-sid′ĭ-te) deficiency of acid; lack of normal acidity.

hypoactive (hi″po-ak′tiv) pertaining to or characterized by hypoactivity.

hypoactivity (hi″po-ak-tiv′ĭ-te) abnormally diminished activity, as of peristalsis.

hypoacusis (hi″po-ah-ku′sis) [hypo- + Gr. *akousis* hearing] slightly diminished auditory sensitivity, with hearing threshold levels above the normal limit so that the impairment is measureable in decibels.

hypoadrenalism (hi″po-ah-dre′nal-izm) abnormally diminished activity of the adrenal gland, as in Addison's disease.

hypoadrenocorticism (hi″po-ah-dre″no-kor′tĭ-sizm) abnormally diminished secretion of the adrenal cortex; see *Addison's disease.*

hypoalbuminemia (hi″po-al-bu″mĭn-e′me-ah) an abnormally low albumin content of the blood.

hypoalbuminosis (hi″po-al-bu″mĭ-no′sis) a condition characterized by an abnormally low level of albumin.

hypoaldosteronemia (hi″po-al″do-stēr″o-ne′me-ah) an abnormally low level of aldosterone in the blood.

hypoaldosteronism (hi″po-al″do-stēr′ŏn-izm) a deficiency of aldosterone in the body, usually associated with hypoadrenalism, and characterized by hypotension and a tendency to excrete excessive sodium. **isolated h.,** a rare endocrine disorder characterized by reduced or absent aldosterone production, with normal production of cortisol and all other adrenal steroids.

hypoaldosteronuria (hi″po-al″do-stēr″o-nu′re-ah) presence of an abnormally low level of aldosterone in the urine.

hypoalgesia (hi″po-al-je′se-ah) hypalgesia.

hypoalimentation (hi″po-al″ĭ-men-ta′shun) insufficient nourishment.

hypoalkaline (hi″po-al′kah-lin) less alkaline than normal.

hypoalkalinity (hi″po-al″kah-lin′ĭ-te) the state of being less alkaline than normal.

hypoalonemia (hi″po-al″o-ne′me-ah) [hypo- + Gr. *hals* salt + *haima* blood + -ia] a deficiency of salts in the blood.

hypoaminoacidemia (hi″po-am″ĭ-no-as″ĭ-de′me-ah) the presence of less than the normal amount of amino acids in the blood.

hypoandrogenism (hi″po-an-dro′jen-izm) a state characterized or caused by deficiency of androgens.

hypoazoturia (hi″po-az″o-tu′re-ah) [hypo- + L. *azotum* nitrogen + -uria] diminished excretion of nitrogenous material in the urine.

hypobaric (hi″po-bār′ik) [hypo- + Gr. *baros* weight] characterized by less than normal pressure or weight; applied to gases under less than atmospheric pressure or to a solution of lower specific gravity than another taken as a standard of reference. See under *solution.*

hypobarism (hi″po-bar′izm) the condition resulting from exposure to ambient gas pressure or atmospheric pressures that are below those within body tissues, fluids, cavities.

hypobaropathy (hi″po-bār-op′ah-the) [hypo- + Gr. *baros* pressure + *pathos* disease] the disturbances experienced in high altitudes due to reduced air pressure; see *high-altitude sickness* and *mountain sickness,* under *sickness.*

hypobetalipoproteinemia (hi″po-ba″tah-lip″o-pro″te-in-e′me-ah) the presence of abnormally low levels of β-lipoprotein in the serum, as in debilitating diseases and malabsorption syndromes. **familial h.,** see *familial lipoprotein deficiency.*

hypobilirubinemia (hi″po-bil″ĭ-ru″bĭ-ne′me-ah) abnormal diminution of bilirubin in the blood.

hypoblast (hi′po-blast) [hypo- + Gr. *blastos* germ] entoderm.

hypoblastic (hi″po-blas′tik) entodermic.

hypobranchial (hi″po-brang′ke-al) [hypo- + Gr. *branchia* gills] located beneath the branchial arches.

hypobromite (hi″po-bro′mīt) any salt of hypobromous acid.

hypobromous acid (hi″po-bro′mus) an unstable acid, HBrO; used as a disinfectant, bleaching agent, and in testing for urea.

hypocalcemia (hi″po-kal-se′me-ah) [hypo- + *calcium* + Gr. *haima* blood + -ia] reduction of the blood calcium below normal; manifestations include hyperactive deep tendon reflexes, Chvostek's sign, muscle and abdominal cramps, and carpopedal spasm.

hypocalcia (hi″po-kal′se-ah) deficiency of calcium.

hypocalcification (hi″po-kal″sĭ-fĭ-ka′shun) diminished calcification. **enamel h.,** an autosomal dominant form of amelogenesis imperfecta due to faulty mineralization of enamel, characterized by a tooth crown that appears normal at eruption but soon assumes a white chalky appearance and gradually undergoes brown discoloration; the affected teeth are soft and rough.

hypocalcipectic (hi″po-kal″sĭ-pek′tik) pertaining to or characterized by hypocalcipexy.

hypocalcipexy (hi″po-kal′sĭ-pek″se) deficient calcium fixation.

hypocalciuria (hi″po-kal″se-u′re-ah) an abnormally diminished amount of calcium in the urine.

hypocapnia (hi″po-kap′ne-ah) [hypo- + Gr. *kapnos* smoke + -ia] deficiency of carbon dioxide in the blood, resulting from hyperventilation and eventually leading to alkalosis.

hypocapnic (hi″po-kap′nik) pertaining to or characterized by hypocapnia.

hypocarbia (hi″po-kar′be-ah) hypocapnia.

hypocellular (hi″po-sel′u-lar) pertaining to or characterized by hypocellularity.

hypocellularity (hi″po-sel″u-lār′ĭ-te) a state of abnormal decrease in the number of cells present, as in bone marrow.

hypocelom (hi″po-se′lom) hypocoelom.

hypochloremia (hi″po-klo-re′me-ah) an abnormally diminished level of chloride in the blood.

hypochloremic (hi″po-klo-re′mik) pertaining to or characterized by hypochloremia.

hypochlorhydria (hi″po-klor-hi′dre-ah) [hypo- + Gr. *chlōros* green + *hydōr* water + -ia] deficiency of hydrochloric acid in the gastric juice. Cf. *achlorhydria.*

hypochloridation (hi″po-klo″rĭ-da′shun) chloride deficiency in the system.

hypochloridemia (hi″po-klo″rid-e′me-ah) hypochloremia.

hypochlorite (hi″po-klo′rīt) [hypo- + Gr. *chlōros* green] any salt of hypochlorous acid; used as a medicinal agent, particularly as a diluted solution of sodium hypochlorite. See *sodium hypochlorite solution, diluted,* under *solution.*

hypochlorization (hi″po-klo″ri-za′shun) reduction of the amount of sodium chloride in the diet.

hypochlorous acid (hi″po-klor′us) an unstable, strongly oxidizing but weak compound, HClO, known only in aqueous solution as a greenish yellow liquid that deteriorates when exposed to light, and used as a bleaching agent and disinfectant; its derivatives and salts (hypochlorites) are used as medicinal agents, particularly as surgical solution of chlorinated soda. See *sodium hypochlorite solution (diluted),* under *solution.*

hypochloruria (hi″po-klo-ru′re-ah) [hypo- + *chloride* + -uria] deficiency of chlorides in the urine.

hypocholesteremia (hi″po-ko-les″tĕ-re′me-ah) hypocholesterolemia.

hypocholesteremic (hi″po-ko-les″tĕ-re′mik) hypocholesterolemic.

hypocholesterinemia (hi″po-ko-les″ter-ĭ-ne′me-ah) hypocholesterolemia.

hypocholesterolemia (hi″po-ko-les″ter-o-le′me-ah) an abnormally diminished amount of cholesterol in the blood.

hypocholesterolemic (hi″po-ko-les″ter-o-le′mik) pertaining to, characterized by, or producing hypocholesterolemia.

hypocholia (hi-po-ko′le-ah) oligocholia.

hypocholuria (hi″po-ko-lu′re-ah) abnormal reduction in the amount of bile in the urine.

hypochondria (hi″po-kon′dre-ah) 1. plural of *hypochondrium*. 2. hypochondriasis.

hypochondriac (hi″po-kon′dre-ak) 1. pertaining to the hypochondrium or to hypochondriasis. 2. a person affected with hypochondriasis.

hypochondriacal (hi″po-kon-dri′ah-kal) affected with hypochondriasis.

hypochondriasis (hi″po-kon-dri′ah-sis) [so called because it was supposed by the ancients to be due to disturbed function of the organs of the upper abdomen] [DSM III-R] a mental disorder characterized by a preoccupation with bodily functions and the interpretation of normal sensations (such as heart beats, sweating, peristaltic action, and bowel movements) or minor abnormalities (such as a runny nose, minor aches and pains, or slightly swollen lymph nodes) as indications of highly disturbing problems needing medical attention. Negative results of diagnostic evaluations and reassurance by physicians only increase the patient's anxious concern about his health, and the patient continues to seek medical attention. Called also *hypochondriacal neurosis*.

hypochondrium (hi″po-kon′dre-um), pl. *hypochon′dria* [*hypo-* + Gr. *chondros* cartilage] NA alternative for *regio hypochondriaca* [*dextra et sinistra*].

hypochondroplasia (hi″po-kon″dro-pla′ze-ah) a common chondrodystrophy resembling achondroplasia but with milder clinical features, which include short stature with a long trunk and short limbs, broad and short fingers, and a normal face; it is transmitted as an autosomal dominant trait.

hypochordal (hi″po-kor′dal) situated ventral to the notochord.

hypochromasia (hi″po-kro-ma′ze-ah) [*hypo-* + Gr. *chrōma* color] 1. the condition of staining less intensely than normal. 2. decrease of hemoglobin in the erythrocytes so that they are abnormally pale in color.

hypochromatic (hi″po-kro-mat′ik) containing an abnormally small number of chromosomes; marked by hypochromatism.

hypochromatism (hi″po-kro′mah-tizm) [*hypo-* + *chromatin*] abnormally deficient pigmentation, especially deficiency of the chromatin in a cell nucleus.

hypochromatosis (hi″po-kro″mah-to′sis) the gradual fading and disappearance of the nucleus (the chromatin) of a cell.

hypochromemia (hi″po-kro-me′me-ah) [*hypo-* + Gr. *chrōma* color + *haima* blood + *-ia*] a condition in which the blood has an abnormally low color index. **idiopathic h.,** idiopathic hypochromic anemia.

hypochromia (hi″po-kro′me-ah) [*hypo-* + Gr. *chrōma* color + *-ia*] 1. abnormal decrease in the hemoglobin content of the erythrocytes. 2. hypochromatism.

hypochromic (hi″po-kro′mik) pertaining to or marked by hypochromia.

hypochromotrichia (hi″po-kro″mo-trik′e-ah) abnormally reduced pigmentation of the hair.

hypochrosis (hi″po-kro′sis) [*hypo-* + Gr. *chrōma* color + *-osis*] anemia in which there is an abnormally small amount of hemoglobin in the blood.

hypochylia (hi″po-ki′le-ah) [*hypo-* + Gr. *chylos* chyle + *-ia*] deficiency of chyle.

hypocinesia (hi″po-si-ne′ze-ah) hypokinesia.

hypocist (hi′po-sist) hypocistis.

hypocistis (hi″po-sis′tis) the juice and extract of various species of the parasitic herb *Cytinus*, as of *C. hypocistis* of southern Europe: astringent.

hypocitremia (hi″po-sĭ-tre′me-ah) [*hypo-* + *citric* acid + Gr. *haima* blood + *-ia*] abnormally low content of citric acid in the blood.

hypocitruria (hi″po-sĭ-troo′re-ah) [*hypo-* + *citric* acid + Gr. *ouron* urine + *-ia*] excretion of urine containing an abnormally small amount of citric acid.

hypocoagulability (hi″po-ko-ag″u-lah-bil′ĭ-te) the state of being less readily coagulated than normal.

hypocoagulable (hi″po-ko-ag′u-lah-b'l) characterized by abnormally decreased coagulability.

hypocoelom (hi″po-se′lom) [*hypo-* + Gr. *koilōma* hollow] the ventral portion of the coelom of any embryonic vertebrate.

Hypocomatina (hi″po-ko″mah-ti′nah) [*hypo-* + Gr. *komē* hair] a suborder of ectocommensal or endocommensal ciliate marine protozoa (order Cyrtophorida, superorder Phyllopharyngidea), characterized by the presence of a densely ciliated ventral body surface, a humped dorsal surface, a cytopharyngeal apparatus not surrounded by nematodesmata that may protrude from the body, an inconspicuous adhesive organelle in a ventral pit, and a macronucleus that is not heteromerous.

hypocomplementemia (hi″po-kom″plĕ-men-te′me-ah) abnormally low levels of complement in the blood.

hypocomplementemic (hi″po-kom″plĕ-men-te′mik) denoting or involving lowered levels of complement in the blood.

hypocondylar (hi″po-kon′dĭ-lar) below a condyle.

hypocone (hi′po-kōn) [*hypo-* + Gr. *kōnos* cone] the distolingual cusp of an upper molar tooth.

hypoconid (hi″po-ko′nid) the distobuccal cusp of a lower molar tooth.

hypoconulid (hi″po-kon′u-lid) the distal, or fifth, cusp of a lower molar tooth; usually found on the mandibular first molar.

hypocorticalism (hi″po-kor′tĭ-kal-izm) hypoadrenocorticism.

hypocorticism (hi″po-kor′tĭ-sizm) hypoadrenocorticism.

hypocotyl (hi″po-kot′il) [*hypo-* + *kotyle* hollow] the part of the axis of a plant embryo or seedling below the point of attachment of the cotyledon and from which the radicle, or primary root, grows.

Hypocreales (hi″po-kre-a′les) a family of ascomycetous fungi.

hypocupremia (hi″po-ku-pre′me-ah) an abnormally diminished concentration of copper in the blood.

hypocyclosis (hi″po-si-klo′sis) [*hypo-* + Gr. *kyklos* circle + *-osis*] insufficiency of accommodation due either to undue rigidity of the crystalline lens (*lenticular h.*) or to weakness of the ciliary muscle (*ciliary h.*).

hypocythemia (hi″po-si-the′me-ah) [*hypo-* + Gr. *kytos* cell + *haima* blood + *-ia*] deficiency in the number of erythrocytes in the blood.

hypocytosis (hi″po-si-to′sis) [*hypo-* + *-cyte* + *-osis*] defect or scantiness of corpuscles in the blood.

hypodactyly (hi″po-dak′tĭ-le) the presence of less than the normal number of fingers or toes.

hypoderm (hi′po-derm) [*hypo-* + *-derm*] tela subcutanea.

Hypoderma (hi″po-der′mah) [*hypo-* + Gr. *derma* skin] a genus of ox-warble flies or heel flies of the family Oestridae whose larvae cause a creeping eruption in man and cattle. **H. bo′vis,** a species whose larvae infest cattle, seriously damaging the hide and interfering with the nutrition of the animal; it sometimes causes a creeping eruption in man. **H. linea′tum,** an ox-warble fly of cattle in the United States.

hypodermatic (hi″po-der-mat′ik) hypodermic.

hypodermatoclysis (hi″po-der-mah-tok′lĭ-sis) hypodermoclysis.

hypodermatomy (hi″po-der-mat′o-me) [*hypo-* + Gr. *derma* skin + *temnein* to cut] incision of the subcutaneous tissue.

hypodermiasis (hi″po-der-mi′ah-sis) infection by *Hypoderma*; see *larva migrans*.

hypodermic (hi″po-der′mik) [*hypo-* + Gr. *derma* skin] applied or administered beneath the skin.

hypodermis (hi″po-der′mis) [*hypo-* + Gr. *derma* skin] 1. tela subcutanea. 2. the outer cellular layer of the body of invertebrates which secretes the cuticular exoskeleton.

hypodermoclysis (hi″po-der-mok′lĭ-sis) [*hypo-* + Gr. *derma* skin + *klyzein* to wash out] introduction into the subcutaneous tissues of fluids, especially physiologic sodium chloride solution, to replace inadequate intake or loss of water and salt during illness or operation.

hypodermolithiasis (hi″po-der″mo-lĭ-thi′ah-sis) [*hypo-* +

Gr. *derma* skin + *lithos* stone + *-iasis*]　the formation or presence of subcutaneous calcareous nodes.

hypodiploid (hi″po-dip′loid)　1. pertaining to or characterized by hypodiploidy.　2. an individual or cell with less than the diploid number of chromosomes.

hypodiploidy (hi″po-dip′loi-de)　the state of having less than the diploid number of chromosomes (< 2n).

hypoploidy (hi′po-ploi-de)　the state of having less than the diploid number of chromosomes (< 2n).

hypodipsia (hi″po-dip′se-ah) [*hypo-* + Gr. *dipsa* thirst + *-ia*] abnormally diminished thirst. See *subliminal thirst*, under *thirst*.

hypodipsic (hi″po-dip′sik)　characterized by abnormally diminished thirst.

hypodontia (hi″po-don′she-ah) [*hypo-* + Gr. *odous* tooth + *-ia*]　partial absence of the teeth. A relatively common congenital condition characterized by absence of one or more teeth because of absence of their anlage, which is seldom associated with other anomalies. Called also *partial anodontia.*

hypodynamia (hi″po-di-na′me-ah) [*hypo-* + Gr. *dynamis* force]　diminished power. **h. cor′dis,** diminished cardiac power.

hypodynamic (hi″po-di-nam′ik)　pertaining to poor ventricular contractility.

hypoeccrisia (hi″po-ek-kris′e-ah) [*hypo-* + Gr. *ekkrisis* excretion + *-ia*]　a state characterized by abnormally diminished excretion.

hypoeccrisis (hi″po-ek′kri-sis)　hypoeccrisia.

hypoeccritic (hi″po-ek-krit′ik)　pertaining to or characterized by hypoeccrisia.

hypoechoic (hi″po-ĕ-ko′ik)　in ultrasonography, giving off few echoes; said of tissues or structures that reflect relatively few of the ultrasound waves directed at them.

hypoelectrolytemia (hi″po-e-lek″tro-li-te′me-ah)　abnormally decreased electrolyte content of the blood.

hypoeosinophilia (hi″po-e″o-sin″o-fil′e-ah)　eosinopenia.

hypoepinephrinemia (hi″po-ep″ĭ-nef″rĭ-ne′me-ah)　an abnormally low level of epinephrine in the blood.

hypoequilibrium (hi″po-e″kwĭ-lib′re-um)　unusual freedom from tendency to vertigo.

hypoergasia (hi″po-er-ga′se-ah) [*hypo-* + Gr. *ergon* work] abnormally decreased functional activity.

hypoergia (hi″po-er′je-ah)　1. hypoergasia.　2. hyposensitivity to allergens.

hypoergic (hi″po-er′jik)　1. less energetic than normal.　2. pertaining to or characterized by hypoergy.

hypoergy (hi″po-er′je)　abnormally diminished reactivity.

hypoesophoria (hi″po-es″o-fo′re-ah)　a tendency of the visual axis to deviate downward and medially when fusion is prevented.

hypoesthesia (hi″po-es-the′ze-ah) [*hypo-* + Gr. *aisthēsis* sensation + *-ia*]　abnormally decreased sensitivity to stimulation. **acoustic h., auditory h.,** hypoacusis. **gustatory h.,** hypogeusia. **olfactory h.,** hyposmia. **tactile h.,** hypopselaphesia.

hypoesthetic (hi″po-es-thet′ik)　pertaining to or characterized by hypoesthesia.

hypoestrinemia (hi″po-es″trĭ-ne′me-ah)　hypoestrogenemia.

hypoestrogenemia (hi″po-es″tro-jĕ-ne′me-ah)　an abnormally diminished amount of estrogen in the blood, as in the menopause.

hypoevolutism (hi″po-e-vol′u-tizm)　a condition characterized by abnormally retarded development.

hypoexophoria (hi″po-ek″so-fo′re-ah)　a tendency of the visual axis to deviate downward and laterally when fusion is prevented.

hypoferremia (hi″po-fĕ-re′me-ah)　deficiency of iron in the blood.

hypoferrism (hi″po-fer′izm) [*hypo-* + L. *ferrum* iron]　deficiency of iron in the system.

hypofertile (hi″po-fer′til)　having a diminished reproductive capacity.

hypofertility (hi″po-fer-til′ĭ-te)　diminished reproductive capacity.

hypofibrinogenemia (hi″po-fi-brin″o-jĕ-ne′me-ah)　abnormally low fibrinogen content of the blood.

hypofunction (hi″po-funk′shun)　diminished function.

hypogalactia (hi″po-gah-lak′she-ah)　deficiency of milk secretion.

hypogalactous (hi″po-gah-lak′tus) [*hypo-* + Gr. *gala* milk] producing a deficient secretion of milk.

hypogammaglobulinemia (hi″po-gam″ah-glob″u-lĭ-ne′me-ah)　a condition characterized by abnormally low levels of all classes of immunoglobulins. Cf. *agammaglobulinemia* and *dysglobulinemia.* See *immunodeficiency.* **acquired h.,** a term used in an early classification of antibody immunodeficiency disorders to refer to hypogammaglobulinemias with onset several years after birth, most of which would now be included in the category of common variable immunodeficiency and many of which now appear to be associated with genetic defects. Cf. *congenital h.* **common variable h.,** see under *immunodeficiency.* **congenital h.,** a term used in an early classification of antibody immunodeficiency disorders to refer to hypogammaglobulinemias with onset in infancy, most of which were cases of X-linked infantile agammaglobulinemia. **physiologic h.,** a normal period of hypogammaglobulinemia seen in all infants at about 5–6 months of age as the level of transplacentally acquired maternal immunoglobulins declines before endogenous immunoglobulin synthesis rises to normal levels. **transient h. of infancy,** prolongation of the normal physiologic hypogammaglobulinemia of infancy caused by delayed development of endogenous immunoglobulin production and associated with increased susceptibility to infections. **X-linked h., X-linked infantile h.,** see under *agammaglobulinemia.*

hypoganglionosis (hi″po-gang″gle-o-no′sis)　deficiency in the number of myenteric ganglion cells in the distal segment of the large bowel, resulting in constipation; it is a variant of congenital megacolon.

hypogastric (hi″po-gas′trik) [L. *hypogastricus*]　1. situated below the stomach.　2. pertaining to the hypogastrium.　3. pertaining to the internal iliac artery.

hypogastrium (hi″po-gas′tre-um) [*hypo-* + Gr. *gastēr* stomach]　NA alternative for *regio pubica.*

hypogastropagus (hi″po-gas-trop′ah-gus) [*hypo* + Gr. *gastēr* belly + *pagos* thing fixed]　conjoined twins united at the hypogastric region.

hypogastroschisis (hi″po-gas-tros′kĭ-sis) [*hypo-* + Gr. *gastēr* belly + *schisis* cleft]　a developmental anomaly in which an abdominal fissure is restricted to the hypogastric region.

hypogenesis (hi″po-jen′ĕ-sis) [*hypo-* + Gr. *genesis* production]　defective embryonic growth or development. **polar h.,** defective development at either extremity of the embryo, resulting in deformity.

hypogenetic (hi″po-jĕ-net′ik)　pertaining to or characterized by hypogenesis.

hypogenitalism (hi″po-jen′ĭ-tal-izm″)　hypogonadism.

hypogeusesthesia (hi″po-gūs″es-the′ze-ah)　hypogeusia.

hypogeusia (hi″po-gu′ze-ah) [*hypo-* + Gr. *geusis* taste]　diminished sensitivity of taste.

hypoglandular (hi″po-glan′du-lar)　marked by abnormally decreased glandular activity.

hypoglossal (hi″po-glos′al) [*hypo-* + Gr. *glōssa* tongue] situated under the tongue.

hypoglucagonemia (hi″po-gloo″kah-gon-e′me-ah)　abnormally reduced levels of glucagon in the blood.

hypoglycemia (hi″po-gli-se′me-ah) [*hypo-* + Gr. *glykys* sweet + *haima* blood + *-ia*]　an abnormally diminished concentration of glucose in the blood, which may lead to tremulousness, cold sweat, piloerection, hypothermia, and headache, accompanied by irritability, confusion, hallucinations, bizarre behavior, and ultimately, convulsions and coma. **factitial h., factitious h.,** apparently spontaneous hypoglycemia in a diabetic, which is in fact caused by the surreptitious injection of insulin. **fasting h.,** hypoglycemia occurring in the fasting state, i.e., after the glucose contents of the intestine have been absorbed; it occurs in such conditions as insulinoma, glycogen storage disease, severe hepatic failure, starvation, malabsorption, hypopituitarism, and adrenocortical insufficiency. **ketotic h.,** episodic hypoglycemia, ketonuria, convulsions, and vomiting occurring in young children in the early morning after carbohydrate deprivation. **leucine-induced h.,** familial infantile hypoglycemia induced by ingestion of leucine (leucine-containing protein), which causes an exaggerated release of insulin in susceptible persons; it is transmitted as an autosomal recessive trait. **mixed h.,** hypoglycemia occurring both during the fasting state and following the ingestion of carbohydrate; it occurs in hypoglycemia of infancy, anterior pituitary and adrenocortical insufficiency, and insulin-secreting tumors of the islet cells of the pancreas. **reactive h.,** hypoglycemia occurring after the ingestion of carbohydrate, with a consequent excessive release of insulin.

hypoglycemic (hi″po-gli-se′mik) 1. pertaining to, characterized by, or producing hypoglycemia. 2. an agent that acts to lower the level of glucose in the blood.

hypoglycemosis (hi″po-gli″sĕ-mo′sis) an abnormally diminished content of glucose in the blood and tissues; see *hypoglycemia.*

hypoglycin, hypoglycine (hi″po-gli′sin; hi″po-gli′sēn) a hypoglycemic principle occurring in two forms (A and B), from the fruit and seed of the akee tree; it inhibits hepatic gluconeogenesis.

hypoglycogenolysis (hi″po-gli″ko-jen-ol′ĭ-sis) depressed glycogenolysis.

hypoglycorrhachia (hi″po-gli″ko-ra′ke-ah) [*hypo-* + Gr. *glykys* sweet + *rhachis* spine + *-ia*] less than the normal content of glucose in the cerebrospinal fluid; usually indicative of meningeal infection.

hypognathous (hi-pog′nah-thus) 1. having a protruding lower jaw. 2. of the nature of a hypognathus.

hypognathus (hi-pog′nah-thus) [*hypo-* + Gr. *gnathos* jaw] a parasitic monster attached to the lower jaw of the autosite.

hypogonadism (hi″po-go′nad-izm) a condition resulting from or characterized by abnormally decreased functional activity of the gonads, with retardation of growth and sexual development. **eugonadotropic h.,** that associated with normal levels of pituitary gonadotropins. **hypergonadotropic h.,** that due to defective development or function of the gonads, with elevated levels of pituitary gonadotropins. **hypogonadotropic h.,** that due to failure of gonadotropin secretion. **primary h.,** hypergonadotropic h. **secondary h.,** hypogonadotropic h., due to pituitary failure.

hypogonadotropic (hi″po-gon″ah-do-trop′ik) relating to or caused by deficiency of gonadotropin.

hypogranulocytosis (hi″po-gran″u-lo-si-to′sis) reduction in the number of granular leukocytes in the blood. Cf. *agranulocytosis.*

hypohepatia (hi″po-he-pat′e-ah) [*hypo-* + Gr. *hēpar* liver] deficient functioning of the liver.

hypohidrosis (hi″po-hi-dro′sis) [*hypo-* + Gr. *hidrōsis* sweating] abnormally diminished perspiration.

hypohidrotic (hi″po-hĭ-drot′ik) pertaining to, characterized by, or causing hypohidrosis; see also *anhidrosis.*

hypohydration (hi″po-hi-dra′shun) a state of decreased water content of the body; dehydration.

hypohydrochloria (hi″po-hi″dro-klo′re-ah) hypochlorhydria.

hypohypnotic (hi″po-hip-not′ik) marked by light sleep.

hypoidrosis (hi″po-id-ro′sis) hypohidrosis.

hypoinsulinemia (hi″po-in″su-lĭ-ne′me-ah) a deficiency of insulin in the blood.

hypoinsulinism (hi″po-in′su-lin-izm″) deficient secretion of insulin by the pancreas, resulting in hyperglycemia.

hypoiododidism (hi″po-i-o′dĭ-dizm) [*hypo-* + *iodide* + *-ism*] deficiency of iodide in the body.

hypoisotonic (hi″po-i″so-ton′ik) less than isotonic; said of a solution having a lesser osmotic power than another.

hypokalemia (hi″po-ka-le′me-ah) abnormally low potassium concentration in the blood; it may result from potassium loss by renal secretion or by the gastrointestinal route, as by vomiting or diarrhea. It may be manifested clinically by neuromuscular disorders ranging from weakness to paralysis, by electrocardiographic abnormalities (depression of the T wave and elevation of the U wave), by renal disease, and by gastrointestinal disorders.

hypokalemic (hi″po-ka-le′mik) 1. pertaining to or characterized by hypokalemia. 2. an agent that acts to lower the potassium content of the blood.

hypokaliemia (hi″po-kal″e-e′me-ah) hypokalemia.

hypokinemia (hi″po-ki-ne′me-ah) [*hypo-* + Gr. *kinein* to move + *haima* blood + *-ia*] subnormal cardiac output.

hypokinesia (hi″po-ki-ne′ze-ah) [*hypo-* + Gr. *kinēsis* motion + *-ia*] abnormally decreased mobility; abnormally decreased motor function or activity.

hypokinesis (hi″po-ki-ne′sis) hypokinesia.

hypokinetic (hi″po-ki-net′ik) pertaining to or characterized by hypokinesia.

hypolactasia (hi″po-lak-ta′ze-ah) deficiency of lactase activity in the intestines.

hypolarynx (hi″po-lar′inks) the infraglottic compartment of the larynx from the true vocal cords to the first tracheal ring.

hypolemmal (hi″po-lem′al) [*hypo-* + Gr. *lemma* sheath] located beneath a sheath, as the end-plates of motor nerves under the sarcolemma of muscle.

hypolethal (hi″po-le′thal) not sufficient to cause death.

hypoleydigism (hi″po-li′dig-izm) abnormally diminished functional activity of Leydig's interstitial cells.

hypolipemia (hi″po-li-pe′me-ah) an abnormally decreased amount of fat in the blood.

hypolipidemic (hi″po-lip″ĭ-de′mik) promoting the reduction of lipid concentrations in the serum.

hypolipoproteinemia (hi″po-lip″o-pro″te-in-e′me-ah) the presence of abnormally low levels of lipoproteins in the serum, as in hypobetalipoproteinemia and Tangier disease.

hypoliposis (hi″po-li-po′sis) a deficiency of lipids in the blood or tissues. Lipids are transported in the blood as lipoproteins; see *hypolipoproteinemia.*

hypoliquorrhea (hi″po-li″kwo-re′ah) chronic deficiency of cerebrospinal fluid.

hypolymphemia (hi″po-lim-fe′me-ah) [*hypo-* + *lymph* + Gr. *haima* blood + *-ia*] abnormal deficiency in the proportion of lymphocytes in the blood.

hypomagnesemia (hi″po-mag″nĕ-se′me-ah) an abnormally low magnesium content of the blood plasma, manifested chiefly by neuromuscular hyperirritability. It may result from malabsorption, dehydration, alcoholism, or renal disease.

hypomania (hi″po-ma′ne-ah) [*hypo-* + Gr. *mania* madness] an abnormality of mood resembling mania (persistent elevated or expansive mood, hyperactivity, inflated self-esteem, etc.) but of lesser intensity.

hypomanic (hi″po-ma′nik) pertaining to hypomania.

hypomastia (hi-po-mas′te-ah) [*hypo-* + Gr. *mastos* breast + *-ia*] abnormal smallness of the mammary glands.

hypomelancholia (hi″po-mel″an-ko′le-ah) [*hypo-* + Gr. *melancholia* melancholia] mild melancholia.

hypomelanosis (hi″po-mel″ah-no′sis) [*hypo-* + *melanosis*] a deficiency of melanin in the tissues, especially in the skin. Cf. *amelanosis, depigmentation,* and *hypopigmentation.* **idiopathic guttate h.,** a common condition of unknown etiology manifested by small, sharply demarcated, irregular hypopigmented spots that appear chiefly on the sun-exposed areas of the extremities in individuals over the age of 30. Called also *leukopathia punctata reticularis symmetrica.* **h. of Ito,** incontinentia pigmenti achromians.

hypomenorrhea (hi″po-men″o-re′ah) [*hypo-* + Gr. *mēn* month + *rhein* to flow] uterine bleeding of less than the normal amount occurring at regular intervals, the period of flow being of the same or less than usual duration.

hypomere (hi′po-mēr) 1. the ventrolateral portion of a myotome, innervated by an anterior ramus of a spinal nerve. 2. the lateral plate of mesoderm that develops into the walls of the body cavities.

hypometabolic (hi″po-met″ah-bol′ik) pertaining to hypometabolism.

hypometabolism (hi″po-mĕ-tab′o-lizm) [*hypo-* + *metabolism*] abnormally decreased utilization of any substance by the body in metabolism; low metabolic rate.

hypometria (hi″po-me′tre-ah) [″a deficiency″; by analogy with Gr. *eumetria, hypermetria*] a condition in which voluntary muscular movement falls short of reaching the intended goal.

hypomicron (hi″po-mi′kron) submicron.

hypomineralization (hi″po-min″er-al-i-za′shun) deficiency of mineral elements in the body.

hypomnesis (hi″pom-ne′sis) [*hypo-* + Gr. *mnēmē* memory] defective memory.

hypomodal (hi″po-mo′dal) in statistics, relating to the values or items falling below the mode of the frequency distribution.

hypomorph (hi′po-morf) [*hypo-* + Gr. *morphē* form] a mutant gene that shows only a partial reduction in the activity it influences. Cf. *hypermorph.*

hypomotility (hi″po-mo-til′ĭ-te) deficient movement in any part.

hypomyotonia (hi″po-mi″o-to′ne-ah) [*hypo-* + Gr. *mys* muscle + *tonos* tension + *-ia*] deficient muscular tonicity.

hypomyxia (hi″po-mik′se-ah) [*hypo-* + Gr. *myxa* mucus + *-ia*] decreased secretion of mucus.

hyponasality (hi″po-na-zal′ĭ-te) a quality of voice in which there is a complete lack of nasal emission of air and nasal resonance, so that the speaker sounds as if he has a cold. Called also *denasality.*

hyponatremia (hi″po-nah-tre′me-ah) deficiency of sodium in the blood; salt depletion. **depletional h.,** that in which there is a low level of sodium and of body fluids (dehydration). **dilutional h.,** that in which there is a low level of serum sodium but a high level of body fluids (edema). **hyperlipemic h.,** apparent hyponatremia (when expressed per unit of plasma) due to a high concentration of lipids combined with proteins in the blood plasma.

hyponatruria (hi″po-nah-troo′re-ah) an abnormally low level of sodium in the urine.

hyponeocytosis (hi″po-ne″o-si-to′sis) [*hypo-* + Gr. *neos* new + *-cyte* + *-osis*] leukopenia with immature forms of leukocytes present in the blood.

hyponitremia (hi″po-ni-tre′me-ah) a low level of nitrogen in the blood, sometimes associated with protein malnutrition.

hyponoia (hi″po-noi′ah) [*hypo-* + Gr. *nous* mind + *-ia*] sluggish mental activity.

hyponychial (hi″po-nik′e-al) subungual; beneath a nail.

hyponychium (hi″po-nik′e-um) [*hypo-* + Gr. *onyx* nail] [NA] the thickened epidermis underneath the free distal end of the nail.

hyponychon (hi-pon′ĭ-kon) [*hypo-* + Gr. *onyx* nail] ecchymosis beneath the nail.

hypo-orchidism (hi″po-or′ki-dizm) defective activity of the testes.

hypo-orthocytosis (hi″po-or″tho-si-to′sis) [*hypo-* + Gr. *orthos* regular + *-cyte* + *-osis*] leukopenia in which the proportion of the various forms of leukocytes is normal.

hypo-osmolality (hi″po-os″mo-lal′ĭ-te) a decrease in the osmolality of the body fluids.

hypo-ovarianism (hi″po-o-va′re-an-izm) deficient endocrine activity of the ovaries.

hypopallesthesia (hi″po-pal″es-the′ze-ah) [*hypo-* + *pallesthesia*] abnormally decreased sensibility to vibrations.

hypopancreatism (hi″po-pan′kre-ah-tizm″) diminished pancreatic activity.

hypopancreorrhea (hi″po-pan″kre-o-re′ah) abnormally diminished secretion from the pancreas.

hypoparathyroidism (hi″po-par″ah-thi′roid-izm) the condition produced by greatly reduced function of the parathyroids possibly due to autoimmune disease or genetic factors, or by the removal of those bodies. The lack of parathyroid hormone leads to a fall in plasma calcium level—which may result in increased neuromuscular excitability and, ultimately, tetany—followed by a rise in plasma phosphate level, resulting in a decrease in bone resorption and consequent increased density of bone. There may also be dermatologic, ophthalmologic (cataracts), psychiatric, and dental symptoms, and associated primary failure of other endocrine glands, e.g., the adrenal cortex.

hypopepsia (hi″po-pep′se-ah) [*hypo-* + Gr. *pepsis* digestion + *-ia*] impairment of digestion, due to hypochlorhydria.

hypopepsinia (hi″po-pep-sin′e-ah) deficiency in the pepsin secretion of the stomach.

hypoperfusion (hi″po-per-fu′zhun) decreased blood flow

through an organ, as in circulatory shock; if prolonged it may result in permanent cellular dysfunction and death.

hypoperistalsis (hi″po-per″ĭ-stal′sis) abnormally sluggish peristalsis.

hypopexia (hi″po-pek′se-ah) [*hypo-* + Gr. *pēxis* fixation + *-ia*] the fixation by a tissue of a deficient amount of a substance.

hypopexy (hi′po-pek″se) hypopexia.

hypophalangism (hi″po-fah-lan′jizm) less than the usual number of phalanges of a finger or toe.

hypophamine (hi-pof′ah-min) the substance once thought to be the active principle of the posterior lobe of the pituitary gland. **alpha h.,** oxytocin. **beta h.,** vasopressin.

hypopharyngeal (hi″po-fah-rin′je-al) pertaining to the hypopharynx.

hypopharyngoscope (hi″po-fah-ring′go-skōp) an instrument for inspecting the lower part of the pharynx.

hypopharyngoscopy (hi″po-far″in-gos′ko-pe) examination of the lower part of the pharynx.

hypopharynx (hi″po-far′inks) that division of the pharynx which lies below the upper edge of the epiglottis and opens into the larynx and esophagus.

hypophonesis (hi″po-fo-ne′sis) [*hypo-* + Gr. *phōnēsis* sounding] diminished intensity of the sound in auscultation or percussion.

hypophonia (hi″po-fo′ne-ah) [*hypo-* + Gr. *phōnē* voice + *-ia*] defective speech due to lack of phonation and resulting in whispering.

hypophoria (hi″po-fo′re-ah) [*hypo-* + *phoria*] heterophoria in which there is downward deviation of the visual axis of an eye when visual fusional stimuli are eliminated. When both eyes are affected, it is called *cataphoria.*

hypophosphatasia (hi″po-fos″fah-ta′ze-ah) [*hypo-* + *phosphatase* + *-ia*] a genetic metabolic disorder resulting from serum and bone alkaline phosphatase deficiency leading to hypercalcemia, ethanolamine phosphatemia, and ethanolamine phosphaturia. Clinical manifestations include severe skeletal defects resembling vitamin D–resistant rickets, failure of the calvarium to calcify, dyspnea, cyanosis, vomiting, constipation, renal calcinosis, failure to thrive, disorders of movement, beading of the costochondral junction, and rachitic bone changes (bowing). There are three clinical types based upon age of onset and the severity of the symptoms. Two are autosomal recessive: *infantile,* the severest, lethal in over 50 per cent of the cases; *childhood,* whose first symptom is usually the spontaneous loss of the deciduous teeth; and *adult,* the mildest form, is autosomal dominant. See *pseudohypophosphatasia.*

hypophosphatemia (hi″po-fos″fah-te′me-ah) [*hypo-* + *phosphate* + *-emia*] an abnormally decreased amount of phosphates in the blood; manifestations include hemolysis, lassitude, weakness, and convulsions. It may be found in hyperparathyroidism, rickets, osteomalacia, and several renal tubular abnormalities, including the Fanconi syndrome. **familial h.,** an X-linked dominant disorder of phosphate metabolism, that may be associated with vitamin D–resistant rickets (q.v.).

hypophosphatemic (hi″po-phos″fah-te′mik) pertaining to or characterized by hypophosphatemia.

hypophosphaturia (hi″po-fos″fah-tu′re-ah) an abnormally decreased amount of phosphate in the urine.

hypophosphite (hi″po-fos′fīt) any salt of hypophosphorous acid.

hypophosphoremia (hi″po-fos″fo-re′me-ah) hypophosphatemia.

hypophosphorous acid (hi″po-fos-for′us) a strong monobasic acid, H_3PO_2, used as a reducing agent.

hypophrenia (hi″po-fre′ne-ah) [*hypo-* + Gr. *phrēn* mind + *-ia*] mental retardation.

hypophrenic (hi″po-fren′ik) [*hypo-* + Gr. *phrēn* diaphragm, mind] 1. below the diaphragm. 2. mentally retarded.

hypophrenium (hi″po-fre′ne-um) a peritoneal space between the diaphragm and the transverse colon.

hypophyseal (hi″po-fiz′e-al) hypophysial.

hypophysectomize (hi″po-fiz-ek′to-mīz) to remove the hypophysis, or pituitary gland.

hypophysectomy (hi-pof″ĭ-sek′to-me) [*hypophysis* + Gr. *ek-*

tomē excision] surgical removal or destruction of the hypophysis, or pituitary gland.

hypophyseoportal (hi″po-fiz″e-o-por′tal) hypophysioportal.

hypophyseoprivic (hi″po-fiz″e-o-priv′ik) hypophysioprivic.

hypophyseotropic (hi″po-fiz″e-o-trop′ik) hypophysiotropic.

hypophysial (hi″po-fiz′e-al) pertaining to a hypophysis, especially to the hypophysis cerebri, or pituitary gland.

hypophysioportal (hi″po-fiz″e-o-por′tal) pertaining to the portal system of the hypophysis (pituitary gland). Also spelled *hypophyseoportal*.

hypophysioprivic (hi″po-fiz″e-o-prīv′ik) pertaining to deficiency of hormone secretion by the hypophysis (pituitary gland).

hypophysiotropic (hi″po-fiz″e-o-trop′ik) acting on the hypophysis (pituitary gland), as a hypothalamic hypophysiotropic hormone.

hypophysis (hi-pof′ĭ-sis) [*hypo-* + Gr. *phyein* to grow] [NA] the pituitary gland (see under *gland*), a neural and epithelial body of dual origin located at the base of the brain in the sella turcica. **h. cer′ebri,** see *pituitary gland,* under *gland.* **pharyngeal h.,** a small median residual collection of adenohypophysial glandular tissue situated in the mucoperiosteum of the roof of the nasopharynx; it develops from Rathke's pouch in the embryo. Called also *pars pharyngea lobi anterioris hypophyseos* and *pharyngeal pituitary.*

hypophysitis (hi-pof″ĭ-si′tis) inflammation of the hypophysis.

hypopiesia (hi-po-pi-e′se-ah) abnormally low blood pressure occurring independently of any discoverable organic disease.

hypopiesis (hi″po-pi-e′sis) [*hypo-* + Gr. *piesis* pressure] abnormally low pressure, as abnormally low blood pressure.

hypopietic (hi″po-pi-et′ik) pertaining to, characterized by, or causing hypopiesis.

hypopigmentation (hi″po-pig″men-ta′shun) [*hypo-* + *pigmentation*] abnormally diminished pigmentation, resulting from decreased melanin production. Cf. *amelanosis, depigmentation,* and *hypomelanosis.*

hypopigmenter (hi″po-pig-men′ter) an agent that reduces pigmentation of the skin; a bleach.

hypopinealism (hi″po-pin′e-al-izm″) presumed defective functional activity of the pineal body.

hypopituitarism (hi″po-pĭ-tu′ĭ-tah-rizm″) diminution or cessation of anterior pituitary function due to surgical removal of the pituitary gland, to ablation by irradiation, or to spontaneous causes, as in chromophobe adenoma and postpartum necrosis (Sheehan's syndrome). It leads to hormonal deficiency—varying with the degree of dysfunction—of the following: (*a*) gonadotropins, with consequent regression of secondary sex characteristics and decrease in libido (secondary hypogonadism); (*b*) somatotropin, which in children results in pituitary dwarfism; (*c*) thyrotropin (secondary hypothyroidism; see *hypothyroidism*); (*d*) corticotropin, resulting in symptoms similar to those in hypoadrenalism (secondary hypoadrenocorticism).

hypoplasia (hi″po-pla′ze-ah) [*hypo-* + Gr. *plasis* formation + *-ia*] incomplete development or underdevelopment of an organ or tissue; it is less severe in degree than aplasia. **cartilage-hair h.,** an autosomal recessive disorder originally described in an Amish population but which has been seen in other groups, characterized by bone dysplasia, resulting in short-limbed dwarfism, fine, sparse, light-colored hair, and neutropenia with defective cell-mediated immunity. **enamel h.,** a form of amelogenesis imperfecta characterized by incomplete formation of the dental enamel. It may be transmitted as an X-linked or autosomal dominant trait, or be associated with vitamin A, C, or D deficiency, measles, chickenpox, scarlet fever, congenital syphilis (Hutchinson's teeth), prematurity, birth injuries, Rh incompatibility, trauma, local infection, or Morquio's disease. Small grooves, pits, and fissures on the enamel surface may be seen in mild cases, deep horizontal rows of pits in severe cases; or absence of enamel in extreme cases, associated with yellow, reddish, or brown discoloration of the teeth. Called also *hypoplastic e.* **focal dermal h.,** a hereditary disorder found exclusively in females, transmitted as an X-linked

dominant trait, characterized typically by linear areas of dermal-hypoplasia with herniation of underlying tissue through the defects, telangiectasia, linear or reticular areas of hyper- or hypopigmentation, localized superficial fatty deposits in the skin, papillomas of mucous membranes of periorificial skin, and anomalies of the extremities, including syndactyly, adactyly, and oligodactyly. Called also *Coltz's syndrome.* **oligomeganephronic renal h.,** oligomeganephronia. **h. of right ventricle,** a defective development of the right ventricular myocardium, which may be paper-thin (parchment heart); there may be right-sided heart failure. **thymic h.,** DiGeorge syndrome. **Turner's h.,** see under *tooth.*

hypoplastic (hi″po-plas′tik) marked by hypoplasia.

hypoplasty (hi″po-plas″te) hypoplasia.

hypoploid (hi′po-ploid) [*hypo-* + *-ploid*] the aneuploid, nearly always fatal condition in which there is less than the normal diploid number of chromosomes, e.g., 45 chromosomes in man, the 2n−1 state.

hypopnea (hi″po-ne′ah) [*hypo-* + Gr. *pnoia* breath] abnormal decrease in the depth and rate of the respiratory movements.

hypopneic (hi″po-ne′ik) pertaining to or characterized by hypopnea.

hypoponesis (hi″po-po-ne′sis) [*hypo-* + Gr. *ponēsis* toil, exertion] dysponesis in which there is insufficient action-potential output from the motor and premotor areas of the cortex.

hypoporosis (hi″po-po-ro′sis) [*hypo-* + Gr. *pōros* callus + *-osis*] deficient formation of callus after fracture.

hypoposia (hi″po-po′ze-ah) [*hypo-* + Gr. *posis* drinking + *-ia*] abnormally diminished ingestion of fluids.

hypopotassemia (hi″po-po″tah-se′me-ah) hypokalemia.

hypopotassemic (hi″po-po″tah-se′mik) hypokalemic.

hypopotentia (hi″po-po-ten′she-ah) [*hypo-* + L. *potentia* power] a condition of diminished power, especially of diminished electrical activity of the cerebral cortex.

hypopraxia (hi″po-prak′se-ah) [*hypo-* + Gr. *praxis* action + *-ia*] abnormally diminished activity.

hypoprosody (hi″po-pros′o-de) diminution of the normal variation of stress, pitch, and rhythm of speech.

hypoproteinemia (hi″po-pro″tĭ-ne′me-ah) abnormal decrease in the amount of protein in the blood, sometimes resulting in edema and fluid accumulation in serous cavities. **prehepatic h.,** hypoproteinemia occurring as a result of prolonged ingestion of faulty low-protein diet.

hypoproteinia (hi″po-pro″tēn′e-ah) a subnormal protein status of the body.

hypoproteinic (hi″po-pro″tēn′ik) pertaining to or characterized by hypoproteinia.

hypoproteinosis (hi″po-pro″tĭ-no′sis) deficiency of proteins or protein foods.

hypoprothrombinemia (hi″po-pro-throm″bĭ-ne′me-ah) deficiency of prothrombin (coagulation Factor II) in the blood; called also *Factor II deficiency.*

hypopselaphesia (hi″pop-sel″ah-fe′ze-ah) [*hypo-* + Gr. *psēlaphēsis* touch + *-ia*] diminution or dullness of the tactile sense; tactile hypoesthesia.

hypopteronosis cystica (hi″po-ter-on′o-sis sis′tĭ-kah) [*hypo-* + Gr. *pteron* feather] a condition observed in birds, known commonly as "lumps," in which a cyst forms when the growth of the feather shaft is confined within the follicle.

hypoptyalism (hi″pop-ti′al-izm) [*hypo-* + Gr. *ptyalon* spittle] abnormally decreased secretion of saliva, as in xerostomia. Called also *hyposalivation* and *hyposialosis.*

hypopus (hi-po′pus) a stage in the development of the grain mites (Acaridae) between the first and the second nymph stages.

hypopyon (hi-po′pe-on) [*hypo-* + Gr. *pyon* pus] an accumulation of pus in the anterior chamber of the eye.

hyporeactive (hi″po-re-ak′tiv) pertaining to or characterized by a less than normal response to stimuli.

hyporeflexia (hi″po-re-flek′se-ah) weakening of the reflexes.

hyporeninemia (hi″po-re″nin-e′me-ah) low levels of renin in the blood.

hyporeninemic (hi″po-re″nin-e′mik) characterized by low levels of renin in the blood.

hyporrhea (hi″po-re′ah) [*hypo-* + Gr. *rhoia* flow] slight hemorrhage.

hyposalemia (hi″po-sah-le′me-ah) [*hypo-* + L. *sal* salt + Gr. *haima* blood + *-ia*] abnormally decreased concentration of salt in the blood.

hyposalivation (hi″po-sal″ĭ-va′shun) hypoptyalism.

hyposarca (hi″po-sar′kah) anasarca.

hyposcleral (hi″po-skle′ral) under the sclerotic coat of the eye.

hyposecretion (hi″po-se-kre′shun) diminished secretion as of a gland.

hyposensitive (hi″po-sen′sĭ-tiv) 1. exhibiting abnormally decreased sensitivity. 2. having the specific or general ability to react to a specific allergen reduced by repeated and gradually increasing doses of the offending substance.

hyposensitivity (hi″po-sens″ĭ-tiv′ĭ-te) the condition of being hyposensitive.

hyposensitization (hi″po-sen″sĭ-ti-za′shun) the act or process of making hyposensitive; desensitization.

hyposexuality (hi″po-seks″u-al′ĭ-te) abnormally decreased sexual desire.

hyposialosis (hi″po-si″ah-lo′sis) hypoptyalism.

hyposkeocytosis (hi″po-ske″o-si-to′sis) [*hypo-* + Gr. *skaios* left + *-cyte* + *-osis*] hyponeocytosis.

hyposmia (hi-poz′me-ah) [*hypo-* + Gr. *osmē* smell + *-ia*] diminished sensitivity of smell.

hyposmolarity (hi-poz″mo-lar′i-te) abnormally decreased osmolar concentration.

hyposmosis (hi″pos-mo′sis) decreased speed of osmosis.

hyposomatotropism (hi″po-so″mat-o-tro′pizm) a condition of deficient secretion of somatotropin (growth hormone), resulting in short stature (pituitary dwarfism).

hyposomia (hi″po-so′me-ah) [*hypo-* + Gr. *sōma* body + *-ia*] inadequate bodily development.

hyposomnia (hi″po-som′ne-ah) insomnia.

hypospadia (hi″po-spa′de-ah) hypospadias.

hypospadiac (hi″po-spa′de-ak) a person affected with hypospadias.

hypospadias (hi″po-spa′de-as) [*hypo-* + Gr. *spadōn* a rent] a developmental anomaly in the male in which the urethra opens on the underside of the penis or on the perineum. **balanic h., balanitic h.,** the commonest type of hypospadias, in which the urethral orifice opens at the site of the frenum, which may be rudimentary or absent; the normal site of the urinary meatus is represented on the glans penis as a blind pit. Called also *glandular h.* **female h.,** a developmental anomaly in the female in which the urethra opens into the vagina. **glandular h.,** balanic h. **penile h.,** hypospadias in which the urethral opening lies between the glandular sulcus and the junction of the penis and scrotum. **penoscrotal h.,** hypospadias in which the urethral orifice is at the junction of the penis and scrotum; it may be associated with congenital chordee. **perineal h.,** hypospadias with anomalous development of the genitalia, the rudimentary penis often being engulfed by an overlying bifid scrotum. The extreme form is called *pseudovaginal h.* **pseudovaginal h.,** see *perineal h.*

hyposphresia (hi″pos-fre′ze-ah) [*hypo-* + Gr. *osphrēsis* smell + *-ia*] hyposmia.

hyposplenism (hi″po-splen′izm) a condition characterized by diminished functioning of the spleen.

hypostasis (hi-pos′tah-sis) [*hypo-* + Gr. *stasis* halt] poor or stagnant circulation in a dependent part of the body or organ, as in venous insufficiency.

hypostatic (hi″po-stat′ik) 1. pertaining to, caused by, or associated with hypostasis. 2. abnormally static; said of certain inherited traits which are liable to be suppressed by other traits.

hyposteatolysis (hi″po-ste″ah-tol′ĭ-sis) inadequate hydrolysis of fats during ingestion.

hyposthenia (hi″pos-the′ne-ah) [*hypo-* + Gr. *sthenos* strength + *-ia*] an enfeebled state; weakness.

hypostheniant (hi″pos-the′ne-ant) reducing the strength; debilitant.

hyposthenic (hi″pos-then′ik) pertaining to or character-

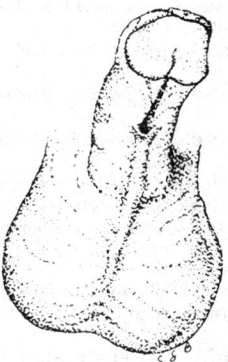

Hypospadias with chordee.

ized by hyposthenia.

hyposthenuria (hi″pos-thĕ-nu′re-ah) a condition characterized by inability to form urine of high specific gravity. **tubular h.,** hyposthenuria occurring as a result of injury to the epithelial cells of the renal tubules.

Hypostomatia (hi″po-sto-ma″she-ah) [*hypo-* + Gr. *stoma* mouth] a subclass of protozoa (class Kinetofragminophorea, phylum Ciliophora) having a nonpolar cytostome on the ventral surface; a cylindrical or dorsoventrally flattened body, often with reduced somatic ciliature; a cytopharyngeal apparatus typically of the cyrtos type; and an oral area that may be sunk into a ciliated atrium. Some species are astomatous. They are free living or ectocommensals or endocommensals, chiefly of invertebrates. The subclass comprises four superorders: Nassulidea, Phyllopharyngidea, Rhynchodea, and Apostomatidea.

hypostome (hi″po-stōm) [*hypo-* + Gr. *stōma* mouth] any of several structures, parts, or organs found in association with the mouth in various organisms; e.g., the rodlike piercing mouth part, sometimes with spines or teeth, used by certain ticks and mites to thrust into and hold firmly onto the tissues of a prey or host.

hypostomia (hi″po-sto′me-ah) [*hypo-* + Gr. *stōma* mouth + *-ia*] a developmental anomaly characterized by abnormal smallness of the mouth, the slit being vertical instead of horizontal.

hypostomial (hi″po-sto′me-al) pertaining to ciliate protozoa of the subclass Hypostomatia.

hypostosis (hip″os-to′sis) [*hypo-* + Gr. *osteon* bone + *-osis*] deficient development of bone.

hypostypsis (hi″po-stip′sis) [*hypo-* + Gr. *stypsis* contraction] moderate astringency.

hypostyptic (hi″po-stip′tik) moderately or mildly styptic.

hyposulfite (hi″po-sul′fit) thiosulfate.

hyposuprarenalism (hi″po-su″prah-re′nal-izm) hypoadrenalism.

hyposympathicotonus (hi″po-sim-path″ĭ-ko-to′nus) a decreased tone of the sympathetic nervous system.

hyposynergia (hi″po-sĭ-ner′je-ah) [*hypo-* + *synergia*] defective coordination.

hyposystole (hi″po-sis′to-le) [*hypo-* + *systole*] (obs.) abnormal diminution of the systole.

hypotaxia (hi″po-tak′se-ah) [*hypo-* + Gr. *taxis* arrangement + *-ia*] the emotional rapport between subject and hypnotist at the beginning of hypnosis.

hypotelorism (hi″po-tel′o-rizm) [*hypo-* + Gr. *tēlouros* distant] abnormally decreased distance between two organs or parts. **ocular h., orbital h.,** a condition characterized by abnormal decrease in the intraorbital distance, consistently present in trigonocephaly.

hypotension (hi″po-ten′shun) abnormally low blood pressure; seen in shock but not necessarily indicative of it. See also *blood pressure,* under *pressure.* **chronic orthostatic h., chronic idiopathic orthostatic h., idiopathic orthostatic h.,** Shy-Drager syndrome. **orthostatic h.,** a fall in blood pressure associated with dizziness, syncope, and blurred vision occurring upon standing or when standing motionless in a fixed position; it can be acquired or idiopathic, transient or chronic, and occur alone or secondary to a disorder of the central nervous system, such as the Shy-Drager syndrome (see under *syndrome*). Called also *postural h.* and *postural syncope.* **postural h.,** orthostatic h. **vascular h.,** severe hypotension from dilatation of the blood vessels.

hypotensive (hi″po-ten′siv) 1. characterized by or causing diminished tension or pressure, as abnormally low blood pressure. 2. a person with abnormally low blood pressure.

hypotensor (hi″po-ten′sor) a substance that lowers the blood pressure; a hypotensive agent.

hypothalamic (hi″po-thah-lam′ik) of or involving the hypothalamus.

hypothalamotomy (hi″po-thal″ah-mot′o-me) [*hypothalamus* + Gr. *temnein* to cut] production of lesions in the posterolateral part of the hypothalamus; done in the treatment of psychotic disorders.

hypothalamus (hi″po-thal′ah-mus) [*hypo-* + *thalamus*] [NA] the ventral part of the diencephalon that forms the floor and part of the lateral wall of the third ventricle. Anatomically, it includes the preoptic area, optic tract, optic chiasm, mamillary bodies, tuber cinereum, infundibulum, and neurohypophysis, but for physiological purposes the neurohypophysis is considered a distinct structure. In general, the hypothalamus may be divided into four regions: *dorsal,* consisting of the nucleus of the lenticular ansa; *anterior,* consisting of the lateral and medial preoptic nuclei, the supraoptic and paraventricular nuclei, and the anterior hypothalamic nucleus; *intermediate,* consisting of the arcuate and tuberal nuclei, the lateral hypothalamic area, the ventromedial, dorsomedial, and dorsal hypothalamic nuclei, and the posterior periventricular and the infundibular nuclei; and *posterior,* consisting of the lateral and medial nuclei of the mamillary body and the posterior hypothalamic nucleus. The hypothalamic nuclei comprise that part of the corticodiencephalic mechanism that activates, controls, and integrates the peripheral autonomic mechanisms, endocrine activity, and many somatic functions, e.g., a general regulation of water balance, body temperature, sleep, and food intake, and the development of secondary sex characteristics. The hypothalamus secretes vasopressin and oxytocin, which are stored in the pituitary, as well as many releasing factors (hypophyseotropic hormones) by means of which it exerts control over functions of the adenohypophysis portion of the pituitary gland.

hypothenar (hi-poth′ĕ-nar) [*hypo-* + Gr. *thenar* palm] 1. [NA] the fleshy eminence on the palm along the ulnar margin; called also *eminentia hypothenaris* [NA alternative] and *hypothenar eminence.* 2. relating to this eminence.

hypothermal (hi″po-ther′mal) [*hypo-* + Gr. *thermē* heat] pertaining to or characterized by reduced body temperature.

hypothermia (hi″po-ther′me-ah) [*hypo-* + Gr. *thermē* heat + *-ia*] a low body temperature, as that due to exposure in cold weather or a state of low temperature of the body induced as a means of decreasing metabolism of tissues and thereby the need for oxygen, as used in various surgical procedures, especially on the heart, or in an excised organ being preserved for transplantation. **endogenous h.,** abnormally reduced body temperature resulting from physiologic causes, due to hypofunction of the central nervous system (diencephalon) or of the endocrine system, e.g., the thyroid gland.

hypothermic (hi″po-ther′mik) pertaining to or exhibiting reduced body temperature, pertaining to hypothermia.

hypothermy (hi″po-ther′me) hypothermia.

hypothesis (hi-poth′ĕ-sis) a supposition that appears to explain a group of phenomena and is advanced as a basis for further investigation; a proposition that is subject to proof or to an experimental or statistical test. See also *theory.* **alternative h.,** the hypothesis that is compared with the null hypothesis in a statistical test. **biogenic amine h.,** the hypothesis that depression is associated with deficiency of catecholamines, especially norepinephrine, at functionally important receptor sites in the brain and that elation is associated with excess of such amines. **cardionector h.,** the hypothesis that there are two pacemakers or cardionectors in the heart; one, the atrionector, controls the atria, and the other, the ventriculonector, controls the ventricles. **Dreyer and Bennett h.,** see *recombinational germline*

theory, under *theory.* **Gad's h.,** the arterial and portal venous communications in the portal canal meet at an acute angle, leaving a wedge-shaped valve between them at their junction. **gate h.,** gate theory. **insular h.,** the hypothesis that diabetes mellitus is due to disordered function of the pancreatic islets. **jelly roll h.,** a theory explaining the formation of nerve myelin, which states that it consists of successive layers of the plasma membrane of a Schwann cell wrapped spirally around the axon in a jelly roll fashion. **lattice h.,** a theory of the nature of the antigen-antibody reaction which postulates reaction between multivalent antigen and divalent antibody to give an antigen-antibody complex of a lattice-like structure. **Lyon h.,** all X chromosomes in somatic cells in excess of one are inactivated (in the form of sex chromatin) on a random basis in all mammalian cells at an early stage of embryogenesis. In effect, then, the normal human female is a mosaic for heterozygous X-linked genes, since the paternal X chromosome is inactivated in some cells and the maternal one in the remainder. Hence, females heterozygous for an X-linked disorder often exhibit some stigmata for the condition. See also *lyonization.* **Makeham's h.,** the assumption that death is due to two co-existing causes: (1) chance, which is constant; (2) inability to withstand destruction, which progresses geometrically. **null h.,** the hypothesis that the effect under investigation does not exist. For example, in determining whether a drug has a particular effect, an experiment is designed to compare that drug treatment with a control treatment; the null hypothesis would be, "the drug has no effect." If after the experiment is completed the difference between the results in the drug treatment group and the control treatment group are so large that they should not be attributable to chance errors in random sampling, the null hypothesis is rejected and the drug is said to have an effect. **one gene–one enzyme h.,** see *one gene–one polypeptide chain h.* **one gene–one polypeptide chain h.,** a gene is the DNA sequence that codes for the production of one polypeptide chain; formerly referred to as the one gene–one enzyme or one gene–one protein hypothesis. Antibody genes are an exception; separate genes for variable and constant regions are rearranged to code for a single polypeptide. **sliding-filament h.,** the stretching of individual muscle fibers raises the number of tension-developing bridges that can be formed between the sliding contractile protein elements (actin and myosin) and thus augments the force of the next muscle contraction. **Starling's h.,** the direction and rate of fluid transfer between blood plasma in the capillary and fluid in the tissue spaces depend on the hydrostatic pressure on each side of the capillary wall, on the osmotic pressure of protein in plasma and in tissue fluid, and on the properties of the capillary wall as a filtering membrane. **unitarian h.,** the theory that antibody is a single species of modified serum globulin regardless of the overt consequences of its reaction with homologous antigen, e.g., agglutination, precipitation, complement fixation, etc. **wobble h.,** a hypothesis proposed by F. H. C. Crick to explain how a specific transfer RNA (tRNA) molecule can translate different codons in a messenger RNA (mRNA) template. It states that the third base of the tRNA anticodon does not have to pair with a complementary codon (as do the first two bases) but can form base pairs with several mRNA codons.

hypothrepsia (hi″po-threp′se-ah) malnutrition.

hypothrombinemia (hi″po-throm″bĭ-ne′me-ah) a deficiency of thrombin in the blood.

hypothymia (hi″po-thi′me-ah) [*hypo-* + Gr. *thymos* spirit + *-ia*] abnormal diminution of emotional tone; diminution of feeling tone.

hypothymic (hi″po-thi′mik) marked by hypothymia.

hypothymism (hi″po-thi′mizm) abnormally deficient thymus activity.

hypothyrea (hi″po-thi′re-ah) hypothyroidism.

hypothyreosis (hi″po-thi″re-o′sis) hypothyroidism.

hypothyroid (hi″po-thi′roid) marked by or due to hypothyroidism.

hypothyroidea (hi″po-thi-roi′de-ah) hypothyroidism.

hypothyroidism (hi″po-thi′roid-izm) deficiency of thyroid activity. In adults, it is most common in women and is characterized by decrease in basal metabolic rate, tiredness and lethargy, sensitivity to cold, and menstrual disturbances. If untreated, it progresses to full-blown myxedema. In infants, severe hypothyroidism leads to cretinism. In juveniles, the manifestations are intermediate, with less severe mental and developmental retardation and only mild symptoms of the adult form. When due to pituitary deficiency of thyrotropin secretion it is called secondary hypothyroidism.

hypothyrosis (hi″po-thi-ro′sis) hypothyroidism.

hypotonia (hi″po-to′ne-ah) [*hypo-* + Gr. *tonos* tone + *-ia*] a condition of diminished tone of the skeletal muscles; diminished resistance of muscles to passive stretching. **benign congenital h.**, a condition marked by signs of weakness and floppiness in babies, due to nonprogressive weakness of skeletal muscles from birth. **h. o′culi,** low intraocular pressure.

hypotonic (hi-po-ton′ik) a biological term denoting a solution which, when bathing body cells, causes a net flow of water across the semipermeable cell membrane into the cell. Also, denoting a solution having less tonicity than another solution, e.g., the blood, with which it is compared.

hypotonicity (hi″po-to-nis′ĭ-te) the state or quality of being hypotonic.

hypotonus (hi-pot′o-nus) hypotonia.

hypotony (hi-pot′o-ne) hypotonia.

hypotoxicity (hi″po-tok-sis′ĭ-te) [*hypo-* + Gr. *toxikon* poison] the state or quality of possessing mitigated or diminished toxicity.

hypotrichiasis (hi″po-trĭ-ki′ah-sis) congenital alopecia.

Hypotrichida (hi″po-trik′ĭ-dah) [*hypo-* + Gr. *thrix* hair] an order of ciliate protozoa (subclass Spirotricha, class Polyhymenophorea) having a dorsoventrally flattened, highly mobile body dominated by compound ciliary structures; unique cursorial type of locomotion; cirri on the ventral surface; and widely spaced rows of short bristle-like cilia on the dorsal surface. It comprises two suborders: Stichotrichina and Sporadotrichina.

hypotrichosis (hi″po-trĭ-ko′sis) [*hypo-* + Gr. *thrix* hair + *-osis*] presence of less than the normal amount of hair.

hypotrichous (hi-po′trĭk-us) [*hypo-* + Gr. *thrix* hair] having cilia principally on the ventral surface; characteristic of ciliate protozoa of the order Hypotrichida.

hypotrophy (hi-pot′ro-fe) [*hypo-* + Gr. *trophē* nutrition] abiotrophy.

hypotropia (hi″po-tro′pe-ah) [*hypo-* + Gr. *tropos* a turning + *-ia*] strabismus in which there is permanent downward deviation of the visual axis of an eye.

hypotryptophanic (hi″po-trip-to-fan′ik) caused by deficiency of tryptophan in the diet.

hypotympanotomy (hi″po-tim″pah-not′o-me) surgical opening of the hypotympanum.

hypotympanum (hi″po-tim′pah-num) a space in the middle ear, below the lower edge of the sulcus tympanicus.

hypouremia (hi″po-u-re′me-ah) an abnormally low level of urea in the blood.

hypouresis (hi″po-u-re′sis) oliguria.

hypouricemia (hi″po-u″rĭ-se′me-ah) deficiency of uric acid in the blood, along with xanthinuria, due to deficiency of xanthine oxidase, the enzyme required for conversion of hypoxanthine to xanthine and of xanthine to uric acid.

hypouricuria (hi″po-u″rĭ-ku′re-ah) deficiency of uric acid in the urine.

hypourocrinia (hi″po-u″ro-krin′e-ah) [*hypo-* + Gr. *ouron* urine + *krinein* to secrete + *-ia*] deficient secretion of urine.

hypovaria (hi″po-va′re-ah) hypo-ovaria.

hypovarianism (hi″po-va′re-an-izm) hypo-ovarianism.

hypovenosity (hi″po-ve-nos′ĭ-te) incomplete development of the venous system in any area.

hypoventilation (hi″po-ven″tĭ-la′shun) a state in which there is a reduced amount of air entering the pulmonary alveoli.

hypovitaminosis (hi″po-vi″tah-min-o′sis) a condition due to a deficiency of one or more essential vitamins; see specific vitamins.

hypovolemia (hi″po-vo-le′me-ah) [*hypo-* + *volume* + Gr. *haima* blood + *-ia*] abnormally decreased volume of circulating fluid [plasma] in the body.

hypovolemic (hi″po-vo-le′mik) pertaining to or characterized by hypovolemia.

hypovolia (hi″po-vo′le-ah) diminished water content or volume, as of extracellular fluid.

hypoxanthine (hi″po-zan′thēn) 6-oxypurine, a purine base, $C_5H_4N_4O$, being an intermediate product of uric acid synthesis, formed from adenylic acid and itself a precursor of xanthine.

hypoxanthine guanine phosphoribosyltransferase (hi″po-zan′thēn gwan′ēn fos″fo-ri″bo-sil-trans′fer-ās) hypoxanthine phosphoribosyl transferase.

hypoxanthine guanine phosphoribosyltransferase (HGPRT, HPRT) deficiency Lesch-Nyhan syndrome.

hypoxanthine oxidase (hi″po-zan′thēn ok′sĭ-dās) xanthine oxidase.

hypoxanthine phosphoribosyltransferase (HPRT) (hi″po-zan′thēn fos″fo-ri″bo-sil-trans′fer-ās) [EC 2.4.2.8] an enzyme of the transferase class that catalyzes the reaction hypoxanthine (of guanine) + 5-phospho-α-D-ribose 1-diphosphate = inosine 5′-monophosphate (or guanosine 5′-monophosphate) + pyrophosphate. The reaction acts as a salvage mechanism for recovery of preformed purines, especially in the central nervous system. Deficiency of the enzyme, an X-linked recessive trait, results in Lesch-Nyhan syndrome. Called also *hypoxanthine guanine phosphoribosyltransferase.*

hypoxemia (hi″pok-se′me-ah) [*hypo-* + *oxygen* + Gr. *haima* blood + *-ia*] deficient oxygenation of the blood; hypoxia.

hypoxia (hi-pok′se-ah) reduction of oxygen supply to tissue below physiological levels despite adequate perfusion of the tissue by blood. Cf. *anoxia.* **anemic h.,** hypoxia due to reduction of the oxygen-carrying capacity of the blood as a result of a decrease in the total hemoglobin or an alteration of the hemoglobin constituents. **histotoxic h.,** that due to impaired utilization of oxygen by tissues, as in cyanide poisoning. **hypoxic h.,** that due to insufficient oxygen reaching the blood, as at decreased barometric pressures at high altitudes. **stagnant h.,** that due to failure to transport sufficient oxygen because of inadequate blood flow, as in heart failure.

hypoxic (hi-pok′sik) pertaining to or characterized by hypoxia.

hypoxidosis (hi-pok″sĭ-do′sis) impaired cell function due to reduced supply of oxygen.

HypRho-D (hi′pro-de) trademark for a preparation of $Rh_0(D)$ immune serum globulin.

hypsarhythmia (hip″sah-rith′me-ah) see *hypsarrhythmia.*

hypsarrhythmia (hip″sah-rith′me-ah) [*hyps-* + *arrhythmia*] Gibbs' term for an electroencephalographic abnormality sometimes observed in infants, with random, high-voltage slow waves and spikes that arise from multiple foci and spread to all cortical areas. The disorder is usually characterized by spasms or quivering spells (myoclonus), and is commonly associated with mental retardation.

hypsi- [Gr. *hypsi* aloft] a combining form meaning high.

hypsibrachycephalic (hip″se-brak″e-sĕ-fal′ik) [*hypsi-* + Gr. *brachys* broad + *kephalē* head] having the head broad and high.

hypsicephalic (hip″se-sĕ-fal′ik) [*hypsi-* + Gr. *kephalē* head] having a vertical index over 75.

hypsicephaly (hip″se-sef′ah-le) oxycephaly.

hypsiconchous (hip″se-kong′kus) [*hypsi-* + Gr. *konchē* shell] having an orbital index over 85.

hypsiloid (hip′sĭ-loid) [Gr. *hypsiloeidēs*] shaped like a capital Greek letter upsilon (Υ) . Cf. *hyoid.*

hypsistaphylia (hip″sĭ-stah-fil′e-ah) [*hypsi-* + Gr. *staphylē* uvula + *-ia*] a condition characterized by an unusually high-arched, narrow palate.

hypsistenocephalic (hip″se-sten″o-sĕ-fal′ik) [*hypsi-* + Gr. *stenos* narrow + *kephalē* head] having a high, curved vertex, cheek bones prominent, and jaws prognathic.

hyps(o)- [Gr. *hypsos* height] a combining form denoting relationship to height.

hypsocephalous (hip″so-sef′ah-lus) [*hypso-* + Gr. *kephalē* head] having a high vertex; having a breadth-height index of the head of over 75.

hypsochrome (hip′so-krōm) [*hypso-* + Gr. *chrōma* color] an atom or group whose introduction into a compound shifts the compound's absorption maximum to a shorter wavelength; cf. *bathochrome*.

hypsochromy (hip″so-kro′me) a shift of the absorption band toward higher frequencies (shorter wavelengths), with lightening of color.

hypsodont (hip′so-dont) [*hypso-* + Gr. *odous* tooth] having prism-shaped teeth with high crowns, as in many herbivorous mammals.

hypsokinesis (hip″so-ki-ne′sis) [*hypso-* + Gr. *kinēsis* motion] a backward swaying, retropulsion, or falling when in erect posture, seen in cases of paralysis agitans and other forms of the amyostatic syndrome.

hypsonosus (hip-so′no-sus) [*hypso-* + Gr. *nosos* disease] mountain sickness; balloon sickness.

hypsotherapy (hip″so-ther′ah-pe) [*hypso-* + *therapy*] the therapeutic use of high altitude.

hypurgia (hi-pur′je-ah) [L.; Gr. *hypourgiai* medical services] the sum of the minor or subsidiary factors that make for recovery in any particular case.

hyrtenal (her′tĭ-nal) a terpene aldehyde, $(CH_3)_2C{:}C_6H_7{\cdot}{\cdot}CHO$, from the tropical tree *Hernandia peltata*.

Hyrtl's loop (anastomosis), recess, sphincter (hēr′tlz) [Jozsef *Hyrtl*, eminent anatomist at Prague and Vienna, 1810–1894] see under *loop* and *sphincter*, and see *recessus epitympanicus*.

hysteralgia (his″tĕ-ral′je-ah) [*hystero-* + *-algia*] metralgia or metrodynia.

hysteratresia (his″ter-ah-tre′ze-ah) atresia of the uterus.

hysterectomy (his″tĕ-rek′to-me) [*hystero-* + Gr. *ektomē* excision] the operation of excising the uterus, performed either through the abdominal wall (*abdominal h.*) or through the vagina (*vaginal h.*). **abdominal h.,** excision of the uterus through an incision in the abdominal wall. **cesarean h.,** cesarean section followed by removal of the uterus. **complete h.,** total h. **partial h.,** subtotal h. **radical h.,** hysterectomy with pelvic lymphadenectomy and wide lateral excision of parametrial and paravaginal supporting structures; called also *Wertheim's operation* or, when done by the vaginal route, *Schauta's operation.* **subtotal h., supracervical h., supravaginal h.,** hysterectomy in which the cervix is left in place. **total h.,** hysterectomy in which the uterus and cervix are completely excised; called also *panhysterectomy.* **vaginal h.,** excision of the uterus through the vagina.

hysteresis (his″tĕ-re′sis) [Gr. *hysterēsis* a lagging behind] a time lag in the occurrence of two associated phenomena, as between cause and effect. **protoplasmic h.,** a postulated cause of cell senescence: the colloidal state of the protoplasm is altered, becoming less dispersed, with loss of water and electrical charge.

hystereurynter (his″ter-u-rin′ter) [*hystero-* + Gr. *eurynein* to widen] an instrument for dilating the os uteri: a metreurynter.

hystereurysis (his″ter-u′rĭ-sis) dilation of the os uteri.

hysteria (his-tēr′e-ah) [Gr. *hystera* uterus + *-ia*] a now somewhat nebulous term used to refer to (1) classic hysteria or Briquet's syndrome, a disease of females characterized by multiple somatic complaints that do not appear to result from physical illness and by a chronic fluctuating course, many patients exhibiting "conversion symptoms" mimicking neurological disease (seizures, paralysis, dyskinesia, anesthesia, blindness, aphonia) or "dissociative" phenomena (amnesia, fugue), and which once was considered a physical disorder (it was attributed by the ancient Greeks to displacement of the uterus, hence the name); (2) hysterical neurosis, classified as conversion type or dissociative type according to the predominant symptoms, a conception of hysteria as a neurotic disorder; (3) anxiety hysteria (q.v.); (4) hysterical personality, a personality type, characterized by excitability, emotional overreaction, self-dramatization, and acting out, often seen in association with classic hysteria; and (5) a term of opprobrium applied to any excitable behavior in females. DSM III does not use the term hysteria; disorders of this type are classified as somatoform disorders or dissociative disorders, the former comprising somatization disorder (classic hysteria), conversion disorder (conversion hysteria), and psychogenic pain disorder, and the latter (equivalent to the dissociative type of hysterical neuroses) comprising psychogenic amnesia, psychogenic fugue, multiple personality, and depersonalization disorder. Hysterical personality has been renamed histrionic

personality disorder. **anxiety h.,** Freud's term for phobias, reflecting his view that the same defense mechanisms, repression and displacement, and the same unconscious conflicts involving infantile sexuality are involved in both hysteria and phobias. **canine h.,** fright disease. **conversion h.,** see *hysteria*. **dissociative h.,** see *hysteria*. **fixation h.,** hysteria in which the symptoms are based on those of an organic disease, as the persistence of a nervous cough after pertussis. **h. ma′jor,** la grande hystérie of Charcot, hysteria with dramatic epileptiform attacks involving intense emotional display.

hysteric (his-ter′ik) 1. pertaining to or characterized by hysteria. 2. a person affected with hysteria.

hysterical (his-ter′ĭ-kal) characterized by hysteria.

hystericism (his-ter′ĭ-sizm) a tendency toward hysteria.

hysterics (his-ter′iks) popular term for an uncontrollable emotional outburst.

hysteriform (his-ter′ĭ-form) having the appearance of hysteria.

hyster(o)- [Gr. *hystera* uterus] a combining form denoting relationship to the uterus, or to hysteria; see also *metr(o)-*.

hysterobubonocele (his″ter-o-bu-bon′o-sēl) an inguinal hernia containing the uterus.

hysterocarcinoma (his″ter-o-kar″sĭ-no′mah) endometrial carcinoma.

hysterocele (his′ter-o-sēl″) [*hystero-* + Gr. *kēlē* hernia] hernia of the uterus.

hysterocleisis (his″ter-o-kli′sis) [*hystero-* + Gr. *kleisis* closure] surgical closure of the ostium uteri.

hysterocolpectomy (his″ter-o-kol-pek′to-me) [*hystero-* + Gr. *kolpos* vagina + *ektomē* excision] surgical removal of the uterus and vagina.

hysterocolposcope (his″ter-o-kol′po-skōp) [*hystero-* + Gr. *kolpos* vagina + *skopein* to examine] an electrically lighted device for viewing the interior of the uterus.

hysterocystic (his″ter-o-sis′tik) pertaining to the uterus and the bladder.

hysterocystocleisis (his″ter-o-sis″to-kli′sis) [*hystero-* + Gr. *kystis* bladder + *kleisis* closure] the operation of turning the cervix uteri into the bladder and suturing it; done for the relief of vesicouterovaginal fistula or for ureterouterine fistula. Called also *Bozeman's operation.*

hysterodynia (his″ter-o-din′e-ah) [*hystero-* + Gr. *odynē* pain] metralgia or metrodynia.

hysteroepilepsy (his″ter-o-ep′ĭ-lep″se) hysteria with attacks imitating epileptic seizures.

hysterogram (his′ter-o-gram) a roentgenogram of the uterus.

hysterograph (his′ter-o-graf) [*hystero-* + Gr. *graphein* to record] an apparatus for measuring the strength of uterine contractions in labor.

hysterography (his″tĕ-rog′rah-fe) [*hystero-* + Gr. *graphein* to record] 1. graphic recording of the strength of uterine contractions in labor. 2. roentgenography of the uterus after instillation of a contrast medium. Called also *metrography* and *uterography.*

hysteroid (his′ter-oid) [*hystero-* + Gr. *eidos* form] resembling hysteria.

hysterolith (his′ter-o-lith″) [*hystero-* + Gr. *lithos* stone] a uterine calculus.

hysterolysis (his″tĕ-rol′ĭ-sis) [*hystero-* + Gr. *lysis* dissolution] the operation of loosening the uterus from its attachments or adhesions.

hysterometer (his″tĕ-rom′ĕ-ter) [*hystero-* + Gr. *metron* measure] an instrument for measuring the uterus.

hysterometry (his″tĕ-rom′ĕ-tre) [*hystero-* + Gr. *metron* measure] the measurement of the dimensions of the uterus.

hysteromyoma (his″ter-o-mi-o′mah) uterine leiomyoma.

hysteromyomectomy (his″ter-o-mi″o-mek′to-me) [*hystero-* + *myoma* + Gr. *ektomē* excision] excision of a uterine leiomyoma.

hysteromyotomy (his″ter-o-mi-ot′o-me) [*hystero-* + Gr. *mys* muscle + *tomē* a cutting] incision of the uterus.

hysteropathy (his″tĕ-rop′ah-the) [*hystero-* + Gr. *pathos* disease] any uterine disease or disorder.

hysteropexy (his′ter-o-pek-se) [*hystero-* + Gr. *pēxis* fixation] the fixation of a displaced uterus by a surgical operation. It may be done by ventrofixation, shortening of the round ligaments, shortening of the sacrouterine ligaments, or shortening of the endopelvic fascia It is called *abdominal* or *vaginal*, depending on whether the uterus is fastened to the abdominal wall or to the vagina.

hysteroptosia (his″ter-op-to′ze-ah) metroptosis.

hysteroptosis (his″ter-op-to′sis) metroptosis.

hysterorrhaphy (his-ter-or′ah-fe) [*hystero-* + Gr. *rhaphē* suture] 1. hysteropexy. 2. the operation of suturing of the lacerated uterus.

hysterorrhexis (his″ter-o-rek′sis) metrorrhexis.

hysterosalpingectomy (his″ter-o-sal″pin-jek′to-me) [*hystero-* + Gr. *salpinx* tube + *ektomē* excision] excision of the uterus and uterine tubes.

hysterosalpingography (his″ter-o-sal″ping-gog′rah-fe) [*hystero-* + Gr. *salpinx* tube + *graphein* to record] roentgenography of the uterus and uterine tubes after the injection of opaque material. Called also *uterosalpingography*, *uterotubography*, *hysterotubography*, *metrosalpingography*, *metrotubography*.

hysterosalpingo-oophorectomy (his″ter-o-sal-ping″go-o″of-o-rek′to-me) excision of the uterus, uterine tubes, and ovaries.

hysterosalpingostomy (his″ter-o-sal″ping-gos′to-me) [*hystero-* + Gr. *salpinx* tube + *stomoun* to provide with an opening or mouth] the operation of forming an anastomosis between the uterus and the distal portion of the uterine tube after excision of a strictured or obstructed portion of the tube.

hysteroscope (his′ter-o-skōp″) [*hystero-* + Gr. *skopein* to examine] an endoscope used in direct visual examination of the canal of the uterine cervix and the cavity of the uterus.

hysteroscopy (his″ter-os′ko-pe) inspection of the interior of the uterus with an endoscope.

hysterospasm (his′ter-o-spazm″) spasm of the uterus.

hysterostat (his′ter-o-stat) [*hystero-* + Gr. *statikos* stopping] a mechanical intrauterine device for holding sealed sources of ionizing radiation (radium, cesium-137, etc.) in order to give planned patterns of irradiation.

hysterothermometry (his″ter-o-ther-mom′ĕ-tre) uterothermometry.

hysterotome (his″ter-o-tōm) [*hystero-* + Gr. *tomē* a cutting] an instrument for incising the uterus.

hysterotomy (his″ter-ot′o-me) [*hystero-* + Gr. *temnein* to cut] incision of the uterus, usually for delivery of a fetus. **abdominal h.,** incision of the uterus through the wall of the abdomen. **vaginal h.,** incision of the uterus through the vagina.

hysterotrachelectasia (his″ter-o-tra″kel-ek-ta′se-ah) surgical dilation of the cervix and uterus.

hysterotrachelectomy (his″ter-o-tra″kel-ek′to-me) cervicectomy.

hysterotracheloplasty (his″ter-o-tra′kel-o-plas″te) plastic repair of the cervix uteri; tracheloplasty.

hysterotrachelorrhaphy (his″ter-o-tra″kel-or′ah-fe) [*hystero-* + Gr. *trachēlos* neck + *rhaphē* suture] suture of the cervix uteri.

hysterotrachelotomy (his″ter-o-tra″kel-ot′o-me) [*hystero-* + Gr. *trachēlos* neck + *tomē* a cutting] incision of the cervix uteri.

hysterotubography (his″ter-o-tu-bog′rah-fe) hysterosalpingography.

hysterovagino-enterocele (his″ter-o-vaj″ĭ-no-en′ter-o-sēl) [*hystero-* + *vagina* + Gr. *enteron* intestine + *kēlē* hernia] hernia containing the uterus, vagina, and intestine.

Hytakerol (hi-tak′er-ol) trademark for preparations of dihydrotachysterol.

Hyzyd (hiz′id) trademark for a preparation of isoniazid.

Hz hertz.

I

I chemical symbol for *iodine;* symbol for *inosine* (in nucleotides).

I symbol for *intensity* (of radiant energy) and *ionic strength.*

ι iota, the ninth letter of the Greek alphabet.

-ia [L. and Gr. noun-forming suffix] a word termination denoting a state or condition.

IAEA International Atomic Energy Agency.

IAHA immune adherence hemagglutination assay.

iamatology (i″am-ah-tol′o-je) [Gr. *iama, iamatos* remedy + *-logy*] the study or science of remedies.

-iasis a word termination meaning a process or the condition resulting therefrom, particularly a morbid condition. See *-sis.*

iatraliptic (i″ah-trah-lip′tik) [Gr. *iatreia* cure + *aleiphein* to anoint] pertaining to the application of remedies by inunction and friction.

iatraliptics (i″ah-trah-lip′tiks) treatment by inunction and friction.

iatric (i-at′rik) [Gr. *iatrikos*] pertaining to medicine or to a physician.

-iatric [Gr. *iatrikos* pertaining to a physician, from *iatros* physician] a combining form denoting relationship to medical treatment.

-iatrics [*-iatric*] a combining form denoting medical treatment.

iatr(o)- [Gr. *iatros* physician] a combining form denoting relationship to a physician or to medicine.

Iatrobdella (i″at-ro-del′ah) (obs.) *Hirudo.*

iatrochemical (i-at″ro-kem′ĕ-kal) pertaining to iatrochemistry.

iatrochemistry (i-at″ro-kem′is-tre) [*iatro-* + *chemistry*] a school of medicine active from 1525 to 1660; it theorized that life, health, and disease were the result of chemical balances, and that disease was to be treated chemically. Its most famous members were Paracelsus, J.B. van Helmont, and de la Boë Sylvius.

iatrogenesis (i-at″ro-jen′ĕ-sis) [*iatro-* + Gr. *genesis* production] the creation of additional problems or complications resulting from treatment by a physician or surgeon.

iatrogenic (i-at″ro-jen′ik) [*iatro-* + Gr. *gennan* to produce] resulting from the activity of physicians. Originally applied to disorders induced in the patient by autosuggestion based on the physician's examination, manner, or discussion, the term is now applied to any adverse condition in a patient occurring as the result of treatment by a physician or surgeon, especially to infections acquired by the patient during the course of treatment. Cf. *nosocomial.*

iatrology (i″ah-trol′o-je) [*iatro-* + *-logy*] the science of medicine.

iatromathematical (i-at″ro-math″ĕ-mat′ĭ-kal) iatrophysical.

iatromechanical (i-at″ro-mĕ-kan′ĭ-kal) iatrophysical.

iatrophysical (i-at″ro-fiz′ĭ-kal) an Italian school of medicine active in the 17th century; the school opposed iatrochemistry and, inspired by the earlier experiments of Harvey and Sanctorius, combined medicine, physics, and mechanics. René Descartes was an early exponent of iatrophysics, and his posthumous De homine (1662) was the first modern textbook on physiology.

iatrophysics (i-at″ro-fiz′iks) [*iatro-* + Gr. *physikos* natural] 1. the physics of medicine or of medical and surgical treatment. 2. the treatment of diseases by physical or mechanical means; physiatrics.

-iatry [Gr. *iatreia* healing, from *iatros* physician] a word termination denoting medical treatment.

I.B. inclusion body.

IBF immunoglobulin-binding factor.

Ibn Rushd see *Averroes.*

Ibn Sinā see *Avicenna.*

Ibn Zuhr see *Avenzoar.*

ibogaine (i-bo′gah-ēn) an alkaloid, $C_{20}H_{26}N_2O$, from the root of *Tabernanthe iboga* Baill. (Apocynaceae) that has antidepressant and euphoric properties; it is isomeric with tabernanthine.

ibufenac (i-bu′fĕ-nak) chemical name: 4-(2-methylpropyl)-benzeneacetic acid; an analgesic and anti-inflammatory, $C_{13}H_{18}O_2$, formerly used in the treatment of rheumatic conditions.

ibuprofen (i-bu′pro-fen) [USP] a nonsteroidal anti-inflammatory agent that is a propionic acid derivative; used for treatment of osteoarthritis and rheumatoid arthritis.

IC inspiratory capacity; irritable colon.

-ic 1. a suffix meaning pertaining to or characteristic of, e.g., acidic. 2. in chemistry, a suffix used to indicate an ion or acid exhibiting the higher of two oxidation states, the other being indicated by the suffix -ous.

ICD International Classification of Diseases (of the World Health Organization); intrauterine contraceptive device.

ice (īs) any of the six solid forms of water; but usually the common low-density form melting at 0° C. at 1 atmosphere. **Dry I.**, trademark for carbon dioxide snow.

Iceland disease (īs′land) benign myalgic encephalomyelitis.

Iceland moss (īs′land maws′) see under moss.

ich (ik) white spot disease, def. 3.

ichnogram (ik′no-gram) [Gr. ichnos a footprint + gramma mark] a footprint, in ink on paper.

ichor (i′kor) [Gr. ichōr] a thin, serous, or sanious fluid from a sore or wound.

ichoremia (i″kor-e′me-ah) [ichor + Gr. haima blood + -ia] septicemia.

ichoroid (i′ko-roid) [ichor + Gr. eidos form] resembling ichor or pus.

ichorous (i′kor-us) of the nature of a serum or ichor.

ichorrhea (i-ko-re′ah) [ichor + Gr. rhoia flow] a copious discharge of ichorous fluid or sanies.

ichorrhemia (i″ko-re′me-ah) [ichor + Gr. haima blood + -ia] septicemia.

ichthammol (ik′tham-mol) [USP] a reddish brown to brownish black viscous fluid, with a strong, characteristic odor, obtained by the destructive distillation of certain bituminous schists, sulfonation of the distillate, and neutralization of the product with ammonia; used as a local skin anti-infective. Called also ammonium ichthyosulfonate and ammonium sulfoichthyolate.

ichthyism (ik′the-izm) ichthyotoxism.

ichthyismus (ik″the-iz′mus) [Gr. ichthys fish] ichthyotoxism.

ichthy(o)- [Gr. ichthys fish] a combining form denoting relationship to fish.

ichthyoacanthotoxin (ik″the-o-ah-kan″tho-tok′sin) [ichthyo- + Gr. akantha thorn + toxikon poison] the venom secreted by venomous fishes, in connection with stings, spines, or "teeth."

ichthyoacanthotoxism (ik″the-o-ah-kan″tho-tok′sizm) intoxication resulting from injuries produced by the stings, spines, or "teeth" of venomous fishes.

ichthyocolla (ik″the-o-kol′ah) [ichthyo- + Gr. kolla glue] a form of gelatin prepared from the swimming-bladders of the Russian sturgeon, Acipenser huso; used as an adhesive and clarifying agent. Called also isinglass.

ichthyohemotoxin (ik″the-o-he″mo-tok′sin) [ichthyo- + Gr. haima blood + toxikon poison] a toxic substance found in the blood of certain fish.

ichthyohemotoxism (ik″the-o-he″mo-tok′sizm) intoxication caused by the ingestion of ichthyohemotoxin, characterized by gastrointestinal and neurological disturbances.

ichthyoid (ik′the-oid) [ichthyo- + Gr. eidos form] resembling a fish; shaped like a fish.

Ichthyol (ik′the-ol) trademark for a preparation of ichthammol.

ichthyology (ik″the-ol′o-je) that branch of zoology specializing in the study of fishes.

ichthyolsulfonate (ik″the-ol-sul′fo-nāt) a salt of ichthyolsulfonic acid, a derivative of ichthammol.

ichthyootoxin (ik″the-o″o-tok′sin) [ichthyo- + Gr. ōon egg + toxikon poison] a toxic substance derived from the roe of certain fish; see also ichthyootoxism.

ichthyootoxism (ik″the-o″o-tok′sizm) intoxication caused by the ingestion of toxic fish roe, characterized by gastrointestinal and neurological disturbances.

ichthyophagia (ik″the-o-fa′je-ah) [ichthyo- + Gr. phagein to eat + -ia] the practice of subsisting on fish.

ichthyophagous (ik″the-of′ah-gus) eating or subsisting on fish.

ichthyophthiriasis (ik″the-o-thǐ-ri′ah-sis) [ichthyo- + Gr. phtheir louse + -iasis] white spot disease, def. 3.

Ichthyophthirius (ik″the-o-thi′re-us) [ichthyo- + Gr. phtheir louse] a genus of histophagous protozoa (suborder Ophryoglenina, order Hymenostomatida). I. multifiliis causes white spot disease in marine and freshwater fishes, which may result in great economic loss.

ichthyosarcotoxin (ik″the-o-sar″ko-tok′sin) [ichthyo- + Gr. sarx, sarkos flesh + toxikon poison] the poison found in the flesh of poisonous fishes, excluding toxins which may result from bacterial contamination.

ichthyosarcotoxism (ik″the-o-sar″ko-tok′sizm) fish poisoning; intoxication characterized by various gastrointestinal and neurological disturbances, resulting from the ingestion of the flesh of poisonous fishes, excluding ordinary bacterial food poisoning. See, for example, ciguatera, elasmobranch, gymnothorax, and scombroid poisoning, under poisoning.

ichthyosiform (ik″the-o′sǐ-form) resembling ichthyosis.

ichthyosis (ik″the-o′sis) [ichthy- + -osis] a group of cutaneous disorders characterized by increased or aberrant keratinization, resulting in noninflammatory scaling of the skin. Many different metaphors have been used to describe the appearance and texture of the skin in the various types and stages of ichthyosis, e.g., alligator, collodion, crocodile, fish, and porcupine skin. Most ichthyoses are genetically determined, while some may be acquired and develop in association with various systemic diseases or be a prominent feature in certain genetic syndromes. The term is commonly used alone to refer to i. vulgaris. **i. congen′ita, congenital i.,** ichthyosis present at birth. See also collodion baby, under baby, and harlequin fetus, under fetus. **i. hys′trix,** a localized form of epidermolytic hyperkeratosis having the appearance of linear epidermal nevi. **lamellar i.,** a congenital, chronic form of ichthyosis present at birth, inherited as an autosomal recessive trait, in which the affected infant is born encased in a collodionlike membrane (see collodion baby, under baby) that is soon shed, the skin then becoming covered with large, coarse scales with involvement of all of the flexures as well as the palms and soles. Universal erythroderma and pruritus are characteristic, and ectropion of variable degree is usually present. Formerly called nonbullous congenital ichthyosiform erythroderma. **i. linea′ris circumflex′a,** a congenital autosomal recessive disorder present at birth, and characterized by the presence of generalized erythroderma and scaling associated with migratory, polycyclic lesions with a peripheral double-edged scale and hyperkeratosis of the flexural areas, and hyperhidrosis of the palms and soles. **i. palma′ris et planta′ris,** palmoplantar keratoderma. **i. sim′plex,** i. vulgaris. **i. u′teri,** a condition marked by the transformation of the columnar epithelium of the endometrium into stratified squamous epithelium. **i. vulga′ris,** the most common form of ichthyosis, inherited as an autosomal dominant trait, having an onset sometime after the first year of life, especially near puberty. It is characterized by the presence of prominent fine scaling principally on the extensor surfaces of the extremities and back, with the flexures being spared and the abdomen and face being relatively spared; accentuated marking and creases on the palms and soles; and, possibly, atopy. Called also i. simplex. **X-linked i.,** a chronic form of ichthyosis affecting only males, transmitted as an X-linked recessive trait, that may be present at birth or appear in early infancy. It is characterized by the presence of prominent, very adherent scales, often brown, especially on the neck, extremities, trunk, and buttocks. Corneal opacities that do not interfere with vision are a frequent associated finding; these may occur in minor form in heterozygotic female carriers. The condition is always associated with a deficiency of the microsomal enzyme steroid sulfatase.

ichthyotic (ik″the-ot′ik) pertaining to or characterized by ichthyosis.

ichthyotoxic (ik″the-o-tok′sik) caused by the toxic principle of fish.

I J K

ichthyotoxicology (ik″the-o-tok″sĭ-kol′o-je) [*ichthyo-* + Gr. *toxikon* poison + *-logy*] the science of poisons derived from certain fish, their cause, detection, and effects, and the treatment of conditions produced by them.

ichthyotoxicum (ik″the-o-tok′sĭ-kum) [*ichthyo-* + Gr. *toxikon* poison] an obsolete term proposed (1889) to designate a toxic substance found in eel serum.

ichthyotoxin (ik″the-o-tok′sin) [*ichthyo-* + *toxin*] a general term applied to any type of toxic substance derived from fish.

ichthyotoxism (ik″the-o-tok′sizm) [*ichthyo-* + *toxin* + *-ism*] a general term applied to intoxication caused by any toxic substance derived from fish.

ick (ik) white spot disease, def. 3.

I.C.N. International Council of Nurses.

icosanoic acid (i″ko-sah-no′ik) arachidic acid.

I.C.R.P. International Commission on Radiological Protection.

I.C.R.U. International Commission on Radiological Units and Measurements.

I.C.S. International College of Surgeons.

ICSH interstitial cell–stimulating hormone (luteinizing hormone).

I.C.T. insulin coma therapy.

ictal (ik′tal) [L. *ictus* stroke] pertaining to, characterized by, or caused by a stroke or an acute epileptic seizure.

icterepatitis (ik″ter-ep″ah-ti′tis) icterohepatitis.

icteric (ik-ter′ik) pertaining to or affected with jaundice.

icteritious (ik″ter-ish′us) icteric.

icter(o)- [L. *icterus*, q.v.] a combining form meaning affected with or pertaining to jaundice.

icteroanemia (ik″ter-o-ah-ne′me-ah) a disease marked by the development of icterus and anemia, with splenic enlargement, urobilinuria, and a hemolysis associated with fragility of the red blood corpuscles. Called also *hemolytic icteroanemia* and *Widal's syndrome*.

icterogenic (ik″ter-o-jen′ik) [*icterus* + Gr. *gennan* to produce] causing icterus.

icterogenicity (ik″ter-o-jĕ-nis′ĭ-te) ability to cause icterus.

icterohematuria (ik″ter-o-hem″ah-tu′re-ah) jaundice associated with hematuria. **i. of sheep,** a form caused by *Babesia ovis*, which is transmitted by *Rhipicephalus bursa*.

icterohematuric (ik″ter-o-hem″ah-tu′rik) pertaining to icterohematuria; marked by jaundice and hematuria.

icterohemoglobinuria (ik″ter-o-he″mo-glo″bĭ-nu′re-ah) combined jaundice and hemoglobinuria.

icterohepatitis (ik″ter-o-hep″ah-ti′tis) inflammation of the liver with marked jaundice.

icteroid (ik′ter-oid) [*icterus* + Gr. *eidos* form] resembling jaundice.

icterus (ik′ter-us) [L.; Gr. *ikteros*] jaundice. **chronic familial i.,** hereditary spherocytosis. **congenital familial i.,** hereditary spherocytosis. **congenital hemolytic i.,** hereditary spherocytosis. **epidemic catarrhal i.,** a mild form of infectious hepatitis. **i. gra′vis,** massive hepatic necrosis. **i. gra′vis neonato′rum,** severe jaundice in the newborn, usually a form of isoimmunization with Rh factor; called also *erythroleukoblastosis*. See also *kernicterus*. **i. me′las** ["black jaundice"] (*obs.*), Winckel's disease. **i. neonato′rum,** the jaundice sometimes seen in newborn children. **nuclear i.,** kernicterus. **i. prae′cox,** mild jaundice developing within the first 24 hours of life (before physiologic jaundice normally occurs), due to incompatibility of the ABO blood group system between mother and infant; it usually clears rapidly and spontaneously, only occasionally resulting in hemolytic disease. **i. typhoi′des,** acute yellow atrophy; see under *atrophy*.

ictus (ik′tus), pl. *ic′tus* [L. "stroke"] a seizure, stroke, blow, or sudden attack; see also *seizure*. **i. cor′dis,** the heart beat. **i. epilep′ticus,** an epileptic attack. **i. paralyt′icus,** a paralytic stroke. **i. san′guinis,** stroke due to cerebral hemorrhage. **i. so′lis,** a sunstroke.

ICU intensive care unit.

ID intradermal; inside diameter.

ID₅₀ median infective dose, being that amount of patho-genic microorganisms which will produce infection in 50 per cent of the test subjects.

Id. abbreviation for L. *i′dem*, the same.

id¹ (id) [L. *id*, from Ger. *es* it] in psychoanalytic theory, the innate, totally unconscious, primitive aspect of the personality dominated by the pleasure principle and harboring instinctive impulses that seek immediate personal pleasure, gratification, or satisfaction. Cf. *ego* and *superego*.

id² (id) [-id] a sterile cutaneous eruption, general or local, occurring as an allergic reaction (id reaction) to an agent causing a primary infection elsewhere.

-id 1. [Gr. *eidos* form, shape] a word termination meaning having the shape of, or resembling. 2. see *id*, def. 2.

-idae [Gr. *-idai*, pl. of *-ides* patronymic ending] in zoology, a word termination denoting a family.

IDD insulin-dependent diabetes.

-ide a suffix signifying a binary chemical compound, such as a chloride, sulfide, or carbide.

idea (i-de′ah) [Gr. "form"] a mental impression or conception. **autochthonous i.,** a persistent idea, arising from the unconscious, that seems to the patient to have been put into his mind by a foreign influence. **compulsive i.,** an idea which intrudes, recurs, and persists despite reason and will, and which impels toward some inappropriate act. **dominant i.,** a morbid or other impression that controls or colors every action and thought. **fixed i.,** a morbid impression or belief which stays in the mind and cannot be changed by reason; called also *idée fixe*. **imperative i.,** compulsive i. **i. of reference, referential i.,** the assumption by a patient that the words and actions of others refer to himself or the projection of the causes of his own imaginary difficulties upon someone else; called also *delusion of reference*.

ideal (i-de′al) having some relation to ideas, impressions, or imaginations; a standard of perfection. **ego i.,** the component of the superego comprising the internalized image of what one desires to become and toward the attainment of which the ego strives, formed through conscious or unconscious identification with or emulation of one who plays a significant role or has a place of esteem in the life of the developing child.

idealization (i-de″al-i-za′shun) a conscious or unconscious mental mechanism in which the individual overestimates an admired aspect or attribute of another person.

ideation (i″de-a′shun) the formation of a mental concept or image.

ideational (i″de-a′shun-al) relating to ideation.

idée (e-da′) [Fr.] idea. **i. fixe** (e-da′fēks′), fixed idea.

identification (i-den″tĭ-fĭ-ka′shun) an unconscious defense mechanism by which a person patterns himself after another person. **cosmic i.,** identification of one's self with the universe, as in schizophrenic delusions of omnipotence.

identity (i-den′tĭ-te) the aggregate of characteristics by which an individual is recognized by himself and others. **core gender i.,** gender i. **ego i.,** a sense of unity and continuity of one's own personality. **gender i.,** a person's concept of himself as being male and masculine or female and feminine, or ambivalent, usually based on the physical characteristics, parental attitudes and expectations, and psychological and social pressures to which the individual is subjected. It is the private experience of gender role. Cf. *gender role*, under *role*.

ideogenetic (i″de-o-jĕ-net′ik) related to mental processes in which images of sense impressions are used, rather than ideas that are ready for verbal expression.

ideogenous (i″de-oj′ĕ-nus) ideogenetic.

ideoglandular (i″de-o-glan′du-lar) arousing glandular activity as a result of some recollection or thought.

ideokinetic (i-de″o-ki-net′ik) ideomotor.

ideology (i″de-ol′o-je, id″e-ol′o-je) [Gr. *idea* + *-logy*] 1. the science of the development of ideas. 2. the body of ideas characteristic of an individual or of a social unit.

ideometabolic (i″de-o-met-ah-bol′ik) producing metabolic activity as a result of mental action, normal or other.

ideometabolism (i″de-o-mĕ-tab′o-lizm) metabolism produced by mental influence.

ideomotion (i″de-o-mo′shun) motion or muscular action

which is neither reflex nor volitional, but is induced by some dominant idea.

ideomotor (i″de-o-mo′tor) aroused by an idea or thought; said of involuntary motion so aroused.

ideomuscular (i″de-o-mus′ku-lar) producing involuntary muscular action as a result of some ideation, memory, or hallucination.

ideovascular (i″de-o-vas′ku-lar) producing vascular change as a result of some ideation, memory, or hallucination.

idi(o)- [Gr. *idios* one's own, separate] a combining form meaning one's own, separate, or self-produced.

idioagglutinin (id″e-o-ah-gloo′tĭ-nin) [*idio-* + *agglutinin*] an agglutinin that originates independently of any transfer or artificial means in the animal in which it is formed.

idiochromatin (id″e-o-kro′mah-tin) [*idio-* + *chromatin*] chromatin concerned in reproduction; the chromatin bearing the ids.

idiochromidia (id″e-o-kro-mid′e-ah) [*idio-* + *chromidia*] that part of the chromidia or extranuclear chromatin which takes part in the reproduction of the cell. Cf. *trophochromidia*.

idiochromosome (id″e-o-kro′mo-sōm) any sex chromosome.

idiocy (id′e-o-se) the condition of being an idiot; profound mental retardation. **amaurotic i., amaurotic familial i.,** a term for several lipidoses differing biochemically in clinical manifestation; the congenital form may be lethal within less than one month from birth; a disialoganglioside, G (D3), is present in tissue, and there is a three-fold concentration of cholesterol in the brain. The *infantile type* is Tay-Sachs disease. The *late infantile type* begins between three and four years of age, shows no racial or ethnic preference, no fundus changes, cherry-red spot, or optic atrophy; called also *Jansky-Bielschowsky disease*. The *juvenile type* is a neuronal ceroid lipofuscinosis with onset between five and ten years, a prolonged course, and death during late adolescence; it is relatively common among Scandinavians, and shows a "salt and pepper" pigmentary degeneration (atypical retinitis pigmentosa), then cerebellar ataxia, polymyoclonia, and dementia; called also *Batten disease, Vogt-Spielmeyer disease,* and *neuronal ceroid lipofuscinosis*. The *adult type* begins in the late teens or twenties, has the same biochemical defect and clinical progression as the juvenile type, and may be the same entity. Called also *Kufs disease.* See also *lipidosis* and *cerebromacular degeneration,* under *degeneration.* **athetosic i.,** athetosis. **Aztec i.,** microcephalic i. **cretinoid i.,** cretinism with gross mental retardation. **Kalmuk i.,** mongolian i. **microcephalic i.,** severe mental retardation associated with microcephaly. **mongolian i.,** a name formerly applied to the marked mental retardation associated with *Down syndrome.* **moral i.,** see under *insanity.* **spastic amaurotic axonal i.,** infantile neuroaxonal dystrophy. **xerodermic i.,** De Sanctis-Cacchione syndrome.

idiogenesis (id″e-o-jen′e-sis) [*idio-* + Gr. *genesis* production] the spontaneous origin of disease.

idioglossia (id″e-o-glos′e-ah) [*idio-* + Gr. *glōssa* tongue + *-ia*] imperfect articulation, with the utterance of meaningless vocal sounds.

idioglottic (id″e-o-glot′ik) pertaining to idioglossia.

idiogram (id′e-o-gram″) [*idio-* + *-gram*] a diagrammatic representation of a chromosome complement, based on measurement of the chromosomes of a number of cells. Cf. *karyotype.*

idioheteroagglutinin (id″e-o-het″er-o-ah-gloo′tĭ-nin) [*idio-* + Gr. *heteros* other + *agglutinin*] a heteroagglutinin normally present in the blood.

idioheterolysin (id″e-o-het-er-ol′ĭ-sin) a heterolysin normally present in the blood.

idiohypnotism (id″e-o-hip′no-tizm) [*idio-* + *hypnotism*] spontaneous or self-induced hypnotism.

idio-imbecile (id″e-o-im′bĕ-sil) (*obs.*) a grade of mental retardation between idiot and imbecile.

idioisoagglutinin (id″e-o-i″so-ah-gloo′tĭ-nin) an isoagglutinin normally present in the blood, and not produced by artificial means.

idioisolysin (id″e-o-i-sol′ĭ-sin) a lysin normally present

which lyses the cells of other members of the same species as the animal in which it is formed.

idiolalia (id″e-o-la′le-ah) a condition marked by the use of invented language.

idiolog (id′e-o-log) a word that has meaning only to the user.

idiologism (id″e-ol′o-jizm) the utterance of words that are meaningless to anyone but the speaker.

idiolysin (id″e-ol′ĭ-sin) [*idio-* + *lysin*] a lysin, normally present in the blood and not produced by artificial means, that lyses the cells of the animal in which it is formed.

idiomere (id′e-o-mēr) chromomere (def. 1).

idiomuscular (id″e-o-mus′ku-lar) [*idio-* + L. *musculus* muscle] pertaining to the muscular tissue apart from any nerve stimulus; a term applied to certain muscular contractions which occur in degenerated muscles only.

idiopathetic (id″e-o-pah-thet′ik) idiopathic.

idiopathic (id″e-o-path′ik) of the nature of an idiopathy; self-originated; of unknown causation.

idiopathy (id″e-op′ah-the) [*idio-* + Gr. *pathos* disease] a morbid state of spontaneous origin; one neither sympathetic nor traumatic.

idioreflex (id″e-o-re′fleks) [*idio-* + *reflex*] a reflex brought about by a cause within the same organ.

idioretinal (id″e-o-ret′ĭ-nal) pertaining to the retina alone; a term applied to a visual sensation occurring without any visual stimulus.

idiosome (id′e-o-sōm″) [*idio-* + Gr. *sōma* body] 1. a supposed ultimate element of living matter. 2. the centrosome of a spermatocyte, together with surrounding Golgi apparatus and mitochondria.

idiospasm (id′e-o-spazm) a spasm of a limited area or region.

idiosyncrasy (id″e-o-sin′krah-se) [*idio-* + Gr. *synkrasis* mixture] 1. a habit or quality of body or mind peculiar to any individual. 2. an abnormal susceptibility to some drug, protein, or other agent which is peculiar to the individual.

idiosyncratic (id″e-o-sin-krat′ik) pertaining to or characterized by idiosyncrasy.

idiot (id′e-ot) [Gr. *idiōtēs* a person not in public life, a nonexpert or layman] (*obs.*) a person with the lowest grade of feeblemindedness (q.v.), equivalent to the modern classification "profound mental retardation." **mongolian i.,** former name for a person affected with Down's syndrome. **i.-savant** (e′dyo sah-vahn′) Fr. "learned idiot", a person who is severely mentally retarded in some respects, yet has a particular mental faculty that is developed to an unusually high degree, as memory, mathematics, or music.

idiotope (id′ĭ-o-tōp″) idiotypic determinant; an antigenic determinant on a variable domain of an immunoglobulin molecule. Cf. *allotope.*

idiotopy (id′e-o-top″e) [*idio-* + Gr. *topos* place] the position and relation of the parts of an organ among themselves.

idiotrophic (id″e-o-trof′ik) [*idio-* + Gr. *trophē* nutrition] capable of selecting its own nourishment.

idiotropic (id″e-o-trop′ik) [*idio-* + Gr. *tropos* a turning] introspective; egocentric.

idiotype (id′e-o-tīp′) a set of one or more idiotopes that distinguish a clone of immunoglobulin-producing cells from other clones. Idiotypes occur in the variable domains of immunoglobulin molecules and may be within, near to, or outside of the antigen-binding site; antibodies to idiotypes located within or near to the antigen-binding site will prevent the immunoglobulin from combining with antigen.

idiotypic (id″e-o-tip′ik) pertaining to idiotypes.

idiovariation (id″e-o-var″e-a′shun) a mutation or change in the germ plasm, the cause of which is unknown.

idioventricular (id″e-o-ven-trik′u-lar) relating to or affecting the cardiac ventricle alone, as idioventricular rhythm.

idiozome (id′e-o-zōm) idiosome.

iditol (i′dĭ-tol) a hexahydric alcohol, $CH_2OH(CHOH)_4CH_2OH$, a reduction product of the hexose known as idose.

L–iditol dehydrogenase (i′dĭ-tol de-hi′dro-jĕ-nās) [EC 1.1.1.14] an enzyme of the oxidoreductase class that catalyzes the reaction L-iditol + NAD^+ = L-sorbose + NADH. The enzyme occurs in significant quantities only in the liver. Increased activity in serum is used as an indicator of parenchymal liver damage. Called also *sorbitol dehydrogenase.*

IDL intermediate-density lipoprotein.

idose (i′dōs) an aldohexose.

idoxuridine (i-doks-ur′ĭ-dēn) [USP] chemical name: 2′-deoxy-5-iodouridine. An analog of pyrimidine, $C_9H_{11}IN_2O_5$, occurring as a white crystalline powder, which inhibits viral DNA synthesis; used as an antiviral agent in the treatment of herpes simplex keratitis, applied topically to the conjunctiva. Abbreviated IDU.

IDU idoxuridine.

iduronate-2-sulfatase (īd″u-ron′āt sul′fah-tās) [EC 3.1.6.13] an enzyme of the hydrolase class that catalyzes the hydrolysis of the 2-sulfate groups on L-iduronate units of dermatan sulfate, heparan sulfate, and heparin. The reaction is important in the metabolism of mucopolysaccharides. Deficiency of the enzyme, transmitted as an X-linked recessive trait, results in Hunter's syndrome (mucopolysaccharidosis II). Called also *iduronic sulfatase* and *sulfoiduronate sulfatase.*

iduronic sulfatase (īd″u-ron′ik sul′fah-tās) iduronate-2-sulfatase.

L-iduronidase (īd″u-ron′ĭ-dās) [EC 3.2.1.76] an enzyme of the hydrolase class that catalyzes the hydrolysis of α-L-iduronosidic linkages in desulfated heparin. It is important in the degradation of dermatan and heparan sulfates. Genetic deficiency of the enzyme, transmitted as an autosomal recessive trait, leads to mucopolysaccharidosis I.

α-L-iduronidase deficiency mucopolysaccharidosis I.

IEP immunoelectrophoresis.

IFN interferon.

ifosfamide (i-fos′fah-mīd) chemical name: *N*,3-bis(2-chloroethyl)tetrahydro-2*H*-1,3,2-oxazaphosphorin-2-amine 2-oxide; an antineoplastic, $C_7H_{15}Cl_2N_2O_2P$.

Ig immunoglobulin. The five classes are designated IgM, IgG, IgA, IgD, IgE. Subclasses are designated by numerical suffixes, e.g., IgG1.

ignatia (ig-na′she-ah) [L.] the poisonous dried ripe seed of *Strychnos ignatii;* it contains several alkaloids, the principal ones being strychnine and brucine, and has been used as a bitter tonic.

ignipuncture (ig′nĭ-punk″chur) [L. *ignis* fire + *punctura* puncture] therapeutic puncture with hot needles.

ignis (ig′nis) [L.] fire. **i. inferna′lis** ["infernal fire"], ergotism.

ignisation (ig″ni-za′shun) [L. *ignis* fire] hyperthermia produced by exposure to artificial sources of heat.

ignotine (ig′no-tin) carnosine.

IGT impaired glucose tolerance.

I.H. infectious hepatitis.

II-para secundipara.

III-para tertipara.

IL interleukin.

Il chemical symbol for *illinium,* former name for promethium.

il- see *in-.*

I.L.A. International Leprosy Association.

Ile isoleucine.

ileac (il′e-ak) 1. of the nature of ileus. 2. pertaining to the ileum.

ileadelphus (il″e-ah-del′fus) iliopagus.

ileal (il′e-al) pertaining to the ileum.

ileectomy (il″e-ek′to-me) [ileum + Gr. *ektomē* excision] surgical removal of the ileum.

ileitis (il″e-i′tis) inflammation of the ileum. **distal i.,** Crohn's disease affecting the ileum. **regional i., terminal i.,** Crohn's disease affecting the ileum.

ile(o)- [L. *ileum*] a combining form denoting relationship to the ileum.

ileocecal (il″e-o-se′kal) pertaining to the ileum and cecum.

ileocecostomy (il″e-o-se-kos′to-me) surgical creation of an opening between the ileum and the cecum; also, the opening so established.

ileocecum (il″e-o-se′kum) the ileum and cecum considered as one organ.

ileocolic (il″e-o-kol′ik) pertaining to the ileum and colon.

ileocolitis (il″e-o-ko-li′tis) inflammation of the ileum and colon. **tuberculous i.,** tuberculous inflammation of the ileum and colon. **i. ulcero′sa chron′ica,** a chronic form characterized by fever, rapid pulse, anemia, diarrhea, and right iliac pain.

ileocolonic (il″e-o-ko-lon′ik) ileocolic.

ileocolostomy (il″e-o-ko-los′to-me) [ileo- + colon + Gr. *stoma* mouth] surgical creation of an opening between the ileum and colon; also, the opening so established.

ileocolotomy (il″e-o-ko-lot′o-me) [ileo- + colon + Gr. *temnein* to cut] surgical incision of the ileum and colon.

ileocystoplasty (il″e-o-sis′to-plas″te) [ileo- + Gr. *kystis* bladder + *plassein* to form] surgical reconstruction of the bladder, incorporating an isolated loop of the ileum as part of the bladder wall.

ileocystostomy (il″e-o-sis-tos′to-me) surgical creation of an opening between the urinary bladder and ileum.

ileoileostomy (il″e-o-il″e-os′to-me) [ileo- + ileo- + Gr. *stoma* mouth] surgical creation of an opening between two parts of the ileum; also, the opening so established.

ileoproctostomy (il″e-o-prok-tos′to-me) [ileo- + Gr. *prōktos* rectum + *stoma* mouth] anastomosis of the ileum and rectum.

ileorectal (il″e-o-rek′tal) pertaining to or communicating with the ileum and rectum, as an ileorectal fistula.

ileorectostomy (il″e-o-rek-tos′to-me) ileoproctostomy.

ileorrhaphy (il″e-or′ah-fe) [ileo- + Gr. *rhaphē* suture] operative repair of the ileum.

ileosigmoid (il″e-o-sig′moid) pertaining to the ileum and the sigmoid.

ileosigmoidostomy (il″e-o-sig″moi-dos′to-me) [ileo- + sigmoid flexure + Gr. *stoma* mouth] surgical creation of an opening between the ileum and the sigmoid colon; also, the opening so established.

ileostomy (il″e-os′to-me) [ileo- + Gr. *stoma* mouth] surgical creation of an opening into the ileum, usually by establishing an ileal stoma on the abdominal wall.

ileotomy (il″e-ot′o-me) [ileo- + Gr. *temnein* to cut] incision of the ileum.

ileotransversostomy (il″e-o-trans″vers-os′to-me) surgical creation of an opening between the ileum and the transverse colon.

Iletin (il′ĕ-tin) trademark for preparations of insulin. **Lente I.,** trademark for preparations of insulin zinc suspension. **NPH I.,** trademark for preparations of insulin isophane suspension. **protamine, zinc & I.,** trademark for preparations of protamine zinc insulin suspension. **regular I.,** trademark for preparations of insulin injection (regular insulin). **Semilente I.,** trademark for preparations of prompt insulin zinc suspension. **Ultralente I.,** trademark for preparations of extended zinc insulin suspension.

ileum (il′e-um) [L.] [NA] the distal portion of the small intestine, extending from the jejunum to the cecum; called also *intestinum ileum.* **duplex i.,** congenital duplication of the ileum.

ileus (il′e-us) [L.; Gr. *eileos,* from *eilein* to roll up] obstruction of the intestines. **adynamic i.,** ileus resulting from inhibition of bowel motility, which may be produced by numerous causes, most frequently by peritonitis. **dynamic i., hyperdynamic i.,** spastic i. **mechanical i.,** ileus due to mechanical causes, such as hernia, adhesions, volvulus, etc. **meconium i.,** ileus in the newborn due to blocking of the bowel with thick meconium; a manifestation of fibrocystic disease (mucoviscidosis). **occlusive i.,** mechanical i. **paralytic i., i. paralyt′icus,** adynamic i. **spastic i.,** ileus due to persistent contracture of a bowel segment; see *Ogilvie's syndrome,* under *syndrome.* **i. subpar′ta,** ileus due to pressure of the gravid uterus on the pelvic colon.

Ilex (i′leks) a genus of aquifoliaceous shrubs and tree, including the hollies. **I. verticillata.** (L.) Gray (*Prinos verticillatus*), the black alder, or winterberry, has a tonic and astringent bark.

ilia (il′e-ah) [L.] plural of *ilium.*

iliac (il′e-ak) [L. *iliacus*] pertaining to the ilium.

iliadelphus (il″e-ah-del′fus) iliopagus.

ilicin (il′ĭ-sin) a bitter antiperiodic compound derived from holly, *Ilex aquifolium*.

Ilidar (il′ĭ-dar) trademark for a preparation of azapetine phosphate.

ili(o)- [L. *ilium*] a combining form denoting relationship to the ilium or iliac region.

iliococcygeal (il″e-o-kok-sij′e-al) pertaining to the ilium and coccyx.

iliocostal (il″e-o-kos′tal) [*ilio-* + L. *costa* rib] connecting or pertaining to the ilium and ribs.

iliofemoral (il″e-o-fem′or-al) pertaining to the ilium and femur.

iliohypogastric (il″e-o-hi″po-gas′trik) pertaining to the ilium and hypogastrium.

ilioinguinal (il″e-o-in′gwĭ-nal) pertaining to the iliac and inguinal regions.

iliolumbar (il″e-o-lum′ber) pertaining to the iliac and lumbar regions, or to the flank and loin.

iliolumbocostoabdominal (il″e-o-lum″bo-kos″to-ab-dom′ĭ-nal) pertaining to the iliac, lumbar, costal, and abdominal regions.

iliometer (il″e-om′ĕ-ter) [*iliac* spines + Gr. *metron* measure] an instrument for determining the relative heights of the iliac spines and their relative distance from the center of the spinal column.

iliopagus (il″e-op′ah-gus) [*ilio-* + Gr. *pagos* thing fixed] symmetrical conjoined twins united in the iliac region.

iliopectineal (il″e-o-pek-tin′e-al) pertaining to the ilium and pubes.

iliopelvic (il″e-o-pel′vik) pertaining to the iliac region or muscle and to the pelvis.

iliopsoas (il″e-o-so′as) see Table of *Musculi*.

iliopubic (il″e-o-pu′bik) iliopectineal.

iliosacral (il″e-o-sa′kral) pertaining to the ilium and the sacrum.

iliosciatic (il″e-o-si-at′ik) pertaining to the ilium and the ischium.

iliospinal (il″e-o-spi′nal) pertaining to the ilium and the spinal column.

iliothoracopagus (il″e-o-tho″rah-kop′ah-gus) [*ilium* + Gr. *thōrax* chest + *pagos* thing fixed] symmetrical conjoined twins fused from the pelvis to the thorax.

iliotibial (il″e-o-tib′e-al) pertaining to or extending between the ilium and tibia.

iliotrochanteric (il″e-o-tro-kan-ter′ik) pertaining to the ilium and a trochanter.

ilioxiphopagus (il″e-o-zi-fop′ah-gus) symmetrical conjoined twins fused from the pelvis to the xiphoid process.

ilium (il′e-um), pl. *il′ia* [L.] NA alternative for *os ilii*. See illustration accompanying *skeleton*. The expansive superior portion of the hip bone (os coxae); it is a separate bone in early life. See illustration accompanying *skeleton*. Called also *os ilii* [NA].

ill (il) 1. not well; sick. 2. a disease or disorder. **föhn i.,** the headache, weariness, and depression reported to be felt when the föhn (a special wind from the south in Central Europe) blows. **joint i.,** navel i. **leg i.,** foot rot; see under *rot*. **louping i.,** encephalomyelitis primarily affecting sheep in Great Britain and Ireland, caused by a virus which is transmitted by the tick, *Ixodes ricinus*. **navel i.,** generalized septicemia affecting foals, lambs, and calves, usually characterized by omphalophlebitis and the formation of abscesses in the joints resulting in polyarthritis; it is due to infection through the open navel by various organisms, including species of *Staphylococcus*, *Streptococcus*, *Shigella*, *Escherichia*, and *Pasteurella*, and has a high mortality rate. Called also *joint i.* **quarter i.,** blackleg. **thorter i.,** gid.

illacrimation (il″ak-rĭ-ma′shun) epiphora.

illaqueation (il″ak-we-a′shun) [L. *illaqueare* to ensnare] the cure of an ingrowing eyelash by drawing it out with a loop.

Illicium (il-is′e-um) [L.] a genus of magnoliaceous trees and shrubs whose fruit, Chinese anise, is the source of anise oil. The leaves of *I. religiosum*, or sikimi, are the source of sikimin.

illinition (il-ĭ-nish′un) [L. *illinire* to smear] the application of an ointment or liniment with rubbing.

illinium (il-lin′e-um) [University of *Illinois*] former name of the element *promethium*.

illness (il′ness) a condition marked by pronounced deviation from the normal healthy state; sickness. **compressed-air i.,** decompression sickness. **emotional i.,** a colloquialism roughly equivalent to "mental disorder," but not usually applied to organic mental disorders or mental retardation. **high-altitude i.,** see under *sickness*. **manic-depressive i.,** bipolar disorder. **mental i.,** see under *disorder*. **psychosomatic i.,** see under *disorder*. **radiation i.,** see under *sickness*.

illumination (ĭ-lu″mĭ-na′shun) [L. *illuminatio*] the lighting up of a part, cavity, organ, or object for inspection. **axial i.,** the transmission or reflection of light along the axis of a microscope. **central i.,** axial i. **contact i.,** illumination of the eye by means of an instrument which is pressed directly to the cornea and conjunctiva. **critical i.,** the focusing of light precisely upon an object inspected. **dark-field i., dark-ground i.,** the throwing of peripheral rays of light upon a microscopical object from the side, the center rays being blocked out: the object appears bright upon a dark background. See under *microscope*, and see *ultramicroscope*. **direct i.,** the throwing of light upon a microscopical object from above or from the direction of observation. **focal i.,** 1. the throwing of light upon the focus of a lens or mirror. 2. illumination of an object by focusing a source of light on it through an optical system. **Köhler i.,** an improved method of illumination by adjustment of the substage Abbe condenser, for obtaining the best image detail in microscopical work. **lateral i., oblique i.,** illumination in which the object is illuminated by oblique light. **through i.,** the tranmission of light through an object, or from the direction opposite to that of observation.

illuminator (ĭ-lu″mĭ-na′tor) the source of light for viewing an object. **Abbe's i.,** see under *condenser*.

illuminism (ĭ-lu′min-izm) a hallucinatory state characterized by conversations with supernatural beings.

illusion (ĭ-lu′zhun) [L. *illusio*] a false or misinterpreted sensory impression; a false interpretation of a real sensory image. Cf. *delusion*.

illusional (ĭ-lu′zhun-al) pertaining to or characterized by illusions.

illutation (il″u-ta′shun) [L. *in* in + *lutum* mud] treatment by mud baths.

Ilopan (il′o-pan) trademark for a preparation of dexpanthenol.

Ilosone (il′o-sōn) trademark for a preparation of erythromycin estolate.

Ilotycin (i″lo-ti′sin) trademark for preparations of erythromycin.

Ilozyme (il′o-zīm) trademark for a preparation of pancrelipase.

I.M. intramuscularly (by intramuscular injection).

im- 1. see *in-*. 2. a prefix in chemical names indicating the bivalent group =NH.

ima (i′mah) [L.] lowest.

imafen hydrochloride (im′ah-fen) chemical name: 2,3,5,6-tetrahydro-5-phenyl-1*H*-imidazo[1,2-*a*]imidazole monohydrochloride; an antidepressant, $C_{11}H_{13}N_3 \cdot HCl$.

image (im′ij) [L. *imago*] a picture or conception with more or less likeness to an objective reality. See also *imaging*. **accidental i.,** afterimage. **body i.,** a three-dimensional concept of one's self, recorded in the cortex by the perception of ever-changing postures of the body and constantly changing with them. **direct i., erect i.,** virtual i. **eidetic i.,** an unusually vivid, elaborate, and exact mental image of objects previously seen or imagined. **false i.,** the one formed by the deviating eye in strabismus. **heteronymous i.,** the two images seen when the eyes are focused on a point beyond the object; cf. *crossed diplopia*. **homonymous i.,** the two images seen when the eyes are focused on a point nearer than the object; cf. *direct diplopia*. **incidental i.,** the impression of an image which remains on the retina after the object has been removed. **inverted i.,** real i. **memory i.,** a sensation or sense perception as it is pictured in the memory. **mental i.,** any concept corresponding to an object appreciated by the senses. **mirror**

i., 1. the image of light made visible by the reflecting surface of the cornea and lens when illuminated through the slit lamp. 2. an identical reproduction of an object except for transposition of right and left relations, as appears in the reflection of an object in a mirror. **motor i.,** the organized cerebral model of the possible movements of the body. **negative i.,** after-image. **optical i.,** one formed by the reflection of refraction of rays of light. **Purkinje-Sanson mirror i's,** reflected images formed on the anterior surface of the cornea and the anterior and posterior surfaces of the crystalline lens. The images on the two anterior surfaces are virtual and noninverted, and the image on the posterior surface is real and inverted. Useful in the study of the movement of the lens surfaces in accommodation and, formerly, in the evaluation of cataract. **radioisotope i.,** a quasi-pictorial representation of the distribution of radioactive materials in the body. **real i.,** one formed where the emanating rays are collected, in which the object is pictured as being inverted. **retinal i.,** the representation formed upon the retina of an object seen. **Sanson's i's,** Purkinje i's. **sensory i.,** a representation formed by means of one or more of the sense organs. **specular i.,** mirror i., def. 1. **virtual i.,** a picture from projected light rays that are intercepted before focusing, as by a plane mirror; it cannot be received on a screen, and it has the same orientation as the object. Called also *direct* or *erect i.*

imagines (ĭ-maj'ĭ-nēz) [L.] plural of *imago*.

imaging (im'ah-jing) the production of clarity, contrast, and detail in images, especially in radiological and ultrasound images. **electrostatic i.,** a method of visualizing deep structures of the body, in which an electron beam, rather than x-rays, is passed through the patient and the emerging beam (unabsorbed electrons) strikes an electrostatically charged vacuum-packed plate, dissipating the charge according to the strength of the beam. A record (e.g., a film) is then made from the plate. **magnetic resonance i. (MRI),** a method of visualizing soft tissues of the body by applying an external magnetic field that makes it possible to distinguish between hydrogen atoms in different environments; cf. *nuclear magnetic resonance,* under *resonance.*

imago (ĭ-ma'go), pl. *ima'goes,* or *imag'ines* [L.] 1. the final or adult stage of an insect. Cf. *larva, pupa.* 2. in psychoanalysis, an idealized, unconscious mental image of a key person in one's early life.

imagocide (ĭ-ma'go-sīd) [*imago* + L. *caedere* to kill] an agent that destroys adult insects, especially adult mosquitoes.

imapunga (im-ah-pung'ah) a disease occurring to a limited extent among African cattle; closely related in pathology to African horse sickness.

imbalance (im-bal'ans) [*im-* + L. *bilanx* a balance with two pans] inability to stand upright; lack of balance between muscles. **autonomic i.,** autonomic ataxia; any disturbance of the autonomic nervous system. **binocular i.,** inequality in some aspect of binocular vision, such as aniseikonia, anisometropia, heterophoria, or strabismus. **sympathetic i.,** vagotonia. **vasomotor i.,** autonomic i.

imbecile (im'bĕ-sil) [L. *imbecillus* weak, feeble] (*obs.*) a person with the intermediate grade of feeblemindedness (q.v.), equivalent to the modern classifications "moderate" and "severe mental retardation."

imbecility (im'bĕ-sil'ĭ-te) [L. *imbecillitas*] the condition of being an imbecile; moderate or severe mental retardation. **moral i.,** see under *insanity.* **phenylpyruvic i.,** an obsolete term for the mental retardation due to untreated phenylketonuria.

imbed (im-bed') embed; see *embedding.*

imbibition (im'bĭ-bish'un) [L. *imbibere* to drink] 1. the absorption of a liquid. 2. insudation. **hemoglobin i.,** absorption by the tissue of free hemoglobin.

imbricated (im'brĭ-kāt''ed) [L. *imbricatus; imbrex* tile] overlapping like tiles or shingles.

imbrication (im'brĭ-ka'shun) the overlapping of apposing surfaces, like shingles on a roof.

ImD$_{50}$ the immunizing dose of vaccine or antigen sufficient to protect 50% of the animals in a particular test group.

Imerslund-Graesbeck syndrome (e'mer-slund grās'bek) [Olga *Imerslund,* 20th century Scandinavian physician; Ralph *Graesbeck,* Finnish biochemist, born 1930] familial megaloblastic anemia.

Imhoff tank (im'hof) [Karl *Imhoff,* German engineer, 1876–1965] digestion tank; see under *tank.*

imidamine (im''id-am'in) antazoline.

imidazole (im''id-az'ōl) a base, found combined with alanine in histidine.

$$\begin{array}{c} HC-N \\ \parallel \quad H \!\!>\!\! CH \\ HC-N \end{array}$$

imidazolylethylamine (im''id-az''o-lil-eth''il-am'in) histamine.

imide (im'id) any compound containing the bivalent group, $=NH$, to which are attached only acid radicals.

imido- (ĭ-me'do) a prefix denoting the presence in a compound of the bivalent group $=NH$ attached to two acid radicals.

imidocarb hydrochloride (ĭ-mid'o-karb) chemical name: N,N'-bis[3-(4,5-dihydro-1H-imidazol-2-yl)phenyl] urea dihydrochloride; an antiprotozoal effective against *Babesia,* $C_{19}H_{20}N_6O \cdot 2HCl.$

imidogen (ĭ-me'do-jen) the bivalent radical $=NH.$

iminazole (im''in-az'ōl) imidazole.

imino- (ĭ-me'no) a prefix used to denote the presence of the bivalent group $>NH$ attached to nonacid radicals.

iminoglycinuria (ĭ-me''no-gli''sin-u're-ah) a benign hereditary disorder of renal tubular reabsorption of glycine and imino acids (proline and hydroxyproline), marked by excessive levels of all three substances in the urine.

iminourea (ĭ-me''no-u-re'ah) guanidine.

imipramine hydrochloride (ĭ-mip'rah-mēn) [USP] chemical name: 10,11-dihydro-N,N-dimethyl-5H-dibenz[b,f]azepine-5-propanamine monohydrochloride. A tricyclic antidepressant, $C_{19}H_{24}N_2 \cdot HCl,$ occurring as a white to off-white, crystalline powder; used especially in the treatment of endogenous depression and in childhood enuresis, administered orally.

Imlach's fat plug (im'laks) [Francis *Imlach,* Scottish physician, 1819–1891] see under *plug.*

immature (im''ah-tūr') [L. *in* not + *maturus* mature] unripe or not fully developed.

immediate (ĭ-me'de-it) [L. *in* not + *mediatus* mediate] direct; with nothing intervening; occurring without delay.

immedicable (ĭ-med'ĭ-kah-b'l) beyond the hope of cure.

immersion (ĭ-mer'shun) [L. *immersio*] 1. the placing or plunging of a body into a liquid. 2. the use of the microscope with the object and object glass both covered with a liquid. **homogeneous i.,** the employment in microscopy of a liquid of nearly the same refractive power as the cover glass. **oil i.,** the covering of the microscopical objective and the object with oil. **water i.,** the covering of the microscopical objective and the object with water.

immiscible (ĭ-mis'ĭ-b'l) not susceptible to being mixed.

immobility (im''mo-bil'ĭ-te) 1. the state of being immovable. 2. chronic hydrocephalus of cattle.

immobilization (im-mo''bil-i-za'shun) the act of rendering immovable, as by a cast or splint.

immobilize (im-mo'bil-īz) [L. *in* not + *mobilis* movable] to render incapable of being moved, as by a cast or splint.

immune (ĭ-mūn') [L. *immunis* free, exempt] 1. protected against infectious disease by either specific or nonspecific mechanisms. 2. pertaining to the immune system and immune responses.

immunifacient (ĭ-mu''nĭ-fa'shent) (*obs.*) producing immunity; said of diseases, such as diphtheria and typhoid, which for a time after infection produce immunity against themselves.

immunifaction (ĭ-mu''nĭ-fak'shun) (*obs.*) immunization.

immunity (ĭ-mu'nĭ-te) [L. *immunitas*] the condition of being immune; the protection against infectious disease conferred either by the immune response generated by immunization or previous infection or by other nonimmunologic factors (*innate i.*). **acquired i.,** immunity involving the functioning of the immune system acquired by natural infection or vaccination (active immunity) or transfer of antibody or lymphocytes from an immune donor (passive immunity). Cf. *innate i.* **active i.,** acquired immunity attributable to the presence of antibody or of immune lymphoid cells formed in response to antigenic stimulus. **adoptive**

i., passive immunity of the cell-mediated type conferred by the administration of sensitized lymphocytes from an immune donor. **antibacterial i.,** immunity against the action of bacteria, i.e., the ability to resist infection by bacteria. **antitoxic i.,** immunity against toxins, attributable to the presence of specific antitoxin(s) in the immune individual. **antiviral i.,** immunity against viruses. **artificial i.,** acquired (active or passive) immunity produced by deliberate exposure to an antigen, as in vaccination. **cell-mediated i. (CMI) cellular i.,** immunity mediated by T lymphocytes either through release of lymphokines or through exertion of direct cytotoxicity, transmissible by transfer of lymphocytes but not serum; it comprises delayed hypersensitivity reactions, systemic response to viral and microbial infections, contact dermatitis, granulomatous reactions, allograft rejection, and graft-versus-host reactions. Called also *T cell–mediated i.* Cf. *humoral i.* **community i.,** herd i. **concomitant i.,** infection i. **cross i.,** immunity produced by inoculation with an agent (e.g., a bacterium or virus) that is different from, but closely related to, the agent causing the disease. **familial i.,** genetic i. **genetic i.,** innate i. **herd i.,** the resistance of a group to attack by a disease because of the immunity of a large proportion of the members and the consequent lessening of the likelihood of an affected individual coming into contact with a susceptible individual. **humoral i.,** immunity mediated by antibodies. Cf. *cell-mediated i.* **infection i.,** the development of resistance to reinfection even though the original infection persists, an apparent paradox. Called also *concomitant i.* **inherent i.,** innate i. **inherited i.,** innate i. **innate i.,** immunity based on the genetic constitution of the individual, e.g., immunity of man to canine distemper. Called also *familial i., genetic i., inherent i., inherited i.,* and *native i.* **intrauterine i.,** passive immunity acquired by the fetus as a consequence of the passage of maternal IgG antibodies from an immune mother through the placenta into the fetal circulation. **local i.,** immunity confined to a particular tissue or organ. **maternal i.,** passively transferred humoral immunity from the mother to the offspring, across the placenta before birth in primates, from the colostrum via the intestines in ungulates, and from the egg yolk in birds. **native i.,** innate i. **natural i.,** immunity mediated by cells capable of immune activity without being stimulated by immunization and without antigen specificity, e.g., the activity of NK cells against virus infection and tumor cells. **nonspecific i.,** immunity that does not involve the recognition of antigen by lymphocytes and the mounting of a specific immune response; e.g., the protection afforded by lysozyme, interferon, the cells involved in natural immunity, and anatomical barriers to infection. **passive i.,** immunity acquired by transfer of antibody or lymphocytes from an immune donor. **species i.,** resistance of members of a particular species to a disease; immunity enjoyed by members of a particular species and determined by their genetic constitution. **specific i.,** immunity against a particular disease, e.g., scarlet fever, or against a particular antigen. **T cell–mediated i. (TCMI),** cell-mediated i. **tissue i.,** local i.

immunization (im″u-ni-za′shun) the induction of immunity; see *active i.* and *passive i.* **active i.,** stimulation of the immune system to confer protection against disease, e.g., by administration of a vaccine or toxoid. **passive i.,** the conferring of specific immune reactivity on previously nonimmune individuals by the administration of sensitized lymphoid cells or serum from immune individuals.

immunize (im′u-nīz) to render immune.

immunoadjuvant (im″u-no-aj′ĕ-vent) a nonspecific stimulator of the immune response, e.g., BCG vaccine or Freund's complete and incomplete adjuvants.

immunoadsorbent (im″u-no-ad-sor′bent) a preparation of antigen or antibody in an insoluble form used to bind homologous antibody or antigen, respectively, and remove it from a mixture of substances.

immunoadsorption (im″u-no-ad-sorp′shun) the use of an immunoadsorbent to effect a chemical separation of antigen or antibody, as in immunoassays or in affinity chromatography.

immunoassay (im″u-no-as′a) any of several methods for the quantitative determination of chemical substances that utilize the highly specific binding between an antigen or hapten and homologous antibodies, including radioimmunoassay, enzyme immunoassay, and fluoroimmunoassay.

enzyme i., any of several immunoassay methods that use an enzyme covalently linked to an antigen or antibody as a label, the two most common being ELISA (enzyme-linked immunosorbent assay) and EMIT (enzyme multiplied immunoassay technique). Abbreviated EIA.

immunobiology (im″u-no-bi-ol′o-je) that branch of biology dealing with immunologic effects on such phenomena as infectious disease, growth and development, recognition phenomena, hypersensitivity, heredity, aging, cancer, and transplantation.

immunoblast (im″u-no-blast′) lymphoblast.

immunoblastic (im″u-no-blas′tik) pertaining to or involving immunoblasts (lymphoblasts).

immunochemical (im″u-no-kem′ĭ-kal) pertaining to immunochemistry.

immunochemistry (im″u-no-kem′is-tre) 1. the study of the chemical basis of immunological phenomena. 2. the application of antibodies as chemical reagents.

immunochemotherapy (im″u-no-ke″mo-ther′ah-pe) a combination of immunotherapy and chemotherapy.

immunocompetence (im″u-no-kom′pĕ-tens) the ability or capacity to develop an immune response (i.e., antibody production and/or cell-mediated immunity) following exposure to antigen; called also *immunologic competence.*

immunocompetent (im″u-no-kom′pĕ-tent) exhibiting immunocompetence.

immunocomplex (im″u-no-kom′pleks) immune complex.

immunocompromised (im″u-no-kom′pro-mīzd) having the immune response attenuated by administration of immunosuppressive drugs, by irradiation, by malnutrition, or by some disease processes (e.g., cancer).

immunoconglutinin (im″u-no-kon-gloo′tĭ-nin) an autoantibody, usually of the immunoglobulin M class, that is specific for activated C3 and C4 components of complement. It is found in low titer in most normal sera and in increased levels in certain infectious diseases, in autoimmune disease, and after immunization with many antigens. Not to be confused with *conglutinin.* Called also *immune conglutinin.*

immunocyte (im″u-no-sīt′) a cell of the lymphoid series which can react with antigen to produce antibody or to become active in cell-mediated immunity or delayed hypersensitivity reactions; called also *immunologically competent cell.*

immunocytoadherence (im″u-no-si″to-ad-hēr′ens) the formation of rosettes by the binding of red cells bearing a homologous antigen to lymphocytes bearing surface immunoglobulin (B cells); used to identify B cells.

immunocytochemistry (im″u-no-si″to-kem′is-tre) the application of immunochemical techniques, e.g., immunoperoxidase staining, to cytochemistry.

immunodeficiency (im″u-no-dĕ-fish′en-se) a deficiency of immune response or a disorder characterized by deficient immune response; classified as antibody (B cell), cellular (T cell), combined deficiency, or phagocytic dysfunction disorders (see accompanying table). *Antibody immunodeficiencies* are marked by hypo- or dysgammaglobulinemia and recurrent bacterial otitis media and sinopulmonary infections, while *cellular immunodeficiencies* are marked by recurrent infections with low-grade or opportunistic pathogens, by graft-versus-host reactions following blood transfusions, and by severe disease following immunization with live vaccines. *Phagocytic dysfunction disorders* may be extrinsic (e.g., suppression of the number of phagocytes by immunosuppressive agents, or dysfunction caused by corticosteroids) or intrinsic (related to enzyme deficiencies); they are marked by bacterial or, sometimes, fungal infections, which range from mild recurrent skin infection to fatal systemic infection. See also *acquired immune deficiency syndrome,* under *syndrome.* **combined i.,** deficiency of lymphoid cells that mediate both antibody (B-lymphocytes) and cellular (T-lymphocytes) immunity. **common variable i., common variable unclassifiable i.,** a heterogeneous group of disorders characterized by hypogammaglobulinemia, decreased antibody production in response to antigenic challenge, and recurrent pyogenic infections, and often associated with hematologic and autoimmune disorders. Most patients have normal numbers of circulating B cells but lack plasma cells, and are thus thought to have an intrinsic defect of B cell differentiation. Many also have T cell defects and exhibit cutaneous energy to recall antigens. Called also *acquired,* or *common*

PRIMARY IMMUNODEFICIENCY DISORDERS, DISEASES AND SYNDROMES

Antibody (B Cell) Deficiency Disorders
  X-linked infantile agammaglobulinemia (Bruton's disease)
  Common, variable, unclassifiable immunodeficiency
  Transient hypogammaglobulinemia of infancy
  Selective IgA deficiency
  Immunodeficiency with hyper-IgM
  Selective IgM deficiency
  Selective deficiency of IgG subclasses
  Kappa light chain deficiency
  Secretory component deficiency
  Specific antibody deficiency with normal immunoglobulins
  X-linked lymphoproliferative syndrome (Duncan's syndrome)
Cellular (T Cell) Deficiency Disorders
  Thymic hypoplasia (DiGeorge syndrome)
  Chronic mucocutaneous candidiasis
  Cellular immunodeficiency with purine nucleoside phosphorylase deficiency
  Acquired immunodeficiency syndrome (AIDS)
Combined (B Cell and T Cell) Deficiency Disorders
  Severe combined immunodeficiency (SCID)
    Autosomal recessive SCID
    SCID with adenosine deaminase deficiency
    X-linked recessive SCID
    Reticular dysgenesis

Cellular immunodeficiency with immunoglobulins (Nezlof syndrome)
Immunodeficiency with thrombocytopenia and eczema (Wiskott-Aldrich syndrome)
Ataxia-telangiectasia
Immunodeficiency with short-limbed dwarfism
Immunodeficiency with thymoma
Transcobalamin II deficiency
Episodic lymphopenia with lymphotoxin
Phagocytic Dysfunction Disorders
  Chédiak-Higashi syndrome
  Chronic granulomatous disease
  Job syndrome
  Lazy leukocyte syndrome
  Deficiency disorders
    Alkaline phosphatase deficiency
    Glucose-6-phosphate dehydrogenase deficiency
    Myeloperoxidase deficiency
    Tuftsin deficiency
  Elevated IgE with defective chemotaxis, eczema, and recurrent infection
  Leukocyte movement disorders

variable, agammaglobulinemia or *hypogammaglobulinemia*. **i. with hyper-IgM,** a rare syndrome characterized by elevated immunoglobulin M levels and decreased levels of G and A immunoglobulins, associated with recurrent pyogenic infections, and possibly caused by failure of IgM-producing cells to switch to production of IgC and IgA. Most cases appear to exhibit X-linked recessive inheritance. Called also *i. with elevated* (or *increased*) *IgM*. **severe combined i., (SCID),** a group of rare congenital disorders characterized by gross impairment of both humoral and cell-mediated immunity manifested by lack of antibody formation in response to antigenic challenge, absence of delayed hypersensitivity, and inability to reject transplants of foreign tissue. In most cases all classes of immunoglobulins are nearly or completely absent, and there is marked lymphocytopenia. Blood transfusions can result in graft-versus-host (GVH) disease and routine vaccinations in fatal infection. Unless immune function is restored by a histocompatible bone marrow or fetal tissue transplant or the patient is kept in gnotobiotic isolation, death from opportunistic infection usually occurs before the first birthday. Four major forms are distinguished. *Swiss-type agammaglobulinemia,* the first form to be described (1958), is marked by nearly complete absence of lymphocytes and immunoglobulin and by autosomal recessive inheritance. One form is associated with a specific metabolic defect, adenosine deaminase (ADA) deficiency (see *adenosine deaminase*). In another form B cells are present at normal levels but antibody response is absent owing to lack of T cells; and the pattern of inheritance may be either autosomal recessive or X-linked. The last form, *reticular dysgenesis,* is due to a hematopoietic stem cell defect that results in absence of granulocytes and macrophages as well as lymphocytes. Formerly called *leukopenic agammaglobulinemia* and *thymic alymphoplasia.* **i. with short-limbed dwarfism,** short-limbed dwarfism marked by short, pudgy hands, redundant skin, and hyperextensible joints of the hands and feet associated with immunodeficiency, which may be either antibody or cellular or combined. **i. with thymoma,** an immunodeficiency disorder in which thymoma, usually of the benign spindle-cell type, is associated with hypogammaglobulinemia; deficiencies of cell-mediated immunity, such as eosinopenia, hypoplastic or aplastic anemia, or autoimmune diseases, may occur also. Removal of the thymoma does not cure the immunodeficiency, and patients suffer from recurrent severe infections.

immunodepression (im″u-no-dĕ-presh′un) immunosuppression.

immunodepressive (im″u-no-dĕ-pres′iv) immunosuppressive.

immunodermatology (im″u-no-der″mah-tol′o-je) the study of immunologic phenomena as they affect skin disorders and their treatment or prophylaxis.

immunodeviation (im″u-no-de″ve-a′shun) split tolerance, def. 2.

immunodiagnosis (im″u-no-di″ag-no′sis) diagnosis based on blood serum reactions to antigens; serodiagnosis.

immunodiffusion (im″u-no-dĭ-fu′zhun) any technique involving diffusion of antigen or antibody through a semisolid medium, usually agar or agarose gel, resulting in a precipitin reaction. Precipitin lines or bands form where the concentration of an antigen and antibody are serologically equivalent. **radial i. (RID),** single radial diffusion.

immunodominance (im″u-no-dom′ĭ-nans) the degree to which a subunit of an antigenic determinant is involved in binding or reacting with specific antibody.

immunodominant (im″u-no-dom′ĭ-nant) denoting the subunits of the antigenic determinant group that most influence the specificity of the induced antibodies.

immunoelectrophoresis (ĭ-mu″no-e-lek″tro-fo-re′sis) a technique combining protein electrophoresis and double immunodiffusion; proteins are separated by agarose gel electrophoresis; then specific antisera are placed in a trough cut parallel to the protein track, and the proteins and antibodies are allowed to diffuse through the gel, the proteins diffusing radially from their electrophoretic placement and the antibodies diffusing perpendicularly from the trough, resulting in a distinct elliptical precipitin arc for each protein detectable by the antisera. Abbreviated IEP. **counter i.,** counterimmunoelectrophoresis. **countercurrent i.,** counterimmunoelectrophoresis. **crossed i.,** a combination of protein electrophoresis and rocket immunoelectrophoresis; protein antigens are separated by agarose gel electrophoresis; then a strip containing the separated antigens is cut out and placed in a trough in a gel containing antiserum, and an electric field perpendicular to the trough is applied, producing a "rocket" precipitin pattern for each antigen. **rocket i.,** one-dimensional single electroimmunodiffusion; a technique in which antigen is placed in a row of wells in an agar plate containing antiserum and an electric field perpendicular to the line of wells is applied; this drives the antigen through the gel, forming a spike or "rocket" precipitin pattern trailing away from each well. The length of the rocket is proportional to the amount of antigen placed in the well. Called also *Laurell technique.*

immunoferritin (im″u-no-fer′ĭ-tin) an antibody labeled with ferritin; when combined with antigen, the antigenic determinant sites are visible under the electron microscope.

immunofiltration (im″u-no-fil-tra′shun) the purification of antigen or antibody using an immunoadsorbent.

immunofluorescence (im″u-no-floo″o-res′ens) any immunohistochemical method using antibody labeled with a fluorescent dye; called *direct* if a specific antibody or antiserum is conjugated with a fluorochrome and used as a specific fluorescent stain and *indirect* if the fluorochrome is attached to an antiglobulin, and a tissue constituent is stained using

THE HUMAN IMMUNOGLOBULINS

| | Polypeptide Chains | | | | | | | | |
| | H Chains | | | | | L Chains | | Other | |
Immunoglobulin classes	μ IgM	γ IgG	α IgA	δ IgD	ϵ IgE	κ all	λ all	J IgM, IgA	SC* IgA
Subclasses or subtypes	1,2	1–4	1,2	—	—		1–4		
Allotypes	—	Gm(1)–(25)	Am(1)–(2)	—	—	Km(1)–(3)	—		
Mol. wt. (thousands)	70	50	55	62	70	23	23	15	70
Carbohydrate (%)	15	4	10	18	18			8	16

| | Immunoglobulins | | | | | |
| | Serum | | | | | Secretory |
	IgM $(\mu_2L_2)_5$J	IgG γ_2L_2	IgA α_2L_2 or $(\alpha_2L_2)_n$J†	IgD δ_2L_2	IgE ϵ_2L_2	IgA $(\alpha_2L_2)_2$J, SC
Molecular formula						
Mol. wt. (thousands)	900	150	155,325,580	180	190	400
Sedimentation coefficient (S)	19	7	7,10,14	7	8	—
Electrophoretic mobility	fast γ to β	γ	fast γ to β	fast γ	fast γ	—
Serum concentration (mg/dl)	25–200	700–1500	40–350	1–40	<0.06	—
Serum half-life (days)	5	23	6	3	2	—

*Secretory component
†n = 2 or 3

an unlabeled specific antibody and the labeled antiglobulin, which binds the unlabeled antibody.

immunogen (im'u-no-jen) a substance capable of inducing an immune response, in most contexts synonymous with antigen; in some contexts immunogen is used to draw a distinction with substances capable of reacting only with antibody (antigens or haptens) or to denote a form of an antigen that induces an immune response as opposed to a tolerogen, a form that induces tolerance.

immunogenetic (ĭ-mu''no-jĕ-net'ik) pertaining to immunogenetics.

immunogenetics (im''u-no-jĕ-net'iks) [immuno- + genetics] the study of the genetics of the immune response, e.g., the study of immune response genes, or the association of HLA antigens with disease susceptibility, or the generation of antibody diversity.

immunogenic (im''u-no-jen'ik) producing immunity; evoking an immune response.

immunogenicity (im''u-no-jĕ-nis'ĭ-te) the property that endows a substance with the capacity to provoke an immune response, or the degree to which a substance possesses this property.

immunoglobulin (im''u-no-glob'u-lin) any of the structurally related glycoproteins that function as antibodies (μB cell antigen receptors; divided into five classes (IgM, IgG, IgA, IgD, and IgE) on the basis of structure and biologic activity. The basic structural unit of the immunoglobulin molecule, referred to as a monomer, is a Y-shaped molecule composed of two heavy (H) chains and two light (L) chains (see accompanying illustration). IgD, IgG, and IgE occur only as monomers; IgM and IgA may occur as monomers or polymers. The polymeric forms contain an additional polypeptide called the J chain, and secretory IgA contains another structure called the secretory component (SC). Each chain consists of a variable region (V_H or V_L) and a constant region (C_H or C_L), which are coded for by different genes. Parts of the V_H and V_L regions make up the antigen-binding site, one on each "arm" (Fab region) of the monomer. An individual can make about 10^4 different V_H regions and 10^3 V_L regions, which combine to make about 10^7 different antigen-binding sites, each with a distinct antigenic specificity. Parts of the C_H regions make up the "body" (Fc region) of the monomer, which contains various sites responsible for the biological activity of the molecule. In any one immunoglobulin molecule, all of the H chains are identical, as are the L chains. The C_H region determines both the heavy chain class to which the H chain belongs and the immunoglobulin class to which the molecule belongs. The H chain classes are denoted by the Greek letters (μ, δ, γ, ϵ, and α) corresponding to the Latin letters of the immunoglobulin classes, e.g., μ to IgM. There are two types of light chains (denoted κ and λ) either of which may combine with any of the heavy chains and thus occur in any of the immunoglobulin classes. In human immunoglobulins, three of the classes (IgM, IgG, and IgA) have subclasses; i.e., there are several similar but distinct C_H region genes in these classes. In addition, the λ light chain type has subtypes. The subclasses (subtypes) are denoted by numerical suffixes,

e.g., IgG1 and γ1 subclasses and λ2 subtype. Immunoglobulins (monomeric IgM and IgD) first appear on the surface of B cells as antigen receptors. When a cell is activated by contact with antigen and differentiates into a plasma cell, the cell continues to produce the same L chain and V_H region of the H chain, but gene rearrangement may occur to attach this V_H region to a different C_H region (class switching). Thus the secreted immunoglobulin may be of any class but has the same antigenic specificity as the antigen receptors of the parent B cell. In addition to the effects produced solely by the binding of antigen by antibody, e.g., viral neutralization or the inability of some bacteria to invade mucosal surfaces when coated by antibody, certain classes of antibodies can trigger other processes when bound to antigen: IgM and IgG activate the classic complement pathway, IgA and IgG activate the alternative pathway, and IgM, IgG1, and IgG3 act as opsonins, triggering phagocytosis of the bound antigens by macrophages and neutrophils. IgE has the unique function of mediating immediate hypersensitivity (q.v.) reactions; it binds to specific receptors on basophils and mast cells and triggers the release of mediators on contact with antigen. IgG is the only class transferred across the placenta, providing the fetus and neonate with protection against infection. See also *immunoglobulin genes*, under *gene*, *homology region*, under *region*, and *allotype*, *idiotype*, and *isotype*. **monoclonal i.**, see *M component*. **secretory i. A**, secretory IgA; the predominant immunoglobulin in secretions (oral, nasal, bronchial, urogenital, and intestinal mucous secretions and tears, saliva, and milk), a dimer containing the J chain and the secretory component (SC). **thyroid-binding inhibitory i's (TBII)**, see *thyroid-stimulating i*. **thyroid-stimulating i's (TSI)**, circulating IgG antibodies with the ability to mimic TSH (thyroid-stimulating hormone, thyrotropin) by binding to the TSH receptor of thyroid cells and activating adenylate cyclase, thus causing an increase in the level of the intracellular second messenger cyclic AMP, which results in the release of thyroid hormones; thought to be responsible for most cases of Graves' disease. Called also *human thyroid adenylate cyclase stimulators* (HTACS). Formerly called long-acting thyroid stimulator (LATS). **TSH-binding inhibitory i's (TBII)**, proteins present in the serum of patients with Graves' disease that inhibit the binding of TSH (thyrotropin) to its receptors in human thyroid tissues. Called also *TSH-displacing antibody*.

immunoglobulinopathy (im''mu-no-glob''u-lin-op'ah-the) gammapathy.

immunohematology (ĭ-mu''no-hem''ah-tol'o-je) that branch of hematology which studies antigen-antibody reactions and analogous phenomena as they relate to the pathogenesis and clinical manifestations of blood disorders.

immunohistochemical (im''u-no-his''to-kem'ĭ-kal) denoting the application of antigen-antibody interactions to histochemical techniques, as in the use of immunofluorescence.

immunohistofluorescence (im''u-no-his-to-floo''o-res'ens) histofluorescence accomplished by injection of antibody labeled with fluorochrome.

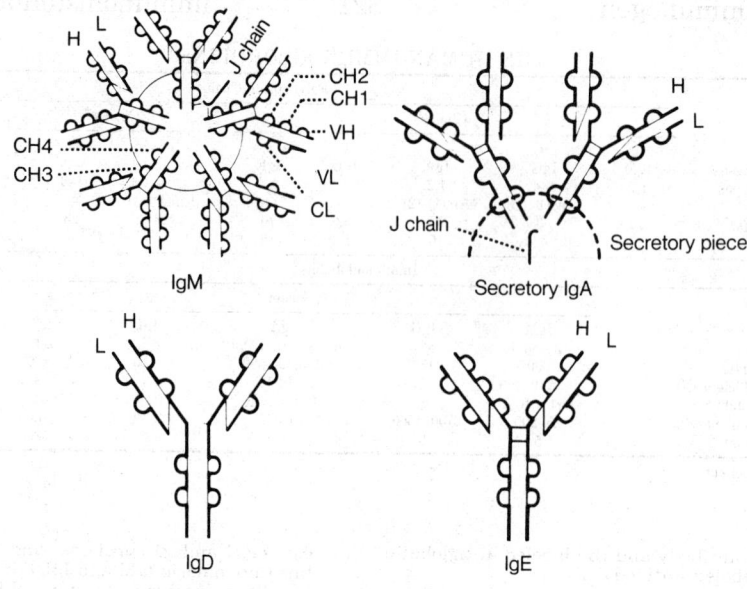

Structure of Immunoglobulin G and A Subclasses

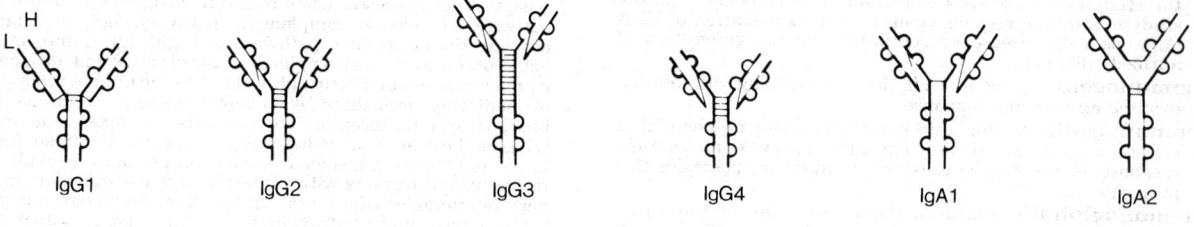

Molecular structure of the five classes of immunoglobulins. Schematic representation of the basic four polypeptide chain, monomeric unit structure of immunoglobulin molecules. Heavy (H) chains determine *class*. Those in IgG are gamma, in IgM are mu, in IgA are alpha, in IgD are delta, and in IgE are epsilon. The two *types* of light (L) chains (kappa and lambda) are shared by all five immunoglobulin classes, although only one type is present in any individual molecule. Both heavy and light chains have looped structures referred to as domains or regions. Heavy chains possess one variable (VH) region, and three constant (CH1, CH2, CH3) regions, except in the case of IgM and IgE, which contain one variable (VH) and four constant regions (CH1, CH2, CH3, CH4). Light chains contain one variable (VL) and one constant (CL) region each. The heavy and light chains are fastened together by disulfide bonds as well as by noncovalent forces. The disulfide bonds differ in number at the *hinge* (inter H chain) region according to immunoglobulin subclass. Antigen-binding sites are located in the variable (amino-terminus) regions of each immunoglobulin monomer. IgM and dimeric or multimeric IgA molecules have J chains that are associated with the ability of these molecules to form polymers. Secretory IgA contains a secretory piece which is produced by epithelial cells and is believed to protect the molecule from enzymatic cleavage in the hinge region. Serum IgA2 has no heavy to light chain disulfide bonds, whereas IgA1 has a classic structure.

immunoincompetent (im″u-no-in-kom′pĕ-tent) lacking the ability or capacity to develop an immune response to antigenic challenge.

immunologic, immunological (im″u-no-loj′ik, im″u-no-loj′ĭ-kal) pertaining to immunology.

immunologist (im″u-nol′o-jist) a person who makes a special study of immunology.

immunology (im″u-nol′o-je) that branch of biomedical science concerned with the response of the organism to antigenic challenge, the recognition of self and not self, and all the biological (*in vivo*), serological (*in vitro*), and physical chemical aspects of immune phenomena. It encompasses the study of the structure and function of the immune system (basic immunology); immunization, organ transplantation, blood banking, and immunopathology (clinical immunology); laboratory testing of cellular and humoral immune function (laboratory immunology); and the use of antigen-antibody reactions in other laboratory tests (serology and immunochemistry).

immunomodulation (im″u-no-mod″u-la′shun) adjustment of the immune response to a desired level, as in immunopotentiation, immunosuppression, or induction of immunologic tolerance.

immunomodulator (im″u-no-mod′u-la″tor) an agent that specifically or nonspecifically augments or diminishes immune responses, i.e., an adjuvant, immunostimulant, or immunosuppressant.

immunoparasitology (im″u-no-par″ah-si-tol′o-je) immunology as applied to the interaction of animal parasites and their hosts.

immunopathogenesis (im″u-no-path″o-jen′ĕ-sis) a process in which the course of a disease is altered or affected by an immune response (either the cellular [T-cell] or humoral [B-cell] response) or by the products of an immune reaction, such as the antigen-antibody-complement complexes deposited in renal glomeruli.

immunopathologic (im″u-no-path′o-loj′ik) pertaining to immunopathology.

immunopathology (im″u-no-pah-thol′o-je) 1. that branch of biomedical science concerned with immune responses to disease, with immunodeficiency diseases, and with diseases with an immunological etiology or pathogenesis. 2. the structural and functional manifestations associated with immune responses to disease or with diseases having an immunologic etiology.

immunoperoxidase (im″u-no-per-ok′sĭ-das) pertaining to immunocytochemical methods using antibody coupled to the enzyme peroxidase to stain tissue constituents; frequently used to identify tissue antigens to aid diagnosis in surgical pathology.

immunophysiology (im″u-no-fiz″e-ol′o-je) the physiology of immunological processes.

immunopotency (im″u-no-po′ten-se) the immunogenic capacity of an individual antigenic determinant on an antigen molecule to initiate antibody synthesis.

immunopotentiation (im″u-no-po-ten″she-a′shun) enhancement of the immune response by use of an adjuvant or immunostimulant.

immunopotentiator (im″u-no-po-ten′she-a-tor) an agent that specifically or nonspecifically enhances or augments the immune response, such as an adjuvant, BCG vaccine, or transfer factor.

immunoprecipitation (im″u-no-pre-sip″ĭ-ta′shun) precipitation resulting from interaction of specific antibody and antigen. See *precipitin reaction,* under *reaction.*

immunoproliferative (im″u-no-pro-lif′er-ah-tiv) a term used to refer to the uncontrolled proliferation of lymphoid cells, as in immunoproliferative disorders.

immunoprophylaxis (im″u-no-pro″fĭ-lak′sis) the prevention of disease by the use of vaccines or therapeutic antisera.

immunoradiometric (im″u-no-ra″de-o-met′rik) pertaining to immunoradiometry or to immunoradiometric assay.

immunoradiometry (im″u-no-ra″de-om′ĕ-tre) the use of radiolabelled antibody (in the place of radiolabelled antigen) in radioimmunoassay techniques.

immunoreactant (im″u-no-re-ak′tant) a substance that participates in an immune reaction, e.g., an antigen or antibody. **glucagon i's,** enteroglucagon.

immunoreaction (ĭ-mu″no-re-ak′shun) the reaction that takes place between an antigen and its antibody or between an antigen and an immunocyte sensitized to it.

immunoreactive (im″u-no-re-ak′tiv) exhibiting immunoreaction.

immunoreactivity (im″u-no-re″ak-tiv′ĭ-te) the quality or state of being immunoreactive. **glucagon-like i.,** enteroglucagon.

immunoregulation (im″u-no-reg″u-la′shun) control of the immune response by mechanisms such as suppressor and contrasuppressor lymphocyte circuits and the immunoglobulin idiotype–anti-idiotype network.

immunoresponsiveness (im″u-no-re-spon′siv-ness) the capacity to react immunologically.

immunoselection (im″u-no-sĕ-lek′shun) the survival of certain cell lines attributable to their having the least surface antigenicity and thus the least susceptibility to antibody and/or immune lymphoid cells.

immunosorbent (im″u-no-sor′bent) immunoadsorbent.

immunostimulant (im″u-no-stim′u-lant) an agent capable of stimulating immune responses, usually used to refer to agents other than adjuvants.

immunostimulation (im″u-no-stim″u-la′shun) stimulation of an immune response, e.g., by use of BCG vaccine.

immunosuppressant (im″u-no-sŭ-pres′ant) an agent capable of suppressing immune responses.

immunosuppression (im″u-no-sŭ-presh′un) the prevention or diminution of the immune response, as by irradiation or by administration of antimetabolites, antilymphocyte serum, or specific antibody; called also *immunodepression.*

immunosuppressive (im″u-no-sŭ-pres′iv) 1. pertaining to or inducing immunosuppression. 2. immunosuppressant.

immunosurveillance (im″u-no-ser-va′lens) immune surveillance.

immunotherapy (ĭ-mu″no-ther′ah-pe) a general term encompassing active and passive immunization, treatment with immunopotentiators and immunosuppressants, hyposensitization for allergic disorders, bone marrow transplantation, and thymus implantation.

immunotoxin (im′u-no-tok″sin) a hybrid molecule formed by coupling an entire toxin or the A chain of a toxin to an antibody or antigen molecule; the resulting molecule has the specificity of the antibody or antigen and the toxicity of the toxin.

immunotransfusion (ĭ-mu″no-trans-fu′zhun) transfusion of blood from donors previously immunized by the bacteria infecting the patient, or from the specific infection or of blood from persons recently recovered from the specific infection.

Imodium (ĭ-mo′de-um) trademark for a preparation of loperamide hydrochloride.

IMPA incisal mandibular plane angle.

impact (im′pakt) [L. *impactus*] a sudden and forcible collision.

impacted (im-pakt′ed) [L. *impactus*] driven firmly in; closely or firmly lodged in position, as an impacted tooth.

impaction (im-pak′shun) [L. *impactio*] the condition of being firmly lodged or wedged. In obstetrics, the indentation of any fetal parts of one twin onto the surface of its co-twin, so that the simultaneous partial engagement of both twins is permitted. **ceruminal i.,** an accumulation of cerumen in the external auditory canal. **dental i.,** the condition in which a tooth is blocked by a physical barrier, usually other teeth, so that it is prevented from erupting. See also *impacted tooth,* under *tooth.* **fecal i.,** a collection of putty-like or hardened feces in the rectum or sigmoid. **food i.,** forceful wedging of food into the peridontium by occlusal forces, which may occur interproximally or in relation to the vestibular or oral tooth surfaces. It is a common contributing factor in gingival and periodontal disease.

impalpable (im-pal′pah-b'l) [L. *in* not + *palpare* to feel] impossible of being detected by touch; extremely fine, or small.

impaludation (im″pal-u-da′shun) the application of malariotherapy.

impar (im′par) [L. "unequal"] [NA] a general anatomical term meaning unpaired; having no fellow; azygous.

imparidigitate (im-par″ĭ-dij′ĭ-tāt) [L. *impar* unequal + *digitus* finger] perissodactylous.

impatency (im-pa′ten-se) the condition of being closed or obstructed.

impatent (im-pa′tent) not open; closed or obstructed.

impedance (im-pēd′ans) the opposition to the flow of an alternating current, which is the vector sum of ohmic resistance plus additional resistance, if any, due to induction, to capacity, or to both. Its symbol is Z. The resistance due to the inductive and condenser characteristics of a circuit is called reactance. In mechanics, the resistance to an applied force. **acoustic i.,** an expression of the opposition to passage of sound waves, being a function of the density and elasticity of a substance.

imperception (im″per-sep′shun) defective power of perception.

imperforate (im-per′fo-rāt) [L. *imperforatus*] not open; abnormally closed, as imperforate anus.

imperforation (im-per′fo-ra′shun) the state of being abnormally closed.

imperialine (im-pe′re-al-in) a crystalline alkaloid, $C_{27}H_{43}NO_3$, from the bulbs of the liliaceous plant *Fritillaria imperialis*.

impermeable (im-per′me-ah-b'l) [L. *in* not + *per* through + *meare* to move] not permitting passage, as of fluid.

impervious (im-per′ve-us) [L. *impervius*] impenetrable; not affording a passage.

impetiginization (im″pe-tij″ĭ-ni-za′shun) the development of impetigo upon an area previously affected with some other skin disease.

impetiginous (im″pe-tij′ĭ-nus) [L. *impetiginosus*] pertaining to or of the nature of impetigo.

impetigo (im″pĕ-ti′go) [L.] 1. a contagious pyoderma caused by direct inoculation of group A streptococci or *Staphylococcus aureus* into superficial cutaneous abrasions or compromised skin, most commonly seen in children, usually located on the face, especially about the nose and mouth, and characterized by the presence of discrete fragile vesicles surrounded by an erythematous border that become pustular and rupture to discharge a thin, amber-colored seropurulent fluid that dries and forms a thick yellowish crust; the pustules may spread peripherally with central healing, evolving into annular, circinate, or gyrate patterns. Called also *i. contagiosa, i. vulgaris,* and *streptococcal i.* 2. i. bullosa. **Bockhart's i.,** a superficial folliculitis, usually caused by *Staphylococcus aureus,* marked by the formation of small purulent pustules at the orifices of the pilosebaceous glands, and affecting especially the scalp and the extremities. Called also *superficial pustular perifolliculitis.* **i. bullo′sa,** a highly contagious, usually localized pyoderma caused by *Staphylococcus aureus,* especially affecting newborns but seen also in older children and adults, characterized by the eruption on otherwise normal-appearing skin of flaccid bullae with erythematous rims that contain a thin fluid, varying from slightly turbid to frankly purulent, followed by spontaneous rupture of the lesions and formation of a thin, varnish-like crust, and sometimes spreading to involve large areas of the skin. Called also *impetigo, i. contagiosa bullosa, i. neonatorum, staphylococcal i.,* and formerly *pemphigus neonatorum.* **i. contagio′sa,** impetigo, def. 1. **i. contagio′sa bullo′sa,** i. bullosa. **i. herpetifor′mis,** a rare, acute, severe dermatosis, generally considered to be a form of pustular psoriasis precipitated by pregnancy, associated with hypocalcemia and sometimes tetany and high fetal and maternal mortality, and characterized by the development of crops of pruritic sterile pustules that resolve with desquamation, each crop of lesions being accompanied by fever, lethargy, and prostration. **i. neonato′rum,** i. bullosa. **staphylococcal i.,** bullous i. **streptococcal i.,** impetigo, def. 1. **i. vulga′ris,** impetigo, def. 1.

impilation (im″pi-la′shun) rouleau formation; see under *formation.*

Implacentalia (im″plas-en-ta′le-ah) in former classifications, a division of the class Mammalia, comprising the mammals that do not have a placenta, such as the monotremes.

implant¹ (im-plant′) to insert or graft an object or material, such as an alloplastic or radioactive material, a drug capsule, or tissue, into the body of a recipient.

implant² (im′plant) 1. an object or material, such as an alloplastic or radioactive material or tissue, partially or totally inserted or grafted into the body for prosthetic, therapeutic, diagnostic, or experimental purposes. See also *graft* and *insert.* **dental i.,** a prosthetic device of alloplastic material implanted into the oral tissues beneath the mucosal or periosteal layer or within the bone to provide support and retention to a partial or complete denture. **endodontic i.,** a metallic implant extending through the root canal of a tooth into the periapical bone structure, thereby lengthening the root of a pulpless tooth. **endometrial i's,** fragments of endometrial mucosa transferred through the oviducts and implanted on the uterus, ovaries, or pelvic peritoneum. **endosseous i.,** a dental implant, usually of metal or, less commonly, of ceramic or polymeric material, consisting of a blade, screw, pin, or vent, which is inserted into the jaw bone through the alveolar or basal bone, either directly or through the root canal and the apex of a tooth, with a post protruding through the mucoperiosteum into the oral cavity to serve as an abutment for dentures or orthodontic appliances, or to serve in fracture fixation. Called also *endosteal i.* **endosteal i.,** endosseous i. **intraperiosteal i.,** a frame fabricated to conform to the shape of the bone, implanted beneath the outer or fibrous layer of the periosteum and resting firmly on the bone, with a post protruding into the oral cavity to serve as an abutment for dentures; used most commonly for upper fixed bridges and in the treatment of cleft palate. **magnet i.,** denture magnet. **osseointegrated i.,** an endosseous (intraosseous) implant containing pores into which osteoblasts and supporting connective tissue can migrate. Metallic, ceramic, and polymeric materials have been used. **subperiosteal i.,** a metal frame implanted under the periosteum and resting on the bone, with a post protruding into the oral cavity, being firmly bound by the mucoperiosteum; used most commonly as an abutment for upper fixed bridges and in the treatment of cleft palate.

implantation (im″plan-ta′shun) [L. *in* into + *plantare* to set] 1. attachment of the blastocyst to the epithelial lining of the uterus, its penetration through the epithelium, and, in humans, its embedding in the compact layer of the endometrium, occurring six or seven days after fertilization of the ovum. 2. the insertion of an organ or tissue, such as skin, nerve, or tendon, in a new site in the body. 3. the insertion or grafting into the body of biological, living, inert, or radioactive material. **central i.,** superficial i. **circumferential i.,** superficial i. **eccentric i.,** embedding of the blastocyst within a recess of the uterine cavity. **hypodermic i.,** the placing of a medicine in the subcutaneous tissue. **interstitial i.,** complete embedding of a blastocyst within the endometrium. **nerve i.,** the operation of inserting and attaching a nerve into the sheath of another nerve. **periosteal i.,** surgical insertion of a normal tendon into the periosteum of a bone at the insertion of a paralyzed tendon, to take its place. **superficial i.,** embedding of the blastocyst so that the blastocyst, and later the chorionic sac, come to occupy the uterine cavity. **teratic i.,** the partial blending of an imperfect with a nearly perfect fetus.

implantodontics (im″plan-to-don′tiks) the branch of dentistry dealing with the implantation of artificial devices and materials into the oral hard and soft tissues for prosthetic, therapeutic, or diagnostic purposes. Called also *dental* or *oral implantology* and *implantodontology.*

implantodontist (im″plan-to-don′tist) 1. a dentist who specializes in the practice of implantodontics. 2. implantologist.

implantodontology (im-plan″to-don′tol′o-je) implantodontics.

implantologist (im″plan-tol′o-jist) 1. a specialist in implantology. 2. implantodontist.

implantology (im″plan-tol′o-je) the science dealing with the study and practice of inserting implants into the body. **dental i., oral i.,** implantodontics.

implosion (im-plo′zhun) in behavior therapy, a form of desensitization for the treatment of phobias and related disorders; the patient is repeatedly exposed, in imagination or real life, to emotionally distressing stimuli while the therapist makes verbal interpretation of the psychological meaning of the stimuli in order to intensify the patient's emotional arousal. Cf. *flooding* and *systematic desensitization*. The term *implosion* has also been used synonymously with *flooding*.

impotency (im′po-ten″se) impotence.

impotentia (im″po-ten′she-ah) [L.] impotence. **i. co-eun′di**, inability of the male to perform the sexual act. **i. erigen′di**, inability to have an erection of the penis. **i. generan′di**, inability to reproduce.

impregnate (im-preg′nāt) [L. *impregnare*] 1. to render pregnant; to fertilize. 2. to saturate or charge with.

impregnation (im″preg-na′shun) [L. *impregnatio*] 1. the act of fecundation or of rendering pregnant. 2. the process or act of saturation; or a saturated condition.

impressio (im-pres′se-o), pl. *impressio′nes* [L.] an impression, indentation, or concavity; [NA] a general term for an indentation produced in the surface of one organ by pressure exerted by another. **i. cardi′aca hep′atis** [NA], cardiac impression of the liver: a depression on the superior part of the mediastinal (medial) surface of the liver, corresponding to the position of the heart. **i. cardi′aca pulmo′nis** [NA], cardiac impression of the lung: the indentation on the medial surface of either lung produced by the heart and pericardium. **i. col′ica hep′atis** [NA], colic impression of the liver: a variable concavity in the right lobe of the liver, where it is in contact with the right flexure of the colon. **impressio′nes digita′tae** [NA], digitate or digital impressions: poorly defined depressions on the inner surface of the cranium, corresponding to the gyri of the brain. Called also *gyrate impressions* and *i. gyrorum* [NA alternative]. **i. duodena′les hep′atis** [NA], duodenal impression of the liver: a concavity on the right lobe of the liver where it is in contact with the descending part of the duodenum. **i. esopha′gea hep′atis**, NA alternative for *i. oesophagea hepatis.* **i. gas′trica hep′atis** [NA], gastric impression of the liver: a large concavity in the left lobe of the liver where it is in contact with the anterior surface of the stomach. **i. gas′trica re′nis**, a concavity on the anterior surface of the left kidney where it is in contact with the stomach. **i. gyro′rum**, NA alternative for *i. digitatae.* **i. hepat′ica re′nis**, an impression on the anterior surface of the left kidney where it is in contact with the liver. **i. ligamen′ti costoclavicula′ris** [NA], impression of the costoclavicular ligament: the point on the inferior surface of the clavicle where the costoclavicular ligament is attached; called also *tuberositas costalis claviculae* and *costal tuberosity of clavicle.* **i. meningea′lis**, see *foveolae granulares.* **i. muscula′ris re′nis**, a depression on the posterior surface of the kidney where it is in contact with the psoas muscle. **i. oesopha′gea hep′atis** [NA], esophageal impression of liver: a concavity on the left hepatic lobe corresponding to the position of the abdominal part of the esophagus; called also *i. esophagea hepatis* [NA alternative]. **i. petro′sa pal′lii**, a shallow groove on the base of the brain corresponding to the superior angle of the petrous portion of the temporal bone. **i. rena′lis hep′atis** [NA], renal impression of the liver: the concavity on the right lobe of the liver where it is in contact with the right kidney. **i. suprarena′lis hep′atis** [NA], suprarenal impression of the liver: a small concavity on the right lobe of the liver, superior to the renal impression, caused by contact with the right suprarenal gland. **i. trigemina′lis os′sis tempora′lis** [NA], **i. trigem′ini os′sis tempora′lis**, trigeminal impression of the temporal bone: the shallow impression in the floor of the middle cranial fossa on the petrous part of the temporal bone, lodging the semilunar ganglion of the trigeminal nerve.

impression (im-presh′un) [L. *impressio*] 1. a slight indentation or depression; see *impressio.* 2. a negative copy or the impressed reverse of the surface of an object. 3. an effect produced upon the mind, body, or senses by some external stimulus or agent. 4. dental i. **anatomic i.**, an impression of the form of a dental arch or portion thereof that records the structures in a passive or unstrained form, making possible a static relationship of a prosthesis produced from such an impression. **angular i. for gasserian ganglion**, impressio trigemini ossis temporalis. **basilar i.**, a developmental deformity of the occipital bone and upper end of the cervical spine, in which the latter appears to have pushed the floor of the occipital bone upward; called also *platybasia* and *basilar invagination.* **bridge i.**, an impression made for the purpose of constructing or assembling a fixed restoration, fixed partial denture, or bridge. **cardiac i.**, an impression made by the heart on another organ; see *impressio cardiaca hepatis* and *impressio cardiaca pulmo-*

nis. **cardiac i. of liver**, impressio cardiaca hepatis. **cardiac i. of lung**, impressio cardiaca pulmonis. **cleft palate i.**, an impression of the upper jaw made in patients with cleft palate, to be used in the prosthetic repair of the defect. **colic i. of liver**, impressio colica hepatis. **complete denture i.**, 1. one made of the entire edentulous arch of the maxilla or mandible, for the purpose of construction of a complete denture. 2. a negative registration of the entire denture-bearing area of the maxilla or mandible. 3. a negative registration of the entire denture-bearing and border seal areas of the edentulous mouth. **i. of costoclavicular ligament**, impressio ligamenti costoclavicularis. **deltoid i. of humerus**, tuberositas deltoidea humeri. **dental i.**, an imprint or negative likeness of the teeth and/or edentulous areas, made in plastic material that becomes hardened or set while in contact with the tissue, which is later filled with plaster of Paris or artificial stone to produce a facsimile of the oral structures present. **digastric i.**, fossa digastrica. **digital i's, digitate i's**, impressiones digitatae. **direct bone i.**, an impression of denuded bone used in the construction of dental implants. **duodenal i. of liver**, impressio duodenalis hepatis. **esophageal i. of liver**, impressio oesophagea hepatis. **final i.**, secondary i. **gastric i.**, an impression made by the stomach on another organ; see *impressio gastrica hepatis* and *impressio gastrica renis.* **gastric i. of liver**, impressio gastrica hepatis. **gyrate i's**, impressiones digitatae. **hydrocolloid i.**, a denture impression made of a hydrocolloid material. **lower i.**, mandibular i. **mandibular i.**, an impression of the mandibular jaw and related tissues and dental structures. **maxillary i.**, an impression of the maxillary jaw and related tissues and dental structures; called also *upper i.* **meningeal i.**, see *foveolae granulares.* **partial denture i.**, a negative copy of the partially edentulous dental arch or its section made for the purpose of constructing a partial denture. **preliminary i., primary i.**, primary i. **primary i.**, an impression of the edentulous mouth that usually lacks fine details of the tissue and is often used for construction of a secondary impression. Called also *preliminary i.* **renal i. of liver**, impressio renalis hepatis. **rhomboid i. of clavicle**, impressio ligamenti costoclavicularis. **secondary i.**, an impression made by using an impression material in a tray, produced by the primary impression method for the reproduction of fine details of an edentulous mouth. Called also *final i.* **sectional i.**, a dental impression that is made in sections. **suprarenal i. of liver**, impressio suprarenalis hepatis. **trigeminal i. of temporal bone**, impressio trigemini ossis temporalis. **upper i.**, maxillary i.

impressiones (im-pres″e-o′nēz) [L.] plural of *impressio.*

imprinting (im′print-ing) rapid learning of species-specific behavior patterns that occurs with exposure to the proper stimulus at a sensitive period of early life.

impulse (im′puls) 1. a sudden pushing force. 2. a sudden uncontrollable determination to act. 3. a nerve impulse. **apex i., apical i.**, a cardiac impulse usually caused by left ventricular contraction and characterized by a relatively localized outward movement beginning synchronously with the first heart sound. **cardiac i.**, 1. the palpable or recorded movement of the chest wall caused by the heartbeat. 2. excitation wave; see under *wave.* **episternal i.**, an aortic impulse felt at the episternal (suprasternal) notch. **irresistible i.**, an impulse to commit a criminal act that cannot be resisted because mental disease has destroyed the person's freedom of will and power to choose between right and wrong. The "irresistible impulse test" that a person is not criminally responsible if the act was due to an irresistible impulse is still used in some states. **left parasternal i's**, cardiac impulses categorized according to their location along the upper, mid, or lower left sternal border. An *upper left parasternal impulse* is usually caused by a systolic expansion of a dilated pulmonary artery; a *mid* to *lower left parasternal impulse* usually occurs as a result of a right ventricular contraction, and is characterized by an outward movement beginning synchronously with the first heart sound, but is sometimes caused by mitral incompetence. **nerve i., neural i.**, the electrochemical process propagated along nerve fibers. **right parasternal i's**, cardiac impulses categorized according to their location along the upper, mid, or lower right sternal border.

impulsion (im-pul′shun) blind obedience to internal

drives, without regard for acceptance by others or pressure from the superego; seen in children and in adults with weak psychic organization.

Imuran (im′u-ran) trademark for a preparation of azathioprine.

IMV intermittent mandatory ventilation; see under *ventilation.*

IMViC, imvic a mnemonic indicating the tests used in classifying coliform bacteria, namely indole, methyl red, Voges-Proskauer, and citrate.

In chemical symbol for *indium.*

in-¹ [L. *in* in, into] a prefix meaning in or into; occurs as *il*-before *l*, *im*-before *b*, *m*, or *p*, and *ir*- before *r*.

in-² [L. *in*- not] a prefix meaning not; occurs as *il*- before *l*, *im*- before *b*, *m*, or *p*, and *ir*- before *r*.

I.N.A. International Neurological Association.

inacidity (in″ah-sid′ĭ-te) anacidity.

inactivate (in-ak′tĭ-vāt) to render inactive; to destroy the activity of.

inactivation (in-ak″tĭ-va′shun) the destruction of biological activity, as of a virus or enzyme, by the action of heat or other physical or chemical means. **complement i.,** any method of destroying the complement activity of serum, such as heat inactivation or treatment with hydrazine. **heat i.,** any destruction of biological activity by heating, such as the destruction of complement activity in serum by heating to 56° C for 30 minutes. **X-i.,** lyonization.

inactivator (in-ak′tĭ-va″tor) an agent that renders another inactive. **anaphylatoxin i. (AI),** a serum carboxypeptidase that destroys the anaphylatoxin activity of C3a, C4a, and C5a by removing C-terminal arginyl or lysyl residues. **C3b i. (C3b INA),** factor I.

inactose (in-ak′tōs) an optically inactive plant sugar.

inadequacy (in-ad′ĕ-kwah-se) [L. *in* not + *adaequare* to make equal] inability to perform an allotted function; insufficiency; incompetence.

inalimental (in″al-ĭ-men′tal) [L. *in* not + *alimentum* food] not nutritious; not serviceable as food.

inanimate (in-an′ĭ-māt) [L. *in* not + *animatus* alive] 1. without life. 2. lacking in animation.

inanition (in″ah-nish′un) [L. *inanis* empty] a condition characterized by marked weakness, extreme weight loss, and a decrease in metabolism resulting from prolonged (usually weeks to months) and severe insufficiency of food.

inappetence (in-ap′ĕ-tens) [L. *in* not + *appetere* to desire] lack of desire or appetite.

Inapsine (in-ap′sēn) trademark for a preparation of droperidol.

inarticulate (in″ar-tik′u-lāt) [L. *in* not + *articulatus* joined] not having joints; disjointed; not uttered like articulate speech.

in articulo mortis (in ar-tik′u-lo mor′tis) [L.] at the very point of death.

inassimilable (in″ah-sim′ĭ-lah-b′l) [L. *in* not + *assimilable*] not susceptible of being utilized as nutriment.

inaxon (in-ak′son) [Gr. *is, inos* fiber + *axōn* axis] a nerve cell whose axon breaks up into terminal filaments at a considerable distance from the cell. Cf. *dendraxon.*

inborn (in′born) congenitally formed or acquired during intrauterine life; see also *inborn error,* under *metabolism.*

inbreeding (in′brēd-ing) the mating of closely related individuals, or of individuals having closely similar genetic constitutions.

incallosal (in″kah-lo′sal) characterized by absence of the corpus callosum, and usually associated with mental retardation.

incandescent (in″kan-des′ent) [L. *incandescens* glowing] glowing with heat and light; emitting light on being heated.

incarcerated (in-kar′ser-āt″ed) [L. *incarceratus* imprisoned] imprisoned; constricted; subjected to incarceration.

incarceration (in-kar″ser-a′shun) [L. *in* in + *carcer* prison] unnatural retention or confinement of a part, as may occur in hernia.

incarnatio (in″kar-na′she-o) [L., from *in* in + *caro*, gen. *carnis* flesh] ingrowth. **i. un′guis,** unguis incarnatus; ingrowth of a toenail; ingrown toenail.

incarnative (in-kar′nah-tiv) [L. *incarnare* to invest in flesh]

1. promoting the formation of granulations. 2. an agent that promotes granulations.

incasement (in-kās′ment) the act of surrounding or state of being surrounded, as with a case. See *preformation.*

incertae sedis (in-ser′te se′dis) [L.] of uncertain position; said of taxa that are of uncertain classification.

incest (in′sest) sexual intercourse or other sexual activity between persons so closely related that marriage between them is legally or culturally prohibited.

inch (inch) a unit of linear measure, one-twelfth of a foot, or one thirty-sixth of a yard, being the equivalent of 2.54 cm.

inchacao (in-chah-kah′o) [Brazilian] beriberi.

incidence (in′sĭ-dens) [L. *incidere* to occur, to happen] 1. the rate at which a certain event occurs, e.g., the number of new cases of a specific disease occurring during a certain period (see *incidence rate,* under *rate*). Cf. *prevalence.* 2. the arrival of radiant energy at a surface.

incident (in′sĭ-dent) [L. *incidere* to fall upon] falling or striking upon, as incident radiation.

incineration (in-sin″ĕ-ra′shun) [L. *in* into + *cineres* ashes] the act of burning to ashes; cremation.

incipient (in-sip′e-ent) beginning to exist; coming into existence.

incisal (in-si′zal) cutting.

incised (in-sīzd′) [L. *incisus*] cut; made by cutting.

incision (in-sizh′un) [L. *incidere* (*in* + *caedere*), to cut open, to cut through] 1. a cut, or a wound produced by cutting with a sharp instrument. 2. the act of cutting. **Battle's**

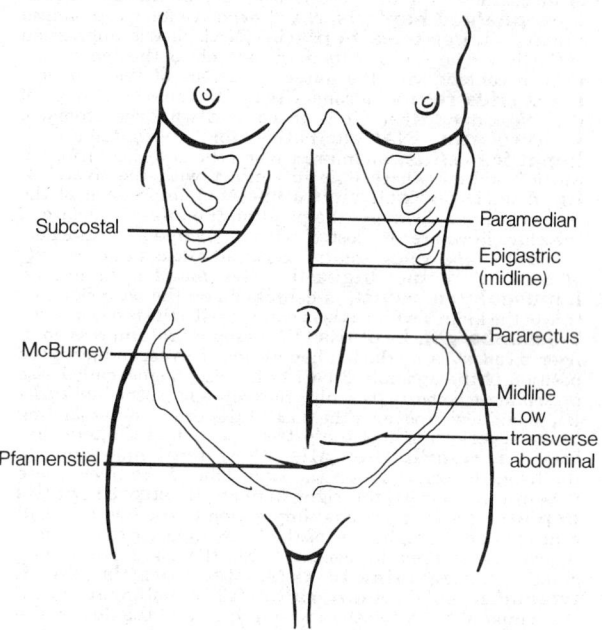

Various abdominal incisions.

i., Battle-Jalaguier-Kammerer i., Kammerer-Battle i. **Bevan's i.,** one along the outer border of the rectus muscle, for operations in the upper abdominal quadrants. **celiotomy i.,** an incision made through the abdominal wall to give access to the peritoneal cavity. **Chernez i.,** an abdominal incision in the surgical approach to the female reproductive organs. **Deaver's i.,** incision through the anterior sheath of the right rectus muscle, the muscle then being retracted medially. **Dührssen's i's,** incisions made in the cervix uteri to facilitate delivery. **epigastric i.,** see illustration. **Fergusson's i.,** an incision for excision of the upper jaw; it runs along the junction of the nose with the cheek, around the ala of the nose to the median line, and descends to bisect the upper lip. Called also *Fergusson's operation.* **gridiron i.,** McBurney's i. **Kammerer-Battle i.,** a vertical abdominal incision through the skin and superficial fascia, vertical division of the anterior layer of the rectal sheath, with retraction of the rectus muscle medialward, and vertical division of the posterior layer of the sheath nearer the median line, together with the subserous areolar tissue and peritoneum. **Kocher's i.,** a subcostal incision that, when made on the right, provides exposure of the gallbladder and common bile duct and, when made on the left, provides exposure for splenectomy or splenorenal venous anastomosis. **low transverse abdominal i.,** see illustration. **Maylard i.,** an abdominal incision in the surgical approach to the female reproductive organs. **McBurney's i.,** an abdominal incision parallel to the fibers of the external oblique muscle, about one-third the distance along a line from the anterior superior iliac spine to the umbilicus, half the incision being above and the remainder below this point. The skin and subcutaneous fat are incised down to the external oblique muscle, the fibers of which are split; the underlying internal oblique and transversus abdominalis are then split and separated. **midline i.,** see illustration. **Munro Kerr i.,** a transverse incision of the lower uterine segment for cesarean section. **Nagamatsu i.,** in renal surgery, an extrapleural retroperitoneal dorsolumbar approach to the kidney that provides an osteoplastic flap of the lower rib cage. **paramedian i.,** see illustration. **pararectus i.,** see illustration. **paravaginal i.,** incision of the vagina and perineum in order to secure enlargement of the vulvovaginal outlet, and thereby permit easy access to the vagina in cancer operations and, rarely, to facilitate childbirth; called also *Schuchardt's i.* and *vaginoperineotomy.* **Pfannenstiel's i.,** a curved abdominal incision, the convexity being directed downward, just above the symphysis, passing through skin, superficial fascia, and aponeurosis, exposing the pyramidalis and rectus muscles, which are separated from each other in the midline, the peritoneum then being opened vertically. See illustration. **relief i.,** one made to relieve tension in tissue. **Rockey-Davis i.,** an incision similar to McBurney's incision, except that the skin incision is transverse rather than vertical. **Schuchardt's i.,** paravaginal i. **subcostal i.,** see illustration. **Warren's i.,** an incision following the thoracomammary fold, permitting access to any part of the breast.

incisive (in-si′siv) [L. *incisivus*] 1. having the power or quality of cutting. 2. pertaining to the incisor teeth.

incisolabial (in-si″zo-la′be-al) denoting the incisal and labial surfaces of an anterior tooth.

incisolingual (in-si″zo-ling′gwahl) denoting the incisal and lingual surfaces of an anterior tooth.

incisoproximal (in-si″zo-prok′sĭ-mal) denoting the incisal and proximal surfaces of an anterior tooth.

incisor (in-si′zer) [L. *incidere* to cut into] 1. adapted for cutting. 2. any of the four anterior teeth in either jaw; a tooth that is mesial to the canines. See under *tooth.* **central i., first i.,** the two incisor teeth (see under *tooth*) in each jaw which are located closer to the midline of the body. **Hutchinson's i's,** see under *tooth.* **lateral i.,** the second incisor tooth on either side of the midline of each jaw, located distal to the central incisor and mesial to the canine. **medial i.,** central i. **second i.,** lateral i. **shovel-shaped i's,** large upper medial incisor teeth that are concave on the lingual side; called also *hawk-bill i's.* **winged i.,** a rotation deformity of a maxillary incisor tooth in which the distal edge of the tooth protrudes labially.

incisura (in-si-su′rah), gen. and pl. *incisu′rae* [L., from *incidere* to cut into] a cut, notch, or incision; [NA] a general term for an indention or depression, chiefly on the edge of a bone or other structure. Called also *incisure* and *notch.* **i. acetab′uli** [NA], incisure of acetabulum: a notch in the inferior portion of the lunate surface of the acetabulum. **i. angula′ris gas′tris** [NA], angular notch of stomach: the lowest point on the lesser curvature of the stomach, marking the junction of the cranial two-thirds and caudal one-third of the stomach. Called also *gastric notch* and *i. angularis ventriculi* [NA alternative]. **i. angula′ris ventric′uli,** NA alternative for *i. angularis gastris.* **i. ante′rior au′ris** [NA], anterior incisure of the ear: a depression between the crus of the helix and the tragus; called also *auricular notch.* **i. ap′icis cor′dis** [NA], incisure of apex of heart: a slight notch found at the site where the anterior and posterior interventricular sulci become continuous and cross the right margin of the heart. **i. cardi′aca gas′tris** [NA], cardiac incisure of stomach: a notch at the junction of the esophagus and the greater curvature of the stomach.

Called also *cardiac notch of stomach* and *i. cardiaca ventriculi* [NA alternative]. **i. cardi′aca pulmo′nis sinis′tri** [NA], cardiac incisure of left lung: a notch in the anterior border of the left lung; called also *cardiac notch of left lung.* **i. cardi′aca ventric′uli,** NA alternative for *i. cardiaca gastris.* **incisu′rae cartilag′inis mea′tus acus′tici** [NA], two vertical fissures in the anterior part of the cartilage of the external acoustic meatus; called also *Santorini's fissures.* **i. cerebel′li ante′rior,** a wide notch on the anterior surface of the cerebellum, occupied by the inferior colliculi and superior cerebellar peduncles; called also *anterior cerebellar notch.* **i. cerebel′li poste′rior,** a notch between the cerebellar hemispheres posteriorly, containing the falx cerebelli; called also *posterior cerebellar notch.* **i. clavicula′ris ster′ni** [NA], clavicular incisure of the sternum: an oval surface on each side of the cranial border of the manubrium of the sternum, where it articulates with the clavicle; called also *clavicular notch of sternum.* **incisu′rae costa′les ster′ni** [NA], costal incisures of the sternum: the facets on the sternum, seven on each lateral edge, for articulation with the costal cartilages; called also *costal notches of sternum.* **i. ethmoida′lis os′sis fronta′lis** [NA], ethmoidal incisure of frontal bone: a space between the orbital parts of the frontal bone, in which the ethmoid bone is lodged; called also *ethmoid notch of frontal bone.* **i. fastig′ii,** a transverse furrow on the ventricular surface of the cerebellar lamina of the developing cerebellum. **i. fibula′ris tib′iae** [NA], fibular incisure of tibia: a depression on the lateral surface of the lower end of the tibia, which articulates with the lower end of the fibula; called also *fibular notch.* **i. fronta′lis** [NA], frontal incisure: a notch located in the supraorbital margin of the frontal bone medial to the supraorbital notch or foramen, for transmission of branches of the supraorbital nerve and vessels; frequently converted into a foramen (*foramen frontale*) by a bridge of osseous tissue; called also *frontal notch.* **i. interarytenoi′dea laryn′gis** [NA], interarytenoid incisure of larynx: the posterior portion of the aditus laryngis between the two arytenoid cartilages; called also *interarytenoid notch.* **i. interloba′ris hep′atis,** i. ligamenti teretis. **i. interloba′ris pulmo′nis,** an incisure separating adjacent lobes of a lung; see *fissura obliqua pulmonis* and *fissura horizontalis pulmonis dextri.* **i. intertrag′ica** [NA], the intertragic incisure: the notch at the lower part of the pinna of the ear between the tragus and the antitragus; called also *intertragic notch.* **i. ischiad′ica ma′jor** [NA], greater incisure of ischium: the large notch on the posterior border of the hip bone, where the posterior borders of the ilium and the ischium become continuous. Called also *greater ischial incisure* or *notch, greater notch of ischium, greater sciatic notch,* and *i. ischialis major* [NA alternative]. **i. ischiad′ica mi′nor** [NA], lesser incisure of ischium: the notch on the posterior border of the ischium just inferior to the ischiadic spine. Called also *i. ischialis minor* [NA alternative], *lesser ischial incisure* or *notch, lesser notch of ischium,* and *lesser sciatic notch.* **i. ischia′lis ma′jor,** NA alternative for *i. ischiadica major.* **i. ischia′lis mi′nor,** NA alternative for *i. ischiadica minor.* **i. jugula′ris os′sis occipita′lis** [NA], jugular incisure of occipital bone: a notch on the anterior surface of the jugular process of the occipital bone, forming the posterior wall of the jugular foramen; called also *jugular notch of occipital bone.* **i. jugula′ris os′sis tempora′lis** [NA], jugular incisure of temporal bone: a prominent depression on the inferior surface of the petrous part of the temporal bone. It forms the anterior and lateral wall of the jugular foramen and lodges the superior bulb of the internal jugular vein in its lateral part and the glossopharyngeal, vagus, and accessory nerves in its medial part; called also *jugular notch of temporal bone.* **i. jugula′ris ster′ni** [NA], jugular incisure of sternum: the notch on the upper border of the sternum between the clavicular notches; called also *jugular notch of sternum.* **i. lacrima′lis maxil′lae** [NA], lacrimal incisure of maxilla: an indentation on the posterior border of the frontal process of the maxilla, that lodges the lacrimal sac; called also *lacrimal notch of maxilla.* **i. ligamen′ti te′retis** [NA], a notch in the inferior border of the liver, occupied by the ligamentum teres in the adult; called also *i. umbilicalis, umbilical notch* or *incisure,* and *notch of the ligamentum teres.* **i. mandib′ulae** [NA], incisure of mandible: a deep notch on the upper edge of the ramus of the mandible between the condyle and the coronoid process; called also *mandibular notch.* **i. mastoi′dea os′sis tempora′lis**

[NA], mastoid incisure of temporal bone: a deep groove on the medial surface of the mastoid process of the temporal bone, which gives origin to the posterior belly of the digastric muscle; called also *mastoid notch.* **i. nasa'lis maxil'lae** [NA], nasal incisure of maxilla: the large notch in the anterior border of the maxilla that forms the lateral and inferior margins of the anterior nasal aperture; called also *nasal notch of maxilla.* **i. pancre'atis** [NA], a notch at the junction of the left half of the head of the pancreas and the neck of the pancreas; called also *pancreatic notch.* **i. parieta'lis os'sis tempora'lis** [NA], parietal incisure of temporal bone: the notch found on the upper margin of the temporal bone where the squamous and parietomastoid sutures meet; called also *parietal notch of temporal bone.* **i. perone'a tib'iae,** i. fibularis tibiae. **i. preoccipita'lis** [NA], preoccipital incisure: a notch near the posterior end of the inferolateral border of the cerebral hemisphere. A line joining it to the parietooccipital sulcus serves to delineate the parietal and temporal lobes from the occipital lobe; called also *preoccipital notch.* **i. radia'lis ul'nae** [NA], radial incisure of ulna: the cavity on the outer side of the coronoid process, articulating with the rim of the head of the radius; called also *radial notch (of ulna).* **i. Rivi'ni,** i. tympanica [Rivini]. **i. Santori'ni,** 1. incisura anterior auris. 2. see *incisurae cartilaginis meatus acustici.* **i. scap'ulae** [NA], incisure of scapula: a notch, converted into a foramen by a ligament, on the upper border of the scapula at the base of the coracoid process; called also *scapular notch.* **i. semiluna'ris tib'iae,** i. fibularis tibiae. **i. semiluna'ris ul'nae,** i. trochlearis ulnae. **i. sphenopalati'na os'sis palati'ni** [NA], sphenopalatine incisure of palatine bone: a notch between the orbital and sphenoid processes of the palatine bone; it is converted into a foramen by the undersurface of the sphenoid bone; called also *sphenopalatine notch of palatine bone.* **i. supraorbita'lis** [NA], supraorbital incisure: a palpable notch in the frontal bone at the junction of the medial one-third and lateral two-thirds of the supraorbital margin, for transmission of the supraorbital nerve and vessels to the forehead. In life it is bridged by fibrous tissue, which is sometimes ossified, forming a bony aperture (*foramen supraorbitale*). Called also *supraorbital notch.* **i. tempora'lis,** a slight fissure between the uncus of the parahippocampal gyrus and the apex of the temporal lobe. **i. tento'rii cerebel'li** [NA], incisure of tentorium of cerebellum: an opening at the anterior part of the cerebellum, formed by the free, internal border of the tentorium and the dorsum sellae of the sphenoid, and occupied chiefly by the mesencephalon; called also *tentorial notch.* **i. termina'lis au'ris** [NA], terminal incisure of the ear: a deep notch separating the lamina tragi and cartilage of the external acoustic meatus from the main auricular cartilage. **i. thyroi'dea infe'rior** [NA], inferior thyroid incisure: a notch at the lower part of the anterior border of the thyroid cartilage; called also *inferior thyroid notch.* **i. thyroi'dea supe'rior** [NA], superior thyroid incisure: a deep notch in the upper portion of the anterior border of the thyroid cartilage; called also *superior thyroid notch.* **i. trag'ica,** i. intertragica. **i. trochlea'ris ul'nae** [NA], a large concavity on the anterior surface at the proximal end of the ulna, formed by the olecranon and coronoid processes, for articulation with the trochlea of the humerus; called also *i. semilunaris ulnae* and *trochlear notch of ulna.* **i. tympan'ica [Rivi'ni]** [NA], tympanic notch: a defect in the upper portion of the tympanic part of the temporal bone, between the greater and lesser tympanic spines, which is filled in by the pars flaccida of the tympanic membrane. **i. ulna'ris ra'dii** [NA], ulnar incisure of radius: a concavity on the medial side of the distal extremity of the radius, articulating with the head of the ulna; called also *ulnar notch (of radius).* **i. umbilica'lis,** i. ligamenti teretis. **i. vertebra'lis infe'rior** [NA], inferior vertebral incisure: the indentation found below each pedicle of a vertebra which, with the indentation located above the pedicle of the vertebra below, forms the intervertebral foramen; called also *inferior vertebral notch.* **i. vertebra'lis supe'rior** [NA], superior vertebral incisure: the indentation found above each pedicle of a vertebra which, with the indentation located below the corresponding pedicle of the vertebra above, forms the intervertebral foramen; called also *superior vertebral notch.*

incisurae (in″si-su're) [L.] genitive and plural of *incisura.*

incisure (in-si'zhūr) a cut, notch, or incision; called also

incisura [NA]. **i. of acetabulum,** incisura acetabuli. **i. of apex of heart,** incisura apicis cordis. **i. of calcaneus,** sulcus tendinis musculi flexoris hallucis longi calcanei. **cardiac i. of left lung,** incisura cardiaca pulmonis sinistra. **cardiac i. of stomach,** incisura cardiaca gastris. **clavicular i. of sternum,** incisura clavicularis sterni. **costal i's of sternum,** incisurae costales sterni. **cotyloid i.,** incisura acetabuli. **digastric i. of temporal bone,** incisura mastoidea ossis temporalis. **i. of ear, anterior,** incisura anterior auris. **i. of ear, terminal,** incisura terminalis auris. **ethmoidal i. of frontal bone,** incisura ethmoidalis ossis frontalis. **falciform i. of fascia lata,** margo falciformis hiatus saphenus. **fibular i. of tibia,** incisura fibularis tibiae. **frontal i.,** incisura frontalis. **humeral i. of ulna,** incisura trochlearis ulnae. **iliac i., lesser,** incisura ischiadica minor. **interarytenoid i. of larynx,** incisura interarytenoidea laryngis. **interclavicular i.,** incisura jugularis sterni. **intertragic i.,** incisura intertragica. **ischial i., greater, i. of ischium, greater,** incisura ischiadica major. **ischial i., lesser, i. of ischium, lesser,** incisura ischiadica minor. **jugular i. of occipital bone,** incisura jugularis ossis occipitalis. **jugular i. of sternum,** incisura jugularis sterni. **jugular i. of temporal bone,** incisura jugularis ossis temporalis. **lacrimal i. of maxilla,** incisura lacrimalis maxillae. **i's of Lanterman, i's of Lanterman-Schmidt,** channels of cytoplasm in the myelin sheath of neurons that lead back to the Schwann cell body; they appear as oblique lines or slashes in the sheath. Called also *Lanterman's clefts* and *Schmidt-Lanterman i's.* **lateral i. of sternum,** incisura clavicularis sterni. **i. of mandible,** incisura mandibulae. **mastoid i. of temporal bone,** incisura mastoidea ossis temporalis. **maxillary i., inferior,** margo lacrimalis maxillae. **nasal i. of frontal bone,** margo nasalis ossis frontalis. **nasal i. of maxilla,** incisura nasalis maxillae. **obturator i. of pubic bone,** sulcus obturatorius ossis pubis. **palatine i.,** fissura pterygoidea. **palatine i. of Henle,** incisura sphenopalatina ossis palatini. **parietal i. of temporal bone,** incisura parietalis ossis temporalis. **patellar i. of femur,** facies patellaris femoris. **peroneal i. of tibia,** incisura fibularis tibiae. **popliteal i.,** fossa intercondylaris femoris. **preoccipital i.,** incisura preoccipitalis. **pterygoid i.,** fissura pterygoidea. **radial i. of ulna,** incisura radialis ulnae. **Rivinus' i.,** incisura tympanica [Rivini]. **i. of scapula,** incisura scapulae. **Schmidt-Lanterman i's,** i's of Lanterman. **semilunar i.,** incisura scapulae. **semilunar i., greater, of ulna,** incisura trochlearis ulnae. **semilunar i., lesser, of ulna,** incisura radialis ulnae. **semilunar i. of mandible,** incisura mandibulae. **semilunar i. of radius,** incisura ulnaris radii. **semilunar i. of scapula,** incisura scapulae. **semilunar i. of sternum,** incisura clavicularis sterni. **semilunar i. of sternum, superior,** incisura jugularis sterni. **semilunar i. of tibia,** incisura fibularis tibiae. **semilunar i. of ulna,** incisura trochlearis ulnae. **sigmoid i. of mandible,** incisura mandibulae. **sigmoid i. of ulna,** incisura trochlearis ulnae. **sphenopalatine i. of palatine bone,** incisura sphenopalatina ossis palatini. **sternal i.,** incisura jugularis sterni. **supraorbital i.,** incisura supraorbitalis. **suprascapular i.,** incisura scapulae. **i. of talus,** sulcus tendinis musculi flexoris hallucis longi tali. **i. of tentorium of cerebellum,** incisura tentorii cerebelli. **thoracic i.,** angulus infrasternalis thoracis. **thyroid i., inferior,** incisura thyroidea inferior. **thyroid i., superior,** incisura thyroidea superior. **trochlear i. of ulna,** incisura trochlearis ulnae. **ulnar i. of radius,** incisura ulnaris radii. **umbilical i.,** incisura ligamenti teretis. **vertebral i., greater, vertebral i., inferior,** incisura vertebralis inferior. **vertebral i., lesser, vertebral i., superior,** incisura vertebralis superior.

incitogram (in-si'to-gram) the neural conditions which organize and initiate efferent impulses.

inclinatio (in″kli-na'she-o), pl. *inclinatio'nes* [L., from *inclinare* to lean] inclination. **i. pel'vis** [NA], pelvic inclination: the angle between the plane of the superior aperture of the minor pelvis and the horizontal plane, when the body is in the erect position; called also *pelvic incline.*

inclination (in″kli-na'shun) [L. *inclinare* to lean] 1. a deviation from the horizontal or vertical; a sloping or leaning.

2. deviation of the long axis of a tooth from the perpendicular line. 3. deviation of a portion of the surface of a tooth from the general plane of that surface. 4. description of the angles with the surface of a tooth at which the walls of a cavity may be cut, or of the relation of the opposing walls to each other, as *outward inclination, inward inclination,* etc. 5. inclination of enamel rods from a line perpendicular to the surface of a tooth. **condylar guidance i., condylar guide i.,** the angle of inclination of the condylar guidance to an accepted horizontal plane. **lateral condylar i.,** the direction of the lateral condyle path. **lingual i.,** deviation of a tooth from the vertical, in the direction of the tongue. **pelvic i., i. of pelvis,** inclinatio pelvis.

inclinationes (in″klĭ-na″she-o′nēz) [L.] plural of *inclinatio.*

incline (in′klīn) inclination. **pelvic i., i. of pelvis,** inclinatio pelvis.

inclinometer (in″klĭ-nom′ĕ-ter) [*inclination* + *-meter*] an instrument for determining ocular inclinations, angles, and directions of the visual axes.

inclusion (in-klu′zhun) [L. *inclusio*] 1. the act of enclosing or condition of being enclosed. 2. anything that is enclosed; often used alone to refer to cell inclusions. **cell i.,** a usually lifeless, often temporary, constituent of the cytoplasm of a cell, such as an accumulation of proteins, fats, carbohydrates, pigments, secretory granules, crystals, or other insoluble components. **dental i.,** 1. a tooth so surrounded with bony material that it is unable to erupt. 2. a cyst of oral soft tissue or bone. **fetal i.,** a partially developed embryo enclosed within the body of its twin. **Guarnieri's i's,** see under *body.* **intranuclear i's,** inclusion bodies. **leukocyte i's,** Döhle's inclusion bodies. **Walthard's i's,** see under *islet.*

incoagulability (in″ko-ag″u-lah-bil′ĭ-te) the state of being incapable of coagulation.

incoagulable (in″ko-ag′u-lah-b'l) not susceptible to coagulation.

incoherent (in″ko-hēr′ent) [L. *in* not + *cohaerere* to cling together] without proper sequence; incongruous.

incompatibility (in″kom-pat″ĭ-bil′ĭ-te) the quality of being incompatible. See also *histoincompatibility.* **chemical i.,** the quality of not being miscible with another given substance without a chemical change. **physiologic i.,** the quality of not being administrable with another given remedy on account of their antagonistic pharmacologic effects. **therapeutic i.,** opposition in therapeutic effect between two or more medicines.

incompatible (in″kom-pat′ĭ-b'l) [L. *incompatibilis*] not suitable for combination or simultaneous administration; mutually repellent. See also *histoincompatible.*

incompetence (in-kom′pe-tens) [L. *in* not + *competens* sufficient] 1. physical or mental inadequacy or insufficiency. 2. the legal status of a person determined by the court to be unable to manage his own affairs. **aortic i.,** see under *regurgitation.* **i. of the cardiac valves,** see *valvular regurgitation,* under *regurgitation.* **ileocecal i.,** inability of the ileocecal valve to prevent the flow of material from the colon to the ileum. **relative i.,** inadequate closure of a cardiac valve associated with dilatation of the corresponding ventricle of the heart. **valvular i.,** see *valvular regurgitation,* under *regurgitation.*

incompetency (in-kom′pe-ten″se) incompetence.

incompetent (in-kom′pe-tent) 1. lacking competence; unable to perform the required functions. 2. an individual who is unable to perform the required functions of everyday living. 3. a person determined by the court to be unable to manage his own affairs.

incompressible (in″kom-pres′ĭ-b'l) not susceptible of being squeezed together.

incontinence (in-kon′tĭ-nens) [L. *incontinentia*] 1. inability to control excretory functions, as defecation (fecal i.) or urination (urinary i.). 2. immoderation or excess. **active i.,** incontinence in which the bowels or bladder are emptied involuntarily, but at regular intervals and in the normal way. **fecal i., i. of the feces,** failure of voluntary control of the anal sphincters, with involuntary passage of feces and flatus. **intermittent i.,** loss of control of the urine on a sudden movement or on pressure on the bladder, due to interruption of the voluntary path above the lumbar center. **overflow i.,** urinary incontinence due to pressure of retained

urine in the bladder after the bladder has contracted to its limits, with dribbling of urine; called also *paradoxical i.* **paradoxical i.,** overflow i. **paralytic i.,** fecal and urinary incontinence caused by relaxation of the sphincters from destruction of the lumbar centers. **passive i.,** incontinence of urine in which the bladder is full and cannot be emptied in the normal way, but the urine dribbles away from mere pressure. **rectal i.,** fecal i. **stress i.,** involuntary discharge of urine due to anatomic displacement which exerts an opening pull on the bladder orifice, as in straining or coughing. **urinary i., i. of urine,** failure of voluntary control of the vesical and urethral sphincters, with constant or frequent involuntary passage of urine.

incontinent (in-kon′tĭ-nent) 1. unable to control excretory functions; see *incontinence.* 2. immoderate.

incontinentia (in-kon″tĭ-nen′she-ah) [L.] incontinence. **i. al′vi,** fecal incontinence. **Bloch-Sulzberger i. pigmen′ti,** i. pigmenti. **Naegeli's i. pigmen′ti,** Franceschetti-Jadassohn syndrome. **i. pigmen′ti,** a male-lethal X-linked dominant syndrome with onset at birth or shortly thereafter, characterized by the presence of brown or slate-brown bands, whorls, swirls, or splatter-like hyperpigmented cutaneous lesions, preceded by vesiculobullous and verrucous inflammatory changes, often associated with developmental anomalies involving other structures, such as the hair, eyes, and skeletal and central nervous systems. Called also *Bloch-Sulzberger i. pigmenti* and *Bloch-Sulzberger syndrome.* Cf. *Franceschetti-Jadassohn syndrome.* **i. pigmen′ti achro′mians,** a congenital neurocutaneous syndrome, not present at birth but appearing in early life, characterized by the presence of peculiar whorled, linear, and splatter-like patterns of hypopigmentation, and often associated with other abnormalities, including hair loss and ocular, musculoskeletal, and mental disturbances. It is unrelated to incontinentia pigmenti. Called also *hypomelanosis of Ito.* **i. uri′nae,** urinary incontinence.

incoordination (in″ko-or″dĭ-na′shun) [L. *in* not + *coordination*] lack of the normal adjustment of muscular motions; failure of organs to work harmoniously.

incorporation (in-kor″po-ra′shun) [L. *in* into + *corpus* body] 1. the union of one substance with another, or with others, in a composite mass. 2. in psychoanalytic theory, a primitive unconscious defense mechanism in which aspects of another person are assimilated into the self through a figurative process of symbolic oral ingestion.

incostapedial (ing″ko-sta-pe′de-al) pertaining to the incus and stapes.

increment (in′kre-ment) [L. *incrementum*] addition, or increase; the amount by which a given quantity or value is increased.

incretion (in-kre′shun) an internal secretion; (*obs.*) a hormone.

incross (in′kros) [*in-* (def. 1) + *cross* (def. 2)] the mating of individuals homozygous for the same gene; cf. *intercross.*

incrustation (in″krus-ta′shun) [L. *in* on + *crusta* crust] 1. the formation of a crust. 2. a crust, scale, or scab.

incubate (in′ku-bāt) [L. *incubare* to lie in or on; to watch over jealously] 1. to place in an optimal situation for development, as by provision of the proper temperature and humidity for the growth of living cells, such as ova, microorganisms, or tissue cells. 2. to maintain a culture or a reaction mixture at a fixed temperature. 3. material which has been incubated.

incubation (in″ku-ba′shun) [L. *incubatio*] 1. the development of the embryo in the eggs of oviparous animals. 2. the maintenance of an environment with controlled temperature, humidity, and oxygen for the development of an infant, especially of a premature one. 3. the development of an infectious disease from the entrance of the pathogen to the appearance of clinical symptoms (see also under *period,* and cf. *decubation*). 4. the development of microorganisms or other cells in an appropriate medium under controlled environmental conditions, especially of temperature, to permit optimum growth. 5. the process of maintaining reaction mixtures at a given temperature for specified time periods for the development of chemical or enzymatic reactions.

incubator (in′ku-ba-ter) 1. an apparatus for maintaining a premature infant in an environment of proper temperature and humidity. 2. an apparatus for maintaining a constant and suitable temperature for the development of eggs, cultures of microorganisms, or other living cells.

incubus (in′ku-bus) [L.] 1. a nightmare. 2. a heavy mental burden.

incudal (ing′ku-dal) [L. *incus* anvil] pertaining to the incus.

incudectomy (ing″ku-dek′to-me) [L. *incus* anvil + Gr. *ektomē* excision] surgical removal of the incus.

incudiform (ing-ku′dĭ-form) anvil-shaped.

incudomalleal (ing″ku-do-mal′e-al) pertaining to the incus and malleus.

incudostapedial (ing″ku-do-sta-pe′de-al) pertaining to the incus and stapes.

incurable (in-ku′rah-b'l) not susceptible of being cured.

incurvation (in″kur-va′shun) [L. *incurvare* to bend in] a condition of being bent in.

incus (ing′kus) [L. "anvil"] [NA] the middle of the three ossicles of the ear, which, with the stapes and malleus, serves to conduct vibrations from the tympanic membrane to the inner ear. See Plate accompanying *ear*. Called also *anvil*.

incyclophoria (in-si″klo-fo′re-ah) [L. *in* toward + *cyclophoria*] cyclophoria in which the upper pole of the vertical axis of the eye deviates toward the midline of the face, or toward the nose; called also *negative* or *minus cyclophoria*. Cf. *excyclophoria*.

incyclotropia (in-si″klo-tro′pe-ah) [L. *in* toward + *cyclotropia*] cyclotropia in which the upper pole of the vertical axis of the eye deviates toward the midline of the face, or toward the nose; called also *negative* or *minus cyclotropia*.

in d. abbreviation for L. *in di′es*, daily.

indacrinic acid (in″da-krin′ik) INN for indacrinone.

indacrinone (in″da-kri′nōn) a uricosuric diuretic.

indanedione (in″dān-di′ōn) any of a group of synthetic anticoagulants derived from 1,3-indanedione, including phenindione, chemically different from the coumarin (q.v.) drugs but similar to them in structure and actions, i.e., they impair the hepatic synthesis of the vitamin K–dependent coagulation factors (prothrombin, Factors VII, IX, and X).

Indecidua (in″de-sid′u-ah) a division of the class Mammalia, comprising the mammals without a decidua, including whales and ungulates.

indenization (in-den″i-za′shun) innidiation.

indentation (in″den-ta′shun) [L. *indentatio; dens* tooth] 1. a condition of being notched; a notch, pit, or depression. 2. the act of indenting, as with the finger.

Inderal (in′der-al) trademark for a preparation of propranolol hydrochloride.

Inderide (in′der-īd) trademark for preparations of propranolol hydrochloride with hydrochlorothiazide.

index (in′deks), pl. *indexes* or *in′dices* [L.] 1. [NA], the second digit of the hand, or forefinger; the finger adjacent to the thumb; called also *digitus secundus* (II) *manus* [NA alternative]. 2. a dimensionless quantity, usually a ratio of two measurable quantities having the same dimensions, or such a ratio multiplied by 100. 3. a core or mold used in dentistry to record or maintain the relative position of a tooth or teeth to one another and/or to a cast, to ensure reproduction in the dental prosthesis of their original position. **absorbancy i.** absorptivity. **ACH i.,** an index for nutritional condition of children based on measurements of arm girth, chest depth, and hip width. **air velocity i.** (*obs.*), the ratio between the maximal breathing capacity and the vital capacity. **altitudinal i.,** the relation of the cranial height to the cranial length; called also *height i.* and *length-height i.* **alveolar i.,** gnathic i. **antitryptic i.,** a number representing the increased viscosity of a solution of casein treated with trypsin to which the blood serum of a cancer patient has been added, as compared with the viscosity after the same procedure in which the blood serum is normal. **Arneth i.,** see under *count*. **auricular i.,** the relation of the width to the height of the auricle of the ear. **auriculoparietal i.,** the ratio of the breadth of the skull between the auricular points to its greatest breadth. **auriculovertical i.,** the ratio of the height of the skull above the auricular point to its greatest height. **Ayala i.,** see under *quotient*. **baric i.,** 100 times the body weight divided by the cube of the stature. **basilar i.,** the ratio of the distance between the basion and the alveolar point to the total length of the skull. **Becker-Lennhoff i.,** Lenn-

hoff's i. **biochemical racial i.,** the ratio of the percentage of persons having agglutinogen A in their erythrocytes to the percentage having agglutinogen B, or the ratio of persons of blood group II to those of blood group III. **body build i.,** body weight divided by the square of the stature. **Bouchard's i.** (of adiposity or emaciation), the weight in kilograms divided by the height in decimeters; in a normal adult male each decimeter of height weighs 4200 gm. **brachial i.,** 100 times the length of the forearm divided by the length of the upper arm. **Broders' i.,** an index of malignancy based on the fact that the more undifferentiated or embryonic the cells of a tumor, the more malignant the tumor. Grade 1 contains one fourth undifferentiated cells; Grade 2, one half undifferentiated cells; Grade 3, three fourths undifferentiated cells; Grade 4, all cells undifferentiated. **Brugsch i.,** chest circumference × 100 divided by body length. **calcium i.,** the relative amount of calcium in the blood compared with that in a 1:6000 solution of calcium oxide. **cardiac i.,** the minute cardiac output per square meter of body surface; a normal average is 2.8 liters. **cardiothoracic i.,** the size of the heart in relation to the size of the chest, being the greatest transverse diameter of the heart shadow as compared with the greatest transverse diameter of the chest shadow on radioscopy. **I.-Catalogue,** Index-Catalogue of the Library of the Surgeon General's Office, published from 1880 to 1950; replaced by Current List of Medical Literature published to 1959; in 1960 replaced by Index Medicus. **centromeric i.,** the ratio of the length of the shorter arm of a mitotic chromosome to the total length of the chromosome. **cephalic i.,** 100 times the maximal head breadth divided by the maximal head length. **cephalo-orbital i.,** 100 times the capacity of the cranium divided by the capacity of the two orbits. **cephalorhachidian i.,** cerebrospinal i. **cephalospinal i.,** the ratio of the area of the foramen magnum in square meters and the cranial capacity in cubic centimeters. **cerebral i.,** the ratio of the greatest transverse to the greatest anteroposterior diameter of the cranial cavity. **cerebrospinal i.,** the figure obtained by multiplying the final cerebrospinal pressure by the quantity of fluid withdrawn in spinal puncture and then dividing by the initial pressure. **chemotherapeutic i.,** therapeutic i. **color i.,** an outmoded concept for an expression of the relative amount of hemoglobin contained in a red blood corpuscle compared with that of a normal individual of the patient's age and sex; divide the percentage of hemoglobin by the percentage of erythrocytes. **Colour I.,** a publication of the Society of Dyers and Colourists and the American Association of Textile Chemists and Colorists containing an extensive list of dyes and dye intermediates. Each chemically distinct compound is identified by a specific number, the C.I. number, avoiding the confusion of trivial names used for dyes in the dye industry. **coronofrontal i.,** the ratio of the greatest frontal to the greatest coronal breadth of the head. **cranial i.,** 100 times the maximal breadth of the skull divided by its length. **Cumulated I. Medicus,** an annual publication of the National Library of Medicine, comprising the twelve monthly issues of the Index Medicus. **degenerative i.,** the percentage of neutrophils exhibiting toxic granulation (basophilic granules probably representing phagosomes or autophagic vacuoles). **dental i.,** a craniometric index obtained by multiplying the dental length by 100 and dividing the product by the basinasal length. Called also *Flower's i.* **effective temperature i.,** an index indicating the warmth due to air temperature, air movement, and humidity. **endemic i.,** the percentage of persons in any locality affected with an endemic disease. **erythrocyte indices** see *MCH, MCHC,* and *MCV.* **facial i.,** the relation of the length of the face to its width, obtained by multiplying by 100 the bizygomatic width and dividing the product by the distance from the ophryon to the alveolar point. **femorohumeral i.,** 100 times the length of the upper arm divided by the length of the thigh. **Flower's i.,** dental i. **forearm-hand i.,** 100 times the length of the hand divided by the length of the forearm. **Fourmentin's thoracic i.,** the number obtained by multiplying the transverse diameter of the thorax by 100 and dividing by the anteroposterior diameter. **gnathic i.,** the degree of prominence of the upper jaw, expressed as a percentage of the distance from basion to nasion. Called also *alveolar i.* **habitus i.,** 100 times the sum of the chest girth and the abdominal girth divided by the stature. **hair i.,** the figure obtained by dividing the least diameter of the cross section of a hair by its greatest diameter and multiplying by 100; a high index indicates an approximately round shape; a low index indicates an ovoid cross section. **hand i.,** 100 times the breadth of the hand divided by the length of the hand. **hematopneic i.,** a figure denoting the intensity of blood oxygenation. **hemorenal i., hemorenal salt i.,** the ratio of the amount of inorganic salts in the urine to that in the blood, obtained by dividing the electric resistance of the blood by that of the urine. **Hench-Aldrich i.,** see under *test*. **icteric i., icterus i.** (*obs.*) a measure of the degree of icterus in serum based on comparison of the serum absorbance at 460 nm with that of a standard potassium dichromate solution. **intermembral i.,** 100 times the length of the entire arm divided by the length of the entire leg. **juxtaglomerular i.,** semiquantitative estimation of the degree of granulation of juxtaglomerular cells, obtained by a counting method and expressed as a ratio to the number of glomeruli. **Kaup i.,** weight divided by length of the body squared. **length-breadth i.,** the breadth of the skull expressed as a percentage of its length. **length-height i.,** the height of the skull expressed as a percentage of its length. **Lennhoff's i.,** the number obtained by dividing 100 times the distance from the sternal notch to the symphysis pubis by the greatest circumference of the abdomen. **Livi's i.,** $100 \times \sqrt[3]{P;6}$, in which P = body weight in grams × body length in centimeters. **lower leg-foot i.,** 100 times the length of the foot divided by the length of the lower leg. **maxilloalveolar i.,** the distance between the two most lateral points on the external surface of the upper alveolar margin, usually opposite the middle of the second permanent molar teeth, divided by the maxilloalveolar length. **I. Medicus,** a monthly publication of the National Library of Medicine in which the world's leading biomedical literature is indexed by author and subject; see also *Cumulated I. Medicus*. **metacarpal i.,** the average of the figures obtained by dividing the lengths of the right second, third, fourth, and fifth metacarpal bones by their respective breadths at the exact midpoint; stated to range normally between 5.4 and 7.9. A value above 8.4 is diagnostic of arachnodactyly. **mitotic i.,** the ratio of the number of cells in a population undergoing mitosis to the number not undergoing mitosis. **morphological i.,** the volume of the trunk divided by the length of the limbs. **morphologic face i.,** 100 times the distance from the nasion to the gnathion divided by the bizygomatic breadth. **nasal i.,** 100 times the maximal breadth of the nasal aperture divided by the nasion-nasospinale height. **nucleoplasmic i.,** the relation of the size of the nucleus of a cell to that of the cytoplasm, expressed numerically by the quotient of the nuclear volume divided by the difference between the volume of the cell and the nuclear volume. **obesity i.,** body weight divided by body volume. **opsonic i.,** a measure of opsonic activity determined by the ratio of the number of microorganisms phagocytized by normal leukocytes in the presence of serum from an individual infected by the microorganism, to the number phagocytized in serum from a normal individual. **orbital i. (of Broca),** 100 times the height of the opening of the orbit, divided by its width. **palatal i., palatine i., palatomaxillary i.,** a numerical expression of the ratio of various proportions of the palate obtained by multiplying the palatal breadth by 100 and dividing the product by the palatal length. See also *brachystaphyline* and *leptostaphyline*. **parasite i.,** the percentage of individuals in a population whose blood smears show the presence of malarial parasites. **phagocytic i.,** any arbitrary measure of the ability of neutrophils to ingest native or opsonized particles determined by various assays; it reflects either the average number of particles ingested or the rate at which particles are cleared from the blood or culture medium. **physiognomonic upper face i.,** 100 times the distance from the nasion to the stomion divided by the bizygomatic breadth. **Pignet i.,** see under *formula*. **Pirquet's i.** (of nutritional status), multiply the weight in grams by 10, divide this product by the sitting height in centimeters and extract the cube root of this quotient. A result lower than 0.945 indicates faulty nutrition. See also *pelidisi*. **ponderal i.,** an index of body mass determined by dividing the height in inches by the cube root of the weight in pounds. **Quarterly Cumulative I. Medicus,** a former publication of the American Medical Association, in which was indexed most of the medical literature in the world; replaced by Cumulated I. Medicus.

radiohumeral i., 100 times the maximal length of the radius divided by the maximal length of the humerus. **refractive i.,** the refractive power of a medium compared with that of air, which is assumed to be 1. Symbol n, or n_D. **Röhrer's i.** (of the state of nutrition), multiply the weight in grams by 100 and divide the product by the cube of the height in centimeters. **sacral i.,** 100 times the breadth of the sacrum divided by the length. **salivary urea i.,** see *Hench-Aldrich test*, under *tests*. **short increment sensitivity i. (SISI),** tones of 1- to 5-decibel increments in intensity and lasting 0.5 second are superimposed on a continuous (carrier) tone of the same frequency at random intervals, the carrier tone being 20 decibels above the speech reception threshold; only patients with cochlear damage can detect these increments. **spleen i., splenic i.,** the percentage of individuals in the population having enlarged spleens; used in malaria surveys. **splenometric i.,** an index of the amount of malarial infection; obtained by multiplying the spleen rate by the average enlarged spleen. **stimulation i. (SI),** see *lymphocyte proliferation test*, under *tests*. **therapeutic i.,** originally, the ratio of the maximum tolerated dose to the minimum curative dose; now defined, so as to account for variability of individual response, as the ratio of the median lethal dose (LD_{50}) to the median effective dose (ED_{50}). It is used in assessing the safety of a drug. Called also *chemotherapeutic i.* **thoracic i.,** the ratio of the anteroposterior diameter of the thorax to the transverse diameter. **tibiofemoral i.,** 100 times the length of the lower leg divided by the length of the thigh. **tibioradial i.,** 100 times the length of the forearm divided by the length of the lower leg. **trunk i.,** 100 times the bi-acromial breadth divided by the sitting suprasternale height. **ureosecretory i.,** see *Ambard's formula*, under *formula*. **uricolytic i.,** the percentage of uric acid oxidized to allantoin before being secreted. **vertical i.,** 100 times the height of the skull divided by the length of the skull. **vital i.,** the ratio of births to deaths within a given time in a population; called also *birth-death ratio*. **xanthoproteic i.,** see *Mulder's test* (def. 2), under *tests*. **zygomaticoauricular i.,** the ratio between the zygomatic and auricular diameters of the skull.

indican (in′dĭ-kan) 1. a yellow indoxyl glycoside, C_6H_4·NH·CH:C·O·$C_6H_{11}O_5$, from plants that yield indigo. On hydrolysis it yields glucose and indoxyl. 2. potassium indoxyl sulfate, $C_6H_4NH·CH·CO·SO_2·OK$, formed by decomposition of trytophan in the intestines, absorbed, conjugated, and excreted in the urine.

indicanemia (in″dĭ-kan-e′me-ah) [*indican* + Gr. *haima* blood + *-ia*] the presence of indican in the blood.

indicanmeter (in″dĭ-kan-me′ter) an instrument for estimating the amount of indican in the urine.

indicanorachia (in″dĭ-kan-o-ra′ke-ah) the presence of indican in the spinal fluid.

indicant (in′dĭ-kant) 1. indicating. 2. a symptom which indicates the true diagnosis or treatment.

indicanuria (in″dĭ-kan-u′re-ah) [*indican* + *-uria*] the presence in the urine of indican in excessive quantity.

indicarmine (in″dĭ-kar′min) indigotindisulfonate sodium.

indicatio (in″dĭ-ka′she-o) [L., from *indicare* to point out] indication. **i. causa′lis,** an indication as to the treatment of a disease afforded by its cause. **i. curati′va, i. mor′bi,** an indication as to treatment afforded by the nature of the morbid processes observed. **i. symptomat′ica,** an indication as to disease afforded by the symptoms that may arise.

indication (in″dĭ-ka′shun) [L. *indicatio*] a sign or circumstance which points to or shows the cause, pathology, treatment, or issue of an attack of disease; that which points out; that which serves as a guide or warning.

indicator (in′dĭ-ka″ter) [L.] 1. the index finger (index [NA]). 2. the extensor muscle of the index finger (musculus extensor indicis [NA]). 3. any substance which, when added in small quantities, shows the appearance or disappearance of a chemical individual by a conspicuous change of color or the attainment of a certain pH. **anaerobic i.,** a dilute solution of methylene blue is decolorized in the absence of oxygen. **Andrade's i.,** a solution of acid fuchsin in water, decolorized to a yellow color by sodium hydroxide, and added to peptone-water sugar culture medium. An acid-producing organism cultivated in this broth turns the medium magenta red. **dew point i.,** an instrument for measuring relative humidity or moisture content of a gas by measuring its dew point. **radioactive i.,** see under *tracer.* **redox i.,** a pigment which indicates by a change of color the change in pH. **Schneider's i.,** an index designed to reflect cardiovascular fitness, based mainly on heart rate during and after mild exercise.

indicophose (in′dĭ-ko″fōz) an indigo-colored phose.

Indiella (in″de-el′ah) former name for the genus *Madurella.*

indifférence (ahn-de″fa-rahns′) [Fr.] indifference. **belle i.** (bel″ahn-de″fa-rahns′) [Fr. "beautiful indifference"], an inappropriately complacent attitude toward their condition and symptoms shown by individuals who have a conversion disorder.

indifferent (in-dif′er-ent) [L. *indifferens*] not tending one way or another; neutral; having no preponderating affinity.

indigenous (in-dij′ĕ-nus) [L. *indigenus*] native, or not exotic; native to a particular place or country.

indigestible (in″di-jes′tĭ-b'l) [*in*- neg. + *digestible*] not susceptible of being digested.

indigestion (in″di-jes′chun) lack or failure of digestion; commonly used to denote vague abdominal discomfort after meals. **acid i.,** hyperchlorhydria. **fat i.,** inability to digest fat; steatorrhea. **gastric i.,** indigestion taking place in or due to some disorder of the stomach. **intestinal i.,** imperfect performance of the digestive function of the intestine. **nervous i.,** nervous dyspepsia. **sugar i.,** defective ability to digest sugar, resulting in fermentative diarrhea.

indigitation (in-dij″ĭ-ta′shun) [L. *in* into + *digitus* finger] intussusception (def. 1), or invagination.

indiglucin (in″dĭ-gloo′sin) a sweet substance obtained together with indigo on the decomposition of plant indican.

indigo (in′dĭ-go) [Gr. *Indikon* Indian dye] a blue dyeing material from various leguminous and other plants (*Indigofera tinctoria,* etc.), being the aglycone of indican; also made synthetically. It is sometimes found in the sweat and the urine, where it is derived from urinary indican (indoxyl sulfate).

indigogen (in′dĭ-go-jen) a crystalline principle from indigo.

indigopurpurine (in″dĭ-go-pur′pu-rin) a purple pigment occasionally found in the urine.

indigotin (in″dĭ-go′tin) a neutral, tasteless, dark blue powder, $C_{16}H_{10}N_2O_2$, the principal ingredient of commercial indigo; called also *indigo blue.*

indigotindisulfonate sodium (in″dĭ-go″tin-di-sul′fo-nāt) [USP] chemical name: 2-(1,3-dihydro-3-oxo-5-sulfo-2H-indol-2-ylidene)-2, 3-dihydro-3-oxo-1H-indole-5-sulfonic acid disodium salt. A dye, $C_{16}H_8N_2Na_2O_8S$, occurring as a dusky, purplish blue powder or blue granules; used as a diagnostic aid for determining renal function, administered intravenously. Called also *indigo carmine, indicarmine,* and *soluble indigo blue.*

indirect (in″di-rekt′) [L. *indirectus*] 1. not immediate or straight. 2. acting through an intermediary agent.

indirubin (in″di-roo′bin) a red pigment occasionally found in the urine.

indirubinuria (in″di-roo″bin-u′re-ah) the presence of indirubin in the urine.

indiscriminate (in″dis-krim′ĭ-nāt) [L. *in* not + *discrimen* distinction] affecting various parts without distinction.

indisposition (in″dis-po-zish′un) the condition of being slightly ill; a slight illness.

indium (in′de-um) [L. *indicum* indigo] a metallic element; atomic number, 49; atomic weight, 114.82; symbol, In; named from its blue line in the spectrum. It is used in semiconductor research and in bearing alloys.

individuation (in″dĭ-vid″u-a′shun) 1. the process of developing individual characteristics. 2. differential regional activity in the embryo occurring in response to organizer influence.

Indocin (in′do-sin) trademark for a preparation of indomethacin.

Indoklon (in-dok′lon) trademark for flurothyl. See also under *therapy.*

indolaceturia (in″do-las″ĕ-tu′re-ah) the presence of indolacetic acid in the urine; excessive amounts of 5-

OH-indoleacetic acid, the urinary metabolite of serotonin, may be excreted when carcinoid tumors are present.

indolamine (in-dol′ah-mēn) [*indole* + *amine*] any derivative, of indole, e.g., serotonin or melatonin.

indole (in′dōl) a heterocyclic compound, M.W. 117.14, obtained from coal tar, and produced by the decomposition of tryptophan in the intestine, being partly responsible for the peculiar odor of the feces. It is also found in cultures of *Vibrio cholerae* and other bacteria; a color test for its production is used in classifying enteric bacteria.

indolent (in′do-lent) [L. *in* not + *dolens* painful] causing little pain, as an *indolent* tumor; slow growing, as an indolent lesion.

indologenous (in″do-loj′ĕ-nus) [*indole* + Gr. *gennan* to produce] causing the formation of indole.

indoluria (in″dōl-u′re-ah) the presence of indole in the urine.

indomethacin (in″do-meth′ah-sin) [USP] a nonsteroidal anti-inflammatory agent; used in the treatment of rheumatoid arthritis, osteoarthritis, ankylosing spondylitis, and acute gouty arthritis.

indophenol (in″do-fe′nol) any one of a series of dyes which are nitrogen derivatives of quinone.

indoprofen (in″do-pro′fen) chemical name: 2-(1,3-dihydro-1-oxo-2H-isoindol-2-yl)-α-methylbenzeneacetic acid; an analgesic and anti-inflammatory, $C_{17}H_{15}NO_3$.

indoramin (in-dor′ah-min) chemical name: *N*-[1-[2-(1H-indol-3-yl)ethyl] - 4 - piperidyl] benzamide; an antihypertensive, $C_{22}H_{25}N_3O$.

indoxyl (in-dok′sil) [Gr. *indikon* indigo + *oxys* sharp] an oxidation product of indole, $C_6H_4 \cdot C(OH){:}CH \cdot NH$, formed by decomposition from tryptophan, and excreted in the urine as indican (potassium indoxyl sulfate).

indoxylemia (in-dok″sil-e′me-ah) [*indoxyl* + *-emia*] the presence of indoxyl in the blood.

indoxyl-sulfate (in-dok′sil-sul′fāt) a compound found in the urine in some cases in which great putrefactive changes are occurring in the intestine.

indoxyluria (in″dok-sil-u′re-ah) [*indoxyl* + *-uria*] the presence of an excess of indoxyl in the urine.

indriline hydrochloride (in′drĭ-lēn) chemical name: *N,N*-dimethyl-1-phenyl-1H-inden-1-ethylamine hydrochloride; a central nervous system stimulant, $C_{19}H_{21}N \cdot HCl$.

induced (in-dūst′) [L. *inducere* to lead in] 1. produced artificially. 2. produced by induction.

inducer (in-dūs′er) in molecular genetics, a molecule that causes a cell or organism to accelerate synthesis of the enzyme or sequence of enzymes involved in the metabolism of the inducing compound. The inducer often acts by antagonizing the action of a corresponding repressor.

inductance (in-duk′tans) that property of a circuit by virtue of which a magnetic field is associated with the circuit when the circuit is carrying current. The unit of inductance, or "self-induction," is the henry.

induction (in-duk′shun) [L. *inductio*] 1. the act or process of inducing or causing to occur, especially the production of a specific morphogenetic effect in the developing embryo through the influence of evocators or organizers, or the production of anesthesia or unconsciousness by use of appropriate agents. 2. the appearance of an electric current or of magnetic properties in a body because of the presence of another electric current or magnetic field nearby. **autonomous i.,** induction in which the inductor forms no part of the portion produced. **complementary i.,** induction in which the inductor forms a part of the portion produced. **enzyme i.,** in bacterial genetics, the synthesis of certain enzymes in response to the presence of the substrate (or of an analogue). In inducible enzyme systems, genes coding for the enzymes involved in metabolism of the substrate, linked in an operon, are expressed only in the presence of the substrate. **somatic i.,** the production of new characters through the influence of the soma on the germ cells. **Spemann's i.,** the stimulating and directing effect shown by certain tissues on neighboring tissues or parts in early development of the embryo. **spinal i.,** that process by which one reflex lowers the threshold of another reflex which otherwise cannot be penetrated.

inductogram (in-duk′to-gram) roentgenogram.

inductor (in-duk′ter) a tissue elaborating a chemical substance which acts to determine the growth and differentiation of embryonic parts. Cf. *activator* (def. 2) and *organizer.*

inductorium (in″duk-to′re-um) an apparatus for generating currents of induced electricity; as in physiological experiments.

inductotherm (in-duk′to-therm) an apparatus for producing high body temperature by electric induction.

inductothermy (in-duk′to-ther″me) the production of artificial fever by electric induction.

indulin (in′du-lĭn) a coal tar dye, used as a histologic stain.

indulinophil (in″du-lin′o-fil) 1. an element easily stainable with indulin. 2. indulinophilic.

indulinophilic (in″du-lin-o-fil′ik) [*indulin* + Gr. *philein* to love] stainable with indulin.

indurated (in′du-rāt″ed) [L. *indurare* to harden] hardened; rendered hard.

induration (in″du-ra′shun) [L. *induratio*] 1. the quality of being hard; the process of hardening. 2. an abnormally hard spot or place. **black i.,** the hardening and pigmentation of lung tissue seen in pneumonia. **brawny i.,** inflammatory hardening and thickening of tissues. **brown i.,** 1. a deposit of altered blood pigment in the lung in pneumonia. 2. marked increase of the connective tissue of the lung and excessive pigmentation, due to long-continued congestion from valvular heart disease or to anthracosis. **cyanotic i.,** a congested, dense, and purple state of the kidney in which the blood current is slowed and the transudation of fluid through the glomeruli is impeded. **fibroid i.,** cirrhosis. **Froriep's i.,** myositis fibrosa. **granular i.,** cirrhosis. **gray i.,** an induration of lung tissue in or after pneumonia, without pigmentation. **laminate i.,** a thin layer of round-cell infiltration of the corium in chancre. **parchment i.,** laminate i. **penile i.,** Peyronie's disease. **phlebitic i.,** indurated cellulitis. **plastic i.,** sclerosis of the corpora cavernosa of the penis. **red i.,** interstitial pneumonia in which the lung is red and congested.

indurative (in′du-ra″tiv) pertaining to or marked by induration.

indusium griseum (in-du′ze-um gris′e-um) [L.] [NA] a thin layer of gray substance on the dorsal aspect of the corpus callosum; called also *supracallosal gyrus* and *gyrus supracallosus.*

-ine a suffix indicating an alkaloid, an organic base, or a halogen.

inebriant (in-e′bre-ant) [L. *inebriare* to make drunk] 1. an inebriating agent. 2. inebriating.

inebriation (in-e″bre-a′shun) [L. *inebriatio*] the condition of being drunk.

inebriety (in″ĕ-bri′ĕ-te) [L. *in* intensive + *ebrietas* drunkenness] habitual drunkenness.

inelastic (in″e-las′tik) lacking elasticity.

Inermicapsifer (in-er″mĭ-kap′sĭ-fer) a genus of tapeworms, family Linstowiidae, parasitic in hyraxes and rodents in Africa; *I. arvicanthidis* has been found in humans in Cuba and Central America.

inert (in-ert′) having no action; not reacting with other elements, as inert gases.

inertia (in-er′she-ah) [L.] inactivity; inability to move spontaneously. **colonic i.,** weak muscular activity of the colon, leading to distention of the organ and constipation. **immunological i.,** specific depression of immunity in a mother toward the histocompatibility antigens of a fetus, or in a fetus toward those of the mother; it does not include immunologic tolerance. **i. u′teri,** sluggishness of the uterine contractions during labor.

in extremis (in ek-stre′mis) [L. "at the end"] at the point of death.

Inf. abbreviation for L. *infun′de,* pour in.

infancy (in′fan-se) the early period of life; see *infant.*

infant (in′fant) [L. *infans; in* neg. + *fans* speaking] a young child; considered to designate the human young from birth or from the termination of the newborn period (the first four weeks of life) to the time of assumption of erect posture (12 to 14 months); it is regarded by some to extend to the end of the first 24 months. **floppy i.,** see under *syndrome.*

immature i., one weighing 500 to 999 grams (17 ounces to 2.2 pounds) at birth, usually before the twenty-eighth week of gestation, and having an extremely poor chance of survival. **mature i.,** one weighing 2500 grams (5.5 pounds) or more at birth, usually at or near full term, and having an optimum chance of survival. **newborn i.,** the human young during the first two to four weeks after birth. **postmature i., post-term i.,** an infant born at any time after the beginning of the forty-second week (288 days) of gestation. **premature i.,** one usually born after the twenty-seventh week and before full term, and arbitrarily defined as an infant weighing 1000 to 2499 grams (2.2 to 5.5 lbs.) at birth, having poor to good chance of survival, depending on the weight. In countries where adults are smaller than in the United States, the upper limit is 2250 grams (5 lbs.). Other criteria such as crown-heel length (less than 47 cm.) and occipitofrontal diameter (less than 11.5 cm.) have also been used. **preterm i.,** an infant born at any time before the thirty-seventh completed week (259 days) of gestation. **term i.,** an infant born anytime from the beginning of the thirty-eighth week (260 days) to the end of the forty-first week (287 days) of gestation.

infanticide (in-fan′tĭ-sīd) [L. *infans* infant + *caedere* to kill] the taking of the life of an infant.

infanticulture (in-fan′tĭ-kul″tūr) puericulture.

infantile (in′fan-tīl) [L. *infantilis*] pertaining to an infant or to infancy.

infantilism (in′fan-tĭ-lizm″, in-fan′tĭ-lizm) a condition in which the characters of childhood persist into adult life; it is marked by mental retardation, underdevelopment of the sexual organs, and often, but not always, by dwarfism. Cf. *progeria.* **Brissaud's i.,** infantile myxedema. **cachetic i.,** infantilism due to chronic infection or poisoning. **celiac i.,** infantilism resulting from the infantile form of nontropical sprue (celiac disease); see under *sprue.* **dysthyroidal i.,** infantilism due to defective thyroid activity. **hepatic i.,** infantilism associated with hepatic cirrhosis. **Herter's i.,** the infantile form of nontropical sprue; see under *sprue.* **hypophysial i.,** a type of dwarfism, with retention of infantile characteristics, due to undersecretion of the growth hormone and the gonadotropic hormones of the anterior pituitary gland (adenohypophysis); called also *pituitary infantilism, pituitary dwarfism, Levi-Lorain dwarfism,* and *ateleiosis.* **intestinal i.,** the infantile form of nontropical sprue; see under *sprue.* **Levi-Lorain i., Lorain's i.,** hypophysial i. **lymphatic i.,** infantilism associated with lymphatism. **myxedematous i.,** cretinism. **pancreatic i.,** a form caused by defective pancreatic action. **partial i.,** arrested development of a single part or tissue. **pituitary i.,** hypophysial i. **regressive i.,** reversion to an infantile state after body growth has been completed. **renal i.,** renal osteodystrophy. **sexual i.,** retardation of sexual development, as in adiposogenital dystrophy. **symptomatic i.,** infantilism due to general defective development of tissues. **toxemic i.** (*obs.*), the infantile form of nontropical sprue; see under *sprue.* **universal i.,** general dwarfishness in stature with absence of the secondary sexual characteristics.

infantorium (in″fan-to′re-um) a hospital for the newborn and young infants.

infarct (in′farkt) [L. *infarctus*] an area of coagulation necrosis in a tissue due to local ischemia resulting from obstruction of circulation to the area, most commonly by a thrombus or embolus. See also *infarction.* **anemic i.,** an area of necrosis in a tissue produced by sudden arrest of circulation in a vessel; called also *pale i.* and *white i.* **bilirubin i's,** masses of crystals of bilirubin in the pyramids of the kidneys, especially in the newborn. **bland i.,** an uninfected infarct. **bone i.,** an area of bone tissue which has become necrotic as a result of loss of its arterial blood supply. **Brewer's i's,** dark-red, wedge-shaped areas, resembling infarcts, seen on section of a kidney in pyelonephritis. **calcareous i.,** a deposit of calcium salt in the tissues. **cystic i.,** an infarct enclosed in a membrane. **embolic i.,** one caused by an embolus. **hemorrhagic i.,** an infarct that is red in color owing to the oozing of red corpuscles into the dead area; called also *red i.* **pale i.,** anemic i. **red i.,** hemorrhagic i. **septic i.,** one in which the tissues have been invaded by pathogenic organisms. **thrombotic i.,** one caused by a thrombus. **uric acid i.,** a deposit of uric acid crystals in the renal tubules of the newborn. **white i.,** anemic i.

infarctectomy (in″fark-tek′to-me) surgical removal of an infarct.

infarction (in-fark′shun) [L. *infarcire* to stuff in] 1. the formation of an infarct. 2. an infarct. **anterior myocardial i.,** infarction localized to the left ventricular free wall between the interventricular groove and the lateral margin of the anterior papillary muscle; it is characterized electrocardiographically by abnormal Q waves in V_3 or V_4. **anteroinferior myocardial i.,** one involving features of both anterior and inferior myocardial infarction. **anterolateral myocardial i.,** one involving features of both anterior and lateral myocardial infarction. **anteroseptal myocardial i.,** one involving features of both anterior and septal myocardial infarction. **atrial i.,** the formation of an infarct in a cardiac atrium, which may be due to coronary artery occlusion, periarteritis nodosa, obliterating endarteritis of the small branches of coronary arteries, or other conditions. **cardiac i.,** myocardial i. **cerebral i.,** an ischemic condition of the brain, producing a persistent focal neurological deficit in the area of distribution of one of the cerebral arteries. **Freiberg's i.,** Köhler's bone disease, def. 2. **inferior myocardial i.,** one localized in the region between the lateral border of the posterior papillary muscle and the posterior septum; it is characterized electrocardiographically by abnormal Q waves in lead II, III, or aV_F. **inferolateral myocardial i.,** one involving features of both inferior and lateral myocardial infarction. **intestinal i.,** occlusion of an artery or arteriole in the wall of the intestine, resulting in the formation of an area of coagulation necrosis. **lateral myocardial i.,** infarction in the region between the lateral margin of the anterior papillary muscle and the lateral margin of the posterior papillary muscle; it is marked electrocardiographically by abnormal Q waves in V_5 or V_6. **mesenteric i.,** coagulation necrosis of the intestines due to a decrease in blood flow in the mesenteric vasculature; it may be caused by occlusion of the mesenteric arteries or by cardiogenic abnormalities or hypovolemia (*nonocclusive mesenteric i.*). **myocardial i.,** gross necrosis of the myocardium, as a result of interruption of the blood supply to the area, as in coronary thrombosis. **posterior myocardial i.,** one localized in the basal third

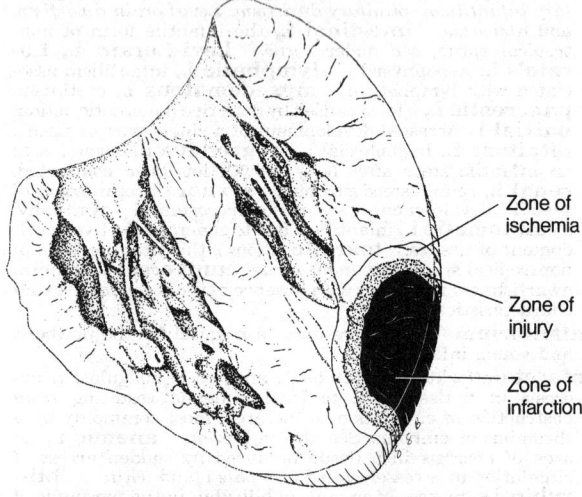

Zone of ischemia

Zone of injury

Zone of infarction

Myocardial infarction shown in cross-section of heart (ventricles only).

of the posteroinferior heart wall; it is characterized electrocardiographically by abnormal R waves in V_1 or V_2. **pulmonary i.,** localized necrosis of lung tissue caused by obstruction of the arterial blood supply, most often due to pulmonary embolism. Clinical manifestations range from the nonexistent to pleuritic chest pain, dyspnea, hemoptysis, and tachycardia. **septal myocardial i.,** one localized to the interventricular septum and characterized electrocardiographically by abnormal Q waves in V_1 or V_2. **transmural myocardial i.,** one involving the entire thickness of the heart wall.

infaust (in′fowst) [L. *infaustus* unlucky] unfavorable.

infectible (in-fek′tĭ-b'l) capable of being infected.

infection (in-fek′shun) 1. invasion and multiplication of microorganisms in body tissues, which may be clinically inapparent or result in local cellular injury due to competitive metabolism, toxins, intracellular replication, or antigen-antibody response. The infection may remain localized, subclinical, and temporary if the body's defensive mechanisms are effective. A local infection may persist and spread by extension to become an acute, subacute, or chronic clinical infection or disease state. A local infection may also become systemic when the microorganisms gain access to the lymphatic or vascular system. 2. an infectious disease. Cf. *infestation.* **airborne i.,** an infection that is contracted by inhalation of microorganisms or spores suspended in air on water droplets or dust particles. Microorganisms are often rendered airborne as a result of a sneeze or cough. Cf. *droplet nuclei,* under *nucleus.* **apical i.,** infection situated at the apex of the root of a tooth. **colonization i.,** an infection characterized by the attachment and subsequent growth of the invading microorganism on or within tissue. **cross i.,** infection transmitted between individuals infected with different pathogenic microorganisms. **cryptogenic i.,** infection whose pathogenesis is unclear or undefinable, as salmonella arteritis with no preceding salmonella infection elsewhere. **droplet i.,** see *droplet nuclei,* under *nuclei.* **dust-borne i.,** airborne infection by pathogens which have become affixed to particles of dust and are transmitted by that means. **ectogenous i.,** exogenous i. **endogenous i.,** infection due to reactivation of organisms present in a dormant focus, as occurs in tuberculosis, histoplasmosis, coccidioidomycosis, etc. **exogenous i.,** infection caused by organisms not normally present in the body but which have gained entrance from the environment. **germinal i.,** transmission of infection to the child by means of the ovum or sperm of the parent. **iatrogenic i.,** see *iatrogenic.* **inapparent i.,** an infection with no clinical symptoms that is unnoticed by the affected individual; cf. *subclinical i.* **latent i.,** 1. a phase during the course of some established infections during which the pathogenic microorganisms are dormant and manifestations of disease that may have been recognizable earlier are no longer detectable, as in latent syphilis. 2. infection in which the etiologic agent has not yet produced or does not produce symptoms. **mass i.,** infection produced by a large number of pathogenic organisms in the circulation. **mixed i.,** infection of an organ or tissue by more than one microorganism, as in wound infections, abscesses, pneumonia, and rarely meningitis and endocarditis; mixtures of every type occur, e.g., bacterial and viral, bacterial and fungal, and protozoan and viral. Called also *polyinfection.* **nosocomial i.,** see *nosocomial.* **opportunistic i.,** infection by an organism that does not ordinarily cause disease but that, under certain circumstances (e.g., impaired immune responses), becomes pathogenic. **pyogenic i.,** an infection caused by pus-producing microorganisms, commonly species of *Staphylococcus* and *Streptococcus.* The most numerous white blood cells responding immunologically to a pyogenic infection are the polymorphonuclear leukocytes. **Salinem i.,** a form of leptospirosis occurring in Salinem and caused by *Leptospira interrogans* serogroup *pyrogenes;* called also *Salinem fever.* **secondary i.,** infection by a microorganism following an infection by another kind of microorganism. **subclinical i.,** infection in which symptoms and signs are not detectable by clinical examination or laboratory tests; this may occur in an early stage(s) of the infection, with symptoms and signs becoming manifest later during the course of the infection, or the symptoms and signs may never become apparent. Cf. *inapparent i.* **vector-borne i.,** infection caused by microorganisms transmitted from one host to another by a carrier, such as a mosquito, louse, fly, or tick. **Vincent's i.,** acute necrotizing ulcerative gingivitis. **water-borne i.,** infection caused by microorganisms which may be transmitted through water and acquired through ingestion, bathing, or other means.

infectiosity (in-fek″she-os′ĭ-te) the degree of infectiousness of a microorganism.

infectious (in-fek′shus) caused by or capable of being communicated by infection, as an infectious disease; infective. Cf. *communicable, contagious,* and *infestation.*

infectiousness (in-fek′shus-nes) the state or quality of being infectious.

infective (in-fek′tiv) [L. *infectivus*] infectious; capable of producing infection; pertaining to or characterized by the presence of pathogens.

infectivity (in″fek-tiv′ĭ-te) infectiousness.

infecundity (in″fe-kun′dĭ-te) [L. *infecunditas*] sterility or barrenness.

inferent (in′fer-ent) afferent.

inferior (in-fēr′e-or) [L. "lower"; neut. *inferius*] situated below, or directed downward; [NA] a term used in reference to the lower surface of an organ or other structure, or to the lower of two (or more) similar structures.

inferiority (in-fēr″e-or′ĭ-te) the condition of being inferior. **constitutional psychopathic i., psychopathic i.** (*obs.*), see *antisocial personality disorder,* under *personality.*

inferolateral (in″fer-o-lat′er-al) [L. *inferus* low + *latus* side] situated below and to one side.

inferomedian (in″fer-o-me′de-an) [L. *inferus* low + *medius* middle] situated in the middle of the under side.

inferonasal (in″fer-o-na′zal) [L. *inferus* low + *nasal*] in ophthalmology, that quadrant of the eye or of the visual field inferior to the horizontal meridian of the eye and medial to the vertical meridian.

inferoposterior (in″fer-o-pos-tēr′e-or) situated below and behind.

inferotemporal (in″fer-o-tem′por-al) [L. *inferus* low + *temporal*] in ophthalmology, that quadrant of the eye or of the visual field inferior to the horizontal meridian of the eye and lateral to the vertical meridian.

infertile (in′fer-til) not fertile; exhibiting infertility.

infertilitas (in″fer-til′ĭ-tas) [L.] infertility.

infertility (in″fer-til′ĭ-te) [L. *in* not + *fertilis* fruitful, prolific] diminished or absent capacity to produce offspring; the term does not denote complete inability to produce offspring as does *sterility.* Called also *relative sterility.* **primary i.,** infertility occurring in patients who have never conceived. **secondary i.,** infertility occurring in patients who have previously conceived.

infestation (in-fes-ta′shun) parasitic attack or subsistence on the skin and its appendages, as by insects, mites, or ticks; sometimes used to denote parasitic invasion of the tissues or organs, as by helminths because helminths are larger than bacteria, viruses, and protozoa, and unlike the case with infection by those organisms, do not multiply within the body.

infibulation (in-fib-u-la′shun) [L. *infibulare* to buckle together] the act of buckling, or fastening as if with buckles, especially the chiefly abandoned practice of fastening the prepuce or labia minora together with clasps, stitches, or other devices to prevent coitus. Cf. *pharaonic circumcision,* under *circumcision.*

infiltrate (in-fil′trāt) 1. to penetrate the interstices of a tissue or substance. 2. material deposited by infiltration. **Assmann's tuberculous i.,** see under *focus.*

infiltration (in″fil-tra′shun) [L. *in* into + *filtration*] the diffusion or accumulation in a tissue or cells of substances not normal to it or in amounts in excess of the normal. Also, the material so accumulated. Cf. *degeneration.* **adipose i.,** fatty i. **calcareous i.,** a deposit of lime and magnesium salts in the tissues. **calcium i.,** a deposit of calcium salts within the tissues of the body. **cellular i.,** the migration and accumulation of cells within the tissues. **epituberculous i.,** a collateral hyperemia and inflammatory infiltration surrounding a tuberculous focus. **fatty i.,** 1. a deposit of fat in the tissues, especially between the cells. 2. the presence of fat vacuoles in the cytoplasm of cells, as occurs in fatty change in the liver, myocardium, and kidneys. **gelatinous i.,** gray i. **glycogen i.,** abnormal accumulations of glycogen within the cytoplasm of cells, as occurs in diabetes mellitus and the glycogen storage diseases. **gray i.,** a condition of the lungs in acute tuberculosis in which, after death, they assume a gray appearance; called also *gelatinous i.* **inflammatory i.,** that formed by an inflammatory exudation penetrating the interstices of a tissue. **lymphocytic i. of skin,** a manifestation of cutaneous lymphoid hyperplasia, occurring most often in men, characterized by the appearance of asymptomatic, single or multiple, firm, reddish papules or plaques that expand peripherally to form circinate lesions, sometimes with central clearing; the lesions may be induced or aggravated by light exposure. **paraneural i.,** paraneural anesthesia.

sanguineous i., infiltration with extravasated blood. **serous i.,** the abnormal presence of lymph in a tissue. **tuberculous i.,** the formation of a group or of groups of tuberculous cells and bacilli in a tissue. **urinous i.,** extravasation of urine into a tissue.

infirm (in-firm′) [L. *infirmis; in* not + *firmus* strong] weak; feeble, as from disease or old age.

infirmary (in-fir′mah-re) [L. *infirmarium*] a hospital or place where sick or infirm persons are maintained or treated; commonly used to denote a space or a building set aside for the care of members of a group or community; a dispensary.

infirmity (in-fir′mĭ-te) [L. *infirmitas*] 1. a feeble or weak state of the body or mind. 2. a disease or condition producing weakness.

inflammagen (in-flam′ah-jen) an irritant that elicits both edema and the cellular response of inflammation. Cf. *edemagen.*

inflammation (in″flah-ma′shun) [L. *inflammatio; inflammare* to set on fire] a localized protective response elicited by injury or destruction of tissues, which serves to destroy, dilute, or wall off (sequester) both the injurious agent and the injured tissue. It is characterized in the acute form by the classical signs of pain (dolor), heat (calor), redness (rubor), swelling (tumor), and loss of function (functio laesa). Histologically, it involves a complex series of events, including dilatation of arterioles, capillaries, and venules, with increased permeability and blood flow; exudation of fluids, including plasma proteins; and leukocytic migration into the inflammatory focus. **acute i.,** inflammation, usually of sudden onset, characterized by the classical signs (see *inflammation*), in which the vascular and exudative processes predominate. **adhesive i.,** that which promotes the adhesion of contiguous surfaces. **atrophic i.,** a form which results in atrophy and deformity. **catarrhal i.,** a form which affects principally a mucous surface, and which is marked by a copious discharge of mucus and epithelial debris. **chronic i.,** inflammation of slow progress and marked chiefly by the formation of new connective tissue; it may be a continuation of an acute form or a prolonged low-grade form, and usually causes permanent tissue damage. **cirrhotic i.,** atrophic i. **croupous i.,** a fibrinous inflammation leading to the formation of a false membrane. **diffuse i.,** one that is both interstitial and parenchymatous or is spread over a large area. **disseminated i.,** one that has a number of distinct foci. **exudative i.,** one in which the prominent feature is an exudate. **fibrinous i.,** one that is characterized by an exudate of coagulated fibrin. **fibroid i.,** atrophic i. **focal i.,** one that is confined to a single spot or to a few limited spots. **granulomatous i.,** an inflammation, usually chronic, characterized by the formation of granulomas; see also *granuloma.* **hyperplastic i.,** one which leads to the formation of new connective tissue fibers. **hypertrophic i.,** inflammation marked by increase in the size of the elements composing the affected tissue. **interstitial i.,** one that primarily affects the stroma of an organ. **metastatic i.,** one that is reproduced in a distant part by the conveyance of infectious material through the blood vessels and lymph organs. **necrotic i.,** inflammation attended by death of the affected tissue. **obliterative i.,** inflammation of the lining membrane of a cavity or vessel, producing adhesions between the surfaces and consequent obliteration of the lumen. **parenchymatous i.,** one that primarily affects the essential tissue elements of an organ. **plastic i., productive i., proliferous i.,** hyperplastic i. **pseudomembranous i.,** an acute inflammatory response to a powerful necrotizing toxin, such as the diphtheria toxin, characterized by the formation on a mucosal surface, most often in the pharynx, larynx, respiratory passages, and intestinal tract, of a false membrane composed of precipitated fibrin, necrotic epithelium, and inflammatory white cells. **purulent i.,** suppurative i. **sclerosing i.,** atrophic i. **seroplastic i.,** inflammation accompanied by both serous and plastic exudation. **serous i.,** one which produces an exudation of serum. **simple i.,** that in which there is no flow of pus or other product of inflammation. **specific i.,** one that is due to a particular microorganism. **subacute i.,** a condition intermediate between chronic and acute inflammation, exhibiting some of the characteristics of each. **suppurative i.,** one characterized by the formation of pus. **toxic i.,** one that is caused by a poison, such as a bacterial product. **traumatic i.,** one that is caused by an injury. **ulcera-**

tive i., that in which necrosis on or near the surface leads to loss of tissue and creation of a local defect (ulcer).

inflammatory (in-flam'ah-to″re) pertaining to or characterized by inflammation.

inflation (in-fla'shun) [L. *in* into + *flare* to blow] 1. distention with air, gas, or a fluid. 2. the act of distending with air or with a gas.

inflator (in-fla'tor) an instrument for inflating any organ for therapeutic or diagnostic purposes.

inflection, inflexion (in-flek'shun) [L. *inflexio; in* in + *flectere* to bend] the act of bending inward or the state of being bent inward, as of a limb.

inflorescence (in″flo-res'ens) the structure or arrangement of the flowers of a plant.

influenza (in″flu-en'zah) [Ital. "influenza"] an acute viral infection involving the respiratory tract, occurring in isolated cases, in epidemics, or in pandemics striking many continents simultaneously or in sequence. It is marked by inflammation of the nasal mucosa, the pharynx, and conjunctiva, and by headache and severe, often generalized myalgia. Fever, chills, and prostration are common. Involvement of the myocardium and of the central nervous system occur infrequently. A necrotizing bronchitis and interstitial pneumonia are prominent features of severe influenza and account for the susceptibility of patients to secondary bacterial pneumonia due to *Streptococcus pneumoniae, Haemophilus influenzae,* and *Staphylococcus aureus.* The incubation period is one to three days and the disease ordinarily lasts for three to ten days. Influenza is caused by a number of serologically distinct strains of virus, designated A (with many subgroups), B, and C. Called also *flu* and *grippe* (grip). See also *influenza virus,* under *virus.* **i. A,** the most common variety of influenza caused by the type A strain of influenza virus; epidemics of this form occur at two- to three-year intervals. The causative strain is subject to wide variations in antigenic type, called antigenic shift, and outbreaks of influenza A caused by such antigenic types have been called *Asian i., Spanish i., Russian i.,* and so on. See *influenza virus,* under *virus.* **Asian i.,** a pandemic of influenza A occurring in 1957, thought to originate in China. **avian i.,** Newcastle disease. **i. B,** a variety of influenza caused by the type B strain of influenza virus; epidemics of this form occur at four- to five-year intervals. See *influenza virus,* under *virus.* **i. C,** a variety of influenza occurring sporadically and caused by the type C strain of influenza virus. See *influenza virus,* under *virus.* **endemic i.,** infection with influenza virus occurring continuously within a population, i.e., between epidemics, either sporadically and not recognized as influenza or as a clinically inapparent infection. **equine i.,** a highly contagious febrile respiratory disease of horses caused by two immunologically distinct strains of influenza virus A. **feline i.,** a name loosely applied to any of a group of highly contagious viral infections of the respiratory tract in cats. **goose i.,** infectious avian serositis in geese. **Hong Kong i.,** a pandemic of influenza A occurring in 1968, thought to originate in Hong Kong. **laryngeal i.,** influenza in horses in which pharyngitis is the chief symptom. **Russian i.,** a pandemic of influenza A occurring in 1978, thought to originate in the U.S.S.R. **Spanish i.,** a name given to the acute influenza-like disease, a pandemic of which passed over Europe and America during the summer and autumn of 1918. **swine i.,** a highly contagious disease of hogs caused by simultaneous infection with *Haemophilus influenzae* and a virus.

influenzal (in″flu-en'zal) pertaining to influenza.

infolding (in-fōld'ing) 1. the folding inward of a layer of tissue, as in the formation of the neural tube in the embryo. 2. the enclosing of redundant tissue by suturing together the walls of the organ on either side of it.

informosome (in-for'mo-sōm) a name suggested for the combination of mRNA and protein found in the cytoplasm of eukaryotic cells.

infra- [L. *infra* beneath] a prefix meaning below or beneath.

infra-axillary (in″frah-ak'sĭ-lar″e) below the axilla.

infrabulge (in'frah-bulj) the surfaces of a tooth gingival to the height of contour, or sloping cervically; the surface of the crown of a tooth cervical to the clasp guideline or surveyed height of contour, being the retention area of a tooth. Cf. *suprabulge.*

infraciliature (in″frah-sil'ĭ-ah-chur) [*infra-* + *cilium*] the basal bodies and kinetodesmata of ciliate protozoa considered collectively.

infraclass (in'frah-klas) a taxonomic category sometimes established, subordinate to a subclass and superior to an order.

infraclavicular (in″frah-klah-vik'u-lar) beneath a clavicle.

infraclusion (in″frah-kloo'zhun) malocclusion in which a tooth has failed to erupt fully and reach the line of occlusion and is out of contact with the opposing tooth. Called also *infraversion.*

infraconstrictor (in″frah-kon-strik'tor) the inferior constrictor of the pharynx.

infracortical (in″frah-kor'tĭ-kal) beneath the cortex, as of the brain.

infracostal (in″frah-kos'tal) [*infra-* + L. *costa* rib] below a rib or below the ribs.

infracotyloid (in″frah-kot'ĭ-loid) beneath the cotyloid cavity or acetabulum.

infraction (in-frak'shun) [L. *in* into + *frac'tio* break] incomplete fracture of a bone without displacement of the fragments. **Freiberg's i.,** osteochondrosis of the head of the second metatarsal bone.

infradentale (in″frah-den-ta'le) an osteometric landmark, being the highest anterior point on the gingiva between the mandibular central incisors.

infradian (in″frah-de'an, in-fra'de-an) [*infra-* + L. *dies* day] pertaining to the rhythmic repetition of certain phenomena in living organisms occurring in cycles of less frequency than circadian, that is, less frequently than once a day. Cf. *circadian* and *ultradian.*

infradiaphragmatic (in″frah-di″ah-frag-mat'ik) below the diaphragm.

infraduction (in″frah-duk'shun) [*infra-* + *duction*] 1. the downward rotation of an eye around its horizontal axis. 2. the downward rotation of one eye independent of the other by a baseup prism in testing for vertical divergence. See also *infravergence* and *infraversion.* Called also *deorsumduction* and *subduction.*

infraglenoid (in″frah-gle'noid) below the fossa of the glenoid cavity.

infraglottic (in″frah-glot'ik) below the glottis.

infrahyoid (in″frah-hi'oid) below the hyoid bone.

inframamillary (in″frah-mam'ĭ-lar″e) below the nipple.

inframammary (in″frah-mam'ah-re) below the mammary gland.

inframandibular (in″frah-man-dib'u-lar) beneath the lower jaw.

inframarginal (in″frah-mar'jĭ-nal) situated below a margin or border.

inframaxillary (in″frah-mak'sĭ-lar″e) beneath the upper jaw (maxilla).

infranuclear (in″frah-nu'kle-ar) below a nucleus.

infraorbital (in″frah-or'bĭ-tal) lying under or on the floor of the orbit.

infrapatellar (in″frah-pah-tel'ar) below the patella.

infrapsychic (in″frah-si'kik) below the psychic level; automatic.

infrared (in-frah-red') denoting thermal radiation of wavelength greater than that of the red end of the visible spectrum, between the red waves and the radio waves, having wavelengths between 0.75 and 1000 μm. Infrared rays emanating from tissues are the basis of thermography. **far i., long-wave i.,** infrared radiation of the longest wavelength, i.e., furthest from the visible spectrum (wavelength about 3.0 to 1000 μm.). **near i., short-wave i.,** infrared radiation of the shortest wavelength, i.e., closest to the visible spectrum (wavelength about 0.75 to 3.0 μm.).

infrascapular (in″frah-skap'u-lar) beneath the scapula.

infrasonic (in″frah-son'ik) below the frequency range of the waves normally perceived as sound by the human ear.

infraspinous (in″frah-spi'nus) beneath the spine of the scapula.

infrasternal (in″frah-ster'nal) below the sternum.

infrastructure (in″fra-struk'chur) substructure, def. 2. **implant i.,** see under *substructure.*

infratemporal (in″frah-tem′po-ral) below the temporal fossa.

infratentorial (in″frah-ten-to′re-al) beneath the tentorium of the cerebellum.

infratonsillar (in″frah-ton′sĭ-lar) below the faucial tonsil.

infratracheal (in″frah-tra′ke-al) beneath the trachea.

infratrochlear (in″frah-trok′le-ar) beneath the trochlea.

infratubal (in″frah-tu′bal) beneath a tube.

infraturbinal (in″frah-tur′bĭ-nal) the inferior turbinate bone.

infraumbilical (in″frah-um-bil′ĭ-kal) beneath the umbilicus.

infravergence (in″frah-ver′jens) [infra- + vergence] disjunctive reciprocal movement of the eyes in which one eye rotates downward while the other one remains still; called also *deorsumvergence*.

infraversion (in″frah-ver′zhun) [infra- + version] 1. infraclusion. 2. the downward deviation of one eye. 3. conjugate downward rotation of both eyes; called also *deorsumversion*.

infriction (in-frik′shun) [L. in on + frictio rubbing] the rubbing of medicaments upon the skin.

infundibula (in″fun-dib′u-lah) [L.] plural of *infundibulum*.

infundibular (in″fun-dib′u-lar) of the nature of or resembling an infundibulum or funnel.

infundibulectomy (in″fun-dib″u-lek′to-me) excision of the infundibulum of the heart. **Brock's i.,** resection of the interior portion of the hypertrophied outflow tract of the right ventricle to assist in relief of pulmonary stenosis in tetralogy of Fallot.

infundibuliform (in″fun-dib′u-lĭ-form″) [L. *infundibulum* funnel + *forma* form] shaped like a funnel.

infundibuloma (in″fun-dib-u-lo′mah) a tumor of the infundibulum hypothalami.

infundibulopelvic (in″fun-dib″u-lo-pel′vik) pertaining to an infundibulum and a pelvis, as of the kidney.

infundibulum (in″fun-dib′u-lum), pl. *infundib′ula* [L. "funnel"] 1. a funnel-shaped passage; [NA] a general term for such a structure. Often used alone to refer to the infundibulum hypothalami, to the median eminence, and to the infundibular stem. 2. NA alternative for *conus arteriosus*. 3. the deep, often tubular or funnel-shaped part of the buccal cavity seen in certain protozoa, especially peritrichous ciliates. **crural i., i. crura′le,** canalis femoralis. **ethmoidal i. of cavity of nose,** i. ethmoidale cavi nasi. **ethmoidal i. of ethmoid bone,** infundibulum ethmoidale ossis ethmoidalis. **i. ethmoida′le ca′vi na′si** [NA], a passage connecting the cavity of the nose with the anterior ethmoidal cells and the frontal sinus. **i. ethmoida′le os′sis ethmoida′lis** [NA], a variable sinuous passage extending upward from the middle nasal meatus through the ethmoidal labyrinth, communicating with the anterior ethmoidal cells and often with the frontal sinus. **i. of fallopian tube,** i. tubae uterinae. **i. of heart,** conus arteriosus. **i. hypothal′ami** [NA], **i. of hypothalamus,** a hollow, funnel-shaped mass in front of the tuber cinereum, which extends to the neurohypophysis. Called also *hypophyseal* or *neural stalk, infundibular stalk* or *stem,* and *pituitary stalk.* See also *pituitary gland,* under *gland.* **infundibula of kidney,** calices renales minores. **i. na′si, i. of nose,** 1. infundibulum ethmoidale cavi nasi. 2. infundibulum ethmoidale ossis ethmoidalis. **i. pulmo′nis, i. pulmo′num,** any of the ductuli alveolares. **infundib′ula re′num,** calices renales minores. **i. tu′bae uteri′nae** [NA], infundibulum of uterine tube: the funnel-like dilation at the distal end of the uterine tube. **i. of urinary bladder,** fundus vesicae urinariae. **i. of uterine tube,** i. tubae uterinae.

infusible (in-fu′zĭ-b'l) incapable of being melted.

infusion (in-fu′zhun) 1. [L. *infusio;* from *in* into + *fundere* to pour] the steeping of a substance in water to obtain its medicinal principles. 2. [L. *infusum,* gen. *infusi*] the product of the process of steeping a drug for the extraction of its medicinal principles. 3. the therapeutic introduction of a fluid other than blood, as saline solution, into a vein. NOTE—An *infusion* flows in by gravity, an *injection* is forced in by a syringe, an *instillation* is dropped in, an *insufflation* is blown in, and an *infection* slips in unnoticed. **amni-**

otic fluid i., a complication of labor in which rupture of the uterine venous sinuses permits the entrance of amniotic fluid into the maternal circulation. **cold i.,** the product of steeping a drug in cold water. **meat i.** (for bacteriological use), fresh lean meat free from fat is ground and extracted with water; the mixture is infused overnight in the refrigerator, gradually raised to the boiling point, and filtered. **saline i.,** administration, either subcutaneously or intravenously, of saline solution.

infusodecoction (in-fu″so-de-kok′shun) a mixture of the infusion and the decoction of a substance.

Infusoria (in″fu-so′re-ah) [L. pl., so called because found in *infusions,* after exposure to air] former name for Ciliophora.

infusum (in-fu′sum) [L.] an infusion, def. 2.

ingesta (in-jes′tah) [L. pl., *in* into + *gerere* to carry] food and drink taken into the stomach.

ingestant (in-jes′tant) a substance that is or may be taken into the body by way of the mouth, or through the digestive system.

ingestion (in-jes′chun) the act of taking food, medicines, etc., into the body, by mouth.

ingestive (in-jes′tiv) pertaining to or affecting an ingestion.

ingluvies (in-gloo′ve-ēz) [L.] 1. the craw or crop of birds. 2. the first stomach (rumen) of ruminant animals.

Ingrassia's process (apophysis), wings (in-grah′se-ahs) [Giovanni Filippo *Ingrassia,* Italian anatomist, 1510–1580] see *ala minor ossis sphenoidalis,* and see *wings of sphenoid bone,* under *wing.*

ingravescent (in″grah-ves′ent) [L. *in* upon + *gravesci* to grow heavy] gradually increasing in severity.

ingrowth (in′grōth) an inward growth; something that grows inward or into. **epithelial i.,** a complication of intraocular surgery, most often cataract extraction, or of penetrating wounds of the cornea where wound healing is poor, in which epithelium proliferates through the wound into the anterior chamber, causing obstruction of the trabecula, and sometimes pupillary block, resulting in glaucoma.

inguen (ing′gwen), pl. *in′guina* [L.] [NA] the groin; the junctural region between the abdomen and the thigh.

inguina (ing′gwĭ-nah) [L.] plural of *inguen.*

inguinal (ing′gwĭ-nal) [L. *inguinalis*] pertaining to the inguen, or groin.

inguinoabdominal (ing″gwĭ-no-ab-dom′ĭ-nal) pertaining to the groin and the abdomen.

inguinocrural (ing″gwĭ-no-kroo′ral) pertaining to the groin and the thigh.

inguinodynia (ing″gwĭ-no-din′e-ah) pain in the groin.

inguinolabial (ing″gwĭ-no-la′be-al) pertaining to the groin and labium.

inguinoscrotal (ing″gwĭ-no-skro′tal) pertaining to the groin and the scrotum.

INH trademark (from *isonicotine hydrazine*) for preparations of isoniazid.

inhalant (in-ha′lant) a substance that is or may be taken into the body by way of the nose and trachea, or through the respiratory system. **antifoaming i.,** an agent inhaled as a vapor to prevent the formation of foam in the respiratory passages of a patient with pulmonary edema.

inhalation (in″hah-la′shun) [L. *inhalatio*] 1. the drawing of air or other substances into the lungs; see also under *anesthesia* and *therapy.* 2. any drug or solution of drugs administered (as by means of nebulizers or aerosols) by the nasal or oral respiratory route for local or systemic effect. **isoproterenol sulfate i.** [USP], a solution of isoproterenol hydrochloride in purified water made isotonic by the addition of sodium chloride; used as a bronchodilator administered by inhalation as an aerosol.

inhale (in-hāl′) [L. *inhalare*] to take into the lungs by breathing.

inhaler (in-ha′ler) 1. an apparatus for administering vapor or volatilized remedies or anesthetics by inhalation. 2. an apparatus to prevent dust, smoke, noxious gases, or the like from entering the lungs, or to enable a person with affected lungs to breathe cold or damp air with less danger and discomfort. **Allis' i.,** an apparatus for administering ether, chloroform, or other highly volatile liquid anesthetics by the drop method. **ether i.,** an apparatus for administering the vapor of ether as an anesthetic. **H. H. i.,** an oxygen inhaler used in treating gassed patients; named from the inventors, Henderson and Haggard. **Junker i.,** a bottle-like inhaler formerly used for administration of chloroform (1867).

inherent (in-hēr′ent) [L. *inhaerens* sticking fast] implanted by nature; intrinsic; innate.

inheritance (in-her′ĭ-tans) [L. *inhereditare* to appoint an heir] 1. the acquisition of characters or qualities by transmission from parent to offspring. 2. that which is transmitted from parent to offspring. See also the entries of and subentries to *character* (def. 2) and *gene*. **alternative i.,** inheritance in which the characters are inherited from one parent. **codominant i.,** see under *gene*. **complemental i.,** inheritance of characters dependent on the presence of two independent pairs of nonallelic genes (complementary genes), both of which must be present before a given character can be expressed. **cytoplasmic i.,** extrachromosomal i. **dominant i.,** see under *gene*. **extrachromosomal i.,** the inheritance of traits controlled by genes on the DNA of mitochondria in the ooplasm. The genes are thus inherited entirely from the mother, and the inheritance is nonmendelian. Called also *cytoplasmic i., maternal i.,* and *mitochondrial i.* See also *mitochondrial chromosome*. **holandric i.,** inheritance carried only by males, as by genes on the Y chromosome. **homochronous i.,** the inheritance of characteristics which appear in the offspring at the same age as they appeared in the parent. **homotropic i.,** the alleged inheritance of acquired characteristics. **intermediate i.,** inheritance in which the phenotype of the heterozygote is intermediate between that of the two homozygous types. Contrast *codominant gene*. **maternal i.,** the transmission of characters that are dependent on peculiarities of the egg cytoplasm produced, in turn, by nuclear genes. **mendelian i.,** see *Mendel's law*, under *law*. **mitochondrial i.,** extrachromosomal i. **monofactorial i.,** the acquisition of a characteristic or quality, the transmission of which depends on a single gene. **multifactorial i.,** inheritance determined by multiple factors, genetic and possibly nongenetic (environmental), each with only a minor effect. See also *polygenic i.* **polygenic i., quantitative i.,** inheritance determined by many genes at different loci, with small additive effects. See also *multifactorial i.* **quasidominant i.,** inheritance in which there is direct transmission, generation to generation, of a recessive trait; thus, although it is produced by the mating of a recessive homozygote with a heterozygote, the proportion of affected offspring resembles that in dominant inheritance. **recessive i.,** see under *gene*. **sex-linked i.,** see under *gene*.

inhibin (in-hib′in) a postulated nonsteroid testicular factor, believed to be a peptide, elaborated by the Sertoli cells of the seminiferous tubules and thought to inhibit pituitary production of follicle-stimulating hormone.

inhibit (in-hib′it) to retard, arrest, or restrain.

inhibition (in″hĭ-bish′un) [L. *inhibēre* to restrain, from *in* in + *habēre* to hold] 1. arrest or restraint of a process. 2. in psychoanalysis, the conscious or unconscious restraining of an impulse or desire. **allogenic i.,** injury to cells in vitro as a consequence of contact with lymphocytes that are of a different genotype. **allosteric i.,** inhibition of an enzyme by binding of an inhibitor at an allosteric site, thus altering the affinity of the enzyme for its substrate or changing the rate of turnover at separate catalytic sites. **competitive i.,** inhibition of enzyme activity in which the inhibitor (substrate analogue) reversibly combines with catalytic sites, thus competing with the substrate for binding on the enzyme. The inhibition is reversible since it can be overcome by increasing the substrate concentration. Similarly, the reversible binding of a physiologic antagonist to a receptor site for a hormone or neurotransmitter. **contact i.,** the inhibition of cell division and cell motility in normal animal cells when in close contact with each other. **endproduct i.,** feedback i. **enzyme i.,** inhibition of enzyme activity, as in competitive or endproduct inhibition. **feedback i.,** inhibition of the initial steps of a process by an endproduct of the reaction. **hemagglutination i. (HI, HAI),** see under *tests*. **noncompetitive i.,** inhibition of enzyme activity by a substance that combines with the enzyme at a site other than that utilized by the substrate, causing a change in enzyme configuration and a decrease in activity. Similarly, the inhibition of a hormone or neurotransmitter by binding of a

physiologic antagonist to a receptor at a site other than the active center. **proactive i.,** the interference of earlier learning in the retention of new learning; cf. *retroactive i.* **reciprocal i.,** the inhibition of one group of muscles on excitation of their antagonists, a phenomenon resulting from reciprocal innervation (q.v.). **retroactive i.,** the interference of new learning in the recall of earlier learning; cf. *proactive i.* **selective i.,** competitive i. **uncompetitive i.,** inhibition of an enzyme by a substance that binds reversibly to the enzyme-substrate complex. The enzyme-substrate-inhibitor complex cannot yield the normal product until the inhibitor is released. **Wedensky i.,** a partial block to conduction in a nerve may transmit impulses at low frequencies but not at higher frequencies.

inhibitive (in-hib′ĭ-tiv) inhibitory.

inhibitor (in-hib′ĭ-tor) 1. any substance that interferes with a chemical reaction, growth, or other biological activity. 2. a chemical substance that inhibits an enzyme reaction. See also *inhibition*. 3. a mechanical device for curing mouth breathing. **angiotensin converting enzyme (ACE) i's,** competitive inhibitors of dipeptidyl carboxypeptidase, kininase II; used for treatment of hypertension, usually in conjunction with a diuretic. They are effective in both renovascular and essential low-renin hypertension. **C1 i. (C1 INH),** an inhibitor of C1, the activated esterase formed from C1; see *complement*. **carbonic anhydrase i.,** an agent that inhibits carbonic anhydrase either in the kidney, causing increased excretion of bicarbonate, sodium, and water; or in the eye, causing decreased production of aqueous humor and lowered intraocular pressure; used for glaucoma and rarely for edema and epilepsy. **C1 esterase i.,** C1 i. **cholesterol i.,** an agent that suppresses the production of cholesterol or decreases the level of cholesterol in the blood. **cholinesterase i.,** anticholinesterase. **membrane attack complex i. (MAC INH),** S protein. **mitotic i.,** a substance that slows or arrests the process of mitosis, e.g., colchicine. **monoamine oxidase i. (MAOI),** any of a group of antidepressant drugs that have the ability to block the oxidative deamination of monoamines. It is thought that by inhibiting monoamine oxidase activity the inhibitors increase the level of catecholamines in the central nervous system, which would have been otherwise neutralized by the enzyme, and that these increased concentrations are responsible for their antidepressant effects.

inhibitory (in-hib′ĭ-tor″e) [L. *inhibere* to restrain] restraining or arresting any process; effecting a stay or arrest, partial or complete.

inhomogeneity (in-ho″mo-jě-ne′ĭ-te) lack of normal homogeneity.

inhomogeneous (in″ho-mo-je′ne-us) lacking homogeneity.

iniac (in′e-ak) pertaining to the inion.

iniad (in′e-ad) toward the inion.

inial (in′e-al) iniac.

iniencephalus (in″e-en-sef′ah-lus) a fetus exhibiting iniencephaly.

iniencephaly (in″e-en-sef′ah-le) [Gr. *inion* occiput + *enkephalos* brain] a developmental anomaly characterized by enlargement of the foramen magnum, and absence of the laminal and spinal processes of the cervical, dorsal, and sometimes lumbar vertebrae, with vertebrae reduced in number and irregularly fused, the brain and much of the cord occupying a single cavity.

inio- (in′e-o) [Gr. *inion* occiput] a combining form denoting relationship to the occiput.

iniodymus (in″e-od′ĭ-mus) [*inio-* + Gr. *didymos* twin] iniopagus.

inion (in′e-on) [Gr. "the back of the head"] [NA] the most prominent point of the external occipital protuberance.

iniopagus (in″e-op′ah-gus) [*inio-* + Gr. *pagos* thing fixed] conjoined symmetrical twins fused at the occiput.

iniops (in′e-ops) [*inio-* + Gr. *ōps* eye] a double-faced monster with the posterior face undeveloped.

initial (ĭ-nish′al) [L. *initialis*, from *initium* beginning] pertaining to the very first stage of any process.

initis (in-i′tis) [Gr. *is, inos* fiber] inflammation of the substance of a muscle.

injectable (in-jek′tah-b′l) 1. capable of being injected. 2. a substance that may be injected.

injected (in-jekt′ed) 1. introduced by injection. 2. congested.

injectio (in-jek′she-o), pl. *injectio′nes* [L.] injection.

injection (in-jek′shun) [L. *injectio*, from *inicere* to throw into] 1. the act of forcing a liquid into a part, as into the subcutaneous tissues, the vascular tree, or an organ. Cf. *infusion* (def. 3). 2. a substance so forced or administered. Officially, in pharmacy, a solution of a medicament suitable for injection. See also under specific substances. 3. the condition of being injected; congestion. **adrenal cortex i.,** a preparation containing a mixture of the endocrine principles derived from the cortex of adrenal glands; formerly used in treatment of adrenal insufficiency. **anatomical i.,** an injection into the vessels or organs of the cadaver, designed to facilitate dissection or demonstration. **circumcorneal i.,** dilatation of the ciliary and conjunctival blood vessels close to the limbus, and diminishing toward the periphery. **coarse i.,** an anatomical injection that fills only the larger vessels. **dextrose i.,** a sterile solution of dextrose in water for injection; used as a fluid and nutrient replenisher. **endermic i.,** intracutaneous i. **epifascial i.,** one made upon the surface of a fascia, particularly the fascia lata. **ethiodized oil i.** [USP], see under *oil*. **fine i.,** an anatomical injection that fills even the smallest vessels. **fructose i.,** a sterile solution of fructose in water, used as a fluid and nutrient replenisher. **gaseous i.,** injection of gas or air for therapeutic purposes as in collapse therapy; for diagnostic purposes, as in ventriculography; or for facilitating anatomical demonstrations. **gelatin i.,** a preservative injection of which gelatin is the base. **hypodermic i.,** an injection made into the subcutaneous tissues; called also *subcutaneous i.* **intracutaneous i., intradermal i., intradermic i.,** one made into the corium or substance of the skin. **intramuscular i.,** an injection into the substance of a muscle. **intrathecal i.,** injection of a substance through the theca of the spinal cord into the subarachnoid space. **intravascular i.,** an injection made into a vessel. **intravenous i.,** an injection made into a vein. **iodinated I 125 albumin i.** [USP], a sterile, buffered isotonic solution containing not less than 10 mg. of radioiodinated normal human albumin per liter, and adjusted to provide not more than 1 millicurie of radioactivity per milliliter, used as a diagnostic aid in determining blood volume and cardiac output. **iodinated I 131 albumin i.** [USP], a sterile aqueous suspension of albumin human iodinated with ^{131}I and denatured to produce aggregates of controlled particle size; each ml. contains 300 μg to 3.0 mg. of aggregated albumin with specific activity of 200 microcuries to 1.2 millicuries per mg. **iron dextran i.** [USP], a sterile colloidal solution of ferric hydroxide in complex with partially hydrolyzed dextran of low molecular weight, in water for injection; used as a hematinic. **iron sorbitex i.** [USP], a sterile solution of a complex of iron, sorbitol, and citric acid that is stabilized with the aid of dextrin and an excess of sorbitol; used as a hematinic. **jet i.,** injection of a drug in solution through the intact skin by an extremely fine jet of the solution under high pressure. **opacifying i.,** the injection of a radiopaque substance into the vessels or into some body cavity for diagnostic radiological study. **paraperiosteal i.,** the production of local anesthesia by deposition of a local anesthetic solution close to the periosteum; the solution is then free to diffuse through the cortical bony plate and anesthetize the larger terminal nerve fibers. **parathyroid i.** [USP], a sterile solution of water-soluble principles of the parathyroid glands, administered intramuscularly to maintain the level of calcium in the blood; called also *parathyroid extract.* **parenchymatous i.,** one made into the substance of an organ. **posterior pituitary i.** [NF], a sterile solution in water of the principles from the posterior lobe of the pituitary of domestic animals that are used for food by man; used as an oxytocic, in the treatment of diabetes insipidus, and to stimulate intestinal peristalsis. **preservative i.,** an injection that serves to protect a cadaver or specimen from decay. **protamine sulfate i.** [USP], a sterile isotonic solution prepared from the sperm or from the mature testes of fish belonging to the genus *Oncorhynchus, Salmo,* or *Trutta;* used to counteract the action of heparin. **protein hydrolysate i.** [USP], a sterile solution of amino acids and short-chain peptides, used as a fluid and nutrient replenisher. **Ringer's i.** [USP], a sterile solution of sodium chloride, potassium chloride, and calcium chloride in water for injection, given as a fluid and

electrolyte replenisher by intravenous infusion. **Ringer's i., lactated** [USP], a sterile solution of calcium chloride, potassium chloride, sodium chloride, and sodium lactate in water for injection, given as a fluid and electrolyte replenisher by intravenous infusion. **sclerosing i.,** the injection into a blood vessel of material (e.g., sodium citrate) which will tend to obliterate the vessel; used in varicose veins, angioma, etc. **sodium chloride i.** [USP], a sterile isotonic solution of sodium chloride in water for injection, used as a fluid and electrolyte replenisher and as an irrigating solution. It is also used as a vehicle for the injection of medications. **sodium pertechnate Tc 99m i.** [USP], a sterile solution containing radioactive technetium (^{99m}Tc) in the form of sodium pertechnate and sufficient sodium chloride to make the solution isotonic. **sodium radiochromate i.,** sodium chromate Cr 51 i. **subcutaneous i.,** hypodermic i. **technetium Tc 99m albumin aggregated i.** [USP], see under *technetium*. **vasopressin i.** [USP], a sterile solution in water for injection of the water-soluble, pressor principle of the posterior lobe of the pituitary of healthy domestic animals that are used as food by man; used as an antidiuretic.

injector (in-jek′tor) [L. *injicere* to inject] an instrument used in making injections.

injury (in′ju-re) [L. *injuria; in* not + *jus* right] harm or hurt; a wound or maim. Usually applied to damage inflicted to the body by an external force. **birth i.,** impairment of body function or structure due to adverse influences to which the infant has been subjected at birth. **blast i.,** see *blast,* def. 3. **deceleration i.,** an injury sustained by sudden deceleration in the movement of the body, as in a motor vehicle accident; the brain is especially liable to such trauma. **egg-white i.,** biotin deficiency; see *biotin.* **Goyrand's i.,** pulled elbow. **steering-wheel i.,** injury to the chest and sometimes contusion of the heart in motorists, caused by being thrown forward against the steering wheel. **whiplash i.,** a nonspecific term applied to injury to the spine and spinal cord at the junction of the fourth and fifth cervical vertebrae, occurring as the result of rapid acceleration or deceleration of the body. Because of their greater mobility, the four upper vertebrae act as the lash, and the lower three act as the handle of the whip.

inlay (in′la) 1. material, such as bone or skin, inserted into a tissue defect. 2. a dental restoration made outside of a tooth to correspond with the form of a prepared cavity and then cemented into the tooth. **epithelial i.,** a method of securing epithelialization of an unhealed deep wound. A mold of the wound cavity is taken and covered with a Thiersch graft of epidermis, the whole being inserted into the wound cavity, and the edges then approximated with sutures. The mold is removed after ten days, leaving the cavity completely epithelialized. Called also *Esser's operation.* See also under *onlay.*

inlet (in′let) an avenue of ingress. **pelvic i.,** the superior aperture of the minor pelvis, bounded by the crest and pecten of the pubic bones, the arcuate lines of the ilia, and the anterior margin of the base of the sacrum; called also *apertura pelvis superior* [NA].

I.N.N. International Nonproprietary Names, the nonproprietary designation recommended by the World Health Organization for any pharmaceutical preparation. Such names are selected according to general principles set forth by the World Health Organization, and lists are published periodically in the *WHO Chronicle.*

innate (in′nāt) [L. *in* in + *nasci* to be born] inborn; hereditary; congenital.

innervation (in″er-va′shun) [L. *in* into + *nervus* nerve] 1. the distribution or supply of nerves to a part. 2. the supply of nervous energy or of nerve stimulus sent to a part. **double i.,** innervation of a structure by two kinds of nerve fibers, e.g., sympathetic and parasympathetic. **reciprocal i.,** the innervation of muscles around the joints, where the motor centers are so connected in pairs that when one is excited the center of the corresponding antagonist is inhibited.

innidiation (ĭ-nid″e-a′shun) [L. *in* into + *nidus* nest] the development of cells in a part to which they have been carried by metastasis; called also *colonization* and *indenization.*

innocent (in′o-sent) [L. *innocens; in* not + *nocere* to harm] not malignant; benign; not tending of its own nature to a fatal issue. See *innocent bystander,* under *bystander.*

innocuous (ĭ-nok′u-us) harmless.

innominatal (ĭ-nom″ĭ-na′tal) pertaining to the innominate (brachiocephalic) artery or to the innominate (hip) bone.

innominate (ĭ-nom′ĭ-nāt) [L. *innominatus* nameless; *in* not + *nomen* name] not having a name; nameless. The term has been applied to certain structures better identified by their descriptive names, as the innominate (brachiocephalic) artery and the innominate (hip) bone.

Innovar (in′o-var) a trademark for a preparation of droperidol and fentanyl citrate in a 50:1 ratio; used as a neuroleptanalgesic.

innoxious (ĭ-nok′shus) [L. *in* not + *noxius* harmful] not injurious; not hurtful.

innutrition (in″nu-trish′un) want of nutrition.

in(o)- [Gr. *is*, gen. *inos* fiber] a combining form denoting relationship to a fiber, or fibrous material.

inoblast (in′o-blast) [*ino-* + Gr. *blastos* germ] any connective tissue cell in the formative stage.

inoccipitia (in-ok″sĭ-pit′e-ah) absence or deficiency of the occipital lobe of the brain.

inochondritis (in″o-kon-dri′tis) [*ino-* + Gr. *chondros* cartilage + *-itis*] inflammation of a fibrocartilage.

inocula (ĭ-nok′u-lah) [L.] plural of *inoculum*.

inoculability (ĭ-nok″u-lah-bil′ĭ-te) the quality or state of being inoculable.

inoculable (ĭ-nok′u-lah-b'l) 1. susceptible of being inoculated; transmissible by inoculation. 2. not immune against a disease transmissible by inoculation.

inoculate (ĭ-nok′u-lāt) to communicate a disease by inserting its etiologic agent; to implant microbes or infective materials in or on culture media; to introduce immune serum, vaccines of various kinds, and other antigenic materials for preventive, curative, or experimental purposes.

inoculation (ĭ-nok″u-la′shun) [L. *inoculatio*, from *in* into + *oculus* bud] introduction of microorganisms, infective material, serum, and other substances into tissues of living plants and animals, or culture media; introduction of a disease agent, e.g., vaccine virus, into a healthy individual to produce a mild form of the disease followed by immunity. **protective i.,** the injection of a biological preparation, e.g., a vaccine or an antiserum, to protect against a disease; vaccination against a disease.

inoculum (ĭ-nok′u-lum), pl. *inoc′ula* [L.] the substance used in inoculation.

inocyte (in′o-sīt) [*ino-* + *-cyte*] a cell of fibrous tissue.

inogen (in′o-jen) [*ino-* + Gr. *gennan* to produce] a hypothetical substance of the muscular tissue, the sudden breaking up of which was once supposed to cause muscular contraction.

inogenesis (in″o-jen′ĕ-sis) the formation of fibrous tissue.

inogenous (in-oj′ĕ-nus) produced from or producing fibrous tissue.

inoglia (in-og′le-ah) [*ino-* + Gr. *glia* glue] fibroglia.

inohymenitis (in″o-hi″mĕ-ni′tis) [*ino-* + Gr. *hymēn* membrane + *-itis*] inflammation of any fibrous membrane.

inolith (in′o-lith) [*ino-* + Gr. *lithos* stone] a fibrous concretion.

inomyositis (in″o-mi″o-si′tis) fibromyositis.

inoperable (in-op′er-ah-b'l) not suitable to be operated upon.

inophragma (in″o-frag′mah) [*ino-* + Gr. *phragmos* a fencing in] ground membrane; a name given to the Z band and M band (q.v. under *band*) because they continue uninterruptedly as transverse membranes through all the adjoining fibrils of a muscle fiber. See *mesophragma* and *telophragma*.

inorganic (in″or-gan′ik) [*in-* not + *organic*] 1. having no organs. 2. not of organic origin. 3. pertaining to substances not of organic origin. 4. in chemistry, denoting substances not derived from hydrocarbons.

inorganic pyrophosphatase (in″or-gan′ik pi′ro-fos′fah-tās) [EC 3.6.1.1] an enzyme of the hydrolase class that catalyzes the reaction pyrophosphate + H_2O = 2 orthophosphate. The enzyme is present in all cells and regulates the concentration of endogenous pyrophosphate. Inorganic pyrophosphatase may be identical with alkaline phosphatase in some tissues.

inosclerosis (in″o-skle-ro′sis) [*ino-* + Gr. *sklēros* hard] sclerosis or induration by increase of fibrous tissue.

inoscopy (in-os′ko-pe) [*ino-* + Gr. *skopein* to examine] the diagnosis of disease by artificial digestion and examination of the fibers or fibrinous matter of the sputum, blood, effusions, etc.

inosculate (in-os′ku-lāt) [L. *in* into + *osculum* little mouth] to unite or communicate by means of small openings or anastomoses.

inosculation (in-os″ku-la′shun) the establishment of communication, by means of small openings or anastomoses, applied especially to establishment of such communication between already existing blood vessels or other tubular structures that come in contact.

inose (in′ōs) inositol.

inosemia (in″o-se′me-ah) [*ino-* + Gr. *haima* blood + *-ia*] 1. an excess of fibrin in the blood. 2. the presence of inose (inositol) in the blood.

inosinate (in-o′sĭ-nāt) a salt of inosinic acid.

inosine (in′o-sēn) a nucleoside, xanthine β-D-ribofuranoside. **i. monophosphate (IMP)** a nucleotide, inosine 5′-monophosphate, formed by deamination of adenosine monophosphate AMP; it is also an intermediate in the formation of AMP.

inosine phosphorylase (in′o-sin, -sēn fos-for′ĭ-lās) purine-nucleoside phosphorylase.

inosinic acid (in″o-sin′ik) inosine monophosphate.

inosite (in′o-sīt) inositol.

inositis (in″o-si′tis) [*ino-* + *-itis*] inflammation of fibrous tissue.

inositol (in-o′sĭ-tol) 1. any of the stereoisomeric forms of inositol, especially *myo*-inositol (see def. 2). 2. chemical name: *myo*- inositol. A sugar-like vitamin of the B complex, $C_6H_{12}O_6$, which is found in many plant and animal tissues and has been synthesized. It is concerned in the growth of yeast, promotes growth of several species of bacteria, and is curative of mouse alopecia, and may have lipotropic activity; called also *antialopecia factor* and *meso-inositol*. **i. niacinate,** a peripheral vasodilator, $C_{42}H_{30}N_6O_{12}$.

inosituria (in″o-si″tol-u′re-ah) inosituria.

inosituria (in″o-si-tu′re-ah) [*inosite* + *-uria*] the occurrence of inositol in the urine, as in diabetes inositus; called also *inosuria*.

inostosis (in″os-to′sis) the re-formation of bony tissue to replace such tissue which has been destroyed.

inosuria (in″o-su′re-ah) 1. an excess of fibrin in the urine. 2. inosituria.

inotagma (in″o-tag′mah) [*ino-* + Gr. *tagma* arrangement] a linear arrangement of the contractile structural elements of a muscle cell.

inotropic (in″o-trop′ik) [*ino-* + Gr. *trepein* to turn or influence] affecting the force or energy of muscular contractions. **negatively i.,** weakening the force of muscular contraction. **positively i.,** increasing the strength of muscular contraction.

inotropism (in-ot′ro-pizm) the quality of influencing the contractility of muscle fibers.

in ovo (in o′vo) [L.] in the egg; referring specifically to various experimental procedures involving the use of chick embryos.

inquest (in′kwest) [L. *in* into + *quaerere* to seek] a legal inquiry before a coroner or medical examiner, and usually a jury, into the manner of a death.

inquiline (in′kwĭ-līn) [L. *inquilinus* a lodger] an organism that lives within the body of another, but does not derive its nourishment from the host.

insalivation (in″sal-ĭ-va′shun) [L. *in* in + *saliva* spittle] the saturation of the food with saliva in mastication.

insalubrious (in″sah-lu′bre-us) not salubrious; not conducive to health.

insane (in-sān′) [L. *in* not + *sanus* sound] mentally deranged. See *insanity*.

insanitary (in-san′ĭ-ter-e) not in a good sanitary condition; not conducive to good health; unclean.

insanity (in-san′ĭ-te) [L. *insanitas*, from *in* not + *sanus* sound] mental derangement or disorder, a legal rather than a medical term denoting a condition due to which a person lacks criminal responsibility for a crime and therefore cannot be convicted of it. **affective i.** (*obs.*), mood disorder. **alcoholic i.** (*obs.*), see under *psychosis*. **alternating i.** (*obs.*), circular psychosis. **circular i.** (*obs.*), see under *psychosis*. **climacteric i.** (*obs.*), involutional melancholia. **communicated i.** (*obs.*), folie à deux. **cyclic i.** (*obs.*), circular psychosis. **doubting i.** (*obs.*), insanity characterized by morbid doubt, suspicion, and indecision. **impulsive i.**, a compelling tendency to acts of violence. **manic-depressive i.** (*obs.*), bipolar disorder. **moral i.**, a 19th century concept corresponding roughly to antisocial personality disorder; a disorder of emotions and habits without impairment of the intellectual faculties in which the moral sense (concern for the rights and feelings of others) is stunted (*moral imbecility*) or absent (*moral idiocy*). Called also *moral oligophrenia* and *pathomania*. **simultaneous i.** (*obs.*), folie à deux. **toxic i.** (*obs.*), see under *psychosis*.

inscriptio (in-skrip′she-o), pl. *inscriptio′nes* [L., from *inscribere* to write on] 1. inscription. 2. intersectio. **i. tendin′ea**, intersectio tendinea. **inscriptio′nes tendin′eae mus′culi rec′ti abdom′inis,** intersectiones tendineae musculi recti abdominis.

inscription (in-skrip′shun) [L. *inscriptio*] 1. a mark, or line. 2. that part of a prescription which contains the names and amounts of the ingredients. **tendinous i.**, intersectio tendinea. **tendinous i′s of rectus abdominis muscle,** intersectiones tendineae musculi recti abdominis.

inscriptiones (in-skrip″she-o′nēz) [L.] plural of *inscriptio*.

insect (in′sekt) any individual of the class Insecta.

Insecta (in-sek′tah) [L. from *in* + *sectum* cut] a class of the Arthropoda whose members are characterized by division into three parts: head, thorax, and abdomen; there are three orders of medical interest, Hemiptera, Diptera, and Siphonaptera.

insectarium (in″sek-ta′re-um) a place for breeding and raising insects.

insecticide (in-sek′tĭ-sīd) [L. *insectum* insect + *caedere* to kill] any substance selectively poisonous to insects.

insectifuge (in-sek′tĭ-fūj) [*insect* + L. *fugare* to put to flight] a preparation that repels insects.

Insectivora (in″sek-tiv′o-rah) [*insect* + L. *vorare* to devour] an order of small, terrestrial mammals, including moles, shrews, etc., which feed primarily on invertebrates, especially on insects.

insectivore (in-sek′tĭ-vōr) an individual of the order Insectivora.

insectivorous (in″sek-tiv′o-rus) subsisting on insects.

insemination (in-sem″ĭ-na′shun) [L. *inseminatus* sown, from *in* into + *semen* seed] the deposit of seminal fluid within the vagina or cervix. **artificial i.**, introduction of semen into the vagina or cervix by artificial means. **donor i.**, **heterologous i.**, artificial insemination in which the semen used is that of a man other than the woman's husband; called also A.I.D. **homologous i.**, artificial insemination in which the husband's semen is used; called also A.I.H.

insenescence (in″sĕ-nes′ens) the process of growing old.

insensible (in-sen′sĭ-b′l) [L. *in* not + *sensibilis* appreciable] 1. not appreciable by or perceptible to the senses. 2. devoid of consciousness or of sensibility.

insert (in′sert) [L. *inserere* to graft, insert] 1. to put in, introduce, or implant something into another thing. 2. something that is inserted. **intramucosal i.**, **mucosal i.**, a nonreactive metal stud, consisting of a base, cervix, and head, attached to a prosthesis that is inserted into a small pocket of oral mucosa through a hole in the mucosa made immediately prior to fitting the denture; most commonly used for added retention of complete upper dentures.

insertio (in-ser′she-o) [L.] insertion. **i. velamento′sa,** velamentous insertion.

insertion (in-ser′shun) [L. *inserere* to join to] 1. the place of attachment, as of a muscle to the bone which it moves. 2. in genetics, a rare nonreciprocal translocation (q.v.) involving three breaks in which a segment is removed from one chromosome and then inserted into a broken region of a nonhomologous chromosome. **parasol i.**, insertion of the umbilical cord in the placenta, in which the vessels of the cord separate before they join the placenta and resemble the ribs of a parasol. **velamentous i.**, attachment of the umbili-

cal cord to the membranes, with the vessels coursing for a long or short distance between the amnion and the chorion to the body of the placenta.

insheathed (in-shēthd′) enclosed within a sheath.

insidious (in-sid′e-us) [L. *insidiosus* deceitful, treacherous] coming on in a stealthy manner; of gradual and subtle development.

insight (in′sīt) 1. in psychiatry, the patient's awareness and understanding of the origins and meaning of his attitudes, feelings, and behavior and of his disturbing symptoms; self-understanding. 2. in problem solving, the sudden perception of the appropriate relationships of things that results in a solution.

in situ (in si′tu) [L.] in the natural or normal place; confined to the site of origin without invasion of neighboring tissues.

insolation (in″so-la′shun) [L. *insolare* to expose to the sun; *in* in + *sol* sun] 1. treatment by exposure to the sun's rays; the sun bath. 2. sunstroke. **asphyxial i.,** sunstroke with low temperature, cold skin, and feeble pulse. **hyperpyrexial i.,** thermic fever with very high temperature, coma, and congested skin.

insoluble (in-sol′u-b′l) [L. *insolubilis*, from *in* not + *solvere* to dissolve] not susceptible of being dissolved.

insomnia (in-som′ne-ah) [L. *in* not + *somnus* sleep + -*ia*] inability to sleep; abnormal wakefulness.

insomniac (in-som′ne-ak) an individual exhibiting insomnia.

insomnic (in-som′nik) characterized by insomnia; unable to sleep.

insonate (in-so′nāt) to expose to ultrasound waves.

insorption (in-sorp′shun) the movement of a substance into the blood; said of such movement from the contents of the gastrointestinal tract into the circulating blood.

inspersion (in-sper′zhun) [L. *inspersio; in* upon + *spargere* to sprinkle] the act of sprinkling, as with a powder.

inspirate (in′spĭ-rāt) inhaled gas (or air).

inspiration (in″spĭ-ra′shun) [L. *inspirare*, from *in* in + *spirare* to breathe] the act of drawing air into the lungs.

inspirator (in′spĭ-ra″tor) [L.] (*obs.*) a form of inhaler or respirator.

inspiratory (in-spi′rah-to″re) pertaining to or subserving inspiration.

inspirometer (in″spi-rom′ĕ-ter) [*inspire* + Gr. *metron* measure] an apparatus for measuring the amount of air inspired.

inspissated (in-spis′āt-ed) [L. *inspissatus*, from *in* intensive + *spissare* to thicken] being thickened, dried, or rendered less fluid.

inspissation (in″spis-sa′shun) [L. *inspissatio*] 1. the act or process of rendering dry or thick by the evaporation of readily vaporizable parts. 2. the condition of being rendered less thin by evaporation.

inspissator (in-spis′a-tor) an apparatus for inspissating fluids, such as blood serum.

instar (in′stahr) [L. "a form"] any stage of an arthropod between molts.

instep (in′step) the dorsal part of the arch of the foot.

instillation (in″stil-la′shun) [L. *instillatio*, from *in* into + *stillare* to drop] administration of a liquid drop by drop.

instillator (in′stil-la″tor) an instrument for performing instillations.

instinct (in′stinkt) [L. *instinctus; in* on + *stinguere* to prick] a complex of unlearned responses that is characteristic of species. **aggressive i.**, death i. **death i.**, Freud's concept of an unconscious drive toward dissolution and death, in opposition to the life instinct. **ego i.**, any instinct that is not sexual, particularly the self-preservative instincts. **herd i.**, the instinct or urge to be one of a group and to conform to the standards of that group in conduct and opinion. **life i.**, Freud's concept of all the constructive tendencies of the organism aimed at maintenance and perpetuation of the individual and species, in opposition to the death instinct. **mother i.**, the complex behavior in a mother which accomplishes the care of the young; whether such an instinct exists in human females is questioned. **sexual i.**, life i.

instinctive (in-stink′tiv) of the nature of an instinct; performed apparently without the exercise of the reason.

instrument (in′stroo-ment) [L. *instrumentum; instruere* to furnish] any tool, appliance, or apparatus.

instrumental (in″stroo-men′tal) pertaining to or performed by instruments.

instrumentarium (in″stroo-men-ta′re-um) the instruments or equipment required for any particular operation or purpose; the physical adjuncts with which a physician combats disease.

instrumentation (in″stroo-men-ta′shun) the use of instruments; work performed with instruments. **Harrington i.,** a system of metal hooks and rods inserted surgically in the posterior elements of the spine to provide distraction and compression in treatment of scoliosis and other deformities.

insuccation (in″sŭ-ka′shun) [L. *insuccare* to soak in; *in* into + *succus* juice] the thorough soaking of a drug before preparing an extract from it.

insudation (in″su-da′shun) [*in-* + L. *sudare* to sweat] 1. the accumulation, as in the kidney or the arterial (intimal) wall, of substances derived from the blood. 2. the substance so accumulated.

insufficiency (in″sŭ-fish′en-se) [L. *insufficientia,* from *in* not + *sufficiens* sufficient] the condition of being insufficient or inadequate to the performance of the allotted duty. **active i.,** the inability of a muscle to act owing to the abnormal (or other) approximation of its insertion to its origin. **adrenal i.,** hypoadrenalism. **aortic i.,** see under *regurgitation.* **cardiac i.,** insufficiency of the heart muscle; see also *heart failure.* **coronary i.,** decrease in flow of blood through the coronary blood vessels. **i. of the externi,** insufficient power in the externi muscles of the eye, so that they are overbalanced by the interni, producing esophoria. **i. of the eyelids,** a condition in which the eyes are closed only by a conscious effort. **gastric i., gastromotor i.,** inability of the stomach to empty itself; myasthenia gastrica. **hepatic i.,** inability of the liver properly to perform its functions. **ileocecal i.,** inability of the ileocecal valve to prevent backflow of contents from the cecum into the ileum. **i. of the interni,** insufficient power in the interni muscles of the eye, so that they are overbalanced by the externi, producing exophoria. **mitral i.,** see under *regurgitation.* **muscular i.,** the inability of a muscle to do its normal work by a normal contraction. **myocardial i.,** insufficiency of the heart muscle; see also *heart failure.* **parathyroid i.,** hypoparathyroidism. **placental i.,** inability of the placenta to properly perform its functions, which compromises the fetal environment so that the fetus is in jeopardy. **pulmonary i.,** see *pulmonic regurgitation,* under *regurgitation.* **renal i.,** a state of disordered function of the kidneys verifiable by quantitative tests. See also *renal failure,* under *failure.* **thyroid i.,** hypothyroidism. **tricuspid i.,** see under *regurgitation.* **uterine i.,** weakness of the contractile power of the uterus, due to muscular atony. **i. of the valves, valvular i.,** see under *regurgitation.* **velopharyngeal i.,** inability to achieve velopharyngeal closure, due to muscular dysfunction, deficiency of the soft palate, or superior constrictor muscle, cleft palate, or other disorders, often resulting in defective speech. **venous i.,** inadequacy of the venous valves and impairment of venous return (venous stasis) from the legs, often with edema and sometimes with stasis ulcers at the ankle. **vertebrobasilar i.,** transient ischemia of the brain stem and cerebellum due to stenosis of the vertebral or basilar artery, resulting in attacks of such symptoms as vertigo, diplopia, nystagmus, muscle weakness, and dysarthria.

insufflation (in″sŭ-fla′shun) [L. *in* into + *sufflatio* a blowing up] 1. the act of blowing a powder, vapor, gas, or air into a body cavity. Cf. *infusion* (def. 3). 2. finely powdered or liquid drugs carried into the respiratory passages by such devices as aerosols. **cranial i.,** the forcing of air into the subdural space and the cerebral ventricles. **endotracheal i.,** introduction of air into the trachea through a tube passed into the larynx; employed to inflate the lungs during intrathoracic operations. **i. of the lungs,** the act of blowing air into the lungs for the purpose of artificial respiration. **perirenal i.,** the injection of air around the kidneys for the purpose of roentgen visualization of the adrenal glands. **presacral i.,** the injection of gas, usu-

ally carbon dioxide, around the kidneys through a needle inserted into the retrorectal space for the purpose of roentgen visualization of the entire retroperitioneal space, with delineation of renal and adrenal areas. **tubal i.,** see *Rubin's test,* under *test.*

insufflator (in′sŭ-fla″tor) an instrument used in performing insufflation.

insula (in′su-lah), gen. and pl. *in′sulae* [L. "island"] NA alternative for *lobus insularis.* **insulae of Peyer,** folliculi lymphatici aggregati. **i. of Reil,** lobus insularis.

insulae (in′su-le) [L.] genitive and plural of *insula.*

insular (in′su-lar) pertaining to an island, especially to the insula or to the islands of Langerhans.

insularine (in′su-lar-in) a yellow amorphous alkaloid, $C_{37}H_{38}O_6N_2$, from *Cissampelos insularis.*

Insulatard NPH (in′su-lah-tard) trademark for preparations of isophane insulin suspension.

insulation (in″sŭ-la′shun) [L. *insulare* to make an island of] 1. the surrounding of a space or body with material designed to prevent the entrance or escape of radiant or electrical energy. 2. the material so used.

insulator (in′su-la″tor) any substance or appliance of such nonconducting properties that it can be used to secure insulation.

insulin (in′su-lin) [L. *insula* island + *-in*] a protein hormone (molecular weight 5734) secreted by the beta cells of the pancreatic islets that serves as a hormonal signal of the fed state; it is secreted in response to elevated blood levels of glucose, amino acids, fatty acids, and ketone bodies and promotes the efficient storage and utilization of these fuel molecules by controlling the transport of metabolites and ions across cell membranes and regulating various intracellular biosynthetic pathways. Insulin promotes the entry of glucose, fatty acids, and amino acids into cells; promotes glycogen, protein, and lipid synthesis; and inhibits gluconeogenesis, glycogen degradation, protein degradation, and lipolysis. Insulin secretion is also influenced by several gastrointestinal hormones and by autonomic nervous activity. Insulin is formed from a single polypeptide chain (proinsulin) that is cleaved by specific proteases at two points; the two end pieces (the A and B chains) held together by two disulfide bridges, make up insulin; the middle piece (the connecting peptide or C-peptide) is also secreted but has no physiologic activity. Relative insulin deficiency is the cause of most cases of diabetes mellitus. Exogenous insulin is used for control of diabetes; various preparations differ in regard to source (bovine, porcine, a mixture of the two, or human), rapidity of onset and duration of action and degree of purification (most preparations contain some proinsulin and other antigenic components). **extended i. zinc suspension** [USP], a long-acting insulin with an approximate time of onset of 7 hours and duration of action of 36 hours, consisting of bovine or porcine insulin in the form of large zinc-insulin crystals. **globin i.,** see *globin zinc i.* **globin zinc i. injection** [USP], an intermediate-acting insulin; with an approximate time of onset of 2 hours and duration of action of 18 hours, consisting of bovine or porcine insulin reacted with zinc chloride and globin I (from bovine hemoglobin) to form a protein complex from which insulin is slowly released; now rarely used. **i. injection** [USP], regular insulin; a rapid-acting insulin with an approximate time of onset of 1 hour and duration of action of 6–8 hours, consisting of crystalline bovine or porcine insulin dissolved in a clear fluid. Called also *regular i.* **isophane i. suspension** [USP], an intermediate-acting insulin with an approximate time of onset of 2 hours and duration of action of 24 hours, consisting of bovine or porcine insulin reacted with zinc chloride and protamine to form a protein complex with a ratio of free and bound insulin, providing action intermediate between regular insulin and protamine zinc insulin. Called also *NPH i.* **Lente i.,** trademark for preparations of insulin zinc suspension. **NPH i.** [*N*eutral *P*rotamine *H*agedorn], isophane i. suspension. **prompt i. zinc suspension** [USP], a rapid-acting insulin with an approximate time of onset of 1 hour and duration of action of 14 hours, consisting of bovine or porcine insulin modified by the addition of zinc chloride to produce a suspension of amorphous insulin. **protamine zinc i. suspension** [USP], a long-acting insulin with an approximate time of onset of 7 hours and duration of action 36 hours, consisting of bovine or porcine insulin reacted with zinc chloride and protamine to form a protein complex from which insulin is slowly released. **regular i.,** i. injection. **Semilente i.,** trademark for preparations of prompt insulin zinc suspension. **three-to-one i.,** a combination of regular insulin and protamine zinc insulin, having the activity of three parts of the former and one part of the latter. **Ultralente i.,** trademark for preparations of extended insulin zinc suspension. **i. zinc suspension** [USP], an intermediate-acting insulin with an approximate time of onset of 2 hours and duration of action of 24 hours, consisting of a stable mixture of prompt and extended insulin zinc suspensions yielding a 7:3 ratio of crystalline to amorphous insulin.

insulinase (in′su-lin-ās) (obs.) an enzyme previously reported in body tissues that destroys or inactivates insulin; this effect is probably due to several nonspecific proteases.

insulinemia (in″su-lĭ-ne′me-ah) [*insulin* + Gr. *haima* blood + *-ia*] the presence of insulin in the blood.

insulinlipodystrophy (in″su-lin-li″po-dis′tro-fe) the local disappearance of fat at the sites of injection in diabetic patients on insulin treatment.

insulinogenesis (in″su-lin-o-jen′ĕ-sis) the formation and release of insulin by the islands of Langerhans.

insulinogenic (in″su-lin″o-jen′ik) pertaining to, characterized by, or promoting insulinogenesis.

insulinoid (in′su-lin-oid″) 1. resembling insulin. 2. any substance with hypoglycemic properties like those of insulin.

insulinoma (in″su-lin-o′mah) a tumor of the beta cells of the islets of Langerhans; although usually benign, such tumors are among the most important causes of hypoglycemia.

insulinopenic (in″su-lin-o-pe′nik) diminishing, or pertaining to a decrease in, the level of circulating insulin; said of most forms of diabetes mellitus characterized by clear-cut deficiency of insulin production.

insulism (in′su-lizm) hyperinsulinism.

insulitis (in″su-li′tis) cellular infiltration of the islands of Langerhans, a reaction similar to that observed in autoimmune diseases.

insulogenic (in″su-lo-jen′ik) insulinogenic.

insuloma (in″su-lo′mah) [L. *insula* island (of Langerhans) + *-oma*] insulinoma.

insult (in′sult) [L. *insultus* attack] injury or trauma; attack.

insusceptibility (in″sŭ-sep″tĭ-bil′ĭ-te) the quality of not being susceptible; immunity.

intake (in-tāk′) the substances, or the quantities thereof, taken in and utilized by the body. **caloric i.,** the caloric ingested or otherwise taken into the body. **fluid i.,** the fluid taken into the body by drinking or parenterally.

Intal (in′tal) trademark for a preparation of cromolyn sodium.

integration (in″tĕ-gra′shun) 1. assimilation; anabolic action or activity. 2. the combining of different acts so that they cooperate toward a common end; coordination. 3. constructive assimilation into the personality of knowledge and experience. 4. in bacterial genetics, assimilation of genetic material from one bacterium (donor) into the chromosome of another (recipient). **biological i.,** the acquisition of functional coordination during embryonic development through humoral and nervous influences.

integrator (in′tĕ-gra″tor) an instrument for measuring body surfaces.

integument (in-teg′u-ment) [L. *integumentum*] 1. a covering or investment. 2. integumentum commune. **common i.,** integumentum commune.

integumentary (in-teg-u-men′tar-e) 1. pertaining to or composed of skin. 2. serving as a covering, like the skin.

integumentum (in-teg″u-men′tum) [L., from *in* on + *tegere* to cover] [NA] 1. a covering or investment. 2. i. commune. **i. commu′ne** [NA], common integument: the covering of the body, or skin, including its various layers and their appendages; in humans, it comprises the epidermis, dermis, subcutaneous tissue, hair, nails, cutaneous glands, the breast, and mammary glands. Called also *integument* and *integumentum.*

in tela (in te′lah) [L.] in tissue; relating especially to stained histological preparations.

intellect (in′te-lekt) [L. *intellectus*, from *intelligere* to understand] the mind, thinking faculty, or understanding.

intellectualization (in″tĕ-lek″chu-al-ĭ-za′shun) an unconscious defense mechanism in which reasoning is used to avoid confronting an objectionable impulse and thus to defend against anxiety.

intelligence (in-tel′ĭ-jens) [L. *intelligere* to understand] the ability to comprehend or understand; see also under *quotient.*

intemperance (in-tem′per-ans) [L. *in* not + *temperare* to moderate] excess or lack of self-control in respect of food and drink; immoderate indulgence in the use of alcoholic drinks.

intensification (in-ten″sĭ-fi-ka′shun) [L. *intensus* intense + *facere* to make] 1. the act of making anything intense. 2. the process of becoming intense.

intensimeter (in″ten-sim′ĕ-ter) Fürstenau's device for measuring the intensity of roentgen rays; it is based on the variation of electric resistance of a selenium cell under influence of irradiation at different intensities.

intensionometer (in-ten″se-o-nom′ĕ-ter) an ionometric instrument for measuring the intensity of roentgen rays. Two series of plates, separated by an air gap that serves as the dielectric, are connected to opposite terminals in a closed chamber. An electric circuit is completed when the air becomes ionized by the roentgen rays, and the difference in electric potential is registered by deflection of a galvanometer needle.

intensity (in-ten′sĭ-te) [L. *intensus* intense; *in* on + *tendere* to stretch] the condition or quality of being intense; a high degree of tension, activity, or energy. **i. of electric field,** the force exerted on a unit charge in an electric field. **luminous i.,** the light-giving power of a source of light. Cf. *candle power.* **i. of roentgen rays,** the roentgen-ray energy passing per unit time through unit area normal to the direction of propagation.

intensive (in-ten′siv) [L. *in* on + *tendere* to stretch] of great force or intensity; see also *intensive care unit,* under *unit.*

intention (in-ten′shun) [L. *intentio,* from *in* upon + *tendere* to stretch] a manner of healing; see under *healing.*

inter- [L. *inter* between] a prefix meaning between or among.

interaccessory (in″ter-ak-ses′o-re) connecting the accessory processes of the vertebrae.

interacinar (in″ter-as′ĭ-nar) situated between acini.

interacinous (in″ter-as′ĭ-nus) interacinar.

interaction (in″ter-ak′shun) the quality, state, or process of (two or more things) acting on each other. **drug i.,** the action of one drug upon the effectiveness or toxicity of another (or others).

interalveolar (in″ter-al-ve′o-lar) between alveoli.

interangular (in″ter-ang′gu-lar) situated or occurring between two or more angles.

interannular (in″ter-an′u-lar) [*inter-* + L. *annulus* ring] situated between two rings or constrictions.

interarticular (in″ter-ar-tik′u-lar) [*inter-* + L. *articulus* joint] situated between articular surfaces.

interarytenoid (in″ter-ar″e-te′noid) between the arytenoid cartilages.

interatrial (in″ter-a′tre-al) situated between the atria of the heart.

interauricular (in″ter-aw-rik′u-lar) interatrial.

interbrain (in′ter-brān) diencephalon.

intercalary (in-ter′kah-ler″e) [L. *intercalarius; inter-* + *calare* to call] inserted or placed between; interposed.

intercalate (in-ter′kah-lāt) [L. *intercalare*] to insert between.

intercalatum (in″ter-kah-la′tum) (obs.) substantia nigra.

intercanalicular (in″ter-kan″ah-lik′u-lar) between canaliculi.

intercapillary (in″ter-kap′ĭ-lār-e) among or between capillaries.

intercarotic (in″ter-kah-rot′ik) between the carotid arteries.

intercarotid (in″ter-kah-rot′id) intercarotic.

intercarpal (in″ter-kar′pal) between the carpal bones.

intercartilaginous (in″ter-kar″tĭ-laj′ĭ-nus) connecting or situated between two or more cartilages.

intercavernous (in″ter-kav′er-nus) between two cavities.

intercellular (in″ter-sel′u-lar) situated between the cells of any structure.

intercentral (in″ter-sen′tral) situated between or connecting two or more nerve centers.

intercerebral (in″ter-ser′ĕ-bral) connecting or situated between the two cerebral hemispheres.

interchange (in′ter-chānj″) translocation.

interchondral (in″ter-kon′dral) intercartilaginous.

intercilium (in″ter-sil′e-um) [*inter-* + L. *cilium* eyelash] the space between the eyebrows.

interclavicular (in″ter-klah-vik′u-lar) [*inter-* + L. *clavicula* clavicle] situated between the clavicles.

interclinoid (in″ter-kli′noid) pertaining to or passing between the clinoid processes.

intercoccygeal (in″ter-kok-sij′e-al) situated between the segments of the coccyx.

intercolumnar (in″ter-ko-lum′nar) [*inter-* + L. *columna* column] situated between columns or pillars.

intercondylar (in″ter-kon′dĭ-lar) situated between two condyles.

intercondyloid (in″ter-kon′dĭ-loid) intercondylar.

intercondylous (in″ter-kon′dĭ-lus) intercondylar.

intercostal (in″ter-kos′tal) [*inter-* + L. *costa* rib] situated between the ribs.

intercostohumeral (in″ter-kos-to-hu′mer-al) pertaining to an intercostal space and the humerus.

intercourse (in′ter-kōrs) [L. *intercursus* running between] mutual exchange. **sexual i.,** coitus.

intercricothyrotomy (in″ter-kri″ko-thi-rot′o-me) [*inter-* + *cricothyroid* + Gr. *temnein* to cut] incision of the larynx through the cricothyroid membrane; inferior laryngotomy.

intercristal (in″ter-kris′tal) between two crests.

intercritical (in″ter-krit′ĭ-kal) denoting the period between attacks, as of gout.

intercross (in′ter-kros) [*inter-* + *cross* (def. 2.)] the mating of individuals heterozygous for the same gene; cf. *incross.*

intercrural (in″ter-kru′ral) between two crura.

intercurrent (in″ter-kur′ent) [L. *intercurrens,* from *inter-* + *currere* to run] breaking into and modifying the course of an already existing disease.

intercuspation (in″ter-kus-pa′shun) the fitting together of cusps of opposing teeth in occlusion; the cusp-to-fossa relationship of the upper and lower posterior teeth to each other.

intercusping (in″ter-kusp′ing) the occlusion of the cusps of the teeth of one jaw with the depressions in the teeth of the other jaw.

interdeferential (in″ter-def″er-en′shal) between the two ductus deferentes.

interdental (in″ter-den′tal) [*inter-* + L. *dens* tooth] situated between the proximal surfaces of adjacent teeth in the same dental arch. See also *interocclusal* and *interproximal.*

interdentale (in″ter-den-ta′le) a craniometric landmark located between the right and left central incisors, in the midline on the tip of the alveolar septum.

interdentium (in″ter-den′she-um) the interproximal space; see under *space.*

interdigit (in″ter-dij′it) the space between any two contiguous fingers or toes.

interdigital (in″ter-dij′ĭ-tal) [*inter-* + L. *digitus* finger] situated between two adjacent fingers or toes.

interdigitate (in″ter-dij′ĭ-tāt) [*inter-* + L. *digitus* finger] to interlock and interrelate, as the fingers of clasped hands.

interdigitation (in″ter-dij″ĭ-ta′shun) [*inter-* + L. *digitus* digit] 1. an interlocking of parts by finger-like processes. 2. any one of a set of finger-like processes.

interface (in′ter-fās) in chemistry, the surface of separation or boundary between two phases of a heterogeneous system. **dineric i.,** the interface between two immiscible liquids.

interfacial (in″ter-fa′shal) pertaining to an interface.

interfascicular (in″ter-fah-sik′u-lar) [*inter-* + L. *fasciculus* bundle] situated between fasciculi.

interfemininium (in″ter-fĕ-min′e-um) [L.] (*obs.*) the space between the thighs, or the inside of the thighs.

interfemoral (in″ter-fem′o-ral) between the thighs.

interfemus (in″ter-fe′mus) [L.] interfemininium.

interference (in″ter-fēr′ens) [*inter-* + L. *ferire* to strike] 1. opposition or hampering of an action or procedure. 2. the process in which two or more light, sound, or electromagnetic waves of the same frequency combine to reinforce or cancel each other, the amplitude of the resulting wave being equal to the sum of the amplitudes of the combining waves. 3. an interplay of two intrinsic pacemakers in the heart, one or the other dominating the rhythm. See also *interference dissociation,* under *dissociation.* 4. any premature contact point along the occlusal surface of the teeth that prevents maximum contact, function, and proper alignment in full occlusion. See also *deflective occlusal contact,* under *contact.* **cuspal i.,** deflective occlusal contact. **occlusal i's,** occlusal contacts hampering or hindering smooth, gliding, harmonious jaw movements with the teeth maintaining contact. **proactive i.,** see under *inhibition.* **retroactive i.,** see under *inhibition.*

interfering (in″ter-fēr′ing) brushing; the striking or rubbing of the fetlock of a horse by the opposite foot.

interferometer (in″ter-fēr-om′ĕ-ter) an instrument for measuring lengths or movements by means of the phenomena caused by the interference of two rays of light, or of sound (acoustic i.).

interferometry (in″ter-fēr-om′ĕ-tre) the use of the interferometer for measuring distances or movements.

interferon (in″ter-fēr′on) any of a family of glycoproteins that exert virus-nonspecific but host-specific antiviral activity by inducing the transcription of cellular genes coding for antiviral proteins that selectively inhibit the synthesis of viral RNA and proteins. Interferons also have immunoregulatory functions (inhibition of B cell activation and antibody production enhancement of T cell activity, and enhancement of NK cell cytotoxic activity) and can inhibit the growth of nonviral intracellular parasites. Production of interferon can be stimulated by viral infection, especially by the presence of double-stranded RNA, by intracellular parasites (chlamidiae, rickettsiae), by protozoa (*Toxoplasma*) and by bacteria (streptococci, staphylococci) and bacterial products (endotoxins). Interferons have been divided into three distinct types (α, β, and γ) associated with specific producer cells and functions, but all animal cells are able to produce interferons, and certain producer cells (leukocytes and fibroblasts) produce more than one type (both interferon-α and interferon-β). Abbreviated IFN. **i.-α (IFN-α),** the major interferon produced by virus-induced leukocyte cultures; the primary producer cells are null lymphocytes, and the major activities are antiviral activity and activation of NK cells. It is used in the experimental treatment of hairy cell leukemia and other selected neoplasia. Called also *leukocyte i.* **i.-β (IFN-β),** the major interferon produced by double-stranded RNA–induced fibroblast cultures; the primary producer cells are fibroblasts, epithelial cells, and macrophages, and the major activity is antiviral activity. Called also *epithelial, fibroblast,* or *fibroepithelial i.* **epithelial i., fibroblast i., fibroepithelial i.,** i.-β. **i.-γ (IFN-γ),** the major interferon produced by immunologically stimulated (by mitogens or antigens) lymphocyte cultures; the primary producer cells are T lymphocytes, and the major activity is immunoregulation. IFN-γ has been implicated in aberrant expression of class II histocompatibility antigens by tissue cells (such as thyroid cells) that do not normally express them, leading to autoimmune disease. Called also *immune i.* **immune i.,** i.-γ. **leukocyte i.,** i.-α. **type I i.,** i.-α and i.-β. **type II i.,** i.-γ.

interfibrillar (in″ter-fi′bril-ar) [*inter-* + L. *fibrilla* small fiber] between or among fibrils.

interfibrillary (in″ter-fi′brĭ-lār″e) interfibrillar.

interfibrous (in″ter-fi′brus) between fibers.

interfilamentous (in″ter-fil″ah-men′tus) between filaments.

interfilar (in″ter-fi′lar) [*inter-* + L. *filum* thread] between or among the fibrils of a reticulum.

interfrontal (in″ter-fron′tal) between the halves of the frontal bone.

interfurca (in″ter-fur′kah), pl. *interfur′cae* [*inter-* + L. *furca* fork] the area lying between and at the base of divided tooth roots.

interfurcae (in″ter-fur′se) [L.] plural of *interfurca.*

interganglionic (in″ter-gang″gle-on′ik) [inter- + ganglion] between ganglia.

intergemmal (in″ter-jem′al) [inter- + L. gemma bud] between taste buds or other buds.

interglobular (in″ter-glob′u-lar) [inter- + L. globulus globule] between or among globules, as of the dentin.

intergluteal (in″ter-gloo′te-al) between the buttocks.

intergonial (in″ter-go′ne-al) between the tips of the two angles of the mandible.

intergradation (in″ter-grah-da′shun) [inter- + L. gradus step] the interbreeding of two subspecies of the same species in the environmental area where they meet (primary i.) or of closely related species whose ranges overlap before isolating mechanisms are fully developed (secondary i.).

intergrade (in′ter-grād) [inter- + L. gradus a step] a step or stage between two other stages. **sex i.,** an individual showing characteristics between the typical male and female condition. See intersex and hermaphroditism.

intergranular (in″ter-gran′u-lar) between the granule cells of the brain.

intergyral (in″ter-ji′ral) between cerebral gyri or convolutions.

interhemicerebral (in″ter-hem″ĭ-ser′ĕ-bral) intercerebral.

interhemispheric (in″ter-hem″ĭ-sfer′ik) intercerebral.

interictal (in″ter-ik′tal) occurring between attacks or paroxysms.

interior (in-tēr′e-or) [L. "inner"; neut. interius] 1. situated inside; inward. 2. an inner part or cavity.

interischiadic (in″ter-is″ke-ad′ik) between the two ischia.

interkinesis (in″ter-ki-ne′sis) [inter- + Gr. kinēsis motion] a period intervening between the first and second divisions in meiosis, similar to the interphase in mitosis.

interlabial (in″ter-la′be-al) [inter- + L. labium lip] between the lips, or between any two labia.

interlamellar (in″ter-lah-mel′ar) [inter- + L. lamella layer] situated between lamellae.

interleukin (in″ter-loo′kin) a generic term for a group of protein factors produced by macrophages and T cells in response to antigenic or mitogenic stimulation and affecting primarily T cells. **i.-1 (IL-1),** a macrophage-produced interleukin that induces the production of interleukin-2 by T cells that have been stimulated by antigen or mitogen; at least two types exist, designated α and β. IL-1 or a similar protein is also produced by epithelial cells and stimulates fibroblast proliferation and release of proteolytic enzymes (e.g., collagenase) and prostaglandins in inflammatory processes. IL-1 also appears to be identical to endogenous pyrogen. Formerly called lymphocyte-activating factor (LAF). **i.-2 (IL-2),** an interleukin produced by T cells in response to antigenic or mitogenic stimulation and the signal carried by interleukin-1. It stimulates the proliferation of T cells bearing specific receptors for IL-2, which are only expressed by antigenically stimulated T cells. IL-2 also seems to induce production of interferon-γ. It is used as an anticancer drug in the treatment of a wide variety of solid malignant tumors. Formerly called T-cell growth factor (TCGF). **i.-3 (IL-3),** a lymphokine produced by antigen- or mitogen-activated T lymphocytes, which stimulates proliferation of hematopoietic as well as lymphoid stem cells; a colony-stimulating factor for all bone marrow progenitor cells. IL-3 supports the growth and differentiation of early hematopoietic and lymphoid stem cells as well as that of more mature hematopoietic cells, including granulocytes, macrophages, and mast cells.

interligamentary (in″ter-lig″ah-men′tah-re) between or among ligaments.

interligamentous (in″ter-lig″ah-men′tus) interligamentary.

interlobar (in″ter-lo′bar) [inter- + L. lobus lobe] situated or occurring between lobes.

interlobitis (in″ter-lo-bi′tis) interlobular pleurisy.

interlobular (in″ter-lob′u-lar) [inter- + L. lobulus lobule] situated or occurring between lobules.

interlocking (in″ter-lok′ing) a complication of labor in twin births in which the inferior surface of the chin of one twin is hooked to that of its co-twin above or below the pelvic inlet. When this condition occurs in the true pelvis, it is called compaction.

intermalleolar (in″ter-mah-le′o-lar) between the malleoli.

intermamillary (in″ter-mam′ĭ-lār″e) between the nipples.

intermammary (in″ter-mam′ah-re) between the breasts.

intermarriage (in″ter-mar′ij) [inter- + L. maritare to wed] 1. the marriage of persons related by blood or consanguinity. 2. the marriage of persons of different racial, ethnic, social, or religious groups.

intermaxilla (in″ter-mak-sil′ah) the intermaxillary bone.

intermaxillary (in″ter-mak′sĭ-lār″e) situated between the two maxillae.

intermediary (in″ter-me′de-ār″e) [inter- + L. medius middle] 1. performed or occurring in a median stage; neither early nor late; intermediate. 2. an intermediate stage.

intermediate (in″ter-me′de-it) [inter- + L. medius middle] 1. placed between; intervening; resembling, in part, each of two extremes. 2. a substance formed in a chemical process that is essential to the formation of the end product of the process.

intermedin (in″ter-me′din) melanocyte-stimulating hormone; so called because in amphibia, reptiles, and fish, it is secreted by the pars intermedia of the pituitary gland.

intermediolateral (in″ter-me″de-o-lat′er-al) both intermediate and lateral.

intermedius (in″ter-me′de-us) intermediate; [NA] a term denoting the middle of three structures, one of which is situated closer to and the other farther from the midline of the body or part.

intermembranous (in″ter-mem′brah-nus) situated or occurring between membranes.

intermeningeal (in″ter-mĕ-nin′je-al) situated or occurring between the meninges.

intermenstrual (in″ter-men′stroo-al) [inter- + menstrual] occurring between the menstrual periods.

intermenstruum (in″ter-men′stroo-um) the interval between two menstrual periods.

intermetacarpal (in″ter-met″ah-kar′pal) [inter- + metacarpal] situated between the metacarpal bones.

intermetameric (in″ter-met″ah-mer′ik) between two metameres.

intermetatarsal (in″ter-met″ah-tar′sal) situated or occurring between the metatarsal bones.

intermission (in″ter-mish′un) [L. intermissio; inter between + mittere to send] an interval; a period of temporary cessation, as between two occurrences or paroxysms.

intermitotic (in″ter-mi-tot′ik) pertaining to or occurring during the interval between successive mitoses.

intermittent (in″ter-mit′ent) [L. intermittens; inter between + mittere to send] occurring at separated intervals; having periods of cessation of activity.

intermolecular (in″ter-mo-lek′u-lar) between molecules.

intermural (in-ter-mu′ral) [inter- + L. murus wall] situated between the walls of organs.

intermuscular (in″ter-mus′ku-lar) situated between muscles.

intern (in′tern) 1. [Fr. interne] a graduate of a medical or dental school serving and residing in a hospital preparatory to being licensed to practice medicine or dentistry. Cf. resident. 2. [Fr. interner] to confine within certain geographical or physical boundaries.

internal (in-ter′nal) [L. internus] situated or occurring within or on the inside; many anatomical structures formerly called internal are now correctly termed medial.

internalization (in-ter″nal-ĭ-za′shun) the mental process whereby certain attributes, attitudes, or standards of others are unconsciously taken as one's own.

internarial (in″ter-na′re-al) [inter- + L. nares nostrils] situated between the nares.

internasal (in″ter-na′zal) situated between the nasal bones.

internatal (in″ter-na′tal) [inter- + L. nates buttocks] between the buttocks or gluteal prominences.

International Nonproprietary Names see I.N.N.

interne (in-tern′) [Fr.] intern.

interneuron (in″ter-nu′ron) any neuron, in a chain of

neurons, which is situated between the primary afferent (sensory) neuron and the final motoneuron. Also, any neuron whose processes are entirely confined within a specific area, as within the olfactory lobe, and which synapse with neurons extending into that area.

internist (in-ter′nist) a physician who specializes in the diagnosis and medical, as opposed to surgical and obstetrical, treatment of diseases of adults.

internodal (in″ter-no′dal) between two nodes.

internode (in′ter-nōd) [inter- + L. nodus knot] a space between two nodes. **i. of Ranvier,** the segment of a nerve fiber between two nodes of Ranvier.

internodular (in″ter-nod′u-lar) between two nodules.

internship (in′tern-ship) the position or term of service of an intern in a hospital.

internuclear (in″ter-nu′kle-ar) 1. pertaining to or affecting structures between nuclei, as internuclear ophthalmoplegia. 2. between the nuclear layers of the retina.

internuncial (in″ter-nun′she-al) [L. internuncius a go-between] serving as a medium of communication between nerve cells or centers; see interneuron.

internus (in-ter′nus) internal; [NA] a term denoting something situated nearer to the center of an organ or a cavity.

interocclusal (in″ter-ŏ-kloo′zal) situated between the occlusal surfaces of opposing teeth of the mandibular and maxillary arches. See also interdental and interproximal.

interoceptive (in″ter-o-sep′tiv) Sherrington's term for the internal surface field of distribution of receptor organs; see receptor (def. 3), exteroceptive, and proprioceptive.

interoceptor (in″ter-o-sep′tor) any one of the sensory nerve terminals which are located in and transmit impulses from the viscera; see receptor (def. 3), exteroceptor, and proprioceptor.

interofection (in″ter-o-fek′shun) the responses of the body to changes in the internal environment of the body effected by the sympathetic system.

interofective (in″ter-o-fek′tiv) affecting the interior of the organism; a term applied by Cannon to the autonomic nervous system.

interoinferiorly (in″ter-o-in-fēr′e-or″le) inwardly and in a downward position or direction.

interolivary (in″ter-ol′ĭ-vār″e) situated between the olivary bodies of the brain.

interorbital (in″ter-or′bĭ-tal) [inter- + L. orbita orbit] situated between the orbits.

interosseal (in″ter-os′e-al) [inter- + L. os bone] 1. situated between bones. 2. pertaining to the interossei muscles.

interosseous (in″ter-os′e-us) [L. interosseus; inter between + os bone] between bones.

interpalpebral (in″ter-pal′pe-bral) between the eyelids.

interparietal (in″ter-pah-ri′ĕ-tal) [inter- + L. paries wall] 1. intermural. 2. situated between the parietal bones.

interparoxysmal (in″ter-par″ok-siz′mal) occurring between paroxysms.

interpediculate (in″ter-pĕ-dik′u-lāt) between the pedicles of a vertebra, as interpediculate distance.

interpeduncular (in″ter-pĕ-dunk′u-lar) [inter- + L. pedunculus peduncle] situated between two peduncles, as between two cerebellar peduncles.

interphalangeal (in″ter-fah-lan′je-al) [inter- + L. phalangeal] situated between two contiguous phalanges.

interphase (in′ter-fāz) the interval between two successive cell divisions, during which the chromosomes are not individually distinguishable and the normal physiological processes proceed. Formerly called resting phase.

interphyletic (in″ter-fi-let′ik) [inter- + phyletic] intermediate in form between two types of cell.

interpial (in″ter-pi′al) situated between the two layers of the pia mater.

interplant (in′ter-plant) [inter- + L. plantare to set] an embryonic part isolated by transference to an indifferent environment provided by another embryo.

interpleural (in″ter-ploor′al) between two layers of the pleura, as between the visceral and the parietal pleura.

interpolar (in″ter-po′lar) [inter- + L. polus pole] situated between two poles.

interpolation (in-ter″po-la′shun) the determination of intermediate values in a series on the basis of observed values.

interposition (in″ter-po-zish′un) the act of placing between; the condition of being interposed.

interpositum (in″ter-poz′i-tum) [L.] interposed; see under velum.

interpretation (in-ter″prĕ-ta′shun) in psychotherapy, the therapist's explanation of the latent or hidden meanings of what the patient says, does, or experiences, in terms which are understandable to him.

interprotometamere (in″ter-pro″to-met′ah-mēr) [inter- + Gr. prōtos first + meta across + meros part] the structure between the primary segments of the embryo.

interproximal (in″ter-prok′sĭ-mal) between adjoining surfaces, as the space between adjacent teeth. See also interdental and interocclusal.

interpubic (in″ter-pu′bik) [inter- + L. pubes] between the pubic bones.

interpupillary (in″ter-pu′pĭ-lar″e) between the pupils.

interradial (in″ter-ra′de-al) situated between rays.

interrenal (in″ter-re′nal) [inter- + renal] between the kidneys.

interrupted (in″ter-rupt′ed) [L. interruptus; inter between + ruptus broken] not continuous; marked by intermissions or breaches of continuity.

interscapilium (in″ter-skah-pil′e-um) [L.] the space between the scapulae.

interscapular (in″ter-skap′u-lar) [inter- + L. scapula shoulder blade] situated between the scapulae.

interscapulum (in″ter-skap′u-lum) the interscapilium.

intersciatic (in″ter-si-at′ik) between the two ischia.

intersectio (in″ter-sek′she-o), pl. intersectio′nes [L., from inter between + secare to cut] [NA] a general term denoting a cutting across, or between; a site at which one structure cuts across another. **i. tendin′ea,** tendinous intersection: a fibrous band that crosses the belly of a muscle and more or less completely divides it into two parts; called also inscriptio tendinea. **intersectio′nes tendin′eae mus′culi rec′ti abdom′inis** [NA], tendinous intersections of rectus abdominis muscle: three or more fibrous bands that cross the front of the rectus abdominis muscle, fusing with the anterior layer of its sheath; called also inscriptiones tendineae musculi recti abdominis.

intersection (in″ter-sek′shun) a site at which one structure cuts across another. **tendinous i.,** intersectio tendinea.

intersectiones (in″ter-sek″she-o′nēz) [L.] plural of intersectio.

intersegment (in″ter-seg′ment) 1. any one of a series of segments, like the angiotomes, etc. 2. a metamere.

intersegmental (in″ter-seg-men′tal) between segments.

interseptal (in″ter-sep′tal) between two septa.

interseptum (in″ter-sep′tum) [L.] the diaphragm.

intersex (in′ter-seks) 1. intersexuality. 2. an individual who shows intermingling, in varying degrees, of the characters of each sex, including physical form, reproductive organs, and sexual behavior. See also hermaphrodite and pseudohermaphrodite. **female i.,** a female pseudohermaphrodite: an individual who shows one or more contradictions of the morphological criteria of sex but who has only female gonadal tissue and shows sex chromatin in the somatic cells (XX chromosomal constitution). **male i.,** a male pseudohermaphrodite: an individual who shows one or more contradictions of the morphological criteria of sex but who has only male gonadal tissue and shows no sex chromatin in the somatic cells (usually XY chromosomal constitution). **true i.,** a true hermaphrodite: an individual who shows one or more contradictions of the morphological criteria of sex and possesses both male and female gonadal tissue; the chromatin test may be either positive or negative (XX or XY chromosomal constitution or mosaicism).

intersexual (in″ter-seks′u-al) pertaining to or characterized by intersexuality.

intersexuality (in″ter-seks″u-al′ĭ-te) the intermingling, in varying degrees, of the characters of each sex, including physical form, reproductive organs, and sexual behavior, in one individual, as a result of any one of several errors in embryonic development. See also *intersex, hermaphroditism,* and *pseudohermaphroditism.*

interspace (in'ter-spās) a space between two similar structures. **dineric i.,** the surface between two liquid phases.

interspinal (in-ter-spi'nal) between two spinous processes.

interspinous (in''ter-spi'nus) interspinal.

intersternal (in''ter-ster'nal) between parts of the sternum.

interstice (in-ter'stis) [L. *interstitium*] a small interval, space, or gap in a tissue or structure.

interstitial (in''ter-stish'al) [L. *interstitialis; inter* between + *sistere* to set] pertaining to or situated between parts or in the interspaces of a tissue.

interstitium (in''ter-stish'ĭ-um) [L.] 1. interstice. 2. interstitial tissue.

intertarsal (in''ter-tar'sal) situated between the tarsal bones.

intertransverse (in''ter-trans-vers') [*inter-* + L. *transversus* turned across] situated between or connecting the transverse processes of the vertebrae.

intertriginous (in''ter-trij'ĭ-nus) affected with or of the nature of intertrigo.

intertrigo (in''ter-tri'go) [*inter-* + L. *terere* to rub] a superficial dermatitis occurring on apposed skin surfaces, such as the axillae, creases of the neck, intergluteal fold, groin, between the toes, and beneath pendulous breasts, with obesity being a predisposing factor, caused by moisture, friction, warmth, and sweat retention, and characterized by erythema, maceration, burning, itching, and sometimes erosions, fissures, and exudations and secondary infections. Called also *eczema intertrigo.* **i. labia'lis,** perlèche.

intertrochanteric (in''ter-tro''kan-ter'ik) [*inter-* + *trochanter*] situated in or pertaining to the space between the greater and the lesser trochanter.

intertubercular (in''ter-tu-ber'ku-lar) between tubercles.

intertubular (in''ter-tu'bu-lar) [*inter-* + L. *tubulus* tubule] situated between or among tubules.

interureteral (in''ter-u-re'ter-al) interureteric.

interureteric (in''ter-u''rĕ-ter'ik) [*inter-* + *ureter*] situated between the ureters.

intervaginal (in''ter-vaj'ĭ-nal) situated between sheaths.

interval (in'ter-val) [*inter-* + L. *vallum* rampart] the space between two objects or parts; the lapse of time between two recurrences or paroxysms. **atrioventricular i.,** the P–R interval; the time between atrial and ventricular systole. **auriculoventricular i.,** atrioventricular i. **cardioarterial i.,** the time between the apex beat and arterial pulsation; abbreviated c.-a. i. **confidence i.,** a type of statistical interval estimate for an unknown parameter: a range of values believed to contain the parameter, with a predetermined degree of confidence. Its endpoints (confidence limits) are statistics computed from sample data and it has a stated probability (the confidence coefficient) of containing the parameter. **focal i.,** the distance from the anterior to the posterior focal point; called also *Sturm's i.* **lucid i.,** a brief period of remission of symptoms in a psychosis, or a brief return to consciousness after loss of consciousness in head injury. **postsphygmic i.,** see under *period.* **P–R i.,** the portion of the electrocardiogram between the onset of the P wave (atrial activity) and the QRS complex (ventricular activity). **presphygmic i.,** see under *period.* **QRST i., Q–T i.,** the duration of ventricular electrical activity. **reference i.,** see under *value.* **Sturm's i.,** focal i. **tolerance i.,** an interval estimate that has a specified probability of covering a specified fraction of the parent population.

intervalvular (in''ter-val'vu-lar) between valves.

intervascular (in''ter-vas'ku-lar) between blood vessels.

intervention (in''ter-ven'shun) the act or fact of interfering so as to modify. **crisis i.,** 1. an immediate, short-term, psychotherapeutic approach, the goal of which is to help resolve a personal crisis within the individual's immediate environment. 2. the procedures involved in responding to an emergency.

interventricular (in''ter-ven-trik'u-lar) [*inter-* + L. *ventriculum* ventricle] situated between ventricles.

intervertebral (in''ter-ver'tĕ-bral) [*inter-* + *vertebra*] situated between two contiguous vertebrae; see under *disk.*

intervillous (in''ter-vil'us) [*inter-* + L. *villus* tuft] situated between or among villi.

intestinal (in-tes'tĭ-nal) [L. *intestinalis*] pertaining to the intestine.

intestine (in-tes'tin) [L. *intesti'nus* inward, internal; Gr. *enteron*] the portion of the alimentary canal extending from the pyloric opening of the stomach to the anus; called also *bowel* and *gut.* See *intestinum.* **blind i.,** caecum (def. 2). **empty i.,** jejunum. **iced i.,** peritonitis chronica fibrosa encapsulans. **jejunoileal i.,** intestinum tenue mesenteriale. **large i.,** the distal portion of the intestine; see *intestinum crassum* [NA]. **mesenterial i.,** intestinum tenue mesenteriale. **segmented i.,** colon. **small i.,** the proximal portion of the intestine; see *intestinum tenue* [NA]. **straight i.,** rectum.

intestino-intestinal (in-tes''tĭ-no-in-tes'tĭ-nal) pertaining to two different portions of the intestine, as the intestino-intestinal reflex.

intestinum (in''tes-ti'num), pl. *intesti'na* [L., from *intestinus* inward, internal] intestine: the portion of the alimentary canal extending from the pyloric opening of the stomach to the anus: it is a membranous tube, comprising the intestinum tenue and the intestinum crassum, whose function is to complete the processes of digestion, to provide the body (through absorption) with water, electrolytes, and nutrients, and to move along and store fecal wastes until they are expelled. **i. cae'cum,** caecum (def. 2). **i. cras'sum** [NA], the large intestine: the distal portion of the intestine, about five feet long, extending from its junction with the small intestine to the anus; it comprises the cecum, colon, rectum, and anal canal. **i. il'eum,** ileum. **i. jeju'-num,** jejunum. **i. rec'tum,** rectum. **i. ten'ue** [NA], the small intestine: the proximal portion of the intestine, smaller in caliber than the large intestine, and about twenty feet long, extending from the pylorus to the cecum; it comprises the duodenum, jejunum, and ileum. **i. ten'ue mesenteria'le** the portion of the small intestine which has a mesentery, comprising the jejunum and ileum.

intima (in'tĭ-mah) [L.] [NA] a general term denoting an innermost structure; see *tunica intima vasorum.*

intimal (in'tĭ-mal) pertaining to the inner layer of the blood vessels (tunica intima vasorum).

intimitis (in''tĭ-mi'tis) inflammation of the tunica intima of an artery or vein.

Intocostrin (in''to-kos'trin) trademark for a preparation of tubocurarine chloride.

intolerance (in-tol'er-ans) [L. *in* not + *tolerare* to bear] inability to withstand; sensitivity, as to a drug. **disaccharide i.,** an inborn error of metabolism due either to a deficiency in the intestinal mucosal enzymes responsible for the hydrolysis of dietary saccharides and starch or sometimes to inability to absorb the final products of hydrolysis. The unabsorbed substrate accumulates in intestinal lumen, causing the clinical symptoms of abdominal fullness, bloating, and distension, nausea, cramps, and diarrhea. Homozygotes have severe enzyme deficiency and lifelong symptoms; heterozygotes have mild enzyme deficiency and mild symptoms as infants, but no symptoms as adults. Disaccharide intolerance occurs in three types: *I,* called also *congenital sucrose-isomaltose malabsorption* or *deficiency, congenital sucrose intolerance,* and *intestinal sucrose-α-dextrinase deficiency; II,* called also *congenital lactose intolerance* or *malabsorption;* and *III,* which affects about 10 per cent of non-Mediterranean Caucasians and most Blacks, Asians, and Mediterraneans, and is called also *adult* or *intestinal lactase deficiency.* Called also *intestinal disaccharidase deficiency* and *small-intestinal disaccharidase deficiency.* **drug i.,** the state of reacting to the normal pharmacologic doses of a drug with the symptoms of overdosage. **hereditary fructose i.,** an autosomal recessive disorder of carbohydrate metabolism due to deficient fructose-1-phosphate aldolase; it occurs in infants soon after the introduction of fructose in the diet, and is characterized by hypoglycemia and its clinical manifestations, associated with various other symptoms, including fructosuria, fructosemia, anorexia, vomiting, failure to thrive, jaundice, splenomegaly, and an aversion to fructose-containing foods. If the condition is left untreated, death may occur. See also *essential fructosuria,* under *fructosuria.* **lactose i.,** inability to digest lactose. It occurs with loss of lactase from the brush border of the intestinal mucosa in most black, Oriental, and Mediterranean adults, but much less often in Caucasians, and is characterized by abdominal discomfort, flatulence, and diarrhea after ingestion of milk. A congenital form, inherited as an autosomal recessive trait, is due to absence of or a defect in lactase and is characterized by diarrhea, vomiting, and failure to thrive. Called also *disaccharide intolerance* and *lactase deficiency.* **lactose i., congenital,** 1. disaccharide i. II. 2. a severe autosomal dominant disorder with vomiting, dehydration, failure to thrive, disacchariduria (including lactosuria and aminoaciduria), and cataracts. **lysine i., congenital,** hyperlysinemia. **lysinuric protein i.,** a hereditary disorder of metabolism transmitted as an autosomal recessive trait, involving a defect in dibasic amino acid transport and resulting in a lack of sufficient ornithine to support activity of ornithine transcarbamylase, an intramitochondrial urea cycle enzyme, in the liver. It is characterized by growth retardation, episodic hyperammonemia, seizures, mental retardation, hepatomegaly, muscle weakness, and osteopenia and is treated by citrulline supplementation. **sucrose i., congenital,** see *disaccharide i.*

intorsion (in-tor'shun) [L. *in* toward + *torsio* twisting] inward rotation of the upper pole of the vertical meridian of each eye; called also *adtorsion* and *conclination.* Cf. *extorsion.*

intorter (in'tor-ter) [L. *intorquere* to twist] an internal rotator.

intoxication (in-tok"sĭ-ka'shun) [L. *in* intensive + Gr. *toxikon* poison] 1. poisoning; the state of being poisoned. 2. a state of impaired mental or physical functioning resulting from ingestion of alcohol; inebriation, simple drunkenness: 3. [DSM III-R] an organic brain syndrome characterized by the presence in the body of an exogenous psychoactive substance that produces a substance-specific syndrome of effects on the central nervous system (e.g., disturbances of perception, wakefulness, attention, thinking, judgment, emotional control, or psychomotor behavior) that leads to maladaptive behavior such as belligerence or impaired social or occupational functioning. **acid i.,** acidosis of a severe grade. **alcohol idiosyncratic i.** [DSM III-R], maladaptive behavioral change, usually belligerence, produced by ingestion of amounts of alcohol insufficient to cause intoxication in most persons. Called also *pathological i.* **alkaline i.,** alkalosis of a severe grade. **bongkrek i.,** poisoning from bongkrek, a native Javanese dish, prepared by means of molds from copra press cake. When the fermentation process is faulty, severe poisoning occurs, with vomiting, profuse perspiration, muscle cramps, and coma. Called also *tempeh poisoning.* **intestinal i.,** autointoxication. **pathological i.,** alcohol idiosyncratic i. **roentgen i.,** radiation sickness. **water i.,** the condition induced by the undue retention of water with sodium depletion; it is marked by lethargy, nausea, vomiting, and mild mental aberrations, and in severe cases by convulsions and coma.

intra- [L. *intra* within] a prefix meaning within, into, or during.

intra-abdominal (in"trah-ab-dom'ĭ-nal) within the abdomen.

intra-acinous (in"trah-as'ĭ-nus) within an acinus.

intra-appendicular (in"trah-ap'en-dik'u-lar) within the appendix.

intra-arachnoid (in"trah-ah-rak'noid) within or underneath the arachnoid.

intra-arterial (in"trah-ar-te're-al) within an artery or arteries.

intra-articular (in"trah-ar-tik'u-lar) [*intra-* + L. *articulus* joint] within a joint.

intra-atomic (in"trah-ah-tom'ik) within an atom.

intra-atrial (in"trah-a'tre-al) within an atrium.

intra-aural (in"trah-aw'ral) within the ear.

intra-auricular (in"trah-aw-rik'u-lar) intra-atrial.

intrabronchial (in"trah-brong'ke-al) situated or occurring within a bronchus.

intrabuccal (in"trah-buk'al) within the mouth or within the cheek.

intracanalicular (in"trah-kan"ah-lik'u-lar) within canaliculi.

intracapsular (in"trah-kap'su-lar) within a capsule.

intracardiac (in"trah-kar'de-ak) within the heart.

intracarpal (in"trah-kar'pal) within the wrist.

intracartilaginous (in"trah-kar"tĭ-laj'ĭ-nus) within a cartilage; endochondral.

intracavitary (in"trah-kav'ĭ-tār"e) within a cavity, as that of the cervix or of the uterus.

intracelial (in"trah-se'le-al) within one of the body cavities.

intracellular (in"trah-sel'u-lar) [*intra-* + L. *cellula* cell] situated or occurring within a cell or cells.

intracephalic (in"trah-sĕ-fal'ik) within the brain.

intracerebellar (in"trah-ser"ĕ-bel'ar) situated within the cerebellum.

intracerebral (in"trah-ser'ĕ-bral) situated within the cerebrum.

intracervical (in"trah-ser'vĕ-kal) situated within the canal of the cervix uteri.

intrachondral (in"trah-kon'dral) endochondral.

intrachondrial (in"trah-kon'dre-al) endochondral.

intrachordal (in"trah-kor'dal) within the notochord.

intracisternal (in"trah-sis-ter'nal) within a cistern, especially the cisterna cerebellomedularis.

intracolic (in"trah-kol'ik) within the colon.

intracordal (in"trah-kor'dal) [*intra-* + L. *cor* heart] within the heart.

intracorporal (in"trah-kor'po-ral) intracorporeal.

intracorporeal (in"trah-kor-po're-al) situated or occurring within the body.

intracorpuscular (in"trah-kor-pus'ku-lar) occurring within corpuscles.

intracostal (in"trah-kos'tal) on the inner surface of the rib.

intracranial (in"trah-kra'ne-al) situated within the cranium.

intracrureus (in"trah-kroo-re'us) the internal part of the musculus vastus intermedius.

intractable (in-trak'tah-b'l) resistant to cure, relief, or control.

intracutaneous (in"trah-ku-ta'ne-us) within the skin; intradermal.

intracystic (in"trah-sis'tik) within a cyst.

intracytoplasmic (in"trah-si"to-plaz'mik) within the cytoplasm of a cell.

intrad (in'trad) [*intra-* + *-ad*] (*obs.*) within; inward in direction.

intradermal (in"trah-der'mal) 1. within the dermis. 2. intracutaneous.

intraductal (in"trah-duk'tal) situated or occurring within the duct of a gland.

intraduodenal (in"trah-du"o-de'nal) within the duodenum.

intradural (in"trah-du'ral) within or beneath the dura.

intraepidermal (in"trah-ep"ĭ-der'mal) within the epidermis.

intraepiphyseal (in"trah-ep"ĭ-fiz'e-al) within an epiphysis.

intraepithelial (in"trah-ep"ĭ-the'le-al) situated among the cells of the epithelium.

intraerythrocytic (in"trah-ĕ-rith"ro-sit'ik) located or occurring within the erythrocyte.

intrafascicular (in"trah-fah-sik'u-lar) within a fascicle.

intrafat (in"trah-fat') situated in or introduced into fatty tissue, as the subcutaneous tissue.

intrafetation (in"trah-fe-ta'shun) the development of a fetus within another fetus.

intrafilar (in"trah-fi'lar) [*intra-* + L. *filum* thread] situated within a reticulum.

intrafissural (in"trah-fish'u-ral) within a cerebral fissure.

intrafistular (in"trah-fis'tu-lar) within a fistula.

intrafollicular (in"trah-fo-lik'u-lar) within a follicle.

intrafusal (in"trah-fu'zal) [*intra-* + L. *fusus* spindle] pertaining to the striated fibers within a muscle spindle.

intragalvanization (in"trah-gal'van-i-za'shun) the galvanization of the inner surface of any organ.

intragastric (in"trah-gas'trik) situated or occurring within the stomach.

intragemmal (in″trah-jem′al) [*intra-* + L. *gemma* bud] situated within a bud, as a taste bud.

intragenic (in″trah-jen′ik) within a gene.

intraglandular (in″trah-glan′du-lar) within a gland.

intraglobular (in″trah-glob′u-lar) within a globe or globule, as within an erythrocyte.

intragyral (in″trah-ji′ral) within a cerebral gyrus.

intrahepatic (in″trah-hĕ-pat′ik) within the liver.

intrahyoid (in″trah-hi′oid) within the hyoid bone.

intraictal (in″trah-ik′tal) occurring during an attack or seizure.

intraintestinal (in″trah-in-tes′tĭ-nal) within the intestine.

intrajugular (in″trah-jug′u-lar) within the jugular foramen, process, or vein.

intralamellar (in″trah-lah-mel′ar) within lamellae.

intralaryngeal (in″trah-lah-rin′je-al) within the larynx.

intralesional (in″trah-le′zhun-al) occurring in or introduced directly into a localized lesion.

intraleukocytic (in″trah-lu″ko-si′tik) within a leukocyte.

intraligamentous (in″trah-lig″ah-men′tus) within a ligament.

intralingual (in″trah-ling′gwal) within the tongue.

Intralipid (in″trah-lip′id) trademark for an intravenous fat emulsion containing 10 per cent soybean oil stabilized with egg-yolk phospholipids; used to prevent or correct deficiency of essential fatty acids and to provide calories in high density form during total parenteral nutrition.

intralobar (in″trah-lo′bar) within a lobe.

intralobular (in″trah-lob′u-lar) within a lobule.

intralocular (in″trah-lok′u-lar) within the loculi of a structure.

intraluminal (in″trah-lu′mĭ-nal) within the lumen of a tube, as of a blood vessel.

intramammary (in″trah-mam′ah-re) within the breast.

intramarginal (in″trah-mar′jĭ-nal) within a margin.

intramastoiditis (in″trah-mas″toi-di′tis) inflammation of the mastoid antrum and cells of the mastoid process.

intramatrical (in″trah-mat′re-kal) within a matrix.

intramedullary (in″trah-med′u-lār″e) 1. within the spinal cord. 2. within the medulla oblongata. 3. within the marrow cavity of a bone.

intramembranous (in″trah-mem′brah-nus) within a membrane.

intrameningeal (in″trah-mĕ-nin′je-al) within the meninges.

intramolecular (in″trah-mo-lek′u-lar) within the molecule.

intramural (in″trah-mu′ral) [*intra-* + L. *murus* wall] within the wall of an organ.

intramuscular (in″trah-mus′ku-lar) [*intra-* + L. *musculus* muscle] within the substance of a muscle.

intramyocardial (in″trah-mi″o-kar′de-al) within the myocardium.

intranarial (in″trah-na′re-al) within the nares.

intranasal (in″trah-na′zal) [*intra-* + L. *nasus* nose] within the nose.

intranatal (in″trah-na′tal) occurring during birth.

intraneural (in″trah-nu′ral) within or into a nerve.

intranuclear (in″trah-nu′kle-ar) within a nucleus, as a cell nucleus.

intraocular (in″trah-ok′u-lar) within the eye.

intraoperative (in″trah-op″er-ah′tiv) occurring during the course of a surgical operation.

intraoral (in″trah-o′ral) within the mouth.

intraorbital (in″trah-or′bĭ-tal) within the orbit.

intraosseous (in″trah-os′e-us) within a bone.

intraosteal (in″trah-os′te-al) intraosseous.

intraovarian (in″trah-o-va′re-an) within the ovary.

intraovular (in″trah-o′vu-lar) within an ovum.

intraparenchymatous (in″trah-par″en-kim′ah-tus) within the parenchyma of an organ.

intraparietal (in″trah-pah-ri′ĕ-tal) [*intra-* + L. *paries* wall] 1. intramural. 2. situated in the parietal region of the brain.

intrapartum (in″trah-par′tum) occurring during childbirth, or during delivery.

intrapelvic (in″trah-pel′vik) within the pelvis.

intrapericardial (in″trah-per″ĭ-kar′de-al) within the pericardium.

intraperineal (in″trah-per″ĭ-ne′al) within the tissues of the perineum.

intraperitoneal (in″trah-per″ĭ-to-ne′al) within the peritoneal cavity.

intrapial (in″trah-pe′al) within or beneath the pia mater.

intraplacental (in″trah-plah-sen′tal) within the placenta.

intrapleural (in″trah-ploor′al) within the pleura.

intrapontine (in″trah-pon′tīn) [*intra-* + L. *pons*] within the substance of the pons.

intraprostatic (in″trah-pros-tat′ik) within the prostate gland.

intraprotoplasmic (in″trah-pro″to-plaz′mik) within the protoplasm.

intrapsychic (in-trah-si′kik) occurring inside the mind; taking place within the mind.

intrapulmonary (in″trah-pul′mo-ner″e) situated in the substance of the lung.

intrapyretic (in″trah-pi-ret′ik) [*intra-* + Gr. *pyretos* fever] during the stage of fever.

intrarachidian (in″trah-rah-kid′e-an) intraspinal.

intrarectal (in″trah-rek′tal) within the rectum.

intrarenal (in″trah-re′nal) within the kidney.

intraretinal (in″trah-ret′ĭ-nal) within the retina.

intrascleral (in″trah-skle′ral) within the sclera.

intrascrotal (in″trah-skro′tal) within the scrotum.

intrasellar (in″trah-sel′ar) within the sella turcica.

intraspinal (in″trah-spi′nal) situated or occurring within the vertebral column.

intrasplenic (in″trah-sple′nik) within the spleen.

intrasternal (in″trah-ster′nal) within the sternum.

intrastitial (in″trah-stish′al) within the cells or fibers of a tissue.

intrastromal (in″trah-stro′mal) within the stroma of an organ.

intrasynovial (in″trah-sĭ-no′ve-al) within the synovial cavity of a joint.

intratarsal (in″trah-tar′sal) within or on the inner side of the tarsus.

intratesticular (in″trah-tes-tik′u-lar) within the testis.

intrathecal (in″trah-the′kal) within a sheath; see also under *injection*.

intrathenar (in″trah-the′nar) situated between the thenar and hypothenar eminences.

intrathoracic (in″trah-tho-ras′ik) endothoracic.

intratonsillar (in″trah-ton′sĭ-lar) within a tonsil.

intratrabecular (in″trah-trah-bek′u-lar) within a trabecula.

intratracheal (in″trah-tra′ke-al) endotracheal.

intratubal (in″trah-tu′bal) situated or occurring within a tube, especially within a uterine tube.

intratubular (in″trah-tu′bu-lar) within the tubules of an organ.

intratympanic (in″trah-tim-pan′ik) within the tympanic cavity.

intraureteral (in″trah-u-re′ter-al) within the ureter.

intraurethral (in″trah-u-re′thral) within the urethra.

intrauterine (in″trah-u′ter-in) within the uterus.

intravaginal (in″trah-vaj′ĭ-nal) within the vagina.

intravasation (in-trav″ah-za′shun) the entrance of foreign material into a blood vessel.

intravascular (in″trah-vas′ku-lar) [*intra-* + L. *vasculum* vessel] within a vessel or vessels.

intravenation (in″trah-ve-na′shun) the entrance or injection of foreign matter into a vein.

intravenous (in″trah-ve′nus) within a vein or veins.

intraventricular (in″trah-ven-trik′u-lar) within a ventricle.

intraversion (in″trah-ver′zhun) in orthodontics, malocclusion in which the teeth or other maxillary structures are too near the median plane. Cf. *extraversion, def 2.*

intravertebral (in″trah-ver′te-bral) intraspinal.

intravesical (in″trah-ves′e-kal) [*intra-* + L. *vesica* bladder] situated within the bladder.

intravillous (in″trah-vil′us) situated within a villus.

intravital (in″trah-vi′tal) occurring during life.

intra vitam (in′trah vi′tam) [L.] during life.

intravitelline (in″trah-vi-tel′in) within the vitellus or yolk.

intravitreous (in″trah-vit′re-us) into or within the vitreous.

intrazole (in′trah-zōl) chemical name: 1-(4 chlorobenzoyl)-3-(1*H*-tetrazol-5-yimethyl)-1*H*-indole; an anti-inflammatory, $C_{17}H_{12}ClN_5O$.

intrinsic (in-trin′sik) [L. *intrinsecus* situated on the inside] situated entirely within or pertaining exclusively to a part.

intriptyline hydrochloride (in-trip′tĭ-lēn) chemical name: 4-(5*H*-dibenzo[*a,d*]cyclohepten-5-ylidene)-*N,N*-dimethyl-2-butynylamine hydrochloride; an antidepressant, $C_{21}H_{19}N·HCl$.

intro- [L. *intro* within] a prefix meaning into or within.

introducer (in″tro-du′ser) an intubator.

introfier (in′tro-fi″er) a liquid which has the property of lowering the interfacial tension of emulsions.

introflexion (in″tro-flek′shun) a bending inward.

introgastric (in″tro-gas′trik) [*intro-* + Gr. *gastēr* stomach] conveyed or leading into the stomach.

introgression (in″tro-gresh′un) [*intro-* + L. *gressus* course] the incorporation of a gene from one complex into another as a result of hybridization.

introitus (in-tro′ĭ-tus) pl. *intro′itus* [L., from *intro* within + *ire* to go] [NA] a general term for the entrance to a cavity or space. **i. oesoph′agi,** the entrance into the esophagus. **i. pel′vis,** apertura pelvis superior. **i. vagi′nae,** ostium vaginae.

introjection (in″tro-jek′shun) [*intro-* + L. *jacēre* to throw] an immature unconscious defense mechanism in which loved or hated external objects are absorbed into the self; anxiety is diminished by reducing the possibility of loss in the case of a loved object, or by internally controlling aggression on the part of a hated object.

intromission (in″tro-mish′un) [*intro-* + L. *mittere* to send] the insertion of one part or instrument into another, as of the penis into the vagina.

intron (in′tron) a noncoding intervening sequence in a gene; almost all eukaryotic genes contain several introns separating the coding sequences (exons). After the 5′ cap and polyA tail are added to a primary mRNA transcript, the introns are removed and the exons spliced together by enzymes that recognize short sequences that identify exon-intron junctions, resulting in a mature mRNA that is ready for translation (protein synthesis). Called also *intervening sequence.*

Intropin (in′tro-pin) trademark for a preparation of dopamine hydrochloride.

introspection (in″tro-spek′shun) [*intro-* + L. *spicere* to look] the contemplation or observation of one's own thoughts and feelings; self-analysis.

introsusception (in″tro-sus-sep′shun) [*intro-* + L. *suscipere* to receive] intussusception.

introversion (in″tro-ver′zhun) [*intro-* + L. *versio* a turning] 1. the turning outside in, more or less completely, of an organ. 2. the turning inward to the self of one's interest, with lack of interest in the external world. 3. intraversion.

introvert (in′tro-vert) 1. a person whose interest is turned inward to the self. 2. to turn one's interest inward to the self.

intrusion (in-troo′zhun) in orthodontic therapy, a technique of depressing a tooth back into the occlusal plane or an effort to prevent its eruption or elongation during the correction of an excessive overbite. Called also *tooth depression.* Cf. *extrusion, def. 3.*

intubate (in′tu-bāt) to treat by intubation.

intubation (in″tu-ba′shun) [L. *in* into + *tuba* tube] the insertion of a tube into a body canal or hollow organ, as into the trachea or stomach. **endotracheal i.,** insertion of a tube into the trachea for administration of anesthesia, maintenance of an airway, aspiration of secretions, ventilation of the lungs, or prevention of entrance of foreign material into the tracheobronchial tree. **nasal i.,** insertion of a tube into the respiratory or gastrointestinal tract through the nose. **nasotracheal i.,** insertion of a tube through the nose into the trachea to serve as an airway. **oral i.,** insertion of a tube into the respiratory or gastrointestinal tract through the mouth. **orotracheal i.,** insertion of a tube through the mouth into the trachea to serve as an airway.

intubationist (in-tu-ba′shun-ist) one who performs an intubation.

intubator (in′tu-ba-tor) an instrument used in intubation.

intumesce (in-tu-mes′) to swell up.

intumescence (in-tu-mes′ens) [L. *intumescentia*] 1. a swelling, normal or abnormal. 2. the process of swelling.

intumescent (in-tu-mes′ent) [L. *intumescens*] swelling or becoming swollen.

intumescentia (in-tu-mě-sen′she-ah), pl. *intumescen′tiae* [L.] [NA] a general term for an enlargement or swelling. **i. cervica′lis** [NA], the enlargement of the cervical spinal cord at the level of attachment of the nerves to the upper limbs. **i. lumba′lis,** i. lumbosacralis. **i. lumbosacra′lis** [NA], the enlargement of the lumbar spinal cord, at the level of attachment of the nerves to the lower limbs; called also *i. lumbalis.* **i. tympan′ica** [NA], a pseudoganglion on the tympanic branch (nerve) of the glossopharyngeal nerve; called also *ganglion tympanicum* [NA alternative], *tympanic ganglion, tympanic ganglion of Valentin,* and *Valentin's pseudoganglion.*

intussusception (in″tus-sus-sep′shun) [L. *intus* within + *suscipere* to receive] a receiving within; specifically: (1) the prolapse of one part of the intestine to the lumen of an immediately adjoining part (Treves, 1899). There are four varieties: *colic,* involving segments of the large intestine; *enteric,* involving only the small intestine; *ileocecal,* in which the ileocecal valve prolapses into the cecum, drawing the ileum along with it; and *ileocolic,* in which the ileum prolapses through the ileocecal valve into the colon. (2) In

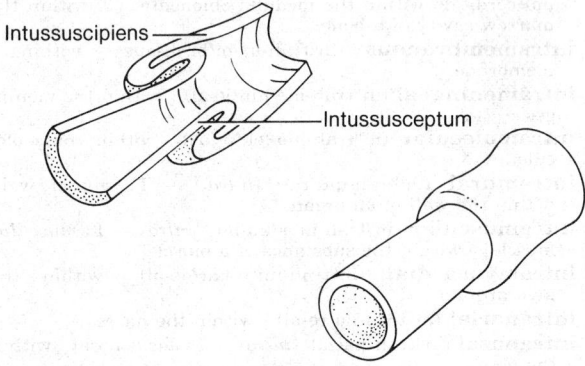

Intussuscipiens —
— Intussusceptum

Intussusception.

physiology, the reception into an organism of matter, such as food, and its transformation into new protoplasm. **agonic i., postmortem i.,** intussusception occurring in the death agony. **retrograde i.,** the invagination of a distal part of the bowel into a proximal part.

intussusceptum (in″tus-sus-sep′tum) [L.] the portion of intestine that has been invaginated within another part in intussusception.

intussuscipiens (in″tus-sus-sip′e-ens) [L.] the portion of intestine into which another portion has invaginated in intussusception.

Inula (in′u-lah) [L.] a genus of composite flowers. *I. helenium* L. yields alantic acid. Its rhizome contains inulin. The root has numerous uses in folk medicine.

inulase (in′u-lās) β-2,1-fructan fructanohydrolase, an enzyme occurring in *Aspergillus niger, Penicillium glaucum, Saccharomyces fragilis,* and other fungi, and in higher plants, which changes inulin into fructose with one D-glucose molecule per molecule of inulin.

inulin (in′u-lin) a vegetable starch, $(C_6H_{10}O_5)_4$, an indigestible polysaccharide occurring in the rhizome of certain plants (Compositae). It is a polymer of fructofuranose, yields fructose on hydrolysis, and is used in a test for determining renal function.

inulinase (in′u-lin-ās) inulase.

inuloid (in′u-loid) a colorless compound, $C_6H_{10}O_5$, resembling inulin, but more soluble.

inunction (in-ungk′shun) [L. *in* into + *unguere* to anoint] 1. the act of anointing or of applying an ointment with friction. 2. an ointment made with lanolin as a menstruum.

inunctum (in-ungk′tum) inunction, def. 2. **i. men′tholis compos′itum,** compound menthol ointment.

in utero (in u′ter-o) [L.] within the uterus.

InV [abbreviation of a patient's name] see *Km allotypes,* under allotype.

in vacuo (in vak′u-o) [L.] in a vacuum.

invaginate (in-vaj′ĭ-nāt) to infold one portion of a structure within another portion.

invagination (in-vaj′ĭ-na′shun) [L. *invaginatio,* from *in* within + *vagina* sheath] 1. the state of being or the process of becoming invaginated. 2. in embryology, a process by which (*a*) one region of a hollow, single-walled, spherical blastula caves in to form and line a new cavity in the now cup-shaped, double-walled gastrula, or (*b*) an ever-deepening pit develops into a diverticulum or tube from the surface into the tissues below. 3. intussusception. **basilar i.,** basilar impression.

invalid (in′vah-lid) [L. *invalidus; in* not + *validus* strong] 1. not well and strong. 2. a person who is disabled by illness or infirmity.

invasin (in-va′zin) hyaluronidase.

invasion (in-va′zhun) [L. *invasio; in* into + *vadere* to go] 1. the attack or onset of a disease. 2. the simple harmless entrance of bacteria into the body or their deposition in the tissues, as distinguished from infection. 3. the infiltration and active destruction of surrounding tissue, a characteristic of malignant tumors.

invasive (in-va′siv) 1. having the quality of invasiveness. 2. involving puncture or incision of the skin or insertion of an instrument or foreign material into the body; said of diagnostic techniques.

invasiveness (in-va′siv-nes) 1. the ability of a pathogenic microorganism to enter and spread throughout the tissues of the body. 2. the ability to infiltrate and actively destroy surrounding tissue; said of malignant tumors.

inventory (in′ven-tor′′e) a comprehensive list of personality traits, aptitudes, and interests. **Millon clinical multiaxial i. (MGMI),** a self-report inventory designed to produce a profile of the personality style and structure underlying mental disorders. **Minnesota Multiphasic Personality I. (MMPI),** a self-report psychiatric test designed to appraise the major clinical syndromes of mental disorder.

invermination (in-ver′′mĭ-na′shun) infestation of the body by vermin.

Inversine (in-ver′sēn) trademark for a preparation of mecamylamine hydrochloride.

inversion (in-ver′zhun) [L. *inversio; in* into + *vertere* to turn] a turning inward, inside out, upside down, or other reversal of the normal relation of a part. In psychiatry, a term used by Freud for homosexuality. In genetics, a chromosomal aberration caused by the inverted reunion of a chromosome segment after breakage of a chromosome at two points, resulting in a change in sequence of genes or nucleotides; e.g., the sequence *abcdefg* may be inverted to *abfedcg.* It may be paracentric (on one side of the centromere) or pericentric (including the centromere). **carbohydrate i.,** hydrolysis of disaccharides or polysaccharides to monosaccharides. **chromosome i.,** see under *aberration.* **sexual i.,** homosexuality. **thermic i.,** the state in which the body temperature is highest in the morning. **i. of uterus,** a turning of the uterus inside out, whereby the fundus is forced through the cervix and protrudes into or outside of the

vagina. **visceral i.,** the more or less complete right and left transposition of the viscera; see *situs inversus viscerum.*

inversus (in-ver′sus) [L., past participle of *invertere* to invert] opposite to, or inverted from, the normal; see *situs inversus viscerum.*

invert (in′vert) a homosexual.

invertase (in-ver′tās) β-fructofuranosidase.

Invertebrata (in-ver′′tĕ-bra′tah) a former division of the animal kingdom, including all forms that have no spinal column.

invertebrate (in-ver′tĕ-brāt) 1. any animal that has no spinal column; a nonvertebrate animal. 2. having no spinal column.

invertor (in-ver′tor) a muscle that turns a part inward.

invertose (in′ver-tōs) invert sugar, a levorotatory mixture of glucose and fructose obtained by the hydrolysis of dextrorotatory sucrose.

invest (in′vest) to surround, envelop, or embed in an investment material.

investing (in-vest′ing) 1. the act or process of covering or enveloping wholly or in part an object, such as a denture, tooth, wax form, or crown with a refractory investment material before curing, soldering, or casting. 2. the covering or enveloping of a tissue or part by another tissue, such as a fascia. **i. the pattern,** surrounding the wax pattern with an investment material, such as a mix of a plaster, for low temperature casting, or a mix consisting of dental stone and a silica refractory for high temperature casting; the investment hardens to form a mold into which casting materials are poured. **vacuum i.,** subjecting the water-investment mixture to a vacuum during the investing procedure in order to remove air bubbles from the mixture.

investment (in-vest′ment) 1. any tissue, such as fascia, that envelops or covers other tissues or parts. 2. a material applied as a soft paste to a pattern that hardens to form a mold for casting.

inveterate (in-vet′er-āt) [L. *inveteratus; in* intensive + *vetus* old] chronic and confirmed; long established and of difficult cure.

inviscation (in′′vis-ka′shun) [L. *in* among + *viscum* slime] the mixing of the food with the mucous secretion of the mouth in mastication.

in vitro (in ve′tro) [L.] within a glass; observable in a test tube; in an artificial environment.

in vivo (in ve′vo) [L.] within the living body.

involucre (in′vo-lu′′ker) an involucrum.

involucrum (in′′vo-lu′krum), pl. *involu′cra* [L.; *in* in + *volvere* to wrap] a covering or sheath, such as contains the sequestrum of a necrosed bone.

involuntary (in-vol′un-ter′′e) [L. *involuntarius; in* against + *voluntas* will] performed independently of the will; contravolitional.

involuntomotory (in-vol′′un-to-mo′tor-e) pertaining to motion that is not voluntary.

involute (in′vo-lūt) [L. *in* into + *volvere* to roll] 1. to return to normal size after enlargement. 2. to regress; to change to an earlier or to a more primitive condition. See *involution.*

involution (in′′vo-lu′shun) [L. *involutio; in* into + *volvere* to roll] 1. a rolling or turning inward. 2. one of the movements involved in the gastrulation of many animals. 3. a retrograde change of the entire body or in a particular organ, as the retrograde changes in the female genital organs that result in normal size after delivery. 4. the progressive degeneration occurring naturally with advancing age, resulting in shriveling of organs or tissues. **senile i.,** the progressive degeneration that occurs naturally with advancing age, resulting in the shriveling of organs or tissues.

involutional (in′′vo-lu′shun-al) pertaining to, due to, or occurring in involution.

Io chemical symbol for *ionium.*

iobenzamic acid (i′′o-ben-zam′ik) chemical name: *N*-(3-amino-2,4,6-triiodobenzoyl)-*N*-phenyl-β-alanine; a diagnostic radiopaque medium (cholecystography), $C_{16}H_{13}I_3N_2O_3$.

iocarmic acid (i′′o-kar′mik) chemical name: 3,3′-[(1,6-di-oxo-1,6-hexanediyl)diimino]diimino]bis[2, 4, 6- triiodo- 5- [(methylamino)carbonyl]benzoic acid]; a radiopaque medium, $C_{24}H_{20}N_4O_8$. See *iocarmate meglumine.*

iocetamic acid (i-o-se-tam′ik) [USP] a water-insoluble iodinated radiographic contrast medium that after oral administration is absorbed from the gastrointestinal tract, conjugated with glucuronic acid in the liver, and excreted in the bile; it is used for oral cholecystography.

iodamide (i-o′dah-mīd) chemical name: 3-(acetylamino)-5-[(acetylamino)methyl]-2,4,6-triiodobenzoic acid; a diagnostic radiopaque medium, $C_{12}H_{11}I_3N_2O_4$.

iodate (i′o-dāt) any salt of iodic acid; the IO_3^- anion.

iod-Basedow (i″ōd-baz′ĕ-do) jodbasedow.

iodemia (i″o-de′me-ah) [iodine + Gr. haima blood + -ia] the presence of iodides in the blood.

iodic acid (i-o′dik) a strong inorganic acid, HIO_3, which is a highly corrosive oxidizing agent.

iodide (i′o-dīd) any binary compound of iodine; the I^- anion. Dietary iodine is reduced to iodide and absorbed in the intestines; it is taken up from the bloodstream by the thyroid gland and incorporated into thyroid hormones.

iodide peroxidase (i′o-dīd pĕ-rok′sĭ-dās) [EC 1.11.1.8] an enzyme of the oxidoreductase class that catalyzes the reaction iodide H_2O_2 = iodine + $2H_2O$. The iodine formed in the reaction iodinates tyrosines in thyroglobulin, a step in the synthesis of thyroxine. A defect in the enzyme, an autosomal recessive trait, prevents formation of organic iodine and results in familial goiter. Called also thyroid peroxidase.

iodimetry (i″o-dim′ĕ-tre) [iodine + Gr. metron measure] 1. the estimation of the quantity of iodine in a mixture or compound. 2. in quantitative analysis, the procedure used to determine an oxidizing agent consisting of the quantitative oxidation of potassium iodide to free iodine, and then titration with sodium thiosulfate.

iodinate (i-o′dĭ-nāt) to combine or compound with iodine.

iodination (i″o-din-a′shun) the incorporation or addition of iodine in a compound.

iodine (i′o-dīn) [Gr. ioeides violet-like, from the color of its vapor] 1. a halogen element of a peculiar odor and acrid taste; symbol, I; atomic number, 53; atomic weight, 126.904. It is a nonmetallic element, occurring in heavy, grayish black plates or granules. Iodine is essential in nutrition, being especially necessary for the synthesis of thyroid hormones (thyroxine and triiodothyronine), which regulate the metabolic rate in all cells. 2. [USP] a preparation of iodine used as a topical anti-infective (see also under solution). Iodine, usually in the form of iodides, is used in the treatment of hyperthyroidism. **butanol-extractable i.,** iodine that can be separated from the plasma proteins by extraction with certain organic solvents, such as butanol; it serves as a measure of thyroid hormone levels in the blood. Abbreviated BEI. **imidecyl i.,** a topical anti-infective compound, consisting of a mixture of 2-alkyl-(C_7H_{15} to $C_{17}H_{35}$)-1-(carboxymethyl)-1 - (2 - hydroxyethyl) - 2 - imidazolinium chloride; 3,6,9,12,15,18,21,24,27,30,33,36,39 - tridecaoxadopentacontan-1-ol; and iodine. **povidone i.,** see povidone-iodine. **protein-bound i.,** iodine firmly bound to protein in the blood serum, determination of which constitutes a now infrequently used test of thyroid function. **radioactive i.,** radioiodine.

iodinophil (i″o-din′o-fil) [iodine + Gr. philein to love] 1. any cell or other element readily stainable with iodine. 2. iodinophilous.

iodinophilous (i″o-din-of′ĭ-lus) readily stainable with iodine.

iodipamide (i″o-dip′ah-mīd) a water-soluble iodinated radiographic contrast medium used for intravenous cholangiography and cholecystography. Available as iodipamide [USP] and iodipamide meglumine [USP]. **i. meglumine, i. methylglucamine,** the meglumine salt of iodipamide, $(C_7H_{17}NO_5)_2 \cdot C_{20}H_{14}I_4N_2O_6$; used as a radiopaque medium in cholangiography and cholecystography, administered intravenously. **i. sodium,** the sodium salt of iodipamide, $C_{20}H_{12}I_6N_2Na_2O_6$, used as a radiopaque medium in cholangiography and cholecystography, administered intravenously.

iodism (i′o-dizm) chronic poisoning by iodine or iodine compounds; it is marked by coryza, ptyalism, frontal headache, emaciation, weakness, and eruptions on the skin.

iodize (i′o-dīz) to impregnate with iodine or to put under its influence; to incorporate iodine or one of its compounds.

iodoacetic acid (i-o″do-ah-se′tik) a compound, ICH_2-COOH, used in biochemical studies; it alkylates free thiol groups but not disulfide bridges.

iodobrassid (i-o″do-bras′sid) chemical name: ethyl diiodobrassidate; used in iodide therapy and as a radiopaque medium.

iodochlorhydroxyquin (i-o″do-klōr″hi-drok′se-kwin) [USP] chemical name: 5-chloro-7-iodo-8-quinolinol. An antiamebic, antibacterial, and antifungal agent with antieczematic and antipruritic properties, C_9H_5ClINO, occurring as a voluminous, spongy, yellowish white to brownish yellow powder. It is used in the treatment of amebic dysentery, and as a local anti-infective in a wide range of dermatoses, including all types of eczema, and in vaginitis due to Trichomonas vaginalis, Candida albicans, Trichophyton, or mixed bacteria; administered orally, topically, or intravaginally. Called also clinoquinol.

iodocholesterol (i-o″do-ko-les′ter-ol) a radioisotope, [131]I-19-iodocholesterol, used in visualization of the adrenal glands by the photoscintillation scanner.

iododerma (i-o″do-der′mah) [iodine + Gr. derma skin] any skin eruption or lesion resulting from iodism.

iodoform (i-o′do-form) [iodine + formyl] chemical name: triiodomethane. A greenish yellow powder or crystals, CHI_3, having a strong, penetrating odor, containing about 96 per cent of iodine, and soluble in chloroform and ether and somewhat in alcohol and water: used as a topical anti-infective, applied to the skin.

iodoformism (i′o-do-form″izm) poisoning by iodoform.

iodoformum (i″o-do-for′mum) iodoform.

iodogenic (i″o-do-jen′ik) [iodine + Gr. gennan to produce] yielding or producing iodine.

iodoglobulin (i″o-do-glob′u-lin) an iodine-containing globulin (protein).

iodogorgoric acid (i-o″do-gor′gor-ik) diiodotyrosine.

iodohippurate sodium (io″do-hip′u-rāt) chemical name: o-iodohippurate sodium. An iodine-containing compound, $C_9H_7INNaO_3$, administered orally, intravenously, or by retrograde injection as a radiopaque medium in pyelography. When labeled with radioactive iodine 131, it may be used as a diagnostic aid in determination of renal function.

iodolography (i″o-do-log′rah-fe) roentgenologic visualization of an organ or part after the injection into it of iodized oil.

iodometric (i″o-do-met′rik) pertaining to iodometry.

iodometry (i″o-dom′ĕ-tre) [iodine + Gr. metron measure] estimation of the quantity of a chemical by titration with iodine.

iodopanoic acid (i-o″do-pah-no′ik) iopanoic acid.

iodophenol (i″o-do-fe′nol) 1. a mono-iodophenol, $OH \cdot C_6H_5I$. 2. a preparation of iodine, phenol, and glycerin: antiseptic.

iodophil (i′o-do-fil) iodinophil.

iodophilia (i″o-do-fil′e-ah) [iodine + Gr. philein to love + -ia] the reaction shown by leukocytes in certain conditions when treated with iodine or iodides. Normal leukocytes are colored bright yellow, but in certain pathologic conditions, as toxemia and severe anemia, the polymorphonuclears show diffuse brownish coloration. When the staining affects the leukocytes themselves, it is termed intracellular; when only the particles around the leukocytes are affected, it is extracellular.

iodophor (i-o′do-fōr) a compound consisting of iodine combined with a carrier, such as polyvinylpyrrolidone, used in veterinary medicine as a preoperative skin disinfectant.

iodophthalein sodium (i″o-do-thal′e-in) chemical name: disodium salt of tetraiodophenolphthalein; used as a radiopaque medium in cholecystography.

iodopsin (i″o-dop′sin) [Gr. iōdēs violet colored + opsis vision] a photosensitive violet retinal pigment found in the retinal cones of some animals and important for color vision; called also visual violet.

iodopyracet (i-o″do-pi′rah-set) chemical name: 3,5-diiodo-4-oxo-1(4H)-pyridineacetic acid compound with 2,2′-iminodiethanol (1:1). A radiopaque medium, $C_{11}H_{16}I_2N_2O_5$, used especially in urography; administered intravenously or intramuscularly.

iodoquinol (i-o″do-kwin′ol) [USP] chemical name: 5,7-diiodo-8-quinolinol. An amebicide, $C_{15}H_{13}I_2NO_4$, occurring as a light yellowish to tan, microcrystalline powder; used in the treatment of intestinal amebiasis, administered orally, and in *Trichomonas vaginalis* vaginitis, administered intravaginally. It has also been used topically in fungal and bacterial skin infections and in seborrheic dermatitis. Called also *diiodohydroxyquin*.

iodosulfate (i″-do-do-sul′fāt) a combination of a base with iodine and sulfuric acid.

iodotherapy (i″-do-do-ther′ah-pe) [*iodine* + Gr. *therapeia* treatment] treatment, usually of a goiter, with iodine or the iodides.

iodothyroglobulin (i″-do-do-thi″ro-glob′u-lin) thyroglobulin.

iodothyronine (i″-do-do-thi′ro-nēn) a nonspecific term for iodinated thyronines, including the thyroid hormones triiodothyronine and tetraiodothyronine (thyroxine).

iodotyrosine (i″-do-do-ti′ro-sēn) any iodinated derivative of tyrosine.

iodotyrosine dehalogenase (i″-do-do-ti′ro-sēn de-hal′o-jĕ-nās) iodotyrosine deiodinase.

iodotyrosine deiodinase (i″-do-do-ti′ro-sēn de-i′o-dĭ-nās) an enzyme that catalyzes the removal of iodine from monoiodotyrosine and diiodotyrosine. The reaction is a step in the conservation of iodine by the thyroid. Congenital deficiency of the enzyme results in severe loss of iodine, resulting in hypothyroidism and goiter. Called also *iodotyrosine dehalogenase*.

iodoventriculography (i″-do-do-ven-trik″u-log′rah-fe) ventriculography with iodine contrast medium.

iodovolatilization (i″-do-do-vol″ah-til-i-za′shun) the liberation of free iodine by living epidermal cells in the iodogenic layer of certain brown algae or kelp. It accumulates in the algae as potassium iodide and has been used as a commercial source of iodine.

iodoxamic acid (i″-do-dox-am′ik) chemical name: 3,3′-[1,16-dioxo-4,7,10,13-tetraoxohexadecane-1,16-diyl)diimino]-bis[2,4,6-triiodobenzoic acid]; a radiopaque medium, $C_{26}H_{26}$-$I_6N_2O_{10}$, used in cholecystography.

iodum (i-o′dum), gen. *io′di* [L.] iodine.

ioduria (i″-o-du′re-ah) the presence of iodides in the urine.

ioglicic acid (i″-o-glis′ik) chemical name: 3-(acetylamino)-2,4,6-triiodo-5-[[[2-(methylamino)-2-oxoethyl]amino]carbonyl]benzoic acid; a radiopaque medium, $C_{13}H_{12}$-$I_3N_3O_5$.

ioglycamic acid (i″-o-gli-sam″ik) chemical name: 3,3′-[oxobis(1-oxo-2,1 ethanediyl)]bis[2,4,6-triiodobenzoic acid]. An acid, $C_{18}H_{10}I_6N_2O_7$, the meglumine and sodium salts of which are used as diagnostic radiopaque media in cholecystography.

ion (i′on) [Gr. *iōn* going] an atom or radical having a charge of positive (cation) or negative (anion) electricity owing to the loss (positive) or gain (negative) of one or more electrons. Substances that form ions are called electrolytes. See *ionic theory*, under *theory*. **dipolar i.,** zwitterion. **gram i.,** the weight in grams of an ion numerically equal to the atomic or molecular weight of the ion. **hydrogen i.,** the nucleus of the hydrogen atom or a hydrogen atom that has lost its electron, H^+; it bears a positive charge equivalent to the negative charge of the electron and is called a proton. **hydronium i.,** the hydrated form, H_3O^+, in which the proton (hydrogen ion, H^+) exists in aqueous solution; a combination of H^+ and H_2O.

Ionamin (i-o′nah-min) trademark for a preparation of phentermine.

ionic (i-on′ik) pertaining to an ion or to ions.

ionium (i-o′ne-um) [*ion*] a radioactive isotope of thorium, of atomic weight 230.5; it emits both alpha and gamma rays.

ionization (i″-on-ĭ-za′shun) 1. any process by which a neutral atom gains or loses electrons, thus acquiring a net charge, as the dissociation of a substance in solution into ions or ion production by the passage of radioactive particles. 2. iontophoresis. **avalanche i.,** the multiplicative process in which a single charged particle, accelerated by a strong electric field, produces additional charged particles through collision with neutral gas molecules; called also *Townsend i*. **Townsend i.,** avalanche i.

ionize (i′on-īz) to separate into ions.

ionocolorimeter (i″-o-no-kol″or-im′ĕ-ter) an apparatus for measuring the ionic acidity of a solution.

ionogen (i-on′o-jen) [*ion* + Gr. *gennan* to form] a substance that can be ionized.

ionogenic (i-on″o-jen′ik) forming or supplying ions.

ionometer (i″o-nom′ĕ-ter) an instrument for the measurement of the intensity or quantity of radiation from an ionizing radiation source.

ionometry (i″o-nom′ĕ-tre) roentgenometry.

ionone (i′on-ōn) [Gr. *ion* violet] an odoriferous derivative of orris root, $C_{13}H_{20}O$, prepared commercially from citral and used as a perfume.

ionophore (i′on-o-fōr″) any molecule, as of a drug, that increases the permeability of cell membranes to a specific ion.

ionophose (i′o-no-fōz) [Gr. *ion* violet + *phose*] a violet phose.

ionoscope (i-on′o-skōp) an instrument for detecting alkaline or acid impurity in nitrous oxide.

ionosphere (i-on′o-sfēr) the region of the atmosphere characterized by the formation of ions by the action of solar radiations upon the atmospheric constituents.

ionotherapy (i″o-no-ther′ah-pe) 1. [*ion* + *therapy*] iontophoresis. 2. [Gr. *ion* violet + *therapy*] treatment by means of ultraviolet rays.

ion-protein (i-on-pro′te-in) a protein molecule combined with an inorganic ion.

iontherapy (i″on-ther′ah-pe) iontophoresis.

iontophoresis (i-on″to-fo-re′sis) the introduction by means of the electric current, of ions of soluble salts into the tissues of the body, often for therapeutic purposes; a form of electro-osmosis. Called also *iontherapy*.

iontophoretic (i-on″to-fo-ret′ik) pertaining to iontophoresis.

iontoquantimeter (i-on″to-quan-tim′ĕ-ter) [*ion* + *quantimeter*] ionometer.

iontoradiometer (i-on″to-ra″de-om′ĕ-ter) ionometer.

IOP intraocular pressure.

iopamidol (i″o-pam′ĭ-dol) a nonionic, water-soluble radiopaque medium used in myelography.

iopanoic acid (i″o-pah-no′ik) [USP] an iodinated radiographic contrast medium that after oral administration is absorbed from the duodenum, conjugated with glucuronic acid in the liver, and secreted in the bile; it is used for oral cholecystography and cholangiography.

iophendylate (i″o-fen′dĭ-lāt) [USP] chemical name: iodo-*ι*-methylbenzene decanoic acid. A radiopaque medium, C_{19}-$H_{29}IO_2$, occurring as a colorless to pale yellow, viscous liquid; used in myelography, administered intrathecally or by special injection.

iophenoxic acid (i″o-fen-ok′sik) chemical name: *α*-ethyl-3-hydroxy-2,4,6-triiodobenzenepropanoic acid. A compound, $C_{11}H_{11}I_3O_3$, used as a radiopaque medium in cholecystography. Called also *triiodoethionic a*.

iopydol (i-o-pi′dōl) chemical name: 1-(2,3-dihydroxypropyl)-3,5-diiodo-4(1*H*)-pyridinone; a radiopaque medium for bronchography, $C_8H_9I_2NO_3$.

iopydone (i-o-pi′dōn) chemical name: 3,5-diiodo-4(1*H*)-pyridinone; a radiopaque medium for bronchography, C_5H_3-I_2NO.

ioseric acid (i″o-ser′ik) chemical name: 3-[[[1-(hydroxymethyl)-2-(methylamino)-2-oxoethyl]amino]carbonyl]-2,4,6-triiodo-5-[(methoxy-acetyl)amino] benzoic acid; a radiopaque medium, $C_{15}H_{16}I_3N_3O_7$.

iosulamide meglumine (i″o-sul′ah-mīd) chemical name: 3,3′-[sulfonylbis[(1-oxo-3, 1-propanediyl) imino]]bis[5-(acetylethylamino)-2,4,6-triiodobenzoic acid] compound with 1-deoxy-1-(methylamino)-D-glucitol(1:1); a radiopaque medium, $C_{28}H_{28}I_6N_4O_{10}S \cdot C_7H_{17}NO_5$.

iosumetic acid (i″o-soo-met′ik) chemical name: 4-[ethyl-[2,4,6-triiodo-3-(methylamino)-phenyl]amino]-4-oxobutanoic acid; a radiopaque medium, $C_{13}H_{15}I_3N_2O_3$.

iota (i′o-tah) [I, *ι*] the ninth letter of the Greek alphabet.

iotacism (i-o′tah-sizm) [Gr. *iōta* letter I] excessive use of the sound of the Greek letter iota (English e, as in be) in speaking.

iotetric acid (i″o-tet′rik) chemical name: benzoic acid, 3,3′-[(1,14-dioxo3,6,9,12-tetraoxatetradecane-1,14-diyl)diimino]bis[2,4,6-triiodobenzoic acid]; a radiopaque medium, C_{24}-$H_{22}I_6N_2O_{10}$.

iothalamate (i″o-thal′ah-māt) a water-soluble iodinated radiographic contrast medium used for angiography, angiocardiography, excretory urography, retrograde urography, and contrast enhancement of computed tomographic brain images. Available as *iothalamate meglumine* [USP], *iothalamate sodium* [USP], or a mixture of the two salts. **i. meglumine,** a radiopaque medium, $C_{18}H_{26}I_3N_2O_9$, available in solution, consisting of iothalamic acid in water for injection, prepared with the aid of meglumine; used intra-arterially in cerebral angiography and peripheral arteriography and intravenously in excretory urography and peripheral pyelography. **i. sodium,** a radiopaque medium, $(C_{11}H_8I_3N_2Na-O_4)$, available in solution, consisting of iothalamic acid in water for injection, prepared with the aid of sodium hydroxide; used intra-arterially or intravenously in angiocardiography and aortography.

iothalamic acid (i″o-thal′ah-mik) [USP] the free acid of iothalamate, used in the preparation of certain radiopaque media.

iothiouracil (i″o-thi″o-u′rah-sil) chemical name: 5-iodo-2-thiouracil; a thyroid inhibitor.

iotroxic acid (i″o-trok′sik) chemical name: 3,3′-[oxybis-[2,1-ethanediyloxy(1-oxo-2,1-ethanediyl)imino]]bis[2,4,6-triiodobenzoic acid]; a radiopaque medium, $C_{22}H_{18}I_6N_2O_9$.

I.P. intraperitoneally; isoelectric point.

I.P.A.A. International Psychoanalytical Association.

I-para primipara.

ipecac (ip′ĕ-kak) [USP] the dried rhizome and roots of *Cephaelis ipecacuanha* (Brotero) Rich. (Rubiaceae) (Rio or Brazilian i.) or of *C. acuminata* Karsten (Cartagena, Nicaragua, or Panama i.). Originally introduced as a remedy for dysentery, it has been replaced by its alkaloid emetine for that purpose, and is now used in syrup as an emetic, particularly in cases of poisoning. It also has expectorant properties. **powdered i.** [USP], ipecac reduced to a very fine powder; used in the preparation of ipecac syrup.

ipodate (i′po-dāt) 3-[[(dimethylamino)methylene]amino]-2,4,6-triiodobenzenepropanoic acid, $C_{12}H_{13}I_3N_2O_2$. **i. calcium** [USP], the calcium salt of ipodate, $C_{24}H_{24}CaI_6N_4O_4$, occurring as a white to off-white, fine, crystalline powder; used as a radiopaque medium in cholecystography, administered orally. **i. sodium** [USP], the sodium salt of ipodate, $C_{12}H_{12}I_3N_2NaO_2$, occurring as a white to off-white fine, crystalline powder; used as a radiopaque medium in cholecystography, administered orally.

ipomea (i″po-me′ah) the dried root of *Ipomoea orizabensis,* used as a cathartic; called also *Mexican scammony* and *orizaba jalap root.*

Ipomoea (i″po-me′ah) a genus of herbs and shrubs of the family Convolvulaceae, comprising some 300 species. Some species, e.g., *I. orizabensis* Ledenois, contain cathartic resins; others, e.g., *I. violacea* L., possess psychotomimetic indole alkaloids, such as lysergic acid amide.

IPPB intermittent positive pressure breathing; see under *breathing.*

Ipral (ip′ral) trademark for preparations of probarbital.

ipratropium bromide (ĭ-prah-tro′pe-um) chemical name: (+)-(endo,syn)-3-(3-hydroxy-1-oxo-2-phenylpropoxy)-8-methyl-8-(1-methylethyl)-8-azoniabicyclo[3,2,1]octane bromide; a bronchodilator, $C_{20}H_{30}BrNO_3$.

iprindole (ĭ-prin′dōl) chemical name: 6,7,8,9,10,11-hexahydro-*N,N*-dimethyl-5*H*- cylooct[*b*]indole- 5- propanamine; an antidepressant, $C_{19}H_{28}N_2$.

iproniazid (i″pro-ni′ah-zid) chemical name: 4-pyridinecarboxylic acid 2-(1-methylethyl)hydrazine; a monoamine oxidase inhibitor, antidepressant, and antitubercular, $C_9H_{13}-N_3O$.

ipronidazole (i-pro-nīd′ah-zōl) chemical name: 1-methyl-2-(1-methylethyl)-5-nitro-1*H*-imidazole; an antiprotozoal, $C_7-H_{11}N_3O_2$, effective against *Histomonas.*

iproxamine hydrochloride (ĭ-proks′ah-mēn) chemical name: 4-[2-(dimethylamino)ethoxy]-2-methyl-5-(1-methylethyl)phenyl 1-methylethyl ester hydrochloride; a vasodilator, $C_{18}H_{29}NO_4 \cdot HCl$.

ipsi- [L. *ipse* self] a combining form meaning the same.

ipsilateral (ip″sĭ-lat′er-al) [L. *ipse* self + *latus* side] situated on, pertaining to, or affecting the same side, as opposed to contralateral.

IPSP inhibitory postsynaptic potential.

IPV poliovirus vaccine inactivated.

I.Q. intelligence quotient; see under *quotient.*

Ir chemical symbol for *iridium.*

ir- see *in-.*

IRC inspiratory reserve capacity.

Ircon (ir′kon) trademark for a preparation of ferrous fumarate.

iridal (i′rĭ-dal) iridic.

iridalgia (i″rĭ-dal′je-ah) [*irid-* + *-algia*] pain in the iris.

iridauxesis (ir″id-awk-se′sis) [*irid-* + Gr. *auxēsis* increase] thickening of the iris.

iridectome (ir″ĭ-dek′tōm) [*irid-* + Gr. *ektemnein* to cut out] a cutting instrument for use in iridectomy.

iridectomesodialysis (ir″ĭ-dek″to-me″so-di-al′ĭ-sis) [*irid-* + *ectomy* + *meso-* + *dialysis*] surgical formation of an artificial iris by excision and separation of adhesions around the inner edge of the iris.

iridectomize (ir″ĭ-dek′to-mīz) to remove part of the iris by excision.

iridectomy (ir″ĭ-dek′to-me) [*irid-* + *ectomy*] surgical excision of a full-thickness piece of the iris; called also *corectomy.* **basal i.,** iridectomy at the base of the iris close to its attachment to the ciliary body. **complete i.,** surgical excision of a whole radial section of the iris from the root to, and including, the margin. Called also *sector i.* and *total i.* **optic i., optical i.,** excision of part of the iris as a means of enlarging an abnormally small pupil and improving vision. **peripheral i.,** a surgical treatment for narrow–angle glaucoma, and consisting of a full-thickness excision of a portion of the periphery or root of the iris, the pupillary border and sphincter muscle being left intact. Called also *basal i., buttonhole i.,* and *stenopeic i.* **preliminary i., preparatory i.,** iridectomy performed before removal of the lens in cataract surgery. **sector i.,** complete i. **stenopeic i.,** peripheral i. **therapeutic i.,** iridectomy performed for the cure of disease of the eye.

iridectropium (ir″ĭ-dek-tro′pe-um) ectropion uveae.

iridemia (ir″ĭ-de′me-ah) [*irid-* + Gr. *haima* blood + *-ia*] hemorrhage from the iris.

iridencleisis (ir″ĭ-den-kli′sis) [*irid-* + Gr. *enklein* to lock in] the surgical creation of a permanent drain by incarceration of a slip of the iris within a corneal or limbal incision to act as a wick through which the aqueous is filtered from the anterior chamber to the subconjunctival tissues; done to reduce intraocular pressure.

iridentropium (ir″ĭ-den-tro′pe-um) entropion uveae.

irideremia (ir″ĭ-der-e′me-ah) [*irid-* + Gr. *erēmia* want of, absence] congenital absence of the iris.

irides (i′rĭ-dēz, ir′ĭ-dēz) [Gr.] plural of *iris.*

iridescence (ir″ĭ-des′ens) [L. *iridescere* to gleam like a rainbow] the condition of gleaming with bright and changing colors.

iridescent (ir″ĭ-des′ent) [Gr. *iris* rainbow] having a rainbow-like display of colors in reflected light, as in mother-of-pearl; said of a colony of microorganisms.

iridesis (i-rid′ĕ-sis) [*iris* + *-desis*] the operation of repositioning the pupil by bringing a sector of the iris through a corneal or limbal incision and fixing the sector with a suture.

iridiagnosis (i″rĭ-di-ag-no′sis) iridodiagnosis.

iridial (i-rid′e-al) iridic.

iridian (i-rid′e-an) iridic.

iridic (i-rid′ik) pertaining to the iris.

iridium (ĭ-rid′e-um, i-rid′e-um) [L. *iris* rainbow, from the tints of its salts] a very hard white metal; symbol, Ir; atomic number, 77; atomic weight, 192.2.

iridization (ir″ĭ-di-za′shun) the subjective perception of iridescent halos about lights, occurring in glaucoma.

irid(o)- [Gr. *iris,* gen *iridos* rainbow] a combining form meaning iridescent, or denoting relationship to the iris.

iridoavulsion (ir″ĭ-do-ah-vul′shun) complete tearing away of the iris from its periphery.

iridocapsulitis (ir″ĭ-do-kap-su-li′tis) inflammation of the iris and the capsule of the lens.

iridocele (i-rid′o-sēl) [*irido-* + *-cele*] hernial protrusion of a part of the iris through the cornea.

iridochoroiditis (ir″ĭ-do-ko″roi-di′tis) inflammation of the iris and the choroid.

iridocoloboma (ir″ĭ-do-kol″o-bo′mah) [*irido-* + Gr. *kolobōma* mutilation] congenital fissure or coloboma of the iris.

iridoconstrictor (ir″ĭ-do-kon-strik′tor) [*irido-* + *constrictor*] a muscle element or an agent that causes constriction of the pupil of the eye.

iridocorneosclerectomy (ir″ĭ-do-kor″ne-o-skle-rek′to-me) surgical excision of a portion of the iris, cornea, and sclera for glaucoma.

iridocyclectomy (ir″ĭ-do-si-klek′to-me) [*irido-* + *cyclo-* + *ectomy*] surgical removal of a portion of the iris and of the ciliary body.

iridocyclitis (ir″ĭ-do-si-kli′tis) [*irido-* + *cyclitis*] inflammation of the iris and of the ciliary body; anterior uveitis. **heterochromic i.,** unilateral low-grade iridocyclitis, leading to depigmentation of the iris of the affected eye; called also *heterochromic uveitis.*

iridocyclochoroiditis (ir″ĭ-do-si″klo-ko″roi-di′tis) [*irido-* + *cyclo-* + *choroiditis*] inflammation of the iris, ciliary body, and choroid coat.

iridocystectomy (ir″ĭ-do-sis-tek′to-me) [*irido-* + *cyst-* + *ectomy*] an operation to establish an artificial pupil in an eye in which the iris adheres to the residual lens capsule, accomplished by excising a portion of the iris and lens capsule; through a corneal incision.

iridocyte (i-rid′o-sīt) [*irido-* + *-cyte*] one of the cells in the scales of fishes that contains crystals of guanine capable of producing iridescence.

iridodesis (ir″ĭ-dod′ĕ-sis) iridesis.

iridodiagnosis (ir″ĭ-do-di″ag-no′sis) [*irido-* + *diagnosis*] diagnosis of disease by the appearance of the iris, its color, markings, changes, etc.

iridodialysis (ir″ĭ-do-di-al′ĭ-sis) [*irido-* + *dialysis*] separation or loosening of the iris from its root at the ciliary body, either from trauma or from surgical accident.

iridodiastasis (ir″ĭdo-di-as′tah-sis) [*irido-* + Gr. *diastasis* separation] a defect of the peripheral border of the iris, but not affecting the pupillary margin, producing the clinical appearance of more than one pupil.

iridodilator (ir″ĭ-do-di-la′tor) [*irido-* + *dilator*] 1. the dilator muscle of the pupil. 2. an agent that causes dilation of the pupil of the eye.

iridodonesis (ir″ĭ-do-do-ne′sis) [*irido-* + Gr. *donēsis* tremor] abnormal tremulousness of the iris on movements of the eye, occurring in subluxation of the lens, depriving the iris of this support.

iridokeratitis (ir″ĭ-do-ker″ah-ti′tis) [*irido-* + *keratitis*] inflammation of the iris and cornea.

iridokinesia (ir″ĭ-do-ki-ne′ze-ah) iridokinesis.

iridokinesis (ir″ĭ-do-ki-ne′sis) [*irido-* + *kinesis*] the contraction and expansion of the iris.

iridokinetic (ir″ĭ-do-ki-net′ik) pertaining to iridokinesis.

iridoleptynsis (ir″ĭ-do-lep-tin′sis) [*iris* + Gr. *leptynsis* attenuation] thinning or atrophy of the iris.

iridology (ir″ĭ-dol′o-je) [*irido-* + *-logy*] the study of the iris, particularly of its color, markings, changes, etc., as associated with disease.

iridomalacia (ir″ĭ-do-mah-la′she-ah) [*irido-* + *malacia*] softening of the iris.

iridomesodialysis (ir″ĭ-do-me″so-di-al′ĭ-sis) [*irido-* + *meso-* + *dialysis*] surgical loosening of adhesions around the inner edge of the iris.

iridomotor (ir″ĭ-do-mo′tor) pertaining to movements of the iris; affecting contraction or dilation of the pupil of the eye.

iridoncus (ir″ĭ-dong′kus) [*irid-* + Gr. *onkos* bulk] tumor or swelling of the iris.

iridoparalysis (ir″ĭ-do-pah-ral′ĭ-sis) iridoplegia.

iridopathy (ir″ĭ-do-dop′ah-the) [*irido-* + Gr. *pathos* disease] disease of the iris.

iridoperiphakitis (ir″ĭ-do-per″e-fa-ki′tis) [*irido-* + Gr. *peri* around + *phakitis*] inflammation of the capsule of the crystalline lens.

iridoplegia (ir″ĭ-do-ple′je-ah) [*irido-* + *-plegia*] paralysis of the sphincter of the iris, with lack of contraction or dilation of the pupil. **accommodation i.,** failure of the pupil to contract when an accommodative effort is made. **complete i.,** paralysis of the sphincter of the pupil, with failure to react to any stimulus. **reflex i.,** failure of the pupil to contract under the influence of light or when skin is stimulated. **sympathetic i.,** failure of the pupil to dilate when the skin is stimulated.

iridoptosis (ir″ĭ-dop-to′sis) [*irido-* + *ptosis*] prolapse of the iris.

iridopupillary (ir″ĭ-do-pu′pĭ-ler″e) pertaining to the iris and the pupil.

iridorhexis (ir″ĭ-do-rek′sis) [*irido-* + *rhexis*] 1. rupture of the iris. 2. the tearing away of the iris.

iridoschisis (ir″ĭ-dos′kĭ-sis) [*irido-* + Gr. *schisis* splitting] splitting of the mesodermal stroma of the iris into two layers so that the anterior section separates and disintegrates into fibrils, the unattached ends of which float freely in the anterior chamber.

iridosclerotomy (ir″ĭ-do-skle-rot′o-me) [*irido-* + *sclero-* + *-tomy*] incision of the sclera and of the edge of the iris in treatment of glaucoma.

iridosteresis (ir″ĭ-do-ste-re′sis) [*irido-* + Gr. *sterēsis* loss] the absence or loss or removal of part or all of the iris.

iridotasis (ir″ĭ-dot′ah-sis) [*irido-* + Gr. *tasis* stretching] the operation of stretching the iris in treatment of glaucoma.

iridotomy (ir″ĭ-dot′o-me) [*irido-* + *-tomy*] incision of the iris, as in creating an artificial pupil.

iridovirus (ir″ĭ-do-vi′rus) any of a group of large, morphologically similar DNA viruses, which infect the larvae of various insects, giving an iridescent appearance to the infected insect; called also *iridescent virus.*

I.R.I.S. International Research Information Service.

Iris (i′ris) a genus of perennial iridaceous herbs. The roots of several species, *I. florentina* L., *I. germanica* L., and *I. pallida* L., are the source of orris. *I. versicolor* L. (blue flag), a plant indigenous to America, is the source of a substance formerly used as a purgative, emetic, and diuretic. Some species, e.g., *I. missouriensis* Nutt., have been reported to be poisonous to livestock due to an irritant principle in the leaves and rootstalks that causes gastroenteritis.

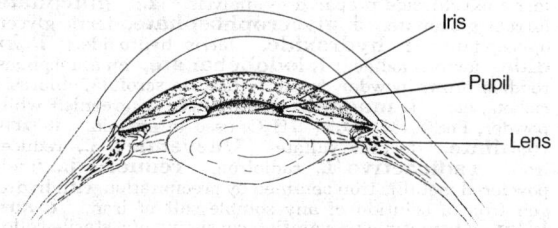

Iris, showing relation to the lens and pupil.

iris (i′ris), pl. *i′rides* [Gr. "rainbow, halo"] 1. [NA] the circular pigmented membrane behind the cornea, perforated by the pupil; the most anterior portion of the vascular tunic of the eye, it is made up of a flat bar of circular muscular fibers surrounding the pupil, a thin layer of smooth muscle fibers by which the pupil is dilated, thus regulating the amount of light entering the eye, and posteriorly two layers of pigmented epithelial cells. 2. the rhizome of *Iris versicolor*, formerly used as a purgative, emetic, and diuretic. **i. bombé,** a condition in which the iris is bowed forward by the collection of aqueous humor between the iris and lens in total posterior synechia. **detached i.,** iridodialysis. **Florentine i.,** 1. *Iris florentina* L. 2. orris. **tremulous i.,** iridonesis. **umbrella i.,** i. bombé.

irisin (i′rĭ-sin) a fructose polysaccharide, $(C_6H_{10}O_5)_n$, from *Iris pseudo-acorus*; it is an aperient and cholagogue.

irisopsia (i″ris-op′se-ah) [Gr. *iris* rainbow + *-opsia*] a visual defect in which objects appear surrounded by rings of colored light.

iritic (i-rit′ik) pertaining to or of the nature of iritis.

iritis (i-ri′tis) [*iris* + *-itis*] inflammation of the iris, usually marked by pain, congestion in the ciliary region, photophobia, contraction of the pupil, and discoloration of the iris. **i. catamenia′lis,** iritis recurring before each menstrual period. **diabetic i.,** iritis marked by the deposit of glycogen in diabetic patients. **follicular i.,** iritis marked by multiple small nodules the size of a pinhead. **gouty i.,** painful iritis occurring in gouty patients; uratic iritis. **i. papulo′sa,** iritis with papules in the iris; usually syphilitic. **plastic i.,** a variety in which the exudate consists of fibrinous matter which forms new tissue. **purulent i.,** iritis in which the exudate is purulent. **serous i.,** iritis in which the exudate consists of serum. **spongy i.,** iritis with a fibrinous exudate, forming a spongy mass in the anterior chamber. **sympathetic i.,** iritis occurring in sympathetic ophthalmoplegia. **uratic i.,** gouty i.

iritoectomy (i″ri-to-ek′to-me) [*iris* + *ectomy*] surgical excision of iritic deposits of after-cataract, together with iridectomy, to form an artificial pupil.

iritomy (i-rit′o-me) iridotomy.

irium (ir′e-um) sodium lauryl sulfate.

iron (i′ern) [A. S. *iren*; L. *ferrum*] a metallic element found in certain minerals, in nearly all soils, and in mineral waters: atomic number 26; atomic weight, 55.847; specific gravity, 7.85–7.88; symbol, Fe. Iron is an essential constituent of hemoglobin, cytochrome, and other components of respiratory enzyme systems. Its chief functions are in the transport of oxygen to tissues (hemoglobin) and in cellular oxidation mechanisms. Depletion of iron stores may result in iron-deficiency anemia (see under *anemia*). Iron is used to build up the blood in anemia. The compounds of iron are astringent and styptic. **i. acetate,** a compound, $Fe(C_2H_3O_2)_3$, used as an astringent. **alcoholized i.,** pulverized i. **i. and ammonium citrate,** see *ferric ammonium citrate,* under *ammonium.* **i. and ammonium sulfate,** see *ferric* and *ferrous ammonium sulfates,* under *ammonium.* **i. and ammonium tartrate,** see *ferric ammonium tartrate,* under *ammonium.* **i. arsenate,** ferrous arsenate. **i. arsenite,** ferric arsenite. **available i.,** that portion of iron in the food which can be separated from the total iron content by digestive processes. **i. carbonate,** ferrous carbonate. **i. chloride,** either of the binary compounds $FeCl_2$ or $FeCl_3$. **i. choline citrate,** ferrocholinate. **i. citrate,** ferric citrate. **i. citrate green,** a complex ferric ammonium citrate used for intramuscular and subcutaneous injection. **dialyzed i.,** an aqueous solution of ferric oxychloride prepared by dialysis. **i. gluconate,** ferrous gluconate. **i. glycerophosphate,** ferric glycerophosphate. **i. hydroxide,** ferric hydroxide. **i. iodide,** ferrous iodide. **i. iodobehanate,** an amorphous, reddish brown powder, formerly used in scrofula, chlorosis, rickets, etc. **i. magnesium sulfate,** a greenish white powder, $FeSO_4 \cdot MgSO_4 + 7H_2O$, used in anemia. **i. protosulfate,** ferrous sulfate. **Quevenne's i.,** reduced iron. **radioactive i.,** radioiron. **reduced i.,** finely powdered metallic iron obtained by precipitation with hydrogen from a solution of any soluble salt of iron. **i. sorbitex,** a hematinic preparation consisting of a sterile colloidal solution of a complex of trivalent iron, sorbitol, and citric acid, stabilized with dextrin and sorbitol. **i. subcarbonate,** an amorphous, brownish powder, consisting mainly of iron hydroxide. **i. subsulfate,** ferric subsulfate. **i. succinate,** a green-gray substance said to be useful in cholelithiasis. **i. sulfate,** ferrous sulfate.

irotomy (i-rot′o-me) iridotomy.

irradiate (i-ra′de-āt) 1. to treat with roentgen rays or other form of radioactivity. 2. to apply ionizing radiation for therapeutic or diagnostic purposes.

irradiation (i-ra″de-a′shun) [L. *in* into + *radiare* to emit rays] 1. treatment by photons, electrons, neutrons, or other ionizing radiations. 2. the dispersion of nervous impulse beyond the normal path of conduction. 3. the application of rays, such as ultraviolet rays, to a substance to increase its vitamin efficiency. 4. a phenomenon in which, owing to the difference in the illumination of the field of vision, objects appear to be much larger than they really are. **interstitial i.,** therapeutic irradiation by the insertion into tissues of radioactive sources in fluid form, e.g., colloidal radioactive gold (^{198}Au), or in solid form, e.g., metallic needles or seeds. **Medinger-Craver i.** (*obs.*), whole-body i. **ultraviolet blood i.,** a treatment involving removal of blood from a patient, exposing it to ultraviolet light, and returning it to the patient's circulation; abbreviated UBI. **whole-body i.,** exposure of the entire body to ionizing radiation from external radiation sources.

irreducible (ir″re-dūs′i-b'l) not susceptible to reduction, as a fracture, dislocation, or chemical substance.

irregular (ir-reg′u-lar) [L. *in* not + *regula* rule] not in conformity with the rule of nature; not recurring at regular intervals.

irregularity (ir-reg″u-lar′i-te) the quality of not conforming with the rule of nature, or of not occurring at regular intervals. **i. of pulse,** arrhythmia.

irrespirable (ir″re-spir′ah-b'l) not possible of being breathed, or not possible of being breathed with safety.

irreversibility (ir″re-ver″si-bil′i-te) the quality of being incapable of being reversed. **i. of conduction,** the principle that the pathway for every reflex permits passage of the nerve impulse in one direction only.

irreversible (ir″re-ver′si-b'l) incapable of being reversed.

irrigate (ir′i-gāt) to wash out, as a wound; lavage.

irrigation (ir″i-ga′shun) [L. *irrigatio; in* into + *rigare* to carry water] 1. washing by a stream of water or other fluid; see also *lavage.* 2. a liquid used for irrigation. **acetic acid i.** [USP], a sterile aqueous solution, containing, in each 100 ml., 237.5 to 262.5 mg. of glacial acetic acid; used to irrigate the bladder in the treatment of urinary infections with cystitis. **aminoacetic acid i.** [USP], a sterile aqueous solution, containing 95 to 105 per cent of the labeled amount of aminoacetic acid; used to irrigate body cavities. **Ringer's i.** [USP], a sterile solution containing, in each 100 ml., 820–900 mg. of sodium chloride, 25–35 mg. of potassium chloride, and 30–36 mg. of calcium chloride in water for injection; used as a topical physiological salt solution. Called also *Ringer's mixture* and *Ringer's solution.* **sodium chloride i.** [USP], a sterile aqueous solution, containing 0.85 to 0.95 per cent of sodium chloride; used to irrigate wounds and body cavities and as an enema to flush the colon and promote evacuation. Called also *sodium chloride solution.*

irrigator (ir′i-ga″tor) [L. "waterer"] an apparatus for performing irrigation.

irrigoradioscopy (ir″i-go-ra″de-os′ko-pe) roentgenoscopy of the intestines during the introduction of a contrast enema.

irrigoscopy (ir″i-gos′ko-pe) irrigoradioscopy.

irritability (ir″i-tah-bil′i-te) [L. *irritabilitas,* from *irritare* to tease] 1. the quality of being irritable, or of responding to stimuli. 2. abnormal responsiveness to slight stimuli. **i. of the bladder,** a condition in which the presence of a small amount of urine in the bladder produces a desire to urinate. **chemical i.,** responsiveness to a stimulus that acts by producing a chemical change in the tissues. **electric i.,** responsiveness of nerve or muscle to the stimulus of an electric current passed through it. **faradic i.,** the property of responding by muscular contraction to faradic current. **galvanic i.,** the property of muscle by which it responds to a galvanic current. **mechanical i.,** responsiveness to a mechanical stimulus. **muscular i.,** the normal contractile quality of muscular tissue. **myotatic i.,** the power of a muscle to contract in response to stretching. **nervous i.,** 1. the ability of a nerve to transmit impulses. 2. morbid excitability of the nervous system. **specific i.,** see under *law.* **i. of the stomach,** a condition of the stomach in which vomiting is caused by normal amounts of digestible food. **tactile i.,** a condition of cells that repels foreign particles; negative chemotaxis.

irritable (ir′i-tah-b'l) [L. *irritabilis; irritare* to tease] 1. capable of reacting to a stimulus. 2. abnormally sensitive to a stimulus.

irritant (ir′i-tant) [L. *irritans*] 1. giving rise to irritation. 2. an agent that produces irritation. **primary i.,** an agent that produces irritation, especially of the skin, on the first exposure to it.

irritation (ir″i-ta′shun) [L. *irritatio*] 1. the act of stimulating. 2. a state of overexcitation and undue sensitivity. **cerebral i.,** the second stage of brain concussion. **direct i.,** irritation due to direct stimulation of a part. **functional i.,** that which is attended with functional derangement without organic lesion; also overexcitability due to excessive functional activity.

irritative (ir′i-ta″tiv) dependent on or caused by irritation.

Irukandji sting (ir″u-kan′je) [*Irukandji,* an aboriginal tribe in the vicinity of Cairns, Queensland, Australia] see under *sting.*

IRV inspiratory reserve volume.

I.S. intercostal space.

Isambert's disease (e-zahm-bārz′) [Emile *Isambert*, French physician, 1827–1876] see under *disease*.

isamoxole (i″sah-moks′ōl) chemical name: *N*-butyl-2-methyl-*N*-(4-methyl-2-oxazolyl)propanamide; an antiasthmatic, $C_{12}H_{20}N_2O_2$.

isatin (i′sah-tin) a crystalline compound, $C_8H_5O_2N$, in the form of yellowish red crystals, soluble in alcohol and ether, slightly soluble in water: used as a reagent.

isauxesis (is″awk-se′sis) [Gr. *isos* equal + *auxēsis* increase] growth of a part or parts at the same rate as the growth of the whole.

ischemia (is-ke′me-ah) [Gr. *ischein* to suppress + *haima* blood + *-ia*] deficiency of blood in a part, due to functional constriction or actual obstruction of a blood vessel. **myocardial i.,** deficiency of blood supply to the heart muscle, due to obstruction or constriction of the coronary arteries. **i. ret′inae,** anemia of the retina; it may occur after profuse hemorrhage in another part of the body or result from arterial embolism or poison.

ischemic (is-kem′ik) pertaining to, or affected with, ischemia.

ischesis (is-ke′sis) [Gr. *ischein* to suppress] retention or suppression of a discharge.

ischia (is′ke-ah) [L.] plural of *ischium*.

ischiadelphus (is″ke-ah-del′fus) [ischio- + Gr. *adelphos* brother] ischiodidymus.

ischiadic (is″ke-ad′ik) 1. sciatic. 2. ischial.

ischial (is′ke-al) pertaining to the os ischii (ischium); ischiadic; ischiatic; sciatic.

ischialgia (is″ke-al′je-ah) [ischio- + -*algia*] pain in the os ischii (ischium); ischiodynia.

ischiatic (is″ke-at′ik) [L. *ischiaticus*] 1. sciatic. 2. ischial.

ischiectomy (is″ke-ek′to-me) surgical removal or excision of the ischium.

ischi(o)- [Gr. *ischion* hip] a combining form denoting relationship to the os ischii (ischium), or to the hip.

ischioanal (is″ke-o-a′nal) [ischio- + *anus*] pertaining to ischium and anus.

ischiobulbar (is″ke-o-bul′bar) [ischio- + L. *bulbus* bulb] pertaining to the os ischii (ischium) and the bulb of the urethra.

ischiocapsular (is″ke-o-kap′su-lar) [ischio- + L. *capsula* capsule] pertaining to the ischium and the capsular ligament of the hip joint.

ischiocele (is′ke-o-sēl″) [ischio- + Gr. *kēlē* hernia] sciatic hernia.

ischiococcygeal (is″ke-o-kok-sij′e-al) pertaining to the ischium and coccyx.

ischiococcygeus (is″ke-o-kok-sij′e-us) [ischio- + Gr. *kokkyx* coccyx] 1. musculus coccygeus. 2. the posterior part of the levator ani.

ischiodidymus (is″ke-o-did′ĭ-mus) [ischio- + Gr. *didymos* twin] symmetrical conjoined twins united at the pelvis.

ischiodymia (is″ke-o-dim′e-ah) [ischio- + Gr. *didymos* twin + -*ia*] the condition of symmetrical conjoined twins united at the pelvis.

ischiodynia (is″ke-o-din′e-ah) [ischio- + Gr. *odynē* pain] ischialgia.

ischiofemoral (is″ke-o-fem′o-ral) [ischio- + *femur*] pertaining to the ischium and femur.

ischiofibular (is″ke-o-fib′u-lar) pertaining to the ischium and the fibula.

ischiomelus (is″ke-om′ĕ-lus) [ischio- + Gr. *melos* limb] a monster with an extra limb attached at the base of the spine.

ischionitis (is″ke-o-ni′tis) inflammation of the tuberosity of the ischium.

ischiopagia (is″ke-o-pa′je-ah) the condition exhibited by an ischiopagus.

ischiopagus (is-ke-op′ah-gus) [ischio- + Gr. *pagos* thing fixed] conjoined twins fused at the ischia, the axes of the two bodies extending in a straight line but in opposite directions.

ischiopagy (is″ke-op′ah-je) ischiopagia.

ischiopubic (is″ke-o-pu′bik) pertaining to the ischium and pubis.

ischiorectal (is″ke-o-rek′tal) pertaining to the ischium and rectum.

ischiosacral (is″ke-o-sa′kral) pertaining to the ischium and sacrum.

ischiothoracopagus (is″ke-o-tho″rah-kop′ah-gus) iliothoracopagus.

ischiovaginal (is″ke-o-vaj′ĭ-nal) pertaining to the ischium and vagina.

ischiovertebral (is″ke-o-ver′te-bral) pertaining to the ischium and the vertebral column.

ischium (is′ke-um), pl. *is′chia* [L.; Gr. *ischion* hip] NA alternative for os ischii. See illustration accompanying *skeleton*.

isch(o)- [Gr. *ischein* to suppress] a combining form denoting relationship to suppression or deficiency.

ischogyria (is″ko-ji′re-ah) [ischo- + *gyrus*] a condition in which the cerebral convolutions have a jagged appearance, as in bulbar sclerosis.

ischuretic (is″ku-ret′ik) pertaining to ischuria.

ischuria (is-ku′re-ah) [ischo- + Gr. *ouron* urine + -*ia*] suppression or retention of the urine. **i. paradox′a,** a condition in which the bladder is overdistended with urine, although the patient continues to urinate. **i. spas′tica,** ischuria caused by spasm of the sphincter urinae.

I.S.C.P. International Society of Comparative Pathology.

iseiconia (īs″i-ko′ne-ah) iso-iconia.

iseiconic (īs″i-kon′ik) iso-iconic.

iseikonia (īs″i-ko′ne-ah) iso-iconia.

isethionate (is″-eth-i′o-nāt) USAN contraction for 2-hydroxyethanesulfonate.

isethionic acid (is″eth-i-o′nik) trivial name for 2-hydroxyethanesulfonic acid, $HOCH_2CH_2SO_3H$.

I.S.G.E. International Society of Gastro-Enterology.

I.S.H. International Society of Hematology.

Ishihara's test (ish″ĭ-hah′rahz) [Shinobu *Ishihara*, Japanese ophthalmologist, 1879–1963] see under *tests*.

isinglass (i′sin-glas) ichthyocolla. **Japanese i.,** agar.

island (i′land) a cluster of cells or an isolated piece of tissue. See also *islet*. **blood i's,** aggregations of mesenchyme cells in the angioblast of the early embryo, which develop into vascular endothelium and blood corpuscles. **i's of Calleja,** discrete collections of pyramidal and polymorphic cells in the caudal part of the anterior perforated substance (olfactory tubercle). **cartilage i's,** see *intrachondrial bone*, under *bone*. **i's of Langerhans,** pancreatic islets. **olfactory i's,** i's of Calleja. **i's of pancreas,** pancreatic islets. **Pander's i's,** reddish yellow cords of corpuscular matter in the splanchnopleure of the embryo which develop into blood and blood vessels. **i. of Reil,** insula.

islet (i′let) a cluster of cells or an isolated piece of tissue; see also *island*. **blood i's,** see under *island*. **Calleja's i's,** see under *island*. **i's of Langerhans,** pancreatic islets. **pancreatic i's,** irregular microscopic structures scattered throughout the pancreas and comprising its endocrine portion. In man, they are composed of at least three types of cells: the *alpha cells*, which secrete the hyperglycemic factor glucagon; the *beta cells*, which are the most abundant and secrete insulin; and the *delta cells*, which secrete somatostatin. Degeneration of the beta cells, whose secretion (insulin) is important in carbohydrate metabolism, is the major cause of diabetes mellitus. Called also *islands* or *islets of Langerhans* and *islands of pancreas*. **Walthard's i's,** microscopic inclusions of the germinal epithelium of the ovary, found either in contact with the serosal covering or just below it; they have been implicated in the development of Brenner tumors. Called also *Walthard's cell rests* or *inclusions*.

-ism [Gr. *-ismos* noun-forming suffix] a word termination denoting (*a*) a state or condition, particularly a disease state resulting from a specific cause, e.g., alcoholism, (*b*) a process, (*c*) the result of an action, or (*d*) a doctrine or principle, e.g., determinism.

I.S.M. International Society of Microbiologists.

Ismelin (is′me-lin) trademark for a preparation of guanethidine sulfate.

iso- [Gr. *isos* equal] a prefix or combining form meaning equal, alike, or the same. In immunology, it indicates *from a genetically identical individual* (as an isograft) or existing in alternate forms in the same species (as an isoantigen). In chemistry it denotes a structural isomer; used in trivial names of alkanes to indicate a one-carbon branch next to the end of the chain, e.g., isohexane is 2-methylpentane; an isoalkyl radical has its free valence at the end of the chain opposite the branch, i.e., isohexyl is 4-methylpentyl.

I.S.O. International Standards Organization.

isoadrenocorticism (i″so-ah-dre″no-kōr′tĭ-sizm) euadrenocorticism.

isoagglutination (i″so-ah-gloo″tĭ-na′shun) agglutination of cells from members of a species by agglutinins originating in genetically dissimilar members of the same species.

isoagglutinin (i″so-ah-gloo′tĭ-nin) an agglutinin from members of a species that agglutinates cells of genetically different members of the same species.

isoallele (i″so-ah-lēl′) [iso- + *allele*] an allelic gene that is considered as being normal but can be distinguished from another allele by its differing phenotypic expression when in combination with a mutant allele.

isoallelism (i″so-ah-le′lizm) [iso- + *allele*] the presence of more than one kind of normal allele at a locus.

isoalloxazine (i″so-ah-lok′sah-zēn) an isomer of alloxazine from which riboflavins and other flavins are derived.

isoamylamine (i″so-am″il-am′in) a liquid ptomaine, $(CH_3)_2CHCH_2CH_2NH_2$, obtainable from stale yeast, cod liver oil, and other sources, especially the distillation of horn with potassium hydroxide. Leucine by the loss of CO_2 becomes isoamylamine.

isoamylethylbarbituric acid (i″so-am″il-eth″il-bahr″bĭ-tu′rik) amobarbital.

isoamyl nitrite (i″so-am″il ni-trīt) amyl nitrite.

isoandrosterone (i″so-an-dro′stēr-ōn) epiandrosterone.

isoantibody (i-so-an′tĭ-bod″e) an antibody produced by one individual that reacts with antigens (isoantigens) of another individual of the same species; called also *alloantibody*.

isoantigen (i″so-an′tĭ-jen) an antigen that exists in alternative (allelic) forms in a species, and thus induces an immune response when one form is transferred (as by blood transfusion or tissue graft) to members of the species who lack it. Typical isoantigens are the blood group antigens. Called also *alloantigen*.

isobar (i′so-bar) [iso- + Gr. *baros* weight] 1. one of two or more chemical species with the same atomic weight but different atomic numbers. 2. a line on a map or chart depicting the boundaries of an area of constant atmospheric pressure.

isobaric (i″so-bār′ik) [iso- + Gr. *baros* weight] see under *solution*.

isobolism (i-sob′o-lizm) [iso- + Gr. *ballein* to throw] the tendency of motor nerve fibers to undergo maximal excitation on stimulation.

isobornyl thiocyanoacetate (i″so-bor″nil thi″o-si″ah-no-as′e-tāt) chemical name: terpinyl thiocyanoacetate; used as a pediculicide.

isobucaine hydrochloride (i″so-bu′kān) [USP] chemical name: 2-methyl-2-[(2-methylpropyl)amino]-1-propanol benzoate (ester) hydrochloride. A local anesthetic, $C_{15}H_{23}-NO_2 \cdot HCl$, occurring as a white, crystalline solid; used in combination with epinephrine in dentistry.

isobutamben (i″so-bu-tam′ben) chemical name: 4-aminobenzoic acid 2-methylpropyl ester; a topical anesthetic, $C_{11}H_{15}NO_2$.

isobutanol (i″so-bu′tah-nol″) isobutyl alcohol.

isobutyric acid (i″so-bu-tēr′ik) trivial name for 2-methylpropanoic acid, $(CH_3)_2CHCHCOOH$.

isocaloric (i″so-kah-lo′rik) containing or providing the same number of calories; equicaloric.

isocarboxazid (i″so-kar-bok′sah-zid) [USP] chemical name: 5-methyl-3-isoxazolecarboxylic acid 2-(phenylmethyl)-hydrazide. A monoamine oxidase inhibitor, $C_{12}H_{13}N_3O_2$, occurring as a white or nearly white, crystalline powder; used as an antidepressant, administered orally.

isocarveol (i″so-kar′ve-ol) pinocarveol.

isocellobiose (i″so-sel″o-bi′ōs) a disaccharide once considered to be formed in the degradation of cellulose; now recognized as a mixture of cellobiose with oligosaccharides.

isocellular (i″so-sel′u-lar) [iso- + L. *cellula* cell] composed of cells of the same kind and size.

isocenter (i′so-sen″ter) a point at which there is a maximum or minimum of the radiation dose, i.e., the center of the surrounding isodose curves.

isocholesterin (i″so-ko-les′ter-in) isocholesterol.

isocholesterol (i″so-ko-les′ter-ol) a compound found with cholesterol in wool; apparently a mixture of C_{30} trimethyl cholestanes.

isochromatic (i″so-kro-mat′ik) [iso- + Gr. *chrōma* color] of the same color throughout.

isochromatophil (i″so-kro-mat′o-fil) [iso- + Gr. *chrōma* color + *philein* to love] staining equally with the same dye.

isochromosome (i″so-kro′mo-sōm) [iso- + *chromosome*] an abnormal chromosome having a median centromere and two identical arms, probably formed by the transverse, rather than the normal longitudinal separation of the centromere of the replicating chromosome.

isochronal (i-sok′ro-nal) isochronous.

isochronia (i-so-kro′ne-ah) 1. a condition of correspondence between processes with respect to their time, rate, or frequency. 2. the condition of having the same chronaxy as between a muscle and its nerve.

isochronic (i″so-kron′ik) isochronous.

isochronism (i-sok′ro-nizm) isochronia.

isochronous (i-sok′ro-nus) [iso- + Gr. *chronos* time] performed in equal times; said of motions and vibrations occurring at the same time and being equal in duration.

isochroous (i-sok′ro-us) [iso- + Gr. *chroa* color] isochromatic.

isocitrate (i″so-sĭ-trāt) a fully dissociated (ionized) salt of isocitric acid.

isocitrate dehydrogenase (NAD⁺) (i″so-sĭ′trāt de-hi′-dro-jĕ-nās) [EC 1.1.1.41] an enzyme of the oxidoreductase class that catalyzes the reaction isocitrate + NAD^+ = 2-ketoglutarate + CO_2 + NADH. It occurs in cell mitochondria. The enzyme requires Mg^{2+} or Mn^{2+}; it is activated by ADP, citrate, and Ca^{2+}, and inhibited by NADH, NADPH, and ATP. The reaction is the key rate-limiting step of the citric acid (tricarboxylic) cycle.

isocitrate dehydrogenase (NADP⁺) (i″so-sĭ′trat de-hi′-dro-jĕ-nās) [EC 1.1.1.42] an enzyme of the oxidoreductase class that catalyzes the reaction isocitrate + $NADP^+$ = 2-ketoglutarate + CO_2 + NADPH. It requires Mg^{2+} or Mn^{2+}. The enzyme occurs in all tissues. There are two distinct isozymes, the cytoplasmic and the mitochondrial. The reaction is significant in maintaining the level of reducing equivalents within the cell.

isocitric acid (i″so-sit′rik) a structural isomer of citric acid, $HOOC-CH_2-CH(COOH)-CH(OH)-COOH$, that is an intermediate in the citric (tricarboxylic) acid cycle (q.v.).

isocolloid (i-so-kol′oid) a colloid having the same composition in both phases—the disperse phase and the dispersion medium.

isoconazole (i″so-ko′nah-zōl) chemical name: 1-[2-(2,4-dichlorophenyl)-2-[(2,6-dichlorophenyl)methoxyethyl]-1*H*-imidazole; an antibacterial and antifungal, $C_{18}H_{14}Cl_4N_2O$.

isocoria (i″so-ko′re-ah) [iso- + Gr. *korē* pupil] equality in size of the two pupils.

isocortex (i″so-kor′teks) neopallium.

isocreatinine (i″so-kre-at′ĭ-nin) a base similar to creatinine reported to have been found in the muscle of fish.

Isocrin (i′so-krin) trademark for a preparation of oxyphenisatin acetate.

isocyanide (i″so-si′ah-nīd) one of a class of organic cyanides characterized by their disagreeable odor and formed by heating silver cyanide with alkyl iodides; called also *carbylamine*.

isocyclic (i″so-si′klik) [iso- + Gr. *kyklos* circle] homocyclic.

isocytolysin (i″so-si-tol′ĭ-sin) [iso- + *cytolysin*] a cytolysin that acts on the cells of animals of the same species as that from which it is derived.

isocytosis (i″so-si-to′sis) [iso- + *-cyte* + *-osis*] equality of the size of cells, especially red blood corpuscles.

isodactylism (i-so-dak'til-izm) [*iso-* + Gr. *daktylos* finger + *-ism*] a condition in which the fingers are of relatively even length.

isodesmosine (i"so-des'mo-sēn) one of two unusual amino acids found in elastin, the other being desmosine.

isodiametric (i"so-di"ah-met'rik) [*iso-* + Gr. *dia* through + *metron* measure] having the same diameter in all directions.

isodispersoid (i"so-dis-per'soid) isocolloid.

isodontic (i"so-don'tik) [*iso-* + Gr. *odous* tooth] having all the teeth of the same size and shape.

isodose (i'so-dōs) a radiation dose of equal intensity to more than one body area; see also under *curve*.

isodulcite (i"so-dul'sīt) rhamnose.

isodynamic (i"so-di-nam'ik) [*iso-* + Gr. *dynamis* power] exhibiting equal force or power.

isodynamogenic (i"so-di-nam"o-jen'ik) [*iso-* + Gr. *dynamis* power + *gennan* to produce] producing equal force or power.

isoeffect (i"so-ĕ-fekt') an effect midway between two reference points; see under *line*.

isoelectric (i"so-e-lek'trik) [*iso-* + *electric*] showing no variation in electric potential.

isoenergetic (i"so-en"er-jet'ik) exhibiting equal energy.

isoenzyme (i"so-en'zīm) isozyme. **Regan i.,** an isoenzyme of alkaline phosphatase, apparently identical to placental alkaline phosphatase, found in the serum of some patients with cancer of the female reproductive organs, breast, or lung.

isoetharine (i-so-eth'ah-rēn) chemical name: 4-[(1-hydroxy-2-[(1-methylethyl)amino]-butyl]-1,2-benzenediol. An adrenergic, $C_{13}H_{21}NO_3$, used as a bronchodilator in the treatment of bronchial asthma and bronchospasm, administered by inhalation. Its hydrochloride and mesylate salts are prepared in conformance with USP standards.

isoflupredone acetate (i"so-floo"pre-dōn) chemical name: 21-(acetyloxy)-9-fluoro-11β,17-dihydroxypregna-1,4-diene-3,20-dione; an anti-inflammatory, $C_{23}H_{29}FO_6$.

isoflurane (i"so-floo'rān) chemical name: 1-chloro-2,2,2-trifluoroethyl difluoromethyl ether, a potent inhalational ar.esthetic, an isomer of enflurane with similar properties, used for induction and maintenance of general anesthesia.

isoflurophate (i"so-flūr'o-fāt) [USP] nonproprietary drug name for diisopropyl flurophosphate (DFP), a potent irreversible anticholinesterase agent; used topically to produce miosis, decrease intraocular pressure, and potentiate accommodation in treatment of open-angle glaucoma and accommodative convergent strabismus.

isogame (i-sog'ah-me) isogamy.

isogamete (i"so-gam'ēt) [*iso-* + *gamete*] a gamete of the same size as the gamete with which it unites; cf. *heterogamete* and *homogamete*.

isogametic (i"so-gah-met'ik) characterized by the production of gametes of the same size.

isogamety (i"so-gam'e-te) production by an individual of one sex of gametes identical with respect to the sex chromosome.

isogamous (i-sog'ah-mus) pertaining to isogamy.

isogamy (i-sog'ah-me) [*iso-* + Gr. *gamos* marriage] reproduction resulting from the union of two cells (gametes) that are identical in size and structure, as occurs in protozoa. See also *heterogamy* and *homogamy*.

isogeneic (i"so-jĕ-ne'ik) syngeneic.

isogeneric (i"so-jĕ-ner'ik) of the same kind; pertaining to or obtained from individuals of the same genus.

isogenesis (i"so-jen'ĕ-sis) [*iso-* + Gr. *genesis* production] similarity in the processes of development.

isogenous (i-soj'ĕ-nus) developed from the same cell.

isograft (i'so-graft) syngraft.

isohemagglutination (i"so-hem"ah-gloo"tĭ-na'shun) agglutination of erythrocytes caused by a hemagglutinin from another individual of the same species.

isohemagglutinin (i"so-hem"ah-gloo"tĭ-nin) a hemagglutinin that agglutinates the erythrocytes of other individuals of the same species.

isohemolysin (i"so-he-mol'ĭ-sin) [*iso-* + *hemolysin*] a hemolysin that acts on the blood of animals of the same species as that from which it is derived.

isohemolysis (i"so-he-mol'ĭ-sis) hemolysis of the blood corpuscles of an animal by the lysins in serum from another animal of the same species.

isohemolytic (i"so-he"mo-lit'ik) pertaining to or characterized by isohemolysis.

isohydric (i"so-hi'drik) a term applied to the series or cycle of chemical reactions in the erythrocyte in which carbon dioxide is taken up and oxygen released without the production of an excess of hydrogen.

isoiconia (i"so-i-ko'ne-ah) [*iso-* + Gr. *eikōn* image] a condition in which the image of an object is the same in both eyes.

isoiconic (i"so-i-kon'ik) marked by isoiconia.

isoimmunization (i"so-im"u-ni-za'shun) development of antibodies against an antigen derived from a genetically dissimilar individual of the same species; see also *isoantigen*. **Rh i.,** development of antibodies against Rh antigens, the antigen involved in almost all cases being the Rh_0 antigen (D antigen). Rh isoimmunization of Rh-negative women may occur after transfusion of Rh-positive blood or during pregnancy with an Rh-positive fetus, when the mother is exposed to fetal blood during delivery, amniocentesis, miscarriage, or abortion, and may result in the development of erythroblastosis fetalis in any subsequent pregnancy with an Rh-positive fetus. See also $Rh_0(D)$ *immune globulin*, under *globulin*.

isokreatinin (i"so-kre-at'ĭ-nin) a ptomaine from decaying fish, crystallizable in a yellow powder, $C_4H_7N_3O$.

isolactose (i"so-lak'tōs) a disaccharide formed by the action of lactase on glucose and galactose.

isolate (i'so-lāt) 1. to separate from other persons, materials, or objects. 2. in microbiology, to obtain from a source such as a clinical specimen a pure strain that may have been part of a mixed primary culture. 3. a population that has been obtained by isolation (such as bacteria or other cells obtained in pure culture), or a group of individuals prevented by geographic, ecologic, or social barriers from interbreeding with others of their kind, and thus differentiated by the accumulation of new characteristics.

isolation (i"so-la'shun) 1. the process of isolating, or the state of being isolated. 2. the physiologic separation of a part, as by tissue culture or by interposition of inert material. 3. the extraction and purification of a chemical substance of unknown structure from a natural source. 4. the separation of infected individuals from those uninfected for the period of communicability of a particular disease; cf. *quarantine* (def. 1). 5. the successive propagation of a growth of microorganisms until a pure culture is obtained. 6. in psychiatry, a defense mechanism in which the emotions connected with an idea, impulse, or memory are repressed; the idea or impulse enters consciousness detached from its unacceptable feeling. Called also *isolation of affect*.

isolator (i"so-la'tor) anything that isolates. **surgical i.,** a large, clear, plastic bag with man-sized pockets that is attached to the patient's body during surgical procedures to prevent contamination by infective agents; the pockets, in which the nurses and surgeons stand, have plastic helmets, earphones and microphones for communication, and closed sleeves leading into the bag through which the surgeons work.

isolecithal (i"so-les'ĭ-thal) [*iso-* + *lekithos* yolk] having yolk evenly distributed throughout the cytoplasm of the ovum.

isoleucine (i"so-lu'sin) an amino acid, ethylmethyl-alpha-aminopropionic acid, $CH_3(C_2H_5) \cdot CHCH(NH_2) \cdot COOH$, produced by the hydrolysis of fibrin and other proteins; essential for optimal growth in infants and for nitrogen equilibrium in human adults.

isoleucyl (i"so-loo'sil) the acyl radical of isoleucine.

isoleukoagglutinin (i"so-lu"ko-ah-glu'tĭ-nin) a leukocyte agglutinin.

isologous (i-sol'o-gus) characterized by an identical genotype; see *isograft*.

isolysergic acid (i"so-li-sur'jik) one of the main cleavage products of the alkaline hydrolysis of the alkaloids characteristic of ergot, and the parent compound of the ergotinine group of alkaloids.

isolysin (i-sol′ĭ-sin) a lysin that acts on the cells of animals of the same species as that from which it is derived.

isolysis (i-sol′ĭ-sis) lysis of cells by isolysins.

isolytic (i″so-lit′ik) pertaining to isolysis.

isomaltase (i″so-mawl′tās) oligo-1,6-α-glucosidase.

isomaltose (i″so-mawl′tōs) an isomeric form of maltose formed by treating glucose with strong acids or by the action of maltase on glucose; it occurs in beer, urine, blood, honey, liver, and other natural substances. Called also *brachiose* and *dextrinose.*

isomastigote (i″so-mas′tĭ-gōt) [iso- + Gr. *mastix* lash] having two equal and similar flagella at the anterior pole.

isomer (i′so-mer) [iso- + Gr. *meros* part] any compound exhibiting, or capable of exhibiting, isomerism. An isomer may be structural or stereochemical; see *isomerism.*

isomerase (i-som′er-ās) [EC 5] a class of enzymes that catalyze geometric or structural changes within a molecule to form a single product. The reactions do not involve a net change in the concentration of compounds other than the substrate and the product. The class includes epimerases, isomerases, mutases, and racemases.

isomeric (i″so-mer′ik) pertaining to or exhibiting isomerism.

isomeride (i-som′er-īd) isomer.

isomerism (i-som′ĕ-rizm) [iso- + Gr. *meros* part] the relationship that exists between two or more different chemical compounds that have the same molecular formula; the compounds are *isomers* (of each other) and are *isomeric* (to each other). Isomerism is divided into two broad classes: *structural isomerism* and *stereoisomerism* (q.v.). **chain i.,** a type of structural isomerism in which the compounds differ

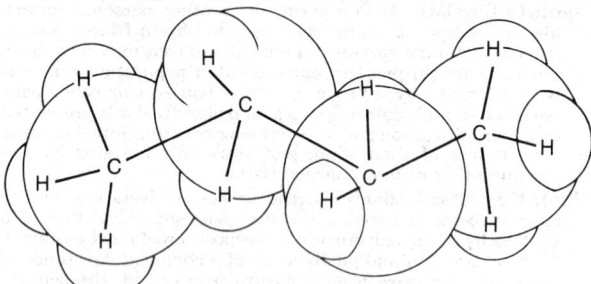

Normal butane

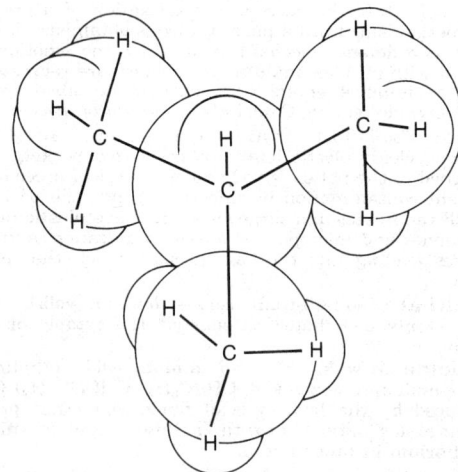

Isobutane

Chain isomerism.

in regard to the linkages in the basic chain of carbon atoms; see illustration. **cis-trans i.,** geometric i. **configurational i.,** stereoisomerism. **conformational i.,** the relationship between stereoisomers that differ only by rotations about single bonds (conformers). **constitutional i.,**

structural i. **functional group i.,** a type of structural isomerism dependent upon the presence of different functional groups, such compounds being of distinct chemical types, e.g., ethyl alcohol, C_2H_5OH, and dimethyl ether, CH_3OCH_3. **geometric i.,** an old division of stereoisomerism that contains isomers that differ in the arrangement of substituents of a rigid structure, such as double-bonded carbon atoms or a ring. The *cis* isomer has two referenced groups on the same side of the ring or double bond; the *trans* isomer on opposite sides. Geometric isomers are thus diastereomers. Called also *cis-trans i.* **optical i.,** an old division of stereoisomerism that contains isomers that differ in the arrangement of substituents at one or more asymmetric carbon atoms, thus some but not necessarily all are optically active, e.g., *d*-, *l*-, and *meso*-tartaric acid. Some optical isomers are enantiomers (the *d* and *l* forms); some are diastereomers (the *d* and *meso* forms). **position i.,** a type of structural isomerism in which the position occupied by an atom or group differs with reference to the same fundamental carbon chain; for example, *n*-propyl chloride, $CH_3CH_2CH_2Cl$, and isopropyl chloride, $CH_3CHClCH_3$. **spatial i.,** stereoisomerism. **stereochemical i.,** stereoisomerism. **structural i.,** the relationship between two or more isomers that have different structures (the same atoms linked in different ways) in contrast to stereoisomerism in which the isomers have the same structure but different configurations (the same linkages but different spatial arrangements). Called also *constitutional i.* **substitution i.,** position i.

isomerization (i-som″er-i-za′shun) the process whereby any isomer, whether structural or stereochemical, is converted into another, usually requiring special conditions of temperature, pressure, or catalysts.

isometheptene hydrochloride (i″so-meth′ep-tēn) chemical name: *N*,1,5-trimethyl-4-hexenylamine hydrochloride. An adrenergic, $C_9H_{20}ClN$, used as an antispasmodic for the urinary and gastrointestinal tracts and as a vasodilator in the treatment of migraine; administered intramuscularly.

isometric (i″so-met′rik) [iso- + Gr. *metron* measure] 1. maintaining, or pertaining to, the same measure or length; of equal dimensions. 2. not isotonic.

isometropia (i″so-mĕ-tro′pe-ah) [iso- + Gr. *metron* measure + -*opia*] equality in the refraction of the two eyes.

isometry (i-som′ĕ-tre) equality of dimension.

isomorphic (i″so-mor′fik) isomorphous.

isomorphism (i″so-mor′fizm) the quality of being isomorphous.

isomorphous (i″so-mor′fus) [iso- + -*morphous*] having the same form. In genetics, denoting genotypes of polyploid organisms which produce similar gametes even though containing genes in different combinations on homologous chromosomes.

isomuscarine (i″so-mus′kah-rin) a basic substance formed by oxidizing choline; it is isomeric with muscarine, but has different physiologic properties.

isomylamine hydrochloride (i″so-mil′ah-mēn) chemical name: 1-(3-methylbutyl)-cyclohexanecarboxylic acid 2-(diethylamino)ethyl ester hydrochloride; a smooth muscle relaxant, $C_{18}H_{35}NO_2 \cdot HCl$.

isonaphthol (i″so-naf′thol) betanaphthol.

isonephrotoxin (i″so-nef′ro-tok′sin) [iso- + *nephrotoxin*] a nephrotoxin which acts on cells of the animals of the same species from which it is derived.

isoniazid (i″so-ni′ah-zid) [USP] chemical name: 4-pyridinecarboxylic acid hydrazide. An antibacterial, $C_6H_7N_3O$, occurring as colorless or white crystals or white, crystalline powder; used as a tuberculostatic, administered orally and intramuscularly.

isonicotinoylhydrazine (i″so-nik″o-tin″o-il-hi′drah-zēn) isoniazid.

isonicotinylhydrazine (i″so-nik″o-tin″il-hi′drah-zēn) isoniazid.

isonipecaine (i″so-nip′e-kān) meperidine hydrochloride.

isonitril (i″so-ni′tril) isocyanide.

iso-oncotic (i″so-on-kot′ik) having the same oncotic pressure.

iso-osmotic (i″so-oz-mot′ik) isosmotic.

Isopaque (i″so-pāk′) trademark for preparations of metrizoate sodium.

Isoparorchis trisimilitubis (i″so-par-or′kis tri-sim″ĭ-li-tu′bis) a fluke, commonly parasitic in the air bladder of fish in India and China and sometimes found in man.

isopathy (i-sop′ah-the) [*iso-* + Gr. *pathos* disease] the treatment of disease by means of products of the disease or with material from the organ affected, e.g., smallpox by giving minute doses of variolous matter, disease of the liver by giving extract of liver, etc.

isopentenyl-diphosphate δ-isomerase (i″so-pen″tĕ-nil-di-fos′fāt i-som′er-ās) [EC 5.3.3.2] an enzyme of the isomerase class that catalyzes the reaction isopentenyl diphosphate = dimethylallyl diphosphate. The reaction is a step in the biosynthesis of cholesterol and other isoprenoid compounds.

isophagy (i-sof′ah-je) [*iso-* + Gr. *phagein* to eat] autolysis.

isophoria (i″so-fo′re-ah) [*iso-* + *phoria*] equality in the tension of the vertical muscles of each eye; absence of hyperphoria and of hypophoria.

Isophrin (i′so-frin) trademark for a preparation of phenylephrine hydrochloride.

isopia (i-so′pe-ah) [*iso-* + *-opia*] equality of vision in the two eyes.

isoplassont (i″so-plas′ont) [*iso-* + Gr. *plassein* to form] either of two things which have certain features in common.

isoplastic (i″so-plas′tik) [*iso-* + *plastic*] taken from another animal of the same species or from another inbred strain within the same species; said of tissue transplants or grafts.

isoprecipitin (i″so-pre-sip′ĭ-tin) a precipitin that is active against antigens of animals of the same species (but of dissimilar genetic makeup) as the animal in which it is formed.

isopregnenone (i″so-preg′ne-nōn) dydrogesterone.

isoprenaline (i″so-pren′ah-lēn) isoproterenol.

isoprene (i′so-prēn) the basic building unit of terpenes, C_5H_8.

isopropamide iodide (i″so-pro′pah-mīd) [USP] chemical name: γ-(aminocarbonyl)-*N*-methyl-*N*,*N*-bis(1-methylethyl)-γ-phenylbenzenepropanaminium iodide. A long-acting quaternary anticholinergic, $C_{23}H_{33}IN_2O$, used in the treatment of peptic ulcer and other gastrointestinal disorders marked by hyperacidity and hypermotility, administered orally.

isopropanol (i″so-pro′pah-nol) isopropyl alcohol.

isopropyl (i″so-pro′pil) the univalent radical, $(CH_3)_2CH$. **i. alcohol, i. rubbing alcohol,** see under *alcohol.* **i. meprobamate,** carisoprodol. **i. myristate** [NF], a compound of isopropyl alcohol and saturated high molecular weight fatty acids, principally myristic acid, occurring as a clear, oily liquid; used as an emollient in pharmaceutical preparations.

isopropylarterenol (i″so-pro″pil-ar″tĕ-re′nol) isoproterenol.

isopropyl-benzanthracene (i″so-pro″pil-benz-an″thrah-sēn) a carcinogenic hydrocarbon, 6-isopropyl-1,2-benzanthracene.

isoproterenol (i″so-pro″tĕ-re′nol) chemical name: 4-[1-hydroxy-2-[(1-methylethyl)amino]ethyl]-1,2-benzenediol. A synthetic adrenergic, $C_{11}H_{17}NO_3$, derived from norepinephrine, having powerful bronchodilator and cardiac stimulant actions. **i. hydrochloride** [USP], the hydrochloride salt of isoproterenol, $C_{11}H_{17}NO_3 \cdot HCl$, occurring as a white to practically white, crystalline powder; used chiefly as a bronchodilator in the treatment of bronchial asthma, administered by oral inhalation, sublingually, and parenterally. It may also be used in the management of shock, treatment and prevention of cardiac standstill and arrhythmias, and treatment of bronchospasm during anesthesia. **i. sulfate** [USP], the sulfate salt of isoproterenol, $(C_{11}H_{17}NO_3)_2 \cdot H_2SO_4 \cdot 2H_2O$, having the appearance, actions, and uses as the hydrochloride salt; administered by oral inhalation.

isopter (i-sop′ter) [*iso-* + Gr. *optēr* observer] a line depicting the area in the field of vision in which the visual acuity is the same.

isopyknic (i″so-pik′nik) [*iso-* + Gr. *pyknos* thick] of equal density or thickness; see under *centrifugation.*

isopyknosis (i″so-pik-no′sis) [*iso-* + *pyknosis*] the state of being of uniform density; applied especially to a state of uniform condensation observed in comparison of different chromosomes, or of different regions of the same chromosome.

isopyknotic (i″so-pik-not′ik) pertaining to or characterized by isopyknosis.

Isordil (i′sor-dil) trademark for preparations of isosorbide dinitrate.

isorhodeose (i″so-ro′de-ōs) a sugar, *d*-glucomethylose or 6-deoxy-D-glucose, $CH_3(CHOH)_4CHO$, from cinchona bark.

isoriboflavin (i″so-ri″bo-fla′vin) a compound, dichlororibityl isoalloxazine, which can produce riboflavin deficiency.

isorrhea (i″so-re′ah) [*iso-* + Gr. *rhein* to flow] the maintenance of a relatively constant body fluid volume and composition; water and solute intake is balanced by an equivalent output of the substances from the body.

isorrheic (i″so-re′ik) pertaining to or characterized by isorrhea.

isorrhopic (i″so-rop′ik) [*iso-* + Gr. *rhopē* momentum] of equal value.

isorubin (i″so-ru′bin) new fuchsin.

isoscope (i′so-skōp) [*iso-* + *-scope*] an apparatus for observing the changes of position of the horizontal and vertical lines in the movements of the eyeball.

isosensitization (i″so-sen″sĭ-ti-za′shun) allosensitization.

isoserine (i″so-se′rin) a compound, $CH_2NH_2 \cdot CHOH \cdot COOH$, isomeric with serine.

isosexual (i″so-seks′u-al) [*iso-* + *sexual*] pertaining to or characteristic of the same sex.

isosmotic (i″sos-mot′ik) having the same osmotic pressure.

isosmoticity (i″sos-mo-tis′ĭ-te) the state or quality of being isosmotic.

isosorbide (i″so-sor′bīd) a bicyclic ether derivative of glucitol; used as an osmotic diuretic to reduce intraocular pressure. **i. dinitrate,** the dinitric acid ester of isosorbide, $C_6H_8N_2O_8$, occurring as a white, crystalline powder, having coronary and peripheral vasodilating properties; used in the treatment of coronary insufficiency and angina pectoris, administered sublingually and orally.

Isospora (i-sos′po-rah) [*iso-* + *spore*] a genus of coccidian protozoa (suborder Eimeriina, order Eucoccidiida) characterized by the presence of two sporocysts in each oocyst and four sporozoites in each sporocyst; found in birds, amphibians, reptiles, and mammals, including man. **I. bel′li,** a species that parasitizes the small intestine of man; infection (coccidiosis) is usually asymptomatic but may result in a severe watery mucous diarrhea. **I. bigem′ina,** a form found in dogs and cats, closely resembling *I. hominis;* called also *Coccidium bigeminum.* **I. fe′lis,** a species causing intestinal coccidiosis in cats. **I. hom′inis,** see *Sarcocystis bovihominis* and *Sarcocytis suihominis.* **I. laca′zei,** a species causing intestinal coccidiosis in passerine birds. **I. rivol′ta,** a species causing intestinal coccidiosis in dogs and cats. **I. su′is,** a species that may cause coccidiosis in swine.

isospore (i′so-spōr) [*iso-* + Gr. *sporos* spore] 1. an isogamete of organisms that reproduce by spores. 2. an asexual spore produced by a homosporous organism.

isosporiasis (i-sos″po-ri′ah-sis) infection with *Isospora.* See *coccidiosis.*

isosporous (i-sos′po-rus) having isospores.

isostere (i′so-stēr) a compound resembling another compound in electron arrangement but differing in chemical structure.

isosthenuria (i″sos-thĕ-nu′re-ah) [*iso-* + Gr. *sthenos* strength + *ouron* urine + *-ia*] the excretion of urine with the same osmolality as that of plasma.

isothebaine (i″so-the′ba-in) chemical name: 1-hydroxy-2-11-dimethoxyaporphine. An alkaloid, $C_{19}H_{21}O_3N$, from *Papaver orientalis.*

isotherapy (i″so-ther′ah-pe) [*iso-* + Gr. *therapeia* treatment] isopathy.

isotherm (i′so-therm) a line on a map or chart depicting the boundaries of an area in which the temperature is the same.

isothermal (i″so-ther′mal) [*iso-* + Gr. *thermē* heat] isothermic.

isothermic (i″so-ther′mik) having the same temperature.

isothermognosis (i″so-ther″mo-no′sis) [*iso-* + Gr. *thermē* heat + *gnōsis* recognition] disordered sense perception in which pain, cold, and heat stimuli are all perceived as heat.

isothiazine hydrochloride (i″so-thi′ah-zēn) ethopropazine hydrochloride.

isothiocyanate (i″so-thi″o-si′ah-nāt) an ester of isothiocyanic acid R—N=C=S.

isothiocyanic acid (i″so-thi″o-si-an′ik) the molecular species H—N=C=S, that occurs in equilibrium with thiocyanic acid.

isothipendyl (i″so-thi′pen-dil) chemical name: 10-(2-dimethylamino-2-methylethyl)-10*H*-pyrido[3,2-*b*][1,4]benzothiazine. A compound, $C_{16}H_{19}N_3S$, used as an antihistaminic.

isothromboagglutinin (i″so-throm″bo-ah-gloo′ti-nin) a platelet isoagglutinin.

isotone (i′so-tōn) one of several nuclides having the same number of neutrons, but differing in the number of protons in their nuclei.

isotonia (i″so-to′ne-ah) [*iso-* + Gr. *tonos* tone] 1. a condition of equal tone, tension, or activity. 2. equality of osmotic pressure between two elements of a solution or between two different solutions.

isotonic (i″so-ton′ik) [*iso-* + Gr. *tonos* tone] a biological term denoting a solution in which body cells can be bathed without a net flow of water across the semipermeable cell membrane. Also, denoting a solution having the same tonicity as some other solution with which it is compared, such as physiologic salt solution and the blood serum.

isotonicity (i″so-to-nis′ĭ-te) the quality of being isotonic.

isotope (i′so-tōp) [*iso-* + Gr. *topos* place] a chemical element having the same atomic number as another (i.e., the same number of nuclear protons) but possessing a different atomic mass (i.e., a different number of nuclear neutrons). **radioactive i.**, radioisotope. **stable i.**, an isotope that does not transmute into another element with emission of corpuscular or electromagnetic radiations.

isotopology (i″so-to-pol′o-je) the scientific study of isotopes, and of their uses and applications.

isotoxic (i″so-tok′sik) pertaining to an isotoxin.

isotoxin (i″so-tok′sin) [*iso-* + *toxin*] a toxin that is poisonous to other animals of the same species.

isotransplant (i″so-trans′plant) [*iso-* + *transplant*] isograft.

isotransplantation (i″so-trans″plan-ta′shun) the transplanting of an isograft.

isotretinoin (i″so-tret′ĭ-noin) 13-*cis*-retinoic acid, used systemically for treatment of severe cystic and conglobulate acne; it inhibits the secretion of sebum and alters the lipid composition of the skin surface.

Isotricha (i-sot′rĭ-kah) [*iso-* + Gr. *thrix, trichos* hair] a genus of ciliate protozoa (suborder Trichostomatina, order Trichostomatida) found in the stomachs of ungulates, and characterized by the presence of an apical cytostome and by dense longitudinal rows of cilia over the entire body surface. Species include *I. prostoma* and *I. intestinalis*.

isotrimorphism (i″so-tri-mor′fizm) [*iso-* + Gr. *treis* three + *morphē* form] isomorphism between the three forms of two trimorphous substances.

isotrimorphous (i″so-tri-mor′fus) pertaining to or characterized by isotrimorphism.

isotron (i′so-tron) an apparatus for separating isotopes electromagnetically.

isotropic (i″so-trop′ik) [*iso-* + Gr. *tropos* a turning] 1. similar in all directions with respect to a property, as in a cubic crystal or a piece of glass. 2. being singly refractive.

isotropy (i-sot′ro-pe) the quality or condition of being isotropic.

isotype (i′so-tīp) an immunoglobulin heavy or light chain class or subclass characterized by antigenic determinants (isotypic markers) in the constant region. Every normal individual expresses all of the isotypes of its species. Cf. *allotype* and *idiotype*.

isotypic (i″so-tip′ik) pertaining to isotypes.

isotypical (i″so-tip′ĭ-kal) [*iso-* + *typical*] of the same type.

isouretin (i″so-u-re′tin) formamidoxim, $NH_2CH:NOH$, a compound isomeric with urea.

isovaleric acid (i″so-vah-lār′ik) trivial name for 3-methylbutanoic acid, $(CH_3)_2CHCH_2COOH$; isovaleryl coenzyme A

is an intermediate in leucine catabolism; free isovaleric acid is released in isovaleric acidemia.

isovaleric acid CoA dehydrogenase deficiency isovaleric acidemia.

isovalericacidemia (i″so-vah-ler″ik-as″ĭ-de′me-ah) isovaleric acidemia.

isovaleryl-CoA dehydrogenase (i″so-val′er-il de-hi′dro-jĕ-nās) [EC 1.3.99.10] an enzyme of the oxidoreductase class that catalyzes the reaction 3-methylbutanoyl-CoA + ubiquinone = 3-methylcrotonoyl-CoA + ubiquinol. It is a flavoprotein (FAD). The reaction is a step in the use of leucine as a fuel. Deficiency of the enzyme, an autosomal recessive trait, results in isovaleric acidemia.

isoxepac (i-soks′ĕ-pak) chemical name: 6,11-dihydro-11-oxo-dibenz[*b,e*]-oxepin-2-acetic acid; an anti-inflammatory, $C_{16}H_{12}O_4$.

isoxicam (i-soks′ĭ-kam) chemical name: 4-hydroxy-2-methyl-*N*-(5-methyl-3-isoxazolyl)-2*H*-1,2-benzothiazine-3-carboxamide 1,1-dioxide; an anti-inflammatory, $C_{14}H_{13}N_3$-O_5S.

isoxsuprine hydrochloride (i-sok′su-prēn) [USP] chemical name: 4-hydroxy-α-[1-[(1-methyl-2-phenoxyethyl)-amino]ethyl] benzenemethanol hydrochloride. An adrenergic, $C_{18}H_{23}NO_3$·HCl, occurring as a white, crystalline powder, used as a vasodilator in the treatment of cerebral vascular insufficiency and of peripheral vascular diseases such as arteriosclerosis obliterans, thromboangiitis obliterans, and Raynaud's disease. It is administered orally or intramuscularly.

isozyme (i′so-zīm) one of various structurally related forms of an enzyme, each having the same mechanism but with differing chemical, physical, or immunological characteristics. For example, lactate dehydrogenase, a tetramer, exists as five isozymes arising from different combinations of its two kinds of subunits. Called also *isoenzyme*.

issue (is′u) a discharge of pus, blood, or other matter; a suppurating lesion emitting such a discharge.

IST insulin shock therapy.

isthmectomy (is-mek′to-me) [*isthmus* + Gr. *ektomē* excision] excision of an isthmus, particularly the isthmus of the thyroid gland affected with goiter.

isthmi (is′mi) [L.] plural of *isthmus*.

isthmian (is′me-an) isthmic.

isthmic (is-mik) pertaining to an isthmus.

isthmitis (is-mi′tis) inflammation of the isthmus of the fauces.

isthmoparalysis (is″mo-pah-ral′ĭ-sis) isthmoplegia.

isthmoplegia (is″mo-ple′je-ah) [*isthmus* + Gr. *plēgē* stroke] paralysis of the isthmus faucium.

isthmospasm (is′mo-spazm″) spasm of an isthmus, as of the isthmus of a uterine tube or of the fauces.

isthmus (is′mus), pl. *isth′mi* [L., from Gr *isthmos*] a narrow connection between two larger bodies or parts; [NA] a general term for such a connecting structure or region. **anterior i. of fauces**, i. faucium. **i. of aorta, i. aor′tae** [NA], **aortic i.**, a narrowed portion of the aorta, especially noticeable in the fetus, at the point where the ductus arteriosus is attached. **i. of auditory tube**, i. tubae auditivae. **i. of cartilage of auricle, i. cartilag′inis au′ris** [NA], a bridge of cartilage connecting the cartilage of the external acoustic meatus with the main part of the cartilage of the auricle of the external ear. **i. of cingulate gyrus**, i. gyri cinguli. **i. of eustachian tube**, i. tubae auditivae. **i. of fallopian tube**, i. tubae uterinae. **i. of fauces, i. fau′cium** [NA], the constricted aperture between the cavity of the mouth and the pharynx. **i. glan′dulae thyroi′deae** [NA], isthmus of thyroid gland: the band of tissue connecting the lobes of the thyroid gland. **i. gy′ri cingula′tus**, NA alternative for *i. gyri cinguli*. **i. gy′ri cin′guli** [NA], isthmus of cingulate gyrus: the constricted portion of the cingulate gyrus, connecting with the parahippocampal gyrus in the region of the splenium of the corpus callosum; called also *i. gyri cingulatus* [NA alternative]. **Haller's i.**, fretum halleri. **i. of His**, i. rhombencephali. **Krönig's i.**, a narrow, ribbon-like area of resonance extending over the shoulder and connecting the larger areas of resonance on the chest and back, overlying the apex of the lung (Krönig's fields). **i. of limbic lobe**, i. gyri cinguli. **oropharyngeal i., pharyngo-oral i.**, faucium. **i. prosta′tae** [NA], **i. of prostate,** the commissure on the base of the prostate, between the right and the left lateral lobe. **i. rhombenceph′ali** [NA], **i. of rhombencephalon,** a narrow segment of the brain in the fetus, forming the plane of separation between the rhombencephalon and the cerebrum; called also *i. of His.* **i. of thyroid gland,** i. glandulae thyroideae. **i. tu′bae auditi′vae** [NA], isthmus of auditory tube: the narrowest part of the auditory tube, at the junction of the pars ossea and the pars cartilaginea of the tube. **i. tu′bae uteri′nae** [NA], the narrow part of the uterine tube at its junction with the uterus. **i. ure′thrae,** a constricted part of the urethra, at the junction of the cavernous with the membranous urethra. **i. u′teri** [NA], **i. of uterus,** the constricted part of the uterus between the cervix and the body. **i. of Vieussens,** limbus fossae ovalis.

I.S.U. International Society of Urology.

Isuprel (i′su-prel) trademark for a preparation of isoproterenol.

isuria (i-su′re-ah) [Gr. *isos* equal + *ouron* urine + *-ia*] excretion of urine at a uniform rate.

I.T.A. International Tuberculosis Association.

Itard's catheter (e-tarz′) [Jean Marie Gaspard *Itard,* French otologist, 1774–1838] see under *catheter.*

Itard-Cholewa sign (e-tar′ ko-la′vah) [J. M. G. *Itard;* Erasmus Rudolph *Cholewa,* German physician, born 1845] see under *sign.*

itate (i′tāt) a substance in milk which oxidizes nitrite to nitrate.

itch (ich) 1. marked by itching, or pruritus. 2. any of various skin disorders in which itching is a characteristic. See also *pruritus.* 3. scabies. **Aujeszky's i.,** pseudorabies. **bakers′ i.,** any of several inflammatory dermatoses of the hands, especially chronic monilial paronychia, occurring with special frequency in bakers. **barbers′ i.,** 1. sycosis barbae. 2. tinea barbae. 3. pseudofolliculitis. **clam diggers′ i.,** cercarial dermatitis. **copra i.,** a dermatitis affecting those who unload coconuts, caused by the mite *Tyrophagus castellani.* **Cuban i.,** variola minor. **dew i.,** ground i. **dhobie mark i.,** allergic contact dermatitis caused by oleoresins in the marking fluid (bhilawanol oil) used on laundry by the native washermen (dhobie) of India. **grain i.,** a self-limited, wheal-like, pruritic eruption caused by the mite *Pyemotes ventricosus,* which parasitizes the larvae of various insects that infest straw, grain, and other plants, and affecting those coming in contact with host plants. Called also *acarodermatitis urticarioides, prairie i.,* and *straw i.* **grocers′ i.,** a vesicular dermatitis caused by *Glycyphagus domesticus,* found in stored hides, dried fruits, and grain, or *Tyrophagus castellanei* or *T. longior,* found in copra and cheese, respectively. **ground i.,** the itching eruption caused by the entrance into the skin of the larvae of *Necator americanus* or *Ancylostoma duodenale* (see *hookworm disease,* under *disease*). Called also *uncinarial dermatitis.* **jock i.,** tinea cruris. **mad i.,** pseudorabies. **prairie i.,** grain i. **seven-year i.,** scabies. **straw i.,** grain i. **swimmers′ i.,** cercarial dermatitis. **winter i.,** an itching of the skin occurring in cold weather, unassociated with structural lesions; called also *pruritus hiemalis.*

itching (ich′ing) pruritus.

-ite 1. [Gr. *-itēs* noun and adjective suffix] a suffix denoting a mineral or a rock, or a part of a body or of an organ. 2. [F., alteration of *-ate*] in chemistry, a suffix denoting a salt or ester of an acid with a name ending in *-ous,* e.g., phosphite. Cf. *-ate.*

iter (i′ter) [L.] a way or tubular passage. **i. ad infundib′ulum,** the passage from the third ventricle of the brain to the infundibulum. **i. chordae anterius,** an opening in the anterior part of the middle ear for exit of the chorda tympani nerve from the tympanic cavity; called also *Huguier's canal.* **i. chordae posterius,** an opening in the posterior part of the middle ear for entrance of the chorda tympani nerve into the tympanic cavity. **i. den′tium,** the area through which a permanent tooth makes its appearance. **i. e ter′tio ad quar′tum ventric′ulum,** aqueductus cerebri. **i. of Sylvius,** aqueductus mesencephali.

iteral (i′ter-al) pertaining to an iter.

iteroparity (it″er-o-par′ĭ-te) [L. *iterare* to repeat + *parere* to bear] the state, in an individual organism, of reproducing repeatedly, or more than once in a lifetime.

iteroparous (it″er-op′ah-rus) reproducing more than once in a lifetime.

-ites [Gr. *-itēs,* a masculine adjectival termination agreeing with *hydrōps* dropsy (understood)—e.g., tympanites, the windy dropsy] a word termination indicating edema of the part denoted by the word stem to which it is attached.

ithycyphos (ith″e-si′fōs) ithyokyphosis.

ithylordosis (ith″e-lor-do′sis) [Gr. *ithys* straight + *lordōsis* bending forward] lordosis without any lateral curvature.

ithyokyphosis (ith″e-o-ki-fo′sis) [Gr. *ithys* straight + *kyphos* humped + *-osis*] backward projection of the spinal column.

-itides plural of *-itis.*

-itis, pl. *-it′ides* [*-itis,* a feminine adjectival termination agreeing with Gr. *nosos* disease (understood)] a word termination denoting inflammation of the part indicated by the word stem to which it is attached.

Ito-Reenstierna test (e′to rēn-stēr′nah) [Hayazo *Ito,* Japanese pathologist, born 1865; John *Reenstierna,* Swedish dermatologist, born 1882] see under *tests.*

ITP idiopathic thrombocytopenic purpura.

Itrumil (it′roo-mil) trademark for a preparation of iothiouracil.

I.U. immunizing unit; international unit.

IUCD intrauterine contraceptive device.

IUD intrauterine contraceptive device.

I.V. intravenously (by intravenous injection).

ivermectin (i-ver-mek′tin) a semisynthetic macrocyclic lactone, used as an antiparasitic.

ivory (i′vo-re) [L. *ebur, eburneus*] 1. the bonelike substance (modified dentin) of the tusks of elephants or of such large mammals as the walrus. 2. dentin (dentinum [NA]).

Ivy's method (i′vēz) [Andrew Conway *Ivy,* Chicago, physiologist, born 1893] see *bleeding time,* under *time.*

Iwanoff's (Iwanow's) cysts (e-wan′ofs) [Wladimir P. *Iwanoff* (Iwanow), Russian ophthalmologist, born 1861] see *Blessig's cysts,* under *cyst.*

Ixodes (iks-o′dēz) [Gr. *ixōdes* like bird-lime] a genus of ticks that are parasitic on man and other animals. **I. bicor′nis,** *Rhipicentor bicornis.* **I. canisu′ga,** the British dog tick, a species commonly infesting dogs in Britain; also found in Western Europe and North America. **I. cavipal′pus,** an African tick that infests monkeys and children. **I. dam′mini,** a species that is the vector of Lyme arthritis. **I. fre′quens,** a species that infests cattle, horses, and man in Japan. **I. hexag′onus,** a species that infests wild and domestic carnivores in Europe and Africa. **I. holocy′clus,** a tick, particularly of marsupials, but which causes a tick paralysis in young cattle in New South Wales, and may be the vector of North Queensland tick typhus. **I. pacif′icus,** a common deer and cattle tick of California, which may bite man, and is thought to be a possible vector of tularemia. **I. persulca′tus,** the taiga tick, vector of Russian spring-summer encephalitis. **I. pilo′sus,** a species infesting many animals in South Africa; formerly thought to cause paralysis in sheep. **I. pu′tus,** a species that infests the nests of many marine birds. **I. ra′sus,** a species that attacks a variety of insectivores, rodents, ungulates, carnivores, and occasionally man and other primates in Africa. **I. rici′nus,** the castor bean tick, which is parasitic on cattle, sheep, and wild animals, and transmits the agents of gallsickness, malignant jaundice in dogs, tularemia, louping ill, and Russian spring-summer encephalitis. **I. rubicun′dus,** a species that may cause a tick paralysis in sheep, goats, and cattle in West Africa. A single human case has been reported. **I. scapula′ris,** the black-legged tick of the Eastern United States, which may inflict a painful bite in man. **I. spinipal′pus,** a species that infests rabbits and squirrels in British Columbia, and may transmit Powassan virus.

ixodiasis (iks″o-di′ah-sis) any disease or lesion due to the bite of ticks; infestation with ticks.

ixodic (ik-sod′ik) caused by ticks.

Ixodidae (iks-od′ĭ-de) a family of the superfamily Ixodoidea, comprising the hard ticks, distinguished from the soft-bodied ticks (Argasidae) by the presence of a scutum. It includes the following genera: *Amblyomma, Anocenter, Aponomma, Boophilus, Dermacentor, Haemaphysalis, Hyalomma, Ixodes, Margaropus, Rhipicentor,* and *Rhipicephalus.*

Ixodides (iks-od′ĭ-dēz) the ticks, a suborder of Acarina, including the superfamily Ixodoidea, which comprises the families Ixodidae, or hard ticks, and Argasidae, or soft ticks.

Ixodiphagus (iks″o-dif′ah-gus) a genus of hymenopterans. **I. caucur′tei,** a hymenopteran parasite of ticks of the family Ixodidae.

ixodism (iks′o-dizm) ixodiasis.

Ixodoidea (iks″o-doi′de-ah) a superfamily of the suborder Ixodides, which embraces the families Argasidae, or soft ticks, and Ixodidae, or hard ticks.

Izar's reagent (i′zarz) [Guido *Izar,* Italian pathologist, born 1883] see under *reagent.*

-ize [Gr. *-izein* verb-forming suffix] a word termination meaning (*a*) to cause to be, (*b*) to cause to acquire some quality, (*c*) to become, (*d*) to become similar to, (*e*) to subject to an action or treatment.

J

J symbol for *joule.*

jaagsiekte, jaagziekte (yahg-sēk′tĕ; yahg-zēk′tĕ) [Afrikaans *jag* hunt + *siekte* sickness] pulmonary adenomatosis (def. 2).

Jaboulay's amputation (operation), button (zhah″-boo-lāz′) [Mathieu *Jaboulay,* French surgeon, 1860–1913] see *interpelviabdominal amputation,* and see under *button.*

Jaccoud's fever, sign (zhah-kōōz′) [Sigismond *Jaccoud,* French physician, 1830–1913] see under *fever* and *sign.*

jacket (jak′et) an enveloping structure or garment, especially a covering for the trunk or for the upper part of the body; see also under *crown.* **Minerva j.,** a plaster-of-Paris jacket that includes both the trunk and the head, with the ears and face left free; used for fractures of the cervical spine and after operations for torticollis. **plaster-of-Paris j.,** a casing of plaster of Paris enveloping the body for the purpose of correcting deformities. **porcelain j.,** a jacket crown of porcelain. **Risser j.,** a combination of plaster, turnbuckles, and hinges, extending from the chin and occiput to one knee, sometimes including one arm as far as the elbow; used in scoliosis. **strait j.,** see *straitjacket.*

jackscrew (jak′skroo) a threaded device used in orthodontic appliances for the separation or approximation of teeth or jaw segments.

Jackson appliance (crib) (jak′son) [Victor Hugo *Jackson,* American dentist, 1850–1929] see under *appliance.*

Jackson's law, etc. (jak′sunz) [John Hughlings *Jackson,* London neurologist, 1835–1911] see under *law, rule, sign,* and *syndrome.*

Jackson's membrane (veil) [Jabez North *Jackson,* surgeon in Kansas City, 1868–1935] see under *membrane.*

Jackson's safety triangle, sign [Chevalier *Jackson,* American laryngologist, 1865–1958] see under *triangle,* and see *asthmatoid wheeze,* under *wheeze.*

Jackson's sign [James *Jackson,* Jr., Boston physician, 1810–1834] see under *sign,* def. 3.

jacksonian epilepsy (jak-so′ne-an) [John Hughlings *Jackson*] see under *epilepsy.*

Jacob (zhah-kob′), François. French biologist, born 1920; co-winner with André Michael Lwoff and Jacques Lucien Monod, of the Nobel prize in medicine and physiology for 1965, for discoveries concerning the genetic control of enzymes and virus synthesis.

Jacob's membrane, ulcer (ja′kubz) [Arthur *Jacob,* Irish ophthalmologist, 1790–1874] see *layer of rods and cones,* under *layer,* and see under *ulcer.*

jacobine (ja′ko-bin) a poisonous alkaloid, $C_{18}H_{25}O_6N$, from the composite-flowered plant *Senecio jacobea;* it may cause necrosis of the liver.

Jacobson's canal, etc. (ja′kub-sunz) [Ludwig Levin *Jacobson,* Danish anatomist, 1783–1843] see under *canal, cartilage, nerve, organ, plexus,* and *sulcus.*

Jacobson's retinitis [Julius *Jacobson,* German ophthalmologist, 1828–1889] syphilitic retinitis.

Jacobsthal's test (yak′obz-talz) [Erwin Wolfgang Jakob *Jacobsthal,* Hamburg bacteriologist, born 1879] see under *tests.*

Jacquet's dermatitis (erythema) (zhak-āz′) [Leonard Marie Lucien *Jacquet,* French dermatologist, 1860–1914] diaper dermatitis.

jactatio (jak-ta′she-o) [L., from *jactare* to toss about] jactitation. **j. cap′itis noctur′na,** rhythmic rolling of the head of a child just before falling asleep.

jactation (jak-ta′shun) jactitation.

jactitation (jak″tĭ-ta′shun) [L. *jactitatio; jactitare* to toss] the tossing to and fro of a patient in acute disease.

jaculiferous (jak″u-lif′er-us) [L. *jaculum* dart + *ferre* to bear] bearing prickles.

Jadassohn's anetoderma, sebaceous nevus, test (yah′das-ōnz) [Josef *Jadassohn,* German dermatologist in Bern, 1863–1936] see under *anetoderma* and *nevus,* and see *irrigation test,* under *tests.*

Jadassohn-Pellizari anetoderma (yah′dah-sōn-pel″ĭ-zar′e) [Josef *Jadassohn;* Pietro *Pellizari,* Italian dermatologist, 1823–1892] see under *anetoderma.*

Jadelot's lines (furrows) (zhad-lōz′) [Jean François Nicolas *Jadelot,* physician in Paris, 1791–1830] see under *line.*

Jaeger's test types (ya′gerz) [Edward *Jaeger* von Jastthal, Austrian oculist, 1818–1884] see under *test types.*

Jaffé's reaction, test (zhah-fāz′) [Max *Jaffé,* German physiologic chemist, 1841–1911] see under *reaction* and *tests.*

jagsiekte, jagziekte (yahg-sēk′tĕ; yahg-zēk′tĕ) jaagsiekte.

Jakob's disease (yak′obz) [Alfons Maria *Jakob,* German psychiatrist, 1884–1931] Creutzfeldt-Jakob syndrome.

Jakob-Creutzfeldt disease (yak′ob-kroits′felt) [Alfons Maria *Jakob;* Hans Gerhard *Creutzfeldt,* German psychiatrist, 1885–1964] Creutzfeldt-Jakob disease.

Jaksch's disease, test (yaksh) [Rudolf von *Jaksch,* physician in Prague, 1855–1947] see *anemia pseudoleukemica infantum,* and see under *Jaksch's test,* under *tests.*

jalap (jal′ap) [Sp. *jalapa,* from *Jalapa,* a city of Mexico] the dried tuberous root of *Exogonium purga* (Hayne) Lindl. Convolvulaceae; its resins possess cathartic properties.

jamais vu (zhah′mĕ voo) [Fr. "never seen"] the sensation that familiar surroundings are strangely unfamiliar; the illusion that one has never seen anything like that before.

Janet's disease, test (zhah-nāz′) [Pierre Marie Felix *Janet,* French physician, 1859–1947] see *psychasthenia,* and see under *tests.*

Janeway's lesion, spots (jān′wāz) [Edward Gamaliel *Janeway,* American physician, 1841–1911] see under *lesion.*

Janeway's sphygmomanometer (jān′wāz) [Theodore Caldwell *Janeway,* American physician, 1872–1917] see under *sphygmomanometer.*

janiceps (jan′ĭ-seps) [L. *Janus* a two-faced god + *caput* head] a double monster with one head and two opposite faces. **j. asym′metros,** a janiceps with one imperfect and one more complete face. **j. parasit′icus,** a double monster in which there is partial duplication of the head in the frontal plane.

Janošík's embryo (yan′o-siks) [Jan *Janošík,* Prague anatomist, 1856–1927] see under *embryo.*

Jansen's disease, test [W. Murk *Jansen,* Dutch orthopedic surgeon, 1867–1935] see *metaphyseal dysostosis,* under *dysostosis,* and see under *tests.*

Jansen's operation (yan′senz) [Albert *Jansen,* German otologist, 1859–1933] see under *operation.*

Jansky's classification (jan′skēz) [Ján *Janský,* Czech psychiatrist, 1873–1921] see under *classification.*

Janthinobacterium (jan″thĭ-no-bak-te′re-um) [L. *janthinus* violet colored + *bacterium*] a genus of gram-negative, aerobic, rod-shaped bacteria of uncertain affiliation, made up of motile flagellated organisms that produce violet colonies, found in soil and water. The type species is *J. li'vidum.*

Janthinosoma (jan"thĭ-no-so'mah) a genus of mosquitoes; it is often considered to be a subgenus of the genus *Psorophora.* **J. lut'zi,** a species which transports the eggs of botflies (*Dermatobia*) glued to its abdomen. **J. postica'ta,** a species which also transports the eggs of the botfly.

Jaquet's apparatus (zhah-kāz') [Alfred *Jaquet,* Swiss pharmacologist, 1865–1937] see under *apparatus.*

jar (jar) a wide-mouthed, glass or earthenware container. **bell j.,** a glass vessel, closed at top, open at bottom, used in laboratory vacuum experiments. **Leyden j.,** a glass jar partially covered inside and out with tinfoil or other metal, used as a condenser or collector of electricity.

jararaca (jah"rah-rak'ah) a venomous pit viper, *Bothrops jararaca,* of tropical and southern South America.

Jarcho's pressometer (jahr'kōz) [Julius *Jarcho,* New York obstetrician, 1882–1963] see under *pressometer.*

jargon (jar'gon) the technical or specialized language used in a profession or other field of activity.

jargonaphasia (jar"gon-ah-fa'ze-ah) a speech defect in which several words are run into one.

Jarisch-Herxheimer reaction (yah'rish-herks'hĭm-er) [Adolf *Jarisch,* Austrian dermatologist, 1850–1902; Karl *Herxheimer,* German dermatologist, 1861–1944] see under *reaction.*

Jarjavay's muscle (zhar'zah-vaz) [Jean François *Jarjavay,* French physician, 1815–1868] see under *muscle.*

Jarotzky's (Jarotsky's) treatment (yar-ot'skēz) [Alexander *Jarotzky,* Moscow physician, born 1866] see under *treatment.*

Jatropha (jat'ro-fah) [Gr. *iatros* physician + *trophē* nourishment] a genus of tropical euphorbiaceous plants. Various species possess purgative, stomachic, febrifuge, and astringent properties. Common to Mexico and South America. *J. curcas* L. and *J. multifida* L. (physic nut) produce seeds containing a purgative oil and a potentially toxic phytotoxin.

jaundice (jawn'dis) [Fr. *jaunisse,* from *jaune* yellow] a syndrome characterized by hyperbilirubinemia and deposition of bile pigment in the skin, mucous membranes and sclera with resulting yellow appearance of the patient; called also *icterus.* **acholuric j.,** jaundice without bilirubinuria, associated with elevated unconjugated bilirubin that is not excreted by the kidney; seen in hemolytic disease and other forms of unconjugated hyperbilirubinemia. **acholuric familial j.,** hereditary spherocytosis. **anhepatic j., anhepatogenous j.,** yellow appearance of the skin and mucous membranes not caused by liver disease. **black j.,** Winckel's disease. **breast milk j.,** elevated unconjugated bilirubin in some breast-fed infants due to the presence of 5-β-pregnane-3-α-20-β-diol, which inhibits glucuronyl transferase conjugating activity. **Budd's j.** (obs.), massive hepatic necrosis. **catarrhal j.** (obs.), infectious hepatitis. **cholestatic j.,** jaundice resulting from an abnormality in the flow of bile, usually accompanied by elevation of serum alkaline phosphatase, retention of bile salts (with resulting pruritus) and varying hypercholesterolemia. The cholestasis may be *extrahepatic,* due to obstruction caused by a stone, stricture, or neoplasm, or *intrahepatic,* which may be due to liver cell disease (e.g., hepatitis), or altered permeability and/or obstruction of the intrahepatic biliary system (as in drug reactions or hepatic infiltrative disease). **chronic acholuric j.,** hereditary spherocytosis. **Crigler-Najjar j.,** see under *syndrome.* **epidemic j.,** hepatitis A. **familial acholuric j.,** hereditary spherocytosis. **hemolytic j.,** hemolytic anemia. **hepatocellular j.,** jaundice caused by injury to or disease of the liver cells. **hepatogenic j., hepatogenous j.,** that which is due to some disease or disorder of the liver. **homologous serum j., human serum j.,** hepatitis B. **infectious j., infective j.,** 1. infectious hepatitis. 2. Weil's syndrome. **latent j.,** hyperbilirubinemia without yellow staining of the tissues. **leptospiral j.,** Weil's syndrome. **malignant j.,** massive hepatic necrosis. **malignant j. of dogs,** canine babesiosis. **mechanical j.,** obstructive j. **j. of the newborn,** icterus neonatorum. **nonhemolytic j.,** jaundice caused by an abnormality in the metabolism of bilirubin, and resulting in an excessive accumulation of unconjugated bilirubin in the blood. The various forms include *Crigler-Najjar syndrome, Dubin-Johnson syndrome, Gilbert syndrome, physiologic jaundice of newborn, hyperbilirubinemia of premature infant,* and *Rotor's syndrome.* **nonhemolytic j., congenital,** Crigler-Najjar syndrome. **nonhemolytic j., congenital familial,** Crigler-Najjar syndrome. **nonhemolytic j., familial,** Gilbert syndrome. **nuclear j.,** kernicterus. **obstructive j.,** that which is due to an impediment to the flow of the bile from the liver cells to the duodenum. **occult j.** (obs.), latent j. **physiologic j.,** mild icterus neonatorum lasting the first few days after birth. **picric acid j.,** jaundice due to picric acid poisoning; seen in munition workers and in malingering soldiers who deliberately ingest picric acid. **post-arsphenamine j.,** jaundice following the administration of arsphenamine. **regurgitation j.,** jaundice attributed to escape of bile from the bile canaliculi into the blood stream and marked by urobilinogen in the urine. **retention j.,** a form of jaundice due to inability of the liver to dispose of the bilirubin provided by the circulating blood. **Schmorl's j.,** kernicterus. **spirochetal j.,** Weil's syndrome. **toxemic j., toxic j.,** jaundice produced by poisons, such as phosphorus, arseniuretted hydrogen, picric acid, snake venom, etc.

Javal's ophthalmometer (zhah-valz') [Louis Emile *Javal,* French oculist, 1839–1907] see *ophthalmometer.*

jaw (jaw) either of the two bony structures (mandible and maxilla) in the head of vertebrates, bearing the teeth (in dentate species) and enabling carnivores to seize their prey and others to bite and chew food. **bird-beak j.,** the condition produced by protrusion of the upper jaw; called also *parrot j.* **big j.,** actinomycosis in cattle. **cleft j.,** a cleft between the median nasal and maxillary processes through the alveolus. Called also *gnathoschisis.* **crackling j.,** noise (crepitation) in the normal or diseased temporomandibular joint associated with jaw movement. **drop j.,** the paralytic stage of rabies in a dog, in which the jaw drops. **Hapsburg j.,** a mandibular prognathous jaw, often accompanied by a thick overdeveloped lower lip (Hapsburg lip), as seen in many members of the Hapsburg family. **lower j.,** mandibula. **lumpy j.,** actinomycosis in cattle. **parrot j.,** bird-beak j. **phossy j.,** phosphonecrosis. **pig j.,** an abnormal protrusion of the upper jaw of the horse, with hypertrophy of the teeth. **pipe j.,** a painful condition of the jaws caused by carrying a tobacco pipe in the mouth. **rubber j.,** a softened condition of the jaw in animals, caused by resorption and replacement of the bone by fibrous tissue, occurring in association with renal osteodystrophy; osteoporosis. **upper j.,** maxilla.

Jaworski's corpuscles (bodies), test (yah-wor'skēz) [Walery *Jaworski,* Polish physician, 1849–1924] see under *corpuscle* and *tests.*

Jeanselme's nodules (zhah-selmz') [Antoine Edouard *Jeanselme,* French dermatologist, 1858–1935] see under *nodule.*

jecorize (jek'o-rīz) [L. *jecur* liver] to impart to a food the therapeutic qualities of cod liver oil, as by treating milk with ultraviolet ray.

Jectofer (jek'to-fer) trademark for a preparation of iron sorbitex.

Jefferson fracture (jef'er-son) [Sir Geoffrey *Jefferson,* English neurosurgeon, b. 1886] see under *fracture.*

Jeffersonia (jef"er-so'ne-ah) [named for T. *Jefferson,* 1743–1826] a genus of berberidaceous herbs. The root of *J. diphylla* (L.) Pers., of North America, is tonic, diuretic, and expectorant; emetic in large doses.

Jefron (jef'ron) trademark for a preparation of polyferose.

jejunal (jě-joo'nal) pertaining to the jejunum.

jejunectomy (jě"joo-nek'to-me) [*jejuno-* + Gr. *ektomē* excision] excision of the jejunum.

jejunitis (jě"joo-ni'tis) inflammation of the jejunum.

jejun(o) [L. *jejunum,* q.v.] a combining form denoting relationship to the jejunum.

jejunocecostomy (jě-joo"no-se-kos'to-me) [*jejuno-* + *cecum* + Gr. *stoma* opening] the formation of an anastomosis between the jejunum and cecum; also, the anastomosis so formed.

jejunocolostomy (jĕ-joo″no-ko-los′to-me) [*jejuno-* + *colon* + Gr. *stoma* mouth] the formation of an anastomosis between the jejunum and the colon; also, the anastomosis so formed.

jejunoileal (jĕ-joo″no-il′e-al) pertaining to the jejunum and ileum; connecting the proximal jejunum with the distal ileum.

jejunoileitis (jĕ-joo″no-il″e-i′tis) inflammation of the jejunum and ileum together.

jejunoileostomy (jĕ-joo″no-il″e-os′to-me) [*jejuno-* + *ileum* + Gr. *stoma* mouth] the formation of an anastomosis between the proximal jejunum and the terminal ileum; also, the anastomosis so formed.

jejunojejunostomy (jĕ-joo″no-jĕ″joo-nos′to-me) the operative formation of an anastomosis between two portions of the jejunum; also, the anastomosis so formed.

jejunorrhaphy (jĕ″joo-nor′ah-fe) [*jejuno-* + Gr. *rhaphē* suture] operative repair of the jejunum.

jejunostomy (jĕ″joo-nos′to-me) [*jejuno-* + Gr. *stomoun* to provide with an opening, or mouth] the surgical creation of a permanent opening between the jejunum and the surface of the abdominal wall; also, the opening so established.

jejunotomy (jĕ″joo-not′o-me) [*jejuno-* + Gr. *temnein* to cut] surgical incision of the jejunum.

jejunum (jĕ-joo′num) [L. "empty"] [NA] that portion of the small intestine which extends from the duodenum to the ileum; called also *intestinum jejunum.*

Jellinek's sign (symptom) (yel′ĭ-neks) [Stefan *Jellinek,* physician in Vienna, born 1871] see under *sign.*

jelly (jel′e) [L. *gelatina*] a soft substance which is coherent, tremulous, and more or less translucent; generally, a colloidal semisolid mass. **cardiac j.,** a gelatinous substance present between the endothelium and myocardium of the embryonic heart, that transforms into the connective tissue of the endocardium. **contraceptive j.,** a nongreasy jelly for introduction into the vagina to prevent conception. **cyclomethycaine sulfate j.** [USP], a preparation containing 90 to 110 per cent of the labeled amount of cyclomethycaine sulfate in a water-soluble, viscous base; used as a local anesthetic, applied topically. **glycerin j.** [NF], a compound of gelatin, arsenic trioxide, and glycerin, used as a reagent; called also *glycerogelatin.* **lidocaine hydrochloride j.** [USP], a preparation containing 95 to 105 per cent of the labeled amount of lidocaine hydrochloride in a suitable, water-soluble, sterile, viscous base; used as a local anesthetic, applied topically to the mucous membranes. **mineral j.,** petrolatum. **petroleum j.,** petrolatum. **pramoxine hydrochloride j.** [USP], a preparation containing 94 to 106 per cent of the labeled amount of pramoxine hydrochloride; used as a local anesthetic, applied topically. **Wharton's j.,** the soft, jelly-like, homogeneous intercellular substance of the umbilical cord; it gives the reaction for mucin and contains thin collagenous fibers which increase in number with the age of the fetus.

Jendrassik's maneuver (yen-drah′siks) [Ernst *Jendrassik,* physician in Budapest, 1858–1921] see under *maneuver.*

Jenner (jen′er), Edward. An English physician (1749–1823), who developed the process of producing immunity to smallpox by inoculation (vaccination) with cowpox (vaccinia) vaccine.

Jenner's stain (jen′erz) [Louis Leopold *Jenner,* London physician, 1866–1904] see *Table of Stains and Staining Methods.*

jennerian (jen-ne′re-an) named for Edward *Jenner.*

jennerization (jen″er-i-za′shun) production of immunity to a disease by inoculation of an attenuated form of the virus producing the disease.

Jensen's classification (yen′senz) [Sigurd Orla-*Jensen,* Danish bacteriologist, born 1870] see under *classification.*

Jensen's sarcoma (tumor), (yen′senz) [Carl Oluf *Jensen,* Danish veterinary pathologist, 1864–1934] see under *sarcoma.*

jerk (jerk) a sudden reflex or involuntary movement. **Achilles j., ankle j.,** triceps surae j. **biceps j.,** biceps reflex. **crossed j.,** adduction of the leg when attempt is made to elicit the quadriceps jerk on the opposite side. **elbow j.,** involuntary flexion of the elbow on striking the tendon of the biceps or triceps muscle. **jaw j.,** jaw reflex. **knee j.,** quadriceps j. **quadriceps j.,** a twitchlike con-

traction of the quadriceps muscle, elicited by sharply tapping the patellar ligament; called also *knee j.* **tendon j.,** see under *reflex.* **triceps surae j.,** a twitchlike contraction of the triceps surae muscle, elicited by sharply tapping the muscle or the Achilles tendon; called also *ankle j.*

Jesionek lamp (yes-e′o-nek) [Albert *Jesionek,* Giessen dermatologist, 1870–1935] see under *lamp.*

jessur (jes′er) native Bengal name for Russell's viper.

Jewett nail (joo′et) [Eugene Lyon *Jewett,* American surgeon, born 1900] see under *nail.*

jigger (jig′ger) chigoe.

Jobert's fossa, (zho-bārz′) [Antoine Joseph *Jobert* de Lamballe, French surgeon, 1799–1867] see under *fossa.*

Job's syndrome (jŏb) [*Job,* a patriarch of the Old Testament] see under *syndrome.*

Jocasta complex (jo-kas′tah) see under *complex.*

Jochmann's test (yōk′manz) [Georg *Jochmann,* Berlin internist, 1874–1915] 1. Müller-Jochmann test. 2. antitrypsin test. See under *tests.*

jodbasedow (i″ōd-baz′ĕ-do) [Ger.] iodine-induced hyperthyroidism.

Joest's bodies (yests) [Ernst *Joest,* Dresden veterinary pathologist, 1873–1926] see under *body.*

Joffroy's reflex, sign (zhof-rwhahz′) [Alexis *Joffroy,* French physician, 1844–1908] see under *reflex* and *sign.*

Johne's bacillus, disease (yo′nez) [Heinrich Albert *Johne,* German pathologist, 1839–1910] see *Mycobacterium paratuberculosis* and under *disease.*

johnin (yo′nin) a filtrate of cultures of Johne's bacillus (*Mycobacterium paratuberculosis*), similar to tuberculin, used to produce a skin reaction (johnin reaction) in testing cattle for Johne's disease.

Johnson's test (john′sonz) [Sir George *Johnson,* English physician, 1818–1896] see under *tests.*

Johnson-Stevens disease (john′son-ste′venz) [Frank Chambliss *Johnson,* 1894–1934; Albert Mason *Stevens,* 1884–1945, American pediatricians] Stevens-Johnson syndrome.

joint (joint) [L. *junctio* a joining, connection] an articulation: the place of union or junction between two or more bones of the skeleton, especially a junction that admits of more or less motion of one or more bones. See also *articulatio* [NA]. For English names of specific joints not included here, see under *articulation.* **amphidiarthrodial j.,** amphidiarthrosis. **ankle j.,** articulatio talocruralis. **arthrodial j.,** plane j. **ball-and-socket j.,** spheroidal j. **biaxial j.,** one permitting movement in two of the assumed three mutually perpendicular axes, or having two degrees of freedom, as the ellipsoidal joint. **bicondylar j.,** articulatio bicondylaris. **bilocular j.,** a joint in which the synovial cavity is divided into two compartments by an interarticular cartilage, as the temporomandibular joint. **bleeders' j.,** hemorrhage into a joint in persons with a hemorrhagic diathesis. **Budin's j.,** a band of cartilage seen at birth between the squamous and the two condylar portions of the occipital bone. **carpal j's,** 1. articulationes carpi. 2. see *articulationes intercarpales.* **cartilaginous j.,** one in which the components are connected by cartilage; called also *junctura cartilaginea* [NA]. **cartilaginous j's,** articulationes cartilagineae. **Charcot's j.,** neuropathic arthropathy. **Chopart's j.,** articulatio tarsi transversa. **Clutton's j.,** painless symmetrical hydrarthrosis, especially of the knee joints, seen in congenital syphilis. **cochlear j.,** a form of hinge joint which permits some rotation or lateral motion, as the knee joint. **coffin j.,** the second interphalangeal joint of the foot of a horse. **composite j., compound j.,** a joint in which several bones articulate; articulatio composita [NA]. **condylar j., condyloid j.,** one in which an ovoid head of one bone moves in an elliptical cavity of another, permitting all movements except axial rotation, as the metacarpophalangeal joints; articulatio condylaris [NA]. **Cruveilhier's j.,** articulatio atlanto-occipitalis. **diarthrodial j.,** synovial j. **dry j.,** one affected with chronic villous arthritis. **elbow j.,** the joint between the arm and forearm; see *articulatio cubiti* [NA]. **ellipsoidal j.,** a biaxial joint resembling a ball-and-socket joint, but with the articulating surfaces much longer in one direction than in the direction at right angles, the circumference of the joint thus resembling an ellipse, as the radiocarpal joint; articulatio ellipsoidea [NA]. **enarthrodial j.,** spheroidal j.

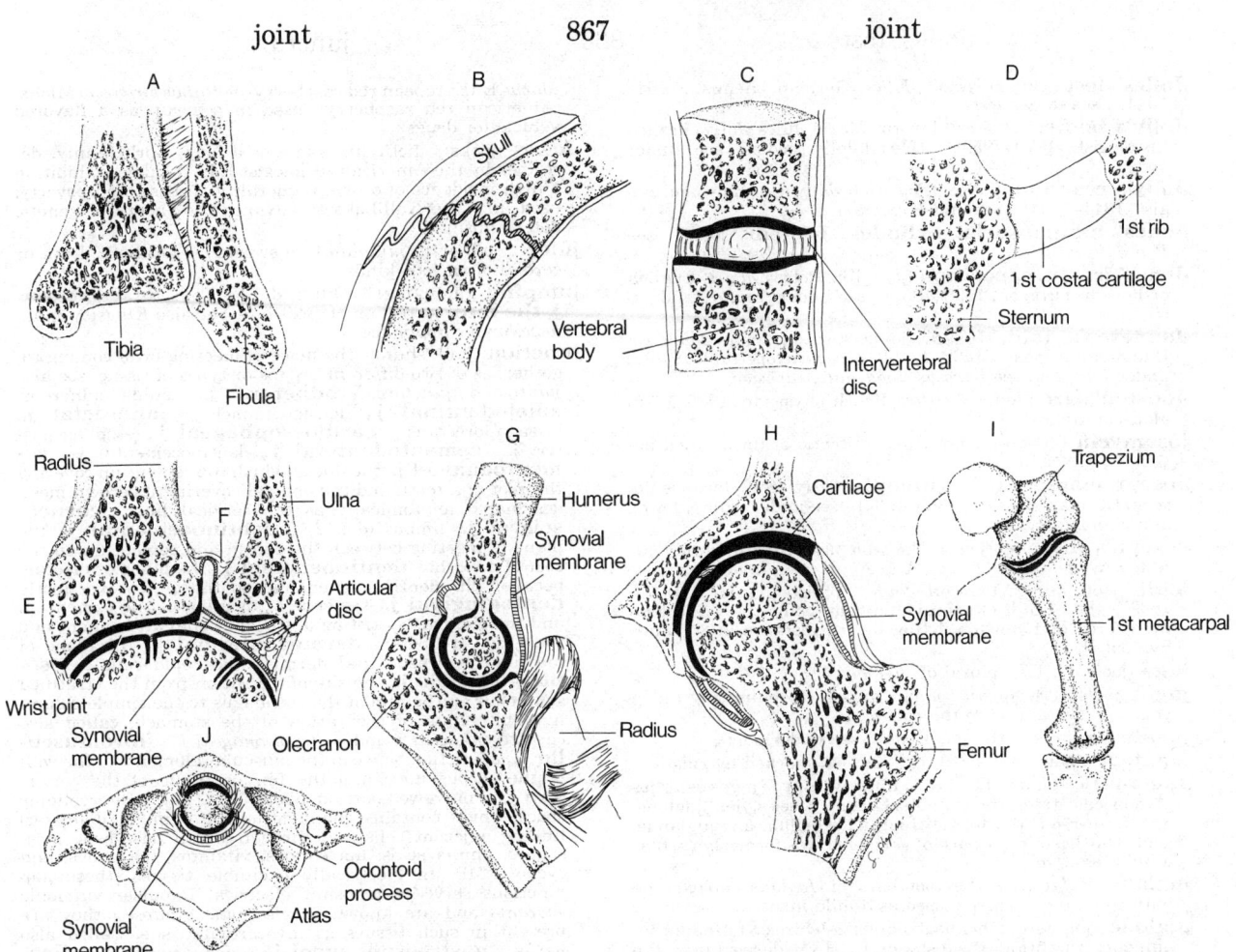

Various kinds of joints. *Fibrous* —A, syndesmosis (tibiofibular); *B*, suture (skull). *Cartilaginous: C*, symphysis (vertebral bodies); *D*, synchondrosis (1st rib and sternum). *Synovial: E*, condyloid (wrist); *F*, gliding (radioulnar); *G*, hinge or ginglymus (elbow); *H*, ball and socket (hip); *I*, saddle (carpometacarpal of thumb); *J*, pivot (atlantoaxial).

facet j's, the articulations of the vertebral column. **false j.,** pseudarthrosis. **fibrocartilaginous j.,** one in which the participating elements are united by fibrocartilage, usually separated from the bones by thin plates of hyaline cartilage; called also *symphysis.* **fibrous j's,** articulationes fibrosae. **flail j.,** one showing abnormal mobility. **freely movable j.,** synovial j. **fringe j.,** one affected with chronic villous arthritis. **ginglymoid j.,** ginglymus. **gliding j.,** plane j. **hemophilic j.,** bleeders' j. **hinge j.,** ginglymus. **hip j.,** the joint formed at the head of the femur and the acetabulum of the hip bone; called also *articulatio coxae* [NA] and *articulation of the hip.* Loosely called *hip.* **immovable j.,** fibrous j. **intercarpal j's,** 1. articulationes intercarpales. 2. see *articulationes carpi.* **irritable j.,** a joint subject to attacks of inflammation without discoverable cause. **knee j.,** the compound joint between the femur, patella, and tibia; see *articulatio genus* [NA]. **ligamentous j.,** syndesmosis. **Lisfranc's j.,** articulationes tarsometatarsales. **j's of Luschka,** a series of jointlike structures at the lateral edges of the vertebral bodies from vertebra C3 to T1, forming small spurlike lips at the upper surface, covered with cartilage, and containing a capsule filled with fluid. They are considered by some to be true diarthrodial joints, and by others to be degenerative spaces of the intervertebral disks filled with extracellular fluid and lined by a membrane formed by fibrocytes. They are frequent sites of spur formation. **manubriosternal j.,** see *symphysis manubriosternalis* and *synchondrosis manubriosternalis.* **midcarpal j.,** the joint between the scaphoid, lunate, and cuneiform bones and the second row of the carpal bones; called also *articulatio mediocarpea* [NA]. **mixed j.,** one combining features of different types of joints. **multiaxial j.,** spheroidal j. **open j.,** a veterinary term for a joint in which

the surface of the bones is exposed, as a result of inflammation and sloughing of the tissues. **peg-and-socket j.,** gomphosis. **pivot j.,** a uniaxial joint in which one bone pivots within a bony or an osseoligamentous ring; articulatio trochoidea [NA]. **plane j.,** a type of synovial joint in which the opposed surfaces are flat or only slightly curved; called also *articulatio plana* [NA], *gliding j.,* and *arthrodial j.* **polyaxial j.,** spheroidal j. **rotary j.,** pivot j. **saddle j.,** a joint having two saddle-shaped surfaces at right angles to each other; articulatio sellaris [NA]. **scapuloclavicular j.,** articulatio acromioclavicularis. **sellar j.,** saddle j. **shoulder j.,** articulatio humeri. **simple j.,** a joint in which only two bones articulate; articulatio simplex [NA]. **socket j. of tooth,** gomphosis. **spheroidal j.,** a type of synovial joint in which a spheroidal surface on one bone ("ball") moves within a concavity ("socket") on the other bone, as in the hip joint. Called also *articulatio spheroidea* [NA] and *ball-and-socket j.* **spiral j.,** cochlear j. **stifle j.,** the articulation in quadrupeds corresponding with the knee joint of man, consisting actually of two joints, that between the femur and tibia, and that between the femur and patella. **synarthrodial j's,** articulationes fibrosae. **synovial j.,** a special form of articulation permitting more or less free movement; called also *diarthrodial j.* and *diarthrosis.* See *articulationes synoviales.* **tarsal transverse,** articulatio tarsi transversa. **through j.,** synovial j. **trochoid j.,** pivot j. **uniaxial j.,** one permitting movement in only one of the assumed three mutually perpendicular axes, or having only one degree of freedom, as a hinge joint and the interphalangeal joints. **unilocular j.,** a synovial joint having only one cavity. **von Gies j.,** a chronic syphilitic chondro-osteoarthritis. **wrist j.,** articulatio radiocarpalis.

Jolles' test (yol′ez) [Adolf *Jolles*, German chemist, 1864–1944] see under *tests*.

Jolly's bodies (zho-lēz′) [Justin Marie Jules *Jolly*, French histologist, 1870–1953]   Howell-Jolly bodies; see under *body*.

Jolly's reaction (yo′lēz) [Friedrich *Jolly*, German neurologist, 1844–1904]   see under *reaction*.

Jones' albumosuria, cylinder, protein (jōnz)   see *Bence Jones*.

Jones' fracture, position (jōnz) [Sir Robert *Jones*, English orthopedic surgeon, 1858–1933]   see under *fracture* and *position*.

Jonnesco's fold, fossa (jo-nes′kōz) [Thoma *Jonnesco*, Rumanian surgeon, 1860–1926]   see *parietoperitoneal fold*, under *fold*, and see *recessus duodenalis superior*.

Jonston's arc [Johns *Jonston*, Polish physician, 1603–1675] alopecia areata.

josamycin (jo″sah-mi′sin)   an antibiotic of unspecified action, $C_{42}H_{69}NO_{15}$.

Joseph clamp, knife, rhinoplasty (yo′sef) [Jacques *Joseph*, German surgeon, 1865–1934]   see under *clamp, knife*, and *rhinoplasty*.

Joseph's disease (jo′sefs) [*Joseph* an Azorean family affected by the disease]   see *Azorean disease*, under *disease*.

joule (jool) [James Prescott *Joule*, English physicist, 1818–1889]   the SI unit of energy and heat, being the work done by a force of 1 newton acting over a distance of 1 meter. Symbol, J.

juga (joo′gah) [L.]   plural of *jugum*.

jugal (joo′gal) [L. *jugalis; jugum* yoke]   1. connecting like a yoke.   2. pertaining to the cheek.

jugale (joo-ga′le)   the jugal point; see under *point*.

jugate (joo′gāt)   1. locked together.   2. marked by ridges.

Juglans (joo′glans) [L. "Jove's nut," walnut]   a genus of juglandaceous trees; the walnuts. Certain species yield juglone, and *J. cinerea* L. (butternut tree) yields juglans and juglandic acid. The dried inner bark of *J. cinerea* was formerly used as a mild laxative.

juglans (joo′glans)   the root bark of *Juglans cinerea*, the butternut tree, formerly used as a mild laxative.

juglone (jug′lōn)   chemical name: 5-hydroxy-1,4-naphthoquinone. An antibiotic substance, $C_{10}H_6O_3$, derived from the leaves of certain species of *Juglans* and from walnut shells, which has antihemorrhagic properties and is active against certain fungi.

jugomaxillary (joo″go-mak′sĭ-lār″e)   pertaining to the zygomatic bone and the maxilla.

jugular (jug′u-lar) [L. *jugularis: jugulum* neck]   1. pertaining to the neck.   2. a jugular vein.

jugulation (jug″u-la′shun) [L. *jugulare* to cut the throat of] the sudden and rapid arrest of disease by therapeutical measures.

jugum (joo′gum), pl. *ju′ga* [L. "a yoke"] [NA]   a general term for a depression or ridge connecting two structures. **ju′ga alveola′ria mandib′ulae** [NA], depressions on the anterior surface of the alveolar process of the mandible, between the ridges caused by the roots of the incisor teeth. **ju′ga alveola′ria maxil′lae** [NA], the depressions on the anterior surface of the alveolar process of the maxilla, between the ridges caused by the roots of the incisor teeth. **ju′ga cerebra′lia os′sium cra′nii,** cerebral ridges of cranial bones: variable ridges on the inner surface of the cranium, corresponding to the sulci of the brain.   **j. sphenoida′le** [NA], the portion of the body of the sphenoid bone that connects the lesser wings.

juice (joos′) [L. *jus* broth]   any fluid from an animal or plant tissue; see also *succus*.   **appetite j.,** gastric juice secreted during eating and varying in character with the appetite for the food which is being eaten.   **cancer j.,** a milky juice obtained from cancerous tissue, and containing cancer cells.   **cherry j.,** liquid expressed from the fresh ripe fruit of *Prunus cerasus* L. (Rosaceae) used as an ingredient in preparing flavored vehicles for pharmaceuticals and liqueurs.   **gastric j.,** succus gastricus.   **intestinal j.,** succus entericus.   **pancreatic j.,** succus pancreaticus.   **press j.,** liquid obtained by submitting finely ground tissue to great pressure.   **raspberry j.,** the liquid expressed from the fresh ripe fruit of varieties of *Rubus*

idaeus L. (European red raspberry) or *Rubus strigosus* Michx. (American red raspberry); used in a syrup as a flavored vehicle for drugs.

Jukes (jooks)   fictitious name of a New York family, described by the American sociologist R.L. Dugdale, exhibiting a high incidence of crime, immorality, disease, and poverty; used, like the Kallikaks to advance the theory of genetic determinism.

julep (joo′lep) [L. *julapium*]   a sweetened alcoholic drink or cordial of various kinds.

jumping (jump′ing)   Gilles de la Tourette's syndrome. **j. the bite,** correction of cross-bite. See also *Kingsley appliance*, under *appliance*.

junction (junk′shun)   the place of meeting or of coming together, as of two different organs or types of tissue; see also *joint* and *junctura*.   **adherent j.,** zonula adherens. **amelodentinal j.,** dentinoenamel j.   **anorectal j.,** linea anorectalis.   **cardioesophageal j.,** esophagogastric j.   **cementodentinal j.,** dentinocemental j.   **cementoenamel j.,** the line at which the cementum covering the root of a tooth and the enamel covering its crown meet, designated anatomically as the cervical line.   **corneoscleral j.,** limbus (def. 2).   **dentinocemental j.,** the plane of meeting between the dentin and cementum on the root of a tooth.   **dentinoenamel j.,** the plane of meeting between the dentin and enamel on the crown of a tooth. **dentogingival j.,** the zone of meeting of the cementum and the gingiva, consisting of the epithelial attachment and the gingival fibers.   **dermoepidermal j.,** the plane of meeting between the dermis and epidermis.   **esophagogastric j.,** the site of transition from the stratified squamous epithelium of the esophagus to the simple columnar epithelium of the cardia of the stomach; called also *cardioesophageal j.* and *gastroesophageal j.*   **fibromuscular j.,** a junction between the muscular elements of the wall of the corpus uteri and the fibrous tissue of the cervix. **gap j.,** a narrowed portion (about 3μm.) of the intercellular space which contains channels (about 2μm. in diameter) linking adjacent cells and through which pass ions, most sugars, amino acids, nucleotides, vitamins, hormones, and cyclic AMP. In electrically excitable tissues, these gap junctions serve to transmit electrical impulses via ionic currents and are known as *electronic synapses;* they are present in such tissues as myocardial tissue. Called also *nexus*.   **gastroesophageal j.,** esophagogastric j.   **ileocecal j.,** the junction of the ileum and cecum, located at the lower right side of the abdomen and fixed to the posterior abdominal wall.   **intermediate j.,** zonula adherens. **manubriogladiolar j.,** synchondrosis sternalis.   **mucocutaneous j.,** the site of transition between skin and mucous membrane.   **mucogingival j.,** a sharply scalloped, generally indistinct line running parallel with the free margin, separating the gingival tissue from that of the oral mucosa; visible under the microscope. Called also *mucogingival line*.   **myoneural j.,** neuromuscular j.   **neuromuscular j.,** the site of apposition of a motor nerve fiber and a skeletal muscle fiber that it innervates, the discoid expansion of the terminal branch of the axon forming the motor end plate, and the opposed region of the surface of the muscle fiber forming the sole plate; the neurotransmitter at the synapse is acetylcholine, which is released from the axon terminal when the nerve is excited, diffuses across the synaptic cleft, and reversibly binds to receptor molecules on the muscle fiber surface, causing the initiation of an action potential that propagates along the muscle fiber causing it to contract. Called also *myoneural j.*   **occluding j.,** zonula occludens.   **osseous j's,** the sites of union of different bones; called also *articulationes* [NA].   **sclerocorneal j.,** limbus (def. 2).   **tendinous j's,** conexus intertendineus. **tight j.,** an intercellular junction at which adjacent plasma membranes are joined tightly together by interlinked rows of integral membrane proteins, which create a seal impermeable to intercellular passage of molecules.   **ureteropelvic j.,** junction of the ureter and the kidney at the pelvis of the kidney.   **ureterovesical j.,** the junction of the bladder and ureter; called also *ureterotrigonal complex*.

junctional (junk′shun-al)   pertaining to a junction.

junctura (junk-tu′rah), pl. *junctu′rae* [L. "a joining"]   a general term used in anatomical nomenclature to designate the site of union between different structures; see also *articulatio* and *joint*.   **junctu′rae cartilagin′eae** articulones cartilagineae.   **junctu′rae cin′guli mem′bri**

inferio'ris, articulationes cinguli membri inferioris. **junctu'rae cin'guli mem'bri superio'ris** articulationes cinguli membri superioris. **junctu'rae colum'nae vertebra'lis, thora'cis, et cra'nii,** the articulations of the vertebral column, thorax, and cranium. See *articulationes synoviales cranii, articulationes vertebrales,* and *articulationes thoracis.* **juncturae fibro'sae,** articulationes fibrosae. **j. lumbosacra'lis,** articulatio lumbrosacralis. **junctu'rae mem'bri inferio'ris li'beri,** articulationes membri inferioris liberi. **junctu'rae mem'bri superio'ris li'beri** articulationes membri superioris liberi. **j. os'sium,** a joint; see also *articulatio.* **junctu'rae os'sium,** NA alternative for *articulationes;* see *articulatio.* **j. sacrococcyg'ea** articulatio sacrococcygea. **juncturae synovia'les,** articulationes synoviales. **junctu'rae ten'dinum,** connexus intertendineus. **junctu'rae zygapophysea'les,** articulationes zygapophyseales.

juncturae (junk-tu're) [L.] genitive and plural of *junctura.*

Jung (yoong), Carl Gustav. Swiss psychiatrist (1875–1961), founder of the school of analytic psychology, which postulates a collective unconscious of mankind.

Jung's muscle (yoongz) [Karl Gustav *Jung,* Swiss anatomist, 1794–1864] musculus pyramidalis auriculae.

Jungbluth's vasa propria (vessels) (yoong'bloots) [Hermann *Jungbluth,* German physician] see *vasa propria of Jungbluth,* under *vas.*

juniper (joo'nĭ-per) 1. any of the trees or shrubs of the genus *Juniperus.* 2. the dried ripe fruit of *Juniperus communis* L., or common juniper tree, formerly used as a diuretic; the fruit is used for flavoring certain alcoholic beverages. Called also *juniper berries.*

Juniperus (joo-nip'er-us) a genus of coniferous trees and shrubs of the family Cupressaceae, including *J. communis* L., the juniper tree, and *J. sabina* L., the evergreen shrub or savin.

Junker inhaler (apparatus, bottle) (junk'er) [Ferdinand Ethelbert *Junker,* English physician of 19th century] see under *inhaler.*

jurisprudence (joor"is-proo'dens) [L. *juris prudentia* knowledge of law] the scientific study or application of the principles of law and justice. **dental j.,** the application of the principles of law and justice as they relate to the practice of dentistry, to the obligations of the practitioner to his patient, and to the relations of dentists to each other and to society in general. This term and *forensic dentistry* are sometimes used as synonyms, but some authorities consider the first a branch of law and the second a branch of dentistry. See also *medical j.* and *forensic dentistry.* **medical j.,** the application of the principles of law as they relate to the practice of medicine, to the obligations of the practitioner to his patient, and to the relations of physicians to each other and to society in general. This term and *forensic medicine* are sometimes used as synonyns, but some authorities consider the first a branch of law and the second a branch of medicine.

juscul. abbreviation for L. *jus'culum,* soup or broth.

justo major (jus'to ma'jor) see *pelvis aequabiliter justo major.*

justo minor (jus'to mi'nor) see *pelvis aequabiliter justo minor.*

jute (joot) the fibers of tropical herbs or undershrubs of *Corchorus capsularis* L. (Tiliaceae), formerly used in surgical dressings.

juvantia (joo-van'she-ah) [L. pl.] adjuvant and palliative medicines or appliances.

juvenile (joo'vĕ-nīl) 1. pertaining to youth or childhood; young or immature. 2. a youth or child; a young animal. 3. a cell or organism intermediate between the immature form and the mature form.

juxta- [L. *juxta* near, close by] a combining form meaning situated near or adjoining.

juxta-articular (juks"tah-ar-tik'u-lar) [L. *juxta* near + *articulus* joint] situated near a joint or in the region of a joint.

juxtaepiphyseal (juks"tah-ep-ĭ-fiz'e-al) [*juxta-* + *epiphysis*] near to or adjoining an epiphysis.

juxtaglomerular (juks"tah-glo-mer'u-lar) [*juxta-* + *glomerulus*] near to or adjoining a glomerulus of the kidney, as juxtaglomerular cells.

juxtangina (juks-tan'jĭ-nah) [L. "almost quinsy"] inflammation involving the muscles of the pharynx.

juxtaposition (juks"tah-po-zish'un) [*juxta-* + L. *positio* place] apposition.

juxtapyloric (juks"tah-pi-lor'ik) [*juxta-* + *pylorus*] situated near the pylorus or the pyloric part of the stomach (see *pars pylorica ventriculi*).

juxtaspinal (juks-tah-spi'nal) [*juxta-* + *spine*] close to the spinal column.

juxtavesical (juks"tah-ves'ĭ-kal) [*juxta-* + *vesical*] situated near or adjoining the urinary bladder.

K

K chemical symbol for *potassium* [L. *kalium*]; symbol for *kelvin.*

k symbol for *kilo-.*

K symbol for equilibrium constant (K_a acid ionization constant, K_b base ionization constant, K_d dissociation constant, K_{sp} solubility product).

k symbol for *Boltzmann's constant.*

κ kappa, the tenth letter of the Greek alphabet; symbol for one of the two types of immunoglobulin light chains.

Ka. kathode (cathode).

kabure (kah-boo're) a skin disease in Japan, probably caused by the burrowing of the cercariae of *Schistosoma japonica* in the skin.

Kader's operation (kah'ders) [Bronislaw *Kader,* Polish surgeon, 1863–1937] see under *operation.*

Kaes' feltwork, line (kiz) [Theodor *Kaes,* German neurologist, 1852–1913] see under *feltwork* and *line.*

Kaes-Bekhterev layer [Theodor *Kaes;* Vladimir Mikhailovich *Bekhterev,* Russian neurologist, 1857–1927] Bekhterev's layer.

KAF conglutinogen activating factor (factor I).

Kafocin (ka-fo'sin) trademark for a preparation of cephaloglycin.

Kahler's disease, law (kah'lerz) [Otto *Kahler,* Austrian physician, 1849–1893] see *multiple myeloma,* and see under *law.*

kahweol (kah'we-ol) [Turkish *galweh* coffee] a white crystalline lipid which forms the principal part of the unsaponifiable fraction of coffee.

kain(o)- see *cen(o)-* (def. 1).

kaiserling (ki'zer-ling) 1. Kaiserling's solution. 2. a specimen preserved in Kaiserling's solution.

Kaiserling's method, solution (fixative) (ki'zer-lings) [Karl *Kaiserling,* German pathologist, 1869–1942] see under *method* and *solution.*

kak- for words beginning thus, see also those beginning *cac-.*

kakke (kahk'ka) [Japanese] beriberi.

kakodyl (kak'o-dil) cacodyl.

kakosmia (kak-oz'me-ah) [Gr. *kakos* bad + *osmē* smell + *-ia*] cacosmia.

kakotrophy (kak-ot'ro-fe) cacotrophy.

kala-azar (kah'lah ah-zar') [Hindi, "black fever"] the classic form of visceral leishmaniasis.

kaladana (kal-ah-da'nah) the dried seeds of *Ipomoea nil* L.; used in India and China for its purgative and anthelmintic properties.

kalafungin (kah-lah-fun'jin) an antifungal antibiotic substance produced by *Streptomyces tanashiensis* strain *kala.*

kalagua (kah-lah′gwah) a drug used in South America in the treatment of tuberculosis.

kalemia (kah-le′me-ah) [L. *kalium* potassium + Gr. *haima* blood + *-ia*] the presence of potassium in the blood; see *hyperkalemia*.

kali (ka′li, kah′le) [Ger.] potash. **k. arsenico′sum,** potassium arsenite solution; see under *solution*.

kaliemia (ka-le-e′me-ah) kalemia.

kaligenous (ka-lij′e-nus) [*kalium* + Gr. *gennan* to produce] producing potash.

kalimeter (ka-lim′ĕ-ter) alkalimeter.

kaliopenia (ka″le-o-pe′ne-ah) [L. *kalium* potassium + Gr. *penia* poverty] hypokalemia.

kaliopenic (ka″le-o-pe′nik) pertaining to, characterized by, or producing kaliopenia.

kalium (ka′le-um), gen. *ka′lii* [L., from Ar. *gily* saltwort] potassium.

kaliuresis (ka″le-u-re′sis) [L. *kalium* potassium + Gr. *ourēsis* a making water] the excretion of potassium in the urine.

kaliuretic (ka″le-u-ret′ik) 1. pertaining to, characterized by, or promoting kaliuresis. 2. an agent that promotes kaliuresis.

kallak (kal′ak) [Eskimo for disease of the skin] a pustular dermatitis occurring in the Eskimos.

kallidin (kal′ĭ-dĭn) lysyl-bradykinin, a decapeptide kinin produced by the action of tissue and glandular kallikreins on LMW (low-molecular-weight) kininogen and having physiologic effects similar to those of bradykinin. Formerly the term was applied to both nona- and decapeptides; bradykinin was called *kallidin I* or *kallidin-9,* and Lys-bradykinin was called *kallidin II* or *kallidin-10.*

Kallikak (kal′ĭ-kak) [Gr. *kallos* beauty + *kakos* bad] fictitious name of a New Jersey family, described by the American sociologist H.H. Goddard, having two branches, one consisting of highly intelligent and successful individuals, the other exhibiting a high incidence of mental deficiency, immorality, and criminality; used to advance the theory that these traits are genetically determined.

kallikrein (kal″ĭ-kre′in) a proteolytic enzyme (serine protease) found in blood plasma, lymph, urine, saliva, pancreatic juice, and other exocrine secretions that cleaves kininogens to form kinins (bradykinin, kallidin) and activates plasminogen. **plasma k.** [EC 3.4.21.34], an enzyme of the hydrolase class that hydrolyzes Lys-Arg and Arg-Ser bonds in kininogen to produce bradykinin. It is formed from prekallikrein by coagulation Factor XII or XIIa (activated Hageman factor). It also activates coagulation Factors XII and VII and plasminogen. It is found in blood plasma. **tissue k.** [EC 3.4.21.35], an enzyme of the hydrolase class that hydrolyzes Met-Lys and Arg-Ser bonds in kininogen to produce lysyl-bradykinin (kallidin). It and closely related forms are found in lymph, pancreatic juice, urine, and saliva.

kallikreinogen (kal″ĭ-kri′no-jin) prekallikrein.

Kalmia (kal′me-ah) a genus of ericaceous shrubs, the leaves of which have been used in syphilis, diarrhea, and chronic inflammatory disorders, and are thought to possess cardiac and sedative properties; *K. latifolia* L. (mountain laurel) and other related species yield the poisonous principle andromedotoxin.

Kalmuk idiocy (kal′mook) [*Kalmuk,* a Mongolian people in Asia and Russia] severe mental retardation associated with Down's syndrome.

kaluresis (kal″u-re′sis) kaliuresis.

kaluretic (kal″u-ret′ik) kaliuretic.

kamala (kam′ah-lah) the glands and hairs of the capsules of *Mallotus philippinensis* Muell.-Arg. (Euphorbiaceae), an East Indian shrub; it has been used as a purgative and is used in veterinary medicine as a teniacide. Called also *rottlera.*

Kaminer's reaction (kam′ĭ-ner) [Gisa *Kaminer,* Vienna physician, 1883–1941] Freund's reaction.

kanamycin (kan″ah-mi′sin) chemical name: *O*-3-amino-3-deoxy-α-D-glucopyranosyl-(1→6)-*O*-[6-amino-6-deoxy-α-D-glucopyranosyl-(i→4)]-2-deoxy-D-streptamine. A water-soluble antibiotic derived from *Streptomyces kanamyceticus,* first isolated in Japan in 1957; it is effective against some gram-positive, many gram-negative, and some acid-fast bacteria. **k. sulfate** [USP], the sulfate salt of kanamycin, $C_{18}H_{36}N_4O_{11} \cdot H_2SO_4$, occurring as a white, crystalline pow-

der; used especially in the treatment of infections due to gram-negative bacteria, such as *Klebsiella, Aerobacter,* some *Proteus* species, *Serratia,* and *Escherichia coli,* and has been used in the treatment of pulmonary tuberculosis, administered orally, intramuscularly, and intravenously.

Kanavel's sign (kan-a′velz) [Allen Buchner *Kanavel,* Chicago surgeon, 1874–1938] see under *sign.*

Kanner's syndrome (kah′nerz) [Leo *Kanner,* Austrian-born American child psychiatrist, born 1894] autistic disorder.

Kantrex (kan′treks) trademark for preparations of kanamycin.

kanyemba (kan″e-em′bah) an acute rectitis of unknown cause, reported from South America and Northern Rhodesia.

Kaochlor (ka′o-klōr) trademark for a preparation of potassium chloride.

kaolin (ka′o-lin) [USP] a native hydrated aluminum silicate, powdered and freed from gritty particles by elutriation. A soft white or yellowish white powder with a claylike taste, used as an adsorbent and in kaolin mixture with pectin. Called also *argilla, bolus alba,* and *China clay.*

kaolinosis (ka″o-lin-o′sis) pneumoconiosis caused by inhaling particles of kaolin.

Kaon (ka′on) trademark for preparations of potassium gluconate.

Kaplan's test (kap′lanz) [David M. *Kaplan,* New York physician, born 1870] see under *tests.*

Kaposi's sarcoma, varicelliform eruption (kah′po-shēz) [Moritz *Kaposi* (Moritz Kaposi Kohn), Austrian dermatologist, 1837–1902] see under *eruption* and *sarcoma.*

kappa (kap′ah) [K, κ] the tenth letter of the Greek alphabet.

Kappadione (kap″pah-di′ōn) trademark for a preparation of menadiol sodium diphosphate.

Kappeler's maneuver (kap′ĕ-lerz) [Otto *Kappeler,* German surgeon, 1841–1909] see under *maneuver.*

kara-kurt (kah′rah-koort″) the venomous Russian spider *Latrodectus lugubris.*

karaya (kar′a-ah) see under *gum.*

Karotomorpha (kah-ro″to-mor′fah) a genus of parasitic protozoa (order Proteromonadida, class Zoomastigophorea) found in the intestine of frogs and toads.

Karroo syndrome (kah-roo′) [*Karroo,* region of South Africa] see under *syndrome.*

Kartagener's syndrome (triad) (kar-tag′ĕ-nerz) [Manes *Kartagener,* Swiss physician, born 1897] see under *syndrome.*

karyapsis (kar″e-ap′sis) [*karyo-* + Gr. *hapsis* joining] union of nuclei in a conjugating cell.

karyenchyma (kar″e-en′kĭ-mah) [*karyo-* + Gr. *enchymos* juicy] karyolymph.

kary(o)- [Gr. *karyon* nut, kernel] a combining form denoting relationship to a nucleus; see also words beginning *cary(o)-.*

karyochrome (kar′e-o-krōm″) [*karyo-* + Gr. *chrōma* color] a nerve cell the nucleus of which is deeply stainable, while the body is not; its nucleus is larger than that of a cytochrome, and there are varieties designated by Greek letters.

karyochylema (kar″e-o-ki-le′mah) karyolymph.

karyoclasis (kar″e-ok′lah-sis) karyoklasis.

karyoclastic (kar″e-o-klas′tik) karyoklastic.

karyocyte (kar′e-o-sīt) [*karyo-* + *-cyte*] a nucleated cell.

karyogamic (kar″e-o-gam′ik) [*karyo-* + Gr. *gamos* marriage] pertaining to or characterized by union of nuclei.

karyogamy (kar″e-og′ah-me) [*karyo-* + Gr. *gamos* marriage] the union of the nuclei of cells following plasmogamy in fertilization.

karyogenesis (kar″e-o-jen′ĕ-sis) [*karyo-* + Gr. *genesis* production] the development of the nucleus of a cell.

karyogenic (kar″e-o-jen′ik) forming the nucleus of a cell; pertaining to karyogenesis.

karyokinesis (kar″e-o-ki-ne′sis) [*karyo-* + Gr. *kinesis* motion] the phenomena involved in division of the nucleus, usually an early stage in the process of cell division, or mitosis. **asymmetrical k.,** mitosis in which the chromosomes divide unequally and into dissimilar masses. **hyperchromatic k.,** mitosis in which the number of chromosomes is abnormally large. **hypochromatic k.,** mitosis in which the number of chromosomes is abnormally small.

karyokinetic (kar″e-o-ki-net′ik)   pertaining to or of the nature of karyokinesis.

karyoklasis (kar″e-ok′lah-sis) [*karyo-* + Gr. *klasis* breaking] the breaking down of the cell nucleus or nuclear membrane.

karyoklastic (kar″e-o-klas′tik)   1. breaking down cell nuclei. 2. arresting mitosis.

karyolymph (kar′e-o-limf″) [*karyo-* + *lymph*]   the liquid part of a cell nucleus, as contrasted with the chromatin and linin.

karyolysis (kar″e-ol′ĭ-sis) [*karyo-* + Gr. *lysis* dissolution]   a form of necrobiosis in which the nucleus of a cell swells and gradually loses its chromatin.

karyolytic (kar″e-o-lit′ik)   producing or pertaining to karyolysis; destroying cell nuclei.

karyomastigont (kar″e-o-mas′tĭ-gont) [*karyo-* + Gr. *mastigoun* to whip]   a condition characteristic of certain flagellate protozoa in which the mastigont system is associated with a nucleus. Cf. *akaryomastigont*.

karyomegaly (kar″e-o-meg′ah-le) [*karyo-* + Gr. *megale* great]   abnormal enlargement of the nucleus of a cell, not caused by polyploidy.

karyomere (kar′e-o-mēr″)   1. chromomere (def. 1).   2. a vesicle containing only a small portion of the typical nucleus, usually following abnormal mitosis.

karyometry (kar″e-om′ĕ-tre) [*karyo-* + Gr. *metron* measure]   measurement of a cell nucleus.

karyomicrosome (kar″e-o-mi′kro-sōm) [*karyo-* + *microsome*]   nucleomicrosome.

karyomitosis (kar″e-o-mi-to′sis)   division of the nucleus of a cell preceding mitosis.

karyomitotic (kar″e-o-mi-tot′ik)   pertaining to karyomitosis.

karyomorphism (kar″e-o-mor′fizm) [*karyo-* + Gr. *morphe* form]   the shape of a cell nucleus.

karyon (kar′e-on) [Gr. *karyon* nucleus]   the nucleus of a cell.

karyophage (kar′e-o-fāj″) [*karyo-* + Gr. *phagein* to eat]   a protozoan that exercises phagocytic action on the nucleus of the cell it infects.

karyoplasm (kar′e-o-plazm″) [*karyo-* + Gr. *plasma* plasm]   the nucleoplasm, or protoplasm of the nucleus of a cell.

karyoplasmic (kar″e-o-plaz′mik)   pertaining to karyoplasm.

karyoplast (kar′e-o-plast)   the nucleus of a cell.

karyoplastin (kar″e-o-plas′tin)   the substance of a mitotic spindle; the parachromatin.

karyopyknosis (kar″e-o-pik-no′sis)   shrinkage of a cell nucleus, with condensation of the chromatin into a solid, structureless mass or masses.

karyopyknotic (kar″e-o-pik-not′ik)   pertaining to, characterized by, or causing karyopyknosis.

karyoreticulum (kar″e-o-re-tik′u-lum) [*karyo-* + *reticulum*]   the fibrillar part of the karyoplasm as distinguished from the fluid part of karyolymph.

karyorrhectic (kar″e-o-rek′tik)   pertaining to, characterized by, or causing karyorrhexis.

karyorrhexis (kar″e-o-rek′sis) [*karyo-* + Gr. *rhexis* a breaking]   rupture of the cell nucleus in which the chromatin disintegrates into formless granules which are extruded from the cell.

karyosome (kar′e-o-sōm″) [*karyo-* + Gr. *soma* body]   any of the condensed irregular clumps of chromatin dispersed in the chromatin network of a cell; called also *net knot, false nucleolus, chromatin nucleolus, chromatin reservoir*, and *chromocenter*.

karyostasis (kar″e-os′tah-sis) [*karyo-* + Gr. *stasis* halt]   the so-called resting stage of the nucleus between mitotic divisions.

karyotheca (kar″e-o-the′kah) [*karyo-* + Gr. *theke* sheath]   nuclear membrane.

karyotin (kar′e-o-tin)   chromatin.

karyotype (kar′e-o-tīp) [*karyo-* + *type*]   the full chromosome set of the nucleus of a cell; by extension, the photomicrograph of chromosomes arranged according to a standard classification. Cf. *idiogram*, and see illustration accompanying *chromosome*.

karyotypic (kar″e-o-tip′ik)   pertaining to or representative of the karyotype.

karyozoic (kar″e-o-zo′ik) [*karyo-* + Gr. *zōon* animal]   existing in or inhabiting the nuclei of cells, as do certain protozoa.

Kasabach-Merritt syndrome (kas′ah-bok-mer′it) [Haig Haigouni *Kasabach*, American physician, 1898–1943; Katharine Krom *Merritt*, American pediatrician, born 1896]   see under *syndrome*.

kasai (kah-si′)   a syndrome occurring in the Congo, characterized by anemia, depigmentation of the skin, and edema, all of which may be secondary to iron deficiency.

kasal (ka′sal)   chemical name: basic sodium aluminum phosphate; a food additive, $Na_8Al_2(OH)_2(PO_4)_4$, with about 30 per cent dibasic sodium phosphate.

kat   symbol for katal.

kat-, kata- [Gr. *kata* down]   a prefix meaning down, lower, under, against, along with, very. For words beginning thus, see also those beginning *cat-, cata-*.

katachromasis (kat″ah-kro′mah-sis)   the process by which the daughter chromosomes reconstruct the daughter nuclei.

katadidymus (kat″ah-did′ĭ-mus) [*kata-* + Gr. *didymos* twin]   a twin monster divided above, but single toward the podalic pole (monstra duplicia katadidyma—Förster).

katal (kat′al)   a unit of measurement proposed to express activities of all catalysts, including enzymes, being that amount of a catalyst, such as an enzyme, which catalyzes a reaction rate of 1 mole of substrate per second. Symbol kat.

katathermometer (kat″ah-ther-mom′ĕ-ter)   a pair of alcoholic thermometers, one with a dry bulb and one with a wet bulb. They are heated to 110° F and exposed to the air, and the time is noted that it takes each bulb to fall from 100° to 90° F. From this the temperature as it affects the body can be deduced.

Katayama (kat″ah-yah′mah)   *Oncomelania*.

Katayama's test (kat″ah-yah′mahz) [Kunika *Katayama*, Japanese physician, 1856–1931]   see under *tests*.

katharometer (kath″ah-rom′ĕ-ter)   an instrument for electrometric determination of basal metabolic rates.

kathisophobia (kath″ĭ-so-fo′be-ah)   intense, irrational fear of sitting down.

katine (ka′tin)   an alkaloid, d-norpseudoephedrine, $C_9H_{13}NO$, from *Catha edulis* Forsk. (Celastraceae); it acts on the nervous system like cocaine, but has no local anesthetic properties, and is used as an appetite depressant and mild euphoriant. The leaves are used as tea and masticatory in Ethiopia, East and South Africa, and Yemen.

kation (kat′i-on)   cation.

katolysis (kah-tol′ĭ-sis) [Gr. *kato* below + *lysis* dissolution]   the incomplete or intermediate conversion of complex chemical bodies into simpler compounds; applied especially to digestive processes.

katophoria (kat″o-for′re-ah)   cataphoria.

katotropia (kat″o-tro′pe-ah)   cataphoria.

Katz (kats), Sir Bernard.   German-born British physiologist, born 1911; co-winner, with Julius Axelrod and Ulf Svante von Euler, of the Nobel prize for medicine or physiology in 1970 for his discovery of the manner of electrical impulse transmission from nerves to muscles.

Katz formula [Johann Rudolf *Katz*, German colloid chemist, 1880–1938]   see under *formula*.

katzenjammer (kats′en-yam′er) [Ger.]   the symptoms of headache, nausea, possibly cerebral edema, and functional neuritis, following ingestion of alcohol; hangover.

Kay Ciel (ka′sēl)   trademark for preparations of potassium chloride.

Kayexalate (ka-ek′sah-lāt)   trademark for a preparation of sodium polystyrene sulfonate.

Kayser's disease (ki′zers) [Bernhard *Kayser*, German ophthalmologist, 1869–1954]   hepatolenticular degeneration.

Kayser-Fleischer ring (ki′zer flīsh′er) [Bernhard *Kayser*; Bruno *Fleischer*, Munich physician, 1848–1904]   see under *ring*.

Kazanjian forceps, operation (kah-zan′ge-an) [Varaztad Hovhannes *Kazanjian*, Armenian-born plastic and maxillofacial surgeon, born 1879] see under *forceps* and *operation*.

Kb in genetics, kilobase (1000 base pairs).

KBr Potassium bromide.

kc. kilocycle.

KC₂H₃O₂ potassium acetate.

kCi kilocurie.

KCl potassium chloride.

KClO₃ potassium chlorate.

K₂CO₃ potassium carbonate.

kc.p.s. kilocycles per second.

KCT kathodal (cathodal) closing tetanus.

Ke an antigenic marker distinguishing human immunoglobulin λ light chain subtypes. Called also *Kern*.

Kearns-Sayre syndrome (kerns sār) [Thomas P. *Kearns*, American ophthalmologist, born 1922; George P. *Sayre*, American pathologist, born 1911] see under *syndrome*.

kebocephaly (keb″o-sef′ah-le) cebocephaly.

ked (ked) the sheep tick, *Melophagus ovinus*.

keel (kēl) a septicemic enteritis of ducklings caused by *Salmonella anatum*.

Keen's operation, sign (kēnz) [William Williams *Keen*, Philadelphia surgeon, 1837–1932] see *omphalectomy*, and see under *sign*.

Keflex (kef′leks) trademark for a preparation of cephalexin.

Keflin (kef′lin) trademark for a preparation of cephalothin sodium.

Kefzol (kef′zōl) trademark for a preparation of cefazolin sodium.

Kehrer's reflex (kār′erz) [Ferdinand *Kehrer*, German neurologist, born 1883] see under *reflex*.

Keith's bundle, node (kēths) [Sir Arthur *Keith*, London anatomist, 1866–1955] see under *bundle*, and see *sinoatrial node*, under *node*.

Keith's low ionic diet [Norman M. *Keith*, American physician, born 1885] see under *diet*.

Keith-Flack node [Sir Arthur *Keith*; Martin William *Flack*, physiologist in London, 1882–1931] sinoatrial node.

kelectome (ke′lek-tōm) [Gr. *kēlē* tumor + *ektomē* excision] a device used in removing specimens of tissue from tumors.

Kelene (kel′ēn) trademark for a preparation of ethyl chloride.

Kelling's test (kel′ings) [Georg *Kelling*, German physician, born 1866] see under *tests*.

Kelly's operation (kel′ēz) [Joseph Dominic *Kelly*, otolaryngologist in New York, born 1888] arytenoidopexy.

Kelly's operation, sign, speculum (kel′ēz) [Howard Atwood *Kelly*, American surgeon, 1858–1943] see under *operation* (def. 1), *sign*, and *speculum*.

keloid (ke′loid) [Gr. *kēlē* tumor + *eidos* form] a sharply elevated, irregularly-shaped, progressively enlarging scar due to the formation of excessive amounts of collagen in the corium during connective tissue repair. **acne k.,** dermatitis papillaris capillitii. **k. of gums,** fibromatosis gingivae.

kelosomus (ke-lo-so′mus) celosomus.

kelotomy (ke-lot′o-me) [Gr. *kēlē* a rupture + *temnein* to cut] herniotomy.

kelp (kelp) any of various large brown marine algae of the genus *Laminaria*, which are widely used as food in the Orient, and are the source of alginates.

kelvin (kel′vin) [after Lord *Kelvin*] the SI unit of thermodynamic temperature equal to 1/273.15 of the absolute temperature of the triple point of water. See also *absolute temperature*, under *temperature*, and *Kelvin scale*, under *scale*. Abbreviated K.

Kelvin scale (kel′vin) [Lord *Kelvin* (William Thompson), British physicist, 1824–1907] see under *scale*.

Kemadrin (kem′ah-drin) trademark for a preparation of procyclidine hydrochloride.

Kempner diet (kemp′ner) [Walter *Kempner*, American physician, born 1903] see under *diet*.

Kenacort (ken′ah-kort) trademark for preparations of triamcinolone.

Kenalog (ken′ah-log) trademark for preparations of triamcinolone acetonide.

Kendall (ken′dal), Edward Calvin. American biochemist, 1886–1972; co-winner, with Philip Showalter Hench and Tadeus Reichstein, of the Nobel prize for medicine or physiology in 1950 for his research on the hormones of the adrenal cortex.

Kendall's method (ken′dalz) [Edward Calvin *Kendall*] see under *method*.

Kendall's rank correlation coefficient (tau) (ken′dalz) [Maurice George *Kendall*, British statistician, born 1907] see under *coefficient*.

Kennedy's syndrome (ken′ĕ-dēz) [Foster *Kennedy*, New York neurologist, 1884–1952] see under *syndrome*.

Kenny's treatment (ken′e) [Sister Elizabeth *Kenny* of Brisbane, Australia, later in U.S.A., 1886–1952] see under *treatment*.

ken(o)- [Gr. *kenos* empty] a combining form denoting empty; see also words beginning *cen(o)-*.

kenotoxin (ke′no-tok-sin) [*keno-* + *toxin*] the toxin of fatigue; produced in muscle by muscular contractions.

Kent's bundle (kents) [Albert Frank Stanley *Kent*, English physiologist, 1863–1958] see under *bundle*.

Kent-His bundle [A. F. S. *Kent*; Wilhelm *His*, Jr.] bundle of His.

kentrokinesis (ken″tro-ki-ne′sis) centrokinesia.

kentrokinetic (ken″tro-ki-net′ik) centrokinetic.

Kepone (ke′pōn) trademark for a polychlorinated ketone, $C_{10}Cl_{10}O$, used as an insecticide; workers exposed to this nonbiodegradable compound have suffered neurologic symptoms, such as tremors and slurred speech.

Kerandel's sign (symptom) (ker″an-delz′) [Jean François *Kerandel*, French colonial physician, 1873–1934] see under *sign*.

keraphyllocele (ker″ah-fil′o-sēl) [Gr. *keras* horn + *phyllon* leaf + *kēlē* tumor] keratoma, def. 2.

kerasin (ker′ah-sin) a cerebroside, $C_{48}H_{93}O_8N$, obtained from brain tissue; it yields galactose, sphingosine, and lignoceric acid on hydrolysis.

keratalgia (ker″ah-tal′je-ah) [*kerat-* + *-algia*] pain in the cornea.

keratan sulfate (ker′ah-tan) a glycosaminoglycan found in the cornea, in cartilage, and in the nucleus pulposus and also as the accumulation product in Morquio's syndrome. It is a linear chain of repeating disaccharide units, each containing one residue of D-galactose (Gal) and one of N-acetyl-D-glucosamine 6-sulfate (GlcNAc) linked by glycosidic bonds that are alternately 1→3 and 1→4, so that the formula for the repeating unit is (1→3)-β-Gal-(1→4)-β-GlcNAc. There are two forms, *keratan sulfate I* and *keratan sulfate II*, which differ in carbohydrate content; both also contain fucose, sialic acid, and mannose; keratan sulfate II also contains N-acetyl-D-galactosamine. Called also *keratosulfate*.

keratansulfaturia (ker″ah-tan-sul″fah-too′re-ah) Morquio syndrome.

keratectasia (ker″ah-tek-ta′ze-ah) [*kerat-* + Gr. *ektasis* extension] protrusion of a thinned, scarred cornea; called also *corneal ectasia*.

keratectomy (ker″ah-tek′to-me) [*kerat-* + *ectomy*] excision of a portion of the cornea, usually done for anterior staphyloma.

keratic (ker-at′ik) 1. pertaining to keratin. 2. horny. 3. pertaining to the cornea.

keratin (ker′ah-tin) a scleroprotein which is the principal constituent of epidermis, hair, nails, horny tissues, and the organic matrix of the enamel of the teeth. It is a very insoluble protein, contains high amounts of sulfur as cystine, and also yields tyrosine and leucine on decomposition. Its solution in glacial acetic acid or ammonia is sometimes used in coating pills when the latter are desired to pass through the stomach unchanged. **false k.,** pseudokeratin.

keratinase (ker′ah-tĭ-nās) an enzyme of the hydrolase class that hydrolyzes keratin. The enzyme, produced by ringworm of the foot (*Trichophyton mentagrophytes*) [EC 3.4.24.10] cleaves preferentially at hydrophobic residues. The enzyme produced by *Streptomyces* [EC 3.4.99.11] cleaves preferentially at Ser-His, Leu-Val, Phe-Tyr, and Lys-Ala.

keratinization (ker″ah-tin″i-za′shun) the development of or conversion into keratin.

keratinize (ker′ah-tin-īz) to make, or become, keratinous.

keratinocyte (kĕ-rat′ĭ-no-sīt) the epidermal cell which synthesizes keratin; constituting 95 per cent of the epidermal cells and, with the melanocyte, forming the binary cell system of the epidermis. In its various successive stages it is known as basal cell, prickle cell, and granular cell. Called also *malpighian cell*.

keratinoid (ker′ah-tin-oid) a form of keratin-coated tablet not soluble in the stomach, but readily soluble in the intestine.

keratinosome (kĕ-rat′ĭ-no-sōm″) [*keratin* + Gr. *sōma* body] one of the spherical lamellar granules that are formed in the upper spinous and granular layers of the skin near the Golgi apparatus and migrate into the cytoplasm, ultimately fusing with the plasma membrane to discharge their contents (bipolar phospholipids, glycoproteins, and acid phosphates) into the intracellular space; this extruded material is thought to function as a barrier to penetration by foreign substances. Called also *membrane-coating granule* and *Odland body*.

keratinous (ke-rat′ĭ-nus) containing or of the nature of keratin.

keratitis (ker″ah-ti′tis) [*kerat-* + *-itis*] inflammation of the cornea. Cf. *keratoconjunctivitis* and *keratopathy*. **acne rosacea k.**, rosacea k. **actinic k.**, a form due to the action of ultraviolet light. **aerosol k.**, keratitis following direct exposure of the eye to chemical sprays from aerosol cans, including hair spray, insecticides, etc. **alphabet k.**, striate k. **anaphylactic k.**, interstitial keratitis in one eye, caused by an antibody-antigen reaction to an intracorneal injection of protein in the second eye after sensitization from intracorneal injection of protein into the first eye. **annular k.**, marginal k. **k. arbores′cens**, dendriform k. **artificial silk k.**, keratitis occurring among workers in artificial silk manufacture; it is marked by blurring of vision with the appearance of haloes around lights. **aspergillus k.**, keratitis due to infection from the *Aspergillus* fungus. **band k., band-shaped k., k. bandelette**, ribbon-like k. **k. bullo′sa**, the formation of large or small bullae or blebs upon the cornea. **catarrhal ulcerative k.**, a mild form of keratitis secondary to conjunctivitis. **deep k.**, interstitial k. **deep pustular k.**, k. pustiliformis profunda. **dendriform k., dendritic k.**, herpetic keratitis resulting in a branching ulceration of the cornea. **desiccation k.**, lagophthalmic k. **Dimmer's k.**, k. nummularis. **disciform k., k. discifor′mis**, keratitis with the formation of a round or oval, disklike opacity of the cornea. **epithelial diffuse k.**, keratitis possibly due to vitamin B_2 deficiency, generally associated with uveitis, and characterized by minute gray epithelial flecks. **epithelial punctate k.**, superficial punctate k. **exfoliative k.**, keratitis that may occur with exfoliative dermatitis in a hypersensitive reaction to arsenic and marked by extensive denudation of the corneal epithelium. **exposure k.**, lagophthalmic k. **fascicular k.**, keratitis attended by the formation of a band of blood vessels. **k. filamento′sa**, keratitis with twisted filaments of mucoid material on the surface of the cornea; called also *filamentary keratopathy*. **furrow k.**, dendriform k. **herpetic k.**, 1. keratitis, commonly with dendritic ulceration (*dendriform* or *dendritic k.*), due to infection with herpes simplex virus. 2. keratitis occurring in herpes zoster ophthalmicus. **hypopyon k.**, suppurative keratitis associated with purulent infiltration and hypopyon; see *ulcus serpens corneae*. **infectious bovine k.**, see under *keratoconjunctivitis*. **interstitial k.**, a chronic variety of keratitis with deep deposits in the substance of the cornea, which becomes hazy throughout and has a ground-glass appearance. The disease is associated with congenital syphilis, and occurs in children before the fifteenth year. Called also *parenchymatous k., deep k.,* and *k. profunda*. **lagophthalmic k.**, that which accompanies lagophthalmos; it is due to exposure of the eyeball to the air. **lattice k.**, bilateral hereditary dystrophy of the cornea with the formation of interwoven filamentous lesions. **marginal k.**, phlyctenular keratitis in which the papules are arranged around the margin of the cornea; called also *annular k.* **metaherpetic k.**, keratitis occurring as a result of recurrent herpesvirus infection of the cornea, characterized by shallow ulceration of an anesthetic cornea, accompanied by parenchymatous infiltration and often by persistent iridocyclitis

and secondary glaucoma. **mycotic k.**, keratomycosis. **neuroparalytic k.**, keratitis characterized by dryness and fissuring of the corneal epithelium as a result of an injury to the trifacial nerve which prevents proper closing of the eyelids; called also *trophic k.* **neurotrophic k.**, keratitis due to loss of corneal sensation. **k. nummula′ris**, a slowly developing benign type of keratitis marked by corneal deposits forming circular areas with sharply defined edges surrounded by a halo of less dense character; called also *Dimmer's k.* **parenchymatous k.**, interstitial k. **k. petri′ficans**, keratitis with calcareous changes. **phlyctenular k.**, see under *keratoconjunctivitis*. **k. profun′da**, interstitial k. **k. puncta′ta lepro′sa**, a keratitis consisting of scattered, minute, white spots, occurring in leprosy. **k. puncta′ta profun′da**, deep punctate k. **k. puncta′ta, punctate k.**, an old term for the formation of cellular and fibrinous deposits (keratic precipitates) on the posterior surface of the cornea, occurring after injury or iridocyclitis and giving an appearance of fine drops of dew. **k. puncta′ta subepithelia′lis**, a form with gray areas on the cornea under Bowman's membrane, with an intact superficial epithelium. **punctate k., deep**, a rare keratitis occurring in hereditary or acquired syphilitic iritis and marked by sharply defined, pinhead-sized, grayish opacities in the substantia propria; called also *k. punctata profunda*. **punctate k., superficial**, a keratitis often associated with epidemic keratoconjunctivitis and characterized by many small circular epithelial erosions. **purulent k.**, severe keratitis characterized by a large ulcer with pus in the anterior chamber and purulent disintegration of the cornea. **k. pustulifor′mis profun′da**, a painful keratitis marked by deep-seated yellow intracorneal spots, hypopyon, and purulent iritis; called also *deep pustular k.* **reaper's k.**, suppurative keratitis due to the wounding of the cornea by the awn of some grain, as barley. **reticular k.**, familial degeneration of the cornea with reticular areas. **ribbon-like k.**, the formation of a transverse film on the cornea. **rosacea k.**, severe keratitis due to involvement of the cornea in rosacea, sometimes leading to ulceration; called also *acne rosacea k.* **sclerosing k.**, keratitis associated with scleritis, leading to hyperplasia. **scrofulus k.**, phlyctenular keratitis. **secondary k.**, keratitis due to disease of some other part of the eye. **serpiginous k.**, ulcus serpens corneae. **k. sic′ca**, keratoconjunctivitis sicca. **striate k.**, keratitis marked by parallel and intersecting lines on the corneal epithelium; called also *alphabet k.* Cf. *striate keratopathy*. **suppurative k.**, keratitis attended with, or associated with, suppuration. **trachomatous k.**, pannus trachomatosus. **trophic k.**, neuroparalytic k. **vascular k.**, keratitis accompanied by the formation of blood vessels beneath the conjunctiva and outer layers of the cornea. **vesicular k.**, keratitis with the development of small vesicles on the surface. **xerotic k.**, dryness of the cornea; a condition that precedes keratomalacia. **zonular k.**, ribbon-like k.

kerat(o)- [Gr. *keras*, gen. *keratos* horn] a combining form denoting relationship to horny tissue, or to the cornea.

keratoacanthoma (ker″ah-to-ak″an-tho′mah) [*kerato-* + *acanthoma*] a benign, usually self-limited epithelial tumor closely resembling squamous cell carcinoma clinically and histopathologically, occurring in three clinical forms: *Solitary* and *multiple* forms, which are clinically and histologically identical, primarily affect white males, the former type occurring after the age of 45 on sunlight-exposed surfaces of the skin, especially the face, neck, back of the hands, and arms, and the latter type presenting in adolescence or early adulthood and having a more general distribution, including unexposed skin. Both forms are manifested by a firm, erythematous papule that grows rapidly to form a dome-shaped, skin-colored nodule with a keratin-filled umbilicated center, which slowly involutes, leaving a small focus of scarring. The *eruptive* form usually presents in middle life, equally involving both sexes, as a generalized papular eruption of numerous dome-shaped, skin-colored papules, often sparing the palms and soles. Many cases of multiple keratoacanthoma (called also *multiple self-healing squamous epithelioma*) are autosomal dominants (see *self-healing squamous epithelioma*, under *epithelioma*), but no hereditary role has been shown in solitary and eruptive forms, although a viral etiology has been postulated.

keratocele (ker′ah-to-sēl″) [*kerato-* + *-cele*] hernia of the innermost layer of the cornea (Descemet's membrane).

keratocentesis (ker″ah-to-sen-te′sis) [*kerato-* + *centesis*] aqueous paracentesis.

keratoconjunctivitis (ker″ah-to-kon-junk″tĭ-vi′tis) [*kerato-* + *conjunctivitis*] inflammation of the cornea and conjunctiva. **epidemic k.,** a highly infectious disease characterized by relatively little ocular exudate, development of round subepithelial corneal opacities in association with the keratitis, and often swelling of regional lymph nodes; systemic symptoms, especially headache, may also be present. Adenovirus type 8 has been repeatedly isolated from patients with the disease. Called also *shipyard k., viral k.,* and *Sanders' disease.* **flash k.,** keratoconjunctivitis caused by exposure to a welding arc or other source of ultraviolet rays. **infectious bovine k.,** a general term for a group of diseases among cattle, sheep, and goats; the diseases are characterized by keratitis and conjunctivitis and are different, distinct clinical syndromes. **phlyctenular k.,** a form marked by the formation of a small, gray, circumscribed lesion, or phlyctenule, at the corneal limbus; it has been associated with malnutrition, tuberculosis, and staphylococcus sensitivity. Called also *phlyctenular keratitis, phlyctenular ophthalmia,* and *strumous ophthalmia.* See also *phlyctenulosis.* **shipyard k.,** epidemic k. **k. sic′ca,** a condition marked by hyperemia of the conjunctiva, lacrimal deficiency, thickening of the corneal epithelium, itching and burning of the eye, and often reduced visual acuity. Cf. *Sjögren syndrome.* **viral k.,** epidemic k.

keratoconus (ker″ah-to-ko′nus) [*kerato-* + Gr. *kōnos* cone] a noninflammatory, usually bilateral protrusion of the cornea, the apex being displaced downward and nasally. It occurs most commonly in females at about puberty. The cause is unknown, but hereditary factors may play a role. Called also *conical cornea.*

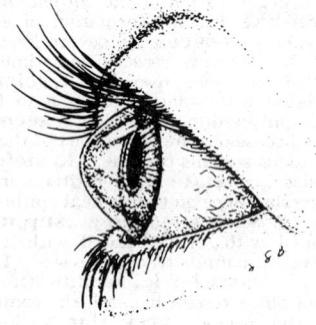

Keratoconus.

keratocyte (ker′ah-to-sīt″) [*kerato-* + -*cyte*] one of the flattened connective tissue cells between the lamellae of fibrous tissue composing the cornea.

keratoderma (ker″ah-to-der′mah) [*kerato-* + Gr. *derma* skin] 1. a horny skin or covering. 2. hypertrophy of the horny layer of the skin. Called also *keratodermia.* Cf. *hyperkeratosis* (def. 1), *keratoma* (def. 1), *keratosis, tyloma,* and *tylosis.* **k. blennorrha′gicum,** a cutaneous manifestation of Reiter's disease, most often involving the palms, soles, toes, and glans penis, and characterized by the presence of erythematous macules that vesiculate, become purulent, and develop thick keratotic coverings; the lesions are sometimes indistinguishable from those of pustular psoriasis. The disorder was formerly thought to be associated with gonorrhea. Called also *keratosis blennorrhagica.* **k. climacter′icum,** an acquired form of palmoplantar keratoderma occurring in women about the time of menopause, which may be associated with fissuring of the thickened patches. **k. palma′re et planta′re,** palmoplantar k. **palmoplantar k.,** a group of mostly inherited disorders characterized by the excessive formation of keratin, localized or diffuse, on the palms and soles, sometimes with painful lesions resulting from fissuring of the skin, which may occur alone or may accompany or be part of another disorder. Called also *hyperkeratosis of the palms and soles, ichthyosis palmaris et plantaris, k. palmare et plantare,* and *keratosis palmaris et plantaris.* **palmoplantar k., diffuse,** an autosomal

dominant disorder characterized by the presence of well-demarcated, usually bilateral and symmetrical, confluent areas of scaling on the palms and soles, sometimes involving adjacent skin of the hands and feet, which is usually present early but may appear later in life. Striate and punctate variants have also been reported; the latter may be associated with focal gingival hyperkeratosis. Called also *Unna-Thost disease* or *syndrome.* See also *Howell-Evans syndrome,* under *syndrome.*

keratodermatocele (ker″ah-to-der′mah-to-sēl) [*kerato-* + *dermato-* + Gr. *kēlē* hernia] keratocele.

keratodermia (ker″ah-to-der′me-ah) [*kerato-* + Gr. *derma* skin + -*ia*] keratoderma.

keratoectasia (ker″ah-to-ek-ta′ze-ah) kerectasis.

keratogenesis (ker″ah-to-jen′ĕ-sis) the formation or production of horny material.

keratogenetic (ker″ah-to-jĕ-net′ik) pertaining to keratogenesis.

keratogenous (ker″ah-toj′ĕ-nus) [*kerato-* + Gr. *gennan* to produce] giving rise to a growth of horny material.

keratoglobus (ker″ah-to-glo′bus) megalocornea.

keratohelcosis (ker″ah-to-hel-ko′sis) [*kerato-* + Gr. *helkōsis* ulceration] ulceration of the cornea.

keratohemia (ker″ah-to-he′me-ah) [*kerato-* + Gr. *haima* blood + -*ia*] the presence of deposits of blood in the cornea.

keratohyalin (ker″ah-to-hi′ah-lin) 1. a substance in the granules in the granular layer of the epidermis, the origin and chemistry of which is unclear, but which may be involved in the process of keratinization. See also *keratohyaline granules,* under *granule.* 2. a substance found in granules in the Hassall corpuscles of the thymus.

keratohyaline (ker″ah-to-hi′ah-līn) 1. both horny and hyaline. 2. pertaining to keratohyalin or to the keratohyalin granules or the keratohyaline layer (stratum granulosum epidermidis). 3. keratohyalin.

keratoid (ker′ah-toid) [*kerato-* + Gr. *eidos* form] resembling horn or corneal tissue.

keratoiditis (ker″ah-toi-di′tis) keratitis.

keratoiridocyclitis (ker″ah-to-ir″ĭ-do-sik-li′tis) [*kerato-* + *irido-* + *cyclitis*] inflammation of the cornea, iris, and ciliary body.

keratoiridoscope (ker″ah-to-i-rid′o-skōp) [*kerato-* + *irido-* + -*scope*] a form of compound microscope for examining the eye.

keratoiritis (ker″ah-to-i-ri′tis) [*kerato-* + Gr. *iris* iris + -*itis*] inflammation of the cornea and iris. **hypopyon k.,** hypopyon keratitis.

keratoleptynsis (ker″ah-to-lep-tin′sis) [*kerato-* + Gr. *leptynsis* attenuation] removal of the anterior portion of the cornea and covering of the denuded area with bulbar conjunctiva.

keratoleukoma (ker″ah-to-lu-ko′mah) [*kerato-* + *leukoma*] a white opacity of the cornea.

keratolysis (ker″ah-tol′ĭ-sis) [*kerato-* + Gr. *lysis* dissolution] softening and dissolution or peeling of the horny layer of the epidermis. **pitted k., k. planta′re sulca′tum,** a superficial bacterial infection of the skin of worldwide distribution usually involving the weight-bearing portions of the soles of the feet, and characterized by the formation of shallow asymptomatic discrete round pits, some of which become confluent and form fissures; the specific etiologic agent is unknown. Called also *cracked heels.*

keratolytic (ker″ah-to-lit′ik) 1. pertaining to, characterized by, or producing keratolysis. 2. an agent that promotes keratolysis.

keratoma (ker″ah-to′mah), pl. *keratomas* or *kerato′mata* [*kerato-* + -*oma*] 1. a callus or callosity. Cf. *hyperkeratosis* (def. 1), *keratoderma, keratosis, tyloma,* and *tylosis.* 2. a horny tumor on the inner surface of the wall of a horse's hoof. Called also *keraphyllocele.* **k. heredita′rium mu′tilans,** an autosomal dominant, progressive, dystrophic form of palmoplantar keratoderma, beginning in childhood, characterized by a stellate pattern of hyperkeratosis on the backs of the hands and feet, linear keratoses on the elbows and knees, and annular ainhum-like constriction of the digits, and sometimes associated with scarring alopecia and deafness. Called also *progressive dystrophic hyperkeratosis* and

Vohwinkel's syndrome. **k. planta′re sulca′tum,** pitted keratolysis. **k. seni′le,** actinic keratosis.

keratomalacia (ker″ah-to-mah-la′she-ah) [*kerato-* + *malacia*] a usually bilateral condition associated with vitamin A deficiency. It begins with xerotic spots (Bitôt's spots) on the conjunctiva, while the cornea becomes xerotic and insensitive (xerotic keratitis); as the condition progresses, the haze increases until finally the entire cornea becomes soft, and colliquative necrosis occurs.

keratomata (ker″ah-to′mah-tah) plural of *keratoma.*

keratome (ker′ah-tōm) [*kerato-* + *-tome*] a knife for incising the cornea.

keratometer (ker″ah-tom′ĕ-ter) [*kerato-* + *-meter*] an instrument for measuring the curves of the cornea; called also *ophthalmometer.*

keratometric (ker″ah-to-met′rik) pertaining to keratometry, or to measurements made with a keratometer.

keratometry (ker″ah-tom′ĕ-tre) [*kerato-* + *-metry*] measurement of the anterior curvature of the cornea with a keratometer; called also *ophthalmometry.*

keratomileusis (ker″ah-to-mĭ-loo′sis) [*kerato-* + Gr. *smileusis* carving] keratoplasty in which a slice of the patient's cornea is removed, shaped to the desired curvature on a lathe after freezing, and then sutured back on the remaining cornea to correct optical error.

keratomycosis (ker″ah-to-mi-ko′sis) [*kerato-* + Gr. *mykēs* fungus + *-osis*] fungous infection of the cornea. **k. lin′guae,** black tongue.

keratonosus (ker″ah-ton′o-sus) [*kerato-* + Gr. *nosos* disease] any disease of the cornea.

keratonyxis (ker″ah-to-nik′sis) [*kerato-* + *nyxis*] aqueous paracentesis.

keratopathy (ker″ah-top′ah-the) [*kerato-* + *-pathy*] a noninflammatory disease of the cornea. **band k., band-shaped k.,** a degenerative condition in which a gray band develops axially from the limbus at the level of Bowman's membrane into the exposed part of the cornea in the palpebral aperture. **bullous k.,** corneal degeneration marked by recurring epithelial blebs or bullae that rupture, expose corneal nerves, and cause great pain; it occurs in glaucoma, iridocyclitis, and Fuchs' epithelial dystrophy. **climatic k.,** bilateral, symmetrical corneal degeneration due to extreme heat or cold; called also *Labrador k.* **filamentary k.,** keratitis filamentosa. **Labrador k.,** climatic k. **lipid k.,** deposits of fat in an area of previous corneal vascularization. **striate k.,** corneal stromal edema causing a network of lines, which is a common, temporary occurrence after cataract surgery. Cf. *striate keratitis.* **vesicular k.,** corneal epithelial edema with formation of vacuoles. Cf. *vesicular keratitis.*

keratophakia (ker″ah-to-fa′ke-ah) [*kerato-* + Gr. *phakos* lentil, lens] a form of keratoplasty in which a slice of donor's cornea is shaped to a desired curvature and inserted between layers of the recipient's cornea to change its curvature.

keratoplasty (ker′ah-to-plas″te) [*kerato-* + *-plasty*] plastic surgery of the cornea; corneal grafting. **autogenous k.,** autokeratoplasty. **lamellar k.** a transplant of the anterior half of the cornea with the anterior chamber remaining intact. **optic k.,** transplantation of corneal material to replace scar tissue which interferes with vision. **penetrating k.,** a transplant of a section of full-thickness cornea. **refractive k.,** that in which a section of cornea is removed from the patient or a donor, shaped to the desired curvature, and inserted either between (keratophakia) layers of or on (keratomileusis) the patient's cornea to change its curvature and correct optical errors. **tectonic k.,** transplantation of corneal material to replace tissue which has been lost.

keratoprotein (ker″ah-to-pro′te-in) [*kerato-* + *protein*] the protein of the horny tissues of the body, such as the hair, nails, and epidermis.

keratorhexis, keratorrhexis (ker″ah-to-rek′sis) [*kerato-* + *rhexis*] rupture of the cornea.

keratoscleritis (ker″ah-to-skle-ri′tis) inflammation of the cornea and sclera.

keratoscope (ker′ah-to-skōp″) [*kerato-* + *-scope*] a device consisting of alternate black or white concentric circles and used for examining corneal curvature; called also *Placido's disk.*

keratoscopy (ker″ah-tos′ko-pe) the examination of the cornea; more especially the study of the reflections of light from its anterior surface.

keratosis (ker″ah-to′sis), pl. *kerato′ses* [*kerato-* + *-osis*] any horny growth, such as a wart or callosity, usually either an actinic keratosis or a seborrheic keratosis. Cf. *hyperkeratosis* (def. 1), *keratoderma, keratoma* (def. 1), *tyloma,* and *tylosis.* **actinic k.,** a sharply outlined, red or skin-colored, flat or elevated, verrucous or keratotic growth, which may develop into a cutaneous horn, and may give rise to a squamous cell carcinoma; it usually affects the middle-aged or elderly, especially those of fair complexion, and is caused by excessive exposure to the sun. Called also *solar k;* formerly called *keratoma senile* and *senile k.* **arsenic k., arsenical k.,** a cutaneous manifestation of chronic arsenic poisoning, after use for medicinal purposes or other exposure, which may occur years after arsenic ingestion, characterized by the development of discrete hyperkeratotic papules, chiefly located on the palms and soles, and sometimes associated with premalignant and malignant epidermal lesions on other skin areas. **k. blennorrha′gica,** keratoderma blennorrhagicum. **k. follicula′ris,** a slowly progressive autosomal dominant disorder of keratinization characterized by pinkish to tan or skin-colored papules on the seborrheic areas of the body that coalesce to form plaques, which may become crusted and secondarily infected; over time, the lesions may become darker and may fuse to form papillomatous and warty malodorous growths. Called also *Darier's disease* and *Darier-White disease.* **k. follicula′ris contagio′sa,** a widespread, symmetrical eruption of the skin resembling keratosis follicularis, most often involving the back of the neck, shoulders, and extensor surfaces of the extremities, which occurs in children, and is apparently an infectious disease. Called also *Brooke's disease* and *epidemic acne.* **k. lin′guae,** leukoplakia. **k. obtu′rans,** a condition characterized by a mass of epidermic scales and cerumen obstructing the external auditory meatus. **k. palma′ris et planta′ris,** palmoplantar keratoderma. **k. pharyn′gea,** a condition characterized by projection of numerous white horny masses from the tonsils and from the orifices of the lymph follicles in the wall of the pharynx. **k. pila′ris,** a condition in which hyperkeratosis is limited to the hair follicles, usually on the extensor surfaces of the thighs and arms, but occurring anywhere, with discrete follicular papules which re-form after removal. **k. puncta′ta,** a form of hyperkeratosis in which the lesions are localized in multiple points on the palms and soles; it is transmitted as an autosomal dominant. **roentgen k.,** premalignant keratotic lesions occurring at the site of severe chronic radiodermatitis. **seborrheic k., k. seborrhe′ica,** a common benign, noninvasive tumor composed of basaloid cells, usually occurring in middle life, sometimes rapidly in crops, commonly presenting as soft, friable plaques that show slight to marked pigmentation and are most often located on the face, trunk, and extremities. Called also *seborrheic wart* and *verruca seborrheica.* See also *Leser-Trélat sign,* under *sign.* **senile k., k. seni′lis,** actinic k. **solar k.,** actinic k. **stucco k.,** a condition seen especially in men over the age of 40 who have dry skin, characterized by the presence of multiple superficial, gray to light brown, flat keratotic lesions with a "stuck-on" appearance on the dorsa of the feet and hands, ankles, instep, and forearms; thought by some authorities to be a variant of seborrheic keratosis. **k. suprafollicula′ris** (*obs.*), k. pilaris. **tar k.,** a keratosis caused by exposure to tar, in which keratotic foci develop, sometimes followed by the formation of keratoacanthomas or intraepidermal, squamous, or basal cell carcinoma.

keratosulfate (ker″ah-to-sul′fāt) keratan sulfate.

keratotic (ker″ah-tot′ik) pertaining to, characterized by, or promoting keratosis.

keratotome (ker-at′o-tōm) keratome.

keratotomy (ker″ah-tot′o-me) [*kerato-* + *-tomy*] surgical incision of the cornea. **delimiting k.,** incision of the cornea in ulcus serpens by a cut tangential to the advancing border of the ulcer and made to emerge at a corresponding point in the other side. **radial k.,** an operation in which a series of incisions is made in the cornea from its outer edge toward its center in spoke-like fashion; done to flatten the cornea and thus to correct myopia.

keratotorus (ker″ah-to-to′rus) [*kerato-* + L. *torus* a protuberance] a vaultlike protrusion of the cornea.

Kerckring's (Kerkring's) center (ossicle), folds (valves) (kerk′ringz) [Theodorus *Kerckring*, Dutch anatomist, 1640–1693] see under *center* and *fold*.

kerectasis (ke-rek′tah-sis) [Gr. *keras* cornea + *ektasis* distention] a uniform bulging or protrusion of the cornea.

kerectomy (ke-rek′to-me) keratectomy.

kerion (ke′re-on) [Gr. *kērion* honeycomb] a nodular, boggy, exudative, circumscribed tumefaction which is covered with pustules, occurring in association with tinea infections, usually tinea barbae and tinea capitis.

Kerkring see *Kerckring*.

kerma (ker′mah) [*k*inetic energy *r*eleased in *ma*terial] a unit of quantity that represents the kinetic energy transferred to charged particles by the uncharged particles per unit mass of an irradiated medium.

kermes (ker′mēz) [Arabic, Persian] the *Coccus ilicis*, an insect found on the leaves of various oaks, chiefly on *Quercus coccifera* (kermes-oak). It furnishes a red pigment which is used as a dyestuff.

Kern see *Ke*.

kernel (ker′nel) that part of an atom left after removal of the valence electrons.

kernicterus (ker-nik′ter-us) [Ger. "nuclear jaundice"] a condition with severe neural symptoms, associated with high levels of bilirubin in the blood. It is characterized by deep yellow staining of the basal nuclei, globus pallidus, putamen, and caudate nucleus, as well as the cerebellar and bulbar nuclei, and gray substance of the cerebrum, and is accompanied by widespread destructive changes. It is commonly a sequela of icterus gravis neonatorum. Called also *bilirubin encephalopathy*.

Kernig's sign (ker′nigz) [Vladimir Mikhailovich *Kernig*, Russian physician, 1840–1917] see under *sign*.

keroid (ker′oid) keratoid.

kerosene, kerosine (ker′o-sēn) a colorless volatile liquid distilled from petroleum; it is used as a reagent and in insecticides.

kerril (ker′il) a venomous sea snake, *Kerilia jerdoni*, of the Indian Ocean.

Keshan disease (ke′shan) [*Keshan* a province of China] see under *disease*.

Kesling appliance, spring (kes′ling) [Harold D. *Kesling*, American orthodontist, born 1901] see under *appliance* and *spring*.

Ketaject (ket′ah-jekt) trademark for a preparation of ketamine hydrochloride.

ketal (ke′tal) a derivative formed by a combination of a ketone with an alcohol.

Ketalar (ket′ah-lar) trademark for a preparation of ketamine hydrochloride.

ketamine hydrochloride (kēt′ah-mēn) [USP] chemical name: 2-(2-chlorophenyl)-2-(methylamino)cyclohexanone hydrochloride. A rapid-acting general anesthetic, $C_{13}H_{16}ClNO \cdot HCl$, occurring as a white, crystalline powder; administered intramuscularly and intravenously.

ketazocine (ket-a′zo-sēn) chemical name: $(2\alpha,6\alpha,11S^*)$-3-(cyclopropylmethyl)3,4,5,6- tetrahydro- 8- hydroxy-6, 11-dimethyl- 2,6 -methano- 3 -benzazocin-1(2*H*)- one; an analgesic, $C_{18}H_{23}NO_2$.

ketazolam (ke-ta′zo-lam) chemical name: 11-chloro-8, 12b-dihydro - 2, 8 - dimethyl - 4*H* [1, 3] oxazino[3,2-*d*]-[1,4]benzodiazepine; a minor tranquilizer, $C_{20}H_{17}ClN_2O_3$.

ketene (ke′tēn) a colorless gas of penetrating odor, carbomethane, $H_2C\text{:}CO$; also any one of several derivatives from it. It combines with water to form acetic acid.

kethoxal (ke-thoks′al) chemical name: 3-ethoxy-1,1-dihydroxy-2-butanone; an antiviral agent, $C_6H_{12}O_4$.

ketimine (ke′tĭ-min) a compound in which the oxygen of a ketone is replaced by the imino group.

ketipramine fumarate (ke-tip′rah-mēn) chemical name: 5-[3-(dimethylamino)propyl]-5,11-dihydro-10*H*-dibenz[*b,f*]azepin- 10 - one; an antidepressant, $C_{19}H_{22}N_2O \cdot C_4H_4O_4$.

keto- a prefix which denotes possession of the carbonyl group, :C:O, in a structure in which the other two bonds to carbon are attached to hydrocarbon moieties.

keto acid (ke′to) a carboxylic acid containing a carbonyl group, e.g., α-ketoglutaric acid.

keto acid decarboxylase (ke′to as′id de″kar-bok′sĭ-lās) branched-chain α-keto acid dehydrogenase.

keto acid decarboxylase deficiency maple syrup urine disease.

ketoacidemia (ke″to-as″id-e′me-ah) the presence of keto acids in the blood. **branched-chain k.,** maple syrup urine disease.

ketoacidosis (ke″to-ah″sĭ-do′sis) acidosis accompanied by the accumulation of ketone bodies (ketosis) in the body tissues and fluids, as in diabetic acidosis.

ketoaciduria (ke″to-as″ĭ-du′re-ah) the presence of keto acids in the urine. **branched-chain k.,** maple syrup urine disease.

3-ketoacyl-CoA thiolase (ke″to-as′il ko′a thi′o-lās) acetyl-CoA acyltransferase.

keto-aldehyde (ke″to-al′de-hīd) see under *aldehyde*.

ketoaminoacidemia (ke″to-ah-me″no-as″ĭ-de′me-ah) maple syrup urine disease.

β-ketobutyric acid (ke″to-bu-tēr′ik) acetoacetic acid.

ketoconazole (ke″to-kon′ah-zōl) a broad-spectrum antifungal agent, given orally, that has been reported effective in the treatment of a variety of extensive, chronic cutaneous fungal infections.

Keto-Diastix (ke″to-di′ah-stiks) trademark for a reagent strip designed for the determination of ketones and glucose in urine.

ketogenesis (ke″to-jen′ĕ-sis) [*ketone* + Gr. *genesis* production] the production of ketone (acetone) bodies.

ketogenetic (ke″to-je-net′ik) forming ketone bodies.

ketogenic (ke″to-jen′ik) forming or capable of being converted into ketone bodies. Metabolic sources are fatty acids and some of the amino acids of protein.

α-ketoglutarate (ke″to-gloo′tah-rāt) an anionic form of α-ketoglutaric acid.

α-ketoglutarate dehydrogenase (ke″to-gloo′tah-rāt de-hi′dro-jĕ-nās) [EC 1.2.4.2] an enzyme of the oxidoreductase class that catalyzes the reaction α-ketoglutarate + lipoamide = S-succinyldihydrolipoamide + CO_2. The enzyme requires thiamine diphosphate and is a component of the multienzyme α-ketoglutarate dehydrogenase complex. Called also *oxoglutarate dehydrogenase (lipoamide)* in formal EC nomenclature. See also under *complex*.

α-ketoglutarate glyoxylate carboligase (ke″to-gloo′-tah-rāt gli-ok′sĭ-lāt kar″bo-li′-gās) an enzyme that catalyzes the reaction glyoxylate + α-ketoglutarate = α-hydroxy-β-ketoadipate + CO_2. The reaction requires thiamine pyrophosphate. Deficiency of the enzyme, an autosomal recessive trait, causes primary hyperoxaluria type I.

α-ketoglutaric acid (ke″to-gloo-tar′ik) 2-oxopentanedioic acid, 2-oxoglutaric acid, an intermediate in the tricarboxylic acid cycle (q.v.); α-ketoglutarate is also produced from glutamate in amino group transfer reactions and by oxidative deamination.

ketoheptose (ke″to-hep′tōs) a ketone sugar containing seven carbon atoms: $C_7H_{14}O_7$.

ketohexokinase (ke″to-hek″so-ki′nās) [EC 2.7.1.3] an enzyme of the transferase class that catalyzes the reaction ATP + D-fructose = ADP + D-fructose 1-phosphate. Genetic deficiency of the enzyme leads to essential fructosuria. Called also *fructokinase*.

ketohexose (ke″to-hek′sōs) a hexose which contains a ketone group. Cf. *aldohexose*.

ketohydroxyestrin (ke″to-hi-drok″se-es′trin) estrone.

α-ketoisovalerate dehydrogenase (ke″to-i″so-val′er-āt de-hi′dro-jĕ-nās) [EC 1.2.4.4] an enzyme of the oxidoreductase class that catalyzes the reaction 3-methyl-2-ketobutanoate + lipoamide = S-(2-methylpropanoyl) dihydrolipoamide + CO_2. It also acts on 2-ketoisocaproate and 2-keto-3-methylvalerate. The enzyme is a part of the branched-chain α-keto acid dehydrogenase complex, and the reaction is a step in the use of the branched-chain amino acids leucine, isoleucine, and valine as fuels. See also *maple syrup urine disease*.

ketol (ke′tol) a ketonic alcohol.

ketol-isomerase (ke″tol-i-som′er-ās) [EC 5.3.1] an enzyme of the transferase class, that catalyzes the interconversion aldose = ketose.

ketolysis (ke-tol′ĭ-sis) [*ketone* + Gr. *lysis* dissolution] the cleavage of ketone bodies.

ketolytic (ke″to-lit′ik) pertaining to, characterized by, or promoting ketolysis.

ketone (ke′tōn) any of a large class of organic compounds containing the carbonyl group, C=O, whose carbon atom is joined to two other carbon atoms, that is, with the carbonyl group occurring within the carbon chain. See also under *body*. **dimethyl k.,** acetone.

ketonemia (ke″to-ne′me-ah) [*ketone* + Gr. *haima* blood + *-ia*] an excess of ketone bodies in the blood, as in starvation and diabetes mellitus.

ketonic (ke-to′nik) pertaining to or developed from a ketone.

ketonization (ke″to-ni-za′shun) conversion into a ketone.

ketonuria (ke″to-nu′re-ah) [*ketone* + Gr. *ouron* urine + *-ia*] ketone bodies in the urine, as in diabetes mellitus.

ketonurine (ke″tōn-u′rin) the urine excreted after administration of a ketogenic diet.

ketoplasia (ke″to-pla′se-ah) the formation of ketone bodies.

ketoplastic (ke″to-plas′tik) [*ketone* + Gr. *plassein* to form] pertaining to, characterized by, or promoting the formation of ketone bodies.

ketoprofen (ke″to-pro′fen) a non-steroidal anti-inflammatory agent that is a propionic acid derivative.

β-keto-reductase (ke″to-re-duk′tās) 1. 3-hydroxyacyl CoA dehydrogenase. 2. the enzymatic activity in fatty acid synthase that reduces 3-ketoacyl groups on the carrier protein to the 3-hydroxyacyl derivative using NADPH.

ketose (ke′tōs) a ketone derivative of a polyatomic alcohol (any sugar which contains a ketone group).

ketoside (ke′to-sīd) any glycoside which yields a ketose on hydrolysis.

ketosis (ke-to′sis) a condition characterized by an abnormally elevated concentration of ketone bodies in the body tissues and fluids; it is a complication of diabetes mellitus and starvation.

ketosteroid (ke-to′ste-roid) a steroid that possesses ketone groups on functional carbon atoms. The 17-ketosteroids, usually denoting urinary metabolites of androgens secreted by the human adrenal cortex and gonads, have a ketone group on the 17th carbon atom. They are found in the urine of normal men and women and in excess in certain adrenal cortical and ovarian tumors. The principal ketosteroids are androsterone, epiandrosterone, etiocholanolone, dehydroepiandrosterone, and a few 11-oxygenated 17-ketosteroids. Abbreviated 17-KS.

ketosuria (ke″to-su′re-ah) the presence of ketose in the urine.

keto-tetrahydrophenanthrene (ke″to-tet″rah-hi″dro-fe-nan′thrēn) 1-keto-1,2,3,4-tetrahydrophenanthrene, a carcinogenic substance.

ketotetrose (ke″to-tet′rōs) a ketose that contains 4 carbon atoms.

3-ketothiolase (ke″to-thi′o-lās) acetyl-CoA acyltransferase.

3-ketothiolase deficiency a genetic aminoacidopathy due to an enzyme deficiency in the sixth, last, step of isoleucine catabolism and characterized by episodes of ketoacidosis and urinary excretion of several intermediates in the isoleucine pathway.

β-ketothiolase (ke″to-thi′o-lās) acetyl-CoA acyltransferase.

ketotic (ke-tot′ik) pertaining to, characterized by, or causing ketosis.

ketotransferase (ke″to-trans′fer-ās) transketolase.

ketourine (ke″to-u′rin) ketonurine.

ketoxime (ke-tok′sīm) the oxime derivative of a ketone.

keV, kev, kilo electron volt.

key (ke) 1. an instrument for opening a lock, or a device for making or breaking an electric circuit; by extension, any tool for revealing specific information. **torquing k.,** an orthodontic instrument used to facilitate the engaging of rectangular arch wires into the edgewise brackets.

keynote (ke′nōt) in homeopathy, the characteristic property of a drug which indicates its use in treating a similar symptom of disease.

Key-Retzius connective tissue sheath, foramen (ke′ret′ze-us) [Ernst Axel Henrik *Key*, Swedish physician, 1832–1901; Magnus Gustaf *Retzius*, Swedish histologist, 1842–1919] see *connective tissue sheath of Key and Retzius*, under *sheath*, and see *apertura lateralis ventriculi quarti*.

kg kilogram.

KHCO₃ potassium bicarbonate.

khellin (kel′in) chemical name: 4,9-dimethoxy-7-methyl-5H-furo[3,2-g][1]benzopyran-5-one. An active principle, $C_{14}H_{12}O_5$, from the fruit of *Ammi visnaga* Lam., an umbelliferous plant of Eastern Mediterranean regions; an antihypertensive and vasodilator.

Khorana (ko-rah′nah), Har Gobind. Indian-born American chemist, born 1922; co-winner, with Robert William Holley and Marshall Warren Nirenberg, of the Nobel prize for medicine or physiology in 1968 for discovery of the process by which enzymes determine a cell's function in a genetic environment.

KI potassium iodide.

kibisitome (ki-bis′ĭ-tōm) [Gr. *kibisis* pouch + *-tome*] cystitome.

kidney (kid′ne) [L. *ren*; Gr. *nephros*] either of the two organs in the lumbar region that filter the blood, excreting the end-products of body metabolism in the form of urine, and regulating the concentrations of hydrogen, sodium, potassium, phosphate, and other ions in the extracellular fluid. Called also *ren* [NA]. Each kidney is about four inches long, two inches wide, and one inch thick, and weighs from four to six ounces. The kidney is of characteristic shape, and presents a notch on the inner, concave, border, known as the *hilus*, which communicates with the cavity or sinus of the kidney and through which the vessels, nerves, and ureter pass. The kidney consists of a *cortex* and a *medulla*. The medullary substance forms pyramids, whose bases are in the cortex and whose apices, which are called *papillae*, project into the calices of the kidney. The renal pyramids number from 10 to 15. The parenchyma of each kidney is composed of about one million *renal tubules* (nephrons, the functional unit of the kidney), held together by a little connective tissue. Each tubule begins blindly in a renal corpuscle, consisting of a glomerulus and its capsule, situated within the cortex. After a neck or constriction below the capsule, it becomes the proximal convoluted tubule, Henle's loop, distal convoluted tubule, arched collecting tubule, and then the straight collecting tubule, which opens at the apex of a renal papilla. The straight collecting tubules converge as they descend, forming groups in the center, known as *medullary rays*. **abdominal k.,** an ectopic kidney situated above the iliac crest with the hilus adjacent to the second lumbar vertebra. **amyloid k.,** one marked by deposition of amyloid, usually concentrated in small blood vessels and capillaries; called also *Rokitansky's k.* **arteriosclerotic k.,** one characterized by sclerotic changes of intrarenal arteries and large arterioles. **artificial k.,** a popular name for an extracorporeal device employed to remove from the blood, while it is being circulated outside the body, elements which are usually excreted in the urine; see *hemodialyzer.* Intracorporeal artificial kidneys are under development, in which intestinal or pulmonary tissue is used as the filtration membrane. **atrophic k.,** one that is diminished in size because of inadequate circulation and/or loss of nephrons. **cake k.,** a solid, irregularly lobed organ of bizarre shape, usually situated in the pelvis toward the midline, developed as result of fusion of the two renal anlagen. **cicatricial k.,** a shriveled, irregular, and scarred kidney, resulting from suppurative pyelonephritis. **clump k.,** cake k. **congested k.,** large red k. **contracted k.,** an atrophic kidney which may be scarred and granular. **crush k.,** lower nephron nephrosis. **cyanotic k.,** passive congestion of the kidney. **cystic k.,** a kidney containing one or more cysts. **definite k.,** metanephros. **disk k.,** a disk-shaped organ produced by fusion of both poles of the contralateral kidney anlagen. **doughnut k.,** an anomalous organ resulting from bipolar fusion of the renal anlagen before rotation begins, both kidneys being on the same level. **fatty k.,** a kidney affected with fatty degeneration. **flea-bitten k.,** a kidney which has small, randomly scattered petechiae on its surface, sometimes seen in bacterial

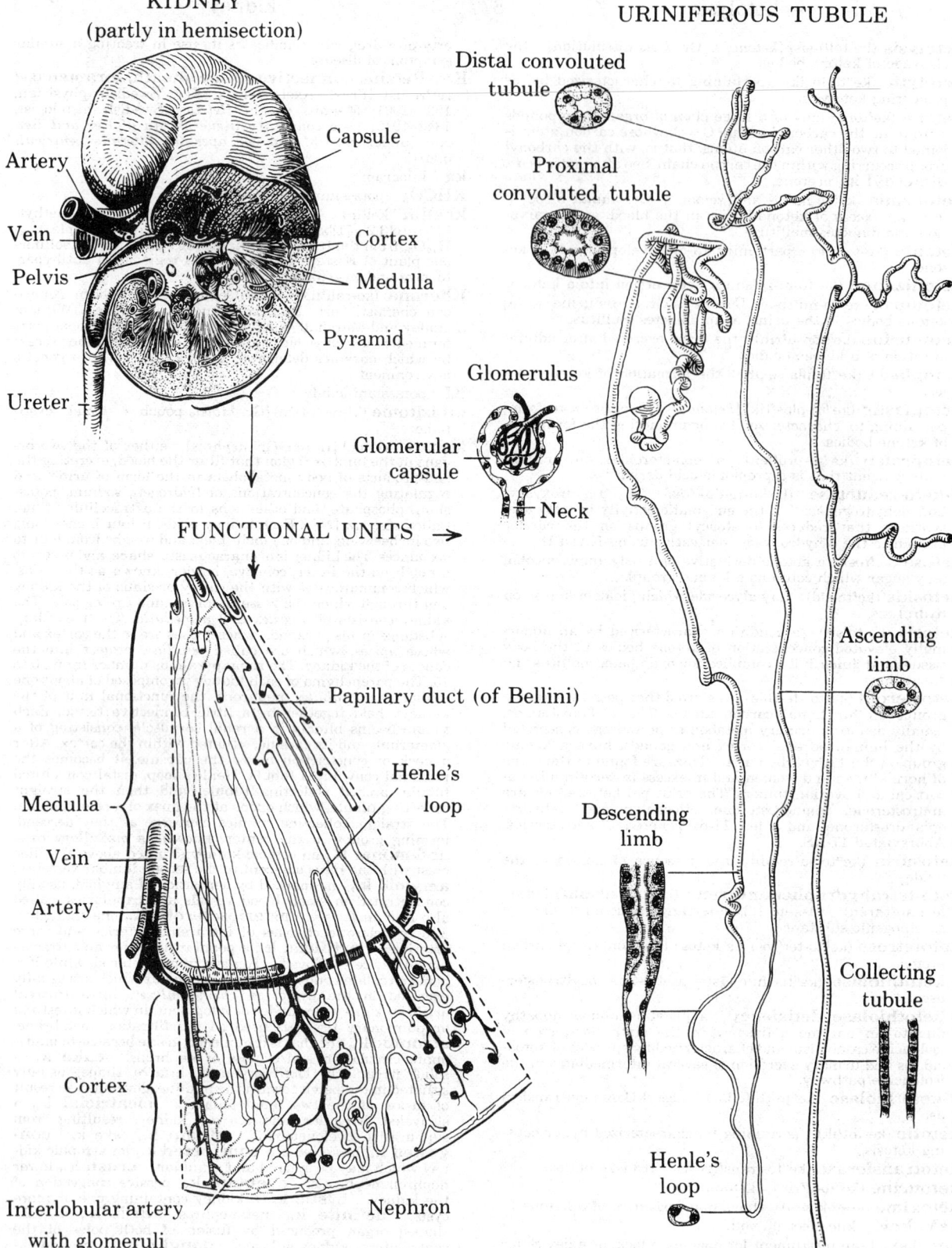

KIDNEY
(partly in hemisection)

Artery

Vein

Pelvis

Ureter

Capsule

Cortex

Medulla

Pyramid

FUNCTIONAL UNITS →

Medulla

Vein

Artery

Cortex

Interlobular artery
with glomeruli

Papillary duct (of Bellini)

Henle's
loop

Nephron

URINIFEROUS TUBULE

Distal convoluted
tubule

Proximal
convoluted tubule

Glomerulus

Glomerular
capsule

Neck

Ascending
limb

Descending
limb

Collecting
tubule

Henle's
loop

PLATE 21 — STRUCTURE OF THE KIDNEY

endocarditis. **floating k.**, hypermobile k. **Formad's k.**, an enlarged and deformed kidney, sometimes seen in chronic alcoholism. **fused k.**, a single anomalous organ developed as a result of fusion of the renal anlagen. **Goldblatt k.**, one in which the blood flow is obstructed, resulting in renal hypertension. **head k.**, pronephros. **hind k.**, metanephros. **horseshoe k.**, an anomalous organ developed as a result of fusion of the corresponding poles of the renal anlagen. **hypermobile k.**, one that is freely movable. **lardaceous k.**, amyloid k. **large red k.**, a congested, edematous kidney which may result from inflammation, impaired venous circulation, or urinary obstruction; called also *congested k.* **lumbar k.**, an ectopic kidney situated opposite the sacral promontory in the iliac fossa, anterior to the iliac vessels. **lump k.**, cake k. **medullary sponge k.**, sponge k. **middle k.**, mesonephros. **mortar k.**, putty k. **movable k.**, hypermobile k. **mural k.**, a kidney located in a pocket of peritoneum in the abdominal wall. **myelin k.**, a kidney infiltrated with myelin, producing minute whitish specks or streaks on its surface. **myeloma k.**, renal changes occurring in multiple myeloma, due to filtration of large amounts of Bence Jones protein; they include tubular atrophy with the presence of intraluminal casts and multinucleated giant cells in tubular walls and interstitium, and they result in renal failure. **pelvic k.**, an ectopic kidney situated opposite the sacrum and below the aortic bifurcation. **polycystic k.**, see *polycystic disease of the kidneys*, under *disease*. **primordial k.**, pronephros. **putty k.**, one containing caseous material trapped by stricture of the ureter by tuberculous granulations in renal tuberculosis. **Rokitansky's k.**, amyloid k. **Rose-Bradford k.**, a form of fibrotic kidney of inflammatory origin found in young subjects. **sacciform k.**, a distended kidney; nephrectasia. **sigmoid k.**, a deformed and fused kidney, the upper pole of one kidney being fused with the lower pole of the other. **sponge k.**, a rare congenital condition, anatomically characterized by multiple small cystic dilatations of the collecting tubules of the medullary portion of the renal pyramids, giving the organ a spongy, porous feeling and appearance. It is usually asymptomatic, but there may be calculus formation within the cysts, hematuria, renal colic, or recurrent renal infection. **supernumerary k.**, a kidney in addition to the two usually present, developed as the result of splitting of the nephrogenic blastema, or from separate metanephric blastemas into which partially or completely reduplicated ureteral stalks enter to form separate capsulated kidneys. In some cases the separation of the reduplicated organ is incomplete (*fused supernumerary k.*). **thoracic k.**, an ectopic kidney that partially or completely protrudes above the diaphragm into the posterior mediastinum. **wandering k.**, hypermobile k. **waxy k.**, amyloid k.

Kielland's (Kjelland) forceps (kel'andz) [Christian *Kielland*, Norwegian obstetrician and gynecologist, 1871–1941] see under *forceps*.

Kienböck disease, etc. (kēn'bek) [Robert *Kienböck*, Austrian roentgenologist, 1871–1953] see under *disease, dislocation, phenomenon,* and *unit.*

Kienböck-Adamson points (kēn'bek-ad'am-son) [Robert *Kienböck*; Horatio George *Adamson*, London dermatologist, 1865–1955] see under *point.*

Kiernan's spaces (kēr'nanz) [Francis *Kiernan*, English physician, 1800–1874] see under *space.*

Kiesselbach's area (space) (ke'sel-bahks) [Wilhelm *Kiesselbach*, German laryngologist, 1839–1902] see under *area.*

kiestein (ki-es'te-in) · kyestein.

kil (kil) a white, sticky, soapy clay from the Black Sea region; when sterilized, it is employed as an ointment base for use in skin diseases.

Kilian's line (kil'e-anz) [Hermann Friedrich *Kilian*, German gynecologist, 1800–1863] see under *line.*

killeen (kil'lēn) chondrus.

Killian's operation (kil'e-anz) [Gustav *Killian*, German laryngologist, 1860–1921] see under *operation.*

Killian's test (kil'e-anz) [John Allen *Killian*, biochemist in New York, born 1891] see under *tests.*

Killian-Freer operation (kil'e-an frēr) [Gustav *Killian*; Otto *Freer*, American laryngologist, 1857–1932] see under *operation.*

kilo- [Fr., from Gr. *chilioi* thousand] a combining form used in naming units of measurement to indicate a quantity one thousand (10^3) times the unit designated by the root with which it is combined. Symbol, k.

kilobase (kil'o-bās) a unit used in designating the length of a nucleic acid sequence; e.g., 7 kb indicates a sequence 7000 nucleotides long.

kilocalorie (kil'o-kal"o-re) large calorie; see under *calorie.*

kilocurie (kil"o-cu're) a unit of radioactivity, being one thousand (10^3) curies, or the quantity of radioactive material in which the number of nuclear disintegrations is 3.7×10^{13} per second. Abbreviated kCi.

kilocycle (kil'o-si"kl) a unit of 1000 (10^3) cycles, e.g., 1000 cycles per second, applied to the frequency of electromagnetic waves. Abbreviated kc.

kilogram (kil'o-gram) a unit of mass (weight) of the metric system, being 1000 (10^3) grams, or the equivalent of 2.204623 pounds avoirdupois and of 2.679229 pounds apothecaries' weight. Abbreviated kg.

kilohertz (kil'o-hertz) one thousand (10^3) hertz (cycles per second). Abbreviated kHz.

kilometer (kil'o-me"ter, kĭ-lom'ĕ-ter) [Fr. *kilométre*] a unit of linear measurement of the metric system, being 1000 (10^3) meters, or the equivalent of 3280.83 feet, or about five-eighths of a mile. Abbreviated km.

kilounit (kil"o-u'nit) a quantity equivalent to one thousand (10^3) units.

kilovolt (kil'o-vōlt) a unit of electrical pressure or electromotive force, being 1000 (10^3) volts. Symbol, kV.

Kimberley horse disease (kim'ber-le) [Kimberley, a district in northeastern Western Australia] see under *disease.*

Kimmelstiel-Wilson syndrome (kim'el-stēl wil'son) [Paul *Kimmelstiel*, German pathologist in the United States, 1900–1970; Clifford *Wilson*, English physician, born 1906] intercapillary glomerulosclerosis.

Kimpton-Brown tube (kimp'ton brown') [Arthur Ronald *Kimpton*, Boston surgeon, born 1881] see under *tube.*

kinanesthesia (kin"an-es-the'ze-ah) [Gr. *kinēsis* motion + *anesthesia*] loss of power of perceiving the sensation of movement, due to derangement of deep sensibility.

kinase (ki'nās) 1. [EC 2.7] a subclass of the transferase class of enzymes, comprising those that catalyze the transfer of a high-energy phosphate group from a donor compound (e.g., ATP or GTP) to an acceptor compound (alcohol, carboxyl, nitrogenous group, or another phosphate group). 2. an enzyme that converts an inactive or precursor form of an enzyme to the active form.

kine-, kin(o)- [Gr. *kinein* to move] a combining form denoting relationship to movement. For words beginning *kine-*, see also words beginning *cine-*.

kinematics (kin"ĕ-mat'iks) [Gr. *kinēma* motion] that phase of mechanics which deals with the possible motions of a material body.

kinemia (ki-ne'me-ah) cardiac output; see under *output.*

kinemic (ki-ne'mik) [*kine-* + Gr. *haima* blood] pertaining to kinemia.

kineplastics (kin"ĕ-plas'tiks) kineplasty.

kineplasty (kin'ĕ-plas"te) [Gr. *kinein* to move + *plassein* to form] plastic amputation; amputation in which the stump is so formed as to be utilized for motor purposes.

kinesalgia (kin"ĕ-sal'je-ah) [*kinesio-* + *-algia*] pain on muscular exertion.

kinescope (kin'ĕ-skōp) [*kine-* + Gr. *skopein* to examine] an instrument for measuring ocular refraction, in which the patient observes a fixed object through a slit in a moving disk.

kinesia (ki-ne'se-ah) kinetosis.

kinesialgia (ki-ne"se-al'je-ah) kinesalgia.

kinesiatrics (ki-ne"se-at'riks) [*kinesio-* + Gr. *iatrikē* surgery, medicine] kinesitherapy.

kinesics (ki-ne'siks) the study of body movement as a part of the process of communication.

kinesi-esthesiometer (ki-ne"se-es-the"ze-om'ĕ-ter) [*kinesio-* + Gr. *aisthēsis* perception + *metron* measure] an instrument for estimating or measuring the sense of motion.

kinesimeter (kin″ĕ-sim′ĕ-ter) [*kinesio-* + Gr. *metron* measure] 1. an instrument for the quantitative measurement of movements. 2. an instrument for exploring the surface of the body to test cutaneous sensibility.

kinesi(o)- [Gr. *kinēsis* movement] a combining form denoting relationship to movement.

kinesiodic (ki-ne″se-od′ik) kinesodic.

kinesiology (ki-ne″se-ol′o-je) [*kinesio-* + *-logy*] the sum of what is known regarding human motion; the study of motion of the human body.

kinesiometer (ki-ne″se-om′ĕ-ter) kinesimeter.

kinesioneurosis (ki-ne″se-o-nu-ro′sis) [*kinesio-* + *neurosis*] a functional nervous disorder characterized by motor disturbances, such as spasms or tics.

kinesiotherapy (ki-ne″se-o-ther′ah-pe) kinesitherapy.

kinesis (ki-ne′sis) [Gr.] 1. movement, e.g., the activity of an organism in response to a stimulus; the direction of the response is not controlled by the direction of the stimulus (in contrast to a taxis). 2. a word termination denoting movement or motion, e.g., cytokinesis.

kinesitherapy (ki-ne″sĕ-ther′ah-pe) [*kinesio-* + Gr. *therapeia* cure] the treatment of disease by movements or exercise.

kinesodic (kin″ĕ-sod′ik) [*kinesio-* + Gr. *hodos* way] conducting or pertaining to the conduction of motor impulses.

kinesthesia (kin″es-the′ze-ah) [*kine-* + Gr. *aisthēsis* perception + *-ia*] the sense by which movement, weight, position, etc., are perceived; commonly used to refer specifically to the perception of changes in the angles of joints.

kinesthesiometer (kin″es-the″ze-om′ĕ-ter) [*kinesthesia* + Gr. *metron* measure] an instrument for testing kinesthesia.

kinesthesis (kin″es-the′sis) kinesthesia.

kinesthetic (kin″es-thet′ik) pertaining to kinesthesia or the muscular sense.

kinetia (ki-ne′she-ah) plural of *kinety*.

kinetic (kĭ-net′ik) [Gr. *kinētikos*] pertaining to or producing motion.

kineticist (ki-net′ĭ-sist) a specialist in kinetics.

kinetics (kĭ-net′iks, ki-net′iks) [Gr. *kinētikos* of or for putting in motion] the branch of dynamics that pertains to the turnover, or rate of change, of a specific factor (e.g., erythrocytes—erythrokinetics, leukocytes—leukokinetics, or iron—ferrokinetics), commonly expressed as units of amount per unit time. **chemical k.,** the study of the rates and mechanisms of chemical reactions.

kinetin (ki-ne′tin) a highly potent plant-growth factor, 6-furfurylaminopurine, which promotes cytokinesis in tobacco callus tissue.

kinetism (kin′ĕ-tizm) the ability to perform or initiate muscular action.

kinet(o)- [Gr. *kinētos* movable] a combining form denoting relationship to motion.

kinetocardiogram (ki-ne″to-kar′de-o-gram) the graphic record obtained by kinetocardiography; called also *precordial cardiogram*.

kinetocardiography (ki-ne″to-kar″de-og′rah-fe) the technique of graphically recording the slow vibrations of the anterior chest wall in the region of the heart, the vibrations representing the absolute motion of the heart at a given point on the chest.

kinetochore (ki-ne′to-kōr) [*kineto-* + Gr. *chora* space] a structure beside the centromere and to which the spindle fibers are attached.

kinetocyte (ki-ne′to-sīt) [*kineto-* + *-cyte*] a term once applied to one of the round or oval bodies about the size of a blood platelet, as forming a fourth element in the blood, where it moves actively among the corpuscles; called also *Edelmann's cell*.

kinetodesma (ki-ne″to-des′mah), pl. *kinetodesma′tah* [*kineto-* + Gr. *desmos* band, ligament] one of a bundle of fine, striated fibrils, each of which arises close to the base of a basal body and runs anteriorly parallel to and just beneath the surface of certain ciliate protozoa; the kinetodesmata serve to connect the basal bodies in longitudinal rows. Called also *kinetodesmos*.

kinetodesmata (ki-ne″to-des-mah′tah) plural of *kinetodesma*.

kinetodesmos (ki-ne″to-des′mos) kinetodesma.

kinetofragment (ki-ne″to-frag′ment) a group of somatic kinetids, not always completely covered with cilia, occurring in the region of the cytosome or oral area in certain ciliate protozoa, many of which are in the class Kinetofragminophorea. See also *frange* and *pseudomembranelle*.

Kinetofragminophorea (ki-ne″to-frag″min-o-for′e-ah) [*kineto-* + L. *fragmen* piece + Gr. *phōros* bearing] a class of ciliate protozoa (phylum Ciliophora), characterized by the presence of isolated kineties in the oral region of the body (kinetofragments) bearing cilia but not compound ciliary organelles; a cytostome and cytopharyngeal apparatus are often present. It comprises four subclasses: Gymnostomatia, Vestibuliferia, Hypostomatia, and Suctoria.

kinetogenic (ki-ne″to-jen′ik) [*kineto-* + Gr. *gennan* to produce] causing or producing movement.

kinetographic (ki-ne″to-graf′ik) [*kineto-* + Gr. *graphein* to record] recording graphically the movements of parts and features.

kinetonucleus (ki-ne″to-nu′kle-us) [*kineto-* + *nucleus*] kinetoplast.

kinetoplasm (ki-ne′to-plazm) [*kineto-* + Gr. *plasma* something formed] the most highly contractile portion of the cytoplasm of a cell; the energy plasm: the term is applied to the chromatophilic elements in the nervous tissue.

kinetoplast (ki-ne′to-plast) [*kineto-* + Gr. *plassein* to form] a large rod-shaped or cylindrical, DNA-rich, independently replicating cytoplasmic organelle located in close association with the basal body (with which it may seem to be fused) and found within the elongated mitochondrion of protozoa of the order Kinetoplastida. Called also *kinetonucleus*.

kinetoplastid (ki-ne″to-plas′tid) pertaining or relating to protozoa of the order Kinetoplastida.

Kinetoplastida (ki-ne″to-plas′tĭ-dah) an order of flagellate protozoa (class Zoomastigophorea, subphylum Mastigophora), many species of which are free living, although most are parasites of plants, invertebrates, and vertebrates. Kinetoplastids have one or two flagella arising from a depression in the cell body and usually contain a conspicuous kinetoplast located near the flagellar basal bodies. The order comprises two suborders: Bodonina and Trypanosomatina. Called also *Protomastigida* and *Protomonadina*.

kinetoscope (ki-ne′to-skōp) [*kineto-* + Gr. *skopein* to examine] an apparatus designed to make serial photographs depicting body motions.

kinetoscopy (ki″nĕ-tos′ko-pe) serial photography which exhibits the motions of the limbs or features; used in diagnosis of disorders of gait and in the study of muscle action.

kinetosis (ki″ne-to′sis), pl. *kineto′ses* [*kineto-* + *-osis*] any disorder caused by unaccustomed motion; see *motion sickness*.

kinetosome (ki-ne′to-sōm) [*kineto-* + Gr. *sōma* body] basal body.

kinetotherapy (ki-ne″to-ther′ah-pe) kinesitherapy.

kinety (ki-ne′te), pl. *kine′tia*, *kineties* [Gr. *kinētos* movable] a longitudinal unit comprised of cilia, basal bodies, and kinetodesmata in the infraciliature of ciliate protozoa. Called also *kinety system*.

King unit (king) [Earl Judson *King*, Toronto biochemist, 1901–1962] see under *unit*.

kingdom (king′dum) [A.S. *cyningdom*] classically, one of the three categories into which natural objects are usually classified: the *animal kingdom*, including all animals; the *plant kingdom*, including all plants; and the *mineral kingdom*, including all objects and substance without life. A fourth kingdom, the *Protista*, has been added and includes all single-celled organisms.

Kingella (king-el′lah) [Elizabeth O. *King*, American bacteriologist] a genus of gram-negative, aerobic or facultatively anaerobic, rod-shaped bacteria of the family Neisseriaceae, found as natural inhabitants of the human oropharynx. The organisms are potential human pathogens. **K. denitri′ficans,** a usually nonpathogenic species isolated from the upper respiratory tract and genital tract specimens. **K. indolog′enes,** a species isolated from eye infections. **K. kin′gae,** a species that has been isolated from blood, bone, joint, and throat infections and from cultures of normal mucous membranes.

Kingsley appliance (plate), splint (king′sle) [Norman William *Kingsley*, American dentist, 1829–1913]　see under *appliance* and *splint*.

kinic acid (kin′ik)　quinic acid.

kinin (ki′nin)　the generic term for polypeptides related in amino acid sequence and physiological activity to bradykinin and kallidin. **C2 k.**, see under *complement*.

kininase (ki′nin-ās)　an enzyme that destroys the activity of circulating kinins. **k. I,** arginine carboxypeptidase. **k. II,** dipeptidyl carboxypeptidase I.

kininogen (ki′nin-o-jen″)　either of two plasma α_2-globulins that are kinin precursors. HMW (high-molecular-weight) kininogen (mol. wt. 100,000–250,000) is split by plasma kallikrein to produce bradykinin; LMW (low-molecular-weight) kininogen (mol. wt. 50,000–75,000) is split by tissue kallikrein to produce lysyl-bradykinin (kallidin).

kink (kink′)　a bend or twist. **ileal k., Lane's k.,** the term once applied to sharp twists in the distal ileum caused by Lane's bands; such twists were thought to result in chronic partial obstruction of the ileum.

kino (ki′no)　the dried juice of *Pterocarpus marsupium* Roxb. (Leguminosae), of southern Asia, and of various other trees; it has been used as an astringent because of its high content of kinotannic acid.

kin(o)- [Gr. *kinein* to move]　see *kine-*.

kinocentrum (ki″no-sen′trum)　centrosome.

kinocilia (ki″no-sil′e-ah) [L.]　plural of *kinocilium*.

kinocilium (ki″no-sil′e-um), pl. *kinocil′ia*.　A motile, protoplasmic filament on the free surface of a cell. Cf. *stereocilium*.

kinohapt (ki′no-hapt) [*kino-* + Gr. *haptein* to touch]　an esthesiometer for making several tactile stimulations at definite intervals of time or space.

kinology (ki-nol′o-je)　kinesiology.

kinomometer (ki″no-mom′ĕ-ter) [*kino-* + Gr. *metron* measure]　an instrument for estimating the degree of motion in fingers and wrist.

kinoplastic (ki″no-plas′tik)　pertaining to kinoplasm.

Kinorhyncha (kin″o-rin′kah) [*kino-* + Gr. *rhynchos* snout]　a class of small marine animals of the phylum Aschelminthes, which have a cuticle divided into segments and a retractible spiny head. In some systems of classification, they are considered to be a separate phylum.

kinosphere (ki′no-sfēr) [*kino-* + *sphere*]　aster.

kinotoxin (ki″no-tok′sin) [*kino-* + *toxin*]　a fatigue toxin.

kinovin (kin-o′vin)　quinovin.

kinship (kin′ship) [A.S. *cynscip*]　a group of individuals of varying degrees of descent from a common ancestor.

kion(o)-　for words beginning thus, see those beginning *ciono-*.

kiotome (ki′o-tōm) [Gr. *kiōn* column + *temnein* to cut]　a knife for amputating the uvula.

kiotomy (ki-ot′o-me)　the use of the kiotome; amputation of the uvula.

Kirchner's diverticulum (kĕrk′nerz) [Wilhelm *Kirchner*, Würzburg otologist, 1849–1936]　see under *diverticulum*.

Kirk's amputation (kirks) [Major General Norman Thomas *Kirk*, former Surgeon General of U.S. Army, 1888–1960]　see under *amputation*.

Kirschner wire (kērsh′ner) [Martin *Kirschner*, German surgeon, 1879–1942]　see under *wire*.

Kirstein's method (ker′stīnz) [Alfred *Kirstein*, German physician, 1863–1922]　see under *method*.

Kisch's reflex (kish′ez) [Bruno *Kisch*, German physiologist, 1890–1966]　Kehrer's reflex.

kitasamycin (kit″ah-sah-mi′sin)　an antibiotic substance produced by *Streptomyces kitasatoensis*, active against most gram- positive and some gram-negative bacteria, as well as certain other pathogenic microorganisms. Called also *leucomycin*.

Kitasatoa (ki″tah-sah-to′ah) [*Kitasato*, Japanese bacteriologist]　a genus of bacteria of the family Actinoplanaceae, order Actinomycetales, consisting of soil organisms that produce club-shaped sporangia, each containing a chain of motile spores.

Kitasato's filter (ke-tah-sah′tōz) [Shibasaburo *Kitasato*, Japanese bacteriologist, 1852–1931]　see under *filter*.

kitol (ki′tol) [Gr. *kētos* sea monster, big fish]　a substance from whale oil which yields vitamin A on heating.

Kittel's treatment (kit′elz) [M. J. *Kittel*, German physician, 20th century]　see under *treatment*.

k.j.　knee jerk.

Kjeldahl's method (test) (kel′dahlz) [Johan Gustav Christoffer *Kjeldahl*, Danish chemist, 1849–1900]　see under *method*.

Kjelland (kel′land)　see *Kielland*.

kl　kiloliter.

Klapp's creeping treatment (klaps) [Rudolf *Klapp*, surgeon in Berlin, 1873–1949]　see under *treatment*.

Klebs-Löffler bacillus (klebz′ lef′ler) [Theodor Albrecht Edwin *Klebs*, German physiologist, 1834–1934; Friederich A. J. *Löffler*, German bacteriologist, 1852–1915]　*Corynebacterium diphtheriae*.

Klebsiella (kleb″se-el′lah) [Theodor Albrecht Edwin *Klebs*, German bacteriologist, 1834–1913]　a genus of bacteria of the family Enterobacteriaceae, made up of small, gram-negative, facultatively anaerobic, nonmotile rods, usually occurring singly. The organisms, widely distributed in nature, are commonly found in the human intestinal tract. They are a frequent cause of nosocomial urinary and pulmonary infections and of wound infections. **K. friedlän′deri,** *K. pneumoniae.* **K. oxyto′ca,** a species similar to *K. pneumoniae* except that it is indole positive, found in the mammalian intestinal tract and human clinical specimens and a cause of urinary tract infections in humans. **K. ozae′nae,** *K. pneumoniae ozaenae.* **K. plantic′ola,** a species that is both indole positive and ornithine positive, found mainly in botanic, aquatic, and soil isolates. **K. pneumo′niae,** an encapsulated species found in soil, water, and grain, in the intestinal tract of humans and animals, and in association with infections of the urinary and respiratory tracts. It is the etiologic agent of acute bacterial pneumonia (*Friedländer's pneumonia*). Called also *K. friedländeri* and, formerly, *Bacillus pneumoniae*. **K. pneumo′niae ozae′nae,** a species occurring in ozena and other chronic respiratory diseases. **K. pneumo′niae rhinosclero′matis,** a species found in patients with rhinoscleroma and their contacts. **K. rhinoscleroma′tis,** *K. pneumoniae rhinoscleromatis.* **K. terrige′na,** a species similar to *K. pneumoniae* except that it ferments glucose at 5° C and 10° C; isolated from aquatic and soil samples.

Klebsielleae (kleb″se-el′le-e)　in some systems of classification, a tribe of gram-negative, facultatively anaerobic, rod-shaped bacteria of the family Enterobacteriaceae, made up of the genera *Klebsiella, Enterobacter, Pectobacterium,* and *Serratia*.

kleeblattschädel (kla″blat-sha′del) [Ger.]　cloverleaf skull; a congenital anomaly in which there is intrauterine synostosis of multiple or all cranial sutures. See under *syndrome*.

Kleine-Levin syndrome (klīnĕ lev′in) [Willi *Kleine*, German psychiatrist, 20th century; Max *Levin*, American neurologist, born 1901]　see under *syndrome*.

klept(o)- [Gr. *kleptein* to steal]　combining form denoting relationship to theft or stealing.

kleptolagnia (klep″to-lag′ne-ah) [*klepto-* + *lagneia* lust]　sexual gratification produced by theft.

kleptomania (klep″to-ma′ne-ah) [*klepto-* + Gr. *mania* madness] [DSM III-R] an uncontrollable impulse to steal, the objects taken usually having a symbolic value of which the subject is unconscious, rather than an intrinsic value.

kleptomaniac (klep″to-ma′ne-ak)　an individual exhibiting kleptomania.

Klieg eye (klēg) [named from *Kliegl*, the manufacturer of electric lamps used in motion picture making]　see under *eye*.

Klimow's test (klim′ofs) [Ivan Alex. *Klimow*, Russian physician, born 1865]　see under *tests*.

Kline's test (klīn) [Benjamin S. *Kline*, American pathologist, 1886–1968]　see under *tests*.

Klinefelter's syndrome (klīn′fel-terz) [Harry Fitch *Klinefelter*, Jr., American physician, born 1912]　see under *syndrome*.

Klippel's disease (klĭ-pelz′) [Maurice *Klippel*, French neurologist, 1858–1942]　arthritic general pseudoparalysis.

Klippel-Feil sign, syndrome (klĭ-pel′fīl) [Maurice *Klippel*; André *Feil*, French physician, born 1884] see under *sign* and *syndrome*.

kliseometer (klis″e-om′ĕ-ter) cliseometer.

klismaphilia (kliz″mah-fil′e-ah) love of enemas; a paraphilia in which sexual excitement depends on the use of enemas.

Kloeckera (kle′ker-ah) a genus of ascomycetous yeasts of the family Saccharomycetaceae. **K. apicula′tus,** a species from fermenting fruit; its oval cells are joined at the ends. Called also *Saccharomyces apiculatus.*

Klossiella (klŏs″e-el′ah) a genus of coccidian protozoa (suborder Adeleina, order Eucoccidiida) parasitic in the renal cells of mammals, such as the mouse and guinea pig, characterized by the presence of an oocyst with many spores, each producing many sporozoites.

Klumpke's paralysis (kloomp′kez) [Madame A. *Klumpke* Dejerine, Parisian neurologist, 1859–1927, wife of Joseph Jules Dejerine] see under *paralysis.*

Klumpke-Dejerine paralysis, syndrome (kloomp′kĕ-dezh″er-ēn′) [Madame A. *Klumpke* Dejerine; Joseph Jules *Dejerine*, French neurologist, 1849–1917] Klumpke's paralysis.

Klüver-Bucy syndrome (kle′ver bu′se) [Heinrich *Klüver*, American neurologist, born 1897; Paul Clancy *Bucy*, American neurologist, born 1904] see under *syndrome.*

Kluyvera (kli′ver-ah) [A.J. *Kluyver,* Dutch microbiologist] a genus of gram-negative, facultatively anaerobic, rod-shaped bacteria of the family Enterobacteriaceae, occurring in human clinical specimens. It is an occasional opportunistic pathogen, causing respiratory and urinary infections. The type species is *K. ascorba′ta.*

Km symbol for the *Michaelis constant;* see *Michaelis-Menten equation* under *equation.*

Km see under *allotype.*

km kilometer.

KMnO₄ potassium permanganate.

Knapp's forceps, operation, streaks (striae) (naps) [Herman Jakob *Knapp,* New York ophthalmologist, 1832–1911] see under *forceps, operation,* and *streak.*

Knapp's test (knaps) [Karl *Knapp,* German chemist of the 19th century] see under *tests.*

kneading (nēd′ing) a movement in massage consisting of grasping and pressing of muscles.

knee (ne) 1. the site of articulation between the thigh (femur) and leg; called also *genu* [NA]. 2. any structure bent like the knee. **k. of aquaeduc′tus fallo′pii,** geniculum canalis facialis. **back k.,** genu recurvatum. **beat k.,** a subcutaneous cellulitis over the kneecap. **big k.,** 1. bursitis over the knee in cattle. 2. a tumor of the bony parts of the knee joint in horses. **Brodie's k.,** a chronic synovitis of the knee joint in which the affected parts acquire a soft and pulpy consistency. **capped k.,** distention of the synovial bursa over the knee joint of horses or cattle. **football k.,** a swollen, relaxed, somewhat tender condition of the knee seen in football players. **hooped k.,** the presence of exostoses in the knee of a horse. **housemaid's k.,** inflammation of the bursa in front of the patella, with fluid accumulating within it. **in k.,** genu valgum. **k. of internal capsule,** genu capsulae internae. **knock k.,** genu valgum. **locked k.,** inability to extend the leg fully as a result of tear of the medial semilunar cartilage. **out k.,** genu varum, or bowleg. **rugby k.,** Schlatter's disease. **septic k.,** a suppurating knee joint. **sprung k.,** forward bending of the knee of a horse, due to shortening of the flexor tendons. **trick k.,** popular term for a knee joint susceptible to locking in position, most often due to longitudinal splitting of the medial meniscus.

knee-gall (ne′gawl) distension of the carpal sheath at the back of the knee joint in the horse.

kneippism (nīp′izm) [Rev. Father Sebastian *Kneipp,* 1821–1897, who introduced the practice] a system of hydrotherapy involving applications of cold water, as cold bathing, walking barefoot in the morning dew, etc.

Knemidokoptes (ne″mĭ-do-kop′tēz) a genus of mites. *K. gal′linae,* the depluming mite, causes depluming of fowls. *K. mu′tans* causes scaly legs in fowl and cage birds.

knife (nīf) a cutting instrument of various shapes and sizes. **Blair k.,** a knife with a long sharp blade used to cut skin grafts. **buck k.,** a periodontal knife with spear-shaped cutting points, used for interdental incision during gingivectomy. **button k.,** a small knife used for the cutting of cartilage. **cataract k.,** a knife for cutting the cornea in operations for cataract. **cautery k.,** a knife connected with an electric battery, so that the tissues may be seared while being cut, in order to prevent bleeding. **electric k.,** a knife-shaped electrode or steel needle which cuts by causing dissolution of tissue when activated by a high-frequency current. **Goldman-Fox k.,** any of a group of knives designed for incision and contouring of gingival tissues in periodontal surgery. **Graefe's k.,** a slender knife used in linear extraction of cataract. **Humby k.,** a knife with a roller attached, used for cutting skin grafts of varying thickness; the distance between the roller and the blade of the knife can be varied by means of a calibration device. **Joseph k.,** a double-bladed knife used in corrective rhinoplasty. **Kirkland k.,** a periodontal knife that consists of a thin, flattened blade attached to the handle by an angulated shank, the outer edge being elliptical and the inner straight; used for primary gingivectomy. **Liston's k.,** a long-bladed amputation knife. **Merrifield's k.,** a periodontal knife with a long narrow triangular blade; used in gingivectomy. **Ramsbotham's sickle k.,** a sickle-shaped knife used for intrauterine decapitation of a fetus.

knismogenic (nis″mo-jen′ik) [Gr. *knismos* tickling + *gennan* to produce] producing a tickling sensation.

knitting (nit′ing) the physiological process of repair of a fractured bone.

KNO₃ potassium nitrate.

knob (nob) a bulbous mass or protuberance. **surfers' k's,** see under *nodule.* **synaptic k's,** end-feet.

knock (nok) a sound as of a blow against a firm surface. **pericardial k.,** a clear, metallic clicking sound heard over the precordium in certain cases of penetrating chest wounds in the neighborhood of the pericardium; ascribed to emphysema of the mediastinal connective tissue or to free air in the interstitial connective tissue of the lung. Cf. *clicking pneumothorax,* under *pneumothorax.*

knock-knee (nok′ne) genu valgum.

Knoepfelmacher's butter meal (knep′fel-mahk′erz) [Wilhelm *Knoepfelmacher,* pediatrist in Vienna, born 1866] see under *meal.*

knot (not) 1. an intertwining of the ends or parts of one or more threads, sutures, or strips of cloth so they cannot easily

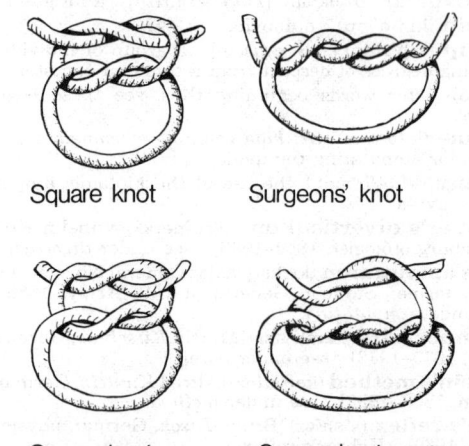

Square knot   Surgeons' knot

Granny knot   Square knot

be separated. 2. in anatomy, a knoblike swelling or protuberance, as a node. **clove-hitch k.,** a knot consisting of two contiguous loops that are applied around an object, the ends of the cord being toward each other; used for making traction on a part for the reduction of dislocations. **double k.,** a knot in which the ends of the cord are twisted around each other twice. **enamel k.,** a small dense group of epithelial cells in the stellate reticulum of a developing tooth, which disappears before enamel formation begins. **false k.,** 1. a local bulge on the umbilical cord caused by protuberant vessels. Cf. *true k.* 2. granny k.

friction k., double k. **granny k.,** a double knot in the second loop of which the end of one cord is over, and the other under, its fellow, so that the loops do not lie in the same line and the knot will not hold. **Hensen's k.,** primitive k. **net k.,** karyosome. **primitive k.,** a mass of cells at the cranial end of the primitive streak, related to the organization of an embryo. **protochordal k.,** primitive k. **reef k.,** square k. **square k.,** a double knot in which the free ends of the second knot lie in the same plane as the ends of the first knot. **stay k.,** a knot made with two or more ligatures, each being tied with the first half of a square knot; then all the ends of one side are taken in one hand, and all the ends on the other side in the other hand, and tied as if they formed one single thread. **surfers' k's,** see under *nodule*. **surgeons' k., surgical k.,** a knot in which the thread is passed twice through the first loop to prevent slippage. **syncytial k's,** protuberances of syncytium along the chorionic villi. **true k.,** a simple knot produced in the looped umbilical cord during pregnancy. Cf. *false k.*

knuckle (nuk″l) the dorsal aspect of any phalangeal joint, especially of the metacarpophalangeal joints of the flexed fingers. By extension sometimes applied to any anatomical structure of similar appearance, such as an extruded loop of intestine in hernia. **aortic k.,** the hump or knuckle formed by the aortic arch as seen in radiographs in anteroposterior projections.

knuckling (nuk′ling) a condition in which the fetlock joint of a horse is pushed upward and forward, due to shortening of the tendons behind.

Kobelt's tubes, tubules (ko′belts) [George Ludwig *Kobelt,* German physician, 1804–1857] see under *tube* and *tubule.*

Kober's test (ko′berz) [Philip Adolph *Kober,* American chemist, born 1884] see under *tests.*

Kobert's test (ko′bārts) [Eduard Rudolf *Kobert,* German chemist, 1854–1918] see under *tests.*

KOC kathodal (cathodal) opening contraction.

Koch (kōk), Robert. German physician and bacteriologist, 1843–1910; winner of the Nobel prize for medicine or physiology in 1905 for his work and discoveries concerning tuberculosis.

Koch's bacillus, etc. (kōks) [Robert *Koch*] see under *bacillus, phenomenon, postulate, reaction,* and *tuberculin.*

Koch's node (kōks) [Walter *Koch,* German surgeon, born 1880] atrioventricular node.

Koch-Weeks bacillus (kōk-wēks) [Robert *Koch*; John Elmer *Weeks,* New York ophthalmologist, 1853–1949] *Haemophilus aegyptius.*

Kocher (kōk′er), Emil Theodor. Swiss surgeon, 1841–1917; winner of the Nobel prize for medicine or physiology in 1909 for his work on the physiology and pathology of the thyroid gland and for thyroidectomy for treatment of goiter.

Kocher's forceps, etc. (kōk′erz) [Emil Theodor *Kocher*] see under *forceps, incision, maneuver, operation, reflex,* and *sign.*

kocherization (kōk″er-i-za′shun) Kocher maneuver.

Koeberlé's forceps (ke″ber-lāz′) [Eugène *Koeberlé,* French surgeon, 1828–1915] hemostatic forceps.

Koebner's phenomenon (keb′nerz) [Heinrich *Koebner,* German dermatologist, 1838–1904] see under *phenomenon.*

Koenecke's reaction, test (ke-nek′ez) see under *tests.*

Kogoj's pustule (ko-goiz) [Franjo *Kogoj,* Yugoslavian physician, born 1894] see *spongiform pustule of Kogoj,* under *pustule.*

KOH potassium hydroxide.

koha (ko′hah) a Japanese drug derived from cyanine; given intravenously it is said to stimulate the formation of leukocytes and of new tissue and thus hasten wound healing.

Köhler's bone disease (ka′lerz) [Alban *Köhler,* German physician, 1874–1947] see under *disease.*

Kohlrausch's folds (valves) (kōl′rowsh-ez) [Otto Ludwig Bernhard *Kohlrausch,* German physician, 1811–1854] plicae transversales recti.

Kohn's pores (kōnz) [Hans *Kohn,* German pathologist, born 1866] interalveolar pores; see under *pore.*

Kohnstamm's phenomenon (kōn′stahmz) [Oscar Felix *Kohnstamm,* German physician, 1871–1917] after-movement.

koil(o)- [Gr. *koilos* hollow] a combining form meaning hollow or concave.

koilonychia (koi″lo-nik′e-ah) [*koilo-* + *onyx* nail + *-ia*] dystrophy of the fingernails, sometimes associated with iron deficiency anemia, in which they are thin and concave, with the edges raised; called also *spoon nail.*

koilorrhachic (koi″lo-rak′ik) [*koilo* + Gr. *rhachis* spine] having a vertebral column in which the lumbar curvature is concave anteriorly. Cf. *kyphosis, kyrtorrhachic,* and *orthorrhachic.*

koilosternia (koi″lo-ster′ne-ah) [*koilo-* + *sternum* + *-ia*] funnel chest.

koin(o)- see *cen(o)-,* def. 3.

koinonia (koi-no′ne-ah) [Gr. *koinōnia* community] associated or common action, as of like cells in the same tissue.

kojic acid (ko′jik as′id) a pyrone formed from sugars by a variety of microorganisms, especially species of *Aspergillus;* it has antibiotic and antifungal properties.

Kolantyl (ko-lan′til) trademark for a preparation of alumina and magnesia.

Kölliker's column, etc. (kel′ĭ-kerz) [Rudolf Abert von *Kölliker,* eminent Swiss anatomist, histologist, and zoologist, professor at Zurich and Würzburg, 1817–1905] see under *column, granule, membrane,* and *nucleus.*

Kollmann's dilator (kol′manz) [Arthur *Kollmann,* Leipzig urologist, born 1858] see under *dilator.*

Kolmer test (kōl′mer) [John A. *Kolmer,* American pathologist, 1886–1962] see under *tests.*

Kolmogorov-Smirnov test (kol-mŏ′go-rov smēr′nov) [Andrei Nicolaievich *Kolmogorov,* Russian mathematician, born 1903; Nicolai Vasilievich *Smirnov,* Russian mathematician, born 1900] see under *tests.*

kolp- for words beginning thus, see those beginning *colp-.*

kolypeptic (ko″le-pep′tik) [Gr. *kōlyein* to hinder + *peptikos* peptic] hindering or checking digestion.

kolytic (ko-lit′ik) [Gr. *kōlyein* to hinder] *(obs.)* inhibited, withdrawn, schizoid.

Konakion (kon″ah-ki′on) trademark for a preparation of phytonadione (vitamin K₁).

König's rods (ken′igz) [Charles Joseph *König,* German otologist, born 1868] see under *rod.*

König's syndrome (ken′igz) [Franz König, German surgeon, 1832–1910] see under *syndrome.*

konimeter (ko-nim′ĕ-ter) konometer.

koniocortex (ko″ne-o-kor′teks) [Gr. *konis* dust + *cortex*] the granular cortex of sensory areas of the brain.

koniology (ko″ne-ol′o-je) coniology.

konometer (ko-nom′ĕ-ter) [Gr. *konis* dust + *metron* measure] an apparatus for counting the number of dust particles in the air.

Konsyl (kon′sil) a brand of psyllium hydrophilic muciloid.

koomis (koo′mis) koumiss.

kophemia (ko-fe′me-ah) [Gr. *kōphos* deaf] word deafness.

kopiopia (ko″pe-o′pe-ah) copiopia.

Koplik's spots (sign) (kop′liks) [Henry *Koplik,* New York pediatrician, 1858–1927] see under *spot.*

Kopp's asthma (kops) [Johann Heinrich *Kopp,* German physician, 1777–1858] thymic asthma.

kopr- for words beginning thus, see also those beginning *copr-.*

kopratin (kop′rah-tin) [Gr. *kopros* dung] the chemical substance which produces the so-called pyridine-hemochromogen spectrum in the pyridine test for blood. It is produced from alpha-hematin by putrefaction.

koprosterin (kop″ro-ste′rin) coprostanol.

Korányi's auscultation (percussion), sign (ko-ran′yēz) [Baron *Korányi,* Hungarian physician, 1828–1913] see under *auscultation* and *sign.*

Korányi's treatment (ko-ran′yēz) [Baron Alexander von *Korányi* (Sandor), Hungarian physician, 1866–1944] see under *treatment.*

Korányi-Grocco triangle (ko-ran′ye-grok′o) [Baron F. von *Korányi*; Pietro *Grocco,* physician in Florence, 1857–1916] see *Grocco's sign (def. 1),* under *sign.*

Kornberg (korn′berg), Arthur. American physician and biochemist, born 1918; co-winner, with Severo Ochoa, of the

Nobel prize for medicine or physiology in 1959 for discovering the mechanisms in the biological synthesis of deoxyribonucleic acid and ribonucleic acid.

koro (ko'ro) a culture-specific acute delusional syndrome occurring among the Malay people and southern Chinese in which the patient believes that his penis is shrinking and may disappear into his abdomen and that if this happens he will die (a belief widespread in this culture).

koronion (ko-ro'ne-on), pl. *koro'nia* [Gr. *korōnē* crow, crown] coronion.

koroscopy (ko-ros'ko-pe) retinoscopy.

Korotkoff's method, sounds, test (ko-rot'kofs) [Nicolai Sergeevich *Korotkoff*, Russian physician, 1874–1920] see under the nouns.

Korsakoff's (Korsakov's) syndrome (psychosis) (kor-sak'ofs) [Sergei Sergeevich *Korsakoff*, Russian neurologist, 1854–1900] see under *syndrome*.

Körte-Ballance operation (ker'te-bal'ans) [Werner *Körte*, Berlin surgeon, 1853–1937; Sir Charles Alfred *Ballance*, British surgeon, 1856–1936] see under *operation*.

kosam (ko'sam) a small evergreen shrub, *Brucea sumatrana* Roxb. (Simaroubaceae), of southeastern Asia and Australia, whose seeds are sometimes used locally in the treatment of diarrhea, dysentery, and uterine hemorrhage.

Koshevnikoff's (Koschewnikow's, Kozhevnikov's) disease, epilepsy (ko-shev'ne-kofs) [Alexei Jakovlevich *Koshevnikoff*, Russian neurologist, 1836–1902] epilepsia partialis continua.

Kossel (kos'el), Albrecht. German physiologist, 1853–1927; winner of the Nobel prize for medicine or physiology in 1910 for his contributions to cellular chemistry through his work on proteins, including nucleic substances.

Kossel's test (kos'elz) [Albrecht *Kossel*] see under *tests*.

Kostmann's syndrome (kōst'mahnz) [Rolf *Kostmann*, Swedish physician, born 1909] infantile genetic agranulocytosis.

koumiss (koo'mis) [Tartarian] a fermented alcoholic drink prepared from cow's milk; originally from mare's milk by the Tartars. **kefir k.,** milk fermented with kefir fungi.

Kovalevsky's canal (ko"val-ev'skēz) [Alexander Onufrievich *Kovalevsky*, Russian embryologist, 1840–1901] neurenteric canal.

Kowarsky's test (ko-var'skēz) [Albert *Kowarsky*, German physician of the 20th century] see under *tests*.

Koyter's muscle (koi'terz) [Volcherus *Koyter*, Dutch anatomist, 1534–1600] musculus corrugator supercilii.

K.P. keratitic precipitates; see *keratitis punctata*, under *keratitis*.

K-Phos (ka'fos) trademark for a preparation of monobasic potassium phosphate.

K₃PO₄ normal ortho- or tribasic potassium phosphate.

Kr chemical symbol for *krypton*.

Krabbe's disease (leukodystrophy) (krab'ēz) [Knud H. *Krabbe*, Danish neurologist, 1885–1961] see under *disease*.

Kraepelin (kra'pĕ-lin), Emil. German psychiatrist, 1856–1926; the father of descriptive psychiatry. He differentiated manic-depressive psychosis from dementia praecox (schizophrenia) and described the basic schizophrenic subtypes: catatonic, hebephrenic, and paranoid. Modern classifications of the psychoses are still essentially kraepelinian.

krait (krāt) an extremely venomous elapid snake of the genus *Bungarus;* see table accompanying *snake*.

Krameria (krah-me're-ah) [J. G. H. and W. H. *Kramer*, German botanists] a genus of leguminous shrubs and herbs. The dried roots of *K. triandra* R. et P., or Peruvian rhatany, and of *K. argentea* Mart., or Brazilian rhatany, were formerly used as an astringent because of their high content of krameric acid.

Kraske's operation (kras'kēz) [Paul *Kraske*, German surgeon, 1851–1930] see under *operation*.

kratom (krah'tom) a masticatory containing the leaves of *Mitragyna speciosa* Korth. (Rubiaceae), which is chewed or smoked like opium in Thailand.

kratometer (kra-tom'ĕ-ter) a prism-refracting instrument for use in orthoptic training.

krauomania (kraw"o-ma'ne-ah) a tic marked by rhythmic movements, such as balancing, head rotation, etc.

kraurosis (kraw-ro'sis) [Gr. *krauros* brittle] a dry, shriveled condition of a part, especially of the vulva (see *k. vulvae*).
k. vul'vae, an atrophic disease affecting the female external genitalia, most often of older women, resulting in drying and shriveling of the parts, and marked by leukoplakic patches on the mucosa, itching, dyspareunia, dysuria, and soreness. It occurs most commonly as a result of lichen sclerosus et atrophicus of the vulva, but may be associated with other types of genital atrophy. Called also *leukokraurosis, leukoplakic vulvitis,* and *Breisky's disease.*

Krause's bulbs, etc. (krow'zez) [Wilhelm Johann Friedrich *Krause*, German anatomist, 1833–1910] see under *bulb, corpuscle, line, membrane,* and *suture.*

Krause's ligament, valve (krow'zez) [Karl Friedrich Theodor *Krause*, German anatomist, 1797–1868] see *ligamentum transversum perinei*, and see *Béraud's valve*, under *valve.*

Krause's operation (krow'zez) [Fedor Victor *Krause*, German surgeon, 1857–1937] see under *operation.*

Krause-Wolfe graft (krowz-wolf) [Fedor *Krause;* John Reissberg *Wolfe*, Scotch ophthalmologist, 1824–1904] see under *graft.*

kreatin (kre'ah-tin) creatine.

krebiozen (krĕ-bi'o-zen) a substance identified as creatine by the Food and Drug Administration, isolated from the blood of horses injected with *Actinomyces bovis*, claimed to be effective in the treatment of cancer; its sale is banned in the United States.

Krebs (krebz), Sir Hans Adolf. German-born British biochemist, 1900–1981; co-winner, with Fritz Albert Lipmann, of the Nobel prize for medicine or physiology in 1953 for the discovery of the citric acid cycle.

Krebs cycle (krebz) [Sir Hans Adolf *Krebs*] tricarboxylic acid cycle; see under *cycle.*

Krebs' leukocyte index (krebz) [Carl *Krebs*, Copenhagen pathologist, born 1892] see under *index.*

kre(o)- for words beginning thus, see also those beginning *cre(o)-.*

kreotoxicon (kre"o-tok'sĭ-kon) the substance in poisonous meat that produces the toxic symptoms; see *meat poisoning*, under *poisoning.*

kreotoxin (kre"o-tok'sin) any basic poison generated in a flesh food by a plant microorganism; see *meat poisoning*, under *poisoning.*

kreotoxism (kre"o-tok'sizm) [Gr. *kreas* meat + *toxikon* poison] meat poisoning; see under *poisoning.*

kresofuchsin (kres"o-fōōk'sin) a blue-gray powder used as a stain in histology; its aqueous solution is red, the alcoholic solution blue.

kresol (kres'ol) cresol.

Kretschmann's space (krech'mahnz) [Friedrich *Kretschmann*, German otologist, 1858–1934] see under *space.*

Kretschmer types (krech'mer) [Ernst *Kretschmer*, German psychiatrist, 1888–1964] see under *type.*

Kretz's granules (krets'ez) [Richard *Kretz*, German pathologist, 1865–1920] see under *granule.*

Kreysig's sign (kri'zigs) [Friedrich Ludwig *Kreysig*, physician in Dresden, 1770–1839] Heim-Kreysig sign; see under *sign.*

krimpsiekte (krimp-zēk'te) a disease of cattle in South Africa caused by poisoning with the plant *Cotyledon wallachii.*

Krishaber's disease (krēs"hab-ārz') [Maurice *Krishaber*, Hungarian physician in France, 1836–1883] see under *disease.*

Kristeller's method (expression, technique) (kris'tel-er) [Samuel *Kristeller*, Berlin gynecologist, 1820–1900] see under *method.*

Krogh (krōg), Schack August Steenberg. Danish physiologist, 1874–1949; winner of the Nobel prize for medicine or physiology in 1920 for his discovery of the capillary motor regulating mechanism.

Kromayer's burn, lamp (kro'mi-erz) [Ernst Ludwig Franz *Kromayer*, German dermatologist, 1862–1933] see under *burn* and *lamp.*

Krompecher's carcinoma, tumor (krōm'pek-erz) [Edmund *Krompecher*, pathologist in Budapest, 1870–1926] rodent ulcer; see under *ulcer.*

kromskop (krōm′skŏp) [German, from Gr. *chrōma* color + *skopein* to examine]   an apparatus used for color photography of pathological specimens.

Kronecker's center, puncture (kro′nek-erz) [Karl Hugo *Kronecker*, Swiss pathologist, 1839–1914]   see *cardioinhibitory center*, under *center*, and see under *puncture*.

Krönig's field (area), isthmus (kra′nigz) [Georg *Krönig*, physician in Berlin, 1856–1911]   see under *field* and *isthmus*.

Krönlein's hernia, operation (krän′linz) [Rudolf Ulrich *Krönlein*, surgeon in Zurich, 1847–1910]   see *inguino-properitoneal hernia*, under *hernia*, and see under *operation*.

Krukenberg's spindle, tumor (kroo′ken-bergz) [Friedrich Ernst *Krukenberg*, German pathologist, 1871–1946]   see under *spindle* and *tumor*.

Krukenberg's veins (kroo′ken-bergz) [Adolph *Krukenberg*, German anatomist, 1816–1877]   venae centrales hepatis.

Kruse's brush (kroo′zez) [Walther *Kruse*, German bacteriologist, 1864–1943]   see under *brush*.

kryoscopy (kri-os′ko-pe)   cryoscopy.

krypt(o)-   for words beginning thus, see also those beginning *crypt(o)-*.

krypton (krip′ton) [Gr. *kryptos* hidden]   an inert gaseous chemical element found in the atmosphere; atomic number, 36; atomic weight, 83.80; symbol, Kr.

KSC   kathodal (cathodal) closing contraction.

K₂SO₄   potassium sulfate.

KST   kathodal (cathodal) closing tetanus.

K.U.B.   kidney, ureter, and bladder.

kubisagari, kubisgari (koo-bis″ah-gah′re, koo′bis-gah′re)   a form of Gerlier's disease (paralytic vertigo) endemic in Japan (Gerlier-Nakano, 1884).

Kufs' disease (koofs) [H. *Kufs*, German psychiatrist, 1871–1955]   see under *disease*.

Kuhlmann's test (kool′manz) [Frederick *Kuhlmann*, American psychologist, 1876–1941]   see under *tests*.

Kuhn's mask (koonz) [Ernst *Kuhn*, Prussian physician, 1873– 1920]   see under *mask*.

Kuhn's tube (koonz) [Franz *Kuhn*, Berlin surgeon, 1866 –1929]   see under *tube*.

Kühne's methylene blue (ke′nez) [Heinrich *Kühne*, German histologist]   see *methylene blue*.

Kühne's muscular phenomenon, terminal plates, spindle (ke′nez) [Wilhelm Friedrich (Willy) *Kühne*, German physiologist, 1837–1900]   see *Porret's phenomenon*, under *phenomenon*, see under *plate*, and see *muscle spindle*, under *spindle*.

Kuhnt's illusion (koonts) [Hermann *Kuhnt*, German ophthalmologist, 1850–1925]   see under *illusion*.

Kulchitsky's cells (kool-chits′kēz) [Nicolai K. *Kulchitsky*, Russian histologist, 1856–1925]   see under *cell*.

Kulenkampff's anesthesia (koo′len-kahmpfs) [Dietrich *Kulenkampff*, German surgeon, born 1880]   see under *anesthesia*.

Külz's cast (cylinder), test (kiltsez) [Rudolph Eduard *Külz*, German physician, 1845–1895]   see *coma casts*, under *cast*, and see under *tests*.

kumiss (koo′mis)   koumiss.

Kümmell's disease (spondylitis) (kim′elz) [Hermann *Kümmell*, surgeon in Hamburg, 1852–1937]   see under *disease*.

Kümmell-Verneuil disease (kim′el-ver″na′e) [Hermann *Kümmell*; Aristide August Stanislas *Verneuil*, French surgeon, 1823–1895]   Kümmell's disease.

kumyss (koo′mis)   koumiss.

Kunkel's syndrome (kung′kel) [Henry George *Kunkel*, American physician, born 1916]   lupoid hepatitis.

Küntscher nail (kint′sher) [Gerhard *Küntscher*, German surgeon, 1902–1972]   see under *nail*.

Kupffer's cells (koop′ferz) [Karl Wilhelm von *Kupffer*, German anatomist, 1829–1902]   see under *cell*.

kupramite (ku′prah-mīt)   a gas mask adsorbent for ammonia fumes.

Kupressoff's center (koo-pres′ofs) [J. *Kupressoff*, Russian physician of the 19th century]   micturition center; see under *center*.

Kurloff's (Kurlov's) bodies (koor′lofs) [Mikhail Georgievich *Kurloff*, Russian physician, 1859–1932]   see under *body*.

Kurthia (ker′the-ah) [Heinrich *Kurth*, German bacteriologist, 1860–1901]   a genus of coryneform bacteria, consisting of gram-positive, regular, unbranched rods with rounded ends, occurring in chains and of pleomorphic forms. They have been isolated from human feces in mild cases of food poisoning and under normal conditions and from meats and meat products, and are found in the intestinal contents of chickens and in manure, stagnant water, and milk. It contains a single species, *K. zopfii*. Called also *Proteus zenkeri*.

kurtosis (kur-to′sis) [Gr. "convexity"]   the degree of peakedness or flatness of a probability distribution, relative to the normal distribution with the same variance. See *leptokurtic* and *platykurtic*.

kuru (koo′roo)   a chronic, progressive, uniformly fatal nervous system disorder characterized by a long incubation period and transmissible to subhuman primates. It is found only among the Fore and neighboring peoples of New Guinea and is thought to be associated with cannibalism. The chief symptoms are truncal and limb ataxia, a shivering-like tremor, and dysarthria, but strabismus and extrapyramidal symptoms may also be found. Pathologically, the brain shows the changes of the spongiform encephalopathies: neuronal loss, astrogliosis, and status spongiosus; amyloid plaques are also present in about two thirds of the cases.

Kusnezovia (kus″nĕ-zo′ve-ah) [S.I. *Kusnezov*, Russian microbiologist]   a genus of budding bacteria found in mud, of uncertain status, made up of coccoid cells connected by filaments and encrusted with manganese and oxalic acid. The type species is *K. polymor′pha*.

Küss' experiment (kes) [Emil *Küss*, German physiologist, 1815–1871]   see under *experiment*.

Kussmaul's aphasia, etc. (koos′mowlz) [Adolph *Kussmaul*, German physician, 1822–1902]   see under *aphasia*, *paralysis*, *pulse*, *respiration*, and *sign*, and see *periarteritis nodosa*, def. 1.

Kussmaul-Kien respiration (koos′mowl kēn) [Adolf *Kussmaul*; Alphonse M. J. *Kien*, German physician of the 19th century]   air hunger; see under *hunger*.

Kussmaul-Landry paralysis (koos′mowl lan′dre) [Adolf *Kussmaul*; Jean Baptiste Octave *Landry*, French physician, 1826–1865]   acute febrile polyneuritis.

Kussmaul-Maier disease (koos′mowl mi′er) [Adolf *Kussmaul*; Rudolf *Maier*, German physician, 1824–1888]   periarteritis nodosa, def. 1.

Küstner's law, sign (kist′nerz) [Otto Ernst *Küstner*, gynecologist in Breslau, 1850–1931]   see under *law* and *sign*.

Kutrol (ku′trol)   trademark for a preparation of urogastrone.

kV.   kilovolt.

kVp   kilovolts peak.

kW.   kilowatt.

kwashiorkor (kwash-e-or′kor) [local name in Gold Coast, Africa, "displaced child"]   a syndrome produced by severe protein deficiency, characterized by retarded growth, changes in skin and hair pigment, edema, and pathologic changes in the liver, including fatty infiltration, necrosis, and fibrosis. Other findings are peevish mental apathy, atrophy of the pancreas, gastrointestinal disorders, anemia, low serum albumin, and dermatoses. The skin may exhibit darkened, thickened patches on limbs and back which may desquamate, leaving pink, almost raw surfaces of a pellagroid appearance. First reported from Africa, kwashiorkor is now known to occur throughout the world, but mainly in the tropics and subtropics, and is now considered to be related to marasmus. **marasmic k.,** a condition in which there is deficiency of both calories and protein, with severe tissue wasting, loss of subcutaneous fat, and usually dehydration.

kwaski   see under *shakes*.

Kwell (kwel)   trademark for preparations of lindane.

kW.-hr.   kilowatt-hour.

kyan(o)-   for words beginning thus, see also those beginning *cyano-*.

kyestein (ki-es′te-in)   a film sometimes seen on stale urine, formerly thought a sign of pregnancy.

kyllosis (kil-lo′sis) [Gr. *kyllōsis* a crippling] clubfoot, or other deformity of the foot.

kymatism (ki′mah-tizm) myokymia.

kymocyclograph (ki″mo-si′klo-graf) an apparatus for recording movement.

kymogram (ki′mo-gram) a tracing or other graphic record made by a kymograph.

kymograph (ki′mo-graf) [Gr. *kyma* wave + *graphein* to record] an instrument for recording variations or undulations, arterial or other.

kymography (ki-mog′rah-fe) the use of the kymograph. **roentgen k.,** roentgenkymography.

Kynex (ki′neks) trademark for preparations of sulfamethoxypyridazine.

kynocephalus (ki″no-sef′ah-lus) [Gr. *kyōn* dog + *kephalē* head] a human fetus with a head resembling that of a dog.

kynurenic acid (ki″nu-ren′ik) 4-hydroxyquinaldic acid, an intermediate in tryptophan metabolism; it is dehydroxylated to quinaldic acid, which is excreted.

kynurenin (ki″nu-re′nin) kynurenine.

kynureninase (kin″u-ren′ĭ-nās) [EC 3.7.1.3] an enzyme of the hydrolase class that catalyzes the reaction L-kynurenine + H_2O = anthranilate + L-alanine. The enzyme is a pyridoxal-phosphate protein. The reaction occurs in the metabolism of tryptophan.

kynurenine (ki-nu′rĕ-nēn) [Gr. *kyon* dog + L. *ren* kidney] a crystalline nitrogenous base, first isolated from dog urine; $NH_2C_6H_4CO \cdot CH_2CH(NH_2)COOH$ (3-anthraniloylalanine), a metabolite of tryptophan found in microorganisms and in the urine of normal animals, and a precursor of kynurenic acid. It is also an intermediate in the conversion of tryptophan to niacin, a member of the vitamin B complex.

kynurenine 3-hydroxylase (kin′u-rĕ-nēn hi-drok′sĭ-lās)

kynurenine 3-monooxygenase.

kynurenine 3-monooxygenase (kin′u-rĕ-nēn mo″no-ok′sĭ-jĕ-nās) [EC 1.14.13.9] an enzyme of the oxidoreductase class that catalyzes the reaction L-kynurenine + NADPH + O_2 = 3-hydroxy-L-kynurenine + NADP + H_2O. The enzyme is a flavoprotein. The reaction is a step in the metabolism of tryptophan. Called also *kynurenine 3-hydroxylase.*

kyphos (ki′fos) [Gr. "a hump"] the convex prominence of the spine in kyphosis.

kyphoscoliosis (ki″fo-sko″le-o′sis) [*kyphosis* + *scoliosis*] backward and lateral curvature of the spinal column, as in vertebral osteochondrosis (Scheuermann's disease).

kyphosis (ki-fo′sis) [Gr. *kyphōsis* humpback] abnormally increased convexity in the curvature of the thoracic spine as viewed from the side; hunchback. Cf. *lordosis* and *scoliosis.* **k. dorsa′lis juveni′lis, juvenile k., Scheuermann's k.,** see *osteochondrosis.*

kyphotic (ki-fot′ik) affected with or pertaining to kyphosis.

kyrin (ki′rin) a peptide obtained by Siegfried by the partial hydrolysis of proteins and assumed to be a fundamental protein unit.

Kyrle's disease (kir′les) [Joseph *Kyrle*, Austrian dermatologist, 1880–1926] see under *disease.*

kyrtorrhachic (ker″to-rak′ik) [Gr. *kyrtos* curved, convex + *rhachis* spine] having a vertebral column in which the lumbar curvature is convex anteriorly. Cf. *koilorrhachic* and *orthorrhachic.*

kysth(o)- [Gr. *kysthos* vagina] a combining form formerly used to denote relationship to the vagina; for words beginning thus, see those beginning colp(o)-.

kyt(o)- [Gr. *kytos* hollow vessel] for words beginning thus, see those beginning cyt(o)-.

L

L symbol for *lambert, liter,* and *lumbar vertebrae* (L-1 through L-5).

L symbol for *inductance.*

L. 1. an abbreviation for *Latin, Lactobacillus, left, light sense, libra* (pound, balance), *liter, length, limes* (boundary), *lumbar* (in vertebral formulas), and *coefficient of induction.* 2. Ehrlich's symbol for *lethal* (fatal).

L- a chemical prefix (small capital L) that specifies the relative configuration of an enantiomer, the mirror image being specified as D-. Carbohydrates having the same configuration as L-glyceraldehyde at the asymmetric carbon atom most distant from the carbonyl functional group are designated as L. Amino acids having the same configuration as L-serine at the α carbon are designated as L. See D- for further explanation.

l SI symbol for *liter.*

l- [abbreviation for *levo* (left or counterclockwise)] a chemical prefix indicating an enantiomer that rotates the plane of polarization of a beam of light in the counterclockwise direction, the other enantiomer being specified as *d-* (for *dextro*). See note at *d-.*

Λ the Greek capital letter lambda.

Lg- (el-sub-je) see L-; this chemical prefix (with the subscript *g*) is occasionally used to emphasize that the rules of carbohydrate nomenclature are being employed. The subscript refers to the standard monosaccharide, glyceraldehyde. Opposed to Dg-.

Ls- (el-sub-es) see L-; this chemical prefix (with the subscript *s*) is used where needed in amino acid nomenclature to avoid possible confusion with carbohydrate nomenclature, as in Ls-threonine. The subscript refers to the standard amino acid, serine. Opposed to Ds-.

λ lambda, the eleventh letter of the Greek alphabet; symbol for *wavelength, decay constant,* and one of the two types of immunoglobulin light chains.

L. & A. light and accommodation (reaction of pupils).

La chemical symbol for *lanthanum.*

lab [Ger.] rennin.

Labarraque's solution (lab″ah-raks′) [Antoine Germain *Labarraque,* French chemist, 1777–1850] see under *solution.*

Labbé's triangle, vein (lab-āz′) [Léon *Labbé,* French surgeon, 1832–1916] see under *triangle,* and see *vena anastomotica superior.*

label (la′b'l) something that identifies; an identifying mark, tag, etc. **radioactive l.,** see under *tracer.*

labetalol (la-bet′ah-lol) a beta and alpha blocker used in treatment of hypertension.

labetalol hydrochloride (lah-bet′ah-lol) chemical hydroxy-5-[2- hydroxy-5-[1-hydroxy-2-[(1-methyl-3-phenylpropyl) amino] ethyl]benzamide monohydrochloride; a beta-adrenergic blocking agent with some alpha-adrenergic blocking activity, $C_{19}H_{24}N_2O_3 \cdot HCl$, used in the treatment of hypertension; administered orally or intravenously.

labia (la′be-ah) [L.] plural of *labium.*

labial (la′be-al) [L. *labialis*] pertaining to a lip, or labium. In dental anatomy, used to refer to the labial surface of a tooth; see *labial surface,* under *surface.*

labialism (la′be-ah-lizm″) defective speech, with use of labial sounds.

labially (la′be-al-e) toward the lips.

labichorea (la″be-ko-re′ah) labiochorea.

Labidognatha (lab″ĭ-dog′nah-thah) a suborder of spiders (order Araneae), including the medically important families, Theridiidae and Loxoscelidae.

labile (la′bil) [L. *labilis* unstable, from *labi* to glide] 1. gliding; moving from point to point over the surface; unstable; fluctuating. 2. chemically unstable. **heat l.,** thermolabile.

lability (lah-bil′ĭ-te) the quality of being labile. In psychiatry, emotional instability; rapidly changing emotions.

labio- [L. *labium* lip] a combining form denoting relationship to a lip, especially to the lips of the mouth.

labioalveolar (la″be-o-al-ve′o-lar) 1. pertaining to the lip and dental alveoli. 2. pertaining to the labial side of a dental alveolus.

labioaxiogingival (la″be-o-ak″se-o-jin′jĭ-val) pertaining to or formed by the labial, axial, and gingival walls of a tooth cavity preparation.

labiocervical (la″be-o-ser′vĭ-kal) 1. pertaining to the labial surface of the neck of an anterior tooth. 2. labiogingival.

labiochorea (la″be-o-ko-re′ah) [L. *labium* lip + *chorea*] a choreic stiffening of the lips in speech, with stammering.

labioclination (la″be-o-klĭ-na′shun) deviation of an anterior tooth from the vertical, in the direction of the lips.

labiodental (la″be-o-den′tal) 1. pertaining to the lips and teeth. 2. a speech sound produced by the contact of the lips and teeth, such as *f* and *v*.

labiogingival (la″be-o-jin′jĭ-val) pertaining to or formed by the labial and gingival walls of a tooth cavity. Called also *labiocervical*.

labioglossolaryngeal (la″be-o-glos″o-lah-rin′je-al) [L. *labium* lip + Gr. *glōssa* tongue + *larynx*] pertaining to the lips, tongue, and larynx.

labioglossopharyngeal (la″be-o-glos″o-fah-rin′je-al) pertaining to the lips, tongue, and pharynx.

labiograph (la′be-o-graf″) [L. *labium* lip + Gr. *graphein* to record] an instrument for recording the motions of the lips in speaking.

labioincisal (la″be-o-in-si′zal) pertaining to or formed by the labial and incisal surfaces of a tooth.

labiolingual (la″be-o-ling′gwal) 1. pertaining to the lips and the tongue. 2. pertaining to the labial and lingual surfaces of an anterior tooth.

labiologic (la″be-o-loj′ik) pertaining to labiology.

labiology (la″be-ol′o-je) the study of the movements of the lips.

labiomental (la″be-o-men′tal) pertaining to the lip and chin.

labiomycosis (la″be-o-mi-ko′sis) [L. *labium* lip + Gr. *mykēs* fungus] any disease of the lips due to a fungus, such as thrush.

labionasal (la″be-o-na′zal) pertaining to the lip and nose.

labiopalatine (la″be-o-pal′ah-tin) pertaining to the lip and palate.

labioplacement (la″be-o-plās′ment) displacement of a tooth toward the lip.

labioplasty (la′be-o-plas″te) [L. *labium* lip + Gr. *plassein* to mold] cheiloplasty.

labiotenaculum (la″be-o-te-nak′u-lum) [L. *labium* lip + *tenaculum*] an instrument for holding the lip.

labioversion (la″be-o-ver′zhun) displacement of a tooth labially from the line of occlusion.

labium (la′be-um) pl. *la′bia* [L.] a fleshy border or edge; used in anatomical nomenclature as a general term to designate such a structure. In the plural, often used alone to designate the *labia majora* and *minora pudendi*. Called also *lip*. See also *limbus* and *margo*. **l. ante′rius orific′ii exter′ni u′teri**, l. anterius ostii uteri. **l. ante′rius os′tii pharyn′gei tu′bae auditi′vae**, the anterior lip of the pharyngeal opening of the auditory tube. **l. ante′rius os′tii u′teri** [NA], anterior lip of ostium of uterus: the anterior projection of the cervix into the vagina; it is shorter and thicker than the posterior lip. Called also *l. anterius orificii externi uteri*. **l. cer′ebri**, an edge of a deep sulcus, e.g., the lips of the calcarine sulcus. **l. exter′num cris′tae ili′acae** [NA], the outer margin or external lip of the iliac crest. **l. infe′rius o′ris** [NA], the lower lip: the fleshy margin of the inferior border of the mouth. **l. infe′rius val′vulae co′li**, the inferior lip of the valve between the ileum and cecum. **l. inter′num cris′tae ili′acae** [NA], the inner margin or internal lip of the iliac crest. **l. latera′le lin′eae as′perae fem′oris** [NA], lateral lip of rough line of femur: the distinct outer part of the linea aspera that becomes continuous with the gluteal tubers tuberosity and ends at the greater trochanter above and with the lateral supracondylar line below. **l. lim′bi tympan′icum lam′inae spira′lis** [NA], the tympanic lip of the limb of the spiral lamina: the lower border of the internal spiral sulcus, formed by the lower extremity of the limbus laminae spiralis; called also *l. tympanicum laminae*

spiralis. **l. lim′bi vestibula′re lam′inae spira′lis** [NA], the vestibular lip of the limb of the spiral lamina: the upper border of the internal spiral sulcus, formed by the upper extremity of the limbus laminae spiralis; called also *crista spiralis*, *l. vestibulare laminae spiralis*, and *spiral crest*. **l. ma′jus puden′di** [NA], pl. *la′bia majo′ra puden′di*, the greater lip of the pudendum: an elongated fold running downward and backward from the mons pubis in the female, one on either side of the median pudendal cleft. **l. mandibula′re**, l. inferius oris. **l. maxilla′re**, l. superius oris. **l. media′lis lin′eae as′perae fem′oris** [NA], medial lip of rough line of femur: the distinct inner part of the linea aspera that becomes continuous with the intertrochanteric line above and the medial supracondylar line below. **l. mi′nus puden′di** [NA], pl. *la′bia mino′ra puden′di*, lesser lip of the pudendum: a small fold of skin located on either side, between the labium majus and the opening of the vagina. **la′bia o′ris** [NA], the lips: the fleshy upper and lower margins of the mouth. **l. poste′rius orific′ii exter′ni u′teri**, l. posterius ostii uteri. **l. poste′rius os′tii pharyn′gei tu′bae auditi′vae**, the posterior lip of the pharyngeal opening of the auditory tube. **l. poste′rius os′tii u′teri** [NA], posterior lip of ostium of the uterus: the posterior projection of the cervix into the vagina; called also *l. posterius orificii externi uteri*. **l. supe′rius o′ris** [NA], the upper lip: the fleshy margin of the superior border of the mouth. **l. supe′rius val′vulae co′li**, the superior lip of the valve between the ileum and cecum. **l. tympan′icum lam′inae spira′lis**, l. limbi tympanicum laminae spiralis. **l. ure′thrae**, either lateral margin of the external urinary meatus. **l. vestibula′re lam′inae spira′lis**, l. limbi vestibulare laminae spiralis. **l. voca′le**, a projection at each side of the rima glottidis.

labor (la′bor) [L. "work"] the function of the female organism by which the product of conception is expelled from the uterus through the vagina to the outside world. Labor may be divided into four stages: The first (the stage of dilatation) begins with the onset of regular uterine contractions and ends when the os is completely dilated and flush with the vagina, thus completing the birth canal. The second stage (stage of expulsion) extends from the end of the first stage until the expulsion of the infant is completed. The third stage (placental stage) extends from the expulsion of the child until the placenta and membranes are expelled. The fourth stage denotes the hour or two after delivery, when uterine tone is established. Called also *childbirth*, *confinement*, *delivery*, *parturition*, and *travail*. See also *labor pains*, under *pain*. **artificial l.**, induced l. **atonic l.**, labor protracted because of atony of the uterus. **complicated l.**, labor in which cephalopelvic disproportion, hemorrhage, or some other untoward event occurs. **delayed l.**, postponed l. **dry l.**, labor in which the amniotic fluid escapes before the onset of uterine contractions. **false l.**, see *false pains*. **immature l.**, labor taking place between the sixteenth and the twenty-eighth week of pregnancy. **induced l.**, labor brought on by mechanical or other extraneous means, usually by the intravenous infusion of oxytocin. **instrumental l.**, labor in which birth of the baby is facilitated by the use of instruments. **mimetic l.**, see *false pains*. **missed l.**, retention of a dead fetus in the uterus beyond the period of normal gestation. **multiple l.**, labor in which two or more infants are born. **obstructed l.**, labor hindered by some mechanical obstruction, such as a contraction in some region of the parturient canal or a tumor. **postmature l., postponed l.**, labor occurring two weeks or more after the expected date of confinement. **precipitate l.**, labor which occurs with undue rapidity. **premature l.**, expulsion of a viable infant before the normal end of gestation, usually applied to interruption of pregnancy between the twenty-eighth and the thirty-seventh week. **premature l., habitual**, delivery occurring in at least three successive pregnancies at about the same stage of development and prior to completion of the full gestation period. **prolonged l., protracted l.**, labor prolonged beyond the ordinary 18-hour limit. **spontaneous l.**, labor in which no artificial aid is required.

laboratorian (lab″o-rah-to′re-an) a person who devotes himself to laboratory work, as distinguished from a clinician.

laboratory (lab′o-rah-to″re) [L. *laboratorium*] a place equipped for performing experimental work or investigative procedures, for the preparation of drugs, chemicals, etc. **clinical l.**, a laboratory for examination of materials derived from the human body for the purpose of providing information on diagnosis, prevention, or treatment of disease.

Laborde's forceps, method, sign (test) (lah-bordz′) [Jean Baptiste Vincent *Laborde,* French physician, 1830–1903] see under *forceps* and *method,* and see *Cloquet's needle sign,* under *sign.*

labra (la′brah) [L.] plural of *labrum.*

labrale (lah-bra′le) an anthropometric landmark on the border of the lip. **l. infe′rius,** the lowest point, in the midsagittal plane, on the vermilion border of the lower lip. **l. supe′rius,** the highest point, in the midsagittal plane, on the vermilion border of the upper lip.

labrocyte (lab′ro-sīt) [Gr. *labros* greedy + *-cyte*] a mast cell.

labrum (la′brum), pl. *la′bra* [L.] 1. [NA] a general term for an edge, brim, or lip. 2. any liplike part or structure, such as the shelflike projection of the head that anteriorly covers the mandibles of and forms the roof of the mouth of arthropods. **l. acetabula′re** [NA], acetabular lip: a ring of fibrocartilage attached to the rim of the acetabulum of the hip bone, increasing the depth of the cavity; called also *l. glenoidale articulationis coxae.* **l. articula′ris** [NA], articular lip: a prominent fibrocartilaginous rim around the periphery of certain joints, such as the acetabulum of the hip bone and the glenoid cavity of the scapula; see also *l. acetabulare* and *l. glenoidale.* **l. glenoida′le** [NA], glenoid lip: a ring of fibrocartilage attached to the rim of the glenoid cavity of the scapula, increasing the depth of the cavity; called also *l. glenoidale articulationis humeri.* **l. glenoida′le articulatio′nis cox′ae,** l. acetabulare. **l. glenoida′le articulatio′nis hu′meri,** l. glenoidale.

laburinine (lah-bu′rĭ-nēn) cytisine.

labyrinth (lab′ĭ-rinth) [Gr. *labyrinthos*] a system of intercommunicating cavities or canals, especially that constituting the internal ear (auris internus [NA]). **bony l.,** the bony part of the internal ear; called also *labyrinthus osseus* [NA] or *osseus l.* **cochlear l.,** labyrinthus cochlearis. **cortical l.,** a network of tubules and blood vessels in the cortex of the kidney. **endolymphatic l.,** labyrinthus membranaceus. **l. of ethmoid, ethmoidal l.,** labyrinthus ethmoidalis. **Ludwig's l's,** spaces between Bertin's columns and the cortical arches. **membranous l.,** labyrinthus membranaceus. **nonacoustic l.,** statokinetic l. **olfactory l.,** labyrinthus ethmoidalis. **osseous l.,** bony l. **perilymphatic l.,** spatium perilymphaticum. **statokinetic l.,** the vestibule and semicircular canals; called also *nonacoustic l.* **vestibular l.,** labyrinthus vestibularis.

labyrinthectomy (lab″ĭ-rin-thek′to-me) [*labyrinth* + Gr. *ektome* excision] excision of the labyrinth of the ear.

labyrinthi (lab″ĭ-rin′thi) [L.] genitive and plural of *labyrinthus.*

labyrinthine (lab″ĭ-rin′thīn) pertaining to a labyrinth.

labyrinthitis (lab″ĭ-rin-thi′tis) inflammation of the labyrinth; otitis interna. **circumscribed l.,** that due to erosion of the bony wall of a semicircular canal with exposure of the membranous labyrinth.

labyrinthodont (lab″ĭ-rin′tho-dont) [Gr. *labyrinthos* labyrinth + *odontos* tooth] an extinct amphibian in which the enamel of the tooth was completely invaginated into the dentin; labyrinthodonts were the first terrestrial vertebrates and the ancestors of modern amphibians and reptiles.

Labyrinthomorpha (lab″ĭ-rin″tho-mor′fah) [*labyrinth* + Gr. *morphe* form] a phylum of naked protozoa, saprobic and parasitic on algae, mostly in marine and estuarine waters, occurring as fusiform protoplasmic masses grouped in a network formed by ramifying and anastomosing filopodia, and sometimes having a flagellate stage. It comprises one class: Labyrinthulea.

labyrinthotomy (lab″ĭ-rin-thot′o-me) [*labyrinth* + Gr. *temnein* to cut] surgical incision into the labyrinth.

Labyrinthulea (lab″ĭ-rin-thu′le-ah) a class of parasitic aquatic protozoa (phylum Labyrinthomorpha) with characters of the phylum. It comprises one order: Labyrinthulida.

Labyrinthulida (lab″ĭ-rin-thu′lĭ-dah) an order of parasitic aquatic protozoa (class Labyrinthulea, phylum Labyrinthomorpha) with characters of the class.

labyrinthus (lab″ĭ-rin′thus), gen. and pl. *labyrin′thi* [L., from Gr. *labyrinthos*] 1. [NA] a general term for a system of in-

tercommunicating cavities or canals. 2. the internal or inner ear (auris interna [NA]). Called also *labyrinth.* **l. cochlea′ris** [NA], cochlear labyrinth: the part of the membranous labyrinth that includes the perilymphatic space and the cochlear duct. **l. ethmoida′lis** [NA], the ethmoidal labyrinth: either of the paired lateral masses of the ethmoid bone, consisting of numerous thin-walled cellular cavities, the ethmoidal cells. **l. membrana′ceus** [NA], the membranous labyrinth: a system of communicating epithelial sacs and ducts, including the endolymphatic duct, utricle, saccule, and semicircular ducts, lodged within and attached at certain points to the wall of the osseous labyrinth but separated from the major portion of the bony labyrinth by the perilymphatic space, and containing endolymph; it is divided into vestibular and cochlear parts (see *l. vestibularis* and *l. cochlearis*). **l. os′seus** [NA], bony or osseous labyrinth: a layer of dense bone in the petrous portion of the temporal bone, in which the membranous labyrinth is lodged; it consists of three parts: the vestibule, the semicircular canals, and the cochlea. **l. vestibula′ris** [NA], vestibular labyrinth: the part of the membranous labyrinth that includes the utricle and saccule lodged within the vestibule and the semicircular ducts lodged eccentrically in the corresponding canals.

lac (lak), gen. *lac′tis,* pl. *lac′ta* [L.] 1. milk. 2. any milklike medicinal preparation. 3. a resinous material collected from various tropical trees, secreted by an insect, *Laccifer lacca* Kerr (Coccidae), and used in the preparation of shellac. **l. femini′num,** the secretion of the human mammary gland. **l. fermen′tum,** koumiss. **l. sulfu′ris,** precipitated sulfur. **l. vacci′num,** cow's milk.

Laccifer (lak′sĭ-fer) a genus of insects, including *L. lacca* Kerr (Coccidae), which is the source of lac and shellac.

lacerable (las′er-ah-b′l) capable of becoming lacerated.

lacerated (las′er-āt″ed) [L. *lacerare* to tear] torn; mangled; wounded by a jagged instrument.

laceration (las″er-a′shun) [L. *laceratio*] 1. the act of tearing. 2. a torn, ragged, mangled wound.

lacertofulvin (lah-ser″to-ful′vin) [L. *lacertus* lizard + *fulvus* yellow] a yellow coloring matter from the skin of certain reptiles.

lacertus (lah-ser′tus) [L., "lizard," because of a fancied resemblance] [NA] a general term for certain fibrous attachments of muscles. **l. cor′dis,** see *trabeculae carneae cordis.* **l. fibro′sus mus′culi bicip′itis bra′chii,** aponeurosis musculi bicipitalis brachii. **l. me′dius Weitbrech′tii,** **l. me′dius Wrisber′gii,** ligamentum longitudinale anterius. **l. mus′culi rec′ti latera′lis bul′bi** [NA], the check ligament of the lateral rectus muscle, which is attached to the lateral palpebral ligament.

Lachesis (lak′ĕ-sis) [L.; Gr. *Lachesis* one of the three Fates] a genus of venomous snakes of Central and South America. *L. mu′ta* is the bushmaster, or suruçucu.

Lachnospira (lak″no-spi′rah) [Gr. *lachnos* woolly hair + Gr. *speira* coil] a genus of gram-negative anaerobic bacteria of the family Bacteroidaceae, made up of curved, rod-shaped cells found in the rumen of cattle. The type species is *L. multipa′ris.*

lachry- for words beginning thus, see those beginning *lacri-.*

lacinia (lah-sin′e-ah) [L. "fringe"] (*obs.*) fimbria, def. 1.

lacmus (lak′mus) [Ger. *Lackmus*] litmus.

lacrima (lak′rĭ-mah), pl. *lacrimae* [L.] see *tears.*

lacrimae (lak′rĭ-me) [L.] plural of *lacrima;* the watery secretion of the lacrimal glands. See *tears.*

lacrimal (lak′rĭ-mal) pertaining to the tears.

lacrimation (lak″rĭ-ma′shun) [L. *lacrimatio*] the secretion and discharge of tears.

lacrimator (lak″rĭ-ma″tor) a substance which increases the flow of tears, such as certain gases.

lacrimatory (lak′rĭ-mah-to″re) causing a flow of tears.

lacrimonasal (lak″rĭ-mo-na′zal) pertaining to the lacrimal sac and the nose.

lacrimotome (lak′rĭ-mo-tōm) [*lacrima* + *-tome*] a knife for incising the lacrimal sac or duct.

lacrimotomy (lak″rĭ-mot′o-me) [*lacrima* + *-tomy*] incision of the lacrimal sac or duct.

lacta (lak′tah) [L.] plural of *lac.*

lactacidemia (lak-tas″ĭ-de′me-ah) [*lactic acid* + Gr. *haima* blood + -ia] an excess of lactic acid in the blood, as after violent exercise.

lactacidin (lak-tas′ĭ-din) a food preservative composed of lactic and salicylic acids.

lactacidogen (lak″tah-sid′o-jen) [*lactic acid* + Gr. *gennan* to produce] a term used by Embden to designate the hexose phosphate precursor of lactic acid in muscle contraction.

lactaciduria (lak-tas″ĭ-du′re-ah) [*lactic acid* + Gr. *ouron* urine + -ia] the presence of lactic acid in the urine.

lactagogue (lak′tah-gog) [L. *lac* milk + Gr. *agōgos* leading] galactagogue.

lactalbumin (lak″tal-bu′min) an albumin found in milk and resembling serum albumin.

lactam (lak′tam) a cyclic amide formed from aminocarboxylic acids by the elimination of water. They are isomeric with lactims, which are enol forms of lactams.

$$
\begin{array}{cc}
-C{=}O & -C-OH \\
| & \| \\
-NH & -N \\
\text{Lactam} & \text{Lactim}
\end{array}
$$

β-**lactamase** (lak′tah-mās) [EC 3.5.2.6] an enzyme of the hydrolase class that catalyzes the reaction *β*-lactam + H_2O = substituted *β*-amino acid. The activity comprises a group of enzymes of varying specificity, acting on penicillins and cephalosporins. The reaction hydrolyzes the *β*-lactam ring of penicillin to form penicilloic acid, which lacks antibiotic activity. The enzyme is produced by certain species of *Staphylococcus*, *Bacillus*, and *Clostridium*, rendering them resistant to many of the penicillins. Called also *cephalosporinase* and *penicillinase*.

lactamide (lak-tam′id) the amide of lactic acid, $CH_3\cdot CHOH\cdot CONH_2$.

Lactarius (lak-ta′re-us) a genus of fungi of the order Agaricales, series Homobasidiomycetidae, having white spores, and including both edible and poisonous species. When they are cut or broken, a white or milk-like substance is discharged. *L. delicio′sus*, an edible species, is the source of lactaroviolin.

lactaroviolin (lak″tah-ro-vi′o-lin) chemical name: 1-formyl-4-methyl-7-isopropenylazalone. A pigment, $C_{15}H_{14}O$, isolated from the fungus *Lactarius deliciosus*.

lactase (lak′tās) [EC 3.2.1.108] an enzyme of the hydrolase class that catalyzes the reaction lactose + H_2O = D-glucose + D-galactose. The enzyme occurs in the brush border of the intestinal mucosa. It is a complex that also cleaves the terminal sugar residues from glycosly-*N*-acylsphingosine. A defect in or absence of the enzyme causes lactose intolerance. **adult l. deficiency,** disaccharide intolerance III. **l. deficiency,** lactose intolerance. **intestinal l. deficiency,** disaccharide intolerance III.

lactate (lak′tāt) 1. the anionic form of lactic acid; a salt of lactic acid. 2. to secrete milk. **ferrous l.,** greenish white crystals or powder, $Fe(C_3H_5O_3)_2$, used orally as a hematinic. **lactic acid l.,** a substance formed by concentration by the boiling of lactic acid; used in the preparation of sodium lactate.

L-lactate dehydrogenase (LDH) (lak′tāt de-hi′dro-jĕnās) [EC 1.1.1.27] an enzyme of the oxidoreductase class that catalyzes the reaction (S)-lactate + NAD^+ = pyruvate + NADH. The reaction is the final step in glycolysis (white fibers). The reverse reaction is the first step in the combustion of lactate (heart, red fibers) or its conversion to glucose (liver). The enzyme occurs in the cytoplasm of nearly all cells. It is a tetramer containing M(muscle) and H (heart) subunits; it exists as five distinct isozymes (M_4, M_3H, M_2H_2, MH_3, H_4). Identification of isozyme types in serum is used for clinical diagnosis.

lactation (lak-ta′shun) [L. *lactatio*, from *lactare* to suckle] 1. the secretion of milk. 2. the period of the secretion of milk. 3. suckling.

lactational (lak-ta′shun-al) pertaining to lactation.

lacteal (lak′te-al) [L. *lacteus* milky] 1. pertaining to milk. 2. any of the intestinal lymphatics that transport chyle; so called because during absorption they are white from absorbed fat. Called also *chyliferous vessels* and *lacteal vessels*.

lactenin (lak′tĕ-nin) a bacteriostatic substance in milk.

lactescence (lak-tes′ens) [L. *lactescere* to become milky] resemblance to milk; milkiness.

lactic (lak′tik) pertaining to milk.

lactic acid (lak′tik) a metabolic intermediate involved in many biochemical processes; it is the end product of glycolysis, which provides energy anaerobically in skeletal muscle during heavy exercise, and it can be oxidized aerobically in the heart for energy production or can be converted back to glucose (gluconeogenesis) in the liver. Moderate elevations of blood lactate occur during heavy exercise; severe elevations (lactic acidosis) can occur in diabetes mellitus and in genetic deficiencies of enzymes involved in gluconeogenesis. Lactate is also the end product of fermentation in several bacterial species.

lacticemia (lak″tĭ-se′me-ah) the presence of lactic acid in the blood.

lactiferous (lak-tif′er-us) [L. *lac* milk + *ferre* to bear] producing or conveying milk.

lactifuge (lak′tĭ-fūj) [L. *lac* milk + *fugare* to expel] 1. checking or stopping the secretion of milk. 2. an agent that checks the secretion of milk.

lactigenous (lak-tij′ĕ-nus) [L. *lac* milk + Gr. *gennan* to produce] producing or secreting milk.

lactigerous (lak-tij′er-us) [L. *lac* milk + *gerere* to carry] lactiferous.

lactim (lak′tim) see under *lactam*.

lactin (lak′tin) lactose, or milk sugar.

lactinated (lak′tĭ-nāt″ed) prepared with lactose.

lactivorous (lak-tiv′o-rus) [L. *lac* milk + *vorare* to devour] feeding or subsisting upon milk.

lact(o)- [L. *lac*, gen. *lactis* milk] a combining form denoting relationship to milk or to lactic acid.

Lactobacillaceae (lak″to-bas″il-la′se-e) a family of bacteria made up of gram-positive, asporogenous, straight or curved rods occurring singly or in chains. Formerly called *Lactobacteriaceae*.

Lactobacilleae (lak″to-bah-sil′e-e) in former systems of classification, a tribe of bacteria of the family Lactobacillaceae, made up of straight or curved rods occurring singly or in chains, the organisms of which have been assigned to the genera *Lactobacillus* and *Eubacterium*.

lactobacilli (lak″to-bah-sil′i) [L.] plural of *lactobacillus*.

Lactobacillus (lak″to-bah-sil′lus) [*lacto-* + L. *bacillus* small rod] a genus of bacteria of the family Lactobacillaceae, occurring as large, gram-positive, asporogenous, rod-shaped organisms. They are anaerobic or microaerophilic and occur widely in nature and in the human mouth, vagina, and intestinal tract. In the oral cavity, they are found associated with dental caries but have no known etiologic role. They are separable into two groups, the homofermentative group producing only lactic acid, and the heterofermentative group producing other end-products of fermentation. **L. acidoph′ilus,** a homofermentative lactobacillus producing the fermented product, acidophilus milk. **L. bif′idus,** *Bifidobacterium bifidum*. **L. bulgar′icus,** a homofermentative lactobacillus producing the fermented product known as Bulgarian or bulgaricus milk.

lactobacillus (lak″to-bah-sil′us), pl. *lactobacil′li*. An organism of the genus *Lactobacillus*.

Lactobacteriaceae (lak″to-bak-te″re-a′se-e) a former name of a family of bacteria now called *Lactobacillaceae*.

lactobutyrometer (lak″to-bu″tĭ-rom′ĕ-ter) [*lacto-* + *butyrometer*] an instrument for measuring the proportion of cream in milk.

lactocele (lak′to-sēl) galactocele.

lactochrome (lak′to-krōm) [*lacto-* + Gr. *chrōma* color] riboflavin.

lactoconium (lak-to-ko′ne-um) [*lacto-* + Gr. *konis* dust] one of the small particles, of unknown nature, seen with the ultramicroscope in the milk of animals.

lactocrit (lak′to-krit) [*lacto-* + Gr. *kritēs* judge] an instrument for estimating the amount of fat in milk.

lactodensimeter (lak″to-den-sim′ĕ-ter) lactometer.

lactofarinaceous (lak″to-far″ĭ-na′shus) composed of milk and farinaceous foods; said of a diet.

lactoferrin (lak′to-fer″in) an iron binding protein found in the specific granules of neutrophils where it apparently exerts an antimicrobial activity by withholding iron from ingested bacteria and fungi, it also occurs in many secretions and exudates (milk, tears, mucus, saliva, bile, etc.)

lactoflavin (lak′to-fla″vin) [lacto- + L. flavus yellow] riboflavin.

lactogen (lak′to-jen) any substance that enhances lactation, the principal one being prolactin. **human placental l.,** a polypeptide hormone secreted by the placenta that disappears from the circulation immediately after delivery. It has lactogenic, luteotropic, and growth-promoting activity, is immunologically similar to human growth hormone, and inhibits maternal insulin activity during pregnancy. Called also chorionic somatomammotropin and placental growth hormone. Abbreviated hPL.

lactogenesis (lak″to-jen′ĕ-sis) the secretion of milk by the mammary glands.

lactogenic (lak″to-jen′ik) stimulating the production of milk.

lactoglobulin (lak″to-glob′u-lin) a globulin occurring in milk.

lactometer (lak-tom′ĕ-ter) [lacto- + Gr. metron measure] an instrument for ascertaining the specific gravity of milk.

lactone (lak′tōn) 1. an aromatic liquid, $C_{10}H_8O_4$, prepared by distillation from lactic acid. 2. a cyclic organic compound in which the chain is closed by ester formation between a carboxyl and a hydroxyl group in the same molecule.

lacto-ovovegetarian (lak″to-o″vo-vej″ĕ-ta′re-an) a vegetarian who includes eggs and dairy products in his diet.

lactophenin (lak″to-fe′nin) a bitter, crystalline powder, $C_6H_4(OC_2H_5)\cdot NH\cdot CO\cdot CH(OH)CH_3$, derived from phenetidin and lactic acid, soluble in 500 parts of cold and in 55 parts of boiling water; formerly used as an analgesic and antipyretic.

lactophosphate (lak″to-fos′fāt) [lacto- + L. phosphas phosphate] any salt of lactic and phosphoric acids.

lactoprotein (lak″to-pro′te-in) a protein derived from milk.

lactorrhea (lak″to-re′ah) galactorrhea.

lactosazone (lak″to-sa′zōn) the phenylosazone of lactose. It is a yellow crystalline substance made by treating lactose with phenylhydrazine and acetic acid. The crystals melt at 200° C. and may be used in identifying lactose.

lactoscope (lak′to-skōp) [lacto- + Gr. skopein to examine] a device showing the proportion of cream in milk.

lactose (lak′tōs) [L. saccharum lactis] [USP] 4-O-β-D-galactopyranosyl-D-glucose. A white crystalline sugar (disaccharide), $C_{12}H_{22}O_{11}$, obtained from milk which on hydrolysis with acids or certain enzymes yields glucose and galactose; used as a tablet and capsule diluent. It is also used as an osmotic laxative and diuretic, and in infant feeding formulas. Lactose, a constituent of milk, is not tolerated in many persons after weaning, owing to reduced lactase activity. Called also lactin and milk sugar. **beta l.,** a disaccharide obtained by allowing a solution of lactose to crystallize above 93.5° C.; it is sweeter and more soluble than lactose.

lactoside (lak′to-sīd) a glycoside whose sugar constituent is lactose. **ceramide l.,** lactosyl-N-acylsphingosine, the major sphingolipid accumulated in lactosylceramidosis. It has also been isolated from human epidermoid carcinoma. Called also cytolipin H.

lactosidosis (lak″to-si-do′sis), pl. lactosido′ses. The accumulation of lactoside in tissues. **ceramide l.,** lactosylceramidosis.

lactosum (lak-to′sum) lactose.

lactosuria (lak″to-su′re-ah) [lactose + Gr. ouron urine + -ia] the presence of lactose in the urine, observed frequently during lactation.

lactosyl ceramidase (lak″to-sil-ser-am′ĭ-dās) [EC 3.2.1] any of the enzymes of the hydrolase class that catalyze the hydrolysis of O-glycosyl bonds in lactosyl ceramides. See also galactosylceramidase (lactosyl ceramidase I) and β-galactosidase (lactosyl ceramidase II).

lactosylceramide (lak-to″sil-ser′ah-mīd) ceramide lactoside. See ceramide lactoside, under lactoside.

lactosylceramide galactosyl hydrolase (lak″to-sil-ser′ah-mīd gah-lak″to-sil hi′dro-lās) lactosyl ceramidase.

lactosylceramidosis (lak-to″sil-ser″ah-mi-do′sis) [lactosyl-ceramide + -osis] a sphingolipidosis marked by an accumulation in the viscera and nervous system of lactosylceramide

because of deficient lactosylceramide galactosyl hydrolase. Clinically, retarded psychomotor development is evident by 25 months. Called also lactosyl ceramidosis, ceramide lactosidosis, and neutral β-galactosidase deficiency.

lactotherapy (lak″to-ther′ah-pe) [lacto- + therapy] treatment by milk diet; called also galactotherapy.

lactotoxin (lak″to-tok′sin) a toxic substance formed in milk.

lactotrope (lak′to-trōp) lactotroph.

lactotroph (lak′to-trōf) an acidophilic cell of the anterior pituitary that secretes prolactin; called also mammotroph.

lactotrophin, lactotropin (lak″to-tro′fin; lak″to-tro′pin) prolactin.

lactovegetarian (lak″to-vej″ĕ-ta′re-an) 1. pertaining to, consisting of, or subsisting on milk (or other dairy products) and vegetables. 2. a vegetarian who uses dairy products in addition to vegetables in his diet.

lactoylglutathione lyase (lak″to-il-gloo-tah-thi′ōn li′ās) [EC 4.4.1.5] an enzyme of the lyase class that catalyzes the reaction (R)-S-lactoylglutathione = glutathione + methylglyoxal. The reaction converts methylglyoxal to lactic acid. Formerly called glyoxalase I.

Lactuca (lak-tu′kah) [L.] a genus of composite-flowered plants, including L. sati′va L., common lettuce, and L. viro′sa L., the inspissated juice of which was formerly used as a sedative and hypnotic.

lactulose (lak′tū-lōs) chemical name: 4-O-β-D-galactopyranosyl-D-fructose. A synthetic disaccharide, $C_{12}H_{22}O_{11}$, used as a cathartic and to enhance excretion or formation of ammonia in the treatment of portosystemic encephalopathy, including the stages of hepatic precoma and coma.

lacuna (lah-ku′nah), gen. and pl. lacu′nae [L.] 1. a small pit or hollow cavity; [NA] a general term for such a compartment within or between other body structures. Called also lake. 2. a defect or gap, as in the field of vision (scotoma). **absorption l.,** resorption l. **Blessig's l.,** see Blessig's cysts. **blood l.,** any one of the blood-filled spaces in the trophoblast of the embryo that serve hemotrophic nutrition. **bone l.,** a small cavity within the bone matrix containing an osteocyte and from which slender canaliculi radiate and penetrate the adjacent lamellae to anastomose with the canaliculi of neighboring lacunae, thus forming a system of cavities interconnected by minute canals. Called also osseous l. **cartilage l.,** any of the small cavities within the cartilage matrix, containing a chondrocyte, or cartilage cell. **cerebral lacunae,** small areas of cerebral ischemic infarction resulting from occlusion of branches of the middle cerebral, posterior cerebral, and basilar arteries; seen in association with hypertension and arteriosclerosis. **great l. of urethra,** fossa navicularis urethrae. **Howship l.,** rebsorption l. **intervillous l.,** one of the blood spaces of the placenta in which the fetal villi are found; called also trophoblastic l. **lateral lacunae, lacu′nae latera′les** [NA], venous meshworks within the dura mater on either side of the superior sagittal sinus; arachnoidal granulations project into them. **l. mag′na,** fossa navicularis urethrae. **lacunae of Morgagni,** lacunae urethrales in the male urethra. **lacu′nae Morga′gnii ure′thrae mulie′bris,** glandulae urethrales urethrae femininae. **l. of muscles, l. musculo′rum** [NA], a compartment beneath the inguinal ligament for the passage of the iliopsoas muscle and femoral nerve, separated from the lacuna vasorum by the iliopectineal arch. **osseous l.,** bone l. **parasinoidal l's,** lacunae laterales. **l. pharyn′gis,** a depression at the pharyngeal end of the auditory tube. **resorption l.,** a pit or concavity found in bones undergoing resorption, frequently containing osteoclasts. Similar lacunae also may be found in eroding surfaces of cementum, in which cementoclasts may or may not be located. Called also absorption l. and Howship's l. **trophoblastic l.,** intervillous l. **lacunae of urethra, urethral lacunae,** lacunae urethrales. **urethral lacunae of Morgagni,** lacunae urethrales in the male urethra. **lacu′nae urethra′les** [NA], urethral lacunae: numerous small depressions or pits in the mucous membrane of the urethra, with their openings usually directed distally. Some contain openings of ducts of the urethral glands. **l. vaso′rum** [NA], **l. of vessels,** a space for the passage of the femoral vessels into the thigh, separated from the lacuna musculorum by the iliopectineal arch.

lacunae (lah-ku′ne) [L.] genitive and plural of *lacuna*.

lacunar (lah-ku′nar) pertaining to or containing lacunae; of the nature of a lacuna.

lacune (lah-kūn′) lacuna.

lacunule (lah-ku′nŭl) [L. *lacunula*] a small lacuna.

lacus (la′kus), pl. *la′cus* [L.] lake. **l. lacrima′lis** [NA], lacrimal lake: the triangular space at the medial angle of the eye, where the tears collect; called also *lacrimal bay* and *lake*.

Ladd-Franklin theory (lad-frangk′lin) [Christine *Ladd-Franklin*, Baltimore physician, 1847–1930] see under *theory*.

Ladendorff's test (lah′den-dorfs) [August *Ladendorff*, German physician of the 19th century] see under *tests*.

Ladin's sign (la′dinz) [Louis Julius *Ladin*, American obstetrician, born 1862] see under *sign*.

lae- for words beginning thus, see also those beginning *le-*.

Laelaps (le′laps) *Echinolaelaps*.

Laënnec's catarrh, etc. (la″en-neks′) [René Théophile Hyacinthe *Laënnec*, distinguished French physician and inventor of the stethoscope, 1781–1826] see under *catarrh, cirrhosis, disease, pearl,* and *sign*.

Laetrile (la′ĕ-tril) trademark for *l*-mandelonitrile-β-glucuronic acid, derived by hydrolysis of amygdalin and oxidation of the resulting *l*-mandelonitrile-β-glucoside; it is alleged to have antineoplastic properties. The term is sometimes used interchangeably with *amygdalin*.

laeve (le′vĕ) [L. *levis* smooth] nonvillous, as the *chorion laeve*.

laev(o)- for words beginning thus, see those beginning *lev(o)-*.

Lafora's bodies, disease, sign (lah-fo′rahz) [Gonzalo Rodríguez *Lafora*, Spanish physician, 1887–1971] see under *body* and *sign*, and see *myoclonus epilepsy*, under *epilepsy*.

Lag. abbreviation for L. *lage′na*, a flask.

lag (lag) 1. the period of time elapsing between the application of a stimulus and the resulting reaction. 2. see *lag phase*, under *phase*. **nitrogen l.,** the time that elapses after the administration of a protein before there appears in the urine an amount of nitrogen equivalent to that administered.

lagena (lah-je′nah) [L. "flask"] 1. a part of the upper extremity of the ductus cochlearis. 2. the curved, flask-shaped organ of hearing in vertebrates lower than mammals.

lageniform (lah-jen′ĭ-form) [L. *lagena* flask + *form*] flask-shaped.

Lagochilascaris minor (lag″o-ki-las′kah-ris mi′nor) a nematode worm found in subcutaneous abscesses of man in Trinidad and Surinam.

lagophthalmos (lag″of-thal′mos) [Gr. *lagōs* hare + *ophthalmos* eye] a condition in which the eye cannot be completely closed.

lagophthalmus (lag″of-thal′mus) lagophthalmos.

Lagrange's operation (lah-grah′zez) [Pierre Félix *Lagrange*, French ophthalmologist, 1857–1928] sclerectoiridectomy.

laiose (li′ōs) a pale yellow substance, $C_6H_{12}O_6$, found in the urine in diabetes mellitus; it is nonfermentable and levorotatory.

lake (lāk) [L. *lacus*] 1. to undergo separation of hemoglobin from the erythrocytes, a phenomenon sometimes occurring in blood. 2. a circumscribed collection of fluid in a hollow or depressed area. See also *lacuna*. **lacrimal l.,** lacus lacrimalis. **marginal l's,** discontinuous venous lacunae, relatively free of villi, near the edge of the placenta, formed by merging of the marginal portions of the intervillous space with the subchorial lake. Called also *marginal sinus*, because it was thought to be circumferentially continuous and important for placental drainage. **subchorial l.,** the portion of the placenta, relatively free of villi, just beneath the chorionic plate; at the edge of the placenta it becomes continuous with irregular channels to form the marginal lakes. Called also *subchorial space*. **venous l.,** small blue-purple sessile, compressible papules or blebs seen most often on the lips, ears, and face of elderly persons, which histologically represent dilated capillaries filled with red blood cells and lined with flattened endothelial cells.

laliatry (lah-li′ah-tre) [Gr. *lalia* talking + *iatria* therapy] the study and treatment of disorders of speech.

lallation (lah-la′shun) [L. *lallatio*] a babbling, infantile form of speech.

Lallemand's bodies (lal-mahz′) [Claude François *Lallemand*, French surgeon, 1790–1854] Bence Jones cylinders.

lalo- [Gr. *lalein* to babble, speak] a combining form denoting relationship to speech.

lalognosis (lal″og-no′sis) [*lalo-* + Gr. *gnōsis* knowledge] the understanding of speech.

lalopathology (lal″o-pah-thol′o-je) [*lalo-* + *pathology*] the branch of medicine which deals with disorders of speech.

lalopathy (lah-lop′ah-the) [*lalo-* + Gr. *pathos* illness] any disorder of speech.

lalophobia (lal″o-fo′be-ah) [*lalo-* + *phobia*] irrational fear of speaking.

laloplegia (lal″o-ple′je-ah) [*lalo-* + Gr. *plēgē* stroke] paralysis of the organs of speech.

lalorrhea (lal″o-re′ah) [*lalo-* + Gr. *rhoia* flow] logorrhea.

Lalouette's pyramid (lal″oo-ets′) [Pierre *Lalouette*, French physician, 1711–1792] see under *pyramid*.

Lamarck's theory (lah-marks′) [Jean Baptiste Pierre Antoine Monet de *Lamarck*, French naturalist, 1744–1829] see under *theory*.

Lamaze method (le-mahz′) [Fernand *Lamaze*, French obstetrician, 1890–1957] see under *method*.

lambda (lam′dah) [the eleventh letter of the Greek alphabet, Λ or λ] the point at the site of the posterior fontanel where the lambdoid and sagittal sutures meet; used as a craniometric landmark.

lambdacism, lambdacismus (lam′dah-sizm; lam-dah-siz′mus) [Gr. *lambdakismos*] 1. the substitution of *l* for *r* in speaking. 2. inability to utter correctly the sound of *l*.

lambdoid (lam′doid) [Gr. *lambda* + *eidos* form] shaped like the Greek letter Λ or λ.

lambert (lam′bert) [Johann Heinrich *Lambert*, German mathematician and physicist, 1728–1777] a unit of brightness, being the brightness of a perfect diffuser emitting one lumen per square centimeter. The unit generally used is one one-thousandth of this and is called a *millilambert*. When the area chosen is one square foot the unit is called a *foot lambert*.

Lambert's cosine law (lam′berts) [Johann Heinrich *Lambert*] see under *law*.

Lamblia (lam′ble-ah) [Vilem Dusan *Lambl*, Bohemian physician, 1824–1895] *Giardia*. **L. intestina′lis,** *Giardia lamblia*.

lambliasis, lambliosis (lam-bli′ah-sis; lam-ble-o′sis) giardiasis.

lame (lām) incapable of normal locomotion; deviation from the normal gait.

lame foliacée (lam′fol-yă-sā′) [Fr. *lame* plate, lamina; *foliacée* foliaceous] the whorled or concentrically laminated connective tissue structures contained in some nevi; called also *foliate lamina*.

lamel (lam′el) lamella, def. 2.

lamella (lah-mel′ah), gen. and pl. *lamel′lae* [L., dim. of *lamina*] 1. a thin leaf or plate, as of bone. 2. a medicated disk or wafer prepared from gelatin, glycerin, and distilled water, and containing a small quantity of an alkaloid, to be inserted under the eyelid. **annulate lamel′lae,** cytoplasmic organelles which consist of parallel arrays of cisternae exhibiting small annuli or circular fenestrae at very regular intervals along their length. **articular l.,** the layer of bone to which an articular cartilage is attached. **basic l.,** circumferential l. **circumferential l.,** one of the layers of bone that underlie the periosteum (*external circumferential l.*) and endosteum (*internal circumferential l.*); called also *basic l.* **concentric l.,** haversian l. **cornoid l.,** a thick column of parakeratotic cells extending outward from a notch in the malpighian layer of the epidermis, and forming the raised border of a lesion of porokeratosis. **enamel lamellae,** imperfectly calcified areas of enamel located generally in the cervical enamel but also found in the interdigitating surface of the premolars and molars; they are foliaceous structures visible only under the microscope and may extend from the surface to the dentinoenamel junctions and beyond. **endosteal l.,** one of the bony plates lying beneath the endosteum. **ground l.,** interstitial l. **haversian l.,** one of the concentric bony plates surrounding a haversian canal. **intermediate l.,** interstitial l. **inter-**

stitial l., one of the bony plates that fill in between the haversian systems; called also *ground l.* or *intermediate l.* **osseous l.,** any one of the thin plates into which bone can be divided. **periosteal l., peripheral l.,** the layer of bone lying next to the periosteum. **posterior border l. of Fuchs,** the fibrillar layer of the dilator muscle of the iris; called also *Henle's membrane.* **triangular l.,** the area above the roof of the third ventricle of the brain occupied by the velum interpositum. **vitreous l.,** lamina basalis.

lamellae (lah-mel′e) [L.] genitive and plural of *lamella.*

lamellar (lah-mel′ar) pertaining to or resembling lamellae.

lamellasome (lah-mel′ah-sōm) [*lamella* + Gr. *sōma* body] an intracytoplasmic membranous inclusion consisting of a series of invaginated lamellae enclosed by a common membrane. Such structures appear to be confined to unicellular blue-green algae.

lamelliform (lah-mel′ĭ-form) resembling lamellae.

lamellipodia (lah-mel″ĭ-po′de-ah), sing. *lamellipodium* [*lamella* + Gr. *pous* foot + *-ia*] delicate sheetlike extensions of cytoplasm which form transient adhesions with the cell substrate and wave gently, enabling the cell to move along the substrate.

lamellipodium (lah-mel″ĭ-po′de-um) singular of lamellipodia.

lamina (lam′ĭ-nah), gen. and pl. *lam′inae* [L.] a thin flat plate, or layer; [NA] a general term for such a structure, or a layer of a composite structure. The term is often used alone to mean the lamina arcus vertebrae. **l. affix′a** [NA], the narrow strip of ependyma overlying the thalamostriate vein and stria terminalis in the central part of the lateral ventricle. **alar l., l. ala′ris** [NA], either of the pair of longitudinal zones of the embryonic neural tube dorsal to the sulcus limitans, from which are developed the dorsal gray columns of the spinal cord and the sensory centers of the brain; called also *alar plate.* **lam′inae al′bae cerebel′li** [NA], white laminae of the cerebellum: the core of white substance that supports a folium of the cerebellar cortex; called also *laminae medullares cerebelli.* **anterior limiting l.,** l. limitans anterior corneae. **l. ante′rior vagi′nae mus′culi rec′ti abdo′minis** [NA], the portion of its sheath lying anterior to the rectus abdominis muscle, formed by aponeuroses of the internal and external oblique above the arcuate line and by the aponeuroses of the internal oblique and transversus, below the arcuate line. **l. ar′cus ver′tebrae** [NA], lamina of the vertebral arch: either of the pair of broad plates of bone flaring out from the pedicles of the vertebral arches and fusing together at the midline to complete the dorsal part of the arch and provide a base for the spinous process. **basal l.,** l. basalis. **basal l. of choroid,** complexus basalis choroideae. **basal l. of ciliary body,** l. basalis corporis ciliaris. **l. basa′lis** [NA], the basal lamina: either of the pair of longitudinal zones of the embryonic neural tube ventral to the sulcus limitans, from which are developed the ventral gray columns of the spinal cord and the motor centers of the brain; called also *basal plate.* **l. basa′lis chorioi′deae,** l. basalis choroideae. **l. basa′lis choroi′deae,** NA alternative for *complexus basalis choroideae.* **l. basa′lis cor′poris cilia′ris** [NA], basal lamina of the ciliary body: the innermost layer of the ciliary body, continuous with the basal lamina of the choroid. **l. basila′ris duc′tus cochlea′ris** [NA], the wall of the cochlear duct, which separates it from the scala tympani; the spiral organ lies against it. Called also *basilar membrane of cochlear duct.* **Bowman's l.,** l. limitans anterior corneae. **l. cartilag′inis cricoi′deae** [NA], lamina of cricoid cartilage: the broad posterior part of the cricoid cartilage. **l. cartilag′inis latera′lis tu′bae auditi′vae** [NA], lateral lamina of cartilage of auditory tube: the smaller of the two laminae that compose the tubal cartilage; it lies in the lateral wall of the auditory tube. **l. cartilag′inis media′lis tu′bae auditi′vae** [NA], medial lamina of cartilage of auditory tube: the larger of the two laminae that compose the tubal cartilage; it lies in the medial wall of the auditory tube. **l. cartilag′inis thyroi′deae [dex′tra/sinis′tra]** [NA], lamina of thyroid cartilage: either of the broad plates that form the sides (right and left) of the thyroid cartilage, converging anteriorly to meet at the midline. **l. choriocapilla′ris,** l. choroidocapillaris. **l. chorioi′dea epithelia′lis thal′ami,** the ependyma lining the superior surface of the thalamus. **l. chori-**

oi′dea epithelia′lis ventric′uli latera′lis, the ependyma lining the lateral ventricle of the cerebrum. **l. chorioi′dea epithelia′lis ventric′uli quar′ti,** the ependyma lining the roof of the fourth ventricle of the cerebrum. **l. choroidocapilla′ris** [NA], the inner layer of the choroid, composed of a single-layered network of small capillaries; called also *choriocapillaris* and *choriocapillaris l.* **l. cine′rea termina′lis** (obs.), l. terminalis hypothalami. **cribriform l.,** fascia cribrosa. **cribriform l. of ethmoid bone,** lamina cribrosa ossis ethmoidalis. **cribriform l. of transverse fascia,** septum femorale. **l. cribro′sa os′sis ethmoida′lis,** cribriform lamina of ethmoid bone: the horizontal plate of the ethmoid bone that forms the roof of the nasal cavity; it is perforated by many foramina (foramina cribrosa ossis ethmoidalis) for the passage of the olfactory nerves. In official anatomical nomenclature [NA], the cribriform lamina and foramina of the ethmoid bone are considered together, and are designated *lamina et foramina cribrosa ossis ethmoidalis.* **l. cribro′sa scle′rae** [NA], the perforated portion of the sclera through which pass the axons of the ganglion cells of the retina; called also *optic foramen of sclera.* **l. of cricoid cartilage,** l. cartilaginis cricoideae. **dental l.,** a horizontal band projecting perpendicularly from the vestibular lamina and extending into the substance of the embryonic gum, assuming a horseshoe-like shape to conform with the dental arches. Called also *l. dentalis* and *dentogingival l.* **dental l., lateral,** a lateral band of cells believed to be functionally and structurally similar to the parent dental lamina, which connects the developing tooth germ to the dental lamina. Called also *lateral enamel strand.* **l. denta′lis,** dental l. **l. denta′ta,** labium limbi vestibulare laminae spiralis. **dentogingival l.,** dental l. **descending l. of sphenoid bone,** processus pterygoideus ossis sphenoidalis. **l. du′ra,** see *bundle bone,* under *bone.* **elastic l., external,** external elastic membrane. **elastic l., internal,** internal elastic membrane. **l. elas′tica ante′rior [Bow′mani],** l. limitans anterior corneae. **l. elas′tica poste′rior [Demour′si, Descem′eti],** l. limitans posterior corneae. **episcleral l., l. episclera′lis** [NA], loose connective and elastic tissue covering the sclera and anteriorly connecting it with the conjunctiva. **epithelial l., l. epithelia′lis** [NA], the layer of ependymal cells covering the choroid plexus. **l. exter′na cra′nii** [NA], **l. exter′na os′sium cra′nii,** outer table of skull: the outer compact layer of bone of the flat bones of the skull. **external l. of peritoneum,** peritoneum parietale. **external l. of pterygoid process,** l. lateralis processus pterygoidei. **l. fibrocartilagin′ea interpu′bica,** discus interpubicus. **foliate l.,** lame foliacée. **l. fus′ca scle′rae** [NA], a thin layer of loose, pigmented connective tissue on the inner surface of the sclera, connecting it with the choroid. **l. granula′ris exter′na cor′ticis cer′ebri** [NA], external granular layer of cerebral cortex: layer II of the cortex cerebri (q.v.), composed of many small pyramidal cells and granule cells with short axons. **l. granula′ris inter′na cor′ticis cer′ebri** [NA], internal granular layer of cerebral cortex: layer IV of the cerebral cortex, composed of many densely packed granule cells with short axons and some small pyramidal cells, and transversed by a stria of horizontally arranged fibers (external or outer band or line of Baillarger); it contains neurites derived from cells other layers and areas of the cerebral cortex and subcortical areas. **l. horizonta′lis os′sis palati′ni** [NA], horizontal plate of palatine bone: the horizontal part of the palatine bone, forming the posterior part of the hard palate. **inferior l. of sphenoid bone,** processus pterygoideus ossis sphenoidalis. **l. inter′na cra′nii** [NA], **l. inter′na os′sium cra′nii,** inner table of skull: the inner compact layer of bone of the flat bones of the skull. **internal l. of pterygoid process,** l. medialis processus pterygoidei. **interpubic l., fibrocartilaginous,** discus interpubicus. **labial l.,** the ectodermal plate that on splitting separates lip from gum, thus forming the labial groove. **labiodental l.,** the thickened ectodermal band from which the dental and labial laminae develop. **labiogingival l.,** labial l. **lateral l. of cartilage of auditory tube,** l. cartilaginis lateralis tubae auditivae. **lateral l. of pterygoid process,** l. lateralis processus pterygoidei. **l. latera′lis cartilag′inis tu′bae auditi′vae,** l. cartilaginis lateralis tubae auditivae. **l. latera′lis proces′sus pterygoi′dei** [NA], lateral lamina of the pterygoid process: either of a pair of bony plates projecting downward from the roots of the greater wings of the sphenoid bone and forming the medial wall of the ipsilateral infratemporal fossa; called also *lateral plate of pterygoid process.* **l. lim′itans ante′rior cor′neae** [NA], anterior limiting lamina: a thin layer of the cornea beneath the outer layer of stratified epithelium, composed of condensed stroma, between it and the substantia propria; called also *l. elastica anterior [Bowmani]* and *Bowman's membrane.* **l. lim′itans poste′rior cor′neae** [NA], posterior limiting lamina: a thin hyaline membrane between the substantia propria and the endothelial layer of the cornea; called also *l. elastica posterior [Demoursi, Descemeti]* and *Descemet's membrane.* **limiting l., anterior,** l. limitans anterior corneae. **limiting l., posterior,** l. limitans posterior corneae. **medial l. of cartilage of auditory tube,** l. cartilaginis medialis tubae auditivae. **medial l. of pterygoid process,** l. medialis processus pterygoidei. **l. media′lis cartilag′inis tu′bae auditi′vae,** l. cartilaginis medialis tubae auditivae. **l. media′lis proces′sus pterygoi′dei** [NA], medial lamina of pterygoid process: either of a pair of bony plates projecting downward from the roots of the greater wings of the sphenoid bone and forming the lateral boundary of the ipsilateral posterior aperture of the nasal cavity and the most posterior part of the lateral wall of the nasal cavity. Called also *medial plate of pterygoid process.* **la′minae mediastina′les,** the mediastinal layers of the pleura. **lam′inae medulla′res cerebel′li,** laminae albae cerebelli. **l. medulla′ris latera′lis cor′poris stria′ti** [NA], lateral medullary lamina of corpus striatum: a layer of white substance that separates the lateral globus pallidus from the putamen; called also *external medullary l.* or *stria of corpus striatum.* **l. medulla′ris media′lis cor′poris stria′ti** [NA], medial lamina of corpus striatum: a layer of white substance that divides the medial portion of the lentiform nucleus (globus pallidus) into a larger, lateral, and a smaller, medial part; called also *internal medullary l.* or *stria of corpus striatum.* **lam′inae medulla′res thal′ami interna and externa** [NA], internal and external medullary layers of thalamus: two layers of myelinated nerve fibers in the dorsal thalami. The *internal* layer, which is a vertical sheet of white substance, partially splits anterosuperiorly, and separates the medial and lateral nuclei; it contains the intralaminar nuclei. The *external* layer of white substance covers the lateral surface of the dorsal thalamus, and separates it from the internal capsule. **l. medulla′ris transver′sa cor′poris quadrigem′ini,** stratum album profundum corporis quadrigemini. **medullary l., of corpus striatum, external,** l. medullaris lateralis corporis striati. **medullary l., of corpus striatum, internal,** l. medullaris medialis corporis striati. **medullary l., external,** see *laminae medullares thalami interna et externa.* **medullary l., internal,** see *laminae medullares thalami interna et externa.* **medullary l. of corpus striatum, lateral** l. medullaris lateralis corporis striati. **medullary l., of corpus striatum, medial,** l. medullaris medialis corporis striati. **medullary laminae of thalamus,** laminae medullares thalami interna and externa. **l. membrana′cea tu′bae auditi′vae** [NA], **membranous l. of auditory tube,** the connective tissue lamina that supports the inferior and lateral parts of the auditory tube. **l. mesenter′ii pro′pria,** the proper layer of the mesentery. **l. modi′oli** [NA], a bony plate extending upward toward the cupula as a continuation of the modiolus and of the bony spiral lamina of the cochlea. **l. molecula′ris cor′ticis cer′ebri** [NA], molecular layer of cerebral cortex: layer I of the cortex cerebri (q.v.), which is the most superficial of the six layers, composed chiefly of a stria of tangentially oriented myelinated nerve fibers; this layer also contains dendritic terminals from cells of deeper layers, some cortical afferent fibers, sparsely scattered horizontal cells of Cajal, and various other cell types. Called also *lamina plexiformis corticis cerebri* [NA alternative] and *plexiform* or *zonal layer of cerebral cortex.* **l. multifor′mis cor′ticis cer′ebri** [NA] multiform layer of cerebral cortex: layer VI of the cerebral cortex, composed of various cell types, chiefly containing irregular fusiform cells, the axons of which project into the white substance of the cerebral cortex hemisphere. Called also *fusiform* or *polymorphic layer of cerebral cortex.* **l. muscula′ris muco′sae** [NA], the thin layer of smooth muscle fibers usually found as a part of the tunica mucosa deep to the lamina propria mucosae. **l. muscula′ris muco′sae co′li** [NA], the muscular layer of the tunica mucosa of the colon. **l. mus-**

cula′ris muco′sae esoph′agi, NA alternative for *l. muscularis mucosae oesophagi.* **l. muscula′ris muco′sae gas′tris** [NA], the muscular layer of the tunica mucosa of the stomach; called also *l. muscularis mucosae ventriculi* [NA alternative]. **l. muscula′ris muco′sae intesti′ni cras′si** [NA], the muscular layer of the tunica mucosa of the large intestine. **l. muscula′ris muco′sae intesti′ni rec′ti,** l. muscularis mucosae recti. **l. muscula′ris muco′sae intesti′ni ten′uis** [NA], the muscular layer of the tunica mucosa of the small intestine. **l. muscula′ris muco′sae oesophagi** [NA], the muscular layer of the tunica mucosa of the esophagus. Written also *l. muscularis mucosae esophagi* [NA alternative]. **l. muscula′ris muco′sae rec′ti** [NA], the muscular layer of the tunica mucosa of the rectum. **l. muscula′ris muco′sae ventric′uli,** NA alternative for *l. muscularis mucosae gastris.* **orbital l., l. orbita′lis os′sis ethmoida′lis** [NA], a thin plate of bone laterally bounding the ethmoid labyrinth on either side and forming part of the medial wall of the orbit; called also *l. papyracea.* **palatine l. of maxilla,** processus palatinus maxillae. **l. papyra′cea,** l. orbitalis ossis ethmoidalis. **l. parieta′lis pericar′dii** [NA], the parietal layer of the serous pericardium; it lines the fibrous pericardium. **l. parieta′lis tu′nicae vagina′lis pro′priae tes′tis, l. parieta′lis tu′nicae vagina′lis tes′tis** [NA], parietal layer of tunica vaginalis of testis: the outer layer of the tunica vaginalis of the testis, separated from the visceral layer by a cavity. **periclaustral l.,** capsula extrema. **perpendicular l. of ethmoid bone,** l. perpendicularis ossis ethmoidalis. **l. perpendicula′ris os′sis ethmoida′lis** [NA], perpendicular lamina of ethmoid bone: a thin bony plate that descends from the inferior surface of the cribriform plate of the ethmoid bone and participates in forming the nasal septum; called also *perpendicular plate of ethmoid bone.* **l. perpendicula′ris os′sis palati′ni** [NA], the flat, vertical, bony plate that extends superiorly on either side from the palatine bone; it is surmounted by the orbital and sphenoidal processes. Called also *pars perpendicularis ossis palatini* and *perpendicular plate of palatine bone.* **l. plexifor′mis cor′ticis cer′ebri,** NA alternative for *l. molecularis corticis cerebri.* **posterior limiting l.,** l. limitans posterior corneae. **l. poste′rior vagi′nae mus′culi rec′ti abdo′minis** [NA], the portion of its sheath lying posterior to the rectus abdominis muscle, formed by the transversus abdominis and its aponeurosis at the level of the xiphoid process; below the xiphoid process, to the arcuate line, it is formed by the aponeuroses of the internal oblique and the transversus. **l. pretrachea′lis fas′ciae cervica′lis** [NA], the layer of the cervical fascia that is anterior to the trachea. **l. prevertebra′lis fas′ciae cervica′lis** [NA], the prevertebral fascia: the layer of the cervical fascia that is anterior to the vertebrae; called also *fascia praevertebralis.* **l. profun′da fas′ciae tempora′lis** [NA], the deep portion of the fascia investing the temporal muscle. **l. profun′da mus′culi levato′ris pal′pebrae superi′o′ris** [NA], the deeper of the two layers of the levator palpebrae superioris muscle, the fibers of which are attached to the tarsus superior palpebrae. **proper l. of mesentery,** lamina mesenterii propria. **l. pro′pria membra′nae tym′pani,** the middle fibrous basis of the tympanic membrane, attached, except anterosuperiorly, to the tympanic plate of the temporal bone. **l. pro′pria muco′sae** [NA], proper mucous membrane: the connective tissue coat of a mucous membrane just deep to the epithelium and basement membrane. **l. pyramida′lis exter′na cor′ticis cer′ebri** [NA], external pyramidal layer of cerebral cortex: layer III of the cortex cerebri (q.v.), composed of an inner zone of medium-sized pyramidal cells and an outer zone of larger pyramidal cells and other cells whose dendrites and axons extend beyond this layer. **l. pyramida′lis gangliona′ris cor′ticis cer′ebri,** NA alternative for *l. pyramidalis interna corticis cerebri.* **l. pyramida′lis inter′na cor′ticis cer′ebri** [NA] internal pyramidal lamina of cerebral cortex: layer V of the cerebral cortex (q.v.), composed of the largest pyramidal cells, Martinotti's cells, and Betz's cells, and is traversed by a stria of horizontally arranged fibers (inner or internal line or band of Baillarger); the axons of the pyramidal cells leave this layer as either association, projection, or commissural fibers. Called also *ganglionic layer of cerebral cortex* and *l. pyramidalis ganglionaris corticis cerebri* [NA alternative]. **l. quadrigem′ina,** l. tecti mesencephali. **l. reticula′ris,** the perforated hyaline membrane which covers the organ of Corti. **Rexed's laminae,** an architectural scheme used to classify the structure of the spinal cord, based on the cytological features of the neurons in different regions of the gray substance. It consists of nine laminae (I–IX) that extend throughout the cord, roughly paralleling the dorsal and ventral columns of the gray substance, and a tenth region (lamina X) that surrounds the central canal and consists of the dorsal and ventral commissures and the central gelatinous substance. **rostral l., l. rostra′lis,** the thin terminal part of the rostrum of the corpus callosum passing down in front of the anterior commissure to the anterior perforated substance and the paraterminal gyrus. **l. sep′ti pellu′cidi** [NA], **l. of septum pellucidum,** either of the thin, vertical sheets, separated by a cleftlike space, which constitute the septum pellucidum. **spiral l., bony,** l. spiralis ossea. **spiral l., secondary,** l. spiralis secundaria. **l. spira′lis os′sea** [NA], bony spiral lamina: a double plate of bone winding spirally around the modiolus and dividing the spiral canal of the cochlea incompletely into two parts, the scala tympani and the scala vestibuli; called also *spiral plate.* **l. spira′lis secunda′ria** [NA], secondary spiral lamina: a bony projection on the outer wall of the osseous spiral lamina in the lower part of the first turn of the cochlea. **submucous l. of stomach,** tela submucosa gastris. **l. superficia′lis fas′ciae cervica′lis** [NA], the layer of the cervical fascia that lies deep to the skin. **l. superficia′lis fas′ciae tempora′lis** [NA], the superficial portion of the fascia investing the temporal muscle. **l. superficia′lis mus′culi levato′ris palpe′brae superio′ris** [NA], the superficial of the two layers of the levator palpebrae superioris muscle. **l. suprachorioi′dea, suprachoroid l., l. suprachoroi′dea** [NA], the outermost layer of the choroid, which connects it with the sclera; called also *suprachoroid layer.* **l. supraneuropor′ica,** the part of lamina terminalis caudal to the anterior neuropore of the embryo; it cannot be delimited accurately in human embryos. **tectal l. of mesencephalon,** l. tecti mesencephali. **l. tecta′lis mesenceph′ali,** NA alternative for *l. tecti mesencephali.* **l. tec′ti mesenceph′ali** [NA], **l. of tectum of mesencephalon,** the layer of mingled gray and white substance in the tectum of the mesencephalon, from which arise the superior and inferior colliculi; called also *l. tectalis mesencephali* [NA alternative] and *quadrigeminal plate.* **terminal l. of hypothalamus, l. termina′lis hypothal′ami** [NA], a thin plate derived from the telencephalon extending upward from the optic chiasm and preoptic recess, and forming the anterior wall of the third ventricle of the cerebrum; called also *terminal plate.* **l. of thyroid cartilage, right and left,** l. cartilaginis thyroideae dextra/sinistra. **l. tra′gi** [NA], **l. tra′gica,** the longitudinal curved lamina of cartilage in the tragus of the auricle, at the beginning of the cartilaginous portion of the external acoustic meatus. **vascular l. of choroid,** l. vasculosa choroideae. **vascular l. of stomach,** tela submucosa gastris. **l. vasculo′sa chorioi′deae, l. vasculo′sa choroi′deae** [NA], vascular lamina of choroid: the layer of the choroid between the suprachoroid and choriocapillary layers, containing the largest blood vessels; called also *Haller's membrane.* **l. of vertebra, l. of vertebral arch,** l. arcus vertebrae. **l. viscera′lis pericardii** [NA], visceral layer of pericardium: the inner layer of the serous pericardium; it is in contact with the heart and the roots of the great vessels; called also *epicardium* [NA alternative], and *visceral pericardium.* **l. viscera′lis tu′nicae vagina′lis pro′priae tes′tis, l. viscera′lis tu′nicae vagina′lis tes′tis** [NA], visceral layer of tunica vaginalis of testis: the inner part of the tunica vaginalis of the testis, firmly attached to the testis and epididymis. **l. vi′trea, vitreal l., vitreous l.,** complexus basalis choroideae. **white laminae of cerebellum,** laminae albae cerebelli.

laminae (lam′ĭ-ne) [L.] genitive and plural of *lamina.*

laminagram (lam′ĭ-nah-gram) a roentgenogram of a selected layer of the body made by body-section roentgenography.

laminagraph (lam′ĭ-nah-graf) an x-ray machine for making roentgenograms of a layer of tissue at a selected depth.

laminagraphy (lam″ĭ-nag′rah-fe) [L. *lamina* layer + Gr. *graphein* to record] see *body section roentgenography,* under *roentgenography.*

laminar (lam′ĭ-nar) [L. *laminaris*] made up of, or arranged in, laminae.

Laminaria (lam″ĭ-na′re-ah) a genus of seaweeds, the kelps, various species of which are used as sources of alginates; see *laminarin.* The dried stems of *L. digitata* are used to dilate the uterine cervix in induced abortion.

laminarin (lam″ĭ-na′rin) a polysaccharide from seaweed (*Laminaria*) consisting essentially of β-D-glucose residues. **l. sulfate,** the sulfated form, having antilipemic and anticoagulant properties.

laminectomy (lam″ĭ-nek′to-me) [L. *lamina* layer + Gr. *ektomē* excision] excision of the posterior arch of a vertebra.

laminitis (lam″ĭ-ni′tis) inflammation of a lamina, and especially of the laminae of a horse's foot; see *founder.*

laminogram (lam′ĭ-no-gram) laminagram.

laminography (lam″ĭ-nog′rah-fe) laminagraphy; see *body section roentgenography,* under *roentgenography.*

laminotomy (lam″ĭ-not′o-me) [*lamina* + Gr. *tomē* a cutting] division of the lamina of a vertebra.

lamp (lamp) an apparatus for furnishing heat or light. **annealing l.,** an alcohol lamp for heating and purifying gold foil to be used for filling tooth cavities. **arc l.,** a source of light consisting of gaseous particles from the electrodes of an electric arc which are raised to a temperature of incandescence by an electric current. **carbon arc l.,** a lamp that produces an intense white light from an electric arc between carbon rods; used in artificial light therapy. **cold quartz mercury vapor l.,** an ultraviolet radiation lamp having a low vapor pressure, low amperage, high voltage, and a glow discharge; more than 95 per cent of its emission is in the resonance emission line of mercury vapor at 254 mμ. **diagnostic l.,** a light used for observing subtle shadings in weak fluorescence, for external body examinations, observations of tissue fluorescence, identification of vulvar fluorescence, chromatography, etc. **Eldridge-Green l.,** an arrangement of lights for testing color vision. **Finsen l.,** a carbon arc lamp operating at 50 volts and 50 amperes so constructed that radiation is concentrated on an area 1 inch square; a water-cooled quartz system is used to remove caloric radiation and a compression quartz piece to dehematize the skin. **Finsen-Reya l.,** a modification of the Finsen lamp in which the electrodes are placed at right angles to each other. **Gullstrand's slit l.,** slit l. **Jesionek l.,** a light for giving artificial sunlight baths. **Kromayer's l.,** a small water-cooled mercury vapor lamp with a quartz window that produces ultraviolet radiation. **Lortet l.,** an electric lamp used in Finsen light treatment. **mercury vapor l.,** a lamp in which the arc is struck in mercury and is enclosed in a quartz burner; used in light therapy. There are two types, the air-cooled and water-cooled (*Kromayer's l.*). **quartz l.,** a mercury vacuum lamp made of melted quartz glass embedded in a running water-bath, used for applying ultraviolet light treatment. **Simpson l.,** see under *light.* **slit l.,** one embodying a diaphragm containing a slitlike opening, by means of which a narrow flat beam of intense light may be projected into the eye. It gives intense illumination so that microscopic study may be made of the conjunctive, cornea, iris, lens, and vitreous, the special feature being that it illuminates a section through the substance of these structures. Called also *Gullstrand's slit lamp* and *slit-lamp biomicroscope.* **tungsten arc l.,** an electric arc lamp having tungsten electrodes; it has been used in the treatment of acne, alopecia, etc. **ultraviolet l.,** one which produces ultraviolet rays. **Wood's l.,** see under *light.*

lampas (lam′pas) a swelling and hardening of the mucosa of the hard palate, immediately behind the upper incisors in horses; called also *palatitis.*

Lamprocystis (lam″pro-sis′tis) [Gr. *lampros* bright, brilliant + *kystis* sac, bladder] a genus of aquatic phototrophic bacteria of the family Chromatiaceae, order Rhodospirillale, consisting of spherical motile cells that contain gas vacuoles and fix carbon dioxide in the presence of hydrogen sulfide. Cell suspensions are purple. The type species is *L. roseopersici′na.*

Lampropedia (lam″pro-ped′e-ah) [Gr. *lampros* bright + *pedion* a plain] a genus of gram-negative, aerobic, coccoid bacteria of uncertain affiliation, found in environments rich in organic matter, made up of chemorganotrophic cells. The type species is *L. hyalina.*

lamprophonia (lam″pro-fo′ne-ah) [Gr. *lampros* clear + *phōnē* voice + *-ia*] clearness of voice.

lamprophonic (lam″pro-fon′ik) pertaining to or characterized by lamprophonia.

Lamus (la′mus) a former genus name of predatory insects of the family Reduviidae now placed under the genera *Panstrongylus* and *Triatoma*.

lamziekte (lam′zēk-te) [Dutch "lame-sickness"] a disease of cattle in South Africa secondary to bovine osteophagia; the cattle chew putrefying bones and thus absorb the toxin of *Clostridium botulinum*.

lana (lan′ah), *la′nae*. gen. and pl. [L] wool.

lanatoside C (lah-nat′o-sīd) [NF] an easily absorbed and stable glycoside, $C_{49}H_{76}O_{20}$, obtained from the leaves of *Digitalis lanata*. It occurs as colorless or white, odorless crystals or powder, and is used as a cardiotonic where digitalis is recommended.

lanaurin (lan′aw-rin) a pyrrole pigment found in the sweat and urine of sheep which may color the wool yellow.

lance (lans) [L. *lancea*] 1. lancet. 2. to cut or incise with a lancet.

Lancefield classification (lans′fēld) [Rebecca Craighill *Lancefield*, New York bacteriologist, 1895–1981] see under *classification*.

lanceolate (lan′se-o-lāt) shaped like a lance.

Lancereau-Mathieu disease (lahn″ser-o mat″e-u) [Etienne *Lancereau*; Albert *Mathieu*, physician in Paris, 1855–1917] leptospiral jaundice.

lancet (lan′set) [L. *lancea* lance] a small pointed and two-edged surgical knife. **abscess l.,** a wide-bladed lancet with one convex and one concave edge. **acne l.,** a form with a narrow blade for puncturing the papules of acne. **gingival l., gum l.,** a knife for incising the gingivae. **spring l.,** one the blade of which is held by a spring.

Lancet coefficient (lan′set) [*The Lancet*, a British medical periodical] see under *coefficient*.

lancinating (lan′sĭ-nāt″ing) [L. *lancinas*] tearing, darting, or sharply cutting; see under *pain*.

Lancisi's nerves, stria (lan-che′sēz) [Giovanni Maria *Lancisi*, Italian physician, 1654–1720] see *stria longitudinalis lateralis corporis callosi* and *stria longitudinalis medialis corporis callosi*.

landmark (land′mark) a readily recognizable anatomical structure used as a point of reference in establishing the location of another structure or in determining certain measurements.

Landolt's bodies, operation (lahn-dolts′) [Edmond *Landolt*, ophthalmologist in Paris, 1846–1926] see under *body* and *operation*.

Landouzy's disease, dystrophy (type) (lan-doo′zēz) [Louis Théophile Joseph *Landouzy*, French physician, 1845–1917] see *Weil's syndrome*, under *syndrome*, and see *Landouzy-Dejerine dystrophy*, under *dystrophy*.

Landouzy-Dejerine dystrophy (atrophy, type) (lan-doo′ze-deh″zher-ēn′) [L. T. J. *Landouzy*; Joseph Jules *Dejerine*, French neurologist, 1849– 1917] see under *dystrophy*.

Landouzy-Grasset law (lan-doo′ze-gras-sa′) [L. T. J. *Landouzy*; Joseph *Grasset*, French physician, 1849– 1918] see under *law*.

Landry's paralysis (disease, palsy, syndrome) (lan-drēz′) [Jean Baptiste Octave *Landry*, French physician, 1826–1865] acute febrile polyneuritis.

Landsteiner (land′sti-ner) Karl. Austrian pathologist and immunologist, 1868–1943; winner of the Nobel prize for physiology or medicine in 1930 for his discovery of the human blood groups in 1901.

Landström's muscle (lahnd′stremz) [John *Landström*, Swedish surgeon, 1869–1910] see under *muscle*.

Lane's band, etc. (lānz) [Sir William Arbuthnot *Lane*, English surgeon, 1856–1943] see under *band, disease, kink, operation,* and *plate*.

Langdon Down's disease (lang′don downz) [John *Langdon* Haydon *Down*, British physician, 1828–1896] Down's syndrome.

Lange's solution, test (reaction) (lahng′ez) [Carl *Lange*, German physician, born 1883] see under *solution*, and see *colloidal gold test*, under *tests*.

Langenbeck's amputation, etc. (lahng′en-beks) [Bernhard Rudolf Konrad von *Langenbeck*, German surgeon, 1810–1887] see under *amputation, flap,* and *triangle*.

Langer's axillary arch, lines, muscle (lang′erz) [Carl Ritter von Edenberg von *Langer*, Austrian anatomist, 1819–1887] see under *arch, line,* and *muscle*.

Langerhans' cells, granules, islets, (islands) (lahng′er-hanz) [Paul *Langerhans*, German pathologist, 1847–1888] see under *cell* and *islet*, and see *Birbeck's granules*, under *granule*.

Langhans' cells, layer, stria (lahng′hahnz) [Theodor *Langhans*, German pathologist, 1839–1915] see under *cell*, and see *cytotrophoblast*.

Langley's ganglion, granules, nerves (lang′lēz) [John Newport *Langley*, English physiologist, 1852–1925] see under *ganglion* and *granule*, and see *pilonidal nerves*, under *nerve*.

laniary (lan′e-a″re) [L. *laniare* to tear to pieces] suitable for lacerating, or tearing to pieces; said of canine teeth.

lanolin (lan′o-lin) [L. *lanolinum*; *lana* wool + *oleum* oil] [USP] the purified fatlike substance from the wool of sheep, *Ovis aries*, occurring as a yellowish white mass and mixed with 25 to 30 per cent of water; used as a water-in-oil ointment base. **anhydrous l.** [USP], lanolin that contains not more than 0.25 per cent of water, used as an absorbent ointment base.

lanosterol (lah-nos′ter-ol) a triterpenic sterol, $C_{30}H_{50}O$, formed from squalene; it is the parent steroid in animals, being itself converted in several steps to cholesterol.

Lanoxin (lah-nok′sin) trademark for preparations of digoxin.

Lanterman's incisures (clefts) (lahn″ter-mahnz′) [A.J. *Lanterman*, American anatomist in Strassburg, 19th century] see under *incisure*.

Lanterman-Schmidt incisures (lahn″ter-mahn′-schmit′) [A. J. *Lanterman*; Henry D. *Schmidt*, American anatomist, 1823–1888] incisures of Lanterman.

lanthanic (lan′than-ik) [Gr. *lanthanein* to escape notice, to be concealed] symptom-free; said of a symptomless disease that is undetected, or detected by accident.

lanthanin (lan′thah-nin) oxychromatin.

lanthanum (lan′thah-num) [Gr. *lanthanein* to be concealed] a rare metallic element; symbol, La; atomic number, 57; atomic weight, 138.91.

lanuginous (lah-nu′jĭ-nus) [L. *lanuginosus*] covered with lanugo.

lanugo (lah-nu′go) [L.] [NA] the fine hair on the body of the fetus; called also *down* and *lanugo hair*.

lanum (la′num) [L. *lana* wool] lanolin.

Lanz's point (lahnts) [Otto *Lanz*, surgeon in Amsterdam, 1865–1935] see under *point*.

LAP 1. leukocyte alkaline phosphatase. 2. lyophilized anterior pituitary (tissue).

lapactic (lah-pak′tik) [Gr. *lapaktikos, lapassein* to discharge] pertaining to or effecting a removal; purgative; laxative.

lapar(o)- [Gr. *lapara* flank] a combining form denoting relationship to the loin or flank. Sometimes used loosely in reference to the abdomen.

laparocele (lap′ah-ro-sēl) ventral hernia.

laparocholecystotomy (lap″ah-ro-ko″le-sis-tot′o-me) [*laparo-* + Gr. *cholē* bile + *kystis* bladder + *tomē* a cutting] cholecystectomy.

laparocolectomy (lap″ah-ro-ko-lek′to-me) [*laparo-* + Gr. *kolon* colon + *ektomē* excision] colectomy.

laparocolostomy (lap″ah-ro-ko-los′to-me) [*laparo-* + Gr. *kolon* colon + *stomoun* to provide with an opening, or mouth] surgical creation of a permanent opening into the colon through an incision in the anterolateral wall of the abdomen; colostomy.

laparocolotomy (lap″ah-ro-ko-lot′o-me) [*laparo-* + Gr. *kolon* colon + *tomē* a cutting] colotomy.

laparocystectomy (lap″ah-ro-sis-tek′to-me) [*laparo-* + Gr. *kystis* cyst + *ektomē* excision] removal of a cyst by an abdominal incision.

laparocystidotomy (lap″ah-ro-sis″tĭ-dot′o-me) [*laparo-* + Gr. *kystis* bladder + *tomē* a cutting] suprapubic cystotomy.

laparocystotomy (lap″ah-ro-sis-tot′o-me) [*laparo-* + Gr.

kystis bladder + *tomē* a cutting] laparotomy with removal of the contents of a cyst.

laparoenterostomy (lap″ah-ro-en″ter-os′to-me) [*laparo-* + Gr. *enteron* intestine + *stomoun* to provide with an opening, or mouth] surgical creation of an artificial opening into the intestine through the abdominal wall.

laparoenterotomy (lap″ah-ro-en″ter-ot′o-me) [*laparo-* + Gr. *enteron* intestine + *tomē* a cutting] laparotomy with incision into the intestine.

laparogastroscopy (lap″ah-ro-gas-tros′ko-pe) [*laparo-* + *gastroscopy*] examination of the interior of the stomach through an abdominal incision.

laparogastrostomy (lap″ah-ro-gas-tros′to-me) [*laparo-* + Gr. *gastēr* stomach + *stomoun* to provide with an opening, or mouth] surgical creation of a permanent gastric fistula through the abdominal wall.

laparogastrotomy (lap″ah-ro-gas-trot′o-me) [*laparo-* + Gr. *gastēr* stomach + *tomē* a cutting] incision into the stomach through the abdominal wall.

laparohepatotomy (lap″ah-ro-hep″ah-tot′o-me) [*laparo-* + *hepatotomy*] incision of the liver through the abdominal wall.

laparohysterectomy (lap″ah-ro-his″ter-ek′to-me) [*laparo-* + Gr. *hystera* uterus + *ektomē* excision] removal of the uterus through an opening in the abdominal wall.

laparohystero-oophorectomy (lap″ah-ro-his″ter-o-o″of-ŏ-rek′to-me) [*laparo-* + Gr. *hystera* uterus + *oophorectomy*] laparotomy with removal of the uterus and ovaries.

laparohysterosalpingo-oophorectomy (lap″ah-ro-his″ter-o-sal-ping″go-o″of-ŏ-rek′to-me) removal of the uterus, uterine tubes, and ovaries through an abdominal incision.

laparohysterotomy (lap″ah-ro-his″ter-ot′o-me) [*laparo-* + Gr. *hystera* uterus + *tomē* a cutting] laparotomy with incision of the uterus.

laparoileotomy (lap″ah-ro-il″e-ot′o-me) [*laparo-* + *ileum* + Gr. *tomē* a cutting] laparotomy with incision of the ileum.

laparomonodidymus (lap″ah-ro-mon″o-did′ĭ-mus) [*laparo-* + Gr. *monos* single + *didymos* twin] a monster, double above but single below the pelvis.

laparomyitis (lap″ah-ro-mi-i′tis) [*laparo-* + Gr. *mys* muscle + *-itis*] inflammation of the abdominal or lumbar muscles.

laparomyomectomy (lap″ah-ro-mi″o-mek′to-me) [*laparo-* + Gr. *mys* muscle + *ektomē* excision] surgical removal of a uterine myoma (leiomyoma) through an abdominal incision.

laparonephrectomy (lap″ah-ro-ne̊-frek′to-me) [*laparo-* + Gr. *nephros* kidney + *ektomē* excision] removal of a kidney by an incision in the loin.

laparorrhaphy (lap-ah-ror′ah-fe) [*laparo-* + Gr. *rhaphē* suture] suture or repair of the abdominal wall.

laparosalpingectomy (lap″ah-ro-sal″pin-jek′to-me) [*laparo-* + Gr. *salpinx* tube + *ektomē* excision] removal of a uterine tube through an abdominal incision.

laparosalpingo-oophorectomy (lap″ah-ro-sal- ping″go-o″of-ŏ-rek′to-me) removal of a uterine tube and ovary through an abdominal incision.

laparosalpingotomy (lap″ah-ro-sal″pin-got′o-me) [*laparo-* + Gr. *salpinx* tube + *tomē* a cutting] incision of a uterine tube through an abdominal incision.

laparoscope (lap′ah-ro-skōp″) an instrument comparable to an endoscope which, when inserted into the peritoneal cavity, permits it to be inspected; peritoneoscope.

laparoscopy (lap″ah-ros′ko-pe) [*laparo-* + Gr. *skopein* to examine] examination of the interior of the abdomen by means of a laparoscope.

laparosplenectomy (lap″ah-ro-sple-nek′to-me) [*laparo-* + Gr. *splēn* spleen + *ektomē* excision] laparotomy with excision of the spleen.

laparosplenotomy (lap″ah-ro-sple-not′o-me) [*laparo-* + Gr. *splēn* spleen + *tomē* a cutting] laparotomy to gain access to the spleen, usually for the purpose of draining a cyst or abscess of the spleen.

laparotomaphilia (lap″ah-rot″o-mah-fil′e-ah) [*laparotomy* + Gr. *philein* to love + *-ia*] Munchausen syndrome (q.v.) in which the patient desires abdominal surgery.

laparotome (lap′ah-ro-tōm) a knife used in laparotomy.

laparotomy (lap-ah-rot′o-me) [*laparo-* + Gr. *tomē* a cutting] surgical incision through the flank; less correctly, but more generally, abdominal section at any point to gain access to the peritoneal cavity.

laparotyphlotomy (lap″ah-ro-tif-lot′o-me) [*laparo-* + Gr. *typhlon* cecum + *tomē* a cutting] incision into the cecum through the flank.

Lapicque's constant, law (lah-pēks′) [Louis *Lapicque*, French physiologist, 1866–1952] see under *constant* and *law*.

Lapidus operation (lap′ĭ-dus) [Paul W. *Lapidus*, American orthopedic surgeon, born 1893] see under *operation*.

lapinization (lap″in-i-za′shun) [Fr. *lapin* rabbit] passage of a virus through rabbits as a means of modifying its characteristics.

lapinize (lap′in-īz) to attenuate (as a virus or vaccine) by serial passage through rabbits.

lapis (la′pis, lap′is) [L.] stone. **l. al′bus,** the native silicofluoride of calcium. **l. calamina′ris,** calamine. **l. imperia′lis, l. inferna′lis, l. luna′ris,** silver nitrate.

lapsus (lap′sus) [L., from *labi* to slip or fall] 1. an error, or slip, thought to be revealing of an unconscious wish or association. 2. falling or dropping of a part; ptosis. **l. cal′ami,** an unconsciously motivated slip of the pen. **l. lin′guae,** an unconsciously motivated slip of the tongue. **l. memo′riae,** an unconsciously motivated lapse of memory.

lapyrium chloride (lah-pēr′e-um) chemical name: 1-[2-oxo-2-[[2 -[(1-oxododecyl) oxy] ethyl] amino] ethyl] pyridinium chloride. A surfactant, $C_{21}H_{35}ClN_2O_3$, used in pharmaceutic preparations.

Larat's treatment (lah-raz′) [Jules Louis François Adrien *Larat*, French physician, born 1857] see under *treatment*.

lard (lard) [L. *lardum*] the purified internal fat of the abdomen of the hog. **benzoinated l.,** a preparation of lard containing 1 per cent benzoin; used as a vehicle for medicinal agents and in ointments. Called also *adeps benzoinatus*.

lardacein (lar-da′se-in) a protein found in tissues affected with amyloid degeneration. It is characterized by being insoluble in nearly all reagents, not acted upon by the gastric juice, and not readily subject to putrefaction. It gives a brown color with iodine and sulfuric acid.

lardaceous (lar-da′shus) 1. resembling lard. 2. containing lardacein.

Largon (lar′gon) trademark for a preparation of propiomazine hydrochloride.

larithmics (lah-rith′miks) [Gr. *laos* people + *arithmos* number] the study which deals with population in its quantitative aspects.

Larix (la′riks) [L.] a genus of coniferous trees, the larches. The astringent bark of *L. europaea* D.C. (Pinaceae) has been used in skin diseases and in pectoral complaints.

larixin (la-rik′sin) azaric acid.

larkspur (lark′spur) the dried ripe seeds of *Delphinium ajacis* L. (Ranuncullaceae), used medically as a pediculicide. Listed as poisonous plant due to its content of alkaloids, including delphinine. Called also *staggerweed*.

Larodopa (lar″o-do′pah) trademark for preparations of levodopa.

Larotid (lar′o-tid) trademark for preparations of amoxicillin.

Larrey's amputation (operation), cleft, spaces (lar-rāz′) [Dominique Jean (Baron de) *Larrey*, French surgeon, 1766–1842; the greatest military surgeon of his time, serving in the Napoleonic wars] see under *amputation* and *space*, and see *trigonum sternocostale*.

Larsen's disease (lar′senz) [Christian Magnus Falsen Sinding *Larsen*, Norwegian physician, 1866–1930] see under *disease*.

Larsen-Johansson disease (la′sen-yo-han′son) [C.M.F. Sinding *Larsen*; Sven *Johansson*, Swedish surgeon, born 1880] Larsen's disease.

larva (lar′vah), gen. and pl. lar′vae [L. "ghost"] an independent, motile, sometimes feeding, developmental stage in the life history of an animal. Cf. *imago* (def. 1) and *pupa*. **l. cur′rens,** an extremely rapidly progressive creeping eruption manifested by an urticarial perianal band, which represents autoinoculation of the larvae of *Strongylus sterco-*

ralis that migrate to and mature at the anus in intestinal infections with the parasite. **l. mi′grans, l. mi′grans, cutaneous** a skin disease marked by thin, pruritic, erythematous, serpiginous, papular, or vesicular lines of eruption corresponding to the movements of parasitic larvae beneath the skin. It is most often due to the presence of larvae of the cat and dog hookworm, *Ancylostoma braziliense*, which burrow beneath the skin but cannot complete their migration to the gut (called also *creeping eruption*). The terms *larva migrans* and *creeping eruption* are also applied to similar lesions caused by other parasites such as those seen in gnathostomiasis and cutaneous migratory myiasis (*dermamyiasis, dermatomyiasis*). Called also *sandworm disease*. **l. mi′grans, ocular,** infection of the eye with larvae of roundworms (*Toxocara canis* or *T. cati*), which may lodge in the choroid or retina or migrate to the vitreous; on the death of the larvae, a granulomatous inflammation occurs, the lesion varying from a translucent elevation of the retina, to massive retinal detachment and pseudoglioma. Called also *human toxocariasis*. **l. migrans, visceral,** a condition caused by prolonged migration of larvae of nematodes in human tissues other than skin, characterized by persistent hypereosinophilia, hepatomegaly, and frequently by pneumonitis; commonly caused by *Toxocara canis* or *T. cati*, which do not complete their life cycle in man. See also *l. migrans, ocular*. **rat-tailed l.,** see *Eristalis tenax*.

larvaceous (lar-va′shus) larvate.

larvae (lar′ve) [L.] plural of *larva*.

larval (lar′val) 1. pertaining to larvae. 2. larvate.

larvate (lar′vāt) [L. *larva* mask] masked; concealed: said of a disease or a symptom of disease.

larvicide (lar′vĭ-sīd) [*larva* + L. *caedere* to kill] an agent destructive to insect larvae. **Panama l.,** a mixture of crude carbolic acid, rosin, and caustic soda, heated to a uniform dark colored soap; formerly used in Panama to kill *Anopheles* larvae.

larviphagic (lar″vĭ-fa′jik) larvivorous.

larviposition (lar″vĭ-po-zish′un) the act of depositing larvae (living maggots) in the tissues of a host.

larvivorous (lar-viv′o-rus) [*larva* + L. *vorare* to eat] feeding on or consuming larvae; said especially of fish which ingest mosquito larvae.

laryngalgia (lar″in-gal′je-ah) [*laryngo-* + *-algia*] pain in the larynx.

laryngeal (lah-rin′je-al) of or pertaining to the larynx.

laryngectomee (lar″in-jek′to-me) a person whose larynx has been removed.

laryngectomy (lar″in-jek′to-me) [*laryngo-* + Gr. *ektomē* excision] extirpation of the larynx.

larynges (lah-rin′jēz) [L.] plural of *larynx*.

laryngismal (lar″in-jiz′mal) pertaining to laryngismus.

laryngismus (lar″in-jiz′mus) [L.; Gr. *laryngismos* a whooping] spasm of the larynx. **l. paralyt′icus,** roaring. **l. strid′ulus,** a condition marked by sudden laryngeal spasm, with a crowing inspiration and the development of cyanosis. It occurs in laryngeal inflammations and as an independent disease, especially in connection with rickets. Called also *Miller's* or *Wichmann's asthma*.

laryngitic (lar″in-jit′ik) pertaining to laryngitis.

laryngitis (lar″in-ji′tis) inflammation of the larynx, a condition attended with dryness and soreness of the throat, hoarseness, cough, and dysphagia. **acute catarrhal l.,** a form characterized by aphonia or hoarseness, pain and dryness of the throat, dyspnea, a wheezy cough, and more or less fever. **atrophic l.,** an extreme form of chronic catarrhal laryngitis. **chronic catarrhal l.,** a form of laryngitis due to recurring inflammation or more frequently a sequela of acute catarrhal laryngitis, characterized by atrophy of the glands of the mucous membrane. See also *l. sicca*. **croupous l.,** a condition occurring chiefly in infants or small children and characterized by a resonant barking cough, hoarseness, and stridor. Infection, allergy, a foreign body, or new growths may be the cause. Laryngeal diphtheria was once a common cause but is now relatively rare. **diphtheritic l.,** diphtheria (q.v.) localized to the larynx or trachea, which may be associated with croup. **membranous l.,** laryngitis attended with the formation of a false membrane. **necrotic l.,** calf diphtheria. **phlegmonous l.,** a usually fatal complication of erysipelas, smallpox,

etc. attended with submucous suppuration and edema. **l. sic′ca,** chronic laryngitis in which the usual secretions are gluelike; it often accompanies atrophic rhinitis. **l. stridulo′sa,** laryngismus stridulus. **subglottic l.,** inflammation of the under surface of the vocal cords. **syphilitic l.,** a chronic form due to syphilitic involvement of the larynx. **tuberculous l.,** a chronic form due to tuberculous ulceration of the larynx. **vestibular l.,** viral laryngitis in which edema forms a ring outlining the vestibule of the larynx.

laryng(o)- [L. *larynx*, q.v.] a combining form denoting relationship to the larynx.

laryngocele (lah-ring′go-sēl) [*laryngo-* + Gr. *kēlē* hernia] a congenital anomalous air sac communicating with the cavity of the larynx, which may become manifest as an enlargement seen as a tumor-like lesion on the outside of the neck; the enlargement is increased by intralaryngeal pressure, as from coughing. **ventricular l., l. ventricula′ris,** congenital dilatation or herniation of the sacculus or appendix of the laryngeal ventricle.

laryngocentesis (lah-ring″go-sen-te′sis) [*laryngo-* + Gr. *kentēsis* puncture] surgical puncture of the larynx.

laryngofissure (lah-ring″go-fish′ūr) the operation of opening the larynx by a median incision through the thyroid cartilage, for the removal of cancer of the larynx; median laryngotomy.

laryngogram (lah-ring′go-gram) a roentgenogram of the larynx.

laryngography (lar″ing-gog′rah-fe) [*laryngo-* + Gr. *graphein* to record] 1. the description of the larynx. 2. roentgenography of the larynx after instillation of a radiopaque substance into it.

laryngohypopharynx (lah-ring″go-hi′po-far′inks) the posterior wall of the hypopharynx, the piriform sinus, and areas adjacent to the larynx, considered together.

laryngology (lar″ing-gol′o-je) [*laryngo-* + *-logy*] that branch of medicine which has to do with the throat, pharynx, larynx, nasopharynx, and tracheobronchial tree.

laryngomalacia (lah-ring″go-mah-la′she-ah) [*laryngo-* + Gr. *malakia* softness] flaccidity of the epiglottis and aryepiglottic folds, as in congenital laryngeal stridor.

laryngometry (lar″ing-gom′ĕ-tre) [*laryngo-* + Gr. *metron* measure] measurement of the larynx.

laryngoparalysis (lah-ring″go-pah-ral′ĭ-sis) [*laryngo-* + *paralysis*] paralysis of the larynx.

laryngopathy (lar″ing-gop′ah-the) [*laryngo-* + Gr. *pathos* disease] any disorder of the larynx.

laryngopharyngeal (lah-ring″go-fah-rin′je-al) pertaining to the larynx and pharynx.

laryngopharyngectomy (lah-ring″go-far″in-jek′to-me) excision of the larynx and pharynx.

laryngopharyngeus (lah-ring″go-fah-rin′je-us) the inferior constrictor of the pharynx.

laryngopharyngitis (lah-ring″go-far″in-ji′tis) inflammation of the larynx and pharynx.

laryngopharynx (lah-ring″go-far′inks) [*laryngo-* + *pharynx*] the portion of the pharynx which lies below the upper edge of the epiglottis and opens into the larynx and esophagus (pars laryngea pharyngis [NA]).

laryngophony (lar″ing-gof′o-ne) [*laryngo-* + Gr. *phōnē* voice] the vocal sound as heard in auscultation of the larynx.

laryngophthisis (lar″ing-gof′thĭ-sis) [*laryngo-* + Gr. *phthisis* phthisis] tuberculosis of the larynx.

laryngoplasty (lah-ring′go-plas″te) [*laryngo-* + Gr. *plassein* to mold] plastic surgery of the larynx.

laryngoplegia (lar″ing-go-ple′je-ah) [*laryngo-* + Gr. *plēgē* stroke + *-ia*] paralysis of the larynx.

laryngoptosis (lah-ring″go-to′sis) [*laryngo-* + Gr. *ptōsis* fall] a lowering and mobilization of the larynx as sometimes seen in the aged.

laryngopyocele (lah-ring″go-pi′o-sēl) a laryngocele containing pus.

laryngorhinology (lah-ring″go-ri-nol′o-je) [*laryngo-* + Gr. *rhis* nose + *-logy*] the sum of what is known regarding the larynx and nose and their diseases.

laryngorrhagia (lar″ing-go-ra′je-ah) [*laryngo-* + Gr. *rhēgnynai* to break] hemorrhage from the larynx.

laryngorrhaphy (lar″ing-gor′ah-fe) [*laryngo-* + Gr. *rhaphē* suture] the operation of suturing the larynx.

laryngorrhea (lar″ing-go-re′ah) [*laryngo-* + Gr. *rhoia* flow] excessive secretion of mucus whenever the voice is used.

laryngoscleroma (lah-ring″go-skle-ro′mah) [*laryngo-* + *scleroma*] scleroma of the larynx.

laryngoscope (lah-ring′go-skōp) [*laryngo-* + Gr. *skopein* to examine] an endoscope for use in direct visual examination of the larynx.

laryngoscopic (lar″ing-go-skop′ik) pertaining to laryngoscopy.

laryngoscopist (lar″ing-gos′ko-pist) an expert in laryngoscopy.

laryngoscopy (lar″ing-gos′ko-pe) [*laryngo-* + Gr. *skopein* to examine] examination of the interior of the larynx, especially that performed with the laryngoscope (*direct laryngoscopy*). **direct l.,** direct visual examination of the interior of the larynx performed with a speculum or with a laryngoscope. **indirect l.,** examination of the interior of the larynx by observation of the reflection of it in a laryngeal mirror. **mirror l.,** indirect l. **suspension l.,** examination of the larynx performed with a direct laryngoscope suspended so as to leave both hands of the examiner free.

laryngospasm (lah-ring′go-spazm) [*laryngo-* + Gr. *spasmos* spasm] spasmodic closure of the larynx.

laryngostasis (lar″ing-gos′tah-sis) [*laryngo-* + Gr. *stasis* stoppage] croup.

laryngostat (lah-ring′go-stat) an appliance for holding a source of radioactive material within the larynx.

laryngostenosis (lah-ring″go-stě-no′sis) [*laryngo-* + Gr. *stenōsis* contracture] narrowing or stricture of the larynx.

laryngostomy (lar″ing-gos′to-me) [*laryngo-* + Gr. *stomoun* to provide with an opening, or mouth] surgical creation of an artificial opening into the larynx.

laryngostroboscope (lar″ing-go-strob′o-skōp) [*laryngo-* + Gr. *strophos* whirl + *skopein* to examine] an apparatus for observing the intralaryngeal phenomena with a stroboscopic light.

laryngotome (lah-ring′go-tōm) an instrument used in incising the larynx.

laryngotomy (lar″ing-got′o-me) [*laryngo-* + Gr. *tomē* a cutting] surgical incision of the larynx. **complete l.,** the longitudinal slitting of the entire larynx. **inferior l.,** incision of the larynx through the cricothyroid membrane. **median l.,** incision of the larynx through the thyroid cartilage; laryngofissure. **superior l., subhyoid l.,** incision of the larynx through the thyrohyoid membrane. **thyrohyoid l.,** subhyoid l.

laryngotracheal (lah-ring″go-tra′ke-al) pertaining to the larynx and trachea.

laryngotracheitis (lah-ring″go-tra″ke-i′tis) inflammation of the larynx and trachea. **avian l., infectious l.,** a viral disease of poultry characterized by respiratory distress, gasping, and expectoration of bloody exudate.

laryngotracheobronchitis (lah-ring″go-tra″ke-o-brong-ki′tis) inflammation of the larynx, trachea, and bronchi; the acute form is the most common cause of croup.

laryngotracheobronchoscopy (lah-ring″go-tra″ke-o-bron-kos′ko-pe) endoscopic examination of the larynx, trachea, and bronchi.

laryngotracheoscopy (lah-ring″go-tra″ke-os′ko-pe) peroral laryngoscopy and tracheoscopy.

laryngotracheotomy (lah-ring″go-tra″ke-ot′o-me) [*laryngo-* + *tracheotomy*] incision of the larynx and trachea.

laryngovestibulitis (lah-ring″go-ves-tib″u-li′tis) inflammation of the vestibule of the larynx.

laryngoxerosis (lah-ring″go-ze-ro′sis) [*laryngo-* + Gr. *xērōsis* a drying up] dryness of the larynx.

larynx (lar′inks), gen. *laryn′gis*, pl. *laryn′ges* [L., from Gr.] [NA] the musculocartilaginous structure, lined with mucous membrane, connected to the superior part of the trachea and to the pharynx inferior to the tongue and the hyoid bone; the essential sphincter guarding the entrance into the trachea and functioning secondarily as the organ of voice. It is formed by nine cartilages—the thyroid, cricoid, epiglottis, two arytenoid, two corniculate, and two cuneiform cartilages, connected by ligaments. **artificial l.,** an electromechani-

cal device that enables a laryngectomized person to converse. When the device is placed against the region of the laryngectomy a buzzing sound is produced, which is converted into simulated speech by movements of the organs of articulation (lips, tongue, glottis).

lasalocid (lah-sal′o-sid) chemical name: 6-[7*R*-[5*S*-ethyl-5-(5*R*-ethyltetrahydro-5-hydroxy-6*S*-methyl-2*H*-pyran-2*R*-yl)tetrahydro-3*S*-methyl-2*S*-furanyl]-4*S*-hydroxy-3*R*,5*S*-dimethyl-6-oxononyl]-2-hydroxy-3-methylbenzoic acid; a coccidiostat for use in poultry, $C_{34}H_{54}O_8$.

Lasègue's sign (lah-sāgz′) [Ernest Charles *Lasègue*, French physician, 1816–1883] see under *sign*.

laser (la′zer) [*l*ight *a*mplification by *s*timulated *e*mission of *r*adiation] a device which transforms light of various frequencies into an extremely intense, small, and nearly nondivergent beam of monochromatic radiation in the visible region with all the waves in phase. Capable of mobilizing immense heat and power when focused at close range, it is used as a tool in surgical procedures, in diagnosis, and in physiologic studies. **argon l.,** a laser with ionized argon as the active medium whose beam is in the blue and green visible light spectrum; used for photocoagulation. **carbon-dioxide l.,** a laser with carbon dioxide gas as the active medium that produces infrared radiation at 10,600 nm; used to excise and incise tissue and to vaporize. **dye l.,** a laser with organic dye dissolved in a solvent as the active medium whose beam is in the visible light spectrum; used in photodynamic therapy. **helium-neon l.,** a laser with a mixture of ionized helium and neon gases as the active medium whose beam is in the red visible light spectrum; used as a guiding beam for lasers operating at nonvisible wavelengths. **ion l.,** a laser that uses one of the inert gases (argon, helium, neon, or krypton) as the active medium. **krypton l.,** a laser with krypton ionized by electric current as the active medium whose beam is in the yellow-red visible light spectrum; used for photocoagulation. **neodymium:yttrium-aluminum-garnet (Nd:YAG) l.,** a laser whose active medium is a crystal of yttrium, aluminum, and garnet doped with neodymium ions, and whose beam is in the near infrared spectrum at 1060 nm; used for photocoagulation and photoablation.

Lasiohelea (las″e-o-he′le-ah) a genus of blood-sucking flies of the family Heleidae.

Lasix (la′siks) trademark for preparations of furosemide.

Lassar's paste, betanaphthol paste, plain zinc paste (las′arz) [Oskar *Lassar*, German dermatologist, 1849–1907] see under *paste*.

lassitude (las′ĭ-tūd) [L. *lassitudo* weariness] weakness; exhaustion.

latah (lah′tah) a culture-specific syndrome seen chiefly among the Malays and other people of Southeast Asia, characterized by hypersuggestibility, echolalia, echopraxis, coprolalia, disorganization, and automatic obedience.

Lat. dol. abbreviation for L. *lat′eri dolen′ti*, to the painful side.

latebra (lat′ĕ-brah) [L. "hiding place"] a flask-shaped mass of white yolk extending from the blastodisc to the center of eggs such as those of birds.

latency (la′ten-se) a state of seeming inactivity, as that occurring between the instant of stimulation and the beginning of response; see also *stage*.

latent (la′tent) [L. *latens* hidden] concealed; not manifest; potential; dormant; quiescent.

latentiation (la-ten″she-a′shun) the process of making latent; in pharmacology, the chemical modification of a biologically active compound to affect its absorption, distribution, etc., the modified compound being transformed after administration to the active compound by biological processes.

laterad (lat′er-ad) toward a side or a lateral aspect.

lateral (lat′er-al) [L. *lateralis*] 1. denoting a position farther from the median plane or midline of the body or of a structure. 2. pertaining to a side.

lateralis (lat″er-a′lis) lateral; [NA] a term denoting a structure situated farther from the midplane of the body.

laterality (lat″er-al′ĭ-te) a relationship to one side, such as a tendency, in voluntary motor acts, to use preferentially the organs (hand, foot, ear, eye) of the same side. **crossed l.,** the preferential use, in voluntary motor acts, of contralateral members of the different pairs of organs, as the right eye and the left hand. **dominant l.,** the preferential use, in voluntary motor acts, of ipsilateral members of the different pairs of organs, as the right ear, eye, hand, and foot (dextrality) or of the left ear, eye, hand, and foot (sinistrality).

latericeous (lat″er-ish′us) lateritious.

lateritious (lat″er-ish′us) [L. *lateritius; later* brick] resembling brick dust.

latero- [L. *latus,* gen. *lateris* side] a combining form denoting relationship to the side.

lateroabdominal (lat″er-o-ab-dom′ĭ-nal) pertaining to the side and the abdomen.

laterodeviation (lat″er-o-de″ve-a′shun) deviation or slight displacement to one side.

lateroduction (lat″er-o-duk′shun) [*latero-* + L. *ducere* to draw] movement of an eye to one side.

lateroflexion (lat″er-o-flek′shun) flexion to either side.

lateroposition (lat″er-o-po-zish′un) displacement to one side.

lateropulsion (lat″er-o-pul′shun) [*latero-* + L. *pellere* to drive] an involuntary tendency to go to one side while walking.

laterotorsion (lat″er-o-tor′shun) [*latero-* + *torsion*] turning the eyeball to the left or right on its anteroposterior axis.

lateroversion (lat″er-o-ver′shun) [*latero-* + *version*] a turning to one side, as of the uterus.

latex (la′teks) [L. "fluid"] a viscid, milky juice secreted by some seed plants.

latexed (lat-eksd′) (*obs.*) bent to one side.

latexion (la-tek′shun) (*obs.*) lateral flexion.

Latham's circle (la′thamz) [Peter Mere *Latham,* English physician, 1789–1875] see under *circle.*

lathyrism (lath′ĭ-rizm) a morbid condition resulting from ingestion of the seeds of leguminous plants of the genus *Lathyrus,* which includes many kinds of peas. The toxic ingredient is β-aminopropionitrile, which inhibits the enzyme lysyl oxidase. The disease is characterized by spastic paraplegia, pain, hyperesthesia, and paresthesia. Cf. *lupinosis* and *osteolathyrism.*

lathyritic (lath″ĭ-rit′ik) pertaining to or characterized by lathyrism.

lathyrogen (lath′ĭ-ro-jen) any agent that causes lathyrism.

lathyrogenic (lath″ĭ-ro-jen′ik) capable of producing the symptoms characteristic of lathyrism.

latissimus (lah-tis′ĭ-mus) [L.] widest; [NA] a general term denoting a broad structure, as a muscle.

latrodectism (lat″ro-dek′tizm) [*Latrodectus* + *-ism*] intoxication caused by venom of spiders of the genus *Latrodectus.*

Latrodectus (lat″ro-dek′tus) [L. *latro* robber + Gr. *daknein* to bite] a genus of poisonous spiders. *L. mac′tans,* a species found in the United States, is commonly known as the "black widow." Its bite may cause severe symptoms or even death. *L. bisho′pi* is found in southern Florida; *L. curarien′sis* in Brazil and Argentina; *L. geomet′ricus* in California and southern Florida; *L. hassel′tii* in New Zealand; *L. lugu′bris* (kara-kurt) in Russia; *L. macula′tus* in South Africa; *L. malmigniat′tus* in Europe; and *L. tredecimgutta′tus* in Southern Europe and Asiatic Russia.

LATS long-acting thyroid stimulator.

LATS-p LATS protector.

lattice (lat′is) a framework of regularly placed, intersecting narrow strips, such as the geometrical arrangement of the atoms in a crystal as shown by x-ray analysis.

latus¹ (la′tus) broad, wide.

latus² (la′tus), pl. *la′tera* [L.] [NA] the side; flank.

Latzko's cesarean section (lahts′köz) [Wilhelm *Latzko,* Austrian obstetrician, 1863–1945] see *cesarean section,* under *section.*

laudable (law′dah-bl) [L. *laudabilis*] commendable; healthy; see under *pus.*

laudanum (law′dah-num) opium tincture.

laugh (laf) 1. an act or paroxysm of laughter. 2. to indulge in laughter. **canine l., sardonic l.,** risus sardonicus.

laughter (laf′ter) a series of spasmodic and partly involuntary expirations with inarticulate vocalization, normally indicative of merriment, often a hysteric manifestation or a

reflex result of tickling. **compulsive l., forced l., obsessive l.,** hearty laughter for which there is no occasion.

Laugier's hernia, sign (lo″zhe-āz′) [Stanislas *Laugier,* French surgeon, 1799–1872] see under *hernia* and *sign.*

Laumonier's ganglion (lo-mon″e-āz′) [Jean Baptiste Philippe Nicolas Réné *Laumonier,* French surgeon, 1749–1818] 1. carotid ganglion. 2. inferior carotid ganglion.

Launois-Cléret syndrome (lo-nwah′ kla-rah′) [Pierre-Emile *Launois,* French physician, 1856–1914; M. *Cléret,* French physician of the 20th century] Fröhlich's syndrome.

Laurence-Biedl syndrome (law′rens be′del) [John Zachariah *Laurence,* British ophthalmologist, 1830–1874; Artur *Biedl,* Prague endocrinologist, 1869–1933] see under *syndrome.*

Laurence-Moon-Biedl syndrome [J. Z. *Laurence;* Robert C. *Moon,* American ophthalmologist, 1844–1914; A. *Biedl.*] Laurence-Biedl syndrome.

laureth 9 (law′reth) a spermaticide and surfactant consisting of a mixture of polyethylene glycol monododecyl ethers averaging about 9 ethylene oxide groups per molecule.

lauric acid (law′rik) trivial name for dodecanoic acid, the 22-carbon, straight-chain saturated fatty acid.

laurocerasus (law″ro-ser′ah-sus) [L. *laurus* laurel + *cerasus* cherry] the European cherry laurel, an evergreen cherry tree, *Prunus laurocerasus.*

Lauth's canal, sinus (lowts) [Ernst Alexander *Lauth,* Strasbourg physiologist, 1803–1837] sinus venosus sclerae.

Lauth's ligament (lowts) [Thomas *Lauth,* Strasbourg anatomist and surgeon, 1758–1826] ligamentum transversum atlantis.

Lauth's violet (lawths) [Charles *Lauth,* English chemist, 1836–1913] thionine hydrochloride.

LAV lymphadenopathy-associated virus; see *human immunodeficiency virus,* under *virus.*

lavage (lah-vahzh′) [Fr.] 1. the irrigation or washing out of an organ, such as the stomach or bowel. 2. to wash out, or irrigate. **peritoneal l.,** dialysis by instillation into the peritoneal cavity and subsequent withdrawal of dialysis fluid, for the removal of elements not being excreted by the kidneys. **pleural l.,** irrigation of the pleural cavity.

Lavandula (lah-van′du-lah) [L.] a genus of labiate plants; lavenders. The flowers of *L. officinalis* Chaix (*L. vera* DC.), Labiatae, contain a volatile oil used in fumigation, perfumery, moth repellant, and occasionally as a carminative.

Lavdovski's nucleoid (lav-dov′skēz) [Mikhail Dormidontovich *Lavdovski,* Russian histologist, 1846–1902] centrosome.

Lavema (lah-ve′mah) trademark for preparations of oxyphenisatin.

Laveran (lah-vran′) Charles Louis Alphonse, French physician and parasitologist, 1845–1922; winner of the Nobel prize for medicine or physiology in 1907 for his discoveries of hematozoa, protozoa, and trypanosomes and their role in causing disease, and for his discovery of the malarial parasite *Plasmodium.*

Laveran's bodies, corpuscles (lav-ranz′) [Charles Louis Alphonse *Laveran*] see *Plasmodium.*

laveur (lah-vur′) [Fr.] an instrument for performing lavage or irrigation.

law (law) a uniform or constant fact or principle. **Allen's paradoxic l.,** whereas in normal individuals the more sugar is given the more is utilized, the reverse is true in diabetics. **all-or-none l.,** see *all or none.* **Angström's l.,** the wavelengths of the light absorbed by a substance are the same as those given off by it when luminous. **Aran's l.,** fractures of the base of the skull (except those by contrecoup) result from injuries to the vault, the fractures extending by radiation along the line of shortest circle. **Arndt's l., Arndt-Schulz l.,** weak stimuli increase physiologic activity and very strong stimuli inhibit or abolish activity. **l's of articulation,** a set of rules to be followed in arranging teeth to produce a balanced articulation. **l. of avalanche,** hypothetical law assumed by Ramón y Cajal, that multiple sensations may be aroused in the brain by a simple sensation at the periphery. **l. of average localization,** visceral pain is most accurately localized in the least mobile viscus. **Avogadro's l.,** equal volumes of all perfect gases at the same temperature and pressure contain the same number of molecules or, in the case of monatomic gases, of atoms. **Babinski's l.,** the law of voltaic vertigo that a normal subject inclines to the side of the positive pole; one with disease of the labyrinth falls to the side to which he tends to incline spontaneously. If the labyrinth is destroyed, then there is no reaction. **Baer's l.,** those more general features that are common to all the members of a group of animals are developed in the embryo earlier than the more special features that distinguish the various members of the group. This concept is the predecessor of the recapitulation theory. **Barfurth's l.,** the axis of the tissue in a regenerating structure is at first perpendicular to the cut. **Baruch's l.,** when the temperature of the water used in a bath is above or below that of the skin the effect is stimulating; when both temperatures are the same the effect is sedative. **Bastian's l., Bastian-Bruns l.,** if there is a complete transverse lesion in the spinal cord cephalad to the lumbar enlargement, the tendon reflexes of the lower extremities are abolished. **Beer's l.,** the absorbance (*A*) of a solution is directly proportional to the length of the light path (*b*) and the concentration (*c*); the proportionality constant is termed the absorptivity (*a*); thus $A = abc$. The absorptivity is independent of the concentration and is thus a property of the solute and solvent. Beer's law generally holds only up to a certain concentration above which the relation between concentration and absorbance becomes nonlinear. **Behring's l.,** the blood and serum of an immunized person, when transferred to another subject, will render the latter immune. **Bell's l., Bell-Magendie l.,** the anterior roots of the spinal nerves are motor roots, and the posterior are sensory. **Bergonié-Tribondeau l.,** the sensitivity of cells to radiation varies directly with the reproductive capacity of the cells and inversely with their degree of differentiation. **biogenetic l.,** ontogeny recapitulates phylogeny; see *recapitulation theory,* under *theory.* **Bowditch's l.,** 1. see *all-or-none.* 2. nerves cannot be tired out by stimulation. **Boyle's l.,** at a constant temperature the volume of a perfect gas varies inversely as the pressure, and the pressure varies inversely as the volume. **Breton's l.,** there is a parabolic relation between stimulus and just noticeable difference, expressed by the formula S = (R/C)½. **Bunge's l.,** the secreting cells of the mammary gland in the dog, cat, and rabbit take from the blood plasma mineral salts in the exact proportion in which they are needed for developing and building up the offspring. **Bunsen-Roscoe l.,** the photochemical effect produced is equal to the product of the intensity of the illumination and the duration of exposure. **Camerer's l.,** children of the same weight have the same food requirements regardless of their ages. **Charles' l.,** at a constant pressure the volume of a given mass of perfect gas varies directly with the absolute temperature. **Collin's l.,** in infants and children, if after removal of a neoplasm, metastasis or recurrence does not occur for a period equivalent to the age of the patient plus nine months, the possibility of such occurrence is slight. **l. of conservation of energy,** in any given system the amount of energy is constant; energy is neither created nor destroyed, but only transformed from one form to another. **l. of conservation of matter,** in any chemical reaction atoms are neither created nor destroyed but simply change partners. **l. of contrary innervation,** Meltzer's l. **Cope's l.,** genera with little specialization originate many types of organisms; highly specialized genera produce but few biological variations. **Coulomb's l.,** the force of attraction or repulsion between two electrified bodies is proportional directly to the quantities of electric charge, and inversely as the square of their distance apart. **Courvoisier's l.,** when the common bile duct is obstructed by a stone, dilatation of the gallbladder is rare; when the duct is obstructed in some other way, dilatation is common. **Coutard's l.,** in radiotherapy, the point of origin of a mucous membrane tumor is the last site to heal following irradiation. **Curie's l.,** all substances may be rendered radioactive by the influence of the emanations of radium, and substances thus influenced hold their radioactivity longer when enclosed in some material through which the emanations cannot pass. **Cushing's l.,** increase of intracranial tension causes increase of blood pressure to a point slightly above the pressure exerted against the medulla. **Dalton's l.,** the pressure exerted by a mixture of nonreacting gases is equal to the sum of the partial pressures of the separate components. **Dalton-Henry l.,** when a fluid absorbs a mixture of gases, it will absorb as much of each gas

as it would have absorbed of either gas separately. **l. of definite proportions,** any compound always contains the same kind of elements in the same proportions; called also *Proust's l.* **l. of denervation,** denervation of a structure increases its sensitivity to chemical stimulation. **Descartes' l.,** the sine of the angle of incidence bears a constant relation to the sine of the angle of refraction for two given media. Called also *l. of sines* and *Snell's l.* **Desmarres' l.,** when the visual axes are crossed the images are uncrossed; when the axes are uncrossed (diverging) the images are crossed. Useful in determining presence of esophoria and exophoria, and esotropia and exotropia. See also *direct* and *crossed diplopia.* **l. of diffusion,** any process set up in the nerve centers affects the organism throughout by a process of diffused motion. **Dollo's l.,** phyletic development is irreversible, i.e., reversion to an ancestral peculiarity (atavism) is impossible. **Donders' l.,** the rotation of the eye around the line of sight is not voluntary; when attention is fixed upon a remote object, the amount of rotation is determined entirely by the angular distance of the object from the median plane and from the horizon. **Draper's l.,** only the rays that are absorbed by a photochemical substance will produce a chemical change in it. **DuBois-Reymond's l.,** it is the variation of current density, and not the absolute value of current density at any given moment, that acts as a stimulus to a muscle or motor nerve. **Dulong and Petit's l.,** the atoms of all elements have exactly the same capacity for heat. **Edinger's l.,** a gradual increase in the function of the neuron causes at first increased growth, but if irregular and excessive, then it leads to atrophy and degeneration. **Einstein-Starck l.** (of photochemical equivalence), according to the quantum theory, quanta of light are absorbed at random during irradiation; the absorption of one quantum of light by a molecule (or atom) produces only one activated molecule (or atom). **Einthoven l.,** if electrocardiograms are taken simultaneously with the three leads, at any given instant the potential in lead II is equal to the sum of the potentials in leads I and III. **Elliott's l.,** the activity of epinephrine is due to a stimulation of the endings of the sympathetic nerve. **Ewald's l.,** nystagmus resulting from endolymph currents in a semicircular canal is in a direction parallel with the plane of that canal and opposite to the current; and in the horizontal canals the amount of ocular motor impulse derived from the canals whose hair cells are bent toward the utricle is twice as great as from the other (short end); but in the vertical canals the reverse is true. **l. of excitation,** a motor nerve responds by the contraction of its muscle to the alterations of the strength of an electric current and not to its absolute strength. **l. of facilitation,** when an impulse has passed once through a certain set of neurons to the exclusion of others, it will tend to take the same course on a future occasion, and each time it traverses this path the resistance in the path will be smaller. See also *facilitation* (def. 2). **Fajans' l.,** the product left after the emission of alpha rays has a valence less by two than that of the parent radioactive substance; the product left after the emission of beta rays has a valence greater by one than that of the parent radioactive substance. **Faraday's l.,** in electrolysis the amount of an ion liberated in any given time is proportional to the strength of the current. **Farr's l.,** "subsidence is a property of all zymotic diseases"; the gradually diminishing increase of incidence in an epidemic disease, by virtue of which the epidemic curve first ascends rapidly, then more slowly to a maximum, with a descent more rapid than the ascent. **l. of fatigue (Houghton's),** when the same muscle or group of muscles is kept in constant action until fatigue sets in, the total work done, multiplied by the rate of work, is constant. **Fechner's l.,** the intensity of a sensation produced by a varying stimulus varies directly as the logarithm of that stimulus. **Ferry-Porter l.,** critical fusion frequency is directly proportional to the logarithm of the light intensity. **Fick's first l. of diffusion,** a substance will diffuse through an area at a rate which is dependent upon the difference in concentration of the substance at two given points. **first l. of thermodynamics,** see *l's of thermodynamics.* **Flatau's l.,** the greater the length of the fibers of the spinal cord, the closer are they situated to the periphery. **Flechsig's myelogenetic l.,** myelogenetic l. **Flint's l.,** the ontogeny of an organ is the phylogeny of its blood supply. **Flourens' l.,** stimulation of the semicircular canal causes nystagmus in the plane of that canal. **Froriep's l.,** the skull is developed by the annexation of true vertebrae, the head growing at the expense of the neck. **Galton's l.,** each parent contributes, on an average, one half, or (0.5), of an individual's heritage, each grandparent one fourth, or $(0.5)^2$, each great-grandparent one eighth, or $(0.5)^3$, etc., the occupier of each ancestral place in the nth degree, whatever the value of n, contributing $(0.5)^{n-2}$ of the heritage. **Galton's l. of regression,** average parents tend to produce average children, but the offspring of extreme parents inherit the parental peculiarities in a less marked degree than the latter were manifested in the parents themselves. **gas l.,** see *ideal gas l.* **Gay-Lussac's l.,** Charles' l. **Gerhardt-Semon l.,** various peripheral and central lesions affecting the recurrent laryngeal nerve cause the vocal cord to assume a position between abduction and adduction, the paralysis of the parts being incomplete. **Giraud-Teulon l.,** binocular retinal images are formed at the intersection of the primary and secondary axes of projection. **Godélier's l.,** tuberculosis of the peritoneum is invariably associated with tuberculosis of the pleura. **Golgi's l.,** the severity of a malarial attack depends upon the number of parasites in the blood. **Gompertz l.,** at advanced ages the risk of dying increases geometrically with age: the death rate at age x may be computed by the formula $q_x = q_0 e\, a^x$, where q_x is the death rate at age x, q_0 is the death rate at age 0, and a is a constant. From middle age on, actual death rates closely approximate the curve that corresponds to this formula. **Goodell's l.,** see under *sign.* **Graham's l.,** the rate of diffusion of a gas through porous membranes is in inverse ratio to the square root of their density. **Grasset's l.,** Landouzy-Grasset l. **l. of gravitation,** all bodies attract each other with a force that is directly proportional to their masses and inversely proportional to the square of their distance apart; called also *Newton's l.* **Grotthus' l.,** only those rays of ultraviolet light that are absorbed produce a chemical effect. **Gudden's l.,** the degeneration of the proximal end of a divided nerve is cellulipetal. **Guldberg and Waage's l.,** the velocity of a chemical reaction is proportional to the active masses of the reacting substances; called also *l. of mass action* and *mass l.* **Gull-Toynbee l.,** in otitis media, the lateral sinus and cerebellum are liable to involvement in mastoid disease, and the cerebrum may be attacked when the roof of the tympanum becomes carious. **Gullstrand's l.,** in strabismus, if the patient is made to turn his head while fixing a distant object and the corneal reflex of either eye moves in the direction in which the head is turning, then the movement is toward the weaker muscle. **Haeckel's l.,** ontogeny recapitulates phylogeny; see *recapitulation theory,* under *theory.* **Hanau's l's of articulation,** a set of purely physical laws that must be observed in the formation of the masticatory surfaces of natural dentition or dentures, to assure establishment or production of balanced articulation. **Hardy-Weinberg l.,** the proportions of the three genotypes determined by two alleles (A and a) occurring with a frequency of p and q, respectively, in a randomly mating population will remain constant from one generation to the next: $AA = p^2$, $Aa = 2\,pq$, $aa = q^2$. Mutation, selection, non-random mating, migration, and genetic drift can disturb this equilibrium. **l. of the heart,** the energy set free at each contraction of the heart is a simple function of the length of the fibers composing its muscular walls (Starling). **Heidenhain's l.,** glandular secretion always involves change in the structure of the gland. **Hellin's l., Hellin-Zeleny l.,** one in about 89 pregnancies ends in the birth of twins; one in 89×89, or 7921, of triplets; one in $89 \times 89 \times 89$, or 704,969, of quadruplets. **Henry's l.,** the solubility of a gas in a liquid solution is proportional to the partial pressure of the gas. **Hering's l.,** 1. the principle of bilateral ocular innervation; equal innervation is sent to the muscles of the two eyes so that one eye is never moved independently of the other. 2. the clearness or purity of any conception or sensation depends on the proportion existing between its intensity and the sum total of the intensities of all the simultaneous conceptions and sensations. **Heyman's l.,** the threshold value of a visual stimulus is increased in proportion to the strength of the inhibitory stimulus. **Hilton's l.,** a nerve supplying a joint supplies also the muscles moving the joint and the skin over the insertions of the muscles. **Hoff's l.,** van't Hoff's l. **Hoorweg's l.,** there is a duration of electric discharge above which time is not a factor, and a duration of discharge below which the time is a factor, in the provocation of neuromuscular response. **Horner's l.,** ordinary color

blindness is transmitted from males to males through normal females. **ideal gas l.,** the equation of state for an ideal gas: $PV = nRT$, where P is pressure, V volume, n the number of moles of gas, R the gas constant, and T the absolute temperature. It holds approximately for real gases at low pressures and high temperatures. **l. of independent assortment,** the members of different gene pairs segregate independently during meiosis; see also *Mendel's l.* **l. of initial value,** Wilder's l. of initial value. **inverse square l.,** the intensity of radiation is inversely proportional to the square of the distance between a point source and the irradiated surface. **l. of isochronism,** a nerve and its innervated muscle have identical chronaxie values. **isodynamic l.,** in the production of heat in the body the different foodstuffs are interchangeable in accordance with their heat-producing values. **l. of isolated conduction,** the wave of change or nervous impulse which passes through a neuron is never communicated to other neurons except at the terminals. **Jackson's l.,** the nerve functions that are latest developed are the earliest to be destroyed. **Kahler's l.,** the ascending branches of the posterior roots of the spinal nerves pass within the cord in succession from the root zone toward the mesial plane. **Knapp's l.,** there should be no difference in retinal image size in the correction of spherical axial anisometropia, provided that the lenses are placed at the anterior focal point of the eye. **Koch's l.,** see *Koch's postulates,* under *postulate.* **Küstner's l.,** if an ovarian tumor is left-sided, torsion of its pedicle takes place toward the right; if right-sided, toward the left. **Lambert's cosine l.,** the intensity of radiation on an absorbing surface varies as the cosine of the angle of incidence for parallel rays. **Landouzy-Grasset l.,** in lesion of one cerebral hemisphere the head is turned to the side of the brain lesion if there is paralysis, and to that of the affected muscles if there is spasticity. **Lapicque's l.,** the chronaxy is inversely proportional to the diameter of the nerve fiber. **Laplace's l.,** in hemodynamics, the pressure produced in the ventricles depends not only on the tension developed by the cardiac ventricular muscle in contraction but also on the size and shape of the heart. **Leopold's l.,** when the placenta is inserted upon the posterior wall of the uterus, the oviducts assume directions converging upon the anterior wall; but when the insertion is on the anterior wall during recumbency, the tubes turn backward and become parallel to the axis of the body. **Levret's l.,** the insertion of the cord is marginal in placenta previa. **Listing's l.,** when the eyeball is moved from a resting position, the rotational angle in the second position is the same as if the eye were turned about a fixed axis perpendicular to the first and second position of the visual line. **Lossen's l.,** see under *rule.* **Louis' l.,** 1. pulmonary tuberculosis generally begins in the left lung. 2. tuberculosis of any part is attended by localization in the lungs. **Magendie's l.,** Bell's l. **malthusian l.,** the hypothesis that population tends to outrun the means available to sustain it. **Marey's l.,** as the blood pressure rises, the pulse rate slows. **Mariotte's l.,** Boyle's l. **l. of mass action, mass l.,** Guldberg and Waage's l. **Maxwell-Boltzmann distribution l.,** a method for calculating the relative number of molecules in a given population which possess a given amount of energy. **Meltzer's l.** (*of contrary innervation*), all living functions are continually controlled by two opposing forces: augmentation or action on the one hand, and inhibition on the other. **Mendel's laws, mendelian l.,** the laws of inheritance of single-gene traits that form the basis of the science of genetics, first described by Gregor Mendel in 1865. From experimental crosses of pea plants differing in one or more characteristics determined by single genes, and counting the types of progeny in successive generations, Mendel derived two laws now usually expressed as the law of segregation (the members of a pair of allelic genes segregate from one another and pass to different gametes) and the law of independent assortment (genes that are not alleles are distributed to the gametes independently of one another). **Mendeléeff's l.,** periodic l. **Meyer's l.,** the internal structure of fully developed normal bone represents the lines of greatest pressure or traction and affords the greatest possible resistance with the least possible amount of material. **Minot's l.,** organisms age fastest when young. **Müller's l.,** l. of specific irritability. **Müller-Haeckel l.,** biogenetic l. **l. of multiple variants,** any variation from the normal in the bones of the hand or foot is always multiple. **myelogenetic l.** (of Flechsig), the myelination of the nerve fibers of the developing brain takes place in a definite sequence so that fibers belonging to particular functional systems mature at the same time. **Nernst's l.,** the current required to stimulate muscle action varies as the square root of its frequency. **Neumann's l.,** the molecular heat in compounds of analogous constitution is always the same. **Newland's l.,** a forerunner of the periodic law, in which the chemical elements, arranged in order of their atomic weights, showed a repetition of properties in octaves. **Newton's l.,** l. of gravitation. **Nysten's l.,** rigor mortis affects first the muscles of mastication, next those of the face and neck, then those of the upper trunk and arms, and last of all those of the legs and feet. **Ohm's l.,** the strength of an electric current varies directly as the electromotive force, and inversely as the resistance. **Ollier's l.,** in the case of two parallel bones which are joined at their extremities by ligaments, arrest of growth in one of them involves growth disturbance in the other. **Pajot's l.,** a solid body contained within another body having smooth walls will tend to conform to the shape of those walls; this law governs the rotating movements of the fetus during labor. **Pascal's l.,** pressure applied to a liquid at any point is transmitted equally in all directions. **periodic l.,** if the elements are arranged in the sequence of their atomic numbers, they fall into distinctive periods of 2, 8, 8, 18, 18, and 32 elements; see also *periodic table,* under *table.* Called also *Mendeléeff's l.* **Petit's l.,** Dulong and Petit's l. **Pflüger's l.,** a nerve tract is stimulated when catelectrotonus develops or anelectrotonus disappears, but not under the reverse conditions. **Poiseuille's l.,** the volume flow in a tube is (*a*) directly proportional to the pressure drop along the length of the tube and to the fourth power of the radius of the tube, and (*b*) is inversely proportional to the length of the tube and to the viscosity of the fluid. **Prévost's l.,** in a lateral cerebral lesion the head is turned toward the side involved. **Proust's l.,** l. of definite proportions. **psychophysical l.,** Weber-Fechner l. **Raoult's l.,** 1. (*for freezing points*) the depression of the freezing point for the same type of electrolyte dissolved in a given solvent is proportional to the molecular concentration of the solute. 2. (*for vapor pressures*) (*a*) the vapor pressure of a volatile substance from a liquid solution is equal to the mole fraction of that substance times its vapor pressure in the pure state. (*b*) when a nonvolatile nonelectrolyte is dissolved in a solvent the decrease in vapor pressure of that solvent is equal to the mole fraction of the solute times the vapor pressure of the pure solvent. **l. of reciprocal proportions,** two chemical elements that unite with a third element do so in proportions that are multiples of those in which they unite with each other. **l. of referred pain,** referred pain only arises from irritation of nerves which are sensitive to those stimuli that produce pain when applied to the surface of the body. **l. of refraction,** rays of light passing from a rarer to a denser medium are deflected toward a perpendicular to the surface of incidence, whereas rays passing from a denser to a rarer medium are deflected away from the perpendicular. Cf. *Descartes' l.* **l. of refreshment,** the refreshment of a laboring muscle depends on the rate of supply of arterial blood. **l. of regression,** Galton's l. of regression. **l. of relativity,** simultaneous and successive sensations modify each other. **Ricco's l.,** the relation between intensity and area of illumination: intensity times area equals constant. **Ritter-Valli l.,** the primary increase and secondary loss of irritability in a nerve, produced by a section which separates from the nerve center, travel in a peripheral direction. **Rosa's l.,** the possibilities of phyletic variation in an organism decrease in proportion to the extent of its development. **Rubner's l.,** 1. (*law of constant energy consumption*) the rapidity of growth is proportional to the intensity of the metabolic process. 2. (*law of constant growth quotient*) the same fractional part of the entire energy is utilized for growth; this fractional part is called the "growth quotient." **Schroeder van der Kolk's l.,** the sensory fibers of a mixed nerve are distributed to the parts moved by muscles which are stimulated by the motor fibers of the same nerve. **second l. of thermodynamics,** see *l's of thermodynamics.* **l. of segregation,** see *Mendel's l.* **Semon's l., Semon-Rosenbach l.,** in progressive organic diseases of the motor laryngeal nerves, the abductors of the vocal cords (posterior cricoarytenoids) are the first, and occasionally the only, muscles affected. **Sherrington's l.,** 1. every posterior spinal nerve root supplies a special region of the skin, although

fibers from adjacent spinal segments may invade such a region. 2. when a muscle receives a nerve impulse to contract, its antagonist receives simultaneously an impulse to relax (see *reciprocal innervation*). **l. of similars,** see *homeopathy.* **l. of sines,** *Descartes' l.* **Snell's l.,** Descartes' l. **Spallanzani's l.,** the law that regeneration is more complete in younger individuals than in older ones. **l. of specific irritability,** every sensory nerve reacts to one form of stimulus and gives rise to one form of sensation only, though if under abnormal conditions it be excited by other forms of stimuli, the sensation evoked will be the same. Called also *Müller's l.* **Starling's l.,** 1. the heart output per beat is directly proportional to the diastolic filling. 2. see *l. of the heart.* **Stokes' l.,** a muscle situated above an inflamed membrane is often affected with paralysis. **surface l.,** at constant temperature, the heat production, heat loss, and oxygen consumption in an animal are inversely proportional to the free surface or to the square of a linear dimension. **Talbot's l.,** when complete fusion occurs and the sensation is uniform, the intensity is the same as would occur were the same amount of light spread uniformly over the disk. **Teevan's l.,** fractures of bones occur in the line of extension, and not in the line of compression. **l's of thermodynamics,** *Zeroth law:* two systems in thermal equilibrium with a third system are in thermal equilibrium with each other. *First law:* energy is conserved in any process; i.e., the energy gained (or lost) by a system is exactly equal to the energy lost (or gained) by the surroundings. *Second law:* there is always an increase in entropy in any naturally occurring (spontaneous) process. *Third law:* absolute zero is unattainable. **third l. of thermodynamics,** see *l's of thermodynamics.* **Toynbee's l.,** in cases of brain disease due to otitis, the cerebellum and lateral sinuses are affected from the mastoid, and the cerebrum from the tympanic roof. **Valli-Ritter l.,** see Ritter-Valli l. **van der Kolk's l.,** Schroeder van der Kolk's l. **van't Hoff's l.,** 1. many substances in solution exert an osmotic pressure equal to the gas pressure that they would exert if their molecules were in a gaseous state and occupied a volume equal to that of the solution under the same conditions of temperature and pressure. 2. van't Hoff's rule; see under *rule.* **Virchow's l.,** the cell elements of tumors are derived from normal and preexisting tissue cells. **Waller's l., wallerian l.,** if the sensory fibers of the root of a spinal nerve be divided on the central side of the ganglion, the fibers on the peripheral side of the cut do not degenerate; while those that remain connected with the cord degenerate. **Walton's l.,** l. of reciprocal proportions. **Weber's l.,** the variation of stimulus which causes the smallest appreciable change in sensation maintains an approximately fixed ratio to the whole stimulus. **Weber-Fechner l.,** for a sensation to increase by equal amounts (arithmetical progression), the stimulus must increase by geometrical progression; called also *psychophysical l.* **Weigert's l.,** loss or destruction of elements in the organic world is apt to be followed by overproduction of such elements in the reparative process. **Wilder's l. of initial value,** the more intense the function of a vegetative organ, the weaker its capacity for being excited by stimuli and the stronger its reaction to depressing factors; with extremely high or low initial value, there is marked tendency to paradoxic reactions (reversal of direction of reaction). **Wolff's l.,** a bone, normal or abnormal, develops the structure most suited to resist the forces acting upon it. **Wundt-Lamansky l.,** the line of vision in moving through a vertical plane parallel to the frontal plane moves in straight lines in the vertical and horizontal directions, but in curved paths in all other movements. **zeroth l. of thermodynamics,** see *l's of thermodynamics.*

Lawrence-Seip syndrome (law′rens sīp) [Robert Daniel *Lawrence,* English physician, 1912–1964; Martin Fredrik *Seip,* Norwegian pediatrician, born 1921] lipoatrophic diabetes.

lawrencium (law-ren′se-um) [Ernest Orlando *Lawrence,* American physicist, 1901–1958; builder of the first cyclotron for the production of high-energy particles, and winner of the Nobel prize for physics in 1939] the chemical element of atomic number 103, atomic weight 257, symbol Lw; produced in 1961 by bombardment of californium isotopes of mass 250, 251, and 252.

Lawson Tait see *Tait.*

lawsone (law′sōn) 2-hydroxy-1,4-naphthoquinone, $C_{10}H_6$-

O₃, a principle isolated from the leaves of *Lawsonia inermis* L. (Lythraceae), used as a topical sunscreen agent.

Lawsonia (law-so′ne-ah) a genus of tropical Old World shrubs, including *L. inermis*, the source of lawsone and of henna.

laxation (lak-sa′shun) defecation.

laxative (lak′sah-tiv) [L. *laxativus*] 1. aperient; mildly cathartic. 2. an agent that acts to promote evacuation of the bowel; a cathartic or purgative. **bulk l.,** an agent that acts to promote evacuation of the bowel by increasing the volume of the feces.

laxator (lak-sa′tor) [L. *laxare* to unloose or relax] that which slackens or relaxes. **l. tym′pani ma′jor,** ligamentum mallei anterius. **l. tym′pani mi′nor,** ligamentum mallei laterale.

layer (la′er) a sheetlike mass of tissue of nearly uniform thickness, several of which may be superimposed, one above another, as in the epidermis; called also *lamina* and *stratum*. **abscission l.,** a special layer or zone of thin-walled cells, loosely joined together, extending across the base of the petiole, thus weakening the base of the leaf, permitting the leaf to fall. **adamantine l.,** dental enamel. **ambiguous l.,** the second layer of the cerebral cortex, counting from without; named from the indefinite shapes of many of its cells. **ameloblastic l.,** the inner layer of cells of the enamel organ, created by its invagination, which forms the enamel prisms. **bacillary l.,** l. of rods and cones. **basal l.,** 1. lamina basalis choroideae. 2. stratum basale epidermidis. **basal l. of epidermis,** stratum basale epidermidis. **basement l.,** see under *membrane*. **Bekhterev's l.,** a layer of fibers in the external granular layer of the cerebral cortex. **Bernard's glandular l.,** a layer of cells which line the acini of the pancreas. **blastodermic l.,** germ l. **Bowman's l.,** lamina limitans anterior corneae. **Bruch's l.,** complexus basalis choroideae. **cerebral l. of retina,** pars nervosa retinae. **Chievitz l.,** a transient fiber layer separating the inner and outer neuroblastic layers of the optic cup. **choriocapillary l.,** lamina choroidocapillaris. **circular l. of drumhead,** stratum circulare membranae tympani. **circular l. of muscular tunic of colon,** stratum circulare tunicae muscularis coli. **circular l. of muscular tunic of rectum,** stratum circulare tunicae muscularis recti. **circular l. of muscular tunic of small intestine,** stratum circulare tunicae muscularis intestini tenuis. **circular l. of muscular tunic of stomach,** stratum circulare tunicae muscularis gastris. **circular l. of tympanic membrane,** stratum circulare membranae tympani. **clear l. of epidermis,** stratum lucidum epidermidis. **columnar l.,** mantle l. **compact l.,** stratum compactum. **cortical l.,** the cortex of an organ, as of the brain or kidney. **l's of cranial colliculus,** see *strata grisea et alba colliculi rostralis*. **cutaneous l. of tympanic membrane,** stratum cutaneum membranae tympani. **cuticular l.,** a striate border of modified cytoplasm at the free end of some columnar cells. **deep l. of triangular ligament,** fascia diaphragmatis urogenitalis superior. **Dobie's l.,** Z band; see under *band*. **enamel l., inner,** the inner, concave wall of the enamel organ. **enamel l., outer,** the outer, convex wall of the enamel organ. **ependymal l.,** the innermost layer of the wall of the primitive neural tube, bounding the central canal, which differentiates regionally into the roof plate and the floor plate. **epitrichial l.,** the most superficial layer of the epidermis of the embryo. **fibrous l. of articular capsule,** membrana fibrosa capsulae articularis. **Floegel's l.,** a granular layer in each transparent lateral disk of a muscle fibril. **functional l.,** stratum functionale. **fusiform l. of cerebral cortex,** lamina multiformis corticis cerebri. **ganglion cell l.,** a layer of the pars nervosa retinae, situated between the inner molecular layer and the stratum opticum, or nerve fiber layer, consisting essentially of the ganglion cells of the retina, and containing also the fibers of Müller, neuroglia, and branches of the retinal vessels. **ganglionic l. of cerebellum,** stratum gangliosum cerebelli. **ganglionic l. of cerebral cortex,** lamina pyramidalis interna corticis cerebri. **ganglionic l. of optic nerve,** the layer of the nervous part of the retina that contains the multipolar neurons, the axons of which form the fibers of the optic nerve; see also *retina*. Called also *stratum ganglionare nervi optici* and *ganglionic stratum of retina*. **ganglionic l. of retina,** the layer of the nervous part of retina that contains the

bipolar cells; see also *retina*. Called also *stratum ganglionare retinae* and *ganglionic stratum of retina*. **germ l.,** one of the three primary layers of cells of the embryo (ectoderm, entoderm, or mesoderm), from which the tissues and organs develop. **germinative l., germinative l. of epidermis,** 1. stratum germinativum epidermidis [Malpighii]. 2. stratum basale epidermidis. **germinative l. of nail,** stratum germinativum unguis. **granular l. of cerebellum,** stratum granulosum cerebelli. **granular l. of cerebral cortex, external,** lamina granularis externa corticis cerebri. **granular l. of epidermis,** stratum granulosum epidermidis. **granular l. of follicle of ovary,** stratum granulosum folliculi ovarici vesiculosi. **granular l. of Tomes,** a layer of imperfectly calcified dentin made of small interglobular spaces immediately beneath the dentinocemental junction in the root of a tooth. Called also *Tomes' granular l.* **granule l.,** stratum granulosum cerebelli. **gray l's of cranial colliculus, gray l's of rostral colliculus, gray l. of superior colliculus,** see *strata grisea et alba colliculi rostralis*. **half-value l.,** the thickness of a given substance that will reduce the intensity of a beam of radiation to one half of its initial value; called also *half-value thickness*. Abbreviated *HVL*. **Haller's l.,** that portion of the vascular layer of the choroid which is made up of large vessels. **Henle's l.,** the outer layer of cells of the inner root sheath of a hair follicle, lying between the outer root sheath and Huxley's layer. **Henle's fiber l.,** the outer plexiform layer in the region of the macula retinae; see also *entoretina*. **horny l. of epidermis,** stratum corneum epidermidis. **horny l. of nail,** stratum corneum unguis. **Huxley's l.,** a layer of the inner root sheath of a hair follicle, lying between Henle's layer and the inner sheath cuticle. **inferior l. of pelvic diaphragm,** fascia diaphragmatis pelvis inferior. **Kaes-Bekhterev l.,** Bekhterev's l. **Langhans' l.,** cytotrophoblast. **limiting l., internal,** the basal lamina of the Müller cells in the retina, separating the inner, conical ends of the cells from the vitreous body. Called also *inner* or *internal limiting membrane*. **longitudinal l. of muscular tunic of colon,** stratum longitudinale tunicae muscularis coli. **longitudinal l. of muscular tunic of rectum,** stratum longitudinale tunicae muscularis recti. **longitudinal l. of muscular tunic of small intestine,** stratum longitudinale tunicae muscularis intestini tenuis. **longitudinal l. of muscular tunic of stomach,** stratum longitudinale tunicae muscularis gastris. **malpighian l.,** stratum germinativum. **mantle l.,** middle layer of the wall of the primitive neural tube, containing primitive nerve cells and later forming the gray substance of the central nervous system. **marginal l.,** the outermost layer of the wall of the primitive neural tube, a fibrous mesh into which the nerve fibers later grow, forming the white substance of the central nervous system. **medullary l's of thalamus, internal and external,** laminae medullares thalami interna et externa. **Meynert's l.,** the layer of pyramidal cells in the cortex of the cerebrum. **molecular l. of cerebellum,** stratum moleculare cerebelli. **molecular l. of cerebral cortex,** lamina molecularis corticis cerebri. **molecular l., external, molecular l., outer,** external plexiform l. **molecular l., inner, molecular l., internal,** inner plexiform l. **mucous l.,** stratum germinativum. **mucous l. of tympanic membrane,** stratum mucosum membranae tympani. **multiform l. of cerebral cortex,** lamina multiformis corticis cerebri. **muscular l. of fallopian tube,** tunica muscularis tubae uterinae. **nerve fiber l.,** a layer of the retina, situated between the ganglion cell layer and the internal limiting membrane, consisting essentially of the axons of the ganglion cells which pass through the lamina cribrosa to form the optic nerve. **nervous l. of retina,** pars nervosa retinae. **neuroepidermal l.,** ectoderm. **neuroepithelial l. of retina,** l. of rods and cones. **Nitabuch's l.,** an interrupted sheet of fibrinoid in the placenta at the junction of trophoblast and decidua; called also *Nitabuch's stria* or *zone*. **nuclear l. of cerebellum,** stratum granulosum cerebelli. **nuclear l., external, nuclear l., outer,** the layer of the pars nervosa retinae, situated between the external limiting membrane and the outer molecular layer, consisting essentially of the rod and cone granules (nuclei). **nuclear l., inner, nuclear l., internal,** the layer of the pars nervosa retinae, situated between the inner and outer plexiform layers, consisting essentially of the visual cells. **odonto-**

blastic l., the epithelioid odontoblastic zone, one to five layers thick, which forms the outer surface of the dental pulp adjacent to the dentin, resting on Weil's basal zone. It produces and maintains the dentin. **Ollier's l., osteogenetic l.,** the innermost layer of the periosteum. **palisade l.,** the basal layer of the mucous membrane layer of the tympanic membrane. **Pander's l.,** the splanchnopleural layer of the mesoblast. **papillary l. of corium, papillary l. of dermis,** stratum papillare dermidis. **parietal l. of pelvic fascia,** fascia diaphragmatis pelvis superior. **parietal l. of tunica vaginalis of testis,** lamina parietalis tunicae vaginalis testis. **peripheral l.,** the outer portion of the molecular layer of the cerebral cortex. **perpendicular l. of ethmoid bone,** lamina perpendicularis ossis ethmoidalis. **pigmented l. of ciliary body,** the part of the pigmented layer of the retina that rests on the ciliary body; see also *retina.* Called also *pigmented stratum of ciliary body* and *stratum pigmenti corporis ciliaris.* **pigmented l. of eyeball,** stratum pigmenti bulbi oculi. **pigmented l. of iris,** the part of the pigmented layer of the retina that rests on the posterior surface of the iris; see also *retina.* Called also *pigmented stratum of iris* and *stratum pigmenti iridis.* **pigmented l. of retina,** pars pigmentosa retinae. **piriform neuronal l.,** stratum neuronorum piriformium. **plexiform l. of cerebellum,** stratum moleculare cerebelli. **plexiform l. of cerebral cortex,** lamina molecularis corticis cerebri. **plexiform l., external, plexiform l., outer,** the layer of the pars nervosa retinae, situated between the outer nuclear layer and the inner nuclear layer, consisting essentially of the arborizations of the axons of the rod and cone granules with the dendrites of the bipolar cells. Called also *external* or *outer molecular layer.* **plexiform l., inner, plexiform l., internal,** the layer of the pars nervosa retinae situated between the inner nuclear layer and the ganglion cell layer, consisting primarily of the arborization of the axons of the bipolar cells with the dendrites of the ganglion cells. Called also *inner* or *internal molecular layer.* **polymorphic l. of cerebral cortex,** lamina multiformis corticis cerebri. **prickle cell l.,** stratum epinosum epidermidis. **Purkinje l., Purkinje cell l.,** the layer of Purkinje cells in the cerebellar cortex, between the superficial molecular layer and the subjacent granular layer; considered by some to be the deepest part of the molecular layer. Called also *stratum neuronorum piriformium* [NA] and *piriform neuronal layer.* **pyramidal l. of cerebral cortex, external,** lamina pyramidalis externa corticis cerebri. **radiate l. of tympanic membrane,** stratum radiatum membranae tympani. **Rauber's l.,** the most external of the three layers of cells which form the blastodisc in the young embryo; called also *blastodermic ectoderm* and *primitive ectoderm.* **reticular l. of corium, reticular l. of dermis,** stratum reticulare dermidis. **l. of rods and cones,** the layer of the nervous part of the retina, situated between the pigmented part and the external limiting membrane, comprising the sensitive elements of the retina, the cones, containing a visual pigment, iodopsin, and the rods, containing visual purple, or rhodopsin; see also *retina.* Called also *neuroepithelial layer* or *stratum of retina* and *stratum neuroepitheliale retinae.* **Rohr's l.,** see under *stria.* **l's of rostral colliculus,** see *strata grisea et alba colliculi rostralis.* **Sattler's l.,** that portion of the vascular layer of the choroid which is made up of medium-sized vessels. **sclerotogenous l., skeletogenous l.,** the layer of mesoderm cells surrounding the notochord of the embryo and developing into the axial skeleton. **second half-value l.,** the additional thickness of material needed to reduce the intensity of a radiation beam from one half to one fourth of its original value. Cf. *half-value l.* **somatic l.,** the external layer of the lateral mesoderm after the coelomic split occurs; the inner component of somatopleure of the embryo. **spinous l. of epidermis,** stratum spinosum epidermidis. **splanchnic l.,** the internal layer of the lateral mesoderm after the coelomic split occurs; the component of splanchnopleure outside the entoderm of the embryo. **spongy l.,** stratum spongiosum. **subcallosal l.,** the layer of nerve fibers on the lower side of the corpus callosum. **subendocardial l.,** the layer of loose fibrous tissue uniting the endocardium and myocardium. **subendothelial l.,** a middle, fibrous layer of the tunica intima of typical blood vessels, located between the endothelium and internal elastic membrane. **subepicardial l.,** the layer of loose connective tissue uniting the epicardium and myocardium. **submantle l.,** a layer of interglobular dentin usually situated just below the cover (mantle) dentin. **submucous l.,** tela submucosa. **submucous l. of bladder,** tela submucosa vesicae urinariae. **submucous l. of colon,** tela submucosa coli. **submucous l. of pharynx,** tela submucosa pharyngis. **submucous l. of small intestine,** tela submucosa intestini tenuis. **submucous l. of stomach,** tela submucosa ventriculi. **subodontoblastic l.,** Weil's basal l. **subserous l.,** tela subserosa. **subserous l. of peritoneum,** tela subserosa peritonei. **superficial l. of fascia of perineum,** fascia perinei superficialis. **superficial l. of triangular ligament,** fascia diaphragmatis urogenitalis inferior. **l's of superior colliculus,** see *strata grisea et alba colliculi rostralis.* **superior l. of pelvic diaphragm,** fascia diaphragmatis pelvis superior. **suprachorioid l.,** lamina suprachoroidea. **synovial l. of articular capsule,** membrana synovialis capsulae articularis. **Tomes' granular l.,** granular l. of Tomes. **trophic l.,** the entoderm. **vegetative l.,** the entoderm. **vertical l. of ethmoid bone,** lamina perpendicularis ossis ethmoidalis. **visceral l. of pelvic fascia,** fascia pelvis visceralis. **visceral l. of pericardium,** lamina visceralis pericardii. **visceral l. of tunica vaginalis of testis,** lamina visceralis tunicae vaginalis testis. **Waldeyer's l.,** the vascular layer of the ovary. **Weil's basal l.,** a clear, relatively cell-free layer, located just inside the odontoblastic layer and overlying the cell-rich zone of the dental pulp, which is visible during the inactive phase of dentinogenesis. It is made up of delicate fibrils embedded in the ground substance; in dentinogenesis the fibrils are incorporated into the matrix. Called also *subodontoblastic l.* and *Weil's basal zone.* **white l's of cerebellum,** laminae albae cerebelli. **white l's of rostral colliculus, white l's of superior colliculus, white l's of cranial colliculus,** see *strata grisea et alba colliculi rostralis.* **Zeissel's l.,** a layer in the stomach wall between the tunica muscularis mucosae and the tela submucosa. **zonal l., of cerebral cortex,** lamina molecularis corticis cerebri. **zonal l. of quadrigeminal body,** stratum zonale corporis quadrigemini. **zonal l. of thalamus,** stratum zonale thalami.

lazar (laz′ar) [*Lazarus,* the leper of the Bible] (*obs.*) 1. leper; leprosy patient. 2. of or pertaining to leprosy, as lazar house (leprosarium).

lazaretto (laz″ah-ret′o) 1. a hospital for contagious diseases. 2. a quarantine station.

lb. abbreviation for L. *li′bra,* pound.

LCAT lecithin-cholesterol acyltransferase.

LD lethal dose.

LD₅₀ median lethal dose; a dose that is lethal for 50 per cent of the test subjects.

L.D.A. left dorsoanterior (position of the fetus).

LDH lactate dehydrogenase.

LDL low-density lipoproteins.

L-dopa see *dopa.*

L.D.P. left dorsoposterior (position of the fetus).

LE 1. left eye. 2. lupus erythematosus; see also under *cell.*

leaching (lēch′ing) lixiviation.

lead¹ (led) [L. *plumbum*] a soft, grayish blue metal with poisonous salts; symbol, Pb; atomic number, 82; atomic weight, 207.19. See also under *poisoning.* **l. acetate** [USP], colorless crystals, masses, or granules, $Pb(C_2H_3O_2)_2 \cdot 3H_2O$, used as a reagent and astringent. **l. arsenate,** a mixture of arsenate of soda and acetate of lead, $PbHAsO_4$, in water, used as an insecticide, and in veterinary medicine to kill tapeworms. **black l.,** graphite. **l. chloride,** a compound, $PbCl_2$, used as a reagent and pigment. **l. chromate,** a lemon-yellow powder, $PbCrO_4$, used in stains; called also *chrome yellow.* **l. monoxide,** a binary compound, PbO, called *litharge* when crystalline and *massicot* when amorphous; used as a reagent. **l. nitrate,** a sweetish crystalline agent, $Pb(NO_3)_2$, used as a reagent. **l. oleate,** a white powder, $Pb(C_{18}H_{33}O_2)_2$, used in varnishes. **l. oxide,** see *l. monoxide* and *l. tetroxide.* **radioactive l.,** radiolead. **red l.,** lead tetroxide. **l. subacetate,** a basic acetate of lead. **sugar of l.,** l. acetate. **tetraethyl l.,** a highly poisonous organic lead compound, $Pb(C_2H_5)_4$, used as an antiknock agent in internal combustion motors; it can be absorbed through the skin and may cause mental symptoms and death. Called also *ethyl gas.* **l. tet-**

roxide, a red powder, Pb₃O₄, which may be used like the monoxide. **white l.,** a basic lead carbonate.

lead² (lēd) any of the conductors connected to the electrocardiograph. Also any of the records made by the electrocardiograph, varying with the part of the body from which the current is led off. It is customary to use three peripheral leads: lead I, right arm and left arm; lead II, right arm and left leg; lead III, left arm and left leg; and at least six leads from the precordial region. Called also *derivation.* **aVF l.,** a unipolar lead in which the positive terminal is on the left leg. **aVL l.,** a unipolar lead in which the positive terminal is on the left arm. **aVR l.,** a unipolar lead in which the positive terminal is on the right arm. **bipolar l.,** an array involving two electrodes placed at different body sites. **esophageal l.,** one attached to an electrode inserted within the esophagus. **limb l's,** any of the three leads customarily used in electrocardiography. **precordial l's,** leads in which one electrode is placed on the chest and the other is connected to one or more extremities. Such leads are indicated as follows: CR = chest + right arm; CL = chest + left arm; CF = chest and left leg; V = chest + junction of leads from right and left arms and left leg (sometimes called *Wilson l's*). Subscript numbers 1 to 6 indicate at which points on the chest the lead is taken. **unipolar l.,** an array of

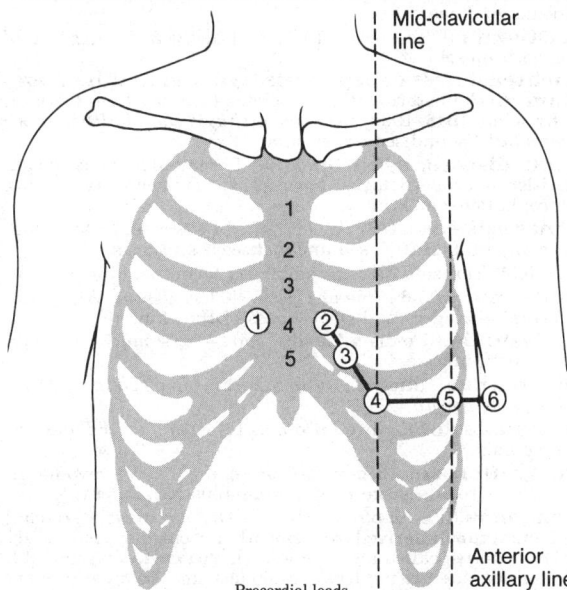

Precordial leads.

two electrodes, only one of which transmits potential variation. **V l's,** precordial leads further designated by a subscript numeral (V₁ to V₆) according to the position along the intercostal spaces. **Wilson's l's,** see *precordial l's.*

leaflet (lēf'let) a structure resembling a small leaf, especially a cusp of a heart valve.

learning (ler'ning) a relatively long-lasting adaptive behavioral change occurring as a result of experience. **insight l.,** the highest form of learning, characterized by the ability to evaluate and combine previous experiences to solve a problem or achieve a desired goal. **latent l.,** that which occurs without reinforcement, becoming apparent only when a reinforcement or reward is introduced.

leash (lēsh) a bundle of cordlike structures, as nerves, blood vessels, fibers, etc.

leben (leb'en) [Arabic] a fermented drink of Egypt made from the milk of cows, buffaloes, and goats.

Leber's congenital amaurosis, etc. (la-berz') [Theodor *Leber,* German ophthalmologist, 1840–1917] see under *amaurosis, atrophy, corpuscle, disease,* and *plexus.*

Lebistes (lĕ-bis'tēz) a genus of small fish, the guppy. **L. reticula'tus,** a species of top-feeding minnows, commonly known as "millions," cultivated in the Barbados to eliminate mosquito larvae.

Leboyer method (technique) (lĕ-boi-ya') [Frederick *Leboyer,* French obstetrician] see under *method.*

lecanopagus (lek"an-op'ah-gus) [Gr. *lekanē* basin + *pagos*

thing fixed] symmetrical conjoined twins fused at the pelvis.

Lecat's gulf (lĕ-kahz') [Claude Nicolas *Lecat,* French surgeon, 1700–1768] the hollow of the bulbous portion of the urethra.

leche de higuerón (la'cha da ēg"a-ron') [Sp. milk of fig] the sap or latex of wild fig trees e.g, *Ficus anthelmintica* Mart. (Moraceae), of Central and South America, used as a vermifuge.

lechopyra (lek"o-pi'rah) [Gr. *lechō* parturient woman + *pyr* fever] puerperal fever.

lecithal (les'ĭ-thal) [Gr. *lekithos* yolk] having a yolk. Used as a word termination, affixed to a word stem descriptive of the state of the yolk substance, as *centrolecithal, isolecithal,* etc. See also entries under *ovum.*

lecithalbumin (les"ĭ-thal'bu-min) a compound of albumin and lecithin, found in the stomach, liver, kidney, lungs, and spleen.

lecithid (les'ĭ-thid) a compound of lecithin with venom hemolysin. **cobra l.,** a hemolytic compound formed by cobra toxin and the lecithin of the blood.

lecithin (les'ĭ-thin) phosphatidylcholine.

lecithinase (les'ĭ-thin-ās) phospholipase. **l. A,** phospholipase A₁ and phospholipase A₂. **l. B,** lysophospholipase. **l. C,** phospholipase C. **l. D,** phospholipase D.

lecithin-cholesterol acyltransferase (LCAT) (les'ĭ-thin ko-les'ter-ol as"il-trans'fer-ās) phosphatidylcholin-esterol acyltransferase. **familial l. deficiency,** an autosomal recessive disorder due to failure of LCAT to esterify plasma cholesterol; cholesterol accumulates in the plasma and tissues, causing corneal opacities, anemia, and often proteinuria. Called also *Norum-Gjone disease.*

lecithinemia (les"ĭ-thĭ-ne'me-ah) the presence of lecithin in the blood.

lecith(o)- [Gr. *lekithos* yolk] a combining form denoting relationship to the yolk of an egg or ovum.

lecithoblast (les'ĭ-tho-blast") [*lecitho-* + Gr. *blastos* germ] the primitive entoderm of a two-layered blastodisc.

lecithoprotein (les"ĭ-tho-pro'te-in) a compound of the protein molecule with a lecithin; lecithoproteins occur in all cells.

lecithovitellin (les"ĭ-tho-vi-tel'in) lecithin-phosphoprotein; a saline extract of egg yolks used in egg-yolk agar to test for bacterial lecithinase.

lectin (lek'tin) any of a group of hemagglutinating proteins found primarily in plant seeds, which bind specifically to the branching sugar molecules of glycoproteins and glycolipids on the surface of cells. Certain lectins selectively cause agglutination of erythrocytes of certain blood groups and of malignant cells but not their normal counterparts; others stimulate the proliferation of lymphocytes.

lectotype (lek'to-tīp) in bacteriology, a culture taken from the original material to serve as a type culture when the original investigator did not designate a type.

ledbänder (led'ben-der) [Ger.] Büngner's bands; see under *band.*

Le Dentu's suture (lĕ-den-tūz') [Jean François-Auguste *Le Dentu,* Paris surgeon, 1841–1926] see under *suture.*

Lederberg (led'er-berg), Joshua. American biochemist, born 1925; co-winner, with George Wells Beadle and Edward Lawrie Tatum, of the Nobel prize for medicine or physiology in 1958 for discoveries concerning genetic recombination and the organization of the genetic material of bacteria.

Ledercillin (led"er-sil'lin) trademark for preparations of penicillin G procaine.

Lederer's anemia (disease) (led'er-erz) [Max *Lederer,* Brooklyn pathologist, 1885–1952] see under *anemia.*

Leduc's current (lĕ-dooks') [Stéphane Armand Nicolas *Leduc,* French physicist, 1853–1939] see under *current.*

Lee's ganglion (lēz) [Robert *Lee,* English physician, 1793–1877] cervical ganglion of the uterus; see under *ganglion.*

leech (lēch) [L. *hirudo*] 1. any of the annelids of the class Hirudinea, especially *Hirudo medicinalis.* Some species, the bloodsuckers, may become temporarily parasitic upon animals, including man. Leeches were formerly used extensively for drawing blood. See also *hirudin* and *leeching* (def. 1). 2. to apply leeches. 3. (*obs.*) a physician. **American l.,**

Macrobdella decora. **artificial l.,** an apparatus for drawing blood by artificial suction. **horse l.,** see *Limnatis* and *Haemopis.* **land l.,** *Haemadipsa.* **medicinal l.,** *Hirudo medicinalis.*

leeching (lēch′ing) the application of a leech for the withdrawal of blood; formerly used extensively in the treatment of various disorders; called also *hirudinization.*

Leeuwenhoekia australiensis (lu″en-ho′ke-ah aus-tra″le-en′sis) [Anton (Anthony, Antony) van *Leeuwenhoek,* Dutch microscopist, 1632–1723] a mite found at Sydney, New South Wales, which may cause great irritation by burrowing in the skin.

Le Fort fracture, etc. (lĕ for′) [Léon-Clément *Le Fort,* French surgeon, 1829–1893] see under *amputation, fracture, operation, sound,* and *suture.*

left-handed (left-han′ded) using the left hand preferentially, or more skillfully than the right, in voluntary motor acts.

leg (leg) that section of the lower limb between the knee and ankle; in common usage, the entire lower limb (in which case, this section is called the lower leg). Called also *crus* [NA]. **badger l.,** inequality in the length of the legs. **baker l.,** genu valgum. **bandy l.,** genu varum. **Barbados l.,** elephantiasis of the leg. **bayonet l.,** uncorrected backward displacement of the bones of the leg at the knee, followed by ankylosis at the joint. **black l.,** symptomatic anthrax. **bow l.,** genu varum. **elephant l.,** elephantiasis of the leg. **milk l.,** phlegmasia alba dolens. **red l.,** a fatal septicemia in frogs caused by *Aeromonas hydrophila.* **restless l's,** see under *syndrome.* **rider's l.,** strain of the adductor muscles of the thigh in horseback riders. **scaly l.,** an enlarged and encrusted condition of the legs in fowls caused by sarcoptic mites of the genus *Knemidokoptes.* **scissor l.,** deformity with crossing of the legs in walking, due to spasticity of adductor muscles of the thighs. **tennis l.,** the condition resulting from a sudden tear at the musculotendinous junction of the medial belly of the gastrocnemius muscle, usually occurring in older persons participating in tennis and other sports activities. **white l.,** phlegmasia alba dolens.

Legal's disease, test (la-galz′) [Emmo *Legal,* German physician, 1859–1922] see under *disease* and *tests.*

Legg's disease (legz) [Arthur Thornton *Legg,* Boston surgeon, 1874–1939] osteochondritis of the capitular epiphysis of the femur; see *osteochondrosis.*

Legg-Calvé-Perthes disease (leg′-kal-va′-per′tez) [Arthur T. *Legg;* Jacques *Calvé,* French orthopedist, 1875–1954; Georg Clemens *Perthes,* German surgeon, 1869–1927] osteochondritis of the capitular epiphysis of the femur; see *osteochondrosis.*

leghemoglobin (leg″he-mo-glo′bin) a pigment found in leguminous root nodules.

Legionella (le″jun-el′ah) [from the disease first identified at an American Legion convention in Philadelphia in 1976] a genus of gram-negative, aerobic, rod-shaped bacteria of the family Legionellaceae, made up of motile, pleomorphic organisms that require cysteine and iron for growth and cause a pneumonia-like disease in humans (legionellosis). Their normal habitat is lakes, streams, and moist soil, and the mode of spread is the airborne route. The organisms have been frequently isolated from cooling-tower water, evaporative condensers, riparian soil, tap water, shower heads, and treated sewage. The type species is *L. pneumoph′ila.* **L. bozema′nii,** a species isolated from human lung tissue that has been associated with pneumonia. **L. dumof′fii,** a species isolated from human lung tissue and from cooling-tower water that has been associated with pneumonia. **L. fee′leii,** a species isolated from coolant-system waters that has been associated with Pontiac fever. **L. gorma′nii,** a species isolated from riparian soil that has been associated with pneumonia. **L. jorda′nis,** a species isolated from riparian soil and treated sewage. **L. long-beach′ae,** a species isolated from human lung tissue and respiratory secretions that has been associated with pneumonia. **L. micda′dei,** a species isolated from human lung tissue, respiratory secretions, and pleural fluid and from cooling-tower water, shower heads, tap water, and nebulizers of respiratory therapy equipment. It is the causative agent of Pittsburgh pneumonia. Called also *L. pittsburgensis* and *Pittsburgh pneumonia agent.* **L. pittsburgen′sis,** *L. micdadei.* **L. pneumoph′ila,** the causative agent of le-

gionnaires' disease and Pontiac fever. It was the first species of the genus isolated and characterized, and it has been found in human lung tissue, respiratory secretions, pleural fluid, and blood and in numerous environmental sites such as riparian and other soil, and in cooling-tower water, tap water, shower heads, construction and excavation sites, and aerosolized droplets from heat-exchange systems. **L. wads wor′thii,** a species isolated from pleural tissue, a cause of human pneumonia.

legionella (le″jun-el′ah), pl. *legionel′lae.* any microorganism of the genus *Legionella.*

Legionellaceae (le″jun-el-la′se-e) a family of bacteria that contains the single genus *Legionella.*

legionellae (le″jun-el′e) plural of *legionella.*

legionellosis (le″jun-el-o′sis) infection caused by species of the genus *Legionella.*

legume (leg′ūm) the pod or fruit of a leguminous plant, such as peas and beans.

legumelin (leg″u-me′lin) an albumin from lentils, beans, and other leguminous seeds.

legumin (lĕ-gu′min) [L. *legumen* pulse] a globulin from the seeds of various plants, chiefly of the family Leguminosae.

leguminivorous (lĕ-gu″mĭ-niv′o-rus) feeding on legumes (beans and peas).

leiasthenia (li″as-the′ne-ah) [*leio-* + *asthenia*] asthenia of smooth muscle.

Leichtenstern's encephalitis (type), sign (phenomenon) (līk′ten-sternz) [Otto Michael *Leichtenstern,* German physician, 1845–1900] see *hemorrhagic encephalitis,* under *encephalitis,* and see under *sign.*

Leigh disease, syndrome (la) [Archibald Denis *Leigh,* British neuropathologist, born 1915] subacute necrotizing encephalomyelopathy.

Leiner's disease, test (li′nerz) [Karl *Leiner,* Austrian pediatrician, 1871–1930] see under *disease* and *tests.*

leio- [Gr. *leios* smooth] a combining form meaning smooth.

leiodermia (li″o-der′me-ah) [*leio-* + Gr. *derma* skin] abnormal glossiness and smoothness of the skin.

leiodystonia (li″o-dis-to′ne-ah) [*leio-* + *dystonia*] dystonia of smooth muscle.

Leiognathus bacoti (li-og′nah-thus bah-ko′te) *Ornithonyssus bacoti.*

leiomyoblastoma (li″o-mi″o-blas-to′mah) epithelioid leiomyoma.

leiomyofibroma (li″o-mi″o-fi-bro′mah) a leiomyoma in which there is a prominent fibromatous component.

leiomyoma (li″o-mi-o′mah) [*leio-* + Gr. *mys* muscle + *-oma*] a benign tumor derived from smooth muscle, most commonly of the uterus; called also *fibroid.* **bizarre l.,** epithelioid l. **l. cu′tis,** one arising from cutaneous smooth muscle fibers of the arrector pili muscles, presenting as a smooth, firm, painful nodule, often with a translucent or waxy appearance, which may occur singly or in groups. **epithelioid l.,** a relatively rare smooth muscle tumor, usually of the stomach, in which the cells are polygonal rather than spindle-shaped; called also *bizarre l.* and *leiomyoblastoma.* **l. u′teri,** a leiomyoma of the uterus, usually occurring in the third and fourth decades, characterized by the development, most commonly within the myometrium, of multiple, sharply circumscribed, uncapsulated, gray-white tumors, which are firm, usually round, and show a whorled pattern on cut section; called also *fibromyoma uteri, myoma previum,* and, colloquially, *fibroids.* **vascular l.,** angioleiomyoma.

leiomyosarcoma (li″o-mi″o-sar-ko′mah) a sarcoma containing large spindle cells of smooth muscle, most commonly of the uterus or retroperitoneal region.

leip(o)- for words beginning thus, see those beginning *lip(o)-.*

Leishman's cells, stain (lēsh′manz) [Sir William Boog *Leishman,* English army surgeon, 1865–1926] see under *cell* and see *Table of Stains and Staining Methods.*

Leishman-Donovan body (lēsh′man-don′o-van) [Sir William B. *Leishman;* Charles *Donovan,* Irish physician in Sanitary Service in India, 1863–1951] amastigote.

Leishmania (lēsh-ma′ne-ah) [Sir William B. *Leishman*] a genus of flagellate protozoa (suborder Trypanosomatina, order Kinetoplastida) comprising parasites of worldwide distribution, several species of which are pathogenic for humans. The organism have two morphologic stages in their life cycle: amastigote (Leishman-Donovan body), found intracellularly in the vertebrate (i.e., human) host; and promastigote (leptomonad), found in the digestive tract of the invertebrate host (i.e., phlebotomine sandfly) and in cultures. Because all species are morphologically indistinguishable, the organisms have usually been assigned to species and subspecies according to their geographic origin, the clinical syndrome they produce, and their ecologic characteristics, or they have been separated on the basis of their tendency to cause visceral, cutaneous, or mucocutaneous leishmaniasis. In some classifications, leishmanias are placed in four complexes comprising species and subspecies: *L. donovani*, *L. tropica*, *L. mexicana*, and *L. brasiliensis*. **L. aethio′pica**, a species of the *L. tropica* complex infecting rock and tree hydraxes in the highlands of Ethiopia and Kenya; the vector in Ethiopia is *Phlebotomus longipes* and in Kenya it is *P. pedifer*. It causes cutaneous leishmaniasis in humans, most cases of which are self-limited although a few develop into diffuse cutaneous leishmaniasis. Called also *L. tropica aethipica*. **L. brasilien′sis**, *L. braziliensis*. **L. brazilien′sis**, 1. a taxonomic complex comprising the subspecies and species causing the mucocutaneous forms of leishmaniasis: *L. b. braziliensis*, *L. b. guyanensis*, *L. b. panamensis*, and *L. peruviana*, all of which develop in the midgut, foregut, and hindgut of their sandfly vectors. Called also *L. brasiliensis*. 2. *L. braziliensis braziliensis*. **L. brazilien′sis brazilien′sis**, a subspecies of the *L. braziliensis* complex, transmitted by species of *Lutzomyia* and *Psychodopygus*, and causing cutaneous and mucocutaneous leishmaniasis in Brazil, Peru, Ecuador, Bolivia, Venezuela, Paraguay, and Colombia. Called also *L. braziliensis*. **L. brazilien′sis guyanen′sis**, a subspecies of the *L. braziliensis* complex, transmitted chiefly by *Lutzomyia umbratilis* and causing pian bois (forest yaws). **L. brazilien′sis panamen′sis**, a subspecies of the *L. braziliensis* complex, transmitted chiefly by *Lutzomyia trapidoi*, and causing the New World form of cutaneous leishmaniasis in Panama and adjacent areas of Central America and Colombia, which is manifested by one or a few deep, ulcer-like lesions and is sometimes associated with nodular lymphatic metastases. **L. donova′ni**, 1. a taxonomic complex comprising the subspecies causing the visceral forms of leishmaniasis: *L. d. donovani*, *L. d. infantum*, and *L. d. chagasi*, all of which multiply in the reticuloendothelial cells and spread to the lymph nodes and then hematogenously throughout the body. The subspecies can be distinguished only by differences in the epidemiology, clinical features, and response to treatment. 2. *L. d. donovani*. **L. donova′ni chaga′si**, a subspecies of the *L. donovani* complex causing visceral leishmaniasis in Central and South America, usually transmitted by the sandfly *Lutzomyia longipalpis*. **L. donova′ni donova′ni**, a subspecies of the *L. donovani* complex causing the classic form of visceral leishmaniasis in India. It is transmitted by the sandfly *Phlebotomus argentipes*, with humans being the only major reservoir hosts. Called also *L. donovani*. **L. donova′ni infan′tum**, a subspecies of the *L. donovani* complex causing the infantile form of visceral leishmaniasis in the Mediterranean littoral (usual vectors *Phlebotomus perniciosus* and *P. major*), Near and Middle East, (usual vectors *P. papatasii* and *P. caucasicus*), sub-Saharan and East Africa (usual vectors *P. orientalis* and *P. martini*), and China (usual vectors *P. chinensis* and *P. (sergenti)*. Called also *L. infantum*. **L. farcimino′sa**, former name for *Histoplasma farciminosus*. **L. garnha′mi**, a species similar to (or identical with) *L. mexicana amazonensis* isolated from cases of cutaneous leishmaniasis in the region of the Venezuelan Andes. **L. infan′tum**, *L. donovani infantum*. **L. ma′jor**, a species of the *L. tropica* complex, transmitted by *Phlebotomus papatasii*, and causing the rural form of Old World cutaneous leishmaniasis. Called also *L. tropica major*. **L. mexica′na**, a taxonomic complex comprising the species and subspecies causing the New World form of cutaneous leishmaniasis in humans: *L. m. mexicana*, *L. m. amazonensis*, and *L. pifanoi*, which infect chiefly forest rodents and opossums. They develop only in the midgut and foregut of their sandfly vectors. **L. mexica′na amazonen′sis**, a subspecies of the *L. mexicana* complex, transmitted by *Lutzomyia flaviscutellata*, and causing a form of New World cutaneous leishmaniasis in the Amazon region of Brazil and neighboring countries and in Trinidad. A single lesion is usually present but a few cases of diffuse cutaneous leishmaniasis caused by *L. m. mexicana*

have been reported. **L. mexica′na mexica′na**, a subspecies of the *L. mexicana* complex transmitted by *Lutzomyia olmeca* and causing chiclero ulcer. **L. mexica′na pi′fanoi**, *L. pifanoi*. **L. nilot′ica**, *L. tropica*, def. 2. **L. peruvia′na**, a species of the *L. braziliensis* complex found in the Peruvian Andes only at altitudes of 900 to 3000 meters, probably transmitted by *Lutzomyia verrucarum* and *Lutzomyia peruensis*, and causing uta in humans. **L. pi′fanoi**, a species of the *L. mexicana* complex causing diffuse cutaneous leishmaniasis in Venezuela and certain areas of Brazil. Called also *L. mexicana pifanoi*. **L. trop′ica**, 1. a taxonomic complex comprising the species causing the Old World form of cutaneous leishmaniasis: *L. tropica*, *L. major*, and *L. aethiopica*. The species can be differentiated on ecologic, biochemical, and serologic grounds. 2. a species of the *L. tropica* complex causing the urban form of Old World cutaneous leishmaniasis. It is found in Iran, Iraq, and India, transmitted by *Phlebotomus sergenti*; and in southern France, Italy, and certain Mediterranean islands, transmitted by *P. papatasi*. Human to human transmission may also occur. Called also *L. nilotica*, *L. tropica minor*, and *L. tropica tropica*. **L. trop′ica aethio′pica**, *L. aethiopica*. **L. trop′ica ma′jor** *L. major*. **L. trop′ica mi′nor**, *L. tropica*, def. 2. **L. trop′ica trop′ica**, *L. tropica*, def. 2.

leishmania (lēsh-ma′ne-ăh) 1. any protozoan of the genus *Leishmania*. 2. see *amastigote*.

leishmanial (lēsh-ma′ne-ăl) 1. pertaining to or caused by leishmanias. 2. denoting a morphologic stage in the life cycle of trypanosomatid protozoa; see *amastigote*.

leishmaniasis (lēsh″mah-ni′ah-sis) infection caused by *Leishmania*. **American l.,** the New World form of leishmaniasis. **anergic l., anergic cutaneous l.,** diffuse cutaneous l. **canine l.,** the Mediterranean type of visceral leishmaniasis. **cutaneous l.,** an endemic disease characterized by the development of a cutaneous papule(s) that envolves into a nodule, breaks down to form an indolent ulcer, and heals, leaving a depressed scar. The disease has been divided into Old and New World forms. *Old World l.* is divided into three distinct types according to clinical manifestations and epidemiology. The acute, rapidly evolving rural (humid, moist, wet) form, primarily an infection of desert rodents in parts of Asia, Russia, Iran, Iraq, India, and the Middle East, is caused by *Leishmania major*, and is transmitted to humans by *Phlebotomus papatasi*. In this form the lesions tend to be multiple and are accompanied by marked inflammation and crusting. The urban form, which is caused by *L. tropica*, is a natural infection of humans and dogs in large urban areas in the Middle East, the Mediterranean region, India, and Pakistan and is transmitted by *P. sergenti*. A slowly developing single lesion that persists for a year or more is typical of urban leishmaniasis. In the highlands of Kenya and Ethiopia *L. aethiopica*, which infects rock and tree hydraxes, is transmitted by *P. pedifer* (Kenya) and *P. longipes* (Ethiopia) and causes human cutaneous leishmaniasis. The lesions of this form are less inflamed and more chronic (usually lasting several years) than those of the other forms, and they are usually self-limited but sometimes become diffuse. This form has received many names, according to its locality of occurrences, including *Aleppo, Bagdad, Biskra, Jericho*, or *Oriental boil; Bagdad* or *Oriental button;* and *Delhi, Kandahar, Lahore, Natal, Oriental,* or *Penjedeh sore.* The *New World form* (American l.) occurs throughout Central and South America with the exception of Chile and Argentina, and is characterized by lesions that develop and heal similarly to those of the Old World form, but they tend to be less nodular and more ulcerative and destructive; it is caused by the species and subspecies of the *L. mexicana* or *L. braziliensis* complexes. Many varieties of cutaneous leishmaniasis of the New World exist, including *mucocutaneous leishmaniasis*, *chicle* or *chiclero ulcer*, *uta*, and *pian bois*, which differ as to etiologic agent, vector, distribution, pathology, epidemiology, and clinical course and manifestations. **diffuse cutaneous l.,** a rare chronic form of cutaneous leishmaniasis caused by *Leishmania aethiopica* in Ethiopia and Kenya, by *L. pifanoi* in Venezuela, and by protozoa of the *L. braziliensis* and *L. mexicana* complexes in South and Central America, respectively. It is characterized by the local and hematogenous spread from a primary lesion to produce generalized nodular lesions resembling those of lepromatous leprosy in the skin and sometimes involving the nasal mucosa and laryngopharynx. Called also *anergic l., anergic cutaneous l., l. cutanea diffusa,* and *l. tegmentaria diffusa.* **infan**

tile l., the Mediterranean type of visceral leishmaniasis. **lupoid l.,** l. recidivans. **mucocutaneous l.,** chronic, progressive metastatic spread of the lesions of cutaneous leishmaniasis of the New World caused by *Leishmania braziliensis braziliensis* to the nasal, pharyngeal, and buccal mucosa months to years after the appearance of the initial cutaneous lesion, which has usually healed. It is often associated with mutilating destruction of the nasal septum, palate, lips, pharynx, and larynx. Called also *espundia*. **New World l.,** see *cutaneous l.* **Old World l.,** see *cutaneous l.* **post–kala-azar dermal l.,** a condition associated with visceral leishmaniasis, commonly characterized by the appearance of hypopigmented or erythematous macules on the face and sometimes on the extremities and trunk; the facial lesions gradually progress to papules or nodules that resemble those of lepromatous leprosy. It is seen in about 20% of Indian patients, usually occurring years after the treatment of or spontaneous recovery from visceral leishmaniasis, and it may last for as long as 20 years. When the conditions affects patients in East Africa (2%) and China (rare), it usually occurs shortly after or during treatment and usually does not persist. Called also *dermal leishmanoid, leishmanoid,* and *post–kala-azar dermal leishmanoid.* **l. recid'ivans,** a relapsing form of cutaneous leishmaniasis of the Old World, resembling tuberculosis of the skin, in which the ulcer heals incompletely, scarring centrally but spreading peripherally, or heals and recrudesces at the edge of the scar; it may last for many years. Called also *lupoid l.* **rural l.,** see *cutaneous l.* (of Old World). **l. tegmenta'ria diffu'sa,** diffuse cutaneous l. **urban l.,** see *cutaneous l.* (of Old World). **visceral l.,** a chronic, highly fatal if untreated, infectious disease caused by one of three subspecies of *L. donovani* in various regions of the world, which are found in the cells of the reticuloendothelial system throughout the body, especially in the liver, spleen, bone marrow, lymph nodes, and skin. It is commonly characterized by hepatosplenomegaly, irregular fever, chills, vomiting, emaciation, anemia, leukopenia, hypergammaglobulinemia, and an earth-gray color of the skin. According to geographic distribution, the disease is classified into three main types: (1) The classic, or Indian, form (black, cachectic, cachexial, and Dumdum fever; kala-azar; tropical splenomegaly) is caused by *L. d. donovani* and is transmitted by *Phlebotomus argentipes;* humans are the only major reservoir hosts. This form usually affects young adults and older children. (2) The infantile form is caused by *L. d. infantum* and is most commonly seen in children between the ages of 1 and 4. In different locations the infantile form has different reservoir hosts and vectors. In the Mediterranean littoral, major reservoirs are dogs, and the usual vectors are *Phlebotomus perniciosus* and *P. major.* In the Near and Middle East, major reservoirs are foxes and jackals, and the usual vectors are *P. papatasi* and *P. caucasicus.* In China, major reservoirs are dogs, and the usual vectors are *P. chinensis* and *P. sergenti.* In sub-Saharan and East Africa, major reservoirs are rodents, dogs, and perhaps humans. (3) *L. d. chagasi* causes visceral leishmaniasis in humans of all ages in South and Central America. Its major reservoirs are dogs and foxes, and it is transmitted by *Lutzomyia longipalpis.*

leishmanicidal (lēsh″man-ĭ-si′dal) destructive to *Leishmania.*

leishmanid (lēsh′man-id) the early cutaneous nodule of cutaneous leishmaniasis.

leishmanin (lēsh′mah-nin) a suspension of killed leishmania promastigotes; used in a skin test for cutaneous leishmaniasis (see *leishmanin test,* under *tests*).

leishmaniosis (lēsh″man-e-o′sis) leishmaniasis.

leishmanoid (lēsh′mah-noid) 1. like or resembling leishmaniasis. 2. a lesion of post–kala-azar dermal leishmaniasis. **dermal l., post–kala-azar dermal l.,** post–kala-azar dermal leishmaniasis.

Lelaps (le′laps) *Echinolaelaps.* **L. echidni'nus,** *Echinolaelaps echidninus.*

lema (le′mah) [Gr. *lēmē*] sebum palpebrale.

Lembert's suture (lah-bārz′) [Antoine *Lembert,* French surgeon, 1802–1851] see under *suture.*

lemma (lem′ah) [Gr. "rind," "husk"] a collective term for the egg membranes (primary, secondary, and tertiary). Also used as a word termination denoting a sheath, as the neurilemma and oolemma.

lemmoblast (lem′o-blast) a primitive or immature lemmocyte.

lemmoblastic (lem″o-blas′tik) forming or developing into neurilemma tissue.

lemmocyte (lem′o-sīt) [Gr. *lemma* husk + *-cyte*] a cell derived from the neural crest and developing into a neurilemma cell.

lemnisci (lem-nis′i) plural of *lemniscus.*

lemniscus (lem-nis′kus), gen. and pl. *lemnis'ci* [L., from Gr. *lēmniskos* ribbon] a ribbon or band; [NA] a general term for a band or bundle of fibers in the central nervous system. **acoustic l., l. acus'ticus** (obs.), l. lateralis. **lateral l., l. latera'lis** [NA], a tract of longitudinal fibers extending upward through the lateral part of the tegmental substance of the pons, formed chiefly by fibers arising from the opposite cochlear nuclei and the trapezoid body, and ascending to terminate in the inferior colliculus and medial geniculate body. **medial l., l. media'lis** [NA], a tract arising from the internal arcuate fibers of the nuclei gracilis and cuneatus, and crossing to the opposite side in the lower part of medulla oblongata to ascend, first between the two olives, and then through the pars dorsalis pontis just dorsal to the pontine nuclei; it continues through the tegmentum of the midbrain and ends in the ventral posterior part of the thalamus. Each lemniscus carries sensory impulses from the opposite side of the body. Called also *sensory l.* or *l. sensitivus.* **optic l.,** tractus opticus. **l. sensiti'vus, sensory l.,** l. medialis. **spinal l., l. spina'lis** [NA], the part of each spinothalamic tract within the pons and mesencephalon, forming a diffuse bundle between the medial and lateral lemnisci. It carries pain, temperature, and tactile impulses from the opposite side of the body and ends in the ventral posterior part of the thalamus. **trigeminal l., l. trigemina'lis** [NA], fibers conveying sensory impulses from the trigeminal nuclei to the ventral posterior part of the opposite thalamus; they ascend intermingled with the spinal lemniscus and adjacent medial lemniscus. Called also *tractus trigeminothalamicus* [NA alternative] and *trigeminothalmic tract.*

lemon (lem′un) the fruit of *Citrus limon* (Linné) Burmann filius (Rutaceae); the peel contains a volatile oil used as a flavoring agent, and the fruit contains citric and ascorbic acids.

lemoparalysis (le″mo-pah-ral′ĭ-sis) [Gr. *laimos* gullet + *paralysis*] paralysis of the esophagus.

lemostenosis (lem″o-stĕ-no′sis) [Gr. *laimos* gullet + *stenōsis* narrowing] stenosis of the esophagus.

Lempert's fenestration operation (lem′perts) [Julius *Lempert,* American otologist, 1890–1968] see under *operation.*

Lemuroidea (lem″u-roi′de-ah) a suborder of Primates, consisting of the lemurs, animals resembling monkeys but having, usually, a sharp, foxlike muzzle and a tail which is usually long and furry, but never prehensile.

Lenard rays (len-ard′) [Philipp *Lenard,* Hungarian physicist, 1862–1947] see under *ray.*

Lenetran (len′ĕ-tran) trademark for a preparation of mephenoxalone.

length (length) an expression of the longest dimension of an object, or of the measurement between the two ends. **arch l.,** the length of a line segment within the median plane perpendicular to and extending from the line connecting the first premolars to the most labial point on the anterior arch, usually to the point between the maxillary central incisors. Called also *anterior arch l.* **basialveolar l.,** the distance from the basion to the lower end of the intermaxillary suture. **basinasal l.,** the distance from basion to nasion. **crown-heel l.,** an expression of measurement from the crown of the head to the heel in embryos, fetuses, and infants; the equivalent of *standing height* in older individuals. **crown-rump l.,** an expression of measurement from the crown of the head to the breech in embryos, fetuses, and infants; the equivalent of *sitting vertex height* in older individuals. **focal l.,** the distance between a lens and an object from which all rays of light are brought to a focus. **foot l.,** a heel-toe measurement useful in estimating the age of fetuses because the foot dimensions are less subject to artifacts of variation and shrinkage than is the fetus as a whole. **greatest l.,** a dimension used to express the size of very young embryos that have not yet developed the structures permitting measurement of crown-rump length. **sitting l.,** the distance from the crown of the head to the coccyx. **stem l.,** the distance from the vertex to a line joining the ischial tuberosities. **wave l.,** see *wavelength.*

leniquinsin (len″ĭ-kwin′sin) chemical name: *N*-[(3,4-dimethoxyphenyl) methylene] -6,7- dimethoxy- 4 -quinolinamine; an antihypertensive, $C_{20}H_{20}N_2O_4$.

lenitive (len′ĭ-tiv) [L. *lenire* to soothe] 1. demulcent or soothing. 2. a demulcent remedy.

Lennhoff's index, sign (len′hofs) [Rudolf *Lennhoff*, German physician, 1866–1933] see under *index* and *sign.*

Lennox syndrome [William Gordon *Lennox*, American neurologist, 1884–1960] see under *syndrome.*

lenperone (len′per-ōn) chemical name: 4-[4-(4-fluorobenzoyl)-1-piperidinyl]-1-(4-fluorophenyl)-1-butanone; a tranquilizer, $C_{22}H_{23}F_2NO_2$.

lens (lenz) [L. "lentil"] 1. a piece of glass or other transparent substance so shaped as to converge or scatter the rays of light, especially the glass used in appropriate frames or other instruments to increase the visual acuity of the human eye. See also *glasses* and *spectacles.* 2. [NA] the transparent biconvex body of the eye situated between the posterior chamber and the vitreous body, constituting part of the refracting mechanism of the eye. See *eye.* Called also *l. crystallina* or *crystalline l.* **achromatic l.,** one corrected

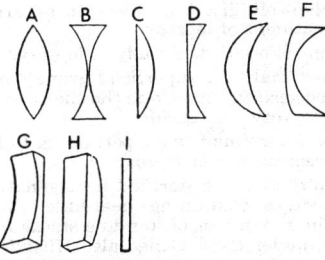

Lenses: *A–F,* Spherical lenses: *A,* biconvex; *B,* biconcave; *C,* planoconvex; *D,* planoconcave; *E,* concavoconvex, periscopic convex, converging meniscus; *F,* convexoconcave, periscopic concave, diverging meniscus; *G, H,* cylindrical lenses, concave and convex; *I,* flat lens.

for chromatic aberration. **acrylic l.,** a plastic lens used to replace the crystalline lens after cataract surgery. **adherent l.,** contact l. **anastigmatic l.,** a lens with spherical surfaces only and no cylindrical ones; called also *stigmatic l.* **aniseikonic l.,** iseikonic l. **aplanatic l.,** one that serves to correct spherical aberration and coma. **apochromatic l.,** one corrected for chromatic and spherical aberration. **astigmatic l.,** cylindrical l. **biconcave l.,** a flat lens that has both surfaces concave; called also *concavoconcave l.* **biconvex l.,** a flat lens that has both surfaces convex. **bicylindrical l.,** one that has both surfaces cylindrical or toroidal. **bifocal l.,** a lens made up of two segments with different refractive powers, ordinarily with the upper for far and the lower segment for near vision; see under *glasses.* **bispherical l.,** one that is spherical on both sides. **Brücke l.,** a combination of a double convex and double concave lens so arranged as to give considerable working distance. **cataract l.,** a powerful lens for glasses to be used after cataract operation. **compound l.,** a lens made up of two or more segments. **concave l.,** a lens with one or both (biconcave) surfaces curved like a section of the interior of a hollow sphere; it diverges the rays of light. Called also *diverging l.* and *minus l.* **concavoconcave l.,** biconcave l. **concavoconvex l.,** one that has one concave surface and one convex; the concave surface is of greater curvature than the convex. Called also *periscopic convex l., converging meniscus l.,* and *positive meniscus l.* **condensing l.,** a large, powerful convex spherical lens to focus available light upon the eye for examination. **contact l.,** a curved shell of glass or plastic applied directly over the globe or cornea to correct refractive errors; called also *adherent l.* **contact l., corneal,** one that rests on the cornea, not on the sclera, and requires no auxiliary liquid; called also *corneal l.* **contact l., gas permeable,** any contact lens that transmits oxygen and carbon dioxide. **contact l., hard,** a contact lens that maintains its shape without support and absorbs little or no

water; called also *hydrophobic contact l.* or *rigid contact l.* **contact l., scleral,** a contact lens covering the cornea and resting on the sclera, with or without an auxiliary liquid between the lens and the cornea. **contact l., soft,** a contact lens that when worn is soft, flexible, and water absorbent; called also *hydrophilic contact l.* **converging l., convex l.,** a lens curved like a section of the exterior of a hollow sphere; it brings light to a focus. Called also *plus l.* **convexoconcave l.,** one that has one convex and one concave surface; the convex surface is of greater curvature than the concave. Called also *periscopic concave l., diverging meniscus l.,* and *negative meniscus l.* **corneal l.,** corneal contact l. **Crookes' l.,** one made from glass rendered opaque to ultraviolet and infrared rays but transparent to visible light. **crossed l.,** a converging lens with minimal spherical aberration. **l. crystalli′na, crystalline l.,** the lens of the eye; see *lens,* def. 2. **cylindrical l.,** a lens used to correct astigmatism, having one plane surface and one cylindrical, or one spherical surface and one toroidal. The meridian along the lens axis has no refractive power, but the meridian at right angles to the axis has maximum refractive power; thus the principal focus is a straight line, not a point. Called also *astigmatic l.* **decentered l.,** one in which the optical axis does not pass through the geometric center. **dispersing l.,** an incorrect name for *concave l.* (diverging l.). **diverging l.,** concave l. **flat l.,** a lens with equal curvature on both sides, as opposed to a meniscus lens. **honey bee l.,** a magnifying eyeglass lens designed to resemble the multifaceted eye of the honeybee. It consists of three or six small telescopes mounted in the upper portion of the spectacles and directed toward the center and right and left visual fields. Prisms are included to provide a continuous, unbroken magnified field of view. **immersion l.,** see under *objective.* **iseikonic l.,** a lens that magnifies but does not refract; it is used to treat aniseikonia because it changes the sizes of the images on the retinas of the eyes. Called also *aniseikonic l.* and *size l.* **meniscus l.,** a crescent-shaped lens with one concave surface and one convex; the surfaces have different degrees of curvature. See *concavoconvex l.* and *convexoconcave l.* **meniscus l., converging,** concavoconvex l. **meniscus l., diverging,** convexoconcave l. **meniscus l., negative,** convexoconcave l. **meniscus l., positive,** concavoconvex l. **meter l.,** a converging lens with a focal length of one meter and a refracting power of one diopter. **minus l.,** concave l. **omnifocal l.,** a lens the power of which increases continuously and regularly in a downward direction, thereby avoiding the discontinuity in field and power which is apparent in bifocal and trifocal lenses. **orthoscopic l.,** one that gives a very flat and undistorted field of vision, especially at the periphery. **periscopic l.,** one with a 1.25D base curve. **periscopic concave l.,** convexoconcave l. **periscopic convex l.,** concavoconvex l. **photochromic l., photosensitive l.,** a light-sensitive lens that darkens in full light and clears in reduced light. **plane l., plano l.,** a lens with no curve and no refracting power; light rays enter and leave parallel. **planoconcave l.,** a lens with one plane and one concave side. **planoconvex l.,** a lens with one plane and one convex side. **plus l.,** convex l. **punktal l.,** a toric lens which is corrected for astigmatism over the entire field of vision. **safety l.,** one that protects the eyes from injury, especially from impact. Impact-resistant lenses may be made by tempering or by using plastic or laminated lenses. Called also *safety glasses.* **size l.,** iseikonic l. **spherical l.,** one that is a segment of a sphere. **spherocylindrical l.,** a lens with one spherical and one cylindrical surface, and functioning as both a simple spherical lens and a simple cylindrical one. **stigmatic l.,** anastigmatic l. **toric l.,** a meniscus lens with a cylindrical curve ground on the outer, convex, surface. **trial l.,** any one of a set of lenses used in testing the vision. **trifocal l.,** a lens made up of three segments with different refractive powers, ordinarily with the upper for distant, the middle for intermediate, and the lower for near vision; see *trifocal glasses,* under *glasses.*

lensometer (lenz-om′ĕ-ter) [*lens* + *-meter*] a device for measuring the optical characteristics of lenses; called also *phacometer.*

Lentard (len′tard) trademark for preparations of insulin zinc suspension.

lenticel (len′tĭ-sel) a lens-shaped gland, especially one of those at the base of the tongue.

lenticonus (len″tĭ-ko′nus) [*lens* + L. *conus* cone] a conical protrusion of the substance of the crystalline lens, covered by capsule or connective tissue, occurring more frequently on the posterior surface, and usually affecting only one eye.

lenticula (len-tik′u-lăh) [L.] nucleus lentiformis.

lenticular (len-tik′u-lar) [L. *lenticularis*] 1. pertaining to or shaped like a lens. 2. pertaining to the crystalline lens. 3. pertaining to the lenticular nucleus.

lenticulo-optic (len-tik″u-lo-op′tik) pertaining to the lenticular nucleus and the optic thalamus.

lenticulostriate (len-tik″u-lo-stri′āt) pertaining to the lenticular nucleus and the corpus striatum.

lenticulothalamic (len-tik″u-lo-thah-lam′ik) relating to the lenticular nucleus and the thalamus.

lentiform (len′tĭ-form) shaped like a lens; see also under *nucleus*.

lentigines (len-tij′ĭ-nēz) [L.] plural of *lentigo*.

lentiginosis (len-tij″ĭ-no′sis) the presence of multiple lentigines. **progressive cardiomyopathic l.,** Moynahan's syndrome, def. 1.

lentiginous (len-tij′ĭ-nus) characterized by multiple lentigines; pertaining to or of the nature of a lentigo.

lentiglobus (len″tĭ-glo′bus) [*lens* + L. *globus* sphere] an exaggerated curvature of the crystalline lens, producing a spherical bulging on its anterior surface.

lentigo (len-ti′go), pl. *lentig′ines* [L. "freckle"] 1. a small, flat, tan to dark brown or black, macular melanosis on the skin resembling a freckle clinically but histologically distinct because of the presence of an increased number of normal-appearing melanocytes along the dermoepidermal junction. Lentigines do not darken on exposure to sunlight, as do freckles. Called also *l. simplex* and *nevus spilus.* 2. nevus spilus. def. 1. **l. malig′na,** see under *melanoma.* **nevoid l.,** 1. a congenital lentigo involving the mucous membranes as well as the skin, occurring in association with various hereditary disorders, including the leopard syndrome and Moynihan's syndrome, and characterized histologically by elongation of rete pegs, an increase in the number of melanocytes with formation of nests, an increase of melanin in both the melanocytes and basal keratinocytes, and melanophages in the upper dermis. Single or multiple lesions may occur, and size and configuration vary widely. Called also *lentigo simplex* and *nevus spilus.* 2. nevus spilus, def. 1. **senile l., l. seni′lis,** a benign, discrete, hyperpigmented macule occurring on chronically sun-exposed skin in adults, especially on the back of the hands and on the forehead. Called also *liver spot* and *solar lentigo.* **l. sim′plex,** 1. lentigo, def. 1. 2. nevoid l., def. 1. **solar l.,** senile l.

lentivirus (len″tĭ-vi′rus) any of a group of retroviruses, including those that cause maedi and visna in sheep.

lentula (len′chu-lah) lentulo.

lentulo (len′chu-lo, len-too′lo) an engine-driven, flexible, spiral, rotating endodontic instrument made of stainless steel wire, used in a handpiece to place cement into the prepared root canal in root canal therapy. Called also *lentula, lentulo paste carrier,* and *paste carrier.*

Leo's test (la′ōz) [Hans *Leo,* German physician, 1854–1927] see under *tests.*

leontiasis (le″on-ti′ah-sis) [Gr. *leōn* lion] the leonine facies of lepromatous leprosy, due to nodular invasion of the subcutaneous tissue of the face, giving it a vaguely leonine appearance. **l. os′sea, l. os′sium,** bilateral and symmetrical hypertrophy of the bones of the face and cranium, giving it a vaguely leonine appearance; called also *megalocephaly.*

Leontodon (le-on′to-don) [Gr. *leōn* lion + *odous* tooth] *Taraxacum.*

Leopold's law (la′o-poldz) [Christian Gerhard *Leopold,* German physician, 1846–1911] see under *law.*

leotropic (le″o-trop′ik) [Gr. *laios* left + *tropos* a turning] running spirally from right to left. Cf. *dexiotropic.*

leper (lep′er) a person afflicted with leprosy; a term now in disfavor.

lepidic (lĕ-pid′ik) [Gr. *lepis* scale] 1. pertaining to scales. 2. pertaining to embryonic layers.

lepid(o)- [Gr. *lepis,* gen. *lepidos* flake or scale] a combining form meaning scale or scaly.

lepidoma (lep″ĭ-do′mah) [*lepido-* + *-oma*] (obs.) a tumor derived from lepidic tissue; an endothelioma or a mesothelioma. **endothelial l.** (*obs.*), an endothelioma of the blood vessels or lymphatics.

Lepidophyton (lep″ĭ-dof′ĭ-ton) [*lepido-* + Gr. *phyton* plant] former name for *Trichophyton concentricum.*

Lepidoptera (lep″ĭ-dop′ter-ah) [*lepido-* + Gr. *pteron* wing] an order of insects including the butterflies and moths.

lepocyte (lep′o-sīt) [Gr. *lepos* rind + *-cyte*] any nucleated cell having a cell wall.

lepra (lep′rah) [Gr. *lepra* the leprosy, which makes the skin scaly] leprosy; (prior to the mid 19th century) psoriasis. See also under *reaction.*

leprechaunism (lep′rĕ-kon″izm) an exceedingly rare and lethal familial condition marked by slow development both physically and mentally, by elfin facies (wide-set eyes and low-set ears, with hirsutism), as suggested by the name, and by severe endocrine disorders, as indicated by enlargement of the clitoris and breasts in females and of the phallus in males. Called also *Donohue's syndrome.*

leprid (lep′rid) cutaneous lesion or lesions of tuberculoid leprosy, being hypopigmented or erythematous macules or plaques showing no evidence of *Mycobacterium leprae* by ordinary methods of examination. Cf. *leproma.*

lepride (lep′rēd) leprid.

leprologist (lep-rol′o-jist) a physician experienced in the study and treatment of leprosy.

leprology (lep-rol′o-je) the study of leprosy.

leproma (lep-ro′mah) a superficial granulomatous nodule rich in *Mycobacterium leprae,* and the characteristic lesion of lepromatous leprosy. Cf. *leprid.*

lepromatous (lep-ro′mah-tus) pertaining to lepromas; see *lepromatous leprosy,* under *leprosy.*

lepromin (lep′ro-min) a purified homogenate of lepromatous skin nodules containing heat-killed *Mycobacterium leprae;* used in a skin test of immune status in leprosy (see *lepromin test,* under *tests*). Called also *Mitsuda antigen.*

leprosarium (lep″ro-sa′re-um) [L.] a hospital or colony for the treatment and isolation of leprosy patients.

leprosary (lep′ro-sār″e) [L. *leprosa′rium*] leprosarium.

leprostatic (lep″ro-stat′ik) 1. inhibiting the growth of *Mycobacterium leprae.* 2. an agent that inhibits the growth of *Mycobacterium leprae.*

leprosy (lep′ro-se) [Gr. *lepros* scaly, scabby, rough] a slowly progressive, chronic infectious disease caused by *Mycobacterium leprae* and characterized by the development of granulomatous or neurotrophic lesions in the skin, mucous membranes, nerves, bones, and viscera. It is manifested by a broad spectrum of clinical symptoms, consisting of two principal, or polar, types, with the *lepromatous* type at one end of the spectrum and the *tuberculoid* type at the other; between these two polar types is the *borderline* type, with two subtypes, *borderline tuberculoid* and *borderline lepromatous.* Called also *Hansen's disease* and *lepra.* See also *lepra reaction,* under *reaction,* and *lepromin test,* under *test.* **borderline l.,** an immunologically unstable form of leprosy transitional between the tuberculoid and lepromatous forms and having clinical and histological features of both types, which may evolve toward the former by reversal reactions or toward the latter by a downgrading reaction. Called also *dimorphous l.* and *intermediate l.* **borderline lepromatous l.,** see *borderline l.* **borderline tuberculous l.,** see *borderline l.* **diffuse l. of Lucio,** Lucio's l. **dimorphous l.,** borderline l. **indeterminate l.,** a frequent early manifestation of leprosy, consisting of a single or few poorly defined anesthetic or hypoanesthetic, hypopigmented or erythematous, histologically uncharacteristic macules in exposed areas of the skin, which may heal spontaneously or progress and evolve into one of the more definitive forms. **intermediate l.,** borderline l. **lazarine l.,** Lucio's l. **lepromatous l.,** the most malignant and infectious polar type of leprosy, characterized principally by widespread dissemination of leprosy bacilli in the tissues, reflecting the poor immune response to infection, and by cutaneous lesions mainly consisting of numerous pale, diffusely and symmetrically distributed macules that if untreated gradually progress to form plaques, nodules (lepromas), and infiltrations, resulting in destructive lesions and deformities; nerve involvement is seen in advanced disease. **Lucio l.,** a form characterized by diffuse lepromatous infiltration of the skin occurring especially in Latin America, particularly in Costa Rica and Mexico. Advanced cases may be complicated by a reactional state (*Lucio's phenomenon*) in which multiple areas of obstructive vasculitis cause dermal necrosis with resultant ulcers that heal with scarring. Called also *diffuse l. of Lucio, lazarine l.*, and *Lucio's phenomenon*. **murine l.**, rat l. **rat l.**, a chronic epizootic disease of wild rats caused by *Mycobacterium lepraemurium*, characterized by lesions containing enormous numbers of acid-fast bacilli closely resembling *M. leprae* in size and shape, which may be transmitted to white rats, mice, and guinea pigs by inoculation of infected tissue; a relationship with human leprosy has not been established. Called also *murine l.* **reactional l.**, see *lepra reaction*, under *reaction*. **tuberculoid l.**, the relatively benign, least infectious, and usually self-limited polar type of leprosy in which, as a result of well-developed cell-mediated immunity to *Mycobacterium leprae*, acid-fast bacilli usually cannot be identified in the lesions. It is characterized by early severe damage to the nerves and by the presence of one to a few typically asymmetric, sharply defined, anesthetic, hypopigmented or erythematous macules or plaques with elevated borders and dry, rough surfaces (leprids). **uncharacteristic l.**, indeterminate l. **water-buffalo l.**, a chronic disease of water buffaloes caused by the acid-fast bacillus *Mycobacterium leprae bubalorum*.

leprotic (lep-rot'ik) pertaining to or affected with leprosy.

leprous (lep'rus) [L. *leprosus*] afflicted with leprosy.

leptandra (lep-tan'drah) [Gr. *leptos* thin + *anēr* anther] the rhizome and rootlets of *Veronica virginica* (L.) Farw. (Scrophulariaceae), used as a cathartic.

leptazol (lep'tah-zol) (Brit.) pentylenetetrazol.

lept(o)- [Gr. *leptos* slender] a combining form meaning slender, thin, or delicate.

leptocephalic (lep''to-sĕ-fal'ik) characterized by leptocephaly.

leptocephalous (lep''to-sef'ah-lus) leptocephalic.

leptocephalus (lep''to-sef'ah-lus) [*lepto-* + Gr. *kephalē* head] a person with an abnormally tall, narrow skull.

leptocephaly (lep''to-sef'ah-le) abnormal tallness and narrowness of the skull.

leptochromatic (lep''to-kro-mat'ik) [*lepto-* + *chromatin*] having a fine chromatin network.

Leptocimex (lep''to-si'meks) *Cimex*. **L. boue'ti,** *Cimex boueti.*

Leptoconops (lep''to-ko'nops) a genus of blood-sucking flies of the family Heleidae.

leptocyte (lep'to-sīt) [*lepto-* + Gr. *kytos* cell] an erythrocyte characterized by a hemoglobinated peripheral border, surrounding a clear area containing a "bull's-eye" center of pigment, as seen in thalassemia.

leptocytosis (lep''to-si-to'sis) the presence of leptocytes in the blood.

leptodactylous (lep''to-dak'tĭ-lus) [*lepto-* + Gr. *daktylos* finger] possessing slender digits.

leptodactyly (lep''to-dak'tĭ-le) abnormal slenderness of the digits.

Leptodera pellio (lep-to'der-ah pel'e-o) *Rhabditis pellio.*

leptodontous (lep''to-don'tus) [*lepto-* + Gr. *odous* tooth] having slender teeth.

leptokurtic (lep''to-kur'tik) [*lepto-* + Gr. *kurtos* convex] pertaining to a probability distribution more heavily concentrated around the mean, i.e., having a sharper, narrower peak, than the normal distribution with the same variance.

leptomeningeal (lep''to-mĕ-nin'je-al) pertaining to the leptomeninges.

leptomeninges (lep''to-mĕ-nin'jēz), sing. *leptomen'inx* [*lepto-* + *meninges*] the pia mater and arachnoid considered together as one functional unit; the pia-arachnoid.

leptomeningioma (lep''to-me-nin''je-o'mah) a tumor of the leptomeninges.

leptomeningitis (lep''to-men''in-ji'tis) [*leptomeninx* + *-itis*] inflammation of the pia and arachnoid of the brain or spinal cord. Leptomeningitis is variously qualified as acute, basilar, cerebrospinal, chronic, epidemic, external, infantile, intracranial, purulent, nonpurulent, serous, tuberculous, etc. Cf. *pachymeningitis*. **l. inter'na,** inflammation of the pia

mater. **sarcomatous l.,** diffuse sarcomatous infiltration of the pia mater.

leptomeningopathy (lep''to-men''in-gop'ah-the) [*leptomeninges* + Gr. *pathos* disease] any disease of the leptomeninges.

leptomeninx (lep''to-men'inks) [*lepto-* + *meninx*] singular of leptomeninges.

Leptomitus (lep-tom'ĭ-tus) former name for the genus *Absidia*.

leptomonad (lep''to-mo'nad) [*lepto-* + *monad*] 1. pertaining to the genus *Leptomonas*. 2. denoting a morphologic stage in the development of certain trypanosomatid protozoa; see *promastigote*. 3. leptomonas.

Leptomonas (lep''to-mo'nas) [*lepto-* + Gr. *monas* unit, from *monos* single] a genus of parasitic protozoa (suborder Trypanosomatina, order Kinetoplastida) found in the digestive tract of various insects, and characterized by having an elongate body with a relatively large nucleus near the center and a long thin flagellum arising from a blepharoplast and a kinetoplast near the anterior end. During their life cycle the organisms pass through promastigote and amastigote stages.

leptomonas (lep''to-mo'nas) 1. any protozoan of the genus *Leptomonas*. 2. see *promastigote*.

Leptomyxida (lep''to-mik'sĭ-dah) [*lepto-* + Gr. *myxa* mucus] an order of ameboid protozoa (class Acarpomyxea, superclass Rhizopoda) typically occurring in thin protoplasmic sheets that are sometimes polyaxial and sometimes cylindrical. Representative genera include *Leptomyxa* and *Rhizamoeba*.

leptonema (lep''to-ne'mah) [*lepto-* + Gr. *nēma* thread] a presynaptic stage of meiosis in which the chromatin is in the form of fine spireme threads.

leptonomorphology (lep''to-no-mor-fol'o-je) the morphology of membranes.

leptopellic (lep''to-pel'ik) [*lepto-* + Gr. *pella* bowl] having a narrow pelvis.

leptophonia (lep''to-fo'ne-ah) [*lepto-* + Gr. *phōnē* voice] weakness or feebleness of the voice.

leptophonic (lep''to-fon'ik) pertaining to or characterized by leptophonia.

leptoprosope (lep-top'ro-sōp) an individual exhibiting leptoprosopia.

leptoprosopia (lep''to-pro-so'pe-ah) [*lepto-* + Gr. *prosōpon* face + *-ia*] narrowness of the face, with slender features, round, open orbits, long nose, narrow nostrils, and small mouth.

leptoprosopic (lep''to-pro-so'pik) pertaining to or characterized by leptoprosopia.

Leptopsylla (lep''to-sil'ah) a genus of fleas. **L. mus'culi,** *L. segnis.* **L. seg'nis,** the common flea of the mouse and rat, being the vector of plague; called also *Ctenopsyllus segnis* and *L. musculi*.

leptorrhine (lep'to-rīn) [*lepto-* + Gr. *rhis* nose] having a nasal index below 48.

leptoscope (lep'to-skōp) [*lepto-* + Gr. *skopein* to examine] an optical apparatus for measuring the thickness of the plasma membrane of a cell.

leptosomatic (lep''to-so-mat'ik) [*lepto-* + Gr. *sōma* body] having a light, thin body.

Leptospira (lep''to-spi'rah) [*lepto-* + Gr. *speira* coil] a genus of bacteria of the family Leptospiraceae, order Spirochaetales, consisting of single, finely coiled, motile, aerobic cells with hooked ends that are visible by darkfield microscopy. **L. austra'lis,** *L. interrogans* serogroup *australia*. **L. autumna'lis,** *L. interrogans* serogroup *autumnalis*. **L. bata'viae,** *L. interrogans* serogroup *bataviae*. **L. biflex'a,** a species that contains saprophytic nonpathogenic strains of the genus found in fresh surface water and seawater, occasionally associated with mammalian infections; Called also *Spirochaeta pseudoicterogenes*. **L. canico'la,** *L. interrogans* serogroup *canicola*. **L. grippotypho'sa,** *L. interrogans* serogroup *grippotyphosa*. **L. hebdom'idis,** *L. interrogans* serogroup *hebdomidis*. **L. hy'os,** an etiologic agent of swineherd's disease. **L. icterohaemorrha'giae,** *L. interrogans* serogroup *icterohaemorrhagiae*. **L. illi'ni,** a species of uncertain status, differentiated from other species by deoxyribonucleic acid base composition. **L. inter'rogans,** the species containing all the pathogenic strains of the genus, i.e., those causing leptospirosis (q.v.), which are divided into serological groups that are in turn separated into serotypes. A wide range of wild and domestic animals serve as animal reservoirs, which shed the organism via the urine. Human infection occurs as a result of direct contact with urine or tissue of an infected animal or indirectly by contact with water, soil, or vegetation contaminated by the urine of an infected animal. **L. inter′rogans** serogroup **austra′-lis,** a serogroup carried by rodents and causing human leptospirosis (cane-field fever). Type A, found in Australia, the United States, Europe, Southeast Asia, and Japan, also causes infection in dogs, cattle, raccoons, opossums, and hedgehogs. Type B, found in Australia, Southeast Asia, and Europe, is not known to cause animal infection. **L. inter′rogans** serogroup **autumna′lis,** a serogroup carried by rodents causing human leptospirosis (e.g., Hasami fever, pretibial fever) and infection in dogs, opossums, raccoons, and cattle in Southeast Asia, Japan, and the United States. **L. inter′rogans** serogroup **bata′viae,** a serogroup carried by rodents and causing human leptospirosis (Weil's syndrome, rice-field fever) and infection in dogs and cats in Southeast Asia, Europe, Africa, and Japan. **L. inter′rogans** serogroup **canic′ola,** a serogroup carried by dogs and causing human leptospirosis (Stuttgard disease) and infection in pigs and cattle in a worldwide distribution. **L. inter′rogans** serogroup **grippotypho′sa,** a serogroup carried by rodents and causing human leptospirosis (mud fever) and infection in cattle, horses, dogs, raccoons, and goats in worldwide distribution. **L. inter′rogans** serogroup **hebdom′idis,** a serogroup carried by field voles and causing human leptospirosis (nanukayami) and infections in dogs and cattle in Japan. **L. inter′rogans** serogroup **ic-terohaemorrha′giae,** a serogroup of worldwide distribution that is carried by rodents and is the major cause of Weil's syndrome (leptospiral jaundice) in humans and yellows in dogs, and also infects pigs, cattle, and horses. **L. inter′rogans** serogroup **pomo′na,** a serogroup carried by pigs, cattle, and rodents and causing pomona fever and swineherd's disease in humans and infection in various animals, e.g., dogs, horses, and skunks; it occurs worldwide. **L. inter′rogans** serogroup **pyrog′enes,** a serogroup carried by rodents and causing human leptospirosis (Salinem infection) in Japan and Southeast Asia. **L. pomo′na,** *L. interrogans* serogroup *pomona.* **L. pyrog′enes,** *L. interrogans* serogroup *pyrogenes.*

Leptospiraceae (lep″to-spi-ra′se-e) a family of bacteria of the order Spirochaetales, consisting of flexible helical cells that are aerobic and utilize long-chain fatty acids or alcohols for growth. It consists of the single genus *Leptospira.*

leptospira (lep″to-spi′rah) an individual organism belonging to the genus *Leptospira.*

leptospiral (lep″to-spi′ral) of, pertaining to, or caused by leptospiras.

leptospire (lep′to-spīr) an individual organism belonging to the genus *Leptospira.*

leptospirosis (lep″to-spi-ro′sis) any of a group of febrile illnesses caused by infection with *Leptospira,* specifically one of the serogroups of *L. interrogans,* which occur in worldwide distribution, being transmitted to man by a wide variety of wild (e.g., opossum, skunk, raccoon, fox) and domestic (e.g., swine, dogs) animals which shed the infective organisms in the urine. Human infection is due to direct contact with the urine or tissue of infected animals or to contact with water, soil, or vegetation contaminated by the urine of infected animals. All serogroups of *L. interrogans* are probably capable of causing any of the clinical syndromes, which vary from a mild carrier state to a fatal disease. The severe forms of leptospirosis, such as Weil's syndrome, usually are characterized by jaundice. Traditionally, different types of leptospirosis have been given different names, depending upon such factors as the clinical features, etiologic serogroup causing the disease, geographic distribution, occupation of those infected, and host. **anicter′ic l.,** benign l. **benign l.,** leptospirosis characterized by the absence of jaundice and by a milder course and symptoms than those in the more severe forms. Marked meningism may occur, and a skin rash may be an outstanding feature. Called also *anicteric l.* and *seven-day fever.* **bovine l., l. of cattle,** a disease of cattle caused primarily by *Leptospira interrogans* serogroup *pomona* and marked by fever, icterus, and anemia, especially in calves. Pregnant animals may abort, and lactating animals may develop mastitis. **canine l.,** see *Stuttgart disease,* under *disease,* and see *yellows.* **equine l.,** a disease

caused by several serogroups of *Leptospira* and characterized by fever, icterus, and depression. Recurrent iridocyclitis and abortion are also associated. **l. icterohaemor-rha′gica,** Weil's syndrome. **swine l.,** a disease of swine most commonly caused by *Leptospira interrogans* serogroup *pomona.* In the acute form, occurring in young pigs, it is marked by fever, icterus, hemorrhages, and death. It may cause abortion in pregnant sows. Transmitted to man, it causes swineherd's disease.

leptospiruria (lep″to-spir-u′re-ah) [*lepto-* Gr. *ouron* urine + *ia*] excretion of *Leptospira* in the urine, due to their invasion of the renal tubules.

leptostaphyline (lep″to-staf′ĭ-lin) [*lepto-* + Gr. *staphylē* bunch of grapes, uvula] pertaining to or characterized by a narrow palate, with a palatal index of 79.9 or less.

leptotene (lep′to-tēn) [*lepto-* + Gr. *tainia* ribbon] the stage of meiosis in which the chromosomes are slender, like threads. See *meiosis.*

leptothricosis (lep″to-thri-ko′sis) leptotrichosis.

Leptothrix (lep′to-thriks) [*lepto-* + Gr. *thrix* hair] a genus of sheathed bacteria, found in fresh or polluted waters and in sludge, made up of gram-negative, rod-shaped cells occurring singly, in pairs, or in chains. The chains are enclosed in sheaths often containing hydrated ferric or manganic oxides. The type species is *L. ochra′cea.*

leptothrix (lep′to-thriks) any microorganism of the genus *Leptothrix.*

Leptotrichia (lep″to-trik′e-ah) [*lepto-* + Gr. *thrix,* gen. *tri-chos* hair] a genus of gram-negative, anaerobic bacteria of the family Bacteroidaceae, found in the human oral cavity, consisting of straight or slightly curved, nonmotile rods with one or both ends rounded or pointed, arranged frequently in pairs or long filaments. **L. bucca′lis,** the single species, isolated frequently from the normal oral cavity and occasionally from the vagina and intestinal tract. It is sometimes associated with oral or urogenital infections. Called also *Fusobacterium plauti-vincenti.*

leptotrichosis (lep″to-trĭ-ko′sis) infection with any species of *Leptothrix.* **l. conjuncti′vae,** Parinaud's oculo-glandular syndrome caused by a leptothrix.

Leptotrombidium (lep″to-trom-bid′e-um) a subgenus of *Trombicula.*

Leptus (lep′tus) [L.] a name for the larval form of mites of the genus *Trombicula* and the subgenus *Eutrombicula.* **L. akamu′shi,** *Trombicula akamushi.* **L. ir′ritans,** *Eutrombicula irritans.*

Lerch's percussion [Otto *Lerch,* physician in New Orleans, born 1894] drop percussion.

lergotrile (ler′go-trīl) chemical name: 2-chloro-6-meth-ylergoline-8-acetonitrile, a prolactin inhibitor, $C_{17}H_{18}ClN_3$. **l. mesylate,** the monomethanesulfonate salt of lergotrile, $C_{17}H_{18}ClN_3 \cdot CH_4O_3S$, which has been used as an antiparkinsonian agent.

Leri's sign (la′rēz) [André *Leri,* French physician, 1875–1930] see under *sign.*

Leriche's disease, syndrome (lě-rēsh′ez) [René *Leriche,* French surgeon, 1879–1955] see *post-traumatic osteoporosis,* under *osteoporosis,* and see under *syndrome.*

Leritine (ler′ĭ-tīn) trademark for preparations of anileridine.

Lermoyez's syndrome (ler″moi-yāz′) [Marcel *Lermoyez,* French otolaryngologist, 1858–1929] see under *syndrome.*

l.e.s. local excitatory state.

lesbian (lez′be-an) [Gr. *Lesbios* of Lesbos, an island off the west coast of Asia Minor, the home of the poetess Sappho and her followers] 1. pertaining to homosexuality between females. 2. a female homosexual.

lesbianism (lez′be-ah-nizm) homosexuality between women; called also *sapphism.*

Lesch-Nyhan syndrome (lesh-ni′an) [Michael *Lesch,* American physician, born 1939; William L. *Nyhan,* Jr., American physician, born 1926] see under *syndrome.*

Leser-Trélat sign (la′zer tre′lah) [Edmund *Leser,* German surgeon, 1853–1916; Ulysse *Trélat,* Jr., French surgeon, 1828–1890] see under *sign.*

Lesgaft's space (triangle) (les′gafts) [Petr Frantsevich *Lesgaft,* Russian physician, 1837–1909] see under *space.*

lesion (le′zhun) [L. *laesio; laedere* to hurt] any pathological or traumatic discontinuity of tissue or loss of function of a part. **Armanni-Ebstein l.,** vacuolization of the renal tubular epithelium in the region of the loop of Henle and the convoluted tubules in diabetes, due to glycogen deposition. **Baehr-Löhlein l.,** Löhlein-Baehr l. **birds' nest l.,** crescentic thickenings or pockets resembling secondary valve structures, below the aortic valve. **Blumenthal l.,** a proliferative vascular lesion in the smaller arteries in diabetics. **Bracht-Wächter l.,** focal collections of lymphocytic and mononuclear cells in the myocardium. **central l.,** any lesion of the central nervous system. **coin l.,** a rounded coinlike tumor. **Councilman l.,** see under *body.* **Duret's l.,** effusion of blood in the region of the fourth ventricle of the cerebrum as a result of slight injury. **Ebstein's l.,** hyaline degeneration and insular necrosis of epithelial cells of the renal tubules in diabetes mellitus. **Ghon's primary l.,** Ghon focus. **gross l.,** a lesion that is visible to the naked eye. **histologic l.,** a microscopic lesion. **impaction l.,** an osteopathic term for a lesion of any spinal joint in which there is present abnormal thickening of the intervertebral disk with approximation of all the bony parts. **indiscriminate l.,** a lesion affecting different parts or systems of the body. **irritative l.,** one that stimulates the functions of the part where it is situated. **Janeway l.,** a small erythematous or hemorrhagic lesion, usually on the palms or soles, in subacute bacterial endocarditis. **local l.,** one in the nervous system giving origin to distinctive local symptoms. **Löhlein-Baehr l.,** a focal glomerular lesion of necrosis and hyalinization occurring in bacterial endocarditis; the process has been described as focal embolic glomerulonephritis. **molecular l.,** a lesion not visible even with the aid of a microscope. **onion scale l.,** the concentric circumvascular fibrosis often found in the spleen and lymph nodes in systemic lupus erythematosus. **organic l.,** structural l. **partial l.,** one that involves only a part of an organ or of the diameter of a conducting tract. **peripheral l.,** a lesion of the nerve endings. **precancerous l.,** a lesion in a tissue in which the cells are likely to become malignant. **primary l.,** the original lesion manifesting a disease, such as chancre in syphilis or tuberculous chancre. **ring-wall l.,** multiple small ring hemorrhages which simulate proliferation of a glial ring; seen in pernicious anemia. **structural l.,** one that produces an obvious change in a tissue. **systemic l.,** one limited to a system or set of organs with a common function. **total l.,** one involving the whole of an organ or of the diameter of a conducting tract. **trophic l.,** a lesion manifested by a disturbance in the nutrition of a part. **wire-loop l.,** thickened capillary walls of some parts of a glomerular tuft in disseminated lupus erythematosus.

Lesser's test (les′erz) [Fritz *Lesser,* Berlin dermatologist, born 1873] see under *tests.*

LET linear energy transfer: the energy dissipation of ionizing radiation over a given linear distance. Highly penetrating radiations, such as gamma rays, cause very low ion concentration and thus have a relatively low LET, beta particles and x-rays have an intermediate LET, and alpha particles have a relatively high LET.

let-down (let′down) the transport of milk from the alveoli of the breast to the ducts; called also *milk l.* See also under *reflex.*

lethal (le′thal) [L. *lethalis,* from *lethum* death] deadly; fatal. See under *dose, equivalent, factor, gene,* etc.

lethality (le-thal′ĭ-te) the capability of an agent or disease of causing death.

lethargy (leth′ar-je) [Gr. *lēthargia* drowsiness] abnormal drowsiness or stupor; a condition of indifference. **African l.,** see under *trypanosomiasis.*

letimide hydrochloride (let′ĭ-mīd) chemical name: 3 - [2 -(diethylamino)ethyl]-2*H*-1,3-benzoxazine-2,4-(3*H*)-dione monohydrochloride; an analgesic, $C_{14}H_{18}N_2O_3 \cdot HCl$.

Letter (let′er) trademark for a preparation of levothyroxine sodium.

Letterer-Siwe disease (let′ter-er si′we) [Erich *Letterer,* German physician, born 1895; Sture August *Siwe,* German physician, 1897–1966] see under *disease.*

Leu leucine.

leucemia (loo-se′me-ah) leukemia.

leucine (loo′sin) [Gr. *leukos* white] chemical name: 2-

amino-4-methylpentanoic acid. An amino acid, $C_6H_{13}NO_2$, or α-aminoisocaproic acid, essential for optimal growth in infants and for nitrogen equilibrium in human adults. It is obtained by the digestion or hydrolytic cleavage of protein.

leucine amino-peptidase (loo′sin am″ĭ-no-pep′tĭ-das) aminopeptidase (cytosol).

leucinethylester (loo″sin-eth″il-es′ter) an oily liquid, $(CH_3)_2 \cdot CH \cdot CH_2CH(NH_2) \cdot CO_2 \cdot C_2H_5$.

leucinimide (loo″sin-im′ĭd) the anhydride of leucine, $C_{12}H_{22}N_2O_2$, a diketopiperazine; it may be produced by evaporation of leucine solutions.

leucinosis (loo″sĭ-no′sis) any condition in which leucine appears in the urine.

leucinuria (loo″sin-u′re-ah) [leucine + Gr. *ouron* urine + *-ia*] the presence of leucine in the urine.

leucitis (loo-si′tis) scleritis.

leuc(o)- see *leuk(o)-.*

leucocyte (loo′ko-sīt) leukocyte.

leucocytosis (loo″ko-si-to′sis) leukocytosis.

Leucocytozoon (loo″ko-si″to-zo′on) [leuco- + cyte + Gr. *zöon* animal] a genus of coccidian protozoa (suborder Haemosporina, order Eucoccidiida) parasitic in wild and domestic birds, causing an acute fatal disease in the latter. Merogony occurs in the hepatocytes and vascular endothelial cells of the host, producing merozoites that invade erythroblasts, erythrocytes, lymphocytes, and monocytes and then develop into gametocytes. Species infecting domestic fowl include: *L. simondi (anseris)* in ducks and geese; *L. smithi* in turkeys; and *L. caulleryi, L. andrewsi,* and *L. sabrazesi* in chickens. All are transmitted by blackflies (*Simulium* spp.) except *L. caulleryi,* which is transmitted by biting midges (*Culicoides* spp.). Written also *Leukocytozoon.* See also *leucocytozoonosis.*

leucocytozoonosis (loo″ko-si″to-zo″o-no′sis) an acute malaria-like protozoal disease of domestic fowl, including chickens, ducks, geese, and turkeys, caused by heavy infection with species of *Leucocytozoon,* and characterized by anemia, leukocytosis, and hepatosplenomegaly, which may result in death.

leucofluorescein (loo″ko-floo″o-res′e-in) fluorescin, produced from fluorescein by reduction with zinc powder in an acid medium.

Leucoium (loo-ko′ĭ-um) [L.; Gr. *leukos* white + *ion* violet] a genus of old world amaryllidaceous plants. *L. aesti′vum* and *L. ver′num* (called snowflake) are common in garden culture: emetic and poisonous.

leucomycin (loo″ko-mi′sin) kitasamycin.

Leuconostoc (loo″ko-nos′tok) [leuko- + *Nostoc* a genus of blue-green algae] a genus of nonpathogenic, gram-positive, saprophytic, facultative anaerobes of the family Streptococcaceae. They are spherical but often lenticular, nonmotile cells, some species of which form dextran. **L. ci-tro′vorum,** *L. cremoris.* **L. cremo′ris,** a species found in milk and dairy products; called also *L. citrovorum.* **L. dextra′nicum,** a dextran-forming species found on fruit and vegetables and in milk and dairy products. **L. lac′-tis,** a species found in milk and dairy products. **L. mesenteroi′des,** a dextran-forming species found in slimy sugar solutions, on fruit and vegetables, and in milk and dairy products. **L. oenos′,** a species found in wine.

leucopterin (loo-kop′ter-in) chemical name: 2-amino-4,6,7-pteridinediol. A colorless pigment, $C_6H_5N_5O_3$, isolated from butterfly wings, especially white wings, and also from xanthopterin by oxidation. See *pterin.*

leucosin (loo′ko-sin) an albumin found in the cereal grains.

Leucothrix (loo′ko-thriks) [leuko- + Gr. *thrix* hair] a genus of gliding bacteria of the family Leucotrichaceae, order Cytophagales, found in water, and made up of short colorless cells growing in long filaments attached to solid substrates. The type species is *L. mu′cor.*

leucotomy (loo-kot′o-me) leukotomy.

Leucotrichaceae (loo″ko-tri-ka′se-e) a family of gliding bacteria of the order Cytophagales, found in water, made up of short cylindrical or ovoid colorless cells in long filaments. It contains the genera *Leucothrix* and *Thiotrix.*

leucovorin (loo″ko-vo′rin) folinic acid. **l. calcium** [USP], the calcium salt of folinic acid, $C_{20}H_{21}CaN_7O_7 \cdot 5H_2O$, occurring as a yellowish white or yellow powder; used as an antidote for folic acid antagonists, e.g., methotrexate, when there is need to reverse the toxic effects of the latter and in the treatment of megaloblastic anemias due to folic acid deficiency, administered intramuscularly.

leucyl (loo'sil)   the acyl radical of leucine.

Leudet's tinnitus (bruit, sign) (led-āz') [Théodor Emile *Leudet*, physician at Rouen, 1825–1887]   see under *tinnitus.*

leu-enkephalin (loo''en-kef'ah-lin)   see *enkephalin.*

leukapheresis (loo''kah-fĕ-re'sis) [*leuk*ocyte + Gr. *aphairesis* removal]   the selective separation and removal of leukocytes from withdrawn blood, the remainder of the blood then being retransfused into the donor.

leukemia (loo-ke'me-ah) [Gr. *leukos* white + *haima* blood + *-ia*]   a progressive, malignant disease of the blood-forming organs, characterized by distorted proliferation and development of leukocytes and their precursors in the blood and bone marrow. Leukemia is classified clinically on the basis of (1) the duration and character of the disease—*acute* or *chronic;* (2) the type of cell involved—*myeloid (myelogenous), lymphoid (lymphogenous),* or *monocytic;* (3) increase or noncrease in the number of abnormal cells in the blood—*leukemic* or *aleukemic (subleukemic).* **acute nonlymphocytic l. (ANLL),** leukemia occurring most commonly after treatment with alkylating agents, including melphalan, cyclophosphamide, and chlorambucil, characterized by pancytopenia, megaloblastic bone marrow, nucleated red cells in the peripheral marrow, and refractoriness to antileukemia treatment, with a short survival time. Most patients have chromosomal abnormalities in marrow cells. **acute promyelocytic l.,** promyelocytic l.   **adult T-cell l.,** a form of leukemia with onset in adulthood, leukemic cells with T-cell properties, frequent dermal involvement, lymphadenopathy and hepatosplenomegaly, and a subacute or chronic course; it is associated with human T-cell leukemia-lymphoma virus.   **aleukemic l., aleukocythemic l.,** leukemia in which the total white blood cell count in the peripheral blood is either normal or below normal; it may be lymphocytic, monocytic, or myelogenous.   **basophilic l.,** a disorder resembling acute or chronic leukemia in which the basophilic leukocytes predominate.   **blast cell l.,** stem cell l.   **bovine l.,** malignant lymphoma of cattle; see under *lymphoma.*   **chronic granulocytic l., chronic myelocytic l.,** a form of leukemia occurring mainly between the age of 25 and 60, usually associated with a unique chromosomal abnormality, in which the major clinical manifestations of malaise, hepatosplenomegaly, anemia, and leukocytosis are related to abnormal, excessive, unrestrained overgrowth of granulocytes in the bone marrow.   **l. cu'tis,** involvement of the skin in leukemia, with tumor-like lesions. See *leukemid.*   **embryonal l.,** stem cell l.   **eosinophilic l.,** a form of leukemia in which the eosinophil is the predominating cell. Although resembling chronic myelocytic leukemia in many ways, this form may follow an acute course despite the absence of predominantly blast forms in the peripheral blood.   **l. of fowls,** an infectious disease of the hematopoietic organs of fowls with atrophy of the bone marrow and changes in the viscera.   **granulocytic l.,** myelocytic l.   **Gross' l.,** a transmissible murine leukemia, first transmitted to newborn C3H mice by inoculation of filtrate of leukemic tissue from AK2 mice, thus demonstrating its viral etiology.   **hairy-cell l.,** leukemia marked by splenomegaly and by an abundance of large, mononuclear abnormal cells with numerous irregular cytoplasmic projections that give them a flagellated or hairy appearance in the bone marrow, spleen, liver, and peripheral blood; called also *leukemic reticuloendotheliosis.* See also *hairy cell,* under *cell.*   **hemoblastic l., hemocytoblastic l.,** stem cell l.   **histiocytic l.,** acute monocytic l.   **leukopenic l.,** aleukemic l.   **lymphatic l., lymphoblastic l., lymphocytic l., lymphogenous l., lymphoid l.,** leukemia associated with hyperplasia and overactivity of the lymphoid tissue, in which the leukocytes are lymphocytes or lymphoblasts.   **lymphosarcoma cell l.,** a form of leukemia characterized by large numbers of lymphosarcoma cells in the peripheral blood; depending on the degree of bone marrow involvement, it may be a variant of lymphosarcoma.   **mast cell l.,** a type of leukemia characterized by the presence of overwhelming numbers of tissue mast cells in the peripheral blood.   **megakaryocytic l.,** hemorrhagic thrombocythemia.   **micromyeloblastic l.,** a form of granulocytic leukemia in which the immature, nucleoli-containing cells are small and are distinguishable from lympho-

cytes only by supravital staining.   **monocytic l.,** leukemia in which the predominating leukocytes are identified as monocytes. The disease is generally divided into two main categories: the Naegeli type, in which many of the cells resemble myeloblasts, or cells of the myeloid series; and the Schilling type, in which the cells more truly resemble monocytes or histiocytes.   **myeloblastic l.,** leukemia in which myeloblasts predominate.   **myelocytic l., myelogenous l., myeloid granulocytic l.,** leukemia arising from myeloid tissue in which the granular, polymorphonuclear leukocytes and their precursors predominate.   **myelomonocytic l.,** the Naegeli type of monocytic leukemia in which the predominant leukocytes resemble cells of the myeloid series.   **Naegeli l.,** see *monocytic l.*   **plasma cell l.,** leukemia in which the predominating cell in the peripheral blood is the plasma cell; whether this is a distinct form of leukemia or a phase of multiple myeloma remains moot.   **plasmacytic l.,** plasma cell l.   **promyelocytic l.,** a subvariety of acute granulocytic leukemia in which the predominant cells are promyelocytes, rather than myeloblasts, often associated with abnormal bleeding secondary to thrombocytopenia, hypofibrinogenemia, and decreased levels of Factor V.   **Rieder cell l.,** a form of myeloblastic leukemia in which the blood contains asynchronously developed cells with immature cytoplasm and a lobulated, indented, comparatively more mature nucleus.   **Schilling's l.,** see *monocytic l.*   **stem cell l.,** a form of leukemia in which the predominating cell is so immature and primitive that its classification becomes exceedingly difficult. Called also *embryonal l., hemoblastic l., hemocytoblastic l.,* and *undifferentiated cell l.*   **subleukemic l.,** aleukemic l.   **undifferentiated cell l.,** stem cell l.

leukemic (loo-ke'mik)   pertaining to or affected with leukemia.

leukemid (loo-ke'mid)   any of the polymorphic skin eruptions associated with leukemia; clinically, they may be nonspecific, i.e., papular, macular, purpuric, etc., but histopathologically they may represent true leukemic infiltrations.

leukemogen (loo-ke'mo-jen)   any substance that causes or produces leukemia.

leukemogenesis (loo-ke''mo-jen'ĕ-sis)   the induction of or development of leukemia.

leukemogenic (loo-ke''mo-jen'ik)   causing leukemia.

leukemoid (loo-ke'moid) [*leukemia* + Gr. *eidos* form]   characterized by blood and sometimes clinical findings resembling true leukemia to such a degree that initial differentiation between the process causing the observed alterations and leukemia becomes extremely difficult.

leukencephalitis (lōōk''en-sef''ah-li'tis) [*leuko-* + *encephalitis*]   inflammation of the white matter of the brain.

Leukeran (loo'ker-an)   trademark for a preparation of chlorambucil.

leukexosis (loo''kek-so'sis)   an aggregation of dead leukocytes in one of the channels of the body.

leukin (loo'kin)   a thermostable, bactericidal substance extracted from polymorphonuclear leukocytes. See *cationic proteins,* under *protein.*

leuk(o)-, leuc(o)- [Gr. *leukos* white]   a combining form meaning white, or denoting relationship to a leukocyte.

leukoagglutinin (loo''ko-ah-gloo'tĭ-nin)   leukocyte agglutinin.

leukoblast (loo'ko-blast) [*leuko-* + Gr. *blastos* germ]   an immature granular leukocyte.   **granular l.,** promyelocyte.

leukoblastosis (loo''ko-blas-to'sis)   a general term for proliferation of leukocytes, including myelosis and lymphadenosis.

leukocidin (loo''ko-si'din) [*leuko-* + L. *caedere* to kill]   a substance that is toxic to leukocytes; specifically, an exotoxin produced by some pathogenic staphylococci and streptococci that destroys leukocytes by lysis of the cytoplasmic granules and is partially responsible for the pathogenicity of the organisms.   **Neisser-Wechsberg l.,** a leukocidin produced by staphylococci that destroys rabbit but not human leukocytes; it is identical with alpha hemolysin.   **Panton-Valentine (P-V) l.,** a leukocidin produced by staphylococci that destroys human and rabbit leukocytes by injuring the cell membrane with subsequent cell degranulation; it is nonhemolytic.

leukocoria (loo′′ko-ko-o′re-ah) leukokoria.

leukocrit (loo′ko-krit) [*leuko-* + Gr. *krinein* to separate] the volume percentage of leukocytes in whole blood.

leukocytal (loo′′ko-si′tal) leukocytic.

leukocyte (loo′ko-sīt) [*leuko-* + Gr. *kytos* cell] 1. any colorless, ameboid cell mass. 2. white blood cell or corpuscle. The varieties of leukocytes may be classified into two main groups: *granular l's* and *nongranular l's* (see below). **agranular l's,** nongranular l's. **basophilic l.,** basophil, def. 2. **endothelial l.,** Mallory's name for the large wandering cells of the circulating blood and the tissues which have notable phagocytic properties; see *endotheliocyte.* **eosinophilic l.,** eosinophil. **granular l's (granulocytes),** leukocytes with abundant granules in the cytoplasm, which are divided into three groups: (1) *Neutrophils,* cells with fine neutrophilic granules in the cytoplasm and an irregular lobed nucleus; see *neutrophil* (def. 1). (2) *Eosinophils,* cells with coarse eosinophilic granules in the cytoplasm and a bilobed nucleus; see *eosinophil.* (3) *Basophils,* cells with coarse basophilic granules in the cytoplasm and a bent nucleus that is partially constricted into two lobes; see *basophil* (def. 2). See also *granulocytic series,* under *series.* **heterophilic l's,** heterophil, def. 1. See also *neutrophil,* def. 1. **hyaline l.,** monocyte. **lymphoid l's,** nongranular l's. **mast l.,** a name sometimes used to designate the circulating blood basophil, which is morphologically and histogenetically different from the tissue mast cell. **motile l.,** a leukocyte that has the power of ameboid movement. **neutrophilic l.,** neutrophil, def. 1. **nongranular l's,** leukocytes without specific granules in their cytoplasm, including the lymphocytes and monocytes. Called also *agranular l's* and *lymphoid l's.* **nonmotile l.,** a leukocyte without the power of ameboid movement. **polymorphonuclear l.,** any of the fully developed, segmented cells of the granulocytic series, especially a neutrophil, whose nuclei contain three or more lobes joined by filamentous connections. See *neutrophil,* def. 1. **polynuclear neutrophilic l.,** neutrophil, def. 1. **transitional l.,** former name for monocyte. **Türk's irritation l.,** Türk's cell; see under *cell.*

leukocythemia (loo′′ko-si-the′me-ah) [*leuko-* + *-cyte* + Gr. *haima* blood + *-ia*] leukemia.

leukocytic (loo′′ko-sit′ik) pertaining to leukocytes.

leukocytoblast (loo′′ko-si′to-blast) [*leukocyte* + Gr. *blastos* germ] leukoblast.

leukocytogenesis (loo′′ko-si′′to-jen′ĕ-sis) [*leukocyte* + Gr. *genesis* production] the formation of leukocytes.

leukocytoid (loo′′ko-si′′toid) [*leukocyte* + Gr. *eidos* form] resembling a leukocyte.

leukocytology (loo′′ko-si-tol′o-je) the study of leukocytes.

leukocytolysin (loo′′ko-si-tol′ĭ-sin) a lysin that leads to disruption of leukocytes.

leukocytolysis (loo′′ko-si-tol′ĭ-sis) [*leukocyte* + Gr. *lysis* dissolution] the breaking down or destruction of leukocytes. **venom l.,** destruction of leukocytes with snake venom.

leukocytolytic (loo′′ko-si′′to-lit′ik) 1. pertaining to, characterized by, or causing leukocytolysis. 2. an agent that causes leukocytolysis.

leukocytoma (loo′′ko-si-to′mah) [*leukocyte* + *-oma*] a tumor-like mass of leukocytes.

leukocytopenia (loo′′ko-si′′to-pe′ne-ah) [*leukocyte* + Gr. *penia* poverty] leukopenia.

leukocytophagy (loo′′ko-si-tof′ah-je) [*leukocyte* + Gr. *phagein* to devour] the ingestion and destruction of leukocytes by histiocytes of the reticuloendothelial system.

leukocytoplania (loo′′ko-si′′to-pla′ne-ah) [*leukocyte* + Gr. *planē* wandering] the wandering of leukocytes or their passage through a membrane.

leukocytopoiesis (loo′′ko-si′′to-poi-e′sis) [*leukocyte* + Gr. *poiein* to make] the production of leukocytes.

leukocytosis (loo′′ko-si-to′sis) a transient increase in the number of leukocytes in the blood, resulting from various causes, as hemorrhage, fever, infection, inflammation, etc. **absolute l.,** increase in the total number of leukocytes in the blood. **agonal l.,** leukocytosis occurring just before death. **basophilic l.,** increase of the basophilic leukocytes in the blood. **mononuclear l.,** mononucleosis.

neutrophilic l., an increase in the number of polymorphonuclear neutrophil leukocytes in the blood. **pathologic l.,** that occurring as the result of some morbid condition, such as infection or trauma. **physiologic l.,** that caused by factors other than disease or trauma. **pure l.,** increase of the polymorphonuclear leukocytes of the blood. **relative l.,** increase in the proportion of any variety of leukocytes in the blood, without increase of the total number of leukocytes. **terminal l.,** agonal l. **toxic l.,** leukocytosis occurring in intoxication with blood poisons.

leukocytotactic (loo′′ko-si′′to-tak′tik) pertaining to or marked by leukotaxis.

leukocytotaxis (loo′′ko-si′′to-tak′sis) leukotaxis.

leukocytotherapy (loo′′ko-si′′to-ther′ah-pe) treatment by the administration of leukocytes.

leukocytotoxicity (loo′′ko-si′′to-tok-sis′ĭ-te) the quality or capability of lysing leukocytes; see *lymphocytotoxicity.*

leukocytotropic (loo′′ko-si′′to-trop′ik) having a selective affinity for leukocytes.

Leukocytozoon (loo′′ko-si′′to-zo′on) *Leucocytozoon.*

leukocyturia (loo′′ko-si-tu′re-ah) [*leukocyte* + Gr. *ouron* urine + *-ia*] the discharge of leukocytes in the urine.

leukoderivative (loo′′ko-de-riv′ah-tiv) any white derivative from a pigment or coloring matter.

leukoderma (loo′′ko-der′mah) [*leuko-* + *derma*] an acquired type of cutaneous depigmentation produced by a specific substance or dermatosis. Called also *leukodermis, leukopathia,* and *leukopathy.* Cf. *piebaldism* and *vitiligo.* **l. acquisi′tum centrif′ugum,** halo nevus. **l. col′li,** syphilitic l. **occupational h.,** leukoderma resulting from contact with or ingestion or inhalation of certain chemicals, e.g., monobenzyl ether of hydroquinone and phenol-containing compounds, in the work place. **postinflammatory l.,** leukoderma occurring after healing of various inflammatory dermatoses or infections, burns, or wounds; it may also been seen after dermabrasion or intralesional steroid injections. **syphilitic l.,** round or oval, ill-defined, depigmented spots surrounded by hyperpigmentation occurring on the anterior region and sides of the neck and on the chest in secondary syphilis. Called also *collar of pearls, collar of Venus, l. colli, melanoleukoderma colli,* and *venereal collar.*

leukodermatous (loo′′ko-der′mah-tus) pertaining to or characterized by leukoderma.

leukodermia (loo′′ko-der′me-ah) leukoderma.

leukodermic (loo′′ko-der′mik) leukodermatous.

leukodextrin (loo′′ko-deks′trin) an intermediate compound formed in the transformation of starch into sugar; achrodextrin.

leukodystrophy (loo′′ko-dis′tro-fe) disturbance of the white substance of the brain. See *leukoencephalopathy.* **globoid l., globoid cell l.,** Krabbe's disease. **hereditary cerebral l.,** Pelizaeus-Merzbacher disease. **Krabbe's l.,** see under *disease.* **metachromatic l.,** an autosomal recessive form of leukoencephalopathy due to defective arylsulfatase or cerebroside sulfatase and characterized by an accumulation of a sphingolipid (sulfatide) in neural and non-neural tissues, with a diffuse loss of myelin in the central nervous system. The *infantile* form usually begins in the third year of life, most commonly before the thirtieth month, with blindness, motor disturbances, rigidity, mental deterioration, and sometimes convulsions; called also *Greenfield's disease* and *diffuse cerebral sclerosis.* The *adult* form begins after 16 years of age, usually with psychiatric disturbances that progress to dementia; the motor and posture disturbances appear late in the course of this form. A *juvenile* form with an onset between four and ten years of age has also been observed. Called also *metachromatic leukoencephalopathy, metachromatic leukoencephaly,* and *sulfatide lipidosis.* **spongiform l.,** Canavan's disease. **sudanophilic l.,** a heterogeneous group of diseases, including adrenoleukodystrophy and Pelizaeus-Merzbacher disease, characterized by myelin destruction, with resulting breakdown products that stain bright red with fat stains.

leukoedema (loo′′ko-e-de′mah) [*leuko-* + *edema*] a disorder of the buccal mucosa resembling early leukoplakia, characterized by the presence of a filmy opalescence of the mucosa in the early stages to a whitish gray cast with a coarsely wrinkled surface in the later stages, associated with intracellular edema of the spinous or malphighian layer.

leukoencephalitis (loo″ko-en-sef″ah-li′tis) [leuko- + Gr. en-kephalos brain + -itis] 1. inflammation of the white substance of the brain. 2. forage poisoning; a noncontagious disease of horses, the lesion of which is softening of the white matter of the brain. It is marked by drowsiness, dimmed vision, unsteady gait, and paralysis of the throat. **acute hemorrhagic l.,** a fatal postinfection or allergic encephalopathy with a fulminating course, characterized by necrosis of the walls of the blood vessels, particularly the venules, resulting in multiple petechial hemorrhages in the white matter of the brain. **l. periaxia′lis concentri′ca,** Baló's disease. **van Bogaert's sclerosing l.,** subacute sclerosing panencephalitis.

leukoencephalopathy (loo″ko-en-sef″ah-lop′ah-the) any of a group of diseases affecting the white matter of the brain, especially of the cerebral hemispheres, and occurring as a rule in infants and children. The term *leukodystrophy* is used to denote such disorders due to defect in the formation and maintenance of myelin in infants and children. **metachromatic l.,** see under *leukodystrophy*. **multifocal progressive l.,** progressive multifocal l. **progressive multifocal l.,** a generally fatal disease probably of viral origin, in which the demyelination is usually found in the white matter but may rarely be seen in the brain stem and cerebellum. It occurs secondary to various neoplastic diseases, including lymphosarcoma and lymphatic or myeloid leukemia. Called also *multifocal progressive l.* **subacute sclerosing l.,** subacute sclerosing panencephalitis.

leukoencephaly (loo″ko-en-sef′ah-le) leukoencephalopathy. **metachromatic l.,** see under *leukodystrophy*.

leukoerythroblastosis (loo″ko-ĕ-rith″ro-blas-to′sis) an anemic condition associated with space-occupying lesions (myelophthisis) of the bone marrow and characterized by a variable number of immature erythroid and myeloid cells in the circulation; called also *leukoerythroblastic anemia*, and *myelopathic* or *myelophthisic anemia*.

leukogram (loo′ko-gram) a diagram or tabulation representing the leukocytes of a specimen of blood.

leukokeratosis (loo″ko-ker″ah-to′sis) [leuko- + keratosis] oral leukoplakia.

leukokinesis (loo″ko-ki-ne′sis) the movement of the leukocytes within the circulatory system.

leukokinetic (loo″ko-ki-net′ik) pertaining to leukokinesis.

leukokinetics (loo″ko-ki-net′iks) [leukocyte + Gr. kinētikos of or for putting in motion] the quantitative, dynamic study of *in vivo* production, circulation, and destruction of leukocytes.

leukokinin (loo″ko-ki′nin) the parent immunoglobulin molecule from which tuftsin is cleaved.

leukokoria (loo″ko-ko′re-ah) [leuko- + Gr. korē pupil + -ia] a condition characterized by appearance of a whitish reflex or mass in the pupillary area behind the lens; called also *cat's eye reflex*.

leukokraurosis (loo″ko-kraw-ro′sis) kraurosis vulvae.

leukolymphosarcoma (loo″ko-lim″fo-sar-ko′mah) lymphosarcoma cell leukemia.

leukolysin (loo-kol′ĭ-sin) leukocytolysin.

leukolysis (loo-kol′ĭ-sis) leukocytolysis.

leukolytic (loo-ko-lit′ik) leukocytolytic.

leukoma (loo-ko′mah) [Gr. leukōma whiteness] a dense white opacity of the cornea. **adherent l.,** a white tumor of the cornea enclosing a prolapsed adherent iris.

leukomaine (loo′ko-mān) [Gr. leukōma whiteness] any one of a large group of basic substances resembling alkaloids, normally present in the tissues, which are products of metabolism and are probably excrementitious. Some of them may become toxic, and many are physiologically active.

leukomainemia (loo″ko-mān-e′me-ah) [leukomaine + Gr. haima blood + -ia] excess of leukomaines in the blood.

leukomainic (loo″ko-mān′ik) pertaining to, caused by, or characterized by a leukomaine.

leukomatous (loo-ko′mah-tus) affected with or of the nature of leukoma.

leukomonocyte (loo″ko-mon′o-sīt) [leuko- + Gr. monos single + -cyte] a lymphocyte.

leukomyelitis (loo″ko-mi″ĕ-li′tis) [leuko- + Gr. myelos marrow + -itis] inflammation of the white substance of the spinal cord.

leukomyelopathy (loo″ko-mi″ĕ-lop′ah-the) [leuko- + Gr. myelos marrow + pathos disease] any disease of the white substance of the spinal cord.

leukomyoma (loo″ko-mi-o′mah) lipomyoma.

leukon (loo′kon) a general term once applied to the circulating leukocytes and the cells from which they arise; it is the counterpart of erythron and thrombon.

leukonecrosis (loo″ko-nĕ-kro′sis) [leuko- + Gr. nekrōsis necrosis] gangrene resulting in the formation of a white slough.

leukonychia (loo″ko-nik′e-ah) [leuko- + Gr. onyx nail + -ia] a whitish discoloration of the nails of unknown cause; it may rarely be total, but is usually partial. Exceptionally, it may occur in transverse streaks (*l. striata*) or bands. Called also *leukopathia unguium*.

leukopathia (loo″ko-path′e-ah) [leuko- + Gr. pathos illness] leukoderma. **l. puncta′ta reticula′ris symmet′rica,** idiopathic guttate hypomelanosis. **l. un′guium,** leukonychia.

leukopathy (loo-kop′ah-the) leukoderma.

leukopedesis (loo″ko-pĕ-de′sis) [leukocyte + Gr. pēdan to leap] the outward passage of leukocytes through intact vessel walls; leukocytic diapedesis.

leukopenia (loo″ko-pe′ne-ah) [leukocyte + Gr. penia poverty] reduction in the number of leukocytes in the blood, the count being 5000 per cu. mm. or less. **basophil l., basophilic l.,** abnormal reduction in the number of basophil leukocytes in the blood. **congenital l.,** congenital neutropenia. **malignant l., pernicious l.,** agranulocytosis.

leukopenic (loo″ko-pe′nik) pertaining to, characterized by, or causing leukopenia.

leukophagocytosis (loo″ko-fag″o-si-to′sis) leukocytophagy.

leukophyl (loo′ko-fil) leukophyll.

leukophyll (loo′ko-fil) [leuko- + Gr. phyllon leaf] a colorless substance in plant tissues which becomes converted into protochlorophyll.

leukophyte (loo′ko-fīt) an alga containing no chlorophyll, i.e., a colorless alga.

leukoplakia (loo″ko-pla′ke-ah) [leuko- + Gr. plax plate + -ia] 1. a white patch on a mucous membrane that will not rub off. 2. oral l. **l. bucca′lis,** the presence of white thickened patches on the mucous membrane of the cheeks. See *oral l.* **l. lingua′lis,** the presence of white thickened patches on the mucous membrane of the tongue. See *oral l.* **oral l.,** a condition marked by white, thick patches on the oral mucosa produced by hyperkeratosis of the epithelium. Histologically, it presents a thickening of the stratified squamous epithelium with hyperkeratosis, hyperplasia, inflammatory infiltration, and degeneration of epithelial cells. It is a benign lesion that provides favorable conditions for the development of epidermoid carcinoma. The etiology is unknown, but tobacco is considered the principal contributing factor. Called also *keratosis linguae, leukokeratosis, psoriasis buccalis,* and *psoriasis linguae.* See also *stomatitis nicotina.* **speckled l.,** see *erythroplasia of Queyrat.* **l. vul′vae,** a sometimes precancerous condition in which there are hypertrophic grayish white infiltrated patches on the vulvar mucosa, characterized chiefly by intense pruritus, although erosion, ulceration, and fissuring are common. When associated with atrophic changes, it is known as *kraurosis vulvae* or *lichen sclerosus et atrophicus.*

leukoplast (loo′ko-plast) leukoplastid.

leukoplastid (loo″ko-plas′tid) [leuko- + Gr. plassein to form] a colorless granule of the plant cells from which the starch-producing elements are formed.

leukopoiesis (loo″ko-poi-e′sis) production of leukocytes.

leukopoietic (loo″ko-poi-et′ik) [leuko cyte + Gr. poiein to make] forming or producing leukocytes.

leukopoietin (loo″ko-poi-e′tin) a hypothetical substance(s) believed to serve as the humoral regulator of leukopoiesis; granulopoietin.

leukoprecipitin (loo″ko-pre-sip′ĭ-tin) a precipitin specific for leukocyte antigens.

leukopsin (loo-kop′sin) [leuko- + Gr. ōps eye] visual white; the colorless matter into which rhodopsin is changed by exposure to white light. It is reconvertible into rhodopsin under proper conditions.

leukorrhagia (loo″ko-ra′je-ah) [*leuko-* + Gr. *rhēgnynai* to break forth] profuse leukorrhea.

leukorrhea (loo″ko-re′ah) [*leuko-* + Gr. *rhoia* flow] a whitish, viscid discharge from the vagina and uterine cavity. **menstrual l., periodic l.,** leukorrhea in place of or along with the menses.

leukorrheal (loo″ko-re′al) pertaining to or marked by leukorrhea.

leukosarcoma (loo″ko-sar-ko′mah) [*leuko-* + *sarcoma*] the development of a leukemic blood picture in patients originally having a well-differentiated, lymphocytic type of malignant lymphoma. The circulating cells contain an ovoid nucleus and nucleoli, and are morphologically different from the mature-type lymphocyte seen in chronic lymphocytic leukemia.

leukosarcomatosis (loo″ko-sar-ko″mah-to′sis) a condition marked by the development of multiple sarcomas composed of leukemic cells.

leukoscope (loo′ko-skōp) [*leuko-* + *-scope*] an instrument that mixes colors to produce white for testing for colorblindness.

leukosis (loo-ko′sis), pl. *leuko′ses.* Proliferation of leukocyte-forming tissue, including myelosis and lymphadenosis. Such proliferation forms the basis of leukemia. **acute l.,** see *Marek's disease,* under *disease.* **avian l.,** a group of transmissible, virus-induced diseases of chickens, characterized by proliferation of immature erythroid, myeloid, or lymphoid cells. Leukemic forms include erythroblastosis and myelosis and, rarely, lymphoblastic leukemia. Solid tumors in visceral organs are seen in cases of lymphoid leukosis, erythroblastosis, and myelocytomatosis. All of the causative viruses are related, and some induce "related neoplasms," such as sarcomas, hemangiomas, nephroblastomas, hepatocarcinomas, and osteopetrosis, a condition marked by thickening of the diaphyses of the long bones. These conditions are now classified as belonging to the leukosis sarcoma group, but were once included, along with Marek's disease, in the avian leukosis complex. Called also, according to the form taken, *avian lymphomatosis, osteopetrosis gallinarum,* and *visceral lymphomatosis.* **avian l. complex,** see *avian l.* **bovine l.,** malignant lymphoma of cattle; see under *lymphoma.* **fowl l.,** avian l. **lymphoid l.,** a form of leukosis involving chiefly the lymphocytes. **myeloblastic l.,** a form involving chiefly the myeloblasts. **myelocytic l.,** a form involving chiefly the myelocytes. **skin l.,** see *Marek's disease,* under *disease.*

leukotactic (loo″ko-tak′tik) pertaining to leukotaxis; having the power of attracting leukocytes.

leukotaxin (loo″ko-tak′sin) leukotaxine.

leukotaxine (loo″ko-tak′sin) a crystalline nitrogenous polypeptide that appears when tissue is injured, that can be recovered from inflammatory exudates, and that promotes leukocytosis and increases capillary permeability and the diapedesis of leukocytes.

leukotaxis (loo″ko-tak′sis) [*leuko-* + Gr. *taxis* arrangement] the cytotaxis of leukocytes; the tendency of leukocytes to collect in regions of injury and inflammation; see also *leukotaxine.*

Leukothrix (loo′ko-thriks) *Leucothrix.*

leukothrombin (loo″ko-throm′bin) a fibrin factor formed by leukocytes in the blood.

leukotome (loo′ko-tōm) [*leuko-* + Gr. *tomē* a cut] a cannula through which a loop of wire is passed to perform the operation of leukotomy or lobotomy.

leukotomy (loo-kot′o-me) the operation of cutting the white matter in the oval center of the frontal lobe of the brain; prefrontal lobotomy. **transorbital l.,** leukotomy performed by way of the orbital plate.

leukotoxic (loo″ko-tok′sik) destructive to leukocytes.

leukotoxicity (loo″ko-tok-sis″ĭ-te) the quality of having a toxic or deleterious effect on leukocytes.

leukotoxin (loo″ko-tok′sin) [*leuko*cyte + *toxin*] a cytotoxin destructive to the leukocytes.

Leukotrichaceae (loo″ko-tri-ka′se-e) Leucotrichaceae.

leukotrichia (loo″ko-trik′e-ah) [*leuko-* + Gr. *thrix* hair + *-ia*] whiteness of the hair in a circumscribed area.

leukotriene (loo″ko-tri′ēn) [from *leuko*cytes + *triene* indicating three double bonds] one of a group of biologically active compounds consisting of straight chain, 20 carbon carboxylic acids with one or two oxygen substituents and three or more conjugated double bonds. They are formed from arachidonic acid by the lipoxygenase pathway, and function as regulators of allergic and inflammatory reactions. Leukotrienes are identified by letters A, B, C, D, and E with subscripts indicating the number of double bonds in the molecule. Some (LTB_4) stimulate the movement of leukocytes; others (LTC_4, LTD_4, and LTE_4) constitute slow reacting substance of anaphylaxis, which causes bronchial constriction and other allergic reactions.

leukourobilin (loo″ko-u-ro-bi′lin) [*leuko-* + *urobilin*] a colorless decomposition product of urobilin.

leukovirus (loo″ko-vi′rus) any of a group of morphologically similar, ether-sensitive, RNA viruses causing leukemia and tumors in animals; the group includes avian leukosis virus, Rous sarcoma virus, and murine leukemia virus.

leuprolide (loo-pro′līd) a gonadotropin releasing hormone analogue used as an antineoplastic.

Levaditi's stain (lev″ah-de′tēz) [Constantin *Levaditi,* Roumanian bacteriologist in Paris, 1874–1928] see *Table of Stains.*

levallorphan tartrate (lev″al-lor′fan) [USP] chemical name: 17-allylmorphinan-3-ol[*R*-(*R*,R**)]-2,3-dihydroxybutanedioate (1:1) (salt). An analogue of levorphanol, $C_{19}H_{25}$-$NO·C_4H_6O_6$, occurring as a white to practically white, crystalline powder, which acts as an antagonist to analgesic narcotics; used in the treatment of respiratory depression produced by narcotic analgesics, administered parenterally.

levamfetamine (le″vam-fet′ah-mēn) chemical name: (−)-α-methylbenzeneethanamine. The levorotatory form of amphetamine, $C_9H_{13}N$, having actions similar to the racemic form but less potent than the racemic or dextrorotatory (dextroamphetamine) forms. See *amphetamine,* def. 1. Spelled also *levamphetamine.* **l. succinate,** the succinate salt of levamfetamine, $C_9H_{13}N·C_4H_6O_4$, used in the treatment of narcolepsy, hyperkinetic behavior disorders, and as an anorexic agent in the treatment of obesity; administered orally.

levamisole hydrochloride (le-vam′ĭ-sōl) chemical name: (*S*)-2,3,5,6-tetrahydro-6-phenylimidazo[2,1-*b*]thiazole monohydrochloride. An oral imidazole used as an anthelmintic, $C_{11}H_{12}N_2S·HCl$, effective against roundworms, hookworms, and strongyloids. It is also an immunopotentiator and has been used (investigatively) to stimulate the immune response in cancer.

levamphetamine (le″vam-fet′ah-mēn) levamfetamine.

levan (lev′an) a homopolysaccharide containing fructose residues in 2,6-fructosidic linkage. It is formed from sucrose by the enzyme levansucrase, which is produced by certain species of *Bacillus* and *Leuconostoc.* Levan increases the adhesion of bacteria to surfaces of the teeth and promotes the formation of dental plaque.

levansucrase (lev″an-su′krās) [EC 2.4.1.10] an enzyme of the transferase class that catalyzes the reaction sucrose + $(2,6-β-D-fructosyl)_n$ = glucosse + $(2,6-β-D-fructosyl)_{n+1}$. The enzyme is produced by certain bacteria. The fructose polymer (levan) formed is a constituent of dental plaque.

levarterenol (lev″ar-tĕ-re′nol) the levorotatory isomer of norepinephrine (q.v.), a much more potent pressor agent than the natural dextrorotatory isomer. **l. bitartrate,** norepinephrine bitartrate.

levator (le-va′tor), pl. *levato′res* [L. *levare* to raise] 1. [NA] a muscle for elevating the organ or structure into which it is inserted; see entries beginning *musculus levator,* in *Table of Musculi.* 2. a surgical instrument used to raise depressed osseous fragments in fractures of the skull and other bones.

levatores (lev″ah-to′rēz) [L.] plural of *levator.*

level (lev′el) 1. relative position, rank, or concentration. 2. a cerebrospinal center for combining or integrating impulses; the first level is spinal, the second is brainstem, the third is cortical. **α l.,** significance l. **confidence l.,** one minus the confidence coefficient; the probability that a confidence interval does not contain the population parameter. Denoted by α. **l's of consciousness,** see *consciousness.* **isoelectric l.,** the level of recorded resting potential of a cell; the baseline of the electrocardiogram. **significance l., l. of significance,** the probability of incorrectly rejecting the null hypothesis when such a hypothesis is tested. Called also α *l.*

levicellular (lev″ĭ-sel′u-lar) [L. *levis* smooth + *cellula* cell] smooth celled.

levidulinose (le-vid′u-lin-ōs) a naturally occurring trisaccharide found in manna; on hydrolysis it yields one molecule of glucose and two molecules of mannose.

levigation (lev″ĭ-ga′shun) [L. *levigare* to render smooth] the grinding to a powder of a hard or moistened substance.

Levin's tube (lĕ-vinz′) [Abraham Louis *Levin*, New Orleans physician, 1880–1940] see under *tube*.

Levinea (le-vi′ne-ah) a proposed genus of gram-negative, facultatively anaerobic, rod-shaped bacteria of the family Enterobacteriaceae. The type species is *L. malona′tica*.

levitation (lev″ĭ-ta′shun) [L. *levis* light] 1. a hallucinatory sensation of floating or rising in the air. 2. a support system for severe burn victims, consisting of a bed in the form of an inflatable chamber containing numerous outlets through which humidified, warm, sterile air is released at a pressure sufficient to raise the patient so that he is supported in a sterile air environment.

lev(o)- [L. *laevus* left] 1. a combining form meaning left, to the left. 2. chemical prefix used to designate the levorotatory enantiomorph of a substance; opposed to *dextro-*. Symbol (−)- (formerly *l*-; sometimes Λ).

levocardia (le″vo-kar′de-ah) [*levo-* + Gr. *kardia* heart] a term denoting the normal position of the heart, used when other viscera are transposed; cf. *dextrocardia*. **isolated l.,** levocardia associated with transposition (situs inversus) of the abdominal viscera, congenital structural anomaly of the heart, and sometimes with absence of the spleen. **mixed l.,** corrected transposition of the great vessels; see under *transposition*.

levocardiogram (le″vo-kar′de-o-gram) [*levo-* + *cardiogram*] a rarely used term denoting that part of the normal electrocardiogram representing electric activity or depolarization potentials of the left ventricle.

levoclination (le″vo-kli-na′shun) [*levo-* + L. *clinatus* leaning] rotation of the upper poles of the vertical meridians of the two eyes to the left. Cf. *dextroclination*.

levocycloduction (le″vo-si″klo-duk′shun) levoduction.

levodopa (le″vo-do′pah) [USP] chemical name: 3-hydroxy-L-tyrosine. The levorotatory isomer of dopa, $C_9H_{11}NO_4$, occurring as a white to off-white crystalline powder; used as an antiparkinsonian agent, administered orally. See *dopa*.

Levo-Dromoran (le″vo-dro′mo-ran) trademark for preparations of levorphanol tartrate.

levoduction (le″vo-duk′shun) movement of either eye to the left.

levofuraltadone (le″vo-fūr-al′tah-dōn) chemical name: (−)-5-(4-morpholinylmethyl)-3-[[(5-nitro-2-furanyl)methylene]amino]-2-oxazolidinone; an antibacterial and antiprotozoal, $C_{13}H_{16}N_4O_6$.

levogram (le″vo-gram) [*levo-* + Gr. *graphein* to record] a rarely used term denoting electrocardiographic tracing showing left axis deviation, indicative of left ventricular hypertrophy.

levogyral (le″vo-ji′ral) [*levo-* + L. *gyrare* to turn] levorotatory.

levogyration (le″vo-ji-ra′shun) levorotation.

Levoid (le′void) trademark for a preparation of levothyroxine sodium.

levomepromazine (le″vo-mĕ-pro′mah-zēn) methotrimeprazine.

levomethadyl acetate (le″vo-meth′ah-dil) chemical name: (−)-β-[2-(dimethylamino)propyl]-α-ethyl-β-phenylbenzeneethanol acetate (ester). A narcotic analgesic, $C_{23}H_{31}NO_2$, used in the treatment of heroin addiction.

levonordefrin (le″vo-nor′dĕ-frin) [USP] chemical name: (−)-4-(2-amino-1-hydroxypropyl)-1,2 benzenediol. An adrenergic, $C_9H_{13}NO_3$, the levo isomer of nordefrin, occurring as a white to buff-colored, crystalline powder; used as a vasoconstrictor in solutions of local anesthetics, especially in dentistry.

Levophed (lev′o-fed) trademark for a preparation of norepinephrine bitartrate.

Levoprome (le′vo-prōm) trademark for a preparation of methotrimeprazine.

levopropoxyphene napsylate (le″vo-pro-pok′sĕ-fēn-nap′sĭ-lāt) [USP] chemical name: [R-($R*,S*$]-α-[2-(dimethylamino)-1-methylethyl]-α-phenylbenzenethanol propanoate (ester) compound with 2-naphthalenesulphonic acid (1:1) monohydrate. The napsylate salt of the levo isomer of propoxyphen, $C_{22}H_{29}NO_2 \cdot C_{10}H_8O_3S \cdot H_2O$, occurring as a white powder; used as an antitussive, administered orally.

levopropylcillin potassium (le″vo-pro″pil-sil′in) chemical name: potassium 3,3-dimethyl-7-oxo-6-(−)-(2-phenoxybutyramido)-4- thia -1- azabicyclo [3.2.0] heptane -2-carboxylate; an antibacterial, $C_{18}H_{21}KN_2O_5S$, effective against gram-positive organism. Called also *propicillin*.

levorotary (le″vo-ro′tah-re) levorotatory.

levorotation (le″vo-ro-ta′shun) a turning to the left.

levorotatory (le″vo-ro′tah-to′re) [*levo-* + L. *rotare* to turn] turning the plane of polarization of polarized light to the left.

levorphanol (lēv-or′fah-nol) see *sodium levothyroxine*, under *sodium*.

levorphanol tartrate (le-vor′fah-nōl) [USP] chemical name: 17-methylmorphinan-3-ol[R-($R*,R*$]-2,3-dihydroxybutanedioate (1:1) (salt) dihydrate. A synthetic narcotic analgesic, $C_{17}H_{23}NO \cdot C_4H_6O_6 \cdot 2H_2O$, occurring as a white, crystalline powder; administered orally and subcutaneously.

levosin (le′vo-sin) a starch occurring in wheat flour, rye, bran, and stubble.

levothyroxine sodium (le″vo-thi-rok′sēn) [USP] chemical name: O-(4-hydroxy-3,5-diiodophenyl)-3,5-diiodo-L-tyrosine monosodium salt hydrate. The monosodium salt of the levo isomer of the thyroid hormone thyroxine, $C_{15}H_{10}I_4$-$NNa_4 x H_2O$, occurring as a light yellow to buff-colored, hygroscopic powder; used for replacement therapy in reduced or absent thyroid function, administered orally.

levotorsion (le″vo-tor′shun) levoclination.

levoversion (le″vo-ver′zhun) an act of turning to the left; in ophthalmology, movement of the eyes to the left.

levoxadrol hydrochloride (le-voks′ah-drōl) chemical name: (−)-2-(2,2-diphenyl-1,3-dioxolan-4-yl)piperidine hydrochloride; a local anesthetic and smooth muscle relaxant, $C_{20}H_{23}NO_2 \cdot HCl$.

Levret's forceps, law, etc. (lev-rāz′) [André *Levret*, French accoucheur, 1703–1780] see under the nouns.

Levugen (lev′u-jen) trademark for a preparation of fructose.

levulan (lev′u-lan) fructosan.

levulin (lev′u-lin) a starchlike compound, $C_6H_{10}O_5$, occurring in certain plant tubers.

levulinic acid (lev″u-lin′ik) trivial name for γ-ketovaleric acid.

levulosan (lev″u-lo′san) fructosan, a fructose (fructofuranose) polysaccharide, e.g., inulin.

levulosazone (lev″u-lo′sa-zōn) fructosazone.

levulose (lev′u-lōs) [L. *laevus* left + *-ose*] fructose.

levulosemia (lev″u-lo-se′me-ah) [*levulose* + Gr. *haima* blood + *-ia*] fructosemia.

levulosuria (lev″u-lo-su′re-ah) [*levulose* + Gr. *ouron* urine + *-ia*] fructosuria.

lewisite (lu′ĭ-sīt) [named for W. Lee *Lewis*, American chemist, 1879–1943] chemical name: dichloro(2-chlorovinyl)arsine. A lethal war gas, $AsCl_2CH:CHCl$. It is a vesicant, lacrimator, and lung irritant.

Lewisohn's method (lu′ĭ-sonz) [Richard *Lewisohn*, New York surgeon, 1875–1961] see under *method*.

Leyden's ataxia, crystals, disease (li′denz) [Ernst Victor von *Leyden*, German physician, 1832–1910] see *pseudotabes*, see *Charcot-Leyden crystals*, under *crystal*, and see under *disease*.

Leyden jar (li′den) see under *jar*.

Leyden-Möbius dystrophy, type (li′den-me′be-us) [E. V. von *Leyden*; Paul Julius *Möbius*, German neurologist, 1853–1910] limb-girdle muscular dystrophy.

Leydig's cells, cylinders, duct (li′digz) [Franz von *Leydig*, German anatomist, 1821–1908] see under *cell* and *cylinder*, and see *ductus mesonephricus*.

leydigarche (li″dig-ar′ke) [*Leydig* cells + Gr. *archē* beginning] the establishment or beginning of gonadal function in the male.

Lf limit flocculation; see *Lf dose*, under *dose*, and *Lf unit*, under *unit*.

L.F.A. left frontoanterior (left mentoanterior, a position of the fetus).

L.F.D. least fatal dose (of a toxin).

L-form L-phase variant; see under *variant*.

L.F.P. left frontoposterior (left mentoposterior, a position of the fetus).

L.F.T. left frontotransverse (left mentotransverse, a position of the fetus).

LH luteinizing hormone.

Lhermitte's sign (lār′mits) [Jean *Lhermitte*, Paris neurologist, 1877–1959] see under *sign*.

LH-RF luteinizing hormone releasing factor.

LH-RH luteinizing hormone releasing hormone; see *gonadotropin releasing hormone*, under *hormone*.

Li chemical symbol for *lithium*.

LIA leukemia-associated inhibitory activity; see under *activity*.

Lib. abbreviation for L. *li′bra*, a pound.

liberomotor (lib″er-o-mo′tor) [L. *liber* free + *motor* mover] pertaining to voluntary and conscious movements or actions.

libidinal (lǐ-bid′ǐ-nal) pertaining to or of the nature of libido; erotic.

libidinous (lǐ-bid′ǐ-nus) [L. *libidinosus*] lustful or salacious.

libido (lǐ-be′do, lǐ-bi′do), pl. *libid′ines* [L.] 1. sexual desire. 2. the energy derived from the primitive impulses. In psychoanalysis the term is applied to the motive power of the sex life; in freudian psychology, to psychic energy in general.

Libman-Sacks disease (syndrome) (lib′man-saks′) [Emanuel *Libman*, New York physician, 1872–1946; Benjamin *Sacks*, New York physician, born 1896] atypical verrucous endocarditis.

LiBr lithium bromide.

libra (li′brah, le′brah), pl. *li′brae* [L.] pound.

library (li′brě-re) [L. *libraria*] in genetics, a set of cloned DNA fragments that together represent the entire genome, or the genes transcribed by a particular tissue. Called also *DNA l.*

Librium (lib′re-um) trademark for preparations of chlordiazepoxide hydrochloride.

lice (līs) plural of *louse*.

Liceida (lǐ-si′dah) an order of ameboid protozoa (subclass Myxogastria, class Eumycetozoa), the organisms of which have a spore mass that is usually light colored and a pseudocapitillium.

license (li′sens) [L. *licere* to be permitted] a permit to perform acts which without it would be illegal.

licentiate (li-sen′she-āt) [L. *licentia* license] one holding a license from an authorized agency entitling him to practice a particular profession.

lichen (li′ken) [Gr. *leichēn* a tree-moss] 1. any of the many thallophytic plants formed by mutualistic combination of an alga and a fungus, the algal component being a green or blue-green alga, and the fungal usually an ascomycete. 2. a name applied to many different kinds of papular skin diseases in which the lesions are typically small, firm papules that are usually set very close together, the specific type being indicated by a modifying term. **l. amyloido′sus,** see under *amyloidosis*. **l. cor′neus hypertro′phicus,** a papular skin eruption of thickened and horny lesions. **l. fibromucinoido′sus,** l. myxedematosus. **l. myxedemato′sus,** a condition resembling myxedema but not associated with thyroid dysfunction, characterized by a fibrocystic proliferation, increased deposition of acid mucopolysaccharides in the skin, and the presence of a circulating paraprotein, usually an immunoglobulin G, which presents as either discrete or generalized lichenoid papules with or without diffuse scleroderma, or as urticaria-like plaques and nodules. Called also *l. fibromucinoidosus, papular mucinosis, papular myxedema,* and *scleromyxedema*. **l. nit′idus,** a usually asymptomatic chronic inflammatory eruption consisting of numerous glistening, flat-topped, discrete, smooth, commonly skin-colored micropapules, located most often on the penis, lower abdomen, inner thighs, flexor aspects of the wrists and forearms, breasts, and buttocks. Widespread involvement may produce confluence of the lesions, with formation of scaly plaques. **l. obtus′us cor′neus,** a papular eruption of thickened,

blunt lesions; probably identical with prurigo nodularis. **l. pila′ris,** l. spinulosus. **l. planopila′ris,** l. planus follicularis. **l. pla′nus,** an inflammatory, pruritic cutaneous disease, sometimes also involving the oral and genital mucosa and nails, which may be acute and widespread or chronic and localized. Lichen planus is characterized by the development of a distinctive eruption consisting typically of angular, umbilicated, flat-topped, violaceous papules that exhibit a shiny fine, but often inconspicuous, scale and whitish lines or puncta (*Wickham's striae*). The lesions may be discrete or coalesce to form plaques, annular lesions, or linear configurations. The disorder may present in many morphological variations, including vesicular or bullous, hypertrophic, atrophic, follicular, erosive and ulcerative, actinic, or erythematous patterns, which usually resolve spontaneously, leaving residual hyperpigmentation and atrophy. Lichen planus–like lesions may also be caused by various drugs and chemical substances. Called also *l. ruber planus*. **l. pla′nus actin′icus,** l. planus tropicum. **l. pla′nus annula′ris,** a variant in which groups of papules form annular configurations, especially on the genitals, lower trunk, and lips, and in the mouth. **l. pla′nus atro′phicus,** a variant characterized by atrophy in the center of preexisting lesions of lichen planus, ultimately leading to atrophic white spots on the skin, which aggregate to form small ivory- or violet-colored patches that may have an erythematous border. **l. pla′nus, bullous,** see *vesiculobullous l. planus*. **l. pla′nus erythemato′sus,** an unusual variant characterized by the presence of soft, nonpruritic, slightly erythematous or purpuric papules. **l. pla′nus follicula′ris,** a variant characterized by the presence of acuminate, keratotic, patchy follicular lesions of the scalp, often leading to local atrophy or alopecia. Called also *l. planopilaris*. **l. pla′nus hypertro′phicus,** a variant characterized by the presence of verrucous plaques covered with scales, which are most often located on the shins but may be found anywhere on the body. Called also *l. planus verrucosus*. **l. pla′nus subtrop′icum,** l. planus tropicum. **l. pla′nus trop′icum,** a variant occurring in the tropics or subtropics, especially on sun-exposed areas of the skin of children and young adults of Oriental extraction, and characterized by papular lesions that may be pigmented, dyschromic, or granuloma annulare–like. Called also *l. planus actinicus* and *l. planus subtropicum*. **l. pla′nus verruco′sus,** l. planus hypertrophicus. **l. pla′nus, vesiculobullous,** a variant in which small vesicles and bullae may occur as part of the general papular eruption, or present de nevo or on uninvolved skin. **l. ru′ber monilifor′mis,** a generalized or localized eruption presenting as either round, dome-shaped, waxy, dark or bright red papules, or as waxy yellow, milia-like papules with a keloidal consistency, often forming a moniliform pattern, sometimes arranged in keloidal bands. Some authorities consider the condition to be a variant of lichen simplex chronicus. Called also *morbus moniliformis*. **l. ru′ber pla′nus,** l. planus. **l. sclero′sus,** l. sclerosus et atrophicus. **l. sclero′sus et atroph′icus,** a chronic, atrophic skin disease characterized by white, angular, flat, well-defined, indurated papules with an erythematous halo and follicular, black, keratotic plugs. It is the most common cause of kraurosis vulvae in females and balanitis xerotica obliterans in males. Called also *white spot disease* and *Csillag's disease*. See also *guttate morphea*, under *morphea*. **l. scrofuloso′rum,** l. scrofulo′sus, a form of tuberculid manifested as an eruption of clusters of lichenoid papules on the trunk of children with tuberculous disease. Called also *tuberculosis cutis lichenoides* and *tuberculosis lichenoides*. **l. sim′plex chron′icus,** an eczematous dermatitis due to repeated itching and rubbing or scratching of the skin, arising spontaneously or initiated by or coexisting with other dermatoses, characterized by sharply demarcated, circumscribed, scaling patches of thickened, furrowed skin, located most commonly on the face, nuchal region, extremities, scrotum, vulva, and perianal region. Called also *circumscribed* or *localized neurodermatitis*. **l. spinulo′sus,** a cutaneous disorder seen chiefly in children, characterized by the presence of discrete groups of minute, filiform, horny spines protruding from acuminate follicular openings, occurring in crops and located especially on the neck, buttocks, abdominal wall, popliteal spaces, and extensor surfaces of the arms. **l. stria′tus,** a self-limited, usually unilateral eruption most commonly seen in children, predominantly located on the extremities and sides of the neck, and typically presenting as discrete, pink, papular or lichenoid lesions with an inconspicuous scale that tend to coalesce and form a continuous or interrupted linear patch. **l. trop′icus,** miliaria rubra. **l. urtica′tus,** papular urticaria.

lichenification (li-ken″ĭ-fĭ-ka′shun) hypertrophy of the epidermis, resulting in thickening of the skin with exaggeration of the normal skin markings, giving the skin a leathery barklike appearance, which is caused by prolonged rubbing or scratching. It may arise on seemingly normal skin, or it may develop at the site of another pruritic cutaneous disorder.

licheniformin (li-ken″ĭ-form′in) a group of antibiotic substances (licheniformin A, B, and C) isolated from *Bacillus subtilis,* resembling subtilin in their properties.

lichenin (li′kĕ-nin) a starchy demulcent polysaccharide, $(C_6H_{10}O_5)_n$, which yields glucose on hydrolysis. It occurs abundantly in Iceland moss, *Cetraria islandica.* Called also *lichen starch* and *moss starch.*

lichenoid (li′ken-oid) [*lichen* + Gr. *eidos* form] resembling the skin lesions designated as lichen.

Lichtheim's aphasia, etc. (likt′hīmz) [Ludwig *Lichtheim,* German physician, 1845–1928] see under *aphasia, disease, plaque, sign, syndrome,* and *tests.*

Lichtheimia (lik-thi′me-ah) former name for the genus *Absidia.*

Li₂CO₃ lithium carbonate.

Licnophorina (lik″no-fo-ri′nah) [Gr. *liknon* winnowing fan + *phoros* bearing] a suborder of ectocommensal ciliate protozoa (order Heterotrichina, subclass Spirotricha) having an hourglass-like shape with a prominent oral disk and large wreath of membranelles; a conspicuous basal disk at the antapical pole that serves as an attachment organelle; and an essentially naked body except for buccal organelles and posterior ciliary rings. They are found chiefly on various marine invertebrates.

licorice (lik′o-ris) glycyrrhiza.

lid (lid) [A.S. *hlid*] an eyelid. **granular l's,** trachoma, def. 1. **tucked l. of Collier,** a retraction of the upper eyelid in cases of ophthalmoplegia due to a supranuclear lesion in the brain stem.

Lida-Mantle (li′dah-man′t'l) trademark for a preparation of lidocaine.

lidamidine (li-dam′ĭ-dēn) an amidinourea with antisecretory and antimotility action in animals that has been investigated as an antidiarrheal.

lidamine (li′dah-mēn) an amidinourea that has been used as an antidiarrheal.

Liddell and Sherrington reflex [Edward George Tandy *Liddell,* British physiologist, born 1895; Sir Charles Scott *Sherrington,* English physiologist, 1857–1952] stretch reflex.

Lidex (li′deks) trademark for preparations of fluocinonide.

lidocaine (li′do-kān) [USP] chemical name: 2-(diethylamino)-N-(2,6-dimethylphenyl)acetamide. A drug, $C_{14}H_{22}$-N_2O, having anesthetic, sedative, analgesic, anticonvulsant, and cardiac depressant activities, occurring as a white or slightly yellow, crystalline powder; used as a local anesthetic, applied topically to the skin and mucous membranes. **l. hydrochloride** [USP], the monohydrated monohydrochloride salt of lidocaine, $C_{14}H_{22}N_2O \cdot HCl \cdot H_2O$, occurring as a white, crystalline powder; used as a cardiac antiarrhythmic, administered intravenously, and to produce local anesthesia by infiltration injection and epidural and peripheral nerve block.

lidofenin (li″do-fen′in) chemical name: N-(carboxymethyl)-N-[2-[(2,6-dimethylphenyl)amino]-2-oxoethyl]glycine; a diagnostic aid for determination of hepatic function, $C_{14}H_{18}$-N_2O_5.

lidofilcon (li″do-fil′kon) either of two hydrophilic contact lens materials, one of which contains 70 percent water (*lidofilcon A*), and the other 79 per cent water (*lidofilcon B*).

lidoflazine (li-do-fla′zēn) chemical name: 4-[4,4-bis-(4-fluorophenyl)butyl]-N-(2,6-dimethylphenyl)-1-piperazineacetamide; a coronary vasodilator, $C_{30}H_{35}F_2N_2O$.

lie (li) the situation of the long axis of the fetus with respect to that of the mother; see *presentation.* **transverse l.,** the situation of the fetus during labor when the long axis of its body crosses the long axis of the maternal body. The shoulder usually presents first, but the arm, trunk, or any

other part of the trunk may be the first to appear. Called also *torso, transverse,* or *trunk presentation.* See table of Positions of the Fetus in Various Presentations, under *position.*

Lieben's test (reaction) (le′benz) [Adolf *Lieben,* Austrian chemist, 1836–1914] see under *tests.*

Lieberkühn's ampulla, crypts, follicles, glands (le′-ber-künz) [Johann Nathaniel *Lieberkühn,* German anatomist, 1711–1756] see under *ampulla,* and see *glandulae intestinales.*

Liebermann-Burchard reaction, test (le′ber-mahn berk′hard) [Carl Theodore *Liebermann,* German chemist, 1842–1914; H. *Burchard,* German chemist, 19th century] see under *reaction* and *test.*

Liebermann's test (le′ber-mahnz) [Leo von Szentlörincz *Liebermann,* Hungarian physician, 1852–1926] see under *tests.*

Liebermeister's furrows, grooves, rule (le′ber-mis″-terz) [Carl von *Liebermeister,* German physician, 1833–1901] see under *furrow, groove,* and *rule.*

Liebig's test, theory (le′bigz) [Baron Justus von *Liebig,* German chemist, 1803–1873] see under *tests* and *theory.*

lien (li′en) [L.] NA alternative for *splen* (spleen). **l. acesso′rius,** splen accessorius. **l. mo′bilis,** floating spleen.

lienal (li-e′nal) pertaining to the spleen; splenic.

lienculus (li-en′ku-lus) an accessory spleen (lien accessorius [NA]).

lienectomy (li″ĕ-nek′to-me) splenectomy.

lienitis (li″ĕ-ni′tis) splenitis.

lien(o)- [L. *lien* spleen] a combining form denoting relationship to the spleen.

lienocele (li-e′no-sēl) splenocele.

lienography (li″e-nog′rah-fe) splenography.

lienomalacia (li-e″no-mah-la′she-ah) splenomalacia.

lienomedullary (li-e″no-med′u-la″re) splenomedullary.

lienomyelogenous (li-e″no-mi″ĕ-loj′ĕ-nus) splenomyelogenous.

lienomyelomalacia (li-e″no-mi″ĕ-lo-mah-la′she-ah) splenomyelomalacia.

lienopancreatic (li-e″no-pan″kre-at′ik) splenopancreatic.

lienopathy (li″e-nop′ah-the) splenopathy.

lienorenal (li-e″no-re′nal) pertaining to the spleen and the kidney.

lienotoxin (li-e″no-tok′sin) [*lieno-* + *toxin*] splenotoxin.

lienteric (li″en-ter′ik) affected by or of the nature of a lientery.

lientery (li′en-ter″e) [Gr. *leienteria; leios* smooth + *enteron* intestine] diarrhea in which the stools contain undigested food.

lienunculus (li″en-ung′ku-lus) a detached mass or exclave of splenic tissue; an accessory spleen.

Liepmann's apraxia (lēp′manz) [Hugo Carl *Liepmann,* Berlin neurologist, 1863–1925] see under *apraxia.*

Liesegang's phenomenon (striae, waves) (le′zĕ-gahng) [Ralph Eduard *Liesegang,* German chemist, 1869–1947] see under *phenomenon.*

Lieskeela (lēs-ke-el′a) [*Lieske,* German microbiologist] a genus of sheathed bacteria, found in water and mud, made up of rod-shaped cells in double, spiral, twisted chains. They are enclosed in a slimy capsule frequently containing ferric hydroxide granules. The type species is *L. bi′fida.*

Lieutaud's triangle (body), uvula (luette) (lu-toz′) [Joseph *Lieutaud,* French physician, 1703–1780] see *trigonum vesicae* and *uvula vesicae.*

LIF left iliac fossa; leukocyte inhibitory factor.

life (līf) [L. *vita;* Gr. *bios* or *zōe*] the aggregate of vital phenomena; a certain peculiar stimulated condition of organized matter; that obscure principle whereby organized beings are peculiarly endowed with certain powers and functions not associated with inorganic matter. Generally, living things share, in varying degrees, the following characteristics: organization, irritability, movement, growth, reproduction, and adaptation. **animal l.,** vegetative life conjoined with the employment of the senses and with spontaneous movements. **intrauterine l., uterine l.,** the period of life spent in the uterus; i.e., embryonic and fetal life. **mean l.,** the average time until decay for a sample of particles of a radionuclide or elementary particle, equal to the reciprocal of the decay constant or 1.443 times the half-life; symbol τ. Called also *lifetime*. **vegetative l.,** that which is manifested in automatic acts requisite for the maintenance of the individual and the propagation of the species.

lifetime (līf′tīm) mean life.

lifibrate (lĭ-fi′brāt) chemical name: bis(4-chlorophenoxy)acetic acid 1-methyl-4-piperidinyl ester; an antihyperlipidemic, $C_{20}H_{21}Cl_2NO_4$.

lig. ligament; ligamentum.

ligament (lig′ah-ment) 1. a band of fibrous tissue that connects bones or cartilages, serving to support and strengthen joints; see *ligamentum*. 2. a double layer of peritoneum extending from one visceral organ to another. 3. cordlike remnants of fetal tubular structures that are nonfunctional after birth. **accessory l.,** any ligament that strengthens or supports another. **accessory l's, plantar,** see *ligamenta plantaria articulationum metatarsophalangealium* and *ligamenta plantaria articulationum interphalangealium pedis*. **accessory l's, volar,** see *ligamenta palmaria articulationum metacarpophalangealium* and *ligamenta palmaria articulationum interphalangealium manus*. **accessory l. of Henle, lateral,** ligamentum laterale articulationis temporomandibularis. **accessory l. of Henle, medial,** ligamentum sphenomandibulare. **accessory l. of humerus,** ligamentum coracohumerale. **accessory l's of metacarpophalangeal joints,** ligamenta collateralia articulationum metacarpophalangearum. **acromioclavicular l.,** ligamentum acromioclaviculare. **acromiocoracoid l.,** ligamentum coracoacromiale. **adipose l. of knee (of Cruveilhier),** plica synovialis infrapatellaris. **alar l's,** ligamenta alaria. **alar l's of knee,** plicae alares. **alveolodental l.,** periodontal l. **annular l., dorsal common,** retinaculum extensorum manus. **annular l., inferior,** ligamentum arcuatum pubis. **annular l., internal,** retinaculum musculorum flexorum pedis. **annular l. of ankle, external,** retinaculum musculorum peroneorum superius. **annular l. of ankle, internal,** retinaculum musculorum flexorum pedis. **annular l. of base of stapes,** ligamentum annulare stapedis. **annular l. of carpus, posterior,** retinaculum extensorum manus. **annular l's of digits of foot,** see *pars annularis vaginae fibrosae digitorum pedis*. **annular l's of digits of hand,** see *pars annularis vaginae fibrosae digitorum manus*. **annular l. of femur,** zona orbicularis articulationis coxae. **annular l's of fingers,** pars annularis vaginae fibrosae digitorum manus. **annular l. of malleolus, external,** retinaculum musculorum extensorum pedis inferius. **annular l. of malleolus, internal,** retinaculum musculorum flexorum pedis. **annular l. of radius,** ligamentum annulare radii. **annular l. of stapes,** ligamentum annulare stapedis. **annular l. of tarsus, anterior,** retinaculum musculorum extensorum pedis inferius. **annular l's of tendon sheaths of fingers,** see *pars annularis vaginae fibrosae digitorum manus*. **annular l's of toes,** pars annularis vaginae fibrosae digitorum pedis. **annular l. of wrist, dorsal posterior,** retinaculum extensorum manus. **anococcygeal l.,** ligamentum anococcygeum. **anterior l. of colon,** tenia omentalis. **anterior l. of head of fibula,** ligamentum capitis fibulae anterius. **anterior l. of head of rib,** ligamentum capitis costae radiatum. **anterior l. of malleus,** ligamentum mallei anterius. **anterior l. of neck of rib,** anterior portion of ligamentum costotransversarium superius. **anterior l. of radiocarpal joint,** ligamentum radiocarpeum palmare. **l. of antibrachium (of Weitbrecht),** chorda obliqua membranae interosseae antebrachii. **apical dental l., apical odontoid l.,** ligamentum apicis dentis axis. **appendiculo-ovarian l.,** a fold of peritoneum extending between the appendix and the broad ligament of the uterus. **Arantius' l.,** ligamentum venosum. **arcuate l's,** ligamenta flava. **arcuate l., lateral,** ligamentum arcuatum laterale. **arcuate l., medial,** ligamentum arcuatum mediale. **arcuate l., median,** l. arcuatum medianum. **arcuate l., pubic,** ligamentum arcuatum pubis. **arcuate l. of diaphragm, external,** ligamentum arcuatum laterale. **arcuate l. of diaphragm, internal,** ligamentum arcuatum mediale. **arcuate l. of diaphragm, lateral,** ligamentum arcuatum laterale. **arcuate l. of knee,** ligamentum popliteum arcuatum. **arcuate l. of pubis, inferior,** ligamentum

arcuatum pubis. **Arnold's l.,** ligamentum incudis superius. **articular l. of vertebrae,** capsula articularis articulationum vertebrarum. **arytenoepiglottic l.,** plica aryepiglottica. **atlantooccipital l., anterior, atlantooccipital l., deep,** membrana atlanto-occipitalis. **atlantooccipital l., lateral,** ligamentum atlanto-occipitale laterale. **atlantooccipital l., posterior,** membrana atlantooccipitalis posterior. **l's of auditory ossicles,** ligamenta ossiculorum auditus. **l's of auricle of external ear,** ligamenta auricularia. **auricular l., anterior,** ligamentum auriculare anterius. **auricular l., posterior,** ligamentum auriculare posterius. **auricular l., superior,** ligamentum auriculare superius. **Barkow's l.,** the anterior and posterior parts of the elbow joint capsule. **Bellini's l.,** a band passing as part of the capsule of the hip joint to the greater trochanter. **Bérard's l.,** the suspensory ligament of the pericardium, extending to the third and fourth thoracic vertebrae. **Berry's l.,** ligamentum thyrohyoideum laterale. **Bertin's l.,** ligamentum iliofemorale. **Bichat's l.,** the lower bundle of the dorsal sacroiliac ligament. **bifurcate l.,** ligamentum bifurcatum. **bifurcate l's, deep,** ligamenta metatarsea plantaria. **bifurcate l's of Arnold, deep,** ligamenta tarsometatarsea plantaria. **Bigelow's l.,** ligamentum iliofemorale. **bigeminate l's of Arnold,** ligamenta tarsometatarsea dorsalia. **l. of Botallo,** ligamentum arteriosum. **Bourgery's l.,** ligamentum popliteum obliquum. **brachiocubital l.,** ligamentum collaterale ulnare. **brachioradial l.,** ligamentum collaterale radiale. **broad l. of liver,** ligamentum falciforme hepatis. **broad l. of lung,** ligamentum pulmonale. **broad l. of uterus,** the peritoneal fold that supports the uterus on either side; called also *ligamentum latum uteri* [NA]. **Brodie's l.,** the transverse humeral ligament. **Burns' l.,** margo falciformis hiatus saphenus. **calcaneocuboid l.,** ligamentum calcaneocuboideum. **calcaneocuboid l., plantar,** ligamentum calcaneocuboideum plantare. **calcaneofibular l.,** ligamentum calcaneofibulare. **calcaneonavicular l.,** ligamentum calcaneonaviculare. **calcaneonavicular l., dorsal,** ligamentum calcaneonaviculare dorsale. **calcaneonavicular l., plantar,** ligamentum calcaneonaviculare plantare. **calcaneotibial l.,** pars tibiocalcaneus ligamenti medialis. **Caldani's l.,** a band passing from the inner border of the coracoid process to the lower border of the clavicle, the first rib, and the tendon of the subclavius. **Campbell's l.,** suspensory l. of axilla. **Camper's l.,** diaphragma urogenitale. **canthal l's,** see *ligamentum palpebrale mediale* and *raphe palpebralis lateralis*. **capitular l., volar,** ligamentum metacarpeum transversum profundum. **capsular l's,** ligamenta capsularia. **capsular l., internal,** ligamentum capitis femoris. **capsular l., pelviprostatic,** fascia prostatae. **Carcassonne's l.,** ligamentum puboprostaticum. **cardinal l.,** part of a thickening of the visceral pelvic fascia beside the cervix and vagina, passing laterally to merge with the upper fascia of the pelvic diaphragm; called also *lateral cervical l.* **carpal l., dorsal,** see *ligamenta intercarpea dorsalia*. **carpal l., radiate,** ligamentum carpi radiatum. **carpometacarpal l's, anterior,** ligamenta carpometacarpalia palmaria. **carpometacarpal l's, dorsal,** ligamenta carpometacarpalia dorsalia. **carpometacarpal l's, palmar,** ligamenta metacarpalia palmaria. **carpometacarpal l's, posterior,** ligamenta carpometacarpalia dorsalia. **carpometacarpal l's, volar,** ligamenta carpometacarpalia palmaria. **Casser's l., casserian l.,** ligamentum mallei laterale. **caudal l. of common integument,** retinaculum caudale. **ceratocricoid l.,** ligamentum ceratocricoideum. **cervical l., anterior,** membrana tectoria. **cervical l., lateral,** cardinal l. **cervical l., posterior,** ligamentum nuchae. **cervical l. of sinus tarsi,** a strong band behind the bifurcate ligament, extending upward to the neck of the talus. **cervicobasilar l.,** membrana tectoria. **check l's of axis,** ligamenta alaria. **chondrosternal l., interarticular,** ligamentum sternocostale intra-articulare. **chondroxiphoid l's,** ligamenta costoxiphoidea. **l. of Civinini,** ligamentum pterygospinale. **Clado's l.,** an occasional peritoneal fold connecting the infundibulopelvic ligament and the mesoappendix. **clavicular l., external capsular,** ligamentum acromioclaviculare. **Cloquet's l.,** vestigium processus vaginalis. **coccygeal l., superior,** ligamentum iliofemorale. **collateral l., fibular,** ligamentum collaterale fibulare. **collateral l.,**

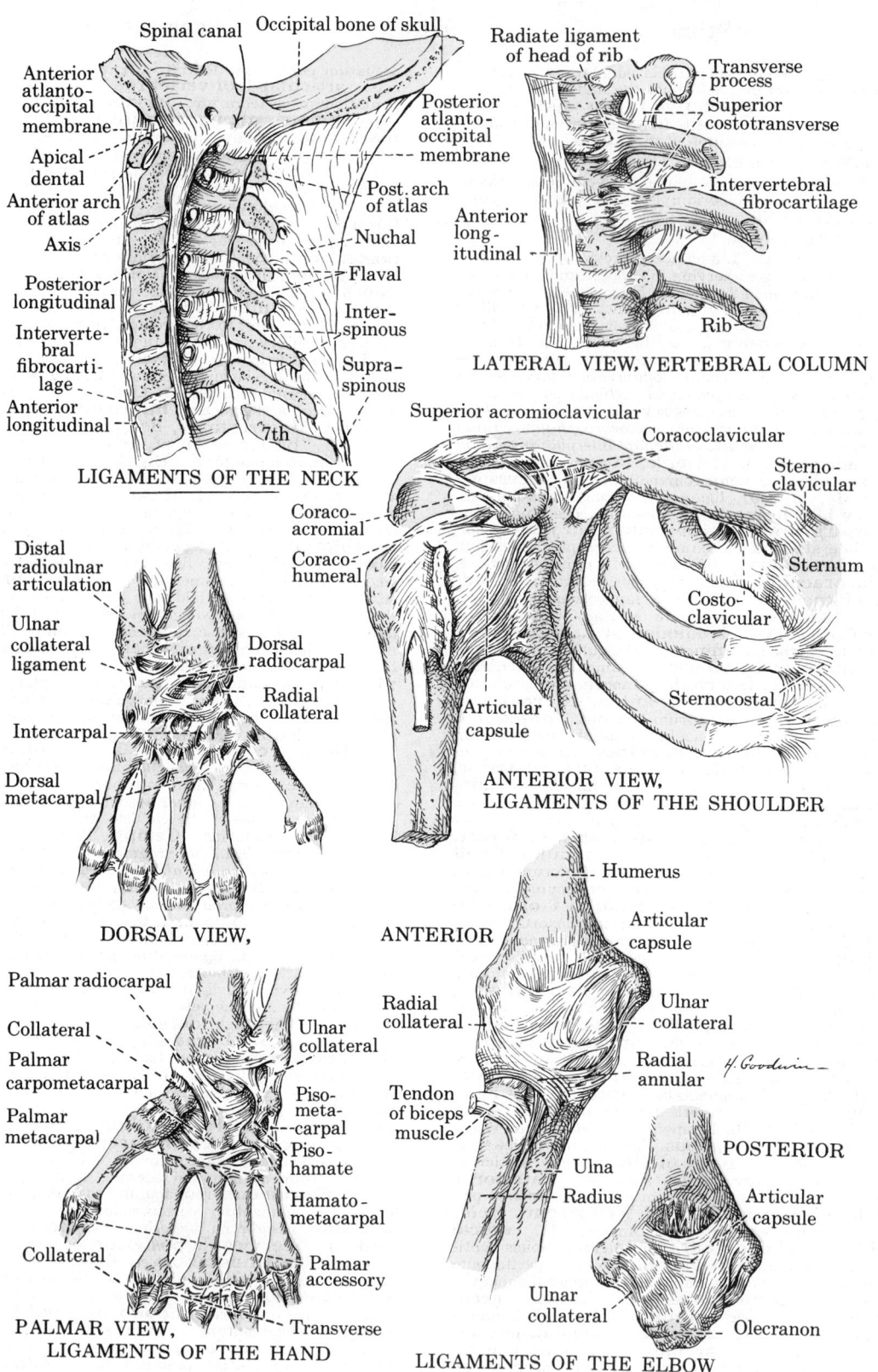

Spinal canal

Occipital bone of skull

Anterior atlanto-occipital membrane

Apical dental

Anterior arch of atlas

Axis

Posterior longitudinal

Intervertebral fibrocartilage

Anterior longitudinal

Posterior atlanto-occipital membrane

Post. arch of atlas

Nuchal

Flaval

Inter-spinous

Supra-spinous

7th

LIGAMENTS OF THE NECK

Radiate ligament of head of rib

Transverse process

Superior costotransverse

Intervertebral fibrocartilage

Anterior long-itudinal

Rib

LATERAL VIEW, VERTEBRAL COLUMN

Distal radioulnar articulation

Ulnar collateral ligament

Intercarpal

Dorsal metacarpal

Dorsal radiocarpal

Radial collateral

DORSAL VIEW,

Superior acromioclavicular

Coracoclavicular

Sterno-clavicular

Coraco-acromial

Coraco-humeral

Costo-clavicular

Sternum

Articular capsule

Sternocostal

ANTERIOR VIEW, LIGAMENTS OF THE SHOULDER

Palmar radiocarpal

Collateral

Palmar carpometacarpal

Palmar metacarpal

Ulnar collateral

Piso-meta-carpal

Piso-hamate

Hamato-metacarpal

Collateral

Palmar accessory

PALMAR VIEW, LIGAMENTS OF THE HAND

Transverse

ANTERIOR

Humerus

Articular capsule

Radial collateral

Ulnar collateral

Radial annular

Tendon of biceps muscle

H. Goodwin

Ulna

Radius

POSTERIOR

Articular capsule

Ulnar collateral

Olecranon

LIGAMENTS OF THE ELBOW

PLATE 22 —ARTICULAR LIGAMENTS

922

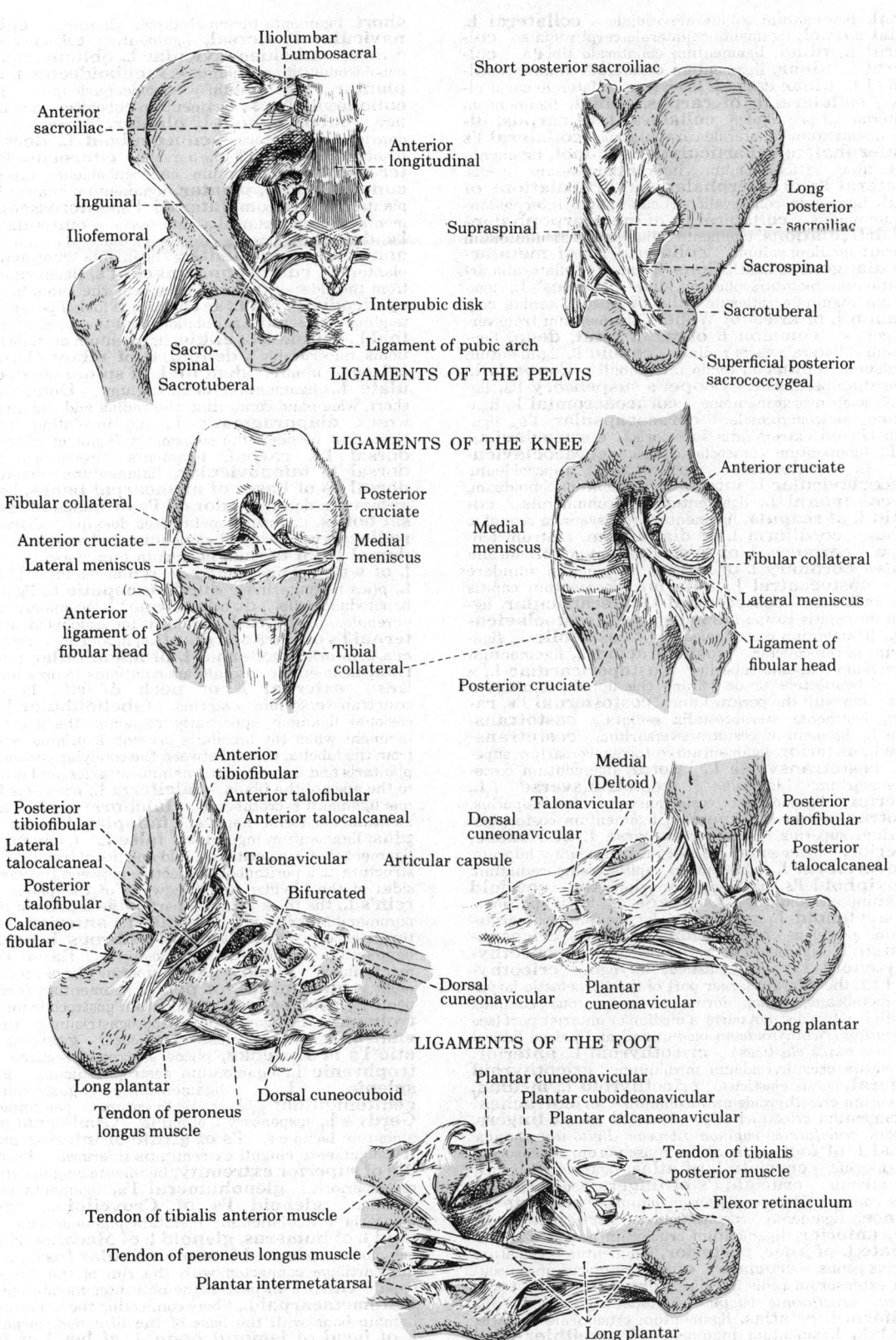

Iliolumbar
Lumbosacral
Anterior
sacroiliac
Anterior
longitudinal
Inguinal
Iliofemoral
Interpubic disk
Sacro-
spinal
Sacrotuberal
Ligament of pubic arch

Short posterior sacroiliac
Long
posterior
sacroiliac
Supraspinal
Sacrospinal
Sacrotuberal
Superficial posterior
sacrococcygeal

LIGAMENTS OF THE PELVIS

LIGAMENTS OF THE KNEE

Fibular collateral
Anterior cruciate
Lateral meniscus
Anterior
ligament of
fibular head
Posterior
cruciate
Medial
meniscus
Tibial
collateral

Anterior cruciate
Medial
meniscus
Fibular collateral
Lateral meniscus
Ligament of
fibular head
Posterior cruciate

Anterior
tibiofibular
Anterior talofibular
Anterior talocalcaneal
Posterior
tibiofibular
Lateral
talocalcaneal
Posterior
talofibular
Calcaneo-
fibular
Talonavicular
Articular capsule
Bifurcated
Dorsal
cuneonavicular
Long plantar
Dorsal cuneocuboid
Tendon of peroneus
longus muscle

Medial
(Deltoid)
Talonavicular
Dorsal
cuneonavicular
Posterior
talofibular
Posterior
talocalcaneal
Plantar
cuneonavicular
Long plantar

LIGAMENTS OF THE FOOT

Plantar cuneonavicular
Plantar cuboideonavicular
Plantar calcaneonavicular
Tendon of tibialis
posterior muscle
Flexor retinaculum
Tendon of tibialis anterior muscle
Tendon of peroneus longus muscle
Plantar intermetatarsal
Long plantar

PLATE 23 —ARTICULAR LIGAMENTS

923

radial, ligamentum collaterale radiale. **collateral l., radial carpal,** ligamenta collaterale carpi radiale. **collateral l., tibial,** ligamentum collaterale tibiale. **collateral l., ulnar,** ligamentum collaterale ulnare. **collateral l., ulnar carpal,** ligamenta collaterale carpi ulnare. **collateral l. of carpus, radial,** ligamentum collaterale carpi radiale. **collateral l. of carpus, ulnar,** ligamentum collaterale carpi ulnare. **collateral l's of interphalangeal articulations of foot,** ligamenta collateralia articulationum interphalangealium pedis. **collateral l's of interphalangeal articulations of hand,** ligamenta collateralia articulationum interphalangealium manus. **collateral l's of metacarpophalangeal articulations,** ligamenta collateralia articulationum metacarpophalangealium. **collateral l's of metatarsophalangeal articulations,** ligamenta collateralia articulationum metatarsophalangealium. **Colles' l.,** ligamentum inguinale reflexum. **l's of colon,** teniae coli. **common l. of knee (of Weber),** ligamentum transversum genus. **common l. of wrist joint, deep,** ligamentum collaterale carpi radiale. **conoid l.,** ligamentum conoideum. **conus l.,** tendo infundibuli. **Cooper's l.,** ligamentum pectineale. **Cooper's suspensory l's,** ligamenta suspensoria mammae. **coracoacromial l.,** ligamentum coracoacromiale. **coracocapsular l's,** ligamenta cinguli extremitatis superioris. **coracoclavicular l.,** ligamentum coracoclaviculare. **coracoclavicular l., external,** ligamentum trapezoideum. **coracoclavicular l., internal,** ligamentum conoideum. **coracohumeral l.,** ligamentum coracohumerale. **coracoid l. of scapula,** ligamentum transversum scapulae superius. **cordiform l. of diaphragm,** centrum tendineum. **coronary l. of liver,** ligamentum coronarium hepatis. **coronary l. of radius,** ligamentum annulare radii. **costocentral l., anterior,** ligamentum capitis costae radiatum. **costocentral l., interarticular,** ligamentum capitis costae intra-articulare. **costoclavicular l.,** ligamentum costoclaviculare. **costocolic l.,** ligamentum phrenicolicum. **costocoracoid l.,** ligamentum transversum scapulae superius. **costopericardiac l.,** a band of connective tissue joining the upper costosternal articulation with the pericardium. **costosternal l's, radiate,** ligamenta sternocostalia radiata. **costotransverse l.,** ligamentum costotransversarium. **costotransverse l., anterior,** ligamentum costotransversarium superius. **costotransverse l., lateral,** ligamentum costotransversarium laterale. **costotransverse l., posterior,** ligamentum costotransversarium superius. **costotransverse l., superior,** ligamentum costotransversarium superius. **costotransverse l. of Krause, posterior,** ligamentum costotransversarium laterale. **costovertebral l.,** ligamentum capitis costae radiatum. **costoxiphoid l's,** ligamenta costoxiphoidea. **cotyloid l.,** labrum acetabulare. **Cowper's l.,** fascia pectinea. **cricoarytenoid l., posterior,** ligamentum cricoarytenoideum posterius. **cricopharyngeal l., cricosantorinian l.,** ligamentum cricopharyngeum. **cricothyroarytenoid l.,** conus elasticus laryngis. **cricothyroid l.,** 1. the inferior, larger part of the fibroelastic laryngeal membrane, which forms a ligamentous complex consisting of two distinct parts: a median or anterior part (see *ligamentum cricothyroideum medianum*) and paired lateral parts (see *conus elasticus*). **cricothyroid l., anterior,** ligamentum cricothyroideum medianum. **cricothyroid l., lateral,** conus elasticus. **cricothyroid l., median,** ligamentum cricothyroideum medianum. **cricotracheal l.,** ligamentum cricotracheale. **crucial l. of fingers,** see *pars cruciformis vaginae fibrosae digitorum manus.* **crucial l. of foot,** retinaculum musculorum extensorum pedis inferius. **cruciate l. of atlas,** ligamentum cruciforme atlantis. **cruciate l's of fingers,** see *pars cruciformis vaginae fibrosae digitorum manus.* **cruciate l's of knee,** ligamenta cruciata genus. **cruciate l. of knee, anterior,** ligamentum cruciatum anterius genus. **cruciate l. of knee, posterior,** ligamentum cruciatum posterius genus. **cruciate l. of leg,** retinaculum musculorum extensorum pedis inferius. **cruciate l's of toes,** see *pars cruciformis vaginae fibrosae digitorum pedis.* **cruciform l. of atlas,** ligamentum cruciforme atlantis. **crural l.,** ligamentum inguinale. **Cruveilhier's l's,** ligamenta palmaria. **cubitoradial l.,** chorda obliqua membranae interosseae antibrachii. **cubitoulnar l.,** ligamentum collaterale ulnare. **cuboideometatarsal l's,**

short, ligamenta tarsometatarsea plantaria. **cuboideonavicular l., dorsal,** ligamentum cuboideonaviculare dorsale. **cuboideonavicular l., oblique,** ligamentum cuboideonaviculare plantare. **cuboideonavicular l., plantar,** ligamentum cuboideonaviculare plantare. **cubonavicular l.,** ligamentum cuboideonaviculare plantare. **cuboscaphoid l., plantar,** ligamentum cuboideonaviculare plantare. **cuneocuboid l., dorsal,** ligamentum cuneocuboideum dorsale. **cuneocuboid l., interosseous,** ligamentum cuneocuboideum interosseum. **cuneocuboid l., plantar,** ligamentum cuneocuboideum plantare. **cuneometatarsal l's, interosseous,** ligamenta cuneometatarsalia interossea. **cuneonavicular l's, dorsal,** ligamenta cuneonavicularia dorsalia. **cuneonavicular l's, plantar,** ligamenta cuneonavicularia plantaria. **cutaneophalangeal l's,** ligamentous fibers from the sides of the phalanges near the joints to the skin. **cysticoduodenal l.,** an anomalous fold of peritoneum extending between the gallbladder and the duodenum. **deltoid l., deltoid l. of ankle,** ligamentum mediale articulationis talocruralis. **deltoid l. of elbow,** ligamentum collaterale ulnare. **dentate l. of spinal cord, denticulate l.,** ligamentum denticulatum. **Denucé's l.,** a short, wide band connecting the radius and the ulna at the wrist. **diaphragmatic l.,** the involuting urogenital ridge that becomes the suspensory ligament of the ovary. **dorsal l's, carpal,** ligamenta intercarpea dorsalia. **dorsal l., talonavicular,** ligamentum talonaviculare. **dorsal l's of bases of metacarpal bones,** ligamenta metacarpea dorsalia. **dorsal l's of bases of metatarsal bones,** ligamenta metatarsea dorsalia. **dorsal l. of radiocarpal joint,** ligamentum radiocarpeum dorsale. **dorsal l's of tarsus,** ligamenta tarsi dorsalia. **dorsal l. of wrist,** retinaculum extensorum manus. **Douglas' l.,** plica rectouterina. **duodenohepatic l.,** ligamentum hepatoduodenale. **duodenorenal l.,** ligamentum duodenorenale. **epihyal l.,** ligamentum stylohyoideum. **external l's of Barkow, plantar,** ligamenta intercuneiformia plantaria. **external l. of mandibular articulation,** ligamentum laterale articulationis temporomandibularis. **external l. of neck of rib,** ligamentum costotransversarium posterius. **fabellofibular l.,** an occasional ligament apparently replacing the short lateral ligament when the fabella is present; it originates directly from the fabella, passes between the condylar portions of the plantaris and lateral gastrocnemius muscles, and is attached to the apex of the fibula. **falciform l.,** processus falciformis ligamenti sacrotuberosi. **falciform l. of liver,** ligamentum falciforme hepatis. **fallopian l., l. of Fallopius,** ligamentum inguinale. **false l.,** 1. any suspensory ligament that is a peritoneal fold and not of true ligamentous structure. 2. a peritoneal connection between the vertex and sides of the bladder and the walls of the pelvis. **Ferrein's l.,** the thick external part of the capsule of the temporomandibular joint. **fibrous l., anterior,** ligamentum sternoclaviculare anterius. **fibrous l. posterior,** ligamentum sternoclaviculare posterius. **flaval l's,** ligamenta flava. **Flood's l.,** the superior glenohumeral ligament. **fundiform l. of penis,** ligamentum fundiforme penis. **gastrocolic l.,** ligamentum gastrocolicum. **gastrohepatic l.,** ligamentum hepatogastricum. **gastrolienal l.,** ligamentum gastrosplenicum. **gastropancreatic l's of Huschke,** plicae gastropancreaticae. **gastrophrenic l.,** ligamentum gastrophrenicum. **gastrosplenic l.,** ligamentum gastrosplenicum. **genitoinguinal l.,** ligamentum genitoinguinale. **Gerdy's l.,** suspensory l. of axilla. **Gimbernat's l.,** ligamentum lacunare. **l's of girdle of inferior extremity,** ligamenta cinguli extremitatis inferioris. **l's of girdle of superior extremity,** ligamenta cinguli extremitatis superioris. **glenohumeral l's,** ligamenta glenohumeralia. **glenoid l's of Cruveilhier,** ligamenta plantaria articulationum metatarsophalangearum. **glenoid l. of humerus, glenoid l. of Macalister,** labrum glenoidale. **glenoid l. of mandibular fossa,** a ring of fibrocartilage connected with the rim of the mandibular fossa. **Günz's l.,** part of the obturator membrane. **hamatometacarpal l.,** fibers connecting the hamulus of the hamate bone with the base of the fifth metacarpal bone. **l. of head of femoral bone, l. of head of femur,** ligamentum capitis femoris. **Helmholtz's l.,** that part of the anterior ligament of the malleus which is attached to the greater tympanic spine. **l's of Helvetius,** ligamenta pylori. **Henle's l.,** falx inguinalis. **Hensing's l.,** a small serous fold from the upper end of the descending colon to the abdominal wall. **hepatic l's,** ligamenta hepatis. **hepatocolic l.,** ligamentum hepatocolicum. **hepatocystocolic l.,** a hepatocolic ligament arising from the gallbladder. **hepatoduodenal l.,** ligamentum hepatoduodenale. **hepatogastric l.,** ligamentum hepatogastricum. **hepatogastroduodenal l.,** omentum minus. **hepatorenal l.,** ligamentum hepatorenale. **hepatoumbilical l.,** ligamentum teres hepatis. **Hesselbach's l.,** ligamentum interfoveolare. **Hey's l.,** margo falciformis hiatus saphenus. **Hueck's l.,** reticulum trabeculare anguli iridocornealis. **Humphry's l.,** ligamentum meniscofemorale anterius. **Hunter's l.,** ligamentum teres uteri. **Huschke's l's,** plicae gastropancreaticae. **hyaloideocapsular l.,** the tissue connecting the vitreous body to the peripheral zone of the lens capsule. **hyoepiglottic l.,** ligamentum hyoepiglotticum. **iliocostal l.,** ligamentum lumbocostale. **iliofemoral l.,** ligamentum iliofemorale. **iliolumbar l.,** ligamentum iliolumbale. **iliopectineal l.,** arcus iliopectineus. **iliopubic l.,** ligamentum inguinale. **iliosacral l's, anterior,** ligamenta sacroiliaca ventralia. **iliosacral l's, interosseous,** ligamenta sacroiliaca interossea. **iliosacral l., long,** ligamentum sacroiliaca dorsalia. **iliotibial l. of Maissiat,** tractus iliotibialis. **iliotrochanteric l.,** a portion of the articular capsule of the hip joint. **inferior l. of epididymis,** ligamentum epididymidis inferius. **inferior l. of neck of rib,** posterior portion of ligamentum costotransversarium posterius. **inferior l. of neck of rib of Henle,** ligamentum costotransversarium. **inferior l. of tubercle of rib,** ligamentum costotransversarium laterale. **infundibulopelvic l.,** ligamentum suspensorium ovarii. **inguinal l.,** ligamentum inguinale. **inguinal l., anterior,** crus mediale anuli inguinalis superficialis. **inguinal l., external,** ligamentum inguinale. **inguinal l., internal,** 1. ligamentum inguinale reflexum. 2. crus mediale anuli inguinalis superficialis. **inguinal l., posterior,** ligamentum interfoveolare. **inguinal l., reflex,** ligamentum inguinale reflexum. **inguinal l. of Blumberg,** ligamentum interfoveolare. **inguinal l. of Cooper,** ligamentum pectineale. **interarticular l.,** any ligament situated within the capsule of a joint. **interarticular l. of articulation of humerus,** caput longum musculi bicipitis brachii. **interarticular l. of head of rib,** ligamentum capitis costae intra-articulare. **interarticular l. of hip joint,** ligamentum capitis femoris. **interarticular sternocostal l.,** ligamentum sternocostale intra-articulare. **intercarpal l's, dorsal,** ligamenta intercarpalia dorsalia. **intercarpal l's, interosseous,** ligamenta intercarpalia interossea. **intercarpal l's, palmar,** ligamenta intercarpalia palmaria. **intercarpal l's, volar,** ligamenta intercarpalia palmaria. **interclavicular l.,** ligamentum interclaviculare. **intercostal l's, external,** see *membrana intercostalis externa.* **intercostal l's, internal,** see *membrana intercostalis interna.* **intercuneiform l's, dorsal,** ligamenta intercuneiformia dorsalia. **intercuneiform l's, interosseous,** ligamenta intercuneiformia interossea. **intercuneiform l's, plantar,** ligamenta intercuneiformia plantaria. **interfoveolar l.,** ligamentum interfoveolare. **intermaxillary l.,** raphe pterygomandibularis. **intermetacarpal l's, anterior, intermetacarpal l's, distal,** see *ligamentum metacarpeum transversum profundum.* **intermetacarpal l's, dorsal,** ligamenta metacarpalia dorsalia. **intermetacarpal l's, interosseous,** ligamenta metacarpalia interossea. **intermetacarpal l's, palmar,** ligamenta metacarpalia palmaria. **intermetacarpal l's, proximal, anterior,** ligamentametacarpalia palmaria. **intermetacarpal l's, proximal, posterior,** ligamenta metacarpalia dorsalia. **intermetacarpal l's, transverse, dorsal,** ligamenta metacarpalia dorsalia. **intermetacarpal l's, transverse, volar,** ligamenta metacarpalia palmaria. **intermetatarsal l's, interosseous,** ligamenta metatarsalia interossea. **intermetatarsal l's, plantar, distal,** see *ligamentum metatarsale transversum profundum.* **intermetatarsal l's, proximal, dorsal,** ligamenta metatarsalia dorsalia. **intermetatarsal l's, proximal, plantar,** ligamenta metatarsalia plantaria. **intermetatarsal l's, transverse, dorsal,** ligamenta metatarsalia dorsalia. **intermetatarsal l's, transverse, plantar,** ligamenta metatarsalia plantaria. **intermuscular l., fibular,** septum

intermusculare anterius cruris. **intermuscular l. of arm, external,** septum intermusculare brachii laterale. **intermuscular l. of arm, internal,** septum intermusculare brachii mediale. **intermuscular l. of arm, lateral,** septum intermusculare brachii laterale. **intermuscular l. of arm, medial,** septum intermusculare brachii mediale. **intermuscular l. of thigh, external,** septum intermusculare femoris laterale. **intermuscular l. of thigh, lateral,** septum intermusculare femoris laterale. **intermuscular l. of thigh, medial,** septum intermusculare femoris mediale. **internal l. of neck of rib,** ligamentum costotransversarium superius. **interosseous l., radioulnar,** membrana interossea antebrachii. **interosseous l's, transverse metacarpal,** ligamenta metacarpea interossea. **interosseous l's of Barkow, internal,** ligamenta intercuneiformia plantaria. **interosseous l's of bases of metacarpal bones,** ligamenta metacarpea interossea. **interosseous l's of bases of metatarsal bones,** ligamenta metatarsea interossea. **interosseous l. of Cruveilhier, costovertebral,** ligamentum capitis costae intra-articulare. **interosseous l. of Cruveilhier, transversocostal,** ligamentum costotransversarium. **interosseous l's of knee,** ligamenta cruciata genus. **interosseous l. of leg,** membrana interossea cruris. **interosseous l. of pubis,** discus interpubicus. **interosseous l. of pubis (of Winslow),** ligamentum transversum perinei. **interosseous l's of tarsus,** ligamenta tarsi interossea. **l's of interphalangeal articulations of foot, plantar,** ligamenta plantaria articulationum interphalangealium pedis. **l's of interphalangeal articulations of hand, palmar,** ligamenta palmaria articulationum interphalangealium manus. **interprocess l.,** a ligament that connects two processes on the same bone. **interpubic l.,** discus interpubicus. **interspinal l's, interspinous l's,** ligamenta interspinalia. **intertarsal l's, dorsal,** ligamenta tarsi dorsalia. **intertarsal l's, interosseous,** ligamenta tarsi interossea. **intertarsal l's, plantar,** ligamenta tarsi plantaria. **intertransverse l's,** ligamenta intertransversaria. **interureteral l.,** plica interureterica. **intervertebral l.,** 1. either of the two longitudinal ligaments of the vertebrae (ligamentum longitudinale anterius and ligamentum longitudinale posterius). 2. one of the disci intervertebrales. **intraarticular l. of head of rib,** ligamentum capitis costae intra-articulare. **ischiocapsular l., ischiofemoral l.,** ligamentum ischiofemorale. **ischioprostatic l.,** diaphragma urogenitale. **ischiosacral l's,** see *ligamentum sacrospinale* and *ligamentum sacrotuberale.* **Krause's l.,** ligamentum transversum perinei. **laciniate l.,** retinaculum musculorum flexorum pedis. **laciniate l., external,** retinaculum musculorum peroneorum superius. **lacunar l., lacunar l. of Gimbernat,** ligamentum lacunare. **lambdoid l.,** retinaculum musculorum extensorum pedis inferius. **lateral l. of ankle joint,** ligamentum laterale articulationis talocruralis. **lateral l. of carpus, radial,** ligamentum collaterale carpi radiale. **lateral l. of carpus, ulnar,** ligamentum collaterale carpi ulnare. **lateral l. of colon,** tenia omentalis. **lateral l's of joints of fingers,** ligamenta collateralia articulationum interphalangearum manus. **lateral l's of joints of toes,** ligamenta collateralia articulationum interphalangearum pedis. **lateral l. of knee,** ligamentum collaterale fibulare. **lateral l's of liver,** see *ligamentum triangulare dextrum hepatis* and *ligamentum triangulare sinistrum hepatis.* **lateral l. of malleus,** ligamentum mallei laterale. **lateral meniscofemoral l.,** ligamentum meniscofemorale posterius. **lateral l's of metacarpophalangeal joints,** ligamenta collateralia articulationum metacarpophalangearum. **lateral l's of metatarsophalangeal joints,** ligamenta collateralia articulationum metatarsophalangearum. **lateral l. of temporomandibular articulation,** ligamentum laterale articulationis temporomandibularis. **lateral l. of temporomandibular joint, external,** ligamentum laterale articulationis temporomandibularis. **lateral l. of temporomandibular joint, internal,** ligamentum sphenomandibulare. **lateral l. of wrist joint, external,** ligamentum collaterale carpi radiale. **lateral l. of wrist joint, internal,** ligamentum collaterale carpi ulnare. **Lauth's l.,** ligamentum transversum atlantis. **l. of left superior vena cava,** plica venae cavae sinistrae. **lienophrenic l.,** ligamentum splenorenale. **lienorenal l.,** a fold of peritoneum connecting the spleen and the left kidney. **Lisfranc's l.,** a fibrous band running from the lower external surface of the medial cuneiform bone to the internal surface of the base of the second metatarsal bone. **Lockwood's l.,** the thickened area of contact between Tenon's capsule and the sheaths of the inferior rectus and inferior oblique muscles. **longitudinal l., anterior,** ligamentum longitudinale anterius. **longitudinal l., posterior,** ligamentum longitudinale posterius. **longitudinal l. of abdomen,** linea alba. **lumbocostal l.,** ligamentum lumbocostale. **l's of Luschka,** ligamenta sternopericardiaca. **Mackenrodt's l.,** plica rectouterina. **l. of Maissiat,** tractus iliotibialis. **Mauchart's l's,** ligamenta alaria. **maxillary l., lateral,** ligamentum laterale articulationis temporomandibularis. **maxillary l., middle,** ligamentum sphenomandibulare. **l. of Mayer,** ligamentum carpi radiatum. **Meckel's l.,** Meckel's band. **medial l. of elbow joint,** ligamentum collaterale ulnare. **medial l. of temporomandibular articulation,** ligamentum me- diale articulationis temporomandibularis. **medial l. of wrist,** ligamentum collaterale carpi ulnare. **meniscofemoral l., anterior,** ligamentum meniscofemorale anterius. **meniscofemoral l., posterior,** ligamentum meniscofemorale posterius. **mesocolic l. of colon,** tenia mesocolica. **metacarpal l's, dorsal,** ligamenta metacarpalia dorsalia. **metacarpal l's, interosseous,** ligamenta metacarpalia interossea. **metacarpal l's, palmar,** ligamenta metacarpalia palmaria. **metacarpal l's, transverse, deep,** ligamenta metacarpalium transversum profundum. **metacarpal l., transverse, superficial,** ligamentum metacarpale transversum superficiale. **metacarpophalangeal l's, anterior, metacarpophalangeal l's, palmar,** ligamenta palmaria. **l's of metacarpophalangeal articulations, palmar,** ligamenta palmaria articulationum metacarpophalangealium. **metatarsal l., anterior,** ligamentum metatarsale transversum profundum. **metatarsal l's, dorsal,** ligamenta metatarsalia dorsalia. **metatarsal l's, interosseus,** ligamenta metatarsalia interossea. **metatarsal l's, lateral,** ligamenta metatarsalia interossea. **metatarsal l's, lateral proper (of Weber), metatarsal l's, lateral (of Weitbrecht),** ligamenta metatarsalia interossea. **metatarsal l's, plantar,** ligamenta metatarsalia plantaria. **metatarsal l., transverse, deep,** ligamentum metatarsale transversum profundum. **metatarsal l., transverse, interosseous,** ligamentum metatarsale interosseum. **metatarsal l., transverse, superficial,** ligamentum metatarsale transversum superficiale. **metatarsophalangeal l's, inferior,** ligamenta plantaria articulationum metatarsophalangealium. **l's of metatarsophalangeal articulations, plantar,** ligamenta plantaria articulationum metatarsophalangealium. **middle l. of neck of rib,** ligamentum costotransversarium. **mucous l.,** plica synovialis. **l. of nape,** ligamentum nuchae. **navicularicuneiform l's, plantar,** ligamenta cuneonavicularia plantaria. **nephrocolic l.,** fasciculi from the fatty capsule of the kidney passing down on the right side to the posterior wall of the ascending colon and on the left side to the posterior wall of the descending colon. **nuchal l.,** ligamentum nuchae. **oblique l. of Cooper, oblique l. of forearm,** chorda obliqua membranae interosseae antebrachii. **oblique l's of knee,** ligamenta cruciata genus. **oblique l. of knee, posterior,** ligamentum popliteum obliquum. **oblique l. of scapula,** ligamentum transversum scapulae superius. **oblique l. of superior radioulnar joint,** chorda obliqua membranae interosseae antebrachii. **obturator l., atlantooccipital,** membrana atlantooccipitalis anterior. **obturator l. of atlas,** see *membrana atlantooccipitalis anterior* and *posterior*. **obturator l. of pelvis,** membrana obturatoria. **occipitoaxial l.,** membrana tectoria. **occipitoodontoid l's,** ligamenta alaria. **odontoid l., middle,** ligamentum apicis dentis axis. **odontoid l's of axis,** ligamenta alaria. **orbicular l. of radius,** ligamentum anulare radii. **ovarian l.,** ligamentum ovarii proprium. **palmar l's,** 1. see *ligamenta palmaria articulationum interphalangealium manus* and *ligamenta palmaria articulationum metacarpophalangealium.* 2. see *aponeurosis palmaria.* **palmar l., transverse, deep,** ligamentum metacarpeum transversum profundum. **palmar l. of carpus,** ligamentum carpi radiatum. **palmar l. of radiocarpal joint,** ligamentum radiocarpeum palmare. **palpebral l., medial,** ligamentum palpebrale mediale. **patellar l.,**

orale posterius. **round l. of acetabulum,** ligamentum capitis femoris. **round l. of Cloquet,** ligamentum capitis costae intraarticulare. **round l. of femur,** ligamentum capitis femoris. **round l. of forearm,** chorda obliqua membranae interosseae antebrachii. **round l. of uterus,** ligamentum teres uteri. **sacciform l.,** capsula articularis radioulnaris distalis. **sacrococcygeal l., anterior,** ligamentum sacrococcygeum anterius. **sacrococcygeal l., dorsal, deep,** ligamentum sacrococcygeum posterius profundum. **sacrococcygeal l., dorsal, superficial,** ligamentum sacrococcygeum posterius superficiale. **sacrococcygeal l., lateral,** ligamentum sacrococcygeum laterale. **sacrococcygeal l., posterior, deep,** ligamentum sacrococcygeum posterius profundum. **sacrococcygeal l., posterior, superficial,** ligamentum sacrococcygeum posterius superficiale. **sacrococcygeal l., ventral,** ligamentum sacrococcygeum anterius. **sacroiliac l's, anterior,** ligamenta sacroiliaca anteriora. **sacroiliac l's, dorsal,** ligamenta sacroiliaca posteriora. **sacroiliac l's, interosseous,** ligamenta sacroiliaca interossea. **sacroiliac l's, posterior,** ligamenta sacroiliaca posteriora. **sacroiliac l's, ventral,** ligamenta sacroiliaca anteriora. **sacrosciatic l., anterior,** ligamentum sacrospinale. **sacrosciatic l., great,** ligamentum sacrotuberale. **sacrosciatic l., internal,** ligamentum sacrospinale. **sacrosciatic l., least,** ligamentum sacrospinale. **sacrospinal l., sacrospinous l.,** ligamentum sacrospinale. **sacrotuberal l., sacrotuberous l.,** ligamentum sacrotuberale. **salpingopharyngeal l.,** plica salpingopharyngea. **Santorini's l.,** ligamentum cricopharyngeum. **Sappey's l.,** the thicker posterior part of the capsule of the temporomandibular joint. **scaphocuneiform l's, plantar,** ligamenta cuneonavicularia plantaria. **l. of Scarpa,** cornu superius marginis falciformis. **Schlemm's l's,** two ligamentous bands strengthening the capsule of the shoulder joint. **scrotal l. of testis,** gubernaculum testis. **serous l.,** ligamentum serosum. **short lateral l.,** a knee ligament attached to the lowest part of the lateral femoral condyle and extending beyond the dorsum of the semilunar cartilage to the apex of the fibula. See also *fabellofibular l.* **short plantar l.,** ligamenta calcaneocuboideum plantare. **sphenoidal l., external,** ligamentum intercuneiformia plantaria. **sphenoideotarsal l's,** ligamenta tarsometatarsea plantaria. **sphenomandibular l.,** ligamentum sphenomandibulare. **spinoglenoid l.,** ligamentum transversum scapulae inferius. **spinosacral l.,** ligamentum sacrospinale. **spiral l. of cochlea,** crista spiralis. **splenogastric l.,** ligamentum gastrosplenicum. **splenophrenic l.,** ligamentum splenorenale. **splenorenal l.,** ligamentum splenorenale. **spring l.,** ligamentum calcaneonaviculare plantare. **stapedial l.,** l. annulare stapedis. **stellate l.,** ligamentum capitis costae radiatum. **sternoclavicular l., anterior,** ligamentum sternoclaviculare anterius. **sternoclavicular l., posterior,** ligamentum sternoclaviculare posterius. **sternocostal l's,** ligamenta sternodiscus interpubicus. **pubocapsular l.,** ligamentum pubofemorale. **pubofemoral l.,** ligamentum pubofemorale. **puboischiadic l. of prostate gland,** fascia diaphragmatis urogenitalis superior. **puboprostatic l.,** ligamentum puboprostaticum. **puborectal l.,** 1. ligamentum puboprostaticum. 2. ligamentum pubovesicale. **pubovesical l.,** ligamentum pubovesicale. **pulmonary l.,** ligamentum pulmonale. **quadrate l.,** ligamentum quadratum. **radial l., lateral,** ligamentum collaterale carpi radiale. **radial l. of cubitocarpal articulation,** ligamentum collaterale carpi radiale. **radiate l.,** ligamentum capitis costae radiatum. **radiate l., lateral,** ligamentum collaterale carpi ulnare. **radiate l. of carpus,** ligamentum carpi radiatum. **radiate l. of head of rib,** ligamentum capitis costae radiatum. **radiate l. of Mayer,** ligamentum carpi radiatum. **radiocarpal l., anterior,** ligamentum radiocarpale palmare. **radiocarpal l., dorsal,** ligamentum radiocarpale dorsale. **radiocarpal l., palmar,** ligamentum radiocarpale palmare. **radiocarpal l., volar,** ligamentum radiocarpale palmare. **rectouterine l.,** musculus rectouterinus. **reflex l. of Gimbernat,** ligamentum inguinale reflexum. **reinforcing l's,** ligaments that serve to reinforce joint capsules. **rhomboid l. of clavicle,** ligamentum costoclaviculare. **rhomboid l. of wrist,** ligamentum radiocarpeum dorsale. **ring l. of hip joint,** zona orbicularis articulationis coxae. **Robert's l.,** ligamentum meniscofemorale posterius. **round l. of acetabulum,** ligamentum capitis femoris. **round l. of Cloquet,** ligamentum capitis costae intraarticulare. **round l. of femur,** ligamentum capitis femoris. **round l. of forearm,** chorda obliqua membranae interosseae antebrachii. **round l. of uterus,** ligamentum teres uteri. **sacciform l.,** capsula articularis radioulnaris distalis. **sacrococcygeal l., anterior,** ligamentum sacrococcygeum anterius. **sacrococcygeal l., dorsal, deep,** ligamentum sacrococcygeum posterius profundum. **sacrococcygeal l., dorsal, superficial,** ligamentum sacrococcygeum posterius superficiale. **sacrococcygeal l., lateral,** ligamentum sacrococcygeum laterale. **sacrococcygeal l., posterior, deep,** ligamentum sacrococcygeum posterius profundum. **sacrococcygeal l., posterior, superficial,** ligamentum sacrococcygeum posterius superficiale. **sacrococcygeal l., ventral,** ligamentum sacrococcygeum anterius. **sacroiliac l's, anterior,** ligamenta sacroiliaca anteriora. **sacroiliac l's, dorsal,** ligamenta sacroiliaca posteriora. **sacroiliac l's, interosseous,** ligamenta sacroiliaca interossea. **sacroiliac l's, posterior,** ligamenta sacroiliaca posteriora. **sacroiliac l's, ventral,** ligamenta sacroiliaca anteriora. **sacrosciatic l., anterior,** ligamentum sacrospinale. **sacrosciatic l., great,** ligamentum sacrotuberale. **sacrosciatic l., internal,** ligamentum sacrospinale. **sacrosciatic l., least,** ligamentum sacrospinale. **sacrospinal l., sacrospinous l.,** ligamentum sacrospinale. **sacrotuberal l., sacrotuberous l.,** ligamentum sacrotuberale. **salpingopharyngeal l.,** plica salpingopharyngea. **Santorini's l.,** ligamentum cricopharyngeum. **Sappey's l.,** the thicker posterior part of the capsule of the temporomandibular joint. **scaphocuneiform l's, plantar,** ligamenta cuneonavicularia plantaria. **l. of Scarpa,** cornu superius marginis falciformis. **Schlemm's l's,** two ligamentous bands strengthening the capsule of the shoulder joint. **scrotal l. of testis,** gubernaculum testis. **serous l.,** ligamentum serosum. **short lateral l.,** a knee ligament attached to the lowest part of the lateral femoral condyle and extending beyond the dorsum of the semilunar cartilage to the apex of the fibula. See also *fabellofibular l.* **short plantar l.,** ligamenta calcaneocuboideum plantare. **sphenoidal l., external,** ligamentum intercuneiformia plantaria. **sphenoideotarsal l's,** ligamenta tarsometatarsea plantaria. **sphenomandibular l.,** ligamentum sphenomandibulare. **spinoglenoid l.,** ligamentum transversum scapulae inferius. **spinosacral l.,** ligamentum sacrospinale. **spiral l. of cochlea,** crista spiralis. **splenogastric l.,** ligamentum gastrosplenicum. **splenophrenic l.,** ligamentum splenorenale. **splenorenal l.,** ligamentum splenorenale. **spring l.,** ligamentum calcaneonaviculare plantare. **stapedial l.,** l. annulare stapedis. **stellate l., anterior,** ligamentum capitis costae radiatum. **sternoclavicular l., anterior,** ligamentum sternoclaviculare anterius. **sternoclavicular l., posterior,** ligamentum sternoclaviculare posterius. **sternocostal l's,** ligamenta sternocostalia radiata. **sternocostal l., interarticular, sternocostal l., intra-articular,** ligamentum sternocostale intra-articulare. **sternocostal l's, radiate,** ligamenta sternocostalia radiata. **sternopericardiac l's,** ligamenta sternopericardiaca. **stylohyoid l.,** ligamentum stylohyoideum. **stylomandibular l., stylomaxillary l., stylomylohyoid l.,** ligamentum stylomandibulare. **subflaval l.,** ligamentum flavum. **subpubic l.,** ligamentum arcuatum pubis. **superficial l. of carpus,** 1. ligamentum radiocarpeum dorsale. 2. ligamentum radiocarpeum palmare. **superior l. of epididymis,** ligamentum epididymidis superius. **superior l. of hip,** ligamentum iliofemorale. **superior l. of incus,** ligamentum incudis superius. **superior l. of malleus,** ligamentum mallei superius. **superior l. of neck of rib, anterior,** the anterior part of the superior costotransverse ligament. **superior l. of neck of rib, external,** the posterior part of the superior costotransverse ligament. **superior l. of pinna,** ligamentum auriculare superius. **suprascapular l.,** ligamentum transversum scapulae superius. **supraspinal l's, supraspinous l's,** ligamenta supraspinalia. **suspensory l., marsupial,** plica synovialis infrapatellaris. **suspensory l. of axilla,** a layer ascending from the axillary fascia and ensheathing the pectoralis minor muscle; so called because traction by it, when the arm is abducted, produces the hollow of the armpit. Called also *Campbell's l.* and *Gerdy's l.* **suspensory l.**

of axis, ligamentum apicis dentis. **suspensory l. of bladder,** plica umbilicalis mediana. **suspensory l's of breast,** ligamenta suspensoria mammae. **suspensory l. of clitoris,** ligamentum suspensorium clitoridis. **suspensory l. of humerus,** ligamentum coracohumerale. **suspensory l. of lens,** zonula ciliaris. **suspensory l. of liver,** ligamentum falciforme hepatis. **suspensory l's of mammary gland,** ligamenta suspensoria mammae. **suspensory l. of ovary,** ligamentum suspensorium ovarii. **suspensory l. of penis,** ligamentum suspensorium penis. **suspensory l. of spleen,** ligamentum phrenicolienale. **sutural l.,** a band of fibrous tissue between the opposed bones of a suture or immovable joint. **synovial l.,** a large synovial fold. **synovial l. of hip,** ligamentum capitis femoris. **talocalcaneal l., interosseous,** ligamentum talocalcaneare interosseum. **talocalcaneal l., lateral,** ligamentum talocalcaneare laterale. **talocalcaneal l., medial,** ligamentum talocalcaneare mediale. **l. of talocrural joint, lateral,** the anterior and posterior talofibular ligaments and the calcaneofibular ligament considered together. **talofibular l., anterior,** ligamentum talofibulare anterius. **talofibular l., posterior,** ligamentum talofibulare posterius. **talonavicular l.,** ligamentum talonaviculare. **talotibial l., anterior,** pars tibiotalaris anterior ligamenti medialis. **talotibial l., posterior,** pars tibiotalaris posterior ligamenti medialis. **tarsal l., anterior,** retinaculum musculorum extensorum pedis inferius. **tarsometatarsal l's, dorsal,** ligamenta tarsometatarsalia dorsalia. **tarsometatarsal l's, plantar,** ligamenta tarsometatarsalia plantaria. **temporomandibular l.,** ligamentum laterale articulationis temporomandibularis. **tendinotrochanteric l.,** a portion of the capsule of the hip joint. **tensor l.,** musculus tensor tympani. **Teutleben's l's,** lateral folds joining the pericardium and diaphragm. **thyroepiglottic l.,** ligamentum thyroepiglotticum. **thyrohyoid l.,** ligamentum thyrohyoideum laterale. **thyrohyoid l., median,** ligamentum thyrohyoideum medianum. **tibiocalcaneal l., tibiocalcanean l.,** pars calcaneus ligamenti medialis. **tibiofibular l.,** syndesmosis tibiofibularis. **tibiofibular l., anterior,** ligamentum tibiofibulare anterius. **tibiofibular l., posterior,** ligamentum tibiofibulare posterius. **tibionavicular l.,** pars tibionavicularis ligamenti medialis. **Toynbee's l.,** musculus tensor tympani. **tracheal l's,** ligamenta annularia tracheae. **transverse l. of acetabulum,** ligamentum transversum acetabuli. **transverse l. of atlas,** ligamentum transversum atlantis. **transverse l. of carpus,** retinaculum flexorum manus. **transverse l. of knee,** ligamentum transversum genus. **transverse l. of leg,** retinaculum musculorum extensorum pedis superius. **transverse l. of little head of rib,** ligamentum capitis costae intraarticulare. **transverse l. of pelvis,** ligamentum transversum perinei. **transverse l. of scapula, inferior,** ligamentum transversum scapulae inferius. **transverse l. of scapula, superior,** ligamentum transversum scapulae superius. **transverse l. of tibia,** retinaculum musculorum extensorum pedis superius. **transverse l's of wrist,** retinaculum flexorum manus. **transverse l's of wrist, dorsal,** ligamenta intercarpea dorsalia. **transverse humeral l.,** a band of fibers bridging the intertubercular groove of the humerus and holding the tendon of the biceps muscle in the groove; called also *Brodie's l.* **transversocostal l., superior,** ligamentum costotransversarium superius. **trapezoid l.,** ligamentum trapezoideum. **l. of Treitz,** musculus suspensorius duodeni. **triangular l. of abdomen,** ligamentum inguinale reflexum. **triangular l. of Colles,** fascia diaphragmatis urogenitalis superior. **triangular l. of linea alba,** adminiculum lineae albae. **triangular l. of liver, left,** ligamentum triangulare sinistrum hepatis. **triangular l. of liver, right,** ligamentum triangulare dextrum hepatis. **triangular l. of pubis, anterior,** ligamentum arcuatum pubis. **triangular l. of scapula,** ligamentum transversum scapulae inferius. **triangular l. of thigh,** ligamentum inguinale reflexum. **triangular l. of urethra,** ligamentum puboprostaticum. **trigeminate l's of Arnold,** ligamenta tarsometatarsea dorsalia. **triquetral l.,** 1. ligamentum cricoarytenoideum posterius. 2. ligamentum coracoacromiale. **triquetral l. of foot,** ligamentum calcaneofibulare. **triquetral l. of scapula,** ligamentum transversum scapulae inferius. **trochlear l.,** ligamentum metacarpeum transversum profundum.

trochlear l's of foot, ligamenta plantaria articulationum metatarsophalangearum. **trochlear l's of hand,** ligamenta palmaria. **trochlear l's of little heads of metacarpal bones,** see *ligamenta metacarpeum transversum profundum.* **true l. of bladder, anterior,** 1. ligamentum puboprostaticum. 2. ligamentum pubovesicale. **tuberososacral l.,** ligamentum sacrotuberale. **tubopharyngeal l. of Rauber,** plica salpingopharyngea. **Tuffier's inferior l.,** that part of the mesentery which is connected with the wall of the iliac fossa. **ulnar l., lateral, ulnar l. of carpus,** ligamentum collaterale carpi ulnare. **ulnocarpal l., palmar,** ligamentum ulnocarpale palmare. **umbilical l., lateral,** ligamentum umbilicale mediale. **umbilical l., medial,** ligamentum umbilicale mediale. **umbilical l., median, umbilical l., middle,** ligamentum umbilicale medianum. **utero-ovarian l.,** ligamentum ovarii proprium. **uteropelvic l's,** expansions of muscular tissue in the broad ligament of the uterus, radiating from the fascia over the obturator internus to the side of the uterus and the vagina. **uterosacral l.,** a part of the thickening of the visceral pelvic fascia beside the cervix and vagina, passing posteriorly in the rectouterine fold to attach to the front of the sacrum; called also *Petit's l.* **vaginal l.,** ligamentum vaginale. **vaginal l's of fingers,** vaginae fibrosae digitorum manus. **vaginal l's of toes,** vaginae fibrosae digitorum pedis. **l. of vaginal sheaths,** ligamentum vaginale. **l's of vaginal sheaths of fingers,** vaginae fibrosae digitorum manus. **l's of vaginal sheaths of toes,** vaginae fibrosae digitorum pedis. **l's of Valsalva,** ligamenta auricularia. **venous l. of liver,** ligamentum venosum. **ven-**

tricular l. of larynx, ligamentum vestibulare. **vertebropleural l.,** membrana suprapleuralis. **l. of Vesalius,** ligamentum inguinale. **vesical l., lateral,** ligamentum umbilicale mediale. **vesicopubic l.,** ligamentum pubovesicale. **vesicoumbilical l.,** ligamentum umbilicale mediale. **vesicouterine l.,** a ligament that extends from the anterior aspect of the uterus to the bladder. **vestibular l.,** ligamentum vestibulare. **vocal l.,** ligamentum vocale. **volar l. of carpus, proper,** retinaculum flexorum manus. **volar l. of wrist, anterior,** retinaculum flexorum manus. **Walther's oblique l.,** ligamentum talofibulare posterius. **Weitbrecht's l.,** chorda obliqua membranae interosseae antebrachii. **Winslow's l.,** ligamentum popliteum obliquum. **Wrisberg's l.,** ligamentum meniscofemorale posterius. **xiphicostal l's of Macalister, xiphoid l's,** ligamenta costoxiphoidea. **Y l.,** ligamentum iliofemorale. **yellow l's,** ligamenta flava. **Zinn's l.,** annulus tendineus communis. **zonal l. of thigh,** zona orbicularis articulationis coxae.

ligamenta (lig″ah-men′tah) [L.] plural of *ligamentum.*

ligamentopexy (lig″ah-men″to-pek′se) ventrosuspension by shortening or suturing the round ligaments of the uterus.

ligamentous (lig″ah-men′tus) pertaining to or of the nature of a ligament.

ligamentum (lig″ah-men′tum), pl. *ligamen′ta* [L. "a bandage," from *ligare* to bind] [NA] a ligament: a band of tissue that connects bones or supports viscera. Some ligaments are distinct fibrous structures; some are folds of fascia or of indurated peritoneum; still others are relics of fetal organs. For names of specific structures, see *Table of Ligamenta.*

TABLE OF LIGAMENTA

Descriptions are given on NA terms, and include anglicized names of specific ligaments.

l. acromioclavicula′re [NA], acromioclavicular ligament: a dense band that joins the superior surface of the acromion and the acromial extremity of the clavicle together, and strengthens the superior part of the articular capsule.

ligamen′ta ala′ria [NA], alar ligaments: two strong bands that pass from the posterolateral part of the tip of the dens of the axis upward and laterally to the condyles of the occipital bone; they limit rotation of the head.

l. annula′re ba′seos stape′dis, l. annulare stapedis.

l. anula′re stape′dis, NA alternative for *l. annulare stapedis.*

ligamen′ta annula′ria digito′rum ma′nus, see *pars anularis vaginae fibrosae digitorum manus.*

ligamen′ta annula′ria digito′rum pe′dis, see *pars anularis vaginae fibrosae digitorum pedis.*

l. annula′re ra′dii, l. anulare radii.

l. anococcyg′eum [NA], anococcygeal ligament: a fibrous band connecting the posterior fibers of the sphincter of the anus to the coccyx.

l. annula′re ra′dii [NA], annular ligament of radius: a strong fibrous band that encircles the head of the radius and holds it in position; it is attached to the anterior and posterior margins of the radial notch of the ulna, forming, with the notch, a complete ring. Called also *l. anulare radii.*

l. annula′re stape′dis [NA], annular ligament of stapes: a ring of fibrous tissue that attaches the base of the stapes to the fenestra vestibuli of the inner ear; called also *l. annulare baseos stapedis* and *l. anulare stapedis* [NA alternative].

ligamen′ta annula′ria tra′cheae [NA], annular ligaments of trachea: circular horizontal ligaments that join the tracheal cartilages together; called also *ligamenta trachealia* and *tracheal ligaments.*

l. a′picis den′tis ax′is [NA], apical dental ligament: a cord of tissue extending from the tip of the dens of the axis to the occipital bone, near the anterior margin of the foramen magnum; it is usually delicate, but is sometimes well developed. Called also *l. apicis dentis epistrophei.*

l. a′picis den′tis epistro′phei, l. apicis dentis axis.

l. arcua′tum latera′le [NA], lateral arcuate ligament: the ligamentous arch, formed by the fascia of the quadratus lumborum muscle, constituting part of the lumbar portion of the diaphragm; called also *arcus lumbocostalis lateralis* [Halleri].

l. arcua′tum media′le [NA], medial arcuate ligament: the ligamentous arch, formed by the fascia of the psoas muscle, constituting part of the lumbar portion of the diaphragm; called also *arcus lumbocostalis medialis* [Halleri].

l. arcua′tum media′num [NA], median arcuate ligament: the ligamentous arch across the front of the aorta, interconnecting the crura of the diaphragm; called also *median arcuate ligament.*

l. arcua′tum pu′bis [NA], arcuate ligament of pubis: a thick archlike band of fibers situated along the inferior margin of the symphysis pubis. Its fibers are attached to the medial borders of the inferior rami of the pubic bones and thus it rounds out and forms the summit of the pubic arch. Called also *inferior pubic ligament.*

l. arterio′sum [NA], a short, thick, strong fibromuscular cord extending from the pulmonary artery to the arch of the aorta; it is the remains of the ductus arteriosus. Called also *l. arteriosum arteriae pulmonalis* and *ligament of Botallo.*

l. arterio′sum arte′riae pulmona′lis, l. arteriosum.

l. atlanto-occipita′le ante′rius, l. atlanto-occipita′lis ante′rior, membrana atlanto-occipitalis anterior.

l. atlanto-occipita′le latera′le [NA], **l. atlanto-occipita′lis latera′lis,** lateral atlanto-occipital ligament: a thickened portion of the articular capsule of the atlanto-occipital joint attached to the jugular processes of the occipital bone and to the base of the transverse process of the atlas.

ligamen′ta auricula′ria [NA], ligaments of auricle: the three ligaments, anterior, superior, and posterior, that help attach the auricle to the side of the head; called also *ligaments of Valsalva.*

ligamen′ta auricula′ria [Valsal′vae], ligamenta auricularia.

l. auricula′re ante′rius [NA], anterior auricular ligament: the auricular ligament that passes from the helix and tragus to the zygoma.

l. auricula′re ante′rius [Valsal′vae], l. auriculare anterius.

l. auricula′re poste′rius [NA], posterior auricular ligament: the auricular ligament that passes from the eminence of the concha to the mastoid part of the temporal bone.

l. auricula′re poste′rius [Valsal′vae], l. auriculare posterius.

l. auricula′re supe′rius [NA], superior auricular ligament: the auricular ligament that passes from the spine of the helix to the superior margin of the bony external acoustic meatus.

l. auricula're supe'rius [Valsal'vae], l. auriculare superius.

l. bifurca'tum [NA], bifurcate ligament: a Y-shaped ligament on the dorsum of the foot, comprising the calcaneonavicular and calcaneocuboid ligaments.

l. calcaneocuboi'deum [NA], calcaneocuboid ligament: the band of fibers connecting the superior surface of the calcaneus and the dorsal surface of the cuboid bone; called also *pars calcaneocuboidea ligamenti bifurcati.*

l. calcaneocuboi'deum planta're [NA], plantar calcaneocuboid ligament: a short, wide, strong band connecting the plantar surfaces of the calcaneus and the cuboid bone, called also *short plantar ligament.*

l. calcaneofibula're [NA], calcaneofibular ligament: a band of fibers arising from the lateral surface of the lateral malleolus of the fibula just anterior to the apex and passing inferiorly and posteriorly to be attached to the lateral surface of the calcaneus.

l. calcaneonavicula're [NA], calcaneonavicular ligament: the band of fibers connecting the superior surface of the calcaneus and the lateral surface of the navicular bone; called also *pars calcaneonavicularis ligamenti bifurcati.*

l. calcaneonavicula're dorsa'le, dorsal calcaneonavicular ligament: the dorsal portion of the calcaneonavicular part of the bifurcate ligament, connecting the dorsal surfaces of the calcaneus and the navicular bone.

l. calcaneonavicula're planta're [NA], plantar calcaneonavicular ligament: a broad, thick band passing from the anterior margin of the sustentaculum tali to the plantar surface of the navicular bone; it bears on its deep surface a fibrocartilage that helps to support the head of the talus.

l. calcaneotibia'le, pars tibiocalcanea ligamenti medialis.

l. cap'itis cos'tae intra-articula're [NA], interarticular ligament of head of rib: a horizontal band of fibers attached to the crest separating the two articular facets on the head of the rib, and to the intervertebral disk, thus dividing the joint of the head of the rib into two cavities. It is lacking in the joints of the first, tenth, eleventh, and twelfth ribs. Called also *interarticular ligament of head of rib* and *l. capituli costae interarticulare.*

l. cap'itis cos'tae radia'tum [NA], radiate ligament of head of rib: fibers that from their attachment on the ventral surface of the head of a rib radiate medially, in a fanlike manner, to attach to the two adjacent vertebrae and to the intervertebral disk between them; called also *l. capituli costae radiatum.*

l. cap'itis fem'oris [NA], ligament of head of femur: a curved triangular or V-shaped fibrous band, attached by its apex to the anterosuperior part of the fovea of the head of the femur and by its base to the sides of the acetabular notch and the intervening transverse ligament of the acetabulum. Called also *l. teres femoris* and *round ligament of femur.*

l. cap'itis fib'ulae ante'rius [NA], anterior ligament of head of fibula: a band of fibers that passes obliquely superiorly from the anterior part of the head of the fibula to the lateral condyle of the tibia.

l. cap'itis fib'ulae poste'rius [NA], posterior ligament of head of fibula: a band of fibers that passes obliquely superiorly from the posterior part of the head of the fibula to the lateral condyle of the tibia.

l. capit'uli cos'tae interarticula're, l. capitis costae intra-articulare.

l. capit'uli cos'tae radia'tum, l. capitis costae radiatum.

ligamen'ta capit'uli fib'ulae, see *l. capitis fibulae anterius* and *l. capitis fibulae posterius.*

ligamen'ta capsula'ria [NA], thickenings of the fibrous membrane of a joint capsule.

l. car'pi dorsa'le, retinaculum extensorum manus.

l. car'pi radia'tum [NA], radiate carpal ligament: a group of about seven fibrous bands which diverge in all directions on the palmar surface of the mediocarpal joint; the majority radiate from the capitate to the scaphoid, lunate, and triquetral bones.

l. car'pi transver'sum, retinaculum flexorum manus.

l. car'pi vola're, transverse reinforcing fibers in the antebrachial fascia over the palmar surface of the wrist.

ligamen'ta carpometacarpa'lia dorsa'lia [NA], **ligamen'ta carpometacar'pea dorsa'lia,** dorsal carpometacarpal ligaments: a series of bands on the dorsal surface of the carpometacarpal articulations, joining the carpal bones to

the bases of the second to fifth metacarpals. The second metacarpal bone is thus joined to the trapezium, trapezoid, and capitate, the third to the capitate, the fourth to the capitate and hamate, and the fifth to the hamate. Called also *posterior carpometacarpal* ligaments.

ligamen'ta carpometacarpa'lia palma'ria [NA], **ligamen'ta carpometacar'pea palma'ria,** palmar carpometacarpal ligaments: a series of bands on the palmar surface of the carpometacarpal articulations, joining the carpal bones to the second to fifth metacarpals. The second metacarpal bone is thus joined to the trapezium, the third to the trapezium, capitate, and hamate, the fourth to the hamate, and the fifth to the hamate. Called also *anterior* or *volar carpometacarpal ligaments.*

l. cauda'le integumen'ti commu'nis, retinaculum caudale.

l. ceratocricoi'deum [NA], ceratocricoid ligament: any of the three (anterior, lateral, or posterior) fibrous bands that serve to attack the capsule of the cricothyroid joint on either side.

ligamen'ta collatera'lia articulatio'num interphalangea'lium ma'nus [NA], **ligamen'ta collatera'lia articulatio'num interphalangea'rum ma'nus,** collateral ligaments of interphalangeal articulations of hand: massive fibrous bands on each side of the interphalangeal joints of the fingers; they are placed diagonally, the proximal ends being near the dorsal, and the distal ends near the palmar margins of the digits. Called also *ligamenta collateralia articulationum digitorum manus.*

ligamen'ta collatera'lia articulatio'num interphalangea'lium pe'dis [NA], **ligamen'ta collatera'lia articulatio'num interphalangea'rum pe'dis,** collateral ligaments of interphalangeal articulations of foot: fibrous bands, one on either side of each of the interphalangeal joints of the toes. Called also *ligamenta collateralia articulationum digitorum pedis.*

ligamen'ta collatera'lia articulatio'num metacarpophalangea'lium [NA], **ligamen'ta collatera'lia articulatio'num metacarpophalangea'rum,** collateral ligaments of metacarpophalangeal articulations: massive, strong fibrous bands on either side of each metacarpophalangeal joint, holding the two bones involved in each joint firmly together.

ligamen'ta collatera'lia articulatio'num metatarsophalangea'lium [NA], **ligamen'ta collatera'lia articulatio'num metatarsophalangea'rum,** collateral ligaments of metatarsophalangeal articulations: strong fibrous bands on either side of each metatarsophalangeal joint, holding the two bones involved in each joint firmly together.

l. collatera'le car'pi radia'le [NA], radial carpal collateral ligament: a short, thick band that passes from the tip of the styloid process of the radius to attach to the scaphoid bone.

l. collatera'le car'pi ulna're [NA], ulnar carpal collateral ligament: a strong fibrous band that passes from the tip of the styloid process of the ulna and is attached to the triquetral and pisiform bones.

l. collatera'le fibula're [NA], collateral fibular ligament: a strong, round fibrous cord on the lateral side of the knee joint, entirely independent of the capsule of the knee joint; it is attached superiorly to the posterior part of the lateral epicondyle of the femur and inferiorly to the lateral side of the head of the fibula just in front of the styloid process.

l. collatera'le radia'le [NA], collateral radial ligament: a large bundle of fibers arising from the lateral epicondyle of the humerus and fanning out to be attached to the lateral side of the annular ligament of the radius.

l. collatera'le tibia'le [NA], collateral tibial ligament: a broad, flat, longitudinal band on the medial side of the knee joint; it is attached superiorly to the medial epicondyle of the femur, inferiorly to the medial surface of the body of the tibia, and in between to the medial meniscus.

l. collatera'le ulna're [NA], collateral ulnar ligament: a triangular bundle of fibers attached proximally to the medial epicondyle of the humerus, distally to the coronoid process of the ulna and the medial surface of the olecranon, and to a ridge running between the two.

l. col'li cos'tae, l. costotransversarium.

l. conoi'deum [NA], conoid ligament: the conical, posteromedial portion of the coracoclavicular ligament, attached inferiorly by its tip to the base of the coracoid process of the scapula and superiorly by its base to the inferior surface of the clavicle.

929

l. coracoacromia′le [NA], coracoacromial ligament: one of three intrinsic ligaments of the scapula, a strong broad triangular band that is attached by its base to the lateral border of the coracoid process and by its tip to the summit of the acromion just in front of the articular facet for the clavicle.

l. coracoclavicula′re [NA], coracoclavicular ligament: a strong band that joins the coracoid process of the scapula and the acromial extremity of the clavicle; it is divided into two parts, the trapezoid and conoid ligaments.

l. coracohumera′le [NA], coracohumeral ligament: a broad band that arises from the lateral border of the coracoid process of the scapula and passes downward and laterally to be attached to the major tubercle of the humerus.

l. corona′rium hep′atis [NA], coronary ligament of the liver: the line of reflection of the peritoneum from the diaphragmatic surface of the liver to the under surface of the diaphragm.

l. costoclavicula′re [NA], costoclavicular ligament: a short, powerful ligament that extends from the superior margin of the first costal cartilage to the inferior surface at the sternal end of the clavicle.

l. costotransversa′rium [NA], costotransverse ligament: short fibers that connect the dorsal surface of the neck of a rib with the anterior surface of the transverse process of the corresponding vertebra; called also *l. colli costae.*

l. costotransversa′rium latera′le [NA], lateral costotransverse ligament: a fibrous band that passes transversely from the posterior surface of the tip of a transverse process of a vertebra to the nonarticular part of the tubercle of the corresponding rib; called also *l. tuberculi costae.*

l. costotransversa′rium supe′rius [NA], superior costotransverse ligament: a strong band of fibers ascending from the crest of the neck of a rib to the transverse process of the vertebra above; it may be divided into a stronger anterior portion and a weaker posterior portion. It is lacking for the first rib.

ligamen′ta costoxiphoi′dea [NA], costoxiphoid ligaments: inconstant strandlike bands that pass obliquely from the anterior surface of the seventh and sometimes from the sixth costal cartilage to the anterior surface of the xiphoid process of the sternum. Some bands may also be present on the posterior surface.

l. cricoarytenoi′deum poste′rius [NA], posterior cricoarytenoid cartilage: the ligament extending from the lamina of the cricoid cartilage to the medial surface of the base and muscular process of the arytenoid cartilage.

l. cricopharyn′geum [NA], cricopharyngeal ligament: a ligament extending from the cricoid lamina to the midline of the pharynx.

l. cricothyroi′deum media′num [NA], median cricothyroid ligament: the median or anterior part of the inferior, larger part of the fibroelastic laryngeal membrane, occurring as a flat band of white tissue continuous medially with the conus elasticus and cranially with the plica vocalis and ligamentum vocale, and connecting the cricoid and thyroid cartilages; called also *anterior cricothyroid ligament.* See also *cricothyroid ligament,* under *ligament.*

l. cricotrachea′le [NA], cricotracheal ligament: a narrow fibrous ring that connects the lower margin of the cricoid cartilage with the upper tracheal cartilage; it is continuous posteriorly with the membranous wall of the trachea.

l. crucia′tum ante′rius ge′nu, l. cruciatum anterius genus.

l. crucia′tum ante′rius ge′nus [NA], anterior cruciate ligament of knee: a strong band that arises from the posteromedial portion of the lateral condyle of the femur, passes anteriorly and inferiorly between the condyles, and is attached to the depression in front of the intercondylar eminence of the tibia. Called also *l. cruciatum anterius genu.*

l. crucia′tum atlan′tis, l. cruciforme atlantis.

l. crucia′tum cru′ris, retinaculum musculorum extensorum pedis inferius.

ligamen′ta crucia′ta digito′rum ma′nus, see *pars cruciformis vaginae fibrosae digitorum manus.*

ligamen′ta crucia′ta digito′rum pe′dis, see *pars cruciformis vaginae fibrosae digitorum pedis.*

ligamen′ta crucia′ta ge′nu, ligamenta cruciata genus.

ligamen′ta crucia′ta ge′nus [NA], cruciate ligaments of knee: strong, thick bundles situated in the knee joint between the condyles of the femur, which together form a somewhat cross-shaped structure; called also *ligamenta cruciata genu.* See *l. cruciatum anterius genus* and *l. cruciatum posterius genus.*

l. crucia′tum poste′rius ge′nu, cruciatum posterius genus.

l. crucia′tum poste′rius ge′nus [NA], posterior cruciate ligament of knee: a strong band that arises from the anterolateral surface of the medial condyle of the femur, passes posteriorly and inferiorly between the condyles, and is inserted into the posterior intercondylar area of the tibia. Called also *l. cruciatum posterius genu.*

l. crucifor′me atlan′tis [NA], cruciform ligament of atlas: a ligament in the form of a cross, of which the transverse ligament of the atlas forms the horizontal bar, and the longitudinal fascicles the vertical bar of the cross; called also *l. cruciatum atlantis.*

l. cuboideonavicula′re dorsa′le [NA], dorsal cuboideonavicular ligament: a fibrous bundle connecting the dorsal surfaces of the cuboid and navicular bones.

l. cuboideonavicula′re planta′re [NA], plantar cuboideonavicular ligament: a fibrous band connecting the plantar surfaces of the cuboid and navicular bones.

l. cuneocuboi′deum dorsa′le [NA], dorsal cuneocuboid ligament: fibers connecting the dorsal surfaces of the cuboid and lateral cuneiform bones.

l. cuneocuboi′deum interos′seum [NA], interosseous cuneocuboid ligament: fibers connecting the central portions of the adjacent surfaces of the cuboid and lateral cuneiform bones, between the articular surfaces.

l. cuneocuboi′deum planta′re [NA], plantar cuneocuboid ligament: a band of fibers connecting the plantar surfaces of the cuboid and lateral cuneiform bones.

ligamen′ta cuneometatarsa′lia interos′sea [NA], **ligamen′ta cuniometatarsea interos′sea,** interosseous cuneometatarsal ligaments: fibrous bands that join the adjacent surfaces of the cuneiform and the metatarsal bones.

ligamen′ta cuneonavicula′ria dorsa′lia [NA], dorsal cuneonavicular ligaments: bands that join the dorsal surface of the navicular bone to the dorsal surfaces of the three cuneiform bones; called also *ligamenta navicularicuneiformia dorsalia.*

ligamen′ta cuneonavicula′ria planta′ria [NA], plantar cuneonavicular ligaments: bands that join the plantar surface of the navicular bone to the adjacent plantar surfaces of the three cuneiform bones; called also *ligamenta navicularicuneiformia plantaria.*

l. deltoi′deum, NA alternative for *l. mediale.*

l. denticula′tum [NA], denticulate ligament: a fold of pia mater of the spinal cord, beginning in a longitudinal line along the spinal cord between the lines of attachment of the anterior and posterior roots. The lateral edge is scalloped and has about 21 pointed processes that extend laterally and fuse with the arachnoid and dura mater. Called also *dentate ligament of spinal cord.*

l. duodenorena′le, duodenorenal ligament: a fold of peritoneum that passes from the duodenum to the right kidney.

l. epididym′idis infe′rius [NA], inferior ligament of epididymis: a strand of fibrous tissue, covered with a reflection of the tunica vaginalis, which connects the lower end of the body of the epididymis with the testis.

l. epididym′idis supe′rius [NA], superior ligament of epididymis: a strand of fibrous tissue, covered with a reflection of the tunica vaginalis, which connects the upper end of the body of the epididymis with the testis.

ligamen′ta extracapsula′ria [NA], ligaments of a joint capsule that are outside the capsule.

l. falcifor′me hep′atis [NA], falciform ligament of the liver: a sickle-shaped sagittal fold of peritoneum that helps to attach the liver to the diaphragm, separates the right and left lobes of the liver, and extends from the coronary ligament of the liver behind to the umbilicus in front; called also *broad ligament of liver.*

ligamen′ta fla′va [NA], yellow ligaments: a series of bands of yellow elastic tissue attached to and extending between the ventral portions of the laminae of two adjacent vertebrae, from the junction of the axis and the third cervical vertebra to the junction of the fifth lumbar vertebra and the sacrum. They assist in maintaining or regaining the erect position and serve to close in the spaces between the arches. Called also *arcuate ligaments,* and *flaval ligaments.*

l. fundifor′me pe′nis [NA], fundiform ligament of penis: a broad elastic band of fascial fibers that arises from the linea alba and from the fibrae intercrurales just above the symphysis pubis and then passes down to the penis, where it divides and passes around the penis and on into the scrotum.

l. gastrocol′icum [NA], gastrocolic ligament: a peritoneal fold, part of the greater omentum, that extends from the greater curvature of the stomach to the transverse colon.

l. gastroliena'le, NA alternative for *l. gastrosplenicum.*

l. gastrophren'icum [NA], gastrophrenic ligament: a fold of peritoneum continuous with the gastrosplenic ligament, extending from right under surface of the diaphragm to the cardiac part of the stomach.

l. gastrosple'nicum [NA], gastrosplenic ligament: a peritoneal fold extending from the greater curvature of the stomach to the hilum of the spleen; called also *l. gastrolienale* [NA alternative] and *gastrolienal* or *splenogastric ligament.*

l. genitoinguina'le [NA], genitoinguinal ligament: the embryonic precursor of the gubernaculum testis.

ligamen'ta glenohumera'lia [NA], glenohumeral ligaments: bands, usually three in number, on the inner surface of the articular capsule of the humerus, attached to the margin of the glenoid cavity and to the anatomical neck of the humerus.

lig'amenta hep'atis [NA], hepatic ligaments: the ligaments of the liver, including the ligamenta coronaria hepatis, falciforme hepatis, triangulare dextrum hepatis, triangulare sinistrum hepatis, and hepatorenale.

l. hepatocol'icum [NA], hepatocolic ligament: an occasional fold of peritoneum, an extension of the lesser omentum to the right, passing from the lower surface of the liver near the gallbladder to the right colic flexure.

l. hepatoduodena'le [NA], hepatoduodenal ligament: a peritoneal fold that passes from the porta hepatis to the superior portion of the duodenum. It is continuous on the left with the gastrohepatic ligament, and on the right it forms one of the borders of the epiploic foramen. It contains the hepatic artery, portal vein, bile duct, nerves, and lymphatics.

l. hepatogas'tricum [NA], hepatogastric ligament: a peritoneal fold, part of the lesser omentum, that passes from the under surface of the liver to the lesser curvature of the stomach.

l. hepatorena'le [NA], hepatorenal ligament: a fold of peritoneum that passes from the back part of the lower surface of the liver to the front of the right kidney and forms the right margin of the epiploic foramen.

l. hyoepiglot'ticum [NA], hyoepiglottic ligament: a triangular elastic band with its base attached to the upper border of the body of the hyoid bone and its tip to the anterosuperior surface of the epiglottis.

l. hyothyreoi'deum latera'le, l. thyrohyoideum laterale.

l. hyothyreoi'deum me'dium, l. thyrohyoideum medianum.

l. iliofemora'le [NA], iliofemoral ligament: a very strong triangular or inverted Y-shaped band that covers the anterior and superior portions of the hip joint. It arises by its apex from the lower part of the anterior inferior iliac spine and is inserted by its base into the intertrochanteric line of the femur.

l. iliolumba'le [NA], iliolumbar ligament: a strong band that passes from the transverse processes of the fourth and fifth lumbar vertebrae to the internal lip of the adjacent portion of the iliac crest.

l. incu'dis poste'rius [NA], posterior ligament of incus: a fibrous band by which the cartilaginous tip of the short crus of the incus is fixed to the fossa incudis.

l. incu'dis supe'rius [NA], superior ligament of incus: a fibrous band that passes from the body of the incus to the roof of the tympanic cavity just back of the superior ligament of the malleus.

l. inguina'le [NA], inguinal ligament: a fibrous band running from the anterior superior spine of the ilium to the spine of the pubis. Called also *inguinal arch* and *arcus inguinalis* [NA alternative].

l. inguina'le [Poupar'ti], l. inguinale.

l. inguina'le reflex'um [NA], reflex inguinal ligament: a triangular band of fibers arising from the lacunar ligament and the pubic bone and passing diagonally upward and medially behind the superficial abdominal ring and in front of the inguinal aponeurotic falx to the linea alba.

l. inguina'le reflex'um [Colle'si], l. inguinale reflexum.

ligamen'ta intercarpa'lia dorsa'lia [NA], **ligamen'ta intercar'pea dorsa'lia,** dorsal intercarpal ligaments: several bands that extend transversely across the dorsal surfaces of the carpal bones, connecting various ones together.

ligamen'ta intercarpa'lia inteross'ea [NA], **ligamen'ta intercar'pea interos'sea,** interosseous intercarpal ligaments: short fibrous bands that join the adjacent surfaces of the various carpal bones.

ligamen'ta intercarpa'lia palma'ria [NA], **ligamen'ta intercar'pea palma'ria,** palmar intercarpal

ligaments: several bands that extend transversely across the palmar surfaces of the carpal bones, connecting various ones together; called also *ligamenta intercarpea volaria* and *volar intercarpal ligaments.*

l. interclavicula're [NA], interclavicular ligament: a flattened band that passes from the superior surface of the sternal end of one clavicle across the superior margin of the sternum to the same position on the other clavicle.

ligamen'ta intercosta'lia, see *membrana intercostalis externa* and *membrana intercostalis interna.*

ligamen'ta intercosta'lia exter'na, see *membrana intercostalis externa.*

ligamen'ta intercosta'lia inter'na, see *membrana intercostalis interna.*

ligamen'ta intercuneifor'mia dorsa'lia [NA], dorsal intercuneiform ligaments: fibrous bands connecting the dorsal surfaces of the three cuneiform bones.

ligamen'ta intercuneifor'mia interos'sea [NA], interosseous intercuneiform ligaments: short fibrous bands that join the adjacent surfaces of the medial and intermediate, and the intermediate and lateral, cuneiform bones.

ligamen'ta intercuneifor'mia planta'ria [NA], plantar intercuneiform ligaments: fibrous bands that join the plantar surfaces of the cuneiform bones.

l. interfoveola're [NA], interfoveolar ligament: a thickening in the transversalis fascia on the medial side of the deep inguinal ring; it is connected above to the transversus muscle and below to the inguinal ligament.

l. interfoveola're [Hesselba'chi], l. interfoveolare.

ligamenta interspina'lia [NA], interspinal ligaments: several fine fibrous membranes that extend from one vertebral spinous process to the next. They extend obliquely from the yellow ligaments ventrally to the supraspinous ligament dorsally, and contain white fibrous and yellow elastic tissue. They are poorly developed or lacking in the cervical region. Called also *interspinous ligaments.*

ligamenta intertransversa'ria [NA], intertransverse ligaments: several poorly developed fibrous bands that extend from one vertebral transverse process to the next. They consist of fine membranes in the lumbar region and of small cords in the thoracic region, and are lacking in the cervical region.

ligamen'ta intracapsula'ria [NA], ligaments within a joint capsule.

l. ischiocapsula're, l. ischiofemorale.

l. ischiofemora'le [NA], ischiofemoral ligament: a broad triangular band on the posterior surface of the hip joint. Its base is attached to the ischium posterior and inferior to the acetabulum; its fibers pass superiorly, laterally, and anteriorly across the capsule, bend over the neck, and in part are inserted into the inner side of the trochanteric fossa of the femur and in part blend into the zona orbicularis. Called also *l. ischiocapsulare* and *ischiocapsular ligament.*

l. lacinia'tum, retinaculum musculorum flexorum pedis.

l. lacuna're [NA], lacunar ligament: a small triangular membrane with its base just medial to the femoral ring; one side is attached to the inguinal ligament and the other to the pectineal line of the pubis.

l. lacuna're [Gimberna'ti], l. lacunare.

l. later'ale articulatio'nis talocrura'lis, lateral ligament of ankle joint: the three ligamentous fasciculi present on the lateral side of the ankle joint (i.e., the *partes tibiocalcanea, tibiotalaris anterior,* and *tibiotalaris posterior*) considered collectively.

l. latera'le articulatio'nis temporomandibula'ris [NA], lateral ligament of temporomandibular articulation: a strong triangular fibrous band that is attached superiorly by its base to the zygomatic process of the temporal bone, passes down on the lateral side of the joint in contact with the capsule, and is inserted by its apex into the lateral and posterior surfaces of the neck of the condyloid process of the mandible. Called also *l. temporomandibulare* and *temporomandibular ligament.*

l. la'tum u'teri [NA], broad ligament of uterus: a broad fold of peritoneum extending from the side of the uterus to the wall of the pelvis; it is divided into the mesometrium, mesosalpinx, and mesovarium.

l. lienorena'le, NA alternative for *l. splenorenale.*

l. longitudina'le ante'rius [NA], anterior longitudinal ligament: a single long, fibrous band in the midline, attached to the ventral surfaces of the bodies of the vertebrae; it extends from the occipital bone and the anterior tubercle of the atlas down to the sacrum.

l. longitudina'le poste'rius [NA], posterior longitudinal ligament: a single mid-line fibrous band attached to the dorsal surfaces of the bodies of the vertebrae, extending from the occipital bone to the coccyx.

l. lumbocosta'le [NA], lumbocostal ligament: a strong fascial band that passes from the twelfth rib to the tips of the transverse processes of the first and second lumbar vertebrae.

l. mal'lei ante'rius [NA], anterior ligament of malleus: a fibrous band that extends from the neck of the malleus just above the anterior process to the anterior wall of the tympanic cavity close to the petrotympanic fissure. Some of the fibers pass through the fissure to the spina angulares of the sphenoid bone.

l. mal'lei latera'le [NA], lateral ligament of malleus: a triangular fibrous band that passes from the posterior portion of the incisura tympanica to the head or neck of the malleus.

l. mal'lei supe'rius [NA], superior ligament of malleus: a delicate fibrous strand passing from the roof of the tympanic cavity to the head of the malleus.

l. malle'oli latera'lis ante'rius, l. tibiofibulare anterius.

l. malle'oli latera'lis poste'rius, l. tibiofibulare posterius.

l. media'le articulatio'nis talocrura'lis, [NA], medial ligament of talocrural articulation: a large fan-shaped ligament on the medial side of the ankle, passing from the medial malleolus of the tibia down onto the tarsal bones. It comprises four parts: pars tibionavicularis, pars tibiocalcanea, pars tibiotalaris anterior, and pars tibiotalaris posterior. Called also *l. deltoideum* [NA alternative] and *deltoid ligament of ankle.*

l. media'le articulatio'nis temporomandibula'ris [NA], the medial ligament of temporomandibular articulation.

l. meniscofemora'le ante'rius [NA], anterior meniscofemoral ligament: a small fibrous band of the knee joint, attached to the posterior area of the lateral meniscus and passing superiorly and medially, anterior to the posterior cruciate ligament, to attach to the anterior cruciate ligament.

l. meniscofemora'le poste'rius [NA], posterior meniscofemoral ligament: a small fibrous band of the knee joint, attached to the posterior area of the lateral meniscus and passing superiorly and medially, posterior to the posterior cruciate ligament, to the medial condyle of the femur.

ligamen'ta metacarpa'lia dorsa'lia [NA], **ligamen'ta metacar'pea dorsa'lia,** dorsal metacarpal ligaments: bands that interconnect the bases of the second to fifth metacarpal bones by passing transversely from bone to bone on their dorsal surfaces; called also *ligamenta basium [ossium metacarpalium] dorsalia.*

ligamen'ta metacarpa'lia interos'sea [NA], **ligamen'ta metacar'pea interos'sea,** interosseous metacarpal ligaments: short, strong fibrous bands situated between the adjacent surfaces of the bases of the second to fifth metacarpal bones, just distal to the articular surfaces; called also *ligamenta basium [ossium metacarpalium] interossea.*

ligamen'ta metacarpa'lia palma'ria [NA], **ligamen'ta metacar'pea palma'ria,** palmar metacarpal ligaments: bands that interconnect the bases of the second to fifth metacarpal bones by passing transversely from bone to bone on their palmar surfaces; called also *ligamenta basium [ossium metacarpalium] volaria.*

l. metacar'peum transver'sum profun'dum [NA], deep transverse metacarpal ligament: a narrow fibrous band that extends across and is attached to the palmar surfaces of the heads of the second to fifth metacarpal bones, joining them together.

l. metacarpa'le transver'sum superficia'le [NA], **l. metacar'peum transver'sum superficia'le,** superficial transverse metacarpal ligament: transverse fibers occupying the intervals between the diverging longitudinal bands of the palmar aponeurosis.

ligamen'ta metatarsa'lia dorsa'lia [NA], **ligamen'ta metatar'sea dorsa'lia,** dorsal metatarsal ligaments: light transverse bands on the dorsal surfaces of the bases of the second to fifth metatarsal bones, similar to the corresponding ligaments on the metacarpal bones; called also *anterior metatarsal l.*

ligamen'ta metatarsa'lia interos'sea [NA], **ligamen'ta metatar'sea interos'sea,** interosseous metatarsal ligaments: bands between the bases of the second to fifth metatarsal bones, similar to the corresponding ligaments of the hand.

ligamen'ta metatarsa'lia planta'ria [NA], **ligamen'ta metatar'sea planta'ria,** plantar metatarsal ligaments: strong transverse bands on the plantar surfaces of the bases of the second to fifth metatarsal bones.

l. metatarsa'le transver'sum profundum [NA], **l. metatar'seum transver'sum profun'dum,** deep transverse metatarsal ligament: a narrow fibrous band that extends across, is attached to the plantar surfaces of, and thus joins together the heads of all the metatarsal bones.

l. metatarsa'le transver'sum superficia'le [NA], **l. metatar'seum transver'sum superficia'le,** superficial transverse metatarsal ligament: fibers that lie in the superficial fascia of the sole of the foot beneath the heads of the metatarsal bones.

ligamen'ta navicularicuneifor'mia dorsa'lia, ligamenta cuneonavicularia dorsalia.

ligamen'ta navicularicuneifor'mia planta'ria, ligamenta cuneonavicularia plantaria.

l. nu'chae [NA], nuchal ligament: a broad, fibrous, roughly triangular sagittal septum in the back of the neck, separating the right and left sides. It extends from the tips of the spinous processes of all the cervical vertebrae to attach to the entire length of the external occipital crest. Caudally it is continuous with the supraspinous ligament.

ligamen'ta ossiculo'rum audi'tus [NA], ligaments of auditory ossicles: the ligaments of the auditory ossicles, comprising the anterior, lateral, and superior ligaments of the malleus, the posterior and superior ligaments of the incus, and the annular ligament of the stapes.

l. ova'rii pro'prium [NA], ovarian ligament: a musculofibrous cord in the broad ligament, joining the ovary to the upper part of the lateral margin of the uterus just below the attachment of the uterine tube; called also *utero-ovarian ligament.*

ligamen'ta palma'ria articulatio'num interphalangea'lium ma'nus [NA], **ligamen'ta palma'ria articulatio'num interphalangea'rum manus,** palmar ligaments of interphalangeal articulations of hand: thick, dense fibrocartilaginous plates on the palmar surfaces of the interphalangeal articulations of the hand, between the collateral ligaments.

ligamen'ta palma'ria articulatio'num metacarpophalangea'lium [NA], **ligamen'ta palma'ria articulatio'num metacarpophalangea'rum,** palmar ligaments of metacarpophalangeal articulations: thick dense fibrocartilaginous plates on the palmar surfaces of the metacarpophalangeal articulation, between the collateral ligaments. Called also *anterior* or *palmar metacarpophalangeal ligaments.*

l. palpebra'le latera'le [NA], lateral palpebral ligament: a ligament that anchors the lateral end of the superior and inferior tarsal plates to the margin of the orbit; called also *canthal ligament.*

l. palpebra'le media'le [NA], medial palpebral ligament: fibrous bands that connect the medial ends of the tarsi to the bones of the orbit, an anterior bundle passing in front of the lacrimal sac and being attached to the frontal process of the maxilla, and a posterior bundle passing behind the lacrimal sac and being attached to the posterior crest of the lacrimal bone.

l. patel'lae [NA], patellar ligament: the continuation of the central portion of the tendon of the quadriceps femoris muscle distal to the patella; it extends from the patella to the tuberosity of the tibia.

l. pectina'tum an'guli iridocornea'lis, NA alternative for *reticulum trabeculare anguli iridocornealis.*

l. pectina'tum i'ridis, reticulum trabeculare anguli iridocornealis.

l. pectinea'le [NA], pectineal ligament: a strong aponeurotic lateral continuation of the lacunar ligament along the pectineal line of the pubis; called also *Cooper's ligament* and *inguinal ligament of Cooper.*

l. phrenicocol'icum [NA], phrenicocolic ligament: a peritoneal fold that passes from the left colic flexure to the adjacent costal portion of the diaphragm.

l. phrenicoliena'le l. splenorenale.

l. phrenicosple'nicum, NA alternative for *l. splenorenale.*

l. pisohama'tum [NA], pisohamate ligament: a fibrous band extending from the pisiform bone to the hook of the hamate bone.

l. pisometacar'peum [NA], pisometacarpal ligament: a fibrous band extending from the pisiform bone to the bases of the fifth, usually the fourth, and sometimes the third metacarpal bone.

ligamen'ta planta'ria articulatio'num interphalangea'lium pe'dis [NA], **ligamen'ta planta'ria articulatio'num interphalangea'rum pe'dis,** plantar ligaments of interphalangeal articulations of foot: thick, dense bands on the plantar surfaces of the interphalangeal articulations of the foot, between the collateral ligaments.

ligamen'ta planta'ria articulatio'num metatarsophalangea'lium [NA], **ligamenta planta'ria articulatio'num metatarsophalangea'rum,** plantar ligaments of metatarsophalangeal articulations: thick, dense bands on the plantar surface of the metatarsophalangeal articulations, between the collateral ligaments. Called also *inferior or plantar metatarsophalangeal ligaments.*

l. planta're lon'gum [NA], long plantar ligament: the longest ligament of the foot, arising from the lower surface of the calcaneus as far back as the lateral and the medial processes, passing forward over the tendon of the peroneus longus, and inserting into the bases of the second through fifth metatarsal bones.

l. poplite'um arcua'tum [NA], arcuate popliteal ligament: a band of variable and ill-defined fibers at the posterolateral part of the knee joint; it is attached inferiorly to the apex of the head of the fibula, arches superiorly and medially over the popliteal tendon, and merges with the articular capsule. Called also *popliteal arch* and *arcuate ligament of knee.*

l. poplite'um obli'quum [NA], oblique popliteal ligament: a broad band of fibers that arises from the medial condyle of the tibia, merges more or less with the tendon of the semimembranosus, and passes obliquely across the back of the knee joint to the lateral epicondyle of the femur. It contains large openings for the passage of vessels and nerves.

l. pterygospina'le [NA], pterygospinal ligament: a band of fibers extending from the upper part of the superior border of the lateral pterygoid plate to the spine of the sphenoid bone; called also *l. pterygospinosum.*

l. pterygospino'sum, l. pterygospinale.

l. pu'bicum supe'rius [NA], superior pubic ligament: fibers that pass transversely across the superior margin of the symphysis pubis; attached to the bones and to the interpubic disk, they extend laterally as far as the pubic tubercle.

l. pubocapsula're, l. pubofemorale.

l. pubofemora'le [NA], pubofemoral ligament: a band that arises from the entire length of the obturator crest of the pubic bone and passes laterally and inferiorly to merge into the capsule of the hip joint, some fibers reaching to the lower part of the neck of the femur. Called also *l. pubocapsulare.*

l. puboprostat'icum [NA], puboprostatic ligament: a thickening of the superior fascia of the pelvic diaphragm in the male that, laterally, extends from the prostate to the tendinous arch of the pelvic fascia and, medially, is a forward continuation of the tendinous arch to the pubis.

l. pubovesica'le [NA], pubovesical ligament: a thickening of the superior fascia of the pelvic diaphragm in the female that, laterally, extends from the neck of the bladder to the tendinous arch of the pelvic fascia and, medially, is a forward continuation of the tendinous arch to the pubis.

l. pubovesica'le latera'le, lateral extension of ligamentum pubovesicale.

l. pubovesica'le me'dium, medial extension of ligamentum pubovesicale.

l. pulmona'le [NA], pulmonary ligament: a vertical pleural fold that extends from the hilus down to the base on the medial surface of the lung, forming the posterior boundary of the impressio cardiaca; called also *broad ligament of lung.*

ligamen'ta pylo'ri, thickened bands of the longitudinal muscular layer of the stomach situated on the anterior and the posterior surfaces of the antrum pyloricum.

l. quadra'tum [NA], quadrate ligament: a fibrous bundle connecting the distal margin of the radial notch of the ulna to the neck of the radius.

l. radiocarpa'le dorsa'le [NA], **l. radiocar'peum dorsa'le,** dorsal radiocarpal ligament: a fibrous band that passes obliquely from the posterior border of the distal extremity of the radius to the dorsal surfaces of the proximal row of carpal bones, especially the triquetral and lunate, and to the dorsal intercarpal ligaments.

l. radiocarpa'le palma're [NA], **l. radiocar'peum palma're,** palmar radiocarpal ligament: several bundles of fibers that pass obliquely from the styloid process and the distal anterior margin of the radius to the lunate, triquetral, capitate, and hamate bones; called also *volar radiocarpal ligament.*

l. sacrococcyg'eum ante'rius [NA], anterior sacrococcygeal ligament: a flat band, homologous with the anterior longitudinal ligament of the vertebral column, that passes from the lower part of the sacrum over onto the anterior part of the coccyx. Called also *l. sacrococcygeum ventrale* [NA alternative] and *ventral sacrococcygeal ligament.*

l. sacrococcyg'eum dorsa'le profun'dum, NA alternative for *l. sacrococcygeum posterius profundum.*

l. sacrococcyg'eum dorsa'le superficia'le, NA alternative for *l. sacrococcygeum posterius superficiale.*

l. sacrococcyg'eum latera'le [NA], lateral sacrococcygeal ligament: a fibrous band, homologous with the intertransverse ligaments, that passes from the transverse process of the first coccygeal vertebra to the lower lateral angle of the sacrum, thus helping to complete the foramen of the fifth sacral nerve.

l. sacrococcyg'eum poste'rius profun'dum [NA], deep posterior sacrococcygeal ligament: the terminal portion of the posterior longitudinal ligament of the vertebral column; it helps to unite the dorsal surfaces of the fifth sacral and the coccygeal vertebrae. Called also *deep dorsal sacrococcygeal ligament* and *l. sacrococcygeum dorsale profundum* [NA alternative].

l. sacrococcyg'eum poste'rius superficia'le [NA], superficial posterior sacrococcygeal ligament: a fibrous band continuous with the supraspinous ligament of the vertebral column; attached cranially to the margin of the sacral hiatus, and diverging as it passes caudally to attach to the dorsal surface of the coccyx. Called also *l. sacrococcygeum dorsale superficiale* [NA alternative] and *superficial dorsal sacrococcygeal ligament.*

l. sacrococcyg'eum ventra'le, NA alternative for *l. sacrococcygeum anterius.*

ligamen'ta sacroili'aca anterio'ra [NA], anterior sacroiliac ligaments: numerous thin fibrous bands passing from the ventral margin of the auricular surface of the sacrum to the adjacent portions of the ilium; called also *ligamenta sacroilica ventralis* [NA alternative] and *ventral sacroiliac ligaments.*

ligamen'ta sacroili'aca dorsa'lia, NA alternative for *ligamenta sacroiliaca posteriora.*

ligamen'ta sacroili'aca interos'sea [NA], interosseous sacroiliac ligaments: numerous short, strong bundles connecting the tuberosities and adjacent surfaces of the sacrum and the ilium.

ligamen'ta sacroili'aca posterio'ra [NA], posterior sacroiliac ligaments: numerous strong bands that pass from the tuberosity of the ilium and the posterior inferior and posterior superior iliac spines to the intermediate sacral crest and adjacent areas of the sacrum. Called also *ligamenta sacroiliaca dorsalia* [NA alternative] and *dorsal sacroiliac ligaments.*

ligamenta sacrospina'lia [NA], sacrospinal ligaments: long vertical fibrous bands attached by the apex to the spine of the ischium and by the base to the lateral margins of the sacrum; they are continuous above with the ligamentum muchae. Called also *supraspinous ligaments.*

l. sacrospino'sum, l. sacrospinale.

l. sacrotubera'le [NA], sacrotuberal ligament: a large, flat band that is attached below to the ischial tuberosity, spreads out as it ascends, and is attached to the lateral margins of the sacrum and the coccyx and to the posterior inferior iliac spine; called also *l. sacrotuberosum.*

l. sacrotubero'sum, l. sacrotuberale.

l. sero'sum, serous ligament: a fold of peritoneum or other serous membrane that helps to hold an organ or part in position and transmits blood vessels and nerves.

l. sphenomandibula're [NA], sphenomandibular ligament: a thin aponeurotic band that extends from the angular spine of the sphenoid bone downward medial to the temporomandibular articulation and attaches to the lingula of the mandible.

l. spira'le coch'leae, NA alternative for *crista spiralis cochleae.*

l. splenorena'le [NA], splenorenal ligament: a peritoneal fold that passes from the diaphragm to the concave surface of the spleen; called also *l. lienorenale* and *l. phrenicosplenicum* [NA alternatives], *l. phrenicolienale,* and *lienophrenic, phrenicosplenic,* or *splenophrenic ligament.*

l. sternoclavicula're, see *l. sternoclaviculare anterius* and *l. sternoclaviculare posterius.*

l. sternoclavicula're ante'rius [NA], anterior sternoclavicular ligament: a thick reinforcing band on the anterior portion of the articular capsule of the sternoclavicular articulation. It is attached superiorly to the anterior and superior parts of the sternal extremity of the clavicle and inferiorly to the anterior surface of the manubrium of the sternum.

l. sternoclavicula're poste'rius [NA], posterior sternoclavicular ligament: a thick reinforcing band on the posterior portion of the articular capsule of the sternoclavicular articulation. It is attached superiorly to the posterior and superior parts of the sternal extremity of the clavicle and inferiorly to the posterior surface of the manubrium of the sternum.

l. sternocosta′le interarticula′re, l. sternocostale intra-articulare.

l. sternocosta′le intra-articula′re [NA], intra-articular sternocostal ligament: a horizontal fibrocartilaginous plate in the center of the second sternocostal joint, which joins the tip of the costal cartilage to the fibrous junction between the manubrium and the body of the sternum, and thus divides the joint into two parts. Called also *interarticular sternocostal ligament* and *l. sternocostale interarticulare.*

ligamen′ta sternocosta′lia radia′ta [NA], radiate sternocostal ligaments: fibrous bands attached to the sternal end of a costal cartilage, radiating from there out onto the ventral part of the sternum.

ligamen′ta sternopericardi′aca [NA], sternopericardiac ligaments: two (superior and inferior) or more fibrous bands that attach the pericardium to the dorsal surface of the sternum.

l. stylohyoi′deum [NA], stylohyoid ligament: a vertical fibroelastic aponeurotic cord attached above to the tip of the styloid process of the temporal bone and below to the lesser horn of the hyoid bone.

l. stylomandibula′re [NA], stylomandibular ligament: an aponeurotic band attached superiorly to the tip of the styloid process of the temporal bone and inferiorly to the angle and posterior margin of the ramus of the mandible.

l. supraspina′le [NA], supraspinal ligament: a single long, vertical fibrous band passing over and attached to the tips of the spinous processes of the vertebrae from the seventh cervical to the sacrum; it is continuous above with the ligamentum nuchae.

l. suspenso′rium clitor′idis [NA], suspensory ligament of clitoris: a strong fibrous band that comes from the external deep investing fascia and attaches the root of the clitoris to the linea alba, symphysis pubis, and arcuate pubic ligament.

ligamen′ta suspenso′ria mam′mae [NA], suspensory ligaments of mammary gland: fibrous processes, extending from the corpus mammae to the corium, homologous with the retinacula cutis of other regions of the body.

l. suspenso′rium ova′rii [NA], suspensory ligament of ovary: the portion of the broad ligament lateral to and above the ovary; it contains the ovarian vessels and nerves and passes upward over the iliac vessels.

l. suspenso′rium pe′nis [NA], suspensory ligament of penis: a strong fibrous band that comes from the external deep investing fascia and attaches the root of the penis to the linea alba, symphysis pubis, and arcuate pubic ligament.

l. talocalcanea′re interos′seum [NA], **l. talocalca′neum interos′seum,** interosseous talocalcaneal ligament: fibrous bands in the sinus tarsi, passing between the opposed surfaces of the calcaneus and the talus.

l. talocalcanea′re latera′le [NA], **l. talocalca′neum latera′le,** lateral talocalcaneal ligament: a fibrous band passing from the lateral surface of the talus to that of the calcaneus.

l. talocalcanea′re media′le [NA], **l. talocalca′neum media′le,** medial talocalcaneal ligament: a fibrous band connecting the medial tubercle of the talus with the sustentaculum tali of the calcaneus.

l. talofibula′re ante′rius [NA], anterior talofibular ligament: one or more fibrous bands that pass from the anterior surface of the lateral malleolus of the fibula to the anterior margin of the lateral articular surface of the talus.

l. talofibula′re poste′rius [NA], posterior talofibular ligament: a strong fibrous horizontal band passing from the posteromedial face of the lateral malleolus of the fibula to the area of the posterior process of the talus.

l. talonavicula′re [NA], talonavicular ligament: a broad, thin fibrous band passing from the dorsal and lateral surfaces of the neck of the talus to the dorsal surface of the navicular bone; called also *l. talonaviculare* [*dorsale*] and *talonavicular dorsal ligament.*

l. talonavicula′re [dorsa′le], l. talonaviculare.

l. talotibia′le ante′rius, pars tibiotalaris anterior ligamenti medialis.

l. talotibia′le poste′rius, pars tibiotalaris posterior ligamenti medialis.

ligamen′ta tar′si dorsa′lia [NA], dorsal ligaments of tarsus: including the bifurcate, the dorsal cuboideonavicular, cuneocuboid, cuneonavicular, and intercuneiform, and the talonavicular ligaments; called also *dorsal intertarsal ligaments.*

ligamen′ta tar′si interos′sea [NA], interosseous ligaments of the tarsus, including the interosseous cuneocuboid, intercuneiform, talocalcaneal ligaments.

ligamen′ta tar′si planta′ria [NA], plantar ligaments of tarsus: the inferior ligaments of the foot, comprising the long plantar and the plantar calcaneocuboid, calcaneonavicular, cuneonavicular, cuboideonavicular, intercuneiform, and cuneocuboid ligaments.

ligamen′ta tarsometarsa′lia dorsa′lia [NA], **ligamen′ta tarsometatar′sea dorsa′lia,** dorsal tarsometatarsal ligaments: fibrous bands passing from the dorsal surfaces of the bases of the metatarsal bones to the dorsal surfaces of the cuboid and the three cuneiform bones.

ligamen′ta tarsometatarsa′lia planta′ria [NA], **ligamen′ta tarsometatar′sea planta′ria,** plantar tarsometatarsal ligaments: fibrous bands passing from the plantar surfaces of the bases of the metatarsal bones to the plantar surfaces of the cuboid and the three cuneiform bones.

l. temporomandibula′re, l. laterale articulationis temporomandibularis.

l. te′res fem′oris, l. capitis femoris.

l. te′res hep′atis [NA], a fibrous cord, the remains of the left umbilical vein, extending from the porta hepatis, where it is attached to the left branch of the portal vein, out through the fissure of the ligamentum teres and the falciform ligament to the umbilicus.

l. te′res u′teri [NA], round ligament of uterus: a fibromuscular band in the female that is attached to the uterus near the attachment of the uterine tube, passing then along the broad ligament, out through the inguinal ring, and into the labium majus.

l. thyreoepiglot′ticum, l. thyroepiglotticum.

l. thyroepiglot′ticum [NA], thyroepiglottic ligament: a fibrous band that attaches the petiolus of the epiglottis to the thyroid cartilage just below the superior notch; called also *l. thyreoepiglotticum.*

l. thyrohyoi′deum latera′le [NA], lateral thyrohyoid ligament: a round elastic cord that forms the posterior margin of the thyrohyoid membrane; it extends from the tip of the superior horn of the thyroid cartilage upward to the tip of the greater horn of the hyoid bone. Called also *l. hyothyreoideum laterale* and *Berry's ligament.*

l. thyrohyoi′deum media′num [NA], median thyrohyoid ligament: the central, thicker portion of the thyrohyoid membrane; its broader upper part is attached to the body of the hyoid bone and its narrow lower end to the superior incisure of the thyroid cartilage. Called also *l. hyothyreoideum medium.*

l. tibiofibula′re ante′rius [NA], anterior tibiofibular ligament: a flat triangular band that passes diagonally, inferiorly, and laterally from the anterior portion of the lateral surface of the distal end of the tibia to the anterior surface of the distal end of the fibula; called also *l. malleoli lateralis anterius.*

l. tibiofibula′re poste′rius [NA], posterior tibiofibular ligament: a fibrous band that passes diagonally, inferiorly, and laterally from the posterior surface of the distal end of the tibia to the adjacent posterior surface of the distal end of the fibula; called also *l. malleoli lateralis posterius.*

l. tibionavicula′re, pars tibionavicularis ligamenti medialis.

ligamenta trachea′lia, NA alternative for *ligamenta annularia tracheae.*

l. transver′sum acetab′uli [NA], transverse ligament of acetabulum: a fibrous band continuous with the acetabular lip of the hip joint, which bridges the acetabular notch and converts it into a foramen.

l. transver′sum atlan′tis [NA], transverse ligament of atlas: the strong horizontal portion of the cruciform ligament of the atlas. It is attached at each end to the lateral masses of the atlas and curves posteriorly around the dens of the axis. It thus divides the atlantal ring into a smaller anterior division for the dens and a larger posterior division for the spinal cord and related structures. Called also *Lauth's ligament.*

l. transver′sum cru′ris, retinaculum musculorum extensorum pedis superius.

l. transver′sum ge′nu, l. transversum genus.

l. transver′sum ge′nus [NA], transverse ligament of knee: a more or less distinct bundle of fibers in the knee joint, joining together the anterior convex margin of the lateral meniscus and the anterior concave margin or anterior end of the medial meniscus; called also *l. transversum genu.*

l. transver′sum pel′vis, l. transversum perinei.

934

l. transver'sum perine'i [NA], transverse perineal ligament: a fibrous band that spans the subpubic angle just behind the deep dorsal vein of the penis, formed by thickening of the anterior boundary of the perineal membrane.

l. transver'sum scap'ulae infe'rius [NA], inferior transverse ligament of scapula: one of three intrinsic ligaments of the scapula, composed of more or less distinct fascial fibers that pass from the lateral border of the spine of the scapula to the adjacent margin of the glenoid cavity, thus converting the notch at the base of the spine into a foramen for the passage of the suprascapular vessels and nerves to the infraspinous fossa.

l. transver'sum scap'ulae supe'rius [NA], superior transverse ligament of scapula: one of three intrinsic ligaments of the scapula, a band of fibers that bridges the scapular notch, thus forming a foramen for the passage of the suprascapular nerve. One end is attached to the base of the coracoid process, the other end to the medial border of the scapular notch.

l. trapezoi'deum [NA], trapezoid ligament: a broad, flat band forming the anterolateral portion of the coracoclavicular ligament; it is attached inferiorly to the superior surface of the coracoid process of the scapula and superiorly to the oblique ridge on the inferior surface of the clavicle.

l. triangula're dex'trum hep'atis [NA], right triangular ligament of liver: the pointed right extremity of the coronary ligament of the liver where the superior and the inferior layer join in their attachment to the diaphragm.

l. triangula're sinis'trum hep'atis [NA], left triangular ligament of liver: a triangular extension of the left extremity of the coronary ligament, which helps to attach the left lobe of the liver to the diaphragm.

l. tuber'culi cos'tae, l. costotransversarium laterale.

l. ulnocarpa'le palma're [NA], **l. ulnocar'peum palma're,** palmar ulnocarpal ligament: bundles of fibers that pass from the styloid process of the ulna to the carpal bones.

l. umbilica'le latera'le, former NA term for *l. umbilicale mediale*.

l. umbilica'le media'le [NA], a fibrous cord, the remains of the obliterated umbilical artery, which is situated in and produces the lateral umbilical fold. Called also *obliterated hypogastric artery, lateral umbilical ligament, l. umbilicale laterale*, and *medial umbilical ligament*.

l. umbilica'le media'le [NA], medial umbilical ligament: a fibrous cord, the remains of the obliterated umbilical artery, which is situated in and produces the lateral umbilical fold. Called also *lateral umbilical ligament* and *umbilicale laterale*.

l. umbilica'le me'dium, l. umbilicale mediale.

l. vagina'lo, vinculum tendinum.

ligamen'ta vagina'lia digito'rum ma'nus, vaginae fibrosae digitorum manus.

ligamen'ta vagina'lia digito'rum pedis, vaginae fibrosae digitorum pedis.

l. ve'nae ca'vae sinis'trae, plica venae cavae sinistrae.

l. veno'sum [NA], venous ligament of liver: a fibrous cord, the remains of the fetal ductus venosus, lying in the fissura ligamenti venosi.

l. veno'sum [Aran'tii], l. venosum.

l. ventricula're, l. vestibulare.

l. vestibula're [NA], vestibular ligament: the membrane that extends from the thyroid cartilage in front to the anterolateral surface of the arytenoid cartilage behind; it lies within the vestibular fold, above the vocal ligament. Called also *l. ventriculare* and *ventricular ligament of larynx*.

l. voca'le [NA], vocal ligament: the elastic tissue membrane that extends from the thyroid cartilage in front to the vocal process of the arytenoid cartilage behind; it lies within the vocal fold, below the vestibular ligament.

---

ligand (li'gand, lig'and) [L. *ligare* to tie or bind] 1. a molecule that binds to another molecule, used especially to refer to a small molecule that binds specifically to a larger molecule, e.g., an antigen binding to an antibody, a hormone or neurotransmitter binding to a receptor, or a substrate or allosteric effector binding to an enzyme. 2. a molecule that donates or accepts a pair of electrons to form a coordinate covalent bond with the central metal atom of a coordination complex.

ligase (li'gās, lig'ās) [EC 6] one of the six main classes of enzymes. These enzymes catalyze the formation of a bond between two substrate molecules, coupled with the hydrolysis of a pyrophosphate bond in ATP or a similar energy donor. Called also *synthetase*.

ligate (li'gāt) to tie or bind with a ligature.

ligation (li-ga'shun) [L. *ligatio*] the application of a ligature. **Barron l.,** treatment of hemorrhoids by binding them at the base with rubber ligatures so that the distal portion sloughs away within several days. **rubber band l.,** Barron l. **teeth l.,** the binding together of teeth with wire, thread, or other material for their stabilization and immobilization as a method of tooth movement in orthodontic therapy or following traumatic injury. **tubal l.,** sterilization of the female by constricting the uterine tubes by means of ligatures; the tubes may, in addition, be severed or crushed.

ligature (lig'ah-chūr) [L. *ligatura*] 1. any substance, such as catgut, cotton, silk, or wire, used to tie a vessel or strangulate a part. 2. see under *wire*. **elastic l.,** a band of rubber used to strangulate hemorrhoids and pedunculated growths. **interlacing l., interlocking l.,** a continuous suture in which the loops interlock. **lateral l.,** a ligature so applied as to check, but not to interrupt, the distal blood flow. **occluding l.,** a ligature that occludes the blood supply to distal tissue. **provisional l.,** one applied at the beginning of an operation, but removed before its termination. **soluble l.,** a ligature of prepared animal membrane which is subsequently absorbed, the time of absorption depending upon the method of preparation and the size of the ligature. **suboccluding l.,** a ligature that obstructs the main blood supply, but leaves unimpaired a portion of tissue capable of establishing capillary anastomosis. **terminal l.,** a ligature applied to the transected end of a vessel. **thread-elastic l.,** an elastic thread used for various forms of orthodontic therapy, such as assisting in eruption of impacted teeth, closing spaces, and rotating teeth.

ligg. ligaments, or ligamenta.

light (līt) the electromagnetic radiation having a velocity of about 3×10^{10} cm. (186,284 miles) per second, and the vibrations in space being at right angles to the direction of transmission. Frequently construed as limited to the range of wavelength between 3900 and 7700 angstroms, which provides the stimulus for the subjective sensation of sight, but sometimes considered as including part of the ultraviolet and infrared ranges as well. **actinic l.,** light rays capable of producing chemical effects. **axial l., central l.,** light whose rays are parallel to each other and to the optic axis. **coherent l.,** light of a single frequency that travels in intense, nearly perfect, parallel rays without appreciable divergence. **cold l.,** a light transmitted through a quartz or plastic structure to dissipate the heat. The lamp may be applied directly to the skin and is used for transillumination of the tissues for cancer diagnosis. **l. difference,** the difference between the two eyes in their sensitivity to light; often abbreviated L.D. **diffused l.,** that which has been scattered by reflection and refraction. **Finsen l.,** light consisting principally of the violet and ultraviolet rays given off by a Finsen lamp; used in the treatment of lupus and similar diseases. **idioretinal l.,** sensation of light that occurs in the complete absence of the electromagnetic waves that ordinarily stimulate the sensation. **infrared l.,** see under *ray*. **intrinsic l.** (of the retina), the dim light always present in the visual field. **Landeker-Steinberg l.,** a light that emits a spectrum similar to that of the sun except that the ultraviolet waves are eliminated; used therapeutically. **l. minimum,** the smallest degree of light perceived by the eye; often abbreviated L.M. **Minin l.,** a therapeutic lamp for the administration of violet and ultraviolet light. **monochromatic l.,** one of the colors of the spectrum into which light is divided by a prism. **neon l.,** a light that contains no ultraviolet and no infrared rays. **oblique l.,** the light that falls obliquely on a surface. **polarized l.,** light the vibrations of which are made over one plane or in circles or ellipses. **reflected l.,** light whose rays have been turned back from an illuminated surface. **refracted l.,** light whose rays have been bent out of their original course by passing through a transparent membrane. **Simpson l.,** an electric arc light with electrodes of tungstate of iron and manganese; formerly used in the treatment of skin lesions. **transmitted l.,** light the rays of which have passed through an object. **Tyndall l.,** the light that is reflected or dispersed by particles suspended in a gas or liquid; see *Tyndall phenomenon,* under *phenomenon.* **ultraviolet l.,** see under *ray.* **white l.,** that produced by a mixture of all wavelengths of electromagnetic energy perceptible as light. **Wood's l.,** ultraviolet radiation from a mercury-vapor source, transmitted through a nickel-oxide filter (Wood's filter or glass), which holds back all but a few violet rays of the visible spectrum and passes ultraviolet wavelengths of about 365 nm.; much used in the diagnosis of fungus infections of the scalp and erythrasma, and also to reveal the presence of porphyrins and fluorescent minerals.

lightening (līt′en-ing) the sensation of decreased abdominal distention produced by the descent of the uterus into the pelvic cavity, occurring from two to three weeks before labor begins.

ligneous (lig′ne-us) woody; having a wooden feeling.

lignocaine (lig′no-kān) lidocaine.

lignoceric acid (lig″no-sēr′ik) trivial name for tetracosanoic acid, the 24-carbon straight-chain saturated fatty acid; it occurs in sphingomyelin.

lignum (lig′num), gen. *lig′ni* [L.] wood. **l. sanc′tum, l. vi′tae,** the heartwood of *Guajacum officinale* Linne or of *G. sanctum* Linne.

ligroin, ligroine (lig′ro-in) a petroleum fraction similar in nature to (and sometimes used synonymously with) petroleum benzin; it is used as an organic solvent. Called also *naphtha.*

Lilienthal's probe (lil′e-en-thalz″) [Howard *Lilienthal,* surgeon in New York, 1861–1946] see under *probe.*

limb (lim) 1. one of the paired appendages of the body used in locomotion or grasping. In man, an arm or a leg with all its component parts; called also *membrum* [NA] and, formerly, *extremitas.* In embryology, the skeleton of each limb is divided into four main parts: the *zonoskeleton,* comprising the scapula and clavicle (as a unit) and the hip bone; the *stylopodium,* comprising the humerus and femur; the *zygopodium,* comprising the radius and ulna and the tibia and fibula; and the *autopodium,* comprising the hand and the foot. 2. a structure or part resembling an arm or leg. **anacrotic l.,** the ascending portion of a tracing of the pulse wave obtained by the manometer or the sphygmograph. **l's of anthelix,** crura anthelicis; see under *crus.* **catacrotic l.,** the descending portion of a tracing of the pulse wave obtained by the manometer or the sphygmograph. **l. of incus, long,** crus longum incudis. **l. of incus, short,** crus breve incudis. **l. of internal capsule, anterior,** crus anterius capsulae internae. **l. of internal capsule, posterior,** crus posterius capsulae internae. **pectoral l.,** the arm (membrum superius), or a homologous part. **pelvic l.,** the lower limb (membrum inferius). **phantom l.,** the sensation, after amputation of a limb, that the absent part is still present; there may also be paresthesias, transient aches, and intermittent or continuous pain perceived as originating in the absent limb. **l. of stapes, anterior,** crus anterius stapedis. **l. of stapes, posterior,** crus posterius stapedis. **thoracic l.,** pectoral l.

limbal (lim′bal) limbic; occurring at the junction of the cornea and conjunctiva.

limberneck (lim′ber-nek) a disease of fowl resulting from ingestion of food contaminated with *Clostridium botulinum,* and characterized by a flaccid paralysis which gives the condition its name.

limbi (lim′bi) [L.] genitive and plural of *limbus.*

limbic (lim′bik) pertaining to a limbus, or margin; forming a border around; see under *system.*

Limbitrol (lim′bĭ-trol) trademark for a combination of amitriptyline and chlordiazepoxide.

limbus (lim′bus), gen. and pl. *lim′bi* [L.] 1. a border, hem, fringe; used in official anatomical nomenclature as a general term for such a structure. See also *labium* and *margo.* 2. [NA] the junctional region between the cornea and the sclera, marked on the outer surface of the eyeball by a slight furrow, the sulcus sclerae; called also *corneoscleral junction* and *sclerocorneal junction.* **l. acetab′uli** [NA], margin of acetabulum: the peripheral margin of the acetabulum to which the labrum acetabulare is attached; called also *border of acetabulum* and *margo acetabuli.* **alveolar l. of man-** dible, arcus alveolaris mandibulae. **alveolar l. of maxilla,** arcus alveolaris maxillae. **l. alveola′ris mandib′ulae,** arcus alveolaris mandibulae. **l. alveola′ris maxil′lae,** arcus alveolaris maxillae. **l. angulo′sus,** linea obliqua cartilaginis thyroideae. **l. chorioi′deus** (*obs.*), that part of the embryonic gyrus fornicatus which forms, in the adult, the choroid plexus of the lateral ventricle. **l. conjuncti′vae,** 1. l. corneae. 2. annulus conjunctivae. **l. of cornea,** see *limbus* (def. 2). **l. foram′inis ova′lis,** the border of the foramen ovale. **l. fos′sae ova′lis** [NA], **l. fos′sae ova′lis [Vieussen′ii],** the prominent rounded margin of the fossa ovalis cordis. **l. lam′inae spira′lis os′seae** [NA], the thickened periosteum of the osseous spiral lamina at the attachment of the vestibular membrane. **l. lu′teus re′tinae,** macula retinae. **l. membra′nae tym′pani,** 1. the thickened margin of the tympanic membrane attached to the tympanic sulcus. 2. annulus fibrocartilagineus membranae tympani. **lim′bi palpebra′les anterio′res** [NA], the rounded anterior edges of the free margin of the eyelids, from which the eyelashes arise. **lim′bi palpebra′les posterio′res** [NA], the sharp posterior edges of the free margin of the eyelids, closely applied to the eyeball. **l. of sclera,** see *limbus* (def. 2). **spiral l.,** l. laminae spiralis osseae. **l. of Vieussens,** l. fossae ovalis.

lime (līm) [L. *calx*] 1. calcium oxide. 2. [USP] a pharmaceutical preparation containing not less than 95 per cent of calcium oxide; used as a pharmaceutical necessity. 3. the acid fruit of *Citrus aurantifolia;* its juice, which contains ascorbic acid, is antiscorbutic and refrigerant. **l. arsenate,** a solution of white arsenic and sal soda in water, used as an insecticide. **barium hydroxide l.,** a mixture of barium hydroxide octahydrate and calcium hydroxide used as a carbon dioxide absorbant in the administration of anesthetic gases and oxygen. **chlorinated l.,** a white or grayish white powder used as a bleaching agent and disinfectant and, formerly, as a topical germicide. **slaked l.,** calcium hydroxide. **soda l.,** a mixture of calcium oxide and sodium hydroxide. **sulfurated l.,** see *calx sulfurata.*

limen (li′men), pl. *lim′ina* [L.] threshold, as of a stimulus; [NA] a general term for the beginning point, boundary, or threshold of a structure. **l. of insula, l. in′sulae** [NA], the point at which the cortex of the insula is continuous, on the inferior surface of the cerebral hemisphere, with the cortex of the frontal lobe. **l. na′si** [NA], the ridge at the junction of the lateral nasal cartilage and the lateral crus of the greater alar cartilage, marking the boundary between the vestibule of the nose and the nasal cavity proper. **l. of twoness,** the distance between two points of contact on the skin necessary for their recognition as giving rise to separate stimuli.

limes (li′mēz) [L. "boundary"] limit; boundary. **l. dose,** see *L + d., L0 d., Lf d.,* and *Lr d.,* under *dose.*

limina (lim′ĭ-nah) [L.] plural of *limen.*

liminal (lim′ĭ-nal) [L. *limen* threshold] barely appreciable to the senses; pertaining to a threshold.

liminometer (lim″ĭ-nom′ĕ-ter) [*limen* + Gr. *metron* measure] an instrument for measuring the strength of a stimulus applied over a tendon and determining the reflex threshold.

limit (lim′it) [L. *limes* boundary] a boundary, as one that confines. **assimilation l.,** the amount of carbohydrate that an organism can metabolize without causing glycosuria; called also *saturation limit.* **audibility l.,** the extremes of frequency beyond which the human ear perceives no sound: lower limit, 8 Hz; upper, 20,000 Hz. **elastic l.,** the extent to which elastic material may be deformed without impairing its ability to return to original dimensions. **l. of flocculation,** a term used in expressing the strength of toxin, toxoid, and antitoxin; see *Lf dose,* under *dose.* **l. of perception,** the minimum visual angle below which perception is impossible: an object to be perceived must subtend a visual angle of four or five minutes, thus making its image on the retina about the size of a retinal cone of 3.3–3.6 microns in diameter. **quantum l.,** minimum wavelength. **saturation l.,** assimilation l.

limitans (lim′ĭ-tanz) [L.] limiting; see *membrana limitans.*

limitation (lim-ĭ-ta′shun) circumscription; the act of limiting, or state of being limited. **eccentric l.,** a circumscribed condition of the visual field, more pronounced at some parts of the periphery than at others. **genetic l.,** the necessity that all cells react in accordance with the standards of the particular species to which they belong.

limit dextrinase (deks′trin-ās) α-dextrinase.

limitrophic (lim″ĭ-trof′ik) controlling nutrition.

Limnatis (lim-na′tis) the land leeches, a genus of the family Gnathobdellidae, class Hirudinea. **L. nilot′ica**, a species of North Africa, middle Europe, and the Near East, where they are commonly used for drawing blood. They sometimes become lodged in the nasal passages, larynx and pharynx of mammals, and when present in large numbers may cause anemia and asphyxia. Called also *Hirudo aegyptiaca*.

limonene (lim′o-nēn) an essential oil found in the peel of oranges and lemons; it is a terpene, $C_3H_5 \cdot C_6H_8 \cdot CH_3$.

limophthisis (li-mof′thĭ-sis) [Gr. *limos* hunger + *phthisis* wasting] wasting from lack of food or starvation.

limosis (li-mo′sis) [Gr. *limos* hunger] abnormal or morbid hunger.

Linacre (lin′ah-ker), Thomas (1460–1524). A noted English physician and classicist, who was physician to Henry VIII and the first president of the Royal College of Physicians of London. He was also renowned for his translations of Greek classics (e.g., Galen) into Latin.

linamarin (lin″ah-mah′rin) a bitter glycoside, $C_{10}H_{17}O_6N$, found in flax, *Linum usitatissimum* L. (Linaceae) and the lima bean, *Phaseolus limensis* Macf. (Leguminosae). Called also *phaseolunatin*.

Lincocin (lin-ko′sin) trademark for a preparation of lincomycin hydrochloride.

lincomycin (lin″ko-mi′sin) chemical name: (2S-*trans*)-methyl- 6,8- dideoxy- 6-[[(1-methyl-4 -propyl-2-pyrrolidinyl) carbonyl] amino] -1- thio -D-*erythro*-α-D-*galacto*-octopyranoside. An antibiotic, $C_{18}H_{34}N_2O_6S$, primarily a gram-positive specific antibacterial, produced by a variant of *Streptomyces lincolnesis*. **l. hydrochloride** [USP], the monohydrated monohydrochloride salt of lincomycin, $C_{18}H_{34}N_2O_6S \cdot HCl \cdot H_2O$, occurring as a white or practically white, crystalline powder; used as an antibacterial, mainly in the treatment of infections due to susceptible strains of streptococci, pneumococci, and staphylococci, administered intramuscularly and intravenously.

lincture (lingk′tūr) an electuary.

linctus (lingk′tus) [L. "a licking"] an electuary.

lindane (lin′dān) [USP] chemical name: 1α,2α,3β,4α, 5α,6β-hexachlorocyclohexane. The gamma isomer of benzene hexachloride, $C_6H_6Cl_6$, occurring as a white, crystalline powder; an insecticide more potent than chlorophenothane (DDT), it is used as a pediculicide and scabicide, applied topically to the skin. Called also *gamma benzene hexachloride*.

Lindau's disease (lin′dowz) [Arvid *Lindau*, Swedish pathologist, 1892–1958] von Hippel-Lindau disease.

Lindau-von Hippel disease (lin′dow-von hip′el) [Arvid *Lindau*; Eugen *von Hippel*, German ophthalmologist, 1867–1939] von Hippel-Lindau disease.

Lindbergh pump [Charles A. *Lindbergh*, American aviator, 1902–1974] see under *pump*.

line (līn) [L. *linea*] 1. a stripe, streak, mark, or narrow ridge. 2. in anthropometry, often an imaginary line connecting different anatomical landmarks. See also *axis* and *plane*, def. 1. **abdominal l.**, any imaginary line projected upon the surface of the abdomen, such as one indicating the boundary of a region. **absorption l's**, dark lines in the spectrum due to absorption of light by the substance (usually an incandescent gas or vapor) through which the light has passed. Cf. *absorption bands*, under *band*. **accretion l's**, incremental l's. **adrenal l.**, Sergent's white adrenal l. **Aldrich-Mees l's**, Mees' l's. **alveolobasilar l.**, a line from the basion to the upper alveolar limit. **l. of Amici**, Z band; see under *band*. **angular l.**, an irregular jagged line dividing the anterior surface of the iris into two regions; called also *collarette*. **anococcygeal l., white**, ligamentum anococcygeum. **anocutaneous l.**, linea anocutanea. **anorectal l.**, linea anorectalis. **arcuate l. of ilium**, linea arcuata ossis ilii. **arcuate l. of occipital bone, external superior**, linea nuchae superior. **arcuate l. of occipital bone, highest**, linea nuchae suprema. **arcuate l. of occipital bone, inferior**, linea nuchae inferior. **arcuate l. of**

occipital bone, superior, linea nuchae superior. **arcuate l. of occipital bone, supreme**, linea nuchae suprema. **arcuate l. of pelvis**, linea terminalis pelvis. **arcuate l. of sheath of rectus abdominis muscle**, linea arcuata vaginae musculi recti abdominis. **atropic l.**, one normal to the place of the axes of rotation of the eye. **auriculobregmatic l.**, a line from the auricular point to the bregma. **axillary l.**, linea axillaris anterior. **axillary l., median**, linea axillaris media. **axillary l., posterior**, linea axillaris posterior. **l's of Baillarger**, see *stria laminaris granularis interna corticis cerebri* and *stria laminae pyramidalis interna corticis cerebri*. **base l.**, 1. one from the infraorbital ridge to the external auditory meatus and the middle line of the occiput. 2. baseline. **base-apex l.**, a line perpendicular to the edge of a prism and bisecting the refracting angle of the prism. **basinasal l.**, a line from the basion to the nasion. Called also *nasobasal l.* **basiobregmatic l.**, a line from the basion to the bregma. **Baudelocque's l.**, see under *diameter*. **Beau's l's**, transverse lines or grooves in the nail plate caused by various systemic and local traumatic factors. **biauricular l.**, a line passing over the vertex from one auditory meatus to the other. **bi-iliac l.**, one joining the most prominent points of the two iliac crests. **bismuth l.**, a thin blue-black line in the marginal gingiva around the teeth, sometimes confined to the gingival papilla, observed in bismuth poisoning. See also *bismuth stomatitis*, under *stomatitis*. **blood l.**, a line of direct descent through several generations. **blue l.**, see *bismuth l.* and *lead l.* **Borsieri's l.**, see under *sign*. **Brödel's white l.**, a longitudinal white line on the anterior surface of the kidney near the convex border. **Brücke's l's**, broad bands alternating with Z bands in the fibrils of the striated muscles. **Bryant's l.**, 1. the vertical side of the iliofemoral triangle. 2. a test line for detecting shortening of the femur. **Burton's l.**, lead l. **calcification l's**, incremental l's. **cell l.**, a group of animal cells derived from a primary culture at the time of first subculture; it is considered to be an *established cell line* when it demonstrates the potential for indefinite subculture *in vitro*. **cement l.**, a name applied to a line, visible in microscopic examination of bone in cross section, marking the boundary of an osteon (haversian system). **cervical l.**, an anatomical landmark determined by the junction of the enamel- and the cementum-covered portions of a tooth (the cementoenamel junction); the dividing line between the crown and root portions of a tooth. **Chaussier's l.**, the median raphe of the corpus callosum. **Chiene's l's**, a set of lines established to aid in localizing the cerebral centers. **Clapton's l.**, a green line on the gums in copper poisoning. **clavicular l.**, one following the course of the clavicles. **cleavage l's**, Langer's l's. **Conradi's l.**, a line from the base of the xiphoid process to the point on the chest at which the apex beat is felt, indicating the upper limit of percussion dullness of the left lobe of the liver. **contour l's**, l's of Owen. **copper l.**, a greenish or red line at the border of the gums in copper poisoning. **Correra's l.**, a line in the roentgenogram of the chest, around the outline of the thorax, and bounding the lung fields. **Corrigan's l.**, a purplish line observed on the gums in copper poisoning. **costoarticular l.**, a line from the sternoclavicular joint to a point on the eleventh rib. **costoclavicular l.**, linea parasternalis. **costophrenic septal l's**, see *Kerley's l's*. **cricoclavicular l.**, a line from the cricoid cartilage of the larynx to the point at which the upward projection of the anterior axillary line intersects the clavicle. **cruciate l.**, eminentia cruciformis. **curved l. of ilium**, linea arcuata ossis ilii. **curved l. of ilium, inferior**, linea glutea inferior. **curved l. of ilium, middle**, linea glutea anterior. **curved l. of ilium, superior**, linea glutea posterior. **curved l. of occipital bone, highest**, linea nuchae suprema. **curved l. of occipital bone, inferior**, linea nuchae inferior. **curved l. of occipital bone, superior**, linea nuchae superior. **curved l. of occipital bone, supreme**, linea nuchae suprema. **Czermak's l's**, spatia interglobularia; see under *spatium*. **Daubenton's l.**, see under *plane*. **dentate l.**, linea anocutanea. **De Salle's l.**, nasal l. **developmental l's**, see under *groove*. **Dobie's l.**, Z band; see under *band*. **l. of Douglas**, linea arcuata vaginae musculi recti abdominis. **Duhot's l.**, a line from the superior iliac spine to the apex of the sacrum. **dynamic l's**, lines on the face, e.g., laugh lines and frown lines, which develop as a result of repetitious right-angled pull on the skin by the muscles of expression; they are considered a sign of aging. **Eberth's l's,** microscopic broken or scalariform lines at the junction of the cardiac muscle cells. **l's of Ebner,** delicate lines indicating periods of rest between daily increments of dentin, which are visible on ground sections of a tooth. Called also *incremental l's of Ebner.* **ectental l.,** the line of junction between the ectoderm and entoderm. **Ellis' l., Ellis-Garland l.,** an S-shaped line on the chest, showing the upper border of pleuritic effusions. **embryonic l.,** the primitive streak in the center of the germinal area. **epiphyseal l.,** 1. linea epiphysialis. 2. a strip of lesser density apparent in the roentgenogram of a long bone, representing the noncalcified portion of the cartilaginous growth plate between the epiphysis and the diaphysis. **established cell l.** see *cell l.* **l's of expression,** relaxed skin tension l's. **facial l.,** a line connecting the nasion with the pogonion, gnathion, or menton. See also under *height.* **Farre's white l.,** the boundary of the insertion of the mesovarium at the hilus of the ovary. **Feiss' l.,** a line from the medial malleolus to the plantar surface of the first metatarsophalangeal joint. **l. of fixation,** a straight line extending through the center of rotation of the eye to the object of vision. **focal l., anterior,** a line whose direction is perpendicular to the meridian of greatest curvature of a refracting surface. **focal l., posterior,** a line whose direction is perpendicular to the meridian of least curvature of a refracting surface. **Fraunhofer's l's,** dark lines of the solar spectrum. **Frommann's l's,** transverse marks on the axon of a medullated nerve fiber, rendered visible by silver nitrate. **fulcrum l.,** an axis that extends from one abutment tooth to another, about which a partial denture can rotate during function. **fulcrum l., retentive,** an imaginary line connecting the retentive points of clasp arms on retaining teeth adjacent to mucosa-borne denture bases, around which a denture tends to rotate when subjected to such forces as the pull of sticky foods. **fulcrum l., stabilizing,** an imaginary line connecting occlusal rests, around which a denture will rotate under masticatory forces. **genal l.,** one of Jadelot's lines, extending from the nasal line near the mouth toward the malar bone. **l. of Gennari,** the name given to the prominent external band of Baillarger (see *stria laminae granularis interna corticis cerebri*) in the region of the calcarine sulcus; because it is so highly visible the region is called the *striate cortex.* Called also *band, stria,* or *stripe of Gennari.* **gingival l.,** 1. a line determined by the level to which the gingiva extends on a tooth; although it tends to follow the curvature of the cervical line, the two rarely coincide. 2. any linear mark visible on the surface of the gingiva, such as the discoloration resulting from the ingestion of lead (lead l.). **gluteal l., anterior,** linea glutea anterior. **gluteal l., inferior,** linea glutea inferior. **gluteal l., posterior,** linea glutea posterior. **Gottinger's l.,** a line along the upper border of the zygomatic arch. **Granger l.,** a curved line seen in the roentgenograms of skulls, indicating the position of the optic groove. **Gubler's l.,** a line connecting the apparent origins of the roots of the fifth nerve. **gum l.,** gingival l. (def. 1.). **Haller's l.,** fissura mediana ventralis medullae spinalis. **Hampton l.,** a significant roentgenologic characteristic associated with the niche of the typical benign gastric ulcer in profile. **Harris l's,** lines of retarded growth seen radiographically at the epiphyses of long bones. **heave l.,** a groove appearing along the costal arch coincidental with forced contraction of the abdominal muscles following the normal passive expiratory movement in an animal with heaves. **Helmholtz's l.,** a line perpendicular to the plane of the axis of rotation of the eyes. **Hensen's l.,** M band; see under *band.* **Hilton's white l.,** a narrow wavy zone, usually not visible macroscopically but palpable on digital examination, that forms the lower border of the pecten, at the level of the interval between the subcutaneous part of the external anal sphincter and the lower border of the internal sphincter; called also *anal intersphincteric groove.* **Holden's l.,** a sulcus below the inguinal fold, crossing the capsule of the hip joint. **hot l.,** see under *H.* **Hudson's l., Hudson-Stähli l.,** pigmented line of the cornea; a linear horizontal brown mark located at about the junction of the middle and lower thirds of the cornea but not reaching the limbus, seen in the normal corneas of 16 per cent of aged individuals. Called also *pigmented l. of the cornea, Stähli's pigment l.* and *superficial l. of the cornea.* **Hueter's l.,** a straight line connecting

the medial epicondyle of the humerus with the top of the olecranon when the arm is extended. **Hunter's l.,** linea alba. **iliopectineal l.,** linea arcuata ossis illii. **imbrication l's of cementum,** incremental l's of cementum. **imbrication l's of Pickerill,** lines formed by ends of rod bundles that overlie one another and are arranged in scalariform fashion on the surface of the crown of a tooth; seen on longitudinal sections of a tooth together with the incremental lines, but forming areas not completely contained in the enamel. Called also *Pickerill's imbrication l's.* See also *incremental l's.* **incremental l's,** lines showing the successive layers deposited in a tissue. In the enamel, they are brown striations visible under transmitted light and colorless in reflected light. They may be observed under the microscope in longitudinal sections as oblique lines running inward from the surface and toward the root and in cross sections as rings similar to those in a tree trunk. Dry dentin often shows a series of somewhat parallel lines caused by imperfectly calcified dentin arranged in layers. Called also *accretion l's, calcification l's, l's of Retzius,* and *Retzius' parallel striae.* See also *l's of Ebner, imbrication l's of Pickerill,* and *neonatal l.* **incremental l's of cementum,** very fine dark lines present in longitudinal sections of a tooth, which follow the contour of the root and border with wider light bands, revealing the cyclic activity of cementogenesis. Called also *imbrication l's of cementum.* **incremental l's of Ebner,** l's of Ebner. **infracostal l.,** planum subcostale. **infrascapular l.,** a horizontal line at the level of the inferior angles of the scapulae. **intercondylar l., intercondyloid l.,** linea intercondylaris femoris. **intermediate l. of iliac crest,** linea intermedia cristae iliacae. **interspinal l.,** planum interspinale. **intertrochanteric l., intertrochanteric l., anterior,** linea intertrochanterica. **intertrochanteric l., posterior,** crista intertrochanterica. **intertuberal l.,** a line drawn between the prominences of the frontal bone. **intertubercular l.,** planum intertuberculare. **intraperiod l's,** see *period l's.* **isoeffect l's,** in radiotherapy, lines on a rectangular graph representing doses of radiation having tumoricidal effects and those having complicating necrotic effects in normal tissues. **isothermal l's,** lines on a map or chart indicating areas of uniform temperature. **Jadelot's l's,** lines of the face in young children, described as being indicative of specific types of disease; the genal, labial, nasal, and oculozygomatic lines. Called also *Jadelot's furrows.* **l. of Kaes,** a thin layer of fibers in the external granular layer of the cerebral cortex. **Kerley's l's,** horizontal linear densities 1 to 2.5 cm. long on chest roentgenograms; they are arranged in stepladder fashion and are believed to represent widening of the interlobular septa, as by edema (in mitral stenosis) or fibrosis (in silicosis). When peripherally situated, particularly at the base of the lungs, they are called *Kerley's B l's,* or *costophrenic septal lines.* When centrally situated, they are called *Kerley's A l's.* **Kilian's l.,** a prominent line on the promontory of the sacrum. **Krause's l.,** Z band; see under *band.* **labial l.,** one of Jadelot's lines, extending laterally from the angle of the mouth; said to indicate disease of the lungs. **Langer's l's,** linear clefts in the skin indicative of direction of the fibers. The lines, which correspond closely to the crease lines in the skin, assume a characteristic pattern in each part of the body but vary with body configuration. Called also *cleavage l's.* **lead l.,** a gray or bluish black line at the gingival margin in lead poisoning, seen especially in patients with poor oral hygiene; it is similar to the bismuth line, but is somewhat more diffuse. Called also *blue l.* and *Burton's line* or *sign.* **lip l.,** a line at the level to which the margin of either lip extends on the teeth. **lip l., high,** the greatest height to which the maxillary lip is raised. **lip l., low,** the lowest position of the lower lip during the act of smiling or voluntary retraction. **lower lung l.,** a horizontal line in roentgenograms of the upper part of the abdomen, running from the lateral chest wall toward the first lumbar vertebra on each side, and representing the lower posterior boundary of the pleural cavity. **magnetic l's of force,** lines indicating direction of force in a magnetic field. **major dense l's, major period l's,** see *period l's.* **mamillary l.,** linea mamillaris. **mammary l.,** milk line. **median l.,** an imaginary vertical line on the body surface, dividing the surface equally into right and left sides. **median l., anterior,** linea mediana anterior. **median l., posterior,** linea mediana posterior. **medioclavicular l.,** linea medioclavicularis. **Mees' l's,** single or multiple transverse white bands on the fingernails; they occur especially in association with arsenic poisoning and in other trace element intoxications, and have been reported in leprosy, septicemia, dissecting aortic aneurysm, and acute and chronic renal failure. Called *Aldrich-Mees l's*. **mesenteric l.**, see *mesenteric triangle*, under *triangle*. **Meyer's l.**, the axial line of the big toe which if extended passes through the center of the heel if shoes have never been worn. **midaxillary l.**, linea axillaris media. **midclavicular l.**, linea mamillaris. **middle l. of scrotum**, raphe scroti. **midspinal l.**, a perpendicular line down the middle of the vertebral column. **midsternal l.**, a line passing through the middle of the sternum from the cricoid cartilage to the xiphoid. **milk l.**, a ridge of thickened epithelium from axilla to groin in the mammalian embryo along which nipples and mammary glands develop, all but one subsequently disappearing in the human. Called also *mammary l.* and *mammary ridge*. **l's of minimal tension**, relaxed skin tension l's. **Monro's l.**, one from the umbilicus to the anterior superior spine of the ilium. **Monro-Richter l.**, one from the umbilicus to the left anterior superior iliac spine. **Morgan's l.**, a secondary crease in the lower eyelids in atopic dermatitis; called also *Dennie's sign*. **Moyer's l.**, a line from the middle of the body of the third sacral vertebra to a point midway between the anterior superior iliac spines. **mucogingival l.**, see under *junction*. **muscular l's of scapula**, lineae musculares scapulae. **mylohyoid l. of mandible, mylohyoidean l.**, linea mylohyoidea mandibulae. **nasal l.**, one of Jadelot's lines, extending from the ala nasi in a semicircle around the mouth. **nasobasal l.**, basinasal l. **nasobasilar l.**, a line through the basion and nasal point. **nasolabial l.**, a line extending from the ala nasi to the angle of the mouth. **Nélaton's l.**, a line from the anterior superior spine of the ilium to the most prominent part of the tuberosity of the ischium. **neonatal l.**, a line seen on longitudinal sections of a tooth, showing a demarcation between the structures present at birth and those deposited postnatally; in cross sections, the lines are seen as rings (neonatal rings), and their variations indicate adaptational changes in tooth formation. See also *l's of Owen*. **nigra l.**, linea nigra. **nipple l.**, linea mamillaris. **nuchal l., highest**, linea nuchae suprema. **nuchal l., inferior**, linea nuchae inferior. **nuchal l., median, nuchal l., middle**, crista occipitalis externa. **nuchal l., superior**, linea nuchae superior. **nuchal l., supreme**, linea nuchae suprema. **oblique l.**, one which follows an oblique course; see terms beginning *linea obliqua*. **oblique l. of femur**, linea intertrochanterica. **oblique l. of fibula**, 1. crista medialis fibulae. 2. margo anterior fibulae. **oblique l. of mandible**, linea obliqua mandibulae. **oblique l. of mandible, internal**, linea mylohyoidea mandibulae. **oblique l. of thyroid cartilage**, linea obliqua cartilaginis thyroideae. **oblique l. of tibia**, linea musculi solei. **l. of occlusion**, the alignment of the occluding surfaces of the teeth in a horizontal plane. **oculozygomatic l.**, one of Jadelot's lines, extending outward from the medial canthus toward the zygoma; said to be a sign of some disorder of the nervous system. **omphalospinous l.**, a line on the abdomen connecting the umbilicus and the anterior superior spine of the ilium; a guide to the location of McBurney's point. **orthostatic l's**, natural furrows on the neck, due to physiologic skin excess required at certain areas for the purpose of flexion and extension. **l's of Owen**, the sweeping bands seen on longitudinal section that outline the growth of the coronal or radicular dentin, representing a lag of several days between calcification phases, each lasting about 4 days. Called also *contour l.* and *Salter's l.* **papillary l.**, linea mamillaris. **pararectal l.**, linea pararectalis. **parasternal l.**, linea parasternalis. **paravertebral l.**, 1. linea paravertebralis. 2. linea vertebralis. **Pastia's l's**, linear striations of hyperpigmentation produced by confluent petechiae in body creases, such as the antecubital fossae and inguinal regions, that occur at the onset of the rash of scarlet fever and persist after desquamation. Called also *Pastia's sign* and *Thomson's sign*. **pectinate l.**, linea anocutanea. **pectineal l.**, 1. linea pectinea femoris. 2. pecten ossis pubis. **pelvic pain l.**, an imaginary line beneath which pain impulses from the bladder neck, prostate, urethra, uterine cervix, and the lower end of the colon are conducted. **period l's**, a series of light and dark lines occurring in a concentric, repeating pattern in mature myelin: the darker

lines (*major dense l's*) represent the apposition of the inner, cytoplasmic surfaces of the Schwann cell plasma membrane; the lighter lines (*intraperiod l's*) bisect the spaces between the darker lines, and represent the apposition of the outer surfaces of the membrane. **Pickerill's imbrication l's**, imbrication l's of Pickerill. **pigmented l. of the cornea**, Hudson's l. **Poirier's l.**, a line running from the nasofrontal angle to a point just above the lambda. **popliteal l. of femur**, linea intercondylaris femoris. **popliteal l. of tibia**, linea musculi solei. **postaxillary l.**, linea axillaris posterior. **Poupart's l.**, an imaginary line on the surface of the abdomen, passing perpendicularly through the midpoint of Poupart's ligament. **preaxillary l.**, linea axillaris anterior. **precentral l.**, a line on the head, extending from a point midway between the inion and glabella downward and forward. **primitive l.**, primitive streak. **pupillary l.**, pupillary axis. **quadrate l.**, a slight ridge sometimes seen passing vertically downward from the middle of the intertrochanteric crest on the posterior surface of the femur. **recessional l's**, lines or markings on the teeth due to the recession, in the formative period of the teeth, of the soft tissue which gives place to the dentin. **Reid's base l.**, base l. (def. 1). **relaxed skin tension l's**, the natural skin lines and creases of the face and neck, which are the preferred lines of incision in facial and cervical surgery; called also *l's of expression* and *l's of minimal tension*. **Retzius' l's**, incremental l's. **Robson's l.**, an imaginary line drawn from the nipple to the umbilicus. **Rolando's l.**, a line on the head marking the position of the fissure of Rolando beneath. **Roser's l.**, Nélaton's l. **rough l. of femur**, linea aspera femoris. **Salter's l's**, l's of Owen. **scapular l.**, linea scapularis. **Schoemaker's l.**, one connecting the point of the trochanter with the anterior superior iliac spine; the extension of this line normally runs above the umbilicus, but runs below the umbilicus when the trochanter is higher than normal. **l's of Schreger**, the dark and light lines visible under reflected light in a ground section of a tooth, which terminate at the dentinoenamel junctions, coinciding with the enamel prism curvatures. The dark bands are known as *diazones*, and the light ones as *parazones*. Called also *Hunter-Schreger bands, Schreger's bands, Schreger's striae*, and *zones of Schreger*. **segmental l's**, developmental grooves. **semicircular l's, supreme**, linea nuchae suprema. **semicircular l. of Douglas**, linea arcuata vaginae musculi recti abdominis. **semicircular l. of frontal bone**, linea temporalis ossis frontalis. **semicircular l. of occipital bone, highest**, linea nuchae suprema. **semicircular l. of occipital bone, middle**, linea nuchae superior. **semicircular l. of occipital bone, superior**, linea nuchae superior. **semicircular l. of parietal bone, inferior**, linea temporalis inferior ossis parietalis. **semicircular l. of parietal bone, superior**, linea temporalis superior ossis parietalis. **semilunar l.**, linea semilunaris. **Sergent's white adrenal l.**, a white line on the abdomen caused by drawing the finger nail across it; seen in cases of deficient adrenal activity. **Shenton's l.**, a curved line seen in the roentgenogram of the normal hip joint, formed by the top of the obturator foramen. **l. of sight**, a straight line from the center of the pupil to the object viewed. **simian l.**, see under *crease*. **Skinner's l.**, Shenton's l. **soleal l. of tibia**, linea musculi solei. **Spieghel's l., spigelian l., Spigelius' l.**, linea semilunaris. **spiral l. of femur**, linea intertrochanterica. **Stähli's l., Stähli's pigment l.**, Hudson's l. **sternal l., sternal l., lateral**, linea sternalis. **subcostal l.**, a transverse line on the surface of the abdomen at the level of the lower edge of the tenth costal cartilage. **subscapular l's**, lineae musculares scapulae. **superficial l. of the cornea**, Hudson's l. **supracondylar l. of femur, lateral**, linea supracondylaris lateralis femoris. **supracondylar l. of femur, medial**, linea supracondylaris medialis femoris. **l. supracondyla′ris latera′lis fem′oris** [NA], lateral supracondylar line of femur: a slight ridge on the lower third of the posterior surface of the femur that is continuous above with the lateral lip of the linea aspera and descends to the lateral epicondyle. **l. supracondyla′ris media′lis fem′oris** [NA], medial supracondylar line of femur: an indistinct ridge on the lower third of the posterior surface of the femur that is continuous above with the medial lip of the linea aspera, being interrupted at its upper end to allow passage of the femoral artery, and descends to the adductor tubercle.

supracrestal l., planum supracrestale. **supraorbital l.,** a line across the forehead, just above the root of the external angular process of the frontal bone. **survey l.,** 1. the line indicating the height of a tooth after the cast has been positioned according to the chosen path of insertion. 2. a line produced on a cast of a tooth by a surveyor scriber, marking the greatest height of contour in relation to the chosen path of insertion of the restoration. 3. a line drawn on a tooth or teeth by means of a surveyor for the purpose of determining the positions of the various parts of a clasp or clasps. Called also *clasp guideline.* **suture l.,** 1. a line of juncture where parts of the body, internal or external, interface or converge. 2. système sécant. **sylvian l.,** a line on the head extending from the external angular process of the frontal bone to a point three fourths of an inch below the most prominent point of the parietal bone. It coincides with the direction of the fissure of Sylvius. **temporal l., inferior,** linea temporalis inferior ossis parietalis. **temporal l., superior,** linea temporalis superior ossis parietalis. **temporal l. of frontal bone,** linea temporalis ossis frontalis. **temporal l. of parietal bone, inferior,** linea temporalis inferior ossis parietalis. **temporal l. of parietal bone, superior,** linea temporalis superior ossis parietalis. **terminal l. of pelvis,** linea terminalis pelvis. **Thompson's l.,** a red line observed on the gingivae in pulmonary tuberculosis. **thyroid red l.,** an erythematous line produced by irritation of the skin on the front of the neck and upper part of the chest in patients with hyperthyroidism. **Topinard's l.,** a line from the glabella to the pogonion. **transverse l's of sacral bone, transverse l. of sacrum,** lineae transversae ossis sacri. **trapezoid l.,** linea trapezoidea. **Trümmerfeld l.,** a zone of metaphyseal degeneration sometimes seen in the bones in infantile scurvy. **Ullmann's l.,** in cases of spondylolisthesis, a line extended upward at a right angle from the anterior edge of the first sacral vertebra to the superior surface of the sacrum, it will pass through the last lumbar vertebra. **umbilicoiliac l.,** a line from the umbilicus to the anterior superior spine of the ilium. **vertebral l.,** linea vertebralis. **vibrating l.,** an imaginary line across the palate that separates its immovable portion, the hard palate, from its movable portion, the soft palate. **Virchow's l.,** a line from the nasion to the lambda. **visual l.,** axis opticus. **Voigt's l's,** a dorsoventral pigmented line of demarcation on the skin, usually extending bilaterally and symmetrically for about 10 cm., along the lateral edge of the biceps muscle; seen in 20 to 26 per cent of blacks and rarely in whites. **Wagner's l.,** a thin whitish line at the junction of the epiphysis and diaphysis of a bone, formed by preliminary calcification. **white l.,** linea alba. **white adrenal l.,** Sergent's white adrenal l. **white l. of ischiococcygeal muscle,** ligamentum anococcygeum. **white l. of pelvic fascia,** arcus tendineus fasciae pelvis. **white l. of pelvis,** arcus tendineus musculi levatoris ani. **white l. of pharynx,** raphe pharyngis. **Wrisberg's l's,** a set of filaments connecting the motor and sensory roots of the trigeminal nerve. **Z l.,** Z band. **l's of Zahn,** laminations visible in antemortem blood clots, caused by alternating layers of gray-white fibrin interspersed with narrow zones of apparent red-blue clot. **Zöllner's l's,** an optical illusion in which long parallel lines seem to converge or diverge owing to their being crossed by a series of short lines parallel to one another but oblique to the long lines and at reverse oblique angles to both adjacent series of intersecting lines, as in a herringbone pattern.

linea (lin′e-ah), gen. and pl. *lin′eae* [L.] a stripe, streak, mark, or narrow ridge; [NA] a general term for a streak or narrow ridge on the surface of some structure. Called also *line.* **l. al′ba** [NA], **l. al′ba abdom′inis,** white line: the tendinous median line on the anterior abdominal wall between the two rectus muscles, formed by the decussating fibers of the aponeuroses of the three flat abdominal muscles. **l. al′ba cervica′lis,** the blending of the fascial sheaths of the sternothyroid and sternohyoid muscles in the median plane of the neck. **lin′eae albican′tes,** see *striae atrophicae.* **l. anocuta′nea** [NA], anocutaneous line: the sinuous line following the level of the anal valves and crossing the bases between them, marking the junction of the zone of the anal canal lined with stratified squamous epithelium and that lined with columnar epithelium; called also *dentate line* or *margin* and *pectinate line.* **l. anorecta′lis** [NA], anorectal line: the site at which the rectum becomes continuous with the anal canal; called also *anorectal*

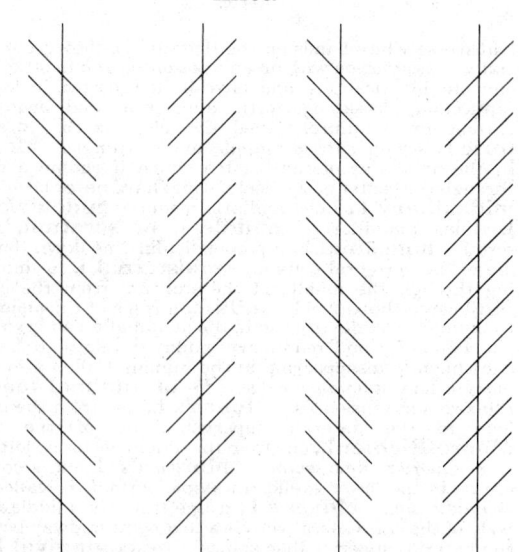

Zöllner's lines.

junction. **l. arcua′ta os′sis il′ii** [NA], arcuate line of ilium: the iliac portion of the terminal line, limiting the ala of the ilium inferiorly on its medial surface. **l. arcua′ta vagi′nae mus′culi rec′ti abdom′inis** [NA], arcuate line of sheath of rectus abdominis muscle: a crescentic line marking the termination of the posterior layer of the sheath of the rectus abdominis muscle, just below the level of the iliac crest; called also *l. semicircularis* [*Douglasi*] and *semicircular line of Douglas.* **l. as′pera fem′oris** [NA], rough line of femur: the broad, thickened ridge that forms the posterior border of the femur and has distinct lateral and medial lips. **lin′eae atroph′icae,** striae atrophicae. **l. axilla′ris ante′rior** [NA], anterior axillary line: an imaginary vertical line continuing the line of the anterior axillary fold with the arm in the anatomical position; called also *l. preaxillaris* [NA alternative] and *preaxillary line.* **l. axilla′ris me′dia** (NA), middle axillary line: an imaginary line halfway between the anterior axillary line and the posterior axillary line, passing through the apex of the axilla; called also *l. medio-axillaris* (NA alternative) and *midaxillary line.* **l. axilla′ris** [NA], axillary line: an imaginary vertical line passing through the middle of the axilla, dividing the body into an anterior and a posterior portion. **l. axilla′ris poste′rior** [NA], posterior axillary line: an imaginary vertical line continuing the line of the posterior axillary fold with the arm in the anatomical position; called also *l. postaxillaris* [NA alternative] and *postaxillary line.* **l. epiphysia′lis** [NA], a plane or plate visible in sections in radiograms, marking the site of recent ossification of an epiphyseal cartilage. **l. glu′tea ante′rior** [NA], anterior gluteal line: the middle of three rough curved lines on the gluteal surface of the ala of the ilium; it begins from the iliac crest about an inch posterior to the anterior superior iliac spine and arches more or less posteriorly to the greater sciatic notch. **l. glu′tea infe′rior** [NA], inferior gluteal line: a rough curved line, often indistinct, on the gluteal surface of the ala of the ilium; it runs from the notch between the anterior superior and anterior inferior iliac spines posteriorly to the anterior part of the greater sciatic notch. **l. glu′tea poste′rior** [NA], posterior gluteal line: a rough curved line on the gluteal surface of the ala of the ilium; it begins from the iliac crest about two inches anterior to the posterior superior iliac spine and runs downward to the greater sciatic notch. **l. iliopectin′ea,** l. arcuata ossis ilii. **l. innomina′ta,** l. terminalis pelvis. **l. intercondyla′ris fem′oris** [NA], **l. intercondyloi′dea fem′oris,** intercondylar line: a transverse ridge separating the floor of the intercondylar fossa from the popliteal surface of the femur, and giving attachment to the posterior portion of the capsular ligament of the knee. **l. interme′dia cris′tae ili′acae** [NA], intermediate line of iliac crest: the area between the inner and outer lips of the iliac crest. **l. intertrochanter′ica** [NA], intertrochanteric line: a line running obliquely downward and medially from the tubercle of the femur, winding around the medial side of the body of the bone.

l. intertrochanter′ica poste′rior, crista intertrochanterica. **l. mamilla′ris** [NA], mamillary line: an imaginary vertical line on the anterior surface of the body, passing through the center of the nipple; called also *l. medioclavicularis* and *midclavicular line.* **l. media′na ante′rior** [NA], anterior median line: an imaginary vertical line on the anterior surface of the body, dividing the surface equally into right and left sides. **l. media′na poste′rior** [NA], posterior median line: an imaginary vertical line on the posterior surface of the body, dividing the surface equally into right and left sides. **l. medio-axilla′ris,** NA alternative for *l. axillaris media.* **l. medioclavicula′ris** [NA], medioclavicular line: an imaginary vertical line on the anterior surface of the body, passing through the midpoint of the clavicle. **lin′eae muscula′res scap′ulae,** muscular lines of scapula: low ridges on the costal surface of the scapula, marking the site of attachment of muscle fibers. **l. mus′culi sol′ei** [NA], soleal line of tibia: a line extending from the fibular facet downward and inward across the posterior surface of the tibia, giving attachment to fibers of the soleus muscle; called also *l. poplitea tibiae* and *popliteal line of tibia.* **l. mylohyoi′dea mandib′ulae** [NA], mylohyoid line of mandible: a ridge on the inner surface of the mandible from the base of the symphysis to the ascending ramus behind the last molar tooth; it affords attachment to the mylohyoid muscle and superior constrictor of the pharynx. **l. ni′gra,** a name given the tendinous mesial line of the abdomen (l. alba) when it has become pigmented in pregnancy. **l. nu′chae infe′rior** [NA], inferior nuchal line: the lowest of the three nuchal lines found on the outer surface of the occipital bone, extending laterally from the middle of the external occipital crest to the jugular process. **l. nu′chae supe′rior** [NA], superior nuchal line: a curved line on the outer surface of the occipital bone, extending from the external occipital protuberance toward the lateral angle, and giving attachment medially to the trapezius muscle and laterally to the sternocleidomastoid muscle. **l. nu′chae supre′ma** [NA], highest or supreme nuchal line: a sometimes indistinct line arching upward from the external occipital protuberance and running toward the lateral angle of the occipital bone: the epicranial aponeurosis attaches to it. **l. obli′qua cartilag′inis thyroi′deae** [NA], oblique line of thyroid cartilage: a line on the external surface of the lamina of the thyroid cartilage, extending between the two thyroid tubercles. **l. obli′qua fib′ulae,** crista medialis fibulae. **l. obli′qua mandib′ulae** [NA], oblique line of mandible: a ridge on the external surface of the body of the mandible extending from the mental tubercle to the anterior border of the ascending ramus on either side. **l. obli′qua tib′iae,** l. musculi solei. **l. pararecta′lis,** pararectal line: an imaginary line corresponding to the lateral margin of the rectus abdominis muscle. **l. parasterna′lis** [NA], parasternal line: an imaginary line on the anterior surface of the body midway between the mamillary line and the border of the sternum. **l. paravertebralis** [NA], 1. paravertebral line; an imaginary line corresponding to the transverse vertebral processes. 2. l. vertebralis. **l. pectin′ea fem′oris** [NA], pectineal line: a line running down the posterior surface of the shaft of the femur, giving attachment to the pectineus muscle. **l. poplite′a tib′iae,** l. musculi solei. **l. postaxilla′ris,** NA alternative for *l. axillaris posterior.* **l. preaxilla′ris,** NA alternative for *l. axillaris anterior.* **l. scapula′ris** [NA], scapular line: an imaginary vertical line on the posterior surface of the body, passing through the inferior angle of the scapula at rest. **l. semicircula′ris [Doug′lasi],** l. arcuata vaginae musculi recti abdominis. **l. semiluna′ris** [NA], **l. semiluna′ris [Spige′li],** semilunar line: a curved line along the lateral border of each rectus abdominis muscle, corresponding to the meeting of the aponeuroses of the internal oblique and transverse abdominal muscles; called also *Spieghel's line* and *Spigelius' line.* **l. spira′lis,** l. intertrochanterica. **l. splen′dens, Macal′ister,** the sheath for the anterior spinal artery formed by the pia mater in the fissura mediana anterior medullae spinalis. **l. sterna′lis** [NA], sternal line: an imaginary verticle line on the ventral surface of the body, corresponding to the lateral border of the sternum. **l. tempora′lis infe′rior os′sis parieta′lis** [NA], inferior temporal line of parietal bone: a curved line on the external surface of the parietal bone, marking the limit of attachment of the temporal muscle. **l. tempora′lis os′sis fronta′lis** [NA], temporal line of frontal bone: a ridge extending upward and backward from the zygomatic process of the frontal bone, dividing into superior and inferior parts that are continuous with corresponding lines on the parietal bone, and giving attachment to the temporal fascia. **l. tempora′lis supe′rior os′sis parieta′lis** [NA], superior temporal line of parietal bone: a curved line on the external surface of the parietal bone, above and parallel to the inferior temporal line, giving attachment to the temporal fascia. **l. termina′lis pel′vis** [NA], terminal line of pelvis: a line on the inner surface of either pelvic bone, extending from the sacroiliac joint to the iliopubic eminence anteriorly, and marking the plane separating the false from the true pelvis. **lin′eae transver′sae os′sis sa′cri** [NA], transverse lines of sacrum: four transverse ridges on the pelvic surface of the sacrum, running between the pairs of pelvic sacral foramina, marking the positions of the former intervertebral disks. **l. trapezoi′dea** [NA], trapezoid line: a ridge extending anterolaterally from the conoid tubercle on the inferior surface of the clavicle, giving attachment to the trapezoid portion of the coracoclavicular ligament. **l. vertebra′lis,** vertebral line: an imaginary vertical line halfway between the scapular and posterior median lines; called also *linea paravertebralis* and *paravertebral line.*

lineae (lin′e-e) [L.] genitive and plural of *linea.*

lineage (lin′e-ij) [L. *linea* line] descent traced down from or back to a common ancestor. **cell l.,** the developmental history of cells as traced from the first division of the original cell or cells.

linear (lin′e-ar) [L. *linearis*] pertaining to or resembling a line.

Lineola (lin-e-o′la) formerly, a genus of spore-forming bacteria now classified in the genus *Bacillus.*

liner (lin′er) material applied to the inside of the walls of a cavity or container, for protection or insulation of the surface. **cavity l.,** a cavity-lining agent used for the protection of the pulp from irritation and to neutralize the free acid of zinc phosphate and silicate cements.

Lineweaver-Burk equation (lin′ we-ver burk) [Hans *Lineweaver,* American chemist, born 1907; Dean *Burk,* American biochemist, born 1904] see under *equation.*

Lineweaver-Burk plot (lin′we-ver burk) [Hans *Lineweaver,* American chemist, born 1907; Dean *Burk,* American biochemist, born 1904] see under *plot.*

lingua (ling′gwah), gen. and pl. *lin′guae* [L.] [NA], the tongue: the movable, muscular organ on the floor of the mouth, subserving the special sense of taste and aiding in mastication, deglutition, and the articulation of sound; called also *glossa.* See *tongue.* **l. frena′ta,** ankyloglossia. **l. geograph′ica,** benign migratory glossitis. **l. ni′gra,** black tongue. **l. plica′ta,** fissured tongue. **l. villo′sa ni′gra,** black tongue.

linguae (ling′gwe) [L.] genitive and plural of *lingua.*

lingual (ling′gwal) [L. *lingualis,* from *lingua,* tongue] pertaining to or toward the tongue; glossal. In dental anatomy, used to refer to the tooth surface directed toward the tongue (oral cavity); see *facies lingualis dentis.*

linguale (ling-gwa′le) the point at the upper end of the symphysis of the lower jaw on its lingual surface.

lingualis (ling-gwa′lis), pl. *lingua′les* [L., from *lingua*] relating to the tongue.

lingually (ling′gwah-le) toward the tongue.

Linguatula (ling-gwat′u-lah) the tongueworms, a genus of the family Linguatulidae, order Porocephalida, which, in the adult form, inhabit the frontal, nasal, and maxillary sinuses of animals, sometimes including man. Their larval form (known as *Pentastoma* and *Porocephalus*) infests the digestive organs and lungs. See *halzoun.* **L. rhina′ria,** L. serrata. **L. serra′ta,** a species whose adult forms are found in the frontal sinuses and nasal passages of canines and felines. Eggs, passed in the nasal discharges of infected animals, may be ingested by cattle, sheep, rabbits, or occasionally man, and on hatching, bore through the intestinal wall and finally become encysted in the viscera.

linguatuliasis (ling-gwat″u-li′ah-sis) invasion of the body by *Linguatula.*

linguatulid (ling-gwat′u-lid) any member of the family Linguatulidae.

Linguatulidae (lin-gwah-tu′li-de) a family of endoparasitic wormlike arthropods of the order Porocephalida, class

Pentostomida, having flattened bodies. Adults are usually found in the nasal passages of felines and canines, and the larvae are found in the viscera of a variety of mammals, including man. It includes the genus *Linguatula*.

linguatulosis (ling-gwat″u-lo′sis) linguatuliasis.

linguiform (ling′gwĭ-form) tongue-shaped.

lingula (ling′gu-lah), gen. and pl. *lin′gulae* [L., dim. of *lingua*] [NA] a general term for a small tongue-like structure. **l. cerebel′li** [NA], **l. of cerebellum,** the most ventral part of the cranial lobe of the cerebellum, where the cranial medullary velum attaches. **l. of left lung,** l. pulmonis sinistri. **l. of lower jaw,** l. mandibulae. **l. of mandible, l. mandib′ulae** [NA], the sharp medial boundary of the mandibular foramen, to which is attached the spheno-mandibular ligament. **l. pulmo′nis sinis′tri** [NA], lingula of left lung: a projection from the lower portion of the upper lobe of the left lung, just beneath the cardiac notch, between the cardiac impression and the inferior margin. See also *culmen pulmonis sinistri.* **l. of sphenoid, sphenoidal l., l. of sphenoida′lis** [NA], a slender ridge of bone on the lateral margin of the carotid sulcus, projecting backward between the body and great wing of the sphenoid bone.

lingulae (ling′gu-le) [L.] genitive and plural of *lingula.*

lingular (ling′gu-lar) pertaining to a lingula.

lingulectomy (ling″gu-lek′to-me) excision of the lingula of the upper lobe of the left lung.

lingu(o)- [L. *lingua* tongue] a combining form denoting relationship to the tongue.

linguoaxial (ling″gwo-ak′se-al) pertaining to or formed by the lingual and axial walls of a tooth cavity.

linguoaxiogingival (ling″gwo-ak″se-o-jin′jĭ-val) pertaining to or formed by the lingual, axial, and gingival walls of a tooth cavity preparation.

linguocervical (ling″gwo-ser′vĭ-kal) 1. pertaining to the lingual surface of the neck of a tooth. 2. linguogingival.

linguoclination (ling″gwo-klĭ-na′shun) lingual inclination.

linguoclusion (ling″gwo-kloo′zhun) lingual occlusion.

linguodental (ling″gwo-den′tal) 1. pertaining to the tongue and the teeth. 2. a speech sound produced by the tongue and teeth, such as *th.*

linguodistal (ling″gwo-dis′tal) pertaining to or formed by the lingual and distal surfaces of a tooth, or the lingual and distal walls of a tooth cavity.

linguogingival (ling″gwo-jin′jĭ-val) pertaining to the tongue and gingiva; pertaining to or formed by the lingual and gingival walls of a tooth cavity.

linguoincisal (ling″gwo-in-si′zal) pertaining to or formed by the lingual and incisal surfaces of a tooth.

linguomesial (ling″gwo-me′ze-al) pertaining to or formed by the lingual and mesial surfaces of a tooth, or the lingual and mesial walls of a tooth cavity.

linguo-occlusal (ling″gwo-ŏ-kloo′zal) pertaining to or formed by the lingual and occlusal surfaces of a tooth.

linguopapillitis (ling″gwo-pap″ĭ-li′tis) [L. *lingua* tongue + *papillitis*] inflammation or ulceration of the papillae of the edges of the tongue.

linguoplacement (ling″gwo-plās′ment) lingual placement.

linguopulpal (ling″gwo-pul′pal) pertaining to or formed by the lingual and pulpal walls of a tooth cavity.

linguoversion (ling″gwo-ver′zhun) displacement of a tooth lingually from the line of occlusion.

liniment (lin′ĭ-ment) [L. *linimentum; linere* to smear] an oily liquid preparation to be used on the skin. **camphor l.,** a preparation of camphor and cottonseed oil used as a local irritant to the skin. **camphor and soap l.,** a preparation of green soap, camphor, rosemary oil, alcohol, and purified water, used as a local irritant to the skin. **chloroform l.,** a preparation of chloroform with camphor and soap liniment used as a local irritant to the skin. **medicinal soft soap l.,** green soap tincture.

linimentum (lin″ĭ-men′tum) [L.] liniment. **l. cam′phorae, l. cam′phorae et sapo′nis,** camphor and soap liniment. **l. chlorofor′mi,** chloroform liniment. **l. sapo′nis mol′lis,** green soap tincture.

linin (li′nin) [L. *linum* thread] the faintly staining substance composing the fine, netlike threads found in the nucleus of a cell, where it bears the chromatin in the form of granules. Cf. *achromatin.*

linitis (lĭ-ni′tis) [Gr. *linon* thread + *-itis*] inflammation of the gastric cellular tissue. **l. plas′tica,** diffuse fibrous proliferation of the submucous connective tissue of the stomach, resulting in thickening and fibrosis so that the organ is constricted, inelastic, and rigid (like a leather bottle). It is almost always a manifestation of adenocarcinoma but is also seen in benign conditions such as gastric syphilis. Called also *Brinton's disease, gastric sclerosis, cirrhosis of the stomach, cirrhotic gastritis,* and *leather bottle stomach.*

linkage (lingk′ij) 1. the connection between different atoms in a chemical compound, or the symbol representing it in structural formulas; see also *bond.* 2. in genetics, the association of genes having loci on the same chromosome, which results in the tendency of a group of such nonallelic genes to be associated in inheritance.

linked (linkt) in genetics, pertaining to linkage (def. 2); see also *X-linked,* under *gene.*

linnaean (lĭ-ne′an) [Carolus *Linnaeus* latinized form of Carl von Linné, Swedish botanist, 1707–1778] pertaining to Linnaeus or to the system of taxonomic classification of living organisms, which was originated by Linnaeus. Written also *linnean.*

linnean (lĭ-ne′an) linnaean.

Linodil (lin′o-dil) trademark for a preparation of inositol niacinate.

Linognathus (lin-og′nah-thus) a genus of insects of the order Anoplura, sucking lice. *L. peda′lis* infests sheep, *L. seto′sus* the dog, *L. sten′opis* the goat. *L. vitu′li* is the long-nosed louse of the ox.

linoleic acid (lin″o-le′ik) 9,12-octadecadienoic acid, a straight chain, unsaturated, eighteen carbon fatty acid, $CH_3-(CH_2)_3(CH_2CH:CH)_2(CH_2)_7COOH$, occurring in many vegetable oils. It is an essential fatty acid that cannot be synthesized by animal tissues and must be obtained in the diet. It is used in the biosynthesis of prostaglandins and cell membranes. Called also *linolic acid.*

linolein (lin-o′le-in) [L. *linum* flax + *oleum* oil] a neutral fat from linseed oil; the triglyceride of linoleic acid.

linolenic acid (lin″o-len′ik) 9,12,15-octadecatrienoic acid, a straight chain, unsaturated, eighteen carbon fatty acid, $CH_3(CH_2CH=CH)_3CH_2(CH_2)_6COOH$. It is an essential fatty acid that cannot be synthesized by animal tissues and must be obtained in the diet. It is used in the formation of prostaglandins.

linolic acid (lin-o′lik) linoleic acid.

linseed (lin′sēd) the dried ripe seed of *Linum usitatissimum* L. (Linaceae), used as a topical demulcent and emollient; called also *flaxseed* and *linum.*

Linstowiidae (lin-sto-wi′ĭ-de) a family of medium-sized or small tapeworms of the order Cyclophyllidea, subclass Cestoda, which parasitize birds, reptiles, and mammals, including man; medically important genera are *Oochoristica* and *Inermicapsifer.*

lint (lint) [L. *linteum,* from *linum,* flax] an absorbent surgical dressing material once made by scraping or picking apart old woven linen, but now a specially finished fabric woven in sheets; called also *patent l.* or *sheet l.*

lintin (lin′tin) a loose fabric of prepared absorbent cotton used in dressing wounds.

linum (li′num), gen. *li′ni* [L. "flax"] linseed.

lio- for words beginning thus, see also those beginning *leio-.*

Li₂O Li_2O lithium oxide.

LiOH lithium hydroxide.

Lioresal (li-ōr′ĕ-sal) trademark for a preparation of baclofen.

liothyronine (li″o-thi′ro-nēn) chemical name: O-(4-hydroxy-3-iodophenyl)-3,5-diiodo-L-tyrosine. The synthetic levo isomer of the thyroid hormone triiodothyronine, $C_{15}H_{12}I_3NO_4$, which is more potent and has a more rapid action than thyroxine. **l. sodium** [USP], the monosodium salt of liothyronine, $C_{15}H_{11}I_3NNaO_4$, occurring as a light tan, crystalline powder; used for thyroid replacement or supplementation in hypothyroidism and simple (nontoxic) goiter, administered orally.

liotrix (li′o-triks) a mixture of liothyronine sodium and levothyroxine sodium in a ratio of 1:4 in terms of weight; used for replacement therapy in conditions in which there is deficient production of thyroid hormones, administered orally.

lip (lip) 1. either the upper or lower fleshy margin of the mouth, together called *labia oris* [NA]. 2. a marginal part; called also *labium*. **acetabular l.,** labrum acetabulare. **anterior l. of cervix of uterus,** labium anterius ostii uteri. **anterior l. of ostium of uterus,** labium anterius ostii uteri. **anterior l. of pharyngeal opening of auditory tube,** labium anterius ostii pharyngei tubae auditivae. **articular l.,** labrum articularis. **cleft l.,** a congenital cleft or defect in the upper lip, usually due to complete or partial failure of migration and deposit of mesoderm around or over the head in the embryo, with consequent failure of the maxillary prominence to merge with the merged medial nasal prominences. It may be unilateral, bilateral, or median (the true harelip), and may be accompanied by maxillary and palatal defects. Called also *cheiloschisis, harelip,* and *stomatoschisis.* **double l.,** redundancy of the submucous tissue and mucous membrane of the lip on either side of the median line. **external l. of iliac crest,** labium externum cristae iliacae. **external l. of linea aspera of femur,** labium laterale lineae asperae femoris. **fibrocartilaginous l. of acetabulum,** labrum acetabulare. **glenoid l.,** labrum glenoidale. **glenoid l. of articulation of hip,** labrum acetabulare. **glenoid l. of articulation of humerus,** labrum glenoidale. **greater l. of pudendum,** labium majus pudendi. **Hapsburg l.,** a thick overdeveloped lower lip that often accompanies a Hapsburg jaw. **inferior l.,** the lower lip (labium inferius oris [NA]). **inferior l. of ileocecal valve,** labium inferius valvulae coli. **internal l. of iliac crest,** labium internum cristae iliacae. **lateral l. of linea aspera of femur,** labium laterale lineae asperae femoris. **lesser l. of pudendum,** labium minus pudendi. **lower l.,** labium inferius oris. **medial l. of linea aspera of femur,** labium mediale lineae asperae femoris. **posterior l. of cervix of uterus,** labium posterius ostii uteri. **posterior l. of ostium of uterus,** labius posterius ostii uteri. **posterior l. of pharyngeal opening of auditory tube,** labium posterius ostii pharyngei tubae auditivae. **rhombic l.,** the lateral boundary of the rhombencephalon during embryonic life. **superior l.,** the upper lip (labium superius oris [NA]). **superior l. of ileocecal valve,** labium superius valvulae coli. **tympanic l. of limb of spiral lamina,** labium tympanicum limbi laminae spiralis. **upper l.,** labium superius oris. **vestibular l. of limb of spiral lamina,** labium vestibulare limbi laminae spiralis.

lipacidemia (lip″as-ĭ-de′me-ah) [lipo- + L. *acidus* acid + Gr. *haima* blood + -ia] the presence of an excess of fatty acids in the blood, as in diabetes mellitus.

lipaciduria (lip″as-ĭ-du′re-ah) [lipo- + L. *acidus* acid + Gr. *ouron* urine + -ia] the presence of fatty acids in the urine.

liparocele (lip-ar′o-sēl) [Gr. *liparos* oily + *kēlē* tumor] a fatty scrotal tumor; also a hernia containing fatty material.

liparodyspnea (lip″ah-ro-disp′ne-ah) the dyspnea of the obese.

liparoid (lip′ah-roid) fatty; resembling fat.

lipase (lip′ās, lī′ās) 1. triacylglycerol lipase. 2. any enzyme that hydrolyzes a fatty acyl group from a neutral fat or phospholipid, producing a fatty acid anion and a diacylglycerol or lysophospholipid. **acid l.,** one with an acid pH optimum. The lysosomal enzyme hydrolyzes cholesteryl esters and triglycerides of low-density lipoproteins. Genetic deficiency of the enzyme causes Wolman's disease. **pancreatic l.,** triacylglycerol lipase.

lipasic (li-pa′sik) 1. pertaining to lipase. 2. lipolytic.

lipasuria (lip″ās-u′re-ah) the presence of lipase in the urine.

lipectomy (lĭ-pek′to-me) [lipo- + Gr. *ektomē* excision] the excision of a mass of subcutaneous adipose tissue, as from the abdominal wall; called also *adipectomy.*

lipedema (lip″ĕ-de′mah) [lipo- + edema] an accumulation of excess fat and fluid in subcutaneous tissues.

lipemia (lĭ-pe′me-ah) [lipo- + Gr. *haima* blood + -ia] an excess of fat or lipid in the blood; hypercholesterolemia; hyperlipemia. **alimentary l.,** that which occurs after the ingestion of food. **l. retina′lis,** a milky appearance of the veins and arteries of the retina, occurring when the lipoids of the blood exceed 5% and in diabetes mellitus and leukemia.

lipid (lip′id) any of a heterogeneous group of fats and fat-like substances characterized by being water-insoluble and being extractable by nonpolar (or fat) solvents such as alcohol, ether, chloroform, benzene, etc. All contain as a major constituent aliphatic hydrocarbons. The lipids, which are easily stored in the body, serve as a source of fuel, are an important constituent of cell structure, and serve other biological functions. Lipids may be considered to include fatty acids, neutral fats, waxes, and steroids. *Compound lipids* comprise the glycolipids, lipoproteins, and phospholipids. **l. A,** the glycolipid component of lipopolysaccharide (q.v.) that is responsible for its endotoxic activity.

lipidase (lip′ĭ-dās) lipase.

lipide (lip′īd) lipid.

lipidemia (lip″ĭ-de′me-ah) hyperlipidemia.

lipidic (lip-id′ik) pertaining to or containing lipids.

lipidol (lip′ĭ-dol) a lipid alcohol; an aliphatic fatty alcohol.

lipidolysis (lip″ĭ-dol′ĭ-sis) the splitting of lipids.

lipidolytic (lip″ĭ-do-lit′ik) pertaining to, characterized by, or causing lipidolysis.

lipidosis (lip″ĭ-do′sis) [lipid + -osis] a term for several of the lysosomal storage diseases in which there is an abnormal accumulation of lipids in the reticuloendothelial cells. Called also *lipid storage disease.* **cerebroside l.,** Gaucher disease. **galactosylceramide l.,** Krabbe disease. **glucosylceramide l.,** Gaucher disease. **hereditary dystopic l.,** Fabry disease. **sphingomyelin l.,** Niemann-Pick disease. **sulfatide l.,** metachromatic leukodystrophy.

lipidtemns (lip′id-temz) a collective name for the products formed by the digestion of fats, namely, glycerin and fatty acids.

lipiduria (lip″ĭ-du′re-ah) [lipid + Gr. *ouron* urine + -ia] the presence of lipids in the urine.

lipin (lip′in) [Gr. *lipos* fat] lipid.

Lipiodol (lip-i′o-dol) trademark for iodized oil used as a contrast medium.

Lipmann (lip′man), Fritz Albert. German-born American biochemist, born 1899; co-winner, with Hans Adolph Krebs, of the Nobel prize for medicine or physiology for 1953 for his discovery of coenzyme A and its importance in intermediary metabolism.

lip(o)- [Gr. *lipos* fat] a combining form denoting relationship to fat or to lipids.

lipoadenoma (lip″o-ad′ĕ-no-mah) lipomatosis of the parenchyma of a gland.

lipoarthritis (lip″o-ar-thri′tis) [lipo- + *arthritis*] inflammation of the fatty tissue of a joint.

lipoatrophy (li″po-at′ro-fe) [lipo- + *atrophy*] 1. atrophy of subcutaneous fat. 2. lipodystrophy. **insulin l.,** localized lipoatrophy occurring at the site of repeated insulin injections.

lipoblast (lip′o-blast) [lipo- + Gr. *blastos* germ] a specialized connective tissue cell which develops into a fat cell.

lipoblastoma (lip″o-blas-to′mah) [lipo- + Gr. *blastos* germ + -oma] a benign fatty tumor composed of a mixture of embryonal lipoblastic cells in a myxoid stroma and mature fat cells; the tumor cells are arranged in lobules and occur most often in children.

lipocaic (lip″o-ka′ik) [lipo- + Gr. *kaiein* to burn] a substance extracted from the pancreas which reputedly prevents the deposition of fat in the livers of animals after pancreatectomy and after other experimental procedures.

lipocardiac (lip″o-kar′de-ak) [lipo- + Gr. *kardia* heart] relating to a fatty heart.

lipocatabolic (lip″o-kat″ah-bol′ik) pertaining to or effecting the destructive metabolism of fat.

lipocele (lip′o-sēl) [lipo- + Gr. *kēlē* tumor] adipocele.

lipocellulose (lip″o-sel′u-lōs) a heterohexosan composed of lipids and cellulose.

lipoceratous (lip″o-ser′ah-tus) adipoceratous.

lipocere (lip′o-sēr) [lipo- + L. *cera* wax] adipocere.

lipochondria (lip″o-kon′dre-ah) [lipo- + Gr. *chondrion* granule] lipid-containing inclusions in the cytoplasm of amphibian eggs.

lipochondroma (lip″o-kon-dro′mah) [lipo- + Gr. *chondros* cartilage + -oma] a tumor composed of mature lipomatous and cartilaginous elements; such lesions are now generally called *benign mesenchymoma.*

lipochrome (lip′o-krōm) [lipo- + Gr. *chrōma* color] any of a group of fat-soluble pigments, including carotene, lutein, lycopene, and xanthophyll, that are synthesized in plants and on ingestion impart a yellow, yellow-orange, or orange-red color to lipid-containing tissues. Called also *carotenoid, chromolipoid, lipochrome pigment, lipofuscin,* and *wear and tear pigment.*

lipochromemia (lip″o-kro-me′me-ah) [lipochrome + Gr. *haima* blood + -ia] the presence of an excess of lipochrome in the blood.

lipochromogen (lip″o-kro′mo-jen) a substance that becomes converted into lipochrome.

lipoclasis (lĭ-pok′lah-sis) [lipo- + Gr. *klasis* breaking] lipolysis.

lipoclastic (lip″o-klas′tik) [lipo- + Gr. *klastikos* breaking up] lipolytic.

lipocorticoid (lip″o-kor′tĭ-koid) a corticoid effective in causing deposition of fat, especially in the liver.

lipocyanine (lip″o-si′ah-nin) [lipo- + Gr. *kyanos* blue] a blue pigment resulting from the action of strong sulfuric acid on lipochrome.

lipocyte (lip′o-sīt) [lipo- + -cyte] 1. a fat cell. 2. a fat-storing cell of the liver.

lipodieresis (lip″o-di-er′ĕ-sis) [lipo- + Gr. *diairesis* a taking] the splitting up or the decomposition of fat.

lipodieretic (lip″o-di-er-et′ik) pertaining to, characterized by, or causing lipodieresis.

lipodystrophia (lip″o-dis-tro′fe-ah) lipodystrophy. **l. intestina′lis,** intestinal lipodystrophy. **l. progressi′va,** partial lipodystrophy.

lipodystrophy (lip″o-dis′tro-fe) [lipo- + dystrophy] 1. any disturbance of fat metabolism. 2. a group of conditions due to defective metabolism of fat, resulting in the absence of subcutaneous fat, which may be congenital or acquired and partial or total. Called also *lipoatrophy* and *lipodystrophia.* **congenital progressive l.,** total l. **generalized l.,** total l. **intestinal l.,** a disease marked by diarrhea with fatty stools, arthritis, emaciation, and loss of strength, and attended with deposit of fat in the intestinal lymphatic tissue; called also *Whipple's disease* and *lipophagia granulomatosis.* **partial l.,** a condition occurring especially in females in the first decade of life, characterized by a symmetrical loss of subcutaneous fat, usually beginning on the face and gradually extending to the chest, neck, back, and upper extremities, giving the lower part of the body an apparent, and possibly real, adiposity of the buttocks, thighs, and legs. Some affected patients develop insulin-resistant diabetes mellitus, triglyceridemia, and renal disease. Called also *Barraquer's* or *Simons' disease, lipodystrophia progressiva, progressive l.,* and *progressive partial l.* **progressive l.,** partial l. **progressive congenital l.,** total l. **total l.,** an autosomal recessive disorder occurring mainly in females, characterized by a generalized loss of subcutaneous fat and extracutaneous adipose tissue, present at birth or appearing later in life, and associated with hepatomegaly, hypoglycemia and insulin-resistant nonketotic diabetes, hyperlipemia, marked elevation of the basal metabolic rate, accelerated somatic growth, advanced bone age, acanthosis nigricans and hirsutism. Called also *congenital generalized, generalized l,* *Lawrence-Seip syndrome, lipoatrophic diabetes,* and *progressive congenital l.*

lipoferous (lĭ-pof′er-us) [lipo- + L. *ferre* to carry] 1. carrying fat. 2. sudanophil.

lipofibroma (lip″o-fi-bro′mah) a lipoma containing areas of fibrosis.

lipofuscin (lip″o-fu′sin) 1. a yellow to brown, granular, iron-negative lipid pigment found particularly in muscle, heart, liver, and nerve cells undergoing slow, regressive change and accumulating in lysosomes with age, being the product of oxidation and polymerization of the membrane lipids of autophagocytosed organelles. 2. lipochrome.

lipofuscinosis (lip″o-fu″sin-o′sis) [lipofuscin + -osis] any disorder due to abnormal storage of lipofuscins. **neuronal ceroid l.,** see *amaurotic idiocy,* under *idiocy.*

lipogenesis (lip″o-jen′ĕ-sis) [lipo- + *genesis*] the formation of fat; the transformation of nonfat food materials into body fat.

lipogenetic (lip″o-jĕ-net′ik) lipogenic.

lipogenic (lip″o-jen′ik) forming, producing, or caused by fat.

lipogenous (lĭ-poj′ĕ-nus) [lipo- + Gr. *gennan* to produce] producing fatness.

lipogranuloma (lip″o-gran-u-lo′mah) [lipo- + *granuloma*] a nodule of lipoid material; a foreign body inflammation of adipose tissue containing granulation tissue and oil cysts.

lipogranulomatosis (lip″o-gran″u-lo-mah-to′sis) a condition of faulty lipid metabolism in which yellow nodules of lipoid matter are deposited in the skin and mucosae, giving rise to granulomatous reactions. **Farber's l.,** see under *disease.*

lipohemarthrosis (lip″o-hem″ar-thro′sis) [lipo- + Gr. *haima* blood + *arthron* joint + -osis] the presence of fat-containing blood in a joint, with intra-articular fracture.

lipohemia (lip″o-he′me-ah) lipemia.

Lipo-Hepin (lip″o-hep′in) trademark for a preparation of heparin sodium.

lipohistiodieresis (lip″o-his″te-o-di-er′ĕ-sis) the disappearance of stored fat from body tissue.

lipohyalin (lip″o-hi′ah-lin) the lipid deposited in the beta cells of the pancreas in association with hyalinization in diabetes.

lipoic acid (lip-o′ik as′id) a bacterial growth factor present in the water-soluble fraction of liver and yeast. It is necessary for the oxidative decarboxylation of pyruvic acid by *Streptococcus fecalis* and for the growth of *Tetrahymena gelii,* and replaces acetate for the growth of *Lactobacillus casei.* It has been variously known as *acetate replacing factor, protogen A,* and *pyruvate oxidation factor.*

lipoid (lip′oid) [lipo- + Gr. *eidos* form] 1. fatlike; resembling fat; adipoid. 2. lipid. **anisotropic l.,** a lipid having doubly refractive properties.

lipoidal (lip-oi′dal) fatlike; resembling fat.

lipoidemia (lip″oi-de′me-ah) lipemia.

lipoidic (lĭ-poi′dik) fatlike; resembling fat.

lipoidolytic (lĭ-poi″do-lit′ik) lipidolytic.

lipoidosis (lip″oi-do′sis) a disturbance of lipid metabolism with abnormal deposit of lipids in the cells. **arterial l.,** atherosclerosis. **cerebroside l.,** Gaucher's disease. **cholesterol l.,** Hand-Schüller-Christian disease. **l. cu′tis et muco′sae,** lipoid proteinosis. **renal l.,** lipid nephrosis.

lipoidproteinosis (lip″oid-pro″te-in-o′sis) a familial disease occurring in the course of latent diabetes, marked by yellowish nodules on the skin and mucosae, keratotic lesions on the extremities, and hoarseness due to faulty lipid metabolism. See under *proteinosis.*

lipoidsiderosis (lip″oid-sid-ĕ-ro′sis) the deposit of iron pigment in lipids.

lipoiduria (lip″oi-du′re-ah) lipiduria.

lipolipoidosis (lip″o-lip″oi-do′sis) the presence of lipoids and neutral fats in the cells.

Lipo-Lutin (li″po-lu′tin) trademark for preparations of progesterone.

lipolysis (lĭ-pol′ĭ-sis) [lipo- + Gr. *lysis* dissolution] the decomposition or splitting up of fat; called also *adipolysis.*

lipolytic (lip″o-lit′ik) pertaining to, characterized by, or causing lipolysis; adipolytic.

lipoma (lĭ-po′mah) [lipo- + -oma] a benign tumor usually composed of mature fat cells. At times the tumor may be composed partly or entirely of fetal fat cells (hibernoma). **l. annula′re col′li,** Madelung's neck. **l. arbores′cens,** a lipoma within a joint having a treelike form. **l. capsula′re,** a fatty tumor due to increase of the fat in the capsule of an organ. **l. caverno′sum,** angiolipoma. **diffuse l.,** diffuse lipomatosis. **l. diffu′sum re′nis,** lipomatous nephritis. **l. doloro′sa,** see *nodular circumscribed lipomatosis,* under *lipomatosis.* **fat cell l., fetal,** hibernoma. **l. fibro′sum,** a lipoma in which there are areas of fibrosis. **intradural l.,** lipoma with components within or beneath the dura mater of the spine or sacrum.

l. myxomato′des, a lipomyxoma. **nevoid l.** (*obs.*), angiolipoma. **l. ossif′icans,** an ossified lipoma. **l. petrif′icans** (*obs.*), a calcified lipoma. **l. petrif′icum ossif′icans** (*obs.*), an ossified lipoma. **l. sarcomato′des,** liposarcoma. **telangiectatic l., l. telangiecto′des,** angiolipoma.

lipomatoid (lĭ-po′mah-toid) resembling a lipoma.

lipomatosis (lip″o-mah-to′sis) a condition characterized by abnormal localized, or tumor-like, accumulations of fat in the tissues. **l. atroph′icans,** localized accumulations of fat in certain tissues, associated with emaciation of the rest of the body; see also *lipodystrophia progressiva.* **congenital l. of pancreas,** Shwachman-Diamond syndrome. **diffuse l.,** abnormal increase of subcutaneous fat in the parts above the pelvis, usually in males. **l. doloro′sa,** lipomatosis in which the adipose deposits are tender or painful. **l. gigan′tea,** a form in which the adipose deposits form large masses. **nodular circumscribed l.,** the formation of multiple circumscribed or encapsulated lipomas which may be distributed symmetrically (multiple symmetrical lipomatosis) or haphazardly or which may form a collar around the neck (Madelung's neck). At times they may be painful (lipoma, or lipomatosis, dolorosa). **renal l., l. re′nis, replacement l. of kidney,** partial replacement of the renal parenchyma (usually an atrophic or hydronephrotic kidney) by adipose tissue. **symmetrical l.,** see *nodular circumscribed l.*

lipomatous (lĭ-po′mah-tus) affected with, or of the nature of, lipoma.

lipomeningocele (lip″o-mĕ-ning′go-sēl) meningocele associated with an overlying lipoma, in spina bifida.

lipomeria (li″po-me′re-ah) [Gr. *leipein* to leave + *meros* a part] monstrosity consisting of the congenital absence of a limb.

lipometabolic (lip″o-met″ah-bol′ik) pertaining to metabolism of fat.

lipometabolism (lip″o-mĕ-tab′o-lizm) [lipo- + *metabolism*] the metabolism of fat; utilization of fat.

lipomicron (lip″o-mi′kron) a microscopic fat particle in the blood.

lipomucopolysaccharidosis (lip″o-mu″ko-pol″e-sak-ah-rĭ-do′sis) mucolipidosis I.

lipomyohemangioma (lip″o-mi″o-hĕ-man″je-o′mah) a hamartoma composed of adipose, muscle, and vascular tissue.

lipomyoma (lip″o-mi-o′mah) a benign mesenchymoma composed of leiomyomatous and lipomatous tissues.

lipomyxoma (lip″o-miks-o′mah) a myxoma containing fatty elements.

liponephrosis (lip″o-nĕ-fro′sis) lipid nephrosis.

liponeurocyte (lip″o-nu′ro-sīt) the name given by Cramer to cells found in the pituitary body of rats.

Liponyssus (lip″o-nis′us) [lipo- + Gr. *nyssein* to pierce] former name for *Ornithonyssus.* **L. baco′ti,** *Ornithonyssus bacoti.* **L. bur′sa,** *Ornithonyssus buarsa.* **L. sylvia′rum,** *Ornithonyssus sylviarum.*

lipopathy (lĭ-pop′ah-the) [lipo + *pathy*] any disorder of lipid metabolism.

lipopectic (lip″o-pek′tik) pertaining to, characterized by, or causing lipopexia.

lipopenia (lip″o-pe′ne-ah) [lipo- + Gr. *penia* poverty] deficiency of lipids in the body.

lipopenic (lip″o-pe′nik) pertaining to, characterized by, or causing lipopenia.

lipopeptid (lip″o-pep′tid) a poorly defined group of fat-like substances composed of amino acids and fatty acids.

lipopexia (lip″o-pek′se-ah) [lipo- + Gr. *pēxis* fixation] the accumulation of fat in the tissues.

lipopexic (lip″o-pek′sik) lipopectic.

lipophage (lip′o-fāj) a cell that ingests or absorbs fat.

lipophagia (lip″o-fa′je-ah) lipophagy. **l. granulomato′sis,** intestinal lipodystrophy.

lipophagic (lip″o-fa′jik) [lipo- + Gr. *phagein* to eat] pertaining to, characterized by, or causing lipophagy; lipolytic.

lipophagy (lĭ-pof′ah-je) the absorption of fat; lipolysis.

lipophanerosis (lip″o-fan″ĕ-ro′sis) the process by which invisible fat in certain cells becomes detectable as small droplets.

lipophil (lip′o-fil) an element that has an affinity for fat.

lipophilia (lip″o-fil′e-ah) [lipo- + Gr. *philein* to love + *-ia*] 1. affinity for fat. 2. a tendency of the obese for fat fixation.

lipophilic (lip″o-fil′ik) having an affinity for fat; pertaining to or characterized by lipophilia.

lipophore (lip′o-fōr) [lipo- + Gr. *phoros* bearing] a pigment cell containing a lipochrome pigment; chromatophore.

lipopolysaccharide (lip″o-pol″e-sak′ah-rīd) 1. a complex of lipid and polysaccharide. 2. a major component of the cell wall of gram-negative bacteria; lipopolysaccharides are endotoxins and important group-specific antigens (O antigens). The lipopolysaccharide molecule consists of three parts. Lipid A, a glycolipid responsible for the endotoxic activity, is covalently linked to a heteropolysaccharide chain having two parts, the core polysaccharide, which is constant within related strains, and the O-specific chain, which is highly variable. Lipopolysaccharide from *Escherichia coli* is a commonly used B-cell mitogen (polyclonal activator) in laboratory immunology. Abbreviated LPS.

lipoprotein (lip″o-pro′te-in; li″po-pro′te-in) any of the lipid-protein complexes in which lipids are transported in the blood; lipoprotein particles consist of a spherical hydrophobic core of triglycerides or cholesteryl esters surrounded by an amphipathic monolayer of phospholipids, cholesterol, and apolipoproteins; the four principal classes are high-density, low-density, and very-low-density lipoproteins and chylomicrons. **familial l. deficiency,** any of three of the disorders of lipoprotein and lipid metabolism. *Abetalipoproteinemia* is caused by defective synthesis of apolipoprotein B (apo B), is characterized by acanthocytosis, hypocholesterolemia, progressive ataxic neuropathy, atypical retinitis pigmentosa with involvement of the macula, and fat malabsorption, and may be treated with vitamin E; called also *acanthocytosis* and *Bassen-Kornzweig* syndrome. *Familial hypobetalipoproteinemia* is clinically ill defined, having the same, or milder, clinical manifestations as abetalipoproteinemia, but genetically distinct from it; called also *acanthocytosis with hypobetalipoproteinemia. Tangier disease* is caused by a decreased synthesis and increased catabolism of the apolipoprotein components A-L and A-II (apo A-I and apo A-II) of HDL; HDL is absent from plasma, and the other lipoproteins are abnormal; cholesteryl esters accumulate in the reticuloendothelial cells. Clinical signs include enlarged, orange tonsils and pharyngeal and rectal mucosa, recurrent peripheral neuropathy, splenomegaly, and corneal infiltration. Called also *analphalipoproteinemia* and *familial high-density lipoprotein (HDL) deficiency.* **familial high-density l. (HDL) deficiency,** Tangier disease; see *familial l. deficiency.* **high-density l. (HDL),** lipoprotein particles having densities of 1.063–1.21 g/ml and diameters of 10-15 nm; divided into two subclasses, HDL_2 and HDL_3 having densities of 1.063–1.125 and 1.125–1.21g/ml (HDL_1 is a minor variant, see *Lp(a) 1*). HDL is thought to be the lipoprotein responsible for transport of cholesterol from extrahepatic tissue to the liver for excretion. It is synthesized by the liver as discoid "nascent" HDL particles lacking a lipid core. A core of cholesteryl esters accumulates as cholesterol is transferred from cell membranes to the HDL particle and then esterified by lecithin-cholesterol acyltransferase (LCAT). HDL is thought to be converted to IDL and then taken up by the liver. Called also (referring to its electrophoretic mobility) *alpha-lipoprotein.* **intermediate-density l. (IDL),** lipoproteins having a density of 1.006–1.019 g/ml; a transitional stage in the conversion of VLDL to LDL. **Lp(a) l.,** a minor lipoprotein having a density of 1.055-1.085 g/ml. High levels of this lipoprotein occur in a few individuals and appear to have an autosomal dominant pattern of inheritance. Called also HDL_1 and *sinking prebeta-lipoprotein.* **low-density l. (LDL),** lipoprotein particles having density of 1.019–1.063 g/ml and diameters of 17–26 nm. LDL is responsible for transport of cholesterol to extrahepatic tissues. It is formed in the circulation as VLDL (and possibly HDL) pass through the IDL stage becoming LDL by gaining and losing specific apolipoproteins. It is taken up and catabolized by both the liver and extrahepatic tissues by specific receptor-mediated endocytosis (see *LDL receptors*, under *receptor.*) Called also (referring to its electrophoretic mobility) *beta-lipoprotein.* **very low-density l. (VLDL),** lipoprotein particles having densities of 0.95–1.006 g/ml and diameters of 28-75 nm. VLDL particles are synthesized by the liver, and their lipid core consists primarily of triglycerides with some cholesteryl esters. The triglycerides are transferred to muscle and adipose tissue by the action of endothelial lipoprotein lipase. As the triglycerides are removed the particles lose most of their apolipoprotein C and become IDL which is either taken up by the liver or becomes LDL. Called also (referring to its electrophoretic mobility) *prebeta-lipoprotein.* **l. X,** an abnormal LDL with a high content of free cholesterol and abnormal protein content that occurs in patients with cholestasis.

lipoproteinemia (lip″o-pro″te-in-e′me-ah)   the presence of excessive lipoproteins in the blood.

lipoprotein lipase (lip″o-pro′te-in lip′ās, li′pās) [EC 3.1.1.34] an enzyme of the hydrolase class that catalyzes the reaction triacyl glycerol + H₂O = diacylglycerol + a fatty acid anion. The enzyme hydrolyzes triacylglycerols in chylomicrons, very-low-density lipoproteins, low-density lipoproteins, and diacylglycerols. It occurs on capillary endothelial surfaces, especially in mammary, muscle, and adipose tissue. Genetic deficiency of the enzyme causes familial hyperlipoproteinemia Type I.

lipoprotein lipase (LPL) deficiency, familial   familial hyperlipoproteinemia, types I and V.

lipoproteinosis (lip″o-pro″te-in-o′sis)   lipoid proteinosis.

liporhodin (lip″o-ro′din) [*lipo-* + Gr. *rhodon* rose]   a red lipochrome.

liposarcoma (lip″o-sar-ko′mah) [*lipo-* + *sarcoma*]   a malignant tumor derived from primitive or embryonal lipoblastic cells which exhibit varying degrees of lipoblastic and/or lipomatous differentiation.

liposis (lĭ-po′sis) [Gr. *lipos* fat + *-osis*]   lipomatosis.

liposoluble (lip″o-sol′u-b'l) [*lipo-* + *soluble*]   soluble in fats.

liposome (lip′o-sōm) [*lipo-* + Gr. *sōma* body]   a spherical particle in an aqueous medium, formed by a lipid bilayer enclosing an aqueous compartment.

lipostomy (li-pos′to-me) [Gr. *leipein* to fail + *stoma* mouth] congenital smallness or absence of the mouth.

Liposyn (lip′o-sin)   trademark for an intravenous fat emulsion containing 10 per cent safflower oil stabilized with egg phospholipids; used to prevent deficiency of essential fatty acids during prolonged total parenteral nutrition.

lipothymia (li″po-thi′me-ah) [Gr. *leipein* to fail + *thymos* mind]   a feeling of faintness; syncope.

lipotroph (lip′o-trof)   any of the acidophilic cells of the anterior lobe of the pituitary gland that contain β-lipotropin; see *corticotroph.*

lipotrophic (lip″o-trof′ik)   pertaining to, characterized by, or causing lipotrophy.

lipotrophy (lĭ-pot′ro-fe) [*lipo-* + Gr. *trophē* nutrition]   increase of bodily fat.

lipotropic (lip″o-trop′ik)   1. acting on fat metabolism by hastening the removal of or decreasing the deposit of fat in the liver.   2. an agent that has such effects.

β-lipotropin (lip″o-tro′pin)   a 91–amino acid polypeptide synthesized by cells of the adenohypophysis which exerts a mild peripheral lipolytic action and promotes darkening of the skin by stimulation of melanocytes. It is the precursor molecule of the melanocyte-stimulating hormones, the endorphins, and the enkephalins.

lipotropism (lĭ-pot′ro-pizm)   the condition of being lipotropic.

lipotropy (lĭ-pot′ro-pe) [*lipo-* + Gr. *tropē* a turning]   lipotropism.

lipovaccine (lip″o-vak′sēn) [*lipo-* + *vaccine*]   a vaccine prepared by suspending microorganisms in vegetable oil for the purpose of delaying absorption of the antigenic substances.

lipovitellin (lip″o-vi-tel′in)   a lipoprotein found in the yolk of eggs.

lipoxanthine (lip″o-zan′thin) [*lipo-* + Gr. *xanthos* yellow]   a yellow lipochrome.

lipoxidase (lĭ-pok′sĭ-dās)   lipoxygenase.

lipoxygenase (lĭ-pok′se-jĕ-nās) [EC 1.13.11.12]   an enzyme of the oxidoreductase class that catalyzes the reaction linoleate + O₂ = 13-hydropcroxyoctadeca-9,11-dienoate. It oxidizes linoleate and other polyunsaturated fatty acids to form hydroperoxides. For related enzymes oxidizing arachi-

donic acid, see *arachidonate 5-lipoxygenase* and *arachidonate 12-lipoxygenase.* Called also *lipoxidase.*

lipoxysm (lip-oks′izm) [Gr. *lipos* fat + *oxys* sharp, acid] poisoning by oleic acid.

lipoyl transacetylase (lĭp′o-il trans-as′ĭ-tĭ-lās)   dihydrolipoamide acetyltransferase.

lippa (lip′ah)   blepharitis ciliaris.

lipping (lip′ing)   1. a wedge-shaped shadow in the roentgenogram of chondrosarcoma between the cortex and the elevated periosteum.   2. the development of a bony overgrowth in osteoarthritis.

lippitude (lip′ĭ-tūd) [L. *lippitudo; lippus* bleareyed]   blepharitis ciliaris.

Lipschütz bodies, ulcer (disease) (lip′shitz) [Benjamin *Lipschütz,* Austrian dermatologist, 1878–1931]   see under *body,* and see *ulcus vulvae acutum.*

lipuria (lĭ-pu′re-ah) [Gr. *lipos* fat + *ouron* urine + *-ia*]   the presence of oil or fat in the urine.

lipuric (lĭ-pu′rik)   pertaining to or characterized by lipuria.

Liq.   abbreviation for *liquor.*

Liquamar (lik′wah-mar)   trademark for a preparation of phenprocoumon.

liquefacient (lik″wĕ-fa′shent) [L. *liquefaciens*]   having the quality to convert a solid material into a liquid, producing liquefaction.

liquefaction (lik″wĕ-fak′shun) [L. *liquefactio; liquere* to flow + *facere* to make]   the conversion of a material into a liquid form.   **gas l.,** the conversion of gas into a liquid form, brought about by cooling and compression, resulting in a decrease of the average kinetic energy of the molecules sufficiently to allow intermolecular forces of attraction to pull the molecules together. Called also *condensation.*

liquefactive (lik″wĕ-fak′tiv)   pertaining to, characterized by, or causing liquefaction.

liquescent (lik-wes′ent) [L. *liquescere* to become liquid] tending to become liquid; becoming liquid.

liquid (lik′wid) [L. *liquidus; liquere* to flow]   1. a substance that flows readily in its natural state.   2. flowing readily; neither solid nor gaseous. See also *fluid, liquor, mixture,* and *solution.*   **Declat's l.,** a solution of carbolate of ammonia for external and internal use in cholera.   **Müller's l.,** see under *fluid.*

liquiform (lik′wĕ-form)   resembling a liquid.

liquogel (lik′wo-jel)   a gel which after melting gives a sol of low viscosity. Cf. *viscogel.*

liquor (lik′er, li′kwor), pl. *liquors, liquo′res* [L.]   1. a liquid, especially an aqueous solution containing a medicinal substance.   2. a general term used in anatomical nomenclature for certain fluids of the body. See also *fluid, liquid,* and *solution.*   **l. am′nii,** amniotic fluid.   **l. cerebrospina′-lis** [NA], cerebrospinal fluid (CSF): the fluid contained within the four ventricles of the brain, the subarachnoid space, and the central canal of the spinal cord; formed by choroid plexuses and brain parenchyma, it circulates through the ventricles into the subarachnoid space and is absorbed into the venous system.   **l. cho′rii,** a fluid which separates the amnion from the chorion in the early stages of gestation.   **l. cotun′nii,** perilymph (perilympha [NA]).   **l. enter′icus,** succus entericus.   **l. follic′uli,** follicular fluid: an albuminous fluid in the vesicular ovarian follicle surrounding the ovum.   **l. gas′tricus,** succus gastricus.   **Morgagni's l.** (obs.), a fluid between the eye lens and its capsule.   **mother l.,** the liquid from which any substance has been separated by crystallization.   **l. pancreat′icus,** succus pancreaticus.   **l. pericar′dii,** pericardial fluid: a fluid found in small amount in the potential space between the parietal and visceral laminae of the serous pericardium.   **l. prostat′icus,** succus prostaticus.   **l. pu′ris,** the fluid portion of pus.   **l. san′guinis,** the fluid portion of the blood; the blood plasma.   **l. of Scarpa, l. scar′pae,** endolymph (endolympha [NA]).   **l. sem′inis,** the fluid portion of the semen.

liquores (li-kwo′rēz) [L.]   plural of *liquor.*

liquorice (lik′er-is)   see *Glycyrrhiza.*

Lisacort (lis′ah-kort)   trademark for a preparation of prednisone.

Lisfranc's amputation, etc. (lis-frahnks′) [Jacques *Lis-*

franc, French surgeon, 1790–1847] see under *amputation*, *joint*, *ligament*, and *tubercle*.

lisping (lisp′ing) parasigmatism.

Lissauer's marginal zone, paralysis, tract, (column) (lis′ow-erz) [Heinrich *Lissauer*, German neurologist, 1861–1891] see under *paralysis* and *zone*, and see *tractus dorsolateralis*.

Lissencephala (lis″en-sef′ah-lah) [Gr. *lissos* smooth + *enkephalos* brain] a group of placental mammals in which the brain is characteristically smooth or is marked by few convolutions, as bats, rodents, etc. Cf. *Gyrencephala*.

lissencephalia (lis″en-sĕ-fa′le-ah) agyria.

lissencephalic (lis″en-sĕ-fal′ik) 1. pertaining to the Lissencephala. 2. having cerebral hemispheres without or with only shallow convolutions, the normal appearance of the brain of many animals (e.g., bats, rodents). Cf. *gyrencephalic*. 3. agyric.

lissencephaly (lis″sen-sef″ah-le) agyria.

lissive (lis′iv) [Gr. *lissos* smooth] relieving muscle spasm without interfering with function.

Lister (lis′ter), Baron Joseph (1827–1912). English surgeon who, following Pasteur's theory that bacteria cause infection, introduced to surgery the principle of antisepsis. In 1865 Lister, using carbolic acid as his antiseptic agent together with heat-sterilized instruments, greatly reduced postoperative mortality.

Listerella (lis″ter-el′ah) *Listeria*.

listerellosis (lis″ter-el-lo′sis) listeriosis.

Listeria (lis-te′re-ah) [Baron Joseph *Lister*] a genus of bacteria of uncertain affiliation closely resembling the organisms of the family Corynebacteriaceae, made up of small, coccoid, gram-positive rods that have a tendency to form chains and palisades. The organisms are found in the feces of animals and man, on vegetation, and in silage. **L. monocytog′enes**, a species widely distributed in nature, which has a striking monocytic action in blood. It produces meningoencephalitis, meningitis, perinatal septicemia, and other disorders in humans, and septicemia and encephalomyelitis in lower animals. Called also *Corynebacterium infantisepticum* and *Corynebacterium parvulum*. See also *listeriosis*.

listerial (lis-ter′e-al) pertaining to or caused by organisms of the genus *Listeria*.

listeriosis (lis-ter″e-o′sis) infection caused by *Listeria monocytogenes*. In humans, in utero infections occur transplacentally and result in abortion, stillbirth, and premature birth; infections acquired during birth cause cardiorespiratory distress, diarrhea, vomiting, and meningitis. Infection in adults produces meningitis, endocarditis, and disseminated granulomatous lesions. Infection in cattle and sheep causes encephalitis and abortion. Nervous signs are common in ruminants, and necrosis of the liver in monogastric animals. Because affected animals tend to move in circles, it is also known as *circling disease*.

listerism (lis′ter-izm) the principles and practice of antiseptic and aseptic surgery.

Listing's law, plane (lis′tingz) [Johann Benedict *Listing*, German physiologist, 1808–1882] see under *law* and *plane*.

Liston's knives, operation (lis′tonz) [Robert *Liston*, Scottish surgeon in London, 1794–1847] see under *knife* and *operation*.

liter (le′ter, li′ter) [Fr. *litre*] a unit of volume in the metric system, equal to 1000 cubic centimeters, or 1 cubic decimeter, or to 1.0567 quarts liquid measure. Abbreviated l or L.

-lith [Gr. *lithos* stone] a word termination denoting a stone or calculus.

lithagogue (lith′ah-gog) [*litho-* + Gr. *agōgos* leading] 1. expelling calculi. 2. a remedy that promotes the expulsion of calculi.

Lithane (lith′ān) trademark for a preparation of lithium carbonate.

lithangiuria (lith″an-je-u′re-ah) [*litho-* + Gr. *angeion* vessel + *ouron* urine + *-ia*] calculous disease of the urinary tract.

litharge (lith′arj) [Gr. *lithargyros*; *lithos* stone + *argyros* silver] see *lead monoxide*.

lithate (lith′āt) a urate.

lithecbole (li-thek′bo-le) [*litho-* + Gr. *ekbolē* expulsion] expulsion of a calculus.

lithectasy (li-thek′tah-se) [*litho-* + Gr. *ektasis* stretching] the extraction of calculi through the mechanically dilated urethra.

lithectomy (li-thek′to-me) lithotomy.

lithemia (li-the′me-ah) [*lithic acid* + Gr. *haima* blood + *-ia*] excess of uric (lithic) acid or its salts in the blood; see *hyperuricemia*.

lithemic (li-the′mik) pertaining to, affected with, or of the nature of lithemia.

lithia (lith′e-ah) see *lithium*.

lithiasic (lith″e-as′ik) pertaining to lithiasis.

lithiasis (li-thi′ah-sis) [*lith-* + *-iasis*] a condition characterized by the formation of calculi and concretions. **appendicular l.**, a condition in which the lumen of the vermiform appendix becomes obstructed with calculi; it is said to run in families, and to be akin to gout and rheumatism. **l. conjuncti′vae**, a condition marked by the formation of white, calcareous concretions in the acini of the meibomian glands. **pancreatic l.**, the presence of calcium concretions in the pancreas, usually associated with pancreatic exocrine (digestive enzymes) and endocrine (insulin) insufficiency, with steatorrhea, weight loss, and diabetes mellitus.

lithic (lith′ik) 1. pertaining to calculus. 2. pertaining to lithium.

lithic acid (lith′ic) uric acid.

lithium (lith′e-um) [Gr. *lithos* stone] a white metal; atomic number, 3; atomic weight, 6.939; symbol, Li; its oxide, lithia, Li_2O, is alkaline; its salts are solvents of uric acid to a certain extent in the test tube: based on this, it was formerly erroneously thought to be indicated in gout and rheumatic conditions. Lithium salts (lithium carbonate) are used in treating the manic phase of manic-depressive disorders. **l. benzoate**, a salt, $C_6H_5 \cdot CO \cdot O \cdot Li$, in a white powder or in scales. **l. bromide**, a white, deliquescent, slightly bitter granular powder, $LiBr \cdot H_2O$, formerly used as a central nervous system depressant. **l. cacodylate**, a salt, $(CH_3)_2AsOLi$, formerly used as an arsenical remedy in gouty and rheumatic conditions and in anemia. **l. caffeine sulfonate**, a salt formerly used in gout and rheumatism and as a diuretic. **l. carbonate** [USP], chemical name: carbonic acid dilithium salt. A white, granular powder, Li_2CO_3, used in the treatment of acute manic states and in the prophylaxis of recurrent affective disorders manifested by depression or mania only, or those in which both mania and depression occur occasionally, administered orally. **l. citrate**, a white crystalline powder, $C_6H_5O_7Li_3 + 4H_2O$. **l. dithiosalicylate**, an amorphous salt formerly used in the treatment of gout and rheumatism. **l. formate**, a salt in colorless needles, $HCOOLi + H_2O$, formerly used in gout and rheumatism. **l. glycerophosphate**, a white powder, $C_3H_5(OH)_2 \cdot PO_2(OLi)_2$, formerly used as a nerve tonic and antilithic. **l. iodate**, a salt, $LiIO_3$, formerly used in gouty and renal disorders. **l. salicylate**, a white crystalline powder, $OH \cdot C_6H_4 \cdot COOLi$, once used in rheumatism.

lith(o)- [Gr. *lithos* stone] a combining form denoting relationship to stone or to a calculus.

lithocenosis (lith″o-sĕ-no′sis) [*litho-* + Gr. *kenōsis* evacuation] the removal from the bladder of the fragments of calculi that have been crushed.

lithocholate (lith″o-ko′lāt) the dissociated from of lithocholic acid.

lithocholic acid (lith″o-ko′lik) a secondary bile acid, 3α-hydroxy-5β-cholanic acid.

lithocholylglycine (lith″o-ko″lil-gli′sēn) a bile salt, the glycine conjugate of lithocholic acid.

lithocholyltaurine (lith″o-ko″lil-taw′rēn) a bile salt, the taurine conjugate of lithocholic acid.

lithoclast (lith′o-klast) [*litho-* + Gr. *klan* to crush] a lithotrite, or stone-crushing forceps.

lithocystotomy (lith″o-sis-tot′o-me) [*litho-* + Gr. *kystis* bladder + *temnein* to cut] an operation for removing a stone from the bladder.

lithodialysis (lith″o-di-al′ĭ-sis) [*litho-* + Gr. *dialyein* to dissolve] 1. the dissolution of calculi in the bladder by injected solvents. 2. the crushing of a calculus in the bladder.

lithogenesis (lith″o-jen′ĕ-sis) [litho- + Gr. *gennan* to produce] the formation of calculi.

lithogenic (lith″o-jen′ik) promoting the formation of calculi.

lithogenous (lĭ-thoj′ĕ-nus) producing or causing the formation of calculi.

lithokelyphopedion (lith″o-kel″ĭ-fo-pe′de-on) [litho- + Gr. *kelyphos* sheath + *paidion* child] a lithopedion in which both the fetus and the membranes are petrified.

lithokelyphos (lith″o-kel′ĭ-fos) [litho- + Gr. *kelyphos* sheath] a dead fetus in which the fetal membranes are calcified.

litholabe (lith′o-lab) [litho- + Gr. *lambanein* to hold] an instrument for holding a vesical calculus in the operation for its removal.

litholapaxy (lĭ-thol′ah-pak″se) [litho- + Gr. *lapaxis* evacuation] the crushing of a calculus in the bladder, followed at once by the washing out of the fragments; called also *lithotripsy*.

lithology (lĭ-thol′o-je) [litho- + -logy] the sum of what is known regarding calculi and their treatment.

litholysis (lĭ-thol′ĭ-sis) [litho- + Gr. *lysis* dissolution] the dissolution of calculi in the bladder.

litholyte (lith′o-līt) [litho- + Gr. *lysis* dissolution] an instrument used to inject calculi solvents into the bladder.

litholytic (lith″o-lit′ik) 1. dissolving stones or calculi. 2. an agent that dissolves calculi.

lithometer (lĭ-thom′ĕ-ter) [litho- + Gr. *metron* measure] an instrument for measuring calculi.

lithomoscus (lith″o-mos′kus) [litho- + Gr. *moschos* calf] lithopedion in cattle.

lithomyl (lith′o-mil) [litho- + Gr. *mylē* mill] an instrument for crushing a stone in the bladder.

lithonephritis (lith″o-nĕ-fri′tis) [litho- + *nephritis*] inflammation of the kidney due to irritation by calculi.

lithonephrotomy (lith″o-nĕ-frot′o-me) [litho- + Gr. *nephros* kidney + *tomē* a cutting] the operative removal of a renal calculus.

lithopedion (lith″o-pe′de-on) [L. *lithopaedium;* from Gr. *lithos* stone + *paidion* child] a dead fetus that has become stony or petrified *in utero;* calcified fetus.

lithoscope (lith′o-skōp) [litho- + Gr. *skopein* to examine] an instrument for examining calculi in the bladder; cystoscope.

Lithostat (lith′o-stat) trademark for a preparation of acetohydroxamic acid.

lithotome (lith′o-tōm) a knife for performing lithotomy.

lithotomist (lĭ-thot′o-mist) one who performs a lithotomy.

lithotomy (lĭ-thot′o-me) [litho- + Gr. *tomē* a cutting] incision of a duct or organ, especially of the bladder, for removal of stone. **bilateral l.,** one performed by a transverse incision across the perineum. **high l.,** suprapubic l. **lateral l.,** one in which the incision is before the rectum and to one side of the raphe. **median l.,** one in which the incision is made on the raphe of the perineum anterior to the anus. **mediolateral l.,** a combination of the median and lateral operations. **perineal l.,** that in which the incision is made in the perineum. **prerectal l.,** median l. **rectal l., rectovesical l.,** one performed by an incision within the dilated rectum. **suprapubic l.,** one performed by an incision above the pubes. **vaginal l., vesicovaginal l.,** one performed by an incision within the vagina.

lithotony (lĭ-thot′o-ne) [litho- + Gr. *teinein* to stretch] the creation of an artificial bladder fistula which is dilated to allow the extraction of a stone.

lithotresis (lith″o-tre′sis) [litho- + Gr. *trēsis* a boring] the drilling or boring of holes in a calculus.

lithotripsy (lith′o-trip″se) [litho- + Gr. *tribein* to rub] litholapaxy. **extracorporeal shock wave l.,** a procedure for treating upper urinary tract stones: the patient is immersed in a large tub of water and a high-energy shock wave generated by a high-voltage spark is focused by an ellipsoid reflector on the stone. The stone disintegrates into particles which are passed in the urine.

lithotriptic (lith″o-trip′tik) pertaining to or producing lithotripsy.

lithotripter (lith″o-trip″ter) lithotriptor.

lithotriptor (lith″o-trip″tor) an instrument for crushing calculi in the bladder.

lithotriptoscope (lith″o-trip′to-skōp) an instrument for performing lithotriptoscopy.

lithotriptoscopy (lith″o-trip-tos′ko-pe) [litho- + Gr. *tripsis* a crushing + *skopein* to examine] the crushing of a vesical calculus under direct visual control.

lithotrite (lith′o-trīt) [litho- + Gr. *tribein* to rub] an instrument for crushing a stone in the bladder.

lithotrity (lĭ-thot′rĭ-te) the crushing of a vesical calculus within the bladder by means of the lithotrite.

lithotroph (lith′o-trōf) [litho- + Gr. *trophē* nutrition] autotroph.

lithous (lith′us) [Gr. *lithos* stone] pertaining to or of the nature of a calculus.

lithoxiduria (lith″ok-sĭ-du′re-ah) [litho- + oxide + Gr. *ouron* urine + -ia] xanthinuria.

lithuresis (lith″u-re′sis) [litho- + Gr. *ourēsis* urination] the passage of gravel through the urethra with the urine.

lithureteria (lith″u-rĕ-te′re-ah) [litho- + Gr. *ourētēr* ureter] calculous disease of the ureter.

lithuria (lith-u′re-ah) excess of uric (lithic) acid or its salts in the urine; see *hyperuricuria.*

litmocidin (lit″mo-si′din) a toxic antibiotic substance obtained from *Nocardia cyaneus.* It is an anthocyanidine derivative and is bacteriostatic and bactericidal for cocci, *Vibrio cholerae,* and tubercle bacilli in vitro. It is a red indicator pigment (acid—red; alkali—blue).

litmus (lit′mus) a pigment prepared from *Roccella tinctoria* and other lichens, used as a test for acidity and alkalinity. It has a pH range of 4.5 to 8.3. Crude fractions are *azolitmin, erythrolitmin* and *erythrolein.* The principal chemically-defined component is a polymer of 7-hydroxy-2-phenoxazone.

Litomosoides carinii (lit″o-mo-soi′dēz kah-rin′e-i) a filarial worm found in the pleural and peritoneal cavities of the cotton rat, *Sigmodon hispidus.*

litre (le′ter) [Fr.] liter.

Litten's diaphragm phenomenon (sign) (lit′enz) [Moritz *Litten,* German physician, 1845–1907] see under *phenomenon.*

litter (lit′er) 1. a stretcher for transporting the sick or wounded. 2. the offspring produced at one birth by a multiparous animal.

Little's area (lit′elz) [James Laurence *Little,* American surgeon, 1836–1885] see *Kiesselbach's area* under *area.*

Little's disease (lit′elz) [William John *Little,* English physician, 1810–1894] see under *disease.*

Littre's crypts, glands, hernia (le′trz) [Alexis *Littre,* French surgeon, 1658–1725] see *glandulae preputiales* and *glandulae urethrales urethrae masculinae,* and see under *hernia.*

littritis (lit-tri′tis) inflammation of the urethral (Littre's) glands.

Litzmann's obliquity (litz′manz) [Karl Konrad Theodor *Litzmann,* German gynecologist, 1815–1890] see under *obliquity.*

livedo (lĭ-ve′do) [L.] a discolored spot or patch on the skin, commonly due to passive congestion; commonly used alone to refer to *l. reticularis.* **l. racemo′sa, l. racemo′sa,** l. reticularis. **l. reticula′ris,** a vascular response to various disorders caused by dilation of the subpapillary venous plexus as a result of increased viscosity of the blood changes in the blood vessels themselves that delay blood flow away from the skin, and clinically characterized by the presence of a reticular cyanotic cutaneous discoloration surrounding pale central areas involving the extremities and trunk, which becomes more intense on exposure to cold and may disappear on warming. It has been classified in three groups: (1) cutis marmorata, (2) idiopathic with or without ulceration, and (3) symptomatic, i.e., that associated with other disorders. Called also *l. racemosa.* **l. reticula′ris, idiopathic,** a persistent form of livedo reticularis most commonly seen in women, characterized by the presence of symmetrical diffuse lesions. Greater changes occur during the winter months, with some patients developing ulcerations on the legs. Other patients develop edema of the feet and ankles during the spring and summer months followed by ulcerations. **l. reticula′ris,**

symptomatic, livedo reticularis occurring in an asymmetrical, patchy distribution in association with and paralleling various disorders, most of which are characterized by changes in the blood viscosity, embolization, or disease of the blood vessel wall. Diseases in which this type of livedo reticularis may be a manifestation include vascular diseases (e.g., arteriosclerosis, vascular calcification with hyperparathyroidism, and arteritis), intravascular occlusion (e.g., thrombocytopenia, cryoglobulinemia, emboli, and caisson disease), and miscellaneous diseases (e.g., tuberculosis, syphilis, and rheumatic fever). **l. telangiectat′ica,** permanent mottling of the skin due to anomaly of the capillaries of the skin.

livedoid (liv′e-doid) pertaining to or resembling livedo.

liver (liv′er) [L. *jecur;* Gr. *hēpar*] 1. a large gland of a dark-red color situated in the upper part of the abdomen on the right side. Called also *hepar* [NA]. Its domed upper surface fits closely against and is adherent to the inferior surface of the right diaphragmatic dome, and it has a double blood supply from the hepatic artery and the portal vein. It comprises thousands of minute lobules (lobuli hepatis), the functional units of the liver (see also *liver acinus,* under *acinus,* and *portal lobule,* under *lobule*). Its manifold functions include the storage and filtration of blood, the secretion of bile, the excretion of bilirubin and other substances formed elsewhere in the body, and numerous metabolic functions, including the conversion of sugars into glycogen, which it stores. It is essential to life. 2. the same gland of certain animals sometimes used as food or from which pharmaceutical products are prepared. **albuminoid l., amyloid l.,** a liver which is the seat of an albuminoid or amyloid degeneration; called also *waxy l.* **biliary cirrhotic l.,** one in which the bile ducts are clogged and distended, the substance of the organ being inflamed; due to biliary cirrhosis. **brimstone l.,** an enlarged liver of a deep-yellow color, seen in some cases of congenital syphilis. **bronze l.,** the bronze-colored liver seen in malaria, which results from deposition of malarial pigment (q.v.). **cirrhotic l.,** one that is the site of cirrhosis. **degraded l.,** a human liver divided into many lobes. **fatty l.,** one affected with fatty infiltration. **floating l.,** wandering l. **foamy l.,** a liver seen post mortem, marked by the presence of numerous gas bubbles. **frosted l.,** perihepatitis chronica hyperplastica. **hobnail l.,** a liver whose surface is marked by nail-like points from cirrhosis. **icing l.,** perihepatitis chronica hyperplastica. **infantile l.,** biliary cirrhosis of children; see under *cirrhosis.* **iron l.,** the condition of the liver in hepatic siderosis. **lardaceous l.,** albuminoid l. **nutmeg l.,** one presenting a mottled appearance when cut. **pigmented l.,** one containing pigment, usually a result of malaria and melanemia, or the Dubin-Johnson syndrome. **polycystic l.,** congenital cystic disease of the liver. **sago l.,** one affected with amyloid degeneration, the acini resembling boiled sago grains, i.e., translucent granules 2 or 3 mm. in diameter. **stasis l.,** the liver in stasis cirrhosis. **sugar-icing l.,** perihepatitis chronica hyperplastica. **wandering l.,** a displaced and movable liver. **waxy l.,** albuminoid l.

livetin (li′vĕ-tin) a protein found in yolk of egg.

Livi's index (le′vēz) [Rodolfo *Livi,* Italian physician, 1856–1920] see under *index.*

livid (liv′id) [L. *lividus,* lead-colored] discolored, as from the effects of contusion or congestion; black and blue.

lividity (lĭ-vid′ĭ-te) [L. *lividitas*] the quality of being livid; discoloration, as of dependent parts, by the gravitation of the blood. **postmortem l.,** livor mortis.

Livierato's sign (le″ve-er-at′ōz) [Panagino *Livierato,* Italian physician, 1860–1936] see under *sign.*

Livingston's triangle (liv′ing-stunz) [Edward Meakin *Livingston,* American surgeon, born 1895] see under *triangle.*

livor (li′vor), pl. *livo′res* [L. "bluish color"] 1. lividity. 2. l. mortis. **l. mor′tis,** discoloration appearing on dependent parts of the body after death, as a result of cessation of circulation, stagnation of blood, and settling of the blood by gravity; called also *postmortem lividity.*

Lixaminol (liks-am′ĭ-nol) trademark for preparations of aminophylline.

lixiviation (liks″iv-e-a′shun) [L. *lixivia* lye] the separation of soluble from insoluble matter by dissolving out the soluble matter and drawing off the solution; called also *leaching.*

lixivium (liks-iv′e-um) [L.] any alkaline filtrate obtained by leaching ashes or other similar powdered substance; lye.

Lizars' operation (li′zarz) [John *Lizars,* Edinburgh surgeon, 1787(?)–1860] see under *operation.*

L.L.L. left lower lobe (of the lung).

L.M. light minimum; linguomesial.

L.M.A. left mentoanterior (position of the fetus).

LMF lymphocyte mitogenic factor.

L.M.P. left mentoposterior (position of the fetus); last menstrual period.

L.M.T. left mentotransverse (position of the fetus).

LNPF lymph node permeability factor.

L.O.A. left occipitoanterior (position of the fetus).

Loa (lo′ah) [a native word in Angola, West Africa] a genus of filarial nematodes. **L. lo′a,** a threadlike worm of West Africa, 1–2 inches long, that inhabits the subcutaneous connective tissue of the body, which it traverses freely. It is seen especially about the orbit and even under the conjunctiva. It causes itching and occasionally edematous swellings (Calabar swellings). The immature forms or microfilariae are diurnal, being found in the peripheral circulation in greatest concentrations during the day. Flies of the genus *Chrysops* are the intermediate hosts and vectors. Formerly called *Filaria loa.*

load (lōd) the quantity of a measurable entity borne, by an object or organism, such as the work (*work l.*) required of an individual, or the body content, as of water, salt, or heat, especially as it varies from normal. **occlusal l.,** the total force exerted on the teeth through the occlusal surfaces during mastication.

loading (lōd′ing) administering sufficient quantities of a substance to test the subject's ability to metabolize it, as in the histidine loading test.

loaiasis (lo″ah-i′ah-sis) loiasis.

lobar (lo′ber) of, pertaining to, or affecting a lobe.

lobate (lo′bāt) [L. *lobatus*] provided with lobes, or disposed in lobes.

lobation (lo-ba′shun) the formation of lobes; the state of having lobes. **renal l.,** the appearance on x-ray films of small notches along the surface of the kidney, indicating the location of renal lobes.

lobe (lōb) [L. *lobus,* from Gr. *lobos*] 1. a more or less well-defined portion of any organ, especially of the brain, lungs, and glands. Lobes are demarcated by fissures, sulci, connective tissue, and by their shape. 2. one of the main divisions of the crown of a tooth, developmentally representing a center of calcification. **anterior l. of hypophysis, anterior l. of pituitary gland,** adenohypophysis. **appendicular l.,** Riedel's l. **azygos l.,** a small accessory or anomalous lobe situated at the apex of the right lung. **caudate l. of cerebrum** (obs.), insula. **caudate l. of liver,** lobus caudatus. **l. of cerebellum, anterior,** lobus rostralis cerebelli. **l. of cerebellum, cranial,** lobus rostralis cerebelli. **l. of cerebellum, middle,** lobus caudalis cerebelli. **l. of cerebellum, posterior,** l. caudalis cerebelli. **cuneate l.,** cuneus. **flocculonodular l.,** lobus flocculonodularis. **frontal l.,** the anterior portion of the pallium; see *lobus frontalis.* **gracile l. of cerebellum,** lobulus paramedianus cerebelli. **hepatic l's,** lobi hepatis. **inferior l. of left lung,** lobus inferior pulmonis sinistri. **inferior l. of right l.,** lobus inferior pulmonis dextri. **lateral l's of prostate gland,** see *lobus prostatae* [*dexter et sinister*]. **limbic l.,** gyrus fornicatus. **linguiform l.,** Riedel's l. **l's of liver,** lobi hepatis. **l. of liver, left,** lobus hepatis sinister. **l. of liver, right,** lobus hepatis dexter. **l's of lung,** see *lung.* **l's of mammary gland,** lobi glandulae mammariae. **median l. of prostate,** l. medius prostatae. **middle l. of right lung,** lobus medius pulmonis dextri. **neural l., neural l. of neurohypophysis, neural l. of pituitary gland,** lobus nervosus neurohypophyseos. **occipital l.,** the posterior portion of the cerebral hemisphere; see *lobus occipitalis.* **olfactory l.,** lobus olfactorius. **optic l's,** corpora quadrigemina. **parietal l.,** the upper central lobe of the pallium; see *lobus parietalis.* **piriform l.,** the piriform area (q.v.); in lower mammals, the lateral exposed portion of the olfactory cerebral cortex. **polyalveolar l.,** a congenital disorder characterized in early infancy by the presence of far more than the normal number of alveoli in a lobe of the lungs; thereafter, normal multiplication of alveoli does not take place and they become enlarged, i.e., emphysematous. **posterior l. of hypophysis, posterior l. of pituitary gland,** neurohypophysis. **prefrontal l.,** the part of the frontal lobe of the brain anterior to the ascending convolution. **l's of prostate,** see *lobus prostatae [dexter et sinister].* **pulmonary l's,** see *lung.* **pyriform l.,** piriform l. **pyramidal l. of thyroid gland,** lobus pyramidalis glandulae thyroideae. **quadrangular l. of cerebellum,** lobulus quadrangularis cerebelli. **quadrate l. of cerebral hemisphere,** precuneus. **quadrate l. of liver,** lobus quadratus hepatis. **renal l's,** lobi renales. **Riedel's l.,** an anomalous tongue-shaped mass of tissue projecting from the right lobe of the liver. **semilunar l., inferior,** lobulus semilunaris inferior. **semilunar l., superior,** lobulus semilunaris superior. **spigelian l.,** lobus caudatus. **superior l. of left lung,** lobus superior pulmonis sinistri. **superior l. of right lung,** lobus superior pulmonis dextri. **temporal l.,** the lower lateral lobe of the cerebral hemisphere; see *lobus temporalis.* **temporosphenoidal l. of cerebral hemisphere** (*obs.*), lobus temporalis. **l's of thymus,** see *lobus thymi [dexter/sinister].* **l's of thyroid gland,** see *lobus glandulae thyroideae [dexter/sinister].* **vagal l.,** visceral l. **vermiform l.** (*obs.*), vermis cerebelli. **visceral l.,** the visceral sensory area of fishes.

lobectomy (lo-bek′to-me) [Gr. *lobos* lobe + *ektomē* excision] excision of a lobe, as of the thyroid, liver, brain, or lung. See also *lobotomy.* **sleeve l.,** excision of a lobe of the lung with removal of a portion of the bronchus and reanastomosis of the resulting ends.

lobelia (lo-be′le-ah) the dried leaves and tops of *Lobelia inflata* L. (Campanulaceae), an herb with properties resembling those of nicotine.

lobeline (lob′e-lin) alpha-lobeline, $C_{22}H_{27}NO_2$, the principal alkaloid of *Lobelia inflata,* an annual herb of eastern United States and Canada, formerly used to restore normal respiration in asphyxia due to traumatic shock. Currently used in certain anti-smoking preparations.

lobendazole (lo-ben′dah-zōl) chemical name: 1*H*-benzimidazol-2-yl-carbamic acid ethyl ester; a veterinary anthelmintic, $C_{10}H_{11}N_3O_2$.

lobi (lo′bi) [L.] genitive and plural of *lobus.*

lobite (lo′bīt) limited to a definite lobe.

lobitis (lo-bi′tis) inflammation of a lobe, especially of a lobe of the lung.

Loboa loboi (lo-bo′ah lo′boi) an as yet uncultured yeast that is the causative agent of keloidal blastomycosis.

lobopodium (lo″bo-po′de-um), pl. *lobopo′dia* [Gr. *lobos* lobe + *pous* foot] a wide, blunt pseudopodium composed of both ectoplasm and endoplasm. Cf. *axopodium, filopodium,* and *reticulopodium.*

Lobosea (lo-bo′se-ah) [Gr. *lobos* lobe] a class of ameboid protozoa (superclass Rhizopoda, subphylum Sarcodina) typically characterized by the presence of lobopodia, although filopodia or reticulopodia sometimes occur. It comprises two subclasses: Gymnamoebia and Testacealobosia.

lobotomy (lo-bot′o-me) incision into a lobe; in psychosurgery, surgical incision of all the fibers of a lobe of the brain. **frontal l., prefrontal l.,** an operation in which, through holes drilled in the skull, the white matter of the frontal lobe is incised with a leukotome passed through a cannula; called also *leukotomy.* **transorbital l.,** see under *leukotomy.*

Lobstein's disease (syndrome), ganglion (lōb′stīnz) [Johann Friedrich Georg Christian Martin *Lobstein,* surgeon in Strasbourg, 1777–1835] see *osteogenesis imperfecta,* and see under *ganglion.*

lobular (lob′u-lar) [L. *lobularis*] of or pertaining to a lobule.

lobulated (lob′u-lāt″ed) made up of or divided into lobules.

lobulation (lob″u-la′shun) the process of becoming or the state of being lobulated. **portal l.,** in the liver, the lobulated pattern of surviving tissue and the areas in which the tissue has been destroyed after occlusion of the hepatic vein.

lobule (lob′ūl) a small lobe; see *lobulus.* **anterior l. of pituitary gland,** lobus anterior hypophyseos. **l. of auricle,** lobulus auriculae. **l. of azygos vein,** an anatomical variation of the structure of the lung that may be apparent on the radiogram; it is produced when the azygos vein arches over the upper part of the lung instead of at the hilus and presses deeply into the lung tissue to form a fissure

that isolates a medial part of the lung. **biventral l.,** lobulus biventer. **central l. of cerebellum,** lobulus centralis cerebelli. **cortical l's of kidney,** lobuli corticales renis. **l's of epididymis,** lobuli epididymidis. **falciform l.** (*obs.*), cuneus. **fusiform l.** (*obs.*), polus temporalis. **hepatic l's,** lobuli hepatis. **l's of liver,** lobuli hepatis. **l's of lung,** segmenta bronchopulmonalia. **l's of mammary gland,** lobuli glandulae mammariae. **l. of pancreas,** lobulus pancreatis. **paracentral l.,** lobulus paracentralis. **paramedian l.,** lobulus gracilis cerebelli. **parietal l., inferior,** lobulus parietalis inferior. **parietal l., superior,** lobulus parietalis superior. **portal l.,** a polygonal mass of liver tissue, larger than a liver acinus, containing portions of three adjacent hepatic lobules, and having a portal vein at its center and a central vein peripherally at each corner. **primary l. of lung,** the anatomical and functional unit of the lung; distal to a terminal bronchiole, it consists of respiratory bronchioles, two or more alveolar ducts, atria, alveolar sacs, and alveoli. See Plate 46. **pulmonary l's,** segmenta bronchopulmonalia. **quadrangular l. of cerebellum,** lobulus quadrangularis cerebelli. **respiratory l.,** primary l. of lung. **secondary l. of lung,** an anatomical subdivision of a pulmonary segment, consisting of several branching primary lobules. **semilunar l., caudal,** lobulus semilunaris caudalis. **semilunar l., cranial,** lobulus semilunaris rostralis. **semilunar l., inferior,** lobulus semilunaris caudalis. **semilunar l., superior,** lobulus semilunaris rostralis. **l's of testis,** lobuli testis. **l's of thymus,** lobuli thymi. **l's of thyroid gland,** lobuli glandulae thyroideae.

lobuli (lob′u-li) [L.] genitive and plural of *lobulus.*

lobulose (lob′u-lōs) divided into lobules.

lobulous (lob′u-lus) lobulose.

lobulus (lob′u-lus), gen. and pl. *lob′uli* [L. dim of *lobus*] a lobule, or small lobe; [NA] a general term for a small lobe or one of the primary divisions of a lobe. **l. auric′ulae** [NA], lobule of auricle: the inferior, dependent part of the auricle below the antitragus, which contains fibrous and fatty tissue but no cartilage. **l. biven′ter** [NA], biventral lobule: the part of the caudal lobe of the hemisphere of the cerebellum between the tonsilla and the caudal semilunar lobule. **l. centra′lis cerebel′li** [NA], central lobule of cerebellum: the portion of the cranial lobe of the cerebellum between the lingula and the culmen, resting on the lingula and the anterior medullary velum. **lob′uli cortica′les re′nis** [NA], cortical lobules of kidney: more or less distinctly marked small polygonal areas on the surface of a kidney; each area corresponds to a medullary ray together with its attached renal corpuscles and tubules. **lob′uli epididym′idis** [NA], lobules of epididymis: the wedge-shaped parts of the head of the epididymis, each comprising a single efferent ductule of the testis; called also *coni epididymidis* [NA alternative]. **lob′uli glan′dulae mamma′riae** [NA], lobules of mammary gland: the smaller subdivisions that make up a lobe of the mammary gland, each drained by a single branch of a lactiferous duct. Called also *lobuli mammae.* See *mammary gland,* under *gland.* **lob′uli glan′dulae thyroi′deae** [NA], lobules of thyroid gland: irregular areas on the surface of the thyroid gland produced by entrance into the gland of fibrous trabeculae from the sheath. **l. gra′cilis cerebel′li** [NA], the portion of the caudal lobe of the hemisphere of the cerebellum between caudal and semilunar and the biventral lobules; called also *l. paramedianus* [NA alternative] and *paramedian lobule.* **lob′uli hep′atis** [NA], hepatic lobules: the small vascular units comprising the substance of the liver, each of which is polygonal in shape with a central vein at its center and portal canals peripherally at the corners. See also *liver acinus,* under *acinus.* **lob′uli mam′mae,** lobuli glandulae mammariae. **l. pancrea′tis,** lobule of pancreas: any of the distinct lobules into which the pancreas is divided by extension of septa of the capsule into the gland. **l. paracentra′lis** [NA], paracentral lobule: a lobe on the medial surface of the cerebral hemisphere, continuous with the precentral and postcentral gyri of the frontal and parietal lobes, and limited below by the cingulate sulcus; it is comprised of sensorimotor cortex, chiefly for the lower limb. **l. paramedia′nus cerebel′li,** NA alternative for *l. gracilis cerebelli.* **l. parieta′lis infe′rior** [NA], inferior parietal lobule: the lobule that forms the posterior part of the lateral portion of the parietal lobe of the cerebrum. It lies below the intraparietal sulcus, above the posterior ramus of the lateral cerebral fissure, and behind the postcentral sulcus. It includes the supramarginal and the angular gyri. In the dominant hemisphere, it is concerned with language mechanisms. **l. parieta'lis supe'rior** [NA], superior parietal lobule: the posterior part of the upper portion of the parietal lobe of the brain; it lies behind the postcentral sulcus, in front of the parietooccipital fissure, and above the intraparietal sulcus. It comprises association areas concerned with general sensory functions. **lob'uli pulmo'num,** segmenta bronchopulmonalia. **l. quadrangula'ris cerebel'li** [NA], quadrangular lobule of cerebellum: the portion of the cranial lobe of the hemisphere of the cerebellum lying between the postcentral and primary fissures, continuous with the culmen; the term *lobulus quadrangularis* was formerly used to designate the portion of the cerebellum continuous with both the declive and the culmen, which was divided into an anterior part and a posterior part (see *l. simplex cerebelli*). Called also *pars anterior lobuli quadrangularis, pars cranialis lobuli quadrangularis,* and *pars rostralis lobuli cerebelli* [NA alternative]. **l. semiluna'ris cauda'lis** [NA], caudal semilunar lobule: that portion of the caudal lobe of the hemisphere of the cerebellum continuous with the tuber vermis; called also *inferior semilunar lobule, lobulus semilunaris inferior* [NA alternative], and, in comparative anatomy, *crus II.* **l. semiluna'ris crania'lis** l. semilunaris rostralis. **l. semiluna'ris infe'rior,** NA alternative for *l. semilunaris caudalis.* **l. semiluna'ris rostra'lis** [NA], rostral semilunar lobule: that part of the hemisphere of the cerebellum continuous with the folium vermis; called also *cranial semilunar lobule, l. semilunaris superior* [NA alternative], *l. semilunaris cranialis,* and, in comparative anatomy, *crus I.* **l. semiluna'ris supe'rior,** NA alternative for *l. semilunaris rostralis.* **l. sim'plex cerebel'li** [NA], the portion of the caudal lobe of the hemisphere of the cerebellum continuous with the declive; called also *pars caudalis lobuli quadrangularis* [NA alternative] and *pars posterior lobuli quadrangularis* [NA alternative]. See also *l. quadrangularis cerebelli.* **lob'uli tes'tis** [NA], lobules of testis: the pyramidal subdivisions of the testicular substance, each with its base against the albuginea and its apex at the mediastinum, and composed largely of tubuli seminiferi. **lob'uli thy'mi** [NA], lobules of thymus: the smaller subdivisions of the lobes of the thymus gland, separated by fibrous trabeculae.

lobus (lo'bus), gen. and pl. *lo'bi* [L.] a lobe; a more or less well defined portion of any organ; [NA] a general term for such subdivisions, especially of the brain, lungs, and various glands, demarcated by fissures, sulci, or connective tissue septa. **l. ante'rior cerebel'li,** NA alternative for *l. cranialis cerebelli.* **l. ante'rior hypophys'eos,** NA alternative for adenohypophysis. **l. cauda'lis cerebel'li** [NA], caudal lobe of cerebellum: the portion of the cerebellum separated from the cranial lobe by the primary fissure and from the flocculonodular lobe by the dorsolateral fissure, comprising the declive, folium vermis, tuber vermis, pyramid, uvula, simple lobule, cranial and caudal semilunar lobules (paramedian and biventral lobules, and tonsils; called also *l. posterior cerebelli* [NA alternative] and *middle* or *posterior lobe of cerebellum.* **l. cauda'tus** [NA], **l. cauda'tus [Spige'li],** caudate lobe of liver: a small lobe of the liver bounded on the right by the inferior vena cava, which separates it from the right lobe, and on the left by the attachment of the gastrohepatic ligament, which separates it from the left lobe. **lo'bi cer'ebri** [NA], lobes of cerebrum: the well defined areas of the cerebral cortex, demarcated by fissures, sulci, and arbitrary lines, including the frontal, temporal, parietal, and occipital lobes. See Plate accompanying *brain.* **l. crania'lis cerebel'li,** l. rostralis cerebelli. **l. flocculonodula'ris** [NA], flocculonodular lobe: a fundamental subdivision of the cerebellum, consisting of paired lateral flocculi, their penduncli, and the nodulus. **l. fronta'lis** [NA], frontal lobe: the anterior portion of the cerebral hemisphere, extending from the frontal pole to the sulcus centralis. **lo'bi glan'dulae mamma'riae** [NA], lobes of mammary gland: the major subdivisions of the secreting portion of the mammary gland, each drained by a single lactiferous duct and further subdivided into lobules (lobuli glandulae mammariae). See *mammary gland,* under *gland.* Called also *lobi mammae.* **l. glan'dulae thyroi'deae [dex'ter/sinis'ter]** [NA],

lobe of thyroid gland: either of the lobes (right or left) of the thyroid gland, closely applied to either side of the trachea, cricoid cartilage, and thyroid cartilage. **lo'bi hep'atis** [NA], the lobes of the liver; see *l. hepatis dexter, l. hepatis sinister, l. quadratus,* and *l. caudatus.* Called also *hepatic lobes.* **l. hep'atis dex'ter** [NA], right lobe of liver: the largest of the four lobes of the liver. Anteriorly, it is separated from the left lobe by the falciform ligament. Posteroinferiorly, it is separated from the caudate lobe by the inferior vena cava and from the quadrate lobe by the gallbladder. Used in the broad sense, the term includes the caudate and quadrate lobes. **l. hep'atis sinis'ter** [NA], left lobe of liver: the smaller of the two main lobes of the liver. Anteriorly, it is separated from the right lobe by the falciform ligament. Posteroinferiorly, it is separated from the caudate and quadrate lobes by the attachment of the gastrohepatic ligament and the ligamentum teres. **l. infe'rior pulmo'nis dex'tri** [NA], the inferior lobe of the right lung. **l. infe'rior pulmo'nis sinis'tri** [NA], the inferior lobe of the left lung. **l. insula'ris** [NA], insular lobe: the portion of the cerebral cortex lying deep in the lateral sulcus, almost surrounded by the circular sulcus, which is covered over and hidden from view by juxtaposition of the opercula; called also *insula* [NA alternative] and *i. of Reil.* **lo'bi mam'mae,** lobi glandulae mammariae. **l. me'dius prosta'tae** [NA], median lobe of prostate: a normal enlargement of the isthmus of the prostate that sometimes occurs. **l. me'dius pulmo'nis dex'tri** [NA], the middle lobe of the right lung. **l. nervo'sus hypophys'eos,** l. nervosus neurohypophyseos. **l. nervo'sus neurohypophys'eos** [NA], neural lobe of neurohypophysis: the major portion of the neurohypophysis; called also *infundibular process, neural lobe of hypophysis* or *pituitary gland,* and *pars nervosa hypophyseos.* See also *pituitary gland,* under *gland.* **l. occipita'lis** [NA], occipital lobe: the posterior portion of the cerebral hemisphere, extending from the posterior pole to the parietooccipital fissure on the medial surface, but continuous with the parietal lobe on the lateral surface. **l. olfacto'rius,** olfactory lobe: a term applied to the olfactory apparatus on the lower surface of the frontal lobe of the brain. It consists of the olfactory bulb, tract, and trigone. **l. parieta'lis** [NA], parietal lobe: the upper central lobe of the cerebral hemisphere, separated from the temporal lobe below by the lateral sulcus, but continuous at the posterior end of that sulcus, and separated from the frontal lobe in front by the central sulcus. Behind, it is continuous with the occipital lobe on the lateral surface, but separated from it by the parietooccipital sulcus on the medial surface. **lo'bi placen'tae,** distinct areas on the uterine surface of the placenta, demarcated by the connective tissue septa. **l. poste'rior cerebel'li,** NA alternative for *l. caudalis cerebelli.* **l. poste'rior hypophys'eos,** NA alternative for neurohypophysis. **l. prosta'tae dex'ter/sinis'ter** [NA], lobe of prostate: either of the paired halves (right and left) of the prostate, separated by a more or less distinct median sulcus; called also *lateral lobes of prostate gland.* **l. pyramida'lis glan'dulae thyroi'deae** [NA], pyramidal lobe of the thyroid gland: an occasional third lobe of the thyroid gland which extends upward from the isthmus across the thyroid cartilage to the hyoid bone; it is the residuum of the thyroid stalk of the fetus. **l. quadra'tus hep'atis** [NA], quadrate lobe of liver: a small lobe of the liver bounded on the right by the gallbladder, which separates it from the right lobe, and on the left by the ligamentum teres, which separates it from the left lobe. **lo'bi rena'les** [NA], renal lobes: the units of the kidney, each consisting of a pyramid and its surrounding cortical substance; the division of the kidney into lobes is more distinctly marked in some animals and in infants than in the human adult. **l. rostra'lis cerebel'li** [NA], rostral lobe of cerebellum: the portion of the cerebellum lying in front of the primary fissure, comprising the lingula, central lobule, culmen, alae of central lobules, and quadrangular lobules; called also *anterior* or *cranial lobe of cerebellum, l. anterior cerebelli* [NA alternative], and *l. cranialis cerebelli.* **l. spige'lii,** l. caudatus. **l. supe'rior pulmo'nis dex'tri** [NA], the superior lobe of the right lung. **l. supe'rior pulmo'nis sinis'tri** [NA], the superior lobe of the left lung. **l. tempora'lis** [NA], temporal lobe: the lower lateral lobe of the cerebral hemisphere, lying below the posterior ramus of the lateral sulcus, lateral to the collateral sulcus, and merging behind with the occipital lobe. **l. thy'mi [dex'ter/sinis'ter]** [NA], lobe of thymus: either of the two chief parts (right or left) of the thymus, which meet in the midline. **l. va′gi,** visceral lobe.

local (lo′kal) [L. *localis*] restricted to or pertaining to one spot or part; not general.

localization (lo″kah-li-za′shun) 1. the determination of the site or place of any process or lesion. 2. restriction to a circumscribed or limited area. 3. prelocalization. **cerebral l.,** the determination of the situation of the various centers of the brain; also the limitation of the various cerebral faculties to a particular center or organ of the brain. **germinal l.,** the location on a blastoderm of prospective organs; see *fate map*, under *map*.

localized (lo′kal-īzd) not general; restricted to a limited region or to one or more spots.

localizer (lo′kal-īz″er) 1. an instrument for locating solid particles in the eyeball by roentgenography. 2. a visual training instrument for establishing correct spatial localization in treating amblyopia ex anopsia.

locator (lo′ka-ter) an instrument or apparatus by which the location of an object is determined. **abutment l.,** a thin resin base made on a diagnostic denture cast into which holes have been cut to predetermine locations of the cuspid teeth and molar teeth on a subperiosteal implant. **Berman-Moorhead l.,** an instrument for locating metallic fragments embedded in body tissues. **electroacoustic l.,** an apparatus that amplifies into an audible click the contact of a probe with a solid object; used in locating foreign objects within the body.

Loc. dol. abbreviation for L. *lo′co dolen′ti,* to the painful spot.

lochia (lo′ke-ah) [Gr. *lochia*] the vaginal discharge that takes place during the first week or two after childbirth. **l. al′ba,** the final vaginal discharge after childbirth, when the amount of blood is decreased and the leukocytes are increased. **l. cruen′ta,** l. rubra. **l. purulen′ta,** l. alba. **l. ru′bra,** the vaginal discharge of almost pure blood immediately after childbirth. **l. sanguinolen′ta,** the thick, maroon-colored vaginal discharge occurring a few days after childbirth. **l. sero′sa,** the serous vaginal discharge occurring about four or five days after childbirth.

lochial (lo′ke-al) pertaining to the lochia.

lochiocolpos (lo″ke-o-kol′pos) [*lochia* + Gr. *kolpos* vagina] distention of the vagina by retained lochia.

lochiocyte (lo′ke-o-sīt″) [*lochia* + *-cyte*] one of the characteristic decidual cells of the lochia.

lochiometra (lo″ke-o-me′trah) [*lochia* + Gr. *mētra* uterus] distention of the uterus by retained lochia.

lochiometritis (lo″ke-o-me-tri′tis) [*lochia* + *metritis*] puerperal metritis.

lochiorrhagia (lo″ke-o-ra′je-ah) [*lochia* + Gr. *rhēgnynai* to burst forth] lochiorrhea.

lochiorrhea (lo″ke-o-re′ah) [*lochia* + Gr. *rhoia* flow] an abnormally profuse discharge of lochia.

lochioschesis (lo″ke-os′kĕ-sis) [*lochia* + Gr. *schesis* retention] retention of the lochia; lochiostasis.

lochiostasis (lo″ke-os′tah-sis) [*lochia* + Gr. *stasis* halt] retention of the lochia; lochioschesis.

lochometritis (lo″ko-me-tri′tis) [Gr. *lochos* childbirth + *metritis*] puerperal metritis.

loci (lo′si) [L.] genitive and plural of *locus.*

Locke's solution (fluid) (loks) [Frank Spiller *Locke*, British physician, 1871–1941] see under *solution.*

lockjaw (lok′jaw) trismus.

Lockwood's ligament (lok′woodz) [Charles Barrett *Lockwood*, English surgeon, 1856–1914] see under *ligament.*

loco (lo′ko) [Sp. "insane"] 1. a name of various leguminous plants of the genera *Astragalus, Hosackia, Sophora,* and *Oxytropis,* poisonous to horses, cattle, and sheep in certain arid regions because of the selenium they contain. 2. locoism. 3. an animal affected with locoism.

locoism (lo′ko-izm) a disease of horses, cattle, and sheep caused by poisoning by loco and marked by locomotor disturbances, trembling, depression, and, in pregnant animals, absorption. Called also *loco disease* and *loco poisoning.*

locomotion (lo″ko-mo′shun) [L. *locus* place + *movere* to move] movement or the ability to move from one place to another. **brachial l.,** brachiation.

locomotive (lo″ko-mo′tiv) pertaining to locomotion.

locomotor (lo″ko-mo′tor) of or pertaining to locomotion; pertaining to or affecting the locomotive apparatus of the body. See under *ataxia.*

locomotorial (lo″ko-mo-to′re-al) pertaining to the locomotorium.

locomotorium (lo″ko-mo-to′re-um) the locomotive apparatus of the body.

locomotory (lo″ko-mo′tor-e) pertaining to locomotion.

Locorten (lo-kor′ten) trademark for a preparation of flumethasone pivalate.

locular (lok′u-lar) pertaining to a loculus.

loculate (lok′u-lāt) divided into loculi.

loculi (lok′u-li) [L.] plural of *loculus.*

Loculoascomycetidae (lok″u-lo-as″ko-mi-se′tĭ-de) a subclass of ascomycetous fungi, including the order Myriangiales.

loculus (lok′u-lus) pl. *loc′uli* [L., dim. of *locus*] 1. a small space or cavity. 2. a local enlargement of the uterus in some mammals, containing an embryo.

locum (lo′kum) [L., accusative of *locus*] place. **l. ten′ens, l. ten′ent,** a practitioner who temporarily takes the place of another.

locus (lo′kus) gen. *lo′ci;* pl. *lo′ci* or *lo′ca* [L. "a place"] [NA] 1. a general anatomical term for a site in the body. 2. in genetics, the position of a gene on a chromosome, different forms of genes (alleles) being found at the same position on homologous chromosomes. **l. caeru′leus, l. ceru′leus,** l. coeruleus. **l. cine′reus,** l. ceruleus. **l. coeru′leus** [NA], a pigmented eminence in the superior angle of the floor of the brain. Written also *l. caeruleus* and *l. ceruleus.* See also usage note at *coeruleus.* **complex l.,** gene complex; see under *gene.* **l. ferrugin′eus,** l. ceruleus. **heteromorphic l.,** a locus that exists in two or more allelic forms. **l. mino′ris resisten′tiae,** a site of lessened resistance; an area, structure, or organ offering little resistance to invasion by microorganisms and/or their toxins. **l. ni′ger** (*obs.*), substantia nigra. **operator l.,** operator gene. **l. ru′ber,** nucleus ruber.

lodoxamide tromethamine (lo-dok′sah-mīd) chemical name: 2,2′-[(2-chloro-5-cyano-1,3-phenylene)diimino]bis[2-oxoacetic acid] compound with 2-amino-2-(hydroxymethyl)-1,3-propanediol (1:2); an antiasthmatic and antiallergic, $C_{11}H_6ClN_3O_6 \cdot 2C_4H_{11}NO_3$.

Loeb's deciduoma, reaction (lēb) [Leo *Loeb,* American pathologist, 1869–1959] see under *deciduoma* and *reaction.*

Loefflerella (lef″ler-el′ah) in former systems of classification, a genus of bacteria, species of which are now assigned to *Pseudomonas.*

loempe (lem′pe) beriberi.

Loevit's cell (le′fits) [Moritz *Loevit,* Prague pathologist, 1851–1918] erythroblast.

Loewi (la′ve) Otto. German-born American physiologist and pharmacologist, 1873–1961; co-winner, with Sir Henry Hallett Dale, of the Nobel prize for medicine or physiology in 1936 for their study of the chemical transmission of nerve impulses.

Loewi's test (reaction, symptom) (la′vēz) [Otto *Loewi*] see under *tests.*

Löffler's agar (culture medium) blood serum, stain (lef′lerz) [Friederich August Johannes *Löffler,* German bacteriologist, 1852–1915] see under *agar, blood serum,* and *Table of Stains.*

Löffler's endocarditis (disease), syndrome (eosinophilia, pneumonia) (lef′lerz) [Wilhelm *Löffler,* Swiss physician, born 1887] see under *endocarditis* and *syndrome.*

logadectomy (log″ah-dek′to-me) [Gr. *logades* the whites of the eyes + *ectomy*] excision of a portion of the conjunctiva.

logaditis (log″ah-di′tis) [Gr. *logades* the whites of the eyes + *-itis*] an obsolete term for inflammation of the sclera.

logagnosia (log″ag-no′ze-ah) [*logo-* + *a* neg. + Gr. *gnōsis* knowledge] aphasia, alogia, or other central word defect.

logagraphia (log″ah-graf′e-ah) [*logo-* + *a* neg. + Gr. *graphein* to write] inability to express ideas in writing.

logamnesia (log″am-ne′ze-ah) [*logo-* + Gr. *amnēsia* forgetfulness] receptive aphasia.

logaphasia (log″ah-fa′ze-ah) [logo- + aphasia] expressive aphasia.

logasthenia (log″as-the′ne-ah) [logo- + asthenia] disturbance of that faculty of the mind which deals with the comprehension of speech.

log(o)- [Gr. logos word] a combining form denoting relationship to words or speech.

logoclonia (log″o-klon′e-ah) [logo- + Gr. klonos tumult + -ia] spasmodic repetition of end syllables of words.

logogram (log′o-gram) the graphic record of the symptoms and signs exhibited by a specific patient, charted by means of the logoscope.

logoklony (log′o-klon″e) logoclonia.

logokophosis (log″o-ko-fo′sis) [logo- + Gr. kōphōsis deafness] word deafness; inability to comprehend spoken language.

logomania (log″o-ma′ne-ah) [logo- + Gr. mania madness] overtalkativeness.

logopathy (log-op′ah-the) [logo- + Gr. pathos illness] any disorder of speech arising from derangement of the central nervous system.

logopedia (log″o-pe′de-ah) logopedics.

logopedics (log-o-pe′diks) [logo- + orthopedics] the science dealing with the study and treatment of speech defects.

logoplegia (log″o-ple′je-ah) [logo- + Gr. plēgē stroke] paralysis of the speech organs.

logorrhea (log″o-re′ah) [logo- + rrhea flow] excessive volubility, with rapid, pressured speech; seen in manic episodes of bipolar disorder.

logoscope (log′o-skōp) [Gr. logos a thought, idea, or word + skopein to regard or view] a device, in slide-rule form, designed to facilitate identification of the diseases in which certain signs and symptoms occur.

logoscopy (lo-gos′ko-pe) the use of a logoscope for determining the differential diagnostic possibilities in a patient exhibiting certain signs and symptoms.

logospasm (log′o-spazm) [logo- + Gr. spasmos spasm] the spasmodic utterance of words.

-logy [Gr. logos word, reason] a word termination meaning the science or study of, or a treatise on, the subject designated by the stem to which it is affixed.

Lohnstein's saccharimeter (lōn′stīnz) [Theodor Lohnstein, German physician, 1866–1918] see under saccharimeter.

loiasis (lo-i′ah-sis) the state of being infected with nematodes of the genus Loa.

loin (loin) the part of the back between the thorax and the pelvis; called also lumbus [NA].

Lolipid (lo-lip′id) trademark for preparations of gemfibrozil.

Lombardi's sign (lom-bar′dēz) [Antonio Lombardi, physician in Naples] see under sign.

lometraline hydrochloride (lo-met′rah-lēn) chemical name: 8-chloro-1,2,3,4-tetrahydro-5-methoxy-N,N-dimethyl-1-naphthalenamine hydrochloride; a tranquilizer and antiparkinsonian agent, $C_{13}H_{18}ClNO \cdot HCl$.

lomofungin (lo-mo-fun′jin) chemical name: 6-formyl-4,7,9-trihydroxy-1-phenazinecarboxylic acid methyl ester; an antifungal antibiotic derived from Streptomyces lomondensis var. lomondensis.

lomosome (lo′mo-sōm) [Gr. lōma hem, fringe + sōma body] a sponge-like structure in fungi contiguous with the hyphal wall as revealed by the electron microscope.

Lomotil (lo′mo-til) trademark for preparations of diphenoxylate hydrochloride and atropine.

lomustine (lo-mus′tēn) chemical name: N-(2-chloroethyl)-N′-cyclohexyl-N-nitrosourea (CCNU), a cytotoxic alkylating agent of the nitrosourea (q.v.) group, used as an antineoplastic primarily for treatment of brain tumors, bronchogenic carcinoma, and Hodgkin's disease.

Lonchocarpus (lon″ko-kar′pus) a genus of leguminous tropical trees and shrubs which furnish rotenone.

Long's formula (coefficient) (longz) [John Harper Long, American physician, 1856–1927] see under formula.

longevity (lon-jev′ĭ-te) [L. longus long + aevum age] the condition or quality of being long lived.

longilineal (lon″jĭ-lin′e-al) built along long, narrow lines; dolichomorphic.

longimanous (lon″jĭ-man′us) [L. longus long + manus hand] having long hands.

longipedate (lon″jĭ-pe′dāt) [L. longus long + pes foot] having long feet.

longiradiate (lon″jĭ-ra′de-āt) having long radiations; a term applied to certain neuroglial cells.

longissimus (lon-jis′ĭ-mus) [L.] longest; [NA] a general term denoting a long structure, as a muscle.

longitudinal (lon″jĭ-tu′dĭ-nal) [L. longitudo length] lengthwise; parallel to the long axis of the body or an organ.

longitudinalis (lon″jĭ-tu″dĭ-na′lis) [L.] lengthwise; [NA] a term denoting a structure that is parallel to the long axis of the body or an organ.

longitypical (lon″jĭ-tip′ĭ-kal) longilineal; dolichomorphic.

longsightedness (long-sīt′ed-nes) hyperopia.

longus (long′gus) [L.] long; [NA] a general term denoting a long structure, as a muscle.

loop (lōōp) 1. a turn or sharp curve in a cordlike structure; see also ansa. 2. an instrument used in microbiology, consisting of a rod-shaped metal handle holding a firm wire, usually platinum or nichrome, formed into a loop at the free end. The standard loop has an inside diameter of 4 mm. It is used for the inoculation of cultures of bacteria and fungi. **capillary l's**, minute endothelial tubes that carry blood in the papillae of the skin. **cervical l.**, peripheral cuboidal cells of the enamel organ that encircle the edge of a developing tooth. **closed l.**, a system in which the input to one or more of the subsystems is affected by its own output. **gamma l.**, a reflex arc consisting of anterior horn cells, whose gamma fibers to the intrafusal bundle cause the bundle to contract, which excites the afferent impulses passing through the posterior root to the anterior horn cells and causes a stretch reflex. Called also Granit l. **Gerdy's interauricular l.**, a small muscular bundle in the interatrial septum of the heart. **Granit l.**, gamma l. **Henle's l.**, a U-shaped turn in the medullary portion of a renal tubule, with a descending limb from the proximal convoluted tubule and an ascending limb to the distal convoluted tubule; see also kidney. **l. of hypoglossal nerve**, ansa cervicalis. **Hyrtl's l.**, an occasional looplike anastomosis between the right and left hypoglossal nerves in the geniohyoid muscle. **lenticular l.**, ansa lenticularis. **Meyer's l.**, one formed by some of the fibers of the optic radiation as they loop around the inferior horn of the lateral ventricle before turning posteriorly. **open l.**, a system in which an input alters the output, but the output has no effect on the input. Cf. closed l. **peduncular l.**, ansa peduncularis. **l's of spinal nerves**, ansae nervorum spinalium. **Stoerck's l.**, the primitive loop in the embryonic uriniferous tubule which develops into a Henle loop and a portion of the proximal convoluted tubule. **subclavian l.**, ansa subclavia. **ventricular l.**, the early, U-shaped loop of the embryonic heart. **l. of Vieussens**, ansa subclavia.

loopful (lōōp′ful) the quantity of liquid that can be held within the loop of wire used in transferring microorganisms to other culture media.

loosening (lu′sen-ing) in psychiatry, a disorder of thinking in which associations of ideas become so shortened, fragmented, and disturbed as to lack logical relationship; often seen in schizophrenia.

L.O.P. left occipitoposterior (position of the fetus).

loperamide hydrochloride (lo-per′ah-mīd) chemical name: 4-(4-chlorophenyl)-4-hydroxy-N,N-dimethyl-α,α-diphenyl-1-piperidinebutanamide monohydrochloride. An antiperistaltic, $C_{29}H_{33}ClN_2O \cdot HCl$, which exerts a direct effect on the muscles of the intestinal wall; used in the treatment of acute nonspecific diarrhea and chronic diarrhea associated with inflammatory bowel disease and to reduce the volume of discharge from ileostomies. It is administered orally.

loph(o)- [Gr. lophos ridge, tuft] a combining form denoting a relationship to a ridge or to a tuft.

lophodont (lof′o-dont) [lopho- + Gr. odous tooth] having cheek teeth on which the cusps have become connected to form ridges, as in elephants and some rodents.

Lophomonadina (lof″o-mo″nah-di′nah) [lopho- + monad] a suborder of multiflagellated parasitic protozoa (order Hypermastigida, class Zoomastigophorea) found in the gut of termites and cockroaches. Representative genera include Lophomonas and Microjoenia.

Lophomonas (lof″o-mo′nas) a genus of multiflagellated parasitic protozoa (suborder Lophomonadina, order Hypermastigida), found in the cockroach colon, and characterized by the presence of one anterior tuft of flagella.

Lophophora (lo-fof′o-rah) [lopho- + Gr. *phoros* bearing] a genus of Mexican cacti. **L. william′sii**, a species whose flowering heads (mescal buttons) are the source of peyote and mescaline.

lophophorine (lo-fof′o-rin) a poisonous alkaloid, $C_{13}H_{17}NO_3$, from *Lophophora williamsii*, having effects similar to those of mescaline.

lophotrichous (lo-fot′rĭ-kus) [lopho- + Gr. *thrix* hair] having two or more flagella at one or both ends; said of a bacterial cell. See *flagellum*.

Lopid (lo′pid) trademark for a preparation of gemfibrozil.

Lopressor (lo-pres′or) trademark for preparations of metoprolol tartrate.

Lopurin (lo-pūr′in) trademark for preparations of allopurinol.

Lorain's infantilism (disease, type) (lo-rān′) [Paul Joseph *Lorain*, Paris physician, 1827–1875] hypophyseal infantilism.

lorajmine hydrochloride (lor-aj′mēn) chemical name: 17-(chloroacetate)ajmalan-17*ajmalan-17R*,21α-diol monohydrochloride; a cardiac depressant with antiarrhythmic action, $C_{22}H_{27}ClN_2O_3 \cdot HCl$.

lorazepam (lor-ah′zĕ-pam) chemical name: 7-chloro-5-(2-chlorophenyl)-1,3-dihydro-3-hydroxy-2*H*-1,4-benzodiazepin-2-one. A benzodiazepine derivative, $C_{15}H_{10}Cl_2N_2O_2$, occurring as a nearly white powder; used as an antianxiety agent, administered orally.

lorbamate (lor-bah′māt) chemical name: 2-(hydroxymethyl)-2-methylpentyl cyclopropanecarbamate carbamate (ester); a muscle relaxant, $C_{12}H_{22}N_2O_4$.

lorcainide hydrochloride (lor-ka′nĭd) chemical name: *N*-(4-chlorophenyl)-*N*-[1-(1-methylethyl)-4-piperidinyl]benzeneacetamide monohydrochloride; an antiarrhythmic cardiac depressant, $C_{22}H_{27}ClN_2O \cdot HCl$.

lordoscoliosis (lor″do-sko″le-o′sis) [*lordosis* + *scoliosis*] lordosis complicated with scoliosis.

lordosis (lor-do′sis) [Gr. *lordōsis*] the anterior concavity in the curvature of the lumbar and cervical spine as viewed from the side. The term is used to refer to abnormally increased curvature (hollow back, saddle back, swayback) and to the normal curvature (normal lordosis). Cf. *kyphosis* and *scoliosis*.

lordotic (lor-dot′ik) pertaining to or characterized by lordosis.

Lorenz (lor′ents) Konrad Zacharias. Austrian zoologist born 1903; co-winner, with Karl von Frisch and Nikolaas Tinbergen, of the Nobel prize for medicine or physiology for 1973, for his pioneer work in ethology, particularly on imprinting and aggression.

Lorenz's operation, osteotomy (lo′rents-ez) [Adolf *Lorenz*, Austrian surgeon, 1854–1946] see under *operation* and *osteotomy*.

Lorfan (lor′fan) trademark for preparations of levallorphan tartrate.

lorica (lo-ri′kah), pl. *lori′cae* [L. "leather cuirass"] a protective rigid encasement or shell, secreted or created by cementing together of various materials, as seen in some invertebrates such as certain protozoa and many rotifers.

loricate (lor′ĭ-kāt) enclosed in a lorica.

Loridine (lor′ĭ-dēn) trademark for a preparation of cephaloridine.

Lossen's rule (law) (los′enz) [Herman Friedrich *Lossen*, Heidelberg surgeon, 1842–1909] see under *rule*.

L.O.T. left occipitotransverse (position of the fetus).

Lot. abbreviation for L. *lo′tio*, lotion.

lotio (lo′she-o) [L., from *lotus*, past participle of *lavare* to wash] lotion. **l. adstrin′gens**, a mixture of sulfuric acid, alcohol, and oil of turpentine. **l. al′ba, l. sulfura′ta**, white lotion.

Lotioblanc (lo″she-o-blangk′) trademark for a preparation of white lotion.

lotion (lo′shun) [L. *lotio*] a liquid suspension or dispersion for external application to the body. **Abercrombie's l.** (*obs.*), an infusion of tobacco. **amphotericin B l.** [USP], a lotion containing 90 to 125 per cent of the labeled amount of amphotericin B and conforming to FDA regulations for antibiotics; used as a topical antifungal. **benzyl benzoate l.** [USP], a watery solution of benzyl benzoate, triethanolamine, and oleic acid; used as a topical scabicide. **benzyl benzoate-chlorophenothane-benzocaine l.**, a watery solution of benzyl benzoate, chlorophenothane, benzocaine, and polysorbate 80; used as a scabicide and pediculicide, applied topically. **betamethasone dipropionate l.** [USP], a lotion containing 90 to 110 per cent of the labeled amount of betamethasone; used as a topical glucocorticoid. **betamethasone valerate l.** [USP], a preparation containing betamethasone valerate equivalent to 95 to 115 per cent of the labeled amount of betamethasone; used as an anti-inflammatory glucocorticoid. **calamine l.** [USP], a preparation of calamine with zinc oxide, glycerin, bentonite magma, and calcium hydroxide solution, used topically as a protectant. **calamine l., phenolated** [USP], a mixture of calamine lotion and liquefied phenol, used topically as a protectant. **dimethisoquin hydrochloride l.** [USP], a preparation containing 90 to 115 per cent of the labeled amount of dimethisoquin hydrochloride; used as a local anesthetic to relieve pain, itching, and burning of the skin. **flurandrenolide l.** [USP], a lotion containing 90 to 110 per cent of the labeled amount of flurandrenolide; used as a topical glucocorticoid. **gamma benzene hexachloride l.**, lindane l. **Goulard's l.**, diluted lead subacetate solution. **hydrocortisone l.** [USP], a preparation containing 90 to 110 per cent of the labeled amount hydroxycortisone; used as a topical anti-inflammatory in steroid-responsive dermatoses. **lindane l.** [USP], a preparation containing 90 to 110 per cent of the labeled amount of gamma benzene hexachloride in a suitable aqueous vehicle; used as a pediculicide and scabicide, applied topically to the skin. Called also *gamma benzene hexachloride l.* **methylbenzethonium chloride l.** [USP], an emulsion containing 0.067 per cent methylbenzethonium chloride; used as a local anti-infective, applied topically to the genitalia, rectum, thighs, and intertriginous areas in the treatment of ammonia dermatitis and in the treatment and prevention of dermatoses caused by contact with urine, feces, and perspiration. **nystatin l.** [USP], a lotion containing 90 to 140 per cent of the labeled amount of nystatin and conforming to FDA regulations for antibiotics; used as a topical antifungal. **selenium sulfide l.** [USP], an aqueous, stabilized suspension containing 90 to 110 per cent of the labeled amount of selenium sulfide; used as a topical antifungal in the treatment of tinea versicolor, as a topical keratolytic, and applied to the scalp to control seborrheic dermatitis and dandruff. **white l.** [USP], a preparation of zinc sulfate, sulfurated potash, and purified water, used as a topical astringent and protectant; called also *lotio alba*.

Lotrimin (lo-trim′in) trademark for preparation of clotrimazole.

Lotusate (lo′tŭ-sāt) trademark for a preparation of talbutal.

Louis's angle, law (loo-ēz′) [Pierre Charles Alexandre *Louis*, French physician, 1787–1872; the founder of medical statistics] see *angulus sterni*, and see under *law*.

loupe (lōōp) [Fr. "magnifying glass"] a convex lens for low magnification of minute objects at very close range; it may be monocular or binocular, held in the hand, set in a headband, or mounted on spectacles.

louse (lows), pl. *lice* [L. *pediculus*] a general name for various parasitic insects; the true lice, which infest mammals, belong to the order Anoplura. Species parasitic upon man are *Pediculus humanus capitis*, the head louse; *P. humanus corporis*, the body or clothes louse; and *Phthirus pubis*, the crab louse, which lives in the hair upon the pubes and other hairy areas of the body, such as the eyelashes, eyebrows, and axillae. The causal organisms of typhus, relapsing fever, trench fever, and possibly plague are transmitted by the bite of lice. **biting l.**, Mallophaga. **body l.**, *Pediculus humanus corporis*. **chicken l.**, *Dermanyssus gallinae*. **clothes l.**, *Pediculus humanus corporis*. **crab l.**, *Phthirus pubis*. **goat l.**, *Linognathus stenopis*. **head l.**, *Pediculus humanus capitis*. **horse l.**, *Trichodectes pilosus*. **pubic l.**, *Phthirus pubis*. **sucking l.**, Anoplura.

lousicide (lows′ĭ-sīd) pediculicide.

Löwe's ring (la′vez) [Karl Friedrich *Löwe*, German optician, 1874–1955] see under *ring*.

Lowe's syndrome (disease) (lōz) [Charles Upton *Lowe*, American pediatrician, born 1921] oculocerebrorenal syndrome.

Löwenberg's canal, forceps, scala (la'ven-bergz) [Benjamin Benno *Löwenberg*, otologist in Vienna and Paris, 1836–1905] see under *canal* and *forceps*, and see *ductus cochlearis*.

Löwenthal's tract (la'ven-talz) [Wilhelm *Löwenthal*, German physician, 1850–1894] see under *tractus tectospinalis*.

lowering (low'er-ing) a decrease. **vapor pressure l.,** the decrease of the vapor pressure of a solution below that of the pure solvent; the percentage change in vapor pressure is equal to the mole fraction of the solute (osmoles of solute per osmoles of solute plus solvent) and is proportional to the osmolality.

Lower's rings, tubercle (lo'erz) [Richard *Lower*, English anatomist, 1631–1691] see *annuli fibrosi cordis* and *tuberculum intervenosum*.

Löwitt's bodies, lymphocytes (la'vits) [Moritz *Löwitt*, German physician, 1851–1918] lymphogonia.

Lowman balance board (lo'man) [Charles LeRoy *Lowman*, American orthopedic surgeon, born 1879] an isosceles triangle board on which the patient walks with feet in supination; for correction of flatfeet.

Lown-Ganong-Levine syndrome (lown gan'ong lě-vīn') [Bernard *Lown*, American cardiologist, born 1921; William F. *Ganong*, American physiologist, born 1924; Samuel A. *Levine*, American cardiologist, 1891–1966] see under *syndrome*.

Louis-Bar syndrome (loo-e' bahr) [Denise *Louis-Bar*, Belgian neuropathologist, 20th century] see *ataxia-telangiectasia*, under *ataxia*.

loxapine (loks'ah-pēn) chemical name: 2-chloro-11-(4-methyl-1-piperazinyl)dibenz[*b,f*][1,4]oxazepine; a tricyclic antipsychotic agent, $C_{18}H_{18}ClN_3O$. **l. succinate,** the succinate salt of loxapine, $C_{18}H_{18}ClN_3O\cdot C_4H_6O_4$, used in the treatment of schizophrenia, administered orally.

loxarthron (loks-ar'thron) [Gr. *loxos* oblique + *arthron* joint] an oblique deformity of a joint without luxation.

loxarthrosis (loks"ar-thro'sis) loxarthron.

loxia (lok'se-ah) torticollis.

Loxitane (loks'ĭ-tān) trademark for preparations of loxapine succinate.

Loxosceles (loks-os'sě-lēz) a genus of six-eyed spiders of the family Loxoscelidae. **L. lae'ta,** the brown spider, which is the causative agent of loxoscelism in Central South America. **L. reclu'sa,** the brown recluse spider, which causes loxoscelism in North America.

Loxoscelidae (loks"os-sel'ĭ-de) a family of spiders (suborder Labidognatha), the false hackled band spinners, which includes the genus Loxosceles.

loxoscelism (lok-sos'sě-lizm) a morbid condition resulting from the bite of the brown spider, *Loxosceles laeta*, or the (brown) recluse spider, *L. reclusa*, beginning with a painful erythematous vesicle and progressing to a gangrenous slough of the affected area; first recognized in South America, a few cases have been diagnosed in North America. **viscerocutaneous l.,** a sometimes fatal condition resulting from the bite of the brown spider, with fever and hematuria occurring, in addition to the local reaction.

loxotomy (lok-sot'o-me) [Gr. *loxos* oblique + *temnein* to cut] oval amputation.

Loxotrema ovatum (lok"so-tre'mah o-va'tum) *Metagonimus yokogawai*.

lozenge (loz'enj) [Fr.] 1. a medicated tablet or disk; a troche. 2. a triangular area of tissue marked for excision in plastic surgery.

L.P.N. licensed practical nurse.

LPS lipopolysaccharide (def. 2).

LRF luteinizing hormone releasing factor; see under *factor*.

L.S.A. left sacroanterior (position of the fetus); Licentiate of Society of Apothecaries.

L.Sc.A. left scapuloanterior (position of the fetus).

L.Sc.P. left scapuloposterior (position of the fetus).

LSD lysergic acid diethylamide.

L.S.P. left sacroposterior (position of the fetus).

L.S.T. left sacrotransverse (position of the fetus).

LT lymphotoxin.

LTB₄, LTC₄, etc. symbols for various leukotrienes; see *leukotriene*.

LTF lymphocyte transforming factor.

LTH luteotropic hormone; see *luteotropin*.

Lu chemical symbol for *lutetium*.

Lubarsch's crystals (loo'barsh-ez) [Otto *Lubarsch*, German pathologist, 1860–1933] see under *crystal*.

lubb (lub) a syllable used to represent, or mimic, the first sound of the heart in auscultation. See *lubb-dupp*.

lubb-dupp (lub-dup') syllables used to represent the combination of the first and second heart sounds. See *lubb* and *dupp*.

Luc's operation (luks) [Henri *Luc*, French laryngologist, 1855–1925] Caldwell-Luc operation.

lucanthone hydrochloride (loo-kan'thōn) chemical name: 1-[[2-(diethylamino)ethyl]amino]-4-methyl-9*H*-thioxanthen-9-one monohydrochloride. An antischistosomal, $C_{20}H_{24}N_2OS\cdot HCl$, occurring as a yellowish orange powder; administered orally.

Lucas' sign (loo'kas) [Richard Clement *Lucas*, English physician, 1846–1915] see under *sign*.

Luciani's triad (loo"che-an'ēz) [Luigi *Luciani*, Italian physiologist, 1842–1919] see under *triad*.

Lucibacterium (loo"sĭ-bak-te're-um) [L. *lux* light + *bacterium*] a genus formerly comprising the vibrios, now assigned to the species *Vibrio harveyi.*

lucid (loo'sid) [L. *lucidus* clear] clear; not obscure; as, *lucid interval.*

lucidification (loo-sid"ĭ-fi-ka'shun) [L. *lucidus* clear + *facere* to make] the clearing up of the protoplasm of cells.

lucidity (loo-sid'ĭ-te) the quality or state of having a clear mind; clearness of the mind.

luciferase (loo-sif'er-ās) [EC 1.13.12.5-8, 1.14.14.3, 1.14.99.21] any one of several enzymes that catalyze the bioluminescent reaction in certain marine crustaceans, fish, bacteria, and insects. The enzyme is a flavoprotein; it oxidizes luciferin to an electronically excited compound that emits energy in the form of light. The color of light emitted varies with the organism. The firefly enzyme is a valuable reagent for measurement of ATP concentration.

luciferin (loo-sif'er-in) a heterocyclic phenol which can be reduced and oxidized. It exists in many forms and is present in certain animals capable of bioluminescence; when acted upon by luciferase, in the presence of ATP and molecular oxygen, it produces light.

lucifugal (loo-sif'u-gal) [L. *lux* light + *fugere* to flee from] avoiding, or being repelled by, bright light.

Lucilia (loo-sil'e-ah) the greenbottle flies, a genus of the family Calliphoridae that have a blue or green metallic iridescence. **L. cupri'na,** *Phaenicia cuprina*. **L. illus'tris,** a species which usually deposits its eggs in carcasses, but is sometimes found in the wool of sheep. **L. regi'na,** *Phormia regina*. **L. serica'ta,** *Phaenicia sericata.*

Lucio leprosy, phenomenon (loo'sho) [R. *Lucio*, Mexican physician, 1810–1866] see under *leprosy* and *phenomenon.*

lucipetal (loo-sip'ĭ-tal) [L. *lux* light + *petere* to seek] seeking, or being attracted to, bright light.

lucium (loo'se-um) a supposed chemical element discovered in 1896, later found to be a mixture of rare earth metals.

Lücke's test (lik'ez) [George Albert *Lücke*, German surgeon, 1829–1894] see under *tests.*

lückenschädel (lik'en-sha"del) [Ger.] a condition marked by defective calcification of the skull bones, combined with meningocele or encephalocele.

lucotherapy (loo"ko-ther'ah-pe) [L. *lux* light + *therapy*] the treatment of disease by rays of light.

Ludloff's sign (lood'lawfs) [Karl *Ludloff*, surgeon in Breslau, 1864–1945] see under *sign.*

Ludwig's angina (lood'vigz) [Wilhelm Friedrich von *Ludwig*, German surgeon, 1790–1865] see under *angina.*

Ludwig's angle (lood'vigz) [Daniel *Ludwig*, German anatomist, 1625–1680] angulus sterni.

Ludwig's ganglion, theory (lood'vigz) [Karl Friedrich Wilhelm *Ludwig*, eminent German physiologist, 1816–1895, one of the greatest teachers of physiology of all time] see under *ganglion* and *theory.*

Luer's syringe (loo′erz) [German instrument maker in Paris, died 1883] see under *syringe.*

lues (loo′ēz) [L. "a plague"] syphilis.

luetic (loo-et′ik) syphilitic.

luetin (loo′ĕ-tin) an extract of a killed culture of several strains of *Treponema pallidum,* formerly used in the skin test for syphilis.

luette (loo-et′) [Fr.] uvula. **Lieutaud's l.,** uvula vesicae.

lug (lug) 1. a projecting part that holds or supports something. 2. the part of a dental casting that projects. **retention l.,** a piece of metal soldered either to an orthodontic band or to an artificial crown to create greater undercut for retention of a dental prosthesis.

Lugol's caustic, solution (loo-golz′) [Jean Guillaume Auguste *Lugol,* physician in Paris, 1786–1851] see under *caustic,* and see *iodine solution, strong,* under *solution.*

L.U.L. left upper lobe (of lungs).

lumbago (lum-ba′go) [L. *lumbus* loin] pain in the lumbar region. **ischemic l.,** pain in the lower back and buttock(s) due to vascular insufficiency, as in terminal aortic occlusion.

lumbar (lum′bar) pertaining to the loins, the part of the back between the thorax and the pelvis.

lumbarization (lum″ber-i-za′shun) a condition in which the first segment of the sacrum is not fused with the second, so that there is one additional articulated vertebra and the sacrum consists of only four segments.

lumbo- [L. *lumbus*] a combining form denoting relationship to the loins.

lumboabdominal (lum″bo-ab-dom′ĭ-nal) pertaining to the loins and abdomen.

lumbocolostomy (lum″bo-ko-los′to-me) [L. *lumbus* loin + *colostomy*] the operation of forming a permanent opening into the colon by an incision through the lumbar region.

lumbocolotomy (lum″bo-ko-lot′o-me) [L. *lumbus* loin + *colotomy*] an incision into the colon through the loin.

lumbocostal (lum″bo-kos′tal) pertaining to the loin and ribs.

lumbocrural (lum″bo-kroo′ral) pertaining to, affecting or extending between the lumbar and crural regions.

lumbodorsal (lum″bo-dor′sal) pertaining to the lumbar and thoracic (formerly called dorsal) regions.

lumbodynia (lum″bo-din′e-ah) [L. *lumbus* loin + Gr. *odynē* pain] lumbago.

lumboiliac (lum″bo-il′e-ak) pertaining to the loin and ilium.

lumboinguinal (lum″bo-ing′gwĭ-nal) pertaining to the loins and the groin.

lumbosacral (lum″bo-sa′kral) pertaining to the loins and sacrum.

lumbrical (lum′brĭ-kal) 1. lumbricoid. 2. a muscle of the hand; see *musculi lumbricales.*

lumbrici (lum-bri′si) [L.] plural of *lumbricus.*

lumbricide (lum′brĭ-sīd) [*lumbricus* + L. *caedere* to kill] an agent that destroys lumbrici (ascarides).

lumbricoid (lum′brĭ-koid) [*lumbricus* + Gr. *eidos* form] 1. pertaining to or resembling the earthworm, especially *Ascaris lymbricoides;* lumbrical. 2. *Ascaris lumbricoides.*

lumbricosis (lum″brĭ-ko′sis) the condition of being infected with lumbrici (ascarides).

Lumbricus (lum-bri′kus) [L. "earthworm"] a genus of annelids, including the earthworm, *L. terres′tris,* which may act as the host of *Metastrongylus elongatus,* the intermediate host of the virus causing swine influenza.

lumbricus (lum-bri′kus), pl. *lumbri′ci* [L.] 1. the ascaris. 2. an earthworm.

lumbus (lum′bus) [L.] [NA] the part of the back between the thorax and the pelvis; called also *loin.*

lumen (loo′men), pl. *lu′mina* [L. "light"] 1. the cavity or channel within a tube or tubular organ. 2. the unit of light flux: it is the flux emitted in a unit solid angle by a uniform point source of one candela. **residual l.,** the remains of Rathke's pouch located between the pars distalis and pars intermedia of the pituitary gland.

lumichrome (loo′mĭ-krōm) chemical name: 7,8-dimethylalloxazine. A product, $C_{12}H_{10}N_4O_2$, of the irradiation decomposition of riboflavin.

lumiflavin (loo″mĭ-fla′vin) chemical name: 7,8,10-trimethylisoalloxazine. A product, $C_{13}H_{12}N_4O_2$, of the luminiferous decomposition of riboflavin.

lumina (loo′min-ah) [L.] plural of *lumen.*

Luminal (loo′mĭ-nal) trademark for preparations of phenobarbital.

luminal (loo′mĭ-nal) pertaining to the lumen of a tubular structure.

luminescence (loo″mĭ-nes′ens) the property of giving off light without showing a corresponding degree of heat.

luminiferous (loo″mĭ-nif′er-us) [L. *lumen* light + *ferre* to bear] conveying light or propagating those vibrations which constitute light.

luminophore (loo′mĭ-no-fōr″) [L. *lumen* light + Gr. *phoros* bearing] a chemical group that gives the property of luminescence to organic compounds.

luminous (loo′mĭ-nus) emitting or reflecting light; glowing with light.

lumirhodopsin (loo″mĭ-ro-dop′sin) a partially split combination of all-*trans* retinal and scotopsin, occurring as rhodopsin if exposed to light.

lumpectomy (lum-pek′to-me) 1. surgical excision of only the palpable lesion in carcinoma of the breast; called also *tylectomy.* 2. surgical removal of a mass.

lumps (lumps) hypopteronosis cystica.

Lumsden's center (lumz′denz) [Thomas William *Lumsden,* British physician, 1874–1953] pneumotaxic center.

lunacy (loo′nah-se) [L. *luna* moon] (*obs.*) insanity; so named because it was supposed to be sometimes due to or affected by the influence of the moon.

lunar (loo′nar) [L. *lunaris; luna* moon, also silver] 1. pertaining to the moon. 2. pertaining to or containing silver, as lunar caustic (silver nitrate).

lunare (loo-na′re) the lunate bone (os lunatum [NA]).

lunate (loo′nāt) [L. *luna* moon] moon-shaped, or crescentic; see *os lunatum.*

lunatic (loo′nah-tik) [L. *lunaticus;* from *luna* moon] (*obs.*) a mentally deranged person.

lunatomalacia (loo-na″to-mah-la′she-ah) osteochondrosis of the semilunar (carpal lunate) bone; see *Kienböck's disease* (def. 1), under *disease.*

lung (lung) [L. *pulmo;* Gr. *pneumōn* or *pleumōn*] the organ of respiration. Either of the pair of organs, right (*pulmo dexter* [NA]) or left (*pulmo sinister* [NA]), that effect the aeration of the blood. The lungs occupy the lateral cavities of the chest, separated from each other by the heart and mediastinal structures. The right lung is composed of superior, middle, and inferior lobes, and the left, of superior and inferior lobes. Each lobe is subdivided into two to five bronchopulmonary segments which are separated by connective tissue septa. Pulmonary disorders may be confined to, or localized in, one or more of these segments. (See under *bronchi lobares, bronchi segmenta,* and *segmenta bronchopulmonalia.*) Each lung consists of an external serous coat (the visceral layer of the pleura), subserous areolar tissue, and lung parenchyma. The latter is made up of lobules, which are bound together by connective tissue. A primary lobule consists of a terminal bronchiole, respiratory bronchioles, and alveolar ducts, which communicate with many alveoli, each alveolus being surrounded by a network of capillary blood vessels. It is between the alveoli and capillaries that gas exchange takes place. See accompanying plates. **arc-welder l.,** siderosis (def. 1). **artificial l.,** oxygenator. **bird-breeder's l.,** pigeon-breeder's l. **black l.,** pneumoconiosis of coal workers. **book l., book-l.,** a lunglike invagination that functions as a gas exchange organ, found on the underside of the abdomen of many arachnids, which opens to the surface by means of a spiracle and contains numerous thin membranous lamellae arranged like book leaves. **brown l.,** byssinosis. **cardiac l.,** chronic congestion of the lung due to mitral stenosis or left ventricular failure; microscopic examination shows evidence of recurring edema, heart failure cells, and vascular changes. **coalminer's l.,** pneumoconiosis of coal workers. **drowned l.,** airless lung, the air passages being filled with exudate. The volume occupied by a drained lung (or lobe) is usually greater than normal, whereas in atelectasis it is less than normal. **eosinophilic l.,** tropical eosinophilia. **farmer's l.,** a pathological condition caused by inhalation of moldy hay

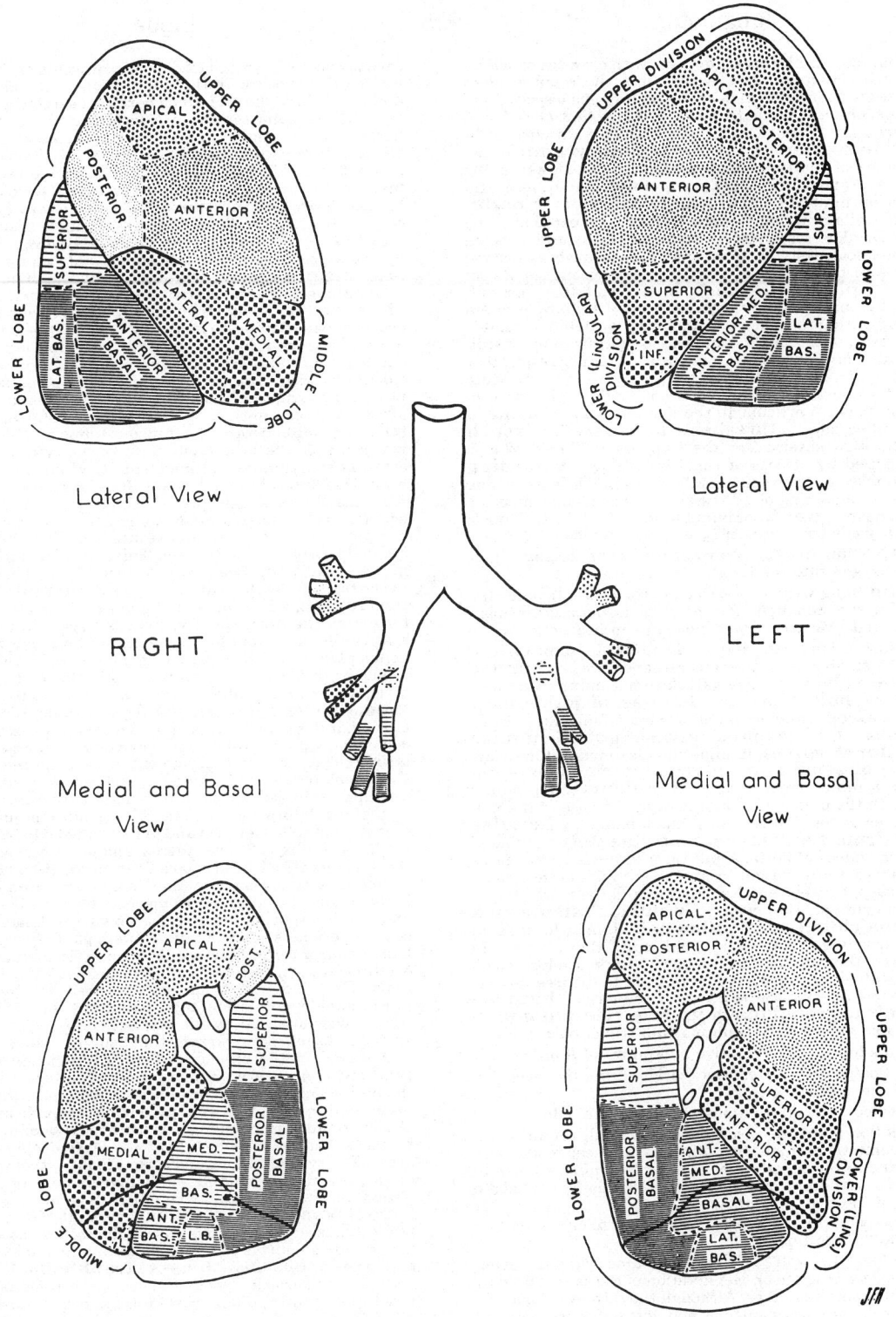

Lateral View

Lateral View

RIGHT

LEFT

Medial and Basal
View

Medial and Basal
View

PLATE 24 —PULMONARY SEGMENTS

Tracheobronchial branching correlated with subdivision of the lungs. Each bronchus is marked the same as the
segment it branches out to supply. The terminology is that suggested by Jackson and Huber.

957

dust, characterized by breathlessness with cyanosis or with a dry cough, anorexia, and weight loss. It is most often associated with inhalation of spores of *Micromonospora faeni* or *Thermoactinomyces vulgaris.* Called also *thresher's l.* and *harvester's l.* **fibroid l.,** a lung affected with chronic fibrosis. **harvester's l.,** farmer's l. **honeycomb l.,** the appearance of multiple small radiolucent shadows on the lung x-ray, representing dilatations of the smaller, less rigid airways or multiple small cysts or cavities. **hyperlucent l.,** unilateral emphysema. **iron l.,** a popular name for the Drinker respirator. **masons' l.,** a lung affected with pneumoconiosis due to the inhalation of dusts associated with this occupation. **miners' l.,** pneumoconiosis of coal workers. **pigeon-breeder's l.,** a respiratory disorder caused by an acquired hypersensitivity to bird excreta following intimate contact with birds; symptoms include chills, fever, and cough. Pulmonary fibrosis may result. Called also *bird-breeder's l.* **shock l.,** adult respiratory distress syndrome. **silo-filler's l.,** a rare form of acute bronchitis affecting individuals who inhale high levels of nitrogen oxides, particularly the dioxide, while working in freshly filled silos. **thresher's l.,** farmer's l. **trench l.,** a condition observed in the trenches in World War I, characterized by attacks of rapid breathing. **vanishing l.,** in emphysema, conversion of the lungs into a delicate, fine network of remaining blood vessels among which no alveolar walls survive. **wet l.,** accumulation of fluid in the lungs; pulmonary edema. **white l.,** pneumonia alba.

lungmotor (lung′mo-tor) an apparatus for forcing air or air and oxygen into the lungs.

lungworm (lung′werm) a parasitic worm that invades the lungs, e.g., the trematode *Paragonimus westermani* in man, the nematode *Metastrongylus elongatus* in hogs, etc.

lunula (loo′nu-lah), gen. and pl. *lu′nulae* [L., dim. of *luna* moon] a small crescent or moon-shaped area. **lunulae of aortic valves,** lunulae valvularum semilunarium aortae. **l. of nail,** l. unguis. **lunulae of pulmonary trunk valves,** lunulae valvularum semilunarium trunci pulmonalis. **l. of scapula,** incisura scapulae. **lunulae of semilunar valves,** lunulae valvularum semilunarium. **lunulae of semilunar valves of aorta,** lunulae valvularum semilunarium aortae. **l. un′guis** [NA], lunula of the nail: the crescentic white area at the base of the nail on a finger or toe. Called also *selene unguium.* **lu′nulae valvula′rum semilunarium aor′tae** [NA], lunulae of semilunar valves of aorta: small thinned areas in the cusps of the valve of the aorta, one located on each side of the nodule of each cusp, between the free margin and the most peripheral segment of the cusp. **lu′nulae valvula′rum semiluna′rium trunci pulmonalis** [NA], lunulae of semilunar valves of pulmonary trunk: small thinned areas in the cusps of the valve of the pulmonary trunk, one located on each side of the nodule of each cusp, close to the free margin and the most peripheral segment of the cusp. **lu′nulae valvula′rum semiluna′rium arte′riae pulmona′lis,** lunulae valvularum semilunarium trunci pulmonalis.

lunulae (loo′nu-le) [L.] genitive and plural of *lunula.*

lupeose (loo′pe-ōs) a tetrasaccharide from the seeds of herbs of the genus *Lupinus.*

lupiform (loo′pĭ-form) [L. *lupus* + *forma* form] lupoid.

lupinosis (loo″pĭno′sis) a morbid, often fatal, condition affecting domestic animals, including cattle, sheep, goats, and horses, due to the ingestion of seeds of leguminous herbs of the genus *Lupinus,* and characterized chiefly by acute atrophy of the liver. Cf. *lathyrism.*

lupoid (loo′poid) [*lupus* + -*oid*] pertaining to or resembling lupus. Called also *lupiform.*

lupus (loo′pus) [L. "wolf" or "pike"] a name originally given to localized destruction or degeneration of the skin caused by various cutaneous diseases. Although the term was formerly used to designate lupus vulgaris and now lupus erythematosus, without a modifier it has no specific meaning. **chilblain l.,** chilblain l. erythematosus. **drug-induced l.,** see *systemic l. erythematosus.* **l. erythemato′sus, (LE),** a group of connective tissue disorders primarily affecting women aged 20 to 40 years, comprising a spectrum of clinical forms in which cutaneous disease may occur with or without systemic involvement. See *cutaneous l. erythematosus* and *systemic l. erythematosus.* **l. erythematosus, chilblain,** a chronic unremitting form of lupus erythematosus, usually involving the fingertips, nose, face, ears, hands,

calves, and heels, and caused by microvascular injury secondary to cold exposure. Initially the lesions resemble chilblains and may mimic those of lupus pernio in sarcoidosis, but they eventually assume the appearance of discoid lupus erythematosus. Called also *chilblain l.* and *l. pernio.* **l. erythemato′sus, cutaneous,** a form of lupus erythematosus in which the skin may be the only organ involved, or it may precede the involvement of other systems. One classification divides the disorder into three clinically distinct types: In the *chronic type,* the basic lesion is discoid in configuration (see *discoid l. erythematosus*). The *subacute type* is characterized by widespread symmetrical, superficial, and nonscarring lesions that may leave self-limited hypopigmentation and telangiectases after resolution (see *systemic l. erythematosus*). The *acute type* is characterized by the development of an acute, edematous, erythematous eruption, presenting either as a malar rash in a "butterfly" distribution, or as an extensive morbilliform eruption that frequently occurs coincidentally with systemic exacerations or sometimes as the presenting symptom of systemic lupus erythematosus, often after sun exposure. **l. erythemato′sus, discoid (DLE),** a chronic form of cutaneous lupus erythematosus in which the skin lesions mimic those of the systemic form but systemic signs are rare, although multisystem manifestations may develop after many years. It is characterized by the presence of discoid skin plaques showing varying degrees of edema, erythema, scaliness, follicular plugging, and skin atrophy surrounded by an elevated erythematous border typically involving the face and scalp, but widespread dissemination may occur. See also *l. erythematosus profundus* and *hypertrophic l. erythematosus.* **l. erythemato′sus, hypertrophic,** a form of discoid lupus erythematosus characterized by the presence of verrucous hyperkeratotic lesions that can be mistaken for keratoacanthoma or hypertrophic lichen planus, which may occur in association with cutaneous lesions with features clinically and histologically suggestive of lichen planus. Called also *l. hypertrophicus.* **l. erythemato′sus, systemic (SLE),** a chronic, remitting, relapsing, inflammatory, and often febrile multisystemic disorder of connective tissue, acute or insidious in onset, characterized principally by involvement of the skin (see *cutaneous l. erythematosus*), joints, kidneys, and serosal membranes. It is of unknown etiology, but it is thought to represent a failure of the regulatory mechanisms of the autoimmune system that sustain self-tolerance and prevent the body from attacking its own cells, cell constituents, and proteins, suggested by the high level of a wide variety of autoantibodies against nuclear and cytoplasmic cellular components seen in affected individuals. The disorder is marked by a wide variety of abnormalities, including arthritis and arthralgias, nephritis, central nervous system manifestations, pleurisy, pericarditis, leukopenia or thrombocytopenia, hemolytic anemia, elevated erythrocyte sedimentation rate, and positive LE-cell preparations. Drug-induced lupus, caused, e.g., by hydralazine, procainamide, esoniazide, D-penicillamine, and chlorpromazine, is characterized by the production of a systemic lupus erythematosus–like syndrome that usually resolves following withdrawal of the offending drug. **l. erythemato′sus profun′dus,** a rare chronic form of cutaneous lupus erythematosus characterized by deep dermal and subcutaneous inflammatory involvement, producing deep, firm nodules, often without surface change, on the head, upper arms, chest, buttocks, and thighs, which heal and leave deeply depressed areas. The typical lesions of discoid lupus erythematosus are often present, and mild systemic involvement often occurs. Called also *LE* or *lupus panniculitis* and *l. profundus.* **l. erythemato′sus tu′midus,** a variant of discoid or systemic lupus erythematosus in which the lesions consist of raised reddish purple or brown plaques, which may resemble erysipelas or cellulitis. **l. hypertroph′icus,** 1. a variant of lupus vulgaris in which the lesions consist of a warty vegetative growth, often crusted or slightly exudative, usually occurring on moist areas near body orifices. 2. hypertrophic l. erythematosus. **l. milia′ris dissemina′tus fa′ciei,** a papular eruption involving the central part of the face of adults that heals spontaneously with scarring. It has been variously considered to be a tuberculid, as a variant of granulomatous rosacea, and as a papular eruption of unknown etiology. **neonatal l.,** a condition that sometimes affects infants born to mothers with systemic lupus erythematosus, characterized most commonly by a rash similar to that seen in discoid lupus and by transiently elevated levels of antinuclear antibodies and LE cells, less commonly by hematologic abnormalities, hepatosplenomegaly, and pericarditis. It is usually benign and self-limited, but the discoid skin lesions may rarely persist. Called also *transient neonatal systemic l. erythematosus.* **l. nephritis,** see under *nephritis.* **l. per′nio,** 1. a cutaneous manifestation of sarcoidosis consisting of violaceous, smooth, shiny plaques on the ears, forehead, nose, fingers, and toes, which is frequently associated with bone cysts. 2. chilblain lupus erythematosus. **l. profun′dus,** l. erythematosus profundus. **transient neonatal systemic l. erythematosus,** neonatal l. **l. tu′midus,** a variant of lupus vulgaris in which the lesions consist of localized, soft edematous patches somewhat resembling keloids. **l. vulga′ris,** the most common, severe, and variable, but rare, form of tuberculosis of the skin, most often involving the face, especially the nasal, buccal, and conjunctival mucosa, predominantly in women. It is typically manifested by the development, usually in normal-appearing skin, of a reddish brown plaque with deeply embedded peripheral nodules, which on diascopic examination have a yellow-brown ("apple-jelly") color, characterized by peripheral extensive and central atrophy and progressive destruction of cartilage in involved sites, and resulting in disfiguring scars, keloids, lymphedema, and functional impairment from contractures. The lesions may also present in other morphological forms, e.g., see *l. hypertrophicus* (def. 1) and *l. tumidus.*

Luria (loor′ĭ-ah), Salvador Edward. Italian-born American biologist, born 1912; co-winner, with Max Delbrück and Alfred Day Hershey, of the Nobel prize for medicine or physiology in 1969 for research on the mechanisms and materials of inheritance of viruses.

Luride (loo′rīd) trademark for a preparation of sodium fluoride.

Luschka's crypts, etc. (lush′kahz) [Hubert von *Luschka,* celebrated German anatomist, 1820–1875] see under *bursa, crypt, duct, gland, muscle,* etc.

luteal (loo′te-al) pertaining to or having the properties of the corpus luteum or its active principle.

lutecium (loo-te′she-um) lutetium.

luteectomy (loo″te-ek′to-me) excision of the corpus luteum.

lutein (loo′te-in) [L. *luteus* yellow] 1. a yellow pigment, or lipochrome, $C_{48}H_{56}O_2$, from the corpus luteum, from fat cells, and from the yolk of eggs. It is closely related to xanthophyll. 2. any lipochrome. **serum l.,** a lipochrome found in blood serum.

luteinic (loo″te-in′ik) 1. pertaining to lutein or to the corpus luteum. 2. pertaining to luteinization.

luteinization (loo″te-in″ĭ-za′shun) the process by which a postovulatory ovarian follicle transforms into a corpus luteum through vascularization, follicular cell hypertrophy, and lipid accumulation, the latter in some species giving the yellow color indicated by the term.

Lutembacher's syndrome (complex, disease) (loo′tem-bak″erz) [René *Lutembacher,* French cardiologist, 1884–1916] see under *syndrome.*

luteohormone (loo″te-o-hor′mōn) progesterone.

luteolysin (loo″te-ol′ĭ-sin) a substance that causes degeneration of corpus luteum. **uterine l.,** prostaglandin F₂α.

luteolysis (loo″te-ol′ĭ-sis) degeneration of corpus luteum.

luteoma (loo″te-o′mah) 1. a granulosa-theca cell tumor in which there has been luteinization of the cells. 2. nodular hyperplasia of ovarian lutein cells sometimes occurring in the last trimester of pregnancy; it may be unilateral or bilateral. Called also *l. of pregnancy* or *pregnancy l.*

luteose (loo″te-ōs) a neutral polysaccharide present in luteic acid.

luteotroph (loo′te-o-trōf) mammotroph.

luteotrophic (loo″te-o-trof′ik) luteotropic.

luteotrophin (loo″te-o-tro′fin) luteotropin.

luteotropic (loo″te-o-trop′ik) stimulating the formation of the corpus luteum; see *luteotropin.*

luteotropin (loo″te-o-tro′pin) a hormone of the anterior pituitary gland which stimulates formation of the corpus luteum in some mammalian species but not man; identical with prolactin. Called also *luteotropic hormone.*

lutetium (loo-te′she-um) the chemical element, atomic number 71, atomic weight 174.97, symbol Lu.

Lutrexin (loo-trek′sin) trademark for a preparation of lututrin.

Lutromone (loo′tro-mōn) trademark for a preparation of progesterone.

lututrin (loo′tu-trin) a protein or polypeptide substance obtained from the corpus luteum of sow ovaries by a process of salting out followed by dialysis; used as a uterine relaxant in treatment of functional dysmenorrhea.

Lutzomyia (loōt″zo-mi′ah) a genus of sandflies of the family Psychodidae, the females of which suck blood. **L. flaviscutella′ta,** the vector of *Leishmania mexicana amazonensis,* the etiologic agent of cutaneous leishmaniasis in Brazil. **L. longipal′pis,** a species believed to transmit kala-azar in South America. **L. nogu′chu,** *Phlebotomus noguchii.* **L. olme′ca,** the vector of *Leishmania mexicana mexicana,* the etiologic agent of chiclero ulcer. **L. peruen′sis,** a probable vector of *Leishmania peruviana,* the etiologic agent of uta. **L. trap′idoi,** a vector of *Leishmania braziliensis panamensis,* the etiologic agent of the New World form of cutaneous leishmaniasis. **L. verruca′rum,** a probable vector of *Leishmania peruviana,* the etiologic agent of uta. **L. umbrati′lis,** the major vector of *Leishmania braziliensis guyanensis,* the etiologic agent of pian bois (forest yaws).

lux (luks) [L. "light"] in SI, the metric unit of illumination, being one lumen per square meter; called also *meter candle.* Cf. *foot-candle.*

luxatio (luk-sa′she-o) [L.] dislocation. **l. cox′ae congen′ita,** congenital dislocation of the hip. **l. erec′ta,** dislocation of the shoulder so that the arm stands straight up above the head. **l. imperfec′ta,** a sprain. **l. perinea′lis,** a form of dislocation of the hip in which the head of the femur lies in the perineum.

luxation (luk-sa′shun) [L. *luxatio*] dislocation. **Malgaigne's l.,** pulled elbow.

luxuriant (luk-su′re-ant) growing freely or excessively.

luxus (luks′us) [L.] excess; see under *consumption* and *heart.*

Luys' body, body syndrome, nucleus (loo-ēz′) [Jules Bernard *Luys,* French physician, 1828–1897] see *pituitary gland,* under *gland,* see *body of Luys syndrome,* under *syndrome,* and see *nucleus subthalamicus.*

Luys' segregator (separator) (loo-ēz′) [Georges *Luys,* French physician, 1870–1953] see under *segregator.*

L.V.H. left ventricular hypertrophy.

L.V.N. licensed vocational nurse.

Lwoff (lwauf), André Michael. French microbiologist and virologist, born 1902; co-winner with François Jacob and Jacques Lucien Monod, of the Nobel prize for medicine or physiology for 1965, for discoveries concerning the genetic control of enzymes and virus synthesis.

lyase (lī-ās) [EC 4] one of the six main classes of enzymes, composed of those that catalyze the cleavage of C–C, C–O, C–N, or other bonds without a hydrolysis or oxidation-reduction. Two molecules are formed, one (or both) of which contains a double bond. The reverse reaction occurs by the addition of a group to a molecule at a double bond. The class includes aldolases, deaminases, decarboxylases, hydrases or dehydratases, and other cleavage or cyclase enzymes. Called also *synthase.*

lycanthropy (li-kan′thro-pe) [Gr. *lykos* wolf + *anthropos* man] a delusion in which the patient believes himself a wolf.

lycetamine (li-se′tah-mēn) chemical name: (S)-2,6-diamino-N-hexadecylhexanamide; a topical antimicrobial, $C_{22}H_{47}N_3O$.

Lychnis githago (lik′is gith-a′go) *Agrostemma githago.*

lycine (li′sin) betaine.

lycopene (li′ko-pēn) the red carotenoid pigment, $C_{40}H_{56}$, of tomatoes and various berries and fruits.

lycopenemia (li″ko-pĕ-ne′me-ah) a variant of carotenemia resulting from the prolonged and excessive ingestion of tomato juice, which contains lycopene.

Lycoperdales (li″ko-per-da′lēs) the puffballs, an order of fungi of the series Gasteromycetes, class Basidiomycetes, including the genera *Calvatia, Lycoperdon,* and *Geaster.*

Lycoperdon (li″ko-per′don) [Gr. *lykos* wolf + *perdesthai* to break wind] a genus of fungi of the order Lycoperdales, class Basidiomycetes; the puffballs. In folk medicine, the dust (spores) is puffed and inhaled to treat nosebleeds.

lycoperdonosis (li″ko-per″do-no′sis) a respiratory disease caused by the inhalation of many spores from mature *Lycoperdon* mushrooms.

Lycopodium (li″ko-po′de-um) [Gr. *lykos* wolf + *pous* foot] a genus of club-mosses which yield lycopodium.

lycopodium (li″ko-po′de-um) a light dry powder formed by the yellow inflammable sporules of *Lycopodium clavatum*, *L. saururus*, and other species; formerly used as a dusting and absorbent powder, and as a coating for pills. The spores are uniform in size and for this reason are used as a measuring unit in microscopy.

lycorine (lik′o-rin) an alkaloid having emetic properties, from the bulbs of the plant *Lycoris radiata;* identical with narcissine.

Lycoris (lik′ŏ-ris) a genus of poisonous, amaryllidaceous plants of China and Japan. *L. radia′ta* Herb. is the source of sekisanine; the bulbs, which contain lycorine, are used in Chinese medicine as an expectorant and emetic.

Lycosa tarentula (li-ko′sah tah-ren′tu-lah) the European tarantula.

lydimycin (lid″ĭ-mi′sin) chemical name: 5-(hexahydro-2-oxo-1*H*-thieno[3,4-*d*]imidazol-4-yl)pentenoic acid; an antifungal antibiotic produced by *Streptomyces lydicus*, $C_{10}H_{14}N_2O_3S$.

lye (li) an alkaline percolate from wood ashes; lixivium. Household lye is a crude mixture of sodium hydroxide with some sodium carbonate.

Lyell's disease, syndrome (li′elz) [Alan *Lyell*, English dermatologist, 20th century] toxic epidermal necrolysis.

lying-in (li″ing-in′) 1. puerperal. 2. the puerperium.

Lyme disease (lim) [from Old Lyme, Connecticut, where the disease was first reported] see under *disease*.

Lymnaea (lim-ne′ah) a genus of pond snails. *L. ollula* and *L. bulimoides* serve as first intermediate hosts of *Fasciola hepatica;* other species are the hosts of schistosome flukes that cause schistosome dermatitis.

lymph (limf) [L. *lympha* water] 1. a transparent, slightly yellow liquid of alkaline reaction, found in the lymphatic vessels and derived from the tissue fluids. It is occasionally of a light-rose color from the presence of red blood corpuscles, and is often opalescent from particles of fat. Under the microscope, lymph is seen to consist of a liquid portion and of cells, most of which are lymphocytes. Lymph is collected from all parts of the body and returned to the blood via the lymphatic system. Called also *lympha* [NA]. See Plate 25. 2. any clear, watery fluid resembling true lymph. **aplastic l.**, lymph that contains an excess of leukocytes and does not tend to become organized; called also *corpuscular l.* **corpuscular l.**, aplastic l. **croupous l.**, inflammatory lymph that tends to the formation of a false membrane. **euplastic l., fibrinous l.**, that which tends to coagulate and become organized. **inflammatory l.**, the lymph produced by inflammation, as in a wound. **intercellular l.**, lymph occupying the intercellular spaces of tissues. **intravascular l.**, the lymph of the lymph vessels. **plastic l.**, inflammatory lymph that has a tendency to become organized. **tissue l.**, lymph derived from the tissues and not from the blood. **vaccine l., vaccinia l.**, (*obs.*) material containing vaccinia virus collected from vaccinial vesicles of calves; used for active immunization against smallpox.

lympha (lim′fah) [L. "water"] [NA] the fluid found in the lymphatic vessels; see *lymph*.

lymphaden (lim′fah-den) [*lymph-* + Gr. *adēn* gland] a lymph node.

lymphadenectasis (lim-fad″ĕ-nek′tah-sis) [*lymph-* + Gr. *adēn* gland + *ektasis* distention] enlargement of a lymph node.

lymphadenectomy (lim-fad″ĕ-nek′to-me) [*lymphaden* + Gr. *ektomē* excision] surgical excision of one or more lymph nodes.

lymphadenhypertrophy (lim-fad″en-hi-per′tro-fe) [*lymphaden* + *hypertrophy*] hypertrophy of a lymph node.

lymphadenia (lim″fah-de′ne-ah) [*lymphaden* + *-ia*] hypertrophy of the lymph nodes. **l. os′sea** (*obs.*), multiple myeloma.

lymphadenitis (lim″fad′ĕ-ni-tis) [*lymphaden* + *-itis*] inflammation of one or more lymph nodes, usually caused by a primary focus of infection elsewhere in the body. **caseous l.**, a chronic disease of sheep and goats caused by *Corynebacterium pseudotuberculosis*, characterized by the formation in the lymph nodes of various organs (e.g., skin, lungs) of abscesses containing caseous material, and may be associated with chronic pneumonia and pleurisy. Called also *pseudotuberculosis*. **mesenteric l.**, a condition clinically resembling acute appendicitis, in which there is inflammation of the mesenteric lymph nodes receiving lymph from the intestine. A septal form, which is frequently fatal, and a milder form, which is self-limited, are caused by *Yersinia* (*Pasteurella*) *pseudotuberculosis*. Called also *mesenteric adenitis*. **nonbacterial regional l.**, cat-scratch disease. **paratuberculous l.**, caseous l. **regional l.**, cat-scratch disease. **tuberculoid l.**, inflammation of the lymph nodes similar to that in tuberculosis lymphadenitis; it may be caused by such disorders as sarcoidosis, regional enteritis, leprosy, syphilis, and several fungal infections. **tuberculous l.**, tuberculosis of the lymph nodes, involving most often the cervical (formerly called *scrofula*) and mediastinal nodes, which may occur as a primary infection or be caused by lymphatic or hematogenous spread from a primary focus of infection elsewhere in the body. Called also *tuberculous lymphadenopathy*. See also *scrofuloderma*.

lymphadenocele (lim-fad′ĕ-no-sēl″) a cyst of a lymph node; called also *adenolymphocele*.

lymphadenocyst (lim-fad′ĕ-no-sist″) a degenerated lymph node caused by occlusion of its incoming lymph vessels. By dilatation of the lymph sinuses it becomes a fine-meshed network.

lymphadenogram (lim-fad′ĕ-no-gram″) a roentgenogram of lymph nodes.

lymphadenography (lim-fad″ĕ-nog′rah-fe) roentgenographic visualization of the lymph nodes, following injection of radiopaque material into a lymphatic vessel.

lymphadenoid (lim-fad′ĕ-noid) [*lymph-* + Gr. *adēn* gland + *eidos* form] resembling the tissue of lymph nodes; lymphadenoid tissue includes the spleen, bone marrow, tonsils, and the lymphatic tissue of the organs and mucous membranes.

lymphadenoleukopoiesis (lim-fad″ĕ-no-lu″ko-poi-e′sis) the production of leukocytes by the lymphadenoid tissue.

lymphadenoma (lim″fad-ĕ-no′mah) hyperplasia of the lymphadenoid tissue; lymphoma. **malignant l.** (*obs.*), malignant lymphoma. **multiple l.** (*obs.*), Hodgkin's disease.

lymphadenomatosis (lim-fad″ĕ-no-mah-to′sis) (*obs.*) generalized malignant lymphoma. **general l. of bones** (*obs.*), multiple myeloma.

lymphadenopathy (lim-fad″ĕ-nop′ah-the) [*lymphaden* + Gr. *pathos* disease] disease of the lymph nodes. **angioimmunoblastic l., angioimmunoblastic l. with dysproteinemia (AILD)**, a systemic disorder resembling lymphoma, characterized by fever, night sweats, weight loss, generalized lymphadenopathy with a pleomorphic cellular infiltrate of lymphocytes, immunoblasts, and plasma cells that alters or effaces the nodal architecture, hepatosplenomegaly, macropapular rash, polyclonal hypergammaglobulinemia, and Coombs-positive hemolytic anemia. It is considered to be a nonmalignant hyperimmune reaction to chronic antigenic stimulation; there is proliferation of B cells accompanied by profound deficiency of T cells. The disease follows a progressive but extremely variable course; some patients have long survival without chemotherapy, whereas others have a rapid course with death due to overwhelming infections. Called also *immunoblastic l.* **dermatopathic l.**, regional lymph node enlargement associated with melanoderma and various diseases in which erythroderma is chronically present, e.g., exfoliative dermatitis and generalized neurodermatitis; called also *lipomelanotic reticulosis*. **immunoblastic l.**, angioimmunoblastic l. **tuberculous l.**, see under *lymphadenitis*.

lymphadenosis (lim-fad″ĕ-no′sis) [*lymphaden* + *-osis*] hypertrophy or proliferation of lymphoid tissue. **aleukemic l.**, a disease marked by diffuse generalized hyperplasia of the lymphadenoid system (lymph glands, spleen, bone marrow, tonsils, and other lymphatic tissues), but without leukemia; see also *pseudoleukemia* and *lymphosarcoma*. **l. benig′na cu′tis**, lymphocytoma cutis.

lymphadenotomy (lim-fad″ĕ-not′o-me) incision into a lymph node.

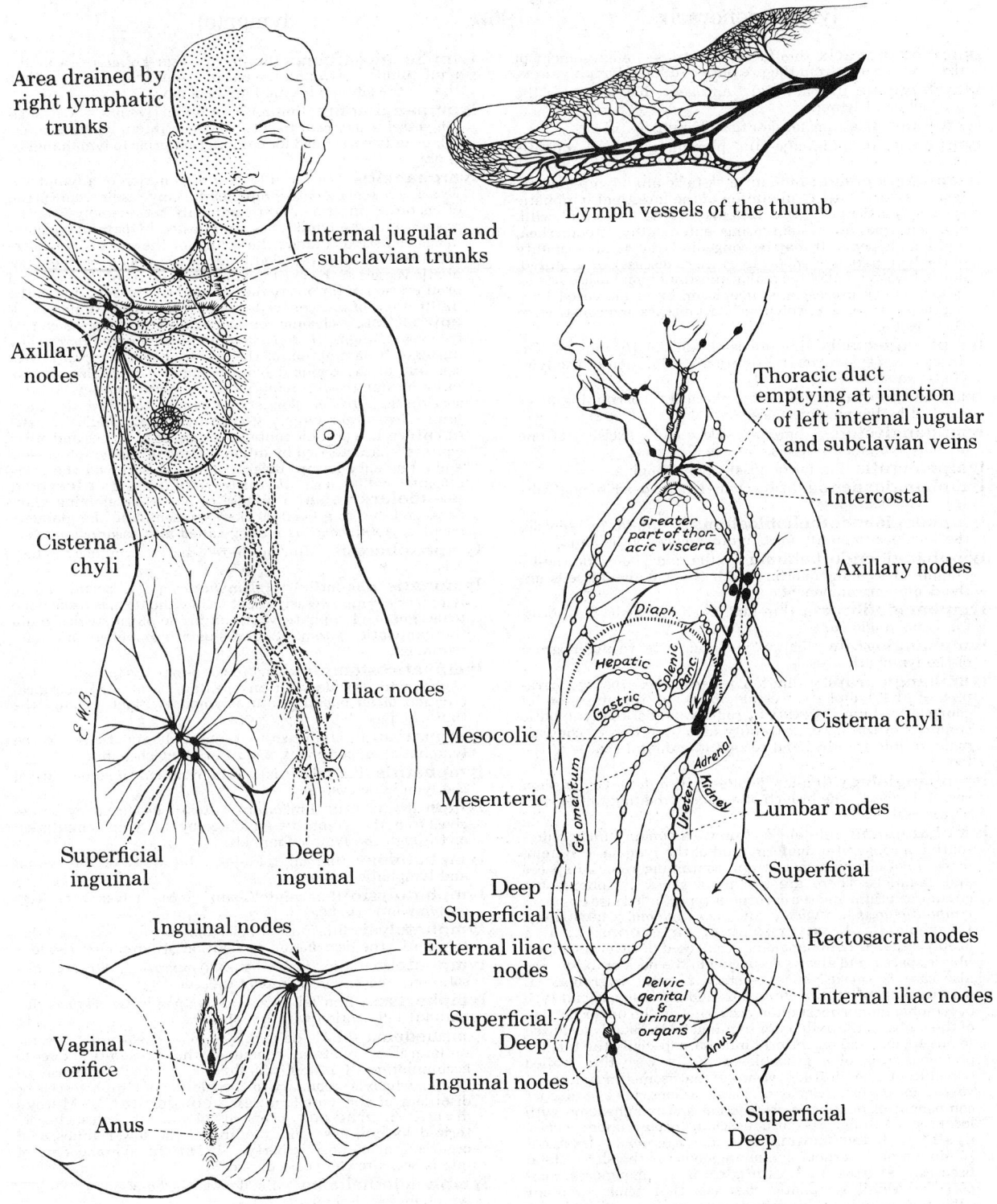

Area drained by right lymphatic trunks

Lymph vessels of the thumb

Internal jugular and subclavian trunks

Axillary nodes

Cisterna chyli

Iliac nodes

Superficial inguinal

Deep inguinal

Thoracic duct emptying at junction of left internal jugular and subclavian veins

Intercostal

Greater part of thoracic viscera

Axillary nodes

Diaph.

Hepatic

Splenic

Panc.

Gastric

Cisterna chyli

Mesocolic

Gt. omentum

Adrenal

Ureter

Kidney

Mesenteric

Lumbar nodes

Deep
Superficial

Superficial

External iliac nodes

Rectosacral nodes

Superficial
Deep

Pelvic genital & urinary organs

Anus

Internal iliac nodes

Inguinal nodes

Superficial
Deep

Inguinal nodes

Vaginal orifice

Anus

PLATE 25 —DIAGRAMMATIC REPRESENTATION OF LYMPHATIC DRAINAGE OF VARIOUS PARTS OF THE BODY

961

lymphadenovarix (lim-fad″ĕ-no-va′riks) enlargement of the lymph nodes from the pressure of dilated lymph vessels.

lymphagogue (lim′fah-gog) an agent that promotes the production of lymph.

lymphangeitis (lim″fan-je-i′tis) lymphangitis.

lymphangial (lim-fan′je-al) pertaining to a lymphatic vessel.

lymphangiectasia (lim-fan″je-ek-ta′ze-ah) lymphangiectasis. **intestinal l.,** dilatation of the intestinal lymphatic system, particularly the lacteals in the intestinal villi, characterized by protein-losing enteropathy, steatorrhea, and lymphopenia. It may be congenital, due to abnormality of the lymphatic system (as in Milroy's disease), or acquired, due to involvement of the major intestinal lymphatic ducts by inflammatory processes or neoplasm, or to increased lymphatic pressure, as in valvular heart disease and constrictive pericarditis.

lymphangiectasis (lim-fan″je-ek′tah-sis) [*lymph-* + Gr. *angeion* vessel + *ektasis* distention] dilatation of the lymphatic vessels.

lymphangiectatic (lim-fan″je-ek-tat′ik) pertaining to or marked by lymphangiectasis.

lymphangiectomy (lim-fan″je-ek′to-me) excision of one or more lymphatic vessels.

lymphangiitis (lim-fan″je-i′tis) lymphangitis.

lymphangioadenography (lym-fan″je-o-ad″ĕ-nog′rah-fe) lymphography.

lymphangioendothelioblastoma (lim-fan″je-o-en″do-the″le-o-blas-to′mah) (*obs.*) lymphangioendothelioma.

lymphangioendothelioma (lim-fan″je-o-en″do-the-le-o′mah) lymphangioma in which the endothelial cells are the dominant component.

lymphangiofibroma (lim-fan″je-o-fi-bro′mah) a fibrosing lymphangioma.

lymphangiogram (lim-fan″je-o-gram) a roentgenogram of the lymphatic vessels.

lymphangiography (lim-fan″je-og′rah-fe) roentgenography of the lymphatic vessels following the injection of contrast medium. **pedal l.,** radiography of the lymphatic channels of the lower extremity after injection of contrast medium into the first and second interdigital spaces of the foot.

lymphangiology (lim-fan″je-ol′o-je) [*lymph-* + Gr. *angeion* vessel + *-logy*] the branch of anatomy relating to the lymphatic vessels.

lymphangioma (lim-fan″je-o′mah) a bengin tumor representing a congenital malformation of the lymphatic system, made up of newly formed lymph-containing vascular spaces and channels. There are two main types: lymphangioma circumscriptium and the cavernous type. Called also *angioma lymphaticum.* Cf. *angioma* and *hemangioma.* **capillary l.,** simple l. **l. caverno′sum, cavernous l.,** 1. a deeply situated lymphangioma, composed of cavernous lymphatic spaces, and always occurring in the neck or axilla. See also *vascular nevus,* under *nevus.* 2. cystic hygroma. **l. circumscrip′tum,** a cutaneous and more superficial type of lymphangioma, most often occurring on the upper portion of the limbs, in the axillary or inguinal folds, usually localized to one region, and on the oral mucosa, especially the tongue, and consisting of a grapelike group of very thin walled translucent lymph-filled vesicles that sometimes have a verrucous surface. Some of these lesions have a deeper component of lymphatic obstruction and lymphedema with localized swelling. See also *vascular nevus,* under *nevus.* **cystic l., l. cys′ticum,** see under *hygroma.* **fissural l.,** simple or cavernous lymphangiomas at the site of fetal fissures. **simple l., l. sim′plex** a lymphangioma composed of small lymphatic channels that tends to occur subcutaneously in the head and neck region as well as in the axilla and sometimes in internal organs. Superficial lesions present as slightly raised or sometimes nodular lesions; deeper lesions are sharply circumscribed, compressible, and gray to pink in color. Called also *capillary l.*

lymphangiomyomatosis (lim-fan″je-o-mi″o-mah-to′sis) a progressive disorder of women of child-bearing age, marked by nodular and diffuse interstitial proliferation of smooth muscle in the lungs, lymph nodes, and thoracic duct.

lymphangiophlebitis (lim-fan″je-o-flĕ-bi′tis) inflammation of the lymph vessels and veins.

lymphangiosarcoma (lim-fan″je-o-sar-ko′mah) a malignant tumor of lymphatic vessels, usually arising in a limb that is the site of chronic lymphedema.

lymphangiotomy (lim-fan″je-ot′o-me) [*lymph-* + Gr. *angeion* vessel + *temnein* to cut] incision into a lymphatic vessel, usually performed for cannulation prior to lymphangiography.

lymphangitis (lim″fan-ji′tis) inflammation of a lymphatic vessel or vessels. Acute lymphangitis may result from spread of bacterial infection (most commonly beta-hemolytic streptococci) into the lymphatics, manifested by painful subcutaneous red streaks along the course of the vessels. **l. carcinomato′sa,** a pseudoinflammatory lesion of the lymphatic vessels of the peritoneum, with edema of the area and proliferation of fibrous tissues around the vessels, due to the infiltration of cancer cells from peritoneal tumors. **l. epizoot′ica,** a chronic contagious disease of horses caused by a yeast fungus, *Histoplasma farciminosus,* and marked by purulent inflammation of the subcutaneous lymphatic vessels and of the regional lymph glands. Called also *pseudofarcy, blastomycosis farciminosus, cryptococcus farcy, lymphosporidiosis, African glanders, Japanese glanders, Japanese farcy, Neapolitan farcy.* **gummatous l.,** cladiosis. **ulcerative l.,** a chronic contagious disease of horses and other equines, characterized by inflammation of the lymph vessels and a tendency toward ulceration of the skin over the parts affected; called also *ulcerative cellulitis.* **l. ulcero′sa pseudofarcino′sa,** a disease of horses resembling glanders, and due to a bacillus closely resembling the glanders bacillus, *Actinobacillus mallei;* called also *pseudoglanders.*

lymphapheresis (lim″fah-fĕ-re′ĕ-sis) lymphocytapheresis.

lymphatic (lim-fat′ik) [L. *lymphaticus*] 1. pertaining to lymph or a lymph vessel; by extension, the term is used alone to designate a lymphatic vessel or, in the plural, to designate the lymphatic system. 2. of a sluggish or phlegmatic temperament.

lymphaticostomy (lim-fat″ĭ-kos′to-me) [*lymphatic* + Gr. *stomoun* to provide with an opening, or mouth] surgical creation of an opening into a lymphatic duct, usually the thoracic duct.

lymphatism (lim′fah-tizm) 1. status lymphaticus. 2. the lymphatic temperament; a slow or sluggish habit.

lymphatitis (lim″fah-ti′tis) inflammation of some part of the lymphatic system.

lymphatogenous (lim″fah-toj′ĕ-nus) produced by or derived from the lymph; disseminated by the lymph circulation or through the lymph channels.

lymphatology (lim″fah-tol′o-je) the study of the lymph and lymphatic system.

lymphatolysin (lim″fah-tol′ĭ-sin) (*obs.*) a lysin that acts on lymphatic tissue.

lymphatolysis (lim″fah-tol′ĭ-sis) [*lymphatic* + Gr. *lysis* dissolution] the destruction or solution of lymphatic tissue.

lymphatolytic (lim″fah-to-lit′ik) [*lymphatic* + Gr. *lysis* dissolution] destroying lymphatic tissue.

lymphectasia (lim″fek-ta′ze-ah) [*lymph-* + Gr. *ektasis* distention] distention with lymph.

lymphedema (lim″fe-de′mah) [*lymph-* + *edema*] chronic unilateral or bilateral edema of the extremities due to accumulation of interstitial fluid as a result of stasis of lymph, which is secondary to obstruction of lymph vessels and disorders of the lymph nodes. **congenital l.,** Milroy's disease. **l. prae′cox,** primarily of young females, characterized by puffiness and swelling of the lower limbs, and occurring at or near puberty. **l. tar′da,** lymphedema of late onset, after 35 years of age.

lymphendothelioma (lim″fen-do-the″le-o′mah) (*obs.*), lymphangioendothelioma.

lymphenteritis (lim″fen-ter-i′tis) enteritis with serous infiltration.

lymphepithelioma (limf″ep-ĭ-the″le-o′mah) lymphoepithelioma.

lymphization (lim″fĭ-za′shun) the formation of lymph.

lymphnoditis (limf″no-di′tis) inflammation of a lymph node; lymphadenitis.

lymph(o)- [L. *lympha* water] a combining form denoting relationship to lymph, lymphoid tissue, lymphatics, or lymphocytes.

lymphoblast (lim′fo-blast) [*lympho-* + Gr. *blastos* germ] the immature, nucleolated precursor of the mature lymphocyte.

lymphoblastic (lim″fo-blas′tik) pertaining to a lymphoblast.

lymphoblastoma (lim″fo-blas-to′mah) [*lymphoblast* + *-oma*] lymphoblastic lymphoma.

lymphoblastosis (lim″fo-blas-to′sis) excess of lymphoblasts in the blood.

lymphocerastism (lim″fo-se-ras′tizm) [*lympho-* + Gr. *kerastos* mixed] the formation of lymphoid cells.

lymphocinesia (lim″fo-si-ne′ze-ah) [*lympho-* + Gr. *kinēsis* motion] lymphokinesis.

lymphocytapheresis (lim″fo-si″tah-fĕ-re′ sis) [*lymphocyte* + Gr. *aphairesis* removal] the selective removal of lymphocytes from withdrawn blood, which is then retransfused into the donor. Called also *lymphapheresis.*

lymphocyte (lim′fo-sīt) [*lympho-* + *-cyte*] any of the mononuclear, nonphagocytic leukocytes, found in the blood, lymph, and lymphoid tissues, that are the body's immunologically competent cells and their precursors. They are divided on the basis of ontogeny and function into two classes, B and T lymphocytes, responsible for humoral and cellular immunity, respectively. In *small lymphocytes,* 7–10 μm in diameter with a round or slightly indented heterochromatic nucleus that almost fills the cell and a thin rim of basophilic cytoplasm that contains few granules. When activated by contact with antigen, small lymphocytes begin macromolecular synthesis, the cytoplasm enlarges until the cells are 10–30 μm in diameter, and the nucleus becomes less completely heterochromatic; they are then referred to as *large lymphocytes* or *lymphoblasts.* These cells then proliferate and differentiate into B and T memory cells and into the various effector cell types, B cells into plasma cells and T cells into helper, cytotoxic, and suppressor cells. Surface markers identifying the lymphocyte types are shown in the accompanying table. See subentries here and under *cell.* **ampli-**

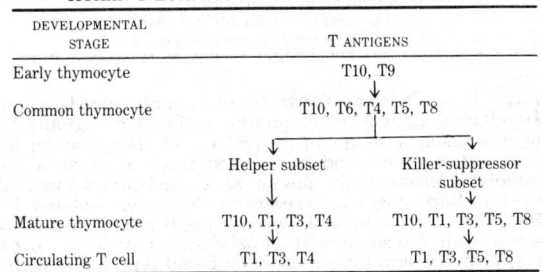

HUMAN T LYMPHOCYTE CELL-SURFACE MARKERS

DEVELOPMENTAL STAGE	T ANTIGENS
Early thymocyte	T10, T9
Common thymocyte	T10, T6, T4, T5, T8
	Helper subset / Killer-suppressor subset
Mature thymocyte	T10, T1, T3, T4 / T10, T1, T3, T5, T8
Circulating T cell	T1, T3, T4 / T1, T3, T5, T8

fier T-l., a T-lymphocyte that modifies a developing immune response by releasing nonspecific signals that other T-lymphocytes (either effector or suppressor cells) respond to. **B l's,** B cells; bursa-dependent lymphocytes and their counterparts in nonavian vertebrates, the cells primarily responsible for humoral immunity, the precursors of antibody-producing cells (plasma cells). In birds B cell maturation takes place in the bursa of Fabricius; the hypothesized analogous tissue in other vertebrates was termed the "bursa-equivalent" tissue. It now appears that B cell maturation occurs primarily in the bone marrow in mammals. B cells are characterized by the presence of surface immunoglobulin, monomeric IgM or IgD, which constitutes the B cell antigen receptors. When stimulated by antigen, a process that requires the cooperation of helper T cells and macrophages, B cells proliferate and differentiate into plasma cells and memory B cells. The entire clone of cells descended from a single activated B cell produces immunoglobulins having the same antigen combining site as that in the antigen receptors of the original cell; thus all of the antibody produced and all of the memory cells are specific for the antigen that induced their formation. **cytotoxic T l's (CTL),** killer cells, killer T cells; differentiated T lymphocytes that can recognize and lyse target cells bearing specific antigens recognized by their antigen receptors. Recognition is MHC restricted; the

foreign antigen is recognized only in association with self MHC antigens. The cytotoxic activity requires firm binding of the killer cell to the target cell and involves the production of holes in the plasma membrane of the target cell, loss of cell content, and osmotic lysis. CTL are important in graft rejection and killing of tumor cells and virus-infected host cells. Murine killer T cells are marked by the Ly-2 and Ly-3 antigens, human cells by the T4 and T8 antigens. **large granular l's,** lymphocytes marked by the presence of large granules visible by light microscopy, responsible for most natural killer cell activity. **Rieder's l.,** a lymphocyte having a nucleus which is lobed and twisted; seen in chronic lymphocytic lymphemia. **T l's,** T cells; thymus-dependent lymphocytes; the cells primarily responsible for cell-mediated immunity. T cells originate from lymphoid stem cells that migrate from the bone marrow to the thymus and differentiate under the influence of the thymic hormones thymopoietin and thymosin. They are characterized by specific surface antigens: the pan-T antigens Thy-1 (murine) and T3 (human) are found on all mature T cells; other markers characterize T cell subsets (see accompanying table). T cell antigen receptors are triggered by antigen only when associated with self MHC antigens, e.g., by antigens processed and presented by macrophages, viral antigens on the surface of host cells, and tumor neoantigens. When activated by antigen, T cells proliferate and differentiate into T memory cells and the various types of regulatory and effector T cells; see *cytotoxic T l's* and *helper, suppressor, contrasuppressor,* and *T_DTH cells* under *cell.* See accompanying table. **thymus-dependent l's,** T l's. **thymus-independent l's,** B l's.

SURFACE MARKERS OF LYMPHOCYTES*

	mIg	Thy-1 / T1, T3	Ly-1 / T4	Ly-2, 3 / T5, T8	FcR	CR
B cells	+	−	−	−	±	±
T cells						
Helper	−	+ / +	+	−	±	−
Killer	−	+ / +	−	+	±	−
Suppressor	−	+ / +	−	+	±	−
Null cells						
K cells	−	−	−	−	+	−
NK cells	−	−	−	−	+	−

*mIg = membrane immunoglobulin; *Thy-1, Ly-1, Ly-2, Ly-3* = mouse T cell surface antigens; *T3, T4, T5, T8* = human T cell surface antigens; *FcR* = Fc receptors; *CR* = complement receptors; ± indicates present only on a subset of cells or on cells of certain maturities.

lymphocytic (lim″fo-sit′ik) pertaining to, characterized by, or of the nature of lymphocytes.

lymphocytoblast (lim″fo-si′to-blast) lymphoblast.

lymphocytoma (lim″fo-si-to′mah) [*lymphocyte* + *-oma*] 1. pseudolymphoma. 2. well-differentiated lymphocytic lymphoma. **l. cu′tis,** a manifestation of cutaneous lymphoid hyperplasia, seen especially in women, characterized by skin lesions ranging from a solitary plaque or nodule to several regionally localized lesions, preferentially involving the facial region and ears, extremities, and areolae of the breasts, to numerous and disseminated lesions. Multiple lesions clinically resemble malignant lymphoma, but some have a tendency toward spontaneous resolution, sometimes with recurrences. Exposure to sunlight, insect bites, and mechanical trauma have been implicated as causative factors. Called also *Bäfverstedt's syndrome, cutaneous lymphoplasia, lymphadenosis benigna cutis, pseudolymphoma of Spiegler-Fendt,* and *Spiegler-Fendt sarcoid.*

lymphocytopenia (lim″fo-si″to-pe′ne-ah) reduction in the number of lymphocytes in the blood.

lymphocytopheresis (lim″fo-si″to-fĕ-re′sis) lymphocytapheresis.

lymphocytopoiesis (lim″fo-si″to-poi-e′sis) [*lymphocyte* + Gr. *poiein* to make] the development of lymphocytes.

lymphocytopoietic (lim″fo-si″to-poi-et′ik) pertaining to or characterized by lymphocytopoiesis.

lymphocytorrhexis (lim″fo-si″to-rek′sis) the rupturing or bursting of lymphocytes.

lymphocytosis (lim″fo-si-to′sis) excess of normal lymphocytes in the blood or in any effusion. **acute infectious l.,** an acute, benign infectious disease of children characterized by an excess of normal small lymphocytes in the blood without lymphadenopathy or splenomegaly, and with varying degrees of clinical expression and constitutional response; called also *Carl Smith disease.*

lymphocytotic (lim″fo-si-tot′ik) pertaining to lymphocytosis.

lymphocytotoxicity (lim″fo-si″to-tok-sis′ĭ-te) the quality or capability of lysing lymphocytes, as that of cytotoxic antibodies in the presence of complement or that of primed histoincompatible cytotoxic T lymphocytes.

lymphocytotoxin (lim″fo-si″to-tok′sin) a toxin that has a specific destructive action on lymphocytes.

lymphoduct (lim′fo-dukt) a lymphatic vessel.

lymphoepithelioma (lim″fo-ep″ĭ-the″le-o′mah) a pleomorphic, poorly differentiated (transitional cell) carcinoma arising from modified epithelium overlying the lymphoid tissue of the nasopharynx; it has a high frequency among young adults of Oriental extraction. Called also *lymphoepithelial carcinoma, Schmincke tumor,* and *Regaud tumor.*

lymphogenesis (lim″fo-jen′ĕ-sis) the production of lymph.

lymphogenous (lim-foj′ĕ-nus) [*lympho-* + Gr. *gennan* to produce] 1. producing lymph. 2. produced from lymph or in the lymphatics.

lymphoglandula (lim″fo-glan′du-lah), pl. *lymphoglan′dulae.* Lymph node (*nodus lymphaticus* [NA]).

lymphogram (lim′fo-gram) a roentgenogram of the lymphatic vessels and lymph nodes.

lymphogranuloma (lim″fo-gran″u-lo′mah) Hodgkin's disease. **l. inguina′le,** l. venereum. **l. malig′num,** Hodgkin's disease. **l. vene′reum,** a sexually transmitted infection, usually occurring in warm climates, due to specific strains of *Chlamydia trachomatis,* characterized by a primary cutaneous or mucosal lesion at the site of infection, which may be a papular, ulcerative, herpetiform, or erosive lesion or urethritis or endocervicitis that heals spontaneously and may go unnoticed, followed by acute unilateral or bilateral lymphadenopathy. The site of the initial infection or primary lesion determines the subsequent manifestations: in men, the primary lesion is usually found on the prepuce, glans, and shaft of the penis, and is most commonly associated with inguinal lymphadenitis, often with draining buboes (the inguinal syndrome); in women, the primary lesion usually involves the posterior vagina and cervix and the labia, and is most often associated with hemorrhagic proctocolitis (anogenitorectal syndrome). Late complications in untreated cases, chiefly seen in women, include locally destructive ulcerations, rectal strictures, rectovaginal fistulas, and genital elephantiasis. Called also *l. inguinale; climatic and tropical, bubo; Durand-Nicolas-Favre, Favre-Nicolas-Durand, fifth veneral, Frei's, Nicolas-Favre,* and *sixth venereal disease; lymphopathia venereum; poradenitis nostras; poradenitis venereum; poradenolymphitis;* and *subacute inguinal poradenitis.*

lymphogranulomatosis (lim″fo-gran″u-lo-mah-to′sis) 1. infectious granuloma of the lymphatic system. 2. a term used by continental writers as a synonym for Hodgkin's disease. See also *pseudoleukemia.* **benign l.,** sarcoidosis. **l. cu′tis,** the cutaneous manifestation of Hodgkin's disease. **l. inguina′lis,** lymphogranuloma venereum. **l. malig′na,** Hodgkin's disease.

lymphography (lim-fog′rah-fe) roentgenography of the lymphatic channels and lymph nodes, following injection of radiopaque material in a lymphatic vessel.

lymphohistiocytic (lim″fo-his″te-o-sit′ik) involving lymphocytes and histiocytes.

lymphohistioplasmacytic (lim″fo-his″te-o-plas″mah-sit′ik) involving lymphocytes, histiocytes, and plasmacytes.

lymphoid (lim′foid) [*lymph* + Gr. *eidos* form] resembling or pertaining to lymph or tissue of the lymphoid system.

lymphoidectomy (lim″foi-dek′to-me) excision of lymphoid tissue, such as adenoids and tonsils.

lymphoidocyte (lim-foi′do-sīt) an embryonic cell considered by some to be the stem cell for all types of blood cells; hemocytoblast.

lymphokentric (lim″fo-ken′trik) [*lympho-* + Gr. *kentron* a stimulant] stimulating the formation of lymphoid cells. Cf. *myelokentric.*

lymphokine (lim′fo-kīn) [*lympho-* + Gr. *kinēsis* movement] a general term for soluble mediators of immune responses

that are not antibodies or complement components and that are released by sensitized lymphocytes on contact with antigen. Cf. *monokine.*

lymphokinesis (lim″fo-ki-ne′sis) [*lympho-* + Gr. *kinēsis* movement] 1. the movement of the endolymph in the semicircular canals. 2. the circulation of lymph in the body.

lymphology (lim-fol′o-je) [*lympho-* + -*logy*] the study of the lymphatic system.

lympholysis (lym-fol′ĭ-sis) lysis of lymphocytes. **cell-mediated l. (CML),** a variation of the mixed lymphocyte culture (MLC) technique that is a functional test of the ability of cytotoxic lymphocytes (CTL) to kill target cells. Lymphocytes from two individuals are cultured together for several days, one population having been prevented from proliferating by treatment with radiation or mitomycin (a "one-way" MLC); they are then cultured for several hours with ^{51}Cr-labeled target cells that are HLA-identical to the stimulator cells. Cytotoxicity is measured as percentage of ^{51}Cr released from specific target cells compared to percentage of ^{51}Cr released from control (nonspecific target) cells.

lympholytic (lim″fo-lit′ik) causing destruction of lymphocytes.

lymphoma (lim-fo′mah) [*lymph-* + -*oma*] any neoplastic disorder of the lymphoid tissue; the term *lymphoma* often is used alone to denote *malignant lymphoma.* **African l.,**

NATIONAL CANCER INSTITUTE FORMULATION OF NON-HODG-KIN'S LYMPHOMAS *(modified)*

Low grade
  Small lymphocytic cell
  Follicular, small cleaved cell
  Follicular, mixed small cleaved and large cell
Intermediate grade
  Follicular, large cell
  Diffuse, small cleaved cell
  Diffuse, mixed small cleaved and large cell
  Diffuse, large cell (cleaved and noncleaved)
High grade
  Diffuse, large cell (immunoblastic)
  Small noncleaved cell (Burkitt and non-Burkitt)
  Lymphoblastic (convoluted and nonconvoluted)

Burkitt's l. **bovine malignant l.,** malignant l. of cattle. **Burkitt's l.,** a form of undifferentiated malignant lymphoma, usually found in central Africa, but also reported from other areas, and manifested most often as a large osteolytic lesion in the jaw or as an abdominal mass. The Epstein-Barr virus, a herpesvirus, has been isolated from Burkitt's lymphoma, and has been implicated as a causative agent. Called also *Burkitt's tumor* and *African l.* **l. cu′tis,** primary skin involvement by B-cell lymphoma without demonstrable systemic disease, most often presenting as a solitary, purple to pink nodule, especially on the head, neck, and face, and usually associated with dissemination to regional lymph nodes and distant hematogenous spread, leading to widespread involvement. **diffuse l.,** malignant lymphoma in which the neoplastic cells diffusely infiltrate the entire lymph node, without any definite organized pattern. Called also *lymphatic sarcoma* and *lymphosarcoma.* **follicular l.,** nodular l. **follicular center cell l.,** B-cell lymphoma comprising four cytologic subtypes (small cleaved, large cleaved, small noncleaved, and large noncleaved) classified on the basis of the similarity of the cell size and nuclear characteristics to those of normal follicular center cells, which seem to retain their ability to form follicles, the degree of which varies with the state of the B-cell transformation. Such tumors are classified on the basis of the predominant cell type. **giant follicle l., giant follicular l.,** nodular l. **granulomatous l.,** Hodgkin's disease. **histiocytic l.,** malignant lymphoma characterized by the presence of large-size tumor cells, resembling histiocytes morphologically but considered to be of lymphoid origin, which are irregular in shape with relatively abundant, frequently acidophilic cytoplasm. It occurs in both nodular and diffuse forms, with the latter being more frequently seen. Called also *reticulum cell sarcoma.* **Hodgkin's l.,** see under *disease.* **Lennert's l.,** malignant lymphoma with a high content of epithelioid histiocytes; bone marrow involvement is common and response to chemotherapy is often poor. **lymphoblastic l.,** a malignant lymphoma composed of a diffuse, relatively uniform proliferation of cells with round or convoluted nuclei and scanty cytoplasm, which are cytologically similar to the lymphoblasts seen in acute lymphocytic leukemia. See also *convoluted T-cell l.* **lymphocytic l., plasmacytoid,** B-cell lymphoma presumably representing a tumor of differentiated interfollicular B lymphocytes that may be functional; those that are secrete identical immunoglobulin molecules. **lymphocytic l., poorly differentiated,** malignant lymphoma in which the neoplastic cells exhibit variability in size, configuration, and degree of differentiation, (which may present a nodular or diffuse histologic pattern) and have distinctive nuclei that are irregular in shape with marked indentations and angularity. **lymphocytic l., well-differentiated,** a diffuse form of malignant lymphoma, representing the neoplastic proliferation of well-differentiated B lymphocytes, with the predominant cell type consisting of compact, small, normal-appearing lymphocytes with dark-staining round nuclei, scanty cytoplasm, and little size variation. The histologic pattern is identical to that of chronic lymphocytic leukemia, and the lymphoma may present with either focal lymph node enlargement or generalized lymphadenopathy and splenomegaly. Called also *lymphocytoma.* **malignant l.,** a group of malignant neoplasms characterized by the proliferation of cells native to the lymphoid tissues, i.e., lymphocytes, histiocytes, and their precursors and derivatives. The group is divided into two major clinicopathologic categories: *Hodgkin's disease* and *non-Hodgkin's lymphoma.* **malignant l. of cattle,** a progressive fatal neoplastic disease of cattle, manifested by enlargement of some or all of the lymph nodes. A C-type virus has been implicated as a causative factor. Called also *bovine malignant l., bovine leukemia, bovine leukosis,* and *bovine lymphomatosis.* **Mediterranean l.,** alpha heavy chain disease; see *heavy chain diseases,* under *disease.* **mixed lymphocytic-histiocytic l.,** malignant lymphoma characterized by the presence of a mixed population of cells, with the smaller cells resembling lymphocytes and the larger ones histiocytes, which usually presents in a nodular histologic pattern but may evolve to a diffuse pattern. **nodular l.,** malignant lymphoma in which the lymphomatous cells are clustered into identifiable nodules within the lymph nodes that somewhat resemble the germinal centers of lymph node follicles. Nodular lymphomas usually occur in older persons, commonly involving many (or all) nodes as well as possibly extranodal sites. Called also *Brill-Symmers'* or *Symmers' disease, follicular l.,* and *giant follicle* or *follicular l.* Cf. *diffuse l.* **non-Hodgkin's l's,** a heterogeneous group of malignant lymphomas, the only common feature being an absence of the giant Reed-Sternberg cells characteristic of Hodgkin's disease. They arise from the lymphoid components of the immune system, and present a clinical picture broadly similar to that of Hodgkin's disease except the disease is initially more widespread, with the most common manifestation being painless enlargement of one or more peripheral lymph nodes. **pleomorphic l.,** undifferentiated l. **small B-cell l.,** B-cell lymphoma representing neoplastic transformation of the small B cells of the follicular mantle, which are blocked from further differentiation, and therefore fail to form follicles or plasma cells. Cf. *well-differentiated lymphocytic l.* **T-cell l's,** a heterogeneous group of lymphoid tumors representing malignant transformation of the T lymphocytes. They have been classified as: small lymphocytic lymphoma, convoluted; cutaneous T-cell lymphomas; and immunoblastic sarcoma of T cells. **T-cell l., convoluted,** T-cell lymphoma essentially identical to the lymphoblastic type, composed of immature intrathymic cells with marked convoluted nuclei. **T-cell l., cutaneous,** a group of lymphomas including a spectrum of disorders, all of which exhibit (1) clonal expansion of malignant T lymphocytes arrested at varying stages of differentiation of cells committed to the series of helper T cells, and (2) malignant infiltration of the skin, which may be the chief or only manifestation of disease. Mycosis fungoides and Sézary syndrome are the best characterized of these disorders. See also *Sézary cell,* under *cell.* **T-cell l., small lymphocytic,** a rare T-cell lymphoma arising from cells that cannot be easily differentiated morphologically from B lymphocytes and may be associated with T-cell chronic lymphocytic leukemia. **U-cell (undefined) l.,** a group of T-cell lymphomas comprising those tumors that cannot be classified into a definite type by either morphologic or currently available immunocytochemical markers. **undifferentiated l.,** malignant lymphoma composed of undifferentiated cells, i.e., cells that do not show morphologic evidence of maturation toward lymphocytes or histiocytes, which vary in size and may include bizarre giant forms. Called also *pleomorphic l.*

lymphomatoid (lim-fo′mah-toid) resembling lymphoma.

lymphomatosis (lim″fo-mah-to′sis) the development of multiple lymphomas in various parts of the body. **avian l., l. of fowl,** avian leukosis involving chiefly the lymphocytes. **bovine l.,** malignant lymphoma of cattle; see under *lymphoma.* **l. granulomato′sa** (obs.), Hodgkin's disease. **neural l.,** see *Marek's disease,* under *disease.* **ocular l.,** see *Marek's disease,* under *disease.* **visceral l.,** see *avian leukosis,* under *leukosis.*

lymphomatous (lim-fo′mah-tus) pertaining to or of the nature of lymphoma.

lymphomyxoma (lim″fo-mik-so′mah) any benign growth consisting of adenoid tissue.

lymphonodi (lim″fo-no′di) [L.] plural of *lymphonodus.*

lymphonoduli (lim″fo-nod′u-li) [L.] plural of *lymphonodulus.*

lymphonodulus (lim″fo-nod′u-lus), pl. *lymphonod′uli* [*lympho-* + L. *nodulus* dim. of *nodus*] a small lymph node. **lymphonod′uli sple′nici,** NA alternative for *folliculi lymphatici splenici.*

lymphonodus (lim″fo-no′dus), pl. *lymphono′di* [*lympho-* + L. *nodis* a knot] nodus lymphaticus.

lymphopathia (lim″fo-path′e-ah) lymphopathy. **l. vene′reum,** lymphogranuloma venereum.

lymphopathy (lim-fop′ah-the) [*lympho-* + Gr. *pathos* disease] any disease of the lymphatic system. **ataxic l.,** a sudden swelling of the lymph nodes sometimes accompanying the pain crises of locomotor ataxia.

lymphopenia (lim-fo-pe′ne-ah) [*lymphocyte* + Gr. *penia* poverty] decrease in the proportion of lymphocytes in the blood.

lymphoplasia (lim″fo-pla′ze-ah) [*lympho-* + Gr. *plasis* formation] the accumulation of lymphoreticular cells in the tissues. **cutaneous l.,** lymphocytoma cutis.

lymphoplasm (lim′fo-plazm) spongioplasm, def. 1.

lymphoplasmapheresis (lim″fo-plaz″mah-fĕ-re′sis) the selective separation and removal of plasma and lympocytes from withdrawn blood, the remainder of the blood then being retransfused into the donor.

lymphoplasty (lim′fo-plas″te) lymphangioplasty.

lymphopoiesis (lim″fo-poi-e′sis) [*lympho-* + Gr. *poiein* to make] 1. the development of lymphatic tissue. 2. lymphocytopoiesis.

lymphopoietic (lim″fo-poi-et′ik) pertaining to, characterized by, or causing lymphopoiesis.

lymphoproliferative (lim″fo-pro-lif′er-ah-tiv) pertaining to or characterized by proliferation of the cells of the lymphoreticular system. The lymphoproliferative disorders comprise a group of malignant neoplasms arising from cells related to the common multipotential, primitive lymphoreticular cell that includes among others the lymphocytic, histiocytic, and monocytic leukemias, multiple myeloma, plasmacytoma, Hodgkin's disease, all lymphocytic lymphomas, and immunosecretory disorders associated with monoclonal gammopathy. An interrelationship with the myeloproliferative (q.v.) disorders is thought to exist. They are called also *lymphoproliferative diseases* or *syndromes.*

lymphoreticular (lim″fo-rĕ-tik′u-lar) pertaining to the cells of the lymphoreticular system. The lymphoreticular disorders are characterized by the proliferation of lymphocytes or lymphoid tissues, and may be either benign (e.g., lymphocytosis or lymphoid hyperplasia) or malignant (e.g., lymphocytic leukemias, multiple myeloma, and nonHodgkin's lymphoma). See also *lymphoproliferative.* They are called also *lymphoreticular diseases* or *syndromes.*

lymphoreticulosis (lim″fo-re-tik″u-lo′sis) proliferation of the reticuloendothelial cells of the lymph nodes. **benign l.,** cat-scratch disease.

lymphorrhage (lim′fo-rij) an accumulation of lymphocytes in a muscle.

lymphorrhagia (lim″fo-ra′je-ah) [*lympho-* + Gr. *rhegnynai* to break out] lymphorrhea.

lymphorrhea (lim″fo-re′ah) [*lympho-* + Gr. *rhoia* flow] a flow of lymph from cut or ruptured lymph vessels.

lymphorrhoid (limf′o-roid) a localized dilatation of a perianal lymph channel, resembling a hemorrhoid; sometimes occurring in lymphogranuloma venereum.

lymphosarcoma (lim″fo-sar-ko′mah) [*lympho-* + *sarcoma*] a diffuse lymphoma. **fascicular l.**, sclerosing l. **sclerosing l.**, a form occurring mainly in childhood, in which the tumor has a fine collagenous stroma and the lymphocytes are arranged in serried rows between the fibers, often giving the tumor a distinctive whorled pattern.

lymphosarcomatosis (lim″fo-sar″ko-mah-to′sis) a condition characterized by the presence of multiple lesions of lymphosarcoma.

lymphosporidiosis (lim″fo-spo-rid″e-o′sis) lymphangitis epizootica.

lymphostasis (lim-fos′tah-sis) [*lympho-* + Gr. *stasis* standing] stoppage of the lymph flow.

lymphotaxis (lim″fo-tak′sis) [*lymphocyte* + Gr. *taxis* arrangement] the property of attracting or repulsing lymphocytes.

lymphotism (lim′fo-tizm) a disordered state associated with the development of adenoid tissue.

lymphotoxin (lim″fo-tok′sin) a lymphokine that effects the lysis of certain target cells, e.g., cultured fibroblasts; abbreviated LT. Three proteins with this activity, α-LT, β-LT, and γ-LT, with molecular weights of 75–100, 45–50, and 25 kilodaltons, have been found in humans. Two other lymphokines, clonal inhibitory factor and proliferation inhibitory factor may be activities exhibited by lymphotoxins at low concentration.

lymphotrophy (lim-fot′ro-fe) [*lympho-* + *-trophy*] nourishment of cells by lymph in tissues lacking sufficient blood supply.

lymphotropic (lim″fo-trop′ik) [*lympho-* + *tropic*] having an affinity for lymphatic tissue.

lymphous (lim′fus) pertaining to or containing lymph.

lymph-vascular (limf-vas′ku-lar) pertaining to or containing lymphatic vessels.

Lynchia maura (lin′ke-ah maw′rah) *Pseudolynchia canariensis.*

Lynen (le′nen), Feodor. German biochemist, 1911–1979; co-winner, with Konrad Bloch, of the Nobel prize for medicine or physiology in 1964, for investigations in biosynthesis of fatty acids and cholesterol.

lynestrenol (lin-es′trĕ-nōl) chemical name: 19-nor-17α-pregn-4-en-20-yn-17-ol; a progestin, $C_{20}H_{28}O$.

Lynoral (lin′or-al) trademark for a preparation of ethinyl estradiol.

lyo- [Gr. *lyein* to dissolve] combining form meaning dissolved or dispersed.

lyochrome (li′o-krōm) [*lyo-* + Gr. *chrōma* color] flavin.

lyogel (li′o-jel) [*lyo-* + *gel*] a gel containing much liquid. Cf. *xerogel.*

Lyon hypothesis (li′on) [Mary Frances *Lyon*, English geneticist, born 1925] see under *hypothesis.*

lyonization (li″on-i-za′shun) [after Mary F. *Lyon*] the process by which or the condition in which all X chromosomes of the cells in excess of one are inactivated on a random basis. Called also *heterochromatinization, heterochromatization,* and *X-inactivation.* See also *Lyon hypothesis,* under *hypo-thesis.*

lyonized (li′o-nīzd) [after Mary F. *Lyon*] denoting the inactivated X chromosome in a cell, according to the Lyon hypothesis.

lyophil (li′o-fil) a lyophilic substance; a material that readily goes into solution.

lyophile (li′o-fīl) 1. lyophil. 2. lyophilic.

lyophilic (li″o-fil′ik) [*lyo-* + Gr. *philein* to love] having an affinity for solution; designating a colloid system in which the solvent and the dispersed particles mutually attract each other and which is quite stable.

lyophilization (li-of″ĭ-li-za′shun) the creation of a stable preparation of a biological substance (blood plasma, serum, etc.), by rapid freezing and dehydration of the frozen product under high vacuum.

lyophilize (li-of′ĭ-līz) to subject to lyophilization.

lyophobe (li′o-fōb) [*lyo-* + *phobia*] a lyophobic substance; a material that does not readily go into or tends to separate out from solution.

lyophobic (li″o-fo′bik) [*lyo-* + Gr. *phobein* to fear] not having an affinity for solution; designating a colloid system in which no attraction exists between the solvent and the dispersed particles and which is unstable.

lyosol (li′o-sol) a sol in which the dispersion medium is a liquid.

lyosorption (li″o-sorp′shun) the selective adsorption of the solvent portion of a solution.

lyotropic (li″o-trop′ik) [*lyo-* + Gr. *tropos* a turning] entering easily into solution; readily soluble.

Lyperosia irritans (li″per-o′se-ah ir′ĭ-tans) *Haematobia irritans.*

Lyponyssus (li″po-nis′us) a genus of mites which sometimes attack man. *L. baco′ti* live normally on rats, *L. bur′sae* on birds.

lypressin (li-pres′in) chemical name: 8-α-lysine vasopressin. A form of vasopressin that contains lysine, $C_{46}H_{65}N_{13}O_{12}S$, as that from pigs. A synthetic preparation is used as an antidiuretic and vasoconstrictor in the treatment of diabetes insipidus due to deficiency of endogenous posterior pituitary antidiuretic hormone (vasopressin), administered by intranasal spray. See also *argipressin.*

lyra (li′rah) [L., Gr. "a stringed instrument resembling the lute"] a name applied to certain anatomical structures because of their fancied resemblance to a lute. **l. Da′vidis** (*obs.*), commissura fornicis.

lyre (līr) lyra. **l. of David** (*obs.*), commissura fornicis.

Lys lysine.

lysate (li′sāt) 1. the material formed by the lysis of cells. 2. a medicinal preparation obtained from an animal organ by means of artificial digestion.

lysatin (lis′ah-tin) a principle derived from casein by Drechsel, later shown to be a mixture of lysine and arginine.

lyse (līz) 1. to cause or produce disintegration of a compound, substance, or cell. 2. to undergo lysis.

lysergic acid (li-sur′jik) a constituent of the ergot alkaloids, $C_6H_4·NH·C_5H_2N(CH_3)(CH:CH·CH_3)·COOH$, obtained by hydrolysis. **l. a. diethylamide, (LSD),** a widely gen produced semisynthetically from ergot alkaloids; it has both sympathomimetic and serotoninergic blocking effects both of which may be involved in the mood changes, sensory distortions, hallucinations, delusions, synesthesia, and depersonalization produced by the drug. LSD use can produce acute panic reactions or precipitate a persistent psychotic state; flashbacks, return of the hallucinatory state triggered by stress or drugs, may also occur.

lysergide (li′ser-jīd) nonproprietary drug name for lysergic acid diethylamide (LSD).

lysidin (lis′ĭ-din) a red crystalline body, methylglyoxalidin, $CH_2·NH·C(CH_3):N·CH_2$; also its yellowish or pinkish, soapy, 50 per cent solution: used as a solvent for uric acid. **l. bitartrate,** a soluble, white, crystalline powder, of one third the solvent power of pure lysidin.

lysimeter (li-sim′ĕ-ter) [Gr. *lysis* dissolution + *metron* measure] an apparatus for determining the solubilities of substances.

lysin (li′sin) [Gr. *lyein* to dissolve] 1. immune lysin, immune cytolysin, an antibody that causes complement-dependent lysis of cells; often used with a prefix indicating the target cells, e.g., hemolysin or bacteriolysin. 2. any substance that causes cell lysis. **beta l.,** beta-lysin. **sperm l.,** a general term for the enzymatic substances of spermatozoa which dissolve egg membranes and permit penetration; these lysins are thought to be produced by the acrosome.

lysine (li′sēn) an amino acid, $NH_2(CH_2)_4·CH(NH_2)·COOH$, or α-ε-diaminocaproic acid, a hydrolytic product of protein first isolated from casein (Drechsel, 1889); essential for optimal growth in infants and for maintenance of nitrogen equilibrium in human adults.

lysine dehydrogenase (li′sēn de-hi′dro-jĕ-nās) [EC 1.4.1.15] an enzyme of the oxidoreductase class that catalyzes the reaction L-lysine + NAD^+ = 1,2-didehydropiperidine-2-carboxylate + NH_3 + NADH. The reaction occurs in the liver and is one of the pathways of lysine degradation (see also saccharopine dehydrogenase [NAD and NADP]). Genetic deficiency of the enzyme causes congenital lysine intolerance.

lysine ketoglutarate reductase (li′sēn ke″to-gloo′tah-rāt re-duk′tās) saccharopine dehydrogenase (NADP).

lysine-ketoglutarate reductase deficiency hyperlysinemia.

L-lysine:NAD oxidoreductase (li′sēn ok″sĭ-do-re-duk′tās) lysine dehydrogenase.

L-lysine:NAD oxidoreductase deficiency hyperlysinemia.

lysinogen (li-sin′o-jen) [*lysin* + Gr. *gennan* to produce] an antigenic substance capable of inducing the formation of lysins.

lysinosis (lis″ĭ-no′sis) [Gr. *lyein* to dissolve + *is, inos* fiber + -*osis*] lung disease due to inhaling cotton fibers, as in mills; lyssinosis.

lysis (li′sis) [Gr. "dissolution; a loosing, setting free, releasing"] 1. destruction, as of cells by a specific lysin. 2. decomposition, as of a chemical compound by a specific agent. 3. mobilization of an organ by division of restraining adhesions. 4. the gradual abatement of the symptoms of a disease; cf. *crisis,* def. 1. **hot-cold l.,** lysis that occurs only if the material is incubated as usual and then allowed to stand overnight at room temperature.

lys(o)- [Gr. *lysis* dissolution] a combining form denoting relationship to lysis or dissolution.

lysocephalin (li″so-sef′ah-lin) a cephalin from which a fatty acid radical has been removed, as by the action of cobra venom.

lysocythin (li″so-si′thin) a substance formed by combination between an animal poison and the body tissues and having a cytolytic action.

Lysodren (li′so-dren) trademark for a preparation of mitotane.

lysogen (li′so-jen) [*lysin* + -*gen*] 1. an agent that induces lysis. 2. lysinogen. 3. a lysogenized bacterium.

lysogenesis (li″so-jen′ĕ-sis) the production of lysis or lysins.

lysogenic (li-so-jen′ik) [*lysin* + Gr. *gennan* to produce] 1. producing lysins or causing lysis. 2. pertaining to lysogeny.

lysogenicity (li″so-jĕ-nis′ĭ-te) [*lyso-* + Gr. *gennan* to produce + -*ity* condition] 1. the ability to produce lysins or cause lysis. 2. the potentiality of a bacterium to produce phage. 3. the specific association of the phage genome, the prophage, with the bacterial genome in such a way that only a few, if any, phage genes are transcribed.

lysogeny (li-soj′e-ne) the phenomenon in which a bacterium is infected by a temperate bacteriophage, the viral DNA is integrated in the chromosome of the host cell and replicated along with the host chromosome for many generations (the lysogenic cycle), and then production of virions and lysis of host cells (the lytic cycle) begins again. The lytic cycle is initiated spontaneously about once in 10,000 cell divisions or may be induced by ultraviolet light or chemical agents.

lysokinase (li″so-ki′nās) a general term for substances of the fibrinolytic system that activate the plasma proactivators.

lysolecithin (li″so-les′ĭ-thin) a lecithin from which the α′ (i.e., terminal) fatty acid radical has been removed, as by the action of phospholipase A; it has strong hemolytic properties and occurs in trace amounts in the pancreas.

lysophosphatide (li″so-fos′fah-tīd) a phosphatide from which one molecule of fatty acid has been split off, as by the action of cobra venom.

lysophosphatidic acid (li″so-fos″fah-tid′ik) glycerol esterified with a fatty acid on the first carbon atom and with phosphoric acid on the third; the second carbon atom has a free hydroxyl group. The name derives from the fact that lysophosphatidyl cholines (lysolecithins) are detergents that can lyse cells.

lysophospholipase (li″so-fos″fo-li′pās   li″so-fos″fo-lip′ās) [EC 3.1.1.5] an enzyme of the hydrolase class that catalyzes the reaction 2-lysophosphatidylcholine + H_2O = glycerophosphocholine + a fatty acid anion. The enzyme is important in the degradation of dietary and intracellular phospholipids.

lysosomal (li″so-so′mal) of or pertaining to a lysosome.

lysosome (li′so-sōm) [*lyso-* + Gr. *sōma* body] one of the minute bodies seen with the electron microscope in many types of cells, containing various hydrolytic enzymes and normally involved in the process of localized intracellular digestion. Injury to a lysosome is followed by release into the cell of the enzymes, which may damage the cell and give rise to wasting and other pathologic aspects of certain diseases, as in muscular dystrophy. **primary l.,** one that has not yet been engaged in digestive activities. **secondary l.,** a primary (or another secondary) lysosome that has fused with a phagosome (or pinosome), bringing hydrolases in contact with the ingested material and resulting in digestion of the material. See also *autophagy* (def. 2) and *heterophagy.*

lysostaphin (li-so-staf′in) an antibacterial enzyme produced by *Staphylococcus staphylolyticus;* it is specifically active against staphylococci.

lysozyme (li′so-zīm) [EC 3.2.1.17] an enzyme of the hydrolase class that catalyzes the hydrolysis of 1,4-β-linkages between N-acetylmuramic acid and N-acetyl-D-glucosamine residues in peptidoglycans, and between N-acetyl-D-glucosamine residues in chitodextrin. The enzyme occurs in saliva, tears, egg white, and many animal fluids and catalyzes the breakdown of some bacterial cell walls.

lysozymuria (li″so-zi-mu′re-ah) urinary excretion of elevated levels of lysozyme.

lyssa (lis′ah) [Gr. "frenzy"; "*the worm* under the tongue of dogs, removed because of the belief that it caused rabies"] 1. former term for *rabies.* 2. septum linguae.

lyssic (lis′ik) pertaining to rabies.

lyss(o)- [Gr. *lyssa* rabies] a combining form denoting relationship to rabies.

lyssoid (lis′oid) [*lysso-* + Gr. *eidos* form] resembling rabies.

lyssophobia (lis″o-fo′be-ah) [*lysso-* + *phobia*] irrational fear of rabies.

Lyster tube (lis′ter) [William J. L. *Lyster,* U. S. Army surgeon, 1869–1947] see under *tube.*

lysyl (li′syl) the acyl radical of lysine.

lysyl hydroxylase (li′sil hi-drok′sĭ-lās) procollagen-lysine, 2-oxoglutarate 5-dioxygenase.

lysyl oxidase (li′sil ok″sĭ dās) an enzyme of the oxidoreductase class that catalyzes the reaction lysine + O_2 = allysine + NH_3 + H_2O. It requires Cu^{2+} and pyridoxal phosphate. The reaction is a step in the formation of covalent cross-links in collagens and elastins. A defect or absence of the enzyme is the cause of *Ehlers-Danlos syndrome V* and of *cutis laxa.*

lyterian (li-te′re-an) indicative of lysis of an attack of disease.

lytic (lit′ik) 1. pertaining to lysis or to a lysin. 2. producing lysis. 3. a word termination denoting lysis of the substance indicated by the stem to which it is affixed.

Lyticum (lit′ĭ-kum) [Gr. *lyticos* dissolving] a genus of bacteria of uncertain affiliation that are parasites of paramecia.

Lytta (lit′ah) a genus of blister beetles; called also *Russian fly.* **L. vesicato′ria,** a species of beetles known as Spanish fly, or blister bug; it is the source of cantharidin. Called also *Cantharis vesicatoria.*

lytta (lit′ah) former term for *rabies.*

lyxose (lik′sōs) an aldopentose, $CH_2OH \cdot (CHOH)_3 \cdot CHO$.

lyze (līz) lyse.

M symbol for *mega-* and *molar* (concentration).

m symbol for *median, meter,* and *milli-*.

μ mu, the twelfth letter of the Greek alphabet; symbol for *mean, micro-, linear attenuation coefficient,* and the heavy chain of IgM.

m- chemical symbol for *meta-*.

M.A. mental age; meter angle; Master of Arts.

Ma symbol for *masurium;* now called *technetium*.

μA microampere.

mA. milliampere.

MAC membrane attack complex.

M.A.C. maximum allowable concentration (of poisons encountered in industry, etc.).

Mac. abbreviation for L. *macerare,* macerate.

Macaca (mah-kak′ah) a genus of Old World monkeys. **M. cynomul′gus,** a species of South American monkeys, much used as laboratory animals. **M. mulat′ta,** a species of monkeys widely used in physiological research.

macaja, macaya (mah-kah′yah) a fixed oil obtained from the fruit of the palm tree, *Acrocomia sclerocarpa*.

McArdle's disease (syndrome) (mah-kar′d′lz) [Brian McArdle, English neurologist of the 20th century] see *glycogen storage disease* (type V), under *disease*.

McBride operation (mak-brīd′) [Earl D. *McBride,* American orthopedic surgeon, born 1891] see under *operation*.

McBurney's incision, etc. (mak-ber′nēz) [Charles *McBurney,* New York surgeon, 1845–1913] see under *incision, operation, point,* and *sign*.

MACC a regimen of methotrexate, Adriamycin (doxorubicin), cyclophosphamide, and CCNU (lomustine), used in cancer chemotherapy.

McCarthy's reflex (mah-kar′thēz) [Daniel J. *McCarthy,* American neurologist, 1874–1958] see under *reflex*.

McClintock (mik-klin′tok) Barbara. American botanist and geneticist, born 1902; winner of the Nobel prize for medicine or physiology in 1983 for her discovery that genes of a corn plant move from one place to another and thus alter future plants.

MacConkey's agar (mah-kon′kēz) [Alfred Theodore *MacConkey,* English bacteriologist, 1861–1931] see under *culture medium*.

Mace (mās) trademark for an aerosol mixture of organic lacrimators.

macerate (mas′er-āt) to soften by wetting or soaking; see *maceration*.

maceration (mas″er-a′shun) [L. *maceratio*] the softening of a solid by soaking. In histology, the softening of a tissue by soaking, especially in acids, until the connective tissue fibers are so dissolved that the tissue components can be teased apart. In obstetrics, the degenerative changes with discoloration and softening of tissues, and eventual disintegration, of a fetus retained in the uterus after its death.

macerative (mas′er-a″tiv) characterized by maceration.

Macewen's operation, sign, triangle (mak-u′enz) [Sir William *Macewen,* surgeon in Glasgow, 1848–1924] see under *operation* and *sign,* and see *suprameatal triangle,* under *triangle*.

McGinn-White sign (mak-gin′ hwit) [Sylvester *McGinn,* American cardiologist, born 1904; Paul Dudley *White,* American cardiologist, 1886–1973] see under *sign*.

Machado-Joseph disease (mah-shah′-do-jo-sef′) [*Machado* and *Joseph,* afflicted families] see under *disease*.

Machaon (mak′ah-on) the older of two brothers, the younger being Podalirius, who were the sons of Aesculapius and were the chief physicians of the Greeks during the Trojan war.

Mache unit (mah′keh) [Heinrich *Mache,* Austrian physicist, 1876–1954] see under *unit*.

machine (mah-shēn′) [L. *machina*] a contrivance or apparatus for the production, conversion, or transmission of some form of energy or force. **heart-lung m.,** a combination blood pump (artificial heart) and blood oxygenator (artificial lung) used in cardiopulmonary bypass for cardiac surgery. **Holtz m.,** an apparatus for developing static electricity. **Van de Graaff m.,** an electrostatic generator of high voltage. **Wimshurst m.,** a machine for the development of static current.

MAC INH membrane attack complex inhibitor.

Mackenrodt's ligament (mahk′en-rōts) [Alwin Karl *Mackenrodt,* German gynecologist, 1859–1925] see *plica rectouterina*.

Mackenzie's disease (mah-ken′zēz) [Sir James *Mackenzie,* Scottish physician, 1853–1925] see *x disease* (def. 1), under *disease*.

Mackenzie's syndrome (mah-ken′zēz) [Sir Stephen *Mackenzie,* London physician, 1844–1909] see under *syndrome*.

Maclagan's thymol turbidity test (mak-lahg′anz) [Noel Francis *Maclagan,* English pathologist, born 1904] see *thymol turbidity test,* under *tests*.

McLean's formula (index) (mak-lānz′) [Franklin C. *McLean,* American pathologist, born 1888] see under *formula*.

MacLean-Maxwell disease (mak-lān′ maks′-wel) [Charles Murray *MacLean,* English physician in West Africa, 1788–1824; James Laidlaw *Maxwell,* Sr., English physician in Formosa, 1836–1921] see under *disease*.

Macleod (mak-lowd′), John James Rickard. Scottish physiologist, 1876–1935; co-winner, with Sir Frederick Grant Banting, of the Nobel prize for medicine and physiology in 1923, for their discovery of insulin.

MacLeod's capsular rheumatism (mak-lowdz′) [Roderick *MacLeod,* Scottish physician, 1795–1852] see under *rheumatism*.

Macleod's syndrome (mak-kloudz′) [William Mathieson *Macleod,* British physician, 1911–1977] see *Swyer-James syndrome,* under *syndrome*.

MacMunn's test (mak-munz′) [Charles Alexander *MacMunn,* British pathologist, 1852–1911] see under *tests*.

McNaughten see *M'Naghten*.

McPheeters' treatment (mak-fe′terz) [Herman Oscar *McPheeters,* American surgeon, born 1891] see under *treatment*.

Macracanthorhynchus (mak″rah-kan″tho-ring′kus) a genus of acanthocephalans. **M. hirudina′ceus,** a species parasitic in swine in the United States; formerly called *Echinorhynchus gigas* and *E. hominis*.

macradenous (mak-rad′ĕ-nus) [*macro-* + Gr. *adēn* gland] having large glands.

macrencephalia (mak-ren′sĕ-fa′le-ah) macrencephaly.

macrencephaly (mak″ren-sef′ah-le) [*macro-* + Gr. *enkephalos* brain] overgrowth of the brain.

macr(o)- [Gr. *makros* large, long] a combining form meaning large, or of abnormal size or length.

macroaggregate (mak″ro-ag′re-gāt) an unusually large aggregate of a substance.

macroaleuriospore (mak″ro-ah-lu′re-o-spōr) a large, usually multicellular, aleuriospore; sometimes used interchangeably with macrocondium.

macroamylase (mak″ro-am′ĭ-lās) serum amylase bound to a globulin. Because the complex formed (M.W. 200,000) is too large for renal clearance, its formation results in elevated levels of plasma amylase.

macroamylasemia (mak″ro-am″il-ah-se′me-ah) the presence of macroamylase in the blood.

macroamylasemic (mak″ro-am″il-ah-se′mik) pertaining to or characterized by macroamylasemia.

macroanalysis (mak″ro-ah-nal′ĭ-sis) chemical analysis using 0.1 to 0.2 gm. of the substance under study.

Macrobdella (mak″ro-del′ah) a genus of leeches of the family Gnathobdellidae. **M. deco′ra,** the American leech, a small species widely distributed in United States and Canada, which is sometimes used in drawing blood.

macrobiota (mak″ro-bi-o′tah) the macroscopic living organisms of a region; the combined macroflora and macro-fauna of a region.

macrobiotic (mak″ro-bi-ot′ik) pertaining to the macrobi-ota, or to macroscopic living organisms.

macroblast (mak′ro-blast) [*macro-* + Gr. *blastos* germ] an abnormally large nucleated red blood cell; a large young normoblast with megaloblastic features. **m. of Naegeli,** proerythroblast.

macroblepharia (mak″ro-blĕ-fa′re-ah) [*macro-* + Gr. *blepharon* eyelid] abnormal largeness of the eyelid.

macrobrachia (mak″ro-bra′ke-ah) [*macro-* + Gr. *brachiōn* arm] abnormal size or length of the arms.

macrocardius (mak″ro-kar′de-us) [*macro-* + Gr. *kardia* heart] a monster with an extremely large heart.

macrocephalia (mak″ro-sĕ-fa′le-ah) macrocephaly.

macrocephalic (mak″ro-se-fal′ik) macrocephalous.

macrocephalous (mak″ro-sef′ah-lus) having an excessively large head.

macrocephalus (mak″ro-sef′ah-lus) megalocephaly.

macrocephaly (mak″ro-sef′ah-le) [*macro-* + Gr. *kephalē* head] excessive size of the head.

macrocheilia (mak″ro-ki′le-ah) [*macro-* + Gr. *cheilos* lip + *-ia*] excessive size of the lips.

macrocheiria (mak″ro-ki′re-ah) [*macro-* + Gr. *cheir* hand + *-ia*] excessive size of the hands.

macrochemical (mak″ro-kem′ĕ-kal) pertaining to macrochemistry.

macrochemistry (mak″ro-kem′is-tre) [*macro-* + *chemistry*] chemistry in which the reactions may be seen with the naked eye. Cf. *microchemistry.*

macrochilia (mak″ro-ki′le-ah) macrocheilia.

macrochiria (mak″ro-ki′re-ah) macrocheiria.

macroclitoris (mak″ro-klit′o-ris) hypertrophy of the clitoris.

macrocnemia (mak″rok-ne′me-ah) [*macro-* + Gr. *knēmē* shin + *-ia*] a condition in which the legs are abnormally large below the knee.

macrocolon (mak″ro-ko′lon) megacolon.

macroconidium (mak″ro-ko-nid′e-um), pl. *macroconidia* [*macro-* + *conidium*] a large, frequently multicelled conidium or exospore; sometimes used interchangeably with macroaleuriospore; see *spore.*

macrocornea (mak″ro-kor′ne-ah) [*macro-* + *cornea*] megalocornea.

macrocrania (mak″ro-kra′ne-ah) abnormal increase in the size of the skull, the facial area being disproportionately small in comparison.

macrocyst (mak′ro-sist) [*macro-* + *cyst*] 1. a large cyst. 2. in mycology, a large spore case; an encysted reproductive cell of certain slime molds. Cf. *microcyst.*

macrocytase (mak″ro-si′tās) a term used by Metchnikoff to describe the proteolytic activity of macrophages.

macrocyte (mak′ro-sīt) [*macro-* + *-cyte*] an abnormally large erythrocyte, i.e., one from 10 to 12 microns in diameter. Cf. *megalocyte* and *gigantocyte.*

macrocytic (mak″ro-sit′ik) pertaining to macrocytes.

macrocythemia (mak″ro-si-the′me-ah) [*macrocyte* + Gr. *haima* blood + *-ia*] a condition in which the erythrocytes are larger than normal.

macrocytosis (mak″ro-si-to′sis) macrocythemia.

macrodactylia (mak″ro-dak-til′e-ah) macrodactyly.

macrodactyly (mak″ro-dak′tĭ-le) [*macro-* + Gr. *daktylos* finger] abnormal largeness of the fingers and toes.

Macrodantin (mak″ro-dan′tin) trademark for a preparation of nitrofurantoin.

macrodont (mak′ro-dont) having large teeth; characterized by macrodontia. Called also *megadont.*

macrodontia (mak″-ro-don′she-ah) [*macro-* + Gr. *odous* tooth] a developmental disorder characterized by increase in the size of the teeth; it may affect a single tooth or all of the teeth, or teeth of normal size may appear to be abnormally large in proportion to abnormally small jaws. Called also *macrodontism, megadontia,* and *megalodontia.*

macrodontic (mak″ro-don′tik) pertaining to or characterized by macrodontia.

macrodontism (mak″ro-don′tizm) macrodontia.

macrodystrophia (mak″ro-dis-tro′fe-ah) [*macro-* + *dys-* + *trophē* nutrition] overgrowth of a part. **m. lipomato′sa progressi′va,** partial gigantism associated with tumor-like overgrowth of adipose tissue.

macroelement (mak″ro-el′ĕ-ment) a chemical element, such as sodium or potassium, that is essential in nutrition and is distributed throughout the tissues in relatively large amounts, as opposed to trace elements.

macroencephaly (mak″ro-en-sef′ah-le) macrencephaly.

macroerythroblast (mak″ro-ĕ-rith′ro-blast) macroblast.

macroesthesia (mak″ro-es-the′ze-ah) [*macro-* + Gr. *aisthēsis* perception + *-ia*] a sensory impression that all things are larger than they really are.

macrofauna (mak″ro-faw′nah) the animal life, visible to the naked eye, which is present in or characteristic of a special location.

macroflora (mak″ro-flo′rah) the plant life, visible to the naked eye, which is present in or characteristic of a special location.

macrogamete (mak″ro-gam′ēt) [*macro-* + *gamete*] the larger, less active female anisogamete.

macrogametocyte (mak″ro-gah-me′to-sīt) [*macro-* + *gametocyte*] macrogamont.

macrogamont (mak″ro-gam′ont) [*macro-* + *gamont*] a gamont that will produce or become a macrogamete. Called also *macrogametocyte.*

macrogastria (mak″ro-gas′tre-ah) [*macro-* + Gr. *gastēr* stomach + *-ia*] (obs.) dilatation of the stomach.

macrogenia (mak″ro-jen′e-ah) [*macro-* + Gr. *genys* jaw] enlargement of the jaw, especially the chin, which may involve only the osseous or soft-tissue components or both the bony and soft tissues.

macrogenitosomia (mak″ro-jen″ĭ-to-so′me-ah) [*macro-* + *genito-* + Gr. *sōma* body + *-ia*] excessive bodily development, with unusual enlargement of the genital organs. **m. pre′cox,** epiphyseal syndrome.

macrogingivae (mak″ro-jin-ji′ve) fibromatosis gingivae.

macroglia (mak-rog′le-ah) neuroglial cells of ectodermal origin, i.e., the astrocytes and oligodendrocytes considered together. Originally, the term was used synonymously with astroglia.

macroglobulin (mak″ro-glob′u-lin) [*macro-* + *globulin*] a plasma globulin with high molecular weight; alpha$_2$-macroglobulin or the IgM M component of Waldenström's macroglobulinemia. α_2**-m.,** see *alpha$_2$-macroglobulin.*

macroglobulinemia (mak″ro-glob′u-lĭ-ne′me-ah) [*macroglobulin* + *-emia*] a condition characterized by increase in macroglobulins in the blood. **Waldenström's m.,** a malignant neoplasm of cells with lymphocytic, plasmacytic, or intermediate morphology, which secrete an IgM M component. There is diffuse infiltration of bone marrow and in many cases also of the spleen, liver, or lymph nodes. The circulating macroglobulin produces symptoms of hyperviscosity syndrome: weakness, fatigue, bleeding disorders, and visual disturbances; peak incidence is in the sixth and seventh decades.

macroglossia (mak″ro-glos′e-ah) [*macro-* + Gr. *glōssa* tongue + *-ia*] excessive size of the tongue.

macrognathia (mak″ro-na′the-ah) [*macro-* + Gr. *gnathos* jaw + *-ia*] a condition characterized by abnormally large jaws. See also *prognathism* and *maxillary protrusion,* under *protrusion.*

macrogol (mak′ro-gol) polyethylene glycol.

macrographia (mak″ro-gra′fe-ah) macrography.

macrography (mak-rog′rah-fe) [*macro-* + Gr. *graphein* to write] the formation in writing of letters that are larger than the normal writing of the individual.

macrogyria (mak″ro-ji′re-ah) [*macro-* + *gyrus*] moderate reduction in the number of sulci of the cerebrum, sometimes with increase in the brain substance, resulting in excessive size of the gyri.

macrolabia (mak″ro-la′be-ah) [*macro-* + L. *labium* lip] macrocheilia.

macrolecithal (mak″ro-les′ĭ-thal) [*macro-* + Gr. *lekithos* yolk] having a large amount of yolk; see under *ovum.*

macroleukoblast (mak″ro-lu′ko-blast) a large leukoblast.

macrolide (mak′ro-līd) 1. a chemical compound characterized by a large lactone ring containing multiple keto and hydroxyl groups. 2. any of a group of antibacterial antibiotics (e.g., erythromycin or oleandomycin) containing a macrolide ring linked glycosidically to one or more sugars. Macrolides are produced by certain species of *Streptomyces* and inhibit protein synthesis by binding to the 50S subunits of 70S ribosomes.

macrolymphocyte (mak″ro-lim′fo-sīt) a large lymphocyte.

macrolymphocytosis (mak-ro-lim″fo-si-to′sis) the presence of an increased number of large lymphocytes.

macromastia (mak″ro-mas′te-ah) [*macro-* + Gr. *mastos* breast + *-ia*] oversize of the breasts or mammae.

macromazia (mak″ro-ma′ze-ah) [*macro-* + Gr. *mazos* breast + *-ia*] macromastia.

macromelia (mak″ro-me′le-ah) enlargement of one or more limbs.

macromelus (mak-rom′e-lus) [*macro-* + Gr. *melos* limb] a fetus with abnormally large or long limbs.

macromere (mak′ro-mēr) [*macro-* + Gr. *meros* part] one of the large blastomeres formed by unequal cleavage of a fertilized ovum, located in the vegetal hemisphere and dividing less rapidly than the micromeres of the animal hemisphere.

macromethod (mak′ro-meth″od) a chemical method in which the substance to be analyzed is used in customary (not minute) quantity. Cf. *micromethod.*

macromolecular (mak″ro-mo-lek′u-lar) having large molecules; pertaining to macromolecules.

macromolecule (mak″ro-mol′ĕ-kūl) a very large molecule having a polymeric chain structure, as in proteins, polysaccharides, and other natural and synthetic polymers.

Macromonas (mak″ro-mo′nas) [*macro-* + Gr. *monas* unit, from *monos* single] a genus of gram-negative chemolithotrophic bacteria of uncertain affiliation, occurring as cylindrical cells that oxidize sulfur compounds and contain sulfur granules. They are found in fresh waters with a low oxygen concentration. The type species is *M. mo′bilis.*

macromonocyte (mak″ro-mon′o-sīt) a very large monocyte.

macromyeloblast (mak″ro-mi′ĕ-lo-blast) a large myeloblast.

macronodular (mak″ro-nod′u-lar) characterized by large nodules.

macronormoblast (mak″ro-nor′mo-blast) a very large nucleated red blood corpuscle; macroblast.

macronucleus (mak″ro-nu′kle-us) [*macro-* + *nucleus*] 1. the larger of two types of nuclei when more than one is present in a cell. 2. in ciliate protozoa, the transcriptively active, polyploid nucleus, much larger than the micronucleus, that governs the organism's vegetative processes and is responsible for its phenotype. Called also *meganucleus, trophic nucleus,* and *trophonucleus.*

macronychia (mak″ro-nik′e-ah) [*macro-* + Gr. *onyx* nail + *-ia*] megalonychia.

macro-orchidism (mak-ro-or′kĭ-dizm) [*macro-* + Gr. *orchis* testicle] abnormal enlargement of the testis.

macropathology (mak″ro-pah-thol′o-je) [*macro-* + *pathology*] the nonmicroscopical pathologic account of any disease or organ.

macrophage (mak′ro-fāj) [*macro-* + Gr. *phagein* to eat] any of the many forms of mononuclear phagocytes found in tissues. Mononuclear phagocytes arise from hematopoietic stem cells in the bone marrow. After passing through the monoblast and promonocyte stages to the monocyte stage, they enter the blood, circulating for about 40 hours. They then enter tissues and increase in size, phagocytic activity, and lysosomal enzyme content and become macrophages. The morphology of macrophages varies among different tissues and between normal and pathologic states, and not all macrophages can be identified by morphology alone. However, most macrophages are large cells with a round or indented nucleus, a well-developed Golgi apparatus, abundant endocytotic vacuoles, lysosomes, and phagolysosomes, and a plasma membrane covered with ruffles or microvilli. Among the functions of macrophages are nonspecific phagocytosis and pinocytosis, specific phagocytosis of opsonized microorganisms mediated by Fc receptors and complement

receptors, killing of ingested microorganisms, digestion and presentation of antigens to T and B lymphocytes, and secretion of a large number of diverse products, including many enzymes (lysozyme, collagenases, elastase, acid hydrolases), several complement components and coagulation factors, some prostaglandins and leukotrienes, and several regulatory molecules (interferon, interleukin-1). Among the cells now recognized as macrophages are histiocytes, Kupffer cells, osteoclasts, microglial cells, synovial type A cells, interdigitating cells, and Langerhans cells (in normal tissues) and epithelioid cells and Langerhans-type and foreign-body-type multinucleated giant cells (in inflamed tissues). **alveolar m.,** one of the rounded, granular, mononuclear phagocytes within the alveoli of the lungs that ingest inhaled particulate matter; called also *alveolar phagocyte* and *dust cell.* **armed m.'s,** those capable of inducing cytotoxicity as a consequence of antigen-binding by cytophilic antibodies on their surfaces or by factors derived from T lymphocytes. **fixed m.,** a quiescent, sessile macrophage similar to a fibroblast in morphology, found in the lymph nodes, spleen, bone marrow, and connective tissue (where it is called a histiocyte). **free m.,** an actively motile macrophage, usually having an ameboid shape and highly ruffled surface, found at sites of inflammation. **inflammatory m.,** free m.

macrophagocyte (mak″ro-fag′o-sīt) a phagocyte of relatively large size.

macrophagus (mak″ro-fal′ah-gus) macrophage.

macrophallus (mak″ro-fal′us) [*macro-* + Gr. *phallos* penis] abnormal largeness of the penis.

macrophthalmia (mak″rof-thal′me-ah) [*macro-* + Gr. *ophthalmos* eye + *-ia*] abnormal enlargement of the eyeball.

macrophthalmous (mak″rof-thal′mus) having abnormally large eyes.

macroplasia (mak″ro-pla′ze-ah) [*macro-* + Gr. *plasis* forming + *-ia*] excessive growth of a part or tissue.

macroplastia (mak″ro-plas′te-ah) macroplasia.

macropodia (mak″ro-po′de-ah) [*macro-* + Gr. *pous* foot + *-ia*] excessive size of the feet.

macropolycyte (mak″ro-pol′e-sīt) a hypersegmented polymorphonuclear leukocyte of greater than normal size. Cf. *polycyte.*

macroprolactinoma (mak″ro-pro-lak″tĭ-no′mah) a prolactin-secreting pituitary adenoma of more than 10 mm in diameter and usually associated with serum prolactin levels exceeding 500 ng per milliliter.

macropromyelocyte (mak″ro-pro-mi′ĕ-lo-sīt) a very large promyelocyte.

macroprosopia (mak″ro-pro-so′pe-ah) [*macro-* + Gr. *prosōpon* face + *-ia*] excessive size of the face.

macropsia (mah-krop′se-ah) [*macro-* + *-opsia*] an illusion in which objects are seen as larger than they actually are.

macrorhinia (mak″ro-rin′e-ah) [*macro-* + Gr. *rhis* nose + *-ia*] excessive size of the nose.

macroscelia (mak″ro-se′le-ah) [*macro-* + Gr. *skelos* leg + *-ia*] excessive size of the legs.

macroscopic (mak″ro-skop′ik) [*macro-* + Gr. *skopein* to examine] visible with the unaided eye or without the microscope.

macroscopical (mak″ro-skop′e-kal) 1. pertaining to macroscopy. 2. macroscopic.

macroscopy (mah-kros′ko-pe) examination with the naked eye.

macrosigmoid (mak″ro-sig′moid) [*macro-* + *sigmoid*] abnormal enlargement of the sigmoid.

macrosis (mah-kro′sis) [*macro-* + *-osis*] increase in size.

macrosmatic (mak″ros-mat′ik) [*macro-* + Gr. *osmasthai* to smell] having the sense of smell strongly or acutely developed.

macrosomatia (mak″ro-so-ma′she-ah) [*macro-* + Gr. *sōma* body] great bodily size. **m. adipo′sa congen′ita,** an obese type of premature development probably dependent on hyperfunction of the adrenal cortex.

macrosomia (mak″ro-so′me-ah) macrosomatia.

macrospore (mak′ro-spōr) [*macro-* + Gr. *sporos* seed] 1. the larger spore form when spores of two sizes are present, as in certain fungi and protozoa. 2. megaspore.

macrostereognosia (mak″ro-ste″re-o-no′se-ah) [*macro-* +

Gr. *stereos* solid + *gnōsis* knowledge + *-ia*] abnormality of perception in which objects felt seem larger than they really are.

macrostomia (mak″ro-sto′me-ah) [*macro-* + Gr. *stoma* mouth + *-ia*] greatly exaggerated width of the mouth, resulting from failure of union of the maxillary and mandibular processes, with extension of the oral orifice toward the ear. The defect may be unilateral or bilateral.

macrostructural (mak″ro-struk′tūr-al) pertaining to gross structure.

macrotia (mak-ro′she-ah) [*macro-* + Gr. *ous* ear] abnormal enlargement of the pinna of the ear.

macrotome (mak′ro-tōm) [*macro-* + Gr. *tomē* cut] an apparatus for cutting large sections of tissue for anatomical study.

macrotooth (mak′ro-tōōth), pl. *macroteeth.* An abnormally large tooth.

macula (mak′u-lah), gen. and pl. *mac′ulae* [L.] 1. a stain, spot, or thickening; [NA] a general term for an area distinguishable by color or otherwise from its surroundings. Often used alone to refer to the macula retinae. 2. a macule: a discolored spot on the skin that is not elevated above the surface. 3. a moderately dense scar of the cornea that can be seen without special optical aids, appreciated as a gray spot intermediate between a nebula and a leukoma. **acoustic maculae, mac′ulae acus′ticae,** see *m. sacculi* and *m. utriculi.* **m. acus′tica sac′culi,** m. sacculi. **m. acus′tica utric′uli,** m. utriculi. **m. adher′ens,** desmosome. **mac′ulae al′bidae,** white spots sometimes seen after death on the serous layer of the peritoneum. **mac′ulae atroph′icae,** white patches resembling scars formed on the skin by atrophy. **mac′ulae ceru′leae,** small grayish blue stainlike, nonpruritic macules located chiefly on the chest, abdomen, thighs, and upper arms in pediculosis pubis, which are especially noticeable in light-skinned individuals. They are probably due to altered blood pigments in infested individuals, or to an excretion product in the louse's saliva that converts bilirubin to biliverdin. Called also *taches bleuâtres.* **cerebral m.,** tache cérébrale. **m. commu′nis,** a thickened area on the wall of the otic vesicle which divides into the macula sacculi and macula utriculi. **mac′ulae cribro′sae** [NA], see *m. cribrosa inferior, m. cribrosa media,* and *m. cribrosa superior.* **m. cribro′sa infe′rior** [NA], the perforated area on the wall of the vestibule through which branches of the vestibulocochlear nerve pass to the posterior semicircular canal. **m. cribro′sa me′dia** [NA], the perforated area on the vestibular wall through which branches of the vestibulocochlear nerve pass to the sacculus. **m. cribro′sa supe′rior** [NA], the perforated area on the vestibular wall through which branches of the vestibulocochlear nerve pass to the utricle and to the anterior and lateral semicircular canals. **m. den′sa,** a zone of compact, heavily nucleated cells, located in the distal renal tubule where it makes contact with the vascular pole of the glomerulus, and closely associated anatomically with the juxtaglomerular cells of the afferent arteriole. **false m.,** the extramacular point on the retina of a squinting eye which receives the same light stimulus as the macula of the fixing eye. **m. fla′va laryn′gis,** a yellowish nodule visible at one end of a vocal cord. **m. fla′va re′tinae,** m. retinae. **m. follic′uli,** follicular stigma. **m. germinati′va,** germinal area. **m. gonorrhoe′ica,** the red, inflamed orifice of the duct of Bartholin's gland in gonorrheal vulvitis; called also *Saenger's m.* **mac′ulae lac′teae,** maculae albidae. **m. lu′tea re′tinae,** m. retinae. **maculae of membranous labyrinth,** see *m. sacculi* and *m. utriculi.* **mongolian m.,** see under *spot.* **m. re′tinae** [NA], an irregular yellowish depression on the retina, about 3 degrees wide, lateral to and slightly below the optic disk; it is the site of absorption of short wavelengths of light, and it is thought that its variation in size, shape, and coloring may be related to variant types of color vision. Called also *m. flava retinae* and *m. lutea retinae.* **m. sac′culi** [NA], a thickening in the wall of the saccule where the epithelium contains hair cells that are stimulated by linear acceleration and deceleration and gravity. The *m. sacculi* and *m. utriculi* together are called *maculae acusticae* or *acoustic maculae.* **Saenger's m.,** m. gonorrhoeica. **mac′ulae tendin′eae,** maculae albidae. **m. utric′uli** [NA], a thickening in the wall of the utricle where the epithelium contains hair cells that are stimulated by linear acceleration and deceleration and

gravity. The *macula sacculi* and the *macula utriculi* together are called *maculae acusticae* or *acoustic maculae.*

maculae (mak′u-le) [L.] genitive and plural of *macula.*

macular (mak′u-lar) pertaining to or characterized by the presence of macules; pertaining to the macula retinae.

maculate (mak′u-lāt) [L. *maculatus* spotted] macular.

macule (mak′ūl) a macula.

maculocerebral (mak″u-lo-ser′e-bral) pertaining to the macula retinae and the brain.

maculopapular (mak″u-lo-pap′u-lar) both macular and papular, as an eruption consisting of both macules and papules; sometimes erroneously used to designate a papule that is only slightly elevated.

maculovesicular (mak″u-lo-vĕ-sik′u-lar) both macular and vesicular.

MacWilliam's test (mak-wil′yamz) [John Alexander *MacWilliam,* British physician, 1857–1937] see under *tests.*

mad (mad) 1. insane. 2. rabid.

madarosis (mad″ah-ro′sis) [Gr. *madaros* bald] loss of the eyelashes or eyebrows. Cf. milphosis.

madder (mad′er) the root of *Rubia tinctoria* L. (Rubiaceae) affording a red dye, mainly alizarin and purpurin.

Maddox prism, rods (mad′oks) [Ernest Edmund *Maddox,* English ophthalmologist, 1860–1933] see under *prism* and *rod.*

Madelung's deformity, neck [Otto Wilhelm *Madelung,* surgeon in Strasbourg, 1846–1926] see under *deformity* and *neck.*

Madurella (mad″u-rel′ah) a genus of imperfect fungi of the family Dematiaceae. *M. gris′ea* and *M. mycetomatis* (*mycetomi*) are etiologic agents of eumycotic mycetoma.

maduromycosis (mah-du″ro-mi-ko′sis) a chronic disease caused by a variety of fungi (e.g., *Madurella mycetomi*) or actinomycetes (e.g., *Nocardia brasiliensis, Streptomyces madurae,* and others), affecting the foot, hands, legs, or other parts, including the internal organs. The most common form is that of the foot, known as *Madura foot.* Following infection through a penetrating wound, the deep tissues become necrosed, sinuses form, and there is marked swelling of the part, in which nodules and vesicles develop. Sinuses discharge pus and penetrate into the bone. The pus contains red, black, or yellow granules which are composed of mycelial filaments of the infecting organism.

maedi (mi′theh) a chronic progressive pulmonary disease of sheep in Iceland, caused by a virus.

MAF macrophage activating factor.

mafenide (maf′en-īd) chemical name: 4-(aminomethyl)-benzenesulfonamide. An antibacterial homologue of sulfanilamide, $C_7H_{10}N_2O_2S$, active against many gram-positive and gram-negative organisms. **m. acetate** [USP], the monoacetate salt of mafenide, $C_7H_{10}N_2O_2S \cdot C_2H_4O_2$, occurring as a white, crystalline powder, having the same antibacterial activity as the base; used as a topical anti-infective for adjunctive therapy of patients with second- and third-degree burns. **m. hydrochloride,** the hydrochloride salt of mafenide, $C_7H_{10}N_2O_2S \cdot HCl$, having antibacterial activity similar to that of the acetate salt; used as a topical anti-infective.

Maffucci's syndrome (mah-fu′chēz) [Angelo *Maffucci,* Italian physician, 1845–1903] see under *syndrome.*

mafilcon A (mah-fil′kon) a hydrophilic contact lens material.

Mag. abbreviation for L. *mag′nus,* large.

magaldrate (mag′al-drāt) [USP] chemical name: aluminum magnesium hydroxide. A chemical combination of aluminum hydroxide and magnesium hydroxide, corresponding approximately to the formula $Al_2H_{14}Mg_4O_{14} \cdot 2H_2O$; used as an oral antacid.

Magan (mag′an) trademark for magnesium salicylate.

magenblase (mah″gen-blah′zĕ) [Ger. "stomach bubble"] in the radiograph of the stomach, a dark area above the light shadow of the opaque meal, marking a collection of gas in the upper part of the stomach.

Magendie's foramen, etc. (ma-jen′dēz) [François *Magendie,* French physiologist, 1783–1855; the pioneer of experimental physiology in France] see under *foramen, law, solution, space,* and *symptom* (*sign*).

Magendie-Hertwig sign (ma-jen′de-hert′vig) [François *Magendie;* Richard *Hertwig,* German zoologist, 1850–1937] skew deviation.

magenstrasse (mah″gen-stras′sĕ) [Ger. "stomach street"] canalis gastricus.

magenta (mah-jen′tah) basic fuchsin. **acid m.,** acid fuchsin. **basic m.,** basic fuchsin. **m. O,** pararosanilin. **m. I,** rosanilin. **m. II,** triaminoditolyphenylmethane chloride, a component of basic fuchsin. **m. III,** new fuchsin.

maggot (mag′ot) a soft-bodied larva of an insect, especially a form living in decaying flesh. The living maggots of the greenbottle fly (*Phaenicia sericata*) and the blackbottle fly (*Phormia regina*) have been used in the treatment of osteomyelitis and other suppurative infections in order to clear away dead tissue and promote healing, this latter effect being due to the allantoin in the secretions of the maggots. **Congo floor m.,** *Auchmeromyia luteola.* **rat-tail m.,** a maggot of a hover-fly of the genera *Eristalis* and *Helophilus;* they cause intestinal and nasal myiasis. **sheep m.,** the maggot of *Phaenicia sericata* and other species of the family Calliphoridae, which invade the tissue of sheep in the British Isles and elsewhere.

magistery (maj′is-ter″e) [L. *magisterium; magister* master] a precipitate; any subtle or masterly preparation.

magistral (maj′is-tral) [L. *magister* master] pertaining to a master; applied to medicines that are prepared in accordance with a physician's prescription.

magma (mag′mah) [Gr. *massein* to knead] 1. a suspension of finely divided material in a small amount of water. 2. a thin, pastelike substance composed of organic material. **bentonite m.** [NF], a preparation of bentonite and purified water used as a suspending agent. **bismuth m.,** milk of bismuth. **dihydroxyaluminum aminoacetate m.** [USP], a white viscous suspension of dihydroxyaluminum aminoacetate in water, yielding an amount of aluminum oxide equivalent to between 28.5 and 35.0 per cent of the labeled amount of dihydroxyaluminum aminoacetate; used as a gastric antacid. **magnesia m.,** milk of magnesia; see under *milk.* **m. reticula′re,** a mesenchymal reticulum within the early chorionic sac.

Magnacort (mag′nah-kort) trademark for a preparation of hydrocortamate.

Magnan's movement, symptom (sign) (mag′nanz) [Valentin Jacques Joseph *Magnan,* alienist in Paris, 1835–1916] see under *movement* and *symptom.*

magnesemia (mag″nes-e′me-ah) the presence of an excess of magnesium in the blood.

magnesia (mag-ne′zhe-ah) [the name of a district in ancient Lydia] magnesium oxide. **m. al′ba,** magnesium carbonate. **m. calcina′ta,** magnesium oxide. **m. carbonata′da,** magnesium carbonate. **citrate of m.,** magnesium citrate. **milk of m.,** see under *milk.* **m. us′ta,** magnesium oxide.

magnesium (mag-ne′ze-um), gen. *magne′sii* [L.] a light, silvery, metallic element; symbol, Mg; atomic number, 12; atomic weight, 24.312; specific gravity, 1.74. Its salts are essential in nutrition, being required for the activity of many enzymes, especially those concerned with oxidative phosphorylation. It is a component of both intra- and extracellular fluids and is excreted in the urine and feces. The serum level is approximately 2 mEq/liter. Deficiency causes irritability of the nervous system with tetany, vasodilation, convulsions, tremors, depression, and psychotic behavior. **m. aluminum silicate** [NF], a colloidal montmorillonoid saponite, in which magnesium has substantially replaced aluminum in the crystal lattice. It is available in Types IA, IB, IC, IIA, IIIA, and IIIB, which differ in viscosity and ratio of aluminum content to magnesium content. Used as a suspending agent for pharmaceuticals. **m. carbonate** [USP], a basic hydrated magnesium carbonate containing the equivalent of 40 to 43.5 per cent of magnesium oxide, used as an antacid. **m. chloride** [USP], colorless, deliquescent flakes or crystals, $MgCl_2 \cdot 6H_2O$, used as an electrolyte replenisher and as a pharmaceutical necessity for hemodialysis and peritoneal dialysis fluids. **m. citrate,** a white, odorless crystalline powder or granules, $Mg_3(C_6H_5O_7)_2 \cdot 14H_2O$, used in solution as a mild cathartic; called also *citrate of magnesia.* **m. hydroxide** [USP], a bulky white powder, $Mg(OH)_2$, used as an antacid and cathartic. **m. oxide** [USP], a bulky (*light m. oxide*) or relatively dense (*heavy m. oxide*) white powder,

containing, after ignition, at least 96 per cent of MgO; used as a sorbent in pharmaceutical preparations, and as an antacid and laxative. **m. peroxide,** a white powder, MgO_2, insoluble in water, but gradually decomposed with the liberation of oxygen; used as an antacid. **m. phosphate** [USP], a bulky, white powder, $Mg_3(PO_4)_2 \cdot 5H_2O$, used as an antacid. **m. salicylate,** the magnesium salt of salicylic acid, used as an antiarthritic. **m. stearate** [NF], a compound of magnesium with varying proportions of stearic and palmitic acids, used as a tablet lubricant in pharmaceutical preparations. **m. sulfate** [USP], small, colorless crystals, usually needle-like, $MgSO_4 \cdot 7H_2O$, used as an anticonvulsant and electrolyte replenisher, administered intramuscularly and intravenously. It is also used as a cathartic and as a local anti-inflammatory. Called also *Epsom salt.* **m. sulfate, exsiccated,** hydrated magnesium sulfate the weight of which has been reduced 25 per cent by drying at 100° C.: an aperient. **m. trisilicate** [USP], a compound of magnesium oxide and silicon dioxide with varying proportions of water, used as a pharmaceutic necessity and antacid.

magnet (mag′net) [L. *magnes;* Gr. *magnēs* magnet] a lodestone; native iron oxide that attracts iron; also a bar of steel or iron that attracts iron and has magnetic polarity. **denture m.,** a magnet made of a nonreactogenic platinum-cobalt alloy or a rare earth element, used for additional retention of dentures. One magnet is implanted into the mandible under the periosteum and the other is attached to the denture, its poles being opposite of those in the mandible. Called also *magnetic implant.* **Grüning's m.,** one made up of a number of steel rods; used in removing metal particles from the eye. **Haab's m.,** a powerful magnet for extracting foreign metallic bodies from the eye. **Hirschberg's m.,** an electromagnet for removing particles of iron from the eye. **permanent m.,** one with permanent magnetic qualities. **temporary m.,** a substance that possesses magnetic properties only during the passage of an electric current or when a permanent magnet is near it.

magnetic (mag-net′ik) pertaining to, derived from, or having the properties of a magnet.

magnetism (mag′nĕ-tizm) magnetic attraction or repulsion. **animal m.,** a hypothetical force or power alleged by Mesmer to be transmitted to his subjects undergoing therapeutic hypnosis. Cf. *mesmerism.*

magnetization (mag″net-i-za′shun) the act or process of rendering an object or substance magnetic.

magnetocardiograph (mag-ne″to-kar′de-o-graf) a cardiograph that generates electrical signals proportional to magnetic pulses emanating from electrical activity in the heart.

magnetoconstriction (mag-ne″to-kon-strik′shun) a change in the dimensions of a body produced by the application of a magnetic field.

magnetoelectricity (mag-ne″to-e″lek-tris′ĭ-te) electricity induced by means of a magnet.

magnetoencephalograph (mag-ne″to-en-sef′ah-lo-graf) an instrument for recording magnetic signals proportional to electroencephalographic waves emanating from electrical activity in the brain.

magnetoinduction (mag-ne″to-in-duk′shun) magnetic induction.

magnetology (mag″nĕ-tol′o-je) that branch of physics which treats of magnetics.

magnetometer (mag″nĕ-tom′ĕ-ter) [*magnetic* + Gr. *metron* measure] an apparatus for measuring magnetic forces.

magneton (mag′nĕ-ton) an ultimate elemental magnetic particle.

magnetotherapy (mag-ne″to-ther′ah-pe) the treatment of disease by magnets or by magnetism.

magnetron (mag′nĕ-tron) an electric vacuum tube for generating extremely short electromagnetic waves (microwaves).

magnetropism (mag-net′ro-pizm) [*magnet* + Gr. *tropē* a turn, turning] a growth response in a nonmotile organism under the influence of a magnet.

magnicellular (mag″nĭ-sel′u-lar) composed of large cells, as opposed to parvicellular.

magnification (mag″nĭ-fi-ka′shun) [L. *magnificatio; magnus* great + *facere* to make] 1. apparent increase in size as under the microscope. 2. the process of making something appear larger, as by use of lenses. 3. the ratio of apparent (image) size to real size.

magnify (mag′nĭ-fi) to cause to appear larger by the use of lenses or suitable mirrors.

magnocellular (mag″no-sel′u-lar) magnicellular.

Magnolia (mag-no′le-ah) [after Pierre *Magnol*, 1638–1715] a genus of magnoliaceous trees.

magnolia (mag-no′le-ah) the bitter aromatic bark of *Magnolia acuminata* L., *M. glauca* L., and *M. tripetala* (Magnoliaceae), once used as a diaphoretic and antifebrile in southern United States.

magnum (mag′num) [L.] great; the os magnum (os capitatum [NA]).

Maher's disease (ma′herz) [James J. E. *Maher*, New York physician, 1857–1931] paracolpitis.

Mahler's sign (mah′lerz) [Richter A. *Mahler*, German obstetrician, 1863–1941] see under *sign*.

ma huang (mah hoo-ang′) the native name for various species of *Ephedra*, including *E. sinica* Stapf., *E. equisetina* Bunge, and *E. vulgaris*, whose stems and leaves furnish ephedrine; used as an herb in parts of Asia, e.g., China.

Maier's sinus (mi′erz) [Rudolf *Maier*, German physician 1824–1888] see under *sinus*.

maim (mām) 1. to disable by a wound; to dismember by violence. 2. a dismemberment or disablement effected by violence.

Maimonides (mi-mon′ĭ-dēz) [Moses ben Maimon, 1135–1204] rabbi, physician, and the greatest of the Jewish philosophers, born in Cordova, Spain. He was the physician to Saladin, under whom he wrote many medical works in Arabic, among them a commentary on the aphorisms of Hippocrates and treatises on asthma, diet, poisons, and hygiene. A prayer attributed to him is considered to rank beside the oath of Hippocrates as an ethical guide to the medical profession.

main (mān) [Fr.] hand. **m. d'accoucheur** (mān″dak-oo-shuhr′), obstetrician's hand; see under *hand*. **m. de tranchées** (mān″dŭ-tran-sha′), trench hand. **m. en crochet** (ma″nong-kro-sha′), a permanently flexed condition of the third and fourth fingers. **m. en griffe** (ma″-nong-grif′), clawhand. **m. en lorgnette** (ma″nong-lor-nyet′), opera-glass hand. **m. en pince** (ma″nong-pins′), cleft hand. **m. en singe** (ma″nong-sēnzh′), monkey hand. **m. en squelette** (ma″nong-skel-et′), skeleton hand. **m. fourché** (mān″foor-sha′), cleft hand. **m. succulente** (mān″suk-u-lent′), a soft, swollen, cyanotic, and cold hand caused by thickening and edema of the subcutaneous tissues; seen in syringomyelia. Called also *Marinesco's sign* or *succulent hand*. See also *Morvan's syndrome* (def. 2), under *syndrome*.

Mainini (mi-ne′ne) see *Galli Mainini*.

maintainer (mān-tān′er) something that keeps or maintains in another thing existence or continuancy. **space m.,** 1. an orthodontic appliance, fixed or removable, used for maintaining the space created by a prematurely lost tooth or the space to be filled by a tooth still to be erupted. See also under *regainer* and *retainer*. 2. separator, def. 2.

maisin (ma′zin) a protein found in the seeds of maize.

Maisonneuve's amputation, bandage, urethrotome (ma″zo-nevz′) [Jules Germain François *Maisonneuve*, French surgeon, 1809–1897] see under *amputation, bandage,* and *urethrotome*.

Maissiat's band (ligament, tract) (ma″se-ahz′) [Jacques Henri *Maissiat*, French anatomist, 1805–1878] tractus iliotibialis.

maize (māz) [L. *mais* maize] Indian corn; a cereal grain, the seed of *Zea mays*.

maizenate (ma′zen-āt) any salt of maizenic acid.

Majocchi's disease (purpura) (mah-yok′ēz) [Domenico *Majocchi*, Italian physician, 1849–1929] purpura annularis telangiectodes.

majoon (mah-joon′) see *ganja*.

makr(o)- for words thus beginning, see those beginning *macr(o)-*.

mal (mahl) [Fr.; L. *malum* ill] disease. **m. de caderas,** 1. a fatal wasting trypanosomiasis associated with weakness, especially of the hindquarters, affecting chiefly South American horses, which is caused by *Trypanosoma equinum*, and transmitted by tabanid flies. 2. a fatal paralytic viral disease affecting South American cattle, caused by the rabies virus, and transmitted by vampire bats. **m. de Cayenne,** elephantiasis. **m. comitial,** epilepsy. **grand m.,** see under *epilepsy*. **haut m.,** grand mal epilepsy. **m. de Meleda,** a chronic, autosomal recessive form of palmoplantar keratoderma occurring in the inhabitants of the island of Meleda off the coast of Dalmatia, Yugoslavia, and also found elsewhere, in which the hyperkeratosis spreads to involve the dorsal aspects of the hands and feet and other areas of the body, and is manifested by erythematous, scaling, malodorous cutaneous lesions that may cause deep fissuring. Called also *Meleda disease*. **m. de mer,** seasickness. **m. morado,** a cutaneous manifestation of onchocerciasis seen in Central America in which the skin has a blue or reddish mauve discoloration, especially on the trunk and upper limbs. **petit m.,** see under *epilepsy*. **m. del pinto,** pinta. **m. rouge,** a syndrome occurring after inhalation or ingestion of calcium cyanamide followed by drinking an alcoholic beverage, marked by intense flushing, rapid pulse and pounding heart, panting respiration, and perception of the taste and smell of acetaldehyde in the exhaled breath, which may be followed by nausea, vomiting, and a precipitous fall in blood pressure; the extent and severity of the symptoms depend on the amount of calcium cyanamide and alcohol in the system. The reactions are due to the inhibition by calcium cyanamide of one or more of the enzymes required for oxidation of acetaldehyde formed from alcohol, resulting in the accumulation of acetaldehyde and the altered vascular reaction to it. A similar syndrome, also due to accumulation of acetaldehyde, occurs on ingestion of disulfiram followed by drinking an alcoholic beverage, but in addition there are impaired taste, unpleasant breath and perspiration, and lessened sexual potency.

mala (ma′lah) [L.] 1. NA alternative for *bucca*, or cheek. 2. the cheek bone.

malabsorption (mal″ab-sorp′shun) impaired intestinal absorption of nutrients; see also under *syndrome*. **congenital lactose m.,** disaccharide intolerance II. **glucose-galactose m., familial,** a disorder of transport clinically identical to disaccharide intolerance but produced by deficient intestinal monosaccharidase. **sucrose-isomaltose m., congenital,** disaccharide intolerance I.

Malacarne's pyramid, space (antrum) (mal″ah-kar′näz) [Michele Vincenzo Giacintos *Malacarne*, Italian surgeon, 1744–1816] see *substantia perforata posterior,* and see under *pyramid*.

malacia (mah-la′she-ah) [Gr. *malakia*] 1. the morbid softening or softness of a part or tissue. Also used with combining forms to denote specific conditions, as osteomalacia. 2. craving for highly spiced food and dishes, as pickles, salads, mustard, etc. **metaplastic m.,** osteitis fibrosa cystica. **myeloplastic m.,** osteogenesis imperfecta. **porotic m.,** softening accompanied by proliferation of connective tissue. **m. traumat′ica,** Kienböck's disease (def. 2.).

malacic (mah-la′sik) marked by malacia or morbid softness.

malac(o)- [Gr. *malakos* soft] a combining form denoting a condition of abnormal softness.

malacoma (mal″ah-ko′mah) [*malaco-* + *-oma*] a morbidly soft part or spot.

malacoplakia (mal″ah-ko-pla′ke-ah) [*malaco-* + Gr. *plax* plaque] the formation of soft patches on the mucous membrane of a hollow organ. **m. vesi′cae,** a soft, yellowish, fungus-like growth on the mucous membrane of the bladder and ureters.

malacosarcosis (mal″ah-ko-sar-ko′sis) [*malaco-* + Gr. *sarx* flesh] softness of muscular tissue.

malacosis (mal″ah-ko′sis) malacia.

malacosteon (mal″ah-kos′te-on) [*malaco-* + Gr. *osteon* bone] osteomalacia.

malacotic (mal″ah-kot′ik) inclined to malacia; soft; said of teeth.

malactic (mah-lak′tik) 1. softening; emollient. 2. an emollient medicine.

maladie (mal″ah-de′) [Fr.] a disease. **m. des jambes** (da-zhamb′), a disease of rice growers in Louisiana, probably beriberi. **m. de plongeurs** (duh-plon-zher′), inflammation and ulceration in divers in the Mediterranean caused by the stings of sea anemones. **m. de Roger,** Roger's disease. **m. du sommeil** (du-so-ma′e), African trypanosomiasis. **m. des tics,** Gilles de la Tourette syndrome.

maladjustment (mal″ad-just′ment) in psychiatry, failure to fit one's inner needs to the evnironment.

malady (mal′ah-de) [Fr. *maladie*] any disease or illness.

malagma (mah-lag′mah) [Gr.] an emollient or cataplasm.

malaise (mal-āz′) [Fr.] a vague feeling of bodily discomfort.

malakoplakia (mal″ah-ko-pla′ke-ah) malacoplakia.

malalignment (mal″ah-līn′ment) displacement out of line, especially displacement of the teeth from their normal relation to the line of the dental arch. Spelled also *malalinement.* See *malocclusion.*

malalinement (mal″ah-līn′ment) malalignment.

malar (ma′lar) [L. *mala* cheek] pertaining to the cheek or cheek bone.

malaria (mah-la′re-ah) [It. "bad air"] an infectious disease endemic in parts of Africa, Asia, Central and South America, and Oceania, on certain Caribbean islands, and in Turkey, caused by obligate intracellular protozoa of the genus *Plasmodium* (*P. falciparum, P. malariae, P. ovale,* and *P. vivax*), and usually transmitted by the bites of infected anopheline mosquitoes. It is characterized by prostration associated with paroxysms of high fever, shaking chills, sweating, anemia, and splenomegaly, with intervals between the attacks being determined by the time required for the development of a new generation of the parasites in the body. After the initial illness, the disease may follow a chronic or relapsing course. Called also *ague, jungle, malarial, marsh,* and *swamp fever,* and *paludism.* See also *transfusion m.* **algid m.,** a severe complication of falciparum malaria manifested by shock, syncope, peripheral vascular failure, hypotension, cold, clammy skin, and gastrointestinal symptoms, diarrhea, and vomiting, which is sometimes followed by coma and death. **benign tertian m.,** vivax m. **bilious remittent m.,** a complication of falciparum malaria mainly involving the liver, characterized by continuous vomiting, epigastric and hepatic tenderness, marked jaundice, and high remittent fever. **bovine m.,** Texas fever. **cerebral m.,** a severe and often fatal complication of falciparum malaria mainly involving the brain, characterized either by the gradual onset of headache, confusion, and psychotic manifestations lapsing into delirium and coma, or by the sudden onset of an abrupt rise in temperature sustained at high levels, convulsions, and coma. **falciparum m.,** malaria due to *Plasmodium falciparum,* in which the febrile paroxysms recur irregularly. It is associated with the highest levels of parasites in the blood and is the most severe form of malaria, and is sometimes fatal. It is the one most likely to be associated with pernicious symptoms, which occur as a result of plugging of capillaries with *P. falciparum*–infected erythrocytes, usually confined to one organ system, including the brain, liver, adrenal gland, gastrointestinal tract, kidneys, and lungs. Called also *malignant tertian m., pernicious m.,* and *subtertian m.* See also *blackwater fever* under *fever.* **hemolytic m.,** blackwater fever. **hemorrhagic m.,** falciparum malaria in which hemorrhage is a prominent symptom. **induced m.,** malaria that is purposely produced by introduction of the causative parasites, as sometimes used in treating neurosyphilis. **malignant tertian m.,** falciparum m. **ovale m.,** malaria caused by *Plasmodium ovale* that is clinically similar to but milder than vivax malaria, and is frequently found in conjunction with infection due to *P. falciparum.* The infected erythrocytes assume an oblong or oval shape on a stained blood film. **pernicious m.,** falciparum m. **quartan m.,** that in which the febrile paroxysms occur every 72 hours, or every fourth day counting the day of occurrence as the first day of each cycle; it is caused by *Plasmodium malariae,* which requires 72 hours for completion of each asexual cycle in the erythrocyte. It is the mildest and most chronic of all human malarial infections. **quotidian m.,** that in which the febrile paroxysms occur daily, due to simultaneous infection with two broods of *Plasmodium vivax,* which complete their 42- to 48-hour cycle on alternate days. See *vivax m.* **subtertian m.,** falciparum m. **tertian m.,** that in which the febrile paroxysms occur every 42 to 47 hours, or every third day counting the day of occurrence as the first day of the cycle. See *ovale m.* and *vivax m.* **transfusion m.,** infection with *Plasmodium falciparum, P. malariae, P. ovale,* or *P. vivax* transmitted directly from a blood donor, by accidental infection of a contaminated needle, or by drug addicts sharing needles.

vivax m., malaria caused by *Plasmodium vivax;* although it is less severe than falciparum malaria, it is the one in which relapses are most likely to occur because of hypnozoite forms in the liver. In vivax malaria the febrile paroxysms often recur ever other day (see *tertian m.*), but they may recur daily (see *quotidian m.*). The infected red cells often appear enlarged on a stained blood film since the parasite tends to infect younger erythrocytes. Called also *benign tertian m.*

malariacidal (mah-la″re-ah-si′dal) destructive to malarial plasmodia; plasmodicidal.

malarial (mah-la′re-al) pertaining or due to malaria.

malariatherapy (mah-la″re-ah-ther′ah-pe) malariotherapy.

malariologist (mah-la″re-ol′o-jist) a person versed in or engaged in the study of malaria.

malariology (mah-la″re-ol′o-je) [*malaria* + *-logy*] the study of malaria.

malariotherapy (mah-la″re-o-ther′ah-pe) treatment of dementia paralytica by infecting the patient with malarial parasites, usually the parasite of tertian malaria (*Plasmodium vivax*) or of quartan malaria (*P. malariae*).

malarious (mah-la′re-us) pertaining to or marked by the presence of malaria.

malaris (mah-la′ris) [L.] malar.

Malassez's disease, rests (mal″ah-sāz′) [Louis Charles *Malassez,* physiologist in Paris, 1842–1909] see under *disease* and *rest.*

Malassezia (mal″ah-se′ze-ah) [Louis Charles *Malassez*] *Pityrosporon.* **M. furfur, M. macfadyani, M. tropica,** *Pityrosporon orbiculare.*

malassimilation (mal″ah-sim″ĭ-la′shun) [L. *malus* ill + *assimilatio* a rendering like] 1. imperfect, faulty, or disordered assimilation. 2. the inability of the gastrointestinal tract to transport to the body fluids one or more ingested nutrients, whether due to faulty digestion (maldigestion) or to impaired intestinal mucosal transport (malabsorption).

malate (ma′lāt, mal′āt) an ionic form of malic acid.

malate dehydrogenase (ma′lāt, mal′āt de-hi′dro-jĕ-nās) [EC 1.1.1.37] an enzyme of the oxidoreductase class that catalyzes the reaction (S)-malate + NAD^+ = oxaloacetate + NADH. The enzyme occurs both in the mitochondria and in the cytosol. The reaction is important in the tricarboxylic acid cycle and in the malate-aspartate electron shuttle. Called also *malate-NAD dehydrogenase.*

malate dehydrogenase (oxaloacetate-decarboxylating) ($NADP^+$) (ma′lāt, mal′at de-hi′dro-jĕ-nās) [EC 1.1.1.40] an enzyme of the oxidoreductase class that catalyzes the reaction (S)-malate + $NADP^+$ = pyruvate + CO_2 + NADPH. The enzyme occurs in mitochondria and in cytosol as two distinct isoenzyme forms. The cytosolic enzyme is a major source of NADPH for fatty acid synthesis. Called also *malate-NADPH dehydrogenase.*

malate-NAD dehydrogenase (ma′lāt, mal′āt de-hi′dro-jĕ-nās) malate dehydrogenase.

malate-NADPH dehydrogenase (ma′lāt, mal′āt de-hi′dro-jĕ-nās) malate dehydrogenase (oxaloacetate-decarboxylating) ($NADP^+$).

malathion (mal″ah-thi′on) chemical name: *O,O*-dimethyl-*S*-(1,2-dicarboxyethyl)dithiophosphate. An organophosphorus compound used as an insecticide.

malaxate (mal′ak-sāt) to knead, as in making pills.

malaxation (mal″ak-sa′shun) [Gr. *malaxis* a softening] an act of kneading.

Malcotran (mal′ko-tran) trademark for a preparation of homatropine methylbromide.

maldevelopment (mal″de-vel′op-ment) abnormal growth or development.

maldigestion (mal″di-jes′chun) impaired digestion.

male (māl) 1. an organism of the sex that begets young or that produces spermatozoa. 2. masculine.

maleate (mal′e-āt) any salt or ester of maleic acid.

maleic acid (mah-le′ik) trivial name for *cis*-butanedioic acid; the *cis* isomer of fumaric acid.

malemission (mal″e-mish′un) failure of the semen to be discharged from the urinary meatus in coitus.

Malerba's test (mah-ler′bahz) [Pasquale *Malerba,* Italian physician, 1849–1917] see under *tests.*

maleruption (mal″ĕ-rup′shun)   faulty eruption of a tooth, so that it is out of its normal position.

malethamer (mal-eth′ah-mer)   a high weight copolymer of ethylene with maleic anhydride, cross-linked with 1 to 2 per cent, by weight, of vinyl crotonate; an antiperistaltic agent.

maleylacetoacetate isomerase (ma′le, mal′e-il-ah-se″-to-as′ĕ-tāt i-som′er-ās) [EC 5.2.1.2]   an enzyme of the isomerase class that catalyzes the reaction 4-maleylacetoacetate = 4-fumarylacetoacetate. The reaction is a step in the use of phenylalanine and tyrosine as fuel.

malformation (mal″for-ma′shun) [L. *malus* evil + *formatio* a forming]   a morphologic defect resulting from an intrinsically abnormal developmental process.   **Arnold-Chiari m.,** see under *deformity.*

malfunction (mal-funk′shun)   dysfunction.

Malgaigne's amputation, etc. (mal-gānz′) [Joseph François *Malgaigne,* French surgeon, 1806–1865]   see under *amputation, luxation,* and *triangle.*

Malherbe's calcifying epithelioma (mahl-ārb′) [Albert *Malherbe,* French surgeon, 1845–1915]   pilomatricoma.

maliasmus (mal″e-as′mus)   glanders, or farcy.

malic acid (mal′ik, ma′lik)   an intermediate in the tricarboxylic acid (Krebs') cycle, formed from fumaric acid and itself oxidized to form oxaloacetic acid; found in apples, pears, and many other fruits; its action is similar to that of tartaric acid, and it is a permitted food additive.

malic enzyme (ma′lik, mal′ik)   malate dehydrogenase (oxaloacetate-decarboxylating) (NADP$^+$).

malignancy (mah-lig′nan-se) [L. *malignare* to act maliciously]   a tendency to progress in virulence; the quality of being malignant.

malignant (mah-lig′nant) [L. *malignans* acting maliciously]   tending to become progressively worse and to result in death. Having the properties of anaplasia, invasion, and metastasis; said of tumors.

malignin (mah-lig′nin)   a protein fragment present in the serum of patients with malignant glial tumors.

mali-mali (mah″le-mah′le)   a form of saltatory spasm endemic in the Philippines.

malingerer (mah-ling′ger-er) [Fr. *malingre* sickly]   an individual who is guilty of malingering.

malingering (mah-ling′ger-ing)   the willful, deliberate, and fraudulent feigning or exaggeration of the symptoms of illness or injury, done for the purpose of a consciously desired end.

malinterdigitation (mal″in-ter-dij″i-ta′shun)   failure of interdigitation of parts which are normally so related.

Mall's formula (mahlz) [Franklin Paine *Mall,* Baltimore anatomist, 1862–1917]   see under *formula.*

malleability (mal″e-ah-bil′ĭ-te)   the quality of being malleable.

malleable (mal′e-ah-b'l) [L. *malleare* to hammer]   susceptible of being beaten out into a thin plate.

malleal (mal′e-al)   mallear.

mallear (mal′e-ar)   pertaining to a malleus (def. 1).

malleation (mal″e-a′shun) [L. *malleare* to hammer]   sharp and swift muscular twitching of the hands.

mallein (mal′e-in) [L. *malleus* glanders]   a concentrate prepared from cultures or extracts of the glanders bacillus, *Pseudomonas mallei,* used in a skin test analogous to the tuberculin test for the diagnosis of glanders.

malleoincudal (mal″e-o-ing′ku-dal)   pertaining to the malleus and incus.

malleolar (mal-e′o-lar)   1. pertaining to a malleolus.   2. mallear.

malleoli (mah-le′o-li) [L.]   genitive and plural of *malleolus.*

malleolus (mah-le′o-lus), gen. and pl. *malle′oli* [L., dim. of *malleus* hammer]   a rounded process, such as the protuberance on either side of the ankle joint; [NA], a general term for such a process.   **external m., m. exter′nus,** m. lateralis.   **m. fib′ulae, fibular m.,** m. lateralis fibulae.   **inner m., internal m., m. inter′nus,** m. medialis.   **lateral m.,** m. lateralis.   **lateral m. of fibula,** m. lateralis fibulae.   **m. latera′lis** [NA], lateral malleolus: the rounded protuberance on the lateral surface of the ankle joint, produced by the m. lateralis fibulae.   **m. latera′lis**

fib′ulae [NA], lateral malleolus of fibula: the process at the outer side of the lower end of the fibula, forming, with the malleolus medialis tibiae, the mortise in which the talus articulates.   **medial m.,** m. medialis.   **medial m. of tibia,** m. medialis tibiae.   **m. media′lis** [NA], medial malleolus: the rounded protuberance on the medial surface of the ankle joint, produced by the m. medialis tibiae.   **m. media′lis tib′iae** [NA], medial malleolus of tibia: the process at the inner side of the lower end of the tibia, forming, with the malleolus lateralis fibulae, the mortise in which the talus articulates.   **outer m.,** m. lateralis.   **radial m., m. radia′lis,** processus styloideus radii.   **m. tib′iae, tibial m.,** m. medialis tibiae.   **ulnar m., m. ulna′ris,** processus styloideus ulnae.

Malleomyces (mal″e-o-mi′sēz) [L. *malleus* glanders + Gr. *mykēs* fungus]   in former systems of classification, a genus of bacteria, species of which have been assigned to the genus *Pseudomonas.*

malleotomy (mal″e-ot′o-me) [*malleus* + Gr. *tomē* a cutting]   1. the operation of dividing the malleus in cases of ankylosis of the ossicles of the middle ear.   2. the operation of separating the malleoli by dividing the ligaments which hold them together.

malleus (mal′e-us) [L. "hammer"]   1. [NA] the largest of the auditory ossicles, and the one attached to the membrana tympani; its club-shaped head articulates with the incus. Called also *hammer.* See Plate accompanying *ear.*   2. glanders.

mallochorion (mal″o-ko′re-on) [Gr. *mallos* wool + *chorion*]   the primitive chorion; so called because of its villi.

Mallophaga (mal-of′ah-gah) [Gr. *mallos* wool + *phagein* to eat]   an order of biting lice, the bird lice, which feed on the feathers and hair of birds and which may attack man and other mammals. It includes the genera *Damalinia, Felicola, Heterodoxus,* and *Trichodectes.* Cf. *Anoplura.*

Mallory's bodies, stain (mal′o-rēz) [Frank Burr *Mallory,* pathologist in Boston, 1862–1941]   see under *body,* and see *Table of Stains.*

mallow (mal′o) [L. *malva*]   any plant of the genus *Malva.* The flowers and leaves of *M. sylvestris* L. and *M. rotundifolia* L. (malvaceae) are demulcent and emollient, and are used in Asia and India for these properties.

malnutrition (mal″nu-trish′un)   any disorder of nutrition; it may be due to unbalanced or insufficient diet or to defective assimilation or utilization of foods.   **malignant m.,** kwashiorkor.   **protein m.,** kwashiorkor.

malocclusion (mal″o-kloo′zhun)   such malposition and contact of the maxillary and mandibular teeth as to interfere with the highest efficiency during the excursive movements of the jaw that are essential for mastication; originally classified by Angle into four major groups, depending on the anteroposterior jaw relationship as indicated by interdigitation of the first molar teeth, but Class IV is not used (see table).   **closed-bite m.,** closed bite.   **open-bite m.,** open bite.

malonal (mal′o-nal)   (*obs.*) barbital.

malonic acid (mah-lon′ik)   propanedioic acid, HOOC-CH$_2$-COOH; malonyl coenzyme A is the source of 2-carbon groups transfered to the growing hydrocarbon chain in fatty acid synthesis.

malonyl (mal′o-nil)   an acyl radical of malonic acid.

malonyl coenzyme A (ma′lo, mal′o-nil ko-en′zīm)   the coenzyme A thioester of malonic acid, formed from acetyl coenzyme A by acetyl-CoA carboxylase. It is an intermediate in fatty acid synthesis.

Malpighi's pyramids, vesicles (mal-pig′ēz) [Marcello *Malpighi,* Italian anatomist, 1628–1694]   see *pyramides renales* and *alveoli pulmonis.*

malpighian bodies, etc. (mal-pig′ĭ-an) [Marcello *Malpighi,* Italian anatomist, 1628–1694]   see under *body, capsule, cell, corpuscle, glomerulus, layer, rete, stigma, tubule,* and *tuft.*

malposed (mal-pōzd′)   not in the normal position.

malposition (mal″po-zish′un) [L. *malus* bad + *positio* placement]   abnormal or anomalous position.

malpractice (mal-prak′tis) [L. *mal* bad + *practice*]   improper or injurious practice; unskillful and faulty medical or surgical treatment.

malpraxis (mal-prak′sis)   malpractice.

malpresentation (mal″prez-en-ta′shun)   a faulty or ab-

ANGLE'S CLASSIFICATION OF MALOCCLUSION

Class I (Neutroclusion). Normal anteroposterior relationship of the jaws, as indicated by correct interdigitation of maxillary and mandibular molars, but with crowding and rotation of teeth elsewhere, i.e., a dental dysplasia or an arch length deficiency.

Class II (Distoclusion). The lower dental arch is posterior to the upper in one or both lateral segments; the lower first molar is distal to the upper first molar.
Division 1. Bilaterally distal with narrow maxillary arch and protruding upper incisors.
Subdivision, unilaterally distal with other characteristics the same.
Division 2. Bilaterally distal with normal or square-shaped maxillary arch, retruded maxillary central incisors, labially malposed maxillary lateral incisors, and an excessive overbite.
Subdivision. Unilaterally distal with other characteristics the same.
Class III (Mesioclusion). The lower arch is anterior to the upper in one or both lateral segments; lower first molar is mesial to upper first molar.
Division. Mandibular incisors are usually in anterior cross-bite.
Subdivision. Unilaterally mesial, with other characteristics the same.
Class IV. The occlusal relations of the dental arches present the peculiar condition of being in distal occlusion upon one lateral half, and in mesial occlusion upon the other half of the mouth.

normal fetal presentation.

malrotation (mal″ro-ta′shun) abnormal or pathologic rotation, as of the vertebral column; failure of normal rotation of an organ, as of the gut, during embryological development.

malt (mawlt) grain, for the most part barley, which has been soaked, made to germinate, and then dried; it contains dextrin, maltose, and diastase. It is nutritive and digestant, aiding in the digestion of starchy foods, and is used in tuberculosis, cholera infantum, and other wasting diseases.

maltase (mawl′tās) α-D-glucosidase.

malthusian law (mal-thu′se-an) [Rev. Thomas Robert *Malthus*, English economist, 1766–1834] see under *law*.

maltobiose (mawl″to-bi′ōs) maltose.

maltodextrin (mawl″to-dek′strin) a dextrin convertible into maltose.

maltoflavin (mawl″to-fla′vin) a flavin or lyochrome malt.

maltol (mawl′tol) a compound, 3-hydroxy-2-methyl-4-pyrone, CH·CH·CO·C(OH):C(CH₃).

maltosazone (mawl″to-sa′zōn) the phenylosazone of maltose, a yellow crystalline substance formed by treating maltose with phenyl hydrazine and acetic acid; the crystals melt at 205° C. and may be used in identifying maltose.

maltose (mawl′tōs) 4-O -[α-D-glucopyranosyl-]D-glucopyranose: a white crystalline disaccharide formed when starch is hydrolyzed by amylase; used as a nutrient and sweetener. Called also *maltobiose*.

maltoside (mawl′to-sīd) acetal of maltose, formed by condensation of an anomeric hydroxyl group with an alcohol; a compound homologous with a glucoside, but in which the sugar is maltose instead of glucose.

maltosuria (mawl″to-su′re-ah) the presence of maltose in the urine.

maltotriose (mawl″to-tri′ōs) a sugar consisting of three glucose molecules, resulting from the action of amylase on starch or glycogen.

malturned (mal-turnd′) turned abnormally; said of teeth twisted on their central axes.

Malucidin (mal″u-si′din) trademark for a yeast extract which has abortifacient activity in the dog, cat, and sheep.

malum (ma′lum) [L.] evil or disease. **m. articulo′rum seni′lis,** a painful, degenerative state of a joint, occurring as a result of aging. **m. seni′le,** a variety of osteoarthritis peculiar to aged persons; see *morbus coxae senilis.* **m. vertebra′le suboccipita′le,** tuberculosis of the atlas and axis.

malunion (mal-ūn′yon) union of the fragments of a fractured bone in a faulty position.

Malva (mal′vah) [L.] see *mallow.*

Maly's test (mah′lēz) [Richard Leo *Maly,* Austrian chemist, 1839–1894] see under *tests.*

mamba (mam′bah) an extremely venomous elapid tree snake of the genus *Dendroaspis.*

mamelon (mam′ĕ-lon) [Fr. "nipple"] 1. one of three tubercles sometimes present on the cutting edge of an incisor tooth. 2. the nipple-like elevation in the umbilicus, considered to be the remains of the solid lower part of the umbilical cord which contained the umbilical arteries and urachus.

mamelonated (mam′ĕ-lon-āt″ed) (*obs.*) mamillated.

mamelonation (mam′ĕ-lo-na′shun) (*obs.*) mamillation.

mamilla (mah-mil′ah), gen. and pl. *mamil′lae* [L., dim. of *mamma,* a breast, teat] 1. the nipple (papilla mammae [NA]). 2. any nipple-like structure. Written also *mamilla.*

mamillae (mah-mil′e) [L.] genitive and plural of *mamilla.*

mamillary (mam′ĭ-ler″e) [L. *mamilla,* dim. of *mamma,* a breast, teat] pertaining to or resembling a nipple.

mamillated (mam″ĭ-lāt′ed) having nipple-like projections.

mamillation (mam″il-la′shun) 1. the condition of being mamillated. 2. a nipple-like elevation or projection.

mamilliform (mah-mil′ĭ-form) [*mamilla* + L. *forma* form] shaped like a nipple.

mamilliplasty (mah-mil′ĭ-plas″te) theleplasty.

mamillitis (mam″ĭ-li′tis) [*mamilla* + *-itis*] inflammation of the mamilla, or nipple; thelitis.

mamma (mam′ah), gen. and pl. *mam′mae* [L.] [NA] the breast: the modified cutaneous, glandular structure on the anterior aspect of the thorax that contains, in the female, the elements that secrete milk for nourishment of the young. See *mammary gland,* under *gland.* **mam′mae acces-so′riae [femini′nae et masculi′nae]** [NA], **accessory mammae,** mammary glands present in excess of the normal number, generally found along the line of the embryonic mammary crest; called also *accessory mammary glands.* **m. areola′ta,** a condition of the breast in which there is bulging of the areola of the nipple. **m. mascu′lina** [NA], the rudimentary mammary gland of the male; called also *m. virilis.* **supernumerary mammae,** mammae accessoriae [femininae et masculinae]. **m. vir′ilis,** m. masculina.

mammae (mam′e) [L.] genitive and plural of *mamma.*

mammal (mam′al) an individual belonging to the class Mammalia.

mammalgia (mah-mal′je-ah) mastalgia.

Mammalia (mah-ma′le-ah) a class of warm-blooded vertebrate animals, including all that possess hair and suckle their young. It includes three major groups: placentals and marsupials, which are viviparous, and monotremes, which are oviparous.

mammalogy (mah-mal′o-je) [*mammal* + *-logy*] the study of mammals.

mammaplasty (mam′ah-plas″te) [L. *mamma* + Gr. *plassein* to shape, form] plastic reconstruction of the breast, as may be performed to augment or reduce its size. **Aries-Pitanguy m.,** an operation to reduce mild to moderate macromastia. **augmentation m.,** plastic reconstruction of the breast, with increase of its volume by insertion of an autogenous or prosthetic material. **Biesenberger m.,** a reduction mammaplasty using transposition of the nipple, consisting in excision of the lateral portion of the mammary gland, with rotation of the remaining glandular pedicle attached to the nipple and formation of a skin brassiere. **Conway m.,** a method of correcting severe macromastia, consisting in partial breast amputation and free transplantation of the nipples and areolae. **reduction m.,** plastic reconstruction of the breast with decrease in its volume by excision of tissue. **Strömbeck m.,** a one-stage breast reduction operation that includes transposition of the nipple in a medial and lateral pedicle.

mammary (mam′er-e) [L. *mammarius*] pertaining to the mamma, or breast.

mammatroph (mam′ah-trōf) mammotroph.

mammectomy (mah-mek′to-me) [*mamma* + Gr. *ektome* excision] excision of the breast; mastectomy.

mammiform (mam′ĭ-form) [*mamma* + L. *forma* form] shaped like the mamma, or breast.

mammilla (mah-mil′ah)   mamilla.

Mammillaria (mam″il-la′re-ah)   a genus of cacti which have numerous sharp spines capable of inflicting painful wounds.

mammillary. (mam′ĭ-ler″e)   mamillary.

mammillated (mam′ĭ-lāt″ed)   mamillated.

mammillation (mam″ĭ-la′shun)   mamillation.

mammilliform (mah-mil′lĭ-form)   mamilliform.

mammillitis (mam″ĭ-li′tis)   mamillitis. **bovine ulcerative m.,** a herpesviral disease affecting milking cows, characterized by ulcerative lesions on the teats and, less frequently, on the udders.

mammiplasia (mam″ĭ-pla′ze-ah)   mammoplasia.

mammitis (mam-i′tis)   mastitis.

mamm(o)- [L. *mamma,* q.v.]   a combining form denoting relationship to the breast, or to a mammary gland; see also words beginning *mast(o)-* and *maz(o)-*.

mammogen (mam′o-jen)   any substance or influence that promotes breast development.

mammogenesis (mam″mo-jen′ĕ-sis)   the development of the mammary glands to the functional state.

mammogram (mam′o-gram)   a roentgenogram of the breast.

mammography (mam-og′rah-fe)   roentgenography of the mammary gland.

mammoplasia (mam″mo-pla′ze-ah) [*mammo-* + Gr. *plasis* formation + *-ia*]   the development of breast tissue; called also *mastoplasia*. **adolescent m.,** the development of breast tissue at adolescence, applied especially to the development and later regression which occurs in males during puberty.

mammoplasty (mam′o-plas″te) [*mammo-* + Gr. *plassein* to shape, form]   mammaplasty.

mammose (mah-mōs′) [L. *mammosus*]   1. having large breasts, or mammae. 2. mamillated.

mammotomy (mam-mot′o-me)   mastotomy.

mammotroph (mam′o-trōf)   one of the acidophils (alpha cells) of the adenohypophysis that stain with an affinity for azocarmine and erythrosin, and are thought to secrete prolactin (luteotropin). Called also *lactotroph* and *luteotroph*.

mammotrophic (mam″o-trof′ik)   mammotropic.

mammotropic (mam″-o-trop′ik) [*mammo-* + Gr. *tropikos* inclined]   having affinity for or a stimulating effect on the mammary gland.

mammotropin (mah-mot′ro-pin)   the lactogenic hormone, prolactin.

Man.   abbreviation for L. *manip′ulus,* a handful.

manaca (man′ah-kah)   the Brazilian plant, *Brunfelsia (Franciscea) hopeana* Benth. (Solanaceae); formerly used in the treatment of syphilis and rheumatism.

Manchester operation (man′ches-ter) [Manchester, England]   see under *operation*.

manchette (man-chet′) [Fr. "a cuff"]   a temporary band around the neck of a spermatozoon.

manchineel (man″kĭ-nēl′)   the *Hippomane mancinella,* a tree of tropical America; it contains a caustic poisonous sap or juice.

Mandelamine (man″del-ah′mēn)   trademark for a preparation of methenamine mandelate.

mandelic acid (man-del′ik, man-de′lik)   an acid with active bacteriostatic properties, used in urinary tract infections, usually as the ammonium or calcium salt. Called also *amygdalic acid* and *phenylglycolic acid*.

mandible (man′dĭ-b'l)   the bone of the lower jaw; see *mandibula*.

mandibula (man-dib′u-lah), gen. and pl. *mandib′ulae* [L., from *mandere* to chew] [NA]   the mandible: the horseshoe-shaped bone forming the lower jaw; the largest and strongest bone of the face, presenting a body and a pair of rami, which articulate with the skull at the temporomandibular joints.

mandibulae (man-dib′u-le) [L.]   genitive and plural of *mandibula*.

mandibular (man-dib′u-lar)   pertaining to the lower jaw bone, or mandible.

mandibulectomy (man-dib″u-lek′to-me)   surgical removal of the mandible.

mandibulopharyngeal (man-dib″u-lo-fah-rin′je-al)   pertaining to the mandible and the pharynx.

Mandragora (man-drag′o-rah) [L.]   a genus of solanaceous plants. *M. officinarum* L. (Solanaceae), the true European or oriental mandrake, has the general properties of belladonna, and was formerly used as a narcotic and sedative. It contains the alkaloids mandragorine, hyoscyamine, and scopolamine.

mandrake (man′drāk)   see *Mandragora*.

mandrel (man′drel)   a shaft in a handpiece that holds a disk, stone, or cup used for grinding or polishing. Called also *mandril*.

mandril (man′dril)   mandrel.

mandrin (man′drin)   a stylet or guide for a catheter.

maneuver (mah-noo′ver)   any dexterous procedure. See also entries under *method, technique,* etc. **Adson's m.,** see under *tests*. **Allen m.,** with the forearm flexed at a right angle, the arm is extended horizontally and rotated externally at the shoulder, the head being rotated to the contralateral shoulder; obliteration of the radial pulse suggests scalenus anticus syndrome. **Bracht's m.** (for breech presentation), the breech is allowed to spontaneously deliver up to the umbilicus. The body and extended legs are held together with both hands maintaining the upward and anterior rotation of the fetal body. When the anterior rotation is nearly complete, the fetal body is held against the mother's symphysis. Maintenance of this position leads to spontaneous completion of delivery. **Brandt-Andrews m.,** a method of expressing the placenta from the uterus in the third stage of labor: the left hand grasps the umbilical cord while the right is placed on the maternal abdomen with the fingers over the anterior uterine surface. The right hand is gently pressed backward and slightly upward as the left applies gentle traction on the cord. **Chassard-Lapiné m.,** the patient sits and bends forward as far as possible. The roentgen rays, directed from above, penetrate the spine and outline the sigmoid loops in a transverse projection. **Credé's m.,** see under *method*. **Engel-Lysholm m.,** a radiologic method of determining the size of the retrogastric organs or masses: the patient takes effervescent powders to fill his stomach with carbon dioxide, and assumes a prone position; a lateral view of the abdomen with a horizontal beam, and a posteroanterior projection with a vertical beam are made. **forward-bending m.,** a method of detecting retraction signs in neoplastic changes in the mammae; the patient bends forward from the waist with chin held up and arms extended toward the examiner. If retraction is present, an asymmetry in the breast is seen. **Fowler m.,** a test for tight intrinsic muscles in ulnar deviation of the digits: in rheumatoid arthritis a heavy, taut ulnar band is demonstrated when the digit is held in its normal axial relationship. **Gowers' m.,** see under *sign* (def. 2). **Halstead m.,** while the examiner exerts downward traction on the upper limb to be tested, the subject rotates his head toward the contralateral shoulder; obliteration of the radial pulse is suggestive of scalenus anticus syndrome. **Heiberg-Esmarch m.** (*obs.*), a pushing forward by the anesthetist of the patient's lower jaw in order to prevent the tongue from slipping backward. **Heimlich m.,** a method of dislodging food or other material from the throat of a choking victim: after wrapping the arms around the victim at the belt line and allowing his upper torso to hang forward, make a fist with one hand and grasp it with the other; with both hands placed against the victim's abdomen slightly above the navel and below the rib cage, forcefully press into the abdomen with a quick upward thrust. If the victim is sitting, stand behind him and perform the same procedure; if he is prone, turn him on his back, kneel astride the torso, place both hands at the location on the victim's abdomen as described above and press forcefully with a sharp upward thrust. The maneuver may be repeated several times if necessary. **Hoguet's m.,** in hernioplasty, conversion of the direct hernial sac to an indirect one by withdrawing the sac from beneath the deep epigastric vessels. **Hueter's m.,** downward and forward pressure on the patient's tongue by the left forefinger of the physician during introduction of a stomach tube. **Jendrassik's m.,** a procedure for emphasizing the patellar reflex: the patient hooks his hands together by the flexed fingers and pulls apart as hard as he can. **Kappeler's m.** (*obs.*), a drawing forward of the patient's lower jaw

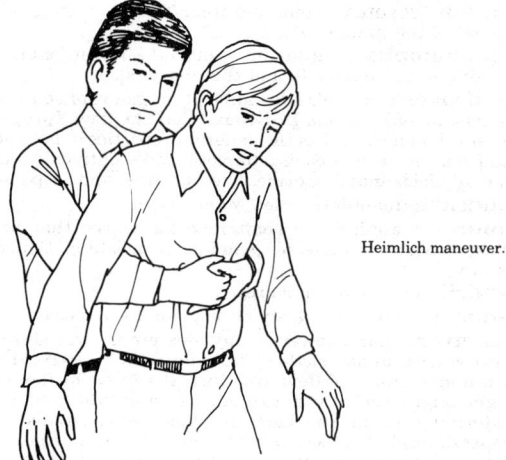

Heimlich maneuver.

by the anesthetist. **Kocher m.,** operative mobilization of the duodenum for exposure of the retroduodenal, intrapancreatic, and intraduodenal portions of the common bile duct. **Leopold's m's,** four maneuvers in palpating the abdomen for ascertaining the position and presentation of the fetus. **Lovset's m.,** extraction of the arms in breech birth by clockwise and counterclockwise rotation of the fetus, after it has been expelled up to the umbilicus. **McDonald m.,** measurement of the contour of the abdomen to calculate the duration of pregnancy; see also under *rule*. **Mauriceau m.,** a method of delivering the aftercoming head in cases of breech presentation. **Müller's m.,** an inspiratory effort with a closed glottis after expiration, used during fluoroscopic examination to cause a negative intrathoracic pressure with engorgement of intrathoracic vascular structures, which is helpful in recognizing esophageal varices, and distinguishing vascular from nonvascular structures. **Müller-Hillis m.,** procedures for ascertaining the relation between the size of the fetal head and the pelvis of the mother. **Munro Kerr m.,** a maneuver for ascertaining the proportion between the head of the fetus and the pelvis of the mother. **Pajot's m.,** for forceps traction along the axis of superior strait; one hand over the lock of the forceps pulls downward towards the floor, while the other hand applies horizontal traction. **Phalen's m.** (for detection of carpal tunnel syndrome), the size of the carpal tunnel is reduced by holding the affected hand with the wrist fully flexed or extended for 30 to 60 seconds, or by placing a sphygmomanometer cuff on the involved arm and inflating to a point between diastolic and systolic pressure for 30 to 60 seconds. **Pinard's m.,** a method of bringing down the foot in breech extraction. **Prague m.,** a method in breech presentation of engaging the head by bringing down the breech and making traction on the head with the finger, which is hooked over the nape of the neck. **Ritgen m.,** delivery of the fetal head by lifting the head upward and forward through the vulva, between pains, by pressing with the tips of the fingers upon the perineum behind the anus. **Saxtorph's m.,** Pajot's m. **Scanzoni m.,** a method of forceps rotation of the fetal head in the posterior position of the occiput. **Schreiber's m.,** rubbing of the inner side of the upper part of the thigh while testing for patellar reflex. **Sellick m.,** the application of pressure to the cricoid cartilage in order to compress the esophagus and prevent passive regurgitation during endotracheal intubation. **Toynbee m.,** pinching the nostrils and swallowing; if the auditory tube is patent, the tympanic membrane will retract medially. **Valsalva's m.,** 1. forcible exhalation effort against a closed glottis; the resultant increase in intrathoracic pressure interferes with venous return to the heart. 2. forcible exhalation effort against occluded nostrils and a closed mouth; the increased pressure in the eustachian tube and middle ear causes the tympanic membrane to move outward. **Van Hoorn's m.,** a maneuver like the Prague maneuver, with the addition of pressure on the fetal forehead from outside. **Wigand's m.,** see under *version*.

manganese (man′gah-nēs) [L. *manganum, manganesium*] a metal resembling iron; symbol, Mn; atomic number, 25; atomic weight, 54.938; specific gravity, 7.2. Manganous salts occur in body tissue in very small amounts and act as an activator of liver arginase and other enzymes. See also *manganese poisoning*, under *poisoning*. **m. butyrate,** a red powder, $(CH_3CH_2CH_2COO)_2Mn$, formerly used in treatment of some skin diseases. **m. glycerophosphate,** a white or pinkish white powder, $C_3H_7MnO_6P$, formerly used as a hematinic and nerve tonic. **m. hypophosphite,** a pink, granular or crystalline powder, $Mn(H_2PO_2)_2 \cdot H_2O$, used as a nutrient and dietary supplement and formerly as a hematinic. **m. sulfate,** a salt, $MnSO_4 + 4H_2O$, used in veterinary medicine in the prevention of perosis in poultry.

manganic (man-gan′ik) pertaining to manganese as a trivalent element.

manganism (man′gah-nizm) manganese poisoning; see under *poisoning*.

manganous (man′gah-nus) pertaining to manganese as a divalent element.

manganum (man′gah-num) [L.] manganese.

mange (mānj) a contagious scabies-like dermatitis occurring in various animals, including cattle, sheep, horses, dogs, cats, foxes, rabbits, rats, and gallinaceous birds, caused by any of several of the mange mites, such as *Chorioptes, Demodex, Knemidokoptes, Notoedres, Otodectes, Psorptes,* and *Sarcoptes,* and known according to the etiologic agent as e.g., chorioptic, demodectic, or sarcoptic mange. Although the distribution, manner of spread, and clinical presentation vary with the host and parasite species, mange is typically characterized by cutaneous burrows produced by the mites; scratching associated with deeper lesions, producing crusts and scabs; alopecia; and epidermal hyperplasia with desquamation. Bacterial infection may occur.

mangosteen (man′gos-tēn) the pericarp of the fruit of *Garcinia mangostana* L. (Guttiferaceae); astringent.

mangostin (man′gos-tin) a yellow, crystalline, xanthone type of pigment, $C_{23}H_{24}O_6$, from mangosteen rind.

mania (ma′ne-ah) [Gr. "madness"] 1. a mood disorder characterized by expansiveness, elation, agitation, hyperexcitability, hyperactivity, and increased speed of thought and speech (flight of ideas); seen in manic bipolar disorder. 2. as a combining form, it signifies obsessive preoccupation with something, as in *dipsomania, erotomania, pyromania,* etc. **acute m.** (*obs.*), mania. **m. à potu,** delirium tremens. **Bell's m.** (*obs.*), hypermania, delirious mania; mania with confusion or disorientation. **doubting m.** (*obs.*), folie du doute. **puerperal m.** (*obs.*), postpartum psychosis with manic features. **religious m.,** mania with abnormal or perverted religious impulses. **unproductive m.,** a condition in which the behavior is that of mania, but the patient's thinking and speech are repressed.

maniac (ma′ne-ak) [L. *maniacus*] one who is affected with mania.

maniacal (mah-ni′ah-kal) affected with mania.

manic (ma′nik) pertaining to or affected with mania.

manic-depressive (ma′nik-de-pres′iv) alternating between attacks of mania and depression, as in bipolar disorder.

manikin (man′i-kin) a model of the body, usually with movable or removable members and parts, used to illustrate anatomy, or for the teaching of nursing and obstetrics, or certain surgical procedures, such as the removal of foreign bodies by bronchoscopy.

maniloquism (mah-nil′o-kwizm) [L. *manus* hand + *loqui* speak] dactylology.

Manip. abbreviation for L. *manip′ulus,* a handful.

maniphalanx (man″i-fa′lanks) [L. *manus* hand + *phalanx*] a phalanx of the hand.

manipulation (mah-nip″u-la′shun) [L. *manipulare* to handle] skillful or dextrous treatment by the hand. In physical therapy, the forceful passive movement of a joint beyond its active limit of motion. **conjoined m.,** manipulation with both hands.

Mann's sign (manz) [John Dixon *Mann,* English physician, 1840–1912] see under *sign*.

Mann-Bollman fistula (man-bol′man) [Frank Charles *Mann,* American physiologist and surgeon, 1887–1962; Jesse Louis *Bollman,* American physiologist, born 1896] see under *fistula*.

Mann-Williamson ulcer (man′wil′yam-son) [Frank C. *Mann;* Carl S. *Williamson,* American surgeon, 1896–1952] see under *ulcer*.

manna (man′ah) [L.] the dried saccharine exudation from the flowering ash tree, *Fraxinus ornus* L. (Oleaceae); its chief constituents are mannitol, mucilage, and sugar, and it has been used as a laxative.

mannan (man′an) a hard, white, insoluble polysaccharide, $(C_6H_{10}O_5)_n$, which yields mannose on hydrolysis; it is found in the vegetable ivory nut, *Phytelephas macrocarpa*, and other plants.

mannans (man′anz) a complex polysaccharide containing mannose $(C_6H_{12}O_6)$ and other moieties, frequently found in the cell walls of fungi, particularly yeasts.

mannerism (man′er-izm) a stereotyped movement or habit peculiar to a given individual.

manninotriose (man″ĭ-no-tri′ōs) a trisaccharide, $C_{18}H_{32}$-O_{16}, from ash manna, which on hydrolysis yields two molecules of galactose and one of glucose.

mannitan (man′ĭ-tan) a modified form of mannitol, having an internal ring formation in the molecule and which tends to revert to mannitol.

mannite (man′īt) mannitol.

mannitol (man′ĭ-tol) a 6-carbon sugar alcohol widely distributed in plants and fungi. *Mannitol* [USP] administered intravenously is used as an osmotic diuretic in the prophylaxis of acute renal failure, in the evaluation of acute oliguria, and for reducing intraocular and cerebrospinal fluid pressure and volume. **m. hexanitrate,** a compound formed by the nitration of mannitol; used as a vasodilator, mainly in urinary insufficiency.

mannitose (man′ĭ-tōs) mannose.

Mannkopf's sign (mahn′kopfs) [Emil Wilhelm *Mannkopf,* German physician, 1836–1918] see under *sign.*

mannocarolose (man″o-kar′o-lōs) a polysaccharide made up of D-mannose units and formed by the growth of *Penicillium charlesii* on culture media containing glucose.

mannohydrazone (man″o-hi′drah-zōn) the phenylhydrazone of mannose. It consists of colorless platelike crystals which melt at 195° C. and may be used in identifying mannose.

mannoketoheptose (man″o-ke″to-hep′tōs) a natural sugar, $CH_2OH·CO(CHOH)_4·CH_2OH$, found in the avocado, *Persea americana* mill. (*P. gratissima* Gaertn) Lauraceae.

mannopyranose (man″o-pi′rah-nōs) mannose in cyclic hemiacetal form.

mannosan (man′o-san) mannan.

mannose (man′ōs) a monosaccharide, $CH_2OH·(CHOH)_4$-CHO: an aldohexose sugar produced by the oxidation of mannitol, similar to dextrose in general properties and conveniently prepared by hydrolyzing the vegetable ivory nut.

mannose-6-phosphate isomerase (man′ōs fos′fāt i-som′er-ās) [EC 5.3.1.8] an enzyme of the isomerase class that catalyzes the reaction D-mannose 6-phosphate = D-fructose 6-phosphate. The reaction is a step in the utilization of a mannose. Called also *phosphomannose isomerase.*

α-mannosidase (man′o-sĭ-dās) [EC 3.2.1.24] an enzyme of the hydrolase class that catalyzes the hydrolysis of terminal, nonreducing α-D-mannose residues in α-D-mannosides. The reaction is a step in the metabolism of N-linked oligosaccharides in glycoproteins. Defect in the enzyme, an autosomal recessive trait, results in mannosidosis.

mannoside (man′o-sīd) a glycoside of mannose.

mannosidosis (man″o-sĭ-do′sis) a lysosomal storage disease due to defective α-D-mannosidase with resultant oligosaccharide accumulation. Clinically, there are coarse facies, upper respiratory congestion and infections, profound mental retardation, hepatosplenomegaly, cataracts, radiographic signs of dyostosis multiplex, and gibbus deformity. Mannosidosis is divided into types I and II for infantile and for juvenile-adult onset, respectively.

mannosocellulose (man-o″so-sel′u-lōs) a variety of polysaccharide from coffee; it is changed by hydrolysis into mannose and dextrose.

Mann-Whitney test (man hwit′ne) [Henry Berthold *Mann,* American mathematician, born 1905; Donald Ransom *Whitney,* American statistician, born 1915] see *rank sum test,* under *tests.*

manometer (mah-nom′ĕ-ter) [Gr. *manos* thin + *metron* measure] an instrument for measuring the pressure or tension of liquids or gases, as the blood, etc. **aneroid m.,** a device that measures pressure by means of an elastic container as compared to that of a vacuum, a true total-pressure-measuring instrument.

manometric (man″o-met′rik) 1. pertaining to or ascertained by the manometer. 2. varying with the pressure.

manoptoscope (man-op′to-skōp) [L. *manus* hand + *opto-* + *-scope*] an apparatus for detecting ocular dominance.

manoscopy (man-os′ko-pe) the measurement of the density of gases.

Man. pr. abbreviation for L. *ma′ne pri′mo,* early in the morning.

manquea (mahn-ka′ah) actinobacillosis of young cattle in South America, marked by the formation of abscesses upon the legs.

mansa (man′sah) the root or rhizome of *Anemonopsis californica* Hook. and Arn. (syn. *Houttuynia californica* Benth. and Hook.), Saururaceae. A perennial herbaceous plant indigenous to southwestern United States and adjacent Mexico, where it is locally used to relieve colds and indigestion, and to purify the blood.

Mansil (man′sil) trademark for preparations of oxamniquine.

Manson's hemoptysis, schistosomiasis (disease) (man′sonz) [Sir Patrick *Manson,* British physician, 1844–1922] see under *hemoptysis* and *schistosomiasis.*

Mansonella (man″son-el′ah) a genus of filarial worms of the family *Dipetalonematidae,* characterized by a rounded, enlarged anterior end and a smooth cuticle, found in Central and South America. **M. ozzar′di,** a filarial nematode parasite of Central and South America and the Caribbean, the cause of mansonellosis in man; transmitted by *Culicoides furens* and *Simulium amazonicum.* **M. per′stans,** a filarial nematode up to 80 mm. long, found in the tropical regions of Central and South America and Africa, transmitted by bites of the small flies of the genus *Culicoides.* The adults inhabit the pleural and peritoneal tissues, while the larval forms (microfilariae) are found in the peripheral blood. Although considered to be nonpathogenic, they have been implicated as the cause of such symptoms as eosinophilia, abdominal and pectoral pain, enlargement of the spleen and liver, and fever followed by urticaria and edema of the lower limbs and scrotum. Called also *Acanthocheilonema perstans, Depetalonema perstans,* and *Filaria perstans.* **M. streptocer′ca,** a filarial worm found in man and chimpanzees in western and central Africa, transmitted by the bite of small flies of the genus *Culicoides.* The microfilariae, which may be found in scarification smears, are sometimes confused with those of *Onchocerca volvulus.* It produces a pruritic rash resembling that of onchocerciasis. Called also *Acanthocheilonema streptocerca* and *Dipetalonema streptocerca.*

Mansonella (man″so-nel′ah) a genus of filarial nematodes.

mansonelliasis (man″so-nel-i′ah-sis) mansonellosis.

mansonellosis (man″so-nel-o′sis) infection with organisms of the genus *Mansonella;* an ill-defined syndrome of headache, coldness of the legs, pruritus, and articular swelling.

Mansonia (man-so′ne-ah) a genus of mosquitoes, several species of which transmit *Brugia malayi.* Some species may also transmit viruses such as those causing equine encephalomyelitis.

Mansonioides (man-so-ne-oi′-dēz) a subgenus of *Mansonia.* **M. annulif′era,** the chief vector of *Wuchereria malayi* in India.

mantle (man′t'l) [L. *mantellum* cloak] an enveloping cover or layer. **brain m.,** pallium. **chordomesodermal m.,** a continuous epithelial sheet composed of notochordal and mesodermal material during gastrulation. **myoepicardial m.,** a layer of visceral mesoderm in the early embryo, surrounding the endocardial tube and developing into the myocardium and epicardium.

Mantoux test (reaction) (man-too′) [Charles *Mantoux,* French physician, 1877–1947] see under *tests.*

manual (man′u-al) [L. *manualis; manus* hand] of or pertaining to the hand; performed by the hand or hands.

manubria (mah-nu′bre-ah) [L.] plural of *manubrium.*

manubrium (mah-nu′bre-um), pl. *manu′bria* [L.] [NA] a general term for a handle-like structure or part; often used alone to designate the manubrium sterni. **m. mal′lei** [NA], **m. of malleus,** the largest process of the malleus; it is attached to the middle layer of the tympanic membrane and has the tendon of the tensor tympani muscle attached to it. **m. ster′ni** [NA], **m. of sternum,** the cranial portion of the sternum, which articulates with the clavicles and the first two pairs of ribs; called also *presternum*.

manudynamometer (man″u-di″nah-mom′ĕ-ter) [L. *manus* hand + Gr. *dynamis* force + *metron* measure] an apparatus for measuring the force of the thrust of an instrument.

manus (ma′nus), pl. *ma′nus* [L.] [NA], the hand: the distal region of the upper limb, including the carpus, metacarpus, and digits. **m. ca′va,** a hand deformed by a deep hollowing of the palm. **m. exten′sa,** backward deviation of the hand. **m. flex′a,** forward deviation of the hand. **m. pla′na,** flattening of the arch formed normally by the proximal row of the carpal bones; flat hand. **m. superexten′sa,** manus extensa. **m. val′ga,** see *radial clubhand* and *ulnar clubhand*, under *clubhand*. **m. va′ra,** see *radial clubhand* and *ulnar clubhand*, under *clubhand*.

manyplies (men′ĭ-plīz″) omasum.

Manz's glands (mahnts′ez) [Wilhelm *Manz*, German ophthalmologist, 1833–1911] see under *gland*.

manzanita (man″zah-ne′tah) [Sp., dim. of *manzana* apple] a small shrub or tree *Arctostaphylos manzanita* Parry (Ericaceae), found in the western part of the United states; the leaves are used by the local Indians as a medicinal tea, astringent, tonic, and diuretic.

MAO monoamine oxidase. See *amine oxidase (flavin-containing)*.

MAOI monoamine oxidase inhibitor.

Maolate (ma′o-lāt) trademark for a preparation of chlorphenesin carbamate.

map (map′) a two-dimensional graphic representation of arrangement in space. **fate m.,** a plan of a blastula or early gastrula stage of an embryo showing areas of prospective significance in normal development. **gene m.,** a map showing the positions of genetic loci on the chromosomes and usually giving some indication of the distance between loci; a *physical map* gives the true distance, usually in kilobases; a *linkage map* gives distances based on recombination frequencies, measured in centimorgans; a *cytologic map* gives the position of loci relative to chromosome bands; *conjugation maps* and *transduction maps*, applicable only to bacteria, give distances based on the time, in minutes, required to transfer the DNA between loci in conjugation or on relative cotransduction frequencies; a *restriction map* is a physical map showing restriction endonuclease cleavage sites.

mapping (map′ing) locating the relative position of genes on chromosomes. Called also *gene m.*

maprotiline (mah-pro′tĭ-lēn) chemical name: N-methyl-9, 10-ethanoanthracene-9(10H)-propanamine; an antidepressant, $C_{20}H_{23}N$.

Maranta (mah-ran′tah) [after B. *Maranta*, physician in Venosa, died 1554] a genus of tropical herbs; the roots of several species afford a starch used as a dusting powder and demulcent.

marantic (mah-ran′tik) [Gr. *marantikos* wasting away] marasmic.

marasmatic (mar″az-mat′ik) marasmic.

marasmic (mah-raz′mik) pertaining to or characterized by marasmus.

marasmoid (mah-raz′moid) [Gr. *marasmos* a dying away + *eidos* form] resembling marasmus.

marasmus (mah-raz′mus) [Gr. *marasmos* a dying away] a form of protein-calorie malnutrition chiefly occurring during the first year of life, characterized by growth retardation and progressive wasting of subcutaneous fat and muscle, but usually with retention of the appetite and mental alertness. Infectious diseases may be precipitating factors. Marasmus is now considered to be related to kwashiorkor. Called also *infantile atrophy, athrepsia, pedatrophy*, and *decomposition* (Finkelstein), *m. infantilis*, and *m. lactanium*. **enzootic m.,** a condition of malnutrition in domestic herbivorous animals due to a deficiency of one or more of the trace elements, especially cobalt and copper. It is marked by progressive emaciation, severe anemia, and finally prostration; similar conditions are *bush sickness* in New Zealand, *pine* or *pining*

in Scotland, and *salt sickness* in Florida. **nutritional m.,** marasmic kwashiorkor.

marble (mar′bl) [L. *marmor*] native crystalline calcium carbonate occurring as a rock.

marbleization (mar″bel-i-za′shun) the state of being veined like marble.

marc (mark) [Fr.] the residue left after maceration of substances used in the preparation of various drugs.

Marcaine (mar-kān′) trademark for a preparation of bupivacaine hydrochloride.

march (march) in neurology, the progression of epileptic activity through the motor cortex, as in jacksonian epilepsy.

Marchand's adrenals (organs) (mar′shandz) [Felix Jacob *Marchand*, German pathologist, 1846–1928] see under *adrenal*, and see *adventitial cell*, under *cell*.

marche à petits pas (marsh-ah-pte′pah) [Fr.] a gait in which the patient takes very short steps: seen in cerebral arteriosclerotic rigidity.

Marchi's balls, etc. (mar′kēz) [Vittorio *Marchi*, Italian physician, 1851–1908] see under *ball, globule, reaction, Table of Stains,* and *tract.*

Marchiafava-Bignami disease (mar″ke-ah-fah′vah-bēn-yah′me) [Ettore *Marchiafava*, Italian pathologist, 1847–1935; Amico *Bignami*, Italian pathologist, 1862–1929] see under *disease.*

Marchiafava-Micheli disease, syndrome (mar″-ke-ah-fah′vah-me-ka′le) [Ettore *Marchiafava*; F. *Micheli*, Italian clinician, 1872–1936] paroxysmal nocturnal hemoglobinuria.

Marcus Gunn (mar′kus gun) see *Gunn.*

marcy (mar′se) a filtrable agent associated with an afebrile type of viral diarrhea.

Maréchal's test (mar″a-shalz′) [Louis Eugène *Maréchal*, French physician of the 19th century] see under *tests.*

Maréchal-Rosin test (mar″a-shal′-ro′zen) [L. E. *Maréchal*; Heinrich *Rosin*, German physician, born 1863] Maréchal's test.

marennin (mah-ren′in) a green pigment from the oysters of Marennes, in France; derived from the chlorophyll of a microorganism that infests them.

Marezine (mar′ē-zēn) trademark for a preparation of cyclizine hydrochloride.

Marfan's sign, syndrome (mar-fahnz′) [Bernard-Jean Antonin *Marfan*, French pediatrician, 1858–1942] see under *sign* and *syndrome.*

marfanoid (mar′fan-oid) having the characteristic symptoms of Marfan's syndrome.

margaric acid (mar-gar′ik) trivial name for heptadecanoic acid, the 17-carbon, straight-chain unsaturated fatty acid.

margarid (mar′gar-id) pearl-like.

margarine (mar′jar-in) [Gr. *margaron* pearl] 1. a food product containing 80 per cent of fat, manufactured primarily from refined cottonseed and soybean oils— sources of vitamin E and essential fatty acids—and fortified to supply a minimum of 15,000 U.S.P. units of vitamin A per pound; called also *oleomargarine*. 2. a (theoretical) trimargarate of propenyl.

margaritoma (mar″gar-ĭ-to′mah) cholesteatoma.

margarone (mar′gar-on) palmitone.

Margaropus (mar-gar′o-pus) a genus of ticks of the family Ixodidae. **M. annula′tus,** *Boophilus annulatus.* **M. winthem′i,** the beady-legged winter horse tick, a species found on horses and other large herbivores in South Africa.

margin (mar′jin) an edge or border, such as the boundary of an organ or other anatomic structure; called also *margo* [NA]. **m. of acetabulum,** limbus acetabuli. **alveolar m. of mandible,** arcus alveolaris mandibulae. **alveolar m. of maxilla,** arcus alveolaris maxillae. **axillary m. of scapula,** margo lateralis scapulae. **cartilaginous m. of acetabulum,** labrum acetabulare. **ciliary m. of iris,** margo ciliaris iridis. **convex m. of testis,** margo anterior testis. **coronal m. of frontal bone,** margo parietalis ossis frontalis. **coronal m. of parietal bone,** margo frontalis ossis parietalis. **crenate m. of spleen, cristate m. of spleen,** margo superior splenis. **dentate m.,** linea anocutanea. **falciform m. of**

fascia lata, **falciform m. of saphenus hiatus,** margo falciformis hiatus saphenus. **falciform m. of white line of pelvic fascia,** arcus tendineus fasciae pelvis. **m. of fibula, anterior,** margo anterior fibulae. **m. of fibula, posterior,** margo posterior fibulae. **m. of foot, fibular, m. of foot, lateral,** margo lateralis pedis. **m. of foot, medial,** margo medialis pedis. **free gingival m., free gum m.,** margo gingivalis. **free m. of eyelid,** the conjunctival-lined portion of each eyelid, about 1 mm. broad, overlying the eyeball; the anterior border of each bears the eyelashes, and the posterior border is closely applied to the eyeball. **free m. of ovary,** margo liber ovarii. **free gum m.,** free gingival m. **frontal m. of parietal bone,** margo frontalis ossis parietalis. **gingival m., gum m.,** margo gingivalis. **m. of humerus, lateral,** margo lateralis humeri. **m. of humerus, medial,** margo medialis humeri. **incisal m.,** margo incisalis. **infraorbital m. of maxilla,** margo infraorbitalis maxillae. **infraorbital m. of orbit,** margo infraorbitalis orbitae. **interosseous m. of fibula,** margo interosseus fibulae. **interosseous m. of tibia,** margo interosseus tibiae. **m. of kidney, lateral,** margo lateralis renis. **m. of kidney, medial,** margo medialis renis. **lacrimal m. of maxilla,** margo lacrimalis maxillae. **lambdoid m. of occipital bone,** margo lambdoideus squamae occipitalis. **lambdoid m. of parietal bone,** margo occipitalis ossis parietalis. **lateral margin of orbit,** margo lateralis orbitae. **m. of lung, anterior,** margo anterior pulmonis. **m. of lung, inferior,** margo inferior pulmonis. **malar m.,** margo zygomaticus alae majoris. **mamillary m.,** margo mastoideus squamae occipitalis. **mastoid m. of occipital bone,** margo mastoideus squamae occipitalis. **mastoid m. of parietal bone,** angulus mastoideus ossis parietalis. **medial m. of orbit,** margo medialis orbitae. **mesovarial m. of ovary,** margo mesovaricus ovarii. **m. of nail, free,** margo liber unguis. **m. of nail, hidden,** margo occultus unguis. **m. of nail, lateral,** margo lateralis unguis. **nasal m. of frontal bone,** margo nasalis ossis frontalis. **obtuse m. of spleen,** margo inferior splenis. **occipital m. of parietal bone,** margo occipitalis ossis parietalis. **occipital m. of temporal bone,** margo occipitalis ossis temporalis. **orbital m.,** margo orbitalis. **m. of pancreas, superior,** margo superior pancreatis. **parietal m. of frontal bone,** margo parietalis ossis frontalis. **parietal m. of great wing of sphenoid bone,** margo parietalis alae majoris. **parietal m. of occipital bone,** margo lambdoideus squamae occipitalis. **parietal m. of parietal bone,** margo sagittalis ossis parietalis. **parietal m. of temporal bone,** margo parietalis ossis temporalis. **m. of parietal bone, anterior, m. of parietal bone, frontal,** margo frontalis ossis parietalis. **m. of parietal bone, sagittal, m. of parietal bone, superior,** margo sagittalis ossis parietalis. **parietofrontal m. of great wing of sphenoid bone,** margo frontalis alae majoris. **pupillary m. of iris,** margo pupillaris iridis. **radial m. of forearm,** margo lateralis antebrachii. **m. of radius, dorsal,** margo posterior radii. **m. of scapula, anterior,** margo lateralis scapulae. **m. of scapula, external,** margo lateralis scapulae. **m. of scapula, lateral,** margo lateralis scapulae. **m. of scapula, superior,** margo superior scapulae. **sphenoidal m. of parietal bone,** angulus sphenoidalis ossis parietalis. **sphenoidal m. of temporal bone,** margo sphenoidalis ossis temporalis. **sphenotemporal m. of parietal bone,** margo squamosus ossis parietalis. **m. of spleen, anterior,** margo superior splenis. **m. of spleen, inferior, m. of spleen, posterior,** margo inferior splenis. **m. of spleen, superior,** margo superior splenis. **squamous m. of great wing of sphenoid bone,** margo squamosus alae majoris. **squamous m. of parietal bone,** margo squamosus ossis parietalis. **straight m. of testis,** margo posterior testis. **supraorbital m. of frontal bone,** margo supraorbitalis ossis frontalis. **supraorbital m. of orbit,** margo supraorbitalis orbitae. **m. of suprarenal gland, inferior,** facies renalis glandulae suprarenalis. **m. of suprarenal gland, medial,** margo medialis glandulae suprarenalis. **m. of suprarenal gland, superior,** margo superior glandulae suprarenalis. **temporal m. of parietal bone,** margo squamosus ossis parietalis. **m. of testis, anterior, m. of testis, external,** margo anterior testis. **m. of testis, internal, m. of testis, posterior,** margo

posterior testis. m. of tibia, anterior, margo anterior tibiae. **m. of tibia, medial,** margo medialis tibiae. **tibial m. of foot,** margo medialis pedis. **m. of tongue, m. of tongue, lateral,** margo linguae. **m. of ulna, anterior,** margo anterior ulnae. **m. of ulna, dorsal, m. of ulna, posterior,** margo posterior ulnae. **ulnar m. of forearm,** margo medialis antebrachii. **m. of uterus, lateral, m. of uterus, right and left,** margo uteri dexter/sinister. **vertebral m. of scapula,** margo medialis scapulae. **volar m. of radius,** margo anterior radii. **volar m. of ulna,** margo anterior ulnae. **zygomatic m. of great wing of sphenoid bone,** margo zygomaticus alae majoris.

marginal (mar′jĭ-nal) [L. *marginalis; margo* margin] pertaining to a margin or border.

margination (mar″jĭ-na′shun) accumulation and adhesion of leukocytes to the epithelial cells of blood vessel walls at the site of injury in the early stages of inflammation.

margines (mar′jĭ-nēz) [L.] plural of *margo.*

marginoplasty (mar-jin′o-plas-te) [*margin* + *-plasty*] surgical restoration of a border, as of the eyelid.

margo (mar′go), pl. *mar′gines* [L.] a margin, edge, or border; [NA] a general term for the edge of a structure. See also *labium* and *limbus.* **m. aceta′buli,** limbus acetabuli. **m. alveola′ris,** see *arcus alveolaris mandibulae* and *arcus alveolaris maxillae.* **m. ante′rior fib′ulae** [NA], anterior margin of fibula: the anterolateral border of the body of the fibula; called also *crista anterior fibulae* and *anterior crest of fibula.* **m. ante′rior hep′atis,** m. inferior hepatis. **m. ante′rior lie′nis,** m. superior splenis. **m. ante′rior pancre′atis** [NA], the anterior margin of the pancreas, which bounds the anterior and inferior surfaces; called also *anterior border of pancreas.* **m. ante′rior pulmo′nis** [NA], anterior margin of lung: the ventral border of either lung, which descends from behind the sternum, a little to the left of the midline, and curves laterally to meet the inferior margin. **m. ante′rior ra′dii** [NA], the edge of the radius that runs obliquely between the radial tuberosity and the styloid process; called also *m. volaris radii, volar margin of radius,* and *anterior border of radius.* **m. ante′rior tes′tis** [NA], anterior margin of testis: the rounded free border of the testis. **m. ante′rior tib′iae** [NA], anterior margin of tibia: the prominent anteromedial margin of the body of the tibia, separating the medial and lateral surfaces; called also *crista anterior tibiae* and *anterior border of tibia.* **m. ante′rior ul′nae** [NA], anterior margin of ulna: the volar border of the ulna, separating the medial and posterior surfaces; called also *m. volaris ulnae* and *volar margin of ulna.* **m. axilla′ris scap′ulae,** m. lateralis scapulae. **m. cilia′ris i′ridis** [NA], ciliary margin of iris: the outer border of the iris, where it is continuous with the ciliary body. **m. dex′ter cor′dis** [NA], right border of heart: the margin of the heart formed by the wall of the profile of the right atrium, running from the apex to the right, and marking the junction of the sternocostal and diaphragmatic cardiac surfaces; seen as a surface except in radiograms and two-dimensional illustrations. Called also *facies dextra cordis* and *right surface of heart.* **m. dorsa′lis ra′dii,** m. posterior radii. **m. dorsa′lis ul′nae,** m. posterior ulnae. **m. falcifor′mis fas′ciae la′tae,** m. falciformis hiatus saphenus. **m. falcifor′mis hia′tus saphe′nus** [NA], falciform margin of saphenous hiatus: the lateral margin of the saphenous hiatus; called also *m. falciformis fasciae latae.* **m. fibula′ris pe′dis,** NA alternative for *m. lateralis pedis.* **m. fronta′lis a′lae mag′nae,** m. frontalis alae majoris. **m. fronta′lis a′lae majo′ris** [NA], frontal margin of great wing of sphenoid bone: a roughened area on the great wing of the sphenoid bone where it articulates with the frontal bone; it is situated at the upper lateral margin of the orbital surface of the great wing where this meets the cerebral and temporal surfaces. Called also *m. frontalis alae magnae.* **m. fronta′lis os′sis parieta′lis** [NA], frontal margin of parietal bone: the edge of the parietal bone that articulates with the frontal bone along the coronal suture. **m. gingiva′lis** [NA], gingival margin: the crest of the free gingiva that surrounds the teeth in a collarlike fashion, separated from the adjacent attached gingiva by the free gingival groove, and forms the wall of the gingival sulcus; called also *gum m.* and *marginal gingiva.* **m. incisa′lis** [NA], incisal margin; the crest of the biting edge of an incisor tooth. **m. infe′rior ce′rebri** [NA], the inferior lateral border of the cerebral hemisphere; called also *m. inferolateralis cerebri.* **m. infe′rior hep′atis** [NA], the anteroinferior edge of the liver, separating the anterior and the visceral surface; called also *m. anterior hepatis* and *inferior border of liver.* **m. infe′rior lie′nis,** NA alternative for *m. inferior splenis.* **m. infe′rior pancre′atis** [NA], the inferior margin of the pancreas, which bounds the inferior and posterior surfaces; called also *m. posterior pancreatis.* **m. infe′rior pulmo′nis** [NA], inferior margin of lung: the border of the lung that extends in a curve behind the sixth costal cartilage, the upper margin of the eighth rib in the axillary line, the ninth or tenth rib in the scapular line, and passes medially to the eleventh costovertebral joint. **m. infe′rior sple′nis** [NA], inferior, or posterior, margin, or border, of spleen: a straight margin of the spleen somewhat less prominent than the superior margin, separating the renal surface from the diaphragmatic surface; called also *m. inferior lienis* [NA alternative] and *m. posterior lienis.* **m. inferolatera′lis cer′ebri,** m. inferior cerebri. **m. inferomedia′lis cer′ebri,** m. medialis cerebri. **m. infraglenoida′lis tib′iae,** the margin of bone that forms the circumference of the condyles of the tibia just inferior to the facies articularis superior. **m. infraorbita′lis maxil′lae** [NA], infraorbital margin of maxilla: the short rounded edge of the maxilla where the orbital surface becomes continuous with the anterior surface. **m. infraorbita′lis or′bitae** [NA], infraorbital margin of orbit: the inferior edge of the entrance to the orbit, formed by the infraorbital process of the zygomatic bone and the infraorbital margin of the maxilla. **m. interos′seus fib′ulae** [NA], a prominent ridge medial to the anterior border of the fibula, connected with a similar ridge on the tibia by a strong, wide fibrous sheet, the interosseous membrane; called also *crista interossea fibulae* and *interosseous border, crest,* or *ridge of fibula.* **m. interos′seus ra′dii** [NA], the prominent medial border of the radius, connected with a similar ridge on the ulna by a strong, wide fibrous sheet, the interossesous membrane; called also *crista interossea radii* and *interosseous border, crest,* or *ridge of radius.* **m. interos′seus tib′iae** [NA], interosseous margin of tibia: the prominent lateral border of the body of the tibia, which separates the posterior and lateral surfaces and gives attachment to the interosseous membrane; called also *crista interossea tibiae* and *interosseous border, crest,* or *ridge of tibia.* **m. interos′seus ul′nae** [NA], the prominent lateral border of the ulna, connected with a similar ridge on the radius by the interosseous membrane; called also *crista interossea ulnae* and *interosseous border, crest,* or *ridge of ulna.* **m. lacrima′lis maxil′lae** [NA], lacrimal margin of maxilla: the posterior border of the frontal process of the maxilla where it articulates with the lacrimal bone; called also *lacrimal border of maxilla.* **m. lamb-doi′deus squa′mae occipita′lis** [NA], lambdoid margin of occipital bone: the edge of the occipital bone that extends from the lateral angle to the superior angle, articulating with the parietal bone to help form the lambdoid suture; called also *lambdoid margin of occipital bone.* **m. latera′lis antebra′chii** [NA], the lateral, or radial, border of the forearm; called also *m. radialis antebrachii* [NA alternative]. **mar′gines latera′les digito′rum pe′dis,** facies laterales digitorum pedis. **m. latera′lis hu′meri** [NA], lateral margin of humerus: the edge of the humerus that extends from posteroinferior part of the greater tubercle to the lateral epicondyle; called also *lateral angle* or *border of humerus.* **m. latera′lis** [lin′guae], m. linguae. **m. latera′lis or′bitae** [NA], the lateral margin of the orbit, formed by the zygomatic process of the frontal bone and the frontal process of the zygomatic bone. **m. latera′lis pe′-dis** [NA], the lateral, or fibular, border of the foot; called also *m. fibularis pedis* [NA alternative]. **m. latera′lis re′nis** [NA], lateral margin of kidney: the convex narrow border of the kidney. **m. latera′lis scap′ulae** [NA], lateral margin of scapula: the thick edge of the scapula, extending from the inferior margin of the glenoid cavity to the inferior angle; called also *m. axillaris scapulae* and *lateral border of scapula.* **m. latera′lis un′guis** [NA], lateral margin of nail: the edge on either side of the nail. **m. latera′lis u′teri,** m. uteri dexter/sinister. **m. li′ber ova′rii** [NA], free margin of ovary: the broad, convex border of the ovary, opposite the mesovarial margin. **m. li′ber un′guis** [NA], the overhanging, distal, free edge of the nail. **m. lin′guae** [NA], margin of tongue: the lateral border of the body of the tongue; called also *m. lateralis* [linguae]. **m. mas-toi′deus squa′mae occipita′lis** [NA], mastoid margin

of occipital bone: the edge of the occipital bone that extends from the jugular process to the lateral angle, articulating with the part of the temporal bone that bears the mastoid process. **m. media′lis antebra′chii** [NA], the medial, or ulnar, border of the forearm; called also *m. ulnaris antebrachii* [NA alternative]. **m. media′lis cer′ebri** [NA], inferior medial margin of the cerebral hemisphere; called also *m. inferomedialis cerebri.* **mar′gines media′les digito′rum pe′dis,** facies mediales digitorum pedis. **m. media′lis glan′dulae suprarena′lis** [NA], medial margin of suprarenal gland: the medial border, which with the superior border divides the anterior from the posterior surface. **m. media′lis hu′meri** [NA], medial margin of humerus: the edge of the humerus that begins at the lesser tubercle above and continues downward to the medial epicondyle; called also *medial angle* or *border of humerus.* **m. media′lis or′bitae** [NA], the medial margin of the orbit, formed above by the bone and below by the lacrimal crest of the frontal process of the maxilla. **m. media′lis pe′dis** [NA], the medial, or tibial, border of the foot; called also *m. tibialis pedis* [NA alternative]. **m. media′lis re′nis** [NA], medial margin of kidney: the concave border of the kidney, which contains the hilus. **m. media′lis scap′ulae** [NA], the thin edge of the scapula extending from the superior to the inferior angle; called also *m. vertebralis scapulae* and *vertebral border* or *margin of scapula.* **m. media′lis tib′iae** [NA], medial margin of tibia: the border that extends between the medial condyle and medial malleolus of the tibia, separating the medial and posterior surfaces; called also *medial angle* or *border of tibia.* **m. mesova′ricus ova′rii** [NA], mesovarial margin of ovary: the border of the ovary that is attached to the broad ligament by means of the mesovarium. **m. nasa′lis os′-sis fronta′lis** [NA], nasal margin of frontal bone: the articular surface, on each nasal part of the frontal bone, that articulates with the nasal bones and with the frontal processes of the maxilla. **m. na′si,** the lower, free, margin of the ala nasi and septum nasi that surrounds the external naris. **m. occipita′lis os′sis parieta′lis** [NA], occipital margin of parietal bone: the edge of the parietal bone that articulates with the occipital bone at the lambdoid suture. **m. occipita′lis os′sis tempora′lis** [NA], occipital margin of temporal bone: the border of the petrous part of the temporal bone that articulates with the occipital bone along the occipitomastoid suture. **m. occul′tus un′guis** [NA], the proximal, buried edge of the nail. **m. orbita′lis** [NA], orbital margin: the border of the orbit, formed mainly by the frontal and zygomatic bones and the maxilla. **m. pal′pebrae,** see *free margin of eyelid.* **m. parieta′lis a′lae majo′ris** [NA], parietal margin of great wing of sphenoid bone: the superior extremity of the squamous margin of the great wing of the sphenoid bone where it articulates with the parietal bone; called also *angulus parietalis ossis sphenoidalis.* **m. parieta′lis os′sis fronta′lis** [NA], parietal margin of frontal bone: the posterior border of the frontal bone, semicircular in shape, which articulates with the parietal bones. **m. parieta′-lis os′sis tempora′lis** [NA], parietal margin of temporal bone: the superior border of the squamous part of the temporal bone where it articulates with the parietal bone; called also *m. parietalis squamae temporalis.* **m. parieta′lis squa′mae tempora′lis,** m. parietalis ossis temporalis. **m. pe′dis latera′lis,** m. lateralis pedis. **m. pe′dis media′lis,** m. medialis pedis. **m. poste′rior fib′ulae** [NA], posterior margin of fibula: the posterolateral margin of the body of the fibula; called also *crista lateralis fibulae* and *posterior border* or *crest of fibula.* **m. poste′rior lie′nis,** m. inferior splenis. **m. poste′rior pancre′atis,** m. inferior pancreatis. **m. poste′rior ra′dii** [NA], the edge of the radius that extends from the posterior part of the radial tuberosity to the middle tubercle; called also *m. dorsalis radii,* and *dorsal margin* or *posterior border of radius.* **m. poste′rior tes′tis** [NA], posterior margin of testis: the border of the testis that is attached to the epididymis and the lower end of the ductus deferens; called also *dorsum of testis.* **m. poste′rior ul′nae** [NA], posterior margin of ulna: the dorsal border of the ulna, separating the posterior and medial surfaces; called also *m. dorsalis ulnae.* **m. pupilla′ris i′ridis** [NA], pupillary margin of iris: the inner edge of the iris, surrounding the pupil. **m. radia′lis antebra′chii,** NA alternative for *m. lateralis antebrachii.* **m. radia′lis antibra′chii,** m. lateralis antebrachii. **m. radia′lis hu′meri,** m. lateralis humeri. **m. sagitta′lis os′sis parieta′lis** [NA], sagittal margin of parietal bone: the edge of the parietal bone that articulates with the other parietal bone along the sagittal suture; called also *parietal* or *superior margin of parietal bone.* **m. sphenoida′lis os′sis tempora′lis** [NA], sphenoidal margin of temporal bone: the anterior border of the temporal bone, articulating with the great wing of the sphenoid bone; called also *m. sphenoidalis squamae temporalis.* **m. sphenoida′lis squa′mae tempora′- lis,** m. sphenoidalis ossis temporalis. **m. squamo′sus a′lae mag′nae,** m. squamosus alae majoris. **m. squamo′sus a′lae majo′ris** [NA], squamous margin of great wing of sphenoid bone: the border of the great wing of the sphenoid bone that articulates with the squama of the temporal bone; called also *m. squamosus alae magnae.* **m. squamo′sus os′sis parieta′lis** [NA], squamous margin of parietal bone: the inferior edge of the parietal bone, which articulates with the sphenoid and temporal bones along the squamous suture. **m. supe′rior cer′ebri** [NA], the superior medial margin of the cerebral hemisphere; called also *m. superomedialis cerebri.* **m. supe′rior glan′dulae suprarena′lis** [NA], the superior margin or border of the suprarenal gland, which with the medial border divides the anterior from the posterior surface. **m. supe′rior lie′nis,** NA alternative for *m. superior splenis.* **m. supe′rior pancre′atis** [NA], the superior border of the pancreas, which bounds the anterior and posterior surfaces. **m. supe′rior scap′ulae** [NA], superior margin of scapula: the thin, short edge of the scapula, extending from the superior angle to the coracoid process; called also *superior border of scapula.* **m. supe′rior sple′nis** [NA], superior, or anterior, margin, or border, of spleen: a somewhat sharp, convex line, sometimes serrated, between the gastric and diaphragmatic surfaces of the spleen; called also *m. anterior lienis* and *m. superior lienis* [NA alternative]. **m. superomedia′lis cer′ebri,** m. superior cerebri. **m. supraorbita′lis or′bitae** [NA], supraorbital margin of orbit: the superior edge of the entrance to the orbit, formed by the supraorbital margin of the frontal bone. **m. supraorbita′lis os′sis fronta′lis** [NA], supraorbital margin of frontal bone: the antero-inferior edge of the frontal bone, bending down laterally to the zygomatic bone and medially to the frontal process of the maxilla; it marks the junction between the squama and the orbital portion of the bone. **m. tibia′lis pe′dis,** NA alternative for *m. medialis pedis.* **m. ulna′ris antebra′chii,** NA alternative for *m. medialis antebrachii.* **m. ulna′ris antibra′chii,** m. medialis antebrachii. **m. ulna′ris hu′meri,** m. medialis humeri. **m. u′teri dex′ter/sinis′ter** [NA], right and left margin of uterus: either border of the uterus (right and left) at the upper portion of which the uterine tube is attached; called also *lateral margin of uterus* and *m. lateralis uteri.* **m. vertebra′lis scap′ulae,** m. medialis scapulae. **m. vola′ris ra′dii,** m. anterior radii. **m. vola′- ris ul′nae,** m. anterior ulnae. **m. zygomat′icus a′lae mag′nae,** m. zygomaticus alae majoris. **m. zygomat′icus a′lae majo′ris** [NA], zygomatic margin of great wing of sphenoid bone: the border on the great wing of the sphenoid bone that separates its temporal and orbital surfaces and articulates with the zygomatic bone; called also *m. zygomaticus alae magnae.*

mariahuana, mariajuana (mah-re-ah-wah′nah) marihuana.

mariculture (mar″ĭ-kul′chur) [L. *mare* sea + culture] the cultivation of sea life to provide nutrients.

Marie's ataxia, etc. (mahrēz′) [Pierre *Marie,* French physician, 1853–1940] see under *ataxia, disease, hypertrophy,* and *sign.*

Marie-Bamberger disease (mah-re′-bahm′ber-ger) [Pierre *Marie;* Eugen *Bamberger,* Austrian physician, 1858–1921] hypertrophic pulmonary osteoarthropathy.

Marie-Strümpell disease, syndrome (mah-re′ strim′- pel) [Pierre *Marie;* Adolf von *Strümpell,* physician in Leipzig, 1853–1925] rheumatoid spondylitis.

Marie-Tooth disease (mah-re′-tooth′) [Pierre *Marie;* Howard Henry *Tooth,* English physician, 1856–1926] progressive neuropathic (peroneal) muscular atrophy.

mariguana (mar″ĭ-hwah′nah) marihuana.

marihuana (mar″ĭ-hwan′ah) [Mexican Sp.] a crude preparation of the leaves and flowering tops of (male or female plants) *Cannabis sativa* L. (Cannabaceae), usually employed in cigarets and inhaled as smoke for its euphoric properties. See *cannabis.*

marijuana (mar″ĭ-hwah′nah) marihuana.

Marinesco's sign, succulent hand (mar″ĭ-nes′kōz) [Georges *Marinesco,* Roumanian neurologist, 1863–1938] main succulente.

marinobufagin (mar″ĭ-no-bu′fah-jin) a cardiac poison, $C_{24}H_{32}O_5$, from the skin of the toad, *Bufo marinus.*

Mariotte's experiment, law, spot (mar″e-ots′) [Edme *Mariotte,* French physicist, 1620–1684] see under *experiment,* and see *Boyle's law,* under *law,* and *blind spot,* under *spot.*

mariposia (mar″ĭ-po′ze-ah) [L. *mare* the sea + Gr. *posis* drinking + -ia] thalassoposia.

maritonucleus (mar″ĭ-to-nu′kle-us) [L. *maritus* married + *nucleus*] the nucleus of the ovum after the sperm cell has entered it.

Marjolin's ulcer (mar″zho-lanz′) [Jean Nicolas *Marjolin,* French surgeon 1780–1850] see under *ulcer.*

mark (mark) a spot, blemish, or other circumscribed area visible on a surface, particularly on the skin or mucous membrane. **beauty m.,** a small pigmented nevus, particularly on the cheek, said to enhance the appearance. **birth m.,** see *birthmark.* **pock m.,** see *pockmark.* **Pohl's m.,** a limited thinning of the shaft of a hair, usually accompanied by interruption of the medulla; it is usually a sign of systemic disease, but may be due to trauma, coronary occlusion, skin disease, or the therapeutic administration of a single substantial dose of an antimetabolite, such as methotrexate or cyclophosphamide. **port-wine m.,** see under *stain.* **strawberry m.,** 1. see under *hemangioma,* def. 1. 2. cavernous hemangioma.

marker (mark′er) something that identifies or that is used to identify. **Amsler's m.,** a form of caliper compass used for marking the point for the application of cautery in Gonin's operation. **cell-surface m.,** an antigenic determinant occurring on the surface of a specific type of cell. **genetic m.,** a genetic polymorphism with a simple mode of inheritance occurring with different frequencies in different populations, and therefore useful in family studies, studies of the distribution of genes in populations, and linkage analysis.

marking (mark′ing) a conspicuous line or spot visible on a surface. **Fontana's m's,** minute transverse folds seen on a divided nerve trunk.

Marlow's test (mar′lōz) [Frank William *Marlow,* Syracuse ophthalmologist, 1858–1942] see under *tests.*

marmoration (mar″mo-ra′shun) [L. *marmor* marble] marbleization.

marmoreal (mar-mo′re-al) resembling marble, as bone in osteopetrosis.

marmot (mar′mot) any of several large terrestrial animals of the squirrel family, members of the genera *Marmota* and *Arctomys,* found in the Northern Hemisphere, such as the hoary marmot, yellow-bellied marmot, and woodchuck or ground-hog of North America and the tarbagan of Asia; they may be natural reservoirs of the plague.

Maroteaux-Lamy syndrome (mah-ro-to′ lah-me′) [Pierre *Maroteaux,* French physician, born 1926; Maurice Emile Joseph *Lamy,* French physician, born 1895] see under *syndrome.*

Marplan (mar′plan) trademark for a preparation of isocarboxazid.

Marriott's method (mar′e-ots) [William McKim *Marriott,* American physician, 1885–1936] see under *method.*

marrow (mar′o) the soft organic material that fills the cavities of the bones (see *medulla ossium*); called also *medulla.* **bone m.,** medulla ossium. **bone m., red,** medulla ossium rubra. **bone m., yellow,** medulla ossium flava. **depressed m.,** bone marrow exhibiting decreased hematopoietic activity. **fat m.,** medulla ossium flava. **gelatinous m.,** bone marrow that has lost its blood cells and its fat and has acquired a gelatinous appearance. **red m.,** medulla ossium rubra. **spinal m.,** the spinal cord (medulla spinalis [NA]). **yellow m.,** medulla ossium flava.

marrowbrain (mar′o-brān) the myelencephalon; def. 1.

Marsh's disease (marsh′ez) [Sir Henry *Marsh,* Irish physician, 1790–1860] Graves' disease.

Marshall's fold, vein (mar'shalz) [John *Marshall*, English anatomist, 1818–1891] see *plica venae cavae sinistrae* and *vena obliqua atrii sinistri.*

Marshall Hall   see *Hall.*

marsupia (mar-su'pe-ah) [L.]   plural of *marsupium.*

marsupial (mar-su'pe-al) [L. *marsupium* a pouch]   a member of the order Marsupialia.

Marsupialia (mar-su″pe-a'le-ah)   an order of the class Mammalia characterized by the possession of an abdominal pouch, or marsupium, in which the young, which are born in a very underdeveloped state, are carried and nourished until their development is complete. It includes the opossums, kangaroos, wallabies, koala bears, and wombats. In some systems of classification, it is considered to be an order of the infraclass or subclass Metatheria, class Mammalia.

marsupialization (mar-su″pe-al-i-za'shun) [L. *marsupium* pouch]   the creation of a pouch; applied especially to surgical exteriorization of a cyst by resection of the anterior wall and suture of the cut edges of the remaining cyst to the adjacent edges of the skin, thereby establishing a pouch of what was formerly an enclosed cyst.

marsupium (mar-su'pe-um), pl. *marsu'pia* [L. "a pouch"]   1. the scrotum.   2. an external abdominal pouch or fold of skin for carrying the young; it contains the mammary glands and occurs in marsupials and the spiny anteaters. Also, a similar structure for carrying eggs and/or the young, as in the male sea horse. **marsu'pia patella'ris,** plicae alares.

Marteilia (mar-ti'le-ah)   a genus of parasitic protozoa (order Occlusosporida, class Stellatosporea) pathogenic in European oysters.

Marteiliida (mar″tĕ-li'ĭ-dah)   Occlusosporida.

martial (mar'shal) [L. *martialis* of Mars, the god of war.]   containing iron; ferruginous or chalybeate.

Martin's bandage, disease (mar'tinz) [Henry Austin *Martin*, American surgeon, 1824–1884]   see under *bandage* and *disease.*

Martinotti's cells (mar″tĭ-not'ēz) [Giovanni *Martinotti*, Bologna pathologist, 1857–1928]   see under *cell.*

masc.   mass concentration.

maschaladenitis (mas″kal-ad″ĕ-ni'tis) [Gr. *maschalē* armpit + *adēn* gland + *-itis*]   inflammation of the glands of the axilla.

maschaloncus (mas″kal-ong'kus)   a tumor of the axilla.

masculation (mas″ku-la'shun)   the development of male characteristics.

masculine (mas'ku-lin) [L. *masculinus*]   pertaining to the male sex, or possessing qualities normally characteristic of the male.

masculinity (mas″ku-lin'ĭ-te)   the possession of masculine qualities.

masculinization (mas″ku-lin-i-za'shun)   the normal induction or development of male sex characters in the male. Also, the induction or development of male secondary sex characters in the female. Called also *virilization.*

masculinize (mas'ku-lĭ-nīz″)   to produce male characteristics (virilism) in a female or to induce normal virilization in a pubertal male.

masculinovoblastoma (mas″ku-lin-o″vo-blas-to'mah)   lipoid cell tumor of ovary; see under *tumor.*

masculonucleus (mas″ku-lo-nu'kle-us)   arsenoblast.

maser (ma'zer) [*m*icrowave *a*mplification by *s*timulated *e*mission of *r*adiation]   a device which produces an extremely intense, small, and nearly nondivergent beam of monochromatic radiation in the microwave region with all waves in phase.

mask (mask) [Fr. *masque*]   1. to cover or conceal, as the masking of the nature of a disorder by the presence of unrelated signs, symptoms, organisms, etc. In audiometry, to obscure or diminish a sound by the presence of another sound of different frequency.   2. a covering for the face, as a bandage, an apparatus for administering oxygen, or a cloth that prevents droplets from the nose and mouth from spreading in the air.   3. in dentistry, to camouflage metal parts of a prosthesis by covering with opaque material.   **BLB m.,** an oxygen-breathing mask for use at high altitudes; it has a combined inspiratory and expiratory valve and a bag for rebreathing (Boothby, Lovelace, Bulbulian). It has also been

used for clinical administration of oxygen.   **Curschmann's m.,** a mask formerly used for inhaling turpentine vapors.   **death m.,** a plaster cast of the face of a dead person.   **ecchymotic m.,** cyanotic discoloration of the head and neck as a result of traumatic asphyxia.   **full-face m.,** a device used in anesthesia to confine the gas to be delivered through the mask into the respiratory tract through the nose or mouth.   **Hutchinson's m.,** a sensation as if the skin of the face were compressed by a mask; often a symptom of tabes dorsalis.   **Kuhn's m.,** a mask worn over the nose and mouth, which, by obstructing the respiration, was reported to produce artificial hyperemia of the pulmonary tissues; formerly used in treating pulmonary tuberculosis.   **meter m.,** an oxygen-breathing mask designed to provide fixed percentage admixtures of air and oxygen.   **Parkinson's m.,** see under *facies.*   **m. of pregnancy,** see *melasma.*   **tabetic m.,** Hutchinson's m. **Wanscher's m.,** a mask for ether anesthesia.

masochism (mas'o-kizm) [Leopold von Sacher-*Masoch*, an Austrian novelist, 1836–1895]   a paraphilia in which sexual gratification is derived from being humiliated or hurt by another. Called sexual masochism in DSM III-R.

masochist (mas'o-kist)   one given to masochism.

masochistic (mas″o-kis'tik)   pertaining to or characterized by masochism.

Mas. pil.   abbreviation for L. *mas'sa pilula'rum,* pill mass.

mass (mas) [L. *massa*]   1. a lump or body made up of cohering particles; see also *massa.*   2. a cohesive mixture suitable for being made up into pills.   3. that characteristic of matter which gives it inertia. The mass of a hypothetical atom of atomic weight 1.000 (a dalton) is 1.648×10^{-24} gm., and the mass of any other atom may be found by multiplying this number by the atomic weight of the atom.   **achromatic m.,** the nonstaining portion of the karyokinetic figure. **appendiceal m., appendix m.,** a palpable mass in the right iliac fossa or right loin due to acute appendicitis, usually with abscess secondary to rupture; occasionally caused by adherent omentum and intestine.   **atomic m.,** the mass of a neutral atom of a nuclide, usually expressed in atomic mass units (amu).   **blue m.,** mercury m.   **body cell m.,** the total weight of the cells of the body, including the cell nucleus, cytoplasm, water, salt, protein, and surrounding membrane, but excluding extracellular water and extracellular solids such as collagen, elastin, and bone matrix, constituting in essence the total mass of oxygen-utilizing, carbohydrate-burning, and energy-exchanging cells of the body; regarded as proportional to total exchangeable potassium in the body.   **electronic m.,** the mass of a negative electron when moving at moderate velocity; it is 8.999×10^{-28} gm. **ferrous carbonate m.,** a soft, dark greenish gray substance containing 36 to 41 per cent of ferrous carbonate; used in anemia.   **fibrillar m. of Flemming,** spongioplasm, def. 1.   **injection m.,** a suspension or solution, usually colored, injected into blood vessels or other tissue spaces to permit their demonstration on dissection or sectioning. **inner cell m.,** an aggregation of cells at one pole of the blastocyst, which is destined to form the embryo proper. **intermediate m.,** adhesio interthalamica.   **intermediate cell m.,** nephrotome.   **lateral m. of atlas,** massa lateralis atlantis.   **lateral m's of ethmoid bone,** see *labyrinthus ethmoidalis.*   **lateral m. of sacrum,** pars lateralis ossis sacri.   **lateral m. of vertebrae,** pediculus arcus vertebrae.   **lean body m.,** that part of the body including all its components except neutral storage lipid; in essence, the fat-free mass of the body.   **mercury m.,** a mixture of mercury oleate, mercury, honey, glycerin, glycyrrhiza, and althea, containing 31–35 per cent of mercury; used in the treatment of pediculosis pubis. Called also *massa hydrargyri, blue mass,* and *blue pill.*   **pill m., pilular m.,** a drug mass of the proper consistency for being made into pills.   **Stent's m.,** a plastic resinous material which sets into a very hard substance; used in surgery for making molds shaped to keep grafts in place. See also *stent.* **tigroid m's,** Nissl's bodies.   **Vallet's m.,** ferrous carbonate m.   **ventrolateral m.,** that portion of the primitive lateral mass of the embryo from which are developed the abdominal, thoracic, and anterior cervical muscles.

massa (mas'ah), gen. and pl. *mas'sae* [L.]   a unified lump or mass of material; [NA] a general term for an accumulation of cells or cohesive tissue. Called also *mass.*   **m. fer'ri carbona'tis,** ferrous carbonate mass.   **m. hydrar'gyri,** mercury mass.   **m. innomina'ta,** paradidymis.   **m. in-**

terme′dia, adhesio interthalamica. **m. latera′lis atlan′tis** [NA], lateral mass of atlas: the thickened lateral portion of the atlas to which the arches are attached and which bears the articulating surfaces and the transverse process. **mas′sae latera′les os′sis ethmoida′lis,** see *labyrinthus ethmoidalis.* **m. latera′lis os′sis sa′cri,** pars lateralis ossis sacri. **m. latera′lis ver′tebrae,** pediculus arcus vertebrae. **m. mol′lis** (*obs.*), adhesio interthalamica.

massae (mas′e) [L.] genitive and plural of *massa.*

massage (mah-sahzh′) [Fr.; Gr. *massein* to knead] the systematic therapeutic friction, stroking, and kneading of the body. **cardiac m.,** rhythmic compression of the heart by pressure applied manually over the sternum (closed cardiac massage) or directly to the heart through an opening in the chest wall (open cardiac massage); done to reinstate and maintain circulation. **Cederschiöld′s m.,** massage by making rhythmic pressure over the parts. **douche m.,** massage combined with the application of a douche. **electrovibratory m.,** massage by means of an electric vibrator. **gingival m.,** the systematic application of frictional rubbing and stroking to the gingiva. **heart m.,** cardiac m. **hydropneumatic m.,** massage by means of air forced through a tube at the end of which is a chamber containing water, the water chamber being applied to the part to be massaged. **tremolo m.,** a variety of mechanical massage. **vapor m.,** treatment of a lung cavity by a medicated and nebulized vapor under interrupted pressure. **vibratory m.,** massage by rapidly repeated light percussion with a vibrating hammer or sound.

Masselon′s spectacles (mas″ĕ-lawz′) [Miche Julien *Masselon,* French ophthalmologist, 1844–1917] see under *spectacles.*

Masset′s test (mas-āz′) [Alfred Auguste *Masset,* French physician, born 1870] see under *tests.*

masseter (mas-se′ter) [Gr. *masētēr* chewer] see *musculus masseter.*

masseteric (mas″e-ter′ik) pertaining to the masseter muscle.

masseur (mah-ser′) [Fr.] 1. a man who performs massage. 2. an instrument for performing massage.

masseuse (mah-suhz′) [Fr.] a woman who performs massage.

massicot (mas′ĭ-kot) lead monoxide, PbO.

massive (mas′iv) having a solid bulky form; heavy; in a mass; complete.

Masson stain (mas-on) [C. L. Pierre *Masson,* Montreal pathologist, 1880–1959] see *Table of Stains.*

massotherapy (mas″o-ther′ah-pe) [Gr. *massein* to knead + *therapy*] the treatment of disease by massage.

MAST [acronym for *m*ilitary or *m*edical *a*nti-*s*hock *t*rousers] see *pneumatic antishock garment,* under *garment.*

mastadenitis (mas″tad-ĕ-ni′tis) [*mast-* + Gr. *adēn* gland + *-itis*] inflammation of the mammary gland; mastitis.

mastadenoma (mas″tad-ĕ-no′mah) [*mast-* + Gr. *adēn* gland + *-oma*] tumor of the breast.

mastalgia (mas-tal′je-ah) [*mast-* + *-algia*] pain in the mammary gland.

mastatrophia (mas″tah-tro′fe-ah) mastatrophy.

mastatrophy (mas-tat′ro-fe) [*mast-* + *atrophy*] atrophy of the mammary gland.

mastauxe (mas-tawk′se) [*mast-* + Gr. *auxē* increase] enlargement of the breast.

mastectomy (mas-tek′to-me) [*mast-* + Gr. *ektomē* excision] excision of the breast; mammectomy. **extended radical m.,** radical mastectomy with removal of the ipsilateral half of the sternum and a portion of ribs two through five with the underlying pleura and the internal mammary lymph nodes. **Halsted m.,** radical m. **Meyer m.,** radical m. **modified radical m.,** total mastectomy with axillary node dissection, but with preservation of the pectoral muscles. **partial m.,** segmental m. **radical m.,** removal of the breast, pectoral muscles, axillary lymph nodes, and associated skin and subcutaneous tissue in treatment of breast cancer. **segmental m.,** removal of only enough breast tissue to ensure that the margins of the resected surgical specimen are free of tumor. **simple m.,** removal of only the breast tissue and nipple and a small portion of the overlying skin. **subcutaneous m.,** excision of breast tissue with preservation of overlying skin, nipple, and areola so that breast form may be reconstructed. **total m.,** simple m.

Master "2-step" exercise test (mas′ter) [Arthur M. *Master,* American physician, 1895–1973] see under *tests.*

Masterone (mas′tĕ-rōn) trademark for a preparation of diomostanolone propionate.

masthelcosis (mas″thel-ko′sis) [*mast-* + Gr. *helkōsis* ulceration] ulceration of the breast or mammary gland.

mastic (mas′tik) [L. *mastiche;* Gr. *mastichē*] a yellowish, hard, resinous exudation obtained from the shrub *Pistacia lentiscus* L. (Anacardiaceae), indigenous to the Mediterranean Islands, especially Chios. It is widely used in Greece as characteristically flavored chewing gum base, and contains about 2 per cent volatile oil and several resin acids. Used in tooth cements as dental liner and in plasters, lacquers, and incense, and pharmaceutically in enteric coatings for tablets.

mastication (mas″tĭ-ka′shun) [L. *masticare* to chew] the process of chewing food in preparation for swallowing and digestion.

masticatory (mas′tĭ-kah-to″re) 1. subserving or pertaining to mastication; affecting the muscles of mastication. 2. a remedy to be chewed but not swallowed.

mastiche (mas′tĭ-kĕ) [L.] mastic.

mastigont (mas′tĭ-gont) [Gr. *mastigoun* to whip] a flagellum; see under *system.*

Mastigophora (mas″tĭ-gof′o-rah) [Gr. *mastix* whip + *phoros* bearing] a subphylum of protozoa (phylum Sarcomastigophora) comprising the flagellates, i.e., all those with one or more flagella in the trophozoite. Mastigophorans have a simple, centrally placed nucleus and reproduce by longitudinal binary fission, and most are free-living but many are parasitic in both invertebrates and vertebrates, including humans. The subphylum comprises two classes; Phytomastigophorea (plantlike protozoa, or phytoflagellates) and Zoomastigophorea (animal-like protozoa, or zooflagellates). Formerly called *Euflagellata* and *Flagellata.*

mastigophoran (mas″tĭ-gof′o-ran) any protozoan of the subphylum Mastigophora; a flagellate; a mastigote.

mastigophorous (mas″tĭ-gof′o-rus) of or pertaining to the subphylum Mastigophora.

mastigote (mas′tĭ-gōt) any protozoan of the subphylum Mastigophora; a flagellate; a mastigophoran.

mastitis (mas-ti′tis) [*mast-* + *-itis*] inflammation of the mammary gland, or breast. **chronic cystic m.,** cystic disease of breast; see under *disease.* **gargantuan m.,** pathologic enlargement of the breasts to a tremendous size. **glandular m.,** parenchymatous m. **interstitial m.,** inflammation of the stroma of the mammary gland. **m. neonato′rum,** a general term applied to an abnormal condition of the breast of the newborn, such as hypertrophy, engorgement and secretion, or inflammation, with or without suppuration. **parenchymatous m.,** inflammation of the secreting elements of the mammary gland. **periductal m.,** inflammation of tissues about the ducts of the mammary gland. **phlegmonous m.,** inflammation of the breast leading to abscess formation. **plasma cell m.,** a morbid condition of the breast characterized by infiltration of the breast stroma with plasma cells and proliferation of the cells lining the ducts, thought by some to be the end-stage of mammary duct ectasia. **puerperal m.,** a form of mastitis occurring after delivery. **retromammary m., submammary m.,** paramastitis. **stagnation m.,** a local engorgement affecting one or more lobules of the breast and forming a painful lump in the organ; it occurs during early lactation. Called also *caked breast.* **suppurative m.,** pyogenic infection of the breast.

mast(o)- [Gr. *mastos* breast] a combining form denoting relationship to the breast or to the mastoid process; see also words beginning *mamm(o)-* and *maz(o)-.*

mastocarcinoma (mas″to-kar″sĭ-no′mah) [*masto-* + *carcinoma*] carcinoma of the breast.

mastoccipital (mas″tok-sip′ĭ-tal) masto-occipital.

mastochondroma (mas″to-kon-dro′mah) [*masto-* + *chondroma*] a chondroma of the breast.

mastochondrosis (mas″to-kon-dro′sis) mastochondroma.

mastocyte (mas′to-sīt) [Ger. *Mast* food + *-cyte*] a mast cell.

mastocytoma (mas″to-si-to′mah) [*masto-* + *cytoma*] a

nodular cutaneous mast cell infiltrate, which is usually present at birth or soon after as a solitary nodule, although three to four lesions may occur. Lesions typical of urticaria pigmentosa may occur later. Called also *mast cell tumor*.

mastocytosis (mas″to-si-to′sis) [*masto-* + *cytosis*] a group of rare diseases characterized by infiltrates of mast cells in the tissues and sometimes other organs. The group includes *diffuse* and *systemic mastocytosis, mastocytoma, urticaria pigmentosa,* and *telangiectasia perstans.* **diffuse m., diffuse cutaneous m.,** a condition in which the entire skin is thickened, lichenified, and leathery in appearance and accompanied by generalized erythroderma and intense pruritus as a result of widespread infiltration with mast cells. In children, it is often associated with systemic mastocytosis. **systemic m.,** a condition in which there are mast cells infiltrates in noncutaneous tissues, occurring with or without cutaneous lesions, and usually involving the liver, spleen, bone, lymph nodes, and gastrointestinal tract. See also *mastocytosis syndrome,* under *syndrome.*

mastodynia (mas″to-din′e-ah) [*masto-* + Gr. *odyně* pain] pain in the breast.

mastogram (mas′to-gram) a roentgenogram of the breast.

mastography (mas-tog′rah-fe) [*masto-* + Gr. *graphein* to write] roentgenography of the breast.

mastoid (mas′toid) [Gr. *mastos* breast + *eidos* form] 1. breast shaped. 2. the mastoid process of the temporal bone. 3. pertaining to the mastoid process.

mastoidal (mas-toi′dal) pertaining to the mastoid process of the temporal bone.

mastoidale (mas″toi-da′le) the lowest point of the mastoid process.

mastoidalgia (mas″toi-dal′je-ah) [*mastoid* + *-algia*] pain in the mastoid region.

mastoidea (mas-toi′de-ah) pars mastoideus ossis temporalis.

mastoidectomy (mas″toi-dek′to-me) [*mastoid* + Gr. *ektomē* excision] excision of the mastoid cells or the mastoid process of the temporal bone.

mastoideocentesis (mas-toi″de-o-sen-te′sis) [*mastoid* + Gr. *kentēsis* puncture] surgical puncture of the mastoid antrum.

mastoideum (mas-toi′de-um) pars mastoideus ossis temporalis.

mastoiditis (mas″toi-di′tis) inflammation of the mastoid antrum and cells. **Bezold's m.,** a form in which the pus has escaped into the digastric groove and deep to the head of the sternocleidomastoid muscle. **m. exter′na,** inflammation of the periosteum of the mastoid process. **m. inter′na,** inflammation of the cells of the mastoid. **sclerosing m.,** mastoiditis attended with hardening and condensation of the bone. **silent m.,** a progressive destructive mastoiditis with mild systemic and local manifestations.

mastoidotomy (mas″toi-dot′o-me) [*mastoid* + Gr. *temnein* to cut] surgical incision of the mastoid process of the temporal bone.

mastomenia (mas″to-me′ne-ah) [*masto-* + Gr. *mēniaia* the menses] vicarious menstruation from the breast.

mastoncus (mas-tong′kus) [*masto-* + Gr. *onkos* bulk] a tumor of the breast or mammary gland.

masto-occipital (mas″to-ok-sip′ĭ-tal) pertaining to the mastoid process and the occipital bone.

mastoparietal (mas″to-pah-ri′ĕ-tal) [*mastoid* + *parietal*] pertaining to the mastoid process and the parietal bone.

mastopathia (mas″to-path′e-ah) mastopathy. **m. cys′tica,** a morbid condition of the mammary gland, with the formation of cysts.

mastopathy (mas-top′ah-the) [*masto-* + Gr. *pathos* disease] disease of the mammary gland. **cystic m.,** mastopathia cystica.

mastopexy (mas′to-pek-se) [*masto-* + Gr. *pēxis* fixation.] mammaplasty performed to correct a pendulous breast.

Mastophora (mas-tof′o-rah) a genus of spiders; called also *Glyptocranium.* **M. gasteracanthoi′des,** the venomous cat-headed spider of Peru, Chile, and Argentina that has been shown to cause necrotic spot among vineyard workers.

mastoplasia (mas″to-pla′ze-ah) mammoplasia.

mastoplasty (mas′to-plas″te) mammaplasty.

mastoptosis (mas″to-to′sis) [*masto-* + Gr. *ptōsis* fall] pendulous breasts.

mastorrhagia (mas″to-ra′je-ah) [*masto-* + Gr. *rhegnynai* to burst forth] hemorrhage from the mammary gland.

mastoscirrhus (mas″to-skir′us) [*masto-* + Gr. *skirros* hardness] hardening, or scirrhus, of the mammary gland.

mastosis (mas-to′sis), pl. *masto′ses* [*mast-* + *-osis*] a general term for pathologic changes in the breast of a degenerative and productive type characterized by enlargement and by the presence of painful nodular tumefactions.

mastosquamous (mas-to-skwa′mus) pertaining to or affecting the mastoid and squama of the temporal bone.

mastostomy (mas-tos′to-me) [*masto-* + Gr. *stomoun* to provide with an opening, or mouth] incision of the breast for drainage.

mastotic (mas-tot′ik) characterized by mastosis.

mastotomy (mas-tot′o-me) [*masto-* + Gr. *tomē* a cutting] surgical incision of a breast.

masturbation (mas″tur-ba′shun) [L. *manus* hand + *stuprare* to rape] self-stimulation of the genitals for sexual pleasure.

Masugi's nephritis (mah-soo′ge) [Matazo *Masugi,* Japanese pathologist] see *nephrotoxic serum nephritis,* under *nephritis.*

Matas' band, operation, test (mat′as) [Rudolph *Matas,* surgeon in New Orleans, 1860–1957] see under *band,* see *endoaneurysmorrhaphy,* and see *tourniquet test* (def. 2), under *tests.*

matching (mach′ing) 1. comparison and selection of objects having similar or identical characteristics. 2. the selection of compatible donors and recipients for transfusion or transplantation. 3. the selection of control and treatment groups in a clinical trial or cases and controls in a case-control study so that they are similar in certain specific characteristics, e.g., age, sex, race, or gene gender, in order to reduce bias caused by comparison of dissimilar groups. **cross m.,** determination of the compatibility of the blood of a donor and that of a recipient before transfusion by placing cells of the donor in the recipient's serum and cells of the recipient in the donor's serum. Absence of agglutination, hemolysis, and cytotoxicity indicates that the two blood specimens are compatible. Cross-matching is also used in determining the compatibility between an organ donor and recipient: donor lymphocytes are placed in a sample of the recipient's serum to detect preformed antibodies that could lead to hyperacute rejection, as of a renal transplant.

maté (mah-ta′) [Spanish American] the dried leaves of *Ilex paraguensis* St. Hil., Aquifoliaceae, a tree grown throughout Brazil, Uruguay, Paraguay, and Argentina as a source of tea. Its several synonyms include, yerba maté, Bartholomew's tea, Paraguay tea, and Jesuit's tea. It contains caffein and tannins, and has been used as a tonic, diuretic, stomachic, stimulant, and laxative (large doses).

mater (ma′ter) [L.] mother. **dura m.** ["hard mother"], see *dura mater.* **pia m.** ["tender mother"], see *pia mater.*

materia (mah-te′re-ah) [L.] matter; see also *materies.* **m. al′ba,** a whitish or cream-colored cheesy mass deposited around the necks of the teeth, composed of food debris, mucin, and dead epithelial cells. **m. den′tica,** that branch of study which deals with medicinal substances used in the practice of dentistry. **m. med′ica,** that branch of medical study which deals with drugs, their sources, preparations, and uses; pharmacology. **m. pec′cans,** materies peccans.

material (mah-te′re-al) substance or elements from which a concept may be formulated, or an object constructed. **baseplate m.,** any dental material used in the construction of a baseplate, including silver, gold, aluminum, platinum, alloys, and plastics. **cross-reacting m. (CRM),** a functionally inactive protein, produced by a mutant structural gene, that reacts with antibody to the normal protein. **dental m.,** any material used in dental practice, particularly a material used in the production of dental bases, restorations, impressions, or prostheses. **genetic m.,** material transmitted from an organism to those of succeeding generations and responsible for the features characteristic of the species, as well as for the heritable difference between individuals of the species. **impression m.,** any material used for making impressions of the teeth and oral structures for the purpose of producing artificial teeth and dentures, including elastic materials, dental plasters, metallic oxide pastes, impression compounds, reversible and irreversible hydrocolloids, silicone base materials, and duplicating compounds. **tissue equivalent m.,** a material whose absorbing and scattering properties for a given radiation simulate as closely as possible those of a given biological tissue, such as bone, fat, or muscle. Water, for example, is usually the best tissue equivalent material for muscle and soft tissue.

materies (mah-te′re-ēz) [L.] matter or substance; see also *materia*. **m. mor′bi** [L. "substance of disease"], the element or principle which causes a disease. **m. pec′cans** [L. "offending substance"], the principle that causes the pathologic changes occurring in disease.

maternal (mah-ter′nal) [L. *maternus; mater* mother] pertaining to the mother.

maternity (mah-ter′nĭ-te) [L. *mater* mother] 1. motherhood. 2. a lying-in hospital.

maternohemotherapy (mah-ter″no-he″mo-ther′ah-pe) [*maternal* + *hemotherapy*] injection of infants with blood from their mothers, formerly used in an attempt to transfer immunity to such diseases as measles and poliomyelitis from mother to child.

Mathieu's disease (mat″e-ūz′) [Albert *Mathieu*, physician in Paris, 1855–1917] leptospiral jaundice.

matico (mah-te′ko) the leaves of *Piper elongatum* Vahl. (*P. angustifolium* R. and P.), Piperaceae, a shrub of South and Central America; formerly used as an astringent and hemostatic. It contains volatile oil, maticin, tannin, and mucilage.

mating (māt′ing) [from Middle low Ger. *mate* companion] pairing of individuals of the opposite sex, especially for reproduction. **assortative m., assorted m., assortive m.,** a nonrandom system of mating in which choice of a mate is influenced by phenotype. Among human beings, *positive assortative mating* occurs, for example, when tall men choose tall women; or short women, short men. *Negative assortative mating* occurs when phenotypically dissimilar mates are chosen, e.g., tall men and short women, or tall women and short men. Nonrandom mating can affect Hardy-Weinberg equilibrium (q.v.) in a population. **backcross m.,** the mating of a heterozygote and a recessive homozygote; useful in revealing, through the phenotypes of the offspring, the genotype of the heterozygous parent. **nonrandom m.,** assortative m. **random m.,** mating in which any sperm (or any pollen grain) has an equal change of fertilizing any egg; thus for any one genotype at any one locus there is a purely random probability of combining with any other genotype at that locus. Called also *panmixis*.

matrass (mat′ras) a glass vessel with a long neck used for treating dry substances in chemical procedures.

matrical (mat′rĭ-kal) of or relating to a matrix.

Matricaria (mat″rĭ-ka′re-ah) [L.] the dried flower heads of the composit plant *Matricaria chamomilla* L. It contains volatile oil, anthemic acid, tannin, and matricarin. Used as a counterirritant externally and as a carminative internally in the form of a tea. Also known as *chamomile tea*.

matrices (ma′trĭ-sēz) plural of *matrix*.

matricial (ma-trish′al) matrical.

matriclinous (mat″rĭ-kli′nus) matroclinous.

matrilineal (ma′trĭ-lin′e-al) [L. *mater* mother + *linea* line] descended through the female line.

matrix (ma′triks) pl. *ma′trices* [L.] 1. the intracellular substance of a tissue or the tissue from which a structure develops. 2. the groundwork on which anything is cast, or that basic material from which a thing develops. 3. a mold or a form for casting. 4. a plastic or metal strip used to support and shape a plastic restorative material. 5. a piece of gold or platinum foil fitted against the sides and bottom of a cavity, used as a mold in which porcelain for an inlay is baked. 6. in a composite restorative resin, the continuous phase (an organic polymer) in which the discrete particles of filler are dispersed. 7. in dental porcelain, feldspar, which provides a glassy matrix in which quartz particles are dispersed. **amalgam m.,** matrix band. **bone m.,** the intercellular substance of bone, consisting of osteocollagenous fibers embedded in an amorphous ground substance and inorganic salts. **capsular m.,** territorial m. **cartilage m.,** the intercellular substance of cartilage, consisting of cells and extracellular fibers embedded in an amorphous ground substance; see also *interterritorial m.* and *territorial m.* **cytoplasmic m.,** the aggregating factor of the basic molecular fabric which ties together the ribosomes, RNA, proteins, small molecules, and water in the cytoplasm. **fluid m.,** Cannon's term for blood and lymph which bathe the cells of the body; see *homeostasis*. **functional m.,** the contiguous and motivating soft tissue organs and tissues in the growth of the craniofacial complex. **hair m.,** the epidermic root of the hair follicle. **interterritorial m.,** a paler-staining region located among the darker territorial matrices. **mitochondrial m.,** the dense substance, generally homogeneous but sometimes finely filamentous or granulated, found in the inner chamber (intercristal space) of mitochondria. **nail m.,** m. unguis. **sarcoplasmic m.,** the liquid substance which fills muscle cells; it contains the soluble enzymes of the cell. **territorial m.,** basophilic material surrounding groups of cartilage cells. **m. un′guis** [NA], the nail matrix: the tissue upon which the deep aspect of the nail rests; called also *nail bed*. The term is also used to denote the proximal portion of the nail bed from which growth chiefly proceeds.

matroclinous (mat″ro-kli′nus) [Gr. *mētēr* mother + *klinein* to incline] inheriting or inherited from the mother; possessing characters inherited from the mother. Cf. *patrocliny*.

matrocliny (mat″ro-kli′ne) the state of being matroclinous.

matt, matte (mat) a term applied to a macroscopic morphology of bacterial colonies that are dull and slightly granular, i.e., neither smooth and glistening nor rough.

matter (mat′er) 1. substance; anything that occupies space. 2. pus. **gelatinous m.,** substantia gelatinosa; see entries beginning thus, under *substantia*. **gray m. of nervous system,** substantia grisea. **radiant m.,** matter in a condition of extreme tenuity or ultragaseous state; gas exhausted to about one millionth of its original density, so that it has lost its original properties and has acquired new, particularly luminous, ones. **white m. of nervous system,** substantia alba.

Matulane (mat′u-lān) trademark for a preparation of procarbazine hydrochloride.

maturant (mach′u-rant) an agent that promotes suppuration.

maturate (mach′u-rāt) 1. to mature. 2. to suppurate.

maturation (mach″u-ra′shun) [L. *maturatio; maturus* ripe] 1. the stage or process of becoming mature or fully developed. The attainment of emotional and intellectual maturity. In biology, a process of cell division during which the number of chromosomes in the germ cells is reduced to one half the number characteristic of the species. 2. suppuration.

mature (mah-chur) [L. *maturus*] 1. to develop to maturity; to ripen. 2. fully developed; ripe.

maturity (mah-chur′rĭ-te) the period of attainment of maximal development.

Matut. abbreviation for L. *matuti′nus,* in the morning.

matutinal (mah-tu′tĭ-nal) [L. *matutinalis*] pertaining to or occurring in the morning.

Mauchart's ligament (mow′karts) [Burkhard David *Mauchart*, German anatomist, 1696–1751] ligamenta aloria.

Maumené's test (mōm-nāz′) [Edme Jules *Maumené*, French chemist, 1818–1891] see under *tests*.

Maunoir's hydrocele (mo′nwarz) [Jean Pierre *Maunoir*, French surgeon, 1768–1861] cervical hydrocele.

Maurer's dots (clefts, spots, stippling) (mow′rerz) [Georg *Maurer*, German physician in Sumatra, born 1909] see under *dot*.

Mauriac's syndrome (mo″re-aks′) [Pierre *Mauriac*, French physician, born 1882] see under *syndrome*.

Mauriceau's lance, maneuver (mo′re-sōz) [François *Mauriceau*, French obstetrician, 1637–1709] see under *lance* and *maneuver*.

Mauthner's cell, fiber, membrane (sheath), test (mowt′nerz) [Ludwig *Mauthner*, Austrian ophthalmologist, 1840–1894] see under *cell, fiber,* and *tests,* and see *axolemma*.

mauvein (mo′ve-in) aniline purple, a violet dye, $C_{27}H_{24}N_4$, used as an indicator, with a pH range of –0.1 to 2.9, being yellow at –0.1 and crimson at 2.9.

Maxibolin (mak-sĭb′o-lin) trademark for a preparation of ethylestrenol.

maxilla (mak-sil′ah), pl. *maxil′las,* gen. and pl. *maxil′lae* [L.]

[NA] the irregularly shaped bone that with its fellow forms the upper jaw; it assists in the formation of the orbit, the nasal cavity, and the palate, and lodges the upper teeth. **inferior m.,** mandible (mandibula [NA]).

maxillae (mak-sĭl′e) [L.] genitive and plural of *maxilla*.

maxillary (mak′sĭ-ler″e) [L. *maxillaris*] pertaining to the maxilla.

maxillectomy (mak″sĭ-lek′to-me) surgical excision of the maxilla.

maxillitis (mak″sĭ-li′tis) inflammation of the maxilla.

maxillodental (mak-sil″o-den′tal) pertaining to the maxilla and the maxillary teeth.

maxilloethmoidectomy (mak″sil-o-eth″moi-dek′to-me) excision of the portion of the maxilla surrounding the maxillary sinus and of the cribriform plate and anterior ethmoid cells.

maxillofacial (mak-sil″o-fa′shal) pertaining to the maxilla and the face.

maxillojugal (mak-sil″o-ju′gal) pertaining to the maxilla and the cheek.

maxillolabial (mak-sil″o-la′be-al) pertaining to the maxilla and the lip.

maxillomandibular (mak-sil″o-man-dib′u-lar) pertaining to the maxilla and the mandible.

maxillopalatine (mak-sil″o-pal′ah-tīn) pertaining to the maxilla and the palate or the palatine bone.

maxillopharyngeal (mak-sil″o-fah-rin′je-al) pertaining to the maxilla and the pharynx.

maxillotomy (mak″sĭ-lot′o-me) surgical sectioning of the maxilla which allows movement of all or a part of the maxilla into the desired position.

maxima (mak′sĭ-mah) [L.] plural of *maximum*.

maximal (mak′sĭ-mal) the greatest possible, allowable, or appreciable; the reverse of *minimal*.

maximum (mak′sĭ-mum), pl. *max′ima* [L. "greatest"] 1. the greatest possible or actual effect or quantity. 2. the acme of a disease or process. 3. largest; utmost. 4. Pirquet's term for the greatest quantity of food which the organism can digest. **tubular m.,** the highest rate in milligrams per minute at which the renal tubules can transfer a substance either from the tubular luminal fluid to the interstitial fluid or from the interstitial fluid to the tubular luminal fluid. Abbreviated T_m.

Maxipen (mak′sĭ-pen) trademark for a preparation of phenethicillin potassium.

Maxitate (mak′sĭ-tāt) trademark for preparations of mannitol hexanitrate.

maxwell (maks′wel) [James Clerk *Maxwell*, British physicist, 1831–1879] the unit of magnetic flux; replaced in SI by the *weber*.

Maxwell's ring, spot (maks′welz) [Patrick William *Maxwell*, Irish ophthalmologist, 1856–1917] see under *ring*, and see *macula retinae*.

Maydl's operation (ma′delz) [Karel *Maydl*, Bohemian surgeon, 1853–1903] see under *operation*.

mayer (ma′er) [Julius Robert von *Mayer*, German physicist, 1814–1878] a unit of heat capacity; it is the capacity of a body that is warmed one degree centigrade by one joule. Abbreviated *my*.

Mayer's hemalum, muchematein (ma′erz) [Paul *Mayer*, German-Italian scientist, 1848–1923] see *Table of Stains*.

Mayer's test (reagent) (ma′erz) [Ferdinand F. *Mayer*, American pharmaceutical chemist of the 19th century] see under *tests*.

mayfly (ma′fli) an insect of the order Ephemeroptera with two, or sometimes one, pair of triangular membranous wings. See *Hexagenia bilineata*.

Mayo's operation, sign (ma′oz) [William James (1861–1939) and Charles Horace (1865–1939) *Mayo*, American surgeons] see under *operation* and *sign*.

Mayo Robson see *Robson*.

maytansine (ma-tan′sēn) an antineoplastic derived from species of *Maytenus*, a genus of tropical American shrubs and trees, $C_{34}H_{46}ClN_3O_{10}$.

maze (māz) a complicated system of intersecting paths used in intelligence tests and in demonstrating learning in experimental animals.

mazindol (ma′zin-dōl) chemical name: 5-(4-chlorophenyl)-2,5-dihydro-3*H*-imidazo[2,1-*a*]isoindol-5-ol. An adrenergic, $C_{16}H_{13}ClN_2O$, having amphetamine-like actions; used as an anorexic in the short-term treatment of exogenous obesity, administered orally.

maz(o)- [Gr. *mazos* breast] a combining form denoting relationship to the breast; see also words beginning *mamm(o)-* and *mast(o)-*.

mazodynia (ma″zo-din′e-ah) mastodynia.

mazopexy (ma′zo-pek″se) mastopexy.

mazoplasia (ma″zo-pla′se-ah) [*mazo-* + Gr. *plassein* to form] degenerative epithelial hyperplasia of the mammary acini.

Mazzini's test (mah-ze′nēz) [Louis Y. *Mazzini*, American serologist, born 1894] see under *tests*.

Mazzoni's corpuscle (mad-zo′nēz) [Vittorio *Mazzoni*, Italian physician, 1880–1940] see under *corpuscle*.

M.B. abbreviation for L. *Medici′nae Baccalau′reus*, Bachelor of Medicine.

m.b. abbreviation for L. *mis′ce be′ne*, mix well.

MBP myelin basic protein.

MBq megabecquerel.

mbundu (em-boon′doo) a West African poison made from roots of trees of genus *Strychnos*.

M.C. abbreviation for L. *Magis′ter Chirur′giae*, Master of Surgery, and for *Medical Corps*.

Mc. megacycle.

mC millicoulomb.

μC microcoulomb.

MCA 3-methylcholanthrene.

MCF macrophage chemotactic factor.

Mcg an antigenic marker distinguishing human immunoglobulin λ light chain subtypes.

mcg. microgram.

MCH mean corpuscular hemoglobin, the average hemoglobin content of an erythrocyte, conventionally expressed in picograms per red cell, obtained by multiplying the blood hemoglobin concentration (in g/dl) by ten and dividing by the red cell count (in millions per ml): MCH = Hb/RBC.

MCHC mean corpuscular hemoglobin contentration, the average hemoglobin concentration in erythrocytes, conventionally expressed in "per cent" meaning grams per deciliter of red cells, obtained by dividing the blood hemoglobin concentration (in g/dl) by the hematocrit (in 1/1): MCHC = Hb/Hct.

μCi hr. microcurie-hour.

MCi megacurie.

mCi millicurie.

μCi microcurie.

mCi-hr millicurie-hour.

μCi-hr microcurie-hour.

MCMI Millon clinical multiaxial inventory.

Mc.p.s. megacycles per second.

MCT mean circulation time.

MCV mean corpuscular volume, the average volume of erythrocytes, conventionally expressed in cubic micrometers or femtoliters (μm^3 = fl) per red cell, obtained by multiplying the hematocrit (in 1/1) by 1000 and dividing by the red cell count (in millions per μl): MCV = Hct / RBC. Automated electronic blood cell counters generally obtain the MCV directly from the average pulse height of the voltage pulses produced during the red cell count. These instruments obtain the hematocrit indirectly from the equation Hct = MCV × RBC.

Md chemical symbol for *mendelevium*.

M.D. abbreviation for L. *Medici′nae Doc′tor*, Doctor of Medicine.

M.D.A. motor discriminative acuity; [L.] mento-dextra anterior (right mentoanterior, a position of the fetus).

M.D.P. [L.] *mento-dextra posterior* (right mentoposterior, a position of the fetus).

M.D.T. [L.] *mento-dextra transversa* (right mentotransverse, a position of the fetus).

Me chemical symbol for *methyl*, or CH_3.

meal (mēl) 1. a portion of food or foods taken at some particular and usually stated or fixed time. Often given with the specific purpose of aiding diagnostic examination. See also *test meal* (under *T*). 2. a coarsely ground substance, prepared from various grains. **bismuth m.,** an opaque meal in which some preparation of bismuth is the opaque constituent. **Boyden m.,** a test meal for the study of gallbladder evacuation in cholecystographic studies, consisting of 3 egg yolks, 3 teaspoonfuls of powdered whole milk, and 1 dessertspoonful of sugar with a drop of vanilla, with water slowly added up to make 200 ml. **butter m.,** a concentrated food containing butter, milk, flour, and sugar. **Knoepfelmacher's butter m.,** a preparation of milk, flour, butter, and sugar, used in child feeding. **liver m.,** a mixture of desiccated beef liver, malted milk, and powdered cinnamon; used for liver diet. **opaque m.,** a light meal, sometimes a glass of buttermilk, which contains some substance opaque to the roentgen rays, so that the outline of the stomach and the intestinal tract can be determined by roentgenography or roentgenoscopy. **Oslo m.** [Carl Schiotz of *Oslo*], a meal for school children consisting of a third of a liter of unskimmed milk, whole-meal bread with margarine and goat's-milk cheese, half an orange, half an apple, and a raw carrot. **retention m.,** a form of test meal which is retained, a specimen of the stomach contents being removed from time to time for analysis. **test m.,** see *test meal*, under *T*.

mean (mēn) [Old French *meien,* from L. *medianus* middle] 1. an average; a number that in some sense represents the central value of a set of numbers. 2. arithmetic m. 3. in probability and statistics, the expected value (mathematical expectation) of a random variable, the limiting value to which the sample mean converges as the sample size is increased indefinitely (if the limit exists). Symbol μ. **arithmetic m.,** the sum of n numbers divided by n. **geometric m.,** the nth root of the product of n numbers. **population m.,** the mean of the probability distribution characterizing a specified population; for a finite population, the arithmetic mean of the population values. Symbol μ. **sample m.,** the arithmetic mean of the observed values of a random sample, conventionally denoted by a barred variable, e.g., $\overline{X}$ (read "X bar"). The sample mean is itself a random variable (statistic) with mean μ and variance σ^2/n, where μ is the population mean, σ^2 is the population variance, and n is the sample size.

measles (me'zelz) 1. a highly contagious infectious disease caused by a paramyxovirus, common among children but also seen in the nonimmune of any age, in which the virus enters the respiratory tract via droplet nuclei and multiplies in the epithelial cells and spreads throughout the reticuloendothelial system, producing lymphoid hyperplasia often accompanied by characteristic Warthin-Finkeldey giant cells. Characteristically, coryza, cervical lymphadenitis, Koplik's spots, palpebral conjunctivitis, photophobia, myalgia, malaise, and a harassing cough with steadily mounting fever precede the skin eruption. The typical rash consists of generalized maculopapular lesions that are at first discrete but gradually become confluent, which initially starts behind the ears and on the face before progressing rapidly down the trunk and onto the extremities. Although measles is usually benign, complications may sometimes occur, including secondary bacterial infections in the form of otitis media, pneumonia, or laryngitis; a rare, fatal giant cell pneumonia, often without a rash, in immunocompromised children; and rarely, subacute sclerosing panencephalitis that may develop years after an initial measles infection. Called also *morbilli* and *rubeola*. 2. cysticercal disease of domestic animals. **atypical m.,** a severe form of measles occurring after exposure to wild measles virus in those who previously received inactivated (killed) measles vaccine, which was only available in the United States from 1963 to 1967, and in some cases live attenuated measles vaccine. It is characterized by fever, headache, myalgia, abdominal symptoms, and cough, followed by an atypical rash, which may be urticarial, vesicular, petechial, or maculopapular, on the wrists and ankles, and spreading to the palms, soles, and trunk before fading, and may be associated with peripheral edema, interstitial pulmonary infiltrates, and pleural effusion. Koplik spots are absent. **black m.,** a rare severe, often fatal, form of measles in which hemorrhage into the skin lesions and mucous membranes is associated with a sudden rise in temperature, convulsions, delirium, stupor, coma, and marked respiratory distress. Called also *hemorrhagic m.* **German m.,** rubella. **hemorrhagic m.,** black m. **pork m.,** a condi-

tion in which pork is infected with the *Cysticercus cellulosae.* **three-day m.,** rubella.

measly (me'zle) containing cysticerci.

measure (mezh'er) [L. *mensurare*] 1. to determine the extent or quantity of a substance. 2. a specific extent or quantity of a substance. 3. a graduated scale by which the dimensions or mass of an object or substance may be determined. See tables of weights and measures (Appendix 3).

meatal (me-a'tal) pertaining to a meatus.

meatome (me'ah-tōm) meatotome.

meatometer (me″ah-tom'ĕ-ter) [L. *meatus* passage + *metrum* measure] an instrument for measuring the urinary meatus.

meatorrhaphy (me″ah-tor'ah-fe) [L. *meatus* + Gr. *rhaphē* suture] suture of the cut end of the urethra to the glans penis after incision for enlarging the meatus.

meatoscope (me-at'o-skōp) [L. *meatus* meatus + Gr. *skopein* to examine] a speculum for examining the urinary meatus.

meatoscopy (me″ah-tos'ko-pe) the inspection of any meatus, especially the urinary meatus. **ureteral m.,** cystoscopic inspection of the vesical orifice of a ureter.

meatotome (me-at'o-tōm) an instrument for performing meatotomy.

meatotomy (me″ah-tot'o-me) [L. *meatus* passage + Gr. *temnein* to cut] incision of the urinary meatus in order to enlarge it.

meatus (mea'tus), pl. *mea'tus* [L., "a way, path, course"] an opening or passage; [NA] a general term for an opening or passageway in the body. **acoustic m., external,** m. acusticus externus. **acoustic m., external, bony,** meatus acusticus externus osseus. **acoustic m., external cartilaginous,** m. acusticus externus cartilagineus. **acoustic m., internal,** m. acusticus internus. **acoustic m., internal, bony,** m. acusticus internus osseus. **m. acus'ticus exter'nus** [NA], external acoustic meatus: the passage of the external ear leading to the tympanic membrane; called also *external auditory m.* **m. acus'ticus exter'nus cartilagin'eus** [NA], cartilaginous external acoustic meatus: the cartilaginous part of the external acoustic meatus, found lateral to the bony part. **m. acus'ticus exter'nus os'seus** [NA], bony external acoustic meatus: the opening in the external surface of the temporal bone, posterior to the condyle of the mandible and anterior to the mastoid air cells. **m. acus'ticus inter'nus** [NA], internal acoustic meatus: the passage through which the facial, intermediate, and vestibulocochlear nerves and the labyrinthine artery pass. **m. acus'ticus inter'nus os'seus** [NA], bony internal acoustic meatus: the opening on the posterior surface of the petrous part of the temporal bone through which the facial, intermediate, and vestibulocochlear nerves, and the labyrinthine artery pass. **m. audito'rius exter'nus,** m. acusticus externus. **m. audito'rius exter'nus cartilagin'eus,** m. acusticus externus cartilagineus. **m. audito'rius exter'nus os'seus,** m. acusticus externus osseus. **m. audito'rius inter'nus,** m. acusticus internus. **m. audito'rius inter'nus os'seus,** m. acusticus internus osseus. **auditory m., external,** m. acusticus externus. **auditory m., external, bony,** m. acusticus externus osseus. **auditory m., external, cartilaginous,** m. acusticus externus cartilagineus. **auditory m., internal,** m. acusticus internus. **auditory m., internal, bony,** m. acusticus internus osseus. **m. con'chae ethmoturbina'lis mino'ris,** m. nasi superior. **m. con'chae maxilloturbina'lis,** m. nasi inferior. **m. con'chae turbina'lis majo'ris,** m. nasi inferior. **fish-mouth m.,** a red, swollen, and everted urinary meatus seen in the first stage of acute gonorrhea. **nasal m., common, bony,** m. nasi communis osseus. **nasal m., inferior,** m. nasi inferior. **nasal m., inferior, bony,** m. nasi inferior osseus. **nasal m., middle,** m. nasi medius. **nasal m., middle, bony,** m. nasi medius osseus. **nasal m., superior,** m. nasi superior. **nasal m., superior, bony,** m. nasi superior osseus. **m. na'si commu'nis,** common meatus of nose: the anterior space on either side of the nasal septum into which the three meatuses open. **m. na'si commun'nis os'seus,** bony common meatus of nose: the space on either side of the nasal septum bounded by the bones of the cranium. **m. na'si infe'rior** [NA], inferior meatus of nose: the space beneath the inferior nasal concha, into which the nasolacrimal duct opens. **m. na'si infe'rior os'seus** [NA], bony inferior meatus of nose: the opening in the cranium overhung by the inferior bony nasal concha. **m. na'si me'dius** [NA], middle meatus of nose: the space beneath the middle nasal concha, with which the anterior ethmoidal cells and frontal and maxillary sinuses communicate. **m. na'si me'dius os'seus** [NA], bony middle meatus of nose: the opening in the cranium overhung by the middle bony nasal concha. **m. na'si supe'rior** [NA], superior meatus of nose: the narrow cavity below the superior nasal concha, with which the posterior ethmoidal cells communicate. **m. na'si supe'rior os'seus** [NA], bony superior meatus of nose: the slender, channel-like opening in the cranium inferior to the superior bony nasal concha. **nasopharyngeal m.,** m. nasopharyngeus. **m. nasopharyn'geus** [NA], nasopharyngeal meatus: the part of the nasal cavity coinciding with the bony nasopharyngeal cavity. **m's of nose,** see *m. nasi communis, m. nasi inferior, m. nasi medius,* and *m. nasi superior.* **m. of nose, bony, common,** m. nasi communis osseus. **m. of nose, common,** m. nasi communis. **m. of nose, inferior,** m. nasi inferior. **m. of nose, inferior, bony,** m. nasi inferior osseus. **m. of nose, middle,** m. nasi medius. **m. of nose, middle, osseous,** m. nasi medius osseus. **m. of nose, superior,** m. nasi superior. **m. of nose, superior, osseous,** m. nasi superior osseus. **m. urina'rius, urinary m.,** the external urethral orifice: the opening of the urethra on the body surface through which urine is discharged. See *ostium urethrae externum feminina* and *ostium urethrae externum masculinae.*

Mebaral (meb'ah-ral) trademark for a preparation of mephobarbital.

mebendazole (mě-ben'dah-zōl) [USP] a versatile anthelmintic agent, which irreversibly inhibits glucose uptake in the parasite, causing immobilization and death; used in the treatment of infections due to *Ascaris lumbricoides, Enterobius vermicularis, Trichuris trichiura,* hookworm species, and *Capillaria philippinensis.*

mebeverine hydrochloride (mě-bev'er-ēn) chemical name: 3,4-dimethoxybenzoic acid 4-[ethyl[2-(4-methoxyphenyl)-1-methylethyl]amino]butyl ester]hydrochloride; a smooth muscle relaxant, $C_{25}H_{35}NO_5 \cdot HCl$.

mebutamate (mě-bu'tah-māt) chemical name: 2-methyl-2-(1-methylpropyl)-1,3-propanediol dicarbamate. A mildly tranquilizing, antihypertensive agent, $C_{10}H_{20}N_2O_4$, occurring as a white, crystalline powder; used alone or in conjunction with diuretics and other hypotensive drugs, administered orally.

mecamine (mek'ah-min) mecamylamine.

mecamylamine hydrochloride (mek"ah-mil'ah-min) [USP] chemical name: N,2,3,3-tetramethylbicyclo [2.2.1]heptan-2-amine hydrochloride. A ganglionic-blocking agent, $C_{11}H_{21}N \cdot HCl$, occurring as a white, crystalline powder; used as an antihypertensive, usually in the treatment of moderate to severe hypertension, administered orally.

meCCNU semustine.

mechanical (me-kan'ĭ-kal) [Gr. *mēchanikos*] 1. pertaining to or accomplished by mechanical or physical forces. 2. performed by means of some artificial mechanism.

mechanicoreceptor (me-kan"ĭ-ko-re-sep'tor) mechanoreceptor.

mechanicotherapeutics, mechanicotherapy (mekan"ĭ-ko-ther"ah-pu'tiks, me-kan"ĭ-ko-ther'ah-pe) mechanotherapy.

mechanics (me-kan'iks) the science dealing with the motions of material bodies, including kinematics, dynamics, and statics. **animal m.,** biomechanics. **body m.,** the application of kinesiology to use of the body in daily life activities and to the prevention and correction of problems related to posture. **developmental m.,** embryological mechanisms as revealed mainly by experimentation.

mechanism (mek'ah-nizm) [Gr. *mēchanē* machine] 1. a machine or machine-like structure. 2. the manner of combination of parts, processes, etc., which subserve a common function. 3. the theory that the phenomena of life are based on the same physical and chemical laws which operate in the inorganic world; opposed to *vitalism.* **countercurrent m.,** the renal mechanism by which urine is concentrated; it is dependent upon the anatomical arrangement of

the loops of Henle and the vasa recta. **defense m.,** an unconscious process that serves to relieve conflict and anxiety arising from one's impulses and drives, e.g., compensation, conversion, denial, rationalization. **double-displacement m.,** ping-pong m. **Duncan m.,** expulsion of the placenta with the maternal, or rough, surface appearing at the vulva. **Frank-Starling m.,** the ventricular response to an increase in either volume load or pressure load by diastolic distention and increased energy release. **m. of labor,** the factors involved in the expulsion of the fetus, placenta, and membranes through the birth canal in labor. **mental m.,** an unconscious process, such as a defense mechanism, memory, perception, or thinking, that is a function of the ego and determines behavior. **oculogyric m.,** the series of nerve centers concerned in movements of the eye. **ping-pong m.,** a process in which one substrate reacts with an enzyme and dissociates into one product, leaving a functional group attached to the enzyme; in a second reaction, the modified enzyme transfers the attached functional group to a second substrate, forming a second product and releasing the enzyme in its original form. Called also *double-displacement m.* **re-entrant m.,** see *re-entry.* **Schultze m.,** expulsion of the placenta with the smooth, glistening, fetal surface appearing at the vulva; this is considered normal and is more common than the Duncan mechanism. **somatic m.,** the structures and organs through which the somatic activities of the body are performed. **splanchnic m.,** the structures and organs through which the visceral activities of the body are performed.

mechanist (mek'ah-nist) one who believes that all phenomena relating to life are based on physical and chemical properties only.

mechan(o)- [Gr. *mēchanē* machine] a combining form meaning mechanical, or denoting relationship to a machine, to physical forces, or to mechanics.

mechanocyte (mek'ah-no-sīt") [*mechano-* + *-cyte*] fibroblast.

mechanogymnastics (mek"ah-no-jim-nas'tiks) gymnastics carried out by means of mechanical apparatus, such as the Zander apparatus.

mechanology (mek"ah-nol'o-je) [*mechano-* + *-logy*] the science of mechanics.

mechanoreceptor (mek"ah-no-re-sep'tor) a receptor that is excited by mechanical pressures or distortions, as those responding to sound, touch, and muscular contractions.

mechanotherapy (mek"ah-no-ther'ah-pe) [*mechano-* + Gr. *therapeia* treatment] the use of mechanical apparatus in the treatment of disease or its results, especially as an aid in performing therapeutic exercises.

mechanothermy (mek"ah-no-ther'me) [*mechano-* + Gr. *thermē* heat] therapeutic heat produced by massage, exercise, etc.

mechlorethamine (mek"lor-eth'ah-mēn) a cytotoxic alkylating agent of the nitrogen mustard group, used primarily for the treatment of disseminated Hodgkin's disease, especially in the MOPP (q.v.) treatment regimen, and in other lymphomas, including mycosis fungoides; common side effects of therapeutic doses are severe nausea and vomiting, bone marrow depression, and gastrointestinal symptoms. Mechlorethamine combines rapidly with water or cellular constituents, reacting completely within a few minutes after administration. It is a powerful vesicant, and care must be taken to avoid accidental contact with skin, eyes, or mucous membranes. Available as *mechlorethamine hydrochloride* [USP]. Called also *HN2* and *nitrogen mustard.*

Mechnikov (mech'nĭ-kov") see *Metchnikoff.*

mecillinam (mě-sil'ĭ-nam) amdinocillin.

mecism (me'sizm) [Gr. *mēkos* length] abnormal lengthening of a part.

mecistocephalic (me-sis"to-sě-fal'ik) [Gr. *mēkistos* tallest + *kephalē* head] having a cephalic index less than 71.

mecistocephalous (me-sis"to-sef'ah-lus) mecistocephalic.

Mecistocirrhus (me-sis"to-sir'us) a genus of nematode parasites found in the fourth stomach of ruminants. **M. digita'tus,** a species found in various ruminants, and in man and swine; called also *Strongylus gibsoni.*

Meckel's band (ligament), cavity (space), ganglion (mek'elz) [Johann Friedrich *Meckel* (the elder), Berlin anatomist, 1714–1774] see under *band,* and see *cavum trigemi-*

nale, ganglion pterygopalatinum, and *ganglion submandibulare.*

Meckel's cartilage (rod), diverticulum, plane, syndrome (mek′elz) [Johann Friedrich *Meckel* (the younger) (grandson of J. F. Meckel, the elder), anatomist in Halle, 1781–1833] see under *cartilage, diverticulum, plane,* and *syndrome.*

meckelectomy (mek″el-ek′to-me) [*Meckel's ganglion* + Gr. *ektomē* excision] surgical removal of Meckel's lesser (the submandibular) ganglion.

meclizine hydrochloride (mek′lĭ-zēn) [USP] chemical name: 1-[(4-chlorophenyl)phenylmethyl]-4-[(3-methylphenyl)methyl]piperazine dihydrochloride monohydrate. An antihistamine, $C_{25}H_{27}ClN_2 \cdot 2HCl \cdot H_2O$, occurring as a white or slightly yellowish, crystalline powder; used as an antiemetic in the management of nausea, vomiting, and dizziness associated with motion sickness, administered orally. Called also *parachloramine.*

meclocycline (mek-lo-si′klēn) chemical name: 7-chloro-4-(dimethylamino)-1,4,4a,5,5a,6,11,12a-octahydro-3,5,10,12,12a-pentahydroxy-6-methylene-1,11-dioxo-2-naphthacenecarboxamide; an antibiotic of unspecified action, $C_{22}H_{21}ClN_2O_8$.

meclofenamate (mĕ-klo″fen-am′āt) the conjugate base of meclofenamic acid; used as *meclofenamate sodium* for treatment of osteoarthritis and rheumatoid arthritis.

meclofenamic acid (mĕ-klo″fen-am′ik) a nonsteroidal anti-inflammatory agent of the fenamate class.

meclofenoxate (mĕ″klo-fen-oks′āt) dimethylaminoethyl para-chlorophenoxyacetate; a drug claimed to aid cellular metabolism in the presence of diminished oxygen concentrations.

Meclomen (mĕ-klo′men) trademark for preparations of meclofenamate sodium.

mecloqualone (mĕ-klo-kwah′lōn) chemical name: 3-(2-chlorophenyl)-2-methyl-4(3H)-quinazolinone; a sedative and hypnotic, $C_{15}H_{11}ClN_2O$.

mecobalamine (me″ko-bal′ah-min) a naturally occurring hematopoietic vitamin found in the blood, $C_{63}H_{91}CoN_{13}O_{14}P$, closely related to cyanocobalamin, in which the cyano radical has been replaced by a methyl radical.

mecocephalic (me″ko-sĕ-fal′ik) [Gr. *mēkos* length + Gr. *kephalē* head] dolichocephalic.

meconate (mek′o-nāt) [Gr. *mēkōn* poppy + *-ate*] any salt of meconic acid.

meconic acid (mĕ-kon′ik) an acid occurring in opium that forms soluble salts with the opiates.

meconiorrhea (mĕ-ko″ne-o-re′ah) [*meconium* + Gr. *rhoia* flow] excessive discharge of meconium.

meconium (mĕ-ko′ne-um) [L.; Gr. *mēkōnion*] 1. a dark green mucilaginous material in the intestine of the full term fetus, being a mixture of the secretions of the intestinal glands and some amniotic fluid. 2. opium.

mecrylate (mĕ-kri′lāt) chemical name: 2-cyano-2-propenoic acid methyl ester; a tissue adhesive for use in surgery, $C_5H_5NO_2$.

mecystasis (mĕ-sis′tah-sis) [Gr. *mēkynein* to lengthen + *stasis* a setting] a state in which a muscle fiber is relatively increased in length, resists stretch, contracts, and relaxes, and manifests the same tension as before elongation.

M.E.D. minimal effective dose; minimal erythema dose.

Medawar (med′ah-war), Peter Brian. Brazilian-born British biologist, born 1915; co-winner, with Sir Frank Macfarlane Burnet, of the Nobel prize for medicine or physiology in 1960 for his discovery of the mechanism of acquired immunological tolerance.

medazepam hydrochloride (mĕ-daz′ĕ-pam) chemical name: 7-chloro-2,3-dihydro-1-methyl-5-phenyl-1H-1,4-benzodiazepine monohydrochloride; a minor tranquilizer, $C_{16}H_{15}ClN_2 \cdot HCl$.

Medex [Fr. *médecin extension* extension of the physician] a program that recruits former military medics for training and practice as physician assistants; abbreviated Mx.

medi (mi′theh) maedi.

media (me′de-ah) [L.] 1. plural of *medium*. 2. middle; see *tunica media.*

mediad (me′de-ad) [L. *medium* middle + *ad* toward] toward a median line or plane.

medial (me′de-al) [L. *medialis*] 1. pertaining to the middle;

closer to the median plane or the midline of a body or structure. 2. pertaining to the middle layer of structures.

medialecithal (me″de-ah-les′ĭ-thal) [*media-* + Gr. *lekithos* yolk] possessing a medium amount of yolk; see under *ovum.*

medialis (me″de-a′lis) medial; [NA] a general term denoting a structure situated nearer to the median plane or the midline of a body or structure.

median (me′de-an) [L. *medianus*] 1. situated in the median plane or in the midline of a body or structure. 2. any value that divides the probability distribution of a random variable in half, i.e., the probability of observing a value above the median and the probability of observing a value below the median are both less than or equal to one half. For a finite population or sample, the median is the middle value of an odd number of values (arranged in ascending order) or any value between the two middle values of an even number of values; in the latter case it is conventional to use the average of the two middle values.

medianus (me″de-a′nus) [L.] median, or situated in the middle; [NA] a general term denoting structures lying in the median plane, that is, in the plane dividing the body into right and left halves.

mediaometer (me″de-ah-om′ĕ-ter) [*media* + *-meter*] an instrument for detecting and measuring refractive errors of the dioptric media.

mediastina (me″de-as-ti′nah) [L.] plural of *mediastinum.*

mediastinal (me″de-as-ti′nal) [L. *mediastinalis*] of or pertaining to the mediastinum.

mediastinitis (me″de-as″tĭ-ni′tis) inflammation of the mediastinum. **fibrous m., indurative m.,** an exuberant inflammatory sclerogenic process of infectious, rheumatic, hemorrhagic, or undetermined origin, which may be associated with fibrous pericarditis and with inflammatory fibrous masses in other parts of the body; it is often accompanied by obstruction of mediastinal structures, especially the superior vena cava, and, less often, the tracheobronchial tree, the esophagus, and other structures.

mediastinography (me″de-as″tĭ-nog′rah-fe) roentgenography of the mediastinum.

mediastinogram (me″de-as-ti′no-gram) a roentgenogram of the mediastinum.

mediastinopericarditis (me″de-as″tĭ-no-per″ĭ-kar-di′tis) adhesive pericarditis in which the adhesions extend from the pericardium to the mediastinum. See also *adhesive pericarditis,* under *pericarditis.*

mediastinoscope (me″de-ah-sti′no-skōp) a specially designed endoscope used in mediastinoscopy.

mediastinoscopic (me″de-as″tĭ-no-skop′ik) pertaining to the mediastinoscope or to mediastinoscopy.

mediastinoscopy (me″de-as″tĭ-nos′ko-pe) examination of the mediastinum by means of an endoscope inserted through an anterior incision in the suprasternal notch, permitting direct inspection and biopsy of tissue in the anterior superior mediastinum.

mediastinotomy (me″de-as″ti-not′o-me) [*mediastinum* + Gr. *tomē* a cutting] the operation of cutting into the mediastinum. Performed from the front, it is *anterior* or *cervical m.;* from the back, *posterior* or *dorsal m.*

mediastinum (me″de-as-ti′num), pl. *mediasti′na* [L.] 1. a median septum or partition. 2. [NA] the mass of tissues and organs separating the two pleural sacs, between the sternum in front and the vertebral column behind, and from the thoracic inlet above to the diaphragm below. It contains the heart and its pericardium, the bases of the great vessels, the trachea and bronchi, esophagus, thymus, lymph nodes, thoracic duct, phrenic and vagus nerves and other structures and tissues. Especially in Great Britain and the United States, the mediastinum is divided into a superior region and an inferior region that comprises anterior, middle, and posterior parts. **anterior m., m. ante′rius** [NA], the division of the mediastinum bounded behind by the pericardium, in front by the sternum, and on each side by the pleura. It contains loose areolar tissue and lymphatic vessels. Called also *cavum mediastinale anterius* or *anterior mediastinal cavity.* **m. cerebel′li** (obs.), falx cerebelli. **m. cer′ebri** (obs.), falx cerebri. **inferior m., m. infe′rius** [NA], the three lower portions of the mediastinum, comprising the *m. anterius, m. medium,* and *m. posterius;* see also *mediastinum* (def. 2). **m. me′dium** [NA], **middle m.,** the division of the mediastinum containing the heart enclosed in its pericardium, the ascending aorta, the superior vena cava, the bifurcation of the trachea into bronchi, the pulmonary arteries and veins, the phrenic nerves, a large portion of the roots of the lungs, and the arch of the azygos vein. Called also *middle mediastinal cavity.* **posterior m., m. poste′rius** [NA], the division of the mediastinum bounded behind by the vertebral column, in front by the pericardium, and on each side by the pleurae. It contains the descending aorta, parts of the greater and lesser azygos and superior intercostal veins, the thoracic duct, the esophagus, the vagus nerves, and the great splanchnic nerves. Called also *cavum mediastinale posterius* or *posterior mediastinal cavity.* **superior m., m. supe′rius** [NA], the division of the mediastinum extending from the pericardium to the root of the neck, and containing the esophagus and the trachea behind, the thymus or its remains in front, and the great vessels related to the heart and pericardium, the thoracic duct, and the vagus nerves in between. Called also *superior* mediastinal cavity. **m. tes′tis** [NA], the partial septum of the testis, formed near its posterior border by fibrous tissue which is continuous with the tunica albuginea; called also *body of Highmore.*

mediastinus (me″de-as-ti′nus) [L.] an assistant physician or surgeon.

mediate (me′de-it) indirect; accomplished by the aid of an intervening medium.

mediation (me″de-a′shun) the act of interposing or serving as an intermediary. **chemical m.,** the concept that excitation in passing from a pre- to a postsynaptic neural element undergoes a necessary chemical step.

mediator (me′de-a″tor) an object or substance by which something is mediated, such as (1) a structure of the nervous system that transmits impulses eliciting a specific response; (2) a chemical substance (transmitter substance) that induces activity in an excitable tissue, such as nerve or muscle; or (3) a substance released from cells as the result of the interaction of antigen with antibody or by the action of antigen with a sensitized lymphocyte.

medicable (med′ĭ-kah-b'l) subject to treatment with reasonable expectation of cure.

medical (med′ĭ-kal) pertaining to medicine or to the treatment of diseases; pertaining to medicine as opposed to surgery.

medicament (med′ĭ-kah-ment, mĕ-dik′ah-ment) [L. *medicamentum*] a medicinal substance or agent.

medicamentosus (med″ĭ-kah-men-to′sus) [L.] medicamentous.

medicamentous (med″ĭ-kah-men′tus) pertaining to, used in, or caused by a drug or drugs.

Medicare (med′ĭ-kār) a program administered by the Social Security Administration which provides medical care for the aged.

medicaster (med′ĭ-kas″ter) a pretender to medical skill; a charlatan or quack.

medicate (med′ĭ-kāt) [L. *medicatus*] to impregnate or imbue with a medicinal substance.

medicated (med′ĭ-kāt″ed) imbued with a medicinal substance.

medication (med″ĭ-ka′shun) [L. *medicatio*] 1. impregnation with a medicine. 2. the administration of remedies. 3. a medicament. **conservative m.,** treatment aimed to build up the vital powers of the patient. **dialytic m.,** treatment by the internal use of artificial mineral waters, i.e., dilute aqueous solutions of salts. **hypodermatic m.,** the introduction of remedial agents beneath the skin. **ionic m.,** iontophoresis. **sublingual m.,** the administration of medicine by placing it beneath the tongue. **substitutive m.,** medication for the purpose of causing an acute nonspecific inflammation to overcome a specific one. **transduodenal m.,** the administration of medicine through a duodenal tube into the intestines without soiling the stomach.

medicator (med′ĭ-ka″tor) an instrument for carrying medicines into a cavity of the body; an applicator.

medicephalic (me″de-sĕ-fal′ik) median cephalic; see under *vein.*

medicinal (me-dis′ĭ-nal) [L. *medicinalis*] 1. having healing qualities. 2. pertaining to a medicine or to healing.

medicine (med′ĭ-sin) [L. *medicina*] 1. any drug or remedy. 2. the art and science of the diagnosis and treatment of disease and the maintenance of health. 3. the treatment of disease by nonsurgical means. **aviation m.,** that branch of medicine which has to do with the physiological, medical, psychological, and epidemiological problems involved in aviation. **clinical m.,** 1. the study of disease by direct examination of the living patient. 2. the last two years of the usual curriculum in a medical college. **comparative m.,** the study of phenomena basic to the diseases of all species. **compound m.,** a medicine containing a mixture of several drugs. **dosimetric m.,** the practice of administering medicines by an exact and determinate system of doses. **emergency m.,** that specialty which deals with acutely ill or injured patients who require immediate medical treatment. **environmental m.,** that which considers the effects of the environment on man, including rapid population growth, changes and extremes in temperature, alterations in atmospheric pressure, water and air pollution, radiation, travel, etc. **experimental m.,** the study of disease based on experimentation in animals. **family m.,** see under *practice.* **folk m.,** the use of home remedies and procedures as handed down by tradition. **forensic m.,** that branch of medicine dealing with the application of medical knowledge to the purposes of law. This term and medical jurisprudence are sometimes used as synonyms, but some authorities consider the first as a branch of medicine and the second as a branch of law. Called also *legal m.* **galenic m.,** an absolute system of practice based upon the teachings of Galen. **geriatric m.,** geriatrics. **group m.,** the practice of medicine by a group of physicians, usually representing various specialties, who are associated together for the cooperative diagnosis, treatment, and prevention of disease. Called also *group practice.* **hermetic m.,** see *spagyric m.* **holistic m.,** a system of medicine which considers man as an integrated whole, or as a functioning unit. **hyperbaric m.,** the treatment of disease in an environment of higher than atmospheric pressure. **internal m.,** that branch of medicine dealing especially with the diagnosis and medical treatment of diseases and disorders of the internal structures of the human body. **ionic m.,** treatment by electrochemical means, as by cataphoresis and iontophoresis. **laboratory animal m.,** that specialty of veterinary medicine which deals with the diagnosis, treatment, and prevention of disease in animals used as subjects in biomedical activities. **legal m.,** forensic m. **neohippocratic m.,** neo-hippocratism. **nuclear m.,** that branch of medicine concerned with the use of radionuclides in the diagnosis and treatment of disease. **oral m.,** dentistry. **patent m.,** a drug or remedy protected by a trademark, available without prescription. **physical m.,** physiatrics. **preclinical m.,** 1. preventive medicine. 2. the first two years of the usual curriculum in a medical college. **preventive m.,** that branch of study and practice which aims at the prevention of disease and the promotion of health. **proprietary m.,** a drug or remedy to which the manufacturing pharmaceutical house has exclusive (proprietary) rights, and which is marketed usually under a name that is registered as a trademark. **psychosomatic m.,** a system of medicine which aims at discovering the exact nature of the relationship of the emotions and bodily function, affirming the principle that the mind and body are one; the simultaneous application of physiologic and psychologic technics in the study and treatment of illness. **rational m.,** practice of medicine based upon actual knowledge; opposed to *empiricism.* **social m.,** phases of preventive medicine and the care of the sick which concern the community as a whole or large groups of persons rather than the individual. **socialized m.,** a system of medical care regulated and controlled by the government, in which the government assumes responsibility for providing for the health needs and hospital care of the entire population, at no direct cost or at a nominal fee to the individual, by means of subsidies obtained by taxation. Called also *state m.* **space m.,** that branch of aviation medicine concerned solely with conditions to be encountered by man in space. **spagyric m.** (obs.), semialchemistic system of practice established by Paracelsus (1493–1541). **sports m.,** the field of medicine concerned with injuries sustained in athletic endeavors, including their prevention, diagnosis, treatment, etc. **state m.,** socialized m. **tropical m.,** medical science as applied to diseases occurring primarily in tropical and subtropical countries. **veterinary m.,** the science of treatment of the diseases of animals.

medicochirurgic (med″ĭ-ko-ki-rur′jik) pertaining to medicine and surgery.

medicodental (med″ĭ-ko-den′tal) pertaining to both medicine and dentistry.

medicolegal (med″ĭ-ko-le′gal) pertaining to medicine and law, or to forensic medicine.

medicomechanical (med″ĭ-ko-me-kan′ĭ-kal) both medicinal and mechanical.

medicophysics (med″ĭ-ko-fiz′iks) physics as applied to medicine.

medicopsychology (med″ĭ-ko-si-kol′o-je) (*obs.*) the science of medicine in its relations with the mind or with mental diseases.

medicosocial (med″ĭ-ko-so′shal) having both medical and social aspects, as, for example, the prevention and treatment of venereal disease.

medicotopographical (med″ĭ-ko-to″po-graf′ĭ-kal) pertaining to topography in its relation to disease.

medicozoological (med″ĭ-ko-zo-o-loj′ĭ-kal) pertaining to zoology in its relation to medicine.

medifrontal (me″dĭ-fron′tal) median and frontal; pertaining to the middle of the forehead.

Medin's disease (ma′dēnz) [Oskar *Medin*, Swedish physician, 1847–1928] see *poliomyelitis*.

mediocarpal (me″de-o-kar′pal) midcarpal.

medioccipital (me″de-ok-sip′ĭ-tal) midoccipital.

mediolateral (me″de-o-lat′er-al) [L. *medius* middle + *lateralis* lateral] pertaining to the middle and to one side.

medionecrosis (me″de-o-ne-kro′sis) necrosis of the tunica media of a blood vessel, often leading to its rupture. **m. of aorta,** Erdheim's cystic medial necrosis.

mediotarsal (me″de-o-tar′sal) [L. *medius* middle + *tarsus*] pertaining to the middle of the tarsus.

mediscalenus (me″de-skah-le′nus) musculus scalenus medius.

medisect (me′dĭ-sekt) [L. *medius* middle + *secare* to cut] to divide or dissect medially.

meditation (med″ĭ-ta′shun) the act of reflecting upon or contemplating; an exercise in contemplation. **transcendental m.,** a technique for attaining a state of physical relaxation and psychological calm by the regular practice of a relaxation procedure which entails the repetition of a mantra.

medium (me′de-um), pl. *mediums* or *me′dia* [L. "middle"] 1. means. 2. a substance which transmits impulses. 3. a substance used in the culture of bacteria; see *culture medium,* under C. 4. a preparation used in treating histologic specimens. **active m.,** the aggregated atoms, ions, or molecules, contained in a laser's optical cavity, in which stimulated emission will occur under the proper excitation. **Bruns' glucose m.,** a mixture of distilled water, glucose, glycerin, and camphorated spirit, used for mounting fresh tissue specimens. **clearing m.,** a substance used for rendering histologic specimens transparent. **contrast m.,** a substance that is introduced into or around a structure and, because of the difference in absorption of x-rays by the contrast medium and the surrounding tissues, allows radiographic visualization of the structure. **culture m.,** a substance used to support the growth of microorganisms or other cells; see *culture medium,* under C. **dioptric media,** refracting media. **disperse m., dispersion m., dispersive m.,** the continuous or external portion of a colloid system in which the particles of the disperse phase are distributed; it is analogous to the solvent in a true solution. Cf. *disperse phase.* **HAT m.,** a tissue culture medium containing hypoxanthine, aminopterin, and thymidine, used in somatic cell fusion experiments. Aminopterin (an antifolate) blocks *de novo* synthesis of purine and thymine nucleotides, but these compounds can be produced from hypoxanthine and thymidine by normal cells possessing the enzymes hypoxanthine phosphoribosyltransferase (HPRT) and thymidine kinase (TK). **mounting m.,** mountant. **nutrient m.,** see *nutrient c.* in Table of Culture Media. **radiolucent m.,** a contrast medium that permits the passage of roentgen rays. **radiopaque m.,** a contrast medium that blocks the passage of roentgen rays. **refracting media,** the transparent tissues and fluids in the eye through which light rays pass and by which they are refracted and brought

to a focus on the retina; the structures include the cornea, aqueous humor, crystalline lens, and vitreous body. Called also *dioptric media.* **separating m.,** any substance which facilitates separation, such as a coating used upon a surface that serves to prevent adherence to it of another surface; in dentistry, a substance applied to the investment surface of a denture flask to protect the resin from the surfaces in the mold space to avoid incorporation of water in the resin from the gypsum and to prevent adherence of the investing material and the resin. **Wickersheimer's m.,** see under *fluid.*

medius (me′de-us) [L.] in the middle; [NA] a term used in reference to a structure lying between two other structures that are anterior and posterior, superior and inferior, or internal and external in position.

MEDLARS (med′larz) [*MED*ical *L*iterature *A*nalysis and *R*etrieval *S*ystem] a computerized bibliographic system of the National Library of Medicine, from which the Index Medicus is produced.

MEDLINE (med′līn) [from *MEDLARS* on-*line*] a computerized bibliographic retrieval system, an on-line segment of MEDLARS.

medorrhea (med″o-re′ah) [Gr. *mēdea* genitals + *rhoia* flow] a urethral discharge.

medrogestone (med-ro-jes′tōn) chemical name: [6,17-dimethylpregna-4,6-diene-3,20-dione]; a progestin, $C_{23}H_{32}O_2$.

Medrol (med′rol) trademark for preparations of methylprednisolone.

medronate disodium (med′ro-nāt) methylenebisphosphonic acid disodium dihydrogen salt; a pharmaceutic aid, $CH_4Na_2O_6P_2$.

medroxyprogesterone acetate (med-rok″se-pro-jes′ter-ōn) [USP] chemical name: 6(α)-17-(acetyloxy)-6-methylpregna-4-ene-3,20-dione. A progestin, $C_{24}H_{34}O_4$, occurring as a white to off-white, crystalline powder; used in the treatment of endometriosis, uterine cancer, habitual and threatened abortion, and menstrual disorders, administered orally or intramuscularly. It has been used in contraceptive products.

medrysone (med′rĭ-sōn) chemical name: 11β-hydroxy-6α-methylpregn-4-ene-3,20-dione. A synthetic glucocorticoid, $C_{22}H_{32}O_3$, occurring as a white to off-white, crystalline powder; used as an anti-inflammatory in allergic and inflammatory eye conditions, such as episcleritis, allergic and vernal conjunctivitis, applied topically to the conjunctiva.

medulla (mĕ-dul′ah), gen. and pl. *medul′lae* [L.] the inmost part; [NA] a general term for the inmost portion of an organ or structure. Called also *marrow.* **adrenal m.,** m. glandulae suprarenalis. **m. of bone,** m. ossium. **m. glan′dulae suprarena′lis** [NA], suprarenal medulla: the inner, reddish brown, soft part of the suprarenal gland; it synthesizes, stores, and releases catecholamines. Called also *substantia medullaris glandulae suprarenalis* and *adrenal medulla.* **m. of kidney,** m. renis. **m. of lymph node,** m. nodi lymphatici. **m. neph′rica,** m. renis. **m. no′di lymphat′ici** [NA], medulla of lymph node: the central part of a lymph node, comprising cords and sinuses; called also *substantia medullaris lymphoglandulae.* **m. oblonga′ta** [NA], the truncated cone of nerve tissue continuous above with the pons and below with the spinal cord; it lies anterior to the cerebellum, and the upper part of its posterior surface forms the floor of the lower part of the fourth ventricle; it contains ascending and descending tracts, and important collections of nerve cells that deal with vital functions, such as respiration, circulation, and special senses. Called also *bulb, bulbus* [NA alternative], and *myelencephalon* [NA alternative]. See also *brain stem,* under B. **m. os′sium,** bone marrow: the soft material filling the cavities of the bones, made up of a meshwork of connective tissue containing branching fibers, the meshes being filled with marrow cells, which consist variously of fat cells, large nucleated cells or myelocytes, and giant cells called megakaryocytes. See *m. ossium flava* and *rubra.* **m. os′sium fla′va** [NA], yellow bone marrow: ordinary bone marrow of the kind in which the fat cells predominate. **m. os′sium ru′bra** [NA], red bone marrow: marrow of developing bone, of the ribs, vertebrae, and many of the smaller bones; it is the site of production of erythrocytes and granular leukocytes. **m. ova′rii [NA], m. of ovary,** the loose fibroelastic tissue and mass of contorted blood vessels that forms the core of the ovary. **m. re′nis** [NA], medulla of kidney: the inner part of the substance of the kidney, composed chiefly of collecting elements and loops of Henle, organized grossly into pyramids; called also *substantia medullaris renis*. **spinal m., m. spina′lis** [NA], the spinal cord: that part of the central nervous system which is lodged in the vertebral canal; it extends from the foramen magnum, where it is continuous with the medulla oblongata, to the upper part of the lumbar region. It ends between the twelfth thoracic and third lumbar vertebrae, often at or adjacent to the disc between the first and second lumbar vertebrae. The spinal cord is composed of an inner core of gray substance in which nerve cells predominate, and an outer layer of white substance in which myelinated nerve fibers predominate, and is enclosed in three protective membranes, or meninges: the dura mater, the arachnoid, and the pia mater. Thirty-one spinal nerves originate from the spinal cord: 8 cervical, 12 thoracic, 5 lumbar, 5 sacral, and 1 coccygeal. It conducts impulses to and from the brain, and controls many automatic muscular activities (reflexes). Called also *chorda spinalis*. See Plate 11, under *brain*. See also *Rexed's laminae*, under *lamina*. **suprarenal m., m. of suprarenal gland,** m. glandulae suprarenalis. **m. thy′mi [NA], m. of thymus,** the central portion of each lobule of the thymus; it contains many more reticular cells and far fewer lymphocytes than does the surrounding cortex.

medullae (mĕ-dul′e) [L.] genitive and plural of *medulla*.

medullary (med′u-lār″e) [L. *medullaris*] pertaining to the marrow or to any medulla; resembling marrow.

medullated (med′u-lāt″ed) myelinated.

medullation (med″u-la′shun) the formation of a medulla or marrow; especially the formation of the medullary sheath around a nerve fiber.

medullectomy (med″u-lek′to-me) [L. *medulla* marrow + Gr. *ektomē* excision] excision of the medulla of an organ, as of the adrenal gland.

medulliadrenal (mĕ-dul″ĭ-ah-dre′nal) medulloadrenal.

medullitis (med″u-li′tis) 1. osteomyelitis. 2. myelitis.

medullization (med″u-li-za′shun) the enlargement of the haversian canals in rarefying osteitis, followed by their conversion into marrow channels; also the replacement of bone by marrow cells.

medulloadrenal (me-dul″o-ah-dre′nal) pertaining to the adrenal medulla.

medulloarthritis (me-dul″o-ar-thri′tis) [L. *medulla* marrow + *arthritis*] inflammation of the marrow spaces of the articular extremities of bones.

medulloblast (mĕ-dul′o-blast) an undifferentiated cell of the embryonic medullary (neural) tube which may develop into either a neuroblast or a spongioblast.

medulloblastoma (mĕ-dul″o-blas-to′mah) a cerebellar tumor composed of undifferentiated neuroepithelial cells; it is highly radiosensitive.

medulloencephalic (mĕ-dul″o-en″sĕ-fal′ik) myeloencephalic.

medulloepithelioma (mĕ-dul″o-ep″ĭ-the″le-o′mah) a rare tumor of the brain composed of primitive neuroepithelial cells lining the tubular spaces.

medullosuprarenoma (mĕ-dul″o-su″prah-re-no′mah) pheochromocytoma.

medullotherapy (mĕ-dul″o-ther′ah-pe) Pasteur's preventive treatment of rabies with emulsions of fixed virus in rabbit spinal cord.

medusa (mĕ-doo-sah) [Gr. *Medusa* one of the three mythological gorgons] a jellyfish; a free-swimming, umbrella-shaped form in the life cycle of certain cnidarians.

medusocongestin (mĕ-du″so-kon-jes′tin) a toxic substance derived from the tentacles of the jelly fish, *Rhizostoma cuvieri*, which, when injected into laboratory animals, causes intense congestion of the splanchnic vessels; believed to be identical with congestin.

Mees′ lines (mēz) [R. A. *Mees*, Dutch scientist, 20th century] see under *line*.

mefenamic acid (me-fe-nam′ik) an analgesic, anti-inflammatory, and antipyretic used to relieve mild to moderate pain from rheumatoid arthritis and dysmenorrhea.

mefenorex hydrochloride (mĕ-fen′o-reks) chemical name: *N*-(3-chloropropyl)-α-methylbenzeneethanamine hydrochloride; an anorexic, $C_{12}H_{18}ClN \cdot HCl$.

mefexamide (mĕ-feks′ah-mīd) chemical name: *N*-[2-(diethylamino)ethyl]-2-(4-methoxyphenoxy)acetamide; a central nervous system stimulant, $C_{15}H_{24}N_2O_3$.

mefloquine (mef′lo-kwin) chemical name: (±)-*R**,*S**)-α-2-piperidinyl-2,8-bis(trifluoromethyl)quinolinemethanol. An antimalarial, $C_{17}H_{16}F_6N_2O$, which has been used in the treatment of drug-resistant falciparum malaria.

mefruside (mef′roo-sīd) chemical name: 4-chloro-*N*¹-[(tetrahydro-2-methyl-2-furanyl)methyl]-1,3-benzenenedisulfonamide; a diuretic, $C_{13}H_{19}ClN_2O_5S_2$.

MEG see *magnetoencephalograph*.

mega- [Gr. *megas* big, great] a combining form meaning large, enlarged, or of abnormally large size; see also words beginning *megal(o)*-. Used in naming units of measurement to indicate a quantity one million (10^6) times the unit designated by the root with which it is combined. Symbol, M.

megabecquerel (meg″ah-bek-rel′) a unit of radioactivity, being one million (10^6) becquerels; abbreviated MBq.

megabladder (meg″ah-blad′er) a condition marked by permanent overdistention of the bladder.

megacalycosis (meg″ah-kal″ĭ-ko′sis) [*mega-* + *calyx* + *-osis*] nonobstructive dilatation of the renal calices due to malformation of the renal papillae.

megacardia (meg″ah-kar′de-ah) [*mega-* + Gr. *kardia* heart] cardiomegaly.

megacaryoblast (meg″ah-kar′e-o-blast″) megakaryoblast.

megacaryocyte (meg″ah-kar′e-o-sīt″) megakaryocyte.

Megace (mĕ-gās′) trademark for a preparation of megestrol acetate.

megacecum (meg″ah-se′kum) [*mega-* + *cecum*] a cecum which is abnormally large.

megacephalic (meg″ah-sĕ-fal′ik) megalocephalic.

megacephalous (meg″ah-sef′ah-lus) megalocephalic.

megacephaly (meg″ah-sef′ah-le) megalocephaly.

megacholedochus (meg″ah-ko-led′o-kus) abnormal dilatation of the common bile duct.

megacolon (meg″ah-ko′lon) an abnormally large or dilated colon; the condition may be congenital or acquired, acute or chronic. **acquired m., acquired functional m.,** colonic enlargement associated with chronic constipation; it may be due to faulty bowel habits and is particularly common in mentally retarded children and adults with chronic mental illness. Called also *idiopathic m.* **acute m.,** toxic m. **aganglionic m.,** congenital m. **congenital m., m. congen′itum,** megacolon due to congenital absence of myenteric ganglion cells in a distal segment of the large bowel. The resultant loss of motor function in this segment causes massive hypertrophic dilatation of the normal proximal colon; the aganglionic segment usually remains narrowed, but may dilate passively. The condition appears soon after birth, is commoner in males, and causes extreme constipation, abdominal distention, sometimes vomiting, and, when severe, growth retardation. Called also *Hirschsprung's disease, aganglionic m.,* and *pelvirectal achalasia*. **idiopathic m.,** acquired m. **toxic m.,** acute dilatation of the colon associated with amebic or ulcerative colitis; the dilatation may precede perforation of the colon. Called also *acute m.*

megacurie (meg″ah-ku′re) a unit of radioactivity, being one million (10^6) curies, or the quantity of radioactive material in which the number of nuclear disintegrations is 3.7×10^{16} per second. Abbreviated MCi.

megacycle (meg′ah-si″k'l) a unit of one million (10^6) cycles, e.g., 1,000,000 cycles per second, applied to the frequency of electromagnetic waves; abbreviated Mc.

megacystis (meg″ah-sis′tis) megalocystis.

megadont (meg′ah-dont) [*mega-* + Gr. *odous* tooth] macrodont.

megadontia (meg″ah-don′she-ah) macrodontia.

megaduodenum (meg″ah-du″o-de′num) an abnormally large or dilated duodenum; it may be congenital or acquired, as in intestinal scleroderma, and is usually due to a disorder of motor function.

megadyne (meg′ah-dīn″) [*mega-* + *dyne*] a million (10^6) dynes.

megaesophagus (meg″ah-ĕ-sof′ah-gus) see *achalasia*.

megagametophyte (meg″ah-gah-me′to-fīt) [*mega-* + Gr. *gametē* wife + *phyton* plant] the female gametophyte in heterosporous plants, developed from the megaspore.

megahertz (meg′ah-hertz) one million (10^6) hertz (cycles per second). Abbreviated MHz.

megakaryoblast (meg″ah-kar′e-o-blast) the earliest cytologically identifiable precursor in the thrombocytic series, which matures to form the promegakaryocyte.

megakaryocyte (meg″ah-kar′e-o-sīt) [*mega-* + Gr. *karyon* nucleus + *-cyte*] the giant cell of bone marrow, a large cell with a greatly lobulated nucleus; mature blood platelets are released from its cytoplasm.

megakaryocytopoiesis (meg″ah-kar″e-o-sīt″o-poi-e′sis) [*megakaryocyte* + Gr. *poiesis* a making] the production of megakaryocytes.

megakaryocytosis (meg″ah-kar″e-o-si-to′sis) the presence of megakaryocytes in the blood or of excessive numbers in the bone marrow.

megalecithal (meg″ah-les′ĭ-thal) [*mega-* + Gr. *lekithos* yolk] macrolecithal.

megalencephalon (meg″al-en-sef′ah-lon) [*megalo-* + Gr. *enkephalos* brain] an abnormally large brain.

megalencephaly (meg″al-en-sef′ah-le) macrencephaly.

megalgia (meg-al′je-ah) [Gr. *megas* large + *-algia*] severe pain, as in muscular rheumatism.

megal(o)- [Gr. *megas*, gen. *megalou* big, great] a combining form meaning large, enlarged, or of abnormally large size; see also words beginning *mega-*.

megaloblast (meg′ah-lo-blast″) [*megalo-* + Gr. *blastos* germ] a large, nucleated, immature progenitor of an abnormal red blood cell series, sequentially following the promegaloblast in development and retaining some of its features; megaloblasts correspond to normoblasts of the normal red cell maturation series and are correspondingly classified as basophilic, polychromatic, and orthochromatic. **m. of Sabin,** pronormoblast.

megaloblastoid (meg″ah-lo-blas′toid) resembling a megaloblast.

megalobulbus (meg″ah-lo-bul′bus) enlargement of the duodenal cap in the roentgenogram.

megalocardia (meg″ah-lo-kar′de-ah) [*megalo-* + Gr. *kardia* heart] cardiomegaly.

megalocaryocyte (meg″ah-lo-kar′e-o-sīt) megakaryocyte.

megalocephalia (meg″ah-lo-sĕ-fa′le-ah) megalocephaly.

megalocephalic (meg″ah-lo-sĕ-fal′ik) pertaining to or characterized by megalocephaly.

megalocephaly (meg″ah-lo-sef′ah-le) [*megalo-* + Gr. *kephalē* head] 1. unusually large size of the head. 2. leontiasis ossium. Called also *megacephaly* and *megacephalia*.

megaloceros (meg″ah-los′ĕ-rus) [*megalo-* + Gr. *keras* horn] a monster having projections from the forehead resembling horns.

megalocheiria (meg″ah-lo-ki′re-ah) [*megalo-* + Gr. *cheir* hand + *-ia*] abnormal largeness of the hands.

megaloclitoris (meg″ah-lo-klit′o-ris) clitoromegaly.

megalocornea (meg″ah-lo-kor′ne-ah) [*megalo-* + *cornea*] a usually bilateral developmental anomaly of the cornea, which is of abnormal size at birth, sometimes reaching a diameter of more than 18 mm. in the adult. It may be inherited as an X-linked recessive or as an autosomal dominant trait. Called also *macrocornea*.

megalocystis (meg″ah-lo-sis′tis) [*megalo-* + Gr. *kystis* bladder] an abnormally enlarged bladder.

megalocyte (meg′ah-lo-sīt″) [*megalo-* + *-cyte*] an extremely large erythrocyte, i.e., one measuring 12 to 25 microns in diameter.

megalocytosis (meg″ah-lo-si-to′sis) macrocythemia.

megalodactylia (meg″ah-lo-dak-til′e-ah) megalodactyly.

megalodactylism (meg″ah-lo-dak′tĭ-lizm) megalodactyly.

megalodactylous (meg″ah-lo-dak′tĭ-lus) exhibiting megalodactyly.

megalodactyly (meg″ah-lo-dak′tĭ-le) [*megalo-* + Gr. *daktylos* finger] abnormal largeness of fingers or toes.

megalodontia (meg″ah-lo-don′she-ah) macrodontia.

megaloenteron (meg″ah-lo-en′ter-on) [*megalo-* + Gr. *enteron* intestine] (*obs.*) enteromegaly.

megaloesophagus (meg″ah-lo-ĕ-sof′ah-gus) see *achalasia*.

megalogastria (meg″ah-lo-gas′tre-ah) [*megalo-* + Gr. *gastēr* stomach + *-ia*] enlargement or abnormally large size of the stomach.

megaloglossia (meg″ah-lo-glos′e-ah) [*megalo-* + Gr. *glōssa* tongue + *-ia*] macroglossia.

megalographia, megalography (meg″ah-lo-gra′fe-ah; meg″ah-log′rah-fe) macrography.

megalohepatia (meg″ah-lo-he-pat′e-ah) [*megalo-* + Gr. *hēpar* liver + *-ia*] hepatomegaly.

megalokaryocyte (meg″ah-lo-kar′e-o-sīt″) megakaryocyte.

megalomania (meg″ah-lo-ma′ne-ah) [*megalo-* + Gr. *mania* madness] unreasonable conviction of one's own extreme greatness, goodness, or power; the ideas in megalomania are known as *delusions of grandeur*.

megalomaniac (meg″ah-lo-ma′ne-ak) an individual exhibiting megalomania.

megalomelia (meg″ah-lo-me′le-ah) [*megalo-* + Gr. *melos* limb + *-ia*] abnormal largeness of the limbs.

megalomicin potassium phosphate (meg″ah-lo-mi′sin) chemical name: megalomicin A compound with potassium dihydrogen phosphate; an antibiotic of unspecified action, $C_{44}H_{80}N_2O_{15} \cdot 2KH_2PO_4$.

megalonychia (meg″ah-lo-nik′e-ah) the condition of having unusually large nails. Called also *macronychia*.

megalopenis (meg″ah-lo-pe′nis) excessive size of the penis.

megalophthalmos (meg″ah-lof-thal′mos) [*megalo-* + Gr. *ophthalmos* eye] abnormally large size of the eyes. **anterior m.,** megalocornea.

megalophthalmus (meg″ah-lof-thal′mus) megalophthalmos.

megalopia (meg″ah-lo′pe-ah) macropsia.

megalopodia (meg″ah-lo-po′de-ah) [*megalo-* + Gr. *pous* foot + *-ia*] excessive size of the feet.

megalopsia (meg″ah-lop′se-ah) macropsia.

Megalopyge (meg″ah-lo-pij′e) a genus of hairy moths whose larvae (caterpillars) have stinging hairs. **M. opercula′ris,** a species whose hairs pierce the skin and cause caterpillar hair poisoning (flannel moth dermatitis).

megalosplanchnic (meg″ah-lo-splank′nik) (*obs.*) having abnormally large viscera.

megalosplenia (meg″ah-lo-sple′ne-ah) [*megalo-* + Gr. *splen* spleen + *-ia*] splenomegaly.

megalospore (meg′ah-lo-spōr″) a macrospore.

Megalosporon (meg″ah-los′po-ron) [*megalo-* + Gr. *sporos* seed] a former genus of fungi made up of large-spored dermatophytes (Sabouraud, 1903). *M. ec′tothrix* included those that form arthrospores on the outside of the hair shaft, and *M. en′dothrix* included those that form arthrospores within the hair shaft. Now included in *Trichophyton*.

megalosporon (meg″ah-los′po-ron), pl. *megalos′pora*. An organism of the genus *Megalosporon*.

megalosyndactyly (meg″ah-lo-sin-dak′tĭ-le) [*megalo-* + *syndactyly*] a condition in which the digits are very large and more or less completely grown together.

megalothymus (meg″ah-lo-thi′mus) an enlarged thymus.

megaloureter (meg″ah-lo-u-re′ter) [*megalo-* + *ureter*] congenital ureteral dilatation without demonstrable cause; called also *congenital* or *primary m.*, megaureter, primary ureteral atony, and ureteral neuromuscular dysplasia. Cf. hydroureter. **congenital m., primary m.,** megaloureter. **reflux m.,** dilatation of the ureter associated with vesicoureteral reflux.

-megaly [Gr. *megas*, gen. *megalou* big, great] a word termination denoting abnormal enlargement of the structure signified by the root to which it is attached, as splenomegaly.

meganucleus (meg″ah-nu′kle-us) (*obs.*) macronucleus.

megaprosopous (meg″ah-pros′o-pus) [*mega-* + Gr. *prosōpon* face] having a large face.

megarectum (meg-ah-rek′tum) a greatly dilated rectum.

Megarhinini (meg″a-rhi′ni-ne) a tribe of tropical non-bloodsucking mosquitoes; they fly by day, feed on flowers, and are usually highly colored. Their large larvae are predaceous and have been used to control the breeding of bloodsucking mosquitoes.

Megarhinus (meg″ah-ri′nus) a genus of large, showy, but harmless mosquitoes of tropical and subtropical countries.

megaseme (meg′ah-sēm) [*mega-* + Gr. *sēma* sign] having an orbital index of 89 or more.

megasigmoid (meg″ah-sig′moid) [*mega-* + *sigmoid*] an enormously dilated sigmoid.

megasoma (meg″ah-so′mah) [*mega-* + Gr. *sōma* body] great size and stature, not amounting to gigantism.

Megasphaera (meg″ah-sfe′rah) [*mega-* + Gr. *sphaira* ball] a genus of bacteria of the family Veillonellaceae, found in the rumen of cattle and sheep and in human feces, made up of gram-negative anaerobic cocci. The type species is *M. elsde′nii.*

megasporangium (meg″ah-spo-ran′je-um), pl. *megasporan′gia* [*mega-* + Gr. *sporos* seed + *angeion* vessel] the sporangium in which megaspores develop.

megaspore (meg′ah-spōr) [*mega-* + Gr. *sporos* seed] 1. macrospore. 2. macroconidium. 3. one of four haploid spores, usually larger than the microspore, formed in the megasporangium from a megaspore mother cell, and from which the megagametophyte, or female gametophyte, develops.

Megatrichophyton (meg″ah-tri″ko-fi′ton) a former genus made up of some large-spored dermatophytes (as *M. equi′num* and *M. megni′ni*); now considered synonymous with *Trichophyton.*

Megatrypanum (meg″ah-trip′ah-num) [*mega-* + Gr. *trypanon* borer] in some systems of classification, a subgenus of stercorarian trypanosomes, including among others the species *Trypanosoma melophagium* and *T. theileri.*

megaunit (meg′ah-u″nit) a quantity one million (10⁶) times that of a standard unit.

megaureter (meg″ah-u-re′ter) megaloureter.

megavitamin (meg″ah-vi′tah-min) a dose of vitamin(s) vastly exceeding the amount recommended for nutritional balance.

megavolt (meg′ah-vōlt) [*mega-* + *volt*] a million (10⁶) volts.

megavoltage (meg″ah-vol′tij) in ionizing radiation therapy, voltage greater than 1 megavolt. Cf. *supervoltage.*

megestrol acetate (mĕ-jes′trōl) chemical name: 17-(acetyloxy)-6-methyl-16-methylene-pregna-4,6-diene-3,20-dione. A synthetic progestin, $C_{25}H_{32}O_4$, occurring as a white, crystalline powder; used as an antineoplastic in adjunctive or palliative management of recurrent or metastatic endometrial carcinoma, administered orally.

Megimide (meg′ĭ-mīd) trademark for a preparation of bemegride.

Méglin's point (ma-glanz′) [J. A. *Méglin*, French physician, 1756–1824] see under *point.*

meglumine (meg′lu-mēn) [USP] chemical name: 1-deoxy-1-(methylamino)-ᴅ-glucitol. A crystalline base, $C_7H_{17}NO_5$, occurring as white to faintly yellowish white, crystals or powder; used in the preparation of certain radiopaque media. Called also *methylglucamine.* See also under *diatrizoate* and *iodipamide.* **m. iothalamate,** a salt of iodothalamic acid, $C_{18}H_{26}I_3N_3O_9$, occurring as a clear, colorless to pale yellow, slightly viscous liquid; used as a diagnostic radiopaque medium for intravascular use in cerebral angiography, excretory urography, and peripheral arteriography.

meglutol (meg′lu-tōl) chemical name: 3-hydroxy-3-methyl pentanedioic acid; an antihyperlipoproteinemic, $C_6H_{10}O_5$.

megohm (meg′ōm) [*mega-* + *ohm*] a million (10⁶) ohms.

megophthalmos (meg-of-thal′mos) [*mega-* + Gr. *ophthalmos* eye] buphthalmos; hydrophthalmos.

megrim (me′grim) migraine.

mehlnährschaden (māl″nahr-shad′en) [Ger.] a nutritional deficiency syndrome similar to kwashiorkor, due to inadequate protein intake and overabundance of carbohydrate; the clinical characteristics include growth failure, preservation of subcutaneous fat with wasting of muscle, edema, and psychomotor abnormalities.

meibomian cyst, foramen, glands, stye (mi-bo′me-an) [Heinrich *Meibom*, German anatomist, 1638–1700] see *chalazion, foramen cecum linguae,* and *glandulae tarsales,* and see under *stye.*

meibomianitis (mi-bo″me-ah-ni′tis) inflammation of the meibomian glands.

meibomitis (mi″bo-mi′tis) meibomianitis.

Meige's disease (mehzh′ez) [Henri *Meige*, French physician, 1866–1940] Milroy's disease.

Meigs' capillaries, test (megz) [Arthur V. *Meigs*, Philadelphia physician, 1850–1912] see under *capillary* and *tests.*

Meigs' syndrome (megz) [Joe Vincent *Meigs*, American surgeon, 1892–1963] see under *syndrome.*

Meinicke test (reaction) (mi′nĭ-ke) [Ernst *Meinicke*, German physician, 1878–1945] see under *tests.*

meio- see *mi(o)-.*

meiogenic (mi″o-jen′ik) [Gr. *meiosis* + *gennan* to produce] promoting or causing meiosis.

meiosis (mi-o′sis) [Gr. *meiōsis* diminution] a special method of cell division, occurring in maturation of the sex cells, by means of which each daughter nucleus receives half the number of chromosomes characteristic of the somatic cells of the species. See illustration. Cf. *mitosis.*

meiotic (mi-ot′ik) pertaining to, characteristic of, or characterized by meiosis.

Meirowsky phenomenon (mi-rof′ske) [Emil *Meirowsky*, German-American dermatologist, 1876–1960] see under *phenomenon.*

Meissner's corpuscles, ganglion, plexus (mīs′nerz) [Georg *Meissner*, German physiologist, 1829–1905] see *corpuscula tactus, plexus submucosus,* and see under *ganglion.*

mel (mel) [L.] 1. honey. 2. a compound of honey with some medicinal agent.

melagra (mel-ag′rah) [Gr. *melos* limb + *agra* seizure] muscular pain in the extremities.

melalgia (mel-al′je-ah) [Gr. *melos* limb + *-algia*] pain in the limbs.

melancholia (mel″an-ko′le-ah) [*melano-* + *cholē* bile] a word used for ages to refer to what is now called depression. In the humoral theory of the ancient Greeks it was the temperament caused by an excess of black bile. In modern psychiatric terminology melancholia is used to refer to especially severe forms of major depression. **m. agita′ta, agitated m.,** agitated depression. **m. atton′ita** (*obs.*), schizophrenia with catatonic stupor. **m. hypochondri′aca, hypochondriacal m.** (*obs.*), concurrent depression and hypochondriasis. **involutional m.,** depression occurring in late middle age in a person with no history of previous mental illness, although premorbid rigid, compulsive, or inhibited personality traits are usually evident. Formerly considered to be a distinct clinical syndrome with characteristic symptomatology, it has been subsumed under the category of major depression in DSM III-R. Called also *involutional psychosis.* **m. sim′plex** (*obs.*), "simple depression" without delusions. **m. stuporo′sa, stuporous m.,** m. attonita.

melancholic (mel″an-kol′ik) characterized by melancholia.

melancholy (mel′an-kol″e) melancholia.

melanemesis (mel″ah-nem′ĕ-sis) [*melano-* + Gr. *emein* to vomit] black vomit.

melanemia (mel″ah-ne′me-ah) [*melano-* + Gr. *haima* blood + *-ia*] the presence of black, pigmentary masses in the blood, as in hemochromatosis.

Melania (mĕ-la′ne-ah) a generic name formerly applied to smaller fresh water operculate snails, now classified under a number of genera of the family Melaniidae (Thiaridae).

melanicterus (mel″ah-nik′ter-us) Winckel's disease.

melaniferous (mel″ah-nif′er-us) [*melanin* + L. *ferre* to bear] containing melanin or other black pigment.

melanin (mel′ah-nin) [Gr. *melas* black] the dark amorphous pigment of the skin, hair, and various tumors, of the choroid coat of the eye and the substantia nigra of the brain. It is produced by polymerization of oxidation products of tyrosine and dihydroxyphenyl compounds, and contains carbon, hydrogen, nitrogen, oxygen, and often sulfur. **artificial m., factitious m.,** a compound resembling melanin, formed when a protein is heated in strong hydrochloric acid; called also *melanoid.*

melanism (mel′ah-nizm) excessive pigmentation or blackening of the integuments or tissues, usually of genetic origin; melanosis. **industrial m.,** the gradual darkening of pop-

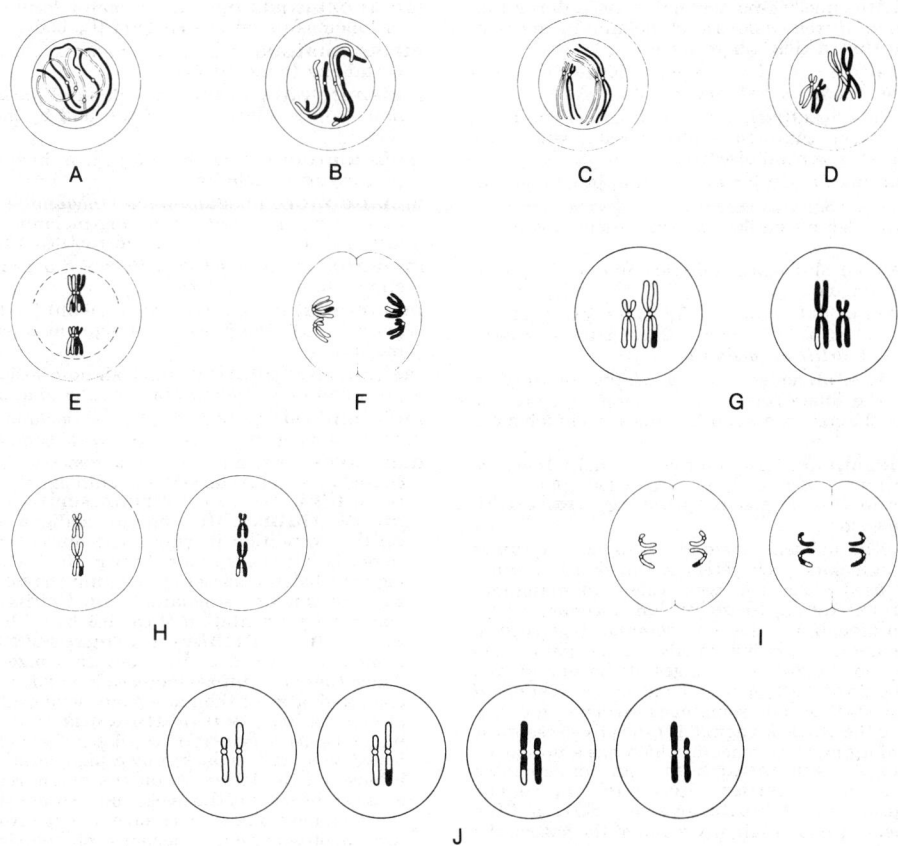

Meiosis (only two of the 23 human chromosome pairs are shown, the chromosomes from one parent in black, those from the other parent in outline). FIRST MEIOTIC DIVISION: *A, leptotene* —first appearance of chromosomes as thin threads; *B, zygotene* —pairing (synapsis) of chromosomes; *C, pachytene* —chromosomal thickening and shortening, the individual chromatids becoming visible; *D, diplotene* —longitudinal separation of chromatids, the centromere remaining intact and a chiasma being formed (NOTE: prophase includes *A* to *D* plus diakinesis [not shown]); *E, metaphase* —movement of chromosomes into the equatorial plane; *F, anaphase* —separation of pairs, one member going to each pole; *G, telophase* —cell division, each of the two daughter cells being haploid. SECOND MEIOTIC DIVISION: *prophase* (not shown)—chromosomes become visible; *H, metaphase* —movement of chromosomes into equatorial plane; *I, anaphase* —division of centromeres, the chromatids going to opposite poles; *J, telophase* —cell division, each daughter cell being haploid.

ulations of organisms living in soot-darkened habitats due to the selective pressure of predators, the darker individuals tending to survive as the conspicuous individuals are eaten, thus favoring the genotype that darkens their color. The peppered moth, *Biston betularia,* has undergone this change. **metallic m.,** argyria.

melanistic (mel″ah-nis′tik)   characterized by melanism.

melan(o) [Gr. *melas,* gen. *melanos* black]   a combining form meaning black, or denoting relationship to melanin.

melanoacanthoma (mel″a-no-ak″an-tho′mah) [*melano-* + *acanthoma*]   a rare, benign epidermal neoplasm composed of keratinocytes pervaded with large dendritic, deeply pigmented melanocytes, which occurs on the head.

melanoameloblastoma (mel″no-ah-mel″o-blas-to′mah) melanotic neuroectodermal tumor.

melanoblast (mel′ah-no-blast″, mě-lan′o-blast) [*melano-* + Gr. *blastos* germ]   a cell originating from the neural crest that differentiates into a melanocyte.

melanoblastoma (mel″ah-no-blas-to′mah) [*melano-* + *blastoma*]   malignant melanoma.

melanoblastosis (mel″ah-no-blas-to′sis)   a condition characterized by the presence of melanoblasts.

melanocarcinoma (mel″ah-no-kar″sĭ-no′mah) [*melano-* + *carcinoma*]   malignant melanoma.

melanocyte (mel′ah-no-sīt, mě-lan′o-sīt)   any of the dendritic clear cells of the epidermis that synthesize tyrosinase and, within their melanosomes, the pigment melanin; the melanosomes are then transferred from melanocytes to keratinocytes.   **dendritic m.,** those having cytoplasmic projections laden with melanosomes to be transferred to keratinocytes.

melanocytic (mel″ah-no-sit′ik)   pertaining to or composed of melanocytes.

melanocytoma (mel″ah-no-si-to′mah)   a neoplasm or hamartoma composed of melanocytes.   **compound m.,** spindle and epithelioid cell nevus.   **dermal m.,** 1. blue nevus. 2. cellular blue nevus.

melanocytosis (mel″ah-no″si-to′sis) [*melanocyte* + *-osis*]   a condition characterized by an excessive number of melanocytes in the tissues.   **oculodermal m.,** nevus of Ota.

melanoderma (mel″ah-no-der′mah) [*melano-* + Gr. *derma* skin]   an abnormally increased amount of melanin in the skin, due either to an increase in the production of melanin by the melanocytes normally present or to an increase in the number of melanocytes, with production of hyperpigmented patches. **parasitic m.,** vagabonds' disease. **senile m.,** pigmentation of the skin in the aged.

melanodermatitis (mel″ah-no-der″mah-ti′tis) dermatitis associated with an increased deposit of melanin in the skin. **m. tox′ica lichenoi′des,** tar melanosis.

melanoflocculation (mel″ah-no-flok″u-la′shun) see *Henry's melanoflocculation test,* under *tests.*

melanogen (mĕ-lan′o-jen)[*melanin* + Gr. *gennan* to produce] a colorless chromogen, convertible into melanin, which may occur in the urine in certain diseases.

melanogenesis (mel″ah-no-jen′ĕ-sis) the production of melanin.

melanogenic (mel″ah-no-jen′ik) causing the production of melanin.

melanoglossia (mel″ah-no-glos′e-ah) [*melano-* + Gr. *glōssa* tongue] black tongue.

melanoid (mel′ah-noid) [*melano-* + Gr. *eidos* form] 1. resembling melanin; of a dark color. 2. a material resembling melanin. See *artificial melanin.*

Melanolestes (mel″ah-no-les′tēz) a genus of insects. **M. pic′ipes,** the "black corsair" or "kissing bug"; its bite much resembles the sting of a wasp, but it is often much more serious.

melanoleukoderma (mel″ah-no-lu″ko-der′mah) [*melano-* + Gr. *leukos* white + *derma* skin] a mottled appearance of the skin, as in chronic arsenic poisoning. **m. col′li,** syphilitic leukoderma.

melanoma (mel″ah-no′mah) [*melano-* + *-oma*] a tumor arising from the melanocytic system of the skin and other organs. When used alone, the term refers to malignant melanoma. **acral-lentiginous m.,** an uncommon type of melanoma, although it is the most common type seen in nonwhite individuals, occurring chiefly on the palms and soles, especially on the distal phalanges of the fingers and toes, often on the tip of the digit or nail fold or bed (*subungual m.* or *melanotic whitlow*), and sometimes involving mucosal surfaces, such as the vulva or vagina. It typically presents as an irregular, enlarging black macule, which has a prolonged noninvasive stage. **amelanotic m.,** an unpigmented malignant melanoma. **benign juvenile m.,** spindle and epithelioid nevus. **Cloudman's m. S91,** a firm, black subcutaneous tumor originally found at the base of the tail of a female DBA mouse, and proven to be transplantable to, and invariably metastatic in, other DBA mice and BALB/c mice. **Harding-Passey m.,** a transplantable, nonmetastasizing melanoma originally found on the ear of a brown mouse. **juvenile m.,** spindle and epithelioid cell nevus. **lenti′go malig′na m.,** a cutaneous malignant melanoma found most often on the sun-exposed areas of the skin, especially the face, which begins as a circumscribed macular patch of mottled pigmentation, showing shades of dark brown, tan, or black (*lentigo maligna* or *melanotic freckle of Hutchinson*), and enlarges by lateral growth before dermal invasion occurs. This type is the slowest growing, has the least tendency to metastasize, and seems to be the least aggressive form of malignant melanoma. Called also *circumscribed precancerous melanosis of Dubreuilh.* **malignant m.,** a malignant neoplasm of melanocytes, arising de novo or from a preexisting benign nevus, which occurs most often in the skin but also may involve the oral cavity, esophagus, anal canal, vagina, leptomeninges, and the conjunctivae or eye. The tumor is classified into four clinical types: *superficial spreading m., lentigo maligna m., acral lentiginous m.,* and *nodular m.* Called also *melanotic carcinoma, melanoblastoma,* and *melanocarcinoma.* **nodular m.,** a type of malignant melanoma arising without a perceptible radial growth phase, most often occurring on the head, neck, and trunk, typically presenting as a uniformly pigmented, elevated, bizarrely colored nodule that enlarges rather rapidly and commonly ulcerates, which may arise de novo or from a preexisting malignant melanoma of a different type. **subungual m.,** acral-lentiginous m. **superficial spreading m.,** the most common type of malignant melanoma, characterized by a period of radial growth atypical of melanocytes in the epidermis, usually associated with a lymphocytic cellular host response that is sometimes accompanied by partial or complete regression of the radial growth phase; deeply invasive growth (vertical growth) is superimposed on the radial phase. It occurs most often on the lower leg or back, usually presenting as a small pigmented macule

to a slightly palpable flat lesion that assumes an irregular outline on enlargement.

melanomatosis (mel″ah-no″mah-to′sis) the formation of melanomas in various parts of the body.

melanomatous (mel″ah-no′mah-tus) characterized by or pertaining to melanoma.

melanonychia (mel″ah-no-nik′e-ah) [*melano-* + Gr. *onyx* nail + *-ia*] blackening of the nail by melanin pigmentation.

melanophage (mel′ah-no-fāj″) a histiocyte laden with phagocytosed melanin.

melanophore (mel′ah-no-fōr″) [*melano-* + Gr. *phoros* bearing] a pigment cell containing melanin, especially such a cell in fishes, amphibians, and reptiles. Cf. *chromatophore.*

melanophorin (mel″ah-nof′o-rin) a principle thought to stimulate melanophores.

melanoplakia (mel″ah-no-pla′ke-ah) [*melano-* + Gr. *plax* plate + *-ia*] the presence of pigmented patches on the oral mucosa.

melanoprecipitation (mel″ah-no-pre-sip″ĭ-ta′shun) the precipitation of melanin pigment; used as a test for malaria.

melanoptysis (mel″ah-nop′tĭ-sis) [*melano-* + Gr. *ptyein* to spit] the expectoration of black sputum, as in anthracosis.

melanosis (mel″ah-no′sis) [*melano-* + *-osis*] a disorder caused by a disturbance in melanin pigmentation; melanism. **m. bul′bi,** m. oculi. **circumscribed precancerous m. of Dubreuilh,** lentigo maligna melanoma. **m. co′li,** a condition in which the mucous membrane of the colon is black or dark brown due to the presence of pigment-laden macrophages within the lamina propria. The pigment is not true melanin. **m. i′ridis, m. of the iris,** abnormal pigmentation of the iris by infiltration of melanoblasts. **m. lenticula′ris progressi′va,** xeroderma pigmentosum. **m. o′culi,** a usually congenital condition in which there is a diffuse increase in pigmentation of the uveal tract and often of the more superficial ocular tissues. Called also *m. bulbi.* **oculocutaneous m.,** see *nevus of Ota,* under *nevus.* **Riehl's m.,** a patchy melanoderma manifested as a light to dark brown pigmentation, which is most intense on the forehead, on the malar regions, behind the ears, on the sides of the neck, and on other sun-exposed areas. It is seen most often in women and may involve an inflammatory photosensitivity, perhaps phototoxic, reaction. **m. scle′rae,** congenital flecks of pigmentation in the sclera. **tar m.,** a dermatosis representing photosensitivity or phototoxicity induced by exposure to tar or other hydrocarbons, usually occupationally, most often involving the face or back of the hands, and characterized by pruritus associated with the development of reticular pigmentation, telangiectases, and small, dark, lichenoid, follicular papules. Called also *melanodermatitis toxica lichenoides.*

melanosome (mel′ah-no-sōm″) any of the granules within the melanocytes that contain tyrosinase and synthesize melanin; they are transferred from the melanocytes to keratinocytes.

melanotic (mel″ah-not′ik) pertaining to or characterized by the presence of melanin.

melanotrichia (mel″ah-no-trik′e-ah) [*melano-* + Gr. *thrix* hair + *-ia*] abnormal hyperpigmentation of the hair. **m. lin′guae,** black tongue.

melanotroph (mel′ah-no-trōf″) a pituitary cell that elaborates melanocyte-stimulating hormone (MSH).

melanotropic (mel″ah-no-trop′ik) [*melanin* + Gr. *tropikos* turning] having an affinity for melanin; influencing the deposit of melanin.

melanthin (mel-an′thin) an amorphous and poisonous glycoside, or saponin, $C_{20}H_{33}O_7$, from the seeds of *Nigella sativa.*

melanuresis (mel″an-u-re′sis) melanuria.

melanuria (mel″an-u′re-ah) [*melano-* + Gr. *ouron* urine + *-ia*] the excretion of darkly stained urine or of urine which turns dark on standing.

melanuric (mel″an-u′rik) pertaining to or marked by melanuria.

melanurin (mel″an-u′rin) a black substance from morbid urine in certain rare cases.

melarsoprol (mel-ar′so-prōl) chemical name: 2-[4-[(4,6-diamino-1,3,5-triazin-2-yl)amino]phenyl]-1,3,2-dithiarsolane-4--methanol. An antiprotozoal effective against *Trypanosoma,* $C_{12}H_{15}AsN_6OS_2$, occurring as a cream-colored powder; used in the treatment of advanced cases of African trypanosomiasis, administered intravenously.

melasma (mĕ-laz′mah) [Gr. *melas* black] hypermelanosis characterized by the development of sharply demarcated blotchy, brown macules usually in a symmetric distribution over the cheeks and forehead and sometimes on the upper lip and neck. It frequently occurs during pregnancy, at menopause, and in those taking oral contraceptives. It is seen occasionally in nonpregnant women who are not taking oral contraceptives and sometimes in men. A similar pattern of facial hyperpigmentation may be associated with chronic liver disease. Called also *chloasma* and *mask of pregnancy*. **m. addison′nii,** Addison's disease. **m. suprarena′le,** Addison's disease.

melatonin (mel″ah-to′nin) 5-methoxy-*N*-acetyl tryptamine, a hormone synthesized by the pineal body, which produces marked lightening of dermal pigmentation in amphibians by stimulating the aggregation of melanosomes in melanophores, and inhibits gonad development and influences estrus in mammals. It is secreted at a rate inversely dependent on environmental lighting, being synthesized and released in response to norepinephrine, whose rate of release, in turn, declines when light activates retinal photoreceptors. Its physiological role in humans is unknown.

Meleda disease (mĕ′la-dah) [*Meleda*, a small island off the Dalmatian coast, where the condition is prevalent, because of intermarriage within the small population] mal de Meleda.

melena (mĕ-le′nah) [Gr. *melaina*, feminine of Gr. *melas* black] 1. the passage of dark, pitchy, and grumous stools stained with blood pigments or with altered blood. 2. black vomit. **m. neonato′rum,** melena of the newborn, due to the extravasation of blood into the alimentary canal. **m. spu′ria,** melena in nurslings in which the blood comes from the fissured nipple of the nursing mother. **m. ve′ra,** true melena.

melenemesis (mel″ĕ-nem′ĕ-sis) [Gr. *melaina* black + *emesis* vomiting] (*obs.*) black vomit.

Meleney's ulcer (chronic undermining ulcer), synergistic gangrene (mĕ-le′nēz) [Frank Lamont *Meleney*, American surgeon, 1889–1963] see under *ulcer* (def. 1), and see *progressive synergistic gangrene*, under *gangrene*.

melengestrol acetate (mel-en-jes′trōl) chemical name: 17 - hydroxy - 6 - methyl - 16 - methylenepregna-4,6-diene-3,20-dione acetate; a progestin and antineoplastic, $C_{25}H_{32}O_4$.

melenic (mĕ-le′nik) marked by melena.

meletin (mel′ĕ-tin) quercetin.

melezitose (mĕ-lez′ĭ-tōs) a trisaccharide, $C_{18}H_{32}O_{16}$, from manna, from the sap of poplars and conifers, which on hydrolysis yields glucose and turanose.

meli-, melit(o)- [Gr. *meli*, gen. *melitos* honey] a combining form meaning sweet, or denoting relationship to honey or to sugar.

melibiase (mel″ĭ-bi′ās) α-galactosidase.

melibiose (mel″ĭ-bi′ōs) chemical name: 6-*O*-α-D-galactopyranosyl-D-glucose. A disaccharide obtained from melitose. On hydrolysis it yields galactose and dextrose.

melicera, meliceris (mel″ĭ-se′rah; mel″ĭ-se′ris) [Gr. *meli* honey + *kēros* wax] 1. a cyst filled with honey-like substance. 2. viscid, syrupy.

melicitose (mĕ-lis′ĭ-tōs) melezitose.

melilotoxin (mel″ĭ-lo-tok′sin) bishydroxycoumarin.

melioidosis (me″le-oi-do′sis) [Gr. *mēlis* a distemper of asses + *eidos* resemblance + *-osis*] a rare infection of humans and animals, clinically resembling glanders, caused by *Pseudomonas pseudomallei*, which occurs worldwide although most cases of disease are seen in Southeast Asia. Human disease, which is usually acquired through contact of a break in the skin with contaminated soil or water, may range from an inapparent dormant infection to localized abscess formation to a relatively benign pneumonia or overwhelming and highly fatal septicemia; late activation of inapparent disease or recrudescence of previous symptoms may occur many years after the initial infection. Formerly called *Whitmore's disease*.

Melissa (mĕ-lis′ah) [Gr. "bee"] a genus of labiate plants. The tops and leaves of *M. officina′lis*, containing tannin and an essential oil, are a cooling stimulant and diaphoretic. Called also *blue, lemon,* or *sweet balm*.

melissic acid (mĕ-lis′ik) trivial name for tricontanoic acid, the 30-carbon, straight-chain unsaturated fatty acid; it occurs in beeswax.

melissotherapy (mĕ-lis″o-ther′ah-pe) [Gr. *melissa* bee + *therapeia* medical treatment] treatment with bee venom; called also *apiotherapy*.

melitis (mĕ-li′tis) [Gr. *mēlon* cheek + *-itis*] inflammation of the cheek.

melit(o)- see *meli-*.

melitoptyalism (mel″ĭ-to-ti′ah-lizm)[*meli-* + Gr. *ptyalon* saliva + *-ism*] the secretion of saliva containing glucose.

melitoptyalon (mel″ĭ-to-ti′ah-lon) glucose occurring in the saliva.

melitose (mel′ĭ-tōs) a crystalline sugar from cottonseed meal and Australian manna, which is obtained from various species of *Eucalyptus*. It is a trisaccharide, $C_{18}H_{32}O_{16}$ + $5H_2O$, which on hydrolysis yields dextrose, fructose, and galactose. Called also *raffinose* and *melitriose*.

melitracen hydrochloride (mel″ĭ-tra′sen) chemical name: 3-(10,10-dimethyl-9(10*H*)-anthracenylidene)-*N,N*-dimethyl-1-propanamine hydrochloride; a tricyclic antidepressant, $C_{21}H_{25} \cdot N\text{-}$ HCl.

melitriose (mĕ-lit′ri-ōs) melitose.

Melittangium (mel″ĭ-tan′je-um) [Gr. *melitta* bee + *angeion* vessel] a genus of gliding bacteria of the family Cystobacteraceae, order Myxobacterales, found in soil and dung from herbivores. The type species is *M. bole′tus*.

melituria (mel″ĭ-tu′re-ah) [*meli-* + Gr. *ouron* urine + *-ia*] the presence of any sugar in the urine. **m. inosi′ta,** inosituria.

melituric (mel″ĭ-tu′rik) pertaining to or affected with melituria.

melizame (mel′ĭ-zām) chemical name: 3-(1*H*-tetrazol-5-yloxy)phenol; a sweetener, $C_7H_6N_4O_2$.

melizitose (mĕ-liz′ĭ-tōs) melezitose.

Melkersson-Rosenthal syndrome (mel′ker-son ro′zen-thal)[Ernst Gustaf *Melkersson*; Curt *Rosenthal*, German psychiatrist, 20th century] Melkersson's syndrome.

Melkersson's syndrome (mel′ker-sonz) [Ernst Gustaf *Melkersson*, Swedish physician, 1898–1932] see under *syndrome*.

Mellaril (mel′ah-ril) trademark for preparations of thioridazine hydrochloride.

mellitum (mĕ-li′tum), pl. *melli′ti* [L.] a pharmaceutical preparation made with honey.

mellituria (mel″ĭ-tu′re-ah) melituria.

mel(o)- [Gr. *melos* limb] a combining form denoting limb.

melodidymus (mel″o-did′ĭ-mus) [Gr. *melos* limb + *didymos* twin] an individual with a supernumerary limb.

melomelus (mĕ-lom′e-lus) [Gr. *melos* limb + *melos* limb] a monster with normal limbs and rudimentary supernumerary limbs.

meloncus (mĕ-long′kus) [Gr. *mēlon* cheek + *onkus* bulk] tumor of the cheek.

melonoplasty (mĕ-lon′o-plas″te) meloplasty.

Melophagus (mĕ-lof′ah-gus) a genus of wingless flies of the family Hippoboscidae. **M. ovi′nus,** a species that is a common ectoparasite of sheep and goats; although not a true tick, it is known as the sheep tick, or sheep ked.

meloplasty (mel′o-plas″te) [Gr. *mēlon* cheek + *plassein* to form] plastic surgery of the cheek.

melorheostosis (mel″o-re″os-to′sis) [Gr. *melos* limb + *rhein* to flow + *osteon* bone] a form of osteosclerosis or hyperostosis extending in a linear track through one of the long bones of an extremity, and consisting of proliferated ivory-like new bone. See *rheostosis*.

melosalgia (mel″o-sal′je-ah) [Gr. *melos* limb + *-algia*] pain in the lower limbs.

meloschisis (mĕ-los′kĭ-sis) [Gr. *mēlon* cheek + *-schisis*] oblique facial cleft.

melotia (mĕ-lo′she-ah) [Gr. *mēlon* cheek + *ous* ear + *-ia*] a developmental anomaly characterized by displacement of the ear onto the cheek.

Melotte's metal (mel-ots′) [George W. *Melotte*, American dentist, 1835–1915] see under *metal*.

melphalan (mel′fah-lan) [USP] a cytotoxic alkylating agent that is the L-phenylalanine derivative of nitrogen mustard, used as an antineoplastic, primarily for treatment of multiple myeloma, but also for carcinoma of the breast and ovarian carcinoma; the major side effect is bone marrow depression. Called also L-*sarcolysin* and L-*phenylalanine mustard* (L-*PAM*).

Meltzer's law, method (anesthesia) (melt′serz) [Samuel James *Meltzer*, American physiologist, 1851–1920] see under *law* and *method*.

MEM macrophage electrophoretic mobility (test).

member (mem′ber) [L. *membrum*] 1. a part of the body distinct from the rest in function or position. 2. a limb. See also *membrum*.

memberment (mem′ber-ment) the manner of arrangement of parts in a body.

membra (mem′brah) [L.] plural of *membrum*.

membrana (mem-brah′nah), gen. and pl. *membra′nae* [L.] a membrane, or thin skin; [NA] a general term for a thin layer of tissue covering a surface, lining a cavity, or dividing a space or organ. **m. abdom′inis,** peritoneum. **m. adamanti′na,** cuticula dentis. **m. adventi′tia,** 1. tunica adventitia. 2. decidua capsularis. **m. agni′na,** amnion. **m. atlanto-occipita′lis ante′rior** [NA], anterior atlanto-occipital membrane: a single midline ligamentous structure that passes from the anterior arch of the atlas to the anterior margin of the foramen magnum, and corresponds in position with the anterior longitudinal ligament of the vertebral column. Called also *anterior* or *deep atlanto-occipital ligament, ligamentum atlanto-occipitale anterius* and *ligamentum atlanto-occipitalis anterior.* **m. atlanto-occipita′lis poste′rior** [NA], posterior atlanto-occipital membrane: a single midline ligamentous structure that passes from the posterior arch of the atlas to the posterior margin of the foramen magnum, and corresponds in position with the ligamenta flava. **m. basa′lis duc′tus semicircula′ris** [NA], basal membrane of semicircular duct: the basement membrane underlying the epithelium of a semicircular duct. **m. basila′ris duc′tus cochlea′ris,** lamina basilaris ductus cochlearis. **m. cadu′ca,** see *membranae deciduae.* **m. capsula′ris,** capsula articularis. **m. choriocapilla′ris,** lamina choroidocapillaris. **m. cricova′lis,** NA alternative for conus elasticus. **membra′nae decid′uae** [NA], decidual or deciduous membranes: the endometrium of the pregnant uterus, all of which, except the deepest layer, is shed at parturition. See subentries under *decidua.* **m. elas′tica laryn′gis,** m. fibroelastica. **m. epipapilla′ris,** an abnormal fibrous membrane on the optic disk. **m. fibroelas′tica laryn′gis** [NA], fibroelastic membrane of larynx: the fibroelastic layer beneath the mucous coat of the larynx, comprising the quadrangular membrane and the conus elasticus; called also *m. elastica laryngis.* **m. fibro′sa cap′sulae articula′ris** [NA], fibrous membrane of articular capsule: the outer of the two layers of the articular capsule of a synovial joint, composed of dense white fibrous tissue; called also *stratum fibrosum capsulae articularis* [NA alternative]. **m. flac′cida,** pars flaccida membranae tympani. **m. fus′ca,** lamina fusca sclerae. **m. germinati′va,** blastoderm. **m. granulo′sa,** layers of cuboidal epithelial cells at the periphery of an ovarian follicle and surrounding the antrum or fluid-filled cavity. **m. granulo′sa exter′na,** the external granular layer of the retina. **m. granulo′sa inter′na,** the internal granular layer of the retina. **m. hyaloi′dea,** m. vitrea. **m. hyothyreoi′dea,** m. thyrohyoidea. **m. intercosta′lis exter′na** [NA], external intercostal membrane: any of the aponeurotic bands parallel with, and perhaps replacing, the fibers of the external intercostal muscles in the spaces between the costal cartilages, from the ventral tips of the ribs medially to the sternum; called also *ligamenta intercostalia externa.* **m. intercosta′lis inter′na** [NA], internal intercostal membrane: any of the aponeurotic bands parallel with, and perhaps replacing, the fibers of the internal intercostal muscles in the spaces between the ribs, from the angles of the ribs medially to the vertebral column; called also *ligamenta intercostalia interna.* **m. interos′sea antebra′chii** [NA], **m. interos′sea antibra′chii,** interosseous membrane of forearm: a thin fibrous sheet that connects the bodies of the radius and ulna, passing from the interosseous margin of the radius to that of the ulna. **m. interos′sea cru′ris,** interosseous membrane of leg: a thin aponeurotic lamina attached to the interosseous margins of the tibia and fibula, deficient for a short distance at

the proximal end of the bones; it separates the muscles on the anterior and posterior parts of the leg. **m. li′mitans,** 1. one of the limiting membranes of the retina; see *external* and *internal limiting membrane* (def. 1), under *membrane.* 2. the limiting membrane of glia fibrils and perivascular feet separating the neural parenchyma from the pia and blood vessels. **m. muco′sa na′si,** tunica mucosa nasi. **m. muco′sa vesi′cae fel′leae,** tunica mucosa vesicae biliaris. **m. nic′titans,** 1. plica semilunaris conjunctivae. 2. nictitating membrane. **m. obturato′ria** [NA], obturator membrane: a strong membrane that fills the obturator foramen except superiorly at the obturator groove, where a deficiency is left, the obturator canal. **m. obturato′ria [stape′dis],** m. stapedis. **m. obtura′trix,** m. obturatoria. **m. perfora′ta,** a term sometimes used to designate the first appearance of dentin in the fetus, manifested as a thick limiting line between the ameloblasts and odontoblasts. **m. perine′i** [NA], membrane of perineum: the triangular fibrous membrane stretched horizontally between the ischiopubic rami, which is attached at its base to the perineal body and as its apex thickens to form the transverse perineal ligament; called also *fascia diaphragmatis urogenitalis inferior, inferior fascia of urogenital diaphragm,* and *perineal membrane.* See also *diaphragma urogenitale.* **m. pituito′sa,** tunica mucosa nasi. **m. pro′pria,** lamina propria mucosae. **m. pro′pria duc′tus semicircula′ris** [NA], proper membrane of semicircular duct: the outer, loose, connective tissue layer of a semicircular duct. **m. pupilla′ris** [NA], pupillary membrane: a mesodermal layer attached to the rim or front of the iris during embryonic development, sometimes persisting in the adult. **m. quadrangula′ris** [NA], quadrangular membrane: the upper part of the fibroelastic membrane of the larynx. **m. reticula′ris duc′tus cochlea′ris** [NA], **m. reticula′ta,** reticular membrane: a netlike membrane over the spiral organ; the free ends of the outer hair cells pass through its apertures. **m. ruyschia′na,** lamina choroidocapillaris. **m. saccifor′mis,** the synovial membrane of the inferior radioulnar articulation. **m. sero′sa,** 1. tunica serosa. 2. the chorion. **m. seroti′na,** decidua basalis. **m. spira′lis duc′tus cochlea′ris,** NA alternative for *paries tympanicus ductus cochlearis.* **m. stape′dis** [NA], stapedial membrane: a membrane filling the arch formed by the crura and base of the stapes; called also *m. obturatoria [stapedis].* **m. statoconio′rum macula′rum** [NA], statoconic membrane of maculae: the gelatinous membrane surmounting the maculae, containing the statoconia, and having special sensory hairs projecting into it. **m. ster′ni** [NA], sternal membrane: the thick fibrous membrane that envelopes the sternum; it is formed by the intermingling of fibers of the radiate sternocostal ligaments, the periosteum, and the tendinous origin of the pectoralis major. **m. succin′gens,** the pleura. **m. suprapleura′lis** [NA], suprapleural membrane: the strengthened portion of the endothoracic fascia attached to the inner part of the first rib and the transverse process of the seventh cervical vertebra. **m. synovia′lis cap′sulae articula′ris** [NA], synovial membrane of articular capsule: the inner of the two layers of the articular capsule of a synovial joint, composed of loose connective tissue and having a free smooth surface that lines the joint cavity. It secretes the synovial fluid. Called also *stratum synoviale capsulae articularis* [NA alternative]. **m. synovia′lis infe′rior,** [NA], inferior synovial membrane: the synovial membrane that lines the articular capsule of the temporomandibular joint below the articular disk. **m. synovia′lis supe′rior** [NA], superior synovial membrane: the synovial membrane that lines the articular capsule of the temporomandibular joint above the articular disk. **m. tecto′ria** [NA], tectorial membrane: a strong fibrous band connected cranially with the basilar part of the occipital bone and caudally with the dorsal surface of the bodies of the second and third cervical vertebrae. It is actually the cranial prolongation of the deeper portion of the posterior longitudinal ligament of the vertebral column. **m. tecto′ria duc′tus cochlea′ris** [NA], tectorial membrane of cochlear duct: a delicate gelatinous mass resting on the spiral organ of the ear and connected with the hairs of the hair cells; called also *Corti's membrane.* **m. ten′sa,** pars tensa membranae tympani. **m. thyrohyoi′dea** [NA], thyrohyoid membrane: a broad fibroelastic sheet attached above to the upper margin of the posterior surface of the hyoid bone and below to the upper border of the thyroid cartilage; called also *m. hyothyreoidea.* **m. tym′pani** [NA], tympanic membrane: the obliquely placed, thin membranous partition between the external acoustic meatus and the tympanic cavity. The greater portion, the pars tensa, is attached by a fibrocartilaginous ring to the tympanic plate of the temporal bone; the much smaller, triangular portion, the pars flaccida, is situated anterosuperiorly between the two mallear folds. Called also *drumhead; drum, eardrum,* and *tympanum* are used loosely as synonyms. **m. tym′pani secunda′ria** [NA], secondary tympanic membrane: the membrane that closes in the fenestra cochlearis; called also *Scarpa's membrane.* **m. versic′olor of Fielding,** tapetum, def. 2. **m. vestibula′ris** [NA alternative], **m. vestibula′ris [Reiss′neri],** paries vestibularis ductus cochleae. **m. vi′brans,** pars tensa membranae tympani. **m. vitelli′na,** vitelline membrane. **m. vi′trea** [NA], vitreous membrane: a delicate boundary layer investing the vitreous body of the eye; called also *m. hyaloidea* or *hyaloid membrane.*

membranaceous (mem″brah-na′shus) [L. *membranaceus*] of the nature of a membrane.

membranae (mem-bra′ne) [L.] genitive and plural of *membrana.*

membranate (mem′brah-nāt) having the character of a membrane.

membrane (mem′brān) a thin layer of tissue which covers a surface, lines a cavity, or divides a space or organ; see also *membrana.* **abdominal m.,** peritoneum. **accidental m.,** false m. **adamantine m.,** cuticula dentis. **alveolocapillary m.,** an exquisitely thin tissue barrier, the mechanism for gas exchange between alveolar air and capillary blood in the lung. **alveolodental m.,** periodontal ligament. **anal m.,** cloacal m. **animal m.,** a thin membranous diaphragm, as of bladder, used as a dialyzer. **aponeurotic m.,** aponeurosis. **arachnoid m.,** arachnoidea. **Ascherson's m.,** the covering of casein enclosing the milk globules. **asphyxial m.,** hyaline m. (def. 2); so called because of its interference with gaseous exchange in the lungs. **atlanto-occipital m., anterior,** membrana atlanto-occipitalis anterior. **atlanto-occipital m., posterior,** membrana atlanto-occipitalis posterior. **basal m. of semicircular duct,** membrana basalis ductus semicircularis. **basement m.,** the delicate layer of extracellular condensation of mucopolysaccharides and proteins underlying the epithelium of mucous membranes and secreting glands. **basilar m. of cochlear duct,** lamina basilaris ductus cochleae. **Bichat's m.,** Henle's fenestrated m. **birth m's,** the amnion and chorion. **Bowman's m.,** a thin layer of the cornea composed of condensed stroma, between the outer layer of stratified epithelium and the substantia propria; called also *lamina limitans anterior corneae* [NA]. **Bruch's m.,** complexus basalis choroideae. **Brunn's m.,** the epithelium of the olfactory region of the nose. **bucconasal m.,** oronasal m. **buccopharyngeal m.,** 1. fascia pharyngobasilaris. 2. oropharyngeal m. **capsular m.,** 1. capsula articularis. 2. a membrane enclosing the central capsule of certain marine planktonic protozoa of the superclass Actinopoda, such as radiolarians, which is perforated to permit communication between the intracapsular cytoplasm and that of the outer cortical layer (*calymma*). **capsulopupillary m.,** membrana pupillaris. **cell m.,** plasma m. **chorioallantoic m.,** chorioallantois. **chromatic m.,** a continuous layer of chromatin substance situated on the internal surface of a nuclear membrane. **cloacal m.,** the thin, temporary barrier between the hindgut and the exterior, formed by the outer and inner germ layers of the embryo; called also *anal m.* and *anal plate.* **complex m.,** a membrane made up of several layers differing in structure. **compound m.,** a membrane, like that of the tympanum, made up of two distinct layers. **Corti's m.,** membrana tectoria ductus cochleae. **costocoracoid m.,** fascia clavipectoralis. **cribriform m.,** fascia cribrosa. **cricothyroid m., cricovocal m.,** conus elasticus. **croupous m.,** a false membrane formed in true croup. **cyclitic m.,** a false membrane which sometimes covers the vitreous body in cyclitis. **Debove's m.,** the delicate layer between the epithelium and the tunica propria of the bronchial, tracheal, and intestinal mucous membranes. **decidual m's, deciduous m's,** membranae deciduae. **Demours' m.** (*obs.*), lamina limitans posterior corneae. **dentinoenamel m.,** a continuous thin membrane laid

down by ameloblasts adjoining the basement membrane separating them from the dentin in an early developing tooth. **Descemet's m.,** a thin hyaline membrane between the substantia propria and the endothelial layer of the cornea; called also *lamina limitans posterior corneae* [NA]. **diphtheritic m.,** a false membrane characteristic of diphtheria and resulting from coagulation necrosis. **drum m.,** membrana tympani. **Duddell's m.** (*obs.*), lamina limitans posterior corneae. **egg m.,** any of several investments surrounding the ovum or egg: if derived from the ovum itself, as the vitelline membrane, it is *primary;* if from the follicular cells, as the zona pellucida, it is secondary; if from the oviduct, as the albumen around rabbit's egg or the albumen and shell of hen's egg, it is *tertiary.* Called also *egg envelope* and, collectively, *lemma.* **elastic m.,** a variety of membrane composed largely of elastic fibers. **elastic m., external,** a fenestrated elastic membrane that constitutes the innermost component of the tunica adventitia of arteries. Called also *external elastic lamina.* **elastic m., internal,** a fenestrated elastic membrane that constitutes the outermost component of the tunica intima of arteries. Called also *internal elastic lamina.* **enamel m.,** 1. cuticula dentis. 2. the inner layer of cells within the enamel organ of the dental germ in the fetus; called also *Hannover's intermediate m.* **endoneural m.,** neurilemma. **endoral m.,** paroral m. **exocoelomic m.,** Heuser's m. **extraembryonic m's,** the trophoblastic parts of the conceptus that provide for the support of the embryo or fetus by attachment, mechanical protection, endocrine action, and the mediation of chemical exchange with the maternal circulation. They include the yolk sac, allantois, amnion, umbilical cord, and chorion, including the placenta. To these, some would add the maternal component, the decidua. Called also *fetal m's.* **false m.,** a morbid pellicle or skinlike layer resembling an organized and living membrane, but made up of coagulated fibrin with bacteria and leukocytes, such as may be formed on mucous membranes in diphtheria. **fenestrated m.,** one of the multiply perforated elastic sheets of the tunica intima and tunica media of arteries. **fertilization m.,** a strong membrane formed around the fertilized ovum in some species of animals by adhesion of part of the contents of the cortical granules to the inner surface of the vitelline membrane; it prevents the entry of additional spermatozoa. **fetal m's,** extraembryonic m's. **fibroelastic m. of larynx,** membrana fibroelastica laryngis. **fibrous m. of articular capsule,** membrana fibrosa capsulae articularis. **Fielding's m.,** tapetum, def. 2. **germinal m.,** blastoderm. **glassy m.,** 1. the basement membrane of a vesicular ovarian follicle which in cross-section appears as a distinct brilliant line and which persists in the ovary long after its follicle has degenerated. Called also *m. of Slavianski.* 2. lamina basalis choroideae. 3. hyaline m., def. 1. **glomerular m.,** the membrane covering a glomerular capillary. **gradocol m's,** thin membranes made of collodion or similar substances and graded as to porosity; used in ultrafiltration and sometimes to estimate the diameters of viruses. **ground m.,** inophragma. **Haller's m.,** lamina vasculosa choroideae. **Hannover's intermediate m.,** enamel m., def. 2. **haptogen m.,** the membrane of protein matter formerly believed to enclose milk globules. **Held's limiting m.,** blood-brain barrier. **Henle's m.,** 1. posterior border lamella of Fuchs; see under *lamella.* 2. formerly, the lamina basalis choroideae. **Henle's elastic m.,** a fenestrated layer between the outer and middle tunics of certain arteries. **Henle's fenestrated m.,** a subendothelial fibroelastic fenestrated layer in the tunica intima of an artery; called also *Bichat's m.* **Heuser's m.,** a delicate sac of mesoblastic tissue that develops as a lining of the blastocyst or chorionic cavity just after implantation, forms the exocoelomic cavity, and quickly disappears; called also *exocoelomic membrane.* **Huxley's m.,** see under *layer.* **hyaline m.,** 1. the membrane between the outer root sheath and the inner fibrous layer of a hair follicle. 2. a layer of eosinophilic hyaline material lining the alveoli, alveolar ducts, and bronchioles, found at autopsy in infants who have died of respiratory distress syndrome of the newborn. Called also *asphyxial membrane* and *vernix membrane.* See *respiratory distress syndrome,* under *syndrome.* **hyaloid m.,** membrana vitrea. **hymenal m.,** hymen. **hyoglossal m.,** a fibrous lamina connecting the under surface of the tongue with the hyoid bone. **hyothyroid m.,** membrana thyrohyoidea. **intercostal m., external,** membrana intercostalis externa. **intercostal m., internal,** membrana intercostalis interna. **interosseous m., radioulnar, interosseous m. of forearm,** membrana interossea antebrachii. **interosseous m. of leg,** membrana interossea cruris. **interspinal m's,** see *ligamentum interspinale.* **intersutural m.,** the pericranium lying between the cranial sutures. **ion-selective m.,** a membrane that is more permeable to particular types of ions than to other types, e.g., K^+-selective glass membrane. Many biological membranes exhibit ion-selective behavior. **Jackson's m.,** a delicate curtain or web of adhesions (regarded by some as a sheet of peritoneum) which may extend from the lateral abdominal wall to the cecum, covering the cecum and producing obstruction of the bowel; called also *Jackson's veil.* **Jacob's m.,** layer of rods and cones. **keratogenous m.,** matrix unguis. **Kölliker's m.,** membrana reticularis ductus cochlearis. **Krause's m.,** Z band; see under *band.* **ligamentous m.,** membrana tectoria. **limiting m.,** a membrane which constitutes the border of some tissue or structure. **limiting m., external,** 1. a thin fenestrated layer of the pars nervosa retinae adjacent to the outer nuclear layer and through which extend the visual rods and cones. 2. a membrane investing the external surface of the embryonic neural tube. Called also *outer limiting m.* **limiting m., inner, limiting m., internal,** 1. internal limiting m. 2. a membrane lining the internal surface of the embryonic neural tube. **limiting m., outer,** external limiting m. **Mauthner's m.,** axolemma. **medullary m.,** endosteum. **mucocutaneous m.,** a membrane that is partly mucous and partly cutaneous, like that of the tympanum. **mucous m.,** tunica mucosa. **mucous m., proper,** lamina propria mucosae. **mucous m. of colon,** tunica mucosa coli. **mucous m. of esophagus,** tunica mucosa esophagi. **mucous m. of gallbladder,** tunica mucosa vesicae biliaris. **mucous m. of mouth,** tunica mucosa oris. **mucous m. of pharynx,** tunica mucosa pharyngis. **mucous m. of rectum,** tunica mucosa recti. **mucous m. of small intestine,** tunica mucosa intestini tenuis. **mucous m. of stomach,** tunica mucosa ventriculi. **mucous m. of tongue,** tunica mucosa linguae. **mucous m. of ureter,** tunica mucosa ureteris. **mucous m. of urinary bladder,** tunica mucosa vesicae urinariae. **Nasmyth's m.,** primary (enamel) cuticle. **nictitating m.,** a transparent fold of skin lying deep to the other eyelids at the mesial side, which may be drawn over the front of the eyeball; the so-called third eyelid, found in reptiles and birds generally and in many mammals. **nuclear m.,** 1. either of the membranes, inner and outer, comprising the nuclear envelope. 2. nuclear envelope. **oblique m. of forearm,** chorda obliqua membranae interosseae antebrachii. **obturator m.,** membrana obturatoria. **obturator m. of atlas, anterior,** membrana atlantooccipitalis anterior. **obturator m. of atlas, posterior,** membrana atlantooccipitalis posterior. **obturator m. of larynx,** membrana thyrohyoidea. **occipitoaxial m., long,** membrana tectoria. **olfactory m.,** the olfactory portion of the mucous membrane lining the nasal fossa. **oral m.,** fascia pharyngobasilaris. **oronasal m.,** a thin epithelial plate separating the nasal pits from the oral cavity of the embryo. **oropharyngeal m.,** a transient embryonic septum at the cranial limit of the foregut, in the depths of the stomodeum; called also *buccopharyngeal m.* **otolithic m.,** membrana statoconiorum macularum. **ovular m.,** vitelline m. **palatine m.,** the membrane covering the roof of the mouth. **pansporoblastic m.,** a surface membrane surrounding the sporoblasts in a pansporoblast; characteristic of microsporidian protozoa of the suborder Pansporoblastina. **paroral m.,** in certain ciliate protozoa, a movable membrane-like sheet(s) formed by fusion of the bases of a longitudinal row of cilia that borders the right side of the buccal cavity; it serves to gather food and push it toward the cytostome. Called also *endoral m.* and *undulating m.* Cf. *membranelle.* **pericolic m., pericolonic m.,** occasional bands of peritoneum extending between the abdominal wall and the serosa of the colon. **peridental m.,** periodontal ligament. **perineal m., m. of perineum,** membrana perinei. **periodontal m.,** see under *ligament.* **periorbital m.,** periorbita. **peritrophic m.,** a delicate, cylindrical sheath of chitin continuously secreted from the posterior edge of the foregut of insects and millipedes that ingest solid food, which surrounds the food as it passes through the midgut. **pharyngeal m., pharyngobasilar m.,** fascia pharyn-

gobasilaris. **pituitary m. of nose,** tunica mucosa nasi. **placental m.,** the semipermeable membrane that separates the fetal from the maternal blood in the placenta. In the human (hemochorial) placenta, it is composed of fetal vascular endothelium, cytotrophoblast, and syncytium, and it becomes thinner as pregnancy progresses. Called also *placental barrier.* **plasma m.,** the structure enveloping a cell, enclosing the cytoplasm, and forming a selective permeability barrier; it consists of lipids, proteins, and some carbohydrates, the lipids thought to form a bilayer in which integral proteins are embedded to varying degrees. Called also *cell m., cytoplasmic m.,* and *plasmalemma.* **platelet demarcation m.,** a more or less tridimensional system of paired membranes that serve to partition the megakaryocyte cytoplasm, each partition containing azurophilic granules and representing a future blood platelet. **pleuropericardial m.,** a membrane in the embryo separating the heart and the lung sac. **pleuroperitoneal m.,** a membrane in the embryo separating the pleural cavity from the peritoneal cavity and developing into a part of the diaphragm. **proligerous m.,** cumulus oophorus. **proper m. of semicircular duct,** membrana propria ductus semicircularis. **prophylactic m.,** pyophylactic m. **pseudoserous m.,** a membrane resembling serous membrane, but differing from it in structure. **pulmonary hyaline m.,** hyaline membrane, def. 2. **pupillary m.,** membrana pupillaris. **pyogenic m.,** a membrane which produces pus. **pyophylactic m.,** a fibrinous membrane lining a pus cavity and tending to prevent reabsorption of injurious materials. **quadrangular m.,** membrana quadrangularis. **Reichert's m.** (*obs.*), lamina limitans anterior corneae. **Reissner's m.,** paries vestibularis ductus cochlearis. **reticular m., reticulated m.,** membrana reticularis ductus cochlearis. **Ruysch's m., ruyschian m.,** lamina choroidocapillaris. **Scarpa's m.,** membrana tympani secundaria. **schneiderian m.,** tunica mucosa nasi. **Schwann's m.,** neurilemma. **semipermeable m.,** a membrane that permits the passage of a solvent, such as water, but prevents the passage of the dissolved substance, or solute. **serous m.,** tunica serosa. **shell m.,** a double fibrous layer lining the shell of the egg of some animals, such as birds. **Shrapnell's m.,** pars flaccida membranae tympani. **m. of Slavianski,** glassy m., def. 1. **slit m.,** one of the exceedingly thin membranes that bridge the slit pores between adjacent pedicels of the podocytes of the renal glomerulus, and close the pores at their bases. **spiral m. of cochlear duct,** membrana spiralis ductus cochlearis. **stapedial m.,** membrana stapedis. **statoconic m. of maculae,** membrana statoconiorum macularum. **sternal m., m. of sternum,** membrana sterni. **striated m.,** see *zona pellucida,* def. 1. **subepithelial m.,** basement membrane. **submucous m.,** tela submucosa. **submucous m. of stomach,** tela submucosa ventriculi. **suprapleural m.,** membrana suprapleuralis. **synaptic m.,** the layer separating the neuroplasm of an axon from that of the body of the nerve cell with which it makes synapsis. **synovial m., inferior,** membrana synovialis inferior. **synovial m., superior,** membrana synovialis superior. **synovial m. of articular capsule,** membrana synovialis capsulae articularis. **tarsal m.,** orbital septum. **tectorial m.,** membrana tectoria. **tectorial m. of cochlear duct,** membrana tectoria ductus cochlearis. **tendinous m.,** aponeurosis. **Tenon's m.,** vagina bulbi. **thyreohyoid m.,** membrana thyrohyoidea. **Traube's m.,** a film of potassium ions formed at the plane of contact of the two liquids, when a solution of potassium ferrocyanide is brought into contact with a solution of a copper salt. **tympanic m.,** the membrane separating the middle from the external ear; see *membrana tympani.* **tympanic m., secondary,** membrana tympani secundaria. **undulating m.,** 1. in certain flagellate protozoa, a delicate finlike cytoplasmic membrane extending from and running along the lateral aspect of the body, the outer margin of which being formed by a flagellum that may continue free beyond the end of the body and the membrane. It serves a locomotor function; vibration of the membrane produces a characteristic undulating movement. 2. paroral m. **unit m.,** the trilaminar structure of the plasma membrane as seen under the electron microscope and postulated to be the same for the membranes of all cells, the cell nucleus, and organelles (mitochondria, etc.). **vascular m. of viscera,** tela submucosa. **vernix m.,** hyaline m. (def. 3); so called because it was originally thought to be the result of aspiration of vernix by the fetus *in utero.* **vestibular m. of cochlear duct,** paries vestibularis ductus cochlearis. **virginal m.,** hymen. **vitelline m.,** the cytoplasmic, noncellular membrane surrounding the eggs of various animals, especially the membrane enveloping the yolk of telolecithal eggs. **vitreous m.,** 1. membrana vitrea. 2. lamina basalis choroidea. 3. lamina limitans posterior corneae. 4. hyaline membrane (def. 1). **Volkmann's m.,** a thin, yellowish membrane, studded with miliary tubercles, lining the fibrous wall of a tubercular abscess. **Wachendorf's m.,** 1. membrana pupillaris. 2. plasma m. **yolk m.,** vitelline m. **Zinn's m.,** zonula ciliaris.

membranectomy (mem″brah-nek′to-me) excision of a membrane.

membranelle (mem″brah-nel′) a triangular or fan-shaped organelle bordering the left side of the buccal cavity or peristomial area in certain ciliate protozoa, formed by fusion of the bases of short, transverse rows (up to three) of cilia; it serves in locomotion and to gather and push food toward the cytostome. Cf. *paroral membrane.* **adoral zone of m's,** serially arranged membranelles (three or more) along the left side of the oral area, typically in a buccal cavity or peristome, in ciliate protozoa.

membraniform (mem-bra′nĭ-form) resembling a membrane.

membranin (mem′brah-nin) a preparation made from the cell wall and/or cell membrane of yeast cells.

membranocartilaginous (mem″brah-no-kar″tĭ-laj′ĭ-nus) 1. developed in both membrane and cartilage. 2. partly cartilaginous and partly membranous.

membranoid (mem″brah-noid) resembling a membrane.

membranolysis (mem″brān-ol′ĭ-sis) disruption of a cell membrane.

membranous (mem′brah-nus) [L. *membranosus*] pertaining to or of the nature of a membrane.

membrum (mem′brum), pl. *mem′bra* [L.] a limb, or member, of the body; [NA] a general term for one of the limbs, that is, the upper (arm, forearm, hand), or lower (thigh, leg, foot). Called also *extremitas* (pl. *extremitates*) or *extremity*. **m. infe′rius** [NA], the lower limb of the body (thigh, leg, and foot); called also *extremitas inferior*. **m. mulie′bre,** clitoris. **m. supe′rius** [NA], the upper limb of the body (arm, forearm, and hand); called also *extremitas superior*. **m. viri′le,** penis.

memory (mem′o-re) [L. *memoria*] that mental faculty by which sensations, impressions, and ideas are recalled. **anterograde m.,** a memory serviceable for events long past, but not able to acquire new recollections. **echoic m.,** that part of the sensory storage system that holds auditory stimuli. **eye m.,** visual memory. **iconic m.,** that part of the sensory storage system that holds visual stimuli. **immunologic m.,** the capacity of the immune system to respond more rapidly and strongly to subsequent antigenic challenge than to the first exposure. Called also *anamnesis.* See *memory cells,* under *cell,* and *primary* and *secondary immune response,* under *response.* **kinesthetic m.,** the memory of movements in the limbs and other parts of the body. **long-term m.,** memory that is retained over long periods of time. **screen m.,** a consciously tolerable memory serving as a "screen" for another memory that may be disturbing or emotionally painful if recalled. **short-term m.,** memory that is lost within a brief period (seconds, minutes, or longer) unless reinforced. **visual m.,** memory for visual impressions.

memotine hydrochloride (mem′o-tēn) chemical name: 3,4-dihydro-1-[(4-methoxyphenoxy)methyl] isoquinoline hydrochloride; an antiviral agent, $C_{17}H_{17}NO_2 \cdot HCl$.

MEN multiple endocrine neoplasia.

menacme (mĕ-nak′me) [Gr. *mēn* month + *akmē* top] 1. the height of menstrual activity. 2. that period of a woman's life which is marked by menstrual activity.

menadiol sodium diphosphate (men″ah-di′ol) [USP] chemical name: 2-methyl-1,4-naphthalenediol bis(dihydrogen phosphate) tetrasodium salt hexahydrate. A synthetic, water-soluble derivative of menadione (vitamin K_3) to which it is converted in the body, $C_{11}H_8N_4O_8P_2 \cdot 6H_2O$, occurring as a white to pink powder, and used as a prothrombinogenic vitamin for the same purposes as menadione (q.v.); administered orally, intravenously, and subcutaneously.

menadione (men″ah-di′ōn) [USP] chemical name: 2-methyl-1,4-naphthalenedione. A synthetic, oil-soluble vitamin K derivative, $C_{11}H_8O_2$, occurring as a bright yellow, crystalline powder; used as a source of vitamin K in the treatment of hemorrhagic conditions associated with hypoprothrombinemia, such as obstructive jaundice, biliary fistula, sprue, celiac disease, and ulcerative colitis, and after prolonged use of salicylates, administered orally and intramuscularly. Called also *menaphthone* and *vitamin K_3*. **m. sodium bisulfite** [USP], a water-soluble derivative of menadione, $C_{11}H_9NaO_5S \cdot 3H_2O$, occurring as a white crystalline powder, having the same actions and uses as menadione; administered intravenously and subcutaneously, and sometimes orally and intramuscularly.

Menagen (men′ah-jen) trademark for a preparation of estrone.

menalgia (men-al′je-ah) [Gr. *mēn* month + -*algia*] pain accompanying menstruation.

menaphthone (men-af′thōn) menadione.

menaquinone (men″ah-kwin′ōn) any of a series of compounds in which the phytyl side chain of phytonadione (vitamin K_1) is replaced by a side chain of prenyl units and which have vitamin K activity; they are synthesized, in particular, by gram-positive bacteria. Called also *farnoquinone* and *vitamin K_2*.

menarchal (mĕ-nar′kal) pertaining to menarche.

menarche (mĕ-nar′ke) [Gr. *mēn* month + *archē* beginning] the establishment or beginning of the menstrual function.

menarcheal, menarchial (mĕ-nar′ke-al) pertaining to or characterized by the establishment of the menstrual function (menarche).

Mendel's law (men′delz) [Gregor Johann *Mendel*, 1822–1884, Austrian monk and naturalist] see under *law.*

Mendel's reflex [Kurt *Mendel*, German neurologist, 1874–1946] see under *reflex.*

Mendel's test [Felix *Mendel*, German physician, 1862–1912] see *Mantoux test,* under *tests.*

Mendel-Bekhterev reflex, sign (men′del-bek- ter′yev) [Kurt *Mendel*; V. M. *Bekhterev*, Russian neurologist, 1857–1927] see under *reflex* and *sign.*

Mendeléeff's (Mendeleev's) law (men″dĕ-la′efs) [Dimitri Ivanovich *Mendeléeff*, Russian chemist, 1834–1907] see *periodic law,* under *law.*

mendelevium (men″dĕ-le′ve-um) [Dimitri Ivanovich *Mendeléeff*] the radioactive chemical element of atomic number 101, atomic weight 256, symbol Md, originally discovered in debris from a thermonuclear explosion in 1952.

mendelian (men-de′le-an) named for Gregor Johann *Mendel*; see under *character,* and see *Mendel's law,* under *law.*

mendelism (men′del-izm) see *mendelian characters,* under *character,* and *Mendel's law,* under *law.*

mendelizing (men′del-īz″ing) exhibiting the simple patterns of inheritance of various contrasting traits elaborated by Gregor Mendel; see *Mendel's laws,* under *law.*

Mendelsohn's test (men′del-sōnz) [Martin Alfred *Mendelsohn*, German physician, 1860–1930] see under *tests.*

Mendocutes (men-dok′u-tēz; men″do-ku′tēz) Mendosicutes.

Mendosicutes (men″do-sik′utēz; men″do-sĭ-ku′tēz) [L. *mendosus* having faults + *cutis* skin] a division of bacteria of the kingdom Procaryotae made up of organisms that usually have a cell wall, although it is lacking in muramic acid, and that have other evidences of an earlier phylogenetic origin (based on ribosomal RNA oligonucleotide analysis). These organisms (the Archaeobacteria) include methanogens, strict halophiles, and thermoacidophiles.

Menest (men′est) trademark for a preparation of esterified estrogens.

Ménétrier's disease (mān″a-tre-ārz′) [Pierre *Ménétrier*, French physician, 1859–1935] giant hypertrophic gastritis.

Menformon (men′for-mon) trademark for a preparation of estrone.

Menge's pessary (meng′gez) [Karl *Menge*, Heidelberg gynecologist, 1864–1945] see under *pessary.*

menhidrosis (men″hid-ro′sis) [Gr. *mēn* month + *hidrōs* sweat] a form of vicarious menstruation consisting of monthly discharge of sweat, sometimes bloody.

menidrosis (men″id-ro′sis) menhidrosis.

Meniere's disease (syndrome) (men″e-ārz′) [Prosper *Meniere*, French physician, 1799–1862. The spelling *Meniere* appears on his birth certificate, *Menière* and *Ménière* on his works. Ménière was the choice of his son] see under *disease.*

meningeal (mĕ-nin′je-al) of or pertaining to the meninges.

meningematoma (mĕ-nin″jem-ah-to′mah) hematoma of the dura mater.

meningeocortical (mĕ-nin″je-o-kor′tĭ-kal) of or pertaining to the meninges and cortex of the brain.

meningeoma (mĕ-nin″je-o′mah) meningioma.

meningeorrhaphy (mĕ-nin″je-or′ah-fe) [Gr. *mēninx* membrane + *rhaphē* suture] suture of the meninges.

meninges (mĕ-nin′jēz) [Gr., pl. of *mēninx* membrane] [NA] the three membranes that envelop the brain and spinal cord: the dura mater, pia mater, and arachnoid.

meninghematoma (mĕ-ninj″hem-ah-to′mah) meningematoma.

meningina (men″in-ji′nah) (*obs.*) pia-arachnoid.

meninginitis (men″in-jin-i′tis) inflammation of the meningina (pia-arachnoid); leptomeningitis.

meningioma (mĕ-nin″je-o′mah) [*meninges* + *-oma* tumor] a hard, slow-growing, usually vascular tumor which occurs mainly along the meningeal vessels and superior longitudinal sinus, invading the dura and skull and leading to erosion and thinning of the skull. **angioblastic m.,** angioblastoma.

meningiomatosis (mĕ-nin″je-o″mah-to′sis) a condition characterized by the formation of multiple meningiomas.

meningism (mĕ-nin′jizm) the symptoms and signs of meningeal irritation associated with acute febrile illness or dehydration without actual infection of the meninges. Called also *Dupré's disease* or *syndrome.*

meningismus (men″in-jis′mus) meningism.

meningitic (men″in-jit′ik) pertaining to or of the nature of meningitis.

meningitides (men″in-jit′ĭ-dēz) plural of *meningitis.*

meningitis (men″in-ji′tis), pl. *meningit′ides* [Gr. *mēninx* membrane + *-itis*] inflammation of the meninges. When it affects the dura mater, the disease is termed *pachymeningitis;* when the arachnoid and pia mater are involved, it is called *leptomeningitis,* or meningitis proper. **acute aseptic m.,** aseptic m. **aseptic m.,** the name given to a mild form of meningitis, most cases of which are caused by viruses; see *viral m.* **m. of the base, basilar m.,** that which affects the meninges at the base of the brain. **benign lymphocytic m.,** viral m. **m. carcinomato′sa,** a misnomer for the condition of widespread carcinomatous infiltration of the meninges; the condition is not inflammatory. **cerebral m.,** inflammation of the meninges of the brain. **cerebrospinal m.,** an inflammation of the membranes of the brain and spinal cord; it may be caused by many different organisms. Abbreviated C.S.M. **eosinophilic m.,** meningitis resulting from infection with *Angiostrongylus cantonensis,* characterized by an increase in lymphocytes and a high percentage of eosinophils in the cerebrospinal fluid; called also *eosinophilic meningoencephalitis.* **epidemic cerebrospinal m.,** an acute infectious disease attended by seropurulent inflammation of the membranes of the brain and spinal cord, and due to infection by the *Neisseria meningitidis.* The disease appears usually in epidemics, and the symptoms are those of acute cerebral and spinal meningitis, in addition to which there is usually an eruption of erythematous, herpetic, or hemorrhagic spots upon the skin. The fulminating or malignant form is known as *Waterhouse-Friderichsen syndrome.* Called also *cerebrospinal fever* and *meningococcal m.* **external m.,** pachymeningitis externa. **gummatous m.,** meningitis during the tertiary stage of syphilis in which there are many small gummata in the membranes. **internal m.,** pachymeningitis interna. **lymphocytic m.,** viral m. **meningococcal m.,** epidemic cerebrospinal m. **Mollaret's m.,** recurrent febrile attacks, malaise, headache, and meningeal signs accompanied by a marked polymorphonuclear inflammatory reaction in the cerebrospinal fluid. **mumps m.,** an aseptic meningitis secondary to mumps. **m. necrotox′ica reacti′va,** a condition marked by areas of focal cerebral softening with symptoms and signs of meningeal irritation suggesting primary inflammatory changes of the cerebral cortex. **occlusive m.,** leptomeningitis of children which leads to the closure of the lateral and median apertures of the fourth ventricle. **m. ossif′icans,** ossification of the cerebral meninges. **otitic m.,** a form that sometimes complicates an attack of otitis media. **parameningococcus m.,** meningitis caused by parameningococcus. **plague m.,** meningitis occurring as a rare complication of bubonic plague as a result of hematogenous spread of the infection from a bubo to involve the meninges, or less often as a primary infection without antecedent bubo formation. Called also *meningeal plague.* **posterior m.,** meningitis of the cerebellar region. **purulent m.,** that which is suppurative. **Quincke's m.,** acute aseptic meningitis. **septicemic m.,** that which is due to septic blood poisoning. **m. sero′sa,** serous m. **m. sero′sa circumscrip′ta,** meningitis giving rise to cystic accumulations of serous fluid which cause symptoms of tumors. **m. sero′sa circumscrip′ta cys′tica,** chronic meningitis with cyst formation. **serous m.,** meningitis with serous exudation into the ventricles and subarachnoid spaces and slight to moderate changes in the spinal fluid. **simple m.,** that in which there is an exudate of fibrin and serum. **spinal m.,** inflammation of the meninges of the spinal cord. **sterile m.,** meningitis in which there is no infection, e.g., that caused by injection of contrast medium to myelography. **m. sympath′ica,** a condition of the cerebrospinal fluid caused by inflammation in the neighborhood of the meninges. It is marked by increase in the pressure of the fluid and increase in its albumin and cellular content. The fluid is sterile and there may be symptoms of meningitis. **torula m., torular m.,** meningitis due to infection with *Cryptococcus neoformans (Torula histolytica).* **tubercular m., tuberculous m.,** a severe meningitis caused by *Mycobacterium tuberculosis.* **viral m.,** meningitis due to various viruses, such as the coxsackieviruses, mumps virus, and the virus of lymphocytic choriomeningitis, characterized by malaise, fever, headache, nausea, cerebrospinal fluid pleocytosis (principally lymphocytic), abdominal pain, stiffness of the neck and back, and a short uncomplicated course. Called also *aseptic m., acute aseptic m., benign lymphocytic m.,* and *lymphocytic m.*

mening(o)- [Gr. *mēninx,* gen. *mēningos* membrane] a combining form denoting relationship to a membrane, especially relationship to the meninges.

meningoarteritis (mĕ-ning″go-ar″ter-i′tis) inflammation of the meningeal arteries.

meningoblastoma (mĕ-ning″go-blas-to′mah) primary malignant melanoma of the meninges.

meningocele (mĕ-ning′go-sēl) [*meningo-* + Gr. *kēlē* hernia] hernial protrusion of the meninges through a defect in the skull (*cranial m.*) or vertebral column (*spinal m.*). **spurious m.,** Billroth's disease, def. 1.

meningocephalitis (mĕ-ning″go-sef″ah-li′tis) meningoencephalitis.

meningocerebritis (mĕ-ning″go-ser″ĕ-bri′tis) [*meningo-* + *cerebritis*] meningoencephalitis.

meningococcemia (mĕ-ning″go-kok-se′me-ah) invasion of the blood stream by meningococci. **acute fulminating m.,** Waterhouse-Friderichsen syndrome.

meningococci (mĕ-ning″go-kok′si) plural of *meningococcus.*

meningococcin (mĕ-ning″go-kok′sin) an antigenic material precipitated from saline suspensions of the meningococcus by means of alcohol. It is applied as a skin test (intradermal) in the detection of meningococcus carriers.

meningococcosis (mĕ-ning″go-kok-ko′sis) infection caused by meningococci.

meningococcus (mĕ-ning″go-kok′us), pl. *meningococ′ci* [*meningo-* + Gr. *kokkos* berry] an individual organism of the species *Neisseria meningitidis.*

meningocortical (mĕ-ning″go-kor′tĭ-kal) pertaining to or affecting the meninges and cortex of the brain.

meningocyte (mĕ-ning′go-sīt) a histiocyte of the meninges.

meningoencephalitis (mĕ-ning″go-en-sef″ah-li′tis) [*meningo-* + Gr. *enkephalos* brain + *-itis*] inflammation of the brain and meninges. Called also *encephalomeningitis.* **eosinophilic m.,** eosinophilic meningitis. **mumps m.,** a usually benign form seen in children, caused by the mumps virus, and characterized by fever, vomiting, nuchal rigidity, lethargy, parotitis, headache, convulsions, abdominal pain, diarrhea, and delirium. **primary amebic m.,** a rare and often fatal acute, febrile, purulent meningoencephalitis caused by usually free-living soil and water amebas of the genera *Naegleria, Acanthamoeba,* or *Hartmannella.* Infection caused by *Naegleria* is generally seen in young persons who swim or bathe in contaminated fresh water, the pathogens gaining access to the central nervous system by penetrating the nasal mucosa and cribriform plate and then following the olfactory bulbs and nerves to the brain and meninges. By contrast, *Acanthamoeba* and *Hartmanella* infections tend to be less fulminant and more benign, are more commonly seen in older presons and in immunocompromised persons, and are sometimes associated with spontaneous recovery; the mode of transmission of these infections is not known, but hematogenous spread from amebic infection at distant sites has been reported. **syphilitic m.,** general paresis.

meningoencephalocele (mě-ning″go-en-sef′ah-lo-sēl″) [*meningo-* + Gr. *enkephalos* brain + *kēlē* hernia] hernial protrusion of the meninges and brain substance through a defect in the skull. Called also *encephalomeningocele.*

meningoencephalomyelitis (mě-ning″go-en-sef″ah-lo-mi″ě-li′tis) [*meningo-* + Gr. *enkephalos* brain + *myelos* marrow + *-itis*] inflammation of the meninges, brain, and spinal cord.

meningoencephalomyelopathy (mě-ning″go-en- sef″ah-lo-mi″ě-lop′ah-the) disease involving the meninges, brain, and spinal cord.

meningoencephalopathy (mě-ning″go-en-sef″ah-lop′-ah-the) noninflammatory disease of the cerebral meninges and the brain. Called also *encephalomeningopathy.*

meningofibroblastoma (mě-ning″go-fi″bro-blas-to′mah) meningioma.

meningogenic (mě-ning″go-jen′ik) [*meningo-* + Gr. *gennan* to produce] arising in the meninges.

meningoma (men″in-go′mah) meningioma.

meningomalacia (mě-ning″go-mah-la′she-ah) [*meningo-* + Gr. *malakia* softness] softening of a membrane.

meningomyelitis (mě-ning″go-mi″ě-li′tis) [*meningo-* + Gr. *myelos* marrow + *-itis*] inflammation of the spinal cord and its membranes.

meningomyelocele (mě-ning″go-mi′ě-lo-sēl″) [*meningo-* + Gr. *myelos* marrow + *kēlē* hernia] hernial protrusion of a part of the meninges and substance of the spinal cord through a defect in the vertebral column.

meningomyeloencephalitis (mě-ning″o-mi″ě-lo-en-sef″ah-li′tis) inflammation of the meninges, spinal cord, and the brain.

meningomyeloradiculitis (mě-ning″go-mi″ě-lo-rah-dik″u-li′tis) inflammation of the meninges, spinal cord, and roots of the spinal nerves.

meningo-osteophlebitis (mě-ning″go-os″te-o-fle-bi′tis) [*meningo-* + Gr. *osteon* bone + *phleps* vein + *-itis*] periostitis with inflammation of the veins of a bone.

meningopathy (men″in-gop′ah-the) [*meningo-* + Gr. *pathos* disease] any disease of the meninges.

meningopneumonitis (mě-ning″go-nu-mo-ni′tis) a disease produced in experimental animals by the injection of the etiologic agent of psittacosis (*Chlamydia psittaci*), and marked by acute meningitis and pneumonitis.

meningorachidian (mě-ning″go-rah-kid′e-an) [*meningo-* + Gr. *rhachis* spine] pertaining to the spinal cord and its membranes.

meningoradicular (mě-ning″go-rah-dik′u-lar) [*meningo-* + L. *radix* root] pertaining to the meninges and the roots of the cranial and spinal nerves.

meningoradiculitis (mě-ning″go-rah-dik″u-li′tis) inflammation of the meninges and roots of the spinal nerves.

meningorecurrence (mě-ning″go-re-kur′ens) syphilitic meningitis induced in a syphilitic patient by antisyphilitic treatment.

meningorrhagia (mě-ning″go-ra′je-ah) [*meningo-* + Gr. *rhēgnynai* to break] hemorrhage from the cerebral or spinal membranes.

meningorrhea (mě-ning″go-re′ah) [*meningo-* + Gr. *rhoia* flow] effusion of blood between or upon the meninges.

meningosis (men″in-go′sis) the membranous attachment of bones to each other.

meningothelioma (mě-ning″go-the″le-o′mah) meningioma.

meningovascular (mě-ning″go-vas′ku-lar) pertaining to the blood vessels of the meninges.

meninguria (men″in-gu′re-ah) [*meningo-* + Gr. *ouron* urine + *-ia*] the occurrence of membranous shreds in the urine.

meninx (me′ninks), pl. *menin′ges* [Gr. *mēninx* membrane] a membrane; especially one of the three membranes enveloping the brain and spinal cord. **m. fibro′sa** (*obs.*), the dura mater. **m. sero′sa** (*obs.*), the arachnoidea. **m. ten′uis** (*obs.*), the pia-arachnoid. **m. vasculo′sa** (*obs.*), the pia mater.

meniscal (mě-nis′kal) of or pertaining to a meniscus.

meniscectomy (men″ĭ-sek′to-me) excision of an intra-articular meniscus, as in the knee joint.

menischesis (men″ĭ-ske′sis) menoschesis.

menisci (men-is′i) plural of *meniscus.*

meniscitis (men″ĭ-si′tis) inflammation of a meniscus of the knee joint.

meniscocyte (mě-nis′ko-sīt) [Gr. *mēniskos* crescent + *-cyte*] a sickle cell.

meniscocytosis (mě-nis″ko-si-to′sis) sickle cell anemia, see under *anemia.*

meniscosynovial (mě-nis″ko-sin-o′ve-al) pertaining to a meniscus and the synovial membrane.

Meniscus (me-nis′kus) [L.; Gr. *mēniskos* crescent] a genus of nonmotile, gram-negative, straight or curved, rod-shaped bacteria that form spiral and ring shapes during growth; they are found in anaerobic marine environments. The type species is *M. glauco′pis.*

meniscus (mě-nis′kus), pl. *menis′ci* [L.; Gr. *mēniskos,* crescent] 1. a crescent-shaped structure appearing at the surface of a liquid column, as in a pipet or buret, made concave or convex by the influence of capillarity. 2. [NA] a general term for a crescent-shaped structure of the body. Often used alone to designate one of the crescent-shaped disks of fibrocartilage attached to the superior articular surface of the tibia. **m. of acromioclavicular joint,** discus articularis articulationis acromioclavicularis. **articular m., m. articula′ris** [NA], a pad, commonly a wedge-shaped crescent of fibrocartilage or dense fibrous tissue, found in some synovial joints; one side forms a marginal attachment at the articular capsule and the other two sides extend into the joint, ending in a free edge. **converging m.,** a concavoconvex lens. **discoid m., discoid lateral m.,** a semilunar lateral meniscus of the knee that has been transformed into a thickened, irregular discoid mass as a result of excess motion of the meniscus, which in turn results from congenital absence of attachment of the posterior horn of the meniscus to the tibial plateau. The excess motion also causes a clicking sound on flexion and extension of the knee. Occasionally, a discoid medial meniscus is observed. Called also *congenital discoid meniscus.* **diverging m.,** a convexoconcave lens. **m. of inferior radioulnar joint,** discus articularis articulationis radioulnaris distalis. **joint m.,** articular m. **Kuhnt's m.,** the lining of the physiologic cup of the optic disk, composed of a thick accumulation of neuroglia. **lateral m. of knee joint, m. latera′lis articulatio′nis ge′nus** [NA], a crescent-shaped disk of fibrocartilage, but nearly circular in form, attached to the lateral margin of the superior articular surface of the tibia; called also *m. lateralis articulationis genu.* **medial m. of knee joint, m. media′lis articulatio′nis ge′nus** [NA], a crescent-shaped disk of fibrocartilage attached to the medial margin of the superior articular surface of the tibia; called also *m. medialis articulationis genu.* **negative m.,** a convexoconcave lens. **positive m.,** a concavoconvex lens. **m. of sternoclavicular joint,** discus articularis articulationis sternoclavicularis. **tactile menisci, menis′ci tac′tus** [NA], small, cup-shaped, tactile nerve endings within the skin, many of which are formed by branches of a single nerve fiber, and each of which is in contact with a single, modified epithelial cell; they are found in the deep epidermis, in hair follicles, and in the hard palate, and function as touch receptors. Called also *Grandy's corpuscles, Grandy-Merkel corpuscles, tactile disks, Merkel's cells, corpuscles,* or *disks,* and *Merkel's tactile cells.* **m. of temporomaxillary joint,** discus articularis articulationis temporomandibularis.

menispermine (men″ĭ-sper′min) a crystalline alkaloid,

$C_{18}H_{24}N_2O_2$, from *Anamirta cocculus* L. Wight & Arn. (Menispermaceae).

Menispermum (men″ĭ-sper′mum) [Gr. *mēnē* moon + *sperma* seed] a genus of plants. The rhizome and roots of *M. canadense* L. (Menispermaceae) (moonseed, or yellow parilla) are tonic and alterative. Because this vine, including the leaves and fruits, resemble a grapevine, children have ingested the fruits and been poisoned, sometimes fatally.

men(o)- [Gr. *mēn* month] a combining form denoting relationship to the menses.

menolipsis (men″o-lip′sis) temporary cessation of the menses.

menometrorrhagia (men″o-met″ro-ra′je-ah) excessive uterine bleeding occurring both during the menses and at irregular intervals.

menopausal (men″o-paw′zal) pertaining to or associated with the menopause.

menopause (men′o-pawz) [*meno-* + Gr. *pausis* cessation] cessation of menstruation in the human female, occurring usually around the age of 50. See also *climacteric*. **artificial m.,** cessation of menstruation produced by artificial means, such as surgical operation or irradiation. **m. prae′ cox,** premature failure of ovulation, possibly due to primary germ cell deficiency, acquired refractoriness to pituitary gonadotropin, or autoimmunization.

menoplania (men″o-pla′ne-ah) [*meno-* + Gr. *planē* deviation] metastasis or aberration of the menses; vicarious menstruation.

menorrhagia (men″o-ra′je-ah) [*meno-* + Gr. *rhēgnynai* to burst forth] excessive uterine bleeding occurring at the regular intervals of menstruation, the period of flow being of greater than usual duration.

menorrhalgia (men″o-ral′je-ah) [*menorrhea* + *-algia*] dysmenorrhea.

menorrhea (men″o-re′ah) [*meno-* + Gr. *rhoia* flow] 1. the normal discharge of the menses. 2. too free or profuse menstruation.

menorrheal (men″o-re′al) pertaining to menorrhea.

menoschesis (mĕ-nos′kĕ-sis, men″o-ske′sis) [*meno-* + Gr. *schesis* retention] retention of the menses.

menostasia, menostasis (men″o-sta′ze-ah; men″o-sta′sis, men-os′tah-sis) amenorrhea.

menostaxis (men″o-stak′sis) [*meno-* + Gr. *staxis* a dropping, dripping] excessively prolonged menstruation.

menotropins (men″o-tro′pins) [USP] an extract of human postmenopausal urine containing both follicle-stimulating hormone and luteinizing hormone. In females, it has the property of stimulating growth and maturation of ovarian follicles. In males, it has the properties of maintaining and stimulating testicular interstitial cells (Leydig tissue) related to testosterone production and of being responsible for full development and maturation of spermatozoa in the seminiferous tubules. Called also *human follicle-stimulating hormone* and *human menopausal gonadotropin*.

menses (men′sēz) [L., pl. of *mensis* month] the monthly flow of blood from the genital tract of women; see *menstruation*.

menstrual (men′stroo-al) [L. *menstrualis*] pertaining to the menses.

menstruant (men′stroo-ant) a person who is menstruating or is capable of menstruating.

menstruate (men′stroo-āt) [L. *menstruare*] to discharge blood from the genital tract at monthly intervals; see *menstruation*.

menstruation (men″stroo-a′shun) the cyclic, physiologic discharge through the vagina of blood and muscosal tissues from the nonpregnant uterus; it is under hormonal control and normally recurs, usually at approximately four-week intervals, in the absence of pregnancy during the reproductive period (puberty through menopause) of the female of the human and a few species of primates. It is the culmination of the menstrual cycle; see illustration accompanying *cycle*. **anovular m., anovulatory m.,** periodic uterine bleeding without preceding ovulation. **delayed m.,** menstruation the first appearance of which is delayed beyond the sixteenth year. **difficult m.,** dysmenorrhea. **infrequent m.,** menstruation occurring less frequently than normal. **nonovulational m.,** anovular m. **profuse m.,** menstruation marked by excessive flow. **regurgitant m.,** a

back flow through the uterine tubes by which epithelial cells and other materials may be discharged through the tubal ostia and deposited on the ovaries and adjacent organs, as in endometriosis. **retrograde m.,** regurgitant m. **scanty m.,** menstruation marked by abnormally slight flow. **supplementary m.,** menstrual discharge from the uterus and also from some other part. **suppressed m.,** failure of the menstrual flow to appear. **vicarious m.,** discharge of blood from an extragenital source at the time a menstrual period is normally expected; thought to result from generally increased capillary permeability related to the menstrual cycle.

menstruous (men′stroo-us) pertaining to menstruation.

menstruum (men′stroo-um) [L. *menstruus* menstruous: it was long believed that the menstrual fluid had a peculiar solvent quality] a solvent medium. **Pitkin m.,** a medium for the administration of heparin, consisting of a mixture of gelatin, dextrose, glacial acetic acid, and water.

mensual (men′su-al) [L. *mensis* month] monthly.

mensuration (men″su-ra′shun) [L. *mensuratio; mensura* measure] the act or process of measuring.

mentagrophyton (men″tah-grof′ĭ-ton) [L. *mentagra* sycosis + Gr. *phyton* plant] a former name for the fungus, *Trichophyton mentagrophytes,* the cause of sycosis barbae and other skin and nail infections.

mental (men′tal) 1. [L. *mens* mind] pertaining to the mind; psychic. 2. [L. *mentum* chin] pertaining to the chin.

mentalis (men-ta′lis) [L.] relating to the chin.

mentality (men-tal′ĭ-te) 1. mental power or capacity. 2. way of thought; mental set.

mentation (men-ta′shun) mental activity.

Mentha (men′thah) [L.] a genus of labiate plants, the mints. **M. canaden′sis,** wild mint. **M. cardia′ca,** Scotch spearmint; see *spearmint*. **M. piperi′ta,** peppermint. **M. pule′gium,** true, or European, pennyroyal. **M. spica′ta, M. vir′idis,** common spearmint.

menthol (men′thol) [USP] chemical name: 5-methyl-2-(1-methylethyl)cyclohexanol. An alcohol, $C_{10}H_{20}O$, obtained from diverse mint oils or prepared synthetically, occurring as colorless, hexagonal crystals, usually needle-like, or in fused masses, or crystalline powder; it may be levorotatory (*l*-menthol), from natural or synthetic sources, or racemic (*dl*-menthol). It is used as a topical antipruritic, and in inhalers for treatment of upper respiratory disorders or added to water for inhalation in acute bronchitis. Called also *peppermint camphor*.

menthyl (men′thil) the monovalent radical, $C_{10}H_{19}$.

menticide (men′tĭ-sīd) [L. *mens* mind + *caedere* to kill] brainwashing.

ment(o)- [L. *mentum* chin] a combining form denoting relationship to the chin. See also words beginning *geni(o)-*.

mentoanterior (men″to-an-te′re-or) [*mento-* + *anterior*] see under *position*.

mentolabial (men″to-la′be-al) [*mento-* + L. *labium* lip] pertaining to the chin and lip.

menton (men′ton) a cranial osteometric landmark, being the lowest point of the mandibular symphysis on the lateral jaw projection as seen on x-ray films.

mentoplasty (men′to-plas″te) [*mento-* + Gr. *plassein* to form] plastic surgery of the chin; surgical correction of deformities and defects of the chin.

mentoposterior (men″to-pos-te′re-or) [*mento-* + *posterior*] see under *position*.

mentotransverse (men″to-trans-vers′) [*mento-* + *transverse*] see under *position*.

mentum (men′tum) [L.] [NA] the chin.

Menyanthes (men″e-an′thēz) [perhaps from Gr. *mēn* month + *anthos* flower] a genus of gentianaceous plants. *M. trifolia′ta* L., or buckbean, is a bitter tonic and has febrifuge properties, and has been used as an emergency food, beer additive, and tea substitute.

meobentine sulfate (me″o-ben′tēn) chemical name: *N*-[(4-methoxyphenyl)methyl]-*N′,N″*-dimethylguanidine sulfate (2:1); an antiarrhythmic cardiac depressant, $(C_{11}H_{17}N_3O_2)\cdot H_2SO_4$.

Meonine (me′o-nīn) trademark for a preparation of racemethionine.

mepacrine hydrochloride (mep'ah-krin) quinacrine hydrochloride.

meparfynol (mĕ-par'fĭ-nōl) chemical name: 3-methyl-1-pentyn-3-ol. A sedative and hypnotic, $C_6H_{10}O$, administered orally. Called also *methylparafynol* and *methylpentynal*.

mepartricin (mĕ-par'trĭ-sin) an antifungal and antiprotozoal; it is a methyl ester of partricin (q.v.), used chiefly in the treatment of vaginal and cutaneous candidiasis, applied topically.

mepazine acetate (mep'ah-zēn) chemical name: 10-[(1-methyl-3-piperidinyl)methyl]-10H-phenothiazine acetate. A tranquilizer, $C_{19}H_{22}N_2S$, used mainly in the treatment of tension and anxiety states, but also used as a pre- or postoperative sedative; administered orally or intramuscularly.

mepenzolate bromide (mĕ-pen'zo-lāt) [USP] chemical name: 3-[(hydroxydiphenylacetyl)oxy]-1,1-dimethyl-piperidinium bromide. An oral anticholinergic, $C_{21}H_{26}Br$-NO_3, occurring as a white or light cream-colored powder; used mainly in disorders in which hypermotility of the colon is a feature.

meperidine hydrochloride (mĕ-per'ĭ-dēn) [USP] chemical name: 1-methyl-4-phenyl-4-piperidinecarboxylic acid ethyl ester. A synthetic narcotic analgesic, $C_{15}H_{21}NO_2 \cdot HCl$, occurring as a fine, white, crystalline powder, used as a preanesthetic medication, postoperative sedative, obstetric analgesic, and when a relatively short duration of analgesia is desired; administered orally in tablets or intramuscularly or subcutaneously. Abuse of this drug may lead to dependence. Called also *isonipecaine* and *pethidine hydrochloride*.

mephenamine (mĕ-fen'ah-mēn) orphenadrine.

mephenesin (mĕ-fen'ĕ-sin) chemical name: 3-(2-methyl-phenoxy)-1,2-propanediol. A skeletal muscle relaxant, C_{10}-$H_{14}O_3$, occurring as a white crystalline powder; administered orally.

mephenoxalone (mef''en-ok'sah-lōn) chemical name: 5-[(o-methoxyphenoxy)methyl]-2-oxazolidinone; a mild tranquilizer and skeletal muscle relaxant, $C_{11}H_{13}NO_4$.

mephentermine sulfate (mĕ-fen'ter-mēn) [NF] chemical name: N,α,α-trimethylbenzeneethanamine sulfate (2:1). An adrenergic, $(C_{11}H_{17}N)_2 \cdot H_2SO_4$, occurring as white crystals or as a crystalline powder; used for its vasopressor effects in the treatment of certain hypotensive states, administered orally, intramuscularly, and intravenously. It is also applied topically to the nasal mucosa as a decongestant.

mephenytoin (mĕ-fen'ĭ-to-in) [USP] chemical name: 5-ethyl-3-methyl-5-phenyl-2,4-imidazolidinedione. An anticonvulsant, $C_{12}H_{14}N_2O_2$, occurring as a white, crystalline powder; used for the control of grand mal, focal, jacksonian, and psychomotor epileptic seizures that are refractory to other drugs, administered orally.

mephitic (mĕ-fit'ik) [L. *mephiticus; mephitis* foul exhalation] emitting a foul odor.

mephitis (mĕ-fi'tis) [L.] a foul exhalation.

mephobarbital (mef''o-bar'bĭ-tal) [USP] chemical name: 5-ethyl-1-methyl-5-phenyl-2,4,6(1H,3H,5H)-pyrimidinetrione. A long-acting barbiturate, $C_{13}H_{14}N_2O_3$, occurring as a white, crystalline powder; used as a sedative in the treatment of anxiety, tension, and apprehension and as an anticonvulsant in grand mal and petit mal epilepsy, administered orally.

Mephyton (mef'ĭ-ton) trademark for preparations of phytonadione (vitamin K_1).

mepivacaine hydrochloride (mĕ-piv'ah-kān) [USP] chemical name: N-(2,6-dimethylphenyl)-1-methyl-2-piperidinecarboxamide monohydrochloride. An analogue of lidocaine, $C_{15}H_{22}N_2O \cdot HCl$, occurring as a white, crystalline solid; used to produce local anesthesia by infiltration injection, peripheral nerve block, and epidural block.

Meprane (me'prān) trademark for preparations of promethestrol dipropionate.

meprednisone (mĕ-pred'nĭ-sōn) [USP] chemical name: 17α,21-dihydroxy-16β-methyl-pregna-1,4-diene-3,11,20-trione. A synthetic glucocorticoid, $C_{22}H_{28}O_5$, occurring as a white to creamy white powder; used in the treatment of inflammatory, allergic, rheumatic, and other corticosteroid-responsive diseases, such as certain endocrine, respiratory, neoplastic, and collagen diseases, administered orally.

meprobamate (mĕ-pro'bah-māt, mep''ro-bam'āt) [USP]

chemical name: 2-methyl-2-propyl-1,3-propanediol. A carbamate derivative, $C_9H_{18}N_2O_4$, occurring as a white powder, having tranquilizing, muscle relaxant, and anticonvulsant actions. It is used as an oral sedative for the relief of anxiety and tension, as an adjunct in the treatment of conditions in which anxiety and tension are manifested, and to promote sleep in anxious tense patients; it is also used in musculoskeletal disorders and as an anticonvulsant in petit mal epilepsy. An intramuscular injection is used as adjunctive therapy in tetanus. **isopropyl m.,** carisoprodol.

Meprospan (mĕ-pro'span) trademark for a preparation of meprobamate.

Meprotabs (mĕ-pro'tabs) trademark for a preparation of meprobamate.

meprylcaine hydrochloride (mep'ril-kān) [USP] chemical name: 2-methyl-2-(propylamino)-1-propanol benzoate (ester) hydrochloride. A local anesthetic, $C_{14}H_{21}NO_2 \cdot HCl$, occurring as a white, crystalline powder; used for infiltration and nerve block anesthesia.

mepyramine maleate (me-pir'ah-mēn) pyrilamine maleate.

mepyrapone (mĕ-pi'rah-pōn) metyrapone.

mEq. milliequivalent.

meq. milliequivalent.

mequidox (mek'wi-doks) chemical name: 3-methyl-2-quinoxalinemethanol 1,4-dioxide; an antibacterial, $C_{10}H_{10}N_2O_3$.

MER the methanol extraction residue of BCG; used in cancer immunotherapy.

meralgia (me-ral'je-ah) [*mero-* (2) + *-algia*] pain in the thigh. **m. paresthet'ica,** a disease marked by paresthesia, pain, and numbness in the outer surface of the thigh, in the region supplied by the lateral femoral cutaneous nerve, due to entrapment of the nerve at the inguinal ligament. Called also *Bernhardt's disturbance of sensation.*

meralluride (mer-al'u-rīd) a mercurial diuretic; also used as *meralluride sodium.*

merbromin (mer-bro'min) chemical name: (2',7'-dibromo-3',6'-dihydroxy-3-oxospiro[isobenzofuran-1(3H),9'[9-H]xanthene]-4'-yl)hydroxomercury disodium salt; a topical antibacterial, $C_{20}H_8Br_2HgNa_2O_6$.

mercaptan (mer-kap'tan) [L. *mercurium captans* seizing or combining with mercury] any compound containing the —SH group bound to carbon.

mercaptide (mer-kap'tid) a compound derived from a mercaptan, with a metal replacing the sulfur hydrogen radical.

mercaptoethanol (mer-kap''to-eth'ah-nol) a reducing agent, $HS \cdot CH_2CH_2 \cdot OH$, that may attack disulfide bonds in proteins, reducing them to sulfhydryl groups, often destroying their physiological activity, e.g., they may inhibit mitosis.

mercaptol (mer-kap'tol) a compound formed from a ketone by introducing two thio-alkyl groups in place of the bivalent oxygen.

mercaptomerin (mer-kap''o-mer'in) a mercurial diuretic, used as *mercaptomerin sodium* [USP].

6-mercaptopurine (mer-kap''to-pūr'ēn) 6-MP; a purine analogue in which sulfur replaces the oxygen atom of purine and which can be incorporated into the nucleotide 6-thioIMP, an analogue of inosine monophosphate (IMP); 6-thioIMP inhibits de novo purine synthesis in two places, by serving as a pseudofeedback inhibitor of the first step in the pathway and also by inhibiting the conversion of IMP to adenine and guanine nucleotides; 6-MP is used as an antineoplastic almost exclusively for treatment of acute granulocytic leukemia, acute lymphocytic leukemia, and chronic granulocytic leukemia. Major side effects are bone marrow depression and occasional severe liver dysfunction. Available as *mercaptopurine* [USP].

mercapturic acid (mer-kap-tūr'ik) a cysteine conjugate of an aromatic compound formed initially as a glutathione conjugate in the liver and excreted in the urine.

Mercier's bar (valve) (mer-se-āz') [Louis Auguste *Mercier,* French urologist, 1811–1882] see *plica interureterica.*

mercocresols (mer''ko-kre'solz) a combination of cresol derivatives and an organic mercury, used for its germicidal, fungicidal, and bacteriostatic properties.

mercupurin (mer-ku'pu-rin) former name for mercurophylline.

mercuramide (mer-kūr'ah-mīd) mersalyl.

mercurammonium (mer-ku"rah-mo'ne-um) a precipitate produced when ammonium hydroxide is added to a solution of a mercuric salt. **m. chloride,** ammoniated mercury.

mercurial (mer-ku're-al) [L. *mercurialis*] 1. pertaining to mercury. 2. a preparation of mercury.

Mercurialis (mer-ku"re-a'lis) a genus of slender herbs of Europe. *M. an'nua* L. (Euphorbiaceae), French mercury, was formerly used as a diuretic and antisyphilitic.

mercurialism (mer-ku're-al-izm") mercury poisoning; see under *poisoning*.

mercurialization (mer-ku"re-al-i-za'shun) the act or process of putting under the influence of mercury.

mercurialized (mer-ku're-al-īzd) treated with mercury; containing mercury.

mercuric (mer-ku'ric) pertaining to mercury as a bivalent element. **m. benzoate,** a white, crystalline, tasteless salt, $(C_6H_5 \cdot CO \cdot O)_2Hg + H_2O$, formerly used in the treatment of syphilis. **m. chloride,** mercury bichloride. **m. cyanide,** a very poisonous salt, $Hg(CN)_2$, formerly used in the treatment of syphilis. **m. iodide, red,** mercury biniodide, HgI_2; formerly used as an antibacterial agent. **m. oxide, yellow,** a yellow to orange-yellow, heavy, impalpable powder, HgO, used as a local anti-infective in ophthalmology. Called also *Pagenstecher's ointment.* **m. oxycyanide,** a white crystalline powder, $Hg(CN)_2 \cdot HgO$, formerly used as an antiseptic and antisyphilitic. **m. salicylate,** a white, tasteless powder, $(OH \cdot C_6H_4 \cdot CO_2)_2Hg$, insoluble in water and alcohol, formerly used in the treatment of syphilis.

Mercurochrome (mer-ku'ro-krōm) trademark for preparations of merbromin.

mercurophylline (mer"ku-ro-fil'lin) a mixture of the sodium salt of 3-[[3-(hydroxymercuri)-2-methoxypropyl]-carbamoyl]-1,2,2- trimethyl($\pm$)cyclopentane carboxylic acid and theophylline in molecular proportions, used as a mercurial diuretic. Formerly called *mercupurin.*

mercurous (mer'ku-rus) pertaining to mercury as a monovalent element. **m. chloride,** calomel. **m. iodide, yellow,** a bright yellow insoluble amorphous powder, HgI; formerly used in the treatment of syphilis.

mercury (mer'ku-re) [L. *mercurius*, or *hydrargyrum*] a metallic element, liquid at ordinary temperatures; quicksilver. Its symbol is Hg; atomic number, 80; atomic weight, 200.59; specific gravity, 13.546. It is insoluble in ordinary solvents, being only partially soluble in boiling hydrochloric acid. It may be dissolved, however, in nitric acid. Mercury forms two sets of compounds—*mercurous,* in which a single atom of mercury combines with a monovalent radical, and *mercuric,* in which a single atom of mercury combines with a bivalent radical. Mercury and its salts have been employed therapeutically as purgatives; as alternatives in chronic inflammations; as antisyphilitics, intestinal antiseptics, disinfectants, and astringents. They are absorbed by the skin and mucous membranes, causing chronic mercury poisoning (see under *poisoning*). Because of toxicity, the use of mercurials is diminishing. The mercuric salts are more soluble and irritant than the mercurous. See also under *mercuric* and *mercurous.* **ammoniated m.** [USP], a topical anti-infective, $HgNH_2Cl$, occurring in white, pulverulent pieces or as a white amorphous powder. **m. bichloride,** an extremely poisonous compound, $HgCl_2$, occurring as odorless, heavy, colorless crystals, as crystalline masses, or as a white powder: formerly used in the treatment of syphilis and now as a disinfectant. Called also *mercuric chloride.* **m. with chalk,** metallic mercury rubbed up with chalk and honey until the particles are very small; used in pediculosis pubis. **m. chloride, mild,** calomel. **French m.,** *Mercurialis annua.* **m. oleate,** a mixture of yellow mercuric oxide and oleic acid: applied locally in parasitic skin diseases. **m. perchloride,** m. bichloride. **m. salicylate,** a basic salt, $Hg \cdot C_6H_3(OH) \cdot COOH$, containing 54 to 59 per cent of mercury; formerly used in syphilis.

Mercuzanthin (mer"ku-zan'thin) trademark for a preparation of mercurophylline.

-mere [Gr. *meros* part] a word termination denoting a segment or a part.

merethoxylline procaine (mer"ĕ-thok'sĭ-lēn) a combination of the organomercurial merethoxylline (dehydro-2-[N-(3'-hydroxymercuri-2'-methoxyethoxy)propylcarba-

mny]phenoxyacetic acid) with theophylline and procaine; used in the treatment of edema secondary to such conditions as congestive heart failure and nephrotic syndrome, administered intramuscularly and subcutaneously.

meridian (mĕ-rid'e-an) an imaginary line on the surface of a spherical body; see also *meridianus.* **m. of cornea,** an imaginary line marking the intersection with its surface of an anteroposterior plane passing through the apex of the cornea. **m's of eyeball,** meridiani bulbi oculi.

meridiani (mĕ-rid"e-a'ni) [L.] plural of *meridianus.*

meridianus (mĕ-rid"e-a'nus), pl. *meridia'ni* [L., from *medius* middle + *dies* day] an imaginary line on the surface of a spherical body, marking the intersection with the surface of a plane passing through its axis. Called also *meridian.* **meridia'ni bul'bi o'culi** [NA], meridians of eyeball: imaginary lines encircling the eyeball, marking the intersection with its surface of planes passing through its anteroposterior axis.

meridional (mĕ-rid'e-o-nal) pertaining to a meridian or made along a meridian; as, *meridional* section.

merisis (mer'ĭ-sis) growth in size due to cell division.

merism (mer'izm) [Gr. *meros* a part] the repetition of parts in an organism so as to form a regular pattern.

meristem (mer'ĭ-stem) [Gr. *merizein* to divide] the undifferentiated embryonic tissue of plants.

meristematic (mer"ĭ-stĕ-mat'ik) pertaining to or composed of meristem.

meristic (mer-is'tik) [Gr. *meristikos* fit for dividing] pertaining to or possessing merism; symmetrical; having symmetrically arranged parts.

meristoma (mer"ĭ-sto'mah) [*meristem* + *-oma*] a tumor of meristem.

Merkel's cells (corpuscles, disks, tactile cells) (mer'-kelz) [Friedrich Sigmund *Merkel,* German anatomist, 1845–1919] menisci tactus.

Merkel's filtrum, muscle (mer'kelz) [Karl Ludwig *Merkel,* German anatomist, 1812–1876] see *filtrum ventriculi* and *musculus ceratocricoideus.*

Merkel-Ranvier cells (mer'kel-rahn-ve-a') [F. S. *Merkel;* Louis Antoine *Ranvier,* French pathologist, 1835–1922] see *Merkel's cells,* under *cell.*

mermithid (mer'mĭ-thid) pertaining to or of the family Mermithidae.

Mermithidae (mer-mith'ĭ-de) a family of nematodes of the superfamily Mermithoidea; the cabbage snakes.

Mermithoidea (mer"mith-oi'de-ah) a superfamily of aphasmids including the cabbage snakes (family Mermithidae), the larvae of which may accidentally occur in the human digestive tract as contaminants of food or water.

mer(o)-[1] [Gr. *meros* part] a combining form meaning part.

mer(o)-[2] [Gr. *mēros* thigh] a combining form denoting relationship to the thigh.

meroacrania (mer"o-ah-kra'ne-ah) [*mero-* (1) + *a* neg. + Gr. *kranion* skull] congenital absence of part of the cranium.

meroblastic (mer"o-blas'tik) [*mero-* (1) + Gr. *blastos* germ] undergoing cleavage in which only part of the ovum participates; partially dividing.

merocoxalgia (me"ro-kok-sal'je-ah) [*mero-* (2) + L. *coxa* hip + *-algia*] pain in the thigh and hip.

merocrine (mer'o-krin) [*mero-* (1) + Gr. *krinein* to separate] partly secreting; denoting that type of glandular secretion in which the secreting cell remains intact throughout the process of formation and discharge of the secretory products; as in the salivary and pancreatic glands. Cf. *apocrine* and *holocrine.*

merocyst (mer'o-sist) [*mero-* (1) + *sist*] a large schizont seen in certain hemosporidian protozoa from which merozoites are released to invade the host's erythrocytes, where they develop into gametocytes.

merocyte (mer'o-sīt) [*mero-* (1) + *-cyte*] supernumerary sperm nucleus in the ovum in cases of polyspermy.

merodiastolic (mer"o-di-ah-stol'ik) [*mero-* (1) + *diastole*] pertaining to a part of the diastole.

merogamy (mĕ-rog'ah-me) microgamy.

merogastrula (mer"o-gas'troo-lah) the gastrula of a meroblastic ovum.

merogenesis (mer″o-jen′ĕ-sis) [*mero*- (1) + Gr. *genesis* production] cleavage of an ovum.

merogenetic (mer″o-jĕ-net′ik) pertaining to merogenesis.

merogenic (mer″o-jen′ik) pertaining to or producing segmentation.

merogonic (mer″o-gon′ik) pertaining to or resulting from merogony.

merogony (mĕ-rog′o-ne) [*mero*-(1) + Gr. *gonos* procreation] 1. the development of a portion only of an ovum; see *andromerogony* and *gynomerogony*. 2. schizogony resulting in the production of merozoites. **diploid m.,** development of a portion of an ovum containing the fused male and female pronuclei. **parthenogenetic m.,** development, as a result of artificial stimulation, of a part of an ovum containing the nucleus.

meromelia (mer″o-me′le-ah) [*mero*-(1) + Gr. *melos* limb + -*ia*] a general term denoting congenital absence of any part of a limb (as in adactyly, hemimelia, and phocomelia), as opposed to amelia, or absence of the entire limb.

meromicrosomia (mer″o-mi″kro-so′me-ah) [*mero*- (1) + *microsomia*] unusual smallness of some part of the body.

meromorphosis (mer″o-mor-fo′sis) [*mero*- (1) + Gr. *morphōsis* a shaping, bringing into shape] incomplete restoration or regeneration of a lost part.

meromyarial, meromyarian (mer″o-mi-a′re-al; mer″o-mi-a′re-an) [*mero*-(1) + Gr. *mys* muscle] designating a type of nematode musculature in which there are only a few muscle cells in a given area, the cells being platymyarial in type.

meromyosin (mer″o-mi′o-sin) a fragment of the myosin molecule isolated by treatment with proteolytic enzymes; there are two types, heavy (H-meromyosin) and light (L-meromyosin). *L-Meromyosin* makes up the major part of the rodlike backbone of the molecule; *H-meromyosin* contains the subfragment responsible for the ATP-ase activity of myosin.

meronecrobiosis (me″ro-nek″ro-bi-o′sis) meronecrosis.

meronecrosis (me″ro-nĕ-kro′sis) [*mero*-(1) + *necrosis*] cellular necrosis.

meront (mer′ont) [*mero*(1)- + *ontos* being] the asexual stage in the development of certain protozoa, especially nonsporozoa, that gives rise to merozoites. See also *schizont* and *segmenter*.

meropia (mĕ-ro′pe-ah) [*mero*-(1) + -*opia*] partial blindness.

merorachischisis (me″ro-rah-kis′kĭ-sis) [*mero*-(1) + Gr. *rhachis* spine + *schisis* fissure] fissure of a part of the spinal cord.

merosmia (mĕ-ros′me-ah) [*mero*-(1) + Gr. *osmē* smell + -*ia*] a disorder of the sense of smell in which certain odors are not perceived.

merostotic (mer″os-tot′ik) [*mero*-(1) + L. *os* bone] pertaining to or affecting only a part of a bone.

merotomy (mĕ-rot′o-me) [*mero*-(1) + Gr. *temnein* to cut] dissection into segments, especially the dissection of a cell.

merozoite (mer″o-zo′ĭt) [*mero*-(1) + Gr. *zōon* animal] a stage in the life cycle of certain sporozoan protozoa resulting from merogony. Called also *schizozoite*.

merozygote (mer″o-zi′gōt) [*mero*-(1) + Gr. *zygotos* yolked together] the partially diploid bacterial zygote that results from the transfer of a portion of the genetic information of a donor cell to the total genetic information of the recipient. See also *heterogenote* and *homogenote*.

Merphenyl (mer′fen-il) trademark for preparations of phenylmercuric compounds.

mersalyl (mer′sah-lil) chemical name: [3-[[2-(carboxymethoxy) benzoyl] amino] - 2 - methoxypropyl] hydroxymercury monosodium salt. A mercurial diuretic, $C_{13}H_{16}HgNNaO_6$, used in combination with theophylline in the treatment of edema secondary to such conditions as cardiorenal diseases, nephrosis, and hepatic cirrhosis, administered intramuscularly and intravenously.

Merseburg triad (mār′zeh-boorg) [*Merseburg*, a town in Germany] see under *triad*.

Merthiolate (mer-thi′o-lāt) trademark for preparations of thimerosal.

Merulius (mĕ-roo′le-us) a genus of fungi of the class Basidiomycetes, order Polyporales. *M. lac′rymans* is the cause of "dry rot" of wood.

merycism (mer′ĭ-sizm) [Gr. *mērykismos* chewing the cud] rumination.

merycismus (mer″ĭ-siz′mus) merycism.

Merzbacher-Pelizaeus disease (merz′bak-er-pa″le-zi′us) [Ludwig *Merzbacher*, German physician in Buenos Aires, born 1875; Friedrich *Pelizaeus*, German neurologist, 1850–1917] familial centrolobar sclerosis.

mesad (me′sad) toward the median line or plane; mesiad.

mesal (me′sal) [Gr. *mesos* middle] mesial.

mesangial (mes-an′je-al) of or pertaining to the mesangium.

mesangiocapillary (mes-an″je-o-kap″ĭ-lar″e) pertaining to or affecting the mesangium and the associated capillaries.

mesangium (mes-an′je-um) the thin membrane which helps to support the capillary loops in a renal glomerulus.

Mesantoin (mĕ-san′to-in) trademark for a preparation of mephenytoin.

mesaortitis (mes″a-or-ti′tis) [*meso*- + *aortitis*] (*obs.*) inflammation of the middle coat of the aorta.

mesaraic (mes″ah-ra′ik) [*meso*- + Gr. *mesaraion* the mesentery] mesenteric.

mesarteritis (mes″ar-ter-i′tis) [*meso*- + Gr. *artēria* artery + -*itis*] inflammation of the middle coat of an artery. **Mönckeberg's m.,** see under *arteriosclerosis*.

mesaticephalic (mes-at″ĭ-se-fal′ik) [Gr. *mesatos* medium + *kephalē* head] mesocephalic.

mesatikerkic (mes-at″ĭ-ker′kik) [Gr. *mesatos* medium + *kerkis* the radius of the arm] having a radiohumeral index of 75–80.

mesatipellic (mes-at″ĭ-pel′ik) [Gr. *mesatos* medium + *pella* bowl] having a transverse diameter of the pelvic inlet almost the same as that of the true conjugated diameter.

mesatipelvic (mes-at″ĭ-pel′vik) mesatipellic.

mesaxon (mes-ak′son) a pair of parallel membranes marking the line of edge-to-edge contact of the sheath cell (Schwann cell) encircling the axon.

mescal (mes-kahl′) [Mex.]. 1. *Lophophora williamsii* (Lemaire) Coult. (Cactaceae). 2. a liquor distilled from pulque, a fermented drink obtained from the juice of species of *Agave* in Mexico and Central America.

mescaline (mes′kah-lin) a poisonous alkaloid, 3,4,5-trimethoxyphenylethylamine, $(CH_3 \cdot O)_3 \, C_6H_2 \cdot CH_2 \cdot CH_2 \cdot NH_2$, in the form of a colorless alkaline oil from the flowering heads (mescal buttons) of *Lophophora williamsii* (Lemaire) Coult. (Cactaceae). It produces an intoxication with delusions of color and music.

mescalism (mes′kah-lizm) intoxication caused by mescal buttons or mescaline.

mesectic (mes-ek′tik) [*mes*- + Gr. *echein* to hold] (*obs.*) taking up (by the blood) a normal amount of oxygen at a given Po_2, i.e., having a normal dissociation curve.

meseclazone (mĕ-sek′lah-zōn) chemical name: 7-chloro-3,3a-dihydro-2-methyl-2*H*,9*H*-isoxazolo[3,2-*b*][1,3]benzoxacine-9-one; an anti-inflammatory, $C_{11}H_{10}ClNO_3$.

mesectoblast (mes-ek′to-blast) ectomesoblast.

mesectoderm (mĕ-sek′to-derm) embryonic migratory cells, derived from the neural crest of the head, that contribute to the formation of the meninges and become pigment cells.

mesencephal (mes-en′sĕ-fal) mesencephalon.

mesencephalic (mes-en″sĕ-fal′ik) pertaining to the mesencephalon.

mesencephalitis (mes″en-sef″ah-li′tis) inflammation of the mesencephalon.

mesencephalohypophyseal (mes″en-sef″ah-lo-hi-po-fiz′-e-al) pertaining to the mesencephalon and the pituitary gland (hypophysis).

mesencephalon (mes″en-sef″ah-lon) [*meso*- + Gr. *enkephalos* brain] 1. [NA] the part of the brain developed from the middle of the three primary vesicles of the embryonic neural tube; it comprises the tectum and the cerebral peduncles; see Plate accompanying *brain*. See also *brain stem*, under *B*. 2. the middle of the three primary brain vesicles in the embryo, lying between the prosencephalon and the rhombencephalon. Called also *midbrain.*

mesencephalotomy (mes"en-sef"ah-lot'o-me) [*mesencephalon* + Gr. *tomē* a cutting] surgical production of lesions in the midbrain, especially in the pain-conducting pathways for the relief of intractable pain.

mesenchyma (mĕ-seng'kĭ-mah) [*meso-* + Gr. *enchyma* infusion] the meshwork of embryonic connective tissue in the mesoderm from which are formed the connective tissues of the body, and also the blood vessels and lymphatic vessels.

mesenchymal (mĕ-seng'kĭ-mal) pertaining to the mesenchyma.

mesenchyme (mes'eng-kīm) mesenchyma.

mesenchymoma (mes"en-ki-mo'mah) a mixed mesenchymal tumor composed of two or more cellular elements not commonly associated, not counting fibrous tissue as one of the elements. **benign m.,** a benign tumor composed of two or more clearly recognizable mesenchymal elements in addition to fibrous tissue. **malignant m.,** a sarcoma composed of two or more cellular elements (excluding fibrous tissue); a mixed cell sarcoma.

mesenterectomy (mes"en-tĕ-rek'to-me) [*mesentery* + Gr. *ektomē* excision] resection of mesentery.

mesenteric (mes"en-ter'ik) [Gr. *mesenterikos*] pertaining to the mesentery.

mesenteriolum (mĕ-sen"ter-i'o-lum) a small mesentery. **m. appen'dicis vermifor'mis, m. proces'sus vermifor'mis,** mesoappendix.

mesenteriopexy (mes"en-ter'e-o-pek"se) [*mesentery* + Gr. *pēxis* fixation] fixation or suspension of the mesentery.

mesenteriorrhaphy (mes"en-ter"e-or'ah-fe) [*mesentery* + Gr. *rhaphē* suture] suture or repair of the mesentery.

mesenteriplication (mes"en-ter"e-pli-ka'shun) [*mesentery* + L. *plicare* to fold] shortening the mesentery by plication.

mesenteritis (mes"en-tĕ-ri'tis) inflammation of the mesentery. **retractile m.,** inflammation of the mesentery producing thickening, sclerosis, and retraction, and occasionally resulting in distortion of intestinal loops.

mesenterium (mes"en-te're-um) [NA] the mesentery: the peritoneal fold attaching the small intestine to the posterior abdominal wall. **m. commu'ne, m. dorsa'le commu'ne** [NA], dorsal common mesentery: the primitive embryonic mesentery, a double-layered median partition formed by association of the splanchnic mesoderm with the entoderm, extending from the roof of the coelom toward the midventral wall, and dividing the coelom into halves; it contains the primitive gut, and encloses the heart, lungs, and liver as they develop.

mesenteron (mes-en'ter-on) [*meso-* + Gr. *enteron* intestine] the midgut.

mesentery (mes'en-ter"e) a membranous fold attaching various organs to the body wall. Commonly used with specific reference to the peritoneal fold attaching the small intestine to the dorsal body wall. Called also *mesenterium* [NA]. **m. of ascending part of colon,** mesocolon ascendens. **caval m.,** a ridge, at the right of the embryonic mesogastrium, in which develops a hepatic segment of the inferior vena cava. **common m., common m., dorsal,** mesenterium dorsale commune. **m. of descending part of colon,** mesocolon descendens. **dorsal m.,** mesenterium dorsale commune. **primitive m.,** mesenterium dorsale commune. **m. of rectum,** mesorectum. **m. of sigmoid colon,** mesocolon sigmoideum. **m. of transverse part of colon,** mesocolon transversum. **ventral m.,** the embryonic mesentery attaching the duodenal region of the early intestine to the ventral body wall. **m. of vermiform appendix,** mesoappendix.

mesentoderm (mĕ-sen'to-derm) the inner layer of an amphibian gastrula not yet separated into mesoderm and entoderm.

mesentomere (mes-en'to-mēr) a blastomere not yet divided into mesomeres and entomeres.

mesentorrhaphy (mes"en-tor'ah-fe) [*mesentery* + Gr. *rhaphē* suture] mesenteriorrhaphy.

mesepithelium (mes"ep-ĭ-the'le-um) mesothelium.

MeSH (mesh) *Me*dical *S*ubject *H*eadings, a thesaurus published by the National Library of Medicine for use in MEDLARS.

mesiad (me'ze-ad) toward the middle; mesad.

mesial (me'ze-al) nearer the center line of the dental arch.

mesially (me'ze-al"e) toward the median line.

mesien (me'ze-en) pertaining to the mesion.

mesi(o)- [Gr. *mesos* in the middle] in dentistry, a combining form denoting relationship to the middle; specifically, the mesial surface of a tooth or the mesial wall of a tooth cavity.

mesiobuccal (me"ze-o-buk'al) pertaining to or formed by the mesial and buccal surfaces of a tooth, or the mesial and buccal walls of a tooth cavity preparation.

mesiobucco-occlusal (me"ze-o-buk"o-ŏ-kloo'zal) pertaining to or formed by the mesial, buccal, and occlusal surfaces of a tooth.

mesiobuccopulpal (me"ze-o-buk"o-pul'pal) pertaining to or formed by the mesial, buccal, and pulpal walls of a tooth cavity.

mesiocervical (me"ze-o-ser'vĭ-kal) 1. pertaining to the mesial surface of the neck of a tooth. 2. mesiogingival.

mesioclination (me"ze-o-kli-na'shun) deviation of a tooth from the vertical, in the direction of the tooth next mesial (anterior) to it in the dental arch.

mesioclusion (me"se-o-kloo'zhun) malocclusion in which the mandibular arch is in an anterior position in relation to the maxillary arch (prognathism). Generally considered as identical with Class III in Angle's classification of malocclusion (see *malocclusion*). Called also *anterior occlusion, anteroclusion,* and *protrusive occlusion.*

mesiodens (me"ze-o-denz), pl. *mesioden'tes* [*mesio-* + Gr. *dens* tooth] the most common supernumerary tooth, appearing singly or in pairs as a small tooth with a cone-shaped crown and a short root between the maxillary central incisors; it may be erupted, impacted, or even inverted.

mesiodentes (me"ze-o-den'tēz) plural of *mesiodens.*

mesiodistal (me"ze-o-dis'tal) pertaining to the mesial and distal surfaces of a tooth.

mesiogingival (me"ze-o-jin'jĭ-val) pertaining to or formed by the mesial and gingival walls of a tooth cavity.

mesioincisodistal (me"ze-o-in-si"zo-dis'tal) pertaining to the mesial, incisal, and distal surfaces of an anterior tooth.

mesiolabial (me"ze-o-la'be-al) pertaining to or formed by the mesial and labial surfaces of a tooth, or the mesial and labial walls of a tooth cavity preparation.

mesiolabioincisal (me"ze-o-la"be-o-in-si'zal) pertaining to or formed by the mesial, labial, and incisal surfaces of a tooth.

mesiolingual (me"ze-o-ling'gwal) pertaining to or formed by the mesial and lingual surfaces of a tooth, or the mesial and lingual walls of a tooth cavity preparation.

mesiolinguoincisal (me"ze-o-ling"gwo-in-si'zal) pertaining to or formed by the mesial, lingual, and incisal surfaces of a tooth.

mesiolinguo-occlusal (me"ze-o-ling"gwo-ŏ-kloo'zal) pertaining to or formed by the mesial, lingual, and occlusal surfaces of a tooth.

mesiolinguopulpal (me"ze-o-ling"gwo-pul'pal) pertaining to or formed by the mesial, lingual, and pulpal walls of a tooth cavity preparation.

mesion (me'se-on) [Gr. *mesos* middle] the plane that divides the body into right and left symmetric halves.

mesio-occlusal (me"ze-o-ŏ-kloo'zal) pertaining to or formed by the mesial and occlusal surfaces of a tooth, or the mesial and occlusal walls of a tooth cavity.

mesio-occlusion (me"ze-o-ŏ-kloo'zhun) mesioclusion.

mesio-occlusodistal (me"ze-o-ŏ-kloo"so-dis'tal) pertaining to the mesial, occlusal, and distal surfaces of a posterior tooth.

mesiopulpal (me"ze-o-pul'pal) pertaining to or formed by the mesial and pulpal walls of a tooth cavity preparation.

mesiopulpolabial (me"ze-o-pul"po-la'be-al) pertaining to or formed by the mesial, pulpal, and labial walls of a tooth cavity preparation.

mesiopulpolingual (me"ze-o-pul"po-ling'gwal) pertaining to or formed by the mesial, pulpal, and lingual walls of a tooth cavity preparation.

mesioversion (me"ze-o-ver'zhun) deviation of a tooth from the vertical, in the direction of the tooth next mesial (anterior) to it in the dental arch.

mesitylene (mes-it′ĭ-lēn)   symmetric trimethylbenzene, C_6-$H_3(CH_3)_3$, from coal tar.

Mesmer (mes′mer), Franz (Friedrich) Anton. An Austrian (1734–1815), who first demonstrated hypnotism in Vienna in about 1775. See *animal magnetism*, under *magnetism*, and see *mesmerism*.

mesmerism (mes′mer-izm) [after Franz A. *Mesmer*, 1734 –1815] 1. the use of animal magnetism and hypnotism as practiced by Mesmer. 2. hypnotism.

mes(o)- [Gr. *mesos* middle] 1. a prefix meaning in the middle, intermediate, or moderate. 2. (always in the form meso-) in chemistry, a prefix signifying inactive or without effect on polarized light even though the molecule has asymmetric carbon atoms, because two halves are mirror images.

meso-aortitis (mes′o-a″or-ti′tis) inflammation of the middle coat of the aorta. **m. syphilit′ica,** inflammation of the middle coat of the aorta due to syphilis.

mesoappendicitis (mes″o-ah-pen″dĭ-si′tis) inflammation of the mesoappendix.

mesoappendix (mes″o-ah-pen′diks) [*meso-* + *appendix*] [NA] the peritoneal fold attaching the appendix to the mesentery of the ileum; called also *mesenteriolum processus vermiformis*.

mesoarial (mes″o-a′re-al) pertaining to the mesovarium.

mesoarium (mes″o-a′re-um) mesovarium.

mesobilin (mes″o-bi′lin) a compound, $C_{33}H_{42}O_6N_4$, occurring in the urine as a derivative of bilirubin via enterohepatic circulation.

mesobilirubin (mes″o-bil″ĭ-roo′bin) a compound, $C_{33}H_{44}$-O_6N_4, formed by the reduction of bilirubin.

mesobilirubinogen (mes″o-bil″ĭ-roo-bin′o-jen) a reduced form of bilirubin, formed in the intestine, which on oxidation forms stercobilin.

mesobiliviolin (mes″o-bil″ĭ-vi′o-lin) an oxidation product of mesobilirubinogen and of stercobilinogen.

mesoblast (mes′o-blast) [*meso-* + Gr. *blastos* germ] mesoderm, especially in the early stages.

mesoblastema (mes″o-blas-te′mah) the cells composing the mesoblast.

mesoblastic (mes″o-blas′tik) pertaining to or derived from the mesoblast.

mesobronchitis (mes″o-brong-ki′tis) [*meso-* + *bronchitis*] inflammation of the middle coat of the bronchi.

mesocardia (mes″o-kar′de-ah) [*meso-* + Gr. *kardia* heart] atypical location of the heart with the apex in the middle line of the thorax.

mesocardium (mes″o-kar′de-um) [*meso-* + Gr. *kardia* heart] that part of the embryonic mesentery which connects the embryonic heart with the body wall in front and the foregut behind. **arterial m.,** that part of the pericardium which encloses the aorta and pulmonary artery. **dorsal m.,** the temporary dorsal mesentery of the heart in the embryo; its site is represented by the transverse sinus of the pericardium. **lateral m.,** pulmonary ridge. **venous m.,** that part of the pericardium which encloses the venae cavae and pulmonary veins. **ventral m.,** a mesentery attaching the heart to the ventral body wall; it is scarcely represented in human development.

mesocarpal (mes″o-kar′pal) midcarpal.

mesocecal (mes″o-se′kal) pertaining to the mesocecum.

mesocecum (mes″o-se′kum) [*meso-* + *cecum*] the occasionally occurring mesentery of the cecum.

mesocephalic (mes″o-sĕ-fal′ik) [*meso-* + Gr. *kephalē* head] 1. pertaining to the mesocephalon. 2. characterized by or pertaining to a skull having an average breadth-length index, with a cephalic index of 75.0 to 79.9.

mesocephalon (mes″o-sef′ah-lon) mesencephalon.

Mesocestoides (mes″o-ses-toi′dēz) a genus of tapeworms of the family Mesocestoididae, whose larvae are often found in the coelom or peritoneum of dogs, cats, mice, snakes, and other vertebrates; the adult form is found in the intestines of carnivorous animals, including man, dogs, cats, racoons, and meat-eating birds.

Mesocestoididae (mes″o-ses-toi′dĭ-de) a family of medium-sized to large tapeworms of the order Cyclophyllidea, subclass Cestoda, which parasitize carnivorous birds and mammals. *Mesocestoides* is the type genus.

mesochondrium (mes″o-kon′dre-um) [*meso-* + Gr. *chondros* cartilage] the matrix in which are embedded the cellular elements of hyaline cartilage.

mesochoroidea (mes″o-ko-roi′de-ah) the middle coat of the choroid.

mesococci (mes″o-kok′si) plural of *mesococcus*.

mesocoelia (mes″o-se′le-ah) (*obs.*) aqueductus cerebri.

mesocolic (mes″o-kol′ik) pertaining to the mesocolon.

mesocolon (mes″o-ko′lon) [*meso-* + Gr. *kolon* colon] [NA] the process of the peritoneum by which the colon is attached to the posterior abdominal wall. It is divided into ascending, transverse, descending, and sigmoid or pelvic portions, according to the segment of the colon to which it gives attachment. **m. ascen′dens** [NA], **ascending m.,** the peritoneum attaching the ascending colon to the posterior abdominal wall, usually obliterated when the ascending colon becomes retroperitoneal. **m. descen′dens** [NA], **descending m.,** the peritoneum attaching the descending colon to the posterior abdominal wall; it is usually absent because the descending colon is ordinarily retroperitoneal. **iliac m.,** m. sigmoideum. **left m.,** m. descendens. **pelvic m.,** m. sigmoideum. **right m.,** m. ascendens. **sigmoid m., m. sigmoi′deum** [NA], the peritoneum attaching the sigmoid colon to the posterior abdominal wall; called also *pelvic m.* **transverse m., m. transver′sum** [NA], the peritoneum attaching the transverse colon to the posterior abdominal wall.

mesocolopexy (mes″o-ko′lo-pek″se) [*mesocolon* + Gr. *pēxis* fixation] suspension or fixation of the mesocolon.

mesocoloplication (mes″o-ko″lo-pli-ka′shun) [*mesocolon* + *plication*] plication of the mesocolon to limit its mobility.

mesocord (mes′o-kord) an umbilical cord adherent to the placenta by a connecting fold of the amnion; more correctly, the connecting fold itself.

mesocornea (mes″o-kor′ne-ah) substantia propria corneae.

mesocranic (mes″o-kra′nik) having a cranial index between 75.0 and 79.9.

mesocuneiform (mes″o-ku′ne-ĭ-form) os cuneiforme intermedius.

mesocyst (mes′o-sist) [*meso-* + Gr. *kystis* bladder] the layer of peritoneum attaching the gallbladder to the liver.

mesocytoma (mes″o-si-to′mah) [*mesocyte* + *-oma*] a connective tissue tumor.

mesoderm (mes′o-derm) [*meso-* + Gr. *derma* skin] the middle layer of the three primary germ layers of the embryo, lying between the ectoderm and the entoderm. From it are derived the connective tissue, bone and cartilage, muscle, blood and blood vessels, lymphatics and lymphoid organs, notochord, pleura, pericardium, peritoneum, kidney, and gonads. Cf. *ectoderm* and *entoderm*. **extraembryonic m.,** that located outside the embryo and belonging to fetal accessory organs. **gastral m.,** that infolded with the entoderm during gastrulation. **head m.,** loose mesoderm, cranial to the somites. **lateral m.,** the lateral sheets of mesoderm within which the embryonic coelom arises. **paraxial m.,** that lying alongside the notochord and neural tube. **peristomal m.,** that derived from the ventral lip of the blastopore or from the primitive streak. **somatic m.,** the outer of the two layers into which the embryonic mesoderm divides; associated with ectoderm to constitute the somatopleure. **splanchnic m.,** the inner of the two layers into which the embryonic mesoderm divides; associated with entoderm to constitute splanchnopleure.

mesodermal (mes″o-der′mal) pertaining to or derived from the mesoderm.

mesodermic (mes″o-der′mik) pertaining to the mesoderm.

mesodermopath (mes″o-der′mo-path) [*mesoderm* + Gr. *pathos* disease] (*obs.*) a person who is constitutionally susceptible to diseases of the tissues derived from embryonic mesoderm, such as heart and kidneys, arteries and veins, joints and muscles.

mesodiastolic (mes″o-di″ah-stol′ik) [*meso-* + *diastole*] pertaining to the middle of the diastole.

mesodont (mes′o-dont) [*meso-* + Gr. *odous* tooth] having a dental index between 42 and 44.

mesodontic (mes″o-don′tik) having medium sized teeth.

mesodontism (mes″o-don′tizm) the state of having medium sized teeth, or a dental index between 42 and 44.

mesoduodenal (mes″o-du″o-de′nal) pertaining to the mesoduodenum.

mesoduodenum (mes″o-du″o-de′num) [meso- + duodenum] the mesenteric fold which in early fetal life encloses the duodenum.

mesoepididymis (mes″o-ep″ĭ-did′ĭ-mis) a fold of tunica vaginalis that sometimes connects the epididymis with the testicle.

mesoesophagus (mes″o-ĕ-sof′ah-gus) the portion of the primitive mesentery which encloses the developing esophagus.

mesogaster (mes″o-gas′ter) [meso- + Gr. gastēr belly] mesogastrium.

mesogastric (mes″o-gas′trik) pertaining to the mesogastrium.

mesogastrium (mes″o-gas′tre-um) [meso- + Gr. gastēr belly] [NA] the portion of the primitive mesentery which encloses the stomach, and from which the greater omentum is developed.

mesoglea (mes″o-gle′ah) [meso- + Gr. gloia glue] the layer between the epidermis and gastrodermis of coelenterates.

mesoglia (mĕ-sog′le-ah) 1. microglia. 2. oligodendroglia.

mesoglioma (mes″o-gli-o′mah) a tumor of the mesoglia; a microglioma or oligodendroglioma.

mesogluteal (mes″o-gloo′te-al) pertaining to the gluteus medius muscle.

mesogluteus (mes″o-gloo′te-us) musculus gluteus medius.

mesognathic (mes″og-na′thik) mesognathous.

mesognathous (mĕ-sog′nah-thus) [meso- + Gr. gnathos jaw] pertaining to or characterized by moderate protrusion of the jaw, with a gnathic index of 98 to 103. Called also mesognathic.

Mesogonimus (mes″o-gon′ĭ-mus) a former name for a genus of flukes, certain species of which are now included in the genera Paragonimus and Heterophyes. **M. heteroph′yes,** Heterophyes heterophyes.

mesohyloma (mes″o-hi-lo′mah) [meso- + Gr. hylē matter + -oma] mesothelioma.

mesohypoblast (mes″o-hi′po-blast) mesentoderm.

mesoileum (mes″o-il′e-um) the mesentery of the ileum.

meso-inositol (mes″o-in-o′sĭ-tol) inositol, def. 2.

mesojejunum (mes″o-je-ju′num) the mesentery of the jejunum.

mesolecithal (mes″o-les′ĭ-thal) [meso- + Gr. lekithos yolk] possessing a moderate amount of yolk.

mesology (mĕ-sol′o-je) ecology.

mesomelic (mes″o-mel′ik) [meso- + Gr. melus limb] pertaining to the midportion of the arm or leg.

mesomere (mes′o-mēr) [meso- + Gr. meros part] 1. a blastomere of size intermediate between a macromere and a micromere. 2. a midzone of the mesoderm between the epimere and hypomere.

mesomeric (mes″o-mer′ik) exhibiting mesomerism.

mesomerism (mĕ-som′er-izm) the existence of organic chemical structures differing only in the position of electons, rather than atoms. For example, the two Kekulé structures for benzene. Such a molecule does not possess one electronic structure part of the time and another structure the rest of the time; the actual electronic state of the molecule is at all times intermediate to the two extremes.

mesometrium (mes″o-me′tre-um) [meso- + Gr. mētra uterus] 1. [NA] the portion of the broad ligament below the mesovarium, composed of the layers of peritoneum that separate to enclose the uterus. 2. the tunica muscularis uteri, or myometrium.

mesomorph (mes′o-morf) an individual having a type of body build in which tissues derived from the mesoderm predominate: there is a relative preponderance of muscle, bone, and connective tissue, usually with heavy, hard physique of rectangular outline, a somatotype classified between ectomorph and endomorph.

mesomorphic (mes″o-mor′fik) pertaining to or characteristic of a mesomorph.

mesomorphy (mes′o-mor″fe) [mesoderm + Gr. morphē form] the condition of being a mesomorph.

mesomucinase (mes″o-mu′sĭ-nās) a testicular mucinolytic enzyme that may play a role in fertilization.

mesomula (mĕ-som′u-lah) an early stage of the embryo, when it consists of an epithelial ectoderm and entoderm enclosing a mass of mesenchyma.

meson (mes′on, me′zon) [Gr. mesos middle] 1. mesion. 2. a subatomic, short-lived particle of a mass less than that of a proton but more than that of an electron, carrying either a positive or a negative electric charge; called also mesotron.

mesonasal (mes″o-na′zal) situated in the middle of the nose.

mesonephric (mes″o-nef′rik) pertaining to the mesonephros.

mesonephroi (mes″o-nef′roi) plural of mesonephros.

mesonephroma (mes″o-ne-fro′mah) a rare malignant tumor of the female genital tract, most often the ovary, formerly considered to be derived from mesonephric rests (Schiller). Two varieties are recognized: (1) clear cell carcinoma, so called because of its histologic resemblance to renal cell carcinoma, and now considered to be of müllerian duct derivation, and (2) an embryonal tumor, variously called infantile embryonal carcinoma, endodermal sinus tumor, and yolk sac tumor, occurring chiefly in children. The latter variety may also arise in the testis.

mesonephron (mes″o-nef′ron) mesonephros.

mesonephros (mes″o-nef′ros), pl. mesoneph′roi [meso- + Gr. nephros kidney] [NA] the excretory organ of the embryo, arising caudad to the pronephric rudiments or the pronephros and using its duct. The mesonephros consists of a long tube in the lower part of the body cavity, running parallel with the spinal axis and joined at right angles by a row of twisting tubes. Called also corpus Wolffi and wolffian body.

meso-omentum (mes″o-o-men′tum) the fold by which the omentum is attached to the abdominal wall.

mesopallium (mes″o-pal′e-um) [meso- + L. pallium cloak] paleopallium.

mesopexy (mes′o-pek″se) mesenteriopexy.

mesophile (mes′o-fīl) an organism which grows best at temperatures between 20° and 45° C.

mesophilic (mes″o-fil′ik) [meso- + Gr. philein to love] fond of moderate temperature; said of bacteria which develop best at temperatures between 20° and 45° C. Cf. psychrophilic and thermophilic.

mesophlebitis (mes″o-fle-bi′tis) inflammation of the middle coat of a vein.

mesophragma (mes″o-frag′mah) [meso- + Gr. phragmos a fencing in] a name given to the M band. Cf. inophragma, and Z band, under band.

mesophryon (mĕ-sof′re-on) [meso- + Gr. ophrys eyebrow] the glabella or its central point.

mesophyll (mes′o-fil) [meso- + Gr. phyllon leaf] the tissue of the inner part of a leaf.

mesopia (mes-o′pe-ah) the condition of having mesopic vision.

mesopic (mes-op′ik) [meso- + Gr. ōpsis sight] pertaining to vision at intermediate levels of illumination, e.g., at twilight.

Mesopin (mes′o-pin) trademark for a preparation of homatropine methylbromide.

mesopneumon (mes″o-nu′mon) [meso- + Gr. pneumon lung] the union of the two layers of the pleura at the hilus of the lung.

mesopneumonium (mes″o-nu-mo′ne-um) (obs.) mesopneumon.

mesoporphyrin (mes″o-por′fĭ-rin) a porphyrin (q.v.) in which two pyrrole rings each have one methyl and one propionate side chain and the other two pyrrole rings each have one methyl and one ethyl side chain.

mesoprosopic (mes″o-pro-sop′ik) [meso- + Gr. prosōpon face] having a face of moderate width.

mesopulmonum (mes″o-pul-mo′num) the portion of the embryonic mesentery that encloses the laterally expanding lung.

mesorachischisis (mes″o-rah-kis′kĭ-sis) [meso- + rachischisis] partial rachischisis; partial fissure of the spinal cord.

mesorchial (mĕ-sor′ke-al) pertaining to the mesorchium.

mesorchium (mes-or′ke-um) [meso- + Gr. orchis testis] [NA] the portion of the primitive mesentery that encloses the fetal testis, represented in the adult by a fold between the testis and epididymis.

mesorectum (mes″o-rek′tum) [*meso-* + *rectum*] the fold of peritoneum connecting the upper portion of the rectum with the sacrum.

mesoridazine (mes″o-rid′ah-zēn) chemical name: 10-[2-(1-methyl-2-piperidinyl)ethyl]-2-(methylsulfinyl)-10*H*-phenothiazine; a metabolite of thioridazine, $C_{21}H_{26}N_2OS_2$. **m. besylate** [USP], **m. benzenesulfonate,** the besylate salt of mesoridazine, $C_{21}H_{26}N_2OS_2 \cdot C_6H_6O_3S$, occurring as a white to pale yellowish powder; an antipsychotic agent, used in the treatment of alcoholism, schizophrenia, psychoneurotic manifestations, and behavioral problems in mental deficiency and chronic brain syndrome, administered orally and intramuscularly.

mesoropter (mes″o-rop′ter) [*meso-* + Gr. *horos* boundary + Gr. *optēr* observer] the normal position of the eyes with their muscles at rest.

mesorrhaphy (mes-or′ah-fe) mesenteriorrhaphy.

mesorrhine (mes′o-rin) [*meso-* + Gr. *rhis* nose] having a nasal index between 48 and 53.

mesosalpinx (mes″o-sal′pinks) [*meso-* + Gr. *salpinx* tube] [NA] the part of the broad ligament of the uterus above the mesovarium, composed of layers that enclose the uterine tube.

mesoscapula (mes″o-skap′u-lah) spina scapula.

mesoseme (mes′o-sēm) [*meso-* + Gr. *sēma* sign] having an orbital index between 83 and 89.

mesosigmoid (mes″o-sig′moid) the peritoneal fold by which the sigmoid flexure is attached to the posterior abdominal wall.

mesosigmoiditis (mes″o-sig″moi-di′tis) inflammation of the mesosigmoid.

mesosigmoidopexy (mes″o-sig-moi′do-pek″se) [*mesosigmoid* + Gr. *pēxis* fixation] suspension or fixation of the mesosigmoid in the treatment of prolapse of the rectum.

mesosome (mes′o-sōm) [*meso-* + Gr. *sōma* body] an invagination of the cell membrane occurring in certain bacteria. Various mesosomes are associated with DNA replication, with cell secretion, and with electron transport of the organism.

mesostaphyline (mes″o-staf′ĭ-lin) [*meso-* + Gr. *staphylē* bunch of grapes, uvula] pertaining to or characterized by a palate with a moderate width, with a palatal index of 80.0 to 84.9.

mesostenium (mes″o-ste′ne-um) mesenterium.

mesosternum (mes″o-ster′num) [*meso-* + Gr. *sternon* sternum] the corpus sterni.

mesostroma (mes″o-stro′mah) the embryonic fibrillar tissue analogous to the vitreous, which develops into Bowman's and Descemet's membranes.

mesosystolic (mes″o-sis-tol′ik) [*meso-* + Gr. *systolē* systole] pertaining to the middle of the systole.

mesotarsal (mes″o-tar′sal) midtarsal.

mesotaurodontism (me″so-taw″ro-don′tism) [*meso-* + Gr. *tauros* bull + *odont-* + *-ism*] taurodontism in which the tooth roots branch only in the middle.

mesotendineum (mes″o-ten-din′e-um) [NA] the delicate connective tissue sheath attaching a tendon to its fibrous sheath.

mesotendon (mes″o-ten′don) mesotendineum.

mesotenon (mes″o-ten′on) mesotendineum.

mesothelial (mes″o-the′le-al) pertaining to the mesothelium.

mesothelioma (mes″o-the″le-o′mah) a malignant tumor derived from mesothelial tissue (peritoneum, pleura, pericardium); it appears as broad sheets of cells, with some regions containing spindle-shaped, sarcoma-like cells and other regions showing adenomatous patterns. Pleural mesotheliomas have been linked to exposure to asbestos.

mesothelium (mes″o-the′le-um) [*meso-* + *epithelium*] [NA] the layer of flat cells, derived from the mesoderm, which lines the coelom or body cavity of the embryo. In the adult, it forms the simple squamous epithelium which covers all true serous membranes (peritoneum, pericardium, pleura).

mesothenar (mes-oth′e-nar) [*meso-* + Gr. *thenar* palm] musculus adductor pollicis.

mesothorium (mes″o-tho′re-um) a disintegration product of thorium, intermediate between thorium and radiothorium

and isotopic with radium. It has radioactive properties and has been used in the treatment of cancer.

mesotron (mes′o-tron) meson, def. 2.

mesotropic (mes″o-trop′ik) situated in the middle of a cavity, as the abdomen.

mesotympanum (mes″o-tim′pah-num) the portion of the middle ear medial to the tympanic membrane.

mesovarium (mes″o-va′re-um) [NA] the portion of the broad ligament of the uterus between the mesometrium and mesosalpinx, which is drawn out to enclose and hold the ovary in place.

Mesozoa (mes″o-zo′ah) [*meso-* + Gr. *zōon* animal] a small group of tiny parasites whose relationships to the Protozoa and Metazoa are uncertain.

messenger (mes′en-jer) an information carrier. **second m.,** cyclic adenosine monophosphate (q.v.) or cyclic guanosine monophosphate; mediators of hormonal action, chiefly located on the plasma membrane of the cell.

mesterolone (mes-ter′o-lōn) chemical name: 17β-hydroxy-1α-methyl-5α-androstan-3-one; an androgen, $C_{20}H_{32}O_2$, with actions and uses similar to those of testosterone.

Mestinon (mes′tĭ-non) trademark for preparations of pyridostigmine bromide.

mestranol (mes′trah-nōl) [USP] chemical name: 3-methyoxy-19-nor-17α-pregna-1,3,5(10)-triene-20-yne-17α-ol. The 3-methyl ether of ethinyl estradiol, $C_{21}H_{26}O_2$, occurring as a white to creamy white, crystalline powder; used as the estrogen component of several progestin-estrogen oral contraceptives.

mesuprine hydrochloride (mes′ŭ-prēn) chemical name: N-[2-hydroxy-5-[1-hydroxy-2-[2-(4-methoxyphenyl)ethyl]amino]propyl]phenyl]methanesulfonamide monohydrochloride; a vasodilator and smooth muscle relaxant, $C_{19}H_{26}N_2O_5S \cdot HCl$.

mesuranic (mes″u-ran′ik) [*meso-* + Gr. *ouranos* palate] having a maxilloalveolar index between 110.0 and 114.9.

mesylate (mes′ĭ-lāt) USAN contraction for methanesulfonate.

Met methionine.

met (met) a unit of measurement of heat production by the body: the metabolic heat produced by a resting-sitting subject, being 50 kilogram calories per square meter of body surface per hour.

meta- [Gr. *meta* after, beyond, over] 1. a prefix indicating (*a*) change, transformation, or exchange or (*b*) after or next. 2. symbol *m*-; in organic chemistry, a prefix indicating a 1,3-substituted benzene ring, e.g., *m*-xylene (1,3-dimethylbenzene) or *m*-nitrophenol (3-nitrophenol). 3. in organic chemistry, a prefix indicating a polymeric acid anhydride, e.g., metaphosphoric acid.

meta-arthritic (met″ah-ar-thrit′ik) occurring as a consequence or result of arthritis.

metabasis (mě-tab′ah-sis) [*meta-* + Gr. *bainein* to go] 1. a change in the manifestations or course of a disease. 2. metastasis, or change in the site of a morbid process from one region of the body to another.

metabiosis (met″ah-bi-o′sis) [*meta-* + Gr. *biōsis* way of life] the dependence of one organism upon another for its existence; commensalism.

metabolic (met″ah-bol′ik) pertaining to or of the nature of metabolism.

metabolimeter (met″ah-bo-lim′ĕ-ter) [*metabolism* + Gr. *metron* measure] an apparatus for measuring basal metabolism.

metabolimetry (met″ah-bo-lim′ĕ-tre) the measurement of basal metabolism.

metabolism (mě-tab′o-lizm) [Gr. *metaballein* to turn about, change, alter] the sum of all the physical and chemical processes by which living organized substance is produced and maintained (anabolism), and also the transformation by which energy is made available for the uses of the organism (catabolism). **ammonotelic m.,** that in which ammonia is the final product of nitrogen metabolism. **basal m.,** the minimal energy expended for the maintenance of respiration, circulation, peristalsis, muscle tonus, body temperature, glandular activity, and the other vegetative functions of the body. The rate of basal metabolism (basal metabolic rate) is measured by means of a calorimeter, in a subject at absolute rest, 14 to 18 hours after eating, and is expressed in calories per hour per square meter of body surface. **endogenous m.,** metabolism of the proteins of the body tissues. **energy m.,** the metabolic processes by which energy is released. **excess m. of exercise,** the amount by which the oxygen consumed or the carbon dioxide eliminated during exercise and recovery exceeds the corresponding amounts during sleep. **exogenous m.,** metabolism of ingested foodstuffs. **inborn error of m.,** a genetically determined biochemical disorder in which a specific enzyme defect produces a metabolic block that may have pathologic consequences at birth (e.g., phenylketonuria) or in later life (e.g., diabetes mellitus); called also *enzymopathy* and *genetotrophic disease.* **intermediary m.,** the various chemical reactions involved in the transformation of food molecules into essential cellular building blocks. **ureotelic m.,** that in which urea is the final product of nitrogen metabolism. **uricotelic m.,** that in which uric acid is the final product of nitrogen metabolism.

metabolite (mĕ-tab'o-līt) any substance produced by metabolism or by a metabolic process. **essential m.,** a necessary constituent of normal metabolic processes.

metabolizable (mĕ-tab'o-līz"ah-b'l) capable of being transformed by metabolism.

metabromsalan (met"ah-brom'sah-lan) chemical name: 3,5-dibromo-2-hydroxy-N-phenylbenzamide. A disinfectant with antibacterial and antifungal activities, $C_{13}H_9Br_2NO_2$, used mainly in medicated soaps.

metabutethamine hydrochloride (met"ah-bu-teth'ah-min) chemical name: 2-[(2-methylpropyl)amino]ethanol 3-aminobenzoate(ester) monohydrochloride. A local anesthetic, $C_{13}H_{21}ClN_2O_2 \cdot HCl$, occurring as a white crystalline solid; used in dentistry to produce infiltration and nerve block anesthesia.

metabutoxycaine hydrochloride (met"ah-bu-tok'se-kān) chemical name: 3-amino-2-butoxybenzoic acid 2-diethylaminoethyl ester hydrochloride. A local anesthetic, $C_{17}H_{28}N_2O_3 \cdot HCl$, used in dentistry.

metacarpal (met"ah-kar'pal) 1. pertaining to the metacarpus. 2. a bone of the metacarpus.

metacarpectomy (met"ah-kar-pek'to-me) excision or resection of a metacarpal bone.

metacarpophalangeal (met"ah-kar"po-fah-lan'je-al) pertaining to the metacarpus and phalanges.

metacarpus (met"ah-kar'pus) [*meta-* + Gr. *karpos* wrist] the part of the hand between the wrist and the fingers, its skeleton being five cylindric bones (metacarpals) extending from the carpus to the phalanges. See also *ossa metacarpi,* under *os²*.

metacele (met'ah-sēl) metacoele.

metacentric (met"ah-sen'trik) [*meta-* + *center* (def. 1)] having the centromere near the middle, so that the arms of the replicating chromosome are approximately equal in length. Cf. *acrocentric* and *submetacentric.*

metacercaria (met"ah-ser-ka're-ah), pl. *metacerca'riae.* The encysted resting or maturing stage of a trematode parasite in the tissues of an intermediate host (mollusks, aquatic arthropods, fishes, or amphibia) or on vegetation. The metacercaria may be the infective or transfer stage to man and other animals.

metacercariae (met"ah-ser-ka're-e) plural of *metacercaria.*

metachemical (met"ah-kem'ĭ-kal) beyond the bounds of chemistry.

metachromasia (met"ah-kro-ma'ze-ah) [*meta-* + Gr. *chrōma* color] 1. a condition in which tissues do not stain true with a given stain. 2. staining in which the same stain colors different tissues in different tints. 3. the change of color produced by staining.

metachromatic (met"ah-kro-mat'ik) [*meta-* + Gr. *chrōmatikos* relating to color] staining differently with the same dye; said of tissues in which different elements take on different colors when a certain dye is applied. By extension, said of dyes by which different tissues are stained differently.

metachromatin (met"ah-kro'mah-tin) the basophil element in chromatin.

metachromatism (met"ah-kro'mah-tizm.) metachromasia.

metachromatophil (met"ah-kro-mat'o-fil) a cell that does not stain in the usual manner with a given stain.

metachromia (met"ah-kro'me-ah) metachromasia.

metachromic (met"ah-kro'mik) metachromatic.

metachromophil (met-ah-kro'mo-fil) [*meta-* + Gr. *chrōma* color + *philein* to love] staining in an abnormal manner with a given stain.

metachromophile (met"ah-kro'mo-fīl) metachromophil.

metachromosome (met"ah-kro'mo-sōm) one of two small chromosomes which conjugate only in the last phase of the spermatocyte division.

metachronous (mĕ-tak'ro-nus) [*meta-* + Gr. *chronos* time] occurring at different times.

metachrosis (met"ah-kro'sis) [*meta-* + Gr. *chrōsis* coloring] change of color in animals.

metachysis (mĕ-tak'ĭ-sis) [*meta-* + Gr. *chysis* effusion] the transfusion of blood.

metacoele (met'ah-sēl) [*meta-* + Gr. *koilia* hollow] 1. (*obs.*) that cavity of the metencephalon which, with the epicoele, makes up the fourth ventricle. 2. metacoeloma.

metacoeloma (met"ah-se-lo'mah) that part of the embryonic coelom which develops into the pleuroperitoneal cavity.

metacone (met'ah-kōn) [*meta-* + Gr. *kōnos* cone] the distobuccal cusp of an upper molar tooth.

metaconid (met"ah-kon'id) the mesiolingual cusp of a lower molar tooth.

metaconule (met"ah-kon'ūl) the small intermediate cusp between the metacone and the protocone of the upper molar teeth of mammals, sometimes also present in man.

metacortandracin (met"ah-kor-tan'drah-sin) prednisone.

metacortandralone (met"ah-kor-tan'drah-lōn) prednisolone.

metacresol (met"ah-kre'sol) one of the three isomeric forms of cresol, and the most strongly antiseptic of the group. **m. acetate,** a compound that has been used in fungus infections. **m. purple, m. sulfonphthalein,** a triphenylmethane compound which is a brilliant indicator, being red at pH 1.2, blue at pH 2.8, yellow at pH 7.4, and purple at pH 9.0.

metacyesis (met"ah-si-e'sis) [*meta-* + Gr. *kyēsis* pregnancy] extrauterine pregnancy.

metaduodenum (met"ah-du'o-de'num) the portion of the duodenum distal to the duodenal papilla, developed embryonically from the midgut.

metafemale (me"tah-fe'māl) [*meta-* + *female*] a sex chromosome abnormality, XXX karyotype, among females; called also *triple-X.*

metagaster (met"ah-gas'ter) [*meta-* + Gr. *gastēr* belly] the permanent intestinal canal of the embryo.

metagastrula (met"ah-gas'troo-lah) [*meta-* + *gastrula*] a gastrula with a cleavage differing from that of the standard type.

metagelatin (met"ah-jel'ah-tin) a substance produced by treating gelatin with oxalic acid.

metagenesis (met"ah-jen'ĕ-sis) [*meta-* + *genesis*] alternation of generations; alternation in regular sequence of asexual with sexual methods of reproduction in the same species, as in certain fungi.

metaglobulin (met"ah-glob'u-lin) a fibrogenous substance occurring in cell protoplasm; fibrinogen.

metagonimiasis (met"ah-go"nĭ-mi'ah-sis) infection with *Metagonimus.*

Metagonimus (met"ah-gon'ĭ-mus) [*meta-* + Gr. *gonimos* productive] a genus of trematodes. **M. ova'tus,** *M. yokogawai.* **M. yokoga'wai,** an intestinal trematode found in the small intestine of man and mammals in Japan, China, Indonesia, Balkans, and Israel.

metahemoglobin (met"ah-he'mo-glo'bin) methemoglobin.

Metahydrin (met"ah-hi'drin) trademark for a preparation of trichlormethiazide.

metaicteric (met"ah-ik-ter'ik) occurring after jaundice.

metainfective (met"ah-in-fek'tiv) occurring after an infection; a term applied to a febrile state occurring during convalescence from an infectious disease.

metakinesis (met″ah-ki-ne′sis) prometaphase.

metal (met′l) [L. *metallum;* Gr. *metallon*] any element marked by luster, malleability, ductility, and conductivity of electricity and heat and which will ionize positively in solution. **alkali m.,** one of a group of monovalent metals including lithium, sodium, potassium, rubidium, and cesium. **alkaline earth m's,** a group of grayish white, malleable metals that are easily oxidized in air, comprising beryllium, magnesium, calcium, strontium, barium, and radium. **Babbitt m.,** an alloy of tin, copper, and antimony; sometimes used in dentistry. **bell m.,** an alloy of copper and tin. **colloidal m.,** a colloidal solution of a metal; see *electrosol.* **fusible m.,** an alloy that melts at a relatively low temperature, as at or around the boiling point of water. Bismuth, lead, and tin are usually the principal constituents. **Melotte's m.,** a soft, fusible alloy consisting of bismuth, lead, and tin; used for dies and counterdies. **Wood's m.,** a metal used in making casts of blood vessels: bismuth, 50 per cent; lead, 25 per cent; tin, 12.5 per cent; cadmium, 12.5 per cent.

metalbumin (met-al-bu′min) [*meta-* + *albumin*] pseudomucin.

metaldehyde (met-al′de-hīd) a crystalline body, a polymer of acetaldehyde, $(CH_3 \cdot CHO)_3$, formerly used as an antiseptic.

metallaxis (met″ah-lak′sis) [Gr. "exchange," "interchange"] the transformation or building over of an organ by pathologic processes.

metallesthesia (met″al-es-the′ze-ah) [*metal* + Gr. *aisthēsis* perception + *-ia*] the recognition of metals by the sense of touch.

metallic (me-tal′ik) 1. pertaining to, consisting of, or of the nature of metal. 2. made of metal.

metallized (met′l-īzd) treated with metals.

metallizing (met′l-īz-ing) making something metallic, as when treating the surface of impression material with metals so that it will conduct electricity before electroplating.

metallocyanide (me-tal″o-si′ah-nīd) a compound of cyanogen with a metal.

metalloenzyme (mĕ-tal″o-en′zīm) an enzyme containing a tightly bound metal atom (e.g., cobalt, copper, iron, molybdenum, or zinc) as an integral part of its structure.

metalloflavoprotein (mĕ-tal″o-fla″vo-pro′tēn) a flavoprotein that contains a bound metal ion as part of its structure, e.g., xanthine oxidase.

Metallogenium (me-tal″o-je′ne-um) [Gr. *metallos* metal + *gennan* to produce] a genus of budding bacteria of uncertain status, found in bottom deposits and plankton in freshwater lakes and ponds, made up of coccoid cells that produce flexible filaments crusted with iron and manganese deposits. The type species is *M. persona′tum.*

metalloid (met′l-oid) [*metal* + Gr. *eidos* form] 1. any element with both metallic and nonmetallic properties, as silicon, boron, or arsenic. 2. any metallic element that has not all the characters of a typical metal. 3. resembling a metal.

metallophilic (mĕ-tal″o-fil′ik) having an affinity for metal-containing stains; said of cells.

metalloporphyrin (me-tal″o-por′fī-rin) a combination of a metal with porphyrin, e.g., heme (iron) and turacin (copper).

metalloscopy (met″′l-os′ko-pe) [*metal* + Gr. *skopein* to examine] observation of the effects of applying metal to the body.

metallotherapy (me-tal″o-ther′ah-pe) [*metal* + Gr. *therapeuein* to heal] the treatment of disease by applying metals to the skin.

metallurgy (met′l-ur″je) [*metal* + Gr. *ergon* work] the science and art of using metals.

metal-sol (met′l-sol″) a colloidal solution of a metal.

metamer (met′ah-mer) a compound exhibiting, or capable of exhibiting, metamerism.

metamere (met′ah-mēr) [*meta-* + Gr. *meros* part] one of a series of homologous segments of the body of an animal. In genetic theory, one of a varying number of common repeating units that make up the repressor segment of a chromosomal locus, the actual number of metameres in a given locus being proportional to the degree of repression of the trait in question.

metameric (met″ah-mer′ik) pertaining to or characterized by metamerism.

metamerism (me-tam′er-ism) 1. a type of structural isomerism in which different radicals of the same chemical type are attached to the same polyvalent element and yet give rise to compounds possessing identical molecular formulas, for example, diethylamine, $(C_2H_5)_2NH$, and methyl propylamine, $CH_3NHC_3H_7$. The term metamerism is seldom used, such compounds being called simply structural isomers of the same chemical type. 2. arrangement into metameres by the serial repetition of a structural pattern. Cf. *antimere.*

Metamine (met′ah-mēn) trademark for preparations of trolnitrate phosphate.

metamonad (met″ah-mo′nad) [*meta-* + *monad*] a group of protozoa comprising all the zooflagellates except those in the orders Choanoflagellida and Kinetoplastida, most of which are symbionts in the insect gut.

metamorphopsia (met″ah-mor-fop′se-ah) [*meta-* + Gr. *morphē* form + *-opsia*] a disturbance of vision in which objects are seen as distorted in shape.

metamorphosis (met″ah-mor′fo-sis) [*meta-* + Gr. *morphōsis* a shaping, bringing into shape] change of shape or structure, particularly a transition from one developmental stage to another, as from larva to adult form. **fatty m.,** any normal or pathologic transformation of fat, including fatty infiltration and fatty degeneration. **ovulational m.,** the developmental changes which occur during ovulation. **platelet m.,** viscous m. **retrograde m., retrogressive m.,** degeneration; more often a retrograde metabolic change. **revisionary m.,** cataplasia. **structural m.,** viscous m. **tissue m.,** any change in tissues, either normal or pathologic. **viscous m.,** the progressive and irreversible aggregation and fusion of blood platelets during the process of coagulation; called also *structural m.* and *platelet m.*

metamorphotic (met″ah-mor-fot′ik) pertaining to or characterized by metamorphosis.

Metamucil (met″ah-mu′sil) trademark for a preparation of psyllium hydrophilic mucilloid.

metamyelocyte (met″ah-mi′ĕ-lo-sīt″) a precursor in the granulocytic series, being a cell intermediate in development between a promyelocyte and the mature, segmented (polymorphonuclear), granular leukocyte, and having an indented (juvenile) nucleus. Called also *juvenile cell* or *form,* and *young form.*

Metandren (mĕ-tan′dren) trademark for preparations of methyltestosterone.

metanephric (met″ah-nef′rik) of or pertaining to the metanephros.

metanephrine (met″ah-nef′rin) chemical name: α-(methylaminomethyl vanillyl alcohol(3-methylepinephrine). A metabolite of epinephrine excreted in the urine and found in certain tissues.

metanephrogenic (met″ah-nef′ro-jen′ik) [*meta-* + Gr. *nephros* kidney + *gennan* to produce] capable of giving rise to the metanephros.

metanephroi (met″ah-nef′roi) plural of *metanephros.*

metanephron (met″ah-nef′ron) metanephros.

metanephros (met″ah-nef′ros), pl. *metaneph′roi* [*meta-* + Gr. *nephros,* kidney] the permanent embryonic kidney, which develops later than and caudal to the mesonephros, from the mesonephric duct and nephrogenic cord.

metaneutrophil (met″ah-nu′tro-fil) [*meta-* + *neutrophil*] staining abnormally with neutral stains.

metanucleus (met″ah-nu′kle-us) [*meta-* + *nucleus*] the egg nucleus during the maturative period.

metapeptone (met″ah-pep′tōn) [*meta-* + *peptone*] a digestive product between dyspeptone and parapeptone.

metaphase (met′ah-fāz) [*meta-* + *phase*] the second stage of cell division (mitosis or meiosis), during which the contracted chromosomes, each consisting of two chromatids, are arranged in the equatorial plane of the spindle prior to separation. See *meiosis* and *mitosis.*

Metaphedrin (met″ah-fed′rin) trademark for a preparation of nitromersol and ephedrine.

Metaphen (met′ah-fen) trademark for preparations of nitromersol.

metaphosphoric acid (me″tah-fos-for′ik) a glassy solid

polymer of phosphoric acid, HO(PO₃)ₓH, soluble in water; used as a reagent for chemical analysis and as a test for albumin in the urine. Called also *glacial phosphoric a.*

metaphrenon (met″ah-fre′non) [Gr. "the part behind the midriff"] (*obs.*) the back, especially the region about the kidneys.

metaphyseal (met″ah-fiz′e-al) pertaining to or of the nature of a metaphysis.

metaphyses (mĕ-taf′ĭ-sēz) plural of *metaphysis.*

metaphysial (met″ah-fiz′e-al) metaphyseal.

metaphysis (mĕ-taf′ĭ-sis), pl. *metaph′yses* [*meta-* + Gr. *phyein* to grow] [NA] the wider part at the extremity of the shaft of a long bone, adjacent to the epiphyseal disk. During development it contains the growth zone and consists of spongy bone; in the adult it is continuous with the epiphysis.

metaphysitis (met″ah-fis-i′tis) inflammation of the metaphysis of a long bone.

metaplasia (met″ah-pla′ze-ah) [*meta-* + Gr. *plassein* to form] the change in the type of adult cells in a tissue to a form which is not normal for that tissue. **myeloid m.,** the occurrence of myeloid tissue in extramedullary sites; specifically, a syndrome characterized by splenomegaly, anemia, the presence of nucleated erythrocytes and immature granulocytes in the circulating blood, and extramedullary hematopoiesis in the liver and spleen. The primary form is also known as *agnogenic myeloid metaplasia, myelosclerosis,* and *myelofibrosis.* The secondary or symptomatic form may be associated with various diseases, including carcinomatosis, tuberculosis, leukemia, and polycythemia vera. **myeloid m., agnogenic,** a condition characterized by foci of extramedullary hematopoiesis, splenomegaly, immature red and white cells in the peripheral blood, and mild to moderate anemia; it is grouped by some hematologists with the myeloproliferative disorders. Called also *aleukemic* or *nonleukemic myelosis,* and *leukoerythroblastic anemia.* **pseudopyloric m.,** gastric metaplasia in which the gastric glands disappear and are replaced by tubules that closely resemble normal pyloric glands. **m. of pulp,** transformation of the usual types of cells normally found in the pulp tissue into entirely different types. **squamous m.,** the transformation of pseudostratified ciliated epithelium into stratified squamous epithelium, as occurs in certain pathologic conditions or may be produced experimentally.

metaplasis (mĕ-tap′lah-sis) the stage in which the organism has attained completed growth.

metaplasm (met′ah-plazm) [*meta-* + Gr. *plasma* something formed] deuteroplasm.

metaplastic (met″ah-plas′tik) 1. pertaining to or characterized by metaplasia. 2. formed by or of the nature of metaplasm (deutoplasm).

metaplexus (met″ah-plek′sus) (*obs.*) the choroid plexus of the fourth ventricle of the brain.

metapneumonic (met″ah-nu-mon′ik) [*meta-* + *pneumonia*] succeeding or following pneumonia.

metapodialia (met″ah-po″de-a′le-ah) [*meta-* + Gr. *pous* foot] a collective term for the bones of the metacarpus and metatarsus.

metapophysis (met″ah-pof′ĭ-sis) [*meta-* + *apophysis*] the mamillary process on the superior articular or prearticular processes of certain vertebrae.

metapore (met′ah-pōr) (*obs.*) apertura mediana ventriculi quarti.

Metaprel (met′ah-prel) trademark for preparations of metaproterenol sulfate.

metaproterenol sulfate (met″ah-pro-ter′ĕ-nol) chemical name: 5-[1-hydroxy-2-[(1-methylethyl)amino]ethyl]-1,3-benzenediol sulfate (2:1) salt. A β-adrenergic, $(C_{11}H_{17}NO_3)_2H_2\cdot SO_4$, similar in chemical structure to isoproterenol but having longer lasting effects; used as a bronchodilator in the treatment of bronchial asthma and for reversible bronchospasm associated with bronchitis and emphysema, administered orally and by inhalation.

metapsyche (met″ah-si′ke) [*meta-* + Gr. *psychē* soul] (*obs.*) the metencephalon.

metapsychology (met″ah-si-kol′o-je) a term applied to various philosophical theories about mental functions and mental "structures" which are justifiable on logical grounds but not verifiable by experiment or observation; in psycho-

analysis such theories concern the topography (id, ego, superego) and economics (quantities of psychic energy or excitation) of mental processes.

metapyrone (met-ah-pi′rōn) metyrapone.

metaraminol (met″ah-ram′ĭ-nol) [USP] chemical name: α-(1-aminoethyl)-3-hydroxybenzenemethanol[*R*-(*R**,*R**)]-2,-3-dihydroxybutanedioate (1:1) (salt). An adrenergic with potent vasopressor activity, $C_9H_{13}NO_2\cdot C_4H_6O_6$; used especially for the prevention and treatment of acute hypotensive states occurring with spinal anesthesia and for adjunctive therapy of hypotension due to hemorrhage, reactions to medications, surgical complication, and shock associated with brain damage due to trauma or tumor, administered intramuscularly and intravenously.

metarchon (met-ar′kon) an agent which, without being toxic, so changes the behavior of a pest that its persistence is diminished, e.g., a confusing sex attractant.

metargon (met-ar′gon) a name given an isotope of argon, atomic weight 38.

metarhodopsin (met″ah-ro-dop′sin) an intermediate compound that is formed as rhodopsin absorbs light and eventually dissociates to opsin and *trans*-retinal; see *retinal,* def. 2.

metarteriole (met″ar-te′re-ōl) an arterial capillary.

metarubricyte (met″ah-roo′brĭ-sīt) orthochromatic normoblast.

metasaccharic acid (met″ah-sak′ah-rik) a dibasic tetrahydroxy acid formed by the oxidation of mannitol; it is $COOH(CHOH)_4COOH$, and in the free state passes into a double lactone.

metasomatome (met″ah-so′mah-tōm) one of the constrictions between successive protovertebrae.

metastable (met′ah-sta″b′l) 1. a condition differing from stable in that, although the substance is stable in small perturbations, it can be transformed to a more stable condition by relatively large perturbations. 2. subject to inevitable change or destruction eventually, but apparently stable owing to slowness of change.

metastases (mĕ-tas′tah-sēz) plural of *metastasis* (def. 2).

metastasis (mĕ-tas′tah-sis) [*meta-* + Gr. *stasis* stand] 1. the transfer of disease from one organ or part to another not directly connected with it. It may be due either to the transfer of pathogenic microorganisms (e.g., tubercle bacilli) or to transfer of cells, as in malignant tumors. The capacity to metastasize is a characteristic of all malignant tumors. 2. Pl. *metastases.* A growth of pathogenic microorganisms or of abnormal cells distant from the site primarily involved by the morbid process. **biochemical m.,** the transportation from the point of production and the deposition in previously normal tissues of abnormal or pathologically produced biochemical substances which bring about immunological or other changes in the tissues. **calcareous m.,** the formation of bone salts in the kidneys and elsewhere in softening of bone. **contact m.,** transfer from one surface to another with which the former is in contact. **crossed m.,** passage of material from the venous to the arterial circulation without going through the lungs. **direct m.,** metastasis in the direction of the blood or lymph stream. **implantation m.,** metastasis brought about by transfer of tumor cells by fluid and their implantation in a distant location. **paradoxical m., retrograde m.,** metastasis taking place in a direction opposite to that of the blood stream. **transplantation m.,** metastasis from one tissue to another.

metastasize (me-tas′tah-sīz) to form new foci of disease in a distant part by metastasis.

metastatic (met″ah-stat′ik) pertaining to or of the nature of metastasis.

metasternum (met″ah-ster′num) [*meta-* + Gr. *sternon* sternum] processus xiphoideus.

Metastrongylidae (met″ah-stron-jil′e-de) a family of nematodes of the superfamily Strongyloidea, comprising the lungworms; it includes the genera *Metastrongylus* and *Angiostrongylus.*

Metastrongylus (met″ah-stron′jĭ-lus) a genus of parasitic nematodes of the family Metastrongylidae. *M. elonga′tus,* a species found in the lungs of hogs, is a host of the swine influenza virus.

metasynapsis (met″ah-sĭ-nap′sis) end-to-end union of the chromosomes in synapsis.

metasyncrisis (met″ah-sin′krĭ-sis) the elimination of waste or morbid matter.

metasyndesis (met″ah-sin-de′sis) metasynapsis.

metatarsal (met″ah-tar′sal) 1. pertaining to the metatarsus. 2. a bone of the metatarsus.

metatarsalgia (met″ah-tar-sal′je-ah) [meta- + Gr. *tarsos* tarsus + -*algia*] pain and tenderness in the metatarsal region.

metatarsectomy (met″ah-tar-sek′to-me) excision or resection of the metatarsus.

metatarsophalangeal (met″ah-tar″so-fah-lan′je-al) pertaining to the metatarsus and the phalanges of the toes.

metatarsus (met″ah-tar′sus) [meta- + Gr. *tarsos* tarsus] the part of the foot between the tarsus and the toes, its skeleton being the five long bones (the metatarsals) extending from the tarsus to the phalanges. See also *ossa metatarsi*, under *os²*. **m. adductoca′vus,** a deformity of the foot in which metatarsus adductus is associated with pes cavus. **m. adductova′rus,** a deformity of the foot in which metatarsus adductus is associated with metatarsus varus. **m. adduc′tus,** a congenital deformity of the foot in which the fore part of the foot deviates toward the midline. **m. atav′icus,** abnormal shortness of the first metatarsal bone. **m. brev′is,** a condition in which the first metatarsal bone is shorter than normal and often abducted. **m. la′tus,** a broadened foot due to spreading of the anterior part of the foot resulting from separation of the heads of the metatarsal bones from each other; called also *broad foot* and *spread foot*, under *foot*. **m. pri′mus va′rus,** angulation of the first metatarsal bone toward the midline of the body, producing an angle sometimes of 20 degrees or more between its base and that of the second metatarsal bone. **m. va′rus,** a congenital deformity of the foot in which its inner border is off the ground with the sole turned inward, the patient walking on the outer border of the foot.

Metatensin (met″ah-ten′sin) trademark for preparations of trichlormethiazide with reserpine.

metathalamus (met″ah-thal′ah-mus) [meta- + *thalamus*] [NA] the part of the diencephalon inferior to the caudal end of the dorsal thalamus, comprising the lateral and medial geniculate bodies.

Metatheria (met″ah-the′rĭ-ah) [meta- + Gr. *thērion* beast, animal] in some systems of classification a subclass of the Mammalia, and in others an infraclass of the subclass Theria, including the pouched mammals or marsupials.

metatherian (met″ah-the′ri-an) any member of the Metatheria.

metathesis (mě-tath′ě-sis) [meta- + Gr. *thesis* placement] 1. the artificial transfer of a morbid process. 2. a chemical reaction in which an element or radical in one compound exchanges places with another element or radical in another compound.

metathetic (met″ah-thet′ik) pertaining to or of the nature of metathesis.

metathrombin (met″ah-throm′bin) [meta- + *thrombin*] the inactive combination of thrombin and antithrombin.

metatroph (met′ah-trōf) a metatrophic organism.

metatrophia (met-ah-tro′fe-ah) 1. atrophy from malnutrition. 2. a change in diet.

metatrophic (met-ah-trof′ik) utilizing organic matter for food. Cf. *paratrophic*.

metatrophy (met-at′ro-fe) [meta- + Gr. *trophē* nutrition] 1. the state of being metatrophic; metatrophic nutrition. 2. metatrophia.

metatypic (met″ah-tip′ik) metatypical.

metatypical (met″ah-tip′e-kal) composed of the elements of the tissue on which it develops, but having those elements arranged in an atypical manner; said of tumors.

metavanadate (met″ah-van′ah-dāt) any salt of vanadic acid. **sodium m.,** a highly poisonous salt, $NaVO_3 \cdot 4H_2O$.

metaxalone (mě-taks′ah-lōn) chemical name: 5-[(3,5-dimethylphenoxy)methyl]-2-oxazolidinone. A smooth muscle relaxant, $C_{12}H_{15}NO_3$, used in the treatment of painful musculoskeletal conditions, administered orally.

metaxenia (met″ah-ze′ne-ah) an improper term for ectogony.

metaxeny (me-tak′sĕ-ne) metoxeny.

Metazoa (met″ah-zo′ah) [meta- + Gr. *zōon* animal] that division of the animal kingdom which embraces all multicellular animals whose cells become differentiated to form tissues. It includes all animals except Protozoa.

metazoa (met″ah-zo′ah) plural of *metazoon*.

metazoal (met″ah-zo′al) 1. belonging to the Metazoa. 2. pertaining to or caused by metazoa.

metazoan (met″ah-zo′an) 1. pertaining to metazoa; metazoal. 2. a metazoon.

metazonal (met″ah-zo′nal) situated after or below a sclerozone.

metazoon (met″ah-zo′on), pl. *metazo′a.* An individual of the Metazoa.

Metchnikoff (mech′nĭ-kof) Elie [Mechnikov, Ilia Llich]. Russian zoologist in Paris, 1845–1916; co-winner, with Paul Ehrlich, of the Nobel prize for medicine or physiology in 1908 for his discovery of phagocytes and phagocytosis.

Metchnikoff's theory (mech′nĭ-kof) [Elie *Metchnikoff* (Ilia Ilich *Mechnikov*)] see under *theory*.

Metchnikovellida (mech″nĭ-ko-vel′ĭ-dah) an order of parasitic protozoa (class Rudimicrosporea, phylum Microspora) having characters of the class.

metecious (me-te′shus) [meta- + Gr. *oikos* house] heterecious.

metencephal (met-en′se-fal) the metencephalon.

metencephalic (met-en″sě-fal′ik) pertaining to the metencephalon.

metencephalon (met″en-sef′ah-lon) [meta- + Gr. *enkephalos* brain] 1. the anterior portion of the rhombencephalon, comprising the cerebellum and the pons; in official anatomical nomenclature [NA], the term *metencephalon* is used as an alternative for *pons*. See Plate accompanying *brain*. 2. the anterior of the two brain vesicles formed by specialization of the rhombencephalon in the developing embryo. Called also *afterbrain* and *epencephalon*.

metencephalospinal (met″en-sef″ah-lo-spi′nal) pertaining to the metencephalon (cerebellum) and the spinal cord.

met-enkephalin (met″en-kef′ah-lin) see *enkephalin*.

meteorism (me′te-ŏ-rizm) [Gr. *meteōrizein* to raise up] tympanites; the presence of gas in the abdomen or intestine.

meteorology (me″te-o-rol′o-je) [Gr. *meteōros* high in the air + -*logy*] the science of the atmosphere and its phenomena; the science of the weather.

meteoropathology (me″te-ĕ-ro-pah-thol′o-je) the pathology of conditions caused by atmospheric conditions.

meteoropathy (me″te-ĕ-rop′ah-the) [Gr. *meteōros* high in the air + *pathos* disease] any disorder due to conditions of climate.

meteororesistant (me″te-ĕ-ro-re-zis′tant) comparatively insensitive to weather conditions.

meteorosensitive (me″te-ĕ-ro-sen′si-tiv) abnormally sensitive to weather conditions.

meteorotropic (me″te-ĕ-ro-trop′ik) responding to influence by meteorological factors; pertaining to or characterized by meteorotropism.

meteorotropism (me″te-ĕ-rot′ro-pizm) the response to influence by meteorological factors noted in certain biological events, such as sudden death, attacks of angina, joint pain, insomnia, and traffic accidents.

metepencephalon (met″ep-en-sef′ah-lon) [meta- + epi- + Gr. *enkephalos* brain] myelencephalon.

meter (me′ter) [Gr. *metron* measure; Fr. *mètre*] 1. the basic unit of linear measure in the metric system, approximately equivalent to 39.37 inches; formerly established as the length of a bar of an alloy of platinum and iridium preserved in a vault at the International Bureau of Weights and Measures, near Paris. Although its dimension is unchanged, it is now defined in terms of the wavelength of a certain line in the spectrum of krypton. Abbreviated m. 2. an apparatus devised to measure the quantity of anything passing through it, such as of a gas, amperes of electric current, etc. **dosage m.,** dosimeter. **light m.,** an instrument for measuring light in foot candles. **peak flow m.,** an instrument for measuring the flow of air in the early part of forced expiration. **rate m.,** a radiation detector whose output is proportional to instantaneous radiation intensity (rate of radioactive emissions).

-meter [Gr. *metron* measure] a word termination denoting an instrument used in measuring.

metergasis (met″er-ga′sis) [*meta-* + Gr. *ergon* work] change of function.

metestrum (mĕ-tes′trum) metestrus.

metestrus (mĕ-tes′trus) [*meta-* + L. *oestrus*] the period of subsiding follicular function or rest following estrus in female mammals.

metformin (met-for′min) chemical name: N,N-dimethylimidodicarbonimidic diamide; an oral hypoglycemic agent, $C_4H_{11}N_5$.

methacholine (meth″ah-ko′lēn) a cholinergic agonist, acetyl-β-methylcholine, having a longer duration of action than acetylcholine and predominantly muscarinic effects; it has vasodilator and cardiac vagomimetic effects but has largely been replaced by other drugs. Available as *methacholine bromide* and *methacholine chloride* [USP]. **m. bromide,** the bromide salt of methacholine, $C_8H_{18}BrNO_2$, occurring as a white, crystalline powder, having actions and uses similar to those of the chloride salt; administered orally. **m. chloride** [USP], the chloride salt of methacholine, $C_8H_{18}ClNO_2$, occurring as colorless or white crystals or as a white, crystalline powder; used as a cholinergic, especially in the treatment of Raynaud's disease, scleroderma, vascular spasm due to cold, and chronic varicose ulcers, administered orally, subcutaneously, and by iontophoresis. Called also *acetyl-betamethylcholine chloride.*

methacrylate (meth-ak′rĭ-lāt) 1. an ester of methacrylic acid. Its methyl and polymethyl esters are the acrylic resins most commonly used in medicine and dentistry. See also *acrylic resin,* under *resin.* 2. an acrylic resin derived from methacrylic acid.

methacrylic acid (meth″ah-kril′ik) an organic acid, 2-methylpropenoic acid, that polymerizes easily to form a ceramic-like mass. Its esters, methyl and polymethyl methacrylate, are used in the manufacture of acrylic resins and plastics.

methacycline (meth″ah-si′klēn) chemical name: 4S-dimethylamino-1,4α,4aα,5α,5aα,6,11,12aα-octahydro-3,5,10,12,12a-penta hydroxy-6-methylene-1,11-dioxo-2-naphthacencarboxamide. A semisynthetic broad-spectrum antibiotic of the tetracycline group, $C_{22}H_{22}N_2O_8$, derived from oxytetracycline. **m. hydrochloride** [USP], the monohydrochloride salt of methacycline, $C_{22}H_{22}N_2O_8 \cdot HCl$, occurring as a yellow to dark yellow crystalline powder; used as an antibacterial, administered orally.

methadone hydrochloride (meth′ah-don) [USP] chemical name: 6-(dimethylamino)-4,4-diphenyl-3-hepanone hydrochloride. A synthetic narcotic, $C_{21}H_{27}NO \cdot HCl$, occurring as colorless crystals or white, crystalline powder, possessing pharmacologic actions similar to those of morphine and heroin and almost equal addiction liability; used as an analgesic and as a narcotic abstinence syndrome suppressant in the treatment of heroin addiction (see also *narcotic blockade,* under *blockade*), administered orally, intramuscularly, and subcutaneously.

methadyl acetate (meth′ah-dil) chemical name: β-[2-(dimethylamino)propyl]-α-ethyl-β-phenylbenzeneethanol; a narcotic analgesic, $C_{23}H_{31}NO_2$. Called also *acetylmethadol.*

methallenestril (meth″al-ĕ-nes′tril) chemical name: β-ethyl-6-methoxy-α,α-dimethyl-2-naphthalenepropionic acid. A synthetic, nonsteroidal, orally effective, estrogenic drug, $C_{18}H_{22}O_3$, occurring as a white, crystalline powder, having uses similar to those of estrogen (q.v.).

methallibure (meth-al′ĭ-būr) chemical name: 1-methyl-6-(1-methylallyl)-2,5-dithiobiurea. A substance, $C_7H_{14}N_4S_2$, used as an anterior pituitary activator in swine.

methamphetamine (meth″am-fet′ah-mēn) chemical name: (S)-N,α-dimethylbenzeneethanamine. A sympathomimetic amine of the amphetamine group, $C_{10}H_{15}N$. Abuse of this drug may lead to dependence; see *amphetamine,* def. 1. **m. hydrochloride,** white crystals or white, crystalline powder, $C_{10}H_{15}N \cdot HCl$, used chiefly for its central stimulant effects in the treatment of mental depression, psychopathic states, narcolepsy, and exogenous obesity, and for its calming effects in hyperkinetic children. It also has pressor effects and is used in various hypotension states, especially in regional and spinal anesthesia and after ganglionic blockade.

methandriol (meth-an′dre-ol) chemical name: 17α-methyl-5-androstene-3β,17β-diol; an anabolic agent.

methandrostenolone (meth-an″dro-sten′o-lōn) [USP] chemical name: 17β-hydroxy-17α-methylandrosta-1,4-dien-3-one. An androgen, $C_{20}H_{28}O_2$, occurring as white to off-white crystals or crystalline powder; used especially in the adjunctive treatment of senile and postmenopausal osteoporosis and in selected cases of pituitary dwarfism, administered orally.

methane (meth′ān) a colorless, odorless, inflammable gas, CH_4, produced by decomposition of organic matter, which may explode when mixed with air or oxygen; it is the first member of a homologous series of saturated hydrocarbons, including butane, ethane, hexane, pentane, and propane. Called also *marsh gas.*

methanesulfonate (meth″ān-sul′fo-nāt) any salt or ester of methanesulfonic acid.

methanesulfonic acid (meth″ān-sul-fon′ik) a corrosive, toxic acid, CH_3SO_2OH, used as a catalyst and as a solvent.

Methanobacteriaceae (meth″ah-no-bak-te″re-a′se-e) a family of methane-producing bacteria, made up of coccoid or rod-shaped, strictly anaerobic cells that obtain energy by the formation of methane. The Methanobacteriaceae are grouped with the archaeobacteria because they lack muramic acid in their cell walls and differ from other bacteria in ribosomal RNA and cell lipid structures. They are found in sewage sludge, mud, and the rumens of cattle and sheep. The family contains the genera *Methanobacterium, Methanococcus,* and *Methanosarcina.*

Methanobacterium (meth″ah-no-bak-te″re-um) [*methane* + Gr. *baktērion* little rod] a genus of methane-producing bacteria of the family Methanobacteriaceae, made up of nonspore-forming, coccoid, rod-shaped organisms that are strictly anaerobic and derive energy by the reduction of carbon dioxide to methane. They are widely distributed, occurring in mud, sewage, and the digestive tracts of animals. The type species is *M. soehnge′nii.*

Methanococcus (meth″ah-no-kok′kus) [*methane* + Gr. *kokkos* berry] a genus of methane-producing bacteria of the family Methanobacteriaceae, made up of spherical cells occurring singly, in pairs, or in masses. They are strict anaerobes that derive energy from the formation of methane from hydrogen, carbon dioxide, and formate. They are found in soils, mud, sewage sludge, and the intestinal tract of animals. The type species is *M. ma′zei.*

methanogen (meth′ah-no-jen″) an anaerobic microorganism that grows in the presence of carbon dioxide and produces methane gas. Methanogens are found in the stomach of cows, in swamp mud, and other environments in which oxygen is not present.

methanogenic (meth″ah-no-jen′ik) producing methane.

methanol (meth′ah-nol) [USP] a clear, colorless, flammable liquid, CH_3OH, with characteristic odor, miscible with alcohol, ether, and water; used as a solvent.

methanolysis (meth″ah-nol′ĭ-sis) alcoholysis of methyl alcohol.

Methanomonadaceae (meth″ah - no - mo″nah - da′se - e) Methylococcaceae.

Methanomonas (meth″ah-no-mo′nas) Methylomonas.

Methanosarcina (meth″ah-no-sar-si′nah) [*methane* + L. *sarcina* bundle] a genus of methane-producing bacteria of the family Methanobacteriaceae, made up of large, spherical, strictly anaerobic cells that derive energy by the formation of methane from acetate and sometimes methanol. They are found in mud and sewage. The type species is *M. metha′nica.*

methantheline bromide (mĕ-than′thĕ-lēn) [USP] chemical name: N,N-diethyl-N-methyl-2-[(9H-xanthene-9-ylcarbonyl)oxy]ethanaminium bromide. A quaternary ammonium anticholinergic, $C_{21}H_{26}BrNO_3$, occurring as a white or nearly white powder; used in conditions requiring inhibition of gastrointestinal and genitourinary motility, in hyperhidrosis, or in control of normal sweating. *Sterile methantheline* is prepared in conformance with USP specifications.

methapyrilene (meth″ah-pīr′ĭ-lēn) chemical name: N,N-dimethyl-N′-2-pyridinyl-N′-(2-thienylmethyl)-1,2-ethanediamine. An antihistaminic, $C_{14}H_{19}N_3S$, which also has moderate sedative action. **m. fumarate** [USP], the fumarate salt of methapyrilene, $(C_{14}H_{19}N_3S)_2 \cdot 3C_4H_4O_4$, occurring as a white, crystalline powder, having actions and uses similar to those of the hydrochloride salt; administered orally. **m. hydrochloride** [USP], the monohydrochloride salt of methapyrilene, $C_{14}H_{19}N_3S \cdot HCl$, occurring as a white, crystalline powder, having the same actions as the base; used in the treatment of allergic manifestations, nausea and vomiting of pregnancy. and insomnia, administered orally.

methaqualone (mĕ-thah′kwah-lōn) [USP] chemical name: 2-methyl-3-(2-methylphenyl)-4(3H)-quinazolinone. A hypnotic and sedative, $C_{16}H_{14}N_2O$, occurring as a white, crystalline powder; administered orally. **m. hydrochloride** [USP], the monohydrochloride salt of methaqualone, $C_{16}H_{14}N_2O \cdot HCl$, having the same appearance, actions, uses, and route of administration as the base.

metharbital (mĕ-thar′bĭ-tal) [USP] chemical name: 5,5-diethyl-1-methyl-2,4,6(1H,3H,5H)pyrimidinetrione. A barbital derivative, $C_9H_{14}N_2O_3$, occurring as a white to nearly white, crystalline powder; used as an anticonvulsant for the control of grand mal, petit mal, myoclonic, and mixed types of epileptic seizures, administered orally.

methazolamide (meth″ah-zo′lah-mīd) [USP] chemical name: N-[5-(aminosulfonyl)-3-methyl-1,3,4-thiadiazol-2(3H)-ylidene]acetamide. A carbonic anhydrase inhibitor, $C_5H_8N_4$-O_3S_2, occurring as a white or faintly yellow, crystalline powder; used chiefly to reduce intraocular pressure in the treatment of glaucoma, administered orally.

methdilazine (meth-di′lah-zēn) [USP] chemical name: 10-[(1-methyl-3-pyrrolidinyl)methyl]-10H-phenothiazine. An antihistaminic, $C_{18}H_{20}N_2S$, occurring as a light tan, crystalline powder; used as an antipruritic in dermatoses of various origins, administered in chewable tablets. **m. hydrochloride** [USP], the monohydrochloride salt of methdilazine, $C_{18}H_{20}N_2S \cdot HCl$, having the same appearance, actions, and uses as the base; administered orally.

methemalbumin (met″hem-al-bu′min) a brownish pigment formed by the binding of albumin with the ferric complex of protoporphyrins (heme), occurring only when the serum has been depleted of unsaturated haptoglobin; it is indicative of intravascular hemolysis. Formerly called *pseudomethemoglobin*.

methemalbuminemia (met″hem-al-bu″min-e′me-ah) the presence of methemalbumin in the blood.

metheme (met′hēm) hematin.

methemoglobin (met-he″mo-glo″bin) a compound formed from hemoglobin by oxidation of the ferrous to the ferric state with essentially ionic bonds. A small amount of methemoglobin is present in the blood normally, but injury or toxic agents convert a larger proportion of hemoglobin into methemoglobin, which does not function reversibly as an oxygen carrier.

methemoglobinemia (met″he-mo-glo″bi-ne′me-ah) [*methemoglobin* + Gr. *haima* blood + *-ia*] the presence of methemoglobin in the blood, resulting in cyanosis. It may be drug-induced or be due to a defect in the enzyme NADH methemoglobin reductase (an autosomal recessive trait) or to an abnormality in hemoglobin M (an autosomal dominant trait).

methemoglobinemic (met″he-mo-glo″bĭ-ne′mik) 1. pertaining to or causing methemoglobinemia. 2. an agent that causes methemoglobinemia.

methemoglobin reductase (NADPH) (met-he″mo-glo′-bin re-duk′tās) NADPH methemoglobin reductase.

methemoglobinuria (met″he-mo-glo-bi-nu′re-ah) [*methemoglobin* + Gr. *ouron* urine + *-ia*] the occurrence of methemoglobin in the urine.

methenamine (meth-en′ah-mēn) [USP] chemical name: 1,3,5,7-tetraazatricyclo[3.3.1.1³,⁷]decane. Colorless, lustrous crystals or a white crystalline powder, $C_6H_{12}N_4$, used as a urinary antibacterial, administered orally. **m. hippurate**, a compound of methenamine and hippuric acid, C_6H_{12}-$N_4 \cdot C_9H_9NO_3$, used orally as a urinary antibacterial. **m. mandelate** [USP], a salt of methenamine and mandelic acid, $C_{14}H_{20}N_4O_3$, occurring as a white crystalline powder; used orally as a urinary antibacterial.

methene (meth′ēn) methylene.

methenolone (mĕ-then′o-lōn) chemical name: 17β-hydroxy-1α-methyl-5α-androst-1-en-3-one; an anabolic steroid, $C_{20}H_{30}O_2$. **m. acetate**, an ester of methenolone $C_{22}H_{32}$-O_3; an anabolic steroid. **m. enanthate**, an ester of methenolone, $C_{27}H_{42}O_3$; an anabolic steroid.

Methergine (meth′er-jin) trademark for preparations of methylergonovine maleate.

methestrol dipropionate (meth′es-trol) promethestrol dipropionate.

methetoin (mĕ-thet′o-in) chemical name: 5-ethyl-1-methyl-5-phenyl-2,4-imidazolidinedione; an anticonvulsant, $C_{12}H_{14}N_2O_2$, which has been used in the treatment of epilepsy.

methexenyl (meth-ek′sē-nyl) hexobarbital.

methicillin sodium (meth″ĭ-sil″in) [USP] chemical name: 6-(2,6-dimethoxybenzamido)-3,3-dimethyl-7-oxo-4-thia-1-azabicyclo[3.2.0]heptane-2-carboxylic acid sodium salt. A semisynthetic penicillin, $C_{17}H_{19}N_2NaO_6S$, occurring as a fine, white, crystalline powder; used intravenously or intramuscularly as an antibacterial in resistant staphylococcal infections. Called also *dimethoxyphenyl penicillin sodium*.

methimazole (meth-im′ah-zōl) [USP] chemical name: 1,3-dihydro-1-methyl-2H-imidazole-2-thione. A thyroid inhibitor, $C_4H_6N_2S$, occurring as a pale buff, crystalline powder; used in the treatment of hyperthyroidism, administered orally. Called also *thiamazole*.

methine (meth′in) methylidyne.

methiodal sodium (meth-i′o-dal) [USP] chemical name: iodomethanesulfonic acid sodium salt. An iodine containing compound, CH_2INaO_3S, occurring as white, crystalline powder; used as a radiopaque medium in urography, administered intravenously.

methionine (mĕ-thi′o-nin) 1. a naturally occurring amino acid, $C_5H_{11}NO_2S$, which is an essential component of the diet, furnishing both methyl groups and sulfur necessary for normal metabolism. 2. racemethionine.

methionine synthase (mĕ thi′o-nēn sin′thās) 5-methyl-tetrahydrofolate-homocysteine methyltransferase.

methionyl (mĕ-thi′o-nil) the acyl radical of methionine.

methisazone (mĕ-this′ah-zōn) chemical name: 2-(1,2-dihydro-1-methyl-2-oxo-3H-indol-3-ylidene)hydrazinecarbothioamide. An antiviral agent, $C_{10}H_{10}N_4OS$, which has been used to provide short-term protection against smallpox and the severe complications of vaccination.

Methium (meth′e-um) trademark for preparations of hexamethonium chloride.

methixene hydrochloride (mĕ-thiks′ēn) chemical name: 1-methyl-3-(9H-thioxanthen-9-yl-methyl)piperidine hydrochloride monohydrate. An anticholinergic, $C_{20}H_{23}NS$--$HCl \cdot H_2O$, occurring as a white, crystalline powder, having a direct spasmolytic effect on smooth muscle; used in the treatment of gastrointestinal hypermotility and spasm associated with functional bowel disease, administered orally.

methocarbamol (meth″o-kar′bah-mol) [USP] chemical name: 3-(2-methoxyphenoxy)-1,2-propanediol 1-carbamate. A skeletal muscle relaxant, $C_{11}H_{15}NO_5$, occurring as a white powder; administered orally, intramuscularly, and intravenously.

Methocel (meth′o-sel) trademark for a preparation of methylcellulose.

method (meth′ud) [Gr. *methodos*] the manner of performing any act or operation; a procedure or technique. See also under *maneuver, stains, tests, treatment*, etc. **Abbott's m.**, treatment of scoliosis by lateral pulling and counterpulling on the spinal column by means of wide bandages and pads until the deformity is overcorrected, and then applying a plaster jacket to produce pressure, counterpressure, and fixation of the spine in its corrected position. **A.B.C. (alum, blood, clay) m.**, a method of deodorizing and precipitating sludge by the addition of alum, charcoal (or some other material), and clay to the raw sewage. **absorption m.**, the separate and selective removal of agglutinins from specific immune sera by the addition of homologous particulate antigen(s) (e.g., bacterial cells or red blood cells) to the immune sera, or by the passage of specific immune sera through columns containing antigen on an insoluble support (immunosorbent) with which the homologous antibody combines and is thereby removed from the serum. **acid hematin m.** (*for hemoglobin*): dilute the blood in tenth normal HCl and compare the color with a standard heme solution or glass standards. **Addis m.**, see under *count* and *tests*. **alkali reserve, m's for**, see *Fridericia's m., Marriott's m., Van Slyke and Cullen's m.* (1), and *Van Slyke and Fitz's m.* **allantoin, m's for**, see *Folin's m.* (15), *Plimmer and Skelton's m., Wiechowski and Handorsky's m.* **Altmann-Gersh m.**, a method of preparing tissue for histologic study by freeze drying. **amino-acid nitrogen, m's for**, see *nitrogen, amino-acid, m's for*. **ammonia nitrogen, m's for**, see *nitrogen, ammonia, m's for*. **Ar-**

nold and Gunning's m. (*for total nitrogen*), a modified form of the Kjeldahl process for urine. **Aronson's m.,** volatilizing formaldehyde gas from the solid polymer, trioxymethylene, by heat. **Askenstedt's m.** (Parker's modification) (*for indican*): precipitate the urine with solid mercuric chloride; oxidize the indican to indigo with Obermeyer's reagent; shake out with chloroform and compare the blue color with a standard solution of indigo. **Austin and Van Slyke's m.** (*for chlorides in whole blood*): lake the blood with distilled water, precipitate the proteins with picric acid, and then proceed as in McLean and Van Slyke's method for chlorides in oxalated plasma. **Autenrieth and Funk's m.** (*for cholesterol*): boil the blood or serum to saponify the fats; extract with chloroform and evaporate the chloroform; make a Liebermann-Burchard test on the residue and compare it with a standard solution of cholesterol. **autoclave m.,** see *Clark-Collip m.* (2). **Baer's m.,** prevention of the re-forming of adhesions by the injection of sterilized oil into an ankylosed joint. **Bang's m.,** 1. estimation of the quantities of the sugar, albumin, urea, etc., in the blood by examination of a few drops only, collected on blotting paper. 2. (*for dextrose*): to an excess of the boiling reagent (an alkaline solution of copper thiocyanate), add the urine and titrate the excess of copper thiocyanate with hydroxylamine sulfate. 3. (*a micromethod for dextrose*): boil the urine with an excess of the reagent ($KHCO_3$, 160 gm.; K_2CO_3, 100 gm.; KCl, 66 gm.; $CuSO_4 \cdot 5H_2O$, 4.4 gm.; and water to 1 liter) and titrate excess of CuCl with a solution of iodine, using starch as an indicator. **Barger's m.,** a method for determining osmotic pressure from vapor pressure. **Barraquer's m.,** phacoerysis. **Bergonié's m.,** see under *treatment*. **beta-hydroxybutyric acid, m's for,** see *Black's m.* and *Van Slyke and Palmer's m.* **Bethea's m.,** see under *sign*. **bile pigments, m's for,** see *Meulengracht's m., Wallace and Diamond's m.,* and see under *tests*. **Bivine's m.,** treatment of strychnine poisoning by administration of chloral hydrate. **Black's m.** (*for beta-hydroxybutyric acid*): evaporate the urine to a small volume, acidify, add plaster of Paris to form a coarse meal, extract the beta-hydroxybutyric acid with ether in a Soxhlet apparatus, evaporate to dryness, take up in water, and determine the amount by a polariscope. **Bloor, Pelkan, and Allen's m.** (*for fatty acids and cholesterol*): extract the lipoids by an alcohol-ether mixture, saponify, extract the cholesterol with chloroform and the soaps with hot alcohol. The cholesterol is then determined colorimetrically, and the fatty acids nephelometrically. **Bock and Benedict's m.** (*for total nitrogen*): it is similar to Folin and Farmer's method, except that the ammonia is distilled instead of aerated over into the acid. **Bogg's m.** (*for protein in milk*): this is a modification of Esbach's method for protein in urine; the protein being precipitated with Bogg's reagent instead of with picric acid. **Brandt-Andrews m.,** see under *maneuver*. **Brehmer's m.,** see under *treatment*. **Breslau's m.,** volatilizing formaldehyde from dilute (8 per cent) solutions to prevent polymerization. **brine flotation m.** (*for concentration of ova*): suspend a portion of the stool in a saturated solution of sodium chloride; let it stand for a time and collect the ova from the surface. **Brunn's m.,** see *Breslau's m.* **calcium m's for,** see *Clark-Collip m.* (1), *Corley and Denis' m., Kramer and Tisdall's m.* (2), *Lyman's m., McCrudden's m.,* and *Shohl and Pedley's m.,* and see under *tests*. **caliper m.,** a method for approximating fat content in the body by measuring the thickness of folds of the skin at stated areas of the body by means of specially designed calipers. **Callahan m.,** 1. a root canal filling method in which the root canal is first flooded with a chloroform-rosin solution and then gutta-percha is dissolved in the solution. 2. a method of tracing and opening up the root canal by destroying the pulp tissue by application of a 50 per cent sulfuric acid solution. **carbon dioxide, m. for,** see *Fridericia's m.* and *Van Slyke and Cullen's m.* (1). **Carrel's m.,** 1. a method of end-to-end suture of blood vessels. 2. see under *treatment*. 3. a method of determining when to make secondary closure of wounds. A loop of material is taken from the wound, spread on a slide, stained, and the number of bacteria counted. **Castaneda's m.** (*for rickettsiae in smears*): (1) a thin smear is made in a phosphate buffer (pH 7.6) and air-dried, (2) stained with methylene blue solution for 3 minutes, (3) counterstained with safranine solution, and (4) washed, blotted, and dried. Rickettsiae appear pale blue; cell nuclei and protoplasm are red. **Cathelin's m.,** introduction of anesthetics into the epidural space through the sacrococcygeal ligament. **Chandler's m.** (*for fibrinogen*): precipitate the fibrinogen with calcium chloride, centrifugalize, and determine the nitrogen in the clot. **Chick-Martin m.,** a method for testing the bactericidal value of disinfectants for water supplies in the presence of organic matter. The procedure originally incorporated 3 per cent human feces. In the revised method, serial dilutions of disinfectant are incubated with a specified quantity of yeast and *Salmonella typhi* for a period of 30 minutes. The effectiveness is expressed by the ratio: effective concentration of phenol divided by effective concentration of test disinfectant (Chick-Martin coefficient). **chlorides, m's for,** see *Austin and Van Slyke's m., Dehn and Clark's m., McLean and Van Slyke's m., Mohr's m., Volhard and Arnold's m., Volhard and Harvey's m.,* and *Whitehorn's m.* **chloropercha m.,** a method of filling a root canal with gutta-percha dissolved in a chloroform-rosin solution; see *Callahan's m.* (def. 1) and *Johnson's m.* **cholesterol, m's for,** see *Autenrieth and Funk's m., Bloor, Pelkan, and Allen's m.,* and *Myers and Wardell's m.,* and see under *tests*. **Ciaccio's m.,** treatment of tissue for the purpose of rendering visible the intracellular lipoids; they are fixed with acid chromate solution and stained with sudan III. **Clark-Collip m.,** 1. (*for calcium in serum*): dilute the serum and add ammonium oxalate; wash the precipitate, dissolve with sulfuric acid, and titrate with potassium permanganate. 2. (*for urea in blood*): to 5 ml. of blood filtrate add 1 ml. of NH_4Cl and heat in autoclave at 150 C. for ten minutes. Make alkaline, distil into acid, and titrate, using methyl red as indicator. **Clausen's m.,** 1. (*for lactic acid in blood*): remove the glucose by adding copper sulfate and calcium hydroxide, filter, and proceed with filtrate as in Clausen's method for lactic acid in urine. 2. (*for lactic acid in urine*): extract the lactic acid from the urine with ether, convert it into acetaldehyde by treatment with sulfuric acid, add sodium bisulfite, and titrate with standard iodine solution. **closed-plaster m.,** treatment of wounds, compound fractures, and osteomyelitis by enclosing the limb in an immobilizing plaster cast. See *Orr treatment* and *Trueta treatment*, under *treatment*. **Converse m.,** reconstruction of the ear lobe by raising a flap of skin below the auricle with a superior base about one third larger than the proposed lobe; a full-thickness skin graft covers the defect at the site of the flap except for the last third of the medial aspect of the pedicle. **Corley and Denis' m.** (*for calcium in tissues*): if there is only a small amount of organic material, it may be removed by washing, aided by nitric acid. With more organic material, add 5 volumes of tenth normal sodium hydroxide and heat in autoclave at 180° C. for two hours. Precipitate as oxalate, dissolve in sulfuric acid, and titrate with potassium permanganate. **Corning's m.,** spinal anesthesia, def. 1. **Corri's m.** (*for lactic acid in tissues*): precipitate the protein with $HgCl_2$, remove the mercury from the filtrate with H_2S, and determine lactic acid by Clausen's method. **Couette m.,** a method for measuring viscosity by calculating the rate of movement of an inner cylinder separated from an outer cylinder by a thin layer of the fluid whose viscosity is being tested. **Coutard's m.,** a method of x-ray irradiation by protracted and fractionated dosage. **creatine, m's for,** see *Folin's m.* (7,8), *Folin, Benedict, and Myers' m., Folin and Wu's m.* (2), and *Meyer's m.* **creatinine, m's for,** see *Folin's m.* (9), *Folin and Wu's m.* (1,2), and *Shaffer's m.,* and see under *tests*. **Credé's m.,** 1. method of expressing the placenta by forcing the uterus down into the pelvis and at the same time squeezing the uterus from all sides so that its contents are expelled. 2. a similar method for expressing urine from the bladder, especially in paralytic bladder. 3. the placing of a drop of 2 per cent solution of silver nitrate in each eye of a newborn child for the prevention of ophthalmia neonatorum. **Cronin m.,** an operation to correct a flat nasal tip with short columella by using bilateral flaps of skin elevated in the floor of the nostrils. **crystallizing oxyhemoglobin, m. for,** see *Reichert's m.* **Cuignet's m.,** skiametry. **cup plate m.,** see *ring test* (def. 1), under *tests*. **Dakin-Carrel m.,** Carrel's treatment; see under *treatment*. **Dehn and Clark's m.** (*for chlorides*): oxidize any interfering organic matter with sodium peroxide and then proceed with Volhard and Arnold's method. **Denis' m.** (*for magnesium in serum*): remove the calcium by the Clark-Collip method, precipitate as magnesium ammonium phosphate, dissolve the precipitate in tenth normal HCl, reduce it with amino-naphthol-sulfonic acid, and compare the blue color with a standard solution of ammonium magnesium phosphate in 0.1 per cent HCl. **Denis and Leche's m.** (*for total sulfate*): add acid and autoclave to decompose protein, then precipitate with barium chloride, dry, and weigh. **Denman's m.,** see under *evolution.* **dextrose, m's for,** see *glucose* (*dextrose*), *m's for.* **Dickinson m.,** a method of controlling postpartum hemorrhage: the entire uterus is grasped through the abdominal wall, lifted out of the pelvis, and compressed against the spinal column. **direct m.,** in ophthalmoscopy, that in which the ophthalmoscope is held close to the eye examined and an erect virtual image is obtained of the fundus. **direct aeration m.** (*for urea in blood*), see *Myers' m.* **direct centrifugal flotation m.,** Lane m. **disk diffusion m.,** see *disk diffusion test,* under *tests.* **Domagk's m.** (*for demonstration of reticuloendothelial cells*): a culture of gram-positive staphylococci in physiologic salt solution is injected into the femoral vein of a rat which is then killed in fifteen to thirty minutes. In formalin-fixed sections stained by cresyl violet or by Gram's stain followed by alum-carmine, Kupffer's cells and other cells of the reticuloendothelial system stand out strikingly. **Douglas' m.,** see under *evolution.* **Duke's m.,** see *bleeding time,* under *time.* **Eggleston's m.,** a method of administering digitalis leaf. **Eicken's m.,** examination of the hypopharynx, with the cricoid cartilage drawn forward. **Ellinger's m.** (*for indican*): precipitate the urine with basic lead acetate and filter. To the filtrate add Obermayer's reagent. Shake out the indigo with chloroform, evaporate off the chloroform, and titrate the residue with potassium permanganate. **Epstein's m.** (*for dextrose*): a modification of the Lewis and Benedict method, making it possible to make the test with very little blood. **ethereal sulfates, m's for,** see *sulfates, ethereal, m's for.* **Fahraeus m.,** the original (1918) method for determination of the erythrocyte sedimentation rate (ESR); no longer used. **fatty acids, m. for,** see *Bloor, Pelkan, and Allen's m.* **Faust's m.,** a method of diagnosing helminth and protozoan infections by centrifugation of washed feces with zinc sulfate of a specific gravity of 1.180, after which eggs and protozoan cysts may be removed from the supernatant layer. **fibrinogen, m. for,** see *Chandler's m.* **Fichera's m.,** see under *treatment.* **Fick m.,** see under *principle.* **Fishberg's m.,** one for determining specific gravity of the urine, which serves as a concentration test of renal function. **Fiske's m.** (*for total fixed base*): remove phosphates with ferric chloride, convert fixed bases into sulfates by heating in H_2SO_4, ignite, take up in water, precipitate sulfates as benzidine sulfate, and titrate with alkali. **Fiske and Subbarow's m.,** 1. (*for acid-soluble phosphorus in blood*): destroy organic matter by heating with sulfuric and nitric acids, precipitate the phosphates as magnesium ammonium phosphate, and reduce the precipitate with para-amino-naphthol-sulfonic acid. Compare the blue color with a standard phosphate solution. 2. (*for inorganic phosphates*): the phosphates are precipitated as ammonium phosphomolybdate. This is then reduced by para-amino-naphthol-sulfonic acid and the blue color compared colorimetrically with a standard solution. **Fitz Gerald m.,** zone therapy. **fixed base, m. for,** see *Fiske's m.* **flash m.,** see *pasteurization.* **flotation m.,** any method for separating cysts and ova from the heavier component of the stool and which depends upon the use of a solution intermediate in density between the parasitic material (which floats) and the bulk of the feces (which remains as sediment after centrifugation). **Folin's m.,** 1. (*for acetone*): aerate the acetone from the urine over into an alkaline hypo-iodite solution of known strength. The acetone is thus changed to iodoform and the excess of iodine is titrated with a standard thiosulfate solution, using starch as an indicator. 2. (*for acetone*): micromethod. Aerate the acetone over into a solution of sodium bisulfite and then determine the amount of nephelometric comparison with a standard acetone solution using Scott and Wilson's reagent. 3. (*for amino acids in blood*): make 10 ml. of protein-free blood filtrate slightly alkaline to phenolphthalein. Add 2 ml. of beta-naphthaquinone solution and place in the dark. The next day add 2 ml. of acetic acid-acetate solution and 2 ml. of 4 per cent thiosulfate solution. Dilute to 25 ml. and compare the blue color with a standard amino-acid solution similarly treated. 4. (*for amino-acid nitrogen in blood*): treat the urine with permutit to remove the ammonia and then with beta-naphtha-quinone sulfonic acid. The red color is compared with a standard amino acid solution. 5. (*for ammonia nitrogen*): sodium carbonate is added to the urine to free the ammonia,

which is aerated into standard acid and titrated. 6. (*for blood sugar*): to 2 ml. of neutral protein-free blood filtrate, add 2 ml. of the Folin copper solution and heat in boiling water bath ten minutes. Cool and add 2 ml. of acid molybdate reagent. Dilute to 25 ml. mark and compare the blue color with a standard glucose solution similarly treated. 7. (*for creatine*): precipitate the proteins of the blood with picric acid and filter. To the filtrate add sodium hydroxide and compare color with a standard solution of creatine. 8. (*for creatine in urine*): change creatine into creatinine by heating at 90° C. for three hours in the presence of third normal HCl. Determine creatinine by picric acid and alkali and deduct the preformed creatinine. 9. (*for creatinine in urine*): to the urine add picric acid and sodium hydroxide and compare the red color with a half normal solution of potassium bichromate. 10. (*for ethereal sulfates*): remove the inorganic sulfates with barium chloride and then the conjugated sulfates after hydrolyzing with boiling dilute hydrochloric acid. 11. (*for inorganic sulfates*): acidify the urine with hydrochloric acid, precipitate with barium chloride, filter, dry, ignite, and weigh. 12. (*for protein in urine*): add acetic acid and heat, wash, dry, and weigh the precipitate. 13. (*for total acidity*): add potassium oxalate to the urine to precipitate the calcium which should otherwise precipitate at the neutral point, and titrate with tenth normal sodium hydroxide, using phenolphthalein as an indicator. 14. (*for total sulfates*): boil the urine for thirty minutes with dilute hydrochloric acid, precipitate with barium chloride, filter, dry, ignite, and weigh. 15. (*for urea and allantoin*): decompose the urea by heating with magnesium chloride and hydrochloric acid, distil off the ammonia, and titrate. **Folin, Benedict, and Myers's m.** (*for creatine in urine*): to 20 ml. of urine add 20 ml. of normal HCl and autoclave at 120° C. for one half hour. Neutralize, add picric acid and alkali, and compare the color with a standard solution of potassium bichromate. **Folin and Wu's m.,** 1. (*for creatinine*): the color produced by the unknown (protein-free blood filtrate or urine) in an alkaline solution of picric acid is compared in a colorimeter with the color produced by a known solution of creatinine or with a standard solution of potassium bichromate. 2. (*for creatine plus creatinine*): the creatine of a protein-free blood filtrate is changed to creatinine by heating with dilute HCl in an autoclave, and the creatinine thus produced together with the preformed is determined colorimetrically after adding an alkaline picrate solution. 3. (*for glucose*): the protein-free blood filtrate is boiled with a dilute alkaline copper tartrate solution, the cuprous oxide is dissolved by adding a phosphomolybdic-phosphoric acid solution, and the blue color produced is compared with the color from sugar solutions of known strength. 4. (*nonprotein nitrogen*): the total nonprotein nitrogen in the protein-free blood filtrate is determined by setting free the nitrogen as ammonia by the Kjeldahl process, nesslerizing this ammonia, and comparing with a standard. 5. (*for protein-free blood filtrate*): lake the blood with distilled water, add sodium tungstate and sulfuric acid, and filter. 6. (*for urea*): change the urea to ammonia by means of urease, and nesslerize. 7. (*for uric acid*): uric acid is precipitated from the protein-free blood filtrate or from urine by silver lactate, treated with phosphotungstic acid, and the blue color compared with the color produced by known amounts of uric acid. **m's for (volatilizing) formaldehyde gas,** see *Aronson's m., Breslau's m., Schlossmann's m.,* and *Trillat's m.* **formol titration, m's of,** see *Malfatti's m.,* and *Sörensen's m.* **Freiburg m.,** twilight sleep; see under *sleep.* **Frey and Gigon's m.** (*for amino-acid nitrogen*): a modified form of Sörensen's method in that the ammonia is aspirated off after adding the barium hydroxide. **Fridericia's m.** (*for alveolar carbon dioxide tension*): the carbon dioxide is absorbed into a solution of potassium hydroxide and the decrease in volume read in percentage in a special apparatus. **Fülleborn's m.** (*for ova in stools*): grind 1 gm. of stool and mix with 20 ml. of a saturated solution of sodium chloride. Allow to stand one hour or more, then float coverglasses on the surface and transfer them, without draining, to slides. **gasometric m.** (*for urea*), see *Stehle's m.* **Gerota's m.,** injection of the lymphatics with a dye, such as prussian blue, which is soluble in chloroform or ether, but not in water. **Girard's m.,** see under *treatment.* **Givens' m.** (*for peptic activity*): varying amounts of diluted gastric juice are added to a series of tubes containing pea globulin, the mixtures are incubated, and the amount of digestion noted. **glucose (dextrose), m's for,** see *Bang's m., Epstein's m., Folin's m.*

(6), *Folin and Wu's m.* (3), *Hagedorn and Jensen's m.*, *Lewis and Benedict's m.*, *Peter's m.*, *Power and Wilder's m.*, *Stammer's m.*, and *Sumner's m.* See also *dextrose test*, under *tests*. **gold number m.**, colloidal gold test. **Gram's m.**, see *Table of Stains*, under *stain*. **Greenwald's m.** (*for nonprotein nitrogen*): the proteins are precipitated by trichloracetic acid, the filtrate is decomposed by sulfuric acid as in the Kjeldahl method, the ammonia is distilled off and the amount titrated with tenth normal sodium hydroxide. **Greenwald and Lewman's m.** (*for titratable alkali of blood*): the protein of the blood is precipitated with an excess of picric acid. Both the free and the total picric acid in the filtrate are then determined. The difference represents the picric acid which is combined with the bases of the blood. **Griffith's m.** (*for hippuric acid*): extract the hippuric acid with ether. Distil off the ether and destroy urea in the residue with sodium hypobromite solution. Determine the nitrogen in the residue by the Kjeldahl method. **Gross's m.** (*for tryptic activity*): add increasing amounts of a trypsin solution to a series of tubes of pure, fat-free casein which have been heated to 40° C. Incubate at 40° C. for fifteen minutes. Test by adding a few drops of acetic acid (dilute) to each tube. A precipitate on acidification indicates that digestion is incomplete or lacking; no precipitate indicates digestion. **guanidine, m's for,** see *Pfiffner and Myers' m.* and *Weber's m.* **Guinard's m.**, see under *treatment*. **Hagedorn and Jensen's m.** (*for sugar in blood*): precipitate the protein with zinc hydroxide. Heat the filtrate with potassium ferricyanide solution and determine the amount of ferricyanide reduced by adding an iodide solution and titrating the iodine set free with sodium thiosulfate. **Hall's m.** (*for total purine nitrogen*): remove phosphates by means of magnesia mixture and precipitate the purine bodies in a specially graduated tube by means of silver nitrate and ammonium hydroxide. After twenty-four hours read the volume of the purine precipitate. **Hamilton's m.** (*in postpartum hemorrhage*): compress the uterus between a fist in the vagina and a hand pressing down the abdominal wall. **Hammerschlag's m.** (*for specific gravity of blood*): prepare a mixture of benzene and chloroform of about 1.050 specific gravity. Into this let fall a drop of blood and add benzene or chloroform until the drop neither rises nor sinks. Then take the specific gravity of the mixture. **Heintz's m.** (*for uric acid*): precipitate the urine by adding hydrochloric acid, filter off the crystals, wash, dry, and weigh. **hemoglobin, m's for,** see *acid hematin m.*, *Dare's m.*, and *Sahli's m.*, and see under *tests*. **Henriques and Sörensen's m.** (*for amino-acid nitrogen by solution of formaldehyde titration*), see *Sörensen's m.* **Herter and Foster's m.** (*for indole in feces, modified by Bergeim*): make the feces alkaline and distil. Make the distillate acid and distil again. To the second distillate add beta-naphtha-quinone sodium monosulfonate and alkali. Extract the blue color with chloroform and compare it with a standard solution of indole containing 0.1 mg. of indole per milliliter. **Heublein m.**, ionizing irradiation of the whole body with low-dose increments protracted for ten to twenty hours per day over several days. **hippuric acid, m'** see *Griffith's m.*, and *Roaf's m.*, and see under *tests*. **Hirschberg's m.**, measurement of the deviation of a strabismic eye by observing the reflection of a candle from the cornea. **holding m.**, see *pasteurization*. **Howard's m.** (*of artificial respiration*): the patient is placed on his back, hands under his head, with a cushion so placed that his head is lower than his abdomen. Manual rhythmical pressure is then applied upward and inward against the lower lateral parts of the chest. **Howell's m.** (*for clotting time of blood*): place 5 ml. of blood in a 21-mm. test tube with suitable precautions. Tilt the tube every two minutes and note time of clotting. **Hunter and Given's m.** (*for uric acid and purine bases*): precipitate and decompose the precipitate as in the Krueger-Schmidt method. Determine the uric acid in an aliquot part and in the remainder destroy the uric acid by oxidation and determine the purine bases as in the Krueger-Schmidt method. **hydrogen ion concentration, m. for,** see *Levy, Rowntree, and Marriott's m.* **indican, m's for,** see *Askenstedt's m.* and *Ellinger's m.*, and see under *tests*. **indole, m's for,** see *Herter and Foster m.*, and see under *tests*. **inorganic phosphates, m. for,** see *phosphates, inorganic, m. for.* **inorganic sulfates, m's for,** see *sulfates, inorganic, m's for.* **iodine, m's for,** see specific methods, including *Kendall's m.*, *Leipert's m.* **iron, m's for,** see *Walker's m.*, *Wolter's m.*, and see under *tests*. **Ivy's m.**, see *bleeding time*, under *time*.

Japanese m., a method for fixing paraffin sections to glass slides with the use of Mayer's albumin. **Johnson m.**, a modification of the Callahan method (def. 1), in which the canal is initially flooded with alcohol, allowing diffusion of the chloroform component of the chloroform-rosin solution; alcohol deep in the dentin facilitates rosin dissolved in the chloroform to be diffused into the dentin. **Kaiserling's m.**, a procedure for preserving the natural colors in museum preparations, employing formaldehyde and potassium acetate. **Karr's m.** (*for urea in blood*): change the urea to ammonium carbonate by means of urease, nesslerize directly, and compare the color with that of a standard urea solution similarly treated. **Kendall's m.** (*for iodine in thyroid tissue*): oxidize the organic matter by fusion in KNO_3 and strong KOH. Acidify, oxidize with bromine, add an excess of KI, and titrate the liberated iodine with sodium thiosulfate. **Kety-Schmidt m.**, a method of measuring perfusion flow of blood through brain tissue. **Kirstein's m.**, inspection of the larynx without a laryngoscope by having the patient incline his head far back and depressing the tongue. **Kjeldahl's m.** (1883), a method of determining the amount of nitrogen in an organic compound. It consists in heating the material to be analyzed with strong sulfuric acid. The nitrogen is thereby converted to ammonia, which is distilled off and caught in tenth normal solution of sulfuric acid. By titration the amount of ammonia is determined, and from this the amount of nitrogen is estimated. **Klüver-Barrera m.**, a histologic staining method in which myelin sheaths are stained blue-green and the cells purple. **Koch and McMeekin's m.** (*for total nitrogen*): destroy organic matter with sulfuric acid and hydrogen peroxide, and nesslerize the resulting solution directly. **Korotkoff's m.**, the auscultatory method of determining blood pressure. **Kramer and Gittleman's m.** (*for sodium in serum*): dry and ash the serum. Take it up in 0.1 per cent HCl and make slightly alkaline with KOH. Precipitate with the pyroantimonate reagent and alcohol, dissolve precipitate in strong HCl, add potassium iodide, and titrate with sodium thiosulfate. **Kramer and Tisdall's m.**, 1. (*for potassium in serum*): precipitate with sodium cobaltinitrite reagent, treat precipitate with acid permanganate solution, then with sodium oxalate, and titrate with standard permanganate. 2. (*for calcium in serum*): precipitate the calcium as oxalate. Wash, dissolve, and titrate with potassium permanganate. **Kristeller's m.**, a method of expelling the fetus in labor. The fetal head should be in the vulva and the abdomen must be sufficiently relaxed so that the assistant may grasp the fundus. The grip on the fundus is made by the fingers of the two hands parallel behind and the thumb in front, the line of force being in the direction of the axis of the inlet. The expression should be done in one or two sustained efforts. **Krogh's m.** (*for urea*): the urea is oxidized by sodium hypobromite to carbon dioxide and nitrogen in an alkaline solution which absorbs the carbon dioxide. The remaining nitrogen is then measured. **Krueger and Schmidt's m.** (*for uric acid and purine bases*): precipitate the uric acid with copper sulfate, decompose the precipitate with sodium sulfite, acidify, concentrate, and let uric acid crystals separate. Determine the nitrogen in them by the Kjeldahl method. Reprecipitate the purine bases with copper sulfate, filter, wash, and determine the nitrogen in the precipitate by the Kjeldahl method. **Kwilecki's m.** (*for albumin*): 10 drops of a 10 per cent solution of ferric chloride are added to the urine before proceeding with the regular method of Esbach. **Laborde's m.**, the making of rhythmic traction movements on the tongue in order to stimulate the respiratory center in asphyxiation. **lactalbumin, m. for,** remove casein from the milk with magnesium sulfate, add Alman's reagent to the filtrate, determine the nitrogen in the precipitate with the Kjeldahl method, and multiply the result by 6.37. **lactic acid, m. for,** see specific methods, including *Clausen's m.* (1), (2), *Corri's m.*, *von Furth and Charnass' m.* See also *lactic acid test*, under *tests*. **Lamaze m.**, a psychoprophylactic method of preparing for delivery, involving education of the prospective mother in the physiology of pregnancy and parturition and in techniques (e.g., breathing exercises and bearing down) to ease delivery. **Lane m.**, a method of diagnosing hookworm infection by centrifugation of 1 ml. of washed feces mixed with brine, the tube being covered with a cover slip on which the eggs can be counted. Called also *direct centrifugal flotation method*, or *D.C.F.* **lateral condensation m.**, a method of filling a root canal in which the main portion of the canal is filled with a primary gutta-percha cone or silver point and sealer cement or paste and the remaining space is packed with auxiliary gutta-percha cones. Spreader sites and pluggers are used to force gutta-percha into the canal laterally and sometimes vertically. Called also *multiple cone m.* **Leboyer m.**, a method of delivery of the infant based upon the theory that the violence associated with birth causes emotional trauma to the infant and that this trauma will affect the child's personality throughout his life. The concepts of this method emphasize that the delivery should be gentle and controlled, without unnecessary intervention; the infant should be handled gently, with the head, neck, and sacrum supported; the infant should not be overstimulated and should be allowed to breathe spontaneously, without painful stimuli, such as spanking. Called also *Leboyer technique.* **Leipert's m.** *(for iodine in blood):* destroy organic matter with chromic-sulfuric acid. Reduce iodic acid to free iodine with arsenous acid, distil off the iodine, and titrate. **Levy, Rowntree, and Marriott's m.** *(for hydrogen ion concentration of blood):* dialyze the blood through a collodion tube against neutral physiologic salt solution; then match the color produced by phenolsulfonphthalein in the dialysate and in solution of known hydrogen ion concentration. **Lewis and Benedict's m.** *(for dextrose):* the proteins of the blood are precipitated by means of picric acid, sodium carbonate is added, and the color of the picramic acid solution is compared with that of a standard glucose solution. **Lewisohn's m.** *(obs.),* a method of indirect transfusion by adding sodium citrate to the blood. **lime m.,** a method of generating or volatilizing formaldehyde gas. Forty per cent formaldehyde, containing 10 per cent of sulfuric acid, is poured over quicklime in a suitable container; $1\frac{1}{2}$ to 2 pounds of lime should be used for each pint of the solution. **Lovset's m.,** see under *maneuver.* **Lyman's m.** *(for calcium):* precipitate the calcium from the protein-free blood filtrate or from urine as calcium oxalate, redissolve in dilute acid and reprecipitate as calcium ricinate, and determine the amount nephelometrically. **McCrudden's m.** *(for calcium and magnesium):* make 200 ml. of urine faintly acid to litmus, add 10 ml. of concentrated hydrochloric acid, precipitate with oxalic acid, filter, ignite, and weigh as calcium oxide, or filter and titrate the precipitate with potassium permanganate. This gives the calcium. For the magnesium, add to the filtrate from the calcium, nitric acid, evaporate to dryness, and heat until the residue fuses. Take up in water, add sodium acid phosphate and ammonia, filter, wash, ignite, and weigh as the pyrophosphate. **McLean and Van Slyke's m.** *(for chlorides):* precipitate the chlorides from oxalated plasma with an excess of silver nitrate and titrate the excess with potassium iodide and starch. **magnesium, m's for,** see *Denis' m.* and *McCrudden's m.* **Malfatti's m.** *(for ammonia nitrogen by solution of formaldehyde titration):* add potassium oxalate to the urine and make neutral to phenolphthalein with tenth normal sodium hydroxide; add the neutral solution of formaldehyde and titrate again. **Marriott's m.** *(for alkali reserve):* the patient rebreathes the air in a bag until its carbon dioxide tension is virtually that of venous blood. This air is then bubbled through a standard bicarbonate solution until the solution is saturated and the color produced is compared with standard color tubes. **Marshall's m.** *(for urea):* the urea is changed into ammonium carbonate by the enzyme urease and the ammonia titrated with tenth normal hydrochloric acid, using methyl orange, as indicator. **Meltzer's m.,** insufflation, through an endotracheal tube, of air containing an anesthetic vapor; employed in thoracic surgery. **Messinger and Huppert's m.** *(for acetone):* the same as the method of Folin and Hart except that the acetone is distilled instead of aspirated. **Mett's m.** *(for peptic activity),* see *Nirenstein and Schiff's m.* **Meulengracht's m.** *(for bile pigment in serum):* the serum is diluted until the yellow color corresponds to that of a standard potassium bichromate solution. **Meyer's m.** *(for creatine):* a modification of Folin and Benedict's method in that the creatine is changed into creatinine after adding hydrochloric acid by digesting in an autoclave. **Moerner-Sjöqvist m.,** see *Sjöqvist's m.* **Mohr's m.** *(for chlorides):* oxidize interfering organic matter by igniting with potassium nitrate. To the solution of the ash add potassium chromate, and titrate with standard silver nitrate until the red silver chromate appears. **Monias and Shapiro's m.,** convert the indican into indigolignon and compare with a standard. **multiple cone m.,** lateral condensation m. **Murphy m.,** 1. suture of an artery by invaginating the

ends over a cylinder in two pieces which can then be removed. 2. continuous proctoclysis; the continuous administration per rectum of saline solution, drop by drop, from an elevated reservoir. Called also *Murphy drip.* **Myers' m.** *(for urea in blood):* change the urea to ammonium carbonate by the action of urease, aerate off the ammonia into an acid solution, and nesslerize; called also *direct aeration m.* **Myers and Wardell's m.** *(for cholesterol):* dry the blood on plaster of Paris and extract the cholesterol with chloroform. Add acetic anhydride and sulfuric acid and compare the color with that of a standard solution of cholesterol similarly treated. **Neumann's m.,** local anesthesia for surgery on the ear by the subperiosteal injection of a solution of cocaine and epinephrine. **Nikiforoff's m.,** a method of fixing blood films by placing them for from five to fifteen minutes in absolute alcohol, pure ether, or equal parts of alcohol and ether. **Nimeh's m.,** a method of determining the size of liver and spleen, based on measurements made on flat films of the hepatic and splenic regions taken separately without any preparation or after retroperitoneal insufflation of carbon dioxide gas. The ventricle diameter is the index of the size of the liver, the broad diameter that of the spleen. **Nirenstein and Schiff's m.** *(for peptic activity):* Mett's tubes are placed in the solution to be tested and incubated for twenty-four hours. The length of the column digested at each end is then determined. **nitrogen, amino acid, m's for,** see *Folin's m.* (4), *Frey and Gigon's m., Sörensen's m., Van Slyke's m.,* and *Van Slyke and Meyer's m.* **nitrogen, ammonia, m's for,** see *Folin's m.* (5), *Malfatti's m.,* and see under *tests.* **nitrogen, nonprotein, m's for,** see *Folin and Denis' m.* (4), *Folin and Wu's m.* (4), and *Greenwald's m.* **nitrogen, purine, m. for,** see *Hall's m.* **nitrogen, total, m's for,** see *Arnold and Gunning's m., Bock and Benedict's m., Koch and McMeekin's m., Taylor and Hulton's m.* **Oberst's m.,** local anesthesia produced by injecting saline solution or distilled water into the subcutaneous connective tissue. **Ogata's m.,** a method of stimulating respiration by stroking the chest. **Ogino-Knaus m.,** the rhythm method of birth control. **optical density m.,** the measuring of growth rates of cells by taking the optical density or turbidity of a dense population and comparing this with optical densities of known dilutions of the sample. **Orr m.,** see under *treatment.* **Orsi-Grocco m.,** palpatory percussion of the heart. **Osborne and Folin's m.** *(for total sulfur in urine):* destroy the organic matter in the concentrated urine and oxidize the sulfur by fusing with sodium peroxide. Precipitate with barium chloride, wash, dry, ignite, and weigh. **ova concentration, m. for,** see *brine flotation m.* **oxalic acid, m. for,** see *Salkowski, Autenrieth, and Barth's m.* **panoptic m.,** see *Giemsa's staining method,* in Table of Stains. **Pap's silver m.,** a method for demonstrating reticulum. **Parker's m.** *(for indican),* see *Askenstedt's m.* **peptic activity, m's for,** see specific methods, including *Givens' m., Nirenstein and Schiff's m.* **Peter's m.** *(for dextrose):* boil the unknown in an excess of the reagent, filter off the reduced copper, and titrate the filtrate with potassium iodide and standard thiosulfate solution. **Pfiffner and Myers' m.** *(for guanidine in blood):* a colorimetric method by the use of an alkaline nitroprusside-ferricyanide reagent. **phenol, m's for,** see *Tisdall's m.* See also *phenol test,* under *tests.* **phosphates, inorganic, m's for,** see *Fiske and Subbarow's m.* (2). **phosphorus, m. for,** see *uranium acetate m.* **phosphorus, acid-soluble, m. for,** see *Fiske and Subbarow's m.* (1). **Plimmer and Skelton's m.** *(for allantoin):* determine the urea and allantoin by Folin's method (15), and the urea alone by Marshall's urease method. The difference is allantoin. **point source m.,** a method of intracavitary irradiation of the bladder wall utilizing a small point source of radiation at the center of a Foley catheter bag inflated with a radiopaque solution containing methylene blue or indigo carmine. **potassium, m. for,** see *Kramer and Tisdall's m.* (1). **Power and Wilder's m.** *(for glucose in urine):* remove interfering substances with mercuric sulfate. To the filtrate add alkaline ferricyanide; heat for ten minutes, cool, and add KI and an acid zinc sulfate solution. Titrate the liberated iodine with standard thiosulfate solution. **Price-Jones m.,** see under *curve.* **protein in milk, m. for,** see *Bogg's m.* **protein-free blood filtrate, m's for,** see *Folin's m.* (6), and *Folin and Wu's m.* (5). **Purdy's m.,** the use of the centrifuge in the determination of the quantity of albumin, chlorides, sulfates, etc. **purine bodies, m's for,** see *Hunter and*

Given's m., Krueger and Schmidt's m., Salkowski's m., Salkowski and Arnstein's m., and Welker's m., and see under tests. **purine, nitrogen, m. for,** see Hall's m. **radioactive balloon m.,** a method of intracavitary irradiation of the bladder wall utilizing a Foley catheter bag filled with a radioactive solution. **Raiziss and Dubin's m.** (for ethereal and inorganic sulfates): oxidize the urine with Benedict's method, precipitate the sulfate with benzidine hydrochloride, as in the method of Rosenheim and Drummond, and titrate with tenth normal potassium permanganate. **Rehfuss' m.,** see under tests. **retrofilling m.,** see retrofilling. **rhythm m.,** a method of preventing conception by restricting coitus to the so-called safe period, avoiding the days just before and after the expected time of ovulation. **Rideal-Walker m.,** a method for testing the bactericidal activity of a disinfectant as compared with that of phenol. Cultures of Salmonella typhi are incubated with serial dilutions of the test compound, with dilutions of phenol as standards. Samples are removed at intervals, transferred to sterile broth, and the resulting cultures incubated and examined for bacterial growth. Activity is expressed as the ratio of effective concentration of test compound divided by that of phenol (phenol coefficient). **Ritchie's formolether m.,** a method whereby feces, fixed in a formol-saline solution, are subjected to extraction with ether to remove fatty materials, and the washed sediment examined for protozoan cysts and helminth ova. **Ritgen's m.,** see under maneuver. **Roaf's m.** (for the preparation of hippuric acid): add 125 gm. of ammonium sulfate and 7.5 gm. of concentrated sulfuric acid to 500 ml. of urine of a horse. Hippuric acid will crystallize out. **Romanovsky's (Romanowsky's) m.,** see Table of Stains. **Rosenheim and Drummond's m.** (for ethereal and inorganic sulfates): precipitate the sulfates with benzidine hydrochloride and titrate the acid in the benzidine sulfate with tenth normal potassium hydroxide. **Ruhemann's uricometer m.** (for uric acid): urine is added in a specially graduated tube to a mixture of carbon bisulfide and iodine solution until the carbon bisulfide is decolorized. **Sahli's m.** (for estimation of hemoglobin): convert the hemoglobin into acid hematin by adding HCl and compare the color with a standard color scale. **Salkowski's m.** (for purine bodies and uric acid): precipitate as silver magnesium salts, decompose the precipitate with hydrogen sulfide, precipitate uric acid by means of sulfuric acid, and the purine bodies as silver salts. **Salkowski and Arnstein's m.** (for purines): precipitate the urine with magnesia mixture and to the filtrate add 3 per cent ammoniacal silver nitrate solution. Wash the precipitate and determine the nitrogen in it by the Kjeldahl method. The uric acid nitrogen is separately determined and deducted. **Salkowski, Autenrieth, and Barth's m.** (for oxalic acid): precipitate the oxalic acid by means of calcium chloride. Dissolve the precipitate in hydrochloric acid, extract the oxalic acid with ether, and reprecipitate it as calcium oxalate. **Satterthwaite's m.,** artificial respiration produced by alternating pressure and relaxation upon the abdomen. **Scherer's m.** (for proteins): precipitate the protein by boiling with dilute acetic acid, wash, dry, and weigh. **Schlossmann's m.,** to prevent polymerization, 10 per cent of glycerin is added to formaldehyde before it is volatilized by heat. **Schüller's m.,** a method of performing artificial respiration by rhythmic raisings of the thorax by means of the fingers hooked under the ribs. **Schweninger's m.,** reduction of obesity by the restriction of fluids in the diet. **Scott and Wilson's m.** (for acetone and acetoacetic acid): distil the acetone into an alkaline solution of basic mercuric cyanide, filter, and titrate the precipitate with potassium thiocyanate. **sectional m., segmentation m.,** a method of filling a root canal in which 2- to 3-mm. cut sections of gutta-percha cones are packed in the canal individually until it is filled. **Shaffer's m.** (for creatinine): Folin's method (9), adapted to very dilute solutions. **Shaffer-Hartmann m.,** a chemical method for determining glucose levels in the blood, utilizing a cupric reagent incorporating potassium iodate and iodide and based on the amount of iodate reduced by the cuprous oxide to iodide, and thus on the amount of reducing sugars present. **Shaffer and Marriott's m.** (for acetone bodies): precipitate the urine with basic lead acetate and ammonia. Distil off the acetone (acetone and diacetic acid). Oxidize the residue with potassium bichromate and distil again (beta-hydroxybutyric acid). Titrate the distillates with standard iodine and thiosulfate solutions. **Shohl and Pedley's m.** (for calcium in urine): oxidize the urine with ammonium persulfate, precipitate the calcium as oxalate, add H_2SO_4 to the precipitate, and titrate with potassium permanganate. **Siffert m.,** a method for computing the volume of the gallbladder by tracing the gallbladder shadow on transparent paper and comparing it with a standard. **silver point (cone) m.,** a method of filling a root canal in which a prefitted silver point is sealed into the apex of the root canal; irregularities in the canal not sealed with the point are obliterated with gutta-percha by lateral condensation or segmentation, or by a root canal paste or sealer. **single cone m.,** a method of filling the root canal of a tooth with a single, well-fitting gutta-percha cone or silver point in conjunction with a sealer cement or paste. **Sippy m.,** see under treatment. **Sjöqvist's m.,** quantitative estimation of the urea in the urine by means of a baryta mixture. **Sluder m.,** removal of the tonsils by means of a tonsil guillotine. **Smellie's m.,** delivery of the aftercoming head with the body of the child resting on the forearm of the obstetrician. **sodium, m. for,** see Kramer and Gittleman's m. **Somogyi m.,** 1. (for blood glucose): a modification of the Shaffer-Hartmann method in which the cuprous oxide reduces an arsenomolybdate reagent, yielding a more stable end product. 2. (for amylase activity): a method based on the disappearance of the blue color given by iodine and amylose (linear fraction of starch) after amylase in serum, urine, etc., is allowed to act on starch. **Sörensen's m.** (for amino acids by solution of formaldehyde titration): titrate the urine for total acidity using phenolphthalein as indicator, add fresh solution of formaldehyde (15 ml. of formalin, 30 ml. of water, and sufficient sodium to make it faintly alkaline to phenolphthalein), and titrate again. **specific gravity, m. for,** see Hammerschlag's m. and Fishberg's m., and see under tests. **split cast m.,** 1. a procedure for placing indexed casts on a dental articulator to facilitate their removal and replacement on the instrument. 2. the procedure of checking the ability of a dental articulator to receive or be adjusted to a maxillomandibular relation record. Called also split cast mounting. **Stammer's m.** (for glucose in blood): precipitate blood proteins by boiling with acid sodium sulfate and treatment with dialyzed iron. In a test tube place 20 ml. of blood filtrate, 2 drops of a 20 per cent solution of sodium hydroxide and 1 ml. of a 0.0075 per cent solution of methylene blue. Boil until the blue color is discharged. The length of time required indicates the amount of sugar present. Time is counted from the beginning of vigorous boiling: thirty-seven seconds indicates 0.3 per cent sugar; sixty seconds, 0.225 per cent; one minute twenty-five seconds, 0.175 per cent; one minute fifty-five seconds, 0.125 per cent; and two minutes forty-five seconds, 0.075 per cent. **Stas-Otto m.,** a method of separating alkaloids and similar amino compounds. **Stehle's m.** (for urea): decompose the urea in a Van Slyke pipet by sodium hypobromite and measure the nitrogen; called also gasometric m. **Stockholm and Koch's m.** (for total sulfur in biological material): the material is disintegrated by heating in strong sodium hydroxide, then oxidized with 30 per cent H_2O_2, and then with nitric acid, and bromine. Precipitate the sulfuric acid with barium, wash, dry, ignite, and weigh. **sugar, m's for,** see glucose (dextrose), m's for. **sulfates, ethereal, m's for,** see Folin's m. (10), Raiziss and Dubin's m., and Rosenheim and Drummond's m. **sulfates, inorganic, m's for,** see Folin's m. (11), Raiziss and Dubin's m., and Rosenheim and Drummond's m. **sulfur, total, m's for,** see Denis and Leche's m., Folin's m. (14), Osborne and Folin's m., and Stockholm and Koch's m. **Sumner's m.** (for sugar in urine): heat 1 ml. of urine and 3 ml. of Sumner's dinitrosalicylic acid reagent, dilute to 25 ml. and compare the color with that of a standard sugar solution similarly treated. **suspension m.,** a method of intracavitary irradiation of the bladder wall by instilling a radioactive solution or suspension directly into the bladder by means of a catheter. **Taylor and Hulton's m.** (for total nitrogen): similar to Folin and Farmer's method except that small amounts of sulfuric acid are used and the ammonia is nesslerized in the original tube without being aerated over into acid. **Thane's m.,** a method of locating the fissure of Rolando. Its upper end is about one-half inch behind the middle of a line uniting the inion and the glabella, and its lower end about one-quarter inch above and one and one-quarter inches behind the external angular process of the frontal bone. **Thézac-Porsmeur m.,** heliotherapy of suppurating wounds by concentrating the sun's rays on the part by means of a large double convex lens mounted on a cylinder of canvas three feet long. **thyroid activity, m. for,** see *thyroid function tests,* under *tests.* **Tisdall's m.** *(for phenols in urine):* extract the phenolic substances from the urine with ether and then shake them from the ether with 10 per cent NaOH. Neutralize and proceed as in the Folin and Denis method (5). **total acidity, m. for,** see *Folin's m.* (13). **total fixed base, m. for,** see *Fiske's m.* **total nitrogen, m. for,** see *nitrogen, total, m.'s for.* **total sulfur, m. for,** see *sulfur, total, m.'s for.* **Tracy and Welker's m.** *(for deproteinizing urine):* a method depending on the use of aluminum hydroxide cream. **Trillat's m.,** volatilization of formaldehyde in an autoclave under pressure to prevent polymerization. **Trueta m.,** see under *treatment.* **tryptic activity, m. for,** see *Gross's m.* **Tswett's m.,** chromatography. **Tuffier's m.** *(obs.),* see *spinal anesthesia* (def. 1), under *anesthesia.* **uranium acetate m.** *(for phosphorus):* add sodium acetate and acetic acid to the urine, heat to boiling, and titrate with a special uranium acetate solution. **urea, m's for,** see *Benedict's m.* (3), *Clark and Collip's m.* (2), *Folin's m.* (15), Folin and Wu's m. (6), *Karr's m., Krogh's m., Marshall's m., Myers' m., Sjöqvist's m., Stehle's m.,* and *Van Slyke and Cullen's m.* (2). See also *urea test,* under *tests.* **urease m's,** see *Marshall's m.* and *Van Slyke and Cullen's m.* (2), and see under *tests.* **uric acid, m's for,** see *Folin and Wu's m.* (7), *Heintz's m., Hunter and Given's m., Krueger and Schmidt's m., Ruheman's m.,* and *Salkowski's m.* See also *uric acid test,* under *tests.* **urobilinogen, m. for,** see *Wallace and Diamond's m.,* and see *urobilin test,* under *tests.* **van Gehuchten's m.,** fixing of a histologic tissue in a mixture of glacial acetic acid 10 parts, chloroform 30 parts, and alcohol 60 parts. **Van Slyke's m.** *(for amino-nitrogen):* the unknown is treated with nitrous acid in a special apparatus and the nitrogen liberated is measured. **Van Slyke and Cullen's m.,** 1. *(for the carbon dioxide in blood, or for the alkali reserve of blood):* freshly prepared oxalated plasma is brought into equilibrium with the carbon dioxide of expired air, acid is then added to a measured amount of the blood, and the carbon dioxide is pumped out and measured. 2. *(for urea):* the urea is changed into ammonium carbonate by means of the enzyme urease, the ammonia is aerated over into standard acid, and the excess titrated. **Van Slyke and Fitz's m.** *(for alkali reserve):* collect the urine for a two-hour period between meals; note amount and determine the ammonia and the titratable acid by Folin's methods. The plasma carbon dioxide capacity (C) may be calculated from the formula $C = 80 - 5\sqrt{D} \div W$, where D = rate of excretion per twenty-four hours, and W = body weight in kilograms. **Van Slyke and Meyer's m.** *(for amino-acid nitrogen):* precipitate the proteins of the blood by means of alcohol and then proceed by Van Slyke's nitrous acid method. **Van Slyke and Palmer's m.** *(for organic acids in urine):* remove carbonates and phosphates and titrate with acid from the turning point for phenolphthalein to the turning point for tropeolin OO. **vertical condensation m.,** a method of filling a root canal by alternately heating and vertically condensing gutta-percha until the apical third of the canal is filled; the coronal portion of the canal is then filled with warmed 2- to 4-mm sections of gutta-percha cones. **Volhard and Arnold's m.** *(for chlorides):* acidify the urine with nitric acid and add a known amount of silver nitrate. Titrate excess of silver nitrate with ammonium sulfocyanate, using ferric thiocyanate as indicator. **Volhard and Harvey's m.** *(for chlorides):* similar to the method of Volhard and Arnold except that the silver chloride is not filtered out, the excess of silver nitrate being titrated in the original mixture. **von Fürth and Charnass' m.** *(for lactic acid in blood):* remove the glucose and convert the lactic acid into acetaldehyde by permanganate. Combine the aldehyde with sodium bisulfite and determine the bound sulfite iodometrically. **Walker's m.** *(for iron in foods):* ignite sample, cool, and dissolve in dilute HNO_3. Filter, filtrate with H_2O_2, add potassium thiocyanate, and compare color with standard iron solution, similarly treated. **Wallace and Diamond's m.** *(for urobilinogen):* add Ehrlich's aldehyde reagent to a series of dilutions of the urine, note the highest dilution which shows a faint pink coloration, and express the result in terms of this dilution. **Wallhauser and Whitehead's m.,** the use of autogenous gland filtrate in the treatment of Hodgkin's disease. **Waring's m.,** a method of sewage disposal by subsurface irrigation; called also *Waring's system.* **Weber's m.** *(for guanidine):* a colorimetric method based on the reaction of guanidine with an alkaline nitro-prusside-ferricyanide reagent. **Welcker's m.,** determination of the total blood volume by bleeding and then washing out the blood vessels. **Welker's m.** *(for purine bodies):* remove the phosphates with magnesia mixture, then precipitate the purine bodies with silver nitrate and ammonium hydroxide. Determine nitrogen in the precipitate by Kjeldahl's method. **Welker and Marsh's m.** *(for clarifying milk):* a method using aluminum hydroxide. **Westergren m.** *(for erythrocyte sedimentation rate [ESR]),* the standard method for ESR, used since 1924; four volumes of whole blood are mixed with one volume of sodium citrate anticoagulant-diluent solution and placed in a Westergren tube, a straight pipette 2.5 mm in internal diameter and graduated in millimeters from 0 to 200, filling to the 0 mark; the tube is left standing undisturbed in a vertical position, and the fall of the level of red cells in exactly one hour is recorded (in mm/hr). **Whipple's m.,** the use of liver in pernicious anemia. **Whitehorn's m.** *(for chlorides in blood):* to the protein-free blood filtrate add nitric acid, then heat, and add an excess of silver nitrate. Titrate excess silver with thiocyanate, using ferric ammonium sulfate as indicator. **Wiechowski and Handorsky's m.** *(for allantoin):* precipitate the urine with phosphotungstic acid, with lead acetate, and with silver acetate to remove chlorides, ammonia, and basic substances. Then add sodium acetate and 0.5 per cent mercuric acetate to precipitate the allantoin, which may be weighed, submitted to a Kjeldahl, or titrated with ammonium thiocyanate. **Wintrobe m.** *(for erythrocyte sedimentation rate [ESR]):* EDTA anticoagulated whole blood is placed in a Wintrobe hematocrit tube, the tube is left standing undisturbed in a vertical position, and the fall of the level of red cells in exactly one hour is recorded (in mm/hr). The volume of packed red cells can then be determined using the same tube. **Wintrobe and Landsberg's m.** *(for the sedimentation rate of red blood cells):* determine the amount of sedimentation after one hour, then centrifuge and measure the volume of the packed red cells. Correct the first reading by the second by means of a table. **Wolter's m.** *(for iron):* add nitric acid to urine, evaporate to dryness, ignite, oxidize the iron with hydrogen peroxide, add potassium iodide and starch, and titrate excess of iodine with one-hundredth normal thiosulfate. **Wynn m.,** a procedure for repair of bilateral cleft lips by means of a long, narrow triangular flap. **Ziehl-Neelsen m.,** see *acid-fast stain* in *Table of Stains.* **Zsigmondy's gold number m.,** colloidal gold test.

methodism (meth′ŏ-dizm) the system of the Methodist school of medicine.

Methodist (meth′ŏ-dist) an ancient Roman medical sect, influenced by Asclepiades, founded (c. 50 B.C.) by Themison, and perfected by Thessalus of Tralles; its most distinguished member was Soranus. Methodists believed in both atomism and solidism.

methodology (meth″ŏ-dol′o-je) the science of method; the science which deals with the principles of procedure in research and study.

methohexital (meth″o-hek′sĭ-tal) [USP] chemical name: (+)- 1-methyl-5-(1-methyl-2-pentynyl)-5-(2-propenyl)-2,4,6 (1H,3H,5H)-pyrimidinetrione. An ultrashort-acting barbiturate, $C_{14}H_{18}N_2O_3$, occurring as a white to faintly yellowish white, crystalline powder; used as a pharmaceutic necessary in the preparation of the sodium salt for injection. **m. sodium** [USP], the monosodium salt of methohexital, $C_{14}H_{17}$-N_2NaO_3, occurring as a white to off-white hygroscopic powder; used as a general anesthetic, administered intravenously.

methomania (meth″o-ma′ne-ah) [Gr. *methē* drunkenness + *mania* madness] *(obs.)* pathologic craving for alcoholic beverages.

methopholine (meth″o-fo′lēn) chemical name: 1-[2-(4-chlorophenyl) ethyl]-1,2,3,4-tetrahydro-6,7-dimethoxy-2-methylisoquinoline; an analgesic, $C_{20}H_{24}ClNO_2$.

methopromazine maleate (meth″o-pro′mah-zēn) methoxypromazine maleate.

methotrexate (meth″o-trek′sāt) [USP] chemical name: N-[4-[[(2,4-diamino-6-pteridinyl)methyl]methylamino]benzoyl]-L-glutamic acid. A folic acid antagonist, $C_{20}H_{22}N_8O_5$, occurring as an orange-brown, crystalline powder; used as an antineoplastic agent in the treatment of acute and meningeal leukemia, gestational choriocarcinoma, mycosis fungoides, carcinomas of the head and neck, breast, testis, and lung, osteosarcomas and carcinomatosis, and as an antipsoriatic agent, administered orally and intramuscularly. It has also been used as an immunosuppressive agent in immunologically mediated disorders.

methotrimeprazine (meth″o-tri-mep′rah-zēn) [USP] chemical name: (–)-2-methoxy-N,N,β-trimethyl-10H-phenothiazine-10-propanamine. An analgesic, $C_{19}H_{24}N_2OS$, occurring as a fine, white, crystalline powder; administered intramuscularly. Called also *levomepromazine*.

methoxamine hydrochloride (mĕ-thok′sah-mēn) chemical name: α-(1-aminoethyl)-2,5-dimethoxybenzenemethanol hydrochloride. An adrenergic, $C_{11}H_{17}NO_3\cdot$HCl, occurring as colorless or white, platelike crystals or white, crystalline powder; used for its vasopressor effect to support, restore, or maintain blood pressure during anesthesia and in the treatment of paroxysmal supraventricular tachycardia, administered intramuscularly and intravenously.

methoxsalen (mĕ-thok′sah-len) [USP] chemical name: 9-methoxy-7H-furo[3,2-g][1]benzopyran-7-one. A psoralen found in *Amni majus* and other plants, $C_{12}H_8O_4$, occurring as white to cream-colored fluffy, needle-like crystals; used orally and topically in conjunction with exposure to ultraviolet light to facilitate repigmentation in idiopathic vitiligo, and to produce a phototoxic reaction in psoriasis. It is also used as a suntan accelerator and sun protectant.

methoxychlor (mĕ-thok′se-klor) chemical name: 1,1′-(2,2,2-trichloroethylidene)bis[4-methoxybenzene]. A chlorinated hydrocarbon insecticide, $C_{16}H_{15}Cl_3O_2$, effective against mosquito larvae and houseflies.

methoxyflurane (meth-ok″se-floo′răn) [USP] chemical name: 2,2-dichloro-1,1-difluroethyl methyl ether, a highly potent inhalational anesthetic agent, used primarily to produce analgesia during the first stage of labor; its use in surgery is limited by a dose-related nephrotoxicity to procedures of short duration; it produces profound analgesia and good muscle relaxation; induction and recovery are slower than with halothane or enflurane.

methoxyl (mĕ-thok′sil) the chemical group, $CH_3\cdot O—$.

methoxyphenamine hydrochloride (mĕ-thok″se-fe-n′ah-mēn) [USP] chemical name: 2-methoxy-N,α-dimethylbenzeneethanamine hydrochloride. An adrenergic, $C_{11}H_{17}NO\cdot$HCl, occurring as a white to off-white, crystalline powder; used mainly as a bronchodilator in the treatment of bronchial asthma, administered orally.

methoxypromazine maleate (mĕ-thok″se-pro′ mah-zēn) chemical name: 2-methoxy-N,N-dimethyl-10H-phenothiazine-10-propanamine maleate; a central depressant, $C_{22}H_{26}N_2O_5S$. Called also *methopromazine maleate*.

8-methoxypsoralen (mĕ-thok″se-sor′ah-len) methoxsalen.

methphenoxydiol (meth″fen-ok″sĭ-di′ol) guaifenesin.

methscopolamine bromide (meth″sko-pol′ah-mēn) [USP] chemical name: [7(S)-(1α,2β,4β,5α,7β)]-7-(3-hydroxy-1-oxo-2-phenylpropoxy)-9,9-dimethyl-3-oxa-9-azoniatricyclo[3.3.1.0²′⁴]nonane bromide. An anticholinergic, the quaternary ammonium derivative of scopolamine hydrobromide, $C_{18}H_{24}$-BrNO$_4$, occurring as white crystals or as a white, crystalline powder, it has an inhibitory effect on gastric secretion and gastrointestinal motility and is used as an adjunct for the treatment of peptic ulcer and gastric disorders associated with spasm, hyperacidity, and hypermotility, administered orally, subcutaneously, and intramuscularly. Called also *scopolamine methylbromide*.

methsuximide (meth-suk′sĭ-mīd) [USP] chemical name: 1,3-dimethyl-3-phenyl-2,5-pyrrolidinedione. An anticonvulsant, $C_{12}H_{13}NO_2$, occurring as a white to grayish white, crystalline powder; used in the treatment of petit mal and psychomotor epilepsy, administered orally.

methyclothiazide (meth″ĭ-klo-thi′ah-zīd) [USP] a thiazide diuretic; used for treatment of hypertension and edema.

methyl (meth′il) [Gr. *methy* wine + *hylē* wood] the chemical group or radical $CH_3—$, sometimes abbreviated Me. **m. amylketone,** a volatile oil, $C_5H_{11}\cdot CO\cdot CH_3$, found in oil of cloves. **m. anthranilate,** chemical name: methyl 2-aminobenzoate. A volatile oil, $NH_2\cdot C_6H_4\cdot CO\cdot O\cdot CH_3$, the

odoriferous constituent or neroli oil, bergamot, jasmine, and other essential oils. **m. benzene,** toluene. **m. chloride,** the hydrochloric acid ester of methyl alcohol, CH_3Cl. When converted by pressure from gas into liquid, it can be used in spray form as a local anesthetic. **m. cyanide,** acetonitrile. **m. ethyl-maleicimid,** a substituted pyrrole, $C_2H_5(C\cdot CO\cdot NH\cdot CO)CCH_3$, obtained from hemoglobin and from chlorophyll. **m. ethyl-pyrrole,** a substituted pyrrole, $CH_3(C:CH\cdot NH:CH:C)C_2H_5$, obtained from, and probably a constituent of, bilirubin. **m. eugenol,** a volatile oil, $C_3H_5\cdot C_6H_3(OCH_3)_2$, found in oil of bay. **m. heptenone,** a volatile oil, $C_8H_{16}O$, found in lemon-grass oil. **m. hydride,** methane. **m. hydroxy-furfurol,** the furfural, $CH_3\cdot C:CH\cdot C(OH):C\cdot CHO$, produced from the hexose in Molisch's test and which produces the color. **m. iodide,** a colorless or brownish liquid, CH_3I, used as a local anesthetic and formerly as a vesicant. **m. isobutyl ketone** [NF], chemical name: 4-methyl-2-pentanone. A transparent, colorless, mobile, volatile liquid, $C_6H_{12}O$; used as an alcohol denaturant in pharmaceutical preparations. **m. methacrylate,** a methyl ester of methacrylic acid, which polymerizes to form polymethyl methacrylate; used in the manufacture of acrylic resins (q.v.) and plastics. **m. salicylate** [NF], salicylic acid methyl ester, a volatile oil with a characteristic wintergreen odor and taste; used as a counterirritant in ointments or liniments for muscle pain and also as a flavoring agent. Called also *betula oil, gaultheria oil, sweet birch oil,* and *wintergreen oil.* **m. sulfonate,** a crystalline, noncaustic, and nonpoisonous antiseptic. **m. telluride,** a gas, $(CH_3)_2Te$, of penetrating odor found in excreta of animals after feeding with telluric and tellurious acids.

α-methylacetoacetyl CoA-β-ketothiolase (meth″il-ah-se″to-as′ĕ-til ke″to-thi′o-lās) acetyl-CoA acyltransferase.

methylal (meth′ĭ-lal) a colorless liquid, $CH_2(OCH_3)_2$, used as a hypnotic and anesthetic and like formaldehyde in certain chemical reactions.

methylamine (meth″il-am′in) a gaseous ptomaine CH_3-NH_2, from decaying fish and from comma-bacillus cultures.

methylarsinate (meth″il-ar′si-nāt) a salt of methylarsinic acid.

methylate (meth′ĭ-lāt) 1. a compound of methyl alcohol and a base. 2. to add a methyl group to a substance.

methylated (meth′ĭ-lāt-ed) containing or combined with a methyl group.

methylation (meth″ĭ-la′shun) treatment with reagent to add a methyl group to a compound.

methylatropine nitrate (meth″il-at′ro-pēn) chemical name: *endo*-(+)-3-(3-hydroxy-1-oxo-2-phenylpropoxy)-8,8-dimethyl-8-azoniabicyclo[3.2.1] octane nitrate (salt). A quaternary ammonium derivative of atropine, $C_{18}H_{25}N_2O_6$, having the same actions and uses as atropine (q.v.), but with much less effect on the central nervous system and with strong ganglionic blocking activity. Called also *atropine methonitrate* and *atropine methylnitrate.*

methylaurin (meth″il-aw′rin) a substance, $C_{23}H_{16}O_3$, derivable from aurin.

methylazoxymethanol (meth″il-az-ok″se-meth′ah-nol) a carcinogen formed after hydrolysis of cycasin by intestinal bacteria.

methylbenzethonium chloride (meth″il-ben″zĕ-tho′ne-um) [USP] chemical name: N,N-dimethyl-N-[2-[2-[methyl-4-(1,1,3,3-tetramethylbutyl)phenoxy]ethoxy]ethyl]benzenemethanaminium chloride monohydrate. A disinfectant quaternary compound, $C_{28}H_{44}ClNO_2\cdot H_2O$, occurring as white crystals, which is bacteriostatic for urea-splitting organisms that may cause ammonia dermatitis. It is applied topically to areas of the skin coming in contact with urine, feces, or perspiration, and is used in a rinse for diapers, bed linen, and undergarments of incontinent adults and children.

methylcellulose (meth″il-sel′u-lōs) [USP] a methyl ether of cellulose, occurring as a white, fibrous powder or granules, supplied in differing degrees of viscosity; used as a suspending and viscosity-increasing agent and tablet excipient in pharmaceutical preparations, administered orally as a cathartic, and applied topically to the conjunctiva to protect the cornea during certain ophthalmic procedures and to lubricate the cornea. **hydroxypropyl m.,** see under *H.*

methylchloroformate (meth″il-klo″ro-for′māt) a lacrimatory gas, $ClCOOCH_3$, used as a warning agent in fumigations with hydrocyanic acid.

3-methylcholanthrene (meth″il-ko-lan′thrēn) a highly carcinogenic polycyclic aromatic hydrocarbon synthesized by pyrolytic degradation of cholic acid, deoxycholic acid, or cholesterol. It is a procarcinogen that requires metabolic activation to exert a mutagenic effect and is widely used in laboratory studies of chemical carcinogenesis. Abbreviated MCA.

methylcreosol (meth″il-kre′o-sol) a phenol, $C_9H_{12}O_2$, obtainable from wood tar creosote.

methylcrotonoyl-CoA carboxylase (meth″il-kroton′o-il kar-bok′sĭ-lās) [EC 6.4.1.4] an enzyme of the ligase class that catalyzes the reaction ATP + 3-methylcrotonoyl-CoA + HCO_3^- = ADP + orthophosphate + 3-methylglutaconyl-CoA. The enzyme is a biotin protein. The reaction is a step in the use of leucine as a fuel. A genetic defect in the enzyme results in β-methylcrotonylglycinuria.

3-methylcrotonyl CoA carboxylase deficiency a genetic aminoacidopathy due to a metabolic block at the third stage of leucine catabolism; clinical manifestations are varied. Called also β-methylcrotonylglycinuria.

β-methylcrotonylglycinuria (meth″il-kro″to-nil-gli″si-nu′re-ah) an autosomal recessive aminoacidopathy due to deficient methylcrotonyl-CoA carboxylase. Increased levels of β-methylcrotonyl acid and β-methylcrotonyl glycine occur in the urine. Those affected may show mental retardation, central nervous system dysfunction, and muscular atrophy.

methylcytosine (meth″il-si′to-sin) a pyrimidine occurring in deoxyribonucleic acid.

methyldichlorarsin (meth″il-di″klor-ar′sin) a lethal and vesicating war gas, CH_3AsCl_2.

methyldihydromorphinone (meth″il-di-hi″dro-mor′fĭ-nōn) metopon (def. 2).

methyldopa (meth″il-do′pah) [USP] chemical name: 3-hydroxy-α-methyl-L-tyrosine. An orally effective antihypertensive, $C_{10}H_{13}NO_4 1\frac{1}{2}H_2O$, occurring as a white to yellowish white, fine powder.

methyldopate hydrochloride (meth″il-do′pāt) [USP] chemical name: 3-hydroxy-α-methyl-L-tyrosine ethyl ester hydrochloride. The ethyl ester hydrochloride of methyldopa, $C_{12}H_{17}NO_4·HCl$, occurring as a white to practically white, crystalline powder; used as an antihypertensive, administered by intravenous infusion.

methylene (meth″ĭ-lēn) the bivalent hydrocarbon radical —CH_2— or CH_2=. Called also *methene*. **m. bichloride,** 1. see *m. chloride.* 2. a mixture of methyl alcohol and chloroform formerly used as an anesthetic agent. **m. blue,** see under *blue.* **m. chloride, m. dichloride,** a volatile anesthetic liquid, CH_2Cl_2, resembling chloroform, formerly used as an anesthetic in minor operations.

5,10-methylenetetrahydrofolate reductase (FADH₂) (meth″il-ēn-tet″rah-hi″dro-fo′lāt re-duk′tās) [EC 1.7.99.5] an enzyme of the oxidoreductase class that catalyzes the reaction 5,10-methylenetetrahydrofolate + FADH₂ = 5-methyltetrahydrofolate + FAD. NAD acts as a secondary electron donor. The reaction is the means by which methyl groups are generated *de novo* for methylation reactions. Deficiency of the enzyme produces homocystinuria II.

methylenetetrahydrofolate (THF) reductase deficiency the most common genetic aminoacidopathy of folate metabolism; the chief biochemical finding is homocystinuria with normal levels of plasma methionine; the chief clinical sign is CNS damage.

methylenophil (meth″ĭ-len′o-fil) 1. an element easily stainable with methylene blue. 2. methylenophilous.

methylenophilous (meth″il-en-of′ĭ-lus) [*methylene* + Gr. *philein* to love] stainable with methylene blue.

methylergonovine maleate (meth″il-er″go-no′vēn) [USP] chemical name: 9,10-didehydro-N-[1-(hydroxymethyl)propyl]-6-methylergoline-8β(S)-carboxamide (Z)-2-butenedioate (1:1) (salt). An oxytocic, $C_{20}H_{25}N_3O_2·C_4H_4O_4$, occurring as a white to pinkish tan, microcrystalline powder; used especially to prevent or combat postpartum hemorrhage and atony, administered orally, intramuscularly, and intravenously.

methylglucamine (meth″il-gloo′kah-mīn) 1. a compound prepared from D-glucose and methylamine, used in the synthesis of pharmaceuticals. 2. meglumine.

methylglyoxalase (meth″il-gli-oks′ah-lās) lactoylglutathione lyase.

methylglyoxalidin (meth″il-gli″oks-al′ĭ-din) lysidin.

methylguanidine (meth″il-gwan′ĭ-din) a poisonous ptomaine, $NH·C(NH)_2NH·CH_3$, from spoiled fish, etc.

methylhexamine (meth″il-heks′ah-mēn) methylhexaneamine.

methylhexaneamine (meth″il-hek-sān′ah-min) chemical name: 1,3-dimethylamylamine. A colorless to pale yellow liquid, $C_7H_{17}N$, readily soluble in alcohol, used for its sympathomimetic action in nasal congestion. Called also *methyhexamine.*

methylhydantoin (meth″il-hi-dan′to-in) a crystalline compound, $CH_3·N·CO·NH·CO·CH_2$, found in fresh meat, and formed by the decomposition of creatine.

methylic (mĕ-thil′ik) containing methyl.

methylidyne (me-thil′ĭ-dīn) the trivalent hydrocarbon radical —CH= or CH≡. Called also *methine.*

methylindol (meth″il-in′dōl) skatole.

methylmalonic acid (meth″il-mah-lon′ik) HOOC-CH(CH₃)-COOH, an intermediate (as methylmalonyl coenzyme A) in the catabolism of certain amino acids and fatty acids with an odd number of carbon atoms; free methylmalonic acid accumulates in methylmalonic acidemia due to a genetic deficiency of enzymes involved in this catabolic pathway.

methylmalonyl-CoA epimerase (meth″il-mal′o-nil ĕ-pim′er-ās) [EC 5.1.99.1] an enzyme of the isomerase class that catalyzes the equilibration of the (R) and (S) isomers of the methylmalonyl CoA according to the formal reaction (R)- 2-carboxy-propanoyl-CoA = (S)-2-carboxypropanoyl-CoA. The reaction occurs in the conversion of propionyl coenzyme A to succinyl coenzyme A. Called also *methylmalonyl-CoA racemase.*

methylmalonyl-CoA mutase (meth″il-mal-o′nil mu′tās) [EC 5.4.99.2] an enzyme of the isomerase class that catalyzes the reaction (R)-2-carboxypropanoyl-CoA = succinyl-CoA. The enzyme requires adenosylcobalamin as a coenzyme. The reaction is a step in the use of isoleucine, threonine, valine, propionate and other odd-chain fatty acids as fuels. Deficiency of the enzyme, an autosomal recessive trait, results in methylmalonic acidemia.

methylmalonyl-CoA racemase (meth″il-mal′o-nil ra′se-mās) methylmalonyl-CoA epimerase.

methylmercaptan (meth″il-mer-kap′tan) a gas, methyl hydrosulfide, $CH_3·SH$, formed in the intestines by the decomposition of proteins; said to impart to the urine the odor noticed after eating asparagus, and to the breath the characterisic odor of fetor hepatis.

methylmorphine (meth″il-mor′fēn) codeine.

Methylococcaceae (meth″il-o-kok-ka′se-e) a family of gram-negative, aerobic, rod-shaped bacteria that utilize one-carbon organic compounds, such as methane or methanol, as a carbon source. The family includes the genera *Methylococcus* and *Methylomonas.* Formerly called *Methanomonadaceae* and *Methylomonadaceae.*

Methylococcus (meth″il-o-kok′us) [*methyl-* + Gr. *kokkos* berry] a genus of gram-negative, aerobic, coccoid bacteria of the family Methylococcaceae, made up of nonmotile cells that utilize methane and methanol as sole sources of carbon and energy. The type species is *M. capsula′tus.*

Methylomonadaceae (meth″il-o-mo″nah-da′se-e) Methylococcaceae.

Methylomonas (meth″il-o-mo′nas) [*methyl-* + Gr. *monas* unit, from *monos* single] a genus of gram-negative, aerobic, rod-shaped bacteria of the family Methylococcaceae, made up of motile cells that utilize methane and methanol as sole sources of carbon and energy. The type species is *M. metha′nica.* Formerly called *Methanomonas.*

methylparaben (meth″il-par′ah-ben) [NF] chemical name: 4-hydroxybenzoic acid methyl ester. An antifungal agent, $C_8H_8O_3$, occurring as small, colorless crystals, or white, crystalline powder; used as a preservative in pharmaceutical preparations.

methylparafynol (meth″il-par″ah-fi′nol) meparfynol.

methylpentynol (meth″il-pen′tĭ-nol) meparfynol.

methylphenidate hydrochloride (meth″il-fen″ĭ-dāt) [USP] chemical name: (R*,R*)-(±)-α-phenyl-2-piperidineacetic acid methyl ester hydrochloride. A central stimulant, $C_{14}H_{19}NO_2 \cdot HCl$, occurring as a white, fine, crystalline powder; used in the treatment of hyperkinetic children, various types of depression, and narcolepsy, administered orally.

methylphenyl levulosazone (meth″il-fen′il lev″u-lo′sa-zōn) the methyl-phenyl-osazone of levulose, CH_2OH (CHOH) $_4C$ [: N·N- $(CH_3) \cdot C_6H_5$]·CHCH·NHN$(CH_3) \cdot C_6H_5$:, homologous with glucosazone.

methylphenylhydrazine (meth″il-fe″nil-hi′drah-zin) a reagent, $C_6H_5N(CH_3)NH_2$, by which ketoses can be distinguished from aldoses, as the former yield osazones, the latter, hydrazones.

methylprednisolone (meth″il-pred″nĭ-so-lōn) [USP] chemical name: 11β,17, 21-trihydroxy-6α-methylpregna-1,4-diene. A synthetic glucocorticoid derived from prednisolone, $C_{22}H_{30}O_5$, with slightly greater anti-inflammatory activity and slightly less sodium-retaining activity than prednisolone; occurring as a white to practically white, crystalline powder, it is administered orally in the treatment of various conditions responsive to the anti-inflammatory actions of glucocorticoids, including rheumatoid arthritis and other collagen diseases, allergic conditions, and certain inflammatory eye diseases, and in acquired hemolytic anemias, lymphoma, and leukemia. **m. acetate** [USP], the 21-acetate ester of methylprednisolone, $C_{24}H_{32}O_6$, occurring as a white or practically white, crystalline powder, having actions and uses similar to those of the base; administered by enema, intra-articular, intramuscular, intralesional, or intracutaneous injection, and applied topically. **m. hemisuccinate** [USP], the hemisuccinate salt of methylprednisolone, $C_{26}H_{34}O_8$, occurring as a white or nearly white hygroscopic solid, having actions and uses similar to those of the base. **m. sodium phosphate,** the 21-phosphate disodium salt of methylprednisolone, $C_{22}H_{29}Na_2O_8P$, having actions similar to those of the base. **m. sodium succinate** [USP], the 21-succinate sodium salt of methylprednisolone, $C_{26}H_{33}NaO_8$, occurring as a white or nearly white, amorphous solid, having actions and uses similar to those of the base; used chiefly for short-term emergency treatment, administered by intramuscular or intravenous injection.

methylpurine (meth″il-pu′rin) see under *purine*.

methylpyrapone (meth″il-pi′rah-pōn) metyrapone.

methylpyridine (meth″il-pi′ri-din) a basic substance, C_5-$H_4(CH_3)N$, oxidized in the body to pyridine-carboxylic acid.

methylquinoline (meth″il-kwin′o-lin) an oily basic substance, $C_9H_6N \cdot CH_3$, from the secretion of the skunk.

methylrosaniline chloride (meth″il-ro-zan′i-lin) gentian violet; see under *violet*.

methyltestosterone (meth″il-tes-tos′ter-ōn) [USP] chemical name: 17β-hydroxy-17α-methylandrost-4-en-3-one. A synthetic androgen derived from cholesterol, $C_{20}H_{30}O_2$, occurring as white or creamy white crystals or crystalline powder, having actions similar to those of testosterone (q.v.); used as replacement therapy for androgen deficiency in males, in the palliation of certain inoperable mammary cancers, and to prevent postpartum breast pain and engorgement in the non-nursing mother, administered orally or sublingually.

5-methyltetrahydrofolate-homocysteine methyltransferase (meth″il-tet″rah-hi″dro-fo′lāt ho″mo-sis′te-in meth″il-trans′fer-ās) [EC 2.1.1.13] an enzyme of the oxidoreductase class that catalyzes the reaction 5-methyltetrahydrofolate + L-homocysteine = tetrahydrofolate + L-methionine. The reaction utilizes methyl groups synthesized *de novo* and transfers them to homocysteine, regenerating methionine. The enzyme requires methylcobalamin as a coenzyme. Decreased enzyme activity, resulting from malabsorption of cobalamin or defective coenzyme synthesis, results in homocystinuria. Called also *homocysteine:tetrahydrofolate methyltransferase*.

methyltheobromine (meth″il-the″o-bro′mēn) caffeine.

methylthionine chloride (meth″il-thi′o-nin) methylene blue.

methylthiouracil (meth″il-thi″o-u′rah-sil) [USP] chemical name: 2,3-dihydro-6-methyl-2-thioxo-4(1H)-pyrimidinone. A thyroid suppressant, $C_5H_6N_2OS$, occurring as a white, crystalline powder; used in the treatment of hyperthyroidism, especially to prepare patients for thyroid surgery

and to maintain those who are poor surgical risks, administered orally. Abbreviated MTU.

methyltransferase (meth″il-trans′fer-ās) [EC 2.1.1] any enzyme of a sub-subgroup of enzymes of the transferase class that catalyzes the transfer of a methyl group from one compound to another. Called also *transmethylase*.

methyluramine (meth″il-u-ram′in) methylguanidine.

methylxanthine (meth″il-zan′thin) any of the methylated derivatives of xanthine, including caffeine, theobromine, and theophylline and their derivatives.

methynodiol diacetate (mĕ-thin″o-di′ōl) chemical name: 11β-methyl-19-norpregn-4-en-20-yne-3β,17α-diol; a progestin, $C_{25}H_{34}O_4$.

methyprylon (meth″ĭ-pri′lon) [USP] chemical name: 3,3-diethyl-5-methyl-2,4-piperidinedione. A hypnotic, $C_{10}H_{17}$-NO_2, occurring as a white, or nearly white, crystalline powder; administered orally.

methysergide (meth″ĭ-ser′jīd) chemical name: 9,10-didehydro-N-[1-(hydroxymethyl)propyl]-1,6-dimethylergoline-8β-carboxamide. A potent serotonin antagonist, $C_{21}H_{27}$-N_3O_2, having direct vasoconstrictor effects. **m. maleate** [USP], the maleate salt of methysergide, $C_{21}H_{27}N_3O_2 \cdot C_4H_4$-$O_4$, occurring as a white to yellowish white or reddish white, crystalline powder, having the same actions as the base; used as an analgesic in the treatment of vascular (migraine) headache in certain patients, administered orally.

metiamide (mĕ-ti′ah-mīd) chemical name: N-methyl-N'-[2-[[(5-methyl-1H-imidazol-4-yl)methyl]thio]ethyl]thiourea; an antagonist to histamine, competing for the H_2 receptor site on cells, $C_9H_{16}N_4S_2$.

metiapine (mĕ-ti′ah-pēn) chemical name: 2-methyl-11-(4-methyl-1-piperazinyl)dibenzo[b,f][1,4]thiazepine; a tranquilizer, $C_{19}H_{21}N_3S$, which has been used in the treatment of schizophrenia.

Meticortelone (met″ĭ-kor′tĕ-lōn) trademark for preparations of prednisolone.

Meticorten (met″ĭ-kor′ten) trademark for a preparation of prednisone.

metizoline hydrochloride (mĕ-tiz′o-lēn) chemical name: 4,5-dihydro-2-[(2-methylbenzo[b]thien-3-yl)methyl]-1H-imidazole monohydrochloride; an adrenergic with vasoconstrictor effects, $C_{13}H_{14}N_2S \cdot HCl$.

metmyoglobin (met-mi″o-glo′bin) a compound formed from myoglobin by oxidation of the ferrous to the ferric state.

metoclopramide hydrochloride (met″o-klo′prah-mīd) chemical name: 4-amino-5-chloro-N-[2-(diethylamino)ethyl]-2-methoxybenzamide monohydrochloride monohydrate; an antiemetic, $C_{14}H_{22}ClN_3O_2 \cdot HCl$.

metocurine iodide (met″o-ku′rēn) [USP] chemical name: 6,6′,6′,12′-tetramethoxy-2,2,2′,2′-tetramethyltubocuraranium diiodide. A skeletal muscle relaxant, $C_{40}H_{48}I_2N_2O_6$, occurring as a white or nearly white, crystalline powder; administered intravenously. Called also *dimethyl tubocurarine iodide*.

metoestrum (met-es′trum) metestrus.

metoestrus (met-es′trus) metestrus.

metogest (met′o-jest) chemical name: 17β-hydroxy-16,16-dimethylestr-4-en-3-one; a hormone, $C_{20}H_{30}O_2$.

metolazone (mĕ-tōl′ah-zōn) a diuretic with the same pharmacologic action as that of thiazide diuretics; used for treatment of hypertension and edema.

metonymy (mĕ-ton′ĭ-me) [*meta*- + Gr. *onyma* name] a disturbance of language seen in schizophrenic disorders in which an inappropriate but related term is used instead of the correct one.

metopagus (mĕ-top′ah-gus) metopopagus.

metopic (me-top′ik) pertaining to the forehead; frontal.

metopimazine (met″o-pim′ah-zēn) chemical name: 1-[3-[2-(methylsulfonyl)-10H-phenothiazin-10-yl]propyl]-4-piperidinecarboxamide; an antiemetic, $C_{22}H_{27}N_3O_3S_2$.

metopion (mĕ-to′pe-on) glabella.

Metopirone (met″o-pi′rōn) trademark for preparations of metyrapone.

metopism (met′o-pizm) the persistence of the frontal suture.

metop(o)- [Gr. *metōpon* forehead] a combining form denoting relationship to the forehead.

metopodynia (met″o-po-din′e-ah) [*metopo-* + Gr. *odynē* pain] frontal headache.

metopon (mĕ-to′pon) 1. [Gr. *metōpon* forehead] (*obs.*) the anterior portion of the frontal lobe of the brain. 2. a morphine derivative, methyldihydromorphinone hydrochloride, used to relieve pain.

metopopagus (met″o-pop′ah-gus) [*metopo-* + Gr. *pagos* thing fixed] a craniopagus in which the fusion is in the region of the forehead.

metoposcopy (met″o-pos′ko-pe) [*metopo-* + Gr. *skopein* to examine] the analysis of character based on shape of the forehead.

metoprine (met′o-prēn) chemical name: 5-(3,4-dichlorophenyl)-6-methyl-2,4-pyrimidinediamine; an antineoplastic, $C_{11}H_{10}Cl_2N_4$.

metoprolol (mĕ-to′pro-lōl)) chemical name: 1-[4-(2-methoxyethyl)phenyl]-3-[(1-methylethyl)amino-2-propanol; an antiadrenergic, $C_{15}H_{25}NO_3$, which is chiefly a beta₁ blocker. Used orally in the treatment of hypertension.

Metorchis (met-or′kis) [*meta-* + Gr. *orchis* testicle] *Pseudamphistomum.*

metoserpate hydrochloride (met″o-ser′pāt) chemical name: 11,17α,18α-trimethoxy-3β,20α-yohimban-16β-carboxylic acid methyl ester monohydrochloride; a veterinary sedative, $C_{24}H_{32}N_2O_5 \cdot HCl$.

metoxenous (mĕ-tok′sĕ-nus) [*meta-* + Gr. *xenos* host] requiring two hosts for the full cycle of existence; said of certain parasites.

metoxeny (mĕ-tok′sĕ-ne) the condition of being metoxenous.

metra (me′trah) [Gr. *metra* womb] uterus.

metralgia (mĕ-tral′je-ah) [*metra-* + *-algia*] pain in the uterus; metrodynia.

metraterm (me′trah-term) [*metra-* + L. *terminus* boundary] the external opening of the uterus in some tapeworms (Diphyllobothriidae).

metratonia (me″trah-to′ne-ah) [*metra-* + Gr. *atonia* atony] uterine atony.

metratrophia (me″trah-tro′fe-ah) [*metra-* + Gr. *atrophia* atrophy] uterine atrophy.

Metrazol (met′rah-zol) trademark for preparations of pentylenetetrazol.

metre (me′ter) meter.

metrechoscopy (met″rĕ-kos′ko-pe) [Gr. *metron* measure + *ēchō* sound + *skopein* to examine] combined mensuration, auscultation, and inspection.

metrectomy (mĕ-trek′to-me) [*metra-* + Gr. *ektomē* excision] hysterectomy.

metrectopia (me″trek-to′pe-ah) [*metra-* + Gr. *ektopos* displaced + *-ia*] uterine displacement.

Metreton (met′rĕ-ton) trademark for a preparation of prednisolone sodium phosphate.

metreurynter (me″troo-rin′ter) [*metra-* + Gr. *eurynein* to stretch] an inflatable bag for dilating the cervical canal of the uterus.

metreurysis (me-troo′ri-sis) dilation of the uterine cervix with the metreurynter.

metria (me′tre-ah) any inflammatory condition of the uterus during the puerperium.

metric (met′rik) [Gr. *metron* measure] 1. pertaining to measures based on the meter; see Appendix 3. 2. having the meter as a basis.

metrifonate (met′ri-fo′nāt) chemical name: (2,2,2-trichloro-1-hydroxyethyl)phosphoric acid dimethyl ester. An organophosphorus insecticide, $C_4H_8Cl_3O_4P$, having potent anticholinesterase activity; used externally as a topical ectoparasiticide and internally as a veterinary anthelmintic; especially effective against *Schistosoma haematobium*. Called also *trichlorfon*.

metriocephalic (met″re-o-sĕ-fal′ik) [Gr. *metrios* moderate + *kephalē* head] having a skull with a vertical index between 72 and 77.

metriphonate (met″ri-fo′nāt) metrifonate.

metritis (mĕ-tri′tis) [*metra-* + *-itis*] inflammation of the uterus. Several varieties are named, according to the part of the organ affected—cervical, corporeal, interstitial, and parenchymatous. **m. dis′secans, dissecting m.,** metritis

characterized by the passage of fragments or large masses of the necrotic uterine wall. **puerperal m.,** infection of the uterus of the puerperal woman.

metrizamide (mĕ-triz′ah-mīd) chemical name: 2-[[3-(acetylamino)-5-(acetylmethylamino)-2,4,6-triiodobenzoyl]amino]-2-deoxy-D-glucose. A radiopaque medium, $C_{18}H_{22}I_3N_3O_8$, used in lumbar myelography; it is water-soluble and is absorbed into the blood stream from the cerebrospinal fluid.

metrizoate sodium (met-ri-zo′āt) chemical name: 3-(acetylamino)-5-(acetylmethylamino)-2,4,6-triiodobenzoic acid monosodium salt; a diagnostic radiopaque medium, $C_{12}H_{10}I_3N_2NaO_4$.

metr(o)- [Gr. *mētra* uterus] a combining form denoting relationship to the uterus; see also *hyster(o)-*.

metrocarcinoma (me″tro-kar″si-no′mah) endometrial carcinoma.

metrocele (me′tro-sēl) [*metro-* + Gr. *kēlē* hernia] hernia of the uterus; hysterocele.

metrocolpocele (me″tro-kol′po-sēl) [*metro-* + Gr. *kolpos* vagina + *kēlē* hernia] hernia of the uterus and the vagina.

metrocystosis (me″tro-sis-to′sis) formation of cysts in the uterus.

metrocyte (me′tro-sīt) [Gr. *mētēr* mother + *-cyte*] a mother cell.

metrodynia (me″tro-din′e-ah) [*metro-* + Gr. *odynē* pain] pain in the uterus; metralgia.

metroendometritis (me″tro-en″do-me-tri′tis) combined inflammation of the uterus and its mucous membranes.

metrofibroma (me″tro-fi-bro′mah) [*metro-* + *fibroma*] leiomyoma of the uterus.

metrogenous (mĕ-troj′ĕ-nus) derived from the uterus.

metrography (mĕ-trog′rah-fe) hysterography.

metroleukorrhea (me″tro-lu″ko-re′ah) leukorrhea of uterine origin.

metrology (mĕ-trol′o-je) [Gr. *metron* measure + *-logy*] the science which deals with measurement.

metrolymphangitis (me″tro-limf″an-ji′tis) inflammation of the uterine lymphatic vessels.

metromalacia (me″tro-mah-la′she-ah) [*metro-* + Gr. *malakia* softness] abnormal softening of the uterus.

metromalacoma (me″tro-mal-ah-ko′mah) metromalacia.

metromenorrhagia (me″tro-men″o-ra′je-ah) metrorrhagia combined with menorrhagia.

metronidazole (me″tro-ni′dah-zōl) [USP] chemical name: 2-methyl-5-nitro-1*H*-imidazole-1-ethanol. An antitrichomonal and antiamebic, $C_6H_9N_3O_3$, occurring as white to pale yellow crystals or crystalline powder; administered orally and intravaginally in *Trichomonas vaginalis* infection in females and orally in male trichomoniasis, and administered orally in intestinal and extraintestinal amebiasis. It is also effective against infections with *Giardia lamblia* and obligate anaerobic bacteria.

metronoscope (mĕ-tron′o-skōp) an instrument for giving exercises in rhythmic reading to correct poorly coordinated ocular movements.

metroparalysis (me″tro-pah-ral′ĭ-sis) paralysis of the uterus.

metropathia (me″tro-path′e-ah) metropathy. **m. hemorrha′gica,** essential uterine hemorrhage.

metropathic (me″tro-path′ik) pertaining to or characterized by uterine disorder.

metropathy (mĕ-trop′ah-the) [*metro-* + Gr. *pathos* suffering] any uterine disease or disorder. **syncytiotrophoblastic m.,** syncytial endometritis.

metroperitoneal (me″tro-per″ĭ-to-ne′al) pertaining to the uterus and peritoneum, or communicating with the uterine and peritoneal cavities, as a metroperitoneal fistula.

metroperitonitis (me″tro-per″ĭ-to-ni′tis) [*metro-* + *peritonitis*] inflammation of the peritoneum about the uterus, or peritonitis resulting from infection after metritis.

metrophlebitis (me″tro-fle-bi′tis) [*metro-* + Gr. *phleps* vein + *-itis*] inflammation of the veins of the uterus.

Metropine (met′ro-pin) trademark for preparations of methylatropine nitrate.

metroplasty (me″tro-plas′te) reconstructive surgery on the uterus.

metropolis (me-trop′o-lis) [Gr. *mētropolis* mother-state, as opposed to her colonies] the area in which a particular species of organisms commonly occurs.

metroptosis (me″tro-to′sis) [*metro-* + Gr. *ptōsis* falling] downward displacement, or prolapse of the uterus.

metrorrhagia (me″tro-ra′je-ah) [*metro-* + Gr. *rhēgnynai* to burst out] uterine bleeding, usually of normal amount, occurring at completely irregular intervals, the period of flow sometimes being prolonged. **m. myopath′ica,** uterine hemorrhage due to insufficient contraction of uterine muscles after parturition.

metrorrhea (me″tro-re′ah) [*metro-* + Gr. *rhoia* flow] a free or abnormal uterine discharge.

metrorrhexis (me″tro-rek′sis) [*metro-* + Gr. *rhēxis* rupture] rupture of the uterus.

metrosalpingitis (me″tro-sal″pin-ji′tis) [*metro-* + Gr. *salpinx* tube + *-itis*] inflammation of the uterus and oviducts.

metrosalpingography (me″tro-sal″ping-gog′rah-fe) hysterosalpingography.

metroscope (me′tro-skōp) hysteroscope.

metrostasis (mĕ-tros′tah-sis) [Gr. *metron* measure + *stasis* a setting] a state in which the length of a muscle fiber is relatively fixed, and at which length it contracts and relaxes.

metrostaxis (me″tro-stak′sis) [*metro-* + Gr. *staxis* a dripping] a slight but persistent escape of blood from the uterus.

metrostenosis (me″tro-ste-no′sis) [*metro-* + Gr. *stenosis* contraction] contraction or stenosis of the cavity of the uterus, as in Asherman's syndrome.

metrotherapy (met″ro-ther′ah-pe) [Gr. *metron* measure + *therapeia* treatment] treatment by measurement, i.e., by demonstrating to the patient his improvement by means of accurate measurements of the increase in the voluntary movements of an impaired joint.

metrotomy (mĕ-trot′o-me) hysterotomy.

metrotubography (me″tro-tu-bog′rah-fe) hysterosalpingography.

-metry [Gr. *metrein* to measure] a word termination denoting the measurement of, or the science of measuring, an object specified by the word stem to which the termination is affixed.

M. et sig. abbreviation for L. *mi′sce et sig′na,* mix and write a label.

Mett's (Mette) method, test tubes (mets) [Emil Ludwig Paul *Mett* (*Mette*) German physician, born 1867] see *Nirenstein and Schiff's method,* under *method,* and see under *tests,* and *tube.*

Metubine (mĕ-tu′bin) trademark for a preparation of metocurine iodide.

meturedepa (met″ūr-ĕ-dĕ′pah) chemical name: [bis(2,2-dimethyl-1-aziridinyl)phosphinyl]carbamic acid ethyl ester; an antineoplastic, $C_{11}H_{22}N_3O_3P$.

Metycaine (met′ĭ-kān) trademark for preparations of piperocaine.

metyrapone (mĕ-tēr′ah-pōn) [USP] an inhibitor of the enzyme steroid 11β-hydroxylase; used in a test of hypothalamic-pituitary function. See *metyrapone test,* under *test.* **m. tartrate,** the tartrate salt of metyrapone, used for the same purpose as the base; administered by intravenous infusion.

metyrosine (mĕ-ti′ro-sēn) chemical name: (−)-α-methyl-L-tyrosine; an antihypertensive, $C_{10}H_{13}NO_3$.

Meulengracht's diet, method (moi′len-grakts) [Einar *Meulengracht,* Danish internist, born 1887] see under *diet* and *method.*

MeV, Mev. megaelectron volt.

mevalonate (mĕ-val′o-nāt) the anionic form of mevalonic acid.

mevalonic acid (mĕ-vah-lon′ik) a precursor of steroids and polyprenyl compounds.

Mexate (meks′āt) trademark for preparations of methotrexate sodium.

mexrenoate potassium (meks-ren′o-āt) chemical name: 17-hydroxy-3-oxo-17α-pregn-4-ene-7α,21-dicarboxylic acid 7-methyl ester monopotassium salt dihydrate; an aldosterone antagonist, $C_{24}H_{33}KO_6 \cdot 2H_2O$.

Meyer's disease (mi′erz) [Hans Wilhelm *Meyer,* Danish physician, 1824–1895] see under *disease.*

Meyer's line, organ, sinus (mi′erz) [Georg Hermann von *Meyer,* anatomist in Zürich, 1815–1892] see under *line, organ,* and *sinus.*

Meyerhof (mi′er-hof), Otto Fritz. German physiologist, 1884–1951; co-winner, with Archibald Vivian Hill, of the Nobel prize for medicine or physiology in 1922 for his studies in cellular oxidation and his discovery of the metabolism of lactic acid in muscles.

Meynert's bundle, etc. (mi′nerts) [Theodor Herman *Meynert,* professor of neurology and psychiatry at Vienna, 1833–1892] see under *bundle, cell, commissure, fasciculus,* and *tract.*

Meynet's nodes (ma-nāz′) [Paul Claude Hyacinthe *Meynet,* French physician, 1831–1892] see under *node.*

mezereon (me-ze′re-on) mezereum.

mezereum (me-ze′re-um) [L.] the dried bark of *Daphne mezereum* L. (Thymelaeaceae), a shrub of Europe; formerly used as a diaphoretic, diuretic, and stimulant. It has long been recognized as a poisonous plant, particularly through ingestion of its berries. The plant parts are acrid and produce vesication when rubbed on the skin.

mezlocillin (mez″lo-sil′in) an antibiotic of unspecified action, $C_{21}H_{25}N_5O_8S_2$.

μF microfarad.

M. flac. abbreviation for L. *membra′na flac′cida* (pars flaccida membranae tympani [NA]).

M. ft. abbreviation for L. *mistu′ra fi′at,* let a mixture be made.

Mg chemical symbol for *magnesium.*

mg. milligram.

mγ milligamma (millimicrogram, micromilligram, or nanogram).

μg. microgram.

μγ microgamma (micromicrogram, or picogram).

MgCl₂ magnesium chloride.

mgm abbreviation for milligram.

MgO magnesium oxide.

MgSO₄ magnesium sulfate.

MHA-TP microhemagglutination assay–*Treponema pallidum.*

MHC major histocompatibility complex.

M.H.D. minimum hemolytic dose.

mho (mo) [*ohm* spelled backwards] siemens.

Mianeh bug [the city of *Mianeh,* Iran] see under *bug.*

mianserin hydrochloride (me-an′ser-in) chemical name: 1,2,3,4,10,14b-hexahydro-2-methyldibenzo[c,f]pyrazino[1,2-a]azepine monohydrochloride; a serotonin inhibitor and antihistaminic, $C_{18}H_{20}N_2 \cdot HCl$.

miasm (mi′azm) miasma.

miasma (mi-az′mah) [Gr. "defilement, pollution"] a supposed noxious emanation from the soil or earth, alleged to be the cause of diseases endemic in certain areas, such as malaria, before the true cause became known. See *tellurism.*

miasmatic (mi″az-mat′ik) pertaining to or caused by miasma.

Mibelli's porokeratosis (me-bel′ez) [Vittorio *Mibelli,* Italian dermatologist, 1860–1910] porokeratosis.

mibolerone (mi-bōl′er-ōn) chemical name: 17β-hydroxy-7α,17-dimethylester-4-en-3-one; an androgenic and anabolic agent, $C_{20}H_{30}O_2$.

mica (mi′kah) [L.] 1. a crumb or grain; a small particle. 2. a group of complex aluminum silicate compounds, some of which can produce pulmonary fibrosis if inhaled in finely divided form in high concentrations over a prolonged period.

micaceous (mi-ka′shus) pertaining to or resembling mica; occurring in silvery gray flakes.

MicaTin (mi′kah-tin) trademark for preparations of miconazole nitrate.

mication (mi-ka′shun) any quick motion, such as winking.

micatosis (mi″kah-to′sis) pneumoconiosis due to inhalation of and tissue reaction to mica particles.

micella (mi-sel′ah) see *micelle.*

micelle (mi-sel′) a colloid particle formed by an aggregation of small molecules.

Michaelis constant, stain (mĭ-ka′lis) [Leonor *Michaelis*, German-born American biochemist, 1875–1949] see under *constant* and *stain*.

Michaelis's rhomboid (mĭ-ka′lis-ez) [Gustav Adolf *Michaelis*, Kiel gynecologist, 1798–1848] see under *rhomboid*.

Michaelis-Gutmann bodies (mĭ-ka′lis gut′man) [Leonor *Michaelis*; C. *Gutmann*, German physician, born 1872] see under *body*.

Michaelis-Menten equation (mĭ-ka′lis men′ten) [Leonor *Michaelis*; Maude Lenore *Menten*, American physician, 1879–1960] see under *equation*.

miconazole nitrate (mĭ-kon′ah-zōl) chemical name: 1-[2-(2,4-dichlorophenyl)-2-[(2,4-dichlorophenyl)methoxy]ethyl]-1*H*-imidazole mononitrate. A synthetic antifungal agent, $C_{18}H_{14}Cl_4N_2O \cdot HNO_3$, used topically in the treatment of tinea pedis, tinea cruris, and tinea corpora due to *Trichophyton rubrum*, *T. mentagrophytes*, and *Epidermophyton floccosum*; of cutaneous candidiasis, and of tinea versicolor; and intravaginally in the treatment of vulvovaginal candidiasis.

micra (mi′krah) plural of *micron*.

micranatomy (mi″kran-at′o-me) [*micro-* + *anatomy*] microscopical anatomy; histology.

micrangiopathy (mi″kran-je-op′ah-the) (*obs.*) microangiopathy.

micrangium (mi-kran′je-um) a capillary.

micranthine (mi-kran′thin) a crystalline alkaloid, $C_{34}H_{32}N_2O_6$, from bark of the tree *Daphnandra micrantha* (Tul.) Benth. (Monimiaceae).

micrencephalia (mi″kren-sĕ-fa′le-ah) micrencephaly.

micrencephalon (mi″kren-sef′ah-lon) [*micr-* + Gr. *enkephalos* brain] 1. a small brain. 2. (*obs.*) the cerebellum.

micrencephalous (mi″kren-sef′ah-lus) having a small brain.

micrencephaly (mi″kren-sef′ah-le) [*micr-* + Gr. *enkephalos* brain] abnormal smallness of the brain.

micr(o)- [Gr. *mikros* small] combining form denoting small size; used in naming units of measurement to indicate one-millionth (10^{-6}) of the unit designated by the root with which it is combined. Symbol, μ.

microabscess (mi″kro-ab′ses) a very small, localized collection of pus. **Munro m.,** a small focal collection of pyknotic polymorphonuclear leukocytes within the parakeratotic portion of the stratum corneum, which is one of the cardinal histologic features of active psoriasis, and also found in other dermatoses such as seborrheic dermatitis and Reiter's disease. Called also *Munro's abscess*. Cf. *spongiform pustule*. **Pautrier's m.,** one of the well-defined collections of mycosis cells located within nonspongiotic intraepidermal vesicles in T-cell lymphoma and mycosis fungoides. Called also *Pautrier's abscess*.

microadenoma (mi″kro-ad″ĕ-no′mah) an adenoma, as of the anterior pituitary gland, less than 10 mm. in diameter.

microadenopathy (mi″kro-ad″ĕ-nop′ah-the) [*micro-* + Gr. *adēn* gland + *pathos* disease] disease of the small lymphatics.

microaerophile (mi″kro-a′er-o-fīl) a microaerophilic microorganism.

microaerophilic (mi″kro-a′er-o-fil′ik) [*micro-* + *aero-* + Gr. *philein* to love] requiring oxygen for growth but at lower concentration than is present in the atmosphere; said of bacteria.

microaerophilous (mi″kro-a′er-of′ĭ-lus) microaerophilic.

microaerotonometer (mi″kro-a′er-o-to-nom′ĕ-ter) an instrument for measuring the volume of gases in the blood.

microaggregate (mi″kro-ag′rĕ-gat) a microscopic collection of particles, as of platelets, leukocytes, and fibrin that occurs in stored blood.

microaleuriospore (mi″kro-ah-lu′re-o-spōr) a small aleuriospore; sometimes used interchangeably with microcondium.

microammeter (mi″kro-am′ĕ-ter) an instrument for measuring currents in the microampere range.

microampere (mi″kro-am′pēr) one-millionth (10^{-6}) ampere. Symbol, μA.

microanalysis (mi″kro-ah-nal′ĭ-sis) [*micro-* + *analysis*] the chemical analysis of minute quantities of material.

microanastomosis (mi″kro-an-as″to-mo′sis) anastomosis between very small tubular structures.

microanatomy (mi″kro-ah-nat′o-me) histology, especially organology.

microaneurysm (mi″kro-an′u-rizm) a microscopic aneurysm, a characteristic feature of thrombotic purpura.

microangiopathic (mi″kro-an″je-o-path′ik) pertaining to or characterized by microangiopathy.

microangiopathy (mi″kro-an″je-op′ah-the) [*micro-* + Gr. *angeion* vessel + *pathos* disease] disease of the small blood vessels. **diabetic m.,** the presence of generalized basement membrane thickening of capillaries throughout many vascular beds, occurring in diabetics. **thrombotic m.,** the formation of thrombi in the arterioles and capillaries; see *thrombotic thrombocytopenic purpura*, under *purpura*.

microangioscopy (mi″kro-an″je-os′ko-pe) capillaroscopy.

microbacteria (mi″kro-bak-te′re-ah) [L.] plural of *microbacterium*.

Microbacterium (mi″kro-bak-te′re-um) a genus of coryneform bacteria of uncertain status, consisting of small diphtheroid, gram-positive, rod-shaped organisms, found in dairy products, and characterized by resistance to heat. **M. fla′vum,** an aerobic species occurring predominantly in dairy products and producing lactic acid without gas in carbohydrate fermentation. **M. lac′ticum,** an aerobic species occurring in the intestinal tract and producing lactic acid without gas in carbohydrate fermentation.

microbacterium (mi″kro-bak-te′re-um), pl. *microbacte′ria* [L.] 1. an organism belonging to the genus Microbacterium. 2. a microorganism.

microbalance (mi′kro-bal′ans) a balance for measuring minute changes in weight.

microbar (mi′kro-bahr) a unit of pressure, being one-millionth (10^{-6}) bar.

microbe (mi′krōb) [*micro-* + Gr. *bios* life] a minute living organism, a microphyte or microzoon; applied especially to those minute forms of life which are capable of causing disease in animals, including bacteria, protozoa, and fungi.

microbial (mi-kro′be-al) of or pertaining to or caused by microbes.

microbian (mi-kro′be-an) 1. pertaining to or of the nature of a microbe. 2. a microbe.

microbic (mi-kro′bik) microbial.

microbicidal (mi-kro″bĭ-si′dal) [*microbe* + L. *caedere* to kill] destructive to microbes.

microbicide (mi-kro′bĭ-sīd) [*microbe* + L. *caedere* to kill] an agent that destroys microbes.

microbioassay (mi″kro-bi″o-as′a) the determination of minute quantities of an active substance or nutrient factor by a biologic method.

microbiological (mi″kro-bi″o-loj′ĭ-kal) pertaining to microbiology.

microbiologist (mi″kro-bi-ol′o-jist) one specializing in microbiology.

microbiology (mi″kro-bi-ol′o-je) [*micro-* + Gr. *bios* life + *-logy*] the science that deals with the study of microorganisms, including algae, bacteria, fungi, protozoa, and viruses.

microbiophotometer (mi″kro-bi″o-fo-tom′ĕ-ter) an instrument for measuring the growth of bacterial cultures by the turbidity of the medium.

microbiota (mi″kro-bi-o′tah) the microscopic living organisms of a region; the combined microflora and microfauna of a region.

microbiotic (mi″kro-bi-ot′ik) pertaining to the microbiota, or to microscopic living organisms.

Microbispora (mi″kro-bi-spo′rah) [*micro-* + L. *bis* twice + Gr. *spora* seed] a genus of bacteria of the family Micromonosporaceae, order Actinomycetales, consisting of soil organisms that form an aerial mycelium bearing paired spores. The type species is *M. ro′sea*.

microblast (mi′kro-blast) [*micro-* + Gr. *blastos* germ] an erythroblast of small size, i.e., 5 μ or less in diameter.

microblepharia (mi″kro-blĕ-fa′re-ah) [*micro-* + Gr. *blepharon* eyelid + *-ia*] a developmental anomaly characterized by abnormal shortness of the vertical dimensions of the eyelids.

microblepharism (mi″kro-blef′ah-rizm) microblepharia.

microblephary (mi″kro-blef′ah-re) microblepharia.

microbody (mi″kro-bod′e) 1. any of the membrane-bound, ovoid or spherical, granular cytoplasmic particles containing enzymes and other substances, which originate in the endoplasmic reticulum of vertebrate liver and kidney cells and other cells, and in protozoa, yeast, and many cell types of higher plants. Two types of microbodies are *peroxisomes* (found in vertebrates) and *glyoxysomes* (found in plants and microorganisms). 2. peroxisome.

microbrachia (mi″kro-bra′ke-ah) [*micro-* + Gr. *brachiōn* arm] abnormal smallness of the arms.

microbrachius (mi″kro-bra′ke-us) [*micro-* + Gr. *brachiōn* arm] a fetus with preternaturally small arms.

microbrenner (mi″kro-bren′er) [*micro-* + Ger. *Brenner* burner] a needle-pointed electric cautery.

microburet (mi″kro-bu-ret′) a buret with a capacity of the order of 0.1 to 10 ml., with graduated intervals of 0.001 to 0.02 ml.

microcalix (mi″kro-kal′iks) a very small renal calix arising by caliceal branching, usually at the side of a calix of normal size. Written also *microcalyx*.

microcalyx (mi″kro-kal′iks) microcalix.

microcardia (mi″kro-kar′de-ah) [*micro-* + Gr. *kardia* heart] smallness of the heart.

microcentrum (mi″kro-sen′trum) [*micro-* + Gr. *kentron* center] centrosome.

microcephalia (mi″kro-sĕ-fa′le-ah) microcephaly.

microcephalic (mi″kro-sĕ-fal′ik) pertaining to or exhibiting microcephaly.

microcephalism (mi″kro-sef′ah-lizm) microcephaly.

microcephalous (mi″kro-sef′ah-lus) microcephalic.

microcephalus (mi″kro-sef′ah-lus) an individual with a very small head.

microcephaly (mi″kro-sef′ah-le) [*micro-* + Gr. *kephalē* head] abnormal smallness of the head, usually associated with mental retardation.

microcheilia (mi″kro-ki′le-ah) [*micro-* + Gr. *cheilos* lip] abnormal smallness of the lips.

microcheiria (mi″kro-ki′re-ah) [*micro-* + Gr. *cheir* hand + *-ia*] abnormal smallness of the hands, as a result of hypoplasia of all the skeletal elements.

microchemical (mi″kro-kem′ĭ-kal) pertaining to microchemistry.

microchemistry (mi″kro-kem′is-tre) [*micro-* + *chemistry*] the study of chemical reactions using quantities invisible to the naked eye; chemistry which deals with minute quantities (a few milligrams) of substances, using apparatus of small size. Cf. *macrochemistry*.

microcinematography (mi″kro-sin″ĕ-mah-tog′rah-fe) [*micro-* + Gr. *kinēma* movement + *graphein* to write] the making of moving picture photographs of microscopic subjects. Called also *microkinematography*. See also *cinemicrography*.

microcirculation (mi″kro-sir″ku-la′shun) the flow of blood in the entire system of finer vessels (100 microns or less in diameter) of the body (the microvasculature).

microclimate (mi″kro-kli′mit) the immediate climatic environment, as that of a vector insect.

microcnemia (mi″kro-ne′me-ah) [*micro-* + Gr. *knēmē* tibia] abnormal shortness of the lower leg.

Micrococcaceae (mi″kro-kok-ka′se-e) [*micro-* + Gr. *kokkos* berry] a family of gram-positive, aerobic or facultatively anaerobic bacteria made up of spherical cells that divide primarily in two or three planes, which sometimes remain in contact after division to form clusters or packets. It includes the genera *Micrococcus, Planococcus, Sarcina,* and *Staphylococcus.*

micrococci (mi″kro-kok′si) plural of *micrococcus.*

Micrococcus (mi″kro-kok′us) a genus of bacteria of the family Micrococcaceae, consisting of spherical, gram-positive, aerobic cells, usually occurring in irregular masses. Saprophytic and nonpathogenic forms are found in soil, water, dust, and dairy products.

micrococcus (mi″kro-kok′us), pl. *micrococ′ci.* 1. an organism of the genus *Micrococcus.* 2. a spherical microorganism of extremely small size.

microcolon (mi″kro-ko′lon) an abnormally small colon.

microcolony (mi″kro-kol″o-ne) a microscopical colony of bacteria.

microconcentration (mi″kro-kon″-sentra′shun) a minute amount of solute, less than 0.05 per cent of the solution.

microconidia (mi″kro-ko-nid′e-ah) plural of *microconidium.*

microconidium (mi″kro-ko-nid′e-um), pl. *microconid′ia.* a small, usually single-celled conidium or exospore; sometimes used interchangeably with microaleuriospore; see *spore.*

microcoria (mi″kro-ko′re-ah) [*micro-* + Gr. *korē* pupil] congenital usually hereditary smallness of the pupil.

microcornea (mi″kro-kor′ne-ah) [*micro-* + *cornea*] a usually bilateral developmental anomaly, in which the cornea is unusually small (less than 11 mm. after one year of age), due to arrest of development. It may be associated with other ocular abnormalities, such as microphthalmia, hydrophthalmia, multiple defects of the anterior chamber, cataract, and glaucoma, and may be inherited as an X-linked recessive or as an autosomal dominant trait.

microcoulomb (mi″kro-koo″lom) a unit of quantity of current electricity, being one one-millionth (10^{-6}) of a coulomb. Symbol, μC.

microcrania (mi″kro-kra′ne-ah) abnormal smallness of the skull, the cranial cavity being reduced in all diameters, and the facial area being disproportionately large in comparison.

microcrith (mi′kro-krith) [*micro-* + *crith*] (*obs.*) the weight of one atom of hydrogen.

microcrystal (mi″kro-kris″tal) an extremely minute crystal.

microcrystalline (mi″kro-kris′tal-īn) [*micro-* + *crystalline*] made up of minute crystals.

microcurie (mi″kro-ku′re) a unit of radioactivity, being one one-millionth (10^{-6}) curie, or the quantity of radioactive material in which the number of nuclear disintegrations is 3.7×10^4 per second. Abbreviated μC.

microcurie-hour (mi″kro-ku″re-owr″) a unit of exposure equivalent to that obtained by exposure for one hour to radioactive material disintegrating at the rate of 3.7×10^4 atoms per second. Abbreviated μC hr.

Microcyclus (mi″kro-si′klus) [*micro-* + Gr. *kyklos* circle] a genus of small, nonmotile, gram-negative, curved, rod-shaped bacteria that form a closed ring during growth. The type species is *M. aqua′ticus.*

microcyst (mi′kro-sist) [*micro-* + *cyst*] 1. a very small cyst. 2. in bacteriology, a type of resting cell developed from the vegetative cells of certain species of Myxobacterales and Nocardiaceae. 3. in mycology, a resting cell produced by certain slime molds. Cf. *macrocyst.*

microcystometer (mi″kro-sis-tom′ĕ-ter) a small portable cystometer.

microcyte (mi′kro-sīt) [*micro-* + *-cyte*] an abnormally small erythrocyte, i.e., one 5 microns or less in diameter.

microcythemia (mi″kro-si-the′me-ah) [*microcyte* + Gr. *haima* blood + *-ia*] a condition in which the erythrocytes are smaller than normal.

microcytosis (mi″kro-si-to′sis) microcythemia.

microcytotoxicity (mi″kro-si″to-tok-sis′ĭ-te) the capability of lysing or damaging cells as detected in procedures (e.g., lymphocytotoxicity procedures) using extremely minute amounts of material, *viz.,* target cells, antibody, and complement.

microdactylia (mi″kro-dak-til′e-ah) microdactyly.

microdactyly (mi″kro-dak′tĭ-le) [*micro-* + Gr. *daktylos* finger] abnormal smallness of the digits.

microdensitometer (mi″kro-dens″ĭ-tom′ĕ-ter) an instrument used in spectroscopy to measure lines in a spectrum by light transmission measurement.

microdermatome (mi″kro-der′mah-tōm) an instrument for cutting very thin skin sections.

microdetermination (mi″kro-de-ter″mĭ-na′shun) a chemical examination in which minute quantities of the substance to be examined are used.

microdissection (mi″kro-di-sek′shun) dissection of tissue or cells under the microscope.

microdont (mi′kro-dont) [*micro-* + Gr. *odous* tooth] having an abnormally small tooth or teeth.

microdontia (mi″kro-don′she-ah) [*micro-* + *odont-* + *-ia*] a developmental disorder characterized by abnormal smallness of the teeth; it may affect a single tooth or all of the teeth, or teeth of normal size may appear abnormally small in proportion to abnormally large jaws. Called also *microdontism.*

microdontic (mi″kro-don′tik) pertaining to or characterized by microdontia.

microdontism (mi″kro-don′tizm) microdontia.

microdosage (mi″kro-do″sij) dosage in small quantities.

microdose (mi′kro-dōs) a very small dose.

microdrepanocytic (mi″kro-drep″ah-no-sit′ik) containing microcytic and drepanocytic elements, as in sickle cell–thalassemia disease.

microdrepanocytosis (mi″kro-drep″ah-no-si-to′sis) sickle cell–thalassemia disease.

microecology (mi″kro-ĕ-kol′o-je) the branch of ecology of parasites concerned with the relationships of the organisms and the environment provided by the hosts.

microecosystem (mi″kro-e″ko-sis′tem) a miniature ecological system, occurring naturally or produced in the laboratory for experimental purposes.

microelectrophoresis (mi″kro-e-lek″tro-fo-re′sis) electrophoresis in which migrating particles are observed by light microscopy.

microelectrophoretic (mi″kro-ĕ-lek″tro-fo-ret′ik) pertaining to microelectrophoresis.

Microellobosporia (mi″kro-el″lo-bos-po′re-ah) [*micro-* + Gr. *ellobos* enclosed in a pod + *spora* seed] a genus of bacteria of the family Streptomycetaceae, order Actinomycetales, consisting of soil organisms forming an aerial mycelium and bearing sporangia, each containing a row of spores. The type species is *M. cine′rea.*

microembolus (mi″kro-em′bo-lus), pl. *microem′boli.* an embolus of microscopic size.

microencephaly (mi″kro-en-sef′ah-le) micrencephaly.

microenvironment (mi″kro-en-vi′ron-ment) the environment at the microscopic or cellular level.

microerythrocyte (mi″kro-ĕ-rith′ro-sīt) microcyte.

microestimation (mi″kro-es″tĭ-ma′shun) microdetermination.

microfarad (mi″kro-far′ad) a unit of electrical capacity, being one one-millionth of a farad (10^{-6} F). Symbol, μF.

microfauna (mi″kro-faw′nah) the animal life, visible only under the microscope, which is present in or characteristic of a special location.

microfibril (mi″kro-fi′bril) an extremely small fibril.

microfilament (mi″kro-fil′ah-ment) any of the submicroscopic filaments composed chiefly of actin, found in the cytoplasmic matrix of almost all cells, often in close association with the microtubules; they are believed by some to have a supportive and cytoskeletal function and/or to mediate movement of the cell and of the organelles within it.

microfilaremia (mi″kro-fil″ah-re′me-ah) the presence of microfilariae in the circulating blood.

microfilaria (mi″kro-fi-la′re-ah) the prelarval stage of Filarioidea in the blood of man and in the tissues of the vector. This term is sometimes incorrectly used as a genus name and is then spelled with a capital M. **m. bancrof′ti,** the microfilaria of *Wuchereria bancrofti.* **m. diur′na,** the microfilaria of *Loa loa.* **m. lo′a,** the microfilaria of *Loa loa.* **m. streptocer′ca,** the microfilaria of *Dipetalonema streptocerca,* found in the subcutaneous tissues. **m. vol′vulus,** the prelarval form of *Onchocerca volvulus,* found in skin snips taken from infected persons.

microfilm (mi′kro-film) 1. a trade term for 16- or 35-millimeter film to be used in high-speed automatic machines for the photographic reproduction, in greatly reduced size, of books, documents, forms, or other record files. 2. to photographically reproduce, in greatly reduced size, on film specially designed for the purpose.

microflora (mi″kro-flo′rah) the entire population of microorganisms present in or characteristic of a special location.

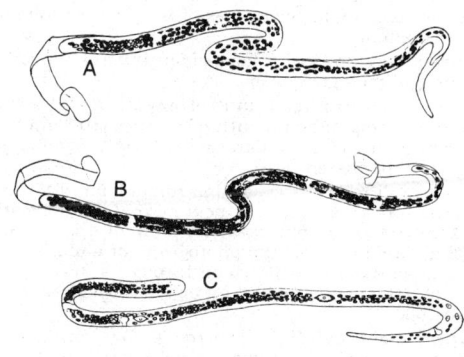

Microfilariae of *A, Wuchereria bancrofti,* 270 × 8.5 μ; *B, Loa loa,* 275 × 7 μ; *C, Onchocerca volvulus,* 320 × 7.5 μ. *A* and *B* have sheaths covering the body.

microfluorometry (mi″kro-floo″or-om′ĕ-tre) cytophotometry.

microgamete (mi″kro-gam′ēt) [*micro-* + *gamete*] the smaller, often flagellated, actively motile male anisogamete.

microgametocyte (mi″kro-gah-me′to-sīt) [*micro-* + *gametocyte*] microgamont.

microgametophyte (mi″kro-gah-me′to-fīt) [*micro-* + Gr. *gametēs* husband + *phyton* plant] the male gametophyte in heterosporous plants, developed from the microspore.

microgamma (mi″kro-gam′mah) picogram.

microgamont (mi″kro-gam′ont) [*micro-* + *gamont*] a gamont that produces microgametes by fission. Called also *microgametocyte.*

microgamy (mi-krog′ah-me) conjugation or fusion when the gametes are smaller than the somatic cells.

microgastria (mi″kro-gas′tre-ah) [*micro-* + Gr. *gastēr* stomach + *-ia*] congenital smallness of the stomach.

microgenesis (mi″kro-jen′ĕ-sis) [*micro-* + Gr. *genesis* production] abnormally small development of a part.

microgenia (mi″kro-jen′e-ah) [*micro-* + Gr. *genys* jaw] underdevelopment of the mental symphysis of the mandible, resulting in an extremely small chin; a similar appearance is caused by malocclusion with excessive prominence of the alveolar structures.

microgenitalism (mi″kro-jen′ĭ-tal-izm) [*micro-* + *genitalism*] smallness of the external genitals.

microglia (mi-krog′le-ah) the small, non-neural, interstitial cells of mesodermal origin that form part of the supporting structure of the central nervous system. They are of various forms and may have slender branched processes. They are migratory and act as phagocytes to waste products of nerve tissue. Called also *Hortega cells, gitter cells, mesoglia,* and *microgliocytes.*

microgliacyte (mi-krog′le-ah-sīt) microgliocyte.

microglial (mi-krog′le-al) of or pertaining to the microglia.

microgliocyte (mi-krog′le-o-sīt) [*microglia* + *-cyte*] the early cell which develops into a microglial cell.

microglioma (mi″kro-gli-o′mah) a tumor composed of microglial cells.

microgliomatosis (mi″kro-gli″o-mah-to′sis) a condition characterized by the formation of tumors containing microglia; called also *reticulum cell sarcoma of the brain.*

microglobulin (mi″kro-glob′u-lin) any globulin, or any fragment of a globulin, of low molecular weight.

β_2-microglobulin (mi″kro-glob′u-lin) see *beta$_2$-microglobulin.*

microglossia (mi″kro-glos′e-ah) [micro- + Gr. glōssa tongue + -ia] undersize of the tongue.

micrognathia (mi″kro-na′the-ah) [micro- + Gr. gnathos jaw + -ia] unusual or undue smallness of the jaws; micromandible or micromaxilla.

microgonioscope (mi″kro-go′ne-o-skōp) [micro- + gonioscope] a magnifying gonioscope.

microgram (mi′kro-gram) a unit of mass (weight) of the metric system, being one-millionth of a gram (10^{-6} gm.), or one one-thousandth of a milligram (10^{-3} mg.). Symbol μg (formerly γ). Abbreviated mcg.

micrograph (mi′kro-graf) 1. an instrument for recording extremely minute movements. It acts by making a greatly magnified record on a photographic film of the minute motions of a diaphragm. 2. the photograph of a minute object or specimen (tissue, etc.) as seen through a microscope. **electron m.,** the photograph of an object through an electron microscope.

micrography (mi-krog′rah-fe) [micro- + Gr. graphein to write] 1. an account of microscopic objects. 2. examination with the microscope.

microgyri (mi″kro-ji′ri) plural of microgyrus.

microgyria (mi″kro-jir′e-ah) [micro- + Gr. gyros + -ia] polymicrogyria.

microgyrus (mi″kro-ji′rus), pl. microgy′ri [micro- + gyrus] an abnormally small, malformed convolution of the brain.

microhematocrit (mi″kro-he-mat′o-krit) the rapid determination of packed cell volume of erythrocytes of an extremely small quantity of blood, by use of a capillary tube and a high speed centrifuge.

microhepatia (mi″kro-he-pat′e-ah) [micro- + Gr. hēpar liver] smallness of the liver.

microhistology (mi″kro-his-tol′o-je) [micro- + histology] microscopical histology.

microincineration (mi″kro-in-sin″er-a′shun) the incineration of minute specimens of tissue or other substance, for identification from the ash of the elements composing it.

microinfarct (mi″kro-in′farkt) a very small infarct due to obstruction of circulation in capillaries, arterioles, or small arteries.

microinjector (mi″kro-in-jek′tor) an instrument for infusion of very small amounts of fluids or drugs into animals or humans.

microinvasion (mi″kro-in-va′zhun) microscopic extension of malignant cells into adjacent tissue in carcinoma in situ.

microinvasive (mi″kro-in-va′siv) exhibiting or pertaining to microinvasion.

Microjoenia (mi″kro-jene-ah) a genus of multiflagellated parasitic protozoa (suborder Lophomonadina, order Hypermastigida), found in the termite gut, and characterized by the presence of longitudinal rows of flagella.

microkinematography (mi″kro-kin″ĕ-mah-tog′rah-fe) microcinematography.

microlaryngoscopy (mi″kro-lār″ing-gos′ko-pe) [micro- + laryngo- + scopy] examination of the interior of the larynx with a laryngoscope with binocular magnification.

microlecithal (mi″kro-les′ĭ-thal) [micro- + Gr. lekithos yolk] containing little yolk; see microlecithal ovum, under ovum.

microlesion (mi″kro-le′zhun) a minute lesion.

microleukoblast (mi″kro-lu′ko-blast) myeloblast.

microliter (mi′kro-le″ter) [Fr. microlitre; micro- + liter] a thousandth part of a milliliter or a millionth part of a liter. Usually abbreviated μl.

microlith (mi′kro-lith) [micro- + Gr. lithos stone] a minute concretion or calculus.

microlithiasis (mi″kro-lĭ-thi′ah-sis) [micro- + lithiasis] the formation of minute concretions in an organ. **m. alveola′ris pulmo′num, pulmonary alveolar m.,** a condition caused by deposition in the alveoli of the lungs of minute calculi, which appear roentgenographically as fine, sandlike mottling.

micrology (mi-krol′o-je) [micro + Gr. logos study] the science dealing with the handling and preparation of materials for microscopic study.

microlymphoidocyte (mi″kro-lim-foi′do-sīt) a small, nongranular, immature lymphoidocyte.

micromandible (mi″kro-man′dĭ-b'l) extreme smallness of the mandible.

micromanipulation (mi″kro-mah-nip″u-la′shun) the performance of surgery, injections, dissections, etc., by means of micromanipulators.

micromanipulator (mi″kro-mah-nip′u-la″tor) an attachment to a microscope for manipulating tiny instruments used in examination and dissection of minute objects under the microscope.

micromanometer (mi″kro-man-om′ĕ-ter) an apparatus for indicating gas or vapor pressure from a very small sample, as of blood, fluid, etc.

micromanometric (mi″kro-man″o-met′rik) relating to gas or vapor pressure from very small samples, as of blood, fluid, etc.

micromastia (mi″kro-mas′te-ah) abnormal smallness of the mamma.

micromaxilla (mi″kro-mak-sil′ah) extreme smallness of the maxilla.

micromazia (mi″kro-ma′ze-ah) [micro- + Gr. mazos breast] micromastia.

micromegalopsia (mi″kro-meg″ah-lop′se-ah) [micro- + megal- + -opsia] the condition in which objects appear too small or too large or too small and too large by turns.

micromelia (mi″kro-me′le-ah) [micro- + Gr. melos limb + -ia] a developmental anomaly characterized by abnormal smallness or shortness of the limbs.

micromelus (mi-krom′e-lus) an individual exhibiting micromelia.

micromere (mi′kro-mēr) [micro- + Gr. meros part] one of the small blastomeres formed by unequal cleavage of a fertilized ovum, located in the animal hemisphere and dividing more rapidly than the macromeres of the vegetal hemisphere.

micrometabolism (mi″kro-mĕ-tab′o-lizm) metabolism as studied by micromethods.

micrometastasis (mi″kro-mĕtas′tah-sis) the spread of cancer cells from the primary tumor to distant sites, where they form microscopic secondary tumors.

micrometeorology (mi″kro-me″te-er-ol′o-je) that branch of meteorology dealing with the effects on living organisms of the extra-organic aspects of the physical environment within a few inches of the surface of the earth.

micrometer[1] (mi-krom′ĕ-ter) [micro- + -meter] an instrument for measuring objects seen through the microscope. **eyepiece m.,** a micrometer that is used in connection with the eyepiece of a microscope. **filar m.,** an eyepiece micrometer in which the micrometer screw acts upon a slide carrying a movable wire: one revolution of the screw moves the wire 1 mm. across the field. **ocular m.,** eyepiece m. **stage m.,** a micrometer fastened to the stage of a microscope.

micrometer[2] (mi′kro-me″ter) one-millionth (10^{-6}) of a meter; symbol μm. Formerly called micron (symbol μ).

micromethod (mi″kro-meth′od) any technique involving use of exceedingly small quantities of material. Cf. macromethod.

micrometry (mi-krom′e-tre) the measurement of microscopic objects.

micromicro- a prefix used in naming units of measurement to indicate one-millionth of one-millionth (10^{-12}) of the unit designated by the root with which it is combined. Now supplanted by the prefix pico-.

micromicrocurie (mi″kro-mi″kro-ku′re) picocurie.

micromolar (mi″kro-mo′lar) denoting a concentration of one micromole per liter. Symbol, μM.

micromolecular (mi″kro-mo-lek′u-lar) composed of small molecules.

Micromonospora (mi″kro-mo-nos′po-rah) [micro- + Gr. monos single + sporos seed] a genus of bacteria of the family Micromonosporaceae, order Actinomycetales; made up of gram-positive, spore-forming, generally aerobic organisms that form a branched mycelium; they occur as saprophytic forms in soil and water. **M. keratolyt′icum,** a species that causes cracked heel disease. See also keratolysis plantare sulcatum. **M. pur′purea,** a species that produces gentamycin.

Micromonosporaceae (mi″kro-mo-nos″po-ra′se-e) a

family of bacteria of the order Actinomycetales, made up of gram-positive, spore-forming soil organisms that form a true mycelium. It contains the genera *Actinobifida, Microbispora, Micromonospora, Micropolyspora, Thermoactinomyces,* and *Thermomonospora.*

Micromyces (mi-krom′ĭ-sēz) [*micro-* + Gr. *mykēs* fungus] in former systems of classification, a genus of bacteria made up of organisms now included in the genus *Mycoplasma.*

micromyelia (mi″kro-mi-e′le-ah) [*micro-* + Gr. *myelos* marrow + *-ia*] abnormal smallness of the spinal cord.

micromyeloblast (mi″kro-mi′ĕ-lo-blast) a small, immature myelocyte, observed in micromyeloblastic leukemia.

micromyelolymphocyte (mi″kro-mi″ĕ-lo-lim′fo-sīt) micromyeloblast.

micron (mi′kron), pl. *mi′crons, mi′cra* [Gr. *mikros* small] one-millionth (10^{-6}) of a meter; no replaced by the SI unit *micrometer* (μm). Symbol μ.

microneedle (mi″kro-ne′d′l) a fine glass needle for use in micrurgy.

microneme (mi″kro-nēm) [*micro-* + Gr. *nēma* thread] any of the electron-dense, convoluted tubular organelles forming part of the apical complex in apicocomplexan protozoa, which are often associated with or give rise to the rhoptries. Called also *sarconeme.*

microneurosurgery (mi″kro-nu″ro-ser′jer-e) surgery conducted under high magnification with miniaturized instruments on microscopic vessels and structures of the nervous system.

micronize (mi′kro-nīz) [Gr. *micron* a small thing] to reduce to a fine powder; to reduce to particles a micron in diameter.

micronodular (mi″kro-nod′u-lar) marked by the presence of small nodules.

micronormoblast (mi″kro-nor′mo-blast) an abnormal red cell precursor in which there has been defective hemoglobin synthesis, characterized by a narrow rim of cytoplasm and a rather overdeveloped, pyknotic nucleus.

micronucleus (mi″kro-nu′kle-us) [*micro-* + *nucleus*] 1. the smaller of two types of nuclei when more than one is present in a cell. 2. in ciliate protozoa, the transcriptively inert, diploid nucleus, much smaller than the macronucleus, that is involved in reproduction.

micronutrient (mi″kro-nu′tre-ent) any essential dietary element required only in small quantities, e.g., trace minerals.

micronychia (mi″kro-nik′e-ah) [*micr-* + Gr. *onyx* nail] abnormal smallness of the nails of fingers or toes.

micro-orchidia (mi″kro-or-kid′e-ah) micro-orchidism.

micro-orchidism (mi″kro-or′kĭ-dizm) [*micro-* + Gr. *orchis* testicle] abnormal smallness of the testis.

microorganic (mi″kro-or-gan′ik) pertaining to a microorganism.

microorganism (mi″kro-or′gan-izm) [*micro-* + *organism*] a microscopic organism; those of medical interest include bacteria, viruses, fungi, and protozoa.

microorganismal (mi″kro-or″gan-iz′mal) pertaining to microorganisms.

microparasite (mi″kro-par′ah-sīt) a parasitic microorganism.

micropathology (mi″kro-pah-thol′o-je) [*micro-* + *pathology*] 1. the sum of what is known regarding minute pathologic changes. 2. the pathology of diseases caused by microorganisms.

micropenis (mi″kro-pe′nis) microphallus.

microperfusion (mi″kro-per-fu′zhun) perfusion of a minute amount of a substance.

microphage (mi′kro-fāj) [*micro-* + Gr. *phagein* to eat] a phagocyte of small size; an actively motile, neutrophilic leukocyte capable of phagocytosis.

microphagocyte (mi″kro-fag′o-sīt) [*micro-* + *phagocyte*] microphage.

microphakia (mi″kro-fa′ke-ah) [*micro-* + Gr. *phakos* lens + *-ia*] abnormal smallness of the crystalline lens.

microphallus (mi″kro-fal′us) [*micro-* + Gr. *phallos* penis] abnormal smallness of the penis.

microphone (mi′kro-fōn) a device for converting an acoustic signal into an electric signal for purposes of amplifi-

cation or transmission. **cardiac catheter-m.,** phonocatheter.

microphonic (mi″kro-fon′ik) 1. serving to amplify sound. 2. cochlear m. **cochlear m's,** the electrical potentials generated in the hair cells of the organ of Corti in response to acoustic stimulation; called also *cochlear potentials.*

microphotograph (mi″kro-fo′to-graf) [*micro-* + *photograph*] a photograph of small size. Cf. *photomicrograph.*

microphthalmia (mi″krof-thal′me-ah) [*micro-* + Gr. *ophthalmos* eye + *-ia*] microphthalmos.

microphthalmos (mi″krof-thal′mus) [*micro-* + Gr. *ophthalmos* eye] a developmental defect causing moderate or severe reduction in size of the eye. Opacities of the cornea and lens, scarring of the retina and choroid, and other abnormalities may also be present. Cf. *nanophthalmos.*

microphthalmoscope (mi″krof-thal′mo-skōp) [*micro-* + *ophthalmoscope*] an instrument for performing fundus microscopy.

microphyte (mi′kro-fīt) [*micro-* + Gr. *phyton* plant] a microscopic vegetable organism. Cf. *microzoon.*

microphytic (mi″kro-fit′ik) (obs.) pertaining to or caused by microphytes.

micropinocytosis (mi″kro-pi″no-si-to′sis) the taking up into a cell of specific macromolecules by invagination of the plasma membrane which is then pinched off, resulting in small vesicles in the cytoplasm.

micropipet (mi″kro-pi-pet′) a pipet for handling small quantities of liquids (up to 1 ml.).

micropituicyte (mi″kro-pi-tu′ĭ-sīt) see pituicyte.

microplasia (mi″kro-pla′ze-ah) [*micro-* + Gr. *plassein* to form] dwarfism.

microplethysmography (mi″kro-pleth″is-mog′rah-fe) [*micro-* + Gr. *plēthysmos* increase + *graphein* to record] the recording of minute changes in the size of a part as produced by the circulation of blood in it.

micropodia (mi″kro-po′de-ah) [*micro-* + Gr. *pous* foot] abnormal smallness of the feet.

micropolariscope (mi″kro-po-lar′ĭ-skōp) a microscope with a polariscope attached.

micropolygyria (mi″kro-pol″e-ji′re-ah) polymicrogyria.

Micropolyspora (mi″kro-pol″e-spo′ra) [*micro-* + Gr. *poly* many + *sporos* seed] a genus of bacteria of the family Micromonosporaceae, order Actinomycaetales, consisting of gram-positive organisms occurring in branching filaments and forming a spore-producing mycelium. **M. fae′ni,** a thermophilic species isolated from compost, hay, and grain that is the principal cause of farmer's lung.

micropore (mi′kro-pōr) [*micro-* + L. *porus* pore] an ultrastructural organelle in the side of the body of apicocomplexan protozoa, consisting of a cytoplasmic ring or cylinder formed by invagination of the outer membrane of the pellicle at the site of a disruption of the inner membrane. Formerly called *micropyle.*

microprecipitation (mi″kro-pre-sip″ĭ-ta′shun) precipitation with a minute amount ($\frac{1}{2}$ to 1 drop or less) of reagent observed under the microscope.

micropredation (mi″kro-pre-da′shun) the derivation by an organism of elements essential for its existence from larger organisms of other species which it does not destroy.

micropredator (mi″kro-pred′ah-tor) [*micro-* + L. *praedator* a plunderer, pillager] an organism, e.g., the mosquito, that derives elements essential for its existence from other species of organisms, larger than itself, without causing their destruction.

microprobe (mi′kro-prōb) a minute probe, as one used in microsurgery. **laser m.,** a laser beam utilized to vaporize a minute area of tissue, as in a biopsy specimen, which is then subjected to emission spectrography.

microprojection (mi″kro-pro-jek′shun) [*micro-* + *projection*] the throwing of the image of a microscopic object on a screen.

microprojector (mi″kro-pro-jek′tor) a projector that fits the viewing stage of a microscope and enlarges the image on an illuminated viewing screen.

microprolactinoma (mi″kro-pro-lak″tĭ-no′mah) a prolactin-secreting pituitary adenoma of less than 10 mm in diameter and usually associated with serum prolactin levels of 100 to 500 ng per milliliter.

microprosopus (mi″kro-pro-so′pus) [*micro-* + Gr. *prosōpon* face] a fetus with a small or undeveloped face.

micropsia (mi-krop′se-ah) [*micro-* + *-opsia*] an illusion in which objects are seen as smaller than they actually are; called also *Lilliputian hallucination.*

microptic (mi-krop′tik) pertaining to or affected with micropsia.

micropuncture (mi′kro-punk″chur) the creation of minute openings by piercing.

micropus (mi-kro′pus) [*micro-* + Gr. *pous* foot] a person with abnormally small feet.

micropyle (mi′kro-pīl) [*micro-* + Gr. *pylē* gate] 1. a minute opening in: (1) the ovum of certain invertebrates, such as arthropods, that permits entrance of a sperm; (2) the apex of the ovule of a seed plant that admits the pollen tube; (3) the covering of a sponge through which geminating cells emerge. 2. former name for *micropore.*

microradiogram (mi″kro-ra′de-o-gram) a picture produced by microradiography.

microradiography (mi″kro-ra″de-og′rah-fe) [*micro-* + *radiography*] a process by which a radiograph of a small or very thin object is produced on fine-grained photographic film under conditions which permit subsequent microscopic examination or enlargement of the radiograph at linear magnifications of up to several hundred and with a resolution approaching the resolving power of the photographic emulsion (about 1000 lines per millimeter).

microrchidia (mi″kror-kid′e-ah) [*micro-* + Gr. *orchis* testicle + *-ia*] micro-orchidism.

microrefractometer (mi″kro-re″frak-tom′ĕ-ter) a refractometer for the discovery of variations in the minute structures, e.g., in blood corpuscles.

microrespirometer (mi″kro-res″pĭ-rom′ĕ-ter) an apparatus for investigating the oxygen utilization of isolated tissues.

microrhinia (mi″kro-rin′e-ah) [*micro-* + Gr. *rhis* nose] abnormal smallness of the nose.

microroentgen (mi″kro-rent′gen) one millionth (10⁶) roentgen; abbreviated μR.

microscelous (mi-kros′kĕ-lus) [*micro-* + Gr. *skelos* leg] short-legged.

Microscilla (mi″kro-sil′ah) in former systems of classification, a genus of bacteria now classified as species of the genera *Vitreoscilla* and *Flexibacter.*

microscler (mi′kro-sklēr) dolichomorphic.

microscope (mi′kro-skōp) [*micro-* + Gr. *skopein* to view] an instrument used to obtain an enlarged image of small objects and reveal details of structure not otherwise distinguishable. **acoustic m.,** one in which very high frequency sound waves (close to one billion cycles per second [one gigahertz]) are focused on the object and the reflected beam is processed electronically and stored for display on a television screen. **beta ray m.,** one which reveals emission of beta particles from a microscopic specimen by means of a scintillator. **binocular m.,** a microscope which has two eyepieces, making possible simultaneous viewing with both eyes. **capillary m.,** an instrument for giving an enlarged image of capillaries, often used for viewing the capillaries of the nail bed. **centrifuge m.,** a microscope built into a high-speed centrifuge, by which a magnified image of a specimen undergoing centrifugal force may be produced. **color-contrast m.,** Rheinberg m. **comparison m.,** an instrument which permits simultaneous viewing of parts of images of two separate specimens, involving two microscopes bridged together with a comparison eyepiece, or one microscope with two body tubes and lens systems. **compound m.,** one that consists of two lens systems, one above the other, in which the image formed by the system nearer the object (objective) is further magnified by the system nearer the eye (eyepiece). **corneal m.,** a specially designed instrument with lens of high magnifying power, for observing minute changes in the cornea and iris. **darkfield m.,** one with a central stop in the condenser, permitting diversion of the light rays and illumination of the object from the side, so that the details appear light against a dark background. See also *ultramicroscope.* **electron m.,** one in which an electron beam, instead of light, forms an image for viewing, allowing much greater magnification and resolution. The image may be viewed on a fluorescent screen or may be photographed. **epic m.,** see *epimicroscope.* **fluorescence m.,** one used for the examination of speci-

mens stained with fluorochromes or fluorochrome complexes, e.g., a fluorescein-labeled antibody, which fluoresces in ultraviolet light. **Greenough m.** (*obs.*), a binocular, biobjective, stereoscopic instrument giving a low-power erect image. **hypodermic m.,** a combination of a fiberoptic probe (housed in a hypodermic needle) and a microscope for examining cell structure in tissue and muscle without a cutaneous incision. **infrared m.,** one in which radiation of 800 mμ or longer wavelength is used as the image-forming energy. **integrating m.,** one in which a special mechanical stage permits recording of the sizes of the components of the specimen. **interference m.,** a microscope for observing the same kind of refractile detail as that observed with the phase microscope, but utilizing two separate beams of light which are sent through the specimen and combined with each other in the image plane. **ion m.,** an electron microscope modified to use ions (e.g., of lithium), instead of electrons. **laser m.,** see *laser microprobe.* **light m.,** one in which the specimen is viewed under visible light. **opaque m.,** one with vertical illumination or with the condenser built around the objective (epimicroscope) for viewing opaque specimens. **operating m.,** a specially designed magnifying instrument employed in the performance of delicate microsurgical procedures, as in operations on the middle ear, on small blood vessels, or on a vocal cord. **phase m., phase-contrast m.,** a microscope that converts variations of the refracting index in the object into variations of intensity in the image. Altering the phase relationship of light passing through and that passing around the object allows details of living cells to be seen without the fixation and staining that is normally necessary. **polarizing m.,** one equipped with a polarizer, analyzer, and means for measurement of the alteration of the polarized light by the specimen. **polarizing m., rectified,** a polarizing microscope corrected for depolarization from curved lens surfaces so that full apertures can be used. **projection x-ray m.,** a microscope using soft x-radiation for high resolution; the images may be photographed or observed directly on a fluorescent viewing screen. **reflecting m.,** one which utilizes mirrors instead of lenses to form the image. **Rheinberg m.,** a darkfield microscope in which the condenser is modified by having a colored instead of an opaque stop, with the annulus in a complementary color. Called also *color-contrast m.* **scanning m., scanning electron m.,** an electron microscope in which a beam of electrons scans over a specimen point by point and builds up an image on the fluorescent screen of a cathode ray tube. **schlieren m.,** one in which light is deviated by the insertion of one or two diaphragms in the optical system, to reveal differences in refractive index in a specimen. **simple m.,** one which consists of a single lens; a magnifying glass. **slit lamp m.,** see *slit lamp,* under *lamp.* **stereoscopic m.,** a binocular biobjective microscope, or a binocular monobjective microscope modified to give a three-dimensional view of the specimen. **stroboscopic m.,** one which utilizes flashing illumination, permitting analysis of motion in the specimen. **trinocular m.,** a binocular microscope with a third eyepiece tube for photomicrography or other use. **ultra-m.,** see *ultramicroscope.* **ultrasonic m.,** one which utilizes the reflection of ultrasonic or mechanical vibration to reveal the detail of the specimen. **ultraviolet m.,** a microscope which utilizes reflecting optics or quartz and other ultraviolet-transmitting lenses, with radiation of less than 400 mμ wavelength as the image-forming energy. **x-ray m.,** one in which a beam of x-rays is used instead of light, the image usually being reproduced on film.

microscopic, microscopical (mi″kro-skop′ik, mi″kro-skop′ĭ-kal) 1. of extremely small size; visible only by the aid of the microscope. 2. pertaining or relating to a microscope or to microscopy.

microscopist (mi-kros′ko-pist) a person skilled in using the microscope.

microscopy (mi-kros′ko-pe) [*micro-* + Gr. *skopein* to examine] examination under or observation by means of the microscope. **clinical m.,** employment of the microscope in making clinical diagnoses. **electron m.,** examination by means of the electron microscope. **fluorescence m.,** microscopy of natural fluorescent materials or of specimens stained with fluorochromes, which emit light when exposed to blue or ultraviolet light. **fundus m.,** examination of the fundus of the eye with an instrument which combines a corneal microscope with an ophthalmoscope. **immuno-**

fluorescence m., fluorescence microscopy using immuno-fluorescence (q.v.) staining methods. **television m.,** projection on a television screen of the image obtained by use of a flying spot, or scanning, microscope, or by use of a television camera over a microscope.

microsecond (mi′kro-sek″und) one-millionth of a second; symbol μs.

microsection (mi″kro-sek′shun) an extremely thin section for examination with the microscope.

microseme (mi′kro-sēm) [micro- + Gr. sēma sign] having an orbital index of 83 or less.

Microsiphonales (mi″kro-si′fo-na′lēz) see Trichomycetes.

microslide (mi′kro-slīd) the slide on which objects for microscopical examination are mounted.

microsmatic (mi″kros-mat′ik) [micro- + Gr. osmasthai to smell] having the sense of smell, but of relatively feeble development, as in man.

microsoma (mi″kro-so′mah) [micro- + Gr. sōma body] a very short but not dwarfish stature.

microsomal (mi″kro-so′mal) of or pertaining to microsomes.

microsome (mi′kro-sōm) [micro- + Gr. sōma body] any of the vesicular fragments of endoplasmic reticulum formed after disruption and centrifugation of cells.

microsomia (mi″kro-so′me-ah) [micro- + Gr. sōma body + -ia] small size of the body. **m. feta′lis,** abnormally small size of the fetus.

microspectrophotometer (mi″kro-spek″tro-fo-tom′ĕ-ter) a system combining a microscope with a spectrophotometer.

microspectroscope (mi″kro-spek′tro-skōp) [micro- + spectroscope] a spectroscope to be used in connection with a microscope for the examination of the spectra of microscopic objects.

microsphere (mi-kro-sfēr′) centrosome.

microspherocyte (mi″kro-sfe′ro-sīt) spherocyte.

microspherocytosis (mi″kro-sfe′ro-si-to′sis) spherocytosis.

microspherolith (mi″kro-sfēr′o-lith) a particle resembling a miniature gallstone in the bile.

microsphygmia (mi-kro-sfig′me-ah) [micro- + Gr. sphygmos pulse + -ia] a pulse that is difficult to perceive by the finger.

microsphygmy (mi″kro-sfig′me) microsphygmia.

microsphyxia (mi″kro-sfik′se-ah) (obs.) microsphygmia.

Microspira (mi″kro-spi′rah) [micro- + Gr. speira coil] in former systems of classification, a genus of bacteria made up of organisms now assigned to the genus Vibrio.

Microspironema (mi″kro-spi″ro-ne′mah) [micro- + Gr. speira coil + nema thread] a genus name once proposed for organisms now included in the genus Treponema.

microsplenia (mi″kro-sple′ne-ah) [micro- + Gr. splēn spleen + -ia] smallness of the spleen.

microsplenic (mi″kro-sple′nik) marked by smallness of the spleen.

Microspora (mi-kros′pŏ-rah) [micro- + spore] a phylum of protozoa found as obligatory intracellular parasites in nearly all major animal groups, being especially common in insects, sometimes causing economically important disease. The spore phase is characterized by the presence of minute unicellular spores, each with an imperforate wall containing one nucleus or a dinucleate sporoplasm and a simple or complex extrusion apparatus with a polar tube or polar cap always present; mitochondria are absent. It comprises two classes: Rudimicrosporea and Microsporea. Called also Cnidospora.

microsporangia (mi″kro-spo-ran′je-ah) plural of microsporangium.

microsporangium (mi″kro-spo-ran′je-um), pl. microsporan′gia [micro- + Gr. sporos seed + angeion vessel] the sporangium in which microspores develop.

microspore (mi″kro-spōr) [micro- + Gr. sporos seed] 1. the smaller spore form when spores of two sizes are present, as in certain fungi and protozoa. 2. in heterogenous plants, one of four haploid spores, usually smaller than the megaspore, formed in the microspangium from a microspore mother cell, and from which the microgametophyte, or male gametophyte, develops. See also pollen.

Microsporea (mi″kro-spor′e-ah) a class of parasitic protozoa (phylum Microspora), the spores of which have a complex extrusion apparatus of Golgi origin, often including a polaroplast and posterior vacuole and a typically filamentous polar tube extending backward from the polar cap and coiling around inside of the three-layered spore wall; a sporocyst may or may not be present. It comprises two orders: Minisporida and Microsporida.

Microsporida (mi″kro-spor′ĭ-dah) [micro- + spore] an order of parasitic protozoa (class Microsporea, phylum Microspora) found in invertebrates, especially arthropods, in lower vertebrates, and rarely in higher vertebrates, which have a tendency toward maximum development and varied specialization of accessory spore organelles accompanied by a reduction of sporocysts. It comprises two suborders: Pansporoblastina and Apansporoblastina. Called also Cnidosporidia and Microsporidia.

microsporidan (mi″kro-spor′ĭ-dan) 1. any protozoan of the phylum Microspora. 2. pertaining to protozoa of the phylum Microspora. 3. microsporidian.

Microsporidia (mi″kro-spo-rid′e-a) Microsporida.

microsporidian (mi″kro-spo-rid′e-an) 1. any protozoan of the order Microsporida. 2. pertaining to protozoa of the order Microsporida. 3. microsporidan.

Microsporon (mi-kros′po-ron) Microsporum.

Microsporum (mi-kros′po-rum) [micro + Gr. sporos seed] a genus of small-spored ectothrix ringworm fungi (dermatophytes) of the Fungi Imperfecti, order Moniliales, family Moniliaceae, which cause various diseases of the skin and hair. As the perfect (sexual) stages are identified, they are classified in the genus Nannizzia. Called also Microsporon. Besides the species listed below, M. cook′ei, M. distor′tum, and M. na′num are pathogenic but have been isolated from man only rarely. **M. audoui′nii,** the most common cause of prepuberal tinea capitis in Europe and of about half the cases in the United States. **M. ca′nis,** a common cause of ringworm in cats and dogs; often transmitted to children, in whom it causes tinea capitis and tinea corporis. It is also probably the cause of a dermatomycosis in horses. **M. feli′neum,** M. canis. **M. ful′vum,** a geophilic species sometimes contracted from soil, which causes tinea corporis or tinea capitis. **M. fur′fur,** Pityrosporon orbiculare. **M. gyp′seum,** a species commonly found in soil; it is a common cause of tinea capitis and tinea corporis in South America, and less frequently in other parts of the world. **M. lano′sum,** M. canis.

microsthenic (mi″kro-sthen′ik) [micro- + Gr. sthenos strength] having feeble muscular power.

Microstix-3 (mi′kro-stiks) trademark for a reagent strip with a chemical test area for recognition of nitrite in urine, which turns pink on contact with nitrite, and two culture areas for semiquantification of bacterial growth after 18–24 hours of incubation; one culture area supports both gram-negative and gram-positive organisms, the other, only gram-negative organisms.

microstomia (mi″kro-sto′me-ah) [micro- + Gr. stoma mouth + -ia] a congenital defect in which the mouth is unusually small.

microstrabismus (mi″kro-strah-biz′mus) [micro- + Gr. strabismos a squinting] strabismus of such slight degree that the deviation is undetectable by the usual methods.

microsurgery (mi′kro-ser″jer-e) dissection of minute structures under the microscope by means of instruments held in the hand, as in microsurgery of the ear and larynx.

microsyringe (mi″kro-sēr′inj) a syringe fitted with a screw-thread micrometer head for the accurate control of minute measurements.

Microtatobiotes (mi″kro-ta″to-bi-o′tēz) [Gr. mikrotatos smallest + biōtes one must live] in former systems of classification, a taxonomic class including the orders Rickettsiales and Virales.

microtechnic (mi″kro-tek′nik) micrology.

microthelia (mi″kro-the′le-ah) [micro- + Gr. thēlē nipple + -ia] unusual smallness of the nipples.

Microthoracina (mi″kro-tho-ras′ĭ-nah) [micro- + thorax] a suborder of often small and laterally flattened ciliate freshwater protozoa (order Nasulida, superorder Nassulidea), characterized by the presence of a frange that has been reduced to three pseudomembranelles and unique trichocysts, and having somatic ciliature that is typically reduced.

microthrombosis (mi″kro-throm-bo′sis) presence of many small thrombi in the capillaries and other small blood vessels of various organs of the body.

microthrombus (mi″kro-throm′bus), pl. *microthrom′bi* [*micro-* + Gr. *thrombos* clot] a small thrombus located in a capillary or other small blood vessel.

microtia (mi-kro′she-ah) [*micro-* + Gr. *ous* ear + *-ia*] gross hypoplasia or aplasia of the pinna of the ear, with a blind or absent external auditory meatus.

microtiter (mi″kro-ti′ter) a titer of minute quantity.

microtome (mi′kro-tōm) [*micro-* + Gr. *tomē* a cut] an instrument for cutting thin slices of tissue for microscopical study. **freezing m.,** a microtome for cutting frozen sections. **rocking m.,** a microtome in which the specimen is held in the end of a lever which passes up and down over a stationary knife. **rotary m.,** one in which a wheel action is translated into a back-and-forth movement of the specimen being sectioned. **sliding m.,** one in which the specimen being sectioned is made to slide on a tract.

microtomy (mi-krot′o-me) [*micro-* + Gr. *temnein* to cut] the cutting of thin sections; called also *histotomy.*

microtonometer (mi″kro-to-nom′ĕ-ter) a small tonometer for measuring the oxygen and carbon dioxide tension in arterial blood.

microtransfusion (mi″kro-trans-fu′zhun) introduction into the circulation of a small quantity of blood of another individual, as sometimes occurs with transplacental passage of a small amount of fetal blood into the maternal circulation.

microtrauma (mi″kro-traw′mah) a slight trauma or lesion; a microscopic lesion.

Microtrombidium akamushi (mi″kro-trom-bid′e-um ak″ah-moo′she) *Trombicula akamushi.*

microtropia (mi″kro-tro′pe-ah) microstrabismus.

microtubule (mi″kro-tu′būl) any of the slender, tubular structures composed chiefly of tubulin, found in the cytoplasmic ground substance of nearly all cells; they are involved in maintenance of cell shape and in the movements of organelles and inclusions, and form the spindle fibers of mitosis. In cilia and flagella, they are constantly arranged with two single microtubules in the center and nine pairs of doublets arrayed around the central two. **subpellicular m.,** any of the microtubules (24 to 26) radiating posteriorly from the polar rings, directly beneath the pellicle, forming part of the apical complex in apicocomplexan protozoa.

Microtus (mi-kro′tus) [*micro-* + Gr. *ous,* *ōtos,* ear] a genus of small rodents distributed throughout the Arctic land areas, commonly called voles or meadow mice. **M. montebel′li,** the field vole, which is probably the host of *Leptospira hebdomidis,* the etiologic agent of nanukayami.

microtus (mi-kro′tus) an individual exhibiting microtia.

microunit (mi′kro-u″nit) one-millionth (10⁻⁶) of a standard unit; abbreviated μU.

microvascular (mi″kro-vas′ku-lar) pertaining to the microvasculature.

microvasculature (mi″kro-vas′ku-lah-tūr) the portion of the vasculature of the body comprising the finer vessels, sometimes described as including all vessels with an internal diameter of 100 microns or less.

microvilli (mi″kro-vil′i) [pl. of L. *microvillus* a tuft of hair] minute cylindrical processes on the free surface of a cell, especially cells of the proximal convolution in a renal tubule and of the intestinal epithelium, which increase the surface size of the cell; see also *brush border,* under *border.*

microvillus (mi″kro-vil′us) a minute process or protrusion from the free surface of a cell; see *microvilli.*

microviscosimeter (mi″kro-vis″ko-sim′ĕ-ter) a viscosimeter for measuring the viscosity of blood plasma, using a small quantity of blood.

microvivisection (mi″kro-viv″ĭ-sek′shun) microdissection.

microvolt (mi′kro-volt) [*micro-* + *volt*] one-millionth of a volt. Symbol, μV.

microvoltometer (mi″kro-vōl-tom′ĕ-ter) an instrument for detecting minute changes of electric potential in the body.

microwatt (mi′kro-wat) [*micro-* + *watt*] one-millionth of a watt. Symbol, μW.

microwave (mi′kro-wāv) a wave typical of electromagnetic radiation between far infrared and radio waves, gener-

ally regarded as extending from 300,000 to 100 megacycles (wavelength of 1 mm. to 30 cm.).

microxycyte (mi-krok′sĭ-sīt) [*micro-* + Gr. *oxys* sharp, acid + *-cyte*] any finely granular oxyphil cell.

microxyphil (mi-krok′sĭ-fil) microxycyte.

microzoa (mi″kro-zo′ah) plural of *microzoon.*

microzoon (mi″kro-zo′on), pl. *microzo′a* [*micro-* + Gr. *zōon* animal] a microscopic animal organism. Cf. *microphyte.*

micrurgic (mi-krur′jik) pertaining to micrurgy.

micrurgy (mi′krur-je) [*micro-* + Gr. *ergon* work] micromanipulative technic in the field of a microscope. See *micromanipulator.*

Micrurus (mi-kroo′rus) a genus of venomous elapid snakes. *M. ful′vius* is the coral, or harlequin, snake. Called also *Elaps.* See table accompanying *snake.*

miction (mik′shun) urination.

micturate (mik′tu-rāt) urinate.

micturition (mik″tu-rish′un) [L. *micturire* to urinate] the passage of urine; urination.

M.I.D. minimum infective dose.

midaflur (mi′dah-floor) chemical name: 2,5-dihydro-2,2,5,5-tetrakis(trifluoromethyl)-1H-imidazol-4-amine; a sedative, $C_7H_3F_{12}N_3$.

Midamor (mi′dah-mor) trademark for preparations of amiloride hydrochloride.

midaxilla (mid″ak-sil′ah) the center of the axilla.

midbody (mid′bod-e) 1. a body or a mass of granules developed in the equatorial region of the spindle during the anaphase of mitosis. 2. the middle region of the trunk.

midbrain (mid′brān) mesencephalon.

midcarpal (mid-kar′pal) between the two rows of bones of the carpus.

middlepiece (mid′′l-pēs) the portion of a spermatozoon between its head and flagellum.

midfoot (mid′foot) the middle portion of the foot, comprising the region of the navicular, cuboid, and cuneiform bones.

midfrontal (mid-fron′tal) pertaining to the middle of the forehead.

midge (mij) a small dipterous insect of the family Chironomidae; many species give painful bites, and some are vectors of *Mansonella ozzardi* and *Dipetalonema perstans.* **owl m.,** *Phlebotomus.*

midget (mij′et) a normal dwarf; an individual who is undersized (shorter than 3 standard deviations below mean height for age in a child) but perfectly formed.

midgut (mid′gut) 1. the region of the embryonic digestive tube into which the yolk sac opens; ahead of it is the foregut and caudal to it is the hindgut. 2. the middle endodermal portion of the alimentary tract of invertebrates, such as arthropods, comprising a stomach and sometimes a midintestine.

Midicel (mid′ĭ-sel) trademark for a preparation of sulfamethoxypyridazine.

midoccipital (mid″ok-sip′ĭ-tal) pertaining to or located in the middle of the occiput.

midpain (mid′pān) intermenstrual pain.

midperiphery (mid″pĕ-rif′er-e) the middle zone of the fundus.

midplane (mid′plān) the median plane of a bilateral structure.

midriff (mid′rif) the diaphragm (diaphragma [NA]); the middle region of the torso; the region between the lower border of the breast and the waistline.

midsection (mid-sek′shun) a cut through the middle of any organ or part.

midsternum (mid-ster′num) mesosternum.

midtarsal (mid-tar′sal) between the two rows of bones of the tarsus.

midtegmentum (mid′′teg-men′tum) the median or central part of the tegmentum.

midwife (mid′wīf) an individual who practices midwifery; see *nurse-midwife.*

midwifery (mid′wi-fer-e) the practice of assisting in childbirth. See *nurse-midwife* and *obstetrics.*

Mierzejewski effect (mēr″ze-yef′ske) [Jan Lucian *Mierzejewski*, Polish neurologist and psychiatrist, 1839–1908] see under *effect*.

Miescher's tube, tubule (me′sherz) [Johann Friedrich *Miescher*, Swiss pathologist, 1811–1887] sarcocyst.

MIF melanocyte-stimulating hormone inhibiting factor; migration inhibiting factor. See under *factor*.

migraine (mi′grān, me′grān) [Fr., from Gr. *hemikrania* an affection of half of the head] an often familial symptom complex of periodic attacks of vascular headache, usually temporal and unilateral in onset, commonly associated with irritability, nausea, vomiting, constipation or diarrhea, and often photophobia; attacks are preceded by constriction of the cranial arteries, usually with resultant prodromal sensory (especially ocular) symptoms, and commence with the vasodilation that follows. **abdominal m.,** migraine in which abdominal symptoms (nausea and vomiting) are prominent. **acute confusional m.,** a rare variant of classical migraine occurring in children, marked by attacks of confusion and disorientation, with agitation manifested as a mixture of apprehension and combativeness; headache may not appear at first but always develops eventually. **fulgurating m.,** violent migraine developing abruptly. **hemiplegic m.,** migraine associated with varying degrees of transient hemiplegia or hemiparesis. **ophthalmic m.,** migraine accompanied by amblyopia or other visual disturbance. **ophthalmoplegic m.,** periodic migraine accompanied by ophthalmoplegia.

migraineur (me″grān-er′) [Fr.] a person who suffers from migraine.

migrainoid (mi′grah-noid) [*migraine* + Gr. *eidos* form] resembling migraine.

migrainous (mi′gra-nus) resembling, or of the nature of migraine.

migration (mi-gra′shun) [L. *migratio*] 1. an apparently spontaneous change of place, as of symptoms. 2. the movement of leukocytes through the walls of the vessels; diapedesis. **anodic m.,** the migration of a negatively charged particle toward the positive pole in an electrical field. **cathodic m.,** the migration of a positively charged particle toward the negative pole in an electric field. **external m.,** the passage of an ovum from the ovary to the oviduct of the opposite side without passing through the uterus. **internal m.,** the passing of an ovum from an ovary into the uterus in the normal way, followed by its entry into the opposite oviduct or, in animals with separate uterine horns, into the opposite horn. **m. of leukocytes,** the passage of white corpuscles through the wall of a vessel; diapedesis. **m. of ovum,** 1. the passage of the ovum into the uterine tube after its discharge from the ovary. 2. the passage of the ovum through the reproductive tract and through the uterine epithelium into the stroma. **retrograde m.,** the passage into the upper urinary tract of foreign bodies introduced through the urethra. **tooth m., pathologic,** drifting of the teeth due to destruction of tooth-supporting structures by periodontal disease or to failure to replace missing teeth. Called also *pathologic tooth wandering.* **tooth m., physiologic,** change of position of the teeth during their growth and development. Called also *physiologic drift.* **transperitoneal m.,** external migration.

Migula's classification (me′goo-lahz) [Walter *Migula*, German naturalist, 1863–1938] see under *classification*.

Mikedimide (mi-ked′ĭ-mīd) trademark for a preparation of bemegride.

mikr(o)- for words beginning thus, see those beginning *micr(o)-*.

Mikulicz's cells, etc. (mik′u-lich″ez) [Johann von *Mikulicz*-Radecki, Polish surgeon, 1850–1905] see under *angle, cell, clamp, disease, drain, operation, pad, pyloroplasty,* and *syndrome.*

mil (mil) contraction of *milliliter.*

milammeter (mil-am′ĕ-ter) milliammeter.

mildew (mil′du) vernacular term for any fungus growing on vegetable or other material; also the condition caused by such a fungus. *Downy* or *powdery mildew* refers to ascomycetous fungi of the *Erysiphe* (order Erysiphales) that cause disease of grapes and other plants.

milenperone (mĭ-len′pĕ-rōn) chemical name: 5-chloro-1-[3-[4-(4-fluorobenzoyl)-1-piperidinyl]propyl]-1,3-dihydro-2*H*-benzimidazol-2-one; a tranquilizer, $C_{22}H_{23}ClFN_3O_2$.

Miles' operation (mīlz) [William Ernest *Miles*, British surgeon, 1869–1947] see under *operation.*

milfoil (mil′foil) see *Achillea.*

milia (mil′e-ah) [L.] plural of *milium.*

Milian's erythema (mēl-yahz′) [Gaston Auguste *Milian*, French dermatologist, 1871–1945] see under *erythema.*

miliaria (mil″e-a′re-ah) [L. *milium* millet] a syndrome of cutaneous changes associated with sweat retention and extravasation of sweat occurring at different levels in the skin; when used alone, it refers to *m. rubra.* **m. al′ba,** m. crystallina. **apocrine m.,** Fox-Fordyce disease. **m. crystalli′na,** miliaria in which the sweat escapes in or just beneath the stratum corneum, producing noninflammatory vesicles which, because of the thinness of the layer covering them, have the appearance of clear droplets. Called also *m. alba* and *sudamina.* **m. profun′da,** miliaria seen in hot humid climates in which the occlusion of the sweat ducts is in the upper cutis; it almost always occurs following a severe episode of miliaria rubra and may lead to heat intolerance as in tropical anhidrotic asthenia. **m. ru′bra,** a condition resulting from obstruction to the ducts of the sweat glands, probably caused in part by prolonged maceration of the skin surface; the sweat escapes into the epidermis, producing pruritic erythematous papulovesicles. The severity of the symptoms fluctuates with the heat load of the individual. Called also *heat rash, lichen tropicus,* and *prickly heat.*

miliary (mil′e-a-re) [L. *miliaris* like a millet seed] 1. resembling a millet seed. 2. characterized by the formation of lesions resembling millet seeds, as in miliary tuberculosis.

Milibis (mil′ĭ-bis) trademark for preparations of glycobiarsol.

milieu (me-lyuh′) [Fr.] surroundings: environment. **m. extérieur** (me-lyuh′ eks-ta″re-ur′), the external environment. **m. intérieur** (me-lyuh′ an-ta″re-ur′) [Fr. "interior environment"], Claude Bernard's term for the blood and lymph which bathe the cells of the body.

Miliolina (mil″ĭ-o-li′nah) [L. *milium* millet seed] a suborder of protozoa (order Foraminiferida, class Granuloreticulosea) having a perforate or imperforate, porcellanous test. Both fossil and recent species are known.

milipertine (mil-ĭ-per′tēn) chemical name: 5, 6 - dimethoxy-3 - [2-[4-(2-methoxyphenyl)-1-piperazinyl]ethyl]-2-methyl-1*H*-indole; a tranquilizer, $C_{24}H_{31}N_3O_3$.

milium (mil′e-um), pl. *mil′ia* [L. "millet seed"] a tiny epidermal cyst presenting as a firm, white to yellow, smooth, globoid, keratin-containing papule lying superficially within the skin, occurring multiply and usually located on the eyelids, cheeks, and forehead, and found in the pilosebaceous follicles in all age groups, including neonates. Milia may arise de novo or in association with various dermatoses and skin traumas. Called also *whitehead.* See also *Epstein's pearls,* under *pearl.* **colloid m.,** a small, discrete, translucent, ivory to yellow, firm papule containing an amorphous colloid material, occurring in profuse eruptions, usually located on the face and dorsum of the hands, during middle age. *Multiple eruptive milia* is a similar condition that presents during childhood, and is transmitted as an autosomal dominant condition.

milk (milk) [L. *lac*] 1. the fluid secretion of the mammary gland forming the natural food of young mammals. 2. any whitish milklike substance, e.g., coconut milk or plant latex. 3. a liquid (emulsion or suspension) resembling the secretion of the mammary gland. **acidophilus m.,** milk fermented with cultures of *Lactobacillus acidophilus;* used in gastrointestinal disorders in attempts to modify the bacterial flora of the intestinal tract. **adapted m.,** milk especially modified so as to adapt it to the child's digestive capacity. **after-m.,** the stripping, or last, milk taken at any one milking. **albumin m.,** specially prepared milk, poor in lactose and salts and rich in casein and fat. **m. of bismuth** [USP], a suspension of bismuth hydroxide and bismuth subcarbonate in water, yielding between 5.2 and 5.8 per cent of bismuth trioxide; used as an astringent and antacid. Called also *bismuth magma.* **bitter m.,** milk that is bitter in taste when first drawn because of bitter herbs in the feed or that later becomes bitter from the growth of certain microorganisms. **blue m.,** milk made blue in color by the action of bacteria, usually *Pseudomonas aeruginosa.* **Budd m., buddeized m.** (*obs.*), milk sterilized by adding hydrogen peroxide and heating so as to decompose the dioxide and liberate the oxygen. **Bulgarian m., bulgaricus m.,**

milk fermented with cultures of *Lactobacillus bulgaricus*. It is thought by some to be therapeutic for intestinal disorders. **cancer m.,** a viscid opaque granular fluid which may be scraped from the surface of a carcinoma which has undergone fatty degeneration. **casein m.,** a prepared milk containing very little salts and sugars and a large amount of fat and casein. **certified m.,** milk whose purity is certified by a committee of physicians or a medical milk commission. **citric acid m.,** milk prepared by adding 4 gm. of dehydrated citric acid to a quart of milk. **condensed m.,** milk which has been partly evaporated and sweetened with sugar. **diabetic m.,** milk containing a small percentage of lactose. **dialyzed m.,** milk from which the sugar has been abstracted by being passed by dialysis through a parchment membrane. **evaporated m.,** milk prepared by evaporation of half its water content. **fat m.,** modified milk that contains as much or more fat than human milk. **fore-m.,** 1. the first milk taken at any one milking. 2. colostrum. **fortified m.,** milk made more nutritious by the addition of cream or white of egg; also vitamin D m. **grade A m.,** milk which may contain not more than 30,000 bacteria per milliliter as delivered. **grade B m.,** milk which may contain not more than 100,000 bacteria per milliliter. **homogenized m.,** milk so treated that the fats become intimately combined with the general body of the milk, the emulsified particles of fat being made so minute that the cream does not separate. **hydrochloric acid m.,** acid milk prepared by adding 5 ml. of tenth normal hydrochloric acid to 100 ml. of cow's milk. **laboratory m.,** milk prepared according to a special formula. **lemon juice m.,** acid milk prepared by adding ¾ oz. (22 ml.) of lemon juice to 1 quart of cow's milk. **litmus m.,** see *litmus milk* c. in *Table of Culture Media.* **m. of magnesia** [USP], a suspension of 7.0 to 8.5 per cent of magnesium hydroxide used as an antacid and cathartic; called also *magnesia magma.* **metallized m.,** milk in which metals (copper, iron, magnesium) are dissolved; used to produce regeneration of hemoglobin. **modified m.,** milk in which the constituents have been made to correspond in amount to the composition of human milk. **perhydrase m.,** milk to which hydrogen dioxide has been added. **protein m.,** a modified milk preparation having a relatively low content of carbohydrate and fat and a relatively high protein content. **red m.,** milk made red by blood, eating of madder root, or the growth of *Erythrobacillus prodigiosus* or other microorganisms. **ropy m.,** milk which has become viscid so that it can be drawn out into threads. It is usually caused by the growth of *Alcaligenes viscolactis* and is eaten as a delicacy in Norway. **Schloss m.,** a modified milk containing the same proportion of salts and fat as human milk. **skimmed m.,** milk from which the cream has been removed. **soft curd m.,** milk the curd of which has been rendered soft and homogeneous by boiling, by the addition of cream or by the addition of sodium citrate. **sour m.,** milk containing lactic acid, produced by the action of lactic acid bacteria. **m. of sulfur,** precipitated sulfur. **uterine m.,** a white milky substance in the gravid uterus of some species, presumably for nourishment of the embryo. **uviol m.,** milk sterilized by the action of ultraviolet rays. **vegetable m.,** synthetic milk made out of vegetables. **vinegar m.,** acid milk prepared by adding vinegar to cow's milk. **vitamin D m.,** cow's milk to which vitamin D has been added either by direct addition, by exposure to ultraviolet light, or by feeding irradiated yeast to the cows. **witch's m.,** milk secreted in the breast of the newborn child; hexenmilch. **yeast m.,** milk from cows which have been fed on irradiated yeast; it has antirachitic potency.

milking (milk′ing) the pressing out of the contents of a tubular part, such as the urethra, by running the finger along it.

milk-leg (milk′leg) postpartum iliofemoral thrombophlebitis.

Milkman's syndrome (milk′manz) [Louis Arthur *Milkman*, American roentgenologist, 1895–1951] see under *syndrome.*

milkpox (milk′poks) variola minor.

milk sick (milk′sik) poisoning by white snake root, *Eupatorium urticaefolium.*

Millar's asthma (mil′arz) [John *Millar*, British physician, 1733–1805] laryngismus stridulus.

Millard's test (mil′ards) [Henry B. *Millard*, American physician, 1832–1893] see under *tests.*

Millard-Gubler syndrome (paralysis) (me-yar′-goob′ler) [Auguste L. J. *Millard*, French physician, 1830–1915; Adolphe Marie *Gubler*, French physician, 1821–1879] see under *syndrome.*

Miller-Abbott tube [T. Grier *Miller*, Philadelphia physician, 1886–1981; William Osler *Abbott*, Philadelphia physician, 1902–1943] see under *tube.*

milli- [L. *mille* thousand] a combining form indicating one thousand (e.g., millipede); used in naming units of measurement to indicate one one-thousandth (10⁻³) of the unit designated by the root with which it is combined. Symbol, m.

milliammeter (mil″e-am′ĕ-ter) an ammeter which registers a current in milliamperes.

milliampere (mil″e-am′pēr) [Fr.] one-thousandth of an ampere. Symbol, mA.

millibar (mil′ĭ-bar) one-thousandth part of a bar.

millicoulomb (mil′ĭ-koo′lom) a unit of quantity of current electricity, being one one-thousandth (10⁻³) of a coulomb. Symbol, mC.

millicurie (mil′ĭ-ku′re) a unit of radioactivity, being one one-thousandth (10⁻³) curie, or the quantity of radioactive material in which the number of nuclear disintegrations is 3.7 × 10⁷ per second. Symbol mCi.

millicurie-hour (mil′ĭ-ku′re-owr″) a unit of cumulated radioactivity equal to the presence of 1 millicurie for 1 hour. Abbreviated mCi-hr.

milliequivalent (mil″ĭ-e-kwiv′ah-lent) the number of grams of a solute contained in one milliliter of a normal solution; abbreviated mEq.

milligamma (mil″ĭ-gam′mah) nanogram; abbreviated μγ.

milligram (mil′ĭ-gram) [*milli-* + *gram*] one-thousandth of a gram. Symbol mg.

Millikan rays (mil′ĭ-kan) [Robert Andrews *Millikan*, American physicist, 1868–1953] cosmic rays.

millilambert (mil″ĭ-lam′bert) one-thousandth of a lambert.

milliliter (mil′ĭ-le″ter) [*milli-* + *liter*] a unit of volume in the metric system, being one one-thousandth (10⁻³) liter. Symbol ml.

millimeter (mil′ĭ-me-ter) a unit of linear measure of the metric system, being one one-thousandth (10⁻³) meter. Symbol mm.

millimicr(o)- a prefix used in naming units of measurement to indicate one-thousandth of one-millionth (10⁻⁹) of the unit designated by the root with which it is combined; now supplanted by the prefix *nan(o)-.*

millimicrocurie (mil″ĭ-mi″kro-ku′re) nanocurie.

millimolar (mil″ĭ-mo′lar) denoting a concentration of 1 millimole per liter. Symbol, mM.

millimole (mil′ĭ-mōl) one-thousandth part of a mole (def. 3); symbol mmol.

milling-in (mil′ing-in) correction of occlusal disharmonies of natural or artificial teeth by the use of abrasives between their occluding surfaces while they are rubbed together in the mouth or on the articulator. See also *grinding-in, occlusal adjustment,* under *adjustment,* and *selective grinding,* under *grinding.*

millions (mil′yunz) a name applied to various small fish that devour mosquito larvae; see *Lebistes reticulatus.*

milliosmol, milliosmole (mil″ĭ-os′mōl) one-thousandth of an osmole. Symbol, mOsm.

millipede (mil′ĭ-pēd) a more or less cylindrical arthropod of the order Chilognatha, class Diplopoda, characterized by having two pairs of short legs on most of its body segments; millipedes may have from 13 to almost 200 pairs of legs.

millirad (mil′ĭ-rad) one-thousandth (10⁻³) rad; abbreviated mrad.

millirem (mil′ĭ-rem) one-thousandth (10⁻³) of a rem; symbol mrem.

milliroentgen (mil′ĭ-rent″gen) one-thousandth (10⁻³) roentgen; abbreviated mr.

millisecond (mil″ĭ-sek′ond) one-thousandth of a second; abbreviated msec; symbol ms.

milliunit (mil′ĭ-u″nit) one-thousandth (10⁻³) of a standard unit; abbreviated mU.

millivolt (mil′ĭ-vōlt) one-thousandth of a volt. Symbol, mV.

Millon's test (reaction, reagent) (mil′onz) [Auguste N. E. *Millon*, French chemist, 1812–1867] see under *tests*.

Mills' disease (milz) [Charles Karsner *Mills*, Philadelphia neurologist, 1845–1931] ascending hemiplegia.

Mills-Reincke phenomenon (milz-rīn′kĕ) [Hiram F. *Mills*, American engineer, 1836–1921; J. J. *Reincke*, German physician, 19th century] see under *phenomenon*.

Milontin (mi-lon′tin) trademark for preparations of phensuximide.

Milpath (mil′path) trademark for a preparation of meprobamate and tridihexethyl chloride.

milphosis (mil-fo′sis) [Gr. *milphōsis*] the falling out of the eyelashes. Cf. *madarosis*.

milrinone (mil′rĭ-nōn) a cardiotonic.

Milroy's disease (edema) (mil′roys) [William Forsyth *Milroy*, American physician, 1855–1942] see under *disease*.

Milton's disease, edema (mil′tonz) [John Laws *Milton*, dermatologist in London, 1820–1898] angioedema.

Miltown (mil′town) trademark for a preparation of meprobamate.

Mima polymorpha (me′mah pol″e-mor′fah) *Acinetobacter calcoaceticus*.

mimbane hydrochloride (mim′bān) chemical name: 1-methylyohimbane monohydrochloride; an analgesic, $C_{20}H_{26}H_2 \cdot HCl$.

mimesis (mi-me′sis) [Gr. *mimēsis* imitation] the simulation of one disease or bodily process by another.

mimetic (mi-met′ik) [Gr. *mimētikos*] marked by simulation of another bodily process or disease. Also used as a word termination indicating simulation of a function, process, etc., designated by the root to which it is affixed, as *sympathomimetic*.

mimic (mim′ik) mimetic.

mimicry (mim′ĭk-re′) [Gr. *mimos* to imitate] an adaptation for survival in which an organism takes on a resemblance to some other organism or a nonliving object.

mimmation (mi-ma′shun) the habitual insertion of the "m" sound in speech in places where it does not belong.

mimosis (mi-mo′sis) mimesis.

min. abbreviation for L. *min′imum*, a minim.

Minamata disease (min″ah-mah′tah) [*Minamata* Bay, Japan] see under *disease*.

Mincard (min′kard) trademark for a preparation of aminometradine.

Minchinia (min-chin′e-ah) a genus of parasitic protozoa (order Balanosporida, class Stellatosporea) found in the epithelial cells of the gills and adjacent tissues of oysters and other aquatic invertebrates, causing disease of great economic importance.

mind (mīnd) [L. *mens;* Gr. *psychē*] the faculty, or function of the brain, by which an individual becomes aware of his surroundings and of their distribution in space and time, and by which he experiences feelings, emotions, and desires, and is able to attend, to remember, to reason, and to decide.

Mindererus, spirit of (min-der-e′rus) [Raymund *Minderer*, German physician, 1570(?)–1621] ammonium acetate solution.

mineral (min′er-al) [L. *minerale*] a nonorganic homogeneous solid substance, usually a constituent of the earth's crust.

mineralocorticoid (min″er-al-o-kor′tĭ-koid) 1. any of the group of C21 corticosteroids, principally aldosterone, predominantly involved in the regulation of electrolyte and water balance through their effect on ion transport in epithelial cells of the renal tubules, resulting in retention of sodium and loss of potassium; some also possess varying degrees of glucocorticoid activity. Their secretion is regulated principally by plasma volume, serum potassium concentration, and angiotensin II, and to a lesser extent by anterior pituitary ACTH. Cf. *glucocorticoid*. 2. of, pertaining to, having the properties of, or resembling a mineralocorticoid.

mingin (min′jin) a nitrogenous compound, $C_{13}H_{18}N_2O_2$, found in small amounts in the urine.

mini- [*mini*ature] a combining form denoting something smaller than is usual for objects in a given class.

minify (min′ĭ-fi) [L. *minus* less] to render less; to diminish. The opposite of magnify.

minilaparotomy (min″e-lap′ah-rot′o-me) [*mini-* + *laparotomy*] a small transperitoneal upper abdominal incision used for liver biopsy, open transhepatic cholangiography, peritoneal lavage, or tubal occlusion.

Mini-Lix (min′ĭ-liks) trademark for a preparation of aminophylline.

minim (min′im) [L. *minimum* least] a unit of capacity (liquid measure), being one-sixtieth part of a fluid dram, or the equivalent of 0.0616 milliliter.

minima (min′ĭ-mah) [L.] plural of *minimum*.

minimal (min′ĭ-mal) [L. *minimus* least] smallest or least; the smallest possible.

minimum (min′ĭ-mum), pl. *min′ima* [L. "smallest"] the smallest amount or lowest limit. **m. audib′ile, m. audible,** auditory threshold. **m. cognosci′bile,** the threshold of visual recognition of complicated shapes or contours. **m. legi′bile,** the threshold of visible recognition of form, as of test letters or numbers. **light m.,** the minimum intensity of light which is visually perceptible in completely darkened surroundings. **m. sensib′ile,** threshold of consciousness. **m. separa′bile,** the least distance that two objects may be apart and still be distinguished as two. **m. visi′bile,** light m.

Minin light (min′in) [A. V. *Minin*, Russian surgeon] see under *light*.

Minipress (min′ĭ-pres) trademark for a preparation of prazosin hydrochloride.

Minisporida (min″ĭ-spor′ĭ-dah) [*mini-* + *spore*] an order of parasitic protozoa (class Microsporea, phylum Microspora) having a general tendency toward minimum development of accessory spore organelles accompanied by maximum development of sporocysts, and characterized by spores without a well-developed polaroplast, usually with a relatively short polar tube, with little or no endospore.

minium (min′e-um) [L.] lead tetroxide.

Minizide (min′ĭ-zīd) trademark for preparations of prazosin hydrochloride with polythiazide.

Minkowski's figure (min-kov′skēz) [Oskar *Minkowski*, Lithuanian physician in Wiesbaden, 1858–1931] see under *figure*.

Minkowski-Chauffard syndrome (min-kov′ske-sho-far′) [Oskar Minkowski; Anatole-Marie-Emile *Chauffard*, French physician, 1855–1932] hereditary spherocytosis.

Minocin (mĭ-no′sin) trademark for preparations of minocycline hydrochloride.

minocycline (mĭ-no-si′klēn) chemical name: 4S,7-bis-(dimethylamino)1,4α,4aα,5,5aα,6,11,12aα-octahydro-3,10,12,12a-tetrahydroxy-1,11-dioxo-2-naphthacenecarboxamide; a semisynthetic broad-spectrum antibiotic of the tetracycline group, $C_{23}H_{27}N_3O_7$. **m. hydrochloride** [USP], the monohydrochloride salt of minocycline, $C_{23}H_{27}N_3O_7 \cdot HCl$, occurring as a yellow, crystalline powder; used in the treatment of a wide variety of infections due to tetracycline-susceptible bacteria and to some tetracycline-resistant organisms, especially staphylococci, administered orally and intravenously.

Minor's disease, sign (me′norz) [Lazar Salomonovich *Minor*, Russian neurologist, 1855–1942] see under *disease* and *sign*.

Minot (mi′nut) George Richards. American physician and pathologist, 1885–1950; co-winner, with William Parry Murphy and George Hoyt Whipple, of the Nobel prize for medicine or physiology in 1934 for their research into the use of liver therapy in pernicious anemia.

Minot-Murphy diet, treatment (mi′nut-mur′fe) [George Richards *Minot* and William Parry *Murphy*] see under *treatment*.

minoxidil (mĭ-noks′ĭ-dil) chemical name: 6-(1-piperidinyl)-2,4-pyrimidinediamine 3-oxide; a potent, long-acting orally effective vasodilator, $C_9H_{15}N_5O$, acting primarily on arterioles, used as an antihypertensive.

mint (mint) see *Mentha*. **mountain m.,** a plant of the genus *Pycnanthemum*. **wild m.,** a fragrant North American plant, *Mentha canadensis*, L. (Labiatae), resembling pennyroyal in its odor and other properties. It is the source of an essential oil with a lemon-like odor used in perfumery.

Mintezol (min′tĕ-zol) trademark for a preparation of thiabendazole.

minuthesis (min-u′thĕ-sis) [Gr. *minuthēsis* a wasting] a decrease in the psychophysical sensitivity of a sense organ due to continuous stimulation of that organ; fatigue.

M.I.O. minimal identifiable odor.

mio-, meio- [Gr. *meiōn* smaller] a combining form meaning less, or denoting relationship to contraction.

miocardia (mi″o-kar′de-ah) [mio- + Gr. *kardia* heart] the contraction of the heart; systole.

Miochol (mi′o-kol) trademark for a preparation of acetylcholine chloride.

miodidymus (mi″o-did′ĭ-mus) [mio- + Gr. *didymos* twin] a fetus with two heads joined at the occiputs.

miolecithal (mi″o-les′ĭ-thal) [mio- + Gr. *lekithos* yolk] containing little yolk; see under *ovum*.

mionectic (mi″o-nek′tik) [Gr. *meionektikos* disposed to take too little] (obs.) taking up (by the blood) less than a normal amount of oxygen at a given PO₂, i.e., the dissociation curve shifts to the right. Cf. *mesectic* and *pleonectic*.

miophone (mi′o-fōn) [mio- + Gr. *phōnē* sound] a microphone for testing the muscles.

miopragia (mi″o-pra′je-ah) [mio- + Gr. *prassein* to perform] decreased functional activity.

miopus (mi′o-pus) [mio- + Gr. *ōps* face] a monster with two fused heads, one face being rudimentary.

miosis (mi-o′sis) [Gr. *meiōsis* diminution] 1. contraction of the pupil. 2. meiosis. 3. that stage of disease during which the intensity of the symptoms diminishes. **irritative m.,** spastic miosis. **paralytic m.,** miosis due to paralysis of the dilator of the iris. **spastic m.,** miosis due to spasm of the sphincter pupillae. **spinal m.,** miosis occurring in spinal diseases.

miotic (mi-ot′ik) 1. pertaining to, characterized by, or producing miosis (def. 1). 2. an agent that causes the pupil to contract. 3. meiotic.

miracidia (mi-rah-sid′e-ah) plural of *miracidium*.

miracidium (mi-rah-sid′e-um), pl. *miracid′ia* [Gr. *meirakidion* a boy, lad, stripling] the first stage larva of a trematode which undergoes further development in the body of a snail.

miraculin (mir-ak′u-lin) a glycoprotein from the fruit of the tropical plant *Synsepalum dulcificum* which, after it is tasted, is able to change the perception of the taste of acids from sour to sweet.

Miradon (mir′ah-don) trademark for a preparation of anisindione.

mire (mēr) [Fr.; L. *mirari* to look at] one of the figures on the arm of an opthalmometer whose images are reflected on the cornea. The measurement of their variations measures the amount of corneal astigmatism.

mirincamycin hydrochloride (mir-in′kah-mi″sin) chemical name: methyl 7-chloro-6,7,8-trideoxy-6-[[4-pentyl-2-pyrrolidinyl)carbonyl]amino]-1-thio-α-threo-α-D-galacto-octapyranoside(2S- cis)-mixture with methyl 7-chloro-6,7,8-trideoxy-6-[[(trans-4-pentyl-2(S)-pyrrolidinyl)carbonyl]amino]-1-thio-L-threo-α-D-galacto- octapyranoside monohydrochloride; an antibacterial and antimalarial, $C_{19}H_{35}ClN_2O_5S \cdot HCl$.

mirror (mir′or) [Fr. *miroir*] a polished surface that reflects sufficient light to yield images of objects in front of it. **concave m.,** one with a concave reflecting surface. **convex m.,** one with a convex reflecting surface. **dental m.,** mouth m. **frontal m., head m.,** a circular mirror strapped to the head of the examiner, used to reflect light into a cavity, especially in connection with nasal, pharyngeal, and laryngeal examinations and to some extent in surgery of these organs. **Glatzel m.,** a flat plate of cold metal held horizontally below and in front of the nose. The patch of moisture deposited on its polished surface indicates the relative functional patency of the two sides of the nose. **mouth m.,** a small mirror, magnifying or nonmagnifying, used to reflect the operating field in the oral cavity, to retract the tissues and tongue, and to protect the tissues from injury during operation. Called also *dental m.* See also *dental reflector,* under *reflector.* **nasographic m.,** Glatzel m. **plane m.,** one with a flat reflecting surface. **van Helmont's m.,** centrum tendineum.

miryachit (mir-e′ah-chit) [Russ.] Gilles de la Tourette's syndrome.

misanthropia, misanthropy (mis″an-thro′pe-ah; mis-an′thro-pe) [miso- + Gr. *anthrōpos* man + -ia] hatred of mankind.

miscarriage (mis-kar′ij) loss of the products of conception from the uterus before the fetus is viable; spontaneous abortion.

misce (mis′e) [L.] mix.

miscegenation (mis″ĕ-jĕ-na′shun) [L. *miscere* to mix + *genus* race] the intermarriage or cohabitation of persons of different races, or the interbreeding of races.

miscible (mis′ĭ-b'l) susceptible of being mixed.

miserere mei (miz″er-a′re ma′e) [L. "have mercy on me"] 1. volvulus. 2. intestinal colic.

mis(o)- [Gr. *misos* hatred] a combining form meaning hatred of.

misogamy (mĭ-sog′ah-me) [miso- + Gr. *gamos* marriage] aversion to marriage.

misogyny (mĭ-soj′ĭ-ne) [miso- + Gr. *gynē* woman] aversion to women.

misonidazole (mi″so-nid′ah-zōl) chemical name: α-(methoxymethyl)-2-nitro-1*H*-imidazole-1-ethanol; an antitrichomonal antiprotozoal, $C_7H_{11}N_3O_4$.

mist. abbreviation for L. *mistu′ra,* a mixture.

mistletoe (mis″'l-to) any of several related parasitic shrubs of the family Loranthaceae that grow on various trees, such as the apple and other deciduous trees, including *Viscum album* L. (*European m.*) and *Phorandendron flavescens* (Pursh.) Nutt. (*American m.*), preparations of which were formerly used for their oxytocic, emmenagogic, cardiac stimulant, and vasodilator properties. Toxic principles in mistletoe include pressor amines, beta-phenylethylamine, and tyramine, and it is the source of the glutinous principle viscin.

mistura (mis-tu′rah) [L.] mixture. **m. cre′tae,** chalk mixture. **m. glycyrrhi′zae compos′ita,** brown mixture. **m. oleobalsam′ica,** oleobalsamic mixture: alcoholic solution of balsam of Peru with aromatic oils and flavoring; used as a skin stimulant. **m. pectora′lis,** expectorant mixture.

MIT monoiodotyrosine.

Mit. abbreviation for L. *mit′te,* send.

mitapsis (mit-ap′sis) [mito- + Gr. *hapsis* joining] the fusion of the chromatin granules in the final stage of cell conjugation.

Mitchell's disease, treatment (mich′elz) [Silas Weir *Mitchell,* Philadelphia neurologist, 1829–1914] see *erythromelalgia,* and see *Weir Mitchell's treatment,* under *treatment.*

Mitchell operation (mich′el) [Charles L. *Mitchell,* American orthopedic surgeon, born ·1901] see under *operation.*

mitchella (mich-el′ah) [John *Mitchell,* American botanist, 18th century] a creeping perennial herb, *Mitchella repens,* L. (Rubiaceae), squaw vine, partridge berry, deerberry, of the U.S. and Canada; used for its diuretic, astringent, and antidiarrheal properties, and formerly as a uterine tonic.

mite (mīt) any arthropod of the order Acarina except the ticks. The mites are minute animals, related to the spiders, usually having transparent or semitransparent bodies; they may be parasitic on man and domestic animals, producing various irritations of the skin (acariasis). Mites important to human and veterinary medicine are *Acarapis, Acarus, Allodermanyssus, Chorioptes, Demodex, Dermanyssus, Eutrombicular, Glycyphagus, Knemidokoptes, Neoschoengastia, Notoedres, Ornithonyssus, Otodectes, Pediculoides, Pneumonyssus, Psoroptes, Rhizoglyphus, Sarcoptes, Tetranychus, Trombicula, Tyrophagus.* **auricular m.,** see *Otodectes.* **beetle m.,** see *Gamasidae.* **bird m., chicken m.,** *Dermanyssus gallinae.* **burrowing m.,** see *Sarcoptes.* **cheese m.,** *Tyrophagus longior.* **clover m.,** *Bryobia praetiosa.* **coolie-itch m.,** *Rhizoglyphus parasiticus.* **copra m.,** *Tyrophagus castellani.* **depluming m.,** *Knemidokoptes gallinae.* **face m.,** *Demodex folliculorum.* **flour m.,** *Tyrophagus farinae.* **follicle m.,** see *Demodex.* **food m.,** *Glycyphagus domesticus.* **fowl m.,** see *Dermanyssus.* **hair follicle m.,** *Demodex folliculorum.* **harvest m.,** see *chigger.* **house dust m.,** *Dermatophagoides pteronyssimus.* **itch m.,** see *Notoedres* and *Sar-*

coptes. **kedani m.,** *Trombicula akamushi.* **louse m.,** *Pyemotes.* **mange m.,** any of various mites that cause mange; see, e.g., *Chorioptes, Demodex, Knemidokoptes, Noto-edres, Otodectes, Psoroptes,* and *Sarcoptes.* **meal m.,** *Tyro-phagus.* **mouse m.,** *Allodermanyssus sanguineus.* **mower's m.,** see *chigger.* **Northern fowl m.,** *Ornithonyssus sylviarum.* **onion m.,** *Acarus rhyzoglypticus hyacinthi.* **poultry m.,** *Dermanyssus gallinae.* **rat m.,** see *Ornithonyssus.* **red m.,** see *chigger.* **scab m.,** see *Psoroptes.* **spider m.,** see *Gamasidae.* **spinning m.,** *Bryobia praetiosa.* **straw m.,** *Pyemotes.* **tropical fowl m.,** *Ornithonyssus bursa.* **tropical rat m.,** *Ornithonyssus bacoti.*

mitella (mi-tel′ah) [L.] an arm sling.

Mithracin (mith′rah-sin) trademark for a preparation of mithramycin.

mithramycin (mith″rah-mi′sin) [USP] an antineoplastic antibiotic, produced by *Streptomyces plicatus* that binds to DNA and inhibits RNA synthesis in a manner similar to dactinomycin; it is used for treatment of advanced testicular carcinoma; major side effects are thrombocytopenia and hemorrhagic diathesis that can be life-threatening. It also has an inhibiting effect on osteoclasts and is used to treat hypercalcemia and hypercalciuria caused by metastatic malignancy or advanced parathyroid carcinoma.

mithridatism (mith′rĭ-da″tizm) [after *Mithridates,* died 63 B.C., king of Pontus, who reportedly took poisons so as to become immunized against them] the acquisition of immunity to the effects of a poison by ingestion of gradually increasing amounts of it.

miticidal (mi″tĭ-si′dal) destructive to mites.

miticide (mi′tĭ-sīd) an agent that is destructive to mites.

mitigate (mit′ĭ-gāt) [L. *mitigara* to soften] to moderate; to render milder.

mitis (mi′tis) [L.] mild.

mit(o)- [Gr. *mitos* thread] a combining form meaning threadlike, or denoting relationship to a thread, or to mitosis.

mitocarcin (mi″to-kar′sin) an antineoplastic antibiotic derived from *Streptomyces* species.

mitochondria (mi″to-kon′dre-ah, mit″o-kon′dre-ah), pl. of *mitochondrion* [*mito-* + Gr. *chondrion* granule] small spherical to rod-shaped components (organelles) found in the cytoplasm of cells, enclosed in a double membrane, with an internal membrane space between the two units, the inner one infolded into the interior of the organelle as a series of projections (cristae). They are the principal sites of the generation of energy (in the form of ion gradients and adenosine triphosphate [ATP] synthesis) resulting from the oxidation of foodstuffs, and they contain the enzymes of the Krebs and fatty acid cycles and the respiratory pathway. Mitochondria also contain RNA and DNA, by means of which they can independently replicate and code for the synthesis of some of their proteins. Called also *chondriosomes.*

mitochondrial (mi″to-kon′dre-al) of or pertaining to mitochondria.

mitochondrion (mi″to-kon′dre-on) singular of *mitochondria.*

mitocromin (mi″to-kro′min) an antineoplastic antibiotic produced by *Streptomyces viridochromogenes.*

mitogen (mi′to-jen) a substance that induces blast transformation; DNA, RNA, and protein synthesis; and proliferation of lymphocytes, e.g., concanavalin A, phytohemagglutinin, pokeweed mitogen, or lipopolysaccharide. **pokeweed m.,** a lectin isolated from pokeweed (*Phytolacca americana*); it is a mitogen that stimulates both B and T lymphocytes. Abbreviated PWM.

mitogenesia (mit″o-jĕ-ne′se-ah) mitogenesis.

mitogenesis (mi″to-jen′ĕ-sis) [*mitosis* + Gr. *genesis* production] the production, or causation, of mitosis in or transformation of a cell.

mitogenetic (mi″to-jĕ-net′ik) pertaining to, inducing, or characterized by mitogenesis.

mitogenic (mi″to-jen′ik) causing or inducing mitosis or cell transformation.

mitokinetic (mit″o-ki-net′ik) [*mito-* + Gr. *kinēsis* motion] a term applied to the force existing in the kinoplasm of a cell which produces the achromatic spindle in karyokinesis.

mitomalcin (mi″to-mal′sin) an antineoplastic antibiotic produced by *Streptomyces malayensis.*

mitome (mi′tōm) a thready network of the protoplasm of a cell; the more solid portion of cell protoplasm.

mitomycin (mi″to-mi′sin) an antineoplastic antibiotic produced by *Streptomyces caespitosus* that acts as a bifunctional or trifunctional alkylating agent causing cross-linking of DNA and inhibition of DNA synthesis and is relatively phase-specific for the late G_1 and early S phases of the cell cycle; it has activity against carcinomas of the stomach, pancreas, colon, rectum, breast, lung, and head and neck, as well as chronic myelogenous leukemia. However, because of its severe toxicity (delayed, cumulative, occasionally fatal bone marrow depression), it is usually used only for palliation in patients who have not responded to other treatment.

mitoplasm (mit′o-plazm) [*mito-* + Gr. *plassein* to form] the chromatic substance of a cell nucleus.

mitoschisis (mĭ-tos′kĭ-sis) [*mito-* + Gr. *schisis* split] karyokinesis.

mitoses (mi-to′sēz) plural of *mitosis.*

mitosin (mit′o-sin) a hormone producing mitosis or follicular maturation.

mitosis (mi-to′sis), pl. *mito′ses* [*mito-* + *-osis*] a method of indirect division of a cell, consisting of a complex of various processes, by means of which the two daughter nuclei normally receive identical complements of the number of chromosomes characteristic of the somatic cells of the species. Mitosis, the process by which the body grows and replaces cells, is divided into four phases. 1. *Prophase:* Formation of paired chromosomes; disappearance of nuclear membrane; appearance of the achromatic spindle; formation of polar bodies. 2. *Metaphase:* Arrangement of chromosomes in the equatorial plane of the central spindle to form the monaster. Chromosomes separate into exactly similar halves. 3. *Anaphase:* The two groups of daughter chromosomes separate and move along the fibers of the central spindle, each toward one of the asters, forming the diaster. 4. *Telophase:* The daughter chromosomes resolve themselves into a reticulum and the daughter nuclei are formed; the cytoplasm divides, forming two complete daughter cells. NOTE: The term *mitosis* is used interchangeably with cell division, but strictly speaking it refers to nuclear division, whereas *cytokinesis* refers to division of the cytoplasm. In some cells, as in many fungi and the fertilized eggs of many insects, nuclear division occurs within the cell unaccompanied by division of the cytoplasm and formation of daughter cells. Cf. *meiosis.* **heterotypic m.,** mitosis in which the halves of bivalent chromosomes move away from each other toward the poles, as occurs in the first, or reductional, division of meiosis. **homeotypic m.,** the ordinary type of cell division in mitosis, as occurs also in the second, or equational, division of meiosis. **multicentric m.,** pluripolar m. **pathologic m.,** atypical, asymmetrical mitosis indicative of malignancy. **pluripolar m.,** cell division that results in the formation of more than two daughter cells.

mitosome (mit′o-sōm) [*mito-* + Gr. *sōma* body] a body formed from the spindle fibers of the preceding mitosis; a spindle remnant.

mitosper (mi′to-sper) an antineoplastic substance derived from *Aspergillus glaucus.*

mitospore (mi′to-spōr) an asexual spore, so called because it is produced by mitosis; when motile it is called a *zoospore.*

mitotane (mi′to-tān) [USP] chemical name: 1-chloro-2-[2,2-dichloro-1-(4-chlorophenyl)ethyl]benzene. An antineoplastic compound, $C_{14}H_{10}Cl_4$, similiar to the insecticides DDT and DDD, and found to cause severe damage to the adrenal cortex, causing a rapid decrease in adrenocorticosteroid production; used for palliation in inoperable adrenocortical carcinoma of both functional and nonfunctional types, administered orally.

mitotic (mi-tot′ik) pertaining to mitosis.

mitral (mi′tral) 1. shaped somewhat like a miter. 2. pertaining to the mitral or bicuspid valve.

mitralism (mi′tral-izm) a tendency toward the development of mitral lesions in the heart.

mitralization (mi″tral-i-za′shun) straightening of the left border and prominence of the pulmonary salient of the cardiac shadow, a configuration commonly seen roentgenographically in mitral stenosis.

Mitsuda antigen, reaction, test (mit′su-dah) [Kensuke *Mitsuda,* Japanese physician, born 1876] see *lepromin,* see under *reaction,* and see *lepromin test,* under *tests.*

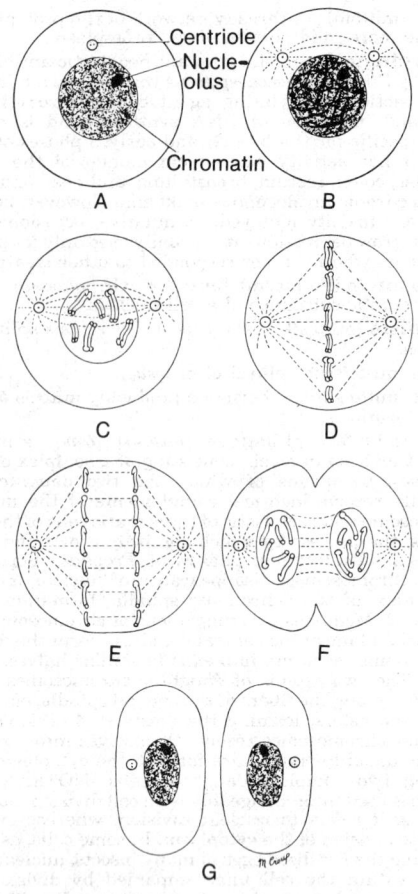

Mitosis shown as occurring in a cell of a hypothetical animal with a diploid chromosome number of six (haploid number three); one pair of chromosomes is short, one pair is long and hooked, and one pair is long and knobbed. *A, Resting stage. B, early prophase:* centriole divided and chromosomes appearing; *C, later prophase* —centrioles at poles, chromosomes shortened and visibly doubled; *D, metaphase* —chromosomes arranged on equator of spindle; *E, anaphase* —chromosomes migrating toward poles; *F, telophase* —nuclear membranes formed; chromosomes elongating; cytoplasmic divisions beginning; *G, daughter cells* —resting phase.

mittelschmerz (mit′el-shmārts) [Ger. *mittel* mid, middle, + *schmerz* pain, suffering] intermenstrual pain.

mittor (mit′or) [L. *mittere* to send] any one of the terminals of a neuron which gives off an impulse or stimulus to the ceptors of an adjoining neuron; see *neuromittor*.

mixed (mikst) affecting various parts at once; showing two or more different characteristics.

mixidine (mik′sĭ-dēn) chemical name: 3,4-dimethoxy-*N*-(1-methyl-2-pyrrolidinylidene)benzeneethanamine; a coronary vasodilator, $C_{15}H_{22}N_2O_2$.

mixoscopia (miks″o-sko′pe-ah) [Gr. *mixis* intercourse + *skopein* to examine] a sexual perversion in which gratification is obtained by the sight of one's love object engaged in sexual intercourse with another.

mixotroph (mik′so-trōf) in bacterial physiology, the ability to use alternative sources for metabolism and energy, as being capable of growth in either the absence or presence of light, or with either organic or inorganic compounds for nutrition.

mixotrophic (mik″so-trof′ik) having the nutritional characters of both animals and plants.

Mixtard (miks′tard) trademark for a mixture of 30 per

cent insulin injection (regular insulin) and 70 per cent isophane insulin suspension.

mixture (miks′chur) [L. *mixtura, mistura*] a combination of different drugs or ingredients, as a fluid resulting from mixing a fluid with other fluids, or with solids, or a suspension of a solid in a liquid. See also under *mistura*. **A.C.E. m.,** a mixture of alcohol, chloroform, and ether. **Agazotti's m.,** a mixture of oxygen and carbon dioxide, formerly used for aviation sickness. **Bagot's m.,** a local anesthetic mixture of cocaine hydrochloride and sparteine sulfate, in boiled water. **Biedert's cream m.,** a food for young infants, containing cream, water, and milk sugar. **brown m.,** a mixture containing glycyrrhiza fluidextract, antimony potassium tartrate, paregoric, alcohol, glycerin, and purified water; used as an expectorant. Formerly called *compound opium* and *glycyrrhiza mixture*. **Castellani's m.,** a mixture for treating yaws, containing tartar emetic, sodium salicylate, potassium iodide, sodium bicarbonate, and water. **Chabaud's m.,** a fixative mixture containing alcohol, phenol, formalin, and acetic acid. **chalk m.,** prepared chalk, with bentonite magma, cinnamon water, and saccharin sodium; used as an antacid. **expectorant m.,** ammonium carbonate 1.75 per cent, fluidextract of senega and squill each 3.5 per cent, camphorated tincture of opium 17.5 per cent, water, and syrup of tolu. **Gregory's m.,** compound powder of rhubarb; see under *powder*. **Gunning's m.,** a mixture used in estimating the nitrogen in the urine, consisting of 15 ml. of concentrated sulfuric acid, 10 gm. of potassium sulfate, and 0.5 gm. of copper sulfate. **kaolin m. with pectin** [NF], a preparation containing kaolin, pectin, powdered tragacanth, benzoic acid, saccharin sodium, glycerin, and peppermint oil in purified water; used as an adsorbent and demulcent. **Mayer's glycerin-albumin m.,** a mixture of equal parts of white of egg and glycerin, with a little camphor or phenol, for affixing paraffin sections to slides. **oleobalsamic m.,** see *mistura oleobalsamica*. **opium and glycyrrhiza m., compound,** former name for *brown mixture*. **pectoral m.,** expectorant mixture. **racemic m.,** racemate. **Ringer's m.,** see under *irrigation*. **Tellyesniczky's m.,** see under *fluid*.

Miyagawanella (mi″yah-ga″wah-nel′ah) [Yoneji *Miyagawa*, Japanese bacteriologist, 1885–1959] *Chlamydia*.

MK monkey lung (cell culture).

M.K.S. abbreviation for *meter-kilogram-second* system, a system of measurements in which the units are based on the meter as the unit of length, the kilogram as the unit of mass, and the second as the unit of time.

ml milliliter.

M.L.A. abbreviation for L. *mento-laeva anterior* (left mentoanterior, a position of the fetus), and for *Medical Library Association*.

MLC mixed lymphocyte culture.

M.L.D. 1. median lethal dose. 2. minimum lethal dose.

M.L.P. abbreviation for L. *mento-laeva posterior* (left mentoposterior, a position of the fetus).

MLR mixed lymphocyte reaction; see *mixed lymphocyte culture*, under *culture*.

M.L.T. abbreviation for L. *mento-laeva transversa* (left mentotransverse, a position of the fetus).

M.M. mucous membranes.

mM millimolar.

mm millimeter.

mm Hg millimeter of mercury, a unit of pressure equal to that exerted by a column of mercury at 0° C one millimeter high at mean sea level. It equals 1/760 atmosphere or 1 torr to within one part in 7 million.

MMPI Minnesota Multiphasic Personality Inventory.

MMR measles-mumps-rubella (vaccine).

mμ millimicron.

mμCi millimicrocurie. See *nanocurie*.

μl microliter.

μM micromolar.

μμCi micromicrocurie. See *picocurie*.

Mn chemical symbol for *manganese*.

M'Naghten (McNaughten) rule (mik-naw′ten) [from *M'Naghten*, a person who in 1843 was acquitted by a British court of murder on the ground of insanity] see under *rule*.

mnemic (ne′mik) mnemonic.

mnemonic (ne-mon′ik) [Gr. *mnēmonikos* pertaining to memory] pertaining to, characterized by, or promoting recollection, or memory.

mnemonics (ne-mon′iks) the cultivation or improvement of memory by special methods or techniques.

M.O. Medical Officer.

Mo chemical symbol for *molybdenum*.

Moban (mo′ban) trademark for a preparation of molindone hydrochloride.

Mobilina (mo″bĭ-li′nah) [L. *mobilis* mobile] a suborder of mobile, usually conical or cylindrical or discoidal and orally and aborally flattened ciliate protozoa (order Peritrichida, subclass Peritrichia), characterized by the presence of a ciliary girdle and a complex thigmotactic apparatus at the aboral end, often with a highly distinctive denticulate ring of "teeth." All species are ectoparasites or endoparasites of freshwater or marine vertebrates and invertebrates, and those found on the gills of fish are pathogenic.

mobility (mo-bil′ĭ-te) [L. *mobilitas*] 1. capability of movement, of being moved, or of flowing freely. 2. rate of movement of a charged particle in an applied electric field. **electrophoretic m.,** 1. the rate of migration (in cm/s) per unit electric field strength (V/cm) of a charged particle in electrophoresis. Symbol, μ. 2. any measure of the rate of migration of an ionic species in electrophoresis, e.g., β electrophoretic mobility, designating the electrophoretic mobility of a beta globulin.

mobilization (mo″bĭ-li-za′shun) the process of making a fixed part or stored substance mobile, as by separating a part from surrounding structures to make it accessible for an operative procedure or by causing release into the circulation for body use of a substance stored in the body. **stapes m.,** surgical correction of immobility of the stapes, in treatment of deafness resulting from otosclerosis.

mobilometer (mo″bil-om′ě-ter) an instrument for measuring the consistency of liquids such as oil, cream, liquid foods, etc.

Möbius' disease, sign, syndrome (me′be-us) [Paul Julius *Möbius*, German neurologist, 1853–1907] see under *disease, sign,* and *syndrome*.

MOCA a regimen of methotrexate, Oncovin (vincristine), cyclophosphamide, and Adriamycin (doxorubicin), used in cancer chemotherapy.

moccasin (mok′ah-sin) a common name applied to several species of snakes, but usually denoting the venomous semiaquatic pit viper *Agkistrodon piscivorus*, or water moccasin, less frequently *A. contortrix*, or Highland moccasin. See table accompanying *snake*.

mocezuelo (mo″se-zwa′lo) [Mexican] trismus neonatorum.

mock-up (mok′up) a full-sized model of an apparatus or other equipment constructed out of substitute materials, used in instruction or for study and improvement of design.

modality (mo-dal′ĭ-te) 1. a homeopathic term signifying a condition which modifies drug action; a condition under which symptoms develop, becoming better or worse. 2. a method of application of, or the employment of, any therapeutic agent; limited usually to physical agents. 3. a specific sensory entity, such as taste.

mode (mōd) [L. *modus* measure, manner] 1. the value at which the peak of the theoretical frequency distribution underlying the sample data occurs; usually referred to as the most frequently occurring value in a statistical sample or population. 2. a relative maximum of the density function of a probability distribution, a value occurring more frequently than values immediately above and below; a distribution with two peaks is bimodal.

model (mod′el) 1. something that represents or simulates something else; a replica. 2. a reasonable facsimile of the body or any of its parts; used for demonstration and teaching purposes. 3. cast, def. 5. 4. to imitate another's behavior; see *modeling*. **animal m.,** any condition found in an animal that is of value in studying a biological phenomenon, e.g., a pathological mechanism of an animal disorder useful in studying human disease.

modeling (mod′el-ing) a behavior modification technique in which the patient is taught to imitate the desired behavior of another.

moderator (mod′er-a-tor) in nuclear chemistry and physics, a substance, such as graphite or beryllium, used to cut down the flux of subatomic particles or radiation by absorption of the same.

Moderil (mod′er-il) trademark for a preparation of rescinnamine.

modification (mod″ĭ-fi-ka′shun) the process or result of changing the form or characteristics of an object or substance. **behavior m.,** see under *therapy*. **racemic m.,** see *racemate*.

modioliform (mo″de-o′lĭ-form) shaped like the hub of a wheel.

modiolus (mo-di′o-lus) [L. "nave," "hub"] [NA] the central pillar or columella of the cochlea; called also *columella cochleae*.

Mod. praesc. abbreviation for L. *mo′do praescrip′to,* in the way directed.

modulation (mod″u-la′shun) [L. *modulare* to measure] the normal capacity of cell adaptability to its environment. **antigenic m.,** alteration or loss of reactivity of cell surface antigens resulting from redistribution of antigenic sites due to the presence of bound antibody.

modulator (mod″u-la′tor) a specific inductor that brings out characteristics peculiar to a definite region.

Moduretic (mod″u-ret′ik) trademark for preparations of amiloride hydrochloride with hydrochlorothiazide.

MODY maturity-onset diabetes of youth.

Moe plate (mo) [John H. *Moe*, American surgeon, born 1905] see under *plate*.

Moebius see *Möbius*.

Moeller's glossitis (me′lerz) [Julius Otto Ludwig *Moeller*, German surgeon, 1819–1887] see under *glossitis*.

Moeller-Barlow disease (me′ler-bar′lo) [J. O. L. *Moeller*; Sir Thomas *Barlow*, London physician, 1845–1945] see under *disease*.

Moenckeberg (menk′ě-berg) see *Mönckeberg*.

Moentjang tina the Malay term in Indonesia for intoxication caused by the use in food of oil obtained from the fruit of the tropical tree *Hernandia sonora* L. (Hernandiaceae). Ordinarily the oil is used only in lamps.

Moerner-Sjöqvist method, test (mer′ner-syek′vist) [Carl Thore *Moerner*, Swedish physician, 1864–1917; John August *Sjöqvist*, Swedish physician, 1863–1934] see *Sjöqvist method*, under *method*.

mogi- [Gr. *mogis* with difficulty] a combining form meaning difficult, or with difficulty.

mogiarthria (moj-e-ar′thre-ah) [*mogi-* + Gr. *arthroun* to utter distinctly + *-ia*] a form of dysarthria in which there is defective coordination of the muscles involved.

mogilalia (moj-e-la′le-ah) [*mogi-* + *lalia* chatter] difficulty in speech; stuttering.

mogiphonia (moj-e-fo′ne-ah) [*mogi-* + Gr. *phōnē* voice] difficulty in making vocal sounds.

Mohr's test (mōrz) [Francis *Mohr*, American pharmaceutical chemist] see under *tests*.

Mohrenheim's fossa, triangle (mo′ren-hīmz) [Baron Joseph Jacob Freiherr von *Mohrenheim*, Austrian surgeon, 1759–1799] fossa infraclavicularis.

Mohs hardness number (mōz) [Friedrich *Mohs*, German mineralogist, 1773–1839] see under *number*.

Mohs' technique (chemosurgery, surgery) (mōz) [Frederic Edward *Mohs*, American surgeon, born 1910] see under *technique*.

moiety (moi′ě-te) [Fr. *moitié*, from L. *medietas, medius,* middle] any equal part; a half; also any part or portion. **carbohydrate m.,** a carbohydrate-derived portion of the structure of a molecule. **corrin m.,** a complex ring system in the vitamin B_{12} molecule, closely related to the porphyrins of the cytochromes.

moist (moist) somewhat wet; damp.

mol (mol) mole, def. 3.

molal (mo′lal) containing one mole of solute per kilogram of solvent. NOTE: *molal* refers to the weight of the solvent, *molar* to the volume of the solution.

molality (mo-lal′ĭ-te) the number of moles of a solute per kilogram of pure solvent. NOTE: *molality* refers to the weight of the solvent, *molarity* to the volume of the solution.

molar (mo′lar) 1. [L. *moles* mass] pertaining to a mass; not molecular. 2. [L. *molaris* belonging to a mill, from *mola* millstone] adapted for grinding; see under *tooth*. 3. a posterior tooth which is used for grinding food and which acts as a major jaw support in the dental arch; see under *tooth*. 4. pertaining to a mole of a substance, such as molar volume, molar mass, or molar absorptivity, i.e., the quantity of some property associated with a mole of the substance. 5. a measure of the concentration of a solute, expressed as the number of moles of solute per liter of solution (symbol M), e.g. 0.25 M = 0.25 moles per liter (mol/l). The latter notation is used in the SI system. **Moon's m's,** see under *tooth*. **mulberry m.,** a malformed first molar characterized by dwarfing of the cusps and hypertrophy of the enamel surrounding the cusp with agglomeration of masses of globules, giving it the appearance of a mulberry; seen in congenital syphilis and certain other diseases. Called also *mulberry tooth.* **sixth-year m.,** one of the permanent first molar teeth, so called because it usually erupts at the age of 6 years immediately posterior to the last molar of the deciduous dentition. **supernumerary m.,** paramolar. **third m.,** dens serotinus. **twelfth-year m.,** one of the permanent second molar teeth, so called because it usually erupts at the age of 12 years.

molariform (mo-lar′ĭ-form) shaped like a molar tooth; showing molarlike characteristics.

molaris (mo-la′ris) [L. "millstone, grinder, molar tooth"] adapted for grinding; molar. **m. ter′tius,** dens serotinus.

molarity (mol-ar′ĭ-te) the number of moles of a solute per liter of solution. Cf. *molality*.

molasses (mo-las′ez) [L. *mellaceus* like honey] a thick, sweet syrup; the residue left after crystallization of sugar; treacle. **sugar-house m.,** that which is left after the refining of sugar. **West India m.,** a variety obtained in making raw sugar.

molc. molar concentration.

mold (mōld) 1. any of a large group of parasitic and saprophytic fungi that cause mold or moldiness and that exist as multicellular filamentous colonies; also, the deposit or growth produced by such fungi. The dimorphic fungi exist, according to environmental conditions, as molds or unicellular (yeast) forms. The common molds are *Mucor, Penicillium, Rhizopus,* and *Aspergillus.* See accompanying plate. 2. a form in which an object is given shape, or cast. 3. an object formed in a mold; also, the shape of a molded object, as the shape of an artificial tooth. 4. the act of molding or shaping. **slime m.,** see *Mycetozoida.* **white m.,** white or slightly woolly patches which form on the surface of meat in cold storage and other products due to the growth of various species of fungi.

molding (mōld′ing) 1. the creation of shape, or fashioning of an object. 2. the shaping of the fetal head in adjustment to the size and shape of the birth canal. **border m.,** the shaping of dental impression material by the manipulation or action of the tissues and structures adjacent to the borders of an impression. Called also *tissue m.* **compression m.,** a method of molding in which compression is used to pack the material in and to express its excess from the mold. **injection m.,** the act or process of forcing a plastic material, such as a softened resin, into the mold space under pressure. **tissue m.,** border m.

mole (mōl) [L. *moles* a shapeless mass] 1. a fleshy mass or tumor formed in the uterus by the degeneration or abortive development of an ovum. 2. a nevocytic nevus; the term is also used to designate a pigmented fleshy growth, and is applied loosely to any blemish of the skin. 3. that amount of a substance (in a system) that contains as many elementary entities (atoms, ions, molecules, or radicals) as there are carbon atoms in 12 grams of carbon-12 (^{12}C), or that amount of a chemical compound whose mass in grams is equivalent to its formula mass (see *gram-molecule,* and see *gram molecular weight,* under *weight*). A mole is considered to be equal to 6.023 × 10²³ (Avogadro's number) elementary entities. Abbreviated mol. **blood m.,** a mass in the uterus made up of blood clots, the placenta, and fetal membranes retained after fetal death. **Breus′ m.,** a pathologic change in the placenta found in abortion consisting of accumulation of masses of intervillous hematomas that project into the chorionic space. **cystic m.,** hydatidiform m. **false m.,** an intrauterine mass formed from a polyp or neoplasm. **fleshy m.,** 1. a blood mole which has assumed a fleshlike appearance. 2. one formed by a dead

ovum in the uterus. **gram m.,** mole, def. 3. **hydatid m., hydatidiform m.,** an abnormal pregnancy resulting from a pathologic ovum, with proliferation of the epithelial covering of the chorionic villi and dissolution and cystic cavitation of the avascular stroma of the villi. It results in a mass of cysts resembling a bunch of grapes. Called also *cystic* or *vesicular m.* **invasive m., malignant m., metastasizing m.,** chorioadenoma destruens. **pigmented m.,** see under *nevus.* **stone m.,** a mole which has undergone a calcareous degeneration. **true m.,** a mole which represents the degenerated ovum itself. **tubal m.,** the mass of blood clot and chorionic villi found after death of the conceptus in a tubal pregnancy. **vesicular m.,** hydatidiform m.

molecular (mo-lek′u-lar) of, pertaining to, or composed of molecules.

molecule (mol′ĕ-kūl) [L. *molecula* little mass] a very small mass of matter; the smallest amount of a substance which can exist alone; an aggregation of atoms; specifically, a chemical combination of two or more atoms which form a specific chemical substance. To break up the molecule into its constituent atoms is to change its character. The number and kind of atoms in a molecule vary with the compound. **cell interaction (CI) m's,** products of cell interaction genes (q.v.). **CI m's,** cell interaction m's. **diatomic m.,** one containing two atoms. **hexatomic m.,** one containing six atoms. **monatomic m.,** one which consists of a single atom. **nonpolar m.,** a molecule in which the electrical potential is symmetrically distributed over the molecule. **polar m.,** a molecule in which the electrical potential is not symmetrically distributed. **tetratomic m.,** a molecule made up of four atoms. **triatomic m.,** one composed of three atoms.

molilalia (mol″ĭ-la′le-ah) mogilalia.

molimen (mo-li′men), pl. *molim′ina* [L. "effort"] a laborious effort made for the performance of any normal body function, especially that manifested by a variety of mild but unpleasant symptoms preceding or accompanying the menstrual period; when such symptoms are severe, the condition is known as premenstrual tension.

molimina (mo-lim′ĭ-nah) plural of *molimen.*

molindone hydrochloride (mo-lin′dōn) chemical name: 3-ethyl-1,5,6,7-tetrahydro-2-methyl-5-(4-morpholinylmethyl)-4*H*-indol-4-one monohydrochloride. A sedative and tranquilizer, $C_{16}H_{24}N_2O_2 \cdot HCl$, occurring as a white, crystalline powder; used in the management of schizophrenia, administered orally.

Mol-Iron (mōl-i′ron) trademark for preparations of ferrous sulfate.

Molisch's test (reaction) (mol′ish-ez) [Hans *Molisch,* chemist in Vienna, 1856–1937] see under *tests.*

Moll's glands (molz) [Jacob Antonius *Moll,* Dutch ophthalmologist, 1832–1914] glandulae ciliares conjunctivales.

mollescuse (mol-les′kūs) [L. *mollis* soft] softening.

Mollicutes (mol″ĭ-ku′tēz) [L. *mollis* soft + *cutis* skin] a class of bacteria of the division Tenericutes, made up of cells bounded by a triple-layered membrane; they differ from other bacteria in lacking a true cell wall. The class comprises the smallest microorganisms capable of growth in a cell-free medium, occurring as pleomorphic, coccoid, or filamentous cells with a tendency to produce myeloid structures. It contains a single order, Mycoplasmatales, and the additional genera *Anaeroplasma* and *Thermoplasma.* Called also *Mycoplasmas.* See also *Mycoplasma,* def. 2.

mollin (mol′in) a glycerinated soft soap with excess of fats, used as a vehicle for medicines to be applied externally.

mollities (mo-lish′e-ēz) [L.] softness; abnormal softening. **m. os′sium,** osteomalacia.

mollusc (mol′usk) mollusk.

Mollusca (mŏ-lus′kah) [L. *molluscus* soft] a phylum of animals containing snails, slugs, mussels, oysters, clams, octopuses, nautiluses, squids, cuttlefish, etc.

molluscacidal (mŏ-lusk″ah-si′dal) destructive to snails and other mollusks.

molluscacide (mŏ-lusk′ah-sīd) an agent that will destroy snails and other mollusks.

molluscicide (mŏ-lus′sĭ-sīd) molluscacide.

molluscous (mŏ-lus′kus) pertaining to molluscum.

molluscum (mŏ-lus′kum) [L. *molluscus* soft] the name

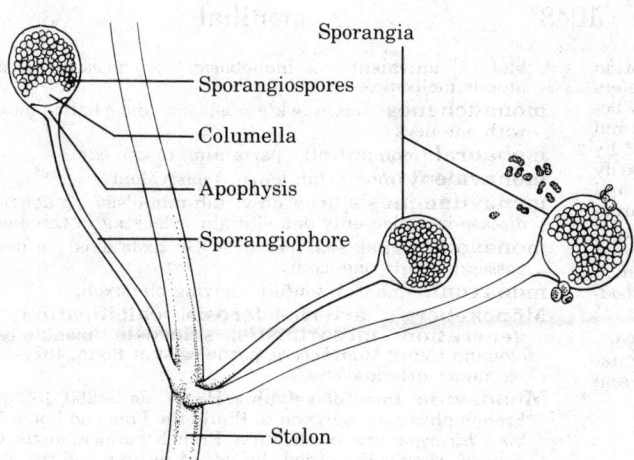

Sporangia
Sporangiospores
Columella
Apophysis
Sporangiophore
Stolon

Sporangia of *Absidia* arising from a stolon.

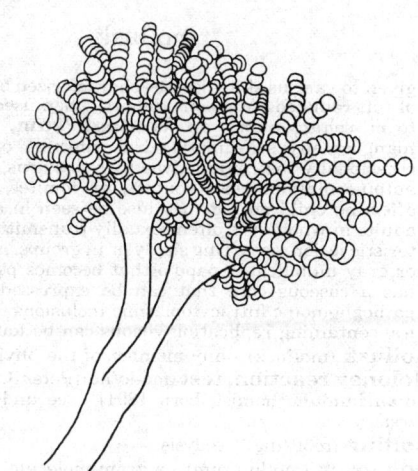

Conidiophores and conidia
of *Aspergillus*.

Conidia
Metula
Conidiophore

Brushlike conidiophores and parallel
chains of conidia of *Penicillium*.

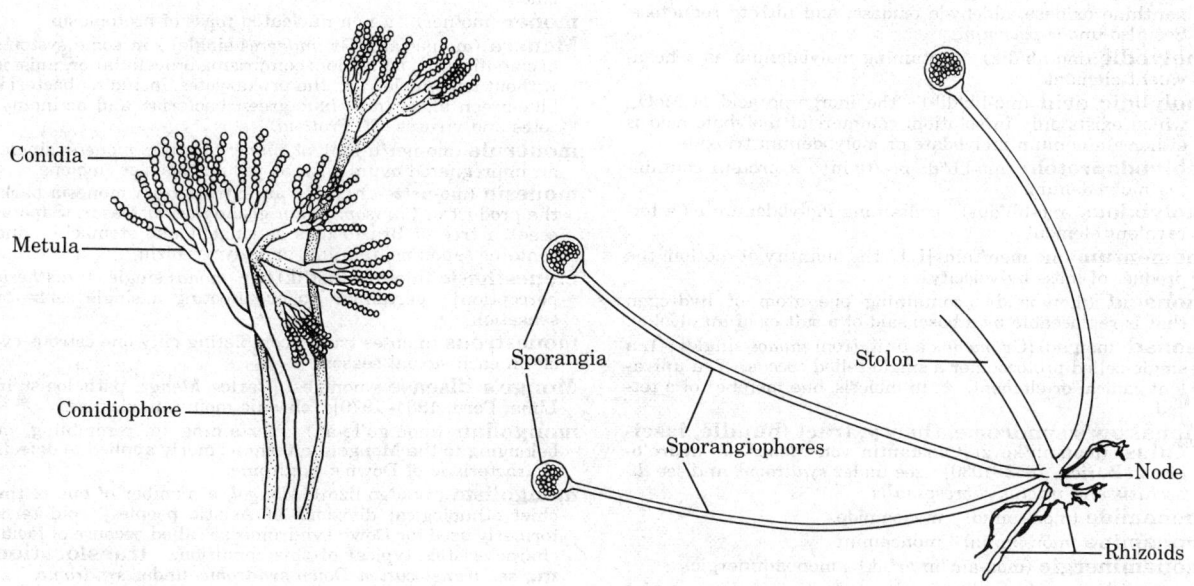

Sporangia
Stolon
Sporangiophores
Node
Rhizoids

Sporangiophores of *Rhizopus* arising from
a node above the rhizoids.

PLATE 26 — CHARACTERISTIC STRUCTURES OF COMMON MOLDS

given to various skin diseases characterized by the formation of soft rounded cutaneous tumors; when used alone it refers to *m. contagiosum*. **m. contagio′sum,** a common, benign, usually self-limited viral infection of the skin and occasionally the conjunctivae by a poxvirus, transmitted by autoinoculation, close contact, or fomites, and primarily affecting children but may also be seen in adolescents and adults in whom it is often sexually transmitted. The characteristic lesion, occurring singly or in groups, is a flesh-colored or gray umbilicated papule that becomes pearly white and has a caseous core that can be expressed and in which pathognomonic intracytoplasmic inclusions (*molluscum bodies*) containing replicating virions can be found.

mollusk (mol′usk) any member of the phylum Mollusca.

Moloney reaction, test (mo-lo′ne) [Peter J. *Moloney*, Canadian immunochemist, born 1891] see under *reaction* and *tests*.

molting (mōlt′ing) ecdysis.

molugram (mol′u-gram) a gram-molecule.

Mol. wt. molecular weight.

molybdate (mo-lib′dāt) any salt of molybdic acid; some are used as tests, especially for the detection of heavy metal ions.

molybdenosis (mo-lib″dĕ-no′sis) chronic molybdenum poisoning; see under *poisoning*.

molybdenum (mo-lib′dĕ-num) [Gr. *molybdos* lead] a hard, silvery-white, metallic element; symbol, Mo; atomic number, 42; atomic weight, 95.94; specific gravity, 10.2. It is an essential trace element, being a component of the enzymes xanthine oxidase, aldehyde oxidase, and nitrate reductase. See also under *poisoning*.

molybdic (mo-lib′dik) containing molybdenum as a hexavalent element.

molybdic acid (mo-lib′dik) the inorganic acid H_2MoO_4, which exists only in solution; commercial molybdic acid is either ammonium molybdate or molybdenum trioxide.

molybdoprotein (mo-lib″do-pro′te-in) a protein containing molybdenum.

molybdous (mo-lib′dus) containing molybdenum as a tetravalent element.

momentum (mo-men′tum) [L.] the quantity of motion; the product of mass by velocity.

monacid (mon-as′id) containing one atom of hydrogen that is replaceable by a base; said of a salt or of an alcohol.

monad (mon′ad) [Gr. *monas* a unit, from *monos* single] 1. a single-celled protozoon or a single-celled coccus. 2. a univalent radical or element. 3. in meiosis, one member of a tetrad.

Monakow's syndrome, theory, tract (bundle, fasciculus) (mon-ah′kovz) [Constantin von *Monakow*, neurologist in Zurich, 1853–1930] see under *syndrome*, and see *diaschisis* and *tractus rubrospinalis*.

monamide (mon-am′id) monoamide.

monamine (mon-am′in) monoamine.

monaminergic (mon-am″in-er′jik) monoaminergic.

monangle (mon′ang-g'l) having only one angle; a dental instrument having only one angulation in the shank connecting the handle, or shaft, with the working portion of the instrument, known as the blade, or nib. Cf. *binangle*, *quadrangle* (def. 2), and *triple-angle*.

Monarda (mo-nar′dah) American horsemint; wild bergamot. The leaves of *Monarda punctata* L. (Labiatae). A herbaceous plant found throughout the midwest and northeast United States and formerly used for its carminative and aromatic stimulant properties.

monarthric (mon-ar′thrik) pertaining to or affecting a single joint.

monarthritis (mon″ar-thri′tis) [*mono-* + *arthritis*] inflammation of a single joint. **m. defor′mans,** arthritis deformans of a single joint.

monarticular (mon″ar-tik′u-lar) monarthric.

monaster (mon-as′ter) [*mono-* + Gr. *aster* star] the single star-shaped figure at the end of the prophase in mitosis.

monathetosis (mon″ath-ĕ-to′sis) [*mono-* + *athetosis*] athetosis of one limb.

monatomic (mon″ah-tom′ik) [*mono-* + Gr. *atomos* indivisi-

ble] 1. univalent. 2. monobasic. 3. consisting of monatomic molecules.

monauchenos (mon-awk′ĕ-nus) a dicephalic monster with one neck.

monaural (mon-aw′ral) pertaining to one ear.

monavalent (mon-av′ah-lent) monovalent.

monavitaminosis (mon″ah-vi″tah-min-o′sis) a deficiency disease in which only one vitamin is lacking in the diet.

monaxon (mon-ak′son) [*mono-* + Gr. *axōn* axis] a neuron possessing only one axon.

monaxonic (mon″ak-son′ik) having one axon.

Mönckeberg's arteriosclerosis, calcification, degeneration, mesarteritis, sclerosis (menk′e-bergz) [Johann Georg *Mönckeberg*, pathologist at Bonn, 1877–1925] see under *arteriosclerosis*.

Mondeville (mon″dĕ-ve′yuh), Henri de (1260–1320) a French physician, surgeon to Philip the Fair and Louis X; in his *Chirurgie*, one of the first French surgical texts from France, Mondeville urged the use of sutures and the avoidance of suppuration in primary healing.

Mondonesi reflex (mon″do-na′ze) [Filippo *Mondonesi*, Italian physician] bulbomimic reflex.

Mondor's disease (mon′dorz) [Henri *Mondor*, French surgeon, 1885–1962] see under *disease*.

monecious (mon-e′shus) monoecious.

monensin (mo-nen′sin) an antibacterial, antifungal, and antiprotozoal antibiotic, $C_{36}H_{62}O_{11}$, produced by *Streptomyces cinnamonensis*, which has been used in veterinary medicine.

moner (mo′ner) a non-nucleated mass of protoplasm.

Monera (mo-ne′rah) [Gr. *monērēs* single] in some systems of classification, a kingdom comprising unicellular organisms without true nuclei, i.e., the prokaryotes, including bacteria, blue-green algae (now blue-green bacteria), and actinomycetes and viruses. Cf. *Protista*.

monerula (mo-ner′u-lah), pl. *moner′ulae* [Gr. *monērēs* single] an impregnated ovum with as yet no cleavage nucleus.

monesia (mo-ne′ze-ah) [L.] an extract from monesia bark, the product of *Chrysophyllum glyciphloeum*, Casar. (Sapotaceae), a tree of Brazil; it is astringent and stomachic, and contains saponins, tannins, and glycyrrhizin.

monesthetic (mon″es-thet′ik) [Gr. *monos* single + *aisthēsis* perception] pertaining to or affecting a single sense or sensation.

monestrous (mon-es′trus) completing only one estrous cycle in each sexual season.

Monge's disease (mon′gez) [Carlos *Monge*, pathologist in Lima, Peru, 1884–1970] chronic mountain sickness.

mongolian (mon-go′le-an) pertaining to, resembling, or belonging to the Mongols; a term formerly applied to defects characteristic of Down's syndrome.

mongolism (mon′go-lizm) [*Mongol*, a member of one of the chief ethnological divisions of Asiatic peoples] old term formerly used for Down syndrome; so called because of facial characteristics typical of this condition. **translocation m.,** see *translocation Down syndrome*, under *syndrome*.

mongoloid (mon′go-loid) [see *mongolism*] 1. pertaining to or resembling the Mongols. 2. an individual with Down's syndrome.

Moniezia (mon″ĭ-e′ze-ah) a genus (family Anoplocephalidae) of tapeworms of cattle, goats, and sheep.

monilated (mon′il-āt″ed) moniliform.

monilethrix (mo-nil′e-thriks) [L. *monile* necklace + Gr. *thrix* hair] a disease condition, inherited as an autosomal dominant trait, in which the hairs exhibit marked multiple constrictions, with a beading effect, and are very brittle, rarely reaching an inch in length before breaking.

Monilia (mo-nil′e-ah) [L. *monile* necklace] 1. a former name for a genus of fungi now called *Candida*. 2. a genus of imperfect fungi of the family Moniliaceae, order Moniliales; its perfect (sexual) stage is *Sclerotinia*.

Moniliaceae (mo-nil″e-a′se-e) a family of colorless or light-colored imperfect fungi of the order Moniliales, which includes the genera *Histoplasma*, *Blastomyces*, *Sporothrix*, *Trichophyton*, *Coccidioides*, *Aspergillus*, *Trichoderma*, *Verticillium*, *Trichothecium*, and *Penicillium*.

monilial (mo-nil′e-al) pertaining to or caused by *Monilia*.

Moniliales (mo-nil″e-a′lēz) an order of imperfect fungi whose conidia are usually borne directly on undifferentiated mycelia, and including the families Cryptococcaceae, Moniliaceae, Dematiaceae, and Tuberculariaceae. Formerly called *Conidiosporales.*

moniliasis (mon-ĭ-li′ah-sis) an infection caused by *Monilia.* See *candidiasis.*

moniliform (mo-nil′ĭ-form) [L. *monile* necklace + *forma* form] shaped like a necklace or string of beads.

Moniliformis (mo-nil″ĭ-for′mis) a genus of acanthocephalans. *M. monilifor′mis* (formerly *Echinorhynchus moniliformis*) is a parasite of rats, mice, and dogs, and a facultative parasite in man.

moniliid (mo-nil′e-id) candidid.

moniliosis (mo-nil″e-o′sis) candidiasis.

Monistat (mo′nĭ-stat) trademark for a preparation of miconazole nitrate.

monitor (mon′ĭ-tor) [L. "one who reminds," from *monere* to remind, admonish] 1. to check constantly on a state or condition, as on the vital signs of a patient under anesthesia and undergoing surgery, or to determine the amount of exposure to radiation. 2. an apparatus used to observe or record such physiological signs as respiration, pulse, and blood pressure in a patient.

monium (mo′ne-um) [Gr. *monos* single] (obs.) a name given an earth metal discovered in 1898, later found to be a mixture of rare earth metals.

Moniz (mo′nēsh) Antonio Caetano de Abreu Friere Egas. Portugese neurosurgeon and diplomat 1874–1955; co-winner, with Walter Rudolf Hess, of the Nobel prize for medicine or physiology in 1949 for his development of cerebral angiography and the introduction of prefrontal lobotomy as a therapy for certain psychoses.

monkey paw (mung′ke-paw) a condition in which the thumb lies in adduction and extension and cannot be opposed so as to touch the tips of the other fingers, owing to weakness of the opposing muscles of the thumb, as in lesion of the median nerve.

monkeypox (mung′ke-poks) a mild, epidemic, exanthematous disease occurring in captive monkeys, which can be transmitted to humans, in whom it causes a disease clinically similar to smallpox.

Monneret's pulse (mon-rāz′) [Jules Auguste Edward *Monneret,* physician in Paris, 1810–1868] see under *pulse.*

mon(o)- [Gr. *monos* single] 1. a combining form meaning one or single, or limited to one part; in chemistry, combined with one atom, group, or radical.

monoamide (mon″o-am′ĭd) an amide containing one amide group.

monoamine (mon″o-am′ēn) an amine molecule containing one amino group, e.g., serotonin, dopamine, and norepinephrine.

monoamine oxidase (mon″o-am′ēn ok′sĭ-dās) amine oxidase (flavin-containing).

monoaminergic (mon″o-am″in-er′jik) of or pertaining to neurons that secrete the monoamine neurotransmitters dopamine, norepinephrine, and serotonin.

monoaminodiphosphatide (mon″o-am″ĭ-no-di-fos′fah-tīd) a phosphatide containing 1 atom of nitrogen and 2 of phosphorus to the molecule.

monoaminomonophosphatide (mon″o-am″ĭ-no-mon″o-fos′fah-tīd) a phosphatide containing 1 atom of nitrogen and 1 of phosphorus to the molecule.

monoamniotic (mon″o-am″ne-ot′ik) having or developing within a single amniotic cavity; said of monozygotic twins.

monoanesthesia (mon″o-an″es-the′ze-ah) [*mono-* + *anesthesia*] anesthesia of a single part or organ.

monoarticular (mon″o-ar-tik′u-lar) monarthric.

monobasic (mon″o-ba′sik) [*mono-* + Gr. *basis* base] having but one base; a term applied to an acid having only one replaceable atom of hydrogen and therefore yielding only one series of salts, as HCl.

monobenzone (mon″o-ben′zōn) [USP] chemical name: 4-(phenylmethoxy)phenol. A melanin-inhibiting agent, $C_{13}H_{12}O_2$, occurring as a white, crystalline powder; used as a depigmenting agent, applied topically to the skin.

monoblast (mon′o-blast) [*mono-* + Gr. *blastos* germ] the earliest precursor in the monocytic series, which matures to develop into the promonocyte; monoblasts have a fine chromatin structure and nucleoli are usually visible. They are not normally seen in the bone marrow or peripheral blood, but may be seen in monocytic anemia.

monoblastoma (mon″o-blas-to′mah) a neoplasm containing monoblasts and monocytes.

monoblepsia (mon″o-blep′se-ah) [*mono-* + Gr. *blepsis* sight + *-ia*] 1. a condition of the vision in which it is more distinct when only one eye is used. 2. a variety of color blindness in which only one color is perceived.

monobrachia (mon″o-bra′ke-ah) [*mono-* + Gr. *brachion* arm + *-ia*] a developmental anomaly characterized by the presence of a single arm.

monobrachius (mon″o-bra′ke-us) an individual exhibiting monobrachia.

monobromated (mon″o-bro′māt-ed) [L. *monobromatus*] having a single atom of bromine in each molecule.

monobromophenol (mon″o-bro″mo-fe′nol) a violet-colored liquid, $OH \cdot C_6H_4Br$, of penetrating odor, soluble in water, alcohol, and ether, formerly used as an external antiseptic.

monocalcic (mon″o-kal′sik) containing one atom of calcium in the molecule.

monocardian (mon-o-kar′de-an) [*mono-* + Gr. *kardia* heart] possessing a heart with a single atrium and ventricle, as that of a shark.

monocelled (mon′o-seld) [*mono-* + *cell*] unicellular; consisting of a single cell.

monocellular (mon″o-sel′u-lar) unicellular.

monocephalus (mon″o-sef′ah-lus) [*mono-* + Gr. *kephalē* head] a monster with one head but with some duplication of its parts. **m. tet′rapus dibra′chius,** a monster with one head, two arms, and partial or complete duplication of the pelvis, with four legs, the pair belonging to one member often being fused in a single limb. **m. tri′pus dibra′chius,** a monster with one head, two arms, and partial duplication of the pelvis, with a median third leg or leg rudiment.

Monocercomonas (mon″o-ser″ko-mo′nas) [*mono-* + *cerco-* + Gr. *monas* unit, from *monos* single] a genus of nonpathogenic parasitic flagellate protozoa (superorder Parabasalidea, order Trichomonadida) found in the digestive tract of many different vertebrates and insects, and characterized by the presence of three flagella, two anterior and one trailing, and an axostyle extending beyond the posterior end of the body, and by the absence of an undulating membrane. Representative species include *M. cuniculi,* found in the cecum of the rabbit; *M. ruminantium,* in the rumen and prepuce of sheep and cattle; and *M. gallinarum,* in the cecum of chickens.

Monocercomonoides (mo″no-ser″ko-mo-noi′dēz) [*mono-* + *cerco-* + Gr. *eidos* form] a genus of parasitic flagellate, nonpathogenic protozoa (order Oxymonadida, class Zoomastigophores) found in insects, amphibians, reptiles, and certain mammals.

monochlorothymol (mon″o-klo″ro-thi′mol) chlorothymol.

monochord (mon′o-kord) [*mono-* + Gr. *chordē* cord] (obs.) an instrument for testing upper tone audition. It consists of a long steel or silver wire fastened at the ends and having an intermediate movable clamp. The tone is produced by longitudinal friction. Called also *Schultze's monochord.*

monochorea (mon″o-ko-re′ah) [*mono-* + *chorea*] chorea affecting but one limb.

monochorial (mon″o-ko′re-al) monochorionic.

monochorionic (mon″o-ko″re-on′ik) [*mono-* + *chorionic*] having or developing in a common chorionic sac; said of monozygotic twins.

monochroic (mon″o-kro′ik) [*mono-* + Gr. *chroa* color] having only one color; monochromatic.

monochromasy (mon″o-kro′mah-se) monochromatism.

monochromat (mon″o-kro′mat) a person affected by monochromatism; called also *achromat.*

monochromatic (mon″o-kro-mat′ik) 1. existing in or having only one color. 2. pertaining to or affected by monochromatism. 3. staining with only one dye at a time. Cf. *polychromatic.*

monochromatism (mon″o-kro′mah-tizm) complete color blindness; inability to discriminate hues, all colors of the spectrum appearing as neutral grays with varying shades of light and dark. Called also *achromatism* and *achromotopsia*. **cone m.,** that in which there is some cone function and normal visual acuity and which is not associated with nystagmus and photophobia. **rod m.,** that in which there is complete absence of cone function and which is accompanied by poor vision, photophobia, and nystagmus.

monochromatophil (mon″o-kro-mat′o-fil) [*mono-* + Gr. *chrōma* color + *philein* to love] 1. stainable with only one kind of stain. 2. any cell or other element that will take only one stain.

monochromophilic (mon″o-kro″mo-fil′ik) stainable with only one kind of stain.

monoclinic (mon″o-klin′ik) [*mono-* + Gr. *klinein* to incline] a term applied to crystals in which the vertical axis is inclined to one lateral axis, but is at right angles to the other.

monoclonal (mon″o-klōn′al) derived from a single cell; pertaining to a single clone.

monocontaminated (mon″o-kon-tam′ĭ-nāt″ed) infected by a single species of microorganism, or by a single type of contaminating agent; see *monoxenic.*

monocontamination (mon″o-kon-tam″ĭ-na′shun) experimental infection of a previously germ-free animal by a single infectious agent. See *monoxenic.*

monocorditis (mon″o-kōr-di′tis) inflammation of one vocal cord.

monocranius (mon″o-kra′ne-us) [*mono-* + Gr. *kranion* cranium] monocephalus.

monocrotic (mon″o-krot′ik) characterized by monocrotism.

monocrotism (mo-nok′ro-tizm) [*mono-* + Gr. *krotos* beat] a simple pulse wave contour having neither an anacrotic nor a dicrotic notch.

monocular (mon-ok′u-lar) [*mono-* + L. *oculus* eye] 1. pertaining to or having but one eye. 2. having but one eyepiece, as in a microscope.

monoculus (mon-ok′u-lus) [*mono-* + L. *oculus* eye] 1. a bandage for covering one eye. 2. a cyclops.

monocyclic (mon″o-si′klik) pertaining to one cycle. In chemistry, having a molecular structure containing only one ring.

monocyesis (mon″o-si-e′sis) [*mono-* + Gr. *kyēsis* pregnancy] pregnancy with a single fetus.

Monocystis (mon″o-sis′tis) [*mono-* + Gr. *kystis* sac, bladder] a genus of parasitic gregarine protozoa (suborder Aseptina, order Eugregarinida) found in the coelom and seminal vessels of the earthworm and related worms.

monocyte (mon′o-sīt) [*mono-* + *-cyte*] a mononuclear phagocytic leukocyte, 13 μ to 25 μ in diameter, with an ovoid or kidney-shaped nucleus, containing lacey, linear chromatin, and abundant gray-blue cytoplasm filled with fine, reddish and azurophilic granules. Formed in the bone marrow from promonocytes, monocytes are transported to tissues, as of the lung and liver, where they develop into macrophages. Formerly called *large mononuclear leukocyte,* and *hyaline* or *transitional leukocyte.* See also *monocytic series,* under *series.*

monocytic (mon″o-sit′ik) 1. pertaining to, characterized by, or of the nature of monocytes. 2. pertaining to the monocytic series; see under *series.*

monocytoid (mon″o-si′toid) resembling a monocyte.

monocytopenia (mon″o-si″to-pe′ne-ah) [*monocyte* + Gr. *penia* poverty] abnormal decrease in the proportion of monocytes in the blood.

monocytopoiesis (mon″o-si″to-poi-e′sis) [*monocyte* + Gr. *poiein* to make] the formation of monocytes.

monocytosis (mon″o-si-to′sis) increase in the proportion of monocytes in the blood.

Monod (mŏ-no′), Jacques Lucien. French biochemist, 1910–1976; co-winner with François Jacob and André Michael Lwoff, of the Nobel prize in medicine or physiology for 1965, for discoveries concerning the genetic control of enzymes and virus synthesis.

monodactylia (mon″o-dak-til′e-ah) monodactyly.

monodactylism (mon-o-dak′til-izm) monodactyly.

monodactyly (mon″o-dak′tĭ-le) [*mono-* + Gr. *daktylos* finger] a developmental anomaly characterized by the presence of only one digit on a hand or foot.

monodal (mon-o′dal) [*mono-* + Gr. *hodos* road] having connection with one terminal of a resonator or of a grounded solenoid, so that the patient is a capacitor for entrance and exit of high frequency currents.

monodermoma (mon″o-der-mo′mah) a tumor that has developed from one germinal layer.

monodiplopia (mon″o-dĭ-plo′pe-ah) [*mono-* + *diplopia*] double vision in one eye only.

Monodontus (mon″o-don′tus) *Bunostomum.*

Monodral bromide (mon′o-dral) trademark for preparations of penthienate bromide.

monoecious (mon-e′shus) [*mono-* + Gr. *oikos* house] having reproductive organs typical of both sexes in a single individual.

monoethanolamine (mon″o-eth″ah-nōl′ah-mēn) chemical name: 2-aminoethanol. An amino alcohol, C_2H_7NO, found in cephalins and phospholipids, and derived metabolically by decarboxylation of serine. The official preparation [NF], occurring as a clear, colorless, moderately viscous liquid, is used as a surfactant in pharmaceutical preparations. A combination of monoethanolamine and oleic acid (known as *ethanolamine oleate*) has been used as a sclerosing agent in the injection treatment of varicose veins. Called also *colamine* and *ethanolamine.*

monofilm (mon′o-film) a monomolecular layer transferred to a prepared plate.

monogamous (mon-og′ah-mus) pertaining to monogamy.

monogamy (mo-nog′ah-me) [*mono-* + Gr. *gamos* marriage] 1. marriage to a single spouse. 2. the animal mating system in which each individual mates with just one partner for the entire breeding season. Cf. *polygamy.*

monoganglial (mon″o-gang′gle-al) affecting a single ganglion.

monogastric (mon″o-gas′trik) [*mono-* + Gr. *gastēr* stomach] having but one belly or stomach.

monogen (mon′o-jen) 1. a univalent chemical element which combines in only one proportion. 2. an antiserum produced by the use of one antigen (i.e., immunogen).

monogenesis (mon″o-jen′ĕ-sis) [*mono-* + *genesis*] 1. the production of only male or female offspring. 2. the theory that all things develop from a single cell.

monogenic (mon-o-jen′ik) pertaining to or influenced by a single gene.

monogerminal (mon″o-jer′mĭ-nal) monozygotic.

monoglyceride (mon″o-glis′er-īd) a compound consisting of one molecule of fatty acid esterified to glycerol.

monograph (mon′o-graf) [*mono-* + Gr. *graphein* to write] an essay or treatise on one subject.

monohybrid (mon″o-hi′brid) [*mono-* + *hybrid*] the offspring of parents differing from each other in that each is homozygous for a different allele at a single locus; thus their offspring will be heterozygous at that locus.

monohydrated (mon″o-hi′drāt-ed) united with a single molecule of water or a single hydroxyl group.

monohydric (mon″o-hi′drik) containing one atom of replaceable hydrogen.

monoinfection (mon″o-in-fek′shun) infection with a single kind of organism.

monoiodotyrosine (mon″o-i-o″do-ti′ro-sēn) an iodinated amino acid that is an intermediate in the thyroidal biosynthesis of thyroxine and triiodothyronine. Abbreviated MIT.

monokaryon (mon″o-ka′re-on) [*mono-* + Gr. *karyon* kernel] a growth stage in the mycelium of fungi, especially Basidiomycetes, in which each cell has one haploid nucleus.

monokaryote (mon″o-kar′e-ōt) a cell having one haploid nucleus.

monokaryotic (mon″o-kar″e-ot′ik) pertaining to the monokaryon or to a monokaryote.

monoketoheptose (mon″o-ke″to-hep′tōs) a natural sugar, $CH_2OH \cdot CO(CHOH)_4 \cdot CH_2OH$, found in the avocado, *Persea gratissima.*

monokine (mon′o-kīn) a general term for soluble mediators of immune responses that are not antibodies or complement components and that are produced by mononuclear phagocytes (monocytes or macrophages). Cf. *lymphokine.*

monolayer (mon″o-la′er) pertaining to or consisting of a single layer, such as a monolayer sheet of cells in cultures used in studies of viruses.

monolene (mon′o-lēn) a clear white, oily hydrocarbon.

monolepsis (mon″o-lep′sis) [*mono*- + Gr. *lēpsis* a taking] the transmission to the offspring of the characters of one parent, to the exclusion of those of the other.

monolocular (mon″o-lok′u-lar) [*mono*- + L. *loculus* cell] having but one cavity or compartment, as a cyst.

monomania (mon″o-ma′ne-ah) [*mono*- + Gr. *mania* madness] a form of mental disorder characterized by preoccupation with one subject or idea.

monomaxillary (mon″o-mak′sĭ-ler″e) pertaining to or affecting one jaw.

monomelic (mon″o-mel′ik) [*mono*- + Gr. *melos* limb] affecting one limb.

monomer (mon′o-mer) a simple molecule of a compound of relatively low molecular weight; a substance consisting of simple unrepeated structural units, but capable of reaction to form a dimer, trimer, polymer, etc. **fibrin m.,** the material resulting from the highly specific and orderly cleavage of fibrinogen by thrombin; through polymerization, these monomers form macromolecular fibrin.

monomeric (mon″o-mer′ik) [*mono*- + Gr. *meros* part] pertaining to, made up of, or affecting a single segment, as distinguished from dimeric, polymeric, etc. In genetics, determined by a gene or genes at a single locus either in the heterozygous or homozygous state.

monometallic (mon″o-mĕ-tal′ik) having one atom of a metal in the molecule.

monomolecular (mon″o-mo-lek′u-lar) pertaining to or involving one molecule.

monomorphic (mon″o-mor′fik) [*mono*- + Gr. *morphē* form] existing in only one form; maintaining the same form throughout all stages of development.

monomorphism (mon″o-mor′fizm) the quality or condition of being monomorphic.

monomorphous (mon″o-mor′fus) composed of lesions all of the same age, form, and shape, as a monomorphous eruption, such as variola.

monomphalus (mon-om′fah-lus) [*mono*- + Gr. *omphalos* navel] a double monster joined at the navel.

monomyoplegia (mon″o-mi′o-ple′je-ah) [*mono*- + Gr. *mys* muscle + *plēgē* stroke] paralysis restricted to a single muscle.

monomyositis (mon″o-mi″o-si′tis) [*mono*- + *myositis*] a myositis of the biceps muscle occurring periodically.

Mononchus (mon-ong′kus) a genus of nematodes living in fresh water or moist soil, reportedly found in human urine, probably representing a case of spurious parasitosis.

mononephrous (mon″o-nef′rus) [*mono*- + Gr. *nephros* kidney] affecting one kidney only.

mononeural (mon″o-nu′ral) pertaining to or receiving branches from a single nerve.

mononeuric (mon″o-nu′rik) [*mono*- + Gr. *neuron* nerve] having only one neuron.

mononeuritis (mon″o-nu-ri′tis) [*mono*- + Gr. *neuron* nerve + *-itis*] disease of a single nerve. **m. mul′tiplex,** simultaneous disease of several peripheral nerves.

mononeuropathy (mon″o-nu-rop′ah-thē) disease affecting a single nerve. **cranial m.,** disease of one of the cranial nerves, as the seventh cranial nerve in Bell's palsy.

mononoea (mon″o-ne′ah) [*mono*- + Gr. *nous* mind] (*obs.*) mental concentration on a single subject, as in monomania.

mononuclear (mon″o-nu′kle-ar) [*mono*- + *nucleus*] 1. having but one nucleus; mononucleate; uninucleated. 2. a cell having a single nucleus, especially a monocyte of the blood or tissues.

mononucleate (mon″o-nu′kle-āt) having a single nucleus; mononuclear.

mononucleosis (mon″o-nu″kle-o′sis) the presence of an abnormally large number of mononuclear leukocytes (monocytes) in the blood. The term is often used alone to refer to infectious mononucleosis. **cytomegalovirus m.,** an infectious disease caused by a cytomegalovirus, in many respects resembling infectious mononucleosis, characterized by fever, splenomegaly, hepatic involvement, and atypical lymphocytes with a negative heterophile test, but without pharyngitis and cervical adenopathy. It may occur sporadi-

cally or may follow multiple blood transfusions. See also *cytomegalic inclusion disease,* under *disease,* and *postperfusion syndrome,* under *syndrome.* **infectious m.,** a common, acute, usually self-limited infectious disease caused by the Epstein-Barr virus, characterized by fever, membranous pharyngitis, lymph node and splenic enlargement, lymphocyte proliferation, and the presence of atypical lymphocytes, and giving rise to various immune reactions, including the development of a transient heterophile and a persistent Epstein-Barr virus antibody response. Potential complications include hepatitis and encephalomeningitis. It affects primarily adolescents and young adults, being spread by saliva transfer and possibly other modes; in children the infection is largely subclinical. Called also *glandular fever,* *Filatov's disease, kissing disease,* and *Pfeiffer's disease.*

post-transfusion m., postperfusion syndrome.

mononucleotide (mon″o-nu′kle-o-tīd″) a product obtained by the digestion or hydrolytic decomposition of nucleic acid. It is a compound of phosphoric acid and a pentoside. The latter is a combination of a pentose (ribose or 2-deoxyribose) with one of the following bases: guanine, adenine, cytosine, uracil, or thymine.

mono-osteitic (mon″o-os″te-it′ik) denoting a type of osteitis which affects a single bone.

mono-ovular (mon″o-ov′u-lar) monovular.

monooxygenase (mon″o-ok′sĭ-jĕ-nās″) an enzyme of the oxidoreductase class that catalyzes the incorporation of one atom from molecular oxygen into a compound while reducing the other atom of oxygen to water. It may make the oxygen acceptor act as the hydrogen donor [EC 1.13.12], or it may use a second compound as the second hydrogen donor in a coupled reaction [EC 1.14.13 to 1.14.18 and 1.14.99]. **unspecific m.,** [EC 1.14.14.1] one that catalyzes the reaction RH + reduced flavoprotein + O_2 = ROH + oxidized flavoprotein + H_2O. The enzyme is a heme-thiolate protein containing cytochrome *P*-450. It acts on a wide range of substrates including xenobiotics, steroids, fatty acids, vitamins and prostaglandins.

monoparesis (mon″o-pah-re′sis) [*mono*- + Gr. *paresis* slackening of strength, paralysis] paresis of a single limb.

monoparesthesia (mon″o-par″es-the′ze-ah) [*mono*- + *paresthesia*] paresthesia of a single limb.

monopathy (mo-nop′ah-the) [*mono*- + Gr. *pathos* disease] a disease affecting a single part.

monopenia (mon″o-pe′ne-ah) monocytopenia.

monophagia (mon″o-fa′je-ah) [*mono*- + Gr. *phagein* to eat + *-ia*] 1. desire for one kind of food only. 2. the eating of only one meal a day.

monophagism (mo-nof′ah-jizm) monophagia.

monophasia (mon″o-fa′ze-ah) [*mono*- + Gr. *phasis* speaking] aphasia with ability to utter but one word or phrase.

monophasic (mon″o-fa′zik) exhibiting only one phase or variation. Cf. *diphasic, triphasic.*

monophenol monooxygenase (mon″o-fe′nol mon″o-ok′sĭ-jĕ-nās″) [EC 1.14.18.1] an enzyme of the oxidoreductase class that catalyzes the reaction L-tyrosine + L-dopa + O_2 = L-dopa + dopaquinone + H_2O. It is a copper protein that also acts on catechol and substituted catechols. The reaction is a step in the formation of melanin pigments from tyrosine. See also *catechol oxidase.*

monophenyl oxidase (mon″o-fen′il ok′sĭ-dās) monophenol monooxygenase.

monophosphate (mon″o-fos′fāt) a salt containing a single phosphate radical.

monophthalmus (mon″of-thal′mus) [*mono*- + Gr. *ophthalmos* eye] a cyclops.

monophyletic (mon″o-fi-let′ik) [*mono*- + Gr. *phylē* tribe] arising or descended from a single cell type.

monophyletism (mon″o-fi′lĕ-tizm) monophyletic theory; see under *theory.*

monophyletist (mon″o-fi′lĕ-tist) an adherent of the monophyletic theory, as in blood origin.

monophyodont (mon″o-fi′o-dont) [*mono*- + Gr. *phyein* to grow + *odous* tooth] having only one set of teeth, and those permanent. Cf. *diphyodont* and *polyphyodont.*

monopia (mon-o′pe-ah) [*mono*- + Gr. *ops* eye + *-ia*] cyclopia.

monoplasmatic (mon″o-plaz-mat′ik) [*mono-* + Gr. *plasma* plasm] made up of a single substance.

monoplast (mon′o-plast) [*mono-* + Gr. *plastos* formed] a single constituent cell.

monoplegia (mon″o-ple′je-ah) [*mono-* + Gr. *plēgē* stroke] paralysis of a limb.

monoplegic (mon″o-ple′jik) pertaining to or characterized by monoplegia.

monopodia (mon″o-po′de-ah) [*mono-* + Gr. *pous* foot + *-ia*] a type of symmelia characterized by the presence of one median foot.

monopodial (mon″o-po′de-al) pertaining to or characterized by monopodia; having a single median foot.

monopoiesis (mon″o-poi-e′sis) the development of monocytes.

monopolar (mon′o-po″lar) monoterminal.

monops (mon′ops) [*mono-* + Gr. *ōps* eye] cyclops.

Monopsyllus (mon″o-sil′us) [*mono-* + Gr. *psylla* flea] a genus of fleas. **M. ani′sus,** the common rat flea of Japan and North China.

monoptychial (mon″o-ti′ke-al) [*mono-* + Gr. *ptychē* fold] arranged in a single layer; said of glands whose cells are arranged on the basement membrane in a single layer. Cf. *polyptychial.*

monopus (mon′o-pus) [*mono-* + Gr. *pous* foot] a fetus having but a single foot or leg.

monorchia (mon-or′ke-ah) monorchism.

monorchid (mon-or′kid) an individual exhibiting monorchism.

monorchidic (mon″or-kid′ik) [*mono-* + Gr. *orchis* testicle] pertaining to or characterized by monorchism; having but one descended testicle.

monorchidism (mon-or′kid-izm) monorchism.

monorchis (mon-or′kis) monorchid.

monorchism (mon′or-kizm) the condition of having only one testis in the scrotum.

Monorchotrema (mon-or″ko-tre′mah) [*mono-* + Gr. *orchis* testicle + *trēma* aperture] a genus of heterophyid flukes found in birds and mammals in the Middle East and Taiwan, and characterized by having only a single testis. They have as invertebrate host an operculate snail, and as first vertebrate host an edible fish.

monorhinic (mon″o-rin′ik) pertaining to or possessing one nasal cavity.

monosaccharide (mon″o-sak′ah-rīd) a simple sugar; a carbohydrate which cannot be decomposed by hydrolysis. The monosaccharides are colorless crystalline substances with a sweet taste and have the same general formula CH_2O. They are classified according to the number of carbon atoms in the chain into diose ($C_2H_4O_2$), triose ($C_3H_6O_3$), tetrose ($C_4H_8O_4$), pentose ($C_5H_{10}O_5$), hexose ($C_6H_{12}O_6$), and heptose ($C_7H_{14}O_7$). Those containing an aldehyde group are termed *aldoses;* those with a ketone group *ketoses.*

monosaccharose (mon″o-sak′ah-rōs) monosaccharide.

monose (mon′ōs) a monosaccharide.

monosexual (mon″o-sek′su-al) showing the traits of one sex only.

monosodium glutamate (mon″o-so′de-um glu′tah-māt) sodium glutamate.

monosome (mon′o-sōm) [*mono-* + Gr. *sōma* body] 1. the unpaired sex chromosome; called also *unpaired allosome.* 2. the single chromosome present in monosomy.

monosomic (mon″o-so′mik) pertaining to or characterized by monosomy.

monosomy (mon′o-so″me) the absence of one chromosome of a homologous pair in the complement of an otherwise diploid cell (2n–1), as seen in the karyotype of Turner syndrome, in which there is only one sex chromosome.

monospasm (mon′o-spazm) [*mono-* + *spasm*] spasm of a single limb or part. Different varieties are distinguished according to the part affected or to the site of the causal lesion; as, brachial, facial, lateral, peripheral, etc.

monospecific (mon″o-spĕ-sif′ik) having an effect only on a particular kind of cell or tissue, or reacting with a single antigen, as a monospecific antiserum.

monospermy (mon′o-sper″me) [*mono-* + Gr. *sperma* seed] fertilization in which only one spermatozoon enters the ovum.

Monosporium (mon″o-spo′re-um) a genus of imperfect fungi, family Moniliaceae, order Moniliales; its perfect (sexual) stage is *Allescheria.* **M. apiosper′mum,** one of the causative organisms of maduromycosis; its perfect stage is *Allescheria boydii.*

Monostoma (mon″o-sto′mah) [Gr. *monos* single + *stoma* mouth] *Paramphistomum.*

Monostomum (mon″o-sto′mum) *Paramphistomum.*

monostotic (mon″os-tot′ik) [*mono-* + Gr. *osteon* bone] pertaining to or affecting a single bone.

monostratal (mon″o-stra′tal) pertaining to a single layer or stratum.

monostratified (mon″o-strat′ĭ-fīd) disposed in a single layer or stratum.

monosubstituted (mon″o-sub′stĭ-tūt″ed) having only one atom in the molecule replaced.

monosymptom (mon″o-simp′tom) [*mono-* + *symptom*] a symptom occurring singly.

monosymptomatic (mon″o-simp′to-mat′ik) expressed by a single symptom.

monosynaptic (mon″o-sĭ-nap′tik) pertaining to or relayed through only one synapse.

Monotard (mon′o-tard) trademark for preparations of insulin zinc suspension.

monoterminal (mon″o-ter′mĭ-nal) the use of one terminal only in giving treatments, the ground acting as the second terminal.

Monothalamida (mon″o-thah-lam′ĭ-dah) [*mono-* + Gr. *thalamos* inner chamber] an order of ameboid protozoa (class Granuloreticulosea, superclass Rhizopoda), the organisms of which have a single-chambered organic or calcareous test, sometimes with foreign matter as a constituent.

monothermia (mon″o-ther′me-ah) [*mono-* + Gr. *thermē* heat] a condition in which the temperature of the body remains the same throughout the day.

monothetic (mon″o-thet′ik) [*mono-* + Gr. *thetikos* fit for placing] denoting a taxonomic group classified on the basis of a single character, as opposed to polythetic.

monothioglycerol (mon″o-thi″o-glis′er-ol) [NF] chemical name: 3-mercapto-1,2-propanediol. A clear, colorless, moderately viscous liquid, C_2H_7NO, used as a preservative in pharmaceutical preparations.

monotic (mon-o′tik) [*mono-* + Gr. *ous* ear] affecting, pertaining to, or possessing a single ear.

monotocous (mo-not′o-kus) [*mono-* + Gr. *tokos* birth] giving birth to but one offspring at a time.

Monotremata (mon″o-tre′mah-tah) the lowest order of mammals, including animals which lay eggs similar to those of reptiles, and nourish their young by a mammary gland which has no nipple, in a shallow pouch developed only during lactation. The only living representatives are the spiny anteater and duck-billed platypus. In some systems of classification, considered to be an order of subclass Prototheria, class Mammalia.

monotreme (mon′o-trēm) a member of the order Monotremata.

monotrichic (mon″o-trik′ik) monotrichous.

monotrichous (mon-ot′rĭ-kus) [*mono-* + Gr. *thrix* hair] having a single polar flagellum; said of a bacterial cell. See *flagellum.*

monotropic (mon″o-trop′ik) [*mono-* + Gr. *tropos* a turning] affecting only one particular kind of bacterium, virus, or tissue. Cf. *polytropic.*

monoureide (mon″o-u′re-id) see *ureide.*

monovalent (mon″o-va′lent) 1. having a valence of one. Called also *univalent.* 2. denoting an antiserum, vaccine, or antitoxin specific for a single antigen or organism.

monovular (mon-ov′u-lar) pertaining to or derived from a single ovum; said of monozygotic twins.

monovulatory (mon-ov′u-lah-to″re) ordinarily discharging only one ovum in one ovarian cycle.

monoxenic (mon″o-zen′ik) [*mono-* + Gr. *xenos* a guest-friend, stranger] associated with a single species of microorganisms; said of otherwise germ-free animals contaminated by a single type of organism.

monoxenous (mo-nok'sĕ-nus) [*mono-* + Gr. *xenos* strange, foreign] homoxenous; requiring only one host in the life cycle; said of certain parasites.

monoxide (mon-ok'sīd) an oxide containing but one atom of oxygen; vernacularly applied to carbon monoxide.

monoxygenase (mon-oks'ĭ-jĕ-nās) monooxygenase.

monozygosity (mon"o-zi-gos'ĭ-te) the state of developing from one zygote.

monozygotic (mon"o-zi-got'ik) pertaining to or derived from one fertilized ovum (zygote), as identical twins.

monozygous (mon"o-zi'gus) monozygotic.

Monro's bursa, foramen, line, sulcus (fissure) (mon-rōz') [Alexander *Monro* (Secundus), Scottish anatomist and surgeon, 1733–1817] see *bursa intratendinea, foramen interventriculare,* and *sulcus hypothalamicus,* and see under *line.*

Monro-Richter line (mon-ro' rik'ter) [Alexander *Monro;* August Gottlieb *Richter,* surgeon in Göttingen, 1742–1812] see under *line.*

mons (monz), gen. *mon'tis,* pl. *mon'tes* [L. "mountain"] [NA] a general term for an elevation, or eminence. **m. pu'bis** [NA], the rounded fleshy prominence over the symphysis pubis. **m. ure'teris,** a papilla-like elevation of the mucosa of the bladder at its junction with the ureter. **m. ven'eris,** m. pubis.

Monsonia (mon-so'ne-ah) a genus of African and Asiatic geraniaceous plants. Some of the species are used in medicine as astringents and for dysentery.

monster (mon'ster) [L. *monstrum*] a fetus or infant with such pronounced developmental anomalies as to be grotesque and usually nonviable. Called also *teras.* **acardiac m.,** acardius. **acraniate m.,** a fetus lacking cranium and a brain as such. **autositic m.,** one capable of independent life, the circulation of which supplies nutrition to a parasitic monster. **celosomian m.,** a celosomus. **compound m.,** one which shows some duplication of body parts. **cyclopic m.,** a cyclops. **diaxial m.,** one which shows duplication of the body axis. **double m.,** one arising from a single ovum but with duplication or doubling of head, trunk, or limbs; see *anadidymus, anakatadidymus,* and *katadidymus.* **emmenic m.,** an infant that menstruates. **endocymic m.,** one which is retained in the uterus and forms the basis of a dermoid tumor. **Gila m.,** a venomous lizard, *Heloderma suspectum,* found especially in Arizona and New Mexico. **hair m.,** one with a heavy hair-coat. **monoaxial m.,** a monster which has a single body axis. **parasitic m.,** an imperfect fetus unable to exist alone and attached to or deriving its nutrition from the circulation of another, more perfectly developed fetus. **polysomatous m.,** a monster consisting of multiple components, each of which shows some of the characteristics of a separate individual. **single m.,** one with a single body but with a defect, malformation, or displacement, or an enlargement or duplication of an organ; see *monstrum.* **sirenoform m.,** a sirenomelus. **triplet m.,** a monster with triplication of body parts. **twin m.,** double m.

monstra (mon'strah) [L.] plural of *monstrum.*

monstricide (mon'stri-sīd) [*monster* + L. *caedere* to kill] destruction of a fetal monster.

monstrosity (mon-stros'ĭ-te) [L. *monstrositas*] 1. great congenital deformity. 2. a monster or teratism.

monstrum (mon'strum), pl. *mon'stra* [L.] a monster. **m. abun'dans,** m. per excessum. **m. defic'iens,** m. per defectum. **m. per defec'tum,** a single monster in which all or part of an organ is missing. **m. per exces'sum,** a single monster in which an organ is enlarged or duplicated. **m. per fab'ricam alie'nam,** a single monster in which an organ is wrongly formed or displaced. **m. sirenofor'me,** a sirenomelus.

Monteggia's dislocation, fracture (mon-tej'ahz) [Giovanni Battista *Monteggia,* Italian surgeon, 1762–1815] see under *dislocation* and *fracture.*

montes (mon'tēz) [L.] plural of *mons.*

Montgomery's cups, follicles, glands, tubercles (mont-gom'er-ēz) [William Fetherstone *Montgomery,* Irish obstetrician, 1797–1859] see under *cup* and *tubercle,* and see *Naboth's follicle,* under *follicle,* and *glandulae areolares.*

monticulus (mon-tik'u-lus), gen. and pl. *montic'uli* [L., dim.

of *mons*] a small eminence. **m. cerebel'li,** the projecting or central part of the superior vermis.

mood (mood) a pervasive and sustained emotion that, when extreme, can color one's whole view of life. Mood is generally used to refer to either elation or depression.

mood-congruent (mood kon-groo'ent) consistent with one's mood. DSM III-R draws a distinction between *mood-congruent psychotic features* (grandiose delusions or related hallucinations during a manic episode or depressive delusions or related hallucinations in a major depressive episode), which may occur in affective disorders, and *mood-incongruent psychotic features* (any other type of delusion or hallucination), which are indicative of a psychotic disorder, e.g., schizophrenic, paranoid, or schizoaffective disorder.

mood-incongruent (mood in"kon-groo'ent) not mood-congruent.

Moon's teeth (molars) (moonz) [Henry *Moon,* 19th century English surgeon] see under *tooth.*

Moore's fracture (moorz) [Edward Mott *Moore,* American surgeon, 1814–1902] see under *fracture.*

Moore's syndrome (moorz) [Matthew T. *Moore,* American neuropsychiatrist, born 1901] abdominal epilepsy.

Moore's test (moorz) [John *Moore,* English physician of the 19th century] see under *tests.*

Mooren's ulcer (moor'enz) [Albert *Mooren,* German oculist, 1828–1899] see under *ulcer.*

Moorhead foreign body locator (moor'hed) [John J. *Moorhead,* New York surgeon, born 1874] Berman-Moorhead locator.

MOPP a regimen of mechlorethamine, Oncovin (vincristine), procarbazine, and prednisone, used in cancer chemotherapy.

Morand's foot, foramen, spur (mor-ahnz') [Sauveur François *Morand,* French surgeon, 1697–1773] see under *foot,* and see *foramen cecum* and *calcar avis.*

morantel tartrate (mo-ran'tel) chemical name: (*E*)-1,4,5,6-tetrahydro-1-methyl-2-[2-(3-methyl-2-thienyl)ethenyl]pyrimidine[*R* - (*R* *,*R* *)]-2,3-dihydroxybutanedioate (1:1); an anthelmintic, $C_{12}H_{16}N_2S \cdot C_4H_6O_6$, which has been used in veterinary medicine.

Morax-Axenfeld bacillus, conjunctivitis, diplococcus (mōr'aks-ak'sen-felt") [Victor *Morax,* ophthalmologist in Paris, 1866–1935; Theodor *Axenfeld,* German ophthalmologist, 1867–1930] see under *conjunctivitis,* and see *Moraxella (Moraxella) lacunata.*

Moraxella (mo"rak-sel'ah) [Victor *Morax,* Swiss ophthalmologist, 1866–1935] a genus of bacteria of the family Neisseriaceae, made up of gram-negative, short, aerobic, oxidase-positive, nonpigmented organisms found as parasites and pathogens on the mucous membranes of mammals. The genus includes two subgenera: *M. (Moraxella)* occurring as rods, and *M. (Branhamella)* occurring as cocci. **M. anatipes'tifer,** a species of uncertain status isolated from septicemic disease in ducks, geese, turkeys, and waterfowl; called also *Pasteurella anatipestifer.* **M. bo'vis,** *M. (Moraxella) bovis.* **M. (Branhamella) catarrha'lis,** a normal inhabitant of the human nasal cavity and nasopharynx, occasionally causing respiratory disease and otitis media; called also *Branhamella catarrhalis* and *Neisseria catarrhalis.* **M. lacuna'ta,** *M. (Moraxella) lacunata.* **M. liquefa'ciens,** *M. (Moraxella) lacunata.* **M. lwof'fii,** *Acinetobacter calcoaceticus.* **M. (Moraxella) bo'vis,** the etiologic agent of pink-eye (epizootic keratoconjunctivitis) in cattle; called also *Haemophilus bovis.* **M. (Moraxella) lacuna'ta,** the etiologic agent of conjunctivitis and corneal infections in humans; called also *diplococcus of Morax-Axenfeld, Haemophilus duplex,* and *Moraxella liquefaciens.*

morbid (mor'bid) [L. *morbidus* sick] 1. pertaining to, affected with, or inducing disease; diseased. 2. unhealthy or unwholesome, as a morbid desire or fear.

morbidity (mor-bid'ĭ-te) a diseased condition or state; the incidence or prevalence of a disease or of all diseases in a population. See *morbidity rate,* under *rate.*

morbidostatic (mor"bĭ-do-stat'ik) checking morbidity; inhibiting the progression of morbid changes, or disease.

morbific (mor-bif'ik) [L. *morbificus; morbus* sickness + *facere* to make] causing disease.

morbigenous (mor-bij'ĕ-nus) producing disease.

morbilli (mor-bil′i) [L.] measles.

morbilliform (mor-bil′ĭ-form) [L. *morbilli* measles + *forma* shape] like measles; resembling the eruption of measles.

morbillous (mor-bil′us) pertaining to measles.

morbus (mor′bus) [L.] disease. **m. cox′ae seni′lis,** hip-joint disease of aged people. **m. monilifor′mis,** lichen ruber moniliformis.

M.O.R.C. Medical Officers Reserve Corps.

morcellation (mor″sel-a′shun) [Fr. *morcellement*] the division of solid tissue (as a tumor) into pieces, followed by its removal piecemeal.

morcellement (mor-sel-maw′) morcellation.

mordant (mor′dant) [L. *mordere* to bite] 1. a substance capable of intensifying or deepening the reaction of a specimen to a stain; the chief mordants are alum, aniline, oil, and phenol. 2. to subject to the action of a mordant preliminary to staining.

Mor. dict. abbreviation for L. *mo′re dic′to,* in the manner directed.

Morel ear, syndrome (mo′rel) [Benoît Augustin *Morel,* French alienist, 1809–1873] see under *ear,* and see *hyperostosis frontalis interna.*

Morelli's test (reaction) (mo-rel′ēz) [F. *Morelli,* Italian physician, died 1918] see under *tests.*

mores (mo′rēz) [L., pl. of *mos,* "manners"] the traditions and habits which are generally regarded as conducive to social welfare.

Moretti's test (mo-ret′ēz) [E. *Moretti,* physician in Milan] see under *tests.*

Morgagni's appendix, etc. (mor-gahn′yēz) [Giovanni Battista *Morgagni,* Italian anatomist and pathologist, 1682–1771; professor at Padua, and the founder of pathological anatomy, whose superb clinicopathological reports were published in 1761 under the title *De sedibus et causis morborum* ("The Seats and Causes of Disease")] see under *appendix, caruncle, column, crypt,* etc.

Morgagni-Adams-Stokes syndrome [Giovanni Battista *Morgagni;* Robert *Adams,* Irish physician, 1791–1875; William *Stokes,* Irish physician, 1804–1878] Adams-Stokes disease.

Morgan (mor′gan), Thomas Hunt. American zoologist, 1866–1945; winner of the Nobel prize for medicine or physiology in 1933 for his research on the fruit fly *Drosophila* in linkage and crossing over, which he used to map the linear arrangement of genes along the chromosome.

morgan see *centimorgan.*

Morgan's bacillus (mor′ganz) [Harry de Reimer *Morgan,* British physician, died 1931] *Proteus morgani.*

Morganella (mor-gah-nel′ah) [H. de R. *Morgan,* British physician, 1863–1931] a genus of gram-negative, facultatively anaerobic, rod-shaped bacteria of the family Enterobacteriaceae, made up of motile, pleomorphic organisms found in fecal material of humans and other mammals. The organisms resemble *Proteus,* except that they do not produce hydrogen sulfide or liquefy gelatin. **M. morga′nii,** the single species of the genus. It is a primary cause of urinary tract infections and is an opportunistic pathogen, causing secondary infections of blood, respiratory tract, and wounds. Called also *Proteus morganii* and *Salmonella morganii.*

morgue (morg) [Fr.] a place where dead bodies may be temporarily kept, for identification or until claimed for burial.

moria (mo′re-ah) [Gr. *mōria* folly] an abnormal tendency to joke.

moribund (mor′ĭ-bund) [L. *moribundus*] in a dying state.

Moringa (mo-rin′gah) a genus of plants. **M. pterygosper′ma,** an East Indian plant, the sajina or horseradish tree, the nuts of which yield an oil that was once used in the treatment of rheumatism and dyspepsia. It is the source of pterygospermin, an antibiotic.

Morison's pouch (mor′ĭ-sunz) [James Rutherford *Morison,* British surgeon, 1853– 1939] see under *pouch.*

Morita therapy (mo-re′tah) [Shomei *Morita,* Japanese physician] see under *therapy.*

Moritz reaction, test (mo′rits) [Friedrich Heinrich Ludwig *Moritz,* German physician, 1861–1938] Rivalta's reaction.

Mörner's body, reagent, test (mer′nerz) [Carl Axel Hampus *Möner,* Stockholm chemist, 1854–1917] see under *rea-*

gent and *tests,* and see *nucleoalbumin,* and *nitroprusside test* (def. 1), under *tests.*

Mornidine (mor′nĭ-dēn) trademark for preparations of pipamazine.

Moro's embrace reflex, test (mo′rōz) [Ernst *Moro,* pediatrist in Heidelberg, 1874–1951] see under *reflex* and *tests.*

moron (mo′ron) [Gr. *mōros* stupid] (*obs.*) a person with the highest grade of feeblemindedness (q.v.), equivalent to the modern classification "mild mental retardation."

moronity (mo-ron′ĭ-te) the condition of being a moron; mild mental retardation.

-morph [Gr. *morphē* form] a word termination denoting relationship to form or shape, especially an individual or substance possessing a certain form, indicated by the preceding root, as *mesomorph.*

morphallactic (mor″fah-lak′tik) pertaining to or characterized by morphallaxis.

morphallaxis (mor″fah-lak′sis) [Gr. *morphē* form + *allaxis* exchange] the renewal of lost tissue or a part by reorganization of the remaining part of the body of an animal.

morphea (mor-fe′ah) [Gr. *morphē* form] a localized form of scleroderma characterized by the presence of one or more supple, nonindurated, rose and violaceous macules followed by the development of yellowish or ivory-colored discrete patches or plaques in which the skin is hard, dry, and smooth. The lesions may remain localized or may become generalized. Called also *circumscribed* or *localized scleroderma.* Cf. *systemic scleroderma.* **generalized m.,** a severe form that may become so extensive as to involve the entire skin, which may lead to progressive disability, contractures of the limbs, and progressive atrophy. **guttate m.,** a form characterized by multiple small, rounded, atrophic macules, sometimes surrounded by a violaceous zone, and arranged in clusters or lines; it is difficult to distinguish from and believed by some authorities to be the same as lichen sclerosus et atrophicus. Called also *white spot disease.* **linear m., m. linea′ris,** see under *scleroderma.*

morpheme (mor′fēm) a meaningful unit of sound.

morphia (mor′fe-ah) morphine.

morphina, pl. and gen. *morphi′nae* [L.] morphine.

morphine (mor′fēn) [L. *morphina, morphinum*] chemical name: 7,8-didehydro-4,5-epoxy-17-methylmorphinan-3,6-diol. The principal and most active narcotic alkaloid of opium (q.v.), $C_{17}H_{19}NO_3$, occurring as a white, crystalline powder or as white, acicular crystals, and having powerful analgesic action and some central stimulant action. In the United States, it is usually used in the form of the sulfate salt, while in Germany and Great Britain, the hydrochloride salt is usually preferred. Abuse of morphine and its salts leads to dependence. **dimethyl m.,** thebaine. **m. hydrochloride,** the trihydrate hydrochloride salt of morphine, $C_{17}H_{19}$-$NO_3 \cdot HCl \cdot 3H_2O$, occurring as colorless, silky crystals or crystalline powder, having the same actions as the base; used as a narcotic analgesic, usually administered orally. It is the form usually preferred in Germany and Great Britain. **m. sulfate** [USP], the pentahydrate sulfate salt of morphine, $(C_{17}H_{19}NO_3)_2 \cdot H_2SO_4 \cdot 5H_2O$, occurring as white, feathery, silky crystals, cubical masses or crystals, or white, crystalline powder, and having the same actions as the base; used as a narcotic analgesic, administered parenterally. It is the form usually preferred in the United States.

morphinic (mor-fin′ik) pertaining to morphine.

morphinism (mor′fin-izm) a pathologic state due to the habitual misuse of morphine; also morphine addiction.

morphinist (mor′fin-ist) a morphine addict.

morphinistic (mor″fi-nis′tik) pertaining to or characteristic of morphinism.

morphinium (mor-fin′e-um) [L.] morphine. **m. sulfate,** morphine sulfate.

morphinization (mor″fin-i-za′shun) subjection to the influence of morphine.

morphium (mor′fe-um) morphine.

morph(o)- [Gr. *morphē* form] a combining form denoting relationship to form or structure.

morphodifferentiation (mor″fo-dif″er-en″she-a′shun) the arrangement of formative cells in the development of tissues or organs, which leads to production of the ultimate shape of the structure.

morphogen (mor'fo-jen) a diffusible substance in embryonic tissue postulated to form a concentration gradient that influences morphogenesis.

morphogenesia (mor″fo-jĕ-ne′se-ah) morphogenesis.

morphogenesis (mor″fo-jen′ĕ-sis) [Gr. *morphē* form + *gennan* to produce] the evolution and development of form, as the development of the shape of a particular organ or part of the body, or the development undergone by individuals who attain the type to which the majority of the individuals of the species approximate.

morphogenetic (mor″fo-jĕ-net′ik) producing growth; producing form or shape.

morphogeny (mor-foj′ĕ-ne) morphogenesis.

morphography (mor-fog′rah-fe) [*morpho-* + Gr. *graphein* to write] a description of organized beings, with special reference to their forms and structure.

morphological (mor″fo-loj′ĭ-kal) pertaining to morphology.

morphology (mor-fol′o-je) [*morpho-* + *-logy*] the science of the forms and structure of organisms; the form and structure of a particular organism, organ, or part.

morpholysis (mor-fol′ĭ-sis) [*morpho-* + Gr. *lysis* dissolution] destruction of form.

morphometry (mor-fom′ĕ-tre) [*morpho-* + Gr. *metron* measure] the measurement of the forms or structures of organisms.

morphon (mor′fon) [Gr. *morphōn* forming] an individual organism or structural unit.

morphophyly (mor-fof′ĭ-le) [*morpho-* + Gr. *phylon* tribe] the branch of phylogenesis dealing with the evolutionary development of form.

morphophysics (mor″fo-fiz′iks) the study of the physical and chemical causes of development.

morphoplasm (mor′fo-plazm) [*morpho-* + Gr. *plasma* anything formed] the substance of the cellular reticulum.

morphosis (mor-fo′sis) [Gr. *morphōsis* a shaping, bringing into shape] the process of formation of a part or organ.

morphotic (mor-fot′ik) pertaining to morphosis or formation; concerned in a formative process.

morpio, morpion (mor′pe-o, mor′pe-on), pl. *morpio′nes* [L.] the crab louse, *Phthirus pubis.*

Morquio's syndrome (disease) (mor-ke′ōz) [Louis *Morquio*, pediatrician in Montevideo, 1867–1935] see under *syndrome.*

Morquio-Ullrich disease (mor-ke′o-ool′rik) [Louis *Morquio*; Otto *Ullrich*, German physician, 1894–1957] Morquio's syndrome.

morrhua (mor′u-ah) [L.] the codfish, *Gadus morrhua*, which furnishes cod liver oil.

morrhuate (mor′u-āt) a salt of morrhuic acid. **m. sodium** [NF], the sodium salts of the fatty acids of cod liver oil; used as a sclerosing agent, especially for the treatment of varicose veins and hemorrhoids, injected in solution into varicosities.

morrhuin (mor′u-in) [L. *morrhua* codfish] a thick oily ptomaine, $C_{19}H_{27}N_3$, from some samples of cod liver oil.

mors (morz), gen. *mor′tis* [L.] death. **m. thy′mica,** sudden death allegedly occurring in thymic asthma and lymphatism (def. 2).

morsal (mor′sal) [L. *morsus* bite] taking part in mastication; a term applied to the masticating surface of a bicuspid or molar.

Mor. sol. abbreviation for L. *mo′re sol′ito,* in the usual way.

morsulus (mor′su-lus) [L., dim. of *morsus* bite] a troche.

morsus (mor′sus) [L.] bite; sting. **m. diab′oli,** the fimbriae at the ovarian extremity of an oviduct. **m. huma′nus,** a bite by a human being.

mortal (mor′tal) [L. *mortalis*] 1. subject to death, or destined to die. 2. fatal; causing or terminating in death.

mortality (mor-tal′ĭ-te) 1. the quality of being mortal. 2. the *mortality rate;* see under *rate.* 3. in life insurance, the ratio of deaths that take place to expected deaths.

mortar (mor′tar) [L. *mortarium*] a bell-shaped or urn-shaped vessel of glass, iron, porcelain, or other material, in which drugs are beaten, crushed, or ground with a pestle.

mortician (mor-tish′an) [L. *mors* death] an undertaker; a person trained to care for the dead.

Mortierella (mor″te-ah-rel′ah) a genus of phycomycetous fungi of the order Mucorales, family Mucoraceae, species of which have been isolated from lesions of mucormycosis.

mortification (mor″tĭ-fi-ka′shun) gangrene or sphacelus; molar death.

Morton's cough (mor′tunz) [Richard *Morton*, English physician, 1637–1698] see under *cough.*

Morton's current (mor′tunz) [William James *Morton*, American neurologist, 1846–1920] see under *current.*

Morton's toe (disease, foot, neuralgia), test (mor′tunz) [Thomas George *Morton*, Philadelphia surgeon, 1835–1903] see under *toe* and *tests.*

mortuary (mor′tu-a″re) [L. *mortuarium* tomb] 1. pertaining to death. 2. a place where dead bodies are kept until burial or cremation.

morula (mor′u-lah) [L. *morus* mulberry] the solid mass of blastomeres formed by cleavage of a fertilized ovum.

morular (mor′u-lar) 1. pertaining to a morula. 2. resembling a mulberry.

morulation (mor″u-la′shun) the process of formation of the morula.

moruloid (mor′u-loid) [L. *morus* mulberry + Gr. *eidos* form] 1. shaped like a mulberry. 2. a bacterial colony in the form of a mulberry-like mass.

Morvan's chorea, disease, syndrome (mor′vanz) [Augustin Marie *Morvan*, French physician, 1819–1897] see under *chorea* and *syndrome* (def. 2), and see *syringomyelia.*

mosaic (mo-za′ik) [L. *mosaicus;* Gr. *mouseion*] a pattern made of numerous small pieces fitted together. (1) *Genetics:* an individual or cell cultures having two or more cell lines that are karyotypically or genotypically distinct but are derived from a single zygote. Cf. *chimera.* (2) *Embryology:* the condition in the fertilized eggs of some species, such as the sea urchin, whereby the cells of early stages have developed cytoplasm which determines the parts that are to develop. (3) *Plant pathology:* a viral disease characterized by mottling of the foliage.

mosaicism (mo-za′ĭ-sizm) in genetics, the presence in an individual of two or more cell lines that are karyotypically or genotypically distinct and are derived from a single zygote. Cf. *chimerism.* **erythrocyte m.,** the mixture of two blood types in each of nonidentical twins as a result of anastomosis of placental blood vessels. **gonadal m.,** mosaicism that results from mosaicism within the gonad so that some of the germ cells are mutants. More than one offspring of a gonadal mosaic for a dominant trait may show the trait although it is not manifested in the parent.

Moschcowitz's disease, test (sign) (mos′ko-witz) [Eli *Moschcowitz*, American physician, 1879–1964] see *febrile pleiochromic anemia,* under *anemia,* and *thrombotic thrombocytopenic purpura,* under *purpura,* and see under *tests.*

Moschcowitz's operation (mos′ko-witz) [Alexis Victor *Moschcowitz*, American surgeon, 1865–1933] see under *operation.*

Mosenthal's test (mo′zen-thalz) [Herman Otto *Mosenthal,* American physician, 1878–1954] see under *tests.*

Mosetig-Moorhof bone wax (filling) (mōs-et′ig-mōr′hof) [Albert von *Mosetig-Moorhof,* German surgeon, 1838–1907] see under *wax.*

mOsm milliosmol.

mosquito (mos-ke′to), pl. *mosquitoes* [Sp. "little fly"] a popular name for gnatlike, bloodsucking and venomous insects of the family Culicidae and of various genera, chiefly *Culex, Aedes, Anopheles, Mansonia, Haemagogus, Psorophora, Theobaldia* and *Chagasia.* **anautogenous m.,** a mosquito that requires a blood meal in the adult stage for the production of viable eggs. **arygamous m.,** a mosquito that requires large or outdoor spaces for breeding. **autogenous m.,** a mosquito that can produce viable eggs without a blood meal. **house m.,** see *Culex pipiens* and *C. quinquefasciatus.* **steyogamous m.,** a mosquito that can breed in captivity in limited spaces. **tiger m.,** *Aedes aegypti.*

mosquitocidal (mos-ke″to-si′dal) destructive to mosquitoes.

mosquitocide (mos-ke′to-sīd) [*mosquito* + L. *caedere* to kill] an agent that is destructive to mosquitoes.

moss (mos) 1. any plant or species of the cryptogamic class *Musci.* 2. material composed of or derived from a plant of the cryptogamic class *Musci.* **Ceylon m.,** a red seaweed, *Gracilaria lichenoides* (L.) Harv. (Gracilariaceae); one of the sources of agar, and also used for food. In China, it is considered to be a pectoral and antidysenteric. **Iceland m.,** *Cetraria,* def. 2. **Irish m., juniper m.,** *Polytrichum juniperinum.* **pearl m., salt rock m.,** chondrus.

Moss' classification (mos'ez) [William Lorenzo *Moss,* American physician, 1876–1957] see under *classification.*

Mosse's syndrome (mos'ez) [Max *Mosse,* Berlin physician, born 1873] see under *syndrome.*

Mosso's ergograph, sphygmomanometer (mos'ōz) [Angelo *Mosso,* Italian physiologist, 1846–1910] see under *ergograph* and *sphygmomanometer.*

Motais' operation (mo-tāz') [Ernest *Motais,* French ophthalmologist, 1845–1913] see under *operation.*

moth (mawth) a lepidopterous insect. **brown-tail m.,** *Euproctis chrysorrhoea.* **flannel m.,** see *Megalopyge.* **io m.,** *Automeris io.* **meal m.,** *Asopia farinalis.* **tussock m.,** *Hemerocampa leucostigma.*

mother (muth'er) [L. *mater*] the female parent. Also, something from which another thing is derived, as a *mother cell.* **m. of vinegar,** a slimy surface film or sediment found in unpasteurized vinegar, caused by *Acetobacter aceti.*

motile (mo'til; mōt'l; mo'tīl) having spontaneous but not conscious or volitional movement.

motilin (mo-til'in) a polypeptide hormone (2698 daltons, 22 amino acids) secreted by the enterochromaffin cells of the gut; it causes increased motility of several portions of the gastrointestinal tract and stimulates pepsin secretion. In human beings, its release is stimulated by the presence of acid and fat in the duodenum; the physiologic role of the hormone in gastrointestinal function is not yet known.

motility (mo-til'i-te) the ability to move spontaneously.

motivation (mo''tĭ-va'shun) in psychology, any of the forces that activate behavior toward satisfying needs or achieving goals.

motive (mo'tiv) in psychology, any state that affects an individual's goal-directed behavior. **achievement m.,** the desire to achieve for the sake of achievement per se. **aroused m.,** one that is actively influencing behavior, or that can be inferred from actual behavior.

motoceptor (mo'to-sep''tor) any muscle sense receptor.

motofacient (mo''to-fa'shent) producing motion; a term applied to that phase of muscular activity by which the muscle produces actual motion, in contradistinction to the *nonmotofacient* phase in which the muscle is contracting without producing motion.

motoneuron (mo''to-nu'ron) motor neuron; a neuron possessing a motor function; an efferent neuron conveying motor impulses. **alpha m's,** neurons of the anterior spinal cord that give rise to the alpha fibers which innervate the skeletal muscle fibers. **gamma m's,** neurons of the anterior spinal cord that give rise to the gamma (fusimotor) fibers which innervate intrafusal fibers of the muscle spindle. **heteronymous m's,** those supplying muscles other than the one from which the afferent impulses originate. **homonymous m's,** those supplying the muscle from which the afferent impulses originate. **lower m's,** peripheral neurons whose cell bodies lie in the ventral gray columns of the spinal cord and whose terminations are in skeletal muscles. **peripheral m's,** neurons in a peripheral reflex arc that receive impulses from interneurons and transmit them to voluntary muscles. **upper m's,** neurons in the cerebral cortex that conduct impulses from the motor cortex to motor nuclei of the cerebral nerves or to the ventral gray columns of the spinal cord.

motor (mo'tor) [L.] 1. a muscle, nerve, or center that effects or produces movement. 2. producing or subserving motion. **m. oc'uli** (*obs.*), the third cranial nerve (nervus oculomotorius [NA]). **plastic m.,** the tissues of an amputation stump used to secure motion in an artificial limb.

motorgraphic (mo''tor-graf'ik) kinetographic.

motoricity (mo''tor-is'ĭ-te) the faculty of performing movement; power of movement.

motorius (mo-to're-us) [L.] a motor nerve.

motorogerminative (mo''tor-o-jer'mĭ-na-tiv) developing into the muscles; said of portions of the mesoderm.

motorpathy (mo-tor'pah-the) [*motor* + Gr. *pathos* disease] treatment of disease by gymnastics.

Motrin (mo'trin) trademark for a preparation of ibuprofen.

MOTT mycobacteria other than tubercle bacilli. See *nontuberculous mycobacteria,* under *mycobacterium.*

Mott's law of anticipation (motz) [Sir Fredrick Walker *Mott,* English neurologist, 1853–1926] see under *law.*

mottling (mot'ling) a condition of spotting with patches of color.

moulage (moo-lahzh') [Fr. "molding"] the making of molds or models in wax or plaster, as of a structure or a lesion; also such a mold or model.

mould (mōld) see *mold.*

moulding (mōld'ing) molding.

mounding (mownd'ing) the rising in a lump of a wasting muscle when struck; called also *myoedema.*

mount (mownt) 1. to fix on or in a support. 2. a support, backing, setting, or the like, on which something may be fixed. 3. to prepare specimens and slides for study.

mountant (mownt'ant) a medium, such as natural resins, polymers, or glycerol, in which objects are embedded for study, especially with the microscope; called also *mounting medium.*

mounting (mownt'ing) the preparation of specimens and slides for study. The chief media used in mounting large specimens are alcohol and glycerin jelly; for microscopic objects on a slide, Canada balsam and glycerin. **split cast m.,** 1. a dental cast with key grooves on its base, mounted on an articulator for the purpose of easy removal and accurate replacement. Split remounting metal plates may be used instead of grooves in casts. 2. see under *method.*

mourning (mor'ning) the normal psychological processes that follow the loss of a loved one; grief is the accompanying emotional state. Four phases have been described: a short phase of numbness and denial, followed by a phase of yearning and protest marked by intense pining for the dead, followed by a phase of disorganization marked by pain and despair, ending in a phase of detachment and reorganization of love relationships that completes the work of mourning.

mouse (mows) 1. a small rodent belonging to the genus *Mus,* frequently used as an experimental animal. 2. a small weight, or movable structure. **C.F.W. m.** (cancer-free *w*hite mouse), one of a strain of mice bred for use in cancer research laboratories. **joint m.,** one of the portions of the fringes in the synovial membrane of joints in osteoarthritis which are changed into cartilage and become free in the joints. Cf. *arthrolith* and *arthrophyte.* **nude m., nu/nu m.,** a mouse homozygous for the *nu* gene; these mice are hairless and congenitally athymic and thus lack T lymphocytes. **NZB (New Zealand black) mice,** an inbred strain of mice that develop an autoimmune disease that closely resembles systemic lupus erythematosus in man. **peritoneal m.,** a free body in the peritoneal cavity, probably representing a small mass of omentum or epiploic appendage which has twisted off and become coated with fibrin, and sometimes appearing as a soft density on the roentgenogram. **pleural m.,** a fibrinous body sometimes seen by x-ray of the chest in the pleural space.

mousepox (mows'poks) infectious ectromelia.

mouth (mowth) [L. *os, oris*] an opening or aperture. Specifically, the anterior or proximal opening of the alimentary canal, which is bounded anteriorly by the lips and which contains the tongue and teeth. Called also *os* [NA]. **Ceylon sore m.,** tropical sprue. **denture sore m.,** denture stomatitis. **dry m.,** xerostomia. **glass-blowers' m.,** swelling of the parotid gland in glass-blowers; see also *parotid pneumatocele,* under *pneumatocele.* **parrot m.,** retraction of the lower jaw in the horse. **sore m.,** orf (contagious ecthyma). **tapir m.,** a condition in which the mouth has something of the appearance of that of a tapir, the orbicular oris muscle being atrophied, and the lips thickened and separated; seen in Landouzy-Dejerine dystrophy. **trench m.,** acute necrotizing ulcerative gingivitis; so called because it occurred in the troops in the trenches in World War I. **white m.,** thrush, def. 1.

mouthwash (mowth'wosh) a solution for rinsing the mouth, e.g., the official [NF] preparation of potassium bicarbonate, sodium borate, thymol, eucalyptol, methyl salicylate, amaranth solution, alcohol, glycerin, and purified water.

movement (mōōv'ment) 1. an act of moving; motion. 2. an act of defecation. **active m.,** voluntary movement produced by the person's own muscles, as opposed to passive m. **ameboid m.,** the movement of an ameba or leukocyte by virtue of the flow of cytoplasm, resulting in the protrusion of a pseudopodium, or a movement similar to it. **angular m.,** a movement which changes the angle between two bones. **associated m.,** a movement of parts which act together, as of the eyes. **automatic m.,** a movement originating within the organism, but not by an act of the will. **Bennett m.,** the lateral shift of the mandibular condyles and articular disks in the direction of the working bite as the lower jaw swings in preparation for mastication. **border m.,** any extreme compass of mandibular movement limited by bone, ligaments, or soft tissues; usually applied to horizontal mandibular movements. **border tissue m's,** movements produced by action of the muscles and other tissues adjoining the borders of a denture. **brownian m., Brownian-Zsigmondy m., brunonian m.,** the dancing motion of minute particles suspended in a liquid, due to thermal agitation. **choreic m's, choreiform m's,** irregular, jerky movements of muscles or groups of muscles. **ciliary m.,** the lashing motion of cilia occurring in certain of the tissues. **circus m.,** 1. a peculiar circular gait; an involuntary rolling or tumbling movement, the result of lesions of the brain and basal nerve centers. 2. a re-entrant mechanism of the excitatory wave in the atrium of the heart; a "circular" path characterized by a gap between the excitatory and refractory tissue, usually resulting in conduction to the ventricle of only a fraction of the impulses. A circus movement is one mechanism of atrial flutter. See also *re-entry.* **contralateral associated m.,** a movement on the paralyzed side in hemiplegia associated with active movement of the corresponding part on the unaffected side. **dystonic m.,** a large slow, amplified athetoid movement. **euglenoid m.,** a wormlike writhing movement, usually nonprogressive, resulting from local expansion and contraction of the body, seen in flagellates with thin pellicles and very plastic bodies, as in certain species of the order Euglenida and certain other protozoa. **excursive m's,** excursion. **fetal m.,** that of a fetus in the uterus usually observable at about 18 weeks in a primigravida and at about 16 weeks in a multipara. **forced m.,** a movement caused by an injury to a motor center or a conducting path. **Frenkel's m's,** a series of movements of precision to be performed by ataxic patients for the purpose of restoring lost coordination. **gliding m.,** a translatory movement in which one surface glides over another, without any angular or rotary movements, being the simplest kind of motion of a joint. **hinge m.,** movement occurring in a single plane, as that occurring in opening or closing of the mouth. **index m.,** a movement of the cephalic part of a body about the fixed caudal part. **intermediary m's, intermediate m's,** mandibular movements between the extremes of mandibular excursions. **jaw m.,** mandibular m. **Magnan's m.,** forward and backward movement of the tongue when it is drawn out; observed in dementia paralytica. Called also *trombone tremor of tongue.* **mandibular m.,** any movement of which the mandible is capable. Called also *jaw m.* **mandibular m., free,** any unhampered movement of the mandible. **mandibular m's, functional,** those movements of the mandible which occur in the performance of some function, as mastication, swallowing, articulation of vocal sounds, and yawning. **masticatory m's,** those movements of the mandible occurring in the mastication of food. **molecular m.,** brownian m. **morphogenetic m.,** a flowing of cell groups concerned with the formation of germ layers or of organ primordia. **nastic m.,** a response of a plant to external stimuli that is independent of the direction from which the stimuli come; some of the so-called sleep movements are nastic movements. **nucleopetal m.,** the movement of a male pronucleus toward the female pronucleus in the fertilized ovum. **opening m.,** a mandibular movement during jaw separation. **opening m., posterior,** the opening movement of the mandible about the terminal hinge axis. **passive m.,** any movement of the body effected by a force entirely outside of the organism; see *passive exercise.* **pendular m.,** one of the movements of the small intestine in digestion, consisting of a gentle swinging to and fro of the different loops; these movements are ascribed to rhythmical contractions of the longitudinal

muscles. See also *segmentation m.* **rapid eye m. (REM),** the rapid conjugate movement of the eyes that occurs during REM sleep. **reflex m.,** an involuntary stereotyped movement provoked by a remote external stimulus acting through a nerve center. **rolling m.,** the rolling of an animal on its long axis. **saccadic m.,** the quick movement of the eye in going from one fixation point to another. **scissors m.,** a movement of the pupillary reflex seen with a retinoscope, resembling the opening and shutting of scissors; it is indicative of irregular astigmatism. **segmentation m.,** one of the movements of the small intestine in digestion, consisting of small, irregular or rhythmic, circular contractions that segment a portion of the intestine into evenly spaced parts somewhat resembling a string of sausages; see also *pendular m.* **sleep m.,** a type of nastic movement in which leaves or plant parts change their position in the late afternoon or evening and return to their original position in the morning. Sleep movement is in no way related to animal sleep. **spontaneous m.,** one originated within the organism. **Swedish m.,** see under *gymnastics.* **synkinetic m's,** minor, unconscious movements that accompany major voluntary movements, such as the facial contortions in severe exertion. **vermicular m's,** the wormlike movements of the intestines in peristalsis.

mover (moo'ver) one that moves. **prime m.,** a muscle that acts directly to bring about a desired movement.

moxa (mok'sah) [Japanese] a tuft of soft, combustible substance to be burned upon the skin, popularly used in the Orient as a cautery and counterirritant.

moxalactam (moks"ah-lak'tam) an antibiotic closely related to the cephalosporins with a wide antibacterial spectrum of activity.

moxazocine (mok-sa'zo-sēn) chemical name: [2R-(2α,6α,11R*)]- 3-(cyclopropylmethyl)-1,2,3,4,5,6-hexahydro-11-methoxy-6-methyl-2,6-methano-3-benzazocin-8-ol; an analgesic and antitussive, $C_{18}H_{25}NO_2$.

moxibustion (mok"sĭ-bus'chun) counterirritation produced by igniting a cone or cylinder of moxa placed on the skin.

moxnidazole (moks-nid'ah-zōl) chemical name: 3-[[1-methyl-5-nitro-1H-imidazol-2-yl]methylene]amino]-5-(4-morpholinylmethyl)-2-oxazolidinone; an antiprotozoal, $C_{13}H_{18}$-N_6O_5, effective against *Trichomonas.*

Moynahan's syndrome (moi'nah-hanz) [E.J. *Moynahan*] see under *syndrome.*

Moynihan's cream, test (moin'yanz) [Berkeley George Andrew *Moynihan* (Lord Moynihan), British surgeon, 1865–1936] see under *cream* and *tests.*

6-MP 6-mercaptopurine.

mp. melting point.

M.P.D. maximum permissible dose; see under *dose.*

M.P.H. Master of Public Health.

MPO myeloperoxidase.

MPS mononuclear phagocyte system.

mR milliroentgen.

μR microroentgen.

μr microroentgen.

M.R.A. Medical Record Administrator.

M.R.A.C.P. Member of Royal Australasian College of Physicians.

mrad millirad.

M.R.C. Medical Reserve Corps.

M.R.C.P. Member of the Royal College of Physicians.

M.R.C.P.E. Member of the Royal College of Physicians of Edinburgh.

M.R.C.P. (Glasg.) Member of the Royal College of Physicians and Surgeons of Glasgow *qua* Physician.

M.R.C.P.I. Member of the Royal College of Physicians of Ireland.

M.R.C.S. Member of the Royal College of Surgeons.

M.R.C.S.E. Member of the Royal College of Surgeons of Edinburgh.

M.R.C.S.I. Member of the Royal College of Surgeons of Ireland.

M.R.C.V.S. Member of the Royal College of Veterinary Surgeons.

M.R.D. minimum reacting dose.

mrem millirem.

MRF melanocyte-stimulating hormone releasing factor.

MRI magnetic resonance imaging.

M.R.L. Medical Record Librarian; now called Medical Record Administrator.

mRNA messenger RNA; see *ribonucleic acid.*

MS multiple sclerosis.

ms millisecond.

μs microsecond.

M.S. Master of Surgery.

msec. millisecond.

MSG monosodium glutamate.

MSH melanocyte-stimulating hormone (see under *hormone*); it occurs in two forms, α-MSH and β-MSH.

MSH-IF melanocyte-stimulating hormone inhibiting factor; see under *factor.*

M.S.L. midsternal line.

M.T. Medical Technologist; membrana tympani.

MTU methylthiouracil.

MTX methotrexate.

M.u. Mache unit.

mU milliunit.

m.u. mouse unit.

μU microunit.

mu (mu) [M, μ] the twelfth letter of the Greek alphabet.

Muc. abbreviation for L. *mucila'go*, mucilage.

mucase (mu'kās) (obs.) mucopolysaccharidase.

Much's granules (mooks) [Hans Christian R. *Much*, German physician, 1880–1932] see under *granule.*

Mucha's disease (moo'kahz) [Viktor *Mucha*, Austrian dermatologist, 1877–1919] acute lichenoid pityriasis.

Mucha-Habermann disease (moo'kah hah'ber-man) [Viktor *Mucha*; Rudolf *Habermann*, German dermatologist, 1884–1941] acute lichenoid pityriasis.

muci- [L. *mucus*] a combining form denoting relationship to mucus, or to mucin.

mucicarmine (mu''sĭ-kar'min) a specific stain for mucin consisting of carmine, aluminum chloride, and distilled water.

muciferous (mu-sif'er-us) [*mucus* + L. *ferre* to bear] muciparous.

mucification (mu''sĭ-fi-ka'shun) the mucus-producing changes in the vaginal epithelium of laboratory animals during the progestational stage of the ovarian cycle.

muciform (mu'sĭ-form) [*mucus* + L. *forma* form] mucoid, def. 1.

mucigen (mu'sĭ-jen) [*mucus* + Gr. *gennan* to produce] the substance from which mucin is derived.

mucigenous (mu-sij'ĕ-nus) muciparous.

mucigogue (mu'sĭ-gog) [*mucus* + Gr. *agōgos* leading] 1. stimulating the secretion of mucus. 2. an agent that stimulates the secretion of mucus.

mucilage (mu'sĭ-lij) [L. *mucilago*] 1. an artificial viscid paste of gum or dextrin used in pharmacy as a vehicle or excipient, or in therapy as a demulcent. 2. a naturally formed viscid principle in a plant, consisting of a gum dissolved in the juices of the plant. **acacia m.,** a preparation of acacia and benzoic acid in purified water, used as a suspending agent for drugs. **tragacanth m.** [NF], a preparation of tragacanth, benzoic acid, and glycerin in distilled water, used as a protective.

mucilaginous (mu''sĭ-laj'ĭ-nus) of the nature of mucilage; slimy and adhesive.

mucilago (mu''sĭ-lah'go) [L.] mucilage. **m. aca'ciae,** acacia mucilage. **m. tragacan'thae,** tragacanth mucilage.

mucilloid (mu'sil-loid) a preparation of a mucilaginous substance. **psyllium hydrophilic m.,** a powdered preparation of the mucilaginous portion of blond psyllium (*Plantago ovata*) seeds used in treatment of simple constipation resulting from lack of bulk.

mucin (mu'sin) a mucopolysaccharide or glycoprotein, the chief constituent of mucus. **gastric m.,** a substance derived from the lining of hog stomachs; formerly used for its protective and lubricating action in the treatment of peptic ulcer.

mucinase (mu'sĭ-nās) (obs.) an enzyme that catalyzes the hydrolysis of mucin. Called also *mucopolysaccharidase.*

mucinoblast (mu-sin'o-blast) [*mucin* + Gr. *blastos* germ] the progenitor of a mucous cell.

mucinogen (mu-sin'o-jen) [*mucin* + Gr. *gennan* to produce] a precursor of mucin.

mucinoid (mu'sĭ-noid) [*mucin* + *-oid*] 1. resembling or pertaining to mucin. Called also *mucoid.* 2. mucoid, def. 3.

mucinolytic (mu''sĭ-no-lit'ik) [*mucin* + Gr. *lysis* dissolution] dissolving or splitting up mucin.

mucinosis (mu''sĭ-no'sis) a condition characterized by abnormal deposits of mucopolysaccharides (mucins) in the skin. The mucinoses have been classified as metabolic (myxedema, diffuse or pretibial; lichen myxedematosus; and gargoylism), secondary or catabolic (degeneration in a variety of neoplasms), and localized (follicular, papular, plaquelike, focal, and the myxoid [synovial] cyst). **follicular m.,** a disease of the pilosebaceous unit, presenting clinically as grouped follicular papules or plaques with associated hair loss, caused by mucinous infiltration of tissues, and usually involving the scalp, face, and neck. It may be primary (idiopathic), occurring most often in children, or it may be secondary to mycosis fungoides or reticulosis. Called also *alopecia mucinosis.* **papular m.,** lichen myxedematosus.

mucinous (mu'sĭ-nus) resembling or marked by the formation of mucin.

mucinuria (mu''sin-u're-ah) [*mucin* + Gr. *ouron* urine + *-ia*] the occurrence of mucin in the urine; it may suggest vaginal contamination.

muciparous (mu-sip'ah-rus) [*mucus* + L. *parere* to produce] producing or secreting mucus. Called also *blennogenic, blennogenous, muciferous,* and *mucigenous.*

mucitis (mu-si'tis) inflammation of the mucous membrane.

Muckle-Wells syndrome (muk'l welz) [Thomas James *Muckle*, Canadian pediatrician of the 20th century; Michael Vernon *Wells*, English physician, 20th century] see under *syndrome.*

muc(o) [L. *mucus*] a combining form denoting relationship to mucus, or to a mucous membrane.

mucocartilage (mu''ko-kar'tĭ-lij) a soft cartilage the cells of which are in a mucuslike matrix.

mucocele (mu'ko-sēl) [*mucus* + Gr. *kēlē* tumor] 1. dilatation of a cavity with accumulated mucous secretion. 2. a mucous polyp. **suppurating m.,** a mucocele whose contents are purulent.

mucoclasis (mu-kok'lah-sis) [*mucus* + Gr. *klasis* a breaking] surgical destruction of the mucous lining of any organ.

mucocolitis (mu''ko-ko-li'tis) former term for irritable bowel syndrome.

mucocolpos (mu''ko-kol'pos) [*mucus* + Gr. *kolpos* vagina] accumulation of mucus in the vaginal canal.

mucocutaneous (mu''ko-ku-ta'ne-us) [*mucus* + *cutaneous*] pertaining to or affecting the mucous membrane and the skin.

mucocyst (mu'ko-sist) [*muco-* + *cyst*] any of the paracrystalline, saccular or rod-shaped, subpellicular cystic organelles seen in certain ciliate protozoa, which contains a mucoid material that is expelled through a pore in the pellicle; its function is uncertain but it may be involved in the formation of cysts or protective coverings. Called also *mucigenic body.*

mucoenteritis (mu''ko-en-ter-i'tis) former term for irritable bowel syndrome.

mucoepidermoid (mu''ko-ep''ĭ-der'moid) composed of mucus-producing and epithelial cells; see under *carcinoma.*

mucofibrous (mu''ko-fi'brus) composed of mucus and fibrous tissue.

mucoflocculent (mu''ko-flok'u-lent) containing threads of mucus.

mucoglobulin (mu''ko-glob'u-lin) one of the class of glycoproteins.

mucoid (mu'koid) [*muc-* + *-oid*] 1. pertaining or relating to, or resembling mucus. Called also *blennoid, muciform,* and *mucous.* 2. mucinoid, def. 1. 3. any of a group of mucus-like proteins of animal origin, differing from mucin in solubility and in the ability to precipitate acetic acid. Called also *mucinoid.* 4. mucous, def. 1.

mucoitin sulfate (mu-ko'ĭ-tin) a sulfur-containing polysaccharide from gastric mucin and from the cornea of the eye.

mucoitin sulfuric acid (mu-ko'ĭ-tin) obsolete name for sulfated mucopolysaccharides (chondroitin sulfate, dermatan sulfate, keratan sulfate, and heparan sulfate).

mucolemma (mu"ko-lem'ah) mucin coat, a noncellular envelope secreted around the rabbit egg and its oolemma by the oviduct; formerly called *albumen layer.*

mucolipid (mu"ko-lip'id) any sphingolipid, such as ganglioside, containing sialic acid (*N*-acetylneuraminic acid).

mucolipidosis (mu"ko-lip"ĭ-do'sis) any of a group of lysosomal storage diseases in which both mucopolysaccharides and lipids accumulate in tissues but without excess of mucopolysaccharides in the urine. **m. I,** a hereditary congenital disorder characterized by mild Hurler-like manifestations with moderate mental retardation, peculiar inclusions in the fibroblasts, and no excess mucopolysacchariduria. Called also *lipomucopolysaccharidosis.* **m. II,** a rapidly progressing disease of young children, characterized histologically by abnormal fibroblasts containing a large number of dark inclusions which fill the central part of the cytoplasm except for the juxtanuclear zone (I-cells), and clinically by severe growth impairment, minimal hepatomegaly, extreme mental and motor retardation, and clear corneas; inherited as an autosomal recessive trait, it is due to deficiency of multiple acid hydrolases. Called also *I-cell disease.* **m. III,** a disorder similar to but milder than mucolipidosis II and thought to be due to the same enzyme deficiency but to a lesser extent. Called also *pseudo-Hurler polydystrophy.* **m. IV,** a form marked by early corneal clouding, psychomotor retardation, and the presence of lysosomal storage bodies; thought to be transmitted as an autosomal recessive trait.

mucolytic (mu"ko-lit'ik) destroying or dissolving mucin; an agent that so acts.

mucomembranous (mu"ko-mem'brah-nus) pertaining to or composed of mucous membrane.

Mucomyst (mu'ko-mist) trademark for a preparation of acetylcysteine.

mucoperichondrial (mu"ko-per"e-kon'dre-al) pertaining to the mucoperichondrium.

mucoperichondrium (mu"ko-per"e-kon'dre-um) perichondrium having a mucosal surface, as that of the nasal septum.

mucoperiosteal (mu"ko-per"e-os'te-al) consisting of mucous membrane and periosteum.

mucoperiosteum (mu"ko-per"e-os'te-um) periosteum having a mucous surface, as in parts of the auditory apparatus.

mucopolysaccharidase (mu"ko-pol"e-sak'ah-ri-dās) an enzyme that catalyzes the hydrolysis of mucopolysaccharides, e.g., N-acetyl galactosaminidase and hyaluronidase.

mucopolysaccharide (mu"ko-pol"e-sak'ah-rīd) a group of polysaccharides which contain hexosamine, which may or may not be combined with protein and which, dispersed in water, form many of the mucins. The major mucopolysaccharides include chondroitin and its sulfate forms (A, B, and C), heparin, and hyaluronic acid. Called also *glycosaminoglycan.*

mucopolysaccharidoses (mu"ko-pol"e-sak"ah-rĭ-do'sēz) plural of mucopolysaccharidosis.

mucopolysaccharidosis (mu"ko-pol"e-sak"ah-rĭ-do'sis) [*mucopolysaccharide* + *-osis*] any disease resulting from defective degradation of the mucopolysaccharide sulfates dermatan sulfate, heparan sulfate, or keratan sulfate or a combination of them, which are then excreted in the urine and accumulate in tissues, affecting the following organs or systems; bony skeleton, joints, liver, spleen, eye, ear, skin, teeth, and the cardiovascular, respiratory, and central nervous systems. Onset is in childhood after at least one year of normal development. Some patients die by ten years of age, others, past their sixties. Specific enzyme assay and prenatal diagnosis are practicable or possible. The prototype for mucopolysaccharidosis is the Hurler syndrome (q.v.). See also *lysosomal storage disease,* under *disease.* **m. I, MPS I,** originally, Hurler's syndrome; it now encompasses any of the forms characterized by defective α-L-iduronidase and by excretion in the urine of dermatan sulfate and heparan sulfate. **m. H, MPS I H,** Hurler syndrome. **m. IH/S, MPS I H/S,** Hurler-Scheie syndrome. **m. IS, MPS I**

S, Scheie syndrome. **m. II, MPS II,** Hunter syndrome. **m. III, MPS III,** Sanfilippo syndrome. **m. IV, MPS IV,** Morquio syndrome. **m. V, MPS V,** former name for Scheie syndrome, now classified as m. IS. **m. VI, MPS VI,** Maroteaux-Lamy syndrome. **m. VII, MPS VII,** Sly syndrome.

mucopolysacchariduria (mu"ko-pol"e-sak"ah-rĭ-du're-ah) an excess of mucopolysaccharides in the urine.

mucoprotein (mu"ko-pro'te-in) a compound present in all connective and supporting tissues, containing mucopolysaccharides as prosthetic groups; they are relatively resistant to denaturation. **Tamm-Horsfall m.,** a substance produced by cells of the ascending limb of the loop of Henle; it is a normal constituent of urine and is the major protein constituent of urinary casts.

mucopurulent (mu"ko-pu'roo-lent) containing both mucus and pus.

mucopus (mu'ko-pus) [*mucus* + *pus*] mucus which has the appearance of pus on account of the presence of leukocytes.

Mucor (mu'kor) [L.] a genus of fungi of the family Mucoraceae, order Mucorales, which form delicate, white tubular filaments and spherical, black sporangia. See *mucormycosis.* **M. corym'bifer,** a species of soil saprophytes frequently found growing on moldy bread and rotting potatoes, and on occasion isolated from otomycosis. **M. muce'do,** a species of common soil saprophytes causing rot of fruit, baked goods, and insects; it is sometimes isolated as a contaminant of the feet and skin, but has not been determined to be pathogenic in humans. **M. pusil'lus,** a species resembling *M. mucedo,* from moist bread. It is pathogenic for rabbits and is occasionally found in cases of otomycosis in man. **M. racemo'sus,** a mold from soil and diseased fruits; it has occasionally been isolated from otomycosis. **M. ramo'sus,** *Absidia ramosa.* **M. rhizopodifor'mis,** *Absidia corymbifera.*

Mucoraceae (mu"ko-ra'se-e) a family of phycomycetes of the order Mucorales, subclass Zygomycetes, in which the thallus is not segmented and ramified; it includes the genera *Absidia, Rhizopus, Mucor,* and *Thamnidium.*

mucoraceous (mu"ko-ra'shus) pertaining to fungi of the order Mucorales.

Mucorales (Mu"kor-a'lēz) an order of phycomycetous fungi of the subclass Zygomycetes made up of bread molds and related fungi, the majority of which are saprophytic; it includes the family Mucoraceae.

mucorin (mu'ko-rin) an albuminous substance prepared from mucoraceous fungi.

mucormycosis (mu"kor-mi-ko'sis) a mycosis due to fungi of the order Mucorales, including species of *Mucor, Absidia,* and *Rhizopus.* It usually occurs as a complication of a chronic debilitating disease, particularly uncontrolled diabetes, most often beginning in the upper respiratory tract or lungs, in which spores germinate and from which mycelial growths metastasize to other organs.

mucosa (mu-ko'sah) [L. "mucus"] a mucous membrane, or tunica mucosa.

mucosal (mu-ko'sal) pertaining to the mucous membrane.

mucosanguineous (mu"ko-sang-gwin'e-us) composed of mucus and blood.

mucosedative (mu"ko-sed'ah-tiv) soothing to the mucous surfaces.

mucoserous (mu"ko-se'rus) pertaining to or producing both mucus and serum.

mucosin (mu-ko'sin) a form of mucin peculiar to the more tenacious varieties of mucus, as that of the nasal and uterine cavities.

mucositis (mu"ko-si'tis) inflammation of a mucous membrane. **m. necrot'icans agranulocyt'ica,** necrotic inflammation of mucous membranes associated with agranulocytosis.

mucosocutaneous (mu-ko"so-ku-ta'ne-us) pertaining to a mucous membrane and the skin.

mucostatic (mu"ko-stat'ik) 1. arresting the secretion of mucus. Called also *blennostatic.* 2. denoting the normal relaxed condition of the tissues of the mucosa of the jaws.

mucosulfatidosis (mu"ko-sul"fah-tīd-o'sis) multiple sulfatase deficiency.

mucotome (mu′ko-tōm) a dermatome for removing mucous membrane for transplantation; see *Castroviejo dermatome*, under *dermatome*.

mucous (mu′kus) [L. *mucosus*] 1. pertaining or relating to, or resembling mucus. 2. covered with mucus. 3. secreting, producing, or containing mucus. 4. mucoid, def. 1.

mucoviscidosis (mu″ko-vis″ĭ-do′sis) cystic fibrosis of the pancreas (q.v. under *fibrosis*); so called because of the abnormally viscous mucoid secretions observed in the disease.

mucro (mu′kro) pl. *mucro′nes* [L. "a sharp point"] the pointed end of a part or organ. **m. ba′seos cartilag′-inis arytaenoi′deae**, processus vocales. **m. cor′dis**, the apex of the heart. **m. ster′ni**, processus xiphoideus.

mucron (mu′kron) [L. *mucro* a sharp point] an anterior anchoring organelle seen in aseptate gregarine protozoa, i.e., those lacking an ectoplasm septum that separates the body of the parasite into anterior (protomerite) and posterior (deuto-merite) segments. Cf. *epimerite*.

mucronate (mu′kro-nāt) [L. *mucro* a sharp point] having a spinelike tip or end.

mucroniform (mu-kron′ĭ-form) spinelike.

Mucuna (mu-ku′nah) [Brazilian] a genus of leguminous plants. The pods of *M. pru′riens*, cowitch or cowage, bear easily detached hairs which may cause unbearable itching; the seeds contain L-dopa.

mucus (mu′kus) [L.] the free slime of the mucous membranes, composed of secretion of the glands, along with various inorganic salts, desquamated cells, and leukocytes.

muffle (muf′′l) a part of a furnace, usually removable or replaceable, in which material may be placed for processing, without exposing it to the direct action of the fire.

Muirhead's treatment (mūr′hedz) [Archibald Laurence *Muirhead*, Omaha pharmacologist, 1863–1921] see under *treatment*.

mulberry (mul′ber-e) any tree of the genus *Morus*. From the juice of the edible fruit a syrup is made which is used as a drink in fevers. The leaves serve as food for the silkworm. See also *molar*.

Mulder's angle (mul′derz) [Johannes *Mulder*, Dutch anatomist, 1769–1810] see under *angle*.

Mulder's test (mul′derz) [Gerardus Johann *Mulder*, Dutch chemist, 1802–1880] see under *tests*.

Mules' operation (mūlz) [Philip Henry *Mules*, English ophthalmologist, 1843–1905] see under *operation*.

muliebria (mu″le-eb′re-ah) [L.] the female genitalia.

muliebrity (mu″le-eb′rĭ-te) [L. *muliebritas*] 1. womanly quality; the sum of the characteristics typical of the female sex. 2. the assumption of female qualities by the male.

Muller (mul′er), Hermann Joseph. American biologist and geneticist, 1890–1967; winner of the Nobel prize for medicine or physiology in 1946 for his research into spontaneous genetic mutation, which led to a technique to induce mutations artificially by x-rays.

Müller (mil′er), Paul Herrmann. Swiss chemist, 1899–1965, noted for synthesis of DDT and discovery of its insecticidal properties; winner of the Nobel prize for medicine or physiology in 1948 for synthesizing DDT and discovering its insecticidal qualities.

muller (mul′er) a kind of pestle, flat at the bottom, used for grinding drugs upon a slab of similar material.

Müller's capsule, duct (canal), maneuver (experiment), tubercle, etc. (mil′erz) [Johannes Peter *Müller*, German physiologist, 1801–1858; one of the most distinguished physiologists of Germany and the founder of scientific medicine in Germany] see *capsula glomeruli* and *ductus paramesonephricus*, and see under *maneuver* and *tubercle*.

Müller's fibers (cells, radial cells), muscle (mil′erz) [Heinrich *Müller*, German anatomist, 1820–1864] see under *fiber* and *muscle*.

Müller's fluid (liquid) (mil′erz) [Hermann Franz *Müller*, German histologist, 1866–1898] see under *fluid*.

Müller's sign [Friedrich von *Müller*, Munich physician, 1858–1941] see under *sign*.

Müller-Haeckel law (mil′er hek′l) [Fritz *Müller*, German naturalist, 1821–1897; Ernst Heinrich *Haeckel*, German biologist, 1834–1919] biogenetic law; see under *law*.

müllerian (mil-e′re-an) named for Johannes Peter *Müller*, as müllerian duct.

müllerianoma (mil-e″re-ah-no′mah) a tumor of müllerian duct origin.

Müllerius (mil-ler′e-us) a genus of nematode lungworms. **M. capilla′ris**, a species of lungworms that is parasitic in sheep and goats.

multangular (mul-tang′gu-lar) having many angles or corners.

multi- [L. *multus* many, much] a combining form meaning many or much; see also words beginning *poly-*.

multiallelic (mul″te-ah-lel′ik) pertaining to or occupied by many alleles at a single gene locus.

multiarticular (mul″te-ar-tik′u-lar) pertaining to or affecting many joints.

multibacillary (mul″tĭ-bas′ĭ-la″re) pertaining to or made up of a number of bacilli.

multicapsular (mul″tĭ-kap′su-lar) having many capsules, as a lamellar (pacinian) corpuscle.

multicell (mul″tĭ-sel) any organ made up of many cells; any group of functionally active cells.

multicellular (mul″tĭ-sel′u-lar) [*multi-* + L. *cellula* cell] 1. composed of many cells. 2. containing many hollow spaces.

multicellularity (mul″tĭ-sel″u-lar′ĭ-te) the state of being composed of many cells; the state of being multicellular.

multicentric (mul″tĭ-sen′trik) [*multi-* + *center*] polycentric.

multicentricity (mul″tĭ-sen-tris′ĭ-te) polycentricity.

Multiceps (mul′tĭ-seps) a genus of tapeworms (family Taeniidae), the bladder worms of which are found in herbivorous animals and the adult forms in carnivorous animals. **M. mul′ticeps**, a species which in the adult stage is parasitic in dogs. Its larval stage (*Coenurus cerebralis*) usually develops in the central nervous system, but sometimes in other organs or tissues, of goats and sheep and occasionally in man, and is productive of gid in sheep. **M. seria′lis**, a species parasitic in dogs, its larval stage developing in rabbits, squirrels, and other rodents; the larvae have rarely been reported from man, generally developing, as in its other intermediate hosts, in the connective tissues.

multicontaminated (mul″tĭ-kon-tam′ĭ-nāt″ed) infected by several different species of microorganisms, or by several different contaminating agents.

multicuspid (mul″tĭ-kus′pid) [*multi-* + *cuspid*] having many cusps, such as a tooth with many cusps. Called also *multicuspidate*.

multicuspidate (mul″tĭ-kus′pĭ-dāt) multicuspid.

multicystic (mul″tĭ-sis′tik) polycystic.

multidentate (mul″tĭ-den′tāt) [*multi-* + L. *dens* tooth] having many teeth or toothlike processes.

multifactorial (mul″tĭ-fak-to′re-al) 1. of or pertaining to, or arising through the action of many factors. 2. in genetics, arising as the result of the interaction of several genes and usually, to some extent, of nongenetic factors. Cf. *polygenic*.

multifid (mul′tĭ-fid) cleft into many parts.

multifidus (mul-tif′ĭ-dus) [L., from *multus* many + *findere* to split] cleft into many parts, as the musculus multifidus.

multifocal (mul″tĭfo′kal) arising from or pertaining to many foci.

multiform (mul′tĭ-form) occurring in several forms; polymorphic.

multiganglionic (mul″tĭ-gang″gle-on′ik) pertaining to, affecting, or possessing many ganglia.

multigesta (mul″tĭ-jes′tah) multigravida.

multiglandular (mul″tĭ-glan′du-lar) pluriglandular.

multigravida (mul″tĭ-grav′ĭ-dah) [*multi-* + L. *gravida* pregnant] a woman who has been pregnant several times. Also written gravida II, III, etc., according to the number of pregnancies. **grand m.**, a woman who has had six or more previous pregnancies.

multihallucalism (mul″tĭ-hal′ŭ-kal-izm) [*multi-* + L. *hallux, hallucis*, great toe + *-ism*] a developmental anomaly characterized by the presence of more than one great toe on one foot.

multihallucism (mul″tĭ-hal′u-sizm) multihallucalism.

multi-infection (mul″tĭ-in-fek′shun) infection with several varieties of organisms.

multilobar (mul″tĭ-lo′bar) having numerous lobes.

multilobular (mul″tĭ-lob′u-lar) [multi- + L. *lobulus* lobule] having many lobules.

multilocular (mul″tĭ-lok′u-lar) [multi- + L. *loculus* cell] having many cells or compartments, as a multilocular cyst.

multimammae (mul″tĭ-mam′e) [multi- + L. *mamma* breast] the condition of having more than two breasts.

multimodal (mul″tĭ-mo-dal) having more than one mode; of a graph, having several maxima (peaks).

multinodular (mul″tĭ-nod′u-lar) composed of many nodules.

multinucleate (mul″tĭ-nu′kle-āt) [multi- + *nucleus*] having several nuclei; said of cells.

multipara (mul-tip′ah-rah) [multi- + L. *parere* to bring forth, produce] a woman who has had two or more pregnancies which resulted in viable fetuses, whether or not the offspring were alive at birth. Also written para II, III, IV, etc., according to the number of offspring. **grand m.,** a woman who has had six or more pregnancies which resulted in viable fetuses.

multiparity (mul″tĭ-par′ĭ-te) 1. the condition of being a multipara. 2. the production of several offspring in one gestation.

multiparous (mul-tip′ah-rus) 1. having had two or more pregnancies which resulted in viable fetuses. 2. producing several ova or offspring at one time.

multiple (mul′tĭ-p'l) [L. *multiplex*] manifold; occurring in or affecting various parts of the body at once.

multiplicitas (mul″tĭ-plis′ĭ-tas) a multiplication; a developmental anomaly characterized by the presence of an abnormal multiplicity of organs, or of a specific organ. **m. cor′dis,** a developmental anomaly characterized by the presence of a number of separate hearts.

multipolar (mul″tĭ-po′lar) [multi- + L. *polus* pole] having more than two poles or processes.

multipollicalism (mul″tĭ-pol′ĭ-kal-izm) [multi- + L. *pollex, pollicis* thumb + -*ism*] a developmental anomaly characterized by the presence of more than one thumb on one hand.

multirooted (mul″tĭ-root′ed) having many roots; said of molar teeth.

multisensitivity (mul″tĭ-sen″sĭ-tiv′ĭ-te) the condition of being sensitive (allergic) to more than one antigen (allergen).

multisynaptic (mul″tĭ-sĭ-nap′tik) polysynaptic.

multiterminal (mul″tĭ-ter′mĭ-nal) having several sets of terminals so that several electrodes may be used.

multituberculate (mul″tĭ-tu-ber′ku-lāt) having many tubercles.

multivalent (mul″tĭ-va′lent) [multi- + L. *valere* to have value] 1. having a valence of two or more. 2. denoting an antiserum, vaccine, or antitoxin specific for more than one antigen or an organism. Called also *polyvalent.*

Multivalvulida (mul″tĭ-val″vu-li′dah) [multi- + *valve*] an order of parasitic protozoa (class Myxosporea, phylum Myxozoa) having a spore wall with three or more valves.

mummification (mum′ĭ-fi-ka′shun) conversion into a state resembling that of a mummy, such as occurs in dry gangrene, or the shriveling and drying up of a dead fetus.

mumps (mumps) an acute infectious disease caused by a paramyxovirus, spread by direct contact, airborne droplet nuclei, fomites contaminated by infectious saliva, and perhaps urine, and usually seen in children under the age of 15, although adults may also be affected. Many cases of mumps are subclinical, but in those that are clinically apparent the principal manifestation is parotitis, usually associated with painful swelling of one or both parotid glands; other salivary glands may also be involved. Infection of other organs may cause complications, chiefly epididymo-orchitis in males, oophoritis in females, meningoencephalitis, and pancreatitis. Called also *epidemic parotitis.* **iodine m.,** swelling of the salivary and lacrimal glands as a toxic reaction to iodine therapy. **m. meningoencephalitis,** see under *meningoencephalitis.*

mumu (mu′mu) a condition characterized by swelling and edema of the spermatic cord, and sometimes swelling of the scrotum, epididymis, and testicle, and by the appearance of a hydrocele; probably an allergic manifestation developing after inoculation by filaria.

Münchausen's syndrome (men-chow′zenz) [named after Baron von *Münchhausen,* a reputed teller of exaggerated tales] see under *syndrome.*

Münchmeyer's disease (minch′mi-erz) [Ernst *Münchmeyer,* German physician, 1846–1880] see under *disease.*

Munk's disease (munks) [Fritz *Munk,* Berlin internist, born 1879] lipid nephrosis.

Munro's point (mun-rōz′) [John Cummings *Munro,* Boston surgeon, 1858–1910] see under *point.*

Munro's microabscess (abscess) (mun-rōz′) [William John *Munro,* English dermatologist, 19th century] see under *microabscess.*

Munro Kerr cesarean section, incision, maneuver (mun-ro′ ker) [John Martin *Munro Kerr,* Scottish gynecologist and obstetrician, 1868–1955] see under *incision, maneuver* and *section.*

mural (mu′ral) [L. *muralis,* from *murus* wall] pertaining to or occurring in the wall of a cavity.

muramic acid (mu-ram′ik) a compound consisting of glucosamine and lactic acid joined by an ether linkage; it occurs naturally as the *N*-acetyl derivative (MurNAc) in peptidoglycan, the characteristic polysaccharide composing bacterial cell walls.

muramidase (mu-ram′ĭ-dās) lysozyme.

Murchison-Pel-Ebstein fever (mur′chĭson-pel-eb′stīn) [Charles *Murchison,* British physician, 1830–1879; Pieter Klaases *Pel,* Dutch physician, 1852–1919; Wilhelm *Ebstein,* German physician, 1836–1912] Pel-Ebstein fever.

Murel (mu′rel) trademark for preparations of valethamate bromide.

Murex (mu′reks) a genus of mollusks. **M. purpu′rea,** a gastropodous mollusk of the Mediterranean from which murexine is obtained.

murexide (mu-rek′sĭd) [L. *murex* purple sea snail] ammonium purpurate, $C_8H_4O_8N_5 \cdot NH_4 \cdot H_2O$, a substance formed in Weidel's test for uric acid; a purple color is produced when uric acid is present. Formerly used as a dye. See also *Weidel's test* (1), under *tests.*

murexine (mu-rek′sin) [L. *murex, muricis* the purple fish or pointed rock + -*ine,* suffix for chemical compounds] chemical name: β-[imidazolyl-(4)]-acrylcholine. A neurotoxic substance derived from the median zone of the hypobranchial gland of gastropods of the genus *Murex* and related species; the substance is called *purpurine* when derived from snails of the genus *Purpura.*

muriate (mu′re-āt) [L. *muria* brine] an obsolete synonym of chloride.

muriatic acid (mu″re-at′ik) former name for hydrochloric acid.

muriform (mu′rĭ-form) [L. *murus* wall + *form*] wall-like, used in bacteriology to describe a spore having both transverse and longitudinal septa.

Murimyces (mu″rĭ-mi′sēz) in former systems of classification, a genus of bacteria species of which have been assigned to the genus *Mycoplasma.*

murine (mu′rin) [L. *mus, muris* mouse] pertaining to or affecting mice or rats.

murivirus (mu″rĭ-vi′rus) [from mild upper respiratory illness + *virus*] former name for rhinovirus.

murmur (mur′mur) [L.] an auscultatory sound, benign or pathologic, particularly a periodic sound of short duration of cardiac or vascular origin. **accidental m.,** a cardiac murmur due to some temporary and unimportant circumstance. **amphoric m.,** a respiratory murmur having a blowing musical character. **anemic m.,** a cardiac murmur heard in anemic patients. **aneurysmal m.,** a vascular murmur heard over an aneurysm. **aortic m.,** a sound generated by blood flowing through a diseased aorta or aortic valve. **apex m.,** one heard at the apex of the heart. **apical diastolic m's,** murmurs at the apex of the heart indicative of mitral stenosis and consisting essentially of low-frequency vibrations, which account for their rumble quality. **arterial m.,** a murmur (bruit) over an artery, sometimes aneurysmal and sometimes constricted. **attrition m.,** the sound produced by the friction of the pericardial surfaces in some cases of pericarditis. **Austin Flint m.,** a presystolic murmur at the apex in aortic regur-

A TABLE OF ENDOCARDIAL MURMURS

TIME OF OCCURRENCE	SITE OF GREATEST INTENSITY	DIRECTION OF TRANSMISSION	SEAT OF LESION	NATURE OF LESION
Systolic.	At cardiac apex.	Along left fifth and sixth ribs—in left axilla—in the back, at inferior angle of left scapula.	Mitral orifice.	Incompetency—Regurgitation.
Systolic.	At junction of right second costal cartilage with sternum.	To junction of right clavicle with sternum—in course of right carotid.	Aortic orifice.	Narrowing—Obstruction.
Systolic.	At ensiform cartilage.	Feebly transmitted.	Tricuspid orifice.	Incompetency—Regurgitation.
Systolic.	At left second intercostal space, close to sternum.	Feebly transmitted.	Pulmonary orifice.	Narrowing—Obstruction.
Diastolic.	At junction of right second costal cartilage with sternum.	To midsternum—in course of sternum.	Aortic orifice.	Incompetency—Regurgitation.
Diastolic.	At left second intercostal space, close to sternum.	In course of sternum.	Pulmonary orifice.	Incompetency—Regurgitation.
(Diastolic) presystolic.	Over body of heart.	To apex of heart.	Mitral orifice.	Narrowing—Obstruction.
(Diastolic) presystolic.	At ensiform cartilage.	Feebly transmitted.	Tricuspid orifice.	Narrowing—Obstruction.

gitation. **basal diastolic m's,** diastolic murmurs at the base of the heart, due to aortic or pulmonic insufficiency. **bellows m.,** to-and-fro sound. **blood m.,** one due to an abnormal, and commonly an anemic, condition of the blood. **brain m.,** a systolic murmur chiefly heard in the temporal region, and principally in cases of rickets. **bronchial m.,** one heard over the large bronchi resembling a laryngeal respiratory murmur. **cardiac m.,** a sound of finite length generated by blood flow through the heart. **cardiopulmonary m., cardiorespiratory m.,** a sound generated within lung tissue and related to movement of the heart. **Carey Coombs m.,** a rumbling mid-diastolic prediastolic apical cardiac murmur occurring in the early stages of rheumatic fever and disappearing after the rheumatic attack abates. **continuous m.,** a humming cardiac murmur extending throughout systole into late diastole or to the end of diastole, and occurring in patent ductus arteriosus, arteriovenous fistulas, rupture of a syphilitic aortic aneurysm into the pulmonary artery, aorticopulmonary septal defect, bronchial artery anastomosis in pulmonary atresia, angioma of lung, and stenosis of a branch of the pulmonary artery. **cooing m.,** musical m. **crescendo m.,** a murmur marked by progressively increasing loudness, e.g., the late diastolic murmur in mitral stenosis with sinus rhythm. **Cruveilhier-Baumgarten m.,** a venous murmur heard at the abdominal wall over veins connecting the portal and caval system. **deglutition m.,** one heard over the esophagus during the act of swallowing. **diamond-shaped m.,** the systolic murmur of aortic stenosis, named for its recorded shape on the phonocardiogram. **diastolic m.,** one occurring during diastole, i.e., after the second sound of the heart. Heard at the apex, it is a sign of mitral obstruction; at the base of the heart, it is due to aortic regurgitation; more rarely to pulmonary regurgitation. **direct m.** (obs.), the sound made by the forward flow of blood related to cardiac obstruction. **Duroziez's m.,** a double murmur over the femoral or other large peripheral artery, due to aortic insufficiency. **ejection m.,** systolic murmurs which occur predominantly in midsystole when ejection volume and velocity of blood flow are at their maximum; heard in aortic or pulmonary stenosis. **Flint's m.,** Austin Flint m. **friction m.,** see under rub. **functional m.,** a cardiac murmur generated within a structurally normal heart. **Gibson m.,** a long rumbling sound occupying most of systole and diastole, usually localized in the second left interspace near the sternum, and usually indicative of patent ductus arteriosus. **Graham Steell's m.,** one caused by pulmonary regurgitation in patients with pulmonary hypertension and mitral stenosis; it is a murmur heard in the third left intercostal space near the border of the sternum and thence propagated down the sternum. **Hamman's m.,** a crunching sound heard over the precordium synchronous with the heart beat; a sign of mediastinal emphysema, it is noted particularly in persons with pneumopericardium and is attributed to agitation of air bubbles by heart action. **heart m.,** cardiac m. **hemic m.,** blood m. **holosystolic m.,** pansystolic m. **hourglass m.,** a cardiac murmur characterized by two periods of maximum loudness joined by a period of decreased loudness. **humming-top m.,** venous hum. **incidental m.,** accidental m. **indirect m.** (obs.), the sound made by the backward flow of blood related to valvular regurgitation. **innocent m.,** functional m. **inorganic m.** (obs.), any cardiac murmur not due to a valvular or other lesion. **machinery m.,** Gibson m. **mitral m.,** cardiac murmur due to disease of the mitral valve. **musical m.,** a cardiac murmur, usually systolic, resulting when the responsible vibrations have a periodic harmonic pattern. **obstructive m.,** direct m. **organic m.,** one due to a structural change in the heart, in a vessel, or in the lung substance. **pansystolic m.,** a cardiac murmur that extends through systole; called also holosystolic m. **pericardial m.,** see pericardial (friction) rub, under rub. **pleuropericardial m.,** a pleural friction sound heard in the pericardial region and resembling a pericardial rub. **prediastolic m.,** one occurring just before and with the diastole. Heard at the apex, it is due to mitral obstruction; at the base of the heart, to aortic regurgitation; more rarely, to pulmonary regurgitation. **presystolic m.,** one occurring shortly before the onset of ventricular ejection, usually attributed to atrial contraction and the acceleration of blood flow through a narrowed atrial ventricular valve. **pulmonic m.,** one due to disease of the valves of the pulmonary artery. **regurgitant m.,** a murmur due to regurgitation of blood through a diseased valvular orifice. **Roger's m.,** bruit de Roger. **sea-gull m.,** a raucous murmur with musical qualities resembling the call of a sea gull, heard occasionally in aortic insufficiency, and attributed specifically to eversion or retroversion of the right aortic cusp. **seesaw m.,** to-and-fro sound. **Steell's m.,** Graham Steell's m. **stenosal m.,** a sound produced in an artery by artificial pressure or by a stenosis. **Still's m.,** a functional cardiac murmur of childhood, occurring in midsystole and usually of maximal intensity at the lower left sternal border. **subclavicular m.,** a sound sometimes produced in the subclavian artery during systole, and due to a stenosis. **systolic m.,** one during systole; usually due to mitral or tricuspid regurgitation, or to aortic or pulmonary obstruction. **to-and-fro m.,** see under sound. **Traube's m.,** gallop rhythm. **tricuspid m.,** a murmur caused by disease of the tricuspid valves. **vascular m.,** a murmur heard over a blood vessel. **venous m.,** a murmur heard over a vein. **vesicular m.,** the normal breath sounds over the lungs.

Murphy (mur′fe), William Parry. American physician, born in 1892, co-winner with George Richards Minot and George Hoyt Whipple, of the Nobel prize for medicine or physiology in 1934, for their work on anemia.

Murphy button, etc. (mur′fe) [John Benjamin Murphy, Chicago surgeon, 1857–1916] see under button, method, percussion, sign, and tests.

Murri's disease (moor′ez) [Augusto Murri, Italian clinician, 1841–1932] intermittent hemoglobinuria.

murrina (moo-re′nah) [Sp.morriña] a severe form of surra seen in horses in Central and South America, which is almost always fatal if untreated. Called also derrengadera.

Mus (mus) [L. "mouse"] a genus of mice. **M. alexan-dri′nus,** *Rattus rattus alexandrinus,* the Egyptian or roof rat. **M. decuma′nus,** *Rattus norvegicus,* the brown rat. **M. mus′culus,** the common house mouse. **M. nor-ve′gicus,** *Rattus norvegicus,* the brown rat. **M. rat′tus rat′tus,** the black rat.

Musca (mus′kah) [L. "fly"] a genus of flies of the family Muscidae which have their mouth parts adapted for suction only. **M. autumna′lis,** the face fly, a species commonly found in Europe, parts of Asia and Africa, and America. **M. domes′tica,** the common house fly. It may act as a mechanical carrier of the microorganisms of typhoid fever, cholera, dysentery, plague, anthrax, tetanus, trachoma, leprosy, and encephalitis, and of pyogenic bacteria, cysts of some

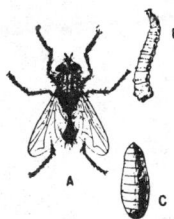

Musca domestica: A, fly; *B,* larva; *C,* pupa.

protozoa, and helminth ova. The larvae may cause myiasis. **M. domes′tica neb′ulo,** a subspecies of *M. domestica* found in India. **M. domes′tica vici′na,** a subspecies of *M. domestica* common in Egypt and India. **M. lute′ola,** see *Auchmeromyia.* **M. sor′bens,** a species of Indonesia, Ethiopia, and Oriental areas, believed to transmit conjunctivitis, trachoma, and other infections. **M. vomito′ria,** *Calliphora vomitoria.*

musca (mus′kah), pl. *mus′cae* [L.] a fly. **mus′cae his-pan′icae,** cantharides. **mus′cae volitan′tes** [L. "flitting flies"], specks seen floating before the eyes; see *floaters.*

muscacide (mus′kah-sīd) [L. *musca* fly + *caedere* to kill] 1. destructive to flies. 2. any agent that destroys flies.

muscae (mus′e) [L.] plural of *musca.*

muscardine (mus′kar-din) a disease of silkworms caused by *Beauvaria bassiana.*

muscarine (mus′kah-rēn) a cholinomimetic alkaloid occurring in the mushrooms *Amanita muscaria* and various species of the genera *Inocybe* and *Cytocybe,* which produce a characteristic toxic syndrome when ingested (see *mushroom poisoning* under *poisoning*). See also *muscarinic* and *muscarinic receptors* under *receptor.*

muscarinic (mus″kah-rin′ik) denoting the effects of muscarine or acetylcholine at muscarinic cholinergic receptors found on parasympathetic autonomic effector cells and also in the central nervous system; parasympathetic effects include a decrease in heart rate and contractility; bronchoconstriction; dilation of arterioles; an increase in motility, tone, and secretion of the stomach and intestines; stimulation of contraction of the urinary bladder; and stimulation of the salivary, lacrimal, and sweat glands. See *muscarinic receptors* under *receptor.*

muscarinism (mus′kar-in-izm) poisoning by muscarine.

muscegenetic (mus″e-jĕ-net′ik) giving rise to muscae volitantes.

muscicide (mus′ĭ-sīd) muscacide.

Muscidae (mus′ĭ-de) a family of flies of the order Diptera. It includes the genera *Fannia, Haematobia, Glossina, Musca, Muscina,* and *Stomoxys.*

Muscina (mŭ-si′nah) the nonbiting stable flies, a genus of the family Muscidae which breeds in dung. It is closely related to the housefly and it also frequents dwellings.

muscle (mus′el) an organ which by contraction produces the movements of an animal organism. Called also *musculus* [NA]. Muscles are of two varieties: *striated,* or *striped,* including all the muscles in which contraction is voluntary and the heart muscle; *unstriated, nonstriated, smooth,* or *organic,* including all the involuntary muscles except the heart, such as the muscular layer of the intestines, bladder, blood vessels, etc. Striated muscles are covered with a thin layer of connective tissue (*epimysium*) from which septa (*perimysium*) pass, dividing the muscle into bundles of fibers,

or *fasciculi.* Each fasciculus contains a number of parallel fibers separated by connective tissue septa (*endomysium*). Each fiber consists of sarcoplasm which is cross-striated or composed of alternate light and dark portions (whence the name *striated muscle*); each contains embedded in it the *myofibrils* and each is surrounded by *sarcolemma.* Smooth muscles are composed of elongated, spindle-shaped, nucleated cells arranged parallel to one another and to the long axis of the muscle, and these cells are often grouped into bundles of varying size. The muscles, bundles, and cells are enclosed in an indifferent connective tissue material much as is found in striated muscles. **abductor m. of great toe,** musculus abductor hallucis. **abductor m. of little finger,** musculus abductor digiti minimi manus. **abductor m. of little toe,** musculus abductor digiti minimi pedis. **abductor m. of thumb, long,** musculus abductor pollicis longus. **abductor m. of thumb, short,** musculus abductor pollicis brevis. **adductor m., great,** musculus adductor magnus. **adductor m., long,** musculus adductor longus. **adductor m., short,** musculus adductor brevis. **adductor m., smallest,** musculus adductor minimus. **adductor m. of great toe,** musculus adductor hallucis. **adductor m. of thumb,** musculus adductor pollicis. **Aeby's m.,** musculus depressor labii inferioris. **agonistic m.,** a muscle opposed in action by another muscle, called the antagonist. **Albinus' m.,** 1. musculus risorius. 2. musculus scalenus medius. **anconeus m.,** musculus anconeus. **anconeus m., lateral,** caput laterale musculi tricipitis brachii. **anconeus m., medial,** caput mediale musculi tricipitis brachii. **anconeus m., short,** caput laterale musculi tricipitis brachii. **antagonistic m.,** a muscle that counteracts the action of another muscle, called the agonist. **antigravity m's,** those muscles that by their tone resist the constant pull of gravity in the maintenance of normal posture. **m. of antitragus,** musculus antitragicus. **appendicular m's,** the muscles of a limb. **arrector m's of hair,** musculi arrectores pilorum. **articular m.,** a muscle that has one end attached to the capsule of a joint; called also *musculus articularis.* **articular m. of elbow,** musculus articularis cubiti. **articular m. of knee,** musculus articularis genus. **aryepiglottic m.,** musculus aryepiglotticus. **arytenoid m., oblique,** musculus arytenoideus obliquus. **arytenoid m., transverse,** musculus arytenoideus transversus. **m's of auditory ossicles,** musculi ossiculorum auditus. **auricular m's,** 1. the extrinsic auricular muscles (anterior, posterior, and superior) that move the auricle and attach it to the skull and scalp. 2. the intrinsic auricular muscles that extend from one part of the auricle to another; see *musculi auricularii.* **auricular m., anterior,** musculus auricularis anterior. **auricular m., posterior,** musculus auricularis posterior. **auricular m., superior,** musculus auricularis superior. **Bell's m.,** the muscular strands between the ureteric orifices and the uvula vesicae, bounding the trigone of the urinary bladder. Called also *ureteric bridge.* **biceps m. of arm,** musculus biceps brachii. **biceps m. of thigh,** musculus biceps femoris. **bipennate m.,** musculus bipennatus. **Bowman's m.,** musculus ciliaris. **brachial m.,** musculus brachialis. **brachioradial m.,** musculus brachioradialis. **bronchoesophageal m.,** musculus bronchoesophageus. **Brücke's m.,** the longitudinal fibers of the ciliary muscle. **buccinator m.,** musculus buccinator. **buccopharyngeal m.,** pars buccopharyngea musculi constrictoris pharyngis superioris. **bulbocavernous m.,** musculus bulbospongiosus. **canine m.,** musculus levator anguli oris. **cardiac m.,** the muscle of the heart, composed of striated muscle fibers. **Casser's m., casserian m.,** ligamentum mallei anterius. **ceratocricoid m.,** musculus ceratocricoideus. **ceratopharyngeal m.,** pars ceratopharyngea musculi constrictoris pharyngis medii. **Chassaignac's axillary m.,** an occasional muscle bundle extending from the lower edge of the latissimus dorsi across the hollow of the axilla to the brachial fascia or to the lower border of the pectoralis minor. **chondroglossus m.,** musculus chondroglossus. **chondropharyngeal m.,** pars chondropharyngea musculi constrictoris pharyngis medii. **ciliary m.,** musculus ciliaris. **coccygeal m's,** those connected with the coccyx, including the musculus coccygeus, musculus sacrococcygeus dorsalis, and musculus sacrococcygeus ventralis; called also *musculi coccygei* [NA]. **coccygeal m.,** musculus coccygeus. **compressor m. of naris,** the transverse part of the nasal muscle; see *partes*

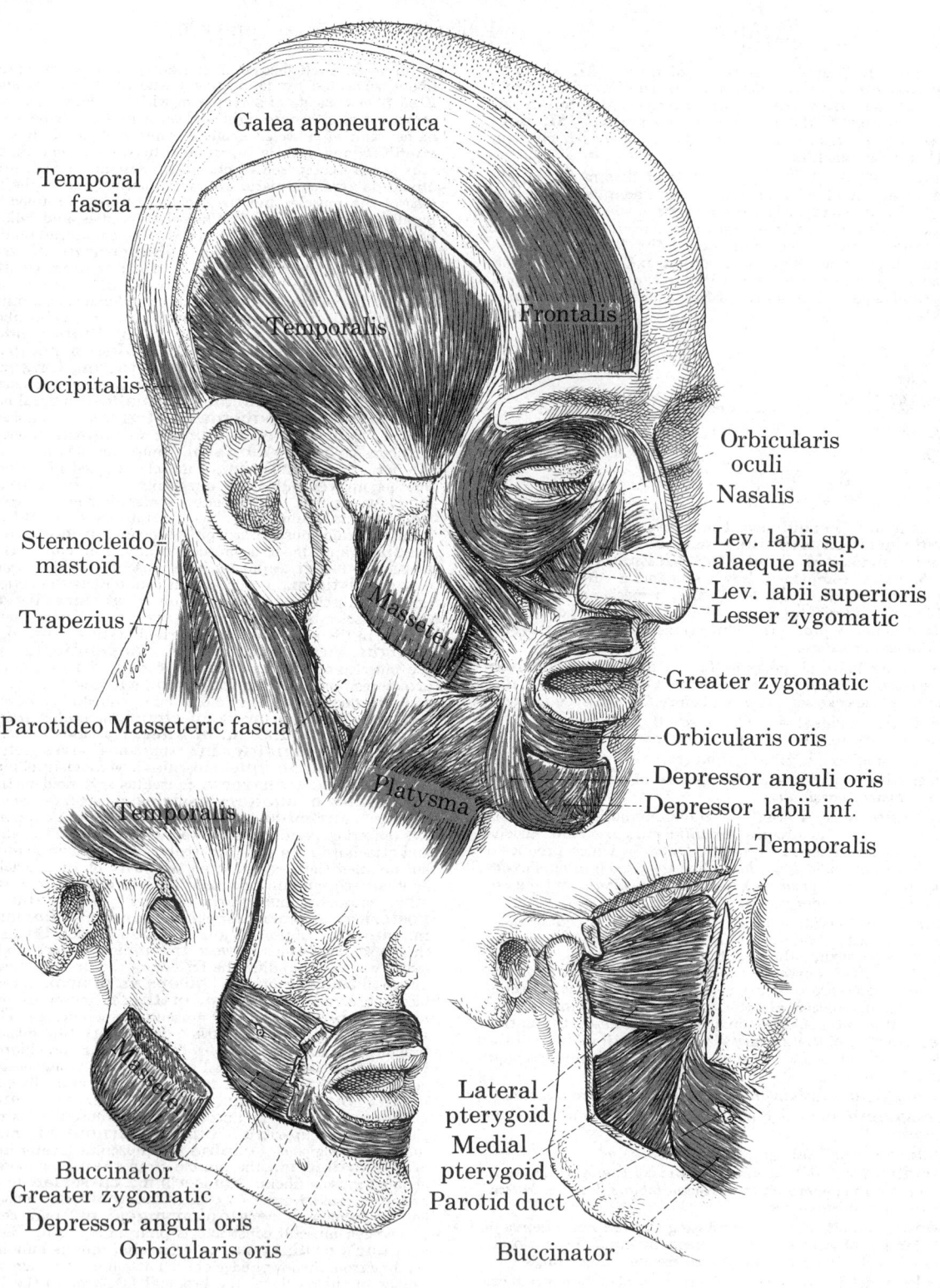

Galea aponeurotica

Temporal
fascia

Temporalis

Frontalis

Occipitalis

Orbicularis
oculi

Nasalis

Sternocleido-
mastoid

Lev. labii sup.
alaeque nasi

Lev. labii superioris

Lesser zygomatic

Trapezius

Masseter

Greater zygomatic

Parotideo Masseteric fascia

Orbicularis oris

Platysma

Depressor anguli oris

Depressor labii inf.

Temporalis

Temporalis

Masseter

Lateral
pterygoid

Medial
pterygoid

Buccinator
Greater zygomatic
Depressor anguli oris
Orbicularis oris

Parotid duct

Buccinator

PLATE 27 — MUSCLES OF THE HEAD AND NECK

1064

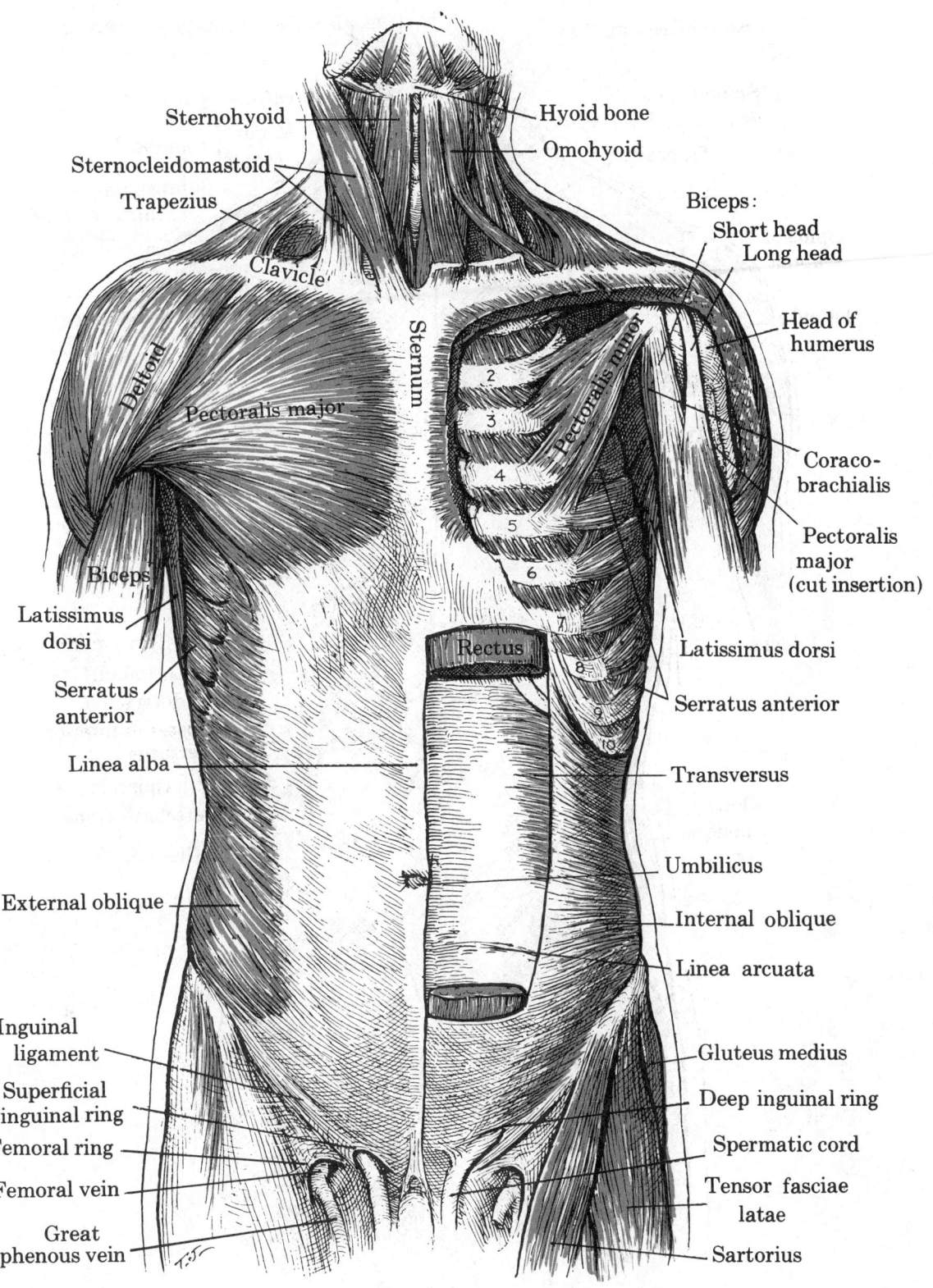

Sternohyoid

Hyoid bone

Sternocleidomastoid

Omohyoid

Trapezius

Biceps:
Short head
Long head

Clavicle

Deltoid

Head of
humerus

Pectoralis major

Sternum

Pectoralis minor

2

3

4

Coraco-
brachialis

5

Pectoralis
major
(cut insertion)

6

Biceps

7

Latissimus dorsi

Rectus

Latissimus
dorsi

8

Serratus anterior

Serratus
anterior

9

10

Transversus

Linea alba

Umbilicus

Internal oblique

External oblique

Linea arcuata

Inguinal
ligament

Gluteus medius

Superficial
inguinal ring

Deep inguinal ring

Femoral ring

Spermatic cord

Femoral vein

Tensor fasciae
latae

Great
saphenous vein

Sartorius

PLATE 28 — MUSCLES OF TRUNK, ANTERIOR VIEW

The left sternocleidomastoid, pectoralis major, external oblique, and a portion of the deltoid have been removed to show underlying muscles. A portion of the rectus abdominis has been cut away to expose the posterior part of its sheath.

1065

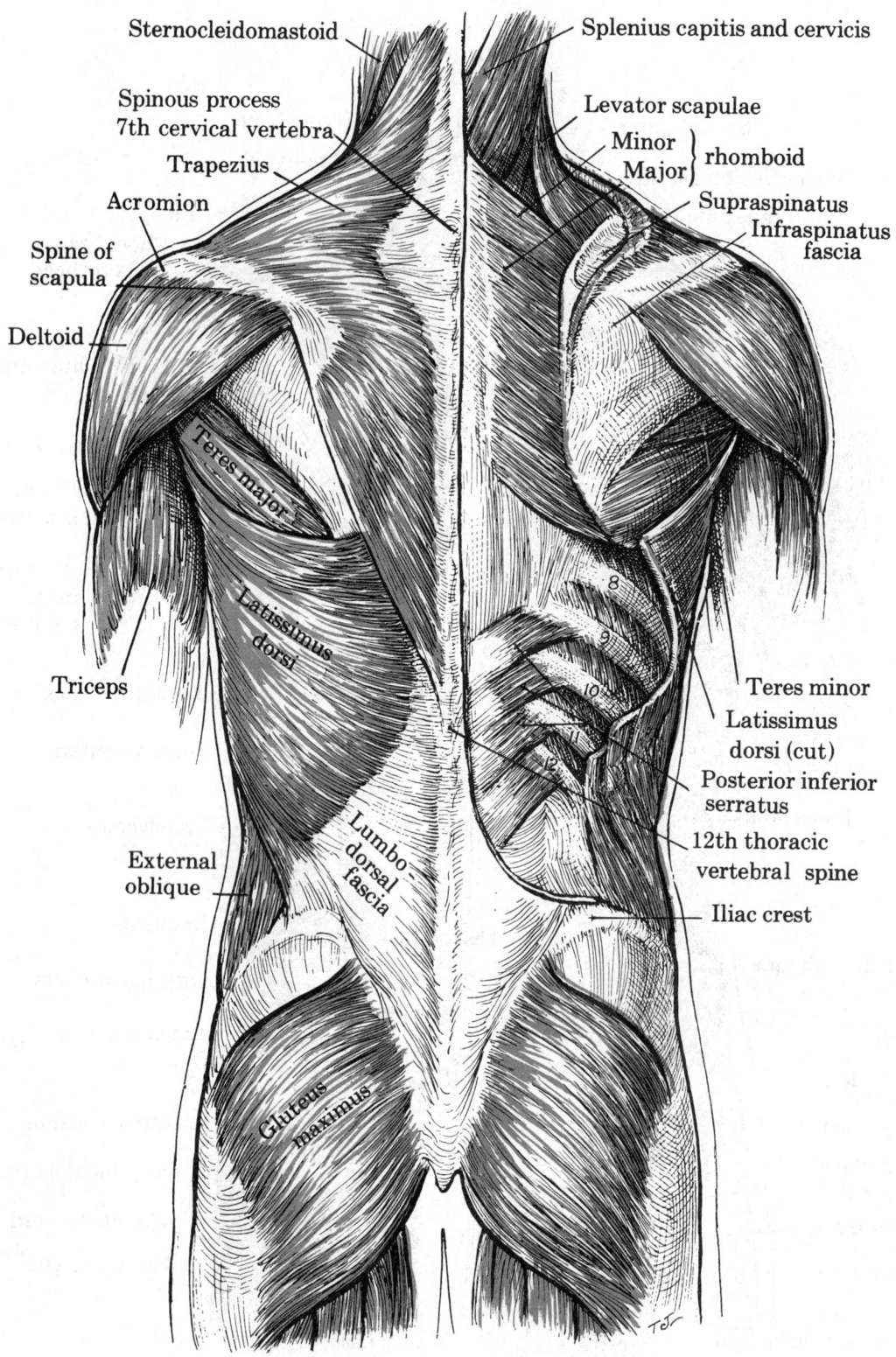

Sternocleidomastoid

Spinous process
7th cervical vertebra

Trapezius

Acromion

Spine of
scapula

Deltoid

Teres major

Latissimus
dorsi

Triceps

External
oblique

Lumbo-
dorsal
fascia

Gluteus
maximus

Splenius capitis and cervicis

Levator scapulae

Minor
Major } rhomboid

Supraspinatus

Infraspinatus
fascia

8

9

10

11

12

Teres minor

Latissimus
dorsi (cut)

Posterior inferior
serratus

12th thoracic
vertebral spine

Iliac crest

PLATE 29 — MUSCLES OF TRUNK, POSTERIOR VIEW

The latissimus dorsi and trapezius on the right side have been cut away to expose the underlying muscles.

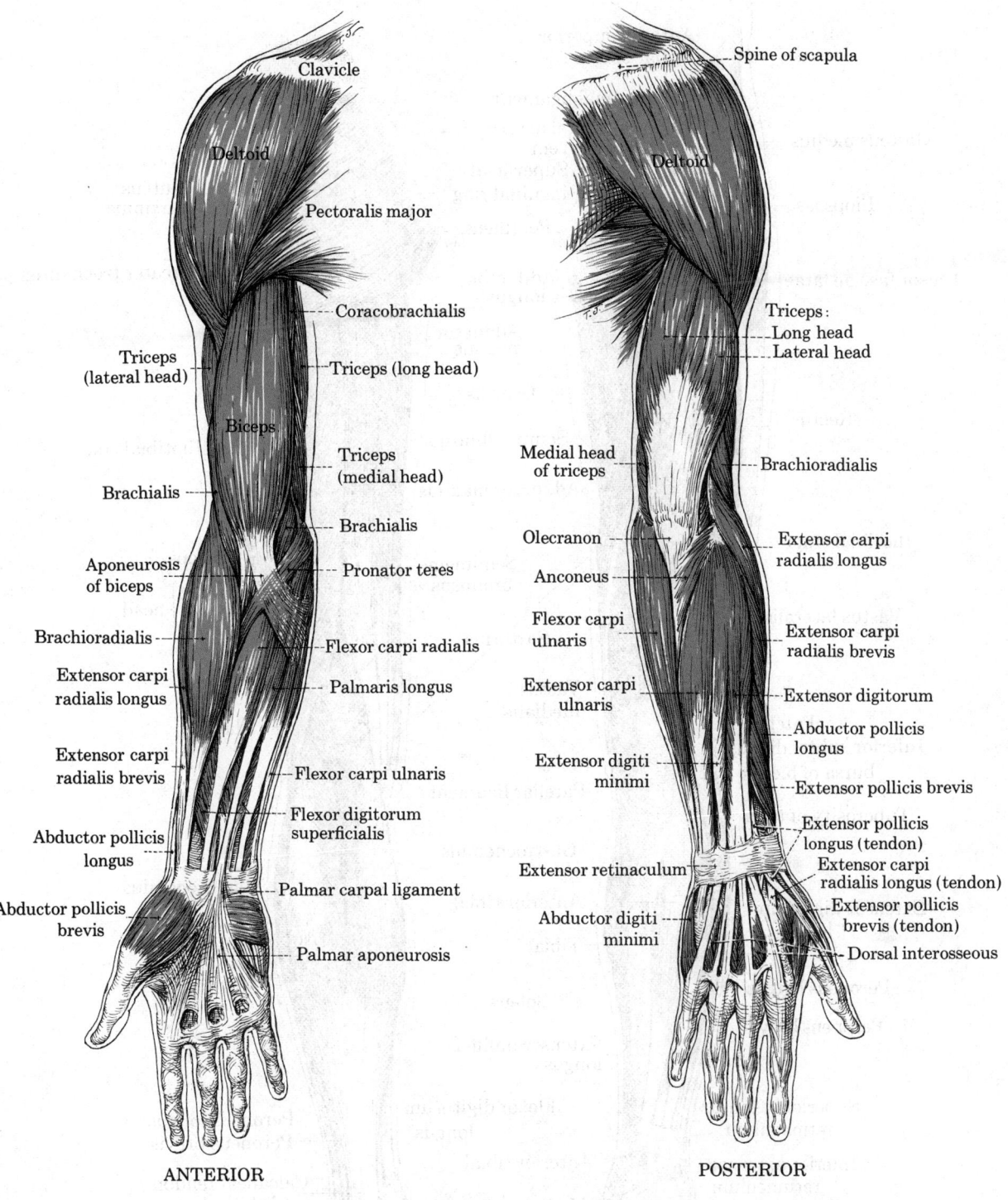

ANTERIOR

POSTERIOR

PLATE 30 — SUPERFICIAL MUSCLES OF THE RIGHT UPPER EXTREMITY

1067

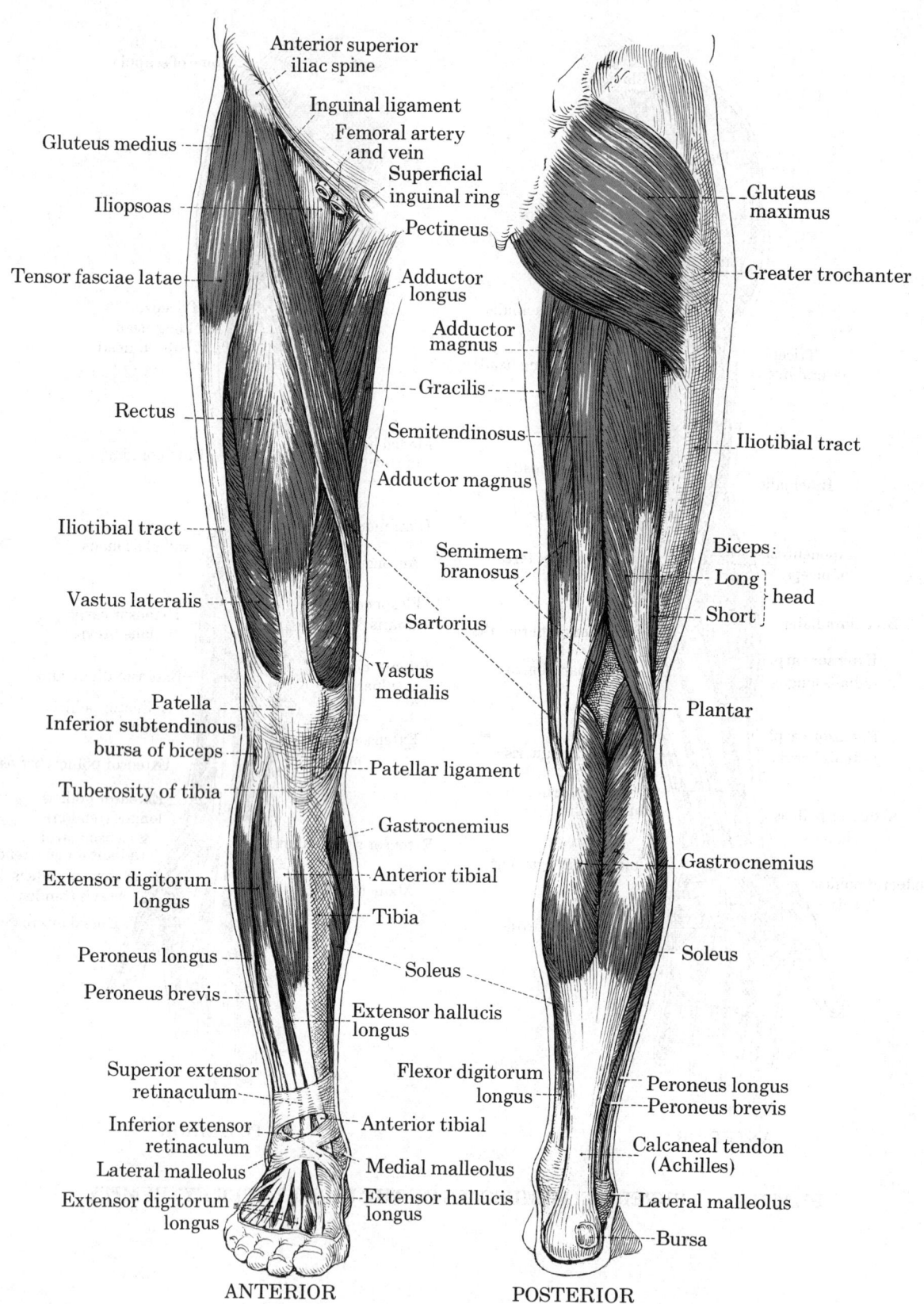

Anterior superior iliac spine	
Inguinal ligament	
Gluteus medius	Femoral artery and vein
	Superficial inguinal ring
Iliopsoas	Pectineus
Tensor fasciae latae	Adductor longus
	Adductor magnus
	Gracilis
Rectus	Semitendinosus
	Adductor magnus
Iliotibial tract	Semimembranosus
Vastus lateralis	Sartorius
	Vastus medialis
Patella	
Inferior subtendinous bursa of biceps	Patellar ligament
Tuberosity of tibia	Gastrocnemius
	Anterior tibial
Extensor digitorum longus	Tibia
Peroneus longus	Soleus
Peroneus brevis	Extensor hallucis longus
Superior extensor retinaculum	Flexor digitorum longus
Inferior extensor retinaculum	Anterior tibial
Lateral malleolus	Medial malleolus
Extensor digitorum longus	Extensor hallucis longus

Gluteus maximus

Greater trochanter

Iliotibial tract

Biceps: Long head / Short

Plantar

Gastrocnemius

Soleus

Peroneus longus
Peroneus brevis

Calcaneal tendon (Achilles)

Lateral malleolus

Bursa

ANTERIOR   POSTERIOR

PLATE 31 — SUPERFICIAL MUSCLES OF THE RIGHT LOWER EXTREMITY

1068

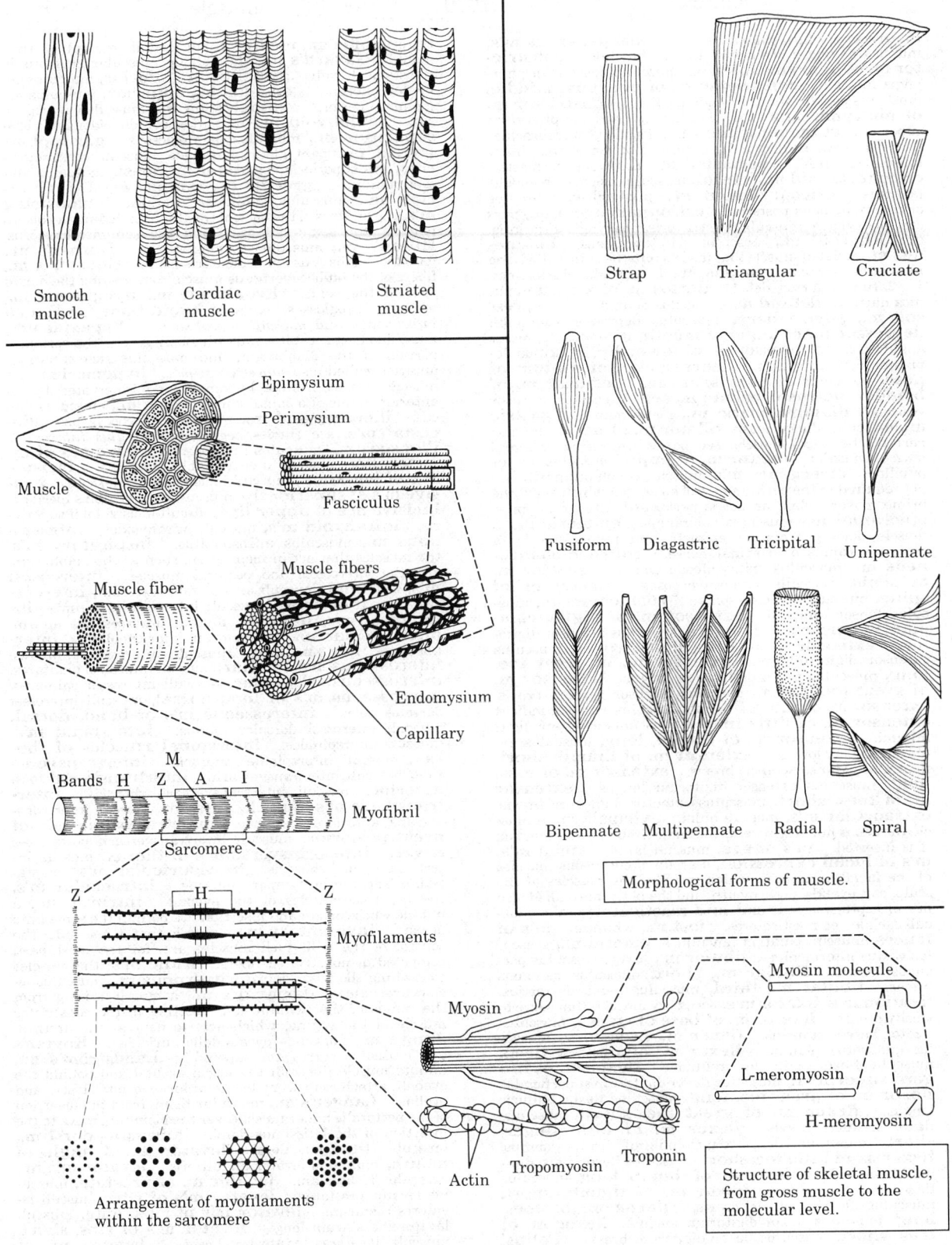

Smooth muscle

Cardiac muscle

Striated muscle

Strap

Triangular

Cruciate

Fusiform

Diagastric

Tricipital

Unipennate

Bipennate

Multipennate

Radial

Spiral

Morphological forms of muscle.

Epimysium

Perimysium

Muscle

Fasciculus

Muscle fibers

Muscle fiber

Endomysium

Capillary

Bands H Z A I
M

Myofibril

Sarcomere

Z H Z

Myofilaments

Arrangement of myofilaments within the sarcomere

Myosin

Actin Tropomyosin Troponin

Myosin molecule

L-meromyosin

H-meromyosin

Structure of skeletal muscle, from gross muscle to the molecular level.

PLATE 32 — TYPES AND STRUCTURE OF MUSCLE

transversa et alaris musculi nasalis. **congenerous m's,** muscles having a common action or function. **constrictor m. of pharynx, inferior,** musculus constrictor pharyngis inferior. **constrictor m. of pharynx, middle,** musculus constrictor pharyngis medius. **constrictor m. of pharynx, superior,** musculus constrictor pharyngis superior. **coracobrachial m.,** musculus coracobrachialis. **Crampton's m.,** the anterior portion of the ciliary muscle in birds. **cremaster m.,** musculus cremaster. **cricoarytenoid m., lateral,** musculus cricoarytenoideus lateralis. **cricoarytenoid m., posterior,** musculus cricoarytenoideus posterior. **cricopharyngeal m.,** pars cricopharyngea musculi constrictoris pharyngis inferioris. **cricothyroid m.,** musculus cricothyroideus. **cutaneous m.,** striated muscle that inserts into the skin; called also *musculus cutaneus.* **dartos m.,** 1. musculus dartos, def. 1. 2. tunica dartos, def. 1. **dartos m. of scrotum,** tunica dartos. **deltoid m.,** musculus deltoideus. **depressor m., superciliary,** musculus depressor supercilii. **depressor m. of angle of mouth,** musculus depressor anguli oris. **depressor m. of lower lip,** musculus depressor labii inferioris. **depressor m. of septum of nose,** musculus depressor septi nasi. **detrusor m. of bladder, detrusor urinae muscle,** musculus detrusor vesicae. **diaphragmatic m.,** diaphragm. **digastric m.,** musculus digastricus. **dilator m. of naris,** the alar part of the nasal muscle; see *partes transversa et alaris musculi nasalis.* **dilator m. of pupil,** musculus dilator pupillae. **emergency m's,** muscles which ordinarily are not required in the performance of an act but which assist the prime movers when an act is performed with great force. **epicranial m.,** musculus epicranius. **epimeric m.,** a muscle derived from an epimere and innervated by a posterior ramus of a spinal nerve. **epitrochleoanconeus m.,** musculus epitrochleoanconaeus. **erector m. of penis,** musculus ischiocavernosus. **erector m. of spine,** musculus erector spinae. **eustachian m.,** musculus tensor tympani. **extensor m. of digits, common, extensor m. of fingers,** musculus extensor digitorum. **extensor m. of fifth digit, proper,** musculus extensor digiti minimi. **extensor m. of great toe, long,** musculus extensor hallucis longus. **extensor m. of great toe, short,** musculus extensor hallucis brevis. **extensor m. of index finger,** musculus extensor indicis. **extensor m. of little finger,** musculus extensor digiti minimi. **extensor m. of thumb, long,** musculus extensor pollicis longus. **extensor m. of thumb, short,** musculus extensor pollicis brevis. **extensor m. of toes, long,** musculus extensor digitorum longus. **extensor m. of toes, short,** musculus extensor digitorum brevis. **extraocular m's,** musculi bulbi. **extrinsic m.,** a muscle that does not originate in the same limb or part in which it is inserted. **m's of eye,** musculi bulbi. **facial m's, m's of facial expression,** a group of cutaneous muscles of the facial structures, which includes the muscles of the scalp, ear, eyelids, nose, mouth, and the platysma; called also *m's of expression.* **facial and masticatory m's,** musculi faciales et masticatores. **fast m.,** white m. **m's of fauces,** musculi palati et faucium. **femoral m.,** musculus vastus intermedius. **fibular m., long,** musculus peroneus longus. **fibular m., short,** musculus peroneus brevis. **fibular m., third,** musculus peroneus tertius. **fixation m's, fixator m's,** accessory muscles that serve to steady a part. **fixator m. of base of stapes,** musculus fixator baseos stapedis. **flexor m., accessory,** musculus quadratus plantae. **flexor m. of fingers, deep,** musculus flexor digitorum profundus. **flexor m. of fingers, superficial,** musculus flexor digitorum superficialis. **flexor m. of great toe, long,** musculus flexor hallucis longus. **flexor m. of great toe, short,** musculus flexor hallucis brevis. **flexor m. of little finger, short,** musculus flexor digiti minimi brevis manus. **flexor m. of little toe, short,** musculus flexor digiti minimi brevis pedis. **flexor m. of thumb, long,** musculus flexor pollicis longus. **flexor m. of thumb, short,** musculus flexor pollicis brevis. **flexor m. of toes, long,** musculus flexor digitorum longus. **flexor m. of toes, short,** musculus flexor digitorum brevis. **Folius' m.,** ligamentum mallei laterale. **frontal m.,** venter frontalis musculi occipitofrontalis. **fusiform m.,** a spindle-shaped muscle; see *musculus fusiformis.* **gastrocnemius m.,** musculus gastrocnemius. **gastrocnemius m., lateral,** caput laterale musculi gastrocnemii. **gas-**

trocnemius m., medial,** caput mediale musculi gastrocnemii. **Gavard's m.,** the oblique muscular elements of the stomach wall. **gemellus m., inferior,** musculus gemellus inferior. **gemellus m., superior,** musculus gemellus superior. **genioglossus m.,** musculus genioglossus. **geniohyoid m.,** musculus geniohyoideus. **glossopalatine m.,** musculus palatoglossus. **glossopharyngeal m.,** pars glossopharyngea musculi constrictoris pharyngis superioris. **gluteal m., least,** musculus gluteus minimus. **gracilis m.,** musculus gracilis. **Guthrie's m.,** musculus sphincter urethrae. **hamstring m's,** the muscles of the back of the thigh, including the biceps femoris, the semitendinosus, and the semimembranosus. **Hilton's m.,** musculus aryepiglotticus. **Horner's m.,** pars lacrimalis musculi orbicularis oculi. **Houston's m.,** fibers of the bulbocavernosus muscle compressing the dorsal vein of the penis. **hyoglossal m., hyoglossus m.,** musculus hyoglossus. **m's of hyoid bone,** see *musculi infrahyoidei* and *musculi suprahyoidei.* **hypaxial m's,** musculus longus capitis, musculus longus colli, the vertebral portion of the diaphragm, and musculus sacrococcygeus anterior; called also *subvertebral m's.* **hypomeric m.,** a muscle derived from a hypomere and innervated by an anterior ramus of a spinal nerve. **iliac m.,** musculus iliacus. **iliococcygeal m.,** musculus iliococcygeus. **iliocostal m's,** see entries beginning *musculus iliocostalis.* **iliopsoas m.,** musculus iliopsoas. **incisive m's of inferior lip,** musculi incisivi labii inferioris. **incisive m's of lower lip,** musculi incisivi labii inferioris. **incisive m's of superior lip,** musculi incisivi labii superioris. **incisive m's of upper lip,** musculi incisivi labii superioris. **infrahyoid m's,** musculi infrahyoidei. **infraspinous m.,** musculus infraspinatus. **inspiratory m's,** the muscles that act in inspiration, such as the diaphragm, and the intercostal and pectoral muscles. **intercostal m's, external,** musculi intercostales externi. **intercostal m's, innermost,** musculi intercostales intimi. **intercostal m's, internal,** musculi intercostales interni. **interfoveolar m.,** ligamentum interfoveolare. **interosseous m's, palmar,** musculi interossei palmares. **interosseous m's, plantar,** musculi interossei plantares. **interosseous m's, volar,** musculi interossei palmares. **interosseous m's of foot, dorsal,** musculi interossei dorsales pedis. **interosseous m's of hand, dorsal,** musculi interossei dorsales manus. **interspinal m's,** musculi interspinales. **interspinal muscles of thorax,** musculi interspinales thoracis. **intertransverse m's,** musculi intertransversarii. **intertransverse m's, anterior,** musculi intertransversarii thoracis. **intertransverse m's of neck, anterior,** musculi intertransversarii anteriores cervicis. **intertransverse m's of neck, posterior,** musculi intertransversarii posteriores cervicis. **intertransverse m's of thorax,** musculi intertransversarii thoracis. **intraauricular m's,** the stapedius and tensor tympani muscles. **intraocular m's,** the intrinsic muscles of the eyeball. **intrinsic m.,** a muscle whose origin and insertion are both in the same limb or part. **involuntary m.,** a muscle that is not under the control of the will; such muscles are, for the most part, composed of nonstriated fibers. **iridic m's,** the muscles controlling the iris. **ischiocavernous m.,** musculus ischiocavernosus. **Jarjavay's m.,** a muscle arising from the ramus of the ischium and inserting in the constrictor muscle of the vagina, which acts to depress the urethra. **Jung's m.,** musculus pyramidalis auriculae. **Koyter's m.,** musculus corrugator supercilii. **Landström's m.,** minute muscle fibers in the fascia around and behind the eyeball, attached in front to the anterior orbital fascia and eyelids. **Langer's m.,** muscular fibers from the insertion of the pectoralis major muscle over the bicipital groove to the insertion of the latissimus dorsi. **latissimus dorsi m.,** musculus latissimus dorsi. **levator m. of angle of mouth,** musculus levator anguli oris. **levator ani m.,** musculus levator ani. **levator m. of prostate,** musculus levator prostatae. **levator m's of ribs,** musculi levatores costarum. **levator m's of ribs, long,** musculi levatores costarum longi. **levator m's of ribs, short,** musculi levatores costarum breves. **levator m. of scapula,** musculus levator scapulae. **levator m. of thyroid gland,** musculus levator glandulae thyroideae. **levator m. of upper eyelid,** musculus levator palpebrae superioris. **levator m. of upper lip,** musculus levator labii superioris. **levator m. of upper lip and ala of** nose, musculus levator labii superioris alaeque nasi. **levator muscle of velum palatini,** musculus levator velum palatini. **lingual m's,** musculi linguae. **longissimus m.,** musculus longissimus. **longissimus m. of back,** musculus longissimus thoracis. **longissimus m. of head,** musculus longissimus capitis. **longissimus m. of neck,** musculus longissimus cervicis. **longissimus m. of thorax,** musculus longissimus thoracis. **longitudinal m. of tongue, inferior,** musculus longitudinalis inferior linguae. **longitudinal m. of tongue, superior,** musculus longitudinalis superior linguae. **lumbrical m's of foot,** musculi lumbricales pedis. **lumbrical m's of hand,** musculi lumbricales manus. **Luschka's m's,** the uterosacral ligaments, which contain muscular tissue. **masseter m.,** musculus masseter. **m's of mastication, masticatory m's,** a group of muscles responsible for movement of the jaws during the process of mastication, including the masseter, temporal and medial and lateral pterygoid muscles. **Merkel's m.,** musculus ceratocricoideus. **mesothenar m.,** musculus adductor pollicis. **Müller's m.,** 1. fibrae circulares musculi ciliaris. 2. musculus orbitalis. **multifidus m's,** musculi multifidi. **multipennate m.,** musculus multipennatus. **mylohyoid m.,** musculus mylohyoideus. **mylopharyngeal m.,** pars mylopharyngea musculi constrictoris pharyngis superioris. **nasal m.,** musculus nasalis. **m's of neck,** musculi colli. **nonstriated m.,** a type of muscle without transverse striations upon its constituent fibers; such muscles are almost always involuntary. Called also *smooth m.* **oblique m. of abdomen, external,** musculus obliquus externus abdominis. **oblique m. of abdomen, internal,** musculus obliquus internus abdominis. **oblique m. of auricle,** musculus obliquus auriculae. **oblique m. of eyeball, inferior,** musculus obliquus inferior bulbi. **oblique m. of eyeball, superior,** musculus obliquus superior bulbi. **obturator m., external,** musculus obturatorius externus. **obturator m., internal,** musculus obturatorius internus. **occipital m.,** venter occipitalis musculi occipitofrontalis. **occipitofrontal m.,** musculus occipitofrontalis. **Ochsner's m.,** an inconstant muscular thickening of the duodenal muscle just distal to the opening of the common bile duct. **ocular m's, oculorotatory m's,** musculi bulbi. **Oddi's m.,** musculus sphincter ductus choledochi, or the combination of this with musculus sphincter ampullae hepatopancreaticae when the ampulla is present. **omohyoid m.,** musculus omohyoideus. **opposing m. of little finger,** musculus opponens digiti minimi. **opposing m. of thumb,** musculus opponens pollicis. **orbicular m.,** a muscle that encircles a body opening, such as the eye or mouth; called also *musculus orbicularis* [NA]. **orbicular m. of eye,** musculus orbicularis oculi. **orbicular m. of mouth,** musculus orbicularis oris. **orbital m.,** musculus orbitalis. **organic m.,** visceral m. **m's of palate and fauces,** musculi palati et faucium. **palatine m's,** musculi palati. **palatoglossus m.,** musculus palatoglossus. **palatopharyngeal m.,** musculus palatopharyngeus. **palmar m., long,** musculus palmaris longus. **palmar m., short,** musculus palmaris brevis. **papillary m's,** musculi papillares. **papillary m. of left ventricle, anterior,** musculus papillaris anterior ventriculi sinistri. **papillary m. of left ventricle, posterior,** musculus papillaris posterior ventriculi sinistri. **papillary m. of right ventricle, anterior,** musculus papillaris anterior ventriculi dextri. **papillary m. of right ventricle, posterior,** musculus papillaris posterior ventriculi dextri. **papillary m's of right ventricle, septal,** musculi papillares septales ventriculi dextri. **pectinate m's,** musculi pectinati. **pectineal m.,** musculus pectineus. **pectoral m., greater,** musculus pectoralis major. **pectoral m., smaller,** musculus pectoralis minor. **m's of pelvic diaphragm,** musculi diaphragmatis pelvis. **penniform m.,** musculus unipennatus. **perineal m's, m's of perineum,** musculi perinei. **peroneal m., long,** musculus peroneus longus. **peroneal m., short,** musculus peroneus brevis. **peroneal m., third,** musculus peroneus tertius. **pharyngopalatine m.,** musculus palatopharyngeus. **Phillips' m.,** a muscular slip from the radial collateral ligament of the wrist and the styloid process of the radius to the phalanges. **piriform m.,** musculus piriformis. **plantar m.,** musculus plantaris. **platysma m.,** see *platysma.* **pleuroesophageal m.,** musculus pleuroesophageus. **popliteal m.,** musculus

popliteus. **postaxial m.,** a muscle on the dorsal side of a limb. **preaxial m.,** a muscle on the ventral side of a limb. **procerus m.,** musculus procerus. **pronator m., quadrate,** musculus pronator quadratus. **pronator m., round,** musculus pronator teres. **psoas m., greater,** musculus psoas major. **psoas m., smaller,** musculus psoas minor. **pterygoid m., external,** musculus pterygoideus lateralis. **pterygoid m., internal,** musculus pterygoideus medialis. **pterygoid m., lateral,** musculus pterygoideus lateralis. **pterygoid m., medial,** musculus pterygoideus medialis. **pterygopharyngeal m.,** pars pterygopharyngea musculi constrictoris pharyngis superioris. **pubicoperitoneal m.,** ligamentum interfoveolare. **pubococcygeal m.,** musculus pubococcygeus. **puboprostatic m.,** musculus puboprostaticus. **puborectal m.,** musculus puborectalis. **pubovaginal m.,** musculus pubovaginalis. **pubovesical m.,** musculus pubovesicalis. **pyloric sphincter m.,** musculus sphincter pyloricus. **pyramidal m.,** musculus pyramidalis. **pyramidal m. of auricle,** musculus pyramidalis auriculae. **quadrate m.,** musculus quadratus. **quadrate m. of lower lip,** musculus depressor labii inferioris. **quadrate m. of sole,** musculus quadratus plantae. **quadrate m. of thigh,** musculus quadratus femoris. **quadrate m. of upper lip,** musculus levator labii superioris. **quadriceps m. of thigh,** musculus quadriceps femoris. **rectococcygeus m.,** musculus rectococcygeus. **rectourethral m.,** musculus rectourethralis. **rectouterine m.,** musculus rectouterinus. **rectovesical m.,** musculus rectovesicalis. **red m.,** the darker-colored muscle tissue of some mammals, composed of small dark fibers rich in mitochondria, myoglobin, and sarcoplasm but with only faint cross-striping; red muscle is designed for slow but repetitive contraction for long periods of time. Called also *slow,* or *tonic, m.* Cf. *white m.* **Reisseisen's m's,** the smooth muscle fibers of the smallest bronchi. **rhomboid m., greater,** musculus rhomboideus major. **rhomboid m., lesser,** musculus rhomboideus minor. **ribbon m's,** musculi infrahyoidei. **rider's m's,** the adductor muscles of the thigh. **Riolan's m.,** 1. ciliary bundle of pars palpebralis musculi orbicularis oculi. 2. musculus cremaster. **risorius m.,** musculus risorius. **rotator m's,** musculi rotatores. **rotator m's, long,** musculi rotatores longi. **rotator m's, short,** musculi rotatores breves. **rotator m's of neck,** musculi rotatores cervicis. **rotator m's of thorax,** musculi rotatores thoracis. **Rouget's m.,** the circular portion of the ciliary muscle. **Ruysch's m.,** the muscular tissue of the fundus uteri. **sacrococcygeal m., anterior,** musculus sacrococcygeus ventralis. **sacrococcygeal m., dorsal,** musculus sacrococcygeus dorsalis. **sacrococcygeal m., posterior,** musculus sacrococcygeus dorsalis. **sacrococcygeal m., ventral,** musculus sacrococcygeus ventralis. **sacrospinal m.,** musculus erector spinae. **salpingopharyngeal m.,** musculus salpingopharyngeus. **Santorini's m.,** musculus risorius. **Santorini's m's, circular,** the nonstriated fibers that encircle the urethra beneath the sphincter urethrae. **sartorius m.,** musculus sartorius. **scalene m., anterior,** musculus scalenus anterior. **scalene m., middle,** musculus scalenus medius. **scalene m., posterior,** musculus scalenus posterior. **scalene m., smallest,** musculus scalenus minimus. **semimembranous m.,** musculus semimembranosus. **semispinal m.,** musculus semispinalis. **semispinal m. of head,** musculus semispinalis capitis. **semispinal m. of neck,** musculus semispinalis cervicis. **semispinal m. of thorax,** musculus semispinalis thoracis. **semitendinous m.,** musculus semitendinosus. **serratus m., anterior,** musculus serratus anterior. **serratus m., posterior, inferior,** musculus serratus posterior inferior. **serratus m., posterior, superior,** musculus serratus posterior superior. **skeletal m's,** striated muscles that are attached to bones and typically cross at least one joint; called also *musculi skeleti.* **slow m.,** red m. **smooth m.,** nonstriated, involuntary muscle. **soleus m.,** musculus soleus. **somatic m's,** musculi skeleti. **sphincter m.,** musculus sphincter. **sphincter m. of anus, external,** musculus sphincter ani externus. **sphincter m. of anus, internal,** musculus sphincter ani internus. **sphincter m. of bile duct,** musculus sphincter ductus choledochi. **sphincter m. of hepatopancreatic ampulla,** musculus sphincter ampullae hepatopancreaticae. **sphincter m. of membranous ure-**

y
w

q

thra, musculus sphincter urethrae. **sphincter m. of pupil,** musculus sphincter pupillae. **sphincter m. of pylorus,** musculus sphincter pyloricus. **sphincter m. of urethra,** musculus sphincter urethrae. **sphincter m. of urinary bladder,** musculus sphincter vesicae urinariae. **spinal m.,** see *musculus spinalis.* **splenius m. of head,** musculus splenius capitis. **splenius m. of neck,** musculus splenius cervicis. **stapedius m.,** musculus stapedius. **sternal m.,** musculus sternalis. **sternocleidomastoid m.,** musculus sternocleidomastoideus. **sternohyoid m.,** musculus sternohyoideus. **sternomastoid m.,** musculus sternocleidomastoideus. **sternothyroid m.,** musculus sternothyroideus. **strap m's,** muscles of the neck, particularly those of the thyroid cartilage and hyoid bone. **striated m., striped m.,** any muscle whose fibers are divided by transverse bands into striations; such muscles are voluntary. See *muscle.* **styloglossus m.,** musculus styloglossus. **stylohyoid m.,** musculus stylohyoideus. **stylopharyngeus m.,** musculus stylopharyngeus. **subclavius m.,** musculus subclavius. **subcostal m's,** musculi subcostales. **suboccipital m's,** musculi suboccipitales. **subscapular m.,** musculus subscapularis. **subvertebral m's,** hypaxial m's. **supinator m.,** musculus supinator. **suprahyoid m's,** musculi suprahyoidei. **supraspinous m.,** musculus supraspinatus. **suspensory m. of duodenum,** musculus suspensorius duodeni. **synergic m's, synergistic m's,** muscles that assist one another in action. **tarsal m., inferior,** musculus tarsalis inferior. **tarsal m., superior,** musculus tarsalis superior. **temporal m.,** musculus temporalis. **temporoparietal m.,** musculus temporoparietalis. **tensor m. of fascia lata,** musculus tensor fasciae latae. **tensor m. of tympanic membrane, tensor m. of tympanum,** musculus tensor tympani. **tensor m. of velum palatini,** musculus tensor veli palatini. **teres major m.,** musculus teres major. **teres minor m.,** musculus teres minor. **thenar m's,** the abductor and flexor muscles of the thumb. **thyroarytenoid m.,** musculus thyroarytenoideus. **thyroepiglottic m.,** musculus thyro-epiglotticus. **thyrohyoid m.,** musculus thyrohyoideus. **thyropharyngeal m.,** pars thyropharyngea musculi constrictoris pharyngis inferioris. **tibial m., anterior,** musculus tibialis anterior. **tibial m., posterior,** musculus tibialis posterior. **m's of tongue,** musculi linguae. **tonic m.,** red m. **tracheal m.,** musculus trachealis. **trachelomastoid m.,** musculus longissimus capitis. **m. of tragus,** musculus tragicus. **transverse m. of abdomen,** musculus transversus abdominis. **transverse m. of auricle,** musculus transversus auriculae. **transverse m. of chin,** musculus transversus menti. **transverse m. of nape,** musculus transversus nuchae. **transverse m. of perineum, deep,** musculus transversus perinei profundus. **transverse m. of perineum, superficial,** musculus transversus perinei superficialis. **transverse m. of thorax,** musculus transversus thoracis. **transverse m. of tongue,** musculus transversus linguae. **transversospinal m.,** musculus transversospinalis. **trapezius m.,** musculus trapezius. **m. of Treitz,** musculus suspensorius duodeni. **triangular m.,** musculus triangularis. **triceps m. of arm,** musculus triceps brachii. **triceps m. of calf,** musculus triceps surae. **twitch m.,** white m. **unipennate m.,** musculus unipennatus. **unstriated m.,** nonstriated m. **m's of urogenital diaphragm,** musculi diaphragmatis urogenitalis. **m. of uvula,** musculus uvulae. **vertical m. of tongue,** musculus verticalis linguae. **vestigial m.,** a muscle that was once well developed but through evolution has become rudimentary. **visceral m.,** muscle fibers associated chiefly with the hollow viscera and largely of splanchnic mesodermal origin; except for the striated fibers in the wall of the heart, they are smooth-muscle fibers bound together by reticular fibers. **vocal m.,** musculus vocalis. **voluntary m.,** any muscle that normally is under the control of the will; such muscles are nearly always composed of striated fibers. **white m.,** the paler-colored muscle tissue of some mammals, composed of fibers with little sarcoplasm and prominent cross-striping and which are paler and of larger diameter than the fibers of red muscle. Called also *fast,* or *twitch, m.* Cf. *red m.* **Wilson's m.,** musculus sphincter urethrae. **yoked m's,** muscles that normally act simultaneously and equally, as in moving the eyes. **zygomatic m., zygomatic m., greater,** musculus zygomaticus major. **zygomatic m., lesser,** musculus zygomaticus minor.

muscle phosphorylase (mus'el fos-for'ĭ-lās) muscle isozyme of glycogen phosphorylase.

musculamine (mus''ku-lam'in) a base isolated from hydrolyzed calf's muscle; it is the same as spermine.

muscular (mus'ku-lar) [L. *muscularis*] 1. pertaining to or composing muscle. 2. having a well-developed musculature.

muscularis (mus''ku-la'ris) [L.] relating to muscles, specifically a muscular coat; see *tunica muscularis.*

muscularity (mus''ku-lar'ĭ-te) the condition or quality of being muscular.

muscularize (mus'ku-lar-īz) to change into muscle tissue.

musculature (mus'ku-lah-chur) the muscular apparatus of the body, or of any part of it.

musculi (mus'ku-li) [L.] genitive and plural of *musculus.*

musculoaponeurotic (mus''ku-lo-ap''o-nu-rot'ik) pertaining to a muscle and its aponeurosis.

musculocutaneous (mus''ku-lo-ku-ta'ne-us) pertaining to or supplying both muscles and skin. Called also *musculodermic.*

musculodermic (mus''ku-lo-der'mik) musculocutaneous.

musculoelastic (mus''ku-lo-e-las'tik) composed of muscular and elastic tissue.

musculointestinal (mus''ku-lo-in-tes'tĭ-nal) pertaining to the muscles and the intestines.

musculomembranous (mus''ku-lo-mem'brah-nus) [L. *musculus* muscle + *membrana* membrane] both muscular and membranous.

Musculomyces (mus''ku-lo-mi'sēz) in former systems of classification, a genus of bacteria made up of organisms now classified as *Mycoplasma.*

musculophrenic (mus''ku-lo-fren'ik) [*muscular + phrenic*] pertaining to or supplying both the diaphragm and the adjoining muscles.

musculoskeletal (mus''ku-lo-skel'ĕ-tal) pertaining to or comprising the skeleton and the muscles, as musculoskeletal system.

musculospiral (mus''ku-lo-spi'ral) [L. *musculus* muscle + *spira* coil] pertaining to muscles and having a spiral direction, as the nervus radialis.

musculospiralis (mus''ku-lo-spi-ra'lis) nervus radialis.

musculotendinous (mus''ku-lo-ten'dĭ-nus) pertaining to or composed of muscle and tendon.

musculotonic (mus''ku-lo-ton'ik) pertaining to muscular contractility.

musculotropic (mus''ku-lo-trop'ik) having a special affinity for or exerting its principal effect upon muscular tissue.

musculus (mus'ku-lus), gen. and pl. *mus'culi* [L., dim. of *mus* mouse, because of a fancied resemblance to a mouse of a muscle moving under the skin] [NA] an organ which by its contraction and relaxation produces movements of certain organs or of the entire animal organism. See *muscle.* For names and description of specific muscles see *Table of Musculi.*

TABLE OF MUSCULI

Descriptions of muscles are given on NA terms, and include anglicized names of specific muscles.

mus'culi abdo'minis [NA], the muscles of the abdomen. **m. abduc'tor dig'iti min'imi ma'nus** [NA], abductor muscle of little finger: *origin,* pisiform bone, flexor carpi ulnaris tendon; *insertion,* medial surface of base of proximal phalanx of little finger; *innervation,* ulnar; *action,* abducts little finger. **m. abduc'tor dig'iti min'imi pe'dis** [NA], abductor muscle of little toe: *origin*, medial and lateral tubercles of calcaneus, plantar fascia; *insertion*, lateral surface of base of proximal phalanx of little toe; *innervation*, superficial branch of lateral plantar; *action*, abducts little toe.

m. abduc′tor dig′iti quin′ti ma′nus, m. abductor digiti minimi manus.

m. abduc′tor dig′iti quin′ti pe′dis, m. abductor digiti minimi pedis.

m. abduc′tor hal′lucis [NA], abductor muscle of great toe: *origin*, medial tubercle of calcaneus, plantar fascia; *insertion*, medial surface of base of proximal phalanx of great toe; *innervation*, medial plantar; *action*, abducts, flexes great toe.

m. abduc′tor pol′licis bre′vis [NA], short abductor muscle of thumb: *origin*, scaphoid, ridge of trapezium, transverse carpal ligament; *insertion*, lateral surface of base of proximal phalanx of thumb; *innervation*, median; *action*, abducts thumb.

m. abduc′tor pol′licis lon′gus [NA], long abductor muscle of thumb: *origin*, posterior surfaces of radius and ulna; *insertion*, radial side of base of first metacarpal bone; *innervation*, posterior interosseous; *action*, abducts, extends thumb.

m. adduc′tor bre′vis [NA], short adductor muscle: *origin*, outer surface of inferior ramus of pubis; *insertion*, upper part of linea aspera of femur; *innervation*, obturator; *action*, adducts, rotates, flexes thigh.

m. adduc′tor hal′lucis [NA], adductor muscle of great toe (2 heads): *origin*, CAPUT OBLIQUUM—bases of second, third, and fourth metatarsals, and sheath of peroneus longus, CAPUT TRANSVERSUM— capsules of metatarsophalangeal joints of three lateral toes; *insertion*, lateral side of base of proximal phalanx of great toe; *innervation*, lateral plantar; *action*, adducts great toe.

m. adduc′tor lon′gus [NA], long adductor muscle: *origin*, crest and symphysis of pubis; *insertion*, linea aspera of femur; *innervation*, obturator; *action*, adducts, rotates, flexes thigh.

m. adduc′tor mag′nus [NA], great adductor muscle (2 parts): *origin*, DEEP PART—inferior ramus of pubis, ramus of ischium, SUPERFICIAL PART—ischial tuberosity; *insertion*, DEEP PART—linea aspera of femur, SUPERFICIAL PART—adductor tubercle of femur; *innervation*, DEEP PART—obturator, SUPERFICIAL PART—sciatic; *action*, DEEP PART—adducts thigh, SUPERFICIAL PART—extends thigh.

m. adduc′tor min′imus, smallest adductor muscle: a name given the anterior portion of the adductor magnus muscle; *insertion*, ischium, body and ramus of pubis; *innervation*, obturator and sciatic; *action*, adducts thigh.

m. adduc′tor pol′licis [NA], adductor muscle of thumb (2 heads): *origin*, CAPUT OBLIQUUM—sheath of flexor carpi radialis, anterior carpal ligament, capitate bone, and bases of second and third metacarpals, CAPUT TRANSVERSUM—lower two-thirds of anterior surface of third metacarpal; *insertion*, medial surface of base of proximal phalanx of thumb; *innervation*, ulnar; *action*, adducts, opposes thumb.

m. ancone′us [NA], anconeus muscle: *origin*, back of lateral epicondyle of humerus; *insertion*, olecranon and posterior surface of ulna; *innervation*, radial; *action*, extends forearm.

m. antitrag′icus [NA], antitragus muscle: *origin*, outer part of antitragus; *insertion*, caudate process of helix and anthelix; *innervation*, temporal and posterior auricular.

mus′culi arrecto′res pilo′rum [NA], arrector muscles of hair: *origin*, papillary layer of skin; *insertion*, hair follicles; *innervation*, sympathetic; *action*, elevate hairs of skin.

m. articula′ris [NA], articular muscle: a muscle that is attached at one end to the synovial capsule of a joint.

m. articula′ris cu′biti [NA], articular muscle of elbow: a few fibers of the deep surface of the triceps brachii that insert into the posterior ligament and synovial membrane of the elbow joint.

m. articula′ris ge′nu, m. articularis genus.

m. articula′ris ge′nus [NA], articular muscle of knee: *origin*, distal fourth of anterior surface of shaft of femur; *insertion*, synovial membrane of knee joint; *innervation*, femoral; *action*, lifts capsule of knee joint.

m. aryepiglot′ticus [NA], aryepiglottic muscle: a name given to an inconstant fascicle of the oblique arytenoid muscle, originating from the apex of the arytenoid cartilage and inserting on the lateral margin of the epiglottis.

m. arytaenoi′deus obli′quus, m. arytenoideus obliquus.

m. arytaenoi′deus transver′sus, m. arytenoideus transversus.

m. arytenoi′deus obli′quus [NA], oblique arytenoid muscle: *origin*, dorsal aspect of muscular process of arytenoid cartilage; *insertion*, apex of opposite arytenoid cartilage; *innervation*, recurrent laryngeal; *action*, closes inlet of larynx.

m. arytenoi′deus transver′sus [NA], transverse arytenoid muscle: *origin*, dorsal aspect of muscular process of arytenoid cartilage; *insertion*, continuous with thyroarytenoid, apex of opposite cartilage; *innervation*, recurrent laryngeal; *action*, approximates arytenoid cartilages.

m. auricula′ris ante′rior [NA], anterior auricular muscle: *origin*, superficial temporal fascia; *insertion*, cartilage of ear; *innervation*, facial; *action*, draws the auricle forward.

m. auricula′ris poste′rior [NA], posterior auricular muscle: *origin*, mastoid process; *insertion*, cartilage of ear; *innervation*, facial; *action*, draws auricle backward.

m. auricula′ris supe′rior [NA], superior auricular muscle: *origin*, galea aponeurotica; *insertion*, cartilage of ear; *innervation*, facial; *action*, raises auricle.

mus′culi auricula′rii [NA], auricular muscles: the intrinsic auricular muscles that extend from one part of the auricle to another, including the helicis major and minor, tragicus, antitragus, transversus auriculae, and obliquus auriculae. See also *auricular muscles* (def. 1), under *muscle*.

m. bi′ceps bra′chii [NA], biceps muscle of arm (2 heads): *origin*, CAPUT LONGUM—upper border of glenoid cavity, CAPUT BREVE—apex of coracoid process; *insertion*, radial tuberosity and fascia of forearm; *innervation*, musculocutaneous; *action*, flexes forearm, supinates hand.

m. bi′ceps fem′oris [NA], biceps muscle of thigh (2 heads): *origin*, CAPUT LONGUM—ischial tuberosity, CAPUT BREVE—linea aspera of femur; *insertion*, head of fibula, lateral condyle of tibia; *innervation*, CAPUT LONGUM—tibial, CAPUT BREVE— peroneal, popliteal; *action*, flexes leg, extends thigh.

m. bipenna′tus [NA], bipennate muscle: a muscle in which the fibers approach the tendon of insertion from a wide area and are inserted through a large segment of its circumference.

m. brachia′lis [NA], brachial muscle: *origin*, anterior surface of humerus; *insertion*, coronoid process of ulna; *innervation*, radial, musculocutaneous; *action*, flexes forearm.

m. brachioradia′lis [NA], brachioradial muscle: *origin*, lateral supracondylar ridge of humerus; *insertion*, lower end of radius; *innervation*, radial; *action*, flexes forearm.

m. bronchoesopha′geus [NA], bronchoesophageal muscle: a name given muscular fasciculi arising from the wall of the left bronchus, reinforcing muscles of the esophagus.

m. bronchooesopha′geus, m. bronchoesophageus.

m. buccina′tor [NA], buccinator muscle: *origin*, buccinator ridge of mandible, alveolar process of maxilla, pterygomandibular ligament; *insertion*, orbicularis oris at angle of mouth; *innervation*, buccal branch of facial; *action*, compresses cheek and retracts angle of the mouth.

m. buccopharyn′geus, pars buccopharyngea musculi constrictoris pharyngis superioris.

mus′culi bul′bi [NA], extraocular muscles: the six voluntary muscles that move the eyeball, including the superior, inferior, middle, and lateral recti, and the superior and inferior oblique muscles.

m. bulbocaverno′sus, m. bulbospongiosus.

m. bulbospongio′sus [NA], bulbocavernous muscle: *origin*, central point of perineum, median raphe of bulb; *insertion*, fascia of penis (clitoris); *innervation*, pudendal; *action*, constricts bulbous urethra (urethra).

m. cani′nus, m. levator anguli oris.

mus′culi cap′itis [NA], the muscles of the head.

m. ceratocricoi′deus [NA], ceratocricoid muscle: a name given a muscular fasciculus arising from the cricoid cartilage and inserted on the inferior cornu of the thyroid cartilage.

m. ceratopharyn′geus, pars ceratopharyngea musculi constrictoris pharyngis medii.

m. chondroglos′sus [NA], chondroglossus muscle: *origin*, medial side and base of lesser cornu of hyoid bone; *insertion*, substance of tongue; *innervation*, hypoglossal; *action*, depresses, retracts tongue.

m. chondropharyn′geus, pars chondropharyngea musculi constrictoris pharyngis medii.

m. cilia′ris [NA], ciliary muscle: *origin*, scleral spur; *insertion*, outer layers of choroid and ciliary processes; *innervation*, oculomotor, parasympathetic; *action*, affects shape of lens in visual accommodation.

mus′culi coccy′gei, coccygeal muscles: the muscles acting upon the coccyx, including the coccygeal and the dorsal and ventral sacrococcygeal muscles.

m. coccyg′eus [NA], coccygeal muscle: *origin*, ischial spine; *insertion*, lateral border of lower part of sacrum, upper coccyx; *innervation*, third and fourth sacral; *action*, supports and raises coccyx.

mus′culi col′li [NA], the muscles of the neck, including the sternocleidomastoid and the longus colli, and the suprahyoid, infrahyoid, and scalene muscles.

m. compres′sor na′ris, pars transversa musculi nasalis.

m. constric′tor pharyn′gis infe′rior [NA], inferior constrictor muscle of pharynx: *origin*, under surfaces of cricoid and thyroid cartilages; *insertion*, median raphe of posterior wall of pharynx; *innervation*, glossopharyngeal, pharyngeal plexus, and external and recurrent laryngeal; *action*, constricts pharynx.

m. constric′tor pharyn′gis me′dius [NA], middle constrictor muscle of pharynx: *origin*, cornua of hyoid and stylohyoid ligament; *insertion*, median raphe of posterior wall of pharynx; *innervation*, pharyngeal plexus of vagus and glossopharyngeal; *action*, constricts pharynx.

m. constric′tor pharyn′gis supe′rior [NA], superior constrictor muscle of pharynx: *origin*, medial pterygoid plate, pterygomandibular raphe, mylohyoid ridge of mandible, and mucous membrane of floor of mouth; *insertion*, median raphe of posterior wall of pharynx; *innervation*, pharyngeal plexus of vagus; *action*, constricts pharynx.

m. coracobrachia′lis [NA], coracobrachial muscle: *origin*, coracoid process of scapula; *insertion*, medial surface of shaft of humerus; *innervation*, musculocutaneous; *action*, flexes, adducts arm.

m. corruga′tor supercil′ii [NA], *origin*, medial end of superciliary arch; *insertion*, skin of eyebrow; *innervation*, facial; *action*, draws eyebrow downward and medially.

m. cremas′ter [NA], cremaster muscle: *origin*, inferior margin of internal oblique muscle of abdomen; *insertion*, pubic tubercle; *innervation*, genital branch of genitofemoral; *action*, elevates testis.

m. cricoarytaenoi′deus latera′lis, m. cricoarytenoideus lateralis.

m. cricoarytaenoi′deus poste′rior, m. cricoarytenoideus posterior.

m. cricoarytenoi′deus latera′lis [NA], lateral cricoarytenoid muscle: *origin*, lateral surface of cricoid cartilage; *insertion*, muscular process of arytenoid cartilage; *innervation*, recurrent laryngeal; *action*, approximates vocal folds.

m. cricoarytenoi′deus poste′rior [NA], posterior cricoarytenoid muscle: *origin*, back of cricoid cartilage; *insertion*, muscular process of arytenoid cartilage; *innervation*, recurrent laryngeal; *action*, separates vocal folds.

m. cricopharyn′geus, pars cricopharyngea musculi constrictoris pharyngis inferioris.

m. cricothyreoi′deus, m. cricothyroideus.

m. cricothyroi′deus [NA], cricothyroid muscle: *origin*, front and side of cricoid cartilage; *insertion*, lamina of thyroid cartilage; *innervation*, superior laryngeal; *action*, tenses vocal folds.

m. crucia′tus [NA], cruciate muscle: a muscle in which the fiber bundles are arranged in the shape of an X.

m. cuta′neus [NA], cutaneous muscle: striated muscle that inserts into the skin.

m. dar′tos [NA], dartos muscle: the nonstriated muscle fibers of the tunica dartos, the deeper layers of which help to form the septum of the scrotum. Called also *dartos* and *dartos muscle.* 2. tunica dartos.

m. deltoi′deus [NA], deltoid muscle: *origin*, clavicle, acromion, spine of scapula; *insertion*, deltoid tuberosity of humerus; *innervation*, axillary; *action*, abducts, flexes, extends arm.

m. depres′sor an′guli o′ris [NA], depressor muscle of angle of mouth: *origin*, lower border of mandible; *insertion*, angle of mouth; *innervation*, facial; *action*, pulls down angle of mouth.

m. depres′sor la′bii inferio′ris [NA], depressor muscle of lower lip: *origin*, anterior portion of lower border of mandible; *insertion*, orbicularis oris and skin of lower lip; *innervation*, facial; *action*, depresses lower lip.

m. depres′sor sep′ti na′si [NA], depressor muscle of nasal septum: *origin*, incisor fossa of maxilla; *insertion*, ala and septum of nose; *innervation*, facial; *action*, contracts nostril and depresses ala.

m. depres′sor supercil′ii [NA], superciliary depressor muscle: a name given a few fibers of the orbital part of the orbicularis oculi muscle that are inserted in the eyebrow, which they depress.

m. detru′sor ve′sicae [NA], detrusor muscle of bladder: the bundles of smooth muscle fibers forming the muscular coat of the urinary bladder, which are arranged in a longitudinal and a circular layer and, on contraction, serve to expel urine; called also *detrusor urinae* and *detrusor urinae muscle.*

musculi diaphrag′matis pel′vis [NA], the muscles of the pelvic diaphragm.

mus′culi diaphrag′matis urogenita′lis [NA], the muscles of the urogenital diaphragm.

m. digas′tricus [NA], digastric muscle: *origin*, VENTER ANTERIOR—digastric fossa on deep surface of lower border of mandible near symphysis, VENTER POSTERIOR—mastoid notch of temporal bone; *insertion*, intermediate tendon on hyoid bone; *innervation*, VENTER ANTERIOR—mylohyoid, VENTER POSTERIOR—digastric branch of facial; *action*, elevates hyoid bone, lowers jaw.

m. dila′tor na′ris, pars alaris musculi nasalis.

m. dila′tor pupil′lae [NA], dilator muscle of pupil: a name given fibers extending radially from the sphincter pupillae to the ciliary margin; *innervation*, sympathetic; *action*, dilates iris.

mus′culi dor′si [NA], dorsal muscles: the muscles of the back.

m. epicra′nius [NA], epicranial muscle: a name given the muscular covering of the scalp, including the occipitofrontalis and temporoparietalis muscles, and the galea aponeurotica.

m. epitrochleoanconae′us, epitrochleoanconeus muscle: an occasional band of fibers originating at the back of the medial condyle of the humerus and inserting on the medial side of the olecranon process, innervated by a branch of the ulnar nerve.

m. erec′tor spi′nae [NA], erector muscle of spine: a name given the fibers of the more superficial of the deep muscles of the back, originating from the sacrum, spines of the lumbar and the eleventh and twelfth thoracic vertebrae, and the iliac crest, which split and insert as the iliocostalis, longissimus, and spinalis muscles (q.v.).

m. exten′sor car′pi radia′lis bre′vis [NA], short radial extensor muscle of wrist: *origin*, lateral epicondyle of humerus, *insertion*, base of third metacarpal bone; *innervation*, radial; *action*, extends and abducts wrist joint.

m. exten′sor car′pi radia′lis lon′gus [NA], long radial extensor muscle of wrist: *origin*, lateral supracondylar ridge of humerus; *insertion*, base of second metacarpal bone; *innervation*, radial; *action*, extends and abducts wrist joint.

m. exten′sor car′pi ulna′ris [NA], ulnar extensor muscle of wrist (2 heads): *origin*, CAPUT HUMERALE—lateral epicondyle of humerus, CAPUT ULNARE—dorsal border of ulna; *insertion*, base of fifth metacarpal bone; *innervation*, deep radial; *action*, extends and adducts wrist joint.

m. exten′sor dig′iti min′imi [NA], extensor muscle of little finger: *origin*, common extensor tendon; *insertion*, tendon of extensor digitorum to little finger; *innervation*, deep radial; *action*, extends little finger.

m. exten′sor dig′iti quin′ti pro′prius, m. extensor digiti minimi.

m. exten′sor digito′rum [NA], extensor muscle of fingers: *origin*, lateral epicondyle of humerus; *insertion*, common extensor tendon of each finger; *innervation*, deep radial; *action*, extends wrist joint and phalanges.

m. exten′sor digito′rum bre′vis [NA], short extensor muscle of toes: *origin*, dorsal surface of calcaneus; *insertion*, extensor tendons of first, second, third, fourth toes; *innervation*, deep peroneal; *action*, extends toes.

m. exten′sor digito′rum commu′nis, m. extensor digitorum.

m. exten′sor digito′rum lon′gus [NA], long extensor muscle of toes: *origin*, anterior surface of fibula, lateral condyle of tibia, interosseous membrane; *insertion*, common extensor tendon of four lateral toes: *innervation*, deep peroneal; *action*, extends toes.

m. exten′sor hal′lucis bre′vis [NA], short extensor muscle of great toe: a name given the portion of the extensor digitorum brevis muscle that goes to the great toe.

m. exten′sor hal′lucis lon′gus [NA], long extensor muscle of great toe: *origin*, front of fibula and interosseous membrane; *insertion*, dorsal surface of base of distal phalanx of great toe; *innervation*, deep peroneal; *action*, dorsiflexes ankle joint, extends great toe.

m. exten′sor in′dicis [NA], extensor muscle of index finger: *origin*, dorsal surface of body of ulna, interosseous membrane; *insertion*, common extensor tendon of index finger; *innervation*, deep radial; *action*, extends index finger.

m. exten'sor in'dicis pro'prius, m. extensor indicis.

m. exten'sor pol'licis bre'vis [NA], short extensor muscle of thumb: *origin,* dorsal surface of radius and interosseous membrane; *insertion,* dorsal surface of proximal phalanx of thumb; *innervation,* deep radial; *action,* extends thumb.

m. exten'sor pol'licis lon'gus [NA], long extensor muscle of thumb: *origin,* dorsal surface of ulna and interosseous membrane; *insertion,* dorsal surface of distal phalanx of thumb; *innervation,* deep radial; *action,* extends, abducts thumb.

mus'culi extremita'tis inferio'ris, musculi membri inferioris.

mus'culi extremita'tis superio'ris, musculi membri superioris.

musculi facia'les et masticato'res [NA], facial and masticatory muscles: the fascial muscles (muscles of facial expression) and the muscles of mastication considered together.

m. fibula'ris bre'vis, NA alternative for *m. peroneus brevis.*

m. fibula'ris lon'gus, NA alternative for *m. peroneus longus.*

m. fibula'ris ter'tius, NA alternative for *m. peroneus tertius.*

m. fixa'tor ba'seos stape'dis, fixator muscle of base of stapes: fibers attaching to the base of the stapes.

m. flex'or accesso'rius, NA alternative for *m. quadratus plantae.*

m. flex'or car'pi radia'lis [NA], radial flexor muscle of wrist: *origin,* medial epicondyle of humerus; *insertion,* base of second metacarpal; *innervation,* median; *action,* flexes and abducts wrist joint.

m. flex'or car'pi ulna'ris [NA], ulnar flexor muscle of wrist (2 heads): *origin,* CAPUT HUMERALE—medial epicondyle of humerus, CAPUT ULNARE—olecranon, ulna, intermuscular septum; *insertion,* pisiform, hook of hamate, proximal end of fifth metacarpal; *innervation,* ulnar; *action,* flexes and adducts wrist joint.

m. flex'or dig'iti min'imi bre'vis ma'nus [NA], short flexor muscle of little finger: *origin,* hook of hamate bone, transverse carpal ligament; *insertion,* medial side of proximal phalanx of little finger; *innervation,* ulnar; *action,* flexes little finger.

m. flex'or dig'iti min'imi bre'vis pe'dis [NA], short flexor muscle of little toe: *origin,* base of fifth metatarsal, plantar fascia; *insertion,* lateral surface of base of proximal phalanx of little toe; *innervation,* lateral plantar; *action,* flexes little toe.

m. flex'or dig'iti quin'ti bre'vis ma'nus, m. flexor digiti minimi brevis manus.

m. flex'or dig'iti quin'ti bre'vis pe'dis, m. flexor digiti minimi brevis pedis.

m. flex'or digito'rum bre'vis [NA], short flexor muscle of toes: *origin,* medial tuberosity of calcaneus, plantar fascia; *insertion,* middle phalanges of four lateral toes; *innervation,* medial plantar; *action,* flexes toes.

m. flex'or digito'rum lon'gus [NA], long flexor muscle of toes: *origin,* posterior surface of shaft of tibia; *insertion,* distal phalanges of four lateral toes; *innervation,* posterior tibial; *action,* flexes toes and extends foot.

m. flex'or digito'rum profun'dus [NA], deep flexor muscle of fingers: *origin,* shaft of ulna, coronoid process; *insertion,* distal phalanges of fingers; *innervation,* ulnar and anterior interosseous; *action,* flexes distal phalanges.

m. flex'or digito'rum subli'mis, m. flexor digitorum superficialis.

m. flex'or digito'rum superficia'lis [NA], superficial flexor muscle of fingers (2 heads): *origin,* CAPUT HUMEROULNARE—medial epicondyle of humerus, coronoid process of ulna, CAPUT RADIALE— oblique line of radius, anterior border; *insertion,* middle phalanges of fingers; *innervation,* median; *action,* flexes middle phalanges.

m. flex'or hal'lucis bre'vis [NA], short flexor muscle of great toe: *origin,* under surface of cuboid, lateral cuneiform; *insertion,* base of proximal phalanx of great toe; *innervation,* lateral and medial plantar; *action,* flexes great toe.

m. flex'or hal'lucis lon'gus [NA], long flexor muscle of great toe: *origin,* posterior surface of fibula; *insertion,* base of distal phalanx of great toe; *innervation,* posterior tibial; *action,* flexes great toe.

m. flex'or pol'licis bre'vis [NA], short flexor muscle of thumb: *origin,* transverse carpal ligament, ridge of trapezium; *insertion,* base of proximal phalanx of thumb; *innervation,* median, ulnar; *action,* flexes and adducts thumb.

m. flex'or pol'licis lon'gus [NA], long flexor muscle of thumb: *origin,* anterior surface of radius and coronoid process of ulna; *insertion,* base of distal phalanx of thumb; *innervation,* anterior interosseous; *action,* flexes thumb.

m. fronta'lis, venter frontalis musculi occipitofrontalis.

m. fusifor'mis [NA], fusiform muscle: a spindle-shaped muscle in which the fibers are approximately parallel to the long axis of the muscle but converge upon a tendon at either end.

m. gastrocne'mius [NA], gastrocnemius muscle (2 heads): *origin,* CAPUT MEDIALE—popliteal surface of femur, upper part of medial condyle, and capsule of knee, CAPUT LATERALE—lateral condyle and capsule of knee; *insertion,* aponeurosis unites with tendon of soleus to form calcaneal tendon (Achilles tendon); *innervation,* tibial; *action,* plantar flexes ankle joint, flexes knee joint.

m. gemel'lus infe'rior [NA], inferior gemellus muscle: *origin,* tuberosity of ischium; *insertion,* greater trochanter of femur; *innervation,* sacral plexus; *action,* rotates thigh laterally.

m. gemel'lus supe'rior [NA], superior gemellus muscle: *origin,* spine of ischium; *insertion,* greater trochanter of femur; *innervation,* sacral plexus; *action,* rotates thigh laterally.

m. genioglos'sus [NA], genioglossus muscle: *origin,* mental spine of mandible; *insertion,* hyoid bone and under surface of tongue; *innervation,* hypoglossal; *action,* protrudes and depresses tongue.

m. geniohyoi'deus [NA], geniohyoid muscle: *origin,* mental spine of mandible; *insertion,* body of hyoid bone; *innervation,* a branch of first cervical nerve through hypoglossal; *action,* elevates, draws hyoid forward.

m. glossopalati'nus, m. palatoglossus.

m. glossopharyn'geus, pars glossopharyngea musculi constrictoris pharyngis superioris.

m. glu'teus max'imus [NA], greatest gluteal muscle: *origin,* lateral surface of ilium, dorsal surface of sacrum and coccyx, sacrotuberous ligament; *insertion,* iliotibial tract of fascia lata, gluteal tuberosity of femur; *innervation,* inferior gluteal; *action,* extends, abducts, and rotates thigh laterally.

m. glu'teus me'dius [NA], middle gluteal muscle: *origin,* lateral surface of ilium between anterior and posterior gluteal lines; *insertion,* greater trochanter of femur; *innervation,* superior gluteal; *action,* abducts thigh.

m. glu'teus min'imus [NA], least gluteal muscle: *origin,* lateral surface of ilium between anterior and inferior gluteal lines; *insertion,* greater trochanter of femur; *innervation,* superior gluteal; *action,* abducts, rotates thigh medially.

m. gra'cilis [NA], gracilis muscle: *origin,* inferior ramus of pubis; *insertion,* medial surface of shaft of tibia; *innervation,* obturator; *action,* adducts thigh, flexes knee joint.

m. hel'icis ma'jor [NA], *origin,* spine of helix; *insertion,* anterior border of helix; *innervation,* auriculotemporal and posterior auricular; *action,* tenses skin of auditory canal.

m. hel'icis mi'nor [NA], *origin,* anterior rim of helix; *insertion,* concha; *innervation,* temporal, posterior auricular.

m. hyoglos'sus [NA], hyoglossal muscle: *origin,* body and greater cornu of hyoid bone; *insertion,* side of tongue; *innervation,* hypoglossal; *action,* depresses and retracts tongue.

m. ili'acus [NA], iliac muscle: *origin,* iliac fossa and base of sacrum; *insertion,* lesser trochanter of femur; *innervation,* femoral; *action,* flexes thigh, trunk on limb.

m. iliococcyg'eus [NA], iliococcygeal muscle: a name given the posterior portion of the levator ani which originates as far forward as the obturator canal and inserts on the side of the coccyx and the anococcygeal body; *innervation,* third and fourth sacral; *action,* helps to support pelvic viscera and resist increases in intra-abdominal pressure.

m. iliocosta'lis [NA], iliocostal muscle: the lateral division of m. erector spinae, which includes the *m. iliocostalis cervicis, m. iliocostalis thoracis,* and *m. iliocostalis lumborum.*

m. iliocosta'lis cer'vicis [NA], iliocostal muscle of neck: *origin,* angles of third, fourth, fifth, and sixth ribs; *insertion,* transverse processes of fourth, fifth, and sixth cervical vertebrae; *innervation,* branches of cervical; *action,* extends cervical spine.

m. iliocosta'lis dor'si, m. iliocostalis thoracis.

m. iliocosta'lis lumbo'rum [NA], iliocostal muscle of loins: *origin,* iliac crest; *insertion,* angles of lower six or seven ribs; *innervation,* branches of thoracic and lumbar; *action,* extends lumbar spine.

m. iliocosta'lis thora'cis [NA], iliocostal muscle of thorax: *origin,* upper borders of angles of six lower ribs; *insertion,* angles of six upper ribs and transverse process of seventh cervical vertebra; *innervation,* branches of thoracic; *action,* keeps thoracic spine erect.

m. iliopso′as [NA], iliopsoas muscle: a compound muscle consisting of iliacus and psoas major.

mus′culi incisi′vi la′bii inferio′ris, incisive muscles of inferior lip: small bundles of muscle fibers, one arising from the incisive fossa of the mandible on each side and passing laterally to the angle of the mouth.

mus′culi incisi′vi la′bii superio′ris, incisive muscles of superior lip: small bundles of muscle fibers, one arising from the incisive fossa of the maxilla on each side and passing laterally to the angle of the mouth.

m. incisu′rae hel′icis [NA], an inconstant muscular slip continuing forward from the m. tragicus to bridge the incisure of the cartilaginous meatus.

m. incisu′rae hel′icis [Santori′ni], m. incisurae helicis.

mus′culi infrahyoi′dei [NA], infrahyoid muscles: the muscles that anchor the hyoid bone to the sternum, clavicle, and scapula, including the sternohyoid, omohyoid, sternothyroid, and thyrohyoid muscles.

m. infraspina′tus [NA], infraspinous muscle: *origin,* infraspinous fossa of scapula; *insertion,* greater tubercle of humerus; *innervation,* suprascapular; *action,* rotates humerus laterally.

mus′culi intercosta′les exter′ni [NA], external intercostal muscles (11 on each side): *origin,* inferior border of rib; *insertion,* superior border of rib below; *innervation,* intercostal; *action,* draw ribs together in respiration and expulsive movements.

mus′culi intercosta′les inter′ni [NA], internal intercostal muscles (11 on each side): *origin,* inferior border of rib and costal cartilage; *insertion,* superior border of rib and costal cartilage below; *innervation,* intercostal; *action,* draw ribs together in respiration and expulsive movements.

mus′culi intercosta′les in′timi [NA], innermost intercostal muscles: the layer of muscle fibers separated from the internal intercostal muscles by the intercostal nerves.

mus′culi interos′sei dorsa′les ma′nus [NA], dorsal interosseous muscles of hand (4): *origin,* by two heads from adjacent sides of metacarpal bones; *insertion,* extensor tendons of second, third, and fourth fingers; *innervation,* ulnar; *action,* abduct, flex proximal phalanges.

mus′culi interos′sei dorsa′les pe′dis [NA], dorsal interosseous muscles of foot (4): *origin,* surfaces of adjacent metatarsal bones; *insertion,* extensor tendons of second, third, and fourth toes; *innervation,* lateral plantar; *action,* abduct, flex toes.

mus′culi interos′sei palma′res [NA], palmar interosseous muscles (3): *origin,* sides of second, fourth, and fifth metacarpal bones; *insertion,* extensor tendons of second, fourth, and fifth fingers; *innervation,* ulnar; *action,* adduct, flex proximal phalanges.

mus′culi interos′sei planta′res [NA], plantar interosseous muscles (3): *origin,* medial surface of third, fourth, and fifth metatarsal bones; *insertion,* extensor tendons of third, fourth, and fifth toes; *innervation,* lateral plantar; *action,* adduct, flex toes.

mus′culi interos′sei vola′res, musculi interossei palmares.

mus′culi interspina′les [NA], interspinal muscles: short bands of muscle fibers between spinous processes of contiguous vertebrae, including the *musculi interspinales cervicis, musculi interspinales thoracis,* and *musculi interspinales lumborum.*

mus′culi interspina′les cer′vicis [NA], interspinal muscles of neck: paired bands of muscle fibers extending between spinous processes of contiguous cervical vertebrae, innervated by spinal nerves, and acting to extend the vertebral column.

mus′culi interspina′les lumbo′rum [NA], interspinal muscles of loins: paired bands of muscle fibers extending between spinous processes of contiguous lumbar vertebrae, innervated by spinal nerves, and acting to extend the vertebral column.

mus′culi interspina′les thora′cis [NA], interspinal muscles of thorax: paired bands of muscle fibers extending between spinous processes of contiguous thoracic vertebrae, innervated by spinal nerves, and acting to extend the vertebral column.

mus′culi intertransversa′rii [NA], intertransverse muscles: small muscles passing between the transverse processes of continguous vertebrae, including the lateral and medial intertransverse muscles of the loins, the intertransverse

muscles of the thorax, and the anterior and posterior intertransverse muscles of the neck.

mus′culi intertransversa′rii anterio′res, musculi intertransversarii thoracis.

mus′culi intertransversa′rii anterio′res cer′vicis [NA], anterior intertransverse muscles of neck: small muscles passing between the anterior tubercles of adjacent cervical vertebrae, innervated by spinal nerves, and acting to bend the vertebral column laterally.

mus′culi intertransversa′rii latera′les, musculi intertransversarii laterales lumborum.

mus′culi intertransversa′rii latera′les lumbo′rum [NA], small muscles passing between the transverse processes of adjacent lumbar vertebrae, innervated by spinal nerves, and acting to bend the vertebral column laterally.

mus′culi intertransversa′rii media′les musculi intertransversarii mediales lumborum.

mus′culi intertransversa′rii media′les lumbo′rum [NA], small muscles passing from the accessory process of one lumbar vertebra to the mamillary process of the contiguous lumbar vertebra, innervated by spinal nerves, and acting to bend the vertebral column laterally.

mus′culi intertransversa′rii posterio′res, musculi intertransversarii posteriores cervicis.

mus′culi intertransversa′rii posterio′res cer′vicis [NA], posterior intertransverse muscles of neck: small muscles, divided into medial and lateral parts, passing between the posterior tubercles of adjacent cervical vertebrae, innervated by spinal nerves, and acting to bend the vertebral column laterally.

mus′culi intertransversa′rii thora′cis [NA], intertransverse muscles of thorax: poorly developed muscle bundles extending between the anterior tubercles of adjacent thoracic vertebrae, innervated by spinal nerves, and acting to bend the vertebral column laterally.

m. ischiocaverno′sus [NA], ischiocavernous muscle: *origin,* ramus of ischium; *insertion,* crus penis (crus clitoridis); *innervation,* perineal; *action,* maintains erection of penis (clitoris).

mus′culi laryn′gis [NA], the intrinsic and extrinsic muscles of the larynx.

m. latis′simus dor′si [NA], *origin,* spines of thoracic and lumbar vertebrae, thoracolumbar fascia, iliac crest, lower ribs, inferior angle of scapula; *insertion,* crest of intertubercular sulcus of humerus; *innervation,* thoracodorsal; *action,* adducts, extends, and rotates humerus medially.

m. leva′tor an′guli o′ris [NA], levator muscle of angle of mouth: *origin,* canine fossa of maxilla; *insertion,* orbicularis oris and skin at angle of mouth; *innervation,* facial; *action,* raises angle of mouth.

m. leva′tor a′ni [NA], levator ani muscle: a name applied collectively to important muscular components of the pelvic diaphragm, including the pubococcygeus (levator prostatae and pubovaginalis), the puborectalis, and the iliococcygeus muscles.

mus′culi levato′res costa′rum [NA], levator muscles of ribs (12 on each side): originating from the transverse processes of the seventh cervical and first to eleventh thoracic vertebrae and inserting medial to the angle of a lower rib (see *musculi levatores costarum breves* and *musculi levatores costarum longi*); innervated by intercostal nerves and aiding in elevation of the ribs in respiration.

mus′culi levato′res costa′rum bre′ves [NA], short levator muscles of ribs: the levatores costarum muscles of each side that insert medial to the angle of the rib next below the vertebra of origin.

mus′culi levato′res costa′rum lon′gi [NA], long levator muscles of ribs: the lower levatores costarum muscles of each side, which have fascicles extending down to the second rib below the vertebra of origin.

m. leva′tor glan′dulae thyreoi′deae, m. levator glandulae thyroideae.

m. leva′tor glan′dulae thyroi′deae [NA], levator muscle of thyroid gland: an inconstant muscle originating on the isthmus or pyramid of the thyroid gland and inserting on the body of the hyoid bone.

m. leva′tor la′bii superio′ris [NA], levator muscle of upper lip: *origin,* lower orbital margin; *insertion,* muscle of upper lip; *innervation,* facial nerve; *action,* raises upper lip.

m. leva′tor la′bii superio′ris alae′que na′si [NA], levator muscle of upper lip and ala of nose: *origin,* nasal process of maxilla; *insertion,* cartilage of ala nasi and upper lip; *innervation,* infraorbital branch of facial; *action,* raises upper lip and dilates nostril.

m. leva′tor pal′pebrae superio′ris [NA], levator muscle of upper eyelid: *origin*, upper border of optic foramen; *insertion*, tarsal plate of upper eyelid; *innervation*, oculomotor; *action*, raises upper lid.

m. leva′tor prosta′tae [NA], levator muscle of prostate: a name applied to a part of the anterior portion of the pubococcygeus muscle, which is inserted in the prostate and the tendinous center of the perineum; innervated by sacral and pudendal nerves, it supports and compresses the prostate and is involved in control of micturition.

m. leva′tor scap′ulae [NA], levator muscle of scapula: *origin*, transverse processes of four upper cervical vertebrae; *insertion*, medial border of scapula; *innervation*, third and fourth cervical; *action*, raises scapula.

m. leva′tor ve′li palati′ni [NA], *origin*, apex of petrous portion of temporal bone and cartilaginous part of auditory tube; *insertion*, aponeurosis of soft palate; *innervation*, pharyngeal plexus of vagus; *action*, raises soft palate.

mus′culi lin′guae [NA], muscles of tongue: the extrinsic and intrinsic muscles that move the tongue; called also lingual muscles.

m. longis′simus [NA], longissimus muscle: the largest element of the m. erector spinae, which includes the *m. longissimus capitis*, *m. longissimus cervicis*, and *m. longissimus thoracis*.

m. longis′simus cap′itis [NA], longissimus muscle of head: *origin*, transverse processes of four or five upper thoracic vertebrae, articular processes of three or four lower cervical vertebrae; *insertion*, mastoid process of temporal bone; *innervation*, branches of cervical; *action*, draws head backward, rotates head.

m. longis′simus cer′vicis [NA], longissimus muscle of neck: *origin*, transverse processes of four or five upper thoracic vertebrae; *insertion*, transverse processes of second to sixth cervical vertebrae; *innervation*, lower cervical and upper thoracic; *action*, extends cervical vertebrae.

m. longis′simus dor′si, m. longissimus thoracis.

m. longis′simus thora′cis [NA], longissimus muscle of thorax: *origin*, transverse and articular processes of lumbar vertebrae and thoracolumbar fascia; *insertion*, transverse processes of all thoracic vertebrae, nine or ten lower ribs; *innervation*, lumbar and thoracic; *action*, extends thoracic vertebrae.

m. longitudina′lis infe′rior lin′guae [NA], inferior longitudinal muscle of tongue: *origin*, under surface of tongue at base; *insertion*, tip of tongue; *innervation*, hypoglossal; *action*, changes shape of tongue in mastication and deglutition.

m. longitudina′lis supe′rior lin′guae [NA], superior longitudinal muscle of tongue: *origin*, submucosa and septum of tongue; *insertion*, margins of tongue; *innervation*, hypoglossal; *action*, changes shape of tongue in mastication and deglutition.

m. lon′gus cap′itis [NA], long muscle of head: *origin*, transverse processes of third to sixth cervical vertebrae; *insertion*, basal portion of occipital bone; *innervation*, branches from first, second, and third cervical; *action*, flexes head.

m. lon′gus col′li [NA], long muscle of neck: *origin*, SUPERIOR OBLIQUE PORTION—transverse processes of third to fifth cervical vertebrae, INFERIOR OBLIQUE PORTION—bodies of first to third thoracic vertebrae, VERTICAL PORTION—bodies of three upper thoracic and three lower cervical vertebrae; *insertion*, SUPERIOR OBLIQUE PORTION—tubercle of anterior arch of atlas, INFERIOR OBLIQUE PORTION—transverse processes of fifth and sixth cervical vertebrae, VERTICAL PORTION— bodies of second to fourth cervical vertebrae; *innervation*, anterior cervical; *action*, flexes and supports cervical vertebrae.

mus′culi lumbrica′les ma′nus [NA], lumbrical muscles of hand: *origin*, tendons of flexor digitorum profundus; *insertion*, extensor tendons of four lateral fingers; *innervation*, median and ulnar; *action*, flex metacarpophalangeal joint and extend middle and distal phalanges.

mus′culi lumbrica′les pe′dis [NA], lumbrical muscles of foot: *origin*, tendons of flexor digitorum longus; *insertion*, extensor tendons of four lateral toes; *innervation*, medial and lateral plantar; *action*, flex proximal phalanges.

m. masse′ter [NA], masseter muscle: *origin*, PARS SUPERFICIALIS—zygomatic process of maxilla and lower border of zygomatic arch, PARS PROFUNDA—lower border and medial surface of zygomatic arch; *insertion*, PARS SUPERFICIALIS—angle and ramus of mandible, PARS PROFUNDA—upper half of ramus and lateral surface of coronoid process of mandible; *innervation*, mandibular division of trigeminal; *action*, raises mandible, closes jaws.

mus′culi mem′bri inferio′ris [NA], the muscles acting on the thigh, leg, and foot.

mus′culi mem′bri superio′ris [NA], the muscles acting on the arm, forearm, and hand.

m. menta′lis [NA], *origin*, incisive fossa of mandible; *insertion*, skin of chin; *innervation*, facial; *action*, wrinkles skin of chin.

musculi multif′idi [NA], *origin*, sacrum, sacroiliac ligament, mamillary processes of lumbar, transverse processes of thoracic, and articular processes of cervical vertebrae; *insertion*, spines of contiguous vertebrae above; *innervation*, dorsal branches of spinal nerves; *action*, extends, rotates vertebral column.

m. multipenna′tus [NA], multipennate muscle: a muscle in which the fiber bundles converge to several tendons.

m. mylohyoi′deus [NA], mylohyoid muscle: *origin*, mylohyoid line of mandible; *insertion*, body of hyoid bone and median raphe; *innervation*, mylohyoid branch of trigeminal; *action*, elevates hyoid bone, supports floor of mouth.

m. mylopharyn′geus, pars mylopharyngea musculi constrictoris pharyngis superioris.

m. nasa′lis [NA], nasal muscle: *origin*, maxilla; *insertion*, PARS ALARIS—ala of nose, PARS TRANSVERSA—by aponeurotic expansion with fellow of opposite side; *innervation*, facial; *action*, PARS ALARIS—aids in widening nostril, PARS TRANSVERSA—depresses cartilage of nose.

m. obli′quus auric′ulae [NA], oblique muscle of auricle: *origin*, cranial surface of concha; *insertion*, cranial surface of auricle above concha; *innervation*, posterior auricular and temporal.

m. obli′quus cap′itis infe′rior [NA], inferior oblique muscle of head: *origin*, spinous process of axis; *insertion*, transverse process of atlas; *innervation*, dorsal branches of spinal nerves; *action*, rotates atlas and head.

m. obli′quus cap′itis supe′rior [NA], superior oblique muscle of head: *origin*, transverse process of atlas; *insertion*, occipital bone; *innervation*, dorsal branches of spinal nerves; *action*, extends and moves head laterally.

m. obli′quus exter′nus abdom′inis [NA], external oblique muscle of abdomen; *origin*, lower eight ribs at costal cartilages; *insertion*, crest of ilium, linea alba through rectus sheath; *innervation*, lower intercostal; *action*, flexes and rotates vertebral column, compresses abdominal viscera.

m. obli′quus infe′rior bul′bi [NA], inferior oblique muscle of eyeball: *origin*, orbital plate of maxilla; *insertion*, sclera; *innervation*, oculomotor; *action*, rotates eyeball upward and outward.

m. obli′quus infe′rior oc′uli, m. obliquus inferior bulbi.

m. obli′quus inter′nus abdom′inis [NA], internal oblique muscle of abdomen: *origin*, inguinal ligament, iliac crest, lumbar aponeurosis; *insertion*, lower three or four costal cartilages, linea alba, conjoined tendon to pubis; *innervation*, lower intercostal; *action*, flexes and rotates vertebral column, compresses abdominal viscera.

m. obli′quus supe′rior bul′bi [NA], superior oblique muscle of eyeball: *origin*, lesser wing of sphenoid above optic foramen; *insertion*, sclera; *innervation*, trochlear; *action*, rotates eyeball downward and outward.

m. obli′quus supe′rior oc′uli, m. obliquus superior bulbi.

m. obtura′tor exter′nus, m. obturatorius externus.

m. obtura′tor inter′nus, m. obturatorius internus.

m. obturato′rius exter′nus [NA], external obturator muscle: *origin*, pubis, ischium, and superficial surface of obturator membrane; *insertion*, trochanteric fossa of femur; *innervation*, obturator; *action*, rotates thigh laterally.

m. obturato′rius inter′nus [NA], internal obturator muscle: *origin*, pelvic surface of hip bone, margin of obturator foramen, ramus of ischium, inferior ramus of pubis, internal surface of obturator membrane; *insertion*, greater trochanter of femur; *innervation*, first, second, and third sacral; *action*, rotates thigh laterally.

m. occipita′lis, venter occipitalis musculi occipitofrontalis.

m. occipitofronta′lis [NA], occipitofrontal muscle: *origin*, VENTER FRONTALIS—galea aponeurotica, VENTER OCCIPITALIS—highest nuchal line of occipital bone; *insertion*, VENTER FRONTALIS—skin of eyebrows and root of nose, VENTER OCCIPITALIS—galea aponeurotica; *innervation*, VENTER FRONTALIS—temporal branch of facial, VENTER OCCIPITALIS—posterior auricular branch of facial; *action*, VENTER FRONTALIS—raises eyebrows, VENTER OCCIPITALIS—draws scalp backward.

mus′culi oc′uli, musculi bulbi.

m. omohyoi′deus [NA], omohyoid muscle, comprising two bellies (superior and inferior) connected by a central tendon that is bound to the clavicle by a fibrous expansion of the cervical fascia; *origin*, superior border of scapula; *insertion*, lateral border of hyoid bone; *innervation*, upper cervical through ansa cervicalis; *action*, depresses hyoid bone.

m. oppo′nens dig′iti min′imi [NA], opposing muscle of little finger: *origin*, hook of hamate bone, transverse carpal ligament; *insertion*, medial aspect of fifth metacarpal; *innervation*, eighth cervical through ulnar; *action*, rotates, abducts fifth metacarpal.

m. oppo′nens dig′iti quin′ti ma′nus, m. opponens digiti minimi.

m. oppo′nens pol′licis [NA], opposing muscle of thumb: *origin*, ridge of trapezium, transverse carpal ligament; *insertion*, radial side of first metacarpal; *innervation*, sixth and seventh cervical through median; *action*, flexes and opposes thumb.

m. orbicula′ris [NA], orbicular muscle: a muscle that encircles a body opening, such as the eye or mouth.

m. orbicula′ris oc′uli [NA], orbicular muscle of eye; the oval sphincter muscle surrounding the eyelids, consisting of three parts: *origin*, PARS ORBITALIS—medial margin of orbit, including frontal process of maxilla, PARS PALPEBRALIS—medial canthus, medial palpebral ligament, PARS LACRIMALIS—posterior lacrimal crest; *insertion*, PARS ORBITALIS—near origin after encircling orbit, PARS PALPEBRALIS— lateral canthus, PARS LACRIMALIS—joins palpebral portion; *innervation*, facial; *action*, closes eyelids, wrinkles forehead, compresses lacrimal sac.

m. orbicula′ris o′ris [NA], orbicular muscle of mouth, comprising a *pars labialis*, fibers restricted to the lips, and a *pars marginalis*, fibers blending with those of adjacent muscles; *innervation*, facial; *action*, closes and protrudes lips.

m. orbita′lis [NA], orbital muscle: *origin*, orbital periosteum; *insertion*, fascia of inferior orbital fissure; *innervation*, sympathetic fibers; *action*, protrudes eye.

mus′culi ossiculo′rum audi′tus [NA], muscles of auditory ossicles: the two muscles of the middle ear, the tensor tympani and the stapedius.

mus′culi os′sis hyoi′dei, muscles of the hyoid bone; see *musculi infrahyoidei* and *musculi suprahyoidei*.

mus′culi pala′ti [NA], palative muscles: the intrinsic and extrinsic muscles that act upon the soft palate.

mus′culi pala′ti et fau′cium [NA], muscles of palate and fauces: the intrinsic and extrinsic muscles that act upon the soft palate (*musculi palati* [NA]) and the adjacent pharyngeal wall.

m. palatoglos′sus [NA], palatoglossus muscle: *origin*, under surface of soft palate; *insertion*, side of tongue; *innervation*, pharyngeal plexus of vagus; *action*, elevates tongue, constricts fauces.

m. palatopharyn′geus [NA], palatopharyngeal muscle: *origin*, soft palate; *insertion*, aponeurosis of pharynx, dorsal border of thyroid cartilage; *innervation*, pharyngeal plexus of vagus; *action*, aids in deglutition.

m. palma′ris bre′vis [NA], short palmar muscle: *origin*, palmar aponeurosis; *insertion*, skin of medial border of hand; *innervation*, ulnar; *action*, tenses palm of hand.

m. palma′ris lon′gus [NA], long palmar muscle: *origin*, medial epicondyle of humerus; *insertion*, transverse carpal ligament, palmar aponeurosis; *innervation*, median; *action*, flexes wrist joint.

mus′culi papilla′res [NA], papillary muscles: conical muscular projections from the walls of the cardiac ventricles, attached to the cusps of the atrioventricular valves by the chordae tendineae. There is an anterior and a posterior papillary muscle in each ventricle, as well as a group of small papillary muscles on the septum in the right ventricle.

m. papilla′ris ante′rior ventric′uli dex′tri [NA], anterior papillary muscle of right ventricle: the papillary muscle arising from the sternocostal wall of the right ventricle.

m. papilla′ris ante′rior ventric′uli sinis′tri [NA], anterior papillary muscle of left ventricle: the papillary muscle arising from the anterior wall of the left ventricle.

m. papilla′ris poste′rior ventric′uli dex′tri [NA], posterior papillary muscle of right ventricle: the papillary muscle arising from the diaphragmatic wall of the right ventricle.

m. papilla′ris poste′rior ventric′uli sinis′tri [NA], posterior papillary muscle of left ventricle: the papillary muscle arising from the posterior wall of the left ventricle.

mus′culi papilla′res septa′les ventric′uli dex′tri [NA], septal papillary muscles of right ventricle: several small papillary muscles in the right ventricle of the heart, arising from the interventricular septum.

mus′culi pectina′ti [NA], pectinate muscles: small ridges of muscle fibers projecting from the inner walls of the auricles of the heart and extending in the right atrium from the auricle to the crista terminalis.

m. pectin′eus [NA], pectineal muscle: *origin*, iliopectineal line, spine of pubis; *insertion*, femur distal to lesser trochanter; *innervation*, obturator and femoral; *action*, flexes, adducts thigh.

m. pectora′lis ma′jor [NA], greater pectoral muscle: *origin*, clavicle, sternum, six upper ribs, aponeurosis of obliquus externus abdominis. These origins are reflected in the subdivision of the muscle into clavicular, sternocostal, and abdominal parts; *insertion*, crest of intertubercular groove of humerus; *innervation*, anterior thoracic; *action*, adducts, flexes, rotates arm medially.

m. pectora′lis mi′nor [NA], smaller pectoral muscle: *origin*, third, fourth, and fifth ribs; *insertion*, coracoid process of scapula; *innervation*, anterior thoracic; *action*, draws shoulder forward and downward.

mus′culi perinea′les, NA alternative for *musculi perinei.*

mus′culi perine′i [NA], the muscles participating in formation of the perineum; called also *musculi perineales* [NA alternative] and *perineal muscles.*

m. perone′us bre′vis [NA], short peroneal muscle: *origin*, lateral surface of fibula; *insertion*, base of fifth metatarsal bone; *innervation*, superficial peroneal; *action*, abducts, plantar flexes foot. Called also *m. fibularis brevis* [NA alternative] or *short fibular muscle.*

m. perone′us lon′gus [NA], long peroneal muscle: *origin*, lateral condyle of tibia, lateral surface of fibula; *insertion*, medial cuneiform, first metatarsal; *innervation*, superficial peroneal; *action*, abducts, everts, plantar flexes foot. Called also *m. fibularis longus* [NA alternative] or *long fibular muscle.*

m. perone′us ter′tius [NA], third peroneal muscle: *origin*, medial surface of fibula; *insertion*, fifth metatarsal; *innervation*, deep peroneal; *action*, everts, dorsiflexes foot. Called also *m. fibularis tertius* [NA alternative] or *third fibular muscle.*

m. pharyngopalati′nus, m. palatopharyngeus.

m. pirifor′mis [NA], piriform muscle: *origin*, ilium, second to fourth sacral vertebrae; *insertion*, upper border of greater trochanter; *innervation*, first and second sacral; *action*, rotates thigh laterally.

m. planta′ris [NA], plantar muscle: *origin*, lateral condyle of femur; *insertion*, posterior part of calcaneus; *innervation*, tibial; *action*, plantar flexes foot.

m. pleuroesopha′geus [NA], pleuroesophageal muscle: a bundle of smooth muscle usually connecting the esophagus with the left mediastinal pleura.

m. pleurooesopha′geus, m. pleuroesophageus.

m. poplite′us [NA], popliteal muscle: *origin*, lateral condyle of femur; *insertion*, posterior surface of tibia; *innervation*, fourth and fifth lumbar and first sacral; *action*, flexes leg, rotates leg medially.

m. proce′rus [NA], procerus muscle: *origin*, skin over nose; *insertion*, skin of forehead; *innervation*, facial; *action*, draws eyebrows down.

m. prona′tor quadra′tus [NA], *origin*, anterior surface and border of distal third or fourth of ulna; *insertion*, distal fourth of shaft of radius; *innervation*, anterior interosseous; *action*, pronates hand.

m. prona′tor te′res [NA], (2 heads): *origin*, CAPUT HUMERALE—medial epicondyle of humerus, CAPUT ULNARE— coronoid process of ulna; *insertion*, lateral surface of radius; *innervation*, median; *action*, pronates hand.

m. prostat′icus, substantia muscularis prostatae.

m. pso′as ma′jor [NA], greater psoas muscle: *origin*, lumbar vertebrae and fascia; *insertion*, lesser trochanter of femur; *innervation*, second and third lumbar; *action*, flexes trunk, flexes and rotates thigh medially.

m. pso′as mi′nor [NA], smaller psoas muscle: *origin*, last thoracic and first lumbar vertebrae; *insertion*, iliopectineal eminence; *innervation*, first lumbar; *action*, flexes trunk on pelvis.

m. pterygoi′deus exter′nus, m. pterygoideus lateralis.
m. pterygoi′deus inter′nus, m. pterygoideus medialis.
m. pterygoi′deus latera′lis [NA], lateral pterygoid muscle (2 heads): *origin*, UPPER HEAD—lateral surface of greater wing of sphenoid and infratemporal crest; LOWER HEAD—lateral surface of lateral pterygoid plate; *insertion*, neck of condyle of mandible, temporomandibular joint capsule; *innervation*, man-

dibular division of trigeminal; *action*, protrudes mandible, opens jaws, moves mandible from side to side.

m. pterygoi′deus media′lis [NA], medial pterygoid muscle: *origin*, lateral pterygoid plate, tuberosity of maxilla; *insertion*, medial surface of ramus and angle of mandible; *innervation*, mandibular division of trigeminal; *action*, closes jaws.

m. pterygopharyn′geus, pars pterygopharyngea musculi constrictoris pharyngis superioris.

m. pubococcyg′eus [NA], pubococcygeal muscle: a name applied to the anterior portion of the levator ani, originating in front of the obturator canal; *insertion*, anococcygeal ligament and side of coccyx; *innervation*, third and fourth sacral; *action*, helps support pelvic viscera and resist increases in intraabdominal pressure.

m. puboprostat′icus [NA], puboprostatic muscle: a name applied to smooth muscle fibers contained within the medial puboprostatic ligament, which pass from the prostate anteriorly to the pubis.

m. puborecta′lis [NA], puborectal muscle: a name applied to a portion of the levator ani having a more lateral origin from the pubic bone, and continuous posteriorly with the corresponding muscle of the opposite side; *innervation*, third and fourth sacral; *action*, helps support pelvic viscera and resist increases in intraabdominal pressure.

m. pubovagina′lis [NA], pubovaginal muscle: a name applied to a part of the anterior portion of the pubococcygeus muscle, which is inserted into the urethra and vagina; innervated by the sacral and pudendal nerves, it is involved in control of micturition.

m. pubovesica′lis [NA], pubovesical muscle: a name applied to smooth muscle fibers extending from the neck of the urinary bladder to the pubis.

m. pyramida′lis [NA], pyramidal muscle: *origin*, front of pubis, anterior pubic ligament; *insertion*, linea alba; *innervation*, last thoracic; *action*, tenses abdominal wall.

m. pyramida′lis auric′ulae [NA], pyramidal muscle of auricle: a prolongation of the fibers of the tragicus to the spina helicis.

m. quadra′tus [NA], quadrate muscle: a square-shaped muscle.

m. quadra′tus fem′oris [NA], quadrate muscle of thigh: *origin*, upper part of lateral border of tuberosity of ischium; *insertion*, quadrate tubercle of femur; *innervation*, last lumbar and first sacral; *action*, adducts, rotates thigh laterally.

m. quadra′tus la′bii inferio′ris, m. depressor labii inferioris.

m. quadra′tus la′bii superio′ris, m. levator labii superioris.

m. quadra′tus lumbo′rum [NA], *origin*, crest of ilium, thoracolumbar fascia, lumbar vertebrae; *insertion*, twelfth rib, transverse processes of four upper lumbar vertebrae; *innervation*, first and second lumbar and twelfth thoracic; *action*, flexes lumbar vertebrae laterally.

m. quadra′tus plan′tae [NA], quadrate muscle of sole: *origin*, calcaneus and plantar fascia; *insertion*, tendons of flexor digitorum longus; *innervation*, lateral plantar; *action*, aids in flexing toes. Called also *m. flexor accessorius* [NA alternative] or *accessory flexor muscle*.

m. quad′riceps fem′oris [NA], quadriceps muscle of thigh: a name applied collectively to the rectus femoris, vastus intermedius, vastus lateralis, and vastus medialis, inserting by a common tendon that surrounds the patella and ends on the tuberosity of the tibia, and acting to extend the leg upon the thigh. See individual components.

m. rectococcyg′eus [NA], rectococcygeal muscle: smooth muscle fibers originating on the anterior surface of the second and third coccygeal vertebrae and inserting on the posterior surface of the rectum, innervated by autonomic nerves, and acting to retract and elevate the rectum.

m. rectourethra′lis [NA], rectourethral muscle: a band of smooth muscle fibers extending from the perineal flexure of the rectum to the membranous urethra in the male.

m. rectouteri′nus [NA], rectouterine muscle: a band of fibers running between the cervix of the uterus and the rectum, in the rectouterine fold.

m. rectovesica′lis [NA], rectovesical muscle: a band of fibers in the male, connecting the longitudinal musculature of the rectum with the external muscular coat of the bladder.

m. rec′tus abdom′inis [NA], *origin*, pubis; *insertion*, xiphoid process, cartilages of fifth, sixth, and seventh ribs; *innervation*, branches of lower thoracic; *action*, flexes lumbar vertebrae, supports abdomen.

m. rec′tus cap′itis ante′rior [NA], *origin*, lateral mass of atlas; *insertion*, basilar process of occipital bone; *innervation*, first and second cervical; *action*, flexes, supports head.

m. rec′tus cap′itis latera′lis [NA], *origin*, upper surface of transverse process of atlas; *insertion*, jugular process of occipital bone; *innervation*, first and second cervical; *action*, flexes, supports head.

m. rec′tus cap′itis poste′rior ma′jor [NA], *origin*, spinous process of axis; *insertion*, occipital bone; *innervation*, suboccipital and greater occipital; *action*, extends head.

m. rec′tus cap′itis poste′rior mi′nor [NA], *origin*, tubercle on dorsal arch of atlas; *insertion*, occipital bone; *innervation*, suboccipital and greater occipital; *action*, extends head.

m. rec′tus fem′oris [NA], *origin*, anterior inferior iliac spine, rim of acetabulum; *insertion*, patella, tubercle of tibia; *innervation*, femoral; *action*, extends leg, flexes thigh.

m. rec′tus infe′rior bul′bi [NA], *origin*, circumference of optic foramen; *insertion*, under side of sclera; *innervation*, oculomotor; *action*, adducts, rotates eyeball downward and medially.

m. rec′tus infe′rior oc′uli, m. rectus inferior bulbi.

m. rec′tus latera′lis bul′bi [NA], *origin*, lateral margin of optic foramen, margin of superior orbital fissure; *insertion*, lateral side of sclera; *innervation*, abducens; *action*, abducts eyeball.

m. rec′tus latera′lis oc′uli, m. rectus lateralis bulbi.

m. rec′tus media′lis bul′bi [NA], *origin*, circumference of optic foramen; *insertion*, medial side of sclera; *innervation*, oculomotor; *action*, adducts eyeball.

m. rec′tus media′lis oc′uli, m. rectus medialis bulbi.

m. rec′tus supe′rior bul′bi [NA], *origin*, upper border of optic foramen; *insertion*, upper aspect of sclera; *innervation*, oculomotor; *action*, adducts, rotates eyeball upward and medially.

m. rec′tus supe′rior oc′uli, m. rectus superior bulbi.

m. rhomboi′deus ma′jor [NA], greater rhomboid muscle: *origin*, spinous processes of second, third, fourth, and fifth thoracic vertebrae; *insertion*, medial margin of scapula; *innervation*, dorsal scapular; *action*, retracts, elevates scapula.

m. rhomboi′deus mi′nor [NA], lesser rhomboid muscle: *origin*, spinous processes of seventh cervical to first thoracic vertebrae, lower part of ligamentum nuchae; *insertion*, medial margin of scapula at root of the spine; *innervation*, dorsal scapular; *action*, adducts, elevates scapula.

m. riso′rius [NA], risorius muscle: *origin*, fascia over masseter; *insertion*, skin at angle of mouth; *innervation*, buccal branch of facial; *action*, draws angle of mouth laterally.

mus′culi rotato′res [NA], rotator muscles: a series of small muscles deep in the groove between the spinous and transverse processes of the vertebrae, including the *musculi rotatores cervicis*, *musculi rotatores thoracis*, and *musculi rotatores lumborum*.

mus′culi rotato′res bre′ves, short rotator muscles: a name given the musculi rotatores that insert on the lamina of the vertebra next above the vertebra of origin.

mus′culi rotato′res cer′vicis [NA], rotator muscles of neck: *origin*, transverse processes of cervical vertebrae; *insertion*, base of spinous process of suprajacent vertebrae; *innervation*, spinal nerves; *action*, extend vertebral column and rotate it toward the opposite side.

mus′culi rotato′res lon′gi, long rotator muscles: a name given the musculi rotatores that cross one or two segments of the vertebral column and insert into the spine of the vertebra next above.

mus′culi rotato′res lumbo′rum [NA], *origin*, transverse processes of lumbar vertebrae; *insertion*, base of spinous process of suprajacent vertebrae; *innervation*, spinal nerves; *action*, extend vertebral column and rotate it toward the opposite side.

mus′culi rotato′res thora′cis [NA], rotator muscles of thorax: *origin*, transverse processes of thoracic vertebrae; *insertion*, base of spinous process of suprajacent vertebrae; *innervation*, spinal nerves; *action*, extend vertebral column and rotate it toward the opposite side.

m. sacrococcyg′eus ante′rior, m. sacrococcygeus ventralis.

m. sacrococcyg′eus dorsa′lis [NA], dorsal sacrococcygeal muscle: a muscular slip passing from the dorsal aspect of the sacrum to the coccyx.

m. sacrococcyg′eus poste′rior, m. sacrococcygeus dorsalis.

m. sacrococcyg′eus ventra′lis [NA], ventral sacrococcygeal muscle: a musculotendinous slip passing from the lower sacral vertebrae to the coccyx.

m. sacrospina′lis, m. erector spinae.

m. salpingopharyn′geus [NA], salpingopharyngeal muscle: *origin,* auditory tube near its orifice; *insertion,* posterior part of palatopharyngeus; *innervation,* pharyngeal plexus of vagus; *action,* raises nasopharynx.

m. sarto′rius [NA], sartorius muscle: *origin,* anterior superior iliac spine; *insertion,* medial side of proximal end of tibia; *innervation,* femoral; *action,* flexes thigh and leg.

m. scale′nus ante′rior [NA], anterior scalene muscle: *origin,* transverse processes of third to sixth cervical vertebrae; *insertion,* tubercle of first rib; *innervation,* second to seventh cervical; *action,* raises first rib. Called also *m. scalenus anticus.*

m. scale′nus me′dius [NA], middle scalene muscle: *origin,* transverse processes of second to sixth cervical vertebrae; *insertion,* first rib; *innervation,* second to seventh cervical; *action,* raises first rib.

m. scale′nus min′imus [NA], smallest scalene muscle: a band occasionally found between the m. scalenus anterior and the m. scalenus medius.

m. scale′nus poste′rior [NA], posterior scalene muscle: *origin,* tubercles of fourth to sixth cervical vertebrae; *insertion,* second rib; *innervation,* second to seventh cervical; *action,* raises first and second ribs.

m. semimembrano′sus [NA], semimembranous muscle: *origin,* tuberosity of ischium; *insertion,* medial condyle of tibia; *innervation,* tibial; *action,* flexes leg, extends thigh.

m. semispina′lis [NA], a muscle composed of fibers extending obliquely from the transverse processes of the vertebrae to the spines, except for the semispinalis capitis; it includes the *m. semispinalis capitis, m. semispinalis cervicis,* and *m. semispinalis thoracis.*

m. semispina′lis cap′itis [NA], *origin,* transverse processes of five or six upper thoracic and four lower cervical vertebrae; *insertion,* occipital bone; *innervation,* suboccipital, greater occipital, and branches of cervical; *action,* extends head.

m. semispina′lis cer′vicis [NA], *origin,* transverse processes of five or six upper thoracic vertebrae; *insertion,* spinous processes of second to fifth cervical vertebrae; *innervation,* branches of cervical; *action,* extends, rotates vertebral column.

m. semispina′lis dor′si, m. semispinalis thoracis.

m. semispina′lis thora′cis [NA], *origin,* transverse processes of sixth to tenth thoracic vertebrae; *insertion,* spinous processes of two lower cervical and four upper thoracic vertebrae; *innervation,* spinal nerves; *action,* extends, rotates vertebral column.

m. semitendino′sus [NA], semitendinous muscle: *origin,* tuberosity of ischium; *insertion,* upper part of medial surface of tibia; *innervation,* tibial; *action,* flexes leg, extends thigh.

m. serra′tus ante′rior [NA], *origin,* eight or nine upper ribs; *insertion,* medial border of scapula; *innervation,* long thoracic; *action,* draws scapula forward; rotates scapula to raise shoulder in abduction of arm.

m. serra′tus poste′rior infe′rior [NA], *origin,* spines of two lower thoracic and two or three upper lumbar vertebrae; *insertion,* inferior border of four lower ribs; *innervation,* ninth to twelfth thoracic; *action,* lowers ribs in expiration.

m. serra′tus poste′rior supe′rior [NA], *origin,* ligamentum nuchae, spinous processes of upper thoracic vertebrae; *insertion,* second, third, fourth, and fifth ribs; *innervation,* upper four intercostal; *action,* raises ribs in inspiration.

mus′culi skel′eti [NA], skeletal muscles: striated muscles that are attached to bones and typically cross at least one joint.

m. so′leus [NA], soleus muscle: *origin,* fibula, popliteal fascia, tibia; *insertion,* calcaneus by tendo calcaneus; *innervation,* tibial; *action,* plantar flexes ankle joint.

m. sphinc′ter [NA], sphincter muscle: a ringlike muscle that closes a natural orifice; called also *sphincter.*

m. sphinc′ter ampul′lae hepatopancreat′icae [NA], muscle fibers investing the hepatopancreatic ampulla.

m. sphinc′ter a′ni exter′nus [NA], external sphincter muscle of anus: *origin,* tip of coccyx and surrounding fascia; *insertion,* tendinous center of perineum; *innervation,* inferior rectal and fourth sacral; *action,* closes anus.

m. sphinc′ter a′ni inter′nus [NA], internal sphincter muscle of anus: a thickening of the circular lamina of the tunica muscularis at the caudal end of the rectum.

m. sphinc′ter duc′tus chole′dochi [NA], an annular sheath of muscle that invests the bile duct within the wall of the duodenum.

m. sphinc′ter pupil′lae [NA], sphincter muscle of pupil: circular fibers of the iris, innervated by the oculomotor nerve (parasympathetic), and acting to contract the pupil.

m. sphinc′ter pylo′ri, m. sphincter pyloricus.

m. sphinc′ter pylo′ricus [NA], pyloric sphincter muscle: a thickening of the circular muscle of the stomach around its opening into the duodenum; called also *m. sphincter pylori, pyloric sphincter,* and *sphincter muscle of pylorus.*

m. sphinc′ter ure′thrae [NA], sphincter muscle of urethra: *origin,* ramus of pubis; *insertion,* median raphe behind and in front of urethra; *innervation,* pudendal; *action,* compresses the membranous part of the urethra. Called also *m. sphincter urethrae membranaceae.*

m. sphinc′ter ure′thrae membrana′ceae, m. sphincter urethrae.

m. sphinc′ter vesi′cae urina′riae, sphincter muscle of urinary bladder: a circular layer of fibers surrounding the internal urethral orifice, innervated by the vesical nerve, and acting to close the internal orifice of the urethra.

m. spina′lis [NA], the medial division of the erector spinae, including the *m. spinalis capitis, m. spinalis cervicis,* and *m. spinalis thoracis.*

m. spina′lis cap′itis [NA], *origin,* spines of upper thoracic and lower cervical vertebrae; *insertion,* occipital bone; *innervation,* spinal nerves; *action,* extends head.

m. spina′lis cer′vicis [NA], *origin,* spinous processes of fifth, sixth, and seventh cervical and two upper thoracic vertebrae; *insertion,* spinous processes of axis and sometimes of second to fourth cervical vertebrae; *innervation,* branches of cervical; *action,* extends vertebral column.

m. spina′lis dor′si, m. spinalis thoracis.

m. spina′lis thora′cis [NA], *origin,* spinous processes of two upper lumbar and two lower thoracic; *insertion,* spines of upper thoracic vertebrae; *innervation,* branches of spinal nerves; *action,* extends vertebral column.

m. sple′nius cap′itis [NA], *origin,* lower half of ligamentum nuchae, spines of seventh cervical and three upper thoracic vertebrae; *insertion,* occipital bone; *innervation,* middle and lower cervical; *action,* extends, rotates head.

m. sple′nius cer′vicis [NA], *origin,* spinous processes of third to sixth thoracic vertebrae; *insertion,* transverse processes of two or three upper cervical vertebrae; *innervation,* dorsal branches of lower cervical; *action,* extends, rotates head and neck.

m. stape′dius [NA], stapedius muscle: *origin,* interior of pyramid of tympanic cavity; *insertion,* posterior surface of neck of stapes; *innervation,* stapedial branch of facial; *action,* dampens stapedial movement.

m. sterna′lis [NA], sternal muscle: a band occasionally found parallel to the sternum on the sternocostal origin of the pectoralis major.

m. sternocleidomastoi′deus [NA], sternocleidomastoid muscle (2 heads): *origin,* sternum and clavicle; *insertion,* mastoid process and superior nuchal line of occipital bone; *innervation,* accessory nerve and cervical plexus; *action,* flexes vertebral column, rotates head.

m. sternohyoi′deus [NA], sternohyoid muscle: *origin,* manubrium sterni; *insertion,* body of hyoid bone; *innervation,* upper cervical; *action,* depresses hyoid bone and larynx.

m. sternothyreoi′deus, m. sternothyroideus.

m. sternothyroi′deus [NA], sternothyroid muscle: *origin,* manubrium sterni; *insertion,* thyroid cartilage; *innervation,* upper cervical; *action,* depresses thyroid cartilage.

m. styloglos′sus [NA], styloglossus muscle: *origin,* styloid process; *insertion,* margin of tongue; *innervation,* hypoglossal; *action,* raises and retracts tongue.

m. stylohyoi′deus [NA], stylohyoid muscle: *origin,* styloid process; *insertion,* body of hyoid bone; *innervation,* facial; *action,* draws hyoid and tongue upward.

m. stylopharyn′geus [NA], stylopharyngeal muscle: *origin,* styloid process; *insertion,* thyroid cartilage and pharyngeal constrictors; *innervation,* pharyngeal plexus, glossopharyngeal; *action,* raises and dilates pharynx.

m. subcla′vius [NA], subclavius muscle: *origin,* first rib and its cartilage; *insertion,* lower surface of clavicle; *innervation,* fifth and sixth cervical; *action,* depresses lateral end of clavicle.

mus′culi subcosta′les [NA], subcostal muscles: *origin,* inner surface of ribs: *insertion,* inner surface of first, second, third rib below; *innervation,* intercostal; *action,* raise ribs in inspiration.

mus′culi suboccipita′les [NA], suboccipital muscles: the muscles situated just below the occipital bone, including the recti capitis posteriores major and minor, the oblique capitis inferior and superior, the recti capitis anterior and lateral, the splenius capitis, and the longus capitis muscles.

m. subscapula′ris [NA], subscapular muscle: *origin*, subscapular fossa of scapula; *insertion*, lesser tubercle of humerus; *innervation*, subscapular; *action*, rotates humerus medially.

m. supina′tor [NA], supinator muscle: *origin*, lateral epicondyle of humerus, ulna, elbow joint fascia; *insertion*, radius; *innervation*, deep radial; *action*, supinates hand.

mus′culi suprahyoi′dei [NA], suprahyoid muscles: the muscles that attach the hyoid bone to the skull, including the digastric, stylohyoid, mylohyoid, and geniohyoid muscles.

m. supraspina′tus [NA], supraspinous muscle: *origin*, supraspinous fossa of scapula; *insertion*, greater tubercle of humerus; *innervation*, suprascapular; *action*, abducts humerus.

m. suspenso′rius duode′ni [NA], suspensory muscle of duodenum: a flat band of smooth muscle originating from the left crus of the diaphragm, and continuous with the muscular coat of the duodenum at its junction with the jejunum.

m. tarsa′lis infe′rior [NA], inferior tarsal muscle: *origin*, inferior rectus muscle; *insertion*, tarsal plate of lower eyelid; *innervation*, sympathetic; *action*, widens palpebral fissure.

m. tarsa′lis supe′rior [NA], superior tarsal muscle: *origin*, m. levator palpebrae superioris; *insertion*, tarsal plate of upper eyelid; *innervation*, sympathetic; *action*, widens palpebral fissure.

m. tempora′lis [NA], temporal muscle: *origin*, temporal fossa and fascia; *insertion*, coronoid process of mandible; *innervation*, mandibular division of trigeminal; *action*, closes jaws.

m. temporoparieta′lis [NA], temporoparietal muscle: *origin*, temporal fascia above ear; *insertion*, galea aponeurotica; *innervation*, temporal branches of facial; *action*, tightens scalp.

m. ten′sor fas′ciae la′tae [NA], tensor muscle of fascia lata: *origin*, iliac crest; *insertion*, iliotibial band of fascia lata; *innervation*, superior gluteal; *action*, flexes, rotates thigh medially.

m. ten′sor tym′pani [NA], tensor muscle of tympanic membrane: *origin*, cartilaginous portion of auditory tube; *insertion*, manubrium of malleus; *innervation*, mandibular division of trigeminal; *action*, tenses tympanic membrane.

m. ten′sor ve′li palati′ni [NA], *origin*, scaphoid fossa of sphenoid, wall of auditory tube; *insertion*, aponeurosis of soft palate, horizontal part of palatine bone; *innervation*, mandibular division of trigeminal; *action*, tenses soft palate, opens auditory tube.

m. te′res ma′jor [NA], teres major muscle: *origin*, inferior angle of scapula; *insertion*, crest of intertubercular sulcus of humerus; *innervation*, subscapular; *action*, adducts, extends, rotates arm medially.

m. te′res mi′nor [NA], teres minor muscle: *origin*, lateral margin of scapula; *insertion*, greater tuberosity of humerus; *innervation*, axillary; *action*, rotates arm laterally.

mus′culi thora′cis [NA], the muscles of the thorax.

m. thyreoarytaenoi′deus [exter′nus], m. thyroarytenoideus.

m. thyreo-piglot′ticus, m. thyroepiglotticus.

m. thyreohyoi′deus, m. thyrohyoideus.

m. thyreopharyn′geus, pars thyropharyngea musculi constrictoris pharyngis inferioris.

m. thyroarytenoi′deus [NA], thyroarytenoid muscle: *origin*, lamina of thyroid cartilage; *insertion*, muscular process of arytenoid cartilage; *innervation*, recurrent laryngeal; *action*, relaxes, shortens vocal folds.

m. thyroepiglot′ticus [NA], thyroepiglottic muscle: *origin*, lamina of thyroid cartilage; *insertion*, epiglottis; *innervation*, recurrent laryngeal; *action*, closes inlet to larynx.

m. thyrohyoi′deus [NA], thyrohyoid muscle: *origin*, thyroid cartilage; *insertion*, greater cornu of hyoid bone; *innervation*, upper cervical; *action*, raises and changes form of larynx.

m. tibia′lis ante′rior [NA], anterior tibial muscle: *origin*, tibia, interosseous membrane; *insertion*, medial cuneiform and first metatarsal; *innervation*, deep peroneal; *action*, dorsiflexes and inverts foot.

m. tibia′lis poste′rior [NA], posterior tibial muscle: *origin*, tibia, fibula, interosseous membrane; *insertion*, bases of metatarsals and tarsals, except talus; *innervation*, posterior tibial; *action*, plantar flexes and inverts foot.

m. trachea′lis [NA], tracheal muscle: a transverse layer of smooth fibers in the dorsal portion of the trachea; *insertion*, tracheal cartilages; *innervation*, autonomic fibers; *action*, lessens caliber of trachea.

m. trag′icus [NA], muscle of tragus: a short, flattened vertical band on the lateral surface of the tragus, innervated by the auriculotemporal and posterior auricular nerves.

m. transversospina′lis [NA], a general term including the semispinalis and multifidus muscles and the rotatores.

m. transver′sus abdom′inis [NA], transverse muscle of abdomen: *origin*, cartilages of six lower ribs, thoracolumbar fascia, iliac crest, inguinal ligament; *insertion*, linea alba through rectus sheath, conjoined tendon to pubis; *innervation*, lower intercostals, iliohypogastric, ilioinguinal; *action*, compresses abdominal viscera.

m. transver′sus auric′ulae [NA], transverse muscle of auricle: *origin*, cranial surface of auricle; *insertion*, circumference of auricle; *innervation*, great auricular and posterior auricular; *action*, retracts helix.

m. transver′sus lin′guae [NA], transverse muscle of tongue: *origin*, median septum of tongue; *insertion*, dorsum and margins of tongue; *innervation*, hypoglossal; *action*, changes shape of tongue in mastication and deglutition.

m. transver′sus men′ti [NA], transverse muscle of chin: superficial fibers of the depressor anguli oris which turn back and cross to the opposite side.

m. transver′sus nu′chae [NA], transverse muscle of nape: a small muscle often present, passing from the occipital protuberance to the posterior auricular muscle; it may be either superficial or deep to the trapezius.

m. transver′sus perine′i profun′dus [NA], deep transverse muscle of perineum: *origin*, inferior ramus of ischium; *insertion*, median raphe of perineum; *innervation*, pudendal; *action*, draws back central point of perineum.

m. transver′sus perine′i superficia′lis [NA], superficial transverse muscle of perineum: *origin*, tuberosity of ischium; *insertion*, central tendon of perineum; *innervation*, perineal branch of pudendal; *action*, tenses central point of perineum.

m. transver′sus thora′cis [NA], transverse muscle of thorax: *origin*, mediastinal surface of sternum and of xiphoid process; *insertion*, cartilages of second to sixth ribs; *innervation*, intercostal; *action*, narrows chest.

m. trape′zius [NA], trapezius muscle: *origin*, occipital bone, ligamentum nuchae, spinous processes of seventh cervical and all thoracic vertebrae; *insertion*, clavicle, acromion, spine of scapula; *innervation*, accessory nerve and cervical plexus; *action*, rotates scapula to raise shoulder in abduction of arm, draws scapula backward.

m. triangula′ris [NA], triangular muscle: a muscle that is triangular in shape.

m. tri′ceps bra′chii [NA], triceps muscle of arm (3 heads): *origin*, CAPUT LONGUM—infraglenoid tubercle of scapula, CAPUT LATERALE—posterior surface of humerus, lateral border of humerus, lateral intermuscular septum, CAPUT MEDIALE—posterior surface of humerus below radial groove, medial border of humerus, medial intermuscular septa; *insertion*, olecranon of ulna; *innervation*, radial; *action*, extends forearm, adducts and extends arm.

m. tri′ceps su′rae [NA], the gastrocnemius and soleus considered together.

m. unipenna′tus [NA], unipennate muscle: a muscle in which the fiber bundles approach the tendon of insertion from only one direction and are inserted through only a small segment of its circumference.

m. u′vulae [NA], muscle of uvula: *origin*, posterior nasal spine of palatine bone and aponeurosis of soft palate; *insertion*, uvula; *innervation*, pharyngeal plexus of vagus; *action*, raises uvula.

m. vas′tus interme′dius [NA], *origin*, anterior and lateral surfaces of femur; *insertion*, patella, common tendon of quadriceps femoris; *innervation*, femoral; *action*, extends leg.

m. vas′tus latera′lis [NA], *origin*, capsule of hip joint, lateral aspect of femur; *insertion*, patella, common tendon of quadriceps femoris; *innervation*, femoral; *action*, extends leg.

m. vas′tus media′lis [NA], *origin*, medial aspect of femur; *insertion*, patella, common tendon of quadriceps femoris; *innervation*, femoral; *action*, extends leg.

m. ventricula′ris, a name applied to fibers of the thyroarytenoid muscle running into the vestibular folds.

m. vertica′lis lin′guae [NA], vertical muscle of tongue: *origin*, dorsal fascia of tongue; *insertion*, sides and base of tongue; *innervation*, hypoglossal; *action*, changes shape of tongue in mastication and deglutition.

m. vis′cerum, a term applied to muscle of a body organ.

m. voca′lis [NA], vocal muscle: *origin*, thyroid cartilage; *insertion*, vocal process of arytenoid cartilage; *innervation*, recurrent laryngeal; *action*, shortens vocal folds.

m. zygomat′icus, m. zygomaticus major.

m. zygomat′icus ma′jor [NA], greater zygomatic muscle: *origin*, zygomatic bone in front of temporal process;

insertion, angle of mouth; *innervation*, facial; *action*, draws angle of mouth backward and upward.

m. zygomat′icus mi′nor [NA], lesser zygomatic muscle: *origin*, zygomatic bone near maxillary suture; *insertion*, orbicularis oris and levator labii superioris; *innervation*, facial; *action*, draws upper lip upward and laterally.

---

mushroom (mush′rōŏm) the fruiting body of any of a variety of basidiomycetous, fleshy fungi of the order Agaricales, especially one that is edible; poisonous species are popularly called *toadstools*. Called also *basidiocarp*. See also *agaric*.

musicogenic (mu″zĭ-ko-jen′ĭk) caused or produced by musical sounds.

musicotherapy (mu″zĭ-ko-ther′ah-pe) [Gr. *mousikē* music + *therapeia* treatment] the treatment of disease by music.

Musset's sign (mu-sāz′) [Louis Charles Alfred de *Musset*, French poet, 1810–1857, who died of aortic insufficiency] see under *sign*.

mussitation (mus″ĭ-ta′shun) [L. *mussitare* to mutter] the moving of the lips with no utterance of articulate sounds.

Mussy see *Guéneau de Mussy*.

must (must) [L. *mustum*] the unfermented juice of grapes and other fruit.

mustard (mus′tard) [L. *sinapis*] 1. a plant of the genus *Brassica*. 2. the ripe seeds of *Brassica nigra* (L.) Koch (Cruciferae) (black mustard) and of *B. alba* (L.) Rabenh. (Cruciferae) (white mustard). When mustard seeds are crushed and moistened, volatile oils are liberated. These oils give mustard its counterirritant, stimulant, and emetic properties. **black m., brown m.**, *Brassica nigra* (L.) Koch, a source of mustard oil and allyl isothiocyanate, and used internally as an emetic and externally as a counterirritant. See *mustard plaster*, under *plaster*. **nitrogen m.**, mechlorethamine hydrochloride; see also *nitrogen m's*. **nitrogen m's**, a group of cytotoxic alkylating agents (q.v.) having the general formula R—N(CH$_2$CH$_2$Cl$_2$; they are homologous with the vesicant war gas dichloroethyl sulfide (mustard gas). Those used as antineoplastic and immunosuppressive agents include mechlorethamine (nitrogen mustard), cyclophosphamide, uracil mustard, melphalan, and chlorambucil. **L-phenylalanine m.**, melphalan. **uracil m.** [USP], a cytotoxic alkylating agent that is the uracil derivative of nitrogen mustard, used as an antineoplastic. **white m., yellow m.**, *Brassica alba* (L.) Rabenh.; it is a source of mustard oil and acrynyl isothiocyanate, and used the same as black mustard (q.v.).

Mustard operation (mus′tard) [William Thornton *Mustard*, Canadian surgeon, born 1914] see under *operation*.

Mustargen (mus′tar-jen) trademark for a preparation of mechlorethamine hydrochloride.

mutacism (mu′tah-sizm) 1. the improper pronunciation of the sounds of mute letters. 2. mytacism.

mutagen (mu′tah-jen) [*muta*tion + *gen*esis] a chemical or physical agent that induces or increases genetic mutations by causing changes in DNA.

mutagenesis (mu″tah-jen′ě-sis) [*mutation* + *genesis*] 1. the production of change. 2. the induction of genetic mutation.

mutagenic (mu″tah-jen′ĭk) 1. causing change. 2. inducing genetic mutation.

mutagenicity (mu″tah-jě-nis′ĭ-te) the property of being able to induce genetic mutation.

Mutamycin (mu″tah-mi′sin) trademark for a preparation of mitomycin.

mutant (mu′tant) [L. *mutare* to change] 1. a gene or organism that has undergone genetic mutation. 2. produced by mutation.

mutarotase (mu″tah-ro′tās) aldose 1-epimerase.

mutarotation (mu″tah-ro-ta′shun) a change in the optical activity of a freshly prepared solution of a pure compound that occurs because of the formation of diastereoisomers of the original compound having different optical activity, e.g., the equilibrium of the α and β anomers of glucose. When equilibrium is reached the optical activity is different from that of the pure material.

mutase (mu′tās) [EC 5.4] one of a subclass of enzymes of the isomerase class that catalyzes the intramolecular shifting of a chemical group (acyl, phospho, amino, or other group) from one position to another.

mutation (mu-ta′shun) [L. *mutatio*, from *mutare* to change] 1. a change in form, quality, or some other characteristic. 2. in genetics, a permanent transmissible change in the genetic material, usually in a single gene. Also, an individual exhibiting such a change. Called also (in classical genetics) a *sport*. **allelic m's**, see *multiple alleles*, under *allele*. **amber m.**, see *nonsense m*. **auxotrophic m.**, a mutation resulting in the inability of bacteria to grow on minimal media. **biochemical m.**, nutritional m. **chromosomal m.**, a mutation affecting large regions of a chromosome and caused by breakage, e.g., by *deletion*, by *inversion*, in which a section of chromosome is inserted in reverse order, and by *translocation*, in which a piece of one chromosome attaches to another. See also *genomic m*. and *point m*. **clear plaque m.**, a mutation resulting in clear plaque formation by a temperate phage that usually makes turbid plaques on bacterial lawns. **cold-sensitive m.**, a conditional mutation producing a gene functional at high temperatures and nonfunctional at low. **conditional m.**, a mutation affecting an organism's phenotype under restrictive growth conditions but not under permissive growth conditions; the wild type is expressed equivalently under both growth conditions. See also *temperature-sensitive m*. **conditional lethal m.**, a mutation lethal only under certain environmental or genetic conditions; see also *lethal m*. **constitutive m.**, a mutation resulting in the formation of a product in the absence of the inducer, either by modifying an operator so that the repressor cannot combine with it or by modifying the regulator so that no repressor is formed. **forward m.**, a point mutation proceeding from the normal wild type to the mutant; cf. *reverse m*. **frameshift m.**, mutation resulting from an addition or subtraction that is not an exact multiple of 3 base pairs in a coding sequence. From the point of mutation onwards, base triplets (codons) are read out of phase; the reading frame of the gene is changed, and a completely different set of amino acids is made into protein. Called also *reading frameshift m*. **genomic m.**, a mutation affecting the number of chromosomes present, e.g., aneuploidy, in which the genome gains or loses one or more chromosomes, and polyploidy, in which the overall chromosome number is doubled or tripled. See also *chromosomal m*. and *point m*. **germinal m.**, a mutation in a germ cell; it generally does not affect the phenotype of the individual in which it first occurs but can be transmitted to offspring. See also *somatic m*. **homoeotic m.**, a mutation interfering with the correct interpretation of positional information. **induced m.**, a genetic mutation caused by external factors which are experimentally or accidentally produced; see also *spontaneous m*. **lethal m.**, a mutation that destroys a gene's ability to produce an active form of an indispensable protein; see also *conditional lethal m*. **missense m.**, one that changes a codon so that it codes for a different amino acid; cf. *nonsense m*. **natural m.**, spontaneous m. **nonsense m.**, a mutation in which one of the three terminator codons in the mRNA (UAG, *amber*; UAA, *ochre*; UGA, *umber* or *opal*), used to signal the end of a polypeptide, appears in the middle of a genetic message, causes premature termination of transcription, and releases incomplete, generally nonfunctional polypeptides from the ribosome. See also *missense m*. **nutritional m.**, a mutation affecting an organism's ability to produce a molecule, e.g., an amino acid, essential for growth; called also *biochemical m*. **ochre m.**, see *nonsense m*. **opal m.**, see *nonsense m*. **point m.**, a mutation resulting from a change in a single base pair in the DNA molecule, caused by the substitution of one nucleotide for another. See also *chromosomal m*. and *genomic m*. **reading frameshift m.**, frameshift m. **reverse m.**, a point mutation reverting from the mutant to the normal wild type; cf. *forward m.* **silent m.,** a mutation that has no detectable phenotypic effect. **somatic m.,** a mutation in a somatic cell, not in a germ cell; it may affect the phenotype in which it occurs since it provides the basis for mosaicism, but generally the mutation will not be transmitted to offspring. Somatic mutations have been proposed as causes of aging and cancer. See also *germinal m.* **spontaneous m's,** mutations occurring at a low but measurable rate in all organisms, presumably because of the inherent rates of error in the replication and transmission of a genome. Called also *natural m.* See also *induced m.* **suppressor m.,** see *suppression,* def. 3. **temperature-sensitive (t-s) m.,** a conditional mutation resulting in an abnormality at one temperature, but not at others; see also *cold-sensitive m.* **umber m.,** see *nonsense m.* **visible m.,** a mutation affecting a morphological trait and for which screening is done by inspection.

mutational (mu-ta′shun-al) pertaining to mutation.

mute (mūt) [L. *mutus*] 1. unable to speak. 2. one who cannot speak. **deaf m.,** see *deaf-mute.*

mutein (mu′te-in) [from *mutant-protein*] a name suggested for a protein arising as a result of a mutation; it is analogous to the wild-type protein but does not necessarily have the same enzymological, immunological, or physicochemical properties.

mutilation (mu″tĭ-la′shun) [L. *mutilatio*] the act of depriving an individual of a limb, member, or other important part; deprival of an organ; castration.

Mutisia (mu-tiz′e-ah) a genus of plants. **M. vici aefo′lia,** a composite-flowered plant of South America, used there as a sedative and in various diseases of the heart, respiratory organs, and nervous system.

mutism (mu′tizm) [L. *mutus* unable to speak, inarticulate] inability or refusal to speak. **akinetic m.,** a state in which the individual makes no spontaneous movement or sound. **deaf m.,** inability to speak as a result of deafness and never having heard spoken words. **elective m.** [DSM III-R], a mental disorder of childhood characterized by continuous refusal to speak in social situations by a child who is able and willing to speak to selected persons.

mutualism (mu′tu-al-izm″) symbiosis in which both populations (or individuals) gain from the association and are unable to survive without it.

mutualist (mu′tu-al-ist) any organism or species associated with another in a relationship which is beneficial to both.

muzolimine (mu-zo′lĭ-mēn) chemical name: 5-amino-2-[1-(3,4-dichlorophenyl)ethyl]-2,4-dihydro-3*H*-pyrazol-3-one; a diuretic and antihypertensive, $C_{11}H_{11}Cl_2N_3O$.

M.V. abbreviation for L. *Med′icus Veterina′rius,* veterinary physician.

Mv chemical symbol for *mendelevium.*

mV millivolt.

μV microvolt.

μW microwatt.

Mx Medex.

My. myopia.

my. mayer.

myalgia (mi-al′je-ah) [*my-* + *algia*] pain in a muscle or muscles. **m. abdom′inis,** pain in the abdominal wall. **m. cap′itis,** pain in the scalp muscles; cephalalgia or headache. **m. cervica′lis,** torticollis. **epidemic m.,** see under *pleurodynia.* **lumbar m.,** lumbago.

Myambutol (mi-am′bu-tol) trademark for a preparation of ethambutol hydrochloride.

Myanesin (mi-an′ĕ-sin) trademark for a preparation of mephenesin.

myasis (mi-a′sis) myiasis.

myasthenia (mi″as-the′ne-ah) [*my-* + Gr. *astheneia* weakness] muscular debility; any constitutional anomaly of muscle. **angiosclerotic m.,** intermittent claudication. **m. gas′trica,** weakness and loss of tone in the muscular coats of the stomach; atony of the stomach. **m. gra′vis, m. gra′vis pseudoparalyt′ica,** a disorder of neuromuscular function due to the presence of antibodies to acetylcholine receptors at the neuromuscular junction; clinically there is fatigue and exhaustion of the muscular system with a tendency to fluctuate in severity and without sensory distur-

bance or atrophy. The disorder may be restricted to a muscle group or become generalized with severe weakness and, in some cases, ventilatory insufficiency. It may affect any muscle of the body, but especially those of the eye, face, lips, tongue, throat, and neck. **m. laryn′gis,** disability of the phonatory laryngeal muscles from overuse, debilitating conditions, or age. **neonatal m.,** a transient (a week to a month) myasthenia affecting offspring of myasthenic women, characteristically marked by difficulty in sucking and swallowing.

myasthenic (mi″as-then′ik) pertaining to or characterized by muscular weakness

myatonia (mi″ah-to′ne-ah) [*my-* + *a* neg. + Gr. *tonos* tension] amyotonia. **m. congen′ita,** amyotonia congenita.

myatony (mi-at′o-ne) myatonia.

myatrophy (mi-at′ro-fe) [*my-* + *atrophy*] atrophy of a muscle; muscular atrophy.

myautonomy (mi″aw-ton′o-me) [*my-* + Gr. *autos* self + *nomos* law] a condition in which muscular contraction aroused by stimulation is so long delayed that it appears to occur independently of the stimulation.

mycelial (mi-se′le-al) pertaining to a mycelium.

mycelian (mi-se′le-an) mycelial.

mycelioid (mi-se′le-oid) having the radiate filamentous appearance of mold colonies.

mycelium (mi-se′le-um), pl. *myce′lia* [*myc-* + Gr. *hēlos* nail] the mass of threadlike processes (hyphae) constituting the fungal thallus.

mycete (mi′sēt) [Gr. *mykēs* fungus] a fungus, def. 1.

mycethemia (mi″sě-the′me-ah) [*myceto-* + Gr. *haima* blood + *-ia*] the presence of fungi in the blood.

mycetism (mi′sě-tizm) mycetismus.

mycetismus (mi″sě-tiz′mus) poisoning caused by a fungus, as that resulting from ingestion of poisonous mushrooms. **m. cer′ebris,** a hallucinogenic intoxication following the ingestion of any of several species of mushrooms. **m. cholerifor′mis,** a serious and often fatal intoxication caused by ingestion of *Amanita phalloides, A. verna,* and probably other *Amanita* species which produce phalloidin; it is characterized by abdominal pain, vomiting, diarrhea, bloody stools, protein and casts in the urine, malaise, and cyanosis. **m. gastrointestina′lis,** a mild form of mycotoxicosis marked by nausea which may be followed by vomiting and diarrhea; it is caused by the ingestion of the orange jack-o-lantern mushroom (*Clitocybe illudens*) and many other species. **m. nervo′sus,** mushroom poisoning caused by ingestion of *Amanita patherina* and *A. muscaria,* which elaborate muscarine, a parasympathetic stimulant; it is marked by such symptoms as tearing, sweating, salivation, persistent peristalsis, retching and vomiting, contraction of the pupil and ciliary muscles, acute excitement, delirium, and coma. **m. sanguina′rius,** mushroom poisoning marked by hemoglobinuria, abdominal distress, and jaundice, caused by ingestion of *Helvella esculenta* and other *Helvella* species.

mycet(o)- see *myc(o)-.*

mycetogenic, mycetogenous (mi″sě-to-jen′ik; mi″sě-toj′ě-nus) [*myceto-* + Gr. *gennan* to produce] caused by fungous growths.

mycetoma (mi″sě-to′mah) [*myceto-* + *-oma*] 1. a chronic, initially localized, slowly progressive, destructive infection of the cutaneous and subcutaneous tissues, fascia, and bone caused by a diverse group of agents that includes certain of

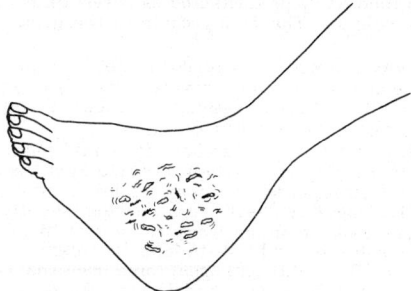

Mycetoma affecting the foot (Madura foot).

PRINCIPAL ETIOLOGIC AGENTS OF MYCETOMA

AGENT	GRAIN COLOR
Actinomycotic	
Actinomyces israelii	white to yellow
Nocardia asteroides	white (when present)
Nocardia brasiliensis	white
Nocardia caviae	white to yellow
Nocardia farcinica[a]	white to yellow
Actinomadura madurae	white to yellow or pink
Actinomadura pellitieri	red
Streptomyces somaliensis	yellow to brown
Eumycotic	
Pseudallescheria boydii	white
Madurella grisea[b]	black
Madurella mycetomatis	black
Acremonium kiliense	white
Acremonium recifei	white
Leptosphaeria senegalensis	black
Pyreochaeta romeroi[b]	black

[a]Believed by some to be within the species limits of *Nocardia asteroides*.
[b]Believed to be related if not identical.

the actinomycetes (*actinomycotic m.*) or true fungi (*eumycotic m.*), acquired as a result of traumatic implantation of the etiologic fungus or bacterium from an exogenous source, and usually involving the foot (Madura foot) or leg, although the hand or any other site may be inoculated. The primary lesion is a tumefaction accompanied by the formation of granulomas, suppurating abscesses, and multiple sinuses from which are discharged grains or granules of various colors that represent microcolonies of the etiologic pathogen. Called also *maduromycosis*. See also accompanying illustration and table. **actinomycotic m.,** that caused by infection with certain actinomycetes; called also *actinomycetoma*. See accompanying table. **eumycotic m.,** that caused by infection with certain true fungi; called also *eumycetoma*. See accompanying table.

Mycetozoa (mi-se″to-zo′ah) [*myceto-* + Gr. *zōon* animal] see Mycetozoida.

Mycetozoida (mi″se-to-zoi′dah) [*myceto-* + Gr. *zōon* animal] in former systems of classification, an order comprising multinucleate rhizopod protozoa occurring as large protoplasmic masses, which in more current classifications have been assigned to the classes Acrasea, Eumyceta, Eumycetozoa, and Plasmodiaphorea. These organisms have also been considered by some to be closely related to the lower fungi and classified in the order Myxomycetes (slime fungi or molds), and by others to be more closely related to the protozoa and classified in the order Mycetozoa (slime animals).

mycid (mi′sid) dermatophytid.

Mycifradin (mi-sif′rah-din) trademark for preparations of neomycin sulfate.

myc(o)-, mycet(o)- [Gr. *mykēs*, gen. *mykētos* fungus] a combining form denoting relationship to fungus.

mycobacteria (mi″ko-bak-te′re-ah) plural of *mycobacterium*.

Mycobacteriaceae (mi″ko-bak-te″re-a′se-e) a family of bacteria, order Actinomycetales, made up of slightly curved or straight, rod-shaped, gram-positive, aerobic, mesophilic cells, sometimes branching. The organisms are found in soil, water, and dairy products and as parasites in humans and lower animals. The family contains the genus *Mycobacterium*.

mycobacteriosis (mi″ko-bak-te″re-o′sis) any tuberculosis-like disease caused by mycobacteria other than *Mycobacterium tuberculosis*; these include Group I–IV mycobacteria. Called also *atypical tuberculosis*.

Mycobacterium (mi″ko-bak-te′re-um) [*myco-* + Gr. *baktērion* little rod] a genus of bacteria of the family Mycobacteriaceae, order Actinomycetales, occurring as gram-positive, aerobic, mostly slow-growing, slightly curved or straight rods, sometimes branching and filamentous, and distinguished by acid-fast staining. It contains many species, including the highly pathogenic organisms that cause tuberculosis (*M. tuberculosis*) and leprosy (*M. leprae*). **M. absces′sus,** *M. chelonei*. **M. africa′num,** a species re-

sembling *M. bovis* and *M. tuberculosis* that is the cause of human disease in tropical Africa. **M. a′quae,** *M. gordonae*. **M. a′vium–intracellula′ re,** a complex of slow-growing, nonphotochromogenic organisms that cause tuberculosis in birds and swine and are associated with human pulmonary disease, lymphadenitis in children, and serious systemic disease in AIDS patients. **M. bal′nei,** *M. marinum*. **M. borstelen′se,** *M. chelonei*. **M. bo′vis,** a virulent species, isolated originally from tuberculous tubercles in cattle, that causes tuberculosis in humans and lower animals. In humans, the disease is usually acquired by children from infected milk. An attenuated strain of *M. bovis* is used to prepare BCG vaccine. **M. brunen′se,** *M. avium–intracellulare*. **M. bu′ruli,** *M. ulcerans*. **M. chelo′nei,** a rapid-growing, nonphotochromogenic species that is an opportunist pathogen, found in soil and recovered from sputum and soft tissue abscesses throughout the body. It produces synovial lesions, gluteal abscesses, and gross lesions in various organs. Called also *M. abscessus* and *M. borstelense*. **M. flaves′cens,** a scotochromogenic species isolated from drug-treated tuberculous guinea pigs but considered nonpathogenic for humans. **M. fortu′itum,** a rapid-growing, nonphotochromogenic species that is potentially pathogenic, producing lesions of lung, bone, or soft tissue following trauma. It has been found in soil and in injection sites of humans, cattle, and cold-blooded animals. Called also *M. ranae*. **M. gas′tri,** a nonpathogenic species found in soil and gastric and sputum specimens obtained from humans. **M. gi′ae,** *M. fortuitum*. **M. gordo′nae,** a nonpathogenic, scotochromogenic species found in tap water and soil and in human sputum and gastric lavage. **M. haba′na,** *M. simiae*. **M. haemo′philum,** a nonphotochromogenic, pathogenic species that requires hemin for growth; associated with skin lesions in immunosuppressed patients. **M. intracellula′re,** see *M. avium–intracellulare*. **M. kansas′ii,** a slow-growing, photochromogenic species. It is the etiologic agent of a tuberculosis-like disease in humans and is frequently isolated from human pulmonary secretions or tubercles. Called also *M. luciflavum*. See also *photochromogen*. **M. lep′rae,** the causative agent of human leprosy, not yet cultivated in vitro, isolated from suspect lesions as acid-fast bacilli. They typically occur in intracellular clumps or rounded masses or in groups of bacilli side by side. **M. lepraemu′rium,** a noncultivable species resembling *M. leprae* in size and shape, which causes a chronic epizootic disease in wild rats; see also *rat leprosy*, under *leprosy*. **M. littora′le,** *M. xenopi*. **M. lucifla′vum,** *M. kansasii*. **M. malmoen′se,** a slow-growing, nonphotochromogenic species associated with pulmonary disease in humans. **M. maria′num,** *M. scrofulaceum*. **M. mari′num,** a moderate-growing, photochromogenic species found in aquariums, diseased fish, and swimming pools. It is the cause of cutaneous lesions and granulomas (swimming pool granuloma) in humans. Called also *M. balnei* and *M. platypoecilus*. **M. micro′ti,** a species producing generalized tuberculosis in field mice and also infecting guinea pigs, rabbits, and calves. It is not virulent for humans and has been used for the preparation of experimental vaccines. Called also *vole bacillus* and *M. tuberculosis* var. *muris*. **M. minet′ti,** *M. fortuitum*. **M. moel′leri,** *M. phlei*. **M. nonchromoge′nicum,** a slow-growing, nonphotochromogenic, nonpathogenic species found in soil. **nontuberculous mycobacteria,** mycobacteria other than *M. tuberculosis* or *M. bovis*. They are divided into four groups (Runyon groups) based on pigmentation and rate of growth, each group consisting of several species. Group I refers to slow-growing photochromogens; group II to slow-growing scotochromogens; group III to slow-growing nonphotochromogens; and group IV to rapidly growing mycobacteria. Called also *anonymous* or *atypical mycobacteria*. **M. paraffi′nicum,** *M. scrofulaceum*. **M. paratuberculo′sis,** the causative agent of Johne's disease, a chronic enteritis of cattle, sheep, and goats; nonpathogenic for man. Called also *Johne's bacillus*. **M. phle′i,** a rapid-growing, photochromogenic, nonpathogenic species found in grasses and soil. Called also *M. moelleri* and *timothy bacillus*. **M. platypoe′cilus,** *M. marinum*. **M. ra′nae,** *M. fortuitum*. **M. scrofula′ceum,** a slow-growing, scotochromogenic species found in human secretions, particularly pus from suppurating cervical lymphadenitis in children. It also occurs in human sputum and gastric lavage, sometimes in association with pulmonary disease. Called also *M. marianum* and *M. paraffinicum*. **M. si′miae,** a slow-growing, photochromogenic species that is sometimes pathogenic. **M. smeg′matis,** a rapid-growing, nonpathogenic, nonphotochromogenic species originally isolated from human smegma and found also in soil and water. Called also *smegma bacillus.* **M. szul′gai,** a slow-growing, pathogenic species that behaves as a scotochromogen at 37° C. and as a photochromogen at 25° C. It is associated with pulmonary infections but may be found in nonpulmonary sites. **M. ter′rae,** a slow-growing, nonpathogenic, nonpigmented species found in soil, water, and human sputum and gastric lavage specimens. **M. trivia′le,** a slow-growing, nonpathogenic, nonpigmented species isolated from sputum and gastric washings. **M. tuberculo′sis,** a slow-growing, nonphotochromogenic, pathogenic species that is the causative agent of tuberculosis in man, other primates, dogs, guinea pigs, and hamsters. Infection in man is commonly pulmonary, but strains of low virulence have also been isolated from cases of lupus erythematosus, scrofuloderma, and urogenital tuberculosis. Called also *tubercle bacillus* and *M. tuberculosis* var. *hominis.* **M. tuberculo′sis** var. **a′vium,** *M. avium–intracellulare.* **M. tuberculo′sis** var. **bo′vis,** *M. bovis.* **M. tuberculo′sis** var. **hom′inis,** *M. tuberculosis.* **M. tuberculo′sis** var. **mu′ris,** *M. microti.* **M. ul′cerans,** a slow-growing, nonphotochromogenic species that causes chronic skin lesions in humans (Buruli ulcer). **M. vac′cae,** a rapid-growing, scotochromogenic, nonpathogenic species, widely distributed in nature and found in cattle. **M. xeno′pi,** a slow-growing, scotochromogenic species occurring usually harmlessly in human secretions but occasionally associated with chronic pulmonary disease. Called also *M. littorale.*

mycobacterium (mi″ko-bak-te′re-um), pl. *mycobacte′ria.* an organism of the genus *Mycobacterium.* **anonymous mycobacteria, atypical mycobacteria,** nontuberculous mycobacteria. **Group I–IV mycobacteria,** nontuberculous mycobacteria.

mycobactin (mi″ko-bak′tin) a complex lipophilic compound found in the cell envelope of certain species of *Mycobacterium;* it is also required for growth by at least one species. Mycobactin chelates iron and facilitates iron transport into the cell.

Mycocandida (mi″ko-kan′dĭ-dah) *Candida.*

mycocidin (mi″ko-si′din) an antibiotic substance extracted from a mold (Aspergillaceae); active in vivo against *Mycobacterium tuberculosis.*

Mycococcus (mi″ko-kok′us) a genus of bacteria of uncertain taxonomic status, formerly classified in the family Mycobacteriaceae.

Mycoderma (mi″ko-der′mah) [*myco-* + Gr. *derma* skin] a former genus of imperfect fungi of the order Moniliales, family Moniliaceae, most species of which are now included in the genus *Candida.* **M. ace′ti,** a name formerly given a combination of yeasts, which together with bacteria, such as *Acetobacter aceti,* grow on the surface of fermenting fluids and produce acetic acid from fermentation of alcohol. **M. dermati′tidis,** *Blastomyces dermatitidis.* **M. immi′te,** *Coccidioides immitis.*

mycoderma (mi″ko-der′mah) [Gr. *mykos* mucus + *derma* skin] mucous membrane (tunica mucosa [NA]).

mycodermatitis (mi″ko-der″mah-ti′tis) candidiasis.

mycoflora (mi″ko-flo′rah) the number and varieties of fungi present in or characteristic of a specific location.

mycohemia (mi″ko-he′me-ah) [*myco-* + Gr. *haima* blood + *-ia*] the presence of fungi in the blood.

mycolic acids (mi-ko′lik) α-alkyl, β-hydroxy substituted long chain fatty acids found in the cell walls of bacteria in the genera *Mycobacterium, Nocardia,* and *Corynebacterium;* they may be responsible for the acid-fast staining properties of these organisms.

mycologist (mi-kol′o-jist) a person specializing in mycology; a student of mycology.

mycology (mi-kol′o-je) [*myco-* + *-logy*] the science and study of fungi.

mycomyringitis (mi″ko-mir″in-ji′tis) [*myco-* + L. *myringa* membrana tympani + *-itis*] myringomycosis.

mycopathology (mi″ko-pah-thol′o-je) the scientific study of the pathologic changes caused by fungi.

mycophage (mi″ko-fāj) [*myco-* + Gr. *phagein* to eat] a virus that infects fungi and may cause their lysis.

mycophagy (mi-kof′ah-je) ingestion of mushrooms and other fungi.

Mycoplasma (mi″ko-plaz′mah) [*myco-* + Gr. *plasma* anything formed or molded] a genus of bacteria of the family Mycoplasmataceae, order Mycoplasmatales, class Mollicutes, made up of highly pleomorphic, gram-negative cells that are spherical to ovoid shaped, bounded by a single triple-layered membrane but lacking a true cell wall. Cholesterol, or another sterol, is required for growth. The genus includes the species causing pleuropneumonia in cattle (*M. mycoides*) and the species comprising the pleuropneumonia-like organisms (PPLO). The organisms are parasites and pathogens, widely distributed on the mucous membranes of humans, animals, and birds. Mycoplasmas are also common contaminants of animal cell cultures. Formerly called *Asterococcus.* **M. bucca′le,** a common inhabitant of the oropharynx of nonhuman primates. Called also *M. orale type 2.* **M. ca′nis,** a nonpathogenic species commonly found in the throat and respiratory and genital tracts of dogs. **M. fau′cium,** a species found occasionally in the oropharynx of humans and frequently in the oropharynx of nonhuman primates. Called also *M. orale type 3.* **M. fermen′tans,** a species occasionally isolated from the mucosa of the genital tract and oropharynx of humans. **M. gallisep′ticum,** a pathogen for poultry, causing respiratory disease, encephalitis, and infectious arthritis in chicken and turkeys. **M. granula′rum,** *Acholeplasma granularum.* **M. hom′inis,** a common parasitic inhabitant of the vagina and cervix and a potential human pathogen, causing infections of the male and female reproductive tracts. It has also been associated with respiratory disease and pharyngitis. **M. hyoarthrino′sa,** a species of uncertain status, reported to cause arthritis in swine. **M. hyorhi′nis,** a common parasite of the nasal cavity in swine; a possible cause of pneumonia and arthritis in swine. **M. laidlaw′ii,** *Acholeplasma laidlawii.* **M. mycoi′des,** the type species of *Mycoplasma,* which is the etiologic agent of contagious pleuropneumonia (def. 2) in cattle and goats. Called also *Bovimyces pleuropneumoniae.* **M. ora′le,** a species found in the upper respiratory tract of humans and primates. Called also *M. orale type 1* and *M. pharyngis.* **M. ora′le type 1,** *M. orale.* **M. ora′le type 2,** *M. buccale.* **M. ora′le type 3,** *M. faucium.* **M. pharyn′gis,** *M. orale.* **M. pneumo′niae,** a species causing inapparent infections and mild respiratory tract disease. It is also an etiologic agent of primary atypical pneumonia. Called also *Eaton agent.* **M. saliva′rium,** a nonpathogenic species found as part of the normal flora of the human oral cavity and upper respiratory tract.

mycoplasma (mi″ko-plaz′mah), pl. *mycopla′smas, mycoplas′mata.* a bacterium of the class Mollicutes. **T-strain m.,** *Ureaplasma urealyticum.*

mycoplasmal (mi″ko-plaz′mal) of, pertaining to, or caused by *Mycoplasma.*

Mycoplasmas (mi″ko-plaz′mahz) Mycoplasmatales.

Mycoplasmataceae (mi″ko-plaz″mah-ta′se-e) a family of bacteria of the order Mycoplasmatales, class Mollicutes, made up of organisms that require a sterol for growth. It contains the genera *Mycoplasma* and *Ureaplasma.*

Mycoplasmatales (mi″ko-plaz″mah-ta′les) an order of bacteria of the class Mollicutes, the members of which are bounded by a triple-layered membrane but lack a rigid cell wall. The order is made up of the families Acholeplasmataceae, Mycoplasmataceae, and Spiroplasmataceae, and two genera of uncertain status, *Anaeroplasma* and *Thermoplasma.* Called also *Mycoplasmas.*

mycoplasmosis (mi″ko-plaz-mo′sis) infection with *Mycoplasma.*

mycoprecipitin (mi″ko-pre-sip′ĭ-tin) [*myco-* + *precipitin*] a precipitin which will precipitate extracts of yeast and fungi.

mycopus (mi′ko-pus) mucus containing pus.

mycorrhiza (mi″ko-ri′zah) [*myco-* + Gr. *rhiza* root] a growth occurring as a result of the symbiotic relationship between certain fungi and the roots of plants and trees; it is most frequently found in poor soil, and is associated with the absorption of minerals and nitrogenous material.

mycose (mi′kōs) [*myc-* + *-ose*] a sugar from ergot and also from trehala manna, $C_{12}H_{22}O_{11}$ + $2H_2O$; trehalose.

mycoside (mi′ko-sīd) a glycolipid that contains mycolic acid and a polysaccharide moiety. A distinctive mycoside found in the cell walls confers immunologic cross-reactivity on cells of *Corynebacterium, Mycobacteria,* and *Nocardia.*

mycosis (mi-ko′sis) [*myco-* + *-osis*] any disease caused by a fungus. **m. fungoi′des,** a chronic or rapidly progressive form of cutaneous T-cell lymphoma (formerly thought to be of fungal origin), which in some cases evolves into generalized lymphoma with a tendency for nodal, hematogenous, and visceral involvement. It may be divided generally into three successive stages: *premycotic,* associated with intensely pruritic erythematous, eczematous, or psoriasiform eruptions; *infiltrated plaques,* or *mycotic,* characterized by the presence of abnormal mononuclear cells (*Sézary cells*)*;* and mushroom-like *tumors* that often ulcerate. The tumor stage (*d'emblée type*) may develop without preceding lesions or prodromal symptoms. Called also *granuloma fungoides.* **m. fungoi′des d'emblée,** see *m. fungoides.* **Gilchrist's m.,** North American blastomycosis. **m. leptoth′rica,** a benign condition of the tonsil and pharynx produced by *Leptotrichia buccalis.* **Posada m.,** coccidioidomycosis. **splenic m.,** siderotic splenomegaly.

mycostasis (mi-kos′tah-sis) [*myco-* + Gr. *stasis* stoppage] prevention of the growth or multiplication of fungi.

mycostat (mi′ko-stat) an agent that inhibits the growth of fungi.

Mycostatin (mi″ko-stat′in) trademark for a preparation of nystatin.

mycosterol (mi-kos′ter-ol) zymosterol.

mycotic (mi-kot′ik) pertaining to a mycosis; caused by fungi.

mycoticopeptic (mi-kot″ĭ-ko-pep′tik) (*obs.*) both mycotic and peptic.

Mycotoruloides (mi″ko-tor″u-loi′dēz) *Candida.*

mycotoxicosis (mi″ko-tok″sĭ-ko′sis) 1. poisoning caused by a fungal or bacterial toxin. 2. poisoning resulting from ingestion of fungi, such as that caused by the fungus *Claviceps purpurea* (ergotism).

mycotoxin (mi″ko-tok′sin) a fungal toxin.

mycotoxinization (mi″ko-tok″sin-i-za′shun) inoculation with a fungal toxin.

mycteric (mik-ter′ik) [Gr. *myktēr* nostril] pertaining to the nasal cavities.

mycteroxerosis (mik″ter-o-ze-ro′sis) [Gr. *myktēr* nostril + *xēros* dry] dryness of the nostrils.

mydaleine (mi-da′le-in) [Gr. *mydaleos* damp, mouldy] a poisonous ptomaine from putrefied viscera. Poisoning by it is attended with salivation, dilatation of the pupils, rise of temperature followed by a fall, and arrest of the heart in diastole.

mydatoxine (mi″dah-tok′sin) [Gr. *mydan* to be damp + *toxin*] a deadly ptomaine, $C_9H_{13}NO_2$, from decaying flesh; also obtained from human intestines kept for a long time at a low temperature.

Mydriacyl (mĭ-dri′ah-sil) trademark for a preparation of tropicamide.

mydriasis (mĭ-dri′ah-sis) [Gr.] 1. physiologic dilatation of the pupil. 2. morbid dilatation of the pupil. 3. dilatation of the pupil effected by a drug. **alternating m.,** varying inequality of the pupils, mydriasis occurring first on one side, then on the other; called also *bounding* or *springing m.* **bounding m.,** alternating mydriasis. **paralytic m.,** that caused by paralysis of the oculomotor nerve. **spasmodic m., spastic m.,** that due to spasm of the dilator of the iris or to overaction of the sympathetic. **spinal m.,** that due to lesion of the ciliospinal center of the spinal cord. **springing m.,** alternating m.

mydriatic (mid″re-at′ik) 1. dilating the pupil. 2. any drug that dilates the pupil.

myectomy (mi-ek′to-me) [*my-* + Gr. *ektomē* excision] excision of a portion of muscle.

myectopia (mi-ek-to′pe-ah) [Gr. *mys* muscle + *ektopos* displaced + *-ia*] displacement of a muscle.

myectopy (mi-ek′to-pe) myectopia.

myelacephalus (mi″el-ah-sel′ah-lus) [*myel-* + *a* neg. + Gr. *kephalē* head] the lowest grade of acephalous monster, being only slightly above a fetus amorphus.

myelalgia (mi″ĕ-lal′je-ah) [*myel-* + *-algia*] pain in the spinal cord.

myelapoplexy (mi″el-ap′o-plek-se) [*myel-* + *apoplexy*] hematomyelia.

myelasthenia (mi″el-as-the′ne-ah) [*myel-* + *asthenia*] neurasthenia due to some cause which affects the spinal cord.

myelatelia (mi″el-ah-te′le-ah) [*myel-* + Gr. *ateleia* imperfection] imperfect development of the spinal cord.

myelatrophy (mi″el-at′ro-fe) [*myel-* + *atrophy*] atrophy of the spinal cord.

myelauxe (mi″el-awks′e) [*myel-* + Gr. *auxē* increase] morbid increase in size of the spinal cord.

myelemia (mi″ĕ-le′me-ah) [*myel-* + Gr. *haima* blood + *-ia*] myelocytosis.

myelencephalitis (mi″ĕ-len-sef″ah-li′tis) inflammation of the brain and spinal cord.

myelencephalon (mi″ĕ-len-sef′ah-lon) [*myel-* + Gr. *enkephalos* brain] 1. NA alternative for *medulla oblongata;* see Plate accompanying *brain.* 2. the posterior of the two brain vesicles formed by specialization of the rhombencephalon in the developing embryo.

myelencephalospinal (mi″ĕ-len-sef″ah-lo-spi′nal) pertaining to the myelencephalon and spinal cord.

myeleterosis (mi″ĕ-let″er-o′sis) [*myel-* + Gr. *heterōsis* alteration] morbid alteration of the spinal cord.

myelin (mi′ĕ-lin) [Gr. *myelos* marrow] 1. the substance of the cell membrane of Schwann's cells that coils to form the myelin sheath (see under *sheath*); it has a high proportion of lipid to protein and serves as an electrical insulator. Called also *white substance of Schwann.* 2. any one of a certain group of lipid substances found in various normal and pathologic tissues and differing from fats in being doubly refractive. 3. a monoaminomonophosphatide found in small quantities in the brain.

myelinated (mi′ĕ-lĭ-nāt″ed) having a myelin sheath.

myelination (mi″ĕ-lĭ-na′shun) myelinization.

myelinic (mi″ĕ-lin′ik) pertaining to or of the nature of myelin.

myelinization (mi″e-lĭ-ni-za′shun) the act of furnishing with or taking on myelin.

myelinoclasis (mi″ĕ-lin-ok′lah-sis) [*myelin* + Gr. *klasis* a breaking] destruction of myelin; demyelination. **acute perivascular m.,** acute disseminated encephalomyelitis. **central pontine m.,** central pontine myelinolysis. **postinfection perivenous m.,** postinfection encephalomyelopathy.

myelinogenesis (mi″ĕ-lin″o-jen′ĕ-sis) myelinization.

myelinogenetic (mi″ĕ-lin″o-jĕ-net′ik) producing myelin; producing myelinization.

myelinogeny (mi″ĕ-lĭ-noj′ĕ-ne) [*myelin* + Gr. *gennan* to produce] the development of the myelin of nerve fibers; the myelinization of nerve fibers.

myelinolysis (mi″ĕ-lin-ol′ĭ-sis) destruction of myelin; demyelination. **central pontine m.,** a rare form of massive demyelination of the pons occurring in alcoholics; called also *central pontine myelinoclasis.*

myelinopathy (mi″ĕ-lĭ-nop′ah-the) any disease of the myelin; degeneration of the white matter of the brain.

myelinosis (mi″ĕ-lĭ-no′sis) a form of fatty necrosis in which myelin is formed.

myelinotoxic (mi″ĕ-lin-o-tok′sik) having a deleterious effect on myelin; causing demyelination.

myelinotoxicity (mi″ĕ-lin-o-tok-sis′ĭ-te) the property of being myelinotoxic.

myelitic (mi″ĕ-lit′ik) pertaining to myelitis.

myelitis (mi″ĕ-li′tis) [Gr. *myelos* marrow + *-itis*] 1. inflammation of the spinal cord (see *leukomyelitis, poliomyelitis*). The symptoms of myelitis vary with the location of the lesion, and include pain in the back, girdle sensation, hyperesthesia, formication, anesthesia, motor disturbances, paralysis, increase of the reflexes, paralysis of the sphincters, decubitus ulcers and, in later stages, spasmodic contractions of the paralyzed limbs. In practice, the term is also used to denote noninflammatory lesions of the spinal cord; see *myelopathy.* 2. inflammation of the bone marrow; see *osteomyelitis.* **acute m.,** any acute inflammatory disease of the spinal cord. **apoplectiform m.,** see under *myelopathy.* **ascending m.,** see under *myelopathy.* **bulbar m.,** that which involves the medulla oblongata. **cavitary m.,** syringomyelitis. **central m.,** inflammation affecting chiefly the gray substance of the spinal cord. **chronic m.,** a slowly progressing inflammation of the spinal cord. **compression m.,** see under *myelopathy.* **concussion m.,** see under *myelopathy.* **cornual m.,** that which affects the horns of gray matter of the spinal cord. **descending m.,** see under *myelopathy.* **diffuse m.,** inflammation involving large and variously placed sections of the spinal cord. **disseminated m.,** a form with several distinct foci in the spinal cord. **focal m.,** see under *myelopathy.* **foudroyant m.,** central m. **funicular m.,** see under *myelopathy.* **hemorrhagic m.,** see under *myelopathy.* **interstitial m.,** sclerosing myelopathy. **neuro-optic m.,** neuromyelitis optica. **parenchymatous m.,** see under *myelopathy.* **periependymal m.,** myelitis surrounding the central canal of the spinal cord. **sclerosing m.,** see under *myelopathy.* **systemic m.,** see under *myelopathy.* **transverse m.,** see under *myelopathy.* **traumatic m.,** see under *myelopathy.* **m. vaccin′ia,** that which sometimes follows vaccination.

myel(o)- [Gr. *myelos* marrow] a combining form denoting relationship to marrow, to the spinal cord, or to myelin.

myeloarchitecture (mi″ĕ-lo-ar′kĭ-tek″tūr) 1. the arrangement of nerve fibers in the cerebral and cerebellar cortices. 2. the organization of the nerve tracts in the spinal cord and brain stem.

myeloblast (mi′ĕ-lo-blast″) [*myelo-* + Gr. *blastos* germ] an immature cell found in the bone marrow and not normally in the peripheral blood; it is the most primitive precursor in the granulocytic series, which matures to develop into the promyelocyte and eventually the granular leukocyte. Myeloblasts have fine, evenly distributed chromatin, several nucleoli, and a nongranular basophilic cytoplasm. Called also *granuloblast.*

myeloblastemia (mi″ĕ-lo-blas-te′me-ah) [*myeloblast* + Gr. *haima* blood + *-ia*] presence of myeloblasts in the blood.

myeloblastoma (mi″ĕ-lo-blas-to′mah) [*myeloblast* + *-oma*] a focal malignant tumor, observed in acute myelogenous leukemia, composed of myeloblasts and lacking green coloration.

myeloblastomatosis (mi″ĕ-lo-blas″to-mah-to′sis) the presence of multiple myeloblastomas.

myeloblastosis (mi″ĕ-lo-blas-to′sis) the presence of an excess of myeloblasts in the blood.

myelocele (mi′ĕ-lo-sēl) [*myelo-* + Gr. *kēlē* hernia] protrusion of the substance of the spinal cord through a defect in the bony spinal canal.

myeloclast (mi′ĕ-lo-klast) [*myelo-* + Gr. *klan* to break] a cell which splits up myelin sheaths.

myelocoele (mi-el′o-sēl) [*myelo-* + Gr. *koilia* cavity] (*obs.*) the central canal of the spinal cord.

myelocone (mi′ĕ-lo-kōn) [*myelo-* + Gr. *konis* dust] a fatty matter from the brain.

myelocyst (mi′ĕ-lo-sist) [*myelo-* + *cyst*] a benign cyst developed from rudimentary medullary canals.

myelocystic (mi″ĕ-lo-sis′tik) both myeloid and cystic in structure.

myelocystocele (mi″ĕ-lo-sis′to-sēl) [*myelo-* + Gr. *kēlē* hernia] myelomeningocele.

myelocystomeningocele (mi″ĕ-lo-sis″to-mĕ-ning′go-sēl) myelomeningocele.

myelocyte (mi′ĕ-lo-sit) [*myelo-* + *-cyte*] 1. a precursor in the granulocytic series, being a cell intermediate in development between a promyelocyte and a metamyelocyte; in this stage, differentiation into specific cytoplasmic granules has begun. 2. any cell of the gray matter of the nervous system.

myelocythemia (mi″ĕ-lo-si-the′me-ah) [*myelocyte* + Gr. *haima* blood + *-ia*] excess of myelocytes in the blood.

myelocytic (mi″ĕ-lo-sit′ik) relating to or of the nature of myelocytes.

myelocytoma (mi″ĕ-lo-si-to′mah) chronic myelocytic leukemia; myeloma, def. 1.

myelocytomatosis (mi″ĕ-lo-si″to-mah-to′sis) 1. (*obs.*) a form of leukosis in which the myelocytes are chiefly involved. 2. a disease of fowl that is included in the avian leukosis complex, marked by the presence of tumors composed of myeloid cells. There may also be an increase of immature myeloid cells in the circulating blood.

myelocytosis (mi″ĕ-lo-si-to′sis) the presence of an excessive number of myelocytes in the blood; myelosis.

myelodysplasia (mi″ĕ-lo-dis-pla′se-ah) [*myelo-* + *dys-* + Gr. *plassein* to form] defective development of any part (especially the lower segments) of the spinal cord.

myeloencephalic (mi″ĕ-lo-en″sĕ-fal′ik) pertaining to the spinal cord and the brain.

myeloencephalitis (mi″ĕ-lo-en-sef″ah-li′tis) [*myelo-* + Gr. *enkephalos* brain + *-itis*] inflammation of the spinal cord and brain. **eosinophilic m.,** a complex of neurologic symptoms produced by invasion of the central nervous system by *Gnathostoma spinigerum,* including severe nerve root pain, followed by paralysis of extremities and sudden sensorial impairment, accompanied by eosinophilic pleocytosis and bloody or xanthochromic spinal fluid. **epidemic m.,** epidemic polioencephalitis.

myelofibrosis (mi″ĕ-lo-fi-bro′sis) replacement of the bone marrow by fibrous tissue, occurring in association with a myeloproliferative disorder or secondary to another, unrelated condition; called also *myelosclerosis.* See also *myeloid metaplasia,* under *metaplasia.* **osteosclerosis m.,** myelosclerosis, def. 2.

myelofugal (mi″ĕ-lof′u-gal) [*myelo-* + L. *fugare* to flee] moving away from the spinal cord.

myelogenesis (mi″ĕ-lo-jen′ĕ-sis) 1. the development of the nervous system, especially of the brain and spinal cord. 2. the deposition of myelin around the axon.

myelogenic (mi″ĕ-lo-jen′ik) myelogenous.

myelogenous (mi″ĕ-loj′ĕ-nus) [*myelo-* + Gr. *gennan* to produce] produced in the bone marrow.

myelogeny (mi″ĕ-loj′ĕ-ne) the maturation of the myelin sheaths of nerve fibers in the development of the central nervous system.

myelogone (mi′ĕ-lo-gōn″) a white blood cell of the myeloid series having a reticulate violaceous nucleus, well-stained nucleolus, and a deep blue rim of cytoplasm.

myelogonic (mi″ĕ-lo-go′nik) characterized by the presence of myelogones.

myelogonium (mi″ĕ-lo-go′ne-um) myelogone.

myelogram (mi′ĕ-lo-gram) 1. a roentgenogram of the spinal cord. 2. a graphic representation of the differential count of cells found in a stained preparation of bone marrow.

myelography (mi″ĕ-log′rah-fe) [*myelo-* + Gr. *graphein* to write] roentgenography of the spinal cord after injection of a contrast medium into the subarachnoid space. **oxygen m.,** myelography in which oxygen is used as the contrast medium.

myeloid (mi′ĕ-loid) [*myelo-* + Gr. *eidos* form] 1. pertaining to, derived from, or resembling bone marrow. 2. pertaining to the spinal cord. 3. having the appearance of myelocytes, but not derived from bone marrow.

myeloidin (mi″ĕ-loi′din) [*myelin* + Gr. *eidos* form] a substance resembling myelin, occurring in the pigmented cells of the retina.

myeloidosis (mi″ĕ-loi-do′sis) the development of myeloid tissue, especially hyperplastic development of such tissue.

myelokentric (mi″ĕ-lo-ken′trik) [*myeloid* + Gr. *kentron* stimulus] stimulating the formation of myeloid cells. Cf. *lymphokentric.*

myelolipoma (mi″ĕ-lo-lĭ-po′mah) a rare benign tumor of the adrenal gland, several centimeters in diameter, composed in varying proportions of adipose tissue, lymphocytes, and primitive myeloid cells, probably a developmental abnormality.

myelolysis (mi″ĕ-lol′ĭ-sis) [*myelin* + Gr. *lysis* dissolution] the dissolution of myelin.

myelolytic (mi″ĕ-lo-lit′ik) pertaining to, characterized by, or causing myelolysis.

myeloma (mi″ĕ-lo′mah) [*myelo-* + *-oma*] a tumor composed of cells of the type normally found in the bone marrow; see *multiple m.* **endothelial m.,** Ewing's tumor. **giant cell m.,** giant cell tumor of bone. **indolent m.,** a variant of multiple myeloma in which the tumor cells are hypoproliferative; an M component and bone marrow plasmacytosis are present, but significant bone marrow destruction, hypercalcemia, or Bence-Jones proteinuria are absent. **localized m.,** solitary m. **multiple m.,** a disseminated malignant neoplasm of plasma cells characterized by multiple bone marrow tumor foci and secretion of an M component (a monoclonal immunoglobulin or immunoglobulin fragment), associated with widespread osteolytic lesions appearing radiographically as punched-out defects, and resulting in bone pain, pathologic fractures, hypercalcemia, and normochromic normocytic anemia; spread to extraosseous sites occurs frequently in advanced disease. Depression of immunoglobulin levels results in increased susceptibility to infection. Bence Jones proteinuria is present in many cases and occasionally results in systemic amyloidosis. Renal failure, resulting from calcium nephropathy or extensive cast formation, occurs in about 20 per cent of cases. Called also *plasma cell m.* **plasma cell m.,** multiple m. **solitary m.,** a variant of multiple myeloma in which there is a single localized tumor focus. Called also *localized m.*

myelomalacia (mi″ĕ-lo-mah-la′she-ah) [*myelo-* + Gr. *malakia* softening] morbid softening of the spinal cord.

myelomatoid (mi″ĕ-lo′mah-toid) resembling myeloma.

myelomatosis (mi″ĕ-lo-mah-to′sis) multiple myeloma.

myelomenia (mi″ĕ-lo-me′ne-ah) [*myelo-* + Gr. *mēn* month] menstrual hemorrhage into the spinal cord, associated with plaques of endometriosis in the spinal canal.

myelomeningitis (mi″ĕ-lo-men″in-ji′tis) [*myelo-* + *meningitis*] inflammation of the spinal cord and its membranes.

myelomeningocele (mi″ĕ-lo-mĕ-ning′go-sēl) [*myelo-* + *meningocele*] hernial protrusion of the cord and its meninges through a defect in the vertebral canal.

myelomere (mi′ĕ-lo-mēr) [*myelo-* + Gr. *meros* part] one of the segments of the developing brain and spinal cord.

myelomyces (mi″ĕ-lom′ĭ-sēz) [*myelo-* + Gr. *mykēs* fungus] medullary carcinoma.

myelon (mi′ĕ-lon) [Gr. *myelos* marrow] (*obs.*) the spinal cord (medulla spinalis [NA]).

myeloneuritis (mi″ĕ-lo-nu-ri′tis) inflammation of both spinal cord and peripheral nerves.

myelonic (mi″ĕ-lon′ik) pertaining to the myelon; myeloid.

myelo-opticoneuropathy (mi″ĕ-lo-op″tĭ-ko-nu-rop′ah-the) a disorder affecting the spinal cord and optic nerve. **subacute m.,** a clinical syndrome reported from Japan affecting the spinal cord, optic nerve, and peripheral nerves, preceded by diarrhea. Symptoms include paresthesia in both lower limbs, gait disturbances, visual disturbances, abnormalities of deep tendon reflexes, and psychic disorders. The hydroxyquinolones (especially Clioquinol), taken for gastrointestinal disorders, have been implicated as an etiologic factor. Abbreviated SMON.

myelopathic (mi″ĕ-lo-path′ik) pertaining to or characterized by myelopathy.

myelopathy (mi″ĕ-lop′ah-the) [*myelo-* + Gr. *pathos* disease] 1. a general term denoting functional disturbances and/or pathological changes in the spinal cord; the term is often used to designate nonspecific lesions, in contrast to inflammatory lesions (myelitis). 2. pathological changes in the bone marrow. **apoplectiform m.,** myelopathy in which paralysis comes on suddenly. **ascending m.,** myelopathy that progresses cephalad along the spinal cord. **compression m.,** myelopathy due to pressure on the spinal cord, as from a tumor. **concussion m.,** myelopathy due to spinal concussion. **descending m.,** myelopathy that progresses caudad along the spinal cord. **focal m.,** myelopathy affecting a small area only, or several small areas. **funicular m.,** myelopathy involving the white matter of the spinal cord, especially the posterior funiculus; it is characteristic of pernicious anemia. **hemorrhagic m.,** myelopathy associated with hemorrhage. **interstitial m.,** sclerosing m. **parenchymatous m.,** myelopathy in which the proper nerve substance of the spinal cord is chiefly affected. **sclerosing m.,** myelopathy marked by hardening of the spinal cord and overgrowth of the glia; called also *interstitial m.* **spondylotic cervical m.,** myelopathy secondary to encroachment of cervical spondylosis upon a congenitally small cervical spinal canal. **systemic m.,** myelopathy which affects distinct tracts or systems in the spinal cord. **transverse m.,** myelopathy which extends across the spinal cord. **traumatic m.,** myelopathy which follows injury to the spinal cord.

myeloperoxidase (MPO) (mi″ĕ-lo-per-ok′sĭ-dās) an enzyme of the oxidoreductase class that catalyzes the reaction $H_2O_2 + Cl^- = H_2O + OCl^-$. The enzyme is a hemoprotein found in the azurophil granules of neutrophils and mononuclear phagocytes. It has the green color seen in pus. The reaction produces hypochlorites with potent antimicrobial activity. Deficiency of the enzyme, an autosomal recessive trait, is usually asymptomatic.

myeloperoxidase (MPO) deficiency an autosomal recessive trait characterized by the complete absence of MPO in azurophil granules of neutrophils and monocytes; the deficiency is usually clinically insignificant.

myelopetal (mi″ĕ-lop′ĕ-tal) [*myelo-* + L. *petere* to seek for] moving toward the spinal cord.

myelophage (mi′ĕ-lo-fāj″) [*myelo-* + Gr. *phagein* to eat] a macrophage which digests or breaks down myelin.

myelophthisis (mi″ĕ-lof′thĭ-sis) [*myelo-* + Gr. *phthisis* wasting] 1. wasting of the spinal cord. 2. reduction of the cell-forming functions of the bone marrow; see *aleukia haemorrhagica.*

myeloplaque (mi′el-o-plak) myeloplax.

myeloplast (mi′ĕ-lo-plast″) [*myelo-* + Gr. *plastos* formed] any leukocyte of the bone marrow.

myeloplax (mi′el-o-plaks″) [*myelo-* + Gr. *plax* plate] any multinuclear giant cell of the bone marrow.

myeloplegia (mi′ĕ-lo-ple′je-ah) [*myelo-* + Gr. *plēgē* stroke] spinal paralysis.

myelopoiesis (mi″ĕ-lo-poi-e′sis) [*myelo-* + Gr. *poiein* to form] the formation of bone marrow or the cells that arise from it. **ectopic m., extramedullary m.,** the formation of myeloid tissue outside the bone marrow.

myelopore (mi′ĕ-lo-pōr) [*myelo-* + Gr. *poros* opening] a canal or opening in the spinal cord.

myeloproliferative (mi″ĕ-lo-pro-lif′er-ah-tiv) pertaining to or characterized by medullary and extramedullary proliferation of bone marrow constituents, including erythroblasts, granulocytes, megakaryocytes, and fibroblasts. The myeloproliferative disorders comprise a group of usually neoplastic diseases, which may be related histogenetically by a common multipotential stem cell, that includes among others acute and chronic granulocytic leukemias, acute and chronic myelomonocytic leukemias, polycythemia vera, myelofibrosis, myeloid metaplasia, essential thrombocythemia, and erythroleukemia. An interrelationship with the lymphoproliferative (q.v.) disorders is thought to exist. They are called also *myeloproliferative diseases* or *syndromes.*

myeloradiculitis (mi″ĕ-lo-rah-dik″u-li′tis) [*myelo-* + L. *radiculus* rootlet + *-itis*] inflammation of the spinal cord and the posterior nerve roots.

myeloradiculodysplasia (mi″ĕ-lo-rah-dik″u-lo-dis-pla′ze-ah) developmental abnormality of the spinal cord and spinal nerve roots.

myeloradiculopathy (mi″ĕ-lo-rah-dik″u-lop′ah-the) disease of the spinal cord and spinal nerve roots.

myelorrhagia (mi″ĕ-lo-ra′je-ah) [*myelo-* + Gr. *rhēgnynai* to burst forth] hematomyelia.

myelosarcoma (mi″ĕ-lo-sar-ko′mah) a sarcomatous growth made up of myeloid tissue or bone marrow cells.

myelosarcomatosis (mi″ĕ-lo-sar-ko″mah-to′sis) myelomatosis.

myeloschisis (mi″ĕ-los′kĭ-sis) [*myelo-* + Gr. *schisis* cleft] a developmental anomaly characterized by a cleft spinal cord, owing to failure of the neural plate to form a complete tube or to rupture of the neural tube after closure.

myeloscintogram (mi″ĕ-lo-sin′to-gram) the graphic record of particles counted by a scintillation counter after injection into the subarachnoid space of a solution containing a radioactive isotope.

myelosclerosis (mi″ĕ-lo-skle-ro′sis) 1. sclerosis of the spinal cord. 2. a condition characterized by obliteration of the normal marrow cavity by the formation of small spicules of bone, the pathogenesis possibly being similar to that of myelofibrosis; called also *osteosclerosis myelofibrosis.* 3. myelofibrosis.

myelosis (mi″ĕ-lo′sis) 1. the proliferation of marrow tissue which produces the blood changes of myelocytic leukemia; myelocytosis. 2. the formation of a tumor of the spinal cord. **aleukemic m.,** agnogenic myeloid metaplasia; see also *pseudoleukemia.* **chronic nonleukemic m.,** agnogenic myeloid metaplasia. **erythremic m.,** a malignant blood dyscrasia regarded as one of the myeloproliferative disorders and characterized by progressive anemia, megaloblastic erythroid hyperplasia, myeloid dysplasia, hepatosplenomegaly, and hemorrhagic phenomena. Called also *Di Guglielmo's disease* or *syndrome*. Cf. *erythroleukemia*. **funicular m.,** myelosis marked by degenerative foci in the white substance of the spinal cord. **nonleukemic m.,** agnogenic myeloid metaplasia.

myelospasm (mi′ĕ-lo-spazm) [*myelo-* + *spasm*] (obs.) spasm due to disease of the spinal cord.

myelospongium (mi″ĕ-lo-spon′je-um) [*myelo-* + Gr. *spongos* sponge] the network from which the neuroglial tissue is developed: it pervades the embryonic neural tube, and is composed of the spongioblasts and their branching processes.

myelosuppression (mi″ĕ-lo-soo-presh′un) suppression of bone marrow activity, resulting in reduction in the number of platelets, red cells, and white cells.

myelosuppressive (mi″ĕ-lo-sŭ-pres′iv) 1. inhibiting bone marrow activity, resulting in decreased production of blood cells and platelets. 2. an agent having such properties.

myelosyphilis (mi″ĕ-lo-sif′ĭ-lis) syphilis of the spinal cord.

myelosyphilosis (mi″ĕ-lo-sif″ĭ-lo′sis) any syphilitic affection of the spinal cord.

myelotherapy (mi″ĕ-lo-ther′ah-pe) [*myelo-* + *therapy*] the therapeutic use of bone marrow.

myelotome (mi′el-o-tōm) [*myelo-* + Gr. *tomē* a cut] 1. an instrument for making sections of the spinal cord. 2. an instrument used for cutting the spinal cord squarely across in removing the brain in postmortem examinations.

myelotomy (mi″ĕ-lot′o-me) the operation of severing tracts in the spinal cord. **commissural m.,** longitudinal division of the spinal cord, to sever crossing sensory fibers and produce localized analgesia.

myelotoxic (mi″ĕ-lo-tok′sik) [*myelo-* + Gr. *toxikon* poison] 1. destructive to bone marrow. 2. arising from diseased bone marrow.

myelotoxicity (mi″ĕ-lo-toks-is′ĭ-te) the quality of being myelotoxic.

myenteric (mi″en-ter′ik) pertaining to the myenteron; see also under *plexus* and *reflex*.

myenteron (mi-en′ter-on) [*my-* + Gr. *enteron* intestine] the muscular coat of the intestine.

myesthesia (mi″es-the′ze-ah) [*my-* + Gr. *aisthēsis* perception] muscle sensibility; sensibility to impressions coming from the muscles.

myiasis (mi′yah-sis) [Gr. *myia* fly + *-iasis*] a condition caused by infestation of the body by fly maggots. **creeping m.,** larva migrans caused by fly larvae. **cutaneous m.,** see *larva migrans*. **dermal m.,** see *larva migrans*. **m. dermato′sa,** infection of the skin with the larvae of flies. **intestinal m.,** the presence of living fly larvae in the intestines. **m. linea′ris,** larva migrans caused by fly larvae. **nasal m.,** myiasis produced by living fly larvae in the nasal passages. **traumatic m.,** maggot infestation of wounds or ulcers.

myiocephalon (mi″yo-sef′ah-lon) iridocele.

myiocephalum (mi″yo-sef′ah-lum) iridocele.

myiodesopsia (mi″yo-des-op′se-ah) [Gr. *myiōdes* flylike + *-opsia*] the appearance of muscae volitantes.

myiosis (mi-yo′sis) myiasis.

myitis (mi-i′tis) [*my-* + *-itis*] inflammation of a muscle; myositis.

myk(o)- for words beginning thus, see those beginning *myc(o)-*.

Mylaxen (mi-lak′sin) trademark for a preparation of hexafluorenium bromide.

Myleran (mil′er-an) trademark for a preparation of busulfan.

Mylicon (mi′lĭ-kon) trademark for preparations of simethicone.

my(o)- [Gr. *mys*, gen. *myos* muscle] a combining form denoting relationship to muscle.

myoadenylate deaminase (mi″o-ad′en-il-āt, mi″o-ah-den′il-āt de-am′ĭ-nās) muscle adenylate deaminase. See *isoenzyme A* under *AMP deaminase*.

myoadenylate (AMP) deaminase deficiency a mild autosomal recessive disorder, due to defective AMP deaminase in the purine nucleotide cycle, and characterized clinically by fatigue, cramps, and myalgia after exercise.

myoalbumin (mi″o-al-bu′min) an albumin constituting about one per cent of the protein of muscle.

myoarchitectonic (mi″o-ar″ke-tek-ton′ik) [*myo-* + *architectonic*] pertaining to the structure of muscle.

myoasthenia (mi″o-as-the′ne-ah) amyosthenia.

myoatrophy (mi″o-at′ro-fe) myatrophy.

myoblast (mi′o-blast) [*myo-* + Gr. *blastos* germ] an embryonic cell which becomes a cell of the muscle fiber.

myoblastic (mi″o-blas′tik) pertaining to a myoblast.

myoblastoma (mi″o-blas-to′mah) a benign circumscribed tumor-like lesion of soft tissue; see *granular cell tumor*, under *tumor*. **granular cell m.,** see under *tumor*.

myoblastomyoma (mi″o-blas″to-mi-o′mah) myoblastoma.

myobradia (mi″o-bra′de-ah) [*myo-* + Gr. *bradys* slow + *-ia*] a slow, sluggish reaction of muscle to electric stimulation.

myocardiac (mi″o-kar′de-ak) myocardial.

myocardial (mi″o-kar′de-al) pertaining to the muscular tissue of the heart; see also under *infarction*.

myocardiogram (mi″o-kar′de-o-gram) a tracing made by the myocardiograph.

myocardiograph (mi″o-kar′de-o-graf″) [*myo-* + Gr. *kardia* heart + *graphein* to record] an instrument for making a tracing of the movements of the heart muscles.

myocardiolysis (mi″o-kar″de-ol′ĭ-sis) local necrosis of the myocardial fibers due to arterial obstruction, in which the fibers are replaced by scar tissue and often, especially when complicated by thrombosis, leading to gross infarction.

myocardiopathy (mi″o-kar″de-op′ah-the) any noninflammatory disease of the muscular walls (myocardium) of the heart. **alcoholic m.,** a form attributed to ingestion of large amounts of alcohol over an extended period of time, characterized chiefly by enlargement of the heart and myocardial degenerative changes, particularly evident on electron microscopy. **chagasic m.,** myocardiopathy with saccular apical ventricular aneurysm associated with Chagas' disease.

myocardiorrhaphy (mi″o-kar″de-or′ah-fe) suture of wounds of the myocardium.

myocardiosis (mi″o-kar″de-o′sis) myocardosis.

myocarditic (mi″o-kar-dit′ik) pertaining to myocarditis.

myocarditis (mi″o-kar-di′tis) [*myo-* + Gr. *kardia* heart + *-itis*] inflammation of the myocardium; inflammation of the muscular walls of the heart. **acute bacterial m.,** acute myocarditis due to bacterial infection. **acute isolated m.,** acute interstitial myocarditis of unknown etiology, marked by sudden onset, absence of endocarditis or pericarditis, and frequently by a fatal outcome; called also *Fiedler's m.* and *idiopathic m.* **chronic m.,** chronic myocardial inflammatory disease; often used loosely to indicate any myocardial deficiency. **diphtheritic m.,** acute myocarditis leaving no permanent damage, occurring in diphtheria. **fibrous m.,** chronic interstitial m. **Fiedler's m.,** acute isolated m. **fragmentation m.,** fragmentation of the myocardium. **giant cell m.,** a granulomatous form of myocarditis in which large discrete foci form, each containing many lymphocytes and macrophages, and sometimes multinucleate giant cells not unlike those found in tuberculosis; called also *tuberculoid myocarditis*. **idiopathic m.,** acute isolated m. **interstitial m.,** myocarditis affecting chiefly the interstitial fibrous tissue. **parenchymatous m.,** myocarditis affecting chiefly the muscle substance itself. **rheumatic m.,** a common sequela of rheumatic fever characterized histologically by perivascular granulomata known as Aschoff bodies or nodules. **toxic m.,** myocarditis due to poisoning by drugs or to toxins of infecting organisms reaching the heart through the blood stream, as in diphtheria. **tuberculoid m.,** giant cell m. **tuberculous m.,** tuberculosis of the myocardium.

myocardium (mi″o-kar′de-um) [*myo-* + Gr. *kardia* heart] [NA] the middle and thickest layer of the heart wall, composed of cardiac muscle.

myocardosis (mi″o-kar-do′sis) a general term for disorders of the myocardium which are not inflammatory, but which may result from hypertension, coronary sclerosis, and hyperthyroidism.

myocele (mi′o-sēl) [*myo-* + Gr. *kēlē* hernia] hernia of muscle; protrusion of a muscle through its ruptured sheath.

myocelialgia (mi″o-se″le-al′je-ah) [myo- + Gr. *koilia* belly + -*algia*] pain in the abdominal muscles.

myocelitis (mi″o-se-li′tis) [myo- + Gr. *koilia* belly + -*itis*] inflammation of the muscles of the abdomen.

myocellulitis (mi″o-sel″u-li′tis) myositis conjoined with cellulitis.

myoceptor (mi′o-sep″tor) [myo- + L. *capere* to take] end-plate.

myocerosis (mi″o-se-ro′sis) [myo- + Gr. *kēros* wax] waxy degeneration of muscle.

myochorditis (mi″o-kor-di′tis) [myo- + Gr. *chordē* cord + -*itis*] inflammation of the muscles of the vocal cords.

myochrome (mi′o-krōm) [myo- + Gr. *chrōma* color] any member of a group of muscle pigments; see *cytochrome* (def. 1) and *myohematin*.

Myochrysine (mi″o-kri′sin) trademark for a preparation of gold sodium thiomalate.

myocinesimeter (mi″o-sin″ĕ-sim′ĕ-ter) myokinesimeter.

myoclonia (mi″o-klo′ne-ah) any disorder characterized by myoclonus. **m. epilep′tica,** myoclonus epilepsy. **m. fibrilla′ris mul′tiplex,** myokymia. **fibrillary m.,** the twitching of the fibrils of a muscle; see *fibrillation,* def. 2. **pseudoglottic m.,** hiccup.

myoclonic (mi″o-klon′ik) relating to or marked by myoclonus.

myoclonus (mi-ok′lo-nus) [myo- + Gr. *klonos* turmoil] shocklike contractions of a portion of a muscle, an entire muscle, or a group of muscles, restricted to one area of the body or appearing synchronously or asynchronously in several areas. **m. mul′tiplex,** paramyoclonus multiplex. **palatal m.,** a condition characterized by a rapid, rhythmic, up-and-down movement of one or both sides of the palate, often accompanied by ipsilateral synchronous clonic movements of muscles of the face, tongue, pharynx, and diaphragm. Called also *palatal nystagmus.*

myocoele (mi′o-sēl) [myo- + Gr. *koilia* cavity] the cavity within a myotome (def. 2).

myocolpitis (mi″o-kol-pi′tis) [myo- + Gr. *kolpos* vagina + -*itis*] inflammation of the muscular layers of the vaginal wall.

myocomma (mi″o-kom′ah) [myo- + Gr. *komma* cut] 1. a myotome or muscle segment, as in a fish. 2. the septum between two adjacent myotomes.

myocrismus (mi″o-kris′mus) [myo- + Gr. *krizein* to creak] a sound heard on auscultation over a contracting muscle.

myoctonine (mi-ok′to-nin) [myo- + Gr. *kteinein* to kill] a poisonous alkaloid, $C_{36}H_{42}N_2O_{10}$, from *Aconitum lycoctonum.*

myoculator (mi-ok′u-la″tor) [myo- + L. *oculus* eye] an ocular instrument, on the principle of the orthoptoscope, which allows fusion and movement laterally, vertically, and in rotation. Cf. myoscope.

myocyte (mi′o-sīt) [myo- + -*cyte*] a cell of the muscular tissue. **Anichkov's m.,** a myocyte found in Aschoff's bodies, having a serrated bar of chromatin in its nucleus; called also *cardiac histiocyte.*

myocytolysis (mi″o-si-tol′ĭ-sis) disintegration of muscle fibers. **focal m. of heart,** a miliary lesion characterized by loss of muscular syncytium, preservation of stroma, absence of inflammatory reaction, and eventual necrosis.

myocytoma (mi″o-si-to′mah) a tumor made up of myocytes or muscle cells.

myodegeneration (mi″o-de-jen″er-a′shun) [myo- + *degeneration*] degeneration of muscle.

myodemia (mi″o-de′me-ah) [myo- + Gr. *dēmos* fat] fatty degeneration of muscle.

myodesopsia (mi″o-des-op′se-ah) myiodesopsia.

myodiastasis (mi″o-di-as″tah-sis) [myo- + Gr. *diastasis* separation] separation of a muscle.

myodiopter (mi″o-di-op′ter) the force of ciliary muscle contraction necessary to raise the refraction of the emmetropic eye by 1 diopter from a state of rest.

myodynamic (mi″o-di-nam′ik) relating to muscular force.

myodynamics (mi″o-di-nam′iks) the physiology of muscular action.

myodynamometer (mi″o-di″nah-mom′ĕ-ter) [myo- + Gr. *dynamis* power + *metron* measure] a device for testing the power of the muscles.

myodynia (mi″o-din′e-ah) [myo- + Gr. *odynē* pain] pains in a muscle; myalgia.

myodystonia (mi″o-dis-to′ne-ah) [myo- + *dys-* + Gr. *tonos* tension + -*ia*] disorder of muscular tone.

myodystony (mi″o-dis′to-ne) myodystonia.

myodystrophia (mi″o-dis-tro′fe-ah) muscular dystrophy; myotonia atrophica. **m. feta′lis,** amyoplasia congenita.

myodystrophy (mi″o-dis′tro-fe) myodystrophia.

myoedema (mi″o-ĕ-de′mah) [myo- + Gr. *oidēma* swelling] 1. edema of a muscle. 2. mounding.

myoelastic (mi″o-e-las′tik) composed of elastic fibers associated with smooth muscle cells.

myoelectric, myoelectrical (mi″o-e-lek′trik; mi″o-e-lek′trĭ-kal) pertaining to the electric or electromotive properties of muscle.

myoendocarditis (mi″o-en″do-kar-di′tis) combined myocarditis and endocarditis.

myoepithelial (mi″o-ep″ĭ-the′le-al) pertaining to or composed of myoepithelium.

myoepithelioma (mi″o-ep″ĭ-the″le-o′mah) [*myoepithelium* + -*oma*] a benign tumor predominantly composed of myoepithelial cells; a pure myoepithelial neoplasm is rare.

myoepithelium (mi″o-ep″ĭ-the′le-um) [myo- + *epithelium*] tissue composed of myoepithelial cells.

myofascitis (mi″o-fah-si′tis) [myo- + *fascitis*] inflammation of a muscle and its fascia, particularly of the fascial insertion of muscle to bone.

myofibril (mi″o-fi′bril) a muscle fibril, one of the slender threads which can be rendered visible in a muscle fiber by maceration in certain acids. They run parallel with the long axis of the fiber, and are composed of numerous myofilaments (q.v.).

myofibrilla (mi″o-fi-bril′ah), pl. *myofibril′lae.* A myofibril.

myofibrillae (mi″o-fi-bril′e) plural of *myofibrilla.*

myofibrillar (mi′o-fi′bril-ar) relating to a myofibril.

myofibroblast (mi″o-fi′bro-blast) an atypical fibroblast combining the ultrastructural features of a fibroblast and a smooth muscle cell; it has a highly irregular nucleus, a large amount of rough endoplasmic reticulum, and a dense collection of myofilaments.

myofibroma (mi″o-fi-bro′mah) a tumor containing both muscular and fibrous elements; fibroid leiomyoma.

myofibrosis (mi″o-fi-bro′sis) [myo- + L. *fibra* fiber] replacement of muscle tissue by fibrous tissue. **m. cor′dis,** myofibrosis of the heart.

myofibrositis (mi″o-fi″bro-si′tis) inflammation of the perimysium; perimysiitis.

myofilament (mi″o-fil′ah-ment) [myo- + *filament*] any of the numerous ultramicroscopic threadlike structures occurring in bundles in the myofibrils of striated muscle fibers. The thick filaments are composed of myosin, the thin ones of actin; together they are responsible for the contractile properties of muscle.

myofunctional (mi″o-funk′shun-al) 1. pertaining to muscular function. 2. pertaining to the use of muscles as an adjunct in orthodontic therapy.

myogelosis (mi″o-jĕ-lo′sis) [myo- + L. *gelare* to freeze] an area of hardening in a muscle, especially in the gluteus muscle.

myogen (mi′o-jen) [myo- + Gr. *gennan* to produce] an albumin-like protein, constituting 10 per cent of the protein of muscle; it is spontaneously coagulable, passing first into soluble myogen fibrin, and then into myosin fibrin. Cf. *myosin.*

myogenesis (mi″o-jen′ĕ-sis) the development of muscle tissue, especially its embryonic development.

myogenetic (mi″o-jĕ-net′ik) pertaining to myogenesis.

myogenic (mi″o-jen′ik) giving rise to or forming muscle tissue.

myogenous (mi-oj′ĕ-nus) originating in muscle tissue.

myoglia (mi-og′le-ah) [myo- + Gr. *glia* glue] a fibrillar substance formed by muscle cells, and present only during early embryogenesis of muscle fibers; called also *border fibrils.*

myoglobin (mi″o-glo′bin) the oxygen-transporting pigment of muscle, a conjugated protein resembling a single subunit of hemoglobin, being composed of one globin polypeptide chain and one heme group (containing one iron atom); it combines with oxygen released by erythrocytes, stores it, and transports it to the mitochondria of muscle cells, where it generates energy by combustion of glucose to carbon dioxide and water.

myoglobinuria (mi″o-glo″bin-u′re-ah) the presence of myoglobin in the urine, as in deficiency of muscle phosphorylase, in crush injuries, and after vigorous and prolonged exercise in susceptible persons. **idiopathic m.,** Meyer-Betz disease. **spontaneous m.,** Meyer-Betz disease.

myoglobulin (mi″o-glob′u-lin) [myo- + globulin] a globulin found in muscle serum.

myoglobulinuria (mi″o-glob″u-lin-u′re-ah) the presence of myoglobulin in the urine.

myognathus (mi-og′nah-thus) [myo- + Gr. gnathos jaw] a monster with a supernumerary lower jaw attached to the normally placed lower jaw.

myogram (mi′o-gram) [myo- + Gr. gramma writing] the record or tracing made by a myograph.

myograph (mi′o-graf) [myo- + Gr. graphein to record] an apparatus for recording the effects of a muscular contraction.

myographic (mi′o-graf′ik) pertaining to a myograph or to myography.

myography (mi-og′rah-fe) [myo- + Gr. graphein to record] 1. the use of the myograph. 2. a description of the muscles. 3. roentgenography of muscle tissue after injection of an opaque medium.

myohematin (mi″o-hem′ah-tin) [myo- + hematin] Mac-Munn's name for the cytochrome of muscle tissue, an iron-containing catalyst of tissue oxidation; see cytochrome, def. 1.

myohemoglobin (mi″o-he″mo-glo′bin) myoglobin.

myohypertrophia (mi″o-hi″per-tro′fe-ah) muscular hypertrophy. **m. kymoparalyt′ica,** a muscular dystrophy, with paralysis, described by Oppenheim (1914).

myoid (mi′oid) [my- + -oid] 1. resembling or like a muscle. 2. a substance resembling muscle. **visual cell m.,** the basophilic inner region of the inner segment of the dendritic process of a retinal rod or cone, lying between the ellipsoid and the soma, and containing agranular endoplasmic reticulum and free ribosomes.

myoidem (mi-oi′dem) myoedema.

myoidema (mi″oi-de′mah) myoedema.

myoideum (mi-oi′de-um) myoid tissue.

myoidism (mi-o-id′izm) [myo- + Gr. idios own] idiomuscular contraction.

myo-inositol (mi″o-in-o′sĭ-tol) inositol, def. 2.

myoischemia (mi″o-is-ke′me-ah) [myo- + ischemia] local deficiency of blood supply in muscle.

myokerosis (mi″o-ke-ro′sis) [myo- + Gr. kēros wax] myocerosis.

myokinase (mi″o-ki′nās) adenylate kinase.

myokinesimeter (mi″o-kin″ĕ-sim′ĕ-ter) [myokinesis + Gr. metron measure] an apparatus for measuring muscular contraction aroused by stimulation by an electric current.

myokinesis (mi″o-ki-ne′sis) [myo- + Gr. kinēsis motion] movement of muscles, especially displacement of muscle fibers in operation.

myokinetic (mi″o-ki-net′ik) 1. pertaining to or characterized by myokinesis. 2. pertaining to the motion or kinetic function of muscle, as contrasted with the myotonic or tonic function.

myokinin (mi″o-kin′in) a base, $C_{11}H_{28}N_2O_3$, found in muscle.

myokymia (mi″o-kim′e-ah) [myo- + Gr. kyma wave] a benign condition marked by brief spontaneous tetanic contractions of motor units or groups of muscle fibers, usually adjacent groups of fibers contracting alternately. Called also myoclonia fibrillaris multiplex.

myolemma (mi″o-lem′ah) [myo- + Gr. lemma sheath] the sarcolemma.

myolin (mi′o-lin) the supposed material of the muscular fibrils.

myolipoma (mi″o-li-po′mah) [myo- + Gr. lipos fat + -oma] myoma (leiomyoma) containing fatty or lipomatous elements; called also benign mesenchymoma.

myologia (mi″o-lo′je-ah) myology; in NA terminology, my-

ologia encompasses the nomenclature relating to the muscles and to the bursae and synovial sheaths.

myology (mi-ol′o-je) [myo- + Gr. logos treatise] the scientific study of muscles, and the body of knowledge relating thereto.

myolysis (mi-ol′ĭ-sis) [myo- + Gr. lysis dissolution] disintegration or degeneration of muscle tissue. **m. cardiotox′ica,** degeneration of the heart muscle due to systemic intoxication, as in infectious diseases.

myoma (mi-o′mah), pl. myomas or myo′mata [myo- + -oma] a tumor made up of muscular elements. **ball m.,** one that is spherical. **m. levicellula′re** (obs.), leiomyoma. **m. pre′vium,** leiomyoma uteri. **m. sarcomato′des,** leiomyosarcoma. **m. striocellula′re,** rhabdomyoma. **m. telangiecto′des,** vascular leiomyoma, a tumor consisting of a coil of blood vessels surrounded by a network of muscular fibers; angiomyoma.

myomagenesis (mi″o″mah-jen′ĕ-sis) the production or causation of myoma (leiomyoma).

myomalacia (mi″o-mah-la′she-ah) [myo- + Gr. malakia softening] morbid softening of a muscle.

myomata (mi-o′mah-tah) plural of myoma.

myomatectomy (mi″o-mah-tek′to-me) myomectomy, def. 1.

myomatosis (mi″o-mah-to′sis) the formation of multiple myomas (leiomyomas).

myomatous (mi-o′mah-tus) pertaining to or of the nature of a myoma (leiomyoma).

myomectomy (mi″o-mek′to-me) [myoma + Gr. ektomē excision] 1. surgical removal of a myoma (leiomyoma). 2. myectomy.

myomelanosis (mi″o-mel″ah-no′sis) [myo- + Gr. melanōsis blackening] melanosis, or black pigmentation of a portion of the muscular substance.

myomere (mi′o-mēr) [myo- + Gr. meros part] myotome, def. 2.

myometer (mi-om′ĕ-ter) [myo- + Gr. metron measure] an apparatus for measuring muscle contraction.

myometritis (mi″o-mĕ-tri′tis) [myo- + Gr. mētra womb + -itis] inflammation of the muscular substance, or myometrium, of the uterus.

myometrium (mi-o-me′tre-um) [myo- + Gr. mētra uterus] the smooth muscle coat of the uterus which forms the main mass of the organ. NA alternative term for tunica muscularis uteri.

myomohysterectomy (mi″o-mo-his″ter-ek′to-me) [myoma + Gr. hystera uterus + ektomē excision] surgical removal of a myomatous uterus.

myomotomy (mi″o-mot′o-me) incision into a myoma.

myon (mi′on) [Gr. mys muscle + on neuter ending] a muscular unit.

myonecrosis (mi″o-nĕ-kro′sis) necrosis, or death of, individual muscle fibers. **clostridial m.,** gas gangrene.

myoneme (mi′o-nēm) [myo- + Gr. nēma thread] any of various fibrillar organelles, known or believed to have contractile properties, commonly seen in the cytoplasm of stalked ciliate protozoa, but also occurring in certain nonciliates and certain nonprotozoans.

myoneural (mi″o-nu′ral) [myo- + Gr. neuron nerve] pertaining to both muscle and nerve; said of the nerve terminations in muscles.

myoneuralgia (mi″o-nu-ral′je-ah) [myo- + -neuralgia] muscular neuralgia.

myoneurasthenia (mi″o-nu″ras-the′ne-ah) [myo- + neurasthenia] (obs.) weakness of the muscular system in neurasthenia.

myoneure (mi′o-nūr) [myo- + Gr. neuron nerve] a nerve cell which supplies a muscle.

myonosus (mi-on′o-sus) [myo- + Gr. nosos disease] myopathy.

myonymy (mi-on′ĭ-me) [myo- + Gr. onoma name] nomenclature of the muscles.

myopachynsis (mi″o-pah-kin′sis) [myo- + Gr. pachynsis thickening] hypertrophy of muscle.

myopalmus (mi″o-pal′mus) muscle twitching.

myoparalysis (mi″o-pah-ral′ĭ-sis) [myo- + paralysis] paralysis of a muscle.

myoparesis (mi″o-par′ĕ-sis) muscle weakness.

myopathia (mi″o-path′e-ah) myopathy. **m. cor′dis,** myocardosis. **m. infraspina′ta,** a condition marked by the sudden development of pain in the shoulder with tenderness in the infraspinatus muscle.

myopathic (mi″o-path′ik) of the nature of a myopathy.

myopathy (mi-op′ah-the) [myo- + -pathy] any disease of a muscle. **alcoholic m.,** myopathy affecting alcoholics, commonly characterized by acute myoglobinuria and sometimes by proximal limb weakness. **centronuclear m.,** myotubular m. **distal m.,** an autosomal dominant form of muscular dystrophy, appearing in two types. The first has *onset in infancy,* does not progress past adolescence, and is not incapacitating. The second, *late distal hereditary m.,* sets in usually after 40, does not affect lifespan and first affects the small muscles of the hands and feet and then spreads proximally. Called also *distal muscular dystrophy* and *Gowers type muscular dystrophy.* **myotubular m.,** myopathy characterized by myofibers resembling those of early fetal muscle, i.e., with the nucleus located centrally and surrounded by a halo of apparently empty space; called also *centronuclear m.* **nemaline m.,** a congenital myofibrillar abnormality in which small threadlike or rod-shaped bodies are scattered through the muscle fibers; it is marked by hypotonia and proximal muscle weakness; called also *rod m.* **ocular m.,** progressive external ophthalmoplegia. **rod m.,** nemaline m.

myope (mi′ōp) [Gr. *myein* to shut + *ōps* eye] a nearsighted person; one affected with myopia.

myopericarditis (mi″o-per″ĭ-kar-di′tis) myocarditis combined with pericarditis.

myophage (mi′o-fāj) a phagocyte which destroys the contractile substance of muscle.

myophagism (mi-of′ah-jizm) [myo- + Gr. *phagein* to eat] the atrophy, or wasting away, of muscular tissue.

myophone (mi′o-fōn) [myo- + Gr. *phōnē* voice] a device which renders audible the sound of a muscular contraction.

myopia (mi-o′pe-ah) [Gr. *myein* to shut + -opia] that error of refraction in which rays of light entering the eye parallel to the optic axis are brought to a focus in front of the retina, as a result of the eyeball being too long from front to back (*axial m.*) or of an increased strength in refractive power of the media of the eye (*index m.*). Called also *nearsightedness,* because the near point is less distant than it is in emmetropia with an equal amplitude of accommodation. **curvature m.,** a form due to changes or increases in the curvature of the refracting surfaces of the eye, especially of the cornea. **index m.,** a form due to variations in the index of refraction of the media of the eye. **malignant m., pernicious m.,** progressive myopia, associated with grave disease of the choroid and leading to retinal detachment and blindness. **primary m.,** simple m. **prodromal m.,** a condition marked by the return of the ability to do close work without eyeglasses; sometimes seen in incipient cataract. **progressive m.,** myopia that continues to increase abnormally rapidly in adult life. **simple m.** 1. that myopia due to normal growth of the healthy eyeball. It stops increasing at maturity and may be corrected to normal visual acuity. 2. myopia without astigmatism.

myopic (mi-op′ik) pertaining to or affected with myopia; nearsighted.

myoplasm (mi′o-plazm) [myo- + Gr. *plasma* something formed] the contractile part of the muscle cell, or myofibril.

myoplastic (mi″o-plas′tik) [myo- + Gr. *plassein* to form] performed by the plastic use of muscle; said of operations.

myoplasty (mi′o-plas″te) plastic surgery on muscle; an operation in which portions of partly detached muscle are utilized, especially in the field of defects or deformities.

myopolar (mi″o-po′lar) [myo- + *polar*] applied to a muscle between the electrodes of a battery.

myoprotein (mi″o-pro′te-in) a protein obtained from muscle tissue.

myopsis (mi-op′sis) myiodesopsia.

myoreceptor (mi″o-re-sep′tor) a proprioceptor occurring in skeletal muscle.

myorrhaphy (mi-or′ah-fe) [myo- + Gr. *rhaphē* suture] suture of divided muscle; myosuture.

myorrhexis (mi″o-rek′sis) [myo- + Gr. *rhēxis* rupture] the rupture of a muscle.

myosalgia (mi″o-sal′je-ah) myalgia.

myosalpingitis (mi″o-sal″pin-ji′tis) [myo- + *salpingitis*] inflammation of the muscular tissue of the oviduct.

myosalpinx (mi″o-sal′pinks) the muscular tissue of the oviduct.

myosan (mi′o-san) a denatured and insoluble form of myosin.

myosarcoma (mi″o-sar-ko′mah) a malignant tumor derived from myogenic cells.

myoschwannoma (mi″o-shwan-no′mah) schwannoma.

myosclerosis (mi″o-skle-ro′sis) [myo- + Gr. *sklēros* hard] hardening, or sclerosis, of muscle tissue.

myoscope (mi′o-skōp) [myo- + -scope] 1. an instrument for observing muscle contraction. 2. an ocular instrument, on the principle of the orthoptoscope, which allows fusion and movement laterally, vertically, and in rotation. Cf. *myoculator.*

myoseism (mi′o-sīzm) [myo- + Gr. *seismos* shake] jerky, irregular muscular contractions.

myoseptum (mi″o-sep′tum) myocomma.

myoserum (mi″o-se′rum) the juice expressed from muscle.

myosin (mi′o-sin) a globin which is the most abundant protein (68 per cent) in muscle, occurring chiefly in the A band. It is soluble in salt solution, but on long standing it coagulates into an insoluble protein called *myosin fibrin.* Along with actin (q.v.), it is responsible for the contraction and relaxation of muscle. Myosin has enzymatic properties, acting as an ATP-ase. It is the main constituent of the thick filaments of muscle fibers. Cf. *myogen* and *actomyosin.* **vegetable m.,** a substance resembling myosin, from seeds of various plants.

myosin ATPase [EC 3.6.1.32] an enzyme of the hydrolase class that catalyzes *in vitro* the reaction ATP + H_2O = ADP + orthophosphate. The myosin is bound to actin for full activity. In the absence of actin, ATPase activity is low and requires calcium. Physiologically, the reaction is the overall result of a cycle of muscular contraction and relaxation. See *adenosine triphosphatase.* Called also *actomyosin.*

myosinogen (mi″o-sin′o-jen) [myosin + Gr. *gennan* to produce] myogen.

myosinuria (mi″o-sin-u′re-ah) [myosin + Gr. *ouron* urine + -ia] the presence of myosin in the urine.

myosis (mi-o′sis) miosis.

myositic (mi″o-sit′ik) pertaining to myositis.

myositis (mi″o-si′tis) [Gr. *myos* of muscle + -itis] inflammation of a voluntary muscle. **acute disseminated m.,** primary multiple m. **acute progressive m.,** a rare disease in which the inflammation gradually involves the whole muscular system and ends in death by asphyxia and pneumonia. **m. a frigo′re,** muscular rheumatism resulting from cold or chilling. **m. fibro′sa,** a type in which there is a formation of connective tissue within the muscle substance. **infectious m., interstitial m.,** inflammation of the connective and septal elements of muscular tissue. **multiple m.,** polymyositis. **orbital m.,** see under *pseudotumor.* **m. ossif′icans,** myositis which is characterized by bony deposits or by ossification of muscles. **m. ossif′icans circumscrip′ta,** a form marked by the formation of a muscular osteoma, such as rider's bone. **m. ossif′icans progressi′va,** a progressive disease, beginning in early life, in which the muscles are gradually converted into bony tissue; called also *progressive ossifying m.* **m. ossif′icans traumat′ica,** myositis ossificans due to injury. **parenchymatous m.,** that which affects the essential substance of a muscle. **primary multiple m.,** an acute febrile disease characterized by edema and inflammation of the skin and muscles in various parts of the body; called also *acute disseminated m.* and *pseudotrichinosis.* **progressive ossifying m.,** myositis ossificans progressiva. **m. purulen′ta,** myositis due to bacteremia and associated with suppuration and gangrene. Cf. *pyomyositis.* **rheumatoid m.,** fibrositis. **m. sero′sa,** muscle inflammation characterized by a serous exudation. **spontaneous bacterial m.,** pyomyositis. **trichinous m.,** that which is caused by the presence of trichinae.

myospasia (mi″o-spa′ze-ah) clonic contraction of muscle; paramyoclonus.

myospasm (mi'o-spazm) [*myo-* + Gr. *spasmos* spasm] spasm of a muscle.

myospasmia (mi"o-spaz'me-ah) disease characterized by uncontrollable muscular spasm.

myosteoma (mi-os"te-o'mah) [*myo-* + Gr. *osteon* bone + *-oma*] osteogenic sarcoma of soft parts.

myosthenic (mi"os-then'ik) [*myo-* + Gr. *sthenos* strength] pertaining to strength of muscle.

myosthenometer (mi"o-sthen-om'ĕ-ter) [*myo-* + Gr. *sthenos* strength + *metron* measure] an instrument for measuring the power of muscle groups.

myostroma (mi"o-stro'mah) [*myo-* + *stroma*] the stroma or framework of muscle tissue.

myostromin (mi"o-stro'min) a protein occurring in muscle stroma.

myosuria (mi"o-su're-ah) [*myo-* + Gr. *ouron* urine + *-ia*] myosin in the urine.

myosuture (mi"o-su'tūr) [*myo-* + L. *sutura* sewing] the suture of a muscle; myorrhaphy.

myosynizesis (mi"o-sin"i-ze'sis) [*myo-* + Gr. *synizēsis* a sinking down] adhesion of muscles.

myotactic (mi"o-tak'tik) [*myo-* + L. *tactus* touch] pertaining to the proprioceptive sense of muscles.

myotasis (mi-ot'ah-sis) [*myo-* + Gr. *tasis* stretching] stretching of muscle.

myotatic (mi"o-tat'ik) [*myo-* + Gr. *teinein* to stretch] performed or induced by stretching or extending a muscle.

myotenontoplasty (mi"o-ten-on'to-plas"te) tenomyoplasty.

myotenositis (mi"o-ten"o-si'tis) [*myo-* + Gr. *tenōn* tendon + *-itis*] inflammation of a muscle and its tendon.

myotenotomy (mi"o-ten-ot'o-me) [*myo-* + *tenotomy*] surgical division of the tendon of a muscle.

myothermic (mi"o-ther'mik) [*myo-* + Gr. *thermē* heat] pertaining to temperature changes in muscle produced by its activity.

myotic (mi-ot'ik) miotic (def. 2).

myotility (mi"o-til'ĭ-te) muscular contractility.

myotome (mi'o-tōm) [*myo-* + Gr. *tomē* a cut] 1. an instrument for performing myotomy. 2. the muscle plate or portion of a somite that develops into voluntary muscle; called also *myomere*. 3. a group of muscles innervated from a single spinal segment.

myotomic (mi"o-tom'ik) pertaining to or derived from a myotome.

myotomy (mi-ot'o-me) [*myo-* + Gr. *tomē* a cutting] the cutting or dissection of a muscle or of muscular tissue.

Myotonachol (mi"o-tōn'ah-kol) trademark for preparations of bethanechol chloride.

myotone (mi'o-tōn) myotonus.

myotonia (mi"o-to'ne-ah) [*myo-* + Gr. *tonos* tension] increased muscular irritability and contractility with decreased power of relaxation; tonic spasm of muscle. **m. acquis'ita,** tonic muscular spasm developed after injury or in consequence of disease; called also *Talma's disease.* **m. atro'phica,** myotonic dystrophy; see under *dystrophy.* **m. congen'ita, m. heredita'ria,** congenital genetic disease characterized by tonic spasm and rigidity of certain muscles when an attempt is made to move them after a period of rest or when mechanically stimulated. The stiffness disappears as the muscles are used. There are autosomal dominant and autosomal recessive forms. **m. dystro'-phica,** myotonic dystrophy. **m. neonato'rum,** tetanism.

myotonic (mi"o-ton'ik) 1. pertaining to or characterized by myotonia. 2. pertaining to the tonic function of muscle, as contrasted with the myokinetic or motion function.

myotonoid (mi-ot'o-noid) [*myo-* + Gr. *tonos* tension + *eidos* form] resembling myotonia; said of reactions in muscle which are marked by slow contraction or relaxation.

myotonometer (mi"o-to-nom'ĕ-ter) [*myotonia* + Gr. *metron* measure] an instrument for measuring muscular tonus.

myotonus (mi-ot'o-nus) tonic spasm of a muscle or of a group of muscles.

myotony (mi-ot'o-ne) myotonia.

myotrophic (mi'o-tro"fik) 1. increasing the weight of muscle. 2. pertaining to myotrophy.

myotrophy (mi-ot'ro-fe) [*myo-* + Gr. *trophē* nutrition] nutrition of muscle.

myotropic (mi"o-trop'ik) [*myo-* + Gr. *tropos* a turning] having an affinity for muscle, as myotropic organisms.

myotube (mi'o-tūb) myotubule.

myotubular (mi"o-tu'bu-lar) relating to a myotubule.

myotubule (mi"o-tu'būl) a developing muscle fiber with a centrally, rather than peripherally, located nucleus.

myovascular (mi"o-vas'ku-lar) [*myo-* + *vascular*] pertaining to a muscle and its blood vessels.

myrcene (mer'sēn) an essential oil from the oil of bay; it is an olefinic terpene, $C_{10}H_{16}$, used in perfumery and pharmaceuticals as an odorant.

myria- [Gr. *myrios* numberless] a combining form meaning a great number.

Myriangiales (mir"e-an"je-a'lēz) an order of ascomycetous fungi (subclass Loculoascomycetaceae), in which the asci are formed in locules scattered throughout the ascocarp (fruiting body). They are usually parasites of higher plants, although a few are insect parasites; the order includes the family Piedraiaceae.

myriapod (mir'e-ah-pod) a member of the Myriapoda; a centipede or millipede.

Myriapoda (mir"e-ap'o-dah) [*myria-* + Gr. *pous* foot] a superclass of arthropods, including the classes Chilopoda (centipedes) and Diplopoda (millipedes).

myrica (mir-i'kah) the dried bark of the root of *Myrica cerifera* L. (Myriaceae), bayberry or wax myrtle, formerly used internally as an emetic and astringent, and externally in the treatment of indolent ulcers.

myricin (mir'i-sin) [L. *myrica* myrtle] 1. a crystallizable principle, $C_{30}H_{61} \cdot C_{16}H_{31}O_2$, from yellow wax (beeswax). 2. a medicinal concentration prepared from *Myrica cerifera*, or wax myrtle; used like myrica.

myricyl (mir'i-sil) the radical, $C_{30}H_{61}$, occurring in beeswax and other waxes.

myringa (mĭ-ring'gah) [L. "membrane," from Gr. *mēninx*] the membrana tympani.

myringectomy (mir"in-jek'to-me) [*myringo-* + *ektomē* excision] surgical removal of the membrana tympani.

myringitis (mir"in-ji'tis) [*myringa* + *-itis*] inflammation of the membrana tympani. **m. bullo'sa, bullous m.,** a form of viral otitis media in which serous or hemorrhagic blebs appear on the membrana tympani and often on the adjacent wall of the auditory meatus.

myring(o)- [L. *myringa*, q.v.] a combining form denoting relationship to the membrana tympani.

myringodectomy (mĭ-ring"go-dek'to-me) myringectomy.

myringodermatitis (mĭ-ring"go-der"mah-ti'tis) [*myringo-* + Gr. *derma* skin] inflammation of the outer layer of the membrana tympani, with the formation of blebs.

myringomycosis (mĭ-ring"go-mi-ko'sis) [*myringo-* + Gr. *mykēs* fungus] disease of the membrana tympani caused by a fungus; otomycosis. **m. aspergilli'na,** infection of the membrana tympani by an aspergillus; see *otomycosis.*

myringoplasty (mĭ-ring'go-plas"te) [*myringo-* + Gr. *plassein* to form] surgical restoration of a perforated tympanic membrane by grafting. See also *tympanoplasty.*

myringorupture (mĭ-ring"go-rup'chur) rupture of the membrana tympani.

myringostapediopexy (mĭ-ring"go-stah-pe'de-o-pek"se) fixation of the pars tensa of the membrana tympani to the head of the stapes.

myringotome (mĭ-ring'go-tōm) a knife for use in operating upon the membrana tympani.

myringotomy (mir"in-got'o-me) [*myringo-* + Gr. *tomē* a cutting] tympanocentesis.

myrinx (mi'rinks) membrana tympani.

myristate (mēr'is-tāt) tetradecanoate: the ionic form of myristic acid, a naturally occurring fatty acid. **isopropyl m.,** see under *isopropyl.*

myristic acid (mĭ-ris'tik) trivial name for tetradecanoic acid, the 14-carbon, straight-chain unsaturated fatty acid.

Myristica (mĭ-ris'tĭ-kah) [L.; Gr. *myrizein* to anoint] a genus of trees of tropical countries. *M. fragrans* Houtt. (Myristicaceae), the nutmeg tree, is the source of myristica. *M. ocuba* is the source of ocuba wax.

myristica (mĭ-ris′tĭ-kah)   nutmeg; the dried ripe seed of *Myristica fragrans* Houtt. (Myristicaceae) deprived of its seed coat and arillode and with or within a coating of lime. It is the source of nutmeg oil, which is used as a flavoring agent in pharmaceutical preparations. It has stimulating aromatic, carminative, and psychomimetic properties.

myristicene (mĭ-ris′tĭ-sēn)   a fragrant eleopten, $C_{10}H_{14}$, from nutmeg (myristica) oil.

myristicol (mĭ-ris′tĭ-kol)   a stearopten, or camphor, $C_{10}H_{16}O$, from nutmeg (myristica) oil.

myristin (mĭ-ris′tin)   chemical name: glyceryl trimyristate, $C_3H_5(C_{14}H_{27}O_2)_3$, found in spermaceti and many vegetable oils and fats, especially coconut oil and fixed nutmeg (myristica) oil.

myrrh (mur)   the oleo-gum-resin obtained from species of East Indian and African trees, e.g., *Commiphora abyssinica* (Berg) Eng. (Burseraceae); it has been used as a carminative and a topical oral stimulant.

myrrholin (mur′o-lin)   a mixture of myrrh and fat in equal parts, used as a vehicle for the administration of creosote.

myrtenol (mur′tĕ-nol)   a terpene alcohol, $(CH_3)_2C:C_6H_7\cdot CH_2OH$, from the volatile oil distilled from the leaves of *Myrtus communis* L. (Myrtaceae).

myrtiform (mur′tĭ-form) [L. *myrtiformis*; *myrtus* myrtle + *forma* shape]   shaped like the leaf or berry of the myrtle.

Myrtus (mur′tus) [L.; Gr. *myrtos*]   a genus of myrtaceous trees. **M. commu′nis**, L. (Myrtaceae), the Old World myrtle, a species affording leaves which are antiseptic and astringent.

Mysoline (mi′so-lēn)   trademark for preparations of primidone.

mysophilia (mi″so-fil′e-ah) [Gr. *mysos* uncleanness of body or mind + Gr. *philein* to love]   paraphilia involving the use of filth or excretions.

mysophobia (mi″so-fo′be-ah) [Gr. *mysos* uncleanness of body or mind + *phobia*]   irrational fear of dirt and contamination.

mysophobic (mi″so-fo′bik)   pertaining to or characterized by mysophobia.

mystin (mis′tin)   a milk preservative, consisting of formaldehyde and sodium nitrite.

mytacism (mi′tah-sizm) [Gr. *mytakismos*]   too free use of *m* sounds in utterance.

Mytelase (mi′tĕ-lās)   trademark for a preparation of ambenonium chloride.

mythophobia (mith″o-fo′be-ah) [Gr. *mythos* myth + *phobia*]   irrational fear of myths or of stating an untruth.

myxadenitis (miks″ad-ĕ-ni′tis) [*myxo-* + Gr. *adēn* gland + *-itis*]   inflammation of a mucous gland. **m. labia′lis**, see *cheilitis glandularis*.

myxadenoma (miks″ad-ĕ-no′mah) [*myxo-* + *adenoma*]   an epithelial tumor with the structure of a mucous gland; mucinous adenoma.

myxameba (mik″sah-me′bah) [*myx-* + *ameba*]   a uninucleate, naked, free-living ameboid cell without either cilia or flagella produced from a spore, which aggregates and fuses with other myxamebas to form a plasmodium or aggregates without fusion to form a pseudoplasmodium.

myxangitis (miks″an-ji′tis) [*myxo-* + Gr. *angeion* vessel + *-itis*]   inflammation of the ducts of mucous glands.

myxangoitis (miks″an-go-i′tis)   myxangitis.

myxasthenia (miks″as-the-ne′ah) [*myxo-* + Gr. *astheneia* weakness]   deficiency in the secretion of mucus.

myxedema (mik″sĕ-de′mah) [*myxo-* + Gr. *oidēma* swelling]   a condition characterized by a dry, waxy type of swelling, with abnormal deposits of mucin in the skin (mucinosis) and other tissues, and associated with primary hypothyroidism. The edema is of the nonpitting type, and the facial changes are strikingly distinctive, with swollen lips and a thickened nose. The term myxedema is sometimes used interchangeably with adult hypothyroidism. Cf. *lichen myxedematosus*. **circumscribed m.**, pretibial m. **congenital m.**, cretinism. **infantile m.**, myxedema beginning during infancy in association with hypothyroidism developing after birth. **nodular m.**, pretibial m. **operative m.**, myxedema developing subsequent to surgical removal of the thyroid gland. **papular m.**, lichen myxedematosus.

pituitary m., myxedema associated with hypothyroidism occurring as a consequence of deficient secretion of thyrotropic hormone by the anterior pituitary gland. **pretibial m.**, localized myxedema associated with preceding hyperthyroidism and exophthalmos, occurring typically on the anterior (pretibial) surface of the legs, the mucin deposits appearing as both plaques and papules; called also *infiltrative dermopathy*. **secondary m.**, pituitary m.

myxedematoid (mik″sĕ-dem″ah-toid) [*myxedema* + Gr. *eidos* form]   resembling myxedema.

myxedematous (mik″sĕ-dem′ah-tus)   pertaining to or characterized by myxedema.

Myxidium (mik-sid′e-um)   a genus of parasitic protozoa (suborder Bipolarina, order Bivalvulida) found in fishes, amphibians, and reptiles.

myxiosis (mik″se-o′sis)   a discharge of mucus.

myx(o)- [Gr. *myxa* mucus]   combining form denoting relationship to mucus, or to slime.

myxoadenoma (mik″so-ad″ĕ-no′mah)   myxadenoma.

Myxobacterales (mik″so-bak-tĕ-ra′lēz) [*myxo-* + Gr. *baktērion* little rod]   an order of gliding bacteria found in soil, decomposing plant material, and animal dung; made up of unicellular aerobic rods that are cylindrical with rounded or tapered ends. It consists of the families Archangiaceae, Cystobacteraceae, Myxococcaceae, and Polyangiaceae.

myxoblastoma (mik″so-blas-to′mah)   myxoma.

Myxobolus (mik″so-bo′lus) [*myxo-* + *bolus*]   a genus of parasitic protozoa (suborder Platysporina, order Bivalvulida) pathogenic in carp and other fish.

myxochondrofibrosarcoma (mik″so-kon″dro-fi″bro-sar-ko′mah)   malignant mesenchymoma.

myxochondroma (mik″so-kon-dro′mah)   chondroma with a stroma resembling primitive mesenchymal tissue.

myxochondrosarcoma (mik″so-kon″dro-sar-ko′mah)   malignant mesenchymoma.

Myxococcaceae (mik″so-kok-ka′se-e)   a family of gliding bacteria of the order Myxobacterales, found in soils, made up of slender, straight or tapered cells with rounded ends that produce myxospores. It contains the genus *Myxococcus*.

Myxococcus (mik″so-kok′us) [*myxo-* + *coccus*]   a genus of gliding bacteria of the family Myxococcaceae, order Myxobacterales, found in decaying plant material and soil. The type species is *M. ful′vus*.

myxocystitis (mik″so-sis-ti′tis) [*myxo-* + *cystitis*]   inflammation of the mucosa of the bladder.

myxocystoma (mik″so-sis-to′mah)   myxoma with cystic degeneration.

myxocyte (mik′so-sīt) [*myxo-* + *cyte*]   one of the characteristic cells of mucous tissue.

myxoenchondroma (mik″so-en″kon-dro′mah)   a chondroma in which some of the elements have undergone mucous degeneration.

myxoendothelioma (mik″so-en″do-the″le-o′mah)   angioendothelioma with myxomatous degeneration.

myxofibroma (mik″so-fi-bro′mah)   a fibroma containing myxomatous tissue.

myxofibrosarcoma (mik″so-fi″bro-sar-ko′mah)   fibrosarcoma with myxomatous areas.

Myxogastria (mik″so-gas′tre-ah) [*myxo-* Gr. *gastēr* stomach]   a subclass of ameboid protozoa (class Eumycetozoea, superclass Rhizopoda), characterized by the occurrence of a major trophic stage consisting of a multinucleate plasmodium and by the presence of multispored fruiting bodies. It includes five orders: Echinosteliida, Liceida, Physarida, Stemonitida, and Trichiida.

myxoglioma (mik″so-gli-o′mah)   a glioma which has undergone myxomatous degeneration.

myxoglobulosis (mik″so-glob″u-lo′sis) [*myxo-* + *globule* + *-osis*]   a cystic condition of the appendix marked by the presence in the cysts of globoid bodies of mucinous character.

myxoid (mik′soid) [*myxo-* + Gr. *eidos* form]   resembling mucus.

myxoinoma (mik″so-in-o′mah)   myxofibroma.

myxolipoma (mik″so-li-po′mah)   lipoma with foci of myxomatous degeneration.

myxoma (mik-so′mah), pl. *myxomas* or *myxo′mata* [*myxo-* + *-oma*]   a tumor composed of primitive connective tissue cells and stroma resembling mesenchyme. **atrial m.,** a benign gelatinous growth usually pedunculated and usually arising from the interatrial septum of the heart in the region of the fossa ovalis; symptoms may include effort dyspnea, loss of weight, fatigue, low-grade fever, polyneuritis, nausea, and palpitations, and sometimes sudden syncopal attacks related to obstruction. **cystic m.,** one that has undergone cystic degeneration. **enchondromatous m.,** one containing cartilage in the intercellular substance. **erectile m.,** an angioma with myxomatous areas. **m. fibro'sum,** myxo-fibroma. **infectious m.,** myxomatosis cuniculi. **lipomatous m.,** a lipoma with myxomatous degeneration. **odontogenic m.,** an uncommon tumor of the jaw, apparently arising from the mesenchymal portion of the tooth germ, and possibly produced by myxomatous degeneration of an odontogenic fibroma. **m. sarcomato'sum,** myxosarcoma. **vascular m.,** a myxoma containing many blood vessels.

myxomatosis (mik″so-mah-to′sis) 1. a condition marked by the development of multiple myxomas. 2. myxomatous degeneration. **m. cunic'uli, infectious m.,** an infectious, highly fatal, febrile disease of rabbits caused by a virus, and characterized by edematous swelling of the mucous membranes and the presence of myxoma-like tumors of the skin.

myxomatous (mik-so′mah-tus) of the nature of a myxoma.

Myxomycetes (mik″so-mi-se′tēz) [myxo- + Gr. mykēs fungus] see Mycetozoida.

myxomyoma (mik″so-mi-o′mah) a myoma with myxomatous degeneration.

myxopapilloma (mik″so-pap″ĭ-lo′mah) myxoma combined with papilloma.

myxopoiesis (mik″so-poi-e′sis) [myxo- + Gr. poiēsis a making, creation] the formation of mucus.

myxorrhea (mik″so-re′ah) [myxo- + Gr. rhoia flow] a flow of mucus; blennorrhea. **m. intestina'lis,** a flow of mucus from the bowel occurring in nervous individuals under mental strain.

myxosarcoma (mik″so-sar-ko′mah) a sarcoma containing myxomatous tissue.

myxosarcomatous (mik″so-sar-ko′mah-tus) relating to or affected with myxosarcoma.

Myxosoma (mik″so-so′mah) [myxo- + Gr. soma body] a genus of parasitic protozoa (suborder Platysporina, order Bivalvulida), characterized by the presence of a mucoid envelope around the spore. It includes *M. cerebralis,* a pathogen of salmid fishes, in which it causes whirling disease.

myxosporan (mik″so-spor′an) any protozoan of the class Myxosporea.

myxospore (mik′so-spōr) a type of resting cell in the fruiting body of a bacterium of the order Myxobacterales.

Myxosporea (mik″so-spor′e-ah) [myxo- + spore] a class of histozoic or celozoic parasitic protozoa (phylum Myxozoa) found in cold-blooded vertebrates, having spores with one or two sporoplasms and one to six (typically two) polar capsules, each capsule with a coiled polar tube, the probable function of which is anchorage to the host's tissues. The spore membrane usually has two, sometimes up to six, valves. It comprises two orders: Bivalvulida and Multivalvulida.

myxovirus (mik″so-vi′rus) a general name for a large group of viruses, including the viruses of influenza, parainfluenza, mumps, and Newcastle disease; the viruses are characterized by an RNA nucleocapsid in a loose membrane, and they typically agglutinate erythrocytes. Myxoviruses have been divided into paramyxoviruses and orthomyxoviruses.

Myxozoa (mik″so-zo′ah) [myxo- + Gr. zōon animal] a phylum of chiefly histozoic or celozoic parasitic protozoa having spores of multicellular origin, with one or more polar capsules and one, two, or three, rarely more, valves, and usually found in fishes but also in amphibians and reptiles. It comprises two classes: Myxosporea and Actinosporea.

myxozoan (mik″so-zo′an) 1. any protozoan of the phylum Myxozoa. 2. pertaining to protozoa of the phylum Myxozoa.

myzesis (mi-ze′sis) [Gr. myzan to suck] sucking.

Myzomyia (mi″zo-mi′yah) [Gr. myzan to suck + myia fly] a subgenus of anopheline mosquitoes, several species of which act as the carriers of malarial parasites.

Myzorhynchus (mi″zo-ring′kus) [Gr. myzan to suck + rhynchos snout] a subgenus of anopheline mosquitoes, several species of which are the carriers of malarial parasites. *M. (Anopheles) barbiros'tris,* a species which transmits malaria and filariasis in the Orient. *M. palu'dis,* an African species. *M. pseudopic'tus,* a European species. *M. sinen'sis,* a Japanese species.

N

N 1. chemical symbol for *nitrogen.* 2. symbol for *normal* (solution); the expressions 2N, N/2 or 0.5N, N/10 or 0.1N, N/50 or 0.02N, N/200 or 0.005N, N/1000 or 0.001N denote the strength of a solution in comparison with the normal, respectively double normal, half-normal, tenth-normal, fiftieth-normal, two-hundredth-normal, and thousandth-normal. 3. symbol for *newton.*

n symbol for *nano-.*

υ nu, the thirteenth letter of the Greek alphabet; symbol for *frequency* and *neutrino.*

NA abbreviation for *Nomina Anatomica.*

N.A. numerical aperture.

Na chemical symbol for *sodium* (L. *natrium*).

nabidrox (nab′ĭ-droks) chemical name: (+)-3-(1,1-dimethylheptyl)-6aβ,7,8,9,10aα-hexahydro-6,6-dimethyl-6H-dibenzo[b,d]pyran-1,9-diol; an antihypertensive, $C_{24}H_{38}O_3$.

nabilone (nab′ĭ-lōn) chemical name: trans-(+)-3-(1,1-dimethylheptyl)-6,6a,7,8,10,10a-hexahydro-1-hydroxy-6,6-dimethyl-9H-dibenzo[b,d]pyran-9-one; a synthetic cannabinoid, $C_{24}H_{36}O_3$, which acts as a minor tranquilizer and antiemetic.

$Na_2B_4O_7 \cdot 10H_2O$ borax.

Naboth's follicles (cysts, glands, ovules, vesicles) (na′bōths) [Martin *Naboth,* Leipzig anatomist, 1675–1721] see under *follicle.*

nabothian (nah-bo′the-an) described by or named in honor of Martin *Naboth.* See under *follicle.*

NaBr sodium bromide.

NaCl sodium chloride.

NaClO sodium hypochlorite.

$NaClO_3$ sodium chlorate.

Na_2CO_3 sodium carbonate.

$Na_2C_2O_4$ sodium oxalate.

nacreous (na′kre-us) [Fr. *nacre* mother of pearl] having a grayish-white, translucent color, with a pearl-like luster; said of bacterial colonies.

Nacton (nak′ton) trademark for a preparation of poldine methylsulfate.

NAD nicotinamide-adenine dinucleotide.

N.A.D. no appreciable disease.

NAD^+ the oxidized form of NAD.

NADH the reduced form of NAD.

NADH cytochrome b_5 reductase (si′to-krōm re-duk′tās) cytochrome b_5 reductase.

NADH dehydrogenase (ubiquinone) (de-hi′dro-jen-ās u-bik′win-ōn) [E.C. 1.6.5.3] an enzyme complex of the inner mitochondrial membrane that catalyzes the reaction $NADH + ubiquinone = NAD^+ + ubiquinol$. It is a flavoprotein (FAD) bound with an iron-sulfide protein and is associated with the pumping of protons and resultant phosphorylation of ADP to ATP. The reaction is part of the terminal electron transport scheme by which oxygen is utilized for fuel combustion.

NADH-methemoglobin reductase (met-he′mo-glo-bin re-duk′tās) an enzyme of the oxidoreductase class that catalyzes the reaction 2 methemoglobin (Fe^{3+}) + NADH = 2 hemoglobin (Fe^{2+}) + NAD^+. Cytochrome b_5 serves as the intermediate electron carrier. The enzyme occurs in erythrocytes and may be identical with the cytochrome-b_5 reductase [EC 1.6.2.2] found on the endoplasmic reticulum. Deficiency of the enzyme is rare and generally asymptomatic.

NADH oxidase (ok'sĭ-dās) an oxidoreductase of neutrophils catalyzing the reaction NADH + O_2 = H_2O_2 + NAD^+. It contains FAD.

nadide (na'dīd) chemical name: adenosine 5'-(trihydrogen diphosphate)5'→5'-ester with 3-(aminocarbonyl)-1-β-D-ribofuranosylpyridinium, hydroxide inner salt; an alcohol and narcotic antagonist, $C_{21}H_{27}N_7O_{14}P_2$, it is the naturally occurring coenzyme nicotinamide-adenine dinucleotide.

nadolol (na-do'lol) chemical name: cis-5-[3-[(1,1-dimethylamino)amino] - 2 - hydroxypropoxy] - 1,2,3,4-tetrahydro-2,3-naph- thalenediol; an antiadrenergic(β-receptor),$C_{17}H_{27}NO_4$.

NADP nicotinamide-adenine dinucleotide phosphate.

NADP$^+$ the oxidized form of NADP.

NADPH the reduced form of NADP.

NADPH-cytochrome reductase (si''to-krōm re-duk'tās) NADPH-ferrihemoprotein reductase.

NADPH-ferrihemoprotein reductase (fer''e-he''mo-pro'tēn re-duk'tās) [EC 1.6.2.4] an enzyme of the oxidoreductase class that catalyzes the reaction NADPH + 2 ferricytochrome = $NADP^+$ + 2 ferrocytochrome. It is a flavoprotein monooxygenase found in the endoplasmic reticulum, serving in the transfer of electrons from NADPH to cytochrome P-450. Called also *cytochrome P-450 reductase*.

NADPH methemoglobin reductase (met-he''mo-glo''bin re-duk'tās) an enzyme of the oxidoreductase class that catalyzes the reaction 2 methemoglobin (Fe^{3+}) + NADPH = 2 hemoglobin (Fe^{2+}) + $NADP^+$. Methylene blue can act as an intermediate electron carrier. The enzyme is found in erythrocytes; its physiological significance is uncertain.

NADPH oxidase (ok'sĭ-dās) an enzyme of the oxidoreductase class that catalyzes the reaction NADPH + 2 O_2 = $NADP^+$ + 2 O_2^-. The reaction is a part of the respiratory burst in neutrophils, eosinophils, and mononuclear phagocytes. It produces superoxide anion as an oxidant in the phagocyte microbicidal system. A genetic defect in the enzyme system leads to chronic granulomatous disease.

Naegeli's leukemia (na'gĕ-lēz) [Otto *Naegeli*, Swiss hematologist, 1871–1937] see *monocytic leukemia*, under *leukemia*.

Naegeli's syndrome (na'gĕ-lēz) [Oskar *Naegeli*, Swiss dermatologist, 1885–1959] Franceschetti-Jadassohn syndrome.

Naegleria (na-gle're-ah)[F.P.O. *Nagler*, Australian bacteriologist, 20th century] a genus of free-living protozoa (order Schizopyrenida, subclass Gymnamoeba) found in fresh water, soil, and sewage, which have both an ameboid and a flagellate stage in their life cycle; in the latter stage, two flagella are present. Certain species, especially *N. fowleri*, are capable of facultative parasitism, and some strains are highly pathogenic and may cause a highly fatal primary amebic meningoencephalitis. Infection is usually acquired by swimming in water contaminated with the organisms.

naegleriasis (nāg''ler-ri'ah-sis) infection with *Naegleria*.

naepaine (ne'pān) chemical name: 2-n-pentylaminoethyl p-aminobenzoate. Dimorphic crystals, $C_{14}H_{22}N_2O_2$, with a bitter taste and soluble in water; its hydrochloride is a local anesthestic for ocular use.

NaF sodium fluoride.

nafcillin (naf-sil'in) chemical name: 6-(2-ethoxy-1-naphthamido)-3,3-dimethyl-7-oxo-4-thia-1-azabicyclo-[3.2.0]heptane-2-carboxylate. A semisynthetic, acid- and penicillinase-resistant penicillin whose sodium salt [USP], $C_{21}H_{21}N_2$-NaO_5S, a white to yellowish white powder, is used as an antibacterial in severe staphylococcal infections caused by penicillinase-positive organisms.

nafenopin (nah-fen'o-pin) chemical name: 2-methyl-2-[4-(1,2,3,4-tetrahydro-1-naphthalenyl)phenoxy]propanoic acid; an antihyperlipidemic, $C_{20}H_{22}O_3$.

Naffziger's operation, syndrome (naf'zig-erz) [Howard Christian *Naffziger*, American surgeon, 1884–1961] see under *operation*, and see *scalenus syndrome*, under *syndrome*.

nafomine malate (naf'o-mēn) chemical name: hydroxybutanedioic acid compound with O-[(2-methyl-1-naphthyl)methyl]hydroxylamine (1:1); a muscle relaxant, $C_{12}H_{13}NO$·- $C_4H_6O_5$.

nafoxidine hydrochloride (naf-oks'ĭ-dēn) chemical name: 1- [2- [4- (3,4- dihydro- 6-methoxy -2-phenyl- 1-naphthalenyl)phenoxy] ethyl]pyrrolidine hydrochloride; an antiestrogen, $C_{29}H_{31}NO_2 \cdot HCl$, which has been used in the treatment of breast cancer.

nafronyl oxalate (naf'fro-nil) chemical name: tetrahydro-α-(1-naphthalenylmethyl)-2-furanpropanoic acid 2-(diethylamino)ethyl ester ethanedioate (1:1); a vasodilator, C_{24}-$H_{33}NO_3 \cdot C_2H_2O_4$, which has been used in the treatment of peripheral and cerebral vascular disorders.

naftalofos (naf'tah-lo''fos) chemical name: 2-[(diethoxyphosphinyl)oxy]-1H-benz[de]isoquinoline-1,3(2H)-dione; a veterinary anthelmintic, $C_{16}H_{16}NO_6P$.

nagana (nah-gah'nah) [Zulu, from *ngana* feeble, weak] a general term for tsetse fly–transmitted animal infections caused by trypanosomes, including *Trypanosoma brucei*, *T. congolense*, *T. simiae*, *T. suis*, *T. vivax*, and *T. uniforme* in various parts of Africa, and affecting especially domestic animals, including cattle, horses, sheep, goats, dogs, pigs, and camels. The disease may be acute or chronic and the pathogenicity and symptoms are determined by many factors, such as the trypanosome involved and the species infected. Anemia, fever, and emaciation are associated with infection in many species, corneal opacities occur in horses and dogs, and cattle may abort.

naganol (nag'ah-nol) suramin sodium.

Nagel's test (nah'gelz)[Willibald A. *Nagel*, German physiologist, 1870–1911] see under *tests*.

Nägele's obliquity, pelvis, rule (na'gĕ-lēz) [Franz Karl *Nägele*, German obstetrician, 1777–1851] see under *obliquity*, *pelvis*, and *rule*.

Nageotte bracelets, cell (nazh-yot') [Jean *Nageotte*, Paris histologist, 1866–1948] see under *bracelet* and *cell*.

Nagler effect (nahg'ler) [Joseph *Nagler*, Vienna radiologist] see under *effect*.

Nagler's reaction (test) (nag'lerz) [F. P. O. *Nagler*, Australian bacteriologist, 20th century] see under *reaction*.

NaHCO$_3$ sodium bicarbonate.

NaH$_2$PO$_4$ monosodium acid phosphate (sodium biphosphate).

Na$_2$HPO$_4$ disodium acid phosphate (sodium phosphate).

naiad (ni'ad) [Gr. *nan* to flow] an aquatic, gill-breathing nymph (q.v.) of certain arthropods.

nail (nāl) 1. [L. *unguis*; Gr. *onyx*] the horny cutaneous plate on the dorsal surface of the distal end of a finger or toe; see *unguis*. 2. a rod of metal, bone, or other material used for

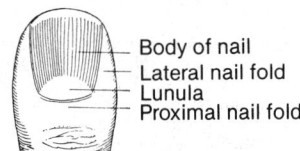

    — Body of nail
    — Lateral nail fold
    — Lunula
    — Proximal nail fold

Parts of the nail.

fixation of the ends or the fragments of fractured bones. **eggshell n.,** a fingernail which has become thin and curved upward at its anterior edge. **hippocratic n.,** see *hippocratic fingers*, under *finger*. **ingrown n.,** aberrant growth of a toenail, with one or, less often, both lateral margins pushing deeply into the adjacent soft tissues. Called also *ingrowing toenail, onychocryptosis, onyxis,* and *unguis incarnatus*. **Jewett n.,** a nail for internal fixation of a trochanteric fracture; the nail is fastened to a plate for fixing the head and neck of the bone to the shaft. **Küntscher n.,** a tubular metal nail for the intramedullary fixation of fractures. **Neufeld n.,** a device for internal fixation of intertrochanteric fracture of the femur, the V nail section being set at an angle of about 130 degrees to the plate portion. **parrot beak n.,** a curvation of the fingernail like that of a parrot's beak. **pitted n's,** nails with surface pits, usually under 1 mm. in diameter, most often seen in psoriasis, frequently in alopecia areata, and sometimes unexplained. **racket n.,** thumbnails that are much shorter than they are wide; rarely, other fingers may be affected. In the commonest form, the distal phalanges of affected digits are shortened as well. **reedy n.,** a fingernail marked by longitudinal furrows. **Smith-Petersen n.,** a flanged nail for fixing the head of the femur in fracture of the femoral neck. **spoon n.,** depression of the central portion of the fingernail, with raising of the edges at the sides. **turtle-back n.,** a fingernail which is greatly distorted, being more convex than normal. **watch-crystal n.,** a nail convex lengthwise as well as crosswise, and often as broad as it is long, seen in pulmonary osteoarthropathy and pachydermoperiostosis.

nailing (nāl′ing) the operation of fixing or fastening of a fractured bone with a nail. **intramedullary n., marrow n., medullary n.,** the fixation of a fractured long bone by insertion of a steel rod into the marrow cavity of the bone.

Nairobi eye, sheep disease (ni-ro′be) [*Nairobi,* the capital of Kenya, in East Africa] see under *disease* and *eye.*

naja (nah′jah) [Arabic] the cobra di capello, *Naja naja* (*N. tripudians*), a common cobra of India; also a homeopathic preparation of its venom. See *cobra.*

Nakayama's reagent, test (nak-ah-yah′mah) [M. *Nakayama,* Japanese chemist] see under *reagent* and *tests.*

nalbuphine hydrochloride (nal′bu-fēn) chemical name: 17-(cyclobutylmethyl)-4,5α-epoxymorphinan-3,6α,14-triol hydrochloride; an analgesic and narcotic antagonist, $C_{21}H_{27}NO_4 \cdot HCl$.

Nalfon (nal′fon) trademark for a preparation of fenoprofen calcium.

nalidixate sodium (nal-ĭ-diks′āt) chemical name: 1-ethyl-1,4-dihydro - 7 - methyl - 4 - oxo - 1,8 - naphthyridine-3-carboxylate sodium salt monohydrate; an antibacterial, $C_{12}H_{11}N_2NaO_3H_2O$.

nalidixic acid (nal-i-dik′sik) [USP] a synthetic antibacterial agent used orally in the treatment of urinary infections caused by gram-negative organisms, especially those caused by *Proteus* species.

Nalline (nal′lēn) trademark for a preparation of nalorphine.

nalmexone hydrochloride (nal-meks′ōn) chemical name: 4,5α-epoxy-3,14-dihydroxy-17-(3-methyl-2-butenyl)-morphinan-6-one hydrochloride; an antagonist and narcotic antagonist, $C_{21}H_{25}NO_4 \cdot HCl$.

nalorphine (nal′or-fēn, nal-or′fēn) chemical name: 17-allyl-7,8-didehydro-4,5α-epoxymorphinan-3,6-α-diol. A drug structurally related to morphine, $C_{19}H_{21}NO_3$, which acts as an antagonist to morphine and related narcotics. Called also *allorphine* and *antorphine.* **n. hydrochloride** the hydrochloride salt of nalorphine, $C_{19}H_{21}NO_3 \cdot HCl$, occurring as a white or practically white, crystalline powder; used as a narcotic antagonist, chiefly to counteract respiratory depression due to narcotic overdosage, administered intravenously. It is also used to diagnose narcotic addiction; withdrawal symptoms occur following its subcutaneous administration to addicts.

naloxone hydrochloride (nal-oks′ōn) chemical name: 17-allyl-4,5α-epoxy-3,14-dihydroxymorphinan-6-one hydrochloride. A narcotic antagonist structurally related to oxymorphone, $C_{19}H_{21}NO_4HCl$, occurring as a white to slightly off-white powder; used as an antidote to narcotic overdosage, and as an antagonist for pentazocine overdosage, administered parenterally.

naltrexone (nal-treks′ōn) chemical name: 17-(cyclopropylmethyl)-4,5α-epoxy-3,14-dihydroxymorphinan-6-one; a narcotic antagonist, $C_{20}H_{23}NO_4$.

name (nām) a word or words used to designate a unique entity and distinguish it from others. **British Approved N.,** see *BAN.* **generic n.,** 1. in chemistry, a name applied to a class of compounds, e.g., alkane or halide. 2. nonproprietary n. 3. in biology, the name applied to a genus. **International Nonproprietary n.,** see INN. **nonproprietary n.,** a short name coined for a drug or chemical not subject to proprietary (trademark) rights and recommended or recognized by an official body, e.g., a USAN, INN, or BAN. **proprietary n.,** a brand name or trademark under which a proprietary product is marketed. See *proprietary.* **systematic n.,** in chemical nomenclature, a name of a substance based on the chemical structure of a compound. **trivial n.,** in chemical nomenclature, a name of a substance that does not reflect its chemical structure; many trivial names are semisystematic, e.g., the *-ol* in glycerol indicates that it is an alcohol. **United States Adopted n.,** see *USAN.*

nandrolone (nan′dro-lōn) chemical name: 17β-hydrox-yestr-4-en-3-one. An anabolic steroid, $C_{18}H_{26}O_2$, differing from testosterone in not having a methyl group attached to carbon 10 of the steroid nucleus. Called also *norandrostenolone.* **n. cyclotate,** an ester of nandrolone, $C_{28}H_{38}O_3$. **n. decanoate** [USP], an ester of nandrolone, $C_{28}H_{44}O_3$, occurring as a fine, white to creamy white, crystalline powder, having the properties of other anabolic steroids and a long duration of action; used mainly as adjunctive therapy in senile and postmenopausal osteoporosis and in the treatment of severe growth retardation in children, administered intramuscularly. **n. phenpropionate** [USP], an ester of nandrolone, $C_{27}H_{34}O_3$, having a moderate duration of action and the appearance, properties, uses, and mode of administration of the decanoate ester.

nanism (na′nizm) [L. *nanus* dwarf] dwarfism or marked undersize from whatever cause. **mulibrey n.,** a rare autosomal recessive disorder marked by dwarfism and constrictive pericarditis; called mulibrey to denote defects of *mu*scle, *li*ver, *br*ain, and *ey*es. Affected infants have a triangular face often with hypocephaloid skull, muscular hypotonia, squeaky voice, and yellowish dots and pigment dispersion in the ocular fundus. **pituitary n.,** hypophysial infantilism. **renal n.,** infantile renal osteodystrophy. **senile n.,** progeria. **symptomatic n.,** nanism with defective ossification, dentition, and sexual development.

Nannizzia (nah-niz′ĭ-ah) a genus of ascomycetous fungi (family Gymnoascaceae, order Eurotiales), in which the hyphae around the gymnothecium are verticillately branched and composed of cells with shallow constrictions; it contains the perfect (sexual) stages of *Microsporum.*

nann(o)- see *nano-.*

Nannocystis (nan″no-sis′tis) [*nanno-* + Gr. *kystis* sac, bladder] a genus of gliding bacteria of the family Polyangiaceae, order Myxobacterales, found in soil. The type species is *N. ex′edens.*

Nannomonas (nan″no-mo′nas) [*nanno-* + Gr. *monas* unit] in some systems of classification, a subgenus of salivarian trypanosomes, including *Trypanosoma congolense, T. dimorphon,* and *T. simiae.*

nan(o)- [Gr. *nanos* dwarf] a combining form designating small size; used in naming units of measurement to indicate one-billionth (10^{-9}) of the unit designated by the root with which it is combined. Symbol, n.

nanocephalia (nan″o-sĕ-fa′le-ah) nanocephaly.

nanocephalous (na″no-sef′ah-lus) [*nano-* + Gr. *kephalē* head] having a small head; pertaining to nanocephaly.

nanocephaly (na″no-sef′ah-le) abnormal smallness of the head.

nanocormia (na″no-kor′me-ah) [*nano-* + Gr. *kormos* trunk + *-ia*] a developmental anomaly characterized by abnormal smallness of the body, or trunk.

nanocurie (na″no-ku′re) a unit of radioactivity, being 10^{-9} curie, or the quantity of radioactive material in which the number of nuclear disintegrations is 3.7×10, or 37, per second. Abbreviated nCi. Called also *millimicrocurie.*

nanogram (na′no-gram) a unit of mass (weight) of the metric system, being one one-billionth (10^{-9}) gram; abbreviated ng. Called also *millimicrogram.*

nanoid (na′noid) [*nano-* + Gr. *eidos* form] dwarfish; resembling a dwarf.

nanoliter (na″no-le′ter) a unit of capacity equal to one-billionth (10^{-9}) of a liter; abbreviated nl. Called also *millimicroliter.*

nanomelia (na″no-me′le-ah) [*nano-* + Gr. *melos* limb + *-ia*] a developmental anomaly characterized by abnormal smallness of the limbs.

nanomelous (na-nom′ĕ-lus) pertaining to or characterized by nanomelia.

nanomelus (na-nom′ĕ-lus) an individual exhibiting nanomelia.

nanometer (na″no-me′ter) a unit of linear measure equal to one-billionth of a meter, 10^{-9} meter; abbreviated nm.

nanophthalmia (nan″of-thal′me-ah) nanophthalmos.

nanophthalmos (nan″of-thal′mus) [*nan-* + Gr. *ophthalmos* eye] microphthalmos in an eye that is otherwise normal. A nanophthalmic eye is very hyperopic and prone to angle-closure glaucoma.

Nanophyetus salmincola (na-no′fi-e-tus sal-min′ko-lah) *Troglotrema salmincola.*

nanoplankton (na″no-plank′ton) plankton of extremely minute size.

nanosecond (na″no-sek′ond) one-billionth (10^{-9}) of a second; abbreviated ns. or nsec.

nanosoma (na″no-so′mah) nanosomia.

nanosomia (na″no-so′me-ah) [nano- + Gr. *sōma* body + -ia] dwarfism; nanism.

nanounit (na″no-u′nit) one-billionth (10^{-9}) of a standard unit; abbreviated nU.

nanous (na′nus) dwarfish; stunted.

nanukayami (nah″nu-kah-yah′me) a leptospirosis marked by fever and jaundice, first reported in Japan and caused by *Leptospira interrogans* serogroup *hebdomidis;* the animal host is the field vole, *Microtus montebelli.* Called also *nanukayami disease* or *fever, akiyami, seven-day fever, autumn fever,* and *gikiyami.*

nanus (na′nus) [L.; Gr. *nanos*] a dwarf.

NaOH sodium hydroxide.

NAP nasion, point A, pogonion; see *angle of convexity.*

napelline (na-pel′in) [L. *napellus* aconite] an analgesic alkaloid, $C_{22}H_{33}O_3N$, from aconite.

napex (na′peks) the region of the scalp just below the occipital protuberance.

naphazoline hydrochloride (naf-az′o-lēn) [USP] chemical name: 4,5-dihydro-2-(1-naphthalenyl)-1H-imidazole monohydrochloride. An adrenergic, $C_{14}H_{14}N_2 \cdot HCl$, occurring as a white, crystalline powder; used as a vasoconstrictor, applied topically to the nasal or ocular mucous membranes.

naphtalin (naf′tah-lin) naphthalene.

naphtalinum, naphthalinum (naf″tah-li′num; naf″-thah-li′num) [L.] naphthalene.

naphtha (naf′thah) [L., from Arabic] 1. petroleum benzin. 2. ligroin. **n. ace′ti, vinegar n.,** ethyl acetate. **wood n.,** methanol.

naphthalene (naf′thah-lēn) [L. *naphthalinum*] a silvery, crystalline hydrocarbon, $C_{10}H_8$, from coal tar oil. It is insoluble in cold water, but soluble in hot water, alcohol, ether, chloroform, and benzene. Formerly used as an antiseptic in diarrhea of typhoid fever.

naphthamine (naf′thah-min) methenamine.

naphthol (naf′thol) a crystalline, antiseptic substance, $C_{10}H_7 \cdot OH$, from coal tar, occurring in two forms, the α (alphanaphthol) and β (betanaphthol). **α-n., alpha-n.,** see *alphanaphthol.* **β-n., beta-n.,** see *betanaphthol.*

naphtholate (naf″tho-lāt′) a naphthol compound in which a base takes the place of hydrogen in the hydroxyl.

naphtholism (naf′thol-izm) naphthol poisoning.

naphthoresorcine (naf″tho-re-sor′sin) a principle in transparent crystals derived from naphthol and resorcinol.

naphthyl (naf′thil) the radical, $C_{10}H_7$. **n. alcohol,** naphthol. **n. benzoate,** benzonaphthol. **n. lactate,** lactol. **n. phenol,** naphthol.

naphthylpararosaniline (naf″thil-par″ah-ro-san′ĭ-lin) a dye, isamine blue, which has been used experimentally in the treatment of malignant tumors.

naphtol (naf′tol) naphthol.

napiform (na′pĭ-form) [L. *napus* turnip + *forma* shape] having the shape or form of a turnip.

N.A.P.N.E.S. National Association for Practical Nurse Education and Services.

naprapath (nap′rah-path) a practitioner of naprapathy.

naprapathy (nah-prap′ah-the) [Czech *napravit* to correct + Gr. *pathos* disease] a system of therapy employing manipulation of connective tissue (ligaments, muscles, and joints) and dietary measures; said to facilitate the recuperative and regenerative processes of the body.

Naprosyn (nah-pro′sin) trademark for a preparation of naproxen.

naproxen (nah-proks′en) [USP] a nonsteroidal anti-inflammatory agent that is a propionic acid derivative; used for treatment of osteoarthritis and rheumatoid arthritis. Also available as *naproxen sodium.*

naproxol (nah-proks′ol) chemical name: (+)-6-methoxy-α-methyl-2-naphthaleneacetic acid. An anti-inflammatory, antipyretic, and analgesic, occurring as a white to off-white, crystalline powder; used in the treatment of rheumatoid arthritis, administered orally.

napsylate (nap′sĭ-lāt) USAN contraction for 2-naphthalenesulfonate.

Naqua (nak′wah) trademark for a preparation of trichlormethiazide.

Naquival (nak′wĭ′val) trademark for a preparation of trichlormethiazide with reserpine.

naranol hydrochloride (nar′ah-nōl) chemical name: 8,-9,10,11,11a,12-hexahydro-8,10-dimethyl-7aH-naphtho[1′,2′:-5,6]pyrano[3,2-c]pyridin-7a-ol; a tranquilizer, $C_{18}H_{21}NO_2 \cdot HCl$.

narasin (nar′ah-sin) chemical name: α4.1.5.3]5-[2-(5-ethyltetrahydro-5-hydroxy-6-methyl-2-H-pyran-2-yl)-15-hydroxy-2,10,12-trimethyl-1,6,8-trioxadispiro[4.1.5.3]pentadec-13-en-9-yl]-2-hydroxy-1,3-dimethyl-4-oxoheptyl]tetrahydro-3,5-dimethyl-2H-pyran-2-acetic acid; a veterinary coccidiostate and growth stimulant, $C_{43}H_{72}O_{11}$.

Narcan (nar′kan) trademark for a preparation of naloxone hydrochloride.

narcism (nar′sizm) narcissism.

narcissine (nar-sis′in) a crystalline alkaloid, $C_{16}H_{17}NO_4$, having emetic properties, from the bulbs of many different plants, including the daffodil, *Narcissus pseudonarcissus* L. (Amaryllidaceae); identical with lycorine.

narcissism (nar′sĭ-sizm) [from *Narcissus,* a character in Greek mythology who fell in love with his own image reflected in water] self-love. In psychoanalytic theory, *primary n.* is the early infantile phase of object relationship development, when the child has not differentiated himself from the outside world and regards all sources of pleasure as originating within himself; in *secondary n.,* the libido, once attached to external love objects, is redirected back to the self.

narcissistic (nar″sĭ-sis′tik) pertaining to or characterized by narcissism.

narco- [Gr. *narkē* numbness] a combining form denoting relationship to stupor, to a stuporous state, or to narcosis.

narcoanalysis (nar″ko-ah-nal′ĭ-sis) a form of psychotherapy that utilizes the slow intravenous administration of barbiturates in order to release suppressed or repressed thoughts, i.e., to disinhibit communication of affect-laden and unacceptable ideas.

narcoanesthesia (nar″ko-an″es-the′ze-ah) [narco- + anesthesia] (obs.) anesthesia by the production of a stuporous condition by the hypodermic injection of scopolamine and morphine.

narcohypnia (nar″ko-hip′ne-ah) [narco- + Gr. *hypnos* sleep + -ia] numbness felt on waking from sleep.

narcohypnosis (nar″ko-hip-no′sis) hypnotic suggestions made while the patient is under the influence of a narcotic drug.

narcolepsy (nar″ko-lep″se) [narco- + Gr. *lepsis* a taking hold, a seizure] recurrent, uncontrollable, brief episodes of sleep, often associated with hypnagogic hallucinations, cataplexy, and sleep paralysis; called also *Gelineau's syndrome* and *paroxysmal sleep.*

narcoleptic (nar″ko-lep′tik) pertaining to, characterized by, or producing narcolepsy. By extension, sometimes used to denote an individual who exhibits narcolepsy.

narcoma (nar-ko′mah) a stuporous state produced by narcotics.

narcose (nar′kōs) stuporous; in a state of stupor.

narcosine (nar′ko-sēn) noscapine.

narcosis (nar-ko′sis) [Gr. *narkōsis* a benumbing] a nonspecific and reversible depression of function of the central nervous system marked by stupor or insensibility produced by drugs. **basal n., basis n.,** narcosis marked by complete unconsciousness, amnesia, and analgesia; see *preanesthesia.* **insufflation n.,** insufflation anesthesia. **intravenous n.,** phlebonarcosis. **medullary n.,** narcosis produced by injection of a local anesthetic into the medullary subarachnoid space. **Nussbaum's n.,** general narcosis by the use of ether or chloroform after an injection of morphine.

narcostimulant (nar″ko-stim′u-lant) having both narcotic and stimulant properties.

narcosynthesis (nar″ko-sin′thĕ-sis) narcoanalysis.

narcotic (nar-kot′ik) [Gr. *narkōtikos* benumbing, deadening] 1. pertaining to or producing narcosis. 2. an agent that produces insensibility or stupor, applied especially to the opioids, i.e., to any natural or synthetic drug that has morphine-like actions.

narcotico-acrid (nar-kot″ĭ-ko-ak′rid) both narcotic and acrid.

narcotico-irritant (nar-kot′ĭ-ko-ir′ĭ-tant) both narcotic and irritant.

narcotile (nar′ko-tīl) ethyl chloride.

narcotine (nar′ko-tēn) noscapine.

narcotism (nar′ko-tizm) (obs.) 1. narcosis. 2. addiction to narcotics.

narcotize (nar′ko-tīz) to put under the influence of a narcotic.

narcous (nar′kus) narcose

Nardil (nar′dil) trademark for a preparation of phenelzine sulfate.

nares (na′rēz) [L., pl. of na′ris, q.v.] [NA] the external orifices of the nose; called also nostrils. See naris.

naris (na′ris), pl. na′res [L.] one of the openings of the nasal cavity. **anterior n., external n.,** either of the external orifices of the nose (nares [NA]). **internal nares,** see cavum nasi. **posterior nares,** the openings between the nasal cavity and the nasopharynx (choanae [NA]).

Narone (nar′ōn) trademark for a preparation of dipyrone.

nasal (na′zal) [L. nasalis] pertaining to the nose.

nasalis (na-za′lis) [L., from nasus nose] relating to the nose.

nascent (nas′ent, na′sent) [L. nascens] 1. just born; just coming into existence. 2. just liberated from a chemical combination, and hence more reactive because uncombined.

nasioiniac (na″ze-o-in′e-ak) pertaining to the nasion and the inion.

nasion (na′ze-on) [L. nasus nose] [NA] a cephalometric landmark located where the intranasal and nasofrontal sutures meet; it corresponds roughly to the depression at the root of the nose just below the level of the eyebrows.

nasitis (na-zi′tis) [L. nasus nose + -itis] inflammation of the nose.

Nasmyth's membrane (nas′miths) [Alexander Nasmyth, Scottish dental surgeon in London, died 1847] primary (enamel) cuticle.

NAS-NRC National Academy of Sciences–National Research Council.

Na₂SO₄ sodium sulfate.

Na₂S₂O₃ sodium thiosulfate.

nas(o)- [L. nasus nose] a combining form denoting relationship to the nose.

nasoantral (na″zo-an′tral) pertaining to the nose and the maxillary antrum (sinus).

nasoantritis (na″zo-an-tri′tis) inflammation of the nose and antrum of Highmore.

nasoantrostomy (na″so-an-tros′to-me) surgical formation of a nasoantral window for drainage of an obstructed maxillary sinus.

nasobronchial (na″zo-brong′ke-al) pertaining to the nasal cavities and the bronchi.

nasociliary (na″zo-sil′e-a″re) pertaining to or affecting the eyes, brow, and root of the nose, as the nasociliary nerve.

nasofrontal (na″zo-frun′tal) pertaining to the nasal and frontal bones.

nasogastric (na″zo-gas′trik) pertaining to the nose and stomach, as in (nasogastric) aspiration of the stomach's contents.

nasolabial (na″zo-la′be-al) [naso- + L. labium lip] pertaining to the nose and lip.

nasolacrimal (na″zo-lak′rĭ-mal) pertaining to the nose and lacrimal apparatus.

nasomanometer (na″zo-mah-nom′ĕ-ter) a manometer for measuring intranasal pressure.

nasonnement (na″zon-maw′) [Fr.] a nasal quality of voice.

naso-oral (na″zo-o′ral) pertaining to or involving the nose and mouth.

nasopalatine (na″zo-pal′ah-tīn) [naso- + palatine] pertaining to the nose and palate.

nasopharyngeal (na″zo-fah-rin′je-al) pertaining to the nasopharynx.

nasopharyngitis (na″zo-far″in-ji′tis) inflammation of the nasopharynx.

nasopharyngolaryngoscope (na″zo-fah-ring″go-lah-ring′go-skōp) a flexible fiberoptic endoscope for examining the nasopharynx and larynx.

nasopharyngoscope (na″zo-fah-rin′go-skōp) a lighted, telescopic endoscope for use in examination of the nasopharynx and the pharyngeal end of the auditory tube.

nasopharynx (na″zo-far′inks) [naso- + pharynx] the part of the pharynx which lies above the level of the soft palate (pars nasalis pharyngis [NA]).

nasorostral (na″zo-ros′tral) pertaining to the rostrum of the nose.

nasoscope (na′zo-skōp) [naso- + Gr. skopein to examine] an electrically lighted instrument for inspecting the nasal cavity.

nasoseptal (na″zo-sep′tal) pertaining to the nasal septum.

nasoseptitis (na″zo-sep-ti′tis) inflammation of the nasal septum.

nasosinusitis (na″zo-si″nu-si′tis) inflammation of the accessory sinuses of the nose.

nasospinale (na″zo-spi-na′le) the point at which a horizontal line tangential to the lower margins of the nasal aperture is intersected by the midsagittal plane.

nasoturbinal (na″zo-tur″bĭ-nal) pertaining to the nose and turbinate bone.

Nassellarida (nas″el-lar′ĭ-dah) an order of marine planktonic protozoa (class Polycystinea, superclass Actinopoda), characterized by the presence of a capsular membrane with pores located at a single pole and a one-piece, often basket-shaped skeleton.

Nassulida (na-soo′lĭ-dah) an order of free-living ciliate protozoa (superorder Nassulidea, subclass Hypostomatia), characterized by the presence of individualized parts of the hypostomial frange that are limited to the left side of the ventral surface of the body, sometimes being reduced to a few pseudomembranelles; and by a distinct preoral suture. It comprises two suborders: Nassulina and Microthoracina.

Nassulidea (na″soo-lid′e-ah) a superorder of free-living, often cylindrical ciliate protozoa (subclass Hypostomatia, class Kinetofragminophorea) most often found in fresh water, and characterized by the presence of a hypostomial frange of many parts that runs obliquely across the anterior end of the ventral surface of the body or is reduced to a few adoral pseudomembranelles (sometimes in an oral atrium); complete somatic ciliature that is less abundant on the ventral than on the dorsal surface; and a cyrtos comprising many nematodesmata.

Nassulina (na-soo′lĭ-nah) a suborder of often large, cylindrical, and completely ciliated protozoa (order Nassulida, superorder Nassulidea), the best known forms of which are found in freshwater habitats, feeding on filamentous algae, and characterized by the presence of a frange of variable composition, always distinct from the suture line.

nastic (nas′tik) of or pertaining to a response of leaves or plant parts to external stimuli that is independent of the direction of origin of such stimuli; see under movement.

nasus (na′sus) [L.] [NA] the specialized structure of the face that serves as the organ of the sense of smell and as part of the respiratory system; called also nose. See n. externa and cavitas nasi. **n. exter′nus** [NA] the external nose: the part of the nose that protrudes on the face; made up of an osteocartilaginous framework, covered externally by muscles and skin and lined internally by mucous membrane; it has two apertures that open into the nasal cavity and is separated into two halves by the nasal septum.

natal (na′tal) 1. [L. natus birth] pertaining to birth. 2. [L. nates buttocks] pertaining to the buttocks; pygal.

natality (na-tal′ĭ-te) [L. natalis pertaining to birth] birth rate.

nataloin (na-tal′o-in) an aloin or glycosidal bitter principle, $C_{25}H_{28}O_{11}$, derived from Natal aloes.

natamycin (nat″ah-mi′sin) chemical name: pimaricin, a polyene antibiotic, $C_{33}H_{47}NO_{13}$, used in topical treatment of fungal keratitis, blepharitis, and conjunctivitis.

nates (na′tēz) [L., pl. of natis] [NA] the prominences formed by the gluteal muscles on the lower part of the back; called also buttocks and clunes.

Nathans (na'thanz) Daniel. American microbiologist, born 1928; co-winner, with Werner Arber and Hamilton Othanel Smith, of the Nobel prize for medicine or physiology in 1978 for his application of restriction enzymes to molecular genetics.

natimortality (na″tǐ-mor-tal'ǐ-te) [L. *natus* birth + *mortality*] (obs.) the stillbirth rate; the number of stillbirths in a specified year divided by the number of still and live births. Now called *fetal death rate*.

National Formulary a book of standards for certain pharmaceuticals and preparations that are not included in the USP. It is revised every five years, and recognized as a book of official standards by the Pure Food and Drugs Act of 1906. Abbreviated NF.

natis (na'tis) [L. "rump"] see *nates*.

native (na'tiv) [L. *nativus*] normal to a location; unaltered from its natural state.

Natolone (nat'o-lōn) trademark for a preparation of pregnenolone.

natremia (nah-tre'me-ah) [L. *natrium* sodium + Gr. *haima* blood + *-ia*] hypernatremia.

natrium (na'tre-um), gen. *na'trii* [L., from Gr. *nitron* sodium carbonate] sodium.

natriuresis (na″tre-u-re'sis) [L. *natrium* sodium + Gr. *ourēsis* a making water] the excretion of abnormal amounts of sodium in the urine.

natriuretic (na″tre-u-ret'ik) 1. pertaining to, characterized by, or promoting natriuresis. 2. an agent that promotes natriuresis.

natron (na'tron) native sodium carbonate; also soda or sodium hydroxide.

natrum (na'trum) sodium.

natruresis (nat″roo-re'sis) natriuresis.

natruretic (nat″roo-ret'ik) natriuretic.

natural (nat'u-ral) [L. *naturalis*, from *natura* nature] neither artificial nor pathologic.

Naturetin (nat″u-re'tin) trademark for preparations of bendroflumethiazide.

naturopath (na'tūr-o-path″) a practitioner of naturopathy.

naturopathic (na″tūr-o-path'ik) pertaining to naturopathy.

naturopathy (na″tūr-op'ah-the) a drugless system of therapy, making use of physical forces such as air, light, water, heat, massage, etc.

Nauheim bath, treatment (now'hīm) [Bad-*Nauheim*, a town and watering place in Hesse, Germany] see under *bath*, and see *Schott's treatment*, under *treatment*.

Naumanniella (naw-man″ne-el'lah) [Einar *Naumann*, Swedish limnologist] a genus of gram-negative chemolithotrophic bacteria of the family Siderocapsaceae, made up of rod-shaped cells surrounded by a capsule containing deposits of iron compounds. They are found in iron-containing water. The type species is *N. neusto'nica*.

nausea (naw'se-ah) [L.; Gr. *nausia* seasickness] an unpleasant sensation, vaguely referred to the epigastrium and abdomen, and often culminating in vomiting. **n. epidem'ica,** an epidemic disease, probably viral gastroenteritis, marked by nausea, vomiting, giddiness, and diarrhea. **n. gravida'rum,** the morning sickness of pregnancy.

nauseant (naw'se-ant) 1. inducing nausea. 2. an agent that causes nausea.

nauseate (naw'se-āt) to affect with nausea.

nauseous (naw'shus, naw'se-us) pertaining to or producing nausea.

Navane (nav'ān) trademark for preparations of thiothixene.

navel (na'vel) the umbilicus. **blue n.,** Cullen's sign. **enamel n.,** in the cap stage of odontogenesis, a slight indentation in the outer dental epithelium of a developing tooth, in the end of the enamel cord; a temporary structure that disappears before enamel formation begins.

navicula (nah-vik'u-lah) [L.] frenulum labiorum pudendi.

navicular (nah-vik'u-lar) [L. *navicula* boat] boat-shaped, as the navicular bone.

navicularthritis (nah-vik″u-lar-thri'tis) inflammation of the navicular joint of the horse's forefoot.

Nb chemical symbol for *niobium*.

N.B.S. National Bureau of Standards.

NBT nitroblue tetrazolium; see under *tests*.

NCF neutrophil chemotactic factor.

NCI National Cancer Institute.

nCi nanocurie.

N.C.M.H. National Committee for Mental Hygiene.

N.C.N. National Council of Nurses.

NCRP National Committee on Radiation Protection and Measurements.

Nd chemical symbol for *neodymium*.

N.D.A. National Dental Association.

NDV Newcastle disease virus.

Ne chemical symbol for *neon*.

nealogy (ne-al'o-je) [Gr. *neaēs* young + *-logy*] the study of the early infant stages of animals.

near-sight (nēr'sīt) myopia.

nearsighted (nēr'sīt-ed) myopic.

nearsightedness (nēr'sīt-ed-nes) myopia.

nearthrosis (ne″ar-thro'sis) [Gr. *neos* new + *arthron* joint] 1. a false joint; pseudarthrosis. 2. an artificial joint inserted in total joint replacement.

Nebcin (neb'sin) trademark for a preparation of tobramycin sulfate.

nebenkern (na″ben-kern) [Ger. *neben* near, beside + *kern* kernel, nucleus] 1. a name given to several structures of the cell, but especially to the paranucleus. 2. a large mitochondrial mass around the axial filament in the flagellum of the spermatozoon; it is formed by coalescence of smaller mitochondria during spermatogenesis.

nebramycin (neb″rah-mi'sin) a complex of antibacterial antibiotic substances produced by *Streptomyces tenebrarius,* consisting of eight components, one of which, factor 6 (known as *tobramycin*), is used clinically.

nebula (neb'u-lah), gen. and pl. *ne'bulae* [L. "mist"] 1. a slight corneal opacity or scar that can be seen only by oblique illumination; it seldom interferes with vision. 2. cloudiness in urine. 3. an oily preparation for use in an atomizer.

nebularine (neb-u-lār'in) chemical name: 9-β-D-ribofuranosyl-9*H*-purine. An antibiotic substance, $C_{10}H_{12}N_4O_4$, isolated from the juice of the fungus *Clitocybe nebularis,* which has tuberculostatic and antimitotic activity, and in high dilutions preferentially inhibits growth of some cancer cells.

nebulization (neb″u-li-za'shun) [L. *nebula* mist] 1. conversion into a spray. 2. treatment by a spray.

nebulizer (neb'u-līz″er) an atomizer; a device for throwing a spray.

Necator (ne-ka'tor) [L. "murderer"] a genus of nematode parasites of the family Ancylostomidae. **N. america'nus,** the American or New World hookworm, a nematode parasite resembling, but shorter and more slender than, *Ancylostoma duodenale.* It is characterized by its buccal cavity containing four plates, four pharyngeal lancets, and a dorsal conic tooth. Infection by this parasite produces hookworm disease. Called also *Ancylostoma americanum* and *Uncinaria americana.* See also *hookworm disease,* under *disease.*

necatoriasis (ne-ka″to-ri'ah-sis) the state of being infected with worms of the genus *Necator.* See *hookworm disease,* under *disease.*

necessity (ne-ses'ǐ-te) something necessary or indispensable. **pharmaceutic n., pharmaceutical n.,** a substance having slight or no value therapeutically, but used in the preparation of various pharmaceuticals, including preservatives, solvents, ointment bases, and flavoring, coloring, diluting, emulsifying, and suspending agents; called also *pharmaceutic* or *pharmaceutical aid.*

neck (nek) a constricted portion, such as the part connecting the head and trunk of the body (collum [NA]), or the constricted part of an organ, as of the uterus (cervix uteri) or other structure (e.g., collum dentis). **anatomical n. of humerus,** collum anatomicum humeri. **n. of ankle bone,** collum tali. **bull n.,** marked edema of the anterior neck and submandibular region associated with massive cervical lymphadenopathy, which may occur in severe (malignant) pharyngeal diphtheria. **n. of condyloid pro-**

cess of mandible, collum mandibulae. **dental n.,** cervix dentis. **n. of dorsal head of spinal cord,** cervix cornus dorsalis medullae spinalis. **false n. of humerus,** collum chirurgicum humeri. **n. of femur,** collum ossis femoris. **n. of fibula,** collum fibulae. **n. of gallbladder,** collum vesicae biliaris. **n. of glans penis,** collum glandis penis. **n. of hair follicle,** collum folliculi pili. **n. of humerus,** collum anatomicum humeri. **lateral n. of vertebra,** pediculus arcus vertebrae. **Madelung's n.,** diffuse symmetrical lipomas of the neck. **n. of malleus,** collum mallei. **n. of mandible,** collum mandibulae. **n. of pancreas,** a constricted portion marking the junction of the head and body of the pancreas. **n. of posterior horn of spinal cord,** cervix cornus dorsalis medullae spinalis. **n. of radius,** collum radii. **n. of rib,** collum costae. **n. of scapula,** collum scapulae. **n. of spermatozoon,** the portion of the tail of a spermatozoon beginning immediately behind the head and extending to the anterior centriole. See illustration under *spermatozoon*. **surgical n. of humerus,** collum chirurgicum humeri. **n. of talus,** collum tali. **n. of tooth,** cervix dentis. **true n. of humerus,** collum anatomicum humeri. **turkey gobbler n.,** submental vertical skin folds due to aging. **n. of urinary bladder,** cervix vesicae. **uterine n., n. of uterus,** cervix uteri. **n. of vertebra, n. of vertebral arch,** pediculus arcus vertebrae. **webbed n.,** pterygium colli. **wry n.,** torticollis.

necklace (nek′las) an encircling band around the neck. **Casal's n.,** an area of erythema and pigmentation around the neck in pellagra; called also *Casal's collar*.

necrectomy (nek-rek′to-me) [*necro-* + Gr. *ektomē* excision] excision of necrotic tissue.

necrencephalus (nek″ren-sef′ah-lus) [*necro-* + Gr. *enkephalos* brain] softening of the brain.

necr(o)- [Gr. *nekros* dead] a combining form denoting relationship to death or to a dead body, cells, or tissue.

necrobacillosis (nek″ro-bas″ĭ-lo′sis) infection with Schmorl's bacillus, *Fusobacterium necrophorum*, which causes diphtheria with abscesses in cattle, gangrenous dermatitis in horses, areas of necrosis in hogs and cattle, and abscesses and areas of necrosis in rabbits. See also *calf diphtheria*, under *diphtheria*, and *Schmorl's disease*, under *disease*.

necrobiosis (nek″ro-bi-o′sis) [*necro-* + Gr. *biōsis* life] swelling, basophilia, and distortion of collagen bundles in the dermis, sometimes with obliteration of normal structure, but short of actual necrosis, characteristic especially of granuloma annulare and necrobiosis lipoidica diabeticorum. Cf. *gangrene* and *necrosis*. **n. lipoi′dica,** a degenerative disease of dermal connective tissue characterized by the development of erythematous papules or nodules in the pretibial area, sometimes found elsewhere on the body, that extend to form shiny, waxy, yellowish red plaques, which are covered with telangiectatic vessels and have a violet-red border and a scaly, atrophic and depressed center. More than half of affected patients have diabetes; the clinical appearance, genetic background for diabetes, and histopathologic findings are similar in both diabetic and nondiabetic patients. See also *diabetic dermopathy*, under *dermopathy*, and *granulomatosis disciformis progressiva et chronica*. **n. lipoi′dica diabetico′rum,** see *n. lipoidica*.

necrobiotic (nek″ro-bi-ot′ik) pertaining to or characterized by necrobiosis.

necrocytosis (nek″ro-si-to′sis) [*necro-* + Gr. *kytos* cell + *-osis*] death and decay of cells.

necrocytotoxin (nek″ro-si″to-tok′sin) a toxin that produces death of cells.

necrogenic (nek″ro-jen′ik) [*necro-* + Gr. *gennan* to produce] productive of necrosis or death.

necrogenous (nĕ-kroj′ĕ-nus) originating or arising from dead matter.

necrologic (nek″ro-loj′ik) pertaining to necrology.

necrologist (nĕ-krol′o-jist) an expert in necrology.

necrology (nĕ-krol′o-je, ne-krol′o-je) [*necro-* + *-logy*] the statistics or records of deaths.

necrolysis (nĕ-krol′ĭ-sis) [*necro-* + Gr. *lysis* dissolution] separation or exfoliation of tissue due to necrosis. **toxic epidermal n.,** an exfoliative skin disease seen primarily in adults, occurring as a severe cutaneous reaction to various etiologic factors, including primarily drugs but also infections (viral, bacterial, and fungal), neoplastic disease, graft-versus-host reaction, and chemical exposures. It is characterized histopathologically by full-thickness epidermal necrosis, resulting in subepidermal separation and bulla formation along with dermal inflammatory changes, and clinically by widespread loss of the skin, leaving raw, denuded areas that make the skin surface look scalded. Called also *Lyell's disease* or *syndrome, nonstaphylococcal scalded skin syndrome*, and *toxic bullous epidermolysis*. Cf. *staphylococcal scalded skin syndrome*.

necromania (nek″ro-ma′ne-ah) [*necro-* + Gr. *mania* madness] pathological preoccupation with dead bodies.

necrometer (nĕ-krom′ĕ-ter) [*necro-* + Gr. *metron* measure] an instrument for measuring the organs of the dead body.

necromimesis (nek″ro-mi-me′sis) [*necro-* + Gr. *mimēsis* imitation] a delusion of being dead, or the feigning of death.

necronectomy (nek″ro-nek′to-me) [*necro-* + Gr. *ektomē* excision] necrectomy.

necrophagous (nĕ-krof′ah-gus) [*necro-* + Gr. *phagein* to eat] devouring or subsisting on dead bodies.

necrophilia (nek″ro-fil′e-ah) sexual attraction to or sexual contact with dead bodies.

necrophilic (nek″ro-fil′ik) 1. pertaining to or characterized by necrophilia. 2. showing preference for dead tissue, as necrophilic bacteria.

necrophilism (nĕ-krof′ĭ-lizm) [*necro-* + Gr. *philein* to love] necrophilia.

necrophilous (nĕ-krof′ĭ-lus) 1. necrophilic. 2. pertaining to or characterized by necrophilia.

necrophily (nĕ-krof′ĭ-le) necrophilia.

necrophobia (nek″ro-fo′be-ah) [*necro-* + *phobia*] 1. irrational fear of death. 2. irrational fear of dead bodies.

necropneumonia (nek″ro-nu-mo′ne-ah) [*necro-* + Gr. *pneumōn* lung + *-ia*] gangrene of the lung.

necropsy (nek′rop-se) [Gr. *nekros* dead + *opsis* view] examination of a body after death; see *autopsy*.

necrosadism (nek″ro-sa′dism) [Gr. *nekros* dead + *sadism*] mutilation of a corpse for the purpose of exciting or gratifying sexual feelings.

necroscopy (nĕ-kros′ko-pe) [Gr. *nekros* dead + *skopein* to examine] necropsy.

necrose (nek′rōs) to become necrotic or to undergo necrosis.

necroses (nĕ-kro′sēz) [Gr.] plural of *necrosis*.

necrosin (nek′ro-sin) a substance liberated by injured cells, which produces the signs of inflammation, central necrosis, lymphatic blockade, injury to vascular endothelium, and swelling of collagen.

necrosis (nĕ-kro′sis), pl. *necro′ses* [Gr. *nekrōsis* deadness] the sum of the morphological changes indicative of cell death and caused by the progressive degradative action of enzymes; it may affect groups of cells or part of a structure or an organ. **arteriolar n.,** arteriolonecrosis. **aseptic n.,** increasing sclerosis and cystic changes in the head of the femur which sometimes follow traumatic dislocation of the hip. A similar condition sometimes develops in the head of the humerus after shoulder dislocation. **avascular n.,** that due to deficient blood supply. **bacillary n.,** necrobacillosis. **Balser's fatty n.,** gangrenous pancreatitis with omental bursitis and disseminated patches of necrosis of the fatty tissues; pancreatitis with fat necrosis. **bridging n.,** septa of confluent necrosis bridging adjacent central veins of hepatic lobules and portal triads characteristic of subacute hepatic necrosis. **caseous n.,** cheesy n. **central n.,** that which affects the central portion of a cell or of a bone or a lobule of the liver. **cerebrocortical n.,** a highly fatal condition due to abnormal utilization of thiamine or to anoxia, affecting calves and ewes and marked by circling movements, staggering gait, excitement, and convulsions. **cheesy n.,** necrosis in which the tissue is soft, dry and cheesy, thus resembling cottage cheese; it is seen mostly in tuberculosis and syphilis. Called also *caseous n.* **coagulation n.,** necrosis of a portion of some organ or tissue, with the formation of fibrous infarcts, in which a relatively small part seems to have been deprived of the afflux of blood by the plugging of its vessels with coagula. **colliquative n.,** necrosis in which the necrotic material becomes softened and liquefied. **cystic medial n.,** Erdheim's cystic medial n. **dry n.,** that in which the necrotic tissue becomes dry.

embolic n., coagulation necrosis of an infarct following embolism. **epiphyseal ischemic n.,** degeneration and eventual replacement of the osseous nucleus of an epiphysis, which collapses under pressure and causes distortion of the surrounding healthy tissue; attributed to interference with the blood supply of the epiphysis. It may affect the femur, tibia, tarsal navicular head, humerus, etc. Called also *osteochondrosis* (q.v.). **Erdheim's cystic medial n.,** changes in the medial layer of the aorta, consisting of degeneration and necrosis of elastic and muscle fibers, mucoid infiltration, and cyst formation, often resulting in dissecting aneurysm; called also *medionecrosis of aorta.* **exanthematous n.,** an acute necrotizing process involving the gingivae, jaw bones, and contiguous soft tissues, which primarily affects children; it resembles gangrenous stomatitis, except that there is slight odor, a tendency to be self-limited, a low mortality rate, and a normal leukocyte count. **fat n.,** a condition in which the neutral fats in the cells of adipose tissue are split into fatty acids and glycerol; it usually affects subcutaneous fat depots, particularly in the female breast, as a result of trauma, and forms a focal area felt on percussion as a firm circumscribed mass. Called also *steatonecrosis.* **focal n.,** the presence of small foci of necrosis often seen in the course of an infection. **gangrenous n.,** cell death caused by a combination of ischemia and superimposed bacterial infection, combining the features of coagulation and colliquative necrosis. **gangrenous pulp n.,** necrosis of the pulp tissue due to ischemia with superimposed bacterial infection, representing an advanced stage of untreated pulpitis. Called also *pulp gangrene.* See also *necrotic pulp,* under *pulp.* **hyaline n.,** Zenker's degeneration. **ischemic n.,** coagulation n. **labial n. of rabbits,** a fatal necrobacillosis of rabbits that begins in the lower lip and extends down to the thorax. **liquefaction n.,** colliquative n. **massive hepatic n.,** massive necrosis of the liver, a rare complication of viral hepatitis (fulminant hepatitis) that may also result from exposure to hepatotoxins or from drug hypersensitivity. A lobe or the entire liver shrinks, becoming a soft, flabby, yellow-brown to green mass with a wrinkled capsule; there is confluent necrosis of hepatocytes, often with fatty change. Mortality is 60 to 90 per cent. Formerly called *acute parenchymatous hepatitis, acute yellow atrophy, Budd's jaundice, icterus gravis, malignant jaundice,* and *Rokitansky's disease.* **medial n.,** medionecrosis. **mercurial n.,** necrosis due to mercury poisoning. **moist n.,** that in which the dead tissue becomes wet and soft. **mummification n.,** dry gangrene. **Paget's quiet n.,** a process of local necrosis and sequestrum formation in the superficial layers of the shaft of a long bone with a minimal amount of suppuration around the sequestrum and without sinus formation. **peripheral n.,** necrosis of the peripheral portions of a liver lobule as in puerperal eclampsia. **phosphorus n.,** necrosis of the jaw, sometimes associated with deposition of new subperiosteal bone, occurring in workers exposed to yellow phosphorus fumes. Called also *phosphonecrosis* and *phossy jaw.* **piecemeal n.,** destruction of hepatocytes at the interface between liver parenchyma and connective tissue associated with lymphocytic infiltration, characteristic of chronic active hepatitis and primary biliary cirrhosis. **postpartum pituitary n.,** necrosis of the pituitary during the postpartum period, often associated with shock and excessive uterine bleeding during delivery, and leading to variable patterns of hypopituitarism; called also *Sheehan's syndrome.* **pressure n.,** necrosis due to insufficient local blood supply as in decubitus ulcers. **n. progre'diens,** progressive sloughing. **progressive emphysematous n.,** gas gangrene. **radiation n.,** death of tissue caused by radiation. **radium n.,** necrosis of the jaw bone occurring in workers in radium plants. **n. of renal papillae, renal papillary n.,** an accompaniment of acute pyelonephritis, most often seen in diabetics, characterized by necrosis of the renal papillae of one or both kidneys, with sharp demarcation between necrotic and living tissue; called also *necrotizing papillitis* and *necrotizing renal papillitis.* **septic n.,** necrosis resulting from bacterial infection. **simple n.,** degeneration of the protoplasm and nucleus of the cells of a tissue without change in the appearance of the tissue. **subacute hepatic n.,** a clinical entity comprising a small group of viral hepatitis cases characterized by bridging necrosis and having an increased incidence of progression to liver failure, chronic active hepatitis, or cirrhosis. Called also *subacute* or *subchronic atrophy of liver*

and *submassive hepatic n.* **subcutaneous fat n.,** adiponecrosis subcutanea neonatorum. **submassive hepatic n.,** subacute hepatic n. **superficial n.,** that which affects only the outer layers of a bone. **syphilitic n.,** necrosis caused by syphilis. **total n.,** that which affects all parts of a bone. **n. ustilagin'ea,** dry gangrene from ergotism. **Zenker's n.,** see under *degeneration.*

necrospermia (nek″ro-sper′me-ah) [Gr. *nekros* dead + *sperm* + *-ia*] a condition in which the spermatozoa of the semen are dead or motionless.

necrospermic (nek″ro-sper′mik) pertaining to or characterized by necrospermia.

necrotic (ne-krot′ik) pertaining to or characterized by necrosis.

necrotizing (nek′ro-tīz″ing) causing necrosis.

necrotomy (ne-krot′o-me) [Gr. *nekros* + *tome* a cutting] 1. dissection of a dead body. 2. the excision of a sequestrum. **osteoplastic n.,** removal of a sequestrum from a bone after first lifting a flap of the bone, which is replaced after the operation.

necrotoxin (nek″ro-tok′sin) a toxin that kills tissue cells, e.g., the exotoxins secreted by species of *Clostridium* and by *Staphylococcus aureus.*

necrozoospermia (nek″ro-zo″o-sper′me-ah) necrospermia.

Necturus (nek-tu′rus) a genus of salamanders having large external gills; employed in physiologic research.

NED no evidence of disease.

needle (ne′d′l) [L. *acus*] 1. a sharp instrument for suturing or puncturing. 2. to puncture with a needle, as in discission of the lens for treatment of cataract. **Abrams' n.,** a biopsy needle designed to reduce the danger of introducing air into tissues, as in pleural biopsy. **aneurysm n.,** one with a handle, used in ligating blood vessels. **aspirating n.,** a long, hollow needle for removing fluid from a cavity. **cataract n.,** one used in removing a cataract. **Chiba n.,** fine n. **Cope's n.,** a blunt-ended hooklike needle with a concealed cutting edge and snare, used in biopsy of the pleura, pericardium, peritoneum, and synovium. **Deschamps' n.,** one with the eye near the point, and a long handle attached; used in ligating deep-seated arteries. **discission n.,** a special form of cataract needle. **fine n.,** a very thin, highly flexible steel needle with a narrow inner core used to cannulate very small bile ducts to perform percutaneous transhepatic cholangiography (*fine needle transhepatic cholangiography*). Called also *skinny n.* **Hagedorn's n's,** surgical needles which are flat from side to side, and have a straight cutting edge near the point and a large eye. **hypodermic n.,** a short, slender, hollow needle used in injecting drugs beneath the skin. **knife n.,** a slender knife with a needle-like point, used in discission of a cataract and other ophthalmic operations, as in goniotomy and goniopuncture. **ligature n.,** a slender steel needle with a long handle and an eye in its curved end, used for passing a ligature underneath an artery. **Menghini n.,** a needle that does not require rotation to cut loose the tissue specimen in a biopsy of the liver. **Reverdin's n.,** a surgical needle having an eye which can be opened and closed by means of a slide. **Silverman n.,** an instrument for taking tissue specimens, consisting of an outer cannula, an obturator, and an inner split needle with longitudinal grooves in which the tissue is retained when the needle and cannula are withdrawn. **skinny n.,** fine n. **stop n.,** a needle with a shoulder that prevents it from being inserted beyond a certain distance. **swaged n.,** one permanently attached to the suture material. **Vim-Silverman n.,** a needle used in needle biopsy.

Neef's hammer (nāfs) [Christopher Ernst *Neef,* German physician, 1782–1849] see under *hammer.*

Neelsen (nēl′sen) see *Ziehl-Neelsen.*

neencephalon (ne″en-sef′ah-lon) [Gr. *neos* new + *enkephalos* brain] the cerebral cortex and its dependencies; the phylogenetically newer part of the brain.

NEFA nonesterified fatty acids.

nefluorophotometer (ne-floo″o-ro-fo-tom′e-ter) fluoronephelometer.

nefopam hydrochloride (nef′o-pam) chemical name: 3,4,5,6-tetrahydro-5-methyl-1-phenyl-1*H*-2,5-benzoxazocine hydrochloride; an analgesic and muscle relaxant, $C_{17}H_{19}NO \cdot HCl.$

Negatan (neg′ah-tan) trademark for a preparation of negatol.

negation (ne-ga′shun) refusal or denial; see *delusion of negation.*

negativism (neg′ah-tiv-izm″) resistance or opposition to advice, suggestions, or commands; e.g., in catatonic schizophrenia the patient may lower his arms if asked to raise them or may resist efforts to move them.

negatol (neg′ah-tol) a colloidal product obtained by reacting meta-cresol sulfonic acid with formaldehyde; used as a parasiticide, germicide, and bacteriostatic, for topical application to the cervix.

negatoscope (neg′ah-to-skōp) an apparatus for showing radiographic negatives.

negatron (neg′ah-tron) the negative electron; see *positron* and *electron.*

NegGram (neg′gram) trademark for preparations of nalidixic acid.

Negri bodies (na′gre) [Adelchi *Negri,* Italian physician, 1876–1912] see under *body.*

Negro's phenomenon (na′grōz) [Camillo *Negro,* Italian neurologist, 1861–1927] see *cogwheel phenomenon,* under *phenomenon.*

neighborwise (na′bor-wīz) descriptive of the plastic behavior of transplanted embryonic cells or tissue in a manner appropriate to its new and strange location. Cf. *selfwise.*

Neill-Mooser bodies, reaction [Mather Humphrey *Neill,* American physician, 1882–1930; Herman *Mooser,* Swiss pathologist, born 1891] see under *body* and *reaction.*

Neisser's diplococcus, syringe (ni′serz) [Albert Ludwig Siegmund *Neisser,* German physician, 1855–1916] see *Neisseria gonorrhoeae* and under *syringe.*

Neisser-Wechsberg phenomenon (ni″ser-veks′berg) [Max *Neisser,* German physician, 1869–1938; Friedrich *Wechsberg,* German physician, 1873–1929] see *complement deviation,* under *deviation.*

Neisseria (nīs-se″re-ah) [Albert Ludwig Siegmund *Neisser,* German physician, 1855–1916] a genus of bacteria of the family Neisseriaceae, consisting of gram-negative, oxidase-positive cocci characteristically coffee-bean–shaped and paired. The organisms are aerobic or facultatively anerobic and are part of the normal flora of the oropharynx, nasopharynx, and genitourinary tract. The genus includes the gonococcus, the several meningococcus types, pigmented forms occasionally associated with meningitis, and a number of saprophytic or parasitic but nonpathogenic species. **N. catarrha′lis,** *Moraxella* (*Branhamella*) *catarrhalis.* **N. flaves′cens,** a species characterized by the production of yellow pigmented colonies. It is sometimes found in the body fluids of patients with meningitis and septicemia. **N. gonorrhoe′ae,** the specific etiologic agent of gonorrhea, occurring typically as pairs of flattened cells, found primarily in purulent venereal discharges. Called also *diplococcus of Neisser.* **N. lactam′ica,** a species that ferments lactose, found frequently in throat and nasopharyngeal cultures of infants and young children; it occasionally causes endocarditis and meningitis in humans. **N. meningi′tidis,** a prominent cause of meningitis and the specific etiologic agent of epidemic cerebrospinal meningitis. The species is differentiated serologically into four main groups (A, B, C, D) and several provisional groups; group C is the most important pathogen. Called also *meningococcus.* **N. muco′sa,** a species that produces mucoid colonies that are often adherent; it is found in the human nasopharynx and is occasionally pathogenic, causing pneumonia. Called also *Diplococcus mucosus.* **N. sic′ca,** a species characterized by dry grayish or slimy white or yellow colonies, which is part of the normal flora of the human nasopharynx, saliva, and sputum. **N. subfla′va,** a species that produces smooth, yellow-pigmented colonies, found in the human nasopharynx and occasionally in cerebrospinal fluid in cases of meningitis.

Neisseriaceae (nīs-se″re-a′se-e) a family of gram-negative, aerobic cocci and rod-shaped bacteria occurring singly or in pairs, short chains, or masses. The organisms are parasitic or saprophytic, and some produce pigment. The family includes four genera: *Acinetobacter, Kingella, Moraxella,* and *Neisseria.*

neisserial (nīs-se′re-al) of, relating to, or caused by *Neisseria.*

nekr(o)- for words beginning thus, see those beginning *necr(o)-.*

nekton (nek′ton) [Gr. *nēktos* swimming] collective term for marine organisms that swim actively, as contrasted with plankton.

Nélaton's catheter, etc. (na-lah-tawz′) [Auguste *Nélaton,* French surgeon, 1807–1873] see under *catheter, line, operation, probe,* and *sphincter.*

Nema (ne′mah) trademark for a preparation of tetrachloroethylene.

nema (ne′mah) [Gr. *nēma* thread] a nematode.

nemathelminth (nem″ah-thel′minth) [*nemato-* + Gr. *helmins* worm] a worm of the phylum Nemathelminthes.

Nemathelminthes (nem″ah-thel-min′thēz) in some systems of classification, a phylum including the Acanthocephala and Nematoda.

nemathelminthiasis (nem″ah-thel′min-thi′ah-sis) infection by nematodes, or roundworms.

nematicide (nĕ-mat′ĭ-sīd) nematocide.

nematization (nem″ah-ti-za′shun) infection with nematodes, or roundworms.

nemat(o)- [Gr. *nēma* thread, gen. *nēmatos*] a combining form denoting relationship to a nematode, or to a threadlike structure.

nematoblast (nem′ah-to-blast″) [Gr. *nēma* thread + *blastos* germ] spermatid.

Nematocera (nem″ah-tos′er-ah) [Gr. *nēma* thread + *keras* horn] a suborder of Diptera characterized by having antennae of many segments and comprising the gnats, mosquitoes, midges, black flies, craneflies, gallflies, etc.

nematocide (nem′ah-to-sīd″) [*nemato-* + L. *caedere* to kill] 1. destructive to nematode worms. 2. an agent that destroys nematodes.

nematocyst (nem′ah-to-sist) a minute stinging structure, found in the cnidoblasts of jellyfish and other coelenterates, used for anchorage, for defense, and for the capture of prey.

Nematoda (nem″ah-to′dah) [Gr. *nēma* thread + *eidos* form] a class of tapered cylindrical helminths, the roundworms, of the phylum Aschelminthes, many species of which are parasites. They are characterized by longitudinally oriented muscles and by a triradiate esophagus. In some systems of classification, they are considered to be a separate phylum. Sometimes called *Nemathelminthes,* or a class under that phylum.

nematode (nem′ah-tōd) a roundworm; any individual belonging to the class Nematoda.

nematodesma (ne″mah-to-dez′mah), pl. *nematodesma′ta* [*nemato-* + Gr. *desmos* band, ligament] a bundle of parallel microtubules serving to support the cytostome and cytopharyngeal apparatus and associated organelles of certain ciliate protozoa; also seen in certain flagellate groups. Called also *trichite.*

nematodiasis (nem″ah-to-di′ah-sis) infection by a nematode parasite.

Nematodirus (nem″ah-to′di-rus) a genus of nematode parasites belonging to the family Trichostrongylidae, found in the duodenum of ruminants.

nematoid (nem′ah-toid) resembling a thread; pertaining to a nematode parasite.

nematologist (nem″ah-tol′o-jist) a specialist in nematology.

nematology (nem″ah-tol′o-je) the branch of zoology which deals with nematode worms.

Nematomorpha (nem″ah-to-mor′fah) [Gr. *nēma* thread + *morphē* form] a class of long, slender, cylindrical worms of the phylum Aschelminthes, commonly called "hairworms," "horse hairs," or "hair eels," which are parasitic as juveniles. In some systems of classification, they are considered to be a separate phylum. Called also *Gordiacea.*

nematosis (nem″ah-to′sis) the condition of being infected with nematodes, or roundworms.

nematospermia (nem″ah-to-sper′me-ah) [*nemato-* + Gr. *sperma* sperm] spermatozoa having elongated tails.

Nembutal (nem′bu-tal) trademark for preparations of sodium pentobarbital.

Nemertea (nem-er′te-ah) Rhynchocoela.

nemertean (nem-er-te'an) 1. pertaining to the Nemertea. 2. any individual of the Nemertea. See *Rhynchocoela.*

Nemertina (nem-er-ti'nah) Rhynchocoela.

nemic (nem'ik) pertaining to nematodes, or roundworms.

Nencki's test (nents'kēz) [Marcellus von *Nencki,* Polish physician, 1847–1901] see under *tests.*

ne(o)- [Gr. *neos* new] 1. a combining form meaning new or recent, or denoting an immature form. 2. in chemistry, a prefix denoting a new chemical compound related in some way to an older one, to whose name it is added.

Neo-Antergan (ne''o-an'ter-gan) trademark for a preparation of pyrilamine maleate.

neoantigen (ne''o-an'tĭ-jen) a new antigen acquired by a tumor cell line in the process of neoplastic transformation, e.g., a viral antigen in tumors induced by viruses, a normal cellular constituent altered by mutation, or an oncofetal antigen produced by activation of repressed genes.

neoarsphenamine (ne''o-ars-fen'ah-mēn) chemical name: [5-[(3-amino-4-hydroxyphenol) arseno]-2-hydroxyani-lino]methanol sulfoxylate sodium. A modified soluble compound of arsphenamine, $C_{13}H_{13}As_2N_2NaO_4S$, formerly used as an antisyphilitic.

neoarthrosis (ne''o-ar-thro'sis) nearthrosis.

neobiogenesis (ne''o-bi''o-jen'ĕ-sis) [neo- + biogenesis] biopoiesis.

Neobiotic (ne''o-bi-ot'ik) trademark for a preparation of neomycin sulfate.

neoblastic (ne''o-blas'tik) [neo- + Gr. *blastos* germ] originating in or of the nature of new tissue.

Neo-Calglucon (ne''o-kal'gloo-kon) trademark for a preparation of calcium glubionate.

neocerebellum (ne''o-ser''ĕ-bel'um) [neo- + cerebellum] [NA] a term applied originally to the cerebellar hemispheres; now applied specifically to those parts whose afferent inflow is predominantly supplied by corticopontocerebellar fibers, including in man the caudal lobe, excluding the pyramid and uvula. Cf. *archaeocerebellum* and *palaeocerebellum.*

neocinchophen (ne''o-sin'ko-fen) chemical name: ethyl ester of 6-methylcinchopher. Yellow needles, $C_{19}H_{17}NO_2$, which have been used as an analgesic, antipyretic, and uricosuric.

neocinetic (ne''o-si-net'ik) neokinetic.

Neo-Cobefrin (ne''o-cob'ĕ-frin) trademark for a preparation of levonordefrin.

neocortex (ne''o-kor'teks) [neo- + cortex] [NA] the newer, six-layered portion of the cortex cerebri (q.v.), showing stratification and organization characteristic of the most highly evolved type of cerebral tissue. Called also *homotypical cortex, isocortex, neopallium,* and *nonolfactory cortex.* Cf. *allocortex.*

neocytosis (ne''o-si-to'sis) the presence of immature cell forms in the blood.

neodarwinism (ne''o-dar'win-izm) the concept that species evolve by natural selection only, thus ruling out the inheritance of acquired traits; see *darwinism.*

Neodecadron trademark for preparations of dexamethasone sodium phosphate.

neodiathermy (ne''o-di'ah-ther''me) short wave diathermy.

Neo-Diloderm (ne''o-di'lo-derm) trademark for a preparation of dichlorisone containing neomycin sulfate.

neodymium (ne''o-dim'e-um) a rare element of atomic number, 60; atomic weight, 144.24; symbol, Nd.

neoencephalon (ne''o-en-sef'ah-lon) neencephalon.

neofetal (ne''o-fe'tal) pertaining to the transitional period between the embryonic and fetal stages of the developing human young.

neofetus (ne''o-fe'tus) the embryo at about the eighth week of intrauterine life.

neoformation (ne''o-for-ma'shun) a new growth or neoplasm.

neoformative (ne''o-for'mah-tiv) concerned in the formation of new tissue.

neogala (ne-og'ah-lah) [neo- + Gr. *gala* milk] the first milk developed after childbirth; see also *colostrum.*

neogenesis (ne''o-jen'ĕ-sis) [neo- + Gr. *genesis* production] a form of tissue regeneration that is slower than anagenesis.

neogenetic (ne''o-jĕ-net'ik) pertaining to neogenesis.

neogermitrine (ne''o-jer'mĭ-trēn) an alkaloid having antihypertensive properties, isolated from green hellebore (*Veratrum viride*).

neoglottic (ne''o-glot'ik) pertaining to a neoglottis.

neoglottis (ne''o-glot'is) a surgically constructed glottis created by suturing the pharyngeal mucosa over the superior end of the transected trachea above the primary tracheostoma and making a permanent stoma in the mucosa; it is created to permit phonation after laryngectomy. Called also *pseudoglottis.*

neoglycogenesis (ne''o-gli''ko-jen'ĕ-sis) gluconeogenesis.

Neogregarinida (ne''o-greg''ah-ri'nĭ-dah) [neo- + L. *gregarius* crowding together] an order of parasitic protozoa (subclass Gregarinia, class Sporozoea) found in the malpighian tubules, intestine, hemocoelom, or fat tissues of insects, which reproduce by merogony, with each spore producing eight sporozoites.

Neohetramine (ne''o-he'trah-min) trademark for a preparation of thonzylamine hydrochloride.

neo-hippocratism (ne''o-hip-pok'rah-tizm) a school of medicine which trends toward a humanistic view of disease focused on the individual patient and scientific observation by the physician, representing a return to the hippocratic theory and practice, with emphasis on observational and bedside medicine.

Neo-Hombreol (ne''o-hom'bre-ol) trademark for preparations of testosterone propionate.

neohymen (ne''o-hi'men) [neo- + Gr. *hymēn* membrane] a false membrane.

neokinetic (ne''o-ki-net'ik) [neo- + Gr. *kinētikos* pertaining to movement] a term applied to the nervous motor mechanism regulating voluntary muscular control. It is associated with the motor area of cerebral cortex, and receives its name because of the fact that it was developed more recently than the older paleokinetic system. Cf. *archeokinetic* and *paleokinetic.*

neolalia, neolalism (ne''o-lal'e-ah; ne''o-lal'izm) [neo- + Gr. *lalia* babble] speech into which many neologisms are incorporated, as in schizophrenia.

neologism (ne-ol'o-jizm) [neo- + Gr. *logos* word] a newly coined word; in psychiatry, a new word whose meaning may be known only to the person using it and may be related to his conflicts.

Neoloid (ne'o-loid) trademark for a preparation of castor oil.

neomembrane (ne''o-mem'brān) a false membrane.

neomin (ne'o-min) neomycin.

neomorph (ne'o-morf) [neo- + Gr. *morphē* form] a part or organ recently acquired in the course of evolution.

neomorphism (ne''o-mor'fizm) the development of new form in the course of evolution.

neomycin (ne'o-mi''sin) a broad-spectrum antibacterial antibiotic produced by the growth of *Streptomyces fradiae,* effective against a wide range of gram-negative organisms, including *Escherichia coli, Aerobacter aerogenes, Proteus vulgaris, Salmonella* and *Shigella* species, *Pseudomonas aeruginosa,* and *Mycobacterium tuberculosis,* and most gram-positive bacteria. **n. palmitate,** the palmitate salt of neomycin; used topically as an antibacterial in the treatment of superficial skin infections, burns, wounds, and ulcers. **n. sulfate** [USP], the sulfate salt of neomycin, occurring as a white to slightly yellow powder or cryodesiccated solid; used in the treatment of urinary tract, eye, skin, ear, and enteric infections due to susceptible bacteria and for preoperative disinfection, administered orally, intramuscularly, and topically.

neon (ne'on) [Gr. *neos* new] an inert gaseous element discovered in the air in 1898; symbol, Ne; atomic weight, 20.183; atomic number, 10.

neonatal (ne''o-na'tal) [neo- + L. *natus* born] pertaining to the first four weeks after birth.

neonate (ne'o-nāt) 1. newly born. 2. a newborn infant.

neonatologist (ne''o-na-tol'o-jist) a physician whose primary concern is in the specialty of neonatology.

neonatology (ne''o-na-tol'o-je) the art and science of diagnosis and treatment of disorders of the newborn infant.

neopallium (ne″o-pal′le-um) [neo- + L. *pallium* cloak] neocortex.

neopathy (ne-op′ah-the) [neo- + Gr. *pathos* disease] (*obs.*) 1. a new disease. 2. a new condition or complication of disease in a patient.

neophrenia (ne″o-fre′ne-ah) [neo- + Gr. *phrēn* mind] Kahlbaum's term for mental disorder occurring in early youth; no longer in use.

neoplasia (ne″o-pla′ze-ah) the formation of a neoplasm, i.e., the progressive multiplication of cells under conditions that would not elicit, or would cause cessation of, multiplication of normal cells. **multiple endocrine n. (MEN),** a group of rare disorders of autonomous hyperfunction of more than one endocrine gland. In *Type I* (MEN I), called also Wermer's syndrome, there are tumors of the pituitary, parathyroid glands, and pancreatic islet cells in association with a high incidence of peptic ulcer; the Zollinger-Ellison syndrome may occur in affected families. *Type II* (MEN II), called also Sipple's syndrome, is characterized by medullary carcinoma of the thyroid, pheochromocytoma, often bilateral and multiple, and parathyroid hyperplasia. *Type III* (MEN III), called also mucosal neuroma syndrome, resembles Type II except that parathyroid hyperplasia is rare, the mean survival time is shorter, a marfanoid body habitus may occur, and there may be disfiguring neuromas of the lips, buccal mucosa, and tongue, ganglioneuromas of the gastrointestinal tract, thickened corneal nerves, and cafe-au-lait spots, neuromas, or neurofibromas of the skin. All forms are transmitted as autosomal dominant traits with varying penetrance. Called also *multiple endocrine adenomatosis, pluriglandular adenomatosis, polyendocrine adenomatosis,* and *polyendocrinoma.*

neoplasm (ne′o-plazm) [neo- + Gr. *plasma* formation] any new and abnormal growth; specifically a new growth of tissue in which the growth is uncontrolled and progressive (see neoplasia). Malignant neoplasms are distinguished from benign in that the former show a greater degree of anaplasia and have the properties of invasion and metastasis. Called also *tumor.* **histoid n.,** a neoplasm whose structure resembles that of the tissues in which it is situated. **organoid n.,** a neoplasm whose structure resembles that of some organ of the body.

neoplastic (ne″o-plas′tik) pertaining to or like a neoplasm; pertaining to neoplasia.

neoplastigenic (ne″o-plas″tĭ-jen′ik) tending to produce neoplasms.

Neopsylla (ne-op′sil-ah) a genus of fleas.

neoquassin (ne″o-kwas′in) a crystalline principle, $C_{24}H_{30}$-O_6, from *Quassia amara* L. (Simarubaceae); it is a phenanthropyran derivative which forms quassin on oxidation.

Neorickettsia (ne″o-rĭ-ket′se-ah) [neo- + *rickettsia*] a genus of bacteria of the tribe Ehrlichieae, family Rickettsiaceae, order Rickettsiales. It includes a single species, *N. helminthoeca,* the etiologic agent of salmon poisoning (q.v.) in dogs, wolves, jackals, and foxes. The organism is found in the salmon fluke, *Troglotrema salmincola,* a parasite of various fish, especially salmon and trout, and is transmitted by ingestion of raw infected fish.

Neoschoengastia (ne″o-shān-gas′te-ah) a genus of mites of the family Trombiculidae. **N. america′na,** a species of mites which infest chickens in the southern United States.

neostibosan (ne″o-sti′bo-san) a pentavalent antimony compound, used as an antileishmanial. Called also *ethylstibamine.*

neostigmine (ne″o-stig′mēn) an anticholinesterase agent used for the symptomatic treatment of myasthenia gravis, for prevention and treatment of postoperative stasis and atony of the gastrointestinal tract or urinary bladder, and for reversal of the effects of nondepolarizing neuromuscular blocking agents (e.g., tubocurarine) after surgery. Available as *neostigmine bromide* [USP] and *neostigmine methylsulfate* [USP]. **n. bromide** [USP], the bromide salt of neostigmine, $C_{12}H_{19}$-BrN_2O_2, occurring as a white, crystalline powder; used as a cholinergic in the symptomatic control of myasthenia gravis, and to produce miosis in certain forms of glaucoma, administered orally and applied to the conjunctiva. **n. methylsulfate** [USP], the methylsulfate salt of neostigmine, C_{13}-$H_{22}N_2O_6S$, occurring as a white crystalline powder; used as a cholinergic in the prevention and treatment of postoperative distention and urinary retention, as a screening test for

pregnancy, in the treatment of delayed menstruation, in the symptomatic treatment of myasthenia gravis, as a diagnostic test for myasthenia gravis, and as an antidote for curare principles, administered intravenously and subcutaneously.

neostomy (ne-os′to-me) [neo- + Gr. *stoma* mouth] surgical creation of an artificial opening into an organ or between two organs.

neostriatum (ne″o-stri-a′tum) [neo- + *striatum*] the later developed portion of the corpus striatum represented by the caudate nucleus and the putamen; called also *striatum.* Cf. *paleostriatum.*

Neo-Synephrine (ne″o-sĭ-nef′rin) trademark for preparations of phenylephrine hydrochloride.

neoteny (ne-ot′ĕ-ne) [neo- + Gr. *teinein* to extend] 1. the tendency to remain in the larval state, although gaining sexual maturity. 2. the retention in an adult organism of some of its ancestor's larval characteristics.

neothalamus (ne″o-thal′ah-mus) [Gr. *neos* new + *thalamus*] new thalamus; the phylogenetically new part of the thalamus, i.e., the part connected to the neocortex. Cf. *paleothalamus.*

Neothylline (ne″o-thil′lin) trademark for preparations of dyphylline.

Neotoma (ne-ot′o-mah) a genus of rodents of western North America, including the wood or pack rats. **N. lep′ida,** the desert wood rat, from which *Brucella neotome* has been isolated.

Neotrizine (ne″o-tri′zēn) trademark for preparations of trisulfapyrimidenes.

neotype (ne′o-tīp) a strain of bacteria that replaces a type culture which no longer exists, and that agrees with the original description of the taxon and is accepted by international agreement.

neovascularization (ne″o-vas″ku-lar-ĭ-za′shun) 1. new blood vessel formation in abnormal tissue or in abnormal positions. 2. revascularization.

nepenthic (ne-pen′thik) [Gr. *nēpenthēs* free from sorrow] pertaining to or inducing peace and forgetfulness.

Nepeta (nep′ĕ-tah) a genus of Eurasian mints that includes *Nepeta cataria,* L. (Labiatae), or catnip; see *cataria.*

nepetalactone (nep″ĕ-tah-lak′tōn) the chief constituent, $C_{10}H_{14}O_2$, of the aromatic volatile oil from the leaves and tops of catnip (*Nepeta cataria*), which is an attractant to cats.

nephel(o)- [Gr. *nephelē* cloud or mist] a combining form denoting relationship to clouds or cloudiness.

nephelometer (nef″ĕ-lom′e-ter) an instrument that measures the turbidity of a solution by measuring the amount of light that is scattered at an angle from a beam of light passing through the solution. Cf. *turbidimeter.*

nephelometry (nef″ĕ-lom′ĕ-tre) [nephelo- + Gr. *metron* measure] measurement of the concentration of a suspension by means of a nephelometer.

nephradenoma (nef″rad-ĕ-no′mah) [nephr- + *adenoma*] adenoma of the kidney.

nephralgia (nĕ-fral′je-ah) [nephr- + -algia] pain in a kidney.

nephralgic (nĕ-fral′jik) pertaining to or characterized by nephralgia.

Nephramine (nef′rah-mēn) trademark for a crystalline solution of eight essential amino acids but no peptides; it is used as a component of total parenteral nutrition in renal failure.

nephrapostasis (nef″rah-pos′tah-sis) [nephr- + Gr. *apostasis* suppuration] abscess or suppurative inflammation of a kidney.

nephratonia (nef″rah-to′ne-ah) [nephr- + a neg. + Gr. *tonos* tension + -ia] atony of the kidney.

nephratony (nĕ-frat′o-ne) nephratonia.

nephrauxe (nef-rawk′se) [nephr- + Gr. *auxē* increase] nephromegaly.

nephrectasia (nef″rek-ta′ze-ah) [nephr- + Gr. *ektasis* distention + -ia] distention of the kidney; sacciform kidney.

nephrectasis (nĕ-frek′tah-sis) nephrectasia.

nephrectasy (nĕ-frek′tah-se) nephrectasia.

nephrectomize (nĕ-frek′to-mīz) to deprive of one or both kidneys by surgical removal.

nephrectomy (nĕ-frek′to-me) [nephr- + Gr. *ektomē* excision]

excision of a kidney. **abdominal n., anterior n.,** nephrectomy through an incision in the abdominal wall. **lumbar n.,** nephrectomy through an incision in the loin. **paraperitoneal n.,** the surgical removal of a kidney by a cut through the side along the twelfth rib. **posterior n.,** lumbar nephrectomy.

nephredema (nef″rĕ-de′mah) renal congestion; nephremia.

nephrelcosis (nef″rel-ko′sis) [*nephr-* + Gr. *helkōsis* ulceration] ulceration of the kidney.

nephremia (nĕ-fre′me-ah) [*nephr-* + Gr. *haima* blood + *-ia*] congestion of the kidney; nephredema.

nephric (nef′rik) pertaining to the kidney; renal.

nephridium (nĕ-frid′e-um) the excretory organ of the embryo; the embryonic tube whence the kidney is developed.

nephritic (nĕ-frit′ik) 1. pertaining to or affected with nephritis. 2. pertaining to the kidneys. 3. a drug or agent useful in kidney disease.

nephritides (nĕ-frit′ĭ-dēz) plural of *nephritis*, used as a collective term, to include all types of nephritis.

nephritis (nĕ-fri′tis), pl. *nephrit′ides* [Gr. *nephros* kidney + *-itis*] inflammation of the kidney; a focal or diffuse proliferative or destructive process which may involve the glomerulus, tubule, or interstitial renal tissue. See also *glomerulonephritis*. Cf. *nephrosis*. **acute n.,** nephritis in an acute and active stage with clinical manifestations usually including edema, weight gain, proteinuria, microhematuria, and cylindruria. When involvement is primarily glomerular, gross hematuria is common. **arteriosclerotic n.,** nephrosclerotic nephritis which may result primarily from the aging process, with hyaline changes of the large and small arterioles, or from hypertension, with hyaline and/or muscular changes of the small arterioles in the glomerular hilum. Renal damage occurs primarily through ischemic atrophy of the tubules with resultant focal or diffuse interstitial fibrosis. **azotemic n.,** nephritis which has resulted in anatomic and functional impairment leading to nitrogen retention. **bacterial n.,** nephritis caused by microorganisms. **Balkan n.,** a very slowly progressive interstitial nephritis occurring in several well-defined areas of Yugoslavia, Rumania, Bulgaria, and Greece; called also *Balkan nephropathy*. **capsular n.,** a form said to affect especially Bowman's capsules. **n. caseo′sa, caseous n.,** cheesy n. **cheesy n.,** a chronic suppurative form with caseous deposits. **chloro-azotemic n.,** nonedematous renal failure with acidosis. **chronic n.,** active and slowly progressive parenchymal renal disease, usually with a predominantly glomerular lesion. **congenital n.,** nephritis existing at birth, as in congenital syphilis. **croupous n.,** acute n. **degenerative n.,** nephrosis. **n. doloro′sa,** nonspecific involvement of the kidney characterized by painful thickening of the renal capsule due to inflammation of indeterminate etiology, as in some forms of perinephritis. **dropsical n.,** nephrotic syndrome. **exudative n.,** nephritis with exudation of the blood serum. **fibrolipomatous n.,** perinephritis in which the perirenal fat has become enmeshed in fibrous tissue proliferation with scarring. **fibrous n.,** interstitial n. **glomerular n.,** that which principally affects the glomeruli; see *glomerulonephritis*. **glomerulo-capsular n.,** a term sometimes used to describe glomerulopathy involving primarily the epithelial cells of Bowman's capsules. **n. gravida′rum,** nephritis or other glomerulopathies complicating pregnancy. **hemorrhagic n.,** glomerulopathy associated with gross hematuria. **hydremic n., hydropigenous n.,** nephrotic syndrome; glomerulopathy with hypoproteinemia, massive proteinuria, and edema. **indurative n.,** a condition marked by atrophy and gross scarring of the kidney due to glomerular, tubular, or interstitial renal disease. **interstitial n.,** primary or secondary disease of the renal interstitial tissue resulting from arterial, arteriolar, glomerular, or tubular disease which destroys individual nephrons, or from toxic involvement of interstitial cells and tubules due to systemic diseases such as gout, to drug exposure (as in phenacetin abuse), or to mercury poisoning. Clinically, it may be manifested primarily by loss of concentrating capacity, mineral wasting, proteinuria, and abnormal urine sediment. It may be seen in an acute form, particularly after specific bacterial infection, and may result in acute papillary necrosis. More commonly, the process is a chronic one with progressive renal atrophy and diminution of renal function.

interstitial n., acute, nephritis in which the inflammatory changes are usually confined to the interstitial tissue. It almost always occurs as a secondary complication of a systemic infection, especially one due to beta-hemolytic streptococci, although it may possibly have an allergic etiology. The kidneys may be normal in size and appearance, or enlarged, soft, and pale or mottled red or gray. Other signs include a thickened cortex, focal or diffuse interstitial infiltration of leukocytes, and tubular degeneration. **Lancereaux's n.,** interstitial nephritis allegedly resulting from rheumatic disease. **lipomatous n.,** fatty replacement of renal nephrons associated with, but not causative of, a primary disease process; called also *lipomatosis renis, lipoma diffusum renis*. **lupus n.,** glomerulonephritis (diffuse, focal, or membranous) associated with systemic lupus erythematosus, marked by deposition of antigen-antibody complexes in the mesangium and basement membrane, by hematuria, and either by a fulminating course, with uremia and death in a few weeks, or by a chronic progressive course; hypertension is rare until late in the course of the disease. **Masugi n.,** nephrotoxic serum n. **nephrotoxic serum n.,** an animal model of antibody-mediated glomerulonephritis produced by injection of heterologous antibody against renal antigens. It occurs in two phases. The heterologous phase, occurring within a few hours, consists of the inflammatory response triggered by the nephrotoxic antibody binding to antigens in the glomerular basement membrane (GBM) and resembles anti-GBM antibody disease. The *autologous phase*, occurring 4-6 days later, consists of the host response to the foreign antibody and does not correspond to a human disease. **parenchymatous n.,** renal parenchymal disease of specific or unknown etiology. **parenchymatous n., chronic,** chronic disease of the renal parenchyma of specific or nonspecific etiology, usually manifested as a diffuse glomerular, tubular, or interstitial fibrosis. **pneumococcus n.,** nephritis from infection with pneumococci, occurring usually as a complication of pneumonia or empyema. **potassium-losing n.,** persistent urinary potassium losses in the presence of hypokalemia. It may be seen in metabolic alkalosis, adrenocortical hormone excess, or in intrinsic renal disease (e.g., renal tubular acidosis or juxtaglomerular cell hyperplasia). Called also *potassium-losing nephropathy*. **n. of pregnancy,** n. gravidarum. **productive n.,** nephritis with the development of serous exudate and hypertrophy of the connective tissue stroma. **n. re′pens,** a condition in which the patient has advanced renal insufficiency and raised blood pressure but without an antecedent history of acute nephritis. **salt-losing n.,** intrinsic renal disease causing abnormal urinary sodium loss in persons ingesting normal amounts of sodium chloride; it usually affects the renal medulla (e.g., medullary cystic disease, polycystic kidney disease, pyelonephritis) and results in vomiting, dehydration, hypotension, and sudden death. Called also *Thorn's syndrome*. **saturnine n.,** a form due to chronic lead poisoning. **scarlatinal n.,** acute nephritis due to scarlet fever. **subacute n.,** parenchymatous n., chronic. **suppurative n.,** a form accompanied by abscess of the kidney. **suppurative n., acute,** a form due to septic infection, generally from operations on the genitourinary tract (then called *surgical kidney*), and marked by the development of multiple abscesses. **suppurative n., chronic,** is caused by infection with the tubercle bacillus; in this disease cavities are found in the kidney, filled with puslike, cheesy masses and tubercle bacilli. **syphilitic n.,** a form of nephritis occurring in tertiary syphilis. **tartrate n.,** acute nephritis produced by the subcutaneous injection of racemic tartaric acid. **transfusion n.,** a nephropathy following blood transfusion from a donor whose blood is incompatible with that of the recipient. **trench n.,** war n. **tubal n., tubular n.,** a variety that affects principally the tubules. **tuberculous n.,** see *interstitial nephritis*. **vascular n.,** nephrosclerosis. **war n.,** an acute diffuse glomerulonephritis affecting soldiers under war conditions.

nephritogenic (nĕ-frit″o-jen′ik) giving rise to inflammation of the kidney, or nephritis.

nephr(o)- [Gr. *nephros* kidney] combining form denoting relationship to the kidney.

nephroabdominal (nef″ro-ab-dom′ĭ-nal) pertaining to the kidney and the abdominal wall.

nephroangiosclerosis (nef″ro-an″je-o-skle-ro′sis) hypertension with renal lesions of arterial origin.

nephroblastoma (nef″ro-blas-to′mah)　Wilms' tumor.

nephrocalcinosis (nef″ro-kal″si-no′sis) [*nephro-* + *calcium* + *-osis*]　a condition characterized by precipitation of calcium phosphate in the tubules of the kidney, with resultant renal insufficiency.

nephrocapsectomy (nef″ro-kap-sek′to-me) [*nephro-* + L. *capsula* capsule + Gr. *ektomē* excision]　excision of the renal capsule; decapsulation of the kidney.

nephrocardiac (nef″ro-kar′de-ak)　pertaining to the kidney and the heart.

nephrocele (nef′ro-sēl) [*nephro-* + Gr. *kēlē* hernia]　hernial protrusion of a kidney.

nephrocolic (nef″ro-kol′ik) [*nephro-* + *colic*]　1. pertaining to the kidney and the colon.　2. renal colic.

nephrocoloptosis (nef″ro-ko″lop-to′sis) [*nephro-* + Gr. *kolon* colon + *ptōsis* fall]　downward displacement of the kidney and colon.

nephrocystanastomosis (nef″ro-sist″ah-nas″to-mo′sis) [*nephro-* + Gr. *kystis* bladder + *anastomōsis* an opening]　the surgical formation of a communication between the kidney and the urinary bladder.

nephrocystitis (nef″ro-sis-ti′tis) [*nephro-* + Gr. *kystis* bladder + *-itis*]　inflammation of the kidney and bladder.

nephrocystosis (nef″ro-sis-to′sis) [*nephro-* + *cyst* + *-osis*]　development of cysts in the kidney.

nephroerysipelas (nef″ro-er″ĭ-sip′ĕ-las)　erysipelas complicated with acute nephritis.

nephrogastric (nef″ro-gas′trik)　pertaining to the kidney and the stomach; renogastric.

nephrogenic (nef″ro-jen′ik) [*nephro-* + Gr. *gennan* to produce]　forming kidney tissue.

nephrogenous (nĕ-froj′ĕ-nus)　originating or arising in the kidney.

nephrogram (nef′ro-gram)　a roentgenogram of the kidney.

nephrography (nĕ-frog′rah-fe) [*nephro-* + Gr. *graphein* to write]　roentgenography of the kidney.

nephrohemia (nef″ro-he′me-ah) [*nephro-* + Gr. *haima* blood + *-ia*]　congestion of the kidney.

nephrohydrosis (nef″ro-hi-dro′sis)　hydronephrosis.

nephrohypertrophy (nef″ro-hi-per′tro-fe) [*nephro-* + *hypertrophy*]　hypertrophy of the kidney.

nephroid (nef′roid) [*nephro-* + Gr. *eidos* form]　kidney-shaped, or resembling a kidney.

nephrolith (nef′ro-lith) [*nephro-* + Gr. *lithos* stone]　a renal calculus; gravel in a kidney.

nephrolithiasis (nef″ro-lĭ-thi′ah-sis)　a condition marked by the presence of renal calculi.

nephrolithotomy (nef″ro-lĭ-thot′o-me) [*nephrolith* + Gr. *tomē* a cutting]　the removal of renal calculi by incision through the kidney.

nephrologist (nĕ-frol′o-jist)　an expert in nephrology.

nephrology (nĕ-frol′o-je) [*nephro-* + *-logy*]　scientific study of the kidney, its anatomy, physiology, and pathology.

nephrolysis (nĕ-frol′ĭ-sis) [*nephro-* + Gr. *lysis* dissolution]　1. solution of kidney substance.　2. the operation of separating the kidney from paranephric adhesions.

nephrolytic (nef″ro-lit′ik)　pertaining to, characterized by, or producing nephrolysis.

nephroma (nĕ-fro′mah) [*nephr-* + *-oma*]　a tumor of kidney tissue; a tumor of the kidney.　**embryonal n.,** Wilms' tumor.

nephromalacia (nef″ro-mah-la′she-ah) [*nephro-* + Gr. *malakia* softness]　softening of the kidney.

nephromegaly (nef″ro-meg′ah-le) [*nephro-* + Gr. *megas* great]　enlargement of the kidney.

nephromere (nef′ro-mēr) [*nephro-* + Gr. *meros* part]　nephrotome.

nephron (nef′ron) [Gr. *nephros* kidney + *on* neuter ending]　the anatomical and functional unit of the kidney, consisting of the renal corpuscle, the proximal convoluted tubule, the descending and ascending limbs of Henle's loop, the distal convoluted tubule, and the collecting tubule. See illustration accompanying *kidney*.　**lower n.,** the thick segment of the ascending limb of Henle's loop and the parts distal to it.

nephroncus (nef-rong′kus) [*nephr-* + Gr. *onkos* mass]　nephroma.

nephronophthisis (nef″ron-of′thĭ-sis) [*nephron* + Gr. *phthisis* wasting]　wasting disease of the kidney substance.　**familial juvenile n.,** a progressive hereditary disease of the kidneys characterized clinically by anemia, polyuria, and renal loss of sodium, progressing to chronic renal failure; pathologically, there is tubular atrophy, interstitial fibrosis, glomerular sclerosis, and medullary cysts. Called also *medullary cystic disease.*

nephroparalysis (nef″ro-pah-ral′ĭ-sis) [*nephro-* + *paralysis*]　paralysis of the kidney.

nephropathia (nef″ro-path′e-ah)　nephropathy.

nephropathic (nef″ro-path′ik)　pertaining to, characterized by, or producing nephropathy.

nephropathy (nĕ-frop′ah-the) [*nephro-* + Gr. *pathos* disease]　disease of the kidneys.　**analgesic n.,** that due to renal damage associated with massive intake of analgesics containing phenacetin.　**Balkan n.,** see under *nephritis*.　**dropsical n.,** hypochloruric n.　**gouty n.,** any of a group of kidney diseases associated with the abnormal production and excretion of uric acid.　**hypazoturic n.,** kidney disease with retention of nitrogen.　**hypochloruric n.,** kidney disease with sodium chloride retention.　**IgA n.,** IgA glomerulonephritis.　**membranous n.,** see under *glomerulonephritis*.　**reflux n.,** childhood pyelonephritis in which the renal scarring results from vesicoureteric reflux, with radiological appearance of intrarenal reflux.

nephropexy (nef′ro-pek″se) [*nephro-* + Gr. *pēxis* fixation]　the fixation or suspension of a floating kidney.

nephrophagiasis (nef″ro-fah-ji′ah-sis) [*nephro-* + Gr. *phagein* to eat]　the devouring of the kidney by certain parasites.

nephrophthisis (nĕ-frof′thĭ-sis) [*nephro-* + Gr. *phthisis* wasting]　1. nephrotuberculosis.　2. nephronophthisis.

nephropoietic (nef″ro-poi-et′ik) [*nephro-* + Gr. *poiein* to make]　forming kidney tissue.

nephropoietin (nef″ro-poi-e′tin)　a substance thought to exist in the blood serum, in embryonic kidney, and in kidneys undergoing regeneration and to stimulate the formation of kidney tissue.

nephroptosia (nef″rop-to′se-ah)　nephroptosis.

nephroptosis (nef″rop-to′sis) [*nephro-* + Gr. *ptōsis* falling]　downward displacement of the kidney.

nephropyelitis (nef″ro-pi″ĕ-li′tis) [*nephro-* + *pyelitis*]　pyelonephritis.

nephropyelography (nef″ro-pi″ĕ-log′rah-fe)　radiography of the kidney and renal pelvis.

nephropyelolithotomy (nef″ro-pi″ĕ-lo-lĭ-thot′o-me) [*nephro-* + Gr. *pyelos* pelvis + *lithos* stone + *tomē* a cut]　removal of a calculus from the renal pelvis by an incision through the kidney substance.

nephropyeloplasty (nef″ro-pi′ĕ-lo-plas″te) [*nephro-* + Gr. *pyelos* pelvis + *plassein* to form]　plastic operation on the pelvis of the kidney.

nephropyosis (nef″ro-pi-o′sis) [*nephro-* + Gr. *pyōsis* suppuration]　suppuration of the kidney.

nephrorosein (nef″ro-ro′ze-in)　a urinary pigment identified spectroscopically.

nephrorrhagia (nef″ro-ra′je-ah) [*nephro-* + Gr. *rhēgnynai* to burst forth]　hemorrhage from the kidney.

nephrorrhaphy (nef-ror′ah-fe) [*nephro-* + Gr. *rhaphē* suture]　the operation of suturing the kidney.

nephroscleria (nef″ro-skle′re-ah)　nephrosclerosis.

nephrosclerosis (nef″ro-skle-ro′sis) [*nephro-* + Gr. *sklērōsis* hardening]　sclerosis or hardening of the kidney; the condition of the kidney due to renovascular disease.　**arteriolar n.,** nephrosclerosis involving chiefly the arterioles; it is frequently associated with hypertension, and characterized by insidious onset, cylindruria, edema, hypertrophy of the heart, degeneration of the renal tubules, and fibrotic thickening of the glomeruli (glomerulonephritis), resulting in renal insufficiency, congestive heart failure, and cerebral hemorrhage. Called also *intercapillary n.* and *glomerulosclerosis.*　**benign n.,** arteriolar nephrosclerosis commonly occurring in patients sixty years of age or older, and frequently associated with benign hypertension and hyaline arteriolosclerosis; in younger persons, it may occur in diabetics with a predisposition to arteriosclerosis and in those who have hypertension resulting from an apparent underlying disease, such as pheochromocytoma. Called also *hyaline arteriolar n.* **hyaline arteriolar n.,** benign n. **hyperplastic arteriolar n.,** malignant n. **intercapillary n.,** arteriolar n. **malignant n.,** an uncommon form of arteriolar nephrosclerosis affecting all the vessels of the body, especially the small arteries and arterioles of the kidneys, and frequently associated with malignant hypertension and hyperplastic arteriolosclerosis. It may occur in the absence of previous history of hypertension, or may be superimposed on benign hypertension or primary renal disease, especially glomerulonephritis, benign nephrosclerosis, and pyelonephritis. Called also *hyperplastic arteriolar n.* and *Fahr-Volhard disease.* **senile n.,** nephrosclerosis which is just a part of the arteriosclerosis common in old age.

nephroscope (nef′ro-skōp) an instrument inserted into an incision in the renal pelvis for viewing the inside of the kidney, equipped with three channels for telescope, fiberoptic light input, and irrigation.

nephroscopy (nĕ-fros′ko-pe) visualization of the kidney by means of the nephroscope.

nephroses (nĕ-fro′sēz) plural of *nephrosis.*

nephrosis (nĕ-fro′sis), pl. *nephro′ses* [*nephr-* + *-osis*] any disease of the kidney, especially any disease of the kidneys characterized by purely degenerative lesions of the renal tubules—as opposed to nephritis—and marked by edema (noninflammatory), albuminuria, and decreased serum albumin (the nephrotic syndrome). **acute n.,** nephrosis marked by scanty urine but with little edema or albuminuria. **amyloid n.,** chronic nephrosis with amyloid degeneration of the median coat of the arteries and the glomerular capillaries; amyloid kidney. **avian n.,** infectious bursal disease. **cholemic n.,** renal disease associated with various types of hepatic or biliary dysfunction, especially those in which there is obstructive jaundice. **chronic n.,** renal disease characterized by chronic degeneration of the renal epithelium. **Epstein's n.,** a type of chronic tubular nephritis resulting from systemic metabolic disorder, occurring usually in young persons and in women, and frequently associated with hypothyroidism or other endocrine disturbance. **glycogen n.,** nephrosis associated with glycogen vacuolation within the proximal convoluted tubules and the loops of Henle. **hydropic n.,** vacuolar n. **hypokalemic n.,** vacuolar n. **infectious avian n.,** infectious bursal disease. **larval n.,** a condition in which the renal lesions are slight and manifested clinically by albuminuria. **lipid n., lipoid n.,** nephrosis characterized by edema, albuminuria, and changes in the protein and lipids of the blood and the accumulation of globules of cholesterol esters in the tubular epithelium of the kidney. **lower nephron n.,** a condition of renal insufficiency leading to uremia, due to necrosis of the cells of the lower nephron, blocking the tubular lumens of this region. The condition is seen after severe injuries, especially crushing injury to muscles (*crush syndrome*). **necrotizing n.,** renal disease characterized by necrosis of tubular epithelium of the kidney. **osmotic n.,** vacuolar n. **toxic n.,** nephrosis caused by some toxic agent, most frequently and typically by bichloride of mercury. **vacuolar n.,** renal disease in which injury of the renal tubules is associated with vacuolization of the proximal convoluted tubules and sometimes of the loops of Henle and collecting tubules, presumed to be caused by disturbances in the normal osmotic relationships within the cells. These changes are seen in various clinical situations, as following the administration of hypertonic solutions, in diseases resulting in marked alterations in fluid balance, and in severe hypokalemia. Called also *hydropic n., hypokalemic n.,* and *osmotic n.*

nephrosonephritis (nĕ-fro″so-nĕ-fri′tis) [*nephrosis* + *nephritis*] renal disease with nephrotic and nephritic components. **hemorrhagic n., Korean hemorrhagic n.,** epidemic hemorrhagic fever.

nephrosonography (nef″ro-so-nog′rah-fe) ultrasonic scanning of the kidney.

nephrospasis (nef″ro-spas′is) [*nephro-* + Gr. *span* to draw] movable kidney in which the natural supports of the organ are so weakened that the organ hangs by its pedicle.

nephrostolithotomy (nĕ″fro-sto-lĭ-thot′o-me) [*nephro-* + Gr. *lithos* stone + Gr. *tomē* a cutting] removal of renal calculi through a nephrostomy tube inserted through the abdominal wall into the renal pelvis.

nephrostoma (nĕ-fros′to-mah) [*nephro-* + Gr. *stoma* mouth] one of the funnel-shaped and ciliated orifices of excretory tubules that open into the coelom in the embryo, best seen in lower vertebrates.

nephrostome (nef′ro-stōm) nephrostoma.

nephrostomy (nĕ-fros′to-me) [*nephro-* + Gr. *stomoun* to provide with an opening, or mouth] the creation of a fistula leading directly into the pelvis of the kidney.

nephrotic (nĕ-frot′ik) pertaining to, resembling, or caused by nephrosis.

nephrotome (nef′ro-tōm) one of the segmented divisions of the mesoderm connecting the somite with the lateral plates of unsegmented mesoderm; it is the source of much of the urogenital system. Called also *intermediate cell mass* and *middle plate.*

nephrotomogram (nef″ro-to′mo-gram) the sectional radiograph of the kidney obtained by nephrotomography.

nephrotomography (nef″ro-to-mog′rah-fe) radiologic visualization of the kidney by tomography after intravenous introduction of contrast medium as a bolus or by infusion.

nephrotomy (nĕ-frot′o-me) [*nephro-* + Gr. *tomē* a cutting] a surgical incision into the kidney. **abdominal n.,** nephrotomy performed through an incision into the abdomen. **anatrophic n.,** incision into the kidney between its vascular segments, to minimize bleeding and parenchymal injury and to prevent atrophy. **lumbar n.,** nephrotomy performed through an incision in the loin.

nephrotoxic (nef″ro-tok′sik) toxic or destructive to kidney cells.

nephrotoxicity (nef″ro-tok-sis′ĭ-te) the quality of being toxic or destructive to kidney cells.

nephrotoxin (nef″ro-tok′sin) [*nephro-* + Gr. *toxikon* poison] a toxin which has a specific destructive effect on kidney cells.

nephrotropic (nef″ro-trop′ik) having a special affinity for or exerting its principal effect upon kidney tissue.

nephrotuberculosis (nef″ro-tu-ber″ku-lo′sis) [*nephro-* + *tuberculosis*] disease of the kidney due to *Mycobacterium tuberculosis.*

nephroureterectomy (nef″ro-u″re-ter-ek′to-me) [*nephro-* + *ureterectomy*] excision of a kidney and a whole or part of the ureter.

nephroureterocystectomy (nef″ro-u-re″ter-o-sis-tek′to-me) [*nephro-* + Gr. *ourētēr* ureter + *kystis* bladder + *ektomē* excision] excision of the kidney, ureter, and a portion of the bladder wall.

nephrozymosis (nef″ro-zi-mo′sis) zymotic or fermentative disease of the kidney.

nephrydrosis (nef″rĭ-dro′sis) [*nephro-* + Gr. *hydōr* water + *-osis*] hydronephrosis.

nephrydrotic (nef″rĭ-drot′ik) pertaining to nephrydrosis.

nepiology (nep″e-ol′o-je) [Gr. *nēpio* infant + *-logy*] (*obs.*) the department of pediatrics treating of young infants.

Neptazane (nep′tah-zān) trademark for a preparation of methazolamide.

neptunium (nep-tu′ne-um) [from planet Neptune] a radioactive element of atomic number 93 and atomic weight 237, occurring in certain earths and obtained by splitting the uranium atom with neutrons. It is unstable and changes into plutonium. Symbol Np.

nequinate (nĕ-kwin′āt) chemical name: 6-butyl-1,4-dihydro-4-oxo-7-(phenylmethoxy)-3-quinolinecarboxylic acid methyl ester; a coccidiostat for poultry, $C_{22}H_{23}NO_4$.

Nerium (ne′rĭ-um) a genus of evergreen apocynaceous shrubs of the Mediterranean region and Asia. *N. odorum* (*N. indicum*) is the sweet-scented oleander; *N. oleander* L. is the common oleander.

Nernst equation, potential (nernst) [Walther Hermann *Nernst,* German physical chemist, 1864–1941] see under *equation* and *potential.*

nerol (ne′rol) an essential oil, $(CH_3)_2C{:}CH \cdot CH_2 \cdot CH_2 \cdot C{-}(CH_3){:}CH \cdot CH_2OH$, a constituent of orange flower oil.

neroli (ner′o-le) an essential oil distilled from orange blossoms; orange flower oil.

nerval (ner′val) (*obs.*) neural.

nerve (nerv) [L. *nervus;* Gr. *neuron*] a cordlike structure, visible to the naked eye, comprising a collection of nerve fibers which convey impulses between a part of the central nervous system and some other region of the body. Called also *nervus* [NA]. A nerve consists of a connective tissue sheath (epineurium) enclosing bundles (funiculi or fasciculi) of nerve fibers, each bundle being surrounded by its own sheath of connective tissue (perineurium), the inner surface of which is formed by a membrane of flattened mesothelial cells. Very small nerves may consist of only one funiculus derived from the parent nerve. Within each such bundle, the individual nerve fibers, which are microscopic in size, are surrounded by interstitial connective tissue (endoneurium). An individual nerve fiber (an axon with its covering sheath) consists of formed elements in a matrix of protoplasm (axoplasm), the entire structure being enclosed in a thin membrane (axolemma). Each nerve fiber is enclosed by a cellular sheath (neurilemma), from which it may or may not be separated by a lipid layer (myelin sheath) derived from neurilemmal cells. **abducent n.,** nervus abducens. **accelerator n's,** the cardiac sympathetic nerves, which, when stimulated, accelerate the action of the heart. **accessory n., accessory n., spinal,** nervus accessorius. **accessory n., vagal,** ramus internus nervi accessorii. **acoustic n.,** nervus vestibulocochlearis. **afferent n.,** any nerve that transmits impulses from the periphery toward the central nervous system, as a sensory nerve; cf. *efferent n.* **alveolar n., inferior,** nervus alveolaris inferior. **alveolar n's, superior,** nervi alveolaris superior. **ampullar n., anterior,** nervus ampullaris anterior. **ampullar n., inferior,** nervus ampullaris posterior. **ampullar n., lateral,** nervus ampullaris lateralis. **ampullar n., posterior,** nervus ampullaris posterior. **ampullar n., superior,** nervus ampullaris anterior. **anabolic n.,** any nerve, such as the vagus, the stimulation of which serves to promote the anabolic processes. **anal n's, inferior,** nervi rectales inferiores. **Andersch's n.,** nervus tympanicus. **anococcygeal n's,** nervi anococcygei. **Arnold's n.,** ramus auricularis nervi vagi. **articular n.,** any mixed peripheral nerve that supplies a joint and its associated structures. See also *nervus et ramus articulares.* **auditory n.,** nervus vestibulocochlearis. **auricular n's, anterior,** nervi auriculares anteriores. **auricular n., great,** nervus auricularis magnus. **auricular n., internal,** ramus posterior nervi auricularis magni. **auricular n., posterior,** nervus auricularis posterior. **auricular n. of vagus n.,** ramus auricularis nervi vagi. **auriculotemporal n.,** nervus auriculotemporalis. **autonomic n.,** any nerve of the autonomic nervous system. Called also *visceral n.* See also *nervus et ramus autonomici.* **axillary n.,** nervus axillaris. **Bell's n.,** nervus thoracicus longus. **Bock's n.,** ramus pharyngeus ganglii pterygopalatini. **buccal n., buccinator n.,** nervus buccalis. **cardiac n., cervical, inferior,** nervus cardiacus cervicalis inferior. **cardiac n., cervical, middle,** nervus cardiacus cervicalis medius. **cardiac n., cervical, superior,** nervus cardiacus cervicalis superior. **cardiac n., inferior,** nervus cardiacus cervicalis inferior. **cardiac n., middle,** nervus cardiacus cervicalis medius. **cardiac n., superior,** nervus cardiacus cervicalis superior. **cardiac n's, supreme,** rami cardiaci cervicales superiores nervi vagi. **cardiac n's, thoracic,** nervi cardiaci thoracici. **caroticotympanic n's,** nervi caroticotympanici. **carotid n's, external,** nervi carotici externi. **carotid n., internal,** nervus caroticus internus. **cavernous n's of clitoris,** nervi cavernosi clitoridis. **cavernous n's of penis,** nervi cavernosi penis. **celiac n's,** rami coeliaci nervi vagi. **centrifugal n.,** efferent n. **centripetal n.,** afferent n. **cerebral n's,** nervi craniales. **cervical n's,** the eight pairs of nerves arising from the cervical segments of the spinal cord; see *nervi cervicales* [NA]. **cervical n., descending,** radix inferior ansae cervicalis. **cervical n., transverse,** nervus transversus colli. **chorda tympani n.,** see *chorda tympani.* **ciliary n's, long,** nervi ciliares longi. **ciliary n's, short,** nervi ciliares breves. **circumflex n.,** nervus axillaris. **clunial n's, inferior,** nervi clunium inferiores. **clunial n's, middle,** nervi clunium medii. **clunial n's, superior,** nervi clunium superiores. **coccygeal n.,** either of the thirty-first pair of spinal nerves, arising from the coccygeal segment of the spinal cord; called also *nervus coccygeus.* **cochlear n.,** pars cochlearis nervi vestibulocochlearis. **n. of Cotunnius,** nervus nasopalatinus. **cranial n's,** the twelve pairs of nerves connected with the brain; see *nervi craniales* [NA]. **cranial n., eighth,** nervus vestibulocochlearis. **cranial n., eleventh,** nervus accessorius. **cranial n., fifth,** nervus trigeminus. **cranial n's, first,** see *nervi olfactorii.* **cranial n., fourth,** nervus trochlearis. **cranial n., ninth,** nervus glossopharyngeus. **cranial n., second,** nervus opticus. **cranial n., seventh,** nervus facialis. **cranial n., sixth,** nervus abducens. **cranial n., tenth,** nervus vagus. **cranial n., third,** nervus oculomotorius. **cranial n., twelfth,** nervus hypoglossus. **crotaphitic n.,** nervus maxillaris. **cubital n.,** nervus ulnaris. **cutaneous n.,** any mixed peripheral nerve that supplies a region of the skin. See also *nervus et ramus cutanei.* **cutaneous n. of abdomen, anterior,** ramus cutaneus anterior [pectoralis et abdominalis] nervorum intercostalium. **cutaneous n. of arm, lateral, inferior,** nervus cutaneus brachii lateralis inferior. **cutaneous n. of arm, lateral, superior,** nervus cutaneus brachii lateralis superior. **cutaneous n. of arm, medial,** nervus cutaneus brachii medialis. **cutaneous n. of arm, posterior,** nervus cutaneus brachii posterior. **cutaneous n. of calf, lateral,** nervus cutaneus surae lateralis. **cutaneous n. of calf, medial,** nervus cutaneus surae medialis. **cutaneous n. of foot, dorsal, intermediate,** nervus cutaneus dorsalis intermedius. **cutaneous n. of foot, dorsal, lateral,** nervus cutaneus dorsalis lateralis. **cutaneous n. of foot, dorsal, medial,** nervus cutaneus dorsalis medialis. **cutaneous n. of forearm, dorsal,** nervus cutaneus antebrachii posterior. **cutaneous n. of forearm, lateral,** nervus cutaneus antebrachii lateralis. **cutaneous n. of forearm, medial,** nervus cutaneus antebrachii medialis. **cutaneous n. of forearm, posterior,** nervus cutaneus antebrachii posterior. **cutaneous n. of thigh, lateral,** nervus cutaneus femoris lateralis. **cutaneous n. of thigh, posterior,** nervus cutaneus femoris posterior. **Cyon's n.,** a depressor nerve, the branch of the vagus nerve in the rabbit, stimulation of which results in lowering of the blood pressure. **dental n., inferior,** nervus alveolaris inferior. **depressor n.,** 1. a nerve that lessens the activity of an organ. 2. an inhibitory nerve whose stimulation depresses a motor center. **diaphragmatic n.,** nervus phrenicus. **digastric n.,** ramus digastricus nervi facialis. **digital n's, dorsal, radial,** nervi digitales dorsales nervi radialis. **digital n's, dorsal, ulnar,** nervi digitales dorsales nervi ulnaris. **digital n's of foot, dorsal,** nervi digitales dorsales pedis. **digital n's of lateral plantar nerve, plantar, common,** nervi digitales plantares communes nervi plantaris lateralis. **digital n's of lateral plantar nerve, plantar, proper,** nervi digitales plantares proprii nervi plantaris lateralis. **digital n's of lateral surface of great toe and of medial surface of second toe, dorsal,** nervi digitales dorsales hallucis lateralis et digiti secundi medialis. **digital n's of medial plantar nerve, plantar, common,** nervi digitales plantares communes nervi plantaris medialis. **digital n's of medial plantar nerve, plantar, proper,** nervi digitales plantares proprii nervi plantaris medialis. **digital n's of median nerve, palmar, common,** nervi digitales palmares communes nervi mediani. **digital n's of median nerve, palmar, proper,** nervi digitales palmares proprii nervi mediani. **digital n's of radial nerve, dorsal,** nervi digitales dorsales nervi radialis. **digital n's of ulnar nerve, dorsal,** nervi digitales dorsales nervi ulnaris. **digital n's of ulnar nerve, palmar, collateral,** nervi digitales palmares proprii nervi ulnaris. **digital n's of ulnar nerve, palmar, common,** nervi digitales palmares communes nervi ulnaris. **digital n's of ulnar nerve, palmar, proper,** nervi digitales palmares proprii nervi ulnaris. **dorsal n. of clitoris,** nervus dorsalis clitoridis. **dorsal n. of penis,** nervus dorsalis penis. **dorsal n. of scapula,** nervus dorsalis scapulae. **efferent n.,** any nerve that carries impulses from the central nervous system toward the periphery, as a motor nerve; cf. *afferent n.* **eighth n.,** nervus vestibulocochlearis. **eleventh n.,** nervus accessorius. **encephalic n's,** nervi craniales. **esodic n.,** afferent n. **ethmoidal n., anterior,** nervus ethmoidalis anterior. **ethmoidal n., posterior,** nervus ethmoidalis posterior. **exciter n.,** a nerve that transmits impulses resulting in an increase in functional activity. **excitoreflex n.,** a visceral nerve that produces reflex action. **exodic n.,** efferent n. **n. of external acoustic meatus,** nervus meatus acustici

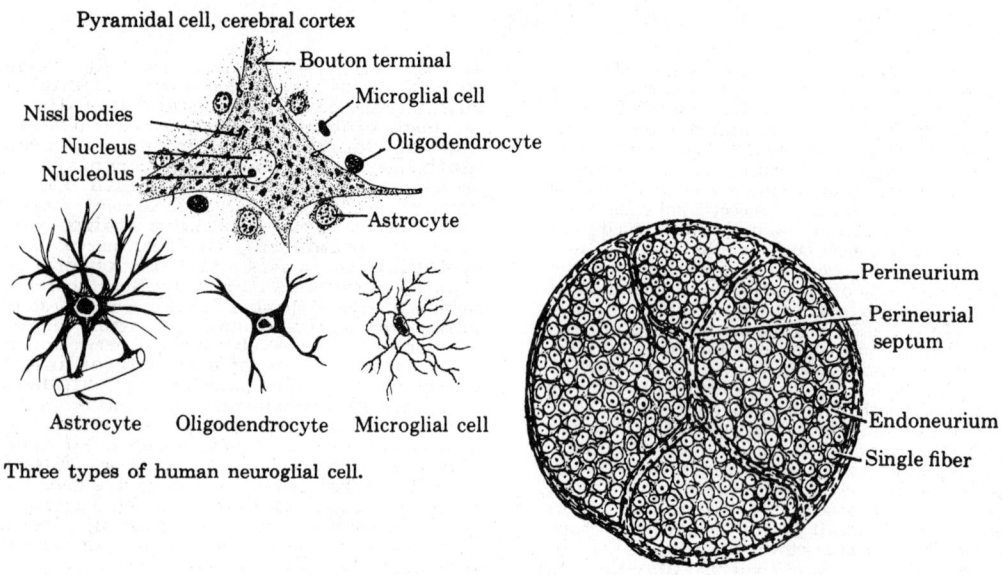

Pyramidal cell, cerebral cortex

Bouton terminal
Microglial cell
Nissl bodies
Oligodendrocyte
Nucleus
Nucleolus
Astrocyte

Astrocyte   Oligodendrocyte   Microglial cell

Three types of human neuroglial cell.

Perineurium
Perineurial septum
Endoneurium
Single fiber

Transverse section of a nerve.

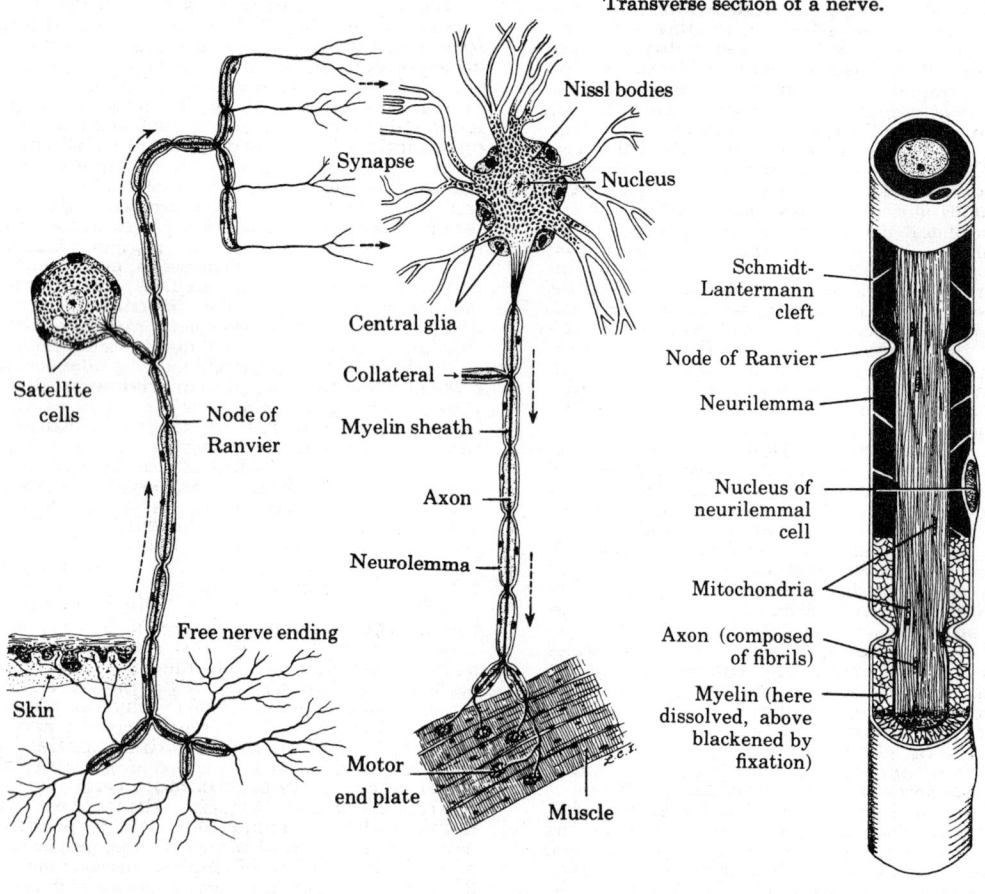

Synapse

Nissl bodies
Nucleus

Satellite cells

Node of Ranvier

Central glia
Collateral →
Myelin sheath
Axon
Neurolemma

Skin

Free nerve ending

Motor end plate
Muscle

Schmidt-Lantermann cleft
Node of Ranvier
Neurilemma
Nucleus of neurilemmal cell
Mitochondria
Axon (composed of fibrils)
Myelin (here dissolved, above blackened by fixation)

SENSORY NEURON   MOTOR NEURON

Diagrammatic representation of two types of neurons.

Longitudinal section of a nerve fiber (Leeson and Leeson).

PLATE 33 — STRUCTURE OF NERVE TISSUE

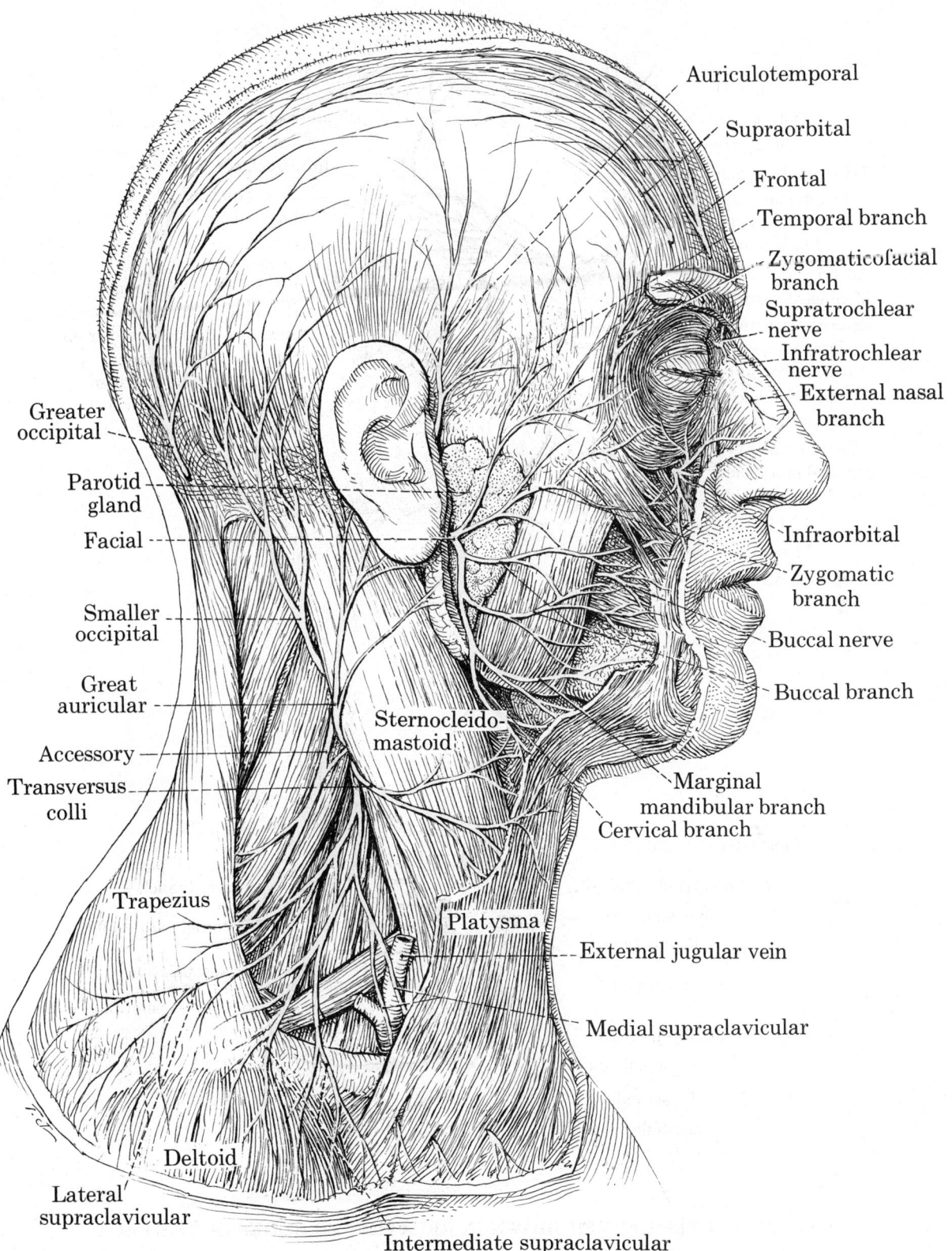

Auriculotemporal

Supraorbital

Frontal

Temporal branch

Zygomaticofacial
branch

Supratrochlear
nerve

Infratrochlear
nerve

External nasal
branch

Greater
occipital

Parotid
gland

Facial

Smaller
occipital

Great
auricular

Accessory

Transversus
colli

Trapezius

Sternocleido-
mastoid

Infraorbital

Zygomatic
branch

Buccal nerve

Buccal branch

Marginal
mandibular branch

Cervical branch

Platysma

External jugular vein

Medial supraclavicular

Deltoid

Lateral
supraclavicular

Intermediate supraclavicular

PLATE 34 — SUPERFICIAL NERVES AND MUSCLES OF THE HEAD AND NECK

Portions of the parotid gland and platysma are shown cut away.

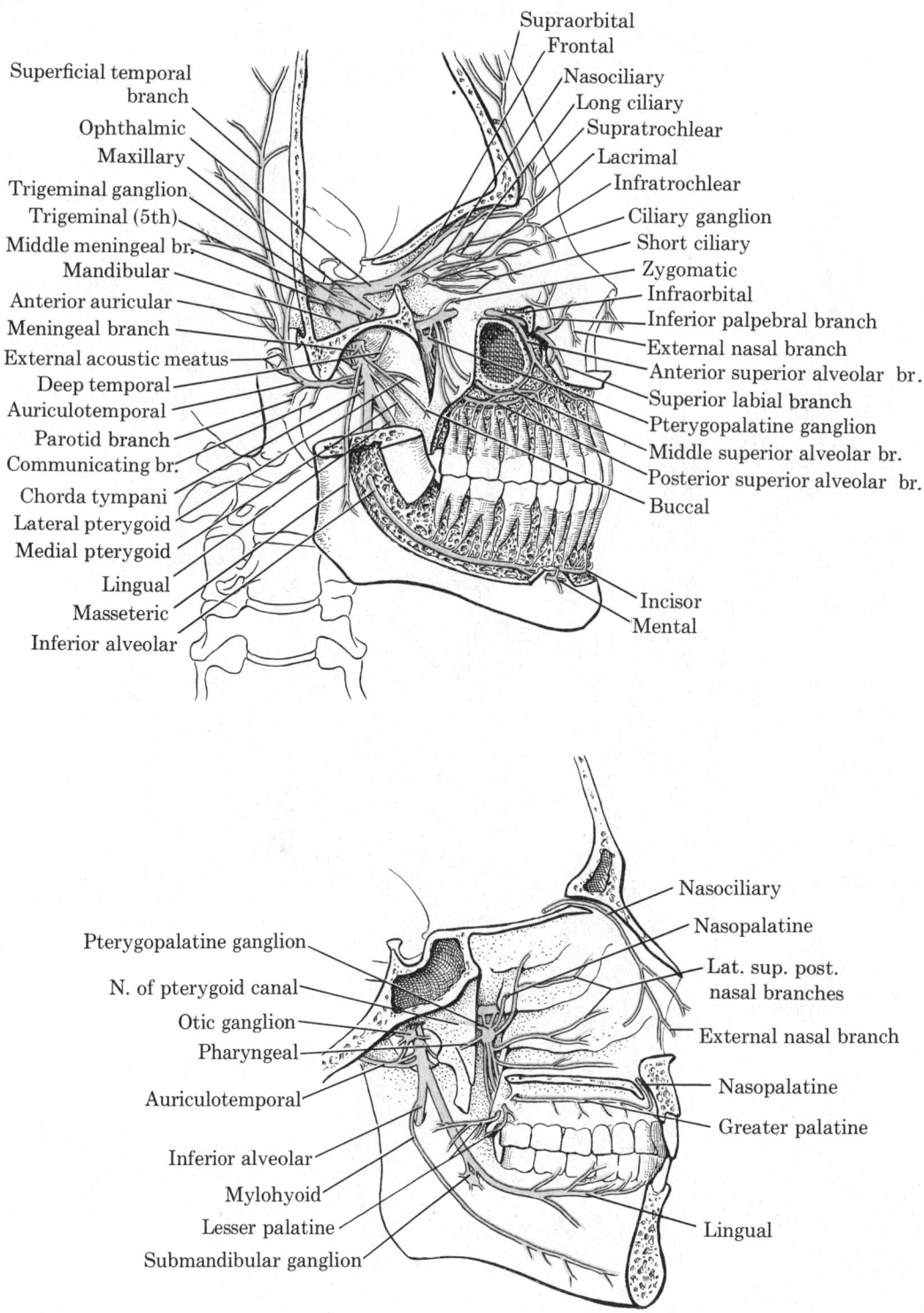

Supraorbital
Frontal
Nasociliary
Long ciliary
Supratrochlear
Lacrimal
Infratrochlear
Ciliary ganglion
Short ciliary
Zygomatic
Infraorbital
Inferior palpebral branch
External nasal branch
Anterior superior alveolar br.
Superior labial branch
Pterygopalatine ganglion
Middle superior alveolar br.
Posterior superior alveolar br.
Buccal
Incisor
Mental

Superficial temporal branch
Ophthalmic
Maxillary
Trigeminal ganglion
Trigeminal (5th)
Middle meningeal br.
Mandibular
Anterior auricular
Meningeal branch
External acoustic meatus
Deep temporal
Auriculotemporal
Parotid branch
Communicating br.
Chorda tympani
Lateral pterygoid
Medial pterygoid
Lingual
Masseteric
Inferior alveolar

Nasociliary
Nasopalatine
Lat. sup. post. nasal branches
External nasal branch
Nasopalatine
Greater palatine
Lingual

Pterygopalatine ganglion
N. of pterygoid canal
Otic ganglion
Pharyngeal
Auriculotemporal
Inferior alveolar
Mylohyoid
Lesser palatine
Submandibular ganglion

PLATE 35 — DEEP NERVES SHOWN IN RELATION TO BONES OF THE FACE

1112

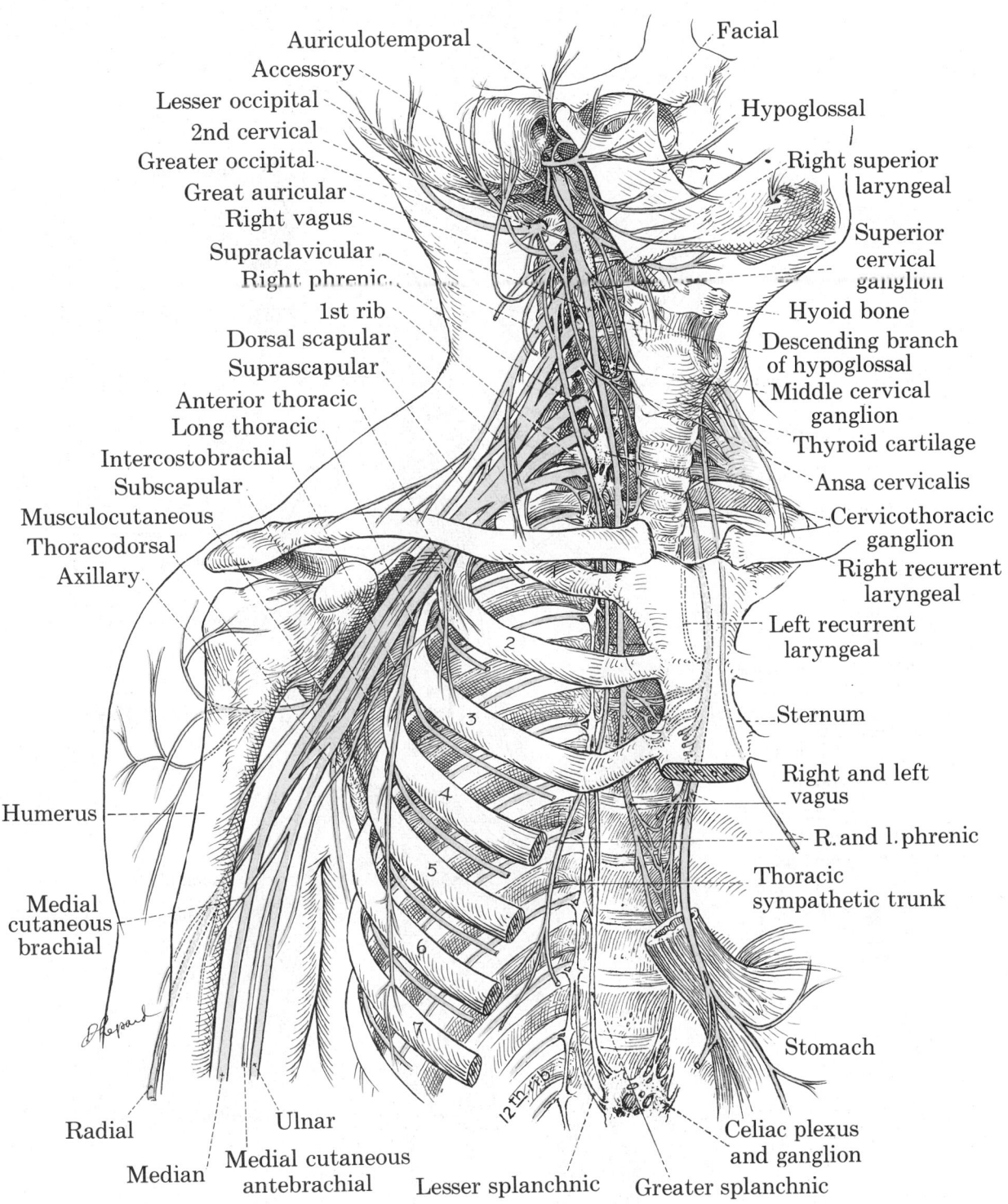

Auriculotemporal

Accessory

Facial

Lesser occipital

Hypoglossal

2nd cervical

Greater occipital

Right superior
laryngeal

Great auricular

Right vagus

Superior
cervical
ganglion

Supraclavicular

Right phrenic

Hyoid bone

1st rib

Descending branch
of hypoglossal

Dorsal scapular

Middle cervical
ganglion

Suprascapular

Anterior thoracic

Thyroid cartilage

Long thoracic

Ansa cervicalis

Intercostobrachial

Cervicothoracic
ganglion

Subscapular

Musculocutaneous

Right recurrent
laryngeal

Thoracodorsal

Axillary

Left recurrent
laryngeal

Sternum

Humerus

Right and left
vagus

R. and l. phrenic

Medial
cutaneous
brachial

Thoracic
sympathetic trunk

Stomach

Radial

Median

Ulnar

Medial cutaneous
antebrachial

Lesser splanchnic

Celiac plexus
and ganglion

Greater splanchnic

PLATE 36 — DEEP NERVES OF THE NECK, AXILLA, AND UPPER THORAX

The sympathetic nerves are uncolored.

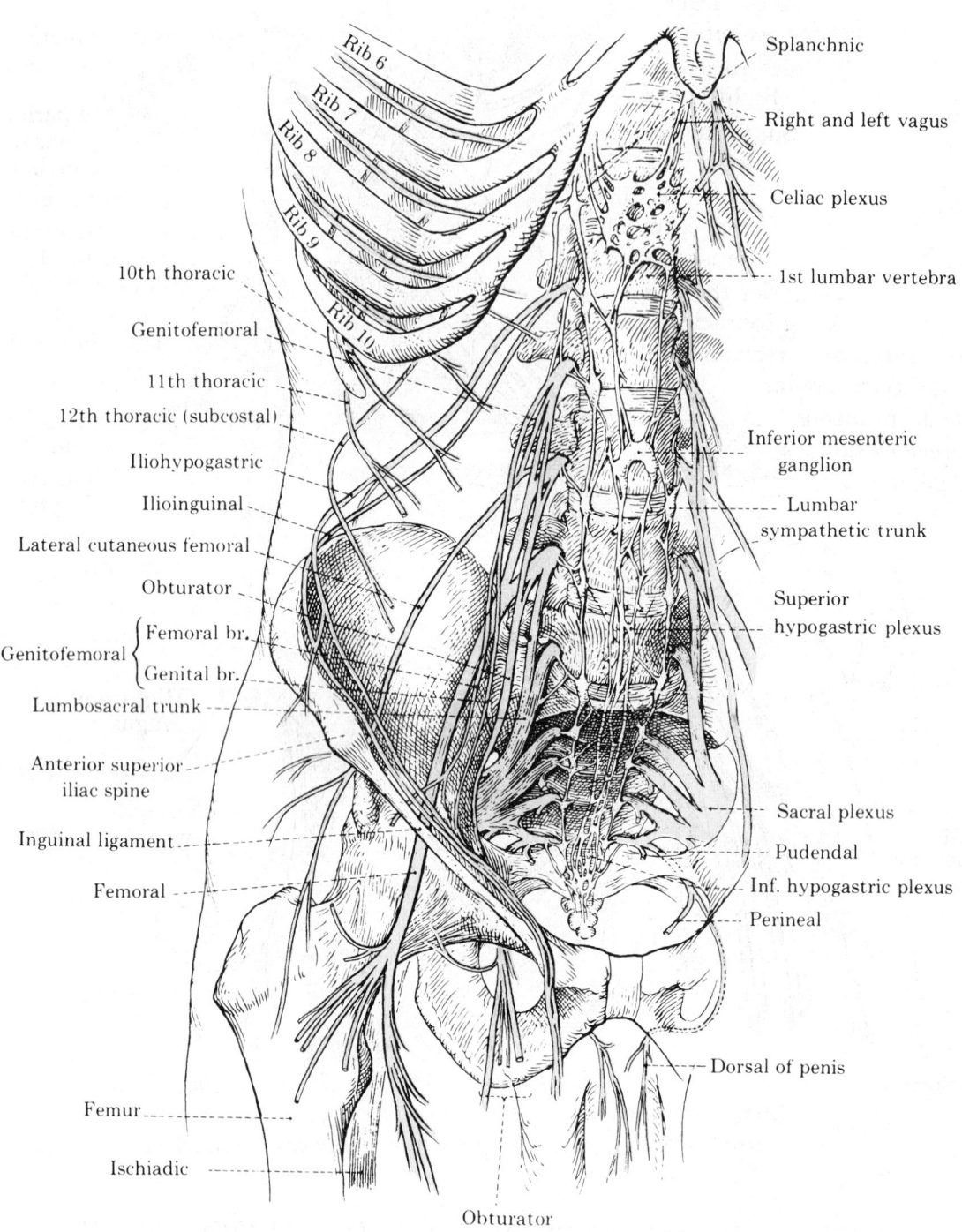

Splanchnic

Right and left vagus

Celiac plexus

Rib 6

Rib 7

Rib 8

Rib 9

1st lumbar vertebra

10th thoracic

Genitofemoral

Rib 10

11th thoracic

12th thoracic (subcostal)

Inferior mesenteric
ganglion

Iliohypogastric

Ilioinguinal

Lumbar
sympathetic trunk

Lateral cutaneous femoral

Obturator

Superior
hypogastric plexus

Genitofemoral { Femoral br.

Genital br.

Lumbosacral trunk

Anterior superior
iliac spine

Sacral plexus

Inguinal ligament

Pudendal

Inf. hypogastric plexus

Femoral

Perineal

Dorsal of penis

Femur

Ischiadic

Obturator

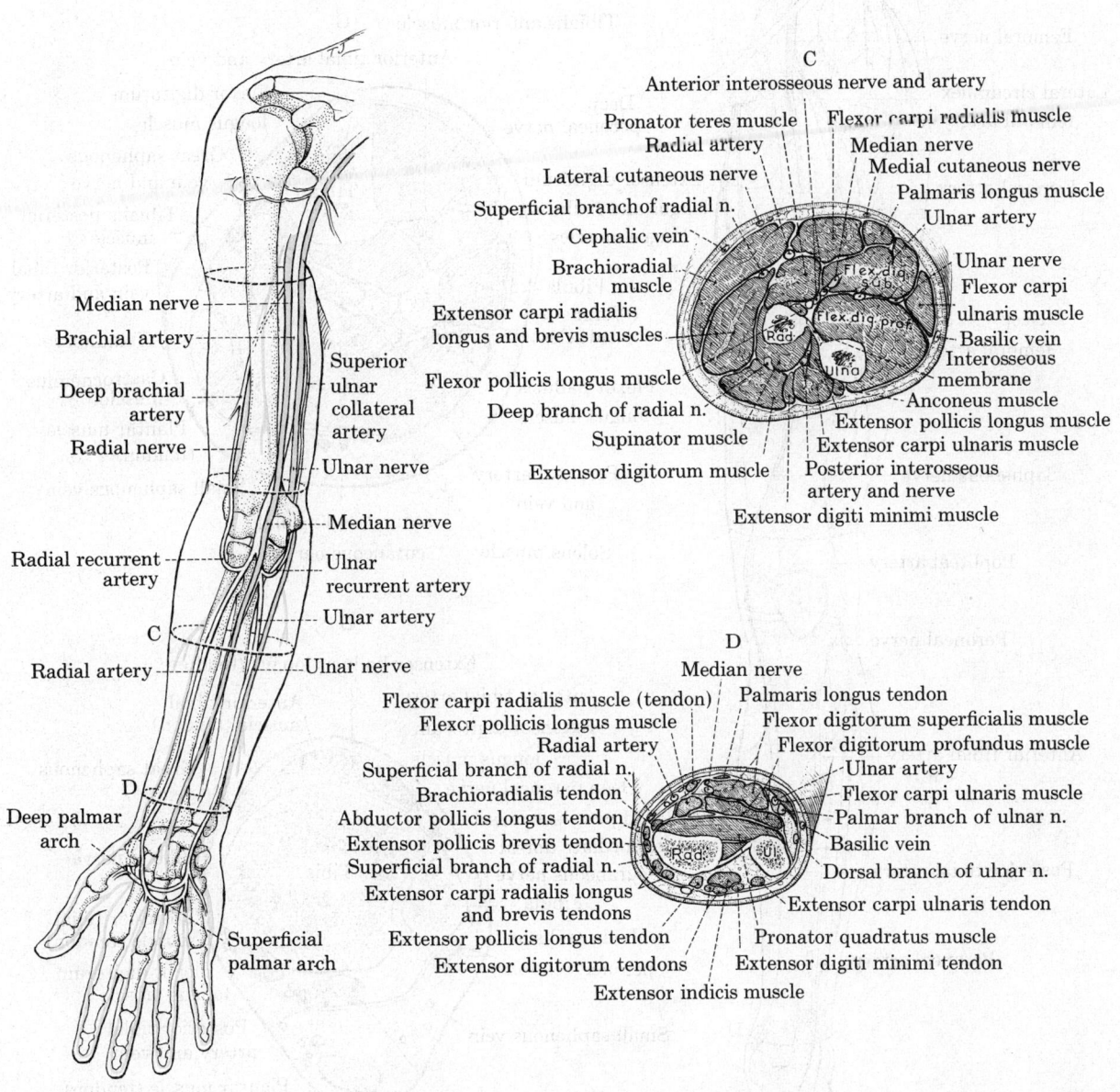

C

Anterior interosseous nerve and artery
Pronator teres muscle
Radial artery
Lateral cutaneous nerve
Superficial branch of radial n.
Cephalic vein
Brachioradial muscle
Extensor carpi radialis longus and brevis muscles
Flexor pollicis longus muscle
Deep branch of radial n.
Supinator muscle
Extensor digitorum muscle

Flexor carpi radialis muscle
Median nerve
Medial cutaneous nerve
Palmaris longus muscle
Ulnar artery
Ulnar nerve
Flexor carpi ulnaris muscle
Basilic vein
Interosseous membrane
Anconeus muscle
Extensor pollicis longus muscle
Extensor carpi ulnaris muscle
Posterior interosseous artery and nerve
Extensor digiti minimi muscle

Flex.dig. subl.
Flex.dig. prof.
Rad.
Ulna

Median nerve
Brachial artery
Deep brachial artery
Radial nerve
Radial recurrent artery
C
Radial artery
D
Deep palmar arch
Superficial palmar arch

Superior ulnar collateral artery
Ulnar nerve
Median nerve
Ulnar recurrent artery
Ulnar artery
Ulnar nerve

D

Median nerve
Flexor carpi radialis muscle (tendon)
Flexor pollicis longus muscle
Radial artery
Superficial branch of radial n.
Brachioradialis tendon
Abductor pollicis longus tendon
Extensor pollicis brevis tendon
Superficial branch of radial n.
Extensor carpi radialis longus and brevis tendons
Extensor pollicis longus tendon
Extensor digitorum tendons

Palmaris longus tendon
Flexor digitorum superficialis muscle
Flexor digitorum profundus muscle
Ulnar artery
Flexor carpi ulnaris muscle
Palmar branch of ulnar n.
Basilic vein
Dorsal branch of ulnar n.
Extensor carpi ulnaris tendon
Pronator quadratus muscle
Extensor digiti minimi tendon
Extensor indicis muscle

Rad.
Ul.

PLATE 38 — NERVES OF THE RIGHT UPPER EXTREMITY

Front view shows principal nerves and arteries (uncolored) in relation to the bones, C and D are cross sections made at levels indicated on drawing at left.

1115

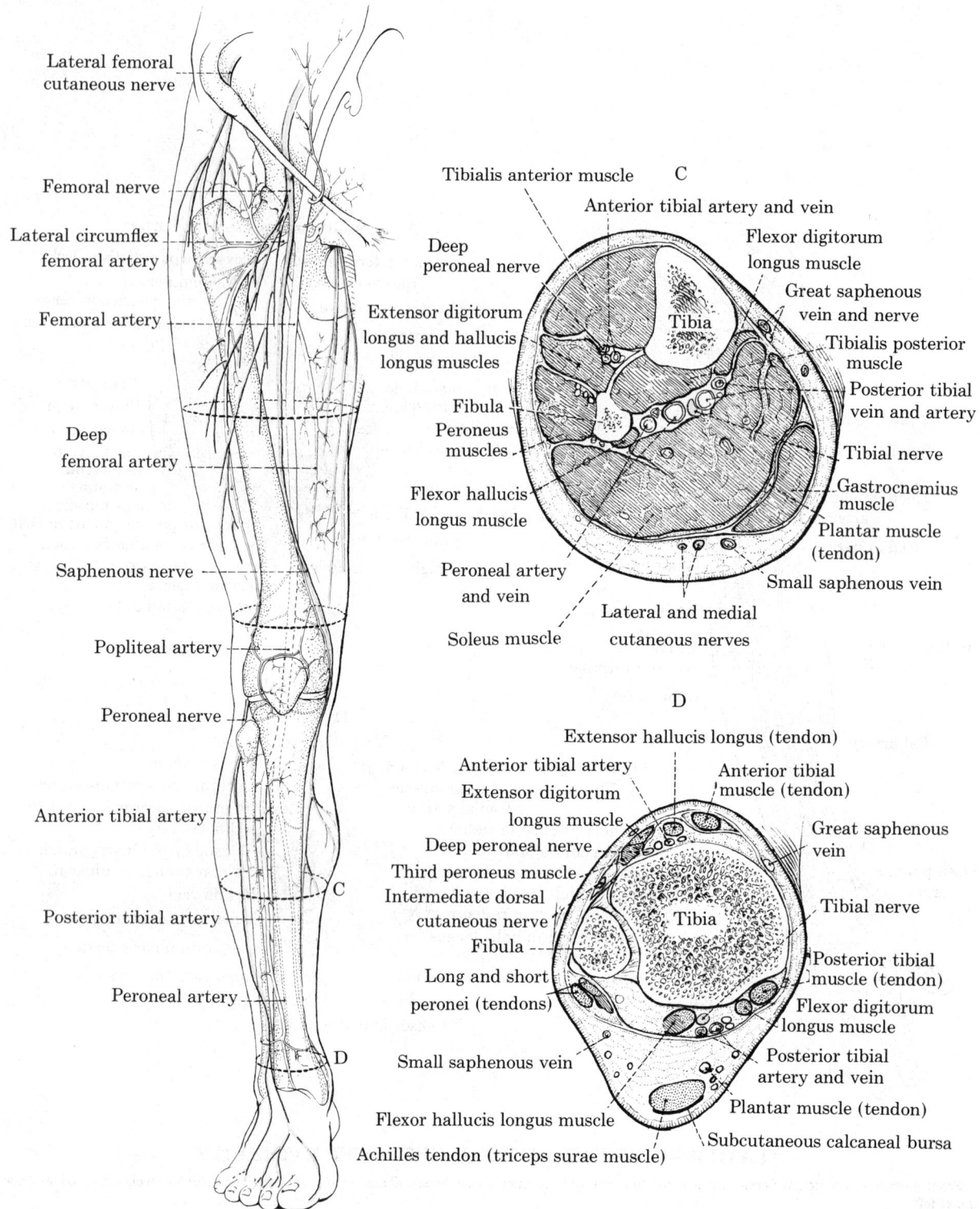

Lateral femoral
cutaneous nerve

Femoral nerve

Lateral circumflex
femoral artery

Femoral artery

Deep
femoral artery

Saphenous nerve

Popliteal artery

Peroneal nerve

Anterior tibial artery

Posterior tibial artery

Peroneal artery

C

D

C

Tibialis anterior muscle

Anterior tibial artery and vein

Deep
peroneal nerve

Extensor digitorum
longus and hallucis
longus muscles

Flexor digitorum
longus muscle

Great saphenous
vein and nerve

Tibia

Tibialis posterior
muscle

Posterior tibial
vein and artery

Fibula
Peroneus
muscles

Flexor hallucis
longus muscle

Tibial nerve

Gastrocnemius
muscle

Plantar muscle
(tendon)

Small saphenous vein

Peroneal artery
and vein

Soleus muscle

Lateral and medial
cutaneous nerves

D

Extensor hallucis longus (tendon)

Anterior tibial artery

Anterior tibial
muscle (tendon)

Extensor digitorum
longus muscle

Deep peroneal nerve

Third peroneus muscle

Intermediate dorsal
cutaneous nerve

Great saphenous
vein

Tibial nerve

Fibula

Tibia

Long and short
peronei (tendons)

Posterior tibial
muscle (tendon)

Flexor digitorum
longus muscle

Small saphenous vein

Posterior tibial
artery and vein

Flexor hallucis longus muscle

Plantar muscle (tendon)

Achilles tendon (triceps surae muscle)

Subcutaneous calcaneal bursa

PLATE 39 — NERVES OF RIGHT LOWER EXTREMITY

Front view shows principal nerves and arteries (uncolored) in relation to the bones. *C* and *D* are cross sections made at levels indicated on drawing at left.

externi. **facial n.,** nervus facialis. **facial n., temporal,** see *rami temporales nervi facialis.* **femoral n.,** nervus femoralis. **fibular n., common,** nervus fibularis communis. **fibular n., deep,** nervus fibularis profundus. **fibular n., superficial,** nervus fibularis superficialis. **fifth n.,** nervus trigeminus. **first n's,** see *nervi olfactorii.* **fourth n.,** nervus trochlearis. **frontal n.,** nervus frontalis. **furcal n.,** the fourth lumbar nerve, so called because its fibers pass to the lumbar and sacral plexuses. **fusimotor n's,** those with a special type of nerve ending that innervates intrafusal fibers of the muscle spindle. **gangliated n.,** any nerve of the sympathetic nervous system. **gastric n's,** truncus vagalis anterior and truncus vagalis posterior. **genitofemoral n.,** nervus genitofemoralis. **glossopharyngeal n.,** nervus glossopharyngeus. **gluteal n., inferior,** nervus gluteus inferior. **gluteal n's, inferior,** nervi clunium inferiores. **gluteal n's, middle,** nervi clunium medii. **gluteal n's, superior,** nervus gluteus superior. **hemorrhoidal n's, inferior,** nervi rectales inferiores. **Hering's n.,** ramus sinus carotici nervi glossopharyngei. **hypogastric n.,** nervus hypogastricus [dexter/sinister]. **hypoglossal n.,** nervus hypoglossus. **iliohypogastric n.,** nervus iliohypogastricus. **ilioinguinal n.,** nervus ilio-inguinalis. **infraoccipital n.,** nervus suboccipitalis. **infraorbital n.,** nervus infraorbitalis. **infratrochlear n.,** nervus infratrochlearis. **inhibitory n.,** a nerve that transmits impulses resulting in a decrease in functional activity. **intercostal n's,** rami ventrales nervorum thoracicorum. **intercostobrachial n's,** nervi intercostobrachiales. **intermediary n., intermediate n.,** nervus intermedius. **interosseous n. of forearm, anterior,** nervus interosseus antebrachii anterior. **interosseous n. of forearm, posterior,** nervus interosseus antebrachii posterior. **interosseous n. of leg,** nervus interosseus cruris. **ischiadic n.,** nervus ischiadicus. **Jacobson's n.,** nervus tympanicus. **jugular n.,** nervus jugularis. **labial n's, anterior,** nervi labiales anteriores. **labial n's, posterior,** nervi labiales posteriores. **lacrimal n.,** nervus lacrimalis. **n's of Lancisi,** stria longitudinalis lateralis corporis callosi and stria longitudinalis medialis corporis callosi. **Langley's n's,** pilomotor n's. **laryngeal n., inferior,** nervus laryngeus inferior. **laryngeal n., recurrent,** nervus laryngeus recurrens. **laryngeal n., superior,** nervus laryngeus superior. **laryngeal n., superior, internal,** ramus internus nervi laryngei superioris. **lingual n.,** nervus lingualis. **longitudinal n's of Lancisi,** stria longitudinalis lateralis corporis callosi and stria longitudinalis medialis corporis callosi. **lumbar n's,** the five pairs of nerves arising from the lumbar segments of the spinal cord; see *nervi lumbales.* **lumboinguinal n.,** ramus femoralis nervi genitofemoralis. **n. of Luschka,** 1. ramus meningeus nervorum spinalium. 2. nervus ethmoidalis posterior. **mandibular n.,** nervus mandibularis. **masseteric n.,** nervus massetericus. **maxillary n.,** nervus maxillaris. **median n.,** nervus medianus. **medullated n.,** myelinated n. **meningeal n.,** ramus meningeus medius nervi maxillaris. **mental n.,** nervus mentalis. **mixed n.,** nervus mixtus. **motor n.,** nervus motorius. **motor n. of tongue,** nervus hypoglossus. **musculocutaneous n.,** nervus musculocutaneus. **musculocutaneous n. of foot,** nervus peroneus superficialis. **musculocutaneous n. of leg,** nervus peroneus profundus. **musculospiral n.,** nervus radialis. **myelinated n.,** a nerve, especially a peripheral nerve, whose fibers (axons) are encased in a myelin sheath, which in turn is enclosed by a neurilemma. Called also *medullated n.* Cf. *unmyelinated n.* **mylohyoid n.,** nervus mylohyoideus. **nasociliary n.,** nervus nasociliaris. **nasopalatine n.,** nervus nasopalatinus. **ninth n.,** nervus glossopharyngeus. **nonmedullated n.,** unmyelinated n. **obturator n.,** nervus obturatorius. **obturator n., accessory,** nervus obturatorius accessorius. **obturator n., internal,** nervus obturatorius internus. **occipital n., greater,** nervus occipitalis major. **occipital n., internal** (obs.), nervus occipitalis major. **occipital n., least,** nervus occipitalis tertius. **occipital n., lesser,** nervus occipitalis minor. **occipital n., third,** nervus occipitalis tertius. **oculomotor n.,** nervus oculomotorius. **olfactory n's,** nervi olfactorii. **ophthalmic n.,** nervus ophthalmicus. **optic n.,** nervus opticus. **pain n.,** a sensory nerve whose function is the conduction of stimuli which produce the sensation of pain. **palatine**

n., anterior, nervus palatinus major. **palatine n., greater,** nervus palatinus major. **palatine n's, lesser,** nervi palatini minores. **palatine n., medial, palatine n., middle,** see *nervi palatini minores.* **palatine n., posterior,** see *nervi palatini minores.* **parasympathetic n.,** any of the nerves of the parasympathetic nervous system; see *parasympathetic system,* under *system.* **parotid n's,** rami parotidei nervi auriculotemporalis. **pectoral n., lateral,** nervus pectoralis lateralis. **pectoral n., medial,** nervus pectoralis medialis. **perineal n's,** nervi perineales. **peripheral n.,** any nerve outside the central nervous system (outside the brain and spinal cord). **peroneal n., accessory deep,** nervus peroneus profundus accessorius. **peroneal n., common,** nervus fibularis communis. **peroneal n., deep,** nervus fibularis profundus. **peroneal n., superficial,** nervus fibularis superficialis. **petrosal n., deep,** nervus petrosus profundus. **petrosal n., greater,** nervus petrosus major. **petrosal n., lesser,** nervus petrosus minor. **petrosal n., middle, superficial,** nervus petrosus minor. **phrenic n.,** nervus phrenicus. **phrenic n's, accessory,** nervi phrenici accessorii. **phrenicoabdominal n's,** rami phrenicoabdominales nervi phrenici. **pilomotor n's,** the nerves that supply the arrectores pilorum muscles. **piriform n.,** nervus piriformis. **plantar n., lateral,** nervus plantaris lateralis. **plantar n., medial,** nervus plantaris medialis. **pneumogastric n.,** nervus vagus. **popliteal n., external,** nervus peroneus communis. **popliteal n., internal,** nervus tibialis. **popliteal n., lateral,** nervus peroneus communis. **popliteal n., medial,** nervus tibialis. **presacral n.,** plexus hypogastricus superior. **pressor n.,** any afferent nerve whose irritation stimulates a vasomotor center and increases intravascular tension. **pterygoid n., external,** nervus pterygoideus lateralis. **pterygoid n., internal,** nervus pterygoideus medialis. **pterygoid n., lateral,** nervus pterygoideus lateralis. **pterygoid n., medial,** nervus pterygoideus medialis. **n. of pterygoid canal,** nervus canalis pterygoidei. **pterygopalatine n's,** nervi pterygopalatini. **pudendal n.,** nervus pudendus. **pudic n.,** nervus pudendus. **n. of quadrate muscle of thigh,** nervus musculi quadrati femoris. **radial n.,** nervus radialis. **radial n., deep,** ramus profundus nervi radialis. **radial n., superficial,** ramus superficialis nervi radialis. **rectal n's, inferior,** nervi rectales inferiores. **recurrent n.,** nervus laryngeus recurrens. **recurrent n., ophthalmic,** ramus tentorii nervi ophthalmici. **saccular n.,** nervus saccularis. **sacral n's,** the five pairs of nerves arising from the sacral segments of the spinal cord; see *nervi sacrales.* **saphenous n.,** nervus saphenus. **Scarpa's n.,** nervus nasopalatinus. **sciatic n.,** nervus ischiadicus. **sciatic n., small,** nervus cutaneus femoris posterior. **scrotal n's, anterior,** nervi scrotales anteriores. **scrotal n's, posterior,** nervi scrotales posteriores. **second n.,** nervus opticus. **secretory n.,** any efferent nerve whose stimulation increases glandular activity. **sensory n.,** nervus sensorius. **seventh n.,** nervus facialis. **sinus n.,** ramus sinus carotici nervi glossopharyngei. **sinu-vertebral n.,** ramus meningeus nervorum spinalium. **sixth n.,** nervus abducens. **somatic n's,** the motor and sensory nerves that supply skeletal muscle and somatic tissues. **spermatic n., external,** ramus genitalis nervi genitofemoralis. **spinal n's,** the thirty-one pairs of nerves arising from the spinal cord; see *nervi spinales.* **splanchnic n's,** the nerves of the blood vessels and viscera, especially the visceral branches of the thoracic, abdominal (lumbar), and pelvic parts of the sympathetic trunks. **splanchnic n., greater,** nervus splanchnicus thoracicus major. **splanchnic n., inferior, splanchnic n., lesser,** nervus splanchnicus thoracicus minor. **splanchnic n., lowest,** nervus splanchnicus thoracicus imus. **splanchnic n's, lumbar,** nervi splanchnici lumbales. **splanchnic n's, pelvic,** nervi splanchnici pelvini. **splanchnic n's, sacral,** nervi splanchnici sacrales. **stapedial n., stapedius n.,** nervus stapedius. **stylohyoid n.,** ramus stylohyoideus nervi facialis. **stylopharyngeal n.,** ramus musculi stylopharyngei nervi glossopharyngei. **subclavian n.,** nervus subclavius. **subcostal n.,** nervus subcostalis. **sublingual n.,** nervus sublingualis. **submaxillary n's,** rami glandulares ganglii submandibularis. **suboccipital n.,** nervus suboccipitalis. **subscapular n's,** nervi subscapulares. **sudomotor n's,** the nerves that innervate the sweat glands. **supraclavicular n's,** nervi supraclaviculares. **supraclavicular n's, anterior,** nervi supraclaviculares mediales. **supraclavicular n's, intermediate,** nervi supraclaviculares intermedii. **supraclavicular n's, lateral,** nervi supraclaviculares laterales. **supraclavicular n's, medial,** nervi supraclaviculares mediales. **supraclavicular n's, middle,** nervi supraclaviculares intermedii. **supraclavicular n's, posterior,** nervi supraclaviculares laterales [posteriores]. **supraorbital n.,** nervus supraorbitalis. **suprascapular n.,** nervus suprascapularis. **supratrochlear n.,** nervus supratrochlearis. **sural n.,** nervus suralis. **sympathetic n.,** 1. truncus sympatheticus. 2. one of the nerves of the sympathetic nervous system; see *sympathetic system,* under *system.* **temporal n's, deep,** nervi temporales profundi. **temporal n's, subcutaneous,** rami temporales superficiales nervi auriculotemporalis. **n. of tensor tympani, n. of tensor tympani muscle,** nervus musculi tensoris tympani. **n. of tensor veli palatini, n. of tensor veli palatini muscle,** nervus musculi tensoris veli palatini. **tenth n.,** nervus vagus. **terminal n's,** nervi terminales. **third n.,** nervus oculomotorius. **thoracic n's,** the twelve pairs of spinal nerves arising from the thoracic segments of the spinal cord; see *nervi thoracici.* **thoracic n., long,** nervus thoracicus longus. **thoracic splanchnic n., greater,** nervus splanchnicus thoracicus major. **thoracic splanchnic n., lesser,** nervus splanchnicus thoracicus minor. **thoracic splanchnic n., lowest,** nervus splanchnicus thoracicus imus. **thoracodorsal n.,** nervus thoracodorsalis. **tibial n.,** nervus tibialis. **Tiedemann's n.,** a name given a plexus of sympathetic nerve fibrils surrounding the central artery of the retina. **tonsillar n's,** rami tonsillares nervi glossopharyngei. **transverse n. of neck,** nervus transversus colli. **trigeminal n.,** nervus trigeminus. **trochlear n.,** nervus trochlearis. **trophic n.,** a nerve that aids in regulating nutrition. **twelfth n.,** nervus hypoglossus. **tympanic n.,** nervus tympanicus. **ulnar n.,** nervus ulnaris. **unmyelinated n.,** a nerve whose fibers (axons) are not encased in a myelin sheath, and which may or may not be enclosed by a neurilemma. Called also *nonmedullated n.* Cf. *myelinated n.* **utricular n.,** nervus utricularis. **utriculoampullar n.,** nervus utriculoampullaris. **vaginal n's,** nervi vaginales. **vagus n.,** nervus vagus. **vascular n's,** nervi vasorum. **vasoconstrictor n.,** a nerve whose stimulation causes contraction of the blood vessels. **vasodilator n.,** a nerve whose

stimulation causes dilation of the blood vessels. **vasomotor n.,** any nerve concerned in controlling the caliber of vessels, whether as a vasodilator or a vasoconstrictor. **vasosensory n.,** any nerve supplying sensory fibers to the vessels. **vertebral n.,** nervus vertebralis. **vestibular n.,** nervus vestibularis. **vestibulocochlear n.,** nervus vestibulocochlearis. **vidian n.,** nervus canalis pterygoidei. **vidian n., deep,** nervus petrosus profundus. **visceral n.,** autonomic n. **n. of Willis,** nervus accessorius. **Wrisberg's n.,** 1. nervus intermedius. 2. nervus cutaneus brachii medialis. **zygomatic n.,** nervus zygomaticus. **zygomaticofacial n.,** ramus zygomaticofacialis nervi zygomatici. **zygomaticotemporal n.,** ramus zygomaticotemporalis nervi zygomatici.

nervi (ner′vi) [L.] genitive and plural of *nervus.*

nervimotility (ner″vĭ-mo-til′ĭ-te) susceptibility to nervimotion.

nervimotion (ner″vĭ-mo′shun) motion effected through the agency of a nerve.

nervimotor (ner″vĭ-mo′tor) pertaining to a motor nerve.

nervimuscular (ner″vĭ-mus′ku-lar) pertaining to the nerve supply of muscles.

nervomuscular (ner″vo-mus′ku-lar) nervimuscular.

nervone (ner′vōn) a cerebroside, $C_{48}H_{91}O_8N$, isolated from nerve tissue.

nervonic acid (ner-von′ik) trivial name for *cis*-15-tetracosenoic acid, the Δ^{15}-monounsaturated, 24-carbon straight-chain fatty acid; it occurs in sphingomyelin and cerebrosides.

nervous (ner′vus) [L. *nervosus*] 1. pertaining to a nerve or to nerves. 2. unduly excitable.

nervous breakdown (ner′vus brāk′down) a nonspecific, popular name for any type of mental disorder that interferes with the affected individual's normal activities, often implying sudden onset.

nervousness (ner′vus-nes) excessive excitability and irritability, with mental and physical unrest.

nervous system see under *system.*

nervus (ner′vus), gen. and pl. *ner′vi* [L.] [NA] a nerve: a cordlike structure, visible to the naked eye, comprising a collection of nerve fibers which convey impulses between a part of the central nervous system and some other region of the body. See also *nerve.* For names and description of specific nerves, see *Table of Nervi.*

TABLE OF NERVI

Descriptions are given on NA terms, and include anglicized names of specific nerves.

n. abdu′cens [NA], abducens nerve (6th cranial): *origin,* a nucleus in the pons, beneath the floor of the fourth ventricle, emerging from the brain stem anteriorly between the pons and medulla oblongata; *distribution,* lateral rectus muscle of eye; *modality,* motor.

n. accesso′rius [NA], accessory nerve (11th cranial); *origin,* by cranial roots from the side of the medulla oblongata, and by spinal roots from the side of the spinal cord (from the upper three or more cervical segments); the roots unite to form the trunk of the accessory nerve, which divides into an internal branch (cranial portion) and an external branch (spinal portion); *distribution,* the internal branch to the vagus and thereby to the palate, pharynx, larynx, and thoracic viscera; the external branch branches to the sternocleidomastoid and trapezius muscles; *modality,* parasympathetic and motor.

n. acus′ticus, n. vestibulocochlearis.

n. alveola′ris infe′rior [NA], inferior alveolar nerve: *origin,* mandibular nerve; *branches,* mylohyoid, inferior dental, mental, and inferior gingival nerves; *distribution*—see individual branches, in this table; *modality,* motor and general sensory.

ner′vi alveola′res superio′res [NA], superior alveolar nerves: a term denoting collectively the dental branches arising from the maxillary and infraorbital nerves, viz., *rami alveolares superiores anteriores nervi infraorbitalis, ramus alveolaris superior medius nervi infraorbitalis,* and *rami alveolares superiores posteriores nervi maxillaris.*

n. ampulla′ris ante′rior [NA], anterior ampullar nerve: the branch of the vestibular nerve that innervates the ampulla of the anterior semicircular duct, ending around the hair cells of the ampullary crest.

n. ampulla′ris infe′rior, n. ampullaris posterior.

n. ampulla′ris latera′lis [NA], lateral ampullar nerve: the branch of the vestibular nerve that innervates the ampulla of the lateral semicircular duct, ending around the hair cells of the ampullary crest.

n. ampulla′ris poste′rior [NA], posterior ampullar nerve: the branch of the vestibular nerve that innervates the ampulla of the posterior semicircular duct, ending around the hair cells of the ampullary crest.

n. ampulla′ris supe′rior, n. ampularis anterior.

nervi ana′les inferio′res, NA alternative for *nervi rectales inferiores.*

ner′vi anococcyg′ei [NA], anococcygeal nerves: *origin,* coccygeal plexus; *distribution,* sacrococcygeal joint, coccyx, skin over the coccyx; *modality,* general sensory.

n. articula′ris, articular nerve.

ner′vi auricula′res anterio′res [NA], anterior auricular nerves: *origin,* auriculotemporal nerve; *distribution,* skin of anterosuperior part of external ear; *modality,* general sensory.

n. auricula′ris mag′nus [NA], great auricular nerve: *origin,* cervical plexus—C2–C3; *branches,* anterior and posterior rami; *distribution,* skin over parotid gland and mastoid process, and both surfaces of auricle; see individual branches under *ramus; modality*, general sensory.

n. auricula'ris poste'rior [NA], posterior auricular nerve: *origin*, facial nerve; *branches*, occipital ramus; *distribution*, auricularis posterior and occipitofrontalis muscles and skin of external acoustic meatus; *modality*, motor and general sensory.

n. auriculotempora'lis [NA], auriculotemporal nerve: *origin*, by two roots from the mandibular nerve; *branches*, anterior auricular nerve, nerve of external acoustic meatus, parotid branches, branch to tympanic membrane, and branches communicating with facial nerve; its terminal branches are superficial temporal to the scalp; *distribution*—see individual branches, in this table and under *ramus; modality*, general sensory.

n. axilla'ris [NA], axillary nerve: *origin*, posterior cord of brachial plexus (C5-C6); *branches*, lateral superior brachial cutaneous nerve and muscular rami; *distribution*, deltoid and teres minor muscles, skin on back of arm; *modality*, motor and general sensory.

n. bucca'lis [NA], buccal nerve: *origin*, mandibular nerve; *distribution*, skin and mucous membrane of cheeks, gums, and perhaps the first two molars and the premolars; *modality*, general sensory.

n. buccinato'rius, n. buccalis.

n. cana'lis pterygoi'dei [NA], nerve of pterygoid canal: *origin*, union of deep and greater petrosal nerves; *distribution*, pterygopalatine ganglion and branches; *modality*, parasympathetic and sympathetic. Called also *radix facialis*.

n. cardi'acus cervica'lis infe'rior [NA], inferior cervical cardiac nerve: *origin*, cervicothoracic ganglion; *distribution*, heart via cardiac plexus; *modality*, sympathetic (accelerator) and visceral afferent (chiefly pain).

n. cardi'acus cervica'lis me'dius [NA], middle cervical cardiac nerve: *origin*, middle cervical ganglion; *distribution*, heart; *modality*, sympathetic (accelerator) and visceral afferent (chiefly pain).

n. cardi'acus cervica'lis supe'rior [NA], superior cervical cardiac nerve: *origin*, superior cervical ganglion; *distribution*, heart; *modality*, sympathetic (accelerator).

n. cardi'acus infe'rior, n. cardiacus cervicalis inferior.

n. cardi'acus me'dius, n. cardiacus cervicalis medius.

n. cardi'acus supe'rior, n. cardiacus cervicalis superior.

ner'vi cardi'aci thora'cici [NA], thoracic cardiac nerves: *origin*, second through fourth or fifth thoracic ganglia of sympathetic trunk; *distribution*, heart; *modality*, sympathetic (accelerator) and visceral afferent (chiefly pain).

ner'vi caroticotympan'ici [NA], caroticotympanic nerves: *origin*, internal carotid plexus; *branches*, together with tympanic nerve, they form the tympanic plexus; *distribution*, tympanic region and parotid gland; *modality*, sympathetic.

n. caroticotympan'icus infe'rior, n. caroticotympan'icus supe'rior, see *nervi caroticotympanici*.

ner'vi carot'ici exter'ni [NA], external carotid nerves: *origin*, superior cervical ganglion; *distribution*, cranial blood vessels and glands via the external carotid plexus; *modality*, sympathetic.

n. carot'icus inter'nus [NA], internal carotid nerve: *origin*, superior cervical ganglion; *distribution*, cranial blood vessels and glands via internal carotid plexus; *modality*, sympathetic.

ner'vi caverno'si clitor'idis [NA], cavernous nerves of clitoris: *origin*, uterovaginal plexus; *distribution*, erectile tissue of clitoris; *modality*, parasympathetic, sympathetic, and visceral afferent.

n. caverno'sus clitor'idis ma'jor, ner'vi caverno'si clitor'idis mino'res, see *nervi cavernosi clitoridis*.

ner'vi caverno'si pe'nis [NA], cavernous nerves of penis: *origin*, prostatic plexus; *distribution*, erectile tissue of penis; *modality*, sympathetic, parasympathetic, and visceral afferent.

n. caverno'sus pe'nis ma'jor, ner'vi caverno'si pe'nis mino'res, see *nervi cavernosi penis*.

ner'vi cerebra'les, nervi craniales.

ner'vi cervica'les [NA], cervical nerves: the eight pairs of nerves that arise from the cervical segments of the spinal cord and, except for the last pair, leave the vertebral column above the correspondingly numbered vertebra. The ventral branches of the upper four, on either side, unite to form the cervical plexus, and those of the lower four, together with the ventral branch of the first thoracic nerve, form most of the brachial plexus.

ner'vi cilia'res bre'ves [NA], short ciliary nerves: *origin*, ciliary ganglion; *distribution*, smooth muscle and tunics of eye;

modality, parasympathetic, sympathetic, and general sensory.

ner'vi cilia'res lon'gi [NA], long ciliary nerves: *origin*, nasociliary nerve, from ophthalmic nerve; *distribution*, dilator pupillae, uvea, cornea; *modality*, sympathetic and general sensory.

ner'vi clu'nium inferio'res [NA], inferior clunial nerves: *origin*, posterior femoral cutaneous nerve; *distribution*, skin of lower part of buttock; *modality*, general sensory.

ner'vi clu'nium me'dii [NA], middle clunial nerves: *origin*, plexus formed by lateral branches of dorsal rami of first four sacral nerves behind the sacrum and coccyx; *distribution*, ligaments of sacrum and skin over posterior part of buttock; *modality*, general sensory.

ner'vi clu'nium superio'res [NA], superior clunial nerves: *origin*, lateral branches of dorsal rami of upper lumbar nerves; *distribution*, skin of upper part of buttock; upper gluteal region; *modality*, general sensory.

n. coccyg'eus [NA], coccygeal nerve: one of the pair of nerves that arise from the coccygeal segment of the spinal cord.

n. coch'leae, pars cochlearis nervi vestibulocochlearis.

n. cochlea'ris [NA], cochlear nerve: the part of the vestibulocochlear nerve concerned with hearing, consisting of fibers that arise from the bipolar cells in the spiral ganglion and have their receptors in the spiral organ of the cochlea. Called also *pars cochlearis nervi octavi* and *pars cochlearis nervi vestibulocochlearis*.

ner'vi crania'les [NA], cranial nerves: the twelve pairs of nerves that are connected with the brain, including the nervi olfactorii (I), and the opticus (II), oculomotorius (III), trochlearis (IV), trigeminus (V), abducens (VI), facialis (VII), vestibulocochlearis (VIII), glossopharyngeus (IX), vagus (X), accessorius (XI), and hypoglossus (XII). Called also *cerebral nerves, nervi cerebrales, encephalic nerves,* and *nervi encephalici* [NA alternative].

n. cuta'neus, cutaneous nerve.

n. cuta'neus antebra'chii latera'lis [NA], lateral cutaneous nerve of forearm: *origin*, continuation of musculocutaneous nerve; *distribution*, skin over radial side of forearm and sometimes an area of skin of dorsum of hand; *modality*, general sensory.

n. cuta'neus antebra'chii media'lis [NA], medial cutaneous nerve of forearm: *origin*, medial cord of brachial plexus (C8, T1); *branches*, anterior and ulnar; *distribution*, skin of front, medial, and posteromedial aspects of forearm; *modality*, general sensory.

n. cuta'neus antebra'chii poste'rior [NA], posterior cutaneous nerve of forearm: *origin*, radial nerve; *distribution*, skin of dorsal aspect of forearm; *modality*, general sensory.

n. cuta'neus antibra'chii dorsa'lis, n. cutaneous antebrachii posterior.

n. cuta'neus bra'chii latera'lis infe'rior [NA], inferior lateral cutaneous nerve of arm: *origin*, radial nerve; *distribution*, skin of lateral surface of lower part of arm; *modality*, general sensory.

n. cuta'neus bra'chii latera'lis supe'rior [NA], superior lateral cutaneous nerve of arm: *origin*, axillary nerve; *distribution*, skin of back of arm; *modality*, general sensory.

n. cuta'neus bra'chii media'lis [NA], medial cutaneous nerve of arm: *origin*, medial cord of brachial plexus (T1); *distribution*, skin on medial and posterior aspects of arm; *modality*, general sensory.

n. cuta'neus bra'chii poste'rior [NA], posterior cutaneous nerve of arm: *origin*, radial nerve in the axilla; *distribution*, skin on back of arm; *modality*, general sensory.

n. cuta'neus col'li, n. transversus colli.

n. cuta'neus dorsa'lis interme'dius [NA], intermediate dorsal cutaneous nerve: *origin*, superficial peroneal nerve; *branches*, dorsal digital nerves of foot; *distribution*, skin of front of lower third of leg and dorsum of foot, and skin and joints of adjacent sides of third and fourth, and of fourth and fifth toes; *modality*, general sensory.

n. cuta'neus dorsa'lis latera'lis pe'dis [NA], lateral dorsal cutaneous nerve: *origin*, continuation of sural nerve; *distribution*, skin and joints of lateral side of foot and fifth toe; *modality*, general sensory.

n. cuta'neus dorsa'lis media'lis [NA], medial dorsal cutaneous nerve: *origin*, superficial peroneal nerve; *distribution*, skin and joints of medial side of foot and big toe, and adjacent sides of second and third toes; *modality*, general sensory.

n. cuta'neus fem'oris latera'lis [NA], lateral cutaneous nerve of thigh: *origin*, lumbar plexus—L2–L3; *distribution*, skin of lateral and front aspects of thigh; *modality*, general sensory.

n. cuta′neus fem′oris poste′rior [NA], posterior cutaneous nerve of thigh: *origin*, sacral plexus—S1–S3; *branches*, inferior clunial nerves and perineal rami; *distribution*, skin of buttock, external genitalia, and back of thigh and calf; *modality*, general sensory.

n. cuta′neus su′rae latera′lis [NA], lateral cutaneous nerve of calf: *origin*, common fibular nerve; *distribution*, skin of lateral side of back of leg, rarely may continue as the sural nerve; *modality*, general sensory.

n. cuta′neus su′rae media′lis [NA], medial cutaneous nerve of calf: *origin*, tibial nerve; usually joins peroneal communicating branch of common peroneal nerve to form the sural nerve; *distribution*, may continue as the sural nerve; *modality*, general sensory.

ner′vi digita′les dorsa′les hal′lucis latera′lis et dig′iti secun′di media′lis [NA], dorsal digital nerves of lateral surface of great toe and of medial surface of second toe: *origin*, medial terminal division of deep peroneal nerve; *distribution*, skin and joints of adjacent sides of great and second toes; *modality*, general sensory.

ner′vi digita′les dorsa′les ner′vi radia′lis [NA], dorsal digital nerves of radial nerve: *origin*, superficial branch of radial nerve; *distribution*, skin and joints of back of thumb, index finger, and part of middle finger, as far distally as the distal phalanx; *modality*, general sensory.

ner′vi digita′les dorsa′les ner′vi ulna′ris [NA], dorsal digital nerves of ulnar nerve: *origin*, dorsal branch of ulnar nerve; *distribution*, skin and joints of medial side of little finger, dorsal aspects of adjacent sides of little and ring fingers and of ring and middle fingers; *modality*, general sensory.

ner′vi digita′les dorsa′les pe′dis [NA], dorsal digital nerves of foot: *origin*, intermediate dorsal cutaneous nerve; *distribution*, skin and joints of adjacent sides of third and fourth, and of fourth and fifth toes; *modality*, general sensory.

ner′vi digita′les palma′res commu′nes ner′vi media′ni [NA], common palmar digital nerves of median nerve: *number*, four; *origin*, lateral and medial divisions of median nerve; *branches*, proper palmar digital nerves; *distribution*, thumb, index, middle, and ring fingers, and first two lumbrical muscles—see individual branches, in this table; *modality*, motor and general sensory.

ner′vi digita′les palma′res commu′nes ner′vi ulna′ris [NA], common palmar digital nerves of ulnar nerve: *number*, two; *origin*, superficial branch of ulnar nerve; *branches*, proper palmar digital nerves; *distribution*, little and ring fingers—see individual branches, in this table; *modality*, general sensory.

ner′vi digita′les palma′res pro′prii ner′vi media′ni [NA], proper palmar digital nerves of median nerve: *origin*, common palmar digital nerves; *distribution*, first two lumbrical muscles, skin and joints of both sides and palmar aspect of thumb, index, and middle fingers, radial side of ring finger, and back of distal aspect of these digits; *modality*, general sensory and motor.

ner′vi digita′les palma′res pro′prii ner′vi ulna′ris [NA], proper palmar digital nerves of ulnar nerve: *origin*, the lateral of the two common palmar digital nerves from the superficial branch of the ulnar nerve; *distribution*, skin and joints of adjacent sides of fourth and fifth fingers; *modality*, general sensory.

ner′vi digita′les planta′res commu′nes ner′vi planta′ris latera′lis [NA], common plantar digital nerves of lateral plantar nerve: *number*, two; *origin*, superficial branch of lateral plantar nerve; *branches*, the medial nerve gives rise to two proper plantar digital nerves; *distribution*, the lateral one to the musculus flexor digiti minimi brevis pedis and to skin and joints of lateral side of sole and little toe; the medial one to adjacent sides of fourth and fifth toes—see individual branches, in this table; *modality*, motor and general sensory.

ner′vi encephal′ici, NA alternative for *nervi craniales*.

ner′vi digita′les planta′res commu′nes ner′vi planta′ris media′lis [NA], common plantar digital nerves of medial plantar nerve: *number*, four; *origin*, medial plantar nerve; *branches*, muscular and proper plantar digital nerves; *distribution*, flexor hallucis brevis muscle and first lumbrical muscles, skin and joints of medial side of foot and big toe, and adjacent sides of first and second, second and third, and third and fourth toes—see individual branches, in this table; *modality*, motor and general sensory.

ner′vi digita′les planta′res pro′prii ner′vi planta′ris latera′lis [NA], proper plantar digital nerves of lateral plantar nerve: *origin*, common plantar digital nerves; *distribution*, flexor digiti minimi brevis muscle, skin and joints of

lateral side of sole and little toe, and adjacent sides of fourth and fifth toes; *modality*, motor and general sensory.

ner′vi digita′les planta′res pro′prii ner′vi planta′ris media′lis [NA], proper plantar digital nerves of medial plantar nerve: *origin*, common plantar digital nerves; *distribution*, skin and joints of medial side of first toe, and adjacent sides of first and second, second and third, and third and fourth toes; the nerves extend to the dorsum to supply nail beds and tips of toes; *modality*, general sensory.

ner′vi digita′les vola′res commu′nes ner′vi media′ni, nervi digitales palmares communes nervi mediani.

ner′vi digita′les vola′res commu′nes ner′vi ulna′ris, nervi digitales palmares communes nervi ulnaris.

ner′vi digita′les vola′res pro′prii ner′vi media′ni, nervi digitales palmares proprii nervi mediani.

ner′vi digita′les vola′res pro′prii ner′vi ulna′ris, nervi digitales palmares proprii nervi ulnaris.

n. dorsa′lis clitor′idis [NA], dorsal nerve of clitoris: *origin*, pudendal nerve; *distribution*, transversus perinei profundus and sphincter urethrae muscles, corpus cavernosum clitoridis, and skin, prepuce, and glans of clitoris; *modality*, general sensory and motor.

n. dorsa′lis pe′nis [NA], dorsal nerve of penis: *origin*, pudendal nerve; *distribution*, transversus perinei profundus and sphincter urethrae muscles, corpus cavernosum penis, and skin, prepuce, and glans of penis; *modality*, general sensory and motor.

n. dorsa′lis scap′ulae [NA], dorsal nerve of scapula: *origin*, brachial plexus—ventral ramus of C5; *distribution*, rhomboid muscles and occasionally the levator scapulae muscle; *modality*, motor.

ner′vi encephal′ici, NA alternative for *nervi craniales*.

ner′vi erigen′tes, NA alternative for *nervi splanchnici pelvini*.

n. ethmoida′lis ante′rior [NA], anterior ethmoidal nerve: *origin*, continuation of nasociliary nerve, from ophthalmic nerve; *branches*, internal, external, lateral, and medial rami; *distribution*, mucosa of upper and anterior nasal septum, lateral wall of nasal cavity, skin of lower bridge and tip of nose; *modality*, general sensory.

n. ethmoida′lis poste′rior [NA], posterior ethmoidal nerve: *origin*, nasociliary nerve, from ophthalmic nerve; *distribution*, mucosa of posterior ethmoid cells and of sphenoidal sinus; *modality*, general sensory.

n. facia′lis [NA], facial nerve (7th cranial), consisting of two roots: a large motor root, which supplies the muscles of facial expression, and a smaller root, the nervus intermedius (q.v.). *Origin*, inferior border of pons, between olive and inferior cerebellar peduncle; *branches* (of motor root), stapedius and posterior auricular nerves, parotid plexus, digastric, temporal, zygomatic, buccal, lingual, marginal mandibular, and cervical rami, and a communicating ramus with the tympanic plexus; *distribution*—see individual branches, in this table and under *ramus*; *modality*, motor, parasympathetic, general sensory, special sensory. See also *n. intermediofacialis*.

n. femora′lis [NA], femoral nerve: *origin*, lumbar plexus—L2–L4; descending behind the inguinal ligament to the femoral triangle; *branches*, saphenous nerve, muscular and anterior cutaneous rami; *distribution*, the skin of the thigh and leg, the muscles of the front of the thigh, and the hip and knee joints—see individual branches, in this table and under *ramus*; *modality*, general sensory and motor.

n. fibula′ris commu′nis [NA], common fibular nerve: *origin*, sciatic nerve in lower part of thigh; *branches and distribution*, supplies short head of biceps femoris muscle (while still incorporated in sciatic nerve), gives off lateral sural cutaneous nerve and fibular communicating branch as it descends in popliteal fossa, supplies knee and superior tibiofibular joints and tibialis anterior muscle, and divides into superficial and deep fibular nerves; *modality*, general sensory and motor. Called also *n. peroneus communis* [NA alternative] or *common peroneal nerve*.

n. fibula′ris profun′dus [NA], deep fibular nerve: *origin*, a terminal branch of common fibular nerve; *branches and distribution*, winds around the neck of the fibula and descends on the interosseous membrane to the front of the ankle; muscular branches given off to the tibialis anterior, extensor hallucis longus, extensor digitorum longus, and third peroneal muscles, and a twig to the ankle joint; a lateral terminal division supplies the extensor digitorum brevis muscle and tarsal joints; the medial terminal division, or digital branch, divides into dorsal digital nerves for the skin and joints of the adjacent sides of the big and second toes; *modality*, general sensory and motor. Called also *n. peroneus profundus* [NA alternative] or *deep peroneal nerve.*

n. fibula′ris superficia′lis [NA], superficial fibular nerve: *origin,* a terminal branch of common fibular nerve; *branches and distribution,* descends in front of the fibula, supplies peroneus longus and brevis muscles and, in the lower part of the leg, divides into the muscular rami, medial and intermediate dorsal cutaneous nerves—see also individual branches, in this table and under *ramus; modality,* general sensory and motor. Called also *n. peroneus superficialis* [NA alternative] or *superficial peroneal nerve.*

n. fronta′lis [NA], frontal nerve: *origin,* ophthalmic division of trigeminal nerve; enters the orbit through the superior orbital fissure; *branches,* supraorbital and supratrochlear nerves; *distribution,* chiefly to the forehead and scalp—see individual branches, in this table; *modality,* general sensory.

n. genitofemora′lis [NA], genitofemoral nerve: *origin,* lumbar plexus—L1–L2; *branches,* genital and femoral rami; *distribution—* see individual branches, under *ramus; modality,* general sensory and motor.

n. glossopharyn′geus [NA], glossopharyngeal nerve (9th cranial): *origin,* several rootlets from lateral side of upper part of medulla oblongata, between the olive and the inferior cerebellar peduncle; *branches,* tympanic nerve, pharyngeal, stylopharyngeal, tonsillar, and lingual rami, ramus to the carotid sinus, and a ramus communicating with the auricular ramus of the vagus nerve; *distribution,* it has two enlargements (superior and inferior ganglia) and supplies the tongue, pharynx, and parotid gland—see individual branches, in this table and under *ramus; modality,* motor, parasympathetic, and general, special, and visceral sensory.

n. glu′teus infe′rior [NA], inferior gluteal nerve: *origin,* sacral plexus—L5–S2; *distribution,* gluteus maximus muscle; *modality,* motor.

n. glu′teus supe′rior [NA], superior gluteal nerve: *origin,* sacral plexus—L4–S1; *distribution,* gluteus medius and minimus muscles, tensor fasciae latae, and hip joint; *modality,* motor and general sensory.

ner′vi haemorrhoida′les inferio′res, nervi rectales inferiores.

ner′vi haemorrhoida′les me′dii, former term for branches of the middle rectal plexus.

ner′vi haemorrhoida′les superio′res, former term for branches of the superior rectal plexus.

n. hypogas′tricus [dex′ter/sinis′ter] [NA], hypogastric nerve: a nerve trunk situated on either side (right and left), interconnecting the superior and inferior hypogastric plexuses.

n. hypoglos′sus [NA], hypoglossal nerve (12th cranial): *origin,* several rootlets in the anterolateral sulcus between the olive and the pyramid of the medulla oblongata; it passes through the hypoglossal canal to the tongue; *branches,* lingual rami; *distribution,* styloglossus, hypoglossus, and genioglossus muscles and intrinsic muscles of the tongue; *modality,* motor.

n. iliohypogas′tricus [NA], iliohypogastric nerve: *origin,* lumbar plexus—L1 (sometimes T12); *branches,* lateral and anterior cutaneous rami; *distribution,* the skin above the pubis and over the lateral side of the buttock, and occasionally the pyramidalis; *modality,* motor and general sensory.

n. ilio-inguina′lis [NA], ilioinguinal nerve: *origin,* lumbar plexus—L1 (sometimes T12); accompanies the spermatic cord through the inguinal canal; *branches,* anterior scrotal or labial rami; *distribution,* skin of scrotum or labia majora, and adjacent part of thigh; *modality,* general sensory.

n. infraorbita′lis [NA], infraorbital nerve: *origin,* continuation of the maxillary nerve, entering the orbit through the inferior orbital fissure, and occupying in succession the infraorbital groove, canal, and foramen; *branches,* middle and anterior superior alveolar, inferior palpebral, internal and external nasal, and superior labial rami; *distribution—*see individual branches, under *ramus; modality,* general sensory.

n. infratrochlea′ris [NA], infratrochlear nerve: *origin,* nasociliary nerve from ophthalmic nerve; *branches,* palpebral rami; *distribution,* skin of root and upper bridge of nose and lower eyelid, conjunctiva, lacrimal duct; *modality,* general sensory.

ner′vi intercosta′les, NA alternative for rami ventrales nervorum thoracicorum.

ner′vi intercostobrachia′les [NA], intercostobrachial nerves: *origin,* second and third intercostal nerves; *distribution,* skin on back and medial aspect of arm; *modality,* general sensory.

n. intermediofacia′lis, NA alternative for the nervus facialis and the nervus intermedius considered together; so

called because they are two radices of the same cranial nerve and, even though they usually occur as separate trunks, they form a common trunk.

n. interme′dius [NA], intermediate nerve: the smaller root of the facial nerve, lying between the main root and the vestibulocochlear nerve; it joins the main root at, or merges with, the geniculate ganglion at the geniculum of the facial nerve; *branches,* chorda tympani and greater petrosal nerve; *distribution,* lacrimal, nasal, palatine, submandibular, and sublingual glands, and anterior two-thirds of tongue; *modality,* parasympathetic and special sensory. See also *n. intermediofacialis.*

n. interos′seus [antebra′chii] ante′rior [NA], anterior interosseous nerve of forearm: *origin,* median nerve; *distribution,* flexor pollicis longus, flexor digitorum profundus, and pronator quadratus muscles, wrist and intercarpal joints; *modality,* motor and general sensory.

n. interos′seus antebra′chii poste′rior [NA], posterior interosseous nerve of forearm: *origin,* continuation of deep branch of radial nerve; *distribution,* abductor pollicis longus, extensors of the thumb and second finger, and wrist and intercarpal joints; *modality,* motor and general sensory.

n. interos′seus [antebra′chii] dorsa′lis, n. interosseus antebrachii posterior.

n. interos′seus [antebra′chii] vola′ris, n. interosseus antebrachii anterior.

n. interos′seus cru′ris [NA], interosseous nerve of leg: *origin,* tibial nerve; *distribution,* interosseous membrane and tibiofibular syndesmosis; *modality,* general sensory.

n. ischiad′icus [NA], sciatic nerve, the largest nerve of the body: *origin,* sacral plexus—L4–S3; it leaves the pelvis through the greater sciatic foramen; *branches,* divides into the tibial and common peroneal nerves, usually in lower third of thigh; *distribution—*see individual branches, in this table; *modality,* general sensory and motor. Called also *n. sciaticus* [NA alternative].

n. jugula′ris [NA], jugular nerve: a branch of the superior cervical ganglion which communicates with the vagus and glossopharyngeal nerves.

ner′vi labia′les anterio′res [NA], anterior labial nerves: *origin,* ilioinguinal nerve; *distribution,* skin of anterior labial region of labia majora, and adjacent part of thigh; *modality,* general sensory.

ner′vi labia′les posterio′res [NA], posterior labial nerves: *origin,* pudendal nerve; *distribution,* labium majus; *modality,* general sensory.

n. lacrima′lis [NA], lacrimal nerve: *origin,* ophthalmic division of trigeminal nerve, entering the orbit through the superior orbital fissure; *distribution,* lacrimal gland, conjunctiva, lateral commissure of eye, and skin of upper eyelid; *modality,* general sensory.

n. laryn′geus infe′rior [NA], inferior laryngeal nerve: *origin,* recurrent laryngeal nerve, especially the terminal portion of this nerve; *distribution,* intrinsic muscles of larynx, except cricothyroid; communicates with the internal laryngeal nerve; *modality,* motor.

n. laryn′geus recur′rens [NA], recurrent laryngeal nerve: *origin,* vagus nerve (chiefly the cranial part of the accessory nerve); *branches,* inferior laryngeal nerve and tracheal, esophageal, and inferior cardiac rami; *distribution—*see individual branches, in this table and under *ramus; modality,* parasympathetic, visceral afferent, and motor.

n. laryn′geus supe′rior [NA], superior laryngeal nerve: *origin,* inferior ganglion of vagus nerve; *branches,* external, internal, and communicating rami; *distribution,* inferior constrictor of the pharynx, cricothyroid muscle, and mucous membrane of back of tongue and larynx—see individual branches, under *ramus; modality,* motor, general sensory, visceral afferent, and parasympathetic.

n. lingua′lis [NA], lingual nerve: *origin,* mandibular nerve, descending to the tongue, first medial to the mandible and then under cover of the mucous membrane of the mouth; *branches,* sublingual nerve, lingual ramus, ramus to the isthmus of the fauces, and rami communicating with the hypoglossal nerve and chorda tympani; *distribution—*see individual branches, in this table and under *ramus; modality,* general sensory.

ner′vi lumba′les [NA], lumbar nerves: the five pairs of nerves that arise from the lumbar segments of the spinal cord, each pair leaving the vertebral column below the correspondingly numbered vertebra. The ventral branches of these nerves participate in the formation of the lumbosacral plexus. Called also *nervi lumbares* [NA alternative].

ner′vi lumba′res, NA alternative for *nervi lumbales.*

n. lumboinguina′lis, ramus femoralis nervi genitofemoralis.

n. mandibula′ris [NA], mandibular nerve, one of three terminal divisions of the trigeminal nerve, passing through the foramen ovale to the infratemporal fossa. *Origin,* trigeminal ganglion; *branches,* meningeal ramus, masseteric, deep temporal, lateral and medial pterygoid, buccal, auriculotemporal, lingual, and inferior alveolar nerves; *distribution,* extensive distribution to muscles of mastication, skin of face, mucous membrane of mouth, and teeth— see individual branches, in this table and under *ramus; modality,* general sensory and motor.

n. masseter′icus [NA], masseteric nerve: *origin,* mandibular division of trigeminal nerve; *distribution,* masseter muscle and temporomandibular joint; *modality,* motor and general sensory.

n. masticato′rius, former term for radix motoria nervi trigemini.

n. maxilla′ris [NA], maxillary nerve, one of the three terminal divisions of the trigeminal nerve, passing through the foramen rotundum, and entering the pterygopalatine fossa. *Origin,* trigeminal ganglion; *branches,* meningeal ramus, zygomatic nerve, posterior superior alveolar rami, infraorbital nerve, pterygopalatine nerves, and, indirectly, the branches of the pterygopalatine ganglion; *distribution,* extensive distribution to skin of face and scalp, mucous membrane of maxillary sinus and nasal cavity, and teeth—see individual branches, in this table and under *ramus; modality,* general sensory.

n. mea′tus acus′tici exter′ni [NA], nerve of external acoustic meatus: *origin,* auriculotemporal nerve; *distribution,* skin lining external acoustic meatus, and tympanic membrane; *modality,* general sensory.

n. mea′tus audito′rii exter′ni, n. meatus acustici externi.

n. media′nus [NA], median nerve: *origin,* lateral and medial cords of brachial plexus—C6–T1; *branches,* anterior interosseous nerve of forearm, common palmar digital nerves, and muscular and palmar rami, and a communicating branch with the ulnar nerve; *distribution,* ultimately, skin on front of lateral part of hand, most of flexor muscles of front of forearm, most of short muscles of thumb, and elbow joint and many joints of hand—see individual branches, in this table and under *ramus; modality,* general sensory.

n. menin′geus me′dius, ramus meningeus medius nervi maxillaris.

n. menta′lis [NA], mental nerve: *origin,* inferior alveolar nerve; *branches,* mental and inferior labial rami; *distribution,* skin of chin, and lower lip; *modality,* general sensory.

n. mix′tus [NA], mixed nerve: a nerve composed of both sensory (afferent) and motor (efferent) fibers.

n. moto′rius [NA], motor nerve: a peripheral efferent nerve that stimulates muscle contraction.

n. musculi quadra′ti fem′oris [NA], nerve of quadrate muscle of thigh: *origin,* ventral branches of ventral rami of L4–L5; *distribution,* gemellus inferior, anterior quadratus femoris muscle, hip joint; *modality,* general sensory and motor. Called also *n. quadratus femoris.*

n. mus′culi tenso′ris tym′pani [NA], nerve of tensor tympani muscle: *origin,* mandibular nerve via nerve to medial pterygoid muscle and otic ganglion; *distribution,* tensor tympani muscle; *modality,* motor. Called also *nerve of tensor tympani* and *n. tensoris tympani.*

n. mus′culi tenso′ris ve′li palati′ni [NA], nerve of tensor veli palatini muscle: *origin,* mandibular nerve via nerve to medial pterygoid muscle and otic ganglion; *distribution,* tensor veli palatini muscle; *modality,* motor. Called also *nerve of tensor veli palatini* and *n. tensoris veli palatini.*

n. musculocuta′neus [NA], musculocutaneous nerve: *origin,* lateral cord of brachial plexus—C5–C7; *branches,* lateral cutaneous nerve of forearm, and muscular rami; *distribution,* coracobrachialis, biceps, brachialis muscles, the elbow joint, and skin of radial side of forearm; *modality,* general sensory and motor.

n. mylohyoi′deus [NA], mylohyoid nerve: *origin,* inferior alveolar nerve; *distribution,* mylohyoid muscle, anterior belly of digastric muscle; *modality,* motor.

n. nasocilia′ris [NA], nasociliary nerve: *origin,* ophthalmic division of trigeminal nerve; *branches,* long ciliary, posterior ethmoidal, anterior ethmoidal, and infratrochlear nerves, and a communicating branch to the ciliary ganglion; *distribution*—see individual branches, in this table; *modality,* general sensory.

n. nasopalati′nus [NA], nasopalatine nerve: *origin,* pterygopalatine ganglion; *distribution,* mucosa and glands of most of nasal septum and anterior part of hard palate; *modality,* parasympathetic and general sensory.

n. obturato′rius [NA], obturator nerve: *origin,* lumbar plexus—L3–L4; *branches,* anterior, posterior, and muscular rami; *distribution,* adductor muscles and gracilis muscle, skin of medial part of thigh, and hip and knee joints—see individual branches, under *ramus; modality,* general sensory and motor.

n. obturato′rius accesso′rius [NA], accessory obturator nerve: *origin,* ventral branches of ventral rami of L3–L4; *distribution,* pectineus muscle, hip joint, obturator nerve; *modality,* general sensory and motor.

n. obturato′rius inter′nus [NA], internal obturator nerve: *origin,* ventral branches of ventral rami of L5, S1–S2; *distribution,* posterior gemellus superior, obturator internus muscle; *modality,* general sensory and motor.

n. occipita′lis ma′jor [NA], greater occipital nerve: *origin,* medial branch of dorsal ramus of C2; *distribution,* semispinalis capitis muscle and skin of scalp as far forward as the vertex; *modality,* general sensory and motor.

n. occipita′lis mi′nor [NA], lesser occipital nerve: *origin,* superficial cervical plexus—C2–C3; *distribution,* ascends behind the auricle and supplies some of the skin on the side of the head and on the cranial surface of the auricle; *modality,* general sensory.

n. occipita′lis ter′tius [NA], third occipital nerve: *origin,* medial branch of dorsal ramus of C3; *distribution,* skin of upper part of back of neck and head; *modality,* general sensory.

n. octa′vus [L. "eighth nerve"], n. vestibulocochlearis.

n. oculomoto′rius [NA], oculomotor nerve (3rd cranial): *origin,* brain stem, emerging medial to cerebral peduncles and running forward in the cavernous sinus; *branches,* superior and inferior rami; *distribution,* entering the orbit through the superior orbital fissure, the branches supply the levator palpebrae superioris, all extrinsic eye muscles except the lateral rectus and superior oblique, and carry parasympathetic fibers for the ciliary muscle and sphincter pupillae; *modality,* motor and parasympathetic.

ner′vi olfacto′rii [NA], olfactory nerves (1st cranial): the nerves of smell, consisting of about 20 bundles which arise in the olfactory epithelium and pass through the cribriform plate of the ethmoid bone to the olfactory bulb.

n. ophthal′micus [NA], ophthalmic nerve, one of the three terminal divisions of the trigeminal nerve. *Origin,* trigeminal ganglion; *branches,* tentorial rami, frontal, lacrimal, and nasociliary nerves; *distribution,* eyeball and conjunctiva, lacrimal gland and sac, nasal mucosa and frontal sinus, external nose, upper eyelid, forehead, and scalp—see individual branches, in this table and under *ramus; modality,* general sensory.

n. op′ticus [NA], optic nerve (2nd cranial): the nerve of sight, consisting chiefly of axons and central processes of cells of the ganglionic layer of the retina, which leave the orbit through the optic canal, join the optic chiasm (the medial ones crossing over to the opposite side), and continue as the optic tract.

ner′vi palati′ni, see *n. palatinus major* and *nervi palatini minores.*

n. palati′nus ante′rior, n. palatinus major.

n. palati′nus ma′jor [NA], greater palatine nerve: *origin,* pterygopalatine ganglion; *branches,* posterior inferior [lateral] nasal branches; *distribution,* emerges through the greater palatine foramen and supplies the palate; *modality,* parasympathetic, sympathetic, and general sensory.

n. palati′nus me′dius, see *nervi palatini minores.*

ner′vi palati′ni mino′res [NA], lesser palatine nerves: *origin,* pterygopalatine ganglion; *distribution,* emerge through the lesser palatine foramen and supply the soft palate and tonsil; *modality,* parasympathetic, sympathetic, and general sensory.

n. palati′nus poste′rior, see *nervi palatini minores.*

n. pectora′lis latera′lis [NA], lateral pectoral nerve: *origin,* lateral cord of brachial plexus or anterior divisions of upper and middle trunks (C5–C7); *distribution,* usually several nerves supplying the musculus pectoralis minor and acromioclavicular and shoulder joints; *modality,* motor and general sensory.

n. pectora′lis media′lis [NA], medial pectoral nerve: *origin,* medial cord or lower trunk of brachial plexus (C8, T1); *distribution,* usually several nerves supplying the musculus pectoralis major and pectoralis minor; *modality,* motor.

ner′vi perinea′les [NA], perineal nerves: *origin,* pudendal nerve in the pudendal canal; *branches,* muscular branches and posterior scrotal or labial nerves; *distribution,* muscular branches supply the bulbospongiosus, ischiocavernosus, superficial transversus perinei muscles and bulb of the penis and, in part, the sphincter ani externus and levator ani; the scrotal (labial) nerves supply the scrotum or labium majus; *modality,* general sensory and motor.

ner'vi perine'i, nervi perineales.

n. perone'us commu'nis, NA alternative for *n. fibularis communis.*

n. perone'us profun'dus, NA alternative for *n. fibularis profundus.*

n. perone'us profun'dus accesso'rius, the accessory deep peroneal nerve: the branch of the superficial peroneal nerve to the musculus peroneus brevis, often prolonged to the lateral malleolus and ending in twigs to the musculus extensor digitorum brevis and adjacent joints.

n. perone'us superficia'lis, NA alternative for *n. fibularis superficialis.*

n. petro'sus ma'jor [NA], greater petrosal nerve: *origin,* intermediate nerve via geniculate ganglion; *distribution,* running forward from the geniculate ganglion, it joins the deep petrosal nerve of the pterygoid canal, and reaches lacrimal, nasal, and palatine glands and nasopharynx, via pterygopalatine ganglion and its branches; *modality,* parasympathetic and general sensory.

n. petro'sus mi'nor [NA], lesser petrosal nerve: *origin,* tympanic plexus; *distribution,* parotid gland via otic ganglion and auriculotemporal nerve; *modality,* parasympathetic.

n. petro'sus profun'dus [NA], deep petrosal nerve: *origin,* internal carotid plexus; *distribution,* joins greater petrosal nerve to form nerve of pterygoid canal, and supplies lacrimal, nasal, and palatine glands via pterygopalatine ganglion and its branches; *modality,* sympathetic.

n. petro'sus superficia'lis ma'jor, n. petrosus major.

n. petro'sus superficia'lis mi'nor, n. petrosus minor.

n. phren'icus [NA], phrenic nerve: *origin,* cervical plexus—C4–C5; *branches,* pericardiac and phrenicoabdominal rami; *distribution,* pleura, pericardium, diaphragm, peritoneum, and sympathetic plexuses; *modality,* general sensory and motor.

ner'vi phren'ici accesso'rii [NA], accessory phrenic nerves: an inconstant contribution of the fifth cervical nerve to the phrenic nerve; when present, they run a separate course to the root of the neck or into the thorax before joining the phrenic nerve.

n. pirifor'mis [NA], piriform nerve: *origin,* dorsal branches of ventral rami of S1–S2; *distribution,* anterior piriform muscle; *modality,* general sensory and motor.

n. planta'ris latera'lis [NA], lateral plantar nerve: *origin,* the smaller of terminal branches of tibial nerve; *branches,* muscular, superficial, and deep rami; *distribution,* lying between first and second layers of muscles of sole, it supplies the quadratus plantae, abductor digiti minimi, flexor digiti minimi brevis, adductor hallucis, interossei, and second, third, and fourth lumbrical muscles, and gives off cutaneous and articular twigs to lateral side of sole and fourth and fifth toes—see individual branches, under *ramus; modality,* general sensory and motor.

n. planta'ris media'lis [NA], medial plantar nerve: *origin,* the larger of the terminal branches of tibial nerve; *branches,* common plantar digital nerves and muscular rami; *distribution,* abductor hallucis, flexor digitorum brevis, flexor hallucis brevis, and first lumbrical muscles, and cutaneous and articular twigs to the medial side of the sole, and to the first to fourth toes—see individual branches, in this table and under *ramus; modality,* general sensory and motor.

n. presacra'lis, NA alternative for *plexus hypogastricus superior.*

n. pterygoi'deus exter'nus, n. pterygoideus lateralis.

n. pterygoi'deus inter'nus, n. pterygoideus medialis.

n. pterygoi'deus latera'lis [NA], lateral pterygoid nerve: *origin,* mandibular nerve; *distribution,* lateral pterygoid muscle; *modality,* motor.

n. pterygoi'deus media'lis [NA], medial pterygoid nerve: *origin,* mandibular nerve; *distribution,* medial pterygoid, tensor tympani, and tensor veli palatini muscles; *modality,* motor.

ner'vi pterygopalati'ni [NA], pterygopalatine nerves: the two nerves which connect the maxillary nerve to the pterygopalatine ganglion; they are the sensory roots of the ganglion.

n. puden'dus [NA], pudendal nerve: *origin,* sacral plexus— S2–S4; *branches,* enters the pudendal canal, gives off

the inferior rectal nerve, and then divides into the perineal nerve and dorsal nerve of the penis (clitoris); *distribution,* muscles, skin, and erectile tissue of perineum—see individual branches; *modality,* general sensory, motor, and parasympathetic. Called also *pudic nerve.*

n. quadra'tus fem'oris n. musculi quadrati femoris.

n. radia'lis [NA], radial nerve: *origin,* posterior cord of brachial plexus—C6–C8, and sometimes C5 and T1; *branches,* posterior cutaneous and inferior lateral cutaneous nerves of arm, posterior cutaneous nerve of forearm, muscular, deep, and superficial rami; *distribution,* descending in the back of arm and forearm, it is ultimately distributed to skin on back of arm, forearm, and hand, extensor muscles on back of arm and forearm, and elbow joint and many joints of hand—see individual branches, in this table and under *ramus; modality,* general sensory and motor.

n. et ra'mus articula'res [NA], any mixed (afferent or efferent) peripheral nerve or any of its branches that supply a joint and its associated structures.

n. et ra'mus autono'mici [NA], any of the parasympathetic and sympathetic nerves and nerve branches of the autonomic nervous system. Called also *n. et ramus viscerales* [NA alternative].

n. et ra'mus cuta'nei [NA], any mixed (afferent or efferent) peripheral nerve or any of its branches that innervate a region of the skin.

n. et ra'mus muscula'res [NA], any mixed (afferent or efferent) peripheral nerve or any of its branches that supply a muscle and its associated structures.

n. et ra'mus viscera'les, NA alternative for *n. et ramus autonomici.*

ner'vi recta'les inferio'res [NA], inferior rectal nerves: *origin,* pudendal nerve, or independently from sacral plexus; *distribution,* sphincter ani externus muscle, skin around anus, and lining of anal canal up to pectinate line; *modality,* general sensory and motor. Called also *inferior anal nerves* and *nervi anales inferiores.*

n. recur'rens, n. laryngeus recurrens.

n. saccula'ris [NA], saccular nerve: the branch of the pars vestibularis nervi octavi that innervates the macula of the saccule.

ner'vi sacra'les [NA], sacral nerves: the five pairs of nerves that arise from the sacral segments of the spinal cord; the ventral branches of the first four pairs participate in the formation of the sacral plexus.

n. saphe'nus [NA], saphenous nerve: *origin,* termination of femoral nerve, descending first with femoral vessels and then on medial side of leg and foot; *branches,* infrapatellar and medial crural cutaneous rami; *distribution,* knee joint, subsartorial and patellar plexuses, skin on medial side of leg and foot—see individual branches, under *ramus; modality,* general sensory.

ner'vi scrota'les anterio'res [NA], anterior scrotal nerves: *origin,* ilioinguinal nerve; *distribution,* skin of anterior scrotal region; *modality,* general sensory.

ner'vi scrota'les posterio'res [NA], posterior scrotal nerves: *origin,* perineal nerves; *distribution,* skin of scrotum; *modality,* general sensory.

n. sensoria'lis, n. sensorius.

n. senso'rius [NA], sensory nerve: a peripheral afferent nerve that conducts impulses from a sense organ to the spinal cord or brain; called also *n. sensorialis.*

n. spermat'icus exter'nus, ramus genitalis nervi genitofemoralis.

ner'vi sphenopalati'ni, nervi pterygopalatini.

ner'vi spina'les [NA], spinal nerves: the thirty-one pairs of nerves that arise from the spinal cord and pass out between the vertebrae, including the eight pairs of cervical, twelve of thoracic, five of lumbar, five of sacral, and one pair of coccygeal nerves.

n. spino'sus, former term for ramus meningeus nervi mandibularis.

n. splanch'nicus i'mus, n. splanchnicus thoracicus imus.

ner'vi splanch'nici lumba'les [NA], lumbar splanchnic nerves: *origin,* lumbar ganglia or sympathetic trunk; *distribution,* upper nerves join celiac and adjacent plexuses, middle ones go to intermesenteric and adjacent plexuses, and lower ones descend to superior hypogastric plexus; *modality,* preganglionic sympathetic and visceral afferent. Called also *n. splanchnici lumbares* [NA alternative].

n. splanch'nici lumba'res, NA alternative for *n. splanchnici lumbales.*

n. splanch'nicus ma'jor, n. splanchnicus thoracicus major.

n. splanch'nicus mi'nor, n. splanchnicus thoracicus minor.

ner'vi splanch'nici pelvi'ni [NA], pelvic splanchnic nerves: *origin,* sacral plexus—S3–S4; *distribution,* leaving the sacral plexus, they enter the inferior hypogastric plexus and supply the pelvic organs; *modality,* preganglionic parasympathetic and visceral afferent. Called also *nervi erigentes* [NA alternative].

ner'vi splanch'nici sacra'les [NA], sacral splanchnic nerves: *origin,* sacral part of sympathetic trunk; *distribution,* pelvic organs and blood vessels via inferior hypogastric plexus; *modality,* preganglionic sympathetic and visceral afferent.

n. splanch'nicus thora'cicus i'mus [NA] lowest thoracic splanchnic nerve: *origin,* last ganglion of sympathetic trunk or lesser splanchnic nerve; *distribution,* aorticorenal ganglion and adjacent plexus; *modality,* sympathetic and visceral afferent. Called also *lowest splanchnic nerve* and *n. splanchnicus imus.*

n. splanch'nicus thora'cicus ma'jor [NA], greater thoracic splanchnic nerve: *origin,* thoracic sympathetic trunk and fifth through tenth thoracic ganglia; *distribution,* descending through the diaphragm or its aortic openings ends in celiac ganglia and plexuses, with a splanchnic ganglion commonly occurring near the diaphragm; *modality,* preganglionic sympathetic and visceral afferent. Called also *greater splanchnic nerve* and *n. splanchnicus major.*

n. splanch'nicus thora'cicus mi'nor [NA], lesser thoracic splanchnic nerve: *origin,* ninth and tenth thoracic ganglia of sympathetic trunk; *branches,* renal ramus; *distribution,* pierces the diaphragm, joins the aorticorenal ganglion and celiac plexus, and communicates with the renal and superior mesenteric plexuses; *modality,* preganglionic sympathetic and visceral afferent. Called also *lesser splanchnic nerve* and *n. splanchnicus minor.*

n. stape'dius [NA], stapedius nerve: *origin,* facial nerve; *distribution,* stapedius muscle; *modality,* motor.

n. subcla'vius [NA], subclavian nerve: *origin,* upper trunk of brachial plexus—C5; *distribution,* subclavius muscle and sternoclavicular joint; *modality,* motor and general sensory.

n. subcosta'lis [NA], subcostal nerve: *origin,* ventral ramus of twelfth thoracic nerve; *distribution,* skin of lower abdomen and lateral side of gluteal region, parts of transversus, oblique, and rectus muscles, and usually the pyramidalis muscle, and adjacent peritoneum; *modality,* general sensory and motor.

n. sublingua'lis [NA], sublingual nerve: *origin,* lingual nerve; *distribution,* sublingual gland and overlying mucous membrane; *modality,* parasympathetic and general sensory.

n. suboccipita'lis [NA], suboccipital nerve: *origin,* dorsal ramus of first cervical nerve; *distribution,* emerges above posterior arch of atlas and supplies muscles of suboccipital triangle and semispinalis capitis muscle; *modality,* motor.

n. subscapula'ris [NA], subscapular nerve: *origin,* posterior cord of brachial plexus—C5; *distribution,* usually two or more nerves, upper and lower, supplying subscapularis and teres major muscles; *modality,* motor.

ner'vi supraclavicula'res [NA], supraclavicular nerves: a term denoting collectively the common trunk, which is a branch of the cervical plexus (C3–C4) and which emerges under cover of the posterior border of the sternocleidomastoid muscle and divides into the nervi supraclaviculares intermedii, nervi supraclaviculares laterales, and nervi supraclaviculares mediales.

ner'vi supraclavicula'res anterio'res, nervi supraclaviculares mediales.

ner'vi supraclavicula'res interme'dii [NA], intermediate supraclavicular nerves: *origin,* cervical plexus—C3–C4; *distribution,* descends in the posterior triangle, crosses the clavicle, and supplies the skin over pectoral and deltoid region; *modality,* general sensory.

ner'vi supraclavicula'res latera'les [posterio'res] [NA], lateral supraclavicular nerves: *origin,* cervical plexus—C3–C4; *distribution,* descends in the posterior triangle, crosses the clavicle, and supplies the skin of superior and posterior parts of shoulder; *modality,* general sensory. Called also *nervi supraclaviculares posteriores* [NA alternative].

ner'vi supraclavicula'res media'les [NA], medial supraclavicular nerves: *origin,* cervical plexus—C3–C4; *distribution,* descends in posterior triangle, crosses the clavicle, and supplies the skin of medial infraclavicular region; *modality,* general sensory.

ner'vi supraclavicula'res me'dii, nervi supraclaviculares intermedii.

ner'vi supraclavicula'res posterio'res, NA alternative for *nervi supraclaviculares laterales.*

n. supraorbita'lis [NA], supraorbital nerve: *origin,* continuation of frontal nerve, from ophthalmic nerve; *branches,* lateral and medial rami; *distribution,* leaves orbit through supraorbital notch or foramen, and supplies the skin of upper eyelid, forehead, anterior scalp (to vertex), mucosa of frontal sinus; *modality,* general sensory.

n. suprascapula'ris [NA], suprascapular nerve: *origin,* brachial plexus—C5–C6; *distribution,* descends through suprascapular and spinoglenoid notches and supplies acromioclavicular and shoulder joints, and supraspinatus and infraspinatus muscles; *modality,* motor and general sensory.

n. supratrochlea'ris [NA], supratrochlear nerve: *origin,* frontal nerve, from ophthalmic nerve; *distribution,* leaves orbit at medial end of supraorbital margin and supplies the forehead and upper eyelid; *modality,* general sensory.

n. sura'lis [NA], sural nerve: *origin,* medial sural cutaneous nerve and peroneal communicating branch of common peroneal nerve; *branches,* lateral dorsal cutaneous nerve and lateral calcaneal rami; *distribution,* skin on back of leg, and skin and joints on lateral side of heel and foot—see individual branches, in this table and under *ramus; modality,* general sensory.

ner'vi tempora'les profun'di [NA], deep temporal nerves, usually two in number, anterior and posterior: *origin,* mandibular nerve; *distribution,* temporal muscles; *modality,* motor.

n. tempora'lis profun'dus ante'rior, the anterior of the two deep temporal nerves.

n. tempora'lis profun'dus poste'rior, the posterior of the two temporal nerves.

n. tenso'ris tym'pani, n. musculi tensoris tympani.

n. tenso'ris ve'li palati'ni, n. musculi tensoris veli palatini.

n. tento'rii, ramus tentorii nervi ophthalmici.

ner'vi termina'les [NA], terminal nerves: nerve filaments, collectively termed the nervus terminalis, found in the pia mater between the olfactory bulb and the crista galli, and passing through the cribriform plate to the nasal mucosa; ganglion cells occur along their course.

ner'vi thoraca'les, nervi thoracici.

n. thoraca'lis lon'gus, n. thoracicus longus.

ner'vi thora'cici [NA], thoracic nerves: the twelve pairs of spinal nerves that arise from the thoracic segments of the spinal cord, each pair leaving the vertebral column below the correspondingly numbered vertebra. They innervate the body wall of the thorax and upper abdomen.

n. thora'cicus lon'gus [NA], long thoracic nerve: *origin,* brachial plexus—ventral rami of C5–C7; *distribution,* descends behind brachial plexus to serratus anterior muscle; *modality,* motor.

n. thoracodorsa'lis [NA], thoracodorsal nerve: *origin,* posterior cord of brachial plexus—C7–C8; *distribution,* latissimus dorsi muscle; *modality,* motor.

n. tibia'lis [NA], tibial nerve: *origin,* sciatic nerve in lower part of thigh; *branches,* interosseous nerve of leg, medial cutaneous nerve of calf, sural, and medial and lateral plantar nerves, and muscular and medial calcaneal rami; *distribution,* while still incorporated in the sciatic nerve, it supplies the semimembranosus and semitendinosus muscles, long head of biceps, and adductor magnus muscle; it supplies the knee joint as it descends in the popliteal fossa and, continuing into the leg, supplies the muscles and skin of the calf and sole of the foot, and the toes—see individual branches, in this table and under *ramus; modality,* general sensory and motor.

n. transver'sus col'li [NA], transverse nerve of neck: *origin,* cervical plexus—C2–C3; *branches,* superior and inferior rami; *distribution,* skin on side and front of neck; *modality,* general sensory.

n. trigem'inus [NA], trigeminal nerve (5th cranial), which emerges from the lateral surface of the pons as a motor and a sensory root, together with some intermediate fibers. The sensory root expands into the trigeminal ganglion, which contains the cells of origin of most of the sensory fibers, and from which the three divisions of the nerve arise. See *n. mandibularis, n. maxillaris,* and *n. ophthalmicus.* The trigeminal nerve is sensory in supplying the face, teeth, mouth, and nasal cavity, and motor in supplying the muscles of mastication.

n. trochlea'ris [NA], trochlear nerve (4th cranial): *origin,* the fibers of each trochlear nerve (one on either side) decussate across the median plane and emerge from the back of the brain stem below the corresponding inferior colliculus; *distribution*, runs forward in lateral wall of cavernous sinus, traverses the superior orbital fissure, and supplies superior oblique muscle of eyeball; *modality*, motor.

n. tympan′icus [NA], tympanic nerve: *origin*, inferior ganglion of glossopharyngeal nerve; *branches*, helps form tympanic plexus; *distribution*, mucous membrane of tympanic cavity, mastoid air cells, auditory tube, and, via lesser petrosal nerve and otic ganglion, the parotid gland; *modality*, general sensory and parasympathetic.

n. ulna′ris [NA], ulnar nerve: *origin*, medial and lateral cords of brachial plexus—C7–T1; *branches*, muscular, dorsal, palmar, superficial, and deep rami; *distribution*, ultimately to skin on front and back of medial part of hand, some flexor muscles on front of forearm, many short muscles of hand, elbow joint, many joints of hand—see individual branches, under *ramus*; *modality*, general sensory and motor.

n. utricula′ris [NA], utricular nerve: the branch of the vestibular nerve that innervates the macula of the utricle.

n. utriculoampulla′ris [NA], utriculoampullar nerve: a nerve that arises by peripheral division of the vestibular nerve, and supplies the utricle and ampullae of the semicircular ducts.

ner′vi vagina′les [NA], vaginal nerves: *origin*, uterovaginal plexus; *distribution*, vagina; *modality*, sympathetic and parasympathetic.

n. va′gus [NA], vagus nerve (10th cranial): *origin*, by numerous rootlets from lateral side of medulla oblongata in the groove between the olive and the inferior cerebellar peduncle; *branches*, superior and recurrent laryngeal nerves, meningeal, auricular, pharyngeal, cardiac, bronchial, gastric, hepatic, celiac, and renal rami, pharyngeal, pulmonary, and esophageal plexuses, and anterior and posterior trunks; *distribution*, descending through the jugular foramen, it presents a superior and an inferior ganglion, and continues through the neck and thorax into the abdomen. It supplies sensory fibers to the ear, tongue, pharynx, and larynx, motor fibers to the pharynx, larynx, and esophagus, and parasympathetic and visceral afferent fibers to thoracic and abdominal viscera—see individual branches, in this table and under *ramus*; *modality*, para-

sympathetic, visceral afferent, motor, general sensory.

ner′vi vaso′rum [NA], nerves of veins: the nerve branches that supply the adventitia of the blood vessels.

n. vertebra′lis [NA], vertebral nerve: *origin*, cervicothoracic and vertebral ganglia; *distribution*, ascends with vertebral artery and gives fibers to spinal meninges, cervical nerves, and posterior cranial fossa; *modality*, sympathetic.

ner′vi vesica′les inferio′res plex′us puden′di, former term for a few small nerves to the bladder, thought to arise from the pudendal plexus (pudendal nerve).

ner′vi vesica′les inferio′res plex′us vesica′lis, former term for the nerves reaching the vesical plexus by way of the inferior vesical artery.

ner′vi vesica′les superio′res plex′us vesica′lis, former term for the nerves reaching the vesical plexus by way of the superior vesical artery.

n. vestibula′ris [NA], vestibular nerve: the posterior part of the vestibulocochlear nerve, which is concerned with equilibration. It consists of fibers arising from bipolar cells in the vestibular ganglion, and divides peripherally into a rostral and a caudal part, with receptors in the ampullae of the semicircular canals, the utricle, and the saccule. Called also *pars vestibularis nervi octavi* and *pars vestibularis nervi vestibulocochlearis*.

n. vestibulocochlea′ris [NA], vestibulocochlear nerve (8th cranial), which emerges from the brain between the pons and the medulla oblongata, at the cerebellopontine angle and behind the facial nerve. It divides near the lateral end of the internal acoustic meatus into two functionally distinct and incompletely united components, the vestibular nerve and the cochlear nerve, and is connected with the brain by corresponding roots, the vestibular and the cochlear roots. Called also *n. acusticus*, *n. octavus*, and *acoustic nerve*.

n. zygomat′icus [NA], zygomatic nerve: *origin*, maxillary nerve, entering the orbit through the inferior orbital fissure; *branches*, zygomaticofacial and zygomaticotemporal rami; *distribution*, communicates with the lacrimal nerve and supplies the skin of the temple and adjacent part of the face—see individual branches, under *ramus*; *modality*, general sensory.

Nesacaine (nes′ah-kān) trademark for preparations of chloroprocaine hydrochloride.

nesidiectomy (ne-sid″e-ek′to-me) [Gr. *nēsidion* islet + *ektomē* excision] excision of the pancreatic islets.

nesidioblast (ne-sid′e-o-blast″) [Gr. *nēsidion* islet + *blastos* germ] any one of the cells that build up the islet cells of the pancreas.

nesidioblastoma (ne-sid″e-o-blas-to′mah) an islet-cell tumor of the pancreas.

nesidioblastosis (ne-sid″e-o-blas-to′sis) diffuse proliferation of the islet cells of the pancreas.

Nessler's reagent (solution, test) (nes′lerz) [A. *Nessler*, German chemist, 1827–1905] see under *reagent*.

nesslerization (nes″ler-i-za′shun) treatment with Nessler's reagent.

nesslerize (nes′ler-īz) to treat with Nessler's reagent.

nest (nest) a small mass of cells foreign to the area in which it is found. **birds′ n's,** endocardial pockets. **Brunn's epithelial n's,** solid or branched clusters of cells occurring in the healthy ureter. **cancer n's,** masses of concentrically arranged cells seen in cancerous growths. **cell n.,** a mass of closely packed epithelial cells surrounded by a stroma of connective tissue. **swallow's n.,** nidus avis.

net (net) a meshlike structure of interlocking fibers or strands; see also under *network*. **achromatic n.,** the network within the cell which does not stain with dyes. **chromidial n.,** a network of chromatin staining material in the cytoplasm of certain cells; it has the properties of active nuclear material. **nerve n.,** a nonsynaptic protoplasmic network of nerve fibers; a form of free nerve fiber ending characteristic of connective tissue, consisting of a network of thin threads. **Trolard's n.,** plexus venosus canalis hypoglossi.

nethalide (neth′ah-līd) pronethalol.

Netherton's syndrome (neth′er-tonz) [Earl Weldon *Neth-*

erton, American dermatologist, born 1893] see under *syndrome*.

netilmicin sulfate (net″il-mi′sin) chemical name: (2S-cis)-4- O -[3-amino-6-(aminomethyl)-3,4-dihydro-2H-pyran-2-yl]-2-deoxy-6- O -[3-deoxy-4- C-methyl-3-(methylamino)-β-L-arabinopyranosyl]-N^1-ethyl-d-streptamine, sulfate (2:5) salt; an antibacterial, $(C_{21}H_{41}N_5O_7)_2 \cdot 5H_2SO_4$.

nettle (net′l) any plant of the genus *Urtica*, having leaves covered with stinging hairs that secrete a poisonous and irritating fluid.

network (net′werk) a meshlike structure of interlocking fibers or strands; see also under *net*. **cell n.,** mitome. **Chiari's n.,** a network of fine fibers which sometimes extend across the interior of the right atrium of the heart from the thebesian and eustachian valves to the crista terminalis. **Gerlach's n.,** an apparent (but not real) interlacement of the dendritic processes of the ganglion cells of the spinal cord. **n. of Gesvelst,** a reticular appearance sometimes seen on the myelin sheath of a nerve, perhaps artificial. **idiotype–anti-idiotype n.,** a B-cell regulatory mechanism. Activation of a B cell results in a clone of plasma cells producing immunoglobulin of a single idiotype, which because it was previously present in very small quantities, can be recognized as "nonself" and results in the production of anti-idiotypic antibodies directed against its idiotypic determinants. There can also be anti-anti-idiotypic antibodies directed against the second antibodies, antibodies directed against them, and so forth. These antibodies react with antigen receptors on B cells and T helper and suppressor cells, as well as with circulating antibodies, to enhance or suppress production of the initial antibody by various mechanisms. **neurofibrillar n.,** the network formed by the neurofibrils of a nerve cell. **peritarsal n.,** a set of lymphatics in the eyelid. **Purkinje's n.,** rami subendocardiales. **subpapillary n.,** rete subpapillare. **venous n.,** rete venosum.

neu (nu) neurilemma.

Neubauer's artery (noi′bow-erz) [Johann Ernst *Neubauer*, German anatomist, 1742–1777] arteria thyroidea.

Neubauer-Fischer test (noi′bow-er-fish′er) [Otto *Neubauer*, Munich physician, born 1874] see *glycyltryptophan test*, under *tests*.

Neuberg ester (noi′berg) [Carl *Neuberg*, German biochemist, 1877–1956] see *fructose-6-phosphate*.

Neufeld nail (nu′feld) [Alonzo John *Neufeld*, American orthopedic surgeon, born 1906] see under *nail*.

Neufeld's reaction (test) (noi′felts) [Fred *Neufeld*, German bacteriologist, 1861–1945] see under *reaction*.

Neumann's cells, sheath (noi′manz) [Ernst *Neumann*, German pathologist, 1834–1918] see under *cell* and *sheath*.

Neumann's law [Franz Ernst *Neumann*, German physicist, 1798–1895] see under *law*.

Neumann's method [Heinrich *Neumann*, otologist in Vienna, 1873–1939] see under *method*.

neurad (nu′rad) toward a neural axis or aspect.

neuragmia (nu-rag′me-ah) [*neur-* + Gr. *agmos* break] the tearing of a nerve trunk.

neural (nu′ral) [L. *neuralis*; Gr. *neuron* nerve] 1. pertaining to a nerve or to the nerves. 2. situated in the region of the spinal axis, as the neural arch; cf. *hemal*.

neuralgia (nu-ral′je-ah) [*neur-* + *-algia*] paroxysmal pain which extends along the course of one or more nerves. Many varieties of neuralgia are distinguished according to the part affected or to the cause, as brachial, facial, occipital, supraorbital, etc., or anemic, diabetic, gouty, malarial, syphilitic, etc. **cardiac n.** (*obs.*), angina pectoris. **cervicobrachial n.**, pain in the neck radiating to the arm, due to compression of nerve roots of the cervical spinal cord. **cervico-occipital n.**, neuralgia in the upper cervical nerves, especially the posterior division of the second cervical nerve. **cranial n.**, neuralgia along the course of a cranial nerve. **n. facia′lis ve′ra**, geniculate n. **Fothergill's n.**, trigeminal n. **geniculate n.**, Ramsay Hunt syndrome, def. 1. **glossopharyngeal n.**, neuralgia affecting the petrosal and jugular ganglia of the glossopharyngeal nerve, marked by severe paroxysmal pain originating on the side of the throat and extending to the ear. Occasionally attacks are associated with cardiac slowing or arrest, and syncope. **hallucinatory n.**, a mental impression of pain without any actual peripheral stimulus. **Harris' migrainous n.**, migrainous neuralgia. **Hunt's n.**, Ramsay Hunt syndrome, def. 1. **idiopathic n.**, neuralgia of unknown etiology, unaccompanied by any structural change. **intercostal n.**, neuralgia of the intercostal nerves. **mammary n.**, neuralgic pain in the breast. **mandibular joint n.**, vertex and occipital pain, otalgia, glossodynia, and pain about the nose and eyes, associated with disturbed function of the temporomandibular joint. **migrainous n.**, a migraine variant characterized by attacks of unilateral excruciating pain over the eye and forehead, with temperature elevation, lacrimation, and rhinorrhea; attacks last 15 to 30 minutes and tend to occur in clusters. Because attacks identical to the spontaneous attacks may be induced in sufferers by subcutaneous injection of histamine diphosphate, it is also known as *histamine cephalalgia* or *headache.* Called also *cluster headache*, and *Horton's headache* or *syndrome.* **Morton's n.**, see under *toe*. **nasociliary n.**, pain in the eyes, brow, and root of the nose. **otic n.**, geniculate n. **peripheral n.**, pain along the course of a peripheral sensory nerve. **postherpetic n.**, persistent burning pain and hyperesthesia along the distribution of a cutaneous nerve following an attack of herpes zoster; it may last for a few weeks or many months. **red n.**, erythromelalgia. **reminiscent n.**, a mental impression of neuralgic pain persisting after the actual pain has ceased. **sciatic n.**, sciatica. **Sluder's n.**, neuralgia of the sphenopalatine ganglion, causing a burning and boring pain in the area of the superior maxilla and a radiation of the pain into the neck and shoulder. Called also *sphenopalatine n.* **sphenopalatine n.**, Sluder's n. **stump n.**, neuralgia at the site of an amputation. **supraorbital n.**, neuralgia of the supraorbital nerve. **trifacial n.**, trigeminal n. **trigeminal n.**, excruciating episodic pain in the area supplied by the trigeminal nerve, often precipitated by stimulation of well-defined trigger points. Called also *Fothergill's n.*, *trifocal n.*, and *tic douloureux.* **vidian n.**, neuralgia affecting the vidian nerve (nervus canalis pterygoidei). **visceral n.**, neurasthenic pain in the pelvic region.

neuralgic (nu-ral′jik) pertaining to or of the nature of neuralgia.

neuralgiform (nu-ral′jĭ-form) resembling neuralgia.

neuraminic acid (nu″rah-min′ik) 3,5-dideoxy-5-amino-nonulosonic acid, a 9-carbon amino sugar; its *N*-acyl derivatives (sialic acids) occur in many glycoproteins and polysaccharides.

neuraminidase (nūr-ah-min′ĭ-dās) sialidase.

neuranagenesis (nu″ran-ah-jen′ĕ-sis) [*neur-* + Gr. *anagennan* to regenerate] regeneration or renewal of nerve tissue.

neurapophysis (nu″rah-pof′ĭ-sis) [*neur-* + *apophysis*] the structure forming either side of the neural arch; also the part supposedly homologous with this structure in a so-called cranial vertebra.

neurapraxia (nu″rah-prak′se-ah) [*neur-* + Gr. *apraxia* absence of action] failure of conduction in a nerve in the absence of structural changes, due to blunt injury, compression, or ischemia; return of function normally ensues. Called also *axonapraxia*. Cf. *axonotmesis* and *neurotmesis*.

neurarchy (nu′rar-ke) [*neur-* + Gr. *archē* rule] the control of the cerebrospinal system over the body.

neurarthropathy (nu″rar-throp′ah-the) neuroarthropathy.

neurasthenia (nu″ras-the′ne-ah) [*neur-* + Gr. *astheneia* debility] (*obs.*) a term introduced by Beard in 1869 to refer to a syndrome of chronic mental and physical weakness and fatigue, which was supposed to be caused by exhaustion of the nervous system. Called also *Beard's disease*, *neurasthenic neurosis*, and *nervous exhaustion* or *prostration.* **acoustic n.**, neurasthenia marked by hearing loss of varying degrees. **traumatic n.**, neurasthenia following shock or injury.

neurasthenic (nu″ras-then′ik) pertaining to or affected with neurasthenia.

neuratrophia (nu″rah-tro′fe-ah) [*neur-* + Gr. *atrophia* atrophy] impaired nutrition of the nervous system.

neuratrophic (nu″rah-trof′ik) 1. characterized by atrophy of the nerves. 2. a person affected with atrophy of the nerves.

neuratrophy (nu-rat′ro-fe) neuratrophia.

neuraxial (nu-rak′se-al) pertaining to the neuraxis.

neuraxis (nu-rak′sis) [*neur-* + *axis*] 1. an axon. 2. the central nervous system.

neuraxon (nu-rak′son) [*neur-* + Gr. *axōn* axis] an axon.

neure (nūr) neuron, def. 1.

neurectasia (nu″rek-ta′ze-ah) [*neur-* + Gr. *ektasis* stretching] neurotony.

neurectomy (nu-rek′to-me) [*neur-* + Gr. *ektomē* excision] the excision of a part of a nerve.

neurectopia (nu″rek-to′pe-ah) [*neur-* + Gr. *ektopos* out of place + *-ia*] displacement of a nerve or abnormal situation of a nerve.

neurectopy (nu-rek′to-pe) neurectopia.

neurenteric (nu″ren-ter′ik) [*neur-* + Gr. *enteron* intestine] pertaining to the neural tube and archenteron of the embryo, applied especially to the canal interconnecting them.

neurepithelial (nūr″ep-ĭ-the′le-al) neuroepithelial.

neurepithelium (nūr″ep-ĭ-the′le-um) neuroepithelium.

neurergic (nu-rer′jik) [*neur-* + Gr. *ergon* work] pertaining to or dependent on nerve action.

neurexeresis (nūr″ek-ser′ĕ-sis) [*neur-* + Gr. *exairein* to extract] operation of tearing out (avulsion) of a nerve.

neuriatry (nu-ri′ah-tre) [*neur-* + Gr. *iatreia* medication] the treatment of nervous diseases.

neuridine (nu′rĭ-dēn) a base isolated from fresh human brain, identical with spermine.

neurilemma (nu″rĭ-lem′mah) [*neur-* + Gr. *eilēma* covering] the thin membrane spirally enwrapping the myelin layers of certain, especially peripheral, myelinated nerve fibers or the axons of certain unmyelinated nerve fibers. Called also *neurolemma*, *Schwann's membrane*, *sheath of Schwann*, and *endoneural membrane.*

neurilemmal (nu″rĭ-lem′al) pertaining to a neurilemma.

neurilemmitis (nu″rĭ-lem-mi′tis) inflammation of the neurilemma.

neurilemmoma (nu″rĭ-lem-mo′mah) neurilemoma.

neurilemoma (nu″rĭ-lĕ-mo′mah) [neur- + Gr. *eilēma* a closely adhering sheath + *-oma*] a tumor of a peripheral nerve sheath (neurilemma). **acoustic n.,** acoustic neuroma.

neurility (nu-ril′ĭ-te) the sum of the attributes and functions of nerve tissue.

neurimotility (nu″rĭ-mo-til′ĭ-te) nervimotility.

neurimotor (nu″rĭ-mo′tor) nervimotor.

neurine (nu′rin) a poisonous ptomaine, vinyl trimethyl ammonium hydroxide, $CH_2:CHN(CH_3)_3OH$, found in decaying fish, fungi, and in the brain and in many other normal tissues.

neurinoma (nu″rĭ-no′mah) [neur- + Gr. *is* fiber + *-oma*] schwannoma. **acoustic n.,** acoustic neuroma.

neurite (nu′rīt) an axon.

neuritic (nu-rit′ik) pertaining to or affected with neuritis.

neuritis (nu-ri′tis) [neur- + *-itis*] inflammation of a nerve, a condition attended by pain and tenderness over the nerves, anesthesia and paresthesias, paralysis, wasting, and disappearance of the reflexes. In practice, the term is also used to denote noninflammatory lesions of the peripheral nervous system; see *neuropathy*. **adventitial n.,** that which affects the sheath of a nerve. **alcoholic n.,** see under *neuropathy*. **ascending n.,** see under *neuropathy*. **brachial n.,** neuralgic amyotrophy. **central n.,** parenchymatous n. **descending n.,** see under *neuropathy*. **dietetic n.,** beriberi. **disseminated n.,** polyneuritis. **endemic n.,** beriberi. **fallopian n.,** neuritis of the facial nerve in the fallopian canal. **Gombault's n.,** progressive hypertrophic interstitial neuropathy. **interstitial n.,** inflammation of the connective tissue of a nerve trunk. **interstitial hypertrophic n.,** progressive hypertrophic interstitial neuropathy. **intraocular n.,** neuritis of the retinal part of the optic nerve. **jake n.,** Jamaica ginger paralysis. **latent n.,** degeneration of the fibers of a nerve without corresponding clinical phenomena. **lead n.,** n. saturnina. **leprous n.,** a form associated with true leprosy. **malarial n.,** a form associated with malaria. **malarial multiple n.,** inflammation involving many nerves, and associated with malaria. **n. mi′grans, migrating n.,** neuritis affecting first one nerve and then another. **multiple n.,** polyneuritis. **n. mul′tiplex endem′ica,** beriberi. **n. nodo′sa,** a form characterized by the formation of nodes on the nerves. **optic n.,** inflammation of the optic nerve; it may affect the part of the nerve within the eyeball (*neuropapillitis*) or the portion behind the eyeball (*retrobulbar n.*). **orbital optic n.,** retrobulbar n. **parenchymatous n.,** neuritis affecting principally the axons and myelin of the peripheral nerves; called also *central n.* **periaxial n.,** segmental (demyelination) neuropathy. **peripheral n.,** inflammation of the nerve endings or of terminal nerves. **porphyric n.,** neuritis occurring as a manifestation of acute intermittent porphyria. **postfebrile n.,** that which mostly follows an attack of severe exanthematous disease. **postocular n.,** retrobulbar n. **pressure n.,** a form due to compression of the nerve. **n. puerpera′lis traumat′ica,** neuritis occurring in parturient women as a result of injury at childbirth. **radiation n.,** radioneuritis. **radicular n.,** neuritis involving the spinal roots of the nerves; radiculitis. **retrobulbar n.,** inflammation in that portion of the optic nerve which is posterior to the eyeball. **rheumatic n.,** a form associated with rheumatic symptoms. **n. saturni′na,** neuritis due to plumbism. **sciatic n.,** sciatica. **segmental n.,** segmental (demyelination) neuropathy. **senile n.,** a form occurring in aged persons, and affecting chiefly the nerves of the extremities. **serum n.,** see under *neuropathy*. **shoulder-girdle n.,** neuralgic amyotrophy. **syphilitic n.,** neuritis due to syphilis. **tabetic n.,** neuritis associated with tabes dorsalis. **toxic n.,** that which is due to some poison. **traumatic n.,** that which follows and is caused by an injury.

neur(o)- [Gr. *neuron* nerve] combining form denoting relationship to a nerve or nervous, or to the nervous system.

neuroallergy (nu″ro-al′er-je) allergy in nervous tissue.

neuroamebiasis (nu″ro-am″e-bi′ah-sis) neuritis due to amebiasis.

neuroanastomosis (nu″ro-ah-nas″to-mo′sis) surgical formation of an anastomosis between nerves.

neuroanatomy (nu″ro-ah-nat′o-me) [neuro- + *anatomy*] that branch of neurology which is concerned with the anatomy of the nervous system.

neuroarthropathy (nu″ro-ar-throp′ah-the) [neuro- + Gr. *arthron* joint + *pathos* disease] any disease of joint structures associated with disease of the central or peripheral nervous system.

neuroastrocytoma (nu″ro-as″tro-si-to′mah) [neuro- + *astrocytoma*] a glioma composed mainly of astrocytes, closely resembling an astrocytoma and most commonly found in the floor of the third ventricle and the temporal lobes, although it may arise in almost any part of the central nervous system.

neurobehavioral (nu″ro-be-hāv′u-ral) relating to neurologic status as assessed by observation of behavior.

neurobiologist (nu″ro-bi-ol′o-jist) a specialist in neurobiology.

neurobiology (nu″ro-bi-ol′o-je) the biology of the nervous system, including its anatomy, physiology, biochemistry, and so on.

neurobiotaxis (nu″ro-bi″o-tak′sis) [neuro- + *biotaxis*] the theory that nerve cell bodies have a tendency during development to migrate in the direction from which they habitually receive their stimuli.

neuroblast (nu′ro-blast) [neuro- + Gr. *blastos* germ] any embryonic cell which develops into a nerve cell or neuron; an immature nerve cell.

neuroblastoma (nu″ro-blas-to′mah) sarcoma of nervous system origin, composed chiefly of neuroblasts and affecting mostly infants and children up to 10 years of age. Most of such tumors arise in the autonomic nervous system (sympathicoblastoma) or in the adrenal medulla. When there is metastasis from the adrenal medulla to the cranium or to the liver, it is known as *Hutchinson's type* or *Pepper's syndrome*, respectively.

neurocanal (nu″ro-kah-nal′) [neuro- + *canal*] the vertebral canal (canalis vertebralis).

neurocardiac (nu″ro-kar′de-ak) [neuro- + Gr. *kardia* heart] pertaining to the nervous system and the heart.

neurocentral (nu″ro-sen′tral) pertaining to the centrum and the two lateral masses of a developing vertebra.

neurocentrum (nu″ro-sen′trum) one of the embryonic vertebral elements from which the spinous processes of the vertebrae develop.

neuroceptor (nu′ro-sep″tor) [neuro- + L. *capere* to take] one of the terminal elements of a dendrite which receives the stimulus from the neuromittor of the adjoining neuron; called also *ceptor*.

neuroceratin (nu″ro-ser′ah-tin) neurokeratin.

neurochemistry (nu″ro-kem′is-tre) that branch of neurology which is concerned with the chemistry of the nervous system.

neurochitin (nu″ro-ki′tin) [neuro- + Gr. *chitōn* frock, skin, membrane] the substance that forms the framework support of nerve fibers.

neurochondrite (nu″ro-kon′drīt) [neuro- + Gr. *chondros* cartilage] one of the embryonic cartilaginous elements which develop into the neural arch of a vertebra.

neurochorioretinitis (nu″ro-ko″re-o-ret″ĭ-ni′tis) [neuro- + *chorioretinitis*] inflammation of the optic nerve, choroid, and retina.

neurochoroiditis (nu″ro-ko″roi-di′tis) inflammation of the choroid coat and optic nerves.

neurocirculatory (nu″ro-cir′cu-lah-to″re) pertaining to the nervous and circulatory systems, as neurocirculatory asthenia.

neurocladism (nu-rok′lah-dizm) [neuro- + Gr. *klados* branch] the formation of new branches by the process of a neuron; especially the force by which, in regeneration of divided nerves, the newly formed axons of the proximal stump become attracted by the peripheral stump so as to form a bridge between the two ends. Called also *odogenesis*.

neuroclonic (nu″ro-klon′ik) [neuro- + Gr. *klonos* spasm] characterized by nervous spasms.

neurocommunications (nu″ro-kŏ-mu″nĭ-ka′shunz)

the branch of neurology dealing with the transfer and integration of information within the nervous system.

neurocranial (nu″ro-kra′ne-al) pertaining to the neurocranium.

neurocranium (nu″ro-kra′ne-um) the portion of the cranium which encloses the brain.

neurocrine (nu′ro-krīn) [*neuro-* + Gr. *krinein* to separate] 1. denoting an endocrine influence on or by the nerves. 2. pertaining to neurosecretion.

neurocrinia (nu″ro-krin′e-ah) endocrine influence on the nerves.

neurocristopathy (nu″ro-kris-top′ah-the) [*neuro-* + L. *crista* crest + *-pathy*] any disease arising from maldevelopment of the neural crest.

neurocutaneous (nu″ro-ku-ta′ne-us) pertaining to the nerves and the skin; pertaining to the cutaneous nerves. See also *phakomatosis*.

neurocyte (nu′ro-sīt) [*neuro-* + *-cyte*] a nerve cell of any kind; a neuron.

neurocytology (nu″ro-si-tol′o-je) that branch of neurology which is concerned with the cellular components of the nervous system.

neurocytolysin (nu″ro-si-tol′ĭ-sin) a constituent of the venom of certain snakes (rattler, coral, cobra), which lyses nerve cells.

neurocytoma (nu″ro-si-to′mah) a brain tumor consisting of undifferentiated cells of nervous origin, i.e., cells resembling medullary neural epithelium; called also *neuroepithelioma* and *medulloepithelioma*.

neurodealgia (nu-ro″de-al′je-ah) [Gr. *neurōdēs* nervelike + *-algia*] pain in the retina.

neurodeatrophia (nu-ro″de-ah-tro′fe-ah) [Gr. *neurōdēs* nervelike + *atrophia*] retinal atrophy.

neurodegenerative (nu″ro-de-jen′er-a-tiv) relating to or marked by nervous degeneration.

neurodendrite (nu″ro-den′drīt) [*neuro-* + Gr. *dendritēs* of a tree] dendrite.

neurodendron (nu″ro-den′dron) dendrite.

neuroderm (nu′ro-derm) the neural ectoderm; that portion of the ectoderm which develops into the neural tube.

neurodermatitis (noo″ro-der″mah-ti′tis) [*neuro-* + *dermatitis*] an extremely variable eczematous dermatosis presumed to be a cutaneous response to prolonged vigorous scratching, rubbing, or pinching to relieve intense pruritus, having the potential to produce polymorphic lesions at the same or different times, and varying in severity, course, and morphologic expression in different individuals. It is believed by some authorities to be a psychogenic disorder. The term is also used to refer to *lichen simplex chronicus* (circumscribed n.) and sometimes to *atopic dermatitis* (disseminated n.). **exudative n., nummular n.,** nummular eczema.

neurodiagnosis (nu″ro-di″ag-no′sis) [*neuro-* + *diagnosis*] the diagnosis of diseases of the nervous system.

neurodin (nu-ro′din) acetyl para-oxyphenylurethane, $C_6H_4(OCOCH_3)NH \cdot COOC_2H_5$, used as an antineuralgic and antipyretic.

neurodynamic (nu″ro-di-nam′ik) [*neuro-* + Gr. *dynamis* force] relating to nervous energy.

neurodynia (nu″ro-din′e-ah) [*neuro-* + Gr. *odynē* pain] pain in a nerve or in nerves.

neuroectoderm (nu″ro-ek′to-derm) the portion of the ectoderm of the early embryo which gives rise to the central and peripheral nervous systems, including some glial cells.

neuroectodermal (nu″ro-ek″to-der′mal) pertaining or relating to the neuroectoderm.

neuroeffector (nu″ro-ef-fek′tor) of or relating to the junction between a neuron and the effector organ it innervates.

neuroelectricity (nu″ro-e″lek-tris′ĭ-te) the electrical signals, currents, or voltages generated by the nervous system.

neuroencephalomyelopathy (nu″ro-en-sef″ah-lo-mi″ĕ-lop′ah-the) [*neuro-* + Gr. *enkephalos* brain + *myelos* marrow + *pathos* disease] disease involving the brain, spinal cord, and nerves. **optic n.,** neuromyelitis optica.

neuroendocrine (nu″ro-en′do-krin) pertaining to neural and endocrine influence, and particularly to the interaction between the nervous and endocrine systems and to hormones

elaborated in the nervous system and ultimately secreted by an endocrine gland, as vasopressin.

neuroendocrinology (nu″ro-en″do-kri-nol′o-je) the study of the interactions of the nervous system and endocrine system.

neuroenteric (nu″ro-en-ter′ik) neurenteric.

neuroepidermal (nu″ro-ep″ĭ-der′mal) [*neuro-* + *epidermis*] pertaining to or giving origin to the nervous and epidermal tissues.

neuroepithelial (nu″ro-ep″ĭ-the′le-al) pertaining to or composed of neuroepithelium.

neuroepithelioma (nu″ro-ep″ĭ-the″le-o′mah) neurocytoma.

neuroepithelium (nu″ro-ep″ĭ-the′le-um) [*neuro-* + *epithelium*] 1. simple columnar epithelium made up of cells specialized to serve as sensory cells for the reception of external stimuli, as the sensory cells of the cochlea, vestibule, nasal mucosa, and tongue. 2. the epithelium of the ectoderm, from which the central nervous system is developed. **n. of ampullary crest, n. cris′tae ampulla′ris** [NA], the specialized epithelium of the ampullary crest of the labyrinth, containing receptor cells from some of which sensory hairs project into the cupula. **n. of maculae, n. macula′rum** [NA], the specialized epithelium of the maculae of the labyrinth, containing receptor cells from some of which sensory hairs project into the statoconic membrane.

neurofiber (noo″ro-fi′ber) [*neuro-* + L. *fibra* fiber] nerve fiber. **afferent n′s,** see under *fiber*. **association n′s,** see under *fiber*. **commissural n′s,** see under *fiber*. **efferent n′s,** see under *fiber*. **postganglionic n′s,** see under *fiber*. **preganglionic n′s,** see under *fiber*. **projection n′s,** see under *fiber*. **somatic n′s,** see under *fiber*. **tangential n′s,** see under *fiber*. **visceral n′s,** see under *fiber*.

neurofibra (noo″ro-fi′brah), pl. *neurofi′brae* [L.] nerve fiber. **neurofi′brae afferen′tes** [NA], afferent fibers. **neurofi′brae associatio′nes** [NA], association fibers. **neurofi′brae commissura′les** [NA], commissural fibers. **neurofi′brae efferen′tes** [NA], efferent fibers. **neurofi′brae postgangliona′res** [NA], postganglionic fibers. **neurofi′brae pregangliona′res** [NA], preganglionic fibers. **neurofi′brae projectio′nes** [NA], projection fibers. **neurofi′brae somat′icae** [NA], somatic fibers. **neurofi′brae tangentia′les** [NA], tangential fibers. **neurofi′brae viscera′les** [NA], visceral fibers.

neurofibrae (noo″ro-fi′bre) [L.] plural of *neurofibra*.

neurofibril (nu″ro-fi′bril) any of the delicate interlacing threads coursing through the cytoplasm of the body of a neuron and extending from one dendrite into another or into the axon; with the electron microscope, it can be seen to be formed by aggregations of neurofilaments and neurotubules.

neurofibrilla (nu″ro-fi-bril′ah), pl. *neurofibril′lae*. A neurofibril.

neurofibrillae (nu″ro-fi-bril′e) plural of *neurofibrilla*.

neurofibrillar (nu″ro-fi-bril′ar) pertaining to neurofibrils.

neurofibroma (nu″ro-fi-bro′mah) [*neuro-* + *fibroma*] a tumor of peripheral nerves caused by abnormal proliferation of Schwann cells.

neurofibromatosis (nu″ro-fi″bro-mah-to′sis) a familial condition characterized by developmental changes in the nervous system, muscles, bones and skin and marked superficially by the formation of multiple pedunculated soft tumors (neurofibromas) distributed over the entire body associated with areas of pigmentation. Called also *multiple neuroma*, *neuromatosis*, and *von Recklinghausen's disease*.

neurofilament (nu″ro-fil′ah-ment) one of the slender, fibrillar elements which, along with the neurotubules, forms a neurofibril; they seem to correspond to the microfilaments occurring in many cells outside the nervous system, and in addition to a cytoskeletal function, they may be involved in intracellular transport of metabolites.

neurogangliitis (nu″ro-gang″gle-i′tis) inflammation of a neuroganglion.

neuroganglion (nu″ro-gang′gle-on) a ganglion, or mass of nervous matter.

neurogastric (nu″ro-gas′trik) involving the nerves of the stomach.

neurogen (nu′ro-jen) the chemical substance by means of which the primary organizer causes the development of the neural plate.

neurogenesis (nu″ro-jen′ĕ-sis) [neuro- + Gr. *genesis* production] the development of nervous tissue.

neurogenetic (nu″ro-jĕ-net′ik) pertaining to neurogenesis.

neurogenic (nu″ro-jen′ik) [neuro- + Gr. *gennan* to produce] 1. forming nervous tissue, or stimulating nervous energy. 2. originating in the nervous system.

neurogenous (nu-roj′ĕ-nus) arising in the nervous system; arising from some lesion of the nervous system.

neuroglia (nu-rog′le-ah) [neuro- + Gr. *glia* glue] the supporting structure of nervous tissue (Virchow, 1854). It consists of a fine web of tissue made up of modified ectodermal elements, in which are enclosed peculiar branched cells known as *neuroglial cells* or *glial cells.* The neuroglial cells are of three types: astrocytes and oligodendrocytes (collectively macroglia, which are of ectodermal origin, and microglia, said to be of mesodermal origin. Astrocytes and oligodendrocytes appear to play a role in myelin formation, transport of material to neurons, and maintenance of the ionic environment of neurons. Called also *bind web* and *glia.* **interfascicular n.,** oligodendroglia of white matter along the myelin sheaths. **peripheral n.,** the neurilemma, Schwann cells, and satellite cells of the peripheral nervous system.

neuroglial, neurogliar (nu-rog′le-al, nu-rog′le-ar) pertaining to the neuroglia.

neurogliocyte (nu-rog′le-o-sīt″) [neuroglia + -cyte] a cell of the neuroglia.

neurogliocytoma (nu-rog″le-o-si-to′mah) a tumor composed of neuroglial cells; a glioma.

neuroglioma (nu″ro-gli-o′mah) [neuro- + glioma] a tumor made up of neuroglial tissue. **n. gangliona′re,** ganglioneuroma.

neurogliomatosis (nu″ro-gli″o-mah-to′sis) neurogliosis.

neurogliosis (nu-rog″le-o′sis) a condition marked by diffuse formation of neurogliomas.

neuroglycopenia (nu″ro-gli″ko-pe′ne-ah) [neuro- + Gr. *glykys* sweet + *penia* poverty] chronic hypoglycemia of a degree sufficient to impair brain function, resulting in personality changes and intellectual deterioration.

neurogram (nu′ro-gram) [neuro- + Gr. *gramma* mark] residua of past cerebral activities which make up the brain disposition and thus take part in the formation of personality.

neurography (nu-rog′rah-fe) [neuro- + Gr. *graphein* to write] a treatise on or description of the nerves.

neurohistology (nu″ro-his-tol′o-je) the histology of the nervous system.

neurohormonal (nu″ro-hor′mo-nal) both neural and hormonal.

neurohormone (nu′ro-hor″mōn) a hormone stimulating the neural mechanism.

neurohumor (nu″ro-hu′mor) a chemical substance formed in a neuron and able to activate or modify the function of a neighboring neuron, muscle, or gland.

neurohumoral (nu″ro-hu′mor-al) pertaining to the neurohumors.

neurohumoralism (nu″ro-hu′mor-al-izm) the theory that the action of the autonomic nerves on peripheral organs is produced through the medium of chemicals (neurohumors) which are liberated at the endings of activated nerves.

neurohypophyseal (nu″ro-hi″po-fiz′e-al) neurohypophysial.

neurohypophysectomy (nu″ro-hi″po-fiz-ek′to-me) [neuro- + hypophysectomy] surgical removal of the neural lobe of the pituitary gland.

neurohypophysial (nu″ro-hi″po-fiz′e-al) pertaining to the neurohypophysis.

neurohypophysis (nu″ro-hi-pof′ĭ-sis) [neuro- + Gr. *phyein* to grow] [NA] the posterior (neural) lobe of the pituitary gland (hypophysis) [NA], as distinguished from the anterior (glandular) lobe (adenohypophysis). It is the storage site for vasopressin, oxytocin, and neurophysins. Called also *lobus posterior hypophyseos* [NA alternative]. See also *pituitary gland,* under *gland.*

neuroid (nu′roid) [neuro- + Gr. *eidos* form] resembling a nerve.

neuroimmunologic (nu″ro-im″u-no-loj′ik) pertaining to neuroimmunology.

neuroimmunology (nu″ro-im″u-nol′o-je) that branch of science which deals with the interaction of the nervous and immune systems in health and disease, as in the effects of autonomic nervous activity on the immune response and the role of antibodies in myasthenia gravis.

neuroinidia (nu″ro-ĭ-nid′e-ah) deficient nutrition of nerve cells.

neurokeratin (nu″ro-ker′ah-tin) [neuro- + Gr. *keras* horn] a variety of keratin said to form the supporting network of the myelin sheath of medullated nerve fibers.

neurokinet (nu″ro-kin′et) [neuro- + Gr. *kinein* to move] an apparatus for stimulating the nerve by percussion.

neurokyme (nu′ro-kīm) a nervous process in general.

neurolabyrinthitis (nu″ro-lab″ĭ-rin-thi′tis) inflammation of the nervous structures of the labyrinth.

neurolathyrism (nu″ro-lath′ĭ-rizm) lathyrism.

neurolemma (nu″ro-lem′ah) neurilemma.

neurolemmitis (nu″ro-lĕ-mi′tis) neurilemmitis.

neurolemmoma (nu″ro-lĕ-mo′mah) neurilemoma.

neuroleptanalgesia (nu″ro-lep″tan-al-je′ze-ah) [neuro- + Gr. *lepsis* a taking hold + *analgesia*] a state of quiescence, altered awareness, and analgesia produced by the administration of a combination of a narcotic analgesic and a neuroleptic agent.

neuroleptanalgesic (nu″ro-lep″tan-al-je′zik) 1. pertaining to or producing neuroleptanalgesia. 2. an agent that produces neuroleptanalgesia.

neuroleptanesthesia (nu″ro-lep″tan-es-the′ze-ah) [neuro- + Gr. *lepsis* a taking hold + *anesthesia*] a state of neuroleptanalgesia and unconsciousness, produced by the combined administration of a narcotic analgesic and a neuroleptic agent, together with the inhalation of nitrous oxide and oxygen.

neuroleptanesthetic (nu″ro-lep″tan-es-thet′ik) 1. pertaining to or producing neuroleptanesthesia. 2. an agent that produces neuroleptanesthesia.

neuroleptic (nu″ro-lep′tik) [neuro- + Gr. *lepsis* a taking hold, a seizure] a term coined to refer to the effects on cognition and behavior of antipsychotic drugs, which produce a state of apathy, lack of initiative, and limited range of emotion and in psychotic patients cause a reduction in confusion and agitation and normalization of psychomotor activity. See *antipsychotic.*

neurolipomatosis (nu″ro-lĭ-po″mah-to′sus) a condition characterized by the formation of subcutaneous multiple fat deposits, with pressure on the nerves resulting in tenderness, pain, and paresthesias. **n. doloro′sa,** adiposis dolorosa.

neurologia (nu″ro-lo′je-ah) neurology.

neurologic (nu-ro-loj′ik) pertaining to neurology or to the nervous system.

neurologist (nu-rol′o-jist) an expert in neurology or in the treatment of disorders of the nervous system.

neurology (nu-rol′o-je) [neuro- + -logy] that branch of medical science which deals with the nervous system, both normal and in disease. **clinical n.,** that specialty concerned with the diagnosis and treatment of disorders of the nervous system.

neurolues (nu″ro-loo′ēz) neurosyphilis.

neurolymph (nu′ro-limf) (obs.) the cerebrospinal fluid.

neurolymphomatosis (nu″ro-lim″fo-mah-to′sis) lymphoblastic infiltration of a nerve. **n. gallina′rum,** Marek's disease.

neurolysin (nu-rol′ĭ-sin) a cytolysin which has a specific destructive action upon nerve cells.

neurolysis (nu-rol′ĭ-sis) [neuro- + Gr. *lysis* dissolution] 1. release of a nerve sheath by cutting it longitudinally. 2. the operative breaking up of perineural adhesions. 3. the relief of tension upon a nerve obtained by stretching. 4. exhaustion of nervous energy. 5. destruction or dissolution of nerve tissue.

neurolytic (nu″ro-lit′ik) destructive of nerve substance.

neuroma (nu-ro′mah) [neuro- + -oma] a tumor or new growth largely made up of nerve cells and nerve fibers; a tumor growing from a nerve. **acoustic n.,** a progressively enlarging, benign tumor within the auditory canal arising from the eighth cranial (acoustic) nerve; the symptoms, which vary with the size and location of the tumor, may include hearing loss, headache, disturbances of balance and gait, facial numbness or pain, and tinnitus. It may be unilateral or bilateral. Called also *acoustic neurilemoma* or *neurinoma,* and *schwannoma.* **amputation n.,** traumatic neuroma occurring after amputation of an extremity or part. **amyelinic n.,** one containing only nonmedullated nerve fibers. **n. cu′tis,** neuroma seated in the skin. **cystic n.,** a false neuroma, or a neuroma which has become cystic. **false n.,** one which does not contain nerve elements. **fascicular n., medullated n.,** a neuroma made up of myelinated nerve fibers. **ganglionar n., ganglionated n., ganglionic n.,** one made up of nerve cells. **malignant n.,** sarcoma of a nerve structure, usually spindle celled. **multiple n.,** see *neuromatosis* and *neurofibromatosis.* **myelinic n.,** one that contains myelinated nerve fibers. **nevoid n.,** neuroma telangiectodes. **plexiform n.,** a neuroma made up of contorted nerve trunks; called also *Verneuil's n.* **n. telangiecto′des,** one which contains an excess of blood vessels; called also *nevoid n.* **traumatic n.,** an unorganized bulbous or nodular mass of nerve fibers and Schwann cells produced by hyperplasia of nerve fibers and their supporting tissues after accidental or purposeful sectioning of the nerve. **true n.,** a neuroma made up of nerve tissue. **Verneuil's n.,** plexiform n.

neuromalacia (nu″ro-mah-la′she-ah) [*neuro-* + Gr. *malakia* softening] morbid softening of the nerves.

neuromalakia (nu″ro-mah-la′ke-ah) neuromalacia.

neuromatosis (nu″ro-mah-to′sis) a disease condition characterized by the presence of many neuromas; see also *neurofibromatosis.*

neuromatous (nu-rom′ah-tus) affected with or of the nature of neuroma.

neuromechanism (nu″ro-mek′ah-nizm) the structure and arrangement of the nervous system in relation to function.

neuromeningeal (nu″ro-men-in′je-al) pertaining to or affecting nervous tissue and the meninges.

neuromere (nu′ro-mēr) [*neuro-* + Gr. *meros* part] 1. any of the series of transitory segmental elevations in the wall of the neural tube of the developing embryo; also commonly used to refer to such elevations in the wall of the mature rhombencephalon. 2. a part of the spinal cord to which a pair of dorsal roots and a pair of ventral roots are attached. Called also *neural segment.*

neuromimesis (nu″ro-mi-me′sis) [*neuro-* + *mimesis*] hysterical simulation of organic disease.

neuromimetic (nu″ro-mi-met′ik) 1. eliciting a response in effector organs that simulates that elicited by nervous impulses. 2. an agent that elicits such a response. 3. pertaining to neuromimesis.

neuromittor (nu″ro-mit′or) [*neuro-* + L. *mittere* to send] one of the terminal elements at the peripheral end of a neuron which transfers a stimulus to the neuroceptor of the adjoining neuron. Called also *mittor.*

neuromodulation (nu″ro-mod″u-la′shun) electrical stimulation of a peripheral nerve, the spinal cord, or the brain for relief of pain; it may be done transcutaneously or with an implanted stimulator.

neuromotor (nu″ro-mo′tor) involving both nerves and muscles; pertaining to nervous impulses to muscles.

neuromuscular (nu″ro-mus′ku-lar) pertaining to muscles and nerves.

neuromyal (nu″ro-mi′al) [*neuro-* + Gr. *mus* a muscle] neuromuscular.

neuromyasthenia (nu″ro-mi″as-the′ne-ah) [*neuro-* + *myasthenia*] muscular weakness associated with emotional lability. **epidemic n.,** a disease somewhat resembling poliomyelitis, usually occurring in epidemics, characterized by headache, muscle pain, cervical lymphadenopathy, fever, and sometimes paralysis, but without atrophy and with hyperreflexia rather than hyporeflexia. Called also *benign myalgic encephalomyelitis* and *Iceland* (or *Icelandic*) *disease.*

neuromyelitis (nu″ro-mi″ĕ-li′tis) [*neuro-* + Gr. *myelos* marrow + *-itis*] inflammation of nervous and medullary substance; myelitis attended with neuritis. **n. op′tica,** com-
bined demyelination of the optic nerve and the spinal cord; it is marked by diminution of vision and possibly blindness, flaccid paralysis of the extremities, and sensory and genitourinary disturbances. Called also *Devic's disease,* optic neuroencephalomyelopathy, neuro-optic myelitis, and ophthalmoneuromyelitis.

neuromyic (nu″ro-mi′ik) [*neuro-* + Gr. *mys* muscle] neuromuscular.

neuromyon (nu″ro-mi′on) [*neuro-* + Gr. *mys* muscle] (*obs.*) the neural elements in a muscle.

neuromyopathic (nu″ro-mi″o-path′ik) pertaining to or affecting the nervous system and muscle, including the heart.

neuromyositis (nu″ro-mi″o-si′tis) [*neuro-* + *myositis*] neuritis complicated with myositis.

neuron (nu′ron) [Gr. nerve] 1. any of the conducting cells of the nervous system. A typical neuron consists of a cell body, containing the nucleus and the surrounding cytoplasm (perikaryon); several short radiating processes (dendrites); and one long process (the axon), which terminates in twiglike branches (telodendrons) and may have branches (collaterals) projecting along its course. The axon together with its covering or sheath forms the nerve fiber. See illustration accompanying *nerve.* Called also *nerve cell.* 2. (*obs.*) axon. 3. (*obs.*) the central nervous system. **afferent n.,** a neuron which conducts a nervous impulse from a receptor to a center. **bipolar n.,** a neuron having two processes, one projecting from each end of the cell body. **central n.,** a neuron which belongs entirely to the central nervous system. **connector n.,** one whose dendrites and axon both synapse with other neurons. **correlation n.,** a neuron which takes part in the function of correlating various stimuli into the appropriate response; see *correlation.* **efferent n.,** a neuron which conducts a nervous impulse from a center to an organ of response. **Golgi type I n's,** pyramidal neurons with very long axons, which leave the gray matter of the central nervous system, traverse the white matter, and terminate in the periphery; called also *Golgi cells.* **Golgi type II n's,** stellate neurons with short axons that do not pass out of the gray matter in which the cell body lies, and are especially numerous in the cerebral and cerebellar cortices and in the retina. Called also *Golgi cells* and *cells of van Gehuchten.* **intercalary n., internuncial n.,** interneuron. **long n.,** axon, def. 1. **motor n.,** any neuron possessing a motor function; an efferent neuron conveying motor impulses. See *motoneuron.* **multiform n.,** multipolar n. **multipolar n.,** a neuron with several to many processes; such neurons vary in shape, depending on the arrangement of the processes, with pyramidal and stellate (star) shapes being common. Called also *polymorphic n.* **peripheral sensory n.,** a neuron forming the first part of a peripheral reflex arc; situated outside the central nervous system, it has a peripheral branch which enters the central nervous system. Together with the interneurons and the peripheral motor neuron it forms a peripheral reflex arc. **polymorphic n.,** multipolar n. **postganglionic n's,** neurons whose cell bodies are situated in the autonomic ganglia and whose purpose is to relay impulses beyond the ganglia. **preganglionic n's,** neurons whose cell bodies lie in the central nervous system and whose efferent fibers terminate in the autonomic ganglia. **premotor n.,** a neuron not connected directly with muscle, but serving as a connecting center to command excitation in one or more motor neurons. **projection n.,** one which serves for the transmission of nervous impulses, whether motor or sensory, between the cerebral cortex and the lower centers. **pseudounipolar n.,** a unipolar neuron which was originally bipolar but whose two processes fused during development to form a single process that bifurcates at a distance from the cell body. **pyramidal n.,** see under *cell.* **sensory n.,** any neuron possessing a sensory function; an afferent neuron conveying sensory impulses. See illustration accompanying *nerve.* **short n.,** a local process from a nerve cell or brain cell reaching only to a nearby gray mass. **unipolar n.,** a neuron with one process only; see also *pseudounipolar n.*

neuronagenesis (nu″rōn-ah-jen′ĕ-sis) [*neuron* + *a* neg. + Gr. *gennan* to produce] lack of development of neurons.

neuronal (nu′ro-nal) pertaining to a neuron or neurons.

neuronatrophy (nu″ron-at′ro-fe) Southard and Solomon's term for any nervous disease due to sclerosis of neurons.

neurone (nu′rōn) neuron.

neuronephric (nu″ro-nef′rik) pertaining to the nervous and renal systems.

neuronevus (nu″ro-ne′vus) [*neuro-* + *nevus*] a nevocytic nevus in which the nevus cells differentiate into neural-like structures, and may clinically resemble neurofibroma or may have the clinical aspect of a giant hairy pigmented nevus. Called also *neural* or *neuroid nevus*.

neuronic (nu-ron′ik) pertaining to or affecting a neuron.

neuronin (nu′ro-nin) the principal protein of the axon of a nerve.

neuronist (nu′ro-nist) (*obs.*) an adherent of the neuron theory.

neuronitis (nu″ro-ni′tis) a term applied by Foster Kennedy to a disorder of unknown origin involving the more proximal part of the peripheral nervous system, characterized by breakdown of nerve fibers, sometimes in association with inflammatory-cell reaction. Currently seldom used, it was in the past one of numerous synonyms used for *acute febrile polyneuritis*.

neuronophage (nu-ron′o-fāj) [*neuron* + Gr. *phagein* to eat] a phagocyte which destroys nerve cells.

neuronophagia (nu″ron-o-fa′je-ah) the destruction of nerve cells by phagocytic action.

neuronophagy (nu″ron-of′ah-je) neuronophagia.

neuronosis (nu″ro-no′sis) [*neuron* + Gr. *nosos* disease] any disease of nervous origin.

neuronotropic (nu-ron″o-trōp′ik) [*neuron* + Gr. *tropein* to turn] having a special affinity for neurons.

neuronymy (nu-ron′ĭ-me) [*neuron* + Gr. *onoma* name] the systematic naming of the parts of the nervous system.

neuro-ophthalmology (noo″ro-of″thal-mol′o-je) [*neuro-* + *ophthalmology*] the field of specialization dealing with portions of the nervous system related to the eye.

neuro-otology (nu″ro-o-tol′o-je) that part of otology dealing especially with portions of the nervous system related to the ear.

neuropacemaker (nu″ro-pās′māk-er) an implant device that relieves pain due to nerve injury.

neuropapillitis (nu″ro-pap″ĭ-li′tis) optic neuritis.

neuroparalysis (nu″ro-pah-ral′ĭ-sis) paralysis due to disease of a nerve or nerves.

neuroparalytic (nu″ro-par″ah-lit′ik) pertaining to or characterized by neuroparalysis.

neuropathic (nu″ro-path′ik) pertaining to or characterized by neuropathy.

neuropathogenesis (nu″ro-path″o-jen′ĕ-sis) development of disease of the nervous system.

neuropathogenicity (nu″ro-path″o-jĕ-nis′ĭ-te) the quality of producing or the ability to produce pathologic changes in nerve tissue.

neuropathology (nu″ro-pah-thol′o-je) the branch of medicine dealing with morphological and other aspects of disease of the nervous system.

neuropathy (nu-rop′ah-the) a general term denoting functional disturbances and/or pathological changes in the peripheral nervous system. The etiology may be known (e.g., *arsenical n.*, *diabetic n.*, *ischemic n.*, *traumatic n.*) or unknown. *Encephalopathy* and *myelopathy* are corresponding terms relating to involvement of the brain and spinal cord, respectively. The term is also used to designate noninflammatory lesions in the peripheral nervous system, in contrast to inflammatory lesions (neuritis). **alcoholic n.**, neuropathy due to thiamine deficiency in chronic alcoholism; called *polyneuritis potatorum*. **ascending n.**, that which progresses from the feet upwards to affect the thigh, hip, trunk, etc. **descending n.**, that which starts proximately (shoulder, hip) and spreads distally toward the limb extremities (hands, feet). **diabetic n.**, a chronic, symmetrical sensory polyneuropathy affecting first the nerves of the lower limbs and often affecting autonomic nerves; pathologically, there is segmental demyelination of the peripheral nerves. An uncommon, acute form is marked by severe pain, weakness, and wasting of proximal and distal muscles, peripheral sensory impairment, and loss of tendon reflexes. With autonomic involvement there may be orthostatic hypotension, nocturnal diarrhea, retention of urine, impotence, and small diameter of the pupils with sluggish reaction to light. **entrapment n.**, any of a group of neuropathies, including the carpal tunnel syndrome, tarsal tunnel syndrome, and meralgia paresthetica, in which a peripheral nerve is injured by compression in its course through a fibrous or osseofibrous tunnel or at a point where it abruptly changes its course through deep fascia over a fibrous or muscular band. **hereditary sensory radicular n.**, a dominantly inherited disorder characterized by signs of radicular sensory loss in both the upper and lower extremities; shooting pains; chronic, indolent, trophic ulceration of the feet; and sometimes deafness. The pathologic findings are primary degeneration of the dorsal root ganglia together with evidence of degeneration of the olivary nuclei, optic nerves, and cerebellum. **periaxial n.**, segmental (demyelination) n. **progressive hypertrophic interstitial n.**, a condition characterized by hyperplasia of the interstitial connective tissue, causing thickening of peripheral nerve trunks and posterior roots, and by sclerosis of the posterior columns of the spinal cord. It is a slowly progressive familial disease beginning in early life, marked by atrophy of distal parts of the legs, and by diminution of tendon reflexes and of sensation. Called also *Dejerine-Sottas disease* or *atrophy*, and *interstitial hypertrophic neuritis*. **segmental (demyelination) n.**, neuropathy in which there is loss of myelin segments; called also *periaxial n.* **serum n.**, **serum sickness n.**, a neurologic disorder, usually involving the cervical nerves or brachial plexus, occurring two to eight days after the injection of foreign protein, e.g., an antiserum or antitoxin of animal origin, and characterized by local pain followed by sensory disturbances and paralysis. Called also *serum neuritis*.

neuropeptide (nu″ro-pep′tīd) any of the molecules composed of short chains of amino acids (endorphins, enkephalins, vasopressin, etc.) found in brain tissue, often localized in axon terminals at synapses; they are classified as putative neurotransmitters, although some are also hormones.

neurophage (nu′ro-fāj) neuronophage.

neuropharmacological (nu″ro-fahr″mah-ko-loj′ĭ-k'l) pertaining to neuropharmacology.

neuropharmacology (nu″ro-fahr″mah-kol′o-je) that branch of pharmacology dealing especially with the action of drugs upon various parts and elements of the nervous system.

neurophilic (nu″ro-fil′ik) neurotropic.

neurophonia (nu″ro-fo′ne-ah) [*neuro-* + Gr. *phōnē* voice + *-ia*] a form of nervous disorder in which the patient utters peculiar cries, sometimes like those of certain animals.

neurophthalmology (noo″rof-thah-mol′o-je) neuro-ophthalmology.

neurophthisis (nu-rof′thĭ-sis) [*neuro-* + Gr. *phthisis* wasting] wasting of nerve tissue.

neurophysin (nu″ro-fi′sin) any of a group of soluble proteins (molecular weights 9500–10,500) secreted in the hypothalamus that serve as binding ("carrier") proteins for vasopressin and oxytocin and play a role in transport of these hormones in the hypothalamicohypophysial portal tract and their storage in the posterior pituitary.

neurophysiology (nu″ro-fiz″e-ol′o-je) [*neuro-* + *physiology*] the physiology of the nervous system.

neuropil (nu′ro-pīl) [*neuro-* + Gr. *pilos* felt] a dense feltwork of interwoven cytoplasmic processes of nerve cells (dendrites and axons) and of neuroglial cells in the central nervous system and in some parts of the peripheral nervous system.

neuropile (nu′ro-pīl) neuropil.

neuropilem (nu-ro-pi′lem) neuropil.

neuroplasm (nu′ro-plazm) [*neuro-* + Gr. *plasma* something formed] the undifferentiated basophilic protoplasm of a nerve cell.

neuroplasmic (nu″ro-plaz′mik) of or relating to neuroplasm.

neuroplasty (nu′ro-plas″te) [*neuro-* + Gr. *plassein* to form] plastic surgery of a nerve.

neuroplexus (nu″ro-plek′sus) a plexus of nerves.

neuropodia (nu″ro-po′de-ah) plural of *neuropodium*.

neuropodion (nu″ro-po′de-on) neuropodium.

neuropodium (nu″ro-po′de-um), pl. *neuropo′dia* [*neuro-* + Gr. *pous* foot] a bulbous termination of an axon in one type of synapse.

neuropore (nu′ro-pōr) [*neuro-* + Gr. *poros* pore]   the open anterior end (foramen anterius) or the open posterior end (foramen posterius) of the neural tube of the early embryo. These openings gradually close as the tube develops, the timing of each closure being so precise that they are used to define horizons XI and XII.   **anterior n.,** the embryonic opening in the anterior portion of the forebrain, which closes at the 20-somite stage, marking the end of Streeter's horizon XI.   **posterior n.,** the embryonic opening at the posterior end of the neural tube, which closes by about the 25-somite stage.

neuropotential (nu″ro-po-ten′shal)   nerve energy; nerve potential.

neuroprobasia (nu″ro-pro-ba′se-ah) [*neuro-* + Gr. *pro* forward + *basis* walking]   advance along the nerves; said of the action of certain viruses.

neuropsychiatrist (nu″ro-si-ki′ah-trist)   a physician who specializes in neuropsychiatry.

neuropsychiatry (nu″ro-si-ki′ah-tre)   the branch of medicine which includes both neurology and psychiatry.

neuropsychic (nu″ro-si′kik) [*neuro-* + Gr. *psychē* soul]   pertaining to the nerve center concerned in mental processes.

neuropsychopathy (nu″ro-si-kop′ah-the) [*neuro-* + Gr. *psychē* soul + *pathos* disease]   a disease condition of the nerves and mind.

neuropsychopharmacology   (nu″ro-si″ko-fahr″mah-kol′o-je)   psychopharmacology.

neuropsychosis (nu″ro-si-ko′sis) [*neuro-* + *psychosis*]   (*obs.*) psychosis.

neuroradiology (nu″ro-ra″de-ol′o-je)   radiology of the nervous system.

neurorecidive (nu″ro-res″ĭ-dēv′)   neurorelapse.

neurorecurrence (nu″ro-re-kur′ens)   neurorelapse.

neurorelapse (nu″ro-re-laps′)   a peculiar outburst of neurosyphilis precipitated by insufficient treatment with arsphenamine, and characterized by various nervous symptoms; called also *neurorecidive* and *neurorecurrence.*

neuroretinitis (nu″ro-ret″ĭ-ni′tis)   inflammation of the optic nerve and retina.

neuroretinopathy (nu″ro-ret″ĭ-nop′ah-the) [*neuro-* + *retina* + *-pathy*]   a disease of the optic disk and retina.   **hypertensive n.,** swelling of the optic disk and formation of serous and fibrinous precipitates in the retina, occurring in severe hypertension.

neuroroentgenography   (nu″ro-rent″gen-og′rah-fe)   neuroradiology.

neurorrhaphy (nu-ror′ah-fe) [*neuro-* + Gr. *rhaphē* stitch]   the suturing of a cut nerve.

neurosarcocleisis (nu″ro-sar″ko-kli′sis) [*neuro-* + Gr. *sarx* flesh + *kleisis* closure]   an operation performed for neuralgia, done by relieving pressure on the affected nerve by partial resection of the bony canal through which it passes, and transplanting the nerve into soft tissues.

neurosarcoma (nu″ro-sar-ko′mah)   a sarcoma with neuromatous elements.

neuroscience (nu″ro-si′ens)   any of the branches of science dealing with the embryology, anatomy, physiology, biochemistry, pharmacology, etc., of the nervous system.

neuroscientist (nu″ro-si′en-tist)   an expert in any of the branches of the neurosciences.

neurosclerosis (nu″ro-skle-ro′sis) [*neuro-* + Gr. *sklēros* hard]   the hardening of the substance of a nerve or nerve center.

neurosecretion (nu″ro-se-kre′shun) [*neuro-* + *secretion*]   1. the secretory activities of nerve cells, as the secretion of releasing hormones, vasopressin, neurotransmitters, etc.   2. the product of such activities; a neurosecretory substance.

neurosecretory (nu″ro-se-kre′to-re) [*neuro-* + *secretory*]   pertaining to neurosecretion.

neurosegmental (nu″ro-seg-men′tal) [*neuro-* + *segmental*]   of or pertaining to a pair of spinal dorsal and ventral roots or to the area which they supply.

neurosensory (nu″ro-sen′so-re)   pertaining to a sensory nerve.

neuroses (nu-ro′sēz)   plural of *neurosis.*

neurosis (nu-ro′sis), pl. *neuro′ses* [*neur-* + *-osis*]   1. a functional mental disorder in which reality testing is intact (as opposed to psychosis, in which reality testing is impaired) and ego-dystonic symptoms, such as obsessions, anxiety attacks, phobias, and somatoform conversion symptoms, are prominent.   2. in psychoanalytic theory, the specific etiological process that gives rise not only to neuroses as defined above but also to personality disorders (called character neuroses to emphasize this) and some psychotic disorders. Unconscious conflicts involving opposing wishes or forbidden infantile wishes give rise to an unconscious anticipation of danger (experienced as anxiety) in situations that activate a conflict, and anxiety serves as a signal to trigger unconscious defense mechanisms, the operation of which is visible to the conscious mind and to observers in the form of neurotic symptoms or pathological personality traits.   **actual n.** (*obs.*), Freud's term for a neurosis caused by sexual excitement without adequate gratification (in which he included neurasthenia and anxiety neurosis), as opposed to psychoneurosis (hysteria, obsessions, phobias) originating in childhood experiences.   **anxiety n.,** neurosis characterized by prominent anxiety, sometimes extending to panic and frequently associated with somatic symptoms, not associated with a specific object or activity (as in phobias).   **association n.** (*obs.*), a condition in which an abnormal mental experience tends to be reproduced, with all its original mental and physical phenomena, when an idea related to the original experience is brought into the mind.   **cardiac n.,** neurocirculatory asthenia.   **character n.,** character or personality disorder; see *neurosis.*   **combat n.,** a term applied to psychiatric combat casualties, especially to those with premorbid neurotic problems aggravated by combat stress. Cf. *combat fatigue.*   **compensation n.,** a factitious disorder in which neurotic symptoms are voluntarily produced in order to obtain insurance, pension, or other monetary compensation.   **compulsion n.,** neurosis marked by compulsions: obsessive-compulsive disorder.   **conversion n.,** see under *disorder.*   **depersonalization n.,** see under *disorder.*   **depressive n.,** dysthymia.   **experimental n.,** a state produced in an experimental animal, usually by exposure to frustration or conflict, that resembles human neuroses.   **hypochondriacal n.,** hypochondriasis.   **hysterical n.,** hysteria considered as a neurosis; see *hysteria* and *conversion disorder* (hysterical neurosis, conversion type), *dissociative disorders* (hysterical neurosis, dissociative type), and *somatization disorder,* under *disorder.*   **neurasthenic n.,** neurasthenia.   **obsessional n.,** neurosis marked by obsessions; obsessive-compulsive disorder.   **obsessive-compulsive n.,** see under *disorder.*   **occupational n.,** (*obs.*), a psychogenic inhibition or symptom that interferes with work.   **pension n.,** compensation n.   **phobic n.,** see *phobia.*   **transference n.,** a phenomenon, occurring in most psychoanalyses, in which the patient undergoes, with the analyst as the object, an intense repetition of childhood conflicts, reexperiencing impulses, feelings, and fantasies that originally developed in relation to the parents.   **traumatic n.,** (*obs.*), neurosis resulting from physical or psychological trauma.   **vegetative n.,** acrodynia.   **war n.,** a general term applied to psychiatric disabilities developing during service in a war zone.

neuroskeletal (nu″ro-skel′ĕ-tal)   pertaining to the nervous tissues and the skeletal muscular tissue.

neuroskeleton (nu″ro-skel′ĕ-ton) [*neuro-* + Gr. *skeleton* skeleton]   endoskeleton.

neurosome (nu′ro-sōm) [*neuro-* + Gr. *sōma* body]   1. the body of a nerve cell.   2. any of a set of minute particles in the ground substance of the protoplasm of the neurons.

neurospasm (nu′ro-spazm) [*neuro-* + Gr. *spasmos* spasm]   the nervous twitching of a muscle.

neurosplanchnic (nu″ro-splangk′nik)   pertaining to the cerebrospinal and sympathetic nervous systems; neurovisceral.

neurospongioma (nu″ro-spon″je-o′mah)   glioma.

neurospongium (nu″ro-spon″je-um) [*neuro-* + Gr. *spongos* sponge]   1. the fibrillar component of neurons.   2. a meshwork of nerve fibers, especially the inner reticular layer of the retina.

Neurospora (nu-ros′po-rah)   a genus of ascomycetous fungi (family Sordariaceae, order Sphaeriales) comprising the bread molds, which are capable of converting tryptophan to nicotinic acid, and are extensively used in genetic and enzyme research.

neurostatus (nu″ro-sta′tus) the state or condition of neural symptoms in a case history.

neurosthenia (nu″ro-sthe′ne-ah) [*neuro-* + Gr. *sthenos* strength + *-ia*] (*obs.*) excessive nervous energy and excitement.

neurosurgeon (nu″ro-sur′jun) a physician who specializes in neurosurgery.

neurosurgery (nu″ro-sur′jer-e) surgery of the nervous system. **functional n.,** that designed (*a*) to restore normal conductivity in malfunctional nerve fibers or to improve blood flow in nerve tissue, or (*b*) to alleviate mental illness.

neurosuture (nu″ro-su′tūr) neurorrhaphy.

neurosyphilis (noo″ro-sif′ĭ-lus) [*neuro-* + *syphilis*] the central nervous system manifestations of tertiary syphilis, which may be divided into two groups: asymptomatic and symptomatic; the latter includes meningovascular and parenchymatous neurosyphilis (see *general paresis,* under *paresis,* and *tabes dorsalis*). **asymptomatic n.,** neurosyphilis diagnosed when there is a positive VDRL test in the cerebrospinal fluid in the absence of the signs and symptoms of neurologic disease. **meningovascular n.,** neurosyphilis characterized by focal or widespread cerebrovascular disease; the former commonly produces hemiplegia or selective neuropathy, and the latter severe headache, mental changes, and convulsions. Called also *meningovascular syphilis.* **parenchymatous s.,** a form in which there is widespread parenchymal damage; called also *parenchymatous syphilis.* See *general paresis,* under *paresis,* and *tabes dorsalis.* **paretic n.,** general paresis. **tabetic n.,** tabes dorsalis.

neurotagma (nu″ro-tag′mah) [*neuro-* + Gr. *tagma* arrangement] a linear arrangement of the structural elements of a nerve cell.

neurotendinous (nu″ro-ten′dĭ-nus) pertaining to both nerve and tendon.

neurotensin (nu″ro-ten′sin) a tridecapeptide first isolated from the bovine hypothalamus that induces vasodilatation and hypotension; it is present in the intestine and brain of man and is postulated to be a neurotransmitter.

neuroterminal (nu″ro-ter′mĭ-nal) an end organ of a peripheral nerve.

neurothele (nu″ro-the′le) [*neuro-* + Gr. *thele* nipple] a sensory papilla of the corium.

neurotic (nu-rot′ik) 1. pertaining to or characterized by neurosis. 2. a person affected with a neurosis.

neuroticism (nu-rot′ĭ-sizm) neurosis; the condition of being neurotic.

neurotigenic (nu-rot″ĭ-jen′ik) producing a neurosis.

neurotization (nu″rot-ĭ-za′shun) the regeneration of a nerve after its division.

neurotmesis (nu″rot-me′sis) [*neuro-* + Gr. *tmēsis* cutting apart] partial or complete severance of a nerve, with disruption of the axon and its myelin sheath and the connective tissue elements; regeneration does not occur. Cf. *axonotmesis* and *neurapraxia.*

neurotology (nu″ro-tol′o-je) neuro-otology.

neurotome (nu′ro-tōm) [*neuro-* + Gr. *tomē* a cut] 1. a needle-like knife for dissecting the nerves. 2. neuromere (def. 2).

neurotomography (nu″ro-to-mog′rah-fe) tomography of the central nervous system.

neurotomy (nu-rot′o-me) [*neuro-* + Gr. *temnein* to cut] 1. the dissection or anatomy of the nerves. 2. the surgical cutting of a nerve. **radiofrequency n.,** interruption of spinal nerve roots by coagulation with radiofrequency waves. **retrogasserian n.,** see under *rhizotomy.*

neurotonia (nu″ro-to′ne-ah) instability of tonus of the vegetative nervous system.

neurotonic (nu″ro-ton′ik) [*neuro-* + *tonic*] having a tonic effect upon the nerves.

neurotony (nu-rot′o-ne) [*neuro-* + Gr. *teinein* to stretch] the stretching of a nerve, chiefly to relieve pain; called also *nerve stretching.*

neurotoxic (nu″ro-tok′sik) poisonous or destructive to nerve tissue.

neurotoxicity (nu″ro-tok-sis′ĭ-te) the quality of exerting a destructive or poisonous effect upon nerve tissue.

neurotoxin (nu″ro-tok′sin) a toxin that is poisonous to or destroys nerve tissue, especially the exotoxins secreted by *Clostridium botulinum, C. tetani, Corynebacterium diphtheriae,* and *Shigella dysenteriae.*

neurotransducer (nu″ro-trans-du′ser) a neuron that synthesizes and releases hormones which serve as the functional link between the nervous system and the pituitary gland.

neurotransmission (nu″ro-trans-mish′un) the process by which a neurotransmitter is released, crosses the synapse, and affects the action of the target cell.

neurotransmitter (nu″ro-trans′mit-er) any of a group of substances that are released on excitation from the axon terminal of a presynaptic neuron of the central or peripheral nervous system and travel across the synaptic cleft to either excite or inhibit the target cell. Among the many substances that have the properties of a neurotransmitter are acetylcholine, norepinephrine, epinephrine, dopamine, glycine, γ-aminobutyrate, glutamic acid, substance P, enkephalins, endorphins, and serotonin. **false n.,** an amine, e.g., octopamine, that can be stored in and released from presynaptic vesicles but that has little effect on postsynaptic receptors.

neurotrauma (nu″ro-traw′mah) [*neuro-* + *trauma*] mechanical injury of a nerve.

neurotrophasthenia (nu″ro-tro″fas-the′ne-ah) [*neuro-* + Gr. *trophē* nutrition + *astheneia* weakness] defective nutrition of the nervous system.

neurotrophic (nu″ro-trof′ik) pertaining to neurotrophy.

neurotrophy (nu-rot′ro-fe) [*neuro-* + Gr. *trophē* nutrition] the nutrition and maintenance of tissues as regulated by nervous influence.

neurotropic (nu″ro-trop′ik) having a selective affinity for nervous tissue, or exerting its principal effect on the nervous system; polioclastic; polioencephalotropic.

neurotropism (nu-rot′ro-pizm) [*neuro-* + Gr. *tropē* a turn, turning] 1. the quality of having a special affinity for nervous tissue. 2. the alleged tendency of regenerating nerve fibers to grow toward specific portions of the periphery.

neurotropy (nu-rot′ro-pe) neurotropism.

neurotrosis (nu″ro-tro′sis) [*neuro-* + Gr. *trōsis* wound] neurotrauma.

neurotubule (nu″ro-too′būl) [*neuro-* + *tubule*] any of the long, straight, parallel tubules within neurons, which along with the neurofilaments, form neurofibrils; they seem to correspond to the microtubules occurring in many cells outside the nervous system.

neurovaccine (nu″ro-vak′sin) vaccine virus prepared by growing the virus in the brain of a rabbit.

neurovaricosis (nu″ro-var″ĭ-ko′sis) [*neuro-* + *varicose* + *-osis*] a varicose state of the fibers of a nerve.

neurovariola (nu″ro-vah-ri′o-lah) neurovaccine.

neurovascular (nu″ro-vas′ku-lar) pertaining to both nervous and vascular elements; pertaining to the nerves that control the caliber of blood vessels.

neurovegetative (nu″ro-vej′ĕ-ta″tiv) pertaining to the vegetative (autonomic) nervous system.

neurovirulence (nu″ro-vir′u-lens) the competence of an infectious agent to produce pathologic effects on the nervous system.

neurovirulent (nu″ro-vir′u-lent) capable of producing pathologic effects on the nervous system.

neurovirus (nu″ro-vi′rus) a vaccine virus which has been modified by passing into nervous tissue.

neurovisceral (nu″ro-vis′er-al) neurosplanchnic.

neurula (nu′roo-lah) [*neuro-* + dim. *-ula*] the early embryo during the development of the neural tube from the neural plate, marking the first appearance of the nervous system; the next stage after the gastrula, and occurring 19 to 26 days after fertilization.

neurulation (nu″roo-la′shun) formation, in the early embryo, of the neural plate, followed by its closure with development of the neural tube.

neururgic (nu-rer′jik) [*neuro-* + Gr. *ergon* work] pertaining to nerve action.

Neusser's granules (noi′serz) [Edmund von *Neusser,* Austrian physician, 1852–1912] see under *granule.*

neutral (nu′tral) [L. *neutralis; neuter,* neither] in chemistry, neither acid nor basic.

neutralism (nu′tral-izm) the absence of interaction between coexisting organisms of different species.

neutrality (nu-tral′ĭ-te) the state of being neutral.

neutralization (nu″tral-ĭ-za′shun) the act or process of rendering neutral. **viral n.,** the process by which antibody alone or antibody plus complement neutralizes the infectivity of a virus. The antibody may coat the virus forming a stable complex or may cause conformational changes in viral structural proteins on binding; either process may interfere with binding of the virion to cellular receptor sites and entry into the cell. Enveloped viruses may be lysed by complement.

neutralize (nu′tral-īz) to render neutral.

neutramycin (nu-trah-mi′sin) an antibacterial substance produced by *Streptomyces rimosus.*

Neutrapen (nu′trah-pen) trademark for a lyophilized preparation of penicillinase.

Neutra-Phos-K (nu″trah-fos′ka) trademark for a preparation of potassium phosphate.

neutrino (nu-tre′no) an elementary (subatomic) particle that has no electric charge and no rest mass, and that very rarely reacts with matter; it is a product of beta decay.

neutroclusion (nu″trŏ-kloo′zhun) malocclusion characterized by irregularities of individual teeth, but with normal mesiodistal or normal anteroposterior relation of the mandibular to the maxillary dental arch. Generally regarded as identical with class I in Angle's classification of malocclusion.

neutrocyte (nu′tro-sīt) a neutrophilic leukocyte; see *neutrophil,* def. 1.

neutrocytopenia (nu″tro-si″to-pe′ne-ah) neutropenia.

neutrocytosis (nu″tro-si-to′sis) neutrophilia.

neutroflavine (nu″tro-fla′vin) acriflavine.

neutron (nu′tron) an electrically neutral or uncharged particle of matter existing along with protons in the atoms of all elements except the mass 1 isotope of hydrogen. **epithermal n.,** a neutron having an energy level of a few hundredths electron volt to 100 electron volts. **fast n.,** a neutron having an energy level exceeding 10^5 electron volts. **intermediate n.,** a neutron having an energy level of 100 to 100,000 electron volts. **slow n.,** 1. thermal n. 2. any neutron having an energy level up to 100 electron volts. **thermal n.,** a neutron having an energy level of about 0.025 electron volt; called also *slow n.*

neutropenia (nu″tro-pe′ne-ah) [*neutrophil* + Gr. *penia* poverty] a decrease in the number of neutrophilic leukocytes in the blood; see *agranulocytosis.* **chronic benign n. of childhood,** a condition observed in children in which granulocytopenia and, often, recurrent infections may be present for a considerable time, with subsequent spontaneous remission. **chronic hypoplastic n.,** a syndrome of extreme chronicity, repeated infections of skin and oral cavity, moderate splenomegaly, and bone marrow markedly deficient in granulocyte precursors. **congenital n.,** a condition occurring in infants, characterized by absence of neutrophils from the peripheral blood; called also *congenital aleukia* and *congenital leukopenia.* **cyclic n.,** periodic n. **familial benign chronic n.,** a familial type of peripheral neutropenia, probably transmitted by an autosomal dominant gene. **hypersplenic n.,** primary splenic n. **idiopathic n.,** agranulocytosis. **Kostmann n.,** a severe congenital condition of virtual absence of neutrophils from the blood; most patients die of infection before reaching adulthood. **malignant n.,** idiopathic n. **neonatal n., transitory,** a short-lived neutropenia, observed in the newborn, which may be of the isoimmune type. **periodic n.,** a chronic form of neutropenia characterized by its regular recurrences in association with malaise, fever, stomatitis, and various types of infections. **peripheral n.,** decrease in the number of neutrophils in the circulating blood. **primary splenic n.,** a syndrome characterized by splenomegaly, profound leukopenia and neutropenia, susceptibility to infection, occasionally anemia and thrombocytopenia, and hypercellular bone marrow.

neutrophil (nu′tro-fil) [L. *neuter* neither + Gr. *philein* to love] 1. a granular leukocyte having a nucleus with three to five lobes connected by slender threads of chromatin, and cytoplasm containing fine inconspicuous granules; neutrophils have the properties of chemotaxis, adherence to immune complexes, and phagocytosis; called also *polymorphonuclear, polynuclear,* or *neutrophilic leukocytes.* Their coun-

terparts in nonhuman mammals are heterophils. 2. any cell, structure, or histologic element readily stainable by neutral dyes. **filamented n.,** a neutrophil having two or more lobes connected by a filament of chromatin. **giant n.,** macropolycyte. **juvenile n.,** a metamyelocyte. **nonfilamented n.,** a neutrophil whose lobes are connected by thick strands of chromatin. **rod n., stab n.,** a neutrophil whose nucleus is not divided into segments.

neutrophilia (nu″tro-fil′e-ah) increase in the number of neutrophils in the blood; it is the most common form of leukocytosis and may result from many causes, among them acute infections, intoxications, hemorrhage, and rapidly growing malignant neoplasms.

neutrophilic (nu″tro-fil′ik) 1. stainable by neutral dyes. 2. neither anthropophilic nor zoophilous; said of certain mosquitoes.

neutropism (nu′tro-pizm) neurotropism.

neutrotaxis (nu″tro-tak′sis) [*neutrophil* + Gr. *taxis* arrangement] the attractive or repellent influence exerted by neutrophilic leukocytes.

nevi (ne′vi) [L.] plural of *nevus.*

nev(o)- [L. *naevus* mole] a combining form denoting relationship to a nevus, or mole.

nevoblast (ne″vo-blast) [*nevo-* + *blast*] a neural crest–derived cell postulated to be the precursor of the nevus cell.

nevocyte (ne″vo-sit) [*nevo-* + *-cyte*] nevus cell.

nevocytic (ne-vo-sit′ik) pertaining to or composed of nevus cells.

nevoid (ne′void) resembling a nevus.

nevolipoma (ne″vo-lĭ-po′mah) [*nevo-* + *lipoma*] a nevus containing a large amount of fibrofatty tissue. Called also *fatty nevus* and *nevus lipomatosus.*

nevoxanthoendothelioma (ne″vo-zan″tho-en″do-the″le-o′mah) [*nevo-* + *xantho-* + *endothelioma*] juvenile xanthogranuloma.

Nevskia (nev′ske-ah) [*Neva,* a river in Russia] a genus of appendaged bacteria, made up of rod-shaped cells that produce slime stalks at right angles to the cell axis and aggregate in colonies on the surface of fresh waters. The type species is *N. ramo′sa.*

nevus (ne′vus), pl. *ne′vi* [L. *naevus*] 1. any congenital lesion of the skin; a birthmark. 2. a circumscribed stable malformation of the skin and occasionally of the oral mucosa, which is not due to external causes and therefore presumed to be of hereditary origin. The excess (or deficiency) of tissue may involve epidermal, connective tissue, adnexal, nervous, or vascular elements; a cutaneous hamartoma. **achromic n.,** n. depigmentosus. **amelanotic n.,** a nevocytic nevus that contains no pigment. Cf. *n. depigmentosus.* **n. ane′micus,** a congenital disorder typically characterized by the presence of pale, round, well-defined macules with irregular borders that may have a normal amount of melanin or may lack melanin but are not totally amelanotic. Studies suggest that the disorder is due to a functional incapacity of the blood vessels to dilate as a result of increased sensitivity to catecholamines. **n. araneus,** vascular spider. **bathing trunk n.,** see *giant congenital pigmented n.* **Becker's n.,** a nevus occurring mostly in males in the second to third decade of life consisting of epidermal melanosis, presenting as segmental, uniform, light hyperpigmentation, followed several years later by the growth of long dark hairs from the lesions; the lesions usually have the same pattern of distribution as those of the nevus unius lateris (q.v.). Called also *n. spilus tardus* and *pigmented hairy epidermal n.* **blue n.,** a benign nevus, usually solitary, representing a localized proliferation of dermal melanocytes, which is manifested by a dark blue to black, moderately firm, rounded, sharply defined nodular tumor composed of spindle-shaped melanocytes with slender cytoplasmic processes, occurring often in association with melanin-laden macrophages in a sclerotic dermis. Called also *dermal melanocytoma* and *Jadassohn-Tieche n.* Cf. *cellular blue n.* **blue rubber bleb n.,** a type of congenital nevus, transmitted as an autosomal dominant trait, characterized by the presence of bluish hemangiomas with soft elevated nipple-like centers on the cutaneous surface and similar lesions scattered throughout the gastrointestinal tract and sometimes on the mucous membranes, and sometimes associated with pain, regional hyperhidrosis, and gastrointestinal bleeding. **cellular n.,** nevocytic nevus. **cellular blue n.,** a large blue or blue-black, multilobulated, well-circumscribed nodular tumor, usually congenital, having a tendency to occur on the buttocks and sacrococcygeal region. It is characterized histologically by deeply pigmented, dendritic, spindle-shaped melanocytes alternating with cellular islands of spindle cells with ovoid nuclei and abundant pale cytoplasm in the dermis and subcutaneous. These nevi have a low incidence of malignant transformation to melanoma, in which case they show cellular pleomorphism, mitotic figures, and evidence of invasion into the deep dermis. Called also *dermal melanocytoma.* Cf. *blue n.* **chromatophore n. of Naegeli,** Franceschetti-Jadassohn syndrome. **n. comedon′icus,** a rare epidermal nevus thought to represent a developmental abnormality of the pilosebaceous apparatus, characterized by the presence of aggregations of dilated keratin-filled hair follicles, producing large cutaneous patches studded with comedo-like lesions that are usually unilateral and generally localized to areas such as the trunk, an upper extremity, or the neck, sometimes in a linear or zosteriform pattern. The condition is occasionally associated with other lesions such as ichthyosis, nevoid cell carcinoma, vascular nevi, and cataracts. **compound n.,** a nevocytic nevus composed of fully formed nests of nevus cells in the epidermis as well as newly forming ones in the dermis. Cf. *intradermal n.* and *junction n.* **connective tissue n.,** any of a group of variable-appearing hamartomas involving various components of the connective tissue, usually present at birth or soon thereafter, which may be inherited or acquired, and may be associated with other diseases. They may present clinically as single or multiple nodules, papules, or plaques, or in various combinations of these lesions, but individual lesions usually appear as a plaque composed of firm, flat, closely set, white to ivory or yellow-brown papules, often having a cobblestonelike surface. Called also *juvenile elastoma, n. elasticus,* and *n. elasticus of Lewandowsky.* **n. depigmento′sus,** a developmental anomaly of melanization producing long bands or streaks of hypopigmentation on the skin, especially on the trunk and extremities, usually unilaterally. Called also *achromic n.* Cf. *amelanotic n.* **dermal n.,** intradermal n. **dysplastic n.,** an acquired atypical nevus with an irregular border, indistinct margin, and mixed coloration, often occurring in large numbers, that is characterized by intraepidermal melanocytic dysplasia and often is a precursor of malignant melanoma. **n. elas′ticus,** 1. pseudoxanthoma elasticum. 2. connective tissue n. **n. elas′ticus of Lewandowsky,** connective tissue n. **epidermal n., epithelial n.,** a circumscribed congenital developmental anomaly resulting in faulty production of mature or nearly mature cutaneous structures, occurring as a result of overproduction of surface or adnexal epithelium. Such nevi vary widely in presentation and are commonly hyperkeratotic. **fatty n.,** nevolipoma. **n. flam′meus,** a common congenital vascular malformation involving mature capillaries, presenting as a sharply demarcated, flat, irregularly shaped patch, ranging in color from faint pink to orange (*salmon patch*) to dark red–purple (*port-wine stain*), and usually found on the face and neck. The paler varieties tend to involute during childhood, while the darker ones usually are persistent. See also *capillary hemangioma* (def. 1), under *hemangioma,* and *vascular nevus,* under *nevus.* **n. fuscoceru′leus acromiodeltoi′deus,** n. of

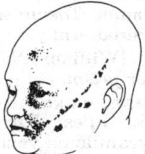

Nevus flammeus.

Ito. **n. fuscoceru′leus ophthalmomaxilla′ris,** n. of Ota. **giant congenital pigmented n., giant hairy n., giant pigmented n.,** any of a group of large darkly pigmented hairy nevi, present at birth, usually bilaterally symmetric, and having a predilection for the chest, upper back, and shoulders; the area usually covered by bathing trunks; and distal upper and lower extremities. These nevi have been shown to be associated with other cutaneous and subcutaneous lesions, neurofibromatosis and other developmental anomalies, and leptomeningeal melanocytosis, and they also exhibit a predisposition to the development of

malignant melanoma. **halo n.,** a pigmented lesion (usually a compound or intradermal nevocytic nevus but sometimes a neuronevus, blue nevus, or malignant melanoma) surrounded by an annular depigmented area. Called also *leukoderma acquisitum centrifugum, Sutton's disease,* and *Sutton's n.* **hepatic n.,** hemorrhagic infarct of the liver. **intradermal n.,** a nevocytic nevus, clinically indistinguishable from compound nevus, in which the nests of nevus cells lie exclusively within the dermis. Called also *dermal n.* Cf. *compound n.* and *junction n.* **n. of Ito,** a mongolian spot–like lesion having the same features as nevus of Ota except for localization to the areas of distribution of the posterior supraclavicular and lateral cutaneous brachial nerves, to involve the shoulder, side of the neck, supraclavicular areas, and upper arm. Called also *n. fusceruleus acromiodeltoideus.* **Jadassohn-Tièche n.,** blue n. **junction n., junctional n.,** a nevocytic nevus in which the nests of nevus cells are confined to the dermoepidermal junction, which usually presents clinically as a small, discrete flat or slightly raised macule. Cf. *compound n.* and *intradermal n.* **n. lipomato′sus,** nevolipoma. **l. lipomato′sus cuta′neus superficia′lis,** a connective tissue nevus, usually congenital, characterized histologically by the presence of ectopic, mature adipocytes in the dermis, and clinically by multiple or single soft, skin-colored to yellowish papules, nodules, and plaques, usually located on the lower trunk, gluteal region, or thigh. **melanocytic n.,** a usually pigmented nevus, acquired or hereditary, caused by a disorder of melanocytes. **neural n., neuroid n.,** neuronevus. **nevocellular n.,** nevocytic n. **nevocytic n., nevus cell n.,** an acquired or inherited tumor composed of nests (*theques*) of nevus cells, usually presenting as tan to deep brown small macules or papules with well-defined, rounded borders, although the clinical appearance is quite variable. Based on the histologic pattern and location of the nevus cells, these nevi are classified as compound, intradermal, and junction. Called also *cellular n.* and *nevocellular n.* **nuchal n.,** nevus flammeus situated on either side of the posterior midline between the occipital protuberance and the tip of the spine of the fifth cervical vertebra, with the long axis up and down. Called also *Unna's n.* **n. of Ota, Ota's n.,** a persistent mongolian spot–like lesion, usually present at birth, involving the conjunctiva and skin about the eye supplied by the first and second branches of the trigeminal nerve as well as the sclera, ocular muscles, retrobulbar fat, periosteum, and buccal mucosa, usually unilaterally. The skin lesions are manifested as macular bluish or gray-brown patchy areas of pigmentation that grow slowly and become deeper in color. Called also *oculodermal melanocytosis* and *n. fusceruleus ophthalmomaxillaris.* **pigmented n., n. pigmento′sus,** a nevus containing melanin; the term is usually restricted to nevocytic nevi, or moles, but may be applied to other pigmented nevi, e.g., nevus spilus and Becker's nevus. **pigmented hairy epidermal n.,** Becker's n. **port-wine n.,** see under *stain.* **sebaceous n., n. seba′ceus, n. seba′ceus of Jadassohn,** a hamartoma occurring as a solitary lesion on the scalp and, less often, the face, persisting throughout life and characterized by progressive clinical and histological changes with age. It presents in children as a yellowish to pale brown, waxy-appearing patch, which is alopecic when on the scalp, with a relatively smooth surface, and is associated with hypoplastic sebaceous glands and hair follicles. After puberty, the lesion becomes thickened and verrucous, often with closely set papillomatous projections, and is associated with abundant and hyperplastic sebaceous glands, some of which open directly to the surface, a papillary epidermal hyperplasia, and ectopic apocrine glands in the deep dermis. In later life, some lesions develop new nodular proliferations, which have a tendency for the development of other adnexal tumors, both benign and malignant, and basal cell carcinoma. **spider n.,** vascular spider. **n. spi′lus,** a smooth-surfaced, tan to brown, macular, epidermal, melanocytic nevus, which is speckled with smaller, darker macules. **n. spi′lus tar′dus,** Becker's n. **spindle and epithelioid cell n.,** a benign compound nevus occurring most often in children before puberty, composed of spindle and epithelioid cells located mainly in the dermis, sometimes in association with large atypical cells and multinucleate cells, and having a close histopathological resemblance to malignant melanoma. The tumor presents as a smooth to slightly scaly, round to oval, raised, firm papule or nodule, ranging in color from pink-tan to purplish red, often with surface telangiectasia. Called also *benign juvenile melanoma, compound melanocytoma, juvenile melanoma,* and *Spitz n.* **Spitz n.,** spindle and epithelioid cell n. **n. spongio′sus al′bus muco′sae,** white sponge n. **stellar n.,** vascular spider. **strawberry n.,** 1. see under *hemangioma,* def. 1. 2. vascular n. 3. cavernous hemangioma. **Sutton's n.,** halo n. **n. uni′us lat′eris,** a verrucous epidermal nevus, ranging from flesh-colored to yellowish brown, but sometimes more deeply pigmented, and occurring in a linear, unilaterally distributed pattern; on the extremities, the lesions usually follow the long axis and may be arranged in continuous or broken spiral streaks, bands, or patches, and on the trunk, they usually have a transverse orientation, as if along the distribution of the intercostal nerves. **Unna's n.,** nuchal n. **vascular n., n. vascula′ris, n. vasculo′sus,** a localized overgrowth of blood vessels characterized by areas of flat or elevated erythema of various sizes resulting from an overgrowth of dilated but otherwise normal thin-walled vessels. According to one classification, nonacquired vascular spider, nevus flammeus, strawberry hemangioma, cavernous hemangioma, and lymphangioma circumscriptum are all types of vascular nevi. Called also *strawberry hemangioma* or *mark* and strawberry n. Cf. *capillary hemangioma,* def. 1. **white sponge n.,** a benign, congenital, autosomal dominant disorder, in which there is an exuberant, extensive, and spongy whiteness of the mucus membranes, especially of the oral mucosa, which produces gray-white, soft, and sometimes friable lesions with fissures and folds; it reaches maximal severity at adolescence or early adulthood without further progression. Called also *familial white folded mucosal dysplasia* and *n. spongiosus albus mucosae.*

newborn (nu′born) 1. recently born. 2. a recently born infant.

Newcastle disease (nu′kas-el) [*Newcastle,* a seaport on the Tyne River in Northeast England] see under *disease.*

newton (nu′ton) [Sir Isaac *Newton,* English mathematician, physicist, and astronomer, 1643–1727] the SI unit of force which, when applied in a vacuum to a body having a mass of one kilogram, accelerates it at the rate of one meter per second. Symbol, N.

Newton's law, rings (nu′tonz) [Sir Isaac *Newton,* English mathematician, physicist, and astronomer, 1643–1727] see under *law* and *ring.*

nexeridine hydrochloride (nek-ser′ĭ-dēn) chemical name: 1-[2-(dimethylamino)-1-methylethyl]-2-phenylcyclohexanol acetate (ester) hydrochloride; an analgesic, $C_{19}H_{29}NO_2 \cdot HCl$.

nexin (neks′in) a substance which serves as a connecting link between the outer pairs of microtubules in cilia and flagella.

nexus (nek′sus), pl. *nex′us* [L. "bond"] 1. a bond, especially one between members of a series or group. 2. gap junction.

Nezelof's syndrome (nez′ĕ-lofs) [C. *Nezelof,* French pediatrician, born 1922] see under *syndrome.*

NF National Formulary.

N.F.L.P.N. National Federation for Licensed Practical Nurses.

ng. nanogram.

NGF nerve growth factor.

NH₃ ammonia.

NH₄Br ammonium bromide.

N.H.C. National Health Council.

NH₄Cl ammonium chloride.

NH₄CNO ammonium cyanate.

(NH₂)₂CO urea.

(NH₄)₂CO₃ ammonium carbonate.

(NH₄)HS ammonium hydrosulfide.

N.H.L.I. National Heart and Lung Institute.

N.H.M.R.C. National Health and Medical Research Council.

NH₄NO₃ ammonium nitrate.

NH₄O·CO·NH₂ ammonium carbamate.

N.H.S. National Health Service (British).

(NH₄)₂·SO₂ ammonium sulfate.

NH₂-terminal (ter′min-al) N-terminal.

Ni chemical symbol for *nickel.*

niacin (ni′ah-sin) [USP] nicotinic acid, a B complex vitamin that is a constituent of the redox coenzymes nicotinamide adenine dinucleotide (NAD) and nicotinamide adenine dinucleotide phosphate (NADP). Niacin and niacinamide are used for the prophylaxis and treatment of pellagra. Niacin, but not niacinamide, also acts as a vasodilator and to reduce plasma cholesterol and has been used for these effects.

niacinamide (ni″ah-sin′ah-mīd) [USP] nicotinamide, a B complex vitamin used in the prophylaxis and treatment of pellagra.

NIAID National Institute of Allergy and Infectious Diseases.

nialamide (ni-al′ah-mīd) chemical name: 4-pyridinecarboxylic acid 2-[3-oxo-3-[(phenylmethyl)amino]propyl]hydrazide. A monoamine oxidase inhibitor, $C_{16}H_{18}N_4O_2$, occurring as a white, crystalline powder; it has been used orally as an antidepressant.

NIAMD National Institute of Arthritis and Metabolic Diseases.

Niamid (ni′ah-mid) trademark for a preparation of nialamide.

nib (nib) the working part of a dental condenser, which corresponds to the blade in an excavating or cutting instrument. Called also *condenser point.*

nibroxane (ni-broks′ān) chemical name: 5-bromo-2-methyl-5-nitro-1,3-dioxane; a topical antimicrobial, $C_5H_8BrNO_4$.

Nicalex (nik′ah-leks) trademark for a preparation of aluminum nicotinate.

niccolum (nik′o-lum), gen. *nic′coli* [L.] nickel.

nicergoline (ni-ser′go-lēn) chemical name: 10-methoxy-1,6-dimethylergoline-8β-methanol 5-bromo-3-pyridinecarboxylate (ester); a vasodilator, $C_{24}H_{26}BrN_3O_3$.

niche (nich) [Fr. "recess"] a defect in an otherwise even surface, especially a depression or recess in the wall of a hollow organ as seen on a roentgenogram, or such a depression in an organ visible to the naked eye. **Barclay's n.,** a deformity of the duodenal cap in a duodenal ulcer, seen as a projection on the radiogram. **ecologic n.,** the place of an organism within its community or ecosystem. **enamel n.,** either of two depressions between the lateral dental lamina and the developing tooth germ, one pointing distally (*distal enamel n.*) and the other mesially (*mesial enamel n.*). **Haudek's n.,** see under *sign.* **n. of round window,** fossula fenestrae cochleae.

NICHHD National Institute of Child Health and Human Development.

nickel (nik′el) [L. *niccolum*] a silver-white metallic element: symbol, Ni; specific gravity, 8.9; atomic number, 28; atomic weight, 58.71. **n. carbonyl,** a volatile liquid, Ni(CO)₄, used in industry, which may produce serious pulmonary edema and dyspnea.

nicking (nik′ing) localized constrictions in the retinal blood vessels seen in arterial hypertension.

niclosamide (nĭ-klo′sah-mīd) chemical name: 5-chloro-N-(2-chloro-4-nitrophenyl)-2-hydroxybenzamide. An anthelmintic, $C_{13}H_8Cl_2N_2O_4$, occurring as a pale yellow, crystalline powder, effective against the tapeworms *Diphyllobothrium latum, Hymenolepsis nana, Taenia saginata,* and the adults of *T. solium;* administered orally.

Nicol prism (nik′ol) [William *Nicol,* Scottish physicist, 1768–1851] see under *prism.*

Nicolas-Favre disease (ne-ko-lah fav′r) [Joseph *Nicolas,* born 1868; Maurice Jules *Favre,* French physician, 1876–1954] lymphogranuloma venereum.

Nicolle (ne-kol′) Charles Jules Henri. French physician and microbiologist, 1866–1936; winner of the Nobel prize for medicine or physiology in 1928 for his demonstration of the transmission of typhus by the body louse.

Niconyl (ni′ko-nil) trademark for a preparation of isoniazid.

Nicorette (nik′o-ret″) trademark for a chewing gum containing nicotine polacrilex.

Nicotiana (nik″o-she-a′nah) [Jean *Nicot* de Villemain, 1530–1600, who introduced tobacco chewing to Catherine de Medici] a genus of solanaceous annual plants, native to tropical America, from which tobacco is derived, mainly from *N. tabacum* L. and its varieties.

nicotinamide (nik″o-tin′ah-mīd) niacinamide. **n. adenine dinucleotide (NAD),** a coenzyme composed of ribosylnicotinamide 5′-phosphate (NMN) coupled to adenosine 5′-phosphate (AMP) by pyrophosphate linkage. It is found widely in nature and is involved in numerous enzymatic reactions in which it serves as an electron carrier by being alternately oxidized (NAD⁺) and reduced (NADH). Formerly called also *coenzyme I* (*CoI*) and *diphosphopyridine nucleotide* (*DPN*). **n. adenine dinucleotide phosphate (NADP),** a coenzyme composed of ribosylnicotinamide 5′-phosphate (NMN) coupled by pyrophosphate linkage to the 5′-phosphate adenosine 2′,5′-bisphosphate. It serves as an electron carrier in a number of reactions, being alternately oxidized (NADP⁺) and reduced (NADPH). Formerly called also *coenzyme II* and *triphosphopyridine nucleotide* (*TPN*). **n. mononucleotide (NMN),** ribosylnicotinamide 5′-phosphate; a nucleotide containing covalently linked nicotinamide and ribose 5-phosphate. It is a constituent of NAD and NADP.

nicotine (nik′o-tēn, nik′o-tin) [L. *nicotiana* tobacco] chemical name: β-pyridyl-α-N-methylpyrrolidine. A very poisonous colorless, soluble fluid alkaloid, $C_{10}H_{14}N_2$, with a pyridine-like odor and a burning taste, obtained from tobacco or produced synthetically. It is used as an agricultural insecticide and, in veterinary medicine, as an external parasiticide and is used in pharmacological and physiological studies for its neurological effects (see *nicotinic*). **n. polacrilex,** nicotine bound to an ion exchange resin; used in nicotine chewing gum as an aid to smoking cessation.

nicotinic (nik″o-tin′ik) denoting the effect of nicotine and other drugs in initially stimulating and subsequently, in high doses, inhibiting neural impulses at autonomic ganglia and the neuromuscular junction.

nicotinic acid (nik″o-tin′ik) niacin.

nicotinism (nik′o-tin-izm″) poisoning by nicotine, characterized by stimulation and subsequent depression of the central and autonomic nervous systems, with death due to respiratory paralysis.

nicotinolytic (nik″o-tin-o-lit′ik) [*nicotine* + Gr. *lysis* dissolution] destroying or suppressing the toxic action of nicotine.

β-nicotyrine (nik-o′ti-rin) chemical name: 3-(1-methyl-2-pyrryl)pyridine. An alkaloid, $C_{10}H_{10}N_2$, from tobacco, which occurs as an oily liquid with a characteristic odor, and has insecticidal properties.

nicoumalone (ni-koo′mah-lōn) acenocoumarin.

Nicozide (nik′o-zīd) trademark for preparations of isoniazid.

nictation (nik-ta′shun) nictitation.

nictitation (nik″tĭ-ta′shun) [L. *nictitare* to wink] the act of winking.

nidal (ni′dal) pertaining to a nidus.

nidation (ni-da′shun) [L. *nidus* nest] implantation of the conceptus in the endometrium.

NIDD non–insulin-dependent diabetes.

nidi (ni′di) [L.] plural of *nidus*.

NIDR National Institute of Dental Research.

nidus (ni′dus), pl. *ni′di* [L. "nest"] 1. the point of origin or focus of a morbid process. 2. nucleus, def. 2. **n. a′vis,** a depression in the cerebellum between the posterior velum and the uvula, the location of the tonsil of the cerebellum. **n. hirun′dinis,** n. avis.

Niemann's disease (splenomegaly) (ne′man) [Albert *Niemann*, German pediatrician, 1880–1921] Niemann-Pick disease.

Niewenglowski's ray (nya-ven-glov′ske) [Gaston Henri *Niewenglowski*, French scientist, 19th century] see under *ray*.

nifedipine (ni-fed′ĭ-pēn) chemical name: 1,4-dihydro-2,6-dimethyl-4-(2-nitrophenyl)pyridinedicarboxylic acid dimethyl ester. A coronary vasodilator, $C_{17}H_{18}N_2O_6$, used in the treatment of coronary insufficiency and angina of effort.

nifungin (ni-fun′jin) an antifungal polypeptide derived from *Aspergillus giganteus*.

nifuradene (ni-fūr′ah-dēn) chemical name: 1-[[(5-nitro-2-furanyl)methylene]amino]-2-imidazolidinone; an antibacterial, $C_8H_8N_4O_4$.

nifuraldezone (ni-fūr-al′de-zōn) chemical name: 5-nitro-2-furaldehyde semioxamazone; an antibacterial, $C_7H_6N_4$.

nifuratel (ni-fūr′ah-tel) chemical name: 5-[(methylthio)-methyl]-3-[[(5-nitro-2-furanyl) methylene] amino]-2-oxazolidinone; an antibacterial, antifungal, and antitrichomonal, $C_{10}H_{11}N_3O_5S$.

nifuratrone (ni-fūr′ah-trōn) chemical name: N-(2-hydroxyethyl)-α-(5-nitro-2-furyl)nitrone; an antibacterial, $C_7H_8N_2O_5$.

nifurdazil (ni-fūr′dah-zil) chemical name: 1-(2-hydroxyethyl)-3-[[(5-nitro-2-furanyl)methylene]amino]-2-imidazolidinone; an antibacterial, $C_{10}H_{12}N_4O_5$.

nifurimide (ni-fūr′ĭ-mīd) chemical name: (±)-4-methyl-1-[[(5-nitro-2-furanyl)methylene]amino]-2-imidazolidinone; an antibacterial, $C_9H_{18}N_4O_4$.

nifurmerone (ni-fūr′mer-ōn) chemical name: 2-chloro-1-(5-nitro-2-furanyl)ethanone; an antifungal agent, $C_6H_4ClNO_4$.

nifuroxime (ni″fūr-ok′sēm) chemical name: 5-nitro-2-furancarboxaldehyde oxime. A fungicide, $C_{13}H_8Cl_2N_2O_4$, occurring as a colorless to pale yellow, somewhat viscous liquid; used in combination with furazolidone (an antibacterial and antiprotozoal agent) in the treatment of bacterial, candidal, and trichomonal vaginitis due to susceptible organisms, administered intravaginally.

nifurpirinol (ni″fūr-pēr′ĭ-nōl) chemical name: 6-[2-(5-nitro-2-furanyl)ethenyl]-2-pyridinemethanol; an antibacterial, $C_{12}H_{10}N_2O_4$.

nifurquinazol (ni-fūr-kwin′ah-zōl) chemical name: 2,2′[[2-(5-nitro-2-furanyl)-4-quinazolinyl]imino]bisethanol; an antibacterial, $C_{16}H_{16}N_4O_5$.

nifursemizone (ni″fūr-sem′ĭ-zōn) chemical name: 1- ethyl-2- [(2-nitro-2-furanyl) methylene] hydrazine- carboxamide. An antiprotozoal, $C_8H_{10}N_4O_4$, effective against *Histomonas;* used in poultry.

nifursol (ni′fūr-sōl) chemical name: 2-hydroxy-3,5-dinitrobenzoic acid [(5-nitro-2-furanyl)methylene]hydrazide. An antiprotozoal, $C_{12}H_7N_5O_9$, effective against *Histomonas;* used in poultry.

nifurtimox (ni-fūr′tĭ-mox) an antitrypanosomal, $C_{10}H_{13}N_3O_5S$, used in the treatment of acute and chronic Chagas' disease.

nightmare (nīt′mār) a terrifying dream; an anxiety attack during dreaming, accompanied by mild autonomic reactions.

nightshade (nīt′shād) a plant of the genus *Solanum*. **deadly n.,** belladonna leaf.

NIGMS National Institute of General Medical Sciences.

nigra (ni′grah) [L. "black"] the substantia nigra.

nigral (ni′gral) pertaining to the substantia nigra.

nigricans (ni′grĭ-kans) [L.] blackish.

nigrities (ni-grish′e-ēz) [L.] blackness. **n. lin′guae,** black tongue.

nigrosin (ni′gro-sin) an aniline dye, $C_{36}H_{27}N_3$, having a special affinity for ganglion cells, used to stain tissues from the central nervous system for study under the microscope.

nigrostriatal (ni″gro-stri-a′tal) projecting from the substantia nigra to the corpus striatum; said of a bundle of nerve fibers.

NIH National Institutes of Health.

nihilism (ni′hil-izm) [L. *nihil* nothing + -*ism*] 1. an attitude of skepticism regarding traditional values and beliefs. 2. a delusion of nonexistence of the self or of the world. **therapeutic n.,** skepticism regarding the therapeutic value of drugs or treatment procedures.

nikethamide (nĭ-keth′ah-mīd) chemical name: N,N-diethyl-3-pyridinecarboxamide. A central and respiratory stimulant, $C_{10}H_{14}N_2O$, occurring as a colorless to pale yellow, somewhat viscous liquid; used to counteract respiratory and central nervous system depression and circulatory failure, administered intramuscularly and intravenously.

Nikiforoff's method (ne″ke-for′ofs) [Mikhail *Nikiforoff*, Russian dermatologist, 1858–1915] see under *method*.

Nikolsky's sign (nĭ-kol′skēz) [Petr Vasilyevich *Nikolsky*, Russian dermatologist, 1858–1940] see under *sign*.

Nilevar (ni′lĕ-var) trademark for preparations of norethandrolone.

nimazone (nim′ah-zōn) chemical name: 3-(4-chlorophenyl)-4-imino-2-oxo-1-imidazolideneacetonitrile; an anti-inflammatory, $C_{11}H_8ClN_4O$.

Nimeh's method (ne′mez) [William *Nimeh*, Lebanese gastroenterologist, born 1891] see under *method.*

NIMH National Institute of Mental Health.

nimidane (nim′ĭ-dān) chemical name: 4-chloro-*N*-1,3-dithietan- 2-ylidene-2-methylbenzeneamine; a veterinary acaricide, $C_9H_8ClNS_2$.

nimiety (nĭ-mi′ĕ-te) [L. *nimis* overmuch + *-ety* state or condition of] (*obs.*) repletion or excess, as that degree of repletion or excess of water which, beyond satiety, elicits aversion to the ingestion of fluids.

NINDB National Institute of Neurological Diseases and Blindness.

Ninhydrin (nin-hi′drin) trademark for a preparation of triketohydrindene hydrate.

niobium (ni-o′be-um) [named for *Niobe*, of Greek mythology, who was turned into stone] the chemical element, atomic number, 41; atomic weight, 92.906; symbol, Nb. It was formerly called *columbium.*

Nionate (ni′o-nāt) trademark for a preparation of ferrous gluconate.

NIOSH National Institute of Occupational Safety and Health.

niperyt (ni′per-it) pentaerythritol tetranitrate.

nipple (nip′'l) the pigmented projection on the anterior surface of the mammary gland, surrounded by the areola; it gives outlet to milk from the breast. Called also *papilla mammae* [NA], *mamilla,* and *thelium.* Also, any similarly shaped structure.

Nippostrongylus (nip″o-stron′jĭ-lus) a genus of hookworms of the family Trichostrongylidae. **N. mu′ris,** a species occurring in rats.

Nipride (nip′rid) trademark for a preparation of sodium nitroprusside.

Nirenberg (nir′en-berg) Marshall Warren. American biochemist, born 1927; co-winner, with Robert William Holley and Har Gobind Khorana, of the Nobel prize for medicine or physiology in 1968 for their interpretation of the genetic code and its function in protein synthesis.

niridazole (nĭ-rid′ah-zōl) chemical name: 1-(5-nitro-2-thiazolyl)-2-imidazolidinone; an antischistosomal, $C_6H_8N_4O_3S$, occurring as a yellow, crystalline powder; it is also used in the treatment of intestinal and extraintestinal amebiasis and in dracunculiasis, administered orally.

nisbuterol mesylate (nis-bu′tĕ-rōl) chemical name: (+)-4-methoxy benzoic acid 2-(acetyloxy)-4-[2-[(1,1-dimethylethyl)amino]-1-hydroxy ethyl]phenyl ester methanesulfonate (salt); a bronchodilator, $C_{22}H_{27}NO_6 \cdot CH_4O_3S$.

Nisentil (ni′sen-til) trademark for a preparation of alphaprodine.

nisin (ni′sin) a polypeptide antibiotic produced by *Streptococcus lactis* and occurring naturally in certain cheeses. Nisin is active against certain streptococci, *Mycobacterium tuberculosis,* and several other bacteria.

nisobamate (ni-so-bah′māt) chemical name: 2-(hydroxymethyl)-2,3-dimethylpentyl isopropylcarbamate carbamate(ester); a minor tranquilizer, sedative, and hypnotic, $C_{13}H_{26}N_2O_4$.

nisoxetine (nĭ-soks′ĕ-tēn) chemical name: (+)-γ-(2-methoxyphenoxy)-*N*-methylbenzenepropanamine; an antidepressant, $C_{17}H_{21}NO_2$.

Nissen operation (nis′n) [Rudolph *Nissen*, German surgeon, born 1896] see *fundoplication.*

Nissl bodies (granules, substance), degeneration, method of staining (nis′'l) [Franz *Nissl,* neurologist in Heidelberg, 1860–1919] see under *body, degeneration,* and *Table of Stains.*

nisterime acetate (ni-stēr′ēm) chemical name: 17β-(acetyloxy)-2α-chloro-5α-androstan-3-one 3-[*O*-(4-nitrophenyl)-oxime]; an androgen, $C_{27}H_{35}ClN_2O_5$.

nisus (ni′sus) [L., from *niti* to strive] an effort, strong tendency, or molimen.

nit (nit) the egg of a louse.

Nitabuch's layer (stria, zone) (ne′tah-books) [Raissa *Nitabuch,* German physician of 19th century] see under *layer.*

nitarsone (ni-tar′sōn) chemical name: (4-nitrophenyl) arsonic acid; an antiprotozoal, $C_6H_6AsNO_5$, effective against *Histomonas;* used in poultry.

nitavirus (ni″tah-vi′rus) [*nuclear inclusion type A*] a name suggested, but not generally accepted, for herpesviruses that induce formation of single homogeneous eosinophilic inclusion bodies occupying most of the central area of the nucleus of the infected cells, and clearly separated from the marginated chromatin (A-type inclusions).

niter (ni′ter) nitre.

nithiamide (ni-thi′ah-mīd) chemical name: *N*-(5-nitro-2-thiazolyl)acetamide; a veterinary antibiotic, $C_5H_5N_3O_3S$; used to treat blackhead (histomoniasis) in turkeys. Called also *acintrazole* and *aminitrozole.*

niton (ni′ton) radon.

nitramine (ni-tram′in) a nitro derivative of an amine.

nitramisole hydrochloride (ni-tram′ĭ-sōl) chemical name: (±)-2,3,5,6-tetrahydro-6-(3-nitrophenyl)-imidazo[2,1-*b*]thiazole monohydrochloride; an anthelmintic, $C_{11}H_{11}N_3O_2S \cdot HCl$.

nitratase (ni′trah-tās) nitrate reductase.

nitrate (ni′trāt) any salt or ester of nitric acid or the NO_3^- anion; organic nitrates, e.g., nitroglycerin, are used as coronary vasodilators in the treatment of angina pectoris.

nitrate reductase (ni′trāt re-duk′tās) [EC 1.7.99.4] an enzyme of the oxidoreductase class that catalyzes the reaction nitrite + acceptor = nitrate + reduced acceptor. The enzyme occurs in certain oxidative bacteria that grow under anaerobic conditions by using nitrate as an electron acceptor. A test for nitrate reduction in a bacterial culture is useful in identification of Enterobacteriaceae, mycobacteria, and certain anaerobic bacteria. Called also *nitratase.*

nitrazepam (ni-trah′zĕ-pam) chemical name: 1,3-dihydro-7-nitro-5-phenyl-2*H*-1,4-benzodiazepin-2-one. One of the benzodiazepine tranquilizers, $C_{15}H_{11}N_3O$, used as an anticonvulsant and hypnotic.

nitre (ni′ter) [L. *nitrum;* Gr. *nitron*] potassium nitrate, or saltpeter. **cubic n.,** sodium nitrate.

nitremia (ni-tre′me-ah) azotemia.

nitric (ni′trik) pertaining to or containing nitrogen, applied especially to compounds containing nitrogen with a higher valence than that contained in the nitrous compounds.

nitric acid (ni′trik) a strong mineral acid, HNO_3, a colorless or yellow, hygroscopic, extremely corrosive liquid with a characteristic suffocating odor; it is a strong oxidizing agent that is highly toxic by inhalation and corrosive to skin and mucous membranes. *Fuming nitric acid* contains dissolved oxides of nitrogen and may be yellow to red in color; it is a very strong oxidizing agent.

nitridation (ni-trĭ-da′shun) combination with nitrogen to form a nitride.

nitride (ni′trīd) a binary compound of nitrogen with a metal.

nitrification (ni″trĭ-fĭ-ka′shun) [*nitric acid* + L. *facere* to make] oxidation of the nitrogen in ammonia and organic compounds to nitrites and to nitrates, carried out by soil bacteria of the family Nitrobacteraceae.

nitrifier (ni′trĭ-fi″er) a nitrifying microorganism.

nitrifying (ni′trĭ-fi″ing) oxidizing ammonia to nitrite (nitrosification) and then to nitrate, the first step being carried out by *Nitrosomonas* and *Nitrosococcus* and the second by *Nitrobacter.*

nitrile (ni′tril) an organic compound containing trivalent nitrogen attached to one carbon atom, ·C::N.

nitrite (ni′trīt) any salt or ester of nitrous acid or the NO_2^- anion; organic nitrites, e.g., amyl nitrite, are used as coronary vasodilators in the treatment of angina pectoris.

nitritoid (ni′trĭ-toid) resembling a nitrite or the reaction caused by a nitrite.

nitrituria (ni″trĭ-tu′re-ah) [*nitrite* + Gr. *ouron* urine + *-ia*] the presence of nitrites in the urine.

nitro- (ni′tro) a prefix indicating presence of the group $-NO_2$.

nitro-amine (ni″tro-am′in) nitramine.

nitro-anisol (ni″tro-an′ĭ-sol) a nitro derivative of anisol, $NO_2 \cdot C_6H_4 \cdot O \cdot CH_3$.

Nitrobacter (ni″tro-bak′ter) [*nitro-* + Gr. *baktron* a rod] a genus of bacteria of the family Nitrobacteraceae, occurring as rod-shaped, gram-negative cells that oxidize nitrites to nitrates. They are found in soil and fresh or sea water. The single species is *N. winograd′sky*. Called also *Nitrocystis*.

Nitrobacteraceae (ni″tro-bak″te-ra′se-e) a family of soil bacteria, consisting of gram-negative chemolithotrophic organisms that oxidize ammonia or nitrites, commonly known as the nitrifying bacteria. It includes the genera *Nitrobacter, Nitrococcus, Nitrosococcus, Nitrosolobus, Nitrosomonas, Nitrosospira,* and *Nitrospina*.

nitrobacteria (ni″tro-bak-te′re-ah) plural of *nitrobacterium*.

nitrobacterium (ni″tro-bak-te′re-um), pl. *nitrobacte′ria* [*nitro-* + Gr. *bakterion* little rod] a bacterium that oxidizes nitrites to nitrates, e.g., *Nitrobacter*.

nitrobenzene (ni″tro-ben′zēn) a poisonous benzene derivative, $C_6H_5NO_2$, occurring as a colorless to pale yellow, oily liquid; used in the manufacture of aniline. Called also *nitrobenzol* and *oil of mirbane*.

nitrobenzol (ni″tro-ben′zol) nitrobenzene.

nitroblue tetrazolium (ni′tro-blu tet″rah-zo′le-um) a yellow water-soluble dye that on reduction is converted to a dark blue water-insoluble formazan; see also under *tests*.

nitrocellulose (ni″tro-sel′u-lōs) pyroxylin.

Nitrococcus (ni″tro-kok′us) [*nitro-* + Gr. *kokkos* berry] a genus of bacteria of the family Nitrobacteraceae, occurring as spherical gram-negative cells that oxidize nitrites to nitrates. They are found in the South Pacific. The single species is *N. mo′bilis*.

nitrocycline (ni-tro-si′klēn) chemical name: 4-(dimethylamino) - 1,4,4a,5,5a,6,11,12a - octahydro - 3,10,12,12a - tetrahydroxy - 7 - nitro-1,11-dioxo-2-naphthacenecarboxamide; an antibiotic, $C_{21}H_{21}N_3O_9$.

Nitrocystis (ni″tro-sis′tis) *Nitrobacter*.

nitrofuran (ni-tro-fu′ran) any of a group of antibacterials, including furazolidone, nitrofurazone, nitrofurantoin, and related compounds, which are effective against a wide range of bacteria.

nitrofurantoin (ni″tro-fu-ran′to-in) [USP] chemical name: 1- [[(5-nitro-2-furanyl)methyl]amino]-2,4-imidazolidinedione. A synthetic antibacterial, $C_8H_6N_4O_5$, occurring as lemon-yellow crystals or fine powder, effective against many gram-negative and grampositive organisms, including *Escherichia coli, Staphylococcus pyogenes, Streptococcus pyogenes, Aerobacter aerogenes,* and *Paracolobactrum* species; used in the treatment of urinary tract infections due to susceptible bacteria, administered orally.

nitrofurazone (ni″tro-fu′rah-zōn) [USP] chemical name: 2-[(5-nitro-2-furanyl)methylene]hydrazinecarboxamide. An antibacterial, $C_6H_6N_4O_4$, occurring as a lemon yellow, crystalline powder, effective against a wide variety of gram-negative and gram-positive organisms. It is used topically as a local anti-infective in many skin lesions, including wounds, burns, skin infections, and ulcers; to aid healing and prevent infection of skin grafts; and in the treatment of otitis media and externa, urethritis, and eye infections. It has also been used orally in the treatment of African trypanosomiasis.

nitrogen (ni′tro-jen) [Gr. *nitron* niter + *gennan* to produce] 1. a colorless, gaseous element found free in the air; symbol, N; specific gravity, 0.9713; atomic number, 7; atomic weight, 14.007. It constitutes part of the atmosphere, forming about four fifths of common air. Chemically, it is almost inert, but forms by combination nitric acid and ammonia. Nitrogen is important biologically, being a constituent of protein and nucleic acids and thus present in all living cells. It is a gas unfitted to support respiration; not a poison, but proving fatal if breathed alone, because of the want of oxygen. It is soluble in the blood and body fluids and when released as bubbles of gas by reduction of atmospheric pressure causes serious symptoms. See *decompression sickness*, under *sickness*. 2. [NF] N_2; nitrogen containing not less than 99 per cent, by volume, of N_2. It is used to replace air in pharmaceutical preparations. **amide n.,** that portion of the nitrogen in protein that exists in the form of acid amides. **n. dioxide,** a brownish, irritant gas, NO_2, generated by the decomposition of nitrogen tetroxide or the reaction of metals with concentrated nitric acid. **n. monoxide,** nitrous oxide. **n. mustards,** see under *mustard*. **nomadic n.,** free nitrogen from the air which enters into plant and animal

growth. **nonprotein n.,** the nitrogenous constituents of the blood exclusive of the protein bodies. It consists of the nitrogen of urea, uric acid, creatine, creatinine, amino acids, polypeptides, and an undetermined part known as *rest nitrogen.* **n. pentoxide,** a crystalline compound, N_2O_5, or nitric anhydride, which combines with water to form nitric acid. **n. peroxide,** a poisonous volatile liquid, N_2O_4, decomposing at room temperature to nitrogen dioxide (q.v.). **rest n.,** see *nonprotein n.* **n. tetroxide,** n. peroxide. **urea n.,** see under *urea*.

nitrogenase (ni′tro-jen-ās) an enzyme system of nitrogen-fixing bacteria and blue-green algae that catalyzes the reduction of molecular nitrogen (N_2) to ammonia (NH_3).

nitrogen-fixing (ni′tro-jen-fiks′ing) accomplishing nitrogen fixation (see under *fixation*); said of certain bacteria.

nitrogenization (ni″tro-jen-i-za′shun) the act of impregnating with nitrogen.

nitrogenous (ni-troj′ĕ-nus) containing nitrogen.

nitroglycerin (ni-tro-glis′er-in) chemical name: glyceryl trinitrate. A colorless to yellow liquid, $C_3H_5N_3O_9$, formed by the action of nitric and sulfuric acids on glycerine. It explodes on concussion, but is rendered safe when compounded in tablets with mannitol. The official preparation [USP] is used in medicine chiefly in the prophylaxis and treatment of angina pectoris, administered sublingually.

Nitroglyn (ni′tro-glin) trademark for a preparation of nitroglycerin.

nitrohydrochloric acid (ni″tro-hi″dro-klor′ik) aqua regia.

Nitrol (ni′trol) trademark for preparations of nitroglycerin.

nitromannite (ni″tro-man′īt) mannitol hexanitrate.

nitromersol (ni″tro-mer′sol) [USP] chemical name: 5-methyl- 2- nitro- 7- oxa- 8- mercurabicyclo [4.2.0] octa- 1, 3, 5- triene. A mercurial compound, $C_7H_5HgNO_3$, occurring as brownish yellow to yellow granules or powder; used as a local anti-infective, applied topically to the skin and mucous membranes. It is also used to disinfect surgical and dental instruments.

nitrometer (ni-trom′-ĕ-ter) [*nitrogen* + Gr. *metron* measure] an apparatus for measuring the quantity of nitrogen given off in a reaction.

nitromethane (ni″tro-meth′ān) a nitrated form of methane, CH_3NO_2, which is a powerful explosive.

nitromifene citrate (ni-tro′mĭ-fēn) chemical name: 1- [2-[4-[1-(4-methoxyphenyl)-2-nitro-2-phenylethenyl]phenoxy] ethyl]pyrrolidine 2-hydroxy-1,2,3-propanetricarboxylate (1:1); an antiestrogen, $C_{27}H_{28}N_2O_4 \cdot C_6H_8O_7$.

nitronaphthalene (ni″tro-naf′thah-lēn) a substance, $C_{10}H_7 \cdot NO_2$, whose vapors may cause vesication and opacity of the cornea.

nitronaphthalin (ni″tro-naf′thah-lin) nitronaphthalene.

nitrophenol (ni″tro-fe′nol) an indicator, para-nitrophenylic acid, $C_6H_4(NO_2)OH$, with a pH range of 5 to 7; being colorless at 5 and yellow at 7.

nitropropiol (ni″tro-pro′pe-ol) orthonitrophenylpropiolic acid, $NO_2 \cdot C_6H_4 \cdot C:C \cdot COOH$: used as a test for sugar.

nitroprotein (ni″tro-pro′te-in) a nitrated protein made by treating serum protein with nitric acid.

nitroprusside (ni″tro-prus′īd) a salt of nitroprussic acid; see also under *sodium*.

nitrosaccharose (ni″tro-sak′ah-rōs) nitrated sucrose, an explosive and vasodilator used like nitroglycerin.

nitrosalol (ni″tro-sal′ol) an ester, $C_6H_4(OH)CO_2 \cdot C_6H_4NO_2$, in a yellowish, crystalline powder.

nitrosamine (ni″trōs-ah′mēn) any of a group of *N*-nitroso derivatives of secondary amines ($R_2N—NO$), formed by the combining of nitrates with amines; some nitrosamines show carcinogenic activity.

nitrosate (ni′tro-sāt) to convert into a nitroso compound.

nitrosation (ni″tro-sa′shun) conversion into a nitroso compound.

nitroscanate (ni″tro-skan′āt) chemical name: 1-isothiocyanato-4-(4-nitrophenoxy)benzene; a veterinary anthelmintic, $C_{13}H_8N_2O_3S$.

nitrose (ni′trōs) a term used to include nitric and nitrous acids.

nitrosification (ni-tro″sĭ-fi-ka′shun)   the oxidation of ammonia into nitrites.

nitrosifying (ni-tro″sĭ-fi′ing)   oxidizing ammonia into nitrites; said of certain nitrogen bacteria, especially of the genera *Nitrosomonas* and *Nitrosococcus*.

nitroso- (ni-tro′so)   a prefix indicating presence of the group —N:O.

nitrosobacteria (ni-tro″so-bak-te′re-ah)   plural of *nitrosobacterium*.

nitrosobacterium (ni-tro″so-bak-te′re-um), pl. *nitrosobacte′ria*.   a bacterium that oxidizes ammonia to nitrites, e.g., *Nitrosomonas*.

Nitrosococcus (ni″tro-so-kok′us) [*nitroso-* + Gr. *kokkos* berry]   a genus of bacteria of the family Nitrobacteraceae, occurring as spherical gram-negative cells that oxidize ammonia to nitrite. They are found in soil and sea water. The type species is *N. nitro′sus*.

Nitrosocystis (ni-tro″so-sis′tis) [*nitroso-* + Gr. *kystis* bladder]   a genus of gram-negative, chemolithotrophic nitrifying bacteria of uncertain status, affiliated with the family Nitrobacteraceae.

Nitrosogloea (ni-tro″so-gle′ah)   a genus of gram-negative, chemolithotrophic, nitrifying bacteria of uncertain status.

nitroso-indol (ni-tro″so-in′dol)   a compound which gives a red reaction when indol is treated with sulfuric acid and potassium nitrite.

Nitrosolobus (ni-tro″so-lo′bus) [*nitroso-* + L. *lobus* lobe]   a genus of bacteria of the family Nitrobacteraceae, occurring as pleomorphic and lobate gram-negative cells that oxidize ammonia to nitrite. They are found in soil. The type species is *N. multifor′mis*.

Nitrosomonas (ni-tro″so-mo′nas) [*nitroso-* + Gr. *monas* unit, from *monos* single]   a genus of bacteria of the family Nitrobacteraceae, occurring as ellipsoidal or short, rod-shaped, gram-negative cells that oxidize ammonia to nitrite. They are found in soil and fresh or sea water. The type species is *N. europae′a*.

Nitrospina (ni″tro-spi′nah) [*nitro-* + L. *spina* spine]   a genus of bacteria of the family Nitrobacteraceae, occurring as long, slender, gram-negative rods that oxidize nitrites to nitrates. They are found in the South Atlantic Ocean. The type species is *N. gra′cilis*.

Nitrosospira (ni-tro″so-spi′rah) [*nitroso-* + Gr. *speira* coil]   a genus of bacteria of the family Nitrobacteraceae, occurring as spiral-shaped, gram-negative cells that oxidize ammonia to nitrite. They are found in soil. The type species is *N. brien′sis*.

nitrososubstitution (ni-tro″so-sub″stĭ-tu′shun)   the substitution of the radical nitroxyl for some other radical or atom in a compound.

nitrosourea (ni-tro″so-ūr′e-ah)   any of several chemically related antineoplastic agents including the closely related group carmustine (BCNU), lomustine (CCNU), and semustine (MeCCNU) and also streptozocin, an antibiotic that contains a methylnitrosourea moiety. BCNU, CCNU, and MeCCNU are highly lipid-soluble, cross the blood-brain barrier, and are used against brain tumors; they act by alkylation, carbamoylation, and inhibition of DNA repair; they are not cross resistant with other alkylating agents and are highly effective against resting (G₀) cells; the major side effect is dose-limiting bone marrow suppression. Streptozocin differs from these in that it is not cross resistant with them, is not myelosuppressive, and does not act by carbamoylation.

Nitrostat (ni′tro-stat)   trademark for a preparation of nitroglycerin.

nitrosugars (ni″tro-shug′erz)   a class of substances which have been used in the treatment of angina pectoris.

nitrosyl (ni′tro-sil)   the univalent radical NO.

nitrous (ni′trus)   pertaining to nitrogen in its lowest valency.   **n. oxide** [USP], chemical name: dinitrogen monoxide, N₂O, a colorless, odorless gas that is a weak inhalational anesthetic; it is nonflammable but supports combustion; primarily used in combination with a potent halogenated inhalational anesthetic (halothane or enflurane) to produce general anesthesia; use as a sole agent requires high concentrations that may cause hypoxia. Called also *laughing gas*.

nitrous acid (ni′trus)   a weak acid, HNO₂, existing only in aqueous solution.

Nitrovas (ni′tro-vas)   trademark for a preparation of nitroglycerin.

nitroxanthic acid (ni″tro-zan′thik)   trinitrophenol.

nitroxyl (ni-trok′sil)   the radical NO₂.

nitryl (ni′tril)   nitroxyl.

nivazol (ni′vah-zōl)   chemical name: 2′(4-fluorophenyl)-2′H-pregna-2,4-dien-20-yno[3,2-c]pyrazol-17α-ol; a glucocorticoid, C₂₈H₃₁FN₂O.

nivemycin (niv′ĕ-mi′sin)   neomycin.

nivimedone sodium (nĭ-vi′mĕ-dōn)   chemical name: 5,6-dimethyl-2-nitro-1*H*-indene-1,3(2*H*)-dione ion(1−)sodium monohydrate; an antiallergic agent, C₁₁H₈NNaO₄·H₂O.

NK.   abbreviation for *Nomenklatur Kommission*, a committee of the Anatomical Society of Germany which has revised and given supplementary names to the terminology of anatomy.

nl.   nanoliter.

N.L.N.   National League for Nursing.

Nm.   abbreviation for L. *nux moscha′ta*, nutmeg.

nm.   nanometer.

N.M.A.   National Medical Association.

NMN   nicotinamide mononucleotide.

NMR   nuclear magnetic resonance.

NMRI   Naval Medical Research Institute, part of the National Naval Medical Center.

N-Multistix (mul′tĭ-stiks)   trademark for a reagent strip for testing urine specimens for protein, glucose, ketones, bilirubin, occult blood, urobilinogen, nitrite, and to indicate urinary pH.

nn.   abbreviation for L. *nervi* (nerves).

N.N.D.   *New and Nonofficial Drugs*, former annual publication of the American Medical Association containing descriptions of agents proposed for use in or on the human body in the prevention, diagnosis, or treatment of disease, which have been evaluated by the Council on Drugs of the A.M.A.

NO   nitric oxide.

N₂O   dinitrogen monoxide (nitrous oxide).

No   chemical symbol for *nobelium*.

No.   abbreviation of L. *nu′mero*, "to the number of."

Nobel prize (no-bel′) [Alfred Bernhard *Nobel*, Swedish chemist and engineer, 1833–1896; the inventor of dynamite, under the terms of whose will the prizes were established]   an award usually given annually for outstanding achievement in chemistry, physics, medicine or physiology, literature, and in the interest of world peace. First presented in 1901. An award for achievement in economics has since been added.

nobelium (no-be′le-um) [Alfred Bernard *Nobel*]   the chemical element of atomic number 102, atomic weight 253, symbol No, obtained in 1958 by bombardment of ²⁴⁶Cm with ¹²C ions in a heavy ion linear accelerator.

Noble's position (no′b′lz) [Charles Percy *Noble*, American gynecologist, 1863–1935]   see under *position*.

Nocardia (no-kar′de-ah) [Edmond Isidore Etienne *Nocard*, French veterinarian, 1850–1903]   a genus of bacteria of the family Nocardiaceae, order Actinomycetales, separable into 30 or more species of which a few are pathogenic and the remainder saprophytic forms. They are gram-positive aerobes, found in the soil, with branching filaments that break into bacillary or coccal forms, and produce chains of spores by simple fragmentation of hyphal branches.   **N. asteroi′des,** an acid-fast filamentous actinomycete producing pulmonary infection in man that simulates tuberculosis, which sometimes becomes systemic and may be fatal (see *nocardiosis*). It may also cause actinomycotic mycetoma.   **N. brasilien′sis,** an acid-fast pathogenic species that produces yellow to brown mycelium with branching filaments, found most commonly in the tropics. They are found in soil and cause nocardiosis and actinomycotic mycetoma in man. Called also *Actinomyces brasiliensis*.   **N. ca′viae,** *N. otitidis-caviarum*.   **N. farci′nica,** a species of acid-fast filamentous actinomycetes of uncertain classification, which may be identical to *N. asteroides*; it is the etiologic agent of cattle farcy and a cause of actinomycotic mycetoma. Called also *Streptothrix farcini* and *Streptothrix nocardii*.   **N. lu′tea,** a partially acid-fast species isolated from the lacrimal gland in lacrimycosis. Called also *Actinomyces luteus*.   **N. madu′rae,** *Actinomadura madurae*.   **N. otitidis-cavia′rum,** a species of widespread distribution that is the etiologic agent of nocardiosis and actinomyocotic mycetoma in which the granules secreted in the pus are white. Called also *N. caviae.*

Nocardiaceae (no-kar″de-a′se-e) a family of bacteria of the order Actinomycetales, consisting of the genera *Actinomadura, Nocardia,* and *Nocardiopsis.*

nocardial (no-kar′de-al) pertaining to or caused by *Nocardia.*

nocardiasis (no″kar-di′ah-sis) nocardiosis.

nocardin (no-kar′din) an antibiotic substance from *Nocardia coeliaca,* active against tubercle bacilli.

Nocardiopsis (no-kar″de-op′sis) a genus of soil bacteria of the family Nocardiaceae, order Actinomycetales, consisting of gram-positive, aerobic, nonacid-fast organisms that form filaments. The organisms resemble *Nocardia* but differ in cell wall type and are not resistant to lysozymes. They are potential pathogens, causing abscesses and pulmonary lesions.

nocardiosis (no-kar-de-o′sis) an acute or chronic suppurative infection, usually of the lungs but with a marked tendency to spread to any organ of the body, especially to the brain; abscess formation occurs in any organ, most commonly in the lungs, brain, or skin or subcutaneous tissue. Lung abscesses tend to cavitate with time. The causative agent in most instances is *Nocardia asteroides,* but *N. brasiliensis* and *N. caviae* cause occasional cases.

Nochtia (nok′te-ah) a genus of small nematode worms. **N. noch′ti,** a species of worms found in and apparently causing the production of tumors in the stomachs of Javanese monkeys.

noci- [L. *nocēre* to injure] a combining form denoting relationship to injury or to a noxious or deleterious agent or influence.

nociassociation (no″se-ah-so″se-a′shun) the unconscious discharge of nervous energy under the stimulus of trauma, as in surgical shock.

nociceptive (no″se-sep′tiv) [*noci-* + L. *capere* to receive] receiving injury; said of a receptive neuron for painful sensations.

nociceptor (no″se-sep′tor) a receptor which is stimulated by injury; a receptor for pain. Cf. *beneceptor* and *ceptor* (def. 2). **polymodal n.,** a nociceptor activated by heat, mechanical pressure, or chemical mediators of inflammation; released as a result of tissue injury.

nocifensor (no″se-fen′sor) [*noci-* + L. *fendere* to defend] Sir Thomas Lewis' name for a system of nerves in the skin and mucous membranes which are concerned with local defense against injury.

noci-influence (no″se-in′floo-ens) injurious or traumatic influence.

nociperception (no″se-per-sep′shun) the perception by the system of injurious (traumatic) stimuli.

nocodazole (no-ko′dah-zōl) chemical name: [5-(2-thienyl-carbonyl)-1*H*-benzimidazolecarbamic acid methyl ester; an antineoplastic, $C_{14}H_{11}N_3O_3S$.

Noct. abbreviation for L. *noc′te,* at night.

noctalbuminuria (nok″tal-bu″mĭ-nu′re-ah) [L. *nox* night + *albuminuria*] the presence of excessive amounts of albumin in the urine secreted during the night.

noctambulation (nok″tam-bu-la′shun) [L. *noctambulatio; nox* night + *ambulare* to walk] somnambulism.

noctambulic (nok″tam-bu′lik) pertaining to or marked by somnambulism.

Noctec (nok′tek) trademark for preparations of chloral hydrate.

noctiphobia (nok″te-fo′be-ah) [L. *nox* night + *phobia*] irrational fear of night and darkness.

Noct. maneq. abbreviation for L. *noc′te mane′que,* at night and in the morning.

nocturia (nok-tu′re-ah) [L. *nox* night + Gr. *ouron* urine + *-ia*] excessive urination at night.

nocturnal (nok-tur′nal) [L. *nocturnus*] pertaining to, occurring at, or active at night.

nodal (no′dal) pertaining to a node, particularly the atrioventricular node.

node (nōd) [L. *nodus* knot] a small mass of tissue in the form of a swelling, knot, or protuberance, either normal or pathological. See also *nodule* and *nodus.* **abdominal**

lymph n's, parietal, nodi lymphatici abdominis parietales. **abdominal lymph n's, visceral,** nodi lymphatici abdominis viscerales. **anorectal lymph n's,** nodi lymphatici pararectales. **n. of anterior border of epiploic foramen,** nodus foraminalis. **aortic lymph n's,** lumbar lymph n's. **aortic lymph n's, lateral,** nodi lymphatici aortici laterales. **apical lymph n's,** six to twelve lymph nodes situated at the apex of the axilla medial to the axillary vein, adjacent to the upper border of the pectoralis minor muscle, which receive lymph from all the other axillary lymph nodes and sometimes from the mammary gland; their efferent vessels unite to form the subclavian trunk **appendicular lymph n's,** nodi lymphatici appendiculares. **Aschoff's n., n. of Aschoff and Tawara,** nodus atrioventricularis. **atrioventricular n.,** nodus atrioventricularis. **axillary lymph n's,** nodi lymphatici axillares. **axillary lymph n's, lateral** nodi lymphatici brachiales. **Bouchard's n's,** cartilaginous and bony enlargements of the proximal interphalangeal joints of the fingers in degenerative joint disease. Such nodules in the terminal interphalangeal joints are called *Heberden's nodes.* **brachial lymph n's,** nodi lymphatici brachiales. **bronchopulmonary lymph n's,** nodi lymphatici bronchopulmonales. **buccal lymph n., buccinator lymph n.,** nodus lymphaticus buccinatorius. **caval lymph n's, lateral,** nodi lymphatici cavales laterales. **celiac lymph n's,** nodi lymphatici coeliaci. **central lymph n's,** the three to five large lymph nodes lying under the axillary fascia embedded in the axillary fat, which receive lymph from the preceding three groups (brachial, interpectoral, and subscapular) of axillary lymph nodes and send afferent vessels to the apical lymph nodes. **central superior n's,** nodi superiores centrales. **cervical lymph n's, anterior,** nodi lymphatici cervicales anteriores. **cervical lymph n's, deep anterior,** nodi lymphatici cervicales anteriores profundae. **cervical lymph n's, deep lateral,** nodi lymphatici cervicales laterales profundi. **cervical lymph n's, prelaryngeal,** nodi lymphatici prelaryngeales. **cervical lymph n's, anterior superficial,** nodi lymphatici cervicales anteriores superficiales. **cervical lymph n's, superficial lateral,** nodi lymphatici cervicales laterales superficiales. **Cloquet's n., n. of Cloquet,** the highest of the deep inguinal lymph nodes; called also *Cloquet's gland.* **colic lymph n's, colic lymph n's, intermediate,** nodi lymphatici colici. **colic lymph n's, left,** nodi lymphatici colici sinistri. **colic lymph n's, middle,** nodi lymphatici colici medii. **colic lymph n's, right,** nodi lymphatici colici dextri. **colic lymph n's, terminal,** lymph nodes associated with the main trunks of the superior and inferior mesenteric arteries, being continuous with the corresponding preaortic lymph nodes. **cubital lymph n's,** nodi lymphatici cubitales. **Delphian n.,** a lymph node encased in the fascia in the midline, just anterior to the thyroid isthmus, so called because it is exposed first at surgery and, if diseased, is indicative of disease in the thyroid gland, but not of a specific disease process. **deltoideopectoral n's,** one or two of small lymph nodes situated below the clavicle beside the cephalic vein, between the pectoralis major and deltoid muscles; called also *infraclavicular n's.* **diaphragmatic lymph n's,** nodi lymphatici phrenici superiores. **Dürck's n's,** granulomatous perivascular infiltrations in the cerebral cortex in trypanosomiasis. **epicolic lymph n's,** minute lymph nodes situated on the wall of the bowel and sometimes in the epiploic appendices. **epigastric lymph n's, inferior,** nodi lymphatici epigastrici inferiores. **n. of epiploic foramen,** nodus foraminalis. **Ewald's n.,** sentinel n. **facial lymph n's,** nodi lymphatici faciales. **Flack's n.,** sinoatrial n. **foraminal n.,** nodus foraminalis. **gastric lymph n's, left,** nodi lymphatici gastrici sinistri. **gastric lymph n's, right,** nodi lymphatici gastrici dextri. **gastroepiploic lymph n's, left,** nodi lymphatici gastro-omentales sinistri. **gastroepiploic lymph n's, right,** nodi lymphatici gastro-omentalis dextri. **gastro-omental lymph n's, left,** nodi lymphatici gastro-omentales sinistri. **gastro-omental lymph n's, right,** nodi lymphatici gastro-omentales dextri. **gluteal lymph n's, inferior,** nodi lymphatici gluteales inferiores. **gluteal lymph n's, superior,** nodi lymphatici gluteales superiores. **gouty n.,** a nodule produced by gouty inflammation. **Haygarth's n's,** joint swellings in arthritis deformans. **Heberden's**

n's, small hard nodules, formed usually at the distal interphalangeal articulations of the fingers, produced by calcific spurs of the articular cartilage and associated with interphalangeal osteoarthritis. Heredity is an important etiologic factor. Called also *Heberden's sign*. Cf. *Bouchard's n's*. **hemal n's,** nodes with a rich content of erythrocytes within sinuses, having an organization much like a lymph node but no lymphatic supply, found near large blood vessels along the ventral side of the vertebrae and near the spleen and kidneys in various mammals, especially ruminants; their functions are probably like those of the spleen. The presence of such nodes in man is doubtful. A special type of hemal node is found in the pig; see *hemolymph n's,* def. 2. Called also *hemal glands, hemolymph n's,* and *vascular glands.* **hemolymph n's,** 1. hemal n's. 2. special types of hemal nodes found in the pig, having characteristics midway between those of ordinary lymph nodes and typical hemal nodes, containing both blood and lymphatic vessels, the contents of both of which mix in the sinuses; called also *hemolymph glands.* **Hensen's n.,** primitive knot. **hepatic lymph n's,** nodi lymphatici hepatici. **hilar lymph n's,** nodi lymphatici bronchopulmonales. **ileocolic lymph n's,** nodi lymphatici ileocolici. **iliac circumflex lymph n's,** circumflex iliac lymph n's. **iliac lymph n's,** nodi lymphatici iliaci. **iliac lymph n's, circumflex,** lymph nodes situated along the deep iliac circumflex vessels; called also *iliac circumflex lymph n's.* **iliac lymph n's, common,** nodi lymphatici iliaci communes. **iliac lymph n's, external,** nodi lymphatici iliaci externi. **iliac lymph n's, intermediate common,** nodi lymphatici iliaci communes intermedii. **iliac lymph n's, intermediate external,** nodi lymphatici iliaci externi intermedii. **iliac lymph n's, internal,** nodi lymphatici iliaci interni. **iliac lymph n's, lateral common,** nodi lymphatici iliaci communes laterales. **iliac lymph n's, lateral external,** nodi lymphatici iliaci externi laterales. **iliac lymph n's, medial common,** nodi lymphatici iliaci communes mediales. **iliac lymph n's, medial external,** nodi lymphatici iliaci externi mediales. **iliac lymph n's, promontory common,** nodi lymphatici iliaci communes promontorii. **iliac lymph n's, subaortic common,** nodi lymphatici iliaci communes subaortici. **inguinal lymph n's, deep,** nodi lymphatici inguinales profundi. **inguinal lymph n's, inferior,** nodi lymphatici inguinales inferiores. **inguinal lymph n's, superficial,** nodi lymphatici inguinales superficiales. **inguinal lymph n's, superolateral,** nodi lymphatici inguinales superolaterales. **inguinal lymph n's, superomedial,** nodi lymphatici inguinales superomediales. **intercostal lymph n's,** nodi lymphatici intercostales. **interiliac lymph n's,** nodi lymphatici interiliaci. **interpectoral lymph n's,** nodi lymphatici interpectorales. **jugular lymph n's, lateral,** nodi lymphatici jugulares laterales. **jugulodigastric lymph n.,** nodus lymphaticus jugulodigastricus. **jugulo-omohyoid lymph n.,** nodus lymphaticus jugulo-omohyoideus. **juxtaintestinal n.,** nodi juxta-intestinales. **Keith's n., Keith-Flack n.,** sinoatrial n. **Koch's n.,** nodus atrioventricularis. **lacunar n., intermediate,** nodus lacunaris intermedius. **lacunar n., lateral,** nodus lacunaris lateralis. **lacunar n., medial,** nodus lacunaris medialis. **lumbar lymph n's,** numerous large lymph nodes extending from the aortic bifurcation to the aortic hiatus of the diaphragm, as three parallel chains: left, intermediate, and right. Called also *aortic lymph nodes.* **lumbar lymph n's, intermediate,** nodi lymphatici lumbales intermedii. **lumbar lymph n's, left,** nodi lymphatici lumbales sinistri. **lumbar lymph n's, right,** nodi lymphatici lumbales dextri. **lymph n.,** any of the accumulations of lymphoid tissue organized as definite lymphoid organs, varying from 1 to 25 mm. in diameter, situated along the course of lymphatic vessels (see illustration accompanying *lymph*), and consisting of an outer cortical and an inner medullary part. The lymph nodes are the main source of lymphocytes of the peripheral blood and, as part of the reticuloendothelial system, serve as a defense mechanism by removing noxious agents, such as bacteria and toxins, and probably play a role in antibody production. Called also *nodus lymphaticus* [NA]. **lymph n. of arch of azygos vein,** nodus lymphaticus arcus venae azygos. **lymph n's of upper limb, deep,** nodi lymphatici membri superioris profundi. **lymph n's of upper limb, superficial,** nodi lymphatici membri superioris superficiales. **malar lymph n.,** nodus lymphat-

icus malaris. **mandibular lymph n.,** nodus lymphaticus mandibularis. **mastoid lymph n's,** nodi lymphatici mastoidei. **mediastinal lymph n's, anterior,** nodi lymphatici mediastinales anteriores. **mediastinal lymph n's, posterior,** nodi lymphatici mediastinales posteriores. **mesenteric lymph n's,** nodi lymphatici mesenterici. **mesenteric lymph n's, inferior,** nodi lymphatici mesenterici inferiores. **mesenteric lymph n's, superior,** nodi superiores centrales. **mesocolic lymph n's,** nodi lymphatici mesocolici. **Meynet's n's,** nodules in the capsules of joints and in tendons in rheumatic disorders, especially of children. **milker's n's,** paravaccinia. **nasolabial lymph n.,** nodus lymphaticus nasolabialis. **n. of neck of gallbladder,** nodus cysticus. **obturator lymph n's,** nodi lymphatici obturatorii. **occipital lymph n's,** nodi lymphatici occipitales. **Osler's n's,** small, raised, swollen tender areas, about the size of a pea, characteristically bluish but sometimes pink or red, and sometimes having a blanched center, occurring most commonly in the pads of the fingers or toes, in the thenar or hypothenar eminences, or the soles of the feet; they are practically pathognomonic of subacute bacterial endocarditis. **pancreatic lymph n's,** nodi lymphatici pancreatici. **pancreatic lymph n's, inferior,** nodi lymphatici pancreatici inferiores. **pancreatic lymph n's, superior,** nodi lymphatici pancreatici superiores. **pancreaticoduodenal lymph n's, inferior,** nodi lymphatici pancreaticoduodenales inferiores. **pancreaticoduodenal lymph n's, superior,** nodi lymphatici pancreaticoduodenales superiores. **paracardial lymph n's,** a group of small lymph nodes forming a chain or ring (annulus lymphaticus cardiae [NA]), around the cardiac opening of the stomach. **paracolic lymph n's,** nodi lymphatici paracolici. **paramammary lymph n's,** nodi lymphatici paramammarii. **pararectal lymph n's,** nodi lymphatici pararectales. **parasternal lymph n's,** nodi lymphatici parasternales. **paratracheal lymph n's,** nodi lymphatici paratracheales. **parauterine lymph n's,** nodi lymphatici para-uterini. **paravaginal lymph n's,** nodi lymphatici paravaginales. **paravesicular lymph n's,** nodi lymphatici paravesiculares. **parotid lymph n's, deep,** nodi lymphatici parotidei profundi. **parotid lymph n's, infra-auricular deep,** nodi lymphatici parotidei profundi infra-auriculares. **parotid lymph n's, intraglandular deep,** nodi lymphatici parotidei profundi intraglandulares. **parotid lymph n's, preauricular deep,** nodi lymphatici parotidei profundi preauriculares. **parotid lymph n's, superficial,** nodi lymphatici parotidei superficiales. **Parrot's n.,** see under *sign,* def. 2. **pectoral lymph n's,** nodi lymphatici interpectorales. **pelvic lymph n's, parietal,** nodi lymphatici pelvis parietales. **pelvic lymph n's, visceral,** nodi lymphatici pelvis viscerales. **pericardial lymph n's,** nodi lymphatici pericardiales. **pericardial lymph n's, lateral,** nodi lymphatici pericardiales laterales. **peroneal n.,** nodus fibularis. **phrenic lymph n's, inferior,** nodi lymphatici phrenici inferiores. **phrenic lymph n's, superior,** nodi lymphatici phrenici superioris. **popliteal lymph n's,** nodi lymphatici popliteales. **popliteal lymph n's, superficial,** nodi lymphatici popliteales superficiales. **postaortic lymph n's,** nodi lymphatici postaortici. **postcaval lymph n's,** nodi lymphatici postcavales. **postvesicular lymph n's,** nodi lymphatici postvesiculares. **preaortic lymph n's,** nodi lymphatici pre-aortici. **precaval lymph n's,** nodi lymphatici precavales. **prececal lymph n's,** nodi lymphatici precaecales. **prelaryngeal n.,** a lymph node deep in the neck that helps drain the thyroid gland. **pretracheal n.,** a lymph node deep in the neck that helps drain the thyroid gland. **pretracheal lymph n's,** nodi lymphatici pretracheales. **prevesicular lymph n's,** nodi lymphatici prevesiculares. **primitive n.,** primitive knot. **pulmonary juxtaesophageal lymph n's,** nodi lymphatici juxta-esophageales pulmonales. **pulmonary lymph n's,** nodi lymphatici pulmonales. **pyloric lymph n's,** nodi lymphatici pylorici. **n's of Ranvier,** constrictions occurring on myelinated nerve fibers at regular intervals of about 1 millimeter; at these sites the myelin sheath is absent and the axon is enclosed only by Schwann cell processes. **rectal lymph n's, superior,** nodi lymphatici rectales superiores. **retroaortic lymph n's,** nodi lymphatici postaortici. **retroauricular lymph n's,** nodi lymphatici mastoidei. **retrocecal lymph n's,** nodi lymphatici retrocaecales. **retropharyngeal lymph nodes,** nodi lymphatici retropharyngeales. **retropyloric n's,** nodi retropylorici. **Rosenmüller's n.,** 1. pars palpebralis glandulae lacrimalis. 2. [pl.] nodi lymphatici inguinales profundi. **Rotter's n's,** lymph nodes occasionally found between the pectoralis major and minor muscles which often contain metastases from mammary cancer. **sacral lymph n's,** nodi lymphatici sacrales. **Schmidt's n.,** the medullated interannular segment of a nerve fiber. **Schmorl's n.,** an irregular or hemispherical bone defect in the upper or lower margin of the body of the vertebra. **sentinel n., signal n.,** an enlarged supraclavicular node which is often the first sign of an abdominal tumor; called also *Virchow's n.* or *gland,* and *Troisier's n.* **sigmoid lymph n's,** nodi lymphatici sigmoidei. **singer's n.,** a small white nodule occurring on the vocal cord in chorditis tuberosa. Called also *vocal nodule.* **sinoatrial n., sinuatrial n., sinus n.,** a microscopic collection of atypical cardiac muscle fibers at the superior end of the sulcus terminalis, at the junction of the superior vena cava and right atrium. Called also *nodus sinuatrialis* [NA]. The cardiac rhythm normally takes its origin in this node which is, for that reason, also known as the pacemaker of the heart. **splenic lymph n's,** nodi lymphatici splenici. **submandibular lymph n's,** nodi lymphatici submandibulares. **submental lymph n's,** nodi lymphatici submentales. **subpyloric n's,** nodi subpylorici. **subscapular lymph n's,** the five to seven lymph nodes extending along the subscapular veins at the lower border of the axilla, which drain the skin and muscles of the dorsal posterior shoulder region and lower part of the back of the neck. **supraclavicular lymph n's,** nodi lymphatici supraclaviculares. **suprapyloric n.,** nodus suprapyloricus. **supratrochlear lymph n's,** nodi lymphatici cubitales. **syphilitic n.,** a swelling on a bone due to syphilitic periostitis. **n. of Tawara,** nodus atrioventricularis. **teacher's n.,** singer's n. **thyroid lymph n's,** nodi lymphatici thyroidei. **tibial n., anterior,** nodus tibialis anterior. **tibial n., posterior,** nodus tibialis posterior. **tracheal lymph n's,** nodi lymphatici paratracheales. **tracheobronchial lymph n's, inferior,** nodi lymphatici tracheobronchiales inferiores. **tracheobronchial lymph n's, superior,** nodi lymphatici tracheobronchiales superiores. **triticeous n.,** cartilago triticea. **Troisier's n., Virchow's n.,** signal n. **vesicular lymph n's, lateral,** nodi lymphatici vesiculares laterales. **vital n.,** an old name applied to the respiratory centers.

nodi (no′di) [L.] genitive and plural of *nodus.*

nodose (no′dōs) [L. *nodosus*] having nodes or projections.

nodosity (no-dos′ĭ-te) [L. *nodositas*] 1. the quality or condition of being nodose. 2. a node. **Haygarth's n's,** see under *node.*

nodular (nod′u-lar) 1. like a nodule or node. 2. marked with nodules.

nodulated (nod′u-lāt″ed) marked with nodules.

nodulation (nod′u-la′shun) the presence of nodules.

nodule (nod′ūl) [L. *nodulus* little knot] a small boss or node which is solid and can be detected by touch; see also *nodulus.* **accessory thymic n's,** noduli thymici accessorii. **aggregate n's,** folliculi lymphatici aggregati. **Albini's n's,** gray nodules of the size of small grains, sometimes seen on the free edges of the atrioventricular valves of infants; they are remains of fetal structures. Called also *Cruveilhier's n's.* **n's of aortic valve,** see *noduli valvularum semilunarium.* **apple jelly n's,** minute translucent nodules of a distinctive yellowish or reddish brown color, visible on diascopic examination of the lesions of lupus vulgaris. **n's of Arantius,** see *noduli valvularum semilunarium.* **Aschoff's n's,** Aschoff bodies. **Bianchi's n's,** nodules of aortic valve; see *noduli valvularum semilunarium.* **Bohn's n's,** inclusion cysts along the buccal and lingual aspects of the dental ridges and on the palate away from the raphe, found in newborn infants; considered to be remnants of mucous-gland tissue trapped during fetal development. Called also *Bohn's pearls.* **Bouchard's n's** (obs.), see under *node.* **Busacca n's,** an accumulation of epithelioid cells and lymphocytes occurring in chronic inflammation of the iris, usually on the anterior surface about the region of the ciliary zone. **n. of cerebellum,** nodulus cerebelli. **cortical n's,** nodules of closely packed lymphocytes in the cortical portion of a lymph gland. **Cruveilhier's n's,** Albini's n's. **Dalen-Fuchs n's,** small hemispherical mounds principally composed of epithelioid cells and cells of the retinal epithelium, seen in sympathetic ophthalmia and certain other disorders. **Fraenkel's n's,** typhus nodules of the cutaneous blood vessels. **Gamna n's,** brown or yellow pigmented nodules seen in the spleen in certain cases of enlargement, such as Gamna's disease and siderotic splenomegaly; called also *nodules tabac.* **Gandy-Gamna n's,** Gamna n's. **Hoboken's n's,** dilatations of the outer surface of the umbilical arteries. **Jeanselme's n's,** gummata of tertiary syphilis and of nonvenereal treponemal diseases, located on joint capsules, bursae or tendon sheaths; called also *juxta-articular n's* and *Steiner's tumors.* **juxta-articular n's,** Jeanselme's n's. **n's of Kerckring,** nodules of aortic valve; see *noduli valvularum semilunarium.* **Koeppe n's,** white to gray nodules observed at the pupillary border in chronic inflammation of the iris, and consisting of accumulations of epithelioid cells and lymphocytes. **lentiform n.,** processus lenticularis. **Lutz-Jeanselme n's,** Jeanselme's n's. **lymphatic n's,** a term applied to lymph nodes, as well as to one of the small collections of lymphoid tissue (nodulus lymphaticus [NA]) situated deep to epithelial surfaces, and also to temporary small (about 1 mm. in diameter), dense accumulations of lymphocytes located within the cortex of a lymph node and expressing the cytogenetic and defense functions of the tissue. **lymphatic n's, solitary, of large intestine,** folliculi lymphatici solitarii intestini crassi. **lymphatic n's, solitary, of small intestine,** folliculi lymphatici solitarii intestini tenuis. **lymphatic n's of stomach,** folliculi lymphatici gastrici. **milkers' n's,** paravaccinia. **Morgagni's n's,** nodules of aortic valve; see *noduli valvularum semilunarium.* **pearly n.,** one of the nodules of bovine tuberculosis. **primary n.,** a lymph nodule without a germinal center, or apart from a center. **n's of pulmonary trunk valves,** see *noduli valvularum semilunarium.* **pulp n.,** denticle, def. 2. **rheumatic n's,** small round or oval, mostly subcutaneous nodules made up chiefly of a mass of Aschoff bodies and seen in cases of rheumatic fever. **Schmorl's n.,** a nodule seen in roentgenograms of the spine, due to prolapse of a nucleus pulposus into an adjoining vertebra. **secondary n.,** germinal center. **siderotic n's,** focal fibrotic lesions characterized by the presence of crystals of iron on the degenerated elastic tissue fibers, seen in the spleen in Banti's disease. **singers' n.,** a small white node occurring on the vocal cord in chorditis tuberosa. **Sister Joseph's n.,** a nodule deep in the subcutis in the umbilical area associated with metastasizing intra-abdominal cancer, usually of gastric, ovarian, colorectal, or pancreatic origin. **surfers' n's,** hyperplastic, fibrosing, rarely ulcerated granulomas 1 to 3 cm. in diameter, occurring over bony prominences of the feet and legs of surfers, occurring as a result of repeated trauma from kneeling on surfboards; called also *Malibu disease* and *surfers' knobs* or *knots.* **n's tabac,** Gamna n's. **teachers' n.,** a nodule of the vocal cords in chorditis tuberosa. **triticeous n.,** cartilago triticea. **typhoid n.,** a mass of macrophages and other necrotic cells observed in the liver in typhoid fever. **typhus n's,** minute nodules in the skin, formed by perivascular infiltration of mononuclear cells in typhus. **n. of vermis,** nodulus cerebelli. **vestigial n.,** tuberculum auriculae. **vocal n.,** singer's node. **warm n.,** a nodule in the thyroid gland which shows the same ^{131}I uptake as the rest of the gland; normally not carcinomatous.

noduli (nod′u-li) [L.] genitive and plural of *nodulus.*

nodulous (nod′u-lus) nodose.

nodulus (nod′u-lus), gen. and pl. *nod′uli* [L., dim. of *nodus*] a nodule or small knot; used in anatomical nomenclature as a general term to designate a comparatively minute collection of tissue, and often used alone to designate the nodulus cerebelli. **nod′uli aggrega′ti proces′sus vermifor′mis,** folliculi lymphatici aggregati appendicis vermiformis. **n. cerebel′li,** [NA], nodule of cerebellum: the most ventral part of the caudal surface of the vermis, connected on each side to the caudal medullary velum, and forming the central part of the flocculonodular lobe; called also *nodulus, nodule of vermis* and *n. vermis.* **n. lymphat′icus** [NA], lymphatic nodule: a small collection of lymphoid tissue found in such organs as the gut; called also *folliculus lymphaticus* [NA alternative] and *lymph* or *lymphatic follicle.* See also *lym-*

phatic nodule, under *nodule.* **nod′uli lymphat′ici aggrega′ti [Peyer′i],** folliculi lymphatici aggregati. **nod′uli lymphat′ici bronchia′les,** lymph nodules situated in the lining of the bronchi. **nod′uli lymphat′ici conjunctiva′les,** lymph nodules situated in the conjunctiva. **nod′uli lymphat′ici gas′trici,** folliculi lymphatici gastrici. **nod′uli lymphat′ici laryn′gei,** folliculi lymphatici laryngei. **nod′uli lymphat′ici rec′ti,** folliculi lymphatici recti. **nod′uli lymphat′ici solita′rii intesti′ni cras′si,** folliculi lymphatici solitarii intestini crassi. **nod′uli lymphat′ici solita′rii intesti′ni ten′uis,** folliculi lymphatici solitarii intestini tenuis. **nod′uli lymphat′ici tuba′rii tu′bae auditi′vae,** lymphatic follicles about the pharyngeal end and internally along the median wall of the auditory tube; called also *Gerlach's tonsil.* **nod′uli lymphat′ici vagina′les,** small collections of lymphatic tissue deep to the epithelial surface of the vagina. **nod′uli lymphat′ici vesica′les,** collections of lymphatic tissue in the lining of the urinary bladder. **nod′uli thy′mici accesso′rii** [NA], accessory thymic nodules: portions of thymus tissue that have been detached from the stalk and left behind in the caudal migration of the gland in embryonic development. **nod′uli valvula′rum aor′tae,** former NA term for nodules of aortic valve; see *noduli valvularum semilunarium.* **nod′uli valvula′rum semiluna′rium** [NA], small fibrous tubercles, one at the center of the free margin of each of the three cusps of the valve of the pulmonary trunk (called also *noduli valvularum semilunarium* [ventriculi dextri] and *nodules of pulmonary trunk valve*) and of the aortic valve (called also *noduli valvularum aortae* or *nodules of aortic valve,* and *nodules of Arantius*). **nod′uli valvula′rum semiluna′rium [Aran′tii],** nodules of aortic valve; see *noduli valvularum semilunarium.* **nod′uli valvula′rum semiluna′rium [ventric′uli dex′tri],** see *noduli valvularum semilunarium.* **n. ver′mis,** n. cerebelli.

nodus (no′dus), gen. and pl. *no′di* [L.] a node or knot; used in anatomical nomenclature as a general term to designate a small mass of tissue. **n. arcus ve′nae azygos** [NA], lymph node of arch of azygos vein: a lymph node sometimes present on the azygos vein at the point where it arches over the root of the lung. **n. atrioventricula′ris** [NA], atrioventricular node: a microscopic collection of specialized cardiac muscle fibers (Purkinje's fibers), located beneath the endocardium of the right atrium, and continuous with atrial muscle fibers and with the atrioventricular bundle; it is similar to but somewhat smaller than the nodus sinuatrialis. Called also *Aschoff's, Koch's,* and *Tawara's node.* **n. cor′dis,** see *trigona fibrosa cordis.* **n. curso′rius,** a point in the corpus striatum of some animals, as the rabbit, stimulation of which causes the animal to rush forward. **n. cys′ticus** [NA], cystic node: a hepatic lymph node situated in the curve of the neck of the gallbladder at the junction of the cystic and common hepatic ducts; called *node of neck of gallbladder.* **n. fibula′ris** [NA], fibular node: a lymph node situated along the peroneal artery; called also *peroneal node.* **n. foramina′lis** [NA], foraminal node: a hepatic lymph node situated along the upper part of the common bile duct; called also *node of anterior border of epiploic foramen* and *node of epiploic foramen.* **no′di juxta-intestina′les** [NA], juxtaintestinal nodes: the mesenteric lymph nodes situated close to the wall of the intestine between the branches of the jejunal and ileal arteries. **n. lacuna′ris interme′dius** [NA], intermediate lacunar node: a lymph node situated between the external iliac vessels at the lacuna vasorum. **n. lacuna′ris latera′lis** [NA], lateral lacunar node: a lymph node situated on the lateral aspect of the external iliac vessels at the lacuna vasorum. **n. lacuna′ris media′lis** [NA], medial lacunar node: a lymph node situated on the medial aspect of the external iliac vessels at the lacuna vasorum. **n. ligamentis arterio′si** [NA], node of ligamentum arteriosum: the lowest of anterior mediastinal lymph node situated anterior to the ligamentum arteriosum. **n. lymphat′icus** [NA], one of the accumulations of lymphoid tissue interposed throughout the lymphatic system. See *lymph node,* under *node.* Called also *lymphoglandula* and *lymphonodus.* **no′di lymphat′ici abdom′inis parieta′les** [NA], parietal abdominal lymph nodes: the lymph nodes that drain the abdominal walls, comprising the left, intermediate, and lumbar lymph nodes, inferior phrenic lymph nodes, and inferior epigastric lymph nodes. **no′di lymphat′ici abdom′inis viscera′les**

[NA], visceral abdominal lymph nodes: the numerous lymph nodes that drain the abdominal viscera. **no′di lymphat′ici anorecta′les,** NA alternative for *nodi lymphatici pararectales.* **no′di lymphat′ici aor′tici latera′les** [NA], lateral aortic lymph nodes: two chains (right and left) of the left lumbar group situated on the left side of the aorta that drain the suprarenal glands; kidneys, ureters, testes, ovaries, pelvic viscera (except the intestines), and posterior abdominal wall. **no′di lymphat′ici apica′les** [NA], see *nodi lymphatici axillares.* **no′di lymphat′ici appendicula′res** [NA], appendicular lymph nodes: lymph nodes situated along the appendicular artery and in the mesoappendix that drain into the ileocolic lymph nodes. **no′di lymphat′ici axilla′res** [NA], axillary lymph nodes: the 20 to 30 lymph nodes of the axilla, which receive lymph from all the lymph vessels of the upper limb, most of those of the breast, and the cutaneous vessels from the trunk above the level of the umbilicus; they are divided into groups: brachial or lateral, interpectoral, or pectoral, subscapular, central, and apical. **no′di lymphat′ici brachia′lis** [NA], brachial lymph nodes: four to six axillary lymph nodes lying medial to, and behind, the axillary vein, which drain most of the upper limb; called also *lateral axillary lymph nodes.* **no′di lymphat′ici bronchopulmona′les** [NA], bronchopulmonary lymph nodes: lymph nodes embedded in the root of the lung, mainly at the hilum that drain into the tracheobronchial lymph nodes; called also *hilar lymph nodes* and *nodi lymphatici hilares.* **n. lymphat′icus bucca′lis,** n. lymphaticus buccinatorius. **n. lymphat′icus buccinato′rius** [NA], buccinator lymph node: one of a variable number of facial lymph nodes lying on a line between the angle of the mandible and the mouth, receiving the afferent vessels draining the temporal and infratemporal fossae and nasopharynx; their efferent vessels drain into the superior deep cervical nodes. Called also *buccal lymph node* and *n. lymphaticus buccalis.* **no′di lymphat′ici cava′les latera′les** [NA], lateral caval lymph nodes: the lymph nodes of the right lumbar group situated on the right side of the inferior vena cava. **no′di lymphat′ici cervica′les anterio′res** [NA], anterior cervical lymph nodes: a group of lymph nodes ventral to the larynx and trachea, consisting of superficial vessels on the anterior jugular vein (*nodi cervicales anteriores superficiales*) and deep vessels (*nodi cervicales anteriores profundi*) on the middle cricothyroid ligament as well as ventral to the trachea. **no′di lymphat′ici cervica′les anterio′res profun′di** [NA], deep anterior cervical lymph nodes: a group of numerous large lymph nodes that form a chain along the internal jugular vein, extending from the base of the skull to the root of the neck, situated near the pharynx, esophagus, and trachea; they receive lymph from both superficial and deep structures. **no′di lymphat′ici cervica′les anterio′res superficia′les** [NA], superficial anterior cervical lymph nodes: lymph nodes along the external jugular vein as it emerges from the parotid gland, being superficial to the sternocleidomastoid muscle; they receive afferent vessels from the auricle and parotid region. **no′di lymphat′ici cervica′les latera′les profun′di** [NA], deep lateral cervical lymph nodes: a chain of lymph nodes situated in the posterior cervical triangle; the chain is subdivided into smaller chains of lymph nodes, including lateral and anterior jugular, jugulodigastric, jugulo-omohyoid, supraclavicular and retropharyngeal lymph nodes. **no′di lymphat′ici cervica′les latera′les superficia′les** [NA], superficial lateral cervical lymph nodes: lymph nodes situated along the external jugular vein that send efferent vessels to the deep lateral cervical lymph nodes. **no′di lymphat′ici coeli′aci** [NA], celiac lymph nodes: a few nodes along the celiac trunk, which receive lymph from the stomach, spleen, duodenum, liver, and pancreas. **no′di lymphat′ici col′ici** [NA], colic lymph nodes: lymph nodes situated along the right, middle, and left colic arteries; they are designated *nodi lymphatici colici dextri, medii,* and *sinistri* [NA], respectively. Called also *intermediate colic lymph nodes.* **no′di lymphat′ici cubita′les** [NA], cubital lymph nodes: one or two superficially placed lymph nodes situated above the medial epicondyle, medial to the basilic vein, the efferent vessels of which accompany the basilic vein and join the deep lymph vessels; called also *supratrochlear lymph nodes.* **no′di lymphat′ici epigas′trici infe′riores** [NA], inferior epigastric lymph nodes: lymph nodes along the deep epigastric vessels, receiving lymph from the lower abdominal wall.

no'di lymphat'ici facia'les [NA], facial lymph nodes: lymph nodes situated along the course of the facial artery and vein, which receive afferent vessels draining the eyelids, conjunctiva, nose, cheeks, lips, and gums, and send efferent vessels to the submandibular nodes. **no'di lymphat'ici gas'trici dex'tri** [NA], right gastric lymph nodes: a few nodes along the right gastric artery that receive lymph from the stomach, spleen, duodenum, liver, and pancreas. **no'di lymphat'ici gas'trici sinis'tri** [NA], left gastric lymph nodes: a few nodes along the left gastric artery that receive lymph from the stomach, spleen, duodenum, liver, and pancreas. **no'di lymphat'ici gastroepiplo'ici dex'tri,** nodi lymphatici gastro-omentales dextri. **no'di lymphat'ici gastroepiplo'ici sinis'tri,** nodi lymphatici gastro-omentales sinistri. **no'di lymphat'ici gastro-omenta'les dex'tri** [NA], right gastro-omental lymph nodes: lymph nodes situated in the greater omentum along the pyloric half of the greater curvature of the stomach in association with the right gastroepiploic artery; called also *nodi lymphatici gastroepiploici* and *right gastroepiploic lymph nodes.* **no'di lymphat'ici gastro-omenta'les sinis'tri** [NA], left gastro-omental lymph nodes: lymph nodes situated in the greater omentum in association with the right gastroepiploic; called also *left gastroepiploic lymph nodes* and *nodi lymphatici gastroepiploici sinistri.* **no'di lymphat'ici glutea'les inferio'res** [NA], inferior gluteal lymph nodes: the internal iliac lymph nodes situated along the inferior gluteal artery. **no'di lymphat'ici glutea'les superio'res** [NA], superior gluteal lymph nodes: the internal iliac lymph nodes situated along the superior gluteal artery. **no'di lymphat'ici hepat'ici** [NA], hepatic lymph nodes: a variable number of lymph nodes situated along the proper and common hepatic arteries and the bile ducts that receive lymph from the stomach, spleen, duodenum, liver, and pancreas; two are fairly common: the cystic node and the foraminal node. **no'di lymphat'ici hila'res** [NA], nodi lymphatici bronchopulmonales. **no'di lymphat'ici ileocol'ici** [NA], ileocolic lymph nodes: nodes in the region of the ileocolic junction, draining adjacent structures. **no'di lymphat'ici ili'aci commu'nes** [NA], common iliac lymph nodes: the four to six lymph nodes grouped at the sides and dorsal to the common iliac vessels, comprising five groups: medial, intermediate, lateral, subaortic, and promontory; they receive efferent vessels from the lateral and internal iliac lymph nodes and send efferent vessels to the lateral aortic lymph nodes. **no'di lymphat'ici ili'aci commu'nes interme'dii** [NA], intermediate common iliac lymph nodes: the common iliac lymph nodes situated between the common iliac vessels. **no'di lymphat'ici ili'aci commu'nes latera'les** [NA], lateral common iliac lymph nodes: the common iliac lymph nodes situated on the lateral aspect of the common iliac vessels. **no'di lymphat'ici ili'aci commu'nes media'les** [NA], medial common iliac lymph nodes: the common iliac lymph nodes situated on the medial aspect of the common iliac vessels. **no'di lymphat'ici ili'aci commu'nes promonto'rii** [NA], promontory common iliac lymph nodes: the common iliac lymph nodes situated in front of the sacral promontory. **no'di lymphat'ici ili'aci commu'nes subaor'tici** [NA], subaortic common iliac lymph nodes: the common iliac lymph nodes situated below the bifurcation of the aorta. **no'di lymphat'ici ili'aci exter'ni** [NA], external iliac lymph nodes: the eight to ten nodes along the external iliac vessels, comprising five groups: medial, intermediate, lateral, interiliac, and obturator lymph nodes; they receive afferent vessels from the inguinal lymph nodes, deep part of the abdominal wall below the umbilicus, and some pelvic viscera and send efferent vessels to the common iliac lymph nodes. **no'di lymphat'ici ili'aci exter'ni interme'dii** [NA], intermediate external iliac lymph nodes: the external iliac lymph nodes situated between the external iliac vessels. **no'di lymphat'ici ili'aci exter'ni latera'les** [NA], lateral external iliac lymph nodes: the external iliac lymph nodes situated on the lateral aspect of the external iliac vessels. **no'di lymphat'ici ili'aci exter'ni media'les** [NA], medial external iliac lymph nodes: the external iliac lymph nodes situated on the medial aspect of the external iliac vessels. **no'di lymphat'ici ili'aci inter'ni** [NA], internal iliac lymph nodes: nodes grouped around the origins of the branches of the internal iliac vessels, comprising two groups: superior and inferior gluteal and sacral lymph nodes; they receive afferent vessels from the pelvic viscera, perineum,

and buttocks and send efferent vessels to the common iliac lymph nodes. **no'di lymphat'ici inguina'les inferi-o'res** [NA], inferior inguinal lymph nodes: the lower superficial inguinal lymph nodes situated below the opening of the saphenous vein. **no'di lymphat'ici inguina'les profun'di** [NA], deep inguinal lymph nodes: nodes deep to the fascia lata along the femoral vein; they receive lymph from the deep structures of the lower limb and from the penis or clitoris, and superficial inguinal lymph nodes and drain into the external iliac lymph nodes. **no'di lymphat'ici inguina'les superficia'les** [NA], superficial inguinal lymph nodes: lymph nodes situated in the subcutaneous tissue inferior to the inguinal ligament on either side of the proximal part of the greater saphenous vein, comprising two upper (supermedial and superolateral) groups and one lower (inferior) group; they drain the skin of the lower abdominal wall, penis, scrotum or labia majora, perineum, and buttocks. **no'di lymphat'ici inguina'les superolatera'les** [NA], superolateral inguinal lymph nodes: the upper superficial inguinal nodes situated on the lateral side of the opening of the saphenous vein. **no'di lymphat'ici inguina'les superomedia'les** [NA], superomedial inguinal lymph nodes: the upper superficial inguinal lymph nodes situated on the medial side of the opening of the saphenous vein. **no'di lymphat'ici intercosta'les** [NA], intercostal lymph nodes: lymph nodes in the back of the thorax, along the intercostal vessels. **no'di lymphat'ici interili'aci** [NA], interiliac lymph nodes: the external iliac lymph nodes situated between the external and internal iliac vessels and the obturator artery. **no'di lymphat'ici interpectora'les** [NA], interpectoral lymph nodes: four or five lymph nodes lying along the lateral thoracic veins at the inferior border of the pectoralis minor muscle, which drain the anterior and lateral body walls above the level of the umbilicus and most of the breast; called also *pectoral lymph nodes.* **no'di lymphat'ici jugula'res anterio'res** [NA], anterior jugular lymph nodes: deep lateral cervical lymph nodes that accompany the anterior jugular vein in the lower neck, which drain the skin and muscles of the anterior infrahyoid region of the neck. **no'di lymphat'ici jugula'res latera'les,** lateral jugular lymph nodes: deep lateral cervical lymph nodes situated lateral to the internal jugular vein that empty into the jugular trunk. **n. lymphat'icus jugulodigas'tricus** [NA], jugulodigastric lymph node: one of the deep lateral cervical lymph nodes lying on the internal jugular vein at the level of the greater cornu of the hyoid bone, i.e., just below the posterior belly of the digastric muscle; called also *hauptganglion of Küttner* and *Küttner's ganglion.* **n. lymphat'icus jugulo-omohyoi'deus** [NA], jugulo-omohyoid lymph node: one of the deep lateral cervical lymph nodes lying on the internal jugular vein just above the tendon of the omohyoid muscle. **no'di lymphat'ici juxta-esophagea'les pulmona'les** [NA], pulmonary juxtaesophageal lymph nodes: posterior mediastinal lymph nodes situated on both sides of the esophagus. **no'di lymphat'ici liena'les,** NA alternative for *nodi lymphatici splenici.* **no'di lymphat'ici lingua'les** [NA], deep cervical lymph nodes receiving afferent vessels from the tongue; called also *lymphoglandulae linguales.* **no'di lymphat'ici lumba'les** [NA], lumbar lymph nodes: a chain of nodes alongside the lower abdominal aorta, receiving most of the lymph from the abdominal structures; called also *lymphoglandulae lumbales.* **no'di lymphat'ici lumba'les dex'tri** [NA], right lumbar lymph nodes: the chain of lumbar lymph nodes situated partly in front of the vena cava and partly behind it on the psoas major muscle, comprising three groups: lateral caval, precaval, and postcaval lymph nodes. Called also *nodi lymphatici lumbares dextri* [NA alternative]. **no'di lymphat'ici lumba'les interme'dii** [NA], intermediate lumbar lymph nodes: the chain of lymph nodes that lie in the median plane, between the left and right lumbar lymph nodes. Called also *nodi lymphatici lumbares intermedii* [NA alternative]. **no'di lymphat'ici lumba'les sinis'tri** [NA], left lumbar lymph nodes: the chain of lumber lymph nodes situated at the side of the abdominal aorta on the psoas major muscle, comprising three groups: right and left lateral aortic, preaortic, and postaortic lymph nodes. Called also *nodi lymphatici lumbares sinistri* [NA alternative]. **no'di lymphat'ici lumba'res dex'tri,** NA alternative for *nodi lymphatici lumbales dextri.* **no'di lymphat'ici lumba'res interme'dii,** NA alternative for *nodi lymphatici lumbales intermedii.* **no'di lymphat'ici lum-**

ba′res sinis′tri, NA alternative for *nodi lymphatici lum-bales sinistri.* **n. lymphat′icus mala′ris** [NA], malar lymph node: one of a variable number of facial lymph nodes situated in the region of the zygomatic minor muscle. **n. lymphat′icus mandibula′ris** [NA], mandibular lymph node: one of a variable number of facial lymph nodes situated near the angle of the mandible, into which lymph from some of the superficial tissues of the head and neck is drained. **no′di lymphat′ici mastoi′dei** [NA], mastoid lymph nodes: lymph nodes, two or three on each side, that are superficial to the mastoid attachment of the sternocleidomastoid muscle and deep to the posterior auricular muscle; they drain the nasal fossae and paranasal sinuses, hard and soft palate, middle ear, and nasopharynx and oropharynx. Called also *nodi lymphatici retroauriculares* and *retroauricular lymph nodes.* **no′di lymphat′ici mediastina′les an-terio′res** [NA], anterior mediastinal lymph nodes: nodes along the great vessels of the superior mediastinum and on the anterior part of the diaphragm, receiving lymph from adjacent structures. **no′di lymphat′ici medias-tina′les posterio′res** [NA], posterior mediastinal lymph nodes: a group of lymph nodes situated behind the pericardium in relation to the esophagus and thoracic aorta, which receive lymph from the esophagus, pericardium, diaphragm, and lungs and pass efferent vessels mainly to the thoracic duct and sometimes to the tracheobronchial lymph nodes. **no′di lymphat′ici mem′bri superio′ris profun′di** [NA], deep lymph nodes of the upper limb: the lymph nodes situated internal to the deep fascia of the upper limb, most of which are grouped in the axilla; they accompany the radial, ulnar, interosseous, and brachial arteries and end in the brachial axillary lymph nodes. **no′di lymphat′ici mem′bri superio′ris superficia′les** [NA], superficial lymph nodes of upper limb: the superficially placed lymph nodes of the upper limb (e.g., the cubital lymph nodes) that, except those in the hand and on the back of the forearm, converge toward and accompany the superficial veins. **no′di lymphat′ici mesenter′ici,** mesenteric lymph nodes: nodes that lie at the root of the mesentery, receiving lymph from parts of the small intestine, cecum, appendix, and large intestine; they comprise three groups: the juxtaintestinal, central superior, and inferior mesenteric lymph nodes. **no′di lymphat′ici mesenter′ici inferio′res** [NA], inferior mesenteric lymph nodes: nodes situated along the inferior mesenteric vessels and receiving lymph from the adjacent region; they comprise two groups: the sigmoid and superior rectal lymph nodes. **no′di lymphat′ici mesenter′ici superio′res** nodi superiores centrales. **n. lymphat′icus nasolabia′lis** [NA], nasolabial lymph node: one of a variable number of facial lymph nodes situated near the junction of the superior labial and facial arteries, which drains the upper lip and external nose into the submandibular node. **no′di lymphat′ici obturato′rii** [NA], obturator nodes: the external iliac lymph nodes situated in the obturator canal. **no′di lymphat′ici oc-cipita′les** [NA], occipital lymph nodes: several small nodes near the occipital insertion of the semispinalis capitis muscle; called also *lymphoglandulae occipitales.* **no′di lym-phat′ici pancreat′ici** [NA], pancreatic lymph nodes: nodes found along the pancreatic arteries that drain lymph from the pancreas to the pancreaticosplenic lymph nodes. **no′di lymphat′ici pancreat′ici inferio′res** [NA], inferior pancreatic lymph nodes: lymph nodes associated with the inferior pancreatic artery. **no′di lymphat′ici pan-creat′ici superio′res** [NA], superior pancreatic lymph nodes: lymph nodes associated with the superior pancreatic artery. **no′di lymphat′ici pan-creaticoduodena′les inferio′res** [NA], inferior pancreaticoduodenal lymph nodes: lymph nodes situated along the inferior pancreaticoduodenal artery. **no′di lymphat′ici pancreaticoduodena′les superio′res** [NA], superior pancreaticoduodenal lymph nodes: lymph nodes situated along the superior pancreaticoduodenal artery. **no′di lymphat′ici paracol′ici** [NA], paracolic lymph nodes: lymph nodes situated along the medial borders of the ascending and descending colon and along the mesenteric borders of the transverse and sigmoid colon. **no′di lym-phat′ici paramamma′rii** [NA], paramammary lymph nodes: lymph nodes on the lateral mammary gland that drain into the axillary lymph nodes. **no′di lymphat′ici pararecta′les** [NA], pararectal lymph nodes: lymph nodes situated around the rectum, embedded in its muscular coat; they drain into the inferior mesenteric, sacral, internal iliac,

common iliac, and superficial inguinal nodes. Called also *anorectal lymph nodes* and *nodi lymphatici anorectales* [NA alternative]. **no′di lymphat′ici parasterna′les** [NA], parasternal lymph nodes: nodes located along the course of the internal thoracic artery, which drain the mammary gland, abdominal wall, and diaphragm. **no′di lymphat′ici paratrachea′les** [NA], paratracheal lymph nodes: lymph nodes on either side of the esophagus, extending upward into the neck, which receive lymph from the esophagus, trachea, and tracheobronchial lymph nodes. **no′di lymphat′ici para-uteri′ni** [NA], parauterine lymph nodes: lymph nodes situated around the uterus, consisting of superficial (beneath the peritoneum) and deep (in the substance of the uterine wall) nodes: they drain into the lumbar, external and internal iliac, sacral, and superficial inguinal lymph nodes. **no′di lymphat′ici paravagina′les** [NA], paravaginal lymph nodes: lymph nodes situated around the vagina; they drain into the external and internal iliac, common iliac, and superficial inguinal lymph nodes. **no′di lymphat′ici paravesicula′res** [NA], paravesicular lymph nodes: lymph nodes situated around the urinary bladder, comprising three groups: perivesicular, postvesicular, and lateral vesicular lymph nodes; they drain into the external and internal iliac lymph nodes and, in association with some lymph nodes from the prostrate, into the sacral and common iliac lymph nodes. **no′di lymphat′ici paroti′dei profun′di** [NA], deep parotid lymph nodes: lymph nodes on the lateral wall of the pharynx lying deep to or embedded in the deep substance of the parotid gland, through which lymph drains from the external acoustic meatus, auditory tube, tympanum soft palate, and posterior nasal cavity. **no′di lymphat′ici paroti′dei profun′di infra-auricula′res** [NA], infra-auricular deep parotid lymph nodes: deep parotid lymph nodes situated below the ear. **no′di lymphat′ici paroti′dei profun′di intraglandula′res** [NA], intraglandular deep parotid lymph nodes: deep parotid lymph nodes situated within the substance of the parotid gland. **no′di lym-phat′ici paroti′dei profun′di preauricula′res** [NA], preauricular deep parotid lymph nodes: deep parotid lymph nodes situated in front of the ear. **no′di lymphat′ici paroti′dei superficia′les** [NA], superficial parotid lymph nodes: lymph nodes lying in the subcutaneous tissue of the parotid gland directly in front of the tragus. **no′di lymphat′ici pectora′les** [NA], see *nodi lymphatici axillares.* **no′di lymphat′ici pel′vis parieta′les** [NA], parietal pelvic lymph nodes: the lymph nodes that drain the wall of the pelvis, including the common iliac, external iliac, and internal iliac lymph nodes. **no′di lymphat′ici pel′vis viscera′les** [NA], visceral pelvic lymph nodes: the lymph nodes that drain the pelvic viscera, including the paravesicular, parauterine, paravaginal, and pararectal lymph nodes. **no′di lymphat′ici pericardia′les latera′les** [NA], lateral pericardial lymphatic nodes: lymph nodes accompanying the pericardiacophrenic artery. **no′di lymphat′ici phren′ici inferio′res** [NA], inferior phrenic lymph nodes: parietal lymph nodes accompanying the inferior vessels of the diaphragm. **no′di lym-phat′ici phren′ici superio′res** [NA], superior phrenic lymph nodes: several nodes on the thoracic surface of the diaphragm, receiving lymph from the intercostal spaces, pericardium, diaphragm, and liver; called also *diaphragmatic lymph nodes.* **no′di lymphat′ici poplitea′les** [NA], popliteal lymph nodes: lymph nodes embedded in the fat of the popliteal fossa, comprising superficial and deep groups; their efferent vessels accompany the femoral vessels to the deep inguinal lymph nodes. **no′di lymphat′ici po-plitea′les profun′di** [NA], deep popliteal lymph nodes: the popliteal lymph nodes situated at the sides of the popliteal vessels. **no′di lymphat′ici poplitea′les superficia′les** [NA], superficial popliteal lymph nodes: the popliteal lymph nodes situated at the termination of the small saphenous vein. **no′di lymphat′ici post-aor′tici** [NA], postaortic lymph nodes: lymph nodes of the left lumbar group situated behind the aorta formed by peripheral nodes of the right and left lateral aortic lymph nodes; called also *retroaortic lymph nodes.* **no′di lymphat′-icipostcavales** [NA], postcaval lymph nodes: the lymph nodes of the right lumbar group situated behind the inferior vena cava. **no′di lymphat′ici post vesicula′res** [NA], postvesicular lymph nodes: the paravesicular lymph nodes situated in back of the urinary bladder. **no′di lymphat′ici preaor′tici** [NA], preaortic lymph nodes: lymph nodes of the left lumbar group situated in front of the aorta that drain the abdominal part of the alimentary canal and its derivatives. **no′di lymphat′ici precaeca′les** [NA], **no′di lymphat′ici prececa′les,** prececal lymph nodes: lymph nodes situated in front of the cecum that drain into the anterior ileocolic lymph nodes. **no′di lymphat′ici precava′les** [NA], precaval lymph nodes: the lymph nodes of the right lumbar group situated in front of the inferior vena cava. **no′di lymphat′ici prelaryngea′les** [NA], prelaryngeal lymph nodes: deep anterior cervical lymph nodes situated in front of the larynx that help drain the thyroid gland. **no′di lymphat′ici prepericardia′les** [NA], prepericardial lymph nodes: lymph nodes situated between the pericardium and sternum. **no′di lymphat′ici pretrachea′les** [NA], pretracheal lymph nodes: deep anterior cervical lymph nodes situated in front of the trachea near the inferior thyroid veins. **no′di lymphat′ici prevertebra′les** [NA], prevertebral lymph nodes: lymph nodes situated in back of the thoracic aorta. **no′di lymphat′ici prevesicula′res** [NA], prevesicular lymph nodes: the paravesicular lymph nodes situated in front of the urinary bladder. **no′di lymphat′ici pulmona′les** [NA], pulmonary lymph nodes: nodes located along the larger bronchi within the lung substance, through which lymph from the lung drains; called also *lymphoglandulae pulmonales*. **no′di lymphat′ici pylo′rici** [NA], pyloric lymph nodes: lymph nodes that lie in front of the head of the pancreas, receiving lymph from the pyloric part of the stomach. They are subdivided into three groups: suprapyloric, subpyloric, and retropyloric nodes. **no′di lymphat′ici recta′les superio′res,** superior rectal lymph nodes: lymph nodes situated along the superior rectal artery. **no′di lymphat′ici retroauricula′res,** nodi lymphatici mastoidei. **no′di lymphat′ici retrocaeca′les** [NA], **no′di lymphatici retroceca′les,** retrocecal lymph nodes: lymph nodes situated in back of the cecum that drain into the posterior ileocecal lymph nodes. **no′di lymphat′ici retropharyngea′les** [NA], retropharyngeal lymph nodes: deep lateral cervical lymph nodes, one median and two lateral groups, situated behind the upper part of the pharynx, especially concerned with drainage of the nasal fossae, paranasal sinuses, hard and soft palates, middle ear, nasopharynx, and oropharynx. **no′di lymphat′ici sacra′les** [NA], sacral lymph nodes: the internal iliac lymph nodes situated along the lateral and median sacral vessels; they receive lymph from the rectum and posterior pelvic wall. **no′di lymphat′ici sple′nici** [NA], splenic lymph nodes: lymph nodes in the capsule and larger trabeculae of the spleen that drain into adjacent lymph nodes; called also *nodi lymphatici lienales* [NA alternative]. **no′di lymphat′ici submandibula′res** [NA], submandibular lymph nodes: the three to six nodes alongside the submandibular gland, through which lymph drains from the adjacent skin and mucous membrane. **no′di lymphat′ici submenta′les** [NA], submental lymph nodes: nodes under the chin into which the lymph from some of the superficial tissues of the head and neck is drained. **no′di lymphat′ici subscapula′res** [NA], see *nodi lymphatici axillares.* **no′di lymphat′ici supraclavicula′res** [NA], supraclavicular lymph nodes: the deep lateral cervical lymph nodes situated inferior to the omohyoid muscle, extending into the omoclavicular portion of the posterior triangle of the neck. **no′di lymphat′ici thyroi′dei** [NA], thyroid lymph nodes: deep anterior cervical lymph nodes situated around the thyroid gland. **no′di lymphat′ici trachea′les,** nodi lymphatici paratracheales. **no′di lymphat′ici tracheobronchia′les inferio′res** [NA], inferior tracheobronchial lymph nodes: nodes in the angle of the bifurcation of the trachea, receiving lymph from adjacent structures. **no′di lymphat′ici tracheobronchia′les superio′res** [NA], superior tracheobronchial lymph nodes: nodes between the trachea and the bronchus on either side, receiving lymph from adjacent structures. **no′di lymphat′ici vesicula′res latera′les** [NA], lateral vesicular lymph nodes: the paravesicular lymph nodes situated in relation to the lateral umbilical ligament. **no′di mesocol′ici** [NA], mesocolic lymph nodes: lymph nodes situated in the mesocolon, comprising two groups: paracolic and right middle, and left colic lymph nodes. **no′di retropylo′rici** [NA], retropyloric nodes: pyloric lymph nodes situated in back of the pylorus. **no′di sigmoi′dei** [NA], sigmoid lymph nodes: lymph nodes situated along the sigmoid arteries. **n. sinuatria′lis** [NA], a microscopic collection of atypical cardiac muscle fibers (Purkinje's fibers) at the superior end of the sulcus terminalis, at the junction of the superior vena cava and the right atrium. See *sinoatrial node*, under *node.* **no′di subpylo′rici** [NA], subpyloric nodes: pyloric lymph nodes situated below the pylorus. **no′di superio′res centra′les,** central superior nodes: the mesenteric lymph nodes situated along the upper part of the superior mesenteric artery; called also *nodi lymphatici mesenterici superiores* and *superior mesenteric lymph nodes.* **n. suprapylo′ricus** [NA], suprapyloric node: a pyloric lymph node situated above the duodenum on the right gastric artery. **n. tibia′lis ante′rior** [NA], anterior tibial node: a lymph node situated along the anterior tibial artery. **n. tibia′lis poste′rior** [NA], posterior tibial node: a lymph node situated along the posterior tibial artery.

noematachograph (no-e″mah-tak′o-graf) [Gr. *noēma* thought + *tachys* swift + *graphein* to write] a device for registering the time required in a mental operation.

noematachometer (no-e″mah-tah-kom′ĕ-ter) [Gr. *noēma* thought + *tachys* swift + *metron* measure] a device for measuring the time required in a mental operation.

noematic (no″e-mat′ik) pertaining to thought or the operation of the mind.

noesis (no-e′sis) [Gr. *noēsis* thought] the operation of the intellect; cognition.

noetic (no-et′ik) pertaining to the intellect or to cognition.

noeud (nuh) [Fr.] knot, or node. **n. vital** (nuh ve-tal′) ["vital node"], an old term applied to the respiratory centers.

nogalamycin (no-gal-ah-mi′sin) an antineoplastic antibiotic produced by a variant of *Streptomyces nogalater.*

Noguchi's reagent, test (no-goo′chēz) [Hideyo *Noguchi*, Japanese pathologist in New York, 1876–1928] see under *reagent* and *tests.*

nolinium bromide (no-lin′e-um) chemical name: 2-[(3,4-dichlorophenyl)amino]quinolizinium bromide; an antisecretory and antiulcerative, $C_{15}H_{11}BrCl_2N_2$.

noma (no′mah) [Gr. *nomai* eating sores] 1. a severe gangrenous process occurring predominantly in debilitated and malnourished children, especially in underdeveloped countries, typically beginning as a small vesicle or ulcer on the gingiva that rapidly becomes necrotic and spreads to produce extensive destruction of the buccal and labial mucosa and tissues of the face, which may result in severe disfigurement and even death. Various bacteria have been implicated in the etiology, including fusiform bacilli, *Treponema vincentii,* and *Bacteroides melaninogenicus.* Called also *cancrum oris* and *gangrenous stomatitis.* 2. a condition marked by the presence of gangrenous erosions similar to those of the oral tissues but involving the genitalia; see *erosive balanitis,* under *balanitis,* and *erosive vulvitis,* under *vulvitis.* **n. vul′vae,** erosive vulvitis.

nomadic (no-mad′ik) wandering; unsettled; free.

nomenclature (no′men-kla″tūr, no-men′kla″tūr) [L. *nomen* name + *calare* to call] a classified system of names, as of anatomical structures, organisms, etc. See *Nomina Anatomica.* **binomial n.,** the nomenclature used in scientific classification of living organisms in which each organism is designated by two latinized names (genus and species), both of which must always be used because species names are not necessarily unique. NOTE: The genus name is always capitalized, the species name is not, and both are italicized, e.g., *Escherichia coli.* When a name is repeated the genus name may be abbreviated by its initial, e.g., *E. coli.*

nomifensine maleate (no″mĭ-fen′sēn) chemical name: 1,2,3,4-tetrahydro-2-methyl-4-phenyl-8-isoquinolinamine(Z)-2-butenedioate (1:1). A central nervous system stimulant, $C_{16}H_{18}N_2 \cdot C_4H_4O_4$, used as an antidepressant.

Nomina Anatomica (no′mĭ-nah an-ah-tom′ĭ-kah) [L. "anatomical names"] the official body of anatomical nomenclature, applied specifically to that revised by the International Anatomical Nomenclature Committee appointed by the Fifth International Congress of Anatomists held at Oxford in 1950, and approved by the Sixth International Congress of Anatomists (Paris, 1955) with revisions approved by the Seventh (New York, 1960), Eighth (Wiesbaden, 1965), Tenth (Tokyo, 1975), and Eleventh (Mexico City, 1980) International Congresses of Anatomists. Abbreviated NA.

nom(o)- [Gr. *nomos* custom, law] a combining form denoting relationship to usage or law.

nomogenesis (no″mo-jen′ĕ-sis) [*nomo-* + Gr. *genesis* generation] the theory of evolution according to which the course of evolution is fixed and predetermined by law, no place being left for chance.

nomogram (nom′o-gram) [*nomo-* + *-gram*] a figure consisting of three or more straight or curved lines, each graduated for a different variable and aligned in such a way that a straightedge crossing all of the scales cuts the scales at values of the variable that have a specified mathematical or empirical relationship. Called also *alignment chart* or *nomograph.*

nomograph (nom′o-graf) nomogram.

nomotopic (no″mo-top′ik) [*nomo-* + Gr. *topos* place] occurring at a normal place; occurring normally.

nona (no′nah) [perhaps from It. *nona* ninth (day after the onset of influenza)] a condition resembling lethargic encephalitis which appeared in epidemic form in southern Europe in 1889–1890.

nonacosane (non″ah-ko′sān) an aliphatic hydrocarbon, $C_{29}H_{60}$, extracted from plant waxes.

nonadherent (non″ad-he′rent) not adherent to or connected with adjacent structures.

nonan (no′nan) [L. *nonus* ninth] recurring every ninth day, or at intervals of eight days.

nonantigenic (non″an-tĭ-jen′ik) not antigenic; not eliciting an immune response in a particular animal.

nonapeptide (non″ah-pep′tid) a peptide containing nine amino acids.

non compos mentis (non kom′pos men′tis) [L.] not of sound mind.

nonconductor (non″kon-duk′tor) any substance that does not readily transmit electricity, light, or heat.

nondepolarizer (non″de-po′lar-īz″er) a muscle relaxant that produces striate muscle paralysis by competitive interference with the transmission of nerve impulses from nerve ending to muscle receptor.

nondisjunction (non″dis-junk′shun) failure (*a*) of two homologous chromosomes to pass to separate cells during the first division of meiosis, or (*b*) of the two chromatids of a chromosome to pass to separate cells during mitosis or during the second meiotic division. As a result, one daughter cell has an extra chromosome and the other has one too few. If this happens in meiosis, after fertilization an *aneuploid* individual may develop, e.g., a child with trisomy 21 (Down syndrome).

nonelectrolyte (non″e-lek′tro-līt) a substance which in solution is a nonconductor of electricity.

nonheme (non-hēm) not bound within a porphyrin ring; said of iron so contained within a protein.

nonhomogeneity (non-ho″mo-jĕ-ne′ĭ-te) the lack of homogeneity; the state of not being homogeneous.

nonigravida (no″ne-grav′ĭ-dah) [L. *nonus* ninth + *gravida* pregnant] a woman pregnant for the ninth time. Written gravida IX.

noninfectious (non″in-fek′shus) not infectious; not spread by contact, inhalation, etc.; not able to spread disease.

noninvolution (non″in-vo-lu′shun) failure of a part to return to normal size and condition after enlargement from functional activity, as noninvolution of the uterus after pregnancy.

nonipara (no-nip′ah-rah) [L. *nonus* ninth + *parere* to bring forth, produce] a woman who has had nine pregnancies which resulted in viable offspring. Written para IX.

nonmedullated (non-med′u-lāt″ed) unmyelinated.

nonmetal (non-met′al) any chemical element that is not a metal or a metalloid.

nonmyelinated (non-mi′ĕ-lĭ-nāt″ed) unmyelinated.

Nonne's syndrome, test (non′ez) [Max *Nonne,* Hamburg neurologist, 1861–1959] see *hereditary cerebellar ataxia,* and see *Ross-Jones test,* under *tests.*

Nonne-Apelt reaction (phase, test) (non′ĕ-ah′pelt) [Max *Nonne;* F. *Apelt,* German physician, 1877–1911] see under *reaction.*

Nonne-Milroy-Meige syndrome (non′e-mil′roy mehzh′e) [Max *Nonne;* William Forsyth *Milroy,* American physician, 1855–1942; Henri *Meige,* French physician, 1866–1940] Milroy's disease.

non-neuronal (non″nu-ro′nal) pertaining to or composed of nonconducting cells of the nervous system, e.g., neuroglial cells.

non-nucleated (non-nu′kle-āt″ed) without a nucleus; cf. *anuclear.*

nonocclusion (non″ŏ-kloo′zhun) open bite malocclusion.

nonoliguric (non-ol″ĭ-gu′rik) not pertaining to, characterized by, or conducive to oliguria.

nononcogenic (non″on-ko-jen′ik) not giving rise to tumors or causing tumor formation.

nonopaque (non″o-pāk′) not opaque to roentgen rays; radiolucent.

nonose (non′ōs) [L. *nonus* ninth] a carbohydrate containing nine atoms of carbon in the molecule.

nonoxynol (no-noks′ĭ-nŏl) nonylphenoxypolyethoxyethanol. A group of compounds of the general composition $C_{15}H_{24}O(C_2H_4\ O)_n$, which are assigned numbers according to the approximate value of *n*: nonoxynol 4 is $C_{15}H_{24}O(C_2H_4-O)_4$, or $C_{23}H_{40}O_5$; nonoxynol 9 is $C_{33}H_{60}O_{10}$; nonoxynol 15 is $C_{45}H_{84}O_{16}$; nonoxynol 30 is $C_{75}H_{144}O_{31}$. Nonoxynol 4, 15, and 30 are nonionic surfactants, and nonoxynol 9 is used as a spermaticide. Nonoxynol 10 [NF], in which *n* varies from 6 to 16, is used as a pharmaceutical surfactant.

nonparametric (non″par-ah-met′rik) denoting a statistical procedure that is applicable to a family of probability distributions too large to be characterized by a finite number of parameters. Nonparametric tests are usually less powerful than competing parametric tests, but they are valid in cases where parametric tests are not, e.g., either a *t*-test (parametric) or a rank sum test (nonparametric) can be used to test for a difference between the means of two samples; the *t*-test will usually give a more significant *P* value, but this will be valid only when both populations are approximately normally distributed and have equal variances, whereas the *P* value of the rank sum test is valid whenever the distributions of both populations are continuous and have the same shape.

nonparous (non-par′us) nulliparous.

nonphotochromogen (non″fo-to-kro′mo-jen) a microorganism that does not produce pigment in the presence of light. The term is specifically applied to mycobacteria that do not produce carotenoid pigmentation; included in this group is the common pathogen *Mycobacterium avium–intracellulare.*

nonpolar (non-po′lar) not having poles; not exhibiting dipole characteristics.

non repetat. abbreviation for L. *non repeta′tur,* do not repeat.

nonrotation (non″ro-ta′shun) [*non-* + L. *rotare* to turn] failure of rotation of a part to the proper position. **n. of the intestine,** failure of rotation of the intestine during embryonic development, with the result that the small intestine lies on the right side of the abdomen and the large intestine on the left.

nonsecretor (non″se-kre′tor) an individual possessing A or B type blood whose saliva and other body secretions do not contain the particular (A or B) substance.

nonself (non′self) in immunology, pertaining to foreign antigens. Cf. *self.*

nonseptate (non-sep′tāt) without a septum or septa.

nonspecific (non-spĕ-sif′ik) 1. not due to any single known cause, as to a particular pathogen. 2. not directed against a particular agent, but rather having a general effect, as nonspecific therapy.

nonunion (non-ūn′yun) failure of the ends of a fractured bone to unite.

nonus (no′nus) [L. "ninth"] (*obs.*) the hypoglossal nerve (nervus hypoglossus [NA]); so called because formerly regarded as the ninth cranial nerve.

nonvalent (non-va′lent) [L. *non* not + *valere* to be able] having no chemical valency: not capable of entering into chemical composition; said of argon, helium, and the other inert gases.

nonviable (non-vi′ah-b'l) [L. *non* not + *viable*] not capable of living.

nonyl (no′nil) the monovalent radical C_9H_{19}.

Noonan's syndrome (noo′nanz) [Jacqueline Anne *Noonan,* American cardiologist, 20th century] see under *syndrome.*

Noorden treatment (noor'den) [Carl Harko von *Noorden*, German physician, 1858–1944] oatmeal treatment.

nopalin G (no'pal-in) bluish eosin; see under *eosin*.

N.O.P.H.N. National Organization for Public Health Nursing.

nor- chemical prefix denoting (*a*) a compound (e.g., norleucine) of normal structure (having an unbranched chain of carbon atoms) that is isomeric with one (e.g., leucine) having a branched chain, or (*b*) a compound (e.g., norepinephrine) whose chain or ring contains one less methylene (CH_2) group than does that of its homologue (e.g., epinephrine).

noradrenaline (nor''ah-dren'ah-lin, nor''ah-dren'ah-lēn) norepinephrine.

noradrenergic (nor''ah-dren-er'jik) activated by or secreting norepinephrine.

norandrostenolone (nor-an''dro-sten'o-lōn) nandrolone.

nordefrin hydrochloride (nor-def'rin) chemical name: 4-(2-amino-1-hydroxypropyl)-1,2-benzenediol hydrochloride. An adrenergic agent isomeric with epinephrine, $C_9H_{13}NO_3$, having significant central stimulant action and almost no vasoconstrictor action; the levo-isomer, *levonordefrin* (q.v.), is usually used when vasoconstriction is desired. Called also *homoarterenol hydrochloride*.

norepinephrine (nor''ep-ĭ-nef'rin) one of the naturally occurring catecholamines; a neurohormone released by the postganglionic adrenergic nerves, which is the principal neurotransmitter of adrenergic neurons, having predominately α-adrenergic but some β-adrenergic activity. It is also secreted by the adrenal medulla in response to splanchnic stimulation and is stored in the chromaffin granules, being released predominantly in response to hypotension. Norepinephrine is a powerful vasopressor and is used pharmaceutically in the form of the bitartrate salt. Called also *arterenol* and *noradrenaline*. **n. bitartrate** [USP], the bitartrate salt of norepinephrine, $C_8H_{11}NO_3 \cdot C_4H_6O_6 \cdot H_2O$, occurring as a white or faintly gray, crystalline powder, having the vasoconstrictor actions of the parent compound; used to restore the blood pressure in certain cases of acute hypotension, and as an adjunct in the treatment of cardiac arrest and profound hypotension, administered by intravenous infusion. Called also *levarterenol bitartrate*.

norethandrolone (nor''eth-an'dro-lōn) [NF] chemical name: 17-hydroxy-19-nor-17α-pregn-4-en-3-one. A synthetic androgen, $C_{20}H_{30}O_2$, equal to testosterone in anabolic activity, but having less androgenic activity.

norethindrone (nor-eth'in-drōn) [USP] chemical name: 17β-hydroxy-19-nor-17α-pregn-4-en-20-yn-3-one. A progestin, $C_{20}H_{26}O_2$, occurring as a white to creamy white, crystalline powder, having some anabolic, estrogenic, and androgenic properties; used in the treatment of amenorrhea, abnormal uterine bleeding due to hormonal imbalance, and endometriosis, administered orally. Also used, alone or in combination with an estrogen component, as an oral contraceptive. **n. acetate** [NF], the acetate salt of norethindrone, $C_{22}H_{28}O_3$, having the same appearance, actions, uses, and route of administration as the base.

norethisterone (nor''eth-is'ter-ōn) norethindrone.

norethynodrel (nor''ĕ-thi'no-drel) [USP] chemical name: 17-hydroxy-19-nor-17α-pregn-5(10)-en-20-yn-3-one. A progestin, $C_{20}H_{26}O_2$, occurring as a white or nearly white, crystalline powder; used in combination with an estrogen component as an oral contraceptive, to control endometriosis, for the treatment of hypermenorrhea, and to produce cyclic withdrawal bleeding.

Norflex (nor'fleks) trademark for a preparation of orphenadrine citrate.

norfloxacin (nor-flok'sah-sin) an antibacterial organic acid structurally related to nalidixic acid and effective against penicillin-resistant *Neisseria gonorrhoeae;* administered orally.

norflurane (nor-floor'ān) chemical name: 1,1,1,2-tetrafluoroethane; an inhalation anesthetic, $C_2H_2F_4$.

norgestimate (nor-jes'tĭ-māt) chemical name: (+)-17-(acetyloxy)-13-ethyl-18,19-dinor-17α-pregn-4-en-20-yn-3-one oxime; a progestin, $C_{23}H_{31}NO_3$.

norgestomet (nor-jes'to-met) chemical name: 17-(acetyloxy)-11β-methyl-19-norpregn-4-ene-3,20-dione; a progestin, $C_{23}H_{32}O_4$.

norgestrel (nor-jes'trel) [USP] chemical name: (±)13β-

ethyl-17-hydroxy-18,19-dinor-17α-pregn-4-en-20-yn-3-one. A potent progestin, $C_{21}H_{28}O_2$, occurring as a white or nearly white, crystalline powder; used in combination with an estrogen component as an oral contraceptive.

norhyoscyamine (nor-hi''o-si'ah-mēn) chemical name: 1-tropic acid 3α-nortropanyl ester. An alkaloid, $C_{16}H_{21}NO_3$, from plants of the family Solanaceae, having properties like those of hyoscyamine. Called also *pseudohyoscyamine* and *solandrine*.

Norisodrine (nor-i'so-drin) trademark for preparations of isoproterenol.

norleucine (nor-lu'sin) chemical name: 2-aminohexanoic acid. A nonessential amino acid, $CH_3 \cdot (CH_2)_3 \cdot CH(NH_2) \cdot COOH$, extracted from the leucine fraction of the decomposition of the proteins of nervous tissue. It has been synthesized.

Norlutate (nor-lu'tāt) trademark for a preparation of norethindrone acetate.

Norlutin (nor-lu'tin) trademark for a preparation of norethindrone.

norm (norm) [L. *norma* rule] a fixed or ideal standard.

norma (nor'mah) [L.] an outline established to define the aspects of the cranium; also a norm or typical standard. **n. ante'rior,** n. facialis. **n. basila'ris,** the outline of the inferior aspect of the skull, viewed from above; called also *n. inferior* and *n. ventralis.* **n. facia'lis** [NA], the outline of the skull as viewed from the front; called also *n. anterior* and *n. frontalis.* **n. fronta'lis,** n. facialis. **n. infe'rior,** n. basilaris. **n. latera'lis,** the outline of the skull seen from either side. **n. occipita'lis,** the outline of the skull seen from behind. **n. poste'rior,** n. occipitalis. **n. sagitta'lis,** the outline of a sagittal section through the skull. **n. supe'rior,** n. verticalis. **n. tempora'lis,** n. lateralis. **n. ventra'lis,** n. basilaris. **n. vertica'lis,** the outline of the skull viewed from above; called also *n. superior.*

normal (nor'mal) [L. *norma* rule] 1. agreeing with the regular and established type. 2. in chemistry, (*a*) denoting a solution containing in each 1000 ml. 1 gram equivalent weight of the active substance; (*b*) denoting aliphatic hydrocarbons in which no carbon atom is combined with more than two other carbon atoms; (*c*) denoting salts formed from acids and bases in such a way that no acidic hydrogen of the acid remains nor any of the basic hydroxyl of the base. Abbreviated N, n.

normality (nor-mal'ĭ-te) 1. the state of being normal. 2. the number of gram-equivalent weights of solute per liter of solution.

normalization (nor''mal-i-za'shun) the process of bringing or restoring to the normal standard.

normergic (norm-er'jik) [*norm-* + Gr. *ergon* work] reacting in a normal manner.

normetanephrine (nor-met''ah-nef'rin) α-(aminomethyl)vanillyl alcohol (3-methylnorepinephrine): a metabolite of epinephrine excreted in the urine and found in certain tissues.

norm(o)- [L. *norma* rule] a combining form meaning conforming to the rule; normal or usual.

normoblast (nor'mo-blast) [*normo-* + Gr. *blastos* germ] a nucleated precursor cell in the erythrocyte series; four developmental stages are recognized: the pronormoblast and the basophilic, polychromatic, and orthochromatic normoblasts. **acidophilic n.,** orthochromatic n. **basophilic n.,** a nucleated immature erythrocyte. The cytoplasm in general is similar to that of the earlier pronormoblast but may be even more basophilic, and is usually regular in outline. The nucleus is still relatively large, but the chromatin strands are thicker and more deeply staining, giving a coarser appearance; the nucleoli have disappeared. Called also *prorubricyte, early normoblast,* and *early* or *basophilic erythroblast.* **early n.,** basophilic n. **eosinophilic n.,** orthochromatic n. **intermediate n.,** polychromatic n. **late n.,** orthochromatic n. **orthochromatic n.,** the final stage of the nucleated, immature erythrocyte, before nuclear loss. Typically the cytoplasm is described as acidophilic, but it still shows a faint polychromatic tint. The nucleus is small and initially may still have very coarse, clumped chromatin, as in its precursor, the polychromatic normoblast, but ultimately it becomes pyknotic, and appears as a deeply staining, blue-black, homogeneous structureless mass. The nucleus is often eccentric and is sometimes lobulated. Called also *late,*

acidophilic, oxyphilic, or *eosinophilic normoblast; late, ortho-chromatic, acidophilic, oxyphilic,* or *eosinophilic erythroblast;* and *metarubricyte.* **oxyphilic n.,** orthochromatic n.
polychromatic n., a nucleated, immature erythrocyte in which the nucleus occupies a relatively smaller part of the cell than in its precursor, the basophilic normoblast. The cytoplasm is beginning to acquire hemoglobin and thus is no longer a purely blue color, but takes on an acidophilic tint, which becomes progressively more marked as the cell matures. The chromatin of the nucleus is arranged in coarse, deeply staining clumps. Called also *intermediate n., intermediate* or *polychromatic erythroblast,* and *rubricyte.*

normoblastic (nor″mo-blas′tik) relating to or having the character of a normoblast.

normoblastosis (nor″mo-blas-to′sis) excessive production of normoblasts by the bone marrow.

normocalcemia (nor″mo-kal-se′me-ah) a normal level of calcium in the blood.

normocalcemic (nor″mo-kal-se′mik) pertaining to or characterized by normocalcemia.

normocapnia (nor″mo-kap′ne-ah) a normal tension of carbon dioxide in the blood.

normocapnic (nor″mo-kap′nik) pertaining to or characterized by normocapnia.

normocholesterolemia (nor″mo-ko-les″ter-o-le′me-ah) a normal level of cholesterol in the blood.

normocholesterolemic (nor″mo-ko-les″ter-o-le′mik) pertaining to, characterized by, or tending to produce a normal level of cholesterol in the blood.

normochromasia (nor″mo-kro-ma′ze-ah) [*normo-* + Gr. *chrōma* color] 1. a normal staining reaction in a cell or tissue. 2. normal color of the red blood cells.

normochromia (nor″mo-kro′me-ah) normal color of the red blood cells.

normochromic (nor″mo-kro′mik) having a normal color; having a normal hemoglobin content.

normocrinic (nor″mo-krin′ik) pertaining to normal secretion or to normal endocrine action.

normocyte (nor′mo-sīt) [*normo-* + *-cyte*] an erythrocyte that is normal in size, shape, and color.

normocytic (nor″mo-sit′ik) relating to or having the character of a normocyte.

Normocytin (nor″mo-si′tin) trademark for preparations of concentrated crystalline vitamin B_{12}. See *cyanocobalamin.*

normocytosis (nor″mo-si-to′sis) a normal state of the blood in respect to the erythrocytes.

Normodyne (nor′mo-dīn) trademark for a preparation of labetalol hydrochloride.

normoerythrocyte (nor″mo-ĕ-rith′ro-sīt) normocyte.

normoglycemia (nor″mo-gli-se′me-ah) the state of having the level of glucose in the blood within the normal range.

normoglycemic (nor″mo-gli-se′mik) pertaining to, characterized by, or conducive to normoglycemia.

normokalemia (nor″mo-kah-le′me-ah) a normal level of potassium in the blood.

normokalemic (nor″mo-kah-le′mik) pertaining to, characterized by, or conducive to normokalemia.

normolineal (nor″mo-lin′e-al) built on normal lines.

normomastic (nor″mo-mas′tik) see *Kafka's test,* under *tests.*

normo-orthocytosis (nor″mo-or″tho-si-to′sis) [*normo-* + Gr. *orthos* correct + *-cyte* + *-osis*] a condition of the blood leukocytes in which the total number is increased, but the proportion between the different varieties remains normal.

normoskeocytosis (nor″mo-ske″o-si-to′sis) [*normo-* + Gr. *skaios* left + *-cyte* + *-osis*] a condition of the leukocytes of the blood in which the number is normal, but many immature forms (deviation to the left) are present.

normospermic (nor″mo-sper′mik) producing spermatozoa normal in number and motility.

normosthenuria (nor″mo-sthen-u′re-ah) [*normo-* + Gr. *sthenos* strength + *ouron* urine + *-ia*] 1. the secretion of urine of varying specific gravity within the normal range. 2. normally active urination.

normotension (nor″mo-ten′shun) normal tone, tension, or pressure.

normotensive (nor″mo-ten′siv) 1. characterized by nor-

mal tone, tension, or pressure, as by normal blood pressure. 2. a person with normal blood pressure.

normothermia (nor″mo-ther′me-ah) [*normo-* + Gr. *thermē* heat + *-ia*] a normal state of temperature, especially (*a*) normal body temperature (98.6° F.), or (*b*) that state of normal environmental temperature at which there is neither stimulation nor depression of the activity of the body cells (Herrmann).

normothermic (nor″mo-ther′mik) pertaining to or characterized by normal temperature; neither hyperthermic nor hypothermic.

normotonia (nor″mo-to′ne-ah) normal tone or tension.

normotonic (nor″mo-ton′ik) pertaining to or characterized by normotonia.

normotopia (nor″mo-to′pe-ah) [*normo-* + Gr. *topos* place + *-ia*] (*obs.*) normal location.

normotopic (nor″mo-top′ik) (*obs.*) normally located.

normotrophic (nor″mo-trof′ik) of normal development; exhibiting neither hypertrophy nor hypotrophy.

normouricemia (nor″mo-u″rĭ-se′me-ah) a normal value of uric acid in the blood.

normouricemic (nor″mo-u″rĭ-se′mik) pertaining to or characterized by normouricemia.

normouricuria (nor″mo-u″rĭ-ku′re-ah) a normal amount of uric acid in the urine.

normouricuric (nor″mo-u″rĭ-ku′rik) pertaining to or characterized by normouricuria.

normovolemia (nor″mo-vo-le′me-ah) [*normo-* + *volume* + Gr. *haima* blood + *-ia*] normal blood volume.

normovolemic (nor″mo-vo-le′mik) pertaining to or characterized by normovolemia; having a normal volume of circulating fluid (plasma) in the body.

Norodin (nor′o-din) trademark for a preparation of methamphetamine hydrochloride.

Norpace (nor′pās) trademark for a preparation of disopyramide phosphate.

Norpramin (nor′pram-in) trademark for a preparation of desipramine hydrochloride.

norpseudoephedrine (nor-su″do-ĕ-fed′rēn) a nervous system stimulant, $C_9H_{13}NO$, from the leaves of the shrub *Catha edulis.*

Norris' corpuscles (nor′is-ez) [Richard *Norris,* English physician, 1831–1916] see under *corpuscle.*

norsulfazole (nor-sul′fah-zōl) sulfathiazole.

Northrop (north′rup), John Howard. American chemist, born 1891; co-winner, with James Batcheller Sumner and Wendell Meredith Stanley, of the Nobel prize for chemistry in 1946 for isolation and crystallization of enzymes and for isolating virus proteins in pure form.

nortriptyline hydrochloride (nor-trip′tĭ-lēn) [USP] chemical name: 3-(10,11-dihydro-5*H*-dibenzo[*a,d*]cyclohepten-5-ylidene)-*N*-methyl-1-propanamine hydrochloride. An antidepressant, $C_{19}H_{21}N\cdot HCl$, occurring as a white to off-white powder; administered orally.

nortropinon (nor-tro′pĭ-non) a solid, fusible ketone, $C_6H_{11}NO$, derived from tropin.

nosazontology (nos-az″on-tol′o-je) nosetiology.

noscapine (nos′kah-pēn) chemical name: (*S*)-6,7-dimethoxy-3-(5,6,7,8-tetrahydro-4-methoxy-6-methyl-1,3-dioxolo[4,5-*g*]isoquinolin-5-yl)-1(3*H*)-isobenzofuranone. An alkaloid of opium, $C_{22}H_{23}NO_7$, occurring as a white to nearly white, crystalline powder; used as an antitussive, administered orally. **n. hydrochloride,** the hydrochloride salt of noscapine, $C_{22}H_{23}NO_7\cdot HCl$, having the same appearance, actions, uses, and route of administration as the base.

nose (nōz) [L. *nasus;* Gr. *rhis*] 1. the specialized structure of the face that serves as the organ of the sense of smell and as part of the respiratory system; the term includes both the external nose (*nasus externus*) and the nasal cavity (*cavitas nasi*). Called also *nasus* [NA]. 2. nasus externus. **cleft n.,** a developmental anomaly resulting from incomplete union of the paired nasal primordia. **external n.,** nasus externus. **saddle n., saddle-back n., swayback n.,** concavity of the contour of the bridge of the nose due to collapse of cartilaginous or bony support, or both; it was once most often due to congenital syphilis, but is now more commonly the result of congenital epidermal defect or of leprosy.

nosebrain (nōz'brān) (*obs.*) rhinencephalon, def. 1.

nosegay (nōz'ga) a name applied to an anatomical structure resembling a small bunch of flowers. **Riolan's n.,** the group of muscles that take their origin from the styloid process of the temporal bone.

Nosema (no-se'mah) [Gr. *nosēma* sickness] 1. a genus of intracellular protozoa (suborder Apansporoblastina, order Microsporida) parasitic in invertebrates, and especially pathogenic in insects. 2. *Encephalitozoon.* **N. a'pis,** the etiologic agent of nosema disease of bees. **N. bomby'cis,** the etiologic agent of the disease pébrine in silkworms. **N. cunic'uli,** *Encephalitozoon cuniculi.*

nosematosis (no-se''mah-to'sis) 1. infection with protozoa of the genus *Nosema.* 2. encephalitozoonosis.

nosencephalus (no''sen-sef'ah-lus) [noso- + Gr. *enkephalos* brain] a fetus with a defective cranium and brain.

nosepiece (nōz'pēs) the portion of a microscope nearest to the stage, which bears the objective or objectives, constructed so as to permit change of the objective without disturbing the focus of the instrument. **quick-change n.,** one bearing a single objective, which may be quickly attached to or removed from a microscope. **rotating n.,** one bearing more than one objective, designed to permit the one selected to be rotated into place, with its axis coincident with the optical axis of the microscope.

nosetiology (nos''e-te-ol'o-je) [noso- + Gr. *aitia* cause + -*logy*] the study of the causation of disease.

nosiheptide (no''si-hep'tīd) a veterinary growth stimulant, $C_{51}H_{43}N_{13}O_{12}S_6$.

nos(o)- [Gr. *nosos* disease] a combining form denoting relationship to disease.

nosochthonography (nos''ok-tho-nog'rah-fe) [noso- + Gr. *chthōn* land + *graphein* to write] the geography of epidemic or other diseases; the study of the geographical distribution of diseases; nosogeography.

nosocomial (nos''o-ko'me-al) [nosa- + Gr. *komeion* to take care of] pertaining to or originating in the hospital; said of an infection not present or incubating prior to admittance to the hospital, but generally occurring 72 hours after admittance; the term is usually used to refer to patient disease, but hospital personnel may also acquire nosocomial infection. Cf. *iatrogenic.*

nosogenesis (nos''o-jen'ĕ-sis) pathogenesis.

nosogenic (nos''o-jen'ik) pathogenic.

nosogeny (no-soj'ĕ-ne) [noso- + Gr. *gennan* to produce] pathogenesis.

nosogeography (nos''o-je-og'rah-fe) [noso- + Gr. *gē* earth + *graphein* to write] nosochthonography.

nosography (no-sog'rah-fe) [noso- + Gr. *graphein* to write] a written account or description of diseases.

nosologic (nos''o-loj'ik) pertaining to the classification of disease.

nosology (no-sol'o-je) [noso- + -*logy*] the science of the classification of diseases. Called also *nosonomy* and *nosotaxy.*

nosomania (nos''o-ma'ne-ah) [noso- + Gr. *mania* madness] the incorrect belief of a patient that he has some special disease; hypochondriasis.

nosometry (no-som'ĕ-tre) [noso- + Gr. *metron* measure] the measurement of the morbidity rate.

nosomycosis (nos''o-mi-ko'sis) [noso- + Gr. *mykēs* fungus] a disease caused by a fungus.

nosonomy (no-son'o-me) [noso- + Gr. *nomos* law] nosology.

nosoparasite (nos''o-par'ah-sīt) [noso- + *parasite*] an organism found in conjunction with a disease which it is able to modify, but not to produce.

nosophilia (nos''o-fil'e-ah) [noso- + Gr. *philein* to love] a desire to be sick.

nosophobia (nos''o-fo'be-ah) [noso- + *phobia*] irrational dread of sickness or of some particular disease.

nosophyte (nos'o-fīt) [noso- + Gr. *phyton* plant] a pathogenic plant microorganism.

nosopoietic (nos''o-poi-et'ik) [noso- + Gr. *poiein* to make] causing or producing disease.

Nosopsyllus (nos''o-sil'us) [noso- + Gr. *psylla* flea] a genus of fleas. **N. fascia'tus,** the common rat flea of North America and Europe; it is a vector of murine typhus and probably of plague. Formerly called *Ceratophyllus fasciatus.*

nosotaxy (nos''o-tak''se) [noso- + Gr. *taxis* arrangement] nosology.

nosotoxic (nos''o-tok'sik) producing nosotoxicosis.

nosotoxicity (nos''o-tok-sis'ĭ-te) the quality of being nosotoxic.

nosotoxicosis (nos''o-tok''sĭ-ko'sis) [noso- + *toxicosis*] any disease due to or associated with poisoning.

nosotoxin (nos''o-tok'sin) [noso- + *toxin*] any toxin causing or associated with disease.

nosotrophy (no-sot'ro-fe) [noso- + Gr. *trophē* nourishment] the care and nursing of the sick.

nosotropic (no''so-trop'ik) [noso- + Gr. *tropos* a turning] directed against or opposed to a disease.

nostalgia (nos-tal'je-ah) [Gr. *nostein* to return home + -*algia*] homesickness; longing to return home or to familiar surroundings.

nostomania (nos''to-ma'ne-ah) [Gr. *nostein* to return home + *mania* madness] intense homesickness; irresistible urge to return home.

nostril (nos'tril) one of the external orifices of the nose; called also *anterior* or *external naris.* See nares.

nostrum (nos'trum) [L.] a quack, patent, or secret remedy.

Nostyn (nos'tin) trademark for a preparation of ectylurea.

notalgia (no-tal'je-ah) [Gr. *nōton* back + -*algia*] pain in the back; dorsalgia.

notancephalia (no''tan-sĕ-fa'le-ah) [Gr. *nōton* + *an* neg. + *kephalē* head + -*ia*] congenital absence of the back of the skull.

notanencephalia (no''tan-en-sĕ-fa'le-ah) [Gr. *nōton* back + *an* neg. + *enkephalos* brain + -*ia*] absence of the cerebellum.

notatin (nō'tā-tĭn) (*obs.*) glucose oxidase.

notch (noch) an indentation or depression, especially one on the edge of a bone or other organ. See also *incisura.* **acetabular n.,** incisura acetabuli. **angular n. of stomach,** incisura angularis gastris. **aortic n.,** dicrotic n. **auricular n.,** incisura anterior auris. **cardiac n. of left lung,** incisura cardiaca pulmonis sinistri. **cardiac n. of stomach,** incisura cardiaca gastris. **cerebellar n., anterior,** incisura cerebelli anterior. **cerebellar n., posterior,** incisura cerebelli posterior. **clavicular n. of sternum,** incisura clavicularis sterni. **coracoid n.,** incisura scapulae. **costal n's of sternum,** incisurae costales sterni. **cotyloid n.,** incisura acetabuli. **dicrotic n.,** a small downward deflection in the arterial pulse or pressure contour immediately following the closure of the semilunar valves, sometimes used as a marker for the end of systole or the ejection period. **ethmoidal n. of frontal bone,** incisura ethmoidalis ossis frontalis. **fibular n.,** incisura fibularis tibiae. **frontal n.,** incisura frontalis. **n. of gallbladder,** fossa vesicae felleae. **gastric n.,** incisura angularis gastris. **interarytenoid n.,** incisura interarytenoidea laryngis. **interclavicular n.,** incisura jugularis sterni. **interclavicular n. of occipital bone,** incisura jugularis ossis occipitalis. **interclavicular n. of temporal bone,** incisura jugularis ossis temporalis. **intercondylar n. of femur,** fossa intercondylaris femoris. **interlobar n.,** incisura ligamenti teretis. **intertragic n.,** incisura intertragica. **intervertebral n.,** see *incisura vertebralis inferior* and *incisura vertebralis superior.* **ischial n., greater, n. of ischium, greater,** incisura ischiadica major. **ischial n., lesser, n. of ischium, lesser,** incisura ischiadica minor. **jugular n. of occipital bone,** incisura jugularis ossis occipitalis. **jugular n. of sternum,** incisura jugularis sterni. **jugular n. of temporal bone,** incisura jugularis ossis temporalis. **lacrimal n. of maxilla,** incisura lacrimalis maxillae. **n. of ligamentum teres,** incisura ligamenti teretis. **mandibular n.,** incisura mandibulae. **marsupial n.,** incisura cerebelli posterior. **mastoid n.,** incisura mastoidea ossis temporalis. **nasal n. of maxilla,** incisura nasalis maxillae. **palatine n.,** fissura pterygoidea. **palatine n. of palatine bone,** incisura sphenopalatina ossis palatini. **pancreatic n.,** incisura pancreatis. **parietal n. of temporal bone,** incisura parietalis ossis temporalis. **parotid n.,** the notch between the ramus of the mandible and the mastoid process of the temporal bone. **popliteal n.**, fossa intercondylaris femoris. **preoccipital n.**, incisura preoccipitalis. **presternal n.**, incisura jugularis sterni. **pterygoid n.**, fissura pterygoidea. **radial n., radial n. of ulna**, incisura radialis ulnae. **rivinian n., n. of Rivinus**, incisura tympanica. **sacrosciatic n., greater**, incisura ischiadica major. **sacrosciatic n., lesser**, incisura ischiadica minor. **scapular n.**, incisura scapulae. **sciatic n., greater**, incisura ischiadica major. **sciatic n., lesser**, incisura ischiadica minor. **semilunar n. of mandible**, incisura mandibulae. **semilunar n. of scapula**, incisura scapulae. **Sibson's n.**, an inward bend of the left upward limit of precordial dullness in acute pericardial effusion. **sigmoid n.**, incisura mandibulae. **sphenopalatine n. of palatine bone**, incisura sphenopalatina ossis palatini. **sternal n.**, incisura jugularis sterni. **supraorbital n.**, incisura supraorbitalis. **suprascapular n.**, incisura scapulae. **suprasternal n.**, incisura jugularis sterni. **tentorial n.**, incisura tentorii cerebelli. **thyroid n., inferior**, incisura thyroidea inferior. **thyroid n., superior**, incisura thyroidea superior. **trigeminal n.**, a notch in the superior border of the petrosal portion of the temporal bone, near the apex, for transmission of the trigeminal nerve. **trochlear n. of ulna**, incisura trochlearis ulnae. **tympanic n.**, incisura tympanica. **ulnar n., ulnar n. of radius**, incisura ulnaris radii. **umbilical n.**, incisura ligamenti teretis. **vertebral n., inferior**, incisura vertebralis inferior. **vertebral n., superior**, incisura vertebralis superior.

Notechis (no-tek′is) a genus of extremely venomous snakes of Australia. *N. scuta′tus* is the tiger snake.

notencephalocele (no″ten-sĕ-fal′o-sēl″) [*noto-* + Gr. *enkephalos* brain + *kēlē* hernia] hernial protrusion of the brain from the back of the head.

notencephalus (no″ten-sef′ah-lus) [*noto-* + Gr. *enkephalos* brain] a monster affected with notencephalocele.

Nothnagel's bodies, syndrome, type (nōt′nah- gelz) [Carl Wilhelm Hermann *Nothnagel*, German physician, 1841–1905] see under *body, syndrome,* and *acroparathesia.*

not(o)- [Gr. *nōton* back] a combining form denoting relationship to the back.

notochord (no′to-kord) [*noto-* + Gr. *chordē* cord] the rod-shaped body, composed of cells derived from the mesoblast, below the primitive groove of the embryo, defining the primitive axis of the body; it is the common factor of all species of the phylum Chordata. It is the center of development of the axial skeleton. Called also *chorda dorsalis.*

notochordoma (no″to-kor-do′mah) chordoma.

Notoedres (no″to-ed′rēz) a genus of mites. **N. ca′ti**, an itch mite which causes a very persistent and often fatal mange in cats; it also infests domestic rabbits, and may temporarily infest man.

notogenesis (no″to-jen′ĕ-sis) [*noto-* + Gr. *gennan* to produce] the development of the notochord.

notomelus (no-tom′ĕ-lus) [*noto-* + Gr. *melos* limb] a fetus with accessory limbs on the back.

notomyelitis (no″to-mi″ĕ-li′tis) [*noto-* + *myelitis*] (*obs.*) inflammation of the spinal cord.

not-self (not′self) a term introduced by Burnet and Fenner to denote antigens foreign to an animal against which it will normally mount an immune response.

notum (no′tum) [Gr. *nōton* the back] 1. the dorsal part of the body. 2. the dorsal element of each segment of an arthropod.

noumenal (nu′me-nal) [Gr. *noumenon* a thing thought] pertaining to rational intuition independent of sensory perception.

Novaldin (no-val′din) trademark for preparations of dipyrone.

novobiocin (no″vo-bi′o-sin) chemical name: *N*-[7-[[3-*O*-(aminocarbonyl)-5,5-di-*C*-methyl-4-*O*-methyl-α-L-lyxopyranosyl]oxy]-4-hydroxy-8-methyl-2-oxo-2*H*-1-benzopyran-3-yl]-4-hydroxy-3-(3-methyl-2-butenyl)benzamide. An antibiotic, $C_{13}H_{36}N_2O_{11}$, obtained from *Streptomyces niveus* and other *Streptomyces* species, effective chiefly against staphylococci and other gram-positive organisms. **n. calcium**, the calcium salt of novobiocin, $C_{62}H_{70}CaN_4O_{22} \cdot 2H_2O$, occurring as a white or nearly white, crystalline powder, having the same actions as the base; used in the treatment of infections in children due to susceptible bacteria resistant to other antibi-

otics, administered orally. **n. sodium**, the sodium salt of novobiocin, $C_{31}H_{35}N_2NaO_{11}$, having the same appearance, actions, uses, and mode of administration as the calcium salt; usually used in adults.

Novocain (no′vo-kān) trademark for preparations of procaine hydrochloride.

novoscope (no′vo-skōp) [L. *novus* new + *scope*] Fornai's instrument for auscultatory percussion.

Novrad (nov′rad) trademark for preparations of levopropoxyphene napsylate.

Novy's rat disease (no′vēz) [Frederick George *Novy*, American bacteriologist, 1864–1957] see under *disease.*

noxa (nok′sah), pl. *nox′ae* [L. "harm"] an injurious agent, act, or influence.

noxious (nok′shus) [L. *noxius*] hurtful; not wholesome; pernicious; damaging to tissue.

Np chemical symbol for *neptunium.*

N.P.A. National Perinatal Association.

NPN nonprotein nitrogen.

NPO abbreviation for L. *nil per os,* nothing by mouth.

N.R.C. normal retinal correspondence.

NREM non-rapid eye movements (see under *sleep*).

ns. nanosecond.

nsec. nanosecond.

N.S.N.A. National Student Nurse Association.

N-terminal (ter′min-al) the amino (NH₂) end of a polypeptide chain, conventionally written to the left; called also *NH₂-terminal.*

N.T.P. normal temperature and pressure.

nU. nanounit.

nu (noo) [N, ν] the thirteenth letter of the Greek alphabet.

nubecula (nu-bek′u-lah) [L., dim. of *nubes* cloud] 1. a slight cloudiness of the cornea or of the urine; a nebula. 2. statoconia.

nubility (nu-bil′ĭ-te) [L. *nubilitas;* from *nubere* to marry] marriageableness; fitness to marry; said of the female.

nucha (nu′kah) [L.] [NA] the nape, or scruff, or back of the neck.

nuchal (nu′kal) pertaining to the nucha, or back of the neck.

nucin (nu′sin) [L. *nux, nucis,* nut] juglandic acid.

nucis (nu′sis) [L.] genitive of *nux.*

Nuck's canal, diverticulum, hydrocele (nuks) [Anton *Nuck,* Dutch anatomist, 1650–1692] see *processus vaginalis peritonei* and *hydrocele muliebris.*

nuclear (nu′kle-ar) pertaining to a nucleus.

nuclease (nu′kle-ās) a general term for enzymes of the hydrolase class that split the phosphodiester linkages in nucleic acids to form nucleotides or oligonucleotides. The nucleases are classified in subgroups as exonucleases (EC 3.1.11–16) or endonucleases (EC 3.1.21–31). Important enzymes of the group are ribonucleases and deoxyribonucleases.

nucleated (nu′kle-āt″ed) [L. *nucleatus*] having a nucleus or nuclei.

nuclei (nu′kle-i) [L.] genitive and plural of *nucleus.*

nucleic acid (nu-kle′ik) a high-molecular-weight nucleotide polymer. There are two types: *deoxyribonucleic acid* (DNA) and *ribonucleic acid* (RNA) (q.v.). **infectious n. a.**, viral nucleic acid capable of infecting a cell and inducing the production of viruses.

nucleide (nu′kle-īd) any compound of nucleic acid with a metallic element.

nucleiform (nu′kle-ĭ-form) shaped like a nucleus.

nuclein (nu′kle-in) a decomposition product of nucleoprotein intermediate between native nucleoprotein and nucleic acid (F. Miescher, 1874). It is a colorless, amorphous compound, soluble in dilute alkalis, but insoluble in dilute acids. The nucleins consist of nucleic acid and bases which vary in the different nucleins.

nucleinic acid (noo-kle-in′ik) nucleic acid.

nucle(o)- [L. *nucleus,* q.v.] a combining form denoting relationship to a nucleus.

nucleocapsid (nu″kle-o-kap′sid) a unit of viral structure, consisting of a capsid (protein coat) with the enclosed nucleic acid; some simple viruses are naked nucleocapsids, while in others the nucleocapsids form part of a more complex structure.

nucleochylema (nu″kle-o-ki-le′mah) [*nucleus* + Gr. *chylos* juice] the ground substance of the nucleus of a cell as distinguished from that of the cytoplasm.

nucleochyme (nu′kle-o-kīm) [*nucleus* + Gr. *chymos* juice] karyolymph.

nucleocytoplasmic (nu″kle-o-si″to-plaz′mik) pertaining to the nucleus and the cytoplasm of cells.

nucleofugal (nu″kle-of′u-gal) [*nucleus* + L. *fugere* to flee] moving away from a nucleus.

nucleoglucoprotein (nu″kle-o-gloo″ko-pro′te-in) a combination of a nucleoprotein with a carbohydrate.

nucleohistone (nu″kle-o-his′tōn) a complex nucleoprotein made up of deoxyribonucleic acid (DNA) and a histone, the principal constituent of chromatin.

nucleohyaloplasm (nu″kle-o-hi-al′o-plazm) linin.

nucleoid (nu′kle-oid) 1. resembling a nucleus. 2. a nucleus-like body sometimes seen in the center of an erythrocyte. 3. the nuclear region of a bacterium, consisting of a dense, centrally located, irregularly shaped region containing DNA material without a surrounding nuclear membrane. 4. the genetic material (nucleic acid) of a virus, situated in the center of the virion. **Lavdovski's n.,** centrosome.

nucleokeratin (nu″kle-o-ker′ah-tin) a variety of keratin found in the nervous system.

nucleolar (nu-kle′o-lar) pertaining to a nucleolus.

nucleoli (nu-kle′o-li) [L.] plural of *nucleolus*.

nucleoliform (nu″kle-ol′ĭ-form) resembling a nucleolus.

nucleolin (nu-kle′o-lin) the substance composing the nucleolus of a cell.

nucleolinus (nu″kle-o-li′nus) a deeply staining granule in the nucleolus.

nucleoloid (nu′kle-o-loid) resembling a nucleolus.

nucleololus (nu″kle-ol′o-lus) a minute spot within the nucleolus.

nucleolonema (nu″kle-o″lo-ne′mah) [*nucleolus* + Gr. *nēma* thread] a network of strands formed by organization of a finely granular substance, perhaps containing ribonucleic acid, in the nucleolus of a cell.

nucleoloneme (nu″kle-o′lo-nēm) nucleolonema.

nucleolonucleus (nu″kle-o-lo-nu′kle-us) a nucleololus.

nucleolus (nu-kle′o-lus), gen. and pl. *nucle′oli* [L., dim. of *nucleus*] a rounded refractile body present in the nucleus of most cells, which is the site of synthesis of ribosomal RNA, becoming enlarged during periods of synthesis and atrophied during quiescent periods; it consists of a mixed granular (pars granulosa) and a fibrillar (pars fibrosa) portion. Multiple nucleoli occur in some cells. Called also *micronucleus* and *plasmosome*. **chromatin n., false n., nucleinic n.,** karyosome. **secondary n.,** a mass sometimes seen near a nucleolus, and looking like a separated portion of the latter.

nucleolymph (nu′kle-o-limf″) karyolymph.

nucleomicrosome (nu″kle-o-mi′kro-sōm) [*nucleus* + Gr. *mikros* small + *sōma* body] any of the minute segments of a chromatin fiber.

nucleon (nu′kle-on) 1. a particle of the atomic nucleus, a proton or a neutron. 2. phosphocarnic acid.

nucleonic (nu″kle-on′ik) pertaining to a nucleus.

nucleonics (nu″kle-on′iks) the study of atomic nuclei and their reactions; nuclear physics.

nucleopetal (nu″kle-op′e-tal) [*nucleus* + L. *petere* to seek] moving toward a nucleus.

nucleophagocytosis (noo″kle-o-fag″o-si-to′sis) the engulfing of the nuclei of other cells by phagocytes; see *tart cell*, under *cell*.

nucleophile (nu′kle-o-fil″) an electron donor in chemical reactions involving covalent catalysis in which the donated electrons bond other chemical groups (electrophiles).

nucleophilic (nu″kle-o-fil′ik) having an affinity for nuclei; being or serving as a nucleophile.

nucleophosphatase (nu″kle-o-fos′fah-tās) nucleotidase.

nucleoplasm (nu′kle-o-plazm″) [*nucleus* + *plasma*] the protoplasm composing the nucleus of a cell; karyoplasm. Cf. *cytoplasm*.

nucleoprotamine (nu″kle-o-pro-tam′in) a compound of protamine and nucleic acid found chiefly in fish sperm.

nucleoprotein (nu″kle-o-pro′te-in) a substance composed of a simple basic protein, usually a histone or protamine, combined with a nucleic acid. **deoxyribose n.,** a deoxyribonucleic acid–protein complex. **ribose n.,** a ribonucleic acid–protein complex.

nucleoreticulum (nu″kle-o-re-tik′u-lum) [*nucleus* + *reticulum*] any intranuclear network.

nucleosidase (noo″kle-o-si′dās) [EC 3.2.2] any enzyme of a sub-subclass of enzymes of the hydrolase class that catalyzes the hydrolysis of *N*-glycosyl linkages in a nucleoside to produce a purine or pyrimidine base and a sugar.

nucleoside (nu′kle-o-sīd″) one of the glycosidic compounds into which a nucleotide is split by the action of nucleotidase or by chemical means; it is a combination of a sugar (a pentose) with a purine or a pyrimidine base.

nucleoside monophosphate kinase (noo′kle-o-sīd″ mon″o-fos′fāt ki′nās) [EC 2.7.4] any enzyme of a sub-subclass of enzymes of the transferase class that catalyzes the reaction ATP + nucleoside monophosphate = ADP + nucleoside diphosphate. The reaction is part of the mechanism that regenerates high-energy nucleotides for metabolic processes and conserves the purine-pyrimidine pool. Specific enzymes exist for each nucleoside. See *AMP-kinase*.

nucleoside phosphorylase (noo′kle-o-sīd″ fos-fōr′ĭ-lās) [EC 2.4.2] any enzyme of the pentosyltransferase sub-subclass of enzymes of the transferase class that catalyzes the reaction purine (or pyrimidine) nucleoside + orthophosphate = purine (or pyrimidine) + α-D-ribose 1-phosphate. The reaction is a step in the degradation of nucleic acids and nucleotides. See also *purine nucleoside phosphorylase*.

nucleosin (nu′kle-o-sin) thymopoietin.

nucleosis (nu″kle-o′sis) nuclear proliferation; abnormal increase in the production of nuclei, such as occurs in the subsarcolemmal nuclei of muscle following injury.

nucleosome (nu′kle-o-sōm″) [*nucleus* + Gr. *sōma* body] any of the complexes of histone and DNA in eukaryotic cells, seen under the electron microscope as beadlike bodies on a string of DNA.

nucleospindle (nu″kle-o-spin′d'l) the spindle-shaped body in mitosis.

nucleotherapy (nu″kle-o-ther′ah-pe) [*nuclein* + *therapy*] the treatment of disease with nucleins.

nucleotidase (noo″kle-o-ti′dās) [EC 3.1.3] any enzyme of the phosphomonoesterase sub-subclass of the hydrolase class that catalyzes the reaction nucleotide + H_2O = nucleoside + orthophosphate. See also *5′-nucleotidase*.

5′-nucleotidase (noo″kle-o-ti′dās) [EC 3.1.3.5] an enzyme of the hydrolase class that catalyzes the reaction 5′-ribonucleotide + H_2O = ribonucleoside + orthophosphate. The enzyme occurs in the cytoplasmic membrane and acts on a wide range of 5′-nucleotides. The reaction is part of the main nucleotide degradation pathway.

nucleotide (nu′kle-o-tīd) one of the compounds into which nucleic acid is split by the action of nuclease; the nucleotides are composed of a base (purine or pyrimidine), a sugar (ribose or deoxyribose), and a phosphate group. See *mononucleotide*. **cyclic n's,** nucleotides in which the phosphate group forms a ring, as in AMP and GMP.

nucleotide cyclase (noo″kle-o-tīd si′klās) [EC 4.6.1] any enzyme of a sub-subclass of enzymes of the lyase class that catalyzes the reaction nucleoside triphosphate = cyclic nucleoside monophosphate + pyrophosphate. See also *adenylate cyclase*.

nucleotide polymerase (noo″kle-o-tīd″ pol-im′er-ās) see *DNA-directed DNA polymerase* and *DNA-directed RNA polymerase*.

nucleotidyl (nu″kle-o-tīd′il) a nucleotide residue.

nucleotidylexotransferase (noo″kle-o-tīd″il-ek″so-trans′fer-ās) DNA nucleotidylexotransferase.

nucleotidyltransferase (noo″kle-o-tīd′il-trans′fer-ās) [EC 2.7.7] any enzyme of a sub-subclass of enzymes of the transferase class that catalyzes the transfer of a nucleotidyl group from a nucleoside di- or triphosphate donor group to an acceptor group. See also *DNA-directed DNA polymerase* and *DNA-directed RNA polymerase*.

nucleotoxin (nu″kle-o-tok′sin) 1. a toxin from cell nuclei. 2. any toxin exerting a deleterious effect on cell nuclei.

nucleus (nu′kle-us), gen. and pl. *nu′clei* [L., dim. of *nux* nut] **1.** a cell nucleus: a spheroid body within a cell, consisting of a number of characteristic organelles visible with the optical microscope, a thin nuclear membrane, a nucleolus or nucleoli, irregular granules of chromatin and linin, and a diffuse nucleoplasm. **2.** [NA] a general term used to designate a group of nerve cells ordinarily located within the central nervous system and bearing a direct relationship to the fibers of a particular nerve. **3.** in organic chemistry, the combination of atoms forming the central element or basic framework of the molecule of a specific compound or class of compounds. **4.** see *atomic n.* **n. abdu′cens, n. of abducens nerve,** n. nervi abducentis. **n. accesso′rius, accessory n., accessory oculomotor n.,** n. oculomotorius accessorius. **n. accesso′rius colum′nae ventra′lis medul′lae spina′lis,** NA alternative for *n. nervi accessorii.* **n. of accessory nerve,** n. nervi accessorii. **accessory n. of ventral column of spinal cord,** n. nervi accessorii. **n. accum′bens sep′ti,** a collection of pleomorphic cells in the caudal part of the anterior horn of the lateral ventricle of the olfactory tubercle, lying between the head of the caudate nucleus and the anterior perforated substance. **acoustic nuclei, nuclei of acoustic nerve,** see *nuclei cochleares* and *nuclei vestibulares.* **n. a′lae cine′reae,** n. dorsalis nervi vagi. **ambiguous n.,** n. ambiguus. **ambiguous n. of Quain,** n. nervi hypoglossi. **n. ambig′uus** [NA], ambiguous nucleus: the nucleus of origin of motor fibers of the vagus, glossopharyngeal, and accessory nerves that supply the striated muscles of the larynx and pharynx. It consists of an intermittent cell column in the middle of the lateral funiculus of the medulla oblongata, between the caudal end of the medulla and the level of exit of the glossopharyngeal nerve. **n. amyg′dalae, amygdaloid n.,** corpus amygdaloideum. **n. amygdalifor′mis of J. Stilling,** n. subthalamicus. **amygdaloid n.,** corpus amygdaloideum. **n. an′sae lenticula′ris** [NA], **n. of ansa lenticularis,** a collection of neurons in the ansa lenticularis as it curves around the medial edge of the globus pallidus. **anterior nuclei of thalamus,** nuclei anteriores thalami. **nu′clei anteri o′res thal′ami** [NA], anterior nuclei of thalamus: the three nuclei in the anterior part of the thalamus: the nucleus anteroventralis, nucleus anterodorsalis, and nucleus anteromedialis. Together, they receive connections from the mamillary body and fornix and project fibers to the cingulate body. **n. anterodorsa′lis thal′ami** [NA], see *nuclei anteriores thalami.* **n. anteromedia′lis thalami** [NA], see *nuclei anteriores thalami.* **n anteroventra′lis thal′ami** [NA], see *nuclei anteriores thalami.* **nu′clei arcifor′mes,** nuclei arcuati. **arcuate nuclei of medulla oblongata, nu′clei arcua′ti medul′lae oblonga′tae** [NA], small, irregular areas of gray substance found on the ventromedial aspect of the pyramid of the medulla oblongata. **n. arcua′tus hypothal′ami,** NA alternative for *n. infundibularis hypothalami.* **nu′clei a′reae H H₁, H₂** [NA], the group of nuclei in the ventral thalamus comprising the nucleus of the prerubral field (field H of Forel) and neurons scattered along the thalamic and lenticular fasciculi in fields H₁ and H₂ of Forel. **n. of atom, atomic n.,** the central core of an atom, constituting almost all of its mass but only a small part of its volume, and composed of protons and neutrons, the protons being positively charged and their number (atomic number) being fixed for all the atoms of each element and equal to the number of the orbiting electrons. The neutrons, which bear no charge, may vary in number, accounting for the isotopes of an element. **auditory nuclei, nuclei of auditory nerve,** see *nuclei cochleares* and *nuclei vestibulares.* **auditory n., large cell,** n. vestibularis lateralis. **autonomic n., n. autonom′icus,** n. oculomotorius accessorius. **Balbiani's n.,** yolk n. **basal n.,** nucleus olivaris. **n. basa′lis,** n. olivaris. **basal nuclei, nu′clei basa′les** [NA], specific interconnected groups of masses of gray substance deep in the cerebral hemispheres and in the upper brainstem. Although various subcortical nuclei have been considered to be part of the basal nuclei, in official anatomical nomenclature the term includes the corpus striatum (the nucleus caudatus and nucleus lentiformis being considered together), claustrum, corpus amygdaloideum, capsula externa, capsula extreme, and capsula interna. Called also *basal ganglia.* **Béclard's n.,** a vascular lentil-shaped center of ossification seen in the cartilage of the lower epiphysis of the femur during the latter part of fetal life.

Bekhterev's n., the cranial (superior) vestibular nucleus; see *nuclei vestibulares.* **Blumenau's n.,** the lateral portion of the cuneate nucleus. **n. of Burdach's column,** n. cuneatus. **n. caeru′leus, n. ceruleus, n. coeru′leus,** a compact aggregation of pigmented neurons subjacent to the locus coeruleus. **n. of caudal colliculus,** n. colliculi caudalis. **n. cauda′lis centra′lis** [NA], central caudate nucleus: an unpaired collection of cells in the caudal third of the oculomotor nuclear complex, located in the median raphe somewhat dorsal to the lateral nuclei. **caudate n., n. cauda′tus** [NA], an elongated, arched gray mass closely related to the lateral ventricle throughout its entire extent and consisting of a head, body, and tail. The caudate nucleus and putamen form a functional unit (the neostriatum) of the corpus striatum. **cell n., cellular n.,** see *nucleus,* def. 1. **n. centra′lis latera′lis thal′ami** [NA], lateral central nucleus of thalamus: one of the smaller intralaminar nuclei of the dorsal thalamus, situated in the dorsal part of the internal medullary lamina. **n. centra′lis media′lis thal′ami** [NA], medial central nucleus of thalamus: one of the smaller intralaminar nuclei, situated medially in the internal medullary lamina. **central n. of ventral column of spinal cord, n. ventra′lis colum′nae ventra′lis medul′lae spina′lis** [NA], a group of nerve cells in the gray substance in the central region of the ventral column of the spinal cord. **n. centromedia′nus thal′ami** [NA], centromedian nucleus of thalamus: the largest and most caudal of the intralaminar nuclei of the dorsal thalamus; its main connections are with the corpus striatum. Called also *central medial n. of thalamus* and *n. medialis centralis thalami.* **nu′clei cerebel′li** [NA], nuclei of cerebellum: four accumulations of gray substance embedded in the white substance of the cerebellum, comprising the nucleus dentatus, nucleus emboliformis, nucleus globosus, and nucleus fastigii; called also *intracerebellar nuclei* and *roof nuclei* (q.v.). **n. of cerebellum, dentate,** n. dentatus. **n. of cerebellum, medullary,** corpus medullare cerebelli. **cervical n., cervical n., lateral,** n. lateralis cervicalis. **cholane n.,** a cyclopentanophenanthrene structure forming the basis of the specific compounds, found in the bile acids, the sterols, in toad poisons, in digitalis, strophanthus, ouabain, and other heart aglycones, in the sex hormones, and in some carcinogenic hydrocarbons. **n. cine′reum,** substantia grisea medullae spinalis. **Clarke's n.,** columna thoracica. **cleavage n.,** segmentation n. **cochlear nuclei,** nuclei cochleares. **cochlear n., anterior,** n. cochlearis ventralis. **cochlear n., dorsal,** n. cochlearis dorsalis. **cochlear n., posterior,** n. cochlearis dorsalis. **cochlear n., ventral,** n. cochlearis ventralis. **nu′clei cochlea′res** [NA], cochlear nuclei: the two nuclei, *ventral* and *dorsal,* partly encircling the caudal cerebellar peduncle at the junction of the medulla oblongata and the pons, in which the fibers of the cochlear part of the vestibulocochlear nerve terminate; called also *nuclei of acoustic nerve* and *nuclei nervi cochlearis.* **n. cochlea′ris ante′rior,** NA alternative for *n. cochlearis ventralis.* **n. cochlea′ris dorsa′lis** [NA], dorsal cochlear nucleus: a nucleus of nerve cells on the dorsal aspect of the caudal cerebellar peduncle, which forms an eminence (auditory, or acoustic, tubercle) on the lateral part of the vestibular area of the floor of the fourth ventricle; called also *n. cochlearis posterior* [NA alternative] and *posterior cochlear n.* **n. cochlea′ris poste′rior,** NA alternative for *n. cochlearis dorsalis.* **n. cochlea′ris ventra′lis** [NA], ventral cochlear nucleus: a nucleus of nerve cells on the ventrolateral aspect of the caudal cerebellar peduncle, which receives the larger, ascending branches of the cochlear nerve; called also *anterior cochlear n.* and *n. cochlearis anterior* [NA alternative]. See also *nuclei cochleares.* **nuclei of cochlear nerve,** nuclei cochleares. **n. collic′uli cauda′lis** [NA], nucleus of caudal colliculus: the large oval-shaped group of nerve cells that makes up most of the substance of the caudal colliculus; called also *n. colliculi inferioris* [NA alternative] and *n. of inferior colliculus.* **n. collic′uli inferio′ris,** NA alternative for *n. colliculi caudalis.* **commissural n., n. commissura′lis** [NA], a group of noradrenergic neurons that encloses the dorsolateral aspect of the nucleus of the hypoglossal nerve and approaches the ependymal floor of the fourth ventricle. **compact n.,** a cellular nucleus with an inconspicuous nuclear membrane and minute chromatin granules throughout its substance. **conjugation n.,** fertilization n. **n. cor′poris genicula′ti latera′lis** [NA], nucleus of lateral geniculate body: a nucleus within the lateral geniculate body, composed of a small ventral and a large dorsal part, the latter consisting of six concentrically arranged cell layers which receive crossed and uncrossed fibers of the optic tract and which are connected with the visual cortex. Called also *lateral geniculate n.* and *n. geniculatus lateralis.* **n. cor'poris genicula'ti media'lis** [NA], nucleus of medial geniculate body: a nucleus within the medial geniculate body, composed of ventral and dorsal parts which receive ascending auditory fibers and project to the auditory cortex. Called also *medial geniculate n.* and *n. geniculatus medialis.* **nu'clei cor'poris mamilla'ris media'les et latera'les** [NA], lateral and medial nuclei of mamillary body: the two main nuclei of the mamillary body, lateral and medial, which receive fibers from the basal olfactory areas and the fornix, and project to the thalamus and midbrain via mamillothalamic and mamillotegmental fasciculi. **n. of corpus striatum, intraventricular,** n. caudatus. **nuclei of cranial nerves,** nuclei nervorum cranialium. **cuneate n.,** n. cuneatus. **cuneate n., accessory, cuneate n., lateral,** n. cuneatus accessorius. **n. cunea'tus** [NA], cuneate nucleus: a nucleus in the medulla oblongata at the rostral end of the fasciculus cuneatus, in which the fibers of this fasciculus synapse; the cells project to the thalamus via the medial lemniscus. **n. cunea'tus accesso'rius** [NA], accessory cuneate nucleus: a group of nerve cells lying lateral to the nucleus cuneatus that relay impulses from upper limb fibers in the fasciculus cuneatus to the cerebellum (rostral spinocerebellar tract) via external arcuate fibers and the inferior cerebellar peduncle; called also *lateral cuneate n.* **Darkshevich's n.,** a small nucleus dorsal to the medial longitudinal fasciculus in the central gray matter at the rostral end of the cerebral aqueduct; it is believed to receive fibers from the fasciculus and from the superior colliculus. **daughter n.,** a new cell nucleus formed in mitosis by the diaster. **Deiters' n.,** n. vestibularis lateralis. **dental n.,** pulpa dentis. **dentate n., n. denta'tus** [NA], the largest of the deep cerebellar nuclei, lying in the white matter of the cerebellum just lateral to the emboliform nucleus, and receiving Purkinje cell fibers from the neocerebellum; its axons form most of the cranial cerebellar peduncle and project chiefly to the contralateral red nucleus and thalamus. **diploid n.,** a cell nucleus containing the number of chromosomes typical of the somatic cells of the particular species. **dorsal n.** (of Clarke), **n. dorsa'lis,** columna thoracica. **n. dorsa'lis cor'poris trapezoi'dei** [NA], dorsal nucleus of trapezoid body: a group of nerve cell bodies dorsolateral to the trapezoid body; it receives cochlear fibers and contributes to the formation of the trapezoid body and lateral lemniscus. Called also *n. olivaris superior* or *superior olivary n.* **n. dorsa'lis ner'vi glossopharyn'gei,** dorsal nucleus of glossopharyngeal nerve: the cranial pole of the dorsal nucleus of the vague nerve, which is believed to give some parasympathetic fibers to the glossopharyngeal nerve. Some authorities equate this nucleus with the nucleus salivatorius caudalis (q.v.). **n. dorsa'lis ner'vi va'gi** [NA], dorsal nucleus of vagus nerve: the nucleus of origin of the parasympathetic fibers of the vagus nerve, situated in the trigone of the vague nerve in the floor of the fourth ventricle, lateral to the nucleus of the hypoglossal nerve; called also *dorsal vagal n., n. alae cinereae,* and *n. vagalis dorsalis* [NA alternative]. **dorsolateral n., n. dorsolatera'lis** [NA], dorsally placed cells in the lateral part of the oculomotor nuclear complex; they are very distinct from the ventrally placed cells in the middle third of the complex and have a somatic motor function. **dorsolateral n. of ventral column of spinal cord, n. dorsolatera'lis colum'nae ventra'lis medul'lae spina'lis** [NA], a group of nerve cells in the gray substance of the dorsolateral region of the ventral column of the spinal cord. **dorsomedial n. of ventral column of spinal cord, n. dorsomedia'lis colum'nae ventra'lis medul'lae spina'lis** [NA], a group of nerve cells in the gray substance of the dorsomedial region of the ventral column of the spinal cord. **n. dorsomedia'lis hypothal'ami,** n. hypothalamicus dorsomedialis. **droplet nuclei,** small, pathogen-containing particles of respiratory secretions expelled into the air by coughing, which are reduced by evaporation to small, dry particles that can remain airborne for long periods; one possible mechanism for transmission of infection from one individual to another. Cf. *airborne infection,* under *infection.* **drumstick n.,** see *drumstick,* under D. **Duval's n.,** a collection of multipolar ganglion cells situated ventrolaterally

from the hypoglossal nucleus in the medulla oblongata. **Edinger's n., Edinger-Westphal n.,** n. oculomotorius accessorius. **emboliform n., n. embolifor'mis cerebel'li** [NA], a small mass that lies between the dentate nucleus and globose nucleus and contributes to the cranial cerebellar peduncles. **end nuclei,** terminal nuclei. **entopeduncular n., n. entopeduncula'ris** [NA], a collection of neurons situated in the internal capsule adjacent to the medial edge of the globus pallidus, dorsolateral to the lateral hypothalamic nucleus. **n. facia'lis, n. of facial nerve,** n. nervi facialis. **fastigial n., n. fasti'gii** [NA], the most medial of the deep cerebellar nuclei, near the midline in the roof of the fourth ventricle; it projects to the pons and medulla oblongata, chiefly to the vestibular nuclei. **fertilization n.,** the nucleus produced by fusion of the male and female pronuclei in the fertilized ovum; called also *conjugation n., zygote n.,* and *synkaryon.* **free n.,** a cell nucleus from which the other elements of the cell have disappeared. **n. gelatino'sus,** n. pulposus disci intervertebralis. **geniculate n., lateral,** n. corporis geniculati lateralis. **geniculate n., medial,** n. corporis geniculati medialis. **n. genicula'tus latera'lis,** n. corporis geniculati lateralis. **n. genicula'tus media'lis,** n. corporis geniculati medialis. **germ n., germinal n.,** pronucleus. **gingival n.,** a part of the cerebellum in the third and fourth months of fetal life. **globose n., n. globo'sus cerebel'li** [NA], a deep cerebellar nucleus that lies between the emboliform nucleus and the fastigial nucleus and projects its fibers via the cranial cerebellar peduncle. **n. of glossopharyngeal nerve, dorsal,** n. dorsalis nervi glossopharyngei. **n. of Goll's column,** n. gracilis. **gonad n.,** micronucleus, def. 1. **n. gra'cilis** [NA], a nucleus in the medulla oblongata at the rostral end of the fasciculus gracilis of the cord, in which the fibers of the fasciculus gracilis synapse; the cells project to the thalamus via the medial lemniscus. Called also *Goll's tract.* **gray n.,** substantia grisea medullae spinalis. **nuclei of habenula, nu'clei habenulae, habenular nuclei, nuclei haben'ulae media'lis et latera'lis** [NA], two nerve cell groups, one medial and one lateral, situated deep to the habenular trigone, which receive fibers from the stria medullaris thalami. **haploid n.,** a cell nucleus containing half of the number of chromosomes typical of the somatic cells of a particular species. **hypoglossal n., n. of hypoglossal nerve,** n. nervi hypoglossi. **n. hypoglossa'lis,** NA alternative for *n. nervi hypoglossi.* **hypothalamic n., n. hypothalam'icus** (*obs.*), n. subthalamicus. **hypothalamic n., anterior,** n. hypothalamicus anterior. **hypothalamic n., dorsal,** n. hypothalamicus dorsalis. **hypothalamic n., dorsomedial,** n. hypothalamicus dorsomedialis. **hypothalamic n., posterior,** n. hypothalamicus posterior. **hypothalamic n., ventromedial,** n. hypothalamicus ventromedialis. **n. hypothalam'icus ante'rior** [NA], anterior hypothalamic nucleus: a nucleus of nerve cells in the anterior hypothalamic region. **n. hypothalam'icus dorsa'lis** [NA], dorsal hypothalamic nucleus: a nerve cell nucleus situated in the dorsal portion of the intermediate hypothalamic region. **n. hypothalam'icus dorsomedia'lis** [NA], dorsomedial hypothalamic nucleus: a group of nerve cell bodies found in the dorsal part of the intermediate hypothalamic region. **n. hypothalam'icus poste'rior** [NA], posterior hypothalamic nucleus: a nucleus of nerve cells in the posterior hypothalamic region, above the lateral and medial nuclei of the mamillary body; it has major brain stem connections via periventricular fibers and the dorsal longitudinal fasciculus. Called also *n. posterior hypothalami* and *posterior nucleus of hypothalamus.* **n. hypothalam'icus ventromedia'lis** [NA], ventromedial hypothalamic nucleus: a group of nerve cell bodies found in the ventral portion of the intermediate hypothalamic region; it is involved in diverse functions, e.g., food intake and sexual behavior. Called also *n. ventromedialis hypothalami* and *ventromedial n. of hypothalamus.* **n. of hypothalamus, arcuate,** n. infundibularis hypothalami. **n. of hypothalamus, dorsomedial,** n. hypothalamicus dorsomedialis. **n. of hypothalamus, infundibular,** n. infundibularis hypothalami. **n. of hypothalamus, paraventricular,** n. paraventricularis hypothalami. **n. of hypothalamus, posterior,** n. hypothalamicus posterior. **n. of hypothalamus, supraoptic,** n. supraopticus hypothalami. **n. of hypothalamus, ventromedial,** n. hypothalamicus ventromedialis. **n. of inferior**

colliculus, n. colliculi caudalis. **n. infe′rior ner′vi trigem′ini,** NA alternative for *n. spinalis nervi trigemini.* **inferior n. of trigeminal nerve,** n. spinalis nervi trigemini. **n. infundibula′ris hypothal′ami** [NA], infundibular nucleus of hypothalamus: a nucleus of nerve cells in the posterior hypothalamic region, extending into the median eminence and almost entirely surrounding the base of the infundibulum. Called also *arcuate n. of hypothalamus* and *n. arcuatus hypothalami* [NA alternative]. **n. intercala′tus** [NA], a group of nerve cells between the dorsal nucleus of the vagus nerve and the nucleus of the hypoglossal nerve, forming part of the perihypoglossal nuclear complex; called also *Staderini's n.* **intermediolateral n., n. intermediolatera′lis,** a nucleus situated in the substantia intermedia lateralis of thoracic and upper lumbar levels of the spinal cord, which forms the lateral horn, and whose cells give rise to the preganglionic sympathetic outflow. **intermediomedial n., n. intermediomedia′lis,** a nucleus composed of scattered cells in the substantia intermedia centralis, medial to the nucleus intermediolateralis; it is most prominent in the cervical spinal cord and is thought to be propriospinal in its connections. **n. of internal geniculate body,** n. corporis geniculati medialis. **interpeduncular n., n. interpeduncula′ris** [NA], a nucleus situated between the cerebral peduncles immediately dorsal to the interpeduncular fossa, which receives the fasciculus retroflexus; called also *Ganser's ganglion.* **interstitial n., interstitial n. of Cajal, n. interstitia′lis,** a nucleus at the rostral end of the medial longitudinal fasciculus in the mesencephalic tegmentum; its chief connections are reciprocal with vestibular nuclei and it also projects to the spinal cord. **intracerebellar nuclei,** nuclei cerebelli. **nu′clei intralamina′res thal′ami** [NA], intralaminar nuclei of thalamus: the nuclei within the internal medullary lamina of the thalamus, lying between the dorsal medial nucleus above and the lateral posterior nucleus below, and comprising the centromedian, paracentral, parafascicular, and lateral and medial central nuclei. **Kaiser's nuclei,** longitudinal motor nuclei in the cervical and lumbar enlargements of the cord, between the intermediolateral column and the median column. **Klein-Gumprecht nuclei** (*obs.*), unstainable nuclei seen in degenerating lymphocytes in leukemia. **Kölliker's n.,** substantia intermedia centralis. **laryngeal n.,** the nucleus of origin (nucleus ambiguus) of the nerve fibers going to the larynx. **n. of lateral geniculate body,** n. corporis geniculati lateralis. **n. of lateral lemniscus,** n. lemnisci lateralis. **n. latera′lis cervica′lis,** lateral cervical nucleus: a small group of cells in the lateral funiculus of the first and second cervical segments of the spinal cord, comprising a relay station in a spinocervicothalamic path. **n. latera′lis dorsa′lis thal′ami** [NA], the dorsal lateral nucleus of the ventrolateral nuclei of the thalmus; see *nuclei ventrolaterales thalami.* **n. latera′lis medul′lae oblonga′tae** [NA], a nucleus in the reticular substance of the medulla oblongata, dorsolateral to the olive; it relays spinal impulses to the cerebellum. Called also *lateral reticular n.* **n. latera′lis poste′rior thal′ami** [NA], the posterior lateral nucleus of the ventrolateral nuclei of the thalamus; see *nuclei ventrolateralis thalami.* **nu′clei latera′les thal′ami,** see *nuclei ventrolaterales thalami.* **n. lemnis′ci latera′lis** [NA], nucleus of lateral lemniscus: several diffuse cell groups interposed in the course of the lateral lemniscus through the pons. **n. of lens,** n. lentis. **lenticular n., n. lenticula′ris,** NA alternative for *n. lentiformis.* **n. lentifor′mis** [NA], the part of the corpus striatum somewhat resembling a biconvex lens, divided into an external, larger, lateral part, the putamen, and an internal, smaller, lighter colored medial part (globus pallidus), which is in turn subdivided into a smaller, medial, and a larger, lateral part by the medial medullary lamina; called also *lenticular n.* and *n. lenticularis* [NA alternative]. **n. len′tis** [NA], nucleus of the lens: the harder internal part of the lens of the eye. **n. of Luys,** nucleus subthalamicus. **n. magnocellula′ris,** n. vestibularis lateralis. **nuclei of mamillary body, lateral and medial,** nuclei corporis mamillaris mediales et laterales. **n. of medial geniculate body,** n. corporis geniculati medialis. **n. media′lis centra′lis thal′ami,** n. centromedianus thalami. **n. media′lis dorsa′lis thal′ami** [NA], dorsal medial nucleus of thalamus: the largest of the medial nuclei of the thalamus, having a rostral magnocellular part and a caudolateral parvocellular part, both of which make exten-sive intrathalamic connections with most of the other thalamic nuclei. Called also *dorsomedial n. of thalamus.* **nu′clei media′les thal′ami** [NA], medial nuclei of thalamus: groups of nerve cells lying between the internal medullary lamina laterally and projecting toward the ependymal lining of the third ventricle medially; included are the large nucleus medialis dorsalis and a series of smaller nuclei of uncertain significance and connections. **nuclei of median raphe,** nuclei raphae medullae oblongatae. **nu′clei media′ni thal′ami** [NA], median nuclei of thalamus: small groups of nonspecific nerve cells scattered in the periventricular gray substance, separating the medial part of the thalamus from the ependyma of the third ventricle, and partly forming the interthalamic adhesion; included in the group are the nuclei-paraventriculares anteriores et posteriores, nucleus rhomboidalis, and nucleus reuniens. **n. of medulla oblongata, arcuate,** nuclei arcuati. **n. medulla′ris cerebel′li,** corpus medullare cerebelli. **mesencephalic n. of trigeminal nerve, n. of mesencephalic tract of trigeminal nerve,** n. tractus mesencephalicus nervi trigemini. **n. mesencephal′icus ner′vi trigem′ini** [NA], **n. mesencephal′icus trigemina′lis, n. trac′tus mesencephal′ici ner′vi trigem′ini,** mesencephalic nucleus of trigeminal nerve: a slender column of cells in the lateral part of the central gray matter of the rostral portion of the fourth ventricle and the cerebral aqueduct. It is the only central nervous system site of primary sensory neurons, its cells resembling dorsal root ganglion cells. The peripheral processes of its cells, which form the mesencephalic tract, carry proprioceptive impulses; the central processes have widespread cerebellar and brain stem connections, including the motor nucleus of the trigeminal nerve. Called also *n. of mesencephalic tract of trigeminal nerve* and *trigeminal mesencephalic n.* **Monakow's n.,** the lateral part of the cuneate nucleus. **motor n.,** any collection of cells of the central nervous system giving origin to motor fibers of a nerve. **motor n. of trigeminal nerve, n. moto′rius trigemina′lis, n. moto′rius ner′vi trigem′ini** [NA], the nucleus of origin of the motor fibers of the trigeminal nerve, located in the dorsolateral part of the pons, just medial to the main sensory nucleus and the entering sensory root. **n. ner′vi abducen′tis** [NA], nucleus of abducens nerve: the nucleus of origin of the abducens nerve; it lies in the lower part of the pons and forms the lateral part of the facial colliculus in the floor of the fourth ventricle; fibers of the facial nerve form a complicated loop about the nucleus. Called also *abducens n., n. abducens,* and *n. abducentis.* **n. ner′vi accesso′rii** [NA], nucleus of accessory nerve: an irregularly shaped group of nerve cells formed by the axons of nerve cells entering the spinal part of the accessory nerve; found at the ventral border of the ventral column of the spinal cord in an intermediate or central position. Called also *n. accessorius columnae ventralis medullae spinalis* [NA alternative] and *accessory n. of ventral column of spinal cord.* **nu′clei ner′vi acus′tici,** nuclei nervi vestibulocochlearis. **nu′clei nervo′rum cerebra′lium,** nuclei nervorum cranialium. **nu′clei ner′vi cochlea′ris,** nuclei cochleares. **nu′clei nervo′rum crania′lium** [NA], nuclei of cranial nerves: groups of nerve cells in the central nervous system that give rise to, or transmit or receive impulses from, the motor and sensory components of the cranial nerves. Called also *nuclei nervorum encephalicorum* [NA alternative]. **nu′clei nervo′rum encephalico′rum,** NA alternative for *nuclei nervorum cranialium.* **n. ner′vi facia′lis** [NA], nucleus of facial nerve: the nucleus of origin of the motor fibers of the facial nerve, which innervate the muscles of facial expression; the nucleus lies in the ventrolateral part of the lower pons, and its emerging fibers form a complicated loop about the nucleus of the abducent nerve. The term is also applied collectively to the motor nucleus, the superior salivatory nucleus, and the nucleus of the tractus solitarius. Called also *n. facialis.* **n. ner′vi facia′lis of Arnold,** colliculus facialis. **n. ner′vi glossopharyn′gei** [NA], the nucleus of origin and termination of the glossopharyngeal nerve; located in the medulla oblongata, it comprises the inferior salivatory nucleus, the nucleus ambiguus (rostral part), and the nucleus of the tractus solitarius. **n. ner′vi hypoglos′si** [NA], nucleus of hypoglossal nerve: the nucleus of origin of the hypoglossal nerve, forming a column in the central gray matter of the medial eminence from below the level of the inferior olive to the upper part of the medulla oblongata. Called also *hypoglossal n.* and *n. hypoglossalis* [NA alternative]. **n. ner'vi oculomoto'rii** [NA], nucleus of oculomotor nerve: the nucleus or origin of the fibers of the oculomotor nerve, situated in the tegmentum of the mesencephalon immediately ventral to the central gray matter, where its two cell groups form a complex between the medial longitudinal fasciculi; the complex comprises paired lateral somatic groups, an unpaired median somatic group, and paired dorsal autonomic (parasympathetic) groups. The somatic groups supply the levator palpebrae superioris and all the extrinsic eye muscles except the lateral rectus and superior oblique; the autonomic group supplies the ciliary muscle and sphincter pupillae. Called also *n. oculomotorius* [NA alternative] and *oculomotor n.* **n. ner'vi phren'ici** [NA], nucleus of phrenic nerve: a centrally positioned group of nerve cells in the gray substance of the ventral column of the spinal cord, extending from the third to the seventh cervical segments, which innervate the diaphragm; called also *phrenic n. of ventral column of spinal cord* and *n. phrenicus columnae ventralis medullae spinalis* [NA alternative]. **nu'clei ner'vi trigem'ini**, nuclei of trigeminal nerve: located chiefly in the pons and medulla oblongata, but also in the mesencephalon and upper cervical cord. See *n. mesencephalicus nervi trigemini, n. motorius nervi trigemini, n. pontius nervi trigemini,* and *n. spinalis nervi trigemini.* **n. ner'vi trochlea'ris** [NA], nucleus of trochlear nerve: the nucleus of origin of the motor fibers of the trochlear nerve; it lies in the central gray matter on the dorsal surface of the medial longitudinal fasciculus in the lower part of the mesencephalon. Called also *n. trochlearis* [NA alternative] and *trochlear n.* **n. ner'vi va'gi**, the nucleus of origin and termination of the vagus nerve; situated in the medulla oblongata, it comprises the nucleus dorsalis, the nucleus ambiguus, and the nucleus of the tractus solitarius. **nu'clei ner'vi vestibula'ris**, nuclei vestibulares. **nu'clei ner'vi vestibulocochlea'ris** [NA], vestibulocochlear nuclei: the nuclei of termination of the sensory fibers of the vestibular and cochlear divisions of the eighth cranial nerve, comprising the ventral and dorsal cochlear nuclei and the medial, lateral, superior, and inferior vestibular nuclei. Called also *nuclei nervi acustici.* **n. oculomoto'rius**, NA alternative for *n. nervi oculomotorii.* **n. oculomoto'rius accesso'rius** [NA], **n. oculomoto'rius autonom'icus**, accessory oculomotor nucleus: a collection of small cells located dorsal to the upper part of the somatic groups of the oculomotor nuclear complex, comprising the parasympathetic outflow via the ciliary ganglion to the ciliary muscle and sphincter pupillae of the eye; called also *accessory n., autonomic n., Edinger's or Edinger-Westphal n., n. accessorius,* and *n. autonomicus.* **oculomotor n., n. of oculomotor nerve**, n. nervi oculomotorii. **n. oliva'ris**, n. olivaris caudalis. **n. oliva'ris accesso'rius dorsa'lis** [NA], dorsal accessory olivary nucleus: the band of cells that lies dorsal to the caudal olivary nucleus and projects fibers to the opposite side of the cerebellum, especially to the vermis. Called also *n. olivaris accessorius posterior* [NA alternative] and *posterior accessorius olivary nucleus.* **n. oliva'ris accesso'rius media'lis** [NA], medial accessory olivary nucleus: the band of gray substance that lies medial to the caudal olivary nucleus and projects fibers to the opposite side of the cerebellum, especially to the vermis. **n. oliva'ris accesso'rius poste'rior**, NA alternative for *n. olivaris accessorius dorsalis.* **n. oliva'ris cauda'lis** [NA], caudal olivary nucleus: a folded band of gray substance enclosing a white core (*hilum nuclei olivaris caudalis*), which produces the elevation on the medulla oblongata known as the *oliva*; it is a nuclear complex that receives heavy projections from the spinal cord, mesencephalon, and cerebral cortex, and projects fibers, via the opposite caudal cerebellar peduncle, partly to the vermis, but principally to the neocerebellum. Called also *inferior olivary n., n. olivaris,* and *n. olivaris inferior* [NA alternative]. **n. oliva'ris crania'lis**, see *n. olivaris rostralis.* **n. oliva'ris inferior**, NA alternative for *n. olivaris caudalis.* **n. oliva'ris rostra'lis** [NA], rostral olivary nucleus: a band of gray substance located laterally at the level of the pontomedullary junction superior to the olivary nucleus, the fibers of which form the olivocochlear tract. When at the level of or inside the skull, this nucleus is designated *rostralis,* when it is not, *cranialis.* Called also *n. olivaris superioris* [NA alternative] and *n. of superior olive.* **n. oliva'ris supe'rior**, n. dorsalis corporis trapezoidei. **n. oliva'ris superio'ris**, NA alternative for *n. olivaris rostralis.* **olivary n.**, 1. n. olivaris caudalis. 2. oliva. **olivary n.,**

accessory, olivary n., dorsal accessory, n. olivaris accessorius dorsalis. **olivary n., caudal,** n. olivaris caudalis. **olivary n., inferior,** n. olivaris caudalis. **olivary n., medial accessory,** n. olivaris accessorius medialis. **olivary n., posterior accessory,** n. olivaris accessorius dorsalis. **olivary n., rostral,** n. olivaris rostralis. **olivary n., superior,** 1. n. dorsalis corporis trapezoidei. 2. n. olivaris rostralis. **nuclei of origin, nu'clei ori'ginis** [NA], groups of nerve cells in the central nervous system from which arise the motor, or efferent, fibers of the cranial nerves. **Pander's n.**, n. subthalamicus. **n. paracentra'lis thal'ami** [NA], paracentral nucleus of thalamus: one of the smaller intralaminar nuclei of the dorsal thalamus, situated ventrolateral to the dorsal medial nucleus and medial to the lateral central nucleus. **n. parafascicula'ris thal'ami** [NA], parafascicular nucleus of thalamus: one of the smaller intralaminar nuclei of the dorsal thalamus, situated medial to the centromedian nucleus and ventral to the dorsal medial nucleus. **paramedian n., dorsal,** n. paramedianus dorsalis. **paramedian n., posterior,** n. paramedianus dorsalis. **n. paramedia'nus dorsa'lis** [NA], dorsal paramedian nucleus: a group of nerve cells near the dorsal surface of the medulla oblongata, forming part of the perihypoglossal nuclear complex; called also *n. paramedianus posterior* [NA alternative] and *posterior paramedian n.* **n. paramedia'nus posterior**, NA alternative for *n. paramedianus dorsalis.* **n. parasolita'rius** [NA], **parasolitary n.,** an aggregation of nerve cells situated ventrolateral to the solitary nucleus. **nu'clei parasympath'ici sacra'les** [NA], parasympathetic sacral nuclei: a group of nerve cells in the second through the fourth sacral segments of the spinal cord, located lateral to the central canal and central gelatinous substance, between the bases of the ventral and dorsal gray columns; the cells are the source of the pelvic or sacral outflow of parasympathetic preganglionic fibers. **nu'clei paraventricula'res anterio'res et posterio'res thal'ami** [NA], see *nuclei mediani thalami.* **n. paraventricula'ris hypothal'ami** [NA], paraventricular nucleus of hypothalamus: a sharply defined band of cells in the wall of the third ventricle in the anterior hypothalamic region; many of its cells are neurosecretory in function, secreting oxytocin, which is carried to the posterior lobe of the pituitary gland by the fibers of the paraventriculohypophysial tract. **n. periventricula'ris poste'rior** [NA], posterior periventricular nucleus: a nucleus of nerve cells in the intermediate hypothalamic region, lying in the posterior part of the third ventricle. **Perlia's n.**, a group of cells in the midline of the oculomotor nuclear complex, thought to be associated with ocular convergence. **phenanthrene n.,** cholane n. **n. of phrenic nerve**, n. nervi phrenici. **phrenic n. of ventral column of spinal cord**, n. nervi phrenici. **n. phren'icus colum'nae ventra'lis medul'lae spina'lis**, NA alternative for *n. nervi phrenici.* **polymorphic n.,** a cell nucleus that assumes an irregular form or splits up into more or less completely separated lobes, such as the nuclei in the polymorphonuclear leukocytes (neutrophils). **nuclei of pons, pontine nuclei, nu'clei pon'tis** [NA], masses of nerve cells scattered throughout the ventral part of the pons, in which the longitudinal fibers of the pons terminate, and whose axons in turn cross to the opposite side and form the middle cerebellar peduncle, which projects fibers to the neocerebellum. **pontine n. of trigeminal nerve**, n. pontinus nervi trigemini. **n. ponti'nus ner'vi trigem'ini** [NA], pontine nucleus of trigeminal nerve: the nucleus of termination of afferent fibers of the trigeminal nerve, carrying impulses for sensations of touch and pressure, located in the dorsolateral part of the middle of the pons, just lateral to the entering trigeminal root fibers. Called also *principal sensory n. of trigeminal nerve* and *n. sensorius principalis nervi trigemini.* **n. poste'rior hypothal'ami**, n. hypothalamicus posterior. **posterior periventricular n.**, n. periventricularis posterior. **nu'clei posterio'res thal'ami** [NA], the nuclei forming the posterior end of the dorsal thalamus, comprising the pulvinar and the nuclei of the lateral and medial geniculate bodies; called also *pulvinar thalami.* **preoptic nuclei, lateral and medial**, nuclei preoptici medialis et lateralis. **nu'clei preop'tici media'lis et latera'lis** [NA], medial and lateral preoptic nuclei: a nucleus of nerve cells in the medial and lateral parts of the anterior hypothalamic region. **n. of prerubral field**, groups of neurons scattered along the caudomedial border of the zona incerta in field H of Forel (prerubral field); called also *n. of tegmental field.* See also *nuclei areae H, H₁, H₂.* **pretectal n., n. pretecta′lis** [NA], an indistinct mass of nerve cells in the pretectal area which receive impulses chiefly from the optic tract; they project to the nucleus accessorius of the oculomotor nerve and constitute the midbrain center for the pupillary light reflex. **n. pro′-prius,** a column of large neurons that extends throughout the posterior horn of the spinal cord, ventral to the gelatinous substance. Called also *dorsal funicular column.* **n. pul-po′sus dis′ci intervertebra′lis** [NA], **pulpy n.,** a semifluid mass of fine white and elastic fibers that forms the central portion of an intervertebral disk; it has been regarded

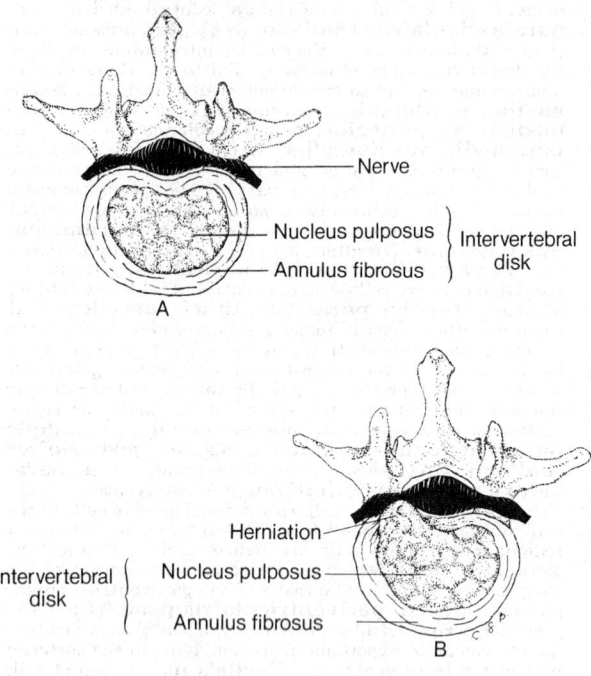

Intervertebral disk in transverse section, showing the nucleus pulposus and the annulus fibrosus. *A,* normal disk; *B,* herniation of the nucleus pulposus.

as the persistent remains of the embryonic notochord. **nu′clei pulvina′res thal′ami** [NA], the nuclei forming the prominent, cushion-like medial portion of the posterior extremity of the thalamus (the pulvinar). **pyramidal n.,** n. olivaris accessorius medialis. **n. radi′cis descen-den′tis ner′vi trigem′ini,** n. tractus mesencephalicus nervi trigemini. **nu′clei ra′phae medul′lae oblon-ga′tae** [NA], **rapheal nuclei,** reticular nuclei aggregated in narrow, vertical sheets along the median plane of the medulla oblongata, pons, and midbrain; some of their constituent cells contain serotonin. Called also *nuclei of median raphe* and *nuclei raphae medianae.* **red n.,** n. ruber. **reproductive n.,** micronucleus, def. 1. **reticular n., lateral,** n. lateralis medullae oblongatae. **n. reticula′-ris tegmen′ti,** a nucleus in the tegmentum of the pons which receives fibers from the cerebral cortex and mesencephalon and which projects fibers to the neocerebellum via the middle cerebellar peduncle. **n. reticula′ris thal′ami** [NA], reticular nucleus of thalamus: a thin layer of cells on the lateral surface of the thalamus, within and lateral to the external medullary lamina. **retrodor-solateral n. of ventral column of spinal cord, n. retrodorsolatera′lis colum′nae ventra′lis medul′lae spina′lis** [NA], a group of nerve cells in the gray substance of the retrodorsolateral region of the ventral column of the spinal cord, which innervates the digital muscles. **n. reu′niens thal′ami** [NA], see *nuclei media-na thalami.* **n. rhomboida′lis thal′ami** [NA], see *nuclei mediana thalami.* **Roller′s n.,** 1. sublingual n. 2.

cells near the hilum of the caudal olivary nucleus. **roof nuclei,** a term sometimes used to refer to the nuclei cerebelli because some of them are situated in close proximity to the roof of the fourth ventricle of the brain. **n. ru′ber** [NA], red nucleus: a distinctive oval nucleus (pink in fresh specimens because of an iron-containing pigment in many of the cells) centrally placed in the upper mesencephalic reticular formation; it receives fibers from the deep cerebellar nuclei and cerebral cortex and projects fibers to the cerebellum, brain stem, spinal cord, and probably to the thalamus. The nucleus is divided into two regions: *pars magnocellularis* and *pars parvocellularis.* **sacral para-sympathetic nuclei,** nuclei parasympathici sacrales. **n. salivato′rius cauda′lis** [NA], caudal salivatory nucleus: the caudal part of the column of scattered cells in the dorsolateral part of the reticular formation in the lower pons and upper medulla oblongata, whose cells compromise the parasympathetic outflow of the glossopharyngeal nerve for the supply of the parotid gland; called also *inferior salivatory n.* and *n. salivatorius inferior* [NA alternative]. See also *n. dorsalis nervi glossopharyngei.* **n. salivato′rius crania′lis** [NA], see *n. salivatorius rostralis.* **n. salivato′rius infe′rior,** NA alternative for *n. salivatorius caudalis.* **n. salivato′rius rostra′lis** [NA], rostral salivatory nucleus: an ill-defined column of scattered cells in the dorsolateral part of the reticular formation of the dorsal pons, whose cells comprise the parasympathetic outflow of the facial nerve for the supply of the lacrimal, nasal, palatine, submandibular, and sublingual glands; it is continuous with the caudal salivatory nucleus. When at the level of or inside the skull, this nucleus is designated *rostralis;* when it is not, *cranialis.* Called also *n. salivatorius superior* [NA alternative] and *superior salivatory n.* **n. salivato′rius supe′rior,** NA alternative for *n. salivatorius rostralis.* **salivatory n., caudal,** n. salivatorius caudalis. **salivatory n., cranial,** see *n. salivatorius rostralis.* **salivatory n., in-ferior,** n. salivatorius caudalis. **salivatory n., rostral, salivatory n., superior,** n. salivatorius rostralis. **n. of Sappey,** n. ruber. **Schwalbe′s n.,** n. vestibularis medialis. **Schwann′s n.,** the nucleus of a Schwann cell. **segmentation n.,** the fertilization nucleus after cleavage has begun. **n. senso′rius infe′rior ner′vi tri gem′ini,** n. tractus spinalis nervi trigemini. **n. sen-so′rius principa′lis ner′vi trigem′ini,** n. pontinus nervi trigemini. **sensory n.,** the nucleus of termination of the afferent (sensory) fibers of a peripheral nerve. **sen-sory n. of trigeminal nerve, lower,** n. tractus spinalis nervi trigemini. **sensory n. of trigeminal nerve, principal,** n. pontinus nervi trigemini. **Setchenow′s (Sechenoff′s) nuclei,** see under *center.* **shadow n.,** a cell nucleus that does not stain and appears as a faint shadow under the microscope. **Siemerling′s n.,** one of the subdivisions of the oculomotor nuclear complex. **n. solita′rius** [NA], solitary nucleus: the nucleus of termination of the visceral afferent fibers of the facial, glossopharyngeal, and vagus nerves, which enter the tractus solitarius. It surrounds the tractus solitarius and its caudal end joins with the caudal end of the corresponding nucleus of the opposite side. Called also *n. of solitary tract* and *n. tractus solitarii.* **solitary n., of solitary tract,** n. solitarius. **soma-tic n.,** macronucleus. **sperm n.,** the male pronucleus. **spherical n.,** n. globosus. **spinal n. of accessory nerve,** n. spinalis nervi accessorii. **n. of spinal tract of trigeminal nerve,** n. spinalis nervi trigemini. **spi-nal n. of trigeminal nerve,** n. spinalis nervi trigemini. **n. spina′lis ner′vi accesso′rii** [NA], spinal nucleus of accessory nerve: the group of cells in the anterior horn of the upper five or six levels of the cervical spinal cord that form the spinal roots of the accessory nerve. **n. spina′lis ner′vi trigem′ini** [NA], spinal nucleus of trigeminal nerve: a column of cells which lies along the medial aspect of the spinal tract, extending from the level of entry of the trigeminal nerve in the pons to the second cervical segment of the spinal cord, where it is continuous with the dorsal gray column. The nucleus has several cytoarchitectonic subdivisions and the fibers of the spinal tract end in it. Called also *inferior n. of trigeminal nerve, n. inferior nervi trigemini* [NA alternative], *n. of spinal tract of trigeminal nerve,* and *n. tractus spinalis nervi trigemini.* **Spitzka′s n.,** Perlia′s n. **Staderini′s n.,** n. intercalatus. **Stilling′s n.,** columna thoracica. **Stilling′s sacral n.,** sacral n. **striate n.,** a term loosely applied to the neostriatum, to a nucleus of the corpus striatum, or to the corpus striatum itself. **n. sub-**

caeru′leus, n. subceru′leus, n. subcoeru′leus, a group of neurons subjacent to the nucleus coeruleus in the parvocellular lateral reticular column of the oral part of the pons. **subependymal n.,** the dorsal cochlear nucleus. **sublingual n.,** a sharply defined nucleus immediately ventral to the nucleus of the hypoglossal nerve, forming part of the perihypoglossal nuclear complex; called also *Roller's n.* **subthalamic n., n. subthalam′icus** [NA], a biconvex mass of gray matter on the medial side of the junction of the internal capsule and the crus cerebri; its chief connections are with the globus pallidus. Called also *n. of Luys, corpus Luysi,* and *Luys' body.* **n. of superior olive,** n. olivaris rostralis. **n. supraop′ticus hypothal′ami** [NA], supraoptic nucleus of hypothalamus: a sharply defined nucleus of nerve cells in the anterior hypothalamic region, immediately above the lateral part of the optic chiasm; many of its cells are neurosecretory in function, secreting antidiuretic hormone, which is carried to the posterior lobe of the pituitary gland by the fibers of the supraopticohypophysial tract; other cells are osmoreceptors which respond to increased osmotic pressure to signal the release of antidiuretic hormone by the posterior lobe of the pituitary gland. **n. taeniaefor′mis,** corpus amygdaloideum. **n. tec′ti,** n. fastigii. **tegmental nuclei,** nuclei tegmenti. **nu′clei tegmenta′les,** nuclei tegmenti. **n. of tegmental field,** n. of prerubral field. **nu′clei tegmen′ti** [NA], tegmental nuclei: several nuclear masses of the reticular formations of the pons and midbrain, especially of the latter, where they are in close approximation to the cranial cerebellar peduncles. Called also *nuclei tegmentales* [NA alternative]. **terminal nuclei, nu′clei terminatio′nis** [NA], groups of nerve cells within the central nervous system upon which the axons of primary afferent neurons of various cranial nerves synapse. **nuclei of thalamus, anterior,** nuclei anteriores thalami. **n. of thalamus, anterodorsal,** see *nuclei anteriores thalami.* **n. of thalamus, anteromedial,** see *nuclei anteriores thalami.* **n. of thalamus, anteroventral,** see *nuclei anteriores thalami.* **n. of thalamus, central medial,** n. centromedianus thalami. **n. of thalamus, centromedian,** n. centromedianus thalami. **n. of thalamus, dorsal medial,** n. medialis dorsalis thalami. **n. of thalamus, dorsomedial,** n. medialis dorsalis thalami. **nuclei of thalamus, intralaminar,** nuclei intralaminares thalami. **nuclei of thalamus, lateral,** see *nuclei ventrolaterales thalami.* **n. of thalamus, lateral central,** n. centralis lateralis thalami. **nuclei of thalamus, medial,** nuclei mediales thalami. **n. of thalamus, medial central,** n. centralis medialis thalami. **nuclei of thalamus, median,** nuclei mediani thalami. **n. of thalamus, parafascicular n.** parafascicularis thalami. **nuclei of thalamus, paraventricular, anterior and posterior,** see *nuclei mediani thalami.* **n. of thalamus, posterior,** n. posterior thalami. **n. of thalamus, reticular,** n. reticularis thalami. **n. of thalamus, rhomboid,** see *nuclei mediani thalami.* **n. of thalamus, ventral,** see *nuclei ventrolaterales thalami.* **nuclei of thalamus, ventrolateral,** nuclei ventrolaterales thalami. **thoracic n.,** columna thoracica. **n. thorac′icus,** NA alternative for *columna thoracica.* **n. of tongue, fibrous,** septum linguae. **n. trac′tus solita′rii,** n. solitarius. **n. trac′tus spina′lis ner′vi trigem′ini,** n. spinalis nervi trigemini. **n. of trapezoid body, dorsal,** n. dorsalis corporis trapezoidei. **n. of trapezoid body, ventral,** n. ventralis corporis trapezoidei. **triangular n., n. triangularis,** n. vestibularis medialis. **trigeminal mesencephalic n.,** n. mesencephalicus nervi trigemini. **nuclei of trigeminal nerve,** nuclei nervi trigemini. **n. trochlea′ris,** NA alternative for *n. nervi trochlearis.* **trochlear n., n. of trochlear nerve,** n. nervi trochlearis. **trophic n.,** macronucleus. **tuberal nuclei, nu′clei tubera′les** [NA], **tuberal nuclei, lateral, nu′clei tu′beris latera′lis,** nerve cell nuclei situated ventrally in the intermediate hypothalamic region, mainly in the lateral hypothalamic area. **n. vaga′lis dorsa′lis,** NA alternative for *n. dorsalis nervi vagi.* **vagoglossopharyngeal n.,** n. ambiguus. **vagal n., dorsal, n. of vagus nerve, dorsal** n. dorsalis nervi vagi. **n. ventra′lis ante′rior thal′ami** [NA], **n. ventra′lis anterolatera′lis thal′ami,** the anterior ventral nucleus of the ventrolateral nuclei of the thalamus; see *nuclei ventrolaterales thalami.* **n. ventra′lis cor′poris trapezoi′dei** [NA], ventral nu-

cleus of trapezoid body: a group of nerve cells intermingled with the fibers of the trapezoid body, medial and ventral to the dorsal nucleus (superior olive); they contribute fibers to the lateral lemniscus. **n. ventra′lis interme′dius thal′ami,** n. ventralis lateralis thalami. **n. ventra′lis latera′lis thal′ami** [NA], the lateral ventral nucleus of the ventrolateral nuclei of the thalamus; called also *n. ventralis intermedius thalami.* See *nuclei ventrolaterales thalami.* **n. ventra′lis media′lis thal′ami** [NA], the medial ventral nucleus of the ventrolateral nuclei of the thalamus; see *nuclei ventrolaterales thalami.* **nu′clei ventra′les posterio′res thal′ami,** the nuclei that form the posterior ventral part of the ventrolateral nuclei of the thalamus, comprising the posterolateral ventral nucleus, which is the terminus of the spinothalamic tract and medial lemniscus and projects to the postcentral gyrus, and the posteromedial ventral nucleus, which is the secondary trigeminal tract and sends axons to the somesthetic area of the postcentral gyrus for the face. **n. ventra′lis posterolatera′lis thal′ami** [NA], the posterolateral ventral nucleus of the posterior ventral nuclei of the thalamus; see *nuclei ventrales posteriores thalami.* **n. ventra′lis posteromedia′lis thal′ami** [NA], the posteromedial ventral nucleus of the posterior ventral nuclei of the thalamus; see *nuclei ventrales posteriores thalami.* **n. ventra′lis thal′ami,** see *nuclei ventrolaterales thalami.* **nu′clei ventrolatera′les thal′ami** [NA], ventrolateral nuclei of thalamus: a large group of nuclei lying between the internal medullary lamina and the internal capsule, divided into a larger ventral portion and a smaller lateral portion. The ventral part comprises anterior ventral, lateral ventral, medial ventral, posterior ventral, posterolateral ventral, and posteromedial ventral nuclei; these nuclei are concerned with relaying impulses to specific areas of the cerebral cortex. The lateral part comprises the posterior lateral and dorsal lateral nuclei; the former has major connections with the cingulate gyrus and the latter has extensive connections with the cerebral cortex. **ventrolateral n. of ventral column of spinal cord, n. ventrolatera′lis colum′nae ventra′lis medul′lae spina′lis** [NA], a group of nerve cells in the gray substance of the ventrolateral region of the ventral column of the spinal cord. **n. ventromedia′lis hypothal′ami,** n. hypothalamicis ventromedialis. **ventromedial n. of ventral column of spinal cord, n. ventromedia′lis colum′nae ventra′lis medul′lae spina′lis** [NA], a group of nerve cells in the gray matter of the ventromedial region of the ventral column of the spinal cord. **n. ventromedia′lis,** ventrally placed cells in the lateral part of the oculomotor nuclear complex; they are very distinct from the dorsally placed cells in the middle third of the complex and have a somatic motor function. **vesicular n.,** a form of cell nucleus, the membrane of which stains deeply, while the central part is rather pale. **vestibular nuclei,** nuclei vestibulares. **vestibular n., caudal,** n. vestibularis caudalis. **vestibular n., cranial,** see *n. vestibularis rostralis.* **vestibular n., inferior,** n. vestibularis caudalis. **vestibular n., lateral,** n. vestibularis lateralis. **vestibular n., rostral,** n. vestibularis rostralis. **vestibular n., superior,** n. vestibularis rostralis. **nu′clei vestibula′res** [NA], vestibular nuclei: the four cellular masses in the floor of the fourth ventricle: *rostral* or *cranial* (superior), *lateral, medial,* and *caudal* (inferior) vestibular nuclei, in which the short ascending and longer descending branches of the pars vestibularis nervi octavi terminate and in which cerebellar projections are received. The nuclei give rise to a widely dispersed special sensory system through projections to motor nuclei in the brain stem and cervical cord via the medial longitudinal fasciculi from all the vestibular nuclei to the cerebellum (chiefly from the caudal and medial nuclei), and to motor cells throughout the spinal cord (from the lateral nucleus). Additional connections of the nuclei provide for conscious perception of, and autonomic reactions to, labyrinthine stimulation. Called also *nuclei of acoustic nerve* and *nuclei nervi vestibularis.* **n. vestibula′ris cauda′lis** [NA], caudal vestibular nucleus: a nucleus of nerve cells that lies lateral to the medial nucleus and between the medial vestibular nucleus and the caudal cerebellar peduncle; called also *inferior vestibular n.* and *n. vestibularis inferior* [NA alternative]. **n. vestibula′ris crania′lis,** see *n. vestibularis rostralis.* **n. vestibula′ris infe′rior,** NA alternative for *n. vestibularis caudalis.* **n. vestibula′ris latera′lis** [NA], lateral vestibular nucleus: a nucleus composed of large multipolar nerve cells that lies immediately cranial to the caudal vestibular nucleus and its upper end becomes continuous with the cranial vestibular nucleus; called also *Deiter's n., large cell auditory n.,* and *n. magnocellularis.* See also *nuclei vestibulares.* **n. vestibula′ris media′lis** [NA], middle vestibular nucleus: a nucleus of nerve cells that lies in the floor of the fourth ventricle and extends upward from the medulla oblongata and pons; called also *n. triangularis, Schwalbe's n.,* and *triangular n.* See also *nuclei vestibulares.* **n. vestibula′ris rostra′lis** [NA], rostral vestibular nucleus: a small nucleus of nerve cells that lies above the lateral vestibular nuclei. When at the level of or inside the skull, this nucleus is designated *rostralis;* when it is not, *cranialis.* Called also *Bekhterev's n., n. vestibularis superior* [NA alternative], and *superior vestibular n.* See also *nuclei vestibulares.* **n. vestibula′ris supe′rior,** NA alternative for *n. vestibularis rostralis.* **vestibulocochlear nuclei,** nuclei nervi vestibulocochlearis. **Voit's n.,** a cerebellar nucleus accessory to the dentate nucleus. **Westphal's n.,** n. accessorius. **yolk n.,** a special area of the cytoplasm of an ovum in which the synthetic activities leading to the accumulation of food supplies in the oocyte are apparently initiated; called also *vitelline body, Balbiani's body,* and *Balbiani's n.* **zygote n.,** fertilization n.

nuclide (nu′klĭd) a species of atom characterized by the atomic number, mass number, and quantum state of its nucleus, and capable of existing for a measurable lifetime (generally greater than 10^{-10} sec.). Thus nuclear isomers are separate nuclides, but promptly decaying excited nuclear states and unstable intermediates in nuclear reactions are not so considered. **radioactive n.,** radionuclide.

nudophobia (nu″do-fo′be-ah) [L. *nudus* unclothed, bare + *phobia*] an abnormal aversion to being unclothed.

Nuel's space (ne-elz′) [Jean Pierre *Nuel,* Belgian oculist, 1847–1920] see under *space.*

nufenoxole (noo″fĕ-nok′sōl) chemical name: 2-[3-(5-methyl-1,3,4-oxidiazol-2-yl)-3,3-diphenylpropyl]-2-azabicyclo[2.2.2]octane; an antiperistaltic, $C_{25}H_{29}N_3O$.

NUG necrotizing ulcerative gingivitis; see *acute necrotizing ulcerative gingivitis.*

Nuhn's glands (noonz) [Anton *Nuhn,* German anatomist, 1814–1889] glandulae linguales anteriores.

nullipara (nuh-lip′ah-rah) [L. *nullus* none + *parere* to bring forth, produce] a woman who has never borne a viable child. Also written para 0.

nulliparity (nul″ĭ-par′ĭ-te) the condition or fact of being nulliparous.

nulliparous (nuh-lip′ah-rus) having never given birth to a viable infant.

nullisomic (nul″ĭ-som′ik) lacking one pair of chromosomes.

number (num′ber) [Fr. *nombre,* from L. *numerus*] a symbol, as a figure or word, expressive of a certain value or of a specified quantity determined by count. **acetyl n.,** the number of milligrams of KOH necessary to neutralize the acetic acid saponified from 1 gram of acetylated fat; it represents the extent to which hydroxyl groups are present. **acid n.,** the number of milligrams of potassium hydroxide necessary to neutralize the free fatty acids in 1 gram of fat; it represents a measure of the amount of free fatty acids in the fat. **atomic n.,** the number of protons in the nucleus of a nuclide; all the atoms of a chemical element have the same atomic number; sometimes indicated by a subscript preceding the symbol of a chemical element (e.g., ^2H). Symbol Z. **Avogadro's n.,** the number of particles in one mole of a substance: 6.0220×10^{23}. **Brinell hardness n.,** a number indicative of the degree of relative hardness of a material, calculated after measuring the diameter of the impression made by a steel ball pressed under a known load into the surface of the material being tested; equal to the load in kilograms divided by the surface area of the indentation in square millimeters. **chromosome n.,** the number of chromosomes present in the somatic cells of an organism; the normal individual receives, at conception, one set of chromosomes (the haploid number, symbol *n*) from each of the gametes forming the zygote, thus acquiring the diploid number (*2n*). In humans, *n* equals 23. **CT n's,** attenuation values determined for each pixel in a CT scan on a scale in which water is 0, compact bone +1000, and air −1000. See *Hounsfield unit* under *unit.* **dibucaine n.,** an expression of the percentage of inhibition of the enzyme cholinesterase in

a serum sample by dibucaine; used to differentiate between normal and abnormal serum cholinesterase phenotypes. Normal or usual is about 80; intermediate is about 60; abnormal or atypical is about 20. Abbreviated DN. **hardness n.,** a number indicative of the degree of relative hardness of materials. See *Brinell, Knoop, Mohs, Rockwell,* and *Vickers hardness n.* and *scleroscope test,* under *test.* **Hehner n.,** the percentage of fatty acids not volatile with steam, obtainable from a fat. **Hittorf n.,** the fraction of the total current passing through an electrolysis cell that is carried by a given ion species; called also *transport n.* **Hübl n.,** iodine n. **hydrogen n.,** the amount of hydrogen that fats can take up; it represents the amount of unsaturated fatty acids present. **iodine n.,** the amount of iodine in grams which 100 grams of the fat can take up; it indicates the amount of unsaturated fatty acids present in the fat. **isotopic n.,** the number which added to twice the atomic number gives the atomic weight. **Knoop hardness n.,** a number indicative of the degree of relative hardness of a material, calculated from the load employed and the length of the long axis of the impression made by the rhomboidal pyramid of a diamond pressed into the surface of the material being tested. It is the test most commonly used in dental practice to test the hardness of teeth. **Loschmidt's n.,** the number of molecules per unit volume of an ideal gas at STP; Avogadro's number divided by 22.4 liters per mole. **mass n.,** the number of nucleons (protons plus neutrons) in the atom of a nuclide; generally indicated by a superscript preceding the symbol of a chemical element (e.g., ^{131}I) to denote a specific isotope. Symbol *A.* **Mohs hardness n.,** a number on an arbitrary mineralogical scale of hardness, in which a mineral will scratch other minerals that are lower on the scale and will in turn be scratched by those higher on the scale. **oxidation n.,** a number assigned to each atom in a molecule or ion that represents the number of electrons theoretically gained (positive oxidation numbers) or lost (negative numbers) in converting the atom to the elemental form. Oxidation numbers are assigned according to the following rules. The oxidation number of atoms in an elemental form is zero, and the oxidation number of a monatomic ion equals the ionic charge. Group I and Group II metals always have oxidation numbers of +1 and +2, respectively. Fluorine always has an oxidation number of −1; oxygen always of −2, except in peroxides and superoxides (where it is −1) and in compounds containing 0-F bonds. Hydrogen always has an oxidation number of +1, except in metal hydrides (where it is −1). Oxidation numbers are assigned to other atoms so that the sum for all atoms in a neutral compound equals zero and the sum for all atoms in a polyatomic ion equals the ionic charge. Called also *oxidation state.* **polar n.,** the number of valences (positive or negative) possessed by an atom in any particular compound. **Polenske n.,** the number of milliliters of tenth normal KOH required to neutralize the insoluble, volatile fatty acids from 5 gm. of the fat. **Reichert-Meissl n.,** the number of milliliters of tenth normal KOH required to neutralize the soluble volatile fatty acids distilled from 5 gm. of fat after it has been saponified with KOH and then made acid with H_3PO_4 or H_2SO_4. **Reynold's n.,** the velocity of flow of a fluid multiplied by the diameter of the vessel and divided by the kinematic viscosity of the circulating fluid. **Rockwell hardness n.,** a number indicative of the degree of relative hardness of materials, determined by measuring the depth of the impression made by a steel or diamond penetrator pressed into the surface of the material being tested. There are a number of Rockwell hardness tests and scales, using various combinations of loads and penetrators; the load and penetrator combination must always be specified when stating a Rockwell hardness number. **saponification n.,** the number of milligrams of potassium hydroxide required to neutralize the fatty acids in 1 gram of a fat or oil; it indicates the average size of the fatty acid molecules or the amount of the lower fatty acids present. **thiocyanogen n.,** the amount of thiocyanogen absorbed by a fat or oil. **transport n.,** Hittorf number. **turnover n.,** the number of molecules of substrate acted upon by one molecule of enzyme per minute. **Vickers hardness n.,** a number indicative of the degree of relative hardness of materials, determined by measuring the long diagonals of indentation made by pressing the pyramidal point of a diamond into the surface of the material being tested; equal to the load in kilograms divided by the area, in square millimeters, of the recovered indentation; called also *diamond pyramid hard-*

ness. **wave n.,** in light waves, the reciprocal of the wavelength expressed as a fraction of a centimeter.

numbness (num′nes) a lack or diminution of sensation in a part.

nummular (num′u-lar) [L. *nummularis*] 1. coin-sized and coin-shaped. 2. made up of round, flat disks. 3. piled, like coins, in a rouleau.

Numorphan (nu-mor′fan) trademark for preparations of oxymorphone hydrochloride.

nunnation (nun-a′shun) [Heb. *nun* letter N] the too frequent use of *n* sounds, or the nasalizing of sounds or words.

Nupercainal (noo″per-kān′al) trademark for a preparation of dibucaine.

Nupercaine (nu′per-kān) trademark for preparations of dibucaine.

N-Uristix (u′rĭ-stiks) trademark for a reagent strip designed for testing for nitrite, glucose, and protein in urine.

nurse (ners) 1. a person who is especially prepared in the scientific basis of nursing and who meets certain prescribed standards of education and clinical competence. 2. to provide services that are essential to or helpful in the promotion, maintenance, and restoration of health and well-being. 3. to breast-feed an infant. See also *nursing.* **charge n.,** one who is in charge of a patient care unit of a hospital or similar health agency; called also *head n.* **clinical n. specialist,** a registered nurse with a high degree of knowledge, skill, and competence in a specialized area of nursing. These skills are made directly available through the provision of nursing care to clients and are indirectly available through guidance and planning of care with other nursing personnel. Clinical nurse specialists hold a master's degree in nursing, preferably with an emphasis in clinical nursing. Called also *n. specialist.* **n. clinician,** a registered nurse, referred to as a *nurse clinician* or as a *nurse practitioner,* who has well-developed competencies in utilizing a broad range of cues. These cues are used for prescribing and implementing both direct and indirect nursing care and for articulating nursing therapies with other planned therapies. Nurse clinicians demonstrate expertise in nursing practice and ensure ongoing development of expertise through clinical experience and continuing education. Generally, minimal preparation for this role is the baccalaureate degree. **community n.,** the name given in Great Britain to a public health nurse, from the fact that such a nurse was placed in charge of each one of the districts into which the city or community was divided. See also *public health n.* **community health n.,** public health n. **district n.,** community n. **dry n.,** a woman who has charge of another's infant but does not breast-feed it. **general duty n.,** a registered nurse, usually one who has not undergone training beyond the basic nursing program, who sees to the general nursing care of patients in a hospital or other health agency. **graduate n.,** a graduate of a school of nursing; often used to designate one who has not been registered or licensed to practice. Called also *trained n.* **head n.,** charge n. **hospital n.,** one employed by a hospital. **licensed practical n.,** a graduate of a school of practical nursing whose qualifications have been examined by a state board of nursing and who has been legally authorized to practice as a licensed practical or vocational nurse (L.P.N. or L.V.N.), under the supervision of a physician or registered nurse. **licensed vocational n.,** see *licensed practical n.* **monthly n.,** a nurse who attends confinement cases. **occupational health n.,** an especially prepared registered nurse employed by an institution to apply nursing principles and procedures for the promotion, restoration, and maintenance of optimal health of its employees as compared to a nurse who performs normal nursing functions in an occupational setting. **office n.,** a registered nurse employed by a physician in his office to perform or to assist him in the performance of certain procedures. **practical n.,** a person who has had practical experience in nursing care but who is not a graduate of any kind of nursing school; not to be confused with a licensed practical nurse. **n. practitioner,** see *n. clinician.* **private n., private duty n.,** one who attends an individual patient, usually on a fee-for-service basis, and who may specialize in a specific class of diseases; called also *special n.* **probationer n.,** a person who has entered a school of nursing and is under observation to determine her fitness for the nursing profession; applied principally to nursing students enrolled in hospital schools of

nursing. **public health n.,** an especially prepared registered nurse employed in a community agency to safeguard the health of persons in the community, giving care to the sick in their homes, promoting health and well-being by teaching families how to keep well, and assisting in programs for the prevention of disease. Called also *community health n.* and *visiting n.* **Queen's n.,** in Great Britain, a district nurse who has been trained at or in accordance with the regulations of the Queen Victoria Jubilee Institute for Nurses. **registered n.,** a graduate nurse who has been legally authorized (registered) to practice after examination by a state board of nurse examiners or similar regulatory authority, and who is legally entitled to use the designation R.N. **school n.,** an especially prepared registered nurse employed in a school system or public health agency to assist in safeguarding the health of students and to teach health practices. **scrub n.,** one who directly assists the surgeon in the operating room. **special n.,** 1. a private nurse. 2. a nurse who specializes in a particular class of cases. **n. specialist,** clinical n. specialist. **student n.,** a person enrolled in a basic program of nursing education. **trained n.,** graduate n. **visiting n.,** see *public health n.* **wet n.,** a woman who breast-feeds the infant of another.

nurse-midwife (ners-mid′wĭf) an individual educated in the two disciplines of nursing and midwifery, who possesses evidence of certification according to the requirements of the American College of Nurse-Midwives. Abbreviated C.N.M. (Certified Nurse-Midwife).

nurse-midwifery (ners-mid′wi-fer-e, ners-mid′wĭf-ĕ-re) the independent management of care of essentially normal newborns and women, antepartally, intrapartally, postpartally, and/or gynecologically, occurring within a health care system which provides for medical consultation, collaborative management, or referral, and is in accord with the functions, standards, and qualifications as defined by the American College of Nurse-Midwives.

nursery (ner′sĕ-re) the department in a hospital where newborn infants are cared for. **day n., day care n.,** an institution devoted to the care of young children during the day.

nursing (ners′ing) the provision, at various levels of preparation, of services that are essential to or helpful in the promotion, maintenance, and restoration of health and well-being or in the prevention of illness, as of infants, of the sick and injured, or of others for any reason unable to provide such services for themselves. Sometimes designated according to the age of the patients being cared for (e.g., pediatric or geriatric nursing), or their particular health problems (e.g., gynecologic, medical, obstetrical, orthopedic, psychiatric, surgical, urological nursing, or the like), or the setting in which the services are provided (e.g., office, school, or occupational health nursing). See also *nurse.*

Nussbaum's narcosis (nōōs′bowmz) [Johann Nepomuk *Nussbaum,* German surgeon, 1829–1890] see under *narcosis.*

Nussbaum's experiment (nōōs′bowmz) [Moritz *Nussbaum,* German histologist, 1850–1915] see under *experiment.*

nut (nut) [L. *nux;* Gr. *karyon*] a seed element, as of various trees, usually enclosed in a coating of variable hardness. **betel n.,** areca.

nutation (nu-ta′shun) [L. *nutatio*] the act of nodding, especially involuntary nodding.

nutatory (nu′tah-tor″e) [L. *nutare* to keep nodding, to sway] pertaining to nodding.

nutgall (nut′gawl) [L. *galla*] an excrescence growing on oak trees, especially species of *Quercus* (e.g., *Q. infectoria* Oliv., Fagaceae), produced by insect eggs and larvae embedded in the plant tissues; it is a source of gallic and tannic acids, which are used in various pharmaceuticals for their astringent properties. Called also *gall, Aleppo gall, Smyrna gall,* and *gallnut.*

nutmeg (nut′meg) myristica.

nutrient (nu′tre-ent) [L. *nutriens*] 1. nourishing; affording nutriment. 2. a nutritious substance; food, or a component of food. **essential n's,** those nutrients (proteins, minerals, carbohydrates, fat, vitamins) necessary for growth, normal functioning, and maintaining life; they must be supplied by food, since they cannot be synthesized by the body. **secondary n.,** a substance that stimulates the intestinal microflora to synthesize other nutrients.

nutrilite (nu′trĭ-līt) a substance that is essential in minute amounts in the nutrition of a microorganism.

nutriment (nu′trĭ-ment) [L. *nutrimentum*] nourishment; nutritious material; food.

nutriology (nu″tre-ol′o-je) the science of nutrition; the study of foods and their use in diet and therapy.

nutrition (nu-trish′un) [L. *nutritio*] 1. the sum of the processes involved in taking in nutriments and assimilating and utilizing them. 2. nutriment. **adequate n.,** see under *diet.* **total parenteral n.,** total parenteral alimentation.

nutritional (nu-trish′un-al) relating to or affecting nutrition.

nutritionist (nu-trish′un-ist) a specialist in food and nutrition.

nutritious (nu-trish′us) [L. *nutritius*] affording nourishment.

nutritive (nu′trĭ-tiv) pertaining to nutrition.

nutriture (nu′trĭ-tūr″) the status of the body in relation to nutrition, generally or in regard to a specific nutrient, such as protein.

nutrix (nu′triks) a wet nurse.

nutrose (nu′trōs) neutral casein sodium; a dry food preparation of milk for the use of invalids.

Nuttallia (nŭ-tal′e-ah) [George H. F. *Nutall*, biologist, Cambridge University, 1862–1937] *Babesia.*

nux (nuks), gen. *nu′cis* [L.] nut. **n. moscha′ta,** myristica. **n. vom′ica,** the dried ripe seed of *Strychnos nux-vomica* L. (Loganiaceae), containing several alkaloids, principally strychnine and brucine. It has been used as a bitter tonic and central nervous system stimulant, and in veterinary medicine it is used as a bitter tonic and in the treatment of inappetence, atony of the rumen, and chronic indigestion.

nyacyne (ni′ah-sīn) neomycin.

nyad (ni′ad) the nymph form of certain arthropods.

nyctalgia (nik-tal′je-ah) [*nycto-* + *-algia*] pain that occurs in sleep only.

nyctalope (nik′tah-lōp) a person affected with nyctalopia.

nyctalopia (nik″tah-lo′pe-ah) [Gr. *nyx* night + *alaos* blind + *-opia*] night blindness; failure or imperfection of vision at night or in a dim light, with good vision only on bright days.

nyctaphonia (nik″tah-fo′ne-ah) [*nycto-* + *aphonia*] loss of voice during the night.

nycterine (nik′ter-īn) [Gr. *nykterinos* by night] 1. occurring at night. 2. obscure.

nycterohemeral (nik″ter-o-hem′er-al) nyctohemeral.

nyct(o)- (nik′to) [Gr. *nyx,* gen. *nyctos* night] a combining form denoting relationship to night or to darkness.

nyctohemeral (nik″to-hem′er-al) [*nycto-* + Gr. *hēmera* day] pertaining to both night and day.

nyctophilia (nik″to-fil′e-ah) [*nycto-* + Gr. *philein* to love] preference for night over day.

nyctophobia (nik″to-fo′be-ah) [*nycto-* + *phobia*] irrational fear of darkness.

nyctophonia (nik″to-fo′ne-ah) [*nycto-* + Gr. *phōnē* voice] loss of voice during the day but not at night.

Nyctotherus (nik-tot′er-us) [Gr. "one who hunts at night"] a genus of endoparasitic, kidney-shaped, usually ciliated protozoa (suborder Clevelandellina, order Heterotrichida) having a lateral cytostome containing cilia and a very large anterior macronucleus. *N. cordiformis* is found in amphibians and *N. ovalis* in the cockroach.

nycturia (nik-tu′re-ah) [*nycto-* + Gr. *ouron* urine + *-ia*] frequent urination during the night, especially the passage of more urine at night than during the day.

N.Y.D. not yet diagnosed.

Nydrazid (ni′dra-zid) trademark for preparations of isoniazid.

nylestriol (ni-les′tre-ōl) chemical name: 3-(cyclopentyloxy)-19-nor-17α-pregna-1,3,5(10)-trien-20-yne-16,17-diol; an estrogen, $C_{25}H_{32}O_3$.

nylidrin hydrochloride (nil′ĭ-drin) [USP] chemical name: 4-hydroxy-α-[1-[(1-methyl-3-phenylpropyl)amino]ethyl] benzenemethanol hydrochloride. A synthetic

adrenergic, $C_{19}H_{25}NO_2 \cdot HCl$, occurring as a white, crystalline powder; used as a peripheral vasodilator, administered orally, intramuscularly, and subcutaneously.

nylon (ni′lon) a synthetic polymerized plastic which in fiber form is used as suture material.

nymph (nimf) [Gr. *nymphē* a bride] a stage in the life cycle of certain arthropods, as the ticks, between the larva and the adult without an intervening stage. A nymph somewhat resembles the adult but is small, sexually immature, and wingless. Cf. *naiad.*

nympha (nim′fah), gen. and pl. *nym′phae* [L., from Gr. *nymphē*] labium minus pudendi. **n. of Krause,** clitoris.

nymphae (nim′fe) [L.] genitive and plural of *nympha.*

nymphectomy (nim-fek′to-me) [*nympha* + Gr. *ektomē* excision] excision of the nymphae.

nymphitis (nim-fi′tis) inflammation of the nymphae.

nympho- (nim′fo) [L. *nympha*] a combining form denoting relationship to the nymphae, or labia minora.

nymphocaruncular (nim″fo-kah-rung′ku-lar) pertaining to the labia minora and the caruncula hymenalis.

nymphohymeneal (nim″fo-hi″mĕ-ne′al) pertaining to the labia minora and the hymen.

nymphomania (nim″fo-ma′ne-ah) [*nympho-* + Gr. *mania* madness] abnormal, excessive, insatiable sexual desire in the female. Cf. *satyriasis.*

nymphomaniac (nim″fo-ma′ne-ak) 1. affected with nymphomania. 2. one who is affected with nymphomania.

nymphoncus (nim-fong′kus) [*nympho-* + Gr. *onkos* mass, bulk] swelling of the nymphae.

nymphotomy (nim-fot′o-me) [*nympho-* + Gr. *tomē* a cutting] surgical incision of the nymphae or clitoris.

Nyssorhynchus (nis″o-ring′kus) [Gr. *nyssa* prick + *rhynchos* snout] a subgenus of anopheline mosquitoes, several species of which act as carriers of the malarial parasite in tropical America.

nystagmic (nis-tag′mik) pertaining to or characterized by nystagmus.

nystagmiform (nis-tag′mĭ-form) nystagmoid.

nystagmograph (nis-tag′mo-graf) [*nystagmus* + *-graph*] an instrument for recording the movements of the eyeball in nystagmus.

nystagmoid (nis-tag′moid) resembling nystagmus.

nystagmus (nis-tag′mus) [Gr. *nystagmos* drowsiness, from *nystazein* to nod] an involuntary, rapid, rhythmic movement of the eyeball, which may be horizontal, vertical, rotatory, or mixed, i.e., of two varieties. **amaurotic n.,** nystagmus in the blind or in those with defects of central vision; called also *ocular n.* **amblyopic n.,** nystagmus due to any lesion interfering with central vision. **ataxic n.,** a unilateral nystagmus occurring in multiple sclerosis and marked by impaired lateral conjugate gaze. **aural n.,** nystagmus due to disturbances in the labyrinth; the eye movements are rhythmic, with a fast and a slow component. **caloric n.,** that induced by irrigating the ears with warm or cold water or air; see *Bárány's symptom* (def. 2), under *symptom.* **central n.,** a jerk nystagmus due to a lesion in the vestibular system. **Cheyne's n., Cheyne-Stokes n.,** a peculiar rhythmical eye movement resembling Cheyne-Stokes respiration in its rhythm. **congenital n., congenital hereditary n.,** nystagmus usually present at birth, usually horizontal and pendular, but occasionally jerky and pendular; the nystagmus may be caused by or associated with optic atrophy, coloboma, albinism, bilateral macular lesions, congenital cataract, severe astigmatism, and glaucoma. **convergence n.,** a rhythmic oscillation of the eyes, consisting of a rapid adduction movement of the eyes relative to each other alternating with a slow adduction movement; usually caused by a tumor of the aqueduct of Sylvius, third ventricle, or midbrain. It is often accompanied by retraction nystagmus. **disjunctive n.,** nystagmus in which the eyes swing toward and away from each other. **dissociated n.,** nystagmus in which the movements in the two eyes are dissimilar. **downbeat n.,** a vertical nystagmus with the fast phase downward, occurring in lesions at the cervicomedullary junction. **electrical n.,** galvanic n. **end-position n.,** nystagmus occurring at extremes of gaze; called also *pseudonystagmus.* **fixation n.,** nystagmus which appears only on gazing fixedly at an object. **gal-**

vanic n., a vestibular nystagmus caused by electrical stimulation of the labyrinth of the inner ear; called also *electrical n.* **gaze n.,** nystagmus made apparent by looking to the right or to the left. **jerk n., jerky n.,** nystagmus which consists of a slow movement in one direction, followed by a rapid return movement in the opposite direction; called also *resilient n.* and *rhythmical n.* **labyrinthine n.,** vestibular n. **latent n.,** nystagmus which occurs only when one eye is covered. **lateral n.,** nystagmus in which the movement of the eyes is from side to side. **miner's n.,** an occupational disease of coal miners consisting of abnormal eye movements associated with other signs and symptoms; it is considered by some to be related to poor lighting and by others as a functional disorder. **ocular n.,** amaurotic n. **opticokinetic n., optokinetic n.,** the normal nystagmus occurring when looking at objects passing across the field of vision, as in viewing from a moving railroad car or automobile. **oscillating n.,** pendular n. **palatal n.,** see under *myoclonus.* **paretic n.,** a false nystagmus occurring when there is a weakness of the ocular muscles. **pendular n.,** nystagmus in which the oscillations of the eyes have an equal rate, amplitude, direction, and type of movement; called also *oscillating n., undulatory n.,* and *vibratory n.* **periodic alternating n.,** a rare form of jerk nystagmus with rhythmic changes in amplitude and direction and with intervals of quiet between periods. **positional n.,** that which occurs, or is altered in form or intensity, on assumption of certain positions of the head. **railroad n.,** optokinetic n. **resilient n.,** jerk n. **retraction n., n. retracto′rius,** 1. a spasmodic backward retraction of the eyeball occurring on attempted movement of the eye; it is a sign of disease of the midbrain. 2. sylvian syndrome. **rhythmical n.,** jerk n. **rotatory n.,** nystagmus in which the movement is about the visual axis. **secondary n.,** nystagmus occurring after the abrupt cessation of rotation of the head, caused by the labyrinthine fluid continuing to move. **see-saw n.,** that in which one eye moves up as the other moves down. **spontaneous n.,** that occurring without specific stimulation of the vestibular system. **undulatory n.,** pendular n. **unilateral n.,** nystagmus manifest in only one eye. **upbeat n.,** a vertical nystagmus with the fast phase upward, occurring in lesions of the vermis cerebelli. **vertical n.,** an up-and-down movement of the eyes. **vestibular n.,** nystagmus due to vestibular disturbance; eye movements are rhythmic, with a slow and a fast component. Called also *labyrinthine n.* **vibratory n.,** pendular n. **visual n.,** nystagmus characterized by smooth pendulum-like movement. **voluntary n.,** rapid rhythmic eye movements, up to 80 a second, that can be produced at will by some normal individuals.

nystagmus-myoclonus (nis-tag′mus-mi-ok′lo-nus) a rare congenital condition in which there is nystagmus together with abnormal involuntary movements of the extremities and trunk.

nystatin (nis′tah-tin) [USP] an antibiotic, $C_{46}H_{77}NO_{19}$, produced by the growth of *Streptomyces noursei,* occurring as a yellow to tan powder, specifically effective against *Candida albicans;* used in the treatment of vaginal, intestinal, oral, or cutaneous candidal infections, administered orally and topically. Called also *fungicidin.*

nystaxis (nis-tak′sis) [Gr.] nystagmus.

Nysten's law (ne-stahz′) [Pierre Hubert *Nysten,* French pediatrician, 1771–1818] see under *law.*

nyxis (nik′sis) [Gr. "pricking"] puncture, or paracentesis.

O chemical symbol for *oxygen.*

o- chemical symbol for *ortho-.*

O₂ symbol for the diatomic form of oxygen; molecular oxygen.

o omicron, the fifteenth letter of the Greek alphabet.

Ω the Greek capital letter omega; symbol for *ohm.*

ω omega, the twenty-fourth letter of the Greek alphabet; symbol for *angular frequency,* or *angular velocity.*

ω- symbol for the carbon atom farthest from the principal functional group, as in ω-oxidation.

OAF osteoclast activating factor.

oak (ōk) a cupuliferous tree of the genus *Quercus.* The bark of all species contains a large proportion of tannin. **poison o.,** the plants *Toxicodendron diversilobum* (T. and G.) Greene (true western poison oak) and *T. quercifolium* (Michx.) Greene (true eastern poison oak). The term is also used loosely to refer to *T. radicans* (L.) Kuntze (poison ivy). All contain toxic urishiol resin, whose major constituent is 3-*n*-pentadicylcatechol, a highly allergenic compound.

OAP a regimen of Oncovin (vincristine), ara-C (cytarabine), and prednisone, used in cancer chemotherapy.

oari(o)- for words beginning thus, see those beginning oophor(o)- and ovari(o)-.

oasis (o-a′sis), pl. **oa′ses** [Gr. "a fertile islet in a desert"] an island or spot of healthy tissue in a diseased area.

oath (ōth) a solemn declaration or affirmation. **o. of Hippocrates, hippocratic o.,** see under *Hippocrates.*

OB. obstetrics.

obcecation (ob″se-ka′shun) incomplete blindness.

obducent (ob-du′sent) [L. *obducere* to draw over, to cover] serving as a cover; covering.

obduction (ob-duk′shun) [L. *obductio*] a medicolegal autopsy.

O'Beirne's sphincter (o-birnz′) [James *O'Beirne,* Irish surgeon, 1786–1862] see under *sphincter.*

obeliac (o-be′le-ak) pertaining to the obelion.

obeliad (o-be′le-ad) toward the obelion.

obelion (o-be′le-on) [Gr., dim. of *obelos* a spit] a point on the sagittal suture where it is crossed by a line which connects the parietal foramina.

Ober's operation, test (sign) (o′berz) [Frank Roberts *Ober,* Boston orthopedic surgeon, 1881–1960] see under *operation* and *tests.*

Obermayer's test (o′ber-mi″erz) [Friedrich *Obermayer,* physiologic chemist in Vienna, 1861–1925] see under *tests.*

Obermüller's test (o′ber-mil-erz) [Kuno *Obermüller,* German physician, born 1861] see under *tests.*

Oberst's method (o′bersts) [Maximilian *Oberst,* German surgeon, 1849–1925] see under *method.*

Obersteiner-Redlich area (zone) (o′ber-sti″ner-red′likh) [Heinrich *Obersteiner,* Austrian neurologist, 1847–1922; Emil *Redlich,* Austrian neurologist, 1866–1930] see under *area.*

obese (o-bēs′) [L. *obesus*] excessively fat.

obesity (o-bēs′ĭ-te) [L. *obesus* fat] an increase in body weight beyond the limitation of skeletal and physical requirement, as the result of an excessive accumulation of fat in the body. **adult-onset o.,** obesity beginning in adulthood and characterized by increase in size (hypertrophy) of adipose cells with no increase in number; called also *hypertrophic o.* **alimentary o.,** exogenous obesity. **endogenous o.,** obesity due to metabolic (endocrine) abnormalities. **exogenous o.,** obesity due to overeating. **hyperinsulinar o.,** obesity due to overactivity of insulin secretion, associated with hypoglycemia and increased appetite. **hyperinterrenal o.,** obesity associated with hyperfunction of the adrenal cortex. **hyperplasmic o.,** obesity due to increase in the body protoplasm, as distinguished from that due to accumulation of fat and water. **hyperplastic-hypertrophic o.,** lifelong o. **hypertrophic o.,** adult-onset o. **hypogonad o.,** obesity associated with hypofunction of the gonads. **hypoplasmic o.,** obesity due to increase of fat and water and marked by decrease of the body protoplasm. **hypothyroid o.,** obesity due to hypothyroidism. **lifelong o.,** obesity beginning in childhood and characterized by an increase both in number (hyperplasia) and in size (hypertrophy) of adipose cells; called also *hyperplastic-hypertrophic o.* **morbid o.,** the condition of weighing two or three, or more, times the ideal weight; so called because it is associated with many serious and life threatening disorders (diabetes mellitus, atherosclerosis, hypertension, pickwickian syndrome, etc.). **simple o.,** exogenous o.

obesogenous (o-bēs-oj′ĕ-nus) producing or causing obesity.

Obesumbacterium (o-be′sum-bak-te′re-um) [L. *obesum* fat + *bacterium*] a genus of gram-negative, facultatively anaerobic, rod-shaped bacteria of the family Enterobacteriaceae, occurring as a brewery contaminant. The type species is *O. pro′teus.*

obex (o′beks) [L. "barrier"] [NA] the ependyma-lined junction of the taeniae of the fourth ventricle of the brain at the inferior angle.

obfuscation (ob″fus-ka′shun) [L. *obfuscatio* a darkening] the act of rendering, or process of becoming, obscure; a darkening.

obidoxime chloride (ŏ-bǐ-doks′ēm) chemical name: 1,1′-(oxydimethylene)bis[4-formylpyridinium]dichloride; a cholinesterase reactivator, $C_{14}H_{16}Cl_2N_4O_3$, which has been used to counter organophosphorus poisoning.

objective (ob-jek′tiv) [L. *objectivus*] 1. perceptible to the external senses. 2. a result for whose achievement an effort is made. 3. the lens or system of lenses in a microscope (or telescope) that is nearest to the object under examination. **achromatic o.,** a microscope objective in which the chromatic aberration is corrected for two colors and the spherical aberration is corrected for one color. **apochromatic o.,** a microscope objective in which the chromatic aberration is corrected for three colors and the spherical aberration is corrected for two colors. **dry o.,** a microscope objective designed to be used without a liquid between its tip and the cover glass over the specimen. **flat field o.,** a microscope objective that provides an image in which all parts of the field are simultaneously in focus. **fluorite o.,** a microscope objective in which some of the lenses are made from fluorite instead of glass. **immersion o.,** a microscope objective designed to have its tip and the cover glass over the specimen connected by a liquid instead of by air. The liquid may be water (water immersion) or a specially prepared oil (oil immersion). **semiapochromatic o.,** a type of microscope objective in which spherical aberration and chromatic aberration are both corrected for two colors.

obligate (ob′lǐ-gāt) [L. *obligatus*] not facultative; necessary; compulsory; capable of survival only under particular conditions, as an obligate aerobe.

oblique (ŏ-blēk, ŏ-blīk) [L. *obliquus*] slanting; inclined; between a horizontal and a perpendicular direction.

obliquity (ob-lik′wǐ-te) the state of being oblique, or slanting. **Litzmann′s o.,** inclination of the fetal head so that the posterior parietal bone presents to the parturient canal; called also *posterior asynclitism.* **Nägele′s o.,** the position of the fetal head in which the anterior parietal bone presents to the parturient canal, the biparietal diameter being oblique in relation to the brim of the pelvis; called also *anterior asynclitism.* **o. of pelvis,** inclination of the pelvis.

obliquus (ob-li′kwus) [L.] oblique.

obliteration (ob-lit″er-a′shun) [L. *obliteratio*] complete removal, whether by disease, degeneration, surgical procedure, irradiation, or otherwise. **cortical o.,** cortical achromia; a condition in which the cerebral cortex is marked by areas in which the ganglion cells have disappeared.

oblongata (ob″long-ga′tah, ob″long-gah′tah) [L.] oblong, sometimes used informally to refer to the medulla oblongata.

oblongatal (ob″long-ga′tal) pertaining to the medulla oblongata.

obnubilation (ob-nu″bǐ-la′shun) clouding of consciousness.

O′Brien akinesia (o-bri′en) [Cecil Starling *O′Brien,* American ophthalmologist, born 1889] see under *akinesia.*

obsession (ob-sesh′un) [L. *obsessio*] a recurrent, persistent thought, image, or impulse that is unwanted and distressing (ego-dystonic) and comes involuntarily to mind despite attempts to ignore or suppress it. Common obsessions involve thoughts of violence, contamination, and self-doubt.

obsessive (ob-ses′iv) pertaining to or characterized by obsession.

obsessive-compulsive (ob-ses′iv-kom-pul′siv) pertaining to obsessions and compulsions, to obsessive-compulsive disorder, or to compulsive personality disorder.

obsolescence (ob″so-les′ens) [L. *obsolescere* to grow old] the cessation or the beginning of the cessation of any physiologic process.

obsolete (ob′so-lēt) [L. *obsoletus,* from *obsolere* to go out of use] indistinct; faded; gone out of use.

obstetric, obstetrical (ob-stet′rik; ob-stet′re-kal) [L. *obstetricius*] pertaining to obstetrics.

obstetrician (ob″stĕ-trish′un) [L. *obstetrix* midwife] one who practices obstetrics.

obstetrics (ob-stet′riks) [L. *obstetricia*] that branch of surgery which deals with the management of pregnancy, labor, and the puerperium.

obstipation (ob″stǐ-pa′shun) [L. *obstipatio*] intractable constipation.

obstruction (ob-struk′shun) [L. *obstructio*] 1. the act of blocking or clogging. 2. the state or condition of being clogged. **false colonic o.,** see *Ogilvie′s syndrome,* under *syndrome.* **intestinal o.,** any hindrance to the passage of the intestinal contents. See also *ileus.*

obstruent (ob′stroo-ent) [L. *obstruens*] 1. causing obstruction or blocking. 2. any agent or agency that causes obstruction.

obtund (ob-tund′) [L. *obtundere*] to render dull or blunt; to render less acute.

obtundent (ob-tun′dent) [L. *obtundens*] 1. having the power to dull sensibility or to soothe pain. 2. a soothing or partially anesthetic medicine.

obturation (ob″tu-ra′shun) the act of closing or occluding; a form of intestinal obstruction. **canal o.,** filling of the entire root canal completely and densely with a nonirritating hermetic sealing agent. Called also *root canal filling.*

obturator (ob′too-ra″tor) [L.] 1. any structure, natural or artificial, that closes an opening. 2. a prosthesis used to close an acquired or congenital opening in the palate (cleft palate). See also *artificial palate,* under *palate,* and *speech-aid prosthesis,* under *prosthesis.*

obtusion (ob-tu′zhun) [L. *obtusio*] blunting of sensation and perception.

occipital (ok-sip′ǐ-tal) [L. *occipitalis*] pertaining to the occiput; located near the occipital bone, as the occipital lobe of the brain.

occipitalis (ok-sip″ǐ-ta′lis) [L.] the posterior part of the occipitofrontalis muscle.

occipitalization (ok-sip″ǐ-tal-i-za′shun) synostosis of the atlas with the occipital bone.

occipitoanterior (ok-sip″ǐ-to-an-te′re-or) having the occiput directed forward toward the pubis (designating the position of the fetus in relation to the maternal pelvis).

occipitoatloid (ok-sip″ǐ-to-at′loid) pertaining to the occipital bone and the atlas.

occipitoaxoid (ok-sip″ǐ-to-ak′soid) pertaining to the occipital bone and the axis.

occipitobasilar (ok-sip″ǐ-to-bas′ǐ-ler) pertaining to the occiput and the base of the skull.

occipitobregmatic (ok-sip″ǐ-to-breg-mat′ik) pertaining to the occiput and the bregma.

occipitocalcarine (ok-sip″ǐ-to-kal′kar-īn) both occipital and calcarine.

occipitocervical (ok-sip″ǐ-to-ser′vǐ-kal) pertaining to the occiput and neck.

occipitofacial (ok-sip″ǐ-to-fa′shal) pertaining to the occiput and the face.

occipitofrontal (ok-sip″ǐ-to-fron′tal) pertaining to the occiput and the forehead.

occipitomastoid (ok-sip″ǐ-to-mas′toid) pertaining to the occipital bone and the mastoid process.

occipitomental (ok-sip″ǐ-to-men′tal) pertaining to the occiput and the chin.

occipitoparietal (ok-sip″ǐ-to-pah-ri′e-tal) pertaining to the occipital and parietal bones or lobes of the brain.

occipitoposterior (ok-sip″ǐ-to-pos-te′re-or) having the occiput directed toward the back, or turned toward the sacrum (designating the position of the fetus in relation to the maternal pelvis).

occipitotemporal (ok-sip″ǐ-to-tem′po-ral) pertaining to the occipital and the temporal bones.

occipitothalamic (ok-sip″ǐ-to-thah-lam′ik) pertaining to the occipital lobe and thalamus.

occiput (ok′sǐ-put) [L.] [NA] the back part of the head; called also *o. cra′nii* and *o. of cranium.*

occlude (ŏ-klōōd′) to fit close together; to close tight, as to bring the mandibular teeth into contact with the teeth in the maxilla; to obstruct or close off.

occluder (ŏ-klōōd′er) a form of dental articulator.

occlusal (ŏ-kloo′zal) 1. pertaining to occlusion. 2. pertaining to the contacting surfaces of opposing teeth or of opposing occlusion rims, or to the masticating surfaces of the premolar and molar teeth.

occlusion (o-kloo′zhun) [L. *occlusio*] 1. the act of closure or state of being closed; an obstruction or a closing off. 2. the trapping of a material, either liquid or gas, within cavities in a solid. 3. the relationship between all of the components of the masticatory system in normal function, dysfunction, and parafunction. See also *bite* and *malocclusion*. 4. momentary complete closure of some area in the vocal tract, causing stoppage of the breath and accumulation of pressure. **abnormal o.**, malocclusion. **acentric o.**, a condition in which the habitual voluntary closure pattern of the mandible does not coincide with centric relation, producing primary premature tooth contacts in the centric path of closure. **anatomic o.**, that in which the arrangement of natural teeth in the same arch and in opposing arches is defined by dental or skeletal landmarks rather than functional criteria. **anterior o.**, mesioclusion. **balanced o.**, that in which the occlusal contact of the teeth on the working side of the jaw is accompanied by the harmonious contact of the teeth of the opposite (balancing) side. The occlusion of artificial teeth may be *mechanically balanced*, as on an articulator, without reference to physiologic considerations, or *physiologically balanced*, functioning in harmony with the temporomandibular joint and the neuromuscular system. **buccal o.**, the position of a posterior tooth when it is outside (buccal to) the line of occlusion. **centric o.**, that in the vertical and horizontal position of the mandible in which the cusps of the mandibular and maxillary teeth interdigitate maximally. Ideally, the lingual cusps of the maxillary bicuspids make contact with the marginal ridges of the mandibular bicuspids and the marginal ridges of the second bicuspid and first molar. The mesial lingual cusps of the maxillary molar occlude in the central fossae of the mandibular molars, while the distal cusps of the maxillary molars occlude on the marginal ridges of the mandibular molars. Similarly, the supporting cusps of the mandibular teeth occlude on the marginal ridges and fossae of the maxillary molars and bicuspids. **coronary o.**, complete obstruction of an artery of the heart, usually from progressive atherosclerosis (sometimes complicated by thrombosis), rarely from embolism, arteritis, or dissecting aneurysm. **distal o.**, the position of a lower tooth when it is distal to its opposite number in the maxilla. Called also *postnormal o.* **eccentric o.**, acentric o. **edge-to-edge o., end-to-end o.**, that in which the anterior maxillary and mandibular teeth meet along their incisal edges when the mandible is in centric position. Called also *edge-to-edge bite* and *end-to-end bite*. **enteromesenteric o.**, obstruction of blood vessels in both the mesentery and the wall of the intestine. **functional o.**, such contact of the maxillary and mandibular teeth as will provide the highest efficiency in the centric position and during all excursive movements of the jaw that are essential to mastication, without producing trauma. **habitual o.**, the consistent relationship of the teeth in the maxilla to those of the mandible when the teeth in both jaws are brought into maximum contact, such relationship varying from individual to individual; the ideal habitual occlusion is centric occlusion, but it is seldom attained without corrective dental treatment. **hyperfunctional o.**, traumatic o. **ideal o.**, perfect interdigitation of the upper and lower teeth. **labial o.**, the position of an anterior tooth when it is outside (labial to) the line of occlusion. **lateral o.**, the occlusion of the teeth when the lower jaw is moved to the right or left of centric position. **lingual o.**, malocclusion in which the tooth is lingual to the line of the normal dental arch. Called also *linguoclusion o.* **mechanically balanced o.**, see *balanced o.* **mesial o.**, the position of a lower tooth when it is mesial to its opposite number in the maxilla. Called also *prenormal o.* **neutral o.**, normal o. **normal o.**, the contact of the upper and lower teeth in the centric relationship. **pathogenic o.**, an occlusal relationship that is capable of producing pathologic changes in the supporting tissues. See also *traumatic o.* **physiologically balanced o.**, see *balanced o.* **posterior o.**, distoclusion. **postnormal o.,**

distal o. **prenormal o.**, mesial o. **protrusive o.**, mesioclusion. **retrusive o.**, distoclusion. **spherical form of o.**, an arrangement of teeth that places their occlusal surfaces on the surface of an imaginary sphere, about 8 inches in diameter, with its center above the level of the teeth; see also *Monson curve*, under *curve*. **terminal o.**, the relationship of opposing occlusal surfaces that provides the maximum natural or planned contact and/or intercuspation. **traumatic o.**, progressive injury to the supporting structure of the teeth as a result of occlusal dysfunction. Called also *hypofunctional o.* See also *traumatogenic o.* **traumatogenic o.**, abnormal occlusion capable of producing injury to the teeth, residual ridges, and periodontal structures. See *traumatic o.* **working o.**, the contact made between the teeth on the side toward which the mandible is moved.

occlusive (ŏ-kloo′siv) pertaining to or effecting occlusion.

occlusocervical (ŏ-kloo″so-ser′vĭ-kal) pertaining to the occlusal surface and the neck of a tooth.

occlusometer (ok″loo-som′ĕ-ter) gnathodynamometer.

occlusorehabilitation (ŏ-kloo″zo-re″hah-bil″ĭ-ta′shun) occlusal rehabilitation.

Occlusosporida (o-kloo″so-spor′ĭ-dah) an order of parasitic protozoa (class Stellatosporea, phylum Ascetospora) having spores with more than one sporoplasm and an uninterrupted spore wall, and characterized by sporulation involving a series of endogenous buddings that produce sporoplasm(s) within sporoplasm(s). *Marteilia* is a representative genus. Called also *Marteiliida.*

occult (ŏ-kult′) [L. *occultus*] obscure; concealed from observation; difficult to understand.

occupancy (ok′u-pan-se) the period of time during which a unit quantity of a substance, administered in a specified way, is present in, or occupies, a part of the body before it is excreted or broken down.

Oceanospirillum (o″she-a″no-spi-ril′um) [L. *oceanus* ocean + *spirillum*] a genus of rigid, helical, gram-negative, aerobic bacteria that are motile with flagella; they are found in seawater and putrid marine mussels. The type species is *O. li′num.*

ocellus (o-sel′us) [L., dim. of *oculus* eye] 1. a small simple eye in insects and other invertebrates. 2. one of the elements of a compound eye of insects. 3. a roundish, eyelike patch of color.

ochlesis (ok-le′sis) [Gr. *ochlēsis* crowding] any disease due to overcrowding.

Ochoa (o-cho′ah), Severo. Spanish-born American physician and biochemist, born 1905; co-winner, with Arthur Kornberg, of the Nobel prize for medicine or physiology in 1959 for discovering the mechanisms in the biological synthesis of deoxyribonucleic acid and ribonucleic acid.

Ochrobium (o-kro′be-um) [Gr. *ōchros* yellow + *bios* life] a genus of gram-negative chemolithotrophic bacteria of the family Siderocapsaceae, made up of ellipsoidal to rod-shaped cells partially surrounded by a marginal thickening heavily impregnated with iron, and contained in a delicate, transparent capsule. The type species is *O. tec′tum.*

ochrometer (o-krom′ĕ-ter) [Gr. *ōchros* paleness + *metron* measure] an instrument for measuring the capillary blood pressure by registering the force necessary to compress a finger by a rubber balloon until blanching of the skin occurs.

Ochromyia (o″kro-mi′yah) Cordylobia.

ochronosis (o″kro-no′sis) [Gr. *ōchros* yellow + *nosos* disease] a peculiar discoloration of certain tissues of the body, caused by the deposit of alkapton bodies as the result of a metabolic disorder. **exogenous o.**, ochronosis allegedly resulting from exposure to some noxious substance in the internal environment, such as phenol, trinitrophenol, or benzene derivatives. **ocular o.**, a condition characterized by symmetrical, semilunar, or V-shaped accumulations of brown or gray pigment in the sclera, midway between the margin of the cornea and the inner or outer canthus. The eyelids and conjunctivae may also be affected.

ochronosus (o″kro-no′sus) ochronosis.

ochronotic (o″kro-not′ik) pertaining to, characterized by, or caused by ochronosis.

Ochsner's muscle, ring, treatment (oks′nerz) [Albert John *Ochsner*, surgeon in Chicago, 1858–1925] see under *muscle, ring,* and *treatment.*

Ocimum (os'ĭ-mum) a genus of herbs, including *O. basilicum* L. (Labiatae), or basil. They are a source of condiment and perfume oil.

ocrylate (ok'rĭ-lāt) a tissue adhesive for use in surgery.

octa- [Gr. *oktō*, L. *octo* eight] a combining form meaning eight.

octabenzone (ok"tah-ben'zōn) chemical name: [2-hydroxy-4-(octyloxy)phenyl]phenylmethanone; an ultraviolet screen, $C_{21}H_{26}O_3$.

octacosane (ok"tah-ko'sān) an aliphatic hydrocarbon, $C_{28}H_{58}$, extracted from plant waxes.

octacosanol (ok"tah-ko-sa'nol) a solid white alcohol, $C_{28}H_{57}OH$, from wheat oil and from the cuticular wax of apples.

octadecanoate (ok"tah-dek"ah-no'āt) systematic name for stearate, denoting that it has eighteen (*octa* eight + *deca* ten) carbon atoms in a straight chain.

octamethyl pyrophosphoramide (ok"tah-meth'il pir"o-fos-for'ah-mīd) chemical name: octamethyldiphosphoramide. A cholinesterase inhibitor, $C_8H_{24}N_4O_3P_2$, used as a systemic insecticide for plants. Called also *schradan*. Abbreviated OMPA.

octamylose (ok-tam'ĭ-lōs) a crystalline amylose, $(C_6H_{10}O_5)_8$.

octan (ok'tan) [L. *octo* eight] recurring every eighth day, or at intervals of seven days.

octane (ok'tān) an oily hydrocarbon, $CH_3(CH_2)_6CH_3$, occurring in petroleum.

octanoic acid (ok"tah-no'ik) systematic name for caprylic acid.

octapeptide (ok"tah-pep'tid) a peptide which on hydrolysis yields eight amino acids.

octarius (ok-ta're-us) [L.; from *octo* eight] a pint; the eighth part of a gallon.

octavalent (ok"tah-va'lent) [L. *octo* eight + *valens* able] having a valence of eight.

octazamide (ok-ta'zah-mīd) chemical name: 5-benzoylhexahydro-1*H*-furo[3,4-c]pyrrole; an analgesic, $C_{13}H_{15}NO_2$.

octet (ok'tet) a group of eight identical or similar objects or entities, as the group of eight electrons (four pairs) in the outer, or valence, shell of an atom, which pairs may or may not be shared with another atom.

octicizer (ok"tĭ-si'zer) chemical name: 2-ethylhexyl diphenyl ester phosphoric acid; a plasticizer for pharmaceuticals, $C_{20}H_{27}O_4P$.

octigravida (ok"tĭ-grav'ĭ-dah) [L. *octo* eight + *gravida* pregnant] a woman pregnant for the eighth time; also written gravida VIII.

Octin (ok'tin) trademark for preparations of isometheptene.

octipara (ok-tip'ah-rah) [L. *octo* eight + *parere* to bring forth, produce] a woman who has had eight pregnancies which resulted in viable offspring; also written para VIII.

octodrine (ok'to-drēn) chemical name: 1,5-dimethylhexylamine; an adrenergic with vasoconstrictor and local anesthetic actions, $C_8H_{19}N$.

octofollin (ok"to-fol'in) benzestrol.

Octomyces (ok"to-mi'sēz) a former genus of yeastlike fungi, now considered to be identical with *Saccharomyces*. **O. etien'nei**, yeastlike fungi of uncertain identity once isolated from a severe pleuropulmonary infection, probably as a contaminant.

octopamine (ok"to-pam'ēn) a sympathomimetic amine thought to result from inability of the diseased liver to metabolize tyrosine; it is called a false neurotransmitter, since it can be stored in presynaptic vesicles, replacing norepinephrine, but has little effect on postsynaptic receptors. It is used as the hydrochloride salt in treatment of hypotension.

octose (ok'tōs) [L. *octo* eight] a monosaccharide having the formula $C_8H_{16}O_8$.

octoxynol 9 (ok-toks'ĭ-nol) [NF] a clear, pale yellow, viscous liquid composed of an anhydrous mixture of mono-*p*-(1,1,3,3-tetramethylbutyl)phenyl]ethers of polyethylene glycols containing 5 to 15 oxyethylene groups in the polyoxyethylene chain, and having an average molecular weight of 647, corresponding to the formula $C_{34}H_{62}O_{11}$; used as a surfactant in pharmaceutical preparations. Called also *octylphenoxy polyethoxyethanol*.

octriptyline phosphate (ok-trip'tĭ-lēn) chemical name: 3-(1a,10b-dihydrodibenzo[*a,e*]cyclopropa[*c*]cyclohepten-6(1-*H*)-ylidene)-*N*-methyl-1-propanamine phosphate(1:1); an antidepressant, $C_{20}H_{21}N \cdot H_3PO_4$.

octylphenoxy polyethoxyethanol (ok"til-fe"nok-se pol"e-eth-ok"se-eth'ah-nol) octoxynol 9.

ocufilcon (ok"u-fil'kon) any of three hydrophilic contact lens materials, designated A, B, or C.

ocular (ok'u-lar) [L. *ocularis*, from *oculus* eye] 1. of, pertaining to, or affecting the eye. 2. eyepiece.

oculentum (ok"u-len'tum), pl. *oculen'ta*. An eye ointment.

oculi (ok'u-li) [L.] genitive and plural of *oculus*.

oculist (ok'u-list) ophthalmologist.

oculistics (ok"u-lis'tiks) the treatment of diseases of the eye.

ocul(o)- [L. *oculus* eye] a combining form denoting relationship to the eye.

oculocephalogyric (ok"u-lo-sef"ah-lo-ji'rik) [*oculo-* + *cephalo-* + Gr. *gyros* ring or circle] pertaining to the movements of the head in connection with vision.

oculocutaneous (ok"u-lo-ku-ta'ne-us) pertaining to or affecting both the eyes and the skin.

oculofacial (ok"u-lo-fa'she-al) pertaining to the eyes and the face.

oculogyration (ok"u-lo-ji-ra'shun) movement of the eye about the anteroposterior axis.

oculogyric (ok"u-lo-ji'rik) pertaining to, characterized by, or causing oculogyration; see also under *crisis*.

oculometroscope (ok"u-lo-met'ro-skōp) [*oculo-* + Gr. *metron* measure + *-scope*] an instrument for performing retinoscopy in which the trial lenses are rotated before the eyes without effort on the part of the examiner.

oculomotor (ok"u-lo-mo'tor) [*oculo-* + L. *motor* mover] pertaining to or effecting movements of the eye.

oculomotorius (ok"u-lo-mo-to're-us) [L.] nervum oculomotorius.

oculomycosis (ok"u-lo-mi-ko'sis) [*oculo-* + *mycosis*] any eye disease caused by a fungus.

oculonasal (ok"u-lo-na'zal) pertaining to the eye and the nose.

oculopathy (ok"u-lop'ah-the) ophthalmopathy.

oculopupillary (ok"u-lo-pu'pĭ-lār-e) pertaining to the pupil of the eye.

oculospinal (ok"u-lo-spi'nal) pertaining to the eye and the spinal cord.

oculozygomatic (ok"u-lo-zi"go-mat'ik) pertaining to the eye and the zygoma.

oculus (ok'u-lus), gen. and pl. *o'culi* [L.] [NA] the organ of vision; see *eye*.

Ocusert (ok'u-sert) trademark for a drug delivery system placed in the cul-de-sac of the eyes and providing a sustained release of pilocarpine.

OD optical density.

O.D. abbreviation for *Doctor of Optometry*; L. *o'culus dex'ter*, right eye; and *outside diameter*; popular term for overdose.

O.D.A. abbreviation for L. *occipito-dextra anterior* (right occipito-anterior, a position of the fetus).

odaxesmus (o"dak-sez'mus) [Gr. *odaxēsmos* an itching] the biting of the tongue or cheek in an epileptic seizure.

odaxetic (o"dak-set'ik) [Gr. *odaxētikos*] causing a biting or itching sensation.

Oddi's muscle (sphincter) (od'ēz) [Ruggero *Oddi*, Italian physician, 1864–1913] see under *muscle*.

odditis (od-di'tis) inflammation of Oddi's muscle.

odogenesis (od"o-jen'ĕ-sis) [Gr. *hodos* pathway + *genesis* formation] neurocladism.

odontalgia (o-don-tal'je-ah) [*odont-* + *-algia*] toothache.

odontalgic (o-don-tal'jik) pertaining to or characterized by toothache.

odontectomy (o"don-tek'to-me) [*odont-* + *ectomy*] excision or removal of a tooth; tooth extraction.

odontiatrogenic (o-don"te-at"ro-jen'ik) [*odont-* + Gr. *iatros* one who heals + *gennan* to produce] occurring as a result of treatment by a dentist.

odontic (o-don′tik) [Gr. *odous* tooth] pertaining to the teeth; dental.

odont(o)- [Gr. *odous*, gen. *odontos* tooth] a combining form denoting relationship to a tooth or to the teeth.

odontoameloblastoma (o-don″to-am″ĕ-lo-blas-to′mah) ameloblastic odontoma.

odontoblast (o-don′to-blast) [*odonto-* + *blast*] one of the columnar connective tissue cells which deposit dentin and form the outer surface of the dental pulp adjacent to the dentin.

odontoblastoma (o-don″to-blas-to′mah) a tumor made up of odontoblasts.

odontobothrion (o-don″to-both′re-on) [*odonto-* + Gr. *bothrion* a small trench] one of the dental alveoli.

odontobothritis (o-don″to-both-ri′tis) alveolitis.

odontoclamis (o-don″to-kla′mis) [*odonto-* + Gr. *klamys* cloak] dental operculum.

odontoclast (o-don′to-klast) [*odonto-* + Gr. *klasis* a breaking] cementoclast.

odontogen (o-don′to-jen) [*odonto-* + *-gen*] the substance which develops into the dentin of the teeth.

odontogenesis (o-don″to-jen′ĕ-sis) [*odonto-* + *genesis*] the development and formation of the teeth. **o. imperfec′ta,** dentinogenesis imperfecta.

odontogenetic (o-don″to-jĕ-net′ik) pertaining to odontogenesis.

odontogenic (o-don″to-jen′ik) 1. forming teeth. 2. arising in tissues which give origin to the teeth.

odontogenous (o″don-toj′ĕ-nus) arising or originating in the teeth, or a dental condition.

odontogram (o-don′to-gram) [*odonto-* + *-gram*] the tracing made by an odontograph.

odontograph (o-don′to-graf) [*odonto-* + *-graph*] an instrument for recording the unevenness of surface of tooth enamel.

odontography (o″don-tog′rah-fe) [*odonto-* + *-graphy*] 1. a description of the teeth. 2. the use of the odontograph. Called also *dentography*.

odontoiatria (o-don″to-i-at′re-ah) [*odonto-* + Gr. *iatreia* cure] dental therapeutics.

odontoid (o-don′toid) [*odonto-* + Gr. *eidos* form] toothlike; resembling a tooth.

odontolith (o-don′to-lith) [*odonto-* + Gr. *lithos* stone] dental calculus.

odontolithiasis (o-don″to-lĭ-thi′ah-sis) [*odonto-* + *lith-* + *-iasis*] a condition marked by the presence of dental calculus.

odontologist (o″don-tol′o-jist) a dentist.

odontology (o″don-tol′o-je) [*odonto-* + *-logy*] 1. the sum of knowledge regarding the teeth. 2. dentistry.

odontolysis (o-don-tol′ĭ-sis) [*odonto-* + Gr. *lysis* dissolution] tooth resorption.

odontoma (o-don-to′mah) [*odonto-* + *-oma*] 1. any tumor of odontogenic origin. 2. a mixed tumor of odontogenic origin, in which both the epithelial and mesenchymal cells exhibit complete differentiation, resulting in the formation of tooth structures. **o. adamanti′num,** ameloblastic o. **ameloblastic o.,** a rare, slow-growing, mixed tumor of odontogenic origin that combines the characteristics of composite odontoma and ameloblastoma, and occurs more commonly on the mandible than on the maxilla. **composite o.,** an odontogenic tumor of the jaws, most commonly of the molar region, composed of both the ectodermal and mesodermal components of the tooth apparatus. A type that consists of calcified dental tissue exhibiting complete differentiation, resulting in the formation of enamel and dentin that bear resemblance to normal tooth structures, is known as *compound composite odontoma*; a type in which calcified dental tissue presents a disorganized mass bearing no similarity to normal tooth structure is known as *complex composite odontoma*. **composite o., complex,** a composite odontoma in which the calcified dental tissues occur in an irregular mass, and there is no morphologic similarity to even rudimentary teeth. **composite o., compound,** a composite odontoma in which the enamel and dentin are laid down so that the structure bears a superficial anatomic resemblance to normal teeth. **coronal o., coronary o.,** odontoma associated with the crown of a tooth, or one formed at the time when the crown of the tooth was developing. **dilated o.,** dens in dente. **embryoplastic o.,** a soft odontoma formed in the period that precedes the formation of the dental tissues. **fibrous o.,** an odontoma containing fibrous elements. **mixed o.,** an odontogenic neoplasm containing different elements of the tooth structure. **radicular o.,** one associated with the root of a tooth, or one formed at the time when the root of the tooth was developing.

odontonomy (o″don-ton′o-me) [*odonto-* + Gr. *onoma* name] the nomenclature of dentistry; a system of terminologies in all branches of dentistry and related fields. Called also *dentonomy*.

odontopathic (o-don″to-path′ik) relating to disease of the teeth.

odontopathy (o″don-top′ah-the) [*odonto-* + Gr. *pathos* illness] any disease of the teeth.

odontoperiosteum (o-don″to-per″e-os′te-um) periodontium, def. 1.

odontophobia (o-don″to-fo′be-ah) [*odonto-* + *phobia*] an irrational fear associated with teeth, as that aroused by the sight of teeth, or abnormal dread of dental operations.

odontoprisis (o-don″to-pri′sis) [*odonto-* + Gr. *prisis* sawing] bruxism.

odontoradiograph (o-don″to-ra′de-o-graf) a roentgenogram of a tooth or of the teeth.

odontoschism (o-don′to-skizm) [*odonto-* + Gr. *schisma* cleft] fissure of a tooth.

odontoscopy (o″don-tos′ko-pe) [*odonto-* + *-scopy*] the taking of dental impressions.

odontoseisis (o-don″to-si′sis) [*odonto-* + Gr. *seisis* a shaking] looseness of the teeth.

odontosis (o″don-to′sis) [*odont-* + *-osis*] the formation or eruption of the teeth.

Odontostomatida (o″don-to-sto″mah-ti′dah) [*odonto-* + Gr. *stoma* mouth] an order of small ciliate protozoa (subclass Spirotricha, class Polyhymenophorea) having a laterally compressed, wedge-shaped body with an armorlike cuirass and often posterior spines, reduced somatic ciliature, a reduced adoral zone of membranelles, and no paroral membrane. They are found chiefly in putrefying organic matter, mostly in fresh water.

odontotheca (o-don″to-the′kah) [*odonto-* + Gr. *thēkē* case] the dental sac.

odontotomy (o″don-tot′o-me) [*odonto-* + Gr. *tomē* a cutting] the operation of cutting into a tooth, especially incision into an occlusal groove.

odontotripsis (o-don″to-trip′sis) [*odonto-* + Gr. *tripsis* rubbing] wearing away of the teeth.

odor (o′dor) [L.] a volatile emanation that is perceived by the sense of smell. **minimal identifiable o.,** the lowest concentration of a substance in air, or in another medium, which still permits its identification by the sense of smell.

odorant (o′dor-ant) any substance capable of eliciting olfactory excitation, i.e., of stimulating the sense of smell.

odoratism (o″dor-a′tizm) osteolathyrism.

odoriferous (o″dor-if′er-us) [*odor* + L. *ferre* to bear] fragrant; emitting an odor.

odorimeter (o″dor-im′ĕ-ter) an instrument for performing odorimetry.

odorimetry (o″dor-im′ĕ-tre) the measurement of olfactory stimuli.

odoriphore (o-dor′ĭ-fōr) osmophore.

odorivector (o″dor-ĭ-vek′tor) a substance which gives off an odor.

odorography (o″dor-og′rah-fe) [*odor* + Gr. *graphein* to write] a description of odors.

O.D.P. abbreviation for L. *occipito-dextra posterior* (right occipitoposterior, a position of the fetus).

O.D.T. abbreviation for L. *occipito-dextra transversa* (right occipitotransverse, a position of the fetus).

odynacusis (o″din-ah-ku′sis) [*odyno-* + Gr. *akousis* hearing] painful hearing.

-odynia [Gr. *odynē* pain] a word ending denoting a painful condition.

odyn(o)- [Gr. *odynē* pain] a combining form meaning pain.

odynometer (o″din-om′ĕ-ter) [*odyno-* + Gr. *metron* measure] an instrument for measuring pain.

odynophagia (od″ĭ-no-fa′je-ah) [*odyno-* + Gr. *phagein* to eat] pain on deglutition.

odynphagia (o″din-fa′je-ah) odynophagia.

oe- for words beginning thus, see also those beginning with *e-*.

Oeciacus (e-si′ah-kus) a genus of insects closely related to the bedbugs (*Cimex*), but distinguished by their hairy bodies covered by long silklike coats; they are found on birds and in their nests. *O. hirudinis* is found on barn swallows in Europe and sometimes invades homes and attacks man, causing a severe irritation; *O. vicarius* is found on swallows in North America.

oedipism (ed′ĭ-pizm) [see *Oedipus complex*] edipism.

Oehler's symptom (e′lerz) [Johannes *Oehler*, German physician, born 1879] see under *symptom*.

oenanthol (e-nan′thol) heptoic aldehyde, CH₃(CH₂)₅CHO; called also *heptanal*.

oersted (er′sted) [Hans Christian *Oersted*, Danish physicist, 1777–1851] the unit of magnetizing force, symbol *H*.

Oertel's treatment (er′telz) [Max Joseph *Oertel*, physician in Munich, 1835–1897] see under *treatment*.

oesophag(o)- for words beginning thus, see those beginning *esophag(o)-*.

oesophagostomiasis (e-sof″ah-go-sto-mi′ah-sis) infection with Oesophagostomum.

Oesophagostomum (e-sof″ah-gos′to-mum) [*Oesophagus* + Gr. *stoma* mouth] a genus of nematode worms of the family Strongylidae, parasitic in the intestines of various animals; the larvae often encyst in the intestinal wall, while the adults are mostly free in the lumen. *Oe. apios′tomum, Oe. bifurcum.* **Oe. bifur′cum,** a parasite that forms tumors in the large intestine of monkeys and occasionally of man in Africa and the Philippines. **Oe. brevicau′dum,** a species found in pigs. **Oe. brump′ti,** *Oe. bifurcum.* **Oe. columbia′num,** the nodular worm, infects sheep and goats in the southern United States; see *nodular disease,* under *disease.* **Oe. denta′tum,** a parasite of the pig. **Oe. infla′tum,** *Oe. radiatum.* **Oe. longicau′dum,** a parasite of pigs. **Oe. radia′tum,** a parasite of cattle. **Oe. stephanos′tomum,** a species, normally parasitic in gorillas; a single human case has been recorded from Brazil. **Oe. su′is,** *Oe. brevicaudum.*

oesophagus (ĕ-sof′ah-gus) [Gr. *oisophagos*, gullet, related to *phagein* to eat] [NA] the esophagus.

Oestreicher's reaction (est′ri-kerz) [A. *Oestreicher*] xanthydrol reaction.

oestriasis (es-tri′ah-sis) infestation with larvae of flies of the genus Oestrus.

Oestridae (es′tri-de) the family of the "bot," "heel," or "warble" flies. They are very hairy diptera with rudimentary mouth parts and with the antennae inserted into round pits. The family includes the following genera: *Gasterophilus, Oestrus, Hypoderma, Dermatobia, Rhinoestrus,* and *Cuterebra.*

oestrone (es′trōn) estrone.

oestrous (es′trus) estrous.

oestrual (es′troo-al) estrual.

oestrum (es′trum) estrus.

oestrus (es′trus) estrus.

Oestrus (es′trus) [Gr. *oistros* gadfly] a genus of botflies of the family Oestridae, which may cause ophthalmomyiasis, called also *Cephalomyia.* **O. hom′inis,** *O. ovis.* **O. o′vis,** a species of botfly whose larvae infest nasal cavities and sinuses of sheep; they may cause ocular myiasis in man.

official (ŏ-fish′al) [L. *officialis; officum* duty] recognized by the current U. S. Pharmacopeia or National Formulary, and meeting the standards established by the respective authority.

officinal (ŏ-fis′ĭ-nal) [L. *officinalis; officina* shop] regularly kept for sale in the shops of druggists.

Ogata's method (o-gah′tahz) [M. *Ogata*, Japanese physician] see under *method.*

Ogen (o′jen) trademark for preparations of estropipate.

Ogston-Luc operation (og′ston-luk′) [Sir Alexander *Ogston*, Scottish surgeon, 1844–1929; Henry *Luc*, French laryngologist, 1855–1925] see under *operation.*

Oguchi's disease (o-goo′chēz) [Chuta *Oguchi*, Japanese ophthalmologist, 1875–1945] see under *disease.*

OH hydroxyl group; (with negative sign) hydroxide ion; a hydroxide.

Ohara's disease (o-hah′rahz) [Hachiro *Ohara*, Japanese physician, born 1882] see under *disease.*

ohm (ōm) [George S. *Ohm*, German physicist, 1787–1854] the SI unit of electrical resistance, being equivalent to that of a column of mercury one square millimeter in cross-section and one hundred and six centimeters long. Symbol Ω.

Ohm's law (ōmz) [George S. *Ohm*, German physicist, 1787–1854] see under *law.*

ohmammeter (ōm′am-me″ter) an ohmmeter and ammeter combined.

ohmmeter (ōm′me-ter) an instrument for measuring electric resistance in ohms.

ohne Hauch (o′nah-houkh) [Ger. "without breath"] see *O antigen,* under *antigen.*

-oid [Gr. *-oeidēs,* from *eidos* form] a word termination denoting resemblance to the thing specified by the stem to which it is affixed, as ovoid.

Oidiomycetes (o-id″e-o-mi-se′tēz) former name for a group of fungi characterized by having mycelial threads and producing small spores by fragmentation.

oidiomycosis (o-id″e-o-mi-ko′sis) [*oidium* + Gr. *mykēs* fungus] infection with fungi of the genus *Oidium.*

oidiomycotic (o-id″e-o-mi-kot′ik) pertaining to oidiomycosis.

Oidium (o-id′e-um) [dim. of Gr. *ōon* egg] 1. a former name for a genus of fungi the species of which are now included in the genera *Candida* and *Geotrichum.* 2. the imperfect (sexual) stage of the powdery mildews (order Erysiphales), causing many plant diseases.

oikosite (oi′ko-sīt) ecosite.

oil (oil) [L. *oleum*] 1. an unctuous, combustible substance which is liquid, or easily liquefiable, on warming, and is soluble in ether but insoluble in water. Such substances, depending on their origin, are classified as animal, mineral, or vegetable oils. Depending on their behavior on heating, they are classified as volatile or fixed. 2. a fat that is liquid at room temperature. **allspice o.,** pimenta o. **almond o.** [NF], a preparation of the fixed oil obtained from the kernels of varieties of *Prunus amygdalus;* used as an emollient and perfume and as an ingredient of rose water ointment. Called also *expressed* or *sweet almond o.,* and *oleum amygdalae expressum.* **almond o., bitter,** the volatile oil obtained from the dried ripe kernels of *Prunus amygdalus* var. *amara* Focke (Rosaceae) or from other kernels containing amygdalin; formerly used as a topical antipruritic; used also in perfumery and liqueurs. **almond o., expressed,** see *almond o.* **almond o., sweet,** see *almond o.* **anise o.** [NF], a volatile oil distilled from the dried, ripe fruit of *Pimpinella anisum* or of *Illicium verum;* used as a flavoring agent for drugs, and has been used as a carminative and expectorant. **apricot kernel o.,** persic o. **arachis o.,** peanut o. **argemone o.,** an oil from *Argemona mexicana* L. (Papaveraceae), the prickly poppy; contamination of mustard oil used for cooking in India, Fiji, and South Africa with argemone oil causes epidemic dropsy. **bay o.,** myrcia o. **Benne o.,** sesame o. **bergamot o.,** a volatile oil obtained by expression from the rind of the fresh fruit of *Citrus bergamia;* used as a perfuming agent and insecticide. **betula o.,** methyl salicylate. **bhilawanol o.,** a fluid obtained from the nut of a tree, *Semecarpus anacardium* (ral tree, bella gutta tree), in India, used by native washermen for marking laundry, and the cause, through induction of eczematous contact sensitization, of dhobie itch. **birch o., sweet,** methyl salicylate. **birch tar o., rectified,** the pyroligneous oil obtained by the dry distillation of the bark and wood of *Betula alba* L. (Betulaceae) and other species of *Betula,* and rectified by steam distillation; used topically in the treatment of eczema and other dermatitides. **cade o.,** juniper tar. **o. of cajuput,** a volatile oil from the fresh leaves and twigs of *Melaleuca leucadendron* L. (Myrtaceae) and other species of *Melaleuca;* used as a stimulant, expectorant, counterirritant, and external parasiticide, and in veterinary medicine as a rubifacient and parasiticide in the treatment of ringworm. **camphorated o.,** camphor liniment. **caraway o.** [NF], a volatile oil distilled from the dried ripe fruit of *Carum carvi,* yielding at least 50 per cent by volume of carvone; used as a flavoring agent for drugs. Called also *oleum cari.* **cardamom o.** [NF], a volatile oil distilled from the seed of *Elettaria cardamomum* (cardamom seed), a perennial herb of the ginger family of tropical Asia; used as a flavoring agent in pharmaceutical preparations. Called also *oleum cardamomi.* **cassia o.,** cinnamon o. **castor o.** [USP], a fixed oil obtained from the seed of *Ricinus communis;* used as a cathartic and as a plasticizer for pharmaceutical preparations, and has been used as a bland emollient to the skin in certain dermatoses. **castor o., aromatic** [USP], a mixture of cinnamon, clove, and castor oils, with saccharin, vanillin, and alcohol, used as a cathartic. **cedar o.,** a volatile oil from cedar wood, used as a clearing agent in microscopical techniques; the thicker fraction is used as the immersion medium with oil-immersion objectives. **chaulmoogra o.,** a fixed oil expressed from the ripe seeds of *Taraktogenos kurzii* King. (Bixaceae), *Hydnocarpus wightiana* Blume, and *H. anthelmintica* Pierre (Flacourtiaceae); formerly used in the treatment of leprosy; ethyl esters of the fatty acids (e.g., ethyl chaulmoograte) obtained from this oil are now so used. **chenopodium o.,** a volatile oil obtained by steam distillation of fresh overground parts of the flowering and fruiting plant of *Chenopodium ambrosiodes,* L. (Chenopodiaceae); it contains 65 per cent of ascaridole, an active anthelmintic principle and was once used as an anthelmintic. **chloriodized o.,** an iodine monochloride addition product of vegetable oil; formerly used as a radiopaque medium in roentgenography of the uterus and uterine tubes, and of the bronchi. **cinnamon o.** [NF], a volatile oil distilled with steam from the leaves and twigs of *Cinnamomum cassia;* used as a flavoring agent for pharmaceuticals and as a carminative. **citronella o.,** a fragrant oil used as an insect repellent. **clove o.** [NF], a volatile oil distilled with steam from clover, the dried flowerbuds of *Eugenia caryophyllus;* used as a flavor in pharmaceutical preparations, and as a topical germicide and analgesic in dentistry. **coconut o.,** the fixed oil obtained by expression or extraction from the kernels of seeds of *Cocos nucifera;* used as an ointment base and edible oil and in soap, chocolate, and candle formulations. **cod liver o.** [USP], the partially destearinated fixed oil obtained from fresh livers of *Gadus morrhua* and other species of the family Gadidae; used as a source of vitamin A and vitamin D. In veterinary medicine, it is also used topically to promote wound-healing and in abscesses, burns, and dermatoses. **cod liver o., nondestearinated** [NF], the entire fixed oil obtained from fresh livers of *Gadus morrhua* and other species of the family Gadidae; used as a source of vitamins A and D. **o. of copaiba,** a volatile oil derived from copaiba, *Copaifera* spp. (Leguminosae), trees indigenous to central South America; it contains aromatic principles and was once used for chronic inflammations of mucous membranes. **coriander o.** [NF], a volatile oil distilled with steam from the dried ripe fruit of *Coriandrum sativum;* used as a flavoring agent. **corn o.** [NF], a refined fixed oil obtained from the embryo of *Zea mays;* used as a solvent and vehicle for various medicinal agents and as a vehicle for injections. It has also been promoted as a source of polyunsaturated fatty acids in special diets. **cottonseed o.** [NF], the fixed oil obtained by expression from the seeds of cultivated varieties of the cotton plant, *Gossypium herbaceum* L. It is widely used in soaps, oleomargarine, lubricants, cosmetics, and salad and cooking oils. In veterinary medicine, used as delousing agent, usually combined with two parts of pine tar for ear ticks of horses, and as a mild emollient and laxative for small animals. **croton o.,** the thick, fixed oil of the seeds of *Croton tiglium,* L. Euphorbiaceae, an Asiatic plant. A drastic purgative and counterirritant, unsafe for human use, it is used as standard irritant in pharmacological research. **o. of dill,** an oil distilled from the dried ripe fruits of *Anethum graveolens* L. (Umbelliferae); used as an aromatic carminative and as a source of carvone. **distilled o.,** volatile o. **drying o.,** a type of fixed oil which thickens and hardens on exposure to the air, especially when spread out in a thin layer, being converted to a solid by absorption and reaction with oxygen. **empyreumatic o.,** a volatile oil formed by the destructive distillation of organic material. **essential o.,** volatile o. **ethereal o.,** 1. a compound of ether with heavy oil of wine. 2. a volatile oil. **ethiodized o.** [USP], an iodine addition product of the ethyl ester of the fatty acids of poppyseed oil, containing 35.2 to 38.9 per cent of organically combined iodine; used as a radiopaque medium in hysterosalpingogra-

phy and lymphography. **eucalyptus o.** [NF], a volatile oil distilled with steam from the fresh leaf of *Eucalyptus globulus* and other species of *Eucalyptus;* used as a flavor in pharmaceutical preparations, and as an expectorant and local antiseptic with mild anesthetic effect. Formerly used as a vermifuge. **expressed o., fatty o.,** fixed o. **fennel o.** [NF], a volatile oil distilled with steam from the dried ripe fruit of *Foeniculum vulgare;* used as a flavoring agent for pharmaceuticals and formerly as a carminative. **fixed o.,** an oil which does not evaporate on warming. Such oils, consisting of a mixture of fatty acids and their esters, are classified as solid (chiefly stearin), semisolid (chiefly palmitin), and liquid (chiefly olein) Fixed oils are also classified as *drying, semidrying,* and *nondrying,* depending on their tendency to solidify when exposed, in a thin film, to air. Called also *expressed o.* and *fatty o.* **flaxseed o.,** linseed o. **gaultheria o.,** methyl salicylate. **gingili o.,** sesame o. **groundnut o.,** peanut o. **Haarlem o.,** juniper tar. **halibut liver o.,** a fixed oil obtained from fresh or suitably preserved livers of halibut species of the genus *Hippoglossus* Linné; used as a source of vitamins A and D. **heavy o.,** an oily product obtained by the action of sulfuric acid on alcohol. **hydnocarpus o.,** chaulmoogra o. **iodized o.,** an iodine addition product of vegetable oil; used as radiopaque medium in roentgenography of the uterus and uterine tubes. **juniper o.,** a volatile oil distilled with steam from the dried ripe fruit of *Juniperus communis;* used to preserve catgut sutures and has been used as a diuretic. **lavender o.** [NF], a volatile oil distilled with steam from the fresh flowering tops of *Lavandula officinalis;* used as a perfume in pharmaceutical preparations and formerly as a carminative and insect repellant. **lavender flowers o.,** lavender o. **lemon o.** [NF], the volatile oil obtained by expression from the fresh peel of the fruit of *Citrus limon;* used as a flavoring agent. **linseed o., raw linseed o.,** the fixed oil obtained from the dried ripe seed of *Linum usitatissimum* (L. Linaceae); used as an emollient in liniments, pastes, and medicinal soaps, and in veterinary medicine as a laxative. Called also *flaxseed o.* **o. of male fern,** an oleoresin from the root of the male fern, *Dryopteris filix-mas* (L.) Schott., Polypodiaceae; it contains about 24 per cent of crude filicin and is used as an anthelmintic. **mineral o.** [USP], a mixture of liquid hydrocarbons obtained from petroleum, with a specific gravity of 0.845–0.905; used as a cathartic and as a solvent and oleaginous vehicle in pharmaceutical preparations. Called also *heavy liquid petrolatum, liquid petrolatum, liquid paraffin, petrolatum liquidum,* and *white mineral o.* **mineral o., light** [USP], **mineral o., light white,** a mixture of liquid hydrocarbons obtained from petrolatum, with a specific gravity of 0.818–0.880; used as a vehicle for drugs and also as a laxative. Called also *light liquid paraffin* and *light liquid petrolatum.* **mineral o., white,** liquid petrolatum. **o. of mirbane,** nitrobenzene. **o. of mustard,** an oil derived from the seeds of species of *Brassica.* Volatile mustard oil is from the seeds of black mustard (see *allyl isothiocyanate).* Used internally as a condiment and emetic and externally as a counterirritant. **myrcia o.,** the volatile oil obtained by distilling the leaves of *Pimenta officinalis* Lindl. (Myrtaceae). It contains 55–65 per cent of eugenol and other related aromatic principles and is used in perfumes and such products as bay rum as an after-shave lotion and rub or liniment. Called also *bay o.* **myristica o.,** nutmeg o. **neroli o.,** orange flower o. **nutmeg o.,** [NF], the volatile oil distilled with steam from the dried kernels of the ripe seeds of *Myristica fragrans* Houtt. (Myristicaceae); used as a flavoring agent in pharmaceutical preparations. Called also *myristica o.* **olive o.** [NF], the fixed oil obtained from the ripe fruit of *Olea europaea;* used as a setting retardant for dental cements and as a topical emollient, and has been used as a laxative. Called also *sweet o.* **orange o.** [NF], the volatile oil obtained by expression from the fresh peel of the ripe fruit of *Citrus sinensis;* used as a flavoring agent in pharmaceuticals. Called also *sweet orange o.* **orange o., bitter,** a volatile oil obtained by expression from the fresh peel of the fruit of *Citrus aurantium* L. (Rutaceae); used as a flavoring agent. **orange o., sweet,** orange o. **orange flower o.** [NF], a volatile oil distilled from the fresh flowers of *Citrus aurantium;* used as a flavoring agent and perfume. Called also *neroli.* **o. of Palma Christi,** castor o. **peach kernel o.,** persic o. **peanut o.** [NF], the refined fixed oil obtained from the seed kernels of one or more of the cultivated varieties of *Arachis hypogaea;* used as a solvent and oleaginous vehicle for drugs, and as a laxative in veterinary medicine. **peppermint o.** [NF], the volatile oil distilled with steam from the fresh overground parts of the flowering plant of *Mentha piperita* L. (Labiate); used as a flavor in pharmaceutical preparations, and as a gastric stimulant and carminative. **persic o.** [NF], an oil expressed from the kernels of varieties of *Prunus armeniaca*, the apricot, or from *P. persica*, the peach; used as a vehicle for drugs. **pimenta o.**, the volatile oil distilled from the fruit of *Pimenta officinalis Lindl.* (Myrtaceae); used as a flavor for pharmaceutical preparations. **pine o.**, the volatile oil obtained by steam distillation of the wood of *Pinus palustris* and of other species of *Pinus;* used as a deodorant and disinfectant. **pine needle o.** [NF], **pine needle o., dwarf,** the volatile oil distilled with steam from the fresh leaf of the dwarf pine, *Pinus mugo* and its variety *pumilio;* used as a perfume and flavoring agent. **ricinus o.,** castor o. **rose o.** [NF], the volatile oil distilled with steam from the fresh flowers of *Rosa gallica* L., *R. damascena* Mill., *R. alba* L., *R. centifolia,* and varieties of these species; used as a perfuming agent in pharmaceuticals. It has also been used as a flavoring agent in ointments and lozenges. Called also *attar of rose.* **rosemary o.,** the volatile oil distilled with steam from the fresh flowering tops of *Rosmarinus officinalis* L.; used as a flavoring or perfuming agent. **safflower o.,** an oily liquid extracted from the seeds of the safflower, *Carthamus tinctorius;* used as a dietary supplement in the management of hypercholesterolemia. **sandalwood o.,** santal o. **santal o.,** a pale yellow, somewhat viscid, oily liquid with characteristic odor and taste of sandalwood, distilled with steam from the dried heartwood of *Santalum album* L. (Santalaceae), or sandalwood; formerly used as a urinary antiseptic. **sassafras o.,** the volatile oil distilled with steam from the root of *Sassafras albidum;* used as a flavoring agent for liquid pharmaceutical preparations and to offset their disagreeable odor. It is also applied to insect bites and stings and has been used as a topical antiseptic, pediculicide, and carminative. It contains safrene and safrol. The oil is also the basis of the soda beverage known as root beer. **savin o.,** an acrid oil from the fresh tops of savin, *Juniperus sabina* L. (Cupressaceae), the chief constituent of which is sabinol; it has been used in folk medicine as an emmenagogue, anthelmintic, and antirheumatic, and is used in perfumery. **sesame o.** [NF], the refined fixed oil obtained from the seed of one or more cultivated varieties of *Sesamum indicum;* it is used as a solvent and oleaginous vehicle for drugs, and has been used internally as a laxative and externally as a skin softener. **spearmint o.** [NF], the volatile oil distilled with steam from the fresh overground parts of *Mentha spicata* L. (Labiatae) (*M. viridis* L.) or *Mentha cardiaca* L., yielding at least 55 per cent by volume of carvone; used as a flavor for pharmaceutical preparations and has been used as a carminative. **o. of spike,** a volatile oil obtained from a broad-leaved variety of lavender, *Lavandula latifolia* Medic. (Labiatae), growing wild in Europe; used in perfumery, and formerly in home remedies as an emmenagogue and abortive. **o. of spruce,** a volatile oil obtained from the hemlock tree, *Tsuga canadensis,* (L.) Carr (Pinaceae); sometimes used in veterinary liniments. **sweet o.,** olive o. **tangan-tangan o.,** castor o. **tar o., rectified,** the volatile oil from *Pinus palustris* Mill. (Pinaceae) and pine tar rectified by steam distillation; used, in veterinary medicine, internally as a stimulant expectorant and externally as an antipruritic, antiseptic, and stimulant for diseases of the skin. Also widely used in disinfecting and deodorizing preparations. **teel o.,** sesame o. **theobroma o.,** cocoa butter. **thyme o.,** the volatile oil distilled from the flowering plant of *Thymus vulgaris;* used as a flavoring agent for drugs, and has been used as a rubefacient, expectorant, counterirritant, antiseptic, and carminative. **turpentine o.,** the volatile oil distilled from an oleoresin obtained from *Pinus palustris* Mill. (Pinaceae) and other species of *Pinus.* Its chief constituent is pinene, which is used in the synthetic production of camphor. It is used as a counterirritant and rubefacient. **turpentine o., rectified,** turpentine oil rectified by use of sodium hydroxide; used as an inhalation expectorant. **o. of vitriol,** sulfuric acid. **volatile o.,** an oil which evaporates readily. The volatile oils occur in aromatic plants, to which they give odor and other characteristics. Most volatile oils consist of a mixture of two or more terpenes or of a mixture of an eleopten with a stearopten. Called also *distilled o., essential o.,* and *ethereal o.* **wheat-germ o.,** oil derived from the

germ of wheat kernels; it is rich in vitamin E. **wintergreen o.,** methyl salicylate. **wormseed o., American,** chenopodium o.

ointment (oint′ment) [L. *unguentum*] a semisolid preparation for external application to the body, and usually containing a medicinal substance. Called also *unguent, unction,* and *salve.* **ammoniated mercury o.** [USP], a preparation of ammoniated mercury, liquid petrolatum, and white ointment, containing 4.5 to 5.5 per cent of $HgNH_2Cl$; used as a topical anti-infective. Called also *white precipitate o.* **anthralin o.** [USP], a preparation of anthralin in a petrolatum or other suitable base; used as a topical antipsoriatic. **bacitracin o.** [USP], a preparation of bacitracin or bacitracin zinc in an anhydrous ointment base, containing not less than 500 U.S.P. units per gram; used as an antibacterial, applied topically to the skin. **bacitracin ophthalmic o.** [USP], a preparation of bacitracin in an anhydrous ointment base, containing not less than 500 U.S.P. units per gram; used as an antibacterial, applied topically to the conjunctiva. **belladonna o.,** a preparation of pilular belladonna extract and diluted alcohol in yellow ointment; used locally as an analgesic. **benzocaine o.** [USP], a preparation of finely powdered benzocaine in white ointment; used as a local anesthetic, applied topically to the skin and mucous membranes. Called also *ethyl aminobenzoate o.* **benzoic and salicylic acids o.** [USP], a preparation of benzoic acid and salicylic acid in a water-soluble base (polyethylene glycol ointment), formerly used topically as an antifungal agent. Called *Whitfield's o.* **betamethasone valerate o.** [USP], a preparation containing betamethasone valerate equivalent to 95 to 120 per cent of the labeled amount of betamethasone; used as an anti-inflammatory glucocorticoid. **blue o.,** mercurial o., mild. **boric acid o.,** a preparation of finely powdered boric acid and liquid petrolatum in white ointment, formerly used extensively for its emollient and protective action in superficial wounds, abrasions, and burns, and for ophthalmic application. **calamine o.,** a preparation containing calamine, yellow wax, anhydrous lanolin, and petrolatum; used as an astringent protective application. **calomel o.,** a preparation of calomel, hydrous wool fat, and white petrolatum, containing 28.5 to 31.5 per cent calomel; has been used to treat various infections and parasitic infestations of the skin. Called also *mild mercurous chloride o.* **candicidin o.** [USP], a semisolid preparation of candicidin in a suitable ointment base, containing 90 to 140 per cent of the labeled amount of candicidin; used as a local antifungal agent in the treatment of vaginal candidiasis, administered intravaginally. **carbolic acid o.,** phenol o. **chloramphenicol ophthalmic o.** [USP], an ointment containing between 90 and 130 per cent of the labeled amount of chloramphenicol; used as an antibacterial, applied topically to the conjunctiva. **chrysarobin o.,** a preparation of chrysarobin, chloroform, and white ointment; used topically in the treatment of psoriasis and other chronic skin diseases. **coal tar o.** [USP], a preparation of coal tar, polysorbate 80, and zinc oxide paste, used as a topical antieczematic and antipsoriatic. **cyclomethycaine sulfate o.** [USP], a preparation containing 90 to 110 per cent of the labeled amount of cyclomethycaine sulfate in a suitable ointment base; used as a topical anesthetic. **dexamethasone sodium phosphate ophthalmic o.** [NF], an ointment containing 90 to 115 per cent of the labeled amount of dexamethasone sodium phosphate; used as an anti-inflammatory glucocorticoid applied to the conjunctiva. **dibucaine o.** [USP], a semisolid preparation of dibucaine in a suitable ointment base, containing 90 to 110 per cent of the labeled amount of dibucaine; used as a local anesthetic, especially for dry, encrusted lesions, applied topically to the skin and mucous membranes. **dimethisoquin hydrochloride o.** [USP], an ointment containing 90 to 110 per cent of the labeled amount of dimethisoquin hydrochloride; used as a local anesthetic, applied topically to the skin to relieve pain, itching, and burning. **diperodon o.** [USP], a preparation containing 90 to 110 per cent of the labeled amount of diperodon in a suitable ointment base; used as a local anesthetic, applied topically to the skin for abrasions, irritations, and pruritus or intrarectally for relief of discomfort associated with hemorrhoids. **erythromycin o.** [USP], a preparation containing 90 to 125 per cent of the labeled amount of erythromycin (the labeled amount being 10 mg. of erythromycin per gm. of ointment) in a suitable ointment base; used as a topical antibacterial in the treatment of superficial infections of the skin due to organisms susceptible to erythromycin. **erythromycin ophthalmic o.** [USP], a preparation containing 90 to 120 per cent of the labeled amount of erythromycin (the labeled amount being 5 mg. of erythromycin per gm. of ophthalmic ointment) in a suitable ointment base; used as a topical antibacterial in the treatment of superficial infections of the conjunctiva and/or cornea due to organisms susceptible to erythromycin. **ethyl aminobenzoate o.**, benzocaine o. **fluocinolone acetonide o.** [USP], an ointment containing 90 to 110 per cent of the labeled amount of fluocinolone acetonide; used as an anti-inflammatory in steroid-responsive dermatoses, applied topically. **flurandrenolide o.** [USP], an ointment containing 85 to 115 per cent of the labeled amount of flurandrenolide; used as a topical anti-inflammatory glucocorticoid in the treatment of steroid-responsive dermatoses. **gentamicin sulfate o.** [USP], a semisolid preparation of gentamicin sulfate in a suitable ointment base, containing 90 to 135 per cent of the labeled amount of gentamicin; used as a topical antibacterial. **gentamicin sulfate ophthalmic o.** [USP], a sterile preparation of gentamicin sulfate in a petroleum base, containing the equivalent of 90 to 135 per cent of the labeled amount of gentamicin; used as an antibacterial, applied topically to the conjunctiva. **hydrocortisone o.** [USP], a semisolid preparation of hydrocortisone in a suitable ointment base, containing 90 to 110 per cent of the labeled amount of hydrocortisone; used as an anti-inflammatory adrenocortical steroid. **hydrocortisone acetate o.** [USP], a preparation containing 1.00 to 1.25 per cent hydrocortisone acetate, equivalent to 0.9 to 1.1 per cent hydrocortisone, used as a topical adrenocortical steroid. **hydrocortisone acetate ophthalmic o.** [USP], a semisolid preparation of hydrocortisone acetate in a suitable ointment base, containing 90 to 110 per cent of the labeled amount of hydrocortisone acetate; used as an anti-inflammatory steroid applied to the conjunctiva. **hydrophilic o.** [USP], a water-in-oil emulsion consisting of methylparaben, propylparaben, sodium lauryl sulfate, propylene glycol, stearyl alcohol, white petrolatum, and purified water; used as an ointment base. **ichthammol o.** [USP], a preparation of ichthammol in anhydrous lanolin and petrolatum, used as a local anti-infective, applied topically to skin. **idoxuridine ophthalmic o.** [USP], a semisolid preparation of idoxuridine in a petrolatum base, containing 0.45 to 0.55 per cent idoxuridine; used as an antiviral agent in the treatment of herpes simplex keratitis, applied topically to the conjunctiva. **iodochlorhydroxyquin o.** [USP], an ointment containing 90 to 110 per cent of the labeled amount of iodochlorhydroxyquin in a suitable ointment base; used as a local anti-infective in the treatment of a wide range of dermatoses, including all types of eczema, applied topically. **iodochlorhydroxyquin and hydrocortisone o.**, an ointment containing 90 to 110 per cent of the labeled amounts of iodochlorhydroxyquin and of hydrocortisone; used for its local anti-infective effect and the anti-inflammatory and antipruritic activity of glucocorticoids in a wide range of dermatoses, applied topically. **isoflurophate ophthalmic o.** [USP], an ointment containing 0.0225 to 0.0275 per cent of isoflurophate in a suitable anhydrous base; used as a cholinergic applied to the conjunctiva in the treatment of glaucoma. **lidocaine o.** [USP], a semisolid preparation of lidocaine in a suitable hydrophilic base, containing 95 to 105 per cent of the labeled amount of lidocaine; used as a local anesthetic, applied topically to the mucous membranes. **mercurial o., diluted,** mercurial o., mild. **mercurial o., mild,** a preparation of mercury and mercury oleate, in solid bases, containing between 9 and 11 per cent mercury, used chiefly as a topical parasiticide. Called also *blue o.* **mercurial o., strong,** a preparation of mercury, mercury oleate, anhydrous lanolin, white wax, and white petrolatum, containing 47.5–52.5 per cent of mercury; used as a topical parasiticide. **mercuric oxide ophthalmic o., yellow,** a mixture of finely powdered yellow mercuric oxide, liquid petrolatum, and white ointment, containing 0.9–1.1 per cent of mercuric oxide, used as a topical anti-infective in the treatment of blepharitis, conjunctivitis, and styes. **mercurous chloride o., mild,** calomel o. **methylbenzethonium chloride o.** [USP], an ointment containing 0.1 per cent methylbenzethonium chloride; used as a local anti-infective, applied topically to the skin of the genitalia, rectum, thighs, and intertriginous areas in the treatment of ammonia dermatitis and in the treatment and prevention of dermatoses caused by contact with urine, feces, and perspira-

tion. **monobenzone o.** [USP], an ointment containing 94 to 106 per cent of the labeled amount of monobenzone; used as a depigmenting agent. **neomycin sulfate o.** [USP], an ointment containing 3.5 mg. of neomycin base per gram, used as a topical antibacterial. **neomycin and polymyxin B sulfates, and bacitracin zinc o.** [USP], an ointment containing 90 per cent of the labeled amounts of neomycin sulfate, polymyxin B sulfate, and zinc bacitracin; used as a local anti-infective agent. **nitrofurazone o.** [USP], an ointment containing 95 to 105 per cent of the labeled amount of nitrofurazone in a suitable water-miscible base; used as a local anti-infective against a wide variety of gram negative and gram positive bacteria in the treatment of many skin lesions, especially second and third degree burns and to aid healing and prevent infection of skin grafts, applied topically. **nystatin o.** [USP], a semisolid preparation of nystatin in a suitable ointment base, containing in each gram, 90,000 to 130,000 units of nystatin activity, the labeled amount being 100,000 units per gram; used as a topical antifungal agent in the treatment of cutaneous candidal infections. **Pagenstecher's o.,** yellow mercuric oxide; see under *mercuric.* **penicillin o.,** a preparation of calcium penicillin, crystalline penicillin, or procaine penicillin in a suitable ointment base, with or without incorporation of a suitable anesthetic. **phenol o.,** a preparation of phenol, glycerin, and white ointment, containing 1.8–2.2 per cent of phenol; used as an antipruritic. Called also *carbolic acid o.* **pine tar o.,** a preparation of pine tar, yellow wax, and yellow ointment, used as a local antiezematic and rubefacient. **polyethylene glycol o.** [NF], a mixture of polyethylene glycol 4000 and polyethylene glycol 400, used as a water-soluble ointment base. **polymyxin B sulfate o.,** a semisolid preparation of polymyxin B sulfate in an anhydrous petrolatum base, containing 90 to 120 per cent of the labeled amount of polymyxin B, the labeled amount being 20,000 polymyxin B units per gram; used as a topical antibacterial agent to treat skin infections from susceptible gram-negative organisms. **resorcinol o., compound** [USP], a preparation of resorcinol, zinc oxide, bismuth subnitrate, juniper tar, yellow wax, petrolatum, anhydrous lanolin, and glycerin, used as a topical antifungal and keratolytic, applied topically. **rose water o.** [USP], a preparation of spermaceti, white wax, almond oil, sodium borate, stronger rose water, purified water, and rose oil, used as an emollient and ointment base. **rose water o., petrolatum,** an ointment prepared with spermaceti, white wax, mineral oil, sodium borate, rose water, purified water, and rose oil. **scarlet red o.,** a preparation of scarlet red, olive oil, anhydrous lanolin, and petrolatum, applied locally as a protective agent. **simple o.,** white o. **sulfacetamide sodium ophthalmic o.** [USP], a sterile ointment containing 95 to 105 per cent of the labeled amount of sulfacetamide sodium; used as an antibacterial in sulfonamide-responsive eye infections, applied topically to the conjunctiva. **sulfisoxazole diolamine ophthalmic s.** [USP], a sterile ointment containing sulfisoxazole diolamine equivalent to 90 to 110 per cent of the labeled amount of sulfisoxazole; used as an antibacterial in the treatment of sulfonamide-responsive eye infections. **sulfur o.** [USP], a mixture of precipitated sulfur, mineral oil, and white ointment, used as a scabicide. **tar o., compound,** a preparation of rectified tar oil, benzoin tincture, zinc oxide, yellow wax, lard, and cottonseed oil, used locally as an antibacterial and irritant. **tetracaine o.** [USP], an ointment containing 5 per cent of tetracaine in a suitable ointment base; used as a local anesthetic, applied topically to the conjunctiva. **tetracaine ophthalmic o.** [USP], a sterile ointment containing 5 per cent tetracaine in white petrolatum; used a local anesthetic, applied topically to the conjunctiva. **triamcinolone acetonide o.** [USP], a semisolid preparation of triamcinolone acetonide in a suitable ointment base, containing 90 to 115 per cent of the labeled amount of triamcinolone acetonide; used as a topical anti-inflammatory in steroid-responsive dermatoses. **triclobisonium chloride o.,** an ointment containing 90 to 110 per cent of the labeled amount of triclobisonium chloride; used as a topical anti-infective agent, primarily in gynecological infections. **undecylenic acid o., compound, 1.** [USP] a preparation containing 5 per cent undecylenic acid and 20 per cent zinc undecylenate in a suitable ointment base; used as a topical antifungal. **2.** a preparation of clove and cinnamon oils, salicylic acid, undecylenic acid, benzoic acid, and white petrolatum, used in podiatry. **white o.** [USP], an oleaginous ointment base prepared from white wax and white petrolatum. **Whitfield's o.**, benzoic and salicylic acid o. **yellow o.** [USP], a mixture of yellow wax and petrolatum, used as an ointment base for drugs. **zinc o.**, zinc oxide o. **zinc oxide o.** [USP], a preparation of zinc oxide and mineral oil in white ointment, used topically as an astringent and protective.

Oken's body (corpus), canal (o'kenz) [Lorenz *Oken*, German physiologist, 1779–1851] see *mesonephros* and *ductus mesonephricus.*

O.L. abbreviation for L. *o'culus lae'vus,* left eye.

Ol. abbreviation for L. *o'leum,* oil.

-ol suffix indicating that the substance is an alcohol or a phenol, i.e., a hydroxyl derivative of a hydrocarbon.

O.L.A. abbreviation for L. *occipito-laeva anterior* (left occipito-anterior, a position of the fetus).

olamine (ol'ah-mēn) USAN contraction for ethanolamine.

Olea (o'le-ah) a genus of small trees or shrubs having oily fruit, including the true wild olive (*O. oleaster*) and the common olive (*O. europaea* L.).

olea[1] (o'le-ah) [L.] olive.

olea[2] (o'le-ah) [L.] plural of *oleum.*

oleaginous (o″le-aj'ĭ-nus) [L. *oleaginus*] oily; greasy; unctuous.

oleander (o″le-an'der) a poisonous evergreen apocynaceous shrub, *Nerium oleander,* whose roots, flowers, seeds, and bark contain a cardiac glycoside.

oleandomycin phosphate (o″le-an′do-mi″sin) a macrolide antibiotic, $C_{35}H_{61}NO_{12} \cdot H_3PO_4$, elaborated by the growth of *Streptomyces antibioticus,* resembling erythromycin in chemical structure, actions, and uses but having weaker antibacterial activity; it has been used chiefly in the treatment of infections due to staphylococci and other gram-positive bacteria resistant to other systemic antibiotics, administered parenterally.

oleandrin (o″le-an'drin) 1. a cardiac glycoside, $C_{30}H_{46}O_8$, from oleander, composed of digitalose and digitaligenin. 2. an alkaloid, $C_{32}H_{48}O_9$, from oleander which is a potent diuretic and has been used in cardiac insufficiency.

oleandrism (o″le-an'drizm) poisoning by oleander.

oleanol (o-le'ah-nol) a white solid alcohol, $C_{18}H_{35}OH$, from the liver oils of fish.

oleaster (o″le-as'ter) 1. the true wild olive, *Olea oleaster.* 2. any plant of the genus *Elaeagnus,* a large shrub or small tree native to Asia and southern Europe, but especially the Russian olive (*E. angustifolia*).

oleate (o'le-āt) 1. any salt or ester of oleic acid. 2. [L. *olea-tum*] a solution of an alkaloid or other basic drug in oleic acid, used as an ointment.

olecranal (o-lek'rah-nal) pertaining to the olecranon.

olecranarthritis (o-lek″ran-ar-thri'tis) [*olecranon* + *arthritis*] inflammation of the elbow joint.

olecranarthrocace (o-lek″ran-ar-throk'ah-se) [*olecranon* + Gr. *arthron* joint + *kakē* badness] tuberculosis of the elbow joint.

olecranarthropathy (o-lek″ran-ar-throp'ah-the) [*olecranon* + Gr. *arthron* joint + *pathos* disease] disease of the elbow joint.

olecranoid (o-lek'rah-noid) resembling the olecranon.

olecranon (o-lek'rah-non) [Gr. *ōlekranon*] [NA] the proximal bony projection of the ulna at the elbow, its anterior surface forming part of the trochlear notch.

olefin (o'le-fin) [*oleo-* + L. *facere* to make] an unsaturated hydrocarbon; alkene.

oleic acid (o-le'ik) trivial name for *cis*-9-octadecenoic acid, the Δ^9-unsaturated, 18-carbon, straight-chain fatty acid; it is liquid at room temperature and occurs in most animal fats and vegetable oils.

olein (o'le-in) glycerotrioleate, $C_3H_5[CH_3(CH_2)_7CH:CH-(CH_2)_7CO \cdot O]_3$, found in various fixed oils and fats; it is a colorless, oily liquid, insoluble in water but freely soluble in ether and alcohol.

olenitis (o-len-i'tis) inflammation of the elbow joint.

ole(o)- [L. *oleum* oil] a combining form denoting relationship to oil.

oleochrysotherapy (o″le-o-kris″o-ther'ah-pe) [*oleo-* + Gr.

chrysos gold + *therapy*] therapeutic administration of gold salts in oily suspensions.

oleocreosote (o″le-o-kre'o-sōt) the oleic acid ester of creosote.

oleodipalmitin (o″le-o-di-pal'mĭ-tin) a fat found in soya bean oil, butter, cocoa fat, etc.

oleodistearin (o″le-o-di-ste'ah-rin) a fat found in the seeds of the Indian mango, *Mangifera indica.*

oleogranuloma (o″le-o-gran″u-lo'mah) paraffinoma.

oleoinfusion (o″le-o-in-fu'zhun) a preparation made by infusing a drug in oil.

oleoma (o″le-o'mah) [*oleo-* + *-oma*] paraffinoma.

oleomargarine (o″le-o-mar'jah-rin) margarine, def. 1.

oleometer (o″le-om'ĕ-ter) [*oleo-* + Gr. *metron* measure] an instrument for testing the purity of oil.

oleonucleoprotein (o″le-o-nu″kle-o-pro'te-in) the caseinogen and fat of milk regarded as forming one complex substance.

oleopalmitate (o″le-o-pal'mĭ-tāt) an oleate and a palmitate of the same base.

oleoperitoneography (o″le-o-per″ĭ-to-ne-og'rah-fe) roentgenography of the peritoneum following the injection of iodized oil.

oleoresin (o″le-o-rez'in) [*oleo-* + *resin*] 1. any natural combination of a resin and a volatile oil such as exudes from pines and other plants. 2. a compound prepared by exhausting a drug by percolation with a volatile solvent, such as acetone, alcohol, or ether, and evaporating the solvent. **aspidium o.**, a thick dark green liquid, an ether extract from aspidium, yielding not less than 24 per cent of crude filicin; used as an anthelmintic in the treatment of intestinal tapeworm infestation. **capsicum o.**, the extract from capsicum obtained by percolation, with either acetone or ether as the menstruum; used as an irritant and carminative.

oleosaccharum (o″le-o-sak'ah-rum) eleosaccharum.

oleostearate (o″le-o-ste'ar-āt) an oleate and a stearate of the same base.

oleosus (o″le-o'sus) [L.] oily; greasy.

oleotherapy (o″le-o-ther'ah-pe) [*oleo-* + *therapy*] treatment with oil, particularly treatment by the injection of oil.

oleotine (o″le-o'tīn) a peptonized fat for use as a butter substitute.

oleovitamin (o″le-o-vi'tah-min) a preparation of fish liver oil or edible vegetable oil containing one or more fat-soluble vitamins or their derivatives. **o. A**, an oily preparation containing the natural or synthetic form of vitamin A. **o. A and D** [USP], an oily preparation containing vitamin A and natural or synthetic vitamin D; used as a dietary supplement. **o. D, synthetic**, a solution of calciferol or of activated 7-dehydrocholesterol in an edible vegetable oil, used as an antirachitic vitamin. **o. D₂**, calciferol. **o. D₃**, 7-dehydrocholesterol, activated.

oleum (o'le-um), gen. *o'lei*, pl. *o'lea* [L.] oil. **o. ae-the'reum**, ethereal oil. **o. amyg'dalae ama'rae**, bitter almond oil. **o. amyg'dalae expres'sum**, almond oil. **o. ane'thi**, oil of dill. **o. arach'idis**, peanut oil. **o. auran'tii**, orange oil. **o. auran'tii ama'ri**, bitter orange oil. **o. auran'tii flo'ris**, orange flower oil. **o. bergamot'tae**, bergamot oil. **o. bet'ulae empyreumat'icum rectifica'tum**, rectified birch tar oil. **o. cardamo'mi**, cardamom oil. **o. ca'ri**, caraway oil. **o. caryophyl'li**, clove oil. **o. chaulmoo'grae**, chaulmoogra oil. **o. chenopo'dii**, chenopodium oil. **o. co'cois**, coconut oil. **o. eucalyp'ti**, eucalyptus oil. **o. gossyp'ii sem'inis**, cottonseed oil. **o. hippoglos'si**, halibut liver oil. **o. jec'oris asel'li**, cod liver oil. **o. junip'eri**, juniper oil. **o. junip'eri empyreumat'icum**, juniper tar. **o. li'ni**, linseed oil. **o. may'dis**, corn oil. **o. men'thae piperi'tae**, peppermint oil. **o. mor'rhuae**, cod liver oil. **o. myr'ciae**, myrcia oil. **o. pi'cis li'quidae rectifica'tum**, **o. pi'cis rectifica'tum**, rectified tar oil. **o. pimen'tae**, pimenta oil. **o. pi'ni**, pine oil. **o. pi'ni pumili-o'nis**, dwarf pine needle oil. **o. ric'ini**, castor oil. **o. ric'ini aromat'icum**, aromatic castor oil. **o. rosmari'ni**, rosemary oil. **o. rus'ci**, rectified birch tar oil. **o. san'tali**, santal oil. **o. ses'ami**, sesame oil. **o. terebin'thinae**, turpentine oil. **o. terebin'thinae**

rectifica′tum, rectified turpentine oil. **o. thy′mi,** thyme oil. **o. tig′lii,** croton oil.

olfact (ol′fakt) a unit of odor, the *minimum perceptible odor,* being the minimum concentration of a substance in solution which can be perceived by a large number of normal individuals, expressed in terms of grams per liter.

olfactie (ol-fak′te) a term applied by Zwaardemaker to a unit of the distance of withdrawal of the tube of his olfactometer at which an odorous substance was recognized, representing the exposed surface area of the odorous or solution-impregnated substance of which the cylinders were made.

olfaction (ol-fak′shun) [L. *olfacere* to smell] the act of smelling; the sense of smell.

olfactism (ol-fak′tizm) a sensation of smell produced by other than olfactory stimuli.

olfactology (ol″fak-tol′o-je) the science of the sense of smell.

olfactometer (ol″fak-tom′ĕ-ter) [L. *olfactus* smell + *metrum* measure] an apparatus for testing the sensitiveness of perception of odors.

olfactometry (ol″fak-tom′ĕ-tre) the study of the sense of smell.

olfactory (ol-fak′to-re) [L. *olfacere* to smell] pertaining to olfaction, or the sense of smell.

olfactus (ol-fak′tus) a unit of acuity of smell. See also under *organum.*

oligakisuria (ol″ĭ-gak″ĭ-su′re-ah) [Gr. *oligakis* few times + *ouron* urine + *-ia*] a condition in which urination occurs at long intervals.

oligemia (ol″ĭ-ge′me-ah) [*oligo-* + Gr. *haima* blood + *-ia*] deficiency in the volume of the blood.

oligemic (ol″ĭ-ge′mik) pertaining to or characterized by oligemia.

olig(o)- [Gr. *oligos* little, few] a combining form meaning (*a*) few, little, or scanty, (*b*) less than normal, or (*c*) deficient. Cf. *pauci–*

oligoamnios (ol″ĭ-go-am′ne-os) [*oligo-* + *amnios*] oligohydramnios.

oligoblast (ol′ĭ-go-blast″) a primitive oligodendrocyte.

oligocardia (ol″ĭ-go-kar′de-ah) [*oligo-* + Gr. *kardia* heart] bradycardia.

oligochromasia (ol″ĭ-go-kro-ma′se-ah) hypochromasia.

oligochromemia (ol″ĭ-go-kro-me′me-ah) [*oligo-* + Gr. *chrōma* color + *haima* blood + *-ia*] insufficiency of hemoglobin in the blood.

oligocystic (ol″ĭ-go-sis′tik) [*oligo-* + Gr. *kystis* sac, bladder] containing only a few cysts.

oligocythemia (ol″ĭ-go-si-the′me-ah) [*oligo-* + *-cyte* + Gr. *haima* blood + *-ia*] reduction in the red cell mass of the blood; called also *oligocytosis.*

oligocythemic (ol″ĭ-go-si-them′ik) relating to or affected with oligocythemia.

oligocytosis (ol″ĭ-go-si-to′sis) oligocythemia.

oligodactyly (ol″ĭ-go-dak′tĭ-le) [*oligo-* + Gr. *daktylos* finger] a developmental anomaly characterized by a smaller than usual number of fingers or toes.

oligodendria (ol″ĭ-go-den′dre-ah) oligodendroglia.

oligodendroblastoma (ol″ĭ-go-den″dro-blas-to′mah) oligodendroglioma.

oligodendrocyte (ol″ĭ-go-den′dro-sīt) [*oligodendro* glia + *-cyte*] see *oligodendroglia.*

oligodendroglia (ol″ĭ-go-den-drog′le-ah) [*oligo-* + Gr. *dendron* dendron + *neuroglia*] 1. the non-neural cells of ectodermal origin forming part of the adventitial structure (neuroglia) of the central nervous system; projections of the surface membrane of each of these cells (oligodendrocytes) fan out and coil around the axon of many neurons to form myelin sheaths in the white matter. With microglia, they form the perineuronal satellites in the gray matter. 2. the tissue composed of such cells.

oligodendroglioma (ol″ĭ-go-den″dro-gli-o′mah) a neoplasm derived from and composed of oligodendrogliocytes in varying stages of differentiation; called also *oligodendroblastoma.*

oligodipsia (ol″ĭ-go-dip′se-ah) [*oligo-* + Gr. *dipsa* thirst + *-ia*] abnormally diminished thirst.

oligodontia (ol″ĭ-go-don′she-ah) [*olig-* + *odont-* + *-ia*] absence of many teeth, usually associated with small size of the existing teeth and other anomalies.

oligodynamic (ol″ĭ-go-di-nam′ik) [*oligo-* + Gr. *dynamis* power] active in very minute quantities; said especially of heavy metal ions (Hg^{2+}, Ag^+) to describe toxic effect on cells and organisms.

oligoencephalon (ol″ĭ-go-en-sef′ah-lon) [*oligo-* + Gr. *enkephalos* brain] micrencephalon (def. 1).

oligogalactia (ol″ĭ-go-gah-lak′she-ah) [*oligo-* + Gr. *gala* milk + *-ia*] deficient secretion of milk.

oligogenic (ol″e-go-jen′ik) [*oligo-* + *gene*] produced by a few genes at most; used in reference to certain hereditary characters.

oligogenics (ol″ĭ-go-jen′iks) [*oligo-* + Gr. *gennan* to produce] limitation of the number of offspring; birth control.

oligoglia (ol″ĭ-gog′le-ah) oligodendroglia.

oligo-1,6-glucosidase (ol″ĭ-go gloo-ko′sĭ-dās) [EC 3.2.1.10] α-dextrinase.

oligohemia (ol″ĭ-go-he′me-ah) oligemia.

oligohydramnios (ol″ĭ-go-hi-dram′ne-os) [*oligo-* + Gr. *hydōr* water + *amnion*] the presence of less than 300 ml. of amniotic fluid at term.

oligohydruria (ol″ĭ-go-hi-droo′re-ah) [*oligo-* + Gr. *hydōr* water + *ouron* urine + *-ia*] abnormally high concentration of the urine.

Oligohymenophorea (ol″ĭ-go-hi″mĕ-no-for′e-ah) [*oligo-* + *hymen* + Gr. *phoros* bearing] a class of ciliate protozoa (phylum Cilophora), characterized by the presence of an oral apparatus that is usually well developed and situated at least partially in a buccal cavity and by oral ciliature that is clearly distinct from the somatic ciliature, consisting of a paroral membrane on the right side and a few compound organelles on the left. Some species are loricate, and colony formation is common in some groups. It comprises two subclasses: Hymenostomatia and Peritrichia.

oligohypermenorrhea (ol″ĭ-go-hi″per-men″o-re′ah) infrequent menstruation with excessive menstrual flow.

oligohypomenorrhea (ol″ĭ-go-hi″po-men″o-re′ah) infrequent menstruation with diminished menstrual flow.

oligolecithal (ol″ĭ-go-les′ĭ-thal) [*oligo-* + Gr. *lekithos* yolk] possessing only a little yolk.

oligomeganephronia (ol″ĭ-go-meg″ah-nĕ-fro′ne-ah) [*oligo-* + Gr. *megas* great + *nephros* kidney] congenital renal hypoplasia in which there is a reduction in the number of lobes and of total number of nephrons, and hypertrophy of the nephrons.

oligomeganephronic (ol″ĭ-go-meg″ah-nef-ron′ik) 1. characterized by a reduced number of and hypertrophy of the nephrons. 2. pertaining to oligomeganephronia.

oligomenorrhea (ol″ĭ-go-men″o-re′ah) [*oligo-* + Gr. *mēn* month + *rhoia* flow] markedly diminished menstrual flow; relative amenorrhea.

oligometallic (ol″ĭ-go-mĕ-tal′ik) containing only small quantities of metals.

oligomorphic (ol″ĭ-go-mor′fik) [*oligo-* + Gr. *morphē* form] passing through only a few forms of growth; said of microorganisms.

oligonecrospermia (ol″ĭ-go-nek″ro-sper′me-ah) [*oligo-* + Gr. *nekros* dead + *sperma* sperm + *-ia*] a condition of the spermatic fluid in which there is diminution of the number of spermatozoa, some of which are dead.

oligonitrophilic (ol″ĭ-go-ni″tro-fil′ik) [*oligo-* + *nitrogen* + Gr. *philein* to love] absorbing nitrogen from the air and from media containing combined nitrogen; said of microorganisms.

oligonucleotide (ol″ĭ-go-nu′kle-o-tīd) [*oligo-* + *nucleotide*] a polymer made up of a few (2–10) nucleotides. In molecular genetics, a short sequence synthesized to match a region where a mutation is known to occur, and then used as a probe (oligonucleotide probe).

oligo-ovulation (ol″ĭ-go-ov″u-la′shun) maturation and discharge of fewer than the normal number of ova from the ovaries.

oligopeptide (ol″ĭ-go-pep′tīd) the structure formed by the linkage of a few amino acids.

oligophosphaturia (ol″ĭ-go-fos″fah-tu′re-ah) deficiency in the excretion of phosphates in the urine.

oligophrenia (ol″ĭ-go-fre′ne-ah) [*oligo-* + Gr. *phrēn* mind + *-ia*] (*obs.*) mental retardation. **moral o.**, see under *insanity*. **phenylpyruvic o.** (*obs.*), the mental retardation of untreated phenylketonuria. **polydystrophic o.**, Sanfilippo's syndrome.

oligophrenic (ol″i-go-fren′ik) pertaining to oligophrenia.

oligopnea (ol″ĭ-gop-ne′ah) [*oligo-* + Gr. *pnoia* breath] hypoventilation.

oligoposia (ol″ĭ-go-po′ze-ah) [*oligo-* + Gr. *posis* drinking + *-ia*] abnormally diminished ingestion of fluids.

oligoposy (ol″ĭ-gop′o-se) oligoposia.

oligopyrene, oligopyrous (ol″ĭ-go-pi′rēn; ol″ĭ-go-pi′rus) [*oligo-* + Gr. *pyrēn* stone of fruit] deficient in nuclear or chromatin material.

oligosaccharide (ol″ĭ-go-sak′ah-rīd) a carbohydrate which on hydrolysis yields a small number (from two to four or as many as ten, according to various authorities) of monosaccharides. Cf. *polysaccharide*.

oligospermatism (ol″ĭ-go-sper′mah-tizm) oligospermia.

oligospermia (ol″ĭ-go-sper′me-ah) [*oligo-* + Gr. *sperma* seed + *-ia*] deficiency in the number of spermatozoa in the semen.

oligosynaptic (ol″ĭ-go-sin-ap′tik) [*oligo-* + *synaptic*] involving a few synapses in series and therefore a sequence of only a few neurons; called also *paucisynaptic*. Cf. *polysynaptic*.

Oligotrichida (ol″lĭ-go-trik′ĭ-dah) [*oligo-* + Gr. *thrix* hair] an order of free-swimming, mainly pelagic ciliate protozoa (subclass Spirotricha, class Polyhymenophorea) having an ovoid to elongate, sometimes tailed body; a thickened pellicle with a perilemma external to the cell membrane in many species; reduced somatic ciliature; and an extensive adoral zone of membranelles, often with one part inside the body and another on the body surface. It comprises two suborders: Oligotrichina and Tintinnina.

Oligotrichina (o″lĭ-go-trĭ-ki′nah) a suborder of mostly marine ciliate protozoa (order Oligotrichida, subclass Spirotricha), characterized by somatic ciliature commonly reduced to a few short cirruslike bristles, and by a prominent bipartile adoral zone of membranelles, forming an open or closed ring, with the perioral region used in locomotion.

oligotrophia (ol″ĭ-go-tro′fe-ah) [*oligo-* + Gr. *trophē* nourishment + *-ia*] a state of poor (insufficient) nutrition.

oligotrophic (ol″ĭ-go-trof′ik) pertaining to, characterized by, or conducive to poor (insufficient) nutrition.

oligotrophy (ol″ĭ-go-got′ro-fe) oligotrophia.

oligozoospermatism (ol″ĭ-go-zo″o-sper′mah-tizm) oligospermia.

oligozoospermia (ol″ĭ-go-zo″o-sper′me-ah) oligospermia.

oliguresis (ol″ĭ-gu-re′sis) oliguria.

oliguria (ol″ĭ-gu′re-ah) [*oligo-* + Gr. *ouron* urine + *-ia*] secretion of a diminished amount of urine in relation to the fluid intake. Called also *hypouresis* and *oligouresis*.

oliguric (ol″ĭ-gu′rik) pertaining to or characterized by oliguria.

olisthe (o-lis′the) olisthy.

olisthy (o-lis′the) [Gr. *olisthanein* to slip] a slipping, as the slipping of the bones of a joint from their normal relation in the joint.

oliva (o-li′vah), gen. and pl. *oli′vae* [L.] [NA] a rounded elevation, lateral to the upper part of each pyramid of the medulla oblongata, between the ventrolateral and dorsolateral sulci. It is produced by an irregular mass of gray substance (*nucleus olivaris caudalis*) located just beneath its surface. Called also *ventral olive, inferior olive*, and *olivary body* or *nucleus*. **o. cerebella′ris**, nucleus dentatus.

olivae (o-li′ve) [L.] genitive and plural of *oliva*.

olivary (ol′ĭ-ver″e) [L. *olivarius*] shaped like an olive, as the olivary nucleus.

olive (ol′iv) [L. *oliva*] 1. the tree *Olea europaea* L. (Oleaceae), and its fruit. The latter affords a fixed oil (*olive oil, sweet oil*), which consists chiefly of olein and palmitin, and is employed as a food, as a mild laxative, and as an application to wounds, bruises, etc. Used also in soap manufacture, sulfonated oils, and cosmetics, and in pharmaceutical formulations. 2. a rounded elevation, lateral to the upper part of each pyramid of the medulla oblongata; see *oliva*. **infe-**

rior **o.**, oliva. **spurge o.**, mezereum. **superior o.**, nucleus dorsalis corporis trapezoidei.

Oliver's sign (ol′ĭ-verz) [William Silver *Oliver*, English physician, 1836–1908] tracheal tugging.

Oliver's test (ol′ĭ-verz) [George *Oliver*, English physician, 1841–1915] see under *tests*.

olivifugal (ol″ĭ-vif′u-gal) [*olive* + L. *fugere* to flee] moving or conducting away from the oliva.

olivipetal (ol″ĭ-vip′e-tal) [*olive* + L. *petere* to seek] passing or conducting toward the oliva.

olivopontocerebellar (ol″ĭ-vo-pon″to-ser″ĕ-bel′ar) pertaining to the olivae, the middle peduncles, and the cortex of the cerebellum.

Ollier's disease, law, layer (ol″e-āz′) [Léopold Louis Xavier Edouard *Ollier*, French surgeon, 1830–1900] see *enchondromatosis*, and under *law* and *layer*.

Ollier-Thiersch graft (ol″e-a′tērsh′) [L.L.X.E. *Ollier*; Karl *Thiersch*, German surgeon, 1822–1895] see under *graft*.

Ol. oliv. abbreviation for L. *o′leum oli′vae*, olive oil.

olophonia (ol″lo-fo′ne-ah) [Gr. *oloos* destroyed, lost + *phōnē* voice + *-ia*] defective speech due to malformed vocal organs.

O.L.P. abbreviation for L. *occipito-laeva posterior* (left occipitoposterior, a position of the fetus).

Olpitrichum (ol-pĭ-trik′um) a genus of imperfect fungi of the order Moniliales, family Monidiaceae, which contains species of the former genera *Oidium* and *Acladium;* they are found in soil, and are sometimes isolated from infected wounds.

Olshausen's operation (ols′how-zenz) [Robert von *Olshausen*, obstetrician in Berlin, 1835–1915] see under *operation*.

Olshevsky tube (ol-shev′ske) [Dimitry E. *Olshevsky*, American physician, born 1900] see under *tube*.

O.L.T. abbreviation for L. *occipito-laeva transversa* (left occipitotransverse, a position of the fetus).

o.m. abbreviation for L. *om′ni ma′ne*, every morning.

-oma [Gr. *ōma*, noun-forming suffix] a word termination meaning tumor or neoplasm of the part indicated by the stem to which it is attached.

omacephalus (o″mah-sef′ah-lus) [Gr. *ōmos* shoulder + *a* neg. + *kephalē* head] a fetus with a deficient head and no upper extremities.

omagra (o-ma′grah) [Gr. *ōmos* shoulder + *agra* seizure] gout in the shoulder.

omalgia (o-mal′je-ah) [Gr. *ōmos* shoulder + *-algia*] pain in the shoulder.

omarthritis (o″mar-thri′tis) [Gr. *ōmos* shoulder + *arthron* joint + *-itis*] inflammation of the shoulder joint.

omasitis (o″mah-si′tis) inflammation of the omasum.

omasum (o-ma′sum) [L.] the third division of the stomach of ruminant animals; called also *manyplies* and *psalterium*.

Ombrédanne's operation (ahm-bra-danz′) [Louis Ombrédanne, Paris surgeon, 1871–1956] see under *operation*.

ombrophore (om′bro-fōr) [Gr. *ombros* rain + *phoros* bearer] an apparatus for applying a douche bath of water containing carbon dioxide.

omeire (o-mi′re) a native drink of southwest Africa, made by permitting milk to ferment.

omenta (o-men′tah) [L.] plural of *omentum*.

omental (o-men′tal) pertaining to the omentum.

omentectomy (o″men-tek′to-me) [*omentum* + Gr. *ektomē* excision] excision of all or a portion of the omentum.

omentitis (o″men-ti′tis) inflammation of the omentum.

omentofixation (o-men″to-fik-sa′shun) omentopexy.

omentopexy (o-men′to-pek″se) [*omentum* + Gr. *pēxis* fixation] in general, an operation in which omentum is fastened to other tissue, especially one in which omentum is used as a circulatory bridge to reduce congestion or provide vascular nutrition.

omentoplasty (o-men′to-plas″te) [*omentum* + Gr. *plassein* to form] the use of omental grafts to cover raw surfaces in abdominal surgery.

omentoportography (o-men″to-por-tog′rah-fe) roentgenography of the hepatic portal veins after injection of a contrast medium into the gastroepiploic vein in the base of the omentum.

omentorrhaphy (o″men-tor′ah-fe) [*omentum* + Gr. *rhaphē* suture] suture or repair of the omentum.

omentotomy (o″men-tot′o-me) [*omentum* + Gr. *temnein* to cut] incision of the omentum.

omentovolvulus (o-men″to-vol′vu-lus) volvulus of the omentum.

omentum (o-men′tum), pl. *omen′ta* [L. "fat skin"] a fold of peritoneum extending from the stomach to adjacent organs in the abdominal cavity; see *omentum majus* and *omentum minus*. **colic o., gastrocolic o.**, o. majus. **gastrohepatic o.**, o. minus. **gastrosplenic o.**, ligamentum gastrolienale. **greater o.**, o. majus. **lesser o.**, 1. ligamentum hepatogastricum. 2. omentum minus. **o. ma′jus** [NA], greater omentum: a prominent peritoneal fold suspended from the greater curvature of the stomach and passing inferiorly a variable distance in front of the intestines; it is attached to the anterior surface of the transverse colon. **o. mi′nus** [NA], lesser omentum: a peritoneal fold joining the lesser curvature of the stomach and the first part of the duodenum to the porta hepatis. **pancreaticosplenic o.**, a fold of peritoneum connecting the tail of the pancreas and the visceral surface of the spleen. **splenogastric o.**, ligamentum gastrolienale.

omentumectomy (o-men″tum-ek′to-me) [*omentum* + Gr. *ektomē* excision] omentectomy.

omicron (om′ĭ-kron) [O, o] the fifteenth letter of the Greek alphabet.

omitis (o-mi′tis) [*omo-* + -*itis*] inflammation of the shoulder.

ommatidium, (om″ah-tid′e-um), pl. *ommatid′ia* [Gr. dim. of *omma* eye] one of the units of the compound eye of arthropods, itself complete with all the functional and structural elements of the eye (including lens, retina, photoreceptor cells).

Ommaya reservoir (ŏ-mi′yah) [Ayub Khan *Ommaya*, Pakistani neurosurgeon in the United States, born 1930] see under *reservoir*.

ommochrome (om′o-krōm) [Gr. *omma* eye + *chrōma* color] a product of tryptophan metabolism which gives rise to pigments, particularly the eye pigments of certain animals; it is apparently not involved in the visual processes.

Omn. bih. abbreviation for L. *om′ni biho′ra*, every two hours

Omn. hor. abbreviation for L. *om′ni ho′ra*, every hour.

Omnipen (om′nĭ-pen) trademark for preparations of ampicillin.

omnivorous (om-niv′o-rus) [L. *omnis* all + *vorare* to eat] subsisting upon both plants and animals.

Omn. noct. abbreviation for L. *om′ni noc′te*, every night.

om(o)- [Gr. *ōmos* shoulder] a combining form denoting relationship to the shoulder.

omocephalus (o″mo-sef′ah-lus) [*omo-* + Gr. *kephalē* head] a fetus with no arms and an incomplete head.

omoclavicular (o″mo-klah-vik′u-lar) pertaining to the shoulder and the clavicle.

omodynia (o″mo-din′e-ah) [*omo-* + Gr. *odynē* pain] pain in the shoulder.

omohyoid (o″mo-hi′oid) pertaining to the shoulder and the hyoid bone.

omophagia (o″mo-fa′je-ah) [Gr. *ōmos* raw + *phagein* to eat] the eating of raw food.

omoplata (o″mo-plat′ah) [Gr. *ōmoplatē* the shoulder-blade] the scapula.

omosternum (o″mo-ster′num) the interarticular cartilage at the joint between the sternum and clavicle.

OMPA octamethyl pyrophosphoramide.

omphalectomy (om″fah-lek′to-me) [*omphalo-* + Gr. *ektomē* excision] excision of the umbilicus.

omphalelcosis (om″fal-el-ko′sis) [*omphalo-* + Gr. *helkōsis* ulceration] ulceration of the umbilicus.

omphalic (om-fal′ik) [Gr. *omphalikos*] pertaining to the umbilicus.

omphalitis (om″fah-li′tis) [*omphalo-* + -*itis*] inflammation of the umbilicus. **o. of birds**, infection of the yolk sac with bacteria normally found in the alimentary tract and on the skin of the hen, leading to death of the embryos and chicks, occurring up to ten days after hatching; called also *mushy chick disease*.

omphal(o) [Gr. *omphalos* navel] a combining form denoting relationship to the umbilicus.

omphaloangiopagous (om″fah-lo-an″je-op′ah-gus) [*omphalo-* + Gr. *angeion* vessel + *pagos* thing fixed] allantoidoangiopagous.

omphaloangiopagus (om″fah-lo-an″je-op′ah-gus) allantoidoangiopagus.

omphalocele (om″fah-lo-sēl″) [*omphalo-* + Gr. *kēlē* hernia] protrusion, at birth, of part of the intestine through a large defect in the abdominal wall at the umbilicus, the protruding bowel being covered only by a thin transparent membrane composed of amnion and peritoneum.

omphalochorion (om″fah-lo-ko′re-on) the structure formed by fusion of the yolk sac with the chorion; a choriovitelline placenta.

omphalodidymus (om″fah-lo-did′ĭ-mus) [*omphalo-* + Gr. *didymos* twin] gastrodidymus.

omphalogenesis (om″fah-lo-jen′ĕ-sis) [*omphalo-* + Gr. *genesis* formation] development of the umbilicus or yolk sac in the embryo.

omphaloma (om″fah-lo′mah) [*omphalo-* + -*oma*] a tumor of the umbilicus.

omphalomesaraic (om″fah-lo-mes-ah-ra′ik) omphalomesenteric.

omphalomesenteric (om″fah-lo-mes″en-ter′ik) pertaining to the umbilicus and mesentery.

omphaloncus (om″fah-long′kus) [*omphalo-* + Gr. *onkos* mass, bulk] omphaloma.

omphalopagus (om″fah-lop′ah-gus) [*omphalo-* + Gr. *pagos* thing fixed] monomphalus.

omphalophlebitis (om″fah-lo-fle-bi′tis) [*omphalo-* + Gr. *phleps* vein + -*itis*] 1. inflammation of the umbilical veins. 2. a condition characterized by markedly suppurative lesions of the umbilicus in young animals, due to infection through the umbilicus; see *navel ill*, under *ill*.

omphalorrhagia (om″fah-lo-ra′je-ah) [*omphalo-* + Gr. *rhēgnynai* to burst forth] hemorrhage from the umbilicus.

omphalorrhea (om″fah-lo-re′ah) [*omphalo-* + Gr. *rhoia* flow] an effusion of lymph at the navel.

omphalorrhexis (om″fah-lo-rek′sis) [*omphalo-* + Gr. *rhēxis* rupture] rupture of the umbilicus.

omphalosite (om′fah-lo-sīt″) [*omphalo-* + Gr. *sitos* food] an underdeveloped member of allantoidoangiopagous twins, which is joined to the more developed member (autosite) by the vessels of the umbilical cord.

omphalotomy (om″fah-lot′o-me) [*omphalo-* + Gr. *tomē* a cutting] the cutting of the umbilical cord.

omphalus (om′fah-lus) [Gr. *omphalos*] the umbilicus.

Om. quar. hor. abbreviation for L. *om′ni quadran′te ho′ra*, every quarter of an hour.

o.n. abbreviation for L. *om′ni noc′te*, every night.

onanism (o′nah-nizm) [*Onan*, son of Judah] 1. coitus interruptus. 2. masturbation.

onaye (o-nah′ye) an exceedingly virulent poison from the seeds of *Strophanthus hispidus*.

onch(o)- see *onco-* (2).

Onchocerca (ong″ko-ser′kah) [Gr. *onkos* tumor + *kerkos* tail] a genus of nematode parasites of the superfamily Filarioidea. The adults live and breed in subcutaneous fibroid nodules; the young (the microfilariae) are carried by the lymph and are found chiefly in the skin, subcutaneous connective tissues, and eyes. **O. caecu′tiens**, *O. volvulus*. **O. cervica′lis**, a species found in the cervical ligament of horses and mules. **O. gibso′ni**, a species that infects the subcutaneous tissues of cattle and zebra, producing nodular swellings on the flanks, knees, and shoulders. **O. volvulus**, a common parasite of humans breeding in fast-flowing rivers and streams in southern Mexico, Guatemala, northern South America, equatorial Africa, particularly West Africa. It is the etiologic agent of human onchocerciasis and is transmitted by the bites of blackflies (buffalo gnats) of the genus *Simulium*, in which the parasite passes part of its life cycle. Formerly called *Filaria volvulus* and *O. caecutiens*.

onchocerciasis (on″ko-ser-ki′ah-sis) [*oncho-* + Gr. *kerkos* tail + *iasis*] the state of being infected with worms of the genus *Onchocerca*. Human infection is caused by *O. volvulus*, with heavy infestations usually being characterized by: firm, generally freely movable, nontender subcutaneous nodules (onchocercomas) containing tangled masses of adult worms; a persistent dermatitis manifested by an intensely pruritic papular rash, which may be associated with edema, lichenification, thickening, wrinkling, and atrophy of the skin, areas of leukoderma giving the skin a spotted appearance, and lymphadenitis; and ocular lesions, directly or indirectly related to the invasion and local death of the microfilariae of *O. volvulus*, which may progress to optic neuritis, optic atrophy, and blindness. Called also *onchocercosis* and *volvulosis*. The condition is also known by many local and regional names (e.g., craw-craw and Robles' disease) and by various names descriptive of the manifestations of the disease (e.g., *coast erysipelas, mal morado, river blindness* or *blinding filarial disease*, and *sowdah*).

onchocercoma (ong″ko-ser-ko′mah) [*oncho-* + Gr. *kerkos* tail + *-oma*] one of the dermal or subcutaneous nodules containing *Onchocerca volvulus* in human onchocerciasis.

onchocercosis (ong″ko-ser-ko′sis) onchocerciasis.

Onciolo (on-si′o-lah) a genus of acanthocephalous parasites. **O. ca′nis,** a species found in the intestines of dogs in Texas and Nebraska.

onc(o)- 1. [Gr. *onkos* mass, bulk] a combining form denoting relationship to a tumor, swelling, or mass. 2. [Gr. *onkos* barb, hook] a combining form denoting relationship to a barb or hook.

Oncocerca (ong″ko-ser′kah) *Onchocerca*.

oncocyte (on′ko-sit″) a large epithelial cell with an extremely acidophilic and granular cytoplasm, containing vast numbers of mitochondria; such cells undergo neoplastic transformation.

oncocytic (on″ko-sit′ik) composed of or containing oncocytes.

oncocytoma (ong″ko-si-to′ma) [*oncocyte* + *-oma*] Hürthle cell tumor; see under *tumor*.

oncodnavirus (on-kod′nah-vi″rus) [*onco-* + *DNA* + *virus*] any DNA virus that causes cancer.

oncofetal (on″ko-fe′tal) see under *antigen*.

oncogene (ong′ko-jēn) a gene found in the chromosomes of tumor cells whose activation is associated with the initial and continuing conversion of normal cells into cancer cells.

oncogenesis (ong″ko-jen′ĕ-sis) [*onco-* + Gr. *genesis* production, generation] the production or causation of tumors.

oncogenetic (ong″ko-jĕ-net′ik) pertaining to or characterized by oncogenesis.

oncogenic (ong″ko-jen′ik) giving rise to tumors or causing tumor formation; said especially of tumor-inducing viruses. Cf. *tumorigenic*.

oncogenicity (ong″ko-jĕ-nis′ĭ-te) the quality or property of being able to cause tumor formation.

oncogenous (ong-koj′ĕ-nus) arising in or originating from a tumor.

oncoides (ong-koi′dēz) [*onco-* + Gr. *eidos* form] turgid swelling; intumescence.

oncology (ong-kol′o-je) [*onco-* + *-logy*] the sum of knowledge concerning tumors; the study of tumors.

oncolysate (on-kol′ĭ-sāt) any agent that lyses or destroys tumor cells.

oncolysis (ong-kol′ĭ-sis) [*onco-* + Gr. *lysis* dissolution] the lysis or destruction of tumor cells.

oncolytic (ong″ko-lit′ik) pertaining to, characterized by, or causing oncolysis.

oncoma (ong-ko′mah) [Gr. *onkōma*] a swelling; tumor.

Oncomelania (ong″ko-mĕ-la′ne-ah) a genus of snails species of which transmit schistosomiasis japonica; formerly called *Katayama*.

oncometer (ong-kom′ĕ-ter) an instrument for measuring oncotic pressure.

oncornavirus (on-kor′nah-vi″rus) [*onco-* + *RNA* + *virus*] any RNA virus that causes cancer.

oncosis (ong-ko′sis) [*onco-* + *-osis*] a morbid condition characterized by the development of tumors.

oncosphere (ong′ko-sfēr) [Gr. *onkos* barb + *sphaira* sphere] the larva of the tapeworm contained within the external embryonic envelope and armed with six hooks; it may be found in the feces.

oncotherapy (ong″ko-ther′ah-pe) [*onco-* + *therapy*] the treatment of tumors.

oncothlipsis (ong″ko-thlip′sis) [*onco-* + Gr. *thlipsis* pressure] pressure caused by a tumor.

oncotic (ong-kot′ik) pertaining to, caused by, or marked by swelling; see also under *pressure*.

oncotomy (ong-kot′o-me) [*onco-* + Gr. *temnein* to cut] the incision of a tumor or swelling.

oncotropic (ong″ko-trop′ik) [*onco-* + Gr. *tropos* a turning] having a special affinity or attraction for tumor cells.

Oncovin (on′ko-vin) trademark for a preparation of vincristine sulfate.

oncovirus (on′ko-vi″rus) [*onco-* + *virus*] any virus that causes cancer.

ondometer (on-dom′ĕ-ter) an apparatus for measuring the frequency of the oscillations in high frequency currents.

-one a suffix used in chemistry to indicate (*a*) quintivalent nitrogen, and (*b*) a compound having two hydrocarbon radicals attached to the carbonyl group; a ketone.

oneiric (o-ni′rik) pertaining to or characterized by dreaming.

oneirism (o-ni′rizm) an abnormal dreamlike state of consciousness.

oneir(o)- [Gr. *oneiros* dream] a combining form denoting relationship to a dream.

oneirodynia (o-ni″ro-din′e-ah) [*oneiro-* + Gr. *odynē* pain] nightmare.

oneirogenic (o″ni-ro-jen′ik) producing a dreamlike state; capable of causing dreams.

oneirogmus (o″ni-rog′mus) [Gr. *oneirōgmos* an effusion during sleep] emission of semen accompanying dreams.

oneiroid (o′ni-roid) resembling a dream.

oneirology (o″ni-rol′o-je) [*oneiro-* + *-logy*] the science of dreams.

oneirophrenia (o-ni″ro-fre′ne-ah) [*oneiro-* + Gr. *phrēn* mind + *-ia*] a form of schizophrenia characterized by clouding of consciousness.

oneiroscopy (o″ni-ros′ko-pe) [Gr. *oneiroskopilkos* of the interpretation of dreams] analysis of dreams for the purpose of diagnosing the patient's mental state.

onium (o′ne-um) a term applied to a cation in which nitrogen has its maximum covalency, as in the ammonium ion NH_4^+. The compounds include betaines, cholines, and amine oxides.

onkinocele (on-kin′o-sēl) [Gr. *onkos* swelling + *is* fiber + *kēlē* hernia, tumor] a swollen condition of a tendon sheath.

onlay (on′la) a graft applied or laid on the surface of an organ or structure. **epithelial o.,** an epithelial graft, the edges of which are not completely approximated to the edges of the wound, thus permitting new epithelium to grow out around the margin; see also under *inlay*.

onobaio (o″no-ba′yo) a powerful arrow poison from Obok, in Africa; it has a depressant action on the heart.

onomatology (on″o-mah-tol′o-je) [Gr. *onoma* name + *-logy*] the science of names and nomenclature.

onomatomania (on″o-mat″o-ma′ne-ah) [Gr. *onoma* name + *mania* madness] an irresistible impulse to repeat certain words.

onomatophobia (on″o-mat″o-fo′be-ah) [Gr. *onoma* name + *phobia*] irrational fear of hearing a particular word or name.

onomatopoiesis (on″o-mat″o-poi-e′sis) [Gr. *onoma* name + *poiein* to make] the formation of meaningless words that imitate sounds.

ontogenesis (on″to-jen′ĕ-sis) ontogeny.

ontogenetic (on″to-jĕ-net′ik) ontogenic.

ontogenic (on″to-jen′ik) pertaining to ontogeny.

ontogeny (on-toj′ĕ-ne) [Gr. *ōn* existing + *gennan* to produce] the development of the individual organism. Cf. *phylogeny*.

onyalai, onyalia (o″ne-al′a-e; o″ne-a′le-ah) a nutritional disorder occurring among the blacks in various parts of Africa, and marked by the formation, on the palatal and buccal mucous membrane, of blebs containing semicoagulated blood and without signs of constitutional disorder. It is a form of thrombopenic purpura.

onychatrophia (o″nik-ah-tro′fe-ah) [onych- + atrophia] atrophy of the nail(s).

onychatrophy (on″ik-at′ro-fe) onychatrophia.

onychauxis (on″ĭ-kawk′sis) [onych- + Gr. auxein to increase] simple hypertrophy of the nail(s) without deformity. Called also hyperonychia. Cf. onychogryphosis.

onychectomy (on″ĭ-kek′to-me) [onych- + Gr. ektomē excision] excision of a nail or nail bed, or of the claws of animals.

onychia (o-nik′e-ah) [onych- + -ia] inflammation of the matrix of the nail resulting in shedding of the nail. Called also onychitis. See also paronychia.

onychitis (on″ĭ-ki′tis) [onych- + -itis] onychia.

onych(o)- [Gr. onyx, gen. onychos nail] a combining form denoting relationship to the nails.

onychoclasis (on″ĭ-kok′lah-sis) [onycho- + Gr. klasis breaking] breaking of the nail.

onychocryptosis (on″ĭ-ko-krip-to′sis) [onycho- + Gr. kryptein to conceal] ingrown nail.

onychodystrophy (on″ĭ-ko-dis′tro-fe) [onycho- + dystrophy] dystrophia unguium.

onychogenic (on″ĭ-ko-jen′ik) [onycho- + Gr. gennan to produce] producing or forming nail substance.

onychogram (o-nik′o-gram) a tracing made by the onychograph.

onychograph (o-nik′o-graf) [onycho- + Gr. graphein to write] an instrument for observing and recording the nail pulse and capillary circulation.

onychogryphosis (on″ĭ-ko-grĭ-fo′sis) [onycho- + gryposis] hypertrophy of the nail(s), producing a hooked or incurved clawlike deformity. Called also onychogryposis. Cf. onychauxis.

onychogryposis (on″ĭ-ko-grĭ-po′sis) onychogryphosis.

onychoheterotopia (on″ĭ-ko-het″er-o-to′pĭ-ah) [onycho- + heterotopia] a condition in which the nails are abnormally situated.

onycholysis (on″ĭ-kol′ĭ-sis) [onycho- + Gr. lysis dissolution] separation of the nail plate from the nail bed, usually beginning at the free margin and progressing proximally.

onychomadesis (on″ĭ-ko-mah-de′sis) [onycho- + Gr. madēsis loss of hair] periodic separation of the proximal portions of the nail plate from the matrix and bed with subsequent shedding of the nails. Called also defluvium unguium and onychoptosis.

onychomalacia (on″ĭ-ko-mah-la′she-ah) [onycho- + malacia] softening of the nail(s).

onychomycosis (on″ĭ-ko-mi-ko′sis) [onycho- + mycosis] fungal infection of the nail plate, usually caused by species of Epidermophyton, Microsporum, and Trichophyton, and producing nails that are opaque, white, thickened, friable, and brittle. Called also ringworm of nails and tinea unguium.
dermatophytic o., tinea unguium.

onycho-osteodysplasia (on″ĭ-ko-os″te-o-dis-pla′ze-ah) [onycho- + Gr. osteon bone + dysplasia] a hereditary syndrome with dystrophy of the nails, absence or hypoplasia of the patella, hypoplasia of the lateral side of the elbow joint, and bilateral iliac horns; called also arthro-onychodysplasia and nail-patella syndrome.

onychopathic (on″ĭ-ko-path′ik) pertaining to onychopathy or any disease of the nails.

onychopathology (on″ĭ-ko-pah-thol′o-je) [onycho- + pathology] the pathology of diseases of the nails.

onychopathy (on″ĭ-ko-kop′ah-the) [onycho- + Gr. pathos disease] disease or deformity of the nail(s). Called also onychosis.

onychophagia (on″ĭ-ko-fa′je-ah) [onycho- + Gr. phagein to eat + -ia] the habit of biting the nails. Called also onychophagy.

onychophagy (on″ĭ-kof′ah-je) [onycho- + Gr. phagein to eat] onychophagia.

onychoptosis (on″ĭ-kop-to′sis) [onycho- + Gr. ptōsis falling] onychomadesis.

onychorrhexis (on″ĭ-ko-rek′sis) [onycho- + Gr. rhēxis a breaking] longitudinal striation of the nail plate associated with brittleness and breakage of the nail(s).

onychoschizia (on″ĭ-ko-skiz′e-ah) [onycho- + Gr. schizein to divide + -ia] splitting or lamination of the nail plate, usually in the horizontal plane at the free edge.

onychosis (on″ĭ-ko′sis) [onycho- + -osis] onychopathy.

onychotillomania (on″ĭ-ko-til″o-ma′ne-ah) compulsive picking at the nails.

onychotomy (on″ĭ-kot′o-me) [onycho- + Gr. tomē a cutting] incision of a nail.

O'nyong-nyong (o-nyong′nyong) an acute, nonfatal febrile disease due to an alphavirus, transmitted by anopheline mosquitoes, occurring in Uganda, Kenya, Tanzania, Malawi, and Senegal, and clinically resembling dengue and chikungunya; it is characterized by lymphadenitis, joint pains, and an extremely pruritic morbilliform skin rash. Called also O'nyong-nyong fever.

onyx (on′iks) [Gr. "nail"] 1. a fingernail or toenail; see unguis [NA]. 2. a variety of hypopyon.

onyxis (o-nik′sis) ingrown nail.

oo- [Gr. ōon egg] a combining form denoting relationship to an egg or ovum; see also words beginning ovo-.

ooblast (o′o-blast) [oo- + Gr. blastos germ] a primitive cell from which an ovum ultimately is developed.

oocenter (o″o-sen′ter) ovocenter.

oocephalus (o″o-sef′ah-lus) [oo- + Gr. kephalē head] an individual characterized by an egg-shaped head.

Oochoristica (o″o-ko-ris′tĭ-kah) a large genus of tapeworms, family Linstowiidae, which are parasitic in birds, reptiles, and mammals.

oocinesia (o″o-sĭ-ne′ze-ah) ookinesis.

oocyan (o″o-si′an) a blue-green pigment from the shells of birds' eggs; it is a dehydro bilirubin.

oocyanin (o″o-si′ah-nin) [oo- + Gr. kyanos blue] a bluish coloring matter from birds' eggs.

oocyesis (o″o-si-e′sis) [oo- + Gr. kyēsis pregnancy] ovarian pregnancy.

oocyst (o′o-sist) [oo- + cyst] the encysted or encapsulated zygote in the life cycle of sporozoan protozoa, which by the process of sporogony develops into a sporozoite or a sporocyst containing sporozoites.

oocyte (o′o-sīt) [oo- + -cyte] a developing egg cell in one of two stages: The primary oocyte (one that has begun but not completed the first maturation division) is derived from an oogonium by differentiation near the time of birth. The secondary oocyte (one in the period between the first and second maturation division) is derived from a primary oocyte shortly before ovulation by a division that splits off the first polar body. Ovulation follows. If fertilized, the secondary oocyte divides into an ootid and the second polar body; otherwise it perishes.

oocytin (o″o-si′tin) a substance, obtained from spermatozoa, leukocytes, and red blood cells, that will cause the formation of fertilization membranes in ova.

oogamous (o-og′ah-mus) pertaining or relating to or produced by oogamy; heterogamous.

oogamy (o-og′ah-me) 1. the fertilization of a large nonmotile egg by a small, motile male gamete or sperm, as seen in certain algae. 2. the conjugation of two dissimilar gametes; heterogamy.

oogenesis (o″o-jen′ĕ-sis) [oo- + Gr. genesis production] the process of formation of the female gametes (ova).

oogenetic (o″o-jĕ-net′ik) pertaining to oogenesis.

oogenic (o″o-jen′ik) producing ova.

oogonium (o″o-go′ne-um), pl. oogo′nia [oo- + Gr. gonē generation] 1. an ovarian egg during fetal development; it is derived from primordial germ cell, multiplies rapidly, then becomes encapsulated in primordial follicle cells and, near time of birth, becomes a primary oocyte by entering into prophase of first maturation division. 2. in certain fungi and algae, the female gametangium containing one or more eggs (oospheres).

ookinesis (o″o-kĭ-ne′sis) [oo- + Gr. kinēsis motion] the mitotic movements of the egg during maturation and fertilization.

ookinete (o″o-ki′nēt, o″o-kĭ-net′) [oo- + Gr. kinetos movable] the motile, worm-shaped zygote of certain protozoa, such as *Plasmodium*, which is found in the insect vector.

oolemma (o″o-lem′ah) [oo- + Gr. *lemma* sheath] zona pellucida, def. 1.

Oomycetes (o″o-mi-se′tēz) [oo- + Gr. *mykēs* fungus] a subclass of phycomycetous fungi having sporangia of different kinds and cell walls made up of cellulose, in which reproduction takes place sexually by biflagellate spores; it includes the order Saprolegniales.

oophagia (o″o-fa′je-ah) oophagy.

oophagy (o-of′ah-je) [Gr. *ōophagein* to eat eggs] the eating of eggs; said of insects whose diet consists largely of eggs.

oophoralgia (o″of-or-al′je-ah) [oophor- + -algia] pain in an ovary.

oophorectomize (o″of-o-rek′to-mīz) to deprive of the ovaries by surgical removal.

oophorectomy (o″of-o-rek′to-me) [oophor- + Gr. *ektomē* excision] the removal of an ovary or ovaries; called also *ovariectomy*.

oophoritis (o″of-o-ri′tis) [oophor- + -itis] inflammation of an ovary. **o. parotid′ea**, oophoritis occurring in association with infection by the virus causing mumps.

oophor(o)- [Gr. *ōophoros* bearing eggs] a combining form denoting relationship to the ovary.

oophorocystectomy (o-of″o-ro-sis-tek′to-me) [oophoro- + cyst + Gr. *ektomē* excision] excision of an ovarian cyst.

oophorocystosis (o-of″o-ro-sis-to′sis) [oophoro- + cyst + -osis] the formation of ovarian cysts.

oophorogenous (o-of″o-roj′ĕ-nus) derived from the ovary.

oophorohysterectomy (o-of″o-ro-his″ter-ek′to-me) [oophoro- + Gr. *hystera* uterus + *ektomē* excision] surgical removal of the uterus and ovaries.

oophoroma (o-of″o-ro′mah) seldom used term for malignant tumor of the ovary. **o. follicula′re**, Brenner tumor.

oophoron (o-of′o-ron) [Gr. *ōon* egg + *pherein* to bear] an ovary (ovarium [NA]).

oophoropathy (o-of″o-rop′ah-the) [oophoro- + Gr. *pathos* disease] any disease of the ovaries.

oophoropexy (o-of′o-ro-pek″se) [oophoro- + Gr. *pēxis* fixation] ovariopexy.

oophoroplasty (o-of′o-ro-plas″te) plastic surgery of the ovary.

oophorosalpingectomy (o-of″o-ro-sal″pin-jek′to-me) [oophoro- + Gr. *salpinx* tube + *ektomē* excision] salpingo-oophorectomy.

oophorosalpingitis (o-of″o-ro-sal″pin-ji′tis) salpingo-oophoritis.

oophorostomy (o-of″o-ros′to-me) [oophoro- + Gr. *stomoun* to provide with an opening or mouth] the making of an opening into an ovarian cyst for drainage purposes.

oophorotomy (o-of″o-rot′o-me) [oophoro- + Gr. *tomē* a cutting] incision of the ovary.

oophorrhagia (o-of″o-ra′je-ah) [oophoro- + Gr. *rhēgnynai* to burst forth] severe hemorrhage from an ovary.

oophyte (o′o-fīt) [oo- + Gr. *phyton* plant] any member of the generation in the life history of mosses, ferns, etc., in which the sexual organs are produced.

ooplasm (o′o-plazm) the cytoplasm of the egg.

ooporphyrin (o″o-por′fir-in) protoporphyrin contained in egg shells.

oorhodein (o″o-ro′de-in) [oo- + Gr. *rhodon* rose] a red coloring matter from birds' eggs.

oosperm (o′o-sperm) [oo- + Gr. *sperma* seed] the recently fertilized ovum.

oosphere (o′o-sfēr) 1. an unfertilized female gamete of certain fungi. 2. the large, nonmotile, fertile gamete of certain algae and fungi.

Oospora (o-os′po-rah) [oo- + Gr. *sporos* seed] a genus of imperfect fungi of the family Moniliaceae, order Moniliales, which is associated with disease of citrus trees and potatoes. **O. catena′ta**, **O. frag′ilis**, species of uncertain classification which were once isolated from black tongue, probably as a contaminant. **O. lac′tis**, *Geotrichum candidum*. **O. tozeu′ri**, *Madurella mycetomi*.

oosporangium (o″o-spo-ran′je-um) the female element in the sexual formation of oospores.

oospore (o′o-spōr) [oo- + *spore*] 1. the final developmental stage after fusion of sexually differentiated gametes in certain fungi. 2. the thick-walled, resting zygote formed from a fertilized oosphere.

oosporosis (o″o-spo-ro′sis) (obs.) infection with an oospore; e.g., in chronic bronchitis.

ootheca (o″o-the′kah) [oo- + Gr. *thēkē* case] 1. an egg case, such as is found in some lower animals. 2. an ovary.

oothec(o)- [Gr. *ōon* egg + *thēkē* case] for words beginning thus, see those beginning *oophor(o)* and *ovari(o)*-.

ootherapy (o″o-ther′ah-pe) ovotherapy.

ootid (o′o-tid) a ripe ovum; one of four cells derived from the two consecutive divisions of the primary oocyte, and corresponding to the spermatids derived from division of the primary spermatocyte. In mammals, the second maturation division is not completed unless fertilization occurs; hence the ootid has male as well as female pronuclear (haploid) elements.

ootype (o′o-tīp) [oo- + Gr. *typos* impression] in some trematodes, a dilated portion of the uterus into which the oviduct opens and where the ovum is fertilized, provided with the yolk, and invested with a shell.

ooxanthine (o″o-zan′thin) [oo- + Gr. *xanthos* yellow] a yellow pigment found in egg shells.

oozooid (o″o-zo′oid) [oo- + Gr. *zōo-eidēs* like an animal] an individual developed from an ovum, that is, as a result of sexual reproduction. Cf. *blastozooid*.

opacification (o-pas″ĭ-fĭ-ka′shun) 1. the development of opacity, as of the cornea or lens. 2. the rendering of a tissue or organ opaque to radiation by introduction of a contrast medium.

opacity (o-pas′ĭ-te) [L. *opacitas*] 1. the condition of being opaque. 2. an opaque spot or area. See also *cataract*.

opalescent (o″pal-es′ent) showing a milky iridescence, like an opal.

opalescin (o″pal-es′in) an albuminoid derivable from milk; its solutions are opalescent.

opalgia (o-pal′je-ah) [Gr. *ōps* face + -algia] facial neuralgia.

Opalina (o″pah-li′nah) [L. *opalus* opal] a genus of ciliate parasitic protozoa (order Opalinida, class Opalinata) found as endocommensals in the colon of frogs and toads. The life cycle of *O. ranarum* involves asexual reproduction in adult frogs and sexual reproduction in tadpoles.

Opalinata (o″pah-li-na′tah) a subphylum of parasitic, flat, leaflike, multinucleate protozoa (phylum Sarcomastigophora) found as endocommensals in anurans and less often in fish, salamanders, and reptiles. They have cilia arranged in multiple oblique longitudinal rows over the entire body surface, but differ from the Ciliophora in that they possess only one type of nucleus (i.e., no differentiated micronuclei and macronuclei) and they reproduce sexually. It comprises one class: Opalinatea.

Opalinatea (o″pah-lĭ-na′te-ah) a class of parasitic ciliated protozoa (subphylum Opalinata, phylum Mastigophora) with characters of the subphylum. It comprises one order: Opalinida.

opaline (o′pah-lēn) [L. *opalus* opal] having the appearance of an opal.

opalinid (o″pah-lin′id) 1. pertaining or referring to protozoa of the subphylum Opalinata. 2. any protozoan of the subphylum Opalinata.

Opalinida (o″pah-lin′ĭ-dah) an order of ciliated parasitic protozoa (class Opalinatea, subphylum Opalinata) with characters of the class. *Opalina* is a representative genus.

opalisin (o-pal′ĭ-sin) an opalescent protein, obtainable from human milk.

opaque (o-pāk′) [L. *opacus* dark] impervious to light rays, or by extension to roentgen rays or other electromagnetic radiations; neither transparent nor translucent.

open (o′pen) 1. exposed to the air; not covered by unbroken skin. 2. interrupted (as a circuit) so that an electric current cannot pass. 3. not obstructed or closed.

opening (o′pen-ing) an aperture, orifice, or open space; see also *ostium*. **o. in adductor magnus muscle**, hiatus tendineus. **aortic o.**, ostium aorticum. **aortic o. in diaphragm**, hiatus aorticus. **o. of aqueduct of cochlea, external**, apertura externa canaliculi cochleae.

o. of bladder, ostium urethrae internum. **cardiac o.,** ostium cardiacum. **o. of coronary sinus,** ostium sinus coronarii. **cutaneous o. of male urethra,** ostium urethrae externum masculinae. **duodenal o. of stomach,** ostium pyloricum. **esophageal o. in diaphragm,** hiatus esophageus. **o. of Hunter's canal, inferior,** hiatus tendineus. **ileocecal o.,** ostium ileocaecale. **o. to lesser sac of peritoneum,** foramen epiploicum. **o. for lesser superficial petrosal nerve,** apertura superior canaliculi tympanici. **nasal o. of facial skeleton,** apertura piriformis. **orbital o., o. of orbital cavity, anterior,** aditus orbitae. **ovarian o. of uterine tube,** ostium abdominale tubae uterinae. **o. of pelvis, inferior,** apertura pelvis inferior. **o. of pelvis, superior,** apertura pelvis superior. **pharyngeal o. of auditory tube,** ostium pharyngeum tubae auditoriae. **piriform o.,** apertura piriformis. **o. of pulmonary trunk,** ostium trunci pulmonalis. **pyloric o.,** ostium pyloricum. **o. of sacral canal, inferior,** hiatus sacralis. **saphenous o.,** hiatus saphenus. **semilunar o. of ethmoid bone,** hiatus semilunaris. **o. for smaller superficial petrosal nerve,** apertura superior canaliculi tympanici. **o. of sphenoidal sinus,** apertura sinus sphenoidalis. **o. of stomach, anterior,** ostium pyloricum. **tendinous o.,** hiatus tendineus. **thoracic o., inferior, thoracic o., lower,** apertura thoracis inferior. **thoracic o., superior, thoracic o., upper,** apertura thoracis superior. **tympanic o. of auditory tube,** ostium tympanicum tubae auditivae. **o. for tympanic branch of glossopharyngeal nerve,** apertura inferior canaliculi tympanici. **o. of tympanic canal, superior,** apertura superior canaliculi tympanici. **uterine o. of uterine tube,** ostium uterinum tubae uterinae. **o. for vena cava,** foramen venae cavae. **o. of vermiform appendix,** ostium appendicis vermiformis. **vesicourethral o.,** ostium urethrae internum.

operable (op′er-ah-b'l) subject to being operated upon with a reasonable degree of safety; appropriate for surgical removal.

operant (op′ĕ-rant) in psychology, any response that is not elicited by specific external stimuli but that recurs at a given rate in a particular set of circumstances. See also *conditioning.*

operate (op′er-āt) 1. to perform an operation. 2. an individual that has undergone a specific experimental surgical procedure, in contrast to the normal control.

operation (op″er-a′shun) [L. *operatio*] any act performed with instruments or by the hands of a surgeon; a surgical procedure. **Abbe o.,** attachment of a triangular, full-thickness flap from the median portion of the lower lip to fill a defect in the upper lip. **Abbe's o.,** 1. a lateral intestinal anastomosis made with rings of catgut. 2. division of an esophageal stricture by string friction. 3. (*obs.*) intracranial resection of the second and third divisions of the fifth nerve for trigeminal neuralgia. **Adams' o.,** 1. subcutaneous intracapsular division of the neck of the femur for ankylosis of the hip. 2. subcutaneous division of the palmar fascia at various points for Dupuytren's contracture. 3. excision of a wedge-shaped piece from the eyelid for relief of ectropion. **Akin o.,** resection of the medial prominence of the first metatarsal head and cuneiform osteotomy of the proximal phalanx of the great toe, done for hallux valgus. **Albee's o.,** operation for ankylosis of the hip, consisting of cutting off the upper surface of the head of the femur and freshening a corresponding point on the acetabulum, and permitting the two freshened surfaces to rest in contact. **Albee-Delbet o.,** an operation for fracture of the neck of the femur, done by drilling a hole through the trochanter and the neck and head of the femur and inserting a bone peg in this hole. **Albert's o.,** excision of the knee to secure ankylosis for the cure of flail joint. **Alexander's o., Alexander-Adams o.,** shortening of the round ligaments to repair displacement of the uterus. **Alouette's o.,** see under *amputation.* **Ammon's o.,** 1. blepharoplasty by a flap from the cheek. 2. dacryocystotomy. 3. for epicanthus: resection of a spindle-shaped piece of skin over the bridge of the nose, undermining the flaps of the epicanthal fold and closing with sutures. **Amussat's o.,** a long transverse incision for exposure of the colon. **Anagnostakis' o.,** an operation for entropion; also an operation for trichiasis. **Aries-Pitanguy o.,** see under

mammaplasty. **Asch o.,** an operation for deflection of the nasal septum by reinserting resected pieces of cartilage and holding them in place with a splint; of historical interest. **Babcock's o.,** extirpation of the saphenous vein by inserting a long probe with an acorn tip and drawing out the vein by invagination; done for eradication of varicose veins. **Baldy's o., Baldy-Webster o.,** Webster's o. **Barkan's o.,** goniotomy. **Barker's o.,** 1. an excision of the hip joint by an anterior cut. 2. a special method of excising the astragalus by an incision extending from just above the external malleolus forward and inward to the dorsum of the foot. **Barraquer's o.,** phacoerysis. **Barsky's o.,** an operation for repair of a cleft hand with a missing central ray and a deep central V-shaped cleft, consisting in closing the cleft, bringing the ring and index fingers closer together, and correcting the associated syndactyly, if present. **Barton's o.,** an operation for ankylosis consisting of sawing through the bone and removing a V-shaped piece. **Basset's o.,** a method of dissecting the inguinal glands in operation for cancer of the vulva. **Bassini's o.,** repair of inguinal hernia, with high ligation of the sac, reinforcement of the floor of the canal, and placement of the spermatic cord under the external oblique anastomosis. **Battle's o.,** an operation for appendicitis in which the rectus muscle is temporarily retracted. **Beer's o.,** a flap method for cataract. **Belsey Mark IV o.,** an operation for gastroesophageal reflux performed through a thoracic incision; the fundus is wrapped 270 degrees around the circumference of the esophagus, leaving its posterior wall free. **Berger's o.,** interscapulothoracic amputation. **Berke o.,** an operation for ptosis of the upper eyelid, consisting of (1) a modification of the Blaskovics operation, with resection of the levator muscle through a skin incision and excision of excess muscle, or (2) a modification of the Motais operation, with suspension of the ptotic lid from the superior rectus muscle. **Bevan's o.,** an operation for an undescended testicle, by which the testicle is brought down permanently into the scrotum. **Bier's o.,** see under *amputation.* **Biesenberger's o.,** see under *mammaplasty.* **Bigelow's o.,** litholapaxy. **Billroth's o.,** 1. partial resection of the stomach with anastomosis of the severed end of the duodenum to the end of the resected stomach (Billroth I), or with anastomosis of the resected stomach to the jejunum (Billroth II). 2. excision of the tongue by making a transverse incision below the symphysis of the jaw and joining it by two incisions, one on each side, parallel to the body of the mandible, with preliminary ligation of the lingual arteries. **Blair-Brown o.,** repair of a cleft lip by the use of a lateral flap one-half the length of the lip. **Blalock-Hanlon o.,** a palliative operation for transposition of the great vessels, consisting in the creation of an interatrial septal defect. **Blalock-Taussig o.,** the anastomosis of the subclavian artery to the pulmonary artery in order to shunt some of the systemic circulation into the pulmonary circulation; performed as palliative treatment of congenital cardiac anomalies (tetralogy of Fallot). **Blaskovics o.,** an operation for ptosis of the upper eyelid, consisting of excision of the levator muscle and the tarsus through a conjunctival approach. **Bozeman's o.,** hysterocystocleisis. **Bricker's o.,** the surgical creation of an ileal conduit with a flat stoma for the collection of urine; the flat contour is achieved by suturing the ileal mucosa to the skin. **Brock's o.,** transventricular closed valvotomy. **Brophy's o.,** one for cleft palate (with or without cleft lip), consisting of the forcible approximation of the freshened palate margins, which are held in position by special sutures supported by lead plates. **Browne o.,** a urethroplasty for hypospadias repair, in which an intact strip of epithelium is left on the ventral surface of the penis to form the roof of the urethra, and the floor of the urethra is formed by epithelialization from the lateral wound margins. **Brunschwig's o.,** a technique of pancreatoduodenectomy. **Buck's o.,** cuneiform excision of the patella and the ends of tibia and fibula. **(von) Burow's o.,** a method of excising triangles of skin at the base of the pedicle of a skin flap to facilitate advancement. **Caldwell-Luc o.,** 1. the operation of opening into the maxillary sinus by way of an incision into the supradental fossa opposite the premolar teeth, usually done to remove tooth roots or abnormal tissue from the sinus. 2. in compound zygomaticomaxillary fractures, the packing of the maxillary sinus by approaching the antrum through the canine fossa of the maxilla above the tooth apices, thus allowing reduction of displaced fragments of the zygoma by upward and outward pressure. Called also *Luc's o.* **Carpue's o.**, the Indian method of rhinoplasty. **Cecil's o.,** 1. a two-stage urethroplasty for hypospadias repair, with construction of a new urethral segment buried in the scrotum, followed by separation of the new urethra from the scrotum. 2. a three-stage urethroplasty for repair of urethral stricture, with excision of the strictured area through an incision on the ventral surface of the penis, followed by the steps of the operation used for hypospadias repair. **Chopart's o.**, see under *amputation.* **Colonna's o.,** 1. a reconstruction operation for intracapsular fracture of the femoral neck. 2. capsular arthroplasty of the hip. **Commando's o.**, an operation for management of oral cancer, consisting in resection of the primary lesion and the regional lymphatic nodes. **Conway o.**, see under *mammaplasty.* **cosmetic o.**, one intended to remove or correct a deformity in an esthetically acceptable manner. **Cotte's o.**, removal of the presacral nerve. **Cotting's o.**, operation for ingrowing toenail, consisting in cutting off the side of the toe down to and including the ingrowing edge of the nail. **Daviel's o.**, extraction of cataract through a corneal incision without cutting the iris. **Denis Browne o.,** Browne o. **Denonvilliers' o.**, plastic correction of a defective ala nasi by transferring a triangular flap from the adjacent side of the nose. **Dieffenbach's o.**, plastic closure of triangular defects by displacing a quadrangular flap toward one side of the triangle. **Dittel's o.**, enucleation of an enlarged prostate through an external incision; of historical interest. **Doléris' o.**, an operation for retrodeviation of the uterus by shortening the round ligaments and fixing them on either side by an opening in the rectus muscle just above the spine of the ilium. **Duhamel o.**, the treatment of congenital megacolon (Hirschsprung's disease) by a modification of the pull-through procedure and establishment of a longitudinal anastomosis between the proximal ganglionated segment of colon and the rectum, leaving the latter *in situ.* **Dührssen's o.**, vaginofixation of the uterus. **Duplay's o.**, a method of urethroplasty for repair of hypospadias, employing a buried skin strip. **Dupuy-Dutemps o.**, blepharoplasty of the lower lid with tissue from the opposing lid. **Dupuytren's o.**, see under *amputation.* **Elliot's o.**, a method of trephining the sclerocornea for the relief of increased tension in glaucoma. **Emmet's o.**, 1. a method of repairing a lacerated perineum. 2. trachelorrhaphy, or suture of the edges of a lacerated cervix uteri. 3. surgical creation of a vesicovaginal fistula to secure drainage of the bladder in cystitis. **equilibrating o.**, tenotomy of the direct antagonist of a paralyzed eye muscle. **Esser's o.**, epithelial inlay; see under *inlay.* **Estes' o.**, implantation of an ovary into a uterine cornu; performed for sterility when the tubes are absent. **Estlander's o.** 1. resection of one or more ribs in empyema so as to allow the chest wall to collapse and close the abnormal cavity; of historical interest. 2. rotation of a triangular flap from the side of the lower lip to fill a defect in the lateral upper lip. **Eversbusch's o.**, an operation for ptosis of the upper eyelid, consisting of resection of the levator muscle through a skin incision. **exploratory o.**, surgical incision into an area of the body followed by inspection and palpation of organs and tissues to determine the cause of unexplained symptoms. **Fergusson's o.**, see under *incision.* **Finney's o.**, see under *pyloroplasty.* **flap o.**, any operation involving the raising of a flap of tissue. In periodontics, an operation to secure greater access to granulation tissue and osseous defects, consisting of detachment of the gingivae, the alveolar mucosa, and/or a portion of the palatal mucosa. See also under *amputation.* **Fothergill o.**, Manchester o. **Franco's o.**, suprapubic cystotomy. **Frank's o.**, Ssabanejew-Frank o. **Frazier-Spiller o.**, division of the sensory root of the gasserian ganglion for relief of trigeminal neuralgia. **Fredet-Ramstedt o.**, pyloromyotomy. **Freund's o.**, resection of cartilages of the chest wall to restore elasticity and improve respiratory mechanics; of historical interest. **Freyer's o.**, a method of performing suprapubic enucleation of the hypertrophied prostate; of historical interest. **Frost-Lang o.**, insertion of a gold ball to take the place of an enucleated eyeball. **Fukala's o.**, removal of the lens of the eye for the treatment of marked myopia. **Fuller's o.**, perineal incision and drainage of the seminal vesicles; of historical interest. **Gifford's o.**, delimiting keratotomy. **Gigli's o.**, lateral section of the os pubis by means of Gigli's wire saw; done in difficult labor. **Gilliam's o.**, an opera-

tion for retroversion of the uterus by drawing a loop of each round ligament through the abdominal wall and fixing the loops to the abdominal fascia. **Gillies o.,** 1. operation for correction of ectropion utilizing a split-thickness skin graft and a mold. 2. a technique for reducing fractures of the zygoma and zygomatic arch through an incision in the temporal region above the hairline. **Glenn o.**, an operation for congenital cyanotic heart disease, consisting of anastomosis of the superior vena cava to the right pulmonary artery. **Gonin's o.**, treatment of retinal detachment by thermocautery of the fissure in the retina performed through an opening in the sclera. **Graefe's o.**, removal of the cataractous lens by a scleral cut, with laceration of the capsule and iridectomy. **Gritti's o.**, see under *amputation.* **Grondahl-Finney o.**, esophagogastroplasty in which the orifice between the esophagus and stomach is enlarged. **Guyon's o.**, see under *amputation.* **Halsted's o.**, 1. an operation for inguinal hernia with transposition of the spermatic cord above the external oblique aponeurosis. 2. radical mastectomy. **Hancock's o.**, see under *amputation.* **Hartmann's o.**, see under *procedure.* **Hartley-Krause o.** excision of the gasserian ganglion and its roots to relieve trigeminal neuralgia; of historical interest. **Haultain's o.**, a modification of the Huntington operation (q.v.) for replacement of a chronically inverted uterus, involving a posterior incision in the uterus through the cervical ring. **Heath's o.**, division of the ascending rami of the lower jaw with a saw for ankylosis, performed within the oral cavity; rarely done. **Heine's o.**, cyclodialysis in glaucoma. **Heineke-Mikulicz o.**, see under *pyloroplasty.* **Heller's o.**, cardiomyotomy for relief of obstruction of the esophagogastric junction. **Herbert's o.**, displacement of a wedge-shaped flap of sclera in order to form a filtering cicatrix in glaucoma. **Hey's o.**, see under *amputation.* **Hibbs' o.**, a spinal fusion operation done by fracturing the spinous processes of the vertebrae and pressing the tip of each downward to rest in the denuded area caused by the fracture of its elbow below. **Hochenegg's o.**, total excision of the rectum with preservation of the anal sphincter; of historical interest. **Hoffa's o.**, Hoffa-Lorenz o., Lorenz's o. **Holth's o.**, excision of the sclera by punch operation. **Horsley's o.** excision of an area of motor cortex for relief of athetoid and convulsive movements of an upper extremity; of historical interest. **Huggins' o.**, orchiectomy performed for cancer of the prostate. **Hunter's o.** litigation of an artery in the proximal side of an aneurysm, above the first collateral; of historical interest. **Huntington's o.**, transabdominal repair of a chronically inverted uterus. It is done by grasping the invaginated portion of the uterus with forceps; as the uterus is pulled up, additional forceps are placed sequentially lower down, and upward traction is applied. After the uterus is in place, the position is maintained by packing through the vagina. **Indian o.**, see under *rhinoplasty.* **interposition o.**, Watkins' o. **interval o.**, an operation performed during the interval between two acute attacks of a disease, as in appendicitis. **Irving's sterilization o.**, a method of tubal ligation in which the uterine tubes are ligated and severed. **Italian o.**, see *taglia cotian rhinoplasty,* under *rhinoplasty.* **Jaboulay's o.**, interpelviabdominal amputation. **Kader's o.**, gastrostomy by which the feeding tube is introduced through a valvelike flap which closes on withdrawal of the tube. **Kasai o.**, portoenterostomy. **Kazanjian's o.**, 1. a technique of surgical extension of the buccal vestibular sulcus of edentulous ridges to increase their height and to improve denture retention. 2. the use of extraskeletal fixation for support in compound zygomaticomaxillary fractures: a small hole is drilled through the infraorbital rim, and a stainless steel wire is inserted with both ends brought out through the wound, where they are twisted together into a loop or hook. Rubber band traction between the suspension wire and an outrigger on a head cap provides support for the zygomatic fragments. **Keller o.**, sagittal resection of the medial prominence of the first metatarsal head and excision of the base of the proximal phalanx of the great toe; done for hallux valgus. **Kelly's o.**, 1. [Howard A. *Kelly*] an operation for correction of urinary incontinence (usually due to stress) in women, in which the site of the internal urethral sphincter is identified by means of a balloon catheter, and the connective tissue between the vagina and the urethra and the floor of the bladder are sutured to form a wide shelf of firm tissue to support the urethra and bladder. 2. [J. D. *Kelly*] arytenoidopexy. **Killian's o.**, excision of the anterior wall of the frontal sinus, removal of the diseased tissue, and formation of a permanent communication with the nose. **Killian-Freer o.,** submucous resection of the nasal septum, including the septal cartilage, vomer, and perpendicular plate of the ethmoid. **King's o.,** arytenoidopexy. **Knapp's o.** (for cataract), the formation of a peripheral opening in the capsule behind the iris, without iridectomy. **Kocher's o.,** 1. a method of excising the ankle joint by a cut below the outer malleolus, division of the peroneal tendons, removal of the diseased tissues, and suture of the divided tendons. 2. a method of reducing a subcoracoid dislocation of the humerus. 3. excision of the tongue through an incision extending from the symphysis of the jaw to the hyoid bone and thence to the mastoid process. 4. see under *maneuver.* 5. a method of pylorectomy. **Körte-Ballance o.,** anastomosis of the facial and hypoglossal nerves. **Kraske's o.,** removal of the coccyx and part of the sacrum for access to a carcinoma of the rectum. **Krause's o.** extradural excision of the gasserian ganglion for trigeminal neuralgia; of historical interest. **Krimer's o.,** uranoplasty in which mucoperiosteal flaps from each side of the palatal cleft are sutured together at the median line. **Krönlein's o.,** resection of the outer wall of the orbit for the removal of an orbital tumor without excising the eye. **Küstner o.,** replacement of an inverted uterus through an incision made in the cervix and uterus along the posterior surface. **Lagrange's o.,** sclerectoiridectomy. **Landolt's o.,** the formation of a lower eyelid with a double pedicle or bridge flap of eyelid skin taken from the upper lid. **Lane's o.,** the operation of dividing the ileum near the cecum, closing the distal portion and anastomosing the proximal end with the upper part of the rectum or lower part of the sigmoid, thus eliminating the colon from the fecal current. **Lapidus o.,** Silver o., with wedge resection and fusion of the innermost cuneometatarsal joint and establishment of a bridge between the bases of the first and second metatarsals; done for hallux valgus. **Larrey's o.,** see under *amputation.* **Latzko's o.,** 1. see *cesarean section, Latzko's,* under *section.* 2. a method of repairing a vesicovaginal fistula by using mucosa denuded from the posterior wall of the vagina as a flap to cover the fistula. **Le Fort's o., Le Fort-Neugebauer o.,** the operation of uniting the anterior and posterior vaginal walls along the middle line for the repair of prolapse of the uterus. **Lempert's fenestration o.,** an operation for otosclerosis, consisting of drilling a small window into the lateral semicircular canal and then placing a flap of skin over the fistula. **Lisfranc's o.,** see under *amputation.* **Liston's o.,** an operation for excision of the upper jaw. **Lizars' o.,** excision of the upper jaw by a curved incision extending from the angle of the mouth to the malar bone. **Lorenz's o.,** an operation for congenital dislocation of the hip, consisting in reduction of the dislocation, and keeping the head of the femur fixed against the rudimentary acetabulum until a socket is formed. **Lowsley's o.,** an operation for repair of simple epispadias, consisting in closing the glandular cleft urethra, splitting the glans, and burying the repaired urethra deep in the soft tissue so that the orifice will be positioned at the normal site. **Luc's o.,** Caldwell-Luc o. **McBride o.,** resection of the medial prominence of the first metatarsal head, medial capsulorrhaphy, resection of the fibular sesamoid, and transfer of the adductor tendon to the neck of the first metatarsal; done for hallus valgus. **McBurney's o.,** an operation for inguinal hernia: the sac is exposed, ligated, and cut off at the internal ring; the skin is turned in and stitched to the underlying tendinous and ligamentous structures. **Macewen's o.,** an operation for the radical cure of hernia by closing the internal ring with a pad made of the hernial sac. **McGill's o.,** suprapubic transvesical prostatectomy; of historical interest. **Madlener o.,** a method of sterilization in the female, in which the middle portion of the fallopian tube is crushed with a clamp, which is then replaced with a ligature of nonabsorbable material. **magnet o.,** removal of a fragment of steel or iron from the eyeball by means of a powerful magnet. **major o.,** a surgical procedure of major magnitude and risk. **Manchester o.,** an operation for uterine prolapse comprising dilation and curettage, anterior repair, amputation of the vaginal portion of the cervix, shortening of the cardinal ligaments, and posterior colpoperineorrhaphy. **Marshall-Marchetti-Krantz o.,** an operation for the correction of stress incontinence, the anterior portion of the urethra, vesical neck, and bladder being sutured to the posterior surface of

the pubic bone. **mastoid o.,** mastoidectomy. **Matas' o.,** endoaneurysmorrhaphy. **Maydl's o.,** 1. colostomy in which the colon is drawn out through the wound and maintained in position by placing a glass rod beneath it until adhesions have formed; of historical interest. 2. insertion of the ureters into the rectum for exstrophy of the bladder; of historical interest. **Mayo's o.,** 1. excision of the pyloric end of the stomach, followed by closure of both duodenum and stomach and the construction of an independent posterior gastrojejunostomy. 2. for umbilical hernia; the hernial mass is excised and the abdominal aponeuroses are overlapped transversely; of historical interest. 3. subcutaneous removal of varicose veins with a long-handled stripper terminating in a small ring angled with the shaft of the instrument. **Meller's o.,** an operation for excision of the tear sac. **Mikulicz's o.,** 1. removal of the sternocleidomastoid muscle for torticollis. 2. Heineke-Mikulicz pyloroplasty. 3. tarsectomy in which the heel, os calcis, and astragalus are removed, the articular surfaces of the tibia, fibula, cuboid, and scaphoid are excised, and the foot brought into line with the leg; called also *Vladimiroff's o.* 4. enterectomy in stages, including exteriorization of the section of intestine to be resected, usually the colon; resection of the exteriorized loop; elimination of the fecal fistula by crushing the spur between the two barrels of the anastomosis; and closure of the fecal fistula. **Miles' o.,** abdominoperineal resection for cancer of the lower sigmoid and rectum, which includes permanent colostomy, removal of the pelvic colon, mesocolon, and adjacent lymph nodes, and wide perineal excision of the rectum and anus. **Millin-Read o.,** an operation for the correction of stress incontinence employing the suprapubic approach. **minor o.,** a surgical operation which is not serious in its magnitude or risk. **Mitchell o.,** Silver o., with distal osteotomy of the first metatarsal; done for hallux valgus. **Moschcowitz's o.,** an operation for the repair of a femoral hernia by the inguinal approach. **Motais' o.,** an operation for ptosis, consisting of transplanting the middle portion of the tendon of the superior rectus muscle of the eyeball into the upper lid. **Mules' o.,** evisceration of the eyeball, with insertion of an artificial vitreous. **Mustard o.,** creation of an intra-atrial baffle using pericardial tissue to correct the anatomic defect in transposition of the great vessels. **Naffziger's o.,** excision of the superior and lateral walls of the orbit for exophthalmos. **Nissen o.,** fundoplication. **Ober's o.,** medial subtalar syndesmotomy for clubfoot. **Olshausen's o.,** the operation of fixing or suturing the uterus to the abdominal wall for the cure of retroversion. **Ombrédanne's o.,** transscrotal orchiopexy. **open o.,** an operation in which the tissues and organs are exposed to view through a surgical incision. **Partsch's o.,** a technique for marsupialization of dental cyst. **Patey's o.,** modified radical mastectomy. **Péan's o.,** 1. (*obs.*) vaginal hysterectomy bit by bit. 2. hip joint amputation in which the vessels are ligated as the operation goes on. **Phelps' o.,** an open and direct incision through the sole and inner side of the foot, done for talipes. **Phemister o.,** use of an onlay graft of cancellous bone without internal fixation, for treatment of a stable but ununited fracture. **plastic o.,** one in which the shape of a part or the character of its covering is altered by transplantation of tissue, etc. **Polya's o.,** anastomosis of the transected end of the stomach to the side of the jejunum following subtotal gastrectomy. **Pomeroy's o.,** a method of sterilization in the female, in which the fallopian tube is picked up about two inches from the uterine cornua, a chronic catgut ligature tied around the loop without crushing it, and the tied loop is then resected. **Potts' o.,** anastomosis between the aorta and the pulmonary artery as palliative treatment of congenital pulmonary stenosis. **radical o.,** one involving extensive resection of tissue for the complete extirpation of disease. **Ramstedt's o.,** Fredet-Ramstedt o. **Rastelli's o.,** an operation to correct such cardiac anomalies as transposition of the great vessels (with pulmonary stenosis), truncus arteriosus, and pulmonary arterial atresia, in which a graft is used to carry blood from the right ventricle to the pulmonary artery. **Regnoli's o.,** excision of the tongue through a median opening below the lower jaw, reaching from the chin to the hyoid bone. **Ridell o.,** obliteration of the frontal sinus by removal of the anterior wall and floor and sometimes posterior walls of the sinus; for treatment of malignant tumors. **Roux-en-Y o.,** see under *anastomosis.* **Saemisch's o.,** transfixion of the cornea and of the base of the ulcer for the cure of hypopyon. **Scanzoni's** o., see under *maneuver*. **Schauta's o.**, radical hysterectomy by the vaginal route. **Schede's o.**, 1. resection of the thorax for chronic empyema. 2. an operation for varicose veins of the leg, done by a circular incision, rolling one cuff up and another down, so as to reach and remove the varices. 3. excision of the necrosed part of a bone, all dead bone and diseased tissue being scraped away, and the cavity permitted to fill with blood clot, the latter being kept moist and aseptic with a cover of gauze and rubber tissue, and eventually becoming organized. **Scheie's o.**, 1. scleral cauterization with peripheral iridectomy for treatment of glaucoma. 2. a technique for needling and aspiration of cataract. **Schönbein's o.**, staphyloplasty in which a flap of mucous membrane from the posterior wall of the pharynx is stitched to the velum palati, shutting off the nose from the mouth. **Sédillot's o.**, 1. a method of staphylorrhaphy. 2. a flap operation for restoring the upper lip. **Senning o.**, surgical creation of two interatrial channels for crossing the systemic and pulmonary venous circulations in transposition of the great vessels. **Serre's o.**, an operation for correction of skin contractures that distort the angle of the mouth, involving switching of a skin and subcutaneous tissue flap from one lip to another. **Silver o.**, resection of the medial prominence of the first metatarsal head, medial capsulorrhaphy of the first metatarsophalangeal joint, and sectioning of the adductor tendon; done for hallux valgus. **Sistrunk o.**, a surgical procedure for removal of thyroglossal cysts and sinuses. **Smith's o.**, extraction of an immature cataract with an intact capsule. **Soave o.**, the treatment of congenital megacolon (Hirschsprung's disease) by endorectal pull-through, with normal colon connected to the anus through a rectum denuded of mucosa. **Spinelli's o.**, the operation of splitting the anterior wall of the prolapsed inverted uterus, reversing the organ, and restoring it to the correct position. **Ssabanejew-Frank o.**, a method of performing gastrostomy by pulling a cone of the stomach through an incision in the left rectus muscle and suturing it to the skin. **Stacke's o.**, the removal of the mastoid and the contents of the tympanum, so that the antrum, attic, tympanum, and meatus form a single cavity. **State o.**, the treatment of congenital megacolon (Hirschsprung's disease) by end-to-end anastomosis of the colon from above the aganglionic segment to the upper part of the rectum. **Stein o.**, an operation for reconstruction of the lower lip with flaps taken from the upper lip. **Stokes's o.**, Gritti-Stokes amputation. **Strömbeck o.**, see under *mammaplasty*. **Sturmdorf's o.**, conical excision of the diseased endocervix. **Swenson's o.**, an operation for congenital megacolon (Hirschsprung's disease), consisting in removal of the rectum and the aganglionic segment of the bowel, with preservation of the anal sphincters, by the pull-through surgical technique. **Syme's o.**, see under *amputation*. **tagliacotian o.**, see under *rhinoplasty*. **Talma's o.**, omentopexy in treatment of ascites; of historical interest. **Tanner's o.**, an operation for bleeding esophageal varices in which the terminal end of the esophagus, the cardia, and the proximal portion of the stomach are freed of all external vascular and ligamentous connections, and the stomach is transected below the cardia. **Teale's o.**, see under *amputation*. **Thiersch's o.**, removal of thin split-thickness skin grafts by means of a razor, skin-graft cutting knife, or a dermatome. **Torek o.**, 1. an operation for an undescended testicle. 2. an operation for the excision of the thoracic part of the esophagus; of historical interest. **Torkildsen's o.**, ventriculocisternostomy. **Toti's o.**, dacryocystorhinostomy. **Trendelenburg' o.**, 1. excision of varicose veins. 2. ligation of the great saphenous vein for varicose veins. 3. synchondroseotomy. 4. transthoracic pulmonary embolectomy. **van Hook's o.**, ureteroureterostomy. **Vineberg o.**, implantation of the internal mammary artery into the myocardium to enhance the growth of collateral circulation. **Vladimiroff o.**, Mikulicz's o., def. 3. **Voronoff's o.**, transplantation into man of the testes of an anthropoid ape, in the hope of rejuvenating the recipient. **Waters' o.**, a form of extraperitoneal cesarean section. **Waterston o.**, anastomosis between the ascending aorta and right pulmonary artery as palliative treatment of congenital pulmonary stenosis. **Watkins' o.**, an operation for prolapse and procidentia uteri in which the bladder is separated from the anterior wall of the uterus so that the uterus is left in a position to support the entire bladder. Called also *interposition o.* **Webster's o.**, for retrodisplacement of the uterus: the round ligaments

are passed through the perforated broad ligaments and fixed to the back of the uterus. **Wertheim's o.**, radical hysterectomy; removal of the uterus, tubes, parametrium, tissues surrounding the upper vagina, and pelvic lymphatics. **Whipple's o.**, radical pancreatoduodenectomy with removal of the distal third of the stomach, the entire duodenum, and the head of the pancreas, with gastrojejunostomy, choledochojejunostomy, and pancreatic jejunostomy. **White's o.**, castration for hypertrophy of the prostate. **Whitehead's o.**, treatment of hemorrhoids by excision. **Whitman's o.**, 1. an operation for arthroplasty of the hip joint. 2. a method of astragalectomy. **Witzel's o.**, see under *gastrostomy*. **Wölfler's o.**, anterior gastrojejunostomy for pyloric obstruction; of historical interest. **Young's o.**, 1. an operation for penile epispadias, with formation of a new urethral tube. 2. perineal prostatectomy. **Ziegler's o.**, V-shaped iridectomy for forming an artificial pupil.

operative (op′er-ah-tiv, op′rah-tiv, op′ĕ-ra″tiv) [L. *operativus*] 1. pertaining to an operation. 2. effective; not inert.

operator (op′er-a-tor) [L. "worker"] 1. one who performs an operation, or operates a mechanical device. 2. operator gene.

opercula (o-per′ku-lah) [L.] plural of *operculum*.

opercular (o-per′ku-lar) pertaining to an operculum.

operculectomy (o-per″ku-lek′to-me) the surgical removal of a mucosal flap partially or completely covering an unerupted tooth.

operculitis (o-per″ku-li′tis) pericoronitis.

operculum (o-per′ku-lum), pl. *oper′cula* [L.] 1. a lid or covering structure, such as the mucus plug obstructing the cervix of the gravid uterus in various animals. 2. one of the opercula of the insula; see *pars opercularis gyri frontalis inferioris*, *o. frontoparietale*, and *o. temporale*. **cartilaginous o.**, discus articularis articulationis temporomandibularis. **dental o.**, the hood of gingival tissue overlying the crown of an erupting tooth; called also *odontoclamis* and *tooth hood*. **frontal o., o. fronta′le**, pars opercularis gyri frontalis inferioris. **frontoparietal o., o. frontoparieta′le** [NA], the part of the inferior frontal gyrus behind the ascending branch of the lateral sulcus, together with the lower ends of the precentral and postcentral gyri, plus the anterior and lower part of the inferior parietal lobule, all covering over a part of the insular lobe (insula). **opercula of insula**, the areas of the cerebral cortex overlapping the insular lobe (insula) of the cerebral hemisphere forming part of the lips of the lateral sulcus, and separated by the rami of the lateral sulcus; see *pars opercularis gyri frontalis inferioris*, *o. frontoparietale*, and *o. temporale*. **occipital o.**, a part of the occipital lobe of the brain demarcated by the sulcus lunatus, when the latter structure is present. **temporal o., o. tempora′le** [NA], the parts of the superior temporal gyrus and transverse temporal gyri that cover over a part of the insular lobe (insula). **trophoblastic o.**, the plug of trophoblast that helps close the gap in the endometrium made by the implanting blastocyst.

operon (op′er-on) [L. *opera* work + Gr. *-on* neuter ending] in genetic theory, a segment of a chromosome comprising an operator gene and the closely linked structural gene or genes whose action it controls; the operon codes for single messenger RNA molecules and acts as a unit of genetic transcription and genetic regulation.

ophiasis (o-fi′ah-sis) [Gr. *ophis* snake] a form of alopecia areata of long duration, involving the temporal and occipital margins of the scalp in a continuous band.

Ophidia (o-fid′e-ah) [Gr. *ophidion* serpent] a suborder of Reptilia which embraces the snakes.

ophidiasis (o″fĭ-di′ah-sis) ophidism.

ophidic (o-fid′ik) pertaining to, caused by, or derived from snakes.

ophidism (o′fĭ-dizm) poisoning by snake venom.

Ophiophagus hannah (o″fe-of′ah-gus han′ah) the king cobra of India; see *cobra*.

ophiotoxemia (o″fe-o-tok-se′me-ah) [Gr. *ophis* snake + *toxemia*] poisoning by snake venom.

ophitoxemia (o″fe-tok-se′me-ah) ophiotoxemia.

Ophryoglenina (of″re-o-glĕ-ni′nah) [Gr. *ophrys* eyebrow + *glēnē* socket] a suborder of large, chiefly freshwater, histophagous ciliate protozoa (order Hymenostomatida, subclass

Hymenostomatia), characterized by a polymorphous life cycle and an oral apparatus including three ciliary organelles on the left and an associated watchglass organelle on the right. Several species cause disease in marine and freshwater fish, resulting in great economic loss. *Ichthyophthirius* is a representative genus.

ophryon (of′re-on) [Gr. *ophrys* eyebrow + *on* neuter ending] the middle point of the transverse supraorbital line.

ophryosis (of″re-o′sis) [Gr. *ophrys* eyebrow] spasm of the eyebrow.

Ophthaine (of′thān) trademark for a preparation of proparacaine hydrochloride.

ophthalmagra (of″thal-mag′rah) [*ophthalm-* + Gr. *agra* seizure] sudden pain in the eye.

ophthalmalgia (of″thal-mal′je-ah) [*ophthalm-* + *-algia*] pain in the eye.

ophthalmatrophia (of″thal-mah-tro′fe-ah) [*ophthalm-* + Gr. *atrophia* atrophy] atrophy of the eye.

ophthalmectomy (of″thal-mek′to-me) [*ophthalm-* + *ectomy*] the surgical removal of an eye; enucleation of the eyeball.

ophthalmencephalon (of″thal-men-sef′ah-lon) [*ophthalm-* + *encephalon*] the retina, optic nerve, and visual apparatus of the brain.

ophthalmia (of-thal′me-ah) [Gr., from *ophthalmos* eye] severe inflammation of the eye or of the conjunctiva or deeper structures of the eye. **actinic ray o.**, electric o. **Brazilian o.**, keratomalacia. **catarrhal o.**, a severe form of simple conjunctivitis. **caterpillar o.**, o. nodosa. **o. eczemato′sa**, phlyctenulosis. **Egyptian o.**, trachoma, def. 1. **electric o.**, conjunctivitis due to the effect of bright electric light, especially that of a welding arc. **flash o.**, electric o. **gonorrheal o.**, acute and severe purulent ophthalmia due to gonorrheal infection. **granular o.**, trachoma. **hepatic o.**, retinochoroidal degeneration with nyctalopia due to liver disease. **jequirity o.**, a form due to poisoning by jequirity, the poisonous seeds of *Abrus precatorius*. **metastatic o.**, choroiditis due to metastasis or to pyemia. **migratory o.**, sympathetic o. **mucous o.**, catarrhal o. **o. neonato′rum**, any hyperacute purulent conjunctivitis occurring during the first ten days of life, usually contracted during birth from infected vaginal discharge of the mother. Formerly it referred only to ocular gonorrheal infections. **neuroparalytic o.**, keratitis due to lesion of branches of the fifth nerve or of the gasserian ganglion. **o. nivia′lis**, snow blindness. **o. nodo′sa**, inflammation of the conjunctiva produced by caterpillar hairs, and marked by the formation of a round, gray swelling where each hair is embedded. **periodic o.**, a form of recurrent uveitis affecting horses. **phlyctenular o.**, see under *keratoconjunctivitis*. **purulent o.**, a form with a purulent discharge, commonly due to gonorrheal infection. **scrofulous o.**, keratoconjunctivitis associated with tuberculosis. **spring o.**, vernal conjunctivitis. **strumous o.**, phlyctenular keratoconjunctivitis. **sympathetic o.**, granulomatous inflammation of the uveal tract of the uninjured eye (the sympathizing eye) following some weeks after a wound involving the uveal tract of the other eye (the exciting eye). The end result is bilateral granulomatous inflammation of the entire uveal tract. Called also *sympathetic uveitis*. **transferred o.**, sympathetic o. **ultraviolet ray o.**, electric o. **varicose o.**, a variety associated with varicosity of the veins of the conjunctiva.

ophthalmiac (of-thal′me-ak) a person affected with ophthalmia.

ophthalmiatrics (of″thal-me-at′riks) [*ophthalm-* + Gr. *iatrikē* surgery, medicine] the treatment of eye diseases.

ophthalmic (of-thal′mik) pertaining to the eye.

ophthalmitic (of″thal-mit′ik) pertaining to ophthalmitis.

ophthalmitis (of″thal-mi′tis) [*ophthalm-* + *-itis*] inflammation of the eye.

ophthalm(o)- [Gr. *ophthalmos* eye] a combining form denoting relationship to the eye.

ophthalmoblennorrhea (of-thal″mo-blen″o-re′ah) [*ophthalmo-* + *blennorhea*] gonorrheal or purulent ophthalmia.

ophthalmocele (of-thal′mo-sēl) exophthalmos.

ophthalmocopia (of-thal″mo-ko′pe-ah) [*ophthalmo-* + Gr.

kopos weariness] asthenopia, or eyestrain; fatigue of the eyes.

ophthalmodesmitis (of-thal″mo-dez-mi′tis) [*ophthalmo-* + *desmitis*] inflammation of the ocular tendons.

ophthalmodiaphanoscope (of-thal″mo-di-ah-fan′o-skōp) [*ophthalmo-* + *diaphanoscope*] an instrument to examine the interior or the retina of the eye by transillumination.

ophthalmodiastimeter (of-thal″mo-di″as-tim′ĕ-ter) [*ophthalmo-* + *diastema* + *-meter*] an instrument for determining the proper distance at which to place lenses for the two eyes.

ophthalmodonesis (of-thal″mo-do-ne′sis) [*ophthalmo-* + Gr. *donēsis* trembling] a trembling motion of the eyes.

ophthalmodynamometer (of-thal″mo-di″nah-mom′ĕ-ter) [*ophthalmo-* + *dynamo-* + *-meter*] 1. an instrument for measuring the retinal arterial pressure. 2. an instrument for determining the near point of convergence.

ophthalmodynamometry (of-thal″mo-di″nah-mom′ĕ-tre) 1. determination of retinal arterial pressure by ophthalmodynamometer. 2. determination of the near point of convergence by an ophthalmodynamometer.

ophthalmodynia (of-thal″mo-din′e-ah) ophthalmalgia.

ophthalmoeikonometer (of-thal″mo-i″ko-nom′ĕ-ter) [*ophthalmo-* + Gr. *eikōn* image + *-meter*] an instrument used to determine both the refraction of the eye and the relative size and shape of the ocular images.

ophthalmograph (of-thal′mo-graf) [*ophthalmo-* + *-graph*] an instrument for photographing the movements of the eye during reading.

ophthalmography (of″thal-mog′rah-fe) [*ophthalmo-* + *-graphy*] description or photography of the eyes.

ophthalmogyric (of-thal″mo-ji′rik) oculogyric.

ophthalmoleukoscope (of-thal″mo-lu′ko-skōp) [*ophthalmo-* + *leukoscope*] an apparatus for testing color perception by means of colors produced by polarized light.

ophthalmolith (of-thal′mo-lith) [*ophthalmo-* + Gr. *lithos* stone] a lacrimal calculus.

ophthalmologic (of″thal-mo-loj′ik) pertaining to ophthalmology.

ophthalmologist (of″thal-mol′o-jist) a physician who specializes in the diagnosis and medical and surgical treatment of diseases and defects of the eye and related structures.

ophthalmology (of″thal-mol′o-je) [*ophthalmo-* + *-logy*] that branch of medicine dealing with the eye, its anatomy, physiology, pathology, etc.

ophthalmomalacia (of-thal″mo-mah-la′she-ah) [*ophthalmo-* + *malacia*] abnormal softness of the eye.

ophthalmometer (of″thal-mom′ĕ-ter) keratometer.

ophthalmometroscope (of-thal″mo-met′ro-skōp) [*ophthalmo-* + *metro-* + *-scope*] an ophthalmoscope with an attachment for measuring the refraction of the eye.

ophthalmometry (of″thal-mom′ĕ-tre) keratometry.

ophthalmomycosis (of-thal″mo-mi-ko′sis) [*ophthalmo-* + *mycosis*] any disease of the eye caused by a fungus.

ophthalmomyiasis (of-thal″mo-mi′yah-sis) [*ophthalmo-* + *myiasis*] infection of the eye by the larvae of the fly *Oestrus ovis*.

ophthalmomyitis (of-thal″mo-mi-i′tis) [*ophthalmo-* + *myitis*] inflammation of the muscles that move the eyeball.

ophthalmomyositis (of-thal″mo-mi″o-si′tis) [*ophthalmo-* + *myositis*] inflammation of the eye muscles.

ophthalmomyotomy (of-thal″mo-mi-ot′o-me) [*ophthalmo-* + *myotomy*] surgical division of the muscles of the eye.

ophthalmoneuritis (of-thal″mo-nu-ri′tis) inflammation of the ophthalmic nerve.

ophthalmoneuromyelitis (of-thal″mo-nu″ro-mi-ĕ-li′tis) neuromyelitis optica.

ophthalmopathy (of″thal-mop′ah-the) [*ophthalmo-* + *-pathy*] any disease of the eye. **external o.**, any affection of the eyelids, cornea, conjunctiva, or eye muscles. **internal o.**, any affection of the deep or more essential parts of the eye.

ophthalmophacometer (of-thal″mo-fa-kom′ĕ-ter) [*ophthalmo-* + *phacometer*] an ophthalometer used to determine the refractive power of the lens.

ophthalmophantom (of-thal″mo-fan′tom) 1. a model of

the eye used in demonstration. 2. an apparatus for holding animals' eyes for operation.

ophthalmophlebotomy (of-thal″mo-flĕ-bot′o-me) [*ophthalmo-* + *phlebotomy*] phlebotomy to relieve congestion of the conjunctival veins.

ophthalmophthisis (of″thal-mof′thĭ-sis) [*ophthalmo-* + Gr. *phthisis* wasting] ophthalmomalacia.

ophthalmoplasty (of-thal′mo-plas″te) [*ophthalmo-* + *-plasty*] plastic surgery of the eye or of its appendages.

ophthalmoplegia (of-thal″mo ple′je-ah) [*ophthalmo-* + *-plegia*] paralysis of the eye muscles. **basal o.,** ophthalmoplegia due to a lesion at the base of the brain. **exophthalmic o.,** external ocular paresis and exophthalmos of Graves' disease. **external o.,** paralysis of the external ocular muscles. **fascicular o.,** ophthalmoplegia due to lesion in the pons varolii. **internal o.,** paralysis of the iris and ciliary apparatus. **internuclear o.,** a horizontal ocular motor disturbance due to a lesion of the medial longitudinal fasciculus. **nuclear o.,** that which is due to some lesion of the nuclei of the motor nerves of the eye. **orbital o.,** ophthalmoplegia due to lesion in the orbit. **Parinaud's o.,** Parinaud syndrome. **partial o.,** paralysis of either one or two of the eye muscles. **progressive external o.,** a slowly progressing, bilateral myopathy often affecting only the extraocular muscles, but sometimes also the orbicularis oculi. The levators of the upper lids are usually affected first, with ptosis resulting, followed by progressive, total ocular paresis. Called also *ocular myopathy.* **total o., o. tota′lis,** that affecting both the extrinsic and intrinsic muscular apparatus of the eye.

ophthalmoplegic (of-thal″mo-ple′jik) pertaining to ophthalmoplegia.

ophthalmoptosis (of-thal″mop-to′sis) [*ophthalmo-* + *ptosis*] exophthalmos.

ophthalmoreaction (of-thal″mo-re-ak′shun) see *ophthalmic reaction,* under *reaction.*

ophthalmorrhagia (of-thal″mo-ra′je-ah) [*ophthalmo-* + *-rrhagia*] hemorrhage from the eye.

ophthalmorrhea (of-thal″mo-re′ah) [*ophthalmo-* + *-rrhea*] oozing of blood from the eye.

ophthalmorrhexis (of-thal″mo-rek′sis) [*ophthalmo-* + *rhexis*] rupture of the eyeball.

ophthalmoscope (of-thal′mo-skōp) [*ophthalmo-* + *-scope*] an instrument containing a perforated mirror and lenses used to examine the interior of the eye; called also *funduscope.* **binocular o.,** stereo-ophthalmoscope. **direct o.,** one that produces an upright, or unreversed, image of approximately 15 times magnification. **indirect o.,** one that produces an inverted, or reversed, direct image of 2 to 5 times magnification, depending on the dioptic power to the examining lens.

ophthalmoscopy (of-thal-mos′ko-pe) the examination of the interior of the eye with the ophthalmoscope. Called also *funduscopy.* **direct o.,** direct, close-range ophthalmoscopic observation of the fundus; the image is virtual, erect, and magnified. **indirect o.,** ophthalmoscopic examination of the fundus with the interposition of a strong convex lens between the observer and the patient; the image is real and inverted. **medical o.,** ophthalmoscopy performed to diagnose local or systemic diseases such as diabetes mellitus, hypertension, and cerebral tumor. **metric o.,** that performed for the measurement of refraction.

ophthalmospectroscope (of-thal″mo-spek′tro-skōp) an instrument used in ophthalmospectroscopy.

ophthalmospectroscopy (of-thal″mo-spek-tros′ko-pe) [*ophthalmo-* + *spectroscopy*] ophthalmoscopic and spectroscopic examination of the ocular fundus.

ophthalmostasis (of″thal-mos′tah-sis) [*ophthalmo-* + *stasis*] fixation of the eye with the ophthalmostat.

ophthalmostat (of-thal′mo-stat) [*ophthalmo-* + Gr. *histanai* to halt] an instrument for holding the eye steady during operation.

ophthalmostatometer (of-thal″mo-stah-tom′ĕ-ter) exophthalmometer.

ophthalmosteresis (of-thal″mo-stĕ-re′sis) [*ophthalmo-* + Gr. *steresis* privation, loss] loss of an eye.

ophthalmosynchysis (of-thal″mo-sin′kĭ-sis) [*ophthalmo-* + *synchysis*] effusion into the eye.

ophthalmothermometer (of-thal″mo-ther-mom′ĕ-ter)

[*ophthalmo-* + *thermometer*] an apparatus for recording the temperature of the eye.

ophthalmotomy (of″thal-mot′o-me) [*ophthalmo-* + *-tomy*] the operation of incising the eyeball.

ophthalmotonometer (of-thal″mo-to-nom′ĕ-ter) tonometer.

ophthalmotonometry (of-thal″mo-to-nom′ĕ-tre) [*ophthalmo-* + *tono-* + *-metry*] the indirect estimation of intraocular pressure by determining the resistance of the eyeball to indentation by an applied force; called also *tonometry.*

ophthalmotoxin (of-thal″mo-tok′sin) [*ophthalmo-* + *toxin*] 1. a toxin formed on injection of emulsion of the ciliary body. 2. a toxin acting on the eye.

ophthalmotrope (of-thal′mo-trōp) [*ophthalmo-* + Gr. *trepein* to turn] a mechanical eye that moves like a real eye, used for demonstrating the action of the ocular muscles.

ophthalmotropometer (of-thal″mo-tro-pom′ĕ-ter) strabismometer.

ophthalmotropometry (of-thal″mo-tro-pom′ĕ-tre) strabismometry.

ophthalmovascular (of-thal″mo-vas′ku-lar) pertaining to the blood vessels of the eye.

ophthalmoxerosis (of-thal″mo-ze-ro′sis) xerophthalmia.

ophthalmoxyster (of-thal″moks-is′ter) [*ophthalmo-* + *xystēr*] an instrument for scraping the conjunctiva.

Ophthetic (of-thet′ik) trademark for a preparation of proparacaine hydrochloride.

Ophthochlor (of′tho-klōr) trademark for a preparation of chloramphenicol.

-opia [Gr. *ōps* eye] a combining form denoting condition or a defect of the eye, or of vision.

opian (o′pe-an) noscapine.

opianine (o-pi′ah-nin) noscapine.

opiate (o′pe-at) a remedy containing or derived from opium; also any drug that induces sleep.

Opie paradox (o′pe) [Eugene Lindsay *Opie,* American pathologist, 1873–1971] see under *paradox.*

opioid (o′pe-oid) 1. any synthetic narcotic that has opiate-like activities but is not derived from opium. 2. denoting naturally occurring peptides, e.g., enkephalins, that exert opiate-like effects by interacting with opiate receptors of cell membranes.

opiomania (o″pe-o-ma′ne-ah) [*opium* + Gr. *mania* madness] addiction to opium.

opipramol hydrochloride (o-pip′rah-mōl) chemical name: 4-[3-[5*H* - dibenz [*b,f*] azepin - 5 - yl)propyl] - 1 - piperazineethanol dihydrochloride; a tricyclic antidepressant with mild tranquilizing properties, $C_{23}H_{29}N_3O \cdot 2HCl$.

Opisocrostis (o″pĭ-so-kros′tis) a genus of fleas. **O. bru′neri,** a squirrel flea said to be a vector of sylvatic plague.

opisthe (o-pis′the) [Gr. *opisthen* behind] the posterior daughter organism after transverse division of a ciliate protozoan; cf. *proter.*

opisthenar (o-pis′the-nar) [*opistho-* + Gr. *thenar* palm of the hand] the dorsum of the hand.

opisthencephalon (o-pis″then-sef′ah-lon) [*opistho-* + Gr. *enkephalos* brain] the cerebellum.

opisthiobasial (o-pis″the-o-ba′se-al) pertaining to or connecting the opisthion and basion.

opisthion (o-pis′the-on) [Gr. *opisthion* rear, posterior] [NA] a craniometric landmark located at the midpoint of the posterior border of the foramen magnum.

opisthionasial (o-pis″the-o-na′ze-al) connecting the opisthion and nasion.

opisth(o)- [Gr. *opisthen* behind, at the back] a combining form meaning backward or denoting relationship to the back.

opisthocranion (o-pis″tho-kra′ne-on) [*opistho-* + Gr. *kranion* the upper part of the head] a craniometric landmark determined instrumentally to indicate the posterior end of the maximum cranial length measured along the midline of the glabella.

opisthogenia (o-pis″tho-je′ne-ah) defective development of the jaws following ankylosis of the jaw.

opisthognathism (o″pis-thog′nah-thizm) the condition of having receding jaws.

opisthomastigote (o″pis-tho-mas′tĭ-gōt) [*opistho-* + Gr. *mastix* whip] any of the bodies representing the morphologic stage in the life cycle of trypanosomatid protozoa of the genus *Herpetomonas*, in which the kinetoplast and basal body are posterior to the nucleus and the flagellum runs through the body of the cell to emerge anteriorly as a free-flowing structure. Cf. *amastigote, choanomastigote, epimastigote, promastigote,* and *trypomastigote.*

opisthoporeia (o-pis″tho-po-ri′ah) [*opistho-* + Gr. *poreia* walk] involuntary walking backward, as in parkinsonism; retropulsion.

opisthorchiasis (o″pis-thor-ki′ah-sis) infection of the biliary tract by the liver flukes *Opisthorchis felineus* and *O. viverrini.* In heavy infections, local injury to the distal bile capillaries and surrounding liver tissue develops; in severe infections, there may be cirrhosis of the liver with areas of necrosis and fatty degeneration.

Opisthorchis (o″pis-thor′kis) [*opistho-* + Gr. *orchis* testicle] a genus of trematodes or flukes characterized by having the testes near the posterior end of the body. **O. felin′eus,** the Siberian liver fluke found in the liver of cats, dogs, pigs, and man; infection (see *opisthorchiasis*) results from ingestion of infected fish (*Leuciscus rutilis, Idus melanotus,* and related species). **O. nover′ca,** *Amphimerus noverca.* **O. sinen′sis,** the common liver fluke of man in China, Japan, Korea, Taiwan, and Indochina. Adult worms inhabit the bile ducts. Larval development requires two intermediate hosts, the first a snail of the genus *Parafossarulus* or *Bithynia,* the second a freshwater fish of the carp family. Human infection (see *clonorchiasis*) is acquired from the latter host. Called also *Clonorchis sinensis* and *Distoma sinensis.* **O. viverri′ni,** a species found in Thailand in the civet cat and sometimes in man (see *opisthorchiasis*).

opisthorchosis (o″pis-thor-ko′sis) infection with any species of *Opisthorchis.*

opisthotic (o″pis-thot′ik) [*opistho-* + Gr. *ous* ear] situated behind the ear.

opisthotonoid (o″pis-thot′o-noid) resembling opisthotonos.

opisthotonos (o″pis-thot′o-nos) [*opistho-* + Gr. *tonos* tension] a form of spasm in which the head and the heels are bent

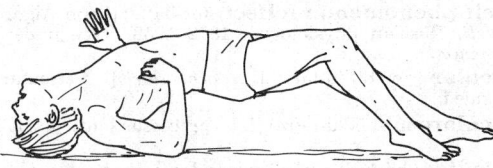

Opisthotonus.

backward and the body bowed forward. **o. feta′lis,** an exaggerated deflection attitude of the fetus during labor, which may persist during the neonatal period, but which gradually changes to a more normal posture.

opisthotonus (o″pis-thot′o-nus) opisthotonos.

Opitz's disease (o′pitz) [Hans *Opitz,* German pediatrician, born 1888] see under *disease.*

opium (o′pe-um) [L.; Gr. *opion*] [*USP*] an air-dried milky exudate obtained by incising the unripe capsules of *Papaver somniferum* L. (Papaveraceae) or its variety, *album,* yielding not less than 9.5 per cent of anhydrous morphine. Called also *crude o.* and *gum o.* Various principles and derivatives of opium, including some 20 alkaloids, notably morphine, codeine, paperavine, and thebaine, are used for their narcotic and analgesic effects. Because it is highly addictive, the production of opium is restricted, and the cultivation of the plants from which it is obtained is prohibited by most nations under an international agreement. **crude o.,** see *opium.* **denarcotized o., o. deodora′tum, deodorized o.,** powdered opium freed from certain nauseating constituents by extraction with purified petroleum benzin. **granulated o., o. granula′tum,** opium reduced to a coarse powder. **gum o.,** see *opium.* **lettuce o.,** the bitter, inspissated juice of various species of lettuce, e.g., *Lactuca sativa* L. (Compositae), formerly used for mild hypnotic and sedative action. **powdered o.** [*USP*], **o. pulvera′tum,** opium dried at a temperature not exceeding 70° C., and reduced to a very fine powder, yielding not less than 10 per cent and not more than 10.5 per cent of anhydrous morphine. It may

contain any of the diluents, except starch, permitted in powdered extracts. See *brown mixture,* under *mixture,* and see *paregoric.*

opobalsamum (o″po-bal′sah-mum) [Gr. *opos* juice + *balsamon* balsam] balsam of Gilead.

opocephalus (o″po-sef′ah-lus) [Gr. *ōps* face + *kephalē* head] a monster with the ears fused to the head, one orbit, no mouth, and no nose.

opodidymus (o″po-did′ĭ-mus) [Gr. *ōps* face + *didymos* twin] a fetus with two fused heads and with the sense organs partially fused.

opodymus (o-pod′ĭ-mus) opodidymus.

opossum (o-pos′um) a marsupial animal, species of which (*Didelphis*) in South America are reservoirs of *Trypanosoma cruzi.*

Oppenheim's disease (syndrome), sign (reflex) (op′en-hīmz) [Hermann *Oppenheim,* neurologist in Berlin, 1858–1919] see *amyotonia congenita,* and see under *sign.*

opponens (o-po′nenz) [L.] opposing; said of an opposing structure, as musculus opponens.

opportunistic (op″or-tu-nis′tik) 1. denoting a microorganism that does not ordinarily cause disease but that, under certain circumstances (e.g., impaired immune responses resulting from other disease or drug treatment), becomes pathogenic. 2. denoting a disease or infection caused by such an organism.

oppositipolar (o-poz″ĭ-ti-po′lar) having two poles on opposite sides of a cell.

-opsia [Gr. *opsis* sight] a combining form denoting a condition or a defect of vision.

opsialgia (op″se-al′je-ah) [Gr. *ōps* face + *-algia*] geniculate neuralgia.

opsin (op′sin) a protein of the retinal rods (scotopsin) and cones (photopsin) that combines with 11-*cis*-retinal to form visual pigments; see *retinal* (def. 2). The opsins are also named according to the color of pigment: iodopsin (violet), porphyropsin (red), rhodopsin (purple), etc.

opsinogen (op-sin′o-jen) (*obs.*) a substance (antigen) with the power to induce the formation of opsonins in the body.

opsinogenous (op″sin-oj′ĕ-nus) able to form opsonins.

opsiometer (op″se-om′ĕ-ter) optometer.

opsiuria (op″se-u′re-ah) [Gr. *opse* late + *ouron* urine + *-ia*] the condition in which more urine is excreted during fasting than during digestion.

opsoclonia, opsoclonus (op″so-klo′ne-ah; op″so-klo′nus) a condition characterized by nonrhythmic horizontal and vertical oscillations of the eyes, observed in various disorders of the brain stem or cerebellum.

opsogen (op′so-jen) opsinogen.

opsomania (op″so-ma′ne-ah) [Gr. *opson* dainty + *mania* madness] a craving for some special food.

opsonic (op-son′ik) pertaining to opsonins.

opsonin (op′so-nin) [Gr. *opsōnein* to buy victuals] any substance that binds to particulate antigens and induces their phagocytosis by macrophages and neutrophils. In current usage the term is used to refer to substances of two types, opsonizing antibodies (IgM, IgG1, and IgG3 immunoglobulins specific for the antigen) and certain complement fragments (C3b, C3d, and C4b), which become bound to the antigen during complement activation), both of which trigger phagocytosis by binding to specific cell-surface receptors, Fc receptors, and C3b receptors on neutrophils and macrophages and C3d receptors on macrophages. **immune o.,** opsonizing antibody; see *opsonin.*

opsonization (op″so-ni-za′shun) the rendering of bacteria and other cells subject to phagocytosis by the action of an opsonin.

opsonize (op′so-nīz) to function as an opsonin.

opsonocytophagic (op″so-no-si″to-faj′ik) denoting the phagocytic activity of blood in the presence of serum opsonins and homologous leukocytes.

opsonometry (op″so-nom′ĕ-tre) (*obs.*) the measurement of opsonocytophagic activity or the opsonic index.

opsonophilia (op″so-no-fil′e-ah) [*opsonin* + Gr. *philein* to love] affinity for opsonins.

opsonophilic (op″so-no-fil′ik) having an affinity for opsonins.

Optef (op'tef) trademark for a preparation of hydrocortisone.

optesthesia (op''tes-the'ze-ah) [opt- + esthesia] visual sensibility; ability to perceive visual stimuli.

optic (op'tik) [Gr. optikos of or for sight] of or pertaining to the eye.

optical (op'tĭ-kal) [L. opticus; Gr. optikos] pertaining to or subserving vision.

optician (op-tish'an) an expert in opticianry.

opticianry (op-tish'an-re) the science of optics as applied to filling and adapting of ophthalmic prescriptions and products.

opticochiasmatic (op''tĭ-ko-ki''az-mat'ik) pertaining to the optic nerves and chiasma.

opticociliary (op''tĭ-ko-sil'e-a-re) pertaining to the optic and ciliary nerves.

opticonasion (op''tĭ-ko-na'se-on) the distance from the posterior edge of the optic foramen to the nasion.

opticopupillary (op''tĭ-ko-pu'pĭ-ler-e) pertaining to the optic nerve and the pupil.

optics (op'tiks) [Gr. optikos of or for sight] the science which treats of light and of vision. **fiber o.,** see fiberoptics.

optimal (op'tĭ-mal) the best; the most favorable.

optimeter (op-tim'ĕ-ter) optometer.

optimum (op'tĭ-mum) [L. "best"] 1. that condition of surroundings which is conducive to the most favorable activity or function. 2. Pirquet's term for the amount of food most desirable under given circumstances.

opt(o)- [Gr. optos seen] a combining form denoting relationship to vision or sight.

optochiasmic (op''to-ki-az'mik) opticochiasmatic.

optogram (op'to-gram) [opto- + -gram] the retinal image formed by the bleaching of the visual purple under the influence of light.

optokinetic (op''to-ki-net'ik) [opto- + kinetic] pertaining to movement of the eyes and of objects in the visual field, as in nystagmus.

optomeninx (op''to-me'ningks) [opto- + Gr. mēninx membrane] the retina.

optometer (op-tom'ĕ-ter) [opto- + -meter] an instrument that measures ocular refraction; called also opsimeter, optimeter, and refractometer.

optometrist (op-tom'ĕ-trist) one trained and licensed to practice optometry.

optometry (op-tom'ĕ-tre) [opto- + -metry] 1. the professional practice of primary eye and vision care for the diagnosis, treatment, and prevention of associated disorders and for the improvement of vision by the prescription of spectacles and by use of other functional, optical, and pharmaceutical means regulated by state law. 2. the use of an optometer.

optomyometer (op''to-mi-om'ĕ-ter) [opto- + myometer] a device used in measuring the power of the extrinsic ocular muscles.

optophone (op'to-fōn) [opto- + Gr. phōne voice] an instrument by means of which light and darkness are made discernible to the blind through their sense of hearing, the light waves being transformed into sound waves.

optotype (op'to-tīp) test type.

Opuntia (o-pun'she-ah) a genus of cacti. O. vulgaris, the prickly pear, is used as a remedy in homeopathic practice.

OPV poliovirus vaccine live oral.

O.R. operating room.

ora[1] (o'rah), gen. and pl. o'rae [L.] an edge or margin. **o. serra'ta re'tinae** [NA], the irregular anterior margin of the pars optica of the retina, lying internal and slightly posterior to the junction of the choroid and the ciliary body.

ora[2] (o'rah) [L.] plural of os, mouth.

Orabilex (or''ah-bi'leks) trademark for a preparation of bunamiodyl.

orad (o'rad) [L. os, oris mouth + ad toward] toward the mouth.

orae (o're) [L.] genitive and plural of ora[1].

Oragrafin (or''ah-graf'in) trademark for a preparation of the calcium or the sodium salt of ipodate.

oral (o'ral) [L. oralis] 1. pertaining to the mouth, taken through or applied in the mouth, as an oral medication or an oral thermometer. 2. see facies lingualis dentis.

orale (o-ra'le) a craniometric landmark, being the point in the midline of the maxillary suture just lingual to the central incisors in the alveolar process.

orality (o-ral'ĭ-te) in psychoanalytic theory, the psychic organization of all the sensations, impulses, and personality traits derived from the oral stage of psychosexual development.

oralogy (o-ral'o-je) [L. oralis pertaining to the mouth + -logy] stomatology.

orange (or'anj) [L. aurantium] 1. the rutaceous tree, Citrus aurantium L., and its yellow, edible fruit (aurantii fructus). There are two varieties, bitter orange (aurantii amara) and sweet orange (aurantii dulcis). The peel of the two varieties is used in making various pharmaceutical preparations. 2. a color between red and yellow. 3. a dye or stain that produces an orange color. **acridine o.,** see under acridine. **ethyl o.,** an indicator with a pH range of 2 to 4. **o. G,** an acid azo dye used as a cytoplasmic stain, $C_6H_5 \cdot N:N \cdot C_{10}H_4$-$(SO_2 \cdot ONa)_2 \cdot OH$. **gold o.,** methyl o. **o. III,** methyl o. **methyl o.** [USP], an orange-yellow powder, the sodium salt of dimethylaminoazobenzene sulfonic acid, used as an indicator with a pH range of 3.2 to 4.4 and a color change from pink to yellow. Called also gold o., helianthin, o. III and Poirrier's o. **o. Poirrier's o.,** methyl o. **victoria o.,** a salt of dinitrocresol used in histology as a stain. **wool o.,** orange G.

orangeophil (or-an'je-o-fil) 1. staining readily with orange dyes. 2. a cell or other histologic element that stains readily with orange dyes. 3. one of the acidophils, or alpha cells (somatotropes), of the adenohypophysis staining readily with orange G; called also alpha acidophil.

orangutan (o-rang'oo-tan'') [Malayan orang a human being + utan (hutan) wild] one of the anthropoid apes, of the family Pongidae, frequently used for laboratory studies because it is susceptible to some of the same diseases as man.

Oranixon (or''ah-nik'son) trademark for a preparation of mephenesin.

Ora-Testryl (o''rah-tes'tril) trademark for a preparation of fluoxymesterone.

Orbeli phenomenon (effect) (or-ba'le) [Leon Algarovich Orbeli, Russian physiologist, 1882–1958] see under phenomenon.

orbicular (or-bik'u-lar) [L. orbicularis] circular, or rounded.

orbiculare (or-bik''u-la're) [L.] processus lenticularis incudis.

orbiculi (or-bik'u-li) genitive and plural of orbiculus.

orbiculus (or-bik'u-lus), gen. and pl. orbic'uli [L., dim. of orbis orb, circle] [NA], a general term denoting a structure shaped like a small circle, or disk. **o. cilia'ris** [NA], the thin part of the ciliary body extending between its crown and the ora serrata retinae; called also ciliary disk and pars plana corporis ciliaris.

orbit (or'bit) the bony cavity that contains the eyeball; see orbita [NA].

orbita (or'bĭ-tah), gen. and pl. or'bitae [L. "mark of a wheel, circuit"] [NA] the orbit: the bony cavity that contains the eyeball and its associated muscles, vessels, and nerves; the ethmoidal, frontal, lacrimal, nasal, palatine, sphenoidal, and zygomatic bones, and the maxilla contribute to its formation.

orbitae (or'bĭ-te) [L.] genitive and plural of orbita.

orbital (or'bĭ-tal) 1. pertaining to the orbit. 2. a region in an atom that may contain either one or two opposite spin electrons; orbitals of various sizes and shapes may occur in a single atom. A set of orbitals is a housing arrangement for electrons.

orbitale (or''bĭ-ta'le) an anthropometric landmark, the lowest point on the inferior margin of the orbit.

orbitalis (or''bĭ-ta'lis) [L.] pertaining to the orbit.

orbitonasal (or''bĭ-to-na'zal) pertaining to the orbit and the nose.

orbitonometer (or''bĭ-to-nom'ĕ-ter) [orb + tonometer] an instrument for measurement of the backward displacement of the eyeball produced by a given pressure exerted against its anterior aspect; called also piezometer.

orbitonometry (or″bĭ-to-nom′ĕ-tre) the measurement of the backward displacement of the eyeball under varying pressures.

orbitopagus (or″bĭ-top′ah-gus) [*orbit* + Gr. *pagos* thing fixed] a twin monster composed of a small fetus attached to the orbit of the autosite.

orbitostat (or′bĭ-to-stat) [*orbit* + Gr. *statos* placed] an instrument for measuring the axis of the orbit.

orbitotemporal (or″bĭ-to-tem′po-ral) pertaining to the orbital and temporal regions.

orbitotomy (or″bĭ-tot′o-me) [*orbit* + *-tomy*] the operation of incising or opening into the orbit through the orbital margin.

orbivirus (or′bĭ-vi″rus) a group of RNA viruses, a subgroup of the diplornavirus.

orcein (or-se′in) a brown coloring matter, $C_{28}H_{24}N_2O_7$, derived from orcin and soluble in alcohol; used as a specific stain for elastic tissue.

orchectomy (or-kek′to-me) orchiectomy.

orchella (or-shel′ah) a histologic stain composed of 5 ml. of acetic acid and 40 ml. each of alcohol and water, colored to a dark red with archil from which excess of ammonia has been driven off.

orchialgia (or″ke-al′je-ah) [*orchi-* + *-algia*] pain in a testis.

orchic (or′kik) orchidic.

orchichorea (or″ke-ko-re′ah) [*orchi-* + *chorea*] a twitching or jerking movement of a testis.

orchidalgia (or″kĭ-dal′je-ah) orchialgia.

orchidectomy (or″kĭ-dek′to-me) orchiectomy.

orchidic (or-kid′ik) pertaining to the testes.

orchiditis (or″kĭ-di′tis) orchitis.

orchid(o)- [Gr. *orchidion*, dim. of *orchis* testis] a combining form denoting relationship to the testes.

orchidoepididymectomy (or″kĭ-do-ep″ĭ-did″ĭ-mek′to-me) [*orchido-* + *epididymis* + Gr. *ektomē* excision] the operation of excising the testis and epididymis.

orchidometer (or″kĭ-dom′ĕ-ter) an instrument for measuring the testis. **Prader o.,** a string of plastic models of testicular shape, marked according to their volume in cubic centimeters; used for measuring the size of the testes in genital development.

orchidoncus (or″kĭ-dong′kus) [*orchido-* + Gr. *onkos* tumor] a tumor of a testis.

orchidopathy (or″kĭ-dop′ah-the) orchiopathy.

orchidopexy (or′kĭ-do-pek″se) orchiopexy.

orchidoplasty (or′kĭ-do-plas″te) orchioplasty.

orchidoptosis (or″kĭ-dop-to′sis) [*orchido-* + Gr. *ptōsis*] downward displacement of the testis, a condition due to varicocele or relaxation of the scrotum.

orchidorrhaphy (or″kĭ-dor′ah-fe) orchiopexy.

orchidotomy (or″kĭ-dot′o-me) orchiotomy.

orchiectomy (or″ke-ek′to-me) [*orchio-* + Gr. *ektomē* excision] excision of one or both testes.

orchiencephaloma (or″ke-en-sef″ah-lo′mah) [*orchio-* + *encephaloma*] embryonal carcinoma.

orchiepididymitis (or″ke-ep″ĭ-did″ĭ-mi′tis) [*orchio-* + *epididymis* + *-itis*] inflammation of a testis and an epididymis.

orchilytic (or″kĭ-lit′ik) [*orchio-* + Gr. *lytikos* dissolving] destroying testicular tissue.

orchi(o)- [Gr. *orchis*, gen. *orchios* testis] a combining form denoting relationship to the testes.

orchiocatabasis (or″ke-o-kah-tab′ah-sis) [*orchio-* + Gr. *katabasis* descent] the descent of the testes.

orchiocele (or′ke-o-sēl″) [*orchio-* + Gr. *kēlē* hernia] 1. hernial protrusion of a testis. 2. scrotal hernia. 3. tumor of a testis.

orchiodynia (or″ke-o-din′e-ah) orchialgia.

orchiomyeloma (or″ke-o-mi″ĕ-lo′mah) [*orchio-* + *myeloma*] plasmacytoma of the testis.

orchioncus (or″ke-ong′kus) [*orchio-* + Gr. *onkos* mass, tumor] tumor of the testis.

orchioneuralgia (or″ke-o-nu-ral′je-ah) [*orchio-* + *neuralgia*] orchialgia.

orchiopathy (or″ke-op′ah-the) [*orchio-* + Gr. *pathos* disease] any disease of the testis.

orchiopexy (or″ke-o-pek′se) [*orchio-* + G. *pēxis* fixation] surgical fixation in the scrotum of an undescended testis.

orchioplasty (or′ke-o-plas″te) [*orchio-* + Gr. *plassein* to form] plastic surgery of the testis.

orchiorrhaphy (or″ke-or′ah-fe) [*orchio-* + Gr. *rhaphē* suture] orchiopexy.

orchioscheocele (or″ke-os′ke-o-sēl″) [*orchio-* + Gr. *oscheon* scrotum + *kēlē* hernia] scrotal tumor with scrotal hernia.

orchioscirrhus (or″ke-o-skir′us) [*orchio-* + Gr. *skirrhos* hard] hardening of the testis.

orchiotomy (or″ke-ot′o-me) [*orchio* + Gr. *temnein* to cut] incision and drainage of a testis.

Orchis (or′kis) the typical genus of orchidaceous plants, so named because certain species bear root or rhizome systems that resemble testicles. Various species are medicinal.

orchis (or′kis) [Gr.] NA alternative for *testis.*

orchitic (or-kit′ik) pertaining to, causing, or affected with orchitis.

orchitis (or-ki′tis) [*orchio-* + *-itis*] inflammation of a testis. The disease is marked by pain, swelling, and a feeling of weight. It may occur idiopathically, or it may be associated with conditions such as mumps, gonorrhea, filarial disease, syphilis, or tuberculosis. **metastatic o.,** an infection brought to the testis by the blood stream, as in mumps. **spermatogenic granulomatous o.,** orchitis in which the normal structure of the testis has been replaced by gray-white granulomatous tissue without evident necrosis; it is thought to be in some way a reaction to spermatozoa. **traumatic o.,** orchitis following trauma, vas ligation, or surgical manipulation, without evidence of previous disease, believed to be due to an infectious process resulting from lowered resistance of the injured tissues to bacteria. **o. variolo′sa,** orchitis occurring in smallpox.

orchitolytic (or″kĭ-to-lit′ik) orchilytic.

orchotomy (or-kot′o-me) orchiotomy.

orcin (or′sin) orcinol.

orcinol (or′sĭ-nol) chemical name: 5-methylresorcinol. An antiseptic principle, $C_7H_8O_2 \cdot H_2O$, mainly derived from various lichens, used as a reagent in various tests; called also *orcin.*

order (or′der) [L. *ordo* a line, row, or series] a taxonomic category subordinate to a class and superior to a family; see *taxon.*

orderly (or′der-le) a male attendant in a hospital who does general work, attending especially to the preoperative preparation (shaving, catheterizing, etc.) of male patients.

ordinate (or′dĭ-nit) [L. *ordinare* to arrange in order] in a two-dimensional coordinate system, the distance of a point from the horizontal (x) axis, measured along a line parallel to the y-axis. Denoted by y. Cf. *abscissa.*

ordure (or′dūr) excrement.

oreoselinum (o″re-o-se-li′num) [L.] an umbelliferous plant of the Old World, *Peucedanum oreoselinum* (L.) Munch. (Umbelliferae); used in homeopathic practice as a diuretic.

Oretic (o-ret′ik) trademark for a preparation of hydrochlorothiazide.

Oreticyl (o-ret′ĭ-sil) trademark for preparations of hydrochlorothiazide with deserpidine.

Oreton (or′e-ton) trademark for preparations of testosterone propionate.

orexia (o-rek′se-ah) [Gr. *orexis*] appetite.

orexigenic (o-rek″sĭ-jen′ik) [Gr. *orexis* appetite + *gennan* to produce] increasing or stimulating the appetite.

orf (orf) contagious ecthyma.

organ (or′gan) [L. *organum;* Gr. *organnon*] a somewhat independent part of the body that performs a special function or functions; see *organum* [NA]. **accessory o's of eye,** structures accessory to the eye, including the ocular muscles and fascia, and the eyebrows, eyelids, conjunctiva, and lacrimal apparatus (organa oculi accessoria [NA]). **acoustic o.,** organum spirale. **Bidder's o.,** an anterior portion, ovarian in character, of the gonad of male toads. **cell o.,** a structural part of a cell having some definite function in its life or reproduction, as a nucleus or a centrosome. **cement o.,** the embryonic tissue that develops into the cement layer of the tooth. **Chievitz's o.,** an embryonic outgrowth behind the parotid gland which may merge into the latter or may disappear. **o. of Corti,** organum spirale. **digestive o's,** those concerned with the ingestion, digestion, and assimilation of food (apparatus digestorius [NA]). **effector o.,** a muscle or gland that contracts or secretes, respectively, in direct response to nerve impulses. **enamel o.,** a circumscribed knoblike mass of ectodermal cells arising from the dental lamina; it produces the enamel cap from which the dental enamel develops. **end o.,** end-organ; see under *E*. **essential o. of thalamus,** some portion of the thalamus, possibly the medial nucleus, which functions as an integrating center in animals with little or no cerebral cortex and functioning in a more or less similar manner in higher forms. **extraperitoneal o.,** organum extraperitoneale. **genital o's,** organa genitalia. **genital o's, external,** see *organa genitalia feminina externa* and *organa genitalia masculina externa*. **genital o's, female,** see *organa genitalia feminina externa* and *organa genitalia feminina interna*. **genital o's, internal,** see *organa genitalia feminina interna* and *organa genitalia masculina interna*. **genital o's, male,** see *organa genitalia masculina externa* and *organa genitalia masculina interna*. **o. of Giraldés,** paradidymis. **Golgi tendon o.,** a mechanoreceptor found in tendons of mammalian muscles; arranged in series with the muscle, it is sensitive to mechanical distortion induced by either passive stretch of the tendon or isometric contraction of the muscle and thus signals muscle tension, being the receptor responsible for the lengthening reaction, or clasp-knife reflex. Called also *tendon spindle*. **gustatory o.,** the organ concerned with the perception of taste; see *organum gustus* [NA]. **intromittent o.,** any male copulatory organ, e.g., the human penis or the claspers seen especially in male insects and cartilaginous fishes, used to transfer sperm to the female reproductive tract. **Jacobson's o.,** organum vomeronasale. **lateral line o's,** a system of sense organs arranged in longitudinal canals in the skin of fishes and amphibians which are sensitive to changes in pressure and current and to vibrations of low frequency and thus aid in localizing objects. **Marchand's o.,** see under *adrenal*. **o's of mastication,** masticatory apparatus. **Meyer's o.,** an area of circumvallate papillae on either side of the posterior part of the tongue. **olfactory o.,** the organ concerned with the perception of odors; see *organum olfactus* [NA]. **parapineal o.,** a median dorsal outgrowth of the pineal body in certain lower vertebrates, such as tailless amphibians, primitive fishes, and lizards, the principal cell type of which is an apparent photoreceptor. In some species, it may specialize to form an extracranial epiphyseal eye. Called also *parietal o*. **parenchymal o., parenchymatous o.,** organon parenchymatosum. **parietal o.,** parapineal o. **primitive fat o.,** brown adipose tissue. **reproductive o's,** organa genitalia. **reproductive o's, female,** see *organa genitalia feminina externa* and *organa genitalia feminina interna*. **reproductive o's, male,** see *organa genitalia masculina externa* and *organa genitalia masculina interna*. **retroperitoneal o.,** organum extraperitoneale. **Rosenmüller's o.,** epoöphoron. **rudimentary o.,** 1. a primordium. 2. an imperfectly or incompletely developed organ. **o. of Ruffini,** brushes of Ruffini. **segmental o.,** the pronephros, mesonephros, and metanephros together. **sense o's, sensory o's,** organa sensuum. See under *organum*. **o. of shock, shock o.,** the organ which reacts in anaphylactic shock; those organs whose responses determine the nature and, to a large extent, the outcome of a given anaphylactic reaction. **o's of special sense,** organa sensuum; see under *organum*. **spiral o.,** organum spirale. **subcommissural o.,** organum subcommissurale. **subfornical o.,** organum subfornicale. **target o.,** an organ that is affected by a specific hormone, as the adrenal cortex by corticotropin. **terminal o.,** the organ situated at either end of a reflex neural arc. **urinary o's,** organa urinaria. **vestibulocochlear o's,** those structures outside the central nervous system which are concerned with vestibular and auditory function; see *organum vestibulocochleare* [NA]. **vestigial o.,** an undeveloped organ that, in the embryo or in some more or less remote ancestor, was well developed and functional. **o. of vision, visual o.,** organum visus. **vomeronasal o.,** organum vomeronasale. **Weber's o.,** utriculus prostaticus. **X o., X-o.,** a secretory mass of cells found in close association with the sinus gland of certain crustaceans, which produces a hormone that influences molting by inhibiting secretion of the molting

hormone produced by the Y organ, and elaborates other hormones that regulate metabolism, reproduction, the distribution of pigment in the compound eyes, and control of body pigmentation. **Y o., Y-o.,** a mass of secretory cells found at the base of the mandibular muscles or in the base of the antennae of certain crustaceans, which produces a hormone that initiates molting; the hormone may be ecdysone or a very similar steroid. **o's of Zuckerkandl,** corpora paraaortica.

organa (or'gah-nah) plural of *organum* [L.] and *organon* [Gr.].

organacidia (or″gan-ah-sid'e-ah) the presence of an organic acid, especially in the stomach.

organella (or″gah-nel'ah), pl. *organel'lae* [L., dim. of *organum*] organelle.

organellae (or″gah-nel'e) [L.] plural of *organella*.

organelle (or″gah-nel') [L. *organella*, dim. of *organum* organ] any of the membrane-bound organized cytoplasmic structures of distinctive morphology and function present in all eukaryotic cells. Organelles include such structures as nucleus, mitochondria, lysosomes, peroxisomes, Golgi apparatus, and endoplasmic reticulum, as well as chloroplasts in plants and cilia, flagella, and the cytopharynx in protozoa. **Lieberkühn's o.,** watchglass o. **watchglass o.,** a lenticular, refractile, subpellicular organelle characteristic of ciliate protozoa of the suborder Ophryoglenina, in which it is found in association with the left wall of the buccal cavity; its function is unknown. Called also *Lieberkühn's o.* and *watchglass body*.

organic (or-gan'ik) [L. *organicus*; Gr. *organikos*] 1. pertaining to an organ or the organs. 2. having an organized structure. 3. arising from an organism. 4. pertaining to substances derived from living organisms. 5. denoting chemical substances containing carbon. 6. pertaining to or cultivated by the use of animal or vegetable fertilizers, rather than synthetic chemicals.

organicism (or-gan'ĭ-sizm) 1. the theory that all disease is caused by organic lesions. 2. the theory that each of the various organs of the body has its own special constitution. 3. holism.

organicist (or-gan'ĭ-sist) one who believes in organicism.

Organidin (or-gan'ĭ-din) trademark for a preparation of iodinated glycerol.

organism (or'gah-nizm) any individual living thing, whether animal or plant. **consumer o's,** the organisms of an ecosystem, plants or animals, that eat other plants or animals. **nitrifying o's,** those nitrogen bacteria which are capable of oxidizing ammonia to nitrites and nitrates. **nitrosifying o's,** those nitrogen bacteria which are capable of oxidizing ammonia to nitrites. **pleuropneumonia-like o's (PPLO),** originally, a group of filtrable microorganisms similar to *Mycoplasma mycoides*, the causative agent of pleuropneumonia in cattle, which have been isolated from man and other animals (e.g., sheep, goats, dogs, rats, mice). They are now classified as bacteria and have been assigned to various species of the genus *Mycoplasma*.

organization (or″gah-ni-za'shun) 1. the process of organizing or of becoming organized. 2. the replacement of blood clots by fibrous tissue. 3. an organized body, group, or structure.

organize (or'gah-nīz) to provide with an organic structure; to form into organs.

organizer (or'gah-nīz″er) a part of an embryo which so influences some other part as to bring about and direct its histological and morphological differentiation. Parts developing as a result of induction, and inducing in their turn are classified as organizers of the second grade, third grade, and so on. Cf. *activator* (def. 2) and *inductor*. **nucleolar o., nucleolus o.,** material responsible for organization of the nucleolus of a cell; it is thought to comprise slender strands of heterochromatin by which satellites are attached to the rest of the chromosome. **primary o.,** the dorsal lip region of the blastopore. **procentriole o.,** deuterosome. **secondary o.,** one of second grade, such as the optic cup, which exerts influence on the lens. **tertiary o.,** one of third grade, such as the tympanic ring, which exerts influence on the tympanic membrane.

organ(o)- [Gr. *organon* organ] a combining form meaning organic, or denoting relationship to an organ.

organochlorine (or″gah-no-klo'rēn) any compound of

chlorine and organic elements, as an organochlorine pesticide, e.g., DDT.

organofaction (or″gah-no-fak′shun) the formation and development of an organ.

organoferric (or″gah-no-fer′ik) containing iron and some organic compound.

organogel (or-gan′o-jel) a gel in which an organic liquid takes the place of water.

organogen (or-gan′o-jen) any of the chemical elements —carbon, hydrogen, oxygen, nitrogen, sulfur, phosphorus, and chlorine—characteristic of organic substances.

organogenesis (or″gah-no-jen′ĕ-sis) [*organo-* + Gr. *genesis* generation] the origin and development of organs.

organogenetic (or″gah-no-jĕ-net′ik) pertaining to organogenesis.

organogenic (or″gah-no-jen′ik) originating in an organ.

organogeny (or″gah-noj′ĕ-ne) organogenesis.

organography (or-gah-nog′rah-fe) [*organo-* + Gr. *graphein* to write] the roentgenologic visualization of the organs of the body.

organoid (or′gah-noid) [*organ* + Gr. *eidos* form] 1. resembling an organ. 2. a structure which resembles an organ. **cytoplasmic o's,** structures present in all cells which are probably able to divide and thus perpetuate themselves, in contrast to lifeless cell inclusions. Organoids include mitochondria, fibrils, Golgi apparatus, and centrosomes.

organoleptic (or″gah-no-lep′tik) [*organo-* + Gr. *lambanein* to seize] 1. making an impression on an organ of special sense. 2. capable of receiving a sense impression.

organology (or-gah-nol′o-je) [*organo-* + *-logy*] the sum of what is known regarding the organs of the body.

organoma (or-gah-no′mah) a tumor composed of organs or definite portions of an organ, or characterized by the presence in it of definite organs, as a dermoid cyst.

organomegaly (or″gah-no-meg′ah-le) [*organo-* + Gr. *megas* large] enlargement of the viscera; visceromegaly.

organomercurial (or″gah-no-mer-ku′re-al) any mercury-containing organic compound, e.g., the diuretic mercaptomerin.

organometallic (or-gah-no-mĕ-tal′ik) consisting of a metal in combination with an organic radical.

organon (or′gah-non), pl. *or′gana* [Gr.] a somewhat independent part of the body that performs a special function; see *organum.* **o. audi′tus,** organum vestibulocochleare. **or′gana genita′lia,** see under *organum.* **or′gana genita′lia mulie′bria,** see *organa genitalia feminina,* under *organum.* **or′gana genita′lia viril′ia,** see *organa genitalia masculina,* under *organum.* **o. gus′tus,** organum gustus. **or′gana o′culi accesso′ria** see under *organum.* **o. olfac′tus,** organum olfactus. **o. parenchymato′sum,** a parenchymatous organ. **or′gana sen′suum,** see under *organum.* **o. spira′le [Cor′tii],** organum spirale. **or′gan uropoët′ica,** see *organa urinaria,* under *organum.* **o. vi′sus,** organum visus. **o. vomeronasa′le [Jacobso′ni],** organum vomeronasale.

organonomy (or″gah-non′o-me) [*organo-* + Gr. *nomos* law] the laws of organic life and of living organisms.

organopathy (or″gah-nop′ah-the) [*organo-* + Gr. *pathos* disease] organic disease.

organopexy (or′gah-no-pek″se) [*organo-* + Gr. *pēxis* fixation] the surgical fixation of an organ, especially of the uterus.

organophilic (or″gah-no-fil′ik) [*organo-* + Gr. *philein* to love] organotropic.

organophilism (or-gah-nof′ĭ-lizm) organotropism.

organophosphate (or″gan-o-fos′fāt) phosphate esterified to organic compounds such as glucose or sorbitol; see *organophosphorus.*

organophosphorus (or″gah-no-fos′fŏ-rus) a compound containing phosphorus bound to an organic molecule; many organophosphorus compounds are powerful acetylcholinesterase inhibitors and are used as insecticides.

organotaxis (or″gah-no-tak′sis) [*organo-* + Gr. *taxis* arrangement] a tendency to selective migration to some particular organ.

organotherapy (or″gah-no-ther′ah-pe) [*organo-* + Gr. *therapeia* therapy] the treatment of disease by the administration of animal endocrine organs or their extracts; called also *Brown-Séquard's treatment.* **heterologous o.,** orga-

notherapy with substances that have no relation to the diseased organ of the patient; an outmoded method. **homologous o.,** organotherapy by extracts of the organs of animals corresponding to the diseased organ of the patient; an outmoded method.

organotrope (or-gan′o-trōp) an organotropic element or agent.

organotrophic (or″gah-no-trof′ik) [*organo-* + Gr. *trophē* nutrition] heterotrophic. 1. relating to the nutrition of organs of the body. 2. deriving energy from the oxidation of organic compounds; said of bacteria.

organotropic (or″gah-no-trop′ik) pertaining to or characterized by organotropism.

organotropism (or-gah-not′ro-pizm) [*organo-* + Gr. *tropē* a turning] the special affinity of chemical compounds or of pathogenic agents for particular tissues or organs of the body.

organotropy (or″gan-ot′ro-pe) organotropism.

organule (or′gan-ūl) an end-organ of sensory receptors, such as a taste bud.

organum (or′gah-num), pl. *or′gana* [L.] [NA] an organ: a somewhat independent part of the body that is arranged according to a characteristic structural plan, and performs a special function or functions; it is composed of various tissues, one of which is primary in function. Called also *organon.* **o. extraperitonea′le** [NA], extraperitoneal organ: any of the abdominal viscera, e.g., the kidneys, lying on the posterior abdominal wall and invested by peritoneum only on the anterior surface; called also *o. retroperitoneale* and *retroperitoneal organ.* **or′gana genita′lia,** genital organs: the various internal and external organs that are concerned with reproduction; see *organa genitalia feminina externa, organa genitalia feminina interna, organa genitalia masculina externa,* and *organa genitalia masculina interna.* see Plate accompanying *system.* **or′gana genita′lia femini′na** [NA], female genital organs: the various organs in the female that are concerned with reproduction, including the ovary, uterine tube, uterus, vagina, labia, and clitoris. Called also *organa genitalia muliebria.* See Plate accompanying *system.* **or′gana genita′lia femini′na exter′na** [NA], external female genital organs: the external genitalia of the female, comprising the pudendum femininum, clitoris, and urethra femininum; called also *partes genitales femininae externae* and *partes genitales externae muliebris.* **or′gana genita′lia femini′na inter′na** [NA], internal female genital organs: the various organs in the female that are concerned with reproduction, including the ovary, uterine tube, uterus, and vagina. Called also *organa genitalia muliebria.* See Plate accompanying *system.* **or′gana genita′lia masculi′na exter′na** [NA], external male genital organs: the external genitalia in the male, comprising the penis, scrotum, and urethra masculina; called also *partes genitales masculinae externae* and *partes genitales externae viriles.* **or′gana genita′lia masculi′na interna** [NA], internal male genital organs: the various organs in the male that are concerned with reproduction, including the testis, epididymis, ductus deferens, seminal vesicle, ejaculatory duct, prostate, bulbourethral gland, and penis; called also *organa genitalia virilia.* See Plate accompanying *system.* **o. gustato′rium,** NA alternative for *o. gustus.* **o. gus′tus** [NA], gustatory organ: the organ of taste, comprising the taste buds, most of which are found within the epithelial covering of the tongue; called also *o. gustatorium* [NA alternative] and *organon gustus.* **or′gana o′culi accesso′ria** [NA], the accessory organs of the eye, including the ocular muscles and fascia, and the eyebrows, eyelids, conjunctiva, and lacrimal apparatus. Called also *adnexa oculi.* See Plate accompanying *eye.* **o. olfacto′rium,** NA alternative for *o. olfactus.* **o. olfac′tus** [NA], olfactory organ: the specialized structures subserving the function of the sense of smell, including the olfactory region of the nasal mucosa containing the bipolar cells of origin of the olfactory nerves, together with the olfactory glands; called also *o. olfactorium* [NA alternative] and *organon olfactus.* **o. retroperitonea′le,** o. extraperitoneale. **or′gana senso′ria,** NA alternative for *organa sensuum.* **or′gana sen′suum** [NA], sense organs: organs that receive stimuli which give rise to sensations, i.e., organs which translate certain forms of energy into nerve impulses that are perceived as special sensations; they are characterized by highly specialized neuroreceptors and relationships, and include the visual, vestibulocochlear, olfactory, and gustatory organs.

Called also *organa sensoria* [NA alternative] and *organs of special sense.* **o. spira'le** [NA], spiral organ: the organ, resting on the basilar membrane in the cochlear duct, that contains the special sensory receptors for hearing; it consists of neuroepithelial hair cells and several types of supporting cells, including the inner and outer pillar cells, inner and outer phalangeal cells, border cells, and Hansen's cells. Called also *organon spirale* [*Cortii*] and *organ of Corti.* **o. subcommissura'le** [NA], subcommissural organ: a group of tall columnar ciliated ependymal cells lining the dorsal aspect of the cerebral aqueduct, situated dorsoventral to the commissure of the epithalamus; they may have neuroendocrine and neurosecretory functions. **o. subfornica'le** [NA], subfornical organ: a group of specialized ependymal cells, similar to those of the subcommissural organ, projecting toward the cavity of the third ventricle from its anterior wall between the columns of the fornix; called also *intercolumnar tubercle.* **or'gana urina'ria** [NA], **or'gana uropoët'ica,** urinary organs: the organs concerned with the production and excretion of urine, including the kidneys, ureters, bladder, and urethra. See Plate accompanying *system.* **o. vestibulocochlea're** [NA], vestibulocochlear organ: a collective term in official anatomical nomenclature applied to those structures outside the central nervous system that are concerned with balance and hearing, and comprising the internal, middle, and external ear. Called also *organon auditus.* See Plate accompanying *ear.* **o. visua'le,** NA alternative for *o. visus.* **o. vi'sus** [NA], organ of vision: a collective term in official anatomical nomenclature applied to those structures outside the central nervous system that are concerned with vision, comprising the eyeball and its fibrous, vascular, and internal tunics, and the accessory organs of the eye. Called also *organon visus o. visuale* [NA alternative], and *visual organ.* See Plate accompanying *eye.* **o. vomeronasa'le** [NA], vomeronasal organ: a short rudimentary canal just above the vomeronasal cartilage, opening in the side of the nasal septum and passing from there blindly upward and backward; called also *organon vomeronasale* [*Jacobsoni*] and *Jacobson's organ.*

orgasm (or'gazm) [Gr. *orgasmos* swelling, or *organ* to swell, to be lustful] the apex and culmination of sexual excitement.

orgotein (or'go-tēn) any of a group of water-soluble congeners derived from red blood cells, liver, and other tissues, of molecular weight about 33,000 with compact conformation maintained by about 4 gram-atoms of divalent metal; produced from beef liver as a copper-zinc mixed chelate having superoxide dismutation activity. Orgotein has anti-inflammatory properties and has been used as an antirheumatic.

Oribasius (or"ĭ-ba'se-us) [325–403 A.D.] a famous physician and medical writer who became physician to the Emperor Julian. His *magnum opus* was an encyclopedia of medicine in seventy volumes, of which only one third survive; these are invaluable for they contain extracts from the works of many important physicians of antiquity (e.g., Dioscorides, Galen, Antyllus).

orientation (o"re-en-ta'shun) 1. awareness of one's environment, with reference to place, time, and people. 2. the relative positions of atoms or groups in chemical compounds.

orifice (or'ĭ-fis) [L. *orificium*] 1. the entrance or outlet of any cavity in the body. 2. any foramen, meatus, or opening. Called also *ostium* [NA] and *orificium.* **abdominal o. of uterine tube,** ostium abdominale tubae uterinae. **aortic o.,** the opening of the aorta in the left ventricle of the heart. **o. of aqueduct of vestibule, external,** apertura externa aqueductus vestibuli. **atrioventricular o., auriculoventricular o.,** see *ostium atrioventriculare dextrum* and *ostium atrioventriculare sinistrum.* **cardiac o.,** ostium cardiacum. **o. of coronary sinus,** ostium sinus coronarii. **duodenal o. of stomach,** ostium pyloricum. **epiploic o.,** foramen epiploicum. **o. of female urethra, external,** ostium urethrae externum feminina. **hymenal o.,** ostium vaginae. **o. of male urethra, external,** ostium urethrae externum masculinae. **o. of maxillary sinus,** hiatus maxillaris. **mitral o.,** ostium atrioventriculare sinistrum. **pharyngeal o. of auditory tube,** ostium pharyngeum tubae auditariae. **pilosebaceous o's,** the openings of the hair follicles, giving egress to the secretion of the sebaceous glands whose ducts open into the follicles, and to the hairs. **pulmonary o.,** the opening of the pulmonary artery in the right ventricle of the heart. **o. of pulp canal,** foramen apicis dentis. **o. of ureter,** ostium ureteris. **o. of urethra, inter-**

nal, ostium urethrae internum. **uterine o. of uterine tube,** ostium uterinum tubae uterinae. **o. of uterus, external,** ostium uteri. **vesicourethral o.,** ostium urethrae internum.

orificia (or"ĭ-fish'e-ah) [L.] plural of *orificium.*

orificial (or"ĭ-fish'al) pertaining to an orifice.

orificium (or"ĭ-fish'e-um), pl. *orific'ia* [L.] an opening or orifice, especially the entrance or outlet of any cavity or tube. Called *ostium* [NA]. **o. exter'num isth'mi, o. exter'num u'teri,** ostium uteri. **o. hy'menis,** ostium vaginae. **o. inter'num isth'mi, o. inter'num u'teri,** the internal orifice of the cervix uteri, opening into the cavity of the uterus. **o. ure'teris,** ostium ureteris. **o. ure'thrae exter'num mulie'bris,** ostium urethrae externum femininae. **o. ure'thrae exter'num vir'ilis,** ostium urethrae externum masculinae. **o. ure'thrae inter'num,** ostium urethrae internum. **o. vagi'nae,** ostium vaginae.

origin (or'ĭ-jin) [L. *origo* beginning] the source or beginning of anything, especially the more proximal, fixed end or attachment of a muscle (as distinguished from its insertion), or the site of emergence of a peripheral nerve from the central nervous system.

Orimune (or'ĭ-mūn) trademark for a preparation of live oral poliovirus vaccine.

Orinase (or'ĭ-nās) trademark for a preparation of tolbutamide.

orinotherapy (o-ri"no-ther'ah-pe) [Gr. *oreinos* pertaining to mountains + *therapeia* treatment] treatment by living in high, mountainous regions.

ormetoprim (or-met'o-prim) chemical name: 5-[(4,5-dimethoxy-2-methylphenyl)methyl]-2,4-pyrimidinediamine; an antibacterial, $C_{14}H_{18}N_4O_2$.

Orn ornithine.

ornidazole (or-nid'ah-zōl) chemical name: α-(chloromethyl)-2-methyl-5-nitro-1*H*-imidazole-1-ethanol; an antiinfective, $C_7H_{10}ClN_3O_3$.

ornithine (or'nĭ-thin, -thēn) an amino acid, α,δ-di aminovalerianic acid, $NH_2(CH_2)_3 \cdot CH(NH_2) \cdot CO_2H$, it is produced in the urea cycle by the splitting off of urea from arginine and is itself converted into citrulline. On decomposition, it gives rise to putrescine.

ornithine aminotransferase (or'nĭ-thēn ah-me"no-trans'fer-ās) [EC 2.6.1.13] an enzyme of the transferase class that catalyzes the reaction L-ornithine + α-ketoglutarate = L-glutamate 5-semialdehyde + L-glutamate. The reaction is important in the degradation of ornithine from excess dietary or tissue arginine. Deficiency of the enzyme, an autosomal recessive trait, may cause atrophy of the retina and blindness. The formal EC name is ornithine-oxo-acid aminotransferase.

ornithine carbamoyl phosphate (OCT) deficiency (or'ni-thin kar-bam'o-il fos'fāt) an X-linked aminoacidopathy involving the biosynthesis of urea; most hemizygous males show complete deficiency and do not survive the neonatal period; heterozygous females show varying degrees of deficiency and age of onset. Characteristic symptoms include hyperammonemia, neurologic abnormalities, and orotic aciduria. Called also *ornithine-transcarbamylase (OTC) d.,* and *hyperammonemia II.*

ornithine carbamoyltransferase (or'nĭ-thēn kar"bahmo"il-trans'fer-ās) [EC 2.1.3.3] an enzyme of the transferase class that catalyzes the reaction carbamoyl phosphate + L-ornithine = orthophosphate + L-citrulline. The enzyme occurs in the liver. The reaction is a part of the urea cycle. Genetic deficiency of the enzyme, an X-linked trait, impairs urea formation and produces hyperammonemia (Type I). Called also *ornithine transcarbamoylase.*

ornithine decarboxylase (or'nĭ-thēn de"kar-bok'sĭ-lās) [EC 4.1.1.17] an enzyme of the lyase class that catalyzes the reaction L-ornithine = putrescine + CO_2. The reaction occurs in the conversion of arginine to spermine and spermidine in mammals, and as a result of bacterial action in decaying meat. The presence of the enzyme is used in identification of species of Enterobacteriaceae and Vibrionaceae.

ornithine-keto-acid aminotransferase (or'nĭ-thēn-ke'to-as'id ah-me"no-trans'fer-ās) ornithine aminotransferase.

ornithine transcarbamoylase (or′nĭ-thēn trans″kar-bah-mo′il-ās) ornithine carbamoyltransferase.

ornithine-transcarbamylase (OTC) deficiency (trans-kar-bam′ĭ-lās) ornithine carbamoyl phosphate d.

Ornithodoros (or″nĭ-thod′o-ros) [Gr. *ornis, ornithos* bird + *doros* bag] a genus of argasid ticks, many species of which are the reservoirs and vectors of the spirochetes (*Borrelia*) of relapsing fevers. The chief vectors are: *O. as′perus* of Asia; *O. duge′si* of Mexico; *O. errat′icus* of Spain and North Africa; *O. gur′neyi* of Australia; *O. herm′si* of western United States; *O. mouba′ta*, the tampan or tampan tick of South Africa; *O. norman′di* of Tunisia; *O. par′keri* of western United States; *O. ru′dis* of Central and South America; *O. savign′yi* of Africa, Arabia, and India; *O. tala′je* of the tropics of North and South America; *O. tartakov′skyi* in Russia; *O. tholoza′ni* in Turkestan, Syria, and Palestine; *O. turica′ta* in Mexico, Texas, Arizona, Colorado, and California; *O. verrucosus* of North Caucasus. **O. coria′ceus**, the pajaroello, a venomous tick of California whose bite causes painful swellings; it is not known to transmit disease.

Ornithonyssus (or″nĭ-tho-nis′us) a genus of mites; formerly called *Liponyssus*. **O. baco′ti**, the rat mite or tropical rat mite; a species whose bite may cause a painful dermatitis (rat-mite dermatitis), and which experimentally transmits murine typhus; formerly called *Leiognathus bacoti* and *Liponyssus bacoti*. **O. bur′sa**, the tropical fowl mite, commonly found on chickens and wild birds or in their nests. **O. sylvia′rum**, the northern fowl mite, commonly a parasite of many domestic and wild fowl.

ornithosis (or″nĭ-tho′sis) [Gr. *ornis, ornithos* bird + *-osis*] a term that has been used in various ways, including: (1) to replace the term psittacosis (originally thought to affect only psittacine birds); (2) to refer to *Chlamydia psittaci* infection in nonpsittacine birds, with the term psittacosis being reserved for infection in psittacines and humans; and (3) to refer to *Chlamydia psittaci* infection in both psittacines and nonpsittacines, with the term psittacosis being reserved for human infection.

oro-[1] [L. *os*, gen. *oris* mouth] a combining form denoting relationship to the mouth.

oro-[2] [Gr. *oros* whey, serum] see *orrho-*.

orodiagnosis (or″o-di″ag-no′sis) (obs.) serum diagnosis.

orofaciodigital (OFD) s., type III, oral-facial-digital s., type III.

orolingual (o″ro-ling′gwal) [*oro-*(1) + L. *lingua* tongue] pertaining to the mouth and tongue.

oromaxillary (o″ro-mak′sĭ-ler″e) pertaining to the mouth and the maxillary region.

oromeningitis (or″o-men″in-ji′tis) orrhomeningitis.

oronasal (o″ro-na′zal) [*oro-*(1) + L. *nasus* nose] pertaining to the mouth and nose.

oropharynx (o″ro-far′inks) [*oro-*(1) + *pharynx*] that division of the pharynx which lies between the soft palate and the upper edge of the epiglottis (pars oralis pharyngis [NA]).

Oropsylla (o″rop-sil′ah) a genus of fleas. **O. idahoen′sis,** a rodent flea of the western United States, implicated in the transmission of sylvatic plague. **O. monta′na,** former name for *Diamanus montanus*. **O. silantew′i,** a flea of the Manchuria marmot or tarbagan, capable of transmitting plague.

orosomucoid (or″ŏ-so-mu′koid) α_1-acid glycoprotein, a glycoprotein occurring in blood plasma.

orotate phosphoribosyltransferase (OPRT) (or′o-tāt fos″fo-ri″bo-sil-trans′fer-ās) [EC 2.4.2.10] an enzyme activity of the transferase class that catalyzes the reaction orotate + 5-phospho-α-D-ribose 1-diphosphate = orotidine 5′-phosphate + pyrophosphate. The reaction is driven by removal of inorganic pyrophosphate and is a step in pyrimidine synthesis. The catalytic sites for this activity and the site for orotidine 5′-phosphate decarboxylase (ODC) activity occur on a single protein. Both activities are absent in hereditary orotic aciduria, type I.

orotic acid (ŏ-rot′ik) uracil-6-carboxylic acid, an intermediate in the biosynthesis of the pyrimidine nucleotides.

oroticaciduria (o-rot″ik-as″ĭ-du′re-ah) orotic aciduria; see under *aciduria*.

orotidine 5′-phosphate decarboxylase (ODC) (o-rot′ĭ-dēn fos′fāt de″kar-bok′sĭ-lās) [EC 4.1.1.23] an enzyme activity of the lyase class that catalyzes the reaction orotidine

5′-phosphate = uridine 5′-monophosphate + CO_2. The reaction occurs in the synthesis of pyrimidine nucleotides. The catalytic sites for this activity and for the orotate phosphoribosyltransferase (OPRT) activity are on a single protein. Deficiency of ODC, an autosomal recessive trait, results in orotic aciduria type II. Called also *orotidylate decarboxylase.*

orotidine 5′-phosphate pyrophosphorylase (o-rot′ĭ-dēn fos′fāt pi″ro-fos-for′ĭ-lās) orotate phosphoribosyltransferase.

orotidylate decarboxylase (o-rot″ĭ dĭ′lāt de″kar-bok′sĭ-lās) orotidine-5-phosphate decarboxylase.

orpanoxin (or″pah-nok′sin) chemical name: 5-(4-chorophenyl)-β-hydroxy-2-furanpropanoic acid; an anti-inflammatory, $C_{13}H_{11}ClO_4$.

orphenadrine (or-fan′ah-drēn) chemical name: *N,N*-dimethyl-2-[(2-methylphenyl)phenylmethoxy] ethanamine. The *ortho*-methyl analogue of diphenhydramine, $C_{18}N_{23}NO$, having anticholinergic, antihistaminic, antispasmodic, and euphoric actions. Called also *mephenamine*. **o. citrate** [USP], the citrate salt of orphenadrine, $C_{18}H_{23}NO \cdot C_6H_8O_7$, occurring as a white, crystalline powder; used as a skeletal muscle relaxant in acute spasm of voluntary muscles, regardless of location, especially post-traumatic, discogenic, and tension spasms, administered orally, intramuscularly, and intravenously. **o. hydrochloride,** the hydrochloride salt of orphenadrine, $C_{18}H_{23}NO \cdot HCl$, occurring as a white, crystalline powder; used in the treatment of parkinsonian and drug-induced extrapyramidal reactions, administered orally.

Orr treatment (method, technic) [Hiram Winnett *Orr*, American orthopedic surgeon, 1877–1956] see under *treatment.*

orrho- [Gr. *orrhos* whey, serum] a combining form denoting relationship to serum.

orrhomeningitis (or″o-men″in-ji′tis) [*orrho-* + *meningitis*] inflammation of a serous membrane.

orrhorrhea (or-o-re′ah) [*orrho-* + Gr. *rhoia* flow] (obs.) a watery or serous discharge.

orris (or′is) 1. any of several species of herbs of the genus *Iris*, especially *I. florentina* L. (Iridaceae). 2. orris root: the peeled, dried, and powdered, fragrant root of *Iris florentina* and other species of *Iris*; used in dentifrices, toilet and dusting powders, perfumery, etc.

Orsi-Grocco (or″se-grok′o) [Francesco *Orsi*, 1828–1890; Pietro *Grocco*, 1857–1916, Italian physicians] see under *method.*

orthesis (or-the′sis), pl. *orthe′ses*. Orthosis.

orthetic (or-thet′ik) orthotic.

orthetics (or-thet′iks) orthotics.

orthetist (or′thĕ-tist) orthotist.

ortho- [Gr. *orthos* straight] 1. a combining form meaning straight, normal, correct, etc. 2. symbol *o*-; in organic chemistry, a prefix indicating a 1,2-substituted benzene ring, e.g., *o*-xylene (1,2-dimethylbenzene) or *o*-nitrophenol (2-nitrophenol). 3. in inorganic chemistry, a prefix indicating the common form of an acid as opposed to dimeric or polymeric anhydrides indicated by the prefixes *pyro-* and *meta-*, respectively.

ortho-acid (or″tho-as′id) an acid containing as many hydroxyl groups as the valence of the acidulous element.

orthoarteriotony (or″tho-ar-te″re-ot′o-ne) [*ortho-* + Gr. *artēria* artery + *tonos* tension] normal arterial pressure.

orthobiosis (or″tho-bi-o′sis) [*ortho-* + Gr. *biōsis* way of life] proper living; living in accordance with all the laws of health.

orthocephalic (or″tho-sĕ-fal′ik) [Gr. *orthos* straight + *kephalē* head] having a head with a vertical index of 70.1 to 75.

orthocephalous (or″tho-sef′ah-lus) orthocephalic.

orthochorea (or″tho-ko-re′ah) [*ortho-* + *chorea*] choreic movements in the erect posture.

orthochromatic (or″tho-kro-mat′ik) 1. normally colored or stained. 2. denoting a photographic emulsion sensitive to all colors except red.

orthochromia (or″tho-kro′me-ah) [*ortho-* + Gr. *chrōma* color + *-ia*] normal hemoglobin content of the erythrocytes.

orthochromophil (or″tho-kro′mo-fil) [*ortho-* + Gr. *chrōma* color + *philein* to love] staining normally with neutral stains.

orthocresol (or″tho-kre′sol) one of the three isomeric forms of cresol.

orthocytosis (or″tho-si-to′sis) [*ortho-* + *-cyte* + *-osis*] the presence of mature cells only in the blood.

orthodactylous (or″tho-dak′tĭ-lus) [*ortho-* + Gr. *daktylos* finger] having straight digits.

orthodentin (or″tho-den′tin) [*ortho-* + *dentin*] straight-tubed dentin, as seen in the teeth of mammals.

orthodeoxia (or″tho-de-ok′se-ah) accentuation of arterial hypoxemia in the erect position, improved by assumption of a recumbent position.

orthodichlorobenzene (or″tho-di-klo″ro-ben′zēn) an insecticide, $C_6H_4Cl_2$, used as a spray.

orthodigita (or″tho-dij′ĭ-tah) [*ortho-* + L. *digitus* finger or toe] the art of correcting deformities of the toes and fingers.

orthodontia (or″tho-don′she-ah) orthodontics.

orthodontic (or″tho-don′tik) pertaining to orthodontics.

orthodontics (or″tho-don′tiks) [*ortho-* + Gr. *odous* tooth] that branch of dentistry concerned with the supervision, guidance, and correction of the growing or mature dentofacial structures. Called also *dentofacial orthopedics* and *orthodontology*. **corrective o.,** that phase of orthodontics which is concerned with the reduction or elimination of an existing malocclusion and its attendant sequelae. **interceptive o.,** that phase of orthodontics which is concerned with elimination of a condition which might lead to the development of malocclusion. **preventive o., prophylactic o.,** that phase of orthodontics concerned with preservation of the integrity of proper occlusion through the use of orthodontic procedures and devices. **surgical o.,** orthodontic therapy involving surgical procedures or orthognathic surgery, including resections and ostectomies, cosmetic surgery, the surgical uncovering of impacted teeth, and positioning and transpositioning of teeth.

orthodontist (or″tho-don′tist) a dentist who specializes in orthodontics.

orthodontology (or″tho-don-tol′o-je) orthodontics.

orthodromic (or″tho-drom′ik) [Gr. *orthodromein* to run straight forward] conducting impulses in the normal direction; said of nerve fibers. Cf. *antidromic.*

orthogenesis (or″tho-jen′ĕ-sis) [*ortho-* + *genesis*] 1. progressive evolution in a given direction, in contrast with variations in several directions. 2. the theory that the course of evolution is fixed and predetermined; monogenesis.

orthogenics (or″tho-jen′iks) eugenics.

orthoglycemic (or″tho-gli-se′mik) [*ortho-* + Gr. *glykys* sweet + *haima* blood] having the normal amount of sugar in the blood.

Orthognatha (or-thog′nah-thah) a suborder of spiders (order Araneae) of temperate and tropical areas of the world; Theraphosidae and Dipluridae are families of medical importance.

orthognathia (or″thog-nath′e-ah) [*ortho-* + Gr. *gnathos* jaw] the branch of oral medicine dealing with the cause and treatment of malposition of the bones of the jaw.

orthognathic (or″thog-na′thik) 1. pertaining to orthognathia. 2. orthognathous.

orthognathous (or-thog′nah-thus) [*ortho-* + Gr. *gnathos* jaw] pertaining to or characterized by minimal protrusion of the mandible or minimal prognathism, with a gnathic index of 98 or less. Called also *orthognathic.*

orthograde (or′tho-grād) [*ortho-* + L. *gradi* to walk] characterized by walking with the body upright; said of bipeds. Cf. *pronograde.*

orthomelic (or″tho-me′lik) [*ortho-* + Gr. *melos* limb] correcting deformities of the limbs.

orthometer (or-thom′ĕ-ter) exophthalmometer.

orthomolecular (or″tho-mo-lek′u-lar) [*ortho-* + *molecular*] relating to or aimed at restoring the optimal concentrations and functions at the molecular level of the substances (e.g., vitamins) normally present in the body.

orthomorphia (or″tho-mor′fe-ah) [*ortho-* + Gr. *morphē* form] the surgical and mechanical correction of deformities.

orthomyxovirus (or″tho-mik″so-vi′rus) a subgroup of the myxoviruses that includes the viruses of human and animal influenza; cf. *paramyxovirus.*

orthoneutrophil (or″tho-nu′tro-fil) orthochromophil.

orthopaedic (or″tho-pe′dik) orthopedic.

orthopaedics (or″tho-pe′diks) orthopedics.

orthopantograph (or″tho-pan′to-graf″) panoramic radiograph.

Orthopantomograph (or″tho-pan′to-mo-graf) trademark for the equipment used in pantomography.

orthopedic (or″tho-pe′dik) [*ortho-* + Gr. *pais* child] pertaining to the correction of deformities of the musculoskeletal system; pertaining to orthopedics.

orthopedics (or″tho-pe′diks) [*ortho-* + Gr. *pais* child] that branch of surgery which is specially concerned with the preservation and restoration of the function of the skeletal system, its articulations and associated structures. **dentofacial o.,** orthodontics. **functional jaw o.,** the use of muscle force to effect changes in jaw position and tooth alignment with a removable orthodontic appliance.

orthopedist (or″tho-pe′dist) an orthopedic surgeon.

orthopercussion (or″tho-per-kush′un) [*ortho-* + *percussion*] percussion in which the distal phalanx of the pleximeter finger is held perpendicularly to the chest wall.

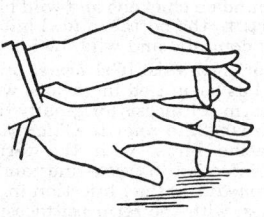

Orthopercussion.

orthophenanthrolene (or′tho-fe-nan′thro-lēn) a white powder, $C_{12}H_8N_2 \cdot H_2O$, used as an indicator.

orthophony (or-thof′o-ne) [*ortho-* + Gr. *phōnē* voice] the direct and correct production of sound.

orthophoria (or″tho-fo′re-ah) [*ortho-* + *phoria*] the absence of heterophoria; the normal condition in which the visual axes remain parallel after the visual fusional stimuli have been partially or entirely eliminated. **asthenic o.,** orthophoria with low relative convergence.

orthophoric (or″tho-for′ik) pertaining to or marked by orthophoria.

orthophosphate (or″tho-fos′fāt) phosphate (as opposed to pyrophosphate, triphosphate, etc.).

orthophosphoric acid (or″tho-fos-for′ik) phosphoric acid (as opposed to pyrophosphoric acid or metaphosphoric acid).

orthophosphoric ester monohydrolase (or″tho-fos-for′ik es′ter mon″o-hi′dro-lās) phosphoric monoester hydrolase.

orthophrenia (or″tho-fre′ne-ah) [*ortho-* + Gr. *phrēn* mind + *-ia*] soundness of mind.

orthopia (or-tho′pe-ah) [*orth-* + *-opia*] the prevention or correction of strabismus.

orthoplessimeter (or″tho-ple-sim′ĕ-ter) an instrument to take the place of the pleximeter finger in orthopercussion.

orthopnea (or″thop-ne′ah) [*ortho-* + Gr. *pnoia* breath] difficult breathing except in an upright position. Cf. *platypnea.* **two-pillow o.,** see under *position.*

orthopneic (or″thop-ne′ik) pertaining to or marked by orthopnea.

orthopod (or′tho-pod) orthopedist.

Orthopoxvirus (or″tho-poks′vi-rus) a genus of poxviruses with nucleic acid homology and serologic cross reactivity that cause generalized infections with a rash in mammals, including vaccinia, cowpox, smallpox, infectious ectromelia, monkeypox, and rabbitpox.

orthopoxvirus (or″tho-poks′vi-rus) an organism of the genus *Orthopoxvirus.*

orthopraxis (or″tho-prak′sis) orthopraxy.

orthopraxy (or'tho-prak-se) [*ortho-* + Gr. *prassein* to make] the mechanical correction of deformities.

orthopsychiatry (or"tho-si-ki'ah-tre) [*ortho-* + *psychiatry*] the branch of psychiatry that deals with the study and practice of maintaining or restoring mental health, using principles from psychology, sociology, social work, and other fields.

Orthoptera (or-thop'ter-ah) [*ortho-* + Gr. *pteron* wing] an order of biting insects which do not undergo metamorphosis; they include the grasshoppers, locusts, crickets, and cockroaches.

orthoptic (or-thop'tik) correcting obliquity of one or both visual axes.

orthoptics (or-thop'tiks) a technique of eye exercises designed to correct the visual axes of eyes not properly coordinated for binocular vision.

orthoptist (or-thop'tist) an expert in orthoptics.

orthoptoscope (or-thop'to-skōp) [*ortho-* + *opto-* + *-scope*] an instrument for orthoptic or exercise treatment in anomalies of the ocular muscles, strabismus or amblyopia.

orthorhombic (or"tho-rom'bik) having three unequal axes intersected at right angles.

orthorrhachic (or"tho-rak'ik) [*ortho-* + Gr. *rhachis* spine] having a vertebral column with practically no curvature in the lumbar region; cf. *koilorrhachic* and *kyrotorrhachic*.

orthoscope (or'tho-skōp) [*ortho-* + *-scope*] an apparatus which neutralizes the corneal refraction by means of a layer of water; it is used in examining the eye.

orthoscopic (or"tho-skop'ik) 1. pertaining to orthoscopy or an orthoscope. 2. having normal, undistorted vision. 3. pertaining to an optical system that produces undistorted images.

orthoscopy (or-thos'ko-pe) examination of the eye by means of the orthoscope.

orthosis (or-tho'sis), pl. *ortho'ses* [Gr. *orthōsis* making straight] an orthopedic appliance or apparatus used to support, align, prevent, or correct deformities or to improve the function of movable parts of the body. **Engen extension o.,** one for extension contracture of the knee or elbow that provides three points of pressure, one over the apex of the deformity and two on the opposite side of the limb at a distance.

orthostatic (or"tho-stat'ik) [*ortho-* + Gr. *statikos* causing to stand] pertaining to or caused by standing erect.

orthostatism (or"tho-stat"izm) an erect standing position of the body.

orthostereoscope (or"tho-ste're-o-skōp) an apparatus for stereoscopic radiography.

orthosympathetic (or"tho-sim"pah-thet'ik) a term applied to the sympathetic (thoracolumbar) division of the autonomic nervous system as contrasted with the parasympathetic (craniosacral) division.

orthotherapy (or"tho-ther'ah-pe) [*ortho-* + *therapy*] treatment of disorders by correction of posture.

orthotic (or-thot'ik) serving to protect or to restore or improve function; pertaining to the use or application of orthoses.

orthotics (or-thot'iks) the field of knowledge relating to orthoses and their use.

orthotist (or'tho-tist) [Gr. *orthōtēr* a restorer or preserver] a person skilled in orthotics and practicing its application in individual cases.

ortho-tolueno-azo-beta-naphthol (or"tho-tol"u-ēn'o-az"o-ba"tah-naf'thol) a poisonous dye used in processing citrus fruits.

orthotonos (or-thot'o-nos) [*ortho-* + Gr. *tonos* tension] tetanic fixation of the head, body, and limbs in a rigid straight line.

orthotonus (or-thot'o-nus) orthotonos.

orthotopic (or"tho-top'ik) [*ortho-* + Gr. *topos* place] occurring at the normal place or upon the proper part of the body; pertaining to a tissue transplant grafted into its normal anatomical position.

orthovoltage (or"tho-vol'tij) in x-ray therapy, voltage in the range of 140 to 400 kilovolts; cf. *supervoltage.*

Orthoxine (or-thok'sēn) trademark for preparations of methoxyphenamine.

orthuria (or-thu're-ah) [*ortho-* + Gr. *ouron* urine + *-ia*] normal frequency of urination.

Ortolani's click (sign) (or-to-lah'nēz) [Marius *Ortolani,* 20th century Italian orthopedic surgeon] see under *click.*

Oryza (o-ri'zah) [L.; Gr. *oryza* rice] a genus of cereal plants; *O. sativa* produces rice.

oryzenin (o-ri'zĕ-nin) [Gr. *oryza* rice] 1. an extractive from rice bran. 2. a glutelin from rice.

O.S. abbreviation for L. *oc'ulus sinis'ter,* left eye.

Os chemical symbol for *osmium.*

os¹ (os), gen. *o'ris,* pl. *o'ra* [L. "an opening, or mouth"] any orifice of the body, [NA] the anterior or proximal opening of the digestive apparatus. See *mouth.* **o. exter'num u'teri,** ostium uteri. **o. of uterus, external,** ostium uteri.

os² (os), gen. *os'sis,* pl. *os'sa* [L.] bone; [NA] a general term which is qualified by the appropriate adjective to designate a specific type of bony structure or a specific segment of the skeleton. **o. acetab'uli,** acetabulum. **o. acromia'le,** a movable joint between the spine of the scapula and the epiphysis of the acromion. **o. acromia'le seconda'rium,** a round structure appearing in the roentgenogram just above the tuberosity of the humerus. **o. basila're,** a term applied to the sphenoid and occipital bones. **o. bre've** [NA], short bone: any bone whose main dimensions are approximately equal. **o. cal'cis,** calcaneus. **o. capita'tum** [NA], capitate bone: the bone in the distal row of carpal bones lying between the trapezoid and hamate bones. **o. carpa'le dista'le pri'mum,** o. trapezium. **o. carpa'le dista'le quar'tum,** o. hamatum. **o. carpa'le dista'le secun'dum,** o. trapezoideum. **o. carpa'le dista'le ter'tium,** o. capitatum. **os'sa carpa'lia,** NA alternative for *ossa carpi.* **os'sa car'pi** [NA], carpal bones: the eight bones of the wrist (carpus), including the o. capitatum, o. hamatum, o. lunatum, o. pisiforme, o. scaphoideum, o. trapezium, o. trapezoideum, and o. triquetrum. Called also *ossa carpalia* [NA alternative]. **o. centra'le** [NA], central bone: an accessory bone sometimes found on the back of the carpus. **o. centra'le tar'si,** o. naviculare. **o. coc'cygis** [NA], coccygeal bone: the small bone caudad to the sacrum in man, formed by union of four (sometimes five or three) rudimentary vertebrae, and forming the caudal extremity of the vertebral column; called also *coccyx* [NA alternative]. **o. coro'nae,** the small pastern bone of the horse. **o. cos'tae,** o. costale. **o. costa'le** [NA], the bony part of a rib; called also *costa* [NA alternative] and *o. costae.* **o. cox'ae** [NA], the hip bone, which comprises the ilium, ischium, and pubis. Called also *o. pelvicum* [NA alternative] and *pelvic bone.* **os'sa crania'lia,** NA alternative for *ossa cranii.* **os'sa cra'nii** [NA], cranial bones: the bones of the cranium, or skull, including the occipital, sphenoidal, temporal, parietal, frontal, ethmoidal, lacrimal, and nasal bones, the concha nasalis, and vomer. Called also *ossa craniales* and *ossa cranialia* [NA alternative]. **o. cuboi'deum** [NA], cuboid bone: a bone on the lateral side of the tarsus between the calcaneus and the fourth and fifth metatarsal bones. **o. cuneifor'me interme'dium** [NA], intermediate cuneiform bone: the intermediate and smallest of the three wedge-shaped tarsal bones located medial to the cuboid and between the navicular and the first three metatarsal bones; called also *o. cuneiforme secundum.* **o. cuneifor'me latera'le** [NA], lateral cuneiform bone: the most lateral of the three wedge-shaped tarsal bones located medial to the cuboid and between the navicular and the first three metatarsal bones; called also *o. cuneiforme tertium.* **o. cuneifor'me media'le** [NA], medial cuneiform bone: the medial and largest of the three wedge-shaped tarsal bones located medial to the cuboid and between the navicular and the first three metatarsal bones; called also *o. cuneiforme primum.* **o. cuneifor'me pri'mum,** o. cuneiforme mediale. **o. cuneifor'me secun'dum,** o. cuneiforme intermedium. **o. cuneifor'me ter'tium,** o. cuneiforme laterale. **os'sa digito'rum ma'nus** [NA], bones of digits of hand: the 14 bones that compose the skeleton of the fingers—two for the thumb and three for each finger. Called also *phalanges digitorum manus* [NA alternative] and *phalanges of fingers.* **os'sa digito'rum pe'dis** [NA], bones of digits of foot: the bones that compose the skeleton of the toes—two for the great toe and often the fifth toe and three for each of the other toes. Called also *phalanges digitorum pedis* [NA alternative] and *phalan-*

ges of toes. **o. epitympan'icum,** a bone of very early fetal life which becomes the posterior portion of the squama that aids in forming the mastoid cells. **o. ethmoida'le** [NA], ethmoid bone: the cubical bone located between the orbits and consisting of the lamina cribrosa, the lamina perpendicularis, and the paired lateral masses. **os'sa facia'les, os'sa facia'lia, os'sa fa'ciei,** facial bones: the bones that constitute the facial part of the skull, including the maxilla, palatine bone, zygomatic bone, mandible, and hyoid bone. **o. fem'orale,** NA alternative for _femur_ (def. 1). **os'sa fonticulo'rum** [NA], sutural bones (ossa suturalia [NA], often present at the fontanelles. **o. fronta'le** [NA], frontal bone: a single bone that closes the front part of the cranial cavity and forms the skeleton of the forehead; it is developed from two halves, the line of separation sometimes persisting in adult life. **o. hama'tum** [NA], hamate bone: the medial bone in the distal row of carpal bones. **o. hyoi'deum** [NA], hyoid bone: a horseshoe-shaped bone situated at the base of the tongue, just above the thyroid cartilage. **o. il'ii** [NA], **o. il'ium,** iliac bone: the expansive superior portion of the os coxae (hip bone); it is a separate bone in early life. Called also _ilium_ [NA alternative]. See illustration accompanying _skeleton._ **o. in'cae,** o. interparietale. **o. incisi'vum** [NA], incisive bone: the portion of the maxilla that bears the incisor teeth. Developmentally it is the premaxilla, which in the human subsequently fuses with the maxilla proper to form the adult bone. In most other vertebrates it persists as an independent bone. **o. innomina'tum,** o. coxae. **o. intercuneifor'me,** an occasionally occurring bone situated between the medial and intermediate cuneiform bones. **o. interme'dium,** o. lunatum. **o. intermetatar'seum,** an occasionally occurring accessory bone situated between the proximal ends of the first and second metatarsal bones. **o. interparieta'le** [NA], interparietal bone: the part of the squama of the occipital bone that lies superior to the highest nuchal line when this portion remains separate throughout life. **o. irregula're** [NA], irregular bone: a bone that is not readily classified as long, short, or flat; e.g., skull and hip bones and vertebrae. **o. is'chii** [NA], the ischial bone: the inferior dorsal portion of the hip bone (os coxae); it is a separate bone in early life. Called also _ischium_ [NA alternative]. See illustration accompanying _skeleton._ **o. lacrima'le** [NA], lacrimal bone: a thin scalelike bone at the anterior part of the medial wall of the orbit, articulating with the frontal and ethmoid bones and the maxilla and inferior nasal concha. **o. lon'gum** [NA], long bone: any bone whose length exceeds its breadth and thickness, as the bones of the limbs. **o. luna'tum** [NA], lunate bone: the bone in the proximal row of carpal bones lying between the scaphoid and triquetral bones. **o. mag'num,** o. capitatum. **o. mastoi'deum,** pars mastoidea ossis temporalis. **os'sa mem'bri inferio'ris** [NA], bones of inferior limb: the os coxae, pelvis, patella, tibia, fibula, tarsus, metatarsus, and digits of the foot. **os'sa mem'bri superio'ris** [NA], bones of superior limb: the humerus, radius, ulna, carpus, metacarpus, and digits of the hand. **os'sa metacarpa'lia,** NA alternative for _ossa metacarpi._ **o. metacarpa'le ter'tium** [NA], the third, or middle, metacarpal bone, which presents the styloid process on the dorsal surface of the radial side of its base. **os'sa metacar'pi** [NA], metacarpal bones: the five cylindrical bones of the hand (metacarpals), which articulate proximally with the bones of the carpus and distally with the proximal phalanges of the fingers; numbered from that articulating with the proximal phalanx of the thumb to the most lateral one articulating with the proximal phalanx of the little finger. Called also _metacarpalia_ [NA alternative]. See also _o. metacarpale tertium._ **os'sa metatarsa'lia,** NA alternative for _ossa metatarsi._ **os'sa metatar'si** [NA], metatarsal bones: the five bones (metatarsals) extending from the tarsus to the phalanges of the toes, being numbered in the same sequence from the most medial to the most lateral. Called also _ossa metatarsalia_ [NA alternative]. **o. multan'gulum ma'jus,** o. trapezium. **o. multan'gulum mi'nus,** o. trapezoideum. **o. nasa'le** [NA], nasal bone: either of the two small, oblong bones that together form the bridge of the nose. **o. navicula're** [NA], navicular bone: the ovoid-shaped tarsal bone that is situated between the talus and the three cuneiform bones; called also _o. naviculare pedis._ **o. navicula're ma'nus,** o. scaphoideum. **o. navicula're pe'dis,** o. naviculare. **o. navicula're ped'is retarda'tum,** see _Köhler's bone disease_ (def. 1), under _dis-_

ease. **o. occipita'le** [NA], occipital bone: a single trapezoid-shaped bone situated at the posterior and inferior part of the cranium, articulating with the two parietal and two temporal bones, the sphenoid bone, and the atlas; it contains a large opening, the foramen magnum. **o. orbicula're,** 1. processus lenticularis incudis. 2. os pisiforme. **os in os,** a radiation-induced injury appearing on roentgenograms as a vertebra within a vertebra. **o. palati'num** [NA], palatine bone: the irregularly shaped bone forming the posterior part of the hard palate, the lateral wall of the nasal fossa between the medial pterygoid plate and the maxilla, and the posterior part of the floor of the orbit. **o. parieta'le** [NA], parietal bone: either of the two quadrilateral bones forming part of the superior and lateral surfaces of the skull, and joining each other in the midline at the sagittal suture. **o. pe'dis,** the coffin bone of the horse. **o. pel'vicum,** NA alternative for _o. coxae._ **o. pe'nis,** baculum. **o. perone'um,** a sesamoid bone sometimes formed in the tendon of the peroneus longus muscle. **o. pisifor'me** [NA], pisiform bone: the medial bone of the proximal row of carpal bones. **o. pla'num,** 1. [NA], flat bone: any bone whose thickness is slight, sometimes consisting of only a thin layer of compact bone, or two layers with intervening spongy bone and marrow; usually bent or curved, rather than flat. 2. Lamina orbitalis ossis ethmoidalis. **o. pneumat'icum** [NA], pneumatic bone: a bone that contains air-filled cavities or sinuses. **o. pri'api,** baculum. **o. pu'bis** [NA], pubic bone: the anterior inferior part of the hip bone (os coxae) on either side, articulating with its fellow in the anterior midline at the pubic symphysis; it is a separate bone in early life; called also _pubis_ [NA alternative]. **o. radia'le,** o. scaphoideum. **o. sacra'le,** NA alternative for _o. sacrum._ **o. sa'crum** [NA], the sacrum: the wedge-shaped bone formed usually by five fused vertebrae that are lodged dorsally between the two hip bones (ossa coxae); called also _os sacrale_ [NA alternative]. **o. scaphoi'deum** [NA], scaphoid bone: the most lateral bone of the proximal row of carpal bones; called also _o. naviculare manus._ **o. sedenta'rium,** tuber ischiadicum. **os'sa sesamoi'dea ma'nus** [NA], the sesamoid bones of the hand. **os'sa sesamoi'dea pe'dis** [NA], the sesamoid bones of the foot. **o. sphenoida'le** [NA], sphenoid bone: a single irregular, wedge-shaped bone at the base of the skull, forming a part of the floor of the anterior, middle, and posterior cranial fossae. **o. subtibia'le,** an occasionally occurring bone found over the tip of the medial malleolus. **os'sa suprasterna'lia** [NA], suprasternal bones: ossicles occasionally occurring in the ligaments of the sternoclavicular articulation. **os'sa sutura'lia** [NA], sutural bones: small irregular bones in the sutures between the bones of the skull, most frequently in the course of the lambdoid suture and often at the fontanelles (_ossa fonticulorum_ [NA]); called also _epactal bones_ and _wormian bones._ **os'sa tarsa'lia,** NA alternative for _ossa tarsi._ **o. tarsa'le dista'le pri'mum,** o. cuneiforme mediale. **o. tarsa'le dista'le quar'tum,** o. cuboideum. **o. tarsa'le dista'le secun'dum,** o. cuneiforme intermedium. **o. tarsa'le dista'le ter'tium,** o. cuneiforme laterale. **os'sa tar'si** [NA], tarsal bones: the seven bones of the ankle (tarsus), including the calcaneus, o. cuboideum, ossa cuneiformia intermedium, laterale, and mediale, o. naviculare, and talus. Called also _ossa tarsalia_ [NA alternative]. **o. tar'si fibula're,** calcaneus. **o. tar'si tibia'le,** talus, def. 1. **o. tempora'le** [NA], temporal bone: one of the two irregular bones forming part of the lateral surfaces and base of the skull, and containing the organs of hearing. **os'sa tho'racis** [NA], thoracic bones: the bones of the thorax, consisting of the thoracic vertebrae, ribs, and sternum. **o. tibia'le exter'num,** a small anomalous bone situated in the angle between the navicular bone and the head of the talus. **o. trape'zium** [NA], trapezium bone: the most lateral bone of the distal row of carpal bones; called also _o. multangulum majus._ **o. trapezoi'deum** [NA], trapezoid bone: the bone in the distal row of carpal bones lying between the trapezium and capitate bones; called also _o. multangulum minus._ **o. trigo'num tar'si** [NA], triangular bone of tarsus: an external tubercle at the back of the talus, sometimes occurring as a separate bone. **o. trique'trum** [NA], triquetral bone: the bone in the proximal row of carpal bones lying between the lunate and pisiform bones; called also _triangular bone._ **o. un'guis,** o. lacrimale. **o. vesalia'num pe'dis,** vesalian bone: the proximal and external part of the tuberosity of the fifth metatarsal bone.

os′sa Wor′mi, ossa suturarum. **o. zygomat′icum** [NA], zygomatic bone: the quadrangular bone of the cheek, articulating with the frontal bone, the maxilla, the zygomatic process of the temporal bone, and the great wing of the sphenoid bone.

osamine (ōs′ah-mēn) a sugar with an amino group replacing one of the hydroxyl groups, e.g., glucosamine.

osazone (o′sa-zōn) any of a series of compounds obtained by heating a sugar with phenylhydrazine and acetic acid; see *glucosazone.*

Osbil (os′bil) trademark for a preparation of iobenzamic acid.

oscedo (os-se′do) [L.] the act of yawning.

oscheal (os′ke-al) [Gr. *oscheon* scrotum] pertaining to the scrotum.

oscheitis (os″ke-i′tis) [oscheo- + -itis] inflammation of the scrotum.

oschelephantiasis (osk″el-ĕ-fan-ti′ah-sis) elephantiasis of the scrotum.

osche(o)- [Gr. *oschē* scrotum] a combining form denoting relationship to the scrotum.

oscheocele (os′ke-o-sēl″) [oscheo- + Gr. *kēlē* hernia, tumor] tumor or swelling of the scrotum.

oscheohydrocele (os″ke-o-hi′dro-sēl) [oscheo- + *hydrocele*] hydrocele in the sac of a scrotal hernia.

oscheolith (os′ke-o-lith) [oscheo- + Gr. *lithos* stone] a concretion in the sebaceous glands of the scrotum.

oscheoma (os″ke-o′mah) [oscheo- + -oma] a tumor of the scrotum.

oscheoncus (os″ke-ong′kus) [oscheo- + Gr. *onkos* mass, bulk] oscheoma.

oscheoplasty (os′ke-o-plas″te) [oscheo- + Gr. *plassein* to mold] plastic surgery of the scrotum.

oschitis (os-ki′tis) oscheitis.

Oscillaria (os″ĭ-la′re-ah) a genus of algae.

oscillation (os″ĭ-la′shun) [L. *oscillare* to swing] a backward and forward motion, like a pendulum; also vibration, fluctuation, or variation. **bradykinetic o.,** slow, recurring, choreiform movements seen in epidemic encephalitis.

oscillator (os′ĭ-la″tor) an apparatus for producing oscillations; an electric circuit designed to generate alternating current at a particular frequency.

oscillo- [L. *oscillare* to swing] a combining form denoting relationship to oscillation.

oscillogram (o-sil′o-gram) the graphic record made by an oscillograph.

oscillograph (o-sil′o-graf) [oscillo- + Gr. *graphein* to write] an instrument for recording electric oscillations. Such an instrument, working on the plan of a string galvanometer, is used in recording the action of the heart.

oscillometer (os″ĭ-lom′ĕ-ter) an instrument for measuring oscillations of any kind, such as changes in the volume of the arteries accompanying the heart beat.

oscillometric (os″ĭ-lo-met′rik) pertaining to oscillometry or the oscillometer.

oscillometry (os″ĭ-lom′ĕ-tre) the use of the string galvanometer or similar apparatus.

oscillopsia (os″ĭ-lop′se-ah) [oscillo- + Gr. *opsis* vision + -ia] oscillating vision, a condition in which objects seem to move back and forth, to jerk, or to wiggle. It occurs in multiple sclerosis.

oscilloscope (ŏ-sil′o-skōp) [oscillo- + Gr. *skopein* to examine] an instrument that displays a visual representation of electrical variations on the fluorescent screen of a cathode-ray tube.

Oscillospira (os″sil-lo-spi′rah) [oscillo- + Gr. *speira* spiral] a genus of endospore-forming, rod-shaped bacteria of uncertain affiliation, formerly classified in the family Oscillospiraceae, found in the alimentary tract of herbivorous animals, and made up of anaerobic, motile cells. The monotype species is *O. guilliermon′di.*

Oscillospiraceae (os″sil-lo-spi-ra′se-e) in former systems of classification, a family of bacteria of the order Caryophanales, including the single genus *Oscillospira.*

oscine (os′in) a substance, $CH_3 \cdot N:C_6H_8:CH \cdot O$, obtained on the decomposition of scopolamine.

Oscinis pallipes (os′ĭ-nis pal′ĭ-pēz) *Hippelatus pallipes.*

oscitate (os′ĭ-tāt) to yawn.

oscitation (os″ĭ-ta′shun) [L. *oscitatio*] the act of yawning.

osculum (os′ku-lum), pl. *os′cula* [L.] a small aperture or minute opening.

-ose a suffix indicating that the substance is a carbohydrate.

Osgood-Haskins test (oz′good-haz′kinz) [Edwin Eugene *Osgood,* American physician, born 1899; Howard Davis *Haskins,* American physician, 1871–1933] see under *tests.*

Osgood-Schlatter disease (oz′good-shlat′er) [Robert Bayley *Osgood,* Boston orthopedist, 1873–1956; Carl *Schlatter,* surgeon in Zurich, 1864–1934] see under *disease.*

-osis [Gr.] a word termination denoting a process, especially a disease or morbid process, and sometimes conveying the meaning of abnormal increase. See also *-sis.*

Osler's disease, nodes, sign, triad (ōs′lerz) [Sir William *Osler,* Canadian-born physician, 1849–1919; successively professor of medicine in McGill University, the University of Pennsylvania, Johns Hopkins University, and the University of Oxford] see *hereditary hemorrhagic telangiectasia,* under *telangiectasia,* see *polycythemia vera,* and see under *node, sign,* and *triad.*

Osler-Vaquez disease (ōs′ler-vak-āz′) [Sir William *Osler;* Louis Henri *Vaquez,* French physician, 1860–1936] polycythemia vera.

Osler-Weber-Rendu disease (os′ler-web′er-ron-duh′) [Sir William *Osler;* Frederick Parkes *Weber,* British physician, 1863–1962; Henri Jules Louis Marie *Rendu,* French physician, 1844–1902] hereditary hemorrhagic telangiectasia.

Oslo meal (breakfast) [*Oslo,* Norway] see under *meal.*

osmate (oz′māt) a salt containing the $OsO_4{}^{2-}$ anion, e.g., potassium osmate K_2OsO_4.

osmatic (oz-mat′ik) [Gr. *osmasthai* to smell] 1. pertaining to the sense of smell. 2. having a sense of smell; applied to a category of animals subdivided further into macrosmatic and microsmatic. Cf. *anosmatic.*

osmazome (oz′mah-zōm) [Gr. *osmē* odor + *zōmos* broth] a principle derivable from muscular fiber which gives the peculiar flavor and odor to roast meats and gravies.

osmesis (oz-me′sis) [Gr. *osmēsis* smelling] the act of smelling.

osmesthesia (oz″mes-the′ze-ah) [osmo- + Gr. *aisthēsis* perception] olfactory sensibility; ability to perceive and distinguish odors.

osmic (oz′mik) containing osmium.

osmic acid (oz′mik) 1. osmium tetroxide. 2. the hypothetical acid, H_2OsO_4, which forms osmate salts.

osmicate (oz′mĭ-kāt) to stain or impregnate with osmic acid.

osmics (oz′miks) [Gr. *osmē* odor] the pure and applied science relating to the olfactory organs and the sense of smell, and to odoriferous organs and substances.

osmidrosis (oz″mĭ-dro′sis) [osmo-(1) + Gr. *hidrōs* sweat] bromhidrosis.

osmification (oz″mĭ-fi-ka′shun) treatment with osmium or osmic acid, as in histologic technic.

osmiophilic (oz″me-o-fil′ik) [osmic acid + Gr. *philein* to love] staining easily with osmium or osmic acid.

osmiophobic (oz″me-o-fo′bik) [osmic acid + *phobia*] resistant to staining with osmium or osmic acid.

osmium (oz′me-um) [Gr. *osmē* odor; so named because of the odor of the vapor, OsO_4, produced by oxidation of the element] 1. a very hard, gray, toxic, and nearly infusible metal; atomic number, 76; atomic weight, 190.2; symbol, Os. 2. a homeopathic trituration of metallic osmium. **o. tetroxide,** colorless or slightly yellow crystals or crystalline granules with a pungent odor, OsO_4, used as a fixative in preparing histologic specimens.

osm(o)-[1] [Gr. *osmē* odor] a combining form denoting relationship to odors.

osm(o)-[2] [Gr. *ōsmos* impulse] a combining form denoting relationship to osmosis.

osmoceptor (oz′mo-sep″tor) osmoreceptor.

osmodysphoria (oz″mo-dis-fo′re-ah) [osmo-(1) + *dys-* + Gr. *pherein* to bear] (obs.) an intense and abnormal dislike of certain odors.

osmol (oz′mōl) osmole.

osmolality (oz″mo-lal′ĭ-te) the concentration of osmotically active particles in solution expressed in terms of osmoles of solute per kilogram of solvent. The osmolality is directly proportional to the colligative properties of solutions: osmotic pressure, boiling point elevation, freezing point depression, and vapor pressure lowering.

osmolar (oz-mo′lar) pertaining to the concentration of osmotically active particles in solution.

osmolarity (oz″mo-lar′ĭ-te) the concentration of osmotically active particles in solution expressed in terms of osmoles of solute per liter of solution.

osmole (oz′mōl) the amount of substance that dissociates in solution to form one mole of osmotically active particles, e.g., 1 mole of glucose, which is unionizable, forms 1 osmole of solute, but 1 mole of sodium chloride forms 2 osmoles of solute. Symbol, Osm. Also written *osmol.*

osmology (oz-mol′o-je) 1. [Gr. *osmē* smell + *-logy*] osphresiology. 2. [Gr. *ōsmos* impulse + *-logy*] that branch of physics that treats of osmosis.

osmolute (oz′mo-lo͞ot″) solute, with reference to the number of osmotically active particles that are present in solution, i.e., the concentration of osmolutes is the osmolality or osmolarity of the solution.

osmometer (oz-mom′ĕ-ter) 1. [Gr. *ōsmos* impulse + *metron* measure] a device for measuring osmotic force. 2. [Gr. *osmē* smell + *metron* measure] an instrument for measuring the acuteness of the sense of smell. **freezing-point o.,** an osmometer using freezing-point depression measurement for analysis of osmotic pressure (number of particles, molecules, or ions) of solutions. **Hepp o.,** an osmometer in which very small quantities of material can be used and a direct reading of the osmotic pressure may be made. **membrane o.,** an osmometer in which diffusion through a semipermeable membrane indicates the osmotic pressure of macromolecules (number of molecules or ions) in a solution.

osmonosology (oz″mo-no-sol′o-je) [*osmo-*(1) + *nosology*] the study of disorders of the sense of smell.

osmophilic (oz″mo-fil′ik) [*osmo-*(2) + Gr. *philein* to love] having an affinity for solutions with a high osmotic pressure.

osmophobia (oz″mo-fo′be-ah) [*osmo-*(1) + *phobia*] irrational fear of odors.

osmophore (oz′mo-fōr) [*osmo-*(1) + Gr. *phoros* bearing] the group of atoms in a molecule of a compound which is responsible for its characteristic odor.

osmoreceptor (oz″mo-re-cep′tor) 1. [*osmo-*(2)] any of a group of specialized neurons in the supraoptic nuclei of the hypothalamus that are stimulated by increased osmolality (chiefly, increased sodium concentration) of the extracellular fluid; their excitation promotes the release of antidiuretic hormone by the posterior pituitary. 2. [*osmo-*(1) +L. *recipere* to receive, accept] a specialized sensory nerve ending sensitive to stimulation giving rise to the sensation of odors.

osmoregulation (oz″mo-reg′u-la′shun) maintenance of osmolarity by a simple organism or body cell with respect to the surrounding medium.

osmoregulatory (oz″mo-reg′u-lah-to″re) pertaining to osmoregulation.

osmoscope (oz′mo-skōp) [*osmo-*(1) + Gr. *skopein* to examine] an apparatus for attachment to the nose for intensifying the sense of smell and enabling the user to make quantitative and qualitative analyses of odor.

osmose (os′mōs) to pass through a membrane by osmosis.

osmosis (oz-mo′sis, os-mo′sis) [Gr. *ōsmos* impulsion] the passage of pure solvent from a solution of lesser to one of greater solute concentration when the two solutions are separated by a membrane which selectively prevents the passage of solute molecules, but is permeable to the solvent.

osmosology (os″mo-sol′o-je) the science of osmosis.

osmostat (os′mo-stat″) the regulatory centers that control the osmolality of the extracellular fluid.

osmotaxis (os″mo-tak′sis) [*osmo-*(2) + Gr. *taxis* arrangement] the movement of cells as affected by the density of the liquid containing them.

osmotherapy (oz″mo-ther′ah-pe) [*osmo-*(2) + *therapy*] treatment by the intravenous injection of hypertonic solutions to produce dehydration.

osmotic (oz-mot′ik) pertaining to or of the nature of osmosis.

osmyl (oz′mil) an odor.

osone (o′sōn) a carbonyl sugar formed by heating an osazone with hydrochloric acid.

osphresi(o)- [Gr. *osphrēsis* smell] a combining form denoting relationship to odors.

osphresiology (os″fre-ze-ol′o-je) [*osphresio-* + *-logy*] the sum of knowledge regarding odors and the sense of smell.

osphresiometer (os″fre-ze-om′ĕ-ter) [*osphresio-* + Gr. *metron* measure] an instrument for measuring the acuteness of the sense of smell.

osphresis (os-fre′sis) [Gr. *osphrēsis* smell] the sense of smell.

osphretic (os-fret′ik) pertaining to the sense of smell.

osphyarthrosis (os″fe-ar-thro′sis) inflammation of the hip joint.

osphyomyelitis (os″fe-o-mi″ĕ-li′tis) [Gr. *osphys* loin + *myelitis*] myelitis of the lumbar region of the spinal cord.

ossa (os′ah) [L.] plural of *os,* bone. See *os².*

ossature (os′ah-tūr) the arrangement of bones in the body or in a part.

ossein (os′e-in) the collagen of bone.

osselet (os′ĕ-let) an exostosis on the inner aspect of a horse's knee or on the lateral aspect of the fetlock.

osseoalbumoid (os″ĕ-o-al′bu-moid) a protein derived from bone after hydration of the collagen.

osseoaponeurotic (os″e-o-ap″o-nu-rot′ik) pertaining to bone and the aponeurosis of a muscle.

osseocartilaginous (os″e-o-kar″tĭ-laj′ĭ-nus) pertaining to or composed of bone and cartilage.

osseofibrous (os″e-o-fi′brus) made up of fibrous tissue and bone.

osseomucin (os″e-o-mu′sin) the homogeneous ground substance which binds together the collagen and elastic fibrils of bony tissue.

osseomucoid (os″e-o-mu′koid) a mucin existing in bone.

osseosonometer (os″e-o-so-nom′ĕ-ter) an instrument used in osseosonometry.

osseosonometry (os″e-o-so-nom′ĕ-tre) [L. *os, ossa* bone + *sonus* sound + Gr. *metron* measure] the measurement of the conduction of sound through bone.

osseous (os′e-us) [L. *osseus*] of the nature or quality of bone; bony.

ossicle (os′sĭ-k'l) [L. *ossiculum*] a small bone. **Andernach's o's,** ossa suturarum. **auditory o's,** the malleus, incus, and stapes, of the middle ear; see *ossicula auditus.* **o's of Bertin,** see *concha sphenoidalis.* **epactal o's,** ossa suturarum. **episternal o's,** ossa suprasternalia. **intercalcar o's,** ossa suturarum. **Kerckring's o.,** see under *center.* **Riolan's o's,** small bones occasionally seen in the suture between the mastoid portion of the temporal bone and the occipital bone. **sphenoturbinal o's,** see *concha sphenoidalis.* **wormian o's,** ossa suturarum.

ossicula (ŏ-sik′u-lah) [L.] plural of *ossiculum.*

ossiculectomy (os″ĭ-ku-lek′to-me) [*ossiculum* + Gr. *ektomē* excision] surgical removal of an ossicle, or of the ossicles, of the ear.

ossiculotomy (os″ĭ-ku-lot′o-me) [*ossiculum* + Gr. *temnein* to cut] surgical incision of the ossicles of the ear.

ossiculum (ŏ-sik′u-lum), pl. *ossic′ula* [L.] [NA] a general term for a small bone, or ossicle. **ossic′ula audi′tus** [NA], auditory ossicles: the malleus, incus, and stapes, the small bones of the middle ear, which transmit the vibrations from the tympanic membrane to the oval window.

ossidesmosis (os″ĭ-des-mo′sis) osteodesmosis.

ossiferous (ŏ-sif′er-us) [L. *os* bone + *ferre* to bear] producing bone.

ossific (ŏ-sif′ik) [L. *os* bone + *facere* to make] forming or becoming bone.

ossification (os″ĭ-fi-ka′shun) [L. *ossificatio*] the formation of bone or of a bony substance; the conversion of fibrous tissue or of cartilage into bone or a bony substance. **cartilaginous o.,** ossification that occurs in and replaces cartilage. **ectopic o.,** a pathological condition in which bone arises in tissues not in the osseous system and in connective tissues usually not manifesting osteogenic properties. **endochondral o.,** cartilaginous o. **intramembranous o.,**

ossification that occurs in and replaces connective tissue, as occurs in the calvaria and in periosteal bone formation. **metaplastic o.,** the development of bony substance in normally soft structures. **perichondral o.,** that which occurs in a layered manner beneath the perichondrium or, later, the periosteum. **periosteal o.,** a type of intramembranous bone formation.

ossifluence (ŏ-sif′lu-ens) softening of bony tissue.

ossiform (os′ĭ-form) resembling bone.

ossifying (os′ĭ-fi″ing) changing or developing into bone.

ossiphone (os′ĭ-fōn) [L. *os, ossa* bone + Gr. *phōnē* voice] an apparatus for enabling deaf persons to hear by transmitting the sound from the instrument through the bony stucture of the body.

ostalgia (os-tal′je-ah) ostealgia.

ostarthritis (os″tar-thri′tis) osteoarthritis.

osteal (os′te-al) bony; osseous.

ostealbumoid (os″te-al′bu-moid) osseoalbumoid.

ostealgia (os″te-al′je-ah) [Gr. *osteon* bone + *-algia*] pain in a bone or in the bones.

osteanabrosis (os″te-an″ah-bro′sis) [*osteo-* + Gr. *anabrōsis* eating up] atrophy of bone.

osteanagenesis (os″te-an″ah-jen′ĕ-sis) osteoanagenesis.

osteanaphysis (os″te-ah-naf′ĭ-sis) [*osteo-* + Gr. *anaphyein* to reproduce] reproduction of bone.

ostearthritis (os″te-ar-thri′tis) osteoarthritis.

ostearthrotomy (os″te-ar-throt′o-me) [*osteo-* + Gr. *arthron* joint + *temnein* to cut] excision of an articular end of a bone.

ostectomy (os-tek′to-me) [*osteo-* + Gr. *ektomē* excision] the excision of a bone or a portion of a bone.

osteectomy (os″te-ek′to-me) ostectomy.

osteectopia (os″te-ek-to′pe-ah) [*osteo-* + Gr. *ektopos* out of place + *-ia*] displacement of a bone.

osteectopy (os″te-ek′to-pe) osteectopia.

ostein (os′te-in) ossein.

osteite (os′te-īt) an independent bony element or center of ossification.

osteitis (os″te-i′tis) [*osteo-* + *-itis*] inflammation of a bone, involving the haversian spaces, canals, and their branches, and generally the medullary cavity, and marked by enlargement of the bone, tenderness, and a dull, aching pain. See also *osteomyelitis.* **acute o.,** osteomyelitis, usually of septic origin. **o. albumino′sa,** osteitis with accumulation of a sticky, albuminous liquid. **alveolar o.,** dry socket. **carious o.,** osteomyelitis. **o. carno′sa,** o. fungosa. **caseous o.,** tuberculous caries of bone. **central o.,** endosteitis. **chronic o.,** central caries or bone abscess; often due to tuberculosis, sometimes syphilitic. **chronic nonsuppurative o.,** sclerosing nonsuppurative osteomyelitis. **o. conden′sans,** condensing o. **o. conden′sans generalisa′ta,** osteopoikilosis. **o. conden′sans il′ii,** a condition marked by an area of dense sclerosis on the iliac side of the sacroiliac joint. **condensing o.,** osteitis with hard deposits of earthy salts in the affected bone; called also *formative o.* and *sclerosing o.* **cortical o.,** periostitis. **o. defor′mans,** a disease of bone marked by repeated episodes of increased bone resorption followed by excessive attempts at repair, resulting in weakened deformed bones of increased mass. There may be bowing of the long bones and deformation of flat bones; pain and pathological fractures are associated. When it affects the bones of the skull, deafness may result. Called also *Paget's disease.* **o. fibro′sa cys′tica, o. fibro′sa cys′tica generalisa′ta,** rarefying osteitis with fibrous degeneration and formation of cysts, and with the presence of fibrous nodules on the affected bones; it is due to marked osteoclastic activity secondary to hyperfunction of the parathyroid gland. Called also *Recklinghausen's* or *von Recklinghausen's disease of bone.* **o. fibro′sa dissemina′ta,** fibrous dysplasia. **o. fibro′sa localisa′ta,** localized fibrous degeneration with weakening and deformity of a bone, as of the patella. **o. fibro′sa osteoplas′tica,** o. fibrosa cystica. **formative o.,** condensing o. **o. fragil′itans,** osteogenesis imperfecta. **o. fungo′sa,** chronic osteitis in which the haversian canals are dilated and filled with granulation tissue. **Garré's o.,** sclerosing nonsuppurative osteomyelitis. **o. granulo′sa,** o. fungosa. **gummatous o.,** a chronic form associated with syphilis. **necrotic o.,** osteomyelitis. **o. ossif′icans,**

condensing o. **parathyroid o.,** o. fibrosa cystica. **pedal o.,** inflammation of the pedal bone of the horse; called also *peditis.* **productive o.,** condensing o. **o. pu′bis,** 1. sclerosis of the pubic bones, in the region of the symphysis, usually observed as an incidental finding in roentgenography of the pelvis. 2. a symptom-producing inflammatory condition of the pubic bones in the region of the symphysis, which may be associated with surgical procedures on pelvic structures or with pregnancy, infection of the urinary tract, degenerative changes, rheumatic disease, or other conditions. **rarefying o.,** a bone disease in which the inorganic matter is lessened and the hard bone becomes cancelled. **sarcomatous o.,** former name for multiple myeloma. **sclerosing o.,** 1. sclerosing nonsuppurative osteomyelitis. 2. condensing osteitis. **secondary hyperplastic o.,** hypertrophic pulmonary osteoarthropathy. **vascular o.,** rarefying osteitis in which the spaces formed become occupied by blood vessels.

ostembryon (os-tem′bre-on) [*osteo-* + Gr. *embryon* fetus] ossification of a fetus.

ostempyesis (os″tem-pi-e′sis) [*osteo-* + Gr. *empyēsis* suppuration] suppuration within a bone.

Ostensin (os-ten′sin) trademark for a preparation of trimethidinium methosulfate.

oste(o)- [Gr. *osteon* bone] a combining form denoting relationship to a bone or to the bones.

osteoacusis (os″te-o-ah-ku′sis) [*osteo-* + Gr. *akousis* hearing] bone conduction.

osteoanagenesis (os″te-o-an″ah-jen′ĕ-sis) [*osteo-* + Gr. *anagenesis*] regeneration of bone.

osteoanesthesia (os″te-o-an″es-the′ze-ah) the insensitiveness of bone.

osteoaneurysm (os″te-o-an′u-rizm) aneurysm in a bone.

osteoarthritis (os″te-o-ar-thri′tis) [*osteo-* + Gr. *arthron* joint + *-itis*] noninflammatory degenerative joint disease occurring chiefly in older persons, characterized by degeneration of the articular cartilage, hypertrophy of bone at the margins, and changes in the synovial membrane. It is accompanied by pain and stiffness, particularly after prolonged activity. Called also *degenerative arthritis, hypertrophic arthritis,* and *degenerative joint disease.* **o. defor′mans, o. defor′mans endem′ica, endemic o.,** Kashin-Beck disease. **o. defor′mans endem′ica,** Kashin-Beck disease. **hyperplastic o.,** hypertrophic pulmonary osteoarthropathy. **interphalangeal o.,** a localized form of arthritis involving the finger joints, characterized by the formation of nodosities (Heberden's nodes) and degenerative changes with intermittent inflammatory episodes, and leading eventually to deformities and ankyloses.

osteoarthropathy (os″te-o-ar-throp′ah-the) [*osteo-* + *arthropathy*] any disease of the joints and bones. **familial o. of fingers,** Thiemann's disease. **hypertrophic o., idiopathic,** pachydermoperiostosis. **hypertrophic o., primary,** pachydermoperiostosis. **hypertrophic pneumic o.,** hypertrophic pulmonary o. **hypertrophic pulmonary o.,** symmetrical osteitis of the four limbs, chiefly localized to the phalanges and the terminal epiphyses of the long bones of the forearm and leg, sometimes extending to the proximal ends of the limbs and the flat bones, and accompanied by a dorsal kyphosis and some affection of the joints. It is often secondary to chronic conditions of the lungs and heart. Called also *hyperplastic pulmonary osteoarthritis, Marie disease* or *syndrome, Marie-Bamberger disease* or *syndrome, pulmonary o.,* and *secondary hypertrophic o.* **pulmonary o.,** hypertrophic pulmonary o. **secondary hypertrophic o.,** hypertrophic pulmonary o.

osteoarthrosis (os″te-o-ar-thro′sis) chronic arthritis of noninflammatory character.

osteoarthrotomy (os″te-o-ar-throt′o-me) ostearthrotomy.

osteoarticular (os″te-o-ar-tik′u-lar) pertaining to or affecting bones and joints.

osteoblast (os′te-o-blast″) [*osteo-* + Gr. *blastos* germ] a cell which arises from a fibroblast and which, as it matures, is associated with the production of bone.

osteoblastic (os″te-o-blas′tik) pertaining to or composed of osteoblasts.

osteoblastoma (os″te-o-blas-to′mah) [*osteoblast* + *-oma*] a benign, painful, rather vascular tumor of bone characterized by the formation of osteoid tissue and primitive bone; called also *giant osteoid osteoma.*

osteocachectic (os″te-o-kah-kek′tik) pertaining to or characterized by osteocachexia.

osteocachexia (os″te-o-kah-kek′se-ah) cachexia due to chronic bone disease; also chronic disease of bone.

osteocampsia (os″te-o-kamp′se-ah) [*osteo-* + Gr. *kamptein* to bend] curvature or bending of a bone, as in rickets.

osteocampsis (os″te-o-kamp′sis) osteocampsia.

osteocartilaginous (os″te-o-kar″tĭ-laj′ĭ-nus) pertaining to or composed of bone and cartilage.

osteocele (os′te-o-sēl) [*osteo-* + Gr. *kēlē* tumor] 1. bony tumor of the testis or scrotum. 2. a hernia containing bone.

osteocementum (os″te-o-se-men′tum) [*osteo-* + *cementum*] a hard bonelike secondary cementum, typically arranged in concentric layers around the root and frequently showing numerous resting lines, such as that occurring in hypercementosis.

osteochondral (os″te-o-kon′dral) pertaining to bone and cartilage; pertaining to a bone and its articular cartilage.

osteochondritis (os″te-o-kon-dri′tis) [*osteo-* + Gr. *chondros* cartilage + *-itis*] inflammation of both bone and cartilage. **calcaneal o.,** Haglund's disease. **o. defor′mans juveni′lis,** osteochondrosis of the capitular epiphysis of the femur; see *osteochondrosis.* **o. defor′mans juveni′lis dor′si,** osteochondrosis of vertebrae; see *osteochondrosis.* **o. dis′secans,** osteochondritis resulting in the splitting of pieces of cartilage into the joint, particularly the knee joint or shoulder joint. **o. ischiopu′bica,** a condition observed in the roentgenogram, consisting of granular looking bodies at the junction of the ischium and os pubis in children. **o. necrot′icans,** a condition marked by necrosis and destruction in the cartilage of the sesamoid bone of the great toe. **o. os′sis metacar′pi et metatar′si,** Thiemann's disease (q.v.) affecting both the fingers and toes.

osteochondrodysplasia (os″te-o-kon″dro-dis-pla′ze-ah) [*osteo-* + *chondro-* + *dys-* + Gr. *plassein* to form] Morquio syndrome.

osteochondrodystrophia (os″te-o-kon″dro-dis-tro′fe-ah) Morquio's syndrome. **o. defor′mans,** Morquio syndrome.

osteochondrodystrophy (os″te-o-kon″dro-dys′tro-fe) Morquio's syndrome. **familial o.,** Morquio's syndrome.

osteochondrofibroma (os″te-o-kon″dro-fi-bro′mah) fibrosing osteochondroma.

osteochondrolysis (os″te-o-kon-drol′ĭ-sis) osteochondritis dissecans.

osteochondroma (os″te-o-kon-dro′mah) [*osteo-* + Gr. *chondros* cartilage + *-oma*] osteoma blended with chondroma, a benign tumor consisting of projecting adult bone capped by cartilage. Called also *chondrosteoma, enchondroma petrificum,* and *osteocartilaginous exostosis.* **fibrosing o.,** a tumor containing the elements of osteoma, chondroma, and fibroma.

osteochondromatosis (os″te-o-kon″dro-mah-to′sis) a condition marked by the presence of multiple osteochondromas. **synovial o.,** a rare condition in which cartilage bodies are formed in the synovial membrane of the joints, tendon sheaths, or bursae, later undergoing secondary calcification and ossification; some of the bodies may become detached and remain as viable, growing structures in the synovial spaces.

osteochondromyxoma (os″te-o-kon″dro-mik-so′mah) osteochondroma blended with myxoma.

osteochondropathia (os″te-o-kon″dro-path′e-ah) osteochondropathy. **o. cretinoi′dea,** Läwen-Roth syndrome.

osteochondropathy (os″te-o-kon-drop′ah-the) [*osteo-* + Gr. *chondros* cartilage + *pathos* disease] any morbid condition affecting both bone and cartilage, or marked by abnormal enchondral ossification. **polyglucose (dextran) sulfate-induced o.,** an experimentally produced disorder of enchondral ossification characterized by a deficient formation of bone matrix in the metaphyses of long bones.

osteochondrophyte (os″te-o-kon′dro-fit) [*osteo-* + Gr. *chondros* cartilage + *phyton* growth] osteochondroma.

osteochondrosarcoma (os″te-o-kon″dro-sar-ko′mah) sarcoma blended with osteoma and chondroma.

osteochondrosis (os″te-o-kon-dro′sis) a disease of the growth or ossification centers in children which begins as a degeneration or necrosis followed by regeneration or recalcification. Called also epiphyseal ischemic necrosis (q.v.). It may affect (1) the CALCANEUS (os calcis), a condition sometimes called *apophysitis;* (2) the CAPITULAR EPIPHYSIS (head) OF THE FEMUR, a condition known as *Legg-Calvé-Perthes disease, Perthes disease, Waldenström's disease, coxa plana,* and *pseudocoxalgia;* (3) the ILIUM; (4) the LUNATE (SEMILUNAR) BONE, known as *Kienböck's disease;* (5) HEAD OF THE SECOND METATARSAL BONE, known as *Freiberg's infraction;* (6) the NAVICULAR (TARSAL SCAPHOID), known as *Köhler's tarsal scaphoiditis;* (7) the TUBEROSITY OF THE TIBIA, called *Osgood-Schlatter disease, Schlatter's disease;* (8) the VERTEBRAE, called *Scheuermann's disease* or *kyphosis, juvenile kyphosis, vertebral epiphysitis,* and *kyphosis dorsalis juvenilis;* (9) *the capitellum of the humerus,* called *Panner's disease.* **o. defor′mans ti-b′iae,** aseptic necrosis of the medial condyle of the tibia, producing lateral bowing of the leg; called also *Blount's disease, nonrachitic bowleg,* and *tibia vara.*

osteochondrous (os″te-o-kon′drus) [*osteo-* + Gr. *chondros* cartilage] composed of bone and cartilage.

osteoclasia (os″te-o-kla′ze-ah) [*osteo-* + Gr. *klasis* a breaking + *-ia*] the absorption and destruction of bone tissue.

osteoclasis (os-te-ok′lah-sis) [*osteo-* + Gr. *klasis* a breaking] the surgical fracture or refracture of bones.

osteoclast (os′te-o-klast″) [*osteo-* + Gr. *klan* to break] 1. a large multinuclear cell associated with the absorption and removal of bone; osteoclasts become highly active in the presence of parathyroid hormone, causing increased bone resorption and release of bone salts (phosphorus and, especially, calcium) into the extracellular fluid. 2. an instrument for use in the surgical fracture or refracture of bones.

osteoclastic (os″te-o-klas′tik) pertaining to or of the nature of an osteoclast; destructive to bone.

osteoclastoma (os″te-o-klas-to′mah) giant cell tumor of bone.

osteoclasty (os′te-o-klas″te) osteoclasis.

osteocomma (os″te-o-kom′ah) [*osteo-* + Gr. *komma* fragment] any of the pieces or members of a series of bony structures, as a vertebra.

osteocope (os′te-o-kōp″) [*osteo-* + Gr. *kopos* pain] a severe pain in a bone or in the bones, generally a symptom of syphilitic bone disease.

osteocopic (os″te-o-kop′ik) pertaining to or characterized by osteocope.

osteocranium (os″te-o-kra′ne-um) [*osteo-* + Gr. *kranion* cranium] the fetal cranium during its stage of ossification.

osteocystoma (os″te-o-sis-to′mah) [*osteo-* + *cystoma*] a bone cyst.

osteocyte (os″te-o-sīt″) an osteoblast that has become embedded within the bone matrix, occupying a flat oval cavity (bone lacuna [q.v.]) and sending, through the canaliculi, slender cytoplasmic processes that make contact with processes of other osteocytes.

osteodentin (os″te-o-den′tin) [*osteo-* + *dentin*] dentin that resembles bone: seen in the teeth of certain fish and pathologically in other lower species, and in man, being produced by rapid formation of secondary dentin, with entrapment of cells.

osteodentinoma (os″te-o-den-tĭ-no′mah) an odontoma composed of bone and dentin.

osteodermia (os″te-o-der′me-ah) [*osteo-* + Gr. *derma* skin + *-ia*] osteoma cutis.

osteodesmosis (os″te-o-des-mo′sis) [*osteo-* + Gr. *desmos* tendon] 1. the formation of bone and tendon. 2. ossification of tendon.

osteodiastasis (os″te-o-di-as′tah-sis) [*osteo-* + Gr. *diastasis* separation] the separation of two adjacent bones.

osteodynia (os″te-o-din′e-ah) [*osteo-* + Gr. *odynē* pain] pain in a bone.

osteodysplasty (os″te-o-dis-plas′te) [*osteo-* + *dys-* + Gr. *plassein* to form] abnormal development of bone. **o. of Melnick and Needles,** a hereditary disorder, transmitted as an autosomal dominant trait, in which there are severe congenital bone abnormalities manifested by striking facies (exophthalmos, full cheeks, micrognathia, and malalignment of the teeth), flaring of the metaphyses of long bones, S-like curvature of the leg bones, irregular constrictions in the ribs, and sclerosis of the base of the skull.

osteodystrophia (os″te-o-dis-tro′fe-ah) osteodystrophy. **o. cys′tica,** osteitis fibrosa cystica. **o. fibro′sa,** osteitis fibrosa cystica.

osteodystrophy (os″te-o-dis′tro-fe) defective bone formation. **Albright's hereditary o.,** pseudohypoparathyroidism. **renal o.,** a condition resulting from chronic disease of the kidneys with onset usually in childhood. It is characterized by impaired renal function, by elevated serum phosphorus and low or normal serum calcium levels, and by stimulation of parathyroid function. The resultant bone disease includes a variable admixture of osteitis fibrosa cystica, osteomalacia, osteoporosis, and sometimes osteosclerosis. If the onset is in childhood, renal dwarfism may result.

osteoectasia (os″te-o-ek-ta′ze-ah) [osteo- + ectasia] bowing of the bones. **familial o.,** hyperostosis corticalis deformans juvenilis.

osteoectomy (os″te-o-ek′to-me) ostectomy.

osteoenchondroma (os″te-o-en″kon-dro′mah) osteochondroma.

osteoepiphysis (os″te-o-ĕ-pif′ĭ-sis) [osteo- + epiphysis] any bony epiphysis.

osteofibrochondrosarcoma (os″te-o-fi″bro-kon″dro-sar-ko′mah) malignant mesenchymoma.

osteofibroma (os″te-o-fi-bro′mah) [osteo- + fibroma] a tumor containing both osseous and fibrous elements.

osteofibromatosis (os″te-o-fi″bro-mah-to′sis) polyostotic form of fibrous dysplasia of bone. **cystic o.,** Jaffe-Lichtenstein disease.

osteofluorosis (os″te-o-floo″o-ro′sis) skeletal changes, usually consisting of osteomalacia and osteosclerosis, caused by the chronic intake of excessive quantities of fluorides. See also *fluorosis,* def. 2.

osteogen (os′te-o-jen″) [osteo- + Gr. *gennan* to produce] the substance composing the inner layer of the periosteum, from which bone is formed.

osteogenesis (os″te-o-jen′ĕ-sis) [osteo- + Gr. *gennan* to produce] formation of bone; the development of the bones. **o. imperfec′ta (OI),** a collagen disorder due to defective biosynthesis of type I collagen and generally characterized by brittle, osteoporotic, easily fractured bones. Other defects that may appear include blue sclerae, wormian bones, lax joints, and dentinogenesis imperfecta. OI is variable in manifestation and severity and has great molecular, genetic, and clinical heterogeneity. There are four major types (I–IV) plus variants of OI. *Type I,* the classic, most common, mildest type, is autosomal dominant; called also *osteogenesis imperfecta with blue sclerae* and *osteogenesis imperfecta tarda. Type II,* the perinatal lethal type, has at least three clinical and genetic subtypes and may be an autosomal dominant trait, an autosomal recessive trait, or an autosomal dominant new mutation. The dominant type is also called *osteogenesis imperfecta congenita, neonatal lethal form;* OI type II, *dominant form;* and *lethal perinatal OI.* The recessive form is also called *osteogenesis imperfecta congenita;* OIC: *Vrolik type of osteogenesis imperfecta;* OI type II, *recessive form;* and *lethal perinatal OI. Type III,* the progressive deforming type, may be autosomal recessive or a new mutation; called also *osteogenesis imperfecta, progressively deforming, with normal sclerae (OI type III). Type IV* is an autosomal dominant form; called also *osteogenesis imperfecta with normal sclerae (OI type IV).* **o. imperfec′ta cys′tica,** a disorder in which the marrow spaces contain myxomatous fibroid tissue, the x-ray showing cystic changes.

osteogenetic (os″te-o-jĕ-net′ik) forming bone; concerned in bone formation.

osteogenic (os″te-o-jen′ik) [osteo- + Gr. *gennan* to produce] derived from or composed of any tissue which is concerned in the growth or repair of bone.

osteogenous (os″te-oj′ĕ-nus) osteogenic.

osteogeny (os″te-oj′ĕ-ne) osteogenesis.

osteogram (os′te-o-gram) a semidiagram of the spine used as a record sheet for the charting of bone lesions.

osteography (os″te-og′rah-fe) [osteo- + Gr. *graphein* to write] a description of the bones.

osteohalisteresis (os″te-o-hah-lis″ter-e′sis) [osteo- + Gr. *hals* salt + *sterein* to deprive] loss or deficiency of the mineral elements of bones.

osteohemachromatosis (os″te-o-hem″ah-kro″mah-to′sis) [osteo- + Gr. *haima* blood + *chrōma* color + *-osis*] a disease of animals marked by discoloration of the bone by blood pigment.

osteohydatidosis (os″te-o-hi″dah-tid-o′sis) hydatid disease of bone.

osteoid (os′te-oid) [osteo- + Gr. *eidos* form] 1. resembling bone. 2. the organic matrix of bone; young bone which has not undergone calcification.

osteolathyrism (os″te-o-lath′ĭ-rizm) a skeletal disorder produced in laboratory animals by diets containing the sweet pea (*Lathyrus odoratus*) or its active principle, β-aminopropionitrile, or other aminonitriles. Characterized, in rats, by hernias, dissecting aortic aneurysms, lameness of the hind logo, okoetoeoe, and kyphoscoliosis and other skeletal deformities, apparently as the result of defective aging of collagen tissue.

osteolipochondroma (os″te-o-lĭ-po″kon-dro′mah) osteochondroma with fatty elements.

osteolipoma (os″te-o-lĭ-po′mah) lipoma with osseous metaplasia.

osteologia (os″te-o-lo′je-ah) osteology; in NA terminology it encompasses the nomenclature relating to the bones.

osteologist (os″te-ol′o-jist) a specialist in osteology.

osteology (os″te-ol′o-je) [osteo- + Gr. *logos* treatise] the scientific study of the bones; applied also to the body of knowledge relating to the bones.

osteolysis (os″te-ol′ĭ-sis) [osteo- + Gr. *lysis* dissolution] dissolution of bone; applied especially to the removal or loss of the calcium of bone.

osteolytic (os″te-o-lit′ik) relating to, characterized by, or promoting osteolysis.

osteoma (os″te-o′mah) [osteo- + -oma] a tumor composed of bone tissue; a hard tumor of bonelike structure developing on a bone (homoplastic o.) and sometimes on other structures (heteroplastic o.). **cavalryman's o.,** osteoma at the insertion of the adductor femoris longus muscle. **compact o.,** o. durum. **o. cu′tis,** a cutaneous ossification manifested by the development of one or more hard, round to irregular, sharply defined tumors of varying size within the dermis or subcutis. Called also *osteodermia* and *osteosis cutis.* **o. du′rum, o. ebur′neum,** a tumor made up of hard bony tissue. **giant osteoid o.,** osteoblastoma. **o. medulla′re,** an osteoma containing marrow spaces. **osteoid o.,** a small, benign but painful, circumscribed tumor of spongy bone occurring especially in the bones of the extremities and vertebrae, most often in young persons. **o. sarcomato′sum,** osteogenic sarcoma. **o. spongio′sum,** osteoma containing cancellated bone.

osteomalacia (os″te-o-mah-la′she-ah) [osteo- + Gr. *malakia* softness] a condition marked by softening of the bones (due to impaired mineralization, with excess accumulation of osteoid), with pain, tenderness, muscular weakness, anorexia, and loss of weight, resulting from deficiency of vitamin D and calcium. **bovine o.,** aphosphorosis. **hepatic o.,** osteomalacia as a complication of cholestatic liver disease, which may lead to severe bone pain and multiple fractures. **infantile o., juvenile o.,** late rickets. **osteogenic o.,** a vitamin D–resistant form seen in association with benign mesenchymal tumors occurring in soft tissues or bone. **puerperal o.,** osteomalacia occurring as a consequence of exhaustion of skeletal stores of calcium and phosphorus by repeated pregnancies and lactation. **renal tubular o.,** osteomalacia occurring as a consequence of acidosis and hypercalciuria, resulting from inability to produce an acid urine or ammonia because of deficient activity of the renal tubules. **senile o.,** softening of bones in old age due to vitamin D deficiency.

osteomalacic (os″te-o-mah-la′sik) pertaining to or characterized by osteomalacia.

osteomalacosis (os″te-o-mal″ah-ko′sis) osteomalacia.

osteomatoid (os″te-o′mah-toid) resembling an osteoma.

osteomatosis (os″te-o-mah-to′sis) the formation of multiple osteomas.

osteomere (os′te-o-mēr″) [osteo- + Gr. *meros* part] one of a series of similar bony structures, such as the vertebrae.

osteometry (os″te-om′ĕ-tre) [osteo- + Gr. *metron* measure] the measurement of bones.

osteomiosis (os″te-o-mi-o′sis) [osteo- + Gr. *meiōsis* diminution] disintegration of bone.

osteomyelitic (os″te-o-mi″ĕ-lit′ik) marked by or characteristic of osteomyelitis.

osteomyelitis (os″te-o-mi″ĕ-li′tis) [*osteo-* + Gr. *myelos* marrow] inflammation of bone caused by a pyogenic organism. It may remain localized or may spread through the bone to involve the marrow, cortex, cancellous tissue, and periosteum. **conchiolin o.,** a condition seen in the workers in mother of pearl, probably due to the inhaled dust being deposited in the bone marrow. Cf. *coniosis.* **Garré's o.,** sclerosing nonsuppurative o. **malignant o.,** former name for multiple myeloma. **salmonella o.,** osteomyelitis due to salmonella organisms; it occurs more frequently than normal in sickle cell disease. **sclerosing nonsuppurative o.,** chronic idiopathic osteomyelitis involving the long bones, particularly the tibia and femur, and characterized by a diffuse inflammatory reaction, increased density and spindle-shaped sclerotic thickening of the cortex, and an absence of suppuration; called also *Garré's disease, osteitis,* or *osteomyelitis,* and *chronic nonsuppurative osteitis.* **typhoid o.,** osteomyelitis occurring in the late convalescent stage of typhoid fever. **o. variolo′sa,** osteomyelitis due to, or occurring as a complication of, smallpox.

osteomyelodysplasia (os″te-o-mi″ĕ-lo-dis-pla′se-ah) [*osteo-* + Gr. *myelos* marrow + *dys-* + *plassein* to form] a condition characterized by thinning of the osseous tissue of bones and increase in size of the marrow cavities, accompanied by leukopenia and fever.

osteomyelography (os″te-o-mi″ĕ-log′rah-fe) roentgen visualization of bone marrow.

osteomyxochondroma (os″te-o-mik″so-kon-dro′mah) osteochondromyxoma.

osteon (os′te-on) [*osteo-* + Gr. *on* neuter ending] the basic unit of structure of compact bone, comprising a haversian canal and its concentrically arranged lamellae, of which there may be 4 to 20, each 3 to 7 microns thick, in a single (haversian) system; such units are directed mainly in the long axis of the bone.

osteone (os′te-ōn) osteon.

osteonecrosis (os″te-o-ne-kro′sis) [*osteo-* + Gr. *nekrōsis* death] death, or necrosis, of bone.

osteoneuralgia (os″te-o-nu-ral′je-ah) [*osteo-* + *neuralgia*] neuralgia of a bone.

osteonosus (os″te-on′o-sus) [*osteo-* + Gr. *nosos* disease] disease of bone.

osteo-odontoma (os″te-o-o″don-to′mah) ameloblastic odontoma.

osteopath (os′te-o-path) a practitioner of osteopathy.

osteopathia (os″te-o-path′e-ah) any disease of a bone; called also *osteopathy.* **o. conden′sans,** myelosclerosis, def. 2. **o. conden′sans dissemina′ta, o. conden′sans generalisa′ta,** osteopoikilosis. **o. hemorrha′gica infan′tum,** Moeller-Barlow disease. **o. hyperostot′ica congen′ita,** melorheostosis. **o. hyperostot′ica mul′tiplex infan′tilis,** diaphyseal dysplasia. **o. stria′ta,** an abnormality apparent only on roentgen examination, and occurring only in cancellous bone; it is characterized by multiple condensations beginning at the epiphyseal line and extending into the diaphysis.

osteopathic (os″te-o-path′ik) pertaining to osteopathy.

osteopathology (os″te-o-pah-thol′o-je) any disease of bone.

osteopathy (os″te-op′ah-the) [*osteo-* + Gr. *pathos* disease] 1. any disease of a bone. 2. a system of therapy founded by Andrew Taylor Still (1828–1917) and based on the theory that the body is capable of making its own remedies against disease and other toxic conditions when it is in normal structural relationship and has favorable environmental conditions and adequate nutrition. It utilizes generally accepted physical, medicinal, and surgical methods of diagnosis and therapy, while placing chief emphasis on the importance of normal body mechanics and manipulative methods of detecting and correcting faulty structure. **alimentary o.,** hunger o. **disseminated condensing o.,** osteopoikilosis. **hunger o.,** disturbances of the skeletal system observed in famine areas, characterized by a reduction in the amount of normally calcified bone, and attributed to dietary deficiencies and associated hormonal dysfunction. **myelogenic o.,** any bone disease due to the impaired relation between the medullary and osseous tissues.

osteopecilia (os″te-o-pĕ-sil′e-ah) [*osteo-* + Gr. *poikilia* spottedness] osteopoikilosis.

osteopedion (os″te-o-pe′de-on) [*osteo-* + Gr. *paidion* child] lithopedion.

osteopenia (os″te-o-pe′nĭ-ah) [*osteo-* + Gr. *penia* poverty] reduced bone mass due to a decrease in the rate of osteoid synthesis to a level insufficient to compensate normal bone lysis. The term is also used to refer to any decrease in bone mass below the normal.

osteopenic (os″te-o-pen′ik) pertaining to osteopenia.

osteoperiosteal (os″te-o-per″ĭ-os′te-al) pertaining to bone and its periosteum.

osteoperiostitis (os″te-o-per″ĭ-os-ti′tis) [*osteo-* + *periostitis*] inflammation of a bone and its periosteum. Called also *periosteitis.* **alveolodental o.,** periodontitis, def. 1.

osteopetrosis (os″te-o-pe-tro′sis) [*osteo-* + Gr. *petra* stone + *-osis*] a rare genetic disease characterized by abnormally dense bone, due to defective resorption of immature bone. The disorder occurs in two forms: a severe autosomal recessive form occurring in utero, infancy, or childhood, and a benign autosomal dominant form occurring in adolescence or adulthood. In the recessive form, the proliferation of bone obliterates the marrow cavity, causing anemia and hepatosplenomegaly, and the nerve foramina of the skull, causing compression of cranial nerves, which may result in deafness and blindness. Fractures are common in both forms. Called also *Albers-Schönberg disease, ivory bones,* and *marble bones.* **o. gallina′rum,** see *avian leukosis,* under *leukosis.*

osteophage (os′te-o-fāj) [*osteo-* + Gr. *phagein* to eat] osteoclast, def. 1.

osteophagia (os″te-o-fa′je-ah) [*osteo-* + Gr. *phagein* to eat] the eating of bone due to a craving for phosphorus.

osteophlebitis (os″te-o-fle-bi′tis) [*osteo-* + Gr. *phleps* vein + *-itis*] inflammation of the veins of a bone.

osteophony (os″te-of′o-ne) [*osteo-* + Gr. *phōnē* voice] the conduction of sounds by bone; bone conduction.

osteophyma (os″te-o-fi′mah) [*osteo-* + Gr. *phyma* growth] a tumor or outgrowth of a bone.

osteophyte (os′te-o-fīt″) [*osteo-* + Gr. *phyton* plant] a bony excrescence or osseous outgrowth.

osteophytosis (os″te-o-fi-to′sis) a condition characterized by the formation of osteophytes.

osteoplaque (os′te-o-plak) a layer of bone.

osteoplast (os′te-o-plast) [*osteo-* + Gr. *plastos* formed] osteoblast.

osteoplastic (os″te-o-plas′tik) 1. osteogenic. 2. pertaining to osteoplasty.

osteoplastica (os″te-o-plas′tĭ-kah) osteitis fibrosa cystica.

osteoplasty (os′te-o-plas″te) [*osteo-* + Gr. *plassein* to form] plastic surgery of the bones.

osteopoikilosis (os″te-o-poi″kĭ-lo′sis) [*osteo-* + Gr. *poikilos* mottled] an autosomal dominant trait in which there are multiple sclerotic foci in the ends of long bones and scattered stippling in round and flat bones, usually without symptoms and diagnosed fortuitously by x-ray examination.

osteopoikilotic (os″te-o-poi″kĭ-lot′ik) pertaining to or characterized by osteopoikilosis.

osteoporosis (os″te-o-po-ro′sis) [*osteo-* + Gr. *poros* passage + *-osis*] reduction in the amount of bone mass, leading to fractures after minimal trauma. **o. circumscrip′ta cra′nii,** demineralization of the bones of the skull, characteristic of the destructive or osteolytic phase of Paget's disease; called also *Schüller's disease.* **o. of disuse,** decrease in bone substance as a result of lack of re-formation of laminae in the absence of functional stress which ordinarily leads to their replacement in new stress lines. **postmenopausal o.,** that occurring in women within 15 to 20 years after menopause, affecting trabecular bone more than cortical bone, and manifested mainly by vertebral fractures of the painful crush type, Colles' fracture, and increased tooth loss. **post-traumatic o.,** loss of bone substance following an injury in which there is damage to a nerve, sometimes due to an increased blood supply caused by the neurogenic insult, or to disuse secondary to pain. **senile o.,** that occurring in men and women over 70, manifested mainly by hip and vertebral fractures of the painless multiple wedge type leading to dorsal kyphosis.

osteoporotic (os″te-o-po-rot′ik) pertaining to or characterized by osteoporosis.

osteopsathyrosis (os″te-op-sath″ĭ-ro′sis) [osteo- + Gr. *psathyros* friable] osteogenesis imperfecta.

osteoradionecrosis (os″te-o-ra″de-o-ne-kro′sis) necrosis of bone following irradiation.

osteorrhagia (os″te-o-ra′je-ah) [osteo- + Gr. *rhēgnynai* to burst out] hemorrhage from bone.

osteorrhaphy (os″te-or′ah-fe) [osteo- + Gr. *rhaphē* suture] the suturing or wiring of bones.

osteosarcoma (os″te-o-sar-ko′mah) [osteo- + *sarcoma*] osteogenic sarcoma. **telangiectatic o.,** an osteogenic sarcoma containing dilated capillaries.

osteosarcomatous (os″te-o-sar-ko′mah-tus) of the nature of osteosarcoma.

osteosclerosis (os″te-o-skle-ro′sis) [osteo- + Gr. *sklērōsis* hardening] the hardening or abnormal density of bone, as in eburnation and condensing osteitis. **o. congen′ita,** achondroplasia. **o. frag′ilis,** osteopetrosis. **o. frag′ilis generalisa′ta,** osteopoikilosis. **o. myelofibrosis,** myelosclerosis, def. 2.

osteosclerotic (os″te-o-skle-rot′ik) pertaining to or characterized by osteosclerosis.

osteoscope (os′te-o-skōp) [osteo- + Gr. *skopein* to examine] an instrument for testing a roentgen ray apparatus by examining a standard preparation of the bones of the forearm.

osteoseptum (os″te-o-sep′tum) [osteo- + *septum*] the bony part of the nasal septum.

osteosis (os″te-o′sis) the formation of bony tissue, especially the infiltration of connective tissue with bone. **o. cu′tis,** see under *osteoma*. **o. ebur′nisans monomel′ica,** melorheostosis. **parathyroid o.,** osteitis fibrosa cystica.

osteosuture (os′te-o-su-tūr) [osteo- + L. *sutura* suture] osteorrhaphy.

osteosynovitis (os″te-o-sin″o-vi′tis) synovitis together with osteitis of the neighboring bones.

osteosynthesis (os″te-o-sin′thĕ-sis) [osteo- + Gr. *synthesis* a putting together] surgical fastening of the ends of a fractured bone by sutures, rings, plates, or other mechanical means.

osteotabes (os″te-o-ta′bēz) [osteo- + L. *tabes* wasting] a disease, chiefly of infants, in which the cells of the bone marrow are destroyed and the marrow disappears.

osteotelangiectasia (os″te-o-tĕ-lan″je-ek-ta′se-ah) [osteo- + *telangiectasia*] telangiectatic osteosarcoma.

osteothrombophlebitis (os″te-o-throm″bo-fle-bi′tis) inflammation extended through intact bone by a progressive thrombophlebitis of small venules, such as sometimes occurs in the mastoid bone.

osteothrombosis (os″te-o-throm-bo′sis) [osteo- + *thrombosis*] thrombosis of the veins of a bone.

osteotome (os′te-o-tōm) [osteo- + Gr. *tomē* a cut] a chisel-like knife for cutting bone.

osteotomy (os″te-ot′o-me) [osteo- + Gr. *temnein* to cut] the surgical cutting of a bone. **angulation o.,** in midhumeral amputation, the bending of a small terminal of the humerus at a right angle to the bone shaft so as to provide a projection that locks the prosthesis to the bone. **block o.,** osteotomy in which a section of bone is removed. **cuneiform o.,** the removal of a wedge of bone. **cup-and-ball o.,** osteotomy in which the distal fragment is pointed and the proximal fragment is recessed. **displacement o.,** surgical division of a bone and shifting of the divided ends to change the alignment of the bone or to alter weight-bearing stresses. **innominate o.,** pelvic osteotomy to deepen the acetabulum in congenital dislocation of the hip. **linear o.,** the sawing or linear cutting of a bone. **Lorenz's o.,** osteotomy of the neck of the femur by a V-shaped cutting of the femur so as to prevent displacement of the shaft. **pelvic o.,** pubiotomy.

osteotribe, osteotrite (os′te-o-trīb″; os′te-o-trīt″) [osteo- + Gr. *tribein* to rub] an instrument for rasping carious bone.

osteotrophy (os″te-ot′ro-fe) [osteo- + Gr. *trophē* nutrition] nutrition of bone.

osteotylus (os″te-ot′ĭ-lus) [osteo- + Gr. *tylos* callus] the callus enclosing the end of a broken bone.

osteotympanic (os″te-o-tim-pan′ik) craniotympanic.

Ostertagia (os″ter-ta′je-ah) [Robert von *Ostertag*, German veterinarian, 1864–1940] a genus of attenuated nematode parasites belonging to the family Trichostrongylus, found mostly in cysts on the wall of the abomasum of cattle and other ruminants.

osthexia, osthexy (os-thek′se-ah; os′thek-se) [Gr. *osteon* bone + *hexis* condition] abnormal ossification.

ostia (os′te-ah) [L.] plural of *ostium*.

ostial (os′te-al) pertaining to an ostium.

ostiary (os′te-a-re) [L. *ostiarius* pertaining to a door] (*obs.*) pertaining to an orifice.

ostitis (os-ti′tis) osteitis.

ostium (os′te-um), pl. *os′tia* [L.] a door, or opening; used in anatomical nomenclature as a general term to designate an opening into a tubular organ, or between two distinct cavities within the body. Called also *orificium, orifice,* and *opening.* **o. abdomina′le tu′bae uteri′nae** [NA], abdominal orifice of uterine tube: the funnel-shaped opening by which the uterine tube communicates with the pelvic cavity. **o. aor′ticum** [NA], the opening between the left ventricle and the aorta. **o. appen′dicis vermifor′mis** [NA], opening of vermiform appendix: the orifice between the vermiform appendix and the cecum. **o. arterio′sum cor′dis,** ostium atrioventriculare sinistrum. **o. atrioventricula′re dex′trum** [NA], the opening between the right atrium and the right ventricle of the heart, guarded by the right atrioventricular valve; called also *o. venosum cordis.* **o. atrioventricula′re sinis′trum** [NA], the opening between the left atrium and the left ventricle of the heart, guarded by the left atrioventricular valve; called also *o. arteriosum cordis* and *mitral orifice.* **o. cardi′acum** [NA], cardiac opening: the orifice between the esophagus and the cardiac part of the stomach. Called also *cardia.* **coronary o.,** either of the two openings in the aortic sinus which mark the origin of the (left and right) coronary arteries. **o. ileocaeca′le** [NA], ileocecal opening: the orifice at the junction of the ileum and cecum, which is rounded at the left (anterior end) and narrow and pointed at the right (posterior) end. It has two flaps or lips, one above and one below, which form the so-called ileocecal valve; in the cadaver the flaps extend into the lumen of the large intestine as thickened folds, but in the living individual the ileum forms a conical or papillary projection (*papilla ileocaecalis*). Called also *o. ileocecale* [NA alternative]. Cf. *o. valvae ilealis.* **o. inter′num u′teri,** o. uterinum tubae uterinae. **persistent o. pri′mum,** an endocardial cushion defect characterized by a cleft in the basal portion of the atrial septum, usually associated with cleft mitral valve. **o. pharyn′geum tu′bae auditi′vae,** o. pharyngeum tubae auditivae. **o. pharyn′geum tu′bae audito′riae** [NA], the pharyngeal opening of the auditory tube, located on each of the lateral walls of the pharynx, behind and below the posterior end of the inferior nasal concha. Called also *o. pharyngeum tubae auditivae* and *pharyngeal orifice of auditory tube.* **o. pri′mum,** an opening in the lowest aspect of the septum primum of the embryonic heart, posteriorly, in the neighborhood of the atrioventricular valve. **o. pylo′ricum** pyloric opening: the orifice between the stomach and the duodenum. **o. secun′dum,** an opening high in the septum primum of the embryonic heart, approximately where the foramen ovale will be later. **o. si′nus corona′rii** [NA], the opening of the coronary sinus, situated between the opening of the inferior vena cava and the atrioventricular opening, the lower part of which is covered by the valve of the coronary sinus. Called also *orifice of coronary sinus.* **sinusoidal o.,** any of the openings of the veins of Vieussens in the chambers of the heart. **sphenoidal o.,** apertura sinus sphenoidalis. **o. trun′ci pulmona′lis** [NA], opening of pulmonary trunk: the opening between the right ventricle (from the conus arteriosus portion) and the pulmonary trunk. **o. tympan′icum tu′bae auditi′vae** [NA], tympanic opening of auditory tube: the opening of the auditory tube on the carotid wall of the tympanic cavity. **o. ure′teris** [NA], the opening of the ureter in the bladder; called also *orificium ureteris.* **o. ure′thrae exter′num femini′nae** [NA], external orifice of female urethra: the opening of the urethra into the vestibule; it is surrounded by a sphincter of striated muscle derived from the bulbocavernosus muscle. Called also *orificium urethrae externum muliebris.* **o. ure′thrae exter′num masculi′nae** [NA], external orifice of male urethra: the slitlike opening of the urethra on the tip of the glans penis; called also *orificium urethrae externum virilis.* **o. ure′thrae inter′num** [NA], internal orifice of urethra: the opening between the bladder and the urethra; called also *orificium urethrae internum.* **o. u′teri** [NA], the external opening of the cervix of the uterus into the vagina; called also *orificium externum uteri* and *external orifice of uterus.* **o. uteri′num tu′bae uteri′nae** [NA], uterine orifice of uterine tube: the point at which the cavity of the uterine tube becomes continuous with that of the uterus. **o. vagi′nae** [NA], the external orifice of the vagina, situated just posterior to the external urethral orifice; called also *orificium vaginae.* **o. val′vae ilea′lis** [NA] opening of ileal valve: the slitlike or oval orifice at the junction of the ileum and cecum, as seen in the cadaver. It has two flaps or lips, one above and one below, that form the so-called ileocecal valve and project at thickened folds into the lumen of the large intestine; in the living individual the ileum forms a conical or papillary projection (*papilla ileocaecalis*). Cf. *o. ileocaecale.* **o. ve′nae ca′vae inferio′ris** [NA], the opening of the inferior vena cava into the right atrium of the heart; it is accompanied by a valve which, in the adult, is usually rudimentary. **o. ve′nae ca′vae superio′ris** [NA], the opening of the superior vena cava into the right atrium of the heart; it is unaccompanied by a valve. **os′tia vena′rum pulmona′lium** [NA], the openings of the pulmonary veins (in the human, usually four) into the left atrium of the heart; they are unaccompanied by valves. **o. veno′sum cor′dis,** ostium atrioventriculare dextrum.

ostomate (os′to-māt)   one who has undergone enterostomy or ureterostomy.

ostomy (os′to-me)   a general term referring to any operation in which an artificial opening is formed between two hollow organs or between one or more such viscera and the abdominal wall for discharge of intestinal contents or of urine.

ostosis (os-to′sis)   osteogenesis.

ostraceous (os-tra′shus) [Gr. *ostrakon* shell]   shaped like or resembling an oyster shell.

ostracosis (os″trah-ko′sis) [Gr. *ostrakon,* shell]   bone change which takes on the consistency of oyster shell.

ostreasterol (os″tre-as′ter-ol)   a solid sterol, $C_{29}H_{48}O$, present in oysters.

ostreotoxismus (os″tre-o-tok-siz′mus) [Gr. *ostreon* oyster + *toxikon* poisoning]   poisoning caused by the eating of contaminated oysters.

Oswaldocruzia (oz-wal″do-kroo′ze-ah) [G. *Oswaldo Cruz,* Brazilian physician, 1872–1917]   a genus of nematode parasites inhabiting the lungs and intestines of reptiles and batrachians.

OT   1. abbreviation for *old term* in anatomy.   2. old tuberculin.

otagra (o-tag′rah)   otalgia.

otalgia (o-tal′je-ah) [Gr. *ōtalgia*]   pain in the ear; earache. **o. denta′lis,** reflex pain in the ear due to dental disease. **geniculate o.,** geniculate neuralgia. **o. intermit′tens,** otalgia of an intermittent type. **reflex o.,** otalgia dependent upon some lesion of the buccal cavity or nasopharynx. **secondary o.,** otalgia dependent on inflammation of the geniculate ganglion. **tabetic o.,** otalgia in tabes dorsalis due to degeneration of the nerve of Wrisberg.

otalgic (o-tal′jik)   1. pertaining to earache.   2. an earache remedy.

OTC   over the counter; applied to drugs not required by law to be sold on prescription only.

OTD   organ tolerance dose; see under *dose.*

otic (o′tik) [Gr. *ōtikos*]   pertaining to the ear; aural.

otiobiosis (o″te-o-bi-o′sis)   otobiosis.

Otiobius (o″te-o′be-us)   Otobius.

otitic (o-tit′ik)   pertaining to otitis.

otitis (o-ti′tis) [*ot-* + *-itis*]   inflammation of the ear, which may be marked by pain, fever, abnormalities of hearing, hearing loss, tinnitus, and vertigo. **aviation o.,** barotitis media. **o. croupo′sa,** that which is associated with the formation of a fibrinous membrane. **o. desquamati′va,** otitis externa or media in which there are overdevelopment and desquamation of the cutaneous or mucous epithelium. **o. diphtherit′ica,** o. crouposa. **o. exter′na,** inflam-

mation of the external auditory canal. **o. exter′na circumscrip′ta,** that which affects a limited area or areas. **o. exter′na diffu′sa,** that which affects the greater part of the meatus. **o. exter′na furunculo′sa,** furuncular o. **furuncular o.,** the formation of furuncles in the external meatus. **o. inter′na,** inflammation of the internal ear; labyrinthitis. **o. labyrin′thica,** labyrinthitis. **o. mastoi′dea,** otitis which involves the mastoid spaces. **o. me′dia,** inflammation of the middle ear; tympanitis. **o. me′dia, adhesive,** otitis media resulting in the formation of adhesions between the tympanic membrane and the bony walls of the middle ear or the ossicles. **o. media, secretory,** a painless accumulation of serous or mucoid fluid in the middle ear, resulting from obstruction of the eustachian tube, and causing conduction hearing loss. **o. media, serous,** that marked by serous effusion into the middle ear. **o. me′dia catarrha′lis acu′ta,** an acute catarrhal form. **o. me′dia catarrha′lis chron′ica,** a chronic catarrhal form of several subvarieties. **o. me′dia purulen′ta acu′ta,** an acute suppurative form. **o. me′dia purulen′ta chron′ica,** otorrhea. **o. me′dia sclerot′ica,** dry catarrh of the middle ear. **o. me′dia sero′sa,** one marked by a serous exudation. **o. me′dia suppurati′va,** suppurative inflammation of the middle ear. **o. me′dia vasomotor′ica,** otitis media of vasomotor origin. **mucosis o., mucosus o.,** otitis media caused by *Streptococcus mucosus.* **o. mycot′ica,** that which is due to parasitic fungi. **parasitic o.,** otoacariasis. **o. sclerot′ica,** that which is marked by hardening of the ear structures.

ot(o)- [Gr. *ous,* gen. *ōtos* ear]   a combining form denoting relationship to the ear.

otoacariasis (o″to-ak″ah-ri′ah-sis) [*oto-* + *acariasis*]   infection of the ears of cats, dogs, and domestic rabbits with the mite *Otodectes;* called also *parasitic otitis.*

otoantritis (o″to-an-tri′tis)   otitis involving the attic of the tympanum and the mastoid antrum.

otobiosis (o″to-bi-o′sis)   infestation by *Otobius.*

Otobius (o-to′be-us) [*oto-* + Gr. *bios* manner of living]   a genus of argasid ticks, the spinous ear ticks. The nymphs of *O. lagophilus* of rabbits and *O. megnini* of cattle and other domestic animals may attack the ears of man.

otoblennorrhea (o″to-blen″o-re′ah) [*oto-* + Gr. *blenna* mucus + *rhoia* flow]   mucous discharge from the ear.

otocariasis (o″to-kah-ri′ah-sis)   otoacariasis.

Otocentor (o″to-sen′tor)   Anocentor. **O. ni′tens,** Anocentor nitens.

otocephalus (o″to-sef′ah-lus) [*oto-* + Gr. *kephalē* head]   an individual exhibiting otocephaly.

otocephaly (o″to-sef′ah-le) [*oto-* + Gr. *kephalē* head]   a congenital malformation characterized by lack of a lower jaw and by ears that are united below the face.

otocerebritis (o″to-ser″ĕ-bri′tis) [*oto-* + *cerebritis*]   inflammation of the brain dependent upon disease of the middle ear.

otocleisis (o″to-kli′sis) [*oto-* + Gr. *kleisis* closure]   closure of the auditory passages.

otoconia (o″to-ko′ne-ah) [*oto-* + Gr. *konis* dust]   statoconia.

otoconite (o-tok′o-nīt)   statoconium; see *statoconia.*

otoconium (o″to-ko′ne-um) [L.]   singular of *otoconia.*

otocranial (o″to-kra′ne-al)   pertaining to the otocranium.

otocranium (o″to-kra′ne-um) [*oto-* + Gr. *kranion* skull]   1. the chamber in the petrous bone that lodges the internal ear. 2. the auditory portion of the cranium; called also *petromastoid.*

otocyst (o′to-sist) [*oto-* + Gr. *kystis* sac, bladder]   1. the auditory vesicle of the embryo.   2. the auditory sac of some of the lower animals.

Otodectes (o″to-dek′tēz) [*oto-* + Gr. *dēktēs* a biter]   a genus of mites; see *otoacariasis.*

otodynia (o″to-din′e-ah) [*oto-* + Gr. *odynē* pain]   otalgia.

otoencephalitis (o″to-en-sef″ah-li′tis) [*oto-* + *encephalitis*]   inflammation of the brain due to an extension from an inflamed middle ear.

otogenic (o″to-jen′ik)   otogenous.

otogenous (o-toj′ĕ-nus) [*oto-* + Gr. *gennan* to produce]   originating within the ear.

otography (o-tog′rah-fe) [*oto-* + Gr. *graphein* to write]   a description of the ear.

otohemineurasthenia (o″to-hem″e-nu″ras-the′ne-ah) [*oto-* + *hemi-* + *neurasthenia*] nervous defect of hearing in one ear.

otolaryngology (o″to-lar″in-gol′o-je) that branch of medicine concerned with medical and surgical treatment of the head and neck, including the ears, nose, and throat.

otolite (o′to-līt) otolith.

otolith (o′to-lith) [*oto-* + Gr. *lithos* stone] 1. see *statoconia*. 2. a calcareous mass in the inner ear of vertebrates or the otocyst of invertebrates.

otolithiasis (o″to-lĭ-thi′ah-sis) the presence of calculi in the ear.

otologic (o″to-loj′ik) pertaining to otology.

otologist (o-tol′o-jist) a physician who specializes in otology.

otology (o-tol′o-je) [*oto-* + *-logy*] that branch of medicine which deals with the medical treatment and surgery of the ear, and its anatomy, physiology, and pathology.

otomastoiditis (o″to-mas″toid-i′tis) mastoiditis combined with otitis.

otomucormycosis (o″to-mu″kor-mi-ko′sis) mucormycosis affecting the ear.

otomyasthenia (o″to-mi″as-the′ne-ah) [*oto-* + Gr. *mys* muscle + *astheneia* weakness] a debilitated state of the ear muscles, interfering with the normal attenuation and selection of sounds.

Otomyces (o″to-mi′sēz) [*oto-* + Gr. *mykēs* fungus] a former name for a genus of fungi which infest the ear; now considered the same as *Aspergillus*. **O. hage′ni, O. purpu′reus**, species of uncertain classification, which were once found in the human ear. *O. purpureus* is probably identical with *Aspergillus nidulans*.

otomycosis (o″to-mi-ko′sis) [*oto-* + Gr. *mykēs* fungus] fungal infection of the external auditory meatus, marked by pruritus and exudative inflammation; there may be secondary bacterial infection. **o. aspergilli′na**, any ear disease caused by the presence of an aspergillus; see *myringomycosis*.

otomyiasis (o″to-mi′yah-sis) infestation of the ear by larvae.

otoneuralgia (o″to-nu-ral′je-ah) [*oto-* + *neuralgia*] neuralgic pain in the ear.

otoneurasthenia (o″to-nu″ras-the′ne-ah) [*oto-* + *neurasthenia*] neurasthenia due to ear disease.

otoneurologic (o″to-nu″ro-loj′ik) pertaining to those portions of the nervous system relating to the ear.

otoneurology (o″to-nu-rol′o-je) neuro-otology.

otopathy (o-top′ah-the) [*oto-* + Gr. *pathos* disease] any disease of the ear.

otopharyngeal (o″to-fah-rin′je-al) pertaining to the ear and pharynx.

otoplasty (o′to-plas″te) [*oto-* + Gr. *plassein* to form] plastic surgery of the ear; the surgical correction of ear deformities and defects.

otopolypus (o″to-pol′ĭ-pus) [*oto-* + *polypus*] a polyp of the ear.

otopyorrhea (o″to-pi″o-re′ah) [*oto-* + Gr. *pyon* pus + *rhein* to flow] a copious purulent discharge from the ear.

otopyosis (o″to-pi-o′sis) [*oto-* + Gr. *pyōsis* suppuration] a suppurative disease of the ear.

otor (o′tor) pertaining to the ear; aural.

otorhinolaryngology (o″to-ri″no-lar″in-gol′o-je) [*oto-* + Gr. *rhis* nose + *larynx* larynx + *-logy*] that branch of medicine concerned with medical and surgical treatment of the head and neck, including the ears, nose, and throat.

otorhinology (o″to-ri-nol′o-je) [*oto-* + Gr. *rhis* nose + *-logy*] that branch of medicine which treats of the nose and ear and their diseases.

otorrhagia (o″to-ra′je-ah) [*oto-* + Gr. *rhēgnynai* to burst forth] hemorrhage from the ear.

otorrhea (o″to-re′ah) [*oto-* + Gr. *rhoia* to flow] a discharge from the ear, especially a purulent one. **cerebrospinal fluid o.**, escape of cerebrospinal fluid through the external auditory meatus due to fracture of the temporal bone.

otosalpinx (o″to-sal′pinks) [*oto-* + Gr. *salpinx* trumpet] the auditory tube (tuba auditiva [NA]).

otosclerosis (o″to-skle-ro′sis) [*oto-* + Gr. *sklērōsis* hardening] a pathological condition of the bony labyrinth of the ear, in which there is formation of spongy bone (otospongiosis), especially in front of and posterior to the footplate of the stapes; it may cause bony ankylosis of the stapes, resulting in conductive hearing loss. Cochlear otosclerosis may also develop, resulting in sensorineural hearing loss.

otosclerotic (o″to-skle-rot′ik) characterized by otosclerosis.

otoscope (o′to-skōp) [*oto-* + Gr. *skopein* to examine] an instrument for inspecting or for auscultating the ear. **Brunton's o.**, an otoscope lighted by means of a funnel attached to the side. **Siegle's o.**, an otoscope which gives a view of the drum membrane when subjected to condensed or rarefied air. **Toynbee's o.**, a tube for insertion into the ear of the patient and of the observer for the purpose of auscultating the patient's ear during politzerization.

otoscopy (o-tos′ko-pe) examination of the ear by means of the otoscope.

otosis (o-to′sis) a false impression of sounds uttered by others.

otospongiosis (o″to-spon″je-o′sis) the formation of spongy bone in the bony labyrinth of the ear; see *otosclerosis*.

ototoxic (o″to-tok′sik) having a deleterious effect upon the eighth nerve, or upon the organs of hearing and balance.

ototoxicity (o″to-toks-is′ĭ-te) the quality of being poisonous to or of exerting a deleterious effect upon the eighth nerve or upon the organs of hearing and balance.

Otrivin (o′trĭ-vin) trademark for preparations of xylometazoline hydrochloride.

Ott's test (ots) [Isaac *Ott*, American physiologist, 1847–1916] see under *tests*.

Otto disease, pelvis (ot′o) [Adolph Wilhelm *Otto*, German surgeon, 1786–1845] see under *disease* and *pelvis*.

O.U. abbreviation for L. *o′culus uter′que*, each eye.

ouabain (wah-ba′in) [USP] chemical name: 3β-[(6-deoxy-α-L-mannopyranosyl)oxy]$1\beta,5\beta,11\alpha,19$-pentahydroxycard-2-0(22)-enolide octahydrate. A cardiac glycoside, $C_{29}H_{44}$-$O_{12} \cdot 8H_2O$, obtained principally from the seeds of *Strophanthus gratus* (Wall & Hock.) Baill. (Apocynaceae), occurring as white crystals or crystalline powder, and having the same actions as digitalis but producing digitalization more rapidly; used in the treatment of acute congestive heart failure, nodal paroxysmal tachycardia, and atrial flutter, administered intravenously. Called also *G-strophanthin* or *strophanthin-G*.

Ouchterlony technique (ok′ter-lo″ne) [Orjan Thomas Gunnarson *Ouchterlony*, Swedish bacteriologist, born 1914] see *immunodiffusion*.

Oudin current, resonator (oo-da′) [Paul *Oudin*, French electrotherapist and roentgenologist, 1851–1923] see under *current* and *resonator*.

oulectomy (oo-lek′to-me) 1. ulectomy, def. 1. 2. gingivectomy.

oulitis (oo-li′tis) gingivitis.

ounce (owns) [L. *uncia*] a measure of weight in both the avoirdupois and the apothecaries' system; abbreviation oz. The ounce avoirdupois is one sixteenth of a pound, or 437.5 grains (28.3495 gm.). The apothecaries' ounce is one twelfth of a pound, or 480 grains (31.103 gm.); symbol ℥. **fluid o.**, a unit of capacity (liquid measure) of the apothecaries' system, being 8 fluiddrams, or the equivalent of 29.57 ml. Abbreviated fl.oz.

-ous 1. a suffix meaning possessing, having, or full of, e.g., cancerous. 2. in chemistry, a suffix used to indicate an ion or acid exhibiting the lower of two oxidation states, the other being indicated by the suffix *-ic*.

outbreeding (owt′brēd-ing) the mating of totally unrelated individuals, which frequently results in the production of offspring that show more vigor, as measured in terms of growth, survival, and fertility, than the parents (heterosis); called also *crossbreeding*.

outlet (owt′let) a means by which something escapes. **pelvic o.**, the lower aperture of the pelvis (apertura pelvis inferior [NA]).

outlier (owt′li-er) in statistics, an observation so distant from the central mass of the data that it is considered an obvious mistake that should be removed from the data whether or not a cause of the deviation can be found.

outpatient (owt′pa-shent) a patient who comes to the hospital, clinic, or dispensary for diagnosis and/or treatment but does not occupy a bed.

outpocketing (owt-pok′et-ing) evagination.

outpouching (owt′powch″ing) the obtrusion of a layer or part to form a pouch; evagination.

output (owt′poot) the yield, or the total of anything produced by any functional system of the body. **cardiac o.,** the effective volume of blood expelled by either ventricle of the heart per unit of time (usually volume per minute); it is equal to the stroke output multiplied by the number of beats per the time unit used in the computation. **energy o.,** the energy a body is able to manifest in work or activity. **stroke o.,** the amount of blood ejected by a ventricle at each beat of the heart. **urinary o.,** the amount of urine excreted by the kidneys.

ova (o′vah) [L.] plural of *ovum.*

oval (o′val) [L. *ovalis*] egg shaped; having the outline of the long section of an egg.

ovalbumin (o″val-bu′min) [L. *ovum* egg + *albumin*] an albumin obtainable from the whites of eggs.

ovalocytary (o″vah-lo-si′ter-e) elliptocytary.

ovalocyte (o′vah-lo-sīt″) elliptocyte.

ovalocytosis (o-val″o-si-to′sis) elliptocytosis.

ovarialgia (o-va″re-al′je-ah) oophoralgia.

ovarian (o-va′re-an) pertaining to an ovary or ovaries.

ovariectomy (o″va-re-ek′to-me) oophorectomy.

ovari(o)- [L. *ovarium* ovary] a combining form denoting relationship to the ovary.

ovariocele (o-va′re-o-sēl″) [ovario- + Gr. *kēlē* hernia] hernial protrusion of an ovary.

ovariocentesis (o-va″re-o-sen-te′sis) [ovario- + Gr. *kentēsis* puncture] surgical puncture of an ovary.

ovariocyesis (o-va″re-o-si-e′sis) [ovario- + Gr. *kyēsis* pregnancy] ovarian pregnancy.

ovariodysneuria (o-va″re-o-dis-nu′re-ah) [ovario- + dys- + Gr. *neuron* nerve + -ia] neuralgic pain in the ovary.

ovariogenic (o-va″re-o-jen′ik) arising in the ovary.

ovariohysterectomy (o-va″re-o-his″ter-ek′to-me) oophorohysterectomy.

ovariopathy (o-va″re-op′ah-the) [ovario- + Gr. *pathos* disease] ovarian disease.

ovariopexy (o-va″re-o-pek′se) [ovario- + Gr. *pēxis* fixation] the operation of elevating and fixing an ovary to the abdominal wall.

ovariorrhexis (o-va″re-o-rek′sis) [ovario- + Gr. *rhēxis* rupture] rupture of an ovary.

ovariosalpingectomy (o-va″re-o-sal″pin-jek′to-me) surgical removal of an ovary and uterine tube.

ovariostomy (o-va″re-os′to-me) oophorostomy.

ovariotestis (o-va″re-o-tes′tis) ovotestis.

ovariotherapy (o-va″re-o-ther′ah-pe) ovotherapy.

ovariotomy (o-va″re-ot′o-me) [ovario- + Gr. *tomē* a cutting] surgical removal of an ovary, or removal of an ovarian tumor. **abdominal o.,** ovariotomy performed through the abdominal wall. **vaginal o.,** ovariotomy performed through the vagina.

ovariotubal (o-va″re-o-tu′bal) pertaining to the ovary and uterine tube.

ovaritis (o″vah-ri′tis) oophoritis.

ovarium (o-va′re-um), pl. *ova′ria* [L.] [NA] the ovary or female gonad: one of the two sexual glands in which the ova are formed. It is a flat oval body along the lateral wall of the pelvic cavity, attached to the posterior surface of the broad ligament. It consists of stroma and ovarian follicles in various stages of maturation, and is covered by a modified peritoneum. **o. masculi′num,** appendix testis.

ovarotherapy (o″vah-ro-ther′ah-pe) ovotherapy.

ovary (o′vah-re) the female gonad: one of the two sexual glands in which the ova are formed; see *ovarium.* **adenocystic o.,** an ovary containing numerous small serous cysts. **oyster o's,** hypertrophied, edematous ovaries usually seen in hydatidiform mole. **polycystic o.,** an ovary containing multiple, small follicular cysts filled with yellow or blood-stained, thin serous fluid; the condition may lead to the full-blown Stein-Leventhal syndrome.

OVD occlusal vertical dimension; see *vertical dimension,* under *dimension.*

overbite (o′ver-bīt) vertical overlap, def. 1. **deep o.,** closed bite. **horizontal o.,** see under *overlap.* **vertical o.,** see *overlap.*

overclosure (o″ver-klo′zhur) the loss of occlusal vertical dimension. **reduced interarch distance o.,** the loss of occlusal or contact vertical dimension.

overcompensation (o″ver-kom″pen-sa′shun) conscious or unconscious exaggerated compensation for a real or imagined physical or psychological deficiency.

overcorrection (o″ver-ko-rek′shun) the use of too powerful lenses in correcting defect of vision.

overdenture (o″ver-den′chur) overlay denture.

overdetermination (o″ver-de-ter″mĭ-na′shun) the concept that in their symbolic meanings dreams and neurotic symptoms are the result of many factors.

overdose (o′ver-dōs″) 1. to administer an excessive dose. 2. an excessive dose.

overdosage (o″ver-do′sij) 1. the administration of an excessive dose. 2. the condition resulting from an excessive dose.

overdrive (o′ver-drīv) in cardiology, the process of increasing the heart rate to overcome ectopic heart rhythms; done by the use of drugs or electrical pacemakers.

overeruption (o″ver-e-rup′shun) supraclusion.

overextension (o″ver-eks-ten′shun) extension, as of a limb, beyond the normal limit.

overflow (o′ver-flo) the continuous escape of a fluid, as of the tears or the urine.

overgrafting (o″ver-graft′ing) the application of a second skin graft over a previously healed graft from which the epithelium has been removed, as a means of reinforcing split thickness grafts.

overgrowth (o′ver-grōth) excessive growth of a part, due either to increase in size of the constituent cells (hypertrophy) or to an increase in their number (hyperplasia).

overhang (o′ver-hang) the extension, over the margins of a tooth cavity, of an excessive amount of filling material.

overhydration (o″ver-hi-dra′shun) a state of excess fluids in the body.

overinflation (o″ver-in-fla′shun) excessive inflation or expansion, as of the lungs; hyperinflation. **nonobstructive pulmonary o.,** compensatory emphysema. **obstructive pulmonary o.,** localized obstructive emphysema.

overjet (o′ver-jet) horizontal overlap.

overjut (o′ver-jut) horizontal overlap.

overlap (o′ver-lap) 1. to cover and extend beyond a certain point. 2. anything that lies or extends over and partially covers something. **horizontal o.,** extension of the incisal or buccal cusp ridges of the maxillary teeth labially or buccally to the incisal margins and ridges of the mandibular teeth when the jaws are in habitual occlusion. Called also *horizontal overbite, overjet,* and *overjut.* **vertical o.,** 1. extension of the incisal ridges of the maxillary anterior teeth below the incisal ridges of the mandibular anterior teeth when the jaws are in centric occlusion. Called also *overbite.* 2. the distance that the teeth lap over their antagonists. 3. the relationship of the maxillary incisors to the mandibular incisors when the incisal edges pass each other in centric occlusion.

overlay (o′ver-la) an increment; a later addition superimposed upon an already existing mass, state, or condition. **emotional o.,** psychogenic o. **psychogenic o.,** the emotionally determined increment to an existing organic symptom or disability.

overreaching (o″ver-rēch′ing) an error of gait in the horse, in which the toe of the hind hoof strikes the heel of the forefoot.

overresponse (o″ver-re-spons′) abnormally intense response or reaction to a stimulus.

overriding (o″ver-rīd′ing) the slipping of either part of a fractured bone past the other.

overstain (o′ver-stān) to stain a tissue excessively, so that certain elements may be properly stained when the excess of stain is washed out.

overstrain (o′ver-strān) an abnormal degree of fatigue brought about by activity; it is intermediate between fatigue and actual exhaustion.

overstress (o′ver-stres) excessive activity resulting in overstrain.

overtoe (o′ver-to) hallux varus in which the great toe overlies its fellows.

overtone (o′ver-tōn) any whole number multiple of a fundamental tone. **psychic o.,** the consciousness of a fringe or halo of associated relations which surrounds every image presented to the mind.

overtransfusion (o″ver-trans-fu′zhun) overloading of the circulation by excessive transfusion of blood or other fluid.

overventilation (o″ver-ven″tī-la′shun) hyperventilation.

overweight (o′ver-wāt) excessive increase in adipose tissue (obese overweight) or in muscle and skeletal tissue (muscular overweight).

ovi- see ovo-.

ovi (o′vi) [L.] genitive of ovum. **o. albu′min** [L.], the white of hens' eggs. **o. vitel′lus** [L.], the yolk of hens' eggs.

ovicide (o′vĭ-sīd) an agent destructive to the ova of certain organisms.

oviducal (o′vĭ-du-kal) pertaining to the oviducts.

oviduct (o′vĭ-dukt) [ovi- + L. ductus duct] 1. a passage through which ova leave the maternal organism or pass to an organ which communicates with the exterior of the body. 2. a uterine tube (tuba uterina [NA]).

oviductal (o″vĭ-duk′tal) pertaining to an oviduct.

oviferous (o-vif′er-us) [ovi- + L. ferre to bear] producing ova.

oviform (o′vĭ-form) [ovi- + L. forma shape] egg-shaped; ovoid.

ovigenesis (o″vĭ-jen′ĕ-sis) [ovi- + Gr. gennan to produce] oogenesis.

ovigenetic (o″vĭ-jĕ-net′ik) oogenetic.

ovigenic (o″vĭ-jen′ik) oogenic.

ovigenous (o-vij′ĕ-nus) oogenic.

ovigerm (o′vĭ-jerm) [ovi- + L. germen a bud] a cell which develops into an ovum.

ovigerous (o-vij′er-us) [ovi- + L. gerere to bear] producing or containing ova.

ovine (o′vīn) [L. ovinus of a sheep] pertaining to, characteristic of, or derived from sheep.

ovinia (o-vin′e-ah) [L. ovis sheep] sheep-pox.

oviparity (o″vĭ-par′ĭ-te) the quality of being oviparous.

oviparous (o-vip′ah-rus) [ovi- + L. parere to bring forth, produce] producing eggs from which the young are hatched outside the body of the maternal organism. Cf. ovoviviparous and viviparous.

oviposition (o″vĭ-po-zish′un) [ovi- + L. ponere to place] the act of laying or depositing eggs.

ovipositor (o″vĭ-pos′ĭ-tor) a specialized organ by means of which many female insects deposit their eggs in various plant structures or in the soil.

ovisac (o′vĭ-sak) [ovi- + L. saccus bag] a graafian follicle (folliculi ovarici vesiculosi [NA]).

ovist (o′vist) one who believes that the undeveloped embryo exists preformed in the ovum. Cf. animalculist.

ovium (o′ve-um) the mature ovum.

ov(o)-, ovi- [L. ovum egg] a combining form denoting relationship to an egg, or to ova. See also words beginning oo-.

ovocenter (o′vo-sen″ter) oocenter.

ovocyte (o′vo-sīt) oocyte.

ovoflavin (o″vo-fla′vin) [L. ovum egg + flavus yellow] riboflavin derived from eggs.

ovogenesis (o″vo-jen′ĕ-sis) oogenesis.

ovoglobulin (o″vo-glob′u-lin) the globulin of white of egg.

ovogonium (o″vo-go′ne-um) oogonium.

ovoid (o′void) [ovo- + Gr. eidos form] egg-shaped.

ovolytic (o″vo-lit′ik) splitting up egg albumin.

ovomucin (o″vo-mu′sin) a glycoprotein from the white of egg.

ovomucoid (o″vo-mu′koid) [ovo- + mucoid] a mucus-like principle derivable from egg white.

ovoplasm (o′vo-plazm) [ovo- + Gr. plasma anything formed] the protoplasm of an unfertilized ovum.

ovotestis (o″vo-tes′tis) an abnormal gonad containing both testicular and ovarian tissue.

ovotherapy (o″vo-ther′ah-pe) therapeutic use of ovarian extract, especially extract from the corpus luteum.

ovotransferrin (o″vo-trans-fer′in) an iron-binding protein in egg white having the same properties as transferrin.

ovoverdin (o″vo-ver′din) [ovo- + Fr. verd green] the green pigment of the chromoprotein of crawfish eggs.

ovovitellin (o″vo-vi-tel′in) vitellin.

ovoviviparity (o″vo-viv″ĭ-par′ĭ-te) the quality of being ovoviviparous.

ovoviviparous (o″vo-vi-vip′ah-rus) [ovo- + L. vivus alive + parere to being forth, produce] bearing living young that hatch from large, yolk-filled eggs inside the body of the maternal organism, the embryo being nourished by food stored in the egg; said of lizards, etc. Cf. oviparous and viviparous.

Ovrette (ov-ret′) trademark for a preparation of norgestrel.

ovula (ov′u-lah) [L.] plural of ovulum.

ovular (o′vu-lar) pertaining to an ovule or an ovum.

ovulation (o″vu-la′shun) the discharge of a secondary oocyte from a vesicular follicle of the ovary. **amenstrual o.,** that which occurs in the absence of menstrual bleeding. **anestrous o.,** that which occurs in animals unaccompanied by other events of estrus. **paracyclic o.,** supplementary o. **supplementary o.,** an extra ovulation in a particular estrous cycle; called also paracyclic o.

ovulatory (ov′u-lah-to″re) pertaining to ovulation.

ovule (o′vūl) [L. ovulum] 1. the ovum within the graafian follicle. 2. any small, egglike structure. 3. the megasporangium enclosed within one or more integuments which, after fertilization, becomes a plant seed. **graafian o's,** folliculi ovarici vesiculosi. **Naboth's o's,** Naboth's follicles. **primitive o., primordial o.,** a rudimentary ovum within the ovary.

ovulogenous (o″vu-loj′ĕ-nus) producing or developing from an ovule or ovum.

ovulum (ov′u-lum), pl. ov′ula [L. dim. of ovum] 1. ovum (def. 2). 2. any small, egglike structure. **ov′ula nabo′thi** ["Naboth's ovules"], Naboth's follicles.

ovum (o′vum), pl. o′va, gen. o′vi [L.] 1. the female reproductive cell which, after fertilization, develops into a new member of the same species (von Baer, 1827); an egg. 2. [NA] the human ovum: a round cell about 0.1 mm. in diameter, produced in the ovary, where there is deposited around it a noncellular covering (oolemma; zona pellucida; zona radiata). It consists of protoplasm which contains some yolk, enclosed by a thin cell wall (vitelline membrane). There is a large nucleus (germinal vesicle), within which is a nucleolus (germinal spot). By extension, the word is also used to designate any early stage of the conceptus, when the embryo itself constitutes a tiny and insignificant part of the whole. **alecithal o.,** one with only a small amount of yolk, or almost no yolk, as in the ova of mammals and many

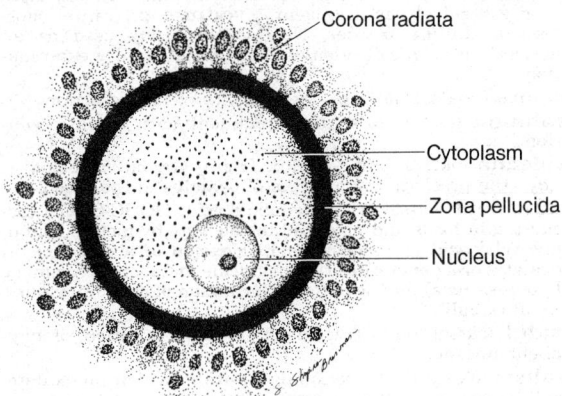

Human ovum.

of the invertebrates; called also *oligolecithal o.* **blighted o.,** a fertilized ovum in which development has become arrested, and abnormality or degeneration is evident. **Bryce-Teacher o.,** a human ovum which was thought to be the youngest known ovum at the time of its study in 1908; now known to be a pathological specimen. **centrolecithal o.,** one in which the yolk is centrally located, and surrounded by a peripheral layer of cytoplasm, as the ova of arthropods. **cleidoic o.,** one which possesses within itself sufficient nutritive material for the production of a complete embryo and so needs to absorb nothing from its environment except oxygen, as a bird's egg. **ectolecithal o.,** one in which the yolk is situated peripherally. **Hertig-Rock ova,** 34 fertilized ova, ranging from 1 to 17 days of age, 21 of which were normal, and 13 abnormal to one degree or another; discovered between 1938 and 1953, they constitute the only series of such early human conceptuses in existence. **holoblastic o.,** one that undergoes total cleavage. **isolecithal o.,** one with yolk evenly distributed throughout the cytoplasm. **macrolecithal o.,** one with much yolk. **Mateer-Streeter o.,** a fertilized ovum about 18 days old, first described in 1920. **medialecithal o.,** one with a medium amount of yolk. **megalecithal o.,** macrolecithal o. **meroblastic o.,** one that undergoes partial cleavage. **microlecithal o.,** miolecithal o. **Miller o.,** a fertilized ovum 10 or 11 days old, first described in 1913. **miolecithal o.,** one containing little yolk. **oligolecithal o.,** alecithal o. **permanent o.,** an ovum ready for fertilization. **Peters' o.,** a fertilized ovum about 13 or 14 days old, first described in 1899. **primitive o., primordial o.,** an egg cell very early in its development. **telolecithal o.,** one in which the yolk is increasingly concentrated toward one pole.

Owen's lines (o′enz) [Sir Richard *Owen*, English anatomist and paleontologist, 1804–1892] see under *line.*

ox- see *oxy-.*

oxacid (oks-as′id) oxo acid.

oxacillin sodium (oks″ah-sil′in) [USP] chemical name: [2S-(2α,5α,6β)]-3,3-dimethyl-6-[[(5-methyl-3-phenyl-4-isoxazolyl)carbonyl]amino]- 7- oxo- 4- thia- 1- azabicyclo [3.2.0] heptane-2-carboxylic acid monosodium salt monohydrate. A semi-synthetic penicillinase-resistant penicillin, $C_{19}H_{18}N_3$-$NaO_5S \cdot H_2O$, occurring as a fine, white, crystalline powder; used primarily in the treatment of infections due to penicillinase-resistant staphylococci, administered orally, intramuscularly, or intravenously.

Oxaine (ok′sān) trademark for a preparation of oxethazaine.

oxalaldehyde (ok″sal-al′dĕ-hīd) glyoxal.

oxalate (ok′sah-lāt) a salt of oxalic acid. **ammonium o.,** odorless crystals or white granules, $(NH_4)_2C_2O_4$, formed by evaporation of the product obtained by the reaction of equivalent amounts of ammonia solution and oxalic acid. **balanced o.,** a mixture of ammonium and potassium oxalates in a 3:2 ratio, used as an anticoagulant in the collection of blood for laboratory examination. **calcium o.,** a salt of oxalic acid which, when formed in high concentrations in the urine, may lead to formation of urinary calculi. **potassium o.,** colorless, odorless crystals, $K_2C_2O_4 \cdot H_2O$, used extensively as a reagent. **sodium o.,** white, odorless, crystalline powder, $Na_2C_2O_4$, formerly used as an anticoagulant in collection of blood for laboratory examination.

oxalated (ok′sah-lāt″ed) treated with oxalate solution.

oxalation (ok″sah-la′shun) treatment with oxalate solution.

oxalemia (ok″sah-le′me-ah) [*oxalate* + Gr. *haima* blood + *-ia*] the presence of an excess of oxalates in the blood.

oxalic acid (ok-sal′ik) ethandioic acid, HOOC-COOH, occurring in foods and produced in the body by metabolism of glyoxylic acid or ascorbic acid; ingestion of a diet rich in oxalates or a genetic disorder of glycine metabolism (primary hyperoxaluria) may lead to the formation of calcium oxalate renal calculi.

Oxalid (ok′sah-lid) trademark for a preparation of oxyphenbutazone.

oxalism (ok′sal-izm) poisoning by oxalic acid or an oxalate.

oxaloacetate (oks″ah-lo-as′ĕ-tāt) an anionic form of oxaloacetic acid.

oxaloacetic acid (ok″sah-lo-ah-se′tik) oxobutanedioic

acid, HOOC-CH_2CO-COOH, an intermediate in the tricarboxylic acid cycle (q.v.); it is convertible to aspartic acid by a transamination reaction.

oxalosis (ok″sah-lo′sis) generalized deposition of calcium oxalate in renal and extrarenal tissues, as may occur in primary hyperoxaluria.

oxaluria (ok″sah-lu′re-ah) hyperoxaluria.

oxaluric acid (ok″sal-ūr′ik) the amide of oxalic acid and urea H_2N-CO-NH-CO-COOH, which occurs in urine.

oxalyl (ok′sah-lil) the divalent group, $(C:O)_2$, formed from oxalic acid by the loss of two hydroxyl groups.

oxalylurea (ok″sah-lil-u′re-ah) 1. oxaluric acid. 2. parabanic acid.

oxamide (ok-sam′id) the diamide of oxalic acid, $NH_2 \cdot CO$-$CO \cdot NH_2$. It will give the biuret reaction.

oxamniquine (oks-am′nĭ-kwin) chemical name: 1,2,3,4-tetrahydro-2-[[(1-methylethyl)amino]methyl]-7-nitro-6-quinolinemethanol. An antischistosomal, $C_{14}H_{21}N_3O_3$, especially effective against *Schistosoma mansoni.*

oxanamide (ok-san′ah-mīd) chemical name: 2-ethyl-3-propyloxiranecarboxamide; a tranquilizer, $C_8H_{15}NO_2$.

oxandrolone (ok-san′dro-lōn) [USP] chemical name: 17β-hydroxy-17-methyl-2-oxa-5α-androstan-3-one. An androgenic steroidal lactone, $C_{19}H_{30}O_3$, which promotes retention of nitrogen, potassium, and phosphorus, and is used to accelerate anabolism and/or to arrest excessive catabolism.

oxantel pamoate (oks′an-tel) chemical name: (*E*)-3-[2-(1,4,5,6-tetrahydro-1-methyl-2-pyrimidinyl)ethenyl]phenol 4,4′-methylenebis[3-hydroxy-2-naphthalenecarboxylate] (2:1) (salt); an anthelmintic effective against *Trichuris*, $(C_{13}$-$H_{16}N_2O)_2 \cdot C_{23}H_{16}O_6$.

oxaprozin (ok″sah-pro′zin) chemical name: 4,5-diphenyl-2-oxazolepropanoic acid; an anti-inflammatory, $C_{18}H_{15}NO_3$.

oxarbazole (ok-sar′bah-zōl) chemical name: 9-benzoyl-2,3,4,9-tetrahydro-6-methoxy-1*H*-carboxole-3-carboxylic acid; an antiasthmatic, $C_{21}H_{19}NO_4$.

oxatomide (ok-sa′to-mīd) chemical name: 1-[3-[4-(diphenylmethyl)-1-piperazinyl]propyl]-1,3-dihydro-2*H*-benzimidazol-2-one; an antiallergic and antiasthmatic, $C_{27}H_{30}N_4O$.

oxazepam (oks-az′ĕ-pam) [USP] chemical name: 7-chloro-1,3-dihydro-3-hydroxy-5-phenyl-2*H*-1,4-benzodiazepin-2-one. One of the benzodiazepine tranquilizers, $C_{15}H_{11}Cl$-N_2O_2, occurring as a creamy white to pale yellow powder. It is used orally as a sedative in the treatment of anxiety, especially in the elderly, and may be used as an adjunct for acute withdrawal symptoms in chronic alcoholics.

oxethazaine (ok-seth′ah-zān) chemical name: 2,2′-(2-hydroxyethylimino)-bis-[*N*-α, α-dimethylphenethyl)-*N*-methylacetamide]. A topical anesthetic, $C_{28}H_{41}N_3O_3$, which has been administered orally to relieve gastric distress.

oxetorone fumarate (ok-set′o-rōn) chemical name: 3-benzofuro[3,2-c][1][benzoxepin-6(12*H*)-ylidene-*N,N*-dimethyl-1-propanamine(*E*)-2-butenedioate (1:1); an analgesic specific in migraine, $C_{21}H_{21}NO_2 \cdot C_4H_4O_4$.

oxfendazole (oks-fen′dah-zōl) chemical name: [5-(phenylsulfinyl)-1*H*-benzimidazol-2-yl]carbamic acid methyl ester; an anthelmintic, $C_{15}H_{13}N_3O_3S$.

oxgall (oks′gawl) see *ox bile extract,* under *extract.*

oxibendazole (ok″sĭ-ben′dah-zōl) chemical name: (5-propoxy-1*H*-benzimidazol-2-yl)carbamic acid methyl ester; a veterinary anthelmintic, $C_{12}H_{15}N_3O_3$.

oxidant (ok′sĭ-dant) the electron acceptor in an oxidation-reduction (redox) reaction.

oxidase (ok′sĭ-dās) [EC 1] an enzyme of the oxidoreductase class that catalyzes the oxidation of a substrate by the addition of oxygen or by the removal of hydrogen or electrons with molecular oxygen acting as the acceptor. **direct o. (oxygenase)** [EC 1.13], one that catalyzes the oxidation of a substrate with reduction of molecular oxygen and its incorporation into the substance oxidized. **indirect o. (peroxidase)** [EC 1.11], one that catalyzes the oxidation of a substrate with reduction of hydrogen peroxide. **primary o.,** direct o.

oxidation (ok′sĭ-da′shun) the act of oxidizing or state of being oxidized. Chemically it consists in the increase of positive charges on an atom or the loss of negative charges. Most biological oxidations are accomplished by the removal of a pair of hydrogen atoms (dehydrogenation) from a molecule. Such oxidations must be accompanied by reduction of an acceptor molecule. *Univalent o.* indicates loss of one electron; *divalent o.*, the loss of two electrons. **beta o.** (β-oxidation), oxidation of a fatty acid at the beta carbon atom, the second carbon from the carboxyl group, with the result that the two end carbons are split off as acetic acid (acetylcoenzyme A) and with the formation of a fatty acid containing two fewer carbon atoms. **biological o.,** the enzymatic process by which food is metabolized, resulting in the release of energy. See also *oxidation.* **coupled o.,** the enzymatic oxidation of two donor molecules, with the incorporation of oxygen into one of the donors. **omega o.,** (ω-oxidation), a minor pathway of fatty acid oxidation in which the ω-carbon is oxidized, forming an α,ω-dicarboxylic acid.

oxidation-reduction (ok″sĭ-da′shun-re-duk′shun) the chemical reaction whereby electrons are removed (oxidation) from atoms of the substance being oxidized and transferred to atoms being reduced (reduction). Called also *redox.*

oxidative (ok′sĭ-da-tiv) referring to the process of oxidation; being capable of an oxidizing reaction.

oxide (ok′sīd) [L. *oxidum*] any compound of oxygen with an element or radical. **arsenous o.,** arsenic trioxide. **diethyl o.,** ether. **stannic o.,** a compound, SnO_2, occurring as a white or slightly grayish powder, found in nature as the mineral cassiterite, or produced through a reaction between tin and concentrated nitric acid at high temperatures. Used as a polishing agent for glass, metals, and especially to produce a high polish on metallic dental restorations. Called also *tin oxide.*

oxidize (ok′sĭ-dīz) to combine or cause to combine with oxygen, or to lose electrons. See *oxidation.*

oxidopamine (oks″ĭ-do′pah-mēn) chemical name: 5-(2-aminoethyl-1,2,4-benzenetriol, $C_8H_{11}NO_3$; an ophthalmic adrenergic.

oxidoreductase (ok″sĭ-do-re-duk′tās) [EC 1] a class of enzymes that catalyze the reversible transfer of electrons from a substrate that is oxidized (hydrogen or electron donor) to a substrate that is reduced (hydrogen or electron acceptor). The class includes dehydrogenases, hydroxylases, oxidases, oxygenases, peroxidases, reductases, and transhydrogenases.

oxidosis (ok″sĭ-do′sis) acidosis.

oxifungin hydrochloride (ok″sĭ-fun′gin) chemical name: 1,2-dihydro-3-(phenoxymethyl)pyrido[3,4-*e*]-1,2,4-triazine monohydrochloride; an antifungal, $C_{13}H_{12}N_4O \cdot HCl$.

oxilorphan (ok″sil-or′fan) chemical name: 17-(cyclopropylmethyl)morphinan-3,14-diol; a narcotic antagonist, $C_{20}H_{27}NO_2$.

oxim, oxime (ok′sim) any of a series of compounds formed by the action of hydroxylamine on an aldehyde or a ketone.

oximeter (ok-sim′ĕ-ter) a photoelectric device for determining the oxygen saturation of the blood. **ear o.,** an oximeter for attachment to the ear, by which oxygen saturation of the blood flowing through the ear can be determined. **intracardiac o.,** an instrument for measuring the concentration of oxygen or dye in blood within the heart; see also *oxygen gas analyzer,* under *analyzer.* **whole blood o.,** an oximeter for determination of oxygen saturation of removed specimens of blood.

oximetry (ok-sim′ĕ-tre) determination of the oxygen saturation of arterial blood by means of bichromate photoelectric colorimetry.

oxiperomide (ok″se-per′o-mīd) chemical name: 1,3-dihydro-1-[1-(2-phenoxyethyl)-4-piperidinyl]-2*H*-benzimidazol-2-one; a dopamine-receptor antagonist, $C_{20}H_{23}N_3O_2$, used as a tranquilizer.

oxiramide (ok-sēr′ah-mīd) chemical name: *cis*-(±)-*N*-[4-(2,6-dimethyl-1-piperidenyl)butyl]-α-phenoxybenzeneacetamide; a cardiac depressant, $C_{25}H_{34}N_2O_2$, with antiarrhythmic activity.

oxisuran (ok″se-sur′an) chemical name: 2-(methylsulfinyl)-1-(1-2-pyridinyl)ethanone; an antineoplastic, $C_8H_9NO_2S$.

oxmetidine mesylate (oks-met′ĭ-dēn″mes′ĭ-lāt) a histamine H_2 receptor antagonist.

oxo- (ok′so) the approved prefix in formal nomenclature for *keto-*, as in *oxoglutarate* for *ketoglutarate.* Terms prefixed with *keto-* are the common forms in the United States.

oxo-acid-lyase (ok″so-as″id-li′ās) [EC 4.1.3] a sub-subclass of enzymes of the lyase class comprising those that cleave a

C—C bond of a 3-hydroxy acid or catalyze the reverse reaction.

oxogestone phenpropionate (ok″so-jes′tōn) chemical name: 20*R*-(1-oxo-3-phenylpropoxy)-19-norpregn-4-3-one; a progestin, $C_{29}H_{38}O_3$.

oxoglutarate dehydrogenase (ok′so-gloo′tah-rāt de-hi′dro-jen-ās) [EC 1.2.4.2] α-ketoglutarate dehydrogenase.

2-oxoglutaric acid (ok″so-gloo-tar′ik) α-ketoglutaric acid.

2-oxoisovalerate dehydrogenase (lipoamide) (ok″-so-i″so-val′er-āt de-hi′dro-jen-ās) [EC 1.2.4.4] α-ketoisovalerate dehydrogenase.

oxolinic acid (ok-so-lin′ik) a synthetic antibacterial used orally for urinary tract infections caused by gram-negative organisms, including *Escherichia coli, Proteus* species, and *Klebsiella* species.

oxonemia (ok″so-ne′me-ah) [L. *oxone* acetone + Gr. *haima* blood + *-ia*] (*obs.*) acetonemia.

oxonium (ok-so′ne-um) containing tetravalent basic oxygen.

oxonuria (ok″so-nu′re-ah) (*obs.*) acetonuria.

oxophenarsine hydrochloride (ok″so-phen-ar′sin) chemical name: 2-amino-arsenophenol hydrochloride. An arsenical, $C_6H_6AsNO_2 \cdot HCl$, with antispirochetal and antitrypanosomal properties; rarely used in the treatment of syphilis and trypanosomiasis, administered intravenously.

5-oxoprolinase (ATP hydrolyzing) (ok″so-pro′lĭ-nās) [EC 3.5.2.9] an enzyme of the hydrolase class that catalyzes the reaction ATP + 5-oxo-L-proline + $2H_2O$ = ADP + orthophosphate + L-glutamate. The reaction is a part of the mechanism of transport of amino acids into tissue cells by the γ-glutamyl cycle. Called also *pyroglutamase.*

5-oxoproline (ok″so-pro′lēn) a ninhydrin-negative, acidic lactam of glutamic acid occurring at the N-terminus of several peptides and proteins. Called also *pyroglutamic acid* or *pyroglutamate.*

5-oxoprolinuria (ok″so-pro″lin-u′re-ah) an inborn error of amino acid metabolism marked by abnormally increased levels of 5-oxoproline in the urine, metabolic acidosis, and an increase in the rate of hemolysis; neurological symptoms may also occur. Called also *pyroglutamic aciduria.*

oxozone (ok′so-zōn) a hypothetical allotropic form of oxygen, O_4, supposed to be present in ozone.

oxpentifylline (oks″ĭ-pin-tif′ĭ-lēn) pentoxifylline.

oxprenolol hydrochloride (oks-pren′o-lōl) chemical name: 1-[(1-methylethyl)amino]-3-[2-(2-propenyloxy)-2-propanol hydrochloride; a beta-adrenergic blocking agent, $C_{15}H_{23}NO_3 \cdot HCl$, having the same actions as propanolol (q.v.)

Oxsoralen (ok-sor′ah-len) trademark for preparations of methoxsalen.

oxtriphylline (oks-trif′ĭ-lēn) [NF] chemical name: 2-hydroxy-*N,N,N*-trimethylethanaminium salt with 3,7-dihydro-1,3-dimethyl-1*H*-purine,2,6-dione. A compound of choline and theophylline, $C_{12}H_{21}N_5O_3$, occurring as a white crystalline powder, having the same actions as the parent compound; used chiefly as a bronchodilator, administered orally. Called also *choline theophyllinate* and *theophylline cholinate.*

oxy-, ox- [Gr. *oxys* keen] a combining form (*a*) meaning sharp, quick, or sour, (*b*) denoting relationship to acid, or (*c*) denoting the presence of oxygen in a compound.

oxyachrestia (ok″se-ah-kres′te-ah) [*oxy-* + *a* neg. + Gr. *chrēsis* use] a condition of defective supply of glucose to the neurons, which is the cause of hypoglycemic coma.

oxyacid (ok″se-as′id) oxo acid.

oxyacoia (ok′se-ah-koi′ah) oxyecoia.

oxybenzene (ok″se-ben′zēn) phenol.

oxybenzone (ok″se-ben′zōn) [USP] chemical name: (2-hydroxy-4-methoxyphenyl)phenylmethanone. A sunscreening agent, $C_{14}H_{12}O_3$, occurring as a white to off-white powder; applied topically to the skin.

oxyblepsia (ok″se-blep′se-ah) [*oxy-* + Gr. *blepsis* vision + *-ia*] unusual acuity of vision.

oxybutynin chloride (ok″se-bu′tĭ-nin) chemical name: 4-(diethylamino) - 2 - butyl-α-phenylcyclohexaneglycolate. An anticholinergic, $C_{22}H_{31}NO_3 \cdot HCl$, which has a direct antispasmodic effect on smooth muscle; used in the treatment of uninhibited neurogenic bladder and reflex neurogenic bladder, administered orally.

oxybutyria (ok″se-bu-tir′e-ah) the presence of hydroxybutyric acid in urine.

oxybutyricacidemia (ok″se-bu-tir″ik-as″ĭ-de′me-ah) oxybutyria.

oxycalorimeter (ok″se-kal-o-rim′ĕ-ter) Benedict's apparatus for determining the caloric value of food by burning a sample in a combustion chamber and measuring the volume of oxygen consumed.

oxycanthine (ok-se-kan′thin) a white alkaloid, $C_{37}H_{40}O_6$-N_2, from the root of *Berberis vulgaris*, the barberry; said to paralyze and irritate the brain and spinal cord.

Oxycel (ok′sĭ-sel) trademark for preparations of oxidized cellulose.

oxycephalia (ok″se-sĕ-fa′le-ah) oxycephaly.

oxycephalic (ok″se-sĕ-fal′ik) pertaining to or characterized by oxycephaly.

oxycephalous (ok″se-sef′ah-lus) oxycephalic.

oxycephaly (ok″se-sef′ah-le) [*oxy-* + Gr. *kephalē* head] a condition in which the top of the head is pointed or conical owing to premature closure of the coronal and lambdoid sutures. Called also *acrocephaly, hypsicephaly, turricephaly, steeple head* or *skull,* and *tower head* or *skull.*

oxychloride (ok″se-klo′rĭd) an element or radical combined with oxygen and chlorine.

oxychlorosene (ok″se-klor′o-sēn) the hypochlorous acid complex of a mixture of the phenyl sulfonate derivatives of aliphatic hydrocarbons, $C_{20}H_{34}O_3S \cdot HOCl$, having actions similar to those of chlorine; used as a topical anti-infective. **o. sodium,** the sodium salt of oxychlorosene, used like the base.

oxycholine (ok″se-ko′lin) muscarine.

oxychromatic (ok″se-kro-mat′ik) [*oxy-* + Gr. *chrōma* color] staining with acid dyes; acidophilic.

oxychromatin (ok″se-kro′mah-tin) [*oxy-* + *chromatin*] that part of the chromatin that stains with acid aniline dyes; called also *lanthanin.*

oxycinesia (ok″se-si-ne′ze-ah) [*oxy-* + Gr. *kinēsis* movement + *-ia*] pain on motion.

oxycodone hydrochloride (ok″se-ko′dōn) chemical name: 4,5α-epoxy-14-hydroxy-3-methoxy-17-methylmorphinan-6-one. A morphine derivative, $C_{18}H_{21}NO \cdot HCl$, used as a narcotic analgesic.

oxycyanide (ox″se-si′ah-nīd) the oxide of any binary compound of cyanogen.

oxydase (ok′se-dās) (obs.) oxidase.

oxydendron (ok″se-den′dron) [*oxy-* + Gr. *dendron* tree] a homeopathic remedy prepared from the leaves of *Oxydendrum arboreum* (L.) DC. (Ericaceae), an ericaceous tree of North America whose leaves are chewed to allay thirst. Formerly used in the treatment of cardiac disorders.

oxydoreductase (ok″sĕ-do-re-duk′tās) oxidoreductase.

oxyecoia (ok″se-e-koi′ah) [*oxy-* + Gr. *akoē* hearing + *-ia*] morbid acuteness of the sense of hearing.

oxyesthesia (ok″se-es-the′ze-ah) [*oxy-* + Gr. *aisthesis* perception + *-ia*] morbid or abnormal acuteness of the senses. Cf. *hyperesthesia.*

oxyetherotherapy (ok″se-e″ther-o-ther′ah-pe) [*oxy-* + *ether* + Gr. *therapeia* medical treatment] treatment by the inhalation of ether vapor which is carried along by a current of oxygen; formerly used in pulmonary infection and in whooping cough.

oxygen (ok′sĭ-jen) [Gr. *oxys* sour + *gennan* to produce] a gaseous element existing free in the air and in combination in most nonelementary solids, liquids, and gases; atomic number, 8; atomic weight, 15.999; symbol, O. Oxygen exists in three isotopes, with atomic weights of 16, 17, and 18 (heavy oxygen). Oxygen constitutes 20 per cent by weight of the atmospheric air; it is the essential agent in the respiration of plants and animals and, although noninflammable, is necessary to support combustion. It forms the characteristic constituent of ternary acids. It is administered by inhalation in some pulmonary and cardiac disorders. **excess o.,** the quantity of oxygen used over and above the resting requirements of the body. **heavy o.,** an isotope of oxygen of atomic weight 18. **high pressure o.,** hyperbaric o. **hyperbaric o.,** high-pressure oxygen, i.e., oxygen under

greater than atmospheric pressure. **molecular o.,** dioxygen, O_2. **singlet o.,** a highly reactive, diamagnetic excited state ($^1O_2$) of dioxygen that rapidly decays with the emission of visible light to the paramagnetic (triplet) ground state. Singlet oxygen is highly reactive and is thought to be involved in the oxidative killing of ingested microorganisms by neutrophils; it is produced spontaneously during the respiratory burst by spontaneous reactions of hydrogen peroxide with superoxide and hypochlorite ions.

oxygenase (ok′sĭ-jĕ-nās″) [EC 1.13] any enzyme of a subclass of enzymes of the oxidoreductase class that catalyzes the oxidation of a substrate with incorporation one or both atoms of oxygen from molecular oxygen into the substance oxidized.

oxygenate (ok′sĭ-jĕ-nāt) to add oxygen to.

oxygenation (ok″sĭ-jĕ-na′shun) the act, process, or result of oxygenating.

oxygenator (ok″sĭ-jĕ-na′tor) a device which mechanically oxygenates venous blood extracorporeally. It is used in combination with one or more pumps for maintaining circulation during open heart surgery and for assisting the circulation in patients seriously ill with some cardiac and pulmonary disorders. **bubble o.,** a device in which pure oxygen is bubbled through an extracorporeal reservoir of blood, either directly or through a filter. **disk o.,** rotating disk o. **film o.,** a device, encased in a container of oxygen, which makes possible the production of a thin film of blood to facilitate the exchange of gases; see *rotating disk o.* and *screen o.* **membrane o.,** a device, usually consisting of a connected series of flat bags made of semipermeable material, such as cellophane, Teflon, or Silastic, encased in a container of oxygen. The exchange of gases between the blood in the bags and the oxygen in the container occurs across the membrane. **pump-o.,** see *pump-oxygenator.* **rotating disk o.,** a type of film oxygenator in which parallel disks in series rotate through an extracorporeal pool of venous blood in a container of oxygen; gaseous exchange occurs between the thin film of blood on the exposed surfaces of the disks and the oxygen in the container. **screen o.,** a type of film oxygenator in which the venous blood is passed over a series of screens in a container of oxygen, gaseous exchange taking place in the thin film of blood produced on the screens.

oxygenic (ok″sĭ-jen′ik) containing oxygen.

oxygeusia (ok″sĭ-gu′se-ah) [*oxy-* + Gr. *geusis* taste + *-ia*] unusual acuteness of the sense of taste.

oxyhematoporphyrin (ok″se-hem″ah-to-por′fĭ-rin) a pigment sometimes found in the urine, closely allied to hematoporphyrin.

oxyheme (ok′se-hēm) heme.

oxyhemochromogen (ok″se-he″mo-kro′mo-jen) heme.

oxyhemocyanine (ok″se-he″mo-si′ah-nin) hematocyanine charged with oxygen.

oxyhemoglobin (ok″se-he″mo-glo′bin) hemoglobin that contains bound O_2, a compound formed from hemoglobin on exposure to alveolar gas in the lungs, with formation of a covalent bond with oxygen and without change of the charge of the ferrous state.

oxyhemogram (ok″se-he′mo-gram) (obs.) a graphic record of the oxygen saturation of the blood as determined by use of the oxyhemograph.

oxyhemograph (ok″se-he′mo-graf) [*oxygen* + Gr. *haima* blood + *graphein* to write] (obs.) an apparatus for determining the oxygen content of the blood, by photoelectric registration of changes in the spectroscopic properties of hemoglobin.

oxyhydrocephalus (ok″se-hi″dro-sef′ah-lus) hydrocephalus in which the top of the head assumes a pointed shape.

oxyhyperglycemia (ok″se-hi″per-gli-se′me-ah) a condition in which there is slight glycosuria and an oral glucose tolerance curve which rises about 180–200 mg. per 100 ml. but returns to fasting values 2½ hours after ingestion of the glucose.

oxyiodide (ok″se-i′o-dīd) an element or radical combined with oxygen and iodine.

oxylalia (ok-se-la′le-ah) [*oxy-* + Gr. *lalein* to talk + *-ia*] rapidity of speech.

Oxylone (ok′sĭ-lōn) trademark for a preparation of fluorometholone.

oxymetazoline hydrochloride (ok″se-met-az′o-lēn) [USP] chemical name: 3-[(4,5-dihydro-1*H*-imidazol-2-yl)-

methyl]-6-(1,1- dimethylethyl)-2,4-dimethylphenol monohydrochloride. An adrenergic, $C_{16}H_{24}N_2O \cdot HCl$, occurring as a white to nearly white, crystalline powder; used topically as a vasoconstrictor to reduce swelling and congestion of the nasal mucosa.

oxymetholone (ok″se-meth′o-lōn) [NF] chemical name: 17β-hydroxy-2-(hydroxymethylene)-17α- methyl-5α-androstan-3-one. An anabolic-androgenic steroid, $C_{21}H_{32}O_3$, occurring as a white to creamy white, crystalline powder; administered orally.

oxymetry (ok-sim′ĕ-tre) oximetry.

Oxymonadida (ok″sĭ-mo nad′ĭ dah) an order of parasitic protozoa (class Zoomastigophorea, subphylum Mastigophora) having one or more karyomastigonts, each containing four flagella typically arranged in two pairs in motile stages, some of which are turned posteriorly and adhere to the body surface. Representative genera include *Monocercomonoides*, *Oxymonas*, and *Pyrsonympha*.

Oxymonas (ok″sĭ-mo′nas) [*oxy-* + Gr. *monas* unit, from *monos* single] a genus of parasitic flagellate protozoa (order Oxymonadida, class Zoomastigophorea) found in the gut of termites and woodroaches.

oxymorphone hydrochloride (ok″se-mor′fōn) [USP] chemical name: $4,5\alpha$-epoxy-3,14-dihydroxy-17-methylmorphinan-6-one hydrochloride. A semisynthetic compound, C_{12}-$H_{19}NO_4 \cdot HCl$, occurring as a white or slightly off-white, odorless powder; used as a narcotic analgesic.

oxymyoglobin (ok″se-mi″o-glo′bin) a compound formed from myoglobin on exposure to atmospheric conditions, with formation of a covalent bond with oxygen and without change of the charge of the ferrous state.

oxymyohematin (ok″se-mi″o-hem′ah-tin) oxidized myohematin from muscle.

oxynervon (ok″se-ner′von) a cerebroside isolated from the brain.

oxyneurine (ok″se-nu′rin) betaine.

oxyntic (ok-sin′tik) [Gr. *oxynō* to make acid] secreting acid, as the parietal (oxyntic) cells.

oxyopia (ok″se-o′pe-ah) [*oxy-* + *-opia*] acuteness of vision.

oxyopter (ok″se-op′ter) [*oxy-* + Gr. *optēr* observer] a unit of measurement of visual acuity, being the reciprocal value of the visual angle expressed in degrees. An oxyopter (1 degree) is equivalent to 60 Snellen units (60′) and corresponds to the counting of fingers at 1 meter.

oxyosis (ok″se-o′sis) [*oxy-* + *-osis*] acidosis.

oxyosmia (ok″se-os′me-ah) [*oxy-* + Gr. *osmē* odor + *-ia*] acuteness of the sense of smell.

oxyosphresia (ok″se-os-fre′ze-ah) [*oxy-* + Gr. *osphrēsis* smell + *-ia*] unusual acuteness of the sense of smell.

oxyparaplastin (ok″se-par″ah-plas′tin) the oxyphil part of paraplastin.

oxypathia (ok″se-pa′the-ah) acuteness of sensation. See *hyperesthesia.*

oxypertine (ok″se-per′tēn) chemical name: 5,6-dimethoxy-2- methyl - 3 - [2 - (4 - phenyl -1 - piperazinyl)ethyl]indole; an antidepressant, $C_{23}H_{29}N_3O_2$.

oxyphenbutazone (ok″se-fen-bu′tah-zōn) [USP] chemical name: 4-butyl-1-(4-hydroxyphenyl)-2-phenyl-3,5-pyrazolidinedione monohydrate. A derivative of phenylbutazone, $C_{19}H_{20}N_2O_3 \cdot H_2O$, having similar toxicity and anti-inflammatory, analgesic, and antipyretic actions; administered orally in the treatment of arthritis, gout, and similar conditions.

oxyphencyclimine hydrochloride (ok″se-fen-si′klĭ-mēn) [USP] chemical name: α - cyclohexyl -α - hydroxybenzeneacetic acid (1,4,5,6 - tetrahydro -1 - methyl -2 - pyrimidinyl)methyl ester monohydrochloride. An anticholinergic, $C_{20}H_{28}N_2O_3 \cdot HCl$, occurring as a white, crystalline powder, having antispasmodic, antisecretory, and antimotility activities; used especially in the treatment of peptic ulcer and spasm of the gastrointestinal tract, administered orally.

oxyphenisatin (ok″se-fĕ-ni′sah-tin) chemical name: 3,3-bis(4-hydroxyphenyl)-1,3-dihydro-$2H$-indol-2-one. A cathartic, $C_{20}H_{15}NO_3$, occurring as a white, crystalline powder; administered as an enema to cleanse the bowel before surgery or colon examination. **o. acetate,** the diacetyl derivative of oxyphenisatin, $C_{24}H_{19}NO_5$, occurring as a white, crystalline powder; used as a cathartic, administered orally.

oxyphenonium bromide (ok″se-fĕ-no′ne-um) chemical name: 2-[cyclohexylhydroxyphenylacetyl)oxy]-*N,N*-diethyl-*N*-methylethanaminium bromide. A quaternary ammonium anticholinergic, $C_{21}H_{34}BrNO_3$, occurring as a white, crystalline powder having antisecretory, antispasmodic, and antimotility activities; used in the treatment of peptic ulcer and other gastrointestinal disorders in which hypermotility and spasm are a feature, administered orally.

oxyphenylethylamine (ok″se-fen″il-eth″il-am′in) tyramine.

oxyphil (ok′se-fil) 1. Hürthle cell. 2. oxyphilic.

oxyphilic (ok″se fil′ik) [*oxy-* + Gr. *philein* to love] stainable with an acid dye; acidophilic.

oxyphilous (oks-if′ĭ-lus) oxyphilic.

oxyphonia (ok″se-fo′ne-ah) [Gr. *oxyphōnia*] an abnormally sharp quality or pitch of the voice.

Oxyphotobacteria (ok″se-fo″to-bak-te′re-ah) [*oxy-* + *photo-* + *bacteria*] a class of bacteria of the division Gracilicutes, kingdom Procaryotae, made up of gram-negative aerobic organisms that derive energy from light (phototrophic metabolism), using water as an electron donor and producing oxygen. The class includes the blue green bacteria (Cyanobacteria) and the green prokaryotic algae (Prochlorophyta).

oxyplasm (ok′se-plazm) the oxyphil part of the cytoplasm.

oxypurine (ok″se-pu′rin) a purine containing oxygen. The oxypurines include hypoxanthine or monoxypurine, xanthine or dioxypurine, and uric acid or trioxypurine.

oxypurinol (ok″se-pūr′ĭ-nol) chemical name: $1H$-pyrazolo[3,4-*d*]pyrimidine-4,6-diol; the active metabolite of allopurinol, a xanthine oxidase inhibitor responsible for much of the activity of allopurinol against gout, $C_5H_4N_4O_2$.

oxyrhine (ok′se-rīn) [*oxy-* + Gr. *rhis* nose] having a sharp-pointed nose.

oxysalt (ok′se-sawlt) any salt of an oxacid.

oxysantonin (ok″se-san′to-nin) a compound formed in the body from ingested santonin.

Oxyspirura (ok″se-spi-roo′rah) a genus of nematode parasites of the superfamily Spiruroidea. **O. manso′ni**, a species found beneath the nictitating membrane of chickens and other fowl in Asia, Africa, Australia, South America, Samoa, and in the United States in Florida, Texas, Louisiana, and Hawaii.

oxytalan (oks-it′ah-lan) a connective tissue fiber found typically in the periodontal membranes of man and certain other animals, including monkeys. It is stained with aldehyde fuchsin after appropriate oxidation. On electron microscopic examination, fibrillar and amorphous components are revealed.

oxytalanolysis (oks-it″ah-lan-ol′ĭ-sis) destruction of oxytalan fibers. **o. calcium** [USP], the calcium salt of oxytetracycline, $C_{44}H_{46}Ca_4O_{18}$, occurring as a yellow to light brown, crystalline powder; used as a antibacterial, administered orally. **o. hydrochloride** [USP], the monohydrochloride salt of oxytetracycline, $C_{22}H_{24}N_2O_9 \cdot HCl$, occurring as a yellow, crystalline powder; used as an antibacterial and antirickettsial, administered orally and by intravenous infusion.

oxytocia (ok-se-to′se-ah) [*oxy-* + Gr. *tokos* birth + *-ia*] rapid labor.

oxytocic (ok-se-to′sik) 1. pertaining to, characterized by, or promoting oxytocia. 2. an agent that hastens evacuation of the uterus by stimulating contractions of the myometrium.

oxytocin (ok″se-to′sin) 1. an octapeptide, one of two hormones formed by the neuronal cells of the hypothalamic nuclei and stored in the posterior lobe of the pituitary, the other being vasopressin. It has uterine-contracting and milk-ejecting actions. Its role in human parturition is not known. 2. the same oxytocic principle obtained synthetically or from the posterior pituitary of domestic animals, prepared in accordance with USP standards; it is administered intramuscularly or by intravenous infusion to induce active labor, increase the force of contractions in labor, contract uterine muscle after delivery of the placenta, control postpartum hemorrhage, and stimulate milk ejection. Often used in veterinary medicine to stimulate the letdown of milk in cows and heifers affected with agalactia. **o. citrate,** the citrate salt of oxytocin, used to initiate or stimulate labor in selected patients, administered buccally.

oxytropism (oks-it′ro-pizm) [oxygen + Gr. *trepein* to turn] response of living cells to the stimulus of oxygen.

oxyuria (ok″se-u′re-ah) oxyuriasis.

oxyuriasis (ok″se-u-ri′ah-sis) infection with *Enterobius vermicularis* (in humans) or with other oxyurids; enterobiasis.

oxyuricide (ok″se-u′ri-sīd) [oxyuris + L. *caedere* to kill] an agent that destroys oxyurids.

oxyurid (ok-se-u′rid) a pinworm, seatworm, or threadworm; any individual organism of the superfamily Oxyuroidea.

oxyurifuge (ok″se-u′ri-fūj) [oxyuris + L. *fugare* to put to flight] an agent that promotes the expulsion of oxyurids.

oxyuriosis (ok″se-u″re-o′sis) oxyuriasis.

Oxyuris (ok″se-u′ris) [Gr. *oxys* sharp + *oura* tail] a genus of intestinal nematode worms of the superfamily Oxyuroidea. **O. e′qui,** the largest known species of pinworm, found in the horse, mainly in the cecum, colon, and rectum. **O. incog′nita,** a name given to certain ova found in human stools; possibly identical with *Heterodera radicicola.* **O. vermicula′ris,** *Enterobius vermicularis.*

oxyuroid (ok-se-u′roid) oxyurid.

Oxyuroidea (ok″se-u″roi-de′ah) the oxyurids: a superfamily of small nematodes, the threadworms or pinworms, characterized by the presence of phasmids and a bulbous esophagus. They are usually found as parasites in the cecum and colon of vertebrates, but may also infect invertebrates, including insects. *Enterobius vermicularis* is the only oxyurid commonly infecting man. In some systems of classification, Oxyuroidea is considered to be an order.

Oz an antigenic marker distinguishing immunoglobulin human λ light chain subtypes.

oz. ounce.

ozena (o-ze′nah) [Gr. *ozaina* a fetid polypus in the nose] an atrophic rhinitis marked by a thick mucopurulent discharge, mucosal crusting, and fetor, often associated with the presence of *Klebsiella pneumoniae* subsp. *ozaenae.* **o. laryn′gis,** a condition of the larynx associated with a foul-smelling discharge usually related to atrophic rhinitis.

ozenous (o′zĕ-nus) pertaining to or of the nature of ozena.

ozolinone (o-zo′lĭ-nōn) ⁻chemical name: (Z)-[3-methyl-4-oxo-5-(1-piperidinyl)-2-thiazolidinylidene]acetic acid; a diuretic, $C_{11}H_{16}N_2O_3S$.

ozonator (o′zo-nāt″or) an instrument for generating ozone.

ozone (o′zōn) [Gr. *ozē* stench] a bluish explosive gas or blue liquid, which is an allotropic and more active form of oxygen, O_3: antiseptic and disinfectant. It is formed when oxygen is exposed to the silent discharge of electricity, and is both irritating and toxic in the pulmonary system. **o.-ether,** a mixture of ethylic ether, hydrogen peroxide, and alcohol, used as an antiseptic and for whooping cough and diabetes.

ozonide (o′zo-nīd) a compound of an olefin and ozone, the union taking place at the double bond.

ozonize (o′zo-nīz) to impregnate with ozone.

ozonometer (o″zo-nom′ĕ-ter) [ozone + Gr. *metron* measure] an instrument for estimating the ozone in the air.

ozonophore (o-zo′no-fōr) [ozone + Gr. *phoros* bearing] 1. one of the granular elements of cell cytoplasm. 2. a red blood cell.

ozonoscope (o-zo′no-skōp) [ozone + Gr. *skopein* to examine] an instrument for studying ozone and its effects.

ozostomia (o″zo-sto′me-ah) [Gr. *ozē* stench + *stoma* mouth + *-ia*] foulness of the breath.

P

P chemical symbol for *phosphorus* or for *phosphate* group (in biochemistry); symbol for *poise* and *peta-*.

P₁ symbol for *parental generation.*

P₂ pulmonic second sound.

p symbol for (1) the short arm of a chromosome or (2) the frequency of the more common allele of a pair.

p- chemical symbol for *para-*.

Π the Greek capital letter pi, used in mathematics to indicate a product; $\Pi_{i=1}^{n} x_i = x_1 \times x_2 \times \ldots \times x_n.$

π pi, the sixteenth letter of the Greek alphabet; mathematical symbol for the ratio of the diameter and circumference of a circle: approximately 3.1415926536.

φ phi, the twenty-first letter of the Greek alphabet.

ψ psi, the twenty-third letter of the Greek alphabet.

PA posteroanterior.

P.A. physician assistant.

Pa 1. chemical symbol for *protactinium.* 2. symbol for *pascal.*

Paas′ disease (pahz) [H. R. *Paas*, German physician] see under *disease.*

PAB, PABA para-aminobenzoic acid; see under *acid;* see *aminobenzoic acid*, under *acid.*

Pabanol (pab′ah-nol) trademark for a preparation of aminobenzoic acid.

pabular (pab′u-lar) pertaining to or of the nature of pabulum.

pabulin (pab′u-lin) the fatty and albuminous products of digestion which appear in the blood after eating.

pabulum (pab′u-lum) [L.] food or aliment.

Pacatal (pak′ah-tal) trademark for a preparation of mepazine.

pacchionian depressions, foramen, granulations (bodies, glands) (pak″e-o′ne-an) [Antonio *Pacchioni*, an Italian anatomist, 1665–1726] see *foveolae granulares, foramen diaphragmatis* [*sellae*], and *granulationes arachnoideales.*

pacemaker (pās′māk-er) an object or substance that influences the rate at which a certain phenomenon occurs; often used alone to indicate the natural cardiac pacemaker or an artificial cardiac pacemaker. In biochemistry, a substance whose rate of reaction sets the pace for a series of interrelated reactions. **artificial p.,** see *cardiac p., artificial.* **asynchronous p.,** an implanted cardiac pacemaker in which the induced ventricular rhythm is independent of the atrium; it is usually set at a fixed rate of ventricular stimulation. **cardiac p.,** the group of cells rhythmically initiating the heart beat, characterized physiologically by a slow loss of membrane potential during diastole. Usually the pacemaker site is the sinoatrial node. **cardiac p., artificial,** a device designed to stimulate, by electrical impulses, contraction of the heart muscle at a certain rate; used particularly in heart block or in absence of normal function of the sinoatrial node; it may be connected from the outside or implanted within the body. Popularly called *pacemaker.* **Chardack-Greatbatch p.,** an implanted asynchronous cardiac pacemaker, with the cardiac electrodes sewn into the myocardium. **cilium p.,** the biological regulator which controls the frequency of the beat of the cilia of cells by determining the rate of contraction and excitation. **demand p.,** an implanted cardiac pacemaker in which the generator stimulus is inhibited for a set interval (refractory period) by a signal derived from depolarization (normal or ectopic), thus minimizing the risk of pacemaker-induced ventricular fibrillation. **ectopic p.,** any biological cardiac pacemaker other than the sinus node. **external p.,** an artificial cardiac pacemaker located outside the body with output wires connected to circular chest electrodes, with a wire sewn directly into the heart, or with an electrode inserted through an intravenous catheter. **fixed-rate p.,** an implanted cardiac pacemaker in which the generator stimulates the heart at a predetermined rate, regardless of the heart's rhythm. **gastric p.,** a saddle-shaped area of the greater curvature of the stomach at the junction of its proximal and middle thirds, where originate electric potentials which regulate the frequency of gastric contractions. **p. of heart,** cardiac p. **implanted p., internal p.,** an artificial cardiac pacemaker implanted into the subcutaneous tissue. **Nathan p.,** a synchronous pacemaker. **radiofrequency p.,** a cardiac pacemaker consisting of an antenna coil cemented to the skin and a subcutaneously implanted receiving coil with an electrode inserted into the ventricular myocardium. Pulses from a lightweight radio transmitter carried by the patient are transmitted to the pacemaker. **synchronous p.,** an implanted cardiac pacemaker that synchronizes the electromechanical events in the atrium with those of the ventricle; the pacemaker stimulates the ventricle when triggered by the P wave from the atrium. **transthoracic p.,** an external cardiac pacemaker connected to the heart by percutaneous pacing wires introduced through a transthoracic needle. **transvenous p.,** an external cardiac pacemaker connected to the heart by an electrode inserted through a catheter introduced into the right ventricle by way of the brachial, subclavian, femoral, or internal jugular vein. **wandering p.,** a condition in which the site of origin of the impulses controlling the heart rate shifts from the head of the sinoatrial node to a lower part of the node or to another part of the atrium.

pachy- [Gr. *pachys* thick] a combining form meaning thick.

pachyblepharon (pak″e-blef′ah-ron) [*pachy-* + Gr. *blepharon* eyelid] a thickening of the eyelid, chiefly near the border.

pachyblepharosis (pak″e-blef″ah-ro′sis) pachyblepharon.

pachycephalia (pak″e-sĕ-fa′le-ah) pachycephaly.

pachycephalic (pak″e-sĕ-fal′ik) pertaining to or characterized by pachycephaly.

pachycephalous (pak″e-sef′ah-lus) pachycephalic.

pachycephaly (pak″e-sef′ah-le) [*pachy-* + Gr. *kephalē* head] abnormal thickness of the bones of the skull, as in acromegaly.

pachycheilia (pak″e-ki′le-ah) [*pachy-* + Gr. *cheilos* lip + *-ia*] thickening of the lips.

pachychromatic (pak″e-kro-mat′ik) [*pachy-* + Gr. *chrōma* color] having thick chromatin threads.

pachydactylia (pak″e-dak-til′e-ah) pachydactyly.

pachydactyly (pak″e-dak′tĭ-le) [*pachy-* + Gr. *daktylos* finger] abnormal enlargement of the fingers and toes.

pachyderma (pak″e-der′mah) [*pachy-* + Gr. *derma* skin] abnormal thickening of the skin. See also *elephantiasis*.

pachydermatocele (pak″e-der-mat′o-sēl) [*pachy-* + Gr. *derma* skin + *kēlē* tumor] plexiform neuroma which attains large dimensions and produces a condition resembling elephantiasis; called also *elephantiasis neuromatosa*.

pachydermatous (pak″e-der′mah-tus) thick-skinned; pertaining or relating to pachyderma. Called also *pachydermic*.

pachydermic (pak″e-der′mik) pachydermatous.

pachydermoperiostosis (pak″e-der″mo-per″e-os-to′sis) [*pachy-* + *dermo-* + *periostosis*] a condition believed to be inherited as an autosomal dominant trait, chiefly characterized by thickening of the skin of the head and distal extremities, deep folds and furrows of the skin of the forehead, cheeks, and scalp (*cutis verticis gyrata*), seborrhea, hyperhidrosis, periostosis of the long bones, digital clubbing, and spadelike enlargement of the hands and feet. It is more prevalent in the male, and is usually first evident during adolescence. Called also *acropachyderma with pachyperiostitis, idiopathic* or *primary hypertrophic osteoarthropathy,* and *Touraine-Solente-Golé syndrome.*

pachyglossia (pak″e-glos′e-ah) [*pachy-* + Gr. *glōssa* tongue + *-ia*] abnormal thickness of the tongue.

pachygnathous (pah-kig′nah-thus) [*pachy-* + Gr. *gnathos* jaw] having a large jaw. See also *macrognathia* and *prognathism.*

pachygyria (pak″e-ji′re-ah) [*pachy-* + *gyrus* + *-ia*] macrogyria.

pachyleptomeningitis (pak″e-lep″to-men″in-ji′tis) [*pachy-* + Gr. *leptos* thin + *mēninx* membrane + *-itis*] inflammation of the dura and pia together.

pachymeninges (pak″e-me-nin′jēz) plural of *pachymeninx.*

pachymeningitis (pak″e-men″in-ji′tis) [*pachy-* + Gr. *mēninx* membrane + *-itis*] inflammation of the dura ma-

ter; the symptoms of the disease resemble those of meningitis. Cf. *leptomeningitis.* **cerebral p.,** inflammation of the dura of the brain. **circumscribed p.,** pachymeningitis limited to a definite area of the dura. **external p.,** inflammation of the outer layers of the dura. **hemorrhagic internal p.,** pachymeningitis associated with dural hematoma. **internal p.,** that which affects the inner layer of the dura. **p. intralamella′ris,** intradural abscess. **purulent p.,** abscess on the dura mater. **serous internal p.,** the so-called external hydrocephalus. **spinal p.,** inflammation of the dura of the spinal column. **syphilitic p.,** that which is caused by syphilis.

pachymeningopathy (pak″e men″in gop′ah tho) [*pachy meninx* + Gr. *pathos* disease] any noninflammatory disease of the dura mater.

pachymeninx (pak″e-me′ninks) pl. *pachymenin′ges* [*pachy-* + Gr. *mēninx* membrane] the dura mater.

pachynema (pak″e-ne′mah) [*pachy-* + Gr. *nēma* thread] a postsynaptic stage of mitosis in which the chromatin is in the form of thick spireme threads.

pachynesis (pak″e-ne′sis) thickening and swelling of a chondriosome.

pachynsis (pah-kin′sis) [Gr.] a thickening, especially an abnormal thickening.

pachyntic (pah-kin′tik) pertaining to or characterized by abnormal thickening.

pachyonychia (pak″e-o-nik′e-ah) [*pachy-* + Gr. *onyx* nail + *-ia*] thickening of the nails. **p. conge′nita,** an autosomal dominant syndrome characterized by increased thickness of the nails that progresses to produce onychogryphosis, hyperkeratosis involving the palms, soles, knees, and elbows, widespread tiny cutaneous horns, leukoplakia of the mucous membranes, and usually hyperhidrosis of the hands and feet, and sometimes associated with the development of bullae on the palms and soles following trauma. Called also *Jadassohn-Lewandowsky syndrome.*

pachyotia (pak″e-o′she-ah) [*pachy-* + Gr. *ous* ear] (*obs.*) marked thickness of the auricles of the ears.

pachyperiostitis (pak″e-per″e-os-ti′tis) periostitis of long bones resulting in abnormal thickness of the bones.

pachyperitonitis (pak″e-per″ĭ-to-ni′tis) [*pachy-* + *peritonitis*] peritonitis with thickening of the affected membrane.

pachypleuritis (pak″e-ploo-ri′tis) [*pachy-* + *pleuritis*] fibrothorax.

pachyrhizid (pak″ir-i′zid) a poisonous glycoside from *Pachyrhizus angulatus,* a plant of various tropical regions.

pachysalpingitis (pak″e-sal″pin-ji′tis) [*pachy-* + Gr. *salpinx* tube + *-itis*] chronic interstitial inflammation of the muscular coat of the oviduct, producing thickening; called also *mural salpingitis* and *parenchymatous salpingitis.*

pachysalpingo-ovaritis (pak″e-sal-ping″go-o″var-i′tis) chronic parenchymatous inflammation of the ovary and oviduct.

pachytene (pak′e-tēn) [Gr. *pachytēs* thickness] in meiosis (q.v.), the stage following synapsis (zygotene) in which the homologous chromosome threads (synaptonemal complex) shorten, thicken, and continue to intertwine, and each of the conjoined (bivalent) chromosomes separate into two sister chromatids, which are held together by a centromere, to form a tetrad. During this phase the chromatids break up and corresponding regions of the nonsister chromatids of the paired chromosomes are exchanged in a process known as crossing over. See also *diplotene, leptotene,* and *zygotene.*

pachyvaginalitis (pak″e-vaj″ĭ-nal-i′tis) [*pachy-* + *vaginalitis*] inflammatory thickening of the tunica vaginalis of the testis.

pachyvaginitis (pak″e-vaj″ĭ-ni′tis) [*pachy-* + *vaginitis*] chronic vaginitis with thickening of the vaginal walls. **cystic p.,** emphysematous vaginitis.

pacing (pās′ing) setting of the pace, or regulation of the rate of. **cardiac p.,** regulation of the rate of contraction of the heart muscle by an artificial cardiac pacemaker. **diaphragm p.,** the production of rhythmic contractions of the diaphragm by electrical stimulation of the phrenic nerve in order to provide ventilatory support in patients with diaphragmatic paralysis.

Pacini's corpuscles (pah-che′nēz) [Filippo *Pacini,* Italian anatomist, 1812–1883] see under *corpuscle.*

pacinian corpuscles (pah-sin′e-an) [named for Filippo *Pacini*] see under *corpuscle*.

pack (pak) 1. treatment by wrapping a patient in blankets or sheets or a limb in towels, wet or dry and either hot or cold; also the blankets, sheets, or towels used for this purpose. 2. a tampon. **cold p.**, blankets, sheets, or towels that have been dipped in cold water, for wrapping the body or an extremity. **dry p.**, dry, hot blankets or towels for wrapping the body or an extremity. **full p.**, one which encloses the entire body. **half p.**, a pack applied from the axillae to below the knees. **hot p.**, hot blankets or towels, wet or dry, for wrapping the body or an extremity. **ice p.**, a folded towel filled with crushed ice, often used in place of an icebag. **Mikulicz p.**, layers of mesh or gutta-percha sewn together at the edges, packed with strips of gauze, often placed in a denuded pelvic area to wall off the unperitonealized surfaces but also used for packing off abdominal viscera to improve operative exposure. **one sheet p.**, a wet pack consisting of only one large sheet. **partial p.**, a wet pack covering only a portion of the body. **periodontal p.**, a surgical dressing applied over the surgical wound following periodontal operations to provide a matrix for the regeneration of tissue and enhance healing processes. **salt p.**, a wet pack utilizing sheets or blankets wrung out after immersion in salt water. **three-quarters p.**, a wet pack extending upward from the toes as far as the axillae. **throat p.**, a moistened gauze pack used as a posterior pharyngeal seal around a non-cuffed endotracheal tube. **wet p., wet-sheet p.**, wet blankets or sheets, hot or cold, for wrapping an extremity or the entire body.

packer (pak′er) an instrument for introducing dressing into the uterus or vagina, or into another body cavity or wound.

packing (pak′ing) 1. the act of filling a wound or cavity with gauze, sponges, pads, or other material. 2. the material used for filling a cavity.

pad (pad) a cushion-like mass of soft material. **abdominal p.**, a pad for the absorption of discharges from abdominal wounds; also for packing off abdominal viscera to improve exposure during surgical procedures. **buccal fat p.**, corpus adiposum buccae. **dinner p.**, a pad placed over the abdomen before a plaster jacket is applied. The pad is then removed, leaving space under the jacket to provide for expansion of the abdomen after eating. **fat p.**, 1. corpus adiposum buccae. 2. a large pad of fat lying behind and below the patella, between the patellar ligament, the head of the tibia, and the femoral condyles; called also *infrapatellar* and *retropatellar fat pad*. **gum p′s**, edentulous segments of the maxilla and the mandible that correspond to the underlying primary teeth. **knuckle p′s**, nodules about the size of a split pea on the dorsal surface of the interphalangeal joints, consisting of new growths of fibrous tissue, with thickening of the dermis and epidermis, and frequently associated with camptodactyly and Dupuytren's contracture; they are probably of genetic origin. **occlusal p.**, a pad which covers the occlusal surface of a tooth. **Passavant's p.**, see under *bar*. **periarterial p.**, see *juxtaglomerular cells*, under *cell*. **retromolar p.**, a mass of tissue, often pear-shaped, located at the distal termination of the mandibular residual ridge, and made up of the retromolar papilla and the retromolar glandular prominence. **sucking p., suctorial p.**, corpus adiposum buccae.

Padgett's dermatome (paj′ets) [Earl Calvin *Padgett*, American surgeon, 1893–1946] see under *dermatome*.

padimate A (pad′ĭ-māt) chemical name: 4-(dimethylamino)benzoic acid pentyl ester; an ultraviolet screen, $C_{14}H_{21}NO_2$.

padimate O (pad′ĭ-mat) chemical name: 4-(dimethylamino)benzoic acid 2-ethylhexyl ester; an ultraviolet screen, $C_{17}H_{27}NO_2$.

pae- for words beginning thus, see also those beginning *pe-*.

Paecilomyces (pe-sil″o-mi′sēz) a genus of soil-inhabiting imperfect fungi of the family Moniliaceae, order Moniliales, morphologically resembling *Penicillium*, and often isolated as contaminants of skin and sputum. See *cladiosis*.

Paederus (pe′der-us) a genus of blistering beetles of South America, Asia, and Africa, from which pederin has been isolated.

paed(o)- see *ped(o)-*[1].

PAF platelet activating factor.

PAF-acether (as-e′ther) see *platelet activating factor*, under *factor*.

Pagenstecher's ointment (pah′gen-stek″erz) [Alexander *Pagenstecher*, German ophthalmologist, 1828–1879] see *yellow mercuric oxide*, under *mercuric*.

Paget's cell, etc. (paj′ets) [Sir James *Paget*, English surgeon, 1814–1899] see under *cell, disease, necrosis*, and *tests*.

pagetic (pah-jet′ik) affected with or relating to Paget's disease (osteitis deformans).

pagetoid (paj′ĕ-toid) resembling or characteristic of Paget disease of the breast or extramammary Paget disease. See under *cell* and *reticulosis*.

Pagitane (paj′ĭ-tān) trademark for a preparation of cycrimine hydrochloride.

pagon (pag′on) [Gr. *pagos* frost] the plant and animal organisms occurring in ice.

pagophagia (pa″go-fa′je-ah) [Gr. *pagos* frost + *phagein* to eat] the ingestion of extraordinary amounts of ice, often related to iron lack.

pagoplexia (pa″go-plek′se-ah) [Gr. *pagos* frost + *plēgē* stroke] frostbite.

-pagus [Gr. *pagos* that which is fixed] a word termination denoting a symmetrical pair of twins conjoined at the site indicated by the stem to which it is affixed, as *craniopagus, pygopagus, thoracopagus*.

PAH, PAHA para-aminohippuric acid; see *aminohippuric acid*.

Pahvant Valley fever, plague (pah′vant) [*Pahvant*, a valley in Utah] tularemia.

pain (pān) [L. *poena, dolor*; Gr. *algos, odynē*] a more or less localized sensation of discomfort, distress, or agony, resulting from the stimulation of specialized nerve endings. It serves as a protective mechanism insofar as it induces the sufferer to remove or withdraw from the source. **bearing-down p.**, pain accompanying uterine contractions during the second stage of labor. **boring p.**, a sensation as of being pierced with a long, slender, twisting object; called also *terebrant p.* **Brodie's p.**, pain induced by folding the skin near a joint affected with neuralgia. **central p.**, pain due to a lesion in the central nervous system. **Charcot's p′s**, rheumatism of a testicle. **dilating p′s**, those of the first stage of labor. **expulsive p′s**, those of the second stage of labor. **false p′s**, ineffective pains which resemble labor pains, but which are not accompanied by effacement and dilatation of the cervix. **fulgurant p′s**, lightning p′s. **gas p′s**, pains caused by distention of the stomach or intestines by accumulations of air or other gases, occurring as a result of ingestion of gas-forming foods. **girdle p.**, a painful sensation as of a cord about the waist. **growing p′s**, recurrent quasirheumatic limb pains peculiar to early youth. **heterotopic p.**, referred pain. **homotopic p.**, pain that is felt at the point of injury. **hunger p.**, pain coming on at the time for feeling hunger for the next meal; it is a symptom of gastric disorder. **intermenstrual p.**, pain occurring during the period between the menses, usually about half way, accompanying extrusion of the ovum. **jumping p.**, a peculiar pain in joint diseases when the bone is laid bare by ulceration of the cartilage. **labor p′s**, the rhythmic pains of increasing severity and frequency, caused by contractions of the uterus during childbirth. **lancinating p.**, a sharp, darting pain. **lightning p′s**, the cutting and intense darting pains of tabes dorsalis; called also *fulgurant p′s* and *shooting p′s*. **middle p.**, intermenstrual pain. **osteocopic p.**, osteocope. **phantom limb p.**, pain felt as though arising in an absent (amputated) limb; see under *limb*. **postprandial p.**, abdominal pain occurring after eating a meal. **premonitory p′s**, mild uterine contractions before the beginning of true labor. **psychic p.**, psychalgia (def. 1). **psychogenic p.**, symptoms of physical pain having psychological origin. **referred p.**, pain felt in a part other than that in which the cause that produced it is situated. **rest p.**, a continuous burning pain of the distal portion of the lower limb, usually the forefoot, which begins or is aggravated after reclining and is relieved by sitting or standing; it is due to ischemia. **root p.**, pain caused by disease of the sensory nerve roots and felt in the cutaneous areas supplied by the affected roots. **shooting p′s**, lightning p′s. **spot p′s**, pains which seem like patches on the integument. **starting p′s**, pain and muscular spasm in the early stages of sleep. **terebrant p., terebrating p.,** boring p. **wandering p.,** a pain which repeatedly changes its location.

paint (pānt) 1. a liquid designed for application to the surface, as of the body or a tooth. 2. to apply a liquid to a specific area as a remedial or protective measure. **antiseptic p.,** a term used to describe immunoglobulin A secreted onto the surfaces of mucous membranes and affording local protection against agents possessing homologous antigens. **Castellani's p.,** carbol-fuchsin solution.

pair (pār) a combination of two related, similar, or identical entities or objects. **base p.,** either of the two pairs —guanine and cytosine, adenine and thymine—of purine-pyrimidine bases joined by hydrogen bonds that make up DNA. In RNA, uracil replaces thymine. **buffer p.,** a buffer system consisting of a weak acid and its conjugate base. **ion p.,** the free electron and the positively charged residual atom that result from the ejection of an orbital electron by ionizing radiation.

pairing (pār'ing) that act or process of joining into pairs. **base p.,** the bonding of purines and pyrimidines in DNA; see under *pair*. **somatic p.,** the close association of homologous pairs of polytene chromosomes, as in meiotic prophase; such chromosomes are considered to be in a permanent prophase.

pajaroello (pah-hah-ro-el'yo) *Ornithodoros coriaceus.*

Pajot's hook, etc. (pahzh-ōz') [Charles *Pajot*, French obstetrician, 1816–1896] see under *hook, law,* and *maneuver.*

pakurin (pak'u-rin) an arrow poison derived from the sap of a tree in Colombia; it has a digitalis-like action on the heart.

Pal's stain (pahlz) [Jacob *Pal*, Vienna clinician, 1863–1936] see *Table of Stains.*

Palade (pal-ād'), George Emil. Rumanian-born American cytologist, born 1912; co-winner, with Albert Claude and Christian René de Duve, of the Nobel prize for medicine or physiology for 1974, for his work on mitochondria, ribosomes, and microsomes in the structural and functional organization of the cell.

palae- for words beginning thus, see those beginning *pale-*.

palaeocerebellum (pa″le-o-ser″e-bel'um) [*palaeo-* + *cerebellum*] [NA] a term applied originally to the phylogenetically older parts of the cerebellum (see *archaeocerebellum*); now applied specifically to those parts whose afferent inflow is predominantly supplied by spinocerebellar fibers, including in man the cranial lobe, excluding the lingula, together with the pyramid and uvula of the caudal lobe. Called also *spinocerebellum,* and spelled also *paleocerebellum* [NA alternative]. Cf. *archaeocerebellum* and *neocerebellum.*

palaeocortex (pa″le-o-kor'teks) [*palaeo-* + L. *cortex* bark, rind, shell] [NA] that portion of the cortex cerebri that, with the archaeocortex, develops in association with the olfactory system, and which is phylogenetically older and less stratified than the neocortex. It is composed chiefly of the piriform cortex and the parahippocampal gyrus. Called also *paleopallium,* and spelled also *paleocortex* [NA alternative].

palata (pah-lah'tah, pah-la'tah) [L.] plural of palatum.

palatal (pal'ah-tal) pertaining to the palate; sometimes used to designate the lingual surface of a maxillary tooth.

palate (pal'at) the partition separating the nasal and oral cavities; see palatum [NA]. **artificial p.,** a prosthetic device used to close a cleft palate; an obturator. **bony p., bony hard p.,** the osseous framework of the hard palate (palatum osseum [NA]). **cleft p.,** congenital fissure of the soft palate alone or both the soft palate and the hard palate, due to faulty fusion. The cleft typically opens through the roof of the mouth into the nasal cavity and extends anteriorly to the premaxilla, where it deviates to the right or left, following the line of fusion. Called also *palatoschisis, palatum fissum, uraniscochasma, uranoschism,* and *uranostaphyloschisis* (cleft of both the hard and the soft palate). **hard p.,** the anterior, rigid portion of the palate; see *palatum durum* [NA]. **pendulous p.,** uvula. **premaxillary p.,** primary p. **primary p.,** that portion of the palate contributed by the median nasal process. **secondary p.,** the palate proper, formed by fusion of the lateral palatine processes. **smoker's p.,** stomatitis nicotina. **soft p.,** the posterior, fleshy part of the palate; see *palatum molle* [NA].

palatine (pal'ah-tīn) [L. *palatinus*] pertaining to the palate.

palatitis (pal″ah-ti'tis) 1. inflammation of the palate. 2. lampas.

palat(o)- [L. *palatum* palate] a combining form denoting relationship to the palate; sometimes used instead of lingu(o)- in terms referring to the lingual surface of maxillary teeth.

palatoglossal (pal″ah-to-glos'al) pertaining to the palate and tongue.

palatognathous (pal″ah-tog'nah-thus) [*palato-* + Gr. *gnathos* jaw] having a cleft palate.

palatograph (pal'ah-to-graf) [*palato-* + Gr. *graphein* to write] an instrument used in palatography.

palatography (pal″ah-tog'rah-fe) the recording of the movements of the palate in speech.

palatomaxillary (pal″ah-to-mak'sĭ-ler'e) pertaining to the palate and the maxilla.

palatomyography (pal″ah-to-mi-og'rah-fe) [*palate* + Gr. *mys* muscle + *graphein* to write] the recording of muscular movements of the palate.

palatonasal (pal″ah-to-na'zal) [*palato-* + L. *nasus* nose] pertaining to the palate and nose.

palatopagus (pal″ah-top'ah-gus) [*palato-* + Gr. *pagos* that which is firmly set] symmetrical twins conjoined at the palate.

palatopharyngeal (pal″ah-to-fah-rin'je-al) pertaining to the palate and pharynx.

palatoplasty (pal'ah-to-plas″te) [*palato-* + Gr. *plassein* to form] plastic reconstruction of the palate, including cleft palate operations.

palatoplegia (pal″ah-to-ple'je-ah) [*palato-* + Gr. *plēgē* stroke] paralysis of the palate.

palatoproximal (pal″ah-to-prok'sĭ-mal) pertaining to the palatal (lingual) and proximal surface of a maxillary tooth.

palatorrhaphy (pal″ah-tor'ah-fe) surgical correction of a cleft palate, the cleft involving the soft palate and the soft tissues over the hard palate; cf. *staphylorrhaphy.*

palatosalpingeus (pal″ah-to-sal-pin'je-us) [*palato-* + Gr. *salpinx* tube] musculus tensor veli palatini.

palatoschisis (pal″ah-tos'kĭ-sis) [*palato-* + Gr. *schisis* cleft] cleft palate.

palatum (pah-lah'tum, pah-la'tum), gen. *pala'ti,* pl. *pala'ta* [L.] [NA] the palate: the partition separating the nasal and oral cavities, consisting anteriorly of a hard bony part and posteriorly of a soft fleshy part. **p. du'rum** [NA], the hard palate: the anterior part of the palate, characterized by an osseous framework, covered superiorly by mucous membrane of the nasal cavity and, on its oral surface, by mucoperiosteum. **p. du'rum os'seum,** p. osseum. **p. fis'sum,** cleft palate. **p. mol'le** [NA], the soft palate: the fleshy part of the roof of the mouth, extending from the posterior edge of the hard palate; from its free inferior border is a projection of variable length, the uvula. Called also *velum palatinum* [NA alternative]. **p. os'seum** [NA], bony palate: the bony part of the anterior two-thirds of the roof of the mouth, formed by the palatine processes of the maxillae and the horizontal plates of the palatine bones. Called also *p. durum osseum* or *bony hard palate.*

paleencephalon (pa″le-en-sef'ah-lon) [*paleo-* + Gr. *enkephalos* brain] the (phylogenetically) old brain; all of the brain except the cerebral cortex and its dependencies.

pale(o)- [Gr. *palaios* old] a combining form meaning old.

paleocerebellar (pa″le-o-ser″e-bel'ar) pertaining to or affecting the paleocerebellum.

paleocerebellum (pa″le-o-ser″e-bel'um) [*paleo-* + *cerebellum*] NA alternative spelling of *palaeocerebellum.*

paleocinetic (pa″le-o-si-net'ik) paleokinetic.

paleocortex (pa″le-o-kor'teks) [*paleo-* + *cortex*] NA alternative spelling for *palaeocortex.*

paleoencephalon (pa″le-o-en-sef'ah-lon) paleencephalon.

paleogenesis (pa″le-o-jen'ĕ-sis) palingenesis, def. 2.

paleogenetic (pa″le-o-jĕ-net'ik) [*paleo-* + Gr. *gennan* to produce] originated in the past; not newly acquired. Said of traits, structures, etc., of species.

paleokinetic (pa″le-o-ki-net'ik) [*paleo-* + Gr. *kinētikos* pertaining to motion] old kinetic; a term applied to the nervous motor mechanism concerned in automatic associated movements. It is under the control of the corpus striatum and represents a primitive (that is, early developed) type of motor control. Cf. *archeokinetic* and *neokinetic*.

paleoneurology (pa″le-o-nu-rol′o-je) the study of the evidence of nervous systems of fossil animals.

paleontology (pa″le-on-tol′o-je) [*paleo-* + Gr. *ōn* existing + *-logy*] the sum of knowledge regarding the early forms of life upon the earth.

paleopallium (pa″le-o-pal′e-um) [*paleo-* + *pallium*] palaeocortex.

paleopathology (pa″le-o-pah-thol′o-je) [*paleo-* + *pathology*] the study of disease in bodies preserved from ancient times, such as mummies.

paleosensation (pa″le-o-sen-sa′shun) [*paleo-* + *sensation*] the sensation of severe pain and marked variations of temperature, as compared with phylogenetically newer sensations such as those of light touch and moderate variations of temperature and the epicritic sensations.

paleostriatal (pa″le-o-stri-a′tal) pertaining to the paleostriatum.

paleostriatum (pa″le-o-stri-a′tum) [*paleo-* + *striatum*] the phylogenetically older part of the corpus striatum represented by the globus pallidus. Cf. *neostriatum*.

paleothalamus (pa″le-o-thal′ah-mus) [*paleo-* + *thalamus*] old thalamus; a term applied occasionally to the phylogenetically older part of the thalamus, i.e., the medial portion which lacks reciprocal connections with the neopallium.

pali-, palin- [Gr. *palin* backward, or again] a combining form meaning again, often denoting pathologic repetition.

palicinesia (pal″e-si-ne′se-ah) palikinesia.

palikinesia (pal″e-ki-ne′se-ah) [*pali-* + Gr. *kinēsis* movement] pathologic repetition of movements.

palilalia (pal″i-la′le-ah) [*pali-* + Gr. *lalein* to babble] a condition characterized by the repetition of a phrase or word with increasing rapidity.

palin- see *pali-*.

palindrome (pal′in-drōm) [Gr. *palindromos* a running back] in genetics, a DNA or RNA sequence that reads the same in both directions.

palindromia (pal″in-dro′me-ah) [Gr. *palindromia* a running back] the recurrence of a disease.

palindromic (pal″in-dro′mik) returning; recurrent.

palinesthesia (pal″in-es-the′ze-ah) [*palin-* + Gr. *aisthēsis* sensation] the rapid termination of the anesthetic state and the restoration to consciousness of a person under general anesthesia: it may be induced by the injection of weak hydrochloric acid; now discontinued because it is ineffective and harmful.

palingenesis (pal″in-jen′ĕ-sis) [*palin-* + *genesis*] 1. the regeneration or restoration of a lost part. 2. the appearance of ancestral characters in successive generations. Cf. *cenogenesis*.

palingraphia (pal″in-gra′fe-ah) [*palin-* + Gr. *graphein* to write] pathologic repetition of letters, words, or parts of words in writing.

palinmnesis (pal″in-ne′sis) [*palin-* + Gr. *-mnēsis* memory] memory for past events or experiences.

palinopsia (pal″in-op′se-ah) [*palin-* + *-opsia*] visual perseveration; the pathologic continuance or recurrence of a visual sensation after the stimulus is gone.

palinphrasia (pal″in-fra′ze-ah) [*palin-* + Gr. *phrasis* speech + *-ia*] pathologic repetition, in speaking, of words or phrases.

paliphrasia (pal″e-fra′ze-ah) palinphrasia.

palisade (pal″i-sād) [Fr. *palissade*, from L. *palus* stake] the arrangement of cells in stained smears of certain bacteria when two or more rods are arranged side by side like pales in a picket fence. The term is used to describe the arrangement of cells in regular rows in tissue sections, a characteristic of certain neoplasms, e.g., schwannoma.

palladium (pah-la′de-um) [L.] 1. a rare, hard, inert metal resembling platinum; symbol, Pd; specific gravity, 12.16; atomic number, 46; atomic weight, 106.4. It is comparatively light in weight and of a neutral color and is used for dentures and orthodontic appliances. 2. a homeopathic preparation of the same metal.

pallanesthesia (pal″an-es-the′ze-ah) [Gr. *pallein* to shake + *anesthesia*] loss of vibration senses; insensibility to the vibrations of a tuning fork.

pallesthesia (pal″es-the′ze-ah) [Gr. *pallein* to shake + *aisthēsis* perception] sensibility to vibrations; the peculiar vibrating sensation felt when a vibrating tuning-fork is placed against a subcutaneous bony prominence of the body. Called also *bone sensibility*.

pallesthetic (pal″es-thet′ik) pertaining to pallesthesia, or vibration sense.

pallhypesthesia (pal″hi-pes-the′ze-ah) [Gr. *pallein* to shake + *hypo* under + *aisthēsis* perception] diminished sensibility to vibrations.

pallial (pal′e-al) pertaining to the pallium.

palliate (pal′e-āt) to reduce the severity of; to relieve.

palliative (pal′e-a′tiv) [L. *palliatus* cloaked] 1. affording relief, but not cure. 2. an alleviating medicine.

pallidal (pal′ĭ-dal) pertaining to the globus pallidum.

pallidectomy (pal″ĭ-dek′to-me) surgical excision of the globus pallidus or extirpation of it by other means (chemopallidectomy).

pallidoansection (pal″ĭ-do-an-sek′shun) surgical section of the globus pallidus and ansa lenticularis.

pallidoansotomy (pal″ĭ-do-an-sot′o-me) production of lesions in the globus pallidus and ansa lenticularis.

pallidofugal (pal″ĭ-dof′u-gal) [*pallidum* + L. *fugere* to flee] conducting impulses away from the globus pallidus.

pallidoidosis (pal″ĭ-doi-do′sis) rabbit syphilis.

pallidotomy (pal″ĭ-dot′o-me) [*pallidum* + Gr. *tomē* a cutting] a stereotaxic surgical technique for producing lesions in the globus pallidus for treatment of extrapyramidal disorders.

pallidum (pal′ĭ-dum) [L. "pale"] globus pallidus. **p. I,** globus pallidus medialis. **p. II,** globus pallidus lateralis.

pallium (pal′e-um) [L. "cloak"] 1. NA alternative for *cortex cerebri*. 2. the cortex cerebri in its entirety, i.e., the mantle of gray substance covering both cerebral hemispheres. 3. the cortex cerebri during its period of development.

pallor (pal′or) [L.] paleness; absence of the skin coloration.

palm (palm) [L. *palma*] 1. the hollow of the hand (palma manus [NA]). 2. any of various, chiefly tropical trees, the palm trees. **handball p.,** contusion of the palm of the hand occurring in handball players.

palma (pal′mah), gen. and pl. **pal′mae** [L.] 1. the palm. 2. the palm tree. **p. ma′nus** [NA], the palm, or flexor surface, of the hand. **pal′mae plica′tae,** the branching folds of the mucosa of the vagina.

palmae (pal′me) [L.] genitive and plural of *palma*.

palmanesthesia (pal″man-es-the′ze-ah) [Gr. *palmos* vibration + *anesthesia*] pallanesthesia.

palmar (pal′mar) [L. *palmaris; palma* palm] pertaining to the palm.

palmaris (pal-ma′ris) palmar; [NA] a general term designating relationship to the palm of the hand.

palmature (pal′mah-tūr) [L. *palma* palm] a webbed state of the fingers.

palmellin (pal-mel′in) a red pigment from the fresh-water alga *Palmella cruenta*.

palmesthesia (pal″mes-the′ze-ah) pallesthesia.

palmesthetic (pal″mes-thet′ik) pallesthetic.

palmital (pal′mĭ-tal) an aldehyde lipid, the aldehyde form of palmitate; see *plasmalogen*.

palmitate (pal′mĭ-tāt) hexadecanote: the ionic form of palmitic acid, the most abundant fatty acid in man.

palmitic acid (pal-mit′ik) trivial name for hexadecanoic acid, the 16-carbon, straight-chain, saturated fatty acid, one of the most prevalent saturated fatty acids in body lipids.

palmitin (pal′mĭ-tin) a crystallizable and saponifiable fat, $C_3H_5(C_{16}H_{31}O_2)_3$, from various fats and oils; glycerol tripalmitate.

palmitoleic acid (pal″mĭ-to-le′ik) trivial name for *cis*-9-hexadecenoic acid, the Δ^9-unsaturated, 16-carbon, straight-chain, fatty acid.

palmitone (pal′mĭ-tōn) a crystalline compound, CH_3-$(CH_2)_{14}\cdot CO\cdot (CH_2)_{14}\cdot CH_3$, obtained when palmitic acid is distilled with lime.

palmus (pal′mus) [Gr. *palmos* a quivering motion] 1. palpitation. 2. saltatory spasm.

palp (palp) a sensory or feeding appendage, especially one of the jointed sensory appendages attached to the mouth of arthropods.

palpable (pal′pah-b′l) perceptible by touch.

palpate (pal′pāt) [L. *palpare* to touch] to examine by the hand; to feel.

palpation (pal-pa′shun) [L. *palpatio*] the act of feeling with the hand; the application of the fingers with light pressure to the surface of the body for the purpose of determining the consistence of the parts beneath in physical diagnosis. **bimanual p.,** examination with both hands. **light touch p.,** light palpation of the surface of the abdomen and thorax with the tip of a finger for the purpose of finding the outlines of the organs.

palpatometry (pal″pah-tom′ĕ-tre) [*palpation* + Gr. *metron* measure] measurement of the amount of pressure that can be borne without causing pain.

palpatopercussion (pal″pah-to-per-kush′un) palpation combined with percussion.

palpebra (pal′pĕ-brah), gen. and pl. *pal′pebrae* [L.] eyelid; either of the two movable folds that protect the anterior surface of the eyeball. **p. infe′rior** [NA], the lower eyelid: the lower of the two movable folds protecting the anterior surface of the eyeball. **p. supe′rior** [NA], the upper eyelid: the upper of the two movable folds protecting the anterior surface of the eyeball. **p. ter′tius,** nictitating membrane.

palpebrae (pal′pĕ-bre) [L.] genitive and plural of *palpebra*.

palpebral (pal′pĕ-bral) pertaining to an eyelid.

palpebralis (pal″pĕ-bra′lis) [L.] pertaining to an eyelid.

palpebrate (pal′pĕ-brāt) [L. *palpebrare* to wink] 1. to wink. 2. having eyelids.

palpebration (pal″pĕ-bra′shun) [L. *palpebratio*] 1. the act of winking. 2. abnormally frequent winking, as from a tic.

palpebritis (pal″pĕ-bri′tis) blepharitis.

palpitation (pal″pĭ-ta′shun) [L. *palpitatio*] a subjective sensation of an unduly rapid or irregular heart beat.

PALS periarterial lymphoid sheath.

palsy (pawl′ze) paralysis. **Bell's p.,** unilateral facial paralysis of sudden onset, due to lesion of the facial nerve and resulting in characteristic distortion of the face. **birth p.,** see under *paralysis*. **brachial p.,** see under *paralysis*. **bulbar p.,** see under *paralysis*. **cerebral p.,** a persisting qualitative motor disorder appearing before the age of three years, due to a nonprogressive damage to the brain. **crossed leg p.,** palsy of the peroneal nerve caused by sitting with one leg crossed over the other. **diver's p.,** decompression sickness. **Erb's p.,** see under *paralysis*. **facial p.,** Bell's p. **hammer p.,** a variety caused by hard work with the hammer. **ischemic p.,** see under *paralysis*. **Klumpke's p.,** see under *paralysis*. **Landry's p.,** acute febrile polyneuritis. **printer's p.,** a condition observed in printers due to chronic antimony poisoning, and marked by neuritis with paralysis, pain in the pubes, and papular eruption. **progressive supranuclear p.,** pseudobulbar paralysis. **pseudobulbar p.,** see under *paralysis*. **radial p.,** see under *paralysis*. **Saturday night p.,** musculospiral paralysis. **scriveners' p.,** writers' cramp. **shaking p.,** paralysis agitans. **spastic bulbar p.,** pseudobulbar paralysis. **tardy median p.,** carpal tunnel syndrome. **Todd's p.,** see under *paralysis*. **transverse p.,** crossed paralysis. **wasting p.,** spinal muscular atrophy.

paludal (pal′u-dal) [L. *palus* marsh] pertaining to or arising from marshes.

paludism (pal′u-dizm) malaria.

Paludrine (pal′u-drin) trademark for a preparation of proguanil hydrochloride.

L-PAM melphalan.

2-PAM pralidoxime.

pamaquine (pam′ah-kwin) chemical name: 6-methoxy-8-(1-methyl-4-diethylamino)butylaminoquinoline. A toxic antimalarial compound, $C_{19}H_{29}N_3O_4$, derived from 8-aminoquinoline, which was discovered in Germany in 1924. It destroys the exoerythrocytic forms of human malarial parasites; now largely replaced by primaquine. Called also *Fourneau 694* or *710*. **p. naphthoate,** the methylenebis-β-hydroxynaphthoate of pamaquine base, $C_{42}H_{45}N_3O_7$, occurring as a yellow to orange yellow powder; now largely replaced as an antimalarial by primaquine.

pamatolol sulfate (pam″ah-to′lōl) chemical name: (+)-[2-[4-[2-hydroxy-3-[(1-methylethyl)amino]propoxy]phenyl]ethyl]carbamic acid methyl ester sulfate (salt); an antiadrenergic (β-receptor), $(C_{16}H_{26}N_2O_4)_2 \cdot H_2SO_4$.

Pamine (pam′ēn) trademark for preparations of methscopolamine bromide.

Pamisyl (pam′ĭ-sil) trademark for preparations of aminosalicylic acid.

pamoate (pam′o-āt) USAN contraction for 4,4′-methylenebis[3-hydroxy-2-naphthoate].

pampiniform (pam-pin′ĭ-form) [L. *pampinus* tendril + *forma* form] shaped like a tendril.

pampinocele (pam-pin′o-sēl) [L. *pampinus* tendril + Gr. *kēlē* tumor] varicocele.

pamplegia (pam-ple′je-ah) [Gr. *pan* all + *plēgē* stroke] total paralysis.

Pan (pan) the genus of primates containing the chimpanzee and gorilla.

pan- [Gr. *pan* all] prefix signifying all.

Panacea (pan″ah-se′ah) [Gr. *Panakeia*] one of two sisters, the other being Hygeia, who were the daughters of Aesculapius.

panacea (pan″ah-se′ah) [Gr. *panakeia*] 1. a universal remedy. 2. an ancient name for a healing herb or its juice.

panagglutinable (pan″ah-gloo″tĭ-nah-b′l) agglutinable with every type of blood serum from the same species, e.g., red blood cells agglutinable with sera of all human blood groups.

panagglutination (pan″ah-gloo″tĭ-na′shun) agglutination (e.g., of red blood cells) by the serum of all blood groups of the same species.

panagglutinin (pan″ah-gloo′tĭ-nin) [*pan-* + *agglutinin*] an agglutinin which agglutinates the red blood cells of all blood groups in the same species.

panangiitis (pan″an-je-i′tis) [*pan-* + Gr. *angeion* vessel + *-itis*] inflammation involving all the coats of the vessel. **diffuse necrotizing p.,** panangiitis with extensive involvement of the blood vessels.

pananxiety (pan″ang-zi′ĕ-te) diffuse, all-pervading anxiety. **analgesic p.,** Morvan's syndrome, def. 2.

panarteritis (pan″ar-tĕ-ri′tis) [*pan-* + *arteritis*] diffuse arterial disease; polyarteritis. See also *periarteritis nodosa*.

panarthritis (pan″ar-thri′tis) [*pan-* + Gr. *arthron* joint] inflammation of all the joints or of all the structures of a joint.

panatrophy (pan-at′ro-fe) [*pan-* + *atrophy*] atrophy affecting several parts; general atrophy.

panautonomic (pan-aw″to-no-mik) pertaining to or affecting the entire autonomic (sympathetic and parasympathetic) nervous system.

panblastic (pan-blas′tik) [*pan-* + Gr. *blastos* germ] pertaining to each of the layers of the blastoderm.

pancarditis (pan″kar-di′tis) [*pan-* + Gr. *kardia* heart] diffuse inflammation of the heart, involving the pericardium, myocardium, and endocardium.

panchrest (pan′krest) [Gr. *panchrēstos* useful for everything] a panacea, or remedy, for every disease.

panchromatic (pan″kro-mat′ik) [*pan-* + *chromatic*] sensitive to all colors; applied to photographic emulsions.

panchromia (pan-kro′me-ah) the condition of staining with various dyes.

Pancoast's suture (pan′kōsts) [Joseph *Pancoast*, American surgeon, 1805–1882] see under *suture*.

Pancoast's syndrome, tumor [Henry Khunrath *Pancoast*, Philadelphia radiologist, 1875–1939] see under *syndrome*, and see *pulmonary sulcus tumor*, under *tumor*.

pancolectomy (pan″ko-lek′to-me) excision of the entire colon with creation of an ileostomy.

pancrealgia (pan″kre-al′je-ah) pancreatalgia.

pancreas (pan′kre-as), gen. *pancre′atis*, pl. *pancre′ata* [L., from Gr. *pankreas*, from *pan* all + *kreas* flesh] [NA] a large, elongated, racemose gland situated transversely behind the stomach, between the spleen and the duodenum. Its right extremity, the *head* (caput) is the larger, and directed downward; the left extremity, or *tail* (cauda), is transverse and terminates close to the spleen. It is subdivided into lobules by septa that extend down into the gland from the thin, areolar tissue that forms an indefinite capsule. The endocrine part (*pars endocrina*) of the pancreas, consisting of the islets of Langerhans, produces and secretes directly into the bloodstream the hormone insulin, which plays a major role in carbohydrate metabolism; and glucagon, which has an effect opposite to insulin. The exocrine part (*pars exocrina*), consisting of secretory units (pancreatic acini), produces and secretes into the duodenum a pancreatic juice, which contains enzymes essential to protein digestion. **aberrant p.,** an exclave of pancreatic tissue occurring most commonly as a firm yellow nodule in the stomach, duodenum, or jejunum, but encountered also in other sites. **p. accesso′rium** [NA], **accessory p.,** an inconstant separate part of the head of the pancreas, usually an unattached uncinate process. **annular p.,** a developmental anomaly in which the pancreas forms a ring entirely surrounding the duodenum. **Aselli's p.,** an assemblage of lymphatic glands at the root of the mesentery, especially in carnivora. **p. divi′sum,** a developmental anomaly in which the pancreas is present as two separate structures, each with its own duct. **dorsal p.,** an embryonic outpocketing from the entodermal lining of the gut on the dorsal wall cephalad to the level of the hepatic diverticulum, which forms much of the pancreas and its functional duct. **lesser p.,** the small, partially detached portion of the pancreas lying dorsad to its head (processus uncinatus pancreatis [NA]); called also *Willis' p.* and *Winslow's p.* **ventral p.,** an embryonic outpocketing from the entodermal lining of the gut on the ventral wall, in the caudal angle between the gut and the hepatic diverticulum, which forms part of the pancreas and the stem of its functional duct. **Willis' p., Winslow's p.,** lesser pancreas.

pancreata (pan-kre′ah-tah) [L.] plural of *pancreas.*

pancreatalgia (pan″kre-ah-tal′je-ah) [*pancreas* + -*algia*] pain in the pancreas.

pancreatectomy (pan″kre-ah-tek′to-me) [*pancreas* + Gr. *ektomē* excision] surgical removal of the pancreas.

pancreatic (pan″kre-at′ik) [L. *pancreaticus*] pertaining to the pancreas.

pancreatic(o)- a combining form denoting relationship to the pancreas, or to the pancreatic duct.

pancreaticoduodenal (pan″kre-at″ĭ-ko-du″o-de′nal) pertaining to the pancreas and duodenum.

pancreaticoduodenostomy (pan″kre-at″ĭ-ko-du″o-denos′to-me) surgical anastomosis of the pancreatic duct, or the divided end of the transected pancreas, with the duodenum.

pancreaticoenterostomy (pan″kre-at″ĭ-ko-en″ter-os′to-me) surgical anastomosis of the pancreatic duct, or the divided end of the transected pancreas, with the intestine.

pancreaticogastrostomy (pan″kre-at″ĭ-ko-gas-tros′to-me) surgical anastomosis of the pancreatic duct, or the divided end of the transected pancreas, with the stomach.

pancreaticojejunostomy (pan″kre-at″ĭ-ko-je″ju-nos′to-me) surgical anastomosis of the pancreatic duct, or the divided end of the transected pancreas, with the jejunum.

pancreaticosplenic (pan″kre-at″ĭ-ko-splen′ik) pertaining to the pancreas and spleen.

pancreatin (pan′kre-ah-tin) [USP] a substance obtained from the pancreas of the hog or the ox, which contains enzymes, chiefly amylase, trypsin, and lipase, and having the same action as do the enzymes of the pancreatic juice; used as a digestive aid in conditions of pancreatic insufficiency, and also to peptonize milk and other foods.

pancreatism (pan′kre-ah-tizm″) activity of the pancreas.

pancreatitis (pan″kre-ah-ti′tis) acute or chronic inflammation of the pancreas, which may be asymptomatic or symptomatic, and which is due to autodigestion of a pancreatic tissue by its own enzymes. It is caused most often by alcoholism or biliary tract disease; less commonly it may be associated with hyperlipemia, hyperparathyroidism, abdominal trauma (accidental or operative injury), vasculitis, or uremia. **acute p.,** a form characterized by sudden onset of abdominal pain, nausea, and vomiting. **acute hemorrhagic p.,** a condition due to autolysis of pancreatic tissue caused by the escape of enzymes into its substance, resulting in hemorrhage into the parenchyma and surrounding tissues. Blood staining of the lateral abdominal wall (Grey Turner's sign) or periumbilical area (Cullen's sign) may result. **calcereous p.,** pancreatitis accompanied by the formation of calculi; pancreatic calcification is usually associated with exocrine insufficiency and diabetes mellitus. **centrilo-**

bar p., pancreatitis located around the branches of the pancreatic duct. **chronic p.,** a form marked usually by chronic abdominal pain and by progressive fibrosis and loss of exocrine (steatorrhea) and endocrine (diabetes mellitus) function; recurrent attacks of acute pancreatitis (*chronic relapsing p.*) are often superimposed. **chronic relapsing p.,** see *chronic p.* **interstitial p.,** pancreatitis in which there is overgrowth of the inter- and intra-acinar connective tissue and frequently a corresponding atrophy of the glandular tissue. **perilobar p.,** fibrosis of the pancreas surrounding collections of atrophic acini. **purulent p.,** purulent inflammation of the pancreas.

pancreat(o)- [L. *pancreas,* q.v.] a combining form denoting relationship to the pancreas.

pancreatoduodenectomy (pan″kre-ah-to-du″o-dĕ-nek′to-me) excision of the head of the pancreas along with the encircling loop of the duodenum.

pancreatoduodenostomy (pan″kre-ah-to-du″o-dĕ-nos′to-me) pancreaticoduodenostomy.

pancreatoenterostomy (pan″kre-ah-to-en″ter-os′to-me) pancreaticoenterostomy.

pancreatogenic (pan″kre-ah-to-jen′ik) pancreatogenous.

pancreatogenous (pan″kre-ah-toj′ĕ-nus) arising in or from the pancreas.

pancreatogram (pan″kre-at′o-gram) the x-ray film produced by pancreatography.

pancreatography (pan″kre-ah-tog′rah-fe) roentgenography of the pancreas performed during surgical exploration, a water-soluble contrast medium being injected into the pancreatic duct and the film being made while the abdomen is open. **endoscopic retrograde p.,** that in which the radiopaque medium is injected into the pancreatic duct at the ampulla of Vater via a cannula introduced through a fiberoptic endoscope. See also *endoscopic retrograde cholangiopancreatography,* under cholangiopancreatography.

pancreatolith (pan″kre-at′o-lith) [*pancreas* + Gr. *lithos* stone] a pancreatic calculus.

pancreatolithectomy (pan″kre-ah-to-lĭ-thek′to-me) [*pancreatolith* + Gr. *ektomē* excision] excision of a calculus from the pancreas.

pancreatolithiasis (pan″kre-ah-to-lĭ-thi′ah-sis) the presence of calculi in the ductal system or parenchyma of the pancreas.

pancreatolithotomy (pan″kre-ah-to-lĭ-thot′o-me) [*pancreatolith* + Gr. *tomē* a cutting] incision of the pancreas for the removal of a calculus.

pancreatolysis (pan″kre-ah-tol′ĭ-sis) pancreolysis.

pancreatolytic (pan″kre-ah-to-lit′ik) pancreolytic.

pancreatomy (pan-kre-at′o-me) pancreatotomy.

pancreatopathy (pan″kre-ah-top′ah-the) [*pancreas* + Gr. *pathos* disease] any disease of the pancreas.

pancreatotomy (pan″kre-ah-tot′o-me) [*pancreas* + Gr. *tomē* a cutting] incision of the pancreas.

pancreatotropic (pan-kre″ah-to-trop′ik) [*pancreas* + Gr. *tropē* a turning] having an affinity for or an influence on the pancreas.

pancreatropic (pan″kre-ah-trop′ik) pancreatotropic.

pancreectomy (pan″kre-ek′to-me) pancreatectomy.

pancrelipase (pan″kre-li′pās) [USP] a standardized preparation of hog pancreas, containing enzymes, principally lipase, with amylase and protease, and having the same actions as those of the pancreatic juice; used as a digestive aid in conditions of pancreatic insufficiency.

pancreolithotomy (pan″kre-o-lĭ-thot′o-me) pancreatolithotomy.

pancreolysis (pan″kre-ol′ĭ-sis) [*pancreas* + Gr. *lysis* dissolution] destruction of pancreatic tissue by pancreatic enzymes.

pancreolytic (pan″kre-o-lit′ik) pertaining to or producing pancreolysis.

pancreopathy (pan″kre-op′ah-the) [*pancreas* + Gr. *pathos* disease] any disease of the pancreas.

pancreoprivic (pan″kre-o-priv′ik) lacking a pancreas.

pancreotherapy (pan″kre-o-ther′ah-pe) therapeutic use of pancreas tissue or of extracts of the pancreas containing digestive enzymes; pancreatic replacement therapy, used in pancreatic insufficiency with malabsorption.

pancreotropic (pan″kre-o-trop′ik) pancreatotropic.

pancreozymin (pan′kre-o-zi″min) a hormone of the duodenal mucosa which stimulates the external secretory activity of the pancreas, especially its production of amylase; identical with cholecystokinin (q.v.).

pancuronium bromide (pan″ku-ro′ne-um) chemical name: 1,1′-[(2β,3α,5α,16β,17β)-3,17-bis(acetyloxy)androstane-2,16-diyl]bis[1-methyl]piperidinium dibromide. A nondepolarizing skeletal muscle relaxant, $C_{35}H_{60}Br_2N_2O_4$, with curariform action; used as an adjunct to anesthesia, and may be used to facilitate mechanical ventilation, administered intravenously.

pancystitis (pan″sis-ti′tis) cystitis involving the entire thickness of the wall of the urinary bladder, as occurs in interstitial cystitis.

pancytopenia (pan″si-to-pe′ne-ah) [*pan-* + *cyto-* + *-penia*] deficiency of all cell elements of the blood; aplastic anemia. **Fanconi's p.,** Fanconi's syndrome, def. 1.

pandemic (pan-dem′ik) [*pan-* + Gr. *dēmos* people] 1. a widespread epidemic of a disease. 2. widely epidemic; distributed or occurring widely throughout a region, country, or continent or globally.

pandemicity (pan″dĕ-mis′ĭ-te) the state of being pandemic.

Pander's islands, layer, nucleus (pan′derz) [Heinrich Christian *Pander,* German anatomist, 1794–1865] see under *island* and *layer,* and see *nucleus subthalamicus.*

pandiculation (pan″dik-u-la′shun) [L. *pandiculari* to stretch one's self] the act of stretching and yawning.

Pándy's test (reaction) (pan′dēz) [Kálmán *Pándy,* Hungarian neurologist, born 1868] see under *tests.*

panel (pan′el) a list of names, a number of individuals participating in a specific discussion or activity, especially a list of names of the medical men who are willing to care for insured persons for a stipulated yearly fee under the system of medical insurance carried on by insurance groups under the supervision of the government in Great Britain, or the list of the insured persons assigned as clients to a physician under the British National Health Insurance Act.

panencephalitis (pan″en-sef″ah-li′tis) encephalitis, probably of viral origin, which produces intranuclear or intracytoplasmic inclusion bodies of type A (Cowdry's classification), which result in parenchymatous lesions affecting the gray and white matter of the brain simultaneously. **Pette-Döring p.,** a form of subacute encephalitis characterized by involvement of both the gray and white matter of the brain, and with a predilection for the basal ganglia. **subacute sclerosing p.,** a rare and devastating form of leukoencephalitis usually affecting children and adolescents. Insidious in onset, it characteristically produces progressive cerebral dysfunction over a course of several weeks or months and death within a year. Pathologically, in addition to the lesions of the white matter, there are demyelination and intranuclear inclusion bodies in nerve cells and oligodendroglia, suggesting a viral etiology. Called also *Dawson's encephalitis, subacute inclusion body encephalitis, subacute sclerosing leukoencephalopathy,* and *van Bogaert's encephalitis* or *sclerosing leukoencephalitis.*

panendography (pan″en-dog′rah-fe) the recording of events observed through a panendoscope.

panendoscope (pan-en′do-skōp) a cystoscope that permits wide-angle viewing of the urinary bladder and urethra. **oral p.,** an illuminated tubular device that permits visual observation and audiovisual recording of the larynx and vocal cords during production of speech sounds.

panendoscopy (pan″en-dos′ko-pe) observation by means of a panendoscope.

panepizootic (pan-ep″ĭ-zo-ot′ik) 1. attacking almost all the animals in a fairly large area; said of disease. 2. a widely diffused and rapidly spreading animal disease.

panesthesia (pan″es-the′ze-ah) [*pan-* + Gr. *aisthēsis* perception] the sum of the sensations experienced.

panesthetic (pan″es-thet′ik) relating to panesthesia.

Paneth's cells (pah′nāts) [Josef *Paneth,* German physician, 1857–1890] see under *cell.*

pang (pang) a sudden, piercing pain. **breast p.,** angina pectoris. **brow p.,** 1. supraorbital neuralgia. 2. hemicrania (def. 1).

pangenesis (pan-jen′ĕ-sis) [*pan-* + *genesis*] Darwin's hypothesis of the inheritance of acquired characteristics. According to the hypothesis true reproductive power lies not in the germ cells, but in the totality of the somatic cells (hence "pangenesis"). The somatic cells generate pangenes that circulate freely in the blood, reproduced by division, and collect in the germ cells, where they combine with and alter earlier pangenes in correspondence to recent changes in the peripheral organs.

panglossia (pan-glos′e-ah) [Gr. *panglōssia*] abnormal or pathologic garrulity.

Pangonia (pan-go′ne-ah) a genus of flies, the zimbs of Ethiopia, which are exceedingly annoying to man and animals.

panhematopenia (pan-hem″ah-to-pe′ne-ah) [*pan-* + Gr. *haima* blood + *penia* poverty] pancytopenia. **primary splenic p.,** a form of hypersplenism of unknown etiology, marked by indiscriminate elimination of all circulating elements of the blood. Whether such an entity exists, as such, is moot, since the hypersplenism may be a manifestation of an underlying systemic disease.

Panheprin (pan-hep′rin) trademark for a preparation of heparin sodium.

panhydrometer (pan″hi-drom′ĕ-ter) [*pan-* + *hydrometer*] an instrument for ascertaining the specific gravity of any liquid.

panhyperemia (pan″hi-per-e′me-ah) [*pan-* + *hyperemia*] general plethora.

panhypogammaglobulinemia (pan-hi″po-gam″ah-glob″u-lin-e′me-ah) [*pan-* + *hypogammaglobulinemia*] hypogammaglobulinemia; deficiency of all immunoglobulin classes.

panhypogonadism (pan-hi″po-go′nad-izm) underdevelopment of all the genital tissues due to abnormally decreased functional activities of the gonads.

panhypopituitarism (pan-hi″po-pĭ-tu″ĭ-tar-izm) generalized hypopituitarism due to absence of or damage to the pituitary gland, which, in its complete form, leads to absence of gonadal function and insufficiency of thyroid and adrenal cortical function. Dwarfism, regression of secondary sex characters and loss of libido, weight loss, fatigability, bradycardia, hypotension, pallor, depression, and many other manifestations may occur. When cachexia is a prominent feature, it is called *hypophysial* or *pituitary cachexia,* and *Simmonds' disease.* **prepubertal p.,** pituitary dwarfism.

panhysterectomy (pan″his-ter-ek′to-me) [*pan-* + Gr. *hystera* uterus + *ektomē* excision] complete removal of the uterus and cervix; total hysterectomy.

panhystero-oophorectomy (pan-his″ter-o-o″of-o-rek′to-me) excision of the body of the uterus, cervix, and ovary.

panhysterosalpingectomy (pan-his″ter-o-sal″pin-jek′to-me) excision of the body of the uterus, cervix, and uterine tube.

panhysterosalpingo-oophorectomy (pan-his″ter-o-sal″ping-go-o″of-o-rek′to-me) excision of the uterus, cervix, uterine tube, and ovary.

panic (pan′ik) acute, extreme anxiety with disorganization of personality and function. **acute homosexual p., homosexual p.,** an acute, extreme anxiety reaction brought on by circumstances that induce the unconscious fear of being homosexual or of succumbing to homosexual impulses.

panimmunity (pan″ĭ-mu′nĭ-te) [*pan-* + *immunity*] immunity to several infections caused by bacteria and viruses.

Panizza's plexus (pan-id′zaz) [Bartolomeo *Panizza,* Professor of anatomy at Pavia, 1785–1867] see under *plexus.*

panleukopenia (pan″lu-ko-pe′ne-ah) a viral disease of cats, characterized by leukopenia and marked by inactivity, refusal of food, diarrhea, and vomiting. Called also *infectious feline agranulocytosis, feline* or *cat enteritis, cat distemper,* and *cat plague.*

panmeristic (pan″mer-is′tik) [*pan-* + Gr. *meros* part] pertaining to the protoplasm of ova, made up of independent units or pangens.

panmixia (pan-mik′se-ah) panmixis.

panmixis (pan-mik′sis) [*pan-* + Gr. *mixis* mixture] random mating, i.e., choice of mate uninfluenced by the genotypes of the mates.

Panmycin (pan-mi′sin)   trademark for preparations of tetracycline.

panmyeloid (pan-mi′ĕ-loid)   pertaining to all the elements of the bone marrow.

panmyelopathia (pan″mi-ĕ-lo-path′e-ah)   panmyelopathy.

panmyelopathy (pan″mi-ĕ-lop′ah-the) [pan- + Gr. *myelos* marrow + *pathos* disease]   a pathologic condition of all the elements of the bone marrow. **constitutional infantile p.,** Fanconi's syndrome, def. 1.

panmyelophthisis (pan-mi″ĕ-lof′thĭ-sis) [pan- + Gr. *myelos* marrow + *phthisis* wasting]   1. aplastic anemia. 2. (*obs.*) aleukia hemorrhagica.

Panner's disease (pan′erz) [Hans Jessen Panner, Danish radiologist, 1871–1930]   see under *disease*.

panneuritis (pan″nu-ri′tis) [pan- + Gr. *neuron* nerve + *-itis*] (*obs.*) multiple or general neuritis.   **p. epidem′ica,** beriberi.

panneurosis (pan″nu-ro′sis)   the occurrence at the same time of all neurotic symptoms, including anxiety, conversion symptoms, obsessions, and phobias.

pannicalgia (pah-nik″u-lal′je-ah)   adiposalgia.

panniculectomy (pah-nik″u-lek′to-me)   surgical excision of the abdominal apron of superficial fat in the obese.

panniculi (pah-nik′u-li) [L.]   genitive and plural of *panniculus.*

panniculitis (pah-nik″u-li′tis) [*panniculus* + *-itis*]   an inflammatory reaction of the subcutaneous fat, which may involve the connective tissue septa between the fat lobes, the septa lobules and vessels, or the fat lobules, characterized by the development of single or multiple cutaneous nodules. **LE p., lupus p.,** lupus erythematosus profundus. **nodular nonsuppurative p.,** relapsing febrile nodular nonsuppurative p.   **relapsing febrile nodular nonsuppurative p.,** a form of panniculitis characterized by recurrent episodes of fever accompanied by crops of single or multiple, erythematous tender or painless subcutaneous nodules on the lower extremities and trunk, which resolve and usually leave a depression in the skin. The condition is most often seen in women, and it may occur alone or it may be associated with numerous other disorders. Called also *Christian-Weber disease, nodular nonsuppurative p.,* and *Weber-Christian p., disease,* or *syndrome.* **subacute nodular migratory p.,** a condition considered by some to be the same as *erythema nodosum migrans,* characterized by the development on the anterior and lateral aspects of the lower extremities, particularly in women, of discrete nodules that spread centrifugally with erythematous borders and central clearing (giving the appearance of migration), which coalesce to form plaques that eventually involute, usually with residual pigmentation.   **Weber-Christian p.,** relapsing febrile nodular nonsuppurative p.

panniculus (pah-nik′u-lus), gen. and pl. *pannic′uli* [L., dim. of *pannus* cloth]   a layer of membrane.   **p. adipo′sus** [NA], the subcutaneous fat: a layer of fat underlying the dermis. Called also *pannus.*   **p. carno′sus,** a thin muscular layer within the superficial fascia of animals with a hairy coat; in man it is represented mainly by the platysma myoides.

pannus (pan′us) [L. "a piece of cloth"]   1. superficial vascularization of the cornea with infiltration of granulation tissue.   2. an inflammatory exudate overlying the lining layer of synovial cells on the inside of a joint, usually occurring in patients with rheumatoid arthritis or related articular rheumatism, and sometimes resulting in fibrous ankylosis of the joint.   3. panniculus adiposus.   **degenerative p., p. degenerati′vus,** a connective-tissue growth between the epithelium of the cornea and Bowman's membrane.   **glaucomatous p.,** degeneration and desquamation of corneal epithelium due to edema in advanced glaucoma.   **phlyctenular p.,** pannus associated with phlyctenular keratitis, the vascularization running all the way around the periphery of the limbus and extending toward the center.   **p. sic′cus,** pannus of the cornea associated with dryness of the cornea and conjunctiva.   **p. trachomato′sus,** pannus occurring secondarily to trachoma, the small fine branching vessels always appearing at the upper limbus and running down under the epithelium into the cornea.

panodic (pah-nod′ik)   panthodic.

panophobia (pan″o-fo′be-ah)   panphobia.

panophthalmia (pan″of-thal′me-ah)   panophthalmitis.

panophthalmitis (pan″of-thal-mi′tis) [*pan-* + *ophthalmitis*]   inflammation of all the structures or tissues of the eye.

panoptic (pan-op′tik) [*pan-* + Gr. *optikos* of or for vision]   rendering everything visible; said of a stain which differentiates all the tissues of a specimen. See *Giemsa's stain,* under *stain.*

panoptosis (pan″op-to′sis) [*pan-* + Gr. *ptōsis* falling]   (*obs.*)   general ptosis of the abdominal organs.

panosteitis (pan″os-te-i′tis) [*pan-* + Gr. *osteon* bone + *-itis*]   inflammation of every part of a bone.

panostitis (pan″os-ti′tis)   panosteitis.

panotitis (pan″o-ti′tis) [*pan-* + Gr. *ous* ear + *-itis*]   an inflammation of all the parts or structures of the ear.

panphobia (pan-fo′be-ah)   fear of everything; a vague morbid dread of some unknown evil.

panplegia (pan-ple′je-ah)   pamplegia.

panproctocolectomy (pan-prok″to-ko-lek′to-me)   excision of the entire rectum and colon, with creation of an ileal stoma.

Pansch's fissure (pansh′ez) [Adolf *Pansch,* German anatomist, 1841–1887]   see under *fissure.*

pansclerosis (pan″skle-ro′sis) [*pan-* + Gr. *sklērōsis* hardening]   complete induration of a part or organ.

panseptum (pan-sep′tum)   the entire nasal septum, including bony and cartilaginous parts.

pansinuitis (pan″si-nu-i′tis)   pansinusitis.

pansinusectomy (pan″si-nus-ek′to-me)   excision of the diseased membrane of all of the paranasal sinuses on one side.

pansinusitis (pan″si-nu-si′tis) [*pan-* + *sinus* + *-itis*]   inflammation involving all of the paranasal sinuses on one side.

panspermatism (pan-sper′mah-tizm)   panspermy.

panspermatist (pan-sperm′ah-tist)   an advocate of panspermy; called also *panspermist.*

panspermia (pan-sper′me-ah) [*pan-* + Gr. *sperma* seed + *-ia*]   1. the doctrine of Anaxagoras and Democritus that the elements were a mixture of all the seeds of things.   2. panspermy.

panspermic (pan-sperm′ik)   pertaining to panspermy.

panspermy (pan-sper′me) [*pan-* + Gr. *sperma* seed]   the 19th-century hypothesis, opposed to spontaneous generation, that the atmosphere is full of invisible germs or reproductive bodies of plants and animals and that these germs penetrate the minutest crevices and develop upon finding a suitable soil or environment. See also *biogenesis* (def. 1). Called also *panspermia, panspermatism,* and *panspermism.*

pansphygmograph (pan-sfig′mo-graf) [*pan-* + Gr. *sphygmos* pulse + *graphein* to record]   a device for recording cardiac, pulse, and chest movements at the same time.

pansporoblast (plan-spor′o-blast) [*pan-* + *spore* + *blast*]   a disporoblastic sporont, i.e., a sporoblast that develops into two or more spores, with or without an enclosing membrane; characteristic of certain protozoa. See *Apansporoblastina* and *Pansporoblastina.*

Pansporoblastina (pan″spor-o″blas-ti′nah)   a suborder of parasitic protozoa (order Microsporida, class Microsporea) in which the sporulation sequence occurs in the host cell within a more or less persistent intracellular sporocyst (with a pansporoblastic membrane); they are often dimorphic, with another sporulation sequence not involving such a membrane. The sporoblasts and spores are usually uninucleate when the membrane is present and dinucleate when it is absent. Representative genera include *Amblyospora, Pleistophora,* and *Thelohania.*

Panstrongylus (pan-stron′jĭ-lus)   a genus of cone-nosed bugs of the family Reduviidae, species of which are vectors of *Trypanosoma.*   **P. genicula′tus,** a vector of *Trypanosoma cruzi* in Panama and Brazil.   **P. infes′tans,** *Triatoma infestans.*   **P. megis′tus,** an important vector of *Trypanosoma cruzi* in Brazil. It frequently bites the face and so is called barbiero by the natives. Formerly called *Triatoma megista.*

pantachromatic (pan″tah-kro-mat′ik) [*pant-* + *achromatic*]   entirely achromatic.

pantalgia (pan-tal′je-ah) [pant- + -algis] pain over the whole body.

pantamorphia (pan″tah-mor′fe-ah) [pant- + Gr. amorphia shapelessness] complete or general deformity.

pantamorphic (pan″tah-mor′fik) formless.

pantanencephaly (pan″tan-en-sef′ah-le) [pant- + an neg. + Gr. enkephalos brain] complete absence of the brain in a fetus.

pantankyloblepharon (pan-tang″kĭ-lo-blef′ah-ron) [pant- + Gr. ankylē noose + blepharon lid] general adhesion of the eyelids to the eyeball and to each other.

pantatrophia (pan″tah-tro′fe-ah) [pant- + Gr. atrophia atrophy] general or complete malnutrition.

pantatrophy (pan-tat′ro-fe) pantatrophia.

Panteric (pan-ter′ik) trademark for a preparation of pancreatin.

pantetheine (pan-tĕ-the′in) a naturally occurring amide of pantothenic acid and β-mercaptoethanolamine; it is an intermediate in the biosynthesis of CoA, a growth factor for Lactobacillus bulgaricus and certain other bacteria, and a cofactor in certain enzyme complexes (e.g., in fatty acid or polypeptide synthesis).

panthenol (pan′thĕ-nōl) chemical name: 2,4-dihydroxy-N-(3-hydroxypropyl)-3,3-dimethylbutanamide. The alcohol derivative of pantothenic acid, $C_9H_{19}NO_4$, which is converted in the body to pantothenic acid, a member of the B-complex vitamins. Called also pantothenyl alcohol and pantothenol. The term is sometimes used to refer to the $D^{(+)}$ form of panthenol; see dexpanthenol.

pantherapist (pan-ther′ah-pist) [pan- + therapist] a practitioner who is ready to draw his information from any and every source.

panthodic (pan-thod′ik) [pan- + Gr. hodos way] radiating in every direction; said of nerve impulses.

Pantholin (pan′tho-lin) trademark for a preparation of calcium pantothenate.

panting (pant′ing) swift and shallow breathing with a fast respiratory frequency and small tidal volume.

pant(o)- [Gr. pas, gen. pantos all] a combining form meaning all, the whole.

pantochromism (pan″to-kro′mizm) [panto- + Gr. chrōma color] the phenomenon of existing in two or more differently colored forms, as a salt.

pantograph (pan′to-graf) [panto- + Gr. graphein to write] an instrument for copying a plane figure to any desired scale.

pantoic acid (pan-to′ik) a constituent of pantothenic acid remaining after cleavage of β-alanine.

pantomographic (pan-to″mo-graf′ik) pertaining to pantomography.

pantomography (pan″to-mog′rah-fe) a method of tomography for visualization of body curved surfaces at any depth. In dentistry, it may be used for roentgenography of the maxillary and mandibular dental arches and their associated structures. Called also panoramic radiography.

pantomorphia (pan″to-mor′fe-ah) [panto- + Gr. morphē form + -ia] 1. general or perfect symmetry. 2. ability to assume various shapes, as an ameba.

pantomorphic (pan″to-mor′fik) able to assume any shape.

Pantopaque (pan-to-pāk′) trademark for a preparation of iophendylate.

pantophobia (pan″to-fo′be-ah) [panto- + phobia] panphobia.

pantoscopic (pan″to-skop′ik) [panto- + Gr. skopein to examine] adapted to view both near and distant objects; a term applied to bifocal lenses.

pantothen (pan′to-then) pantothenic acid.

pantothenate (pan-to′then-āt) a salt of pantothenic acid.

pantothenic acid (pan″to-the′nik) the amide of β-alanine and pantoic acid, a B complex vitamin that is a constituent of coenzyme A; it is distributed ubiquitously in foods and a deficiency syndrome has not been demonstrated in humans except by experimental administration of the pantothenic acid antagonist ω-methylpantothenic acid.

pantothenol (pan″to-the′nōl) 1. panthenol. 2. dexpanthenol.

pantotropic (pan″to-trop′ik) pantropic.

pantoyltaurine (pan″to-il-taw′rēn) a competitive inhibitor of pantothenic acid derived by replacement of the carboxyl group by a sulfonyl group; it is the amide of pantoic acid and taurine. Called also thiopanic acid.

pantropic (pan-trop′ik) [pan- + Gr. tropos a turning] having an affinity for many tissues; capable of attacking derivatives of any of the three embryonic layers.

panturbinate (pan-ter′bĭ-nat) the entire structure of a nasal concha, including bone and soft tissue.

panus (pa′nus) [L. "swelling"] a lymphatic gland inflamed but not suppurating.

panuveitis (pan″u-ve-i′tis) inflammation of the entire uveal tract.

Panwarfin (pan-war′fin) trademark for a preparation of warfarin sodium.

panzerherz (pan′zer-herz) [Ger.] armored heart; see under heart.

panzootic (pan″zo-ot′ik) [pan- + Gr. zōon animal] occurring pandemically among animals.

PAP peroxidase-antiperoxidase; see under technique.

pap (pap) any soft food, as bread soaked in milk.

Pap test (pap) Papanicolaou's test; see under tests.

papain (pah-pa′in, pah-pi′in) [EC 3.4.22.2] an enzyme of the hydrolase class that catalyzes the hydrolysis of proteins and peptides with preferential cleavage at bonds containing arginine, lysine, and glycine residues. The enzyme is obtained from the latex of the papaya, Carica papaya L. (Caricaceae). In medicine, it is used as a protein digestant and as a topical application for enzymatic debridement and promotion of normal healing of surface lesions.

Papanicolaou's stain test (pap″ah-nik″o-la′ōōz) [George Nicolas Papanicolaou, Greek physician, anatomist, and cytologist in the United States, 1883–1962] see Table of Stains, and under tests.

Papaver (pah-pav′er) a genus of herbs of the family Papaveraceae, or poppies. P. somnif′erum, a pink to purplish-pink and purple species, and its variety al′bum, a silvery white species, are the source of opium. The unripe capsules when scarified yield a white latex which when dried is known as crude opium. It contains the opium alkaloids (morphine, codeine, etc.), which are used as narcotics and analgesics. The poppy seeds, devoid of the alkaloids, are used as a condiment on baked products. P. orienta′lis is the source of isothebaine.

papaverine hydrochloride (pah-pav′er-in) [USP] chemical name: 1-[(3,4-dimethoxyphenyl)methyl]-6,7-dimethoxyisoquinoline hydrochloride. The hydrochloride salt of an opium alkaloid, $C_{20}H_{21}NO_4·HCl$, which also may be synthesized, occurring as white crystals or as a white, crystalline powder; used as a smooth muscle relaxant, especially in the treatment of cerebral and peripheral ischemia associated with arterial spasm and myocardial ischemia complicated by arrhythmias, administered orally and intramuscularly.

papaw (pah-paw′) 1. a large herbaceous plant, the papaya, Carica papaya L. (Caricaceae) of Southern United States; also its fruit. The fruit contains papain, a proteolytic enzyme. 2. pawpaw; the tree Asimina triloba (L.) Duval (Annonaceae), which has edible fruit, although ingestion may cause severe skin irritation in sensitive persons.

papaya (pah-pa′yah) papaw, def. 1.

papayotin (pap″a-yo′tin) papain.

paper (pa′per) a substance manufactured in thin sheets, prepared from wood, rags, or other fibrous substance which has first been reduced to a pulp. **alkannin p.,** filter paper dipped in an alcoholic solution of alkannin; alkalis turn it blue, acids red. **amboceptor p.,** filter paper saturated with amboceptor serum; used in the Noguchi test for syphilis. **aniline acetate p.,** filter paper dipped into a mixture of aniline, water, and glacial acetic acid, and then dried. **antigen p.,** filter paper saturated with antigen solution; used in the Noguchi test for syphilis. **articulating p.,** paper strips, coated with ink- or dye-containing wax, used for the marking or locating of occlusal interferences or deflective or interceptive occlusal contacts. **asthma p.,** niter p. **azolitmin p.,** filter paper saturated with a solution of azolitmin; acids turn it from purple to bright red, alkalis turn it blue. **bibulous p.,** a paper which absorbs water readily. **biuret p.,** filter paper previously dipped in Gies' biuret reagent, dried, and cut into strips. **blue litmus p.,** see *litmus p.* **Congo red p.,** wet filter paper with a 0.2 per cent solution of Congo red in water, dried, and cut in strips. **filter p.,** a porous, unsized paper used as a filter. **lacmoid p.,** blotting paper impregnated with lacmoid; used in testing for alkalinity or acidity. **litmus p.,** bibulous paper impregnated with a solution of litmus, dried, and cut into strips. If slightly alkaline the paper is blue, and is used as a test for acids, which turn it red; if slightly acid it is red and alkalis turn it blue. **niter p.,** paper impregnated with potassium nitrate, ignited and used as a moxa or by inhalation in asthma; called also *saltpeter p.* **potassium nitrate p.,** niter p. **red litmus p.,** see *litmus p.* **saltpeter p.,** niter p. **test p.,** paper that is impregnated with litmus or other indicator. **turmeric p.,** paper dyed yellow with turmeric; alkalis turn it brown.

papescent (pah-pes′ent) having the consistence of pap.

papilla (pah-pil′ah), gen. and pl. *papil′lae* [L.] a small nipple-shaped projection, elevation, or structure. **acoustic p.,** organum spirale. **arcuate papillae of tongue,** papillae filiformes. **Bergmeister's p.,** a small mass of neuroglial cells in the center of the embryonic optic disk, surrounding the bulb of the hyaloid artery. Also, a congenital anomaly consisting of a glial veil attached to the anterior aspect of the optic disk, resulting from glial proliferation around the remnants of the posterior part of the hyaloid vessel system. **bile p.,** p. duodeni major. **calciform papillae, capitate papillae,** papillae vallatae. **circumvallate papillae,** papillae vallatae. **clavate papillae,** papillae fungiformes. **papil′lae con′icae** [NA], **conical papillae,** sparsely scattered large elevations on the tongue surface, often considered as a modified type of filiform papillae. **conical papillae of tongue, of Soemmering,** papillae filiformes. **conoid papillae of tongue,** papillae conicae. **p., co′rii** NA alternative for *p. dermatis.* **corolliform papillae of tongue,** papillae filiformes. **dental p., dentinal p., p. den′tis** [NA], a small mass of condensed mesenchymal tissue in the enamel organ, which differentiates into the dentin and dental pulp. **dermal p., p. der′matis,** any of the conical extensions of the collagen fibers, the capillary blood vessels, and sometimes the nerves of the dermis into corresponding spaces among the downward- or inward-projecting rete ridges on the under surface of the epidermis. On the forehead and ear these are less prominent; on the face, neck, and pubes the relations are reversed and "rete pegs" extend inward or downward into spaces among a network of dermal ridges. Called also *p. corii* [NA alternative] *p. of corium,* and *skin p.* **duodenal p., major,** p. duodeni major. **duodenal p., minor,** p. duodeni minor. **p. duode′ni ma′jor** [NA], major duodenal papilla: a small elevation at the site of the opening of the conjoined common bile duct and pancreatic duct into the lumen of the duodenum. Called also *p. duodeni* [Santorini]. See also *p. duodeni minor.* **p. duode′ni mi′nor** [NA], minor duodenal papilla: a small elevation at the site of the opening of the accessory pancreatic duct into the lumen of the duodenum. See also *p. duodeni major.* **p. duode′ni [Santori′ni],** p. duodeni major. **filiform papillae, papil′lae filifor′mes** [NA], threadlike elevations that cover most of the tongue surface. **papil′lae folia′tae** [NA], **foliate papillae,** parallel mucosal folds on the margins of the tongue at the junction of its body and root. **fungiform papillae, papil′lae fungifor′mes** [NA], knoblike projections on the tongue, scattered singly among the filiform papillae. **gingival p., gingiva′lis** [NA], a cone-shaped pad of the interdental gingiva filling the space between two contiguous teeth up to the contact area, as viewed from the labial, buccal, or lingual aspect; called also *interdental p., p. interdentalis* [NA alternative], and *interproximal p.* See also *interdental gingiva,* under *gingiva.* **gustatory papillae,** papillae linguales. **hair p., p.** pili. **p. ilea′lis,** NA alternative for *p. ileocaecalis.* **p. ileocaeca′lis** [NA], **ileocecal p.,** the conical projection formed by the terminal ileum at the junction of the cecum and the ileum and extending into the large intestine, as seen in the living individual; called also *ileal p.* and *p. ilealis* or *p. ileocaecalis* [NA alternatives]. See also *ostium ileocaecale* and *ostium valvulae ilealis.* **p. ileoceca′lis,** NA alternative for *p. ileocaecalis.* **p. incisi′va** [NA], **incisive p.,** a rounded projection at the anterior end of the raphe of the palate. **interdental p.,** gingival p. **p. interdenta′lis,** NA alternative for *p. gingivalis.* **interproximal p.,**

gingival p. **lacrimal p., p. lacrima′lis** [NA], a papilla in the conjunctiva near the medial angle of the eye. **papil′lae lacrima′les,** see *p. lacrimalis.* **lenticular papillae, papil′lae lenticula′res,** a series of papillae of the tongue resembling, but less elevated than, the fungiform papillae. **lingual papillae, papil′lae lingua′les** [NA], the filiform, fungiform, vallate, foliate, and conical papillae of the tongue. **major duodenal p.,** p. duodeni major. **p. mam′mae** [NA], **mammary p.,** nipple of the breast: the pigmented projection on the anterior surface of the mammary gland, surrounded by the areola. The lactiferous ducts open onto it. **medial papillae of tongue.** papillae fungiformes. **minor duodenal p.,** p. duodeni minor. **p. ner′vi op′tici,** discus nervi optici. **papillae of tongue,** papillae fungiformes. **optic p.,** discus nervi optici. **palatine p.,** p. incisiva. **parotid p., p. paroti′dea** [NA], the small papilla marking the orifice of the parotid duct in the mucous membrane of the cheek. **p. pi′li** [NA], hair papilla: the fibrovascular mesodermal papilla enclosed within the hair bulb. **renal papillae, papil′lae rena′les** [NA], the blunted apices of the renal pyramids, which project into the renal sinus. **retromolar p.,** a small papilla of gingival tissue located at the foot of the ramus of the mandible and attached to the most inferior part of the anterior border of the ramus. **p. of Santorini,** p. duodeni major. **simple papillae of tongue,** papillae filiformes. **skin p.,** p. dermatis. **small papillae of tongue,** papillae filiformes. **p. spira′lis,** organum spirale. **sublingual p.,** caruncula sublingualis. **tactile papillae,** corpuscula tactus. **urethral p.,** a slight elevation in the vestibule of the vagina on which is situated the external orifice of the urethra. **papil′lae valla′tae** [NA], **vallate papillae,** the largest papillae of the tongue, 8 to 12 in number, arranged in the form of a V in front of the sulcus terminalis of the tongue. **p. of Vater,** p. duodeni major. **villous papillae of tongue,** papillae filiformes.

papillae (pah-pil′e) [L.] genitive and plural of *papilla.*

papillary (pap′ĭ-ler″e) pertaining to or resembling a papilla, or nipple.

papillate (pap′ĭ-lāt) marked by nipple-like elevations.

papillectomy (pap″ĭ-lek′to-me) [*papilla* + Gr. *ektome* excision] excision of a papilla.

papilledema (pap″il-ĕ-de′mah) choked disk; edema of the optic disk (papilla), most commonly due to increased intracranial pressure, malignant hypertension, or thrombosis of the central retinal vein; called also *choked disk.*

papilliferous (pap″ĭ-lif′er-us) [*papilla* + L. *ferre* to bear] bearing papillae.

papilliform (pah-pil′ĭ-form) [*papilla* + L. *forma* shape] shaped like a papilla.

papillitis (pap″ĭ-li′tis) [*papilla* + *-itis*] inflammation of the optic papilla (disk); see *optic neuritis,* under *neuritis.* **necrotizing p., necrotizing renal p.,** renal papillary necrosis.

papilloadenocystoma (pah-pil″o-ad″ĕ-no-sis-to′mah) papillary cystadenoma.

papillocarcinoma (pah-pil″o-kar″sĭ-no′mah) papillary carcinoma.

papilloma (pap″ĭ-lo′mah) [*papilla* + *-oma*] a benign epithelial neoplasm producing finger-like or verrucous projections from the epithelial surface. Called also *papillary tumor, villoma,* and *villous p.* or *tumor.* **cockscomb p.,** papilloma of the uterine cervix that occurs during pregnancy and regresses following delivery; it is a small, red lesion that projects above the surrounding mucosa and resembles a cockscomb. **cutaneous p.,** acrochordon. **fibroepithelial p.,** a papilloma containing extensive fibrous tissue; fibropapilloma. **hirsutoid p's of penis,** pearly penile papules. **Hopmann's p.,** Hopmann's polyp. **intracanalicular p.,** a warty, nonmalignant growth within the substance of certain glands, especially of the breast. **intracystic p.,** a papilloma formed within a cystic adenoma. **rabbit p.,** a viral disease of rabbits marked by the formation of horny warts. These papillomas were the first mammalian tumors shown to be induced by a virus (by Shope in 1933) and the first to be transmitted by purified viral DNA. Called also *Shope p.* **rabbit oral p.,** a viral disease of wild rabbits, characterized by the appearance of nodules on the lower surface of the tongue. **Shope p.,** rabbit p. **villous p.,** papilloma.

papillomatosis (pap″ĭ-lo″mah-to′sis) the development of multiple papillomas. **confluent and reticulate p.,** a progressive, pruritic papillomatosis, probably a genodermatosis, seen chiefly in girls, especially those at or near puberty, beginning in the intramammary and midback areas as slightly keratotic pigmented papules that increase in size and spread over the trunk and other body areas; centrally located lesions tend to become confluent and peripherally located ones to become reticulate. Called also *Gougerot-Carteaud syndrome.*

papillomatous (pap″ĭ-lo′mah-tus) of the nature of a papilloma.

papillomavirus (pap″ĭ-lo″mah-vi′rus) any of a subgroup of the papovaviruses causing papillomata in humans and in rabbits, cows, dogs, pigs, and various other animals. Cf. *polyomavirus.*

Papillon-Lefèvre syndrome (pap″ĭ-yon′ lĕ-fa′) [M.M. *Papillon,* French dermatologist, 20th century; Paul *Lefèvre,* dermatologist, 20th century] see under *syndrome.*

papilloretinitis (pah-pil″o-ret″ĭ-ni′tis) inflammation of the optic papilla extending to the retina.

papillosphincterotomy (pap″il-lo-sfingk″ter-ot′o-me) surgical division of the sphincter of the major duodenal papilla (Oddi's sphincter).

papillotome (pap″ĭ-lo-tōm″) a cutting instrument for incising the major duodenal papilla.

papillotomy (pap″ĭ-lot′o-me) incision of a papilla, as of the duodenal papilla.

Papin's digester (pah-paz′) [Denis *Papin,* French physicist, 1647–1714] an apparatus for subjecting substances to the action of water at a heat greater than the boiling point.

papovavirus (pap″o-vah-vi′rus) [from *pa*pilloma, *po*lyoma, and *va*cuolating agent + *virus*] any of a group of relatively small, morphologically similar, ether-resistant DNA viruses, many of which are oncogenic or potentially oncogenic; the group includes the papillomaviruses and polyomaviruses.

Pappenheim's stain (pahp′en-hīmz) [Artur *Pappenheim,* German physician, 1870–1916] see *Table of Stains.*

pappose (pap′pōs) having a downy surface.

paprika (pap-re′kah) the fruit of *Capsicum annuum* and a condiment prepared from it; it is rich in vitamin C.

papular (pap′u-lar) [L. *papularis*] consisting of, characterized by, or pertaining to a papule.

papulation (pap″u-la′shun) the production of papules.

papule (pap′ūl) [L. *papula*] a small circumscribed, superficial, solid elevation of the skin. **Gottron's p's,** a cutaneous manifestation pathognomonic of dermatomyositis, consisting of flat-topped violaceous papules on the dorsal aspect of the interphalangeal joints of the hand, which develop central atrophy with hypopigmentation and telangiectasia. Called also *Gottron's sign.* Cf. *Gottron's sign,* def. 1. **moist p., mucous p.,** condyloma acuminatum. **painful piezogenic pedal p's,** piezogenic p's. **pearly penile p's,** numerous white, dome-shaped asymptomatic papules occurring circumferentially around the penile coronal sulcus. Called also *hirsutoid papillomas of penis.* **piezogenic p's,** transitory, noninflammatory, soft, sometimes painful, large papules appearing above the heel on the side of one or both feet, elicited by weight bearing associated with prolonged standing or running, and presumed to result from temporary herniation of fat tissue together with its blood vessels and nerves through connective tissue defects. They disappear when the pressure is removed. Called also *painful fat herniation* and *painful piezogenic pedal p's.* **prurigo p.,** see *prurigo.* **split p's,** fissured papular syphilides sometimes seen at the corners of the mouth.

papuloerythematous (pap″u-lo-er″ĕ-them′ah-tus) marked by papules on an erythematous surface.

papuloid (pap′u-loid) resembling a papule; papular.

papulopustular (pap″u-lo-pus′tu-lar) characterized by the presence of papules and pustules.

papulosis (pap-u-lo′sis) a state marked by the presence of multiple papules. **lymphomatoid p.,** a usually benign, self-healing, recurrent eruption of hemorrhagic papules, clinically quite similar to the lesions of acute lichenoid pityriasis (of which it may be a variant), the lesions of which occur asynchronously primarily on the trunk and extremities, and may involute spontaneously, leaving a macular scar,

or form crusted scales or a central necrotic mass. Histologic features, which may suggest malignancy, include the presence of large clusters of large atypical mononuclear cells with kidney-shaped darkly stained nuclei and large pale histoid cells with large pale-staining ovoid nuclei. **malignant atrophic p.,** an often fatal disease occurring most often in men, characterized by endovasculitis of the skin, gastrointestinal tract, and sometimes other organs, resulting in ischemic infarction of involved tissues. Cutaneous lesions occur in crops of erythematous papules that become umbilicated with characteristic porcelain-white centers with telangiectatic borders, many of which atrophy and leave white scars. Called also *Degos' disease* or *syndrome.*

papulosquamous (pap″u-lo-skwa′mus) both papular and scaly; used to denote a group of dermatoses so characterized, including psoriasis, pityriasis rosea, lichen planus, seborrheic dermatitis, and parapsoriasis.

papulovesicular (pap″u-lo-ve-sik′u-lar) characterized by the presence of papules and vesicles.

papyraceous (pap″ĭ-ra′shus) [L. *papyraceus*] like paper; chartaceous.

par- see *para-*[1].

para (par′ah) [L. *parere* to bring forth, to bear] a woman who has produced viable young regardless of whether the child was living at birth. Used with Roman numerals to designate the number of pregnancies that have resulted in the birth of viable offspring, as *para 0* (none—nullipara), *para I* (one—primipara), *para II* (two—secundipara), *para III* (three—tripara), *para IV* (four—quadripara), etc. The number is not indicative of the number of offspring produced in event of a multiple birth. Cf. *gravida.*

para-[1], **par-** [Gr. *para* to, at, or from the side of] a prefix meaning (a) beside, near, (b) resembling, (c) accessory to, (d) beyond, (e) apart from, (f) abnormal.

para-[2] symbol *p-*; in organic chemistry, a prefix indicating a 1,4-substituted benzene ring, e.g., p-xylene (1,4-dimethylbenzene) or p-nitrophenol (4-nitrophenol).

para-actinomycosis (par″ah-ak″tĭ-no-mi-ko″sis) pseudoactinomycosis.

para-albuminemia (par″ah-al-bu″mĭ-ne′me-ah) bisalbuminemia.

*para-***aminobenzoic acid** *p*-aminobenzoic acid.

para-analgesia (par″ah-an″al-je′ze-ah) analgesia of the lower part of the body, including the lower limbs.

para-anesthesia (par″ah-an″es-the′ze-ah) anesthesia of the lower part of the body and the legs.

para-appendicitis (par″ah-ah-pen″dĭ-si′tis) inflammation of tissues adjacent to the vermiform appendix.

parabanic acid (par″ah-ban′ik) the cyclic anhydride of oxaluric acid, an oxidation product of urea.

Parabasalidea (par″ah-ba″sah-lid′e-ah) a proposed suborder of protozoa (class Zoomastigophorea, subphylum Mastigophora) established to include the closely related orders Trichomonadida and Hypermastigida, all of which are characterized by the presence of an argentophilic parabasal apparatus(es) and typically have at least some basal bodies, with or without flagella.

parabion (par-ab′e-on) parabiont.

parabiont (par-ab′e-ont) [*para-*[1] + Gr. *bioun* to live] one of two or more organisms living in a condition of parabiosis.

parabiosis (par″ah-bi-o′sis) [*para-*[1] + Gr. *biōsis* living] 1. the union of two individuals, as of joined twins, or of experimental animals by surgical operation. 2. temporary suppression of conductivity and excitability in a nerve. **dialytic p.,** the circulation of the blood of two individuals through a dialyzer, separated by a membrane which permits the removal of harmful material from the recipient's blood and the contribution of essential factors from the donor's blood. **vascular p.,** the crossing of the circulation between two individuals by anastomosis of blood vessels.

parabiotic (par″ah-bi-ot′ik) pertaining to or characterized by parabiosis.

parablast (par′ah-blast) [*para-*[1] + Gr. *blastos* germ] that part of the mesoblast from which the blood vessels, lymphatics, etc., are developed.

parablastic (par″ah-blas′tik) pertaining to the parablast.

parablepsia (par-ah-blep′se-ah) [*para-*[1] + Gr. *blepsis* vision + *-ia*] false or perverted vision.

parabulia (par″ah-bu′le-ah) [*para-¹* + Gr. *boulē* will + *-ia*] perversion of the will, as when an individual intends to perform a particular action but halts and substitutes either an opposite action or an unrelated alternative.

paracarbinoxamine (par″ah-kar″bin-ok′sah-min) carbinoxamine.

paracardiac (par″ah-kar′de-ak) beside the heart.

paracarmine (par″ah-kar′min) a staining medium consisting of carminic acid, calcium chloride, and alcohol.

paracasein (par″ah-ka′se-in) the chemical product of the action of rennin on casein; see *casein*.

paracellulose (par″ah-sel′u-lōs) a kind of cellulose found in the pith of plants.

paracelsian (par″ah-sel′se-an) pertaining to or named for Paracelsus.

Paracelsus (par-ah-sel′sus) [Philippus Aureolus Theophrastus Bombastus von Hohenheim] (1493–1541) Swiss physician and alchemist; the "Luther of Medicine," he defied the authority of Galen and Avicenna and condemned all medical teaching not based on experience. His alchemical researches led to the introduction of such substances as lead, sulfur, iron, and arsenic into pharmaceutical chemistry. Although he was far ahead of his time in many of his observations (e.g., on metabolic and on occupational diseases), much of his thinking was made obscure by his mysticism.

paracenesthesia (par″ah-se″nes-the′ze-ah) [*para-¹* + *cenesthesia*] any abnormality of the general sense of well-being.

paracentesis (par″ah-sen-te′sis) [*para-¹* + Gr. *kentēsis* puncture] surgical puncture of the abdominal cavity for the aspiration of peritoneal fluid.

paracentetic (par″ah-sen-tet′ik) pertaining to or accomplished by paracentesis.

paracentral (par″ah-sen′tral) near a center.

paracephalus (par″ah-sef′ah-lus) [*para-¹* + Gr. *kephalē* head] a fetus with a rudimentary or misshapen head, imperfect sense organs, and defective trunk or limbs.

paracerebellar (par″ah-ser″ĕ-bel′ar) pertaining to the lateral part of the cerebellum.

paracervix (par″ah-ser′viks) [*para-¹* + L. *cervix* neck] [NA] the inferior part of the parametrium.

paracetaldehyde (par-as″et-al′de-hīd) paraldehyde.

paracetamol (par-as″et-am′ol) acetaminophen.

parachloralose (par″ah-klo′ral-ōs) a substance, $C_8H_{12}Cl_3O_6$, in iridescent plates, formed by a combination of dextrose and chloral.

parachloramine (par″ah-klōr′ah-men) meclizine.

parachlorophenol (par″ah-klo″ro-fe′nol) [USP] chemical name: 4-chlorophenol. An antibacterial, C_6H_5ClO, occurring as white to pink crystals, effective against most gram-negative organisms; used as a topical anti-infective. **camphorated p.** [USP], a preparation of 33 to 37 per cent parachlorophenol and 63 to 67 per cent camphor; used as a dental anti-infective, applied topically to the root canals and the periapical region.

paracholera (par″ah-kol′er-ah) a disease resembling Asiatic cholera, but caused by an organism other than the *Vibrio cholerae*.

paracholesterin (par″ah-ko-les′ter-in) a form of sterol occurring in vegetable tissue, probably related to sitosterol or phytosterol.

parachordal (par″ah-kor′dal) [*para-¹* + Gr. *chordē* cord] situated beside the notochord; see *parachordal cartilages*, under *cartilage*.

Parachordodes (par″ah-kor-do′dēz) a genus of Gordiacea. A few cases of infection with this worm have been reported. *P. pustilo′sus*, from Italy. *P. tolosa′nus*, from France and from Italy. *P. viola′ceus*, from Italy, one specimen taken from the throat.

parachromatin (par″ah-kro′mah-tin) a chromatophil substance contained in the finer part of the nuclear substance, as in the nucleoplasm of the spindle in karyokinesis.

parachromatism (par″ah-kro′mah-tizm) dichromasy.

parachromatopsia (par″ah-kro″mah-top′se-ah) dichromasy.

paracinesia (par″ah-si-ne′se-ah) parakinesia.

paracinesis (par″ah-si-ne′sis) parakinesia.

paraclinical (par″ah-klin′ĭ-k′l) pertaining to abnormalities (e.g., morphological or biochemical) underlying clinical manifestations (e.g., chest pain or fever).

paracnemis, paracnemidion (par″ak-ne′mis; par″ak-ne-mid′e-on) [*para-¹* + Gr. *knēmē* shin] the fibula.

Paracoccidioides brasiliensis (par″ah-kok-sid″e-oi′dēz brah-sil″e-en′sis) an imperfect fungus of the family Moniliaceae, order Moniliales, which is the etiologic agent of paracoccidioidomycosis. The organisms proliferate multiple budding yeast cells in the tissues, and produce white aerial mycelia and single or double conidia in media at 25° C. or in soil. Called also *Blastomyces brasiliensis*.

paracoccidioidomycosis (par″ah-kok-sid″e-oi″do-mi-ko′sis) an often fatal infection caused by *Paracoccidioides brasiliensis*. The primary infection begins in the lungs and spreads to the mucocutaneous areas, particularly the buccal mucosa, and may extend to the adjacent skin, tonsils, gastrointestinal lymphatics, liver, and spleen. Called also *Almeida's* or *Lutz-Splendore-Almeida disease*, *Brazilian* or *South American blastomycosis*, and *paracoccidioidal granuloma*.

Paracoccus (par″ah-kok′us) [*para-¹* + Gr. *kokkos* berry] a genus of gram-negative coccoid bacteria of uncertain affiliation, found in soil, made up of chemo-organotrophic cells. The type species is *P. denitri′ficans*.

paracolitis (par″ah-ko-li′tis) inflammation of the outer coat of the colon.

Paracolobactrum (par″ah-ko″lo-bak′trum) in former systems of classification, a genus of bacteria made up of nonlactose-fermenting coliform organisms that are now assigned to various other genera.

paracolpitis (par″ah-kol-pi′tis) [*para-¹* + Gr. *kolpos* vagina + *-itis*] inflammation of the tissues around the vagina.

paracolpium (par″ah-kol′pe-um) [*para-* + Gr. *kolpos* vagina] the connective and other tissues that surround the vagina.

paracone (par′ah-kōn) [*para-¹* + Gr. *kōnos* cone] the mesiobuccal cusp of a maxillary tooth of mammals, which normally occludes between the paraconid and hypoconid of the respective lower molar.

paraconid (par″ah-ko′nid) the mesiobuccal cusp of a mandibular molar tooth.

paracortex (par″ah-kor′teks) [*para-¹* + *cortex*] thymus-dependent area.

paracousis (par″ah-koo′sis) paracusis.

paracoxalgia (par″ah-kok-sal′je-ah) a condition marked by pain simulating that of coxitis.

paracresol (par″ah-kre′sol) 1. one of the three isomeric forms or recognized varieties of cresol; see *cresol*. 2. a patented soluble and nearly odorless preparation of cresol: disinfectant.

paracrine (par′ah-krin) [*para-¹* + Gr. *krinein* to separate] 1. denoting a type of hormone function in which hormone synthesized in and released from endocrine cells binds to its receptor in nearby cells and affects their function. 2. denoting the secretion of a hormone by an organ other than an endocrine gland.

paracrystals (par″ah-kris′tals) imperfect crystals, such as the "crystals" of tobacco mosaic virus, which have only two dimensional symmetry instead of three dimensional.

paracusia (par-ah-ku′se-ah) paracusis. **p. a′cris,** intense and incessant acuity of hearing. **p. duplica′ta,** diplacusis. **p. lo′ci,** inability to locate correctly the origin of sounds. **p. willisia′na,** paracusis of Willis.

paracusis (par″ah-ku′sis) any perversion of the sense of hearing. **p. of Willis,** ability to hear best in a loud din (Thomas Willis, 1672).

paracyesis (par″ah-si-e′sis) [*para-¹* + Gr. *kyēsis* pregnancy] (*obs.*) ectopic pregnancy.

paracystic (par″ah-sis′tik) [*para-¹* + Gr. *kystis* bladder] situated near the bladder.

paracystitis (par″ah-sis-ti′tis) [*para-¹* + Gr. *kystis* bladder + *-itis*] inflammation of the tissues around the bladder.

paracystium (par″ah-sis′te-um) [*para-¹* + Gr. *kystis* bladder] the connective and other tissues around the bladder.

paracytic (par″ah-sit′ik) [*para-¹* + *-cyte*] denoting cell elements present in the blood or other part of the organism, but enthetic or not normal to it.

paradental (par″ah-den′tal) 1. having some connection

with or relation to the science or practice of dentistry. 2. periodontal.

paradentitis (par″ah-den-ti′tis) periodontitis.

paradentium (par″ah-den′she-um) periodontium, def. 1.

paradentosis (par″ah-den-to′sis) juvenile periodontitis.

paraderm (par′ah-derm) [para-¹ + Gr. *derma* skin] the part of the vitellus of the ovum that furnishes cells which contribute to the body of the embryo.

paradesmose (par″ah-des′mōs) [para-¹ + Gr. *desmos* band, ligament] the connection between extranuclear centrioles during mitosis in certain protozoa; see *desmose*.

paradidymal (par″ah-did′ĭ-mal) 1. pertaining to the paradidymis. 2. beside the testis.

paradidymis (par″ah-did′ĭ-mis) [para-¹ + Gr. *didymos* testis] [NA] a body made up of a few convoluted tubules in the anterior part of the spermatic cord, considered to be a remnant of the mesonephros; called also *organ of Giraldés′, parepididymis,* and *massa innominata.*

paradimethylaminobenzaldehyde (par″ah-di-meth″il-am″ĭ-no-ben-zal′de-hīd) white or pale yellow crystals or crystalline powder, (CH₃)₂NC₆H₄CHO, used in the preparation of Ehrlich's aldehyde reagent and in the determination of urobilinogen and porphobilinogen.

Paradione (par″ah-di′ōn) trademark for preparations of paramethadione.

paradiphenylbiuret (par″ah-di-fen″il-bi′u-ret) a substance, NH(CO·NH·C₆H₄OH)₂, transformed into benzoic acid in the body.

paradipsia (par″ah-dip′se-ah) [para-¹ + Gr. *dipsa* thirst + -ia] a perverted appetite for fluids, which are ingested without relation to bodily need.

paradox (par′ah-doks) [Gr. *paradoxos* incredible] a statement which seems to be, though it may not be, absurd or self-contradictory. **Opie p.,** necrotizing local anaphylaxis sometimes acts as a specific protective mechanism. **Weber's p.,** the elongation of a muscle which has been so stretched that it cannot contract.

paradoxical (par″ah-dok′se-kal) occurring at variance with the normal rule.

paradysentery (par″ah-dis′en-ter″e) a diarrhea resembling mild dysentery; see *Shigella flexneri.*

paraeccrisis (par″ah-ek′rĭ-sis) [para-¹ + Gr. *ekkrisis* excretion] disordered secretion or excretion.

paraepilepsy (par″ah-ep′ĭ-lep-se) minor focal epilepsy.

paraequilibrium (par″ah-e″kwĭ-lib′re-um) vertigo due to disturbance of the vestibular apparatus of the ear.

paraesophageal (par″ah-ĕ-sof″ah-je′al) alongside, near, or about the esophagus.

parafalx (par″ah-falks′) situated near the falx cerebri or falx cerebelli.

Par. aff. abbreviation for L. *pars affec′ta,* the part affected.

paraffin (par′ah-fin) [L. *parum* little + *affinis* akin] 1. [NF] a purified mixture of solid hydrocarbons obtained from petroleum, occurring as an odorless, tasteless, colorless or white, more or less translucent mass; used as a stiffening agent in pharmaceutical preparations. 2. alkane. **chlorinated p.,** paraffin which has been reacted with chlorine to replace some of the hydrogen atoms with chlorine atoms. **hard p.,** paraffin which has a high melting point. **liquid p.,** mineral oil. **liquid p., light,** light mineral oil. **soft p., white,** white petrolatum. **soft p., yellow,** petrolatum.

paraffinoma (par″ah-fĭ-no′mah) a chronic granuloma produced by prolonged continuous exposure to the irritation of paraffin.

Parafilaria multipapillosa (par″ah-fĭ-la′re-ah mul″te-pap″ĭ-lo′sah) a parasitic worm causing dermatorrhagia parasitica.

Paraflex (par′ah-fleks) trademark for a preparation of chlorzoxazone.

paraflocculus (par″ah-flok′u-lus) [para-¹ + L. *flocculus* tuft] a small lobe of the cerebellar hemisphere located immediately cranial to the flocculus, which sometimes forms a prominent part of the cerebellum; called also *accessory flocculus.*

paraformaldehyde (par″ah-for-mal′de-hīd) a white, crystalline polymer of formaldehyde.

Parafossarulus (par″ah-fos-sar′u-lus) a genus of freshwater snails. **P. manchou′ricus,** a species found throughout the Orient that is the foremost intermediate host of *Opisthorchis sinensis* in Japan and the second most important in China, and also a carrier of *Opisthorchis felineus* and *Echinochasmus perfoliatus.*

parafunction (par″ah-funk″shun) disordered or perverted function.

parafunctional (par″ah-funk′shun-al) characterized by perverted or abnormal function.

paragammacism (par″ah-gam′ah-sizm) [para-¹ + Gr. *gamma,* the Greek letter G] the faulty utterance of *g, k,* and *ch* sounds.

paraganglia (par″ah-gang′gle-ah) plural of *paraganglion.*

paraganglioma (par″ah-gang″gle-o′mah) a tumor of the tissue composing the paraganglia. **medullary p.,** pheochromocytoma. **nonchromaffin p.,** chemodectoma.

paraganglion (par″ah-gang′gle-on), pl. *paragan′glia.* A collection of chromaffin cells, which are derived from neural ectoderm, occurring outside of the adrenal medulla, most commonly near the sympathetic ganglia and in relation to the aorta and its branches. Most, if not all, of the paraganglia secrete epinephrine (or norepinephrine). Called also *chromaffin* or *pheochrome bodies.*

paragelatose (par″ah-jel′ah-tōs) a substance obtained by boiling gelatin.

paragenitalis (par″ah-jen″ĭ-ta′lis) [para-¹ + L. *genitalis* genital] 1. in lower vertebrates, the urinary part of the mesonephros, caudal to the genital part. 2. in higher animals, the paradidymis or paraoophoron.

parageusia (par″ah-gu′se-ah) [para-¹ + Gr. *geusis* taste + -ia] 1. perversion of the sense of taste. 2. a bad taste in the mouth.

parageusic (par″ah-gu′sik) pertaining to or characterized by parageusia.

paragnathus (par-ag′nah-thus) [para-¹ + Gr. *gnathos* jaw] 1. a fetus with a supernumerary jaw. 2. a parasitic fetus attached laterally to the jaw of the autosite.

paragnosis (par″ag-no′sis) [para-¹ + Gr. *gnōsis* knowledge] diagnosis, after death, based on contemporaneous accounts of the diseases which affected historical characters.

paragonimiasis (par″ah-gon″ĭ-mi′ah-sis) the state of being infected with flukes of the genus *Paragonimus.* See individual species.

paragonimosis (par″ah-gon″ĭ-mo′sis) paragonimiasis.

Paragonimus (par″ah-gon′ĭ-mus) [para-¹ + Gr. *gonimos* productive; having generative power] a genus of trematode parasites; they have two invertebrate hosts, the first a snail (*Semisulcospira,* etc.) and the second a crab or crayfish (*Potamon, Eriocheir,* etc.). **P. africa′nus,** a species of the Congo and Cameroons that parasitizes man and carnivores. **P. heterotre′ma,** a species infecting man in Thailand and China. **P. kellicot′ti,** a species closely allied to *P. westermani,* found in cats, dogs, and hogs in the United States. **P. rin′geri,** *P. westermani.* **P. westerman′i,** the lung fluke, an oval or pear-shaped fluke of a pinkish or reddish brown color, found in cysts in the lungs and sometimes in the pleura, liver, abdominal cavity, and elsewhere. It causes the disease known as parasitic or oriental hemoptysis. It occurs especially in Asiatic countries, and infects lower animals as well as man; infection is acquired through ingestion of infected freshwater crabs or crayfish. Called also *Distoma westermani, D. ringeri,* and *D. pulmonale.*

Paragordius (par″ah-gor′de-us) a genus of the class Nematomorpha. Human infection with *P. cinctus, P. tricuspidatus,* and *P. varius* has been reported.

paragrammatism (par″ah-gram′ah-tizm) impairment of speech, with confusion in the use and order of words and grammatical forms.

paragranuloma (par″ah-gran′u-lo′mah) the most benign form of Hodgkin's disease, which is largely confined to the lymph nodes.

paragraphia (par″ah-gra′fe-ah) [para-¹ + Gr. *graphein* to write + -ia] a disorder in which the patient makes mistakes in spelling or writes one word in place of another.

parahemophilia (par″ah-he″mo-fil′e-ah) a hemorrhagic tendency due to deficiency of coagulation Factor V; it varies greatly in intensity and is inherited as an autosomal recessive trait.

parahepatic (par″ah-he-pat′ik) [*para-¹* + Gr. *hēpar* liver] beside the liver.

parahepatitis (par″ah-hep″ah-ti′tis) perihepatitis.

parahormone (par″ah-hor′mōn) [*para-¹* + *hormone*] a substance, not conventionally accepted as a true hormone, which has a hormone-like action in controlling the functioning of some distant organ.

parahypnosis (par″ah-hip-no′sis) [*para-¹* + Gr. *hypnos* sleep] abnormal sleep, as in general anesthesia.

parahypophysis (par″ah-hi-pof′ĭ-sis) an accessory pituitary body.

parakeratosis (par″ah-ker″ah-to′sis) persistence of the nuclei of the keratinocytes into the stratum corneum (horny layer) of the skin. Parakeratosis is normal in the epithelium of true mucous membrane of the mouth and vagina. **p. ostra′cea,** p. scutularis. **p. scutula′ris,** an extremely rare disease of the legs and scalp marked by the formation of hard, cuplike or shieldlike crusts which envelop the hairs and send up incrustations around the hairs. Called also *p. ostracea.* **p. variega′ta,** retiform parapsoriasis.

parakinesia (par″ah-ki-ne′se-ah) [*para-¹* + Gr. *kinēsis* motion + *-ia*] perversion of motor function resulting in strange and unnatural movements. In ophthalmology, irregular action of an individual ocular muscle.

parakinetic (par″ah-ki-net′ik) pertaining to or characterized by parakinesia.

Paral (pah-ral′) trademark for preparations of paraldehyde.

paralalia (par″ah-la′le-ah) [*para-¹* + Gr. *lalia* speech] any disturbance of the faculty of speech, especially the production of a vocal sound different from the one desired, or the substitution in speech of one letter for another. **p. litera′lis,** impairment of the power to utter the sounds of certain letters.

paralambdacism (par″ah-lam′dah-sizm) [*para-¹* + Gr. *lambdakismos*] the faulty utterance of *l* sounds, or the substitution of other sounds for *l.*

paralbumin (par″al-bu′min) [*para-¹* + *albumin*] an albumin or protein substance found in ovarian cysts.

paraldehyde (par-al′dĕ-hīd) [USP] chemical name: 2,4,6-trimethyl-1,3,5-trioxane. A polymerization product of acetaldehyde, $C_6H_{12}O$, occurring as a colorless, transparent liquid and having rapid-acting sedative and hypnotic properties; used to control insomnia, excitement, agitation, delirium, and convulsions, administered rectally and intramuscularly and by intravenous infusion.

paraldehydism (par-al′de-hīd″izm) a condition produced by excessive use of paraldehyde; paraldehyde poisoning.

paralepsy (par′ah-lep″se) psycholepsy.

paralexia (par″ah-lek′se-ah) [*para-¹* + *alexia*] impairment of the power of reading, marked by the transposition of words and syllables into meaningless combinations.

paralexic (par″ah-lek′sik) pertaining to or affected with paralexia.

paralgesia (par″al-je′se-ah) [*para-¹* + Gr. *algesis* sense of pain + *-ia*] any condition marked by abnormal and painful sensations; a painful paresthesia.

paralgesic (par″al-je′sik) pertaining to or affected with paralgesia.

paralgia (par-al′je-ah) paralgesia.

paralinin (par″ah-li′nin) [*para-¹* + *linin*] karyolymph.

parallactic (par″ah-lak′tik) pertaining to parallax.

parallagma (par″ah-lag′mah) [Gr.] displacement of a bone or of the fragments of a broken bone.

parallax (par′ah-laks) [Gr. "change of position"] an apparent displacement of an object due to a change in the observer's position. **binocular p.,** the seeming difference in position of an object as seen separately by one eye and then by the other, the head remaining stationary. **crossed p.,** binocular parallax occurring in exophoria; when one eye is covered, the object viewed seems to move away from the open eye and toward the covered eye. **direct p.,** binocular parallax occurring in esophoria; when one eye is covered, the object viewed seems to move toward the open eye and away from the covered eye. **heteronymous p.,** crossed p. **homonymous p.,** direct p. **ste-**

reoscopic p., binocular p. **uncrossed p.,** direct p. **vertical p.,** binocular parallax occurring in vertical diplopia or heterophoria; the object seen seems to move vertically when each eye is closed in turn.

parallel (par′ah-lel) [L. *parallelus*] 1. pertaining to straight lines or planes that do not intersect. 2. pertaining to electric circuit components connected "in parallel" so that the current flow divides, each branch passing through one component, and rejoins; applied by extension to any similar parallel circuit, e.g., the systemic circulation to the various organs. Cf. *series.*

parallelometer (par″ah-lel-om′ĕ-ter) [*parallel* + *-meter*] an instrument for determining the exact parallel relationships of lines, surfaces, and structures in dental prostheses and casts.

parallergic (par″ah-ler′jik) pertaining to or marked by parallergy.

parallergy (par-al′er-je) a condition in which an allergic state, produced by specific sensitization, predisposes the body to react to other allergens with clinical manifestations that differ from the original reaction.

paralogia (par″ah-lo′je-ah) [*para-¹* + Gr. *logos* reason + *-ia*] evasion. **thematic p.,** evasion limited to one subject, on which the mind dwells insistently.

paralogism (pah-ral′o-jizm) the use of meaningless or illogical language by the psychotic.

paralogy (pah-ral′o-je) anatomical similarity that has no phylogenetic or functional implication.

paralyses (pah-ral′ĭ-sēz) plural of *paralysis.*

paralysis (pah-ral′ĭ-sis), pl. *paral′yses* [*para-¹* + Gr. *lyein* to loosen] loss or impairment of motor function in a part due to lesion of the neural or muscular mechanism; also, by analogy, impairment of sensory function (sensory paralysis). In addition to the types named below, paralysis is further distinguished as *traumatic, syphilitic, toxic,* etc., according to its cause; or as *obturator, ulnar,* etc., according to the nerve, part, or muscle specially affected. For other varieties, see also under *hemiplegia, palsy, paraplegia,* and *paresis.* **abducens p.,** paralysis of the external rectus muscle of the eye due to lesion of the abducens nerve, with internal strabismus and diplopia. **abducens-facial p., congenital,** Möbius' syndrome. **p. of accommodation,** paralysis of the ciliary muscles so as to prevent accommodation of the eye. **acoustic p.,** nerve deafness. **acute ascending spinal p.,** acute febrile polyneuritis. **acute atrophic p.,** see *poliomyelitis.* **acute bulbar p.,** bulbar paralysis usually caused by acute vascular lesions of the brain, most commonly hemorrhage or thrombosis; called also *acute bulbar polioencephalitis.* **acute infectious p.,** epidemic poliomyelitis. **acute wasting p.,** see *poliomyelitis.* **p. ag′itans,** a form of parkinsonism of unknown etiology usually occurring in late life, although a juvenile form has been described. It is a slowly progressive disease characterized by masklike facies, a characteristic tremor of resting muscles, a slowing of voluntary movements, a festinating gait, peculiar posture, and weakness of the muscles. There may be excessive sweating and feelings of heat. Pathologically, there is degeneration within the nuclear masses of the extrapyramidal system and a characteristic loss of melanin-containing cells from the substantia nigra and a corresponding reduction in dopamine levels in the corpus striatum. Called also *Parkinson's disease* and *shaking palsy.* **p. ag′itans, juvenile (of Hunt),** a condition developing in early life, usually familial but occasionally occurring sporadically, marked by increased muscle tonus with the characteristic attitude and facies of paralysis agitans, due to progressive degeneration of the globus pallidus; involvement of the substantia nigra and pyramidal tracts may occur. Called also *paleostriatal syndrome, pallidal atrophy, pallidal syndrome,* and *Ramsay Hunt syndrome.* **alcoholic p.,** paralysis caused by habitual drunkenness. **alternate p., alternating p.,** alternate hemiplegia. **ambiguo-accessorius p.,** Schmidt's syndrome. **ambiguo-accessorius-hypoglossal p.,** Jackson's syndrome. **ambiguohypoglossal p.,** Tapia's syndrome. **ambiguospinothalamic p.,** Avellis' syndrome. **anesthesia p.,** paralysis following anesthesia. **anterior spinal p.,** anterior poliomyelitis. **arsenical p.,** paralysis due to arsenical poisoning. **ascending p.,** spinal paralysis that progresses cephalad. **association p.,** bulbar p. **asthenic bulbar p.,** myasthenia gravis pseudoparalytica.

asthenobulbospinal p., myasthenia gravis. **atrophic spinal p.,** anterior poliomyelitis. **Avellis's p.,** see under *syndrome*. **Bell's p.,** see under *palsy.* **bilateral p.,** diplegia; paralysis on both sides. **birth p.,** paralysis due to injury received at birth. **brachial p.,** paralysis of an arm from lesion of the brachial plexus; see *Erb-Duchenne p.* and *Klumpke-Dejerine p.* **brachiofacial p.,** paralysis affecting the face and an arm. **Brown-Séquard's p.,** 1. Brown-Séquard's syndrome. 2. a flaccid paralysis seen in disorders of the urinary tract. **bulbar p.,** paralysis due to changes in the motor centers of the medulla oblongata; a chronic, usually fatal disease, most commonly affecting persons over 50 years old but also occurring in the course of amyotrophic lateral sclerosis, syringobulbia, and multiple sclerosis. It is marked by progressive paralysis and atrophy of the muscles of the lips, tongue, mouth, pharynx, and larynx, and is due to degeneration of the nerve nuclei of the floor of the fourth ventricle. Called also *labioglossopharyngeal p., labioglossolaryngeal p.,* and *Duchenne's p.* **bulbospinal p.,** myasthenia gravis. **cage p.,** a complex nutritional deficiency sometimes seen in captive primates, which is said to resemble osteomalacia. **central p.,** any paralysis due to a lesion of the brain or spinal cord. **centrocapsular p.,** that which is due to lesions of the internal capsule. **cerebral p.,** any paralysis due to an intracranial lesion; see *cerebral palsy*, under *palsy.* **Chastek p.,** progressive ataxia and paralysis in silver foxes due to thiamine deficiency following the substitution of raw fish for meat in the diet. **circumflex p.,** paralysis of the circumflex nerve. **complete p.,** entire loss of motion, sensation, and function. **compression p.,** paralysis caused by pressure on a nerve, as by a crutch or during sleep. **congenital abducens-facial p.,** Möbius syndrome. **congenital oculofacial p.,** Möbius syndrome. **conjugate p.,** loss of ability to perform some of the parallel ocular movements. **cortical p.,** paralysis dependent upon a lesion of the brain cortex. **crossed p., cruciate p.,** paralysis affecting one side of the face and the opposite side of the body. **crural p.,** that which chiefly affects the thigh or thighs. **crutch p.,** paralysis of one or both arms, due to pressure of the crutch in the axilla. **Cruveilhier's p.,** progressive muscular atrophy. **decubitus p.,** paralysis due to pressure on a nerve from lying for a long time in one position. **Dejerine-Klumpke p.,** Klumpke's p. **diaphragmatic p.,** unilateral paralysis of the diaphragm. **diphtheric p., diphtheritic p.,** a partial paralysis which often follows diphtheria, chiefly affecting the soft palate and throat muscles. **divers' p.,** paralysis occurring in deep-sea divers as a result of too rapid reduction of pressure. **Duchenne's p.,** 1. bulbar paralysis. 2. Erb-Duchenne paralysis. **Duchenne-Erb p.,** Erb-Duchenne p. **epidemic infantile p.,** epidemic poliomyelitis. **Erb's p.,** 1. Erb-Duchenne paralysis. 2. Erb's spastic paraplegia. 3. pseudohypertrophic muscular dystrophy. **Erb-Duchenne p.,** the upper-arm type of brachial paralysis; paralysis of the upper roots of brachial plexus due to destruction of the fifth and sixth cervical roots and characterized by absence of involvement of the small hand muscles. **essential p.,** see *poliomyelitis.* **facial p.,** weakening or paralysis of the facial nerve, as in Bell's palsy. **false p.,** pseudoparalysis. **familial periodic p.,** periodic p. **Felton's p.,** see under *phenomenon.* **Féréol-Graux p.,** see under *palsy.* **flaccid p.,** paralysis with loss of tone of the muscles of the paralyzed part and absence of tendon reflexes. Cf. *spastic p.* **fowl p.,** Marek's disease. **functional p.,** a temporary paralysis which is apparently not caused by a nerve lesion. **p. of gaze,** paralysis due to pathological processes which implicate the supranuclear oculomotor centers or pathways and result in either lateral or vertical gaze paralysis. **general p., general p. of the insane,** see under *paresis.* **ginger p.,** Jamaica ginger p. **glossolabial p., glossopharyngolabial p.,** bulbar p. **Gubler's p.,** Millard-Gubler syndrome. **hereditary cerebrospinal p.,** (hemiplegia, diplegia, paraplegia, or tetraplegia), a hereditary condition which develops usually in early middle life, characterized by gradually developing paralyses which may be manifest in the upper or lower extremities, in the two extremities, or one side, or in all four extremities. **histrionic p.,** paralysis of certain muscles of the face, producing a facial expression of some emotion. **hyperkalemic periodic p.,** see *familial periodic p.* **hypoglossal p.,** paralysis due to a lesion of the hypoglossal nucleus or the hypoglossal nerve at any point.

hypokalemic periodic p., see *familial periodic p.* **hysterical p.,** apparent loss of power of movement in a part, in the absence of an organic neurological cause. **immune p., immunologic p.,** immunologic unresponsiveness induced by administration of large doses of antigen; now called *immunologic tolerance.* **incomplete p.,** partial paralysis or paresis. **Indian bow p.,** paralysis of the thyroarytenoid muscles. **infantile p.,** see *poliomyelitis.* **infantile, cerebral, ataxic p.,** a condition which is dependent upon faulty development of the frontal regions of the brain, is present at birth, affects all extremities, and is not definitely progressive; called also *diataxia infantilis cerebralis* and *cerebral diataxia.* **infantile cerebrocerebellar diplegic p.,** a condition developing in infants, affecting all extremities, and due to combined failure of development or destruction of the reciprocating portions of the cerebrum and the cerebellum. **infantile spastic p.,** cerebral palsy. **infantile spinal p.,** spinal paralytic poliomyelitis. **infectious bulbar p.,** pseudorabies. **ischemic p.,** local paralysis due to an impairment of the circulation, as in certain cases of embolism or thrombosis; called also *Volkmann's ischemic paralysis.* **jake p.,** Jamaica ginger p. **Jamaica ginger p.,** paralysis of the extremities, especially of the legs, following the use of Jamaica ginger as a beverage; called also *jake paralysis, jake neuritis, ginger paralysis, Jamaica ginger polyneuritis.* **juvenile p.,** general paralysis in young persons. **Klumpke's p., Klumpke-Dejerine p.,** the lower-arm type of brachial paralysis; atrophic paralysis of the muscles of the arm and hand, from lesion of the eighth cervical and first dorsal nerves. It often occurs in infants delivered by breech extraction. **Kussmaul's p., Kussmaul-Landry p.,** acute febrile polyneuritis. **labial p., labioglossolaryngeal p., labioglossopharyngeal p.,** bulbar p. **lambing p.,** pregnancy toxemia in ewes. **Landry's p.,** acute febrile polyneuritis. **laryngeal p.,** paralysis of one of the laryngeal muscles. **lead p.,** paralysis caused by lead poisoning, due to a peripheral neuritis, and marked by wrist-drop. **lingual p.,** paralysis of the tongue. **Lissauer's p.,** an apoplectiform type of dementia paralytica. **local p.,** paralysis of one muscle or of a group of muscles. **masticatory p.,** paralysis of the muscles of mastication. **medullary tegmental p's,** paralyses due to lesions of the medullary tegmentum: they include alternate hemiplegia, Tapia's syndrome, syndrome of Babinski-Nageotte, and Cestan's syndrome. **Millard-Gubler p.,** see under *syndrome.* **mimetic p.,** paralysis of the facial muscles. **mixed p.,** combined motor and sensory paralysis. **motor p.,** paralysis of voluntary muscles. **musculospiral p.,** paralysis of the extensor muscles of the wrist and fingers, most often due to compression of the musculospiral (radial) nerve, and, depending upon the site of the nerve injury, sometimes accompanied by weakness of extension of the elbow; called also *radial p.* and *Saturday night palsy.* **myopathic p.,** paralysis due to disease of the muscle itself. **narcosis p.,** paralysis during anesthesia, caused by pressure, cold, curare, etc. **normokalemic periodic p.,** see *familial periodic p.* **p. notario'rum,** writers' cramp. **nuclear p.,** any paralysis due to a lesion in a nucleus of origin. **obstetric p.,** birth p. **ocular p.,** see *amaurosis, cycloplegia,* and *ophthalmoplegia.* **oculofacial p., congenital,** Möbius' syndrome. **oculomotor p.,** paralysis of the oculomotor nerve. **organic p.,** paralysis due to lesion of nerve tissue. **parotitic p.,** paralysis accompanying mumps. **parturient p.,** milk fever, def. 4. **periodic p., familial,** an autosomal dominant trait marked by recurring attacks of rapidly progressive flaccid paralysis; there are three types: *I,* associated with a fall in serum potassium levels (*hypokalemic periodic p.*); *II,* associated with a rise therein (*hyperkalemic periodic p.;* called also *adynamia episodica hereditaria*); and *III,* with normal levels (*normokalemic periodic p.*). **peripheral p.,** loss of power due to some lesion of the nervous mechanism between the nucleus of origin and the muscle. **peroneal p.,** crossed leg palsy. **phonetic p.,** paralysis of the muscles of speech. **postdiphtheric p.,** diphtheric paralysis. **posthemiplegic p.,** residual weakness after a stroke. **posticus p.,** paralysis of the posterior cricothyroid muscle. **Pott's p.,** see under *paraplegia.* **pressure p.,** paralysis, generally temporary, caused by pressure on a nerve trunk. **progressive bulbar p.,** see *bulbar p.* **pseudobulbar p.,** spastic weakness of the muscles innervated by the cranial nerves, i.e., the muscles of the face, pharynx, and tongue, due to bilateral lesions of the corticospinal tract; it is often accompanied by uncontrolled weeping or laughing. Called also *supranuclear p.* and *spastic bulbar palsy*. **pseudohypertrophic muscular p.**, see under *dystrophy*. **radial p.**, 1. musculospiral p. 2. a condition usually affecting horses, but also other domestic animals, in which paralysis of certain muscles of the shoulder and knee occurs as a result of injury to the radial nerve. Called also *dropped elbow*. **Ramsay Hunt p.**, juvenile paralysis agitans. **range p.**, Marek's disease. **reflex p.**, one ascribable to peripheral irritation; in some cases secondary changes occur in the spinal cord, and the paralysis ceases to be truly reflex. **Remak's p.**, paralysis of the extensor muscles of the fingers and wrist; called also *Remak's type*. **rucksack p.**, a disorder of motor and sensory function of the upper extremities as a result of damage to the brachial plexus caused by the wearing of a backpack. **Saturday night p.**, musculospiral p. **sensory p.**, loss of sensation resulting from a morbid process. **serum p.**, peripheral nerve paralysis following administration of serum. **sleep p.**, paralysis occurring at awakening or sleep onset; extension of sleep atonia into the waking state. **spastic p.**, paralysis marked by spasticity of the muscles of the paralyzed part and increased tendon reflexes, due to upper motor neuron lesions. Cf. *flaccid p.* **spastic spinal p.**, lateral sclerosis of the spinal cord. **spinomuscular p.**, paralysis due to lesion of the gray matter of the spinal cord, or the nerves originating therefrom. **supranuclear p.**, pseudobulbar p. **tick p.**, a progressive ascending flaccid motor paralysis which follows the bite of certain ticks (*Dermacentor andersoni.*) in children and in domestic animals in Oregon, British Columbia, and other parts of the world. A similar paralysis sometimes follows the bites of species of *Ixodes, Haemaphysalis,* and *Rhipicephalus.* **Todd's p.**, postepileptic hemiplegia or monoplegia lasting for a few minutes or hours, or occasionally for several days, after the epileptic attack. **trigeminal p.**, paralysis due to a lesion of the trigeminal (fifth) nerve, marked by sensory loss in the face and weakness of the muscles of mastication. **p. vacil'lans**, chorea. **vasomotor p.**, cessation of vasomotor control. **Volkmann's ischemic p.**, ischemic p. **waking p.**, a form of hypnogogic helplessness that follows waking, especially in some cases of narcolepsy. **wasting p.**, spinal muscular atrophy. **Weber's p.**, see under *syndrome*. **writers' p.**, writers' cramp.

paralysor (par'ah-līz''or) paralyzer.

paralyssa (par''ah-lis'ah) paralytic rabies.

paralytic (par''ah-lit'ik) [Gr. *paralytikos*] 1. affected with or pertaining to paralysis. 2. a person affected with paralysis.

paralytogenic (par''ah-lit''o-jen'ik) causing paralysis.

paralyzant (par''ah-līz''ant) 1. causing paralysis. 2. an agent that paralyzes.

paralyze (par'ah-līz) to put into a state of paralysis.

paralyzer (par'ah-līz''er) a substance which hinders or prevents a chemical reaction; an inhibitor.

paramagnetic (par''ah-mag-net'ik) characterized by or exhibiting paramagnetism.

paramagnetism (par''ah-mag'ne-tizm) [*para-¹* + Gr. *magnēs* magnet] the property of being attracted by a magnet, and of assuming a position parallel to that of a magnetic force, but not of becoming permanently magnetized.

paramastigote (par''ah-mas'tǐ-gōt) [*para-¹* + Gr. *mastix* lash] having an accessory flagellum by the side of a larger one.

paramastitis (par''ah-mas-ti'tis) [*para-¹* + Gr. *mastos* mamma + *-itis*] inflammation of the tissues around the mammary gland.

paramastoid (par''ah-mas'toid) near the mastoid process.

paramastoiditis (par''ah-mas'toid-i'tis) inflammation of the temporal bone in mastoiditis.

parameatal (par''ah-me-a'tal) situated near or around a meatus.

paramecia (par''ah-me'she-ah) plural of *paramecium*.

Paramecium (par''ah-me'she-um) [Gr. *paramēkēs* oblong] a genus of ovoid or elongated freshwater protozoa (suborder Peniculina, order Hymenostomatida), some species of which are visible to the naked eye. Certain species have been used as test organisms in cytological, genetic, and other research.

paramecium (par''ah-me'she-um), pl. *parame'cia*. An organism belonging to the genus *Paramecium*.

paramedian (par''ah-me'de-an) [*para-¹* + L. *medianus* median] situated near the midline or midplane.

paramedical (par''ah-med'ǐ-kal) having some connection with or relation to the science or practice of medicine; adjunctive to the practice of medicine in the maintenance or restoration of health and normal functioning. Paramedical workers include physical, occupational, and speech therapists, medical social workers, pharmacists, technicians, and so on.

paramenia (par''ah-me'ne-ah) [*para-¹* + Gr. *mēniaia* menses] disordered or difficult menstruation.

parameniscitis (par''ah-me-nǐ-si'tis) inflammation of the parameniscus.

parameniscus (par''ah-me-nis'kus) the structure or area around the menisci (semilunar fibrocartilages) of the knee.

paramesial (par''ah-me'se-al) [*para-¹* + Gr. *mesos* middle] paramedian.

parameter (pah-ram'ĕ-ter) [*para-¹* + *meter*] 1. an arbitrary constant in a mathematical expression that distinguishes specific cases: a parameter has a definite, fixed value in one case but will have different values in other cases. For example, in the equation of a straight line, $y = mx + b$, m and b are parameters that specify a particular straight line; changing m changes the slope of the line, while changing b changes the point at which the line crosses the y-axis. 2. in statistics, an arbitrary constant that specifies the various members of a family of probability distributions, e.g., the mean and variance of a normal distribution. A parameter is often thought of as the "true value" or "population value" as opposed to the observed value or sample value. 3. a variable whose measure is indicative of a quantity or function that cannot itself be precisely determined by direct methods; e.g., blood pressure and pulse rate are parameters of cardiovascular function, and the level of glucose in blood and urine is a parameter of carbohydrate metabolism.

paramethadione (par''ah-meth''ah-di'ōn) [USP] chemical name: 5-ethyl-3,5-dimethyl-2,4-oxazolidinedione. An anticonvulsant, $C_7H_{11}NO_3$, occurring as a clear, colorless liquid, used especially in the treatment of petit mal epilepsy, administered orally.

paramethasone acetate (par''ah-meth'ah-sōn) [USP] chemical name: 21-(acetyloxy)-6α-fluoro-11β,17-dihydroxy-16α-methylpregna-1,4-diene-3,20-dione. A glucocorticoid, $C_{24}H_{31}FO_6$, occurring as a fluffy, white to creamy white, crystalline powder; used chiefly for its anti-inflammatory and antiallergic actions, administered orally.

parametrial (par''ah-me'tre-al) 1. pertaining to the parametrium. 2. parametric¹.

parametric¹ (par''ah-met'rik) [*para-¹* + Gr. *mētra* uterus] situated near the uterus; parametrial.

parametric² (par''ah-met'rik) [*para-¹* + *meter*] pertaining to or defined in terms of a parameter.

parametritic (par''ah-mĕ-trīt'ik) pertaining to parametritis.

parametritis (par''ah-mĕ-tri'tis) inflammation of the parametrium. **posterior p.**, inflammation of the cellular tissue around the uterosacral ligaments.

parametrium (par''ah-me'tre-um) [*para-¹* + Gr. *mētra* uterus] [NA] the extension of the subserous coat of the supracervical portion of the uterus laterally between the layers of the broad ligament.

paramidoacetophenone (par-am''ǐ-do-as''ĕ-to-fe'nōn) $NH_2 \cdot C_6H_4 \cdot CO \cdot CH_3$; used in Ehrlich's diazo reaction.

paramimia (par''ah-mim'e-ah) [*para-¹* + Gr. *mimēsis* imitation] a condition in which signs are misused in expressing thoughts; the use of wrong or improper gestures in speaking.

paramitome (par''ah-mi'tōm) [*para-¹* + Gr. *mitos* thread] hyaloplasm, def. 1.

paramnesia (par''am-ne'ze-ah) [*para-¹* + *amnesia*] 1. a disturbance of memory in which reality and fantasy are confused. 2. a state in which words are remembered, but are used without a comprehension of their meaning.

Paramoeba (par''ah-me'ba) [*para-¹* + *ameba*] a genus of parasitic or free-living ameboid protozoa (suborder Conopodina, order Amoebida), characterized by the presence of both a nucleus and a nucleus-like body; some authorities consider the latter to be a protistan hyperparasite and not a secondary nucleus. Formerly called *Craigia*.

paramolar (par″ah-mo′lar) [*para-¹* + *molar*] a supernumerary molar, usually a small and rudimentary tooth, most commonly found in the maxilla, situated buccally or lingually to one of the molars or interproximally between the first and second or second and third molars. Called also *supernumerary molar*.

Paramonostomum parvum (par″ah-mo-nos′to-mum par′vum) a trematode infecting ducks and chickens in North America.

paramphistomiasis (par-am″fe-sto-mi′ah-sis) invasion of the body by trematode parasites of the order Paramphistomatoidea, particularly *Watsonius watsoni* and *Gastrodiscoides hominis*.

Paramphistomum (par″am-fis′to-mum) a genus of flukes. **P. cer′vi,** a species found in the rumen and reticulum of sheep, goats, cattle, and other ruminants. Formerly called *Amphistoma conicum* and *Fasciola cervi*.

paramucin (par″ah-mu′sin) a colloid substance found in ovarian cysts, which differs from mucin and pseudomucin in the fact that it reduces Fehling's solution before boiling with acid.

paramusia (par″ah-mu′ze-ah) [*para-¹* + Gr. *mousa* music + *-ia*] perversion or partial loss of the power of correct musical expression.

paramyelin (par″ah-mi′ĕ-lin) a monoaminomonophosphatide from brain substance.

paramyloidosis (par-am″ĭ-loi-do′sis) accumulation of an atypical form of amyloid in tissues.

paramylum (pah-ram′ĭ-lum) a carbohydrate storage compound present in the euglenoids, chemically distinct from both starch and glycogen.

paramyoclonus (par″ah-mi-ok′lo-nus) [*para-¹* + Gr. *mys* muscle + *klonos* turmoil] a condition characterized by myoclonic contractions of various muscles. **p. mul′tiplex,** a condition occurring more often in males than in females, characterized by sudden shocklike contractions affecting first the proximal muscles of the arms and the shoulder girdle, with any muscles of the limbs and trunk being involved later, and finally involving the face and bulbar muscles.

paramyosin (par″ah-mi′o-sin) a muscle protein found in the catch muscle fibers of mollusks and annelids; it has a molecular weight of about 137,000 and shows pronounced symmetry; called also *tropomyosin A*.

paramyosinogen (par″ah-mi″o-sin′o-jen) a protein resembling myosinogen (myogen) derived from muscle plasma.

paramyotone (par″ah-mi′o-tōn) paramyotonus.

paramyotonia (par″ah-mi″o-to′ne-ah) [*para-¹* + Gr. *mys* muscle + *tonos* tension + *-ia*] a disease marked by tonic spasms due to disorder of muscular tonicity, especially a hereditary and congenital affection. **ataxia p.,** muscular spasm with slight ataxia on attempting to move. **p. conge′nita,** an autosomal dominant disorder clinically similar to myotonia congenita, except that the precipitating factor is exposure to cold, the myotonia is aggravated by activity, and only the proximal muscles of the limbs, eyelids, and tongue are affected. Called also *Eulenburg disease*. **symptomatic p.,** temporary stiffness on starting to walk, seen in paralysis agitans.

paramyotonus (par″ah-mi-ot′o-nus) a condition marked by tonic muscular spasm.

Paramyxa (par″ah-mik′sah) [*para-¹* + Gr. *myxa* mucus] a genus of parasitic protozoa (order Paramyxida, class Paramyxea) having characters of the class.

Paramyxea (par″ah-mik′se-ah) a class of parasitic protozoa (phylum Ascetospora) having bicellular spores, each consisting of a parietal cell and one sporoplasm, an uninterrupted spore wall, and no polar tube. It comprises one order: Paramyxida.

Paramyxida (par″ah-mik′sĭ-dah) an order of parasitic protozoa (class Paramyxea, phylum Ascetospora) having characters of the class. *Paramyxa* is a representative genus.

paramyxovirus (par″ah-mik″so-vi′rus) a subgroup of the myxoviruses, including the viruses of human and animal parainfluenza, mumps, and Newcastle disease; it may also include the viruses of measles, canine distemper, rinderpest,

the rubella and pneumonia virus of mice, and the respiratory syncytial virus. Cf. *orthomyxovirus*.

paranalgesia (par″an-al-je′se-ah) analgesia of the lower extremities.

Paranaplasma (par-an″ah-plaz′mah) [*para-¹* + *an-* neg. + *plasma*] in former systems of classification, a genus of bacteria the organisms of which have been assigned to the genus *Anaplasma*.

paraneoplastic (par″ah-ne″o-plas′tik) [*para-¹* + *neoplastic*] pertaining to changes produced in tissue remote from a tumor or its metastases.

paranephric (par″ah-nef′rik) 1. near the kidney. 2. pertaining to the adrenal gland.

paranephritis (par″ah-nĕ-fri′tis) [*para-¹* + Gr. *nephros* kidney + *-itis*] 1. inflammation of the paranephros. 2. inflammation of the connective tissue around and near the kidney. **lipomatous p.,** lipomatous nephritis.

paranephroma (par″ah-nĕ-fro′mah) a tumor of the adrenal gland.

paranephros (par″ah-nef′ros), pl. *paraneph′roi* [*para-¹* + Gr. *nephros* kidney] an adrenal gland.

paranesthesia (par″an-es-the′ze-ah) para-anesthesia.

paraneural (par″ah-nu′ral) [*para-¹* + Gr. *neuron* nerve] beside or alongside a nerve.

parangi (pah-ran′je) Ceylonese name for yaws.

para-nitrosulfathiazole (par″ah-ni″tro-sul″fah-thi′ah-zōl) chemical name: *p*-nitro-*N*-2-thiazolylbenzenesulfonamide. A sulfonamide, $C_9H_7N_3O_4S_2$, occurring as a yellow powder; used as an antibacterial in the treatment of nonspecific ulcerative colitis and of proctitis, administered by rectal injection.

paranoia (par″ah-noi′ah) [Gr. "madness, delirium, a mind 'beside itself,'" from *para-¹* + *noein* to think] a psychotic disorder marked by persistent delusions of persecution or delusional jealousy and behavior like that of the paranoid personality, such as suspiciousness, mistrust, and combativeness. It differs from paranoid schizophrenia, in which hallucinations or formal thought disorder are present, in that the delusions are logically consistent and that there are no other psychotic features. The designation in DSM III-R is delusional (paranoid) disorders, with five types: persecutory, jealous, erotomanic, somatic, and grandiose.

paranoiac (par″ah-noi′ak) 1. a person afflicted with paranoia. 2. pertaining to or characterized by paranoia.

paranoid (par′ah-noid) resembling paranoia.

paranomia (par″ah-no′me-ah) [*para-¹* + Gr. *onoma* name + *-ia*] aphasia characterized by inability to name objects felt (*myotactic p.*) or seen (*visual p.*).

paranormal (par″ah-nor′mal) beyond the normal or natural; said of phenomena such as extrasensory perception.

paranuclear (par″ah-nu′kle-ar) 1. beside a nucleus. 2. pertaining to a paranucleus.

paranucleolus (par″ah-nu-kle′o-lus) a small basophil body in the enclosing sac of the cell nucleus.

paranucleus (par″ah-nu′kle-us) [*para-¹* + *nucleus*] a body resembling the nucleus, sometimes seen in the cell cytoplasm near the nucleus.

paraomphalic (par″ah-om-fal′ik) [*para-¹* + Gr. *omphalos* navel] alongside the umbilicus.

paraoperative (par″ah-op′er-ah-tiv) pertaining to the accessories essential to operative surgery, such as care of instruments and gloves, sterilization, etc.

paraoral (par″ah-o′ral) administered by some other route than by the mouth; said of medication.

paraosmia (par″ah-os′me-ah) parosmia.

parapancreatic (par″ah-pan″kre-at′ik) situated near the pancreas.

paraparesis (par″ah-par′ĕ-sis) [*para-¹* + Gr. *paresis* paralysis] a partial paralysis of the lower extremities.

parapedesis (par″ah-pĕ-de′sis) [*para-¹* + Gr. *pēdēsis* a leaping] passage of body substances into channels not normally conveying them, as of bile pigments into the blood capillaries.

paraperitoneal (par″ah-per″ĭ-to-ne′al) near the peritoneum.

parapertussis (par″ah-per-tus′is) [*para-¹* + *pertussis*] an acute respiratory disease clinically indistinguishable from mild or moderate pertussis, caused by *Bordetella parapertussis.* Cf. *pertussis-like syndrome,* under *syndrome.*

parapestis (par″ah-pes′tis) ambulatory plague.

paraphasia (par″ah-fa′ze-ah) [*para-¹* + *aphasia*] partial aphasia in which the patient employs wrong words, or uses words in wrong and senseless combinations (*choreic p.*). **central p.,** partial aphasia due to a brain lesion. **literal p.,** the replacement of one or more sounds in otherwise correct words. **verbal p.,** the substitution of one correct word or phrase for another, sometimes related in meaning and sometimes completely unrelated.

paraphasic (par″ah-fa′sik) characterized by paraphasia.

paraphasis (pah-raf′ah-sis) an evagination of the membranous roof of the telencephalon in front of the velum transversum in certain vertebrate brains.

paraphemia (par″ah-fe′me-ah) [*para-¹* + Gr. *phēmē* speech + *-ia*] aphasia marked by the employment of the wrong words.

paraphenylenediamine (par″ah-fen″il-ēn-di-am′in) a dye, $C_6H_4(NH_2)_2$, whose hydrochloride dyes the hair black, but may cause delayed contact-type hypersensitivity.

paraphia (par-a′fe-ah) [*para-¹* + Gr. *haphē* touch + *-ia*] a perversion of the sense of touch.

paraphilia (par″ah-fil′e-ah) [*para-¹* + *-philia*] [DSM III-R] a psychosexual disorder characterized by recurrent intense sexual urges and sexually arousing fantasies involving use of a nonhuman object, the suffering or humiliation of oneself or one's partner, or children or other nonconsenting partners; included are exhibitionism, fetishism, frotteurism, pedophilia, sexual masochism, sexual sadism, transvestic fetishism, and voyeurism.

paraphiliac (par″ah-fil′e-ak) 1. pertaining to paraphilia. 2. an individual exhibiting paraphilia; a sexual deviant.

paraphimosis (par″ah-fi-mo′sis) [*para-¹* + Gr. *phimoun* to muzzle + *-osis*] retraction of phimotic foreskin, causing a painful swelling of the glans that, if severe, may cause dry gangrene unless corrected. See also *phimosis.*

paraphobia (par″ah-fo′be-ah) [*para-¹* + *phobia*] a mild phobia.

paraphonia (par″ah-fo′ne-ah) [*para-¹* + Gr. *phōnē* voice + *-ia*] morbid alteration of the voice; partial aphonia. **p. pu′berum,** the change in the male voice at the time of puberty.

paraphora (par-af′o-rah) [*para-¹* + Gr. *pherein* to bear] a slight mental disorder.

paraphrasia (par″ah-fra′ze-ah) [*para-¹* + *aphrasia*] partial aphrasia; speech defect marked by disorderly arrangement of spoken words.

paraphrenia (par″ah-fre′ne-ah) [*para-¹* + Gr. *phrēn* mind + *-ia*] 1. paranoia or paranoid schizophrenia in which there are fantastic, absurd, well-systematized delusions that persist for years without severe personality deterioration; a condition intermediate between paranoia and paranoid schizophrenia. 2. paraphrenitis.

paraphrenic (par″ah-fre′nik) 1. pertaining to or characterized by paraphrenia. 2. an individual exhibiting paraphrenia.

paraphrenitis (par″ah-fre-ni′tis) [*para-¹* + Gr. *phrēn* diaphragm + *-itis*] inflammation of the diaphragm, or, more correctly, of the parts around it.

paraphyseal (par″ah-fiz′e-al) pertaining to the paraphysis.

paraphysis (pah-raf′ĭ-sis) [Gr. "offshoot"] 1. a thin-walled derivative of the roof plate of the telencephalon, present only temporarily in the human embryo and fetus; called also *paraphyseal body.* 2. a sterile thread alongside the spore sac or sexual organs in the hymenial layer of some fungi, especially ascomycetes; also found in mosses and ferns.

parapineal (par″ah-pi′ne-al) pertaining to the parapineal organ of certain lower vertebrates.

paraplasm (par′ah-plazm) [*para-¹* + Gr. *plasma* something formed] 1. hyaloplasm (def. 1). 2. an abnormal growth.

paraplasmic (par″ah-plaz′mik) pertaining to paraplasm.

paraplastic (par″ah-plas′tik) [*para-¹* + Gr. *plassein* to mold] exhibiting a perverted formative power; of the nature of a paraplasm.

paraplastin (par″ah-plas′tin) a substance resembling parachromatin in the cytoplasm and nucleus of a cell.

paraplectic (par″ah-plek′tik) [Gr. *paraplēktikos*] paraplegic.

paraplegia (par″ah-ple′je-ah) [*para-¹* + Gr. *plēgē* stroke + *-ia*] paralysis of the legs and lower part of the body. **alcoholic p.,** paraplegia due to chronic alcoholism, and probably dependent upon peripheral neuritis. **ataxic p.,** subacute combined degeneration of spinal cord; see under *degeneration.* **cerebral p.,** that which is due to a bilateral lesion. **Erb's spastic p., Erb's syphilitic spastic p.,** an uncommon form of meningovascular syphilis marked by progressive spasticity and weakness of the legs, paraplegia, muscular atrophy, paresthesia, increased knee and ankle reflexes, and incontinence. Called also *cerebrospinal syphilis, Erb's paralysis, Erb-Charcot disease,* and *syphilitic paraplegia.* **flaccid p.,** paraplegia with loss of muscle tone of the paralyzed part and absence of tendon reflexes. Cf. *spastic p.* See under *paralysis.* **peripheral p.,** that which is due to a lower motor neuron lesion. **Pott's p.,** that which is due to vertebral caries or spinal tuberculosis; called also *Pott's paralysis.* **reflex p.,** paralysis of the lower limbs due to peripheral irritation of the nerve centers. **senile p.,** a form marked by tonic spasm of the paralyzed muscles, with increased reflex irritability; it is usually caused by transverse lesions of the spinal cord or by anterolateral sclerosis. Called also *tetanoid p.* **spastic p.,** paraplegia marked by spasticity of the muscles of the paralyzed part and increased tendon reflexes, due to damage to the corticospinal tract. Cf. *flaccid p.* **spastic p., congenital,** spastic p., infantile. **spastic p., infantile,** spastic paralysis occurring in early childhood, due to injuries in birth, cerebral hemorrhage before birth, or abnormal development of the brain. **spastic p., primary,** a form of spastic paraplegia said to be due to primary degeneration in the pyramidal tracts. **p. supe′rior,** paralysis of both arms. **syphilitic p.,** Erb's spastic p. **toxic p.,** paraplegia due to poisons in the blood.

paraplegic (par″ah-plej′ik) pertaining to or of the nature of paraplegia; by extension, sometimes used to designate an individual affected with paraplegia.

paraplegiform (par″ah-plej′ĭ-form) resembling paraplegia.

parapleuritis (par″ah-plu-ri′tis) [*para-¹* + Gr. *pleura* side + *-itis*] inflammation in the wall of the chest.

paraplexus (par″ah-plek′sus) [*para-¹* + *plexus*] (*obs.*) the choroid plexus of the lateral ventricle.

parapneumonia (par″ah-nu-mo′ne-ah) a disease resembling pneumonia clinically.

parapophysis (par″ah-pof′ĭ-sis) [*para-¹* + *apophysis*] the lower transverse process of a vertebra (processus transversus vertebrarum [NA]), or its homologue.

parapoplexy (par-ap′o-plek″se) [*para-¹* + *apoplexy*] a condition resembling apoplexy.

Parapoxvirus (pār″ah-poks′vi-rus) a genus of poxviruses with serologic cross reactivity, comprising viruses of ungulates, including orf virus and paravaccinia virus.

parapoxvirus (pār″ah-poks′vi-rus) an organism of the genus *Parapoxvirus.*

parapraxia (par″ah-prak′se-ah) parapraxis.

parapraxis (par″ah-prak′sis) [*para-¹* + Gr. *praxis* doing + *-ia*] a faulty action, as a slip of the tongue or misplacement of an object; attributed by Freud to unconscious motives.

paraproctitis (par″ah-prok-ti′tis) [*paraproctium* + *-itis*] inflammation of the paraproctium; perirectal inflammation.

paraproctium (par″ah-prok′she-um) [*para-¹* + Gr. *prōktos* anus] the tissues that surround the rectum and the anus.

paraprofessional (par″ah-pro-fesh′un-al) 1. a person who is specially trained in a particular field or occupation to assist a professional, such as a physician or some other professional. 2. allied health professional. 3. pertaining to a paraprofessional.

paraprostatitis (par″ah-pros″tah-ti′tis) inflammation of the tissues near the prostate gland.

paraprotein (par″ah-pro′ten) a normal or abnormal plasma protein appearing in large quantities as a result of some pathologic condition, now replaced in most contexts by the term *M component.*

paraproteinemia (par″ah-pro″ten-e′me-ah) plasma cell dyscrasia.

parapsia (par-ap′se-ah) parapsis.

parapsis (par-ap′sis) [*para-¹* + Gr. *hapsis* touch] perversion of the sense of touch; paraphia.

parapsoriasis (par″ah-so-ri′ah-sis) [*para-¹* + *psoriasis*] a group of slowly evolving erythrodermas having common characteristics of chronicity, resistance to treatment, and chronicity. The group includes acute and chronic lichenoid pityriasis and large and small plaque parasoriasis. **acute p.**, acute lichenoid pityriasis. **atrophic p.**, large plaque p. **chronic p.**, chronic lichenoid pityriasis. **p. gutta′ta, guttate p.**, 1. chronic lichenoid p. 2. small plaque p. **large plaque p.**, a chronic, asymptomatic or mildly symptomatic eruption consisting of red-blue, oval, poorly defined, flat, sometimes indurated large plaques with superficial scaling, which preferentially involves the trunk, especially the hips and buttocks, proximal extremities, and breasts in women. It is usually benign, sometimes has a tendency to progress to dermal lymphoma, especially if atrophy and poikiloderma are prominent features. Called also *atrophic p.* and *poikilodermic* or *poikelodermatous p.* See also *retiform p.* **p. lichenoi′des**, retiform p. **p. en plaques**, see *large plaque p.* and *small plaque p.* **poikilodermic p., poikilodermatous p.**, 1. large plaque p. 2. retiform p. **retiform p.**, a chronic eruption consisting of red to brown, scaly lesions with a netlike distribution, intermixed with which are deep red plaques, some exhibiting lichenoid papules, which is histologically similar to large plaque parapsoriasis (considered by some authorities to be a variant) except that atrophy and poikiloderma are prominent features. It is the form of parapsoriasis from which dermal lymphoma is most likely to arise. Called also *p. lichenoides, p. varigata, parakeratosis varigata,* and *poikilodermic* or *poikilodermatous p.* **small plaque p.**, a benign, asymptomatic, chronic eruption consisting of small to moderate sized, red-blue to yellow plaques, occurring chiefly on the trunk and proximal extremities, which have distinct, thin borders and fine, adherent scales, giving the surface a cigarette paper–like appearance. Called also *p. guttata* and *xanthoerythroderma perstans.* **p. variga′ta**, retiform p. **p. variolifor′mis acu′ta**, acute lichenoid pityriasis. **p. variolifor′mis chron′ica**, chronic lichenoid pityriasis.

parapsychology (par″ah-si-kol′o-je) [*para-¹* + *psychology*] the study of psychical effects and experiences which appear to fall outside the scope of physical law, e.g., telepathy and clairvoyance.

parapyknomorphous (par″ah-pik″no-mor′fus) [*para-¹* + Gr. *pyknos* compact + *morphē* form] neither pyknomorphous nor apyknomorphous, but between the two; staining moderately well. Said of certain nerve cells.

parapyle (par′ah-pīl) [*para-¹* + Gr. *pylē* gate] an opening other than the astropyle in the capsular membrane of certain marine planktonic protozoa.

parapyramidal (par″ah-pi-ram′ĭ-dal) beside or near a pyramid.

paraquat (par′a-kwat) a poisonous dipyridilium compound whose dichloride and dimethylsulfate salts are used as contact herbicides. Contact with concentrated solutions causes irritation of the skin, cracking and shedding of the nails, and delayed healing of cuts and wounds. After ingestion of large doses, renal and hepatic failure may develop, followed by pulmonary insufficiency.

paraqueduct (par-ak′we-dukt) (*obs.*) a lateral extension of the cerebral aqueduct.

pararabin (pah-rar′ah-bin) a carbohydrate residuum identified by Reichardt (1875) and obtained by depriving agar of its nitrogen (Bordet-Zung, 1914).

pararectal (par″ah-rek′tal) beside the rectum.

parareducine (par″ah-re-du′sin) [*para-¹* + *reducin*] a leukomaine found in the urine.

parareflexia (par″ah-re-flek′se-ah) any disorder or derangement of the reflexes.

pararenal (par″ah-re′nal) beside the kidney.

pararhizoclasia (par″ah-ri″zo-kla′se-ah) [*para-¹* + Gr. *rhiza* root + *klasis* destruction + *-ia*] inflammatory destruction of the deep layers of the alveolar process and the periodontal ligament around the roots of a tooth. Cf. *perirhizoclasia.*

pararhotacism (par″ah-ro′tah-sizm) [*para-¹* + Gr. *rhō* the Greek letter *r*] imperfect pronunciation of the sound of the letter *r.*

pararosaniline (par″ah-ro-zan′ĭ-lin) a basic dye, triaminotriphenylmethane chloride; generally, the chief constituent of basic fuchsin. **p. pamoate**, chemical name: α-(*p*-aminophenyl)²α-(4-imino-2,5-cyclohexadien-1-ylidene)-*p*-toluidine-4′,4′-methylenebis(3-hydroxy-2-naphthoate) (2:1) dihydrate; an antischistosomal, $[(C_{19}H_{18}N_3)_2 \cdot C_{23}H_{14}O_6] \cdot 2H_2O.$

pararrhythmia (par″ah-rith′me-ah) parasystole.

pararthria (par-ar′thre-ah) [*para-¹* + Gr. *arthron* articulation] disordered or imperfect utterance of speech.

Parasaccharomyces (par″ah-sak″ah-ro-mi′sēz) Candida.

parasacral (par″ah-sa′kral) situated near the sacrum.

Parasal (par′ah-sal) trademark for preparations of aminosalicylic acid.

parasalpingeal (par″ah-sal-pin′je-al) situated beside or in the wall of the fallopian or uterine tube.

parasalpingitis (par″ah-sal″pin-ji′tis) [*para-¹* + Gr. *salpinx* tube + *-itis*] inflammation of the tissues around a fallopian or uterine tube.

parascapular (par″ah-skap′u-lar) near the scapula.

Parascaris (par-as′kar-is) a genus of nematode worms of the family Ascarididae. **P. equo′rum**, a species found in horses.

parascarlatina (par″ah-skar″lah-ti′nah) Duke's disease.

parascarlet (par″ah-skar′let) Duke's disease.

parasecretion (par″ah-se-kre′shun) 1. any disorder or derangement of secretion. 2. hypersecretion. 3. secretion of a hormone by an organ other than an endocrine gland.

parasellar (par″ah-sel′ar) near or around the sella turcica.

parasexual (par″ah-seks′u-al) accomplished by other than sexual means, as by genetic study of *in vitro* somatic cell hybrids rather than by pedigree studies.

parasexuality (par″ah-seks″u-al′ĭ-te) perverted sexuality.

parasigmatism (par″ah-sig′mah-tizm) [*para-¹* + Gr. *sigma* the Greek letter ς] imperfect pronunciation of *s* and *z* sounds. Called also lisping.

parasinoidal (par″ah-si-noi′dal) [*para-¹* + *sinus*] situated along the course of a sinus.

parasite (par′ah-sīt) [Gr. *parasitos*] 1. a plant or animal which lives upon or within another living organism at whose expense it obtains some advantage. See *symbiosis.* 2. the smaller, less complete component of asymmetrical conjoined twins, which is attached to and dependent on the autosite. **accidental p.**, an organism parasitizing an animal other than the usual host, as *Dirofilaria* in man. **allantoic p.**, a twin embryonic parasite in which the weaker member takes its blood supply from the stronger through its umbilical circulation. **animal p.**, any parasite that is a member of the animal kingdom, including many protozoa, helminths, annelids, arthropods, etc. **celozoic p.**, a parasite which lives in a body cavity. **cytozoic p.**, a parasite which lives in body cells, as a plasmodium. **diheteroxenic p.**, a parasite which requires two intermediate hosts. **ectophytic p.**, a plant ectoparasite. **ectozoic p.**, an animal ectoparasite. **endophytic p.**, a plant endoparasite. **entozoic p.**, a parasite which lives in the lumen of the intestine. **eurytrophic p.**, an ectoparasite which can feed on various hosts. **facultative p.**, an organism which may be parasitic upon another but which is capable of independent existence. **hematozoic p.**, a parasite which lives in the blood. **incidental p.**, accidental p. **intermittent p.**, a parasite which lives in its host only at times, being free living during the interval; called also *occasional p.* **karyozoic p.**, a parasite which lives in cell nuclei. **malarial p.**, *Plasmodium.* **obligatory p.**, a parasite which cannot live apart from its host. **occasional p.**, intermittent p. **periodic p.**, a parasite that resides in its host for short periods. **permanent p.**, a parasite which lives in its host from early life until maturity or death. **plant p.**, any parasite of the vegetable kingdom. **specific p.**, one normal to its current host. **spurious p.**, an organism which is parasitic on hosts other than man, but which may pass through the human body without causing harm. **stenotrophic p.**, an ectoparasite which can feed on one host only. **temporary p.**, a parasite which lives free of its host during part of its life cycle. **teratoid p.**, a fetal parasite which appears as a tumor-like mass. **vege-**

table p., any parasite of the vegetable kingdom, such as a fungus.

parasitemia (par″ah-si-te′me-ah) the presence of parasites (especially malarial parasites) in the blood.

parasitic (par″ah-sit′ik) [Gr. *parasitikos*] pertaining to, of the nature of, or caused by a parasite.

parasiticidal (par″ah-sit″ĭ-si′dal) destructive to parasites.

parasiticide (par″ah-sit′ĭ-sīd) [L. *parasitus* a parasite + *caedere* to kill] 1. destructive to parasites. 2. an agent that is destructive to parasites.

parasitifer (par″ah-sit′ĭ-fer) [*parasite* + L. *ferre* to bear] an organism which serves as the host of a parasite.

parasitism (par″ah-si′tizm) 1. symbiosis in which one population (or individual) adversely affects the other, but cannot live without it. 2. infection or infestation with parasites.

parasitization (par″ah-sīt″i-za′shun) infection or infestation with a parasite.

parasitogenic (par″ah-si′to-jen′ik) [Gr. *parasitos* parasite + *gennan* to produce] caused by parasites.

parasitoid (par′ah-si″toid) resembling a parasite.

parasitologist (par″ah-si-tol′o-jist) an expert in parasitology.

parasitology (par″ah-si-tol′o-je) [Gr. *parasitos* parasite + *-logy*] the science or study of parasites and parasitism.

parasitosis (par″ah-si-to′sis) infection or infestation with parasites.

parasitotrope (par″ah-si′to-trōp) parasitotropic.

parasitotropic (par″ah-si′to-trop′ik) [*parasite* + Gr. *trepein* to turn] having special affinity for parasites.

parasitotropism (par″ah-si-tot′ro-pizm) parasitotropy.

parasitotropy (par″ah-si-tot′ro-pe) the affinity of a drug for infective parasites.

parasoma (par″ah-so′mah) paranucleus.

parasomnia (par″ah-som′ne-ah) 1. a state in which there is no response to stimuli, verbal or mental, except that of a reflex nature. 2. abnormal sleep behavior, as sleepwalking, enuresis, or bruxism.

paraspadias (par″ah-spa′de-as) [*para-¹* + Gr. *spadon* a rent] a developmental anomaly in which the urethra opens upon one side of the penis.

paraspasm (par′ah-spazm) [L. *paraspasmus*; Gr. *paraspasmos*] spasm of the corresponding muscles on both sides of the body.

paraspasmus (par″ah-spaz′mus) paraspasm. **p. facia′le,** a painless motor disturbance affecting both sides of the face.

paraspecific (par″ah-spĕ-sif′ik) having curative properties in addition to the specific one.

parasplenic (par″ah-sple′nik) beside the spleen.

parasternal (par″ah-ster′nal) [*para-¹* + Gr. *sternon* sternum] situated beside the sternum.

parasthenia (par″as-the′ne-ah) [*para-¹* + Gr. *sthenos* strength + *-ia*] a condition of organic tissue causing it to function at abnormal intervals.

parastruma (par″ah-stroo′mah) a goiter-like enlargement of a parathyroid gland or glands.

parasuicide (par″ah-soo′ĭ-sīd) an apparent attempt at suicide, as by self-poisoning or self-mutilation, in which death is not the desired outcome.

parasympathetic (par″ah-sim″pah-thet′ik) of or pertaining to that division of the autonomic nervous system made up of the ocular, bulbar, and sacral divisions; see under *system*.

parasympathicotonia (par″ah-sim-path″ĕ-ko-to′ne-ah) vagotonia.

parasympathin (par″ah-sim′pah-thin) a hypothetical product given off when a cranial autonomic nerve is stimulated, and having stimulating action on the parasympathetic nervous system.

parasympatholytic (par″ah-sim″pah-tho-lit′ik) [*parasympathetic* + Gr. *lytikos* dissolving] 1. producing effects resembling those of interruption of the parasympathetic nerve supply to a part. 2. an agent that opposes the effects of impulses conveyed by the parasympathetic nerves. Called also *anticholinergic*.

parasympathomimetic (par″ah-sim″pah-tho-mi- met′ik) [*parasympathetic* + Gr. *mimētikos* imitative] 1. producing

effects resembling those of stimulation of the parasympathetic nerve supply to a part. 2. an agent that produces effects similar to those produced by stimulation of the parasympathetic nerves. Called also *cholinergic*.

parasynanche (par″ah-sin′an-ke) [Gr. *parasynanchē*] inflammation of a parotid gland or of the throat muscles.

parasynapsis (par″ah-sĭ-nap′sis) [*para-¹* + Gr. *synapsis* conjunction] the union of chromosomes side by side during meiosis. Cf. *telosynapsis*.

parasyndesis (par″ah-sin-de′sis) parasynapsis.

parasynovitis (par″ah-sin″o-vi′tis) [*para-¹* + *synovitis*] inflammation of the tissues about a synovial sac.

parasystole (par″ah-sis′to-le) [*para-¹* + Gr. *systolē* contraction] a cardiac irregularity attributed to the interaction of two foci that independently initiate cardiac impulses at different rates; as a rule, one of these foci is the sinoatrial node (the normal pacemaker), and the ectopic focus is usually in the ventricle. Each focus, and thus each rhythm, is protected from the influence of the other.

paratarsium (par″ah-tar′se-um) [*para-¹* + *tarsus*] the side of the tarsus of the foot.

paratenic (par″ah-ten′ik) denoting an intermediate host, sometimes called transfer host, of a parasite that is not essential to (neither hindering nor hastening) the completion of the parasite's life cycle.

paratenon (par″ah-ten′on) [*para-¹* + Gr. *tenōn* tendon] the fatty areolar tissue filling the interstices of the fascial compartment in which a tendon is situated.

paratherapeutic (par″ah-ther″ah-pu′tik) (*obs.*) iatrogenic.

parathion (par″ah-thi′on) chemical name: diethyl-*p*-nitrophenyl thiophosphate. An agricultural insecticide, $C_{10}H_{14}NO_5PS$, highly toxic to humans and animals.

parathormone (par″ah-thor′mōn) parathyroid hormone.

parathymia (par″ah-thi′me-ah) [*para-¹* + Gr. *thymos* spirit] a perverted, contrary, or inappropriate mood.

parathyrin (par″ah-thi′rin) parathyroid hormone.

parathyroid (par″ah-thi′roid) [*para-¹* + *thyroid*] 1. situated beside the thyroid gland. 2. one of the parathyroid glands; see under *gland*. 3. [USP] a sterile preparation of the water-soluble principle(s) of the parathyroid glands; administered parenterally as an antihypocalcemic, especially in the treatment of acute hypoparathyroidism with tetany.

parathyroidal (par″ah-thi-roi′dal) pertaining to the parathyroid glands.

parathyroidectomize (par″ah-thi″roid-ek′to-mīz) to excise the parathyroid gland(s).

parathyroidectomy (par″ah-thi″roi-dek′to-me) [*parathyroid* + Gr. *ektomē* excision] excision of the parathyroid gland(s).

parathyroidin (par″ah-thi-roi′din) an extract of the parathyroid glands that exerts the skeletal, renal, and gastrointestinal actions of parathyroid hormone.

parathyroidoma (par″ah-thi″roi-do′mah) parathyroid adenoma or carcinoma.

parathyropathy (par″ah-thi-rop′ah-the) any disease of the parathyroid glands.

parathyroprival (par″ah-thi″ro-pri′val) pertaining to or caused by absence of the parathyroid glands.

parathyroprivia (par″ah-thi-ro-pri′ve-ah) the condition resulting from the removal of the parathyroid glands.

parathyroprivic (par″ah-thi″ro-priv′ik) parathyroprival.

parathyroprivous (par″ah-thi-rop′rĭ-vus) parathyroprival.

parathyrotrophic (par″ah-thi-ro-trof′ik) parathyrotropic.

parathyrotropic (par″ah-thi-ro-trop′ik) having an affinity for or stimulating the growth or hormonal secretion of the parathyroid glands.

paratonia (par″ah-to′ne-ah) [*para-¹* + Gr. *tonos* tension + *-ia*] a disorder of tone or tension.

paratope (par′ah-tōp) [*para-¹* + Gr. *topos* a place] an antigen-binding site of an antibody molecule. Cf. *epitope*.

paratose (par′ah-tōs) an unusual sugar found to be a polysaccharide somatic antigen of *Salmonella* species.

paratrachoma (par″ah-trah-ko′mah) inclusion conjunctivitis.

paratrophic (par″ah-trof′ik) [*para-¹* + Gr. *trophē* nutrition] requiring living material or complex protein matter for food. Cf. *metatrophic*.

paratrophy (par-at′ro-fe) [*para-¹* + Gr. *trophē* nutrition] dystrophy.

paratuberculosis (par″ah-tu-ber″ku-lo′sis) 1. a disease resembling tuberculosis but not due to *Mycobacterium tuberculosis*. 2. Johne's disease.

paratuberculous (par″ah-tu-ber′ku-lus) having an indirect relation to tuberculosis; due to conditions produced by tuberculosis; pertaining to paratuberculosis.

paratype (par′ah-tīp) any strain of bacteria, other than the holotype, that is specifically stated to be the one on which the original description of the taxon was based.

paratyphlitis (par″ah-tif-li′tis) [*para-¹* + Gr. *typhlos* blind + *-itis*] inflammation of the postperitoneal tissue of the cecum.

paratyphoid (par″ah-ti′foid) [*para-¹* + *typhoid*] 1. see under *fever*. 2. any infection due to any of the *Salmonella* serotypes excepts S. *typhi;* see *enteric fever*, under *fever*, and *salmonellosis*.

paratypic (par″ah-tip′ik) paratypical.

paratypical (par″ah-tip′ĭ-kal) differing from the type.

paraumbilical (par″ah-um-bil′ĭ-kal) alongside the umbilicus.

paraungual (par″ah-ung′gwal) [*para-¹* + L. *unguis* nail] near or beside a nail.

paraurethra (par″ah-u-re′thrah) an accessory urethral canal.

paraurethral (par″ah-u-re′thral) near the urethra.

paraurethritis (par″ah-u″re-thri′tis) inflammation of the tissues near the urethra.

parauterine (par″ah-u′ter-in) alongside the uterus.

paravaccinia (par″ah-vak-sin′e-ah) [*para-¹* + *vaccinia*] an infection due to the paravaccinia virus, a species of the genus *Parapoxvirus* that produces lesions similar to those of cowpox and orf on the udders and teats of milk cows and on the oral mucosa of suckling calves, which begin as small red papules that evolve to vesicles, pustules, and scabbing. Paravaccinia may be transmitted to humans during milking, producing purple nodules on the fingers or adjacent areas; the lesions break down and crust and heal without scarring. It can be retransmitted to uninfected cows. Called also *milker's nodes* or *nodules* and *pseudocowpox*.

paravaginal (par″ah-vaj′ĭ-nal) beside or alongside of the vagina.

paravaginitis (par″ah-vaj′ĭ-ni′tis) inflammation of the tissue about the vagina.

paravenous (par″ah-ve′nus) beside a vein.

paravertebral (par″ah-ver′tĕ-bral) beside the vertebral column.

paravitaminosis (par″ah-vi″tah-mĭ-no′sis) a vitamin deficiency disorder without specific lesions.

paraxial (par-ak′se-al) [*para-¹* + *axis*] situated alongside an axis.

paraxon (par-ak′son) [*para-¹* + *axon*] a collateral branch of an axon.

Parazoa (par-ah-zo′ah) a subdivision of Metazoa comprising the sponges, i.e., multicellular animals having incipient tissues, but no mouth or digestive tract or organ systems. Cf. *Eumetazoa*.

parazone (par′ah-zōn) one of the white bands alternating with the dark bands (diazones) in the layers of enamel prisms and seen in cross-section of a tooth.

parazoon (par″ah-zo′on) [*para-¹* + Gr. *zōon* animal] (*obs.*) an animal organism parasitic upon or within an animal; animal parasite.

parbendazole (par-ben′dah-zōl) chemical name: (5-butyl-1*H*-benzimidazol-2-yl)carbamic acid methyl ester; a veterinary anthelmintic with nematocidal action, $C_{13}H_{17}N_3O_2$.

parconazole hydrochloride (par-ko′nah-zōl) chemical name: *cis*-1-[[2-(2,4-dichlorophenyl)-4-[(2-propynyloxy)methyl]-1,3-dioxolan-2-yl]methyl]-1*H*-imidazole monohydrochloride; an antifungal, $C_{17}H_{16}Cl_2N_2O_3 \cdot HCl$.

Paré (pah-ra′), Ambroise (1510–1590). chief surgeon to three French kings and the greatest surgeon of the 16th century. Paré reformed the treatment of gunshot wounds by abolishing cauterization with boiling oil. He also practiced ligation of arteries after amputation, and re-introduced podalic version into obstetrics. His famous aphorism, *Je le pansay, et Dieu le guarit* ("I dressed him and God healed him"), first appeared in 1585, in the fourth edition of his collected works, which he wrote in French to make more accessible.

parectasia (par″ek-ta′se-ah) parectasis.

parectasis (par-ek′tah-sis) [*para-¹* + Gr. *ektasis* extension] excessive stretching or distention of a part or organ.

parectropia (par″ek-tro′pe-ah) [*para-¹* + Gr. *ek* out + *tropos* a turning] apraxia.

Paredrine (par′ah-drēn) trademark for preparations of hydroxyamphetamine hydrobromide.

paregoric (par″ĕ-gor′ik) [Gr. *parēgorikos* consoling] [USP] a preparation of powdered opium, anise oil, benzoic acid, camphor, diluted alcohol, and glycerin, each 100 ml. of which yields 35–45 mg. of anhydrous morphine; used as an antiperistaltic, especially in the treatment of diarrhea, administered orally. Formerly called *camphorated opium tincture*.

parelectronomic (par″e-lek″tro-nom′ik) giving no response to electromotive stimuli.

parelectronomy (par″e-lek-tron′o-me) [*para-¹* + *electric* + Gr. *nomos* law] a condition in which there is a decrease in strength of an electric current passed through a muscle.

pareleidin (par″el-e′ĭ-din) the keratin of epidermal cells derived from eleidin of the stratum lucidum.

parencephalia (par″en-sĕ-fa′le-ah) [*para-¹* + Gr. *enkephalos* brain + *-ia*] congenital defect of the brain.

parencephalocele (par″en-sef′ah-lo-sēl) [*parencephalon* + Gr. *kēlē* hernia] hernial protrusion of the cerebellum.

parencephalon (par″en-sef′ah-lon) [*para-¹* + Gr. *enkephalos* brain] the cerebellum.

parencephalous (par″en-sef′ah-lus) [*para-¹* + Gr. *enkephalos* brain] having a congenital deformity of the brain.

parenchyma (pah-reng′kĭ-mah) [Gr. "anything poured in beside"] the essential elements of an organ; used in anatomical nomenclature as a general term to designate the functional elements of an organ, as distinguished from its framework, or stroma. **p. glandula′re prosta′tae**, p. prostatae. **p. prosta′tae** [NA], the aggregation of 30 to 50 small compound tubulosaccular or tubuloalveolar glands that make up the bulk of the prostate; called also *p. glandulare prostatae*. **p. tes′tis** [NA], **p. of testis**, the seminiferous tubules, which are located within the lobules of the testis.

parenchymal (pah-reng′kĭ-mal) pertaining to or of the nature of parenchyma.

parenchymatitis (par″eng-kim″ah-ti′tis) inflammation of a parenchyma.

parenchymatous (par″eng-kim′ah-tus) pertaining to or of the nature of parenchyma.

parenchymula (par″eng-kim′u-lah) the embryonic stage next succeeding that called the closed blastula.

Parendomyces (par″en-do-mi′sēz) a former genus of yeastlike fungi, species of which have now been included in the genus *Candida*.

parental (pah-ren′tal) of, pertaining to, or derived from the parents.

parenteral (pah-ren′ter-al) [*para-¹* + Gr. *enteron* intestine] not through the alimentary canal but rather by injection through some other route, as subcutaneous, intramuscular, intraorbital, intracapsular, intraspinal, intrasternal, intravenous, etc.

parepicoele (par-ep′ĭ-sēl) (*obs.*) either of the lateral recesses of the fourth ventricle of the brain.

parepididymis (par″ep-ĭ-did′ĭ-mis) paradidymis.

parepigastric (par″ep-ĭ-gas′trik) near the epigastrium.

paresis (pah-re′sis, par′ĕ-sis) [Gr. "relaxation"] slight or incomplete paralysis. **general p.**, parenchymatous neurosyphilis in which chronic meningoencephalitis causes gradual loss of cortical function, resulting in progressive dementia and generalized paralysis, which generally occurs 10 to 20 years after the initial infection of syphilis. Called also *Bayle's disease, dementia paralytica, general paralysis of the insane, paretic neurosyphilis, polyparesis*, and *syphilitic meningoencephalitis*.

Parest (par′est)   trademark for a preparation of methaqualone hydrochloride.

paresthesia (par″es-the′ze-ah) [*para-¹* + Gr. *aisthēsis* perception]   morbid or perverted sensation; an abnormal sensation, as burning, prickling, formication, etc.   **Berger's p.,** paresthesia in young persons of one or both lower limbs, accompanied by weakness, but without objective symptoms.   **Bernhardt's p.,** meralgia paresthetica.   **visceral p.,** an abnormal sensation referred to some viscus; not a mere excess or defect of a normal visceral sensation.

paresthetic (par″es-thet′ik)   pertaining to or marked by paresthesia.

paretic (pah-ret′ik)   pertaining to or affected with paresis.

parfocal (par-fo′kal) [L. *par* equal + *focus* hearth]   retaining correct focus on changing powers in microscopy.

pargyline hydrochloride (par′gĭ-lēn) [USP]   chemical name: *N*-methyl-*N* -2-propynylbenzylamine hydrochloride. An antihypertensive, $C_{11}H_{13}N \cdot HCl$, occurring as a white or practically white crystalline powder; administered orally.

Parham band (pahr′am) [F. W. *Parham*, New Orleans surgeon, 1856–1927]   see under *band*.

parhormone (par-hor′mōn)   any metabolic substance of the body which influences the functions of other organs or tissue; for example, carbon dioxide.

parica (par″ĭ-kah′)   a narcotic snuff prepared from the leguminous seeds of *Piptadenia* (*Anadenanthera*) species, a tree of Brazil. The seeds contain dimethyltryptamine and related psychotomimetic indole alkaloids. Called also *cohoba*.

paricine (par-ris′in)   a quinoline alkaloid, $C_{16}H_{18}ON_2$, from the bark of *Cinchona succirubra* Parvon. (Rubiaceae), redbark cinchona.

paries (pa′re-ez), pl. *pari′etes* [L.]   a wall; [NA] a general term for the wall of an organ or body cavity.   **p. ante′rior gas′tricus** [NA], the wall of the stomach directed toward the ventral surface of the body. Called also *p. anterior ventriculi* [NA alternative].   **p. ante′rior vagi′nae** [NA], the wall of the vagina that is intimately associated with the posterior wall of the bladder and urethra.   **p. ante′rior ventric′uli,** NA alternative for *p. anterior gastricus*.   **p. carot′icus cavita′tis tympan′icae** [NA], the anterior wall of the tympanic cavity, related to the carotid canal, in which is lodged the internal carotid artery.   **p. exter′nus duc′tus cochlea′ris** [NA], the external wall of the cochlear duct, adjacent to the outer wall of the cochlea.   **p. infe′rior or′bitae** [NA], the inferior wall of the orbit, formed by the orbital surfaces of the maxilla and the zygomatic and palatine bones; called also *floor of orbit*.   **p. jugula′ris cavita′tis tympan′icae** [NA], the floor of the tympanic cavity, which is in intimate relation with the jugular fossa, which lodges the bulb of the internal jugular vein.   **p. labyrin′thicus cavita′tis tympan′icae** [NA], the medial wall of the tympanic cavity.   **p. latera′lis or′bitae** [NA], the lateral wall of the orbit, formed by the orbital surfaces of the great wing of the sphenoid bone, the zygomatic bone, and the zygomatic process of the frontal bone.   **p. mastoi′deus cavita′tis tympan′icae** [NA], the posterior wall of the tympanic cavity, related to the mastoid portion of the temporal bone.   **p. media′lis or′bitae** [NA], the medial wall of the orbit, formed by parts of the maxillary, lacrimal, ethmoid, and sphenoid bones.   **p. membrana′ceus bron′chi** [NA], that part of the wall of the smaller bronchi where the cartilage is deficient.   **p. membrana′ceus cavita′tis tympan′icae** [NA], the outer, or lateral, wall of the tympanic cavity, formed mainly by the tympanic membrane.   **p. membrana′ceus tra′cheae** [NA], the posterior part of the wall of the trachea where the cartilaginous rings are deficient.   **p. poste′rior gas′tricus** [NA], the wall of the stomach directed toward the posterior surface of the body. Called also *p. posterior ventriculi* [NA alternative].   **p. poste′rior vagi′nae** [NA], the wall of the vagina that is intimately associated with the anterior wall of the rectum.   **p. poste′rior ventric′uli,** NA alternative for *p. posterior gastricus*.   **p. supe′rior or′bitae** [NA], the superior wall of the orbit, formed chiefly by the orbital plate of the frontal bone and by the orbital surface of the lesser wing of the sphenoid bone; called also *roof of orbit*.   **p. tegmenta′lis cavita′tis tympan′icae** [NA], the roof of the tympanic cavity, related to part of the petrous portion of the temporal bone.   **p. tympan′icus duc′tus cochlea′ris** [NA], tympanic wall of cochlear duct: the wall of the cochlear duct that separates it from the scala tympani, composed of the osseous spiral laminae and the basilar membrane.   **p. vestibula′ris duc′tus cochlea′ris** [NA], vestibular wall of cochlear duct: the thin anterior wall of the cochlear duct, which separates it from the scala vestibuli; called also *membrana spiralis ductus cochlearis* [NA alternative] or *spiral membrane of cochlear duct*.

parietal (pah-ri′ĕ-tal) [L. *parietalis*]   1. of or pertaining to the walls of a cavity.   2. pertaining to or located near the parietal bone, as the parietal lobe.

parietes (pah-ri′ĕ-tēz) [L.]   plural of *paries*.

parietitis (pah-ri″ĕ-ti′tis)   inflammation of the wall of an organ.

parietofrontal (pah-ri″ĕ-to-fron′tal)   pertaining to the parietal and frontal bones, gyri, or fissures.

parietography (pah-ri″ĕ-tog′rah-fe)   roentgenographic visualization of the walls of an organ.   **gastric p.,** roentgenographic visualization of the stomach wall by special technique, as a means of detecting early gastric neoplasm.

parieto-occipital (pah-ri″ĕ-to-ok-sip′ĭ-tal)   pertaining to the parietal and occipital bones or lobes.

parietosphenoid (pah-ri″ĕ-to-sfe′noid)   pertaining to the parietal and sphenoid bones.

parietosplanchnic (pah-ri″ĕ-to-splank′nik)   parietovisceral.

parietosquamosal (pah-ri″ĕ-to-skwah-mo′sal)   pertaining to the parietal bone and the squamous portion of the temporal bone.

parietotemporal (pah-ri″ĕ-to-tem′po-ral)   pertaining to the parietal and temporal bones or lobes.

parietovisceral (pah-ri″ĕ-to-vis′er-al)   both parietal and visceral; pertaining to the walls of a cavity and the viscera within it.

Parinaud's oculoglandular syndrome (pah-ri-nōz′) [Henri *Parinaud*, French ophthalmologist, 1844–1905]   see under *syndrome*.

pari passu (pa′re pas′u) [L., "at equal pace"]   coincidentally with; to the same proportion or degree.

parity (par′ĭ-te)   1. [L. *parere* to bring forth, produce] para; the condition of a woman with respect to her having borne viable offspring. Cf. *gravidity*.   2. [L. *par* equal] equality; close correspondence or similarity.

Park's aneurysm (parks) [Henry *Park*, English surgeon, 1744–1831]   see under *aneurysm*.

Parker's fluid (park′erz) [George Howard *Parker*, American zoologist, 1864–1955]   see under *fluid*.

Parkinson's disease, facies (sign) (par′kin-sunz) [James *Parkinson*, English physician, 1755–1824]   see *paralysis agitans*, and under *facies*. See also *parkinsonism*.

parkinsonian (par″kin-sōn′e-an)   pertaining to parkinsonism.

parkinsonism (par′kin-sun-izm″)   a group of neurological disorders characterized by hypokinesia, tremor, and muscular rigidity. See *parkinsonian syndrome*, under *syndrome*, and see *paralysis agitans* (Parkinson's disease).   **postencephalitic p.,** parkinsonian syndrome.

Parlodel (par′lo-del″)   trademark for a preparation of bromocriptine mesylate.

Parnate (par′nāt)   trademark for a preparation of tranylcypromine sulfate.

paroccipital (par″ok-sip′ĭ-tal) [*para-¹* + L. *occiput* occiput]   near the occipital bone.

parolivary (par-ol′ĭ-var″e) [*para-¹* + *olivary*]   situated near the olive or olivary nucleus.

paromomycin (par′o-mo-mi′sin)   an aminoglycoside antibiotic, $C_{23}H_{45}N_5O_{14}$, derived from *Streptomyces rimosus* var. *paromomycinus*, which is effective against a wide variety of gram-negative, gram-positive, and acid-fast bacteria.   **p. sulfate** [USP], the sulfate salt of paromomycin, $C_{23}H_{45}N_5O_{14} \cdot xH_2SO_4$, occurring as a creamy white to yellow, amorphous powder; used orally as an antiamebic.

paroniria (par″o-ni′re-ah) [*para-¹* + Gr. *oneiros* dream + *-ia*]   morbid dreaming.

paronychia (par″o-nik′e-ah) [*para-¹* + Gr. *onyx* nail + *-ia*]   inflammation involving the folds of tissue surrounding the nail. Called also *perionychia*. See also *onychia*.   **herpetic p.,** see under *whitlow*.   **p. tendino′sa,** septic inflammation of the sheath of the tendon of a finger.

paronychial (par″o-nik′e-al) pertaining to paronychia; pertaining to the nail folds, as a paronychial wart.

paroöphoric (par″o-o-fo′rik) pertaining to the paroöphoron.

paroophoritis (par″o-of-o-ri′tis) 1. inflammation of the paroophoron. 2. inflammation of the tissues about the ovary.

paroöphoron (par″o-of′o-ron) [*para-* ¹ + Gr. *ōon* egg + *pherein* to bear] [NA] an inconstantly present small group of coiled tubules between the layers of the mesosalpinx, being a remnant of the excretory part of the mesonephros.

parophthalmia (par″of-thal′me-ah) [*para-* ¹ + *ophthalmia*] inflammation of the connective tissue around the eye.

parophthalmoncus (par″of-thal-mong′kus) [*para-* ¹ + *ophthalm-* + *onkos* mass] a tumor situated near the eye.

paropsis (par-op′sis) parablepsia.

parorchidium (par″or-kid′e-um) [*para-* ¹ + Gr. *orchis* testicle] misplacement of a testis or testes.

parorchis (par-or′kis) the epididymis.

parorexia (par″o-rek′se-ah) [*para-* ¹ + Gr. *orexis* appetite] pica.

parosmia (par-oz′me-ah) [*para-* ¹ + Gr. *osmē* smell] any disease or perversion of the sense of smell.

parosphresia (par″os-fre′ze-ah) [*para-* ¹ + Gr. *osphrēsis* smelling + *-ia*] disorder or perversion of the sense of smell.

parosphresis (par″os-fre′sis) parosphresia.

parosteal (par-os′te-al) pertaining to the outer surface of the periosteum.

parosteitis (par″os-te-i′tis) [*para-* ¹ + *osteitis*] inflammation of the tissues around a bone.

parosteosis (par″os-te-o′sis) [*para-* ¹ + Gr. *osteon* bone + *-osis*] ossification of the tissues outside of the periosteum.

parostitis (par″os-ti′tis) parosteitis.

parostosis (par″os-to′sis) parosteosis.

parotic (pah-rot′ik) [*para-* ¹ + Gr. *ous* ear] situated or occurring near the ear.

parotid (pah-rot′id) [*para-* ¹ + Gr. *ous* ear] situated or occurring near the ear, as the parotid gland.

parotidean (pah-rot″ĭ-de′an) pertaining to the parotid gland.

parotidectomy (pah-rot″ĭ-dek′to-me) [*parotid* + Gr. *ektomē* excision] excision of the parotid gland.

parotiditis (pah-rot″ĭ-di′tis) parotitis.

parotidoscirrhus (pah-rot″ĭ-do-skir′us) [*parotid* + Gr. *skirrhos* hardness] hardening of the parotid gland.

parotin (par-o′tin) a proteinaceous factor extractable from human parotid gland, which supposedly has hormonal properties; in rabbits, it promotes mesenchymal growth and calcification of teeth, lowers serum calcium levels, and affects the leukocyte count.

parotitis (par″o-ti′tis) inflammation of the parotid gland. Called also *parotiditis*. **epidemic p.,** mumps. **p. phlegmono′sa,** that associated with suppuration. **postoperative p.,** an acute parotitis due to infection (usually with staphylococci) of the parotid gland following a surgical procedure; it is marked by rapid onset, frequently with severe pain and rapid swelling of the glands, and by trismus, low-grade fever, headache, malaise, and leukocytosis. It affects generally debilitated patients, usually middle-aged or older, suffering from dehydration, suppression of salivary secretion, vomiting, or mouth-breathing. **staphylococcal p.,** postoperative parotitis caused by staphylococci.

parous (par′us) [L. *parere* to bring forth, produce] having borne one or more viable offspring.

parovarian (par″o-va′re-an) 1. situated beside the ovary. 2. pertaining to the parovarium (epoöphoron).

parovariotomy (par″o-va″re-ot′o-me) [*parovarium* + Gr. *tomē* a cutting] incision into the parovarium.

parovaritis (par″o-vah-ri′tis) inflammation of the parovarium (epoophoron).

parovarium (par″o-va′re-um) [*para-* ¹ + L. *ovarium* ovary] epoöphoron.

paroxysm (par′ok-sizm) [Gr. *paroxysmos*] 1. a sudden recurrence or intensification of symptoms. 2. a spasm or seizure.

paroxysmal (par″ok-siz′mal) recurring in paroxysms.

Parpanit (par-pan′it) trademark for a preparation of caramiphen hydrochloride.

Parrot's atrophy of newborn, disease (pseudoparalysis), sign (nodes) (par-ōz′) [Jules Marie *Parrot*, French physician, 1839–1883] see *marasmus*, see *syphilitic pseudoparalysis*, under *pseudoparalysis*, and see under *sign*.

Parry's disease (pār′ēz) [Caleb Hillier *Parry*, English physician, 1755–1822] toxic nodular goiter.

pars (parz), pl. *par′tes* [L.] a division or part; [NA] a general term for a particular portion of a larger area, organ, or structure. **p. abdomina′lis aor′tae** [NA], the continuation of the thoracic part of the aorta, which gives rise to the inferior phrenic, lumbar, median sacral, superior and inferior mesenteric, middle suprarenal, renal, and testicular or ovarian arteries, and celiac trunk. Called *abdominal aorta* and *aorta abdominalis* [NA alternative]. **p. abdomina′lis duc′tus thora′cici** [NA], the abdominal part of the thoracic duct; see *ductus thoracicus*. **p. abdomina′lis esoph′agi,** NA alternative for *p. abdominalis oesophagi*. **p. abdomina′lis et pelvi′na syste′matis autonom′ici,** see *p. abdominalis systematis autonomici* and *p. pelvina systematis autonomici*. **p. abdomina′lis mus′culi pectora′lis majo′ris** [NA], the portion of the pectoralis major muscle originating from the aponeurosis of the obliquus externus abdominis. **p. abdomina′lis oesoph′agi** [NA], the part of the esophagus below the diaphragm, joining the stomach. Written also *p. abdominalis esophagi* [NA alternative]. **p. abdomina′lis syste′matis autonom′ici** [NA], the portion of the autonomic nervous system contained within the abdomen; part of its parasympathetic components (vagus nerves) arise from the medulla oblongata and sacral spinal cord; its sympathetic components from the thoracic and upper lumbar cord. Called also *lumbar part of autonomic nervous system*. **p. abdomina′lis ure′teris** [NA], that portion of the ureter extending from the kidney to the terminal line of the pelvis. **p. ala′ris mus′culi nasa′lis** [NA], see *partes transversa et alaris musculi nasalis*. **p. alveola′ris mandib′ulae** [NA], the superior portion of the body of the mandible, which contains sockets for the teeth. **p. amor′pha,** the spherical, finely granular body surrounded by the nucleolonema of the nucleolus. **p. ana′lis rec′ti,** canalis analis. **p. annula′ris vagi′nae fibro′sae digito′rum ma′nus** [NA], annular ligaments of fingers: a strong transverse band of fibrous tissue in the vagina fibrosa of the fingers, crossing the flexor tendons at the level of the upper half of the proximal phalanx; called also *p. anularis vaginae fibrosae digitorum manus* [NA alternative]. **p. annula′ris vagi′nae fibro′sae digito′rum pe′dis** [NA], annular ligaments of toes: a fibrous band in the toes resembling those of similar name in the fingers; called also *p. anularis vaginae fibrosae digitorum pedis* [NA alternative]. **p. ante′rior commissu′rae anterio′ris cer′ebri,** NA alternative for *p. anterior commissurae rostralis cerebri*. **p. ante′rior commissu′rae rostra′lis cer′ebri** [NA], the smaller anterior part of the rostral commissure of the cerebrum, the fibers of which interconnect the two olfactory bulbs; called also *p. anterior commissurae anterioris cerebri* [NA alternative]. **p. ante′rior dor′si lin′guae,** NA alternative for *p. presulcalis dorsi linguae*. **p. ante′rior fa′ciei diaphragmat′icae hep′atis** [NA], the portion of the diaphragmatic surface of the liver that is directed toward the ventral surface of the body. **p. ante′rior for′nicis vagi′nae** [NA], see *fornix vaginae*. **p. ante′rior lob′uli quadrangula′ris,** lobulus quadrangularis. **p. ante′rior pedun′culi cer′ebri,** NA alternative for *p. ventralis pedunculi cerebri*. **p. anula′ris vagi′nae fibro′sae digito′rum ma′nus,** NA alternative for *p. annularis vaginae fibrosae digitorum manus*. **p. anula′ris vagi′nae fibro′sae digito′rum pe′dis,** NA alternative for *p. annularis vaginae fibrosae digitorum pedis*. **p. ascen′dens aor′tae** [NA], the proximal portion of the aorta, arising from the left ventricle, and giving origin to the right and left coronary arteries before continuing as the arch of the aorta. Called also *aorta ascendens* [NA alternative], and *ascending aorta*. **p. ascen′dens duode′ni** [NA], the terminal part of the duodenum, ending at the duodenojejunal flexure. **p. atlan′tica arte′riae vertebra′lis** [NA], the part of the vertebral artery winding behind the lateral mass of the atlas to lie in a groove on the upper surface of the posterior arch of the atlas; called also *p. atlantis arteriae* *vertebralis* [NA alternative]. **p. atlan′tis arte′riae vertebra′lis,** NA alternative for *p. atlantica arteriae vertebralis.* **p. autonom′ica syste′matis nervo′si** [NA], the autonomic portion of the nervous system concerned with regulation of activity of cardiac muscle, smooth muscle, and glands; called also *autonomic nervous system* (q.v.), *systema nervosum autonomicum* [NA alternative], *systema nervosum sympatheticum,* and *sympathetic nervous system.* See Plate 45. **p. basila′ris os′sis occipita′lis** [NA], a quadrilateral plate of the occipital bone that projects superiorly and anteriorly from the foramen magnum. **p. basila′ris pon′tis,** NA alternative for *p. ventralis pontis.* **p. basolatera′lis cor′poris amygdaloi′dei** [NA], the basolateral part of the amygdaloid body comprising lateral, basal, and accessory basal amygdaloid nuclei. **p. bucca′- lis hypophys′eos,** Rathke's pouch. **p. buccopharyn′gea mus′culi constricto′ris pharyn′gis superio′ris** [NA], buccopharyngeal muscle: the part of the constrictor pharyngis superior muscle arising from the pterygomandibular raphe; called also *musculus buccopharyngeus.* **p. calcaneocuboi′dea ligamen′ti bifurca′ti,** ligamentum calcaneocuboideum. **p. calcaneo navicula′ris ligamen′ti bifurca′ti,** ligamentum calcaneonaviculare. **p. cardi′aca gas′tris** [NA], the part of the stomach immediately adjacent to and surrounding the cardiac opening of the esophagus, distinguished only by the presence of the cardiac glands, and lacking acid (parietal) and pepsin (chief) cells. Called also *cardia* and *p. cardiaca ventriculi* [NA alternative]. **p. cardi′aca ventric′uli,** NA alternative for *p. cardiaca gastris.* **p. cartilagin′ea sep′ti na′si** [NA], cartilaginous part of nasal septum: the plate of cartilage forming the anterior part of the nasal septum; called also *septum cartilagineum nasi.* **p. cartilagin′ea systema′tis skeleta′lis** [NA], the cartilaginous part of the skeletal system; the cartilages of the body. **p. cartilagin′ea tu′bae auditi′vae** [NA], the part of the auditory tube that is chiefly supported by the tubal cartilage; it extends from the pars ossea to the pharyngeal orifice of the auditory tube. **p. cauda′lis lob′uli quadrangula′- ris,** NA alternative for *lobulus simplex cerebelli.* **p. cauda′lis ner′vi vestibula′ris** [NA], the caudal, or inferior branch of the vestibular nerve, the filaments of which end in the ampullary crest of the posterior semicircular ducts and the macula of the saccule. Called also *p. inferior nervi vestibularis* [NA alternative], *p. inferior partis vestibularis nervi octavi,* and *p. inferior partis vestibularis nervi vestibulocochlearis.* **p. caverno′sa arteriae carot′idis inter′nae** [NA], the cavernous part of the internal carotid artery located in the cavernous sinus, and having numerous branches. **p. caverno′sa ure′threa vir′ilis,** p. spongiosa urethrae masculinae. **p. centra′lis syste′matis nervo′si** [NA], the central part of the nervous system, consisting of the brain and spinal cord; called also *central nervous system (CNS)* and *systema nervosum centrale* [NA alternative]. **p. centra′lis ventric′uli latera′lis cer′ebri** [NA], the part of the lateral ventricle found within the parietal lobe of the cerebrum; it communicates with the frontal, occipital, and temporal horns. **p. cephal′ica et cervica′lis syste′matis autonom′ici** [NA], **p. cephal′ica et cervica′lis syste′matis sympath′ici,** the portion of the autonomic nervous system contained in the head and neck. Its sympathetic components arise from the upper thoracic cord, and are relayed by cervical sympathetic ganglia; its parasympathetic components arise from the brain stem via oculomotor, facial, glossopharyngeal, vagus, and accessory nerves, and are relayed by way of ciliary, pterygopalatine, otic, submandibular, and intrinsic ganglia. **p. ceratopharyn′gea mus′culi constricto′ris pharyn′gis me′dii** [NA], ceratopharyngeal muscle: the portion of the constrictor pharyngis medius muscle arising from the greater cornu of the hyoid bone; called also *musculus ceratopharyngeus.* **p. cerebra′lis arte′riae carot′idis inter′nae** [NA], the terminal, cerebral part of the internal carotid artery, which divides into the anterior and middle cerebral arteries in the middle cranial fossa. **p. cervica′lis arte′riae carot′idis inter′nae** [NA], the unbranched, cervical part of the internal carotid artery located in the carotid triangle of the neck. **p. cervica′lis arte′riae vertebra′lis,** NA alternative for *pars transversaria arteriae vertebrae.* **p. cervica′lis duc′tus thora′cici** [NA], the cervical part of the thoracic duct; see *ductus thoracicus.* **p. cervica′lis esoph′agi,** NA alternative for *p. cervicalis oesophagi.* **p. cervica′lis**

medul′lae spina′lis [NA], that part of the spinal cord lodged within the cervical part of the vertebral canal and giving rise to the eight pairs of cervical spinal nerves (*segmenta medullae spinalis cervicalia* [1–8]). **p. cervica′lis oesoph′agi** [NA], the part of the esophagus that is located in the cervical region, related anteriorly to the trachea and the recurrent laryngeal nerves, posteriorly to the longus colli muscle and vertebral column, and laterally to the lobes of the thyroid gland and the commmon carotid arteries. Written also *p. cervicalis esophagi* [NA alternative]. **p. cervica′lis syste′matis sympath′ici,** see *p. cephalica et cervicalis systematis autonomici.* **p. cervica′lis tra′- cheae** [NA], the part of the trachea located in the cervical region, related anteriorly to the jugular venous arch, sternohyoid and sternothyroid muscles, isthmus of thyroid gland, inferior thyroid veins, thymus, arteria thyroidea ima, posteriorly to the esophagus and recurrent laryngeal nerves, and laterally to the lobes of the thyroid gland and common carotid arteries. **p. chondropharyn′gea mus′culi constricto′ris pharyn′gis me′dii** [NA], chondropharyngeal muscle: the portion of the constrictor pharyngis medius muscle arising from the lesser cornu of the hyoid bone; called also *musculus chondropharyngeus.* **p. cilia′ris ret′inae** [NA], the two layers of epithelium lining the basal lamina of the ciliary body. **p. clavicula′ris mus′culi pectora′lis majo′ris** [NA], the portion of the pectoralis major muscle originating from the clavicle. **p. coccyg′ea medul′lae spina′lis** [NA], that part of the spinal cord within the coccygeal part of the vertebral canal and giving rise to the three pairs of coccygeal spinal nerves (*segmenta medullae spinalis coccygea 1–3*). **p. cochlea′- ris ner′vi octa′vi,** **p. cochlea′ris ner′vi vestibulocochlea′ris,** nervus cochlearis. **p. compac′ta** [NA], compact part: the dorsal part of the substantia nigra, medium-sized cells, many of which are pigmented. Cf. *p. reticularis.* **p. convolu′ta lob′uli cortica′lis re′nis** [NA], the part of the renal cortex surrounding the intracortical prolongations of the renal pyramids and composed of convoluted tubules. **p. corneosclera′lis** [NA], the anterior part of the trabecular reticulum of the iridocorneal angle, situated between the venous sinus of the sclera, the scleral spur, and the posterior limiting lamina of the cornea. **par′tes corpo′ris huma′ni** see *regiones et partes corporis,* under *regio.* **p. cortica′lis arteriae cer′ebri me′diae,** NA alternative for *p. terminalis arteriae cerebri mediae.* **p. cortica′lis arte′riae cerebri posterior′- is,** NA alternative for *p. terminalis arteriae cerebri posterioris.* **p. corticomedia′lis cor′poris amygdaloi′dei** [NA], the corticomedial part of the amygdaloid body comprising central, medial, and cortical amygdaloid nuclei, the nucleus of the lateral olfactory stria, and the transitional anterior amygdaloid area; called also *p. olfactoria corporis amygdaloidei* [NA alternative]. **p. costa′lis diaphrag′matis** [NA], the part of the respiratory diaphragm arising from the inner surfaces of the ribs and their cartilages. **p. crania′lis lob′uli quadrangula′ris,** lobulus quadrangularis. **p. cricopharyn′gea mus′culi constricto′ris pharyn′gis inferio′ris** [NA], cricopharyngeal muscle: the portion of the constrictor pharyngis inferior muscle arising from the cricoid cartilage; called also *musculus cricopharyngeus.* **p. crucifor′mis vagi′nae fibro′sae digito′rum ma′nus** [NA], cruciate ligaments of fingers: one of the diagonal bundles of the fascia of the fingers which cross each other on the dorsal surface of each digit at the level of the distal end of the proximal phalanx; called also *ligamenta cruciata digitorum manus.* **p. crucifor′mis vagi′nae fibro′sae digito′rum pe′dis** [NA], cruciate ligaments of toes: one of the bundles of fascial fibers in the toes resembling those of similar name in the fingers; called also *ligamenta cruciata digitorum pedis.* **p. cupula′ris reces′sus epitympan′ici** [NA], cupular space: the part of the epitympanic recess above the head of the malleus. **p. descen′dens aor′tae** [NA], the continuation of the aorta from the arch of the aorta, in the thorax, to the point of its division into the common iliac arteries, in the abdomen. Called also *aorta descendens* [NA alternative] and *descending aorta.* See also *p. abdominalis aortae* and *p. thoracica aortae.* **p. descen′dens duode′ni** [NA], the part of the duodenum between the superior and inferior parts, into which the bile and pancreatic ducts open. **p. dex′tra faci′ei diaphragmat′icae hep′atis** [NA], the portion of the diaphragmatic surface of the liver that is directed toward the right side of the body.

p. dista′lis adenohypophys′eos [NA], **p. dista′lis lo′bi anterio′ris hypophys′eos,** the distal part of the adenohypophysis; see *pituitary gland,* under *gland.* **p. dorsa′lis cor′poris genicula′ti latera′lis** [NA], the dorsal part of the lateral geniculate body; see *nucleus corporis geniculati lateralis.* **p. dorsa′lis cor′poris genicula′ti media′lis** [NA], the medial part of the medial geniculate body; see *nucleus corporis geniculati medialis.* **p. dorsa′lis dienceph′ali,** the dorsal part of the diencephalon, above the hypothalamic sulcus, comprising the epithalamus, dorsal thalamus, and metathalamus. **p. dorsa′lis pedun′culi cer′ebri** [NA], the dorsal part of the cerebral peduncle, which is continuous across the median plane and forms the tegmentum of the mesencephalon; called also *p. posterior pedunculi* [NA alternative] and *posterior part of cerebral peduncle.* **p. dorsa′lis pon′tis** [NA], the tegmental part of the pons, which resembles the medulla oblongata in structure and is continuous with the tegmentum of the mesencephalon. Called also *tegmentum of pons, tegmentum pontis* [NA alternative], and *tegmentum rhombencephali.* **p. endocri′na pancre′atis,** the endocrine part of the pancreas; see *pancreas.* **p. exocri′na pancre′atis,** the exocrine part of the pancreas; see *pancreas.* **p. feta′lis placen′tae** [NA], fetal placenta: the nonmaternal part of the placenta, derived not from the fetus but from the trophoblast that envelops the fetus; from within outward, it consists of amnion, chorionic plate, and chorionic villi. Called also *placenta foetalis.* **p. fibro′sa,** the portion of the nucleolus containing chiefly filaments. **p. flac′cida membra′nae tym′pani** [NA], the small portion of the tympanic membrane, between the mallear folds. **p. fronta′lis cap′sulae inter′nae,** crus anterius capsulae internae. **p. fronta′lis radiatio′nis corpo′ris callo′si,** the frontal part of the radiatio corporis callosi, composed of fibers sweeping forward from the genu into the frontal lobe. **p. functiona′lis,** stratum functionale. **par′tes genita′les exter′nae mulie′bres,** organa genitalia feminina externa. **par′tes genita′les exter′nae vir′iles,** organa genitalia masculina externa. **par′tes genita′les femini′nae exter′nae,** organa genitalia feminina externa. **par′tes genita′les masculi′nae exter′nae,** organa genitalia masculina externa. **p. glossopharyn′gea mus′culi constricto′ris pharyn′gis superio′ris** [NA], glossopharyngeal muscle: the part of the constrictor pharyngis superior muscle arising from the side of the root of the tongue. **p. granulo′sa,** the portion of the nucleolus containing chiefly granules. **p. gris′ea hypothal′ami,** the gray matter, i.e., nuclear masses, of the hypothalamus. **p. horizonta′lis duode′ni** [NA], that part of the duodenum situated between the descending and ascending parts, crossing from right to left ventral to the third lumbar vertebra; called also *p. inferior duodeni* [NA alternative] or *inferior part of duodenum.* **p. horizonta′lis os′sis palati′ni,** lamina horizontalis ossis palatini. **p. ili′aca lin′eae termina′lis,** linea arcuata ossis ilii. **p. infe′rior duode′ni,** NA alternative for p. horizontalis duodeni. **p. infe′rior fos′sae rhomboi′deae,** a space at the lower part of the floor of the fourth ventricle of the brain, between the restiform bodies. **p. infe′rior gy′ri fronta′lis me′dii,** the inferior portion of the middle frontal gyrus. **p. infe′rior ner′vi vestibula′ris,** NA alternative for *p. caudalis nervi vestibularis.* **p. infe′rior par′tis vestibula′ris ner′vi octa′vi,** p. infe′rior par′tis vestibula′ris ner′vi vestibulocochlea′ris, p. caudalis nervi vestibularis. **p. inflex′a,** the bar of a horse's hoof. **p. infraclavicula′ris plex′us brachia′lis** [NA], the part of the brachial plexus that lies in the axilla, below the level of the clavicle. In it arise the medial and lateral pectoral, musculocutaneous, medial brachial cutaneous, medial antebrachial cutaneous, median, ulnar, radial, subscapular, thoracodorsal, and axillary nerves. **p. infraloba′ris** [NA], a tributary to the posterior branch of the right superior pulmonary vein; called also *infralobar vein, intersegmental vein,* and *p. intersegmentalis.* **p. infrasegmenta′lis,** p. intersegmentalis. **p. infundibula′ris lo′bi anterio′ris hypophys′eos,** pars tuberalis adenohypophyseos. **p. insula′ris arte′riae cer′ebri me′diae** [NA], insular part of middle cerebral artery: collectively, the branches of the middle cerebral artery supplying the insula and adjacent areas, comprising the arteriae insulares, arteria frontobasilaris lateralis, and arteriae temporales anterior, media, and posterior. **p. intercartilagin′ea ri′mae glot′tidis** [NA], the part of the

rima glottidis between the arytenoid cartilages; called also *interarytenoid space.* **p. interme′dia bulbo′rum** [NA], a narrow median band spanning the vaginal orifice to unite the bulbi vestibuli vaginae. Called also *commissura bulborum vestibuli vaginae.* **p. interme′dia fos′sae rhomboi′deae,** the middle part of the rhomboid fossa. **p. interme′dia adenohypophys′eos** [NA], **p. interme′dia lo′bi anterio′ris hypophyseos,** the intermediate part of the adenohypophysis; see *pituitary gland,* under *gland.* **p. intermembrana′cea ri′mae glot′tidis** [NA], the part of the rima glottidis between the vocal folds. **p. intersegmenta′lis** [NA], 1. any of the veins lying between and draining adjacent bronchopulmonary segments and supplying a main branch of a right or left pulmonary vein; called also *infrasegmental vein, intersegmental vein,* and *p. infrasegmentalis.* 2. p. intralobaris. **p. interstia′lis tu′bae uteri′nae,** pars uterina tubae uterinae. **p. intracanicula′ris ner′vi op′tici** [NA], the portion of the optic nerve running through the optic canal. **p. intracrania′lis arte′riae vertebra′lis** [NA], the part of the vertebral artery that ascends medially in front of the medulla oblongata where, at about the lower border of the pons, it joins the opposite artery to form the basilar artery. **p. intracrania′lis ner′vi op′tici** [NA], the portion of the optic nerve lying between the optic canal and the optic chiasm. **p. intralamina′ris ner′vi op′tici** [NA], the portion of the intraocular part of the optic nerve that runs through the lamina cribrosa of the sclera. **p. intraocula′ris ner′vi op′tici** [NA], the portion of the optic nerve within the eyeball, separated into postlaminar, intralaminar, and prelaminar parts. **p. intrasegmenta′lis** [NA], any of the small veins lying within a bronchopulmonary segment and draining into one of the main branches of a right or left pulmonary vein; called also *intrasegmental vein.* **p. iri′dica re′tinae** [NA], the two layers of pigmented epithelium lining the posterior part of the iris. **p. labia′lis mus′culi orbicula′ris o′ris** [NA], the part of the orbicular muscle of the mouth whose fibers are restricted to the lips. **p. lacrima′lis mus′culi orbicula′ris oc′uli** [NA], the part of the orbicularis oculi muscle that arises from the posterior lacrimal ridge of the lacrimal bone, to become continuous with the palpebral portion. **p. laryn′gea pharyn′gis** [NA], laryngopharynx: the portion of the pharynx that lies below the upper edge of the epiglottis and opens into the larynx and esophagus. **p. latera′lis ar′cus longitudina′lis pe′dis** [NA], that part of the longitudinal arch of the foot formed by the calcaneus, the cuboid bone, and the lateral two metatarsal bones. **p. latera′lis for′nicis vagi′nae** [NA], see *fornix vaginae.* **p. latera′lis musculo′rum intertransversario′rum posterio′rum cer′vicis** [NA], the lateral part of the posterior intertransverse muscles of the neck. **p. latera′lis os′sis occipita′lis** [NA], lateral part of occipital bone: one of the paired parts of the occipital bone which form the lateral boundaries of the foramen magnum, each being prominently characterized by the presence of one of the occipital condyles. **p. latera′lis os′sis sa′cri** [NA], the part or mass of the sacrum on either side lateral to the dorsal and pelvic sacral foramina; called also *lateral mass of sacrum.* **p. lenticulothalam′icus cap′sulae inter′nae,** p. thalamolenticularis capsulae internae. **p. li′bera colum′nae for′nicis,** the postcommissural component of the columns of the fornix. **p. li′bera mem′bri inferio′ris** [NA], the bones of the thigh, leg, and foot. Called also *skeleton membri inferioris liberi.* **p. li′bera mem′bri superio′ris** [NA], the bones of the arm, forearm, and hand. Called also *skeleton membri superioris liberi.* **p. lumba′lis diaphrag′matis** [NA], the portion of the respiratory diaphragm that arises from the lumbar vertebrae, comprising the right and left diaphragmatic crura, the right crus arising from the upper three or four vertebrae, and the left from the upper two or three. **p. lumba′lis medul′lae spina′lis** [NA], that part of the spinal cord lodged within the lower thoracic part of the vertebral canal (in adults) and giving rise to the five pairs of lumbar spinal nerves (*segmenta medullae spinalis lumbalia* [1–5]). **p. magnocellula′ris nu′clei ru′bri** [NA], in man, the caudal part of the red nucleus, containing a complement of large multipolar cells; the number of these cells is relatively decreased in comparison to the small cells scattered throughout the nucleus; cf. *p. parvocellularis nuclei rubri.* **p. mamilla′ris hypothal′ami,** the mamillary bodies. **p. margina′lis mus′culi orbicula′ris o′ris** [NA], the part of the orbicular muscle of the mouth whose fibers blend with those of adjacent muscles. **p. margina′lis sul′ci cin′guli,** the portion of the cingulate gyrus that turns off at a right angle and is directed toward the dorsal margin of the cerebral hemisphere. **p. mastoi′dea os′sis tempora′lis,** mastoid bone: the posterior portion of the petrous part of the temporal bone, bounded anteriorly by the external acoustic meatus and articulating superiorly with the parietal bone and posteriorly with the occipital bone. **p. media′lis ar′cus longitudina′lis pe′dis** [NA], that part of the longitudinal arch of the foot formed by the calcaneus, talus, and the navicular, cuneiform, and first three metatarsal bones. **p. media′lis musculo′rum intertransversario′rum posterio′rum cer′vicis** [NA], the medial part of the posterior intertransverse muscles of the neck. **p. mediastina′lis faci′ei media′lis pulmo′nis** [NA], the part of the medial surface of each lung that is adjacent to the mediastinum. **p. membrana′cea sep′ti atrio′rum,** p. membranacea septi interventricularis cordis. **p. membrana′cea sep′ti interventricula′ris cor′dis** [NA], the very small, completely membranous area of the interventricular septum of the heart; situated near the root of the aorta, it can be viewed between the opposed margins of the right and posterior semilunar valves of the aorta. Called also *septum membranaceum ventriculorum cordis.* **p. membrana′cea sep′ti na′si** [NA], membranous septum of nose: the anterior inferior part of the nasal septum, beneath the cartilaginous part; it is composed of skin and subcutaneous tissues. Called also *septum membranaceum nasi.* **p. membrana′cea ure′thrae masculi′nae** [NA], **p. membrana′cea ure′thrae viri′lis,** the portion of the male urethra between the pars prostatica and pars spongiosa, and traversing the urogenital diaphragm and the deep perineal space. **p. mo′bilis sep′ti na′si** [NA], mobile part of nasal septum: the part of the nasal septum at the apex of the nose, formed by skin, subcutaneous tissue, and the greater alar cartilages; called also *septum mobile nasi.* **p. muscula′ris sep′ti interventricula′ris cor′dis** [NA], the thick muscular partition forming the greater part of the septum between the ventricles of the heart; called also *septum musculare ventriculorum cordis.* **p. mylopharyn′gea mus′culi constricto′ris pharyn′gis superio′ris** [NA], the part of the constrictor pharyngis superior muscle arising from the mylohyoid ridge of the mandible; called also *musculus mylopharyngeus.* **p. nasa′lis os′sis fronta′lis** [NA], the small, irregularly shaped process that projects downward from the medial part of the squama of the frontal bone to articulate with the nasal bones and the frontal processes of the maxillae. Called also *prefrontal bone* and *nasal process of frontal bone.* **p. nasa′lis pharyn′gis** [NA], nasopharynx: the part of the pharynx that lies above the level of the soft palate. **p. nervo′sa hypophys′eos,** lobus nervosus neurohypophyseos. **p. nervo′sa re′tinae** [NA], nervous, or neural, part of retina: the internal, transparent, light-sensitive portion of the optic nerve part of the retina (cf. *p. pigmentosa*), comprising nine layers seen by light microscopy, named from within outward: internal limiting membrane, nerve fiber layer, ganglion cell layer, inner plexiform layer, inner nuclear layer, outer plexiform layer, outer nuclear layer, outer limiting membrane, and layer of rods and cones; see illustration accompanying *retina.* Called also *cerebral layer* or *stratum of retina, nervous layer,* and *stratum cerebrale retinae.* **p. obli′qua mus′culi cricothyroi′dei** [NA], the fibers of the cricothyroid muscle that are inserted into the inferior horn, caudal margin, and inner surface of the thyroid cartilage. **p. occipita′lis cap′sulae inter′nae,** crus posterius capsulae internae. **p. occipita′lis coro′nae radia′tae,** the part of the corona radiata contained within the occipital lobe. **p. occlu′sa arte′riae umbilica′lis** [NA], the portion of the umbilical artery that atrophies at birth when the placental circulation ceases to become the medial umbilical ligament. **p. olfacto′ria cor′poris amygdaloi′dei,** NA alternative for *p. corticomedialis corporis amygdaloidei.* **p. opercula′ris gy′ri fronta′lis inferio′ris,** [NA], the part of the inferior frontal gyrus lying posterior to the ascending ramus of the lateral sulcus and overlapping the insular lobe (insula) called also *operculum frontale.* **p. op′tica ret′inae** [NA], optic part of retina: the part of the retina that contains receptors sensitive to light, extending posteriorly from the ora serrata on the inner surface of the choroid and continuous at the optic disk with the optic nerve; it consists of an outer pigmented layer (*p.*

pigmentosa) and an inner, multilayered nervous layer (*pars nervosa*). See also *retina.* **p. ora′lis pharyn′gis** [NA], the division of the pharynx lying between the soft palate and the upper edge of the epiglottis; called also *oropharynx.* **p. orbita′lis glan′dulae lacrima′lis** [NA], the main part of the lacrimal gland, limited in front by the orbicularis muscle and the orbital septum; called also *glandula lacrimalis superior.* **p. orbita′lis gy′ri fronta′lis inferio′ris,** [NA], the part of the inferior frontal gyrus lying below the anterior ramus of the lateral sulcus, which curves around the superciliary border to the orbital surface of the frontal lobe of the cerebral hemisphere. **p. orbita′lis mus′culi orbicula′ris oc′uli** [NA], the part of the orbicularis oculi muscle that arises from the medial margin of the orbit and surrounds it and the palpebral part of the muscle, inserting near the site of origin. **p. orbita′lis ner′vi op′tici** [NA], the portion of the optic nerve located between the optic canal and the eyeball. **p. orbita′lis os′sis fronta′lis** [NA], the horizontally placed part of the frontal bone that forms the greater part of the roof of the orbit and of the floor of the anterior cranial fossa; it is separated from its fellow of the other side by the ethmoid incisure. Called also *orbital plate of occipital bone.* **p. os′sea sep′ti na′si** [NA], the bony part of the nasal septum, composed posterosuperiorly of the perpendicular plate of the ethmoid bone and posteroinferiorly of the vomer. **p. os′sea syste′matis skeleta′lis** [NA], the osseous part of the skeletal system; the bones of the body. **p. os′sea tu′bae auditi′vae** [NA], the part of the auditory tube that lies within the temporal bone, extending from the tympanic orifice to the pars cartilaginea of the auditory tube. **p. palpebra′lis glan′dulae lacrima′lis** [NA], the part of the lacrimal gland that projects laterally into the upper eyelid; called also *glandula lacrimalis inferior,* and *Rosenmüller's gland* or *node.* **p. palpebra′lis mus′culi orbicula′ris oc′uli** [NA], palpebral part of orbicularis oculi muscle: the part of the orbicularis oculi muscle that is contained in the eyelids, originating from the medial palpebral ligament and inserting in the lateral canthus. **p. parasympathet′ica syste′matis nervo′si autonom′ici,** NA alternative for *p. parasympathica systematis nervosi autonomici.* **p. parasympath′ica syste′matis nervo′si autonom′ici** [NA], the craniosacral division of the autonomic nervous system, its preganglionic fibers traveling with cranial nerves III, VII, IX, X, and XI, and with the second to fourth sacral ventral roots; it innervates the heart, the smooth muscle and glands of the head and neck, and the thoracic, abdominal, and pelvic viscera. The ganglion cells with which these fibers synapse are in or near the organs innervated. Called also *parasympathetic nervous system* and *p. parasympathetica systematis nervosi autonomici* [NA alternative]. **p. parieta′lis coro′nae radia′tae,** the part of the corona radiata contained in the parietal lobe. **par′tes transver′sa et ala′ris mus′culi nasa′lis** [NA], the two parts of the nasal muscle, *transverse* (compressor muscle of naris, compressor naris) and *alar* (dilator muscle of naris, dilator naris) both of which arise from the maxilla of each side; the former arises just lateral to the nasal notch, the latter from below and medial to the transverse part. **p. parvocellula′ris nu′clei ru′bri** [NA], the complement of small multipolar cells scattered throughout the red nucleus; in man, these cells predominate over the large cells in the caudal part of the nucleus; cf. *pars magnocellula′ris nuclei rubri.* **p. pa′tens arte′riae umbilica′lis** [NA], the proximal, patent section of the fetal umbilical cord, which persists in the adult, although reduced in size. **p. pelvi′na syste′matis autonom′ici** [NA], the portion of the autonomic part of the nervous system contained within the pelvis; it comprises four or five sacral ganglia and is continuous cranially with the abdominal (lumbar) part. **p. pelvi′na syste′matis sympath′ici,** see *p. pelvina systematis autonomici.* **p. pelvi′na ure′teris** [NA], the portion of the ureter that extends from the terminal line of the pelvis to the urinary bladder. **p. peripher′ica syste′matis nervo′si** [NA], the peripheral part of the nervous system, consisting of the nerves and ganglia outside the brain and spinal cord; called also *peripheral nervous system* and *systema nervosum periphericum* [NA alternative]. **p. perpendicula′ris os′sis palati′ni,** lamina perpendicularis ossis palatini. **p. petro′sa arte′riae carot′idis inter′nae** [NA], the petrous part of the internal carotid artery located in the carotid canal. **p. petro′sa os′sis tempora′lis** [NA], petrous portion of temporal bone: a pyramid of dense bone located at the base of the cranium; one of the three parts of the temporal bone, it houses the organ of hearing. **p. pharyn′gea lo′bi anterio′ris hypophys′eos,** pharyngeal hypophysis. **p. pigmento′sa re′tinae** [NA], pigmented part of retina: a layer of pigmented epithelium, the outer of the two parts of the optic part of the retina (cf. *pars nervosa*), extending from the entrance of the optic nerve to the pupillary margin of the iris; see also *retina.* Called also *pigmented layer* or *stratum of retina, stratum pigmenti bulbi oculi,* and *stratum pigmenti retinae.* **p. pla′na cor′poris cilia′ris,** orbiculus ciliaris. **p. plica′ta cor′poris cilia′ris,** corona ciliaris. **p. postcommunica′lis arte′riae cer′ebri anterio′ris** [NA], postcommunical part of anterior cerebral artery: collectively, the branches of the anterior cerebral artery that supply the cortex of the medial parts of the frontal and parietal lobes, comprising arteriae frontobasalis medialis, callosomarginalis (and its rami), paracentralis, precunealis, and parieto-occipitalis. Called also *arteria pericallosa* [NA alternative] and *pericallosal artery.* **p. postcommunica′lis arte′riae cer′ebri posterio′-ris** [NA], postcommunical part of posterior cerebral artery: collectively, the branches of the posterior cerebral artery that supply cerebral peduncles, posterior thalamus, colliculi, and pineal and medial geniculate bodies, and choroid plexuses of lateral and third ventricles, comprising the arteriae posterolaterales and rami thalamici, choroidei posteriores mediales and laterales, and pedunculares. **p. poste′rior commissu′rae anterio′ris cer′ebri,** NA alternative for *p. posterior commissurae rostralis cerebri.* **p. poste′rior commissu′rae rostra′lis cer′ebri** [NA], the posterior part of the rostral commissure of the cerebrum, the fibers of which interconnect the middle and inferior temporal gyri, the parahippocampal gyri, and the amygdaloid bodies of the two sides; called also *p. posterior commissurae anterioris cerebri* [NA alternative]. **p. poste′rior dor′si lin′guae,** NA alternative for *p. postsulcalis dorsi linguae.* **p. poste′-rior faci′ei diaphragmat′icae hep′atis** [NA], the portion of the diaphragmatic surface of the liver that is directed toward the dorsal surface of the body; called also *facies posterior hepatis.* **p. poste′rior for′nicis vagi′nae** [NA], see *fornix vaginae.* **p. poste′rior lob′uli quadrangula′ris,** NA alternative for *lobulus simplex cerebelli.* **p. poste′rior pedun′culi cer′ebri,** NA alternative for *p. dorsalis pedunculi cerebri.* **p. postlamina′ris ner′vi op′tici** [NA], the portion of the intraocular part of the optic nerve located posterior to the lamina cribrosa of the sclera. **p. postsulca′lis dor′si lin′guae** [NA], the part of the dorsum of the tongue posterior to the terminal sulcus. Called also *p. posterior dorsi linguae* [NA alternative]. **p. precommunica′lis arte′riae cer′ebri anterio′ris** [NA], precommunical part of anterior cerebral artery: collectively, the branches of the anterior cerebral artery that supply the thalamus and corpus striatum, comprising arteriae centrales anteromediales, centralis brevis and longa, and communicans anterior, and rami centrales anteromediales. **p. precommunica′lis arte′riae cer′ebri posterio′ris** [NA], precommunical part of posterior cerebral artery: collectively, the branches of the posterior cerebral artery anterior to its point of junction with the posterior communicating branch of the internal carotid artery, comprising the arteriae centrales posterolaterales. **p. prelamina′ris ner′vi op′tici** [NA], the portion of the intraocular part of the optic nerve located anterior to the lamina cribrosa of the sclera. **presulca′lis dor′si lin′guae** [NA], the part of the dorsum of the tongue anterior to the terminal sulcus. Called also *p. anterior dorsi linguae* [NA alternative]. **p. preverte-bra′lis arte′riae vertebra′lis** [NA], the part of the vertebral artery before it ascends through the transverse processes of the upper six cervical vertebrae. **p. profun′da glan′dulae paroti′deae** [NA], that part of the parotid gland located deep to the facial nerve. **p. profun′da mus′culi masse′teris** [NA], the deep portion of the masseter muscle, the fibers of which arise from the medial surface of the zygomatic arch and the fascia over the temporal muscle, and are directed vertically downward. **p. profun′da mus′culi sphinc′teris a′ni exter′ni** [NA], the part of the sphincter ani externus muscle that surrounds the upper part of the anal canal. **p. prostat′ica ure′thrae masculi′nae** [NA], **p. prostat′ica ure′thrae viril′is,** the part of the male urethra that passes through the prostate. **p. pterygopharyn′gea mus′culi constricto′ris pharyn′gis superio′ris** [NA], pterygopharyngeal muscle: the part of the constrictor

pharyngis superioris muscle arising from the caudal part and hamulus of the medial pterygoid plate; called also *musculus pterygopharyngeus.* **p. pylo′rica gas′tris** [NA], the caudal one-third of the stomach, consisting of the pyloric antrum and canal, and distinguished by the presence of the pyloric glands and by the absence of parietal cells; called also *p. pylorica ventriculi* [NA alternative]. **p. pylo′rica ventric′uli,** NA alternative for *p. pylorica gastris.* **p. quadra′ta** [NA], the quadrilateral portion of the medial segment of the left hepatic lobe. **p. radia′ta lob′uli cortica′lis re′nis** [NA], any of the intracortical prolongations of the renal pyramids; called also *processus Ferreini lobuli corticalis renis* and *pyramid of Ferrein.* **p. rec′ta mus′culi cricothyroi′dei** [NA], the fibers of the cricothyroid muscle that are inserted into the caudal margin of the thyroid cartilage. **p. reticula′ris** [NA], the ventral part of the substantia nigra, which contains fewer cells than the pars compacta, only some of which contain a small amount of pigment. **p. retrolentifor′mis cap′sulae inter′nae** [NA], that part of the internal capsule resting on the lateral surface of the thalamus behind the lentiform nucleus, and containing the posterior thalamic radiation. **p. rostra′-lis lob′uli quadrangula′ris** NA alternative for *lobulus quadrangularis.* **p. rostra′lis ner′vi vestibula′ris** [NA], the rostral, or superior, branch of the vestibular nerve, the filaments of which end in the ampullary crests of the anterior and lateral semicircular ducts and the macula of the utricle. Called also *p. superior nervi vestibularis* [NA alternative], *p. superior partis vestibularis nervi octavi,* and *p. superior partis vestibularis nervi vestibulocochlearis.* **p. sacra′lis lin′eae termina′lis,** the sacral part of the terminal line of the pelvis. **p. sacra′lis medul′lae spina′lis** [NA], that part of the spinal cord within the sacral part of the vertebral canal and giving rise to the five pairs of sacral spinal nerves (*segmenta medullae spinalis sacralia* [1–5]). **p. sphenoida′lis arte′riae cer′ebri me′-diae** [NA], sphenoidal part of middle cerebral artery: collectively, the branches of the middle cerebral artery that supply the internal capsule, thalamus, and corpus striatum, comprising the arteriae anterolaterales and rami mediales and laterales. **p. spina′lis ner′vi accesso′rii,** NA alternative for *radices spinales nervi accessorii.* **p. spongio′sa ure′thrae masculi′nae** [NA], the portion of the male urethra found within the corpus spongiosum of the penis; called also *p. cavernosa urethrae virilis.* **p. squamo′sa os′sis tempora′lis** [NA], squamous part of temporal bone: the flat, scalelike, anterior and superior portion of the temporal bone; called also *squama temporalis.* **p. sterna′lis diaphrag′matis** [NA], the portion of the diaphragm that arises from the inner aspect of the xiphoid process of the sternum. **p. sternocosta′lis mus′culi pectora′lis majo′ris** [NA], the portion of the pectoralis major muscle that originates from the sternum and the ribs. **p. subcuta′nea mus′culi sphinc′teris a′ni exter′ni** [NA], the part of the sphincter ani externus muscle that surrounds the lowermost portion of the anal canal. **subendocardial terminal p.,** rami subendocardiales. **p. sublentifor′mis cap′sulae inter′nae** [NA], the part of the internal capsule lying ventral to the back part of the lentiform nucleus, and containing the temporopontile, geniculocalcarine, and auditory radiation fibers. **p. superficia′lis glan′dulae parot′idis** [NA], that part of the parotid gland located superficial to the facial nerve. **p. superficia′lis mus′culi masse′teris** [NA], the superficial portion of the masseter muscle, the fibers of which arise from the anterior part of the zygomatic arch and are directed downward and backward. **p. superficia′lis mus′culi sphinc′teris a′ni exter′ni** [NA], the part of the sphincter ani externus muscle that lies just deep to the pars subcutanea, extending farther toward the rectum. **p. supe′rior duode′ni** [NA], the part of the duodenum adjacent to the pylorus, forming the superior flexure. **p. supe′rior faci′ei diaphragmat′icae hep′atis** [NA], the portion of the diaphragmatic surface of the liver that is directed cranially. **p. supe′rior fos′sae rhomboi′deae,** the superior portion of the rhomboid fossa. **p. supe′rior ganglii vestibula′ris,** NA alternative for *p. rostralis nervi vestibularis.* **p. supe′rior gy′ri fronta′lis me′dii,** the superior portion of the middle frontal gyrus. **p. supe′rior par′tis vestibula′ris ner′vi octa′vi, p. supe′rior par′tis vestibula′ris ner′vi vestibulocochlea′ris** p. rostralis nervi vestibularis. **p. supraclavicula′ris plex′us brachia′lis** [NA], the part of the brachial plexus lying in the cervical region above the level of the clavicle, in which arise the dorsal scapular, long thoracic, and suprascapular nerves, and the nerve to the subclavius muscle. **p. sympathet′ica syste′matis nervo′si autonom′ici,** NA alternative for *p. sympathica systematis nervosi autonomici.* **p. sympath′ica syste′matis nervo′si autonom′ici** [NA], sympathetic nervous system: the portion of the autonomic nervous system that receives its fibers of connection with the central nervous system through the thoracolumbar outflow of visceral efferent fibers. These fibers (preganglionic) arise from cells in the thoracic and upper lumbar levels of the spinal cord, leave by way of ventral roots, and, by way of rami communicantes, enter sympathetic trunks, where some synapse with ganglion cells. The fibers (postganglionic) of these ganglion cells return to spinal nerves by way of rami communicantes to supply the blood vessels, smooth muscle, and glands of the trunk and limbs, or go as visceral branches to the blood vessels, smooth muscles, and glands of the head and neck, and the viscera of the thorax, abdomen, and pelvis. Some preganglionic fibers pass through the sympathetic trunks and synapse in the prevertebral ganglia; postganglionic fibers from those ganglia supply adjacent viscera. Called also *p. sympathetica systematis nervosi autonomici* [NA alternative] and *thoracico-lumbar* or *thoracolumbar division.* **p. tempora′lis radia′tio′nis cor′poris callo′si,** the fibers of the radiatio corporis callosi passing into the temporal lobe. **p. ten′sa membra′nae tym′pani** [NA], the larger portion of the tympanic membrane. **p. termina′lis arte′riae cer′ebri me′diae** [NA] terminal part of middle cerebral artery: collectively, the branches of the middle cerebral artery that supply the lateral surface of the hemisphere, comprising the arteriae sulci centralis, precentralis, and postcentralis, arteriae parietales anterior et posterior, and arteria gyri angularis. Called also *p. corticalis arteriae cerebri mediae* [NA alternative]. **p. termina′lis arte′riae cer′ebri poste′rio′ris** [NA], terminal part of posterior cerebral artery: collectively, the branches of the posterior cerebral artery that supply the cortex of the temporal and parietal lobes, comprising arteriae occipitalis lateralis and medialis and their rami. Called also *pars corticalis arteriae cerebri posterioris* [NA alternative]. **p. thalamolenticula′ris cap′sulae inter′nae** [NA], the part of the posterior limb of the internal capsule adjacent to the thalamus and lentiform nucleus, consisting of fibers of the thalamic radiations and corticospinal, corticorubral, corticoreticular, corticothalamic, and thalamoparietal fibers and the central thalamic radiations. Called also *pars lenticulothalamicus capsulae internae.* **p. thoraca′lis syste′matis autonom′ici** [NA], **p. thoraca′lis syste′matis sympath′ici,** the parts of the autonomic nervous system contained within the thorax; its sympathetic components are derived from the upper thoracic cord, and its parasympathetic components, from the vagus nerves. It also contains preganglionic sympathetic fibers which reach abdominal viscera by way of thoracic splanchnic nerves. **p. thora′cica aor′tae** [NA], the proximal portion of the descending aorta, proceeding from the arch of the aorta, and giving rise to the bronchial, esophageal, pericardiac, and mediastinal branches, and the superior phrenic, posterior intercostal III to XI, and subcostal arteries; it is continuous through the diaphragm with the abdominal aorta. Called also *aorta thoracalis, aorta thoracica* [NA alternative], and *thoracic aorta.* **p. thora′cica duc′tus thora′cici** [NA], the thoracic part of the thoracic duct; see *ductus thoracicus.* **p. thora′cica esoph′agi,** NA alternative for *p. thoracica oesophagi.* **p. thora′cica medul′lae spina′lis** [NA], the part of the spinal cord contained in the upper three-fourths of the thoracic part of the vertebral canal (in the adult), and giving rise to the twelve pairs of thoracic spinal nerves (*segmenta medullae spinalis thoracica* [1–12]). **p. thora′cica oesoph′agi** [NA], the part of the esophagus located in the thoracic region, and related anteriorly to the trachea and pericardium and posteriorly to the vertebral column. Written also *p. thoracica esophagi* [NA alternative]. **p. thorac′ica syste′matis autonom′ici** [NA], the portion of the autonomic part of the nervous system contained within the thorax; its sympathetic components are derived from the upper thoracic cord and its parasympathetic components from the vagus nerves. It also contains preganglionic sympathetic fibers which reach abdominal viscera by way of thoracic splanchnic nerves. **p. thora′cica tra′cheae** [NA], the part of the trachea that lies posteriorly in the superior mediastinum, separated from

the upper four thoracic vertebrae by the esophagus. **p. thyropharyn′gea mus′culi constricto′ris pharyn′gis inferio′ris** [NA], thyropharyngeal muscle: the part of the constrictor pharyngis inferior muscle arising from the thyroid cartilage; called also *musculus thyreopharyngeus.* **p. tibiocalca′nea ligamen′ti media′lis,** p. tibiocalcaneus ligamenti medialis. **p. tibiocalca′neus ligamen′ti media′lis** [NA], the middle portion of the superficial fibers of the medial ligament of the ankle joint; attached superiorly to the medial malleolus of the tibia and inferiorly into nearly the entire length of the sustentaculum tali of the calcaneus. Called also *calcaneotibial ligament, ligamentum calcaneotibiale, p. tibiocalcanea ligamenti medialis,* and *tibiocalcaneal* or *tibiocalcanean ligament.* **p. tibionavicula′ris ligamen′ti media′lis** [NA], the anterior portion of the superficial fibers of the medial ligament of the ankle joint; attached superiorly to the anterior surface of the medial malleolus of the tibia and inferiorly to the navicular bone and the margin of the calcaneonavicular ligament. Called also *ligamentum tibionaviculare* and *tibionavicular ligament.* **p. tibiotala′ris ante′rior ligamen′ti media′lis** [NA], the deeper portion of the medial ligament of the ankle joint; attached superiorly to the medial malleolus of the tibia and inferiorly to the medial surface of the talus. Called also *ligamentum talotibiale anterius* and *anterior talotibial ligament.* **p. tibiotala′ris poste′rior ligamen′ti media′lis** [NA], the posterior portion of the superficial fibers of the medial ligament of the ankle joint; attached superiorly to the posterior part of the medial malleolus of the tibia and inferiorly to the medial surface of the talus. Called also *ligamentum talotibiale posterius* and *posterior talotibial ligament.* **p. transver′sa** [NA], the transverse part of the left branch of the hepatic portal vein. **p. transver′sa mus′culi nasa′lis,** see *partes transversa et alaris musculi nasalis.* **p. transversa′ria arte′riae vertebra′lis** [NA], the part of the vertebral artery in the transverse processes of the upper six cervical vertebrae, which provides spinal and muscular branches; called also *pars cervicalis arteriae vertebralis* [NA alternative]. **p. triangula′ris gy′ri fronta′lis inferio′ris** [NA], the wedge-shaped part of the inferior frontal lobe that lies between the anterior and ascending branches of the lateral sulcus of the cerebral hemisphere. **p. tubera′lis adenohypophys′eos** [NA], **p. tubera′lis lo′bi anterio′ris hypophys′eos,** the tubular part of the adenohypophysis; called also *hypophyseal* or *pituitary stalk* and *p. infundibularis lobi anterioris hypophyseos.* See *pituitary gland,* under *gland.* **p. tympan′ica os′sis tempora′lis** [NA], the curved bony plate, developed from the annulus tympanicus of the fetus, forming the anterior and inferior walls and part of the posterior wall of the external auditory meatus in the adult; called also *tympanic plate.* **p. umbilica′lis** [NA], the part of the left branch of the hepatic portal vein that passes from the hilum of the liver to the umbilicus. **p. uteri′na placen′tae** [NA], uterine placenta: the maternally contributed part of the placenta, derived from the decidua basalis; called also *maternal placenta* and *placenta uterina.* **p. uteri′na tu′bae uteri′nae** [NA], the proximal part of the uterine tube, located within the wall of the uterus. **p. uvea′lis** [NA], the posterior part of the trabecular reticulum of the iridocorneal angle, situated between the scleral spur, the ciliary body, and the anterior iris. **p. vaga′lis ner′vi accesso′rii,** NA alternative for *radices craniales nervi accessorii.* **p. ventra′lis cor′poris genicula′ti latera′lis** [NA], the ventral part of the lateral geniculate body; see *nucleus corporis geniculati lateralis.* **p. ventra′lis cor′poris genicula′ti media′lis** [NA], the ventral part of the lateral geniculate body; see *nucleus corporis geniculati medialis.* **p. ventra′lis dienceph′ali,** the ventral part of the diencephalon, below the hypothalamic sulcus, comprising the ventral thalamus (subthalamus) and the hypothalamus. **p. ventra′lis pedun′culi cer′ebri** [NA], the ventral part of the cerebral peduncle, consisting of a large bundle of nerve fiber tracts (*basis pedunculi cerebri*); called also *anterior part of cerebral peduncle, crus cerebri* [NA alternative] and *p. anterior pedunculi cerebri* [NA alternative]. **p. ventra′lis pon′tis** [NA], the part of the pons connecting the cerebrum, cerebellum, and medulla oblongata. It is a broad, transverse band that arches across the ventral surface of the rostral end of the rhombencephalon and on each side narrows to enter the cerebellum as the middle cerebellar peduncle. It comprises longitudinal fibers originating at the cerebral cortex, transverse fibers, and masses of gray matter, the pontine nuclei. Called also *p. basilaris pontis* [NA alternative]. **p. vertebra′lis facie′i costa′lis pulmo′nis** [NA], the part of the costal surface of each lung related behind to the sides of the vertebral bodies. **p. vertebra′lis facie′i media′lis pulmo′nis,** the part of the medial (mediastinal) surface of each lung adjacent to the vertebral column. See *p. vertebralis faciei costalis pulmonis*. **p. vestibula′ris ner′vi octa′vi, p. vestibula′ris ner′vi vestibulocochlea′ris,** nervus vestibularis.

Parsidol (par′sĭ-dol) trademark for a preparation of ethopropazine hydrochloride.

pars planitis (pars pla-ni′tis) a granulomatous uveitis of the pars plana of the ciliary body.

part (part) [L. *pars* a portion, piece, share] a division or portion. For names of other parts of various anatomical structures, see under *pars*. **broad p. of anterior annular ligament of leg,** retinaculum musculorum extensorum pedis superius. **colic p. of omentum,** omentum majus. **condylar p. of occipital bone,** pars lateralis ossis occipitalis. **exoccipital p. of occipital bone,** pars lateralis ossis occipitalis. **interstitial p. of uterine tube, intramural p. of uterine tube,** pars uterina tubae uterinae. **jugular p. of occipital bone,** pars lateralis ossis occipitalis. **lambdoidal (lower) p. of anterior annular ligament of leg,** retinaculum musculorum extensorum pedis inferius. **lateral p. of occipital bone,** pars lateralis ossis occipitalis. **lumbar p. of autonomic nervous system,** pars abdominalis systematis autonomici. **mamillary p. of temporal bone,** pars mastoidea ossis temporalis. **occipital p. of occipital bone,** squama occipitalis. **parietal p. of pelvic fascia,** fascia diaphragmatis pelvis superior. **pectineal p. of inguinal ligament,** ligamentum lacunare. **presenting p.,** that portion of the fetus which is touched by the examining finger through the uterine cervix and, during labor, is bounded by the girdle of resistance. **squamous p. of occipital bone,** squama occipitalis. **squamous p. of temporal bone,** pars squamosa ossis temporalis. **sternocostal p. of diaphragm,** pars costalis diaphragmatis. **subphrenic p. of esophagus,** pars abdominalis esophagi. **superior p. of anterior annular ligament of leg,** retinaculum musculorum extensorum pedis superius. **tabular p. of occipital bone,** squama occipitalis. **tendinous p. of epicranius muscle,** galea aponeurotica. **third p. of quadriceps femoris muscle,** musculus adductor minimus. **transverse p. of anterior annular ligament of leg,** retinaculum musculorum extensorum pedis superius. **vaginal p. of cervix,** portio vaginalis cervicis. **vertebral p. of diaphragm,** pars lumbalis diaphragmatis. **visceral p. of pelvic fascia,** fascia pelvis visceralis.

Part. aeq. abbreviation for L. *par′tes aequa′les,* equal parts.

partal (par′tal) pertaining to parturition.

partes (par′tēz) [L.] plural of *pars*.

parthenocarpy (par″thĕ-no-kar′pe) the reproduction of fruit without fertilization; it may occur naturally or be artificially induced.

parthenogenesis (par″thĕ-no-jen′ĕ-sis) [Gr. *parthenos* virgin + *genesis* production] a modified form of sexual reproduction by the development of a gamete without fertilization, as occurs in some plants and invertebrates, especially arthropods, as honey bees and wasps, and in certain lizards. It may occur as a natural phenomenon or be induced by chemical, thermal, or mechanical stimulation (*artificial p.*).

parthenophobia (par″thĕ-no-fo′be-ah) [Gr. *parthenos* virgin + *phobia*] irrational fear of girls.

parthogenesis (par″tho-jen′ĕ-sis) parthenogenesis.

particle (par′tĕ-k'l) [L. *particula,* dim. of *pars* part] a tiny mass of material. **alpha p.,** a positively charged particle ejected from the nucleus of a radioactive atom, being a high-speed ionized atom of helium. A stream of these particles constitutes alpha rays. **attraction p.,** a small particle in the center of the centrosome. **beta p.,** an electron emitted from an atomic nucleus during beta decay. **C p.,** a noninfectious RNA virus that is postulated to be a normal inhabitant of all living cells and has been postulated as the single cause of all forms of cancer. **colloid p's,** in colloid chemistry the ultimate particles of a dispersed phase. In lyophilic colloids the particles are larger than a single

molecule, being from 1 to 100 micromicrons in diameter, but not large enough to settle out by gravity; in a lyophobic colloid they may consist of one or more large organic molecules, as of starch or protein. **Dane p.,** an intact hepatitis B virion. **disperse p's,** the dispersed phase of a colloid system; the particles of colloid in a colloid system. **elementary p.,** any of the subatomic particles, including electrons, protons, neutrons, positrons, neutrinos, muons, etc. **elementary p's of mitochondria,** numerous minute, club-shaped granules with spherical heads attached to the inner membrane of a mitochondrion. **high-velocity p's,** nuclear particles, such as electrons, protons, and deuterons, given high speeds in an accelerator. **nuclear p's,** Howell-Jolly bodies. **viral p.,** virion. **X-p.,** a hypothetical particle of matter, believed to arise from the collision of cosmic rays in the upper air. **Zimmermann's elementary p's,** blood platelets.

particulate (par-tik′u-lāt) composed of separate particles.

partinium (par-tin′e-um) an alloy of aluminum and tungsten.

partition (par-tish′un) something that separates or divides into parts. **oropharyngeal p.,** a protective barrier between the oral cavity and the pharynx made of moistened gauze sponges, useful during general anesthesia when a nasal mask is used.

partitioning (par-tish′un-ing) dividing into parts. **gastric p.,** a form of gastroplasty in which a small stomach pouch is formed whose filling signals satiety; used in treatment of morbid obesity. Called also *gastric stapling*.

partricin (par-tri′sin) an antifungal and antiprotozoal produced by *Streptomyces aureofaciens,* consisting of a mixture in a constant ratio (about 1:1) of two polytene substances having very similar structures and biological properties. See also *mepartricin*.

parturient (par-tu′re-ent) [L. *parturiens*] giving birth, or pertaining to childbirth; by extension, a woman in labor.

parturifacient (par″tu-re-fa′shent) [L. *parturire* to have the pains of labor + *facere* to cause] 1. inducing or facilitating childbirth. 2. an agent that induces or facilitates childbirth.

parturiometer (par″tu-re-om′ĕ-ter) [L. *parturitio* childbirth + *metrum* measure] a device used in measuring the expulsive power of the uterus.

parturition (par″tu-rish′un) [L. *parturitio*] the act or process of giving birth to a child; see *labor*.

partus (par′tus) [L.] labor, or childbirth.

Part. vic. abbreviation for L. *parti′tis vi′cibus,* in divided doses.

parulis (pah-roo′lis) [*para-*¹ + Gr. *oulon* gum] an elevated nodule at the site of a fistula draining a chronic periapical abscess. Called also *gumboil* (or *gum boil*).

parumbilical (par″um-bil′ĭ-kal) alongside the navel.

paruria (par-u′re-ah) [*para-*¹ + Gr. *ouron* urine + *-ia*] any disorder of the urine or abnormal state of the urine or its discharge.

parvicellular (par″vĭ-sel′u-lar) [L. *parvus* small + *cellula* cell] composed of small cells.

parvoline (par′vo-lin) an amber-colored liquid poison, $C_9H_{13}N$, from decaying fish or horse flesh.

parvovirus (par″vo-vi′rus) [L. *parvus* small + *virus*] a group of extremely small, morphologically similar, ether-resistant DNA viruses; the group includes the osteolytic hamster viruses and adeno-associated viruses. Called also *picodnavirus*.

parvule (par′vūl) [L. *parvulus* very small] a very small pill, pellet, or granule.

Paryphostomum (par″e-fos′to-mum) a genus of flukes related to *Echinostoma*.

PAS para-aminosalicylic acid; periodic acid-Schiff (see under *reaction*).

pascal (pas-kal′, pas′kal) [after Blaise *Pascal*] the SI unit of pressure, which corresponds to a force of one newton per square meter; symbol, Pa.

Pascal's law (pas-kahlz′) [Blaise *Pascal,* French scientist, 1623–1662] see under *law*.

Paschen's bodies (corpuscles, granules) (pahs′kenz) [Enrique *Paschen,* Hamburg pathologist, 1860–1936] see under *body*.

Paschutin's degeneration (pas-ku′tinz) [Viktor Vasil'evich *Paschutin*, Russian pathologist, 1845–1901] see under *degeneration*.

PASG pneumatic antishock garment.

paspalism (pas′pal-izm) poisoning due to the seeds of a grass, *Paspalum scrobiculatum*, of India.

passage (pas′ij) 1. a channel. 2. an evacuation of the bowels. 3. introduction of infectious material into an experimental animal or culture medium, followed by recovery of the infectious agent. 4. the act of moving from one place to another. 5. the introduction of a catheter, probe, sound, or bougie through a natural channel such as the urethra. **blind p.,** successive transfer of infection through experimental animals, chick embryo, or tissue culture, when overt lesions of disease are not apparent, at least in the earlier members of the series. **false p.,** an unnatural channel or meatus in a body structure, created by trauma or by disease. **serial p.,** the successive transfer of a virus or other infectious agent through a series of experimental animals, tissue culture, or synthetic media with growth occurring in each medium. The process is usually used to attenuate a pathogenic agent.

Passavant's bar (cushion, pad, ridge) (pas′ah-vants) [Philip Gustav *Passavant*, German surgeon, 1815–1893] see under *bar*.

passenger (pas′en-jer) the fetus or any of the fetal membranes during labor.

passer (pas′er) one who or that which conveys something from one place to another. **foil p.,** a pointed or forked instrument used to carry pellets of gold foil through an annealing flame or from the annealing tray to the prepared cavity for compaction. Called also *foil carrier*.

Passiflora (pas″ĭ-flo′rah) [L. *passio* passion + *flos* flower] a genus of twining plants of the warmer parts of America; passion flower. Many species, e.g., *P. incarnata* L. (Passifloraceae), were formerly used medicinally for their sedative and anodyne properties.

passive (pas′iv) [L. *passivus*] neither spontaneous nor active; not produced by active efforts.

passivism (pas′ĭ-vizm) in psychiatry, sexual perversion with submission of the will to the partner.

passivity (pas-siv′ĭ-te) 1. in psychology, an unwillingness, inability, or other failure to take initiative or personal responsibility for routine life events. 2. in dentistry, the condition of rest assumed by the teeth, surrounding tissue, and denture when a removable partial denture is in place but not under masticatory pressure.

Past. abbreviation for *Pasteurella*.

pasta (pas′tah), pl. *pas′tae* [L.] paste.

paste (pāst) [L. *pasta*] a semisolid preparation, generally for external use, of a fatty base, a viscous or mucilaginous base, or a mixture of starch and petrolatum. **dextrinated p.,** a preparation of dextrin, glycerin, and distilled water, used as a vehicle. **Ihle's p.,** an ointment containing resorcin, starch, and zinc oxide in soft paraffin. **Lassar's p.,** zinc oxide and salicylic acid p. **Lassar's betanaphthol p.,** a paste containing betanaphthol, precipitated sulfur, soft soap, and petrolatum. **Lassar's plain zinc p.,** zinc oxide p. **Piffard's p.,** a paste made of copper sulfate, tartrated soda, and caustic soda, used in testing the urine for sugar. **triamcinolone acetonide dental p.** [USP], a preparation containing 90 to 115 per cent of the labeled amount of triamcinolone acetonide in a suitable emollient paste; used in the treatment of steroid-responsive oral inflammatory lesions and ulcerative lesions due to trauma, applied topically. **zinc oxide p.** [USP], a preparation of zinc oxide and starch in white petrolatum, used topically as an astringent and protectant; called also *Lassar's plain zinc paste*. **zinc oxide and salicylic acid p.** [USP], **zinc oxide p. with salicylic acid,** a mixture of zinc oxide paste and salicylic acid, containing 23.5 to 25.5 per cent, by weight, of zinc oxide; used topically as an astringent and local protective. Called also *Lassar's p.* **zipp p.,** see *zipp*.

paster (pās′ter) the portion of a bifocal lens ground for near vision.

pastern (pas′tern) the portion of a horse's foot occupied by the first and second phalanges.

Pasteur (pas-tur′) Louis (1822–1895) French chemist, author of the germ theory of disease, and founder of microbiology, virology, and immunology. Pasteur is famous for disproving spontaneous generation and for his work in stereochemistry, lactic and alcoholic fermentation, microbiology and diseases of wine and beer, diseases of silkworms, anaerobiosis, virulent diseases (anthrax, chicken cholera), and preventive inoculation with attenuated microbes (especially against rabies). Pasteur's work enabled Joseph Lister to develop antiseptic surgery.

Pasteur's effect (reaction), method, theory (pas-terz′) [Louis *Pasteur*] see under *effect, method,* and *theory*.

Pasteur-Chamberland filter (pas-ter′-shahm-ber-lah) [Louis *Pasteur*; Charles Edouard Chamberland, French bacteriologist, 1851–1908] see under *filter*.

Pasteurella (pas″tĕ-rel′ah) [Louis *Pasteur*] a genus of gram-negative, facultatively anaerobic, ovoid to rod-shaped bacteria of the family Pasteurellaceae, made up of nonmotile fermentative organisms. Bipolar staining is common. They are parasitic on humans, wild and domestic animals, and birds, and are potential pathogens, causing abscesses and septicemias in humans and respiratory and septic infections in sheep, cattle, and fowl. **P. aerog′enes,** a species occurring in swine that is a possible cause of abortion in swine and of human wound infections following swine bites. **P. anatipes′tifer,** a species of uncertain affiliation that causes infectious avian serositis. Called also *P. anapestifer* and *Pfeifferella anatipestifer*. **P. haemolyt′ica,** a species that is part of the normal flora of cattle and sheep. It is the etiologic agent of mastitis and respiratory and septic infections in sheep, pneumonia ("shipping fever") in cattle, and a cholera-like disease in fowl. It has also been associated with human infections. **P. multoci′da,** a species that is part of the normal flora of the mouth and respiratory tract of domesticated and wild animals and birds. In animals, it causes hemorrhagic septicemias, pneumonia, local abscesses, and intestinal disease. Human disease usually occurs from a wound infection following a cat or dog bite or scratch, with localized swelling, abscesses, bronchiectasis, pneumonia, meningitis, and septicemia being the common symptoms. Several biotypes and serotypes are recognized. Formerly called *P. septica*. **P. novi′cida,** *Francisella novicida*. **P. pes′tis,** *Yersinia pestis*. **P. pfaf′fii,** a species of uncertain status that is the etiologic agent of an epidemic septicemia in canaries. **P. pneumotro′pica,** a species occurring normally and as an occasional pathogen in rodents; it is of importance as a human pathogen. **P. pseudotuberculo′sis,** former name for *Yersinia pseudotuberculosis*. **P. sep′tica,** *P. multocida*. **P. septicae′miae,** a species of uncertain status that causes septicemia in young geese. **P. tularen′sis,** *Francisella tularensis*. **P. ure′ae,** a species with no known animal host. It has been isolated from human infections of the upper respiratory tract and occasionally from the nasal passages of healthy humans.

Pasteurellaceae (pas″tĕ-rel-a′se-e) a family of facultatively anaerobic, nonmotile, gram-negative, coccoid to rod-shaped bacteria, occurring as parasites in mammals and birds. It contains the genera *Actinobacillus, Haemophilus,* and *Pasteurella*.

Pasteurelleae (pas″ter-el′e-e) in former systems of classification, a tribe of bacteria that included the genus *Pasteurella*.

pasteurellosis (pas″ter-el-lo′sis) infection by microorganisms of the genus *Pasteurella*; see individual species, under *Pasteurella*.

Pasteuria (pas-tu′re-ah) a genus of budding bacteria found in water and in fresh-water crustacea, made up of ovoid or pear-shaped cells, occurring singly or in clusters. The type species is *P. ramo′sa*.

Pasteuriaceae (pas-tu″re-a′se-e) in former systems of classification, a family of bacteria that reproduce by budding. They are now classified in the genera *Pasteuria* and *Planctomyces*.

pasteurization (pas″ter-ĭ-za′shun) [Louis *Pasteur*] the process of heating milk or other liquids, e.g., wine or beer, to destroy microorganisms that would cause spoilage. The milk is held at 62° C. for 30 minutes (LTHM, low temperature holding method, holding method), or heated rapidly to 80° C. and held for 15 to 30 seconds (HTST, high temperature short time, flash method), and then chilled. The procedure kills most pathogenic bacteria while retaining the flavor of the liquid.

pasteurizer (pas′ter-īz″er) an instrument used in effecting pasteurization.

Pastia's lines (sign) (pas′te-ahz) [C. *Pastia*, Rumanian physician, born 1878] see under *sign*.

pastil (pas′til) pastille.

pastille (pas-tēl′) [Fr.] 1. a troche in which the active ingredient is incorporated in a mass of sweetened gum, glycerin, and gelatin base. 2. an aromatic mass to be burnt as a fumigant. 3. A small disk of paper coated with platinocyanide of barium or other substance. The green color changes to brown when exposed to roentgen rays. Formerly used to estimate the amount of x-ray administered and also to test the intensity of ultraviolet radiation.

patch (pach) [L. *pittacium*; Gr. *pittakion*] an area differing from the rest of a surface, in either color or texture, or both, but not elevated above it; a macule more than 3 or 4 cm. in diameter. **Bitot's p's,** see under *spot*. **cotton-wool p's,** see under *spot*. **herald p.,** the solitary lesion that precedes the general eruption in pityriasis rosea. **Hutchinson's p.,** salmon p. (def. 1). **MacCallum's p.,** a sheet of granulation tissue in the deeper layers of the endocardium formed by extensive confluence of Aschoff nodules in the myocardium in rheumatic fever. **mucous p.,** a flat, rounded, grayish white erosion covered by a soggy membrane with an erythematous zone, occurring most often on the oral mucosa, and sometimes on the anogenital mucosa, in early active secondary syphilis. It contains vast numbers of treponemata and is therefore highly contagious. **Peyer's p's,** oval elevated areas of lymphoid tissue on the mucosa of the small intestine, composed of many lymphoid nodules closely packed together (folliculi lymphatici aggregati [NA]). **salmon p.,** 1. a salmon-colored spot in the cornea in syphilis of that structure; called also *Hutchinson's p.* 2. a salmon-colored nevus flammeus, which is usually found over the eyelids, between the eyes, and on the mid forehead, and commonly fades completely. **shagreen p.,** see under *skin*. **smokers' p.,** stomatitis nicotina. **soldiers' p's,** milk spots, def. 1. **white p.,** a white opaque spot on the pericardium or on the capsule of the spleen, due to rubbing against a nodule of a rib in rachitis.

patchouli (pat-shoo′le) a labiate herb of India, *Pogostemon patchouli* Pellet., used chiefly in perfumery and soaps.

patefaction (pat″ĕ-fak′shun) [L. *patefacere* to lay open] the act of laying open.

Patein's albumin (pat-anz′) [Gustav Constant *Patein*, French physician, 1857–1928] acetosoluble albumin.

patella (pah-tel′ah) [L., dim of *patera* a shallow dish] [NA] a triangular sesamoid bone, about 5 cm. in diameter, situated at the front of the knee in the tendon of insertion of the quadriceps extensor femoris muscle. Called also *knee cap.* **p. biparti′ta,** a patella that is divided into two parts. **p. cu′biti,** an anomalous sesamoid bone sometimes occurring over the extensor surface of the elbow joint. **floating p.,** a patella that is separated from the condyles by a large effusion in the knee. **p. parti′ta,** a patella that is divided into two or more parts. **slipping p.,** a patella that is easily movable and readily dislocated.

Patella's disease (pah-tel′ahz) [Vincenzo *Patella*, Italian physician, 1856–1928] see under *disease*.

patellar (pah-tel′ar) [L. *patellarius*] of or pertaining to the patella.

patellectomy (pat″ĕ-lek′to-me) [patella + Gr. *ektomē* excision] excision or removal of the patella.

patelliform (pah-tel′ĭ-form) shaped like the patella.

patellofemoral (pah-tel″o-fem′o-ral) pertaining to the patella and the femur.

patellometer (pat″e-lom′ĕ-ter) [patella + Gr. *metron* measure] an instrument for measuring the patellar reflex.

patency (pa′ten-se) [L. *patens* open] the condition of being wide open.

patent (pa′tent) [L. *patens*] 1. open, unobstructed, or not closed. 2. apparent, evident.

Paterson's syndrome (pat′er-sonz) [Donald Rose *Paterson*, laryngologist in Cardiff (Wales), 1863–1939] Plummer-Vinson syndrome.

Paterson-Brown Kelly syndrome (pat′er-son brown kel′e) [D. R. *Paterson*; Adam *Brown Kelly*, 1865–1941] Plummer-Vinson syndrome.

Paterson-Kelly syndrome (pat′er-son kel′e) [D. R. Paterson; Adam B. *Kelly*] Plummer-Vinson syndrome.

Patey's operation (pa′tēz) [David Howard *Patey*, English surgeon, born 1899] see *modified radical mastectomy*, under *mastectomy*.

path (path) a particular course that is followed, or a route that is ordinarily traversed. In neurology, the set of nerve fibers along which a nervous impulse may move, whether esodic or exodic; particularly the intracranial or intraspinal portion of such a course. See also *pathway*. **condyle p.,** the course followed by the mandibular condyle in the temporomandibular joint during the various movements of the mandible. **copulation p.,** the course taken by the male and female pronuclei as they approach each other in a fertilized ovum. **incisor p.,** the course followed by the incisal edges of the lower anterior teeth in movement of the mandible from the position of normal occlusion to that of edge-to-edge contact with opposing incisors. **p. of insertion,** that direction or path of a removable partial denture that permits the proper relation of the prosthesis to the hard and soft tissues on insertion, on removal, in function, and at rest. Called also *p. of removal*. **ionization p.,** the trail of ion pairs produced by ionizing radiation in its passage through matter; called also *ionization track*. **lateral condyle p.,** the path of the condyle in the glenoid fossa when a lateral mandibular movement is made. **milled-in p's,** 1. the contours carved by various mandibular movements into the occluding surface of an occlusion rim by teeth or studs placed in the opposing occlusion rim. The curves or contours may be carved into wax, modeling plastic, or plaster of Paris. 2. gliding movements of occlusion rims which are composed of materials, including abrasives. **occlusal p.,** the course followed by the occlusal surfaces of the lower teeth in movements of the mandible. **occlusal p., generated,** a registration of the paths of movement of the occlusal surfaces of mandibular teeth on a plastic or abrasive surface attached to the maxillary arch.

pathema (pah-the′mah), pl. *pathemas* or *pathem′ata* [Gr. *pathēma* disease] any disease state or morbid condition.

pathematology (path″ĕ-mah-tol′o-je) [*pathema* + *-logy*] (*obs.*) pathology, especially psychopathology.

pathergia (pah-ther′je-ah) pathergy.

pathergic (path′er-jik) characterized by pathergy.

pathergy (path′er-je) [path- + Gr. *ergon* work] 1. an abnormal reaction to an allergen, either a subnormal reaction or an excessive reaction. 2. the condition of being allergic to numerous antigens; polyvalent allergy.

pathetic (pah-thet′ik) [L. *patheticus*; Gr. *pathētikos*] pertaining to the trochlear nerve.

pathfinder (path′find-er) 1. an instrument for locating strictures of the urethra. 2. root canal probe.

Pathilon (path′i-lon) trademark for a preparation of tridihexethyl chloride.

path(o)- [Gr. *pathos* disease] a combining form denoting relationship to disease.

pathoamine (path″o-am′in) an amine causing disease, or formed as the product of a disease process; a ptomaine.

pathoanatomical (path″o-an″ah-tom′ĭ-kal) pertaining to the anatomy of diseased tissues.

pathoanatomy (path″o-ah-nat′o-me) pathologic anatomy.

pathobiology (path″o-bi-ol′o-je) pathology.

Pathocil (path′o-sil) trademark for a preparation of dicloxacillin sodium.

pathoclisis (path″o-klis′is) a specific elemental sensitivity to specific toxins, or a specific affinity of certain toxins for certain systems of organs.

pathodontia (path″o-don′she-ah) dental pathology.

pathoformic (path″o-for′mik) [patho- + L. *forma* form] pertaining to the beginning of disease; said of symptoms at the beginning of mental disorder.

pathogen (path′o-jen) [patho- + Gr. *gennan* to produce] any disease-producing microorganism.

pathogenesis (path″o-jen′ĕ-sis) [patho- + *genesis*] the development of morbid conditions or of disease; more specifically the cellular events and reactions and other pathologic mechanisms occurring in the development of disease. **drug p.,** the production of symptoms of disease by the use of drugs.

pathogenesy (path″o-jen′ĕ-se) pathogenesis.

pathogenetic (path″o-jĕ-net′ik) pertaining to pathogenesis.

pathogenic (path-o-jen′ik) giving origin to disease or to morbid symptoms.

pathogenicity (path″o-jĕ-nis′ĭ-te) the quality of producing or the ability to produce pathologic changes or disease.

pathogeny (path-oj′ĕ-ne) pathogenesis.

pathognomonic (path″og-no-mon′ik) [patho- + Gr. gnōmonikos fit to give judgment] specifically distinctive or characteristic of a disease or pathologic condition; a sign or symptom on which a diagnosis can be made.

pathognomy (path-og′no-me) [patho- + Gr. gnōmē a means of knowing] the science of the signs and symptoms of disease.

pathognostic (path″og-nos′tik) pathognomonic.

pathography (pah-thog′rah-fe) [patho- + Gr. graphein to write] a history or description of disease.

pathologic (path″o-loj′ik) 1. indicative of or caused by a morbid condition. 2. pertaining to pathology.

pathological (path″o-loj′ĭ-kal) pertaining to pathology; pathologic.

pathologist (pah-thol′o-jist) an expert in pathology. **speech p.,** a person skilled and certified in speech pathology.

pathology (pah-thol′o-je) [patho- + -logy] 1. that branch of medicine which treats of the essential nature of disease, especially of the structural and functional changes in tissues and organs of the body which cause or are caused by disease. 2. the structural and functional manifestations of disease. **cellular p.,** that which regards the cells as starting points of the phenomena of disease and that every cell descends from some preexisting cell (Virchow). **clinical p.,** pathology applied to the solution of clinical problems, especially the use of laboratory methods in clinical diagnosis. **comparative p.,** that which institutes comparisons between various diseases of the human body and those of the lower animals. **dental p.,** the branch of pathology that treats dental changes in disease. Called also pathodontia. See also oral p. **experimental p.,** the study of artificially induced disease processes. **functional p.,** the study of the changes of function due to morbid tissue changes. **general p.,** that which takes cognizance of pathologic conditions which may occur in various diseases and in different organs. **geographical p.,** the study and comparison of variations in morbidity and mortality in different geographic regions to determine the relationship between these variations and environmental conditions found in each region. Called also geopathology. **humoral p.,** see humoralism. **internal p.,** medical p. **medical p.,** that which relates to morbid processes which are not accessible to operative intervention. Cf. surgical p. **oral p.,** the branch of pathology that treats the structural and functional changes in cells, tissues, and organs of the oral cavity that cause or are caused by disease. See also dental p. **plant p.,** the pathology of diseases of plants. **solidistic p.,** that opinion which attributes disease to rarefaction or condensation of the solid tissues. **special p.,** the study of the pathology of particular diseases or organs. **speech p.,** a field of the health sciences dealing with the evaluation of speech, language, and voice disorders and the rehabilitation of patients with such disorders not amenable to medical or surgical treatment. **surgical p.,** the pathology of disease processes which are surgically accessible for diagnosis or treatment. **vegetable p.,** plant p.

pathomaine (path′o-mān) any of the pathogenic cadaveric alkaloids.

pathomania (path-o-ma′ne-ah) [patho- + Gr. mania madness] (obs.) moral insanity.

pathometer (pah-thom′ĕ-ter) an apparatus for recording the incidence of disease in a given locality.

pathometry (pah-thom′ĕ-tre) [patho- + Gr. metrein to measure] (obs.) Sir Ronald Ross' term for the quantitative study of parasitic invasion and infection in individuals or groups of individuals.

pathomimesis (path″o-mi-me′sis) [patho- + Gr. mimēsis imitation] malingering.

pathomimia (path″o-mim′e-ah) malingering.

pathomimicry (path″o-mim′ĭ-kre) malingering.

pathomorphism (path″o-mor′fizm) abnormal morphology.

pathoneurosis (path″o-nu-ro′sis) hysterical symptoms due to a chronic disease process.

pathonomia (path-o-no′me-ah) [patho- + Gr. nomos law] the sum of knowledge regarding the laws of disease.

pathonomy (pah-thon′o-me) pathonomia.

pathophobia (path″o-fo′be-ah) nosophobia.

pathophysiology (path″o-fiz″e-ol′o-je) the physiology of disordered function.

pathopoiesis (path″o-poi-e′sis) [patho- + Gr. poiēsis production] 1. the causation of disease. 2. the tendency of an individual to become diseased.

pathopsychology (path″o-si-kol′o-je) [patho- + psychology] the psychology of mental disease.

pathopsychosis (path″o-si-ko′sis) a psychosis arising from organic diseases, such as brain tumors, encephalitis, etc.

pathosis (pah-tho′sis) [patho- + -osis] a condition of disease; a morbid condition.

pathotropism (pah-thot′ro-pizm) [patho- + Gr. tropos a turning] the tendency of drugs to pass to diseased areas.

pathway (path′wa) a path or course, especially a course followed in the attainment of a specific end. In neurology, the nerve structures through which a sensory impression is conducted to the cerebral cortex (afferent p.) or through which an impulse passes from the brain to the skeletal musculature (efferent p.). See also path. Also used alone to indicate a sequence of reactions which convert one biological material to another (metabolic pathway). **alternative complement p.,** see complement. **amphibolic p.,** a group of metabolic reactions with a dual function, providing small metabolites for further catabolism to end products or for use as precursors in synthetic, anabolic reactions. The tricarboxylic cycle system is an example. See also anabolism and catabolism. **classic complement p.,** see complement. **Embden-Meyerhof p.** (of glucose metabolism), the series of enzymatic reactions in the anaerobic conversion of glucose to lactic acid, resulting in energy in the form of adenosine triphosphate (ATP). **Embden-Meyerhof-Parnas p.,** Embden-Meyerhof p. **Entner-Doudoroff p.,** a series of enzymatic reactions in bacteria that convert glucose to pyruvate by way of the intermediate 2-keto-3-deoxy-6-phosphogluconate, forming ATP. It is the major pathway of glucose metabolism in certain strains of Pseudomonas and Zymomonas. **final common p.,** the motor neurons by which nerve impulses from many central sources pass to a muscle or gland in the periphery. **internuncial p.,** a correlation tract connecting different centers or neurons within the central nervous system. **lipoxygenase p.,** a pathway for the formation of leukotrienes from arachidonic acid. It is initiated by the action of arachidonate 5-lipoxygenase or arachidonate 12-lipoxygenase. The reactions occur in the cytosol of leukocytes, mast cells, platelets, and lung tissue cells. **metabolic p.,** a series of enzymatic reactions that converts one biological material to another. **pentose phosphate p.,** a major branching of the Embden-Meyerhof pathway of carbohydrate metabolism: a pathway of hexose oxidation in which glucose-6-phosphate undergoes two successive oxidations by NADP, the final one being an oxidative decarboxylation to form a pentose phosphate. Called also phosphogluconate p., hexose monophosphate shunt, and pentose shunt. **phosphogluconate p.,** pentose phosphate p. **properdin p.,** alternative complement p., see complement. **reentrant p.,** a mechanism by which a premature or ectopic heart beat is coupled to the normal beat; see reentry.

-pathy [Gr. -patheia, from pathos disease] a word termination denoting a morbid condition, or disease.

patient (pa′shent) [L. patiens] a person who is ill or who is undergoing treatment for disease.

Patrick's test (sign) (pat′riks) [Hugh Talbot Patrick, neurologist in Chicago, 1860–1938] see under tests.

patrilineal (pat″rĭ-lin′e-al) [L. pater father + linea line] descended through the male line.

patroclinous (pat″ro-kli′nus) [Gr. patēr father + klinein to incline] inheriting or inherited from the father; having characters inherited from the father. Cf. matroclinous.

patrogenesis (pat″ro-jen′ĕ-sis) [Gr. patēr father + genesis] androgenesis.

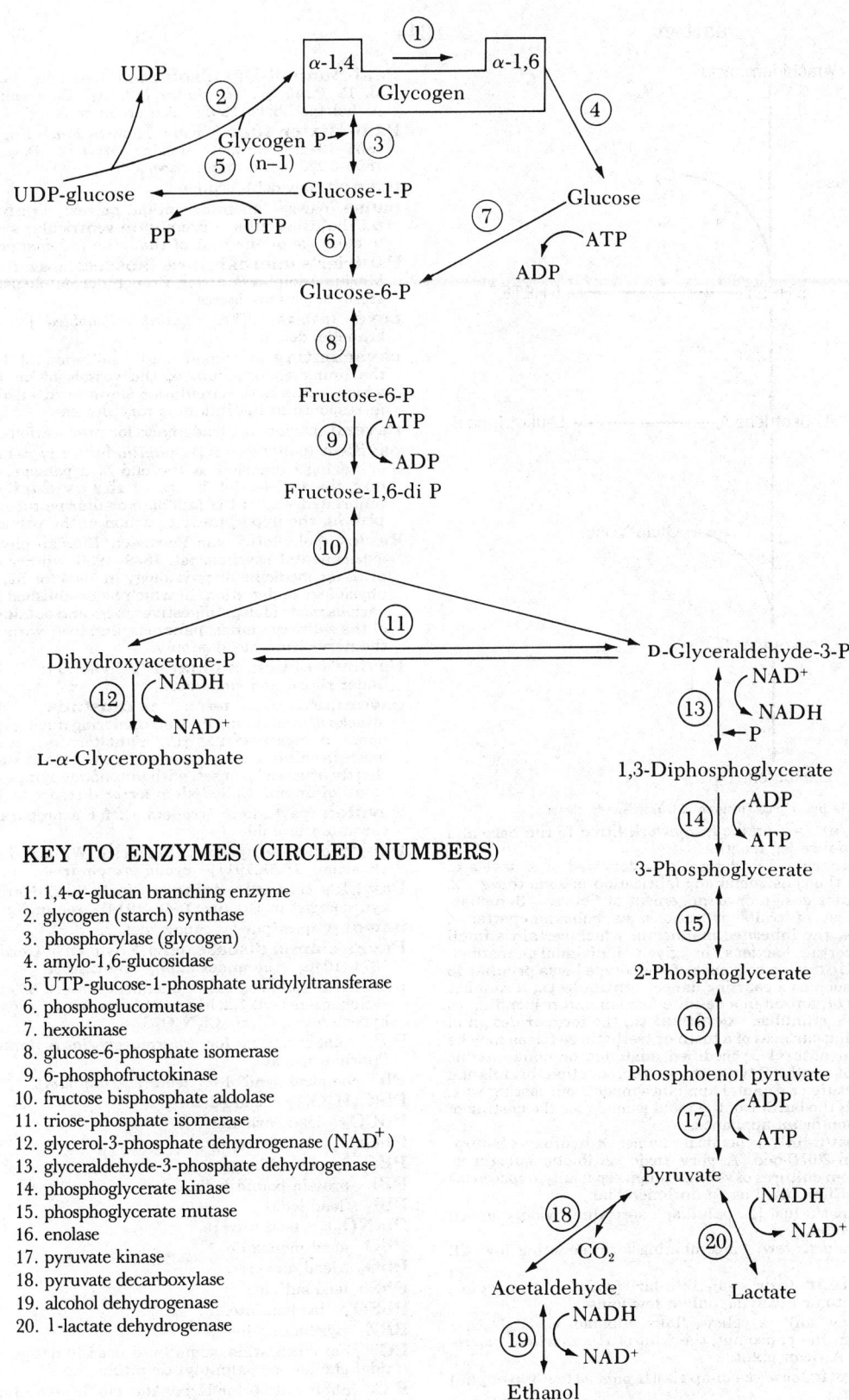

KEY TO ENZYMES (CIRCLED NUMBERS)

1. 1,4-α-glucan branching enzyme
2. glycogen (starch) synthase
3. phosphorylase (glycogen)
4. amylo-1,6-glucosidase
5. UTP-glucose-1-phosphate uridylyltransferase
6. phosphoglucomutase
7. hexokinase
8. glucose-6-phosphate isomerase
9. 6-phosphofructokinase
10. fructose bisphosphate aldolase
11. triose-phosphate isomerase
12. glycerol-3-phosphate dehydrogenase (NAD$^+$)
13. glyceraldehyde-3-phosphate dehydrogenase
14. phosphoglycerate kinase
15. phosphoglycerate mutase
16. enolase
17. pyruvate kinase
18. pyruvate decarboxylase
19. alcohol dehydrogenase
20. l-lactate dehydrogenase

Embden-Meyerhof pathway of glucose metabolism.

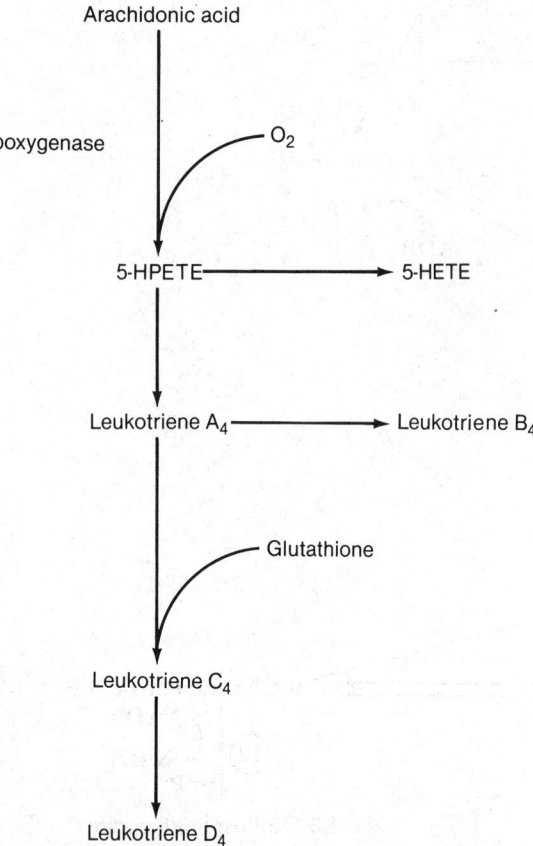

Arachidonic acid

5-Lipoxygenase O_2

5-HPETE ⟶ 5-HETE

Leukotriene A_4 ⟶ Leukotriene B_4

Glutathione

Leukotriene C_4

Leukotriene D_4

The lipoxygenase pathway of leukotriene synthesis.

patten (pat′n) a metallic framework fitted to the base of a shoe to equalize leg length.

pattern (pat′ern) 1. a design to be followed or a device to be used in the construction or fabrication of something. 2. the particular design or arrangement of figures. 3. a characteristic set of traits or actions, as behavior patterns. **action p.,** the inherited manner in which certain stimuli produce certain actions in given individuals; instinct. **fixed action p.,** a sequence of stereotyped acts peculiar to a species, such as a courting dance. **muscle p.,** a number of muscles organized in a definite fashion and responding as a whole to a stimulus. **occlusal p.,** the form or design of the occluding surfaces of a tooth or teeth; these forms may be based upon natural or modified anatomic or nonanatomic concepts of teeth. **wax p.,** a reproduction of missing tooth structure or a dental appliance made from casting wax, from which the outline of the mold is made for the casting of a restoration or an appliance.

patulin (pat′u-lin) chemical name: 4-hydroxy-4*H*-furo-[3,2-*c*]pyran-2(6*H*)-one. A very toxic antibiotic substance, $C_7H_6O_4$, from cultures of various fungi, especially *Aspergillus* and *Penicillium;* used as an antimicrobial.

patulous (pat′u-lus) [L. *patulus*] spreading widely apart; open; distended.

pauci- [L. *paucus* few] a combining form denoting few. Cf. *oligo-.*

pauciarticular (paw″se-ar-tik′u-lar) [*pauci-* + *articular*] pertaining to or involving only a few joints.

paucine (paw′sin) a yellow, flaky alkaloid, $C_{27}H_{39}N_5O_5 \cdot 6\frac{1}{2}H_2O$, from the pauco nut, the fruit of *Pentaclethra macrophylla,* an African plant.

paucisynaptic (paw″se-sin-ap′tik)[L. *paucus* few + *synaptic*] oligosynaptic.

Paul's test, treatment (pawlz) [Gustav *Paul,* Austrian physician, 1859–1935] see under *tests* and *treatment.*

Paul-Bunnell test (pawl buh-nel′) [John Rodman *Paul,* American physician, 1893–1971; Walls Willard *Bunnell,* American physician, born 1902] see under *tests.*

Paul-Bunnell-Davidsohn test (pawl buh-nel′ da′vid-son) [J. R. *Paul;* W. W. *Bunnell;* Israel Davidsohn, American pathologist, born 1895] see under *tests.*

Paul-Mixter tube [Frank Thomas *Paul,* English surgeon, 1851–1941; Samuel Jason *Mixter,* Boston surgeon, 1855–1926] see under *tube.*

paunch (pawnch) rumen.

pause (pawz) an interruption, or rest. **compensatory p.,** the pause after a premature ventricular systole, related to blockage of one beat of the basic pacemaker.

Pautrier's microabscess (abscess) (paw-tre-āz′) [Lucien Marius Adolphe *Pautrier,* French dermatologist, 1876–1959] see under *microabscess.*

pavé (pah-va′) [Fr. *"paved," "cobbled"*] pseudomembranelle, def. 1.

pavementing (pāv′ment-ing) adhesion of leukocytes to the lining endothelium of the vessels of an injured part, which occurs as the circulation slows down within the vessels in response to the inflammatory process.

Paveril (pav′er-il) trademark for preparations of dioxyline.

pavilion (pah-vil′yun) [L. *papilio* butterfly, tent] a dilated or flaring expansion at the end of a passage. **p. of the ear,** the auricle, def. 1. **p. of the oviduct,** the outer, or fimbriated, end of the fallopian or uterine tube. **p. of the pelvis,** the upper, flaring portion of the pelvis.

Pavlov (pahv′lof) Ivan Petrovich. Russian physiologist and experimental psychologist, 1849–1936; winner of the Nobel prize for medicine or physiology in 1904 for his work on the physiology of digestion, in which he established fistulas from various parts of dogs' digestive tracts and obtained secretions of the salivary glands, pancreas, and liver without upsetting the nerves and blood supply.

Pavlov's pouch, stomach (pahv′lovz) [I. P. *Pavlov*] see under *pouch* and *stomach.*

pavor (pa′vor) [L.] terror. **p. diur′nus** [L. "day terrors"], attacks of anxiety in children occurring during the afternoon nap. **p. noctur′nus** [L. "night terrors"], a sleep disturbance in children characterized by extreme anxiety occurring shortly after sleep onset, with autonomic symptoms and poor recall of dream. Called *sleep terror disorder* in DSM III-R.

Pavulon (pav′u-lon) trademark for a preparation of pancuronium bromide.

Pavy's disease (pa′vēz) [Frederick William *Pavy,* English physician, 1829–1911] cyclic proteinuria.

Pawlik's triangle (trigone) (pahv′liks) [Karel J. *Pawlik,* gynecologist in Prague, 1849–1914] see under *triangle.*

pawpaw (paw′paw) papaw, def. 2.

Payr's clamp, disease (pīrz) [Erwin *Payr,* German surgeon, 1871–1946] see under *clamp* and *disease.*

pazoxide (pah-zok′sīd) chemical name: 6,7-dichloro-3-(3-cyclopenten-1-yl)-1,2,4-benzothiadiazine 1,1-dioxide; an antihypertensive, $C_{12}H_{10}Cl_2N_2O_2S$.

P.B. abbreviation for *Pharmacopoeia Britannica,* British Pharmacopoeia.

Pb chemical symbol for *lead* [L. *plumbum*].

Pb($C_2H_3O_2$)$_2$ lead acetate.

PbCO$_3$ lead carbonate.

PbCrO$_4$ lead chromate.

PBG porphobilinogen.

PBI protein-bound iodine.

PbI$_2$ lead iodide.

Pb(NO$_3$)$_2$ lead nitrate.

PbO lead monoxide.

PbO$_2$ lead dioxide.

PbS lead sulfide.

PbSO$_4$ lead sulfate.

PBZ pyribenzamine.

PC phosphocreatine; sometimes used to designate phosphatidyl choline, or palmitoyl carnitine.

P.C. abbreviation for L. *pon′dus civi′le,* avoirdupois weight.

p.c. abbreviation for L. *post ci′bum,* after meals.

PCA passive cutaneous anaphylaxis.

PCB polychlorinated biphenyl; see under *biphenyl.*

PcB abbreviation for *near point of convergence to the intercentral base line.*

P.Cc.   periscopic concave.

PCG   phonocardiogram.

pCi   picocurie.

PCO₂   symbol for *carbon dioxide partial pressure* or *tension*; also written P_{CO_2}, pCO_2, and pCO_2.

PCV   packed cell volume; see under *volume*.

P.Cx.   periscopic convex.

PD   prism diopter; interpupillary distance.

Pd   chemical symbol for *palladium*.

PE   phosphatidylethanolamine.

peak (pēk)   the top or upper limit of a graphic tracing or of any variable.   **Bragg p.,** a peak in the Bragg curve reflecting a sharp increase in the intensity of ionization produced by an ionizing particle just before its velocity falls to zero.   **kilovolts p.,** the highest kilovoltage used in producing a roentgenogram; abbreviated kVp.

Péan's forceps (pa-anz′) [Jules Émile *Péan*, French surgeon, 1830–1898]   see under *forceps*.

pearl (perl)   1. a small calcareous concretion from various species of mollusks, formerly regarded as having curative powers.   2. a small medicated granule, or a glass globule with a single dose of volatile medicine, as amyl nitrite.   3. a rounded mass of tough sputum as seen in the early stages of an attack of bronchial asthma.   **Bohn's p's,** see under *nodule*.   **Elschnig's p's,** see under *body*.   **enamel p.,** enameloma.   **epidermic p's, epithelial p's,** rounded concentric masses of epithelial cells found in certain papillomas and epitheliomas; called also *pearly bodies*.   **Epstein's p's,** small whitish-yellow cysts (*milia*) on each side of the raphe of the hard palate of the newborn.   **gouty p.,** a sodium urate concretion on the cartilage of the ear in gouty persons.   **Laënnec's p's,** soft casts of the smaller bronchial tubes expectorated in bronchial asthma.

pearlash (perl′ash)   impure potassium carbonate in crystals.

Pearson's product-moment correlation coefficient (pēr-sonz′) [Karl *Pearson*, British statistician, 1857–1936]   see under *coefficient*.

peau (po) [Fr.]   skin.   **p. de chagrin** (po″duh shah-gran′) [Fr.], shagreen skin.   **p. d'orange** (po″do-rahnj′) [Fr. "orange skin"], a dimpled condition of the skin, resembling that of an orange.

pebble (peb″l)   a kind of rock crystal from which lenses are sometimes cut.

pébrine (pa-brēn′) [Fr.]   an infectious disease of silkworms caused by *Nosema bombycis*. Cf. *nosema disease*.

pecazine (pe′kah-zēn)   mepazine.

peccant (pek′ant) [L. *peccans* sinning]   unhealthy; causing illness or disease.

peccatiphobia (pek″kah-tĭ-fo′be-ah) [L. *peccata*, sins + *phobia*]   irrational fear of sinning.

pechyagra (pek″e-a′grah) [Gr. *pēchys* forearm + *agra* seizure]   gout of the elbow.

pecil(o)-   for words beginning thus, see those beginning *poikil(o)-*.

Pecquet's cistern (reservoir), duct (pek-āz′) [Jean *Pecquet*, French anatomist, 1622–1674]   see *cisterna chyli* and *ductus thoracicus*.

pecten (pek′ten), pl. *pec′tines* [L.]   1. a comb; applied to certain anatomical structures because of a fancied resemblance to a comb.   2. p. analis.   3. a triangular pleated membrane in the eye of birds, extending forward from the optic disk, which it covers, for a variable distance into the vitreous body.   **p. of anal canal, p. ana′lis** [NA], the zone in the lower half of the anal canal between the anocutaneous line and the anal verge; called also *pecten*.   **p. os′sis pu′bis** [NA], the anterior border of the superior ramus of the pubis, beginning at the pubic tubercle and continuing to the iliopubic eminence; called also *pectineal line*.

pectenine (pek′tĕ-nin)   a poisonous alkaloidal compound from a Mexican cactus, *Cereus pecten*.

pectenitis (pek″tĕ-ni′tis)   inflammation of the pecten of the anus.

pectenosis (pek″tĕ-no′sis)   stenosis of the anal canal caused by a rigid, inelastic ring of tissue of variable width and thickness, between the anal groove and anal crypts, producing pain on defecation, bleeding, and anal irritation.

pectenotomy (pek″tĕ-not′o-me) [*pecten* + Gr. *tomē* a cutting]   surgical correction of pectenosis by incision of the ring of tissue causing it.

pectic (pek′tik)   relating to pectin.

pectic acid (pek′tik)   galacturonic acid.

pectin (pek′tin) [Gr. *pēktos* congealed]   a homosaccharidic polymer of sugar acids of fruit that forms gels with sugar at the proper pH. A purified form [USP] obtained from the acid extract of the inner portion of the rind of citrus fruits or from apple pomace is used as the protective component of various formulations employed in the treatment of diarrhea and as a suspending agent in pharmaceutical preparations. It is also used in the preparation of certain foods, such as jams and jellies.

pectinate (pek′tĭ-nāt) [L. *pecten* comb]   shaped like a comb.

Pectinatus (pek″tĭ-na′tus) [L. *pectinatus* combed]   a genus of gram-negative, anaerobic, slightly curved, rod-shaped bacteria of the family Bacteroidaceae, made up of motile cells with lateral flagella. They are found in spoiled packaged beer. The type species is *P. cerevisii′philus*.

pectineal (pek-tin′e-al) [L. *pecten*, comb, pubes]   pertaining to the os pubis.

pectiniform (pek-tin′ĭ-form) [L. *pecten* comb + *forma* form]   comb-shaped.

pectization (pek″ti-za′shun) [Gr. *pēktikos* curdling]   coagulation or gelatinization; a term used in colloidal chemistry.

Pectobacterium (pek″to-bak-te′re-um)   a genus of gram-negative, facultatively anaerobic, rod-shaped organisms of the family Enterobacteriaceae, made up of plant pathogens. The organisms are not human pathogens but have been occasionally isolated from clinical specimens. Called also *Erwinia*.

pectolytic (pek″to-lit′ik) [*pectin* + Gr. *lytikos* dissolving]   capable of effecting the digestion of pectin.

pectora (pek″to-rah) [L.]   plural of *pectus*.

pectoral (pek′to-ral) [L. *pectoralis*]   1. of, or pertaining to, the breast or chest.   2. relieving disorders of the respiratory tract, as an expectorant.

pectoralgia (pek″to-ral′je-ah) [L. *pectus* breast + *-algia*]   pain in the breast or pectoral muscles.

pectoralis (pek″to-ra′lis) [L., from *pectus*, q.v.]   pertaining to the breast or chest.

pectoriloquy (pek″to-ril′o-kwe) [L. *pectus* breast + *loqui* to speak]   transmission of the sound of spoken words through the chest wall.   **aphonic p.,** the sound of the whispered voice transmitted through a serous, but not through a purulent, exudate within the pleura.   **whispered p., whispering p.,** the transmission of the sound of whispered words through the walls of the chest.

pectorophony (pek″to-rof′o-ne) [L. *pectus* breast + Gr. *phōnē* voice]   exaggeration of the vocal resonance heard on auscultation.

pectose (pek′tōs)   a principle in unripe fruits and plants from which pectin is derived.

pectous (pek′tus)   pertaining to, composed of, or resembling pectin; having a firm, jelly-like consistence.

pectunculus (pek-tung′ku-lus) [L., dim of *pecten* comb]   any one of the series of small longitudinal ridges on the aqueduct of Sylvius.

pectus (pek′tus), gen. *pec′toris*, pl. *pec′tora* [L.]   the breast: the chest or thorax.   **p. carina′tum** [L. "keeled breast"], undue prominence of the sternum; called also *chicken* or *pigeon breast*.   **p. excava′tum** [L. "hollowed breast"], undue depression of the sternum; called also *funnel breast* or *chest*.   **p. gallina′tum,** p. carinatum.   **p. recurva′tum,** p. excavatum.

pedal (ped′al) [L. *pedalis; pes* foot]   pertaining to the foot or feet.

pedarthrocace (pe-dar-throk′ah-se) [Gr. *pais* child + *arthrocace*]   caries of the joints in children.

pedatrophia (pe-dah-tro′fe-ah) [Gr. *pais* child + *atrophia*]   1. marasmus.   2. (obs.) tabes mesenterica.

pederast (ped′er-ast)   one who practices pederasty.

pederasty (ped′er-as″te) [Gr. *pais* boy + *erastēs* lover]   anal intercourse between a man and a boy.

pederin (ped′er-in)   a crystalline toxin, $C_{25}H_{45}NO_9$, isolated from blister beetles of the genus *Paederus*.

pedes (pe′dēz) [L.] plural of *pes*.

pedi- see *ped(o)-*².

Pediaflor (pe′de-ah-floor) trademark for a preparation of sodium fluoride.

pedialgia (ped″e-al′je-ah) [L. *pes* foot + *-algia*] neuralgic pain in the foot.

Pediamycin (pe″de-ah-mi′sin) trademark for preparations of erythromycin ethylsuccinate.

pediatric (pe″de-at′rik) pertaining to pediatrics.

pediatrician (pe″de-ah-trish′un) a physician who specializes in pediatrics.

pediatrics (pe″de-at′riks) [*pedia-* + Gr. *iatrikē* surgery, medicine] that branch of medicine which treats of the child and its development and care and of the diseases of children and their treatment.

pediatrist (pe″de-at′rist) pediatrician.

pediatry (pe′de-at″re) pediatrics.

pedicel (ped′ĭ-sel) a footlike part, especially any of the secondary processes of a podocyte which interdigitate with those of other podocytes in a renal corpuscle; called also *foot process*.

pedicellate, pedicellated (pĕ-dis′ĭ-lāt; ped′ĭ-sel-āt″ed) pediculate; pedunculated.

pedicellation (ped″ĭ-sel-la′shun) the development or possession of a pedicle.

pedicle (ped′ĭ-k′l) [L. *pediculus* little foot] a footlike, stemlike, or narrow basal part or structure, as the stalk by which a nonsessile tumor is attached to normal tissue, or the narrow strip of flap tissue through which it receives its blood supply. **cone p.,** the thick triangular or club-shaped ending of a retinal cone cell, which synapses with the bipolar and horizontal cells in the outer plexiform layer. **p. of lung,** radix pulmonis. **p. of vertebral arch,** pediculus arcus vertebrae.

pedicled (ped′ĭ-k′ld) having a pedicle.

pedicterus (pe-dik′ter-us) [*pedo-* + Gr. *ikteros* jaundice] (obs.) icterus neonatorum.

pedicular (pe-dik′u-lar) [L. *pedicularis*] pertaining to or caused by lice.

pediculate (pe-dik′u-lāt) [L. *pediculatus*] provided with a pedicle; pedunculated.

pediculation (pe-dik″u-la′shun) [L. *pediculatio*] 1. infestation with lice. 2. the formation of a pedicle.

pediculi (pe-dik′u-li) plural of *pediculus*.

pediculicide (pe-dik′u-lĭ-sīd) [*pediculus* + L. *caedere* to kill] 1. destroying lice. 2. an agent that destroys lice.

Pediculidae (ped″ĭ-ku′lĭ-de) a family of lice (order Anoplura) that includes the genera Pediculus and Phthirus, which feed on human blood.

Pediculoides (pe-dik″u-loi′dēz) former name for *Pyemotes*. **P. ventrico′sus,** Pyemotes ventricosus.

pediculosis (pe-dik″u-lo′sis) [*pediculus* + *-osis*] infestation with lice of the family Pediculidae, especially infestation with *Pediculus humanus*. **p. capillit′ii, p. cap′itis,** infestation of the hair of the head by lice. **p. cor′poris,** infestation of the body by lice. **p. inguina′lis,** phthiriasis inguinalis. **p. palpebra′rum,** infestation of the eyelashes by lice. **p. pu′bis,** phthiriasis inguinalis. **p. vestimen′ti, p. vestimento′rum,** infestation of the clothing by lice.

pediculous (pe-dik′u-lus) infested with lice.

Pediculus (pe-dik′u-lus) a genus of sucking lice of the family Pediculidae, order Anoplura, the sucking lice. **P. huma′nus,** a species that feeds on human blood, is a major vector of epidemic typhus, trench fever, and relapsing fever, and causes skin reactions, especially in sensitized persons. It includes two subspecies, *P. humanus capitis* and *P. humanus corporis*. **P. huma′nus cap′itis,** the head louse, found on the scalp hair. **P. huma′nus cor′poris,** the body or clothes louse, which lives on the clothing when feeding is not taking place; called also *P. humanus humanus*, *P. humanus vestimento′rum*, and *P. vestimenti*. **P. huma′nus huma′nus,** *P. humanus corporis*. **P. huma′nus vestimento′rum,** *P. humanus corporis*. **P. inguina′lis, P. pu′bis,** *Phthirus pubis*. **P. vestimen′ti,** *P. humanus corporis*.

pediculus (pe-dik′u-lus), pl. *pedic′uli* [L.] 1. louse. 2. a footlike or stemlike part; called also *pedicle*. **p. ar′cus**

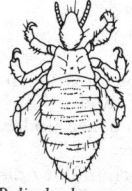

Pediculus humanus.

ver′tebrae [NA], pedicle of vertebral arch: one of the paired parts of the vertebral arch that connect a lamina to the vertebral body; called also *radix arcus vertebrae*. **p. pulmo′nis,** NA alternative for *radix pulmonis*.

pedicure (ped′ĭ-kūr) [L. *pes* foot + *cura* care] 1. professional care and treatment of the feet. 2. a podiatrist.

pedigree (ped′ĭ-gre) [Fr. *pie de grue*, "crane's foot" (from the shape of the stemma)] a table, chart, diagram, or list of an individual's ancestors, used in human genetics in the analysis of inheritance.

pediluvium (ped″ĭ-lu′ve-um) [L. *pes* foot + *luere* to wash] a foot bath.

Pediococcus (pe″de-o-kok′us) [Gr. *pedium* a plane surface + *kokkos* berry] a genus of microaerophilic saprophytic, gram-positive, nonmotile cocci of the family Streptococcaceae. They usually occur in pairs or tetrads, and are found most commonly in fermenting plant products. **P. acidilacti′ci,** a species found in sauerkraut and fermenting mashes. **P. cerevi′siae,** a species found in spoiled beer and brewer's yeast. **P. halophi′lus,** a species found in anchovies and soy mash. **P. pentosa′ceus,** a species occurring commonly in fermenting products, such as pickles, sauerkraut, etc. **P. uri′nae-equi,** a species originally isolated from horse urine, which is often found in brewer's yeast.

pediodontia (pe″de-o-don′she-ah) pedodontics.

pedionalgia (pe″de-o-nal′je-ah) [Gr. *pedion* metatarsus + *-algia* pain] pain in the sole of the foot.

pediphalanx (ped″ĭ-fa′lanks) [L. *pes* foot + *phalanx*] a phalanx of a digit of the foot.

pedistibulum (ped″ĭ-stib′u-lum) [L.] the stapes.

peditis (pe-di′tis) [L. *pes* foot + *-itis*] pedal osteitis.

ped(o)-¹ **paed(o)-** [Gr. *pais*, gen. *paidos* child] a combining form denoting relationship to a child.

ped(o)-², **pedi-** [L. *pes*, gen. *pedis* foot] a combining form denoting relationship to the foot.

pedodontia (pe″do-don′she-ah) pedodontics.

pedodontics (pe-do-don′tiks) [*pedo-*¹ + Gr. *odous* tooth] the branch of dentistry concerned with the diagnosis and treatment of conditions of the teeth and mouth in children.

pedodontist (pe-do-don′tist) a dentist who specializes in pedodontics.

pedodynamometer (ped″o-di-nah-mom′ĕ-ter) [*pedo-*² + *dynamometer*] an instrument for measuring the strength of a leg.

pedogamy (pe-dog′ah-me) [*pedo-*¹ + Gr. *gamos* marriage] endogamy, def. 1.

pedogenesis (pe″do-jen′ĕ-sis) [*pedo-*¹ + Gr. *genesis* reproduction] the production of offspring by young or larval forms.

pedograph (ped′o-graf) [*pedo-*² + Gr. *graphein* to write] an imprint on paper of the weight-bearing surface of the foot, surrounded by a pencil-marked contour of the upper foot.

pedologist (pe-dol′o-gist) a specialist in pedology.

pedology (pe-dol′o-je) [*pedo-*¹ + *-logy*] the systematical study of the life and development of children.

pedometer (pe-dom′ĕ-ter) [*pedo-* + Gr. *metron* measure] 1. an instrument for recording the number of steps taken in walking. 2. (obs.), an instrument for measuring infants.

Pedomicrobium (pe″do-mi-kro′be-um) [Gr. *pedon* soil + *mikros* small + *bios* life] a genus of budding bacteria found in soil, made up of variously shaped cells that produce hyphae from several sites on the cell surface. The type species is *P. ferrugin′eum*.

pedomorphic (pe″do-mor′fik) pertaining to or characterized by pedomorphism.

pedomorphism (pe″do-mor′fizm) [*pedo-*¹ + Gr. *morphē* form + *-ism*] the retention in the adult organism of highly progressive species of bodily characters which at an earlier stage of evolutionary history were actually only infantile.

pedopathy (pe-dop'ah-the) [pedo-² + Gr. *pathos* disease] any disease of the foot.

pedophilia (pe″do-fil′e-ah) [pedo-¹ + -phila] 1. abnormal fondness for children; sexual activity of adults with children. 2. [DSM III-R] a paraphilia in which there are recurrent, intense sexual urges or sexually arousing fantasies of engaging in sexual activity with a prepubertal child.

pedophilic (pe″do-fil′ik) 1. fond of children. 2. pertaining to or characterized by pedophilia.

pedophobia (pe″do-fo′be-ah) [pedo-¹ + *phobia*] irrational fear or dread of children.

pedorthic (pĕ-dor′thik) pertaining to pedorthics.

pedorthics (pĕ-dor′thiks) [pedo-² + Gr. *orthōsis* making straight] the design, manufacture, fit, and modification of shoes and related foot appliances as prescribed for amelioration of painful and/or disabling conditions of the foot and limb.

pedorthist (pe-dor′thist) a person skilled in pedorthics and practicing its application in individual cases.

peduncle (pĕ-dung′k′l) a stemlike connecting part (called also *pedunculus* [NA]); the stalk by which a nonsessile tumor is attached to normal tissue. **cerebellar p., caudal,** pedunculus cerebellaris caudalis. **cerebellar p., cranial,** pedunculus cerebellaris rostralis. **cerebellar p., inferior,** pedunculus cerebellaris caudalis. **cerebellar p., middle,** pedunculus cerebellaris medius. **cerebellar p., pontine,** pedunculus cerebellaris medius. **cerebellar p., rostral,** pedunculus cerebellaris rostralis. **cerebellar p., superior,** pedunculus cerebellaris rostralis. **p's of cerebellum,** pedunculi cerebelli. **cerebral p., p. of cerebrum,** pedunculus cerebri. **p. of flocculus,** pedunculus flocculi. **p. of hypophysis** (obs.), infundibulum hypothalami. **olfactory p.,** in comparative neuroanatomy, the olfactory stalk, especially the region of its attachment to the cerebral hemisphere. **pineal p., p. of pineal body,** habenula, def. 2. **p's of thalamus,** the four two-way radiations of thalamocortical fibers that connect the dorsal thalamus with many parts of the cerebral cortex, which together form a major portion of the internal capsule and the corona radiata: the *anterior* peduncle connects the frontal lobe of the cerebrum with the anterior and medial thalamus; the *superior* connects the precentral and postcentral gyri and adjacent portions of the frontal and parietal lobes of the cerebrum with the ventral and lateral thalamus; the *posterior* connects the occipital and parietal cortex with the posterior and lateral thalamus; and the *inferior* connects the medial geniculate body and posterior thalamus with certain areas of the cortex of the temporal lobe of the cerebrum. Called also *thalamic radiations, radiations of thalamus,* and *stalks of thalamus.* **p. of thalamus, caudal, p. of thalamus, inferior,** pedunculus thalami caudalis.

peduncular (pĕ-dung′ku-lar) pertaining to a peduncle.

pedunculated (pĕ-dung′ku-lāt-ed) provided with a peduncle; opposed to sessile.

pedunculotomy (pĕ-dung″ku-lot′o-me) [L. *pedunculus* + Gr. *tomē* a cutting] incision of a cerebral peduncle, with division of both pyramidal and nonpyramidal fibers, for relief of the tremor of parkinsonism.

pedunculus (pĕ-dung′ku-lus) pl. *pedun′culi* [L.] a stemlike part; [NA] a general term for collections of nerve fibers coursing between different areas in the central nervous system. Called also *peduncle.* **p. cerebella′ris cauda′lis** [NA], caudal cerebellar peduncle: a large bundle of nerve fibers serving to connect the medulla oblongata and spinal cord with the cerebellum (especially the archicerebellum and paleocerebellum) it courses along the lateral border of the fourth ventricle and turns dorsally into the cerebellum. Called also *corpus restiforme, inferior cerebellar peduncle, p. cerebellaris inferior* [NA alternative], and *restiform body.* **p. cerebella′ris crania′lis,** p. cerebellaris rostralis. **p. cerebella′ris infe′rior,** NA alternative for *p. cerebellaris caudalis.* **p. cerebella′ris me′dius** [NA], middle cerebellar peduncle: a large bundle of projection fibers originating in the contralateral pontine nuclei and entering the cerebellum, conveying impulses from the cerebral cortex to the neocerebellum; it is continuous with the pons at the line of attachment of the trigeminal nerve. Called also

pontine cerebellar peduncle and *p. cerebellaris pontinus* [NA alternative]. **p. cerebella′ris ponti′nus,** NA alternative for *p. cerebellaris medius.* **p. cerebella′ris rostra′lis** [NA], rostral cerebellar peduncle: a large bundle of projection fibers arising chiefly in the dentate nucleus of each cerebellar hemisphere (neocerebellum) and ascending to decussate in the mesencephalon; its fibers end mostly in the red nucleus and thalamus. Spinocerebellar fibers to the paleocerebellum lie adjacent to each peduncle. Called also *cranial cerebellar peduncle, p. cerebellaris cranialis,* and *superior cerebellar peduncle.* **p. cerebella′ris supe′rior,** NA alternative for *p. cerebellaris rostralis.* **pedun′culi cerebel′li** [NA], peduncles of cerebellum: three large bundles of projection fibers on each side of the cerebellum that connect it with other parts of the brain and spinal cord; see *p. cerebelli caudalis* (inferior), *pontinus* (middle), and *cranialis* (superior). **p. cerebra′lis,** NA alternative for *p. cerebri.* **p. cer′ebri** [NA], peduncle of cerebrum: either of the two large masses of substance that descend from each cerebral hemisphere, being separated by the interpeduncular fossa until they converge where they enter the pons; they form the ventral part of the mesencephalon. Each peduncle is divided into a ventral part, consisting of a bundle of nerve fiber tracts (basis peduncularis cerebri), and a dorsal part, which is continuous across the median plane, forming the tegmentum of the mesencephalon; the parts are separated by the substantia nigra. The term also has been used to denote the right or left half of the midbrain, each consisting of a ventral part, the crus cerebri, and a dorsal or tegmental part, the tegmentum. Called also *cerebral peduncle* and *p. cerebralis* [NA alternative]. **p. cor′poris callo′si** (obs.), gyrus paraterminalis. **p. cor′poris pinea′lis,** habenula, def. 2. **p. floc′culi** [NA], peduncle of flocculus: a narrow band of afferent and efferent nerve fibers that connects the nodulus of the cerebellum to the flocculus; its dorsal part is continuous with the anterolateral part of the caudal medullary velum, from which most of its fibers are derived. **p. thal′ami cauda′lis** [NA], caudal pedunculus of thalamus: the smallest of the four peduncles of the thalamus, which connects the medial geniculate body of the posterior thalamus with certain areas of the cortex of the temporal lobe of the cerebrum and forms one of the principal components of the ansa peduncularis. Called also *inferior peduncle of thalamus* and *p. thalami inferior* [NA alternative]. **p. thal′ami infe′rior,** NA alternative for *p. thalami caudalis.*

peel (pēl) [L. *pilare* to deprive of hair] the outer rind of a fruit. **bitter orange p.** [NF], the dried rind of unripe but fully grown fruit of *Citrus aurantium* Linné, used as a pharmaceutical flavoring agent. **lemon p.,** the outer, yellow rind of the fresh ripe fruit of *Citrus limon,* used in preparing lemon oil and lemon tincture.

peenash (pe′nash) [India] rhinitis due to the presence of insect larvae in the nose.

PEEP positive end-expiratory pressure; see under *pressure.*

PEG pneumoencephalography.

peg (peg) a projecting structure. **rete p's,** the inward projections of the epidermis into the dermis at the dermoepidermal junction, as seen histologically in vertical sections.

Peganone (peg′ah-nōn) trademark for a preparation of ethotoin.

peglicol 5 oleate (pĕ-gli′kōl) a product obtained by alcoholysis of natural vegetable oils in the presence of polyethylene glycols of molecular weights between 200 and 400, consisting of a mixture of partially mixed esters of glycerin and these polyethylene glycols; the average number of ethylene glycol units is 5. It is used as an emulsifying agent in pharmaceutical preparations. Called also *polyoxyl 5 oleate.*

pegology (pe-gol′o-je) [Gr. *pēgē* fountain + *-logy*] the study of springs, particularly medicinal or mineral springs.

pegoterate (peg″o-ter′āt) a condensation polymer used as a suspending agent in pharmaceutical preparations.

pegoxol 7 stearate (peg-ok′sōl) a mixture of mono- and distearic esters of ethylene glycol and of polyoxyethylene glycol, the latter having an average molecular weight of 450; the average number of ethylene glycol units is 7. It is used as an emulsifying agent in pharmaceutical preparations.

Pel's crises (pelz) [Pieter Klaases *Pel,* Dutch physician, 1852–1919] see under *crisis.*

Pel-Ebstein disease, fever (pyrexia, symptom)

(pel-eb'stīn) [Pieter Klaases *Pel*; Wilhelm *Ebstein*, German physician, 1836–1912] see *Hodgkin's disease*, under *disease*, and see under *fever*.

pelade (pel-ad') [Fr.] alopecia areata.

pelage (pel'ij, pĕ-lahzh') [Fr.] the hairy coat of mammals; the hairs of the body, limbs, and head collectively.

pelagic (pe-laj'ik) [Gr. *pelagios* living in the sea] pertaining to or inhabiting open, offshore waters, as in midocean.

Pelamis (pel'ah-mis) a genus of sea snakes. **P. bico'lor,** a poisonous sea snake of the Indian ocean.

pelargonic acid (pel"ar-gon'ik) trivial name for nonanoic acid, the 9-carbon saturated fatty acid.

Pelecypoda (pel"e-sip'o-dah) [Gr. *pelekys* hatchet + *podos* foot] the bivalves: a class of mollusks which are laterally compressed and have a pair of dorsally hinged lateral shells (valves) and a hatchet-shaped foot for digging; it includes the clams, oysters, and scallops. Called also *Bivalvia.*

Pelger's nuclear anomaly (pel'gerz) [Karel *Pelger*, Dutch physician, 1885–1931] see under *anomaly.*

Pelger-Huët nuclear anomaly (pel'ger-hyoo'et) [Karel *Pelger*; G. J. *Huët*, Dutch physician, born 1879] see under *anomaly.*

pelidisi (pel"ĭ-de'se) [term coined from L. *pondus decies linearis divisus sidentis* (altitudo) meaning weight ten line divided sitting height] the unit of Pirquet's index for determining the nutritive condition of children. It is obtained by dividing the cube root of ten times the weight (in grams) by the sitting height (in centimeters). A pelidisi of 94 or less indicates undernutrition; of 95–100, good nutrition, and of 101 or above, overnutrition.

peliosis (pe"le-o'sis) [Gr. *peliōsis* extravasation of blood] purpura. **p. hep'atis, p. of liver,** mottled blue liver, caused by blood-filled lacunae in the parenchyma.

Pelizaeus-Merzbacher disease (pa"le-zi'us- merz'baker) [Friedrich *Pelizaeus*, German physician, 1850–1917; Ludwig *Merzbacher*, German physician in Buenos Aires, born 1875] familial centrolobar sclerosis.

pellagra (pĕ-la'grah, pĕ-lag'rah) [It. *pelle* skin + *agra* rough] a clinical deficiency syndrome due to deficiency of niacin (or failure to convert tryptophan to niacin) and characterized by dermatitis, inflammation of mucous membranes, diarrhea, and psychic disturbances. The dermatitis occurs on the portions of the body exposed to light or trauma. Mental symptoms include depression, irritability, anxiety, confusion, disorientation, delusions, and hallucinations. **monkey p.,** a condition in caged monkeys manifested by loss of appetite, diarrhea, vomiting, emaciation, and finally death. **p. si'ne pella'gra,** pellagra in which the characteristic dermatitis is not present. **typhoid p.,** pellagra characterized by continued high temperature.

pellagragenic (pĕ-lag"rah-jen'ik) causing pellagra.

pellagral (pĕ-lag'ral) pertaining to or caused by pellagra.

pellagramin (pĕ-lag'rah-min) niacin.

pellagrazein (pel"ah-gra'ze-in) a poisonous ptomaine from damaged maize, formerly regarded as a probable cause of pellagra.

pellagrin (pĕ-la'grin, pĕ-lag'rin) a person affected with pellagra.

pellagrocein (pel"ah-gro'se-in) pellagrazein.

pellagroid (pĕ-lag'roid) a condition resembling pellagra.

pellagrologist (pel"ah-grol'o-jist) one who makes a special study of pellagra.

pellagrology (pel"ah-grol'o-je) the study of pellagra.

pellagrose (pĕ-lag'rōs) pellagrous.

pellagrosis (pel"ah-gro'sis) the dermal syndrome of pellagra characterized by skin pigmentation, erythema, and hyperkeratosis.

pellagrous (pĕ-lag'rus) affected with or of the nature of pellagra.

pellant (pel'ant) [L. *pellere* to drive] depurative.

pellate (pel'āt) to repel or tend to separate.

Pellegrini's disease (pel"a-gre'nez) [Augusto *Pellegrini*, Italian surgeon, born 1877] see under *disease.*

Pellegrini-Stieda disease (pel"a-gre'ne-ste'dah) [A. *Pellegrini*; Alfred *Stieda*, German surgeon, 1869–1945] see *Pellegrini's disease* under *disease.*

pellet (pel'et) a small pill or granule, such as a small rod-

or ovoid-shaped, sterile mass composed of essentially pure steroid hormones, to be implanted under the skin to provide for their slow absorption, or a small pill made from sucrose and impregnated with a medicine, used in homeopathic practice.

pellicle (pel'ĭ-k'l) [L. *pellicula*] 1. a thin skin or film, such as a thin film on the surface of a liquid. 2. in protozoology, a living outer layer of denser cytoplasm containing the peripheral and surface organelles of ciliate protozoa. **brown p.,** a brownish gray to black film formed over a period of time on the surfaces of the teeth, resulting from poor oral hygiene and brushing habits. See also *dental plaque*, under *plaque.*

pellicular, pelliculous (pel-lik'u-lar; pel-lik'u-lus) pertaining to or characterized by a pellicle.

Pellizzi's syndrome (pel-le'zēz) [G. B. *Pellizzi*, Pisa physician] epiphyseal syndrome.

pellote (pa-yo'tah) peyote.

pellucid (pel-lu'sid) [L. *pellucidus*, from *per* through + *lucere* to shine] translucent.

pel(o)- [Gr. *pēlos* mud] a combining form denoting relationship to mud.

Pelobiontida (pel"o-bi-on'tĭ-dah) [pelo- + Gr. *bioun* a living being] an order of large, free-living cylindrical, monopodial, multinucleate ameboid protozoa (subclass Gymnamoebia, class Lobosea) found in soil and water, and characterized by the presence of bacterial and other inclusions and numerous nonmotile cilia. *Pelomyxa* is a representative genus.

Pelodictyon (pe"lo-dik'te-on) [pelo- + Gr. *diktyon* net] a genus of aquatic phototrophic bacteria of the family Chlorobiaceae, order Rhodospirillales, consisting of rod-shaped to ovoid, nonmotile cells that contain gas vacuoles and fix carbon dioxide in the presence of hydrogen sulfide. Cell suspensions are yellow to green. The type species is *P. clathratifor'me.*

peloid (pe'loid) [pelo- + Gr. *eidos* form] mud used for therapeutic purposes, as in packs and baths.

pelology (pĕ-lol'o-je) [pelo- + -logy] the science of mud and similar substances.

Pelomyxa (pel"o-mik'sah) [pelo- + Gr. *myxa* mucus] a genus of protozoa (order Pelobiontida, subclass Gymnamoebida), including *P. carolinesis* (*Chaos chaos*), the giant ameba, which may attain a diameter of 5 mm.

Pelonema (pe"lo-ne'mah) [pelo- + Gr. *nēma* thread] a genus of gliding bacteria of the provisional family Pelonemataceae, found in deep waters and bottom mud, made up of colorless cells in unbranched filaments. The type species is *P. ten'ue.*

Pelonemataceae (pe"lo-ne"mah-ta'se-e) a family of gliding bacteria of uncertain affiliation, made up of cylindrical colorless cells in filaments. It contains the genera *Achroonema, Desmanthos, Pelonema,* and *Peloploca.*

pelopathy (pe-lop'ah-the) pelotherapy.

Peloploca (pĕ-lop'lo-kah) [pelo- + Gr. *plokē* anything twisted] a genus of gliding bacteria of the provisional family Pelonemataceae, found in deep waters and on bottom mud, made up of colorless cells in bundled filaments, sometimes with a gelatinous sheath. The type species is *P. undula'ta.*

Peloplocaceae (pe"lo-plo-ka'se-e) in former systems of classification, a family of gliding bacteria, which are now included in the provisional family Pelonemataceae.

Pelosigma (pe"lo-sig'mah) [pelo- + Gr. *sigmoeidēs*; L. *sigmoides* S-shaped] a genus of nonmotile, gram-negative, curved bacteria made up of S-shaped cells found on mud in fresh or brackish waters. The type species is *P coh'nii.*

pelosine (pe-lo'sin) bebeerine.

pelotherapy (pe"lo-ther'ah-pe) [pelo- + Gr. *therapeia* cure] the therapeutic use of earth or mud.

pelta (pel'tah) [L. "a shield"] a crescent-shaped membranous structure arising from or covering the axostyle of certain parasitic flagellate protozoa, especially trichomonads.

peltate (pel'tāt) [L. *pelta*; Gr. *peltē* shield] shield-shaped.

pelves (pel'vēs) [L.] plural of *pelvis.*

pelvic (pel'vik) pertaining to the pelvis.

pelvicaliceal, pelvicalyceal (pel"ve-kal"ĭ-se-al) pertaining to the renal pelves and calices.

pelvicellulitis (pel"ve-sel"u-li'tis) pelvic cellulitis.

pelvicephalography (pel″ve-sef″ah-log′rah-fe) [*pelvis* + Gr. *kephalē* head + *graphein* to write] roentgenographic measurement of the fetal head and of the birth canal.

pelvicephalometry (pel″ve-sef″ah-lom′ĕ-tre) [*pelvis* + Gr. *kephalē* head + *metron* measure] measurement of the diameters of the head of the fetus in relation to those of the mother's pelvis.

pelvifemoral (pel″ve-fem′o-ral) pertaining to or affecting the pelvis and femur.

pelvifixation (pel″ve-fik-sa′shun) surgical fixation of an organ to the pelvic cavity.

pelvilithotomy (pel″ve-lĭ-thot′o-me) pyelolithotomy.

pelvimeter (pel-vim′ĕ-ter) [*pelvis* + Gr. *metron* measure] an instrument for measuring the diameters and capacity of the pelvis.

pelvimetry (pel-vim′ĕ-tre) the measurement of the dimensions and capacity of the pelvis. **combined p.,** pelvimetry in which measurements are made both within and outside the body. **instrumental p.,** measurement of the pelvis with the pelvimeter. **manual p.,** that which is performed with the hands.

pelviography (pel″ve-og′rah-fe) pelviroentgenography.

pelvioileoneocystostomy (pel″ve-o-il″e-o-ne″o-sis-tos′to-me) anastomosis of renal pelvis to an isolated segment of the ileum, which is then anastomosed to the urinary bladder.

pelviolithotomy (pel″ve-o-lĭ-thot′o-me) pyelolithotomy.

pelvioneostomy (pel″ve-o-ne-os′to-me) ureteropyeloneostomy.

pelvioperitonitis (pel″ve-o-per″ĭ-to-ni′tis) pelvic peritonitis.

pelvioplasty (pel′ve-o-plas″te) pyeloplasty.

pelvioradiography (pel″ve-o-ra″de-og′rah-fe) radiography of the organs of the pelvis; pelviroentgenography.

pelvioscopy (pel″ve-os′ko-pe) [*pelvis* + Gr. *skopein* to examine] 1. the inspection or visual examination of the pelvis or pelvic viscera. 2. pyeloscopy.

pelviostomy (pel″ve-os′to-me) pyelostomy.

pelviotomy (pel″ve-ot′o-me) [*pelvis* + Gr. *tomē* a cutting] 1. the cutting of the pelvic bones. 2. pyelotomy.

pelviperitonitis (pel″ve-per″ĭ-to-ni′tis) pelvic peritonitis.

pelviradiography (pel″ve-ra″de-og′rah-fe) pelviroentgenography.

pelvirectal (pel″ve-rek′tal) pertaining to the pelvis and the rectum.

pelviroentgenography (pel″ve-rent″gen-og′rah-fe) roentgenography of the organs of the pelvis.

pelvis (pel′vis), pl. *pel′ves* [L.; Gr. *pyelos* an oblong trough] [NA] the lower (caudal) portion of the trunk of the body, bounded anteriorly and laterally by the two hip bones and posteriorly by the sacrum and coccyx. The pelvis is divided by a plane passing through the terminal lines into the *false pelvis* (*p. major* [NA]) above and the *true pelvis* (*p. minor* [NA]) below. The upper boundary of the cavity of the pelvis is known as the *inlet, brim,* or *superior strait of the pelvis.* The true pelvis is limited below by the *inferior strait,* or *outlet,* bounded by the coccyx, the symphysis pubis, and the ischium of either side. The outlet of the pelvis is closed by the coccygeus and levator ani muscles and the perineal fascia, which form the *floor of the pelvis.* The inlet and outlet of the pelvis each have three important diameters—an anteroposterior (conjugate), an oblique, and a transverse, the relations of which determine types variously classified by different authors (see entries under *diameter*). The term pelvis is applied also to any basin-like structure, such as the renal pelvis (pelvis renalis [NA]). **android p.,** a pelvis characterized by a wedge-shaped inlet and narrowness of the anterior segment; used as a general designation of a female pelvis showing characters typical of the pelvis in the male. **anthropoid p.,** a female pelvis characterized by a long anteroposterior diameter of the inlet, which equals or exceeds the transverse diameter. **assimilation p.,** a pelvis in which the transverse processes of the last lumbar vertebra are fused with the sacrum (*high-assimilation p.*—including six vertebral segments), or the last sacral vertebra may fuse with the first coccygeal body (*low-assimilation p.*—including only four vertebral segments). **beaked p.,** one with the pelvic bones laterally compressed and their anterior junction pushed forward, as in osteomalacia. **bony p.,** p. ossea. **brachypellic p.,** an oval type of pelvis, the transverse diameter of the inlet

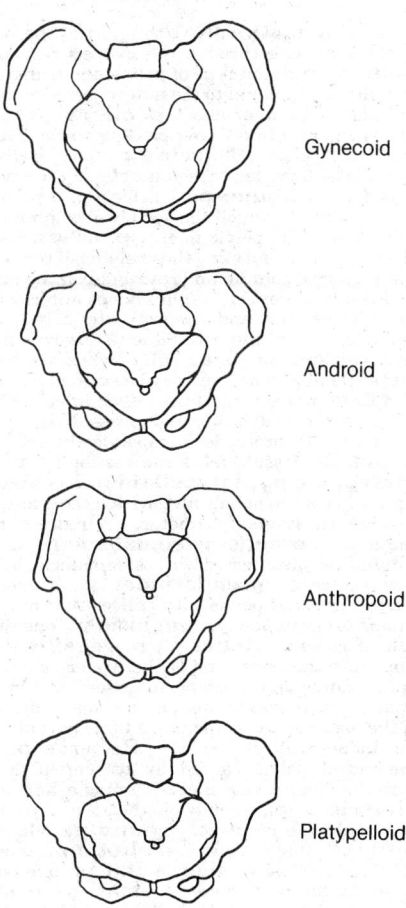

Gynecoid

Android

Anthropoid

Platypelloid

Various types of pelvic inlets.

exceeding the anteroposterior diameter by 1 to 3 cm. **contracted p.,** a pelvis in which there is a diminution of 1.5 to 2 cm. in any important diameter; when all dimensions are proportionally diminished it is a *generally contracted pelvis* (*p. justo minor*). **cordate p., cordiform p.,** one that is somewhat heart shaped. **coxalgic p.,** one deformed in consequence of hip-joint disease. **dolichopellic p.,** an elongated pelvis, the anteroposterior diameter of the inlet being greater than the transverse diameter. **dwarf p.,** a small pelvis seen in several types of dwarfism. **extrarenal p.,** see under *renal p.* **false p.,** p. major. **flat p.,** one in which the anteroposterior dimension is abnormally reduced. **frozen p.,** a condition, due to infection or carcinoma, in which the adnexa and uterus are fixed in the pelvis. **funnel-shaped p.,** a female pelvis with a normal inlet, but a greatly narrowed outlet. **giant p.,** p. justo major. **greater p.,** p. major. **gynecoid p.,** a pelvis having a rounded oval shape with a well rounded anterior and posterior segment; it represents the normal female pelvis. **high-assimilation p.,** see *assimilation p.* **infantile p.,** a generally contracted pelvis characterized by an oval shape, a high sacrum, and marked inclination of the walls. **p. jus′to ma′jor,** a pelvis that is unusually large, with all its dimensions equally increased. **p. jus′to mi′nor,** a pelvis that is unusually small, with all its dimensions equally reduced; see also *contracted p.* **juvenile p.,** infantile p. **kyphoscoliotic p.,** an irregularly contracted pelvis due to rachitic kyphoscoliosis. **kyphotic p.,** one characterized by increase of the conjugate diameter at the brim, with decrease of the transverse diameter at the outlet, due to close proximity of the ischial spines and tuberosities. **large p.,** p. major. **lesser p.,** p. minor. **lordotic p.,** one associated with an anterior curvature in the lumbar region of the vertebral column. **low-assimilation p.,** see *assimila-*

tion p. **p. ma′jor** [NA], the part of the pelvis superior to a plane passing through the ileopectineal lines. **mesati-pellic p.**, a round type of pelvis, the transverse diameter of the inlet being equal to the anteroposterior diameter or being greater by 1 cm. or less. **p. mi′nor** [NA], the part of the pelvis inferior to a plane passing through the iliopectineal lines; see *pelvis*. **Nägele's p.**, one so distorted that the conjugate diameter takes an oblique direction. **p. na′na**, dwarf p. **oblique p.**, Nägele's p. **p. obtec′ta**, a kyphotic pelvis in which the vertebral column extends horizontally across the pelvic inlet. **p. os′sea** [NA], bony pelvis: the ring of bone forming the skeleton of the pelvis, supporting the vertebral column and resting upon the inferior members, and composed of the two hip bones anteriorly and laterally, and the sacrum and coccyx posteriorly. **osteomalacic p.**, deformity of the pelvis due to absorption by the bones of their calcium salts, as a result of which the bones become soft and so flexible that they may be stretched or pushed together and cause narrowing of the pelvic inlet. **Otto p.**, a pelvis in which the acetabulum is depressed, permitting the head of the femur to protrude intrapelvically; see *arthrokatadysis*. **p. ova′lis**, fossula fenestrae vestibuli. **p. pla′na**, flat p. **platypellic p., platypelloid p.**, a pelvis characterized by flattening of the pelvic inlet, with a short anteroposterior and a wide transverse diameter. **Prague p.**, spondylolisthetic p. **pseudo-osteomalacic p.**, a deformed pelvis simulating one affected with osteomalacia, but resulting from other causes. **pseudospider p.**, a congenitally small, long, thin renal pelvis with calices that may simulate renal tumor urographically. **rachitic p.**, one distorted as a result of rickets. **renal p., p. rena′lis** [NA], the expansion from the upper end of the ureter into which the calices of the kidney open; ordinarily lodged within the renal sinus, under certain conditions, as in a long kidney or obstruction of the ureteropelvic junction, a large part of it may be outside the kidney (*extrarenal p.*). **Robert's p.**, a transversely contracted pelvis caused by osteoarthritis affecting both sacroiliac joints, the inlet becoming a narrow wedge. **Rokitansky's p.**, spondylolisthetic p. **p. rotun′da**, fossula fenestrae cochleae. **round p.**, one with an inlet of nearly circular outline. **scoliotic p.**, one deformed as a result of scoliosis. **simple flat p.**, one with a shortened anteroposterior diameter. **small p.**, p. minor. **spider p.**, a renal pelvis which in the pyelogram shows the calices as narrow, string-like extensions, resembling the legs of a spider. **p. spino′sa**, a rachitic pelvis with the crest of the pubis very sharp. **split p.**, one with a congenital separation at the symphysis pubis, often associated with exstrophy of the bladder. **spondylolisthetic p.**, one in which the last, or rarely the fourth or third, lumbar vertebra is dislocated in front of the sacrum, more or less occluding the pelvic brim. Called also *Prague p.* and *Rokitansky's p.* **p. spu′ria**, p. major. **triangular p.**, one with a triangular inlet. **true p.**, p. minor. **p. of ureter**, renal p.

pelvisacral (pel″vĭ-sa′kral) pertaining to the pelvis and the sacrum.

pelvisacrum (pel-vĭ-sa′krum) the pelvis and the sacrum together.

pelviscope (pel′vĭ-skōp) an apparatus for examining roentgenologically the contours of the pelvis.

pelvisection (pel″vĭ-sek′shun) [*pelvis* + L. *sectio* a cutting] a cutting of the pelvis bones, such as pubiotomy and symphysiotomy.

pelvisternum (pel″ve-ster′num) the cartilage of the symphysis pubis.

pelvitomy (pel-vit′o-me) [*pelvis* + Gr. *temnein* to cut] the operation of cutting the pelvis at any point in order to facilitate delivery.

pelvitrochanterian (pel″ve-tro″kan-te′re-an) relating to the pelvis and the great trochanter of the femur.

pelviureteral (pel″ve-u-re′ter-al) relating to the renal pelvis and the ureter.

pelviureteroradiography (pel″ve-u-re″ter-o-ra″de-og′-rah-fe) roentgenography of the ureter and renal pelvis.

pelvoscopy (pel-vos′ko-pe) [*pelvis* + Gr. *skopein* to examine] pelvioscopy.

pelvospondylitis (pel″vo-spon″dĭ-li′tis) inflammation of the pelvic portion of the spine. **p. ossif′icans**, rheumatoid spondylitis.

pelyc(o)- [Gr. *pelyx* bowl] for words beginning thus, see those beginning *pelvi-* and *pyelo-*.

pemerid nitrate (pem′ĕ-rid) chemical name: 4-[3-(dimethylamino)propoxy]-1,2,2,6,6-pentamethylpiperidine dinitrate; an antitussive, $C_{18}H_{32}N_2O\cdot 2HNO_3$.

pemoline (pem′o-lēn) chemical name: 2-imino-5-phenyl-4-oxazolidinone; a central nervous system stimulant, C_9H_8-N_2O_2.

pemphigoid (pem′fĭ-goid) [Gr. *pemphix* blister + *eidos* form] 1. like or resembling pemphigus. 2. a name applied to a group of dermatological syndromes similar to but clearly distinguishable from those of the pemphigus group. The term is often used alone to designate *bullous pemphigoid*. **benign mucosal p., benign mucous membrane p.,** cicatricial p. **bullous p.**, a usually mild, relatively benign, self-limited subepidermal blistering skin disease, sometimes with oral involvement, predominantly affecting the elderly, and characterized clinically by the presence of large, tense bullae that rupture and leave denuded areas, which have a tendency to heal spontaneously. It is characterized histologically by a cleft formation at the dermoepidermal junction, and immunofluorescent studies reveal deposition of complement, usually with immunoglobulin G at the dermoepidermal junction at the level of the lamina lucida of the basement membrane. **bullous p., localized,** a variant of bullous pemphigoid beginning at a localized site, such as on the scalp, trunk, or extremity, especially a lower extremity, and remaining confined to that site throughout the course of the disease. A localized chronic form has been reported. **cicatricial p.**, a benign, chronic, usually bilateral, subepidermal blistering disease chiefly involving the mucous membranes, especially those of the mouth and eye (*ocular pemphigus*), which heals by scarring and may lead to a slowly progressive shrinkage of the affected mucous membranes and connective tissues, and eventually to blindness if untreated. Called also *benign mucosal p.* and *benign mucous membrane p.* **localized chronic p.**, see *localized bullous p.*

pemphigus (pem′fĭ-gus) [Gr. *pemphix* blister] a group of chronic, relapsing, sometimes fatal skin diseases characterized clinically by the development of successive crops of vesicles and bullae, histologically by acantholysis, and immunologically by serum autoantibodies directed against antigens in the intracellular zones of the epidermis. The specific disease is usually indicated by a modifying term, but the term *pemphigus* is often used alone to designate *pemphigus vulgaris*. Cf. *pemphigoid*. **benign familial p.**, a benign, persistently recurrent bullous and vesicular autosomal dominant dermatitis involving chiefly the sides of the neck, axillae, groin, and flexural and apposing surfaces of the body, and characterized by crops of lesions, which may remain localized or become generalized, that rupture, undergo erosion, and become thickly crusted. The histopathologic features are suggestive of keratosis follicularis as well as pemphigus. Called also *Hailey-Hailey disease*. **Brazilian p.**, fogo selvagem. **p. erythemato′sus**, a variant of pemphigus foliaceus, with which it is histologically identical, characterized clinicallly by the development of a lupus erythematosus–like rash on the nose, checks, and ears and seborrhea-like lesions elsewhere on the body; and immunologically by granular deposition of immunoglobulin and complement along the dermoepidermal junction. These findings suggest the coexistence of lupus erythematosus and pemphigus in the same individual. Called also *Senear-Usher syndrome*. **p. folia′ceus**, a superficial, relatively mild and chronic form of pemphigus, usually occurring in the fourth and fifth decades of life, and characterized by the development of small flaccid bullae that rupture and crust and localized or generalized exfoliation. The lesions may be found on the scalp, face, and trunk, or they may spread to become generalized. **ocular p.**, cicatricial pemphigoid involving the conjunctivae. **South American p.**, fogo selvagem. **p. veg′etans**, a variant of pemphigus vulgaris characterized by the development of proliferating verrucous granulations, sometimes with pustules at their periphery, which seemingly arise from denuded bullae, and have a tendency to coalesce into patches. According to some authorities, there are two types: a *Hallopeau type*, which has a more benign course and prognosis; and a *Neumann type*, which closely resembles pemphigus in all respects. **p. veg′etans, benign**, the Hallopeau type of pemphigus vegetans. **p. vulga′ris**, the most common and severe form of pemphigus, usually occurring between the ages of 40 and 60, characterized by the chronic development of flaccid, easily ruptured bullae upon apparently normal skin and mucous membranes, beginning focally but progressing to become generalized, leaving large, weeping, denuded surfaces that become partially crusted over with little or no tendency to heal and that enlarge by confluence. In untreated cases, sepsis, cachexia, and electrolyte imbalance may occur and lead to death. **wildfire p.,** fogo selvagem.

pempidine tartrate (pem′pĭ-dēn) chemical name: 1,2,2,6,6-pentamethylpiperidine tartrate; a ganglion-blocking agent, $C_{10}H_{21}N$, occurring as a white, crystalline powder, which has been used as an antihypertensive.

Penbritin (pen-brit′in) trademark for preparations of ampicillin.

penbutolol sulfate (pen-bu′to-lŏl) (S)-1-(2-cyclopentylphenoxy)-3-[(1,1-dimethylethyl)amino]-2-propanol sulfate (2:1) (salt); an antiadrenergic (β-receptor), $(C_{18}H_{29}NO_2)_2 \cdot H_2SO_4$.

Pende's sign (pen′dēz) [Nicola *Pende*, Italian physician, born 1880] André-Thomas sign.

pendelluft (pen′del-looft″) [Ger. "pendulum breath"] the movement of air back and forth between the lungs, resulting in increased dead space ventilation.

pendular (pen′du-lar) having a pendulum-like movement.

pendulous (pen′joo-lus, pen′dŭ-lus) [L. *pendere* to hang] hanging loosely; dependent.

penectomy (pe-nek′to-me) [*penis* + Gr. *ektome* excision] surgical removal of the penis.

penetrability (pen″ĕ-trah-bil′ĭ-te) the ability of roentgen rays to penetrate matter.

penetrance (pen′ĕ-trans) [L. *penetrare* to enter into] in genetics, the frequency of expression of a genotype. If it is less than 100 per cent, the trait is said to exhibit *reduced penetrance* or *lack of penetrance.* In an individual who has a genotype that characteristically produces an abnormal phenotype but is phenotypically normal, the trait is said to be *nonpenetrant.*

penetrating (pen′ĕ-trāt-ing) [L. *penetrans*] piercing; entering deeply.

penetration (pen″ĕ-tra′shun) [L. *penetratio*] 1. the act of piercing or entering deeply. 2. the focal depth of a lens, or its power of giving a clear definition at various depths.

penetrology (pen″ĕ-trol′o-je) the study of radiant energy.

penetrometer (pen″ĕ-trom′ĕ-ter) 1. step wedge; a device for measuring the penetrability of roentgen rays. 2. an apparatus for registering the resistance of semisolid material to penetration.

penfluridol (pen-floor′ĭ-dōl) chemical name: 1-[4,4-bis(4-fluorophenyl)butyl]-4-[4-chloro-3-(trifluoromethyl)phenyl]-4-piperidinol; a tranquilizer, $C_{28}H_{27}CF_5NO$.

-penia [Gr. *penia* poverty, need] a word termination indicating an abnormal reduction in number of the element denoted by the root to which it is affixed, as leukopenia.

penial (pe′ne-al) penile.

penicidin (pen″ĭ-si′din) patulin.

penicillamine (pen″ĭ-sil-ah-mēn) [USP] chemical name: 3-mercapto-D-valine. A degradation product of penicillin, $C_5H_{11}NO_2S$, occurring as a white or almost white, crystalline powder, which chelates certain heavy metals; used orally to reduce the blood copper level in the treatment of hepatolenticular degeneration and to promote excretion of cystine by forming a more soluble penicillamine-cystine disulfide. It has been used in the treatment of rheumatoid arthritis.

penicilli (pen″ĭ-sil′i) [L.] genitive and plural of *penicillus.*

penicilliary (pen″ĭ-sil′e-er″e) [L. *penicillium,* dim. of *peniculus* a brush] resembling a brush or broom.

penicillic acid (pen″ĭ-sil′ik) an antibiotic substance produced by several species of *Penicillium;* it has antibacterial activity but is also toxic to animal tissues.

penicillin (pen″ĭ-sil′in) any of a large group of natural or semisynthetic antibacterial antibiotics derived directly or indirectly from strains of fungi of the genus *Penicillium* and other soil-inhabiting fungi grown on special culture media, which exert a bacteriocidal as well as a bacteriostatic effect on susceptible bacteria by interfering with the final stages of the synthesis of peptidoglycan, a substance in the bacterial cell wall. The penicillins, despite their relatively low toxicity for the host, are active against many bacteria, especially gram-positive pathogens (streptococci, staphylococci, pneumococci); clostridia; some gram-negative forms (gonococci, meningococci); some spirochetes (*Treponema pallidum* and *T. pertenue*); and some fungi. Certain strains of some target species, e.g., staphylococci, secrete the enzyme penicillinase, which inactivates penicillin and confers resistance to the antibiotic. **aluminum p.,** the aluminum salt of penicillin prepared from extracts of cultures of *Penicillium notatum* or *P. chrysogenum.* **benzyl p. potassium,** potassium p. G. **benzyl p. sodium,** p. G. sodium. **clemizole p.,** the clemizole salt of penicillin G, $C_{16}H_{18}N_2O_4C_{19}H_{20}ClN_3$, the combination of which produces a repository form of penicillin G with antihistaminic properties. **dimethoxyphenyl p. sodium,** methicillin sodium. **p. G,** the most widely used form and the first of the penicillins developed for medicinal use. It is used in the form of the benzathine, potassium, procaine, and sodium salts, principally in the treatment of infections due to penicillin-susceptible gram-positive bacteria, gram-negative cocci, *Treponema pallidum,* and *Actinomyces israeli.* Called also *benzylpenicillin.* **p. G benzathine** [USP], a salt having a long-sustained action, $C_{16}H_{20}N_2 \cdot 2C_{16}H_{18}N_2O_4S \cdot 4H_2O$, obtained by combining penicillin G with *N,N′*-bis(phenylmethyl)-1,2-ethanediamine (2:1), occurring as a white, crystalline powder, and containing 57.9 to 71.6 per cent of penicillin G; administered orally and intramuscularly. **p. G potassium,** a salt $C_{16}H_{17}KN_2O_4S$, occurring as colorless or white crystals, or white, crystalline powder, and containing 80.8 to 94.3 per cent of penicillin G; administered orally and by intravenous injection or infusion. **p. G procaine** [USP], a salt having a long-sustained action, $C_{16}H_{18}N_2O_4S \cdot C_{13}H_{20}N_2H_2O$, obtained by combining penicillin G with procaine (1:1), occurring as white crystals or white, very fine, microcrystalline powder, and containing 51 to 59.6 per cent penicillin G; administered intramuscularly. **p. G sodium,** a salt, $C_{16}H_{17}N_2NaO_4S$, occurring as colorless or white crystals or as a white to slightly yellow, crystalline powder, containing not less than 85 per cent of penicillin G sodium; administered intramuscularly and intravenously. *Sterile penicillin G sodium* [USP] is suitable for parenteral use. **isoxazolyl p.,** a group of semisynthetic penicillins, including oxacillin, cloxacillin, and dicloxacillin, which combine resistance to penicillinase with acid stability and activity against gram-positive bacteria. **p. N,** adicillin. **p. O,** a penicillin produced biosynthetically by adding a precursor to the culture medium; penicillin O and its potassium and sodium salts have actions similar to those of penicillin G and are said to be hypoallergenic. **p. O chloroprocaine,** a salt of 2-chloroprocaine and penicillin O, having actions similar to penicillins G and O. **p. O potassium,** see *p. O.* **p. O sodium,** see *p. O.* **phenoxymethyl p.,** p. V. **potassium phenoxymethyl p.,** p. V potassium. **p. V** [USP], a semisynthetic oral penicillin prepared from cultures of the mold *Penicillium* in the presence of 2-phenoxyethanol with an autolysate of yeast as the source of nitrogen. It is a broad-spectrum antibiotic having pharmacologic and toxic properties similar to those of other penicillins, and is less potent than penicillin G. Called also *phenoxymethyl p.* **p. V benzathine** [USP], an oral penicillin, $(C_{16}H_{18}N_2O_5S)_2C_{16}H_{20}N_2$, occurring as practically white powder. **p. V hydrabamine** [USP], an oral penicillin, $(C_{16}H_{18}N_2O_5S)_2 \cdot C_{42}H_{64}N_2$, occurring as a practically white powder. **p. V potassium** [USP], an oral penicillin, $C_{16}H_{17}KN_2O_5S$, occurring as a white crystalline powder.

penicillinase (pen″ĭ-sil′ĭ-nās) penicillin amido-β-lactam-hydrolase: an enzyme produced by certain bacteria which converts penicillin to an inactive product and thus increases resistance to the antibiotic. A purified preparation from cultures of a strain of *Bacillus cereus* is used in treatment of reactions to penicillin.

penicillin-fast (pen″ĭ-sĭl′in-fast) resistant to the action of penicillin; said of certain strains of bacteria.

penicilliosis (pen″ĭ-sil″e-o′sis) infection with *Penicillium,* usually a pulmonary infection.

Penicillium (pen″ĭ-sil′e-um) [L. *penicillum* brush, roll] a genus of Fungi Imperfecti (family Moniliaceae, order Moniliales) that develop fruiting organs resembling a broom, or the bones of the hand and fingers. When identified, the perfect (sexual) stage is classified with the ascomycetous fungi in the family Eurotiaceae, order Eurotiales. See also *penicillin.* **P. chrysog′enum,** a species from which various penicillins are obtained. **P. citri′num,** a species that produces the antibiotic citrinin. **P. crusta′ceum,** *P. glau′cum.* **P. glau′cum,** a common bluish green mold. **P. nota′tum,** a species that is one of the sources of various penicillins. **P. pat′ulum,** *P. uticale.* **P. utica′le,** one of the species that produces patulin; called also *P. patulum.*

penicilloyl-polylysine (pen″ĭ-sil′oil-pol″ĕ-li′sēn) an agent prepared from polylysine and a penicillenic acid; intradermal injection elicits a wheal and erythema response within 20 minutes in many who are sensitive to penicillin.

penicillus (pen″ĭ-sil′us), gen. and pl. *penicil′li* [L. "brush"] a structure resembling a brush in appearance. **penicil′li arte′riae liena′lis,** NA alternative for *penicilli arteriae splenicae.* **penicil′li arte′riae sple′nicae** [NA], brushlike groups of arterial branches of the lobules of the spleen; called also *penicilli arteriae lienalis* [NA alternative].

Peniculina (pě-nik″u-li′nah) a suborder of large, free-living, monomorphic, mainly freshwater protozoa (order Hymenostomatida, subclass Hymenostomatia), characterized by the presence of explosive fusiform trichocysts and three peniculi, often located deep in the buccal cavity; nematodesmata and preoral and postoral sutures and an oral groove occur often. Many species have algal and gram-negative endosymbionts. *Paramedium* is a representative species.

peniculus (pě-nik′u-lus), pl. *penic′uli* ["little brush"] a modified membrane manifested as a band of fused cilia in the left wall in the buccal cavity of certain ciliate protozoa.

penile (pe′nīl) pertaining to or affecting the penis.

penillamine (pen″il-am′in) chemical name: 2-amino-3-mercapto-3-methylbutanoic acid or β,β-dimethylcysteine. An amine, $C_5H_{11}O_2NS$, derived from penillic acid by the removal of a molecule of carbon dioxide.

penilloaldehyde (pen″ĭ-lo-al′de-hīd) an aldehyde derived from penicillin.

penis (pe′nis) [L.] [NA] the male organ of copulation and of urinary excretion, comprising a root, body, and extremity, or glans penis. The root is attached to the descending portions of the pubic bone by the *crura,* the latter being the extremities of the corpora cavernosa. The body consists of two parallel cylindrical bodies, the *corpora cavernosa,* and beneath them the *corpus spongiosum,* through which the urethra passes. The glans is covered with mucous membrane and ensheathed by the prepuce, or foreskin. The penis is homologous with the clitoris in the female. **clubbed p.,** a condition in which the penis is curved when erect. **concealed p.,** a rudimentary penis concealed beneath the skin of the scrotum, perineum, abdomen, or thigh. **double p.,** an anomaly resulting when the urethral groove completely divides the penile shaft during development of the embryo. **p. mulieb′ris** (obs.), clitoris. **p. palma′tus,** webbed p. **p. plas′tica,** Peyronie's disease. **webbed p.,** a penis that is enclosed by the skin of the scrotum; called also *p. palmatus.*

penischisis (pe-nis′kĭ-sis) [*penis* + Gr. *schisis* splitting] a fissured state of the penis, as epispadias, hypospadias, or paraspadias.

penitis (pe-ni′tis) inflammation of the penis.

Penn seroflocculation reaction [Harry Samuel *Penn,* Russian physician and zoologist in the United States, born 1891] see under *reaction.*

pennate (pen′āt) penniform.

penniform (pen′ĭ-form) [L. *penna* feather + *forma* form] shaped like a feather; looking like a feather.

pennyroyal (pen″e-roi′al) a popular name for various labiate plants, especially *Mentha pulegium* L. (*European p.*) and *M. canadensis* L. (American wild mint); the oil was formerly used as a diaphoretic, aromatic, and emmenagogue.

pennyweight (pen′e-wāt) a unit of weight in the troy system, being 24 grains, or one twentieth of an ounce.

penology (pe-nol′o-je) [Gr. *poinē* penalty + *-logy*] the science of punishment; that branch of criminology which deals with the treatment of criminals.

penoscrotal (pe″no-skro′tal) relating to the penis and the scrotum.

Penrose drain (pen′rōz) [Charles Bingham *Penrose,* Philadelphia gynecologist, 1862–1925] see under *drain.*

pent-, penta- [Gr. *pente* five] a combining form meaning five.

pentabasic (pen″tah-ba′sik) having five replaceable atoms of hydrogen in the molecule.

pentachromic (pen″tah-kro′mik) [*penta-* + Gr. *chrōma* color] 1. pertaining to or exhibiting five colors. 2. able to distinguish only five of the seven colors of the spectrum.

pentacyclic (pen″tah-sik′lik) having a ring of five atoms in the molecule.

pentad (pen′tad) 1. any group of five. 2. a pentavalent element or radical.

pentadactyl (pen″tah-dak′til) [*penta-* + Gr. *daktylos* finger] having five fingers or toes on the hand or foot.

pentaene (pen′tah-ēn) a chemical compound in which there are five conjugated double bonds.

pentaerythritol (pen″tah-ĕ-rith′rĭ-tol) chemical name: 2,2-bis(hydroxymethyl)-1,3-propanediol. An alcohol, $(CH_2OH)_4C$, prepared by treating acetaldehyde with formaldehyde in an aqueous solution of calcium hydroxide; used in synthetic resins and in paints and varnishes. **p. chloral,** petrichloral. **p. tetranitrate,** the nitric acid ester of pentaerythritol, $C_5H_8N_4O_{12}$, having vasodilator action similar to nitroglycerin, occurring as a white, crystalline powder that may explode on percussion. Called also *niperyt, pentaerythrityl tetranitrate, penthrit, pentrinitrol,* and *PTEN.* Diluted p. tetranitrate [USP], a dry mixture of pentaerythritol tetranitrate with lactose, mannitol, or other inert excipients to render it nonexplosive is administered orally in the treatment of angina pectoris.

pentaerythrityl (pen″tah-ĕ-rith′rĭ-til) pentaerythritol. **p. tetranitrate,** pentaerythritol tetranitrate.

pentagastrin (pen″tah-gas′trin) a synthetic pentapeptide consisting of β-alanine and the C-terminal tetrapeptide of gastrin; used as a test of gastric secretory function.

pentalogy (pen-tal′o-je) a combination of five elements or factors, as five concurrent defects or symptoms. **p. of Fallot,** the four defects included in the tetralogy of Fallot, occurring in association with patent foramen ovale or atrial septal defect.

pentamer (pen′tah-mer) a polymer consisting of five monomers; a viral capsomer having five structural units.

pentamethazene (pen″tah-meth′ah-zēn) azamethonium.

pentamethylenediamine (pen″tah-meth″il-ēn-di-am′in) cadaverine.

pentamethylenetetrazol (pen-tah-meth″il-ēn-tet′rah-zol) pentylenetetrazol.

pentamethylmelamine (pen″tah-meth″il-mel′ah-mēn) PMM; an active metabolite of hexamethylmelamine (q.v.) also under investigation as an antineoplastic agent.

pentamidine (pen-tam′ĭ-dēn) chemical name: 4,4′-(pentamethylenedioxy)dibenzamidine; an anti-infective used as the isethionate salt and effective against *Pneumocystis carinii.*

pentane (pen′tān) *n*-pentane; an aliphatic hydrocarbon of the methane series, C_5H_{12}, obtained by distillation of petroleum and occurring as a clear, colorless, flammable liquid. It produces anesthesia when inhaled, ingested, or injected.

pentapeptide (pen″tah-pep′tid) a polypeptide containing five amino acids.

pentapiperide methylsulfate (pen″tah-pi′per-īd) chemical name: 1,1,- dimethyl-4- [(3- methyl- 1-oxo- 2-phenylpentyl)oxy]piperidinium. A synthetic quaternary ammonium anticholinergic, $C_{20}H_{33}NO_8S$, used in the treatment of peptic ulcer and other disorders in which gastrointestinal hypermotility and hypersecretion are features, administered orally. Called also *pentapiperium methylsulfate.*

pentapiperium methylsulfate (pen-tah-pĭ-per′ĭ-um) pentapiperide methylsulfate.

pentapyrrolidinium bitartrate (pen″tah-pir-ro″lĭ-din′e-um) pentolinium tartrate.

pentasomy (pen″tah-so′me) [*penta-* + Gr. *sōma* body] the presence of three additional chromosomes of one type (e.g., 5 X chromosomes) in an otherwise diploid cell (2n + 3).

Pentastoma (pen-tas′to-mah) [*penta-* + Gr. *stoma* mouth] a genus of endoparasitic, wormlike arthropods of the class Porocephalidae. *P. denticulatum* (incorrectly assigned to this genus) is the larva of *Linguatulidae serrata.*

pentastomiasis (pen″tah-sto-mi′ah-sis) infection with pentastomids.

pentastomid (pen-tah-sto′mid) any individual of the class Pentastomida.

Pentastomida (pen″tah-sto′mid-ah) a class of Arthropoda, the tongue worms, consisting of degenerate wormlike parasites, without circulatory or respiratory systems. The adults, otherwise without appendages, possess two pairs of hooks near the mouth. The larvae bear two or three pairs of rudimentary legs. Adults live in the respiratory passages and body cavities of reptiles, birds, and mammals. Two genera, *Armillifer* and *Linguatula*, have been reported on several occasions from man as larval host. It includes the order Porocephalida.

pentatomic (pen″tah-tom′ik) [penta- + atom] 1. containing five atoms. 2. containing five replaceable hydrogen atoms.

Pentatrichomonas (pen″tah-trik″o-mo′nas, pen″tah-trik″o-mon′as) [penta- + tricho- + Gr. monas unit, from monos single] in some systems of classification, a genus of parasitic flagellated protozoa established to include the species of *Trichomonas* having five anterior flagella, i.e., *T. hominis*.

pentavalent (pen″tah-va′lent) having a chemical valence of five; capable of combining with five atoms of hydrogen.

pentazocine (pen-taz′o-sēn) [USP] chemical name: 1,2,3,4,5,6-hexahydro-cis-6,11-dimethyl-3-(3-methyl-2-butenyl)-2,6-methano-3-benzazocin-8-ol. A synthetic analgesic, $C_{27}H_{27}NO$, occurring as a white or very pale tan-colored powder; used in the form of the hydrochloride and lactate salts. **p. hydrochloride** [USP], the hydrochloride salt of pentazocine, occurring as a white crystalline powder; administered orally. **p. lactate** [USP], the lactate salt of pentazocine, administered parenterally.

pentdyopent (pent-di′o-pent) [penta + Gr. dyo two + pente five = 525, referring to the spectroscopic line of the substance] a substance derived from blood pigment, occurring in the urine in certain diseases.

pentene (pen′tēn) amylene.

pentetate calcium trisodium (pen′tĕ-tāt) chemical name: [N,N-bis[2-[bis(carboxymethyl)amino]ethyl]glycinato(5−)]calcinate(3−)trisodium. The calcium trisodium salt of pentetic acid, $C_{14}H_{18}CaN_3Na_3O_{10}$, used as a chelating agent, especially in the treatment of plutonium poisoning. Called also *calcium trisodium pentetate*.

pentetic acid (pen-te′tik) a chelating agent (iron) with the general properties of the edetates.

penthienate bromide (pen-thi′ĕ-nāt) chemical name: 2-[(cyclopentylhydroxy-2-thienylacetyl)oxy]-N,N-diethyl-N-methylethanaminium bromide. A quaternary ammonium anticholinergic, $C_{18}H_{30}BrNO_3S$, used orally, mainly in the treatment of gastric ulcer.

Penthrane (pen′thrān) trademark for a preparation of methoxyflurane.

penthrit (pen′thrit) pentaerythritol tetranitrate.

Pentids (pen′tidz) trademark for preparations of penicillin G potassium.

pentizidone sodium (pen-tiz′ĭ-dōn) chemical name: (R)-4-[(1-methyl-3-oxo-1-butenyl)amino]-3-isoxazolidinone monosodium salt hemihydrate; an antibacterial, $C_8H_{11}N_2NaO_3 \cdot \frac{1}{2}H_2O$.

pentobarbital (pen″to-bar′bĭ-tal) [USP] chemical name: 5-ethyl-5-(1-methylbutyl)-2,4,6 (1H,3H,5H)-pyrimidinetrione. A short- to intermediate-acting barbiturate, $C_{11}H_{17}N_2O_3$, occurring as a white to practically white, fine powder; used as a sedative and hypnotic, administered orally. Called also *pentobarbitone*. **p. sodium** [USP], the sodium salt of pentobarbital, a hypnotic used as a sedative, anticonvulsant, preanesthetic in surgery, an adjunct to anesthesia, and an amnesic in obstetrics.

pentobarbitone (pen″to-bar′bĭ-tōn) pentobarbital.

pentolinium tartrate (pen″to-lin′e-um) chemical name: 1,1′-(1,5-pentanediyl)bis[1-methylpyrrolidinium]. A ganglionic blocking agent, $C_{23}H_{42}N_2O_{12}$, occurring as a white or slightly cream-colored powder; used as an antihypertensive, administered orally, intramuscularly, and subcutaneously.

pentone (pen′tōn) valylene.

pentosan (pen′to-san) any member of a group of pentose polysaccharides having the composition $(C_5H_8O_4)_n$; found in various foods and plant juices. They yield pentose on hydroly-

sis. **methyl p.,** a pentosan which on hydrolysis yields methyl pentoses.

pentosazon (pen″to-sa′zon) a crystalline compound formed by treating a pentose with phenyl hydrazine, sometimes abnormally occurring in the urine.

pentose (pen′tōs) a monosaccharide containing five carbon atoms in a molecule.

pentosemia (pen″to-se′me-ah) the presence of pentose in the blood.

pentosenucleic acid (pen″tōs-noo-kle′ik) ribonucleic acid.

pentoside (pen′to-sid) a compound of a pentose with some other substance. Compounds of pentoses with purine and pyrimidine bases are found in the nucleic acids.

pentosuria (pen″to-su′re-ah) [pentose + Gr. ouron urine + -ia] a benign error of metabolism due to a defect in the activity of the enzyme L-xylulose dehydrogenase, which results in high levels of L-xylulose in the urine. It is transmitted as an autosomal recessive trait. Called also L-xylulosuria.

pentosuric (pen″to-su′rik) affected with pentosuria.

pentosyl (pen′to-sil) a radical of pentose.

Pentothal (pen′to-thol) trademark for preparations of thiopental.

pentoxide (pen-tok′sīd) an oxide containing five atoms of oxygen in a molecule.

pentoxifylline (pen-toks-ĭ′fĭ-lin) chemical name: 2,2-bis[(nitrooxy)methyl]-1,3-propanediol mononitrate (ester); a coronary vasodilator, $C_5H_9N_3O_{10}$.

pentrinitrol (pen-tri-ni′trol) pentaerythritol trinitrate.

Pentritol (pen′trĭ-tol) trademark for a preparation of pentaerythritol tetranitrate.

Pentryate (pen-tri′āt) trademark for preparations of pentaerythritol trinitrate.

pentylenetetrazol (pen″tĭ-lēn-tet′rah-zol) a synthetic camphor-like compound used to induce convulsions in the electroencephalographic evaluation of epilepsy and, formerly, in the treatment of mental disorders (see convulsive therapy, under therapy).

Pen-Vee (pen′ve) trademark for preparations of penicillin V.

Penzoldt's test, reagent (pen′zōldz) [Franz Penzoldt, physician in Erlangen, 1849–1927] see under tests.

Penzoldt-Fischer test (pen′zōld-fish′er) [Franz Penzoldt; Emil Fischer, German chemist, 1852–1919] see under tests.

peonin chloride (pe′o-nin) chemical name: 4′,7-dihydroxy-3,5-di-β-glucosido-3′-methoxyflavylium chloride. A deep purple dye, $C_{28}H_{33}ClO_{16}$, the coloring matter of deep purple peonies; called also peonin.

peotillomania (pe″o-til″o-ma′ne-ah) [Gr. peos penis + tillein to pull + mania madness] a ticlike movement consisting in constant pulling at the penis; called also pseudomasturbation.

peotomy (pe-ot′o-me) [Gr. peos penis + temnein to cut] surgical removal of the penis.

peplomer (pep′lo-mer) a subunit of the peplos, or envelope, of a virion.

peplos (pep′lohs) the lipoprotein envelope possessed by some types of virions, assembled in some cases from subunits called peplomers.

pepo (pe′po) [L. "pumpkin"] pumpkin seed; the dried ripe edible seeds of the pumpkin, Cucurbita pepo L. (Cucurbitaceae); used as an anthelmintic.

pepper (pep′er) [L. piper] black pepper; the dried unripe fruit of Piper nigrum L. (Piperaceae) and other plants of that genus. White pepper is the decorticated ripe fruit of black pepper, and is milder. Pepper contains piperine, an aromatic pungent volatile oil (1–9 per cent), minor alkaloids, fat, protein, and resins; used chiefly as a spice, but it also has diaphoretic, carminative, and gastric secretagogue properties. **cayenne p.,** capsicum.

Pepper's syndrome (type) (pep′erz) [William Pepper, Philadelphia physician, 1874–1947] see under syndrome.

peppermint (pep′er-mint) [USP] the dried leaves and flowering tops of Mentha piperita L. (Labiatae), having carminative, gastric stimulant, and counter-irritant properties; used as an oil, spirit, or water extract as a flavored vehicle for drugs.

pepsic (pep′sik) peptic.

pepsin (pep′sin) a general name for several enzymes of the gastric juice that catalyze the hydrolysis of proteins to form polypeptides. **p. A.,** [EC 3.4.23.1] an enzyme of the hydrolase class that catalyzes the hydrolysis of proteins with preferential cleavage at phenylalanine, tryptophan, tyrosine, and leucine residues. It is secreted by the gastric mucosa in the form of pepsinogen and has an optimum pH of 1.5 to 2.0. **p. B.,** [EC 3.4.23.2] pepsin similar to pepsin A, formed from pig pepsinogen B. A related enzyme is found in human beings. **p. C.,** [EC 3.4.23.3] pepsin similar to pepsin A but highly active with hemoglobin as substrate. Called also *gastricsin*.

pepsinate (pep′sin-āt) to treat or charge with pepsin.

pepsinia (pep-sin′e-ah) the secretion of pepsin; it may be normal, excessive (hyperpepsinia), deficient (hypopepsinia), or totally absent (apepsinia).

pepsiniferous (pep″sin-if′er-us) [*pepsin* + L. *ferre* to bear] producing or secreting pepsin.

pepsinogen (pep-sin′o-jen) a zymogen secreted by chief cells, mucous neck cells, and pyloric gland cells, which is converted into pepsin in the presence of gastric acid or of pepsin itself. Called also *propepsin*.

pepsinuria (pep″sĭ-nu′re-ah) the presence of pepsin in the urine; it may be associated with duodenal ulcer because of the increased volume of gastric secretion.

pepstatin (pep-stat′in) any of the pentapeptide pepsin inhibitors obtained from several species of *Streptomyces*, identified as pepstatin A, B, and C. The A component, $C_{34}H_{63}N_5O_9$, has been used in the treatment of gastric ulcer.

Peptavlon (pep-tav′lon) trademark for a preparation of pentagastrin.

peptic (pep′tik) [Gr. *peptikos*] pertaining to pepsin or to digestion; related to the action of gastric juices.

peptid (pep′tid) peptide.

peptidase (pep′tĭ-dās) [EC 3.4.11-19] any of a sub-subclass of enzymes of the hydrolase class that catalyze the hydrolysis of peptide bonds, and usually restricted to exopeptidases, which attack terminal or penultimate peptide bonds. These enzymes are classified as aminopeptidases, carboxypeptidases, and dipeptidases. Called also *peptide hydrolase*.

peptide (pep′tīd) any member of a class of compounds of low molecular weight which yield two or more amino acids on hydrolysis. Formed by loss of water from the NH_2 and COOH groups of adjacent amino acids, they are known as di-, tri-, tetra- [etc.] peptides, depending on the number of amino acids in the molecule. Peptides form the constituent parts of proteins. **C p.,** the connecting peptide chain that is removed in the cleavage of proinsulin to form insulin. **corticotropin-like intermediate lobe p. (CLIP),** a peptide with a sequence identical to the C-terminal 22 residues of ACTH (adrenocorticotropic hormone, corticotropin), found in the intermediate lobe of the pituitary gland in lower animals; the function, if any, is unknown. **N-formylmethionyl p's,** di- and tripeptides in which the N-terminal amino acid residue is N-formylmethionine (fMet), which are produced by bacteria in protein synthesis (fMet initiates each polypeptide chain in prokaryotes but is often removed after translation) and which are chemotactic for granulocytes and macrophages but not lymphocytes. **vasoactive intestinal p. (VIP),** vasoactive intestinal polypeptide.

peptide hydrolase (pep′tīd hi′dro-lās) peptidase.

peptidergic (pep″tĭ-der′jĭk) having an action resembling that of a peptide hormone.

peptidoglycan (pep″tĭ-do-gli′kan) a high-molecular-weight polymer that forms the tough, rigid structure of bacterial cell walls. It is made up of three parts: (1) a backbone, composed of alternating N-acetylglucosamine and N-acetylmuramic acid; (2) a set of identical tetrapeptide side-chains attached to N-acetylmuramic acid; and (3) a set of identical peptide cross-bridges. The backbone is the same in all bacterial species; however, the tetrapeptide side-chains and the peptide cross-bridges vary from species to species.

peptinotoxin (pep″tĭ-no-tok′sin) a poisonous intestinal product of imperfect stomach digestion.

peptization (pep″ti-za′shun) increase in the degree of dispersion of a colloid solution; the liquefaction of a colloid gel to form a sol.

Peptococcaceae (pep″to-kok-ka′se-e) [Gr. *pepton* digestion + *kokkus* berry] a family of anaerobic, nonmotile, usually gram-positive bacteria, made up of spherical cells occurring singly or in pairs, tetrads, chains, or irregular masses. They are found in the mouth and intestinal and respiratory tracts of man and other animals, in the human female urogenital tract, and in soil. The family includes the genera *Peptococcus*, *Peptostreptococcus*, and *Ruminococcus*.

Peptococcus (pep″to-kok′us) [Gr. *pepton* digestion + *kokkus* berry] a genus of gram-positive, anaerobic, coccoid bacteria of the family Peptococcaceae, occurring singly or in pairs, tetrads, or irregular masses, which are chemo-organotrophic and capable of fermenting protein decomposition products. Part of the normal human flora of the mouth, upper respiratory tract, and large intestine, they also cause infections of soft tissues and bacteremias. The organisms also occur in the lower animals and soil. **P. anaero′bius,** a microaerophilic or obligate anaerobe found in the appendix and the female genital tract, and in cystitis and draining sinus. Called also *Diplococcus magnus*. **P. asaccharolyt′icus,** a species that does not ferment sugars, found in the human large intestine, oral cavity, pleura, uterus, and vagina. **P. constella′tus,** a microaerophilic or obligate anaerobe found in purulent pleurisy and in the tonsils, appendix, nose, throat, gums, and infrequently the skin and vagina. Called also *Diplococcus constellatus*. **P. mag′nus,** a species with large (1–2 μm in diameter) cells that is recovered most frequently from clinical specimens. It is a cause of septic arthritis and soft tissue infections.

peptogenic (pep″to-jen′ik) [Gr. *peptein* to digest + *gennan* to produce] 1. producing pepsin or peptones. 2. promoting digestion.

peptogenous (pep-toj′ĕ-nus) peptogenic.

peptolysis (pep-tol′ĭ-sis) [*peptone* + Gr. *lysis* dissolution] the hydrolysis of peptones.

peptolytic (pep″to-lit′ik) denoting an agent or process that hydrolyzes peptones.

peptone (pep′tōn) [Gr. *pepton* digesting] a derived protein, or a mixture of cleavage products produced by the partial hydrolysis of a native protein either by an acid or by an enzyme. Peptones are readily soluble in water, and are not precipitatable by heat, by alkalis, or by saturation with ammonium sulfate. **beef p.,** a peptone made from beef by treating it with extract of pancreas. **casein p.,** a light-brown powder, soluble in water; a nutrient for convalescents. **gelatin p.,** a peptone formed during the digestion of gelatin with pepsin. **milk p.,** casein p. **venom p.,** a peptone from snake venom.

peptonic (pep-ton′ik) pertaining to or containing peptone.

peptonize (pep′to-nīz) to convert a protein into peptone by the action of an acid or enzyme.

peptonoid (pep′to-noid) a peptone-like substance.

peptonuria (pep″to-nu′re-ah) [*peptone* + Gr. *ouron* urine + *-ia*] the presence of peptones in the urine. **enterogenous p.,** that which is due to disease of the intestine. **hepatogenous p.,** that which is due to disease of the liver. **nephrogenic p.,** that which is due to disease of the kidney. **puerperal p.,** that which occurs during the puerperium. **pyogenic p.,** that which is associated with a suppurative process.

Peptostreptococcus (pep″to-strep″to-kok′us) [Gr. *pepton* digestion + *streptos* twisted + *kokkos* berry] a genus of gram-positive, coccoid bacteria of the family Peptococcaceae, made up of obligately anaerobic, chemo-organotrophic cells. Part of the normal human flora of the mouth, upper respiratory tract, and large intestine, they are also opportunistic pathogens causing soft tissue infections and bacteremias. **P. anaerob′ius,** a species that ferments glucose only, isolated in humans from cases of gangrene, infected wounds, puerperal fever, appendicitis, pleurisy, paranasal sinusitis, and osteomyelitis, and from the intestinal tract, oral cavity, and genital secretions. Called also *Streptococcus foetidus*. **P. lanceola′tus,** a species having large ovoid cells with pointed ends, occurring in short chains and in pairs, which has been isolated from humans in cases of diarrhea, dental infection, vulvovaginitis, and abscesses. Called also *Streptococcus lanceolatus*. **P. mi′cros,** a nonfermentative species having small spheroid cells, isolated from cases of purulent pleurisy, puerperal sepsis, appendicitis, brain and dental abscesses, and actinomycosis. Called also *Streptococcus micros*. **P. par′vulus,** a species with small spherical cells occurring in pairs and short chains, isolated from the human respiratory tract and oral cavity. **P. produc′-**

tus, a species with spherical cells, occurring in chains, isolated from cases of gangrene and pelvic abscesses and from blood and urine.

peptotoxin (pep″to-tok′sin) any toxin or poisonous base developed from a peptone; also a poisonous alkaloid or ptomaine occurring in certain peptones and putrefying proteins.

per- [L. *per* through] 1. a prefix meaning throughout in space or time, or completely or extremely. 2. a prefix used in chemical terms to denote a large amount or to designate combination of an element in its highest valence.

peracephalus (per″ah-sef′ah-lus) [*per-* + *acephalus*] a monster with neither head nor arms, and with a defective thorax.

peracetate (per-as′ĕ-tāt) a salt or derivative of peracetic acid.

peracetic acid (per″ah-se′tik) peroxyacetic acid, CH_3CO-O-OH, a strong oxidizing agent.

peracid (per-as′id) an acid containing more than the usual quantity of oxygen.

peracidity (per″ah-sid′ĭ-te) excessive acidity.

peracute (per″ah-kūt′) [L. *peracutus*] excessively acute or sharp.

Perandren (per-an′dren) trademark for a preparation of testosterone.

Peranema (per″ah-ne′mah) a genus of colorless, predaceous, plantlike, flagellate protozoa (suborder Heteronematina, order Euglenida) that feed on other protozoa, which they ingest through a greatly distensible anterior cytosome.

per anum (per a′num) [L.] through the anus.

perarticulation (per″ar-tik″u-la′shun) [*per-* + L. *articulatio* joint] diarthrosis.

peratodynia (per″at-o-din′e-ah) [Gr. *peran* to pierce + *odynē* pain] (*obs.*) cardialgia or heartburn.

Perazil (per′ah-zil) trademark for preparations of chlorcyclizine hydrochloride.

percentile (per-sen′tĭl, per-sen′til) [*per cent* + *-ile* (by analogy with *quartile, quintile,* etc.)] any one of the 99 values that divide the range of a probability distribution or sample into 100 intervals of equal probability or frequency, e.g., 45 per cent of a population scores below the 45th percentile.

percentual (per-sen′tu-al) pertaining to percentage; figured on the basis of 100.

percept (per′sept) the object perceived; the mental image of an object in space perceived by the senses.

perception (per-sep′shun) [L. *percipere* to take in completely] the conscious mental registration of a sensory stimulus. **depth p.,** the proper recognition of depth or the relative distances to different objects in space. **extrasensory p. (ESP),** knowledge of, or response to, an external thought or objective event by means other than the senses. **facial p.,** see under *vision.* **stereognostic p.,** the recognition of objects by touch.

perceptive (per-sep′tiv) pertaining to perception.

perceptivity (per″sep-tiv′ĭ-te) ability to receive sense impressions.

perceptorium (per″sep-to′re-um) sensorium.

perchloric acid (per-klor′ik) a strong mineral acid and oxidizing agent, $HClO_4$.

perchloride (per-klo′rīd) a chloride that contains more chlorine than the ordinary chloride; an organic compound in which all the hydrogen atoms are substituted by chlorine, as in perchloroethylene (tetrachloroethylene), C_2Cl_4.

perchlormethane (per″klor-meth′ān) carbon tetrachloride.

perchlormethylformate (per″klor-meth″il-for′māt) diphosgene.

perchloroethylene (per-klor″o-eth′ĭ-lēn) tetrachloroethylene.

percine (per′sin) a protamine from the sperm of yellow perch, *Perca flavescens.*

percipient (per-sip′e-ent) 1. pertaining to perception. 2. an individual who perceives or is capable of perception.

percolate (per′ko-lāt) [L. *percolare*] 1. to strain; to submit to percolation. 2. to trickle slowly through a substance. 3. a liquid that has been submitted to percolation.

percolation (per″ko-la′shun) [L. *percolatio*] the extraction of the soluble parts of a drug by causing a liquid solvent to flow slowly through it.

percolator (per′ko-la″tor) a vessel used in percolating drugs.

Percoll (per′col) trademark for a colloidal suspension of silica used in density gradient centrifugation.

percomorph (per′ko-morf) pertaining to Percomorphi, an order of fishes whose liver oil is rich in vitamins A and D.

per contiguum (per kon-tig′u-um) [L.] in contiguity: arranged in such a way that the edges touch.

per continuum (per kon-tin′u-um) [L.] in continuity: without separation or break.

Percorten (per-kor′ten) trademark for preparations of desoxycorticosterone.

percuss (per-kus′) [L. *percutere*] to subject to percussion.

percussible (per-kus′ĭ-b'l) discoverable on percussion.

percussion (per-kush′un) [L. *percussio*] 1. the act of striking a part with short, sharp blows as an aid in diagnosing the condition of the underlying parts by the sound obtained. 2. a method of massage; see *tapotement.* **auscultatory p.,** auscultation of the sound produced by percussion. **bimanual p.,** the usual manner of percussion in which the middle finger of the left hand is placed against the body wall and its nail is struck a quick blow with the end of the bent right middle finger. **coin p.,** see under *tests.* **comparative p.,** percussion of two or more areas in order to compare the sounds obtained. **deep p.,** percussion in which a firm blow is struck in order to obtain a note from a deep-seated tissue. **direct p.,** immediate percussion. **drop p., drop stroke p.,** instrumental percussion in which the plexor is allowed to fall by its own weight on to the pleximeter, the elements considered in the examination being the sound heard, the vibrations felt in the handle of the plexor, and the rebound of the plexor seen. Called also *Lerch's p.* **finger p.,** that in which the fingers of one hand are used as a plexor, and those of the other as a pleximeter. **fist p.,** percussion in which the fist is brought down with a moderate thump over the area to be tested. **Goldscheider's p.,** 1. threshold percussion. 2. orthopercussion. **immediate p.,** that in which no pleximeter is used. **in-**

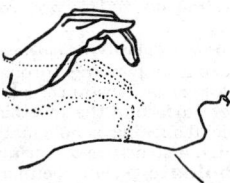

Immediate percussion.

strumental p., that in which a plexor or hammer is used. **Korányi's p.,** see under *auscultation.* auscultatory percussion over the apexes of the lungs in the diagnosis of tuberculosis. **Lerch's p.,** drop p. **mediate p.,** that in which a pleximeter is employed. **Murphy's p.,** piano p. **palpatory p.,** a combination of palpation and percussion, affording tactile rather than auditory impressions. **paradoxical p.,** resonance of the chest combined with abundant rales as in acute edema of the lungs. **pencil p.,** Plesch's p. **piano p.,** percussion by striking the body by the four fingers one after the other, beginning with the little finger; called also *Murphy's p.* **Plesch's p.,** percussion within the intercostal spaces to avoid setting the ribs into vibration, the pleximeter finger with the first interphalangeal joint flexed at a right angle. **pleximetric p.,** mediate p. **respiratory p.,** percussion during respiration so as to bring out the difference in the percussion notes of inspiration and expiration. **slapping p.,** percussion made by a slapping blow: used in comparing the resonance. **strip p.,** percussion which starts from above and progresses downward, thus covering a "strip" of the chest wall. **tangential p.,** percussion with the pleximeter placed vertically on the body, the strokes being applied to the pleximeter in a direction parallel with the surface of the skin. **threshold p.,** percussion performed by tapping lightly with the finger upon a glass rod pleximeter, one end of which, fitted with a rubber cap, rests upon an intercostal space, the rod being held at an angle to the surface of the thorax and parallel to the borders of the organ to be delimited. This method confines the percussion vibrations to a very restricted area. Called also *Goldscheider's p.* **topographic p.,** the demarcation and outlining of a dull area by percussion to determine the boundaries of organs or parts of organs.

percussor (per-kus′or) [L. "striker"] an instrument for use in performing percussion.

percutaneous (per″ku-ta′ne-us) [*per-* + L. *cutis*] performed through the skin, as injection of radiopaque material in radiological examination, or the removal of tissue for biopsy accomplished by a needle.

per cutem [L.] through the skin.

percuteur (per″koo-tūr′) [Fr.] an instrument for therapeutic or diagnostic percussion.

pereirine (per-e′ir-in) [Port. *pereira* brier] a white alkaloid, $C_{19}H_{24}N_2O$, from the bark of *Geissospermum vellosi* Allem. (Apocynaceae), a tree of tropical America; antiperiodic, antipyretic, and tonic.

perencephaly (per″en-sef′ah-le) [Gr. *pēra* pouch + *enkephalos* brain] porencephalia.

perennial (per-en′ĭ-al) [L. *perennis*, from *per* through + *annus* year] lasting through the year or for several years.

perethynol (per-eth′ĭ-nol) (*obs.*) a colloidal suspension prepared from fresh horse heart in chlorethylene and alcohol for Vernes' test for syphilis. See *Vernes' test* (def. 1), under *tests.*

Perez's sign (pa-rāths″) [Jorjen (George) Victor *Perez*, Spanish physician, 1851–1920] see under *sign.*

perfectionism (per-fek′shun-izm) a personality trait characterized by the setting for oneself or others of higher standards of performance than the situation requires.

perfilcon A (per-fil′kon) a hydrophilic contact lens material.

perflation (per-fla′shun) [L. *perflatio*] the act of blowing air into a space in order to force out secretions or other substances.

perforans (per′fo-ranz), pl. *perforan′tes* [L.] penetrating, perforating; a term applied to various muscles, nerves, arteries, and veins that perforate other structures. **p. ma′nus,** musculus flexor digitorum profundus.

perforated (per′fo-rāt″ed) [L. *perforatus*] pierced with holes.

perforation (per″fo-ra′shun) [L. *perforare* to pierce through] 1. the act of boring or piercing through a part. 2. a hole made through a part or substance. **Bezold's p.,** perforation of the inner surface of the mastoid bone. **mechanical p.,** an artificial opening or hole made by boring, piercing, or cutting through a structure or surface, such as the root of a tooth. **pathologic p.,** an opening or hole produced in a tissue surface or structure by a pathologic process, as may occur in internal resorption of a tooth.

perforator (per′fo-ra″tor) an instrument for piercing the bones, and especially for perforating the fetal head.

perforatorium (per″fo-rah-to′re-um) acrosome.

perfrication (per″fri-ka′shun) [L. *perfricare* to rub] rubbing with an ointment or embrocation.

perfrigeration (per-frij″er-a′shun) [*per-* + L. *frigere* to be cold] frostbite.

perfusate (per-fu′zāt) a liquid that has been passed over or through the vessels of an organ or tissue.

perfuse (per-fūz′) to pour over or through.

perfusion (per-fu′zhun) 1. the act of pouring over or through, especially the passage of a fluid through the vessels of a specific organ. 2. a liquid poured over or through an organ or tissue.

pergolide mesylate (per′go-lid mes′ĭ-lāt) a long-acting ergot derivative with dopaminergic properties.

perhexiline maleate (per-heks′ĭ-lēn) chemical name: 2-(2,2-dicylohexylethyl)piperidine (Z)-2-butenedioate. A coronary vasodilator, $C_{19}H_{35}N \cdot C_4H_4O_4$; used in the prophylaxis of angina of effort and has been used to control certain cardiac arrhythmias.

peri- [Gr. *peri* around] a prefix meaning around.

periacinal (per″e-as′ĭ-nal) [*peri-* + L. *acinus* berry] situated around an acinus.

periacinous (per″e-as′ĭ-nus) around an acinus.

Periactin (per″e-ak′tin) trademark for preparations of cyproheptadine hydrochloride.

periadenitis (per″e-ad″ĕ-ni′tis) [*peri-* + Gr. *adēn* gland + *-itis*] inflammation of the tissues around a gland. **p. muco′sa necrot′ica recur′rens,** a recurrent disease of the mucous membranes of unknown etiology, generally considered to be a severe form of recurrent aphthous stomatitis, which is marked by development of deep crateriform ulcers with inflamed borders that leave scars after healing. The mucosa of the lips, cheeks, tongue, palate, and anterior tonsillar pillars are most commonly involved, but the pharynx, larynx, and genitalia may also be affected. Called also *Mikulicz's aphthae, recurring scarring aphthae,* and *Sutton's disease.*

periadventitial (per″e-ad″ven-tish′al) outside the adventitia.

perialienitis (per″e-āl″yen-i′tis) [*peri-* + L. *alienus* foreign + *-itis*] inflammation around a foreign body, as a biliary concretion.

periampullary (per″e-am′pu-lar″e) situated around an ampulla, as around the hepatopancreatic ampulla.

perianal (per″e-a′nal) [*peri-* + L. *anus* anus] located around the anus.

periangiitis (per″e-an″je-i′tis) [*peri-* + Gr. *angeion* vessel + *-itis*] inflammation of the tissue surrounding a blood or lymph vessel.

periangiocholitis (per″e-an″je-o-ko-li′tis) pericholangitis.

periangioma (per″e-an-je-o′mah) [*peri-* + Gr. *angeion* vessel + *-oma*] a tumor which surrounds a blood vessel.

perianth (per′e-anth) [*peri-* + Gr. *anthos* flower] the floral envelope, including the calyx and corolla.

periaortic (per″e-a-or′tik) around the aorta.

periaortitis (per″e-a″or-ti′tis) inflammation of the tissues around the aorta.

periapex (per″e-a′peks) the tissue which surrounds the root apex of a tooth (the periodontal ligament and alveolar bone).

periapical (per″e-ap′ĭ-kal) [*peri-* + L. *apex* tip] situated at or surrounding the apex of a tooth.

periappendicitis (per″e-ah-pen″dĭ-si′tis) [*peri-* + *appendix* + *-itis*] inflammation of the tissues around the vermiform appendix. **p. decidua′lis,** a condition in tubal pregnancy in which, on account of adhesions between the appendix and the fallopian tube, decidual cells are present in the peritoneum of the appendix.

periappendicular (per″e-ap″en-dik′u-lar) around the vermiform appendix.

periapt (per′e-apt) [Gr. *periapton* amulet] a substance worn in the belief that it wards off disease.

periaqueductal (per″e-ak″wĭ-duk′tal) around an aqueduct.

periarterial (per″e-ar-te′re-al) around an artery.

periarteritis (per″e-ar″tĕ-ri′tis) [*peri-* + Gr. *artēria* artery + *-itis*] inflammation of the external coats of an artery and of the tissues around the artery. **p. gummo′sa,** accumulation of gummas on the blood vessels in syphilis. **p. nodo′sa,** 1. classically, a form of systemic necrotizing vasculitis involving the small and medium-sized arteries with signs and symptoms resulting from infarction and scarring of the affected organ system. Called also *arteritis nodosa, Kussmaul's* or *Kussmaul-Maier disease,* and *polyarteritis nodosa.* 2. a group comprising classic periarteritis nodosa, allergic granulomatous angiitis, and many systemic necrotizing vasculitides with clinicopathologic characteristics overlapping the two former disorders. **syphilitic p.,** periarteritis gummosa.

periarthric (per″e-ar′thrik) [*peri-* + Gr. *arthron* joint] around a joint.

periarthritis (per″e-ar-thri′tis) inflammation of the tissues around a joint. **p. of shoulder,** adhesive capsulitis.

periarticular (per″e-ar-tik′u-lar) [*peri-* + L. *articulus* joint] situated around a joint.

periatrial (per″e-a′tre-al) around the atrium of the heart.

periauricular (per″e-aw-rik′u-lar) 1. around the concha of the ear. 2. periatrial.

periaxial (per″e-ak′se-al) [*peri-* + Gr. *axōn* axis] situated around an axis.

periaxillary (per″e-ak′sĭ-ler″e) situated or occurring around the axilla.

periaxonal (per″e-ak′so-nal) [peri- + axon] occurring around an axon.

periblast (per′ĭ-blast) [peri- + Gr. blastos germ] the portion of the blastoderm of telolecithal eggs the cells of which lack complete cell membranes.

peribronchial (per″ĭ-brong′ke-al) situated around a bronchus.

peribronchiolar (per″ĭ-brong-ki′o-lar) situated around the bronchioles.

peribronchiolitis (per″ĭ brong″ke o li′tis) inflammation of the tissues around the bronchioles.

peribronchitis (per″ĭ-brong-ki′tis) a form of bronchitis consisting of inflammation and thickening of the peribronchial tissue.

peribulbar (per″ĭ-bul′bar) surrounding the bulb of the eye.

peribursal (per″ĭ-ber′sal) surrounding a bursa.

pericaliceal (per″ĭ-kal″ĭ-se′al) situated near to or around a renal calix.

pericallosal (per″i-kah-lo′sal) situated around the corpus callosum.

pericalyceal (per″ĭ-kal″ĭ-se′al) pericaliceal.

pericanalicular (per″ĭ-kan″ah-lik′u-lar) occurring around canaliculi.

pericapsular (per″ĭ-kap′su-lar) surrounding a capsule.

pericardectomy (per″ĭ-kar-dek′to-me) pericardiectomy.

pericardiac (per″ĭ-kar′de-ak) pericardial.

pericardial (per″ĭ-kar′de-al) pertaining to the pericardium.

pericardicentesis (per″ĭ-kar″de-sen-te′sis) pericardiocentesis.

pericardiectomy (per″ĭ-kar″de-ek′to-me) [pericardium + Gr. ektomē excision] excision of the pericardium.

pericardiocentesis (per″ĭ-kar″de-o-sen-te′sis) [pericardium + Gr. kentēsis puncture] surgical puncture of the pericardial cavity for the aspiration of fluid.

pericardiolysis (per″ĭ-kar″de-ol′ĭ-sis) [pericardium + Gr. lysis dissolution] the operation of freeing adhesions between the visceral and parietal pericardium.

pericardiomediastinitis (per″ĭ-kar″de-o-me″de-as-tĭ-ni′tis) pericarditis with mediastinitis; inflammation of the pericardium and mediastinum.

pericardiophrenic (per″ĭ-kar″de-o-fren′ik) pertaining to the pericardium and the diaphragm.

pericardiopleural (per″ĭ-kar″de-o-plu′ral) pertaining to the pericardium and the pleura.

pericardiorrhaphy (per″ĭ-kar″de-or′ah-fe) [pericardium + Gr. rhaphē suture] the operation of suturing a wound in the pericardium.

pericardiostomy (per″ĭ-kar″de-os′to-me) [pericardium + Gr. stoma mouth] the operation of making an opening into the pericardium, usually for the drainage of effusions.

pericardiotomy (per″ĭ-kar″de-ot′o-me) [pericardium + Gr. temnein to cut] surgical incision of the pericardium.

pericarditic (per″ĭ-kar-dit′ik) pertaining to pericarditis.

pericarditis (per″ĭ-kar-di′tis) [pericardium + -itis] inflammation of the pericardium. **acute benign p.,** idiopathic p. **acute fibrinous p.,** inflammation of the pericardium marked by fibrinous exudate on the serous membrane. **adhesive p.,** a condition resulting from the presence of dense fibrous tissue between the parietal and visceral layers of the pericardium. There may be complete obliteration of the pericardial cavity, or there may be adhesions extending from the pericardium to the mediastinum (mediastinopericarditis), diaphragm, and chest wall (accretio cordis, accretio pericardii). **amebic p.,** pericarditis occurring as a result of rupture of an amebic abscess of the liver through the diaphragm. **bacterial p.,** pericarditis produced by bacterial infection. **p. calculo′sa,** pericarditis with a calcareous deposit in the pericardium. **carcinomatous p.,** that which is associated with malignant disease of the pericardium. **constrictive p.,** inflammation of the pericardium leading to thickening and sometimes to calcification with impaired diastolic filling, inflow stasis, or constrictive effect. **dry p.,** pericarditis not associated with effusion. **p. with ef-**

fusion, pericarditis associated with the collection of a serous or purulent exudate in the pericardial cavity. **p. epistenocardi′aca,** the symptom complex of stenocardia, fever, pericarditis, and myocardial insufficiency (Sternberg). **p. exter′na et inter′na,** inflammation of the outer and inner surfaces of the pericardium. **external p.,** that which chiefly affects the outer surface of the pericardium. **fibrinous p., fibrous p.,** chronic pericarditis characterized by the formation of fibrous tissue and probably adhesions. **hemorrhagic p.,** that in which there is a bloody exudate. **idiopathic p.,** an acute serofibrinous pericarditis of unknown cause; recurrent attacks are not unusual. Called also acute benign p. **localized p.,** a term usually denoting chronic pericarditis with thickened white or milky epicardial areas. **mediastinal p.,** inflammation of the exterior surface of the pericardium and the mediastinal tissue. **p. oblit′erans, obliterating p.,** an adhesive pericarditis which leads to the obliteration of the pericardial cavity. **purulent p.,** a form characterized by pus formation. **rheumatic p.,** the form associated with active rheumatic heart disease. **serofibrinous p.,** a variety associated with a serous fluid effusion with deposition of fibrin on the pericardial surfaces. **p. sic′ca,** acute fibrinous pericarditis without effusion. **suppurative p.,** purulent p. **tuberculous p.,** a variety caused by tuberculous disease. **uremic p.,** pericarditis occurring as a complication of uremia. **p. villo′sa,** cor villosum.

pericardium (per″ĭ-kar′de-um) [L.; peri- + Gr. kardia heart] 1. [NA] the fibroserous sac that surrounds the heart and the roots of the great vessels, comprising an external layer of fibrous tissue (pericardium fibrosum [NA]) and an inner serous layer (pericardium serosum [NA]). The base of the pericardium is attached to the central tendon of the diaphragm. 2. pericardial sinus. **adherent p.,** a pericardium that is abnormally connected with the heart by dense fibrous tissue, as in adhesive pericarditis. **bread-and-butter p.,** a pericardium having a thick fibrinous deposit on its surfaces. **calcified p.,** a pericardium containing deposits of lime salts. **cardiac p.,** visceral p. **p. fibro′sum [NA], fibrous p.,** the external layer of the pericardium, consisting of fibrous tissue. **parietal p.,** the parietal layer (lamina parietalis) of the serous pericardium, which is in contact with the fibrous pericardium. **p. sero′sum [NA], serous p.,** the inner serous portion of the pericardium consisting of two layers, the lamina parietalis, apposed to the fibrous pericardium, and another layer, the lamina visceralis, or epicardium, which is reflected onto the roots of the great vessels and the heart. The space between the two layers is the cavitas pericardialis. **shaggy p.,** a pericardium coated with a roughened layer of fibrinous exudate. **visceral p.,** the inner layer (lamina visceralis pericardii) of the serous pericardium, which is in contact with the heart and roots of the great vessels; called also epicardium.

pericardotomy (per″ĭ-kar-dot′o-me) pericardiotomy.

pericarp (per′ĭ-karp) [peri- + Gr. karpos fruit] the seed vessel or ripened ovary of a flower.

pericaryon (per″ĭ-kar′e-on) perikaryon.

pericecal (per″ĭ-se′kal) surrounding the cecum.

pericecitis (per″ĭ-sĕ-si′tis) inflammation of the tissues around the cecum.

pericellular (per″ĭ-sel′u-lar) [peri- + L. cellula cell] surrounding a cell.

pericemental (per″ĭ-se-men′tal) pertaining to the pericementum (periodontal ligament).

pericementitis (per″ĭ-se″men-ti′tis) inflammation of the pericementum (periodontal ligament). See periodontitis. **apical p.,** apical abscess. **chronic suppurative p.,** marginal periodontitis.

pericementum (per″ĭ-se-men′tum) [peri- + L. caementum cement] the periodontal ligament.

pericentral (per″ĭ-sen′tral) surrounding a center.

pericentriolar (per″e-sen″tre-o′lar) situated around a centriole.

pericephalic (per″ĭ-sĕ-fal′ik) surrounding the head.

pericholangitis (per″ĭ-ko″lan-ji′tis) [peri- + Gr. cholē bile + angeion vessel + -itis] inflammation of the tissues that surround the bile ducts.

pericholecystitis (per″ĭ-ko″le-sis-ti′tis) inflammation of the tissues around the gallbladder. **gaseous p.,** emphysematous cholecystitis.

perichondrial (per″ĭ-kon′dre-al)   pertaining to or composed of perichondrium.

perichondritis (per″ĭ-kon-dri′tis)   inflammation of the perichondrium.

perichondrium (per″ĭ-kon′dre-um) [*peri-* + Gr. *chondros* cartilage] [NA]   the layer of dense fibrous connective tissue which invests all cartilage except the articular cartilage of synovial joints.

perichondroma (per″ĭ-kon-dro′mah)   a tumor arising from the perichondrium.

perichord (per′ĭ-kord)   the investing sheath of the notochord.

perichordal (per″ĭ-kor′dal) [*peri-* + Gr. *chordē* cord]   situated around the notochord.

perichorioidal (per″ĭ-ko″re-oi′dal)   perichoroidal.

perichoroidal (per″ĭ-ko-roi′dal)   surrounding the choroid coat.

perichrome (per′ĭ-krōm) [*peri-* + Gr. *chrōma* color]   a nerve cell in which the Nissl bodies are arranged in rows beneath the cell membrane. Cf. *arkyochrome, gyrochrome,* and *stichochrome.*

Periclor (pār′ĭ-klōr)   trademark for a preparation of petrichloral.

pericolic (per″ĭ-ko′lik)   around the colon, as pericolic membrane.

pericolitis (per″ĭ-ko-li′tis) [*peri-* + Gr. *kolon* colon + *-itis*]   inflammation around the colon, especially of the peritoneal coat of the colon. **p. dex′tra,** pericolitis affecting the ascending colon. **membranous p.,** a morbid condition resulting from the presence of Jackson's membrane (q.v.). **p. sinis′tra,** inflammation of the surrounding connective tissue and peritoneum of the descending colon.

pericolonitis (per″ĭ-ko″lon-i′tis)   pericolitis.

pericolpitis (per″ĭ-kol-pi′tis) [*peri-* + Gr. *kolpos* vagina + *-itis*]   inflammation of the tissues around the vagina.

periconchal (per″ĭ-kong′kal) [*peri-* + Gr. *konchē* a shell-like cavity]   situated around the concha.

periconchitis (per″ĭ-kong-ki′tis) [*peri-* + Gr. *konchē* a shell-like cavity + *-itis*]   inflammation of the lining of the orbit.

pericorneal (per″ĭ-kor′ne-al)   surrounding the cornea.

pericoronal (per″ĭ-kor′o-nal)   around the crown of a tooth.

pericoronitis (per″ĭ-kor″o-ni′tis) [*peri-* + L. *corona* crown + *-itis*]   inflammation of the gingiva surrounding the crown of a tooth. Called also *operculitis.*

pericoxitis (per″ĭ-kok-si′tis)   inflammation of the tissues about the hip joint.

pericranial (per″ĭ-kra′ne-al)   pertaining to the pericranium.

pericranitis (per″ĭ-kra-ni′tis)   inflammation of the external periosteum of the skull.

pericranium (per″ĭ-kra′ne-um) [*peri-* + Gr. *kranion* cranium] [NA]   the external periosteum of the skull.

pericycle (per″ĭ-si′k'l) [*peri-* + Gr. *kyklos* circle]   a layer of parenchymal cells capable of being transformed into meristem to give rise to the root cambium and cork cambium and to branch roots.

pericystic (per″ĭ-sis′tik)   situated about a cyst.

pericystitis (per″ĭ-sis-ti′tis) [*peri-* + Gr. *kystis* bladder + *-itis*]   inflammation of the tissues around the bladder.

pericystium (per″ĭ-sis′te-um)   the vascular envelope of certain cysts.

pericyte (per′ĭ-sit) [*peri-* + Gr. *kytos* hollow vessel]   one of the peculiar elongated cells with the power of contraction, found wrapped about precapillary arterioles outside the basement membrane; called also *pericyte of Zimmermann* and *Rouget cell.*

pericytial (per″ĭ-si′shal)   situated around a cell.

pericytoma (per″ĭ-si-to′mah)   hemangiopericytoma.

peridectomy (per″ĭ-dek′to-me)   peritectomy.

perideferentitis (per″ĭ-def″er-en-ti′tis)   inflammation of the tissues surrounding the ductus deferens.

peridendritic (per″ĭ-den-drit′ik)   surrounding the dendrites.

peridens (per″ĭ-dens)   a supernumerary tooth appearing elsewhere than in the midline of the dental arch.

peridental (per″ĭ-den′tal)   periodontal, def. 1.

peridentium (per″ĭ-den′she-um)   periodontium, def. 1.

periderm (per′ĭ-derm) [*peri-* + Gr. *derma* skin]   1. the large-celled outer layer of the bilaminar fetal epidermis. In the human it is loosened by the hair which grows beneath it, and generally disappears before birth. Called also *epitrichium.*   2. the cuticle (eponychium and hyponychium), the only part of the periderm which persists after birth.

peridermal (per″ĭ-der′mal)   pertaining to the periderm.

peridesmic (per″ĭ-dez′mik)   around a ligament; pertaining to the peridesmium.

peridesmitis (per″ĭ-dez-mi′tis)   inflammation of the peridesmium.

peridesmium (per″ĭ-dez′me-um) [*peri-* + Gr. *desmion* band]   the areolar membrane which covers the ligaments.

peridia (pĕ-rid′e-ah)   plural of *peridium.*

perididymis (per″ĭ-did′ĭ-mis) [*peri-* + Gr. *didymos* testicle]   the tunica vaginalis testis.

perididymitis (per″ĭ-did″ĭ-mi′tis)   inflammation of the perididymis; called also *vaginitis testis.*

peridium (pĕ-rid′e-um), pl. *perid′ia* [Gr. *pēridion* small leather bag or wallet]   the outer coat or limiting membrane enveloping the fruiting body of certain fungi and protozoa.

peridiverticulitis (per″ĭ-di″ver-tik″u-li′tis)   inflammation of structures around a diverticulum of the intestine.

periductal (per″ĭ-duk′tal)   surrounding a duct, particularly a duct of the mammary gland.

periductile (per″ĭ-duk′tīl)   periductal.

periduodenitis (per″ĭ-du″o-dĕ-ni′tis)   inflammation around the duodenum, a condition marked by a deformed duodenum surrounded and fixed by peritoneal adhesions.

peridural (per″ĭ-du′ral)   around or external to the dura mater.

peridurogram (per″ĭ-du′ro-gram)   the film obtained in peridurography.

peridurography (per″ĭ-du-rog′rah-fe) [*peri-* + *dura* + Gr. *graphein* to write]   roentgenography of the spinal canal and interspaces after injection of a contrast medium in the peridural space.

periencephalitis (per″ĭ-en-sef″ah-li′tis) [*peri-* + Gr. *enkephalos* brain + *-itis*]   inflammation of the surface of the brain; meningitis with cortical encephalitis.

periencephalography (per″e-en-sef″ah-log′rah-fe)   roentgenography of the cerebral meninges.

perienteric (per″e-en-ter′ik)   situated around the intestine.

perienteritis (per″e-en″ter-i′tis) [*peri-* + Gr. *enteron* intestine + *-itis*]   inflammation of the peritoneal coat of the intestine; visceral peritonitis.

perienteron (per″e-en′ter-on) [*peri-* + Gr. *enteron* intestine]   the primitive perivisceral cavity of the embryo.

periependymal (per″e-ep-en′dĭ-mal)   situated around the ependyma.

periepithelioma (per″e-ep″ĭ-the-le-o′mah)   adrenal cortical carcinoma.

periesophageal (per″e-ĕ-sof′ah-je-al)   situated around the esophagus.

periesophagitis (per″e-ĕ-sof″ah-ji′tis)   inflammation of the tissues around the esophagus.

perifascicular (per″e-fah-sik′u-lar)   surrounding a fasciculus of nerve or muscle fibers.

perifistular (per″ĭ-fis′tu-lar)   around a fistula.

perifocal (per″ĭ-fo′kal)   around or surrounding a focus, such as a focus of infection.

perifollicular (per″ĭ-fŏ-lik′u-lar)   surrounding a follicle.

perifolliculitis (per″ĭ-fŏ-lik″u-li′tis)   inflammation around the hair follicles. **p. cap′itis absce′dens et suffo′diens,** a rare chronic suppurative disease of the scalp, usually seen in young adults, especially men, marked by numerous follicular and perifollicular reactions with the formation of nodules that become fluctuant and rupture to produce intercommunicating draining sinuses, which is followed by healing with severe scarring and alopecia. Called also *dissect-*

ing cellulitis of scalp and *folliculitis abscedens et suffodiens.*
superficial pustular p., Bockhart's impetigo.

perigangliitis (per″ĭ-gang″gle-i′tis) inflammation of tissues around a ganglion.

periganglionic (per″ĭ-gang″gle-on′ik) situated around a ganglion.

perigastric (per″ĭ-gas′trik) situated around the stomach; pertaining to the peritoneal coat of the stomach.

perigastritis (per″ĭ-gas-tri′tis) [*peri-* + Gr. *gastēr* stomach + *-itis*] inflammation of the peritoneal coat of the stomach.

perigemmal (per″ĭ-jem′al) surrounding a taste bud or other bud.

periglandular (per″ĭ-glan′du-lar) surrounding a gland or glands.

periglandulitis (per″ĭ-glan″du-li′tis) inflammation of the tissues about a glandule or glandules.

periglial (per″ĭ-gli′al) surrounding the glial cells of the brain.

periglossitis (per″ĭ-glŏ-si′tis) inflammation of the tissues around the tongue.

periglottic (per″ĭ-glot′ik) situated around the tongue.

periglottis (per″ĭ-glot′is) [*peri-* + Gr. *glōtta* tongue] the mucous membrane of the tongue.

perihepatic (per″ĭ-he-pat′ik) [*peri-* + Gr. *hēpar* liver] situated or occurring around the liver.

perihepatitis (per″ĭ-hep″ah-ti′tis) [*peri-* + Gr. *hēpar* liver + *-itis*] inflammation of the peritoneal capsule of the liver and of the tissues around the liver. **p. chron′ica hyperplas′tica,** a disease in which the peritoneal covering of the liver becomes converted into a white mass resembling the icing of a cake; called also *frosted liver, icing liver, sugar-icing liver,* and *zuckergussleber.* **gonococcal p.,** perihepatitis due to extension of gonorrheal infection; see *Fitz-Hugh–Curtis syndrome,* under *syndrome.*

perihernial (per″ĭ-her′ne-al) situated or occurring around a hernia.

perihilar (per″e-hi′lar) around a hilus, e.g., around the pulmonary hilus.

peri-insular (per″e-in′su-lar) surrounding an island, particularly the insula.

peri-islet (per″e-i′let) situated around the islets of Langerhans.

perijejunitis (per″ĭ-je″ju-ni′tis) inflammation around the jejunum.

perikarya (per″ĭ-kar′ĕ-ah) plural of perikaryon.

perikaryon (per″ĭ-kar′e-on), pl. *perikar′ya* [*peri-* + Gr. *karyon* nucleus] the cell body as distinguished from the nucleus and the processes; applied particularly to neurons.

perikeratic (per″ĭ-ker-at′ik) surrounding the cornea.

perikyma (per″ĭ-ki′mah) singular of *perikymata.*

perikymata (per″ĭ-ki′mah-tah), sing. *periky′ma* [*peri-* + Gr. *kyma* wave] the numerous small transverse ridges on the surface of the enamel of permanent teeth, representing overlapping prism groups; continued abrasion erodes the enamel surface, obliterating the perikymata.

perilabyrinth (per″ĭ-lab′ĭ-rinth) the tissue surrounding the labyrinth of the ear.

perilabyrinthitis (per″ĭ-lab″ĭ-rin-thi′tis) inflammation of the tissues around the labyrinth of the ear. It may lead to circumscribed labyrinthitis.

perilaryngeal (per″ĭ-lah-rin′je-al) situated around the larynx.

perilaryngitis (per″ĭ-lar″in-ji′tis) [*peri-* + Gr. *larynx* larynx + *-itis*] inflammation of the tissues around the larynx.

perilemma (per″ĭ-lem′ah) [*peri-* + Gr. *lemma* rind, husk] a living membrane external to the pellicle in certain ciliate protozoa, particularly those of the order Oligotrichida.

perilenticular (per″ĭ-len-tik′u-lar) surrounding the lens of the eye.

perilesional (per″ĭ-le′shun-al) located or occurring around a lesion.

periligamentous (per″ĭ-lig″ah-men′tus) situated around a ligament.

perilobar (per″ĭ-lo′bar) surrounding a lobe.

perilobulitis (per″ĭ-lob-u-li′tis) inflammation of the tissues surrounding the lobules of the lung.

perilymph (per′ĭ-limf) [*peri-* + L. *lympha* lymph] the fluid contained within the space separating the membranous from the osseous labyrinth of the ear; it is entirely separate from the endolymph. Called also *perilympha* [NA].

perilympha (per″ĭ-lim′fah) [NA] the perilymph.

perilymphadenitis (per″ĭ-lim″fad-ĕ-ni′tis) inflammation of the tissues around a lymph gland.

perilymphangeal (per″ĭ-lim-fan′je-al) located around a lymphatic vessel.

perilymphangitis (per″ĭ-lim″fan-ji′tis) inflammation of the tissues around a lymphatic vessel.

perilymphatic (per″ĭ-lim-fat′ik) 1. pertaining to the perilymph. 2. around a lymphatic vessel.

perimastitis (per″ĭ-mas-ti′tis) [*peri-* + Gr. *mastos* breast + *-itis*] inflammation of the connective tissue around the mammary gland.

perimedullary (per″ĭ-med′u-ler″e) surrounding a medulla, as the medulla oblongata or the marrow of a bone.

perimeningitis (per″ĭ-men″in-ji′tis) [*peri-* + Gr. *mēninx* membrane + *-itis*] pachymeningitis.

perimeter (pĕ-rim′ĕ-ter) [*peri-* + *-meter*] 1. a line forming the boundary of a plane figure. 2. an apparatus for determining the extent of the peripheral visual field on a curved surface. **dental p.,** an instrument for measuring the circumference of a tooth.

perimetric (per″ĭ-met′rik) 1. pertaining to a perimeter. 2. around the uterus. 3. pertaining to the perimetrium.

perimetritic (per″ĭ-me-trit′ik) pertaining to or characterized by perimetritis.

perimetritis (per″ĭ-mĕ-tri′tis) [*peri-* + Gr. *mētra* uterus + *-itis*] inflammation of the perimetrium.

perimetrium (per-ĭ-me′tre-um) [*peri-* + Gr. *mētra* uterus] the serous coat of the uterus; NA alternative for *tunica serosa uteri.*

perimetrosalpingitis (per″ĭ-met″ro-sal″pin-ji′tis) inflammation of the uterus and uterine tubes and of surrounding tissues. **encapsulating p.,** perimetrosalpingitis with formation of a membrane about the organs involved.

perimetry (pĕ-rim′ĕ-tre) [*peri-* + *-metry*] determination of the extent of the peripheral visual field by use of a perimeter; cf. perioptometry.

perimolysis (per″ĭ-mol′ĭ-sis) [shortened from *perimylolysis,* q.v.] erosion of the lingual surfaces of the anterior teeth and the occlusal surfaces of the posterior teeth by acid decalcification; commonly seen in anorexia nervosa and also in other conditions involving chronic regurgitation.

perimyelis (per″ĭ-mi′ĕ-lis) [*peri-* + Gr. *myelos* marrow] endosteum.

perimyelitis (per″ĭ-mi″ĕ-li′tis) 1. inflammation of the perimyelis (endosteum). 2. spinal meningitis.

perimyelography (per″ĭ-mi″ĕ-log′rah-fe) [*peri-* + Gr. *myelos* marrow + *graphein* to record] roentgen-ray examination after injecting iodized oil or other contrast fluid into the subarachnoid space of the spinal cord.

perimylolysis (per″ĭ-mĭ-lol′ĭ-sis) [*peri-* + Gr. *mylos* molar + *lysis*] perimolysis.

perimyocarditis (per″ĭ-mi″o-kar-di′tis) [*peri* + *myocarditis*] combined pericarditis and myocarditis.

perimyoendocarditis (per″ĭ-mi″o-en″do-kar-di′tis) pericarditis associated with myocarditis and endocarditis.

perimyositis (per″ĭ-mi″o-si′tis) inflammation of the connective tissue around muscles.

perimysia (per″ĭ-mis′e-ah) plural of perimysium.

perimysial (per″ĭ-mis′e-al) pertaining to the perimysium.

perimysiitis (per″ĭ-mis″e-i′tis) inflammation of the perimysium; myofibrositis.

perimysitis (per″ĭ-mis-i′tis) perimysiitis.

perimysium (per″ĭ-mis′e-um), pl. *perimys′ia* [*peri-* + Gr. *mys* muscle] [NA] the connective tissue demarcating a fascicle of skeletal muscle fibers; called also *internal p.,* or *p. internum.* **p. exter′num,** epimysium. **internal p., p. inter′num,** perimysium.

perinatal (per″ĭ-na′tal) [*peri-* + L. *natus* born] pertaining to or occurring in the period shortly before and after birth; variously defined as beginning with completion of the twentieth to twenty-eighth week of gestation and ending 7 to 28 days after birth.

perinatologist (per″ĭ-na-tol′o-jist) a specialist in perinatology.

perinatology (per″ĭ-na-tol′o-je) [*perinatal* + *-logy*] the branch of medicine (obstetrics and pediatrics) dealing with the fetus and infant during the perinatal period.

perineal (per″ĭ-ne′al) pertaining to the perineum.

perineocele (per″ĭ-ne′o-sēl) [*perineum* + Gr. *kēlē* hernia] a hernia lying between the rectum and the prostate, or between the rectum and vagina; ischiorectal hernia.

perineometer (per″ĭ-ne-om′ĕ-ter) an instrument for measuring the strength of contractions of the perivaginal muscles.

perineoplasty (per″ĭ-ne′o-plas″te) [*perineum* + Gr. *plassein* to shape] plastic surgery of the perineum.

perineorrhaphy (per″ĭ-ne-or′ah-fe) [*perineum* + Gr. *rhaphē* suture] suture of the perineum, performed for the repair of a laceration.

perineoscrotal (per″ĭ-ne-o-skro′tal) pertaining to the perineum and scrotum.

perineotomy (per″ĭ-ne-ot′o-me) [*perineum* + Gr. *temnein* to cut] surgical incision through the perineum.

perineovaginal (per″ĭ-ne″o-vaj′ĭ-nal) pertaining to or communicating with the perineum and vagina, as a perineovaginal fistula.

perineovaginorectal (per″ĭ-ne″o-vaj″ĭ-no-rek′tal) pertaining to the perineum, vagina, and rectum.

perineovulvar (per″ĭ-ne″o-vul′var) pertaining to the perineum and the vulva.

perinephrial (per″ĭ-nef′re-al) pertaining to the perinephrium.

perinephric (per″ĭ-nef′rik) around the kidney.

perinephritic (per″ĭ-nĕ-frit′ik) pertaining to or characterized by perinephritis.

perinephritis (per″ĭ-nĕ-fri′tis) [*peri-* + Gr. *nephros* kidney + *-itis*] inflammation of the perinephrium; it is marked by fever, local pain, and tenderness on pressure.

perinephrium (per″ĭ-nef′re-um) [*peri-* + Gr. *nephros* kidney] the peritoneal envelope and other tissues around the kidney.

perineum (per″i-ne′um) [Gr. *perineos* the space between the anus and scrotum] 1. [NA] the pelvic floor and the associated structures occupying the pelvic outlet; it is bounded anteriorly by the pubic symphysis, laterally by the ischial tuberosities, and posteriorly by the coccyx. 2. the region between the thighs, bounded in the male by the scrotum and anus and in the female by the vulva and anus.

perineural (per″ĭ-nu′ral) surrounding a nerve or nerves.

perineurial (per″ĭ-nu′re-al) pertaining to the perineurium.

perineuritic (per″ĭ-nu-rit′ik) pertaining to or suffering from perineuritis.

perineuritis (per″ĭ-nu-ri′tis) inflammation of the perineurium.

perineurium (per″ĭ-nu′re-um) [*peri-* + Gr. *neuron* nerve] [NA] the connective tissue sheath surrounding each bundle of fibers (fasciculus) in a peripheral nerve.

perinuclear (per″ĭ-nu′kle-ar) situated or occurring around a nucleus.

periocular (per″e-ok′u-lar) situated or occurring around the eye.

period (pe′re-od) [Gr. *periodos* a going around, circuit, period] an interval or division of time; the time for the regular recurrence of a phenomenon. **absolute refractory p.,** the portion of the refractory period when a nerve or muscle fiber cannot respond to a stimulus, as contrasted with the relative refractory period. **child-bearing p.,** the duration of the reproductive ability in the human female, roughly from puberty to menopause. **ejection p.,** sphygmic p. **G₁ p.,** the period in the mitotic cycle from the end of the previous division to the start of DNA synthesis (S period). **G₂ p.,** the period of the mitotic cycle from the end of DNA synthesis (S period) to the beginning of mitosis. **gestational p.,** the duration of pregnancy, which in the human female averages about 266 days. **half-life p.,** see *half-life.* **incubation p.,** 1. the interval of time required for development. 2. the interval of time between the receipt of infection and the onset of the consequent illness or the first symptoms of the illness (*prodromal stage*); called also *latent p.* 3. the interval of time between the entrance into a vec-

tor of an infectious agent and the time at which the vector is capable of transmitting the infection. See also *generation time* (def. 1), under *time.* **isoelectric p.,** the moment in muscular contraction when the electrodes are so related to the contraction wave that no deflection of the galvanometer is produced. **p. of isometric contraction,** presphygmic p. **p. of isometric relaxation,** postsphygmic p. **isovolumic p.,** presphygmic p. **lag p.,** the time which elapses between the introduction of a microorganism into a nutrient medium and the initiation of exponential growth. **latency p.,** 1. see *latent p.* 2. see under *stage.* **latent p.,** a seemingly inactive period, as that between exposure of tissue to an injurious agent and the manifestation of response, or that between the instant of stimulation and the beginning of response. **M p.,** the period of active mitosis. **menstrual p., monthly p.,** the time of menstruation. **postsphygmic p.,** the short interval of ventricular diastole (0.08 second), immediately following the sphygmic period and lasting until the opening of the atrioventricular valves, during which the muscle fibers are relaxing and no blood is entering the ventricles; called also *period of isometric relaxation.* **prefunctional p.,** the time span during morphological and histological development before physiological activity begins. **presphygmic p.,** the first phase of ventricular systole, being the short period (0.04–0.06 second) immediately following closure of the atrioventricular valves and lasting until opening of the semilunar valves, during which the muscle fibers are contracting against the incompressible mass of fluid filling the ventricles; called also *period of isometric contraction* and *isovolumic p.* **prodromal p.,** see under *stage.* **quarantine p.,** the length of time, usually the maximal incubation period of the disease, which must elapse before a person exposed to contagion is regarded as incapable of transmitting or acquiring the disease. See also *quarantine.* **reaction p.,** 1. the stage of rallying from shock after trauma. 2. reaction time, the time that elapses between stimulation and the consequent reaction. **refractory p.,** the period of depolarization of the cell membrane after excitation, during which the nerve or muscle fiber cannot respond to a second stimulus. **relative refractory p.,** the brief period following the absolute refractory period, during which there is repolarization of the cell membrane to the extent that the fiber can respond to a strong stimulus, although the normal resting potential has not been reached. **S p.,** the period of DNA synthesis in the mitotic cycle. **safe p.,** the period during the menstrual cycle when conception is considered least likely to occur; it is approximately the ten days after menstruation begins, and the ten days preceding menstruation. **silent p.,** an interval in the course of a disease in which the symptoms become very mild or disappear for a time. **sphygmic p.,** the second phase of ventricular systole, being the period (0.21–0.30 second) intervening between the opening and closing of the semilunar valves, during which the blood is being discharged into the aortic and the pulmonary arteries; called also *ejection period.* **Wenckebach p.,** a form of partial heart block characterized by progressive lengthening of the P-R interval until ventricular response occurs; such a sequence is usually repetitive.

periodate (per-i′o-dāt) a salt of periodic acid.

periodic (pe″re-od′ik) [Gr. *periodikos*] recurring at regular intervals of time.

periodic acid (per″i-o′dik) a strong mineral acid and oxidizing agent, HIO₄.

periodicity (pe″re-o-dis′ĭ-te) recurrence at regular intervals of time. **filarial p.,** the periodic increase of microfilariae in the peripheral blood: nocturnal periodicity occurs in *Wuchereria bancrofti* infection in most endemic areas and in *Brugia malayi* infection; diurnal periodicity occurs in *Loa loa* infection. **lunar p.,** recurrence synchronized with phases of the moon, as the reproductive phenomena in some lower animals. **malarial p.,** the more or less regular recurrence of paroxysms at intervals of one, two, or three days in malaria; see under *malaria.*

periodontal (per″e-o-don′tal) [*peri-* + Gr. *odous* tooth] 1. pertaining to or occurring around a tooth; peridental. 2. pertaining to the periodontal ligament or periodontium.

periodontia (per″e-o-don′she-ah) 1. plural of *periodontium.* 2. periodontics.

periodontics (per″e-o-don′tiks) [*peri-* + Gr. *odous* tooth] that branch of dentistry dealing with the study and treatment of diseases of the periodontium.

periodontist (per″e-o-don′tist) a dentist who specializes in periodontics.

periodontitis (per″e-o-don-ti′tis) [*peri-* + *odont-* + *-itis*] inflammatory reaction of the tissues surrounding a tooth (periodontium), usually resulting from the extension of gingival inflammation (gingivitis) into the periodontium. Periodontitis has been classified in five clinical types: *prepubertal, juvenile, rapidly progressive, adult,* and *necrotizing ulcerative gingivoperiodontitis.* Called also *alveolodental osteoperiostitis, cementoperiostitis,* and *paradentitis.* **adult p.,** the most common form of periodontitis, usually occurring after the age of 35, and usually manifested by slow progression of tissue destruction, which may ultimately result in loss of the teeth. **apical p.,** inflammatory reaction of the tissues surrounding the root of a tooth. **chronic apical p.,** see *apical* [*granuloma,* under *granuloma.* **juvenile p.,** a rare form of periodontitis that has an onset at puberty, is more common in females, and is manifested by deep periodontal pockets, usually involving the first molars and incisors. It may be associated with rapidly progressive periodontitis in later life. Called also *paradentosis* and *periodontosis.* **marginal p.,** a chronic destructive inflammatory periodontal disease that begins as a simple marginal gingivitis and may migrate along the tooth toward the apex, producing periodontal pockets, usually with pus formation, and destruction of the periodontal and alveolar structures, causing the teeth to become loose. Called also *simple p., chronic suppurative pericementitis, Fauchard's disease, pyorrhea, pyorrhea alveolaris, Riggs' disease,* and *schmutz pyorrhea.* **prepubertal p.,** a rare form of periodontitis, probably having an onset soon after eruption of the primary teeth. It occurs in a localized form that involves only some teeth, and in a generalized form that causes rapid destruction of alveolar bone and may or may not affect the permanent teeth. **rapidly progressive p.,** generalized periodontitis occurring after puberty and before the age of 30 to 35 in those who may or may not have had juvenile periodontitis, characterized by severe and rapid bone destruction, which may progress to abscess formation and tooth loss, or may enter a short or prolonged dormant period. **simple p., p. sim′plex,** marginal p.

periodontium (per″e-o-don′she-um), pl. *periodon′tia* [*peri-* + Gr. *odous* tooth] 1. the tissues that invest or help to invest and support the teeth, including the periodontal ligament, gingivae, cementum, and alveolar and supporting bone. 2. [NA] periodontal ligament. Called also *alveolar periosteum, odontoperiosteum, paradentium,* and *peridontium.* **p. insertio′nis** [NA], free gingiva. **p. protecto′ris** [NA], attached gingiva.

periodontology (per″e-o-don-tol′o-je) [*peri-* + *odont-* + *-logy*] the branch of dentistry that deals with the scientific study of the structures and function of the periodontium in health and disease; broader in scope than *periodontics,* which is limited to the diagnosis, prevention, and treatment of periodontal disease, although the two terms are sometimes used interchangeably.

periodontosis (per″e-o-don-to′sis) juvenile periodontitis.

periomphalic (per″e-om-fal′ik) [*peri-* + Gr. *omphalos* navel] around the umbilicus.

perionychia (per″e-o-nik′e-ah) paronychia.

perionychium (per″e-o-nik′e-um) [*peri-* + Gr. *onyx* nail] the epidermis bordering a nail.

perionyx (per″e-o′niks) [*peri-* + Gr. *onyx* nail] a relic of the eponychium persisting as a band across the root of the nail, seen in the eighth month of fetal life.

perioophoritis (per″e-o-of″o-ri′tis) [*peri-* + Gr. *ōon* egg + *pherein* to bear + *-itis*] inflammation of the tissues around the ovary.

perioophorosalpingitis (per″e-o-of″o-ro-sal″pin-ji′tis) [*peri-* + Gr. *ōon* egg + *pherein* to bear + *salpinx* tube + *-itis*] inflammation of the tissues around the ovary and oviducts.

perioothecitis (per-e-o″o-the-si′tis) perioophoritis.

perioperative (per″e-op′er-ah-tiv) pertaining to the period extending from the time of hospitalization for surgery to the time of discharge.

periophthalmia (per″e-of-thal′me-ah) periophthalmitis.

periophthalmic (per″e-of-thal′mik) situated around the eye.

periophthalmitis (per″e-of″thal-mi′tis) [*peri-* + *ophthalmitis*] inflammation of the tissues around the eye.

periople (per′e-o″p'l) [*peri-* + Gr. *hoplē* hoof] the layer of soft, light-colored horn covering the outer aspect of the hoof in ungulates.

perioptometry (per″e-op-tom′ĕ-tre) [*peri-* + Gr. *optos* visible + *metron* measure] the measurement of the peripheral acuity of vision or of the limits of the visual field; cf. perimetry.

perioral (per″e-o′ral) [*peri-* + L. *os* mouth] situated or occurring around the mouth.

periorbit (per″e-or′bit) periorbita.

periorbita (per″e-or′bi-tah) [*peri-* + L. *orbita* orbit] [NA] the periosteal covering of the bones forming the orbit, or eye socket.

periorbital (per″e-or′bĭ-tal) situated around the orbit, or eye socket.

periorbititis (per″e-or″bĭ-ti′tis) inflammation of the periorbita.

periorchitis (per″e-or-ki′tis) [*peri-* + Gr. *orchis* testis + *-itis*] inflammation of the tunica vaginalis testis. **p. adhaesi′va,** a variety in which the two layers of the tunica vaginalis are more or less adherent. **p. purulen′ta,** periorchitis which goes on to pus formation.

periorchium (per″e-or′ke-um) the parietal layer of the tunica vaginalis.

periost (per′e-ost) periosteum.

periosteal (per″e-os′te-al) pertaining to the periosteum.

periosteitis (per″e-os′te-i′tis) periostitis.

periosteodema (per″e-os″te-o-de′mah) periosteoedema.

periosteoedema (per″e-os″te-o-ĕ-de′mah) edema of the periosteum.

periosteoma (per″e-os-te-o′mah) a morbid bony growth surrounding a bone.

periosteomedullitis (per″e-os″te-o-med″u-li′tis) inflammation of the periosteum and bone marrow.

periosteomyelitis (per″e-os″te-o-mi″ĕ-li′tis) [*peri-* + Gr. *osteon* bone + *myelos* marrow + *-itis*] inflammation of the entire bone, including periosteum and marrow.

periosteophyte (per″e-os′te-o-fīt″) [*periosteum* + Gr. *phyton* growth] a bony outgrowth on the periosteum.

periosteosis (per″e-os″te-o′sis) periostosis.

periosteotome (per″e-os′te-o-tōm) an instrument for cutting the periosteum; also an instrument for separating the periosteum from the bone.

periosteotomy (per″e-os″te-ot′o-me) [*peri-* + Gr. *osteon* bone + *tomē* a cutting] surgical incision or slitting of the periosteum.

periosteous (per″e-os′te-us) pertaining to or of the nature of periosteum.

periosteum (per″e-os′te-um) [*peri-* + Gr. *osteon* bone] [NA] a specialized connective tissue covering all bones of the body, and possessing bone-forming potentialities; in adults, it consists of two layers that are not sharply defined, the external layer being a network of dense connective tissue containing blood vessels, and the deep layer composed of more loosely arranged collagenous bundles with spindle-shaped connective tissue cells and a network of thin elastic fibers. **alveolar p., p. alveola′re,** periodontium, def. 1.

periostitis (per″e-os-ti′tis) inflammation of the periosteum. The condition is generally chronic, and is marked by tenderness and swelling of the bone and an aching pain. Acute periostitis is due to infection, is characterized by diffuse suppuration, severe pain, and constitutional symptoms, and usually results in necrosis. **p. albumino′sa, albuminous p.,** a form accompanied by the exudation of a clear, albuminous liquid into a flattened cavity beneath the periosteum; called also *serous abscess* and *periosteal ganglion.* **diffuse p.,** a noncircumscribed periostitis of the long bones. **hemorrhagic p.,** a form in which blood is extravasated beneath the periosteum. **p. hyperplas′tica,** hypertrophic pulmonary osteoarthropathy. **p. inter′na cra′nii,** inflammation of the endocranium; external pachymeningitis. **precocious p.,** syphilitic osteoperiostitis occurring as an early symptom.

periostoma (per″e-os-to′mah) periosteoma.

periostomedullitis (per″e-os″to-med″u-li′tis) periosteomedullitis.

periostosis (per″e-os-to′sis) the abnormal deposition of periosteal bone; the condition manifested by development of periosteomas. Called also *periosteosis.* **hyperplastic p.,** cortical infantile hyperostosis.

periostosteitis (per″e-os-tos″te-i′tis) osteoperiostitis.

periostotome (per″e-os′to-tōm) periosteotome.

periostotomy (per″e-os-tot′o-me) periosteotomy.

periotic (per″e-o′tik) [*peri-* + Gr. *ous* ear] 1. situated about the ear, especially the internal ear. 2. the petrous and mastoid portions of the temporal bone, at one stage a distinct bone.

periovaritis (per″e-o″vah-ri′tis) perioophoritis.

periovular (per″e-o′vu-lar) surrounding an ovum.

peripachymeningitis (per″ĭ-pak″e-men″in-ji′tis) [*peri-* + Gr. *pachys* thick + *mēninx* membrane + *-itis*] inflammation of the substance between the dura and the bony covering of the central nervous system.

peripancreatic (per″ĭ-pan″kre-at′ik) surrounding the pancreas.

peripancreatitis (per″ĭ-pan″kre-ah-ti′tis) [*peri-* + Gr. *pankreas* pancreas + *-itis*] inflammation of tissues around the pancreas.

peripapillary (per″ĭ-pap′ĭ-ler″e) located around the optic papilla.

peripartum (per″ĭ-par′tum) occurring during the last month of gestation or the first few months after delivery, with reference to the mother.

peripatellar (per″ĭ-pah-tel′ar) around the patella, or knee cap.

peripatetic (per″ĭ-pah-tet′ik) [Gr. *peripatētikos* given to walking about while teaching or disputing] walking about.

peripenial (per″ĭ-pe′ne-al) around the penis.

peripericarditis (per″ĭ-per″ĭ-kar-di′tis) inflammation around the pericardium producing adhesions of the pericardium to the pleura and chest wall.

periphacitis (per″ĭ-fah-si′tis) [*peri-* + *phac-* + *-itis*] inflammation surrounding the capsule of the lens of the eye.

periphakitis (per″ĭ-fah-ki′tis) periphacitis.

peripharyngeal (per″ĭ-fah-rin′je-al) situated around the pharynx.

peripherad (pĕ-rif′er-ad) toward the periphery.

peripheral (pĕ-rif′er-al) pertaining to or situated at or near the periphery; situated away from a center or central structure.

peripheraphose (pĕ-rif′er-ah-fōs) [*periphery* + *aphase*] a subjective sensation of a dark spot in the line of vision, originating in the peripheral ocular mechanism; cf. *peripherophose.*

peripheric (per″ĭ-fer′ik) peripheral.

peripherocentral (pĕ-rif′er-o-sen′tral) both peripheral and central.

peripheroceptor (pĕ-rif′er-o-sep′tor) any of the receptors at the peripheral ends of a sensory peripheral neuron which receive the stimulus.

peripheromittor (pĕ-rif′er-o-mit′or) a terminal mittor placed in connection with the ceptor of a muscle fiber or gland cell which transmits the impulse to the fiber or cell.

peripherophose (pĕ-rif′er-o-fōz) [*periphery* + *phose*] any phose or subjective sensation of light originating in the peripheral ocular mechanism; cf. *peripheraphose.*

periphery (pĕ-rif′er-e) [Gr. *periphereia,* from *peri* around + *pherein* to bear] the outward part or surface or structure; the portion of a system outside the central region.

periphlebitic (per″ĭ-flĕ-bit′ik) pertaining to periphlebitis.

periphlebitis (per″ĭ-flĕ-bi′tis) [*peri-* + Gr. *phleps* vein + *-itis*] inflammation of the tissues around a vein, or of the external coat of a vein. **sclerosing p.,** Mondor's disease.

periphoria (per″ĭ-fo′re-ah) [*peri-* + *-phoria*] cyclophoria.

periphrenitis (per″ĭ-fre-ni′tis) [*peri-* + Gr. *phrēn* diaphragm + *-itis*] inflammation of the diaphragm and structures around it.

Periplaneta (per″ĭ-plah-ne′tah) a genus of roaches. *P. america′na* is the American cockroach; *P. austral′asiae* is the Australian cockroach.

periplasm (per′ĭ-plazm) [*peri-* + Gr. *plasm* something molded] the space between the inner membrane and the wall of a bacterial cell.

periplasmic (per″ĭ-plas′mik) around the plasma membrane; between the plasma membrane and the cell wall of a bacterium.

peripleural (per″ĭ-ploo′ral) surrounding the pleura.

peripleuritis (per″ĭ-ploo-ri′tis) [*peri-* + *pleura* + *-itis*] inflammation of the tissues between the pleura and the chest wall.

periplocin (per″ĭ-plo′sin) a crystallizable glycoside, $C_{36}H_{58}O_{13}$, from a woody vine, *Periploca graeca* L. (Asclepiadaceae); it acts like digitalin as a heart tonic and slower of the pulse.

periplocymarin (per″ĭ-plo-si′mah-rin) a cardiac glycoside, $C_{30}H_{46}O_8$, from the bark and wood of *Periploca graeca* L. (Asclepiadaceae).

periplogenin (per″ĭ-ploj′e-nin) chemical name: $3\beta,5,14$-trihydroxy-5β-card-20(22)-enolide. An aglycone sterol derivative, $C_{23}H_{34}O_5$, from periplocin and periplocymarin.

peripneumonia (per″ĭ-nu-mo′ne-ah) [*peri-* + Gr. *pneumōn* lung + *-ia*] pneumonia; also pleuropneumonia. **p. no′tha,** a variety of acute bronchitis simulating pneumonia.

peripneumonitis (per″ĭ-nu″mo-ni′tis) peripneumonia.

peripolar (per″ĭ-po′lar) situated about a pole or poles.

peripolesis (per″ĭ-po-le′sis) [Gr. *peripolēsis* a going about] the movement of one cell around another; used to refer to the clustering of lymphocytes around macrophages in lymphoid tissue.

periporitis (per″ĭ-por-i′tis) a staphylococcal infection complicating miliaria, with inflammation around the sweat pores, usually affecting infants; called also *periporitis staphylogenes.*

periportal (per″ĭ-por′tal) situated around the portal vein.

periproctic (per″ĭ-prok′tik) [*peri-* + Gr. *prōktos* anus] situated around the anus.

periproctitis (per″ĭ-prok-ti′tis) [*peri-* + Gr. *prōktos* anus + *-itis*] inflammation of the tissues surrounding the rectum and anus.

periprostatic (per″ĭ-pros-tat′ik) situated about the prostate.

periprostatitis (per″ĭ-pros″tah-ti′tis) inflammation of the tissues and structures around the prostate gland.

peripylephlebitis (per″ĭ-pi″le-flĕ-bi′tis) [*peri-* + Gr. *pylē* gate + *phleps* vein + *-itis*] inflammation of the tissue about the portal vein.

peripyloric (per″ĭ-pi-lor′ik) around the pylorus or the pyloric part of the stomach (see *pars pylorica ventriculi*).

periradicular (per″ĭ-rah-dik′u-lar) around or surrounding a root, especially the root of a tooth.

perirectal (per″ĭ-rek′tal) around the rectum.

perirectitis (per″ĭ-rek-ti′tis) periproctitis.

perirenal (per″ĭ-re′nal) [*peri-* + L. *ren* kidney] situated around a kidney.

perirhinal (per″ĭ-ri′nal) [*peri-* + Gr. *rhis* nose] situated about the nose.

perirhizoclasia (per″ĭ-ri″zo-kla′se-ah) [*peri-* + Gr. *rhiza* root + *klasis* destruction] inflammatory destruction of tissues immediately around the root of a tooth, i.e., the pericementum, cementum, and superficial layers of the alveolar process. Cf. *pararhizoclasia.*

perisalpingitis (per″ĭ-sal″pin-ji′tis) [*peri-* + Gr. *salpinx* tube + *-itis*] inflammation of the tissues and peritoneum around a uterine tube.

perisalpingo-ovaritis (per″ĭ-sal-ping″go-o″vah-ri′tis) inflammation involving the ovary and the tissues around the uterine tube.

perisalpinx (per″ĭ-sal′pinks) the peritoneal cover of the upper border of the uterine tube.

perisclerium (per″ĭ-skle′re-um) [*peri-* + Gr. *sklēros* hard] fibrous tissue surrounding ossifying cartilage.

periscopic (per″ĭ-skop′ik) [*peri-* + Gr. *skopein* to examine] affording a wide range of vision; said of microscopical and meniscus lenses.

perisigmoiditis (per″ĭ-sig″moi-di′tis) inflammation of the peritoneal covering of the sigmoid flexure.

perisinuitis (per″ĭ-si″nu-i′tis) perisinusitis.

perisinuous (per″ĭ-sin′u-us) situated around a sinus.

perisinusitis (per″ĭ-si″nŭ-si′tis) inflammation of the tissues around a sinus.

perispermatitis (per″ĭ-sper″mah-ti′tis) inflammation of the tissues about the spermatic cord. **p. sero′sa,** encysted hydrocele of the spermatic cord.

perisplanchnic (per″ĭ-splank′nik) [peri- + Gr. *splanchnon* viscus] around a viscus or the viscera.

perisplanchnitis (per″ĭ-splank-ni′tis) inflammation around the viscera; perivisceritis.

perisplenic (per″ĭ-splen′ik) occurring around the spleen.

perisplenitis (per″ĭ-splĕ-ni′tis) [peri- + Gr. *splēn* spleen + -itis] inflammation of the peritoneal coat of the spleen and of the structures around it. **p. cartilagin′ea,** inflammatory overgrowth of the capsule of the spleen, causing a thickening of cartilaginous hardness.

perispondylic (per″ĭ-spon-dil′ik) around a vertebra.

perispondylitis (per″ĭ-spon″dĭ-li′tis) [peri- + Gr. *spondylos* vertebra + -itis] inflammation of the parts around a vertebra. **Gibney's p.,** a painful condition of the spinal muscles.

Perisporiaceae (per″ĭ-spo″re-a′se-e) Moniliaceae.

Perissodactyla (pĕ-ris″so-dak′tĭ-lah) [Gr. *perissos* odd + *daktylos* finger] an order of ungulates having an odd number of toes, including the horse, tapir, and rhinoceros. Cf. *Artiodactyla.*

perissodactylous (pĕ-ris″so-dak′tĭ-lus) having an odd number of digits on a hand or foot.

peristalsis (per″ĭ-stal′sis) [peri- + Gr. *stalsis* contraction] the wormlike movement by which the alimentary canal or other tubular organs provided with both longitudinal and circular muscle fibers propel their contents. It consists of a wave of contraction passing along the tube for variable distances. **mass p.,** strong usually brief bursts of peristaltic movements, which propel intestinal contents through long stretches of the intestine or colon, often resulting in defecation. **retrograde p.,** reversed p. **reversed p.,** that which impels the contents of the intestine cephalad.

peristaltic (per″ĭ-stal′tik) of the nature of peristalsis.

peristaltin (per″ĭ-stal′tin) a glycoside, $C_{14}H_{18}O_8$, of cascara sagrada.

peristaphyline (per″ĭ-staf′ĭ-līn) [peri- + Gr. *staphylē* uvula] situated around the uvula.

peristasis (pĕ-ris′tah-sis) environment.

peristome (per′ĭ-stōm) [peri- + Gr. *stoma* mouth] 1. in ciliate protozoa, the buccal area and its encircling adoral zone of membranelles. 2. buccal cavity.

peristomial (per″ĭ-sto′me-ah) pertaining or relating to the peristome or to the area around the cytostome of ciliate protozoa.

peristrumitis (per″ĭ-stroo-mi′tis) inflammation extending from an inflamed goiter to the surrounding structures.

peristrumous (per″ĭ-stroo′mus) around or near a goiter.

perisynovial (per″ĭ-sĭ-no′ve-al) around a synovial structure.

perisyringitis (per″ĭ-sir″in-ji′tis) inflammation of tissues around ducts of the sweat glands.

peritectomy (per″ĭ-tek′to-me) [peri- + *ectomy*] excision of a ring of conjunctiva behind the limbus, followed by cauterization of the trench thus made.

peritendineum (per″ĭ-ten-din′e-um) [NA] the connective tissue investing larger tendons and extending as septa between the fibers composing them.

peritendinitis (per″ĭ-ten″dĭ-ni′tis) tenosynovitis. **adhesive p.,** adhesive capsulitis. **p. calca′rea,** a painful condition marked by calcareous deposits in tendons and in peritendinous, capsular, and ligamentous tissues. **p. crep′itans,** tenosynovitis crepitans. **p. sero′sa,** ganglion, def. 2.

peritendinous (per″ĭ-ten′dĭ-nus) around a tendon.

peritenon (per″ĭ-te′non) [peri- + Gr. *tenōn* tendon] the connective tissue structures associated with a tendon.

peritenoneum (per″ĭ-ten″o-ne′um) the loose connective tissue covering the surface of tendons and ligaments and penetrating inside to separate the substance into bundles.

peritenonitis (per″ĭ-ten″o-ni′tis) tenosynovitis.

peritenontitis (per″ĭ-ten″on-ti′tis) tenosynovitis.

perithecium (per″ĭ-the′se-um) [peri- + Gr. *thēkē* case] the flask-shaped fruiting body, with a pore for the escape of spores, enclosing the asci and spores of certain ascomycetous fungi and molds. Cf. *apothecium, cleistothecium,* and *gymnothecium.*

perithelial (per″ĭ-the′le-al) pertaining to the perithelium.

perithelioma (per″ĭ-the″le-o′mah) hemangiopericytoma.

perithelium (per″ĭ-the′le-um) [peri- + Gr. *thēlē* nipple] the layer of connective tissue that surrounds the capillaries and smaller vessels. **Eberth's p.,** a partial layer of cells on the external surface of the capillaries.

perithoracic (per″ĭ-tho-ras′ik) surrounding the thorax.

perithyreoiditis (per″ĭ-thi″re-oid-i′tis) perithyroiditis.

perithyroiditis (per″ĭ-thi″roi-di′tis) inflammation of the capsule of the thyroid body.

peritomist (pĕ-rit′o-mist) one who performs peritomy (circumcision).

peritomy (pĕ-rit′o-me) [peri- + -tomy] 1. surgical incision of the conjunctiva and subconjunctival tissue about the whole circumference of the cornea; usually done as part of enucleation and retinal detachment procedure. 2. circumcision.

peritone(o)- [L. *peritoneum,* q.v.] a combining form denoting relationship to the peritoneum.

peritoneal (per″ĭ-to-ne′al) pertaining to the peritoneum.

peritonealgia (per″ĭ-to″ne-al′je-ah) pain in the peritoneum.

peritonealize (per″ĭ-to-ne′al-īz) to cover with peritoneum.

peritoneocentesis (per″ĭ-to″ne-o-sen-te′sis) [peritoneum + Gr. *kentēsis* puncture] puncture of the peritoneal cavity with a needle for the purpose of obtaining fluid.

peritoneoclysis (per″ĭ-to″ne-o-kli′sis) injection of water or other fluids into the peritoneal cavity.

peritoneography (per″ĭ-to-ne-og′rah-fe) roentgenography of the peritoneum.

peritoneomuscular (per″ĭ-to-ne″o-mus′ku-lar) pertaining to or composed of peritoneum and muscle.

peritoneopathy (per″ĭ-to-ne-op′ah-the) [peritoneum + Gr. *pathos* disease] any disease of the peritoneum.

peritoneopericardial (per″ĭ-to-ne″o-per″ĭ-kar′de-al) pertaining to the peritoneum and pericardium.

peritoneopexy (per″ĭ-to′ne-o-pek″se) [peritoneum + Gr. *pēxis* fixation] fixation of the uterus by the vaginal route.

peritoneoplasty (per″ĭ-to-ne-o-plas″te) [peritoneum + Gr. *plassein* to form] the operation of covering denuded areas of abdominal viscera or of the abdominal cavity with peritoneum; peritonization.

peritoneoscope (per″ĭ-to′ne-o-skōp″) an instrument for performing peritoneoscopy.

peritoneoscopy (per″ĭ-to″ne-os′ko-pe) [peritoneum + Gr. *skopein* to examine] examination of the peritoneal cavity by an instrument inserted through the abdominal wall.

peritoneotome (per″ĭ-to′ne-o-tōm) an area of the peritoneum supplied with afferent nerve fibers by a single posterior root.

peritoneotomy (per″ĭ-to″ne-ot′o-me) [peritoneum + Gr. *tomē* a cutting] incision into the peritoneal cavity.

peritoneovenous (per″ĭ-to-ne″o-ve′nus) communicating with the peritoneal cavity and the venous system; see under *shunt.*

peritoneum (per″ĭ-to-ne′um) [L.; Gr. *peritonaion,* from *peri* around + *teinein* to stretch] [NA] the serous membrane lining the abdominopelvic walls (*parietal p.*) and investing the viscera (*visceral p.*). A strong, colorless membrane with a smooth surface, it forms a double-layered sac that is closed in the male and is continuous with the mucous membrane of the uterine tubes in the female. The potential space between the parietal and visceral peritoneum is called the *peritoneal cavity* (see *cavitas peritonealis* [NA]). **abdominal p.,** p. parietale. **p. of cranium** (obs.), pericranium. **intestinal p.,** p. viscerale. **parietal p., p. parieta′le** [NA], the peritoneum that lines the abdominal and pelvic walls and the undersurface of the diaphragm. **parietal p., anterior,** p. parieta′le anterius. **p. parieta′le ante′rius** [NA], the peritoneum lining the lower anterior abdominal wall. **urogenital p., p. urogenita′le** [NA], the peritoneum lining the urogenital structures in the lower pelvis.

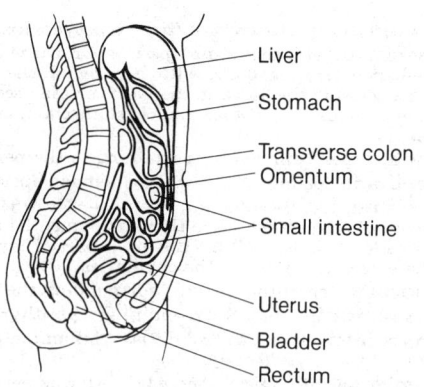

Course of the peritoneum (heavy black line) in a median sagittal section of a female.

- Liver
- Stomach
- Transverse colon
- Omentum
- Small intestine
- Uterus
- Bladder
- Rectum

visceral p., p. viscera'le [NA], a continuation of the parietal peritoneum reflected at various places over the viscera, forming a complete covering for the stomach, spleen, liver, ascending portion of the duodenum, jejunum, ileum, transverse colon, sigmoid flexure, upper end of rectum, uterus, and ovaries; it also partially covers the descending and transverse portions of the duodenum, the cecum, ascending and descending colon, the middle part of the rectum, the posterior wall of the bladder, and the upper portion of the vagina. The peritoneum serves to hold the viscera in position by its folds, some of which form the *mesenteries*, connecting portions of the intestine with the posterior abdominal wall; other folds, the *omenta*, are attached to the stomach; and still others form the *ligaments* of the liver, spleen, stomach, kidneys, bladder, and uterus. The potential space between the visceral and the parietal peritoneum is the peritoneal cavity, which consists of the *pelvic peritoneal cavity* below and the *general peritoneal cavity* above. The general peritoneal cavity communicates by the epiploic foramen with the cavity of the greater omentum, which is also known as the *lesser peritoneal cavity*.

peritonism (per'ĭ-to-nizm) a condition of shock simulating peritonitis, but without inflammation of the peritoneum.

peritonitis (per"ĭ-to-ni'tis) inflammation of the peritoneum; a condition marked by exudations in the peritoneum of serum, fibrin, cells, and pus. It is attended by abdominal pain and tenderness, constipation, vomiting, and moderate fever. **adhesive p.,** that which is characterized by adhesions between adjacent serous surfaces. **benign paroxysmal p.,** familial Mediterranean fever. **bile p., biliary p.,** choleperitoneum. **chemical p.,** peritonitis due to chemical irritation. **p. chron'ica fibro'sa encap'sulans,** a chronic peritonitis marked by the formation on the intestine of a white coating of fibrous tissue undergoing hyaline degeneration; called also *iced intestine* and *zuckergussdarm.* **circumscribed p.,** that which is limited to a portion of the peritoneum. **p. defor'mans,** chronic peritonitis producing shortening of the mesentery so that the intestines are drawn up in loops toward the spine. **diaphragmatic p.,** that which affects the peritoneal surface of the diaphragm. **diffuse p.,** that which is not limited to a portion of the peritoneum. **p. encap'sulans, encysted p.,** that in which a collection of pus or serum is enclosed by adhesions; peritoneal abscess. **fibrocaseous p.,** tubercular peritonitis with fibrous and caseous degeneration. **gas p.,** peritonitis with the accumulation of gas within the peritoneum. **general p.,** inflammation of the greater part of the peritoneum. **hemorrhagic p.,** that which is attended with hemorrhagic effusion. **localized p.,** circumscribed p. **meconium p.,** peritonitis resulting from perforation of the bowel into the peritoneal cavity *in utero* or shortly after birth, resulting in escape of meconium into the peritoneal cavity; it occurs most often as a complication of meconium ileus in fibrocystic disease of the pancreas. **pelvic p.,** perimetritis; peritonitis situated in the pelvis. **perforative p.,** that which is due to a perforation in the digestive tract. **periodic p.,** familial Mediterranean fe-

ver. **puerperal p.,** that which occurs following childbirth. **purulent p.,** peritonitis with the formation of pus. **septic p.,** that which is due to a pyogenic microorganism. **serous p.,** that which is attended by a copious liquid exudation. **silent p.,** asymptomatic peritonitis. **terminal p.,** primary peritonitis in the late stages of a wasting disease. **traumatic p.,** simple acute peritonitis due to trauma. **tuberculous p.,** peritonitis caused by the tubercle bacillus.

peritonization (per"ĭ-to-ni-za'shun) the operation of covering a denuded surface of an abdominal organ or the abdominal wall with peritoneum; peritoneoplasty.

peritonize (per'ĭ-to-nīz) to cover with peritoneum.

peritonsillar (per"ĭ-ton'sĭ-lar) situated around a tonsil.

peritonsillitis (per"ĭ-ton"sĭ-li'tis) inflammation of the peritonsillar tissues.

peritracheal (per"ĭ-tra'ke-al) situated around the trachea.

Peritrate (per'ĭ-trāt) trademark for preparations of pentaerythritol tetranitrate.

peritrich (per'ĭ-trik) 1. any ciliate protozoan of the subclass Peritrichia. 2. peritrichous.

Peritrichia (per"ĭ-trik'e-ah) [peri- + Gr. *thrix* hair] a subclass of typically cone-shaped, ciliate protozoa (class Oligohymenophorea, phylum Ciliophora), characterized by the presence of a prominent oral ciliary field covering the apical end of the body and spiraling counterclockwise into the infundibulum, a paroral membrane and adoral membranelles that become peniculi, and much reduced somatic ciliature. Many are stalked and sedentary, and others are mobile, all with an aboral scopula. The free-swimming larvae have a locomotory posterior ciliary girdle. It comprises one order: Peritrichida.

Peritrichida (per"ĭ-trik'ĭ-dah) an order of ciliate protozoa (subclass Peritrichia, class Oligohymenophorea) having characters of the subclass. It comprises two suborders: Sessilina and Mobilina.

peritrichous (pĕ-rit'rĭ-kus) [peri- + Gr. *thrix* hair] 1. having flagella over the entire surface; said of a bacterial cell; see *flagellum.* 2. having cilia around the cytostome only; said of Ciliophora. Called also *peritrich.*

peritrochanteric (per"ĭ-tro"kan-ter'ik) situated about a trochanter.

perituberculosis (per"ĭ-tu-ber"ku-lo'sis) paratuberculosis.

perityphlic (per"ĭ-tif'lik) [peri- + Gr. *typhlon* cecum] around the cecum; pericecal.

perityphlitis (per"ĭ-tif-li'tis) [peri- + Gr. *typhlon* cecum + -itis] inflammation of the peritoneum surrounding the cecum; appendicitis. **p. actinomycot'ica,** actinomycosis whose principal seat is pericecal.

periumbilical (per"e-um-bil'ĭ-kal) situated around the umbilicus.

periungual (per"e-ung'gwal) around the nail.

periureteral (per"ĭ-u-re'ter-al) around the ureter.

periureteric (per"e-u"re-ter'ik) about the ureter.

periureteritis (per"e-u"re-tĕ-ri'tis) [peri- + Gr. *ourētēr* ureter + -itis] inflammation of the tissues around a ureter.

periurethral (per"e-u-re'thral) occurring around the urethra.

periurethritis (per"e-u"re-thri'tis) [peri- + Gr. *ourēthra* urethra + -itis] inflammation of the tissues around the urethra; spongiitis.

periuterine (per"e-u'ter-in) around the uterus.

perivaginal (per"ĭ-vaj'ĭ-nal) around the vagina.

perivaginitis (per"ĭ-vaj"ĭ-ni'tis) pericolpitis.

perivascular (per"ĭ-vas'ku-lar) situated around a vessel.

perivascularity (per"ĭ-vas"ku-lar'ĭ-te) an infiltrate of cellular elements of mesodermal origin (polymorphonuclear leukocytes, lymphocytes, etc.) in the perivascular spaces, as in those of the cerebral parenchyma.

perivasculitis (per"ĭ-vas"ku-li'tis) inflammation of a perivascular sheath and of the tissues surrounding it.

perivenous (per"ĭ-ve'nus) around a vein.

periventricular (per"ĭ-ven-trik'u-lar) around a ventricle; see also under *system.*

perivertebral (per"ĭ-ver'tĕ-bral) around a vertebra.

perivesical (per″ĭ-ves′ĭ-kal) [peri- + L. vesica bladder] occurring around the bladder.

perivesicular (per″ĭ-vĕ-sik′u-lar) around a seminal vesicle.

perivesiculitis (per″ĭ-vĕ-sik″u-li′tis) inflammation of tissue around the seminal vesicle.

perivisceral (per″ĭ-vis′er-al) occurring around a viscus or the viscera.

perivisceritis (per″ĭ-vis″er-i′tis) inflammation around a viscus or around the viscera.

perivitelline (per″ĭ-vi-tel′ĭn) situated around a vitellus or yolk.

perixenitis (per″ĭ-zĕ-ni′tis) [peri- + Gr. xenos strange + -itis] inflammation occurring around a foreign body in a tissue or organ.

perkeratosis (per″ker-ah-to′sis) hyperkeratosis, def. 3.

Perkinsea (per-kin′se-ah) a class of parasitic homoxenous protozoa (phylum Apicomplexa) having a conoid forming an incomplete cone and flagellated spores with an anterior vacuole. Sexual reproduction does not occur. It comprises one order: Perkinsida.

Perkinsida (per-kin′sĭ-dah) an order of protozoa (class Perkinsea, phylum Apicomplexa) with characters of the class.

perlapine (per′lah-pēn) chemical name: 6-(4-methyl-1-piperazinyl)-11H-dibenz[b,e]azepine; a hypnotic, $C_{19}H_{21}N_3$.

perlèche (per-lesh′) [Fr.] single or multiple fissures and cracks at the corners of the mouth, which may be unilateral or bilateral and in advanced stages may spread to the lips and cheeks. The condition may be due to a primary or superimposed infection with microorganisms such as Candida albicans, staphylococci, or streptococci; poor hygiene; drooling of saliva; overclosure of the jaws in edentulous patients or those with ill-fitting dentures; riboflavin deficiency (see ariboflavinosis); or other causes. Called also angular cheilosis or stomatitis, migrating cheilosis, and intertrigo labialis.

Perlia's nucleus (per′le-ahz) [Richard Perlia, German ophthalmologist, 19th century] see under nucleus.

Perls' test (stain) (perlz) [Max Perls, German pathologist, 1843–1881] see under tests.

perlsucht (perl′sookt) [Ger.] tuberculosis of the mesentery and peritoneum in cattle.

permanganate (per-man′gah-nāt) the MnO_4^{2-} anion, which has a deep purple color in aqueous solution and is a strong oxidizing agent, or a salt containing this ion.

permanganic acid (per″mang-gan′ik) an unstable strong acid and oxidizing agent, $HMnO_4$, existing only in aqueous solution; its salts are permanganates.

permeability (per″me-ah-bil′ĭ-te) the property or state of being permeable; see also osmosis.

permeable (per′me-ah-b'l) [L. per through + meare to pass] not impassable; pervious; permitting passage of a substance.

permease (per′me-ās) a collective term for genetically controlled, stereospecific membrane transport systems occurring in bacterial cells, e.g., the membrane-bound carrier protein (M protein) involved in the transport of β-galactosides across the cell membrane of Escherichia coli.

permeate (per′me-āt″) 1. to penetrate or pass through, as through a filter. 2. the constituents of a solution or suspension that pass through a filter.

permeation (per″me-a′shun) the act of spreading through or penetrating a substance, tissue, or organ, as by a disease process, such as cancer.

Permitil (per′mĭ-til) trademark for a preparation of fluphenazine hydrochloride.

perna (per′nah) a chlorinated naphthalin, which may cause a serious acne in persons handling it.

pernasal (per-na′sal) [L. per through + nasus nose] performed through the nose.

perneiras (pār-na′ras) Brazilian name for beriberi.

perniciosiform (per-nish″e-o′sĭ-form) seemingly pernicious; a term applied to a condition which is apparently, but not actually, pernicious or malignant.

pernicious (per-nish′us) [L. perniciosus] tending to a fatal issue.

pernio (per′ne-o), pl. pernio′nes [L.] chilblain.

pero- [Gr. pēros maimed] a combining form meaning deformed.

perobrachius (pe″ro-bra′ke-us) [pero- + Gr. brachiōn arm] a fetus with deformed arms.

perocephalus (pe″ro-sef′ah-lus) [pero- + Gr. kephalē head] a fetus with a deformed head.

perochirus (pe″ro-ki′rus) [pero- + Gr. cheir hand] a fetus with malformed hands.

perocormus (pe″ro-kor′mus) [pero- + Gr. kormos trunk] perosomus.

perodactylus (pe″ro-dak′tĭ-lus) [pero- + Gr. daktylos finger] a fetus with deformity of fingers or toes, or both, especially absence of one or more digits.

peromelia (per″o-me′le-ah) congenital deformity of the limbs.

peromelus (pe-rom′ĕ-lus) [pero- + Gr. melos limb] a fetus with malformed limbs.

peronarthrosis (per″o-nar-thro′sis) [Gr. peronē anything pointed for piercing or pinning + arthron joint] an articulation in which the surfaces are convex in one direction and concave in the other.

perone (per-o′ne) the fibula.

peroneal (per″o-ne′al) pertaining to the fibula or to the outer side of the leg; fibular.

peroneotibial (per″o-ne″o-tib′e-al) pertaining to the fibula and tibia.

peronia (pe-ro′ne-ah) [Gr. pēros maimed] a developmental malformation or mutilation.

Per. op. emet. abbreviation for L. perac′ta operatio′ne emet′ici, when the action of the emetic is over.

peropus (pe′ro-pus) [pero- + Gr. pous foot] a fetus with malformed legs and feet.

peroral (per-o′ral) [L. per through + os, oris the mouth] performed through or administered through the mouth.

per os (per os) [L.] by mouth.

perosis (pĕ-ro′sis) a disease of chicks marked by bone deformities and associated with deficiency of certain dietary factors, such as choline and manganese.

perosomus (pe″ro-so′mus) [pero- + Gr. sōma body] a fetus with greatly deformed body or trunk.

perosplanchnia (pe″ro-splank′ne-ah) [pero- + Gr. splanchnon viscus + -ia] a developmental anomaly characterized by malformation of the viscera.

perosseous (per-os′e-us) [L. per through + os bone] transmitted through bone.

perotic (pĕ-rot′ik) pertaining to or characterized by perosis.

peroxidase (pe-rok′si-dās) [EC 1.11.1] a sub-subclass of enzymes of the oxidoreductase class that catalyze the oxidation of organic substrates by hydrogen peroxide, which is reduced to water. These enzymes are heme proteins, found frequently in plants and occasionally in animal tissues.

peroxide (pĕ-rok′sīd) that oxide of any element which contains more oxygen than any other. More correctly applied to compounds having such linkage as —O—O—; for instance, hydrogen peroxide, H—O—O—H.

peroxisome (pĕ-roks′ĭ-sōm) 1. any of the microbodies present in vertebrate animal cells, especially liver and kidney cells, which are rich in the enzymes peroxidase, catalase, D-amino acid oxidase, and, to a lesser extent, urate oxidase; their functions are not fully understood, but they participate in metabolic oxidations involving hydrogen peroxide, purine metabolism, cellular lipid metabolism, and gluconeogenesis. Similar structures (glyoxysomes), containing the enzymes of the glyoxylate cycle, are found in certain plants and microorganisms. 2. microbody.

peroxy- a prefix indicating the substitution of —O—O— for —O—, as in peroxyacetic acid.

peroxyacetic acid (per-ok″se-ah-se′tik) peracetic acid.

peroxydol (pĕ-rok′sĭ-dol) sodium perborate.

perphenazine (per-fen′ah-zēn) [USP] chemical name: 4-[3- (2-chloro -10H- phenothiazin -10-yl) propyl] -1-piperazineethanol. A major tranquilizer, $C_{21}H_{26}ClN_3OS$, occurring as a white to creamy white powder; used orally and intramuscularly as an antipsychotic agent, and also used as an antiemetic.

per primam (per pri′mam) [L.] see *per primam intentionem.*

per primam intentionem (per pri′mam in-ten″she-o′nem) [L.] by first intention; see under *healing.*

per rectum (per rek′tum) [L.] by way of the rectum.

Perrin-Ferraton disease (per′an-fer″ah-ton′) [Maurice *Perrin,* Paris surgeon, 1826–1889; Louis *Ferraton,* French surgeon, born 1860] snapping hip.

Perroncito's apparatus (spirals) (per″on-se′tōz) [Aldo *Perroncito,* Italian histologist, 1882–1929] see under *apparatus.*

persalt (per′sawlt) a salt of a peracid; a salt the acid radical of which has a higher valence than the protosalt.

per saltum (per sal′tum) [L.] by a leap or bound; denoting a sudden evolutionary development without intermediate stages.

Persantine (per-san′tēn) trademark for preparations of dipyridamole.

per secundam (per se-kun′dam) [L.] see *per secundam intentionem.*

per secundam intentionem (per se-kun′dam in-ten″she-o′nem) [L.] by second intention; see under *healing.*

perseveration (per-sev″er-a′shun) the persistence or repetition of a response after the causative stimulus has ceased or in response to different stimuli; e.g., a patient answers a question correctly but gives the same answer to succeeding questions; most often associated with organic brain lesions but also seen in schizophrenia.

persister (per-sis′ter) [L. *persistere* persist, from *per* through + *sistere* to stand still] in bacteriology, a microorganism that resists a generally toxic level of a drug but is not genetically resistant.

persona (per-so′nah) [L. "mask"] in jungian psychology, the personality mask or facade presented by a person to the world, as opposed to the *anima,* the inner being.

personality (per″su-nal′ĭ-te) the characteristic way that a person thinks, feels, and behaves; the relatively stable and predictable part of a person's thought and behavior; it includes conscious attitudes, values, and styles as well as unconscious conflicts and defense mechanisms. *Personality traits* are major dispositions to act, feel, and think whose expressive forms are not considered pathological. *Personality types* are categories of both normal and abnormal personality variants; usually they derive from a theory-based typology, such as introvert/extrovert or oral/anal/phallic. *Personality disorders* are specific mental disorders composed of inflexible and maladaptive personality traits that are self-perpetuating, generate subjective distress, and result in significant impairments in social functioning. **affective p. (disorder),** cyclothymia. **alternating p.,** see *multiple p.* **anankastic p.,** obsessive-compulsive p. **antisocial p. (disorder)** [DSM III-R], a personality disorder characterized by continuous and chronic antisocial behavior in which the rights of others are violated; associated personality traits include impulsiveness, egocentricity, inability to tolerate boredom or frustration, irritability and aggressiveness, recklessness, disregard for truth, and inability to maintain consistent, responsible functioning at work, at school, or as a parent. The concept of a personality disorder that predisposes an individual toward criminality has a long history; other terms that have been used are *moral insanity, psychopathic inferiority, constitutional psychopathic inferiority, psychopathic personality,* and *sociopathic personality.* **asthenic p. (disorder)** (*obs.*), a personality disorder characterized by easy fatigability, low energy level, lack of enthusiasm, marked incapacity for enjoyment, and oversensitivity to physical and emotional stress. **avoidant p. (disorder)** [DSM III-R], a personality disorder characterized by social discomfort, hypersensitivity to criticism, and an aversion to activities that involve significant interpersonal contact; there is a proclivity to anxiety, an exaggeration of difficulties, a general timidity, and a desire for affection and acceptance that is restrained for fear of rejection. In previous official classification the diagnosis of schizoid personality disorder or inadequate personality disorder would have been used. **borderline p. (disorder)** [DSM III-R], a personality disorder marked by a pervasive instability of mood, self-image, and interpersonal relationships; impulsive and self-damaging acts are common, as are uncontrolled anger, fears of abandonment, chronic feelings of boredom or emptiness, and recurrent self-mutilating behavior and suicide threats. Borderline personality is often seen in other personality disorders, such as schizotypal, histrionic, narcissistic, or antisocial personality disorder. **compulsive p.,** obsessive-compulsive p. **cycloid p. (disorder),** cyclothymia. **cyclothymic p. (disorder),** cyclothymia. **dependent p. (disorder)** [DSM III-R], a personality disorder marked by feelings of helplessness when alone or when close relationships end, as well as a general preoccupation with fears of being abandoned; other features include difficulty in decision-making without substantial advice and reassurance, low self-esteem, and hypersensitivity to criticism or disapproval. **double p., dual p.,** see *multiple p.* **epileptoid p. (disorder),** intermittent explosive disorder. **explosive p.,** intermittent explosive disorder. **histrionic p. (disorder)** [DSM III-R], a personality disorder marked by excessive emotionality and attention-seeking behavior; there is overconcern with physical attractiveness, sexual seductiveness, intolerance of delayed gratification, and rapid shifting and shallow expression of emotions. Formerly called *hysterical personality.* **hysterical p.,** histrionic p. **inadequate p.,** a diagnostic category referring to persons who are generally ineffectual or inept, socially, intellectually, and physically; it does not correspond to any particular pattern of personality traits and is not included in DSM III or DSM III-R. **multiple p.,** a functional mental disorder characterized by the existence in an individual or two or more distinct personalities, each having unique memories, characteristic behavior, and social relationships that determine the individual's actions when that personality is dominant. Transitions from one personality to another are abrupt. The original personality usually is totally unaware of the other personalities (subpersonalities), experiencing only gaps of time when the others are in control. Subpersonalities may or may not have awareness of the others. **narcissistic p. (disorder)** [DSM III-R], a personality disorder characterized by grandiosity (in fantasy or behavior), a lack of social empathy combined with a hypersensitivity to the judgment of others, interpersonal exploitiveness, a sense of entitlement, and a need for constant signs of admiration. **obsessive p.,** obsessive-compulsive p. **obsessive-compulsive p. (disorder)** [DSM III-R], a personality disorder characterized by an emotionally constricted manner that is unduly conventional, serious, formal, and stingy, by preoccupation with trivial details, rules, order, organization, schedules, and lists, by stubborn insistence on having things one's own way without regard for the effects on others, by excessive devotion to work and productivity to the detriment of interpersonal relationships, and by indecisiveness due to fear of making mistakes. **paranoid p. (disorder)** [DSM III-R], a personality disorder marked by a view of other people as hostile, devious, and untrustworthy and a combative response to disappointments or to events experienced as rebuffs or humiliations. Notable are a questioning of the loyalty of friends, the bearing of grudges, and a tendency to read threatening meanings into benign remarks. It differs from paranoia or paranoid schizophrenia, in which there is delusional or hallucinatory persecution, in that the paranoid personality is overreacting to or misinterpreting real, if minor, slights or setbacks. **passive aggressive p. (disorder)** [DSM III-R], a personality disorder characterized by an indirect resistance to demands for adequate social and occupational performance; anger and opposition to authority and the expectations of others that is expressed covertly by obstructionism, procrastination, stubbornness, dawdling, forgetfulness, and intentional inefficiency. **passive-dependent p.** (*obs.*), dependent p. **psychopathic p.,** antisocial p. **sadistic p. (disorder)** [DSM III-R], a personality disorder marked by a pervasive pattern of cruel, demeaning, and aggressive behavior; satisfaction is gained in intimidating, coercing, and humiliating others; an excitable temper flares readily to argument, belligerence, and the infliction of pain; there is a fascination with violence, social intolerance, and a broad-ranging authoritarianism. **schizoid p. (disorder),** a personality disorder marked by indifference to social relationships and a restricted range of emotional experience and expression. In DSM III-R this category includes persons who lack the capacity for social relationships, are cold and aloof, and are indifferent to praise, criticism, or the feelings of others. In previous classifications schizoid personality included some persons who are now classed as schizotypal or avoidant personalities by DSM III-R criteria. **schizotypal p. (disorder)** [DSM III-R], a personality disorder characterized by marked deficits in interpersonal competence and eccentricities in ideation, appearance, and behavior; ideas of reference are common, as are odd beliefs or magical thinking, a lack of close friends, excessive social anxiety, suspiciousness, and occasional paranoid ideation. In previous official classifications these persons would have been diagnosed as having simple or latent schizophrenia or schizoid personality disorder. Other terms that have been used are borderline, prepsychotic, prodromal, pseudoneurotic, and ambulatory schizophrenia. **seclusive p., shut-in p.,** schizoid p. **self-defeating p. (disorder)** [DSM III-R], a personality disorder marked by feelings of martyrdom, inclination to be drawn to problematic situations or relationships, and failure to accomplish tasks crucial to life objectives; a tendency to engage in excessive self-sacrifice and an inability to enjoy the rewards of success also are notable. **sociopathic p.,** antisocial p. **split p.,** originally, a colloquial equivalent for *schizophrenia,* now more commonly used as an equivalent for *multiple personality.*

personologic (per″son-o-loj′ik) pertaining to personology.

personology (per″sŭ-nol′o-je) the study of personality.

perspiratio (per″spĭ-ra′she-o) [L.] perspiration. **p. insensib′ilis,** insensible perspiration.

perspiration (per″spĭ-ra′shun) [L. *perspira′re* to breathe through] 1. sweating; the functional secretion of sweat. 2. sweat. **insensible p.,** those evaporative losses of water from the moist surfaces of the body (such as the skin and respiratory tree) not due to the secretory activity of glands. **sensible p.,** perspiration due to secretory activity of sweat glands.

persuasion (per-swa′zhun) in psychiatry, a therapeutic approach based on direct suggestion and guidance intended to influence favorably attitudes, behavior, and goals.

persulfate (per-sul′fāt) a salt of persulfuric acid.

persulfide (per-sul′fīd) a sulfide which contains more sulfur than the ordinary sulfide.

persulfuric acid (per″sul-fūr′ik) peroxymonosulfuric acid, H_2SO_5, a strong oxidizing agent.

Perthes' disease, test (per′tēz) [Georg Clemens *Perthes,* German surgeon, 1869–1927] see under *osteochondrosis,* and see *tourniquet test,* under *tests.*

Pertik's diverticulum (per′tiks) [Otto *Pertik,* Hungarian physician, 1852–1913] see under *diverticulum.*

Pertofrane (per′to-frān) trademark for a preparation of desipramine hydrochloride.

per tubam (per tu′bam) [L.] through a tube.

pertubation (per″tu-ba′shun) perflation or insufflation of the uterine tubes to render them patent.

pertucin (per-tu′sin) a bacteriocin produced by *Pseudomonas pertucinogena* that inhibits the growth of *Bordetella pertussis.*

pertussis (per-tus′is) [L. *per* intensive + *tussis* cough] an acute, highly contagious infection of the respiratory tract, most frequently affecting young children, usually caused by *Bordetella pertussis;* a similar illness has been associated with infection by B. *parapertussis* and B. *bronchiseptica.* It is characterized by a *catarrhal stage,* beginning after an incubation period of about two weeks, with slight fever, sneezing, running at the nose, and a dry cough. In a week or two the *paroxysmal stage* begins, with the characteristic paroxysmal cough, consisting of a deep inspiration, followed by a series of quick, short coughs, continuing until the air is expelled from the lungs; the close of the paroxysm is marked by a long-drawn, shrill, whooping inspiration, due to spasmodic closure of the glottis. This stage lasts three to four weeks, after which the *convalescent stage* begins, in which paroxysms grow less frequent and less violent, and finally cease. Called also *whooping cough.* See also *parapertussis,* and see *pertussis-like syndrome,* under *syndrome.*

pertussoid (per-tus′oid) [*pertussis* + Gr. *eidos* form] resembling pertussis.

per vaginam (per vah-ji′nam) through the vagina.

perversion (per-ver′shun) [L. *per* through + *versio* a turning] a turning aside from the normal course; a morbid alteration of function which may occur in emotional, intellectual, or volitional fields. In psychiatry, sexual deviation. **sexual p.,** paraphilia.

pervert (per′vert) a perverted person, especially a person who indulges in unnatural sexual acts (*sexual p.,* or *paraphiliac*).

pervigilium (per″vĭ-jil′e-um) [L.] sleeplessness.

pervious (per′ve-us) [L. *pervius*] permeable.

pes (pes), pl. *pe′des,* gen. *pe′dis* [L.] [NA] the foot: the terminal organ of the lower limb. Used also as a general term to designate a footlike part. **p. abduc′tus,** a deformed foot in which the anterior part is displaced so that it lies laterally to the vertical axis of the leg. **p. adduc′tus,** a deformed foot in which the anterior part is displaced so that it lies medially to the vertical axis of the leg. **p. anseri′nus** [L. "goose's foot"], 1. plexus parotideus nervi facialis. 2. the combined insertion of the tendinous expansions of the sartorius, gracilis, and semitendinosus muscles. **p. ca′vus,** exaggerated height of the longitudinal arch of the foot, present from birth or appearing later because of contractures or disturbed balance of the muscles. **congenital convex p. val′gus,** rocker-bottom foot (def. 1). **p. equinovalgus,** talipes equinovalgus. **equinovarus p.,** talipes equinovarus. **p. febric′itans,** elephantiasis of the foot. **p. gi′gas,** macropodia. **p. hippocam′pi** [NA], a formation of two or three elevations on the rostral end of the ventricular surface of the hippocampus; called also *digitationes hippocampi.* **p. hippocam′pi ma′jor,** hippocampus. **p. hippocam′pi mi′nor,** calcar avis. **p. pedun′culi,** crus cerebri. **p. planoval′gus, p. pla′nus,** flatfoot, a deformed foot in which the position of the bones relative to each other has been altered, with lowering of the longitudinal arch. **p. prona′tus,** a deformed foot in which the outer border of the anterior part is higher than the inner border. **p. supina′tus,** a deformed foot in which the inner border of the anterior part is higher than the outer border. **p. val′gus,** flatfoot. **p. varus,** talipes varus.

pessary (pes′ah-re) [L. *pessarium*] 1. an instrument placed in the vagina to support the uterus or rectum or as a contraceptive device. 2. a medicated vaginal suppository. **cup p.,** a pessary the top of which has a cuplike shape to fit the ostium uteri. **diaphragm p.,** a diaphragm for insertion into the vagina as an occlusive contraceptive. **doughnut p.,** an inflated soft rubber pessary shaped like a doughnut. **Hodge's p.,** a pessary for retrodeviations of the uterus. **lever p.,** a pessary which acts on the principle of the lever. **Menge's p.,** a ring pessary with a fixed crossbar holding a detachable stem. **ring p.,** a round or ring-shaped pessary. **Smith's p.,** a pessary for use in retrodisplacement of the uterus. **stem p.,** a pessary with a stem for introduction into the canal of the cervix uteri.

pessimum (pes′ĭ-mum) a weakened muscular contraction following a strong initial reaction after the stimulation of the neuromuscular system with high-frequency electric current.

pest (pest) plague. **avian p.,** Newcastle disease. **chicken p., fowl p.,** fowl plague.

pesticemia (pes″tĭ-se′me-ah) [L. *pestis* plague + Gr. *haima* blood + *-ia*] septicemic plague.

pesticide (pes′tĭ-sīd) a poison used to destroy pests of any sort; the term includes fungicides, herbicides, insecticides, rodenticides, etc.

pestiferous (pes-tif′er-us) [L. *pestiferus; pestis* plague + *ferre* to bear] causing or propagating a pestilence.

pestilence (pes′tĭ-lens) [L. *pestilentia*] any virulent contagious or infectious epidemic disease; also an epidemic of such a disease.

pestilential (pes″tĭ-len′shal) of the nature of a pestilence; producing an epidemic disease.

pestis (pes′tis) [L.] plague. **p. am′bulans,** ambulatory plague. **p. bubon′ica,** bubonic plague. **p. equo′rum,** African horse sickness. **p. ful′minans, p. ma′jor,** the severe form of bubonic plague. **p. mi′nor,** ambulatory plague. **p. sid′erans,** septicemic plague.

pestle (pes′l) [L. *pestillum*] an implement for pounding drugs in a mortar.

pestology (pes-tol′o-je) the branch of science concerned with pests.

PET positron emission tomography.

peta- a combining form used in naming units of measurement to indicate a quantity one quadrillion (10^{15}) times the unit designated by the root with which it is combined. Symbol, P.

-petal [L. *petere* to seek] a word termination meaning directed or moving toward, the point of reference being indicated by the word stem to which it is affixed, as centripetal (toward a center), corticipetal (toward the cortex).

petalobacteria (pet″ah-lo-bak-te′re-ah) [Gr. *petalon* leaf + *bacteria*] bacteria which become so aggregated as to form thin pellicles.

petechia (pe-te′ke-ah), pl. *pete′chiae* [L.] a pinpoint, non-raised, perfectly round, purplish red spot caused by intradermal or submucous hemorrhage. Cf. *ecchymosis*. **calcaneal petechiae,** black heel.

petechiae (pe-te′ke-e) plural of *petechia*.

petechial (pe-te′ke-al) characterized by or of the nature of petechiae.

Peters' ovum (pa′terz) [Hubert *Peters*, Budapest gynecologist, 1859–1934] see under *ovum*.

Petersen's bag (pa′ter-senz) [C. F. *Petersen*, surgeon in Kiel, 1845–1908] see under *bag*.

pethidine hydrochloride (peth′ĭ-din hi″dro-klo′rĭd) meperidine hydrochloride.

petiolate, petiolated (pet′e-o-lāt; pet′e-o-lāt″ed) having a stalk or petiole.

petiole (pet′e-ōl) a stem, stalk, or pedicle. **epiglottic p.,** petiolus epiglottidis.

petioled (pet′e-ōld) petiolate.

petiolus (pē-ti′o-lus) [L., dim. of *pes* foot] a stem, stalk, or pedicle. **p. epiglot′tidis** [NA], epiglottic petiole: the pointed lower end of the epiglottic cartilage, which is attached to the back of the thyroid cartilage.

Petit's canal, sinus (ptēz) [François Pourfour du *Petit*, French anatomist and surgeon, 1664–1741] see *spatia zonularia* and *sinus aortae*.

Petit's hernia, ligament, triangle (ptēz) [Jean Louis *Petit*, French surgeon, 1674–1750] see under *hernia*, see *uterosacral ligament*, under *ligament*, and see *trigonum lumbare*.

Petit's law (ptēz) [Alexis Therese *Petit*, French physicist, 1791–1820] see *Dulong and Petit's law*, under *law*.

petit mal (pĕ-te′ mahl′) [Fr. "little illness"] see under *epilepsy*.

Petrén's diet (treatment) (pa-trenz′) [Karl Anders *Petrén*, Swedish physician, 1869–1927] see under *diet*.

Pétrequin's ligament (pātr-kanz′) [Joseph Pierre Eléonor *Pétrequin*, Lyons surgeon, 1809–1876] see under *ligament*.

petrichloral (pet″rĭ-klo′ral) chemical name: pentaerythritol chloral. A derivative, $C_{13}H_{16}Cl_{12}O_8$, of chloral with pharmacological properties similar to those of chloral hydrate; used as a hypnotic and sedative.

Petri dish, plate, test (reaction) (pa′tre) [Julius Richard *Petri*, German bacteriologist, 1852–1921] see under *dish*, *plate*, and *tests*.

petrifaction (pet″rĭ-fak′shun) [L. *petra* stone + *facere* to make] conversion into a stonelike substance.

pétrissage (pa″trĭ-sahzh′) [Fr.] foulage.

petroccipital (pet″rok-sip′ĭ-tal) petro-occipital.

petrolate (pet′ro-lāt) petrolatum.

petrolatoma (pet″ro-lah-to′mah) a tumor developing consequent to injection of liquid petrolatum; a discontinued procedure.

petrolatum (pet″ro-la′tum) [L.] [USP] a purified mixture of semisolid hydrocarbons obtained from petroleum; used as an ointment base. It is also used as a protective dressing and soothing application to the skin. Called also *mineral jelly*, *petroleum jelly*, *yellow soft paraffin*, and *petrolate*. **p. al′bum,** white p. **hydrophilic p.** [USP], a mixture of cholesteryl, stearyl alcohol, and white wax, in white petrolatum; used as an absorbent ointment base and topical protectant. **liquid p.,** mineral oil; see under *oil*. **liquid p., heavy,** mineral oil; see under *oil*. **liquid p., light,** light mineral oil; see under *oil*. **p. liq′uidum,** mineral oil; see under *oil*. **p. liq′uidum le′ve,** light mineral oil; see under *oil*. **white p.** [USP], a wholly or nearly decolorized, purified mixture of semisolid hydrocarbons obtained from petroleum; used as an oleaginous ointment base and topical protectant.

petroleum (pĕ-tro′le-um) [L. *petra* stone + *oleum* oil] a thick natural oil obtained from beneath the earth. It consists of a mixture of various hydrocarbons of the paraffin and olefin series. It has been used as an expectorant, diaphoretic, and vermifuge; also in skin diseases, etc.

petrolization (pet″rol-i-za′shun) the spreading of petroleum on water for the purpose of destroying mosquito larvae therein.

petromastoid (pet″ro-mas′toid) 1. pertaining to the petrous portion of the temporal bone and its mastoid process. 2. otocranium (def. 2).

petro-occipital (pet″ro-ok-sip′ĭ-tal) pertaining to the petrous portion of the temporal bone and to the occipital bone.

petropharyngeus (pet″ro-fah-rin′je-us) an occasional muscle arising from the lower surface of the petrous portion of the temporal bone and inserted into the pharynx.

petrosal (pĕ-tro′sal) pertaining to the petrous portion of the temporal bone.

petrosalpingostaphylinus (pet″ro-sal-ping″go-staf″ĭ-li′nus) [Gr. *petra* stone + *salpinx* tube + *staphylē* uvula] musculus levator veli palatini.

petrosectomy (pet″ro-sek′to-me) [*petrous* + Gr. *ektomē* excision] excision of the cells of the apex of the petrous portion of the temporal bone.

petrositis (pet″ro-si′tis) inflammation of the petrous portion of the temporal bone.

petrosomastoid (pĕ-tro″so-mas′toid) petromastoid.

petrosphenoid (pet″ro-sfe′noid) pertaining to the sphenoid bone and the petrous portion of the temporal bone.

petrosphere (pet′ro-sfēr) the solid structure of the earth as distinguished from the atmosphere and the aquasphere.

petrosquamosal (pet″ro-skwah-mo′sal) pertaining to the petrous and squamous portions of temporal bone.

petrosquamous (pet″ro-skwa′mus) petrosquamosal.

petrostaphylinus (pet″ro-staf″ĭ-li′nus) musculus levator veli palatini.

petrous (pet′rus) [L. *petrosus*] resembling a rock; hard; stony.

petrousitis (pet″rus-i′tis) petrositis.

Petruschky's litmus whey, spinalgia (pĕ-trush′kēz) [Johannes *Petruschky*, German bacteriologist, born 1863] see *litmus whey*, under *whey*, and see under *spinalgia*.

Pettenkofer's test, theory (pet′en-kof″erz) [Max Josef von *Pettenkofer*, chemist in Munich, 1818–1901] see under *tests* and *theory*.

pettymorrel (pet″e-mor′rel) *Aralia*.

Petzetaki's test (reaction) (pet″za-tah′kēz) see under *tests*.

Peucetia (pu-se′te-ah) a genus of spiders. **P. vir′idans,** a lynx spider that is capable of producing painful burns of the eye by squirting a corrosive spray.

pexia (pek′se-ah) pexis.

pexic (pek′sik) [Gr. *pēxis* fixation] having the power of fixing substances; said of tissues.

pexin (pek′sin) [Gr. *pēxis* fixation] rennet.

pexis (pek′sis) [Gr. *pēxis*] 1. the fixation of matter by a tissue. 2. surgical fixation, usually by suturing.

-pexy [Gr. *pēxis* a putting together] a word termination meaning fixation.

Peyer's patches (glands, insulae, plaques) (pi′erz) [Johann Conrad *Peyer*, Swiss anatomist, 1653–1712] folliculi lymphatici aggregati.

peyote (pa-o′te) 1. any of several Mexican cacti of the genus *Lophophora*, especially *L. williamsii* or mescal. 2. a stimulant drug from mescal buttons, the flowering heads of *L. williamsii*, used by North American Indians in ceremonies and feasts to produce a state of intoxification marked by feelings of ecstasy. The active euphoric principle is the major alkaloid, mescaline. Called also *peyotl*.

peyotl (pa-o′t'l) peyote.

Peyronie's disease (pa-ron-ēz′) [François de la *Peyronie*, French surgeon, 1678–1747] see under *disease*.

Peyrot's thorax (pa-rōz′) [Jean Joseph *Peyrot*, surgeon in Paris, 1843–1917] see under *thorax*.

Pfannenstiel's incision (pfan′en-stēlz) [Hermann Johann *Pfannenstiel*, gynecologist in Breslau, 1862–1909] see under *incision*.

Pfeiffer's bacillus, phenomenon (reaction) (pfi′erz) [Richard Friedrich Johann *Pfeiffer*, bacteriologist in Breslau,

1858–1945] see *Haemophilus influenzae*, and see under *phenomenon*.

Pfeiffer's disease (pfi'ferz) [Emil *Pfeiffer*, German physician, 1846–1921] infectious mononucleosis.

Pfeifferella (pfi''fer-el'ah) [Richard F. J. *Pfeiffer*] in former systems of classification, a genus of bacteria made up of organisms now classified in various other genera. **P. anatipes'tifer,** *Moraxella anatipestifer.* **P. mal'lei,** *Pseudomonas mallei.*

Pflüger's cords, law, tubes (pfle'gerz) [Edward Friedrich Wilhelm *Pflüger*, physiologist in Bonn, 1829–1910] see under *law*, and see *ovarian tubes*, under *tube*.

Pfuhl's sign (pfoolz) [Adam *Pfuhl*, German physician, 1842–1905] see under *sign*.

PG abbreviation for prostaglandin.

P.G. abbreviation of *Pharmacopoeia Germanica*, German pharmacopeia.

pg. picogram.

PGD$_2$, PGE$_2$, PGF$_2$, α**PGI$_2$,** etc. symbols for various prostaglandins; see *prostaglandin*.

Ph chemical symbol for *phenyl*.

Ph. Pharmacopeia.

pH the symbol relating the hydrogen ion (H$^+$) concentration or activity of a solution to that of a given standard solution. Numerically the pH is approximately equal to the negative logarithm of H$^+$ concentration expressed in molarity. pH 7 is neutral; above it alkalinity increases and below it acidity increases.

PHA phytohemagglutinin (def. 2).

phacitis (fah-si'tis) phakitis.

phac(o)- [Gr. *phakos* lentil, or lentil-shaped object] a combining form denoting relationship (*a*) to a lens, as the crystalline lens, or (*b*) a mole, freckle or mother spot, as in phacomatosis. See also words beginning *phak(o)-*.

phacoanaphylaxis (fak''o-an''ah-fi-lak'sis) [*phaco-* + *anaphylaxis*] hypersensitivity to the protein of the crystalline lens of the eye, induced by escape of material from the lens capsule.

phacocele (fak'o-sēl) [*phaco-* + *-cele*] the dislocation of the eye lens from its proper place; hernia of the eye lens.

phacocyst (fak'o-sist) [*phaco-* + *cyst* (def. 1)] the capsule of the lens (capsula lentis [NA]).

phacocystectomy (fak''o-sis-tek'to-me) [*phacocyst* + *ectomy*] excision of a portion of the capsule of the lens for cataract.

phacocystitis (fak''o-sis-ti'tis) [*phacocyst* + *-itis*] inflammation about the capsule of the crystalline lens; called also *phacohymenitis*.

phacoemulsification (fak''o-e-mul''sĭ-fĭ-ka'shun) [*phaco-* + L. *emulgēre* to milk out] a method of cataract extraction in which the lens is fragmented by ultrasonic vibrations and simultaneously irrigated and aspirated.

phacoerysis (fak''o-er-e'sis) [*phaco-* + Gr. *eryein* to drag away] removal of the lens in cataract by means of suction with an instrument known as an erysiphake; called also *Barraquer's method* or *operation*.

phacoglaucoma (fak''o-glaw-ko'mah) [*phaco-* + *glaucoma*] the structural changes in the lens produced by glaucoma.

phacohymenitis (fak''o-hi''men-i'tis) phacocystitis.

phacoid (fak'oid) [*phaco-* + Gr. *eidos* form] shaped like a lens or a lentil.

phacoiditis (fak''oi-di'tis) phakitis.

phacoidoscope (fah-koi'do-skōp) phacoscope.

phacolysin (fak-kol'ĭ-sin) [*phaco-* + *lysin*] an albumin from the lens of the eye; used in the treatment of early cataract.

phacolysis (fah-kol'ĭ-sis) [*phaco-* + *lysis*] discission of the crystalline lens, followed by extraction.

phacolytic (fak''o-lit'ik) pertaining to or causing dissolution of the crystalline lens.

phacoma (fah-ko'mah) phakoma.

phacomalacia (fak''o-mah-la'she-ah) [*phaco-* + *malacia*] softening of the lens; a soft cataract.

phacomatosis (fak''o-mah-to'sis) phakomatosis.

phacometachoresis (fak''o-met''ah-ko-re'sis) [*phaco-* + Gr. *metachōrēsis* displacement] displacement of the eye lens.

phacometecesis (fak''o-met''ĕ-se'sis) [*phaco-* + Gr. *metoikēsis* migration] phacometachoresis.

phacometer (fah-kom'ĕ-ter) lensometer.

phacopalingenesis (fak''o-pal''in-jen'ĕ-sis) [*phaco-* + *palingenesis* (1)] re-formation of the crystalline lens.

phacoplanesis (fak''o-plah-ne'sis) [*phaco-* + Gr. *planēsis* wandering] abnormal mobility of the eye lens.

phacosclerosis (fak''o-skle-ro'sis) [*phaco-* + *sclerosis*] hardening of the eye lens; a hard cataract.

phacoscope (fak'o-skōp) [*phaco-* + *-scope*] an instrument for viewing accommodative changes of the eye lens; called also *phacoidoscope*.

phacoscopy (fah-kos'ko-pe) the examination of the eye with a phacoscope.

phacoscotasmus (fak''o-sko-taz'mus) [*phaco-* + Gr. *skotasmos* a clouding] the clouding of the lens of the eye.

phacotherapy (fak''o-ther'ah-pe) [*phaco-* + Gr. *therapeia* treatment] heliotherapy.

phacotoxic (fak''o-tok'sik) exerting a deleterious effect upon the crystalline lens.

Phaenicia (fen-ĭ-she'ah) a genus of greenbottle flies of the family Calliphoridae that are metallic green or blue. **P. cupri'na,** a sheep maggot fly of worldwide distribution; its larvae cause various forms of myiasis in humans. Called also *Lucilia cuprina*. **P. serica'ta,** a sheep maggot fly of the British Isles which lays its eggs in wounds of sheep and soiled wool; its larvae have been introduced into infected wounds to facilitate healing. Called also *Lucilia sericata*. See also *maggot*.

phae(o)- for terms beginning thus, see also terms beginning *pheo-*.

Phaeocalpida (fe''o-kal'pĭ-dah) [*pheo-* + Gr. *kalpis* pitcher, urn] an order of marine planktonic protozoa (class Phaeodarea, superclass Actinopoda), characterized by the presence of a skeleton consisting mainly of a small, most often porcellanous and sometimes alveolar shell, usually with many pores, often with one large opening, often with radial spines.

Phaeoconchida (fe''o-kon'chĭ-dah) [*pheo-* + Gr. *konchē* shell] an order of marine planktonic protozoa (class Phaeodarea, superclass Actinopoda) characterized by the presence of a skeleton consisting of two thick, usually hemispherical valves pressed against each other.

Phaeocystida (fe''o-sis'tĭ-dah) [*pheo-* + Gr. *kystis* sac, bladder] an order of marine planktonic protozoa (class Phaeodarea, superclass Actinopoda) either without a skeleton or having one consisting of spicules that are either free or radiating from a common junction point.

Phaeodarea (fe''o-dār'e-ah) [Gr. *phaios* dusky, gray] a class of marine planktonic protozoa (superclass Actinopoda, subphylum Sarcodina), characterized by a skeleton (when present) composed of mixed silica and organic matter, consisting of usually hollow spines and shells; a very thick capsular membrane with an astropyle that functions as a cytopharynx at one pole; two smaller parapyles, which are penetrated by axopodia, usually at the other pole; and a phaeodium in the ectoplasm. It comprises six orders: Phaeocystida, Phaeosphaerida, Phaeocalpida, Phaeogromida, Phaeoconchida, and Phaeodendrida. The classes Phaeodarea and Polycystinea considered together are equivalent to the Radiolaria in former taxonomic classifications.

Phaeodendrida (fe''o-den'drĭ-dah) [*pheo-* + Gr. *dendron* tree] an order of marine planktonic protozoa (class Phaeodarea, superclass Actinopoda) characterized by the presence of a skeleton consisting of two noncontiguous valves, from which arise long, branching spines with ramifications that may produce large external latticed spongious shells.

phaeodium (fe''o-de'um) [*pheo-* + *eidos* form] a prominent aggregation of dark corpuscles and debris associated with the astropyle of certain marine planktonic protozoa, particularly the Phaeodarea. Written also *pheodium*.

Phaeogromida (fe''o-grom'ĭ-dah) [*pheo-* + L. *groma* pole] an order of marine planktonic protozoa (class Phaeodarea, superclass Actinopoda), characterized by the presence of skeleton consisting mainly of a small diatomaceous or alveolar shell with one large opening; the shell is sometimes greatly reduced and may bear spines.

phaeohyphomycosis (fe''o-hi''fo-mi-ko'sis) any opportunistic infection caused by dematiacious fungi.

Phaeosphaerida (fe″o-sfēr′ĭ-dah) [*pheo-* + *sphere*] an order of marine planktonic protozoa (class Phaeodarea, superclass Actinopoda), characterized by the presence of a skeleton consisting mainly of a very large latticed shell with wide polygonal meshes.

phage (fāj) bacteriophage.

phagedena (faj″ĕ-de′nah) [Gr. *phagedaina; phagein* to eat] a progressive and rapidly spreading and sloughing ulceration.

phagedenic (faj″ĕ-den′ik) pertaining to or characterized by phagedena. See under *ulcer.*

phagelysis (fāj′li-sis) [*phage* + Gr. *lysis* dissolution] the destruction or solution of phage; the destructive or solvent action of phage.

-phagia, -phagy [Gr. *phagein* to eat] a word termination denoting a perversion of appetite (pica), such as geophagia, or relationship to eating or swallowing, e.g., aerophagy.

phag(o)- [Gr. *phagein* to eat] a combining form denoting relationship to eating or consumption by ingestion or engulfing.

phagocaryosis (fag″o-kar″e-o′sis) phagokaryosis.

phagocytable (fag′o-sīt″ah-b′l) susceptible to phagocytosis.

phagocyte (fag′o-sīt) [*phago-* + *-cyte*] any cell capable of ingesting particulate matter. The term usually refers to polymorphonuclear leukocytes and mononuclear phagocytes (macrophages and monocytes). These cells ingest microorganisms and other particulate antigens that are coated with antibody or complement (opsonized), a process that is mediated by specific cell-surface receptors (Fc receptors and complement receptors). Other cell types exhibit phagocytosis, but not specific phagocytosis of opsonized particles. **alveolar p's,** see under *macrophage.* **mononuclear p.,** any cell of the monocyte-macrophage lineage; see *mononuclear phagocyte system,* under *system.*

phagocytic (fag″o-sit′ik) exhibiting phagocytosis; pertaining to phagocytosis or phagocytes.

phagocytin (fag″o-si′tin) any of several poorly characterized basic proteins with bactericidal activity found in the granules of neutrophils. See *cationic proteins,* under *protein.*

phagocytize (fag′o-sīt″īz) phagocytose.

phagocytoblast (fag″o-si′to-blast) [*phagocyte* + Gr. *blastos* germ] (*obs.*) a hypothesized phagocyte precursor cell.

phagocytolysis (fag″o-si-tol′ĭ-sis) [*phagocyte* + Gr. *lysis* dissolution] solution or destruction of phagocytes.

phagocytolytic (fag″o-si″to-lit′ik) pertaining to phagocytolysis.

phagocytose (fag″o-si′tōs) to ingest particles by the process of phagocytosis.

phagocytosis (fag″o-si-to′sis) endocytosis of particulate material, such as microorganisms or cell fragments. The material is taken into the cell in membrane-bound vesicles (phagosomes) that originate as pinched off invaginations of the plasma membrane. Phagosomes fuse with lysosomes, forming phagolysosomes in which the engulfed material is killed and digested. See *phagocyte.* **induced p.,** phagocytosis aided by subjecting bacteria to the action of opsonins in the blood. **spontaneous p.,** phagocytosis of bacteria taking place in an indifferent medium, or phagocytosis of nonantigenic particles. **surface p.,** enhanced phagocytosis by macrophages and neutrophils of microorganisms or other particulate antigens that are trapped against surfaces, e.g., other leukocytes, fibrin clots, or tissue surfaces; it does not require opsonins.

phagocytotic (fag″o-si-tot′ik) pertaining to or characterized by phagocytosis.

phagokaryosis (fag″o-kar″e-o′sis) [*phago-* + Gr. *karyon* nucleus + *-osis*] the alleged phagocytic action of the cell nucleus.

phagological (fag″o-loj′ĕ-kal) pertaining to phage.

phagolysis (fah-gol′ĭ-sis) phagocytolysis.

phagolysosome (fag″o-li′so-sōm) the digestive vacuole formed when the membranes of pre-existent lysosomes within the cytoplasm merge with the phagosome; the lysosomes then discharge their hydrolytic enzymes, resulting in digestion of the phagocytized material.

phagolytic (fag″o-lit′ik) phagocytolytic.

phagomania (fag″o-ma′ne-ah) [*phago-* + Gr. *mania* mad-

ness] an insatiable craving for food, or an obsessive preoccupation with the subject of eating.

phagophobia (fag″o-fo′be-ah) [*phago-* + *phobia*] irrational fear of eating.

phagoplasm (fa′go-plasm) [*phago-* + *plasm*] the digestive enzyme-rich cytoplasm of the cytopharyngeal area in certain ciliate protozoa.

phagosome (fag′o-sōm) [*phago-* + Gr. *soma* body] the membrane-bounded vesicle in a phagocyte formed by invagination of the cell membrane and the phagocytized material; called also *phagocytotic vesicle.* See also *phagolysosome.*

phagotroph (fa′go-trōf) a holozoic organism.

phagotrophic (fa″go-trōf′ik) [*phago-* + Gr. *trophē* nutrition] holozoic.

phagotype (fag′o-tīp) phage type; see under *type.*

phakitis (fa-ki′tis) [*phak-* + *-itis*] inflammation of the crystalline lens.

phak(o)- [Gr. *phakos* a lentil, or lentil-shaped object; a spot on the body, a freckle] for words beginning thus, see also those beginning *phac(o)-.*

phakoma (fah-ko′mah) [*phac-* + *-oma*] any of the hamartomas found characteristically in the phacomatoses, such as the herald lesion of tuberous sclerosis, manifested as a refractile, yellowish, multinodular cystic lesion arising from the optic disk or retina, and representing a tumor of glial tissue. Written also *phacoma.* See also *tuber,* def. 3.

phakomatosis (fak″o-mah-to′sis), pl. *phakomato′ses* [*phakoma* + *-osis*] any of a group of congenital and hereditary developmental anomalies having in common selective involvement of the tissues of ectodermal origin (i.e., central nervous system, eye, and skin) and the development of disseminated glial hamartomas (phakomas) in these tissues. The major syndromes in the group are neurofibromatosis, tuberous sclerosis, Sturge-Weber syndrome, von Hippel-Lindau disease, and ataxia-telangiectasia. Called also *neurocutaneous syndrome.* Written also *phacomatosis.*

phalangeal (fah-lan′je-al) pertaining to a phalanx.

phalangectomy (fal″an-jek′to-me) excision of a phalanx of a finger or toe.

phalanges (fah-lan′jēz) plural of *phalanx.*

phalangette (fal″an-jet′) the distal phalanx of a digit. **drop p.,** dropping of the distal phalanx of a finger and loss of power to extend it when the hand is prone.

phalangitis (fal″an-ji′tis) inflammation of one or more phalanges.

phalangization (fal″an-ji-za′shun) surgical separation of the terminal portion of fused digits, without complete extirpation of the connecting web.

phalang(o)- [L. *phalanx,* q.v.] a combining form denoting relationship to a phalanx or to the phalanges.

phalangophalangeal (fah-lan″go-fah-lan′je-al) pertaining to two adjoining phalanges of a finger or toe.

phalangosis (fal″an-go′sis) [*phalanx* + *-osis*] a condition in which the eyelashes grow in rows.

phalanx (fa′lanks), pl. *phalan′ges* [Gr. "a line or array of soldiers"] 1. [NA] any of the bones of the fingers or toes (*ossa digitorum manus* or *ossa digitorum pedis,* respectively). 2. any one of a set of plates (made up of supporting cells, q.v.) disposed in rows which makes up the reticular membrane of the organ of Corti. **Deiters' phalanges,** modified cuticular plates forming the ends of sustentacular epithelial cells of the reticular membrane of the organ of Corti. **phalan′ges digito′rum ma′nus,** NA alternative for *ossa digitorum manus.* **phalan′ges digito′rum pe′dis,** NA alternative for *ossa digitorum pedis.* **phalanges of fingers,** ossa digitorum manus. **p. dista′lis digito′rum ma′nus** [NA], distal phalanx of fingers: any one of the five terminal bones of the fingers, articulating, except in the thumb, with the phalanx media; called also *p. tertia digitorum manus.* **p. dista′lis digito′rum pe′dis** [NA], distal phalanx of toes: any one of the five terminal bones of the toes, articulating, except in the great toe, with the phalanx media; called also *p. tertia digitorum pedis.* **p. me′dia digito′rum ma′nus** [NA], middle phalanx of fingers: any one of the four bones of the fingers (excluding the thumb) situated between the proximal and distal phalanges; called also *p. secunda digitorum manus.* **p. me′dia digito′rum pe′dis** [NA], middle phalanx of toes: any one of the four bones of the toes (excluding the great toe) situated between the proximal and distal phalanges; called also *p. secunda digitorum pedis.* **p. pri′ma digito′rum ma′nus,** p. proximalis digitorum manus. **p. pri′ma digito′rum pe′dis,** p. proximalis digitorum pedis. **p. proxima′lis digito′rum ma′nus** [NA], proximal phalanx of fingers: any one of the five bones of the fingers that articulate with the metacarpal bones and, except in the thumb, with the phalanx media; called also *p. prima digitorum manus.* **p. proxima′lis digito′rum pe′dis** [NA], proximal phalanx of toes: any one of the five bones of the toes that articulate with the metatarsal bones and, except in the great toe, with the phalanx media; called also *p. prima digitorum pedis.* **p. secun′da digito′rum ma′nus,** p. media digitorum manus. **p. secun′da digito′rum pe′dis,** p. media digitorum pedis. **p. ter′tia digito′rum ma′nus,** p. distalis digitorum manus. **p. ter′tia digito′rum pe′dis,** p. distalis digitorum pedis. **phalanges of toes,** ossa digitorum pedis. **ungual p. of fingers,** p. distalis digitorum manus. **ungual p. of toes,** p. distalis digitorum pedis.

Phallales (fah-la′lēz) an order of basidiomycetes of the Gasteromycetes, characterized by the presence of a fetid mucinous substance around the basidiospores that are exposed by an internal stalk which grows and breaks out of the basidiocarp.

phallalgia (fal-al′je-ah) [*phallus* + *-algia*] pain in the penis.

phallanastrophe (fal″an-as′tro-fe) [*phallus* + Gr. *anastrophē* a turning upward] upward distortion of the penis.

phallaneurysm (fal-an′u-rizm) [*phallus* + Gr. *aneurysma* aneurysm] aneurysm of the penis.

phallectomy (fal-ek′to-me) [*phallos* + Gr. *ektomē* excision] penectomy.

phalli (fal′i) genitive and plural of *phallus.*

phallic (fal′ik) [Gr. *phallikos*] pertaining to the phallus, or penis.

phalliform (fal′ĭ-form) [*phallus* + L. *forma* form] shaped like the phallus or penis.

phallin (fal′in) a poisonous hemolytic glycoside from *Amanita phalloides.*

phallitis (fal-i′tis) [*phallus* + *-itis*] inflammation of the penis; penitis.

phall(o)- [Gr. *phallos* penis] a combining form denoting relationship to the penis.

phallocampsis (fal″o-kamp′sis) [*phallo-* + Gr. *kampsis* bending] curvature of the penis when erect.

phallocrypsis (fal″o-krip′sis) [*phallo-* + Gr. *krypsis* hiding] retraction of the penis.

phallodynia (fal″o-din′e-ah) [*phallo-* + Gr. *odynē* pain] pain in the penis.

phalloid (fal′oid) [*phallo-* + Gr. *eidos* form] resembling a penis.

phalloidin, phalloidine (fah-loid′in) a heat-stable, bicyclic hexapeptide poison from the mushroom *Amanita phalloides,* which causes asthenia, vomiting, diarrhea, convulsions, and death.

phalloncus (fal-ong′kus) [*phallo-* + Gr. *onkos* mass] a morbid swelling or tumor of the penis.

phalloplasty (fal′o-plas″te) [*phallo-* + Gr. *plassein* to shape] plastic surgery of the penis.

phallorrhagia (fal″o-ra′je-ah) [*phallo-* + Gr. *rhēgnynai* to burst forth] hemorrhage from the penis.

phallotomy (fal-ot′o-me) [*phallo-* + Gr. *tomē* a cutting] incision of the penis.

Phallus (fal′us) a genus of basidiomycetous fungi of the order Phallales, series Gasteromycetes, including the stinkhorns.

phallus (fal′us), pl. *phal′li* [Gr. *phallos*] 1. the rudiment of embryonic or fetal tissue that develops into the penis or clitoris. 2. the penis or clitoris. 3. the penis or a representation of the penis.

phaner(o)- [Gr. *phaneros* visible] a combining form meaning visible or apparent.

phanerogam (fan′er-o-gam) [*phanero-* + Gr. *gamos* marriage] a true seed-bearing plant.

phanerogenetic (fan″er-o-jĕ-net′ik) phanerogenic.

phanerogenic (fan″er-o-jen′ik) [*phanero-* + Gr. *gennan* to produce] having a known cause. Cf. *cryptogenic.*

phaneroplasm (fan′er-o-plazm) [Gr. *phaneros* visible + *plasm*] membranous organelles and nonmembranous inclusions in the cytoplasm; cf. *cytosol.*

phaneroscope (fan′er-o-skōp) [Gr. *phaneros* visible + *skopein* to examine] (*obs.*) an instrument for illuminating the skin and rendering it translucent for examination.

phanerosis (fan″er-o′sis) [Gr. *phanerōsis*] the act of becoming visible; the setting free of a substance which has previously been undemonstrable owing to its being held in combination. **fat p.,** conversion in the tissues of invisible fatty substances into fat which can be stained and seen.

phanerosterol (fan″er-os′ter-ol) a sterol of one of the higher plants.

Phanodorn (fan′o-dorn) trademark for a preparation of cyclobarbital.

phantasia (fan-ta′ze-ah) fantasy.

phantasm (fan′tazm) [Gr. *phantasma* appearance] an impression or image not evoked by actual stimuli; called also *phantom.*

phantasy (fan″tah-se) [Gr. *phantasia* imagination; the power by which an object is made apparent to the mind] fantasy.

phantogeusia (fan″to-gu′ze-ah) continuous abnormal taste in the mouth, usually metallic or salty.

phantom (fan′tom) [Gr. *phantasma* an appearance] 1. phantasm. 2. a model of the body or of a specific part thereof. 3. in radiology, a device that simulates the conditions encountered when radiation or radioactive material is deposited *in vivo* and permits a quantitative estimation of its effects.

phanurane (fan′u-rān) canrenone.

pha(o)- for words beginning thus, see those beginning *phe(o)-.*

phar., pharm. pharmacy; pharmaceutical; pharmacopeia.

Phar. B. abbreviation for L. *Pharmaciae Baccalaureus,* Bachelor of Pharmacy.

Phar. C. Pharmaceutical Chemist.

pharcidous (fahr′sĭ-dus) [Gr. *pharkis* wrinkled] wrinkled.

Phar. D. abbreviation for L. *Pharmaciae Doctor,* Doctor of Pharmacy.

Phar. G. Graduate in Pharmacy.

Phar. M. abbreviation for L. *Pharmaciae Magister,* Master of Pharmacy.

pharmacal (fahr′mah-kal) pertaining to pharmacy.

pharmaceutic (fahr-mah-su′tik) [Gr. *pharmakeutikos*] pertaining to pharmacy or to drugs.

pharmaceutical (fahr″mah-su′tĭ-kal) 1. pertaining to pharmacy or to drugs. 2. a medicinal drug.

pharmaceutics (fahr″mah-su′tiks) 1. pharmacy (def. 1). 2. pharmaceutical preparations.

pharmaceutist (fahr″mah-su′tist) a pharmacist.

pharmacist (fahr′mah-sist) one who is licensed to prepare and sell or dispence drugs and compounds, and to make up prescriptions; an apothecary, druggist, or (British) chemist.

pharmaco- (fahr″mah-ko) [Gr. *pharmakon* medicine] a combining form denoting relationship to a drug or medicine.

pharmacochemistry (fahr″mah-ko-kem′is-tre) pharmaceutical chemistry.

pharmacodiagnosis (fahr″mah-ko-di″ag-no′sis) [*pharmaco-* + *diagnosis*] the employment of drugs in the diagnosis of disease.

pharmacodynamic (fahr″mah-ko-di-nam′ik) [*pharmaco-* + Gr. *dynamis* power] pertaining to pharmacodynamics.

pharmacodynamics (fahr″mah-ko-di-nam′iks) [*pharmaco-* + Gr. *dynamis* power] the study of the biochemical and physiological effects of drugs and the mechanisms of their actions, including the correlation of actions and effects of drugs with their chemical structure; also, such effects on the actions of a particular drug or drugs.

pharmacoendocrinology (fahr″mah-ko-en″do-kri-nol′o-je) the study of the influence of drugs on the activity of the endocrine glands, and of the effects of hormones on organs and tissues.

pharmacogenetics (fahr″mah-ko-jĕ-net′iks) the scientific study of the relationship between genetic factors and the nature of responses to drugs.

pharmacognostics (fahr″mah-kog-nos′tiks) pharmacognosy.

pharmacognosy (fahr″mah-kog′no-se) [pharmaco- + Gr. gnōsis knowledge] that branch of pharmacology which deals with the biological, biochemical, and economic features of natural drugs and their constituents.

pharmacography (fahr″mah-kog′rah-fe) [pharmaco- + Gr. graphein to write] an account or written description of drugs.

pharmacokinetics (fahr″mah-ko-ki-net′iks) the action of drugs in the body over a period of time, including the processes of absorption, distribution, localization in tissues, biotransformation, and excretion.

pharmacologic (fahr″mah-ko-loj′ik) pertaining to pharmacology or to the properties and reactions of drugs.

pharmacologist (fahr″mah-kol′o-jist) one who makes a study of the actions of drugs.

pharmacology (fahr″mah-kol′o-je) [pharmaco- + -logy] the science that deals with the origin, nature, chemistry, effects, and uses of drugs; it includes pharmacognosy, pharmocokinetics, pharmacodynamics, pharmacotherapeutics, and toxicology.

pharmacomania (fahr″mah-ko-ma′ne-ah) [pharmaco- + Gr. mania madness] uncontrollable desire to take or to administer medicines.

pharmacometrics (fahr″mah-ko-met′riks) [pharmaco- + Gr. metron measure] the comparative evaluation of drug activity, distinguished from bioassay in that substances with different chemical constitutions are compared.

pharmacon (fahr′mah-kon) [Gr. pharmakon] a drug.

pharmaco-oryctology (fahr″mah-ko-or″ik-tol′o-je) [pharmaco- + Gr. oryktos excavated + -logy] the study of mineral drugs.

pharmacopedia, pharmacopedics (fahr″mah-ko-pe′de-ah; fahr″mah-ko-pe′diks) [pharmaco- + Gr. paideia instruction] the science which deals with the properties and preparations of drugs.

pharmacopeia (fahr″mah-ko-pe′ah) [pharmaco- + Gr. poiein to make] an authoritative treatise on drugs and their preparations; a book containing a list of products used in medicine, with descriptions, chemical tests for determining identity and purity, and formulas for certain mixtures of these substances. It also generally contains a statement of average dosage. The first United States pharmacopeia was published on December 15, 1820, printed in both Latin and English, and its 272 pages included 217 drugs which were considered worthy of recognition. See U.S.P.

pharmacopeial (fahr″mah-ko-pe′al) pertaining to or recognized by the pharmacopeia.

pharmacophilia (fahr″mah-ko-fil′e-ah) [pharmaco- + Gr. philein to love] abnormal fondness for drugs; see drug addiction, under addiction.

pharmacophobia (fahr″mah-ko-fo′be-ah) [pharmaco- + phobia] irrational fear of drugs or medicines.

pharmacophore (fahr′mah-ko-fōr″) [pharmaco- + Gr. phoros bearing] the group of atoms in a drug molecule which is responsible for the action of the compound.

pharmacopoeia (fahr″mah-ko-pe′ah) pharmacopeia.

pharmacopsychosis (fahr″mah-ko-si-ko′sis) [pharmaco- + psychosis] any mental disorder due to alcohol, drugs, or poisons.

pharmacoradiography (fahr″mah-ko-ra″de-og′rah-fe) pharmacoroentgenography.

pharmacoroentgenography (fahr″mah-ko-rent″gen-og′rah-fe) roentgenographic examination of a body organ under the influence of a drug which best facilitates such examination.

pharmacotherapeutics (fahr″mah-ko-ther″ah-pu′tiks) [pharmaco- + therapeutics] study of the uses of drugs in the treatment of disease.

pharmacotherapy (fahr″mah-ko-ther′ah-pe) [pharmaco- + therapy] the treatment of disease by medicines.

pharmacy (fahr′mah-se) [Gr. pharmakon medicine] 1. the branch of the health sciences dealing with the preparation, dispensing, and proper utilization of drugs. 2. a place where drugs are compounded or dispensed. **chemical p.,** pharmaceutical chemistry. **galenic p.,** the pharmacy of vegetable medicines.

Pharm.D. abbreviation for Doctor of Pharmacy.

pharyngalgia (far″in-gal′je-ah) [pharyngo- + -algia] pain in the pharynx.

pharyngeal (fah-rin′je-al) [L. pharyngeus] pertaining to the pharynx.

pharyngectasia (far″in-jek-ta′se-ah) pharyngocele.

pharyngectomy (far″in-jek′to-me) [pharyngo- + Gr. ektomē excision] surgical removal of a part of the pharynx.

pharyngemphraxis (far″in-jem-frak′sis) [pharyngo- + Gr. emphraxis stoppage] obstruction of the pharynx.

pharyngeus (far-in-je′us) [L.] pharyngeal.

pharyngism (far′in-jism) pharyngismus.

pharyngismus (far″in-jiz′mus) muscular spasm of the pharynx.

pharyngitic (far″in-jit′ik) affected with or of the nature of pharyngitis.

pharyngitid (fah-rin′ji-tid) a cutaneous eruption occurring in pharyngitis.

pharyngitis (far″in-ji′tis) [pharyngo- + -itis] inflammation of the pharynx. **acute p.,** inflammation with pain in the throat, especially on swallowing, dryness, followed by moisture of the pharynx, congestion of the mucous membrane, and fever; called also catarrhal p. **atrophic p.,** a chronic pharyngitis which leads to wasting of the submucous tissue accompanied by dryness and thickened secretions. **catarrhal p.,** acute p. **chronic p.,** that which results from repeated acute attacks or is due to tuberculosis or syphilis; it is attended with excessive secretion, and in the severe ulcerated varieties by pain and dysphagia. **croupous p.,** membranous p. **diphtheritic p.,** diphtheria (q.v.) involving the pharnyx. **follicular p.,** sore throat with enlargement of the pharyngeal glands. **gangrenous p.,** a form characterized by gangrenous patches. **glandular p.,** follicular p. **granular p.,** a chronic variety in which the mucous membrane becomes granular. **p. herpet′ica,** membranous or aphthous sore throat; a form of acute pharyngitis characterized by the formation of vesicles, which give place to excoriations. **hypertrophic p.,** a chronic form which leads to thickening of the submucous tissues. **p. kerato′sa,** pharyngomycosis. **membranous p.,** pharyngitis with a fibrous exudate leading to the formation of a false membrane. **phlegmonous p.,** acute parenchymatous tonsillitis attended with the formation of abscesses. **plague p.,** pharyngeal plague. **p. sic′ca,** an atrophic pharyngitis in which the throat becomes dry. **p. ulcero′sa,** the formation of ulcers covered by a yellow, membrane-like deposit in the pharynx, with fever, pain, and prostration.

pharyng(o)- (fah-ring′go) [Gr. pharynx pharynx] a combining form denoting relationship to the pharynx.

pharyngocele (fah-ring′go-sēl) [pharyngo- + Gr. kēlē hernia] hernial protrusion of a part of the pharynx; a hernial pouch or other cystic deformity of the pharynx.

pharyngoceratosis (fah-ring″go-ser″ah-to′sis) pharyngokeratosis.

pharyngoconjunctivitis (fah-ring″go-kon-junk″tĭ-vi′tis) inflammation involving the pharynx and conjunctiva, the result of a viral infection.

pharyngodynia (fah-ring″go-din′e-ah) [pharyngo- + Gr. odynē pain] pain in the pharynx.

pharyngoepiglottic (fah-ring″go-ep″ĭ-glot′ik) pertaining to the pharynx and epiglottis.

pharyngoepiglottidean (fah-ring″go-ep″ĭ-glŏ-tid′e-an) pharyngoepiglottic.

pharyngoesophageal (fah-ring″go-e-sof′ah-je″al) pertaining to the pharynx and esophagus.

pharyngoglossal (fah-ring″go-glos′al) pertaining to the pharynx and the tongue.

pharyngoglossus (fah-ring″go-glos′us) the muscular fibers from the superior constrictor of the pharynx to the tongue.

pharyngokeratosis (fah-ring″go-ker″ah-to′sis) keratosis of the pharynx.

pharyngolaryngeal (fah-ring″go-lah-rin′je-al) pertaining to the pharynx and the larynx.

pharyngolaryngitis (fah-ring″go-lar″in-ji′tis) [pharyngo- + Gr. larynx larynx + -itis] inflammation of the pharynx and the larynx.

pharyngolith (fah-ring′go-lith) [*pharyngo-* + Gr. *lithos* stone] a concretion in the walls of the pharynx.

pharyngology (far″ing-gol′o-je) [*pharyngo-* + *-logy*] the sum of what is known regarding the pharynx.

pharyngolysis (far″ing-gol′ĭ-sis) [*pharyngo-* + Gr. *lysis* dissolution] paralysis of the pharynx.

pharyngomaxillary (fah-ring″go-mak′sĭ-ler″e) pertaining to the pharynx and the maxillae.

pharyngomycosis (fah-ring″go-mi-ko′sis) [*pharyngo-* + Gr. *mykēs* fungus + *-osis*] any fungal disease of the pharynx.

pharyngonasal (fah-ring″go-na′sal) pertaining to the pharynx and the nose.

pharyngo-oral (fah-ring″go-o′ral) pertaining to the pharynx and the mouth.

pharyngopalatine (fah-ring″go-pal′ah-tīn) pertaining to the pharynx and the palate.

pharyngoparalysis (fah-ring″go-pah-ral′ĭ-sis) [*pharyngo-* + *paralysis*] paralysis of the pharyngeal muscles.

pharyngopathy (far″ing-gop′ah-the) [*pharyngo-* + Gr. *pathos* disease] disease of the pharynx.

pharyngoperistole (fah-ring″go-pĕ-ris′to-le) [*pharyngo-* + Gr. *peristolē* contracture] narrowing of the pharynx.

pharyngoplasty (fah-ring′go-plas″te) [*pharyngo-* + Gr. *plassein* to form] plastic operation on the pharynx. **Hynes p.,** a technique of pharyngoplasty accomplished by muscle transposition.

pharyngoplegia (far″ing-go-ple′je-ah) [*pharyngo-* + Gr. *plēgē* stroke] paralysis of the muscles of the pharynx.

pharyngorhinitis (fah-ring″go-ri-ni′tis) inflammation of the nasopharynx.

pharyngorhinoscopy (fah-ring″go-ri-nos′ko-pe) examination of the nasopharynx and posterior nares with the rhinoscope.

pharyngorrhagia (far″ing-go-ra′je-ah) [*pharyngo-* + Gr. *rhēgnynai* to break forth] hemorrhage from the pharynx.

pharyngorrhea (far″ing-go-re′ah) [*pharyngo-* + Gr. *rhoia* flow] a discharge of mucus from the pharynx.

pharyngosalpingitis (fah-ring″go-sal″pin-je′tis) inflammation of the pharynx and the eustachian tube.

pharyngoscleroma (fah-ring″go-skle-ro′mah) scleroma of the pharynx.

pharyngoscope (fah-ring″go-skōp) [*pharyngo-* + Gr. *skopein* to examine] an instrument for inspecting the pharynx.

pharyngoscopy (far″ing-gos′ko-pe) direct visual examination of the pharynx.

pharyngospasm (fah-ring′go-spazm) [*pharyngo-* + Gr. *spasmos* spasm] spasm of the pharyngeal muscles.

pharyngostenosis (fah-ring″go-ste-no′sis) [*pharyngo-* + Gr. *stenōsis* narrowing] narrowing of the lumen of the pharynx.

pharyngostoma (fah″ring-gos′to-mah) [*pharyngo* + Gr. *stoma* mouth] the opening formed by pharyngostomy.

pharyngostomy (fah″ring-gos′to-me) [*pharyngo* + Gr. *stomoun* to provide with an opening, or mouth] the surgical creation of an artificial opening into the pharynx.

pharyngotome (fah-ring′go-tōm) a cutting instrument used in pharyngeal surgery.

pharyngotomy (far″ing-got′o-me) [*pharyngo-* + Gr. *tomē* a cutting] surgical incision of the pharynx. **external p.,** pharyngotomy done from the outside. **internal p.,** that which is performed from within the pharynx. **lateral p.,** the opening of the pharynx from one side. **subhyoid p.,** section of the pharynx through the thyrohyoid membrane.

pharyngotonsillitis (fah-ring″go-ton″sĭ-li′tis) inflammation of the pharynx and the tonsil.

pharyngotyphoid (fah-ring″go-ti′foid) enteric fever with angina and sore patches on the tonsils.

pharyngoxerosis (fah-ring″go-ze-ro′sis) [*pharyngo-* + Gr. *xerōsis* dryness] dryness of the pharynx.

pharynx (far′inks) [Gr. "the throat"] [NA] the musculo-membranous passage between the mouth and posterior nares and the larynx and esophagus. The part above the level of the soft palate is the *nasopharynx*, which communicates with the auditory tube. The lower portion consists of two sections—the *oropharynx*, which lies between the soft palate and the upper edge of the epiglottis, and the *hypopharynx*, which lies below the upper edge of the epiglottis and opens into the larynx and esophagus.

phase (fāz) [Gr. *phasis* an appearance] 1. the view that a thing presents to the eye. 2. any one of the varying aspects or stages through which a disease or process may pass. 3. in physical chemistry, any physically or chemically distinct, homogenous, and mechanically separable part of a system, e.g., the ice and steam phases of water. **alpha p.,** the estrous stage of the ovarian cycle. **anal p.,** see under *stage*. **beta p.,** the progestational stage of the ovarian cycle. **cholesteric p.,** a liquid crystal phase that exhibits molecular orientation and arrangement both within and between equispaced planes. **continuous p.,** a phase that is physically continuous; the continuous portion of a colloid system (see *dispersion medium*). **p. of decline,** the stage in the growth of a bacterial culture in which the number of live organisms gradually decreases. **disperse p.,** the internal or discontinuous portion of a colloid system; it is analogous to the solute in a solution. Called also *internal p.* Cf. *dispersion medium*. **erythrocytic p.,** that phase in the life cycle of a malarial plasmodium in which the parasites multiply in the red blood cells. **estrin p.,** proliferative stage. **exponential p.,** logarithmic p. **external p.,** dispersion medium. **genital p.,** see under *stage*. **hematic p.,** a liquid crystal phase that exhibits molecular orientation without periodicity. **internal p.,** disperse p. **lag p.,** the early period following bacterial inoculation into a new medium, a time of stationary population during which the cells adjust to the new environment and synthesize enzymes and intermediates for the subsequent logarithmic phase. **latency p.,** see under *stage*. **logarithmic p.,** the stage in the growth of a bacterial culture when a plot of the logarithm of the number of cells against time gives a straight-upward line. Called also *exponential p.* **meiotic p.,** that stage in meiosis in which the reduction of the chromosomes occurs; called also *reduction p.* **motofacient p.,** see *motofacient*. **negative p.,** the initial lowering of the antibody titer following the injection of corresponding antigen. **nonmotofacient p.,** see *motofacient*. **Nonne-Apelt p.,** see under *reaction*. **oral p.,** see under *stage*. **phallic p.,** see under *stage*. **positive p.,** the rise in antibody titer that follows the negative phase. **postmeiotic p.,** the stage following the reduction of the chromosomes in meiosis. **premeiotic p., prereduction p.,** the stage in meiosis which precedes the reduction of the chromosomes. **reduction p.,** meiotic p. **resting p.,** former term for interphase. **smectic p.,** a liquid crystal phase that exhibits molecular orientation and arrangement in equispaced planes, but no periodicity within the planes. **stance p.,** the element of a forward step in which the foot is in contact with the floor and the leg bears the body weight, comprising heel strike, mid stance, and push-off. **stationary p.,** the stage in the growth of a bacterial culture when the bacteria undergoing division are in equilibrium with those dying, and the number of bacterial cells remains nearly constant. **swing p.,** the element of a forward step in which the foot does not touch the floor and the opposite leg bears the body weight, comprising acceleration, swing through, and deceleration. **synaptic p.,** synapsis.

phaseolamin (fah-se′o-lah′min) an alpha-amylase inhibitor purified from the kidney bean (*Phaseolus vulgaris*); it is the basis of starch-blocker tablets.

phaseolin (fa-se′o-lin) a globulin, $C_{20}H_{18}O_4$, from the kidney bean, *Phaseolus vulgaris*, which has antifungal properties.

phaseolunatin (fa″se-o-lu′nah-tin) linamarin.

phasin, phasein (fa′sin) any of a group of nitrogenous substances found in seeds, bark, and other plant tissues, which agglutinate red blood corpuscles.

phasmid (faz′mid) 1. one of a pair of caudal chemoreceptors occurring in certain nematodes. The class Nematoda is sometimes divided into two subclasses, Phasmidia and Aphasmidia, on the basis of the presence or absence of these organs. 2. a nematode belonging to the Phasmidia. Cf. *aphasmid*.

Phasmidia (faz-mid′e-ah) a subclass of Nematoda comprising those organisms possessing phasmids. The following superfamilies are of medical or veterinary importance. Rhabditoidea, Strongyloidea, Oxyuroidea, Ascarioidea, Spiruroidea, Filarioidea, and Dracunculoidea.

Ph.B. British Pharmacopoeia.

Ph.D. Doctor of Philosophy.

Phe phenylalanine.

phellandrene (fĕ-lan'drēn) chemical name: 5-isopropyl-2-methyl-1,3-cyclohexadiene. A liquid hydrocarbon, $C_{10}H_{16}$, occurring in fennel oil, elemi oil, the oil of water hemlock, and the Australian eucalyptus.

Phelps' operation (felps) [Abel Mix *Phelps*, surgeon in New York, 1851–1902] see under *operation*.

Phe-Mer-Nite (fe'mer-nīt) trademark for preparations of phenylmercuric nitrate.

Phemerol (fe'mer-ol) trademark for preparations of benzethonium.

phemfilcon A (fem-fil'kon) a hydrophilic contact lens material.

Phemister graft, operation (fem'is-ter) [Dallas Burton *Phemister*, American surgeon, 1882–1951] see under *graft* and *operation*.

phemitone (fem'ĭ-tōn) mephobarbital.

phen- see *pheno-*.

phenacaine hydrochloride (fen'ah-kān) [USP] a local anesthetic applied topically to the conjunctiva.

phenacemide (fĕ-nas'ĕ-mīd) [USP] chemical name: *N*-(aminocarbonyl)-benzeneacetamide. An oral anticonvulsant, $C_9H_{10}N_2O_2$, occurring as a white to almost white, fine crystalline powder; used in the treatment of psychomotor, grand mal, and petit mal epilepsy, and in the management of mixed seizures.

phenacetin (fĕ-nas'ĕ-tin) [USP] The ethyl ether of acetaminophen, which is its major active metabolite, an analgesic and antipyretic, $C_{10}H_{13}NO_2$. Formerly called *acetphenetidin* and *acetophenetidin*.

phenacetolin (fen″ah-set'o-lin) a red powder, $C_{16}H_{12}O_2$, used as an indicator: it has a pH range of 5 to 6, being yellow at 5 and red at 6.

phenaglycodol (fen″ah-gli'ko-dol) chemical name: 2-(4-chlorophenyl)-3-methyl-2,3-butanediol. A tranquilizer, $C_{11}H_{15}ClO_2$, occurring as a white, crystalline powder; administered orally.

phenakistoscope (fe″nah-kis'to-skōp) [Gr. *phenakistēs* deceiver + *skopein* to examine] a device consisting of a revolving disk with figures near the center that appear to be in motion when viewed through slots at the periphery of the disk by means of a mirror.

phenanthrene (fe-nan'thrēn) a colorless, crystalline hydrocarbon, $(C_6H_4.CH)_2$.

phenanthrolene (fe-nan'thro-lēn) orthophenanthrolene.

phenantoin (fen'an-to″in) mephenytoin.

phenate (fe'nāt) phenolate.

phenazocine hydrobromide (fĕ-naz'o-sēn) chemical name: 1,2,3,4,5,6-hexahydro-8-hydroxy-6,11-dimethyl-3-phenethyl-2,6-methano-3-benzazocine-8-ol hydrobromide. A synthetic narcotic analgesic, $C_{22}H_{27}NO.HBr$, occurring as a white or nearly white, crystalline powder; administered intramuscularly and intravenously.

phenazone (fen'ah-zōn) antipyrine.

phenazopyridine hydrochloride (fen″ah-zo-pēr'ĭ-dēn) [USP] chemical name: 3-(phenylazo)-2,6-pyridinediamine monohydrochloride. A urinary analgesic, $C_{11}H_{11}N_5.HCl$, occurring as a light or dark red to dark violet, crystalline powder; used orally in cystitis, urethritis, pyelonephritis, and prostatitis. Formerly used as a urinary antiseptic.

phenbutazone sodium glycerate (fen-bu'tah-zōn) chemical name: 4-butyl-3-hydroxy-1,2-diphenyl-3-pyrazolin-5-one sodium salt compound with glycerol (1:1); an anti-inflammatory, $C_{19}H_{19}N_2NaO_2.C_3H_8O_3$.

phencyclidine hydrochloride (fen-si'klĭ-dēn) chemical name: 1-(1-phenylcyclohexyl)piperidine hydrochloride; a potent analgesic and anesthetic, $C_{17}H_{25}N.HCl$, used in veterinary medicine. Abuse of this drug may lead to serious psychological disturbances. Abbreviated PCP.

phene (fēn) [gr. *phainein* to show] advanced stages of the developmental sequence determined by gene action, sometimes with environmental factors, resulting in a special phenotype.

phenelzine sulfate (fen'el-zēn) [USP] chemical name: (2-phenylethyl)hydrazine sulfate. A monoamine oxidase inhibitor, $C_8H_{12}N_2.H_2SO_4$, occurring as a white to yellowish white powder; used as an antidepressant, administered orally.

Phenergan (fen'er-gan) trademark for preparations of promethazine hydrochloride.

phenethicillin (fĕ-neth″ĭ-sil'in) chemical name: 3,3-dimethyl-7-oxo-6-[(1-oxo-2-phenoxypropyl)amino]-4-thia-1-azabicyclo[3.2.0]heptane-2-carboxylic acid. A semisynthetic acid-resistant penicillin, $C_{17}H_{20}N_2O_5S$, which is a methyl analogue of penicillin V. **p. potassium** [USP], the monopotassium salt of phenethicillin, $C_{17}H_{19}KN_2O_5S$, occurring as a white to almost white, fine crystalline powder; used as an antibacterial, especially in certain infections due to susceptible organisms, such as streptococcal infections of the upper respiratory tract, pneumococcal infections of the respiratory tract, staphylococcal infections of skin and soft tissues, and fusospiroketosis. It is administered orally.

phenethylbiguanide (fen-eth″il-bi'gwan-īd) phenformin.

phenetidin (fe-net'ĭ-din) the ethyl ester of para-aminophenol, $NH_2.C_6H_4.OC_2H_5$; used in preparing acetophenetidin. It often appears in the urine after the administration of acetophenetidin.

phenetidinuria (fe-net″ĭ-dĭ-nu're-ah) the presence of phenetidin in the urine.

phenetole (fen'ĕ-tol) ethyl phenyl ether, an oily liquid, $C_6H_5O.C_2H_5$.

phenformin hydrochloride (fen-for'min) chemical name: *N*-(2-phenylethyl)imidodicarbonimidic diamide monohydrochloride; an oral hypoglycemic agent, $C_{10}H_{15}N_5.HCl$, no longer available in the United States.

phengophobia (fen″go-fo'be-ah) photophobia.

phenic acid (fe'nik) phenol (1).

phenidin (fen'ĭ-din) (*obs.*) phenacetin.

phenin (fe'nin) (*obs.*) phenacetin.

phenindamine tartrate (fĕ-nin'dah-mēn) chemical name: 2,3,4,9-tetrahydro-2-methyl-9-phenyl-1*H*-indene[2,1-*c*]pyridine. An antihistaminic, $C_{19}H_{19}N.C_4H_6O_6$, occurring as a creamy white powder; administered orally.

phenindione (fen″in-di'ōn) [USP] chemical name: 2-phenyl-1*H*-indene-1,3,(2*H*)-dione. One of the indanedione anticoagulants, $C_{15}H_{10}O_2$, occurring as creamy white to pale yellow crystals or as a crystalline powder and having a rapid onset and short duration of action; administered orally.

pheniramine maleate (fen-ir'ah-mēn) chemical name: *N*,*N*-dimethyl-γ-phenyl-2-pyridinepropanamine. An antihistaminic, $C_{16}H_{20}N_2.C_4H_4O_4$, occurring as a white crystalline powder; administered orally. Called also *prophenpyridamine maleate*.

phenmetrazine hydrochloride (fen-met'rah-zēn) [USP] chemical name: 3-methyl-2-phenyl morpholine hydrochloride. A central nervous system stimulant, $C_{11}H_{15}NO.HCl$, occurring as a white to off-white crystalline powder, used as an anorexic. Abuse of this drug may lead to habituation; see *amphetamine*.

phen(o)- [Gr. *phainein* to show] 1. a combining form denoting a showing or displaying. 2. in chemistry, a prefix denoting a compound derived from benzene.

phenobarbital (fe″no-bar'bĭ-tal) [USP] chemical name: 5-ethyl-5-phenyl-2,4,6(1*H*,3*H*,5*H*)pyrimidinetrione. A long-acting barbiturate, $C_{12}H_{12}N_2O_3$, occurring as white, glistening, small crystals, or white, crystalline powder; used as a sedative, hypnotic, and anticonvulsant, administered orally. Called also *phenobarbitone* and *phenylethylbarbituric acid*. **p. sodium** [USP], the monosodium salt of phenobarbital, $C_{12}H_{11}N_2NaO_3$, occurring as flaky crystals, or white, crystalline granules, or white powder, having the actions and uses of the base; administered orally, rectally, intravenously, intramuscularly, and subcutaneously.

phenobarbitone (fe″no-bar'bĭ-tōn) phenobarbital.

phenocopy (fe'no-kop″e) [*pheno-* (def. 1) + *copy*] 1. an environmentally induced phenotype mimicking one usually produced by a specific genotype. 2. an individual exhibiting such a phenotype. 3. the simulated trait in a phenocopy.

phenodeviant (fe″no-de've-ant) [*pheno-* (def. 1) + *deviant*] an individual whose phenotype differs significantly from that of the typical phenotype in the population.

phenogenetics (fe″no-jĕ-net′iks) [*pheno-* (def. 1) + *genetics*] the science which attempts to explain the chain of causality between genotype and phenotype.

phenol (fe′nol) 1. [USP] an extremely poisonous, colorless to light pink, crystalline compound, $C_6H_5 \cdot OH$, obtained by the distillation of coal tar, and converted, by the addition of 10 per cent water, into a clear liquid with a peculiar odor and a burning taste. Used as an antimicrobial agent. Called also *carbolic acid, hydroxybenzene, oxybenzene, phenic acid, phenylic acid,* and *phenylic alcohol.* See also under *poisoning.* 2. a generic term for any organic compound containing one or more hydroxyl groups attached to an aromatic or carbon ring. **p. liquefac′tum, liquefied p.** [USP], an aqueous solution of phenol containing not less than 89 per cent by weight of phenol; used as a topical antipruritic. Called also *phenylic alcohol.* **p. red,** phenolsulfonphthalein. **p. salicylate,** phenyl salicylate.

phenolase (fe′no-lās) monophenol monooxygenase.

phenolate (fe′no-lāt) 1. to treat with phenol for purposes of sterilization. 2. a salt formed by union of a base with phenol, in which a monovalent metal, such as sodium or potassium, replaces the hydrogen of the hydroxyl group.

phenolated (fe′no-lāt″ed) charged with phenol.

Phenolax (fe′no-laks) trademark for a preparation of phenolphthalein.

phenolemia (fe″no-le′me-ah) the presence of phenols in the blood.

phenolic (fe-nol′ik) pertaining to or derived from phenol.

phenolization (fe″nol-i-za′shun) treatment by subjection to the action of phenol.

phenologist (fe-nol′o-jist) an expert or specialist in phenology.

phenology (fe-nol′o-je) [Gr. *phainesthai* to appear + *-logy*] a study of the effects of climate upon the life and health of living organisms.

phenolphthalein (fe″nol-thal′e-in) [USP] chemical name: 3,3-bis-(4-hydroxyphenyl)-1(3*H*)-isobenzofuranone. A cathartic and pH indicator, with a range of 8.5 (colorless) to 9.0 (red), $C_{20}H_{14}O_4$.

phenol sulfatase (fe′nol sul′fah-tās) arylsulfatase.

phenolsulfonphthalein (fe″nol-sul″fōn-thal′e-in) [USP] chemical name: 4,4′-(3*H*-2,1-benzoxathiol-3-ylidene)bis(*S, S*-dioxide)phenol. A bright to dark red, crystalline powder, $C_{19}H_{14}O_5S$, administered by intramuscular or intravenous injection as a test of renal function. Called also *phenol red.* Abbreviated PSP.

phenoltetrachlorophthalein (fe″nol-tet″rah-klōr″o-thal′e-in) a coal tar derivative, used intravenously in tests of liver function.

phenoltetraiodophthalein (fe″nol-tet″rah-i″o-do-thal′e-in) phentetiothalein.

phenoluria (fe″nol-u′re-ah) the presence of phenols in the urine.

phenom (fe′nom) in some systems of classification, a group or "cluster" of strains of phenotypically related organisms. Called also *phenon.* See also *numerical taxonomy,* under *taxonomy.*

phenomenology (fe-nom″ĕ-nol′o-je) the study of phenomena; in psychiatry, the theory that behavior is determined by the way the person perceives reality rather than by external reality in objective terms.

phenomenon (fĕ-nom′ĕ-non), pl. *phenom′ena* [Gr. *phainomenon* thing seen] any sign or objective symptom; any observable occurrence or fact. **Anderson's p.,** clumps of red blood cells in the stools of amebic dysentery; seen on microscopic examination. **aqueous-influx p.,** entrance into conjunctival or subconjunctival vessels of clear fluid (aqueous humor), deriving from an aqueous vein during compression of its recipient vessel by a glass rod. Called also *Ascher's positive glass-rod phenomenon.* Cf. *blood-influx p.* **arm p.,** Pool's p., def. 2. **p. of Arthus,** see *Arthus reaction,* under *reaction.* **Ascher's positive glass-rod p.,** aqueous-influx p. **Ascher's negative glass-rod p.,** blood-influx p. **Aschner's p.,** slowing of the pulse following pressure on the eyeball; it is indicative of cardiac vagus irritability. See *oculocardiac reflex,* under *reflex.* **Ashman's p.,** aberrant ventricular activation resulting in a short cardiac cycle following a normal or long cycle; it is associated with supraventricular premature beats and with

atrial fibrillation. **Aubert's p.,** an optical illusion in which a bright vertical line in a dark room tilts to one side when an observer tilts his head to the opposite side. **Austin Flint p.,** Austin Flint murmur; see under *murmur.* **autokinetic visible light p.,** the apparent spontaneous movement of a pin-point source of light as seen by certain susceptible persons when they gaze steadily at it in a completely blacked-out room. **Babinski's p.,** dorsiflexion of the large toe and spreading of the other toes instead of plantar flexion of all the toes when the sole is stimulated; it is a sign of damage to the corticospinal tract. **Becker's p.,** increased pulsation of the retinal arteries in Graves' disease. **Bell's p.,** an outward and upward rolling of the eyeball on the attempt to close the eye; it occurs on the affected side in peripheral facial paralysis (Bell's palsy). **Berry-Dedrick p.,** the transformation of fibroma viruses into myxoma viruses. **blood-influx p.,** filling of conjunctival or subconjunctival vessels with blood during compression by a glass rod of the recipient vessel of an aqueous vein. This and the aqueous-influx phenomenon, depending on minute pressure differences between blood and aqueous humor, differ in glaucomatous eyes and those with normal intraocular pressure. Called also *Ascher's negative glass-rod p.* **Bordet-Gengou p.,** complement fixation. **brake p.,** the tendency of a muscle to maintain itself in its normal resting position; called also *Rieger's p.* **break-off p.,** a state of disconnectedness or unreality experienced by high-altitude pilots. Its symptomatic sensations are apparently indescribable in understandable physical terms, but the condition could be the result of a loss of all the physical sense perceptions. **Chase-Sulzberger p.,** Sulzberger-Chase p. **cheek p.,** in meningitis if pressure is exerted on both cheeks just under the zygomas there is reflex upward jerking of both arms with simultaneous bending of both elbows. **cogwheel p.,** when a hypertonic muscle is passively stretched it resists, and this resistance sometimes takes the form of an irregular jerkiness; called also *Negro's p.* **Collie p.,** when pure neon is enclosed in a glass tube with a globule of mercury and shaken it glows with a bright, orange-red color, and when the globule rolls it appears to be followed by a flame. **Cushing's p.,** a rise in systemic blood pressure as a result of an increase in intracranial pressure. **Dale p.,** see under *reaction.* **Danysz's p.,** decrease of the neutralizing influence of an antitoxin when a toxin is added to it in divided portions instead of all at once. **dawn p.,** the early-morning increase in plasma glucose concentration and thus insulin requirement in a patient with insulin-dependent diabetes mellitus. **Debre's p.,** absence of measles rash at the site of injection of convalescent measles serum which has not prevented the appearance of the eruption. **Dejerine-Lichtheim p.,** Lichtheim sign. **dental p.,** thermal and tactile sensations in the gums with toothache, produced by repeated faradic stimulation of hyperesthetic lines on the body (Calligaris). **Denys-Leclef p.,** phagocytosis taking place in a test tube on mixing therein leukocytes, bacteria, and immune serum specific for the bacteria. **d'Herelle's p.,** Twort-d'Herelle p. **diaphragm p., diaphragmatic p.,** the movement of the diaphragm as seen through the walls of the body; called also *phrenic phenomenon* and *phrenic wave.* **doll's head p.,** an abnormal extraocular muscle manifestation of many ophthalmologic syndromes and conditions: the eyes depress as the head is bent backward. **Doppler p.,** see under *effect.* **Duckworth's p.,** arrest of breathing before stoppage of the heart's action in certain fatal brain conditions. **Erb's p.,** Erb's sign, def. 1. **Erben's p.,** see under *reflex.* **face p., facia′lis p.,** Chvostek's sign. **fall-and-rise p.,** the drop in the number of bacteria that occurs at the beginning of drug treatment and the gradual rise that follows, even while treatment continues. **Felton's p.,** immunologic unresponsiveness or tolerance to pneumococcal polysaccharide induced in mice by administration of large doses of the antigen. **fern p.,** see *ferning.* **Fick's p.,** a fogging of vision, with the appearance of halos around light, occurring in individuals wearing contact lenses. **finger p.** (in hemiplegia), 1. extension of all the fingers or of the thumb and index finger, on pressure against the pisiform bone; called also *Gordon's sign.* 2. Souques' p. **first set p.,** the immunological reaction of the body against a tissue or organ in a host not previously sensitized against the graft antigens. Called also *first-set rejection.* See also *second-set p.* **flicker p.,** see under *flicker.* **Friedreich's p.,** the tympanic note of skodaic resonance in pleuritis with effusion varies in pitch during inspiration and expiration, being raised on inspiration. **Galassi's pupillary p.,** orbicularis pupillary reflex. **Gärtner's p.,** the degree of fulness of the veins of the arm as it is raised to varying heights indicates the degree of pressure in the right atrium. **Gengou p.,** complement fixation. **Gerhardt's p.,** see under *sign*. **glass-rod p., positive,** aqueous-influx p. **glass-rod p., negative,** blood-influx p. **Goldblatt p.,** ischemic tubular atrophy, a characteristic of renovascular hypertension. **Gowers' p.,** see under *sign* (def. 2). **Grasset's p., Grasset-Gaussel p.,** inability of a patient to raise both legs at the same time, though he can raise either alone; seen in incomplete organic hemiplegia. **Gunn's p.,** see under *syndrome*. **Gunn's pupillary p.,** swinging flashlight sign. **halisteresis p.,** selective withdrawal of bone salt from already calcified tissue. **Hamburger p.,** chloride shift. **Hammerschlag's p.,** abnormal fatigability toward continuous sounds of gradually decreasing intensity. **Hata p.,** increase in severity of an infectious disease when a small dose of a chemotherapeutical remedy is given. **Hecht p.,** Rumpel-Leede p. **Hektoen p.,** when antigens are introduced into the animal body in allergic states, there may exist an increased range of new antibody production which may include production of antibodies concerned in previous infections and immunizations. **Hering's p.,** a faint murmur heard with the stethoscope over the lower end of the sternum for a short time after death. **Hertwig-Magendie p.,** skew deviation. **hip-flexion p.,** in paraplegia, when the patient attempts to rise from a lying position, he flexes the hip of the paralyzed side. **Hochsinger's p.,** pressure on the inner side of the biceps muscle produces closure of the fist in tetany. **Hoffmann's p.,** increased excitability to electrical stimulation in the sensory nerves; the ulnar nerve is usually tested. **Holmes' p., Holmes-Stewart p.,** rebound p. **Houssay p.,** hypoglycemia and marked increase in sensitiveness to insulin produced by hypophysectomy in depancreatized experimental animals. **Hunt's paradoxical p.,** in dystonia musculorum deformans, if the examiner attempts forcible plantar flexion of the foot that is in dorsal spasm there is produced increase of the dorsal spasm, but if the patient is ordered to extend the foot he will perform plantar flexion. **jaw-winking p.,** Gunn's syndrome. **Kienböck's p.,** paradoxical diaphragm contraction: the hemidiaphragm on one side rises on inspiration and falls on expiration. **Koch's p.,** if a guinea pig which has been previously infected with tuberculosis organisms is reinjected intracutaneously, the skin over the injected area undergoes necrosis and a superficial ulcer develops. The ulcer heals quickly and infection of regional lymph nodes is retarded. The phenomenon demonstrates development of ability to localize tubercle bacilli. **Koebner's p.,** a cutaneous response seen in certain dermatoses, e.g., psoriasis, lichen planus, and infectious eczematoid dermatitis, manifested by the appearance on uninvolved skin of lesions typical of the skin disease at the site of trauma, on scars, or at points where articles of clothing (e.g., a belt) produce pressure. Called also *isomorphic effect*. **Kohnstamm's p.,** aftermovement. **Kühne's muscular p.,** Porret's p. **LE p.,** the process by which the LE cell is formed. **Leede-Rumpel p.,** Rumpel-Leede p. **Le Grand-Geblewics p.,** a flickering colored light (40–50 per second) observed indirectly is perceived as a constant white light. **Leichtenstern's p.,** see under *sign*. **Lewis' p.,** hydrophagocytosis. **Liacopoulos p.,** nonspecific immunosuppression to an antigen induced by administration of large doses of an unrelated antigen. **Liesegang's p.,** the peculiar periodic formation of a precipitate in concentric banded rings, waves, or spirals, when two electrolytes diffuse into and meet in a colloid gel. **Litten's diaphragm p.,** a movable horizontal depression of the lower part of the sides of the thorax, seen in respiration. **Lucio's p.,** a local exacerbation reaction occurring in diffuse lepromatous leprosy, characterized histologically by ischemic necrosis of the epidermis as a result of necrotizing vasculitis of small blood vessels of the subpapillary plexus, and clinically by the eruption of crops of small erythematous lesions with central necrosis; the eschar may be shed, revealing ulceration, with eventual scar formation. Cf. *erythema nodosum leprosum*. **Lust's p.,** abduction with dorsal flexion of the foot on tapping the external popliteal nerve just below the head of the fibula; indicative of spasmophilia. **Marcus Gunn p.,** see *Gunn's syndrome*, under *syndrome*. **Marcus Gunn pupillary p.,** swinging flashlight sign. **Meirowsky**

p., darkening of existing melanin, perhaps by oxidation, beginning within seconds and complete within minutes to a few hours after exposure to long-wave ultraviolet radiation. See also *tan* (def. 2). **Mills-Reincke p.,** the mortality from all diseases decreases as a result of water purification. **muscle p.,** the tendency of striated muscle to contract in hard lumps upon tapping. **Narsaroff's p.,** the difference in rectal temperature before and after a cold bath gradually decreases as cold baths are repeated. **Negro's p.,** cogwheel p. **Neisser-Wechsberg p.,** complement deviation. **Orbeli p.,** when the response of a nerve-muscle preparation is diminishing because of fatigue, stimulation of the sympathetic nerve increases the height of the contractions. **orbicularis p.,** orbicularis pupillary reflex. **paradoxical diaphragm p.,** one hemidiaphragm moves upward on inspiration and downward on expiration, opposite to the movements on the contralateral side; seen in phrenic nerve paralysis and eventration. **paradoxical p. of dystonia,** Hunt's paradoxical p. **paradoxical pupillary p.,** 1. reversed pupillary reflex. 2. see under *reflex* (def. 2). **peroneal-nerve p.,** Lust's p. **Pfeiffer's p.,** the lysis of *Vibrio cholerae* when injected into the peritoneal cavity of an immunized guinea pig; the term is also used to describe the in vitro lysis of cholera vibrios or other bacteria when incubated with specific antibody and complement. **phi p.,** the perception of the sequential flashing of a stationary row of lights as a moving light. **phrenic p.,** diaphragm p. **Piltz-Westphal p.,** orbicularis pupillary reflex. **Pool's p.,** 1. Schlesinger's sign. 2. contraction of the muscles of the arm following the raising of the arm above the head with the forearm extended, so as to cause stretching of the brachial plexus; seen in postoperative tetany. **Porret's p.,** the passage of a continuous current through a living muscle fiber causes an undulation proceeding from the positive toward the negative pole. **psi p.** [*psyche*], an experience or effect that appears to be produced without physical agency or intermediation. **Purkinje's p.,** as the intensity of illumination decreases and the eye becomes scotopic, the region of maximum visual acuity shifts from red-yellow to blue-green, the reds becoming less luminous, the blues more luminous. Called also *Purkinje's effect* and *shift*. **Queckenstedt's p.,** see under *sign*. **radial p.,** the involuntary dorsal flexion of the wrist which occurs on palmar flexion of the fingers. **Raynaud's p.,** intermittent bilateral attacks of ischemia of the fingers or toes and sometimes of the ears or nose, marked by severe pallor, and often accompanied by paresthesia and pain; it is brought on characteristically by cold or emotional stimuli and relieved by heat, and is due to an underlying disease or anatomical abnormality. When the condition is idiopathic or primary it is termed *Raynaud's disease*. **rebound p.,** a manifestation of loss of coordination between groups of antagonistic muscles of the extremities in cerebellar dysfunction. It may be demonstrated by having the patient extend both arms horizontally, the examiner then tapping both outstretched arms sharply. The normal arm returns to position promptly, whereas the affected arm overshoots the original position and may oscillate several times before achieving it. Or, the patient rests his elbow on a table and tries to flex his arm against the resistance of the examiner. When the resistance is suddenly withdrawn, the affected arm rebounds to the patient's chest, whereas the normal arm flexes only slightly, the flexion being arrested by contraction of antagonistic muscles (the triceps). **reclotting p.,** thixotropy. **release p.,** the unhampered activity of a lower center when a higher inhibiting control is removed. **Rieger's p.,** brake p. **Ritter-Rollet p.,** flexion of the foot upon a gentle electric stimulation, and its extension upon energetic stimulation. **Rumpel-Leede p.,** the appearance of minute subcutaneous hemorrhages below the area at which a rubber bandage is applied not too tightly for ten minutes upon the upper arm; characteristic of scarlet fever and hemorrhagic diathesis. **Rust's p.,** in caries or cancer of the upper cervical vertebrae, the patient supports his head with his hands when rising from or assuming a lying position; see also under *syndrome*. **satellite p.,** the more luxuriant development of a colony of microorganisms when in the neighborhood of a foreign colony, as shown by *Hemophilus influenzae* when contaminated by *Staphylococcus pyogenes* var. *aureus*. **Schellong-Strisower p.,** fall of systolic blood pressure on assuming an erect posture from the lying down position. **Schlesinger's p.,** see under *sign*. **Schramm's p.,** visibility with the cystoscope of a whole or part of the posterior urethra; seen in spinal cord disease. **Schüller's p.,** in hemiplegia due to organic lesion, the patient walks sideward more easily to the affected side than to the healthy side. **Schultz-Charlton p.,** see under *reaction.* **second-set p.,** the accelerated and intensified rejection by the recipient of a second graft of tissue from the same donor as a consequence of the primary immune response (i.e., antibody production and cell-mediated immunity) induced by the first graft. called also *second-set rejection.* **Sherrington p.,** the response of the hind limb musculature on stimulation of a motor nerve which has previously been degenerated. **shot-silk p.,** see under *retina.* **Shwartzman p.,** see under *reaction.* **Simonsen p.,** a graft-versus-host reaction produced by injection of lymphocytes from adult chickens into chick embryos; the principal features are splenomegaly and hemolytic anemia. **Sinkler's p.,** in an extremity with spastic paralysis, sharp flexion of the toe may be followed by flexion of the knee and hip. **Somogyi p.,** a rebound phenomenon occurring in diabetes: overtreatment with insulin induces hypoglycemia, which initiates the release of epinephrine, ACTH, glucagon, and growth hormone, which stimulate lipolysis, gluconeogenesis, and glycogenolysis, which, in turn, result in a rebound hyperglycemia and ketosis. Called also *Somogyi effect.* **Soret p.,** see under *effect.* **Souques' p.,** a phenomenon seen in incomplete hemiplegia, consisting of involuntary extension and separation of the fingers when the arm is raised; called also *finger p.* **springlike p.,** André-Thomas sign. **staircase p.,** treppe. **Staub-Traugott p.,** after a glucose load is administered, subsequent loads, given after a short interval, are disposed of at an accelerated rate. **Straus' p.,** see under *reaction.* **Strümpell p.,** dorsiflexion and supination of the foot on flexing the extended leg against resistance offered by the examiner. **Sulzberger-Chase p.,** abolition of dermal contact hypersensitivity to sensitizing agents, e.g., picryl chloride, produced by prior oral feeding of the agent. **Theobald Smith's p.,** guinea pigs which have been used for standardizing diphtheria antitoxin and have thus been injected with a small dose of blood serum become highly susceptible to the serum and may die very promptly if given a rather large second dose of the same serum a few weeks later. See *anaphylaxis.* **toe p.,** Babinski's reflex. **tongue p.,** a slight blow upon the tongue produces a contraction with the appearance of deep depressions; seen in tetany. Called also *Schultze's sign* and *tongue test.* **Trousseau's p.,** spasmodic contractions of muscles provoked by pressure upon the nerves which go to them; seen in tetany. **Twort-d'Herelle p.,** the phenomenon of transmissible bacterial lysis; bacteriophagia. When to a broth culture of typhoid or dysentery bacilli there is added a drop of filtered broth emulsion of the stool from a convalescent typhoid or dysentery patient, complete lysis of the bacterial culture will occur in a few hours. If a drop of this lysed culture is added to another culture of the bacilli, lysis will take place exactly as in the first. A drop of this culture will then dissolve a third culture, and so on through hundreds of transfers. d'Herelle attributed this phenomenon to the action of an ultramicroscopic parasite of bacteria, which he named the *bacteriophage.* See *bacterial virus,* under *virus.* **Tyndall p.,** the rendering visible of a transverse beam of light through its being broken up by solid particles suspended in a liquid or gas. **Wedensky's p.,** on applying a series of rapidly repeated stimuli to a nerve, the muscle contracts quickly in response to the first stimulus and then fails to respond further; but if the stimuli are applied to the nerve at a slower rate, the muscle responds to all of them. **Wenckebach p.,** the generation of impulses by the sinus node of the heart at a constant rate while the P-R interval grows progressively longer during several beats until an atrial complex is not followed by a ventricular complex. **Westphal's p.,** 1. (A. K. O. *Westphal*) orbicularis pupillary reflex. 2. (C. F. O. Westphal) see under *sign.* **Westphal-Piltz p.,** orbicularis pupillary reflex. **Wever-Bray p.,** cochlear microphonics. **Williams' p.,** the tympanic note of skodaic resonance in pleuritis with effusion varies in pitch with the opening and closing of the patient's mouth.

phenon (fē′non) phenom.

phenopropazine (fe″no-pro′pah-zēn) ethopropazine hydrochloride.

phenothiazine (fe″no-thi′ah-zēn) 1. a greenish, tasteless compound, $C_{12}H_9NS$, prepared by fusing diphenylamine with sulfur; used as a veterinary anthelmintic. Called also *dibenzo-*

thiazine, thiodiphenylamine. 2. any of a group of psychotherapeutic agents (e.g., chlorpromazine) resembling phenothiazine in molecular structure, i.e., all sharing a three-ring structure in which two benzene rings are joined by a sulfur and nitrogen atom. They are potent adrenergic blocking agents, their pharmacologic actions including central nervous system depression, prolongation and potentiation of the effects of narcotic and hypnotic drugs, hypotensive activity, and antispasmodic, antihistaminic, and antiemetic activity.

phenotype (fe′no-tīp) [*pheno-* (def. 1) + *type*] 1. the entire physical, biochemical, and physiological makeup of an individual as determined both genetically and environmentally, as opposed to genotype. 2. the expression of a single gene or gene pair. **Bombay p.,** a rare phenotype produced by the interaction of genes of the ABO blood group and a rare recessive gene at a different locus, resulting in a complete lack of H antigen. Cells of individuals possessing the Bombay phenotype lack A, B, and H antigen, and their serum contains anti-A, anti-B and anti-H antigen.

phenotypic (fe″no-tip′ik) pertaining to or expressive of the phenotype.

Phenoxene (fĕ-nok′sēn) trademark for a preparation of chlorphenoxamine hydrochloride.

phenoxide (fen-ok′sīd) phenolate.

phenoxy- a prefix indicating the presence of the group OC_6H_5, composed of phenyl and an atom of oxygen.

phenoxybenzamine hydrochloride (fĕ-nok″se-ben′-zah-mēn) [USP] chemical name: *N*-(2-chloroethyl)-*N*-(1-methyl-2-phenoxyethyl)benzenemethanamine hydrochloride. A potent α-adrenergic blocking agent, $C_{18}H_{22}ClNO\cdot$HCl, occurring as a white, crystalline powder; used as an antihypertensive, administered orally.

phenozygous (fe″no-zi′gus) [Gr. *phainein* to show + *zygon* yoke] having the cranium much narrower than the face, so that the zygomatic arches are seen when the skull is viewed from above. Cf. *cryptozygous.*

phenprocoumon (fen-pro′koo-mon) [USP] chemical name: 4-hydroxy-3-(1-phenylpropyl)-2*H*-1-benzopyran. One of the synthetic coumarin anticoagulants, $C_{13}H_{16}O_3$, occurring as a fine, white, crystalline powder, having a more rapid onset and longer-acting effects than dicumarol and having a marked cumulative effect; administered orally.

phenpromethamine hydrochloride (fen″pro-meth′-ah-mēn) phenylpropylmethylamine hydrochloride.

phenpropionate (fen-pro′pe-o-nāt″) USAN contraction for 3-phenylpropionate.

phensuximide (fen-suk′sĭ-mīd) [USP] chemical name: 1-methyl-3-phenyl-2,5-pyrrolidinedione. An anticonvulsant, $C_{11}H_{11}NO_2$, occurring as a white to off-white, crystalline powder; used mainly in the treatment of petit mal epilepsy, administered orally.

phentermine (fen′ter-mēn) chemical name: α,α,-dimethylbenzeneethanamine. An adrenergic isomeric with amphetamine, $C_{10}H_{15}N$, occurring as a colorless, oily liquid; used as an anorexic, administered orally as a complex with an ion-exchange resin to produce a sustained action. **p. hydrochloride,** the water-soluble hydrochloride salt of phentermine, $C_{10}H_{15}N\cdot$HCl, occurring as a white, crystalline powder; used as an anorexic, administered orally.

phentolamine (fen-tol′ah-mēn) chemical name: 3-[[(4,5-dihydro -1*H*- imidazol -2- yl)methyl](4 -methylphenyl)amino] phenol. An antiadrenergic, $C_{17}H_{19}N_3O$, which blocks the hypertensive action of epinephrine and norepinephrine and most smooth muscle responses involving alpha-adrenergic cell receptors. **p. hydrochloride** [USP], the monohydrochloride salt of phentolamine, $C_{17}H_{19}N_3O\cdot$HCl, occurring as a white to off-white, crystalline powder, having the same antiadrenergic actions as the base; used mainly in the treatment of peripheral vascular diseases and to prevent and control hypertension due to pheochromocytoma, administered orally. **p. mesylate** [USP], the methanesulfonate salt of phentolamine, $C_{17}H_{19}N_3O\cdot CH_4O_3S$, occurring as a white, crystalline powder, having the same antiadrenergic actions as the base; used mainly in the diagnosis or pheochromocytoma and in the prevention and treatment of cutaneous necrosis and sloughing when extravasation of norepinephrine occurs after intravenous administration, administered intramuscularly and intravenously.

Phenurone (fen′u-rōn) trademark for a preparation of phenacemide.

phenyl (fen′il, fe′nil) the univalent radical, C_6H_5. Symbol Ph. **p. aminosalicylate,** chemical name: 4-amino-2-hydroxybenzoic acid phenyl ester; a tuberculostatic antibacterial, $C_{13}H_{11}NO_3$. **p. carbinol,** benzyl alcohol. **p. hydrate, p. hydroxide,** phenol. **p. mercury acetate** phenylmercuric acetate. **p. mercury nitrate,** phenylmercuric nitrate. **p. salicylate,** a compound occurring in fine white crystals, or as a white crystalline powder, $C_{13}H_{10}O_3$; formerly used as an analgesic, antipyretic, intestinal antiseptic, enteric coating for tablets, and in preparations used in the prevention of sunburn. In veterinary medicine, it is sometimes used internally as an antipyretic and externally as an antiseptic. Called also *salol.*

phenylacetic acid (fen′il-ah-se′tik) an abnormal catabolite of phenylalanine produced by oxidation of phenyllactic acid in phenylketonuria; it is excreted in the urine as the glutamine conjugate.

phenylacetylurea (fen′il-as′′ĕ-til-u-re′ah) phenacemide.

phenylalanine (fen′il-al′ah-nīn) a naturally occurring amino acid, $C_6H_5 \cdot CH_2CH(NH_2)COOH$, discovered in 1879 by Schulze; essential for optimal growth in infants and for nitrogen equilibrium in human adults.

phenylalanine 4-hydroxylase (fen′′il-al′′ah-nīn hi-drok′-sĭ-lās) phenylalanine 4-monooxygenase.

phenylalanine hydroxylase deficiency phenylketonuria.

phenylalanine 4-monooxygenase (fen′′il-al′ah-nēn mon′′o-ok′si-jĕ-nās) [EC 1.14.16.1] an enzyme of the oxidoreductase class that catalyzes the reaction L-phenylalanine + tetrahydrobiopterin + O_2 = L-tyrosine + dihydrobiopterin + H_2O, the reaction synthesizing tyrosine from phenylalanine. Called also *phenylalanine 4-hydroxylase.*

phenylalaninemia (fen′′il-al′′ah-nĭ-ne′me-ah) hyperphenylalaninemia.

phenylalanyl (fen′′il-al′ah-nil) the acyl radical of phenylalanine.

phenylbutazone (fen′′il-bu′tah-zōn) [USP] chemical name: 4-butyl-1,2-diphenyl-3,5-pyrazolidinedione. A congener of aminopyrine and antipyrine, $C_{19}H_{20}N_2O_2$, having analgesic, antipyretic, anti-inflammatory, and mild uricosuric properties; used especially in the treatment of gout, rheumatoid arthritis, ankylosing spondylitis, and other rheumatoid conditions, administered orally. It is given for periods of less than one week because it can cause aplastic anemia and agranulocytosis. Called also *diphe.*

phenylcarbinol (fen′′il-kar′bĭ-nol) benzyl alcohol.

phenylcinchoninic acid (fen′′il-sing′′ko-nin′ik) cinchophen.

phenyldimethylpyrazolon (fen′′il-di-meth′′il-pi-ra′zo-lon) antipyrine.

phenylene (fe′nĭ-lēn) a divalent radical, $= C_6H_4$.

phenylephrine hydrochloride (fen′′il-ef′rin) [USP] chemical name: (S)-3-hydroxy-α-[(methylamino)methyl]benzenemethanol hydrochloride. An adrenergic with strong alpha-receptor stimulant activity, $C_9H_{13}NO_2 \cdot HCl$; used as a vasoconstrictor to decongest nasal and laryngeal mucous membranes, to produce mydriasis without cycloplegia, to maintain blood pressure during spinal and inhalation anesthesia, to treat vascular failure in drug-induced shock, shocklike states, and hypotension, to prolong spinal anesthesia, and to treat supraventricular tachycardia. It is applied topically or administered by intramuscular or intravenous injection or infusion.

phenylethylbarbituric acid (fen′′il-eth′′il-bahr′′bĭ-tu′rik) phenobarbital.

phenylglycolic acid (fen′′il-gli-ko′lik) mandelic acid.

phenylhydrazine (fen′′il-hi′drah-zin) an oily liquid principle, $C_6H_5NH \cdot NH_2$, used as a reagent for sugars, ketones, and aldehydes. Its hydrochloride is also used as a reagent, and has been used as an oral hemolytic in the treatment of polycythemia vera. See also *Kowarsky's test* (def. 1) and *von Jaksch's test* (def. 2), under *tests.*

phenylic (fe-nil′ik) pertaining to phenyl.

phenylic acid (fĕ-nil′ik) phenol (1).

phenylindanedione (fen′′il-in-dān′de-ōn) phenindione.

phenylketonuria (PKU) (fen′′il-ke′′to-nu′re-ah) [*phenyl-* + *ketonuria*] hyperphenylalaninemia, type I: phenylalanine accumulation resulting in mental retardation (phenylpyruvic oligophrenia), neurologic manifestations (including

hyperkinesia, epilepsy, and microcephaly), light pigmentation, eczema, and a mousy odor, unless treated by a diet low in phenylalanine. Called also *PKU1, phenylalanine hydroxylase deficiency, oligophrenia phenylpyruvica, Fφlling disease,* and *classic p.* **atypical p.,** hyperphenylalaninemia, type V. **maternal p.,** an intrauterine development in pregnant women with PKU (the genotype of the conceptus being irrelevant) and, among the surviving non-phenylketonuric (heterozygous) offspring, in severe mental retardation (up to 90 per cent of the children), microcephaly (up to 70 per cent), low birth weight (50 per cent), and random anomalies of the skeletal, cardiac, vascular, intestinal, ocular, hematopoietic, and pulmonary systems. **p. II,** hyperphenylalaninemia, type IV. **p. III,** hyperphenylalaninemia, type V.

phenyllactic acid (fen′′il-lak′tik) an abnormal product of phenylalanine catabolism produced by reduction of phenylpyruvic acid in phenylketonuria and excreted in the urine.

phenylmercuric (fen′′il-mer-ku′rik) denoting a compound containing the radical C_6H_5Hg—, forming various antiseptic, antibacterial, and fungicidal salts. **p. acetate,** chemical name: (aceto-O)phenylmercury. 1. a crystalline salt, $C_8H_8HgO_2$. 2. [NF] a compound with properties similar to those of phenylmercuric nitrate, occurring as a white to creamy white, crystalline powder or as small white prisms or leaflets; used as a bacteriostatic preservative in pharmaceutical preparation, and in solution as a vaginal douche for adjunctive therapy in trichomonal, candidal, bacterial, and mixed infections and nonspecific leukorrhea. It is also widely used as a herbicide, especially for crabgrass. Called also *phenyl mercury acetate.* **p. nitrate,** chemical name: (nitrato- O)phenylmercury. 1. the normal salt, $C_6H_5HgNO_3$, which is converted to the basic compound (see def. 2) in aqueous solution or in moist air. 2. [NF] *basic p. nitrate:* an antibacterial and antifungal compound of phenylmercuric nitrate and its hydroxide, containing 87 to 87.9 per cent of $C_6H_5Hg^+$(phenylmercuric ion), and 62.75 to 63.50 per cent Hg (mercury), occurring as a white, crystalline powder; used as a bacteriostatic preservative in pharmaceuticals, and as an antiseptic for various topical uses. Called also *phenyl mercury nitrate.*

phenylmethanol (fen′′il-meth′ah-nol) benzyl alcohol.

phenylpropanolamine hydrochloride (fen′′il-pro′′pah-nol′- ah-mēn hi′′dro-klo′rīd) [USP] chemical name: (±) (R*,S*)-α-(1-aminoethyl)benzenemethanol hydrochloride. An adrenergic structurally and pharmacologically related to amphetamine and ephedrine, $C_9H_{13}NO \cdot HCl$, occurring as a white, crystalline powder; used as a vasoconstrictor to decongest mucous membranes, applied topically, and to produce bronchodilation in the symptomatic control of allergic manifestations, administered orally. It has also been used as a central nervous system stimulant and as an anorexic.

phenylpropylmethylamine hydrochloride (fen′′il-pro′′- pil-meth′′il-am′ēn) chemical name: N,β-dimethyl-phenethylamine hydrochloride. An adrenergic with chiefly alpha-receptor activity, $C_{10}H_{15}N \cdot HCl$, used mainly as a vasoconstrictor to decongest mucous membranes, applied topically by inhalation. Called also *phenpromethamine hydrochloride.*

phenylpyruvic acid (fen′′il-pi-roo′vik) an abnormal product in phenylketonura, produced by transamination of phenylalanine when the normal catabolic pathway, hydroxylation of phenylalanine to form tyrosine, is blocked.

phenylpyruvicaciduria (fen′′il-pi-ru′′vik-as′′ĭ-du′re-ah) phenylketonuria.

phenylthiocarbamide (fen′′il-thi′′o-kar-bam′id) phenylthiourea.

phenylthiourea (fen′′il-thi′′o-u-re′ah) a compound, C_6H_5-NHCSNH$_2$, used in genetics in dry crystal form or in 5 per cent solution. The ability to taste it is inherited as a dominant trait, the compound being intensely bitter to approximately 70 per cent of the population, and nearly tasteless to the rest. Called also *phenylthiocarbamide* or *PTC.*

phenyltoloxamine citrate (fen′′il-tol-ok′sah-mēn) chemical name: N,N-dimethyl-2-[2-(phenylmethyl)phenoxy]ethanamine citrate. An isomer of diphenhydramine, C_{17}-$H_{21}NO$, used as an antihistaminic, mainly to decongest the nasal mucosa, administered orally.

phenyramidol hydrochloride (fen′′ĭ-ram′ĭ-dol) chemical name: α[(2-pyridylamino)methyl]benzenemethanolmonohydrochloride; an analgesic and skeletal muscle relaxant, $C_{13}H_{14}N_2O$ HCl.

phenytoin (fen′ĭ-to-in) [USP] chemical name: 5,5-diphenyl-2,4-imidazolidinedione. An anticonvulsant and cardiac depressant, $C_{15}H_{12}N_2O_2$, occurring as a white powder; used in the treatment of all forms of epilepsy except petit mal and as an antiarrhythmic, administered orally. Called also *diphenylhydantoin*. **p. sodium** [USP], the monosodium salt of phenytoin, $C_{15}H_{22}N_2NaO_2$, having the same appearance, actions, and uses as the base; administered orally and intravenously.

phe(o)- [Gr. *phaios* dun, dusky] a combining form meaning brown, dun, or dusky. For words beginning thus, see also those beginning *phae(o)-*.

pheochrome (fe′o-krōm) [Gr. *phaios* dusky + *chrōma* color] staining dark with chromium salts; said of certain embryonic cells; chromaffin.

pheochromoblast (fe″o-kro′mo-blast) any of the embryonic structures which develop into pheochrome (chromaffin) cells.

pheochromoblastoma (fe″o-kro″mo-blas-to′mah) pheochromocytoma.

pheochromocyte (fe″o-kro′mo-sīt) [*pheochrome* + Gr. *kytos* hollow vessel] a chromaffin cell.

pheochromocytoma (fe-o-kro″mo-si-to′mah) [*pheochromocyte* + *-oma*] a usually benign, well-encapsulated, lobular, vascular tumor of chromaffin tissue of the adrenal medulla or sympathetic paraganglia. The cardinal symptom, reflecting the increased secretion of epinephrine and norepinephrine, is hypertension, which may be persistent or intermittent. During severe attacks, there may be headache, sweating, palpitation, apprehension, tremor, pallor or flushing of the face, nausea and vomiting, pain in the chest and abdomen, and paresthesias of the extremities.

pheophytin (fe″o-fi′tin) [Gr. *phaios* dusky + *phyton* plant] a brown pigment derived from chlorophyll by removal of magnesium.

pheresis (fĕ-re′sis) [Gr. *aphairesis* removal] any procedure in which blood is withdrawn from a donor, a portion (plasma, leukocytes, etc.) is separated and retained, and the remainder is retransfused into the donor. It includes plasmapheresis, leukapheresis, etc. More properly called *apheresis*.

pheromone (fer′o-mōn) a substance secreted to the outside of the body by an individual and perceived (as by smell) by a second individual of the same species, releasing a specific reaction of behavior in the percipient. **alarm p.,** a mucus secreted by the earthworm on noxious stimulation, which is aversive to other members of the species.

phetharbital (feth-ar′bĭ-tal) chemical name: 5,5-diethyl-1-phenylbarbituric acid. A nonhypnotic barbiturate, $C_{14}H_{16}N_2O_3$, which has been used as an anticonvulsant and in the treatment of unconjugated hyperbilirubinemia.

Ph.G. Graduate in Pharmacy; Pharmacopoeia Germanica (German pharmacopeia).

Φ, φ phi, the twenty-first letter of the Greek alphabet.

phi (fi) [Φ, φ] the twenty-first letter of the Greek alphabet.

phial (fi′al) a vial or small bottle.

phialide (fi′ah-līd) [Gr. *phialis*, dim. of *phiale* a broad flat vessel] 1. a flask-shaped projection from the mycelium of certain fungi that gives rise to endogenous basipetally produced spores. 2. the end cell of a phialophore.

Phialophora (fi″ah-lof′o-rah) a genus of imperfect fungi of the family Dematiaceae, order Moniliales. *P. verrucosa* is a cause of chromomycosis, a chronic subcutaneous fungous infection, and *P. jeanselmi* is an etiologic agent of maduromycosis.

phialophore (fi′ah-lo-fōr) the branch of the mycelium which bears at its tip the phialospores of certain fungi.

phialospore (fi′ah-lo-spōr) a spore which is borne at the end of a phialide or a phialophore.

-phil, -phile [Gr. *philos* loving, dear] a word termination denoting one having an affinity for something.

Philasterina (fil″as-tĕ-ri′nah) [Gr. *philein* to love + *astēr* star, starfish] a suborder of cilate protozoa (order Scuticociliatida, subclass Hymenostomatia), characterized by the presence of a paroral membrane with reduced infraciliature in the anterior and posterior segments, transient scutica, and prominent, rod-shaped mucocysts. They are found especially in brackish or marine habitats.

-phile see *-phil.*

-philia [Gr. *philein* to love] a word termination denoting (*a*) an abnormal craving or attraction or (*b*) an affinity for an object denoted by the word stem to which it is affixed.

philiater (fi-li′ah-ter) [Gr. *philos* fond + *iatreia* healing] a person interested in medical science, particularly a medical student.

-philic [Gr. *philos* loving] a word termination meaning having an affinity for.

Philip's glands (fil′ips) [Sir Robert William *Philip*, Scottish physician, 1857–1939] see under *gland*.

Philippe-Gombault tract (fe-lēp′-gom-bo′) [Claudius *Philippe*, French pathologist, 1866–1903; François Alexis Albert *Gombault*, French neurologist, 1844– 1904] Gombault-Philippe triangle.

phillyrin (fil′ĭ-rin) a crystalline substance, $C_{27}H_{34}O_{11}$, from the leaves and bark of various species of *Phillyrea*, a genus of evergreen shrubs, e.g., *P. latifolia* L. (Oleaceae), which has antimalarial properties.

philter (fil′ter) a substance or object alleged to provoke love or carnal appetite.

philtrum (fil′trum) [Gr. *philtron* love potion] 1. [NA] the vertical groove in the median portion of the upper lip, a part of the prolabium. 2. a philter.

phimosis (fi-mo′sis) [Gr. *phimōsis* a muzzling or closure] constriction of the preputial orifice so that the prepuce cannot be retracted back over the glans. **p. vagina′lis,** atresia of the vagina.

phimotic (fi-mot′ik) pertaining to phimosis.

pHisoHex (fi′so-heks) trademark for an emulsion containing hexachlorophene.

phlebalgia (flĕ-bal′je-ah) [*phleb-* + *-algia*] pain due to varices within or on the surface of a nerve.

phlebanesthesia (fleb″an-es-the′ze-ah) phlebonarcosis.

phlebangioma (fleb″an-je-o′mah) [*phleb-* + *angioma*] a venous aneurysm.

phlebarteriectasia (fleb″ar-te″re-ek-ta′ze-ah) [*phleb-* + Gr. *artēria* artery + *ektasis* extension] general dilatation of veins and arteries.

phlebasthenia (fleb″as-the′ne-ah) [*phleb-* + *a* neg. + Gr. *sthenos* strength + *-ia*] impairment of the vitality of the walls of blood vessels.

phlebectasia (fleb″ek-ta′ze-ah) [*phleb-* + Gr. *ektasis* dilatation + *-ia*] a varicosity; a dilatation of a vein. **p. laryn′gis,** permanent dilatation of the veins of the larynx, especially those of the vocal cords.

phlebectasis (fle-bek′tah-sis) phlebectasia.

phlebectomy (fle-bek′to-me) [*phleb-* + Gr. *ektomē* excision] excision of a vein, or of a part of a vein.

phlebectopia (fleb″ek-to′pe-ah) [*phleb-* + Gr. *ektopos* out of place + *-ia*] displacement of a vein.

phlebectopy (fle-bek′to-pe) phlebectopia.

phlebemphraxis (fleb″em-frak′sis) [*phleb-* + Gr. *emphraxis* stoppage] the stoppage of a vein by a plug or clot.

phlebexairesis (fleb″ek-si′rĕ-sis) [*phleb-* + Gr. *exairesis* a taking out] surgical removal of a vein.

phlebismus (fle-biz′mus) obstruction and consequent turgescence of veins.

phlebitic (flĕ-bit′ik) pertaining to phlebitis.

phlebitis (flĕ-bi′tis) [*phleb-* + *-itis*] inflammation of a vein. The condition is marked by infiltration of the coats of the vein and the formation of a thrombus. The disease is attended by edema, stiffness, and pain in the affected part, and in the septic variety by pyemic symptoms. **adhesive p.,** phlebitis which tends to the obliteration of the vein; called also *plastic p.* and *proliferative p.* **anemic p.,** a form associated with anemia or chlorosis. **blue p.,** phlegmasia cerulea dolens. **chlorotic p.,** anemic p. **gouty p.,** a variety associated with the gouty diathesis, often recurrent, and sometimes occlusive; a causal relation to gout is in question. **p. mi′grans, migrating p.,** recurrent phlebitis in peripheral veins. **obliterating p., obstructive p.,** phlebitis that permanently closes the lumen of a vein. **plastic p.,** adhesive p. **productive p.,** phlebosclerosis. **proliferative p.,** adhesive p. **puerperal p.,** septic inflammation of uterine or other veins following childbirth. **septic p.,** that which is related to a septic process, as in erysipelas, peritonitis, or endometritis. In it the thrombus breaks down and septic emboli are carried to distant parts of the body. Called also *suppurative p.* **sinus p.,** inflammation of a cerebral sinus. **suppurative p.,** septic p.

phleb(o)- [Gr. *phleps, phlebos* vein] a combining form denoting relationship to a vein or veins. See also words beginning *ven(o)-.*

phleboclysis (flĕ-bok'lĭ-sis) [*phlebo-* + Gr. *klysis* injection] injection of fluid into a vein. **drip p., slow p.,** phleboclysis in which the solution is instilled slowly, drop by drop.

phlebofibrosis (fleb″o-fi-bro'sis) fibrosis of the veins, as in phlebosclerosis.

phlebogenous (flĕ-boj'ĕ-nus) originating in a vein.

phlebogram (fleb'o-gram) [*phlebo-* + Gr. *gramma* a writing] 1. roentgenogram of a vein filled with contrast medium. 2. a tracing of the venous pulse made with a phlebograph or sphygmograph.

Jugular venous pulse

Phlebogram: *a,* a positive wave due to contraction of the right atrium; *c,* a venous wave due to contraction of the right ventricle, with downward movement of the tricuspid valve; *x,* a small negative wave due to atrial relaxation; *v,* the early diastolic wave, a positive wave occurring during ventricular contraction and reflecting the filling of the right atrium (also [not shown] the exaggerated positive wave related to reflux of blood through an incompetent atrioventricular valve); *y,* a negative wave due to emptying of the right atrium; *h,* an occasional, late filling wave.

phlebograph (fleb'o-graf) [*phlebo-* + Gr. *graphein* to write] an instrument for recording the venous pulse.

phlebography (flĕ-bog'rah-fe) [*phlebo-* + Gr. *graphein* to write] 1. roentgenography of a vein or veins by use of contrast medium. 2. the graphic recording of the venous pulse. 3. a description of the veins.

phleboid (fleb'oid) [*phlebo-* + Gr. *eidos* form] resembling a vein, or composed of veins.

phlebolith (fleb'o-lith) [*phlebo-* + Gr. *lithos* stone] a calculus or concretion in a vein; a vein stone.

phlebolithiasis (fleb″o-lĭ-thi'ah-sis) [*phlebo-* + Gr. *lithiasis*] a condition characterized by the development of vein stones.

phlebology (flĕ-bol'o-je) [*phlebo-* + *-logy*] the study of the veins and their diseases.

phlebomanometer (fleb″o-mah-nom'ĕ-ter) [*phlebo-* + *manometer*] an instrument for the direct measurement of venous blood pressure (Burch and Winsor).

phlebometritis (fleb″o-mĕ-tri'tis) [*phlebo-* + Gr. *metra* uterus + *-itis*] inflammation of the veins of the uterus.

phlebonarcosis (fleb″o-nar-ko'sis) narcosis produced by intravenous injections.

phlebophlebostomy (fleb″o-flĕ-bos'to-me) [*phlebo-* + Gr. *phleps* vein + *stomoun* to provide with an opening, or mouth] operative anastomosis of vein to vein.

phlebophthalmotomy (fleb″of-thal-mot'o-me) ophthalmophlebotomy.

phlebopiezometry (fleb″o-pi″ĕ-zom'ĕ-tre) [*phlebo-* + Gr. *piesis* pressure + *metron* measure] measurement of the venous pressure.

phleboplasty (fleb'o-plas″te) [*phlebo-* + Gr. *plassein* to form] plastic operation for the repair of a vein.

phleborrhagia (fleb″o-ra'je-ah) [*phlebo-* + Gr. *rhēgnynai* to burst forth] copious hemorrhage from a vein; venous hemorrhage.

phleborrhaphy (flĕ-bor'ah-fe) [*phlebo-* + Gr. *rhaphē* suture] the suturing of a vein.

phleborrhexis (fleb″o-rek'sis) [*phlebo-* + Gr. *rhēxis* rupture] rupture of a vein.

phlebosclerosis (fleb″o-skle-ro'sis) [*phlebo-* + Gr. *sklērōsis* hardening] fibrous thickening of the wall of the veins.

phlebosis (flĕ-bo'sis) abnormal noninflammatory changes in the veins.

phlebostasia (fleb″os-ta'ze-ah) phlebostasis.

phlebostasis (flĕ-bos'tah-sis) [*phlebo-* + Gr. *stasis* stoppage] 1. retardation of the flow of blood in the veins. 2. tempo-

rary sequestration of a portion of the blood from the general circulation by application of tourniquets on an extremity.

phlebostenosis (fleb″o-stĕ-no'sis) [*phlebo-* + Gr. *stenōsis* narrowing] stenosis or constriction of a vein.

phlebothrombosis (fleb″o-throm-bo'sis) [*phlebo-* + *thrombosis*] presence of a clot in a vein, unassociated with inflammation of the wall of the vein. Cf. *thrombophlebitis.*

phlebotome (fleb'o-tōm) a knife or lancet for use in phlebotomy.

phlebotomist (fle-bot'o-mist) one who practices phlebotomy.

phlebotomize (fle-bot'o-mīz) to bleed; to take blood from by phlebotomy.

Phlebotomus (flĕ-bot'o-mus) [*phlebo-* + Gr. *tomos* a cutting] a genus of very small, bloodsucking sandflies of the family Psychodidae, many species of which are vectors of disease-causing organisms. **P. argen'tipes,** the vector of visceral leishmaniasis in India. **P. chinen'sis,** the vector of visceral leishmaniasis in China. **P. lon'gipes,** a vector of *Leishmania aethiopica,* the etiologic agent of diffuse cutaneous leishmaniasis in Kenya and Ethiopia. **P. ma'jor,** a vector of *Leishmania donovani infantum* in the Mediterranean region. **P. marti'ni,** the major vector of visceral leishmaniasis in East Africa. **P. nogu'chi,** a species found in Peru which may transmit *Bartonella bacilliformis,* the etiologic agent of *Carrión's disease;* called also *Lutzomyia noguchii.* **P. orienta'lis,** the vector of visceral leishmaniasis in the Sudan. **P. papatas'ii,** a species that is the vector of the virus of phlebotomus fever, of protozoa of the *Leishmania tropica* complex; and of *L. donovani infantum.* **P. ped'ifer,** a vector of *Leishmania*

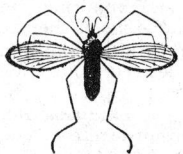

Phlebotomus papatasii.

aethiopica, the etiologic agent of diffuse cutaneous leishmaniasis in Kenya and Ethiopia. **P. pernicio'sus,** a vector of *Leishmania donovani infantum* in the Mediterranean region. **P. sergen'ti,** a vector of *Leishmania tropica,* the etiologic agent of the urban form of Old World cutaneous leishmaniasis. **P. verruca'rum,** a vector of *Bartonella bacilliformis,* the etiologic agent of Carrión's disease.

phlebotomy (flĕ-bot'o-me) [*phlebo-* + Gr. *tomē* a cutting] incision of a vein, as for the letting of blood; needle puncture of a vein for the drawing of blood; venesection. **bloodless p.,** phlebostasis, def. 2.

phlegm (flem) [Gr. *phlegma*] 1. a ropy, viscid, mucous secretion, such as that produced by the mucosa of the respiratory passages and discharged through the mouth. 2. in humoralism, one of the four humors of the body.

phlegmasia (fleg-ma'ze-ah) [Gr. "heat, inflammation"] inflammation or fever. **p. al'ba do'lens,** phlebitis of the femoral vein, occasionally following parturition or an acute febrile illness; it is characterized by swelling of the leg, usually without redness. Called also *leukophlegmasia* and *white leg.* **p. al'ba do'lens puerpera'rum,** postpartum iliofemoral thrombophlebitis. **cellulitic p.,** swelling and inflammation of the leg after childbirth from infection of the connective tissue. **p. ceru'lea do'lens,** an acute fulminating form of deep venous thrombosis, with reactive arterial spasm and pronounced edema of the extremity and severe cyanosis, purpuric areas, and petechiae; called also *blue phlebitis.* **thrombotic p.,** phlegmasia alba dolens.

phlegmatic (fleg-mat'ik) [Gr. *phlegmatikos*] characterized by an excess of the supposed humor called phlegm; hence, heavy, dull, and apathetic.

phlegmon (fleg'mon) [Gr. *phlegmonē*] 1. a spreading, diffuse inflammatory reaction to infection with microaerophilic streptococci, which forms a suppurative or gangrenous and undermining lesion that may extend into deep subcutaneous tissues and muscles, creating multiple small pockets of pus. Called also *phlegmonous cellulitis.* Cf. *cellulitis* and *erysipelas.* 2. a solid, swollen, inflamed mass of pancreatic tissue occurring as a complication of acute pancreatitis, which may subside spontaneously or become secondarily infected and develop into an abscess. Cf. *pseudocyst*, def. 2. **Holz p.,** a chronic cellulitis of the floor of the mouth and neck. **pancreatic p.,** see *phlegmon*, def. 2. **periurethral p.,** an extensive fulminating phlegmon originating in and about the urethra and usually accompanied by massive gangrene of the genital and perigenital tissues; called also *periurethral cellulitis*.

phlegmonosis (fleg″mo-no′us)   phlegmasia.

phlegmonous (fleg′mon-us)   pertaining to or attended by phlegmon; see under *cellulitis*.

phlobaphene (flo′bah-fēn) [Gr. *phloios* bark + *baphē* dye] one of a series of compounds resembling resins and differing from the latter only in that they dissolve in dilute ammonia water. They are derived from tannin by boiling with acids and are characterized by their brown color.

phloem (flo′em) [Gr. *phloios* bark]   a form of vascular tissue in plants which conducts synthesized nutrients, such as glucose, both up and down the stem or root, characterized by the presence of sieve tubes. Cf. *xylem*.

phlogistic (flo-jis′tik) [Gr. *phlogistos*]   inflammatory.

phlogisticozymoid (flo-jis″tĭ-ko-zi′moid)   a hypothetical substance supposed to supply the necessary feeding ground for inflammatory processes.

phlogiston (flo-jis′ton) [Gr. *phlogistos* burnt up, inflammable]   a term and general chemical theory of fire or inflammability proposed by George Ernst Stahl in 1702, warmly defended by Joseph Priestley, denied and disproved by Antoine Laurent Lavoisier (1775), and defunct after 1800. Phlogiston was a material substance present in and compounded with all combustible bodies and was released by combustion, the other structures of the substance being left behind. Liberation of phlogiston thus corresponds to oxidation, and combination with phlogiston, to reduction.

phlog(o)- [Gr. *phlox*, gen. *phlogos* flame]   a combining form denoting relationship to inflammation.

phlogocyte (flo′go-sīt) [*phlogo-* + *-cyte*]   a cell characteristic of tissue in an inflamed state; a plasma cell.

phlogocytosis (flo″go-si-to′sis)   presence of phlogocytes (plasma cells) in the blood.

phlogogen (flo′go-jen)   a body that has the power of causing inflammation.

phlogogenic (flo″go-jen′ik) [*phlogo-* + Gr. *gennan* to produce]   causing inflammation.

phlogogenous (flo-goj′ĕ-nus)   phlogogenic.

phlogotherapy (flog″o-ther′ah-pe) [*phlogo-* + Gr. *therapeia* treatment]   nonspecific therapy; see under *therapy*.

phlogotic (flo-got′ik)   inflammatory.

phlorhizin (flo-ri′zin) [Gr. *phloios* bark + *rhiza* root]   a bitter glycoside, $C_{21}H_{24}O_{10}$ + $2H_2O$, from the root bark of apple, cherry, plum, and pear trees; it causes glycosuria by blocking the tubular reabsorption of glucose.

phlorhizinize (flo-ri′zi-nīz)   to bring under the influence of phlorhizin.

phloridzin (flo-rid′zin)   phlorhizin.

phloridzinize (flo-rid′zi-nīz)   phlorhizinize.

phlorizin (flo-ri′zin)   phlorhizin.

phloroglucin (flo″ro-gloo′sin) [*phlorhizin* + Gr. *glykys* sweet]   chemical name: 1,3,5-trihydroxybenzene. The aglycone of many glycosides, $C_6H_6O_3$, obtained from the bark of apple and other trees, and used as a reagent for pentoses, pentosans, glycuronates, hydrochloric acid in gastric juice, etc. It is an excellent decalcifier of bone specimens. See under *tests*, and see *Günzburg's test*, under *tests*.

phloroglucinol (flo″ro-gloo′sĭ-nol)   phloroglucin.

phlorol (flo′rol)   an oily liquid, $C_6H_5(OC_2H_5)$, derived from creosote; see *phenetole*.

phlorose (flor′ōs)   a sugar formed when phlorhizin is boiled with dilute acids; glucose.

phlorrhizin (flo-ri′zin)   phlorhizin.

phloryl (flo′ril)   a principle obtainable from creosote.

phloxine (flok′sin)   a brick-red acid dye said to have a destructive action on cancer cells.

phlycten (flik′ten)   phlyctena.

phlyctena (flik-te′nah), pl. *phlycte′nae* [Gr. *phlyktaina*]   1. a blister made by a burn.   2. a small vesicle containing lymph seen on the conjunctiva in certain conditions. Called also *phlycten*.

phlyctenar (flik′tĕ-nar)   pertaining to or marked by phlyctenae.

phlyctenoid (flik′tĕ-noid) [*phlycten* + *-oid*]   resembling a phlyctena.

phlyctenosis (flik″tĕ-no′sis) [Gr. *phlyktainōsis*]   (obs.) any phlyctenular disease or lesion.

phlyctenula (flik-ten′u-lah), pl. *phlycten′ulae* [L.]   phlyctenule.

phlyctenular (flik-ten′u-lar)   associated with the formation of phlyctenules or vesicles, or of prominences that look like vesicles.

phlyctenule (flik′ten-ūl) [L. *phlyctaenula*; Gr. *phlyktaina* blister]   a small vesicle, or an ulcerated nodule of the cornea or of the conjunctiva.

phlyctenulosis (flik″ten-u-lo′sis)   the condition marked by the formation of phlyctenules, as phlyctenular keratoconjunctivitis, conjunctivitis, or ophthalmia.   **allergic p.,** phlyctenulosis due to allergy.   **tuberculous p.,** phlyctenulosis due to tuberculous allergy.

phobia (fo′be-ah) [Gr. *phobos* fear + *-ia*]   a persistent, irrational, intense fear of a specific object, activity, or situation (the phobic stimulus), fear that is recognized as being excessive or unreasonable by the individual himself. When a phobia is a significant source of distress or interferes with social functioning, it is considered a mental disorder: phobic disorder (or neurosis). In DSM III phobic disorders are subclassified as agoraphobia, social phobias, and simple phobias. Used as a word termination denoting irrational fear of or aversion to the subject indicated by the stem to which it is affixed.   **simple p.** [DSM III-R], any phobic disorder not involving fear of being alone or of public places (agoraphobia) or fear of embarrassment in social situations (social phobia). Common simple phobias involve fear of animals, particularly dogs, snakes, insects, and mice; fear of closed spaces (claustrophobia); and fear of heights (acrophobia).   **social p.** [DSM III-R], any phobic disorder involving fear and avoidance of social situations in which the individual fears that he will be exposed to possible embarrassment and humiliation, e.g., fears of speaking or performing in public, using public lavatories, or eating in public.

phobic (fo′bik)   of the nature of or pertaining to a phobia.

phobophobia (fo-bo-fo′be-ah) [Gr. *phobos* fear + *phobia*]   irrational fear of one's own fears or of acquiring a phobia.

Phocas' disease (fo-kahz′) [B. Gerasime *Phocas*, French surgeon, 1861–1937]   see under *disease*.

phocomelia (fo″ko-me′le-ah) [Gr. *phōkē* seal + *melos* limb + *-ia*]   a developmental anomaly characterized by absence of the proximal portion of a limb or limbs, the hands or feet being attached to the trunk of the body by a single small, irregularly shaped bone. Cf. *amelia*.

phocomelus (fo-kom′ĕ-lus) [Gr. *phōkē* seal + *melos* limb]   an individual exhibiting phocomelia.

phon (fōn) [Gr. *phōnē* voice]   a unit of the subjective loudness of a sound.

phonacoscope (fo-nak′o-skōp)   the apparatus used in phonacoscopy.

phonacoscopy (fo″nah-kos′ko-pe) [*phon-* + Gr. *skopein* to examine]   combined auscultation and percussion by means of a bell-shaped resonating chamber containing a percussion hammer, which is held on the anterior thoracic wall while the examiner listens at the back of the thorax.

phonal (fo′nal)   pertaining to the voice.

phonarteriogram (fōn″ar-te′re-o-gram″)   a tracing or graphic record of arterial sounds obtained in phonarteriography.

phonarteriographic (fōn″ar-te″re-o-graf′ik)   pertaining to phonarteriography or to a phonarteriogram.

phonarteriography (fōn″ar-te″re-og′rah-fe)   the recording of arterial sounds by means of a phonocardiograph.

phonasthenia (fo″nas-the′ne-ah) [*phon-* + *asthenia*]   weakness of the voice; difficult phonation from fatigue.

phonation (fo-na′shun)   the utterance of vocal sounds.   **subenergetic p.,** hypophonia.   **superenergetic p.,** hyperphonia.

phonatory (fo′nah-to″re)   subserving or pertaining to phonation.

phonautograph (fōn-aw′to-graf) [*phon-* + Gr. *autos* self + *graphein* to write] an apparatus which registers the vibrations of the air caused by the voice.

phoneme (fo′nēm) [Gr. *phōnēma* a sound made, a thing spoken] a speech sound that is the basic unit of spoken language.

phonendoscope (fōn-en′do-skōp) [*phon-* + Gr. *endon* within + *skopein* to examine] a stethoscopic device that intensifies auscultatory sounds.

phonendoskiascope (fōn-en′′do-ski′ah-skōp) a phonendoscope combined with a fluorescent screen for observing the heart movements at the same time as the heart sounds are heard.

phonetic (fo-net′ik) [Gr. *phonētikos*] pertaining to the voice or to articulate sounds.

phonetics (fo-net′iks) the science of vocal sounds; phonology.

phoniatrician (fo′′ne-ah-trish′an) a person who specializes in treating voice and speech defects.

phoniatrics (fo′′ne-at′riks) [*phon-* + Gr. *iatrikē* surgery, medicine] the treatment of voice and speech defects.

phonic (fon′ik, fo′nik) pertaining to the voice.

phonism (fo′nizm) a form of synesthesia in which a sensation of hearing is produced by the effect of something seen, felt, tasted, smelled, or thought of.

phon(o)- [Gr. *phōnē* voice] a combining form denoting relationship to sound, often specifically the sound of the voice.

phonoangiography (fo′′no-an′′je-og′rah-fe) the recording and analysis of arterial bruits to estimate the extent of arterial stenosis.

phonoauscultation (fo′′no-aws′′kul-ta′shun) auscultation in which a tuning-fork is placed over the organ to be examined and its vibrations are listened to through a stethoscope placed over the same organ.

phonocardiogram (fo′′no-kar′de-o-gram) [*phono-* + Gr. *kardia* heart + *gramma* a writing] the graphic record produced by phonocardiography.

phonocardiograph (fo′′no-kar′de-o-graf) the instrument used in phonocardiography. **fetal p.,** an instrument which provides continuous, instantaneous recording of beat-to-beat changes in fetal heart rate.

phonocardiographic (fo′′no-kar′′de-o-graf′ik) pertaining to phonocardiography or to a phonocardiogram.

phonocardiography (fo′′no-kar′′de-og′rah-fe) the graphic representation of heart sounds and murmurs; by extension, the term also includes pulse tracings (carotid, apex, and jugular pulse). **intracardiac p.,** the graphic registration of sounds produced by action of the heart by means of a phonocatheter passed into one of the heart chambers.

phonocatheter (fo′′no-kath′ĕ-ter) a device similar in appearance to a conventional catheter, with a microphone at the tip.

phonocatheterization (fo′′no-kath′′ĕ-ter-i-za′shun) the use of a phonocatheter for the detection of sounds produced by the circulatory system. **intracardiac p.,** the passage of a phonocatheter into a chamber of the heart, for the detection of sounds as an aid in diagnosis of cardiac defects.

phonoelectrocardioscope (fo′′no-e-lek′′tro-kar′de-o-skōp) an instrument incorporating a double beam cathode ray oscilloscope with a fluorescent screen of long afterglow, which permits the simultaneous direct visual recording of two phenomena such as the phonocardiogram and the electrocardiogram, the phonocardiogram and the sphygmogram, or the electrocardiogram and the sphygmogram.

phonogram (fo′no-gram) [*phono-* + Gr. *gramma* mark] a graphic record of a sound, as of a heart sound.

phonology (fo-nol′o-je) [*phono-* + *-logy*] the science which treats of vocal sounds; phonetics.

phonomyoclonus (fo′′no-mi-ok′lo-nus) myoclonus in which a sound is heard on auscultation of an affected muscle, indicating fibrillar contractions.

phonomyogram (fo′′no-mi′o-gram) [*phono-* + Gr. *mys* muscle + *gramma* mark] a tracing of the sound produced by muscle action.

phonomyography (fo′′no-mi-og′rah-fe) the recording of muscle sounds by an oscillograph to which the sounds are transmitted by a microphone placed over the muscle.

phonophobia (fo′′no-fo′be-ah) [*phono-* + *phobia*] irrational fear of sounds or of speaking aloud.

phonopsia (fo-nop′se-ah) [*phono-* + Gr. *opsis* vision + *-ia*] a subjective sensation as of seeing colors, caused by the hearing of sounds.

phonorenogram (fo′′no-re′no-gram) a graphic representation by means of a paper recording of pulsations of the renal artery obtained by use of a phonocatheter passed through a ureter into the pelvis of the kidney.

phonoscope (fo′no-skōp) [*phono-* + Gr. *skopein* to examine] 1. an apparatus for recording photographically the movements of a diaphragm set up by the sounds of the heart. 2. an instrument for auscultatory percussion.

phonoscopy (fo-nos′ko-pe) 1. the delimiting of solid and hollow organs (liver, heart, lungs, etc.) by listening with a stethoscope while percussion is made in the vicinity. 2. the use of the phonoscope.

phonoselectoscope (fo′′no-se-lek′to-skōp) [*phono-* + *select* + Gr. *skopein* to examine] an instrument for auscultation by means of which the lower (normal) range of the pulmonary sounds are eliminated, thus emphasizing the higher-pitched pathologic elements.

phonostethograph (fo′′no-steth′o-graf) an instrument by which the chest sounds are amplified, filtered, and recorded.

-phore [Gr. *phoros* carrying] a word termination denoting a carrier of the object designated by the stem to which it is affixed, as a melanophore.

-phoresis (fo-re′sis) [Gr. *phorēsis* a being carried] a word termination indicating transmission, as electrophoresis.

phoria (fo′re-ah) heterophoria.

phoriascope (fo′re-ah-skōp) [*phoria* + *-scope*] a prism-refracting instrument for use in orthoptic training.

Phormia (for′me-ah) the blackbottle flies, a genus of blue, black, or green flies of the family Calliphoridae. **P. regi′na,** a blowfly which causes a cutaneous myiasis of sheep in the United States and Canada. The larvae have been introduced into infected wounds to facilitate healing. Called also *Lucilia regina*. See also *maggot*.

phoroblast (fo′ro-blast) [Gr. *phoros* carrying + *blastos* germ] fibroblast.

phorocyte (fo′ro-sīt) a connective tissue cell.

phorocytosis (fo′′ro-si-to′sis) proliferation of connective tissue cells.

phorometer (fo-rom′ĕ-ter) [Gr. *phora* movement, range + *-meter*] 1. an instrument to test oculomotor balance. 2. a phoro-optometer.

phorometry (fo-rom′ĕ-tre) use of the phorometer.

phorone (fo′rōn) chemical name: 2,6-dimethyl-2,5- heptadien-4-one. A yellowish, oily, unsaturated ketone, $C_9H_{14}O$, obtained from acetone, camphoric acid, etc.

phoront (fo′ront) [Gr. *phora* producing + *ontos* being] the encysted stage or form in the life cycle of certain ciliate protozoa produced by a tomite and developing into a trophont.

phoro-optometer (fo′′ro-op-tom′ĕ-ter) [Gr. *phora* movement, range + *opto-* + *-meter*] an instrument to test ocular ductions, phorias, refractions, and vergences.

phoroplast (fo′ro-plast) [Gr. *phoros* carrying + *plastos* formed] connective tissue.

Phoroptor (fo-rop′tor) trademark for a phorometer fitted with a battery of cylindrical lenses.

phoroscope (fo′ro-skōp) [Gr. *phora* movement, range + *-scope*] a fixed trial frame for eye testing, with a head rest that may be fastened to the table or the wall.

phorotone (fo′ro-tōn) [Gr. *phora* movement, range + *tonos* tension] an instrument for exercising the muscles of the eye.

phorozoon (fo′′ro-zo′on) [Gr. *phoros* fruitful + *zōon* animal] the asexual stage in the life history of an organism.

phose (fōz) [Gr. *phōs* light] any subjective sensation, as of light or color; see *aphose, centraphose, centrophose, chromophose, peripheraphose, peripherophose,* etc.

phosgene (fos′jēn) a suffocating and highly poisonous war gas, carbonyl chloride, $COCl_2$; called also CG.

phosgenic (fos-jen′ik) [Gr. *phōs* light + *gennan* to produce] producing light.

phosis (fo′sis) the production of a phose.

phosphagen (fos′fah-jen) a group of compounds, including phosphocreatine and phosphoarginine, which occur in tissue and which yield inorganic phosphate with release of energy on cleavage. They are therefore classed as high-energy phosphate compounds.

phosphagenic (fos″fah-jen′ik) producing or forming phosphate.

phosphatase (fos′fah-tās″) [EC 3.1.3.] any of a sub-subclass of enzymes of the hydrolase class that catalyze the release of inorganic phosphate from phosphoric esters. See also *acid phosphatase, alkaline phosphatase.*

phosphate (fos′fāt) [L. *phosphas*] any salt, ester, or anionic form of phosphoric acid. The calcium phosphate mineral hydroxyapatite is the constituent giving hardness to bones and teeth. Phosphate esters (*organic phosphate*) occur in many body constituents: nucleotides and nucleic acids, phospholipids, phosphoproteins, and many small phosphorylated molecules involved in intermediary metabolism. Orthophosphate, usually referred to as *inorganic phosphate* (P_i) is the major intracellular anion. *Inorganic pyrophosphate* (PP_i) also occurs as a product of certain reactions, but it is immediately cleaved by the enzyme inorganic pyrophosphatase, forming orthophosphate. Pyrophosphate esters (*high energy phosphate*) such as adenosine triphosphate (ATP) are a store of chemical energy used to drive chemical syntheses, maintain membrane potentials, and power muscle contraction. Phosphorylation and dephosphorylation of proteins are important control mechanisms. **acid p.,** any phosphate in which only one or two of the three replaceable hydrogen atoms are taken up or replaced. **alkaline p.,** a phosphate of an alkaline metal, as sodium or potassium. **ammoniomagnesium p.,** a double salt of ammonium and magnesium with orthophosphoric acid, $Mg(NH_4)PO_4 \cdot 6H_2O$; closely allied to and often associated with triple phosphate. **arginine p.,** phosphoarginine. **calcium p.,** a compound containing calcium and the phosphate radical (PO_4). **carbamoyl p.,** an important intermediate compound in the formation of pyrimidine and citrulline, the latter being a step in urea formation. **creatine p.,** phosphocreatine. **earthy p.,** a phosphate of any one of the alkaline earth metals. **ferric p.,** a yellowish white powder, $FePO_4 \cdot 4H_2O$, insoluble in water or acetic acid, used as a feed and food supplement, especially to enrich bread, and as a fertilizer. **ferric p., soluble,** ferric phosphate rendered soluble by the presence of sodium citrate; used as a hematinic. **guanidine p.,** phosphoguanidine. **magnesium p., dibasic,** a salt, $MgHPO_4 \cdot 3H_2O$, occurring as a white, crystalline powder; it has been used as a mild saline laxative. **magnesium p., tribasic,** a powdered, white salt, $Mg_3(PO_4)_2 \cdot 5H_2O$, used as a gastric antacid; called also *trimagnesium p.* **normal p.,** any phosphate in which all the replaceable hydrogen atoms in phosphoric acid are replaced. **polyestradiol p.,** a polymeric ester of phosphoric acid and estradiol, used as a palliative in prostatic carcinoma. **stellar p.,** calcium phosphate occurring in star-shaped masses of crystals in urinary sediment. **trimagnesium p.,** magnesium p., tribasic. **triorthocresyl p.,** a poisonous compound, $(CH_3C_6H_4 \cdot O)PO$, contained in Jamaica ginger, ingestion of which causes paralysis. **triose p.,** phosphotriose. **triple p.,** a calcium, ammonium, and magnesium phosphate, sometimes found in the urine.

phosphated (fos′fāt-ed) containing phosphates.

phosphatemia (fos″fah-te′me-ah) [*phosphate* + Gr. *haima* blood + *-ia*] an excess of phosphates in the blood.

phosphatic (fos-fat′ik) pertaining to or containing phosphates.

phosphatidate (fos″fah-ti′dāt) the anionic form of phosphatidic acid.

phosphatide (fos′fah-tīd) phospholipid.

phosphatidic acid (fos″fah-ti′dik) 1,2-diacyl-*sn*-glycerol 3-phosphate, the parent compound of several important phospholipids, e.g., phosphatidylcholine. The fatty acid composition varies, but in most phosphatidyl compounds the 1-acyl group is saturated and the 2-acyl group is unsaturated.

phosphatidosis (fos″fah-tĭ-do′sis), pl. *phosphatido′ses* [*phosphatide* + *-osis*] lipidosis in which the fatty accumulations are phosphatides.

phosphatidylcholine (fos″fa-ti″dil-ko′lēn) a phospholipid in which choline is attached to the phosphate group of phosphatidic acid by an ester linkage; it is a major component of cell membrane and is localized preferentially in the outer surface of the plasma membrane. Abbreviated PC. Also called *lecithin.*

phosphatidylcholine-cholesterol acyltransferase (fos″fah-ti″dil-ko′lēn ko-les′ter-ol as″il-trans′fer-ās) phosphatidylcholine sterol acyltransferase.

phosphatidylcholine-sterol acyltransferase (fos″fah-ti″dil-ko′lēn ste′rol a″sil, as″il-trans′fer-ās) [EC 2.3.1.43] an enzyme of the transferase class that catalyzes the reaction phosphatidylcholine + sterol = 1-acylglycerophosphocholine + sterol ester. The enzyme, secreted by the liver, catalyzes the formation of cholesteryl esters in high-density lipoproteins by transferring long-chain fatty acid residues from phosphatidyl choline to a sterol. The reaction is a step in the synthesis of lipoproteins. Deficiency of the enzyme, an autosomal recessive trait, results in lecithin-cholesterol acyltransferase (LCAT) deficiency. Called also *phosphatidylcholine-cholesterol acyltransferase* and *lecithin-cholesterol acyltransferase.*

phosphatidylethanolamine (fos″fah-ti″dil-eth″ah-nol′ah-mēn) a phospholipid in which ethanolamine is attached to the phosphate group of phosphatidic acid by an ester linkage; it is a major constituent of cell membranes and is localized preferentially in the inner surface of the plasma membrane. Abbreviated PE.

phosphatidylinositol (fos″fah-ti″dil-ĭ-no′sĭ-tol) a phospholipid in which the sugar inositol is attached to the phosphate group of phosphatidic acid by an ester linkage; it is a minor constituent of cell membranes found primarily in the nuclear envelope and the endoplasmic reticulum. Abbreviated PI.

phosphatidylserine (fos″fah-ti″dil-sēr′ēn) a phospholipid in which serine is attached to the phosphate group of phosphatidic acid by an ester linkage; it is an important constituent of cell membranes and is localized preferentially in the inner surface of the plasma membrane. Abbreviated PS.

phosphatoptosis (fos″fah-top-to′sis) [*phosphate* + Gr. *ptōsis* fall] the spontaneous precipitation of phosphates from the urine; phosphaturia.

phosphaturia (fos″fah-tu′re-ah) [*phosphate* + Gr. *ouron* urine + *-ia*] 1. a high percentage of phosphates in any given specimen of urine. 2. ready precipitation of the earthy phosphates from the urine; phosphatoptosis.

phosphene (fos′fēn) [Gr. *phōs* light + *phainein* to show] an objective visual sensation that appears with the eyes closed and in the absence of visual light. **accommodation p.,** the streak of light surrounding the visual field seen in the dark after accommodation.

phosphide (fos′fīd) any binary compound of phosphorus and another element or radical.

phosphine (fos′fēn) 1. hydrogen phosphide, PH_3; a toxic malodorous gas and radical. 2. a coal tar dye extremely destructive to infusorial life; it is used as a stain. Called also *Philadelphia yellow.*

phosphite (fos′fīt) any salt of phosphorous acid.

phosphoarginine (fos″fo-ar′jĭ-nin) an arginine–phosphoric acid compound homologous with phosphocreatine but found in invertebrate muscles.

phosphocreatine (fos″fo-kre′ah-tin) a creatine–phosphoric acid compound, $(OH)_2PO \cdot NH \cdot C(:NH) \cdot N(CH_3) \cdot CH_2 \cdot COOH$, occurring in muscle metabolism, being broken down into creatine and inorganic phosphorus. It is an important storage form of high-energy phosphate, the energy source in muscle contraction. The phosphate group is transferred to ADP on muscle contraction to yield creatine and ATP. Called also *creatine phosphate.*

phosphodiesterase (fos″fo-di-es′ter-ās) [EC 3.1.4] any enzyme of the sub-subclass of enzymes of the hydrolase class that catalyzes the hydrolysis of one of the two ester linkages in a phosphodiester compound.

phosphoenolpyruvate carboxykinase (GTP) (fos″fo-e′nol-pi″roo-vāt kar-bok″se-ki′nās) [EC 4.1.1.32] an enzyme of the lyase class that catalyzes the reaction GTP + oxaloacetate = GDP + phosphoenolpyruvate + CO_2, part of the mechanism of gluconeogenesis in the liver. The enzyme occurs in both the mitochondria and cytosol of mammalian liver. Called also *phosphopyruvate carboxykinase.*

phosphofructaldolase (fos″fo-frukt-al′do-lās) fructose-bisphosphate aldolase.

6-phosphofructokinase (fos″fo-fruk″-, fos″fo-frook″to-ki′nās) [EC 2.7.1.11] an enzyme of the transferase class that catalyzes the reaction ATP + D-fructose 6-phosphate = ADP + D-fructose 1,6-bisphosphate. The reaction is essentially irreversible and is a committed step and a key site of regulation in the Embden-Meyerhof cycle of glucose metabolism. Deficiency of the muscle enzyme, an autosomal recessive trait, is the cause of glycogen storage disease type VII. Called also *phosphohexokinase*.

6-phosphofructo-2-kinase (fos″fo-frook″-, fos″fofruk″-to-ki′nās) [E.C. 2.7.1.105] an enzyme of the transferase class that catalyzes the reaction: fructose 6-phosphate + ATP = fructose 2,6-bisphosphate + ADP. The enzyme occurs in the liver as part of a mechanism for regulating carbohydrate metabolism; it is phosphorylated by the cAMP-dependent protein kinase. Phosphorylation inhibits the enzyme, therefore diminishing the formation of fructose 2,6-bisphosphate, when glucagon or catecholamines are secreted.

phosphoglobulin (fos″fo-glob′u-lin) a phosphoprotein with globulin as the protein moiety.

phosphoglucokinase (fos″fo-gloo″ko-ki′nās) [EC 2.7.1.10] an enzyme of the transferase class that catalyzes the reaction ATP +D-glucose 1-phosphate = ADP +D-glucose 1,6-bisphosphate. The reaction product is a necessary intermediate in the phosphoglucomutase reaction.

phosphoglucomutase (fos″fo-gloo″ko-mu′tās) [EC 5.4.2.2] an enzyme of the isomerase class; it requires the presence of the intermediate α-D-glucose 1,6-bisphosphate to catalyze the reaction α-D-glucose 1-phosphate = α-D-glucose 6-phosphate, a step in the formation and utilization of glycogen.

phosphogluconate dehydrogenase (decarboxylating) (fos″fo-gloo″ko-nāt de-hi′dro-jen-ās) [EC 1.1.1.44] an enzyme of the oxidoreductase class that catalyzes the reaction 6-phospho-D-gluconate + NADP⁺ = D-ribulose 5-phosphate + CO₂ + NADPH. The reaction is a step in the pentose phosphate pathway of glucose metabolism.

phosphoglucoprotein (fos″fo-gloo″ko-pro′te-in) a phosphorus-containing glucoprotein.

phosphoglucose isomerase (fos″fo-gloo′kōs i-som′er-ās) glucosephosphate isomerase.

3-phosphoglyceraldehyde (fos″fo-glis″er-al′dĕ-hīd) a triose phosphate, CH 2 ·O · PO(OH)₂ · CHOH·CHO, which results from the splitting of fructose-1,6-diphosphate in muscle metabolism.

phosphoglycerate (fos″fo-glis′er-āt) a salt of phosphoglyceric acid; it is an intermediate in the metabolic formation of pyruvate, its phosphate group being transferred from the 3-carbon of the glycerate to the 2-carbon.

2-phosphoglycerate (fos″fo-glis′er-at) the anionic form of 2-phosphoglyceric acid.

3-phosphoglycerate (fos″fo-glis′er-at) the anionic form of 3-phosphoglyceric acid.

phosphoglycerate kinase (fos″fo-glis″er-āt ki′nās) [EC 2.7.2.3] an enzyme of the transferase class that catalyzes the reaction ATP + 3-phospho-D-glycerate = ADP + 3-phospho-D-glyceroyl phosphate. The reaction is an important energy-transducing step in carbohydrate metabolism. As written, the reaction drives gluconeogenesis; the reverse reaction generates ATP in the catabolism of glucose. Deficiency of the enzyme, an X-linked trait, causes hemolytic anemia, mental retardation, and behavioral and neurologic abnormalities.

phosphoglycerate mutase (fos″fo-glis″er-āt mu′tās) [EC 5.4.2.1] an enzyme of the isomerase class that catalyzes the reaction 2-phospho-D-glycerate = 3-phospho-D-glycerate, a step in the Embden-Meyerhof pathway. The enzyme requires the presence of a small amount of 2,3-bisphosphoglycerate, which is also an intermediate. Called also *phosphoglyceromutase*.

2-phosphoglyceric acid (fos″fo-glĭ-ser′ik) an intermediate in the Embden-Meyerhof pathway (q.v.) of glucose metabolism.

3-phosphoglyceric acid (fos″fo-glĭ-ser′ik) an intermediate in the Embden-Meyerhof pathway (q.v.) of glucose metabolism.

phosphoglyceride (fos″fo-glis′er-īd) a class of phospholipids, including lecithin and cephalin, consisting of a glycerol backbone, two fatty acid chains, and a phosphorylated alcohol, the common alcohol moieties being choline, ethanolamine, serine, and inositol. Phosphatidic acid is the parent compound. The phosphoglycerides are a major component of cell membranes.

phosphoglyceromutase (fos″fo-glis″er-o-mu′tās) phosphoglycerate mutase.

phosphoguanidine (fos″fo-gwan′ĭ-dēn) a guanidine-phosphoric acid compound which on hydrolysis yields low-energy phosphate linkages.

phosphohexoisomerase (fos″fo-hek″so-i-som′er-ās) glucose-6-phosphate isomerase.

phosphohexokinase (fos″fo-hek″so-ki′nās) 6-phosphofructokinase.

Phospholine (fos′fo-lēn) trademark for a preparation of echothiophate iodide.

phospholipase (fos″fo-lip′ās) any of several enzymes that catalyze the hydrolysis of a phospholipid. They are classified, according to the bond cleaved, as A, B, C, and D.

phospholipase A₁ (fos″fo-lip′ās) [EC 3.1.1.32] an enzyme of the hydrolase class that catalyzes the reaction phosphatidylcholine + H₂O = 2-acylglycerophosphocholine + a fatty acid anion. The enzyme is found in liver lysosomes.

phospholipase A₂ (fos″fo-lip′ās) [EC 3.1.1.4] an enzyme of the hydrolase class that catalyzes the reaction phosphatidylcholine + H₂O = 1-acylglycerophosphocholine + a fatty acid anion. The enzyme is secreted as a proenzyme by the pancreas; the reaction hydrolyzes dietary phospholipids. Called also *lecithinase A*.

phospholipase B (fos″fo-lip′ās) lysophospholipase.

phospholipase C (fos″fo-lip′ās) [EC 3.1.4.3] an enzyme of the hydrolase class that catalyzes the reaction phosphatidylcholine + H₂O = 1,2-diacylglycerol + choline phosphate. The enzyme also acts on sphingomyelin. It is found in liver lysosomes, in the α-toxin of *Clostridium perfringens*, and the β- and γ-toxins of *Clostridium novyi*. Called also *lecithinase C*.

phospholipase D (fos″fo-lip′ās) [EC 3.1.4.4] an enzyme of the hydrolase class that catalyzes the reaction phosphatidylcholine + H₂O = choline + a phosphatidate. The enzyme also acts on other phosphatidyl esters; it occurs in the intestinal mucosa and in brain tissue. Called also *lecithinase D*.

phospholipid (fos″fo-lip′id) any lipid that contains phosphorus, including those with a glycerol backbone (phosphoglycerides and plasmalogens) or a backbone of sphingosine or related substance (sphingomyelins). Phospholipids are the major form of lipid in all cell membranes.

phospholipidemia (fos″fo-lip″ĭ-de′me-ah) the presence of phospholipid in the blood.

phospholipin (fos″fo-lip′in) phospholipid.

phosphomannose isomerase (fos″fo-man′ōs i-som′er-ās) mannose-6-phosphate isomerase.

phosphomevalonate kinase (fos″fo-mev″ah-lon′āt ki′nās) [EC 2.7.4.2] an enzyme of the transferase class that catalyzes the reaction ATP + (*R*)-5-phosphomevalonate = ADP + (*R*)-5-diphosphomevalonate. The reaction occurs in the biosynthesis of cholesterol.

phosphomolybdic acid (fos″fo-mo-lib′dik) a strong acid and oxidizing agent, 24MoO₃2H₃PO₄, used as a protein precipitant and color reagent; alkaloids, xanthine, uric acid, and other substances reduce phosphomolybdic acid to molybdenum blue. It is also used in histology as a mordant.

phosphomonoesterase (fos″fo-mon″o-es′ter-ās) see *acid phosphatase* and *alkaline phosphatase*.

phosphomutase (fos″fo-mu′tās) [EC 5.4.2] any of a subclass of enzymes of the isomerase class that catalyzes the intramolecular transfer of a phosphate group.

phosphonate (fos′fo-nāt) a carbon-phosphate compound. Such compounds may be related to inorganic pyrophosphates in structure but possess stable P—C—P bonds instead of P—O—P bonds; they are stable to both enzymatic and chemical hydrolysis.

phosphonecrosis (fos″fo-nĕ-kro′sis) phosphorus necrosis.

phosphonium (fos-fo′ne-um) the univalent radical, PH₄, forming compounds analogous to those of ammonium.

phosphonuclease (fos″fo-nu′kle-ās) nucleotidase.

phosphopenia (fos″fo-pe′ne-ah) [*phosphorus* + Gr. *penia* poverty] deficiency of phosphorus in the body.

phosphoprotein (fos″fo-pro′tēn) a protein to which one

or more phosphate groups are attached at serine or threonine (rarely tyrosine) residues.

phosphoprotein phosphatase (fos''fo-pro'tēn fos'fa-tās) [EC 3.1.3.16] an enzyme of the hydrolase class that catalyzes the reaction phosphoprotein + n H_2O = protein + n orthophosphate. Enzymes with this activity are involved in digestion and in the regulation of a variety of enzymes undergoing phosphorylation-dephosphorylation cycles.

phosphoptomaine (fos''fo-to'mān) any of a class of toxic compounds found in the blood in phosphorus poisoning.

phosphopyruvate carboxykinase (fos''fo-pi'roo-vāt kar-bok''se-ki'nās) phospho*enol*pyruvate carboxykinase (GTP).

phosphopyruvate carboxylase (fos''fo-pi'roo-vāt kar-bok''sĭ-lās) 1. a plant enzyme [EC 4.1.1.31] involved in photosynthesis. 2. phospho*enol*pyruvate carboxykinase (GTP).

phosphorated (fos'fo-rāt''ed) charged or combined with phosphorus.

phosphorescence (fos''fo-res'ens) the emission of light without appreciable heat; it is characterized by the emission of absorbed light after a delay and at a considerably longer wavelength than that of the absorbed light. Cf. *fluorescence.*

phosphorescent (fos''fo-res'ent) pertaining to or exhibiting phosphorescence.

phosphoretted (fos'fo-ret''ed) phosphorated.

phosphoriboisomerase (fos''fo-ri''bo-i-som'er-ās) ribose-5-phosphate isomerase.

phosphoribosylamine (fos''fo-ri''bo-sil'ah-mēn) an intermediate product in the synthesis of purines formed from phosphoribosylpyrophosphate and glutamine; excessive production is a factor in primary gout.

phosphoribosylpyrophosphate (fos''fo-ri''bo-sil- pi''ro-fos'fāt) an intermediate in the formation of purines and of purine and pyrimidine nucleotides; abbreviated as PRPP.

phosphoribosylpyrophosphate synthetase (fos''fo-ri''bo-sil-pi''ro-fos'fāt sin'thĕ-tās) ribose-phosphate pyrophosphokinase.

phosphoribosyltransferase (fos''fo-ri''bo-sil-trans'fer-ās) [EC 2.4.2] any enzyme of the sub-subclass pentosyltransferase that catalyzes the transfer of ribose 5-phosphate, usually from 5-phospho-α-D-ribose 1-diphosphate, to a purine, pyrimidine, or pyridine to form a 5' nucleotide and inorganic pyrophosphate. These enzymes are important in the biosynthesis of nucleotides.

phosphoric acid (fos-for'ik) a strong mineral acid, H_3PO_4. Phosphoric acid molecules can join by ester linkages to form dimers (*pyrophosphoric acid*) or polymers (*metaphosphoric acid*). For clarity the monomer is specified as *orthophosphoric acid*. Phosphoric acid is an important metabolite; see *phosphate.*

phosphoric acid, diluted (fos-for'ik) [NF] a preparation of phosphoric acid in purified water, containing in each 100 mL, not less than 9.5 g and not more that 10.5 g of phosphoric acid; it is used as a solvent in pharmaceutical preparations and orally as a gastric acidifier.

phosphoric acid, glacial (fos-for'ik) metaphosphoric a.

phosphorism (fos'fo-rizm) chronic phosphorus poisoning; see under *poisoning.*

phosphorized (fos'fo-rīzd) containing phosphorus.

phosphorolysis (fos''fo-rol'ĭ-sis) cleavage of a chemical bond with simultaneous addition of the elements of phosphoric acid to the residues, as in the splitting of the glycosidic bonds of glycogen catalyzed by the enzyme phosphorylase in carbohydrate metabolism. The reaction is analogous to hydrolysis.

phosphoroscope (fos'fōr-o-skōp) an instrument for measuring phosphorescence.

phosphorous (fos'fo-rus) pertaining to or containing phosphorus.

phosphorous acid (fos-for'us) a reducing inorganic acid, H_3PO_3, which readily absorbs oxygen to form phosphoric acid.

phosphorpenia (fos''fōr-pe'ne-ah) phosphopenia.

phosphoruria (fos''fōr-u're-ah) [*phosphorus* + Gr. *ouron* urine + -*ia*] the presence of free phosphorus in the urine.

phosphorus (fos'fŏ-rus) [Gr. *phōs* light + *phorein* to carry] a nonmetallic, allotropic element: poisonous and highly inflammable; symbol, P; atomic number, 15; atomic weight, 30.974. It occurs in three forms—*white* (yellow), *red*, and *black*. It is obtainable from bones, urine, and especially minerals, such as apatite. Ordinary white phosphorus is the kind once used in medicine, and is very inflammable and exceedingly poisonous. Phosphorus is an essential element in the diet; it is a major component of the mineral phase of bone and is abundant in all tissues, being involved in some form in almost all metabolic processes. Free phosphorus causes a fatty degeneration of the liver and other viscera, and the inhalation of its vapor often leads to necrosis of the lower jaw. Therapeutically, it was once used in rickets, osteomalacia, nervous and cerebral diseases, scrofula, and tuberculosis, as a genital stimulant in sexual exhaustion, and as a tonic in conditions of exhaustion. **amorphous p.,** red p. **black p.,** black lustrous crystals, resembling coal, insoluble in organic solvents, produced by heating white phosphorus under very high pressure. **labeled p.,** radioactive p. **ordinary p.,** white p. **radioactive p.,** radiophosphorus. **red p.,** a dark red amorphous powder, which is infusible and insoluble in carbon disulfide, and is not poisonous; called also *amorphous p.* **white p.,** a usually white, sometimes yellow, waxy solid, which is soluble in carbon disulfide, and very inflammable and exceedingly poisonous; it is the form that was once used in medicine in the treatment of various disorders. Called also *ordinary p.* **yellow p.,** white p.

phosphoryl (fos'fōr-il) the trivalent chemical radical ≡P:O.

phosphorylase (fos-for'ĭ-las) 1. any enzyme catalyzing the cleavage of a glycoside with inorganic phosphate, forming the 1-phosphate ester of the sugar. The term is usually qualified by adding the name of the substrate acted upon. 2. in animals, usually glycogen phosphorylase (q.v.); in plants, usually starch phosphorylase. **hepatic p. deficiency,** glycogen storage disease, type VI. **muscle p. deficiency,** glycogen storage disease, type V. **purine nucleoside p.** [EC 2.4.2.1], an enzyme of the purine salvage pathway that catalyzes the formation of purine nucleosides (inosine, guanosine, deoxyinosine, deoxyguanosine) from free purines (hypoxanthine, guanine) via the reaction: purine + ribose (or deoxyribose) 1-phosphate = purine nucleoside + inorganic phosphate. Deficiency of this enzyme results in severe deficiency of cell-mediated immunity with unimpaired humoral immunity, marked by increased susceptibility to viral infection and the development of fulminant infections from live vaccines or graft-versus-host disease from blood transfusion.

phosphorylase kinase (fos-for'ĭ-lās ki'nās) [EC 2.7.1.38] an enzyme of the transferase class that catalyzes the reaction 2 ATP + phosphorylase b = 2 ADP + phosphorylase a. The enzyme catalyzes the activation of glycogen phosphorylase, and is important in the regulation of glycogenolysis. Deficiency of the enzyme in the liver, an autosomal or X-linked recessive trait, is the cause of glycogen storage disease type VIII. Called also *glycogen phosphorylase kinase, phosphorylase b kinase.* **hepatic p. k. deficiency,** glycogen storage disease, type VIII.

phosphorylase phosphatase (fos-for'ĭ-lās fos'fah-tās) [EC 3.1.3.17] an enzyme of the hydrolase class that catalyzes the reaction phosphorylase a + 2 H_2O = phosphorylase b + 2 orthophosphate. The reaction converts active phosphorylase a to inactive phosphorylase b and is important in the regulation of glycogenolysis.

phosphorylation (fos''fōr-ĭ-la'shun) the metabolic process of introducing a phosphate group into an organic molecule. **oxidative p.,** the formation of high-energy phosphate bonds by phosphorylation of ADP to ATP, which is coupled to the transfer of electrons from reduced coenzymes (NADH or $FADH_2$) to molecular oxygen via a chain of electron carriers. Electrons are transferred from NADH to ubiquinone to cytochrome c to O_2 and from $FADH_2$ to cytochrome c to O_2; 3ATP per NADH and 2ATP per $FADH_2$ are produced. The process occurs on the inner membrane of mitochondria. **substrate-level p.,** the formation of high-energy phosphate bonds by phorylation of ADP to ATP (or GDP to GTP) coupled to cleavage of a high-energy metabolic intermediate, e.g., succinyl-CoA in the tricarboxylic acid cycle.

phosphorylysis (fos''fo-ril'ĭ-sis) phosphorolysis.

phosphosugar (fos''fo-shug'ar) a sugar combined with a phosphate; a pentose or hexose phosphate.

phosphotransferase (fos″fo-trans′fer-ās) an enzyme that catalyzes the transfer of a phosphate group, either from one molecule to another [EC 2.7] or within the same molecule [EC 5.4.2].

phosphotriose (fos″fo-tri′ōs) a compound consisting of a 3-carbon sugar combined with a phosphate radical. Two such compounds are formed from hexosediphosphate: 3-phosphoglyceraldehyde and 1-phosphodihydroxyacetone. Called also *triose phosphate*.

phosphotungstate (fos″fo-tung′stāt) a salt of phosphotungstic acid.

phosphotungstic acid (fos″fo-tung′stik) a strong acid and oxidizing agent, 12 $WO_3 \cdot H_3PO_4$, used as a protein precipitant and color reagent; alkaloids, nitrogenous bases, and other substances reduce phosphotungstic acid to tungsten blue. It is also used in histology as a mordant for hematoxylin and other dyes.

phosphovitellin (fos″fo-vi-tel′in) phosvitin.

phosphuresis (fos″fu-re′sis) the urinary excretion of phosphorus (phosphates).

phosphuret (fos′fu-ret) phosphide.

phosphuretic (fos″fu-ret′ik) pertaining to, characterized by, or promoting the urinary excretion of phosphorus (phosphates).

phosphuretted (fos′fu-ret″ed) phosphorated.

phosphuria (fos-fu′re-ah) phosphaturia.

phosvitin (fos-vi′tin) a phosphoprotein isolated from vitellin in egg yolk; called also *phosphovitellin*.

phot (fōt) [Gr. *phōs* light] the C.G.S. unit of illumination, being one lumen per square centimeter.

photalgia (fo-tal′je-ah) [phot- + -algia] ocular pain caused by light.

photallochromy (fo-tal′o-kro″me) [phot- + Gr. *allos* different + *chrōma* color] allotropic change with color alteration due to light, as the change of yellow into red phosphorus.

photaugiaphobia (fo-taw″je-ah-fo′be-ah) [Gr. *phōtaugeia* glare + *phobia*] abnormal intolerance of a glare. ·

photechy (fo′tek-e) [phot- + Gr. *ēchō* echo] the power shown by certain substances of becoming radioactive after having been exposed to radiation.

photerythrous (fo″te-rith′rus) deuteranopic.

photesthesis (fo″tes-the′sis) [phot- + Gr. *aisthēsis* perception] sensitiveness to light.

photic (fo′tik) pertaining to light.

photism (fo′tizm) a visual image; a sensation of color associated with a sensation of hearing, taste, smell, or touch.

phot(o) [Gr. *phōs*, gen. *phōtos* light] combining form denoting relationship to light.

photoablation (fo″to-ab-la′shun) volatilization of tissue by ultraviolet radiation emitted by a laser.

photoactinic (fo″to-ak-tin′ik) giving off both luminous and actinic rays.

photoactive (fo″to-ak′tiv) reacting chemically to sunlight or ultraviolet radiation.

photoallergic (fo″to-al-ler′jik) pertaining to, characterized by, or producing photoallergy.

photoallergy (fo″to-al′er-je) [photo- + allergy] a delayed immunologic type of photosensitivity involving a chemical substance to which the individual has become previously sensitized and radiant energy. See also *photoallergic contact dermatitis*, under *dermatitis*. Cf. *phototoxicity*.

photoautotroph (fo′to-an′to-trōf) a photoautotrophic organism.

photoautotrophic (fo′to-aw″to-trōf′ik) requiring for growth only inorganic compounds with carbon dioxide as the sole source of carbon (autotrophic) and deriving energy from photosynthesis; said of algae and certain photosynthetic bacteria.

photobacteria (fo″to-bak-te′re-ah) [photo- + bacteria] bacteria that derive energy from light by the process of photosynthesis. See also *Anoxyphotobacteria* and *Oxyphotobacteria*.

Photobacterium (fo″to-bak-te′re-um) [photo- + Gr. *baktērion* small rod] a genus of gram-negative, facultatively anaerobic bacteria of the family Vibrionaceae, made up of coccoid or rod-shaped cells. Two species are luminescent cells. They are found in seawater, in the alimentary tract of certain fishes, and on the luminous organs of certain fishes and cephalopods. The type species is *P. phospho′reum*.

photobacterium (fo″to-bak-te′re-um) 1. a bacterium producing luminescent substances. 2. an individual organism of the genus *Photobacterium* or of the division photobacteria.

photobiologic, photobiological (fo″to-bi″o-loj′ik; fo″to-bi″o-loj′ĭ-kal) pertaining to photobiology or to the effect of light on living organisms.

photobiology (fo″to-bi-ol′o-je) [photo- + biology] that department of biology which deals with the effect of light on living organisms, including the study of photosynthesis.

photobiotic (fo″to-bi-ot′ik) [photo- + Gr. *bios* life] living or thriving only in the light; said of certain organisms such as green plants.

photocatalysis (fo″to-kah-tal′ĭ-sis) the promotion or stimulation of a reaction by light.

photocatalyst (fo″to-kat′ah-list) a substance by means of which sunlight is utilized, as chlorophyll in the photosynthesis of carbohydrates by green plants.

photocatalytic (fo″to-kat″ah-lit′ik) promoted or stimulated by light; pertaining to, characterized by, or causing photocatalysis.

photocatalyzer (fo″to-kat′ah-līz″er) photocatalyst.

photoceptor (fo″to-sep′tor) photoreceptor.

photochemical (fo″to-kem′e-kal) pertaining to the chemical properties of light; chemically reactive in the presence of light or other radiation.

photochemistry (fo″to-kem′is-tre) [photo- + chemistry] the branch of chemistry which deals with the chemical properties or effects of light rays or other radiation.

photochemotherapy (fo″to-ke″mo-ther′ah-pe) treatment by means of drugs (e.g., methoxsalen) that react to ultraviolet radiation or sunlight.

photochromogen (fo″to-kro′mo-jen) [photo- + Gr. *chrōma* color + *gennan* to produce] a microorganism whose pigmentation develops as a result of exposure to light, e.g., *Mycobacterium kansasii* (pathogenic for man), which is yellow-orange if grown in the light, and almost colorless if grown in the dark. See also *nontuberculous mycobacteria*, under *mycobacterium*.

photochromogenic (fo″to-kro′mo-jen′ik) pertaining to or characterized by photochromogenicity.

photochromogenicity (fo″to-kro″mo-je-nis′ĭ-te) the property of microorganisms of forming pigment consequent to light exposure; induction occurs within a few minutes in the shorter wavelengths of visible light, pigmentation then occurring within 24 hours if conditions permit continued growth.

photocoagulation (fo″to-ko-ag″u-la′shun) [photo- + coagulation] condensation of protein material by the controlled use of an intense beam of light (e.g., xenon arc light or argon laser); used especially in treatment of retinal detachment and destruction of abnormal retinal vessels, or of intraocular tumor masses.

photoconvulsive (fo″to-kon-vul′siv) photoparoxysmal.

photocutaneous (fo″to-ku-ta′ne-us) [photo- + cutaneous] dermatitis in which the production of which light is an important factor.

photodermatitis (fo″to-der″mah-ti′tis) an abnormal state of the skin in which light is an important causative factor.

photodermatosis (fo″to-der″mah-to′sis) a morbid condition produced in the skin by exposure to light.

photodisruption (fo″to-dis-rup′shun) disruption of tissues by laser-produced rapid ionization of molecules.

photodromy (fo-tod′ro-me) [photo- + Gr. *dromos* running] the phenomenon of moving toward (*positive p.*) or away from (*negative p.*) light; as in the case of particles in suspension.

photodynamic (fo″to-di-nam′ik) [photo- + Gr. *dynamis* power] powerful in the light; said of the action exerted by fluorescent substances in the light.

photodynamics (fo″to-di-nam′iks) the science of the activating effects of light.

photodynesis (fo″to-di-ne′sis) the initiation of cytoplasmic streaming (cyclosis) in plant cells by visible light.

photodynia (fo″to-din′e-ah) [photo- + Gr. *odynē* pain] photalgia.

photodysphoria (fo″to-dis-fo′re-ah) [*photo-* + Gr. *dysphoria* distress] intolerance of light; photophobia.

photoelectric (fo″to-e-lek′trik) pertaining to the electric effects of light or other radiation.

photoelectron (fo″to-e-lek′tron) an electron emitted from a metallic surface when the latter is illuminated with light, especially with light of short wavelength.

photoelement (fo″to-el′e-ment) a galvanic element which is decomposed under the influence of light and produces photoelectricity.

photoerythema (fo″to-er″ĭ-the′mah) erythema due to exposure to light.

photoesthetic (fo″to-es-thet′ik) [*photo-* + Gr. *aisthēsis* perception] pertaining to or having the sensation of light.

photofluorogram (fo″to-floo-or′o-gram) the film produced in photofluorography.

photofluorography (fo″to-floo″or-og′rah-fe) the photographic recording of fluoroscopic images on small films, using a fast lens: a procedure used in mass roentgenography of the chest. Called also *fluororoentgenography*, and sometimes *abreuography*, in honor of Manoel de Abreu, Brazilian physician, who discovered the technique.

photofluoroscope (fo″to-floo-or′o-skōp) a form of fluoroscope used in making either observations or photographs by means of roentgen rays.

photogastroscope (fo″to-gas′tro-skōp) [*photo-* + Gr. *gastēr* stomach + *skopein* to examine] an apparatus for photographing the interior of the stomach.

photogene (fo′to-jēn) after-image.

photogenic (fo″to-jen′ik) 1. produced by light, as photogenic epilepsy. 2. producing or emitting light; phosphorescent.

photogram (fo′to-gram) [*photo-* + Gr. *gramma* mark] the photographic record of a physiologic experiment.

photography (fo-tog′rah-fe) the process of making images on a sensitized material by exposure to light or other radiant energy. **Kirlian p.,** the taking of photographs of ordinarily invisible emanations (an aura or halo) from living organisms, plant and animal, that change in color and size. The object under study, a leaf, fingertip, etc., is placed on a piece of photographic paper or negative film on a metal plate in which a generator induces an electromagnetic field in a dark enclosure.

photohalide (fo″to-hal′ĭd) any halogen salt that is sensitive to light.

photohematachometer (fo″to-hem″ah-tah-kom′ĕ-ter) [*photo-* + Gr. *haima* blood + *tachys* swift + *metron* measure] a device for making a photographic record of the speed of the blood current.

photohenric (fo″to-hen′rik) [*photo-* + *henry*] denoting a change in inductive capacity due to action of light.

photoheterotroph (fo″to-het′er-o-trōf) [*photo-* + Gr. *heteros* other + *trophos* feeder, from *trephein* to nourish] a photoheterotrophic organism.

photoheterotrophic (fo″to-het″er-o-trōf′ik) deriving nourishment from organic compounds and energy from visible light.

photohmic (fo-to′mik) denoting a change in electric resistance produced by light.

photoinactivation (fo″to-in-ak″tĭ-va′shun) inactivation, as of complement, by light.

photokinesis (fo″to-ki-ne′sis) [*photo-* + Gr. *kinētikos* pertaining to motion] a change in the rate of motion in response to light, as an increase or decrease in motility of bacteria with a change in illumination.

photokinetic (fo″to-ki-net′ik) [*photo-* + Gr. *kinētikos* pertaining to motion] pertaining to photokinesis.

photokymograph (fo″to-ki′mo-graf) a camera with a moving film for recording movements as of the string in a string galvanometer; called also a *recording camera*.

photology (fo-tol′o-je) [*photo-* + *-logy*] the branch of physics which treats of light.

photoluminescence (fo″to-lu″mĭ-nes′ens) the quality of being luminescent after being exposed to light.

photolysis (fo-tol′ĭ-sis) 1. chemical decomposition by the action of light. 2. lysis or solution of cells under the influence of light.

photolyte (fo′to-līt) [*photo-* + Gr. *lyein* to dissolve] any substance decomposable by the action of light.

photolytic (fo″to-lit′ik) decomposed by radiant energy.

photoma (fo-to′mah) a flash of light sparks or color with no objective basis.

photomagnetism (fo″to-mag′nĕ-tizm) magnetism induced by the action of light.

photometer (fo-tom′ĕ-ter) [*photo-* + *-meter*] 1. a device for measuring the intensity of infrared, ultraviolet, or visible light. 2. a device for testing the sensitivity of the eye to light by determining the light minimum. **flame p.,** an instrument for analyzing the light emitted by a substance in a flame; commonly used for determination of sodium, potassium, lithium, and calcium in biological materials. **flicker p.,** an instrument in which the frequency of a flickering light can be controlled, for use in performing the flicker test; called also *flicker meter.* **Förster's p.,** photoptometer.

photomethemoglobin (fo″to-met-he″mo-glo′bin) a compound formed by the action of light on methemoglobin.

photometry (fo-tom′ĕ-tre) [*photo-* + *-metry*] the measurement of light. **flicker p.,** see *flicker.*

photomicrograph (fo″to-mi′kro-graf) [*photo-* + Gr. *mikros* small + *graphein* to record] the photograph of a minute object as seen under the light microscope, produced by ordinary photographic methods. Cf. *microphotograph.*

photomicrography (fo″to-mi-krog′rah-fe) the production of photomicrographs.

photomicroscope (fo″to-mi′kro-skōp) a microscope and camera combined for making photomicrographs.

photomicroscopy (fo″to-mi-kros′ko-pe) photography of enlarged pictures of minute objects with the photomicroscope.

photomorphogenesis (fo″to-mor″fo-jen′ĕ-sis) the regulation of form by light, as in the induction of flowering in plants by a minimal period of daylight.

photomyoclonic (fo″to-mi″o-klon′ik) photomyogenic.

photomyogenic (fo″to-mi″o-jen′ik) photomyoclonic; denoting an electroencephalographic response to photic stimulation (brief flashes of light) marked by myoclonus of the facial muscles.

photon (fo′ton) a particle (quantum) of radiant energy.

photoncia (fo-ton′se-ah) [*photo-* + Gr. *onkos* mass] swelling due to the action of light.

photo-onycholysis (fo″to-o″nĭk-ol′ĭ-sis) onycholysis resulting from exposure to sunlight or ultraviolet rays, as after treatment with the tetracyclines, methoxypsoralen, or other photoactive drugs.

photoparoxysmal (fo″to-par″oks-is′mal) photoconvulsive; denoting an abnormal electroencephalographic response to photic stimulation (brief flashes of light), marked by diffuse paroxysmal discharge recorded as spike-wave complexes; the response may be accompanied by minor seizures.

photopathy (fo-top′ah-the) [*photo-* + Gr. *pathos* affection] a pathologic effect produced by light.

photoperceptive (fo″to-per-sep′tiv) [*photo-* + *perceptive*] able to perceive light.

photoperiod (fo″to-pēr′e-od) the period of time per day that an organism is exposed to daylight or to artificial light.

photoperiodic (fo″to-pēr″e-od′ik) pertaining to the photoperiod or to photoperiodism.

photoperiodicity (fo″to-pe″re-o-dis′ĭ-te) photoperiodism.

photoperiodism (fo″to-pe′re-od-izm) the physiologic and behavioral reactions brought about in organisms by changes in the duration of daylight and darkness in a 24-hour period. Called also *photoperiodicity.*

photopharmacology (fo″to-far″mah-kol′o-je) [*photo-* + *pharmacology*] the study of the effects of light and other radiations on drugs and on their pharmacological action.

photophilic (fo″to-fil′ik) [*photo-* + Gr. *philein* to love] thriving in light; said of organisms.

photophobia (fo″to-fo′be-ah) [*photo-* + *phobia*] abnormal visual intolerance of light.

photophobic (fo″to-fo′bik) pertaining to or characterized by photophobia.

photophosphorylation (fo″to-fos″for-ĭ-la′shun) the formation of ATP occurring in chloroplasts during photosynthesis; it is analogous to oxidative phosphorylation. **cyclic p.,** that in which ATP formation is coupled with liberation of the energy arising from a cyclic flow of electrons from the ferredoxin-reducing system back to the chlorophyll.

photophthalmia (fo″tof-thal′me-ah) [phot- + ophthalmia] ophthalmia caused by intense light, such as electric light, rays of welding arc, or reflection from snow (ophthalmia nivialis). **flash p.,** ophthalmia produced by exposure to a welding arc.

photopia (fo-to′pe-ah) day vision; see also *light adaptation.*

photopic (fo-top′ik) pertaining to vision in the light; said of the eye which has become light-adapted.

photoproduct (fo′to-prod″ukt) a substance synthesized in the body by the action of light.

photoprotection (fo″to-pro-tek′shun) the protection of some cells by exposure to light in the near ultraviolet light range prior to exposure to light in the far ultraviolet range.

photopsia (fo-top′se-ah) [photo- + -opsia] an appearance as of sparks or flashes due to retinal irritation.

photopsin (fo-top′sin) the protein moiety of the cones of the retina that combines with retinal to form photochemical pigments.

photopsy (fo-top′se) photopsia.

photoptarmosis (fo″to-tar-mo′sis) [photo- + Gr. *ptarmos* sneezing + -osis] sneezing caused by the influence of light.

photoptometer (fo″top-tom′ĕ-ter) [phot- + opto- + -meter] a device for testing the acuity of vision by determining the smallest amount of light that will render an object just visible; called also *Förster's p.*

photoptometry (fo″top-tom′ĕ-tre) [photo- + opto- + -metry] determination of the flicker fusion threshold. See *flicker.*

photoradiation (fo″to-ra″de-a′shun) photodynamic therapy.

photoradiometer (fo″to-ra″de-om′ĕ-ter) an apparatus for measuring the quantity of roentgen rays penetrating any given surface.

photoreaction (fo″to-re-ak′shun) a chemical reaction produced by the influence of light; a photochemical reaction.

photoreactivation (fo″to-re-ak″tĭ-va′shun) the reversal of the biological effects of ultraviolet radiation on cells by subsequent exposure to visible light; called also *photoreversal.*

photoreception (fo″to-re-sep′shun) [photo- + L. *receptio,* from *recipere* to receive] the process of detecting radiant energy, usually of wavelengths between 370 and 760 nm, being the range of visible light.

photoreceptive (fo″to-re-sep′tiv) sensitive to stimulation by light.

photoreceptor (fo″to-re-sep′tor) a nerve end-organ or receptor sensitive to light.

photorespiration (fo″to-res″pĭ-ra′shun) a process carried out by certain plants, occurring as a result of oxidation of glycolic acid (a product of photosynthesis released by chloroplasts) by glycolic acid oxidase, an enzyme present in the glyoxosomes, ultimately causing an increased output of carbon dioxide.

photoretinitis (fo″to-ret″ĭ-ni′tis) inflammation of the retina due to exposure to intense light, which may result in transient central scotoma.

photoreversal (fo″to-re-ver′sal) photoreactivation.

photoscan (fo′to-skan) a two-dimensional representation (map) of the gamma rays emitted by a radioisotope, revealing its varying concentration in a body tissue, differing only from a scintiscan in that the printout mechanism is a light source exposing a photographic film.

photoscanner (fo″to-skan′ner) the system of equipment used in the making of a photoscan.

photoscope (fo′to-skōp) [photo- + Gr. *skopein* to examine] a kind of fluoroscope.

photoscopy (fo-tos′ko-pe) [photo- + Gr. *skopein* to examine] skiascopy.

photosensitive (fo″to-sen′sĭ-tiv) exhibiting an abnormally heightened reactivity to sunlight.

photosensitivity (fo″to-sen″sĭ-tiv′ĭ-te) [photo- + sensitivity] an abnormal cutaneous response involving the interaction between photosensitizing substances and sunlight or filtered

or artificial light at wavelengths of 280–400 nm. There are two main types: *photoallergy* and *photoxicity.*

photosensitization (fo″to-sen″sĭ-ti-za′shun) the development of abnormally heightened reactivity of the skin to sunlight.

photosensitize (fo″to-sen′sĭ-tīz) [photo- + sensitize] to sensitize a substance or an organism, cell, or tissue to the influence of light.

photostable (fo′to-sta″b'l) unchanged by the influence of light.

photostethoscope (fo″to-steth′o-skōp) a lamp which transforms sounds amplified by a microphone into pulsations of light; used for recording the heartbeats of the fetus.

photosynthesis (fo″to-sin′thĕ-sis) [photo- + Gr. *synthesis* putting together] a chemical combination caused by the action of light; specifically the formation of carbohydrates (with release of molecular oxygen) from carbon dioxide and water in the chlorophyll tissue of plants and blue-green algae under the influence of light. In bacteria, photosynthesis employs hydrogen sulfide, molecular hydrogen, and other reduced compounds in place of water, so that molecular oxygen is not released. See also *light reaction* and *dark reaction,* under *reaction.* Cf. *chemosynthesis.*

phototaxis (fo″to-tak′sis) [photo- + *taxis*] taxis of an organism elicited in response to the source of light stimulus; called also *heliotaxis.*

phototherapy (fo″to-ther′ah-pe) [photo- + *therapy*] the treatment of disease, e.g. bilirubinemia, by exposure to light, especially by variously concentrated light rays.

photothermal (fo″to-ther′mal) pertaining to the heat produced by radiant energy.

photothermy (fo′to-ther″me) [photo- + Gr. *thermē* heat] the heat effects produced by radiant energy.

phototimer (pho′to-tīm″er) a device used in radiology and photography to control the exposure interval by terminating the exposure interval by terminating the exposure when the amount of incident radiation or light reaches a preset quantity.

phototonus (fo-tot′o-nus) [photo- + Gr. *tonos* tension] an irritable state of protoplasm due to the influence of light.

phototoxic (fo″to-tok′sik) [photo- + *toxic*] pertaining to, characterized by, or producing phototoxicity.

phototoxicity (fo″tō-tok-sis′ĭ-te) [photo- + *toxicity*] a nonimmunologic, chemically induced type of photosensitivity. See also *phototoxic dermatitis,* under *dermatitis.* Cf. *photoallergy.*

phototrophic (fo″to-trof′ik) [photo- + Gr. *trophē* nourishment] capable of deriving energy from light, as in certain green plants and bacteria. Cf. *chemotrophic.*

phototropic (fo″to-trop′ik) exhibiting phototropism.

phototropism (fo-tot′ro-pizm) [photo- + Gr. *tropos* a turning] 1. tropism of an organism in response to the source of light stimulus. 2. change of color produced in a substance by the action of light.

phototurbidometric (fo″to-tur-bid″o-met′rik) pertaining to the determination of the turbidity of a solution by optic methods; used in study of the activity of various enzymes.

photovaporization (fo″to-va″por-ĭ-za′shun) laser-produced vaporization of intracellular and extracellular fluids to provide an incision with cauterization of adjacent vessels.

photronreflectometer (fo″tron-re″flek-tom′ĕ-ter) an apparatus for measuring turbidity.

photuria (fo-tu′re-ah) [photo- + Gr. *ouron* urine + -ia] the excretion of urine having a luminous appearance.

Phragmidiothrix (frag-mid′e-o-thriks″) [Gr. *phragma* fence + *eidos* shape + *thrix* hair] a genus of sheathed bacteria found in water, made up of small disk-shaped cells in long unbranched filaments surrounded by a thin sheath and attached to a substrate. The type species is *P. multisepta′ta.*

phragmoplast (frag′mo-plast) [Gr. *phragmos* inclosure + *plastos* formed] the barrel-shaped spindle formed in the equatorial plane during mitosis of plant cells; it precedes the formation of the cell plate.

phren (fren) [Gr. *phrēn*] 1. the diaphragm. 2. the mind, as seat of the intellect, or the heart, as seat of the passions.

phrenalgia (fre-nal′je-ah) [phren- + -algia] pain in the diaphragm.

phrenectomy (fre-nek′to-me) [*phren-* + Gr. *ektomē* excision] the removal of all or a part of the diaphragm.

phrenemphraxis (fren″em-frak′sis) [*phrenic* nerve + Gr. *emphraxis* stoppage] the operation of crushing the phrenic nerve; phrenicotripsy.

phrenetic (frĕ-net′ik) 1. maniacal. 2. a maniac.

phrenic (fren′ik) [L. *phrenicus;* Gr. *phrēn* mind; diaphragm] 1. pertaining to the diaphragm; diaphragmatic. 2. pertaining to the mind.

phrenicectomy (fren″ĭ-sek′to-me) [*phrenic* nerve + Gr. *ektomē* excision] resection of the phrenic nerve; phreniconeurectomy.

phreniclasia, phreniclasis (fren″ĭ-kla′ze-ah; fren″ĭ-kla′sis) [*phrenic* nerve + Gr. *klasis* crushing] crushing of the phrenic nerve with a clamp.

phrenicoexairesis (fren″ĭ-ko-ek-si′re-sis) phrenicoexeresis.

phrenicoexeresis (fren″ĭ-ko-ek-ser′ĕ-sis) [*phrenic* nerve + Gr. *exairesis* a taking out] avulsion of the phrenic nerve.

phreniconeurectomy (fren″ĭ-ko-nu-rek′to-me) [*phrenic* + Gr. *neuron* nerve + *ektomē* excision] excision of a whole or a portion of the phrenic nerve; phrenicectomy.

phrenicotomy (fren″ĭ-kot′o-me) [*phrenic* nerve + Gr. *tomē* a cutting] surgical division of the phrenic nerve and its accessory for the purpose of causing one-sided paralysis of the diaphragm.

phrenicotripsy (fren″ĭ-ko-trip′se) [*phrenic* nerve + Gr. *tripsis* a crushing] crushing of the phrenic nerve; phrenemphraxis.

phrenitis (frĕ-ni′tis) [*phren-* + *-itis*] inflammation of the diaphragm; diaphragmitis.

phren(o)- [Gr. *phrēn* diaphragm, mind] a combining form denoting relationship to the diaphragm, the phrenic nerve, or the mind.

phrenocardia (fren″o-kar′de-ah) [*phren-* + Gr. *kardia* heart] psychogenic palpitations, precordial pain, and dyspnea in anxiety neurosis; neurocirculatory asthenia.

phrenocolic (fren″o-kol′ik) pertaining to or connecting the diaphragm and colon.

phrenodynia (fren″o-din′e-ah) [*phren-* + Gr. *odynē* pain] pain in the diaphragm.

phrenogastric (fren″o-gas′trik) pertaining to the diaphragm and the stomach.

phrenoglottic (fren″o-glot′ik) pertaining to the diaphragm and the glottis.

phrenograph (fren′o-graf) [*phren-* + Gr. *graphein* to write] an apparatus for recording the movements of the diaphragm.

phrenohepatic (fren″o-hĕ-pat′ik) [*phren-* + Gr. *hēpar* liver] pertaining to the diaphragm and the liver.

phrenologist (frĕ-nol′o-jist) a person who practices phrenology.

phrenology (frĕ-nol′o-je) [*phren-* + *-logy*] the study of the mind and character from the shape of the skull.

phrenopericarditis (fren″o-per″ĭ-kar-di′tis) [*phren-* + *pericarditis*] a condition in which the apex of the heart is attached to the diaphragm by adhesions.

phrenoplegia (fren″o-ple′je-ah) [*phren-* + Gr. *plēgē* stroke] paralysis of the diaphragm.

phrenoptosis (fren″op-to′sis) [*phren-* + Gr. *ptōsis* falling] downward displacement of the diaphragm.

phrenosin (fren′o-sin) a cerebroside, probably $C_{48}H_{93}O_9N$, obtained from brain substance; it yields on hydrolysis galactose, sphingosine, and cerebronic acid.

phrenosinic acid (fren″o-sin′ik) cerebronic acid.

phrenospasm (fren′o-spazm) [*phren-* + *spasm*] spasm of the diaphragm.

phrenosplenic (fren″o-splen′ik) pertaining to or connecting the diaphragm and the spleen.

phrenosterol (fren″o-ste′rol) a sterol from brain substance.

phrenotropic (fren″o-trop′ik) [*phreno-* + Gr. *tropē* a turn, turning] exerting its principal effect upon the mind.

phrictopathic (frik″to-path′ik) [Gr. *phriktos* producing a shudder + *pathos* disease] causing a shudder; a term applied to a peculiar sensation caused by irritating a hysterical anesthetic area during recovery.

phronema (fro-ne′mah) [Gr. *phronēma* mind] that portion of the cortex of the brain which is occupied by thought centers or association centers.

phrynin (fri′nin) a poisonous substance obtainable from the skin and secretions of various toads; its properties resemble those of digitalin.

phrynoderma (frin″o-der′mah) [Gr. *phrynē* toad + *derma* skin] follicular hyperkeratosis.

phrynolysin (fri-nol′ĭ-sin) [Gr. *phrynē* toad + *lysis* dissolution] the lysin or toxin from the venom of the fire toad (*Bombinator igneus*).

phthalate (thal′āt) a salt of phthalic acid.

phthalein (thal′e-in) any one of a series of coloring matters formed by the condensation of phthalic anhydride with the phenols; some of them have a purgative action. See *phenolphthalein*. **alpha-naphthol p.,** an indicator used in the determination of hydrogen ion concentration; it has a pH range of 9.3–10.5. **orthocresol p.,** an indicator used in the determination of hydrogen ion concentration; it has a pH range of 8.2–9.8.

phthaleinometer (thal″e-in-om′ĕ-ter) an instrument for use in performing phenolsulfonphthalein tests.

phthalic acid (thal′ik) trivial name for 1,2-benzenedicarboxylic acid.

phthalin (thal′in) any one of a series of colorless compounds formed by reduction of phthalein.

phthalylsulfacetamide (thal″il-sul″fah-set′ah-mīd) [USP] chemical name: 2-[[[4-[(acetylamino)sulfonyl]phenyl] amino]-carbonyl]benzoic acid. A sulfonamide, $C_{16}H_{14}N_2O_5S$, occurring as white or creamy white crystals or a crystalline powder; used as an intestinal antibacterial, administered orally. Called also *phthalylsulfonazole*.

phthalylsulfathiazole (thal″il-sul″fah-thi′ah-zōl) [NF] chemical name: 2-[[[4-[(2-thiazolylamino)sulfonyl]phenyl] amino]carbonyl]benzoic acid. A sulfonamide, $C_{17}H_{13}N_3O_5S_2$, occurring as a white or faintly yellowish white, crystalline powder; used as an intestinal antibacterial, administered orally.

phthalylsulfonazole (thal″il-sul-fon′ah-zōl) phthalylsulfacetamide.

phthiocol (thi′o-kol) chemical name: 2-hydroxy-3-methyl-1,4-naphthoquinone. An antibiotic substance produced by *Mycobacterium tuberculosis* and having some vitamin K activity.

phthioic acid (thi-o′ik as′id) a branched-chain fatty acid occurring in the cell wall of *Mycobacterium tuberculosis*.

phthiriasis (thir-i′ah-sis) [Gr. *phtheiriasis*, from *phtheir* louse] infestation with crab or pubic lice; see *pediculosis*. **p. inguina′lis, pubic p.,** infestation with lice of the species *Phthirus pubis;* it is usually limited to the pubic hairs but may occur on other areas, as the eyelashes.

Phthirus (thir′us) [Gr. *phtheir* louse] a genus of sucking lice of the family Pediculidae, order Anoplura, which feed on human blood. **P. pu′bis,** the pubic or crab louse, which infests the hair of the pubic region and which is sometimes found in other hairy areas of the body, such as the eyebrows, eyelashes, and axillae.

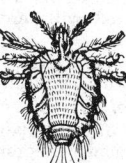

Phthirus pubis.

phthisis (ti′sis) [Gr. *phthisis*, from *phthiein* to decay] 1. a wasting away of the body or a part of the body. 2. tuberculosis especially of the lungs. **aneurysmal p.,** the clinical symptoms of chest pain and cough, at first dry and later productive, sometimes with hemoptysis, produced by aneurysm of the ascending aorta and the aortic arch. **p. bul′bi,** shrinkage and wasting of the eyeball. **p. cor′neae,** the shriveling and disappearance of the cornea after suppurative keratitis. **essential p.** (of the eye), ophthalmomalacia. **ocular p.,** ophthalmomalacia. **p. ven-**

tric′uli (*obs.*), atrophy of the mucous membrane of the stomach and alimentary canal.

phyco- [Gr. *phykos* seaweed] a combining form denoting relationship to seaweed or algae.

phycobilin (fi″ko-bil′in) any of a group of protein-linked pigments including phycoerythrin (red pigment) and phycocyanin (blue pigment), which are found in the red and the blue-green algae.

phycochrome (fi′ko-krōm) [*phyco-* + Gr. *chrōma* color] 1. a blue-green pigment from various fresh-water algae of the simplest type. 2. any of the algae that contain both chlorophyll and a blue pigment; the blue-green algae.

phycochromoprotein (fi″ko-kro″mo-pro′te-in) a colored, conjugated protein, with respiratory function, found in various seaweeds.

phycocyanin (fi″ko-si′an-in) a blue chromoprotein found in blue-green algae.

phycocyanogen (fi″ko-si-an′o-jen) a blue pigment derived from blue-green algae.

phycoerythrin (fi″ko-er′ĭ-thrin) a red chromoprotein found in red algae.

phycologist (fi-kol′o-jist) a specialist in phycology; called also *algologist*.

phycology (fi-kol′o-je) [*phyco-* + *-logy*] the scientific study of algae; algology.

Phycomycetae (fi″ko-mi-se′te) Phycomycetes.

Phycomycetes (fi″ko-mi-se′tēz) [*phyco-* + Gr. *mykēs* fungus] a group of fungi comprising the common water, leaf, and bread molds, and including the classes Chytridiomycetes, Oomycetes, and Zygomycetes. In some classifications, considered to be a class of the Eumycetes, with the subordinate categories as subclasses.

phycomycetosis (fi″ko-mi-sĕ-to′sis) infection with fungi of the group Phycomycetes; see *phycomycosis*. **subcutaneous p.**, subcutaneous phycomycosis.

phycomycetous (fi″ko-mi-se′tus) of or pertaining to fungi of the group Phycomycetes.

phycomycosis (fi″ko-mi-ko′sis) any of a group of acute mycoses caused by fungi of the group Phycomycetes, including species of *Absidia, Mucor, Rhizopus, Hyphomyces, Basidiobolus, Entomophora,* and *Mortierella*; it may involve the sinuses, orbital tissue, central nervous system, lungs, gastrointestinal tract, skin, and subcutaneous tissue. Except in the subcutaneous form, it is characterized by inflammation and vascular thrombosis of the blood vessels of the organ involved. Most infections occur in diabetics; other predisposing factors include primary debilitating disease and therapy with antimetabolites, steroids, or antibiotics. **cerebral p.**, a form affecting the brain, due to extension of rhinophycomycosis through the ophthalmic and carotid arteries, resulting in orbital involvement, infarction of the brain, and meningitis; it usually develops in acidotic diabetics. **p. entomoph′thorae**, rhinophycomycosis. **subcutaneous p.**, a chronic infection caused by *Basidiobolus haptosporus*, in which gradually enlarging nodules (eosinophilic granulomas) form in the subcutaneous tissues of the arms, chest, and trunk. Multiple purulent ulcers may develop. It occurs in Indonesia, central Africa, and India, affecting chiefly children and adolescents. Unlike the other phycomycoses, it is unassociated with any apparent predisposing factors.

phygogalactic (fi″go-gah-lak′tik) [Gr. *pheugein* to avoid + *gala* milk] checking the secretion of milk; galactophygous.

phyla (fi′lah) plural of *phylum*.

phylacagogic (fi-lak″ah-goj′ik) [Gr. *phylakē* a guarding + *agōgos* leading] inducing the formation of phylaxins or protective antibodies.

phylactic (fi-lak′tik) [Gr. *phylaktikos* preservative] serving to protect; pertaining to or producing phylaxis.

phylaxis (fi-lak′sis) [Gr. "a guarding"] protection against infection; the bodily defense against infection.

phyletic (fi-let′ik) pertaining to a phylum, or to phylogeny.

Phyllacanthina (fil″ah-kan-thi′nah) [*phyll-* + Gr. *akantha* thorn, prickle] a suborder of marine protozoa (order Arthracanthida, class Acantharea), usually characterized by the presence of 20 radial spines joined at the cell center by apposition; the bases of the spines have lateral wings.

Phyllanthus (fil-lan′thus) a genus of plants. **P. eng′leri**, a plant of northern Rhodesia known as suicide plant; when the bark or root is smoked it causes death.

phyllidea (fil-id′e-ah) bothridium.

phyll(o)- [Gr. *phyllon* leaf] a combining form denoting relationship to leaves, or to chlorophyll.

Phyllobacterium (fi″lo-bak-te′re-um) [Gr. *phyllos* leaf + *baktērion* small rod] a genus of gram-negative, aerobic, straight, rod-shaped bacteria of the family Rhizobiaceae, which are found in leaf nodules of higher plants.

phyllochlorin (fil″o-klo′rin) a compound of chlorophyll and protein.

phyllode (fil′ode) [Gr. *phyllon* leaf + *eidos* form] resembling a leaf; a term applied to tumors which on section show a lobulated, leaflike appearance.

phylloerythrin (fil″o-er′ĭ-thrin) a derivative of chlorophyll formed in the intestinal canal of ruminant animals and found also in their bile.

phyllolith (fil′o-lith) a small concretion 100 to 200 μ in diameter formed of concentric strata, occurring in cavities in renal tuberculosis.

Phyllopharyngidea (fil″o-far-in-jid′e-ah) [*phyllo-* + *pharynx*] a superorder of ciliate protozoa (subclass Hypostomatia, class Kinetofragminophorea), including free-living, commensal, and parasitic species, and characterized by the presence of a complex cyrtos embedded in foliated or laminated phagoplasm, circumoral ciliature restricted to three short rows of kinetosomes near the oral opening, somatic ciliature only on the ventral surface of the body, and a preoral suture skewed to the left; relatively few but distinctive nematodesmata (often partly recurved with teethlike capitula) are often present. It comprises two orders: Cyrtophorida and Chonotrichida.

phyllopyrrole (fil″o-pir′ol) trimethylethylpyrrole, $(CH_3)_3$-$C_4(NH)C_2H_5$, from bile pigments.

phylloquinone (fil″o-kwin′ōn) phytonadione.

phylloxanthine (fil″o-zan′thin) a compound formed together with phyllocyanic acid by treating chlorophyll with hydrochloric acid.

phylogenesis (fi″lo-jen′ĕ-sis) phylogeny.

phylogenetic (fi″lo-jĕ-net′ik) phylogenic.

phylogenic (fi-lo-jen′ik) pertaining to phylogeny.

phylogeny (fi-loj′ĕ-ne) [Gr. *phylon* tribe + *genesis* generation] the complete developmental history of a race or group of animals. Cf. *ontogeny*.

phylum (fi′lum), pl. *phy′la* [L.; Gr. *phylon* race] a primary or main division of the animal or of the vegetable kingdom, grouping organisms which are assumed to have a common ancestry.

phyma (fi′mah), pl. *phy′mata* [Gr. "a growth"] any skin tumor or cutaneous tubercle, especially a circumscribed swelling on the skin, larger than a tubercle, and produced by exudation into the subcutaneous tissue or the corium.

phymata (fi′mah-tah) [Gr.] plural of *phyma*.

phymatology (fi″mah-tol′o-je) [Gr. *phyma* a growth + *-logy*] the study of tumors, now called oncology.

phymatorhusin (fi″mah-to-roo′sin) [Gr. *phyma* a growth + *rhysis* flow] a dark pigment from hair and melanotic tumors; it is a form of melanin.

phymatorrhysin (fi″mah-to-ris′in) phymatorhusin.

Physalia (fi-sa′le-ah) a genus of hydrozoans, the Portuguese man-of-war, characterized by a large, purple air sac that allows them to float on the surface of the water, and from which many long tentacles of stinging polyps hang. The tentacles are equipped with nematocysts that are able to penetrate the skin of man, causing intense pain; paralysis sometimes results from numerous stings.

physalides (fi-sal′ĭ-dēz) plural of *physalis*.

physaliferous (fis″ah-lif′er-us) [*physalis* + L. *ferre* to bear] physaliphorous.

physaliform (fi-sal′ĭ-form) [*physalis* + L. *forma* shape] resembling bubbles.

physaliphore (fi-sal′ĭ-fōr) [*physalis* + Gr. *phorein* to carry] a globular cavity in certain brood cells of cancers; more correctly, the cell itself which contains such a cavity.

physaliphorous (fis″ah-lif′o-rus) [*physalis* + Gr. *phoros* bearing] containing bubbles or vacuoles.

physalis (fis′ah-lis), pl. *physal′ides* [Gr. *physallis* bubble] 1. a large brood cell from a cancer. 2. a spherical cavity found in certain cells, such as the large brood cells of cancers or the giant cells of sarcoma.

physallization (fis″al-i-za′shun) [Gr. *physallis* bubble] the formation of a permanent froth when a liquid is shaken together with a gas.

Physaloptera (fis″ah-lop′ter-ah) [Gr. *physallis* bubble + *pteron* wing] a genus of nematode worms of the family Spiruroidea, found in the stomach and intestine of man and other vertebrates. **P. caucas′ica,** a species occurring in the Caucasus and in Africa. **P. mor′dens,** *P. caucasica.* **P. ra′ra,** a species found in the stomach of dogs. **P. trunca′ta,** a species found in the proventriculus of chickens and pheasants.

physalopteriasis (fis″ah-lop-ter-i′ah-sis) infection with *Physaloptera.*

Physarida (fi-sahr′ĭ-dah) [G. *physarion* small bellows] an order of ameboid protozoa (subclass Myxogastria, class Eumycetozoa), characterized by the presence of a dark-colored spore mass and a calcareous peridium and capillitium.

physeal (fiz′e-al) pertaining to growth, or to the segment of tubular bone which is concerned mainly with growth (the physis).

physiatrician (fiz″e-ah-trish′an) physiatrist.

physiatrics (fiz″e-at′riks) [*physio-* + Gr. *iatrikē* surgery, medicine] that branch of medicine which deals with the diagnosis, treatment, and prevention of disease with the aid of physical agents, such as light, heat, cold, water, and electricity, or with mechanical apparatus; physical medicine.

physiatrist (fiz″e-at′rist) a physician who specializes in physiatrics.

physiatry (fiz′e-at″re) physiatrics.

physic (fiz′ik) [Gr. *physikos* natural] 1. the art of medicine and of therapeutics. 2. a medicine, especially a cathartic.

physical (fiz′e-kal) [Gr. *physikos*] pertaining to the body, to material things, or to physics.

physician (fĭ-zish′un) 1. an authorized practitioner of medicine, as one graduated from a college of medicine or osteopathy and licensed by the appropriate board. See also *doctor.* 2. one who practices medicine as distinct from surgery. **p. assistant,** one who has been trained in an accredited program and certified by an appropriate board to perform certain of a physician's duties, including history taking, physical examination, diagnostic tests, treatment, certain minor surgical procedures, etc., all under the responsible supervision of a licensed physician. Abbreviated P.A. See also *Medex.* Called also *physician's assistant.* **attending p.,** a physician who attends a hospital at stated times to visit the patients and give directions as to their treatment. **emergency p.,** a specialist in emergency medicine. **family p.,** a medical specialist who plans and provides the comprehensive primary health care of all members of a family, regardless of age or sex, on a continuing basis. **resident p.,** a graduate and licensed physician resident in a hospital.

Physick's operation, pouches (fiz′iks) [Philip Syng *Physick,* American surgeon, 1768–1837] see under *operation* and *pouch.*

physicochemical (fiz″ĭ-ko-kem′ĭ-kal) pertaining to physics and chemistry.

physicotherapeutics, physicotherapy (fiz″ĭ-ko-ther″-ah-pu′tiks; fiz″ĭ-ko-ther′ah-pe) physical therapy.

physics (fiz′iks) [Gr. *physis* nature] the science of the laws and phenomena of nature, but especially of the forces and general properties of matter and energy.

physio- [Gr. *physis* nature] a combining form meaning physical, or denoting relationship to nature or physiology.

physiochemical (fiz″e-o-kem′ĭ-kal) pertaining to physiologic chemistry, or clinical chemistry.

physiochemistry (fiz″e-o-kem′is-tre) physiologic chemistry, or clinical chemistry.

physiogenesis (fiz″e-o-jen′ĕ-sis) embryology.

physiognomy (fiz″e-og′no-me) [*physio-* + Gr. *gnōmōn* a judge] 1. the determination of temperament and character from facial features. 2. physiognosis.

physiognosis (fiz″e-og-no′sis) [*physio-* + Gr. *gnōsis* knowl-edge] diagnosis by means of the facial expression or appearance.

physiologic (fiz″e-o-loj′ik) normal; not pathologic; characteristic of or conforming to the normal functioning or state of the body or a tissue or organ; physiological.

physiological (fiz″e-o-loj′ĭ-kal) pertaining to physiology; physiologic.

physiologicoanatomical (fiz″e-o-loj″e-ko-an″ah-tom′e-kal) pertaining to physiology and anatomy.

physiologist (fiz″e-ol′o-jist) a specialist in the study of physiology.

physiology (fiz″e-ol′o-je) [*physio-* + *-logy*] 1. the science which treats of the functions of the living organism and its parts, and of the physical and chemical factors and processes involved. 2. the basic processes underlying the functioning of a species or class of organism, or any of its parts or processes. **animal p.,** the physiology of animals. **comparative p.,** a study of organ functions in various types of animals, vertebrate and invertebrate, in an effort to find fundamental relations in the physiology of members of the entire animal kingdom. **dental p.,** the study of the function and functional form of the teeth and supporting tissues. **general p.,** the science of the general laws of life and functional activity. **hominal p.,** human physiology. **morbid p., pathologic p.,** the study of disordered function or of function in diseased tissues. **special p.,** the physiology of particular organs. **vegetable p.,** the physiology of plants.

physiolysis (fiz″e-ol′ĭ-sis) [*physio-* + Gr. *lysis* dissolution] natural dissolution and disintegration of tissue.

physiomedicalism (fiz″e-o-med′ĭ-kal-izm) [*physio-* + *medicalism*] a system of medical treatment in which only plant remedies are used, excluding those which are poisonous.

physiometry (fiz″e-om′ĕ-tre) [*physio-* + Gr. *metron* measure] measurement of the physiologic functions of the body by serologic and physiologic methods.

physionomy (fiz″e-on′o-me) [*physio-* + Gr. *nomos* law] the science of the laws of nature.

physiopathic (fiz″e-o-path′ik) [*physio-* + Gr. *pathos* disease] Babinski's term for the nonpsychopathic functional nervous disorders.

physiopathologic (fiz″e-o-path″o-loj′ik) pertaining to both the physiologic and pathologic conditions.

physiopathology (fiz″e-o-pah-thol′o-je) [*physio-* + *pathology*] the science of functions in disease, or as modified by disease.

physiophyly (fiz″e-of′ĭ-le) [*physio-* + Gr. *phylon* tribe] the evolution of bodily functions.

physiotherapeutist (fiz″e-o-ther″ah-pu′tist) physical therapist.

physiotherapist (fiz″e-o-ther′ah-pist) physical therapist.

physiotherapy (fiz″e-o-ther′a-pe) [*physio-* + Gr. *therapeia* cure] physical therapy.

physique (fĭ-zēk′) bodily structure, organization, and development.

physis (fi′sis) [Gr. *phyein* to generate] the segment of tubular bone which is concerned mainly with growth in length of the bone. It consists of four zones: zone of resting cartilage, zone of proliferating cartilage, zone of hypertrophy, and zone of calcification.

physo- [Gr. *physa* air] a combining form denoting relationship to air or gas.

physocele (fi′so-sēl) [*physo-* + Gr. *kēlē* tumor] 1. a tumor filled with gas. 2. a hernial sac filled with gas.

Physocephalus (fi″so-sef′ah-lus) a genus of nematode worms of the superfamily Spiruroidea. **P. sexala′tus,** a species found in the stomach of pigs.

physocephaly (fi″so-sef′ah-le) [*physo-* + Gr. *kephalē* head] emphysematous swelling of the head.

physohematometra (fi″so-hem″ah-to-me′trah) [*physo-* + Gr. *haima* blood + *metra* uterus] the presence of gas and blood within the uterus.

physohydrometra (fi″so-hi″dro-me′trah) [*physo-* + Gr. *hydōr* water + *metra* uterus] the presence of gas and fluid within the uterus.

physometra (fi″so-me′trah) [*physo-* + Gr. *metra* uterus] air or gas in the uterine cavity.

Physopsis (fī-sŏp′sĭs) a subgenus of snails (genus *Bulinus*), several species of which are the intermediate hosts of *Schistosoma haematobium* and other animal schistosomes.

physopyosalpinx (fi″so-pi″o-sal′pinks) [*physo-* + Gr. *pyon* pus + *salpinx* tube] presence of pus and gas in the uterine tube.

Physostigma (fi″so-stig′mah) [*physo-* + Gr. *stigma* stigma] a genus of tropical leguminous plants. The poisonous seed of *P. venenosum* Balf., Calabar bean, a climbing plant of Africa, contains the alkaloid, physostigmine.

physostigmine (fiz″o-stig′mēn) [USP] a cholinergic alkaloid having anticholinesterase activity obtained from the dried ripe seed (Calabar bean) of *Physostigma venenosum;* used topically to produce miosis and decrease of intraocular pressure in glaucoma and parenterally to reverse the central nervous system effects produced by overdosage of anticholinergic drugs (anticholinergic syndrome). Called also *eserine.* Available as *physostigmine* [USP], *physostigmine salicylate* [USP], and *physostigmine sulfate* [USP]. **p. salicylate** [USP], the salicylate salt of physostigmine with the same properties as the alkaloid. **p. sulfate** [USP], the sulfate salt of physostigmine with the same properties as the alkaloid.

physostigminism (fi″so-stig′min-izm) poisoning by physostigmine.

phytagglutinin (fi″tah-gloo′tĭ-nin) a phytotoxin which has the power of agglutinating red blood corpuscles.

phytalbumin (fi″tal-bu′min) [*phyto-* + *albumin*] vegetable albumin.

phytalbumose (fi-tal′bu-mōs) [*phyto-* + *albumose*] an albumose of vegetable origin.

phytanic acid (fi-tan′ik) 3,7,11,15-tetramethylhexadecanoate, a long-chain fatty acid that is an oxidation product of phytol, found in animal fat and dairy products.

phytanic acid α-hydroxylase (fi-tan′ik) an enzyme that catalyzes the conversion of phytanic acid to α-hydroxyphytanic acid. The reaction is stimulated by NADPH and requires molecular oxygen. Defect of the enzyme, an autosomal recessive trait, is the cause of Refsum's disease.

phytase (fi′tās) an enzyme (a hydrolase) of plants that catalyzes the hydrolysis of phytic acid to inositol and phosphoric acid.

6-phytase (fi′tās) [EC 3.1.3.26] an enzyme of the hydrolase class that catalyzes the reaction *myo*-inositol hexakisphosphate + H_2O = 1 L-*myo*-inositol 1,2,3,4,5-pentakisphosphate + orthophosphate. The enzyme, present at a low level in ileal mucosa, hydrolyzes excess dietary phytic acid.

phytate (fi′tāt) an anionic form of phytic acid.

-phyte [Gr. *phyton* plant] a combining form denoting a plant or a pathological growth.

phytic acid (fi′tik) inositol hexaphosphate, a compound occurring in the leaves of plants.

phytin (fi′tin) the calcium-magnesium salt of phytic acid; a form of inositol found in plants, it is used as a dietary supplement.

phyt(o)- [Gr. *phyton* plant] a combining form denoting relationship to a plant or plants.

phytoalexin (fi″to-ah-lek′sin) any of a group of compounds formed in plants in response to fungal infection, physical damage, chemical injury, or a pathogenic process. Phytoalexins inhibit or destroy the invading agent.

phytoanaphylactogen (fi″to-an″ah-fi-lak′to-jen) [*phyto-* + *anaphylactogen*] an antigen of plant origin that is capable of inducing anaphylaxis; called also *phytosensitinogen.*

phytobezoar (fi″to-be′zōr) [*phyto-* + *bezoar*] a gastric concretion composed of vegetable matter such as skins, seeds, and the fibers of fruit and vegetables.

phytochemistry (fi″to-kem′is-tre) [*phyto-* + *chemistry*] the study of plant chemistry, including the chemical processes that take place in plants, the nature of plant chemicals, and the various applications of such chemicals to science and industry.

phytochinin (fi″to-kin′in) a substance isolated from the leaves of certain grasses, said to have an effect on carbohydrate metabolism resembling that of insulin.

phytocholesterol (fi″to-ko-les′ter-ol) phytosterol.

phytochrome (fi′to-krōm) [*phyto-* + Gr. *chrōma* color] a bluish conjugated protein occurring in plants, whose re-

sponse to relative periods of light and darkness regulates photoperiodism (e.g., the flowering cycle); it occurs in two forms, one responding to the red end of the spectrum, the other to far red.

phytodemic (fi″to-dem′ik) [*phyto-* + *epidemic*] an epidemic attack of any disease of plants.

phytodetritus (fi″to-de-tri′tus) detritus produced by the disintegration and decomposition of vegetable organisms. Cf. *zoodetritus.*

phytoflagellate (fi″to-flaj′ĕ-lāt) [*phyto-* + L. *flagellum* whip] a plantlike flagellate protozoan of the class Phytomastigophorea. Cf. *zooflagellate.*

phytogenesis (fi″to-jen′ĕ-sis) [*phyto-* + Gr. *genesis* generation] the origin and development of plants.

phytogenetic, phytogenic (fi″to-jĕ-net′ik; fi″to-jen′ik) phytogenous.

phytogenous (fi-toj′ĕ-nus) [*phyto-* + Gr. *gennan* to produce] derived from a plant, or caused by a vegetable growth.

phytohemagglutinin (fi″to-hem″ah-gloo′tĭ-nin) a lectin isolated from the red kidney bean (*Phaseolus vulgaris*); it is a hemagglutinin that agglutinates mammalian erythrocytes and a mitogen that stimulates predominantly T lymphocytes. Abbreviated PHA.

phytohormone (fi″to-hor′mōn) [*phyto-* + *hormone*] plant hormone; any of the hormones produced naturally in plants and which are active in minute amounts in controlling growth and other functions at a site remote from the place of production. There are three principal types: auxins, cytokinins, and gibberellins.

phytoid (fi′toid) [*phyto-* + Gr. *eidos* form] resembling a plant.

phytol (fi′tol) chemical name: 3,7,11,15-tetramethyl-hexadecen-2-ol-1. An unsaturated aliphatic alcohol, $CH_3[CH-(CH_3)(CH_2)_3]_3C(CH_3){:}CH{\cdot}CH_2OH$, which is related to xanthophyll, to the carotenoids, and to vitamin A, and exists in chlorophyll as an ester; used in the preparation of vitamin E and phytonadione.

Phytomastigophora (fi″to-mas″tĭ-gof′o-rah) Phytomastigophorea.

Phytomastigophorea (fi″to-mas″tĭ-gof″o-re′ah) [*phyto-* + Gr. *mastix* whip + *phoros* bearing] a class comprising all of the plantlike, as opposed to animal-like, protozoa (subphylum Mastigophora, phylum Sarcomastigophora), which are collectively known as the phytoflagellates. Phytomastigophoreans are characterized by the presence of chromatophores and usually one or two emergent flagella, with ameboid forms occurring in some groups. They are mostly free-living and are typically autotrophic. These organisms are sometimes classified with the algae. It comprises 10 orders: Crytomonadida, Dinoflagellida, Euglenida, Chrysomonadida, Heterochlorida, Chloromonadida, Prymnesiida, Volvocida, Prasinomonadida, and Silicoflagellida. Called also *Phytomastigophorea.* Cf. *Zoomastigophorea.*

phytomastigophorean (fi″to-mas″tĭ-gof″o-re′an) a protozoan of the class Phytomastigophorea.

phytomelin (fi″to-mel′in) rutin.

phytomenadione (fi″to-men″ah-di′ōn) phytonadione.

phytomitogen (fi″to-mi′to-jen) a substance of plant origin that induces mitosis in human cells.

Phytomonadina (fi″to-mon-ah-di′nah) an order of protozoa of the class Phytomastigophora, subphylum Mastigophora, comprising plantlike flagellates. In former classifications, it was included, along with the order Protomonadina, in the group Monadina.

phytonadione (fi″to-nah-di′ōn) 1. chemical name: [*R*-[*R**,*R**- (*E*)]]-2-methyl-3-(3,7,-11,15-tetramethyl-2-hexadecenyl)-1,4-naphthalenedione. A fat-soluble vitamin of the K group, $C_{31}H_{46}O_2$, found in green plants or prepared synthetically and having prothrombinogenic properties. 2. [USP] a clear, yellow to amber, very viscous liquid containing 97 to 103 per cent phytonadione; used as a prothrombinogenic agent in the treatment of hypoprothrombinemia due to various causes, administered orally and parenterally. Called also *phylloquinone* and *vitamin K_1.*

phytone (fi′tōn) a peptone made from plant protein.

phytonosis (fi-ton′o-sis) [*phyto-* + Gr. *nosos* disease] any morbid condition due to a plant.

phytoparasite (fi″to-par′ah-sīt) [*phyto-* + *parasite*] any parasitic vegetable organism or species.

phytopathogenic (fi″to-path″o-jen′ik) producing disease in plants.

phytopathology (fi″to-pah-thol′o-je) [*phyto-* + *pathology*] 1. the study of plant diseases and their control. 2. the pathology of morbid conditions caused by schizomycetes and other vegetable parasites.

phytopathy (fi-top′ah-the) [*phyto-* + Gr. *pathos* disease] any disease of plants.

phytophagous (fi-tof′ah-gus) [*phyto-* + Gr. *phagein* to eat] eating vegetable food.

phytopharmacology (fi″to-fahr″mah-kol′o-je) [*phyto-* + *pharmacology*] the study of the effect of drugs on plant growth.

phytophotodermatitis (fi″to-fo″to-der″mah-ti′tis) [*phyto-* + *photo-* + *dermatitis*] phototoxic dermatitis induced by the sequential exposure to certain plants containing psoralen-type photosensitizers and then to sunlight. It is manifested by burning erythema, followed by edema and the development of small vesicles that coalesce into large bullae, and this is followed by intense residual hyperpigmentation in the areas of the skin that come in contact with the psoralen photosensitizer.

phytoplankton (fi″to-plank′ton) [*phyto-* + Gr. *planktos* wandering] the minute plant (vegetable) organisms which, with those of the animal kingdom, make up the plankton of natural waters.

phytoplasm (fi′to-plazm) [*phyto-* + Gr. *plasma* thing formed] vegetable protoplasm.

phytoprecipitin (fi″to-pre-sip′ĭ-tin) a precipitin produced by immunization with protein substances of plant origin.

phytosensitinogen (fi″to-sen″sĭ-tin′o-jen) [*phyto-* + *sensitinogen*] phytoanaphylactogen.

phytosis (fi-to′sis) [*phyto-* + *-osis*] any disease caused by a phytoparasite.

phytosterin (fi-tos′ter-in) [*phyto-* + Gr. *stear* fat] phytosterol.

phytosterol (fi″to-ste′rol) a plant sterol.

phytosterolin (fi″to-ste′rol-in) a glucosidic union of a sterol and glucose.

phytotherapy (fi″to-ther′ah-pe) [*phyto-* + Gr. *therapeia* treatment] treatment by use of plants.

phytotoxic (fi″to-tok′sik) 1. pertaining to a phytotoxin, or plant poison. 2. inhibiting the growth of plants.

phytotoxin (fi″to-tok′sin) an exotoxin produced by certain species of higher plants, notably *Abrus precatorius* (abrin), *Ricinus communis* (ricin), *Croton tiglium* (crotin), and *Robinia pseudacacia* (robin). Phytotoxins are resistant to proteolytic digestion, and are effective when taken by mouth. In the broadest sense a phytotoxin is any toxic substance of plant origin.

phytotrichobezoar (fi″to-tri″ko-be′zōr) [*phyto-* + Gr. *thrix* hair + *bezoar*] a bezoar composed of both plant fibers and hair.

phytotron (fi′to-tron) a laboratory in which virtually any climatic condition can be simulated for plant growth studies.

phytovitellin (fi″to-vi-tel′in) vitellin of vegetable origin.

phytoxylin (fi-tok′sĭ-lin) [*phyto-* + Gr. *xylon* wood] a substance resembling pyroxylin; used in preparing celloidin sections.

PI phosphatidylinositol.

P.I. protamine insulin.

pI the pH of a solution containing a solute at its isoelectric point.

pi (pi) [Π, π] the sixteenth letter of the Greek alphabet.

pia (pi′ah) [L.] 1. tender; soft. 2. pia mater. **p. ma′ter,** see *pia mater,* below.

pia-arachnitis (pi″ah-ar″ak-ni′tis) inflammation of the pia-arachnoid; leptomeningitis.

pia-arachnoid (pi″ah-ah-rak′noid) [*pia* + *arachnoid*] the pia mater and the arachnoid considered together as one functional unit; the leptomeninges.

pia-glia (pi″ah-gli′ah) a membrane formed by the fusion of the pia mater and the marginal glia, and constituting one of the layers of the pia-arachnoid.

pial (pi′al) pertaining to the pia mater.

pia mater (pi′ah ma′ter) [L. "tender mother"] the innermost of the three membranes (meninges) covering the brain and spinal cord, investing them closely and extending into the depths of the fissures and sulci; it consists of reticular, elastic, and collagenous fibers. **p. m. enceph′ali** [NA], the pia mater covering the brain, very thin over the cerebral cortex, and thicker over the brain stem; the blood vessels for the brain ramify within it and, as they enter the brain, are accompanied for a short distance by a pial sheath. **p. m. spina′lis** [NA], the pia mater covering the spinal cord and consisting of collagenous fibers, which also form the denticulate ligament, and reticular fibers, which closely invest the cord, form the various septa, and form an investment for the rootlets.

piamatral (pi″ah-ma′tral) pial.

pian (pe-ahn′) [Fr.] yaws. **p. bois,** a form of cutaneous leishmaniasis of the New World occurring in the forests of the Guianas and northern Brazil, caused by *Leishmania braziliensis guyanensis*, transmitted chiefly by *Lutzomyia umbratilis,* and characterized by the presence of multiple, widespread, deep skin ulcers with nodular lymphatic metastases. Called also *forest yaws.* **hemorrhagic p.,** see *bartonellosis.*

piarachnitis (pi″ar-ak-ni′tis) pia-arachnitis.

piarachnoid (pi″ar-ak′noid) pia-arachnoid.

piarhemia (pi″ar-he′me-ah) [Gr. *piar* fat + *haima* blood + *-ia*] the presence of fat in the blood; lipemia.

piastrinemia (pi-as″trĭ-ne′me-ah) [It. *piastre* coin + Gr. *haima* blood + *-ia*] thrombocythemia.

piblokto (pĭ-blok′to) [Eskimo] a culture-specific syndrome seen chiefly among Eskimo women, marked by attacks of screaming, crying, and running naked through the snow, sometimes with suicidal or homicidal tendencies.

pica (pi′kah) [L. "magpie" (because this bird eats or carries away odd objects)] compulsive eating of nonnutritive substances, such as ice (pagophagia), dirt (geophagia), gravel, flaking paint or plaster, clay, hair (trichophagia), or laundry starch (amylophagia). Pica and unusual food cravings (citta) are common in pregnant women. Pica also occurs in some patients with iron or zinc deficiencies. In children this syndrome, classified with the eating disorders in DSM III-R, is a rare mental disorder with onset typically in the second year of life; it usually remits in childhood but may persist into adolescence.

piceous (pi′se-us) [L. *piceis*] of the nature of or resembling pitch.

pick (pik) any pointed or other sharp device for removing objects from areas that are difficult to access. **apical p.,** see under *elevator.* **crane p.,** an elevator for the removal of root fragments of mandibular molar teeth fractured during extraction. **root p.,** apical elevator.

Pick's bodies, disease (piks) [Arnold *Pick*, Prague psychiatrist, 1851–1924] see under *body* and *disease* (def. 1).

Pick's cell, disease (piks) [Ludwig *Pick*, Berlin physician, 1868–1944] see under *cell,* and *Niemann-Pick disease,* under *disease.*

Pick's disease, syndrome [Friedel *Pick*, Prague physician, 1867–1926] see under *disease* (def. 2), and under *syndrome.*

pickling (pik′ling) 1. the process of cleansing newly cast metallic surfaces and removal of oxides and other impurities from metal objects by immersion in an acid solution. 2. a method of food preservation with the use of organic acid (usually acetic acid), sugar, salt, and spices.

pickwickian syndrome (pik-wik′e-an) [from the description of the fat boy in Dickens' *Pickwick Papers*] see under *syndrome.*

pico- [Sp. *pico* small amount; It. *piccolo* small] a combining form used in naming units of measurement to indicate one-trillionth (10^{-12}) of the unit designated by the root with which it is combined.

picocurie (pi″ko-ku′re) a unit of radioactivity, being one-trillionth (10^{-12}) curie, or the quantity of radioactive material in which the number of nuclear disintegrations is 3.7×10^{-2}, or 0.037, per second. Abbreviated pCi. Called also *micromicrocurie.*

picodnavirus (pi-kod″nah-vi′rus) [*pico-* + *deoxyribonucleic acid* + *virus*] parvovirus.

picogram (pi′ko-gram) a unit of mass (weight) of the metric system, being 10^{-12} gram. Abbreviated pg. Called also *microgamma* and *micromicrogram.*

picopicogram (pi″ko-pi′ko-gram) a unit of mass (weight)

of the metric system, being 10^{-12} picogram, or 10^{-24} gram. Abbreviated ppg.

picornavirus (pi-kor″nah-vi′rus) [pico- + ribonucleic acid + virus] a name applied to one of the extremely small ether-resistant RNA viruses, the group comprising the enteroviruses and the rhinoviruses.

picounit (pi″ko-u′nit) one trillionth part of a unit (10^{-12}).

picrate (pik′rāt) any salt of picric acid.

picric acid (pik′rik) trinitrophenol.

picr(o)- [Gr. pikros bitter] a combining form meaning bitter, or denoting relationship to picric acid.

picrocarmine (pik″ro-kar′min) a stain prepared from picric acid and carmine and used in microscopy. It consists of a mixture of carmine, ammonia, and distilled water, to which is added an aqueous solution of picric acid.

picrogeusia (pik″ro-gu′se-ah) [picro- + Gr. geusis taste + -ia] a pathologic bitter taste.

picrol (pik′rol) chemical name: potassium diiodoresorcin monosulfonate. A colorless and odorless, bitter, antiseptic powder, $(OH)_2 \cdot C_6HI_2 \cdot SO_2OK$, which contains about 53 per cent iodine; used as a substitute for iodoform and corrosive sublimate.

picronigrosin (pik″ro-ni-gro′sin) a solution of picric acid and nigrosin in alcohol, used as a stain.

picropodophyllin (pik″ro-pod″o-fil′in) chemical name: picropodophyllinic acid lactone. A crystalline principle, $C_{22}H_{22}O_8$, from Podophyllum peltatum L. (Berberidaceae): medicinally active. It is obtainable from podophyllotoxin also, and is an isomer of it.

Picrorrhiza (pik″ro-ri′zah) [picro- + Gr. rhiza root] a genus of herbs; the rhizome of P. kurroa Royle (Scrophulariaceae) is tonic and antiperiodic.

picrosaccharometer (pi″kro-sak″ah-rom′ĕ-ter) an instrument used in estimating diabetic sugar.

picrosclerotine (pik″ro-skle′ro-tin) a poisonous alkaloid occurring in ergot of rye.

picrotoxin (pik″ro-tok′sin) [NF] an active principle, $C_{30}H_{34}O_{13}$, obtained from the seed (cocculus indicus) of Anamirta cocculus L. Wight & Arn. (Menispermaceae), and occurring as flexible, shining, prismatic crystals or as a microcrystalline powder; it stimulates all portions of the central nervous system by blocking presynaptic inhibition of neural impulses and has been used as a central and respiratory stimulant in the treatment of poisoning by central nervous system depressant drugs, especially the barbiturates, administered intravenously. Called also cocculin.

picrotoxinism (pik″ro-tok′sĭ-nizm) poisoning by picrotoxin.

PID pelvic inflammatory disease.

piebald (pi′bawld) exhibiting piebaldism.

piebaldism (pi′bawld-izm) a congenital autosomal dominant pigmentary disorder of the skin due to absence of functioning melanocytes and melanin, resulting in patchy areas of depigmentation or hypopigmentation, often occurring in association with white forelock. Called also albinismus circumscriptus and localized or partial albinism. Cf. leukoderma and vitiligo.

piece (pēs) a part or portion. **chief p.**, principal p. **connecting p.**, 1. middle p. 2. the neck of a spermatozoon. **end p.**, 1. end-piece; see under E. 2. the terminal portion of the tail, or flagellum, of a spermatozoon; called also terminal filament. See illustration under spermatozoon. **middle p.**, the portion of the tail of a spermatozoon limited by the anterior centriole and by the annulus; called also connecting p. See also illustration under spermatozoon. **principal p.**, the main portion of the tail of a spermatozoon, beginning at the annulus and gradually tapering toward the end piece; called also chief p. See illustration under spermatozoon. **secretory p.**, see under component.

piedra (pe-a′drah) [Sp.] a fungal infection of the hair shaft characterized by the presence of dark or pale, firm, irregular nodules composed of fungal elements. **black p.**, piedra caused by Piedraia hortae, usually occurring in tropical regions, and characterized by the presence of small black or brown gritty nodules on the shafts of the scalp hair. **white p.**, piedra most commonly involving the hair of the beard, axilla, and groin, caused by Trichosporon cutaneum, usually occurring in tropical regions, and characterized by the presence of white to light brown nodules that are softer

than those seen in the black variety. Called also trichosporosis.

Piedraia (pi″ĕ-dri′ah) a genus of ascomycetous fungi of the family Piedraiaceae, one species of which, P. hortae, is parasitic on hair, forming small black adherent nodules; see black piedra, under piedra.

Piedraiaceae (pi″ĕ-dri-a′se-e) a family of ascomycetous fungi of the order Myriangiales, subclass Loculoascomycetidae, which includes the genus Piedraia.

pier (pēr) intermediate abutment.

Pierre Robin syndrome (pe-yair′ro-ba′) [Pierre Robin, French dentist, 1867–1950] see under syndrome.

Piersol's point (pēr′solz) [George Arthur Piersol, Philadelphia anatomist, 1856–1924] see under point.

piesesthesia (pi-e″zes-the′ze-ah) [Gr. piesis pressure + aisthēsis perception] pressure sensibility; the sense by which pressure stimuli are felt.

piesimeter (pi″e-sim′ĕ-ter) [Gr. piesis pressure + metron measure] an instrument for testing the sensitiveness of the skin to pressure. **Hales' p.**, a glass tube inserted into an artery for the purpose of ascertaining the blood pressure by the height to which the blood rises in the tube.

-piesis [Gr. piesis a pressing or squeezing] a word termination meaning pressure, as in otopiesis.

piezallochromy (pi″e-zal′o-kro-me) [Gr. piesis pressure + allochromy] change of color of a substance caused by crushing.

piezesthesia (pi″e-zes-the′ze-ah) piesesthesia.

piezocardiogram (pi-e″zo-kar′de-o-gram″) a graphic tracing of the changes in pressure caused by pulsation of the heart, often recorded through the esophagus.

piezochemistry (pi-e′zo-kem″is-tre) [Gr. piesis pressure + chemistry] that branch of chemistry which deals with the effect of pressure on chemical phenomena.

piezometer (pi″e-zom′ĕ-ter) [Gr. piezein to press + -meter] 1. piesimeter. 2. orbitonometer.

PIF prolactin inhibiting factor; proliferation inhibitory factor. See under factor.

pifarnine (pĭ-far′nēn) chemical name: 1-(1,3-benzodioxol-5-ylmethyl)-4-(3,7,11-trimethyl-2,6,10-dodecatrienyl) piperazine; a gastric antiulcerative, $C_{27}H_{40}N_2O_2$.

pigment (pig′ment) [L. pigmentum paint] 1. any normal or abnormal coloring matter of the body. 2. a paintlike medicinal preparation to be applied to the skin. **bile p.**, any one of the coloring matters of the bile; they are bilirubin, biliverdin, bilifuscin, biliprasin, choleprasin, bilihumin, and bilicyanin. **blood p.**, any of the pigments derived from hemoglobin; they are heme, hematoidin, hemosiderin, hematoporphyrin, methemoglobin, and hemofuscin. **endogenous p.**, a pigment derived from material normally present in the body. **exogenous p.**, a pigment inhaled or ingested and deposited in the lungs and other tissues. **fatty p.**, lipid p. **hematogenous p.**, a pigment derived from accumulation of hemoglobin derivatives such as hematoidin or hemosiderin. **hepatogenous p.**, bile pigment formed by disintegration of hemoglobin in the liver. **lipid p.**, any of various pigments having lipid characteristics, some of which also contain protein or iron, the most important one being lipofuscin. Called also fatty p. **lipochrome p.**, lipochrome. **malarial p.**, a pigment formed by the malarial parasite from the pigment of the blood and deposited largely in the spleen and liver. **melanotic p.**, melanin. **respiratory p's**, substances, such as hemoglobin, myoglobin, or the cytochromes, which take part in the oxidation processes of the animal body. **wear and tear p's**, lipochromes.

pigmentary (pig′men-ta″re) pertaining to or of the nature of a pigment.

pigmentation (pig″men-ta′shun) 1. the deposition of coloring matter; the coloration or discoloration of a part by a pigment. 2. coloration, especially abnormally increased coloration, by melanin.

pigmented (pig′ment-ed) colored by deposit of pigment.

pigmentogenesis (pig″men-to-jen′ĕ-sis) [pigment + genesis] the production of pigment.

pigmentogenic (pig″men-to-jen′ik) inducing the formation or deposit of pigment.

pigmentolysin (pig″men-tol′ĭ-sin)   a lysin causing destruction of pigment.

pigmentolysis (pig″men-tol′ĭ-sis) [*pigment* + Gr. *lysis* dissolution]   destruction of pigment.

pigmentophage (pig-men′to-fāj) [*pigment* + Gr. *phagein* to eat]   any pigment-devouring cell, especially such a cell of the hair; called also *chromophage*.

pigmentophore (pig-men′to-fōr)   a cell that transports pigment.

Pignet's formula (index, standard) (pēn-yāz′) [Maurice Charles-Joseph *Pignet*, French physician, born 1871]   see under *formula*.

piitis (pi-i′tis)   inflammation of the pia mater.

pikromycin (pik-ro-mi′sin)   proactinomycin A.

Pil.   abbreviation of L. *pilula*, pill, or *pil′ulae*, pills.

Pila (pi′lah)   a genus of freshwater snails. **P. con′ica,** the second intermediate host of *Echinostoma ilocanum* in the Philippines.

pila (pi′lah), pl. *pi′lae* [L.]   a pillar or pillar-like structure, such as a trabecula of spongy bone.

pilae (pi′le) [L.]   genitive and plural of *pila*.

pilar, pilary (pi′lar, pil′a-re) [L. *pilaris*]   pertaining to the hair.

pilaster (pi-las′ter)   a ridge or fluting. **p. of Broca,** linea aspera femoris.

Pilcher bag (pil′cher) [Lewis Stephen *Pilcher*, Brooklyn surgeon, 1845–1934]   see under *bag*.

pile (pīl)   1. [L. *pila* pillar] an aggregation of similar elements for generating electricity. In nucleonics, a chain-reacting fission device for producing slow neutrons and for the preparation of radioactive isotopes. 2. [L. *pila* a ball] a hemorrhoid. **muscular p.,** layers of muscular tissue so arranged as to generate an electric current. **prostatic p.,** enlarged prostate attended by hemorrhage. **sentinel p.,** a hemorrhoid-like thickening of the mucous membrane at the lower end of a fissure of the anus. **thermoelectric p.,** a set of slender metallic bars which, on exposure to heat, generates a current of electricity that moves an index and is made to register delicate changes of temperature. **voltaic p.,** a battery for current electricity made up of a series of metallic disks.

piles (pīlz)   hemorrhoids.

pileus (pi′le-us) [L. "a close fitting felt cap"]   the membrane which sometimes covers a child's head at birth; caul.

pili (pi′li) [L.]   genitive and plural of *pilus*.

pilial (pi′le-al)   pertaining to a pilus or pili.

piliate (pi′le-at)   having pili; said of bacteria.

Pilidae (pil′ĭ-de)   a family of fresh-water snails (order Mesogastropoda) that includes the species *Pila conica*, the second intermediate host of *Echinostoma ilocanum*.

piliform (pi′li-form)   shaped like or resembling hair.

Pilimelia (pi″lĭ-mel′e-ah) [L. *pilus* hair + Gr. *Melia* a mythical water nymph]   a genus of bacteria of the family Actinoplanaceae, order Actinomycetales, consisting of soil organisms producing rod-shaped spores in a parallel chains. The type species is *P. tereva′sa.*

pilimictio (pi″lĭ-mik′she-o)   pilimiction.

pilimiction (pi″lĭ-mik′shun) [L. *pilus* hair + *mictio* micturition]   passing of urine containing hair or hairlike threads of mucus.

pilin (pi′lin)   the protein that composes bacterial pili.

Pilisuctorina (pi″lĭ-suk″to-ri′nah) [*pilus* + L. *suctio*, from *sugere* to suck, suction]   a suborder of protozoa (order Apostomatida, superorder Apostomatidea) associated with various marine crustaceans and perhaps terrestrial mites, the mature forms of which are nonciliated and immobile with migrating immature forms being flattened, ciliated, and without a cytostome.

pill (pil) [L. *pilula*]   a small globular or oval medicated mass to be swallowed. Pills contain, in addition to the active drug, a diluent (or filler) and an excipient to give the mass adhesiveness, firmness, and plasticity, so that the pill can be worked by hand or machine to the desired pillular form. Cf. *tablet.* **A.B.S. p.,** a laxative pill, containing aloin, extract of belladonna, and strychnine. **blue p.,** mercury mass. **chalybeate p's,** ferrous carbonate p's. **compound cathartic p.,** a pill of colocynth, calomel, jalap, and gam-

boge. **enteric p.,** one coated with a substance, such as salol, which will not dissolve in the stomach. **ferrous carbonate p's,** pills containing ferrous sulfate, potassium carbonate, sucrose, tragacanth, althea, glycerin, water; used as a hematinic. **ferruginous p's,** ferrous carbonate p's. **Fothergill's p.** (*obs.*), a pill of calomel, squill, and digitalis. **Guy's p.** (*obs.*), a pill composed of digitalis, squill, extract of hyoscyamus, and mercury mass. **hexylresorcinol p's** [NF], a pill consisting of hexylresorcinol covered with a rupture-resistant coating that disintegrates in the digestive tract; used as an anthelmintic against intestinal nematodes and trematodes. **radio p.,** telemetering capsule.

pillar (pil′ar) [L. *pila*]   a supporting column, usually occurring in pairs. **p. of Corti's organ,** see *pillar cells*, under *cell*. **p's of diaphragm,** see *pars lumbalis diaphragmatis*. **p. of fauces, anterior,** arcus palatoglossus. **p. of fauces, posterior,** arcus palatopharyngeus. **p. of fornix, anterior,** columna fornicis. **p. of fornix, posterior,** crus fornicis. **p's of soft palate,** see *arcus palatoglossus* and *arcus palatopharyngeus*. **Uskow's p's,** two folds of the embryo attached to the dorsolateral portion of the body wall; from these pillars and the septum transversum the diaphragm is formed.

pillet (pil′et)   a little pill, or pellet.

pillion (pil-yon′)   a temporary replacement for an amputated leg.

pil(o)- [L. *pilus* hair]   a combining form denoting relationship to hair, resembling or composed of hair.

pilobezoar (pi″lo-be′zōr)   trichobezoar.

pilocarpine (pi″lo-kar′pēn)   a cholinomimetic alkaloid obtained from leaves of plants of the genus *Pilocarpus* having predominantly muscarinic effects; when applied to the eye, it produces miosis and a transient rise and persistent fall in intraocular pressure; used in the treatment of glaucoma; also administered by iontophoresis to produce sweating in the sweat chloride test for cystic fibrosis. Available as *pilocarpine* [USP], *pilocarpine hydrochloride* [USP], and *pilocarpine nitrate* [USP]. **p. hydrochloride** [USP], the monohydrochloride salt of pilocarpine, $C_{11}H_{16}N_2O_2 \cdot HCl$, with the same properties as the alkaloid. **p. nitrate** [USP], the nitrate salt of pilocarpine, $C_{11}H_{16}N_2 \cdot HNO_3$, having the same actions and uses as the alkaloid.

Pilocarpus (pi″lo-kar′pus) [Gr. *pilos* wool or hair wrought into felt + Gr. *karpos* fruit]   a genus of rutaceous shrubs of tropical America; the leaves of *P. jaborandi* and *P. microphyllus* yield pilocarpine.

pilocystic (pi″lo-sis′tik) [*pilo-* + *cystic*]   hollow, or cystlike, and containing hairs; said of certain dermoid tumors.

pilocytic (pi″lo-si′tik)   composed of fiber-shaped cells.

piloerection (pi″lo-e-rek′shun) [*pilo-* + *erection*]   erection of the hair.

pilojection (pi″lo-jek′shun) [*pilo* + L. *jacere* to throw]   the introduction of one or more hairs into the sac of an aneurysm by means of a pneumatic gun, to furnish the nucleus for a blood clot inside the sac; used in the treatment of intracranial saccular aneurysms.

pilomatricoma (pi″lo-mah-trĭ-ko′mah) [*pilo-* + *matrix* + *-oma*]   a solitary benign calcifying tumor of hair follicle origin manifested as a sharply circumscribed, firm intracutaneous nodule, usually occurring on the face, neck, or upper extremity, and most often presenting before the age of 20. Histological features include a fibrous stroma surrounding nests of basophilic cells and ghost, or shadow, cells. Called also *benign calcified* or *calcified epithelioma, calcifying epithelioma of Malherbe, Malherbe's calcifying epithelioma,* and *pilomatrixoma.*

pilomatrixoma (pi″lo-ma-trik-so′mah)   pilomatricoma.

pilomotor (pi″lo-mo′tor) [*pilo-* + L. *motor* mover]   pertaining to the arrector muscles the contraction of which produces cutis anserina (goose flesh) and the erection of the hairs.

pilonidal (pi″lo-ni′dal) [*pilo-* + L. *nidus* nest]   pertaining to, characterized by, or having a nidus or tuft of hairs.

pilose (pi′lōs) [L. *pilosus*]   hairy; covered with hair.

pilosebaceous (pi″lo-sĕ-ba′shus)   pertaining to the hair follicles and sebaceous glands.

Piltz's reflex, sign (pilts′ez) [Jan *Piltz*, Polish neurologist, 1870–1930]   see *attention reflex of pupil* and *orbicularis pupillary reflex*, under *reflex*.

Piltz-Westphal phenomenon (pilts vest′fahl) [Jan *Piltz;*

A. K. O. *Westphal*, German neurologist, 1863–1941] orbicularis pupillary reflex.

pilula (pil′u-lah), pl. *pil′ulae* [L.] pill.

pilular (pil′u-lar) resembling or pertaining to a pill.

pilule (pil′ūl) [L. *pilula*] a small pill, or pellet.

pilus (pi′lus), gen. and pl. *pi′li* [L.] 1. [NA] any of the filamentous appendages of the skin, consisting of modified epidermal tissue; see *hair*. 2. [pl.] in microbiology, the minute filamentous appendages of certain bacteria; they are considerably smaller and less rigid than flagella and are associated with antigenic properties and sex functions of the cell; called also *fimbria*. **p. annula′tus** (pl. *pi′li annula′ti*), a condition in which the individual hairs appear to be marked by alternating bands of white as a result of some barrier in the hair which prevents passage of light and causes the rays to be reflected back, giving the appearance of white bands. **p. cunicula′tus** (pl. *pi′li cunicula′ti*), burrowing hair. **F p.,** in bacterial genetics, a special sex pilus possessed by (male) F⁺ cells, which carry the F (fertility) plasmid. It forms a connection with a (female) F⁻ cell in bacterial conjugation to allow the transfer of genetic material. **p. incarna′tus** (pl. *pi′li incarna′ti*), ingrown hair. **p. incarna′tus recur′vus** (pl. *pi′li incarna′ti recur′vi*), ingrown hair that has repenetrated the skin after growing from the hair follicle. **pi′li multigem′ini,** multiple hairs growing from the same follicle, as a result of deep division of its base, producing, in effect, a cluster of separate papillae. **p. tor′tus** (pl. *pi′li tor′ti*), twisted hair.

Pima (pim′ah) trademark for a preparation of potassium iodide.

pimelic acid (pĭ-mel′ik) trivial name for hexanedioic acid.

pimelitis (pim″ĕ-li′tis) [*pimelo-* + *-itis*] inflammation of the adipose tissue.

pimel(o)- [Gr. *pimelē* lard] a combining form denoting relationship to fat.

pimeloma (pim″ĕ-lo′mah) [*pimelo-* + *-oma*] a fatty tumor; lipoma.

pimelopterygium (pim″ĕ-lo-ter-ij′e-um) [*pimelo-* + Gr. *pterygion* wing] a fatty outgrowth upon the conjunctiva.

pimelorthopnea (pim″el-or″thop-ne′ah) [*pimelo-* + *orthopnea*] difficulty in breathing while lying down, due to excessive fatness.

pimelosis (pim″ĕ-lo′sis) [*pimelo-* + *-osis*] 1. conversion into fat. 2. fatness, or obesity.

pimeluria (pim″el-u′re-ah) [*pimelo-* + Gr. *ouron* urine + *-ia*] the presence of fat in the urine.

Pimenta (pĭ-men′tah) [Sp. "allspice"] a genus of myrtaceous trees and shrubs of warm regions. The dried fruit of *P. officinalis* Lindl. (*Eugenia pimenta*, DC.), furnishes pimenta and pimenta oil.

pimenta (pĭ-men′tah) the dried, nearly ripe fruit of *Pimenta officinalis* Lindl. (Myrtaceae), once used as an aromatic, stimulant, and carminative; called also *allspice*.

piminodine esylate (pĭ-min′o-dēn) chemical name: 4-phenyl-1-[3-(phenylamino)propyl]-4-piperidinecarboxylic acid ethyl ester monoethanesulfonate. A synthetic narcotic analgesic, $C_{23}H_{30}N_2O_2 \cdot C_2H_6O_3S$, occurring as a colorless, crystalline solid; administered orally, intramuscularly, and subcutaneously.

pimozide (pi′mo-zīd) chemical name: 1-[1-[4,4-bis(4-fluorophenyl)butyl]-4-piperidinyl]-1,3-dihydro-2*H*-benzimidazol-2-one; an antipsychotic, $C_{28}H_{29}F_2N_3O$, used in the treatment of Gilles de la Tourette syndrome and schizophrenia.

Pimpinella (pim″pĭ-nel′ah) [L.] a genus of umbelliferous plants. The roots of *P. saxifraga* L., Burnet saxifrage, are tonic, diuretic, emmenagogue, and carminative, and are the source of pimpinellin. *P. anisum* L. yields anise and anise oil.

pimpinellin (pim″pĭ-nel′in) a bitter, crystallizable principle, $C_{13}H_{10}O_5$, seen in colorless needles, from the root of *Pimpinella saxifraga* L. (Umbelliferae).

pimple (pim′p'l) a papule or pustule, usually of the face, neck, or upper trunk, most often due to acne vulgaris.

pin (pin) 1. a long slender metal rod for the fixation of the ends of fractured bones. 2. a peg or dowel by means of which an artificial crown is fixed to the root of a tooth. **Steinmann p.,** a metal rod for the internal fixation of fractures.

pinacyanole (pin″ah-si′ah-nōl) an aniline dye, $C_{25}H_{25}N_2I$,

used as a tissue stain, and for sensitizing photographic plates for red.

Pinard's maneuver (pe-nahrz′) [Adolphe *Pinard*, French obstetrician, 1844–1934] see under *maneuver*.

pince-ciseaux (pans″se-zo′) [Fr. "forceps-scissors"] a cutting forceps used in iridotomy.

pincement (pans-maw′) [Fr.] the pinching of the flesh in massage.

pincers (pin′serz) 1. forceps (def. 1). 2. the median deciduous incisor teeth in the horse.

pindolol (pin′do-lōl) chemical name: 1-(1*H*-indol-4-yloxy)-3-[(1-methylethyl)amino]-2-propanol; a beta-adrenergic blocking agent, $C_{14}H_{20}N_2O_2$, having the same actions as propranolol (q.v.).

pine (pīn) [L. *pinus*] the name of many coniferous trees, chiefly of the genus *Pinus*. The pines afford turpentine, volatile oils, rosin, pitch, tar, etc. **white p.,** the dried inner bark of *Pinus strobus* L. (Pinaceae), the Eastern white pine; used as an ingredient in compound white pine syrup.

pineal (pin′e-al) [L. *pinealis; pinea* pine cone] 1. pertaining to the pineal body. 2. shaped like a pine cone.

pinealectomy (pin″e-al-ek′to-me) [*pineal* body + Gr. *ektomē* excision] excision of the pineal body.

pinealism (pin′e-al-izm″) the condition due to derangement of the secretion of the pineal body.

pinealoblastoma (pin″e-ah-lo-blas-to′mah) pinealoma in which the pineal cells are not well differentiated. Called also *pineoblastoma*.

pinealocyte (pin′e-ah-lo-sīt″) the principal cell of the pineal body, being an epithelioid cell with pale-staining cytoplasm, prominent nucleoli, and large nuclei that are often irregularly infolded or lobulated; cords of these cells make up the body of the pineal body. Called also *chief cell* and *pineal cell*. See also *interstitial cells*, under *cell*.

pinealocytoma (pin″e-ah-lo-si-to′mah) pinealoma.

pinealoma (pin″e-ah-lo′mah) a rare tumor of the pineal body composed of neoplastic nests of large epithelial cells; symptoms include hydrocephalus, conjugate paralysis of upward gaze, disturbances of gait, and precocious puberty, the last due to the suppression of pineal secretion of melatonin. Called also *pinealocytoma*. **ectopic p.,** pinealoma arising from pineal rests in the midline area, resulting in diabetes insipidus, compression of the optic chiasm, and hypopituitarism.

pinealopathy (pin″e-ah-lop′ah-the) any disease of the pineal gland.

pinene (pi′nēn) a terpene, $C_{10}H_{16}$, found in turpentine and many essential oils; used as a solvent and in the manufacture of camphor. Called also *firpene*. **p. hydrochloride,** bornyl chloride.

pineoblastoma (pin″e-o-blas-to′mah) pinealoblastoma.

pineocytoma (pin″e-o-si-to′mah) pinealoma.

pinguecula (ping-gwek′u-lah), gen. and pl. *pingue′culae* [L. "somewhat fatty"] a yellowish spot of proliferation on the bulbar conjunctiva near the sclerocorneal junction, usually on the nasal side; seen in elderly people.

pinguicula (pin-gwik′u-lah) pinguecula.

piniform (pin′ĭ-form) [L. *pinea* pine cone + *forma* form] conical or cone shaped.

pinkeye (pink′i) acute contagious conjunctivitis.

pinledge (pin′lej) a flat floor or shoulder prepared within the tooth structure, into which pin holes are drilled to accommodate pins in a pin-retained cast restoration.

pinna (pin′nah) [L. "wing"] the projecting part of the ear lying outside of the head (auricula [NA]).

pinnaglobin (pin″ah-glo′bin) a brown respiratory pigment found in the wedge-shaped mollusk *Pinna squamosa*, which contains manganese instead of iron.

pinnal (pin′al) pertaining to the pinna.

pinocarveol (pi″no-kar′ve-ol) a terpene alcohol, $(CH_3)_2C:C_6H_7(OH):CH_2$, from *Eucalyptus globulus;* called also *isocarveol*.

pinocyte (pi′no-, pi″no-sīt) a cell that exhibits pinocytosis.

pinocytic (pin″o-sit′ik) pertaining to a pinocyte or to pinocytosis.

pinocytosis (pi″no-, pin″o-si-to′sis) [Gr. *pinein* to drink + *kytos* cell + *-osis*] the imbibition of liquids by cells, especially the mechanism by which cells ingest extracellular fluid and its contents; it involves the formation of minute incuppings or invaginations (caveolae) by the cell membrane, which close and pinch off to form free, fluid-filled vesicles (*pinosomes*) in the cytoplasm. It is thought to be a method of active transport across the cell membrane.

pinocytotic (pi″no-, pin″no-si-tot′ik)   pertaining to or characterized by pinocytosis.

pinosome (pi′no-, pin′o-sōm) [Gr. *pinein* to drink + *sōma* body]   any of the small fluid-filled vesicles found in the cytoplasm during pinocytosis, formed by invaginations of the cell membrane (caveolae) which pinch off and become free. Called also *pinocytotic vesicle*.

Pinoyella (pi″no-yel′ah)   *Trichophyton*. **P. sim′ii,** *Trichophyton simii*.

Pins' sign (pins) [Emil *Pins*, Vienna physician, 1845–1913]   Ewart's sign.

pint (pīnt)   a measure of capacity (liquid measure), being 16 fluidounces, or the equivalent of 473.17 milliliters; symbol O (L. *octarius*), or abbreviated pt. The imperial pint is equal to 20 fluidounces.

pinta (pēn′tah) [Sp. "painted"]   a form of treponematosis, being a chronic dyschromic dermatosis endemic in certain parts of tropical America and characterized by the presence on the skin of spots, which may be white, coffee colored, blue, red, or violet. It is caused by *Treponema carateum* (the Wassermann reaction is usually positive), and is believed to be transmitted usually by direct person-to-person contact. Results of penicillin therapy are excellent. Called also *mal del pinto* and *carate*.

pintid (pin′tid)   one of the flat erythematous skin lesions constituting the spreading eruption occurring in the second stage of pinta.

pinus (pi′nus) [L.]   the pineal body.

pinworm (pin′werm)   any oxyurid, especially *Enterobius vermicularis*.

pi(o)- [Gr. *piōn* fat]   a combining form denoting relationship to fat. See also words beginning *lip(o)-*.

pioepithelium (pi″o-ep″ĭ-the′le-um) [*pio-* + *epithelium*]   epithelium in which fatty matter is deposited.

pion (pi′on)   a nuclear particle with mass intermediate between an electron and a proton.

pionemia (pi″o-ne′me-ah) [Gr. *pion* fat + *haima* blood + *-ia*]   the presence of fat or oil in the blood; lipemia.

Piophila (pi-of′ĭ-lah)   a genus of flies. **P. ca′sei,** the fly whose larvae are the "cheese skippers" and a common cause of intestinal myiasis.

piorthopnea (pi″or-thop-ne′ah) [*pio-* + Gr. *orthos* upright + *pnoia* breath]   dyspnea when lying down, due to obesity.

pioscope (pi′o-skōp) [*pio-* + Gr. *skopein* to examine]   an instrument for estimating the fat content of milk by comparing its color with the six shades painted on the instrument.

Piotrowski's sign (pe″o-trov′skēz) [Alexander *Piotrowski*, neurologist in Berlin, born in 1878]   see under *sign*.

pipamazine (pi-pam′ah-zēn)   chemical name: 1-[3-(2-chloro-10*H*-phenothiazin-10-yl)propyl]-4-piperidinecarboxamide; an antiemetic, $C_{21}H_{24}ClN_3OS$.

pipamperone (pĭ-pam′pĕ-rōn)   chemical name: 1′-[4-(4-fluorophenyl) -4-oxobutyl]- [1,4′- biperidine] -4′- carboxamide; a tranquilizer that has been used in the treatment of schizophrenia, $C_{21}H_{30}FN_3O_2$.

Pipanol (pip′ah-nol)   trademark for a preparation of trihexyphenidyl hydrochloride.

pipazethate hydrochloride (pĭ-paz′ĕ-thāt)   chemical name: 10*H*-pyrido[3,2-*b*][1,4]benzothiadiazine-10-carboxylic acid 2-(2-piperidinoethoxy)ethyl ester hydrochloride. A non-narcotic antitussive, $C_{21}H_{25}N_3O_3S \cdot HCl$, occurring as a white, crystalline powder; administered orally.

pipecolic acid (pip″e-ko′lik)   homoproline; 2-piperidine carboxylic acid.

pipenzolate bromide (pi-pen′zo-lāt)   chemical name: 1-ethyl-3-[(hydroxydiphenylacetyl)oxy]-1-methylpiperidinium bromide. A synthetic quaternary nitrogen anticholinergic, $C_{22}H_{28}BrNO_3$, occurring as a white, crystalline powder; used mainly for adjunctive therapy in the treatment of peptic ulcer, administered orally.

Piper (pi′per) [L. "pepper"]   a genus of plants producing betel, cubeb, matico, and pepper.

piperacetazine (pip″er-ah-set′ah-zēn) [USP]   chemical name: 1-[10-[3-[4-(2-hydroxyethyl)-1-piperidinyl]propyl]-10-*H*-phenothiazin-2-yl]ethanone. An antipsychotic, $C_{24}H_{30}N_2O_2$ S, occurring as a yellow, granular powder; used in the treatment of various forms of schizophrenia in adults, administered orally.

piperacillin sodium (pi-per′ah-sil″in)   chemical name: [2S- [2α,5α,6β(S*)]]-6-[[[[(4-ethyl-2,3-dioxo-1-piperazinyl)carbonyl]amino]phenylacetyl]amino]-3,3-dimethyl-7-oxo-4-thia-1-azabicyclo[3.2.0]heptane-2-carboxylic acid monosodium salt; an antibacterial, $C_{23}H_{26}N_5NaO_7S$.

piperazidine (pi″per-az′ĭ-dēn)   piperazine.

piperazine (pi′per-ah-zēn) [USP]   a compound NHCH₂-CH₂NHCH₂CH₂; called also *diethylenediamine* and *piperazidine*. Piperazine [USP], piperazine citrate [USP], piperazine edetate calcium, and piperazine phosphate [USP] are used as anthelmintic agents against *Ascaris lumbricoides* and *Enterobius vermicularis*. Piperazine causes a flaccid paralysis of the worm musculature by altering the cell membrane permeability and causing hyperpolarization of the membrane.   **p. citrate** [USP], the citrate salt of piperazine, $(C_4H_{10}N_2)_3 \cdot 2C_6H_8O_7 \cdot xH_2O$, occurring as a white, crystalline powder; used in the treatment of intestinal roundworm and pinworm infections, administered orally.   **p. edetate calcium,** a compound, $C_{14}H_{24}CaN_4O_8 \cdot 2H_2O$, prepared by the reaction of edetate with calcium carbonate and piperazine; used like the citrate salt.   **p. estrone sulfate,** estropipate.   **p. phosphate** [USP], the phosphate salt of piperazine, $C_4H_{10}N_2 \cdot H_3PO_4 \cdot H_2O$, occurring as a white, crystalline powder; used in the treatment of intestinal roundworm and trematode infections.   **p. tartrate,** the tartrate salt of piperazine, $C_8H_{16}N_2O_6$; used like the citrate salt.

piperidione (pi″per-ĭ-di′ōn)   dihyprylone.

piperidolate hydrochloride (pi″per-id′o-lāt) [USP]   chemical name: α-phenylbenzeneacetic acid 1-ethyl-3-piperidinyl ester hydrochloride. A synthetic tertiary anticholinergic, $C_{21}H_{25}NO_2 \cdot HCl$, occurring as a white or cream-colored powder, having the ability to reduce motility of smooth muscle, especially that of the gastrointestinal tract; used as an antispasmodic in functional gastrointestinal disorders, administered orally.

piperine (pi′per-in) [L. *piperinum*]   chemical name: 1-piperoylpiperidine. A crystallizable, slightly soluble alkaloid, $C_5H_{10}N \cdot CO \cdot (CH_3)CH \cdot C_6H_3 \cdot O_2 \cdot CH_2$, from *Piper nigrum* (black pepper), used as an insecticide.

piperism (pi′per-izm) [L. *piper* pepper]   poisoning by pepper.

piperocaine hydrochloride (pi′per-o-kān″)   chemical name: 2-methyl-1-piperidinepropanol benzoate hydrochloride. A local anesthetic, $C_{16}H_{23}NO_2 \cdot HCl$, occurring as small, white crystals or white, crystalline powder; used for topical, infiltration, regional, spinal, and caudal anesthesia.

piperoxan hydrochloride (pi″per-oks′an)   chemical name: 1-[(2,3-dihydro-1,4-benzodioxin-2-yl)methyl] piperidine; an alpha-adrenergic blocking agent, $C_{14}H_{19}NO_2$, formerly used in diagnostic tests for pheochromocytoma and to counteract the effects of epinephrine release before and during surgery for removal of pheochromocytoma.

pipet (pi-pet′)   pipette.

pipette (pi-pet′) [Fr.]   1. a glass or transparent plastic tube used in measuring or transferring small quantities of liquid or gas. 2. to dispense fluid or gas by means of a pipette.

pipitzahoac (pi″zah-ho-ak′) [Mex.]   the root and rhizome of the Mexican plant *Trixis pipitzahuac* Shaffner (*Perezia adnata* Gr., Compositae); used as a cathartic.

Pipizan (pi′pĭ-zan)   trademark for a preparation of piperazine.

pipobroman (pi″po-bro′man) [USP]   chemical name: 1,4-bis(3-bromo-1-oxopropyl)piperazine. An antineoplastic alkylating agent, $C_{10}H_{16}Br_2N_2O_2$, occurring as a white to practically white, crystalline powder; used primarily in the treatment of polycythemia vera, and has been found to be useful in the treatment of chronic granulocytic leukemia, administered orally.

piposulfan (pĭ-po-sul′fan)   chemical name: 1,4-bis[3-[(methylsulfonyl)oxy] -1-oxopropyl]piperazine; an antineoplastic, $C_{12}H_{22}N_2O_8S_2$.

pipotiazine palmitate (pip″o-ti′ah-zēn)   chemical name: 2-[1-[3-[2-[(dimethylamino)sulfonyl]-10*H*-phenothiazine-10-

yl]propyl]-4-piperidinyl]ethyl ester hexanoic acid; a tranquilizer, $C_{40}H_{63}N_3O_4S_2$.

pipoxolan hydrochloride (pĭ-poks'o-lan) chemical name: 5,5-diphenyl-2-[2-(1-piperidinyl)ethyl]-1,3-dioxolan-4-one hydrochloride; a muscle relaxant, $C_{22}H_{25}NO_3HCl$.

pipradrol hydrochloride (pi'prah-drol) chemical name: α,α-diphenyl-2-piperidinemethanol hydrochloride. A central nervous system stimulant, $C_{18}H_{21}NO \cdot HCl$, occurring as small, white crystals or crystalline powder; used mainly as an antidepressant, administered orally.

piprozolin (pip''ro-zo'lin) chemical name: [3-ethyl-4-oxo-5-(1-piperidinyl)-2-thiazolidinylidene] acetic acid ethyl ester; a choleretic, $C_{14}H_{22}N_2O_3S$.

Piptocephalus (pip''to-sef''ah-lus) a genus of molds, some species of which cause alimentary toxic aleukia.

piquizil hydrochloride (pik'wĭ-zil) chemical name: 4-(6,7-dimethoxy-4-quinazolinyl)-1-piperazinecarboxylic acid 2-methyl propyl ester; a bronchodilator, $C_{19}H_{26}N_4O_4 \cdot HCl$.

piqûre (pe-koor') [Fr.] puncture, especially Bernard's (diabetic) puncture.

Piracaps (pi'rah-kaps) trademark for a preparation of tetracycline hydrochloride.

pirandamine hydrochloride (per-an'dah-mēn) chemical name: 1,3,4,9-tetrahydro-*N,N*,1-trimethylindeno[2,1-*c*] pyran-1- ethanamine hydrochloride; a tricyclic antidepressant, $C_{17}H_{23}NO \cdot HCl$.

pirbenicillin sodium (per-ben''ĭ-sil'in) chemical name: [2S-[2α,5α,6β(S')]]-6[[[[[(imino-4-pyridinylmethyl)amino]acetyl]amino]phenylacetyl]amino]-3,3-dimethyl-7-oxo-4-thia-1-azabicyclo[3.2.0]heptane-2-carboxylic acid monosodium salt; an antibacterial, $C_{24}H_{25}N_6NaO_5S$.

pirbuterol hydrochloride (per-bu'ter-ōl) chemical name: α⁶-[[(1,1-dimethylethyl)amino]methyl]-3-hydroxy-2,6-pyridinedimethanol dihydrochloride; a bronchodilator, $C_{12}H_{20}N_2O_3 \cdot 2HCl$.

Pirenella (pi''rĕ-nel'ah) a genus of snails. **P. con'ica,** the host of the intestinal fluke, *Heterophyes heterophyes,* in Egypt.

pirfenidone (per-fen'ĭ-don) chemical name: 5-methyl-1-phenyl-2(1*H*)-pyridinone; an anti-inflammatory and antipyretic, $C_{12}H_{11}NO$.

piriform (pir'ĭ-form) [L. *pirum* a pear + *forma* shape] pear-shaped.

Pirogoff's amputation, angle (pir''o-gofs') [Nikolai Ivanovich *Pirogoff,* Russian surgeon, 1810–1881] see under *amputation,* and see *venous angle,* under *angle.*

pirolate (per'o-lāt) chemical name: 1,4-dihydro-7,8-dimethoxy-4-oxopyrimido[4,5-*b*]quinoline-2-carboxylic acid ethyl ester; an antiasthmatic, $C_{16}H_{15}N_3O_5$.

pirolazamide (per''o-la'zah-mīd) chemical name: hexahydro-α,α-diphenylpyrrolo[1,2-*a*]pyrazine-2(1*H*)-butanamide; a cardiac depressant with antiarrhythmic action, $C_{23}H_{29}N_3O$.

piroplasm (pi'ro-plaz'm) any protozoan of the subclass Piroplasmia. Called also *piroplasmid.*

Piroplasma (pi''ro-plaz'mah) *Babesia.*

Piroplasmia (pi''ro-plaz-me'ah) [L. *pirum* pear + *plasma*] a subclass of heteroxenous parasitic protozoa (class Sporozoea, subphylum Apicocomplexa), occurring as piriform, round, or rod-shaped cells or ameboid cells without a conoid, oocysts, spores, pseudocyts, and flagella, and usually without subpellicular microtubules but with a polar ring and rhoptries. Locomotion is accomplished by flexion, by gliding, or, in sexual stages of certain species, by large axopodium-like organelles (*strahlen*). They are parasitic in the erythrocytes and other circulating and fixed cells of the host, with merogony occurring in vertebrates and sporogony in invertebrates, and producing sporozoites with a single-membraned wall. Ticks are the vectors of most of the piroplasmids. It comprises a single order: Piroplasmida.

piroplasmid (pi''ro-plaz'mid) 1. pertaining or relating to protozoa of the subclass Piroplasmia. 2. piroplasm.

Piroplasmida (pi''ro-plaz'mĭ-dah) an order of protozoa (subclass Piroplasmia, class Sporozoea) having the characters of the subclass. Representative genera include *Babesia, Cytauzoon, Dactylosoma,* and *Theileria.*

piroplasmosis (pi''ro-plaz-mo'sis) babesiosis. **tropical p.,** see under *theileriasis.*

piroxicam (per-ok'sĭ-kam) chemical name: 4-hydroxy-2-methyl-*N*-2-pyridinyl-2*H*-1,2- benzothiazine -3- carboxamide; a nonsteroidal anti-inflammatory agent of the oxicam family having a long plasma half-life; used for once-a-day treatment of rheumatoid arthritis and osteoarthritis.

pirprofen (per-pro'fen) chemical name: 3-chloro-4-(2,5-dihydro-1*H*-pyrrol-1-yl)-α-methylbenzeneacetic acid; an anti-inflammatory, $C_{13}H_{14}ClNO_2$.

Pirquet's reaction (cutireaction, test) (per-kāz') [Clemens Freiherr von *Pirquet,* Austrian pediatrician, 1874–1929] see *cutaneous reaction,* under *reaction.*

piscicide (pis'ĭ-sīd) any substance poisonous to fish.

Piscidia (pĭ-sid'e-ah) [L. *piscis* fish + *caedere* to kill] a genus of leguminous trees; the bark of *P. piscipula* (L.) Sarg. (*P. erythrina* L.), Jamaica dogwood, is a mild anodyne.

piscidin (pĭ-si'din) a neutral principle from *Piscidia piscipula* (L.) Sarg., an anodyne and antispasmodic.

pisiform (pi'sĭ-form) [L. *pisum* pea + *forma* shape] resembling a pea in shape and size.

pisiformis (pi''sĭ-for'mis) [L.] pisiform.

Piskacek's sign (pis'kach-eks) [Ludwig *Piskacek,* Hungarian obstetrician, 1854–1933] see under *sign.*

pistil (pis'til) [L. *pistillus* a pestle] gynecium.

PIT plasma iron turnover.

pit (pit) 1. a hollow fovea or indentation. 2. a pockmark. 3. a small depression or fault in the dental enamel. Considered as belonging to Class I of Black's classification of dental caries (see table accompanying *caries.* See also *fissure,* def. 2. 4. to indent, or to become and remain for a short period of time indented by pressure. 5. a small depression in the nail plate; seen in psoriasis. **anal p.,** the proctodeum. **arm p.,** the axillary fossa. **auditory p.,** a distinct depression appearing in each auditory placode, marking the beginning of the embryonic development of the internal ear. Called also *otic p.* **basilar p.,** a pit in the crown of an incisor tooth above its neck. **coated p's,** small pits in the plasma membrane of many cells that are involved in the receptor-mediated endocytosis of low-density lipoprotein (LDL), insulin, and other ligands. The pits are coated with a protein, clathrin, on the cytoplasmic surface and may be taken into the cell to form vacuoles enclosing the ligands. **costal p.,** fovea costalis inferior. **ear p.,** a slight depression anterior to the helix and superior to the tragus, sometimes leading to a congenital preauricular cyst or fistula. **gastric p's,** foveolae gastricae. **Gaul's p's,** depressions in the corneal epithelium seen in neuroparalytic keratitis. **Herbert's p's,** a characteristic defect left after the healing of a limbal follicle in trachoma. **lens p.,** a pitlike depression in the ectoderm of the fetal head where the lens is developed. **nasal p.,** olfactory p. **oblong p. of arytenoid cartilage,** fovea oblonga cartilaginis arytenoideae. **olfactory p.,** the primordium of a nasal cavity. **otic p.,** auditory p. **postanal p.,** foveola coccygea. **primitive p.,** a depression at the cranial end of the primitive groove; it may open into a neurenteric canal. **pterygoid p.,** see under *fovea.* **p. of the stomach,** the epigastrium or fossa epigastrica. **suprameatal p.,** foveola suprameatica. **triangular p. of arytenoid cartilage,** fovea triangularis cartilaginis arytenoideae.

pitch (pich) [L. *pix*] 1. a dark, lustrous, more or less viscous residue from the distillation of tar and other substances. 2. natural asphalt of various kinds. 3. the quality of sound dependent principally on its frequency. **black p.,** an inflammable substance obtainable from the tar of various species of pine. **Burgundy p.,** an aromatic, oily resin from *Abies* (or *Picea*) *excelsa,* the Norway spruce of Europe, much used in plasters. **Canada p.,** a resin from *Tsuga canadensis,* the hemlock tree, useful in plasters, etc. **liquid p.,** ordinary wood tar. **mineral p.,** bitumen. **naval p.,** black p.

pitchblende (pich'blend) a black mineral containing uranium oxide; from it are obtained radium, polonium, and uranium.

pith (pith) 1. to pierce the spinal cord or brain; see *pithing.* 2. the soft tissue found in plant stems that often disappears so that the stem becomes hollow. 3. the central core of colorless parenchymatous cells in stems and some roots.

pithecoid (pith'e-koid) [Gr. *pithēkos* ape + *eidos* form] apelike.

pithiatism (pith-i'ah-tizm) [Gr. *peithein* to persuade + *iatos* curable] 1. a condition which is caused by suggestion and which renders the patient subject to persuasion. 2. the cure of nervous and mental disorders by persuasion.

pithing (pith′ing) destruction of the brain and spinal cord by thrusting a blunt needle into the spinal canal and cranium; done on animals to destroy sensibility preparatory to experimenting on their living tissues.

pithode (pi′thōd) [Gr. *pithos* wine cask + *eidos* form] the nuclear barrel figure formed in mitosis.

Pithomyces (pith″o-mi′sez) a genus of molds of the class Deuteromycetes. *P. charta′rum* causes facial eczema of ruminants.

Pitocin (pǐ-to′sin) trademark for preparations of oxytocin.

Pitres' sections, sign (pe-tres′) [Jean Albert *Pitres*, physician in Bordeaux, 1848–1927] see under *section* and *sign*.

Pitressin (pǐ-tres′in) trademark for vasopressin injection.

pitting (pit′ting) 1. the formation, usually by scarring, of a small depression. 2. the removal from erythrocytes, by the spleen, of certain structures, such as iron granules, without destruction of the cells. 3. remaining indented for a few minutes after removal of firm finger-pressure, distinguishing fluid edema from myxedema.

pituicyte (pǐ-tu′ǐ-sīt) [*pitui*tary + -*cyte*] any of the dominant and distinctive fusiform cells of the neurohypophysis, which are intermingled with nerve fibers and are regarded as specialized neuroglial cells. According to their morphological appearance on staining with silver, four subtypes are distinguished: adeno-, fibro-, reticulo-, and micropituicytes.

pituita (pǐ-tu′ǐ-tah) [L.] a glutinous mucus.

pituitarigenic (pǐ-tu″ǐ-tār″ǐ-jen′ik) [*pituitary* + Gr. *gennan* to produce] produced by secretions of the pituitary gland.

pituitarism (pǐ-tu′ǐ-tar-izm″) disorder of pituitary function; see *hyperpituitarism* and *hypopituitarism*.

pituitarium (pǐ-tu″ǐ-ta′re-um) [L.] pituitary.

pituitary (pǐ-too′ǐ-tār″e, pǐ-tu′ǐ-tār″e) [L. *pituita* phlegm] 1. pertaining to the pituitary gland. 2. the pituitary gland; see under *gland*. 3. a preparation of some part of the pituitary gland of animals (e.g., cattle, pigs, sheep), used therapeutically. **anterior p.,** the anterior lobe of the pituitary gland; the adenohypophysis or pars distalis. Also a preparation of the dried, partially defatted, powdered anterior lobe of the pituitary gland of hogs, sheep, or cattle. **pharyngeal p.,** see under *hypophysis*. **posterior p.,** 1. the posterior lobe of the pituitary gland; the neurohypophysis or pars nervosa. 2. a powder prepared from the dried posterior pituitary lobe of those domestic animals used for food by man, having the pharmacological actions of its hormones, *oxytocin* and *vasopressin;* used mainly as an antidiuretic in the treatment of diabetes insipidus, administered subcutaneously or by nasal inhalation or topical application to the nasal mucosa. It may be used to stimulate smooth muscle tissue, especially to produce vasoconstriction in the presence of hemorrhage. **whole p.,** a preparation of the dried, partially defatted, powdered whole pituitary gland of domesticated animals.

pituitectomy (pǐ-tu″ǐ-tek′to-me) hypophysectomy.

pituitous (pǐ-tu′ǐ-tus) [L. *pituitosus*] pertaining to mucus or characterized by its secretion.

Pituitrin (pǐ-tu′ǐ-trin) trademark for posterior pituitary injection.

pityriasis (pit″ǐ-ri′ah-sis) [Gr. *pityron* bran + -*iasis*] a name originally applied to a group of skin diseases characterized by the formation of fine, branny scales, but now used only with a modifier. **p. al′ba,** a common skin disorder most often seen in young children and adolescents, usually involving the face, especially the cheeks and the area around the mouth, and characterized by the presence of round or oval, slightly scaling, hypopigmented patches; it usually involutes spontaneously. Called also *erythroderma streptogenes,* *p. maculata,* and *p. simplex.* **lichenoid p., acute, p. lichenoi′des acu′ta,** an acute or subacute, sometimes relapsing, widespread macular, papular, or vesicular eruption that tends to crusting, necrosis, and hemorrhage, which heals, leaving pigmented depressed scars, followed by the development of a new crop of lesions. Occasionally, progression to the chronic lichenoid form may occur. Called also *acute parapsoriasis; Habermann's, Mucha-Habermann,* or *Mucha's disease; parapsoriasis varioliformis acuta;* and *p. lichenoides et varioliformis acuta.* **lichenoid p., chronic, p. lichenoi′des chron′ica,** a chronic brown to

red-brown scaly macular eruption, distributed chiefly over the trunk, characterized histologically by epidermal alterations and a perivascular lymphocytic infiltrate. It may represent progression of the acute lichenoid form or arise de novo. Called also *chronic* or *guttate parapsoriasis, parapsoriasis guttata,* and *parapsoriasis varioliformis chronica.* **p. lichenoi′des et variolifor′mis acu′ta,** acute lichenoid p. **p. lin′guae,** benign migratory glossitis. **p. macula′ta,** p. alba. **p. ro′sea,** a common acute or subacute, self-limited exanthematous disease of unknown etiology, the onset of which is marked by the presence of a solitary erythematous or salmon- or fawn-colored herald plaque, most often seen on the trunk, arms, or thighs, followed by the development of papular or macular lesions, similar to but smaller than the initial lesion, which have vesicular borders subsequently that tend to peel and produce a scaly collarette. **p. rotun′da,** a form of acquired ichthyosis manifested by circular or oval, brown, scaly, sharply demarcated patches on the trunk and extremities, which become worse during the winter and improve in the summer. **p. ru′bra** (Hebra), exfoliative dermatitis. **p. ru′bra pila′ris,** a chronic inflammatory cutaneous disease characterized by tiny acuminate, reddish brown follicular papules topped by central horny plugs in which are embedded hairs, partial or complete; disseminated yellowish pink scaling patches; and often solid confluent hyperkeratosis of the palms and soles with a tendency to fissuring. **p. sic′ca,** dandruff, def. 2. **p. sim′plex,** p. alba. **p. versic′olor,** tinea versicolor.

pityroid (pit′ǐ-roid) [Gr. *pityron* bran + *eidos* form] furfuraceous; branny.

Pityrosporon (pit″ǐ-ros′po-ron) *Pityrosporum.*

Pityrosporum (pit″ǐ-ros′po-rum) a genus of imperfect fungi of the family Cryptococcaceae, which are yeastlike and produce no mycelium; called also *Malassezia.* **P. orbicula′re,** a species which is a customary resident of normal skin, but is capable of causing disease (tinea versicolor) in susceptible hosts; called also *Malassezia furfur, M. macfadyani, M. tropica,* and *Microsporum furfur.* **P. ova′le,** a lipid-dependent species which is abundant in sebaceous areas, such as the skin of the face and scalp, but is not known to be pathogenic.

pivalate (piv′ah-lāt) a salt of pivalic acid; USAN contraction for trimethylacetate.

pivalic acid (pǐ-val′ik) trivial name for trimethylacetic acid, $(CH_3)_3CCOOH$.

pivampicillin hydrochloride (piv-am″pǐ-sil′in) chemical name: 6-[(aminophenylacetyl)amino]-3,3-dimethyl-7-oxo-4-thia-1-azabicyclo[3.2.0]heptane-2-carboxylic acid (2,2-dimethyl-1-oxopropoxy)methyl ester. A derivative of ampicillin, $C_{22}H_{29}N_3O_6S$, having the same broad spectrum of antibacterial activity and uses as ampicillin. Available as *p. hydrochloride, p. pamoate,* and *p. probenate.*

pivot (piv′ut) 1. that on which something turns, such as a dowel or short post. 2. the point of rotation for a removable partial denture. **occlusal p.,** an elevation contrived on the occlusal surface, usually in the molar region, designed to act as a fulcrum and to induce sagittal mandibular rotation.

pix (piks), gen. *pi′cis* [L.] pitch or tar.

pizotyline (pǐ-zo′tǐ-lēn) chemical name: 4-(9,10-dihydro-4*H*-benzo[4,5]cyclohepta[1,2-*b*]thien-4-ylidene)-1-methylpiperidine; an anabolic, antidepressant, and serotonin inhibitor (specific in migraine), $C_{19}H_{21}NS$.

pK the negative logarithm of the ionization constant (K) of an acid; the buffering power of a buffer system is greatest when its pK equals the pH.

PKU phenylketonuria.

placebo (plah-se′bo) [L. "I will please"] any dummy medical treatment; originally, a medicinal preparation having no specific pharmacological activity against the patient's illness or complaint given solely for the psychophysiological effects of the treatment; more recently, a dummy treatment administered to the control group in a controlled clinical trial in order that the specific and nonspecific effects of the experimental treatment can be distinguished—i.e., the experimental treatment must produce better results than the placebo in order to be considered effective. **active p., impure p.,** a substance having pharmacologic properties that are not relevant to the condition being treated.

placement (plās′ment) position or arrangement, as of the teeth. **lingual p.,** displacement of a tooth toward the tongue.

placenta (plah-sen′tah), pl. *placentas* or *placen′tae* [L. "a flat cake"] an organ characteristic of true mammals during pregnancy, joining mother and offspring, providing endocrine secretion and selective exchange of soluble, but not particulate, blood-borne substances through an apposition of uterine and trophoblastic vascularized parts. According to species, the area of vascular apposition may be diffuse, cotyledonary, zonary, or discoid; the nature of apposition may be labyrinthine or villous; the intimacy of apposition may vary according to what layers are lost of those originally interposed between maternal and fetal blood (maternal endothelium, uterine connective tissue, uterine epithelium, chorion, extraembryonic mesoderm, and endothelium of villous capillary). The chorion may be joined by and receive blood vessels from either the yolk sac or the allantois, and the uterine lining may be largely shed with the chorion at birth (deciduate) or may separate from the chorion and remain (nondeciduate). The human placenta is discoid, villous, hemochorial, chorioallantoic, and deciduate. After birth, it weighs about 600 gm. and is about 16 cm. in diameter and 2 cm. thick, discounting a principal functional part, the maternal blood in the intervillous space (which leaks out at birth) into which the chorionic villi dip. The villi are grouped into adjoining cotyledons making about 20 velvety bumps on the side of the placenta facing outward to the uterus; the inner side of the placenta facing the fetus is smooth, being covered with amnion, a thin avascular layer that continues past the edges of the placenta to line the entire hollow sphere of chorion except where it is reflected to cover the umbilical cord, which joins fetus and placenta. The cord usually joins the placenta near the center but may insert at the edge, on the nonplacental chorion, or on an accessory placenta. **accessory p.,** a placenta separate from the main placenta. **p. accre′ta,** abnormal adherence of part or all of the placenta to the uterine wall, with partial or complete absence of the decidua basalis, especially of the spongiosum layer. **adherent p.,** one which adheres closely to the uterine wall. **annular p.,** one which extends around the interior of the uterus like a ring or belt. **battledore p.,** one with marginal insertion of the cord. **bidiscoidal p.,** one consisting of two separate discoidal masses, as in the macaques. **bilobate p., bilobed p.,** a placenta consisting of two lobes. **p. biparti′ta, bipartite p.,** bilobate p. **chorioallantoic p.,** one in which the allantois joins the chorion or provides its major blood supply. **choriovitelline p.,** one in which the yolk sac becomes an intermediary in the fetal-maternal relationship. **p. circumvalla′ta, circumvallate p.,** a placenta in which a dense peripheral ring is raised from the surface and the attached membranes are doubled back over the edge of the placenta. **cirsoid p., p. cirsoi′des,** a placenta the vessels of which appear to be varicose. **deciduate p., deciduous p.,** a placenta or type of placentation in which the decidua or maternal parts of the placenta separate from the uterus and are cast off together with the fetal (or more precisely, trophoblastic) parts. **p. diffu′sa,** a placenta in which placental tissue is distributed over the chorionic membrane, as in swine. **p. dimidia′ta, dimidiate p.,** bilobate p. **discoid p., p. discoi′dea,** a disk-shaped placenta. **Duncan p.,** one that is expelled with the chorionic surface outward; cf. *Schultze's p.* **duplex p.,** bilobate p. **endotheliochorial p.,** one in which syncytial trophoblast embeds maternal vessels bared to their endothelial lining. **epitheliochorial p.,** one in which the uterine epithelial lining is not eroded but merely lies in apposition to the chorion. **p. fenestra′ta,** one which has spots where placental tissue is lacking. **fetal p., p. foeta′lis,** pars fetalis placentae. **fundal p.,** one which is attached to the fundus of the uterus in the normal manner. **furcate p.,** lobed p. **hemochorial p.,** one in which maternal blood comes in direct contact with the chorion. **hemoendothelial p.,** one in which maternal blood comes in contact with the endothelium of chorionic vessels. **horseshoe p.,** a crescentic form of placenta sometimes occurring in twin pregnancy. **incarcerated p.,** retained p. **p. incre′ta,** placenta accreta with penetration of the myometrium. **labyrinthine p.,** one in which maternal blood courses in channeled trophoblast. **lobed p.,** one that is more or less subdivided into lobes. **p. margina′lis, p. margina′ta,** a placenta surrounded by an unusual margin of elevated infarcted tissue. **maternal p.,** the maternally contributed part of the placenta,

derived from the decidua basalis; called also *pars uterina placentae* [NA]. **p. membrana′cea,** a placenta which is abnormally thin and spread out over a large area of the uterine wall. **multilobate p., multilobed p., p. multiparti′ta,** a placenta consisting of more than three lobes. **p. nappifor′mis,** p. circumvallata. **nondeciduate p., nondeciduous p.,** one in which the maternal component remains in the uterus instead of being cast off together with the trophoblastic derivatives. **panduriform p., p. pandurifor′mis,** a placenta composed of two halves side by side, resembling a violin in shape. **p. percre′ta,** placenta accreta with invasion of the myometrium all the way to its peritoneal covering, sometimes resulting in rupture of the uterus. **p. pre′via,** a placenta which develops in the lower uterine segment, in the zone of dilatation, so that it covers or adjoins the internal os; painless hemorrhage in the last trimester, particularly during the eighth month, is the most common symptom. **p. pre′via centra′lis,** placenta previa in which the placenta entirely covers the internal os; called also *complete, total,* or *central placenta previa.* **p. pre′via margina′lis,** placenta previa in which the placenta is just palpable at the margin of the os; called also *lateral* or *marginal placenta previa.* **p. pre′via partia′lis,** placenta previa in which the internal os is partially covered; called also *incomplete* or *partial placenta previa.* **p. reflex′a,** one in which the margin is thickened, appearing to turn back on itself. **p. renifor′mis,** a kidney-shaped placenta. **retained p.,** one which is either adherent or incarcerated by irregular uterine contractions, and which in consequence fails to be expelled after childbirth. **Schultze's p.,** a placenta that is delivered with the gestation sac inside out, the amnion providing a smooth, glistening surface. Cf. *Duncan p.* **p. spu′ria,** an accessory portion having no blood vessel attachment to the main placenta. **p. succenturia′ta, succenturiate p.,** an accessory portion attached to the main placenta by an artery and vein. **syndesmochorial p.,** one in which the lining epithelium of the uterus is the only maternal tissue eroded. **p. tri′loba, trilobate p.,** a placenta having three lobes. **p. triparti′ta, tripartite p.,** trilobate p. **p. trip′lex,** trilobate p. **p. uteri′na, uterine p.,** maternal p. **velamentous p.,** one in which the umbilical cord is attached on the adjoining membranes. **villous p.,** one characterized by the presence of villi which are outgrowths of the chorion. **yolk-sac p.,** choriovitelline p. **zonary p., zonular p.,** 1. annular placenta. 2. a belt-shaped placenta, as occurs in carnivores.

placental (plah-sen′tal) 1. pertaining to the placenta. 2. a mammal whose young receive nourishment *in utero* by means of a placenta.

Placentalia (pla″sen-ta′le-ah) a division of mammals whose embryos are nourished through a placenta; it includes all mammals except marsupials and monotremes.

placentation (plas″en-ta′shun) the process of placenta formation and the result, especially with respect to taxonomically relevant aspects of structure. See *placenta.*

placentin (plah-sen′tin) a defatted desiccation product of beef placenta.

placentitis (plas″en-ti′tis) inflammation of the placenta.

placentogenesis (plah-sen″to-jen′ĕ-sis) [*placenta* + *genesis*] the origin and development of the placenta.

placentogram (plah-sen′to-gram) a film taken in placentography.

placentography (plas″en-tog′rah-fe) radiological visualization of the placenta after the injection of a contrast medium. **indirect p.,** roentgenographic measurement of the space between the placenta and the presenting head of the fetus, for the recognition of placenta previa.

placentoid (plah-sen′toid) resembling the placenta.

placentologist (plas″en-tol′o-jist) a specialist in placentology.

placentology (plas″en-tol′o-je) the scientific study of the development, structure, and functioning of the placenta. **comparative p.,** the scientific study of the development, structure, and functioning of the placenta in different species of animals.

placentolysin (plas″en-tol′ĭ-sin) [*placenta* + Gr. *lysis* dissolution] a lysin formed in the serum of an animal into which have been injected placenta cells from another animal.

It is destructive to the placenta of animals of the species from which the cells were originally taken.

placentoma (plas″en-to′mah) a neoplasm derived from a portion of the placenta retained after an abortion.

placentopathy (plas″en-top′ah-the) any placental disease of the placenta.

Placido's disk (plah-si′dōz) [A. *Placido*, Portuguese ophthalmologist, 1848–1916] see under *disk*.

Placidyl (plas′ĭ-dil) trademark for a preparation of ethchlorvynol.

placode (plak′ōd) [Gr. *plax* plate + *eidos* form] a platelike structure, especially a thickened plate of ectoderm in the early embryo, from which a sense organ develops. **auditory p.,** a thickened epidermal plate located midway alongside the hindbrain in the early embryo, from which the internal ear ultimately develops. Called also *auditory saucer* and *otic p.* **dorsolateral p's,** a series of placodes giving rise to the acoustic and lateral line organs. **epibranchial p's,** a series of placodes located dorsal to the branchial grooves that contribute to adjacent cerebral ganglia. **lens p.,** a thickened area of ectoderm directly overlying the optic vesicle in the early embryo, from which the lens develops. **olfactory p.,** an oval area of thickened ectoderm on either ventrolateral surface of the head of the early embryo, constituting the first indication of the olfactory organ. **otic p.,** auditory p.

placoderm (plak′o-derm) [Gr. *plakos* a tablet or flat plate + *derma* skin] any of the primitive jawed fishes of the class Placodermi.

Placodermi (plak′o-der″mi) a class of primitive jawed fishes of the Paleozoic era, having a bony head shield movably articulated with a thoracic shield; known only from fossils, and believed to be ancestral to both bony and cartilaginous fishes.

placoid (plak′oid) platelike or plaquelike.

plagiocephalic (pla″je-o-se-fal′ik) characterized by plagiocephaly.

plagiocephalism (pla″je-o-sef′ah-lism) plagiocephaly.

plagiocephaly (pla″je-o-sef′ah-le) [Gr. *plagios* oblique + *kephalē* head] an unsymmetrical and twisted condition of the head, resulting from irregular closure of the cranial sutures.

Plagiotomina (pla″je-o″to-mi′nah) [Gr. *plagios* oblique *temno* to cut] a suborder of endocommensal ciliate protozoa (order Heterotrichina, subclass Spirotricha) having a laterally flattened body with an extensive adoral zone of membranelles and two paroral lines in the right side; a subequatorial cytosome; and uniform cilia occurring in cirrilike groups. They are found in oligochetes.

plague (plāg) [L. *plaga*, *pestis*; Gr. *plēgē* stroke] a severe acute or chronic enzootic or epizootic bacterial infection caused by *Yersinia pestis*, which occurs both endemically and epidemically worldwide. It is primarily a disease of urban and sylvatic rodents, transmitted to humans from the natural animal reservoir by the bite of infected fleas, especially the rat flea, or by contact with or ingestion of infected animals. Human-to-human infection usually occurs by inhalation of plague bacilli–laden droplet aerosols. The most common forms are bubonic plague, which presents as acute regional lymphadenitis, pulmonic plague, and septicemic plague; the latter two may occur secondary to the bubonic form or as primary infections. Called also *pest* and *pestis*. **ambulatory p.,** a mild form of bubonic plague, usually occurring only in endemic areas, with lymphadenitis, fever, headache, prostration, and a short course. Called also *parapestis, pestis ambulans,* and *pestis minor.* **avian p.,** fowl p. **black p.,** see *bubonic p.* **Brunswick bird p.,** fowl p. **bubonic p.,** the most common form of plague, typically characterized by abrupt onset of fever, chills, weakness, and headache, followed by pain, tenderness, and lymphadenopathy (buboes) of the regional lymph nodes, most often the inguinal, femoral, axillary, and cervical nodes, associated with a marked hemorrhagic tendency and the development of disseminated intravascular coagulation and necrotic purpura and extensive symmetrical gangrene (which may have led to the epithet "black death," used since the Middle Ages). Hematogenous dissemination may establish suppurative foci throughout the body. Severe complications include pneumonia (see *pulmonic p.*) and septicemia (see *septicemic p.*). Called also *glandular p., pestis bubonica, pestis fulminans,* and *pestis*

major. **canine p.,** black tongue of dogs; it is caused by niacin deficiency. **cat p.,** panleukopenia. **cattle p.,** a viral disease of cattle, which sometimes affects sheep and goats, marked by fever and croupous, ulcerative diphtheritic lesions of the intestinal tract; called also *rinderpest.* **duck p.,** an acute contagious herpesvirus infection of ducks, which may also affect geese and swans. It is characterized by vascular damage, with hemorrhage into the tissues and free blood in the body cavities, exanthematous lesions of the mucosa of the digestive tract, lesions of the lymphoid organs, and retrograde changes in the parenchymatous organs. Called also *duck virus enteritis.* **equine p.,** African horse sickness. **fowl p.,** a viral disease of domestic fowls caused by a highly pathogenic strain of the avian influenza virus; called also *fowl pest.* **glandular p.,** bubonic p. **hemorrhagic p.,** see *bubonic p.* **lung p.,** pleuropneumonia, def. 2. **meningeal p.,** plague meningitis. **Pahvant Valley p.,** tularemia. **pharyngeal p.,** a rare clinical form of plague that may resemble acute tonsillitis, thought to be due to inhalation or ingestion of plague bacilli. Called also *plague pharyngitis.* **pneumonic p.,** that in which there is extensive involvement of the lungs, and the sputum is loaded with the causative organisms. **pulmonic p.,** a rapidly progressive and highly contagious pneumonia in which there is extensive involvement of the lungs and productive cough with mucoid, blood-stained, foamy, plague bacilli–laden sputum. It may occur as a primary infection, transmitted by inhalation of infectious droplet nuclei expelled during coughing; or it may be a secondary complication of bubonic plague due to hematogenous spread of the infection from the buboes to the lungs, which in turn may be associated with human-to-human transmission and cause a primary infection. Called also *plague pneumonia.* **septicemic p.,** acute fulminating, high-density bacteremia occurring in the acute stage of bubonic plague, or as a so-called primary infection that may present and result in death before the appearance of buboes or of pulmonic manifestations. Called also *pesticemia, pestis siderans, plague septicemia,* and *siderating plague.* **siderating p.,** septicemic p. **swine p.,** hemorrhagic septicemia of swine. **sylvatic p.,** plague of the woods, as for example, the plague widely spread and still spreading among the ground squirrels and other wild rodents of the western U.S.A. **white p.,** tuberculosis.

plakins (pla′kinz) substances similar to leukins that can be extracted from blood platelets.

plana (pla′nah) [L.] plural of *planum.*

planarian (plah-nar′i-an) any of the free-living flatworms of the class Turbellaria, which are used extensively in biologic studies of regeneration.

planchet (plan′chet) a metal disk on which radioactive samples are mounted and prepared for determination of radioactivity.

Planck's constant, theory (planks) [Max Karl Ernst Ludwig *Planck*, German physicist, 1858–1947] see under *constant*, and see *quantum theory*, under *theory*.

Planctomyces (plank″to-mi′sēz) [Gr. *planktos* floating + *mykēs* fungus] a genus of appendaged bacteria found in aerobic surface water of lakes, made up of spherical to oblong or pear-shaped cells with long slender stalks that attach to a common substrate site, forming rosettes. They reproduce by budding. The type species is *P. beke′fii.* Called also *Blastocaulis.*

plane (plān) [L. *planus*] 1. a surface such that a straight line connecting any two of its points lies wholly in the surface. In craniotomy and cephalometry, the term plane is sometimes used interchangeably with line because when viewed from the side (lateral projection), as in a radiograph, it appears as a line. 2. a specified level, as the plane of anesthesia. 3. to rub away or abrade; see *planing.* 4. a superficial incision in the wall of a cavity or between tissue layers, especially in plastic surgery, made so that the precise point of entry into the cavity or between the layers can be determined. **Addison's p's,** a series of planes used as landmarks in the topography of the thorax and abdomen. **Aeby's p.,** one passing through the nasion and basion, perpendicular to the median plane of the cranium. **auricular p. of sacral bone,** facies auricularis ossis sacri: **auriculoinfraorbital p.,** Frankfort horizontal p. **axial p.,** one parallel with the long axis of a structure. **axiolabiolingual p.,** one parallel with the long axis of an anterior tooth and passing through its labial and lingual surfaces. **axiomesiodistal p.,** one parallel with the long axis of a tooth and passing through its mesial and distal surfaces. **Baer's p.,** one passing through the upper border of the zygomatic arches. **base p.,** an imaginary plane upon which is estimated the retention of an artificial denture. **bite p.,** 1. biteplane. 2. occlusal p. **Blumenbach's p.,** a plane determined by the base of a skull from which the lower jaw has been removed. **Bolton-nasion p.,** nasion-postcondylare p. **Broadbent-Bolton p.,** nasion-postcondylare p. **Broca's p.,** visual p. **buccolingual**

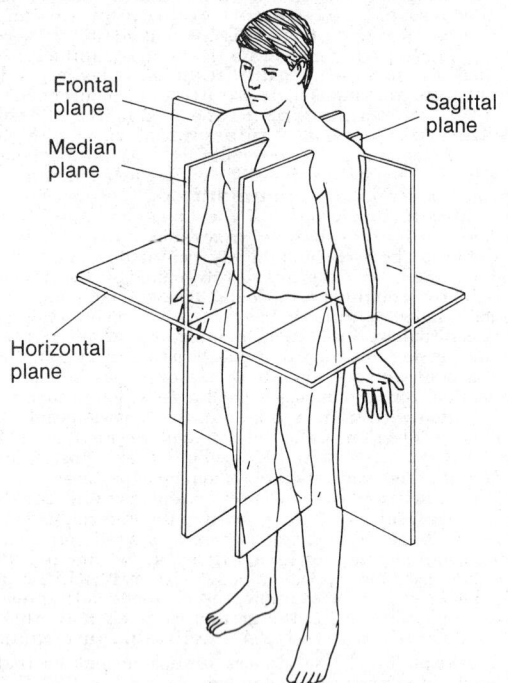

Frontal plane

Sagittal plane

Median plane

Horizontal plane

Planes of the body, with subject in the anatomical position.

p., one passing through the buccal and lingual surfaces of a posterior tooth. **coronal p.,** frontal p. **cove p.,** the ST-T segment of the electrocardiogram in which an inverted T wave is preceded by an isoelectric plateau. **cusp p.,** the small imaginary plane in which buccal cusp tips and lingual cusp tips are located on posterior teeth. **Daubenton's p.,** one passing through the opisthion and the lower edges of the orbits; called also *Daubenton's line.* **eye-ear p.,** Frankfort horizontal p. **facial p.,** any of several planes passing through craniometric or cephalometric landmarks of the face. **Frankfort horizontal p.,** a horizontal plane represented in profile by a line between the lowest point on the margin of the orbit and the highest point on the margin of the auditory meatus. **frontal p.,** any plane passing longitudinally through the body from side to side, at right angles to the median plane, and dividing the body into front and back parts. So called because such a plane roughly parallels the frontal suture of the skull. Called also *coronal p.* because one of these planes passes through the coronal suture. **frontoparallel p.,** any plane parallel to the frontal plane. **guide p., guiding p.,** 1. any plane that guides movement. 2. an orthodontic appliance used to correct crossbite of anterior teeth. 3. two or more vertically parallel surfaces of abutment teeth, so shaped as to direct the path of placement and removal of a partial denture. **Hensen's p.,** one passing through the center of a series of sarcous elements of a muscle fibril. **Hodge's p's,** a series of planes running parallel with the pelvic inlet, the first parallel being in the inlet, the second parallel touching the arch of the pubis and striking the lower part of the second sacral vertebra, the third cutting the spines of the ischia, and the fourth passing through the tip of the coccyx. **horizontal p.,** any plane passing through a body, at right angles to both the median and the frontal plane, and dividing the

body into upper and lower parts; in dentistry, a plane passing through a tooth at right angles to its long axis. Called also *transverse p.* **interparietal p. of occipital bone,** pla-

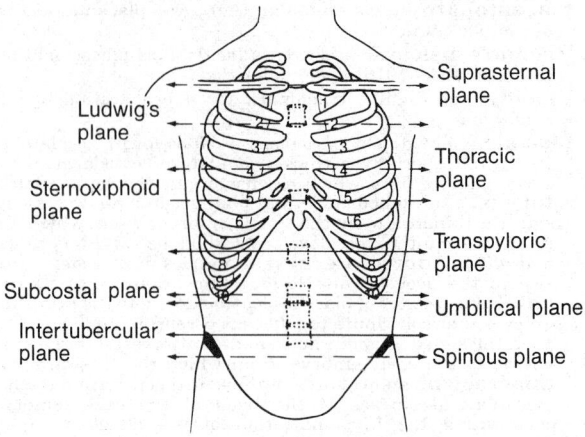

Ludwig's plane

Sternoxiphoid plane

Subcostal plane

Intertubercular plane

Suprasternal plane

Thoracic plane

Transpyloric plane

Umbilical plane

Spinous plane

Planes of the trunk.

num occipitale. **interspinal p.,** planum interspinale. **intertubercular p.,** planum intertuberculare. **labiolingual p.,** one passing through the labial and lingual surfaces of an anterior tooth. **Listing's p.,** a transverse vertical plane perpendicular to the anteroposterior axis of the eye, and containing the center of motion of the eyes; in it lie the transverse and vertical axes of ocular rotation. **Ludwig's p.,** a horizontal plane transecting the trunk at about the level of the joint between the fourth and fifth thoracic vertebrae. **mean foundation p.,** the mean of the various irregularities in form and inclination of the basal seat (denture-supporting tissues). The ideal condition for denture stability exists when the mean foundation plane is most nearly at right angles to the direction of force. **Meckel's p.,** one passing through the auricular and alveolar points. **median p.,** the imaginary plane passing longitudinally through the middle of the body from front to back and dividing it into right and left halves. **median-raphe p.,** the median plane of the head. **mesiodistal p.,** one passing through the mesial and distal surfaces of a tooth. **midpelvic p.,** pelvic p., narrow. **midsagittal p.,** median p. **Morton's p.,** one passing through the most projecting points of the parietal and occipital protuberances. **nasion-postcondylare p.,** one passing at right angles to the median plane, and determined in profile by a line connecting the nasion and postcondylare. **nuchal p.,** planum nuchale. **occipital p.,** planum occipitale. **occlusal p., p. of occlusion,** the hypothetical horizontal plane formed by the contacting surfaces of the upper and lower teeth when the jaws are closed. **orbital p.,** 1. planum orbitale. 2. visual plane. **orbital p. of frontal bone,** pars orbitalis ossis frontalis. **parasagittal p.,** sagittal p. **pelvic p.,** one determined by certain landmarks of the hip bone. **pelvic p., narrow,** an ovoid plane passing through the apex of the pubic arch, the spines of the ischia, and the end of the sacrum. **pelvic p., wide,** an irregularly ovoid plane passing from the middle of the pubis to the junction of the second and third sacral vertebrae, at about the center of the excavation of the pelvis. **pelvic p. of outlet,** a plane passing through the arch of the pubis, the rami of the pubis, the ischial tuberosities, and the tip of the coccyx; see *apertura pelvis inferior.* **popliteal p. of femur,** facies poplitea femoris. **principal p.,** in radiology, the plane which contains the central ray of a radiation beam. **p's of reference,** planes which are referred to as a guide to the location of specific anatomical sites, or of other planes. **p. of regard,** one passing through the center of rotation and the point of fixation in the eye. **sagittal p.,** any vertical plane that passes through the body parallel to the median plane (or to the sagittal suture) and divides the body into left and right portions. **semicircular p. of frontal bone,** facies temporalis ossis frontalis. **semicircular p. of parietal bone,** planum temporale.

semicircular p. of squama temporalis, facies temporalis partis squamosae. **spinous p.,** a horizontal plane transecting the trunk at the level of the anterior superior iliac spine. **sternal p.,** planum sternale. **sternoxiphoid p.,** a horizontal plane transecting the trunk at about the level of the xiphisternal joint. **subcostal p.,** planum subcostale. **supracrestal p.,** planum supracristale. **suprasternal p.,** a horizontal plane transecting the trunk at the level of the jugular notch. **temporal p.,** planum temporale. **thoracic p.,** a horizontal plane transecting the trunk at about the level of the fourth intercostal space. **tooth p.,** any hypothetical plane passing through a tooth. **transpyloric p.,** planum transpyloricum. **transverse p.,** a horizontal plane of the body dividing the body into upper and lower portions, or a plane at right angles to the longitudinal axis of a structure. **umbilical p.,** a horizontal plane transecting the trunk at the level of the umbilicus. **vertical p.,** any plane of the body perpendicular to a horizontal plane and dividing the body into left and right, or front and back portions, as the sagittal and frontal planes. **visual p.,** one passing through the visual axes of the two eyes; called also *Broca's p.* and *orbital p.*

planigram (pla′nĭ-gram) a roentgenogram of a structure at a selected level, made by body section roentgenography.

planigraphy (plah-nig′rah-fe) body section roentgenography; see under *roentgenography.*

planimeter (pla-nim′ĕ-ter) [L. *planus* plane + Gr. *metron* measure] an instrument used in measuring the area of surfaces.

planing (pla′ning) the plastic surgery procedure of abrading disfigured skin to promote reepithelialization with minimal scarring. It may be done by means of sandpaper, emery paper, low- or high-speed wire brushes, etc. (surgical planing; dermabrasion), or by application of caustic substances such as phenol or trichloracetic acid (chemical planing; chemabrasion). **root p.,** smoothing of the root surface of a tooth after sub-gingival scaling or curettage.

planithorax (plan″ĭ-tho′raks) a diagram of the front and back of the chest.

plankton (plank′ton) [Gr. *planktos* wandering] a collective name for the minute free-floating organisms, vegetable and animal, which live in practically all natural waters.

Planobispora (pla″no-bi-spo′rah) [Gr. *planos* wanderer + L. *bis* double + Gr. *spora* seed] a genus of bacteria of the family Actinoplanaceae, order Actinomycetales, consisting of soil organisms bearing sporangia containing a pair of spores formed on aerial mycelia. The type species is *P. longispo′ra.*

planocellular (pla″no-sel′u-lar) made up of flat cells.

Planococcus (plan″o-kok′us) [Gr. *planos* wandering + *kokkus* berry] a genus of bacteria of the family Micrococcaceae, made up of spherical, aerobic, gram-positive, motile cells, occurring singly, in pairs, in threes, or in tetrads. They are found in sea water.

planoconcave (pla″no-kon′kāv) flat on one side and concave on the other; see under *lens.*

planoconvex (pla″no-kon′veks) flat on one side and convex on the other; see under *lens.*

planocyte (pla′no-sīt) [Gr. *plane* wandering + *-cyte*] a wandering cell.

planogram (pla′no-gram) planigram.

planography (plah-nog′rah-fe) planigraphy.

Planomonospora (pla″no-mo-nos′po-rah) [Gr. *planos* wanderer + *monos* single + *spora* seed] a genus of bacteria of the family Actinoplanaceae, order Actinomycetales, consisting of soil organisms that produce motile spores on aerial mycelia. The type species is *P. paronto′spora.*

planorbid (plah-nor′bid) 1. a snail of the family Planorbidae. 2. pertaining to snails of the family Planorbidae.

Planorbidae (plah-nor′bĭ-de) [L. *planus* flat + *orbis* ring + *idae*] a large family of pulmonate fresh-water snails (suborder Basommatophora, order Pulmonata), many species of which are intermediate hosts of pathogenic trematodes; it includes the genera *Biomphalaria, Planorbis* (the type genus), and *Bulinus.*

Planorbis (plan-or′bis) a genus of snails. Several species act as intermediate hosts for *Schistosoma mansoni* and others for *Fasciolopsis buski* and echinostomes.

planotopokinesia (pla″no-top″o-ki-ne′ze-ah) [Gr. *plane*

wandering + *topos* place + *kinēsis* movement] disturbance of the power of orientation in space.

planta pedis (plan′tah pe′dis) [L.] [NA] the undersurface (sole) of the foot. Called also *regio plantaris pedis* [NA alternative].

plantaginis semen (plan-taj′ĭ-nis se′men) [L.] the seed of *Plantago psyllium* L., Plantaginaceae.

Plantago (plan-ta′go) a genus of herbs (family Plantaginaceae), including three species, *P. in′dica* L., *P. ova′ta* Forskal (blond psyllium), and *P. psyllium* L. (Spanish psyllium), whose seeds (plantago, or psyllium seeds) are used as a cathartic. A preparation of the separated mucilaginous outer layers of the seeds of *P. ovata* is used in the preparation of psyllium hydrophilic mucilloid (q.v.).

plantalgia (plan-tal′je-ah) [L. *planta* sole + *-algia*] a painful condition of the sole of the foot.

plantar (plan′tar) pertaining to the sole of the foot.

plantaris (plan-tah′ris) [L.] plantar; [NA] a term designating relationship to the sole of the foot.

plantation (plan-ta′shun) [L. *plantare* to plant] the insertion or application of tissue, such as a tooth, or of other material, in or on the human body. It includes *implantation,* the insertion of similar or other material within the body tissues, as of an artificial or natural tooth into a new socket, or of a therapeutic agent or device; *replantation,* return of body tissue to its original site, as reinsertion of a tooth into the socket from which it was dislodged; and *transplantation,* the insertion or application of tissue derived from another individual, or from a different site in the same individual.

plantigrade (plan′tĭ-grād) [L. *planta* sole + *gradi* to walk] characterized by walking on the full sole of the foot, applied to animals whose entire sole touches the ground, such as the bear and man.

planula (plan′u-lah) a larval coelenterate. **invaginate p.,** the gastrula.

planum (pla′num), pl. *pla′na* [L.] a surface such that a straight line connecting any two of its points lies wholly in the surface. Called also *plane.* Used in anatomical nomenclature to designate a more or less flat surface of a bone or other structure. **p. interspina′le** [NA] a horizontal plane transecting the trunk at the level of the anterior superior iliac spines; called also *interspinal line.* **p. intertubercula′re** [NA] intertubercular plane: a horizontal plane transecting the trunk at the level of the iliac tubercles; called also *intertubercular line.* **p. nucha′le,** nuchal plane: the outer surface of the occipital bone between the foramen magnum and the superior nuchal line. **p. occipita′le,** occipital plane: the outer surface of the occipital bone above the superior nuchal line. **p. orbita′le,** orbital plane: a plane passing through the two orbital points and perpendicular to the Frankfort horizontal plane. **p. poplite′um fem′oris,** facies poplitea femoris. **p. semiluna′tum,** the rounded end of a crista in a semicircular canal. **p. sterna′le,** sternal plane: the anterior surface of the sternum. **p. subcosta′le** [NA], subcostal plane: a horizontal plane transecting the trunk at the level of the lower margins of the tenth costal cartilages; called also *infracostal line.* **p. supracrista′le** [NA] supracrestal plane: a horizontal plane transecting the trunk at the summits of the iliac crests at the level of the fourth lumbar spinous process; called also *supracrestal line.* **p. tempora′le,** temporal plane: the depressed area on the side of the skull below the inferior temporal line. **p. transpylo′ricum** [NA], transpyloric plane: a horizontal plane half way between the superior margins of the manubrium sterni and the symphysis pubis, which usually does not correspond to the level of the pylorus.

planuria (pla-nu′re-ah) [Gr. *planasthai* to wander + *ouron* urine + *-ia*] the discharge of urine from an abnormal site.

plaque (plak) [Fr.] any patch or flat area. **argyrophil p's,** amorphous argyrophilic masses, 40 to 80 microns in diameter, between the neurons of the brain in old people, particularly in the frontal cortex and the hippocampus. **attachment p's,** small regions of increased density along the sarcolemma of skeletal muscles to which myofilaments seem to attach; cf. *dense bodies,* under *body.* **bacterial p.,** dental p. **bacteriophage p.,** a cleared, usually circular, area on a bacterial lawn plate, occurring as a result of lysis of cells by a bacteriophage. **dental p.,** a soft, thin film of food debris, mucin, and dead epithelial cells deposited on the teeth, providing the medium for the growth of various bacteria. The main inorganic components are calcium and phosphorus with small amounts of magnesium, potassium, and sodium; the organic matrix consists of polysaccharides, proteins, carbohydrates, lipids, and other components. Plaque plays an important etiologic role in the development of dental caries and periodontal and gingival diseases and provides the base for the development of materia alba; calcified plaque forms dental calculus. Called also *bacterial p.* **fibromyelinic p's,** areas of overgrowth of medullated fibers and sheaths in areas of incomplete arteriosclerotic necrosis in the cerebral cortex. **fibrous p.,** the lesion of atherosclerosis, a pearly white area within an artery that causes the intimal surface to bulge into the lumen; it is composed of lipid, cell debris, smooth muscle cells, collagen, and, in older persons, calcium. **Hollenhorst p's,** atheromatous emboli containing cholesterol crystals in the retinal arterioles, a warning sign of impending serious cardiovascular disease such as stroke, myocardial infarction, aortic aneurysm, or occlusion of the retinal arterioles. **Hutchinson's p's,** a persistent cutaneous manifestation of sarcoidosis consisting of flat-surfaced, slightly elevated, large, lobulated, nodular plaques, which show a predilection for the cheeks, nose, arms, and buttocks, usually occurring bilaterally and symmetrically. **Lichtheim p's,** areas of degeneration in the cerebral white matter that are seen in pernicious anemia. **Peyer's p's,** Peyer's patches (folliculi lymphatici aggregati). **Randall's p's,** small calcium concretions within the tip of the renal papillae; they may project through the surface and serve as foci for the deposition of urinary salts. **Redlich-Fisher miliary p's,** thickened, dark colored areas in the neuroglia reticulum of the brain, seen in cases of senile psychoses. **senile p's,** microscopic lesions composed of fragmented axon terminals and dendrites surrounding a core of amyloid seen in the cerebral cortex in Alzheimer's disease. **talc p's,** opaque material visible roentgenographically on pleural surfaces in talc miners and processors.

Plaquenil (pla′kwĕ-nil) trademark for a preparation of hydroxychloroquine sulfate.

-plasia [Gr. *plasis* molding, from *plassein* to mold] a combining form denoting development or formation.

plasm (plazm) plasma. **germ p.** (*obs.*), Weismann's term for the reproductive and hereditary substance of individuals which is passed on from the germ cell in which an individual originates in direct continuity to the germ cells of succeeding generations. By it new individuals are produced and hereditary characters are transmitted. Cf. *somatoplasm.*

-plasm [Gr. *plasma* anything formed or molded] a combining form denoting the constituent substance of cells.

plasma (plaz′mah) [Gr. "anything formed or molded"] 1. the fluid portion of the blood in which the particulate components are suspended. *Plasma* is to be distinguished from *serum*, which is the cell-free portion of the blood from which the fibrinogen has been separated in the process of clotting. See *blood plasma.* 2. the lymph deprived of its corpuscles or cells. 3. a glycerite of starch used in preparing ointments. 4. cytoplasm or protoplasm. **antihemophilic human p.,** normal human plasma that has been processed promptly to preserve the antihemophilic properties of the original blood; used for temporary correction of bleeding tendency in hemophilia. **blood p.,** see under *B.* **citrated p.,** blood plasma treated with sodium citrate, which prevents clotting. **muscle p.,** a liquid expressible from muscular tissue; it clots spontaneously. **normal human p.,** sterile plasma obtained by pooling approximately equal amounts of the liquid portion of citrated whole blood from eight or more adult humans, used as a blood volume replenisher. **oxalate p.,** blood plasma to which 1 per cent of ammonium oxalate has been added, to prevent clotting. **peptone p.,** albumose p. **pooled p.,** a mixture of plasma from several donors. **salt p.,** blood plasma to which a neutral salt has been added to prevent clotting. **seminal p.,** the fluid portion of the semen, in which the spermatozoa are suspended. **true p.,** blood plasma drawn direct from the blood without any change in its gas content.

plasmablast (plaz′mah-blast) [*plasma* + Gr. *blastos* germ] the earliest precursor in the plasmacytic series, which matures to form the proplasmacyte and ultimately the mature plasma cell; it may itself be a derivative of the lymphoblast.

plasmacyte (plaz′mah-sīt) [*plasma* + *-cyte*] a plasma cell.

plasmacytic (plaz″mah-sit′ik) pertaining to, characterized by, or of the nature of a plasma cell.

plasmacytoma (plaz″mah-si-to′mah) [*plasmacyte* + *-oma*] 1. plasma cell dyscrasia, a malignant tumor of plasma cells. 2. a discrete, presumably solitary, plasma cell tumor mass. **multiple p. of bone,** multiple myeloma.

plasmacytosis (plaz″mah-si-to′sis) the presence of excess plasma cells in the blood.

plasmagel (plas′mah-jel) a relatively rigid peripheral layer of cytoplasm which is devoid of granules.

plasmagene (plaz′mah-jēn) [*cytoplasm* + *gene*] in human beings, a gene found on the mitochondrial chromosome (q.v.); called also *cytogene.*

plasmahaut (plaz′mah-howt) [Ger.] the superficial layer of the protoplasm of a cell.

plasmal (plas′mal) a long-chain fatty acid aldehyde produced during hydrolysis of plasmalogens.

plasmalemma (plaz″mah-lem′ah) [*plasma* + Gr. *lemma* husk] 1. the plasma membrane. 2. a thin peripheral layer of the ectoplasma in a fertilized egg.

plasmalogen (plaz-mal′o-jen) a term applied to a member of a group of phospholipids, present in platelets, that liberate higher fatty aldehydes (e.g., palmital) on hydrolysis, and may be related to the specialized function of platelets in blood coagulation. Plasmalogens are also found in cell membranes of muscle and of the myelin sheath of nerve fibers.

Plasmanate (plaz′mah-nāt) trademark for a commercial preparation of human plasma protein fraction.

plasmapheresis (plaz″mah-fĕ-re′sis) [*plasma* + Gr. *aphairesis* removal] the removal of plasma from withdrawn blood, with retransfusion of the formed elements into the donor; generally, type-specific fresh frozen plasma or albumin is used to replace the withdrawn plasma. The procedure may be done for purposes of collecting plasma components or for therapeutic purposes.

plasmarrhexis (plaz″mah-rek′sis) [*plasma* + Gr. *rhēxis* rupture] dissolution of the cytoplasm.

plasmatherapy (plaz″mah-ther′ah-pe) the therapeutic use of blood plasma.

plasmatic (plaz-mat′ik) pertaining to or of the nature of the plasma.

plasmatogamy (plaz″mah-tog′ah-me) plasmogamy.

plasmatorrhexis (plaz″mah-to-rek′sis) [*plasma* + Gr. *rhēxis* rupture] the bursting of a cell due to the pressure exerted from within.

plasmatosis (plaz″mah-to′sis) the liquefaction of the substance of a cell.

plasmic (plaz′mik) 1. plasmatic. 2. rich in protoplasm.

plasmid (plaz′mid) [*plasm* + *-id*] an extrachromosomal self-replicating structure found in bacterial cells that carries genes for a variety of functions not essential for cell growth. Plasmids consist of cyclic double-stranded DNA molecules, replicating independently of the chromosomes and transmitting through successive cell divisions genes specifying such functions as antibiotic resistance (R plasmid); conjugation (F plasmid); the production of enzymes, toxins, and antigens; and the metabolism of sugars and other organic compounds. Plasmids can be transferred from one cell to another by conjugation and by transduction. Some plasmids may also become integrated into the bacterial chromosome; these are known as *episomes.* **conjugative p.,** a plasmid that is transferred from one bacterial cell to another during conjugation. **F p.,** a conjugative plasmid found in F+ (male) bacterial cells that leads with high frequency to its transfer and much less often to transfer of the bacterial chromosome. A cell possessing the F plasmid (F+, male) can form a conjugation bridge (F pilus) to a cell lacking the F plasmid (F−, female), through which genetic material may pass from one cell to another. Called also *F (fertility) factor, F element,* and *sex factor.* **F′ p.,** a hybrid F plasmid that contains also a segment of the host chromosome. **oligomeric p.,** a plasmid that contains repeating segments of a determinant, formed by recombination between strands during replication and resulting in gene amplification. **R p.,** a conjugative factor in bacterial cells that promotes resistance to agents such as antibiotics, metal ions, ultraviolet radiation, and bacteriophage. R plasmids are large with two functionally distinct parts: a resistance transfer factor (RTF), consisting of genes for autonomous replication and conjugation; and a resistance determinant (R determinant) containing the genes for resistance (R genes); called also *R factor* and *resistance plasmid.*

plasmin (plaz'min) [EC 3.4.21.7] an enzyme of the hydrolase class that catalyzes the hydrolysis of peptide bonds at the carbonyl end of lysine or arginine residues. The enzyme occurs in plasma as plasminogen, which is physiologically activated by kallikrein or plasma or tissue activators such as urokinase. Plasminogen is activated therapeutically by streptokinase, a streptococcal enzyme. Plasmin converts fibrin to soluble products. Called also *fibrinolysin.*

plasminogen (plaz-min'o-jen) the inactive precursor of plasmin (q.v.).

plasm(o)- [Gr. *plasma,* q.v.] a combining form denoting relationship to plasma, or to the substance of a cell.

plasmocyte (plaz'mo-sīt) [*plasmo-* + *-cyte*] a plasma cell.

plasmocytoma (plas'mo-si-to'mah) plasmacytoma.

plasmodesm, plasmodesma (plaz'mo-dezm; plaz'mo dez'-mah) singular of *plasmodesmata.*

plasmodesmata (plaz'mo-dez'mah-tah), sing. *plas'modesm* or *plasmodes'ma* [*plasmo-* + Gr. *desmos* a band or bond] cytoplasmic bridges found in some plant cells, which pass between the pores in the plasma membranes of adjacent cells and serve to establish continuity between cells.

plasmodia (plaz-mo'de-ah) plural of *plasmodium.*

plasmodial (plaz-mo'de-al) pertaining to plasmodia.

plasmodiblast (plaz-mo'dĭ-blast) syncytiotrophoblast.

plasmodicidal (plaz'mo-dĭ-si'dal) [*plasmodia* + L. *caedere* to kill] destructive to plasmodia.

plasmodicide (plaz-mo'dĭ-sīd) an agent that is destructive to plasmodia.

Plasmodiophora (plaz'mo-di-of'o-rah) [*plasmodium* + Gr. *phōros* bearing] a genus of ameboid protozoa with minute plasmodia (order Plasmodiophorida, class Plasmodiophorea). *P. brassicae* is a plant pathogen, causing a disease of cabbages and other cruciferous plants known as *finger and toe disease.*

Plasmodiophorea (plaz'mo-di'o-fo're-ah) a class of ameboid protozoa (superclass Rhizopoda, subphylum Sarcodina) occurring as obligate intracellular parasites of higher plants, such as the cabbage and potato, certain algae, and certain aquatic fungi, and often causing hypertrophy of infected cells. The organisms are characterized by the presence of minute plasmodia that give rise to zoospores with two unequal anterior flagella in zoosporangia, and they form resting spores in compact sori or clusters with host cells. It includes one order: Plasmodiophorida. See also *Mycetozoida.*

Plasmodiophorida (plaz'mo-di'o-for'ĭ-dah) an order of ameboid protozoa (class Plasmodiophorea, superclass Rhizopoda) with characters of the class. Representative genera include *Plasmodiophora* and *Sorosphaera.*

plasmoditrophoblast (plaz-mo''di-trof'o-blast) syncytiotrophoblast.

Plasmodium (plaz-mo'de-um) [Gr. *plasma* anything formed or molded] the malarial parasite: a genus of coccidian protozoa (suborder Haemosporina, order Eucoccidiida), parasitic in the erythrocytes of mammals, including humans, nonhuman primates, and rodents, birds, and reptiles, mainly lizards. The organisms are transmitted to the bloodstream of humans and other mammals by the bite of female anopheline mosquitoes, in whose saliva the sporozoites are concentrated. From the bloodstream, the sporozoites migrate directly to the liver (exoerythrocytic stage), where they develop and multiply within the parenchymal cells as merozoites, which then burst the hepatocytes and invade erythrocytes. Erythrocytic schizogeny then occurs, with merozoites escaping infected erythrocytes and invading others. Some of the merozoites develop into gametocytes, which are ingested by mosquitoes, beginning the sexual stage, which ends with the development of sporozoites. Avian malaria, caused by many *Plasmodium* species, is transmitted by culicine mosquitoes; the vectors of reptilian malaria are unknown. Species causing infection in various vertebrates other than man include: *P. cnemidophori* and *P. sternoceri* in lizards; *P. bufonis* in the toad *Bufo americanus; P. cathemerium, P. durae, P. gallinacium, P. lophurae, P. relictum, P. rouxi, P. vaughni* in various birds and poultry; *P. brasilianum, P. cynomolgi, P. knowlesi,* and *P. kochi* in various monkeys; and *P. berghei* in rats and mice. **P. falcip'arum,** the species which causes falciparum malaria in man; it is characterized by thin "signet-ring"

forms of trophozoites and the "crescent" form of the gametes. **P. mala'riae,** the species which causes quartan malaria in man. It is characterized by bandlike trophozoites and schizonts with six to twelve merozoites usually arranged in a rosette-like configuration. **P. ova'le,** a species found primarily in East and Central Africa that causes ovale malaria, and is characterized by oval or fimbriated infected red blood cells. **P. vi'vax,** the species causing vivax malaria, characterized by the ameboid activity and irregular form of its trophozoites, and by Schüffner's dots in parasitized red blood cells.

plasmodium (plaz-mo'de-um), pl. *plasmo'dia* [*plasmo-* + Gr. *eidos* form] 1. a protozoan of the genus *Plasmodium.* 2. a multinucleate continuous mass of protoplasm formed by aggregation and fusion of myxamebae; also, a protozoan whose body consists of such a mass. Cf. *pseudoplasmodium.* **exoerythrocytic p.,** a malarial parasite outside a red blood cell; in human malaria this is generally considered to represent the hepatic stage.

plasmogamy (plaz-mog'ah-me) [*plasmo-* + Gr. *gamos* marriage] the union of two or more cells with their nuclei remaining separate; in fertilization, karyogamy follows. Called also *plasmatogamy* and *plastogamy.* Cf. *karyogamy.*

plasmogen (plaz'mo-jen) [*plasmo-* + Gr. *gennan* to produce] the essential part of protoplasm; bioplasm, def. 2.

plasmoid (plas'moid) an abnormal protein cellular element; see also under *humor.*

plasmology (plaz-mol'o-je) [*plasmo-* + *-logy*] the study of the most minute particles or ultimate corpuscles of living matter.

plasmolysis (plaz-mol'ĭ-sis) [*plasmo-* + Gr. *lysis* dissolution] contraction or shrinking of the protoplasm of a plant cell due to the loss of water by osmotic action.

plasmolytic (plaz'mo-lit'ik) tending toward, pertaining to, or characterized by plasmolysis.

plasmolyzability (plaz'mo-līz'ah-bil'ĭ-te) the power of undergoing plasmolysis.

plasmolyzable (plaz'mo-līz'ah-b'l) capable of undergoing plasmolysis.

plasmolyze (plaz'mo-līz) to subject to plasmolysis.

plasmoma (plaz-mo'mah) a tumor made up of plasma cells; plasmacytoma.

plasmon (plaz'mon) [*cytoplasm* + Gr. *-on* neuter ending] the sum total of all non-nuclear extrachromosomal genetic material; in human beings, the mitochondrial chromosome (q.v.). See also *genome.*

plasmonucleic acid (plaz'mo-noo-kle'ik) ribonucleic acid.

plasmoptysis (plaz-mop'tĭ-sis) [*plasmo-* + Gr. *ptyein* to spit] escape of protoplasm from a cell through a ruptured cell wall.

plasmorrhexis (plaz'mo-rek'sis) [*plasmo-* + Gr. *rhēxis* splitting] plasmatorrhexis.

plasmoschisis (plaz-mos'kĭ-sis) [*plasmo-* + Gr. *schisis* fission] the splitting of protoplasm into fragments.

plasmosin (plaz'mo-sin) a protein constituent of cytoplasm.

plasmosome (plaz'mo-sōm) [*plasmo-* + Gr. *sōma* body] 1. the true nucleolus of a cell. 2. [pl.] mitochondria.

plasmotomy (plaz-mot'o-me) [*plasmo-* + Gr. *temnein* to cut] reproduction by the separation from the mother cell of smaller masses of protoplasm, each containing several nuclei.

plasmotrophoblast (plaz'mo-trof'o-blast) syncytiotrophoblast.

plasmotropic (plaz'mo-trop'ik) pertaining to or causing plasmotropism.

plasmotropism (plaz-mot'ro-pizm) [Gr. *plasma* plasm + *tropos* a turning] solution or destruction of erythrocytes in the liver, spleen, or marrow, as contrasted with their destruction in the circulation.

plasome (plaz'ōm) [Gr. *plassein* to form] the hypothetical unit of living protoplasm; see *micelle.*

plasson (plas'on) [Gr. *plassōn* forming] the protoplasm of a cytode, or non-nucleated cell.

-plast [Gr. *plastos* formed] a word termination denoting any primitive organized unit of living matter, e.g. a granule, an organelle, or a cell.

plastein (plas'te-in) the protein synthesized by pepsin from the peptic digestion products of protein.

plaster (plas′ter) [L. *emplastrum*] 1. a gypsum material which hardens when mixed with water, used for immobilizing or making impressions of body parts, as *dental plaster,* or *plaster of Paris.* 2. a pastelike mixture which can be spread over the skin and which is adhesive at body temperature. Plasters may be protectant, counterirritant, etc. **adhesive p.,** see under *tape.* **adhesive p., sterile,** see under *tape.* **dental p.,** a gypsum preparation used for the making of impressions of structures of the mouth; called also *impression p.* **impression p.,** dental p. **mustard p.,** a uniform mixture of powdered black mustard and a solution of suitable adhesive, spread on an appropriate backing material; used as a local irritant. **p. of Paris,** calcium sulfate dihydrate, with about three fourths of the water of crystallization driven off, and reduced to a fine powder; the addition of water produces a porous mass that has been used extensively in making casts and bandages to support or immobilize body parts, and in dentistry for taking dental impressions. **salicylic acid p.** [USP], a uniform mixture of salicylic acid in a suitable base, spread on paper, cotton cloth, or other suitable backing material, containing between 90 and 110 per cent of the labeled amount of salicylic acid; used as a topical keratolytic.

plastic (plas′tik) [L. *plasticus;* Gr. *plastikos*] 1. tending to build up tissues or to restore a lost part. 2. conformable; capable of being molded. 3. a substance produced by chemical condensation or by polymerization. 4. material that can be molded.

plasticity (plas-tis′ĭ-te) 1. the quality of being plastic or conformable. 2. the ability of early embryonic cells to alter in conformity with the immediate environment.

plasticizer (plas′tĭ-si″zer) any of a group of agents added to other organic or synthetic substances to make them soft and flexible.

plastid (plas′tid) [Gr. *plastos* formed] 1. any elementary constructive unit, as a cell. 2. any of the specialized organelles of plant cells that contain pigments (e.g., chlorophyll and carotenoids) or that synthesize and accumulate reserve substances (e.g., starch); they include chloroplasts and amyloplasts.

plastidogenetic (plas-tid″o-jĕ-net′ik) producing plastids or cells.

plastin (plas′tin) 1. linin. 2. spongioplasm (def. 1).

plastiosome (plas′te-o-sōm) [pl.] mitochondria.

plastochondria (plas″to-kon′dre-ah) granular mitochondria.

plastocont (plas′to-kont) chondriocont.

plastodynamia (plas″to-di-na′me-ah) [Gr. *plastos* formed + *dynamis* power] power or ability to develop.

plastogamy (plas-tog′ah-me) [Gr. *plastos* formed matter + *gamos* marriage] plasmogamy.

plastogel (plas′to-jel) a gel possessing great plasticity.

plastokont (plas′to-kont) chondriocont.

plastoquinone (plas″to-kwin′ōn) a quinone occurring in chloroplasts, involved in the transport of electrons during photosynthesis.

plastosome (plas′to-sōm) [Gr. *plastos* formed + *sōma* body] one of the stainable granules or threads of the cytoplasm; [pl.] mitochondria.

plastron (plas′tron) [Fr. "breast-plate"] the sternum and costal cartilages.

-plasty [Gr. *plassein* to form] a word termination denoting plastic surgery.

plate (plāt) [Gr. *platē*] 1. a flat structure or layer, such as a thin layer of bone; see also *lamina, layer,* etc. 2. a dental plate. Sometimes, by extension, incorrectly used to designate a complete denture. 3. a flat vessel, usually a Petri dish, containing sterile solid medium for the culture of microorganisms. 4. to prepare a culture medium in a Petri dish, or to inoculate such a medium with a bacterial culture. **alar p.,** lamina alaris. **anal p.,** cloacal membrane. **auditory p.,** the bony roof of the auditory meatus. **axial p.,** the primitive streak of the embryo. **basal p.,** 1. lamina basalis. 2. the fused parachordal cartilages, precursors of the occipital bone. 3. the portion of the decidua basalis that becomes an integral part of the placenta. **base p.,** see *baseplate.* **bite p.,** a removable orthodontic appliance, generally made of acrylic resin, that makes use of adhesion to the palate to provide part of the anchorage needed for the

desired tooth movement; used to stimulate eruption of the posterior teeth and to decrease the amount of anterior overbite. Written also *biteplate.* **blood p's,** blood platelets. **bone p.,** a metal bar with perforations for the insertion of screws, used to immobilize fractured segments. **cardiogenic p.,** an area of splanchnic mesoderm, at first cephalad and later in the pharyngeal region of the embryo, from which the heart arises. **cell p.,** a thickening midway of the mitotic spindle in plants that forms a dividing septum between the future daughter cells. **chorionic p.,** the inner part of the fetal placenta that gives rise to chorionic villi. **clinoid p.,** the portion of the sphenoid bone behind the sella turcica. **collecting p.,** the electronegative element of a galvanic battery, where the hydrogen and other decomposition products collect. **cortical p.,** the dense outer portion of the alveolar process overlying the spongiosa, being a continuation of the bony plate, which is located on the vestibular and oral aspects of the mandible and maxilla. **cough p.,** a plate of culture medium on which a patient with a respiratory infection, especially pertussis, coughs. **counting p.,** in bacteriology, a plate marked off in square centimeters. A Petri dish culture of microorganisms is placed on the plate and colonies per square centimeter are counted. The number of colonies per plate is calculated by multiplying the average count per square centimeter by 62.5 (the area of a standard Petri dish being 62.5 cm²). **p. of cranial bone, inner,** lamina interna ossis cranii. **p. of cranial bone, outer,** lamina externa ossis cranii. **cribriform p.,** fascia cribrosa. **cribriform p. of ethmoid bone,** lamina cribrosa ossis ethmoidalis. **cuticular p.,** terminal web. **cutis p.,** dermatome, def. 3. **deck p.,** roof p. **dental p.,** a plate of acrylic resin, metal, or other material, which is fitted to the shape of the mouth and serves for the support of artificial teeth. **dermomyotome p.,** the portion of the embryonic somite remaining after migration of the sclerotomic tissue. **die p.,** a plate of metal containing dies for forming the cusps in shell crowns. **dorsal p.,** roof p. **dorsolateral p.,** lamina alaris. **Eggers' p.,** bone plate used for maintaining apposition of bone segments. **end p.,** see *end plate,* under *E.* **epiphyseal p.,** cartilago epiphysialis. **equatorial p.,** the platelike collection of chromosomes at the equator of the spindle in karyokinesis. **ethmovomerine p.,** the central part of the ethmoid bone in the fetus. **floor p.,** the unpaired ventral longitudinal zone of the neural tube, forming the floor of that tube; called also *ventral plate* and *bodenplatte.* **foot p.,** see *footplate.* **frontal p.,** a fetal plate of cartilage between the sides of the ethmoid cartilage and the sphenoid bone. **frontonasal p.,** a fetal plate from which the external nose is developed. **gray p.** (*obs.*), lamina terminalis hypothalami. **growth p.,** cartilago epiphysialis. **horizontal p. of palatine bone,** lamina horizontalis ossis palatini. **jumping the bite p.,** Kingsley appliance. **Kingsley p.,** see under *appliance.* **Kühne's terminal p's,** the motor end-plates of nerves in the muscle spindles. **Lane p's,** steel plates with holes for screws, used in fixing the fragments of a fractured bone. **lateral mesoblastic p.,** the thickened portion of either side of the mesoblast. **lawn p.,** a plate of solid culture medium inoculated by swab or with a liquid inoculum so as to produce a uniform confluent growth of microorganisms, used for assay of bacteriophage. **lingual p.,** a major partial denture connector formed as a lingual bar extended to cover the cingula of the lower anterior teeth. When used on the maxillary arch it is often referred to as a *palatal p.* **medullary p.,** neural p. **mesial p.,** nephrotome. **metaphase p.,** equatorial p. **middle p.,** nephrotome. **Moe p.,** a stainless steel plate for internal fixation of intertrochanteric fractures of the femur. **motor end p.,** see *end plate,* under *E.* **muscle p.,** myotome, def. 2. **nail p.,** 1. stratum corneum unguis. 2. stratum germinativum unguis. **nephrotome p.,** nephrotome. **neural p.,** the thickened plate of ectoderm in the embryo from which the neural tube develops. **notochordal p.,** head process. **oral p.,** fascia pharyngobasilaris. **orbital p. of ethmoid bone,** lamina orbitalis ossis ethmoidalis. **orbital p. of frontal bone,** pars orbitalis ossis frontalis. **palatal p.,** see *lingual p.* **palate p.,** that part of the palatine bone which forms a lateral half of the roof of the mouth. **paper p.,** lamina orbitalis ossis ethmoidalis. **parachordal p.,** basal p., def. 2. **parietal p.,** a thin lamina of the ethmoid bone that forms part of the nasal septum. **perpendicular p. of ethmoid bone,** lamina perpendicularis ossis ethmoidalis. **perpendicular p. of palatine bone,** lamina perpendicularis ossis palatini. **Petri p.,** a Petri dish containing a nutrient medium ready for inoculation with the microorganism to be cultured. **pharyngeal p.,** pharyngeal membrane. **polar p's, pole p's,** platelike bodies at the end of the spindle in certain forms of mitosis. **pour p.,** a bacterial culture poured into a Petri dish from a test tube in which the medium has been inoculated. **prechordal p., prochordal p.,** thickened entoderm, cephalad of the notochord, that combines with ectoderm to become the pharyngeal membrane. **pterygoid p., external,** lamina lateralis processus pterygoidei. **pterygoid p., internal,** lamina medialis processus pterygoidei. **pterygoid p., lateral,** lamina lateralis processus pterygoidei. **pterygoid p., medial,** lamina medialis processus pterygoidei. **quadrigeminal p.,** lamina tecti mesencephali. **reticular p.,** a form of nerve ending in the ciliary body consisting of very fine reticulations of granular nerve fiber. **roof p.,** the unpaired dorsal longitudinal zone of the neural tube, forming the roof of that tube; called also *deck plate, dorsal plate,* and *deckplatte.* **segmental p.,** a plate of mesoblast on either side of the notochord at the posterior end of the embryo, from which the mesoblastic segments are formed. **Sherman p.,** a chrome-cobalt alloy or stainless steel bone plate which can be affixed to a fracture site with screws; often used in open reduction of mandibular fractures. **sole p.,** see *sole plate,* under S. **spiral p.,** lamina spiralis ossea. **spring p.,** a dental prosthesis held in place by the elasticity of the base material which abuts against natural teeth. **Strasburger's cell p.,** midbody, def. 1. **streak p.,** a plate of solid culture medium in which the infectious material is inoculated in streaks across the surface. **subgerminal p.,** a sheet of protoplasm forming the floor of the segmentation cavity of the ovum. **tarsal p's,** see *tarsus superior palpebrae* and *tarsus inferior palpebrae.* **terminal p.,** lamina terminalis hypothalami. **tympanic p.,** pars tympanica ossis temporalis. **urethral p.,** an entodermal plate that gives rise to the terminal portion of the cavernous urethra. **vascular foot p.,** sucker foot. **ventral p.,** floor p. **ventrolateral p.,** lamina basalis. **vertical p. of palatine bone,** lamina perpendicularis ossis palatini. **wing p.,** lamina alaris.

plateau (plah-to′) an elevated and level area. **tibial p.,** either of the bony surfaces of the tibia, internal and external, closest to the condyles of the femur. **ventricular p.,** a nearly level part of the intraventricular curve of blood pressure corresponding to the mid-ejection period of the ventricle.

platelet (plāt′let) a disk-shaped structure, 2 to 4 μm in diameter, found in the blood of all mammals and chiefly known for its role in blood coagulation; platelets, which are formed in the megakaryocyte and released from its cytoplasm in clusters, lack a nucleus and DNA but contain active enzymes and mitochondria. See also under *factor,* and see *thrombocytic series,* under *series.* Called also *blood platelet* and *thrombocyte.* **blood p.,** platelet.

plateletpheresis (plāt″let-fĕ-re′sis) [platelet + Gr. (a)phairesis removal] thrombocytapheresis.

plating (plāt′ing) 1. the act of preparing a bacterial culture on a plate of solid medium in a Petri dish; the preparation of a plate culture. 2. the application of plates to fractured bones for the purpose of holding the fragments in place.

platinic (plah-tin′ik) containing platinum in its higher valency.

platinode (plat′ĭ-nōd) [platinum + Gr. hodos way] the collecting plate of an electric battery.

Platinol (plah′tĭ-nol) trademark for a preparation of cisplatin.

platinosis (plat″ĭ-no′sis) [platinum + -osis] a morbid condition resulting from exposure to soluble platinum salts, with involvement of the upper respiratory tract and allergic manifestations of the skin.

platinous (plat′ĭ-nus) containing platinum in its lower valency.

platinum (plat′ĭ-num) [L.] a heavy, soft, whitish metal, resembling tin: symbol, Pt; atomic number, 78; atomic weight, 195.09; specific gravity, 21.37. It also occurs as a black powder (*p. black*) and a spongy substance (*spongy p.*). Metallic platinum is insoluble except in nitrohydrochloric acid, and is fusible only at very high temperatures; it is therefore used in the manufacture of chemical apparatus. Platinum black and spongy platinum have a strong affinity for oxygen, and act as powerful oxidizing and catalytic agents. **p. chloride,** platinic tetrachloride, a poisonous substance, $PtCl_4 \cdot 5H_2O$, used as a chemical reagent and formerly in syphilis. **p. diamminodichloride,** cisplatin.

cis-**platinum II** cisplatin.

platy- [Gr. *platys* broad] a combining form meaning broad or flat.

platybasia (plat″e-ba′se-ah) [platy- + Gr. basis base (of the skull) + -ia] basilar impression; see under *impression.*

platycelous (plat″e-se′lus) [platy- + Gr. koilos hollow] having vertebrae flat in front, or cephalad, and concave caudad.

platycephalic (plat″e-sĕ-fal′ik) [platy- + Gr. kephalē head] wide headed; having a breadth-height index of less than 70.

platycephaly (plat″e-sef′ah-le) the state of being platycephalic.

platycnemia (plat″ik-ne′me-ah) compression of the tibia from side to side.

platycnemic (plat″ik-ne′mik) [platy- + Gr. knēmē leg] having the tibia compressed from side to side.

platycoria (plat″e-ko′re-ah) [platy- + Gr. korē pupil] a dilated condition of the pupil.

platycrania (plat″e-kra′ne-ah) [platy- + Gr. kranion skull + -ia] artificial flattening of the skull.

platycyte (plat′e-sīt) [platy- + -cyte] a variety of epithelioid cell found in tubercle nodules, intermediate between a leukocyte and a giant cell.

platyglossal (plat″e-glos′al) [platy- + Gr. glōssa tongue] having a broad, flat tongue.

platyhelminth (plat″e-hel′minth) one of the Platyhelminthes.

Platyhelminthes (plat″e-hel-min′thēz) [platy- + Gr. helmins worm] a phylum of acoelomate, dorsoventrally flattened, bilaterally symmetrical animals, commonly known as flatworms, and including the classes Turbellaria, Trematoda, and Cestoidea.

platyhieric (plat″e-hi-er′ik) [platy- + Gr. hieron sacrum] having a wide sacrum; having a sacral index exceeding 100.

platyknemia (plat″ik-ne′me-ah) platycnemia.

platykurtic (plat″e-kur′tik) [platy- + Gr. kurtos convex] (of a probability distribution) having a broader, flatter peak than the normal distribution with the same variance.

platymeria (plat″e-me′re-ah) the condition of being platymeric.

platymeric (plat″e-me′rik) [platy- + Gr. mēros thigh] having a femur that is excessively compressed from front to back.

platymorphia (plat″e-mor′fe-ah) [platy- + Gr. morphē form] having a flat shape; in ophthalmology, a flattened eyeball, resulting in a short anteroposterior axis and hypermetropia.

platymorphic (plat″e-mōr′fik) pertaining to or characterized by platymorphia.

platymyarial, platymyarian (plat″e-mi-a′re-al; plat″e-mi-a′re-an) [platy- + Gr. mys muscle] having all muscle cells lying next to the subcuticula, their sarcoplasm being uncovered on three sides next to the body cavity; said of the muscle arrangement in certain nematodes. Cf. *meromyarial.*

platymyoid (plat″e-mi′oid) [platy- + Gr. mys muscle + eidos form] having the contractile stratum arranged in an even lamina; said of certain muscle cells.

platypellic (plat″e-pel′ik) [platy- + Gr. pella bowl] having a wide pelvis, i.e., a pelvis index below 90.

platypelloid (plat″e-pel′oid) platypellic.

platyphylline (plat″e-fil′in) an alkaloid, $C_{18}H_{27}O_5N$, from *Senecio platyphyllus* D.C. (Compositae) and other species of *Senecio.*

platypnea (plah-tip′ne-ah) [platy- + Gr. pnoia breath] dyspnea induced by assumption of the upright position and relieved by assumption of a recumbent position; the opposite of orthopnea.

platypodia (plat″e-po′de-ah) [platy- + Gr. pous foot + -ia] abnormal flatness of the foot; flatfoot.

Platyrrhina (plat″ĭ-ri′nah) [platy- + Gr. rhis nose] a superfamily of the order Primates (suborder Anthropoidea), characterized by a broad nasal septum and often a prehensile tail, and including the New World monkeys.

platyrrhine (plat′e-rīn) [*platy-* + Gr. *rhis* nose] having a broad nose; having a nasal index exceeding 53.

platysma (plah-tiz′mah) [Gr.] [NA] a platelike muscle that originates from the fascia of the cervical region and inserts in the mandible and the skin around the mouth. It is innervated by the cervical branch of the facial nerve, and acts to wrinkle the skin of the neck and to depress the jaw.

platysmal (plah-tiz′mal) pertaining to the platysma.

platyspondylia (plat″e-spon-dil′e-ah) platyspondylisis.

platyspondylisis (plat″e-spon-dil′ĭ-sis) [*platy-* + Gr. *spondylos* vertebra] congenital flattening of the vertebral bodies.

Platysporina (plat″e-spo-ri′nah) [*platy-* + *spore*] a suborder of parasitic protozoa (order Bivalvulida, class Myxosporea), usually having bilaterally symmetrical spores with two polar capsules at one pole of the spore in a sutural plane. Representative genera include *Myxobolus* and *Myxosoma*.

platystaphyline (plat″e-staf′ĭ-līn) [*platy-* + Gr. *staphylē* palate] having a broad, flat palate.

platystencephalia (plat″e-sten″sĕ-fa′le-ah) platystencephaly.

platystencephalic (plat″e-sten-se-fal′ik) exhibiting or pertaining to platystencephaly.

platystencephalism (plat″e-sten-sef′ah-lizm) platystencephaly.

platystencephaly (plat″e-sten-sef′ah-le) [Gr. *platystatos* widest + *enkephalos* brain + *-ia*] a form of dolichocephalism in which the occiput is very wide and pentagonal, the jaws prognathic; observed among South Africans.

platytrope (plat′e-trōp) [*platy-* + Gr. *trepein* to turn] either of two symmetrical parts on opposite sides of the body; a lateral homologue.

plauracin (plaw′rah-sin) an antibiotic complex produced by *Actinoplanes auranticolor*, the structure of the components of which are not fully confirmed; a veterinary growth stimulant.

Plaut's angina (plowts) [Hugo Carl *Plaut*, German physician, 1858–1928] see *necrotizing ulcerative gingivostomatitis*, under *gingivostomatitis*.

Playfair's treatment (pla′fārz) [William Smoult *Playfair*, British physician, 1836–1903] see under *treatment*.

Plectomycetes (plek″to-mi-se′tēz) a series of ascomycetous fungi of the subclass Euascomycetidae that includes the order Eurotiales; their fruiting body is a cleistothecium or a gymnothecium.

plectron (plek′tron) [Gr. *plēktron* anything to strike with] the hammer form assumed by certain bacilli during sporulation.

plectrum (plek′trum) [L. from Gr. *plēktron* anything to strike with] 1. the uvula. 2. the malleus. 3. the styloid process of the temporal bone.

pledge (plej) a solemn statement of intention. **Nightingale p.,** a statement of principles for the nursing profession, formulated by a committee in 1893 and subscribed to by student nurses at the time of the capping ceremonies.

pledget (plej′et) a small compress or tuft, as of gauze or cotton.

plegaphonia (pleg″ah-fo′ne-ah) [Gr. *plēgē* stroke + *aphonia*] auscultation of the chest during percussion when the larynx or trachea in cases in which the patient cannot or is not allowed to speak. The vibrations produced by the percussion take the place of those of the vocal cords.

-plegia [Gr. *plēgē* a blow, stroke] a word termination meaning paralysis, or a stroke.

pleiades (pli′ah-dēz) [in Greek mythology, seven daughters of Atlas who were placed by Zeus among the stars and form part of the constellation Taurus] a mass of enlarged lymph nodes.

pleio- see *pleo-*.

pleiochloruria (pli″o-klo-roo′re-ah) an excess of chlorides in the urine.

pleiochromia (pli″o-kro′me-ah) [*pleio-* + *chrom-* + *-ia*] (*obs.*) increased coloration, especially increased secretion of bile pigments.

pleiotropia (pli″o-tro′pe-ah) pleiotropy.

pleiotropic (pli″o-trop′ik) pertaining to or characterized by pleiotropy; producing many effects in the phenotype.

pleiotropism (pli-ot′ro-pizm) pleiotropy.

pleiotropy (pli-ot′ro-pe) [*pleio-* + Gr. *tropē* a turning] the quality of a gene to manifest itself in more than one way, i.e., to produce more than one phenotypic expression.

Pleistophora (plīs-tof′o-rah) [Gr. *pleistos* most, very many] a genus of parasitic protozoa (suborder Pansporoblastina, order Microsporida) found in the muscles of tropical freshwater fish.

plektron (plek′tron) [Gr.] plectron.

pleo-, pleio- [Gr. *pleōn* more] a combining form meaning more, excessive, or multiple.

pleocaryocyte (ple″o-kar′e-o-sīt) pleokaryocyte.

pleochroic (ple″o-kro′ik) pleochromatic.

pleochroism (ple-ok′ro-izm) the condition of being pleochromatic.

pleochromatic (ple″o-kro-mat′ik) exhibiting pleochromatism.

pleochromatism (ple″o-kro′mah-tizm) [*pleo-* + Gr. *chrōma* color] the property possessed by some crystals of transmitting one color in one position and the complementary color in a position at right angles to the first.

pleocytosis (ple″o-si-to′sis) presence of a greater than normal number of cells in the cerebrospinal fluid.

pleokaryocyte (ple″o-kar′e-o-sīt) a large nucleated cell found in cachectic disease such as cancer and tuberculosis.

pleomastia (ple″o-mas′te-ah) [*pleo-* + Gr. *mastos* breast + *-ia*] polymastia.

pleomastic (ple″o-mas′tik) polymastic.

pleomazia (ple″o-ma′ze-ah) [*pleo-* + Gr. *mazos* breast + *-ia*] polymastia.

pleomorphic (ple″o-mor′fik) [*pleo-* + Gr. *morphē* form] occurring in various distinct forms; exhibiting pleomorphism.

pleomorphism (ple″o-mor′fizm) the assumption of various distinct forms by a single organism or species; also the property of crystallizing in two or more forms.

pleomorphous (ple″o-mor′fus) pleomorphic.

pleonasm (ple′o-nazm) [Gr. *pleonasmos* exaggeration] an excess in the number of parts.

pleonectic (ple″o-nek′tik) [Gr. *pleonexia* greediness] (*obs.*) taking up more than the average amount of oxygen; said of blood which has a higher than normal O_2 content at a given Po_2. Cf. *mesectic* and *mionectic*.

pleonexia (ple″o-nek′se-ah) [Gr. "greediness"] 1. the condition of being pleonectic. 2. greediness; excessive desire for acquisition of wealth or objects.

pleonosteosis (ple″o-nos″te-o′sis) [*pleo-* + Gr. *osteon* bone + *-osis*] abnormally increased ossification; premature and excessive ossification. **Léri's p.,** a hereditary syndrome resulting from premature ossification of epiphyses of the long bones, with broadening and deformity of the digits, flexion contractures of the fingers, broadening and stiffness of the toes and joints, shortening of stature, limitation of movement, and mongolian facies. Inherited as an autosomal dominant trait, the deformities become apparent during the first few years of life.

pleonotia (ple″o-no′she-ah) [*pleo-* + Gr. *ous* ear] a developmental anomaly characterized by the presence of a supernumerary ear located on the neck.

pleoptics (ple-op′tiks) [*pleo-* + Gr. *optikos* of or for sight] a technique of eye exercises designed to develop fuller vision of an amblyopic eye and assure proper binocular cooperation.

plerocercoid (ple″ro-ser′koid) [Gr. *plēroun* to complete + *kerkos* tail + *eidos* form] the wormlike completed larval stage of certain cestode tapeworms, found in the tissues of vertebrates and invertebrates.

plerosis (ple-ro′sis) the restoration of lost tissue, as after illness.

Plesch's percussion, test (plesh′ez) [Johann *Plesch*, German physician in England, born 1878] see under *percussion* and *tests*.

Plesiomonas (ple″se-o-mo′nas) [Gr. *plēsios* near + *monas* unit, from *monos* single] a genus of gram-negative, facultatively anaerobic bacteria of the family Vibrionaceae, consisting of rod-shaped organisms with polar flagella. They are found in the mammalian intestinal tract and in aquatic animals, and may cause diarrhea in humans. **P. shigelloi′des,** the type species of Plesiomonas, isolated from numerous animal sources and from the human intestinal tract, a cause of infectious diarrhea in humans, especially in tropical and subtropical areas.

plesiomorphism (ple″se-o-mor′fizm) [Gr. *plesios* near + *morphē* form] similarity in form.

plesiomorphous (ple″se-o-mor′fus) pertaining to or characterized by plesiomorphism.

plessesthesia (ples″es-the′ze-ah) [Gr. *plēssein* to strike + *aisthēsis* perception] palpatory percussion; percussion with one hand against a palpating finger of the other hand.

plessigraph (ples′ĭ-graf) [Gr. *plēssein* to strike + *graphein* to write] a form of pleximeter designed to enable the user to mark out the limits of an area.

plessimeter (ples-sim′ĕ-ter) pleximeter.

plessimetric (ples″ĭ-met′rik) pleximetric.

plessor (ples′or) plexor.

plethora (pleth′o-rah) [L.; Gr. *plēthōrē* fullness, satiety] a general term denoting a red florid complexion, or specifically, an excessive amount of blood. **p. hydrae′mica,** increase in amount of blood due to increase in the watery element alone.

plethoric (ple-thor′ik) pertaining to or characterized by plethora.

plethysmogram (ple-thiz′mo-gram) a tracing made by the plethysmograph.

plethysmograph (ple-thiz′mo-graf) [Gr. *plēthysmos* increase + *graphein* to write] an instrument for determining and registering variations in the volume of an organ, part, or limb and in the amount of blood present or passing through it; also used for recording variations in the size of parts and in the blood supply. **body p.,** a device for measuring change in body volume, used especially in measuring pulmonary ventilation. **digital p.,** finger p. **finger p.,** one that registers the change in volume taking place in a single finger. **Franck's p.,** one consisting of an upright glass jar into which the hand and wrist are inserted. **jerkin p.,** a double-layered garment resembling a jerkin, filled with air at slightly positive pressure, used to monitor changes in pressure produced by movements of the chest wall in respiration. **Mosso's p.,** one consisting of a glass tube filled with warm water into which the hand and forearm are placed. The changes in the water level, caused by the changes in volume of the limb, are graphically recorded.

plethysmography (pleth″iz-mog′rah-fe) the recording of the changes in the size of a part as modified by the circulation of the blood in it.

pleura (ploor′ah), gen. and pl. *pleur′ae* [Gr. "rib," "side"] [NA] the serous membrane investing the lungs and lining the thoracic cavity, completely enclosing a potential space known as the pleural cavity. There are two pleurae, right and left, entirely distinct from each other. The pleura is moistened with a serous secretion which facilitates the movements of the lungs in the chest. **cervical p.,** cupula pleurae. **costal p., p. costa′lis** [NA], the part of the parietal pleura

Visceral pleura
Parietal pleura
Right lung
Left lung
Visceral pleura
Pericardium (with two layers)
Heart
Parietal pleura

Pleura; for purposes of illustration, the pleural cavity is shown as an actual space.

lining the rib cage. **diaphragmatic p., p. diaphragmat′ica** [NA], the part of the parietal pleura covering the diaphragm. **mediastinal p., p. mediastina′lis** [NA], a continuation of each pleura, medially, over the lateral face of the mediastinum and the structures within it. **parietal p., p. parieta′lis** [NA], the portion of the pleura lining the walls of the thoracic cavity. **pericardiac p., p. pericardi′aca,** the portion of the mediastinal pleura

covering the pericardium and firmly attached to it. **p. pulmona′lis,** NA alternative for *p. visceralis.* **pulmonary p.,** p. visceralis. **visceral p., p. viscera′lis** [NA], the portion of the pleura investing the lungs and lining their fissures, completely separating the different lobes; called also *p. pulmonalis* [NA alternative] and pulmonary p.

pleuracentesis (ploor″ah-sen-te′sis) thoracentesis.

pleuracotomy (ploor″ah-kot′o-me) [pleura + Gr. *tomē* a cutting] incision into the pleural cavity.

pleurae (ploor′e) [L.] genitive and plural of *pleura.*

pleural (ploor′al) pertaining to the pleura.

pleuralgia (ploor-al′je-ah) [pleur- + -algia] pain in the pleura, or in the side.

pleuralgic (ploor-al′jik) pertaining to or affected with pleuralgia.

pleuramnion (ploor-am′ne-on) an amnion that develops by a process of folding of the somatopleure, a characteristic of many mammals but not man.

pleurapophysis (ploor″ah-pof′ĭ-sis) [pleur- + *apophysis*] a rib, or its homologue; a rib considered as part of a vertebra.

pleurectomy (ploor-ek′to-me) [pleur- + Gr. *ektomē* excision] excision of a portion of the pleura.

pleurisy (ploor′ĭ-se) [Gr. *pleuritis*] inflammation of the pleura, with exudation into its cavity and upon its surface. It may occur as either an acute or a chronic process. In acute pleurisy the pleura becomes reddened, then covered with an exudate of lymph, fibrin, and cellular elements (the *dry* stage); the disease may progress to the second stage, in which a copious exudation of serum occurs (stage of *liquid effusion*). The inflamed surfaces of the pleura tend to become united by adhesions, which are usually permanent. The symptoms are a stitch in the side, a chill, followed by fever and a dry cough. As effusion occurs there is an onset of dyspnea and a diminution of pain. The patient lies on the affected side. **acute p.,** a form marked by sharp, stabbing pain, fever, friction fremitus, and to-and-fro friction sounds, or by rapid development of pleural effusion. **adhesive p.,** that in which exudate forms dense adhesions between the visceral and parietal pleurae, which partially or totally obliterate the pleural space. **blocked p.,** pleurisy in which the exudate is imprisoned in a pocket so that it cannot be aspirated; loculated pleural effusion. **cholesterol p.,** accumulation of cholesterol-containing fluid in the pleural cavity. **chronic p.,** a dry serofibrinous or purulent form, which is long continued. **chyliform p., chyloid p.,** a form in which the effused fluid has a milky appearance. **chylous p.,** pleurisy in which the effusion consists of a turbid milky fluid, with sometimes a high percentage of fat; chylothorax. **circumscribed p.,** pleurisy in which the inflammation is limited to a portion of the pleura. **costal p.,** inflammation of the parietal pleura. **diaphragmatic p.,** parietal inflammation limited to parts near the diaphragm. **diffuse p.,** pleurisy in which the inflammation involves the entire surface of the pleura. **double p.,** inflammation involving the pleurae of both lungs. **dry p.,** a variety with comparatively dry fibrinous exudate, usually chronic. **encysted p.,** a form with adhesions which circumscribe the effused material; loculated pleural effusion. **exudative p.,** pleurisy with effusion. **fibrinous p.,** pleurisy characterized by deposition of large amounts of fibrin in the pleural space. **hemorrhagic p.,** a variety in which there is a bloody exudate. **ichorous p.,** empyema with a thin, offensive pus. **indurative p.,** pleurisy marked by thickening and hardening of the pleura. **interlobular p.,** a variety enclosed between the lobes of the lung. **latent p.,** a form attended with but little pain or inconvenience. **mediastinal p.,** a variety that affects the pleural folds about the mediastinum. **metapneumonic p.,** pleurisy following pneumonia; pneumococcal empyema. **plastic p.,** a form characterized by the deposition of a soft, semisolid exudate in a layer; fibrothorax. **primary p.,** a form not consequent upon pneumonia or any other observed disease. **proliferating p.,** plastic p. **pulmonary p.,** inflammation of the pleura which covers the lungs. **pulsating p.,** a form in which the heart's action conveys a perceptible throbbing to the effused fluid. **purulent p.,** thoracic empyema. **sacculated p.,** pleurisy characterized by an adhesion pocket filled with fluid. **secondary p.,** any pleurisy consequent upon an attack of some other disease. **serofibrinous p.,** one with a watery exudate and deposition of fibrin. **serous p.,** a form characterized by free exudation of fluid. **single p.,** pleurisy involving only one pleural space. **suppurative p.,** thoracic empyema. **typhoid p.,** pleurisy with symptoms of severe prostration. **visceral p.,** pleurisy involving the visceral pleural layer. **wet p., p. with effusion,** pleurisy marked by serous exudation.

pleuritic (ploo-rit'ik) pertaining to or of the nature of pleurisy.

pleuritis (ploo-ri'tis) pleurisy.

pleuritogenous (ploor"ĭ-toj'ĕ-nus) causing pleurisy.

pleur(o)- [Gr. *pleura* rib, side] combining form denoting relationship to the pleura, to the side, or to a rib.

pleurobronchitis (ploor"o-brong-ki'tis) pleurisy and bronchitis combined.

pleurocele (ploor'o-sēl) [*pleuro-* + Gr. *kēlē* hernia] hernia of lung tissue or of pleura.

pleurocentesis (ploor"o-sen-te'sis) [*pleuro-* + *kentēsis* puncture] thoracentesis.

pleurocentrum (ploor"o-sen'trum) [*pleuro-* + Gr. *kentron* center] the lateral element of the vertebral column.

Pleuroceridae (ploor"o-ser'ĭ-de) a family of snails (order Mesogastropoda) that includes the medically important genera *Hua, Semisulcospira,* and *Goniobasis.*

pleurocholecystitis (ploor"o-ko"le-sis-ti'tis) [*pleuro-* + *cholecystitis*] inflammation of the pleura and the gallbladder.

pleurocutaneous (ploor"o-ku-ta'ne-us) pertaining to the pleura and the skin.

pleurodesis (ploo-rod'ĕ-sis) [*pleuro-* + Gr. *desis* binding] the production of adhesions between the parietal and the visceral pleura.

pleurodont (ploor'o-dont) [*pleur-* + Gr. *odous* tooth] having teeth attached by one side on the inner surface of the jaw elements, as in certain lizards.

pleurodynia (ploor"o-din'e-ah) [*pleuro-* + Gr. *odynē* pain] paroxysmal pain in the intercostal muscles due to muscular rheumatism (fibrositis) or irritation of pleural surfaces. **epidemic p.,** an acute, febrile, infectious disease generally occurring in epidemics, most often seen in persons under the age of 20, and usually caused by group B coxsackieviruses and sometimes by group A coxsackieviruses, echoviruses, and other enteroviruses. It is typically characterized by sudden sharp paroxysmal pain located over the rib area of the chest or upper abdomen; relapses occur frequently after asymptomatic periods. Called also *Bornholm, Daae's,* or *Sylvest's disease, devil's grip,* and *epidemic myalgia.*

pleurogenic (ploor"o-jen'ik) pleurogenous.

pleurogenous (ploor-oj'ĕ-nus) [*pleuro-* + Gr. *gennan* to produce] originating in the pleura.

pleurography (ploo-rog'rah-fe) [*pleuro-* + Gr. *graphein* to write] roentgenographic examination of the pleural cavity.

pleurohepatitis (ploor"o-hep"ah-ti'tis) [*pleuro-* + Gr. *hēpar* liver + *-itis*] hepatitis with inflammation of a portion of the pleura near the liver.

pleurolith (ploor'o-lith) [*pleuro-* + Gr. *lithos* stone] a concretion found in the pleura; calcified pleural plaque.

pleurolysis (ploo-rol'ĭ-sis) [*pleuro-* + Gr. *lysis* dissolution] surgical separation of the pleura from its attachments.

pleuromelus (ploor"o-me'lus) [*pleuro-* + Gr. *melos* limb] an individual with a supernumerary limb arising laterally from the thorax.

Pleuronematina (ploor"ro-ne"mah-ti'nah) [*pleuro-* + Gr. *nēma* thread] a suborder of small or very small ciliate protozoa (order Scuticociliatida, subclass Hypostomatia), typically characterized by a paroral membrane that is often prominent, sometimes as a stiff velum, and with the posterior segment serving as a permanent scutica; often conspicuous caudal ciliature; prominent mucocysts; and a cytoproct. They are mostly free-living but some are commensals.

pleuroparietopexy (ploor"o-pah-ri'ĕ-to-pek"se) [*pleuro-* + *parietal* + Gr. *pēxis* fixation] the operation of fixing the visceral pleura to the parietal pleura, thus binding the lung to the chest wall.

pleuropericardial (ploor"o-per-ĭ-kar'de-al) pertaining to both the pleura and the pericardium.

pleuropericarditis (ploor"o-per"ĭ-kar-di'tis) inflammation involving both the pleura and the pericardium.

pleuroperitoneal (ploor"o-per"ĭ-to-ne'al) pertaining to both the pleura and the peritoneum, or communicating with both the pleural and the peritoneal cavity, as a pleuroperitoneal fistula.

pleuropneumonia (ploor"o-nu-mo'ne-ah) 1. pleurisy complicated with pneumonia. 2. a contagious or infectious pneumonia of cattle, combined with pleurisy, caused by *Mycoplasma mycoides;* called also *pleuropneumonia contagiosa bovum* and *lung plague.*

pleuropneumonia-like (ploor"o-nu-mo'nyah-līk) see under *organism.*

pleuropneumonolysis (ploor"o-nu"mo-nol'ĭ-sis) [*pleuro-* + Gr. *pneumōn* lung + *lysis* destruction] division of adhesions between the lung and the parietal pleura.

pleuropulmonary (ploor"o-pul'mo-ner"e) pertaining to the pleura and lungs.

pleurorrhea (ploor"o-re'ah) [*pleuro-* + Gr. *rhoia* flow] a pleural or pleuritic effusion.

pleuroscopy (ploor-os'ko-pe) [*pleuro-* + Gr. *skopein* to examine] examination of the pleural cavity through an endoscope by way of a small incision in the chest wall.

pleurosoma (ploor"o-so'mah) pleurosomus.

pleurosomus (ploor"o-so'mus) [*pleuro-* + Gr. *sōma* body] a fetus with protrusion of the intestine and imperfect development of the arm of one side.

Pleurostomatida (ploo"ro-sto-mat'ĭ-dah) [*pleuro-* + Gr. *stoma* mouth] an order of carnivorous ciliate protozoa (subclass Gymnostomatina, class Kinetofragminophorea), characterized by the presence of a slitlike lateral cytosome and a circumoral infraciliature that includes the anterior parts of only a few somatic kineties and differentiates into left and right components; the body is often large and laterally compressed.

pleurothotonos (ploor"o-thot'o-nos) [Gr. *pleurothen* from the side + *tonos* tension] tetanic bending of the body to one side.

pleurothotonus (ploor"o-thot'o-nus) pleurothotonos.

pleurotin (ploor-o'tin) a toxic antibiotic substance, $C_{20}H_{22}O_5$, obtained from the mushroom *Pleurotus griseus;* it shows activity against staphylococcus (of boils) and tubercle bacillus.

pleurotome (ploor'o-tōm) an area of the lung supplied with afferent nerve fibers by a single posterior spinal root.

pleurotomy (ploor-ot'o-me) [*pleuro-* + Gr. *tomē* a cutting] surgical incision of the pleura.

pleurotyphoid (ploor"o-ti'foid) acute pleurisy followed by and complicated with typhoid fever.

pleurovisceral (ploor"o-vis'er-al) pertaining to the pleura and the viscera.

plexal (plek'sal) pertaining to a plexus.

plexectomy (plek-sek'to-me) [*plexus* + Gr. *ektomē* excision] surgical excision of a plexus.

plexiform (plek'sĭ-form) [L. *plexus* plait + *forma* form] resembling a plexus or network.

pleximeter (plek-sim'ĕ-ter) [Gr. *plexis* stroke + *metron* measure] 1. a plate to be struck in mediate percussion. 2. a diascope; a glass plate used to show the condition of the skin under pressure.

pleximetric (plek"sĭ-met'rik) pertaining to or performed by a pleximeter.

pleximetry (plek-sim'ĕ-tre) the use of the pleximeter.

plexitis (plek-si'tis) inflammation of a nerve plexus.

plexogenic (plek'so-jen"ik) giving rise to a plexus or plexiform structure.

plexometer (plek-som'ĕ-ter) pleximeter.

plexopathy (pleks-op'ah-the) any disorder of a plexus, especially of nerves. **lumbar p.,** neuropathy of the lumbar plexus.

plexor (plek'sor) a hammer used in performing percussion.

plexus (plek'sus), pl. *plexus* or *plexuses* [L. "braid"] a network or tangle; [NA] a general term for a network of lymphatic vessels, nerves, or veins. **annular p.,** a plexus of nerve fibers encircling the corneal margin. **anserine p., p. anseri'nus,** p. parotideus nervi facialis. **aortic p., abdominal,** p. aorticus abdominalis. **aortic p., thoracic,** p. aorticus thoracicus. **p. aor'ticus,** a network of lymphatic vessels about the aorta. **p. aor'ticus**

abdomina′lis [NA], abdominal aortic plexus: an unpaired plexus composed of interconnecting bundles of fibers that arise from the celiac and superior mesenteric plexuses and descend along the aorta. Receiving branches from the lumbar splanchnic nerves, it becomes the superior hypogastric plexus below the bifurcation of the aorta. Branches of the plexus are distributed along the adjacent branches of the aorta. **p. aor′ticus thoraca′lis, p. aor′ticus thora′cicus** [NA], thoracic aortic plexus: a plexus around the thoracic aorta formed by filaments from the sympathetic trunks and vagus nerves, and from which fine twigs accompany branches of the aorta. It is continuous below with the celiac plexus and the plexus of the abdominal aorta. **areolar p.,** p. venosus areolaris. **p. arte′riae cer′ebri anterio′ris,** a thin plexus of sympathetic nerve fibers accompanying the anterior cerebral artery. **p. arte′riae cer′ebri me′diae,** a thin plexus of sympathetic nerve fibers accompanying the middle cerebral artery. **p. arte′riae chorioi′deae,** delicate nerve plexuses accompanying the choroid arteries. **p. arte′riae ovar′icae,** p. ovaricus. **Auerbach's p.,** p. myentericus. **p. auricula′ris poste′rior,** a sympathetic nerve plexus on the posterior auricular artery. **autonomic p's, p. autonom′ici** [NA], extensive networks of nerve fibers and cell bodies associated with the autonomic nervous system; found particularly in the thorax, abdomen, and pelvis, and containing sympathetic, parasympathetic, and visceral afferent fibers. Called also *p. sympathici, visceral p's,* and *p. viscerales* [NA alternative]. **basilar p., p. basila′ris** [NA], a venous plexus of the dura mater situated over the basilar part of the occipital bone and the posterior portion of the body of the sphenoid, extending from the cavernous sinus to the foramen magnum, and communicating with other dural sinuses. **biliary p.,** a network of bile ducts said to be sometimes observable in the liver. **brachial p., p. brachia′lis** [NA], a plexus originating from the ventral branches of the last four cervical spinal nerves and most of the ventral branch of the first thoracic spinal nerves. Situated partly in the neck and partly in the axilla, it is composed successively of ventral branches and trunks (supraclavicular part) which are related to the subclavian artery and which give off the dorsal scapular, long thoracic, subclavius, and suprascapular nerves. The infraclavicular part consists of divisions which lie approximately behind the clavicle and cords and branches in the axilla in relation to the axillary artery. Its branches are medial and lateral pectoral, medial brachial cutaneous, medial antebrachial cutaneous, median, ulnar radial, subscapular, thoracodorsal, and axillary nerves. **cardiac p.,** p. cardiacus. **cardiac p., anterior,** superficial cardiac p. **cardiac p., deep,** the larger part of the cardiac plexus, situated between the aortic arch and the tracheal bifurcation. **cardiac p., great,** deep cardiac p. **cardiac p., superficial,** the part of the cardiac plexus that lies beneath the aortic arch to the right of the ligamentum arteriosum. **p. cardi′acus** [NA], cardiac plexus: the plexus around the base of the heart, chiefly in the epicardium. It is formed by cardiac branches from the vagus nerves and the sympathetic trunks and ganglia, contains visceral afferent fibers, and shows subdivisions related to the arch of the aorta, right and left atria, and right and left coronary arteries. The cardiac plexus is continuous with the right and left pulmonary plexuses. **p. cardi′acus profun′dus,** the deep cardiac plexus. **p. cardi′acus superficia′lis,** the superficial cardiac plexus. **p. carot′icus commu′nis** [NA], common carotid plexus: a nerve plexus on the common carotid artery, formed by branches of the internal and external carotid plexuses and the cervical sympathetic ganglia. **p. carot′icus exter′nus** [NA], external carotid plexus: a nerve plexus located around the external carotid artery, formed by the external carotid nerves from the superior cervical ganglion, and supplying sympathetic fibers which accompany the branches of the external carotid artery. **p. carot′icus inter′nus** [NA], internal carotid plexus: a nerve plexus on the internal carotid artery, formed by the internal carotid nerve, which supplies sympathetic fibers to the branches of the internal carotid artery, to the tympanic plexus, to the nerves in the cavernous sinus and, directly or indirectly, to the cranial parasympathetic ganglia through which they pass. Called also *carotid p.* **carotid p.,** caroticus internus. **carotid p., common,** p. caroticus communis. **carotid p., external,** p. caroticus externus. **carotid p., internal,** p. caroticus internus. **p. caverno′sus,** cavernous plexus: a plexus of sympathetic nerve

fibers related to the cavernous sinus of the dura mater. **p. caverno′sus clitor′idis,** cavernous plexus of clitoris: a plexus of nerve fibers at the root of the clitoris, derived from the vesical plexus and supplying the corpora cavernosa clitoridis. **p. caverno′si concha′rum** [NA], cavernous plexuses of conchae: numerous venous plexuses in the thick mucous membrane of the nasal conchae. **p. caverno′sus pe′nis,** cavernous plexus of penis: a plexus of nerve fibers at the root of the penis, derived from the vesical plexus and supplying the corpora cavernosa penis. **cavernous p.,** p. cavernosus. **cavernous p. of clitoris,** p. cavernosus clitoridis. **cavernous p's of conchae,** p. cavernosi concharum. **cavernous p. of penis,** p. cavernosus penis. **celiac p., p. celia′cus,** p. coeliacus. **cervical p.,** p. cervicalis. **cervical p., posterior,** a plexus in the posterior cervical region, formed by dorsal rami of the first three or four cervical spinal nerves. **p. cervica′lis** [NA], cervical plexus: a nerve plexus formed by the ventral branches of the upper four cervical nerves; arranged as an irregular series of loops, it gives off superficial branches (lesser occipital, greater auricular, transverse cervical, and supraclavicular nerves), and deep branches (phrenic, accessory phrenic, ansa cervicalis, and muscular nerves). **p. cervicobrachia′lis,** the cervical and brachial plexuses together. **choroid p.,** infoldings of blood vessels of the pia mater covered by a thin coat of ependymal cells that form tufted projections into the third, fourth, and lateral ventricles of the brain; they secrete the cerebrospinal fluid. See *p. choroideus ventriculi lateralis, p. choroideus ventriculi quarti,* and *p. choroideus ventriculi tertii.* **choroid p., inferior, choroid p. of fourth ventricle,** p. choroideus ventriculi quarti. **choroid p. of lateral ventricle,** p. choroideus ventriculi lateralis. **choroid p. of third ventricle,** p. choroideus ventriculi tertii. **p. choroi′deus ventric′uli latera′lis** [NA], choroid plexus of lateral ventricle: vascular, fringelike folds of the pia mater in the floor of the pars centralis and the roof of the temporal horn of the lateral ventricle, concerned with production of the cerebrospinal fluid. **p. choroi′deus ventric′uli quar′ti** [NA], choroid plexus of fourth ventricle: vascular fringelike folds of the pia mater in the roof of the posterior part of the fourth ventricle and extending into and through the lateral recesses, concerned with production of the cerebrospinal fluid. **p. choroi′deus ventric′uli ter′tii** [NA], choroid plexus of third ventricle: vascular, fringelike folds of the pia mater in the roof of the third ventricle, concerned with production of the cerebrospinal fluid. **ciliary ganglionic p.,** an autonomic plexus derived from the long and short ciliary nerves, lying on the ciliary muscle, and supplying the dilator and sphincter muscles of the pupil. **coccygeal p., p. coccyg′eus** [NA], a small plexus formed by the ventral branches of the coccygeal and the fifth sacral nerve, and a communication from the fourth sacral nerve, and giving off the anococcygeal nerves. **p. coelia′cus, 1.** [NA] that portion of the prevertebral plexus that lies on the front and sides of the aorta at the origins of the celiac trunk and superior mesenteric and renal arteries. It contains the paired celiac ganglia, the superior mesenteric ganglion (or ganglia), and small unnamed ganglionic masses. Branches of the plexus extend along all of the adjacent arteries; called also *solar p.* **2.** a plexus composed of lymphatic vessel, the superior mesenteric lymph nodes, and the celiac lymph nodes behind the stomach, duodenum, and pancreas. Called also *celiac p.* and *p. celiacus.* **colic p., left,** the part of the inferior mesenteric plexus that accompanies the left colic artery. **colic p., middle,** the part of the superior mesenteric plexus that accompanies the middle colic artery. **colic p., right,** the part of the superior mesenteric plexus that accompanies the right colic artery. **p. corona′rius cor′dis ante′rior,** anterior coronary plexus of heart: a plexus of sympathetic nerve fibers anterior to the heart and related chiefly to the branches of the left coronary artery. **p. corona′rius cor′dis poste′rior,** posterior coronary plexus of heart: a plexus of sympathetic nerve fibers posterior to the heart and related chiefly to the branches of the right coronary artery. **coronary p's, gastric,** p. gastrici. **coronary p. of heart, anterior,** p. coronarius cordis anterior. **coronary p. of heart, posterior,** p. coronarius cordis posterior. **coronary p's of stomach, superior,** p. gastrici. **crural p.,** p. femoralis. **Cruveilhier's p., 1.** posterior cervical plexus. **2.** a form of angioma made up of a knot of varicose veins. **cystic p.,** a nerve plexus near the gallbladder, related to the cystic artery. **deferential p., p. deferentia'lis** [NA], the subdivision of the inferior hypogastric plexus that supplies nerve fibers to the ductus deferens. **dental p., inferior,** p. dentalis inferior. **dental p., superior,** p. dentalis superior. **p. denta'lis infe'rior** [NA], inferior dental plexus: a plexus of nerve fibers from the inferior alveolar nerve, situated around the roots of the lower teeth. **p. denta'lis supe'rior** [NA], superior dental plexus: a plexus of fibers from the superior alveolar nerves, situated around the roots of the upper teeth. **diaphragmatic p.,** p. phrenicus. **enteric p., p. enter'icus** [NA], a plexus of autonomic nerve fibers within the wall of the digestive tube, and made up of the submucosal, myenteric, and subserosal plexuses; it contains visceral afferent fibers, sympathetic postganglionic fibers, parasympathetic preganglionic and postganglionic fibers, and parasympathetic postganglionic cell bodies. **epigastric p.,** p. celiacus. **esophageal p., p. esopha'geus,** NA alternative for *p. oesophageus.* **Exner's p.,** superficial tangential fibers in the molecular layer of the cerebral cortex; called also *molecular p.* **facial p., p. of facial artery,** a nerve plexus along the facial artery. **femoral p., p. femora'lis** [NA], a plexus accompanying the femoral artery, derived chiefly from the aortic plexus by way of the common and external iliac plexuses. **gastric p's, p. gas'trici** [NA], subdivisions of the celiac portion of the prevertebral plexuses, accompanying the gastric arteries and branches and supplying nerve fibers to the stomach. **p. gas'tricus ante'rior,** see *rami gastrici anteriores nervi vagi.* **p. gas'tricus infe'rior,** a plexus of nerve fibers on the greater curvature of the stomach. **p. gas'tricus poste'rior,** see *rami gastrici posteriores nervi vagi.* **p. gas'tricus supe'rior,** a plexus of nerve fibers on the lesser curvature of the stomach. **gastroepiploic p., left,** a nerve plexus near the greater curvature of the stomach. **p. haemorrhoida'lis,** p. venosus rectalis. **p. haemorrhoida'lis me'dius,** see *p. rectales medii.* **p. haemorrhoida'lis supe'rior,** p. rectalis superior. **Heller's p.,** an arterial network in the submucosa of the intestine. **hemorrhoidal p.,** p. venosus rectalis. **hemorrhoidal p., middle,** see *p. rectales medii.* **hemorrhoidal p., superior,** p. rectalis superior. **hepatic p., p. hepat'icus** [NA], a subdivision of the celiac plexus accompanying the hepatic artery to the liver. **Hovius' p.,** a venous plexus in the ciliary region connected with the sinus venosus sclerae. **hypogastric p.,** the hypogastric portion of the prevertebral plexuses; see *p. hypogastricus inferior* and *p. hypogastricus superior.* **hypogastric p., inferior,** p. hypogastricus inferior. **hypogastric p., superior,** p. hypogastricus superior. **p. hypogas'tricus,** 1. see *p. hypogastricus inferior* and *p. hypogastricus superior.* 2. a plexus of lymphatic vessels in the hypogastric region. **p. hypogas'tricus infe'rior** [NA], inferior hypogastric plexus: the plexus formed on each side at the front of the lower part of the sacrum by the junction of the hypogastric and pelvic splanchnic nerves; branches are given off to the pelvic organs. Called also *pelvic p.* and *p. pelvicus* or *p. pelvina* [NA alternative]. **p. hypogas'tricus supe'rior** [NA], superior hypogastric plexus: the downward continuation of the aortic plexus; it lies in front of the upper part of the sacrum, just below the bifurcation of the aorta, receives fibers from the lower lumbar splanchnic nerves, and divides into the right and left hypogastric nerves. Called also *nervus presacralis* [NA alternative] or *presacral nerve.* **ileocolic p.,** the part of the superior mesenteric plexus that accompanies the ileocolic artery. **iliac p's, p. ili'aci** [NA], plexuses derived chiefly from the aortic plexus and accompanying the common iliac arteries. **p. ili'acus exter'nus,** a lymphatic plexus situated about the external iliac vessels. **infraorbital p.,** a nerve plexus situated deep to the levator labii superioris muscle, formed by superior labial branches of the infraorbital nerve and branches of the facial nerve. **inguinal p., p. inguina'lis,** a lymphatic plexus situated near the end of the long saphenous vein and along the femoral artery and vein in the iliopectineal fossa. **intercavernous p.,** a network of venous channels connecting the two cavernous sinuses across both the roof and the floor of the pituitary fossa. **intermesenteric p.,** p. intermesentericus. **intermesenteric p., lumboaortic,** p. aorticus abdominalis. **p. intermesenter'icus** [NA], intermesenteric plexus: the part of the aortic plexus that is located between the origins of the superior and inferior mesenteric arteries. **internal carotid venous p.,** p. venosus ca-

roticus internus. **interradial p.,** Baillarger's lines. **intestinal p., submucous,** p. submucosus. **intramural p.,** a plexus of autonomic intrinsic nerve cells and fibers which are confined entirely to the intestinal and bladder walls, and which take part in or regulate local reflexes and activity. **intrascleral p.,** a network of vessels in the sclera, receiving junctional branches from the sinus venosus sclerae. **ischiadic p.,** p. sacralis. **Jacobson's p.,** p. tympanicus. **jugular p., p. jugula'ris,** a plexus of lymphatic vessels along the internal jugular vein. **laryngeal p.,** a nerve plexus on the outer surface of the inferior constrictor of the pharynx; it is an offshoot of the pharyngeal plexus and is made up of fibers from the sympathetic and external laryngeal nerves. **lateral p.,** p. choroideus ventriculi lateralis. **Leber's p.,** Hovius' p. **lienal p., p. liena'lis,** NA alternative for *p. splenicus.* **lingual p., p. lingua'lis,** a nerve plexus accompanying the lingual artery. **p. lumba'lis,** 1. [NA] lumbar plexus: a plexus formed by the ventral branches of the second to fifth lumbar nerves in the psoas major muscle (the branches of the first lumbar nerve often are included). The lower division of the fourth lumbar nerve joins the fifth, and the lumbosacral trunk thus formed becomes part of the sacral plexus. The branches of the first lumbar nerve are the ilioinguinal and iliohypogastric nerves; branches of the plexus proper are the genitofemoral, lateral femoral cutaneous, obturator, and femoral nerves. Called also *p. lumbaris* [NA alternative]. 2. a lymphatic plexus in the lumbar region. **lumbar p.,** p. lumbalis. **p. lumba'ris,** NA alternative for *p. lumbalis,* def. 1. **lumbosacral p., p. lumbosacra'lis** [NA], a term applied to the lumbar and sacral nerve plexuses together, because of their continuous nature. **lymphatic p., p. lymphat'icus** [NA], an interconnecting network of lymph vessels, i.e., the lymphocapillary vessels, collecting vessels, and trunks, which provides drainage of lymph in a one-way flow. **p. lymphat'icus axilla'ris** [NA], **axillary lymphatic p.,** a plexus of lymph vessels and nodes in the fossa axillaris. **p. mamma'rius,** a plexus of lymph vessels along the internal mammary artery. **p. mamma'rius inter'nus,** a plexus accompanying the internal thoracic artery and its branches. **p. maxilla'ris exter'nus,** p. of facial artery. **p. maxilla'ris inter'nus,** a nerve plexus accompanying the internal maxillary artery. **maxillary p.,** see *p. maxillaris externus* and *p. maxillaris internus.* **Meissner's p.,** p. submucosus. **p. menin'geus,** a nerve plexus accompanying the middle meningeal artery. **mesenteric p., inferior,** p. mesentericus inferior. **mesenteric p., superior,** p. mesentericus superior. **p. mesenter'icus infe'rior** [NA], inferior mesenteric plexus: a subdivision of the aortic plexus accompanying the inferior mesenteric artery. **p. mesenter'icus supe'rior** [NA], superior mesenteric plexus: a subdivision of the celiac plexus accompanying the superior mesenteric artery. **molecular p.,** Exner's p. **myenteric p., p. myenter'icus** [NA], that part of the enteric plexus within the tunica muscularis. **nasopalatine p.,** a nerve plexus near the incisor foramen. **nerve p.,** a plexus made up of intermingled nerve fibers. **p. nervo'rum spina'lium** [NA], plexus of spinal nerves: a plexus formed by the intermingling of the fibers of two or more spinal nerves, such as the brachial or lumbosacral plexus. **nervous p.,** a plexus made up of intermingled nerve fibers. **occipital p., p. occipita'lis,** a nerve plexus accompanying the occipital artery. **p. oesopha'geus** [NA], esophageal plexus: a plexus surrounding the esophagus formed by branches of the left and right vagi and sympathetic trunks and containing also visceral afferent fibers from the esophagus; it is subdivided into anterior and posterior parts; called also *p. esophageus* [NA alternative]. **ophthalmic p., p. ophthal'micus,** a nerve plexus accompanying the ophthalmic artery. **ovarian p., p. ova'ricus,** a subdivision of the aortic plexus, accompanying the ovarian arteries; called also *p. arteriae ovaricae.* **pampiniform p., p. pampinifor'mis** [NA], 1. in the male, a plexus of veins from the testicle and the epididymis, constituting part of the spermatic cord. 2. in the female, a plexus of ovarian veins in the broad ligament. **pancreatic p., p. pancreat'icus** [NA], subdivision of the celiac plexus, accompanying pancreatic arteries. **Panizza's p's,** two plexuses of the lymph vessels in the lateral fossae of the frenum of the prepuce. **parotid p. of facial nerve, p. paroti'deus ner'vi facia'lis** [NA], a plexus formed by anastomosis of the terminal branches of the temporal, zygomatic, buccal, marginal mandibular, and cervical rami of the facial nerve, arising in the parotid gland. **patellar p.,** a plexus of nerve fibers in front of the knee, formed by communications between branches of the saphenous nerves and the femoral cutaneous nerves. **pelvic p.,** p. hypogastricus inferior. **p. pel'vicus, p. pelvi'na,** NA alternatives for *p. hypogastricus inferior.* **periarterial p., p. periarteria'lis** [NA], a network of autonomic and sensory nerve fibers in the adventitia of an artery, some of which follow the course of the artery to reach and innervate other structures and some of which innervate the artery itself. **pericorneal p.,** anastomosing branches of the anterior conjunctival arteries, arranged in a superficial conjunctival and a deep episcleral layer about the cornea. **pharyngeal p.,** p. pharyngeus. **pharyngeal p. of vagus nerve,** p. pharyngeus nervi vagi. **p. pharyngea'lis** [NA], NA alternative for *p. pharyngeus.* **p. pharyn'geus** [NA], pharyngeal plexus: a venous plexus posterolateral to the pharynx, formed by the pharyngeal veins, communicating with the pterygoid venous plexus, and draining into the internal jugular vein. Called also *p. pharyngealis* [NA alternative]. **p. pharyn'geus ascen'dens,** a nerve plexus accompanying the ascending pharyngeal artery. **p. pharyn'geus ner'vi va'gi** [NA], pharyngeal plexus of vagus nerve: a plexus formed chiefly by fibers from branches of the vagus nerves, but also containing fibers from the glossopharyngeal nerves and sympathetic trunks, and supplying motor, general sensory, and sympathetic innervation to the muscles and mucosa of the pharynx and soft palate, except for the tensor veli palatini muscle. **phrenic p., p. phren'icus,** a nerve plexus accompanying the inferior phrenic artery to the diaphragm and suprarenal glands. **popliteal p., p. poplite'us,** a plexus of nerve fibers accompanying the popliteal artery. **presacral p.,** p. venosus sacralis. **prevertebral p's,** autonomic nerve plexuses situated in the thorax, abdomen, and pelvis, anterior to the vertebral column; they consist of visceral afferent fibers, preganglionic parasympathetic fibers, preganglionic and postganglionic sympathetic fibers, and ganglia containing sympathetic ganglion cells, and they give rise to postganglionic fibers. The major plexuses are cardiac, pulmonary, esophageal, celiac, mesenteric, and hypogastric. All are closely related to the aorta; those in the abdomen and pelvis supply adjacent viscera by subdivisions which accompany the branches of the aorta and which are named usually after these branches, but sometimes according to the organ supplied. **primary p.,** a network of capillaries that arise from the superior hypophysial arteries, extend into the median eminence of the hypothalamus, then return to the surface, where they are collected into veins that supply the sinusoids of the adenohypophysis. **prostatic p.,** 1. plexus prostaticus. 2. plexus venosus prostaticus. **prostaticovesical p.,** the plexus venosus vesicalis in the male. **p. prostat'icus** [NA], prostatic plexus: a subdivision of the inferior hypogastric plexus that supplies nerve fibers to the prostate and adjacent organs. **pterygoid p., p. pterygoi'deus** [NA], a network of veins corresponding to the second and third parts of the maxillary artery; situated on the lateral surface of the medial pterygoid muscle and on both surfaces of the lateral pterygoid muscle, and draining into the facial vein. Called also *p. venosus pterygoideus.* **pudendal p., p. puden da'lis,** p. venosus prostaticus. **p. pulmona'lis** [NA], pulmonary plexus: a nerve plexus formed by several strong trunks of the vagus nerve which are joined at the root of the lung by branches from the sympathetic trunk and cardiac plexus. The plexus is often described as having anterior and posterior parts; filaments from each accompany the blood vessels and bronchi into the lungs. **p. pulmona'lis ante'rior,** anterior pulmonary plexus: the smaller portion of the pulmonary plexus, in front of the root of the lung and interconnected with the posterior plexus; see *p. pulmonalis.* **p. pulmona'lis poste'rior,** posterior pulmonary plexus: the larger portion of the pulmonary plexus behind the root of the lung and interconnected with the anterior plexus; see *p. pulmonalis.* **pulmonary p., p.** pulmonalis. **pulmonary p., anterior,** p. pulmonalis anterior. **pulmonary p., posterior,** p. pulmonalis posterior. **pyloric p.,** a nerve plexus that supplies the region of the pylorus. **p. of Raschkow,** a delicate plexus of nerve fibers beneath the odontoblasts in the dental papilla during the formation of dentin. **rectal p's, inferior,** p. rectales inferiores. **rectal p's, middle,** p. rectales medii. **rectal p., supe-**

rior, p. rectalis superior. **p. recta'les inferio'res** [NA], inferior rectal plexuses: a plexus accompanying the inferior rectal artery, derived chiefly from the inferior rectal nerve. **p. recta'les me'dii** [NA], subdivisions of the inferior hypogastric plexus, in proximity with and supplying nerve fibers to the rectum; called also *p. haemorrhoidalis medius.* **p. recta'lis supe'rior** [NA], superior rectal plexus: a plexus accompanying the superior rectal artery to the rectum, derived from the inferior mesenteric and hypogastric plexuses. Called also *p. haemorrhoidalis superior.* **Remak's p.,** former name for p. submucosus. **renal p., p. rena'lis** [NA], a subdivision of the celiac plexus accompanying the renal artery. **sacral p.,** 1. plexus sacralis. 2. plexus venosus sacralis. **sacral p., anterior,** p. venosus sacralis. **sacral lymphatic p.,** p. sacralis medius. **p. sacra'lis** [NA], sacral plexus: a plexus arising from the ventral branches of the last two lumbar nerves (which form the lumbosacral trunk) and the first four sacral nerves. The plexus, which lies in front of the piriformis, has twelve named branches; five supply pelvic structures (the nerves to the piriformis, to levator ani and coccygeus, and to sphincter ani muscles, the pelvic splanchnic nerves and the pudendal nerve); seven supply the buttock and lower limb (superior and inferior gluteal, posterior femoral cutaneous, perforating cutaneous, and sciatic nerves, and nerves to the quadratus femoris and obturator internus muscles). **p. sacra'lis ante'rior,** p. venosus sacralis. **p. sacra'lis me'dius,** a fine network of lymphatic vessels in the hollow of the sacrum. **Santorini's p.,** 1. plexus prostaticus. 2. plexus venosus prostaticus. **Sappey's subareolar p.,** a lymphatic plexus situated beneath the areola of the nipple. **solar p.,** p. celiacus. **spermatic p.,** 1. plexus testicularis. 2. plexus pampiniformis (def. 1). **p. spermat'icus,** p. testicularis. **sphenoid p.** (*obs.*), the upper portion of the internal carotid plexus. **p. of spinal nerves,** p. nervorum spinalium. **splenic p., p. sple'nicus** [NA], a subdivision of the celiac plexus, which accompanies the splenic artery; called also *lienal p.* and *p. lienalis* [NA alternative]. **Stensen's p.,** the venous network around the parotid duct. **stroma p.,** superficial and deep nerve fibrils within the substantia propria of the cornea. **subclavian p., p. subcla'vius** [NA], a sympathetic nerve plexus on the subclavian artery, arising from the cervicothoracic ganglion, contributing fibers to the phrenic nerve and to the branches of the subclavian artery, and continuing to the axillary artery. **submucosal p., p. submuco'sus** [NA], **submucous p.,** the part of the enteric plexus that is situated in the submucosa. **subsartorial p.,** a nerve plexus deep to the sartorius muscle, formed by communications between branches of the medial femoral cutaneous nerve and the saphenous and obturator nerves. **subserosal p., p. subsero'sus** [NA], the part of the enteric plexus situated deep to the serosal surface of the tunica serosa. **subtrapezius p.,** a term occasionally applied to a small plexus situated deep to the trapezius muscle, formed by communications between branches of the accessory nerve and cervical nerves. **supraradial p.,** Bechterew's layer. **suprarenal p., p. suprarena'lis** [NA], a subdivision of the celiac plexus, in proximity with and supplying nerve fibers to a suprarenal (adrenal) gland. **p. sympath'ici,** p. autonomici. **p. tempora'lis superficia'lis,** a plexus of nerve fibers accompanying the superficial temporal artery. **testicular p., p. testicula'ris** [NA], a subdivision of the aortic plexus accompanying the testicular arteries; called also *p. spermaticus.* **p. thyreoi'deus im'par,** p. thyroideus impar. **p. thyreoi'deus infe'rior,** inferior thyroid plexus: a nerve plexus accompanying the inferior thyroid artery to the larynx, pharynx, and thyroid region. **p. thyreoi'deus supe'rior,** superior thyroid plexus: a nerve plexus accompanying the superior thyroid artery to the larynx, pharynx, and thyroid region. **thyroid p., inferior,** p. thyreoideus inferior. **thyroid p., superior,** p. thyreoideus superior. **thyroid p., unpaired,** p. thyroideus impar. **p. thyroi'deus im'par** [NA], unpaired thyroid plexus: a venous plexus investing the surface of the thyroid gland. **tonsillar p.,** a plexus around the tonsil, formed by communications between the middle and posterior palatine nerves and the tonsillar branches of the glossopharyngeal nerve; fibers are supplied to the tonsil, soft palate, and region of the fauces. **Trolard's p.,** p. venosus canalis hypoglossi. **tympanic p., p. tympan'icus** [NA], **p. tympan'icus** [Jacobso'ni], a nerve plexus on the promontory of the middle ear, formed by the tympanic and caroticotympanic nerves. It gives off the lesser petrosal nerve and a branch of the greater petrosal nerve and sends sensory fibers to the mucous membrane of the tympanic cavity, the auditory tube, and the mastoid air cells. **ureteric p., p. ureter'icus** [NA], a plexus supplying the ureter and derived from the renal and hypogastric plexuses. **uterine p.,** 1. the part of the uterovaginal plexus that supplies nerve fibers to the cervix and lower part of the uterus. 2. plexus venosus uterinus. **uterovaginal p., p. uterovagina'lis,** 1. [NA] the subdivision of the inferior hypogastric plexus that supplies nerve fibers to the uterus, ovary, vagina, urethra, and erectile tissue of the vestibule. 2. see *p. venosus uterinus* and *p. venosus vaginalis.* **vaginal p.,** 1. the part of the uterovaginal plexus that supplies nerve fibers to the walls of the vagina. 2. plexus venosus vaginalis. **vascular p.,** p. vasculosus. **p. vasculo'sus** [NA], vascular plexus: a network of intercommunicating blood vessels. **p. veno'sus** [NA], venous plexus: a network of interconnecting veins. **p. veno'sus areola'ris** [NA], areolar venous plexus: a venous plexus in the areola around the nipple, formed by branches of the internal thoracic veins and draining into the lateral thoracic vein. Called also *p. venosus mamillae.* **p. veno'sus cana'lis hypoglos'si** [NA], venous plexus of hypoglossal canal: a venous plexus surrounding the hypoglossal nerve in its canal, and connecting the occipital sinus with the vertebral vein and with the longitudinal vertebral venous sinuses. Called also *rete canalis hypoglossi.* **p. veno'sus carot'icus inter'nus** [NA], internal carotid venous plexus: a venous plexus around the petrosal portion of the internal carotid artery, through which the cavernous sinus communicates with the internal jugular vein. **p. veno'sus foram'inis ova'lis** [NA], venous plexus of foramen ovale: a venous plexus that connects the cavernous sinus through the foramen ovale with the pterygoid plexus and the pharyngeal plexus; called also *rete foraminis ovalis.* **p. veno'sus mamil'lae,** p. venosus areolaris. **p. veno'sus prostat'icus** [NA], prostatic venous plexus: a venous plexus around the prostate gland, receiving the deep dorsal vein of the penis and draining through the vesical plexus and the prostatic veins; called also *p. pudendalis.* **p. veno'sus pterygoi'deus,** p. pterygoideus. **p. veno'sus recta'lis** [NA], rectal venous plexus: a venous plexus that surrounds the lower part of the rectum and drains into the rectal veins; called also *p. haemorrhoidalis.* **p. veno'sus sacra'lis** [NA], sacral venous plexus: the plexus on the pelvic surface of the sacrum that receives the sacral intervertebral veins, anastomoses with neighboring lumbar and pelvic veins, and drains into the middle and lateral sacral veins; called also *p. sacralis anterior.* **p. veno'sus suboccipita'lis** [NA], suboccipital venous plexus: that part of the external vertebral plexus which lies on and in the suboccipital triangle, receives the occipital veins of the scalp, and drains into the vertebral vein. **p. veno'sus uteri'nus** [NA], uterine venous plexus: the venous plexus around the uterus, draining into the internal iliac veins by way of the uterine veins. **p. veno'sus vagina'lis** [NA], vaginal venous plexus: a venous plexus in the walls of the vagina, which drains into the internal iliac veins by way of the internal pudendal veins. **p. veno'sus vertebra'lis exter'nus ante'rior** [NA], anterior external vertebral venous plexus: the venous plexus formed by the anterior external group of veins of the vertebral column that lies on the anterior aspects of the vertebral bodies. **p. veno'sus vertebra'lis exter'nus poste'rior** [NA], posterior external vertebral venous plexus: the venous plexus formed by the posterior external group of veins of the vertebral column that lie on the posterior aspects of the laminae and around the spinous, articular, and transverse processes of the vertebrae. **p. veno'sus vertebra'lis inter'nus ante'rior** [NA], anterior internal vertebral venous plexus: the venous plexus formed by the anterior internal group of veins of the vertebral column that lies on the posterior aspects of the vertebral bodies and intervertebral disks, on either side of the posterior longitudinal ligament. **p. veno'sus vertebra'lis inter'nus poste'rior** [NA], posterior internal vertebral venous plexus: the venous plexus formed by the posterior internal group of veins of the vertebral column that lie on either side of the midline in front of the vertebral arches and ligamenta flava. **p. veno'si vertebra'les exter'ni,** plexuses of veins ramifying external to the bodies of the vertebrae; see *p. venosi vertebrales externi [anterior et posterior].* **p. veno'si vertebra'les exter'ni [an-**

te'rior et poste'rior], see *p. venosus vertebralis externus anterior* and *p. venosus vertebralis externus posterior.* **p. veno'si vertebra'les inter'ni [ante'rior et poste'rior],** see *p. venosus vertebralis internus anterior* and *p. venosus vertebralis internus posterior.* **p. veno'sus vesica'lis** [NA], vesical venous plexus: a venous plexus surrounding the upper part of the urethra and the neck of the bladder, communicating with the vaginal plexus in the female and with the prostatic plexus in the male. **venous p.,** a network of interconnecting veins (p. venosus [NA]). **venous p., areolar,** p. venosus areolaris. **venous p., hemorrhoidal,** p. venosus rectalis. **venous p., prostatic,** p. venosus prostaticus. **venous p., rectal,** p. venosus rectalis. **venous p., sacral,** p. venosus sacralis. **venous p., suboccipital,** p. venosus suboccipitalis. **venous p., uterine,** p. venosus uterinus. **venous p., vaginal,** p. venosus vaginalis. **venous p., vesical,** p. venosus vesicalis. **venous p. of foot, dorsal,** rete venosum dorsale pedis. **venous p. of foramen ovale,** p. venosus foraminis ovalis. **venous p. of hand, dorsal,** rete venosum dorsale manus. **venous p. of hypoglossal canal,** p. venosus canalis hypoglossi. **vertebral p.,** a plexus of veins related to the vertebral column; see terms beginning *p. venosus vertebralis.* **vertebral p's, internal,** see *p. venosus vertebralis internus anterior* and *p. venosus vertebralis internus posterior.* **vertebral p's, external,** see *p. venosus vertebralis externus anterior* and *p. venosus vertebralis externus posterior.* **p. vertebra'lis** [NA], vertebral plexus: a nerve plexus accompanying the vertebral artery, formed by fibers from the vertebral and cervicothoracic ganglia and carrying sympathetic fibers to the posterior cranial fossa via cranial nerves. **vesical p.,** 1. plexus vesicale. 2. plexus venosus vesicalis. **p. vesica'le** [NA], vesical plexus: the subdivision of the inferior hypogastric plexus that supplies sympathetic nerve fibers to the urinary bladder and parts of the ureter, ductus deferens, and seminal vesicle; called also *p. vesicalis.* **p. vesica'lis,** 1. plexus venosus vesicalis. 2. plexus vesicale. **vesicoprostatic p.,** the plexus venosus vesicalis in the male. **vidian p.,** nervus canalis pterygoidei. **visceral p's, p. viscera'les,** NA alternative for *p. autonomici.* **p. viscera'les et vascula'res** [NA], peripheral nerve plexuses through which the viscera and blood vessels receive their innervation.

-plexy [Gr. *plēxis* a stroke] word termination meaning a stroke or seizure.

plica (pli'kah), gen. and pl. *pli'cae* [L.] a fold; [NA] a general term for a ridge or fold, as of peritoneum or other membrane. **pli'cae ala'res** [NA], alar folds: a pair of folds of the synovial membrane of the knee joint; attached to the medial and lateral margins of the articular surface of the patella, they pass posteriorly, converge, and become continuous with the infrapatellar synovial fold. **pli'cae ampulla'res tu'bae uteri'nae,** the folds of the mucous coat lining the ampulla of the uterine tube. **p. aryepiglot'tica** [NA], aryepiglottic fold: a fold of mucous membrane extending on each side between the lateral border of the epiglottis and the summit of the arytenoid cartilage. **p. axilla'ris ante'rior** [NA], anterior axillary fold: the fold of skin and muscle produced by the lower border of the pectoralis major muscle that forms the anterior boundary of the armpit. **p. axilla'ris poste'rior** [NA], posterior axillary fold: the fold of skin and muscle produced by the latissimus dorsi and teres major muscles that form the posterior boundary of the armpit. **pli'cae caeca'les** [NA], cecal folds: the folds of peritoneum on either side of the retrocecal recess, which may connect the cecum to the abdominal wall; called also *plicae cecales* [NA alternative]. **p. caeca'lis vascula'ris** [NA], vascular cecal fold: the fold of peritoneum that covers the anterior cecal vessels, forming the superior ileocecal recess; called also *p. cecalis vascularis* [NA alternative]. **pli'cae ceca'les,** NA alternative for *plicae caecales.* **p. ceca'lis vascula'ris,** NA alternative for *p. caecalis vascularis.* **p. chor'dae tym'pani** [NA], a fold in the mucous membrane of the tympanic cavity overlying the chorda tympani nerve. **pli'cae cilia'res** [NA], ciliary folds: low ridges in the furrows between the ciliary processes. **pli'cae circula'res** [NA], **pli'cae circula'res [Kerk'ringi], pli'cae conniven'tes,** circular folds: the permanent transverse folds of the luminal surface of the small intestine, involving both the mucosa and submucosa. **p. cor'dae utero-inguina'lis,** ligamentum teres uteri. **p. duodena′lis infe′rior** [NA], inferior duodenal fold: a thin fold of peritoneum that bounds the inferior duodenal recess; called also *p. duodenomesocolica* [NA alternative] or *duodenomesocolic fold.* **p. duodena′lis supe′rior** [NA], superior duodenal fold: a fold of peritoneum covering the inferior mesenteric vein and the ascending branch of the left colic artery; called also *p. duodenojejunalis* [NA alternative] or *duodenojejunal fold.* **p. duodenojejuna′lis,** NA alternative for *p. duodenalis superior.* **p. duodenomesocol′ica,** NA alternative for *p. duodenalis superior.* **p. epigas′trica,** p. umbilicalis lateralis, def. 1. **p. epigas′trica peritonae′i,** p. umbilicalis lateralis, def. 2. **epiglottic p.,** a fold of mucous membrane between the tongue and the epiglottis. **p. fimbria′ta** [NA], fimbriated fold: the lobulated fold running backward and outward from the anterior extremity of the frenulum of the tongue. **pli′cae gas′tricae** [NA], gastric folds: the series of folds in the mucous membrane of the stomach; they are oriented chiefly longitudinally and partially disappear when the stomach is distended. **p. gastropancreat′ica** [NA], gastropancreatic fold: a crescentic fold of peritoneum formed by the left gastric artery as it runs from the posterior abdominal wall to the lesser curvature of the stomach; called also *left gastropancreatic* fold. Cf. *p. hepatopancreatica.* **p. glossoepiglot′tica latera′lis,** [NA], lateral glossoepiglottic fold: either of two folds of mucous membrane extending, one on either side, between the base of the tongue and the epiglottis. **p. glossoepiglot′tica media′na,** [NA], median glossoepiglottic fold: a single fold of mucous membrane between the two lateral glossoepiglottic folds, connecting the base of the tongue and the epiglottis. **p. hepatopancreat′ica** [NA], hepatopancreatic fold: a crescentic fold of peritoneum formed by the hepatic artery as it runs forward from the posterior abdominal wall to the lesser omentum; called also *right gastropancreatic fold.* Cf. *p. gastropancreatica.* **p. hypogas′trica,** p. umbilicalis medialis. **p. ileocaeca′lis,** [NA], ileocecal fold: a fold of peritoneum at the left border of the cecum, extending from the ileum above to the appendix below; called also *p. ileocecalis* [NA alternative] or *p. ileoceca′lis,* NA alternative for *p. ileocaecalis.* **p. incu′dis** [NA], incudal fold: a variable fold in the tunica mucosa of the tympanic cavity, passing from the roof of the cavity to the body and short crus of the incus. **p. interarytenoi′dea** [NA], interarytenoid fold: a median fold formed by mucous membrane anterior to the transverse arytenoid muscle as it protrudes into the larynx as the muscle approximates the arytenoid cartilages. **p. interureter′ica** [NA], interureteric fold: a fold of mucous membrane extending across the bladder between the two ureteric orifices; called also *p. ureterica.* **pli′cae i′ridis** [NA], iridial folds: the numerous minute folds on the posterior surface of the iris. **p. lacrima′lis** [NA], **p. lacrima′lis [Has′neri],** lacrimal fold: a fold of mucous membrane at the lower opening of the nasolacrimal duct. **p. longitudina′lis duode′ni** [NA], longitudinal fold of duodenum: a mucosal ridge running longitudinally on the inner surface of the medial wall of the descending part of the duodenum. **p. luna′ta,** p. semilunaris conjunctivae. **p. mallea′ris ante′rior membra′nae tym′pani** [NA], anterior mallear fold of tympanic membrane: the line in the tympanic membrane that extends anteriorly from the mallear prominence and demarks the pars tensa from the pars flaccida; called also *p. malleolaris anterior membranae tympani.* **p. mallea′ris ante′rior tu′nicae muco′sae cavita′tis tympan′icae** [NA], anterior mallear fold of mucous coat of tympanic cavity: a fold in the tunica mucosa of the tympanic cavity, reflected from the tympanic membrane over the anterior process and ligament of the malleus and part of the chorda tympani nerve. **p. mallea′ris poste′rior membra′nae tym′pani** [NA], posterior mallear fold of tympanic membrane: the line in the tympanic membrane that extends posteriorly from the mallear prominence and demarks the pars tensa from the pars flaccida; called also *p. malleolaris posterior membranae tympanicae.* **p. mallea′ris poste′rior tu′nicae muco′sae cavita′tis tympan′icae** [NA], posterior mallear fold of mucous coat of tympanic cavity: a fold of the tunica mucosa of the tympanic cavity, extending from the manubrium of the malleus to the posterior wall of the cavity. **p. malleola′ris ante′rior membra′nae tym′pani,** p. mallearis anterior membranae tympani. **p. malleola′ris poste′rior membra′nae tym′pani,** p. mallearis posterior membranae

tympani. **p. membra′nae tym′pani exter′na ante′rior,** p. mallearis anterior membranae tympani. **p. membra′nae tym′pani exter′na poste′rior,** p. mallearis posterior membranae tympani. **p. ner′vi laryn′gei,** a fold of mucous membrane in the larynx, overlying the laryngeal nerve. **pli′cae palati′nae transver′sae** [NA], transverse palatine folds: four to six transverse ridges on the anterior part of the hard palate. Called also *palatine folds, palatine rugae,* and *rugae palatinae.* **pli′cae palma′tae** [NA], palmate folds: a system of folds on the anterior and posterior walls of the cervical canal of the uterus, consisting of a median longitudinal ridge and shorter elevations extending laterally and upward. **p. palpebronasa′lis** [NA], palpebronasal fold: a vertical fold of skin on either side of the nose, covering the medial canthus of the eye; called also *epicanthus.* **p. paraduodena′lis** [NA], paraduodenal fold: an occasionally found peritoneal fold containing a branch of the left colic artery. **p. pubovesica′lis,** a fold of peritoneum between the pubis and bladder. **p. rec′ti,** see *plicae transversales recti.* **p. rectouteri′na** [NA], **p. rectouteri′na [Doug′lasi],** rectouterine fold: a crescentic fold of peritoneum extending from the rectum to the base of the broad ligament on either side, forming the rectouterine pouch. **p. salpingopalati′na** [NA], salpingopalatine fold: the mucosal fold passing caudally from the auditory tube to the lateral pharyngeal wall. **p. salpingopharyn′gea** [NA], salpingopharyngeal fold: a mucosal fold passing caudally from the posterior lip of the pharyngeal orifice of the auditory tube to the lateral pharyngeal wall. **p. semiluna′ris** [NA], semilunar fold: a curved fold interconnecting the palatoglossal and palatopharyngeal arches and forming the upper boundary of the supratonsillar fossa. **pli′cae semiluna′res co′li** [NA], semilunar folds of colon: crescentic folds in the wall of the large intestine, projecting into the lumen between the haustra. **p. semiluna′ris conjuncti′vae** [NA], semilunar fold of conjunctiva: a fold of mucous membrane at the medial angle of the eye. **p. sigmoi′dea co′li,** see *plicae semilunares coli.* **p. spira′lis** [NA], spiral fold: a spirally arranged elevation in the mucosa of the first part of the cystic duct; called also *valvula spiralis* [*Heisteri*]. **p. stape′dis** [NA], stapedial fold: a mucosal fold that passes from the posterior wall of the tympanic cavity along the tympanic membrane and surrounds the stapes. **p. sublingua′lis** [NA], sublingual fold: the elevation on the floor of the mouth under the tongue, covering part of the sublingual gland and containing its excretory ducts. **p. synovia′lis** [NA], synovial fold: an extension of the synovial membrane from its free inner surface into the joint cavity. **p. synovia′lis infrapatella′ris** [NA], **p. synovia′lis patella′ris,** infrapatellar synovial fold: a large process of synovial membrane, containing some fat, which projects into the knee joint; attached to the infrapatellar adipose body, it passes posteriorly and superiorly to the intercondylar fossa of the femur. **pli′cae transversa′les rec′ti** [NA], transverse folds of rectum: permanent transverse folds in the rectum, usually three in number (two on the left and one on the right), involving the tunica mucosa and tela submucosa, and the circular layer of the tunica muscularis. Called also *Houston's valves.* **p. triangula′ris** [NA], triangular fold: a fold of mucous membrane extending backward from the palatoglossal arch and covering the anteroinferior part of the palatine tonsil. **pli′cae tuba′les tu′bae uteri′nae,** plicae tubariae tubae uterinae. **pli′cae tuba′riae tu′bae uteri′nae** [NA], tubal folds of uterine tube: the folds of the mucous lining of the uterine tube, which are high and complex in the ampulla; called also *plicae tubales tubae uterinae.* **pli′cae tu′nicae muco′sae vesi′cae bilia′ris** [NA], the folds in the mucosa of the gallbladder that bound the polygonal spaces, giving the interior a honeycombed appearance; called also *plicae tunicae mucosae vesicae felleae* [NA alternative]. **pli′cae tu′nicae muco′sae vesi′cae fel′leae,** NA alternative for *plicae tunicae mucosae vesicae biliaris.* **p. umbilica′lis latera′lis,** 1. [NA] lateral umbilical fold: a laterally placed indistinct line on either side of the inferior part of the anterior abdominal wall, overlying the inferior epigastric vessels; called also *p. epigastrica* or *epigastric fold.* 2. [NA] the fold of peritoneum covering the inferior epigastric vessels; called also *plica epigastrica peritonaei.* 3. plica umbilicalis medialis. **p. umbilica′lis me′dia,** p. umbilicalis mediana. **p. umbilica′lis media′lis** [NA], medial umbilical fold: the fold of peritoneum that covers the obliterated umbilical artery; called also *p. umbilicalis lateralis.* **p. umbilica'lis media'na** [NA], median umbilical fold: the fold of peritoneum that covers the median umbilical ligament; called also *p. umbilicalis media.* **p. ura'chi,** umbilicalis mediana. **p. ureter'ica,** p. interureterica. **pli'cae vagi'nae,** rugae vaginales. **p. ve'nae ca'vae sinis'trae** [NA], a fold of visceral pericardium enclosing the remnant of the embryonic left anterior cardinal vein; called also *ligamentum venae cavae sinistrae.* **p. ventricula'ris,** p. vestibularis. **p. vesica'lis transver'sa** [NA], transverse vesical fold: a transverse fold of the peritoneum extending from the bladder onto the pelvic wall when the bladder is empty. **p. vestibula'ris** [NA], vestibular fold: a fold of mucous membrane in the larynx, separating the ventricle from the vestibule; called also *false vocal cord.* **pli'cae villo'sae gas'tris** [NA], villous folds of stomach: a fine network of furrows demarcating the gastric areas; called also *plicae villosae ventriculi* [NA alternative]. **pli'cae villo'sae ventric'uli,** NA alternative for *plicae villosae gastris.* **p. voca'lis** [NA], a fold of mucous membrane in the larynx, forming the inferior boundary of the ventricle, the vocalis muscle being situated deep to it; called also *true vocal cord* and *vocal fold.*

plicae (pli'se) genitive and plural of *plica.*

plicate (pli'kāt) [L. *plicatus*] plaited or folded.

plication (pli-ka'shun) the taking of tucks in any structure to shorten it, or in the walls of a hollow viscus; a folding.

plicidentin (pli″sĭ-den'tin) plicadentin.

plicotomy (pli-kot'o-me) [*plica* + Gr. *tomē* a cutting] surgical division of the posterior fold of the tympanic membrane.

pliers (pli'erz) small tong-jawed pincers for bending metals or holding small objects; various forms are much used in dentistry.

Plimmer's bodies (plim'erz) [Henry George *Plimmer,* English zoologist, 1857–1918] see under *body.*

plint (plint) plinth.

plinth (plinth) a padded table for a patient to sit or lie on while performing therapeutic exercises.

-ploid [Gr. *-ploos* -fold as in *diploos* twofold + *-oid*] a word termination denoting (in adjectives) the condition in regard to degree of multiplication of chromosome sets in the karyotype, or (in nouns) an individual or cell having chromosome sets of the particular degree of multiplication in the karyotype indicated by the root to which it is added, as aneuploid, polyploid.

ploidy (ploi'de) the status of the chromosome set in the karyotype; used also as a word termination denoting the condition in regard to the degree of multiplication of chromosome sets, as aneuploidy, diploidy, haploidy.

plombage (plom-bahzh') [Fr., "sealing, stopping"] the surgical filling of an empty space in the body with inert material, as the filling of part of the chest with polyethylene spheres after removal of ribs in thoracoplasty.

plot (plot) 1. to locate points on a graph. 2. to draw a graph. 3. a graph so produced. **Lineweaver-Burk p.,** a double-reciprocal transformation of the Michaelis-Menten equation (q.v.) in which $1/v$ is graphed as a function of $1/[S]$. This gives a straight line with an *x*-intercept at $-1/K_m$ and a *v*-intercept at $1/V_{max}$. This type of plot is convenient because the graph is also a straight line in the presence of various types of enzyme inhibition. The graphs for different inhibitor concentrations are straight lines with a common *y*-intercept (same K_m) for competitive inhibition, straight lines with a common *x*-intercept (same V_{max}) for noncompetitive inhibition, and parallel straight lines for uncompetitive inhibition (both K_m and V_{max} vary).

plotolysin (plo″to-li'sin) the hemotoxic fraction of plototoxin.

plotospasmin (plo″to-spaz'min) the neurotoxic fraction of plototoxin.

plototoxin (plo″to-tok'sin) a toxic substance derived from the catfish, *Plotosus lineatus,* said to be composed of a hemotoxic fraction (plotolysin) and a neurotoxic fraction (plotospasmin).

PLT 1. primed lymphocyte typing. 2. abbreviation for *psittacosis-l*ymphogranuloma venereum-*t*rachoma (group of organisms); see *Chlamydia.*

plug (plug) a lumpy mass, which closes or obstructs an opening. **copulation p.,** vaginal p. **Dittrich's p's,**

yellowish or gray caseous masses, of varying size, consisting of granular debris, fat globules, fatty acid crystals, and bacteria frequently found in the sputum, or expectorated alone, in cases of putrid bronchitis or bronchiectasis. **Ecker's p.,** a plug of cells in the primitive mouth of the gastrula. **epithelial p.,** a mass of ectodermal cells that temporarily closes the external naris of the fetus. **Imlach's fat p.,** a mass of fatty tissue sometimes found at the mesial angle of the external inguinal ring. **mucous p.,** a plug formed by secretions of the mucous glands of the cervix uteri and closing the cervical canal during pregnancy. **Traube's p's,** Dittrich's p's. **vaginal p.,** a plug consisting of a mass of coagulated sperm and mucus which forms in the vagina of animals after coitus; called also *copulation p.* **yolk p.,** the mass of yolk cells protruding from the blastopore of amphibians at the end of gastrulation.

Plugge's test (plug'ĕz) [Pieter Cornelis *Plugge,* Dutch biochemist, 1847–1897] see under *tests.*

plugger (plug'er) a dental instrument used for packing, condensing, and compacting filling material into a tooth cavity. **amalgam p.,** one for packing and condensing plastic amalgam in a prepared tooth cavity.

plumbage (ploom-bahzh') plombage.

plumbagin (plum-ba'jin) chemical name: 5-hydroxy-2-methyl-1,4-naphthoquinone, $CH_3 \cdot C_{10}H_4(:O)_2 \cdot OH$. A yellow, needle-like irritant substance, obtained from various species of plants of the genus *Plumbago,* e.g., *P. europa* L., which has been used as an abortifacient.

plumbago (plum-ba'go) see *graphite.*

plumbi (plum'bi) [L.] genitive of *plumbum,* lead. **p. ace'tas,** lead acetate. **p. chlo'ridum,** lead chloride. **p. monox'idum,** lead monoxide. **p. ni'tras,** lead nitrate. **p. ox'idum,** lead monoxide.

plumbic (plum'bik) [L. *plumbicus* leaden] pertaining to or containing lead.

plumbism (plum'bizm) lead poisoning; see under *poisoning.*

plumbotherapy (plum″bo-ther'ah-pe) [L. *plumbum* lead + *therapy*] the therapeutic use of lead, especially its salts.

plumbum (plum'bum), gen. *plum'bi* [L.] lead[1].

plumericin (ploo″mer-i'sin) a principle, $C_{15}H_{14}O_6$, isolated from the roots of *Plumeria multiflora* Muell.-Arg., Apocynaceae, which shows *in vitro* activity against fungi and bacteria, including *Mycobacterium tuberculosis.*

Plummer's disease, sign (plum'erz) [Henry Stanley *Plummer,* American physician, 1874–1937] see under *disease* and *sign.*

Plummer-Vinson syndrome (plum'er-vin'son) [Henry Stanley *Plummer;* Porter Paisley *Vinson,* American surgeon, 1890–1959] see under *syndrome.*

plumose (plu'mōs) [L. *plumosus,* Fr. *pluma* feather] feathery; resembling a feather.

plumula (plum'u-lah) a set of delicate cross-furrows occasionally found on the upper wall of the aqueduct of Sylvius.

pluri- [L. *plus,* gen. *pluris* more] a combining form meaning several or more.

pluriglandular (ploor″ĭ-glan'du-lar) [*pluri-* + L. *glandula*] pertaining to, derived from, or affecting several glands.

plurigravida (ploor″ĭ-grav'ĭ-dah) [*pluri-* + L. *gravida* pregnant] multigravida.

plurilocular (ploor″ĭ-lok'u-lar) multilocular.

plurimenorrhea (ploor″ĭ-men'o-re'ah) increased frequency of menstrual periods.

plurinuclear (ploor″ĭ-nu'kle-ar) [*pluri-* + *nucleus*] multinucleate.

pluriorificial (ploor″e-or″ĭ-fish'al) [*pluri-* + L. *orificium* orifice] pertaining to or affecting several orifices of the body.

pluripara (ploo-rip'ah-rah) [*pluri-* + L. *parere* to bear] multipara.

pluriparity (ploor″ĭ-par'ĭ-te) multiparity.

pluripolar (ploor″ĭ-po'lar) multipolar.

pluripotent (ploo-rip'o-tent) pluripotential.

pluripotential (ploor″ĭ-po-ten'shal) pertaining to or characterized by pluripotentiality.

pluripotentiality (ploor″ĭ-po-ten″she-al'ĭ-te) [*pluri-* + L. *potentia* power] possession of the power of developing (as embryonic cells) or acting in any one of several possible ways, or of affecting more than one organ or tissue.

pluriresistant (ploor″ĭ-re-zis′tant) resistant to several drugs.

pluritissular (ploor″ĭ-tis′u-lar) composed of several tissues.

plurivisceral (ploor″ĭ-vis′er-al) [L. *pluri-* + *visceralis*, from *viscus* a body organ] pertaining to or affecting several viscera, or organs.

plutonium (ploo-to′ne-um) [named from the planet *Pluto*] a heavy, metallic, radioactive element of atomic number 94, atomic weight 242, obtained by the addition of neutrons to uranium, thereby changing it into neptunium and then into plutonium. Symbol Pu.

Pm chemical symbol for *promethium*.

P.M.B. polymorphonuclear basophil leukocytes; see *granular leukocytes*, under *leukocyte*.

P.M.E. polymorphonuclear eosinophil leukocytes; see *granular leukocytes*, under *leukocyte*.

P.M.I. point of maximal impulse; see under *point*.

PMM pentamethylmelamine.

P.M.N. polymorphonuclear neutrophil leukocytes; see *granular leukocytes*, under *leukocyte*.

PMR proportionate mortality ratio.

PMSG pregnant mare serum gonadotropin.

P.N. percussion note.

-pnea [Gr. *pnoia* breath] a word termination denoting relationship to breathing.

pneo- [Gr. *pnein* to breathe] a combining form denoting relationship to the breath or to breathing. For words beginning thus, see also those beginning *spiro-* (2).

pneogaster (ne′o-gas″ter) [*pneo-* + Gr. *gaster* the belly] the respiratory tract of the embryo.

pneogram (ne′o-gram) spirogram.

pneograph (ne′o-graf) [*pneo-* + Gr. *graphein* to write] spirograph.

pneometer (ne-om′ě-ter) [*pneo-* + Gr. *metron* measure] spirometer.

pneoscope (ne′o-skōp) [*pneo-* + Gr. *skopein* to examine] a device for determining movements of the chest wall in respiration.

pneuma- see *pneumato-*.

pneumal (nu′mal) pertaining to the lungs.

pneumarthrogram (nu-mar′thro-gram) [*pneumo-* + Gr. *arthron* joint + *gamma* that which is written] a roentgenogram of a joint after it has been injected with air.

pneumarthrography (nu″mar-throg′rah-fe) roentgenography of a joint after it has been injected with air or gas as a contrast medium; called also *pneumoarthrography*.

pneumarthrosis (nu″mar-thro′sis) [*pneumo-* + Gr. *arthron* joint + *-osis*] 1. the presence of gas or air in a joint. 2. the inflation of a joint with air or gas for the purpose of aiding roentgenographical examination.

pneumascope (nu′mah-skōp) spiroscope.

pneumathemia (nu″mah-the′me-ah) [*pneumo-* + Gr. *haima* blood + *-ia*] the presence of air or gas in the blood vessels; air embolism.

pneumatic (nu-mat′ik) [L. *pneumaticus*; Gr. *pneumatikos*] of or pertaining to air or respiration.

pneumatics (nu-mat′iks) the science which deals with the physical properties of gases.

pneumatinuria (nu″mah-tĭ-nu′re-ah) pneumaturia.

pneumatism (noo′mah-tizm) [from Gr. *pneuma* air, breath, spirit] a theory, first associated with Empedocles of Acragas, that combines the folk belief of blood's being the seat of innate heat, and the then current philosophical speculation on pneuma, to establish the heart both as center of the vascular system and as the main organ distributing pneuma, life, and heat by the veins, arteries, and nerves. Pneumatism was rejected by the contemporary, growing Coan School (and therefore by Hippocrates of Cos) and by Aristotle, but was accepted by Erasistratus, Diocles, Athenaeus, and ultimately Galen. Pneumatism reigned till William Harvey.

Pneumatist (noo′mah-tist) an eclectic medical school founded by Athenaeus of Attalia on the principle of pneumatism. Agathinus of Sparta, Archigenes of Apamea, Aretaeus of Cappadocia, Erasistratus, and Antyllus were some of its adherents.

pneumatization (nu″mah-ti-za′shun) the formation of pneumatic cells or cavities in tissue, especially such formation in the temporal bone.

pneumatized (nu′mah-tīzd) filled with air; containing pneumatic cells.

pneumat(o)-, pneuma- [Gr. *pneuma*, gen. *pneumatos* air] combining form denoting relationship to air or gas, or to respiration.

pneumatocardia (nu″mah-to-kar′de-ah) [*pneumato-* + Gr. *kardia* heart] the presence of air in the heart.

pneumatocele (nu-mat′o-sēl) [*pneumato-* + Gr. *kēlē* hernia] 1. hernial protrusion of lung tissue, as through a congenital fissure of the chest. 2. a usually benign, thin-walled, air-containing cyst of the lung, as in staphylococcal pneumonia. 3. a tumor or sac containing gas, especially a gaseous swelling of the scrotum. **p. cra′nii, extracranial p.,** gaseous tumors beneath the scalp after a fracture of the skull that communicates with the paranasal sinuses. **intracranial p.,** pneumocephalus. **parotid p.,** enlargement of the parotid glands as a result of blowing air into the parotid ducts. See also *glass-blowers' mouth*, under *mouth*.

pneumatocephalus (nu″mah-to-sef′ah-lus) pneumocephalus.

pneumatodyspnea (nu″mah-to-disp′ne-ah) [*pneumato-* + *dyspnea*] difficulty in breathing due to emphysema.

pneumatogram (nu-mat′o-gram) spirogram.

pneumatograph (nu-mat′o-graf) spirograph.

pneumatometer (nu″mah-tom′ě-ter) [*pneumato-* + Gr. *metron* measure] a form of spirometer, or instrument for measuring the air inspired and expired.

pneumatometry (nu″mah-tom′ě-tre) the measurement of the air inspired and expired; spirometry.

pneumatophore (nu-mat′o-fōr) [*pneumato-* + Gr. *phoros* bearing] an apparatus consisting of a bag with a tube and mouthpiece, which may be attached to the body; the bag contains oxygen, to be breathed by the wearer in rescue work in mines, etc.

pneumatorrhachis (nu″mah-tor′ah-kis) [*pneumato-* + Gr. *rhachis* spine] the presence of gas in the vertebral canal.

pneumatoscope (nu-mat′o-skōp) [*pneumato-* + Gr. *skopein* to examine] an instrument devised by Gabritschewsky for auscultating the percussion of the thorax from the mouth.

pneumatosis (nu″mah-to′sis) [Gr. *pneumatōsis*] the presence of air or gas in an abnormal situation in the body. **p. cystoi′des intestina′lis, p. cystoi′des intestino′rum,** a condition characterized by the presence of thin-walled, gas-containing cysts in the wall of the intestines; the lesions may be subserosal or submucosal. **intestinal p., p. intestina′lis,** p. cystoides intestinalis. **p. pulmo′num,** pulmonary emphysema.

pneumatotherapy (nu″mah-to-ther′ah-pe) [*pneumato-* + *therapy*] the treatment of disease by rarefied or condensed air.

pneumaturia (nu″mah-tu′re-ah) [*pneumato-* + Gr. *ouron* urine + *-ia*] passage of urine charged with air or gas.

pneumatype (nu′mah-tīp) [*pneuma-* + Gr. *typos* type] a breath picture; a deposition of moisture upon a glass surface or a shiny metal plate from the exhaled air; used in the diagnosis of nasal obstructions.

pneumectomy (nu-mek′to-me) [Gr. *pneumōn* lung + *ektomē* excision] pneumonectomy.

pneumencephalography (nūm″en-sef″ah-log′rah-fe) pneumoencephalography.

pneum(o)- [Gr. *pneuma* breath] a combining form denoting relationship to (*a*) respiration, (*b*) the lungs, (*c*) air, (*d*) pneumonia.

pneumoalveolography (nu″mo-al″ve-o-log′rah-fe) roentgenography of the alveoli of the lungs.

pneumoamnios (nu″mo-am′ne-os) the presence of gas in the amniotic fluid.

pneumoangiogram (nu″mo-an′je-o-gram″) a composite of radiographs obtained by pneumoencephalography and cerebral angiography.

pneumoangiography (nu″mo-an″je-og′rah-fe) roentgenography of the blood vessels of the lungs.

pneumoarthrography (nu″mo-ar-throg′rah-fe) pneumarthrography.

pneumobacillus (nu″mo-bah-sil′us) [*pneumo-* + *bacillus*] *Klebsiella pneumoniae.* **Friedländer's p.,** *Klebsiella pneumoniae.*

pneumobulbar (nu″mo-bul′bar) pertaining to the lungs and to the respiration center in the medulla oblongata.

pneumobulbous (nu″mo-bul′bus) pneumobulbar.

pneumocardial (nu″mo-kar′de-al) pertaining to the lungs and the heart.

pneumocardiograph (nu″mo-kar′de-o-graf) the instrument used in pneumocardiography.

pneumocardiography (nu″mo-kar″de-og′rah-fe) the recording of variations in heart function through sensors that monitor respiratory changes, e.g., changes in thoracic dimensions, in pressure changes in the bronchi, or in temperature differences between inspired and expired air.

pneumocele (nu″mo-sēl) [*pneumo-* + Gr. *kēlē* tumor] pneumatocele.

pneumocentesis (nu″mo-sen-te′sis) [*pneumo-* + Gr. *kentēsis* puncture] pneumonocentesis.

pneumocephalus (nu″mo-sef′ah-lus) [Gr. *pneuma* air + *kephalē* head] the presence of air in the intracranial cavity; intracranial pneumatocele.

pneumocholecystitis (nu″mo-ko″le-sis-ti′tis) emphysematous cholecystitis.

pneumochysis (nu-mok′ĭ-sis) pulmonary edema, or serous infiltration of the lung.

pneumococcal (nu″mo-kok′al) pertaining to or caused by pneumococci.

pneumococcemia (nu″mo-kok-se′me-ah) the presence of pneumococci in the blood.

pneumococci (nu″mo-kok′si) plural of *pneumococcus.*

pneumococcic (nu″mo-kok′sik) pertaining to or caused by pneumococci.

pneumococcidal (nu″mo-kok-si′dal) destroying pneumococci.

pneumococcolysis (nu″mo-kok-kol′ĭ-sis) [*pneumococcus* + Gr. *lysis* dissolution] solubilization of pneumococci.

pneumococcosis (nu″mo-kok-ko′sis) infection with pneumococci.

pneumococcosuria (nu″mo-kok″o-su′re-ah) the presence in the urine of pneumococci or of pneumococcus polysaccharide.

pneumococcus (nu″mo-kok′us), pl. *pneumococ′ci* [*pneumo-* + Gr. *kokkos* berry] an individual organism of the species *Streptococcus pneumoniae.*

pneumocolon (nu″mo-ko′lon) [*pneumo-* + *colon*] the presence of air in the colon, often introduced as an aid to diagnosis.

pneumoconiosis (nu″mo-ko″ne-o′sis) [*pneumo-* + Gr. *konis* dust] a condition characterized by permanent deposition of substantial amounts of particulate matter in the lungs, usually of occupational or environmental origin, and by the tissue reaction to its presence. It may range from relatively harmless forms of anthracosis or siderosis to the destructive fibrosis of silicosis. See *aluminosis, anthracosis, asbestosis, siderosis, silicosis,* etc. **bauxite p.,** rapidly progressive pneumoconiosis leading to extreme pulmonary emphysema, frequently accompanied by pneumothorax, caused by inhalation of bauxite fumes containing fine particles of alumina and silica. Called also *bauxite workers' disease* and *Shaver's disease.* **p. of coal workers,** a form caused by deposition of large amounts of coal dust in the lungs, and typically characterized by centrilobular emphysema; called also *coal-miner's* or *miner's lung, black phthisis,* and *miner's phthisis.* Cf. *anthracosis.* **collagenous p.,** that in which permanent scarring results, due to fibrogenic dust, such as asbestos or silica, or to altered tissue response to nonfibrogenic dust. **noncollagenous p.,** that in which the stromal reaction is minimal, consisting chiefly of reticulin fibers. **rheumatoid p.,** Caplan's syndrome. **p. siderot′ica,** siderosis, def. 1. **talc p.,** pneumoconiosis produced by the inhalation of talc; symptoms include shortness of breath, cough, fatigue, weakness, and weight loss. Prolonged exposure to large quantities of talc may result in pulmonary fibrosis.

pneumocrania (nu″mo-kra′ne-ah) pneumocephalus.

pneumocranium (nu″mo-kra′ne-um) pneumocephalus.

pneumocystic (nu″mo-sis′tik) relating to or caused by *Pneumocystis.*

Pneumocystis (noo″mo-sis′tis) [*pneumo-* + *cyst*] a genus of microorganisms of uncertain status, which are thought by some to be protozoa, probably sporozoa, and by others to be yeastlike fungi. **P. cari′nii,** the causative agent of a highly contagious, epidemic, interstitial plasma cell pneumonia, particularly of infants; see under *pneumonia.*

pneumocystography (nu″mo-sis-tog′rah-fe) cystography following the injection of air into the bladder.

pneumocystosis (nu″mo-sis-to′sis) interstitial plasma cell pneumonia.

pneumocystotomography (nu″mo-sis″to-to-mog′rah-fe) body section roentgenography after inflation of the bladder with air.

pneumocyte (nu-mo-sīt′) pneumonocyte.

pneumoderma (nu″mo-der′mah) [*pneumo-* + Gr. *derma* skin] subcutaneous emphysema.

pneumodograph (nu-mod′o-graf) [*pneumo-* + Gr. *hodos* way + *graphein* to write] an apparatus for registering the degree of respiratory nasal efficiency.

pneumodynamics (nu″mo-di-nam′iks) [*pneumo-* + Gr. *dynamis* force] the dynamics of the respiratory process; the study of the forces exerted in the act of breathing.

pneumoempyema (nu″mo-em″pi-e′mah) empyema marked by the presence of gas; pyopneumothorax.

pneumoencephalitis (nu″mo-en-sef″ah-li′tis) Newcastle disease.

pneumoencephalogram (nu″mo-en-sef′ah-lo-gram) the roentgenogram obtained by pneumoencephalography.

pneumoencephalography (nu″mo-en-sef″ah-log′rah-fe) radiographic visualization of the fluid-containing structures of the brain after cerebrospinal fluid is intermittently withdrawn by lumbar puncture and replaced by air, oxygen, or helium.

pneumoencephalomyelogram (nu″mo-en-sef″ah-lo-mi-el′o-gram) the roentgenogram obtained by pneumoencephalomyelography.

pneumoencephalomyelography (nu″mo-en-sef″ah-lo-mi″e-log′rah-fe) radiographic visualization of the brain and spinal cord after cerebrospinal fluid is removed by lumbar puncture and replaced by gas.

pneumoencephalos (nu″mo-en-sef′ah-los) [*pneumo-* + Gr. *enkephalos* brain] the presence of air or gas in the intracranial cavity.

pneumoenteritis (nu″mo-en″ter-i′tis) [*pneumo-* + Gr. *enteron* intestine + *-itis*] inflammation of the lung and intestine. **p. of calves,** white scours in calves.

pneumoerysipelas (nu″mo-er″ĭ-sip′e-las) (obs.) erysipelas complicated with pneumonia.

pneumofasciogram (nu″mo-fas′e-o-gram) a roentgenogram of tissue after injection of air into the fascial spaces.

pneumogalactocele (nu″mo-gah-lak′to-sēl) [*pneumo-* + Gr. *gala* milk + *kēlē* tumor] a tumor containing gas and milk.

pneumogastric (nu″mo-gas′trik) [*pneumo-* + Gr. *gastēr* stomach] pertaining to the lungs and stomach.

pneumogastrography (nu″mo-gas-trog′rah-fe) [*pneumo-* + *gastrography*] roentgenography of the stomach after the injection of air.

pneumogram (nu′mo-gram) 1. the tracing or graphic record of respiratory movements. 2. a roentgenogram made after the injection of air into the part.

pneumograph (nu′mo-graf) [*pneumo-* + Gr. *graphein* to write] an instrument for registering the respiratory movements.

pneumography (nu-mog′rah-fe) [*pneumo-* + Gr. *graphein* to write] 1. an anatomical description of the lungs. 2. graphic recording of the respiratory movements. 3. roentgenography of a part after injection of a gas. **cerebral p.,** roentgenography of the brain by pneumoencephalography or ventriculography. **retroperitoneal p.,** roentgenography of the abdominal organs after retroperitoneal injection of air or oxygen.

pneumogynogram (nu″mo-gi′no-gram) a roentgenogram of the female reproductive organs after injection of air into the uterus.

pneumohemia (nu″mo-he′me-ah) [*pneumo-* + Gr. *haima* blood + *-ia*] the presence of air or gas in the blood vessels; air embolism.

pneumohemopericardium (nu″mo-he″mo-per″ĭ-kar′de-um) [*pneumo-* + Gr. *haima* blood + *pericardium*] the presence of air or gas and blood in the pericardial cavity.

pneumohemothorax (nu″mo-he″mo-tho′raks) [*pneumo-* + Gr. *haima* blood + *thōrax* chest] the presence of air or gas and blood in the pleural cavity.

pneumohydrometra (nu″mo-hi″dro-me′trah) [*pneumo-* + Gr. *hydōr* water + *mētra* uterus] a collection of gas and fluid in the uterine cavity.

pneumohydropericardium (nu″mo-hi″dro-per″ĭ-kar′de-um) [*pneumo-* + Gr. *hydōr* water + *pericardium*] the presence of air or gas and fluid in the pericardial cavity.

pneumohydrothorax (nu″mo-hi″dro-tho′raks) [*pneumo-* + Gr. *hydōr* water + *thōrax* chest] a collection of air or gas and fluid in the pleural cavity.

pneumokidney (nu″mo-kid″ne) [*pneumo-* + *kidney*] the presence of gas in the kidney pelvis.

pneumokoniosis (nu″mo-ko″ne-o′sis) pneumoconiosis.

pneumolith (nu′mo-lith) [*pneumo-* + Gr. *lithos* stone] a pulmonary calculus or concretion.

pneumolithiasis (nu″mo-lĭ-thi′ah-sis) the presence of concretions in the lungs.

pneumology (nu-mol′o-je) [*pneumo-* + *-logy*] the study of disease of the air passages.

pneumolysis (nu-mol′ĭ-sis) pneumonolysis.

pneumomalacia (nu″mo-mah-la′she-ah) [*pneumo-* + Gr. *malakia* softness] morbid softening of lung tissue.

pneumomassage (nu″mo-mah-sahzh′) [*pneumo-* + *massage*] air massage of the tympanum by the alternate compression and rarefaction of the air in the external auditory canal.

pneumomediastinogram (nu″mo-me″de-as-ti′no-gram) the film produced by pneumomediastinography.

pneumomediastinography (nu″mo-me″de-as″tĭ-nog′rah-fe) roentgenography of the mediastinum after injection of nitrous oxide or oxygen through a needle introduced back of the trachea or behind the manubrium.

pneumomediastinum (nu″mo-me″de-as-ti′num) [*pneumo-* + *mediastinum*] the presence of air or gas in the mediastinum, which may interfere with respiration and circulation, and may lead to such conditions as pneumothorax or pneumopericardium. It may occur spontaneously or as a result of trauma or a pathologic process, or it may be induced deliberately as a diagnostic procedure. Called also *Hamman's disease* or *syndrome* and *mediastinal emphysema*.

pneumomelanosis (nu″mo-mel″ah-no′sis) [*pneumo-* + *melanosis*] the blackening of the lung tissue by inhaled coal dust; see *anthracosis*.

pneumometer (nu-mom′ĕ-ter) pneumatometer.

pneumomycosis (nu″mo-mi-ko′sis) [*pneumo-* + *mycosis*] any fungal disease of the lungs.

pneumomyelography (nu″mo-mi″ĕ-log′rah-fe) [*pneumo-* + Gr. *myelos* marrow + *graphein* to write] roentgen-ray examination after withdrawal of cerebrospinal fluid and injection of air or gas into the spinal canal.

pneumonectasia (nu″mon-ek-ta′ze-ah) pneumonectasis.

pneumonectasis (nu″mo-nek′tah-sis) [*pneumo-* + Gr. *ektasis* extension] emphysema of the lungs; overdistention of lung tissue.

pneumonectomy (nu″mo-nek′to-me) [*pneumono-* + Gr. *ektomē* excision] the excision of lung tissue, especially of an entire lung.

pneumonedema (nu″mo-ne-de′mah) [*pneumo-* + *edema*] edema of the lungs.

pneumonemia (nu″mo-ne′me-ah) [*pneumo-* + Gr. *haima* blood + *-ia*] congestion of the lungs.

pneumonere (nu′mo-nēr) one of the end-buds which cap the primitive bronchi.

pneumonia (nu-mo′ne-ah) [Gr. *pneumōnia*] inflammation of the lungs with consolidation. **abortive p.,** a form with a short and favorable course. **acute p.,** severe pneumonia of rapid onset. **p. al′ba,** a fatal desquamative pneumonia of the newborn resulting from congenital syphilis and characterized by white fatty degeneration of the lungs, which appear pale and virtually airless. Called also *white p.* and *white lung.* **alcoholic p.,** pneumonia associated with alcoholism. **amebic p.,** pneumonia resulting from so-called amebic abscesses in the lung caused by *Entamoeba histolytica.* **anthrax p.,** inhalational anthrax. **apex p., apical p.,** lobar pneumonia limited to the apex of the lung. **p. apostemato′sa,** suppurative p. **aspiration p.,** pneumonia due to the entrance of foreign matter, such as food particles, into the respiratory passages (bronchi). **atypical p.,** primary atypical p. **bacterial p.,** pneumonia caused by bacteria, chief among which are *Streptococcus pneumoniae, S. hemolytica, Staphylococcus aureus,* and *Klebsiella pneumoniae.* **bilious p.,** lobar pneumonia attended with jaundice. **bronchial p.,** bronchopneumonia. **brooder p.,** a pneumonic disease (aspergillosis) of chicks acquired from moldy grain or straw. **Buhl's desquamative p.,** cheesy p. **caseous p.,** cheesy p. **cat p.,** a lung disease of cats probably due to the agent (*Chlamydia*) of psittacosis. **catarrhal p.,** bronchopneumonia. **central p.,** lobar pneumonia beginning in the hilum of a lobe of the lung. **cerebral p.,** pneumonia associated with neurologic symptoms and disturbances of consciousness. **cheesy p.,** pneumonia, usually tuberculous, in which necrotic lung tissue is of semisolid consistency and the cut surface looks like cheese. **chronic p.,** a long-continuing form. **chronic eosinophilic p.,** a chronic interstitial lung disease characterized by cough, dyspnea, malaise, fever, night sweats, weight loss, eosinophilia, and a chest film revealing nonsegmental, nonmigratory infiltrates in the lung periphery. **cold agglutinin p.,** primary atypical p. **congenital aspiration p.,** see *respiratory distress syndrome,* under *syndrome.* **contagious p. of horses,** a condition that may follow equine influenza, characterized by high fever, pneumonia, and necrosis of the lungs. **contusion p.,** pneumonia following an injury. **core p.,** central p. **Corrigan's p.,** Kaufman's p. **croupous p.,** lobar p. **deglutition p.,** aspiration pneumonia due to the entrance of food into the lungs, usually associated with dysphagia. **dermal p.,** a condition produced by injection of virulent pneumococci into the skin of rabbits. **desquamative p.,** chronic pneumonia with hardening of the fibrous exudate and proliferation of the interstitial tissue and epithelium of the lung; called also *parenchymatous p.* **desquamative interstitial p.,** chronic pneumonia of unknown etiology, with desquamation of large alveolar cells and thickening of the walls of distal air passages; it is characterized by dyspnea and often by a nonproductive and harsh cough. **p. dis′secans,** pneumonia interlobularis purulenta. **double p.,** that which affects both lungs. **Eaton agent p.,** mycoplasmal p. **embolic p.,** pneumonia due to embolism of a blood vessel or vessels of the lungs. **ephemeral p.,** that in which the signs of pneumonia disappear after a short period. **ether p.,** pneumonia occurring after anesthesia by ether. **fibrinous p.,** pneumonia characterized by abundant exudation of fibrin into the air passages. **fibrous p.,** a form characterized by an increase in scar tissue during the healing process. **fibrous p., chronic,** interstitial pulmonary fibrosis. **Friedländer's p., Friedländer's bacillus p.,** an acute specific infectious disease characterized by massive mucoid inflammatory exudates in the lung, and caused by *Klebsiella pneumoniae.* **gangrenous p.,** gangrene of the lung. **giant cell p.,** a rare, usually fatal form of interstitial pneumonia caused by the measles virus, affecting children with disease of the reticuloendothelial system (such as leukemia), and marked by the presence of multinucleate giant-cell inclusion bodies; called also *Hecht's p.* **Hecht's p.,** giant cell p. **hypostatic p.,** pneumonia due to dorsal decubitus in weak or aged persons. **indurative p.,** pneumonia associated with dense fibrous scar tissue. **infective p. of goats,** a fatal disease of goats in South Africa. **influenzal p., influenza virus p.,** a severe, usually fatal disease caused by influenza virus and characterized by abrupt onset, high fever, prostration, sore throat, aching pains, and profound dyspnea and anxiety, and by massive pulmonary hemorrhagic edema and consolidation. It may be complicated by bacterial pneumonia, in which case the symptoms of that disease (shaking chills, pleuritic pain, etc.) are superimposed on the primary influenza virus pneumonia. **inhalation p.,** 1. aspiration pneumonia. 2. bronchopneumonia due to the inhalation of irritating vapors. **p. interlobula′ris purulen′ta,** pneumonia in which the lobules are separated from one another. **interstitial p.,** a chronic form of pneumonia with increase of the interstitial tissue and decrease of the proper lung tissue, with induration; called also *chronic fibrous p.* **interstitial plasma cell p.,** a pulmonary disease of infants and debilitated persons, including those receiving cytotoxic drugs, immunosuppressive drugs, cortisone, etc., in which cellular detritus containing plasma cells appears in the lung tissue; it is caused by *Pneumocystis carinii.* Called also *pneumocystis pneumonia.* **intrauterine p.,** pneumonia contracted by the fetus *in utero;* it may result in the death of the fetus or the birth of an infant with fully developed pneumonia. **Kaufman's p.,** acute interstitial pneumonia, a rare fatal form of pneumonia in young infants. **lipid p., lipoid p.,** a pneumonia-like reaction of the lung tissue to the aspiration of oils; called also *oil-aspiration p.* and *pneumonolipoidosis.* **lobar p.,** an acute febrile disease produced by the *Streptococcus pneumoniae,* and marked by inflammation of one or more lobes of the lung, together with consolidation. It is attended with chill, followed by sudden elevation of temperature, dyspnea, rapid breathing, pain in the side, and cough, with blood-stained expectoration. The symptoms abate after a week. It usually begins in the lower lobe, the lung being at first intensely congested (*stage of congestion* or *engorgement*), and afterward becoming red and solid from accumulation of exudate and blood cells in the alveoli (*red hepatization*), and later gray (*gray hepatization*), from degeneration of the exudates, which are finally absorbed. Called also *croupous p., fibrinous p.,* and *lung fever.* **lobular p.,** bronchopneumonia. **Löffler's p.,** Löffler's syndrome. **Louisiana p.,** a form of pneumonia encountered in Louisiana, caused by a strain of *Chlamydia psittaci.* **lymphoid interstitial p.,** lymphocytic interstitial pneumonitis. **p. malleo'sa,** pneumonia caused by or associated with glanders. **massive p.,** lobar pneumonia with extensive solidification of the air cells, or even an entire lung. **metastatic p.,** suppurative pneumonia due to bloodborne infection in bacteremia. **migratory p.,** pneumonia gradually involving one lobe of the lung after another. **mycoplasmal p.,** the most common form of primary atypical pneumonia (q.v.), caused by *Mycoplasma pneumoniae* and occurring most frequently in young adults; called also *Eaton agent p.* **obstructive p.,** that due to obstruction of the air passages, as by bronchogenic carcinoma. **oil-aspiration p.,** lipid p. **parenchymatous p.,** desquamative p. **Pittsburgh p.,** pneumonia resembling legionnaires' disease, caused by *Legionella micdadei,* and occurring as a nosocomial infection in immunosuppressed patients. **plague p.,** pneumonic plague. **plasma cell p.,** interstitial plasma cell p. **pleuritic p.,** pleuropneumonia. **pleurogenetic p., pleurogenic p.,** that which is secondary to pleural disease. **pneumococcal p.,** lobar p. **pneumocystis p., Pneumocystis carinii p.,** interstitial plasma cell p. **primary atypical p.,** a general term applied to an acute infectious pulmonary disease caused by *Mycoplasma pneumoniae,* species of *Rickettsia* and *Chlamydia,* and various viruses, including adenoviruses and parainfluenza virus; it is marked by extensive but tenuous pulmonary infiltration and by fever, malaise, myalgia, sore throat, and a cough which at first is nonproductive but becomes productive and paroxysmal. Called also *atypical p., atypical bronchopneumonia, acute interstitial pneumonitis, cold agglutinin p.,* and *viral p.* **purulent p.,** a form characterized by the expectoration of copious pus. **rheumatic p.,** a rare, usually fatal complication of acute rheumatic fever characterized by extensive pulmonary consolidation and rapidly progressive functional deterioration and by alveolar exudate (with the presence of Masson bodies), interstitial infiltrates, and necrotizing arteritis. **Riesman's p.,** a peculiar form of chronic bronchopneumonia. **secondary p.,** inflammation of the lungs coming on as a complication of some systemic disorder. **septic p.,** pneumonia invasive virulent infectious agents. **staphylococcal p.,** pneumonia caused by infection with *Staphylococcus,* many strains of which are antibiotic-resistant; it has a strong tendency to extend beyond the original site of infection. **streptococcal p.,** pneumonia caused by infection with *Streptococcus* (*s. pneumoniae, s. pyogenes*), usually occurring as a complication of influenza. **superficial p.,** a form which affects only the parts near the pleura. **suppurative p.,** pneumonia with formation of abscesses in the lungs. **terminal p.,** pneumonia developing during some other disease and hastening a fatal termination. **toxemic p.,** infection of the system with pneumococci without marked lung involvement. **traumatic p.,**

inflammation of the lung following physical injury to the thorax. **tuberculous p.,** the simplest form of pulmonary tuberculosis, often the earliest reaction to infection. **tularemic p.,** see *pulmonary tularemia,* under *tularemia.* **typhoid p.,** a form of pneumonia with typhoid symptoms. **unresolved p.,** pneumonia in which the lung signs fail to clear up within the usual period. **vagus p.,** pneumonia associated with injury of the pneumogastric nerve. **varicella p.,** pneumonia developing two to six days after the appearance of varicella (chickenpox) eruption and apparently due to the same virus. Symptoms may be severe, with violent cough, hemoptysis, and severe chest pains. Radiologically, there are numerous nodular densities, which may coalesce, at the base of each lung and, often, enlarged lymph nodes in the hilar region. Small nodular calcifications may persist. **viral p.,** pneumonia caused by a virus, as by adenoviruses, influenza virus, parainfluenza virus, and varicella virus; see also *influenza virus p.* and *primary atypical p.* **wandering p.,** migratory p. **white p.,** p. alba. **woolsorter's p.,** pulmonary anthrax.

pneumonic (nu-mon'ik) [Gr. *pneumonikos*] pertaining to the lung or to pneumonia; see also under *plague.*

pneumonitis (nu″mo-ni'tis) [Gr. *pneumōn* lung + *-itis*] inflammation of the lungs. **acute interstitial p.,** primary atypical pneumonia. **aspiration p.,** aspiration pneumonia. **chemical p.,** pneumonitis caused by the inhalation of chemical irritants; the extent of the injury reflects the concentration of the irritants and the duration of exposure. **cholesterol p.,** pneumonitis characterized by chronic inflammatory changes and deposition of excessive amounts of cholesterol in the tissues. It is often lobar or segmental in distribution and may resemble primary or metastatic tumor. **feline p.,** a fatal pneumonia with conjunctivitis in cats, caused by a strain of *Chlamydia psittaci.* **granulomatous p.,** inflammation of the lung which may result from inhalation of organic dusts by persons who have become sensitized to antigens in the dusts. The term is sometimes used to designate farmer's lung. **hypersensitivity p.,** allergic alveolitis. **lymphocytic interstitial p.,** an insidious, slowly progressive interstitial lung disease of unknown etiology, marked by diffuse peribronchial and interstitial infiltration of the lungs by lymphocytes, plasma cells, and lymphoblasts; in many cases it is associated with immunodeficiency disease or a disorder of immune regulation, occurring frequently in children with the acquired immune deficiency syndrome. Called also *lymphoid interstitial pneumonia.* **malarial p.,** pneumonitis caused by *Plasmodium falciparum,* characterized by cough with bloody sputum and coarse rales; in severe cases thromboses may result from the agglutination of parasitized erythrocytes in small blood vessels of the lung. **mouse p.,** a bronchopneumonia of laboratory mice caused by a strain of *Chlamydia trachomatis.* **pneumocystis p.,** interstitial plasma cell pneumonia. **uremic p.,** pneumonitis associated with uremia; a butterfly or bat-wing configuration of opacities as seen on the chest roentgenogram is indicative of pulmonary edema.

pneumon(o)- [Gr. *pneumon* lung] a combining form denoting relationship to the lungs.

pneumonocele (nu-mon'o-sēl) pneumatocele.

pneumonocentesis (nu-mo″no-sen-te'sis) [*pneumono-* + Gr. *kentesis* puncture] surgical puncture of a lung.

pneumonocirrhosis (nu-mo″no-sĭ-ro'sis) [Gr. *pneumōn* lung + *cirrhosis*] cirrhosis, or hardening, of a lung; pulmonary fibrosis.

pneumonococcus (nu″mo-no-kok'us) pneumococcus.

pneumonoconiosis (nu-mo″no-ko-ne-o'sis) pneumoconiosis.

pneumonocyte (nu-mon'o-sīt) a collective term for the alveolar epithelial cells types I and II alveolar cells) and alveolar phagocytes of the lungs. **granular p.,** type II alveolar cell. **membranous p.,** type I alveolar cell.

pneumonoenteritis (nu-mo″no-en″ter-i'tis) pneumoenteritis.

pneumonoerysipelas (nu-mo″no-er″ĭ-sip'ĕ-las) pneumoerysipelas.

pneumonograph (nu-mon'o-graf) a roentgenogram of the lungs.

pneumonography (nu″mo-nog'rah-fe) [*pneumono-* + Gr. *graphein* to write] roentgenography of the lungs.

pneumonokoniosis (nu-mo″no-ko′ne-o′sis) pneumoconiosis.

pneumonolipoidosis (nu-mo″no-lip″oi-do′sis) [*pneumono-* + Gr. *lipos* fat + *-osis*] see *lipoid pneumonia*, under *pneumonia*.

pneumonolysis (nu″mo-nol′ĭ-sis) [*pneumono-* + Gr. *lysis* dissolution] division of the tissues attaching the lung to the wall of the chest cavity, to permit collapse of the lung; formerly used to treat tuberculosis.

pneumonomelanosis (nu-mo″no-mel″ah-no′sis) [*pneumono-* + Gr. *melas* black + *-osis*] melanosis of the lung tissue.

pneumonometer (nu″mo-nom′ĕ-ter) [*pneumono-* + Gr. *metron* measure] a form of spirometer.

pneumonomoniliasis (nu-mo″no-mo″nĭ-li′ah-sis) moniliasis (candidiasis) of the lungs.

pneumonomycosis (nu-mo″no-mi-ko′sis) pneumomycosis.

pneumonopaludism (nu-mo″no-pal′u-dizm) pneumopaludism.

pneumonopathy (nu″mo-nop′ah-the) [*pneumono-* + Gr. *pathos* disease] any disease of the lung. **eosinophilic p.,** Löffler's syndrome, or other conditions associated with eosinophilic infiltration of the lung parenchyma.

pneumonopexy (nu-mo′no-pek″se) [*pneumono-* + Gr. *pexis* fixation] surgical fixation of the lung to the thoracic wall.

pneumonophthisis (nu″mon-of-thi′sis) pulmonary tuberculosis.

pneumonopleuritis (nu-mo″no-ploo-ri′tis) pneumopleuritis.

pneumonoresection (nu-mo″no-re-sek′shun) surgical resection of a portion of the lung.

pneumonorrhagia (nu-mo″no-ra′je-ah) pneumorrhagia.

pneumonorrhaphy (nu″mo-nor′ah-fe) [*pneumono-* + Gr. *rhaphē* suture] suture of the lung.

pneumonosis (nu″mo-no′sis) [*pneumo-* + Gr. *nosos* disease] any lung disease.

pneumonotherapy (nu-mo″no-ther′ah-pe) treatment of disease of the lung.

pneumonotomy (nu″mo-not′o-me) [*pneumono-* + Gr. *tomē* a cutting] surgical incision of the lung.

Pneumonyssoides (nu″mo-nis-oi′dēz) a genus of mites. *P. cani′num* is found in the sinuses and nasal passages of dogs.

Pneumonyssus (nu″mo-nis′us) a genus of mites. *P. simicola* is found in the lungs of monkeys.

pneumopaludism (nu″mo-pal′u-dizm) [*pneumo-* + L. *palus* swamp] disease of the lungs of malarial origin.

pneumopathy (nu-mop′ah-the) pneumonopathy.

pneumopericardium (nu″mo-per″ĭ-kar′de-um) [*pneumo-* + *pericardium*] the presence of air or gas in the cavity of the pericardium.

pneumoperitoneal (nu″mo-per″ĭ-to-ne′al) pertaining to or characterized by pneumoperitoneum.

pneumoperitoneum (nu″mo-per″ĭ-to-ne′um) [*pneumo-* + *peritoneum*] the presence of gas or air in the peritoneal cavity; it may occur spontaneously, as in subphrenic abscess, or be deliberately introduced as an aid to radiologic examination and diagnosis (*diagnostic p.*).

pneumoperitonitis (nu″mo-per″ĭ-to-ni′tis) [*pneumo-* + *peritonitis*] peritonitis with the accumulation of air or gas in the peritoneal cavity.

pneumopexy (nu″mo-pek″se) pneumonopexy.

pneumophagia (nu″mo-fa′je-ah) [*pneumo-* + Gr. *phagein* to eat + *-ia*] aerophagia.

pneumophonia (nu″mo-fo′ne-ah) a form of dysphonia characterized by a breathy voice.

pneumopleuritis (nu″mo-ploo-ri′tis) inflammation of the lungs and pleura.

pneumoprecordium (nu″mo-pre-kor′de-um) the presence of air in the precordial space.

pneumopreperitoneum (nu″mo-pre-per″ĭ-to-ne′um) the presence of air or gas in the preperitoneal space; it may occur spontaneously or be deliberately introduced as an aid to radiologic examination and diagnosis.

pneumopyelography (nu″mo-pi″ĕ-log′rah-fe) [*pneumo-* + Gr. *pyelos* pelvis + *graphein* to write] pyelography in which oxygen or air, instead of an opaque solution, is injected into the renal pelvis.

pneumopyopericardium (nu″mo-pi″o-per″ĭ-kar′de-um) [*pneumo-* + Gr. *pyon* pus + *pericardium*] the presence of air or gas and pus in the pericardium.

pneumopyothorax (nu″mo-pi″o-tho′raks) [*pneumo-* + Gr. *pyon* pus + *thōrax* thorax] the presence of air and pus in the pleural cavity, usually due to empyema and bronchopleural fistula.

pneumorachicentesis (nu″mo-ra″ke-sen-te′sis) [*pneumo-* + Gr. *rhachis* spine + *kentēsis* puncture] the introduction of air or gas into the spinal canal as a contrast medium for roentgen examination.

pneumorachis (nu″mo-ra′kis) [*pneumo-* + Gr. *rhachis* spine] 1. the presence of a gaseous collection in the spinal cord. 2. the injection of gas into the spinal canal for the facilitation of roentgenological examination.

pneumoradiography (nu″mo-ra″de-og′rah-fe) [*pneumo-* + *radiography*] radiography of a part following the injection of air or oxygen, as in pneumoperitoneum.

pneumoresection (nu″mo-re-sek′shun) pneumonoresection.

pneumoretroperitoneum (nu″mo-re″tro-per″ĭ-to-ne′um) the presence of air or gas in the retroperitoneal space.

pneumoroentgenogram (nu″mo-rent-gen′o-gram) a roentgenogram of a part after the injection of air or gas into it.

pneumoroentgenography (nu″mo-rent″gen-og′rah-fe) roentgenography of a part into which air or gas has been injected.

pneumorrhagia (nu″mo-ra′je-ah) [*pneumo-* + Gr. *rhēgnynai* to burst forth] hemorrhage from the lungs; severe hemoptysis.

pneumosepticemia (nu″mo-sep″tĭ-se′me-ah) pneumonia of an extreme and fatal form associated with septicemia.

pneumoserosa (nu″mo-se-ro′sah) injection of air into a joint cavity for roentgenoscopy.

pneumoserothorax (nu″mo-se″ro-tho′raks) [*pneumo-* + *serum* + Gr. *thōrax* thorax] the presence of gas and serum in the thoracic cavity.

pneumosilicosis (nu″mo-sil″ĭ-ko′sis) the deposition of silica-bearing particles of foreign matter in the lungs; silicosis.

pneumotachograph (nu″mo-tak′o-graf) pneumotachygraph.

pneumotachometer (nu″mo-tak-om′ĕ-ter) a transducer used in measuring expired air flow.

pneumotachygraph (nu″mo-tak′e-graf) [*pneumo-* + Gr. *tachys* swift + *graphein* to write] an instrument for recording the velocity of the respired air.

pneumotaxic (nu″mo-tak′sik) [*pneumo-* + Gr. *taxis* arrangement] relating to the regulation of the rate of respiration; see under *center*.

pneumotherapy (nu″mo-ther′ah-pe) 1. pneumatotherapy. 2. the treatment of diseases of the lungs.

pneumothermomassage (nu″mo-ther″mo-mah-sahzh′) [*pneumo-* + Gr. *thermē* heat + *massage*] the application to the body of hot condensed air that has been medicated.

pneumothorax (nu″mo-tho′raks) [*pneumo-* + Gr. *thōrax* thorax] an accumulation of air or gas in the pleural space, which may occur spontaneously or as a result of trauma or a pathological process, or be introduced deliberately. See *artificial p.* and *diagnostic p.* **artificial p.,** pneumothorax induced intentionally by artificial means; formerly used to allow the lung to collapse in treatment of pulmonary tuberculosis. **clicking p.,** pneumothorax in which the patient is conscious of a clicking sound synchronous with the heart beat. Cf. *precordial knock*, under *knock*. **closed p.,** pneumothorax in which pulmonary air leaks into the pleural cavity through a wound in a lung. **diagnostic p.,** temporary artificial pneumothorax employed for the purpose of clearly demonstrating the parietal or visceral pleura on chest films in order to detect and localize tumors of the pleura. **extrapleural p.,** production of collapse of the lung by formation of an air pocket by stripping the pleural layers from the inner surface of the ribs and intercostal muscle sheaths. **induced p.,** artificial p. **open p.,** pneumothorax in which the pleural cavity is exposed to the atmosphere through an open wound in the chest wall. **pressure p.,** tension p. **tension p.,** closed pneumothorax in which the tissues surrounding the opening into the pleural cavity act as valves, allowing air to enter but not to escape. The resultant positive pressure in the cavity displaces the mediastinum to the opposite side, with consequent embarrassment of respiration. Called also *pressure p.* **therapeutic p.,** artificial p. **valvular p.,** pneumothorax in which an aperture in the pleura has a valvelike action.

pneumotomography (nu″mo-to-mog′rah-fe) body section radiography performed after injection of air or other gas into the region or organ being visualized roentgenographically.

pneumotomy (nu-mot′o-me) pneumonotomy.

pneumotropic (nu″mo-trop′ik) 1. having a selective affinity for pulmonary tissue; exerting its principal effect upon the lungs. 2. having a selective affinity for pneumococci.

pneumotropism (nu-mot′ro-pizm) the predilection of an agent or organism for lung tissue.

pneumotympanum (nu″mo-tim′pah-num) air in the middle ear.

pneumouria (nu″mo-u′re-ah) pneumaturia.

Pneumovax (nu″mo-vaks″) trademark for a pneumococcal vaccine containing capsular polysaccharides (antigens) from 14 types of pneumococci. **P. 23,** trademark for a pneumococcal vaccine containing capsular polysaccharides from 23 types of pneumococci.

pneumoventricle (nu″mo-ven′trĭ-k'l) pneumoventriculi.

pneumoventriculi (nu″mo-ven-trik′u-li) [*pneumo-* + L. *ventriculus* ventricle] presence of air in the cerebral ventricles.

pneumoventriculography (nu″mo-ven-trik″u-log′rah-fe) roentgenography of the cerebral ventricles after the injection of air or gas; see *ventriculography.*

pneusis (nu′sis) [Gr. *pneusis* a blowing] respiration.

PNH paroxysmal nocturnal hemoglobinuria.

P.O. abbreviation for L. *per os,* by mouth, orally.

Po chemical symbol for *polonium.*

POA pancreatic oncofetal antigen.

PO₂ symbol for *oxygen partial pressure (tension);* also written P_{O_2}, pO_2, and pO_2.

Pocill. abbreviation for L. *pocil′lum,* a small cup.

pock (pok) a pustule, especially one of the lesions of smallpox.

pocket (pok′et) a saclike space or cavity. **complex p.,** a spiral type of periodontal pocket involving more than one surface of the tooth, but communicating with the gingival margin only along the surface at which it originates. **compound p.,** a periodontal pocket involving more than one tooth surface, and communicating with the marginal gingiva along each of the involved surfaces. **endocardial p's,** sclerotic thickenings of the mural endocardium, occurring most often on the left ventricular septum below an insufficient aortic valve; called also *regurgitant p's* and *birds' nests.* **gingival p.,** a gingival sulcus deepened by pathological conditions, caused by gingival enlargement with no destruction of the periodontal tissue. Called also *relative p.* **infrabony p., intra-alveolar p.,** intrabony p. **intrabony p.,** intrabony p., a periodontal pocket in which the bottom is apical to the level of the adjacent alveolar bone. **periodontal p.,** a gingival sulcus deepened into the periodontal ligament apically to the original level of the resorbed alveolar crest. **Rathke's p.,** see under *pouch.* **regurgitant p's,** endocardial p's. **relative p.,** gingival p. **Seessel's p.,** see under *pouch.* **simple p.,** a periodontal pocket involving only one tooth surface. **subcrestal p.,** intrabony p. **suprabony p., supracrestal p.,** a periodontal pocket in which the bottom is coronal to the underlying bone. **p's of Zahn,** shallow pockets with miniature leaflets, resembling cusps of the semilunar valve, produced in the endocardium of the left ventricle by the regurgitant aortic stream in the presence of insufficiency of the aortic valve.

pockmark (pok′mark) a depressed scar left by a pustule, especially one left by a lesion of smallpox.

Pocul. abbreviation for L. *poc′ulum,* cup.

poculum (pok′u-lum) [L.] cup. **p. Diog′enis** ["Diogenes' cup"], the concave palm of the hand.

podagra (po-dag′rah) [*pod-* + Gr. *agra* seizure] gouty pain in the great toe.

podagral (pod′ah-gral) pertaining to or characterized by podagra.

podagric (po-dag′rik) podagral.

podagrous (pod′ah-grus) podagral.

podalgia (po-dal′je-ah) [*pod-* + *-algia*] pain in the foot, as from gout or rheumatism.

podalic (po-dal′ik) [Gr. *pous* foot] pertaining to or accomplished by means of the feet; see under *version.*

Podalirius (po″dah-lir′e-us) the younger of two brothers, the older being Machaon, who were the sons of Aesculapius and the chief physicians to the Greeks during the Trojan war.

Podangium (po-dan′je-um) *Melittangium.*

podarthritis (pod″ar-thri′tis) [*pod-* + *arthritis*] inflammation of the joints of the feet.

podedema (pod″e-de′mah) edema of the feet.

podencephalus (pod″en-sef′ah-lus) [*pod-* + Gr. *enkephalos* brain] a fetus whose brain, without a cranium, hangs by a pedicle.

podia (po′de-ah) [L.] plural of *podium.*

podiatric (po″dĭ-at′rik) pertaining to podiatry.

podiatrist (po-di′ah-trist) a specialist in podiatry; formerly called *chiropodist.*

podiatry (po-di′ah-tre) [Gr. *pous* foot + *iatreia* healing] the specialized field that deals with the study and care of the foot, including its anatomy, pathology, medical and surgical treatment, etc. Formerly called *chiropody.*

podium (po′de-um), pl. po′dia [L.] a footlike projection; a sucker foot; see under *foot.*

pod(o)- [Gr. *pous,* gen. *podos* foot] a combining form denoting relationship to the foot.

podocyte (pod′o-sīt) [*podo-* + Gr. *kytos* hollow vessel] a modified epithelial cell of the visceral layer (*capsular epithelium*) of the renal glomerulus, having a small perikaryon and a number of primary and secondary footlike radiating processes (pedicels) which interdigitate with those of other podocytes and which embrace the basal lamina of glomerular capillaries.

pododerm (pod′o-derm) [*podo-* + Gr. *derma* skin] that portion of the skin which is continued downward within the horn capsule of the hoof of an animal.

pododynamometer (pod″o-di″nah-mom′ĕ-ter) a device for determining the strength of the leg muscles.

pododynia (pod″o-din′e-ah) [*podo-* + Gr. *odynē* pain] neuralgic pain of the heel and sole; burning pain without redness in the sole of the foot.

podogram (pod′o-gram) [*podo-* + Gr. *gramma* mark] a print of, or an outline tracing of, the sole of the foot.

podograph (pod′o-graf) [*podo-* + Gr. *graphein* to write] the instrument used in the making of a podogram.

podology (po-dol′o-je) [*podo-* + *-logy*] podiatry.

podophyllin (pod″o-fil′in) see *podophyllum resin,* under *resin.*

podophyllotoxin (pod″o-fil″o-tok′sin) a highly toxic compound, $C_{22}H_{22}O_8$, the main active component of podophyllum; it has cathartic and antineoplastic properties.

podophyllous (po-dof′ĭ-lus) [*podo-* + Gr. *phyllon* leaf] designating the tissues which constitute the sensitive wall of the hoofs of animals.

Podophyllum (pod″o-fil′um) [*podo-* + Gr. *phyllon* leaf] a genus of perennial North American herbs, including *P. peltatum* L. (Berberidaceae), which is the source of podophyllum resin.

podophyllum (pod″o-fil′um) [USP] the dried rhizome and roots of *Podophyllum peltatum* L. (Berberidaceae), yielding not less than 5 per cent of resin (see under *resin*); its main active component is podophyllotoxin. Called also *Indian apple, mandrake, mandrake root, May apple,* and *vegetable calomel.*

podotrochilitis (pod″o-tro-kĭ-li′tis) [*podo-* + Gr. *trochilea* pulley + *-itis*] inflammation of the navicular bone of the horse's foot.

poe- for words beginning thus, see those beginning *pe-.*

poecil(o)- for words beginning thus, see also those beginning *poikil(o)-.*

Poecilia (pe-sil′e-ah) a genus of minnows; called also *Girardinus.* **P. reticula′ta,** a species used, especially in tropical America, to control mosquitoes; they eat the larvae of *Anopheles*. Called also *Girardinus poeciloides*.

pogoniasis (po″go-ni′ah-sis) [Gr. *pōgōn* beard + *-iasis*] 1. excessive growth of the beard. 2. the growth of a beard upon a woman.

pogonion (po-go′ne-on) [Gr., dim. of *pōgōn* beard] a craniometric landmark, being the most anterior point in the contour of the chin in the sagittal plane.

pOH an infrequently used symbol used in expressing the approximate concentration of hydroxide ions in a solution.

Pohl's test (polz) [Julius Heinrich *Pohl*, German pharmacologist, born 1861] see under *tests*.

poi (poi) a Hawaiian food made from the root of the taro plant, *Colocasia esculenta* (L.) Schott., Araceae. It is used as a cereal substitute for allergic infants.

-poiesis [Gr. *poiein* to make] a word termination meaning formation, as in hematopoiesis.

poietin (poi-e′tin) any of the hormones involved in regulation of the numbers of various cell types in the peripheral blood.

poikil(o)- [Gr. *poikilos* spotted, mottled; varied] a combining form meaning mottled, variable, or irregular.

poikiloblast (poi′kĭ-lo-blast″) [*poikilo-* + Gr. *blastos* germ] an abnormally shaped erythroblast.

poikilocarynosis (poi″kĭ-lo-kar″ĭ-no′sis) [*poikilo-* + Gr. *karyon* nucleus + *-osis*] Darier's term for the formation of various types and arrangements of cells which occurs in Bowen's disease.

poikilocyte (poi′kĭ-lo-sīt″) [*poikilo-* + *-cyte*] an erythrocyte showing abnormal variation in shape.

poikilocythemia (poi-kil″o-si-the′me-ah) poikilocytosis.

poikilocytosis (poi″kĭ-lo-si-to′sis) [*poikilocyte* + *-osis*] presence in the blood of erythrocytes showing abnormal variation in shape.

poikiloderma (poi″kĭ-lo-der′mah) a condition characterized by pigmentary and atrophic changes in the skin, giving it a mottled appearance. **p. atroph′icans vascula′re,** p. vasculare atrophicans. **p. of Civatte,** a skin condition seen almost exclusively on sun-exposed areas in middle-aged women, manifested as a reticulated blotchy reddish brown hyperpigmentation and telangiectasia with interspersed atrophic pale puncta localized to the face, neck, and upper chest, and believed to be associated with some type of photosensitivity mechanism. **p. congenita′le,** Rothmund-Thomson syndrome. **p. vascula′re atroph′icans,** a localized or generalized, chronic, slightly scaling, patchy dermatitis characterized by hyper- and hypopigmentation, atrophy, telangiectases, and sometimes bright red papules, and an erythematous cigarette paper–like appearance of the skin resembling radiodermatitis, which usually occurs symmetrically on the breasts, buttocks, and flexural areas. It may be idiopathic or occur as a manifestation of various other dermatoses. It responds to treatment with systemic antibiotics. Called also *p. atrophicans vasculare*.

poikilonymy (poi″kĭ-lon′ĭ-me) [*poikilo-* + Gr. *onoma* name] the mingling of names or terms from different systems of nomenclature.

poikiloploid (poi′kĭ-lo-ploid″) [*poikilo-* + *-ploid*] 1. pertaining to or characterized by poikiloploidy. 2. an individual having different cells with varying numbers of chromosomes.

poikiloploidy (poi′kĭ-lo-ploi″de) the state of having varying numbers of chromosomes in different cells.

poikilosmosis (poi″kil-oz-mo′sis) the processes by which a cell or tissue adjusts the osmolarity of its fluid to that of its immediate environment.

poikilosmotic (poi″kil-oz-mot′ik) pertaining to poikilosmosis.

poikilostasis (poi″kĭ-lo-sta′sis) [*poikilo-* + Gr. *stasis* standing] the maintenance of stability in the body state (internal environment) by behavioral activities involving movement and selection by the whole organism.

poikilotherm (poi-kil′o-therm″) [*poikilo-* + Gr. *thermē* heat] 1. an animal that exhibits poikilothermy; a so-called cold-blooded animal. 2. ectotherm.

poikilothermal (poi″ki-lo-ther′mal) poikilothermic.

poikilothermic (poi″kĭ-lo-ther′mik) 1. pertaining to or characterized by poikilothermy. 2. ectothermic.

poikilothermism (poi″kĭ-lo-ther′mizm) poikilothermy.

poikilothermy (poi″kĭ-lo-ther′me) [*poikilo-* + Gr. *thermē* heat] 1. the exhibition of body temperature which varies with the environmental temperature. 2. the ability of organisms to adapt themselves to variations in the temperature of their environment. Cf. homeothermy (def. 1). 3. ectothermy.

poikilothrombocyte (poi-kil″o-throm′bo-sīt) [*poikilo-* + *thrombocyte*] a blood platelet of abnormal shape.

poikilothymia (poi″kĭ-lo-thi′me-ah) [*poikilo-* + Gr. *thymos* spirit] a mental condition characterized by abnormal variations of mood.

poin (poin) an uncharacterized antibiotic material produced by the fungus *Fusarium sporotrichiella* var. *paoe* Bilai, and cultured from cases involving septic tonsillitis. It is active against staphylococci and streptococci *in vitro*.

point (point) [L. *punctum*] 1. a small area or spot; the sharp end of an object. 2. to approach the surface, like the pus of an abscess, at a definite spot or place. 3. a tapered, pointed endodontic instrument used for exploring the depth of the root canal in root canal therapy; called also *root canal p.* 4. an anthropometric landmark from which measurements are made. 5. an elongated silver or gutta-percha cone used in root canal obturation. **p. A,** subspinale. **absorbent p.,** an endodontic cone of variable width and taper, usually made of paper or a paper product, used to dry or maintain a liquid disinfectant in the root canal of a tooth. Called also *paper p.* **Addison's p.,** the midpoint of the epigastric region. **alveolar p.,** the center of the anterior margin of the alveolar arch. **apophysiary p.,** 1. subnasal point. 2. see *Trousseau's apophysiary points*. **p. Ar,** articulare. **p. of Arrhigi,** an electrode site in electrocardiography, 2 to 3 cm. to the left of the seventh thoracic vertebra. **auricular p.,** the center of the opening of the external auditory meatus; called also *Broca's point*. **p. B,** supramentale. **p. Ba,** basion. **Barker's p.,** a point 1¼ inches above and 1¼ inches behind the middle external auditory meatus, the proper spot to apply the trephine in abscess of the temporosphenoid lobe. **p. Bo,** Bolton p. **Boas' p.,** a tender area to the left of the twelfth thoracic vertebra in patients with gastric ulcer. **boiling p.,** the temperature at which a liquid will boil (at sea level water boils at 100° C., or 212° F.); specifically, the temperature at which the equilibrium vapor pressure of a liquid phase equals the atmospheric pressure. **boiling p., normal,** the temperature at which a liquid boils at one standard atmosphere pressure. **Bolton p.,** a craniometric landmark located at the top of the convex curvature of the retrocondylar fossa, posterior to the condyle and between it and the basal surface of the occipital bone. Called also *point Bo*. **Brewer's p.,** the point of the costovertebral angle, tenderness over which points to kidney infection. **Broadbent registration p.,** the midpoint of the perpendicular from the center of the sella turcica to the Bolton plane. Called also *p. R*. **Broca's p.,** auricular p. **Cannon's p.,** see under *ring*. **cardinal p's,** 1. principal points; points on the optic axis which include the nodal points, the principal foci, and the optic center; may include conjugate focal points of object and image. 2. four points within the pelvic inlet—the two sacroiliac articulations and the two iliopectineal eminences. **Chauffard's p.,** a point of tenderness in gallbladder disease, situated under the right clavicle. **cold rigor p.,** that point of low temperature at which the activity of a cell ceases. **conjugate p.,** conjugate focus. **contact p.,** see under *area*. **convenience p.,** a small depression at the edge of the floor of the prepared cavity, placed there to retain the first piece of direct filling gold during the process of compaction. **p. of convergence,** 1. the point at which the lines of sight cross. 2. the point to which rays of light incline. **corresponding p's,** points upon the two retinae whose impressions unite to produce a single perception. Cf. *disparate p's*. **Cova's p.,** a point at the apex of the costolumbar angle which is tender on pressure in cases of pyelitis of pregnancy. **craniometric p.,** any one of a numerous set of points of reference assumed for use in craniometry. **critical p.,** the temperature at or above which a gas cannot be liquefied by pressure alone. **deaf p.,** one of certain points near the ear where a vibrating tuning-fork cannot be heard. **de Mussy's p.,** a point, exceedingly painful on pressure on the line of the left border of the sternum, at the level of the end of the tenth rib; it is a symptom of diaphragmatic pleurisy. **Desjardins' p.,** a point on the abdomen 5 to 7 cm. from the umbilicus, on a line joining it to the right axilla; it lies over the head of the pancreas. **dew p.,** the temperature of the atmosphere at which the moisture begins to be deposited as dew. **p. of direction,** see *position,* def. 2. **disparate p's,** points on the retina which are not paired exactly. Cf. *corresponding p's.* **p. of dispersion,** in optics, the virtual focus. **p. of divergence,** the conjugate focus from which the light proceeds. **dorsal p.,** in hepatic colic, a point, tender on pressure, situated between the spinous processes of the vertebrae at the border of the right scapula at the level of the fourth and fifth intercostal spaces at a distance of about 2 or 3 cm. from the middle line. Called also *Pauly's p.* **p's douloureux** (pwă doo-loo-ruh′) [Fr.], Valleix's p's. **p. of election,** that point at which any particular surgical operation is done by preference. **Erb's p.,** a point two or three centimeters above the clavicle and beyond the posterior border of the sternomastoid, at the level of the transverse process of the sixth cervical vertebra; stimulation here contracts various arm muscles. **eye p.,** 1. the bright circle seen at the crossing point or nearest the approximation of the rays above the microscopical ocular. 2. See under *spot.* **far p.,** the remotest point at which an object is clearly seen when the eye is at rest; called also *punctum remotum.* **p. of fixation,** 1. the point or object on which one's sight is fixed and through which the axis opticus passes; called also *p. of regard.* 2. the point on the retina, usually the fovea, on which are focused the rays coming from an object directly regarded. **focal p.,** see *focus* (def. 1), and *cardinal p.* (def. 1). **freezing p.,** the temperature at which a liquid begins to freeze; that of pure water is 0° C., or 32° F. **fusion p.,** melting point. **glenoid p.,** the center of the glenoid cavity of the scapula. **Guéneau de Mussy's p.,** see *de Mussy's p.* **gutta-percha p.,** see under *cone.* **Hallé's p.,** a point on the surface of the abdomen corresponding to the point where the ureter crosses the pelvic brim. It is the point of intersection between a horizontal line connecting the anterior superior iliac spines and a vertical line projected upward from the pubic spine. **Hartmann's p., Hartmann's critical p.,** p. of Sudeck. **hinge-axis p.,** a reference point on the skin corresponding with the terminal hinge axis of the mandible. **hysteroepileptogenous p., hysterogenic p.,** a point on which, if pressure be made, a hysteric or hysteroepileptic attack may be produced. **ice p.,** the temperature of equilibrium between ice and air-saturated water under one atmosphere pressure. **identical p's,** corresponding p's. **p. of incidence,** see *refraction,* def. 2. **isobestic p.,** the wavelength at which two intercovertible substances (e.g., oxyhemoglobin and reduced hemoglobin) have the same absorptivity. **isoelectric p.,** the pH of a solution at which a charged molecule does not migrate in an electric field. **isoionic p.,** the pH of a solution at which a specific ion (usually a protein) contains as many negative charges as positive charges. **jugal p.,** the point of the angle formed by the masseteric and maxillary edges of the malar bone (os zygomaticum). **jugomaxillary p.,** the point at the anteroinferior angle of the malar bone (os zygomaticum). **Keen's p.,** a point for puncture of the lateral ventricles; 3 cm. above and 3 cm. behind the external auditory meatus. **Kienböck-Adamson p's,** points and lines to be marked on the scalp to indicate the areas for the application of x-ray therapy in order to produce temporary epilation for the treatment of tinea capitis. **Kocher's p.,** a point for puncture of the lateral ventricles; 2.5 cm. from the midline, 3.5 cm. in front of the bregma. **Krafft p.,** the temperature above which conjugated bile salts form polymolecular aggregates (micelles) of about 3 to 10 nm. in diameter. **lacrimal p.,** the punctum lacrimale; any of the outlets of the lacrimal canaliculi. **Lanz's p.,** a point which indicates the position of the vermiform appendix; it is situated on a line connecting the two anterior superior iliac spines one third of the distance from the right spine. **leak p.,** renal threshold for glucose; see under *threshold.* **McBurney's p.,** a point situated about one-third the distance between the right anterior superior iliac spine and the umbilicus. It corresponds with the normal position of the base of the appendix and is a point of special tenderness in acute appendicitis. **McEwen's p.,** a point above the inner canthus of the eye which is tender in acute frontal sinusitis. **Mackenzie's p.,** a point of tenderness in gallbladder disease in the upper segment of the rectus muscle. **malar p.,** a point on the external tubercle of the malar bone (os zygomaticum). **p. of maximal impulse,** the point on the chest where the impulse of the left ventricle

is felt most strongly, normally in the fifth costal interspace inside the left mamillary line; abbreviated P.M.I. **maximum occipital p.,** the point in the occipital bone situated furthest from the glabella. **median mandibular p.,** a craniometric landmark, being the point on the anteroposterior center of the mandibular ridge in the median sagittal plane, at the site of former mandibular symphysis. **Méglin's p.,** a point where the greater palatine nerve emerges from the great palatine foramen. **melting p.,** the minimum temperature at which a solid begins to liquefy. **mental p.,** pogonion. **metopic p.,** glabella. **motor p.,** 1. the point at which a motor nerve enters a muscle. 2. any point on the skin over a muscle at which the application of galvanic stimulation will cause contraction of a corresponding muscle. **Munro's p.,** a point midway between the umbilicus and the left anterior iliac spine, used for performing abdominal puncture. **Mussy's p.,** see *de Mussy's p.* **nasal p.,** nasion. **near p.,** the nearest point at which the eye can distinctly perceive an object; the nearest point of clear vision; called also *punctum proximum.* **near p., absolute,** the near point for either eye alone with accommodation relaxed. **near p., relative,** the near point for both eyes with the employment of accommodation. **nodal p's,** one of two points on the axis of an optical system so situated that a ray falling on one will produce a parallel ray emerging through the other. **occipital p.,** the posterior point on the occipital bone. **ossification p.,** punctum ossificationis. **ossification p., primary,** punctum ossificationis primarium. **ossification p., secondary,** punctum ossificationis secundum. **painful p's,** Valleix's p's. **paper p.,** absorbent p. **Pauly's p.,** dorsal p. **phrenic-pressure p.,** a point along the phrenic nerve between the sternocleidomastoid and the scalenus anticus on the right side; pressure on the point suggests gallbladder disease. **Piersol's p.,** a point indicating the location of the vesical orifice. **pour p.,** the temperature at which a liquid just begins to flow. **preauricular p.,** a point on the posterior root of the zygomatic arch just in front of the auricular point. **pressure p.,** 1. a point of extreme sensibility to pressure. 2. one of various locations on the body at which digital pressure may be applied for the control of hemorrhage. **pressure-arresting p.,** a point at which pressure arrests spasm. **pressure-exciting p.,** a point at which pressure produces spasm. **principal p's,** cardinal p's, def. 1. **p. R,** Broadbent registration p. **Ramond's p.,** a point of tenderness in gallbladder disease between the heads of the sternocleidomastoid muscle. **reflection p.,** the point from which a ray of light is reflected. **refraction p.,** the point at which a ray of light is refracted. **p. of regard,** p. of fixation (def. 1). **retromandibular tender p.,** a point behind the superior extremity of the inferior maxilla below the lobule of the ear and in front of the mastoid process. Pressure on this point elicits extreme pain in meningitis. **Robson's p.,** the point of greatest tenderness in gallbladder inflammation, situated opposite the junction of the middle and lower third of a line drawn from the right nipple to the umbilicus. **root canal p.,** point, def. 3. **p. SE,** sphenoethmoidal suture (def. 2). **set p.,** see under *S.* **silver p.,** a tapered and elongated silver plug that is cemented into the root canal in endodontic therapy as a root canal filling. Called also *silver cone.* **p. SO,** spheno-occipital synchondrosis (def. 2). **spinal p.,** subnasal p. **stereoidentical p's,** points in space outside of the region within which fusion of double images occurs. **subnasal p.,** the central point of the root of the anterior nasal spine. **subtemporal p.,** the point where the sphenotemporal suture and infratemporal crest intersect. **Sudeck's critical p., p. of Sudeck,** the portion of the rectum between the last sigmoid artery and the bifurcation of the superior hemorrhoidal artery; the former belief that ligation of the latter below this point would lead to gangrene of the rectum has not been borne out by clinical experience. Called also *Hartmann's p.* **supra-auricular p.,** a point at the root of the zygomatic process of the temporal bone, directly above the auricular point. **supraclavicular p.,** a point above the clavicle and outside of the sternomastoid where the application of a stimulus causes contraction of the biceps brachii, deltoideus, brachialis, and brachioradialis muscles. **supranasal p.,** ophryon. **supraorbital p.,** 1. the ophryon. 2. in neuralgia, a tender spot just above the supraorbital notch. **sylvian p.,** a point on the surface of the skull from 29 to 32 mm. behind the external angular process of the frontal bone. **thermal death p.,** the lowest temperature at which a broth culture of microorganisms can be heat-killed in a 10-minute exposure time. **trigger p.,** a particular spot on the body on which pressure or other stimulus will give rise to specific sensations or symptoms. **triple p.,** the temperature and pressure at which three different phases of a substance are in equilibrium. The *triple point of water* (ice, liquid, vapor) is 273.15°K. **Trousseau's apophysiary p's,** points sensitive to pressure along the dorsal and lumbar vertebrae in certain cases of neuralgia. **Valleix's p's,** tender points on the course of certain nerves in neuralgia. **vital p.,** a point in the medulla oblongata, at the respiratory center, puncture of which causes immediate death. **Vogt's p., Vogt-Hueter p.,** a point at the intersection of a horizontal line two fingerbreadths above the zygoma with a vertical line a thumb-breadth behind the ascending sphenofrontal process; here trephination may be performed in traumatic meningeal hemorrhage. **Voillemier's p.,** a point on the linea alba 6.5 cm. below the line which joins the anterior superior iliac spinous processes; here the bladder may be punctured in obese or edematous patients. **p. Z,** a point formed by a line perpendicular to the nasion-menton line through the anterior nasal spine. **Ziemssen's motor p's,** the places of entrance of motor nerves into muscles; they are points of election in the therapeutical application of electricity to muscles.

pointer (point′er) a contusion at a bony eminence. **hip p.,** contusion of the bone of the iliac crest or avulsion of muscle attachments of the iliac crest.

pointillage (pwahn″te-yahzh′) [Fr.] massage with the points of the fingers.

Poirier's glands, line (pwah-re-āz′) [Paul *Poirier*, surgeon in Paris, 1853–1907] see under *gland* and *line*.

poise (poiz; Fr. pwahz) [J. M. *Poiseuille*] the unit of viscosity of a liquid, being number of grams per centimeter per second. The commonly used unit is the *centipoise*, or one one-hundredth of a poise.

Poiseuille's law, space (pwah-zuh′yez) [Jean Leonard Marie *Poiseuille*, physiologist in Paris, 1799–1869] see under *law* and *space*.

poison (poi′zn) [L. *potio* draft] any substance which, when ingested, inhaled or absorbed, or when applied to, injected into, or developed within the body, in relatively small amounts, by its chemical action may cause damage to structure or disturbance of function. See also *toxin*. **acrid p.,** one which produces irritation or inflammation, as the mineral acids, oxalic acid, the caustic alkalis, antimony, arsenic, the salts of copper, some of the compounds of lead, silver nitrate, the salts of zinc, iodine, cantharides, phosphorus, etc. **acronarcotic p., acrosedative p.,** poisons which produce sometimes irritation, sometimes narcotism (or sedation), or both together. They are chiefly derived from the vegetable kingdom. Stramonium and belladonna are examples of the acronarcotic and aconite is an example of the acrosedative poisons. **arrow p.,** a preparation of plant alkaloids used on their arrows by members of certain primitive tribes. **catalyst p.,** a substance firmly bound to the active areas on the surface of a catalyst, which prevents the adsorption of the reactants for the desired chemical reaction. **corrosive p.,** any poison which acts by directly destroying tissue. **fatigue p.,** fatigue toxin. **fugu p.,** tetrodotoxin. **hemotropic p.,** a poison which has a special affinity for erythrocytes. **irritant p.,** acrid p. **microbial p.,** microbial toxin. **mitotic p.,** a toxic principle that interferes with cell division. **muscle p.,** one that interferes with normal action or functioning of muscle. **narcotic p's,** poisons causing stupor or delirium, as opium, hyoscyamus, etc. **paralytic shellfish p.,** gonyaulax p. **puffer p.,** tetrodotoxin. **sedative p's,** those which directly depress the vital centers, as hydrocyanic acid, potassium cyanide, hydrogen sulfide, and other of the poisonous gases. **shellfish p.,** saxitoxin; see *shellfish poisoning*, under *poisoning*. **toot p.,** a poison from *Coriaria sarmentosa*, a plant of New Zealand. **vascular p.,** a poison which acts by affecting the blood vessels. **whelk p.,** a toxic substance which is localized in the salivary gland of whelks, members of the phylum Mollusca, class Gastropoda; its principal ingredient is tetramethylammonium hydroxide. See also under *poisoning*.

poison ivy (poi′zn i′ve) *Rhus.*

poison oak (poi′zn ōk) *Rhus.*

poison sumac (poi′zn soo′mak) *Rhus.*

poisoning (poi′zuh-ning) the morbid condition produced by a poison; see also *intoxication*. **akee p.,** Jamaica vomiting sickness. **antimony p.,** poisoning due to ingestion of antimony compounds, rarely to industrial exposure; the symptoms are similar to those of acute arsenic poisoning, with vomiting a prominent symptom. **arsenic p.,** poisoning due to systemic exposure to inorganic pentavalent arsenic. *Acute arsenic poisoning*, which may result in shock and death, is marked by erythematous skin eruptions, vomiting, diarrhea, abdominal pain, muscular cramps, and swelling of the eyelids, feet, and hands. *Chronic arsenic poisoning*, due to the ingestion of small amounts over a long period of time, is marked by pigmentation of the skin accompanied by scaling, hyperkeratosis of the palms and soles, transverse white lines on the fingernails (Mees' lines), headache, peripheral neuropathy, and confusion. Called also *arsenicalism* and *arsenism*. **blood p.,** septicemia. **bongkrek p.,** see under *intoxication*. **broom p.,** poisoning caused by eating *Cytisus scoparius*, or broom, a leguminous shrub which contains both sparteine and cytisine. **callistin shellfish p.,** poisoning caused by ingestion of gastropods of the genus *Callista*, believed to be due to a choline present in large quantities in the ovaries of the shellfish; called also *esowasure-gai p.* **carbon disulfide p.,** a condition occurring in workers in rubber and viscose products caused by carbon disulfide and marked by weakness, sleeplessness, visual impairment, gastric ulcer, and paralysis. **carbon monoxide p.,** poisoning due to the inhalation of carbon monoxide and the resulting change of oxyhemoglobin to carboxyhemoglobin, which may result in damage to the central nervous system and death. **cheese p.,** tyrotoxicosis. **corncockle p.,** githagism. **cyanide p.,** poisoning due to ingestion or inhalation of cyanides, which are extremely potent, rapid-acting poisons that cause cellular hypoxia by formation of an inactive complex of cytochrome oxidase and cyanide; cyanide is detoxified by the liver enzyme rhodanese, which catalyzes the reaction of cyanide with thiosulfate to form thiocyanide. Sodium thiosulfate and sodium nitrate are used as antidotes; the latter reduces hemoglobin to methemoglobin, which has a greater affinity for cyanide than does cytochrome oxidase. **dural p.,** poisoning in aircraft workers caused by the magnesium in the aluminum-magnesium alloy (Duralumin) used in airplanes. **elasmobranch p.,** a form of ichthyosarcotoxism produced by the ingestion of certain toxic sharks and skates. **ergot p.,** ergotism. **esowasure-gai p.,** Japanese name for callistin shellfish p. **fish p.,** ichthyosarcotoxism. **fluoride p., chronic, fluorine p., chronic,** fluorosis. **food p.,** a group of illnesses, varying in severity from mild and self-limited to life threatening, caused by ingestion of contaminated food or food that is inherently poisonous. Various microorganisms are associated with food poisoning, the most common being pathogenic bacteria or their products (toxins), e.g., *Staphylococcus aureus*, *Bacillus cereus*, *Clostridium botulinum*, *C. perfringens*, *Escherichia coli*, *Vibro cholerae*, *V. parahaemolyticus*, *Shigella* species, *Salmonella* species, and *Yersinia enterocolitica*. Bacterial food poisoning is usually manifested as acute gastroenteritis but may be associated with such syndromes as botulism, typhoid fever, and cholera. Neurologic symptoms can also be caused by food poisoning as a result of ingestion of chemically toxic foods, such as certain mushrooms and berries, or may involve substances such as heavy metals, mercury, or insecticides. **forage p.,** a disease of domestic animals, especially of horses, resulting from ingestion of moldy or fermented food, or from an encephalomyelitic infection; certain forms occurring in Australia are caused by *Clostridium botulinum*. **fugu p.,** tetrodotoxism. **gossypol p.,** poisoning from eating cottonseed cake. **gymnothorax p.,** a form of ichthyosarcotoxism produced by ingestion of certain moray eels of the genus *Gymnothorax*. **heavy metal p.,** poisoning with any of the heavy metals, particularly arsenic, lead, mercury, antimony, cadmium, or thallium. **larkspur p.,** poisoning from the fresh leaves and roots of larkspur, which contain aconite. Ingestion may result in instantaneous death, probably from paralysis of the heart. **lead p.,** poisoning due to the absorption or ingestion of lead or one of its salts. The symptoms include loss of appetite, weight loss, colic, constipation, insomnia, headache, dizziness, irritability, moderate hypertension, albuminuria, anemia, a blue line at the edge of the gums (lead line), encephalopathy (especially in children), and peripheral neuropathy leading to paralysis.

Called also *plumbism.* **loco p.,** locoism. **manganese p.,** a condition usually caused by inhalation of manganese dust; symptoms include mental disorders accompanying a syndrome resembling paralysis agitans, and inflammation throughout the respiratory system. **meat p.,** acute, often severe gastroenteritis, most often caused by meat contaminated with *Bacillus cereus, Clostridium perfringens,* invasive *Escherichia coli, Salmonella, Staphylococcus aureus,* or *Yersinia enterocolitica.* **mercury p.,** acute or chronic disease caused by mercury and its salts. The *acute* form, due to ingestion, is marked by severe abdominalgia, metallic taste in the mouth, vomiting, bloody diarrhea with watery stools, oliguria or anuria (usually at onset), and corrosion and ulceration of the entire digestive tract. The *chronic* form, due to absorption by the skin and mucous membranes, inhalation of vapors, or ingestion of mercury salts, is marked by stomatitis, metallic taste in the mouth, a blue line along the border of the gum, sore hypertrophied gums that bleed easily, loosening of the teeth, erethism, excessive secretion of saliva, tremors, and incoordination. Called also *mercurialism* and *hydrargyism.* **milk p.,** trembles. **molybdenum p.,** poisoning due to ingestion of large amounts of molybdenum, characterized by weakness and diarrhea; no cases of molybdenum poisoning in man have been reported. **mushroom p.,** poisoning resulting from ingestion of poisonous mushrooms, including *Amanita verna, A. phalloides, A. muscaria,* and *A. pantherina.* The clinical course usually begins with nausea, vomiting, abdominal pain, and diarrhea, followed by a period (up to 48 hours) of improvement, and then culminating in signs and symptoms of severe hepatic, renal, and central nervous system damage. Called also *mycetismus.* **mussel p.,** see *gonyaulax poison,* under *poison.* **naphthol p.,** the toxic condition brought on by the excessive or continued use of naphthol, characterized by anemia, jaundice, convulsions, and coma. **nitroaniline p.,** poisoning by nitroaniline, a dye used in paints, paint removers, printing inks, cloth marking inks, and solvents; intense methemoglobinemia is produced. **nutmeg p.,** severe toxic symptoms produced by as little as 1 teaspoonful of powdered nutmeg; narcosis with periods of delirium and excitability may occur within 1 to 6 hours. **O₂ p.,** see under *toxicity.* **paraldehyde p.,** paraldehydism. **parathyroid p.,** the sudden increase in the extent of metastatic calcification of organs, particularly the kidneys, when a high calcium diet is given a hyperparathyroid patient. **phenol p.,** poisoning due to ingestion or absorption through the skin of phenol; the symptoms include colic, weakness, collapse, and local irritation and corrosion. Called also *carbolism.* **phosphorus p.,** a condition resulting from ingestion or inhalation of phosphorus, manifested by toothache and mandibular necrosis (phossy jaw), anorexia, weakness, and anemia. **pitch p.,** a usually fatal disorder of pigs that eat clay pigeons or lick the tarred walls and floors of pigpens, marked by inappetence, depression, weakness, jaundice, anemia. **puffer p.,** tetrodotoxism. **salmon p.,** a hemorrhagic enteritis, particularly affecting canines but which may also affect man and other animals. It is acquired by the ingestion of raw fish, especially salmon and trout, parasitized by the fluke *Troglotrema salmincola,* which serves as a vector of the etiologic agent, *Neorickettsia helminthoeca.* **salt p.,** poisoning of animals, especially pigs and birds, due to ingestion of too much salt in the absence of available water, marked by excessive thirst, diarrhea, and vomiting, often culminating in death. **saturnine p.,** lead p. **sausage p.,** see *allantiasis* and *botulism.* **scombroid p.,** a form of ichthyosarcotoxism caused by the ingestion of a toxic histamine-like substance produced by the action of bacteria on histidine, a normal component of fish flesh. Scombroid fish (tuna, bonito, mackerel, etc.) are particularly susceptible to bacterial decomposition, and when inadequately preserved contaminated fish are eaten the symptoms of the illness, including epigastric pain, nausea, vomiting, headache, dysphagia, thirst, urticaria, and pruritus, develop and usually last for less than 24 hours. **selenium p.,** a form of poisoning of livestock of the North Central Great Plains region of the United States due to the feeding on plants which have absorbed selenium from the soil and characterized by cirrhosis of the liver, anemia, loss of hair, erosions of long bones, emaciation. **shellfish p.,** an acute intoxication caused by ingestion of bivalve mollusks contaminated with the neurotoxin (saxitoxin) secreted by certain dinoflagellates, protozoa that are an important component of marine plankton. One form (*paralytic shellfish p.*) is caused by species of *Gonyaulax,* and is characterized by paresthesias of the mouth, lips, face, and limbs, nausea, vomiting, and diarrhea; in rare severe cases muscle weakness or paralysis and respiratory embarrassment and death may occur. A self-limited milder form (*neurotoxic shellfish p.*) not associated with paralysis is caused by species of *Gymnodinium.* **tempeh p.,** bongkrek intoxication. **tetrachlorethane p.,** a form of poisoning in munition workers caused by inhalation of fumes of tetrachlorethane, and marked by toxic jaundice, headache, anorexia, and gastrointestinal disturbance. **tetraodon p.,** tetrodotoxism. **thallium p.,** poisoning, particularly of children, due to ingestion of thallium compounds, marked by alopecia, by a variety of neurologic and psychic symptoms, including ataxia, restlessness, delirium, hallucinations, delusions, semicoma, blindness, and by liver and kidney damage. **T.N.T. p.,** trinitrotoluene p. **tobacco p.,** tabacosis. **trinitrotoluene p.,** a form of poisoning in munition workers, characterized by dermatitis, gastritis with abdominal pain, vomiting, constipation, flatulence, and blood changes. Abbreviated *T.N.T. p.* **whelk p.,** a form of intoxication characterized by intense headache, dizziness, nausea, and vomiting resulting from the ingestion of whelks, members of the phylum Mollusca, class Gastropoda. See also under *poison.* **zinc p.,** poisoning due to inhalation or ingestion of zinc; the symptoms include colic, diarrhea, vomiting, and fever.

poisonous (poi'son-us) pertaining to, due to, or of the nature of a poison; toxic; venomous.

Poisson distribution (pwah-sawn') [Siméon Denis *Poisson,* French mathematician, 1781–1840] see under *distribution.*

poitrinaire (pwah"tre-nār') [Fr.] a patient with a chronic disease of the chest.

pokeroot (pōk'root) pokeweed.

pokeweed (pōk'wēd) a tall perennial herb, *Phytolacca americana,* of North America; its root has emetic and purgative properties and has been used as an antirheumatic. Mitogen from pokeweed induce lymphocyte transformation and stimulate erythropoiesis. Called also *pokeroot.*

polacrilin (pol-ah-kril'in) methacrylic acid ester with divinylbenzene; a synthetic ion-exchange resin, supplied in the hydrogen or free acid form; a pharmaceutic aid. **p. potassium,** a synthetic ion exchange resin, prepared through polymerization of methacrylic acid and divinylbenzene, and then further neutralized with potassium hydroxide to form the potassium salt of methacrylic acid and divinylbenzene. It is supplied as a pharmaceutical-grade ion-exchange resin in a particle size of 100- to 500-mesh; a tablet disintegrant.

polar (po'lar) [L. *polaris, polus;* Gr. *polos*] 1. of or pertaining to a pole; see also under *compound.* 2. being at opposite ends of a spectrum of manifestations, as polar forms of leprosy.

Polaramine (po-lar'ah-mēn) trademark for preparations of dexchlorpheniramine maleate.

polarimeter (po"lah-rim'ĕ-ter) [*polar* + Gr. *metron* measure] a device for measuring the rotation of plane polarized light; a polariscope.

polarimetry (po"lah-rim'ĕ-tre) measurement of the rotation of plane polarized light by a liquid or solid.

polariscope (po-lar'ĭ-skōp) [*polar* + Gr. *skopein* to examine] an instrument for the measurement of polarized light.

polariscopic (po"lar-ĭ-skop'ik) pertaining to the polariscope or to polariscopy.

polariscopy (po"lar-is'ko-pe) the science of polarized light and the use of the polariscope.

polaristrobometer (po-lar"is-tro-bom'ĕ-ter) a form of polarimeter used for delicate analyses.

polarity (po-lar'ĭ-te) 1. the fact or condition of having poles. 2. the exhibition of opposite effects at the two extremities. 3. the presence of an axial gradient and exhibition by a nerve of both anelectrotonus and catelectrotonus. 4. the orientation of intracellular structures to the tissue as a whole. **dynamic p.,** the specialization of a nerve cell with reference to the flow of impulses.

polarization (po"lar-i-za'shun) 1. the production of that condition in light by virtue of which its vibrations take place all in one plane or else in circles and ellipses. 2. the accumulation of bubbles of hydrogen gas on the negative plate of a galvanic battery, so that the generation of electricity is impeded. **circular p.,** that polarization which causes vibration in circles. **elliptical p.**, that which causes the vibration in ellipses. **plane p.**, the production of polarization such that the light vibrations are all in one plane. **rotatory p.**, circular or elliptical polarization, as distinguished from plane polarization.

polarize (po′lar-īz) 1. to embue with polarity. 2. to put into a state of polarization.

polarizer (po′lah-rīz″er) an appliance for polarizing light.

polarogram (po-lar′o-gram) the curve of current versus voltage obtained in polarography.

polarographic (po″lah-ro-graf′ik) pertaining to polarography.

polarography (po″lar-og′rah-fe) an electrochemical technique for identifying and estimating the concentration of reducible elements by means of the dual measurement of the current flowing through an electrochemical cell (which contains the test solution) and the electrical potential between the two electrodes as the potential is increased at a constant rate by an external voltage source. As the voltage reaches the standard electrode potential of the test substance, there is a sharp increase in current flow. The indicator electrode is usually a dropping mercury electrode.

Polaroid (po′lar-oid) trademark for a sheet (film) polarizer utilizing oriented crystals used as a substitute for Nicol prisms and for reducing glare through lenses and windshields.

polaroplast (po-lar′o-plast) [*polar* + *plast*] an organelle in microsporidans that imbibes water, swells, and exerts pressure to rupture the polar cap and evert the polar tube through which the sporoplasm escapes to infect the host.

poldine methylsulfate (pol′dēn) [USP] chemical name: 2- [(hydroxydiphenylacetyl) oxy] methyl]- 1,1- dimethylpyrrolidinium methyl sulfate. A synthetic quaternary nitrogen anticholinergic, $C_{22}H_{29}NO_7S$, occurring as a creamy white, crystalline powder; used as an adjunct in the treatment of peptic ulcer and gastrointestinal disorders associated with hyperacidity, hypermotility, and spasm, administered orally.

pole (pōl) [L. *polus*; Gr. *polos*] 1. either extremity of an axis, as of the fetal ellipse, or of an organ of the body; called also *polus* or *extremitas*. 2. either one of two points which have opposite physical qualities (electric or other). **animal p.**, the site of an ovum to which the nucleus is approximated, and from which the polar bodies pinch off. Also, in nonmammalian species, the pole of an egg less heavily laden with yolk than the vegetal pole and therefore exhibiting faster cell division. **anterior p. of eyeball**, polus anterior bulbi oculi. **anterior p. of lens**, polus anterior lentis. **antigerminal p.**, vegetal p. **cephalic p.**, the end of the fetal ellipse at which the head of the fetus is situated. **frontal p. of hemisphere of cerebrum**, polus frontalis hemispherii cerebri. **germinal p.**, animal p. **inferior p. of kidney**, extremitas inferior renis. **inferior p. of testis**, extremitas inferior testis. **negative p.**, cathode. **nutritive p.**, vegetal p. **occipital p. of hemisphere of cerebrum**, polus occipitalis hemispherii cerebri. **pelvic p.**, the end of the fetal ellipse at which the breech of the fetus is situated. **positive p.**, anode. **posterior p. of eyeball**, polus posterior bulbi oculi. **posterior p. of lens**, polus posterior lentis. **temporal p. of hemisphere of cerebrum**, polus temporalis hemispherii cerebri. **twin p.**, that part of a spiral-fibered nerve cell from which both the straight and spiral fibers spring. **upper p. of kidney**, extremitas superior renis. **upper p. of testis**, extremitas superior testis. **vegetal p., vegetative p., vitelline p.**, that pole of an ovum at which the greater amount of food yolk is deposited. Cf. *animal p.*

poli (po′li) [L.] genitive and plural of *polus*.

policapram (pol′ĕ-ka′pram) chemical name: poly[imino(1-oxo-1,6-hexanediyl)]: a linear polymer of ε-aminocaproic lactam, $(C_6H_{11}NO)_n$, as microcrystals of colloid dimensions; used as a tablet binder for pharmaceutical preparations.

policeman (po-lēs′man) a glass rod with a piece of rubber tubing on one end, used as a stirring rod and transfer tool in chemical analysis.

policlinic (pol″e-klin′ik) [Gr. *polis* city + *klinē* bed] a city hospital, infirmary, or clinic. Cf. *polyclinic.*

poliencephalitis (pol″e-en-sef″ah-li′tis) polioencephalitis.

poliencephalomyelitis (pol″e-en-sef″ah-lo-mi″ĕ-li′tis) polioencephalomyelitis.

polio (po′le-o) poliomyelitis.

poli(o)- [Gr. *polios* gray] a combining form denoting relationship to the gray matter of the nervous system.

poliocidal (po″le-o-si′dal) neutralizing the poliomyelitis virus.

polioclastic (po″le-o-klas′tik) [*polio-* + Gr. *klastos* breaking] destroying the gray matter of the nervous system; a term applied to the viruses of poliomyelitis, epidemic encephalitis, and rabies; neurotropic.

poliodystrophia (po″le-o-dis-tro′fe-ah) poliodystrophy. **p. cer′ebri**, a rare disease of young children, characterized by neuronal degeneration of the cerebral cortex and elsewhere, accompanied by progressive mental deterioration, motor disturbances, and early death; called also *Alpers' disease.*

poliodystrophy (po″le-o-dis′tro-fe) [*polio-* + *dystrophy*] atrophy of the cerebral gray matter.

polioencephalitis (po″le-o-en-sef″ah-li′tis) [*polio-* + *encephalitis*] 1. inflammatory disease of the gray substance of the brain. 2. cerebral poliomyelitis. **acute superior hemorrhagic p.** (obs.), Wernicke's encephalopathy. **p. acu′ta infan′tum**, an acute variety seen in children under six years of age, and marked by fever, vomiting, and convulsions; it is usually followed by permanent paralysis of the limbs which were affected with convulsions. **acute bulbar p.**, acute bulbar paralysis. **inferior p.**, bulbar paralysis. **posterior p.**, inflammation of the gray matter of the posterior part of the fourth ventricle. **superior hemorrhagic p.** (obs.), Wernicke's encephalopathy.

polioencephalomeningomyelitis (po″le-o-en-sef″ah-lo-mĕ-nin″go-mi″ĕ-li′tis) inflammation of the gray matter of the brain and spinal cord and of the meninges covering it.

polioencephalomyelitis (po″le-o-en-sef″ah-lo-mi″ĕ-li′tis) inflammatory disease of the gray matter of the brain and spinal cord.

polioencephalopathy (po″le-o-en-sef″ah-lop′ah-the) [*polio-* + Gr. *enkephalos* brain + *pathos* disease] disease of the gray matter of the brain.

polioencephalotropic (po″le-o-en-sef″ah-lo-trop′ik) having a special affinity for the gray substance of the brain; neurotropic.

poliomyelencephalitis (po″le-o-mi″el-en-sef″ah-li′tis) [*polio-* + Gr. *myelos* marrow + *enkephalos* brain + *-itis*] poliomyelitis combined with polioencephalitis.

poliomyeliticidal (po″le-o-mi″ĕ-li″tĭ-si″dal) having the power of destroying poliomyelitis virus.

poliomyelitis (po″le-o-mi″ĕ-li′tis) [*polio-* + Gr. *myelos* marrow + *-itis*] an acute viral disease, occurring sporadically and in epidemics, and characterized clinically by fever, sore throat, headache, and vomiting, often with stiffness of the neck and back. In the *minor illness* these may be the only symptoms. The *major illness*, which may or may not be preceded by the minor illness, is characterized by involvement of the central nervous system, stiff neck, pleocytosis in the spinal fluid, and perhaps paralysis. There may be subsequent atrophy of groups of muscles, ending in contraction and permanent deformity. The major illness is called *acute anterior p., infantile paralysis,* and *Heine-Medin disease.* The disease is now largely controlled by vaccines. See also *poliovirus* and *spinal paralytic p.* **acute anterior p.**, see *poliomyelitis.* **acute lateral p.**, spinal paralytic p. **anterior p.**, inflammation of the anterior horns of the gray substance of the spinal cord. **ascending p.**, a paralytic affection which is first manifested in the legs and rapidly ascends cephalad. **bulbar p.**, a serious form of poliomyelitis in which the medulla oblongata is affected, and in which there may be dysfunction of the swallowing mechanism, and respiratory and circulatory distress. **cerebral p.**, poliomyelitis in which the areas most likely to be involved are the brain stem and the motor cortex; called also *polioencephalitis.* **endemic p.**, poliomyelitis occurring sporadically or in a small number of cases, particularly during periods of warm weather, in most countries throughout the world. **epidemic p.**, poliomyelitis occurring in epidemic form. **mouse p., murine p.**, Theiler's disease. **porcine p.**, infectious porcine encephalomyelitis. **postinoculation p.**, acute poliomyelitis appearing within three weeks after some type of inoculation. **post-tonsillectomy p.**, acute poliomyelitis appearing within a short time after tonsillectomy. **postvaccinal p.**, acute poliomyelitis appearing within three weeks after some type of vaccination. **spinal paralytic p.,** the classic form of acute anterior poliomyelitis, in which the appearance of flaccid paralysis, usually of one or more limbs, makes the diagnosis quite definite.

poliomyeloencephalitis (po″le-o-mi″ĕ-lo-en-sef″ah-li′tis) [polio- + Gr. *myelos* marrow + *enkephalos* brain + -*itis*] polioencephalomyelitis.

poliomyelopathy (po″le-o-mi″ĕ-lop′ah-the) [polio- + Gr. *myelos* marrow + *pathos* disease] any disease primarily affecting the gray matter of the spinal cord.

polioneuromere (po″le-o-nu′ro-mēr) [polio- + Gr. *neuron* nerve + *meros* part] one of the primitive segments of the gray matter of the spinal cord.

polioplasm (pol′e-o-plazm″) [polio- + Gr. *plasma* something formed] the internal, granular protoplasm proper of a cell.

poliosis (pol″e-o′sis) [Gr. *polios* gray] circumscribed depigmentation of the hair, particularly of the scalp, occurring in association with or following various pathologic conditions. Cf. *canities.*

poliovirus (po″le-o-vi′rus) the etiologic agent of poliomyelitis, separable, on the basis of specificity of neutralizing antibody, into three serotypes, designated types 1, 2, and 3. Over the years, type 1 has been responsible for about 85 per cent of all paralytic poliomyelitis and for most epidemics, and type 3 for about 10 per cent of paralytic poliomyelitis and for occasional epidemics. Type 2 has been responsible for about 5 per cent of paralytic poliomyelitis. Epidemics caused by poliovirus are now largely controlled by vaccines. **p. mu′ris,** Theiler's virus.

polipropene (pol″ĕ-pro′pēn) chemical name: 1-propene homopolymer; a tablet excipient for pharmaceutical preparations, $(C_3H_6)_n$.

polishing (pol′ish-ing) 1. the creation of a smooth and glossy finish on a surface, as of a denture. 2. [Pl.] material obtained by abrasion of a solid, such as that (rice *polishings* or *perpolitiones oryzae*, a rich source of vitamin B) produced by the milling of rice.

polisography (pol″ĕ-sog′rah-fe) [Gr. *polys* many + *isos* same + *graphein* to write] roentgenography in which several exposures are made in the same film.

Politzer's bag, etc. (pol′it-zerz) [Adam *Politzer,* Hungarian otologist, 1835–1920] see under *bag, cone, speculum,* and *test.*

politzerization (pol″it-zer-i-za′shun) [Adam *Politzer*] inflation of the middle ear by means of a Politzer bag. **negative p.,** displacement of secretion from a cavity through negative pressure produced by means of a Politzer bag.

polkissen (pōl-kis′en) [Ger. "pole cushion"] juxtaglomerular cells.

poll (pōl) the back part of the head, especially that of an animal.

pollakidipsia (pol″ah-kĭ-dip′se-ah) [Gr. *pollakis* often + *dipsa* thirst + -*ia*] a condition characterized by abnormally frequent occurrence of the sensation of thirst.

pollakisuria (pol″ah-kĭ-su′re-ah) pollakiuria.

pollakiuria (pol″ah-ke-u′re-ah) [Gr. *pollakis* often + *ouron* urine + -*ia*] unduly frequent passage of the urine.

polled (pōld) having no horns; said of cattle that have been bred for this inherited trait.

pollen (pol′en) the mass of microspores (male fertilizing elements) of flowering plants. Many pollens, especially the airborne pollens, are allergens; i.e., they produce proteinaceous antigens capable of sensitizing susceptible persons and producing allergic symptoms.

pollenarium (pol″ĕ-na′re-um) a building or room for the collection and storing of pollens.

pollenogenic (pol″ĕ-no-jen′ik) [pollen + Gr. *gennan* to produce] caused by the pollen of plants.

pollenosis (pol″ĕ-no′sis) pollinosis.

pollex (pol′eks), pl. *pol′lices* [L.] [NA] the first digit of the hand, or thumb; called also *digitus primus (I) manus* [NA alternative]. **p. exten′sus,** backward deviation of the thumb. **p. flex′us,** permanent flexion of the thumb. **p. val′gus,** deviation of the thumb toward the ulnar side. **p. va′rus,** deviation of the thumb toward the radial side.

pollicization (pol″is-i-za′shun) [L. *pollex* thumb] the re-

placement or rehabilitation of a thumb, especially surgical construction of a thumb from the index finger or great toe.

pollination (pol″ĭ-na′shun) the transfer of pollen from anther to stigma of a flowering plant.

pollinium (pol″ĭ-ne′um) an aggregation of pollen grains held together by a mucilaginous fluid and transported as a whole during pollination.

pollinosis (pol″ĭ-no′sis) the allergic reaction in the body to the airborne pollen of plants, resulting in the seasonal type of hay fever or rose cold. See *seasonal hay fever,* under *fever.*

pollodic (pol-lo′dik) [Gr. *polloi* many + *hodos* way] panthodic.

pollution (pŏ-lu′shun) [L. *pollutio*] the act of defiling or making impure.

polocyte (po′lo-sīt) [Gr. *polos* pole + -*cyte*] see *polar bodies,* under *body.*

polonium (po-lo′ne-um) [L. *Polonia* Poland] a rare metal resembling bismuth, discovered in 1898 in pitchblende; atomic number, 84; atomic weight, 210; symbol, Po. It is radioactive, but less so than radium.

poloxalene (pol-oks′ah-lēn) a liquid poloxamer, having a molecular weight of approximately 3000; used as a surfactant in pharmaceutical preparations and in the prevention of bloat in ruminants.

poloxalkol (pol-ok′sal-kol) poloxamer 188.

poloxamer (pol-oks′ah-mer) any of a series of nonionic surfactants of the polyoxypropylene-polyoxyethylene copolymer type, having the general formula $HO(C_2H_4O)_a(C_3H_6O)_b(C_2H_4O)_cH$, where $a = c$; the molecular weights of the members of the series vary from about 1000 to more than 16000. The term is used in conjunction with a numerical suffix for individual unique identification of products that may be used as a food, drug, or cosmetic. Poloxamers may be surfactants, emulsifiers, or stabilizers. **p. 182L,** a liquid poloxamer, having an average molecular weight of 2450; used as a food additive and pharmaceutic aid. **p. 188,** a waxy poloxamer, having an average molecular weight of 8350; used as a cathartic, administered orally. Called also *poloxalkol.* **p. 331,** a liquid poloxamer, having an average molecular weight of 3800; used as a food additive.

polster (pōl′ster) a small bulge, as on a vessel wall.

poltophagy (pol-tof′ah-je) [Gr. *poltos* porridge + *phagein* to eat] thorough chewing of the food so that it becomes reduced to a porridge-like mass.

polus (po′lus), gen. and pl. *po′li* [L., from Gr. *polos* axis] a pole: either extremity of an axis; [NA] a general term for the extremity of an organ. **p. ante′rior bul′bi o′culi** [NA], anterior pole of eyeball: the center of the anterior curvature of the eyeball. **p. ante′rior len′tis** [NA], anterior pole of lens: the central point of the anterior surface of the lens. **p. fronta′lis hemisphe′rii cer′ebri** [NA], frontal pole of hemisphere of cerebrum: the most prominent part of the anterior end of each hemisphere of the brain. **p. occipita′lis hemisphe′rii cer′ebri** [NA], occipital pole of hemisphere of cerebrum: the most posterior prominence of the occipital lobe of the cerebral hemisphere. **p. poste′rior bul′bi o′culi** [NA], posterior pole of eyeball: the center of the posterior curvature of the eyeball. **p. poste′rior len′tis** [NA], posterior pole of lens: the central point of the posterior surface of the lens. **p. tempora′lis hemisphe′rii cer′ebri** [NA], temporal pole of hemisphere of cerebrum: the prominent anterior end of the temporal lobe of the brain.

poly (pol′e) colloquial name for a polymorphonuclear leukocyte; see *neutrophil,* def. 1.

poly- [Gr. *polys* many] a combining form meaning many or much.

polyA polyadenylate.

Polya's operation (pōl′yahz) [Jenö (Eugene) *Polya,* Budapest surgeon, 1876–1944] see under *operation.*

polyacid (pol″e-as′id) capable of neutralizing several molecules of an acid radical; said of a base or basic radical.

polyacrylamide (pol″e-ah-kril′ah-mīd) a polymer of acrylamide.

polyadenia (pol″e-ah-de′ne-ah) [poly- + Gr. *adēn* gland + -*ia*] pseudoleukemia.

polyadenitis (pol″e-ad″ĕ-ni′tis) [poly- + Gr. *adēn* gland + -*itis*] inflammation of several or many glands.

polyadenoma (pol″e-ad″ĕ-no′mah) adenoma of many glands.

polyadenomatosis (pol″e-ad″ĕ-no-mah-to′sis) multiple adenomas in a part.

polyadenopathy (pol″e-ad″ĕ-nop′ah-the) any disease affecting several glands at once.

polyadenosis (pol″e-ad″ĕ-no′sis) disorder of several glands, particularly of several endocrine glands.

polyadenous (pol″e-ad′ĕ-nus) [*poly-* + Gr. *adēn* gland] having or affecting many glands.

polyadenylate (pol″e-ah-den′ĭ-lat) a polymer of adenylic acid, e.g., the polyadenylate tail of mRNAs. Abbreviated polyA.

polyalcoholism (pol″e-al′ko-hol-izm) intoxication or poisoning by a mixture of different alcohols.

polyalgesia (pol″e-al-je′se-ah) [*poly-* + Gr. *algēsis* sense of pain + *-ia*] a condition in which a single pin-prick feels as if several had been made.

polyamine (pol″e-am′in) any compound, e.g., spermine and spermidine, containing two or more amine groups.

polyandry (pol″e-an′dre) [*poly-* + Gr. *aner* man] 1. the concurrent marriage of a woman to more than one man, as practiced by certain peoples. 2. an animal mating system seen in polygamous species, in which the female mates with more than one male. 3. union of two or more male pronuclei with a female pronucleus, resulting in polyploidy of the zygote. Cf. *polygyny.*

Polyangiaceae (pol″e-an″je-a′se-e) a family of gliding bacteria of the order Myxobacterales, found in soils and decaying organic matter, made up of cylindrical cells that produce spores in sporangia. It includes the genera *Chondromyces, Nannocystis,* and *Polyangium.*

polyangiitis (pol″e-an″je-i′tis) inflammation involving multiple blood or lymph vessels.

Polyangium (pol″e-an′je-um) [*poly-* + Gr. *angeion* vessel] a genus of gliding bacteria of the family Polyangiaceae, order Myxobacterales, found in soil and tree bark. The type species is *P. vitelli′num.*

polyarteritis (pol″e-ar″tĕ-ri′tis) [*poly-* + *arteritis*] multiple inflammatory and destructive arterial lesions; panarteritis. See also *periarteritis nodosa.* **p. nodo′sa,** periarteritis nodosa, def. 1.

polyarthric (pol″e-ar′thrik) [*poly-* + Gr. *arthron* joint] pertaining to or affecting many joints.

polyarthritis (pol″e-ar-thri′tis) [*poly-* + Gr. *arthron* joint + *-itis*] an inflammation of several joints together. **benign p.,** polyarthritis that is usually mild, but may be severe, though without permanent joint changes; attacks usually occur in winter and last only a few months. **chronic secondary p.,** Jaccoud's syndrome. **chronic villous p.,** chronic inflammation of the synovial membrane of several joints. **p. des′truens,** rheumatoid arthritis. **peripheral p.,** that in which the knees and ankles tend to be involved more commonly than the small joints of the hands or feet; asymmetric involvement is common and the number of joints affected tends to be limited. **p. rheumat′ica acu′ta,** rheumatic fever. **tuberculous p.,** pulmonary hypertrophic osteoarthropathy. **vertebral p.,** disease of the intervertebral substance without caries of the bodies of the vertebrae.

polyarticular (pol″e-ar-tik′u-lar) [*poly-* + L. *articulus* joint] affecting many joints.

polyatomic (pol″e-ah-tom′ik) [*poly-* + Gr. *atomon* atom] composed of several atoms.

polyauxotroph (pol″e-awk′so-trōf) [*poly-* + Gr. *auxein* to increase + *trophē* nourishment] an organism, especially a mutant, which requires multiple growth factors.

polyauxotrophic (pol″e-awk″so-trōf′ik) requiring multiple growth factors; used especially with reference to a single mutation that causes a multiple requirement.

polyavitaminosis (pol″e-a-vi″tah-min-o′sis) [*poly-* + *avitaminosis*] a deficiency disease in which more than one vitamin is lacking in the diet.

polyaxon (pol″e-ak′son) [*poly-* + Gr. *axōn* axis] a nerve cell from the horizontal dendrites of which four or more axons or branches are given off.

polyaxonic (pol″e-ak-son′ik) having several axons.

polyazin (pol″e-az′in) an organic chemical compound whose molecules contain atoms two or more of which are nitrogen.

polybasic (pol″e-ba′sik) [*poly-* + Gr. *basis* base] 1. denoting any acid which has several hydrogen atoms replaceable by a base. 2. denoting any salt of a polybasic acid formed by replacing some or all of its hydrogen atoms by a base.

polyblennia (pol″e-blen′e-ah) [*poly-* + Gr. *blenna* mucus + *-ia*] the secretion of an excessive quantity of mucus.

polybutilate (pol″e-bu′tĭ-lāt) chemical name: poly[oxy-1,4-butanediyloxy(1,6-dioxo-1,6-hexanediyl)]; a surgical suture coating, $(C_{10}H_{16}O_4)_n$.

polycarbophil (pol″e-kar′bo-fil) [USP] a pharmacologically inert, polyacrylic acid cross-linked with divinyl glycol, occurring as white to creamy white granules; used as a gastrointestinal absorbent in the treatment of diarrhea.

polycellular (pol″e-sel′u-lar) multicellular.

polycentric (pol″e-sen′trik) having many centers.

polycentricity (pol″e-sen-tris″ĭ-te) the state or quality of being polycentric.

polycheiria (pol″e-ki′re-ah) [*poly-* + Gr. *cheir* hand + *-ia*] the condition of having more than two hands.

polychemotherapy (pol″e-ke″mo-ther′ah-pe) treatment by the simultaneous administration of several chemotherapeutic agents.

polychloruria (pol″e-klo-roo′re-ah) an increased excretion of chlorine in the urine.

polycholia (pol″e-ko′le-ah) [*poly-* + Gr. *cholē* bile + *-ia*] excessive flow or secretion of bile.

polychondritis (pol″e-kon-dri′tis) inflammation involving many cartilages of the body. **chronic atrophic p., p. chron′ica atro′phicans,** relapsing p. **relapsing p.,** an acquired disease of unknown etiology, having a chronic course and a tendency to recurrence, and marked by inflammatory and degenerative lesions of various cartilaginous structures, including those of the joints, ears, nose, trachea, and bronchi, resulting in such deformities as floppy ear and saddle nose; if the tracheal or bronchial wall collapses, respiratory obstruction may occur. The aorta and the sclera and cornea are also affected. Called also *chronic atrophic p., p. chronica atrophicans,* and *polychondropathia.*

polychondropathia (pol″e-kon″dro-path′e-ah) relapsing polychondritis.

polychondropathy (pol″e-kon-drop′ah-the) relapsing polychondritis.

polychrest (pol′e-krest) [*poly-* + Gr. *chrēstos* useful] 1. useful in many conditions. 2. a remedy useful in many diseases.

polychromasia (pol″e-kro-ma′ze-ah) 1. variation in the hemoglobin content of the erythrocytes of the blood. 2. polychromatophilia.

polychromatia (pol″e-kro-ma′she-ah) polychromatophilia.

polychromatic (pol″e-kro-mat′ik) [*poly-* + Gr. *chrōma* color] exhibiting many colors. Cf. *monochromatic.*

polychromatocyte (pol″e-kro-mat′o-sīt) a cell that is stainable with various stains or colors.

polychromatocytosis (pol″e-kro″mah-to-si-to′sis) polychromatophilia.

polychromatophil (pol″e-kro-mat′o-fil) [*poly-* + Gr. *chrōma* color + *philein* to love] a cell or other element that is stainable with various stains or colors.

polychromatophilia (pol″e-kro″mah-to-fil′e-ah) 1. the quality of being stainable with various stains or tints; affinity for all sorts of stains. 2. a condition in which the erythrocytes, on staining, show various shades of blue combined with tinges of pink.

polychromatophilic (pol″e-kro″mah-to-fil′ik) pertaining to or characterized by polychromatophilia.

polychromatosis (pol″e-kro″mah-to′sis) an excess of abnormally staining erythrocytes in the blood; see *polychromatophilia,* def. 2.

polychromemia (pol″e-kro-me′me-ah) [*poly-* + Gr. *chrōma* color + *haima* blood + *-ia*] increase in the coloring matter of the blood.

polychromic (pol″e-kro′mik) pertaining to or exhibiting many colors.

polychromophil (pol″e-kro′mo-fil) polychromatophil.

polychromophilia (pol″e-kro-mo-fil′e-ah) polychromatophilia.

polychylia (pol″e-ki′le-ah) [*poly-* + Gr. *chylos* chyle + *-ia*] excessive production of chyle.

Polycillin (pol″e-sil′in) trademark for preparations of ampicillin.

polyclinic (pol″e-klin′ik) [*poly-* + Gr. *klinē* bed] a hospital and school where diseases and injuries of all kinds are studied and treated clinically.

polyclonal (pol″e-klōn′al) derived from different cells; of or pertaining to several clones.

polyclonia (pol″e-klo′ne-ah) [*poly-* + Gr. *klonos* clonus + *-ia*] a disease marked by many clonic spasms, resembling tic and chorea, but distinct from either.

polycoria (pol″e-ko′re-ah) 1. [*poly-* + Gr. *korē* pupil + *-ia*] the existence of more than one pupil in an eye. 2. [*poly-* + Gr. *koros* surfeit + *-ia*] the deposit of reserve material in an organ or tissue so as to produce enlargement. **p. spu′ria,** a condition in which the iris contains several openings or holes. **p. ve′ra,** the existence in the eye of several pupils, each with its own sphincter.

polycrotic (pol″e-krot′ik) [*poly-* + Gr. *krotos* beat] having several secondary waves to each pulse beat.

polycrotism (pol-ik′ro-tizm) the fact or quality of being polycrotic.

polycyclic (pol″e-si′klik) [*poly-* + Gr. *kyklos* ring] containing more than one ring or cycle (frequency).

Polycycline (pol″e-si′klēn) trademark for preparations of tetracycline.

polycyesis (pol″e-si-e′sis) [*poly-* + Gr. *kyēsis* pregnancy] multiple pregnancy.

polycystic (pol″e-sis′tik) [*poly-* + Gr. *kystis* cyst] containing or made up of many cysts.

Polycystinea (pol″e-sis-tin′e-ah) [*poly-* + Gr. *kystis* sac, bladder] a class of planktonic marine protozoa (superclass Actinopoda, subphylum Sarcodina), most species of which are characterized by the presence of a siliceous skeleton made up usually of solid elements, consisting of one or more latticed shells with or without radial spines, or of one or more isolated spicules; a capsular membrane composed usually of grossly polygonal plates and containing many pores; and axonemes often originating from an axoplast in the endoplasm. It comprises two orders: Spumellarida and Nassellarida. The classes Polycystinea and Phaeodarea considered together are equivalent to the Radiolaria in former taxonomic classifications.

polycystoma (pol″e-sis-to′mah) a condition in which a part, especially the breast, is riddled with cysts.

polycyte (pol′e-sīt) [*poly-* + Gr. *kytos* cell] a hypersegmented polymorphonuclear leukocyte of normal size. Cf. *macropolycyte.*

polycythemia (pol″e-si-the′me-ah) [*poly-* + Gr. *kytos* cell + *haima* blood + *-ia*] an increase in the total red cell mass of the blood; see *absolute p.* and *relative p.* **absolute p.,** an increase in red cell mass caused by a sustained overactivity of the erythroid component of the bone marrow, which may occur as a compensatory physiologic response to tissue hypoxia (see *secondary p.*), or as the principal manifestation of polycythemia vera. Cf. *relative p.* **appropriate p.,** see *secondary p.* **benign p.,** stress p. **compensatory p.,** see *secondary p.* **p. hyperton′ica,** stress p. **inappropriate p.,** see *secondary p.* **myelopathic p., primary p.,** p. vera. **relative p.,** a decrease in plasma volume without change in red blood cell mass so that the erythrocytes become more concentrated (elevated hematocrit); it may occur as an acute transient condition due to marked loss of body fluid or lowered fluid intake or a combination of both, or it may be a chronic condition associated with a low normal plasma volume and a high normal red cell mass or with other factors (see *stress p.*). Cf. *absolute p.* **p. ru′bra, p. ru′bra ve′ra,** p. vera. **secondary p.,** any absolute increase in the total red cell mass other than polycythemia vera, occurring as a physiologic response to tissue hypoxia. It may be compensatory and *appropriate,* adjusting for general tissue hypoxia, such as that occurring in association with pulmonary disease, alveolar hypoventilation, cardiovascular disease, and prolonged exposure to high altitude or occurring as a result of defective hemoglobin or drugs. Or it may be *inappropriate,* reflecting excessive erythropoietin production due to renal or extrarenal disorders. Called also *erythrocyto-*

sis. **splenomegalic p.,** p. vera. **spurious p.,** 1. relative p. 2. stress p. **stress p.,** chronic relative polycythemia (q.v.) usually affecting white, middle-aged, mildly obese males who are active, anxiety-prone, and hypertensive, occurring without the characteristic symptoms associated with polycythemia vera, i.e., without leukocytosis, splenomegaly, and thrombocytosis. Called also *benign p., Gaisböck's disease* or *syndrome,* and *stress erythrocytosis.* **p. ve′ra,** a myeloproliferative disorder of unknown etiology, characterized by abnormal proliferation of all hematopoietic bone marrow elements and an absolute increase in red cell mass and total blood volume, associated frequently with splenomegaly, leukocytosis, and thrombocythemia. Hematopoiesis is also reactive in extramedullary sites (liver and spleen). In time, myelofibrosis occurs. Called also *erythremia, erythrocythemia, p. rubra, splenomegalic p., myelopathic p., erythrocytosis megalosplenica, Osler's disease, Vaquez's disease,* and *Vaquez-Osler disease.* Cf. *secondary p.*

polydactylia (pol″e-dak-til′e-ah) polydactyly.

polydactylism (pol-e-dak′til-izm) polydactyly.

polydactyly (pol″e-dak′tĭ-le) [*poly-* + Gr. *daktylos* finger + *-ia*] a developmental anomaly characterized by the presence of supernumerary digits (fingers or toes) on the hands or feet.

polydeoxyribonucleotide (pol″e-de-ok″se-ri″bo-nu′kle-o-tīd) a polymer of deoxyribonucleotides; deoxyribonucleic acid.

polydeoxyribonucleotide synthase (ATP) (po″le-de-ok″se-ri″bo-noo″kle-o-tīd sin′the-tās) [EC 6.5.1.1] an enzyme of the ligase class that catalyzes the reaction ATP + (deoxyribonucleotide)$_n$ + (deoxyribonucleotide)$_m$ = AMP + pyrophosphate + (deoxyribonucleotide)$_{n + m}$. The reaction is important in the repair of damaged deoxyribonucleic acids. Called also *DNA ligase, polynucleotide ligase.*

polydipsia (pol″e-dip′se-ah) [*poly-* + Gr. *dipsa* thirst + *-ia*] chronic excessive thirst, as in diabetes mellitus or diabetes insipidus.

polydispersoid (pol″e-dis-per′soid) a colloid in which the disperse phase consists of particles having different degrees of dispersion.

polydysplasia (pol″e-dis-pla′ze-ah) [*poly-* + *dysplasia*] faulty development in several types of tissue or several organs or systems. **hereditary ectodermal p.,** congenital ectodermal defect; see under *defect.*

polydysspondylism (pol″e-dis-spon′dĭ-lizm) malformation of several vertebrae, associated with dwarfed stature, low intelligence, and malformation of the sella turcica.

polydystrophic (pol″e-dis-tro′fik) pertaining to or exhibiting polydystrophy.

polydystrophy (pol″e-dis′tro-fe) dystrophy of several tissues or structures, as may occur in congenital anomalies. **pseudo-Hurler p.,** mucolipidosis III.

polyelectrolyte (pol″e-e-lek′tro-līt) an ion containing more than two charges.

polyembryony (pol″e-em-bri′o-ne) [*poly-* + *embryo*] the production of two or more embryos from the same ovum or seed.

polyendocrine (pol″e-en′do-krīn) pertaining to or affecting several endocrine glands.

polyendocrinoma (pol″e-en″do-kri-no′mah) multiple endocrine neoplasia.

polyendocrinopathy (pol″e-en″do-krĭ-nop′ah-the) a disorder involving several endocrine glands.

polyene (pol-e′ēn) 1. a chemical in which there are several conjugated double bonds. 2. any of a group of polyene antifungal antibiotics (e.g., amphotericin, candicidin, or nystatin) produced by species of *Streptomyces* that damage cell membranes by forming complexes with sterols.

polyergic (pol″e-er′jik) able to act in several different ways.

polyesthesia (pol″e-es-the′ze-ah) [*poly-* + Gr. *aisthēsis* perception + *-ia*] a condition in which a single object seems to be felt in several different places.

polyesthetic (pol″e-es-thet′ik) pertaining to or affecting several senses or sensations.

polyestradiol phosphate (pol″e-es″trah-di′ol, pol″e-estra′de-ol) a polymer of estradiol phosphate having estrogenic activity similar to that of estradiol; used in the palliative therapy of prostatic carcinoma, administered intramuscularly.

polyestrous (pol″e-es′trus) completing two or more estrus cycles in each sexual season.

polyethadene (pol-e-eth′ah-dēn) chemical name: 1,2:3,4-diepoxybutane polymer with ethylenimine; an antacid, $(C_4H_6O_2)_m(C_2H_5N)_n$.

polyethylene (pol″e-eth′ĭ-lēn) polymerized ethylene, $(CH_2—CH_2)_n$, a synthetic plastic material, forms of which have been used in reparative surgery.

polyethylene glycol (pol″e-eth′ĭ-lēn gli′kol) [NF] a generic name for mixtures of condensation polymers of ethylene oxide and water, represented by the general formula $H(OCH_2CH_2)_n$ OH, in which n is greater than or equal to 4. The term is used in combination with a numeric suffix which indicates the approximate average molecular weight. Those with average molecular weights between 200 and 700 are liquid and those above 1000 are waxlike solids: *p. glycol 3000* (*n* varies from 5 to 5.75) is used as a solvent and dispensing agent in pharmaceutical preparations; *p. glycol 400* (*n* varies from 8.2 to 9.1), *p. glycol 600* (*n* varies from 12.5 to 13.9), and *p. glycol 1500* (*n* varies from 29 to 36) are used as ointment and suppository bases; *p. glycol 1540* (*n* varies from 28 to 36) is used as a vehicle in pharmaceutical preparations; *p. glycol 4000* (*n* varies from 68 to 84) and *p. glycol 6000* (*n* varies from 158 to 204) are used as ointment and suppository bases and as tablet excipients. Called also *macrogol*.

polyferose (pol-ĭ-fer′ōs) a chelate complex of iron and a polymerized derivative of sucrose; a hematinic.

Polygala (po-lig′ah-lah) [*poly-* + Gr. *gala* milk] a genus of plants (milkworts) of many species. *P. senega* L. (Polygalaceae), or seneca or senega snakeroot, is found in North America. See *senega*.

polygalactia (pol″e-gah-lak′she-ah) [*poly-* + Gr. *gala* milk] excessive secretion of milk.

polygalin (po-lig′ah-lin) senegenin.

polygamous (po-lig′ah-mus) pertaining to polygamy.

polygamy (po-lig′ah-me) [*poly-* + Gr. *gamos* marriage] 1. the concurrent marriage of a woman or man to more than one spouse. 2. animal mating in which the individual may mate with more than one partner. See also *polyandry* and *polygyny*. Cf. *monogamy*.

polyganglionic (pol″e-gang″gle-on′ik) [*poly-* + Gr. *ganglion* ganglion] 1. having or pertaining to several or many ganglia. 2. affecting several lymphatic glands.

polygene (pol″ĕ-jēn) [*poly-* + *gene*] one of a group of non-allelic genes (multiple factors or cumulative genes) that interact to influence the same character in the same way so that the effect is cumulative.

polygenic (pol″ĕ-jēn′ik) pertaining to or determined by the action of several different genes. Called also *quantitative*. Cf. *multifactorial*.

polyglactin 910 (pol″e-glak′tin) chemical name: 2-hydroxypropanoic acid polymer with hydroxyacetic acid; an absorbable surgical suture material, $(C_3H_4O_2)_m(C_3H_4O_2)_n$.

polyglandular (pol″e-glan′du-lar) pertaining to or affecting several different glands.

polyglycolic acid (pol″e-gli-kol′ik) a polymer of glycolic acid used as an absorbable surgical suture material.

polygnathus (po-lig′nah-thus) [*poly-* + Gr. *gnathos* jaw] a monster in which a parasitic twin is attached to the jaw of the autosite.

Polygonatum (pol″e-go-na′tum) [*poly-* + Gr. *gony* knee] a genus of liliaceous plants. *P. biflorum* (Walt.) Ell., or Solomon's seal, is a perennial herb of eastern North America, tonic, vulnerary, diuretic, emetic, and purgative; in a considerable dose it is a cardiac poison. The starchy rootstock was once used as a food by certain Indians.

polygram (pol′ĕ-gram) a tracing made by a polygraph.

polygraph (pol′ĕ-graf) [*poly-* + Gr. *graphein* to write] an instrument for simultaneously recording various physiological responses as represented by mechanical or electrical impulses, such as respiratory movements, pulse wave, blood pressure, and the psychogalvanic reflex. Such phenomena reflect emotional reactions which are of use in detecting deception. Popularly known as *lie detector*.

polygyny (po-lij′ĭ-ne) [*poly-* + Gr. *gynē* woman] 1. the concurrent marriage of a man to more than one woman, as practiced by certain peoples. 2. an animal mating system

seen in polygamous species, in which the male mates with more than one female. 3. union of two or more female pronuclei with a male pronucleus, resulting in polyploidy of the zygote. Cf. *polyandry*.

polygyria (pol″e-ji′re-ah) [*poly-* + Gr. *gyros* gyrus + *-ia*] a condition in which there is more than the normal number of convolutions in the brain.

polyhedral (pol″e-he′dral) [*poly-* + Gr. *hedra* seat, base] having many faces or sides.

polyhexose (pol″e-hek′sōs) polysaccharide formed by the enzymatic condensation of hexose sugars.

polyhidrosis (pol″e-hid-ro′sis) [*poly-* + Gr. *hidrōs* sweat + *-osis*] hyperhidrosis.

polyhybrid (pol″e-hi′brid) [*poly-* + *hybrid*] a hybrid whose parents differ from each other in more than three characters.

polyhydramnios (pol″e-hi-dram′ne-os) [*poly-* + Gr. *hydōr* water + *amnion* amnion] hydramnios.

polyhydric (pol″e-hi′drik) containing more than two hydroxyl groups.

polyhydruria (pol″e-hi-droo′re-ah) [*poly-* + Gr. *hydōr* water + *ouron* urine + *-ia*] abnormal dilution of the urine.

Polyhymenophorea (pol″e-hi″mĕ-no-for′e-ah) [*poly-* + Gr. *hymen* membrane + *phoros* bearing] a class of often large and commonly free-living ciliated protozoa (phylum Ciliophora) characterized by the presence of a well-developed, conspicuous adoral zone of numerous buccal or peristomial organelles, often extending onto the body surface, with the cytostome at the bottom of a buccal cavity or infundibulum. Cysts and loricae are common in certain species. Somatic ciliature is complete, reduced, or fused into cirri. It comprises one subclass: Spirotrichia.

polyhypermenorrhea (pol″e-hi″per-men″o-re′ah) [*poly-* + Gr. *hyper* over + *menorrhea*] frequent menstruation with abnormally profuse discharge.

polyhypomenorrhea (pol″e-hi″po-men″o-re′ah) [*poly-* + Gr. *hypo* under + *menorrhea*] frequent menstruation with deficient amount of discharge.

polyidrosis (pol″e-id-ro′sis) hyperhidrosis.

polyinfection (pol″e-in-fek′shun) [*poly-* + *infection*] mixed infection.

polyionic (pol″e-i-on′ik) containing several different ions (e.g., potassium, sodium, etc.), as a polyionic solution.

polykaryocyte (pol″e-kar′e-o-sīt) [*poly-* + Gr. *karyon* nucleus + *-cyte*] a giant cell containing several nuclei.

polykinety (pol″e-ki′ne-te) [*poly-* + *kinety*] a row of closely arranged cilia that descends in a counterclockwise spiral into the infundibulum of peritrichous ciliate protozoa.

Polykol (pol′ĕ-kol) trademark for preparations of poloxalkol.

polylecithal (pol″e-les′ĭ-thal) [*poly-* + Gr. *lekithos* yolk] macrolecithal.

polyleptic (pol″e-lep′tik) [*poly-* + Gr. *lambanein* to seize] having many remissions and exacerbations.

polylysine (pol″e-li′sin) a polypeptide composed of lysine molecules in peptide linkage; used with penicillenic acid in the detection of penicillin sensitivity; see *penicilloyl-polylysine*.

polymacon (pol″e-ma′kon) a hydrophilic contact lens material.

polymastia (pol″e-mas′te-ah) [*poly-* + Gr. *mastos* breast] the presence of more than one pair of mammae, or breasts.

Polymastigida (pol″e-mas″tĭ-gi′dah) an order of protozoa of the class Zoomastigophora, subphylum Mastigophora, consisting of small organisms possessing three to eight or more flagella and usually one or two nuclei, although some are multinucleate; they are found in the digestive tract of various arthropods and vertebrates. It includes the genera *Callimastix*, *Enteromonas*, *Eutrichomastix*, *Copromastix*, *Chilomastix*, *Hexamita*, *Giardia*, and *Trichomonas*.

polymastigote (pol″e-mas′tĭ-gōt) a mastigote having several to many flagella.

polymazia (pol″e-ma′ze-ah) polymastia.

polymelia (pol″e-me′le-ah) [*poly-* + Gr. *melos* limb + *-ia*] a developmental anomaly characterized by the presence of supernumerary limbs.

polymelus (po-lim′ĕ-lus) an individual exhibiting polymelia.

polymenia (pol″e-me′ne-ah) polymenorrhea.

polymenorrhea (pol′e-men″o-re′ah) [*poly-* + *menorrhea*] abnormally frequent menstruation.

polymer (pol′ĭ-mer) [*poly-* + Gr. *meros* part] a compound formed by the joining of smaller molecules, referred to as monomers. The term is generally used to refer either to a macromolecule made up of a large number of monomers linked by covalent bonds, e.g., polypeptides, nucleic acids, polysaccharides, and plastics, or to a protein made up of several subunits linked by covalent or noncovalent bonds, e.g., hemoglobin or IgM immunoglobulin. **addition p.,** a compound formed by the repeated combination of smaller molecules (monomers) without the formation of any other products (e.g., polyethylene). **condensation p.,** a compound formed by the repeated reaction of smaller molecules, involving at the same time the elimination of water or other simple compound (e.g., nylon).

polymerase (pol-im′er-ās) any enzyme that catalyzes polymerization, especially of nucleotides to polynucleotides.

polymeria (pol″ĭ-me′re-ah) [*poly-* + Gr. *meros* part + *-ia*] a developmental anomaly characterized by the presence of supernumerary parts or organs of the body.

polymeric (pol″ĭ-mer′ik) exhibiting the characteristics of a polymer.

polymerid (po-lim′er-id) a polymer.

polymerism (po-lim′ĕ-rizm, pol′ĭ-mĕ-rizm) the phenomenon, or process, which results in the formation of a polymer.

polymerization (pol″ĭ-mer″ĭ-za′shun) the act or process of forming a compound (polymer), usually of high molecular weight, by the combination of simpler molecules.

polymerize (pol′ĭ-mer-īz) to subject to or to undergo polymerization.

polymetacarpia (pol″e-met″ah-kar′pe-ah) [*poly-* + *metacarpus* + *-ia*] presence of more than the normal number of metacarpal bones.

polymetaphosphate (pol″e-met″ah-fos′fāt) a phosphate polymer that serves as a phosphate reserve in microorganisms, appearing as a metachromatic granule.

polymetatarsia (pol″e-met″ah-tar′se-ah) [*poly-* + *metatarsus* + *-ia*] presence of more than the normal number of metatarsal bones.

polymethyl (pol″e-meth′il) a chemical substance having two or more CH_3 (methyl) groups. **p. methacrylate,** 1. a polymethyl ester of methacrylic acid, produced by polymerization of methyl methacrylate; used in the manufacture of acrylic resins and plastics. 2. a polymer of methyl methacrylate.

polymicrobial (pol″e-mi-kro′be-al) [*poly-* + *microbe*] characterized by the presence of several species of microorganisms.

polymicrobic (pol″e-mi-kro′bik) polymicrobial.

polymicrogyria (pol″e-mi″kro-ji′re-ah) [*poly-* + Gr. *mikros* small + *gyros* convolution + *-ia*] a malformation of the brain characterized by development of numerous small convolutions (microgyri).

polymicrolipomatosis (pol″e-mi″kro-lip″o-mah-to′sis) [*poly-* + Gr. *mikros* small + *lipomatosis*] lipomatosis marked by the presence in the subcutaneous tissues of numerous small lipomas.

polymicrotome (pol″e-mi′kro-tōm) [*poly-* + *microtome*] a microtome which cuts several sections at once.

Polymnia (po-lim′ne-ah) [Gr.; one of the nine Muses] a genus of composite-flowered plants. *P. uvedalia* L., leafcup or bearsfoot, is anthelmintic, alterative, antispasmodic, and laxative.

polymorph (pol′e-morf) colloquial term for a polymorphonuclear leukocyte; see *neutrophil*, def. 2.

polymorphic (pol″e-mor′fik) [*poly-* + Gr. *morphē* form] occurring in several or many forms; appearing in different forms at different stages of development.

polymorphism (pol″e-mor′fizm) [*poly-* + Gr. *morphē* form] the quality or character of occurring in several different forms. **balanced p.,** a state of equilibrium in which gene frequencies are maintained by a balance between mutation and selection, the heterozygote having an advantage over both homozygotes. **genetic p.,** the occurrence

together in the same population of two or more genetically determined phenotypes in such proportions that the rarest of them cannot be maintained merely by recurrent mutation. **restriction fragment length p. (RFLP),** in molecular genetics, a polymorphism in DNA sequence that can be detected on the basis of differences in fragment lengths of DNA produced by digestion with a specific restriction enzyme.

polymorphocellular (pol″e-mor″fo-sel′u-lar) [*poly-* + Gr. *morphē* form + L. *cellula* cell] having cells of many forms.

polymorphocyte (pol″e-mor′fo-sīt) a cell with a polymorphic nucleus.

polymorphonuclear (pol″e-mor″fo-nu′kle-ar) [*poly-* + Gr. *morphē* form + *nucleus*] 1. having a nucleus deeply lobed or so divided that it appears to be multiple. 2. a polymorphonuclear leukocyte; see *neutrophil*, def. 1. **filament p.,** one whose nuclear segments are joined by the filaments. **nonfilament p.,** one whose nuclear segments are joined by wide bands.

polymorphous (pol″e-mor′fus) polymorphic.

Polymox (pol′ĕ-moks) trademark for preparations of amoxicillin.

polymyalgia (pol″e-mi-al′je-ah) myalgia affecting several muscles. **p. arterit′ica,** p. rheumatica. **p. rheumat′ica,** a syndrome in the elderly characterized by proximal joint and muscle pain, high erythrocyte sedimentation rate, and a self-limiting course; it is frequently associated with temporal arteritis.

polymyarian (pol″e-mi-a′re-an) [*poly-* + Gr. *mys* muscle] having many muscle cells in each quadrant of a cross section, the cells being coelomyarian in type; said of the muscle arrangement in certain nematodes.

polymyoclonus (pol″e-mi-ok′lo-nus) [*poly-* + Gr. *mys* muscle + *klonos* clonus] 1. a fine or minute muscular tremor. 2. polyclonia.

polymyopathy (pol″e-mi-op′ah-the) disease affecting several muscles simultaneously.

polymyositis (pol″e-mi″o-si′tis) [*poly-* + *myositis*] a chronic, progressive inflammatory disease of skeletal muscle, occurring in both children and adults, and characterized by symmetrical weakness of the limb girdles, neck, and pharynx, usually associated with pain and tenderness, and sometimes preceded or followed by manifestations typical of scleroderma, arthritis, systemic lupus erythematosus, or Sjögren's syndrome. It is also sometimes associated with malignancy, and may be accompanied by characteristic skin lesions (see *dermatomyositis*). **trichinous p.,** trichinosis.

polymyxin (pol″e-mik′sin) the generic name for five polypeptide antibiotics (designated A, B, C, D, and E) derived from strains of the soil bacterium *Bacillus polymyxa*, having specific activity against gram-negative bacteria, including *Pseudomonas aeruginosa*, *Proteus vulgaris*, *Escherichia coli*, *Hemophilus influenzae*, *Aerobacter aerogenes*, and *Klebsiella pneumoniae*. The least toxic members of the group are polymyxins B, usually used in the form of the sulfate salt, and E (see *colistin*). **p. B sulfate** [USP], the sulfate salt of the least toxic member of the polymyxin group, occurring as a buff-colored powder; used in the treatment of various systemic, urinary tract, ophthalmic, otic, and cutaneous infections due to susceptible gram-negative bacteria, especially *Pseudomonas aeruginosa*, administered orally, parenterally, and topically.

polynesic (pol″e-ne′sik) [*poly-* + Gr. *nēsos* island] multiple and insular; occurring in many foci.

polyneural (pol″e-nu′ral) [*poly-* + Gr. *neuron* nerve] pertaining to or supplied by several nerves.

polyneuralgia (pol″e-nu-ral′je-ah) neuralgia of several nerves.

polyneuric (pol″e-nu′rik) polyneural.

polyneuritic (pol″e-nu-rit′ik) pertaining to or affected with polyneuritis.

polyneuritis (pol″e-nu-ri′tis) [*poly-* + Gr. *neuron* nerve + *-itis*] inflammation of many nerves at once; multiple, or disseminated, neuritis. **acute febrile p., acute idiopathic p., acute infective p., acute postinfectious p.,** rapidly progressive ascending motor neuron paralysis of unknown etiology, frequently following an enteric or respiratory infection. An autoimmune mechanism following viral infection has been postulated. It begins with paresthesias of the feet, followed by flaccid paralysis and weakness of the legs, ascending to the arms, trunk, and face, and is attended by slight fever, bulbar palsy, absent or lessened tendon reflexes, and an increase in the protein of the cerebrospinal fluid without corresponding increase in cells. Called also *Barré-Guillain syndrome, Guillain-Barré polyneuritis or syndrome, acute ascending spinal paralysis, acute postinfectious polyneuropathy, neuronitis,* and *postinfectious p.* **anemic p.,** polyneuritis seen in subacute combined degeneration of the spinal cord that occurs in pernicious anemia. **p. cerebra′lis menierifor′mis,** symptoms of cochlear, vestibular, facial, and trigeminal nerve irritation occurring in the early period of syphilis; called also *Frankl-Hochwart's disease.* **endemic p., p. endem′ica,** beriberi. **p. gallina′rum,** a form of polyneuritis seen in fowls fed a thiamine-deficient diet. **Guillain-Barré p.,** acute febrile p. **Jamaica ginger p.,** see under *paralysis.* **postinfectious p.,** acute febrile p. **p. potato′rum,** alcoholic neuropathy.

polyneuromyositis (pol″e-nu″ro-mi″o-si′tis) inflammation of the muscles and peripheral nerves, with loss of reflexes, sensory loss, and paresthesias.

polyneuropathy (pol″e-nu-rop′ah-the) [*poly-* + Gr. *neuron* nerve + *pathos* disease] a disease which involves several nerves. **acute postinfectious p.,** acute febrile polyneuritis. **erythredema p.,** acrodynia.

polyneuroradiculitis (pol″e-nu″ro-rah-dik″u-li′tis) [*poly-* + Gr. *neuron* nerve + L. *radix* root + *-itis*] inflammation of the spinal ganglia, the nerve roots, and the peripheral nerves.

polynuclear (pol″e-nu′kle-ar) 1. pertaining to or having several nuclei. 2. polymorphonuclear.

polynucleate (pol″e-nu′kle-āt) having many nuclei.

polynucleated (pol″e-nu′kle-āt″ed) polynuclear.

polynucleolar (pol″e-nu-kle′o-lar) having several nucleoli.

polynucleotidase (pol″e-nu″kle-o′ti-dās) polynucleotide phosphatase.

polynucleotide (pol″e-nu′kle-o-tīd) any polymer of mononucleotides; nucleic acid.

polynucleotide adenylyltransferase (pol″e-noo′kle-o-tīd ad″ĕ-nil-il-trans′fer-ās) [EC 2.7.7.19] an enzyme of the transferase class that catalyzes the reaction *n* ATP + (nucleotide)$_m$ = *n* pyrophosphate + (nucleotide)$_{m+n}$ in the synthesis of ribonucleic acid. Called also *polyadenate nucleotidyltransferase.*

polynucleotide ligase (pol″e-noo′kle-o-tīd li′gās) polydeoxyribonucleotide synthase.

polynucleotide phosphatase (pol″e-noo′kle-o-tīd fos′-fah-tās) an enzyme of the hydrolase class that catalyzes the reaction phosphopolynucleotide + H$_2$O = polynucleotide + orthophosphate. The substrate may be 3′ phosphopolynucleotide (polynucleotide 3′-phosphatase, EC 3.1.3.32) or 5′-phosphopolynucleotide (polynucleotide 5′-phosphatase, EC 3.1.3.33).

polynucleotide phosphorylase (pol″e-noo′kle-o-tīd fos-for′il-ās) polyribonucleotide nucleotidyltransferase.

polyodontia (pol″e-o-don′she-ah) [*poly-* + Gr. *odous* tooth] the presence of supernumerary teeth.

polyol dehydrogenase (pol′e-ol de-hi′dro-jĕ-nās) iditol dehydrogenase.

polyoma (pol″e-o′mah) a tumor caused by an oncogenic virus of broad host range, originally isolated from parotid gland tumors of mice inoculated with Gross leukemia virus.

polyomavirus (pol″e-o-mah-vi′rus) any of a subgroup of the papovaviruses causing neoplastic disease in mice and hamsters; the subgroup includes the K virus and vacuolating virus. Also written *polyoma virus.* Cf. *papillomavirus.*

polyonychia (pol″e-o-nik′e-ah) [*poly-* + Gr. *onyx* nail + *-ia*] the occurrence of supernumerary nails.

polyopia (pol″e-o′pe-ah) [*poly-* + *-opia*] the condition in which one object appears as two or more objects. **binocular p.,** diplopia. **p. monophthal′mica,** a condition in which an object looked at by one eye appears double.

polyopsia (pol″e-op′se-ah) polyopia.

polyopy (pol′e-o″pe) polyopia.

polyorchidism (pol″e-or′kĭ-dizm) a developmental anomaly characterized by the presence of more than two testes.

polyorchis (pol″e-or′kis) [*poly-* + Gr. *orchis* testis] a person with more than two testes.

polyorchism (pol″e-or′kizm) polyorchidism.

polyorrhomeningitis (pol″e-or″o-men″in-ji′tis) (obs.) polyserositis.

polyorrhymenitis (pol″e-or″hi-mĕ-ni′tis) [*poly-* + Gr. *orrhos* serum + *hymēn* membrane + *-itis*] (obs.) polyserositis.

polyostotic (pol″e-os-tot′ik) [*poly-* + L. *os* bone] pertaining to or affecting many bones.

polyotia (pol″e-o′she-ah) [*poly-* + Gr. *ous* ear] the condition of having more than two ears.

polyovular (pol″e-o′vu-lar) pertaining to or produced from more than one ovum, as polyovular twins.

polyovulatory (pol″e-ov′u-lah-to″re) ordinarily discharging several ova in one ovarian cycle.

polyoxyethylene 50 stearate (pol″e-oks″e-eth′ah-lēn) [NF] a mixture of the mono- and distearate esters of mixed polyoxyethylene diols and the corresponding free diols, the average polymer length being equivalent to about 50 oxyethylene units, occurring as a soft, cream-colored, waxy solid; used as a surfactant and emulsifying agent in pharmaceutical preparations. Called also *polyoxyl 50 stearate.*

polyoxyl (pol″e-oks′il) any of various mixtures of the mono- and distearate esters of mixed polyoxyethylene diols and the corresponding free diols. The term is used in combination with an identifying number which indicates the average polymer length in oxyethylene units: *p.* 8 *stearate* and *p.* 40 *stearate* [USP], in which the average polymer lengths in oxyethylene units are equivalent to about 8 and 40, respectively, are used as surfactants in pharmaceutical preparations. **p. 5 oleate,** peglicol 5 oleate. **p. 10 oleyl ether,** see under *ether.* **p. 20 celostearyl ether,** see under *ether.* **p. 50 stearate,** polyoxyethylene 50 stearate.

polyp (pol′ip) [Gr. *polypous* a morbid excrescence] a morbid excrescence, or protruding growth, from mucous membrane; classically applied to a growth on the mucous membrane of the nose, the term is now applied to such protrusions from any mucous membrane. **adenomatous p.,** a benign polypoid adenoma. **cardiac p.,** a ball thrombus or tumor attached by a pedicle to the inside of the heart. **cervical p.,** a common, relatively innocuous tumor of the uterine cervix, usually of the endocervical canal, composed of a loose fibromyxomatous stroma containing mucus-secreting endocervical glands; they vary widely in size and may produce irregular vaginal bleeding. **choanal p's,** nasal polyps that project posteriorly into the nasopharynx. **endometrial p's,** small, sessile, benign projecting masses on the endometrium, composed of an edematous stroma containing cystically dilated glands. **fibrinous p.,** an intrauterine polyp made up of fibrin from retained blood; it may grow from portions of an ovum or from a thrombus at the placental site. **gelatinous p.,** myxoma. **gum p.,** a small pedunculated growth on the gingiva. **Hopmann's p.,** a mass produced by papillary hypertrophy of the nasal mucosa, having something of the appearance of a papilloma. **hydatid p.,** polypus cysticus. **juvenile p's,** small, benign hemispheric hamartomas of the large intestine occurring sporadically in children; histologically, there is an abundant loose fibrovascular stroma containing widely spaced glands; called also *retention p.* **p's of larynx,** smooth, rounded, sessile or pedunculated swellings, occurring on the true vocal cords; caused by edema in the lamina propria of the mucous membrane. **lymphoid p's,** rare, benign tumors of the colon composed of aggregates of lymphoid tissue, usually covered by a fairly regular colonic mucosa. **nasal p's,** focal accumulations of edema fluid in the mucosa of the nose, with hyperplasia of the associated submucosal connective tissue. **retention p's,** juvenile p's.

polypapilloma tropicum (pol″e-pap″ĭ-lo′mah trop′ĭ-kum) yaws.

polyparasitism (pol″e-par′ah-si-tizm) infection or infestation by more than one variety of parasite.

polyparesis (pol″e-pah-re′sis) [*poly-* + Gr. *paresis* slackening] (obs.) general paresis.

polypathia (pol″e-path′e-ah) [*poly-* + Gr. *pathos* disease + *-ia*] the presence of several diseases at once.

polypectomy (pol″ĭ-pek′to-me) [*polyp* + Gr. *ektomē* excision] surgical removal of a polyp.

polypeptidase (pol″e-pep′tĭ-dās) peptidase.

polypeptide (pol″e-pep′tīd) [poly- + peptide] a peptide which on hydrolysis yields more than two amino acids; called tripeptides, tetrapeptides, etc., according to the number of amino acids contained. See peptide. **gastric inhibitory p. (GIP)**, a polypeptide hormone (molecular weight 5165; 43 amino acids) synthesized by K cells in the midzone of the duodenal and jejunal mucosa and released in response to oral glucose, fat, and amino acids; it increases insulin secretion and inhibits gastric secretion and motility. **pancreatic p.**, a hormone (4200 daltons, 36 amino acids) secreted by special endocrine cells in the periphery of the pancreatic islets and the exocrine pancreas and present almost exclusively in the pancreas; it inhibits pancreatic enzyme secretion and gallbladder contraction, but its physiologic role has not been identified. **vasoactive intestinal p. (VIP)**, a peptide hormone (3326 daltons, 28 amino acids) widely distributed throughout the body but found in highest concentrations in the nervous system and gut; it is released locally from nerve endings or endocrine cells. Its primary actions are thought to be as a neurotransmitter, to relax smooth muscles of the circulation, gut, and genitourinary system, to increase secretion of water and electrolytes from the pancreas and gut, and to release hormones from the pancreatic islets, gut, and hypothalamus. It is found in excess in the Verner-Morrison syndrome.

polypeptidemia (pol″e-pep″tĭ-de′me-ah) [polypeptide + Gr. haima blood + -ia] the presence of polypeptides in the blood.

polypeptidorrhachia (pol″e-pep″tĭ-do-ra′ke-ah) [polypeptide + Gr. rhachis spine + -ia] the presence of polypeptides in the spinal fluid.

polyperiostitis (pol″e-per″e-os-ti′tis) inflammation of the periosteum of several bones. **p. hyperesthet′ica**, a chronic disease of the periosteum attended by extreme hyperesthesia of the skin and soft parts.

polyphagia (pol″e-fa′je-ah) [poly- + Gr. phagein to eat] excessive eating; gluttony.

polyphalangia (pol″e-fah-lan′je-ah) side-by-side duplication of one or more of the phalanges of a digit.

polyphalangism (pol″e-fah-lan′jizm) polyphalangia.

polypharmaceutic (pol″e-fahr″mah-su′tik) pertaining to several drugs, especially to the administration of several drugs together.

polypharmacy (pol″e-fahr′mah-se) [poly- + Gr. pharmakon drug] 1. the administration of many drugs together. 2. the administration of excessive medication.

polyphase (pol′e-fāz) [poly- + phase] having several phases; containing colloids of several types.

polyphasic (pol″e-fa′zik) having or existing in many phases; having unlike particles in the disperse phase.

polyphenic (pol″e-fen′ik) see pleiotropism.

polyphenoloxidase (pol″e-fe″nol-ok′sĭ-dās) catechol oxidase.

polyphobia (pol″e-fo′be-ah) [poly- + phobia] irrational fear of many things.

polyphyletic (pol″e-fi-let′ik) [poly- + Gr. phylē tribe] arising or descending from more than one cell type.

polyphyletism (pol″e-fi′lĕ-tizm) polyphyletic theory; see under theory.

polyphyletist (pol″e-fi′lĕ-tist) an adherent of the polyphyletic theory, as in blood origin.

polyphyodont (pol″e-fi′o-dont) [poly- + Gr. phyein to produce + odous tooth] developing several sets of teeth successively throughout life. Cf. diphyodont and monophyodont.

polypi (pol′ĭ-pi) [L.] plural of polypus.

polypiform (po-lip′ĭ-form) resembling a polyp; polypoid.

polypionia (pol″e-pi-o′ne-ah) [poly- + Gr. piōn fat + -ia] obesity.

polyplastic (pol″e-plas′tik) [poly- + Gr. plastos molded] 1. containing many structural or constituent elements. 2. undergoing many changes of form.

Polyplax (pol′e-plaks) a sucking louse of rats and mice. P. miacan′thus, a form found infrequently on rats; P. serra′tus, a louse of rabbits which transmits tularemia; and P. spinulo′sa, the common louse of rats, which transmits murine typhus.

polyplegia (pol″e-ple′je-ah) [poly- + Gr. plēgē stroke + -ia] simultaneous paralysis of several muscles.

polyploid (pol′e-ploid) [poly- + haploid] 1. having more than two full sets of homologous chromosomes. There may be three (triploid), four (tetraploid), five (pentaploid), six (hexaploid), seven (heptaploid), eight (octaploid), etc. 2. an individual or cell having more than two full sets of homologous chromosomes. Polyploid organisms, especially plants, are larger than normal and have larger cells. Affected animals are often abnormal in appearance and usually infertile. Cf. aneuploid.

polyploidy (pol′e-ploi″de) the state of having more than two full sets of homologous chromosomes (see polyploid).

polypnea (pol″ip-ne′ah) [poly- + Gr. pnoia respiration] a condition in which the rate of respiration is increased; hyperpnea.

polypodia (pol″e-po′de-ah) [poly- + Gr. pous foot] the presence of supernumerary feet.

polypoid (pol′e-poid) [polyp + Gr. eidos form] resembling a polyp.

polypoidosis (pol″e-poi-do′sis) a condition of multiple polypoid adenomas or carcinomas; diffuse adenomatosis.

polyporin (pol-ip′o-rin) a mixture of antibiotic substances from species of Polyporus, which is active against some bacteria.

polyporous (pol-ip′o-rus) having many pores.

Polyporus (pol-ip′o-rus) [poly- + Gr. poros pore] basidiomycetous fungi of the order Polyporales, series Hymenomycetes, containing many species, some of which are important pathogens of trees. P. officinalis (larch agaric, purging agaric, white agaric) is the source of agaric acid. See also agaric.

polyposia (pol″e-po′ze-ah) [poly- + Gr. posis + -ia] ingestion of abnormally increased amounts of fluids for long periods of time. Cf. hyperposia.

polyposis (pol″e-po′sis) the development of multiple polyps on a part. **p. co′li**, familial p. **familial p.**, multiple adenomatous polyps with high malignant potential, lining the mucous membrane of the intestine, particularly the colon, beginning at about puberty. It occurs in several autosomal dominant forms: In Gardner's syndrome, colonic polyposis is associated with epidermoid cysts, fibromas, osteomas of the skull, supernumerary teeth, and less commonly ampullary tumors. In Peutz-Jeghers syndrome, mucocutaneous pigmentation (particularly of the lips) is associated with hamartomas of the intestine, particularly the small bowel. In Canada-Cronkhite syndrome, familial polyposis is associated with ectodermal abnormalities. In Turcot syndrome, colonic polyposis is associated with gliomas of the central nervous system. Called also p. coli, familial intestinal p., and multiple familial p. **familial intestinal p.**, familial p. **p. gas′trica**, the presence of multiple polyps on the gastric mucosa, usually associated with atrophic gastritis. **p. intestina′lis**, a condition in which polyps occur in the intestine and rectum. **multiple familial p.**, familial p. **p. ventric′uli**, p. gastrica.

polypotome (po-lip′o-tōm) a cutting instrument for removing polyps.

polypotrite (po-lip′o-trīt) [polyp + L. terere to crush] an instrument for crushing polyps.

polypous (pol′e-pus) of the nature of a polyp; polyp-like.

polypragmasy (pol″e-prag′mah-se) [poly- + Gr. pragma a doing] polypharmacy.

polyptychial (pol″e-ti′ke-al) [poly- + Gr. ptychē fold] arranged in several layers; said of glands whose cells are arranged on the basement membrane in several layers. Cf. monoptychial.

polypus (pol′ĭ-pus), pl. pol′ypi [L., from Gr. polypous, from poly- + pous foot] a polyp. **p. angiomato′des**, a polyp rich in blood vessels. **p. cys′ticus**, a polyp in which the fibrous network is coarse, thus stimulating or actually producing cysts. **p. hydatido′sus**, p. cysticus. **p. telangiecto′des**, a polyp which contains many dilated blood vessels.

polyradiculitis (pol″e-rah-dik″u-li′tis) [poly- + L. radix root + -itis] inflammation of the nerve roots.

polyradiculoneuritis (pol″e-rah-dik″u-lo-nu-ri′tis) [poly- + L. radix root + Gr. neuron nerve + -itis] acute febrile polyneuritis which involves the peripheral nerves, the spinal nerve roots, and the spinal cord.

polyradiculoneuropathy (pol″e-rah-dik″u-lo-nu-rop′-ah-the) Guillain-Barré syndrome.

polyribonucleotide (pol″ĕ-ri′bo-nu′kle-o-tīd) a polymer of ribonucleotides; ribonucleic acid.

polyribonucleotide nucleotidyltransferase (pol″e-ri″bo-noo′kle-o-tīd noo″kle-o-tid′il-trans′fer-ās) [EC 2.7.7.8] an enzyme of the transferase class that catalyzes the reaction RNA_{n+1} + orthophosphate = RNA_n + a nucleoside diphosphate, or the reverse reaction. ADP, IDP, GDP, UDP, and CDP can act as donors in the latter case. This bacterial enzyme was used in research elucidating the genetic code. Called also *polynucleotide phosphorylase*.

polyribosome (pol″e-ri′bo-sōm) a complex made up of ribosomal subunits assembled among themselves by the filaments of messenger RNA containing the genetic information; they play a role in the synthesis of peptides. Called also *ergosome* and *polysome*.

polyrrhea (pol″ĕ-re′ah) [*poly-* + Gr. *rhoia* flow] a copious fluid discharge.

polysaccharide (pol″e-sak′ah-rīd) a carbohydrate which on hydrolysis yields a large number (variously defined as five or more to eleven or more) of monosaccharides. Cf. *oligosaccharide*. **bacterial p's**, polysaccharides found in bacteria and especially in bacterial capsules. **core p.**, the constant part of the heteropolysaccharide chain of lipopolysaccharide. **gastric p.**, the mucopolysaccharide found in gastric mucus. **immune p's**, polysaccharides which can function as specific antigens, such as capsular substances. **O-specific p.**, the variable part of the heteropolysaccharide chain of lipopolysaccharide (q.v.); it is responsible for the antigenic specificity. **pneumococcus p.**, a polysaccharide derived from the capsule of *Streptococcus pneumoniae*. More than 80 immunologically distinct types have been identified which form the basis of pneumococcal typing. The structure of some is known: Type I is a polymer of trisaccharide units containing galacturonic acids; Type 2 is a polymer of glucose; Type 3 is a high molecular weight polymer of glucose and glucuronic acid units (cellobiuronic acid); and Type 8 consists of glucose and glucuronic acid units alternating with glucosyl-galactose residues. **specific p's**, soluble polysaccharides obtained from various microorganisms which in high dilution precipitate specifically the antisera to the corresponding organisms.

polysaccharose (pol″e-sak′ah-rōs) polysaccharide.

polysarcia (pol″e-sar′se-ah) [*poly-* + Gr. *sarx* flesh] corpulence or obesity.

polysarcous (pol″e-sar′kus) corpulent; obese; affected with polysarcia.

polyscelia (pol″e-se′le-ah) [*poly-* + Gr. *skelos* leg + *-ia*] a developmental anomaly characterized by the presence of more than two legs.

polyscelus (pŏ-lis′ĕ-lus) [*poly-* + Gr. *skelos* leg] an individual exhibiting polyscelia.

polyscope (pol″e-skōp) [*poly-* + Gr. *skopein* to examine] diaphanoscope.

polysensitivity (pol″e-sen″sĭ-tiv′ĭ-te) sensitivity to a number of different stimuli.

polysensory (pol″e-sen′so-re) capable of responding to more than one kind of sensory input; said of certain neurons of the cerebral cortex and subcortical regions.

polyserositis (pol″e-se-ro-si′tis) [*poly-* + *serositis*] general inflammation of serous membranes with serous effusion; see also *Concato's disease*. **familial recurrent p.**, familial Mediterranean fever. **periodic p.**, familial Mediterranean fever. **recurrent p.**, familial Mediterranean fever.

polysialia (pol″e-si-a′le-ah) [*poly-* + Gr. *sialon* saliva + *-ia*] ptyalism.

polysinuitis (pol″e-sin″u-i′tis) polysinusitis.

polysinusectomy (pol″e-si″nŭ-sek′to-me) excision of the diseased membrane of several of the paranasal sinuses.

polysinusitis (pol″e-si-nŭ-si′tis) [*poly-* + *sinusitis*] inflammation of several sinuses at once.

polysomatic (pol″e-so-mat′ik) characterized by or pertaining to polysomaty.

polysomaty (pol″e-so′mah-te) [*poly-* + chromos*ome*] the state of having reduplicated chromatin in the nucleus. The term is applied both to the condition of increase in chromosome number resulting from a previous endomitotic cycle (endopolyploidy, def. 3) and to increase in the amount of chromatin per chromosome (polyteny).

polysome (pol′e-sōm) polyribosome.

polysomia (pol″e-so′me-ah) [*poly-* + Gr. *sōma* body + *-ia*] a doubling or tripling of the body of a fetus.

polysomic (pol″e-so′mik) 1. pertaining to or exhibiting polysomy. 2. an individual exhibiting polysomy.

polysomus (pol″e-so′mus) [*poly-* + Gr. *sōma* body] a monster exhibiting polysomia.

polysomy (pol″e-so′me) [*poly-* + chromos*ome*] an excess of a particular chromosome, resulting from meiotic chromosomal nondisjunction. The chromosome may be duplicated three (trisomy), four (tetrasomy), or more times.

polysorbate (pol″e-sor′bāt) a generic name for esters of sorbitol and its anhydrides condensed with polymers of ethylene oxide, used as surfactant agents: *p. 20*, $C_{58}H_{114}O_{26}$, is polyoxyethylene 20 sorbitan monolaurate; *p. 40*, $C_{62}H_{122}$-O_{26}, is polyoxyethylene 20 sorbitan monopalmitate; *p. 60*, $C_{64}H_{126}O_{26}$, is polyethylene 20 sorbitan monostearate; *p. 65*, $C_{100}H_{194}O_{28}$, is polyethylene 20 sorbitan tristearate; *p. 80*, $C_{64}H_{124}O_{26}$, is polyethylene 20 sorbitan monooleate; *p. 85*, $C_{100}H_{188}O_{28}$, is polyethylene 20 sorbitan trioleate. *Polysorbates* 20, 40, 60, and 80 are official in NF.

polyspermia (pol″e-sper′me-ah) [*poly-* + Gr. *sperma* seed + *-ia*] 1. excessive secretion of semen. 2. polyspermy.

polyspermism (pol″e-sper′mizm) polyspermia.

polyspermy (pol″e-sper′me) fertilization of an ovum by more than one spermatozoon. **pathological p.**, entrance of more than one spermatozoon in an ovum when entrance of only one is the rule; usually development is abnormal and the embryo is not viable. **physiological p.**, entrance of more than one spermatozoon in an ovum, occurring normally in certain species, but with only one spermatozoon participating fully in the development of the embryo.

polysplenia (pol″e-sple′ne-ah) the presence of multiple spleens or splenuli.

polystichia (pol″e-stik′e-ah) [*poly-* + Gr. *stichos* row + *-ia*] the presence of two or more rows of eyelashes upon a lid.

polystyrene (pol″e-sti′rēn) a hard, transparent, thermoplastic synthetic resin produced by the polymerization of styrene; used in the construction of denture bases.

polysuspensoid (pol″e-sus-pen′soid) a suspensoid in which the particles are of different degrees of dispersion.

polysynaptic (pol″e-sĭ-nap′tik) involving many synapses in series and therefore a sequence of many neurons; called also *multisynaptic*. Cf. *oligosynaptic*.

polysyndactyly (pol″e-sin-dak′til-e) [*poly-* + *syndactyly*] an association of polydactyly and syndactyly of varying degrees of both the hand and foot.

polysynovitis (pol″e-sin″o-vi′tis) [*poly-* + *synovitis*] general inflammation of the synovial membranes.

polytef (pol′ĕ-tef) a polymer of tetrafluoroethylene, used as a surgical implant material for many prostheses, such as artificial vessels and orbital floor implants and for many applications in skeletal augmentation and skeletal fixation. Also used in industry for many purposes, e.g., as an antistick coating for cooking utensils. Called also *polytetrafluoroethylene* (PTFE). See also *polymer fume fever*, under *fever*.

polytendinitis (pol″e-ten″dĭ-ni′tis) inflammation affecting several tendons.

polytendinobursitis (pol″e-ten″dĭ-no-bur-si′tis) associated bursitis and tendinitis in several parts of the body.

polytene (pol′e-tēn) [*poly-* + Gr. *tainia* (L. *taenia*) band] composed of or containing many strands of chromatin (chromonemata).

polytenosynovitis (pol″e-ten″o-sin″o-vi′tis) inflammation of several or many tendon sheaths at the same time.

polyteny (pol″ĕ-te′ne) reduplication of chromonemata in the chromosome without separation into distinct daughter chromosomes. See also *polysomaty*.

polytetrafluoroethylene (pol″e-tet″rah-floo″o-ro-eth′ĭ-lēn) polytef.

polythelia (pol″e-the′le-ah) [*poly-* + Gr. *thēlē* nipple + *-ia*] the condition of having more than one pair of nipples.

polythelism (pol″e-the′lizm) polythelia.

polythene (pol′e-thēn) polyethylene.

polythetic (pol″e-thet′ik) [poly- + Gr. *thetikos* fit for placing] denoting a taxonomic group classified on the basis of several characters, as opposed to a monothetic group.

polythiazide (pol″e-thi′ah-zīd) [USP] chemical name: 6-chloro-3,4-dihydro-2-methyl-3-[[2,2,2-trifluoroethyl)-thio]-methyl]-2H-1,2,4-benzothiadiazine-7-sulfonamide 1,1-dioxide. An orally effective diuretic and antihypertensive, $C_{11}H_{13}ClF_3N_3O_4S_3$.

polytocous (po-lit′o-kus) [poly- + Gr. *tokos* birth] giving birth to several offspring at one time.

polytomogram (pol″e-tom′o-gram) the record produced by polytomography.

polytomographic (pol″e-to″mo-graf′ik) pertaining to polytomography.

polytomography (pol″e-to-mog′rah-fe) tomography of tissue at several predetermined planes.

polytrichia (pol″e-trik′e-ah) [poly- + Gr. *thrix* hair] hypertrichosis.

polytrichosis (pol″e-trĭ-ko′sis) hypertrichosis.

Polytrichum (po-lit′rĭ-kum) [poly- + Gr. *thrix* hair] a genus of mosses, *P. juniperi′num* Willd. haircap, or juniper moss, is diuretic.

polytrophia (pol″e-tro′fe-ah) [poly- + Gr. *trophē* nourishment] excessive nutrition.

polytrophic (pol″e-trof′ik) pertaining to or characterized by polytrophia.

polytrophy (po-lit′ro-fe) polytrophia.

polytropic (pol″e-trop′ik) [poly- + Gr. *tropē* a turning] affecting many kinds of bacteria, viruses, or tissues. Cf. *monotropic*.

polyunguia (pol″e-ung′gwe-ah) polyonychia.

polyunsaturated (pol″e-un-sach′ĕ-ra-ted) denoting a fatty acid, e.g., linoleic acid, having more than one double bond in its hydrocarbon chain.

polyuria (pol″e-u′re-ah) [poly- + Gr. *ouron* urine + -ia] the passage of a large volume of urine in a given period, a characteristic of diabetes.

polyvalent (pol″e-va′lent) having more than one valence.

polyvinyl (pol″e-vi′nil) a polymerization product of a monomeric vinyl compound, as vinyl chloride.

polyvinylacetate (pol″e-vi′nil-as′ĕ-tāt) a light- and heat-stable resin formed by the polymerization of vinyl acetate.

polyvinylbenzene (pol″e-vi′nil-ben′zēn) polystyrene.

polyvinylchloride (pol″e-vi′nil-klōr′īd) a substance formed by the polymerization of vinyl chloride; a tasteless, odorless, clear hard resin, which changes color on exposure to ultraviolet light or heat.

polyvinylpyrrolidone (pol″e-vi″nil-pir-rol′ĭ-dōn) povidone.

pomade (po-mād′) pomatum.

Pomatiopsis (po-mat″e-op′sis) a genus of amphibious fresh-water snails of the United States; *P. cincinnatien′sis* and *P. lapida′ria* have been shown to be hosts of *Paragonimus kellicotti*.

pomatum (po-ma′tum) [L., from *pomum* apple] a medicated ointment for the hair.

pomegranate (pum-gran′et) [L. *pomum granatum* grained apple] the punicaceous tree, *Punica granatum* L. (Punicaceae), and its fruit. The root and the dried bark of the stem were formerly used as teniacides. Called also *granatum*.

POMP a regimen of prednisone, oncovin (vincristine), methotrexate, and 6-mercaptopurine, used in cancer chemotherapy.

pompholyhemia (pom″fo-le-he′me-ah) [*pompholyx* + Gr. *haima* blood + -ia] the presence of bubbles of gas in the blood, as in decompression sickness.

pompholyx (pom′fo-liks) [Gr. "bubble"] a recurrent eczematous reaction characterized by the development of a vesicular eruption on the palms and soles, particularly along the sides and between the digits, accompanied by pruritus, and a burning sensation and hyperhidrosis. It is a self-limited condition usually lasting a few weeks. Called also *dyshidrotic eczema*, and formerly *cheiropompholyx* and *dyshidrosis*.

pomum (po′mum) [L.] apple. **p. ada′mi** ["Adam's apple"], the prominence in the neck produced by the thyroid cartilage; prominentia laryngea.

ponceau B (pon so′) Biebrich scarlet; see under *scarlet*. **p. 3 B**, scarlet red; see under *red*.

Poncet's disease, operation, rheumatism (pahw-sāz′) [Antonin *Poncet*, French surgeon, 1849– 1913] see under *disease, operation,* and *rheumatism*.

Pond. abbreviation for L. *pon′dere*, by weight.

ponderable (pon′der-ah-b'l) [L. *ponderabilis; pondus* weight] having weight.

ponderal (pon′der-al) [L. *pondus*, weight] pertaining to weight.

Pondimin (pon′dĭ-mēn) trademark for a preparation of fenfluramine hydrochloride.

pondostatural (pon″do-stat′u-ral) pertaining to weight and stature.

ponesiatrics (po-ne″ze-ah′triks) [Gr. *ponēsis* toil, exertion + *iatrikē* surgery, medicine] a system of therapy in which misdirected neurophysiologic reactions are made perceptible (as by the oscilloscope, electromyograph, etc.) and used as a guide in recognizing and correcting such undesirable responses (dysponesis). Called also *effort training*.

Ponfick's shadow (pon′fiks) [Clemens Emil *Ponfick*, German pathologist, 1844–1913] phantom corpuscle; see under *corpuscle*.

Pongidae (pon′jĭ-de) a family of primates, including the anthropoid apes, which together with the family Hominidae (man), constitute the superfamily Hominoidea.

pon(o)- [Gr. *ponos* toil, suffering, pain] a combining form denoting relationship to hard work or to pain.

ponograph (po′no-graf) [pono- + Gr. *graphein* to write] an instrument for estimating and recording sensitiveness to pain.

ponopalmosis (po″no-pal-mo′sis) [pono- + Gr. *palmos* palpitation] (obs.) palpitation on effort; neurocirculatory asthenia.

ponos (po′nos) ["hurt"] the Mediterranean type of visceral leishmaniasis.

pons (ponz), pl. *pon′tes,* gen. *pon′tis* [L. "bridge"] 1. any slip of tissue connecting two parts of an organ; called also *bridge*. 2. [NA] that part of the central nervous system lying between the medulla oblongata and the mesencephalon, ventral to the cerebellum, and consisting of a pars dorsalis and a pars ventralis; called also *bridge of Varolius, metencephalon* [NA alternative], *p. cerebelli,* and *commissura cerebelli.* See Plate accompanying *brain*. See also *brain stem,* under B. **p. cerebel′li,** pons, def. 2. **p. hep′atis,** an occasional projection of fibers partially bridging the longitudinal fissure of the liver. **p. tari′ni,** substantia perforata posterior.

pons-oblongata (ponz″ob-lon-ga′tah) the pons and medulla oblongata considered together.

Ponstel (pon′stel) trademark for a preparation of mefenamic acid.

pontes (pon′tēz) [L.] plural of *pons*.

pontibrachium (pon″te-bra′ke-um) pedunculus cerebellaris medius.

pontic (pon′tik) [L. *pons,* gen. *pontis* bridge] an artificial tooth on a fixed partial denture, which replaces the lost natural tooth, restores its function, and usually occupies the space previously occupied by the natural crown.

ponticular (pon-tik′u-lar) pertaining to the ponticulus (propons).

ponticulus (pon-tik′u-lus), pl. *pontic′uli* [L., dim. of *pons* bridge] propons. **p. auric′ulae,** a point on the eminence of the concha where the posterior auricular muscle is attached. **p. promonto′rii,** a ridge on the median wall of the tympanic cavity connecting the promontory with the pyramid.

pontil (pon′til) pontile; pontine.

pontile (pon′tīl, pon′tēl) pertaining to the pons; pontine.

pontine (pon′tīn, pon′tēn) pertaining to the pons; pontile.

pontis (pon′tis) [L.] genitive of *pons*.

pontobulbar (pon″to-bul′bar) pertaining to, affecting, or regulated by the pons and the region of the medulla oblongata situated dorsad to it.

pontobulbia (pon″to-bul′be-ah) a condition in which cavities exist in the pons and medulla oblongata; syringobulbia.

Pontocaine (pon′to-kān) trademark for preparations of tetracaine.

pontocerebellar (pon''to-ser''ĕ-bel'ar) pertaining to the pons and the cerebellum.

pontomedullary (pon''to-med'u-lār''e) pertaining to the pons and the medulla oblongata.

pontomesencephalic (pon''to-mes''en-sĕ-fal'ik) pertaining to or involving the pons and the mesencephalon.

pontoon (pon-tōōn′) [Fr. ponton; L. ponto boat] a loop or knuckle of the small intestine.

pontopeduncular (pon''to-pĕ-dung'ku-lar) pertaining to, affecting, or communicating with the pons and cerebral peduncles.

pool (pōōl) 1. a common reservoir on which to draw. 2. to mix plasma from several donors. 3. an accumulation, as of blood in any part of the body due to retardation of the venous circulation. **gene p.,** the totality of the genes possessed by all of the members of a population. **metabolic p.,** the entire mass of labile and reactive substances in the body, to which and from which innumerable substances continuously pass; also used in a restricted sense to mean the extracellular pool or the potassium pool.

Pool's phenomenon (pōōlz) [Eugene Hillhouse Pool, New York surgeon, 1874–1949] 1. see under phenomenon. 2. Schlesinger's sign.

Pool-Schlesinger sign (pōōl-shla'zing-er) [E. H. Pool; Hermann Schlesinger, Austrian physician, 1868–1934] Schlesinger's sign.

popin (pop'in) a glycoside of unknown origin which is used in Barbados for amebic dysentery.

poples (pop'lez) [L. "ham"] [NA] the posterior surface of the knee.

popliteal (pop-lit'e-al; pop''lĭ-te'al) [L. poples ham] pertaining to the posterior surface of the knee; see also under ligament.

poppy (pop'e) any member of the poppy or Papaveraceae family. See Papaver.

population (pop''u-la'shun) [L. populatio, from populus people] 1. the individuals collectively constituting a certain category or inhabiting a specified geographic area. 2. in genetics, a stable group of randomly interbreeding individuals. 3. in statistics, the set of objects or individuals from which a random sample is drawn.

POR problem-oriented record; see under record.

poradenia (pōr''ah-de'ne-ah) poradenitis.

poradenitis (pōr''ad-ĕ-ni'tis) [por-(1) + adenitis] a disease of the iliac lymph nodes characterized by the formation of small abscesses. Called also poradenia. **p. nos'tras, subacute inguinal p., p. vene'rea,** lymphogranuloma venereum.

poradenolymphitis (por-ad''ĕ-no-lim-fi'tis) [por-(1) + adeno- + lymphitis] lymphogranuloma venereum.

poral (pōr'al) pertaining to or having pores.

porcelain (por'sĕ-lin) 1. a white, translucent, dense ceramic material produced by fusing under high temperature of a mixture of feldspar, kaolin, quartz, whiting, and other substances. 2. dental p. **dental p.,** a type of porcelain used in dental restorations, either jacket crowns or inlays, artificial teeth, or metal-ceramic crowns. It is essentially a mixture of particles of feldspar and quartz, the feldspar melting first and providing a glass matrix for the quartz.

porcelaneous (por''sĕ-la'ne-us) pertaining to or resembling porcelain.

porcine (por'sīn) [L. porcus a pig, hog] pertaining to, characteristic of, or derived from swine.

pore (pōr) [L. porus; Gr. poros] a small opening; called also porus [NA]. **acoustic p., osseous, external,** porus acusticus externus osseus. **acoustic p., osseous, internal,** porus acusticus internus osseus. **alveolar p's,** openings between adjacent pulmonary alveoli that permit passage of air from one to another; called also pores of Kohn. **biliary p.,** ductus choledochus. **birth p.,** metraterm. **Galen's p.,** canalis inguinalis. **gustatory p.,** porus gustatorius. **interalveolar p's, p's of Kohn,** alveolar p's. **nuclear p's,** small octagonal openings in the nuclear envelope at sites where the two nuclear membranes are in contact, which together with the annuli form the pore complex. See also Plate XI. **slit p's,** small slitlike spaces between the pedicels of the podocytes of the renal glomerulus; called also filtration slits. **sweat p.,** porus sudoriferus. **taste p.,** porus gustatorius.

porencephalia (po''ren-sĕ-fa'le-ah) [por-(1) + Gr. enkephalon brain] 1. the presence of cysts or cavities in the brain cortex communicating by a "pore" with the arachnoid space (Heschl, 1850). 2. the presence of cavities in the brain developed in fetal life or early infancy, whether or not they communicate with the arachnoid space; the cavities are usually the residues of destructive lesions (encephaloclastic p.), but sometimes are the result of maldevelopment (schizencephalic p., schizencephaly). Called also cerebral porosis, perencephaly, and porencephaly.

porencephalic (po''ren-sĕ-fal'ik) pertaining to or characterized by porencephalia. Called also porencephalous.

porencephalitis (po''ren-sef''ah-li'tis) porencephalia associated with an inflammatory process, such as polioencephalitis.

porencephalous (po''ren-sef'ah-lus) porencephalic.

porencephaly (po''ren-sef'ah-le) porencephalia.

porfiromycin (por''fi-ro-mi'sin) chemical name: 6-amino-8- [[(aminocarbonyl)oxy]methyl]-1,1a,2,8,8a,8b- hexahydro-8a-methoxy-1,5-dimethylazirino[2′,3′:3,4]pyrrolo[1,2-a]indole-4,7-dione. An antineoplastic antibiotic with antitumor activity, $C_{16}H_{20}N_4O_5$, derived from Streptomyces ardus; it is the methyl derivative of mitomycin C.

Porges-Hermann-Perutz reaction (por'ges-her'man-pa'root) [Otto Porges, Vienna bacteriologist, born 1879; Otto Hermann, Vienna physician; Alfred Perutz, Austrian dermatologist, born 1885] Perutz reaction.

Porges-Meier test (reaction) [Otto Porges; Georg Meier, German serologist, born 1875] see under tests.

pori (po'ri) [L.] genitive and plural of porus.

Porifera (po-rif'ĕ-rah) [L. porus pore + ferre to bear] the phylum of sponges; the body is perforated with many pores to admit water, from which food is strained.

poriomania (po''re-o-ma'ne-ah) [Gr. poreia walking + mania madness] an irresistible impulse to travel.

porion (po're-on) [Gr. poros pore + -on neuter ending] a craniometric landmark, being the most lateral point on the roof of the bony external auditory meatus, vertically over the middle of the meatus. Called also Po.

por(o)- 1. [L. porus, q.v.] a combining form denoting relationship to a duct, passageway, opening, or pore. 2. [Gr. pōros callus, stone] a combining form denoting relationship to a callus or calculus.

porocephaliasis (po''ro-sef''ah-li'ah-sis) infection with parasites of the order Porocephalida.

Porocephalida (por''o-se-fal'ĭ-dah) an order of the class Pentastomida, wormlike degenerate arthropods, including the families Porocephalidae and Linguatulidae.

Porocephalidae (por''o-sĕ-fal'ĭ-de) a family of the order Porocephalida, class Pentastomida, having cylindrical bodies. Adults are found in the lungs of reptiles, and the larvae are found in various vertebrates, including man. It includes the genera Armillifer, Porocephalus, and Pentastoma.

porocephalosis (po''ro-sef''ah-lo'sis) porocephaliasis.

Porocephalus (po''ro-sef'ah-lus) [poro-(1) + kephalē head] a genus of wormlike arthropods of the order Porocephalida, family Porocephalidae. The species which parasitize man, formerly classified in this genus, are now assigned to other genera. **P. armilla'tus,** Armillifer armillatus. **P. constric'tus,** Armillifer armillatus. **P. denticula'tus,** Pentastoma denticulatum (the larva of Linguatula serrata).

porofocon (por''o-fo'kon) either of two hydrophobic contact lens materials, designated A or B.

porokeratosis (po''ro-ker''ah-to'sis) [poro-(2) + keratosis] a rare, chronic, progressive autosomal dominant skin disorder, seen most often in males, usually first appearing in early childhood, and characterized clinically by the presence of crater-like patches with central atrophy and an elevated thick keratotic border that enlarge to form circinate, serpiginous, or gyrate lesions, and histologically by a cornoid lamella (q.v.). Called also p. of Mibelli. **disseminated superficial actinic p.,** an autosomal dominant skin disorder occurring on sun-exposed skin in individuals over 16 years of age, especially in females, and characterized by the presence of numerous superficial, annular, keratotic, brownish red macules, the centers of which become depressed and the borders form a sharp ridge. **p. of Mibelli,** porokeratosis. **p. palma'ris et planta'ris dissemina'ta,** a distinctive form of porokeratosis inherited as an autosomal dominant trait, in which hundreds of gyrate and annular porokeratotic plaques occur on the soles or palms or both, and later elsewhere.

porokeratotic (po″ro-ker″ah-tot′ik) pertaining to or affected with porokeratosis.

poroma (po-ro′mah) [Gr. *pōrōma* callus] a general term for a neoplasm arising in or from the eccrine pore. **eccrine p.,** a benign tumor arising from the intraepidermal portion of the eccrine sweat duct, often on the palm or sole.

poroplastic (po″ro-plas′tik) both porous and plastic.

porosis (po-ro′sis) 1. [Gr. *pōrōsis* callosity] the formation of the callus in the repair of a fractured bone. 2. [Gr. *pōros* pore] cavity formation. **cerebral p.,** a condition in which there are cavities in the brain substance; porencephalia.

porosity (po-ros′ĭ-te) 1. the condition of being porous. 2. a pore.

porotic (po-rot′ik) pertaining to or characterized by porosis favoring the growth of connective tissue.

porotomy (po-rot′o-me) [Gr. *poros* pore + *tomē* a cutting] meatotomy.

porous (po′rus) penetrated by pores and open spaces.

porphin (por′fin) a cyclic structure of four pyrrole rings connected by methine bridges found in porphyrins.

porphobilinogen (por″fo-bi-lin′o-jen) PBG; the immediate precursor of the porphyrins, a pyrrole ring with acetate, propionate, and methylamine side chains; four molecules of porphobilinogen are condensed to form one molecule of uroporphyrinogen III, which is then converted successively to coproporphyrinogen III, protoporphyrin IX, and heme. Porphobilinogen is produced in excess and excreted in the urine in acute intermittent porphyria.

porphobilinogen deaminase (por″fo-bi-lin′o-jen de-am′-in-ās) [EC 4.3.1.8] an enzyme of the lyase class that catalyzes the reaction 4 porphobilinogen + H_2O = hydroxymethylbilane + $4NH_3$ in the synthesis of porphyrins and heme. Deficiency of the enzyme, an autosomal dominant trait, leads to acute intermittent porphyria. Called also *uroporphyrinogen I synthase*.

porphobilinogen synthase (por″fo-bi-lin′o-jen sin′thās) [EC 4.2.1.24] an enzyme of the lyase class that catalyzes the reaction 2 5-aminolevulinate = porphobilinogen + 2 H_2O in the synthesis of porphyrins. The enzyme is inhibited by minute quantities of lead, and decreased enzyme activity in erythrocytes is an indication of lead poisoning. Called also *aminolevulinate dehydratase*.

porphobilinogenuria (por″fo-bi-lin″o-jen-u′re-ah) the excretion of urine containing porphobilinogen.

porphyran (por′fĭ-ran) a combination of a porphyrin with a metal; a metalloporphyrin.

porphyria (por-fe′re-ah, por-fi′re-ah) [Gr. *porphyra* purple] any of a group of disturbances of porphyrin metabolism, characterized by marked increase in formation and excretion of porphyrins or their precursors. **acute p.,** acute intermittent p. **acute intermittent p.,** hereditary hepatic porphyria manifested by recurrent attacks of abdominal pain, gastrointestinal dysfunction, and neurologic disturbances and by excessive amounts of aminolevulinic acid and porphobilinogen in the urine; it is due to an abnormality of pyrrole metabolism transmitted as an autosomal dominant trait. Called also *acute p., p. hepatica, Swedish genetic p.,* and *pyrroloporphyria.* **congenital erythropoietic p.,** autosomal recessive porphyria in which increased synthesis of uroporphyrinogen I relative to uroporphyrinogen III occurs in bone marrow normoblasts; it is characterized by cutaneous photosensitivity, leading to mutilating skin lesions, by hemolytic anemia and splenomegaly, and by greatly increased urinary excretion of uroporphyrin I (coproporphyrin I excretion is slightly elevated). Erythrodontia and hypertrichosis are invariably present. Called also *congenital photosensitive p., Günther's disease,* and *erythropoietic uroporphyria.* **congenital photosensitive p.,** congenital erythropoietic p. **p. cuta′nea tar′da heredita′ria,** hepatic porphyria resembling variegate porphyria except that abdominal and neurologic symptoms are absent or mild; called also *protocoproporphyria hereditaria.* **p. cuta′nea tar′da symptomat′ica,** a sporadic form of porphyria characterized by chronic skin lesions ranging from slight skin fragility to severe chronic scarring, by hepatomegaly, and by excessive

urinary excretion of uroporphyrin and coproporphyrin; it is usually associated with chronic alcoholism. Called also *urocoproporphyria.* **cutaneous p.,** that characterized by skin manifestations; see *p. cutanea tarda hereditaria* and *symptomatica.* **erythropoietic p., p. erythropoiet′ica,** porphyria in which excessive formation of porphyrin or its precursors occurs in bone marrow normoblasts; it includes congenital erythropoietic porphyria and erythropoietic protoporphyria. **hepatic p.,** porphyria in which the excess formation of porphyrin or its precursors is found in the liver; it includes acute intermittent porphyria, variegate porphyria, and hereditary coproporphyria. **p. hepat′ica,** acute intermittent p. **mixed p.,** variegate p. **South African genetic p.,** variegate p. **Swedish genetic p.,** acute intermittent p. **p. variega′ta, variegate p.,** hereditary hepatic porphyria characterized by chronic cutaneous manifestations, notably extreme mechanical fragility of the skin, particularly areas exposed to sunlight, and by episodes of abdominal pain and neuropathy. There is typically an excess of coproporphyrin and protoporphyrin in the bile and feces. It is transmitted as an autosomal dominant trait. Called also *mixed p.* and *South African genetic p.* See also *p. cutanea tarda hereditaria.*

porphyrin (por′fĭ-rin) any of a group of compounds containing the porphin structure, four pyrrole rings connected by methine (=CH=) bridges in a cyclic configuration, to which a variety of side chains are attached; the nature of the side chains is indicated by a prefix, as uroporphyrin, coproporphyrin, protoporphyrin, etioporphyrin, hematoporphyrin, mesoporphyrin, deuteroporphyrin; structural isomers are indicated by roman numerals. In uroporphyrin and coproporphyrin each pyrrole ring has the same two side chains and there are four isomers; both the type I isomers (which have 4-fold rotational symmetry) and the type III isomers (formed from the type I isomer by interchanging side chains on one ring) occur naturally, but only the type III isomers have functional activity. In protoporphyrin there are fifteen isomers; the naturally occurring one is type IX. Porphyrins occur in the prosthetic groups of hemoglobin, myoglobin, and cytochromes. Cf. *porphyrinogen* and *chlorophyll.*

porphyrinemia (por″fĭ-rin-e′me-ah) the presence of porphyrin in the blood.

porphyrinogen (por″-fĭ-rin′o-jen) a compound formed from the corresponding porphyrin by reduction of the methine bridges connecting the pyrrole rings to methylene (=CH₂=) bridges; as with porphyrins, the nature of the side chains is indicated by a prefix, e.g., uroporphyrinogen and coproporphyrinogen, and the structural isomer by a Roman numeral.

porphyrinopathy (por″fir-in-op′ah-the) any disorder of porphyrin metabolism.

porphyrinuria (por″fĭ-rĭ-nu′re-ah) [*porphyrin* + Gr. *ouron* urine + *-ia*] the presence in the urine of porphyrin (coproporphyrin or uroporphyrin) in excess of the normal amount.

porphyrism (por′fĭ-rizm) porphyria.

porphyrismus (por″fĭ-ris′mus) the triggering action attributed to psychic and emotional disturbances in attacks of acute intermittent porphyria.

porphyrization (por″fĭ-ri-za′shun) pulverization; reduction to a powder: so called because it was performed on a porphyry tablet.

porphyropsin (por″fĭ-rop′sin) a purple pigment in the retinal rods of certain fresh-water fishes.

porphyroxine (por″fĭ-rok′sin) an opium alkaloid, $C_{19}H_{23}O_4N$.

porphyruria (por″fir-u′re-ah) porphyrinuria.

porphyryl (por′fĭ-ril) a name for hemin from which iron has been removed.

Porro's cesarean section (por′ōz) [Edoardo *Porro*, obstetrician in Milan, 1842–1902] see *cesarean section,* under *section.*

porta (por′tah), pl. *por′tae* [L.] an entrance or portal; used in anatomical nomenclature to designate an opening, especially the site of entrance to an organ of the blood vessels and other structures supplying or draining it. **p. hep′atis** [NA], hepatic portal: the transverse fissure on the visceral surface of the liver where the portal vein and hepatic artery enter the liver and the hepatic ducts leave. **p. labyrin′-thi,** fenestra cochleae. **p. lie′nis,** hilum splenicum.

p. of lung, hilus pulmonis. **p. omen′ti, p. of omen-tum,** foramen epiploicum. **p. pulmo′nis,** hilus pulmonis. **p. re′nis,** hilus renalis. **p. of spleen,** hilum splenicum.

portacaval (por″tah-ka′val) pertaining to or connecting the portal vein and the vena cava.

portacid (port-as′id) [Fr. *porte-acid*] a dropper for the local application of an acid.

portal (por′tal) 1. an entrance or gateway; called also *porta*. 2. pertaining to a porta, or entrance, especially to the porta hepatis. **hepatic p.,** porta hepatis. **intestinal p., anterior,** the region of opening of the embryonic foregut into the yolk sac or unclosed midgut. **intestinal p., posterior,** the region of opening of the embryonic hindgut into the yolk sac or unclosed midgut. **velopharyngeal p.,** the opening between the velum palatinum (soft palate) and the pharynx, which must be susceptible to closure by muscular action to permit normal speech and deglutition.

portcaustic (port-kaws′tik) [Fr. *Porte-caustique*] a handle for holding a caustic substance.

porte-aiguille (port″a-gēl′) [Fr.] a surgeon's needle holder.

portepolisher, porte-polisher (pōrt-pol′ish-er) a hand instrument constructed to hold a wooden point, to be used in a dental engine for applying polishing paste to and burnishing teeth.

Porter (por′ter), Rodney Robert. British biochemist, 1917–1985; co-winner, with Gerald Maurice Edelman, of the Nobel prize for physiology or medicine in 1972, for his work on the chemical structure of antibodies, producing the Fc (fragment crystallizable) and the Fab (fragment antigen-binding) portions using pepsin.

Porter's sign (por′terz) [William Henry *Porter*, Dublin physician, 1790–1861] tracheal tugging; see under *tugging*.

Porter's test (por′terz) [William Henry *Porter*, New York physician, 1853–1933] see under *tests*.

Porteus maze test (por′te-us) [Stanley David *Porteus*, psychologist, born 1883] see under *tests*.

portio (por′she-o), pl. **portio′nes** [L.] a part, or division; [NA] a general term for a particular portion of an organ or structure. **p. du′ra pa′ris sep′timi,** nervus facialis (formerly considered as forming one nerve with the portio mollis paris septimi). **p. interme′dia ner′vi acus′tici,** nervus intermedius. **p. ma′jor ner′vi trigem′ini,** radix sensoria nervi trigemini. **p. mi′nor ner′vi trigem′ini,** radix motoria nervi trigemini. **p. mol′lis pa′ris sep′timi,** nervus vestibulocochlearis (formerly considered as forming one nerve with the portio dura paris septimi). **p. supravagina′lis cer′vicis** [NA], the part of the cervix uteri that does not protrude into the vagina. **p. vagina′lis cer′vicis** [NA], the part of the cervix uteri that protrudes into the vagina.

portiones (por″she-o′nēz) [L.] plural of *portio*.

portligature (port-lig′ah-tūr) [Fr. *porte-ligature*] an instrument for applying a ligature in a deep wound.

portoenterostomy (por″to-en″ter-os′to-me) surgical anastomosis of the jejunum to an intrahepatic biliary radicle; done to establish a conduit from the intrahepatic bile ducts to the intestine in biliary atresia or stenosis or common duct tumor. Called also *hepatic p*.

portogram (por′to-gram) a roentgenogram of the portal vein.

portography (por-tog′rah-fe) roentgenography of the portal vein after injection of opaque material. **portal p.,** portography after injection of opaque material into the superior mesenteric vein or one of its branches after laparotomy has been performed. **splenic p.,** portography after percutaneous injection into the substance of the spleen, usually through the ninth intercostal space in the midaxillary line, of opaque material, which passes immediately into the splenic vein, and then into the portal vein, permitting visualization of those two vessels.

portosystemic (por″to-sis-tem′ik) connecting the portal and systemic venous circulation.

portovenogram (por″to-ve′no-gram) portogram.

portovenography (por″to-ve-nog′rah-fe) portography.

porus (po′rus), gen. and pl. **po′ri** [L., from Gr. *poros* passage] a pore; a small opening; [NA] a general term for certain openings in the body. **p. acus′ticus exter′nus** [NA],

the outer end of the external acoustic meatus. **p. acus′ticus exter′nus os′seus** [NA], external osseous acoustic pore: the outer end of the bony external acoustic meatus in the tympanic portion of the temporal bone. **p. acus′ticus inter′nus** [NA], the opening of the internal acoustic meatus. **p. acus′ticus inter′nus os′seus** [NA], internal osseous acoustic pore: the opening into the internal acoustic meatus, found on the posteromedial portion of the internal surface of the petrous part of the temporal bone. **p. gale′ni,** canalis inguinalis. **p. gustato′rius** [NA], gustatory pore: the small opening of a taste bud onto the surface of the tongue. **p. op′ticus,** the opening in the sclera for passage of the optic nerve. **p. sudorif′erus** [NA], sweat pore: the opening of the duct of the sweat gland on the surface of the skin; called also *pore of sweat duct*.

Posada's mycosis (po-sah′dahz) [Alejandro *Posada*, Argentine pathologist, 1870–1902] coccidioidomycosis.

Posada-Wernicke disease (po-sah′dah-ver′nĭ-ke) [Alejandro *Posada*; Robert *Wernicke*, Argentine pathologist of 19th century] coccidioidomycosis.

-posia [Gr. *posis* a drink + *-ia*] a word termination denoting relationship to drinking, or to intake of fluids.

position (po-zish′un) [L. *positio*] 1. a bodily posture or attitude assumed by the patient to achieve comfort in certain conditions, or the particular disposition of the body and extremities to facilitate the performance of certain diagnostic or therapeutic procedures. 2. in obstetrics, the situation of the fetus in the pelvis, determined and described by the relation of a given arbitrary point (point of direction or reference point) in the presenting part to a given arbitrary point in the coronal plane of the maternal pelvis. For the various possible positions see the table. Cf. *presentation*. **Albert's p.,** a semirecumbent position of the patient for

POSITIONS OF THE FETUS IN VARIOUS PRESENTATIONS

CEPHALIC PRESENTATION

1. Vertex—occiput, the point of direction
   - Left occipito-anterior . . . . L.O.A.
   - Left occipitotransverse . . . . L.O.T.
   - Right occipitoposterior . . . . R.O.P.
   - Right occipitotransverse . . . . R.O.T.
   - Right occipito-anterior . . . . R.O.A.
   - Left occipitoposterior . . . . L.O.P.

2. Face—chin, the point of direction
   - Right mentoposterior . . . . R.M.P.
   - Left mento-anterior . . . . L.M.A.
   - Right mentotransverse . . . . R.M.T.
   - Right mento-anterior . . . . R.M.A.
   - Left mentotransverse . . . . L.M.T.
   - Left mentoposterior . . . . L.M.P.

3. Brow—the point of direction
   - Right frontoposterior . . . . R.F.P.
   - Left fronto-anterior . . . . L.F.A.
   - Right frontotransverse . . . . R.F.T.
   - Right fronto-anterior . . . . R.F.A.
   - Left frontotransverse . . . . L.F.T.
   - Left frontoposterior . . . . L.F.P.

BREECH OR PELVIC PRESENTATION

1. Complete Breech—sacrum, the point of direction (feet crossed and thighs flexed on abdomen)
   - Left sacro-anterior . . . . L.S.A.
   - Left sacrotransverse . . . . L.S.T.
   - Right sacroposterior . . . . R.S.P.
   - Right sacro-anterior . . . . R.S.A.
   - Right sacrotransverse . . . . R.S.T.
   - Left sacroposterior . . . . L.S.P.

2. Incomplete breech—sacrum, the point of direction. Same designations as above, adding the qualifications footling, knee, etc.

TRANSVERSE LIE OR SHOULDER PRESENTATION

Shoulder—scapula, the point of direction

Left scapulo-anterior . . . . L.Sc.A.	} Back anterior positions
Right scapulo-anterior . . . . . . R.Sc.A.	
Right scapuloposterior . . . . . . R.Sc.P.	} Back posterior positions
Left scapuloposterior . . . . L.Sc.P.	

roentgenography as a means of determining the diameters of the superior strait of the pelvis. **anatomical p.,** the position of the human body, standing erect, with the palms of the hands turned forward; used as the position of reference in description of site or direction of various structures or parts as established in official anatomical nomenclature. **batrachian p.,** a lying position of infants in which the

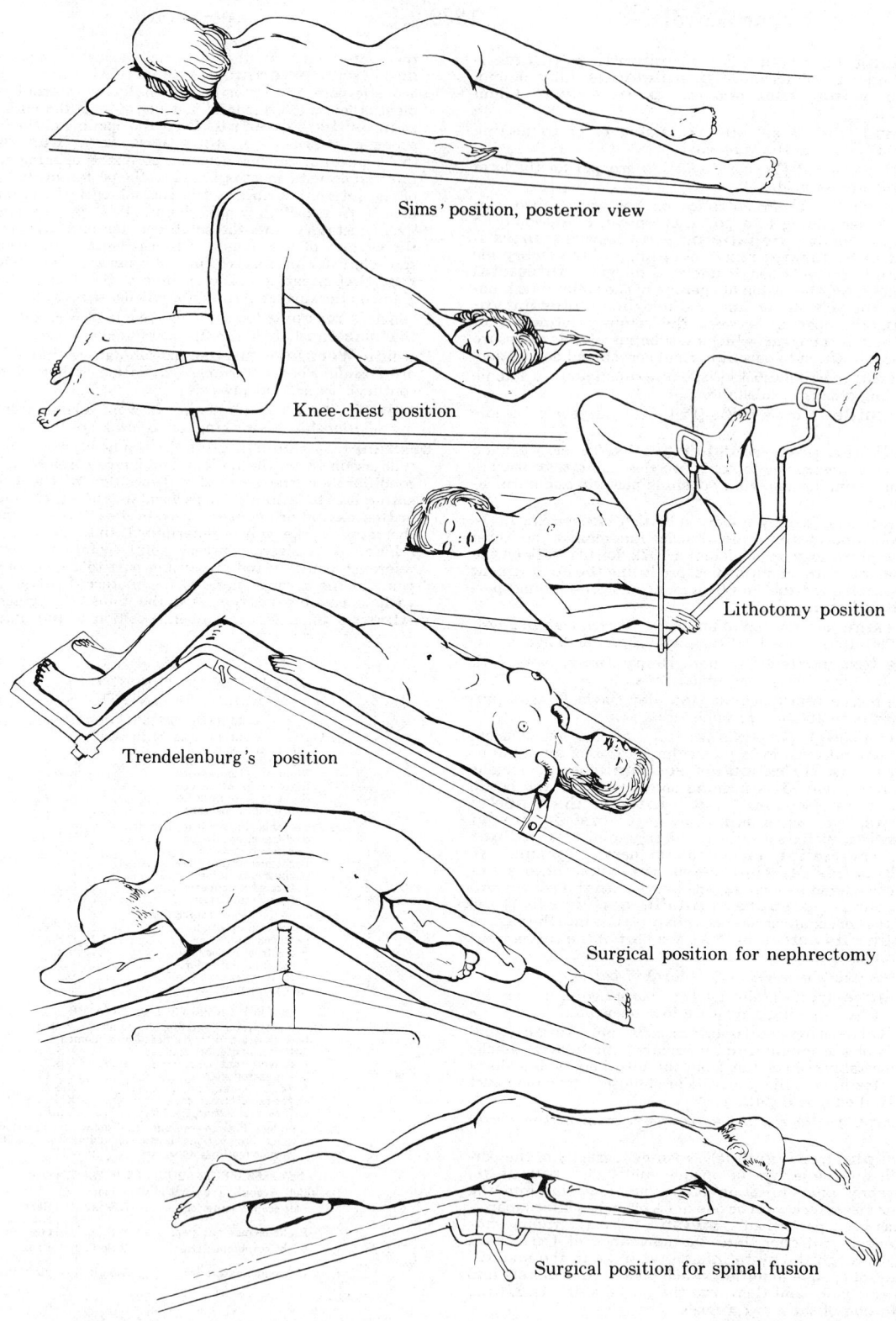

Sims' position, posterior view

Knee-chest position

Lithotomy position

Trendelenburg's position

Surgical position for nephrectomy

Surgical position for spinal fusion

PLATE 40 — VARIOUS POSITIONS USED IN EXAMINATION OR TREATMENT

lower limbs are flexed, abducted, and resting on the bed on their outer aspects, somewhat resembling the legs of a frog. Called also *froglike p.* **Bonner's p.,** flexion, abduction, and outward rotation of the thigh in coxitis. **Bozeman's p.,** one in which the patient is strapped to supports in the knee-elbow position. **Brickner p.,** a position for treating shoulder disability, secured by tying the patient's wrist to the head of the bed with his arm supported on a pillow and raising the head of the bed; thus traction with abduction and external rotation is obtained. **Caldwell p.,** a roentgenographic position with the forehead and nose against the x-ray plate, giving a posteroanterior projection for demonstration of frontal sinuses and the anterior ethmoidal cells. **Casselberry's p.,** a prone position employed after intubation so that the patient may swallow without danger of fluid entering the tube. **centric p.,** the rest position of the mandible, as it is influenced by the muscle tone, while the patient remains standing or is sitting with jaw open, from which the teeth will come into centric occlusion when the jaw is closed. **coiled p.,** the attitude of a patient on his side with hips and knees flexed and thighs drawn up to the body. **decubitus p.,** the position of an individual lying on a horizontal surface, designated, according to the portion of the body resting on the surface, *dorsal decubitus* (lying on the back), *left lateral decubitus* (on the left side), *right lateral decubitus* (on the right side), or *ventral decubitus* (on the abdomen). **Depage's p.,** a prone position with the pelvis raised to form the apex of an inverted V, while the trunk and lower limbs form the branches of the V. **dorsal p.,** the posture of a person lying on his back; called also *supine p.* **dorsal elevated p.,** position of the patient lying on the back, with shoulders and head elevated. **dorsal recumbent p.,** position of patient on back, with lower limbs flexed and rotated outward; used in vaginal examination, application of obstetrical forceps, etc. **dorsal rigid p.,** position on the back with knees flexed and thighs drawn up to the body. **dorsosacral p.,** lithotomy p. **Duncan's p.,** the position of the placenta with its margin presenting at the os for delivery. **eccentric p.,** see under *relation.* **Edebohls' p.,** a dorsal position, the knees and thighs drawn up, legs flexed on the thighs, and thighs flexed on the abdomen, the hips raised, and the thighs abducted; called also *Simon's p.* **Elliot's p.,** position of a patient on the operating table with lower chest elevated by placing a support under the lower costal margin; used in operations on the gallbladder. **emprosthotonos p.,** emprosthotonos. **English p.,** the patient on the left side, the right thigh and knee drawn up; called also *lateral recumbent p.* and *obstetrical p.* **Fowler's p.,** the position in which the head of the patient's bed is raised 18 or 20 inches above the level; the knees are also elevated. **froglike p.,** batrachian p. **frontal anterior p.,** frontoanterior p. **frontal posterior p.,** frontoposterior p. **frontal transverse p.,** frontotransverse p. **frontoanterior p.,** a position of the fetus in cephalic presentation in labor, with its brow directed toward the right (R.F.A.) or left (L.F.A.) anterior quadrant of the maternal pelvis. **frontoposterior p.,** a position of the fetus in cephalic presentation in labor, with its brow directed toward the right (R.F.P.) or left (L.F.P.) posterior quadrant of the maternal pelvis. **frontotransverse p.,** a position of the fetus in cephalic presentation in labor, with its brow directed toward the right (R.F.T.) or left (L.F.T.) iliac fossa of the maternal pelvis. **Fuchs p.,** a roentgenographic position which gives an oblique view of the zygomatic arch projected free of superimposed structures. **genucubital p.,** knee-elbow p. **genufacial p.,** the position of the patient resting on his knees and face. **genupectoral p.,** knee-chest p. **hinge p.,** the position of the condyle in the temporomandibular joint from which an opening by hinge movement is possible beyond the amplitude of rest position. **hinge p., condylar,** the position of the condyles in the glenoid fossa at which hinge axis movement is possible. **hinge p., mandibular,** a position of the mandible that allows the condyles movements on the hinge axis during the opening or closing of the jaws. **hinge p., terminal,** centric relation. **horizontal p.,** the position assumed by a person lying on his back with limbs extended. **jackknife p.,** Kraske p. **Jones' p.,** acute flexion of the forearm for the treatment of fracture of the internal condyle of the humerus. **knee-chest p.,** the position of a patient on his knees with the chest resting on the table. **knee-elbow p.,** the position of a patient resting on knees and elbows with the chest elevated from the table. **kneel-**

ing-squatting p., squatting position with the knees flexed acutely and pressed against the abdomen while the body is held erect; often effective in digital palpation of high rectal lesions. **Kraske p.,** a prone position with the buttocks raised. **lateral recumbent p.,** English p. **lithotomy p.,** the patient in dorsal decubitus with hips and knees flexed and the thighs abducted and externally rotated; called also *dorsosacral p.* **Mayer p.,** a roentgenographic position that gives a unilateral superoinferior view of the temporomandibular joint, external auditory canal, and mastoid and petrous processes; helpful in demonstrating fractures and malformations of the temporomandibular joint and in the study of bony atresia of the external auditory canal. **mentoanterior p.,** a position of the fetus in cephalic presentation in labor, with its chin directed toward the right (R.M.A.) or left (L.M.A.) anterior quadrant of the maternal pelvis. **mentoposterior p.,** a position of the fetus in cephalic presentation in labor, with its chin directed toward the right (R.M.P.) or left (L.M.P.) posterior quadrant of the maternal pelvis. **mentotransverse p.,** a position of the fetus in cephalic presentation in labor, with its chin directed toward the right (R.M.T.) or left (L.M.T.) iliac fossa of the maternal pelvis. **mentum anterior p.,** mentoanterior p. **mentum posterior p.,** mentoposterior p. **mentum transverse p.,** mentotransverse p. **Noble's p.,** position of the patient standing up, leaning forward and supporting the upper body on the arms; used in examining the kidney. **obstetrical p.,** English p. **occipitoanterior p.,** a position of the fetus in cephalic presentation in labor, with its occiput directed toward the right (R.O.A.) or left (L.O.A.) anterior quadrant of the maternal pelvis. **occipitoposterior p.,** a position of the fetus in cephalic presentation in labor, with its occiput directed toward the right (R.O.P.) or left (L.O.P.) posterior quadrant of the maternal pelvis. **occipitosacral p.,** a position of the fetus in cephalic presentation in labor, with the occiput presenting directly behind, or rotated squarely into the hollow of the sacrum. **occipitotransverse p.,** a position of the fetus in cephalic presentation in labor, with its occiput directed toward the right (R.O.T.) or left (L.O.T.) iliac fossa of the maternal pelvis. **occiput anterior p.,** occipitoanterior p. **occiput posterior p.,** occipitoposterior p. **occiput sacral p.,** occipitosacral p. **occiput transverse p.,** occipitotransverse p. **occlusal p.,** a functional position of the jaws in which contact between some or all of the upper and lower teeth occurs when the mandible is closed, *which* it may or may not coincide with centric occlusion. Called also *occlusal relation.* **opisthotonos p.,** opisthotonos. **orthopnea p., orthopneic p.,** the patient assumes an upright or a semivertical position by using two or more pillows to support his head and chest from the recumbent position, or he sits upright in a chair. Used when the patient has difficulty in breathing except in the upright position (orthopnea). **orthotonos p.,** orthotonos. **physiologic rest p.,** rest p. **posterior border p.,** the most posterior position of the mandible at any specific vertical relation to the maxillae. Called also *posterior border jaw relation.* **prone p.,** patient lying face down. **rest p.,** the position of the mandible when its muscles are at rest, the body is in the upright standing or sitting position, and the eyes are focused toward the horizon; the lips are slightly touching and the distance between the upper and lower teeth has a free-way space of about 2 to 5 mm. Called also *physiologic rest p.* and *rest jaw relation.* **Robson's p.,** the patient lying supine with a sand-bag placed beneath the eleventh and twelfth ribs; used in surgery on the biliary tract. **Rose's p.,** one intended to prevent aspiration or swallowing of blood, as from an injured lip: the patient on his back with head hanging over the end of the table in full extension so as to enable the patient to bleed over the margins of the inverted upper incisors. **sacroanterior p.,** a position of the fetus in breech presentation in labor, with its sacrum directed toward the right (R.S.A.) or left (L.S.A.) anterior quadrant of the maternal pelvis. **sacroposterior p.,** a position of the fetus in breech presentation in labor, with its sacrum directed toward the right (R.S.P.) or left (L.S.P.) posterior quadrant of the maternal pelvis. **sacrotransverse p.,** a position of the fetus in breech presentation in labor, with its sacrum directed toward the right (R.S.T.) or left (L.S.T.) iliac fossa of the maternal pelvis. **sacrum anterior p.,** sacroanterior p. **sacrum posterior p.,** sacroposterior p. **sacrum transverse p.,** sacrotransverse p. **scapula anterior p.,** scapuloanterior p. **scapula posterior p.,** scapuloposterior p. **scapuloanterior p.,** a position of the fetus in transverse lie in labor, with its head to the right (R.Sc.A.) or left (L.Sc.A.) of the maternal pelvis, and its back anterior. **scapuloposterior p.,** a position of the fetus in transverse lie in labor, with its head to the right (R.Sc.P.) or left (L.Sc.P.) of the maternal pelvis, and its back posterior. **scorbutic p.,** a pseudoparalytic position characteristic of advanced infantile scurvy, in which the infant lies quietly with the legs flexed at the knees and the hips flexed and externally rotated. **semiaxial p.,** Titterington p. **semiprone p.,** Sims' p. **semireclining p.,** a partly reclining position seen in heart disease, asthma, and pleural effusion. **Simon's p.,** Edebohls' p. **Sims' p.,** the patient lies on the left side with the right knee and thigh flexed and the left arm parallel along the back; for vaginal examination. Called also *semiprone p.* **Stern's p.,** the patient supine with the head lowered over the end of the table, the murmur of tricuspid insufficiency being heard more distinctly. **submentovertex p.,** a roentgenographic position opposite of the verticosubmental position. **supine p.,** dorsal p. **Titterington p.,** a roentgenographic position used to demonstrate fractures of the zygomatic arches, lateral walls of the maxilla, orbital floors, and orbital margins. Called also *semiaxial p.* **trans p.,** trans configuration. **Trendelenburg's p.,** one in which the patient is supine on the table or bed, the head of which is tilted downward 30 to 40 degrees, and the table or bed angulated beneath the knees. See illustration. **tripod p.,** 1. a position assumed by the patient with abdominal weakness or meningeal irritation while sitting in bed, in which he supports himself with his hands in a plane posterior to his pelvis. 2. a sitting position assumed by the patient with respiratory insufficiency, in which his hands are placed anterior to the frontal plane. See also *tripoding.* **Valentine's p.,** the patient supine and the hips flexed by means of a double inclined plane; used in irrigating the urethra. **verticosubmental p.,** a roentgenographic position that gives an axial projection of the mandible, including the coronoid and condyloid processes of the rami, the base of the skull and its foramina, the petrous pyramids, the sphenoidal, posterior ethmoid, and maxillary sinuses, and the nasal septum. **Waters p.,** a roentgenographic position that gives a posteroanterior view of the maxillary sinus, maxilla, orbits, and zygomatic arches; helpful in demonstrating fractures of nasal bones and nasal processes of the maxilla. **Waters p., reverse,** a mento-occipital roentgenographic position used to demonstrate the facial bones when the patient cannot be placed in a prone position; helpful in demonstrating fractures of the orbits, maxillary sinuses, zygomatic bones, and zygomatic arches.

positioner (po-zish′un-er) a resilient elastoplastic removable appliance fitted over the occlusal surfaces of the teeth to obtain limited tooth movement and stabilization, usually at the end of orthodontic treatment. **tooth p.,** see *positioner.*

positive (poz′ĭ-tiv) [L. *positivus*] having a value greater than zero; indicating existence or presence of a condition, organism, etc., as chromatin positive or Wassermann positive; characterized by affirmation or cooperation.

positrocephalogram (poz″ĭ-tro-sef′ah-lo-gram″) [*positron* + Gr. *kephalos* head + *gramma* a mark] a record produced by the emission of positrons by isotopes of arsenic administered to facilitate localization of brain tumors.

positron (poz′ĭ-tron) the positive electron, a particle having the mass of the electron but with a positive electric charge; a free positive electron.

Posner's test (reaction) (pōs′nerz) [Carl *Posner,* Berlin urologist, 1854–1929] see under *tests.*

posologic (po″so-loj′ik) pertaining to doses.

posology (po-sol′o-je) [Gr. *posos* how much + *-logy*] the science of dosage, or a system of dosage.

Possum (pos′um) [*Patient-Operated Selector Mechanism*] trademark for a machine designed for the disabled by which, when breathed into in the correct manner, the individual can operate the telephone, ring bells, turn on the television, switch off a light, type a letter, or perform any of a number of other functions by no movement other than that involved in respiration.

post (pōst) 1. a piece of material firmly secured in an upright position, usually to support something. 2. dowel. **abutment p.,** 1. see under *abutment.* 2. implant p. **im-**

plant p., a constricted part on that portion of the subperiosteal, intraperiosteal, or intraosseous implant protruding into the oral cavity and serving as an abutment for a denture. Called also *abutment p.*

post- [L. *post* after] a prefix meaning after or behind.

postalbumin (pōst″al-bu′min) a serum protein which has an electrophoretic mobility between albumin and alpha-globulin at pH 8.6.

postaurale (pōst″aw-ra′le) a cephalometric landmark, the most posterior point on the helix of the ear.

postauricular (pōst″aw-rik′u-lar) located or performed behind the auricle of the ear.

postaxial (pōst-ak′se-al) situated behind an axis. In anatomical usage, postaxial refers to the medial (ulnar) aspect of the upper limb, and the lateral (fibular) aspect of the lower limb.

postbrachial (pōst-bra′ke-al) on the posterior part of the upper arm.

postbrachium (pōst-bra′ke-um) brachium colliculi inferioris.

postbulbar (pōst-bul′bar) situated behind or distal to a bulb, as behind the medulla oblongata, or distal to the pileus ventriculi (duodenal bulb).

postcapillary (pōst-kap′ĭ-lar′e) a venous capillary.

postcardiotomy (pōst-kar″de-ot′o-me) occurring after or as a consequence of operating on the heart.

postcava (pōst-ka′vah) the vena cava inferior.

postcaval (pōst-ka′val) pertaining to the postcava.

postcentral (pōst-sen′tral) situated or occurring behind a center, as the postcentral gyrus.

postcentralis (pōst″sen-tra′lis) the postcentral fissure.

postcibal (pōst-si′bal) [*post-* + L. *cibum* food] occurring after ingestion of food; postprandial.

post cibum (pōst si′bum) [L.] after meals (after food).

postcisterna (pōst″sis-ter′nah) cisterna cerebellomedullaris.

postcondylare (pōst″kon-dĭ-lah′re) the highest point of the curvature behind the occipital condyle.

postcornu (pōst-kor′nu) cornu posterius ventriculi lateralis.

postcranial (pōst-kra′ne-al) situated posterior or inferior to the cranium, or skull.

postcubital (pōst-ku′bĭ-tal) on the dorsal side of the forearm.

postdiastolic (pōst″di-as-tol′ik) occurring after or following the diastole.

postdicrotic (pōst″di-krot′ik) occurring after the dicrotic elevation of the sphygmogram.

postdormital (pōst-dor′mĭ-tal) pertaining to or occurring during the postdormitum.

postdormitum (pōst-dor′mĭ-tum) the period of increasing consciousness interposed between sound sleep and wakening.

postecdysis (pōst-ek′dĭ-sis) [*post-* + Gr. *ekdysis* a way out] the concluding phase of ecdysis in certain crustaceans and arthropods, during which the endocuticle is secreted and calcification of the skeleton occurs.

postembryonic (pōst″em-bre-on′ik) [*post-* + Gr. *embryon* embryo] occurring after the embryonic stage.

posteriad (pos-te′re-ad) toward the posterior surface of the body.

posterior (pos-tēr′e-or) [L. "behind"; neut. *posterius*] situated in back of, or in the back part of, or affecting the back part of a structure; [NA] a term used in reference to the back or dorsal surface of the body. In lower animals, it refers to the caudal end of the body.

postero- [L. *posterus* behind] a combining form denoting relationship to the posterior part.

posteroanterior (pos″ter-o-an-tēr′e-or) from back to front, or from the posterior (dorsal) to the anterior (ventral) surface. In roentgenology, denoting direction of the beam from the x-ray source to the beam exit surface.

posteroclusion (pos″ter-o-kloo′zhun) distoclusion.

posteroexternal (pos″ter-o-ek-ster′nal) situated on the outer side of a posterior aspect.

posteroinferior (pos″ter-o-in-fēr′e-or) posterior and inferior.

posterointernal (pos″ter-o-in-ter′nal) situated within and toward the back.

posterolateral (pos″ter-o-lat′er-al) situated behind and to one side.

posteromedial (pos″ter-o-me′de-al) situated toward the middle of the back.

posteromedian (pos″ter-o-me′de-an) situated on the midline of the back.

posteroparietal (pos″ter-o-pah-ri′ĕ-tal) situated at the back part of the parietal bone.

posterosuperior (pos″ter-o-soo-pēr′e-or) situated behind and above.

posterotemporal (pos″ter-o-tem′po-ral) situated at the back part of the temporal bone.

posterula (pos-ter′u-lah) [L.] the space between the nasal conchae and the posterior nares.

postexed (pōs-tekst′) bent backward.

postganglionic (pōst″gang-gle-on′ik) situated posterior or distal to a ganglion; said especially of autonomic nerve fibers so located.

postglenoid (pōst-gle′noid) situated behind the glenoid fossa.

postglomerular (pōst″glo-mer′u-lar) located or occurring distal to a glomerulus of the kidney.

posthetomy (pos-thet′o-me) [Gr. *posthē* foreskin + *tomē* a cutting] circumcision.

posthioplasty (pos′the-o-plas″te) [Gr. *posthē* foreskin + *plastos* formed] plastic surgery of the prepuce.

posthitis (pos-thi′tis) [Gr. *posthē* foreskin + *-itis*] inflammation of the prepuce.

postholith (pos′tho-lith) [Gr. *posthē* foreskin + *lithos* stone] a preputial concretion or calculus.

posthumous (pos′tu-mus) [L. *postumus* coming after] occurring after death; born after the father's death.

posthyoid (pōst-hi′oid) situated or occurring behind the hyoid bone.

posthypnotic (pōst″hip-not′ik) following the hypnotic state.

posthypophysis (pōst″hi-pof′ĭ-sis) the posterior part of the hypophysis, or pituitary gland.

posticus (pos-ti′kus) [L.] posterior.

postischial (pōst-is′ke-al) situated behind the ischium.

postmastectomy (pōst″mas-tek′to-me) following mastectomy.

postmastoid (pōst-mas′toid) situated behind the mastoid process of the temporal bone.

postmature (pōst″ma-tūr′) overly developed, as a postmature infant.

postmaturity (pōst″mah-tu′rĭ-te) overdevelopment; the condition of a postmature infant.

postmediastinal (pōst″me-de-as′tĭ-nal) behind the mediastinum; pertaining to the posterior mediastinum.

postmediastinum (pōst″me-de-as-ti′num) mediastinum posterius.

postmeiotic (pōst″mi-ot′ik) [*post-* + Gr. *meioun* to decrease] occurring after or pertaining to the time following meiosis.

postmenopausal (pōst″men-o-paw′zal) occurring after the menopause.

postmenstrua (pōst-men′stroo-ah) the period immediately following cessation of menstrual flow.

postmesenteric (pōst″mes-en-ter′ik) behind or in the posterior part of the mesentery; retromesenteric.

postminimus (pōst-min′ĭ-mus), pl. *postmin′imi* [*post-* + L. *minimus* small] digitus postminimus.

postmiotic (pōst″mi-ot′ik) postmeiotic.

postmitotic (pōst″mi-tot′ik) 1. pertaining to the time following or occurring after mitosis in normally dividing cells. 2. pertaining to cells that stop dividing after reaching maturity, as cells of the mammalian heart or central nervous system.

postmortal (pōst-mor′tal) occurring after death.

post mortem (pōst mor′tem) [L.] after death.

postmortem (pōst-mor′tem) occurring or performed after death; pertaining to the period after death.

postnares (pōst-na′rēs) the posterior naris.

postnarial (pōst-na′re-al) pertaining to the posterior nares.

postnasal (pōst-na′zal) [*post-* + L. *nasus* nose] situated or occurring behind the nose.

postnatal (pōst-na′tal) occurring after birth, with reference to the newborn. Cf. *postpartum.*

postoperative (pōst-op′er-ah-tiv) occurring after a surgical operation.

postpalatine (pōst-pal′ah-tin) behind the palate, or behind the palatine bone.

post partum (pōst par′tum) [L.] after childbirth, or after delivery.

postpartum (pōst-par′tum) occurring after childbirth, or after delivery, with reference to the mother. Cf. *postnatal.*

postpituitary (pōst-pĭ-tu′ĭ-ta-re) pertaining to the posterior lobe of the pituitary body.

postprandial (pōst-pran′de-al) occurring after dinner, or after a meal; postcibal.

postpuberal (pōst-pu′ber-al) postpubertal.

postpubertal (pōst-pu′ber-tal) occurring in or pertaining to the period following puberty.

postpuberty (pōst-pu′ber-te) the period following puberty.

postpubescence (pōst″pu-bes′ens) postpuberty.

postpubescent (pōst″pu-bes′ent) postpubertal.

postrolandic (pōst″ro-lan′dik) situated behind the fissure of Rolando (sulcus centralis).

Post sing. sed. liq. abbreviation for L. *post sin′gulas se′des liq′uidas,* after every loose stool.

postsphenoid (pōst-sfe′noid) the basisphenoid, pterygoid, and alisphenoid bones together; separate bones in infancy, they usually become united with the sphenoid.

postsphygmic (pōst-sfig′mik) occurring after the pulse wave; see under *period.*

postsplenic (pōst-splen′ik) behind the spleen.

poststenotic (pōst″stĕ-not′ik) located or occurring distal to or beyond a stenosed segment.

postsylvian (pōst-sil′ve-an) behind the sylvian fissure (sulcus lateralis).

postsynaptic (pōst″sĭ-nap′tik) situated distal to a synapse, or occurring after the synapse is crossed.

post-traumatic (pōst″traw-mat′ik) occurring as a result of or after injury.

postulate (pos′tu-lāt) [L. *postulatum* demanded] anything assumed or taken for granted. **Koch's p's,** a statement of the kind of experimental evidence required to establish the etiologic relationship of a given microorganism to a given disease. The conditions included are (1) the microorganism must be observed in every case of the disease; (2) it must be isolated and grown in pure culture; (3) the pure culture must, when inoculated into a susceptible animal, reproduce the disease; and (4) the microorganism must be observed in, and recovered from, the experimentally diseased animal.

postural (pos′chur-al) pertaining to posture or position.

posture (pos′chur) [L. *postura*] the attitude of the body. **Drosin's p's,** three postures for eliciting tenderness in appendicitis.

postvaccinal (pōst-vak′sĭ-nal) occurring after or as a consequence of vaccination for smallpox.

postvaccinial (pōst″vak-sin′e-al) occurring after or as a consequence of vaccinia.

postvital (pōst-vi′tal) see *postvital staining,* under *staining.*

postzone (post′zōn) see *zone of antigen excess,* under *zone.*

postzygotic (pōst″zi-got′ik) occurring after the completion of fertilization and formation of the zygote.

potable (po′tah-b'l) [L. *potabilis*] fit to drink; drinkable.

pot AGT potential abnormality of glucose tolerance.

Potain's sign (po-tānz′) [Pierre Carl Edouard *Potain,* French physician, 1825–1901] see under *sign.*

Potamon (pot′ah-mon) a genus of fresh-water crabs; *P. dentricularis, P. dehaani,* and *P. rathbuni* are hosts of the metacercariae of *Paragonimus westermani* in the Orient.

potash (pot′ash) impure potassium carbonate. **caustic p.,** potassium hydroxide. **sulfurated p.** [USP], a mixture of potassium polysulfides and potassium thiosulfate, containing 12.8 per cent of sulfur in combination as sulfide; used as a source of sulfide in pharmaceutic preparations. See *white lotion,* under *lotion.* In veterinary medicine, it is used as a bath for mange. Called also *hepar sulfuris, liver of sulfur,* and *potassa sulfurata.*

potassa (po-tas′ah) [L.] potassium hydroxide. **p. caus′tica,** potassium hydroxide. **p. sulfura′ta,** sulfurated potash.

potassemia (pot″ah-se′me-ah) [*potassa* + Gr. *haima* blood + *-ia*] the presence of an abnormally large amount of potassium in the blood; hyperkalemia.

potassic (po-tas′ik) containing potash.

potassiomercuric (po-tas″e-o-mer-ku′rik) (*obs.*) containing potassium and mercury in its divalent form. **p. iodide,** potassium mercuric iodide.

potassium (po-tas′e-um) [L.] a metallic element of the alkali group, many of whose salts are used in medicine. It is a soft, silver-white metal, melting at 58° F.; atomic number, 19; atomic weight, 39.102; specific gravity, 0.87; symbol, K (L. *kalium*). Potassium is the chief cation of muscle and most other cells (intracellular fluid); see also *sodium-potassium pump,* under *pump.* **p. acetate** [USP], $CH_3 \cdot COOK$, occurring as colorless, monoclinic crystals or white, crystalline powder; used as an electrolyte replenisher and as a urinary and systemic alkalizer, administered by intravenous infusion and orally. Formerly used as a diuretic and expectorant. Called also *diuretic salt* and *sal diureticum.* **p. alum,** see *alum.* **p. arsenite,** a compound formed by the interaction of arsenic trioxide and potassium hydroxide. **p. aspartate and magnesium aspartate,** a mixture of $C_4H_6KNO_4 \cdot \frac{1}{2}H_2O$ and $C_8H_{12}MgN_2O_8 \cdot 4H_2O$; used as a nutrient. **p. bicarbonate** [USP], $KHCO_3$, occurring as colorless, transparent, monoclinic prisms or as a white, granular powder; used as a pharmaceutic necessity in the preparation of Randall's solution, and may be used as an electrolyte replenisher, antacid, and urinary alkalizer. **p. bichromate,** an orange-red, crystalline salt, formerly used as an external astringent, antiseptic, and caustic; in veterinary medicine, it is used as a caustic in the treatment of superficial growths. Called also *p. dichromate.* **p. bismuth tartrate,** bismuth potassium tartrate; see under *bismuth.* **p. bitartrate,** a mild cathartic, $C_4H_5KO_6$, occurring as opaque crystals or a white crystalline powder; administered orally. It is sometimes used in veterinary medicine as a laxative for small animals and as a diuretic for large animals. Called also *cream of tartar.* **p. bromide,** a sedative, KBr, occurring as white, cubical crystals or granular powder; used occasionally for grand mal seizures. See also *bromide.* **p. carbonate,** K_2CO_3, occurring as a white, crystalline or granular powder; formerly used as a systemic alkalizer and diuretic, but now used chiefly in pharmaceutical and chemical manufacturing procedures. **p. chlorate,** an explosive compound, $KClO_3$, occurring as colorless crystals or as white granules or powder, formerly used as an antiseptic for the skin and mucous membranes and in the treatment of hyperthyroidism and thyrotoxicosis. It is sometimes used in veterinary medicine in solution to treat stomatitis and vaginitis. **p. chloride** [USP], KCl, occurring as colorless, elongated, prismatic, or cubical crystals, or white, granular powder; used as an electrolyte replenisher, administered orally or by intravenous infusion. **p. citrate** [USP], $C_6H_5K_3O_7H_2O$, occurring as transparent crystals or as a white, granular powder; used as a systemic alkalizer and as an electrolyte replenisher, diuretic, and expectorant, usually administered orally. It is sometimes used in veterinary medicine as a nonirritating diuretic. **p. cyanide,** an extremely poisonous compound, KCN, occurring as a white granular powder or as fused pieces; formerly used in solution to remove silver nitrate stains from the conjunctiva. **p. dichromate,** p. bichromate. **p. dihydrogen phosphate,** p. phosphate, monobasic. **p. ferricyanide,** deep-red crystals, $K_3Fe(CN)_6$, used in a delicate test for ferrous salts. **p. glucaldrate,** chemical name: potassium diaqua[gluconato(2–)]dihydroxyaluminate(1–); an antacid, $C_6H_{16}AlKO_{11}$. **p. gluconate** [USP], chemical name: D-gluconic acid monopotassium salt. A salt, $C_6H_{11}KO_7$, occurring as a white to yellowish white, crystalline powder or as granules; used as an electrolyte replenisher in the prophylaxis and treatment of hypokalemia, administered orally. **p. glycerophosphate,** a colorless to slightly yellow viscous substance, $K_2C_3H_5(OH)_2PO_4$, formerly used as a tonic. **p. guaiacolsulfonate,** $C_7H_7KO_5S$, occurring as white

crystals or crystalline powder; used as an expectorant. **p. hydroxide** [NF], KOH, white or nearly white, fused masses or small pellets, or flakes, sticks, or other forms; used as an alkalizer in pharmaceutical preparations. Called also *caustic potash, potassa,* and *potassa caustica.* **p. hypophosphite,** a white, crystalline salt, KH_2PO_2, formerly used in the treatment of tuberculosis. **p. iodate,** a compound, KIO_3, occurring as white crystals or crystalline powder, formerly used as a topical antiseptic in the treatment of infections of the mucous membranes. It is added to animal feed as a source of iodine. **p. iodide** [USP], KI, occurring as crystals that are colorless and transparent or somewhat opaque and white, or as a white, granular powder; used as an expectorant, as a source of iodine in thyrotoxic crisis and in the preparation of thyrotoxic patients for thyroidectomy, and as an antifungal in the treatment of lymphocutaneous sporotrichosis; administered orally. **p. mercuric iodide,** a complex, K_2HgI_4, containing about 25.5 per cent of mercury; used as a germicide, and as an ingredient of various reagents. **p. metaphosphate** [NF], KPO_3, a white powder used as a buffering agent in pharmaceutical preparations. **p. nitrate,** KNO_3, occurring as a white granular or crystalline powder or as colorless transparent prisms; formerly used as an oral diuretic. **p. penicillin G,** penicillin G potassium. **p. perchlorate,** $KClO_4$, occurring as colorless crystals or white, crystalline powder; a thyroid inhibitor, it has been used in the treatment of thyrotoxicosis. **p. permanganate** [USP], the potassium salt of permanganic acid, $KMnO_4$, occurring as dark purple crystals, having bactericidal, fungicidal, astringent, and oxidizing properties; used in solution as a topical anti-infective. Because of its oxidizing activity, it is also used in solutions as a gastric lavage for certain poisons. **p. phenoxymethyl penicillin,** penicillin V potassium. **p. phosphate,** K_2HPO_4, occurring as colorless or white, granules or powder; has been used as a cathartic. Called also *dipotassium phosphate.* **p. phosphate, dibasic,** p. phosphate. **p. phosphate, monobasic** [NF], KH_2PO_4, occurring as colorless crystals or as a white, granular or crystalline powder; used as a buffering agent in pharmaceutical preparations. Called also *p. dihydrogen phosphate.* **radioactive p.,** radiopotassium. **p. sodium tartrate** [USP], $C_4H_4KNaO_6 \cdot 4H_2O$, occurring as colorless crystals or as a white crystalline powder; used as a cathartic. Called also *Preston's salt, Rochelle salt,* and *Seignette's salt.* **p. sorbate** [NF], chemical name: 2,4-hexadienoic acid potassium salt. A mold and yeast inhibitor, $C_6H_7O_2$, occurring as white crystals or as a powder; used as a preservative in pharmaceutical preparations. **p. sulfate,** K_2SO_4, occurring as colorless or white crystals or as a white powder or granules, which has an extremely irritant action on the stomach and intestines; has been used as a cathartic. **p. sulfite,** $K_2SO_3 + 2H_2O$, occurring as white crystals or crystalline powder; formerly used as a cathartic and diuretic. **p. sulfocyanate,** p. thiocyanate. **p. tartrate,** $K_2C_4H_4O_6 + \frac{1}{2}H_2O$; occurring as white crystals or granular powder; has been used as a cathartic. **p. tellurate,** K_2TeO, occurring as white crystals; formerly used in tuberculosis. **p. thiocyanate,** KSCN, occurring as colorless, transparent, prismatic crystals; used as a reagent, and formerly as an antihypertensive agent. Called also *p. sulfocyanate.*

Potassium Triplex (po-tas′e-um tri′pleks) trademark for Randall's solution.

potency (po′ten-se) [L. *potentia* power] power; especially (1) the ability of the male to perform sexual intercourse; (2) the power of a medicinal agent to produce the desired effects; (3) the ability of an embryonic part to develop and complete its destiny. **prospective p.,** the total developmental possibilities of which an embryonic part is capable. **reactive p.,** see *competence.*

potentia (po-ten′she-ah) [L.] power.

potential (po-ten′shal) [L. *potentia* power] 1. existing and ready for action but not yet active. 2. the work per unit charge necessary to move a charged body in an electric field from a reference point (usually infinity) to another point. The difference in potential between two points is measured by the work necessary to move a unit positive charge from one to the other. **action p.,** the electrical activity developed in a muscle or nerve cell during activity. It may be elicited by electrical, chemical, or mechanical stimulation, by temperature change, and so on. **after-p.,** the period following termination of the spike potential; it has a negative and positive phase. **after-p., negative,** the period following termination of the spike potential during which there is a lag in the return of the potential of an excitable cell membrane to resting potential. **after-p., positive,** the period following termination of the negative after-potential, during which the potential of an excitable cell membrane is more negative than the resting potential. It is paradoxically called *positive* because it was first detected outside the cell, where the polarity is reversed. **bioelectric p.,** the varying electric potential which accompanies all biochemical processes, as those manifested in the electrocardiogram and the electroencephalogram. **biotic p.,** the maximum rate at which a population can increase when the age ratio is stable and all environmental conditions are ideal. Called also *reproductive p.* **cochlear p.,** see under *microphonics.* **demarcation p.,** the difference in electrical potential between the intact longitudinal surface and the injured end of a muscle or nerve. **electrode p.,** the potential developed by an oxidation-reduction half reaction under prevailing conditions, related to the standard electrode potential by the Nernst equation. **evoked cortical p's,** the various discrete electrical charges in the cerebral cortex which can be produced by stimulation of sense organs or of some point along the ascending pathways to the cerebral cortex. **excitatory postsynaptic p.,** a transient decrease in membrane polarization induced in a postsynaptic neuron when subjected to a volley of impulses over an excitatory afferent pathway; summation of such potentials may cause discharge by the neuron. Abbreviated EPSP. **generator p.,** the depolarization produced in neural receptors in response to specific kinds of physical stimuli; called also *receptor p.* **inhibitory postsynaptic p.,** a transient hyperpolarization of membrane potential induced in a postsynaptic neuron when subjected to a volley of impulses over an inhibitory afferent pathway, resulting in a diminished responsiveness of the neuron. Abbreviated IPSP. **membrane p.,** the electric potential which exists on the two sides of a membrane or across the wall of a cell. **morphogenetic p.,** the degree of strength or ability of an embryonic part to develop into a specific structure. **negative summating p.,** a decrease in voltage difference between the cochlear duct and the vestibule caused by moderate to strong stimulation; it is maintained as long as sound stimulation persists. **Nernst p.,** the voltage produced across a membrane by a concentration gradient of an ion that can diffuse through pores in the membrane while oppositely charged ions cannot pass through the membrane; see *Nernst equation* under *equation.* **pacemaker p.,** the slow diastolic depolarization of cell membranes in the sinoatrial node. **receptor p.,** generator p. **redox p.,** 1. electrode p. 2. for a solution containing several redox couples, the potential of an inert electrode placed in the solution relative to the standard hydrogen electrode; used in bacteriology to characterize the reducing capacity of certain bacterial culture media. It can be estimated using the dyes methylene blue and resazurin, which change color at specific redox potentials. Symbol E_h. **reproductive p.,** biotic p. **resting p.,** the potential difference across the membrane of a normal cell at rest, i.e., the difference in potential between the outside and inside of a cell at rest; cf. *action potential.* **spike p.,** the initial very large change in potential of an excitable cell membrane during excitation. **standard electrode p., standard reduction p.** ($E°$) the electrochemical potential developed by a half-cell under standard conditions (1 atm pressure; specified temperature, usually 25° C; substances in solution at 1 M concentration) compared to the standard hydrogen half-cell, 2 H$^+$ (1 M) + 2ē ⇌ H$_2$ (1 atm), which by definition has an $E°$ of exactly 0 V. **zeta p.,** the electric potential across a solid-liquid interface. The zeta potential at the surface of erythrocytes is the net potential produced by both the negative charges on the cell surface and the positive charges in a cloud of cations that are attracted by the surface charge and form a layer over the surface; it is responsible for a repelling force between erythrocytes that resists agglutination or rouleaux formation.

potentialization, potentiation (po-ten″she-al-i-za′shun, po-ten″she-a′shun) the synergistic action of two drugs, being greater than the sum of the effects of each used alone.

potentiator (po-ten′she-a-tor) an agent that enhances another agent so that the combined effect is greater than the sum of the effects of each one alone.

potentiometer (po-ten″she-om′ĕ-ter) an instrument for the accurate measuring of voltage.

potification (po″tĭ-fĭ-ka′shun) the process of making water fit to drink. Applied to sea water, it is the process of removing sufficient salts to render the remaining fluid safe for drinking.

potion (po′shun) [L. *po′tio* draft] a draft; a large dose of liquid medicine. **Rivière's p.,** an effervescing drink produced by combining a solution of citric acid with one of sodium or potassium bicarbonate.

potocytosis (po″to-si-to′sis) [Gr. *potos* drinking + *kytos* cell + -*osis*] the hypothetical action of cells passing fluids through themselves from one place to another.

potomania (po″to-ma′ne-ah) [Gr. *potos* drinking + *mania* madness] 1. an abnormal desire to drink. 2. delirium tremens.

Pott's aneurysm, disease, etc. (pots) [Sir Percivall *Pott,* English surgeon, 1714–1788] see *aneurysmal varix,* under *varix;* see *tuberculosis of spine;* and see under *abscess, curvature, fracture, paraplegia,* and *tumor.*

Pottenger's sign (pot′en-jerz) [Francis Marion *Pottenger,* American physician, 1869–1961] see under *sign.*

Potter treatment (pot′er) [Caryl Ashley *Potter,* American physician, 1886–1933] see under *treatment.*

Potter version (pot′er) [Irving W. *Potter,* American obstetrician, 1868–1956] see under *version.*

Potts operation [Willis John *Potts,* Chicago surgeon, 1895–1968] see under *operation.*

potus (po′tus) [L. "drink"] a potion. **p. imperia′lis,** imperial drink, a solution of ½ oz. of cream of tartar in 3 pts. of water, sweetened, and flavored with lemon peel.

pouch (powch) a pocket-like space or sac, as of the peritoneum. **abdominovesical p.,** the pouch formed by reflection of the peritoneum from the anterior abdominal wall to the distended bladder. **anal p.,** the expanded end of the hindgut in certain insects. **anterior p. of Tröltsch,** recessus membranae tympani anterior. **branchial p.,** pharyngeal p. **Broca's p.,** a pear-shaped sac in the labium majus, its extremity directed downward and backward, and its smaller one upward, forward, and outward toward the opening of the inguinal canal; composed of elastic fibers, and containing connective tissue and fat. **craniobuccal p., craniopharyngeal p.,** Rathke's p. **p. of Douglas,** excavatio recto-uterina. **enterocoelic p.,** a diverticulum of the enteron of the embryo. **guttural p's,** large mucous sacs in the horse, which are ventral diverticula of the eustachian tube, situated between the base of the cranium and the atlas dorsally and the pharynx ventrally. **Hartmann's p.,** an abnormal sacculation of the neck of the gallbladder. **Heidenhain p.,** a small pocket of the stomach which has been surgically separated from the body of the stomach, and thus vagally denervated, and which drains to the exterior; used in the experimental study of gastric physiology. Cf. *Pavlov p.* **ileocecal p.,** a peritoneal pouch at the ileocecal junction. **laryngeal p.,** sacculus laryngis. **Morison's p.,** a pouch of peritoneum below the liver and to the right of the right kidney and extending downward to the transverse mesocolon. **neurobuccal p.,** Rathke's p. **obturator p.,** paravesical p. **paracystic p.,** the lateral part of the excavatio vesicouterina. **pararectal p.,** the lateral part of the excavatio rectouterina. **paravesical p.,** the lateral part of the uteroabdominal pouch, beside the bladder and in which the obturator canal opens; called also *obturator p.* **Pavlov p.,** a pocket of stomach which has been surgically separated from the body of the stomach by a mucosal septum, but which retains vagal innervation and muscular connection, and which drains to the exterior; used in the experimental study of gastric physiology. Cf. *Heidenhain p.* **perineal p., deep,** spatium perinei profundum. **perineal p., superficial,** spatium perinei superficiale. **pharyngeal p.,** a lateral diverticulum of the pharynx that meets a corresponding groove in the ectoderm, forming a closing plate that may rupture and complete the gill slit condition observed in lower vertebrates. **Physick's p's,** inflamed sacculations between the rectal valves, with mucous discharge. **posterior p. of Tröltsch,** recessus membranae tympani posterior. **Prussak's p.,** recessus membranae tympani superior. **Rathke's p.,** a diverticulum from the embryonic buccal cavity, from which the anterior lobe of the pituitary gland is developed. The lumen of Rathke's pouch persists in adults as small colloid-filled cysts and clefts at the juncture of the pars distalis and the neurohypophysis. Called also *craniobuccal p.* and *neurobuccal p.* **rectouterine p., rectovaginal p.,** excavatio rectouterina. **rectovesical p.,** excavatio rectovesicalis. **Seessel's p.,** a transient outpouching of the embryonic pharynx rostrad of the pharyngeal membrane and caudal to Rathke's pouch. **uteroabdominal p.,** the compartment of the pelvic cavity anterior to the uterus and broad ligaments. **uterovesical p., vesicouterine p.,** excavatio vesico-uterina. **visceral p.,** pharyngeal p. **Willis' p.,** omentum minus. **Zenker's p.,** pulsion diverticulum.

poudrage (poo-drahzh') [Fr.] the application of powder to a surface, as between the visceral and parietal layers of the pericardium or pleura, to promote their fusion. **pleural p.,** the application of an irritating powder on the surfaces of the pleura to promote adhesion.

poultice (pōl'tis) [L. *puls* pap; Gr. *kataplasma*] a soft, moist mass about the consistency of cooked cereal, spread between layers of muslin, linen, gauze, or towels and applied hot to a given area in order to create moist local heat or counterirritation.

pound (pownd) [L. *pondus* weight; *libra* pound] a unit of mass (weight) of both the avoirdupois and the apothecaries' system. The avoirdupois pound contains 16 ounces, or 7000 grains, and is the equivalent of 453.592 gm. The apothecaries' pound contains 12 ounces, or 5760 grains, and is the equivalent of 373.242 gm. Abbreviated lb.

Poupart's ligament, line (poo-parts') [François *Poupart*, French anatomist, 1661–1708] see *ligamentum inguinale,* and see under *line.*

Povan (po'van) trademark for a preparation of pyrvinium pamoate.

poverty (pov'er-te) the absence or scarcity of requisite substance or elements. **p. of movement,** the relative immobility and stationariness of position seen in subjects with parkinsonism; akinesia.

povidone (po'vǐ-dōn) [USP] chemical name: 1-ethenyl-2-pyrrolidinone homopolymer. A synthetic polymer occurring as a white to creamy white, odorless powder, principally consisting of linear 1-vinyl-2-pyrrolidone groups, produced as a series of products having mean molecular weights ranging from about 10,000 to about 700,000; used as a dispersing and suspending agent, and has been used as a tablet binder, coating agent, and viscosity-increasing agent in pharmaceutical preparations. Formerly called *polyvinylpyrrolidone* (*PVP*). See also *povidone-iodine.*

povidone-iodine (po'vǐ-dōn i'o-dīn) [USP], a complex produced by reacting iodine with the polymer povidone, which slowly releases iodine; it occurs as a yellowish brown, amorphous powder and is used as a topical anti-infective. Abbreviated PVP-I.

powder (pow'der) [L. *pulvis*] a substance made up of an aggregation of small particles, as that obtained by the grinding or trituration of a solid drug. **aromatic p.,** powder of cinnamon, ginger, cardamom seed, and myristica. **bleaching p.,** calx chlorinata. **p. of chalk, aromatic,** a preparation of chalk, cinnamon, myristica, clove, cardamom, and sucrose; formerly used as an antacid, stimulant, and astringent. **p. of chalk, aromatic, with opium,** aromatic powder of chalk containing 2.5 per cent of powdered opium. **chalk p., compound,** a powder containing prepared chalk, finely powdered acacia, and sucrose; it is an antacid used in treatment of diarrhea. **chiniofon p.,** chiniofon. **Dalmatian insect p.,** pyrethrum flowers; see under *flower.* **Dover's p.,** ipecac and opium p. **dusting p.,** a fine powder used as a substitute for talc. **dusting p., absorbable,** an absorbable powder prepared by processing cornstarch, with not more than 2 per cent of magnesium oxide; used for dusting surgeons' rubber gloves and other purposes for which talc is used in the hospital. **effervescent p's, compound,** Seidlitz p's. **furazolidone and nifuroxime p.,** a preparation containing 0.09 to 0.11 per cent furazolidone and 0.45 to 0.55 per cent nifuroxime in a suitable, slightly acidified powder base; used in the treatment of candidal, trichomonal, and bacterial vaginitis, administered intravaginally. **glycyrrhiza p., compound,** senna p., compound. **Goa p.,** a bitter, brownish yellow to umber brown powder deposited in irregular interspaces of the wood of *Andira araroba* Aguiar. (Leguminosae), a large leguminous tree common in Brazil. It

is the source of chrysarobin. **impalpable p.,** a powder so fine that its particles cannot be felt as distinct bodies. **iodochlorhydroxyquin p., compound** [USP], a preparation of iodochlorhydroxyquin, boric acid, lactic acid, zinc stearate, and lactose; used as a local anti-infective in the treatment of vaginitis due to *Trichomonas vaginalis, Candida albicans, Trichophyton,* or mixed bacteria, administered by intravaginal sufflation. **ipecac and opium p.,** a pale brown powder prepared by triturating 100 gm. of finely powdered ipecac, 100 gm. of powdered opium, and 800 gm. of coarsely powdered lactose to a very fine, uniform powder; formerly widely used as a sedative and diaphoretic. **p. of jalap, compound,** a mixture of jalap and potassium bitartrate, formerly used in treatment of dropsy. **licorice p., compound, p. of liquorice, compound,** senna p., compound. **methylbenzethonium chloride p.** [USP], a preparation containing 85 to 115 per cent of the labeled amount of methylbenzethonium chloride in a suitable fine powder base, free from grittiness; used topically as a local anti-infective, applied to the skin of the genitalia, rectum, thighs, and intertriginous area in the treatment of ammonia dermatitis and in the treatment and prevention of dermatoses caused by contact with urine, feces, and perspiration. **nystatin topical p.** [USP], a preparation containing 90 to 130 per cent of the labeled amount of nystatin; used as an antifungal. **Persian insect p.,** pyrethrum flowers; see under *flower.* **p. of rhubarb, compound,** a preparation of rhubarb, ginger, and magnesium oxide; formerly used as a laxative antacid. **Seidlitz p's,** a combination of sodium bicarbonate, potassium sodium tartrate, and tartaric acid, used as a cathartic; called also *compound effervescent p's.* See also under *tests.* **senna p., compound,** a weak or dusky yellow powder prepared from fennel oil, finely powdered sucrose, powdered senna, powdered glycyrrhiza, and washed sulfur; used as a laxative. **Sippy p. No. 1,** sodium bicarbonate and calcium carbonate p. **Sippy p. No. 2,** sodium bicarbonate and magnesium oxide p. **sodium bicarbonate and calcium carbonate p.,** a mixture of precipitated calcium carbonate and sodium bicarbonate: antacid; widely used in treatment of peptic ulcer in combination with sodium bicarbonate and magnesium oxide powder. **sodium bicarbonate and magnesium oxide p.,** a mixture of magnesium oxide and sodium carbonate; used as an antacid and laxative. **tolnaftate p.** [USP], a preparation containing 90 to 110 per cent of the labeled amount of tolnaftate; used topically as an antifungal. **triacetin p.,** a preparation containing 90 to 110 per cent of the labeled amount of triacetin in a suitable powder base; used as an antifungal in superficial skin infections, applied topically. **zinc sulfate p., compound,** a preparation of salicylic acid, zinc sulfate, phenol, eucalyptol, menthol, thymol, and boric acid; used as an antiseptic.

power (pow'er) [L. *posse* to have power] 1. capability; potency; the ability to act. 2. a measure of magnification, as of a microscope. **candle p.,** the numerical expression, in international candles, of the luminous intensity of a light source. **carbon dioxide-combining p., CO_2-combining p.,** ability of the blood plasma to combine with carbon dioxide; often, but probably inappropriately, referred to as the alkali reserve. **defining p.,** the ability of a lens to make an object clearly visible. **resolving p.,** the ability of the eye or of a lens to make separately visible small objects that are close together, thus revealing the structure of an object; see also *resolution.*

pox (poks) [variant of *pocks,* from A.S. *pocc* pustule, spot] 1. any eruptive or pustular disease, especially one caused by a virus; see specific entries: *chickenpox, cowpox, horsepox, rabbitpox,* etc. 2. former name for syphilis.

poxvirus (poks-vi'rus) any of a group of relatively large, morphologically similar, and immunologically related DNA viruses, including the viruses of vaccinia (cowpox), variola (smallpox), and those producing pox diseases in lower animals.

P.P. abbreviation for L. *punc'tum prox'imum,* near point of accommodation.

P.P.D. purified protein derivative (tuberculin); see under *tuberculin.*

ppg. picopicogram.

PPLO pleuropneumonia-like organisms; see under *organism.*

ppm. parts per million.

Ppt. precipitate; prepared.

PR prosthion.

P.R. abbreviation for L. *punc'tum remo'tum*, far point of accommodation.

Pr chemical symbol for *praseodymium*.

Pr. presbyopia; prism.

practice (prak'tis) [Gr. *praktikē*] the utilization of one's knowledge in a particular profession, the practice of medicine being the exercise of one's knowledge in the practical recognition and treatment of disease. **contract p.**, the treatment of the members of a specified group for a lump sum, or at so much per member. **family p.**, the medical specialty concerned with the planning and provision of the comprehensive primary health care of all members of a family, regardless of age or sex, on a continuing basis. **general p.**, the provision of comprehensive medical care as a continuing responsibility regardless of age of the patient or of the condition that may temporarily require the services of a specialist. **group p.**, see under *medicine*. **panel p.**, see under *panel*.

practitioner (prak-tish'un-er) one who has complied with the requirements of and who is engaged in the practice of medicine. **nurse p.**, see *nurse clinician*, under *nurse*.

practolol (prak'to-lōl) chemical name: N-[4-[2-hydroxy-3-[(1-methylethyl)amino]propoxy]phenyl]acetamide; a beta-adrenergic blocking agent, $C_{14}H_{22}N_2O_3$, having the same actions as propranolol (q.v.). Its use has been found to be associated with an allergic reaction of the eyes, skin, mucous membranes, and ears.

prae- [L. "before"] a prefix meaning before, in front of; for words beginning thus, see also those beginning *pre-*.

praecox (pre'koks) [L.] premature, early; see *dementia praecox*.

praeputium (pre-pu'she-um) [L.] preputium. **p. clito'ridis**, [NA], the external fold of tissue over the glans clitoris formed by union of the two lateral parts of the labia minora. **p. pe'nis**, preputium penis.

praevia (pre've-ah) [L.] see *praevius*.

praevius (pre've-us) [L., from *prae-* + *via* way] going before, leading the way; see *placenta praevia*, under *placenta*.

pragmatagnosia (prag"mat-ag-no'ze-ah) [Gr. *pragma* object + *agnōsia* absence of recognition] inability to recognize formerly known objects.

pragmatamnesia (prag"mat-am-ne'ze-ah) [Gr. *pragma* object + *amnesia* forgetfulness] loss of power of remembering the appearance of objects.

pragmatic (prag-mat'ik) pertaining to pragmatism; dealing with practical aspects.

pragmatism (prag'mah-tizm) the doctrine that the whole meaning of a conception lies in its practical consequences.

pralidoxime (pral"ĭ-doks'ēm) chemical name: 2-[(hydroxyimino)methyl]-1-methylpyridinium. A cholinesterase reactivator, $C_7H_9N_2O^+$, capable of acting as an antagonist to certain anticholinesterases. Called also *2-PAM*. **p. chloride** [USP], the chloride salt of pralidoxime, $C_7H_9ClN_2O$; used as an antidote in the treatment of poisoning due to organophosphates having anticholinesterase activity and to counteract the effects of overdosage by anticholinesterases used in the treatment of myasthenia gravis, administered orally and by intravenous infusion. **p. iodide**, the iodide salt of pralidoxime, $C_7H_9IN_2O$, having the actions and uses of the chloride salt. **p. mesylate**, the methanesulfonate salt of pralidoxime, $C_8H_{12}N_2O_4S$, having the actions and uses of the chloride salt.

pramoxine hydrochloride (pram-ok'sēn) [USP] chemical name: 4-[3-(4-butoxyphenoxy)propyl]morpholine hydrochloride. A local anesthetic, $C_{17}H_{27}NO_3 \cdot HCl$, occurring as a white to nearly white, crystalline powder; applied topically.

prandial (pran'de-al) [L. *prandium* breakfast] pertaining to a meal, especially dinner.

pranolium chloride (pra-no'le-um) chemical name: 2-hydroxy-N,N-dimethyl-N-(1-methylethyl)-3-(1-naphthalenyloxy)-1-propanaminium chloride; a cardiac depressant with antiarrhythmic actions, $C_{18}H_{26}ClNO_2$.

Prantal (pran'tal) trademark for preparations of diphemanil methylsulfate.

praseodymium (pra"ze-o-dim'e-um, pra"se-o-dim'e-um) a rare earth element; atomic number, 59; atomic weight, 140.907; symbol, Pr.

Prasinomonadida (pra"sĭ-no-mo-nad'ĭ-dah) an order of plantlike flagellate protozoa (class Phytomastigophorea, subphylum Mastigophora) having one, two, four, or eight flagella, grass-green chloroplasts, and a covering of one or more layers of Golgi-derived scales.

P. rat. aetat. abbreviation for L. *pro ratio'ne aeta'tis*, in proportion to age.

pratique (prah-tek') [Fr.] a certificate which releases an incoming vessel from quarantine. It is given by the quarantine officer to the master, and when presented to the collector of the port admits the boat to entry.

Prausnitz-Küstner reaction (test) (prows'nits- kist'ner) [Carl Willy *Prausnitz*, German hygienist, born 1876; Heinz *Küstner*, German gynecologist, born 1897] see under *reaction*.

Praxagoras (prak-sag'o-ras) **of Cos** (c. 340 B.C.) a Greek physician who succeeded Diocles as leader of the Dogmatists. He was apparently the first Greek physician to recognize the difference between arteries (carriers of air) and veins (carriers of blood), and to comment on the pulse.

praxiology (prak"se-ol'o-je) [Gr. *praxis* action + *-logy*] the study of conduct, rather than of thought or consciousness.

praxis (prak'sis) [Gr. "action"] the doing or performance of action; Edinger's term for the execution of pallial impulses. Cf. *gnosis*.

prazepam (prah'zě-pam) chemical name: 7-chloro-1-(cyclopropylmethyl)-1,3-dihydro-5-phenyl-2H-1,4-benzodiazepin-2-one. A benzodiazepine derivative, $C_{19}H_{17}ClN_2O$, used as a muscle relaxant and a tranquilizer in the treatment of conditions in which anxiety is a prominent feature, administered orally.

praziquantel (pra"zĭ-kwon'tel) chemical name: 2-(cyclohexylcarbonyl)-1,2,3,6,7,11b-hexahydro-4H-pyrazino[2,1-a]isoquinolin-4-one; an anthelmintic, $C_{19}H_{24}N_2O_2$, effective against parasitic fluke and tapeworm infections.

prazosin hydrochloride (prah'zo-sin) chemical name: 1-(4-amino-6,7-dimethoxy-2-quinazolinyl)-4-(2-furanylcarbonyl)piperazine monohydrochloride. A quinazoline derivative with vasodilator properties, $C_{19}H_{21}N_5O_4 \cdot HCl$; used as an oral antihypertensive.

pre- [L. *prae* before] a prefix meaning before, in front of.

preadaptation (pre"ah-dap-ta'shun) the acquisition in an ancestral group of certain characters that usually are adaptive to the ancestral mode of life yet at the same time enable a shift in mode of life; for example, lungs in fish ancestral to tetrapods.

preagonal (pre-ag'o-nal) preceding the death agony.

preanesthesia (pre"an-es-the'ze-ah) preliminary anesthesia; light anesthesia or narcosis induced by medication as a preliminary to administration of a general anesthetic.

preanesthetic (pre"an-es-thet'ik) 1. pertaining to or inducing preanesthesia. 2. an agent that induces preanesthesia. 3. occurring before administration of an anesthetic.

preaortic (pre"a-or'tik) in front of the aorta.

preataxic (pre"ah-tak'sik) occurring before or preceding ataxia.

preaurale (pre"aw-ra'le) a cephalometric landmark, the point at which a straight line from the postaurale, perpendicular to the long axis of the auricle, meets the base of the auricle.

preauricular (pre"aw-rik'u-lar) situated in front of the auricle of the ear.

preaxial (pre-ak'se-al) situated or occurring before an axis; in anatomical usage, preaxial refers to the lateral (radial) aspect of the upper limb and the medial (tibial) aspect of the lower limb.

prebacillary (pre-bas'ĭ-ler"e) occurring before the entrance of bacilli into the system, or before they become discoverable.

prebase (pre'bās) that part of the dorsum of the tongue lying in front of the base.

prebeta-lipoprotein (pre"ba"tah-lip"o-pro'te-in) very-low-density lipoprotein. **sinking p.**, Lp(a) lipoprotein.

prebetalipoproteinemia (pre"ba"tah-lip"o-pro'te-ine'me-ah) hyperprebetalipoproteinemia.

prebiotic (pre″bi-ot′ik) denoting the period before the existence of life on earth.

prebladder (pre-blad′er) an extensive cavity formed in front of the orifice of the bladder within the capsule of the prostate.

prebrachium (pre-bra′ke-um) brachium colliculi superioris.

precancer (pre′kan-ser) a condition which tends eventually to become malignant.

precancerosis (pre″kan-ser-o′sis) a precancerous condition; a condition of early cancer.

precancerous (pre-kan′ser-us) pertaining to a pathologic process that tends to become malignant.

precapillary (pre-kap′ĭ-ler″e) a vessel lacking complete coats, intermediate between an arteriole and a true capillary, and containing scattered smooth muscle cells in its wall; these vessels usually have sphincter areas, which control blood flow into capillaries. Called also *metarteriole*.

precarcinomatous (pre″kar-sĭ-nom′ah-tus) preceding the development of carcinoma.

precardium (pre-kar′de-um) [*pre-* + Gr. *kardia* heart] precordium.

precartilage (pre-kar′tĭ-lij) embryonic cartilaginous tissue.

precava (pre-ka′vah) the vena cava superior.

precementum (pre″sĕ-men′tum) cementoid.

precentral (pre-sen′tral) situated in front of a center, as the precentral gyrus.

prechordal (pre-kor′dal) situated in front of the notochord.

precipitable (pre-sip′ĭ-tah-b′l) capable of being precipitated.

precipitant (pre-sip′ĭ-tant) a substance which causes a chemical or mechanical precipitation.

precipitate (pre-sip′ĭ-tāt) [L. *praecipitare* to cast down] 1. to cause a substance in solution to settle down in solid particles. 2. [L. *praecipitatum*] a deposit made or substance thrown down by precipitation. 3. occurring with undue rapidity, as precipitate labor. 4. in immunology, the product of interaction between soluble macromolecular antigen and the homologous antibody, e.g., the antigen-antibody complex formed as a consequence of the reaction of pneumococcus capsular polysaccharide in solution with specific antiserum. **immune p.**, see *precipitate*. **keratic p's**, see under *keratitis punctata.* **keratic p's, mutton-fat,** coalescent precipitates forming translucent rings with opaque centers in the anterior chamber, and occurring in uveitis. **sweet p.,** calomel (mild mercurous chloride). **white p.,** ammoniated mercury.

precipitation (pre-sip″ĭ-ta′shun) [L. *praecipitatio*] the act or process of precipitating. **group p.,** precipitation by a precipitin in a specific antiserum of an antigen common to a group of closely related microorganisms.

precipitin (pre-sip′ĭ-tin) an antibody to antigen that specifically aggregates the macromolecular antigen in vivo or in vitro to give a visible precipitate.

precipitinogen (pre-sip″ĭ-tin′o-jen) the soluble antigen which stimulates the formation of precipitins and is capable of reacting with them in vitro and in vivo.

precipitinoid (pre-sip′ĭ-tin-oid) (*obs.*) a precipitin that has been modified so that it cannot cause precipitation, although it still retains its affinity for the antigen.

precipitogen (pre-sip′ĭ-to-jen) precipitinogen.

precision (pre-sizh′un) 1. the quality of being sharply or exactly defined; for example, a measurement with three significant figures is more precise than a measurement with two. Cf. *accuracy*. 2. in statistics, the extent to which a measurement procedure gives the same results when repeated under identical conditions; the inverse of the variance. Under certain conditions, may be called *reliability*.

preclinical (pre-klin′ĭ-kal) before a disease becomes clinically recognizable.

precocious (pre-ko′shus) developed more than is usual at a given age.

precocity (pre-kos′ĭ-te) unusually early development of mental or physical traits.

precognition (pre″kog-nish′un) [*pre-* + *cognition*] the extrasensory perception of a future event.

precollagenous (pre″kŏ-laj′ĕ-nus) [*pre-* + *collagen*] denoting an incomplete stage in the formation of collagen.

precoma (pre-ko′mah) the neuropsychiatric state preceding coma, as in hepatic encephalopathy.

preconscious (pre-kon′shus) the part of the mind that is not in immediate awareness but can be consciously recalled with effort, one of the systems of Freud's topographic model of the mind. Cf. *conscious* and *unconscious*.

precordia (pre-kor′de-ah) [L. *praecordia*] precordium.

precordial (pre-kor′de-al) pertaining to the precordium.

precordialgia (pre″kor-de-al′je-ah) [*precordia* + *-algia*] pain in the precordium.

precordium (pre-kor′de-um) the region over the heart and lower part of the thorax.

precornu (pre-kor′nu) cornu anterius ventriculi lateralis.

precostal (pre-kos′tal) in front of the ribs.

precritical (pre-krit′ĭ-kal) previous to the occurrence of the crisis.

precuneate (pre-ku′ne-āt) pertaining to the precuneus.

precuneus (pre-ku′ne-us) [*pre-* + L. *cuneus* wedge] [NA] a small, square-shaped convolution on the medial surface of the parietal lobe of the cerebrum, bounded posteriorly by the medial part of the parietooccipital sulcus and anteriorly by the paracentral lobule.

precursor (pre′kur-sor) [L. *praecursor* a forerunner] something that precedes. In biological processes, a substance from which another, usually more active or mature substance is formed. In clinical medicine, a sign or symptom that heralds another.

predation (pre-da′shun) the derivation by an organism of elements essential for its existence from organisms of other species which it consumes and destroys.

predator (pred′ah-tor) [L. *praedator* a plunderer, pillager] an organism that derives elements essential for its existence from organisms of other species, which it consumes and destroys.

predentin (pre-den′tin) the soft fibrillar substance composing the primitive dentin and forming the inner layer of the circumpulpar dentin; called also *dentinoid*.

prediabetes (pre-di″ah-be′tēz) a state of latent impairment of carbohydrate metabolism, in which the criteria for diabetes mellitus are not all satisfied; sometimes controllable by diet alone.

prediastole (pre″di-as′to-le) the interval immediately preceding diastole in the cardiac cycle.

prediastolic (pre″di-ah-stol′ik) 1. pertaining to the beginning of the diastole. 2. occurring just before the diastole.

predicrotic (pre″di-krot′ik) occurring before the dicrotic wave of the sphygmogram.

predigestion (pre″di-jes′chun) the partial artificial digestion of food before its ingestion.

predisposing (pre″dis-pōz′ing) conferring a tendency to disease.

predisposition (pre″dis-po-zish′un) [*pre-* + L. *disponere* to dispose] a latent susceptibility to disease which may be activated under certain conditions, as by stress.

prediverticular (pre-di″ver-tik′u-lar) denoting a condition of thickening of the muscular wall of the colon and increased intraluminal pressure but without herniation of the mucosa, i.e., without evidence of diverticulosis.

prednimustine (pred′nĭ-mus′tēn) an ester of chlorambucil and prednisone, used as an antineoplastic.

prednisolone (pred-nis′o-lōn) [USP] chemical name: 11β17α- 21-trihydroxypregna-1,4-diene-3,20-dione. A synthetic glucocorticoid derived from cortisol, $C_{21}H_{28}O_5$, occurring as a white to practically white, crystalline powder; administered orally in the treatment of various conditions responsive to the anti-inflammatory action of glucocorticoids, including rheumatoid arthritis and other collagen diseases, allergic conditions, neoplastic and gastrointestinal disease, and blood dyscrasias. **p. acetate** [USP], the 21-acetate ester of prednisolone, $C_{23}H_{30}O_4$, occurring as a white to practically white, crystalline powder, having actions and uses similar to those of the base; administered by intra-articular or intramuscular injection. **p. butylacetate,** p. tebutate. **p. sodium phosphate** [USP], the sodium phosphate ester salt of prednisolone, $C_{21}H_{27}Na_2O_8P$, occurring as white or slightly yellow, friable granules or powder, having actions and uses similar to those of the base; administered by intravenous or intramuscular injection when rapid effect is needed, or applied topically to the conjunctiva. **p. sodium succinate for injection** [NF], sterile prednisolone sodium succinate prepared from prednisolone succinate with the aid of sodium carbonate, containing between 90 and 110 per cent of prednisolone; used as a glucocorticoid. **p. succinate** [USP], the succinate ester of prednisolone, $C_{25}H_{32}O_8$, occurring as a fine, creamy white powder with friable lumps, which on solubilization with sodium carbonate produces *prednisolone sodium succinate*, a form administered by intravenous or intramuscular injection when rapid effect is needed. **p. tebutate** [USP], an ester of prednisolone, $C_{27}H_{38}O_6$, occurring as a white to slightly yellow, free-flowing powder that may have some soft lumps; used as a pharmaceutic necessity for the sterile suspension dosage form intended for intra-articular, intrabursal, and soft-tissue injection. Called also *p. butylacetate*.

prednisone (pred′nĭ-sōn) [USP] chemical name: 17α,21-dihydroxypregna-1,4-diene-3,11,20-trione. A synthetic glucocorticoid derived from cortisone, $C_{21}H_{26}O_5$, but having reduced mineralocorticoid activity; it occurs as a white to practically white, crystalline powder and is used orally in the treatment of various conditions responsive to the anti-inflammatory action of glucocorticoids. Called also *deltacortisone*.

predormital (pre-dor′mĭ-tal) pertaining to or occurring in the predormitum.

predormitum (pre-dor′mĭ-tum) the period of waning consciousness interposed between the waking state and sound slumber.

preeclampsia (pre″e-klamp′se-ah) a toxemia of late pregnancy characterized by hypertension, edema, and proteinuria; when convulsions and coma are associated, it is called *eclampsia*.

preelacin (pre-el′ah-sin) a precursor of elacin in the circulating blood.

preepiglottic (pre″ep-ĭ-glot′ik) situated or occurring in front of the epiglottis.

preexcitation (pre-ek″si-ta′shun) 1. premature excitation of a portion of the ventricle occurring in Wolff-Parkinson-White syndrome. It is caused by cardiac impulses transmitted along an accessory pathway not subject to the physiologic delay of the atrioventricular node, and is characterized electrocardiographically by a short P-R interval and a wide QRS interval. 2. Wolff-Parkinson-White syndrome. **ventricular p.,** Wolff-Parkinson-White syndrome.

preformation (pre″for-ma′shun) the theory of early physiologists that the fully formed animal or plant exists in a minute form in the germ cell. Opposed to the theory of *epigenesis*. See *animalculist* and *ovist*.

preformationist (pre″for-ma′shun-ist) a believer in the theory of preformation.

prefrontal (pre-fron′tal) 1. situated in the anterior part of the frontal lobe or region. 2. the central part of the ethmoid bone.

prefunctional (pre-funk′shun-al) denoting the period in embryological development during which the organ rudiments are formed but are incapable of performing their specific functions.

preganglionic (pre″gang-gle-on′ik) situated anterior or proximal to a ganglion; said especially of autonomic nerve fibers so located.

pregenital (pre-jen′ĭ-tal) pertaining to the early stages of psychosexual development (oral and anal), before the genitals have become the dominant influence on sexual behavior.

Pregl's test (pra′g′lz) [Fritz *Pregl*, Austrian chemist, 1869–1930] see under *tests*.

pregnancy (preg′nan-se) [L. *praegnans* with child] the condition of having a developing embryo or fetus in the body, after union of an ovum and spermatozoon. In women duration of pregnancy is about 266 days. Pregnancy is marked by cessation of the menses; nausea on arising in the morning (morning sickness); enlargement of the breasts and pigmentation of the nipples; progressive enlargement of the abdomen. The absolute signs of pregnancy are fetal movements, sounds of the fetal heart, and demonstration of the fetus by x-ray or ultrasound. **abdominal p.,** ectopic pregnancy with development of the fetus in the abdominal cavity. **ampullar p.,** ectopic pregnancy in which the

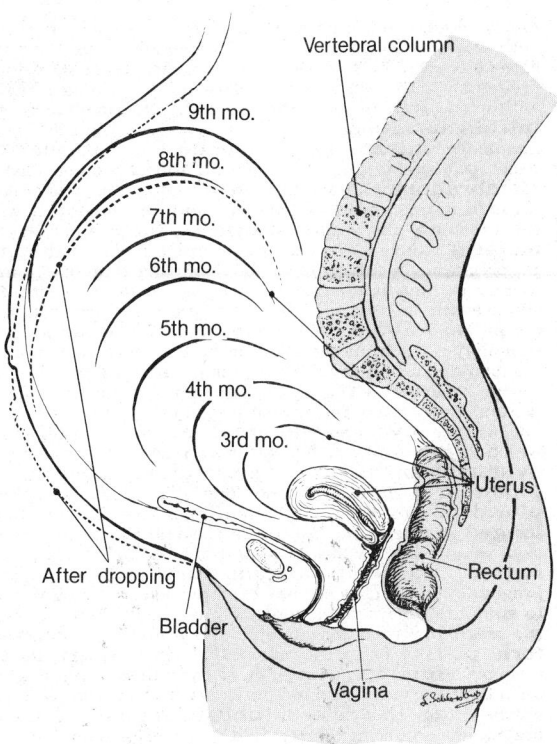

Pregnancy—Uterine levels.

ovum has been arrested in the ampulla of the oviduct. **angular p.,** pregnancy in which the fertilized ovum becomes implanted in the angle or cornu of the uterus. **bigeminal p.,** twin p. **broad ligament p.,** ectopic pregnancy with development of the fertilized ovum in the broad ligament. **cervical p.,** ectopic pregnancy with the development of the ovum within the cervical canal. **combined p.,** simultaneous existence of intrauterine and ectopic pregnancy. **compound p.,** superimposition of an intrauterine pregnancy on a previously existing ectopic pregnancy, generally a lithopedion. **cornual p.,** pregnancy in one of the horns of a bicornate uterus. **ectopic p.,** development of the fertilized ovum outside of the uterine cavity; called also *extrauterine p.* **exochorial p.,** gravid-

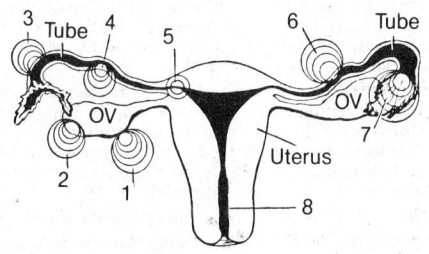

Diagram showing locations of ectopic (extrauterine) pregnancy: (1) primary abdominal; (2) ovarian; (3) ampullar, (4) tubal—rupture into broad ligament; (5) interstitial; (6) tubal—rupture into peritoneal cavity; (7) tubo-ovarian; (8) cervical.

itas exochorialis. **extrauterine p.,** ectopic p. **fallopian p.,** tubal p. **false p.,** absence of the menses and presence of other signs of pregnancy, without occurrence of conception and development of an embryo. It may be due to psychogenic factors, to a tumor or mole, or to endocrine disorders. Called also *pseudocyesis, pseudopregnancy,* and *spurious p.* **gemellary p.,** twin p. **heterotopic p.,** combined p. **hydatid p.,** that which is accompanied by the formation of a hydatid mole. **hysteric p.,** false pregnancy due to psychogenic factors. **incomplete p.,** pregnancy which is interrupted prematurely: abortion (up to the 16th week); immature delivery (16th to 28th week); premature delivery (28th to 36th week). **interstitial p.,** ectopic pregnancy with gestation in that part of the oviduct which is within the wall of the uterus. **intraligamentary p., intraligamentous p.,** ectopic pregnancy within the broad ligament. **intramural p.,** interstitial p. **intraperitoneal p.,** ectopic pregnancy within the peritoneal cavity. **membranous p.,** pregnancy in which the fetus has broken through its membranous envelope and lies in contact with the uterine walls. **mesenteric p.,** tuboligamentary p. **molar p.,** conversion of the ovum into a mole. **multiple p.,** pregnancy resulting in the birth of more than one infant; it may be *monovular* (resulting from the fertilization of a single ovum) or *polyovular* (resulting from the fertilization of more than one ovum). When more than two fetuses co-exist, they may come from one ovum or be the result of combined monovular and polyovular twinning. **mural p.,** interstitial p. **nervous p.,** false pregnancy due to psychogenic factors. **ovarian p.,** ectopic pregnancy occurring within an ovary. **ovario-abdominal p.,** ectopic pregnancy which begins ovarian, but afterward becomes abdominal. **oviductal p.,** tubal p. **parietal p.,** interstitial p. **phantom p.,** false pregnancy due to psychogenic factors. **plural p.,** pregnancy with more than one fetus. **prolonged p.,** pregnancy continuing beyond the normal duration, usually beyond 294 days after the beginning of the last menses. **pseudointraligamentary p.,** an ectopic pregnancy in which a sac has been formed in such a way as to simulate an intraligamentary pregnancy. **sarcofetal p.,** pregnancy with both a fetus and a mole. **sarcohysteric p.,** false pregnancy due to a mole. **spurious p.,** false p. **stump p.,** pregnancy at the stump remaining after a supracervical hysterectomy. **tubal p.,** ectopic pregnancy within an oviduct. **tuboabdominal p.,** ectopic pregnancy occurring partly in the fimbriated end of the oviduct and partly in the abdominal cavity. **tuboligamentary p.,** ectopic pregnancy partly in the tube and partly in the broad ligament. **tubo-ovarian p.,** ectopic pregnancy occurring partly in the ovary and partly in the oviduct. **tubouterine p.,** ectopic pregnancy partly within the uterus and partly in an oviduct. **twin p.,** gestation with development of two fetuses. **uteroabdominal p.,** pregnancy with one fetus in the uterus and another in the abdominal cavity. **utero-ovarian p.,** pregnancy with one fetus in the uterus and another in the ovary. **uterotubal p.,** tubouterine pregnancy.

pregnane (preg′nān) a crystalline saturated steroid hydrocarbon, $C_{21}H_{36}$. 5β-Pregnane, a version of the steroid nucleus, is the form from which several hormones, including progesterone, are derived. 5α-Pregnane, or allopregnane, is the form excreted in the urine.

pregnanediol (preg″nān-di′ol) 5β-pregnane-3α, 20α-diol, a crystalline, biologically inactive dihydroxy derivative of progesterone and its chief urinary metabolite; found especially in urine of women during pregnancy or the secretory phase of the menstrual cycle.

pregnanetriol (preg″nān-tri′ol) a metabolite of 17α-hydroxyprogesterone, normally occurring in small amounts in body fluids and urine, but greatly increased in disorders of the adrenal cortex in which 21-hydroxylation of the steroid nucleus is impaired, as in the most common form of congenital adrenocortical hyperplasia with virilism.

pregnant (preg′nant) [L. *praegnans*] with child; gravid.

pregnene (preg′nēn) $C_{21}H_{34}$, a crystalline unsaturated steroid with one double bond and three methyl groups; the △⁴ and △⁵ pregnene steroid nucleus forms the basis of most of the biologically active androgens and corticosteroids.

pregneninolone (preg″nēn-in′o-lōn) ethisterone.

pregnenolone succinate (preg-nēn′o-lōn) chemical name: (3β-carboxy-1-oxopropoxy)-pregn-5-en-20-one. A glucocorticoid, $C_{25}H_{36}O_5$, which has been used in the treatment of rheumatoid arthritis.

pregonium (pre-go′ne-um) a recess on the lower edge of the body of the mandible in advance of the angle.

prehallux (pre-hal′uks) a supernumerary bone of the foot sometimes found growing from the medial border of the scaphoid.

prehensile (pre-hen′sil) [L. *prehendere* to lay hold of] adapted for grasping or seizing.

prehension (pre-hen′shun) [L. *prehensio*] the act of seizing or grasping.

prehepaticus (pre″he-pat′ĭ-kus) [pre- + Gr. *hēpar* liver] a mass of vascular and connective tissue in the embryo which develops into the interstitial tissue of the liver.

prehormone (pre-hor′mōn) a biosynthetic, usually intraglandular hormone precursor.

prehyoid (pre-hi′oid) in front of the hyoid bone.

prehypophyseal (pre″hi-po-fiz′e-al) pertaining to or derived from the anterior lobe of the pituitary gland (lobus anterior hypophyseos [NA]).

prehypophysial (pre″hi-po-fiz′e-al) prehypophyseal.

prehypophysis (pre″hi-pof′ĭ-sis) the anterior lobe of the pituitary gland.

preictal (pre-ik′tal) [pre- + L. *ictus* stroke] occurring before a stroke or an attack, as before an acute epileptic attack.

preinvasive (pre″in-va′siv) not yet invading other tissues; see *carcinoma in situ*.

preiotation (pre″i-o-ta′shun) [pre- + Gr. *iōta*, the Greek letter ι] the conversion of the initial sound of *i* into *y*.

Preiser's disease (pri′zerz) [Georg Karl Felix *Preiser*, orthopedic surgeon, Hamburg, Germany, 1879–1913] see under *disease*.

Preisz-Nocard bacillus (prīs-no-kard′) [Hugo von *Preisz*, Budapest bacteriologist, 1860–1940; E. I. E. *Nocard*, 1850–1903] *Corynebacterium pseudotuberculosis*.

prekallikrein (pre-kal″ĭ-kre′in) a plasma protein that is the proenzyme of plasma kallikrein. Called also *prokallikrein*.

prelacteal (pre-lak′te-al) preceding the establishment of milk flow; a term applied to the feeding of a newborn baby with carbohydrate-electrolyte solutions to reduce initial weight loss until breast feeding is fully established.

preleukemia (pre-lu-ke′me-ah) a stage of varying duration preceding the development of overt acute myelogenous monocytic or stem-cell leukemia, characterized by bone marrow dysfunction as manifested by anemia, neutropenia, thrombocytopenia, or a combination of these. Splenomegaly, hepatomegaly, or lymphadenopathy may not appear until the onset, often explosive, of the overt leukemia itself.

preleukemic (pre-lu-ke′mik) pertaining to or affected with preleukemia.

prelimbic (pre-lim′bik) situated before a limbus; specifically, anterior to the limbus fossae ovalis.

prelipoid (pre-li′poid) 1. preceding or before the lipoid state. 2. a preliminary stage of lipoid substance.

prelocalization (pre″lo-kal-i-za′shun) the localization in the egg or blastomere of materials which will develop into a particular tissue or organ.

prelocomotion (pre″lo-ko-mo′shun) the movements of a child made with the intention of moving from place to place before motor coordination is sufficently developed to enable it to walk.

premalignant (pre″mah-lig′nant) precancerous.

Premarin (prem′ah-rin) trademark for preparations of conjugated estrogens.

premature (pre-mah-tūr′) [L. *praematurus* early ripe] 1. occurring before the proper time. 2. a premature infant; see under *infant*.

prematurity (pre″mah-tu′rĭ-te) underdevelopment; the condition of a premature infant.

premaxilla (pre″mak-sil′ah) a separate element derived from the median nasal processes in the embryo, which later fuses with the maxilla; see also os *incisivum*.

premaxillary (pre″mak-sĭ-ler″e) 1. situated in front of the maxilla proper. 2. os incisivum. 3. pertaining to the premaxilla or to the os incisivum.

premedical (pre-med′ĭ-kal) preceding and preparing for the regular medical course of study, as premedical education.

premedicant (pre-med′ĭ-kant) a drug used for premedication.

premedication (pre″med-ĭ-ka′shun) preliminary medication, particularly internal medication to produce narcosis prior to inhalation anesthesia.

premeiotic (pre″mi-ot′ik) [pre- + Gr. *meioun* to decrease] occurring before or pertaining to the time preceding meiosis.

premenarchal (pre″mĕ-nar′kal) pertaining to the period

before menstruation is established; occurring prior to the menarche.

premenarche (pre″mĕ-nar′ke) the period before menstruation is established; preceding the menarche.

premenarcheal (pre″mĕ-nar′ke-al) premenarchal.

premenstrua (pre-men′stroo-ah) [L.] plural of *premenstruum.*

premenstrual (pre-men′stroo-al) occurring before menstruation.

premenstruum (pre-men′stroo-um), pl. *premenstrua* [L.] the period immediately preceding occurrence of the menstrual flow.

premitotic (pre″mi-tot′ik) occurring before or pertaining to the time preceding mitosis.

premolar (pre-mo′lar) [pre- + L. *molaris* molar] 1. one of the eight permanent teeth (two on either side of each jaw) anterior to the molars and posterior to the canine teeth; in zoology, those teeth which succeed the deciduous molars regardless of the number to be succeeded. See under *tooth.* 2. situated in front of the molar teeth.

premonitory (pre-mon′ĭ-to-re) [L. *praemonitorius*] serving as a warning.

premonocyte (pre-mon′o-sīt) promonocyte.

premorbid (pre-mor′bid) occurring before the development of disease.

premortal (pre-mor′tal) occurring just before death.

premunition (pre″mu-nish′un) relative immunity; infection immunity; a state of resistance to infection which is established after an acute infection has become chronic and which lasts as long as the infecting organisms remain in the body.

premunitive (pre-mu′nĭ-tiv) pertaining to premunition.

premyeloblast (pre-mi′ĕ-lo-blast″) an early form of a myeloblast.

premyelocyte (pre-mi′ĕ-lo-sīt″) promyelocyte.

prenarcosis (pre″nar-ko′sis) narcosis induced as a preliminary to full general anesthesia or previous to local anesthesia.

prenarcotic (pre″nar-kot′ik) previous to the occurrence of narcosis.

prenares (pre-na′rēz) the nostrils or nares.

prenasale (pre″na-sa′le) a cephalometric landmark, the most projecting point, in the median plane, at the tip of the nose.

prenatal (pre-na′tal) [pre- + L. *natalis* natal] existing or occurring before birth, with reference to the fetus. Cf. *antepartal.*

preoperative (pre-op′er-ah-tiv) preceding an operation.

preoptic (pre-op′tik) situated anterior to the optic chiasma.

preoxygenation (pre-ok″sĭ-jen-a′shun) the prolonged breathing of oxygen before exposure to low atmospheric pressure at high altitudes, as prophylaxis against decompression sickness.

preparation (prep″ah-ra′shun) [L. *praeparatio*] 1. the act or process of making ready. 2. a medicine made ready for use. 3. an anatomic or pathologic specimen made ready and preserved for study. **biomechanical p.,** the procedures involved in exposing, enlarging, cleansing, and shaping the pulp chamber and root canal of a tooth by mechanical means. **cavity p.,** a procedure for establishing in a tooth the biochemically acceptable form necessary to receive and retain a restoration, accomplished by the use of rotary and handcutting instruments. See also *prepared cavity,* under *cavity.* **corrosion p.,** an anatomical preparation made by injecting the parts to be retained and eating away the rest of the tissues with some corrosive substance. **Ehrlich-Hata p.,** arsphenamine. **Hata p.,** arsphenamine. **heart-lung p.,** an animal in which only the heart and lungs are kept alive, the blood from the aorta being diverted into an external system of tubes, simulating the systemic circulation, and back via a reservoir to the right atrium; used in studies of heart function. **impression p.,** a preparation of bacteria on a slide for examination, made by lightly touching a coverglass to a colony.

prepartal (pre-par′tal) [pre- + L. *partus* labor] occurring before, or just previous to, labor.

prepatent (pre-pa′tent) before becoming apparent or manifest; in malariology the term is applied to the period elapsing between infection and appearance of parasites in blood.

preperception (pre″per-sep′shun) in psychology, anticipation of a perception.

preperitoneal (pre″per-ĭ-to-ne′al) situated between the parietal peritoneum and the abdominal wall, or occurring in front of the peritoneum.

preponderance (pre-pon′der-ans) [pre- + L. *pondere* to weigh] the condition of having greater weight, force, or influence. **ventricular p.,** disproportionate hypertrophy between the ventricles of the heart; diagnosed by the electrocardiograph.

prepotency (pre-po′ten-se) [L. *praepotentia*] power superior to that of the other parent in transmitting inheritable characters to the offspring.

prepotent (pre-po′tent) [L. *praepotens*] having superior force; having greater power than the other parent in transmitting inheritable characters to the offspring.

prepotential (pre″po-ten′shal) the slow diastolic depolarization of the cell membranes of the cardiac pacemaker.

preprandial (pre-pran′de-al) before meals.

preprohormone (pre″pro-hor′mōn) a hormone preproprotein.

preproinsulin (pre″pro-in′su-lin) the intraglandular precursor of proinsulin, containing an additional polypeptide sequence at the N-terminal.

preprophage (pre-pro′fāj) [pre- + *prophage*] a postulated stage in the life cycle of a temperate bacteriophage, occurring after infection of a bacterium and before establishment of the prophage.

preproprotein (pre″pro-pro′tēn) a precursor that is cleaved to form a proprotein.

preprosthetic (pre″pros-thet′ik) performed or occurring before insertion of a prosthesis.

preprotein (pre-pro′tēn) a protein precursor that contains a signal peptide sequence, which is a nonpolar sequence at the head of the growing polypeptide chain required for its transfer into the cistern of the endoplasmic reticulum; the signal sequence is then cleaved to form the protein or proprotein.

prepuberal (pre-pu′ber-al) prepubertal.

prepubertal (pre-pu′ber-tal) occurring before puberty; pertaining to the period of accelerated growth preceding gonadal maturity.

prepuberty (pre-pu′ber-te) the period preceding puberty.

prepubescence (pre″pu-bes′ens) prepuberty.

prepubescent (pre″pu-bes′ent) prepubertal.

prepuce (pre′pūs) a covering fold of skin; often used alone to designate the preputium penis. **p. of clitoris,** preputium clitoridis. **p. of penis,** preputium penis. **redundant p.,** a condition in which there is excessive growth of the foreskin, so that it cannot be drawn back over the glans.

preputial (pre-pu′shal) pertaining to the prepuce.

preputiotomy (pre-pu″she-ot′o-me) [*preputium* + Gr. *tomē* a cutting] incision of the preputium penis on the dorsum or side of the penis, to relieve the constriction in phimosis.

preputium (pre-pu′she-um) a covering fold of skin, as the preputium penis. **p. clitor′idis** [NA], a fold formed by the union of the labia minora anterior with the clitoris; called also *prepuce of clitoris.* **p. pe′nis** [NA], the fold of skin covering the glans penis; called also *prepuce of penis* and *foreskin.*

prepyloric (pre″pi-lor′ik) in front of or just proximal to the pylorus or the pyloric part of the stomach (see *pars pylorica ventriculi).*

Presamine (pres′ah-mēn) trademark for a preparation of imipramine hydrochloride.

presby- [Gr. *presbys* old man] a combining form meaning old or denoting relationship to old age.

presbyacusia (pres″be-ah-ku′se-ah) presbycusis.

presbyatrics (pres-be-at′riks) [*presby-* + Gr. *iatrikē* surgery, medicine] geriatrics.

presbycardia (pres″bĭ-kar′de-ah) impaired cardiac function attributed to the aging process, occurring in association with recognizable changes of senescence in the body and in the absence of convincing evidence of other forms of heart disease.

presbycusis (pres″bĕ-ku′sis) [*presby-* + Gr. *akousis* hearing] a progressive, bilaterally symmetrical perceptive hearing loss occurring with age.

presbyesophagus (pres″be-ĕ-sof′ah-gus) a condition characterized by alteration in motor function of the esophagus as a result of degenerative changes occurring with advancing age.

presbyope (pres′be-ōp) one who is presbyopic.

presbyophrenia (pres″be-o-fre′ne-ah) [*presby-* + Gr. *phrēn* mind + *-ia*] senile dementia characterized by amnesia, confabulation, confusion, and disorientation; called also *Wernicke's dementia.*

presbyopia (pres″be-o′pe-ah) [*presby-* + *-opia*] hyperopia and impairment of vision due to advancing years or to old age; it is dependent on diminution of the power of accommodation from loss of elasticity of the crystalline lens, causing the near point of distinct vision to be removed farther from the eye.

presbyopic (pres″be-op′ik) pertaining to presbyopia.

presbytia (pres-bish′e-ah) presbyopia.

presbytism (pres′bĭ-tizm) presbyopia.

prescapula (pre-skap′u-lah) the suprascapular portion of the scapula.

prescapular (pre-skap′u-lar) 1. in front of the scapula. 2. pertaining to the prescapula.

presclerotic (pre″skle-rot′ik) occurring before sclerosis takes place.

prescribe (pre-skrīb′) [L. *praescribere* to write before] to designate in writing a remedy for administration.

prescription (pre-skrip′shun) [L. *praescriptio*] a written direction for the preparation and administration of a remedy. A prescription consists of the heading or *superscription*—that is, the symbol ℞ or the word Recipe, meaning "take"; the *inscription,* which contains the names and quantities of the ingredients; the *subscription,* or directions for compounding; and the *signature,* usually introduced by the sign S. for *sig′na,* "mark," which gives the directions for the patient which are to be marked on the receptacle. **shotgun p.,** an irrational presciption that contains a number of ingredients given with the idea that one or more of them may be effective.

presecretin (pre″se-kre′tin) prosecretin.

presenile (pre-se′nīl) pertaining to a condition resembling senility, but occurring in early or middle life.

presenility (pre″sĕ-nil′ĭ-te) premature old age.

presenium (pre-se′ne-um) the period immediately preceding old age.

present (pre-zent′) [L. *praesentare* to show] to appear or to show, as to appear first at the os uteri (said of various parts of the fetus), or to appear for examination, treatment, etc. (said of a patient).

presentation (pre″zen-ta′shun) [L. *praesentatio*] in obstetrics: (*a*) the relationship of the long axis of the fetus to that of the mother (called also *lie*); (*b*) the presenting part, i.e., that portion of the fetus which is touched by the examining finger through the cervix, or during labor, is bounded by the girdle of resistance. Cf. *position.* **antigen p.,** the activity in which macrophages ingest and partially digest antigens and then present the processed antigen on their surfaces to B and T lymphocytes. The presented antigen is more immunogenic than unprocessed antigen, possibly because it has been broken down into pieces more easily recognized by B and T cells, because it remains on the surface of the presenting cell for a long time, or because it is presented in association with self MHC antigen and thus able to stimulate helper T cells. The principal antigen-presenting cells are dendritic cells in B-dependent areas of lymphoid tissues, interdigitating cells in T-dependent areas, and Langerhans cells in the epidermis. **breech p.,** presentation of the buttocks or feet of the fetus in labor; see also *longitudinal p.* **breech p., complete,** presentation of the buttocks of the fetus in labor, with the feet alongside the buttocks, the fetus being in the same attitude as in vertex presentation, but with polarity reversed. **breech p., double,** complete breech p. **breech p., frank,** presentation of the buttocks of the fetus in labor, with the legs extended against the trunk and the feet lying against the face. **breech p., incomplete,** presentation of the fetus in labor, with one or both feet or one or both knees of the fetus prolapsed into the maternal vagina. **breech**

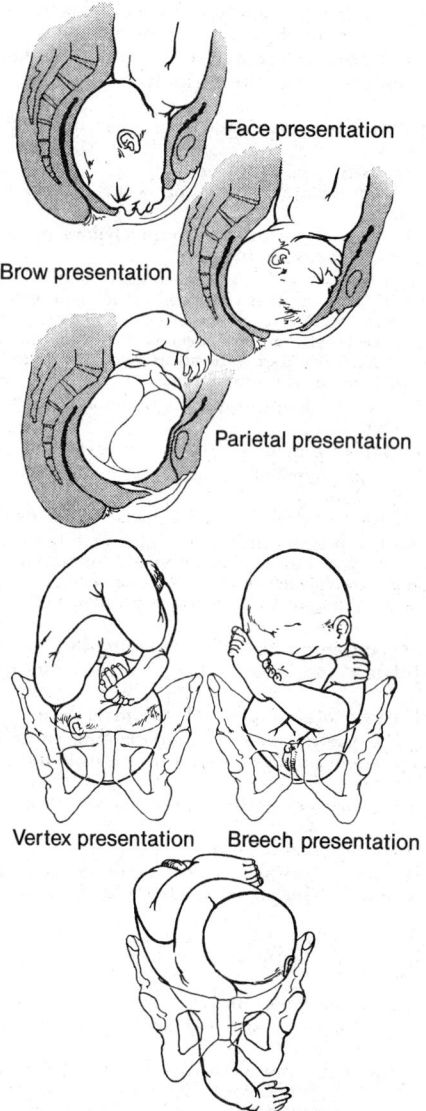

Face presentation

Brow presentation

Parietal presentation

Vertex presentation   Breech presentation

Shoulder presentation

p., single, frank breech p. **brow p.,** presentation of the fetal brow in labor. **cephalic p.,** presentation of any part of the fetal head in labor, including occiput, brow, or face; see also *longitudinal p.* **compound p.,** prolapse of an extremity of the fetus (an arm or leg, or both), alongside the head, or of one or both arms alongside a presenting breech, at the beginning of labor. **face p.,** the presentation of the face of the fetus in labor. **footling p.,** presentation of the fetus in labor with one (single footling) or both feet (double footling) prolapsed into the maternal vagina. **funis p.,** presentation of the umbilical cord in labor. **longitudinal p.,** the situation of the fetus in labor in which the long axis of the fetal body lies parallel to that of the mother. Normally, the head presents first, but sometimes the breech is the first to appear. **oblique p.,** the situation of the fetus in labor in which the long axis of the fetal body lies obliquely to that of the mother; the shoulder presents first.

parietal p., presentation of the parietal portion of the fetal head in labor. **pelvic p.,** breech p. **placental p.,** placenta previa. **polar p.,** longitudinal p. **shoulder p.,** presentation of the fetal shoulder in labor; see also *oblique p.* and *transverse lie*, under *lie*. **torso p.,** transverse lie. **transverse p.,** see under *lie*. **trunk p.,** transverse lie. **vertex p.,** the presentation of the vertex of the fetal head in labor.

preservative (pre-zer′vah-tiv) a substance or preparation added to a product for the purpose of destroying or inhibiting the multiplication of microorganisms.

presomite (pre-so′mīt) [*pre-* + *somite*] referring to embryos before the appearance of somites; in the human, before Horizon IX or 19 days postfertilization.

prespermatid (pre-sper′mah-tid) a secondary spermatocyte.

presphenoid (pre-sfe′noid) the anterior portion of the body of the sphenoid bone.

presphygmic (pre-sfig′mik) occurring before the pulse wave; see under *period*.

prespondylolisthesis (pre-spon″dĭ-lo-lis-the′sis) a congenital defect in the last lumbar vertebra consisting of a bilateral defect in the neural arches at the pedicles.

pressometer (pres-som′ĕ-ter) manometer. **Jarcho p.,** an instrument especially designed for measuring pressure during injection of radiopaque material into the uterus in hysterosalpingography.

pressor (pres′or) tending to increase blood pressure, as a pressor substance.

pressoreceptive (pres″o-re-sep′tiv) sensitive to stimuli due to vasomotor activity, such as blood pressure.

pressoreceptor (pres″o-re-sep′tor) a receptor or nerve ending sensitive to stimuli of vasomotor activity.

pressosensitive (pres″o-sen′sĭ-tiv) pressoreceptive.

pressure (presh′ur) [L. *pressura*] stress or strain, whether by compression, pull, thrust, or shear. **after p.,** a sense of pressure which lasts for a short period after removal of the actual pressure. **arterial p.,** the pressure of the blood within the arteries. **atmospheric p.,** the pressure exerted by the atmosphere; it is about 15 pounds to the square inch at the level of the sea. **back p.,** the pressure caused by the damming back of the blood in a heart chamber and its tributaries, due to an obstructive heart valve or failing myocardium. **biting p.,** occlusal p. **blood p.,** the pressure of the blood on the walls of the arteries, dependent on the energy of the heart action, the elasticity of the walls of the arteries, and the volume and viscosity of the blood. The maximum pressure occurs near the end of the stroke output of the left ventricle of the heart and is termed *maximum* or *systolic* pressure. The minimum pressure occurs late in ventricular diastole and is termed *minimum* or *diastolic* pressure. *Mean blood pressure* is the average of the blood pressure levels. *Basic blood pressure* is the pressure during quiet rest or basal conditions. See also *hypertension* and *hypotension*. **brain p.,** the capillary venous pressure in the brain. **capillary p.,** the blood pressure in the capillaries. **central venous p. (CVP),** the venous pressure as measured at the right atrium, done by means of a catheter introduced through the median cubital vein to the superior vena cava, the distal end of the catheter being attached to a manometer. **cerebrospinal p.,** the pressure or tension of the cerebrospinal fluid, normally 100–150 mm. as measured by the manometer. **diastolic p.,** see *blood p.* **Donders′ p.,** increase of manometric pressure with the instrument placed on the trachea on opening the chest of a dead body; due to collapse of the lung. **endocardial p.,** pressure of blood within the heart. **hydrostatic p.,** the pressure at any level on water at rest due to the weight of the water above it. **intra-abdominal p.,** the pressure between the viscera within the abdominal cavity. **intracranial p.,** the pressure in the space between the skull and the brain, i.e., the pressure of the subarachnoidal fluid. **intraocular p.,** the pressure of the fluids of the eye against the tunics. It is produced by continual renewal of the fluids within the interior of the eye, and is altered in certain pathological conditions (e.g., glaucoma). It may be roughly estimated by palpation of the eye or measured, directly or indirectly, with specially devised instruments, the tonometers. **intrathecal p.,** pressure within a sheath, particularly the pressure of the cerebrospinal fluid within the

subarachnoid membrane. **intraventricular p.,** the pressure within one ventricle of the heart. **mean circulatory filling p.,** a measure of the average (arterial and venous) pressure necessary to cause filling of the circulation with blood; it varies with blood volume and is directly proportional to the rate of venous return and thus to cardiac output. **negative p.,** a pressure less than that of the atmosphere. **occlusal p.,** pressure exerted on the occlusal surfaces of the teeth when the jaws are brought into apposition. Called also *biting p.* **oncotic p.,** the osmotic pressure due to the presence of colloids in a solution; in the case of plasma–interstitial fluid interaction, it is the force that tends to counterbalance the capillary blood pressure. **osmotic p.,** the pressure required to stop osmosis through a semipermeable membrane between a solution and pure solvent; it is proportional to the osmolality of the solution. **osmotic p., effective,** that part of the total osmotic pressure of a solution which governs the tendency of its solvent to pass through a semipermeable bounding membrane or across another boundary. **partial p.,** the pressure exerted by each of the components of a gas mixture. **perfusion p.,** the difference between the arterial and venous pressures at the brain level. **positive p.,** pressure greater than that of the atmosphere. **positive end-expiratory p. (PEEP),** a method of mechanical ventilation in which pressure is maintained to increase the volume of gas remaining in the lungs at the end of expiration, thus reducing the shunting of blood through the lungs and improving gas exchange; done in acute respiratory failure to allow reduction of inspired O_2 concentrations. **pulmonary capillary wedge p.,** intravascular pressure as measured by a catheter introduced into the pulmonary artery; it permits indirect measurement of the mean left atrial pressure. **pulse p.,** the difference between the systolic and diastolic pressures. **selection p.,** an effect produced by a given gene that determines the frequency of a given allele; it may be advantageous for survival (*positive selection pressure*) or disadvantageous (*negative selection pressure*). **solution p.,** the force which tends to bring into solution the molecules of a solid contained in the solvent. **systolic p.,** see *blood p.* **venous p.,** the blood pressure in a vein, usually utilized to reflect filling pressure to the ventricle.

presternum (pre-ster′num) manubrium sterni.

presubiculum (pre″su-bik′u-lum) a modified six-layered cortex situated between the subiculum and the main part of the parahippocampal gyrus.

presumptive (pre-zump′tiv) referring to the expected fate of an embryonic part on the basis of established fate mapping.

presylvian (pre-sil′ve-an) pertaining to the anterior or ascending branch of the sylvian fissure (sulcus lateralis).

presymptom (pre-simp′tom) an indication which is a forerunner of the actual symptoms of a condition.

presymptomatic (pre″simp-to-mat′ik) existing before the appearance of symptoms.

presynaptic (pre″sĭ-nap′tik) situated proximal to a synapse, or occurring before the synapse is crossed.

presystole (pre-sis′to-le) an interval of time just preceding the systole.

presystolic (pre″sis-tol′ik) [*pre-* + *systole*] 1. pertaining to the beginning of the systole. 2. occurring just before the systole.

pretectal (pre-tek′tal) located anterior to the tectum mesencephali.

prethcamide (preth′kah-mīd) a respiratory stimulant composed of equal parts by weight of cropropamide and crotethamide.

prethyroideal, prethyroidean (pre″thi-roi′de-al; pre″-thi-roi-de′an) situated in front of the thyroid gland or thyroid cartilage.

pretuberculosis (pre″tu-ber″ku-lo′sis) tuberculosis in an incipient and occult stage before any symptoms of the disease have appeared.

preurethritis (pre″u-re-thri′tis) inflammation of the vestibule of the vagina around the urethral orifice.

prev AGT previous abnormality of glucose tolerance.

prevalence (prev′ah-lens) [L. *praevalēre* to prevail] the number of cases of a disease that are present in a population at one point in time (see *prevalence rate*, under *rate*). Cf. *incidence*.

preventive (pre-ven′tiv) serving to avert the occurrence of.

preventorium (pre″ven-to′re-um) an institution where persons are confined for the purpose of checking the systemic spread of disease, usually for prophylaxis of children who have been exposed to tuberculosis.

preventriculus (pre″ven-trik′u-lus) the cardiac opening of the stomach (ostium cardiacum [NA]).

prevesical (pre-ves′ĭ-kal) [pre- + L. vesica bladder] situated in front of the bladder.

previable (pre-vi′ah-b′l) not yet viable; said of a fetus incapable of extrauterine existence.

previtamin (pre-vi′tah-min) a precursor of a vitamin. **p. H,** carotene.

Prévost's law, sign (pra-vōz′) [Jean Louis Prévost, Swiss physician, 1838–1927] see under law and sign.

Preyer's reflex, test (pri-erz) [Thierry Wilhelm Preyer, German physiologic chemist and physiologist, 1841–1897] see under reflex and tests.

prezone (pre′zōn) prozone.

prezygapophysis (pre″zi-gah-pof′ĭ-sis) processus articularis superior vertebrarum.

prezygotic (pre-zi-got′ik) occurring before the completion of fertilization.

PRF prolactin releasing factor.

priapism (pri′ah-pizm) [L. priapismus; Gr. priapismos] persistent abnormal erection of the penis, usually without sexual desire, and accompanied by pain and tenderness. It is seen in diseases and injuries of the spinal cord, and may be caused by vesical calculus and certain injuries to the penis. **secondary p.,** priapism caused by obstruction to the outflow of blood through the dorsal vein at the root of the penis.

priapitis (pri″ah-pi′tis) inflammation of the penis.

priapus (pri-ā′-pus) the penis.

Price-Jones curve (method) [Cecil Price-Jones, English physician, 1863–1943] see under curve.

Priessnitz compress (bandage) (prēs′nitz) [Vincenz Priessnitz, a Silesian farmer, 1799–1852] see under compress.

prilocaine hydrochloride (pril′o-kān) [USP] chemical name: N-(2-methyphenyl)-2-(propylamino)propanamide monohydrochloride. A local anesthetic, $C_{13}H_{20}N_2O \cdot HCl$, occurring as a white, crystalline powder; used to produce peripheral nerve block, epidural or caudal block, and infiltration and regional anesthesia.

primaquine phosphate (prim′ah-kwin) [USP] chemical name: N^4-(6-methoxy-8-quinolinyl)-1,4-pentanediamine phosphate (1:2). An antimalarial, $C_{15}H_{21}N_3O \cdot 2H_3PO_4$, occurring as an orange-red crystalline powder, especially effective against exoerythrocytic forms of Plasmodium vivax and P. falciparum; used especially in the treatment of relapsing vivax malaria, administered orally, sometimes in conjunction with other antimalarials.

primary (pri′mer-e; pri′mah-re) [L. primarius principal; primus first] first in order or in time of development; principal.

primate (pri′māt) an individual belonging to the order Primates.

Primates (pri-ma′tēz) [L. primus first] the highest order of mammals, including man, apes, monkeys, and lemurs.

primed (prīmd) immunologically activated by initial exposure to antigen; said of cells of the immune system.

prime mover (prīm′ mov′er) a muscle that acts directly to bring about a desired movement.

primer (prīm′er) a substance which prepares for or facilitates the action of another. **cavity p.,** a substance that enhances adaptation of resin filling materials to cavity walls by inducing wetting between the resinous material and the treated dentin and enamel surfaces.

primeverose (pri-mev′er-ōs) a disaccharide, 6-(β-D-xylosido)-D-glucose, $C_{11}H_{20}O_{10}$, from the cowslip, Primula veris L.

primidone (prim′ĭ-dōn) [USP] chemical name: 5-ethyl-dihydro-5-phenyl-4,6(1H,5H)-pyrimidinedione. An anticonvulsant, $C_{12}H_{14}N_2O_2$, occurring as a white, crystalline powder; used in the treatment of grand mal, focal, and psychomotor epileptic seizures, administered orally. Called also desoxyphenobarbital.

primigravid (pri″mĭ-grav′id) pregnant for the first time.

primigravida (pri″mĭ-grav′ĭ-dah) [L. prima first + gravida pregnant] a woman pregnant for the first time; also written gravida I.

primipara (pri-mip′ah-rah), pl. primip′arae [L. prima first + parere to bring forth, produce] a woman who has had one pregnancy that resulted in a fetus that attained a weight of 500 gm. or a gestational age of 20 weeks, regardless of whether the infant was living at birth, and regardless of whether it was a single or multiple birth. Also written para I or I-para.

primiparity (pri″mĭ-par′ĭ-te) the condition or fact of being a primipara.

primiparous (pri-mip′ah-rus) bearing or having borne but one child.

primite (pri′mīt) [L. primus first] the anterior of a pair of gregarines undergoing syzygy. Cf. satellite, def. 5.

primitiae (pri-mish′e-e) [L. pl., "first things"] that part of the amniotic fluid discharged before the fetus is extruded.

primitive (prim′ĭ-tiv) [L. primitivus] first in point of time; existing in a simple or early form; showing little evolution.

primordial (pri-mor′de-al) [L. primordialis] original or primitive; of the simplest and most undeveloped character.

primordium (pri-mor′de-um), pl. primor′dia [L. "the beginning"] the earliest discernible indication during embryonic development of an organ or part; called also anlage or rudiment.

primverose (prim′ver-ōs) a disaccharide occurring in zein.

Prinadol (prin′ah-dol) trademark for a preparation of phenazocine.

princeps (prin′seps) [L.] principal; chief.

Principen (prin′sĭ-pen) trademark for preparations of ampicillin.

principle (prin′sĭ-p′l) [L. principium] 1. a chemical component. 2. a substance on which certain of the properties of a drug depend. 3. a law of conduct. **active p.,** any constituent of a drug which helps to confer upon it a medicinal property. **antianemia p.,** the constituent in liver (vitamin B_{12}) and certain other tissues that produces the hematopoietic effect in pernicious anemia. **Doppler p.,** see under effect. **Fick p.,** a restatement of the law of conservation of mass used in making indirect measurements, e.g., of cardiac output: the amount of blood traversing the pulmonary capillaries per unit of time is a measure of cardiac output and, because gas diffusion across the pulmonary alveolar walls depends on pulmonary blood flow, the cardiac output (liters per min.) equals O_2 absorption (cc. per minute) divided by the arterial O_2 minus the mixed venous O_2 (cc. per liter). **hematinic p.,** antianemia p. **immediate p.,** any one of the more or less complex substances of definite chemical constitution into which a heterogeneous substance can be readily resolved. **Le Chatelier p.,** if a biological system is subjected to stress, it will act in such a way as to reduce the stress. **organic p.,** immediate p. **pleasure p., pleasure-pain p.,** in psychoanalytic theory, an inborn tendency to avoid pain and seek pleasure through the immediate reduction of tension by either direct or fantasied gratification; cf. reality p. **prothrombin converting p.,** in theoretical hematology, a principle in the plasma that converts prothrombin to thrombin. **proximate p.,** immediate p. **reality p.,** in psychoanalytic theory, the ego functions that modify the demands of the pleasure principle to meet the demands and requirements of the external world. **ultimate p.,** a chemical element.

Pringle's disease (pring′g′lz) [John James Pringle, British dermatologist, 1855–1922] adenoma sebaceum.

Prinos verticellatus (pri′nos ver″tĭ-sil-la′tus) [Gr. prinos oak] Ilex verticellata.

prion (pri′on) a slow infectious particle that lacks nucleic acids; prions are the cause of Creutzfeldt-Jakob disease and scrapie.

Priscoline (pris′ko-lēn) trademark for preparations of tolazoline.

prism (prizm) [Gr. prisma] a solid with a triangular or polygonal cross section. A triangular prism splits up a ray of light into its constituent colors, and turns or deflects light rays toward its base. Prisms are used to correct deviations of the eyes, since they alter the apparent situation of objects. **adamantine p's, enamel p's,** prismata adamantina; see under *prisma*. **Maddox p.,** two prisms with their bases together; used in testing for torsion of the eyeball. **Nicol p.,** two slabs of Iceland spar cemented together and deflecting a ray of light in such a way that it is split in two, one part (the ordinary ray) being totally reflected and the other (polarized ray) passing through. **Risley's p.,** a prism which rotates in a metal frame marked with a scale; used in testing ocular muscles for imbalance.

prisma (priz′mah), pl. *pris′mata* [Gr.] prism. **pris′mata adaman′tina** [NA], adamantine or enamel prisms: the structural units of the tooth enamel, consisting of parallel rods or prisms composed mainly of hydroxyapatite crystals and organic substance and held together with a cement substance, each prism being enveloped in a sheath. Called also *enamel rods.*

prismata (priz′mah-tah) [Gr.] plural of *prisma.*

prismatic (priz-mat′ik) shaped like a prism; produced by a prism.

prismoid (priz′moid) resembling a prism.

prismoptometer (priz″mop-tom′ĕ-ter) [*prism* + *optometer*] an instrument for testing the eye by means of a revolving prism.

prismosphere (priz′mo-sfēr) [*prism* + *sphere*] a prism combined with a globular lens.

prisoptometer (priz″op-tom′ĕ-ter) prismoptometer.

Privine (pri′vēn) trademark for preparations of naphazoline.

PRL, Prl prolactin.

p.r.n. abbreviation for L. *pro re na′ta*, according as circumstances may require.

Pro proline.

pro- [L. and Gr. "before"] 1. a prefix signifying before or in front of. 2. a prefix denoting a precursor, as of an enzyme or hormone.

proaccelerin (pro″ak-sel′er-in) Factor V; see *coagulation factors*, under *factor.*

pro-actinium (pro″ak-tin′e-um) protactinium.

Proactinomyces (pro″ak-tĭ-no-mi′sēz) *Nocardia.*

proactinomycin (pro-ak″tĭ-no-mi′sin) a group of antibiotic substances, designated A, B, and C, from cultures of *Nocardia gardneri*, which acts against gram-positive bacteria.

proactivator (pro-ak′tĭ-va″tor) the inactive precursor form of an activator, or a factor that requires a chemical change, usually by an enzyme, to become an activator, e.g., a substance present in plasma (*plasminogen proactivator*), which is absorbed onto fibrin during clotting and which, when activated, will convert plasminogen to plasmin. **C3 p. (C3PA),** factor B.

proadifen hydrochloride (pro-ad′ĭ-fen) chemical name: α-phenyl-α-propyl-2-(diethylamino)ethyl ester hydrochloride; a nonspecific synergist, $C_{23}H_{31}NO_2 \cdot HCl$.

proagglutinoid (pro″ah-gloo′tĭ-noid) (*obs.*) an agglutinoid that has a stronger affinity for the agglutinogen than has the agglutinin.

proal (pro′al) characterized by forward movement.

proamnion (pro-am′ne-on) that part of the embryonal area at the front and side of the head which remains without mesoderm for some time.

proatlas (pro-at′las) a rudimentary vertebra which in some animals lies in front of the atlas; sometimes seen as an anomaly in man.

proazamine (pro-az′ah-mēn) promethazine.

probability (prob″ah-bil′ĭ-te) [*probabilis* probable, from *pro-bare* to test or examine] the likelihood of occurrence of a specified event; it may be thought of as a number between 0 and 1 that corresponds to the long-run frequency at which an event occurs in a sequence of independent trials under identical conditions. **significance p.,** *P* value.

probacteriophage (pro″bak-te′re-o-fāj″) prophage.

proband (pro′band) [Ger.; from L. *probandus* "the one to be tested"] an affected person ascertained independently of his relatives in a genetic study. Called also *propositus.*

probang (pro′bang) a flexible rod with a ball, tuft, or sponge at one end; used in applying medications to or removing matter from the esophagus or larynx.

Pro-Banthine (pro-ban-thīn′) trademark for preparations of propantheline bromide.

probarbital (pro-bar′bĭ-tal) chemical name 5-ethyl-5-(1-methylethyl)-2,4,6(1*H*,3*H*,5*H*)-pyrimidinetrione. A barbiturate of intermediate duration, $C_9H_{14}N_2O_3$, used as a sedative in the form of its calcium and sodium salts.

probe (prōb) [L. *proba; probare* to test] 1. a slender, flexible instrument designed for introduction into a wound, cavity, or sinus tract for purposes of exploration. 2. in molecular genetics, a radioactive DNA or RNA sequence used to detect the presence of a complementary sequence by molecular hybridization. **Anel's p.,** a delicate probe for the lacrimal puncta and canals. **blood flow p.,** an implanted cuff that fits around a surgically exposed artery or vein to detect blood flow. **blunt p.,** a probe with a blunt end. **Bowman's p.,** one of a set of probes for use on the nasal ducts. **Brackett's p's,** delicate and flexible probes of silver wire for exploring dental fistulas. **bullet p.,** one used for detecting the presence or determining the location of a bullet. **drum p.,** a probe with an attachment which emits a sound when it comes in contact with a foreign body. **electric p.,** one which on contact with a foreign body completes an electric circuit, thereby producing a sound. **eyed p.,** one with a slit near one end through which a ligature or tape may be drawn. **fiberoptic p.,** a flexible probe made up of a bundle of fine glass fibers optically aligned to transmit an image. **lacrimal p.,** one designed for use on the lacrimal passages. **oligonucleotide p.,** see *oligonucleotide.* **periodontal p., pocket p.,** one graduated in millimeters, used to measure the depth and determine the outline of a periodontal pocket and the condition of the crevicular epithelium. **root canal p.,** a slender, flexible, and smooth or edged metal, hand-operated endodontic instrument, usually made of soft iron wire; used for tracing the course of and exploring root canals. Called also *pathfinder, pathfinder broach*, and *smooth broach.* **scissors p.,** a long, delicate pair of scissors that can be used as a probe. **uterine p.,** a probe for uterine exploration. **vertebrated p.,** a flexible probe made up of joined links.

probenecid (pro-ben′ĕ-sid) [USP] a uricosuric agent that acts by inhibiting the carrier-mediated transport of organic acids in the renal tubule, which increases the excretion of uric acid by blocking its tubular reabsorption and decreases the excretion of penicillins and certain other acidic drugs by blocking their tubular secretion; used in the treatment of hyperuricemia of gout and as an adjunct in penicillin therapy.

probit (pro′bit) [contraction of "probability unit"] a normal variate having mean 5 and standard deviation 1. In quantal biological assays, the observed responses are often converted to probits (the fraction responding is converted to the probit that cuts off the same fraction of the area under the normal frequency curve) in order to fit a linear log dose–response curve, a procedure based on the assumption that the response thresholds are normally distributed.

proboscis (pro-bos′is) [*pro-* + Gr. *boskein* to feed, graze] any tubular process or structure of the head or snout of an animal, usually used in feeding.

probucol (pro′bu-kōl) chemical name: 4,4′-[(1-methylethylidene)bis(thio)]bis[2,6-bis(1,1-dimethylethyl)phenol]. An anticholesteremic, $C_{31}H_{48}O_2S_2$, used especially as an adjunct to diet for the reduction of elevated serum cholesterol in primary cholesterolemia, administered orally.

procainamide hydrochloride (pro-kān′ah-mīd) [USP] chemical name: 4-amino-*N*-(2-diethylaminoethyl)benzamide. A cardiac depressant, $C_{13}H_{21}N_3O \cdot HCl$, occurring as a white to tan, crystalline powder; used in the treatment of cardiac arrhythmias, administered orally and intramuscularly, and by intravenous infusion. Called also *procaine amide hydrochloride.*

procaine (pro′kān) chemical name: 4-aminobenzoic acid 2-(diethylamino)ethyl ester; a local anesthetic, $C_{13}H_{20}N_2O_2$. **p. amide hydrochloride,** procainamide hydrochloride. **p. hydrochloride** [USP], the monohydrochloride salt of procaine, $C_{13}H_{20}N_2O_2 \cdot HCl$, occurring as small white crystals or white crystalline powder; used to produce infiltration, epidural, and peripheral nerve block, and spinal anesthesia. **p. penicillin G,** see under *penicillin.*

procallus (pro-kal′us) the granulation tissue formed about the site of fracture of a bone, which develops into callus.

procarbazine hydrochloride (pro-kar′bah-zēn) [USP]

chemical name: *N*-(1-methylethyl-4-[(2-methylhydrazino)-methyl]benzamide monohydrochloride. An antineoplastic, $C_{12}H_{19}N_3O \cdot HCl$, used primarily in combination with mechlorethamine, vincristine, and prednisone (MOPP) in the treatment of advanced Hodgkin's disease; it also has activity against bronchogenic carcinoma, brain tumors, and non-Hodgkin's lymphomas. Major side effects include nausea and vomiting and bone marrow depression.

procarboxypeptidase (pro″kar-bok′se-pep′tĭ-dās) a proenzyme of a carboxypeptidase.

procarcinogen (pro″kar-sin′o-jen) a chemical substance that becomes carcinogenic only after it is altered by metabolic processes.

procaryosis (pro″kar-e-o′sis) prokaryosis.

Procaryotae (pro-kar″e-o′te) [*pro-* + Gr. *karyon* nut, kernel] a kingdom comprising all prokaryotic organisms and consisting of cellular organisms that lack a true nucleus (the bacteria). In one system of classification, the two subdivisions are: Cyanobacteria (blue-green bacteria or Cyanophyceae, [formerly blue-green algae] and the Bacteria (all other bacterin). In another system, the two subdivisions are: the Photobacteria (blue-green bacteria [Cyanobacteria], red or purple bacteria [Rhodospirillaceae and Chromatiaceae], and green bacteria [Chlorobiaceae]) and the Scotobacteria (all other bacteria, rickettsiae, and Mollicutes). More recently the prokaryotes have been arranged in four divisions based on biochemical and phylogenetic analysis and the presence or absence and type of their cell walls: I. Gracilicutes—with thick, gram-negative–type cell walls; II. Fermicutes—with thick, strong, gram-positive–type cell walls; III. Tenericutes—without a cell wall; and IV. Mendosicutes—with faulty cell walls.

procaryote (pro-kar′e-ōt) prokaryote.

procaryotic (pro″kar-e-ot′ik) prokaryotic.

procatarctic (pro″kah-tark′tik) predisposing: said of a cause of disease.

procatarxis (pro″kah-tark′sis) [Gr. *prokatarxis* a first beginning] 1. a predisposing cause. 2. predisposition. 3. the production of a disease partially as a result of predisposition.

procedure (pro-se′jur) [L. *procedere*, from *pro* forward + *cedere* move] a series of steps by which a desired result is accomplished. **Anderson p.,** reconstruction of the hypopharynx and cervical esophagus by the use of bilateral rectangular flaps. **Glenn p.,** see under *operation.* **Gomori-Takamatsu p.,** a method for localizing the alkaline phosphatase enzyme: a tissue secretion is incubated in a buffered solution containing the substrate, glycerophosphate, and calcium ions; hydrolysis of the substrate releases phosphoric acid, and it combines with calcium and precipitates as calcium phosphate. This colorless precipitate is converted to brown cobalt sulfide, which is readily visualized with the microscope. **Hartmann's p.,** resection of a diseased portion of the colon, with the proximal end of the colon brought out as a colostomy and the distal stump or rectum being closed by suture. Bowel continuity can later be restored. Called also *Hartmann's colostomy* or *operation.* **Jannetta p.,** a microsurgical procedure for relief of trigeminal neuralgia: through a small craniotomy, a small nonabsorbable sponge is placed between the root of the trigeminal nerve and blood vessels compressing the nerve. **push-back p.,** see under *technique.* **V-Y p.,** a method of repairing a skin defect in which a V-shaped flap is made proximal to the defect; the flap is transferred to the defect, and the secondary defect thus created is closed to produce a Y-shaped scar.

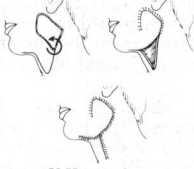

V-Y procedure.

procelous (pro-se′lus) [*pro-* + Gr. *koilos* hollow] concave on the anterior surface; applied to the vertebral centra of certain animals.

procentriole (pro-sen′tre-ol) the immediate precursor of centrioles and ciliary basal bodies; it is developed in proximity to either a preexisting centriole or a deuterosome.

procephalic (pro″sĕ-fal′ik) [*pro-* + Gr. *kephalē* head] pertaining to the anterior part of the head.

procercoid (pro-ser′koid) one of the larval stages of fish tapeworms.

procerus (pro-se′rus) [L.] long; slender.

process (pros′es; pro′ses) [L. *processus*] 1. a prominence or projection, as of bone; for names of specific anatomical structures, see official Latinized terms under *processus.* 2. a series of operations, events, or steps leading to the achievement of a specific result; used also as a verb to designate subjection to such a series designed to produce desired changes in the original material, or achieve other result. **A.B.C. p.,** see under *method.* **accessory p. of sacrum, spurious,** crista sacralis lateralis. **acromial p., acromion p.,** acromion. **acute p. of helix,** spina helicis. **alar p. of sacrum,** crista sacralis lateralis. **aliform p. of sphenoid bone,** ala minor ossis sphenoidalis. **alveolar p.,** that portion of bone in either the maxilla or the mandible which surrounds and supports the teeth. In the maxilla, it is called *processus alveolaris maxillae* (q.v.); in the mandible, *pars alveolaris mandibulae.* **anconeal p. of ulna,** olecranon. **angular p. of frontal bone, external,** processus zygomaticus ossis frontalis. **articular p. of axis, anterior,** facies articularis anterior axis. **articular p. of coccyx, false,** cornu coccygeum. **articular p. of sacrum, spurious,** crista sacralis intermedia. **ascending p's of vertebrae,** see *processus articularis superior vertebrarum.* **axillary p. of mammary gland,** processus lateralis glandulae mammariae. **axiscylinder p.,** axon, def. 2. **basilar p.,** pars basilaris ossis occipitalis. **Beccari p.,** a method of garbage disposal involving bacterial fermentation in closed cells. **p. of Blumenbach,** processus uncinatus ossis ethmoidalis. **calcaneal p. of cuboid bone, calcanean p. of cuboid bone,** processus calcaneus ossis cuboidei. **capitular p.,** the articular process on a vertebra for the head of a rib. **p. of cartilage of nasal septum, posterior,** processus posterior sphenoidalis. **caudate p.,** processus caudatus hepatis. **ciliary p's,** processus ciliares. **Civinini's p. of external pterygoid plate,** processus pterygospinosus. **clinoid p.,** any of three processes of the sphenoid bone; see *processus clinoideus anterior, medius,* and *posterior.* **condyloid p. of vertebrae, inferior,** processus articularis inferior vertebrarum. **condyloid p. of vertebrae, superior,** processus articularis superior vertebrarum. **conoid p.,** tuberculum conoideum. **coracoid p.,** processus coracoideus scapulae. **coronoid p.,** see entries beginning *processus coronoideus.* **cubital p. of humerus,** see *trochlea humeri* and *capitulum humeri.* **Deiters' p.,** axon, def. 2. **dendritic p.,** the branched process of a nerve cell; a dendrite. **dental p.,** processus alveolaris maxillae. **dentoid p. of axis,** dens axis. **descending p's of vertebrae,** see *processus articularis inferior vertebrarum.* **ensiform p. of sphenoid bone,** ala minor ossis sphenoidalis. **ensiform p. of sternum,** processus xiphoideus. **epiphyseal p.,** epiphysis. **ethmoidal p. of Macalister,** crista sphenoidalis. **falciform p. of cerebellum,** falx cerebelli. **falciform p. of cerebrum,** falx cerebri. **falciform p. of fascia lata,** margo falciformis hiatus saphenus. **falciform p. of fascia pelvis,** arcus tendineus fasciae pelvis. **falciform p. of rectus abdominis muscle,** falx inguinalis. **floccular p.,** flocculus, def. 2. **folian p., p. of Folius,** processus anterior mallei. **foot p.,** pedicel. **frontal p., external,** spina nasalis ossis frontalis. **frontonasal p.,** an expansive facial process in the embryo, which develops into the forehead and bridge of the nose. **funicular p.,** the portion of the tunica vaginalis surrounding the spermatic cord. **Gottstein's basal p.,** any attenuated basal process connecting the basilar membrane with an outer hair cell of the organ of Corti. **greater p. of ethmoid bone, hamate p. of ethmoid bone,** processus uncinatus ossis ethmoidalis. **hamular p. of lacrimal bone,** hamulus lacrimalis. **hamular p. of sphenoid bone,** hamulus pterygoideus. **hamular p. of unciform bone,** hamulus ossis hamati. **head p.,** an axial strand of cells in the embryo extending forward from the primitive knot; called also *notochordal plate.* **inframalleolar p. of calcaneus,** trochlea peronealis calcanei. **infundibular p.,** lobus nervosus neurohypophysis. **Ingrassia's p.,** ala minor ossis sphenoidalis. **intercondylar p. of tibia,** eminentia intercondylaris. **internal p. of humerus,** processus supracondylaris humeri. **jugular p. of occipital bone, lateral,** processus paramastoideus ossis occipitalis. **jugular p. of occipital bone, middle,** processus intrajugularis ossis occipitalis. **jugular p. of occipital bone, posterior, of Krause,** processus paramastoideus ossis occipitalis. **lacrimal p.,** a process of the inferior nasal concha that articulates with the lacrimal bone. **lateral p. of calcaneus,** sustentaculum tali. **lateral p. of mammary gland,** processus lateralis glandulae mammariae. **malar p.,** processus zygomaticus maxillae. **mamillary p's of sacrum, oblique,** see crista sacralis intermedia. **mamillary p. of temporal bone,** processus mastoideus ossis temporalis. **mandibular p.,** the ventral process formed by bifurcation of the first branchial arch (mandibular arch) in the embryo, which unites ventrally with its fellow to form the lower jaw. **marginal p. of malar bone,** tuberculum marginale ossis zygomatici. **mastoid p.,** processus mastoideus ossis temporalis. **maxillary p.,** the dorsal process formed by bifurcation of the first branchial arch in the embryo, which joins with the ipsilateral median nasal process in the formation of the upper jaw. **mental p.,** protuberantia mentalis. **nasal p., lateral,** the lateral one of the two limbs of the horseshoe-shaped elevation bounding a nasal pit in the embryo, which participates in formation of the side and wing of the nose. **nasal p., median,** the central one of the two limbs of the horseshoe-shaped elevation bounding a nasal pit in the embryo, which participates with the ipsilateral maxillary process in forming half of the upper jaw. **nasal p. of frontal bone,** pars nasalis ossis frontalis. **nasal p. of inferior turbinate bone,** processus lacrimalis conchae nasalis inferioris. **oblique p. of vertebrae, inferior,** processus articularis inferior vertebrarum. **oblique p. of vertebrae, superior,** processus articularis superior vertebrarum. **occipital p. of occipital bone,** pars basilaris ossis occipitalis. **p. of odontoblast, odontoblastic p.,** one of the slender protoplasmic processes in a dentinal tubule, which is a cytoplasmic extension of the cell body; odontoblastic processes extend from the dentinoenamel junction and cementodentinal junction to the cell bodies of odontoblasts in the dental pulp. Called also dentinal fiber and Tomes' fiber or fibril. **odontoid p. of axis,** dens axis. **olecranon p. of ulna,** olecranon. **olivary p.** (obs.), tuberculum sellae turcicae. **palatine p., lateral,** a shelflike projection developing from each maxillary process region of the upper jaw in the embryo, later fusing with each other and with the nasal septum to form the palate. **palatine p., median,** a shelflike projection developing from each median nasal process in the embryo, which participates with its fellow in forming the premaxillary portion of the upper jaw. **paracondyloid p. of occipital bone, paroccipital p. of occipital bone,** processus paramastoideus ossis occipitalis. **petrosal p., anterior,** lingula sphenoidalis. **petrosal p., middle,** processus clinoideus medius. **petrosal p., posterior superior,** processus clinoideus posterior. **pterygoid p.,** processus pterygoideus ossis sphenoidalis. **Rau's p., ravian p.,** processus anterior mallei. **restiform p. of Henle,** pedunculus cerebellaris inferior. **schizophrenic p.,** process schizophrenia. **small p. of Soemmering,** tuberculum marginale ossis zygomatici. **spinous p.,** a slender, more or less sharp-pointed projection; see spina. **spinous p. of sacrum, spurious,** crista sacralis mediana. **spinous p. of tibia,** 1. eminentia intercondylaris. 2. tuberculum intercondylare mediale. **spinous p. of vertebrae,** processus spinosus vertebrarum. **Stieda's p.,** processus posterior tali. **styloid p. of fibula,** apex capitis fibulae. **sucker p.,** see under foot. **synovial p.,** plica synovialis. **temporal p. of mandible,** processus coronoideus mandibulae. **Todd's p.,** see fibrae intercrurales. **Tomes p.,** 1. (Charles Sissmore Tomes) a finger-like projection of the ameloblast, occurring during the secretory phase of the cell during amelogenesis, which extends from the point of separation of the adjacent cell membrane to the distal free surface. 2. (Sir John Tomes) p. of odontoblast. **transverse p. of sacrum,** crista sacralis lateralis. **transverse p. of vertebrae, accessory,** processus accessorius vertebrarum lumbalium. **trochlear p. of calcaneus,** trochlea peronealis calcanei. **unciform p. of scapula,** processus coracoideus scapulae. **uncinate p. of ethmoid bone,** processus uncinatus ossis ethmoidalis. **uncinate p. of lacrimal bone,** hamulus lacrimalis. **uncinate

p. of pancreas, processus uncinatus pancreatis. **uncinate p. of unciform bone,** hamulus ossis hamati. **uncinate p's of vertebra,** hook-shaped processes on the lateral borders of the superior surface of the bodies of vertebrae C3 to T1; they are frequent sites of formation of spurs (osteophytes), leading to spondylosis uncovertebralis. **ungual p. of third phalanx of foot,** tuberositas phalangis distalis pedis. **vermiform p.,** appendix vermiformis. **xiphoid p.,** the pointed process of cartilage, supported by a core of bone, connected with the lower end of the body of the sternum; called also processus xiphoideus and xiphisternum. **xiphoid p. of sphenoid bone,** ala minor ossis sphenoidalis. **zygomatico-orbital p. of maxilla,** processus zygomaticus maxillae.

processus (pro-ses′us), pl. processus [L.] a process: a prominence or projection; [NA] a general term for such a mass projecting from a larger structure. **p. accesso′rii spu-r′ii,** crista sacralis lateralis. **p. accesso′rius** [NA], accessory process: a small nodule that projects backward from the posterior surface of the transverse process and lateral to and below the mamillary process of a lumbar vertebra. Such a process also occurs on the tenth, eleventh, and twelfth thoracic vertebrae. **p. ala′ris os′sis ethmoida′lis,** ala cristae galli. **p. alveola′ris maxil′lae** [NA], alveolar process of maxilla: the thick parabolically curved ridge that projects downward and forms the free lower border of the maxilla; it is in front of and lateral to the palatine process and it bears the teeth. Called also dental process. **p. ante′rior mal′lei** [NA], **p. ante′rior mal′lei** [Fo′lii], anterior process of malleus: a slender process that arises from the anterior aspect of the neck of the malleus, passes anteriorly and inferiorly to the petrotympanic fissure, and is attached to the petrous portion of the temporal bone by ligamentous fibers. **p. articula′ris infe′rior verte-bra′rum** [NA], inferior articular process of vertebrae: a process on either side of the vertebrae, springing from the inferior surface of the arch near the junction of the lamina and pedicle; it bears a surface that faces anteriorly and inferiorly, articulating with the superior articular process of the vertebra below. Called also zygapophysis inferior [NA alternative]. **p. articula′ris supe′rior os′sis sa′cri** [NA], superior articular process of sacrum: either of two processes projecting backward and medialward from the first sacral vertebra at the junctions between the body and the alae; they articulate with the inferior articular processes of the fifth lumbar vertebra. **p. articula′ris supe′rior vertebra′rum** [NA], superior articular process of vertebrae: a process on either side of the vertebrae, springing from the superior surface of the arch near the junction of the lamina and pedicle; it bears a surface that faces posteriorly and superiorly, articulating with the inferior articular process of the vertebra above. Called also zygapophysis superior [NA alternative]. **p. bre′vis incu′dis,** ligamentum incudis superius. **p. bre′vis mal′lei,** p. lateralis mallei. **p. calca′neus os′sis cuboi′dei** [NA], calcaneal process of cuboid bone: a process projecting posteriorly from the inferomedial angle of the cuboid bone that supports the anterior calcaneus; called also calcanean process of cuboid bone. **p. cauda′tus hep′atis** [NA], caudate process: the right of the two processes seen on the caudate lobe of the liver. **p. cilia′res** [NA], ciliary processes: about 70 meridionally arranged ridges or folds projecting from the crown of the ciliary body; they secrete the aqueous humor into the posterior chamber of the eye. **p. clinoi′deus ante′rior** [NA], anterior clinoid process: the bony process found on the medial extremity of the posterior border of the small wing of the sphenoid bone. **p. clinoi′deus me′dius** [NA], middle clinoid process: either of two small inconstant eminences on the internal surface of the sphenoid bone, one on either side of the anterior part of the hypophyseal fossa. **p. clinoi′deus poste′rior** [NA], posterior clinoid process: either of two tubercles found on the superior angle of either side of the dorsum sellae of the sphenoid bone, and giving attachment to the tentorium of the cerebellum. **p. coch-leariform′mis** [NA], cochleariform process: a small hollow cone of bone at the end of the semicanalis tubae auditivae, just anterior to the vestibular window, with an opening through which the tendon of the tensor tympani passes. **p. condyla′ris mandib′ulae** [NA], **p. condyloi′deus mandib′ulae,** condylar process of mandible: the posterior process on the ramus of the mandible that articulates with the mandibular fossa of the temporal bone. **p. coracoi′-deus scap′ulae** [NA], coracoid process of scapula: a strong curved process that arises from the upper part of the neck of the scapula and overhangs the shoulder joint. **p. coronoi′deus mandib′ulae** [NA], coronoid process of mandible: the anterior part of the upper end of the ramus of the mandible, to which the temporal muscle is attached. **p. coronoi′deus ul′nae** [NA], coronoid process of ulna: a wide eminence at the proximal end of the ulna, forming the anterior and inferior part of the trochlear incisure. **p. costa′lis ver′tebrae** [NA], **p. costa′rius ver′tebrae**, costal process of vertebra: in a cervical vertebra, the part of the transverse process anterior to the transverse foramen. **p. e cerebel′lo ad medul′lam**, pedunculus cerebellaris inferior. **p. e cerebel′lo ad pon′tem**, pedunculus cerebellaris medius. **p. e cerebel′lo ad tes′tes**, pedunculus cerebellaris superior. **p. ethmoida′lis con′chae nasa′lis inferio′ris** [NA], ethmoidal process of inferior nasal concha: a bony projection above and behind the maxillary process of the inferior nasal concha. **p. falcifor′mis ligamen′ti sacrotubero′si** [NA], falciform process of sacrotuberal ligament: a prolongation of the sacrotuberal ligament, continuing forward along the inner border of the ramus of the ischium from the point of attachment of the ligament on the tuber of the ischium. **p. Ferrei′ni lob′uli cortica′lis re′nis**, pars radiata lobuli corticalis renis. **p. fronta′lis maxil′lae** [NA], frontal process of maxilla: a large, strong, irregular process of bone that projects upward from the body of the maxilla, its medial surface forming part of the lateral wall of the nasal cavity. **p. fronta′lis os′sis zygomat′ici** [NA], **p. frontosphenoida′lis os′sis zygomat′ici**, frontal process of zygomatic bone: the strong, upward projecting triangular process of the zygomatic bone lying behind the malar surface and between the orbital and temporal surfaces; it unites above with the zygomatic process of the frontal bone and behind with the great wing of the sphenoid bone. **p. gra′cilis**, p. anterior mallei. **p. of Ingrassia**, ala minor ossis sphenoidalis. **p. intrajugula′ris os′sis occipita′lis** [NA], intrajugular process of occipital bone: a small process that subdivides the jugular notch of the occipital bone into a lateral and a medial part. **p. intrajugula′ris os′sis tempora′lis** [NA], intrajugular process of temporal bone: a small ridge on the petrous part of the temporal bone that separates the jugular notch into a medial and a lateral part, corresponding to similar parts of the jugular notch of the facing occipital bone. **p. jugula′ris os′sis occipita′lis** [NA], jugular process of occipital bone: either of two processes on the occipital bone that project laterally from the occipital condyles and form the posterior boundary of the jugular foramen. **p. lacrima′lis con′chae nasa′lis inferio′ris** [NA], lacrimal process of inferior nasal concha: a process of the inferior nasal concha that articulates with the lacrimal bone. **p. latera′lis glan′dulae mamma′riae** [NA], lateral process of mammary gland: the superolateral part of the mammary gland that extends toward the axilla; called also *axillary process of mammary gland, axillary tail*, and *p. axilla′ris glandulae mammariae* [NA alternative]. **p. latera′lis mal′lei** [NA], lateral process of malleus: a small tapered process that projects laterally from the base of the manubrium mallei and produces the mallear prominence. **p. latera′lis ta′li** [NA], lateral process of talus: a large low process on the lateral surface of the talus, articulating with the lateral malleolus. **p. latera′lis tu′beris calca′nei** [NA], lateral process of tuberosity of calcaneus: a rough process projecting downward from the lower lateral portion of the tuber calcanei. **p. lenticula′ris incu′dis** [NA], lenticular process of incus: a small process on the medial side of the tip of the long limb of the incus, which articulates with the head of the stapes. **p. mamilla′ris** [NA], mamillary process: of vertebrae: a tubercle on each superior articular process of the lumbar vertebrae and on the tenth, eleventh, and twelfth thoracic vertebrae. **p. margina′lis os′sis zygomat′ici**, tuberculum marginale ossis zygomatici. **p. mastoi′deus os′sis tempora′lis** [NA], mastoid process of temporal bone: a conical process projecting forward and downward from the external surface of the petrous part of the temporal bone just posterior to the external acoustic meatus. **p. maxilla′ris con′chae nasa′lis inferio′ris** [NA], maxillary process of inferior nasal concha: a bony process descending from the ethmoid process of the inferior nasal concha. **p. media′lis tu′beris calca′nei** [NA], medial process of tuberosity of calcaneus: a rough process projecting downward from the lower medial portion of the

tuber calcanei. **p. muscula′ris cartilag′inis arytenoi′deae** [NA], muscular process of arytenoid cartilage: the lateral and posterior lower angular projection of the arytenoid cartilage to which the cricoarytenoid muscles are attached. **p. orbita′lis os′sis palati′ni** [NA], orbital process of palatine bone: a pyramidal process on the uppermost part of the palatine bone, one surface of it forming the posterior angle of the floor of the orbit. **p. palati′nus maxil′lae** [NA], palatine process of maxilla: a horizontally arched plate of bone that helps to form the lower part of the maxilla and with its fellow of the opposite side the anterior two-thirds of the hard palate. **p. papilla′ris hep′atis** [NA], papillary process of liver: the left of the two processes seen on the caudate lobe of the liver. **p. paramastoi′deus os′sis occipita′lis** [NA], paramastoid process of occipital bone: a process that in man is represented by a tubercle on the under surface of the jugular process. **p. poste′rior sphenoida′lis** [NA], posterior process of cartilage of nasal septum: a narrow flat strip of cartilage that extends backward and upward along the groove on the upper margin of the vomer and below the perpendicular plate of the ethmoid bone, from the septal cartilage nearly to the sphenoid bone. Called also *p. sphenoidalis septi cartilaginei*. **p. poste′rior ta′li** [NA], posterior process of talus: a backward projection from the posterior portion of the talus, divided into two unequal parts by the sulcus tendinis musculi flexoris hallucis longi tali. **p. pterygoi′deus os′sis sphenoida′lis** [NA], pterygoid process of sphenoid bone: either of two processes on the sphenoid bone descending from the points of junction of the great wings and body of the bone, and each consisting of a lateral and a medial plate. **p. pterygospino′sus** [NA], **p. pterygospino′sus** [Civini′ni], pterygospinous process: a small spine on the posterior edge of the lateral pterygoid plate of the sphenoid bone, giving attachment to the pterygospinous ligament. **p. pyramida′lis os′sis palati′ni** [NA], pyramidal process of palatine bone: a strong process projecting downward, backward, and laterally from the lateral part of the posterior margin of the palatine bone and helping to form the pterygoid fossa. **p. retromandibula′ris glan′dulae parot′idis**, an irregularly wedge-shaped portion of the parotid gland passing medially behind the ramus of the mandible almost to the wall of the pharynx. **p. sphenoida′lis os′sis palati′ni** [NA], sphenoid process of palatine bone: an irregular mass of bone that projects upward and medially from the posterior portion of the superior margin of the perpendicular portion of the palatine bone, and articulates with the body of the sphenoid bone and with the ala vomeris. **p. sphenoida′lis sep′ti cartilagin′ei**, processus posterior sphenoidalis. **p. spino′sus vertebra′rum** [NA], spinous process of vertebrae: a part of the vertebrae projecting backward from the arch, giving attachment to muscles of the back. **p. styloi′deus fib′ulae**, apex capitis fibulae. **p. styloi′deus os′sis metacarpa′lis III** [NA], styloid process of third metacarpal bone: a prominent process projecting proximally from the base of the third metacarpal bone. **p. styloi′deus os′sis tempora′lis** [NA], styloid process of temporal bone: a long spine projecting downward from the inferior surface of the temporal bone just anterior to the stylomastoid foramen, giving attachment to three muscles and two ligaments. **p. styloi′deus ra′dii** [NA], styloid process of radius: a blunt projection from the lateral surface of the distal end of the radius. **p. styloi′deus ul′nae** [NA], styloid process of ulna: the medial, non-articular process on the distal extremity of the ulna. **p. supracondyla′ris hu′meri** [NA], **p. supracondyloi′deus hu′meri**, supracondylar process of humerus: a small inconstant process just proximal to the medial epicondyle of the humerus. **p. tempora′lis os′sis zygomat′ici** [NA], temporal process of zygomatic bone: the posterior blunt process of the zygomatic bone that articulates with the zygomatic process of the temporal bone. **p. transver′sus vertebra′rum** [NA], transverse process of vertebrae: a process on either side of the vertebrae, projecting laterally from the junction between the lamina and the pedicle. **p. trochlea′ris calca′nei**, trochlea peronealis calcanei. **p. uncina′tus os′sis ethmoida′lis** [NA], uncinate process of ethmoid bone: a curved plate of bone that extends inferiorly and posteriorly from the anterior part of the ethmoid labyrinth. **p. uncina′tus pancrea′tis** [NA], uncinate process of pancreas: the left and caudal part of the head of the pancreas, which hooks around behind the pancreatic vessels; called also *Winslow's pancreas*. **p.**

vagina′lis os′sis sphenoida′lis [NA], vaginal process of sphenoid bone: a small plate on the inferior surface of the body of the sphenoid bone on either side, running medially from the medial pterygoid plate to articulate with the ala of the vomer and with the sphenoid process of the palatine bone. **p. vagina′lis peritone′i** [NA], a diverticulum of the peritoneal membrane extending into the inguinal canal, accompanying the round ligament in the female, or the testis in its descent into the scrotum in the male (*processus vaginalis testis*); usually completely obliterated in the female. Called also *canal of Nuck* or *Nuck's diverticulum*. **p. vermifor′mis**, appendix vermiformis. **p. voca′lis** [NA], vocal process: the process of the arytenoid cartilage to which the vocal ligament is attached. **p. xiphoi′deus** [NA], xiphoid process: the pointed process of cartilage, supported by a core of bone, connected with the lower end of the body of the sternum. **p. zygomat′icus maxil′lae** [NA], zygomatic process of maxilla: the rough triangular eminence that articulates with the zygomatic bone and marks the separation of the facies anterior, infratemporalis, and orbitalis. **p. zygomat′icus os′sis fronta′lis** [NA], zygomatic process of frontal bone: a thick, strong process of the frontal bone, situated at the lateral end of the supraorbital margin and articulating with the zygomatic bone, and from which the temporal line starts. **p. zygomat′icus os′sis tempora′lis** [NA], zygomatic process of temporal bone: a long, strong process arising from the lower portion of the squamous part of the temporal bone, passing forward from just above the entrance of the external acoustic meatus to join the zygomatic bone and thus forming the zygomatic arch.

procheilon (pro-ki′lon) [*pro-* + Gr. *cheilon* lip + *-on* neuter ending] the central prominence of the upper border between the skin and the mucous membrane of the upper lip, marking the distal termination of the philtrum (tuberculum labii superioris [NA]).

Prochlorophyta (pro″klo-ro-fi′tah) [*pro-* + *chloro-* + Gr. *phyton* plant] a subgroup of bacteria of the class Oxyphotobacteria, consisting of prokaryotic, unicellular, green, spheroid to ovoid organisms found associated with sea squirts in tropical coastal waters. They contain chlorophyll and are photosynthetic, using water as an electron donor and producing oxygen, and they fix carbon dioxide.

prochlorpemazine (pro″klôr-pem′ah-zēn) prochlorperazine.

prochlorperazine (pro″klôr-per′ah-zēn) [USP] chemical name: 2-chloro-10-[3-(4-methyl-1-piperazinyl)propyl]-10*H*-phenothiazine. A phenothiazine derivative, $C_{20}H_{24}ClN_3S$, occurring as a clear, pale yellow, viscous liquid; used chiefly as an antiemetic, administered rectally. Called also *prochlorpemazine*. **p. edisylate** [USP], the ethanedisulfonate salt of prochlorperazine, occurring as a white to very light yellow, crystalline powder; used as an antiemetic and tranquilizer, administered orally, intramuscularly, and intravenously. **p. maleate** [USP], the maleate salt of prochlorperazine, occurring as a white or pale yellow, crystalline powder; used as an antiemetic and tranquilizer, administered orally.

prochondral (pro-kon′dral) occurring previous to the formation of cartilage.

prochordal (pro-kor′dal) in front of the notochord.

prochorion (pro-ko′re-on) [Gr. *pro-* before + *chorion* skin] an old term for the noncellular covering of the dog egg; it has tufts that are casts of uterine glands producing secretion, but were once mistakenly thought to resemble chorionic villi and to be their predecessors.

prochromatin (pro-kro′mah-tin) the substance composing the true nucleoli; paranuclein.

prochromosome (pro-kro′mo-sōm) a chromosome-like body occurring in resting nuclei.

procidentia (pro″si-den′she-ah) [L.] a prolapse, or falling down, especially prolapse of the uterus to such a degree that the cervix protrudes from the vaginal outlet. See also *prolapse*.

procinonide (pro-sin′o-nīd) chemical name: 6α,9-difluoro-11β-hydroxy-16α,17-[(1-methylethylidene)bis(oxy)]-21-(1-oxopropoxy)pregna-1,4-diene-3,20-dione; an adrenocortical steroid, $C_{27}H_{34}F_2O_7$.

procoagulant (pro″ko-ag′u-lant) 1. tending to favor the occurrence of coagulation. 2. a precursor of a natural substance necessary to coagulation of the blood.

procoelia (pro-se′le-ah) [*pro-* + Gr. *koilia* hollow] (*obs.*) ventriculus lateralis cerebri.

procollagen (pro-kol′ah-jen) the precursor molecule of collagen, synthesized in the fibroblast, osteoblast, etc., and cleaved to form collagen extracellularly.

procollagenase (pro″ko-laj′ĕ-nās) the proenzyme of collagenase.

procollagen-lysine, 2-oxoglutarate 5-dioxygenase (pro-kol′ah-jen li′sēn ok′so-gloo′tah-rāt di-ok′sĭ-jĕ-nās) [EC 1.14.11.4] an enzyme of the oxidoreductase class that catalyzes the reaction procollagen L-lysine + 2-ketoglutarate + O_2 = procollagen 5-hydroxy-L-lysine + succinate + O_2. The enzyme requires Fe^{2+} and ascorbate as cofactors. The reaction, which catalyzes the oxidation of collagen-bound lysine, is a step in the formation of crosslinks and disaccharide prosthetic groups in collagens. Defect in the enzyme, an autosomal recessive trait, results in Ehlers-Danlos syndrome, Type VI. Called also *lysyl hydroxylase*.

procollagen peptidase (pro-kol′ah-jen pep′tĭ-dās) procollagen N-proteinase.

procollagen-proline, 2-oxoglutarate 4-dioxygenase (pro-kol′ah-jen pro′lēn ok″so-gloo′tah-rāt di-ok′sĭ-jĕ-nās) [EC 1.14.11.2] an enzyme of the oxidoreductase class that catalyzes the reaction procollagen L-proline + 2-ketoglutarate + O_2 = procollagen *trans*-4-hydroxy-L-proline + succinate + CO_2 in the biosynthesis of collagens. The enzyme requires ferrous iron and ascorbate. Called also *prolyl hydroxylase*.

procollagen N-proteinase (pro-kol′ah-jen pro′tēn-ās) [EC 3.4.24.14] an enzyme of the hydrolase class that catalyzes the removal of the NH_2-terminal extension in pro α1 and pro α2 chains of procollagen to form altered procollagen in the synthesis of collagen. Deficiency of the enzyme, an autosomal recessive trait, causes Ehlers-Danlos syndrome, Type VII. Called also *procollagen protease, procollagen peptidase*.

proconceptive (pro″kon-sep′tiv) 1. aiding or favoring conception. 2. an agent that facilitates or promotes conception.

proconvertin (pro″kon-ver′tin) Factor VII; see *coagulation factors*, under *factor*.

procreation (pro″kre-a′shun) [L. *procreatio*] the entire process of bringing a new individual into the world.

procreative (pro′kre-a″tiv) concerned in procreation; able to beget.

proctalgia (prok-tal′je-ah) [*proct-* + *-algia*] neuralgia of the lower rectum. **p. fu′gax**, episodic severe pain in the rectum, often awakening the individual at night; it is attributed to spasm of the levator ani and coccygeal muscles.

proctatresia (prok″tah-tre′ze-ah) [*proct-* + *a* neg. + Gr. *trēsis* perforation] imperforation of the anus.

proctectasia (prok″tek-ta′ze-ah) [*proct-* + Gr. *ektasis* dilatation + *-ia*] dilatation of the rectum or of the anus.

proctectomy (prok-tek′to-me) [*proct-* + Gr. *ektomē* excision] surgical removal of the rectum.

proctencleisis (prok″ten-kli′sis) [*proct-* + Gr. *enkleiein* to shut in] constriction, or stenosis, of the lower rectum; a rectal stricture.

procteurynter (prok′tu-rin″ter) [*proct-* + Gr. *eurynein* to widen] a baglike device used in dilating the rectum.

procteurysis (prok-tu′rĭ-sis) dilatation of the rectum by means of a procteurynter.

proctitis (prok-ti′tis) [*proct-* + *-itis*] inflammation of the rectum. **factitial p.**, radiation p. **radiation p.**, proctitis resulting from radiation therapy, as of the cervix or uterus, marked by tenesmus, pain, rectal bleeding, diarrhea, and telangiectasis; it may progress to ulceration. Called also *factitial p.*

proct(o)- [Gr. *prōktos* anus] a combining form designating relationship to the rectum.

proctocele (prok′to-sēl) [*procto-* + Gr. *kēlē* hernia] rectocele.

proctoclysis (prok-tok′lĭ-sis) [*procto-* + Gr. *klysis* a drenching] the slow introduction of large quantities of liquid into the rectum; called also *Murphy drip*. See *Murphy's method* (2d def.), under *method*.

proctococcypexy (prok″to-kok′sĭ-pek″se) [*procto-* + Gr. *kokkyx* coccyx + *pēxis* fixation] fixation of the rectum to the coccyx by sutures.

proctocolectomy (prok″to-ko-lek′to-me) surgical removal of the rectum and colon.

proctocolitis (prok″to-ko-li′tis) coloproctitis.

proctocolonoscopy (prok″to-ko″lon-os′ko-pe) the inspection of the interior of the rectum and lower portion of the colon.

proctocolpoplasty (prok″to-kol′po-plas″te) [procto- + Gr. kolpos vagina + plassein to form] operative repair of a rectovaginal fistula.

proctocystoplasty (prok″to-sis′to-plas″te) [procto- + Gr. kystis bladder + plassein to form] a plastic operation on the rectum and bladder; operative closure of a rectovesical fistula.

proctocystotomy (prok″to-sis-tot′o-me) [procto- + Gr. kystis bladder + tomē a cutting] incision into the bladder from the rectum.

proctodaeum (prok″to-de′um) proctodeum.

proctodeum (prok″to-de′um) [proct- + Gr. hodaios pertaining to a way] an invagination of the ectoderm of the embryo at the point where later the anus is formed; called also anal pit.

proctodone (prok′to-dōn) a hormone said to be secreted by cells of the anterior intestine of insects and to terminate diapause.

proctodynia (prok″to-din′e-ah) [proct- + Gr. odynē pain] pain in or about the anus.

Proctofoam-HC (prok′to-fōm) trademark for an aerosol foam containing 1 per cent hydrocortisone acetate and 1 per cent pramoxine hydrochloride; used to relieve anorectal inflammation, pain, swelling, and pruritus.

proctogenic (prok″to-jen′ik) [procto- + Gr. gennan to produce] derived from the anus or rectum.

proctologic (prok″to-loj′ik) pertaining to proctology.

proctologist (prok-tol′o-jist) a physician who specializes in proctology.

proctology (prok-tol′o-je) [procto- + -logy] the branch of medicine concerned with disorders of the rectum and anus.

proctoparalysis (prok″to-pah-ral′ĭ-sis) [procto- + paralysis] paralysis of the muscles of the anus and rectum.

proctoperineoplasty (prok″to-per″ĭ-ne′o-plas″te) plastic repair of the anus and perineum.

proctoperineorrhaphy (prok″to-per″ĭ-ne-or′ah-fe) proctoperineoplasty.

proctopexy (prok′to-pek″se) [procto- + Gr. pexis fixation] fixation of the rectum to some adjacent tissue or organ by suture.

proctoplasty (prok′to-plas″te) [procto- + Gr. plassein to form] plastic surgery of the rectum.

proctoplegia (prok″to-ple′je-ah) [procto- + Gr. plēgē stroke] proctoparalysis.

proctopolypus (prok″to-pol′ĭ-pus) [procto- + polypus] polyp of the rectum.

proctoptosis (prok″top-to′sis) [procto- + Gr. ptōsis fall] prolapse of the anus.

proctorrhagia (prok″to-ra′je-ah) bleeding from the rectum.

proctorrhaphy (prok-tor′ah-fe) [procto- + Gr. rhaphē seam] surgical repair of the rectum.

proctorrhea (prok″to-re′ah) [procto- + Gr. rhoia flow] a mucous discharge from the anus.

proctoscope (prok′to-skōp) [procto- + Gr. skopein to examine] a speculum or tubular instrument with appropriate illumination for inspecting the rectum. **Tuttle's p.,** a rectal speculum with an electric light at its extremity and an arrangement for inflating the rectal ampulla.

proctoscopy (prok-tos′ko-pe) [procto- + Gr. skopein to examine] inspection of the rectum with a proctoscope.

proctosigmoid (prok″to-sig′moid) the rectum and sigmoid colon.

proctosigmoidectomy (prok″to-sig″moi-dek′to-me) [procto- + sigmoid + Gr. ektomē excision] excision of the anus, rectum, and sigmoid flexure.

proctosigmoiditis (prok″to-sig″moi-di′tis) inflammation of the rectum and sigmoid.

proctosigmoidoscope (prok″to-sig-moid′o-skōp) an instrument for illuminating and viewing the rectum and sigmoid colon.

proctosigmoidoscopy (prok″to-sig″moi-dos′ko-pe) examination of the rectum and sigmoid with the sigmoidoscope.

proctospasm (prok′to-spazm) [procto- + spasm] spasm of the rectum.

proctostasis (prok-tos′tah-sis) [procto- + Gr. stasis stoppage] constipation due to anesthesia of the rectum to the stimulus of defecation.

proctostenosis (prok″to-stĕ-no′sis) [procto- + Gr. stenōsis narrowing] stricture of the rectum.

proctostomy (prok-tos′to-me) [procto- + Gr. stomoun to provide with an opening, or mouth] surgical creation of an artificial opening from the body surface into the rectum.

proctotome (prok′to-tōm) a knife for proctotomy.

proctotomy (prok-tot′o-me) [procto- + Gr. tomē a cutting] incision into the rectum, as for relief of rectal stricture. **external p.,** that done at or below the sphincter. **internal p.,** that done above the sphincter.

procumbent (pro-kum′bent) lying on the face; prone.

procursive (pro-kur′siv) [L. procursivus] characterized by a tendency to run forward.

procurvation (pro″kur-va′shun) [L. procurvare to bend forward] a bending forward, as of the body.

procuticle (pro-ku′tĭ-k'l) [pro- + L. cuticula] the layer of the exoskeleton of certain crustaceans and arthropods beneath the epicuticle, which contains chitin as the principal constituent; it is composed of an endocuticle and an exocuticle.

procyclidine hydrochloride (pro-si′klĭ-dēn) [USP] chemical name: 1-cyclohexyl-1-phenyl-3-pyrrolidino hydrochloride. A synthetic anticholinergic, $C_{19}H_{29}NO\cdot HCl$, occurring as a white crystalline powder; used as a skeletal muscle relaxant in the treatment of parkinsonism, administered orally.

prodigiosin (pro-dij″e-o′sin) chemical name: 2,2′-[3-methoxy-4′-amyl-5′-methyl-5-(2″-pyrryl)]dipyrrylmethene. An antibiotic dye from Serratia marcescens, $C_{20}H_{25}N_3O$, formerly used as an antifungal agent.

prodolic acid (pro-do′lik) an anti-inflammatory.

prodroma (pro-dro′mah), pl. prodro′mata [Gr. prodromē a running forward] prodrome.

prodromal (pro-dro′mal) premonitory; indicating the onset of a disease or morbid state.

prodromata (pro-dro′mah-tah) [Gr.] plural of prodroma.

prodrome (pro′drōm) [L. prodromus; Gr. prodromos forerunning] a premonitory symptom or precursor; a symptom indicating the onset of a disease.

prodromic (pro-dro′mik) prodromal.

pro-drug (pro′drug) [L. pro- before + drug] a compound that, on administration, must undergo chemical conversion by metabolic processes before becoming an active pharmacological agent; a precursor of a drug.

product (prod′ukt) something produced. **cleavage p.,** a substance formed by the splitting of a compound molecule into simpler molecules. **contact activation p.,** a product of the interaction of blood coagulation Factors XII and XI, which functions to activate Factor IX during the formation of intrinsic thromboplastin. **decay p.,** a nuclide, which may be stable or radioactive, resulting from the radioactive disintegration of a radionuclide, being formed either directly or as the result of successive transformations in a radioactive series. Called also daughter. **end p.,** the final product in a chain of metabolic reactions. **fibrinolytic split p's,** fragments of fibrinogen or fibrin degraded by plasmin. **fission p.,** an isotope, usually radioactive, of an element in the middle of the periodic table, produced by fission of a heavy element, such as uranium, under bombardment by high energy particles. **gene p., primary,** the specific protein or polypeptide molecules, frequently enzymes, which depend on the presence of a gene. **spallation p's,** the many different chemical elements produced in small quantities in nuclear fission. **substitution p.,** a chemical product obtained by substituting for one element in a molecule an atom or a radical of some other substance.

productive (pro-duk′tiv) producing or forming; said especially of an inflammation that produces new tissue or of a cough that brings forth sputum or mucus.

proecdysis (pro-ek′dĭ-sis) [pro- + Gr. ekdysis a way out] the period of preparation for the process of ecdysis, during which the new cuticle is laid down and the old one ultimately detached from it.

proemial (pro-e′me-al) [L. *prooemium* a prelude] introductory; serving as an introduction or indication; prodromal; potentially dangerous.

proencephalon (pro″en-sef′ah-lon) prosencephalon.

proencephalus (pro″en-sef′ah-lus) [*pro-* + Gr. *enkephalos* brain] a fetus with a part of the brain protruding from a frontal fissure.

proenzyme (pro-en′zīm) an inactive precursor that can be converted to the active enzyme. Proenzymes, containing extra-long polypeptide chains that block activity, are activated by acid or enzymatic hydrolysis to remove the inhibiting portion. Called also *zymogen.*

proerythroblast (pro″ĕ-rith′ro-blast) pronormoblast.

proerythrocyte (pro″ĕ-rith′ro-sīt) a precursor of an erythrocyte; the term is without standing in any scheme of morphological development.

proestrogen (pro-es′tro-jen) a substance which is without estrogenic activity but which is metabolized in the body to active estrogen.

proestrum (pro-es′trum) proestrus.

proestrus (pro-es′trus) [*pro-* + L. *oestrus*] the period of heightened follicular activity preceding estrus in female mammals.

profadol hydrochloride (pro′fah-dōl) chemical name: 3-(1-methyl-3-propyl-3-pyrrolidinyl)phenol hydrochloride; a narcotic analgesic, $C_{14}H_{21}NO \cdot HCl$.

-profen a suffix indicating an anti-inflammatory agent of the ibuprofen type (propionic acid derivatives).

profenamine (pro-fen′ah-mēn) ethopropazine.

professional (pro-fesh′un-al) 1. pertaining to one's profession or occupation. 2. one who is a specialist in a particular field or occupation. **allied health p.,** a person with special training and licensed when necessary, who works under the supervision of a health professional with responsibilities bearing on patient care. Called also *paraprofessional.*

Professional Standards Review Organization See *PSRO.*

profibrinolysin (pro″fi-brĭ-nol′ĭ-sin) the inactive precursor of fibrinolysin; plasminogen.

Profichet's syndrome (disease) (pro″fe-shāz′) [Georges Charles *Profichet*, French physician, born 1873] see under *syndrome.*

profile (pro′fīl) a simple outline of the shape or form of an object, such as the head or face, viewed from the side. By extension, a graph representing quantitatively a set of characteristics subjected to tests. **antigenic p.,** the total antigenic content and structure of a tissue or cell.

proflavine (pro-fla′vin) chemical name: 3,6-diaminoacridine. An acriflavine derivative, $C_{13}H_{11}N_3$, which is a disinfectant bacteriostatic against many gram-positive bacteria. It has been used in the form of the dihydrochloride and hemisulfate salts as a topical antiseptic, and was formerly used as a urinary antiseptic. Called also *diamino-acridine.*

profluvium (pro-floo′ve-um) [L.] a flowing forth. **p. sem′inis,** a flowing from the vagina of the semen deposited during coitus.

profondometer (pro″fon-dom′ĕ-ter) an apparatus for locating a foreign body by the fluoroscope by obtaining three lines of sight which intersect at the foreign body.

profundaplasty (pro-fun′dah-plas″te) reconstruction of the occluded or stenosed deep femoral artery (profunda femoris artery).

profundoplasty (pro-fun′do-plas″te) profundaplasty.

profundus (pro-fun′dus) [L.] deep; [NA] a term denoting a structure situated deeper than another from the surface of the body.

progamous (prog′ah-mus) [*pro-* + Gr. *gamos* marriage] previous to fertilization of the ovum.

progaster (pro′gas-ter) [*pro-* + Gr. *gastēr* stomach] the archenteron.

progastrin (pro-gas′trin) an inactive precursor of gastrin.

progenia (pro-je′ne-ah) [*pro-* + L. *gena* chin] prognathism.

progenital (pro-jen′ĭ-tal) on the external surface of the genitals.

progenitor (pro-jen′ĭ-tor) [L.] a parent or ancestor.

progeny (proj′ĕ-ne) [L. *progignere* to bring forth] offspring, or descendants.

progeria (pro-je′re-ah) [*pro-* + Gr. *gēras* old age + *-ia*] a syndrome of uncertain genetic inheritance, characterized by precocious senility of striking degree, with death from coronary artery disease frequently occurring before 10 years of age. Cf. *infantilism.* Called also *Hutchinson-Gilford disease* or *syndrome.*

progestagen (pro-jes′tah-jen) progestogen.

progestational (pro″jes-ta′shun-al) 1. a term applied to that phase of the menstrual cycle, just before menstruation, when the corpus luteum is active and the endometrium secreting. 2. denoting a class of pharmaceutical preparations that have effects similar to those of progesterone; used in such disorders as dysfunctional uterine bleeding and recurrent abortion. See also under *agent.*

progesteroid (pro-jes′tĕ-roid) a progesterone-like compound; sometimes used to include progesterone and all other compounds having progestational effects.

progesterone (pro-jes′tĕ-ron) chemical name: pregn-4-ene-3,20-dione. The principal progestational hormone of the body, $C_{21}H_{30}O_2$, liberated by the corpus luteum, adrenal cortex, and placenta, whose function it is to prepare the uterus for the reception and development of the fertilized ovum by transformation of the endometrium from the proliferative to the secretory stage and to maintain an optimal intrauterine environment for sustaining pregnancy. Also [USP], the same principle isolated from pregnant sows or prepared synthetically, occurring as a white or creamy white, crystalline powder, and containing, calculated on the dry basis, between 98 and 102 per cent of progesterone; used, usually in the form of synthetic derivatives, as a progestin in the treatment of functional uterine bleeding, abnormalities of the menstrual cycle, and threatened abortion, administered orally and intramuscularly. Called also *luteohormone* and *progestational hormone.*

progestin (pro-jes′tin) the name originally given (Corner and Allen, 1930) to the crude hormone of the corpora lutea. It has since been isolated in pure form and is now known as *progesterone.* The name progestin is used for certain synthetic or natural progestational agents. See *progestational agents,* under *agent.*

progestogen (pro-jes′to-jen) a term applied to any substance possessing progestational activity.

progestomimetic (pro-jes″to-mi-met′ik) having physiologic activity similar to that of progesterone.

proglossis (pro-glos′is) [Gr. *proglōssis*] the tip or apex of the tongue.

proglottid (pro-glot′id) [*pro-* + *glottis*] one of the segments making up the body of a tapeworm. See *strobilia.*

proglottis (pro-glot′is), pl. *proglot′tides.* Proglottid.

proglumide (pro-gloo′mīd) chemical name: (+)-4-(benzoylamino)-5-(dipropylamino)-5-oxopentanoic acid: an anticholinergic, $C_{18}H_{26}N_2O_4$, reported to have a specific inhibitory effect on gastric secretion.

Proglycem (pro-gli′sem) trademark for a preparation of oral diazoxide.

prognathia (pro-na′the-ah) prognathism.

prognathic (prog-na′thik) prognathous.

prognathism (prog′nah-thizm) [*pro-* + Gr. *gnathos* jaw + *-ism*] a condition marked by abnormal protrusion of the mandible. Called also *caput progeneum, exognathia, progenia,* and *prognathia.*

prognathometer (prog″nah-thom′ĕ-ter) [*prognathous* + Gr. *metron* measure] an instrument or device for measuring the degree of prognathism.

prognathous (prog′nah-thus; prog-na′thus) [*pro-* + Gr. *gnathos* jaw] pertaining to or characterized by protrusion of the lower jaw or prognathism; having projecting jaws; having a gnathic index above 103, the teeth being in mesiocclusion. Called also *prognathic.*

prognose (prog-nōs′) to forecast the course and outcome of a disease.

prognosis (prog-no′sis) [Gr. *prognōsis* foreknowledge] a forecast as to the probable outcome of an attack of disease; the prospect as to recovery from a disease as indicated by the nature and symptoms of the case.

prognostic (prog-nos'tik)   1. affording an indication as to prognosis.   2. a symptom or sign on which a prognosis may be based.

prognosticate (prog-nos'tĭ-kāt)   to forecast the probable outcome of an attack of disease.

prognostician (prog″nos-tish'an)   one who is skilled in prognosis.

progonoma (pro″go-no'mah) [Gr. *pro* before + *gonos* sperm + *-oma*]   a tumor due to misplacement of tissue as the result of fetal atavism to a stage which does not occur in the life history of the species, but which does occur in ancestral forms of the species.   **melanotic p.,** melanotic neuroectodermal tumor.

progranulocyte (pro-gran'u-lo-sīt″)   promyelocyte.

progravid (pro-grav'id) [*pro-* + L. *gravidus* pregnant]   denoting the phase of the endometrium, under the influence of the corpus luteum, during which it is prepared for pregnancy.

progression (pro-gresh'un)   the act of moving or walking forward; the process of spreading or becoming more severe.   **backward p.,** walking backward; an act seen in certain nervous diseases.   **cross-legged p.,** a walk in which the toes are turned in and the foot is placed in front of its fellow.   **metadromic p.,** one of the sequelae of epidemic encephalitis, consisting in the fact that a person who is barely able to walk may have no difficulty in running.

progressive (pro-gres'iv)   advancing; going forward; going from bad to worse; increasing in scope or severity.

proguanil hydrochloride (pro-gwan'il)   chemical name: N-(4-chlorophenyl)-N'-(1-methylethyl)imidodicarbonimidic diamide hydrochloride. An antimalarial, $C_{11}H_{17}Cl_2N_5$, occurring as a white, crystalline powder; used in the prophylaxis and treatment of malaria, administered orally. Seldom used in the United States because of the development of resistance by the malarial parasite to proguanil. Called also *chloroguanide hydrochloride.*

Progynon (pro-jin'on)   trademark for preparations of estradiol.

prohormone (pro-hor'mōn)   a hormone preprotein; a biosynthetic, usually intraglandular hormone precursor, such as proinsulin.

proinsulin (pro-in'su-lin)   a precursor of insulin, with a molecular weight of 8,000 to 10,000; it has minimal hormonal activity and is converted to insulin by removal of the connecting C peptide, leaving the two (A and B)-chain, active insulin molecule.

projection (pro-jek'shun) [*pro-* + L. *jacēre* to throw]   1. a throwing forward, especially the act of referring impressions made on the sense organs to their proper source, so as to locate correctly the objects producing them.   2. the connection between the cerebral cortex and other parts of the nervous system or organs of special sense.   3. the act of extending or jutting out, or a part that juts out.   4. an unconscious defense mechanism in which a person attributes to someone else unacknowledged ideas, thoughts, feelings, and impulses that he finds undesirable or unacceptable in himself.   **eccentric p.,** see *referred sensation,* under *sensation.*   **erroneous p.,** a misjudging of the position of an object, due to weakness or palsy of the eye muscles. Called also *false p.*   **thalamocortical p's,** see under *fiber.*

prokallikrein (pro-kal″ĭ-kre'in)   prekallikrein.

prokaryon (pro-kar'e-on) [*pro-* + Gr. *karyon* nucleus]   1. nuclear material that is scattered in the cytoplasm of the cell, rather than bounded by a membrane; found in some unicellular organisms, such as bacteria.   2. prokaryote.

prokaryosis (pro″kar-e-o'sis) [*pro-* + Gr. *karyon* + *-osis*]   the state of not having a true nucleus, the nuclear membrane being absent and the nuclear material being either scattered in the cytoplasm of the cell or collected in a nucleoid region; a characteristic of bacteria. Cf. *eukaryosis.*

Prokaryotae (pro-kar″e-o'te) [*pro-* + Gr. *karyon* nucleus]   Procaryotae.

prokaryote (pro-kar'e-ōt) [*pro-* + Gr. *karyon* nut, kernel]   any member of the kingdom Procaryotae. Prokaryotes are cellular organisms lacking a true nucleus and nuclear membrane. Their nuclear material consists of a single double-stranded DNA molecule, not associated with basic proteins. The microorganisms, comprising the bacteria and blue-green bacteria (formerly blue-green algae), are predominantly unicellular but may have filamentous, mycelial, or colonial forms. All (except the Mollicutes and Archaeobacteria) have a true cell wall containing peptidoglycan, and all reproduce by cell fission. See also *Procaryotae.* Cf. *eukaryote.*

prokaryotic (pro″kar-e-ot'ik)   pertaining to a prokaryon or to a prokaryote or to prokaryosis.

Proketazine (pro-ke'tah-zēn)   trademark for preparations of carphenazine maleate.

prolabium (pro-la'be-um) [*pro-* + L. *labium* lip]   the prominent central part of the upper lip.

prolactin (pro-lak'tin) [*pro-* + L. *lac* milk]   one of the hormones (molecular weight 23,000; 198 amino acids) secreted by special cells of the anterior pituitary gland that stimulates and sustains lactation in postpartum mammals, the mammary glands having been prepared by other hormones, including estrogens, progesterone, growth hormone, corticosteroids, and insulin; it also stimulates the formation of milk in the crop sac of certain birds, as in pigeons and doves, an action formerly used for bioassay, and shows luteotropic activity in certain mammals. Called also *lactogen* and *lactogenic hormone.*

prolactinoma (pro-lak″tĭ-no'mah)   a pituitary tumor, usually a microadenoma of the mammotropic cells, which secretes prolactin; it is manifested clinically by the galactorrhea-amenorrhea syndrome.

prolamin (pro-lam'in, pro'lah-min)   any one of a group of proteins found in cereals. They are soluble in alcohol (70–80 per cent), but insoluble in water and absolute alcohol. They are also called *alcohol-soluble proteins.*

prolan (pro'lan)   Zondek's term for the gonadotropic principle of human pregnancy urine, responsible for the biologic pregnancy tests. Originally, the response of rodents to pregnancy urine was ascribed to two hormones, *prolan A,* follicle-stimulating, and *prolan B,* luteinizing. It is now known that the gonadotropic principle in human pregnancy is a single entity (chorionic gonadotropin) and differs from the gonadotropic substance of the anterior pituitary. The term prolan has fallen into disuse but is of historic value.

prolapse (pro-laps') [L. *prolapsus; pro* before + *labi* to fall]   1. the falling down, or sinking, of a part or viscus; procidentia.   2. to undergo such displacement.   **anal p., p. of anus,**

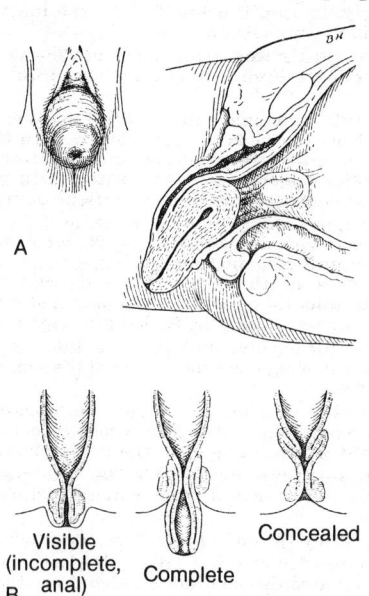

Prolapse of uterus (*A*) and rectum (*B*).

(A)

B   Visible (incomplete, anal)   Complete   Concealed

protrusion of modified anal skin through the anal orifice. **p. of the cord,** premature expulsion of the umbilical cord in labor before the fetus is delivered. **frank p.,** prolapse of the uterus in which the vagina is inverted and hangs from the vulva. **p. of the iris,** protrusion of the iris through a wound in the cornea. **Morgagni's p.,** chronic inflammatory hyperplasia of the mucosa and submucosa of the sacculus laryngis. **rectal p., p. of rectum,** protrusion of the rectal mucous membrane through the anus in varying degree, classified as *incomplete* or *partial* with no displacement of anal sphincter muscle, *complete with displacement* of anal sphincter muscle, *complete with no displacement* of anal muscles but usually with herniation of bowel, and *internal complete* (*concealed*) with intussusception of the rectosigmoid and upper portion of the rectum into the lower rectum. **p. of uterus,** downward displacement of the uterus so that the cervix is within the vaginal orifice (*first-degree p.*), the cervix is outside the orifice (*second-degree p.*), or the entire uterus is outside the orifice (*third-degree p.*).

prolapsus (pro-lap′sus) [L.] prolapse. **p. a′ni,** prolapse of the anus. **p. rec′ti,** prolapse of the rectum. **p. u′teri,** prolapse of the uterus.

prolepsis (pro-lep′sis) the return of a paroxysm before the expected time.

proleptic (pro-lep′tik) occurring prior to the usual time; said of a periodic disease whose paroxysms return at successively shorter intervals.

proleukocyte (pro-lu′ko-sīt) a precursor of a leukocyte; the term is without standing in any current scheme of morphological development.

prolidase (pro′lĭ-dās) proline dipeptidase.

prolidase deficiency a genetic aminoacidopathy caused by defective cleavage of imino acid-containing peptides, and resulting in urinary excretion of imidodipeptide (X-proline). The clinical syndrome shows chronic dermatitis, dysmorphogenesis, mental retardation, and recurrent infection. Called also *hyperimidodipeptiduria.*

proliferate (pro-lif′er-āt) to grow by the reproduction of similar cells.

proliferation (pro-lif″ĕ-ra′shun) [L. *proles* offspring + *ferre* to bear] the reproduction or multiplication of similar forms, especially of cells and morbid cysts. **fibroplastic p.,** an overgrowth of collagenous connective tissue involving many organs of the body, as occurs in systemic lupus erythematosus, scleroderma, and other collagen diseases.

proliferative (pro-lif′er-a-tiv) characterized by proliferation.

proliferous (pro-lif′er-us) proliferative.

prolific (pro-lif′ik) [L. *prolificus*] fruitful; productive.

proligerous (pro-lij′er-us) [L. *proles* offspring + *gerere* to bear] producing offspring.

prolinase (pro′lĭ-nās) prolyl dipeptidase.

proline (pro′lin) an amino acid, 2-pyrrolidine-carboxylic acid, discovered by Fischer in 1901; it is a major constituent of collagen (see *tropocollagen*).

proline dehydrogenase (pro′lēn de-hi′dro-jĕ-nās) [EC 1.5.99.8] an enzyme (a mitochondrial flavoprotein) of the oxidoreductase class that catalyzes the reaction L-proline + ubiquinone + H_2O = (S)-1-pyrroline-5-carboxylate + ubiquinol, which is the initial step in the degradation of proline to glutamate. Deficiency of the enzyme, an autosomal recessive trait, is the cause of hyperprolinemia Type I. Called also *proline oxidase.*

proline dipeptidase (pro′lēn di-pep′tĭ-dās) [EC 3.4.13.9] an enzyme of the hydrolase class that catalyzes the reaction aminoacyl-L-proline + H_2O = amino acid + L-proline. The reaction cleaves C-terminal imino acids from dipeptides. It is important in intestinal absorption of the imino-acid portion of dipeptides. Genetic deficiency causes increased urinary excretion of imino acid-containing dipeptide. See also *prolidase d.* under *deficiency.* Called also *prolidase.*

proline hydroxylase (pro′lēn hi-drok′sĭ-lās) procollagen-proline-2-oxoglutarate 4-dioxygenase.

prolinemia (pro″lĭ-ne′me-ah) hyperprolinemia.

proline-5-oxidase (pro′lēn ok′sĭ-dās) proline dehydrogenase.

prolintane hydrochloride (pro-lin′tān) chemical name: 1-[1-(phenylmethyl)butyl]pyrrolidine hydrochloride; an antidepressant, $C_{15}H_{23}N \cdot HCl$.

Prolixin (pro-lik′sin) trademark for preparations of fluphenazine hydrochloride.

Proloid (pro′loid) trademark for a preparation of thyroglobulin (def. 2).

Proluton (pro-lu′ton) trademark for preparations of progesterone.

prolyl (pro′lyl) the acyl radical of proline.

prolyl dipeptidase (pro′lil di-pep′ti-dās) [EC 3.4.13.8] an enzyme of the hydrolase class that catalyzes the reaction L-prolyl-amino acid + H_2O = amino acid + L-proline. The reaction cleaves N-terminal imino acids from dipeptides. Called also *prolinase.*

prolyl hydroxylase (pro′lil hi-drok′sĭ-lās) procollagen-proline, 2-oxoglutarate 4-dioxygenase.

prolymphocyte (pro-lim′fo-sīt) a developmental form of the lymphocytic series intermediate between the lymphoblast and lymphocyte.

promanide (pro′man-id) glucosulfone sodium.

promastigote (pro-mas′tĭ-gōt) [*pro-* + Gr. *mastix* whip] any of the bodies representing the morphological (leptomonad) stage in the life cycle of certain trypanosomatid protozoa resembling the typical adult form of members of the genus *Leptomonas,* in which the elongate or pear-shaped cell has a central nucleus and at the anterior end a kinetoplast and a basal body from which arises a single long, slender flagellum. Cf. *amastigote, choanomastigote, epimastigote, opisthomastigote,* and *trypomastigote.*

promazine hydrochloride (pro′mah-zēn) [USP] chemical name: *N,N*-dimethyl-10*H*-phenothiazine-10-propanamine monohydrochloride. A phenothiazine derivative, $C_{17}H_{20}N_2S \cdot HCl$, occurring as a white to slightly yellow, crystalline powder; used as an antipsychotic agent, as an antiemetic, and as an analgesic- and anesthetic-potentiating agent, administered orally, intramuscularly, and intravenously.

promegakaryocyte (pro″meg-ah-kar′e-o-sīt″) a precursor in the thrombocytic series, being a cell intermediate between the megakaryoblast and the megakaryocyte.

promegaloblast (pro-meg′ah-lo-blast″) the earliest developmental form in the abnormal red cell maturation sequence occurring in vitamin B_{12} and folic acid deficiencies; it corresponds to the pronormoblast, but differs from it by its larger size, abundant basophilic cytoplasm, and reticulated, unclumped nuclear chromatin. Several nucleoli are usually present.

prometaphase (pro-met′ah-fāz) the phase of mitosis which generally begins with the disintegration of the nuclear membrane. When this has occurred, a more fluid zone is noted in the center of the cell, in which the chromosomes move freely and in apparent disorder, making their way toward the equator.

promethazine hydrochloride (pro-meth′ah-zēn) [USP] chemical name: *N,N,α*-trimethyl-10*H*-phenothiazine-10-ethanamine. A phenothiazine derivative, $C_{17}H_{20}N_2S \cdot HCl$, occurring as a white to faint yellow, crystalline powder, having marked antihistaminic activity as well as sedative and antiemetic actions; used to provide bedtime, surgical, and obstetrical sedation, to potentiate the action of central depressants, and to manage nausea and vomiting associated with surgery, pregnancy, and motion sickness, administered orally, intramuscularly, and intravenously.

promethestrol dipropionate (pro-meth′es-trol) chemical name: 4,4′-(1,2-diethyl-1,2-ethanediyl)bis[2-methylphenol]dipropanoate. An orally effective, synthetic, nonsteroid estrogenic agent, $C_{26}H_{34}O_4$, occurring as a white, crystalline powder, having actions and uses similar to those of diethylstilbestrol (q.v.). Called also *methestrol dipropionate.*

promethium (pro-me′the-um) the radioactive metallic chemical element of atomic number 61, atomic weight 147, and symbol Pm. Formerly called *florentium* and *illinium.*

promine (pro′mēn) a substance widely distributed in animal cells, characterized by its ability to promote cell division and growth. Cf. *retine.*

prominence (prom′ĭ-nens) a protrusion or projection; for names of specific anatomical structures, see under *prominentia.* **Ammon's scleral p.,** a prominence on the globe of the eye of the fetus. **tubal p.,** torus tubarius.

prominentia (prom″ĭ-nen′she-ah), gen. and pl. *prominen′tiae* [L.] a prominence, protrusion, or projection; [NA] a general term for a small protrusion on another structure or part. **p. cana′lis facia′lis** [NA], prominence of facial canal: an elongated elevation on the medial wall of the tympanic cavity, just inferior to the prominence of the lateral semicircular canal and superior and posterior to the vestibular window. **p. cana′lis semicircula′ris latera′lis** [NA], prominence of lateral semicircular canal: a large rounded prominence on the upper portion of the medial wall of the tympanic cavity, between the vestibular window and the mastoid antrum. **p. laryn′gea** [NA], laryngeal prominence: a subcutaneous prominence on the front of the neck produced by the thyroid cartilage of the larynx; called also *Adam's apple*. **p. mallea′ris membra′nae tym′pani** [NA], **p. malleola′ris membra′nae tym′pani**, mallear prominence of tympanic membrane: a small projection at the upper extremity of the stria mallearis, formed by the lateral process of the malleus. **p. spira′lis** [NA], a prominence on the external wall of the cochlear duct, separating the stria vascularis from the external spiral sulcus. **p. styloi′dea** [NA], styloid prominence: an irregular nodule on the posterior portion of the floor of the tympanic cavity, corresponding to the base of the styloid process.

prominentiae (prom″ĭ-nen′she-e) [L.] genitive and plural of *prominentia*.

promitosis (pro″mi-to′sis) a simple form of cell division seen in tumor cells, in which the nucleolus or karyosome divides as in mitosis, the rest of the division simulating amitosis.

promonocyte (pro-mon′o-sīt) a precursor in the monocytic series, being a cell intermediate in development between the monoblast and monocyte.

promontorium (prom″on-to′re-um), pl. *promonto′ria* [L.] promontory, a projecting eminence or process; [NA] a general term for such a structure. **p. faci′ei**, nasus externus. **p. os′sis sa′cri** [NA], promontory of sacrum: the prominent anterior border of the pelvic surface of the body of the first sacral vertebra. **p. tym′pani** [NA], promontory of tympanic cavity: the prominence on the medial wall of the tympanic cavity, formed by the first turn of the cochlea.

promontory (prom′on-to″re) a projecting eminence or process; for names of specific anatomical structures see under *promontorium*.

promoter (pro-mo′ter) a substance in a catalyst which increases the rate of activity of the latter. Cf. *protector*.

promoxolane (pro-mok′so-lān) chemical name: 2,2-diisopropyl-1,3-dioxolane-4-methanol. A liquid, $C_{10}H_{20}O_3$, used as a skeletal muscle relaxant and tranquilizer.

promyelocyte (pro-mi′ĕ-lo-sīt″) a precursor in the granulocytic series, being a cell intermediate in development between a myeloblast and myelocyte, and containing a few, as yet undifferentiated, cytoplasmic granules.

pronate (pro′nāt) to assume or place in a prone position.

pronation (pro-na′shun) [L. *pronatio*] the act of assuming the prone position, or the state of being prone. Applied to the hand, the act of turning the palm backward (posteriorly) or downward, performed by medial rotation of the forearm. Applied to the foot, a combination of eversion and abduction movements taking place in the tarsal and metatarsal joints and resulting in lowering of the medial margin of the foot, hence of the longitudinal arch. Cf. *supination*.

pronatoflexor (pro-na″to-flek′sor) both pronator and flexor.

pronator (pro-na′tor) [L.] a muscle that serves to pronate.

prone (prōn) [L. *pronus* inclined forward] lying face downward; see also *pronation*.

pronephron (pro-nef′ron) pronephros.

pronephros (pro-nef′ros), pl. *pronephroi* [pro- + Gr. *nephros* kidney] the primordial kidney; an excretory structure or its rudiments developing in the embryo before the mesonephros. Its duct is later used by the mesonephros, which arises caudal to it.

Pronestyl (pro-nes′til) trademark for preparations of procainamide hydrochloride.

pronetalol (pro-net′ah-lōl) pronethalol.

pronethalol (pro-neth′ah-lōl) chemical name: α-[(isopropylamino)methyl]-2-naphthalenemethanol; a beta-adrenergic blocking agent, $C_{15}H_{19}NO$, having the same actions as propranolol (q.v.). Called also *nethalide* and *pronetalol*.

prong (prong) a conical projection, such as a conical root of a tooth.

pronograde (pro′no-grād) [L. *pronus* bent downward + *gradi* to walk] characterized by walking with the body approximately horizontal; applied to quadrupeds. Cf. *orthograde*.

pronometer (pro-nom′ĕ-ter) an instrument for measuring the amount of pronation or supination of the forearm.

pronormoblast (pro-nor′mo-blast) the earliest of the im-

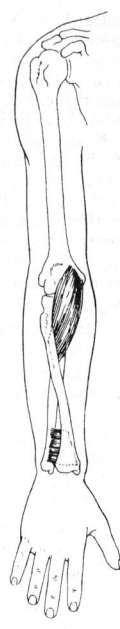

Pronators contracted, forearm and hand pronated.

mature forms recognizable as a normal precursor of the mature erythrocyte. It is round, with a relatively large nucleus which occupies most of the cell and is surrounded by a small amount of cytoplasm. The cytoplasm is of clear deep blue color, often staining slightly unevenly, and showing a pale perinuclear halo. The nucleus is round, and consists of a network of fairly uniformly distributed chromatin strands, giving a finely reticular appearance; it is reddish purple in color and contains several nucleoli. Called also *rubriblast* and *proerythroblast*. See also *normoblast*.

Prontosil (pron′to-sil) trademark for the hydrochloride salt of *p*-[(2,4-diaminophenyl)azo]benzenesulfonamide(sulfamidochrysoidine), $C_{12}H_{13}N_5O_2S \cdot HCl$, occurring as orange-red crystals. The forerunner of the sulfonamide drugs, it was first prepared in 1932 and is no longer used therapeutically. Called also *P. flavum* and *P. rubrum*.

pronucleus (pro-nu′kle-us) the precursor of a nucleus. **female p.**, the haploid nucleus of the fully mature ovum which loses its nuclear envelope and liberates its chromosomes to meet in synapsis with those similarly derived from the male pronucleus. **male p.**, the nuclear material of the head of a spermatozoon, after it has penetrated the ovum and acquired a pronuclear membrane.

proopiomelanocortin (pro-o″pe-o-mel″ah-no-kor′tin) [*pro-* + endogenous *opio*ids + *melano*cyte stimulating hormone + *cort*icotropin + *-in*] the 31,000 dalton prohormone that is the precursor of ACTH (adrenocorticotropic hormone, corticotropin), the lipotropins (LPH's), the melanocyte stimulating hormones (MSH's), and endogenous opioid peptides (endorphins and enkephalins), all of which are produced by posttranslational proteolytic cleavage in cell types that produce these hormones.

pro-otic (pro-ot′ik) [pro- + Gr. *ous* ear] anterior to the ear.

Propadrine (pro′pah-drēn) trademark for preparations of phenylpropanolamine hydrochloride.

propagation (prop″ah-ga′shun) reproduction.

propagative (prop′ah-ga″tiv) pertaining to or concerned in propagation.

propagule (prop′ah-gūl) in ecology, the minimum number of individuals of a species necessary to colonize a habitable island.

propancreatitis (pro-pan″kre-ah-ti′tis) (*obs.*) purulent pancreatitis.

propane (pro′pān) a hydrocarbon of the methane series, $CH_3 \cdot CH_2 \cdot CH_3$, which is a constituent of natural gas and crude petroleum, and occurs as a colorless flammable gas with a characteristic odor.

propanidid (pro-pan′ĭ-did) chemical name: 4-[2-(diethylamino)-2-oxoethoxy]-3-methoxybenzeneacetic acid propyl ester. A short-acting anesthetic, $C_{18}H_{27}NO_5$, derived from eugenol; administered intravenously.

propanolide (pro-pan′o-līd) betapropiolactone.

propantheline bromide (pro-pan′thĕ-lēn) [USP] chemical name: *N*-methyl-*N*-(1-methylethyl)-*N*-[2-[(9*H*-xanthen-9-ylcarbonyl)oxy]ethyl]-2-propanaminium bromide. An anticholinergic, $C_{23}H_{30}BrNO_3$, occurring as white or nearly white crystals, which inhibits gastrointestinal hypermotility and hyperacidity; used especially as adjunctive therapy in the treatment of peptic ulcer, administered orally, intravenously, and intramuscularly.

proparacaine hydrochloride (pro-par′ah-kān) [USP] chemical name: 3-amino-4-propoxybenzoic acid 2-(diethylamino)ethyl ester monohydrochloride. An anesthetic, $C_{16}H_{26}N_2O_3 \cdot HCl$, occurring as a white to off-white, or faintly buff-colored, crystalline powder; applied topically to the conjunctiva.

propatyl nitrate (pro′pah-til) chemical name: 2-ethyl-2-[(nitrooxy)methyl]-1,3-propanediol dinitrate (ester); a coronary vasodilator, $C_6H_{11}N_3O_9$.

propedeutic (pro″pĕ-du′tik) pertaining to preliminary instruction.

propedeutics (pro″pĕ-du′tiks) [Gr. *propaideia* preparatory teaching] preliminary instruction.

propene (pro′pēn) propylene.

propenyl (pro-pe′nil) a three-carbon radical with one double bond between two of the carbons, $CH_3CH{=}CH{-}$.

propepsin (pro-pep′sin) pepsinogen.

propeptone (pro-pep′tōn) hemialbumose.

propeptonuria (pro″pep-to-nu′re-ah) hemialbumosuria.

properdin (pro′per-din) factor P.

properitoneal (pro″per-ĭ-to-ne′al) situated between the parietal peritoneum and the abdominal wall; preperitoneal.

property (prop′er-te) a characteristic quality, ability, capability, or function. **colligative p.,** any of the properties of solutions that depend only on the concentration of osmotically active particles: boiling point elevation, freezing point depression, osmotic pressure, and vapor pressure lowering.

prophage (pro′fāj) [*pro-* + *phage*] the latent stage of a phage in a lysogenic bacterium, in which the viral genome becomes inserted into a specific portion of the host chromosome and is duplicated each cell generation.

prophase (pro′fāz) the first stage in cell reduplication. In mitosis, the stage during which the chromosomes become visible (because of supercoiling of DNA), the cell nucleus starts to lose its identity, and the centrioles begin to migrate. In meiosis, the prophase of the first division consists of five stages: leptotene, zygotene, pachytene, diplotene, and diakinesis. In the second meiotic division, prophase resembles that in mitotic division. See *meiosis* and *mitosis*.

prophenpyridamine (pro″fen-pi-rid′ah-mēn) pheniramine.

prophylactic (pro″fi-lak′tik) [Gr. *prophylaktikos*] 1. tending to ward off disease; pertaining to prophylaxis. 2. an agent that tends to ward off disease.

prophylaxis (pro″fi-lak′sis) [Gr. *prophylassein* to keep guard before] the prevention of disease; preventive treatment. **causal p.,** removal of the cause of a disease. **chemical p.,** the use of chemicals in preventing the transmission of disease, especially venereal disease. **collective p.,** the protection of the community from infection. **dental p.,** oral p. **drug p.,** the use of drugs in the prevention of infection. **gametocidal p.,** the use of drugs, such as primaquine, to destroy the gametocytes of malaria. **individual p.,** the prevention of infection in an individual. **mechanical p.,** prevention of the transmission of venereal disease by mechanical means (e.g., a condom). **oral p.,** cleansing the teeth in the dental office, including removal of plaque, materia alba, calculus, and stains from the exposed and unexposed surfaces of the teeth by scaling and polishing

of the teeth as a preventive measure for the control of local irritational factors. Called also *dental p.*

propicillin (pro″pĭ-sil′in) levopropylcillin potassium.

propiodal (pro-pi′o-dal) chemical name: 2-hydroxy-trimethylene-bis-(trimethylammonium) iodide. A white crystalline powder, $C_9H_{24}I_2N_2O$, formerly used as a source of iodine.

propiolactone (pro″pe-o-lak′tōn) chemical name: 2-oxetanone. A disinfectant, $C_3H_4O_2$, effective against gram-positive, gram-negative, and acid-fast bacteria, fungi, and viruses. It is also used to prepare inactivated vaccines, because it destroys the nucleic acid core of viruses but does not damage the capsid. Called also *beta-propiolactone.*

propiomazine hydrochloride (pro″pe-o-ma′zēn) [USP] chemical name: 1-[10-[2-(dimethylamino)propyl]-10*H*-phenothiazin-2-yl]-1-propanone monohydrochloride. A phenothiazine derivative, $C_{20}H_{24}N_2OS \cdot HCl$, occurring as a yellow powder; used to provide bedtime, perisurgical, and obstetrical sedation and as an antiemetic during labor, administered intramuscularly and intravenously.

propionate (pro′pe-o-nāt) any salt of propionic acid.

propionate carboxylase (pro′pe-o-nāt kar-bok′sĭ-lās) propionyl-CoA carboxylase.

Propionibacteriaceae (pro″pe-on″e-bak-te″re-a′se-e) a family of bacteria closely related to the actinomycetes, consisting of gram-positive, asporogenous, anaerobic or aerotolerant, branching or regular rods or filaments. The organisms are inhabitants of the skin and respiratory and intestinal tracts, and are sometimes found in soft tissue infections. It includes the genera *Eubacterium* and *Propionibacterium.*

Propionibacterium (pro″pe-on″e-bak-te″re-um) [*pro-* + Gr. *piōn* fat + *baktērion* little rod] a genus of bacteria of the family Propionibacteriaceae, made up of nonspore-forming, anaerobic or aerotolerant, gram-positive rods that frequently form configurations resembling letters of the Chinese alphabet. The organisms, found as saprophytes in humans, animals, and diary products, occasionally cause soft tissue infections. **P. ac′nes,** a species that is a normal inhabitant of the skin and a frequent contaminant of anaerobic cultures. It is a potential pathogen associated with chronic infections in the blood and bone marrow. Called also *Corynebacterium acnes* and *Corynebacterium parvum.* **P. freudenreich′ii,** a species isolated from dairy products and important in the manufacture of cheese. Some authorities recognize the subspecies *freudenreichii, globosum,* and *shermanii.* Called also *Bacterium acidi propionici.* **P. granulo′sum,** a species isolated from the intestinal tract and abscesses of humans. Called also *Corynebacterium granulosum.* **P. jense′nii,** a species isolated from dairy products and silage, occasionally found in infections. Called also *Bacterium acidi propionici.*

propionic acid (pro″pe-on′ik) trivial name for propanoic acid, CH_3CH_2COOH, a fermentation product produced by several species of bacteria.

propionicacidemia (pro″pĭ-on″ik-ah″sĭ-de′me-ah) propionic acidemia.

propionitrile (pro″pe-o-ni′tril) ethyl cyanide.

propionyl (pro′pe-o-nil) the acyl radical of propionic acid.

propionyl-CoA carboxylase (pro′pe-o-nil kar-bok′sĭ-lās) [EC 6.4.1.3] an enzyme of the ligase class that catalyzes the reaction ATP + propanoyl-CoA + HCO_3^- = ADP + orthophosphate + (*S*)-methylmalonyl-CoA. The enzyme is a biotin protein and requires Mg^{++}. The reaction is the route by which three-carbon compounds from some amino acids and from odd numbered fatty acids are used as fuels. Defect of the enzyme, an autosomal recessive trait, causes propionic acidemia.

propiram fumarate (pro′pĭ-ram) chemical name: *N*-[1-methyl-2-(1-piperidinyl)ethyl]-*N*-2-pyridinylpropanamide (*E*)-2-butenedioate; an analgesic, $C_{16}N_{25}N_4O \cdot C_3H_4O_4$.

proplasmacyte (pro-plaz′mah-sīt) a precursor in the plasmacytic series, being a cell intermediate between the plasmablast and the plasma cell.

proplasmin (pro-plaz′min) plasminogen.

proplastid (pro-plas′tid) any of the cytoplasmic bodies resembling mitrochondria or chloroplasts, from which plastids are formed.

proplex, proplexus (pro′pleks, pro-plek′sus) (*obs.*) the choroid plexus of the lateral ventricle of the brain.

propons (pro′pons) [L. *pro* before + *pons* bridge] the delicate plates of white substance which pass transversely across the anterior end of the pyramid and just below the pons; called also *ponticulus*.

proporphyrinogen oxidase (pro-por-fĭ-rin′o-jen, pro-por-frin′o-jen ok′sĭ-dās) protoporphyrinogen oxidase.

proportion (pro-por′shun) [L. *proportio*] the relation of one part to another or to the whole. **mutant p.,** in genetics, the proportion of all cases of a given phenotype that arise through new mutation rather than by inheritance. Determined by the mutation rate (q.v.) and the fitness of the mutant phenotype.

propositi (pro-poz′ĭ-ti) [L.] plural of *propositus*.

propositus (pro-poz′ĭ-tus), gen. and pl. *propo′siti* [L. "the one on display"] 1. proband. 2. more specifically the first proband to be ascertained (index case).

propoxycaine hydrochloride (pro-pok′se-kān) [USP] chemical name: 4-amino-2-propoxybenzoic acid 2-(diethylamino)ethyl ester monohydrochloride. A local anesthetic, $C_{16}H_{26}N_2O_3 \cdot HCl$, occurring as a white, crystalline solid; used for infiltration and block anethesia.

propoxyphene (pro-pok′se-fēn) chemical name: (S)-α-[2-(dimethylamino)-1-methylethyl]-α-phenylbenzeneethanol propanoate. An analgesic, $C_{22}H_{29}NO_2$, structurally related to methadone. Called also *dextropropoxyphene*. See also *levopropoxyphene napsylate*. **p. hydrochloride** [USP], the hydrochloride salt of propoxyphene, $C_{22}H_{29}NO_2 \cdot HCl$, occurring as a white, crystalline powder; used as an analgesic to provide relief in mild to moderate pain, administered orally. **p. napsylate,** [USP], the napsylate salt of propoxyphene, $C_{22}H_{29}NO_2 \cdot C_{10}H_8O_3S \cdot H_2O$, occurring as a white powder, used the same as the hydrochloride salt.

propranolol (pro-pran′o-lōl) chemical name: 1-[(1-methylethyl)amino]-3-(1-naphthalenyloxy)-2-propanol. A beta-adrenergic blocking agent, $C_{16}H_{21}NO_2$, which decreases cardiac rate and output, reduces blood pressure, and is effective in the prophylaxis of migraine. **p. hydrochloride,** [USP], the hydrochloride salt of propranolol, $C_{16}H_{21}NO_2 \cdot HCl$, occurring as a white to off-white, crystalline powder. It is used as an antiarrhythmic, and also as an antihypertensive, in the management of hypertrophic aortic stenosis, and in conjunction with an alpha-adrenergic blocking agent in the symptomatic treatment of inoperable pheochromocytoma. It is also effective in the prophylaxis of migraine and in preventing fatal recurrences of cardiac failure. Administered orally or intravenously.

proprietary (pro-pri′ĕ-ta-re) a proprietary medicine; "any chemical, drug, or similar preparation used in the treatment of diseases, if such article is protected against free competition as to name, product, composition, or process of manufacture by secrecy, patent, trademark, or copyright, or by any other means."

proprioception (pro″pre-o-sep′shun) perception mediated by proprioceptors or proprioceptive tissues.

proprioceptive (pro″pre-o-sep′tiv) receiving stimuli within the tissues of the body, as within muscles and tendons. See *proprioceptor*.

proprioceptor (pro″pre-o-sep′tor) sensory nerve terminals which give information concerning movements and position of the body; they occur chiefly in the muscles, tendons, and the labyrinth. See *exteroceptor, interoceptor,* and *receptor,* def. 3.

propriospinal (pro″pre-o-spi′nal) pertaining wholly to the spinal cord; said of ascending and descending nerve fibers that interconnect segments of the spinal cord.

proprotein (pro-pro′tēn) a precursor of a protein that is converted into the active protein by proteolysis or glycosylation.

proptometer (pro-tom′ĕ-ter) exophthalmometer.

proptosis (prop-to′sis) exophthalmos.

propulsion (pro-pul′shun) [pro- + L. *pellere* to thrust] 1. tendency to fall forward in walking. 2. festination.

propyl (pro′pil) the univalent chemical radical, C_3H_7 or $CH_3 \cdot CH_2 \cdot CH_2$. **p. gallate** [NF], chemical name: 3,4,5-trihydroxybenzoic acid propyl ester. An antioxidant, $C_{10}H_{12}O_5$, occurring as a white, crystalline powder having a very slight characteristic odor; used in pharmaceutical preparations.

propylene (prop′ĭ-lēn) chemical name: propene. A gaseous hydrocarbon, $CH_3 \cdot CH:CH_2$, of the olefin series, which has anesthetic properties. **p. glycol** [USP], chemical name: 1,2-propanediol. A clear, colorless, viscous liquid, $C_3H_8O_2$, used as a humectant and solvent in pharmaceutical preparations.

propylhexedrine (pro″pil-hek′sĕ-drēn) [USP] chemical name: *N,α*-dimethyl-2-cyclohexylethylamine. An adrenergic compound, $C_{10}H_{21}N$, occurring as a clear, colorless liquid; used as a vasoconstrictor to decongest nasal mucosa, administered by inhalation.

propyliodone (pro″pil-i′o-dōn) [USP] chemical name: 3,5-diiodo-4-oxo-1(4*H*)-pyridineacetic acid propyl ester. A radiopaque medium, $C_{10}H_{11}I_2NO_3$, occurring as a white to almost white, crystalline powder; used in bronchography, administered intratracheally.

propylparaben (pro″pil-par′ah-ben) [NF] chemical name: 4-hydroxybenzoic acid propyl ester. An antifungal agent, $C_{10}H_{12}O_3$, occurring as small colorless crystals or white powder; used as a preservative in pharmaceutical preparations.

propylthiouracil (pro″pil-thi″o-u′rah-sil) [USP] chemical name: 2,3-dihydro-6-propyl-2-thioxo-4(1*H*)-pyrimidinone. A thyroid inhibitor, $C_7H_{10}N_2OS$, occurring as a white, powdery, crystalline substance; used in the treatment of hyperthyroidism, particularly to prepare patients for thyroid surgery and to maintain those who are poor surgical risks, administered orally.

proquazone (pro′kwah-zōn) chemical name: 7-methyl-1-(1-methylethyl)-4-phenyl-2-(1*H*)-quinazolinone; an anti-inflammatory, $C_{18}H_{18}N_2O$.

pro re nata (pro re na′tah) [L.] according to circumstances. Abbreviated p.r.n.

prorennin (pro-ren′in) prerennin.

prorenoate potassium (pro-ren′o-āt) chemical name: potassium 6,7-dihydro-17-hydroxy-3-oxo-3′*H*-cyclopropa[6,7]-17α-pregna-4,6-diene-21-carboxylate; an aldosterone antagonist, $C_{23}H_{31}KO_4$.

proro- [L. *prōra* prow] a combining form denoting a relationship to a prowlike or projecting anterior part or structure.

Prorocentrum (pro″ro-sen′trum) [*proro-* + L. *centrum* center] a genus of plantlike, marine and freshwater protozoa (order Dinoflagellida, class Phytomastigophorea), which like other dinoflagellates produce discoloration of the water (red tide) when present in vast numbers.

Prorodontina (pro-ro″don-ti′nah) [*proro-* + Gr. *odous* tooth] a suborder of ciliate protozoa (order Prostomatida, subclass Gymnostomatia), most species of which are carnivorous or scavengers, which are characterized by the presence of a round or oval apical or subapical cytosome, sometimes in a shallow atrium; a distinctive brosse typically occurs at or near the oral area and toxicysts are present.

proroxan hydrochloride (pro-rok′san) chemical name: 1-(2,3-dihydro-1,4-benzodioxin-6-yl)-3-(3-phenyl-1-pyrrolidinyl)-1-propanone hydrochloride; an anti-adrenergic (α-receptor), $C_{21}H_{23}NO_3 \cdot HCl$.

prorsad (pror′sad) [L. *prorsum* forward] in a forward direction.

prorubricyte (pro-roo′brĭ-sīt) basophilic normoblast.

proscillaridin (pro-sil-ar′ĭ-din) chemical name: 3β-[(6-deoxy-α-L-mannopyranosyl)oxy]-14-hydroxybufa-4,20,22-trienolide. A cardiac glycoside, $C_{30}H_{42}O_8$, which yields rhamnose on hydrolysis; used as a cardiotonic.

prosecretin (pro″se-kre′tin) the supposed precursor of secretin, thought to be contained in epithelial cells of the duodenum and jejunum and to be converted into secretin on hydrolysis with acids.

prosection (pro-sek′shun) a carefully programmed dissection for demonstration of anatomic structure.

prosector (pro-sek′tor) [L.] one who dissects anatomical subjects for demonstration.

prosencephalon (pros″en-sef′ah-lon) [Gr. *prosō* before + *enkephalos* brain] 1. [NA] the part of the brain developed from the anterior of the three primary vesicles of the embryonic neural tube; it comprises the diencephalon and telencephalon. 2. the most anterior of the three primary brain vesicles in the embryo, later dividing into the telencephalon and the diencephalon. Called also *forebrain*.

prosimian (pro″sim′ĭ-an) [*pro-* + L. *simia* an ape] a primitive living primate or an early ancestral primate.

proso- [Gr. *prosō* forward] a prefix meaning forward, or anterior.

prosocele (pros′o-sēl) prosocoele.

prosocoele (pros′o-sēl) [*proso-* + Gr. *koilia* a hollow] the foremost cavity of the brain; the ventricular cavity of the prosencephalon.

prosodemic (pros″o-dem′ik) [Gr. *prosō* forward + *dēmos* people] pertaining to or denoting a disease transmitted from person to person rather than spread generally (as by a contaminated water supply).

prosody (pros′o-de) [Gr. *prosodos* a solemn procession] the variation in stress, pitch, and rhythm of speech by which different shades of meaning are conveyed.

prosogaster (pros′o-gas″ter) [*proso-* + Gr. *gastēr* stomach] foregut.

prosopagnosia (pros″o-pag-no′se-ah) [*prosop-* + *agnosia*] a form of visual agnosia characterized by an inability to recognize familiar faces, or even one's own face in a mirror, which occurs as a result of bilateral damage to the medioinferior occipital lobes along the medioventral surfaces of the temporal lobes. Called also *prosophenosia*.

prosopalgia (pros″o-pal′je-ah) [*prosopo-* + *-algia*] trigeminal neuralgia.

prosopalgic (pros″o-pal′jik) pertaining to or affected with prosopalgia (trigeminal neuralgia).

prosopantritis (pros″o-pan-tri′tis) [*prosopo-* + Gr. *antron* cavity + *-itis*] inflammation of the frontal sinuses.

prosopectasia (pros″o-pek-ta′ze-ah) [*prosopo-* + Gr. *ektasis* expansion + *-ia*] oversize of the face.

prosophenosia (pros″o-fe-no′se-ah) [*proso-* + Gr. *phainein* to show + *-osis*] prosopagnosia.

prosoplasia (pros″o-pla′se-ah) [*proso-* + Gr. *plassein* to form] 1. abnormal differentiation of tissue. 2. development into a higher level of organization or of function.

prosop(o)- [Gr. *prosōpon* face] a combining form denoting relationship to the face.

prosopoanoschisis (pros″o-po-ah-nos′kĭ-sis) [*prosopo-* + Gr. *ana* up + *schisis* cleft] oblique facial cleft.

prosopodiplegia (pros″o-po-di-ple′je-ah) [*prosopo-* + Gr. *dis* (*di-*) twice + *plēgē* stroke] paralysis of the face and one lower extremity.

prosopodysmorphia (pros″o-po-dis-mor′fe-ah) [*prosopo-* + *dys-* + Gr. *morphē* form + *-ia*] facial hemiatrophy.

prosoponeuralgia (pros″o-po-nu-ral′je-ah) pain in the nerves of the face.

prosopopagus (pros″o-pop′ah-gus) [*prosopo-* + Gr. *pagus* thing fixed] unequal conjoined twins in which the parasite is attached to the face elsewhere than at the jaw.

prosopoplegia (pros″o-po-ple′je-ah) [*prosopo-* + Gr. *plēgē* stroke] facial paralysis.

prosopoplegic (pros″o-po-ple′jik) pertaining to or affected with prosopoplegia (facial paralysis).

prosoposchisis (pros″o-pos′kĭ-sis) [*prosopo-* + Gr. *schisis* cleft] congenital fissure of the face.

prosopospasm (pros′o-po-spazm) [*prosopo-* + *spasm*] spasm of the muscles of the face.

prosoposternodymus (pros″o-po-ster″no-di′mus) [*prosopo-* + Gr. *sternon* sternum + *didymos* twin] a double monster joined face to face and sternum to sternum.

prosopothoracopagus (pros″o-po-tho″rah-kop′ah-gus) [*prosopo-* + Gr. *thōrax* chest + *pagos* thing fixed] conjoined symmetrical twins united in the frontal plane, the fusion extending from the oral region through the thorax.

prostacyclin (pros″tah-si′klin) a prostaglandin, PGI₂, synthesized by endothelial cells lining the cardiovascular system; it is the most potent known inhibitor of platelet aggregation and a powerful vasodilator and thus is a physiologic antagonist of thromboxane A₂; it is unstable in aqueous solution having a half-life of 10 to 15 minutes.

prostaglandin (pros″tah-glan′din) [*prostate gland* + *-in* because they were originally discovered in semen] any of a group of components derived from unsaturated 20-carbon fatty acids, primarily arachidonic acid, via the cyclooxyge-

nase pathway that are extremely potent mediators of a diverse group of physiologic processes (see the specific compounds). The abbreviation for prostaglandin is PG; specific compounds are designated by adding one of the letters A through I to indicate the type of substituents found on the hydrocarbon skeleton and a subscript (1, 2, or 3) to indicate the number of double bonds in the hydrocarbon skeleton e.g., PGE_2. The predominant naturally occuring prostaglandins all have two double bonds and are synthesized from arachidonic acid (5,8,11,14-eicosatetraenoic acid) by the pathway shown in the illustration. The 1 series and 3 series are produced by the same pathway starting with fatty acids having one fewer double bond (8,11,14-eicosatrienoic acid) or one more double bond (5,8,11,14,17-eicosapentaenoic acid) than arachidonic acid. The subscript α or β indicates the configuration at C-9 (α denotes a substituent below the plane of the ring, β, above the plane). The naturally occurring PGF's have the α configuration, e.g., $PGF_{2\alpha}$. All of the prostaglandins act by binding to specific cell-surface receptors causing an increase in the level of the intracellular second messenger cyclic AMP (and in some cases cyclic GMP also). The effect produced by the cyclic AMP increase depends on the specific cell type. In some cases there is also a positive feedback effect. Increased cyclic AMP increases prostaglandin synthesis leading to further increases in cyclic AMP. **p. E₁,** alprostadil. **p. E₂,** dinoprostone. **p. F₂ₐ,** dino-

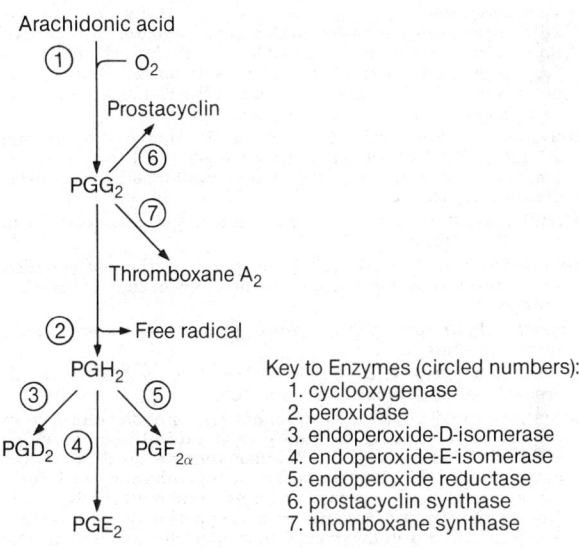

Arachidonic acid

Key to Enzymes (circled numbers):
1. cyclooxygenase
2. peroxidase
3. endoperoxide-D-isomerase
4. endoperoxide-E-isomerase
5. endoperoxide reductase
6. prostacyclin synthase
7. thromboxane synthase

The cyclooxygenase pathway of prostaglandin synthesis.

prost. **p. F₂ₐtromethamine,** dinoprost tromethamine. **PGD₂,** the major prostaglandin produced by mast cells; it is a mediator of immediate hypersensitivity synthesized and released in response binding of IgE to receptors on the mast cell; its effects include vasodilation and contraction of nonvascular smooth muscle. **PGE₁,** the analogue of PGE₂ having one double bond; many of its effects, including vasodilation, are similar to PGE₂, but, unlike PGE₂, it inhibits platelet aggregation; it has been investigated as a vasodilator for use in severe peripheral vascular disease; nonproprietary name *alprostadil.* **PGE₂,** an important stable prostaglandin having many effects; it is produced in the renal medulla, gastrointestinal mucosa, and other tissues and causes renal vasodilation and inhibition of renal tubular sodium resorption, inhibition of gastric secretion, and may cause smooth muscle to either contract or relax, depending on the tissue. It is also released by macrophages and modulates several inflammatory responses; it increases vascular permeability, increases pain sensitivity, is pyrogenic, and suppresses lymphocyte transformation, release of mediators from mast cells, and cell-mediated cytotoxicity. PGE_2 produced by some tumors causes hypercalcemia by stimulation of bone resorption by osteoclasts. It is used as an oxytocic to induce abortion; nonproprietary name, *dinoprostone*. **PGF_2,** a stable prostaglandin formed from PGH_2 or PGD_2; it stimulates the contraction of uterine and bronchial smooth muscle and produces vasoconstriction in some vessels. It is administered as an oxytocic to induce abortion; nonproprietary name, *dinoprost*. **6-keto-PGF_{1a},** an inactive metabolite produced by spontaneous hydrolysis of prostacyclin (PGI_2). **PGG_2,** a prostaglandin cyclic endoperoxide formed from arachidonic acid by incorporation of two oxygen molecules catalyzed by cyclooxygenase; it is an unstable intermediate in the synthesis of other prostaglandins. **PGH_2,** a prostaglandin cyclic endoperoxide formed from PGG_2, by a peroxidase reaction; it is an unstable intermediate that can be converted to several important prostaglandins and thromboxanes. **PGI_2** prostacyclin.

prostaglandin endoperoxide synthase (pros″tah-glan′din en″do-per-ok′sīd sin′thās) [EC 1.14.99.1] an enzyme of the oxidoreductase class that catalyzes three reactions in the synthesis of prostaglandins. Its cyclooxygenase site catalyzes: (1) 5,8,11,14-eicosatetraenoate (arachidonate) + O_2 = 11-hydroperoxyarachidonate and (2) 11-hydroperoxyarachidonate + O_2 = PGG_2 (15-hydroperoxy-$9\alpha,11\alpha$-peroxidoprosta -5(cis)-13(trans)-dienoate. Its peroxidase site catalyzes: (3) PGG_2 = PGH_2 (15-hydroxy-$9\alpha,11\alpha$-peroxidoprosta -5(cis)-13(trans)dienoate. Similar reactions form PGG_1 and PGH_1 from eicosatrienoate and PGG_3 and PGH_3 from eicosapentaenoate.

prostalene (pros′tah-lēn) chemical name: (±)-methyl 7-[(1R^*, 2R^*,3R^*,5S^*)-3,5 -dihydroxy-2-[(E)-3-hydroxy-3-methyl-1-octenyl]cyclopentyl]-4,5-heptadienoate; a prostaglandin, $C_{22}H_{36}O_5$.

Prostaphlin (pro-staf′lin) trademark for preparations of oxacillin sodium.

prostata (pros′tah-tah) [NA] a gland in the male which surrounds the neck of the bladder and part of the urethra; see *prostate*.

prostatalgia (pros″tah-tal′je-ah) [*prostate* + *-algia*] pain in the prostate.

prostatauxe (pros″tah-tawk′se) [*prostate* + Gr. *auxē* increase] enlargement of the prostate.

prostate (pros′tāt) [Gr. *prostates* one who stands before, from *pro* before + *histanai* to stand] a gland in the male which surrounds the neck of the bladder and the urethra. Called also *prostata* [NA]. It consists of a median lobe and two lateral lobes, and is made up partly of glandular matter, the ducts from which empty into the prostatic portion of the urethra, and partly of muscular fibers which encircle the urethra. The prostate contributes to the seminal fluid a secretion containing acid phosphatase, citric acid, and proteolytic enzymes which account for the liquefaction of the coagulated semen.

prostatectomy (pros″tah-tek′to-me) [*prostate* + *ektomē* excision] surgical removal of the prostate or of a part of it. **perineal p.,** removal of the prostate through an incision in the perineum. **retropubic prevesical p.,** removal of the prostate through a suprapubic incision but without entering the urinary bladder. **suprapubic transvesical p.,** removal of the prostate through an incision above the pubis and through the urinary bladder. **transurethral p.,** resection of the prostate by means of a cystoscope passed through the urethra.

prostatelcosis (pros″tat-el-ko′sis) [*prostate* + Gr. *helkōsis* ulceration] ulceration of the prostate.

prostatic (pros-tat′ik) pertaining to the prostate.

prostaticovesical (pros-tat″ĭ-ko-ves′ĭ-kal) pertaining to the prostate and the bladder.

prostaticovesiculectomy (pros-tat″ĭ-ko-ve-sik″u-lek′to-me) excision of the prostate and seminal vesicles.

prostatism (pros′tah-tizm) a symptom complex resulting from compression or obstruction of the urethra, due most commonly to hyperplasia of the prostate; symptoms include

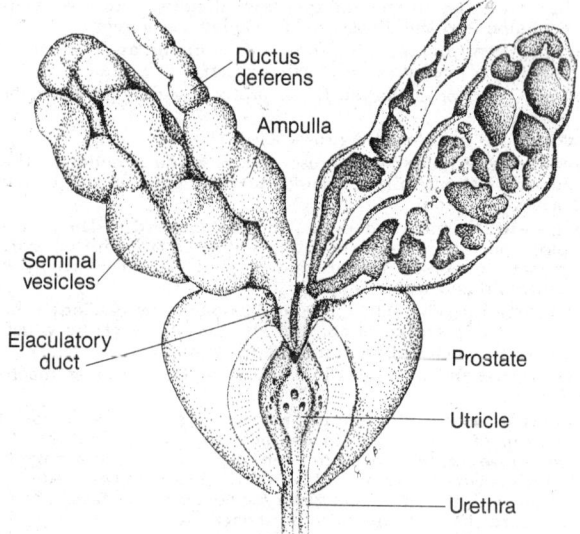

Prostate and seminal vesicles.

diminution in the caliber and force of the urinary stream, hesitancy in initiating voiding, inability to terminate micturition abruptly (with postvoiding dribbling), a sensation of incomplete bladder emptying, and, occasionally, urinary retention. **vesical p.,** a condition of retention of the urine resembling that of prostatic disease, but existing in the absence of any affection of the prostate.

prostatisme (pros′tah-tizm) prostatism. **p. sans prostate,** the symptoms of prostatic obstruction without enlargement of the prostate.

prostatitic (pros″tah-ti′tik) pertaining to prostatitis.

prostatitis (pros″tah-ti′tis) inflammation of the prostate. **allergic p., eosinophilic p.,** a condition seen in patients with certain allergies, characterized by diffuse infiltration of the prostate by eosinophils, with the development of small foci of fibrinoid necrosis. **nonspecific granulomatous p.,** prostatitis characterized histologically by focal or diffuse infiltration of the tissues by peculiar, large, pale macrophages.

prostatocystitis (pros-ta″to-sis-ti′tis) [*prostate* + Gr. *kystis* bladder + *-itis*] inflammation of the neck of the bladder (prostatic urethra) and the bladder cavity.

prostatocystotomy (pros-ta″to-sis-tot′o-me) [*prostate* + Gr. *kystis* bladder + *tomē* a cutting] surgical incision of the bladder and prostate.

prostatodynia (pros″tah-to-din′e-ah) [*prostate* + Gr. *odynē* pain] pain in the prostate.

prostatography (pros″tah-tog′rah-fe) roentgenography of the prostate.

prostatolith (pros-tat′o-lith) a prostatic calculus.

prostatolithotomy (pros-tat″o-lĭ-thot′o-me) incision of the prostate for the removal of calculus.

prostatomegaly (pros″tah-to-meg′ah-le) [*prostate* + Gr. *megalē* great] hypertrophy of the prostate.

prostatometer (pros″tah-tom′ĕ-ter) [*prostate* + Gr. *metron* measure] an instrument for measuring the prostate.

prostatomy (pros-tat′o-me) prostatotomy.

prostatorrhea (pros″tah-to-re′ah) [*prostate* + Gr. *rhoia* flow] a catarrhal discharge from the prostate.

prostatotomy (pros″tah-tot′o-me) [*prostate* + Gr. *tomē* a cutting] surgical incision of the prostate.

prostatotoxin (pros″tah-to-tok′sin) a toxin formed on injection of an extract of the prostate; it is destructive to prostatic cells.

prostatovesiculectomy (pros″tah-to-ve-sik″u-lek′to-me) excision of the prostate and seminal vesicles.

prostatovesiculitis (pros″tah-to-ve-sik″u-li′tis) inflammation of the prostate and seminal vesicles.

prostaxia (pro-stak′se-ah) a stabilized condition of protein dispersion in the body.

prosternation (pro″ster-na′shun) camptocormia.

prostheca (pros-the′kah), pl. *prosthe′cae* [Gr. *prosthēkē* appendage] 1. an appendage of a prokaryotic cell that forms a narrow extension and is enclosed by the cell wall. 2. a movable mandibular appendage in certain insects.

Prosthecochloris (pros-the″ko-klo′ris) [Gr. *prosthēcē* appendage + *chlōros* green] a genus of aquatic phototrophic bacteria of the family Chlorobiaceae, order Rhodospirillales, consisting of spherical to starlike nonmotile cells that do not contain gas vacuoles. The organisms fix carbon dioxide in the presence of hydrogen and sulfide. All suspensions are green. The type species is *P. aestua′rii*.

Prosthecomicrobium (pros-the″ko-mi-kro′be-um) [Gr. *prothēkē* appendage + *mikros* small + *bios* life] a genus of appendaged bacteria found in water, made up of gram-negative cells that produce multiple prosthecae and multiply by transverse fission. The type species is *P. pneumat′icum*.

prostheses (pros-the′sēz) [Gr.] plural of *prosthesis*.

prosthesis (pros-the′sis), pl. *prosthe′ses* [Gr. "a putting to"] an artificial substitute for a missing body part, such as an arm or leg, eye or tooth, used for functional or cosmetic reasons, or both. **antireflux p.,** a ring-shaped device that is placed around the esophagus above the stomach and below the diaphragm for treatment of gastroesophageal reflux and hiatal hernia. **cleft palate p.,** a prosthetic device, such as an obturator, used to correct cleft palate. See also *speech-aid p.,* and *artificial palate,* under *palate*. **dental p.,** a replacement for one or more of the teeth or other oral structure, ranging from a single tooth to a complete denture. See also *bridge* and *denture*. **heart valve p.,** an artificial substitute for a cardiac valve; for various types, see under *valve*. **maxillofacial p.,** a prosthetic replacement for those regions in the maxilla, mandible, and face that are missing or defective because of surgical intervention, trauma, pathology, or development malformations. See also under *prosthetics*. **ocular p.,** 1. an artificial eye; see under *eye*. 2. any other aid to vision, e.g., eyeglasses or occluders. **speech-aid p.,** a device designed to obturate an unrepaired cleft of the hard or soft palate and to perform as a substitute for the structures used for normal speech. Called also *obturator* and *speech bulb*.

prosthetic (pros-thet′ik) serving as a substitute; pertaining to the use or application of prostheses.

prosthetics (pros-thet′iks) the field of knowledge relating to prostheses, their design, use, etc. **dental p., denture p.,** prosthodontics. **facial p.,** maxillofacial p. **maxillofacial p.,** that branch of prosthodontics concerned with anatomic, functional, and cosmetic reconstruction by means of synthetic substitutes of those regions of the maxilla, mandible, and face that have been damaged, absent, or malformed due to illness, injury, congenital defects, or surgical intervention. Called also *facial p*. See also under *prosthesis*.

prosthetist (pros′thĕ-tist) [Gr. *prosthetes* one who adds] a person skilled in prosthetics and practicing its application in individual cases.

prosthion (pros′the-on) [Gr. *prosthios* foremost] a craniometric landmark located at the point of the maxillary alveolar process that projects most anteriorly in the midline of the maxilla; used for measuring upper facial height and in determining the gnathic index.

prosthodontia (pros″tho-don′she-ah) prosthodontics.

prosthodontics (pros″tho-don′tiks) [*prosthesis* + Gr. *odous* tooth] that branch of dentistry pertaining to the restoration and maintenance of oral function, comfort, appearance, and health of the patient by the replacement of missing teeth and contiguous tissues with artificial substitutes. Called also *dental prosthetics, denture prosthetics, prosthetic dentistry,* and *prosthodontia*.

prosthodontist (pros″tho-don′tist) a dentist who specializes in prosthodontics.

Prosthogonimus (pros″tho-gon′ĭ-mus) a genus of trematode parasites. **P. macror′chis,** a species parasitizing chickens, turkeys, pheasants, and other birds.

prosthokeratoplasty (pros″tho-ker′ah-to-plas″te) [*prosthesis* + *kerato-* + *-plasty*] surgical replacement of corneal tissue (as in cataract) by an inert transparent prosthesis.

Prostigmin (pro-stig′min) trademark for preparations of neostigmine.

Prostin E2 (pros′tin) trademark for preparations of dinoprostone.

Prostin F2 Alpha (pros′tin) trademark for preparations of dinoprost tromethamine.

Prostomatina (pro-sto″mah-ti′nah) [*pro-* + Gr. *stoma* mouth] a suborder of ciliate protozoa (order Prostomatida, subclass Gymnostomatia) characterized by the presence of a round apical cytosome, unspecialized circumoral ciliature, and bipolar kineties; no toxicysts are present.

prostration (pros-tra′shun) [L. *prostratio*] extreme exhaustion or powerlessness. **heat p.,** heat exhaustion. **nervous p.,** neurasthenia.

protactinium (pro″tak-tin′e-um) a radioactive metallic chemical element occurring along with radium in pitchblende, carnotite, and other minerals; atomic weight, 231; atomic number, 91; symbol Pa.

protagon (pro′tah-gon) [*prot-* + Gr. *agein* to lead] a crystalline mass, $C_{108}H_{360}N_5PO_{35}$, which separates from an alcoholic extract of brain substance on cooling.

protal (pro′tal) congenital; first; dating from the beginning.

Protalba (pro-tal′bah) trademark for preparations of protoveratrine A.

protalbumose (pro-tal′bu-mōs) a primary proteose.

protaminase (pro-tam′ĭ-nās) carboxypeptidase B.

protamine (pro′tah-min) [*prot-* + *amine*] any of a class of basic proteins of low molecular weight, occurring in combination with nucleic acids in the sperm of salmon and certain other fish and having the property of neutralizing heparin. **p. sulfate** [USP], a purified mixture of simple protein principles obtained from the sperm or testes of suitable species of fish; it has the property of neutralizing heparin, and is used as an antidote to overdosage with heparin, administered intravenously.

Protaminobacter (pro″tah-mi′no-bak′ter) in former systems of classification, a genus of bacteria of the family Pseudomonadaceae.

protan (pro′tan) 1. pertaining to protanomaly or protanopia. 2. a person with protanomaly or protanopia.

protandrous (pro-tan′drus) exhibiting protandry.

protandry (prōt-an′dre) [Gr. *prōtos* first + *aner, andros* man] hermaphroditism in which the male gonad matures before the female gonad; cf. *protogyny*.

protanomal (pro″tah-nom′al) a person with protanomaly.

protanomalous (pro″tah-nom′ah-lus) pertaining to or characterized by protanomaly.

protanomaly (pro″tah-nom′ah-le) [*prot-* + *anomaly*] a type of anomalous trichromasy in which the first, red-sensitive, cones have decreased sensitivity; therefore a greater than normal proportion of lithium red light to thallium green light is required to match a fixed sodium yellow light. Protanomaly is an X-linked trait and affects about 1 per cent of white males.

protanope (pro′tah-nōp) an individual exhibiting protanopia.

protanopia (pro″tah-no′pe-ah) [*prot-* + *an-* neg. + *-opia*] a dichromasy characterized by retention of the sensory mechanism for two hues only (blue and yellow) of the normal 4-primary quota, and lacking that for red and green and their derivatives, with loss of luminance and shift of brightness and hue curves toward the short-wave end of the spectrum, as in twilight vision. Protanopia is an X-linked trait affecting about 1 per cent of males.

protanopic (pro″tah-nop′ik) pertaining to or characterized by protanopia.

protanopsia (pro″tah-nop′se-ah) protanopia.

Protaphane NPH (pro′tah-fān) trademark for preparations of isophane insulin suspension.

Protea (pro′te-ah) [L.] a genus of trees of many species from various wet and warm regions; several species are medicinal, e.g., *P. mellifera* L., Proteaceae, the sugar protea, is made into a syrup used for coughs and pulmonary affections.

protean (pro′te-an) [Gr. *Prōteus* a many-formed deity] 1. assuming different shapes; changeable in form. 2. an insoluble derivative of protein, being the first product of the action of water, dilute acids, or enzymes.

protease (pro′te-ās) proteinase.

protectant (pro-tek′tant) protective.

protective (pro-tek′tiv) [L. *protegere* to cover over] 1. affording defense or immunity. 2. an agent that affords defense against a deleterious influence, such as a substance applied to the skin (*skin p.*) to avoid the effects of the sun's rays (*solar p.*) or other noxious influences; called also *screen*.

protector (pro-tek′tor) a substance in a catalyst which prolongs the rate of activity in the latter. Cf. *promotor*. **LATS p.,** an immunoglobulin found in the serum of patients with Graves' disease that neutralizes the capacity of thyroid tissue to bind LATS (long-acting thyroid stimulator); it interferes with the binding of thyrotropin to the human thyroid cell membrane.

Proteeae (pro-te′e-e) in some systems of classification, a tribe of gram-negative, facultatively anaerobic, rod-shaped bacteria of the family Enterobacteriaceae, made up of the genera *Morganella*, *Proteus*, and *Providencia*.

proteid (pro′te-id) protein.

proteidic (pro″te-id′ik) pertaining to a protein or proteins.

proteidogenous (pro″te-ĭ-doj′ĕ-nus) giving rise to or producing proteins.

protein (pro′tēn, pro′te-in) [Gr. *prōtos* first] any of a group of complex organic compounds which contain carbon, hydrogen, oxygen, nitrogen, and usually sulfur, the characteristic element being nitrogen, and which are widely distributed in plants and animals. Proteins, the principal constituents of the protoplasm of all cells, are of high molecular weight and consist essentially of combinations of α-amino acids in peptide linkages. Twenty different amino acids are commonly found in proteins, and each protein has a unique, genetically defined amino acid sequence which determines its specific shape and function. They serve as enzymes, structural elements, hormones, immunoglobulins, etc., and are involved in oxygen transport, muscle contraction, electron transport, and other activities throughout the body, and in photosynthesis. They may be classified thus: 1. *Simple* or *globular proteins*, including most of the proteins in the body, are generally soluble in water or salt solution and yield only α-amino acids on complete hydrolysis. Based mainly on their chemical properties, this class includes albumins, globulins, histones, and protamines. 2. *Fibrous* or *fibrillar proteins*, the principal structural proteins of the body, are generally insoluble. The major types of this class are collagens, elastins, keratins, and actin and myosin. 3. *Conjugated* or *compound proteins* are those in which the protein molecule is united with a nonprotein molecule or molecules (the prosthetic group) otherwise than as a salt. They include nucleoproteins, mucoproteins, lipoproteins, chromoproteins, phosphoproteins, and metalloproteins. **alcohol-soluble p.,** prolamin. **allosteric p.,** any protein whose biological properties are changed by binding specific small molecules at sites other than the active site. **amyloid A (AA) p.,** see *amyloid*. **amyloid light chain (AL) p.,** see *amyloid*. **bacterial p.,** a protein formed by bacterial activity. **bacterial cellular p.,** a protein that forms part of the substance of a bacterium. **Bence Jones p.,** an abnormal plasma or urinary protein, consisting of monoclonal immunoglobulin light chains, excreted in some plasma cell dyscrasias and characterized by its unusual solubility properties: on heating it precipitates at 50°–60°C and redissolves at 90°–100°C, and on cooling it again precipitates and redissolves. See *M component*, under *component*. **p. C,** a vitamin K–dependent plasma protein that, when activated, inhibits the clotting cascade at the levels of factor V and factor VIII by enzymatic cleavage of the activated forms of these clotting factors; deficiency of protein C results in recurrent venous thrombosis. **C4 binding p.,** a complement system regulatory protein; see *complement*. **carrier p.,** a protein which, when coupled to hapten *in vivo* or *in vitro*, renders the hapten capable of eliciting an immune response. See *hapten*. **cationic p's,** antimicrobial cationic proteins occurring in the primary (azurophilic) granules of neutrophils. They have low molecular weights, are rich in arginine, and appear to inhibit microbial growth. They presumably include the previously characterized substances termed *leukin* and *phagocytin*. **coagulated p.,** an insoluble form which certain proteins assume when denatured at their isoelectric point by heat, alcohol, ultraviolet rays, or other agents. **complete p.,** a protein composed of amino acids in appropriate proportion to each other so that they all can be properly used by the body, and therefore are more valuable for nutrition than is the partial protein (q.v.). **compound p., conjugated p.,** see *protein*. **constitutive p's,** proteins produced in fixed amounts, regardless of the organism's need for them. **cord p's,** the proteins of blood from the umbilical cord. **C-reactive p.,** a globulin that forms a precipitate with the somatic C-polysaccharide of the pneumococcus *in vitro*; its demonstration in the serum is a sensitive indicator of inflammation of infectious or noninfectious origin. Abbreviated *CRP*. **denatured p.,** see *protein denaturation*, under *denaturation*. **derived p.,** derivatives of the protein molecule formed by hydrolytic changes, including proteans, metaproteins, coagulated proteins, proteoses, peptones, and peptides. **encephalitogenic p.,** myelin basic p. **fibrillar p.,** see *protein*. **floating p.,** a protein which does not constitute part of the tissues, but simply circulates in the blood and is then excreted. **globular p.,** see *protein*. **Hektoen, Kretschmer, and Welker p.,** a protein found in urine which resembles Bence Jones protein in solubility, but differs in its crystalline form, in its behavior toward heat, and in its precipitin reactions. **p. hydrolysate,** an artificial digest of protein derived by acid, enzymatic, or other hydrolysis of casein, lactalbumin, fibrin, or other suitable proteins that supply the approximate nutritive equivalent of the source protein in the form of its constituent amino acids; used intravenously as a fluid and nutrient replenisher. **immune p's,** immunoglobulins. **incomplete p.,** partial p. **insoluble p.,** a substance left behind after the other proteins have been extracted from a cell. **iodized p.,** a protein treated with iodine. **iron-sulfur p.,** a group of proteins, including ferredoxins and adrenodoxin, that serve as electron transport proteins; they contain iron-sulfur centers of the form Fe_2S_2-Cys_4 or $Fe_4S_4Cys_4$, where Cys denotes a cysteine residue; the iron atoms undergo reversible transitions between the $+2$ and $+3$ oxidation states. **M p.,** see *permease*. **maintenance p.,** the smallest amount of protein upon which the normal conditions of the body can be maintained. **myelin basic p. (MBP),** a basic protein (M.W. 18,000) that constitutes about 30 per cent of myelin proteins; elevated levels of MBP occur in acute exacerbation of multiple sclerosis and acute cerebral infarction. Immunization of laboratory animals with MPB produces encephalomyelitis by inducing T cell activity that leads to demyelination and lymphoid infiltration. Called also *encephalitogenic p.* **myeloma p.,** a monoclonal immunoglobulin or light chain dimer produced in multiple myeloma or other plasma cell dyscrasias; see *M component*, under *component*. **native p.,** unchanged animal or vegetable protein, especially as it occurs in foods. **partial p.,** a protein having a ratio of amino acids different from that of the average body protein, and therefore less valuable for nutrition than is the complete protein (q.v.). Called also *incomplete p.* **plasma p's,** the hundreds of different proteins present in blood plasma, including carrier proteins (such as albumin, transferrin, and haptoglobin), fibrinogen and other coagulation factors, complement components, immunoglobulins, enzyme inhibitors, precursors of substances such as angiotension and bradykinin, and many other types of proteins. **plasma p. fraction,** see under *fraction*. **racemized p.,** protein so changed by chemical or other agents, usually dilute alkali, that its optical activity is lowered and it becomes more resistant to enzymatic hydrolysis. Acid hydrolysis of a racemized protein shows inactivation (racemization) of several of its constituent amino acids. **p. S,** a vitamin K–dependent plasma protein that inhibits blood clotting by serving as a cofactor for activated protein C. Not to be confused with *S protein*. **S p.,** a complement system regulatory protein; see *complement*. Not to be confused with *protein S*. **serum p's,** proteins of blood serum, i.e., all plasma proteins except fibrinogen. **serum amyloid A (SAA) p.,** see *amyloid*. **silver p., mild,** see under *silver*. **silver p., strong,** see under *silver*. **simple p.,** see *protein*. **staphylococcal p. A,** a protein extracted from the cell wall of *Staphylococcus aureus*, Cowan I strain, that is a specific B cell mitogen in humans. **synthetic p.,** highly complex polypeptides made in the laboratory; they show most of the characteristics of native protein. **Tamm-Horsfall p.,** see under *mucoprotein*. **whole p.,** protein which has not been split.

proteinaceous (pro″te-in-a′shus) pertaining to or of the nature of a protein.

proteinase (pro′tēn-ās) any enzyme that catalyzes the

splitting of interior peptide bonds in a protein; an endopeptidase. The proteinases are classified as serine-proteinases [EC 3.4.21], cysteine-proteinases [EC 3.4.22], aspartic-proteinases [EC 3.4.23] and metalloproteinases [EC 3.4.24] according to the composition of the active center of catalysis.

proteinemia (pro″te-in-e′me-ah)   an excess of protein in the blood. **Bence Jones p.,** the presence of monoclonal immunoglobulin light chains in serum. **broad-beta p.,** see under *disease.* **floating-beta p.,** broad-beta disease.

protein-glutamine γ-glutamyltransferase (pro′tēn gloo″tah-mēn gloo″tah-mil-trans′fer-ās) [EC 2.3.2.13] an enzyme of the transferase class that creates crosslinks within and between fibrin molecules, transferring the glutamyl portion of glutamine side chains to the amino group of lysine side chains: protein-glutamine + lysine-protein = protein-glutamyl lysine-protein + NH_3. The resultant polymerization of fibrin is an important part of blood clotting. Called also *coagulation Factor XIII$_a$, glutaminyl-peptide-γ-glutamyltransferase,* and *transglutaminase.*

proteinic (pro″te-in′ik)   pertaining to protein.

protein kinase (pro′tēn ki′nās) [EC 2.7.1.37] an enzyme of the transferase class that catalyzes the reaction ATP + protein = ADP + phosphoprotein. The reaction phosphorylates the serine, threonine, or tyrosine groups in enzymes and other proteins. Specific protein kinases regulate enzymes catalyzing key reactions in processes such as glycogen turnover, cholesterol biosynthesis, and amino acid transformations. Others create the casseins secreted in milk.

proteinochrome (pro″te-in′o-krōm) [*protein* + Gr. *chrōma* color] any one of a series of coloring matters formed by the action of bromine or chlorine on tryptophan.

proteinochromogen (pro″te-in-o-kro′mo-jen) former name for tryptophan; so called because it gave a red color with bromine.

proteinogen (pro″te-in′o-jen) Northrop's name for the hypothetical mother substance of all proteins.

proteinogenous (pro″te-in-oj′ĕ-nus) formed by or from a protein.

proteinology (pro″te-in-ol′o-je) [*protein* + *-logy*] the scientific study of proteins or of the protein status of the body.

proteinosis (pro″te-in-o′sis) the accumulation of excess protein in the tissues. **lipoid p.,** an autosomal recessive disorder of lipid metabolism characterized by the deposition of hyaline material in the skin and mucosa of the mouth, pharynx, hypopharynx, and larynx, resulting in prolonged hoarseness, often from birth, due to infiltration of the vocal cords. Skin lesions are first manifested as recurrent pustules or bullae on the face and distal exposed surfaces of the arms and legs, which heal and leave white varioliform scars, and later by waxy yellow ivory papules, nodules, or verrucoid plaques primarily located on the face, eyelids, nape, hands, fingers, elbows, and knees. Called also *hyalinosis cutis et mucosae, lipoproteinosis,* and *Urbach-Wiethe disease.* **pulmonary alveolar p.,** a chronic lung disease characterized by dyspnea, productive cough, chest pain, weakness, weight loss, and hemoptysis, and by the filling of the distal alveoli with a bland, eosinophilic, probably endogenous, proteinaceous material that prevents ventilation of affected areas. **tissue p.,** see *amyloidosis.*

proteinotherapy (pro-te″in-o-ther′ah-pe) (*obs.*) treatment of disease by the parenteral injection of foreign protein.

proteinphobia (pro″te-in-fo′be-ah) [*protein* + Gr. *phobein* to be affrighted by + *-ia*] morbid aversion to protein foods.

proteinuria (pro″te-in-u′re-ah) [*protein* + Gr. *ouron* urine + *-ia*] the presence of an excess of serum proteins in the urine; called also *albuminuria.* **accidental p.,** adventitious p. **p. of adolescence,** cyclic p. **adventitious p.,** that which is not due to a kidney disease; called also *accidental* or *false p.* **athletic p.,** functional proteinuria occurring in athletes; effort p. **Bence Jones p.,** the presence in the urine of Bence Jones protein. **cardiac p.,** proteinuria caused by cardiac disease. **colliquative p.,** proteinuria which is at first mild, but increases suddenly and markedly during convalescence; it is seen in several systemic and renal diseases. **cyclic p.,** a term once used to denote the appearance at stated times each day of a small amount of protein in the urine; it is observed principally in young persons (p. of adolescence). Called also *recurrent p.* and *Pavy's disease.* **dietetic p., digestive p.,** that produced by the use of certain foods. **effort p.,** functional protein-

uria occurring as a result of vigorous and prolonged exercise of the lower limbs; called also *athletic p.* **emulsion p.,** proteinuria in which the turbidity does not disappear on filtration, heating, or adding acid; seen in puerperal eclampsia. **enterogenic p.,** that due to intestinal decomposition. **essential p.,** a form of functional proteinuria which is not associated with or followed by renal disease; it includes effort and orthostatic proteinuria. **false p.,** adventitious p. **febrile p.,** proteinuria due to fever. **functional p.,** any proteinuria which is not truly pathologic, such as the transient proteinurias of pregnancy or of adolescence; also known variously as *intermittent, paroxysmal, physiologic,* and *transient p.* **globular p.,** proteinuria due to renal excretion of red blood cells and dependent on blood in the urine. **gouty p.,** functional proteinuria, with excessive secretion of uric acid. **hematogenous p., hemic p.,** a variety due to abnormal condition of the blood, as in some intoxications. **intermittent p.,** functional p. **intrinsic p.,** true p. **light-chain p.,** increased urinary excretion of light-chain fragments of immunoglobulins, as in Fanconi syndrome. **lordotic p.,** postural proteinuria due to lordotic deformity of the spine. **mixed p.,** true proteinuria occurring concurrently with adventitious proteinuria. **nephrogenous p.,** that caused by renal disease; called also *renal p.* **orthostatic p.,** a form of functional proteinuria, usually seen between the ages of ten and twenty, which occurs on standing erect and disappears on lying down. **overflow p.,** that due to hemoglobin, myoglobin, or immunoglobulin loss into the urine, not usually associated with glomerular or tubular disease. **palpatory p.,** temporary proteinuria produced by bimanual palpation of the kidneys. **paroxysmal p.,** functional p. **physiologic p.,** functional p. **postrenal p.,** proteinuria which has arisen at some point beyond the uriniferous tubule, such as the renal pelvis, ureter, bladder, prostate, or urethra. **postural p.,** proteinuria related to body position, as orthostatic and lordotic proteinuria. **p. praetuberculo′sa,** that occurring in the incipient stage of pulmonary tuberculosis. **prerenal p.,** proteinuria due primarily to a disease other than one of the kidney, such as heart disease, liver disease, fever, hyperthyroidism. **pseudo-p.,** adventitious p. **pyogenic p.,** that due to the absorption of pus cells or exudates, as in pneumonia, septic processes, etc. **recurrent p.,** cyclic p. **regulatory p.,** proteinuria or the transitory elimination of protein after excessive physical exercise, etc. **renal p.,** nephrogenous p. **residual p.,** persistence of protein in the urine after an attack of acute nephritis. **serous p.,** true p. **transient p.,** functional p. **true p.,** that which is characterized by the discharge with the urine of some of the protein elements of the blood; called also *intrinsic p.* and *serous p.*

proteinuric (pro″te-in-u′rik) pertaining to or marked by proteinuria.

proteoclastic (pro″te-o-klas′tik) [*protein* + Gr. *klasis* breakage] splitting up proteins or the protein molecule.

proteoglycan (pro″te-o-gli′kan) any of a group of substances found primarily in the matrix of connective tissues and in synovial fluid, vitreous humor, and mucous secretions in which many glycosaminoglycan chains are covalently attached to a protein core like bristles on a bottle brush. Because of charge repulsion, the highly acidic glycosaminoglycan chains spread out over a large volume filled with water, making proteoglycan solutions highly viscous lubricants.

Proteoglypha (pro″te-og′lĭ-fah) Proteroglypha.

proteolipid (pro″te-o-lip′id) a combination of a peptide or protein with a lipid, having the solubility characteristics of lipids. Cf. *lipoprotein.*

proteolipin (pro″te-o-lip′in) proteolipid.

proteolysis (pro″te-ol′ĭ-sis) [*protein* + Gr. *lysis* dissolution] the splitting of proteins by hydrolysis of the peptide bonds with formation of smaller polypeptides; the process may be catalyzed by proteolytic enzymes, by acids, or by bases.

proteolytic (pro″te-o-lit′ik) 1. pertaining to, characterized by, or promoting proteolysis. 2. an enzyme that promotes proteolysis.

proteometabolic (pro″te-o-met″ah-bol′ik) pertaining to proteometabolism.

proteometabolism (pro″te-o-mě-tab′o-lism) the metabolism of protein.

Proteomyces (pro″te-o-mi′sēz)   Trichosporon.

proteopectic (pro″te-o-pek′tik)   proteopexic.

proteopepsis (pro″te-o-pep′sis) [*protein* + Gr. *pepsis* digestion] the digestion of protein.

proteopeptic (pro″te-o-pep′tik)   digesting protein; pertaining to the digestion of protein.

proteopexic (pro″te-o-pek′sik)   fixing protein within the organism.

proteopexy (pro′te-o-pek″se) [*protein* + Gr. *pēxis* fixation] the fixation of proteins within the organism.

proteose (pro′te-ōs) [*protein* + *-ose*] a secondary protein derivative or a mixture of split products formed by a hydrolytic cleavage of the protein molecule more complete than that which occurs with the primary protein derivatives, but not so complete as that which forms amino-acids. The *primary* proteoses are precipitated by half saturation with ammonium sulfate, the *secondary*, by full saturation.

proteosuria (pro″te-o-su′re-ah) [*proteose* + Gr. *ouron* urine + *-ia*] the presence of proteose in the urine.

proteotherapy (pro″te-o-ther′ah-pe)   (*obs.*) proteinotherapy.

proter (pro′ter) [Gr. *proteros* front] the anterior daughter organism after transverse division of a ciliate protozoan; cf. *opisthe.*

Proteroglypha (pro″ter-o-glif′ah) a group of venomous snakes that have small stationary fangs which are grooved rather than hollow and so must be held in the wound if the poison is to reach the deeper tissues. Examples are the Indian cobra and the Sonoran coral snake. Called also *Ankyloproglypha* and *Proteoglypha.*

Proteromonadida (pro″ter-o″mo-nad′ĭ-dah) an order of parasitic protozoa (class Zoomastigophora, subphylum Mastigophora) having one or two pairs of flagella, a single mitochondrion, and a Golgi apparatus encircling a band-shaped rhizoplast passing from kinetosomes near the surface of the nucleus to mitochondrion. Representative genera include *Karotomorpha* and *Proteromonas.*

Proteromonas (pro″ter-o-mo′nas) a genus of parasitic protozoa (order Proteromonadida, class Zoomastigophorea) commonly found in the intestines of reptiles and amphibians.

proteuria (pro″te-u′re-ah) [*protein* + Gr. *ouron* urine + *-ia*] proteinuria.

proteuric (pro″te-u′rik)   proteinuric.

Proteus (pro′te-us) [Gr. *Prōteus* a many-formed ocean deity] a genus of gram-negative, facultatively anaerobic, rod-shaped bacteria of the family Enterobacteriaceae, made up of actively motile, pleomorphic organisms. Colonies exhibit the swarming phenomenon. The organisms are found in fecal material, especially in patients treated with oral antibiotics, and are potential pathogens, associated with urinary tract infections, bacteremia, and abdominal and wound infections. **P. hydroph′ilus,** *Aeromonas hydrophila.* **P. incon′stans,** a former species that has been classified as a separate genus, *Providencia. P. inconstans* subgroup A comprises *Providencia alcalifaciens; P. inconstans* subgroup B comprises *Providencia stuartii.* **P. melanovog′enes,** *Aeromonas hydrophila.* **P. mirab′ilis,** the species most frequently isolated from human clinical material, also found in soil and sewage. It is a leading cause of urinary tract infections. **P. morga′nii,** *Morganella morgani.* **P. myxofa′ciens,** a species found as a pathogen of gypsy moth larvae, not present in human clinical specimens. **P. pen′neri,** a species found in human clinical specimens. It ferments maltose, but is negative for ornithine decarboxylase and indole. **P. rettge′ri,** *Providencia rettgeri.* **P. vulga′ris,** a widespread species found in fecal matter, sewage, and soil. It is a common cause of cystitis and pyelonephritis and is associated with eye and ear infections, pleuritis, peritonitis, and suppurative abscesses. The species has many serotypes. The Ox antigens (Ox-2, Ox-19, Ox-K) react with antibodies formed in rickettsial infections and are used in the Weil-Felix reaction for the diagnosis of typhus, scrub typhus, and Rocky Mountain spotted fever. See plate accompanying *bacterium.* **P. zen′keri,** *Kurthia zopfi.*

proteus (pro′te-us), pl. *pro′tei.* an organism of the genus *Proteus.*

prothallus (prō-thăl′us) the independent, free living gametophyte generation of ferns and related lower vascular plants.

prothipendyl hydrochloride (pro-thi′pen-dil) chemical name: *N,N*-dimethyl-10*H*-pyrido[3,2-*b*][1,4]benzothiazine-10-propanamine hydrochloride monohydrate; an antihistaminic and sedative, $C_{16}H_{19}N_3S \cdot HCl \cdot H_2O$.

prothrombin (pro-throm′bin) [*pro-* + Gr. *thrombos* clot + *-in* chemical suffix] Factor II; see *coagulation factors,* under *factor.*

prothrombinase (pro-throm′bin-āse) thromboplastin. **extrinsic p.,** extrinsic thromboplastin. **intrinsic p.,** intrinsic thromboplastin.

prothrombinogenic (pro-throm″bĭ-no-jen′ik) promoting the production of prothrombin (Factor II).

prothrombinopenia (pro-throm″bĭ-no-pe′ne-ah) hypoprothrombinemia.

prothyl (pro′thil)   protyl.

prothymocyte (pro-thi′mo-sīt) a term applied to the lymphoid precursor cell of thymocytes.

protide (pro′tīd)   protein.

protidemia (pro″tĭ-de′me-ah)   proteinemia.

protinium (pro-tin′e-um)   protium.

protiodide (pro-ti′o-did) that one of the series of iodides of the same base which contains the smallest amount of iodine.

protirelin (pro-ti′re-lin)   thyrotropin releasing hormone.

protist (pro′tist) any member of the kingdom Protista; a single-celled organism. **eukaryotic p.,** the higher protists, comprising those organisms having a true nucleus. See *Protista.* **higher p.,** eukaryotic p's. **lower p.,** prokaryotic p's. **prokaryotic p.,** the lower protists, comprising those organisms lacking a true nucleus. See *Monera.*

Protista (pro-tis′tah) [Gr. *prōtista* the very first, from *prōtos* first] in some systems of classification, a kingdom comprising both animal-like and plantlike unicellular organisms with distinct nuclei, i.e., the eukaryotes, including protozoa, algae (except blue-green algae or bacteria), and certain intermediate forms. In some other systems, Protista includes only the protozoa. Cf *Monera.*

protistologist (pro″tis-tol′o-jist)   a microbiologist.

protistology (pro″tis-tol′o-je) [*Protista* + *-logy*] microbiology.

protium (pro′te-um) the mass one isotope of hydrogen, symbol ¹H; ordinary, or light, hydrogen. See *hydrogen.* Cf. *deuterium* and *tritium.*

prot(o)- [Gr. *prōtos* first] 1. a combining form meaning first or primitive. 2. in chemistry, a prefix denoting the member of a series of compounds with the lowest proportion of the element or radical to which it is affixed.

proto-actinium (pro″to-ak-tin′e-um)   protactinium.

protoalbumose (pro″to-al′bu-mōs)   a primary proteose.

protoanemonin (pro″to-ah-nem′o-nin) chemical name: 5-methylene-2-oxodihydrofuran. An antibiotic substance, $C_5H_4O_2$, from the flowering herb, *Anemone pulsatilla,* active against certain gram-positive and gram-negative bacteria. Its mechanism of action is not well understood.

protobe (pro′tōb)   protobios.

protobiology (pro″to-bi-ol′o-je) [*proto-* + Gr. *bios* life + *-logy*] the science which deals with the forms of life more minute than bacteria, such as viruses.

protobios (pro″to-bi′os) [*proto-* + Gr. *bios* life] a name proposed by d'Herelle for the bacteriophage (protobios bacteriophagus).

protoblast (pro′to-blast) [*proto-* + Gr. *blastos* germ] 1. a cell with no cell wall; an embryonic cell. 2. the nucleus of an ovum. 3. a blastomere from which a particular organ or part develops.

protoblastic (pro″to-blas′tik)   pertaining to a protoblast.

protobrochal (pro″to-bro′kal) [*proto-* + Gr. *brochos* mesh] denoting the first stage in the development of an ovary.

Protocalliphora (pro″to-kah-lif′o-rah) a genus of flies whose larvae feed on nesting birds.

protocaryon (pro″to-kar′e-on) [*proto-* + Gr. *karyon* nucleus] a cell nucleus formed of a single karyosome in a network of linin.

protocatechuic acid (pro″to-kat″ĕ-choo′ik) 3,4-dihydroxybenzoic acid, a catabolite of epinephrine.

protochloride (pro″to-klo′rid) that one of a series of chlorides of the same element which contains the least amount of chlorine.

protochlorophyll (pro″to-klo′ro-fil) a substance in plant tissue which is changed by the action of light into chlorophyll.

protochondral (pro″to-kon′dral) pertaining to the protochondrium or to centers of condrification.

protochondrium (pro″to-kon′dre-um) [*proto-* + Gr. *chondros* cartilage] the basophil substance developed from precartilage which constitutes the intermediate stage in cartilage formation.

Protociliata (pro″to-sil″e-a′tah) [*proto-* + *ciliate*] in former systems of classification, a subclass of ciliate protozoa, the members of which have been assigned to the subphylum Opalinata.

Protococcidiida (pro″to-kok″sĭ-di′ĭ-dah) [*proto-* + Gr. *kokkos* berry] an order of parasitic protozoa (subclass Coccidia, class Sporozoea) found in invertebrates, the life cycle of which involves gametogony and sporogony.

protocol (pro′to-kol) 1. an explicit, detailed plan of an experiment. 2. the original notes made on a necropsy, experiment, or case of disease.

protocone (pro′to-kōn) [*proto-* + Gr. *kōnos* cone] the principal mesiolingual cusp of the upper molar of man and certain mammals, such as the opossum and dog.

protoconid (pro″to-ko′nid) [*proto-* + Gr. *kōnos* cone + *-id*] the mesiobuccal cusp of the lower molars of primitive mammals and man, being greatly modified in many higher mammals and completely disappearing in some.

protocooperation (pro″to-co-op″er-a′shun) 1. symbiosis in which both populations (or individuals) gain from the association but are able to survive without it. 2. the tendency of animals to cluster in groups and thereby to mutually facilitate the survival of individual organisms.

protocoproporphyria (pro″to-kop″ro-por-fir′e-ah) porphyria with an excess of protophyrin and coproporphyrin in the bile and feces; see *porphyria cutanea tarda hereditaria*.

protodiastolic (pro″to-di″ah-stol′ik) pertaining to early diastole, i.e., immediately following the second heart sound.

protoduodenum (pro″to-du-o-de′num) the first or proximal portion of the duodenum, extending from the pylorus to the duodenal papilla, and developed embryonically from the foregut.

protoelastose (pro″to-e-las′tōs) hemielastin.

protofibril (pro″to-fi′bril) the first elongated unit appearing in the process of formation of any type of fiber.

protogaster (pro′to-gas″ter) [*proto-* + Gr. *gastēr* stomach] archenteron.

protoglobulose (pro″to-glob′u-lōs) a primary product formed in the digestion of globulin.

protogonocyte (pro″to-go′no-sīt) [*proto-* + *gonocyte*] one of the two cells resulting from division of the impregnated ovum and, in certain lower forms, constituting the primordial germ cell from which all gametes derive.

protogonoplasm (pro″to-go′no-plazm) [*proto-* + Gr. *gonē* seed + *plasma* anything formed or molded] (*obs.*) idiochromidia.

protogynous (pro-toj′ĭ-nus) exhibiting protogyny.

protogyny (pro-toj′ĭ-ne) [*proto-* + Gr. *gyne* woman] hermaphroditism in which the female gonad matures before the male gonad. Cf. *protandry*.

protoheme (pro″to-hēm) a heme (q.v.) in which the porphyrin is protoporphyrin, e.g., protoheme IX found in hemoglobin.

protohemin (pro″to-he′min) protoheme in which the iron atom is oxidized to the +3 oxidation state.

protohydrogen (pro″to-hi′dro-jen) protium.

protoiodide (pro″to-i′o-dīd) protiodide.

protokylol hydrochloride (pro″to-ki′lol) chemical name: 4-[2-[[2-(1,3-benzodioxol-5-yl)-1-methylethyl]amino]-1-hydroxyethyl]-1,2-benzenediol hydrochloride. An adrenergic, $C_{18}H_{21}NO_5$, occurring as a white crystalline powder; used as a bronchodilator for the treatment of bronchospasm associated with bronchial asthma, pulmonary emphysema, bronchitis, and bronchiectasis, administered orally.

Protomastigida (pro″to-mas-tij′ĭ-dah) [*proto-* + Gr. *mastix* whip] Kinetoplastida.

protomerite (pro″to-me′rīt) [*proto-* + Gr. *meros* part] the smaller anterior portion of the body of certain gregarine protozoa, separated from the posterior nucleus-containing

portion (deutomerite) by an ectoplasmic septum. See also *epimerite*.

protometer (pro-tom′ĕ-ter) exophthalmometer.

Protomonadina (pro″to-mo″nah-di′nah) [*proto-* + Gr. *monas* unit] Kinetoplastida.

proton (pro′ton) [Gr. *prōtos* first + *-on* neuter ending] 1. (*obs.*) the primitive rudiment of a part; a primordium or anlage. 2. an elementary particle of positive charge which forms the nucleus of the ordinary hydrogen atom of mass 1; protons, along with the neutrons, form the nucleus of atoms of all other elements. The proton is the unit of positive electricity, being equivalent to the electron in charge and approximately to the hydrogen ion in mass.

protonephron (pro″to-nef′ron) pronephros.

protonephros (pro″to-nef′ros) pronephros.

protoneuron (pro″to-nu′ron) [*proto-* + Gr. *neuron* nerve] 1. the first neuron in a peripheral reflex arc. 2. a unit of the nerve net of low metazoa that lacks polarization.

protonitrate (pro″to-ni′trāt) that one of several nitrates of the same base which contains the least amount of nitric acid.

proto-oncogene (pro″to-ong′ko-jēn) a normal gene that with slight alteration by mutation or other mechanism becomes an oncogene.

Protopam (pro′to-pam) trademark for preparations of pralidoxime.

protopathic (pro″to-path′ik) [*proto-* + Gr. *pathos* disease] primary; idiopathic. See *protopathic sensibility*, under *sensibility*.

protopecten (pro″to-pek′ten) pectose.

protophyllin (pro″to-fil′in) chlorophyll hydride, a colorless substance which is changed into chlorophyll by the action of air or carbon dioxide.

Protophyta (pro″to-fi′tah) [*proto-* + Gr. *phyton* plant] in former systems of classification, the lowest division of the plant kingdom, consisting of the algae and variously defined to include also the blue-green algae, yeasts, fungi, lichens, bacteria, or viruses.

protophyte (pro′to-fīt) [*proto-* + Gr. *phyton* plant] a unicellular plant or vegetable organism; an individual of the division Protophyta.

protophytology (pro″to-fi-tol′o-je) the scientific study of the simplest forms of plants (protophytes).

protopine (pro′to-pin) 1. an alkaloid, $C_{20}H_{19}NO_5$, from *Eschscholtzia californica*, the California poppy, and many other plants; it is an anodyne and hypnotic. 2. a poisonous alkaloid from various species of perennial herbs of the genus *Dicentra*.

protoplasia (pro-to-pla′se-ah) primary formation of tissue.

protoplasm (pro′to-plazm) [*proto-* + Gr. *plasma* plasm] the viscid, translucent, polyphasic colloid with water as the continuous phase that makes up the essential material of all plant and animal cells. It is composed mainly of nucleic acids, proteins, lipids, carbohydrates, and inorganic salts. The protoplasm surrounding the nucleus is known as the *cytoplasm* and that composing the nucleus is the *nucleoplasm*. **functional p.,** kinoplasm. **granular p.,** protoplasm having granular inclusions, including those in the planeroplasm. **superior p.,** endoplasmic reticulum.

protoplasmatic (pro″to-plaz-mat′ik) protoplasmic.

protoplasmic (pro″to-plaz′mik) pertaining to or consisting of protoplasm.

protoplast (pro′to-plast) [*proto-* + *-plast*] 1. the type or model of some organic being. 2. a bacterial, yeast, or fungal cell that results after complete removal of the rigid cell wall, which forms a membrane-bound cell into a spherical shape that is dependent for its integrity on an isotonic or hypertonic medium. Cf. *spheroplast*.

protoporphyria (pro″to-por-fir′e-ah) an autosomal dominant disorder, a form of erythropoietic porphyria, characterized by increased levels of protoporphyrin in the erythrocytes, plasma, liver, and feces and a wide variety of photosensitive skin changes, ranging from a burning or pruritic sensation to erythema, plaquelike edema, and wheals. Called also *erythropoietic p.* and *erythrohepatic p.* **erythrohepatic p., erythropoietic p.,** an autosomal dominant porphyria with erythropoietic and hepatic lesions, characterized biochemically by increased levels of free protoporphyrin in erythrocytes and usually by elevated plasma and fecal protoporphyrin. Clinical manifestations include pruritus, erythema, and edema after exposure of skin to sunlight; liver failure occurs in some cases.

protoporphyrin (pro″to-por′fĭ-rin) a porphyrin (q.v.) in which two pyrrole rings each have one methyl side chain and one propionate side chain and the other two pyrrole rings each have one methyl side chain and one vinyl side chain. The naturally occurring isomer protoporphyrin IX is produced by oxidative decarboxylation of two side chains and oxidation of the methylene bridges of coproporphyrinogen III; it combines with the Fe^{2+} ion to form protoheme IX, the heme prosthetic group of hemoglobin and myoglobin.

protoporphyrinogen oxidase (pro″to-por″fĭ-rin′o-jen, pro″to-por-frin′o-jen ok′si-dās) [EC 1.3.3.4] an enzyme of the oxidoreductase class that catalyzes the reaction protoporphyrinogen-IX + O_2 = protoporphyrin-IX + H_2O. The reaction is a final step in heme and porphyrin synthesis. Genetic deficiency, an autosomal dominant trait, is a cause of variegate porphyria.

protoporphyrinuria (pro″to-por″fĭ-rin-u′re-ah) [*protoporphyrin* + Gr. *ouron* urine + *-ia*] the presence of protoporphyrin in the urine.

protoproteose (pro″to-pro′te-ōs) a primary proteose.

protosalt (pro′to-sawlt) that one of a series of salts of the same base which contains the smallest amount of the substance combining with the base.

protospasm (pro′to-spazm) [*proto-* + Gr. *spasmos* spasm] a spasm which begins in a limited area and extends to other parts; the earlier and minor spasm of jacksonian epilepsy.

Protospirura (pro″to-spi-roo′rah) a genus of nematode parasites. **P. grac′ilis,** a species found in cats.

Protosteliia (pro″to-stĕ-li′e-ah) [*proto-* + Gr. *stechelo* stem] a subclass of protozoa (class Eumycetozoea, superclass Rhizopoda), characterized by a trophic stage varying from single amebae to plasmodia, with or without flagellate cells, and fruiting bodies consisting of one to several spores on a narrow, hollow stalk. It includes one order: Protosteliida.

Protosteliida (pro″to-stĕ-li′ĭ-dah) an order of ameboid protozoa with characters of the subclass (subclass Protosteliia, class Eumycetozoea). *Ceratiomyxa* is a representative genus.

protostoma (pro″to-sto′mah) blastopore.

Protostomatida (pro″to-sto-mat′ĭ-dah) [*proto-* + Gr. *stoma* mouth] an order of often large, commonly carnivorous ciliate protozoa (subclass Gymnostomatia, class Kinetofragminophorea), characterized by the presence of an apical or subapical cytostome; circumoral infraciliature involving anterior parts of all somatic kineties; and a typical polypoid independent macronucleus. It comprises four suborders: Archistomatina, Prostomatina, Prorodontina, and Haptorina.

protostome (pro′to-stōm) [*proto-* + Gr. *stoma* mouth] an individual of the Protostomia.

Protostomia (pro″to-sto′me-ah) a series of the Eucoelomata, including the mollusks, annelids, and arthropods, in all of which the mouth arises from the blastopore.

Protostrongylus (pro″to-stron′jĭ-lus) a genus of lung worms. **P. rufes′cens,** a species that infects sheep, goats, deer, and domestic rabbits.

protosulfate (pro″to-sul′fāt) that one of several sulfates of the same base which contains the smallest proportion of sulfate ion.

Prototheca (pro″to-the′kah) [*proto-* + Gr. *thēkē* sheath] a genus of ubiquitous yeastlike organisms generally considered as achloric algae, occurring as a spheroid, ovoid, or elliptical cell containing several thick-walled autospores. *P. wickerhamii* and *P. zopfii* are the species involved in human and animal infection (see *protothecosis*).

protothecosis (pro″to-the-ko′sis) [*proto-* + *theca* + *-osis*] an infection caused by organisms of the genus *Prototheca*, especially *P. wickerhamii* or *P. zopfii*, varying from cutaneous and subcutaneous lesions to systemic invasion involving several internal organs, which may occur as an opportunistic infection or as a result of traumatic implantation of the pathogen into the tissues.

Prototheria (pro″to-the′rĭ-ah) [*proto-* + Gr. *thērion* beast, animal] in some systems of classification, a subclass of the

Mammalia, including the order Monotremata, the egg-laying mammals.

prototroph (pro′to-trōf) [*proto-* + Gr. *trophē* nourishment] a prototrophic organism.

prototrophic (pro″to-trof′ik) having the same growth factor requirements as the ancestral or prototype strain; said of microbial mutants.

prototropy (pro-tot′ro-pe) proton tautomerism. Cf *anionotropy.*

prototype (pro′to-tīp) [*proto-* + Gr. *typos* type] 1. the original type or form after which other types or forms are developed. 2. in microbiology, the standard reference strain to which other strains are compared.

protoveratrine (pro″to-ver′ah-trēn) an ester alkaloid obtained from the liliaceous plants *Veratrum album* L. and *V. viride* Aiton, occurring in two forms, designated A and B, both of which possess antihypertensive properties. Protoveratrine A is said to be more active than the B form; the two are usually administered in combination.

protovertebra (pro″to-ver′te-brah) 1. somite. 2. the caudal half of a somite that forms most of a vertebra.

protoxide (pro-tok′sid) that one of a series of oxides of the same metal which contains the smallest amount of oxygen.

Protozoa (pro″to-zo′ah) [*proto-* + Gr. *zoon* animal] a subkingdom (formerly a phylum) comprising the simplest organisms of the animal kingdom, consisting of unicellular organisms that range in size from submicroscopic to macroscopic; most are free living, but some lead commensalistic, mutualistic, or parasitic existences. According to newer classifications, Protozoa is divided into seven phyla: Sarcomastigophora, Labyrinthomorphorpha, Apicomplexa, Microspora, Acetospora, Myxozoa, and Ciliophora. Cf. *Metazoa.*

protozoa (pro″to-zo′ah) plural of *protozoon.*

protozoacide (pro″to-zo′ah-sīd) destructive to protozoa; an agent destructive to protozoa.

protozoal (pro″to-zo′al) protozoan, def. 2.

protozoan (pro″to-zo′an) 1. any individual of the protozoa; protozoon. 2. of or pertaining to the protozoa; protozoal.

protozoiasis (pro″to-zo-i′ah-sis) any disease caused by protozoa.

protozoology (pro″to-zo-ol′o-je) the study of protozoa.

protozoon (pro″to-zo′on), pl. *protozo′a* [*proto-* + Gr. *zōon* animal] protozoan, def. 1.

protozoophage (pro″to-zo′o-fāj) [*protozoa* + Gr. *phagein* to eat] a cell which has a phagocytic action on protozoa.

protozoosis (pro″to-zo-o′sis) protozoiasis.

protraction (pro-trak′shun) [L. *protrahere* to drag forth] 1. drawing out or lengthening. 2. extension or protrusion. 3. a condition in which the teeth or other maxillary or mandibular structures are situated anterior to their normal position. **mandibular p.,** 1. the protrusive movement of the mandible initiated by the lateral and medial pterygoid muscles acting simultaneously. Cf. *mandibular retraction.* 2. a facial anomaly in which the gnathion lies anterior to the orbital plane. **maxillary p.,** a facial anomaly in which the subnasion is anterior to the orbital plane.

protractor (pro-trak′tor) [*pro-* + L. *trahere* to draw] an instrument for extracting bits of bone, bullets, or other foreign material from wounds.

protransglutaminase (pro-tranz″gloo-tam′ĭ-nās) the proenzyme of protein-glutamine γ-glutamyltransferase (transglutaminase).

protriptyline hydrochloride (pro-trip′tĭ-lēn) [USP] chemical name: *N* - methyl - 5*H* - dibenzo [*a,d*] cyclohepten-5-propylamine hydrochloride; a tricyclic antidepressant, $C_{19}H_{21}N \cdot HCl$, occurring as a white to yellowish powder; administered orally.

protrusio (pro-troo′ze-o) [L.] the state of being thrust forward; projection. **p. acetab′uli,** arthrokatadysis.

protrusion (pro-troo′zhun) [L. *protrudere* to push forward] the state of being thrust forward or laterally, as in masticatory movements of the mandible. **bimaxillary p.,** the projection of both the maxilla and the mandible beyond normal limits in relation to the cranial base. **bimaxillary dentoalveolar p.,** the positioning of the entire dentition forward with respect to the facial profile. **intrapelvic p.,** arthrokatadysis.

protrypsin (pro-trip′sin) a substance convertible into trypsin.

protuberance (pro-tu′ber-ans) [pro- + L. *tuber* bulge] a projecting part, or prominence; an apophysis, process, or swelling. For names of specific anatomical structures not included here, see under *protuberantia*. **p. of chin,** protuberantia mentalis. **laryngeal p.,** prominentia laryngea. **occipital p., transverse,** torus occipitalis. **palatine p.,** torus palatinus. **tubal p.,** torus tubarius.

protuberantia (pro-tu″ber-an′she-ah) [L.] protuberance: a projecting part, or prominence. **p. menta′lis** [NA], mental protuberance: a more or less distinct and triangular prominence on the anterior surface of the body of the mandible, on or near the median line. **p. occipita′lis exter′na** [NA], external occipital protuberance: a prominence at the center of the outer surface of the squama of the occipital bone which gives attachment to the ligamentum nuchae. **p. occipita′lis inter′na** [NA], internal occipital protuberance: the projection of bone at the midpoint of the cruciform eminence, on the internal surface of the squama of the occipital bone, sometimes presenting as a ridge (*crista occipitalis interna* [NA]).

protyl, protyle (pro′til) [proto- + Gr. *hylē* matter] a theoretical substance from which all the chemical elements were formerly supposed to be derived.

Provell (pro-vel′) trademark for a preparation of protoveratrines A and B.

proventriculus (pro″ven-trik′u-lus) [pro- + L. *ventriculus,* dim. of *venter* belly] 1. the glandular first portion of the stomach of birds, in which food from the crop is mixed with peptic enzymes and passed to the gizzard. 2. the portion of the foregut in certain invertebrates, e.g., some insects, which may function as a gizzard or as a valve into the stomach.

Provera (pro-ver′ah) trademark for preparations of medroxyprogesterone acetate.

provertebra (pro-ver′tĕ-brah) protovertebra.

Providencia (prŏ″vĭ-den′se-ah) [*Providence,* Rhode Island] a genus of gram-negative, facultatively anaerobic, motile, rod-shaped bacteria of the family Enterobacteriaceae, occurring in normal urine and feces. The organisms are potential pathogens associated with urinary tract and secondary tissue infections. It was formerly classified as a species of the genus *Proteus* (*P. inconstans*). **P. alcalifa′ciens,** a species that does not ferment trehalose or *myo*-inositol; isolated especially from stools of children with diarrhea. Called also *Proteus inconstans* subgroup A. **P. rett′geri,** a species isolated from human clinical specimens and from chicken feces, a possible cause of nosocomial infections. Called also *Proteus rettgeri*. **P. stuar′tii,** a species that ferments trehalose and *myo*-inositol. It causes nosocomial infections and is a major agent in burn infections. Called also *Proteus inconstans* subgroup B.

provirus (pro-vi′rus) the genome of an animal virus integrated (by crossing over) into the chromosome of the host cell, and thus replicated in all of its daughter cells.

provisional (pro-vizh′un-al) formed or performed for temporary purposes; temporary.

provitamin (pro-vi′tah-min) a precursor of a vitamin; a substance from which the animal organism can form vitamin. Provitamin A is carotene. Ergosterol has been spoken of as provitamin D.

provocative (pro-vok′ah-tiv) stimulating the appearance of a sign, reflex, reaction, or therapeutic effect.

Prowazek's bodies (pro-vaht′seks) [Stanislas Joseph Matthias von *Prowazek,* zoologist in Hamburg, 1875–1915] see under *body*.

Prowazek-Greeff bodies (pro-vaht′sek-grāf) [S. J. M. von *Prowazek;* Carl Richard *Greeff,* German ophthalmologist, 1862–1938] trachoma bodies.

proxazole (prok′sa-zōl) chemical name: N,N-diethyl-3-(1-phenylpropyl)-1,2,4-oxadiazole-5-ethanamine; a smooth muscle relaxant, analgesic, and anti-inflammatory, $C_{17}H_{25}N_3O$. **p. citrate,** the citrate salt of proxazole having the same actions as the base.

proxemics (prok-se′miks) the study of the effects of spatial distance between persons interacting with each other, and of their orientation toward each other.

proximad (prok′sĭ-mad) toward the proximal end or in a proximal direction.

proximal (prok′sĭ-mal) [L. *proximus* next] nearest; closer to any point of reference: opposed to *distal*.

proximalis (prok″sĭ-ma′lis) proximal; [NA] a term denoting proximity to the point of origin or attachment of an organ or part.

proximate (prok′sĭ-māt) [L. *proximatus* drawn near] immediate or nearest.

proximoataxia (prok″sĭ-mo-ah-tak′se-ah) ataxia affecting the proximal part of an extremity, as the arm, forearm, thigh, or leg.

proximobuccal (prok″sĭ-mo-buk′al) pertaining to the proximal and buccal surfaces of a posterior tooth.

proximoceptor (prok″sĭ-mo-sep′tor) contiguous receptor.

proximolabial (prok″sĭ-mo-la′be-al) pertaining to the proximal and labial surfaces of an anterior tooth.

proximolingual (prok″sĭ-mo-ling′gwal) pertaining to the proximal and lingual surfaces of a tooth.

prozonal (pro′zo-nal) 1. situated before a sclerozone. 2. pertaining to a prozone.

prozone (pro′zōn) [pro- + *zone*] in an agglutination or precipitation reaction, the zone of relatively high antibody concentrations within which no reaction occurs. As the antibody concentration is lowered below the prozone, the reaction occurs. This phenomenon may be due simply to antibody excess (see *precipitin reaction,* under *reaction*), or it may be due to blocking antibody or to nonspecific inhibitors in serum. Called also *prezone*.

PRPP phosphoribosylpyrophosphate.

PRU peripheral resistance unit.

prual (proo′al) a very violent poison from the root of the tropical flowering vine, *Coptosapelta flavescens;* used as a dart poison.

pruinate (proo′ĭ-nāt) [L. *pruina* hoarfrost] having the appearance of being covered with hoarfrost.

Prulet (pru′let) trademark for a preparation of oxyphenisatin acetate.

Prunella (proo-nel′ah) a genus of labiate plants. *P. vulgaris* L. (heal-all or self-heal) is astringent and tonic.

prunin (proo′nin) a concentration prepared from the wild black cherry, *Prunus serotina* Ehrh. (Rosaceae), formerly used in thoracic and nervous diseases.

Prunus (proo′nus) [L. "plum-tree"] a genus of rosaceous trees and shrubs, including the plums, cherries, sloes, apricots, and peaches, whose fruits are used for making liqueurs. **P. america′na,** Marsh., American wild plum or river plum. **P. amyg′dalus** Batsch., almond. **P. armenia′ca,** apricot. **P. commu′nis** L., almond. **P. domes′tica** L., garden plum. **P. laurocer′asus** L., cherry laurel. **P. per′sica,** peach. **P. serot′ina** Ehrh., a large American cherry tree with dark bark and thick oval leaves; called also *wild cherry*. **P. spino′sa** L., a species of plum, the sloe, or blackthorn sloe. **P. virginia′na** L., the choke cherry of North America; its bark has sedative, pectoral, and astringent qualities and its fruit is highly astringent.

pruriginous (proo-rij″ĭ-nus) of the nature of or tending to cause prurigo.

prurigo (proo-ri′go) [L. "the itch"] a name applied to several itchy skin eruptions of unknown cause, in which the characteristic lesion (prurigo papule) is dome-shaped with a small transient vesicle on top, followed by crusting and lichenification; specific types are usually indicated by a modifying term. **p. ag′ria,** a severe, chronic pruriginous dermatosis characterized chiefly by hard excoriated prurigo papules and lichenification. Called also *p. ferox*. **Besnier's p., p. of Besnier,** atopic dermatitis. **Besnier p. of pregnancy,** p. gestationis of Besnier. **p. chron′ica multifor′mis,** a pruriginous dermatosis characterized by the presence of prurigo papules, patches of lichenification and eczematization, enlarged regional lymph nodes, and eosinophilia. **p. estiva′lis,** a papular dermatosis regarded as a form of polymorphous light eruption, usually occurring in childhood during the summer months, and sometimes improving or resolving after puberty. Called also *summer p. of Hutchinson*. **p. fe′rox,** p. agria. **p. gestatio′nis of Besnier,** an extremely pruritic condition of unknown etiology occurring in the third trimester of pregnancy characterized by the development of tiny crust-covered excoriated papules mainly on the extensor surfaces of the limbs but also found on the upper trunk and other areas of the body, and leaving postinflammatory residua on resolution of the lesions. It tends to clear after delivery and to recur with subsequent pregnancies. Called also *Besnier's p. of pregnancy*. **p. of Hebra,** p. mitis. **melanotic p.,** a form associated with primary biliary cirrhosis in women, characterized by reticulated hyperpigmentation and intense itching. **p. mi′tis,** an extremely pruritic, chronic pruriginous dermatosis beginning in early childhood, characterized by excoriations, lichenification, and eczematization that become progressively more pronounced, and accompanied by enlarged glands and associated constitutional symptoms. The condition may be the same as papular urticaria. Called also *p. of Hebra.* **nodular p.,** a chronic, intensely pruritic form of neurodermatitis, usually occurring in women, located chiefly on the extremities, especially on the anterior thighs and legs, and characterized by the presence of single or multiple, pea-sized or larger, firm, and erythematous or brownish nodules that become verrucous or fissured. **p. sim′plex,** a form in which the prurigo papules are present in various stages of development, especially on the trunk and extensor surfaces of the extremities in middle-aged persons, and usually occur in crops. **summer p. of Hutchinson,** 1. p. estivalis. 2. hydroa vacciniforme.

pruritic (proo-rit′ik) pertaining to or characterized by pruritus.

pruritogenic (proo″rĭ-to-jen′ik) capable of causing or tending to cause pruritus.

pruritus (proo-ri′tus) [L. from *prurire* to itch] 1. itching; an unpleasant cutaneous sensation that provokes the desire to rub or scratch the skin to obtain relief. 2. any of various conditions marked by itching, the specific site or type being indicated by a modifying term. See also *itch.* **p. a′ni,** intense chronic itching in the anal region. **p. hiema′lis,** xerotic eczema. **p. scro′ti,** intense itching in the scrotal area. **senile p., p. seni′lis,** an itching in the aged, possibly due to dryness of the skin occurring as a result of decreased sweat and sebum secretion, or bathing too frequently, or both. **uremic p.,** generalized itching associated with chronic renal failure and not attributable to other internal or skin disease. **p. vul′vae,** intense itching of the external genitals of the female, as in kraurosis vulvae.

Prussak's fibers, pouch, space (proo′sahks) [Alexander *Prussak*, Russian otologist, 1839–1897] see under *fiber*, and see *recessus membranae tympani superior.*

prussiate (prus′e-āt) cyanide.

prussic acid (prus′ik) hydrocyanic acid.

Prymnesiida (prim″nĕ-si′ĭ-dah) an order of plantlike flagellate protozoa (class Phytomastigophorea, subphylum Mastigophora) having two equal or subequal flagella with one flagella-like appendage between them and golden-brown chloroplasts; they are covered by delicate organic scales, which in certain species calcify and form coccoliths. *Coccolithus* is a representative genus.

PS phosphatidylserine.

p.s. abbreviation for *per second.*

psalis (sa′lis) [Gr. "arch"] the fornix of the cerebrum (fornix cerebri [NA]).

psalterial (sal-te′re-al) pertaining to the psalterium.

psalterium (sal-te′re-um) [L.; Gr. *psaltērion* harp] 1. commissura fornicis. 2. the omasum.

Psalydolytta (sal″ĭ-do-lit′tah) a genus of blister beetles. *P. fusca* and *P. substrigata* of Africa produce a severe vesicular dermatitis.

Psamminida (sah-min′ĭ-dah) [Gr. *psammos* sand] an order of testaceous ameboid protozoa (class Xenophyophorea, superclass Rhizopoda) having a more or less rigid body.

psamm(o)- [Gr. *psammos* sand] a combining form meaning sandlike or denoting relation to sand.

psammocarcinoma (sam″o-kar″sĭ-no′mah) [psammo- + carcinoma] carcinoma containing calcareous matter.

psammoma (sam-o′mah) [psammo- + -oma] a tumor, especially a meningioma, that contains psammoma bodies; formerly sometimes called *Virchow's psammoma.*

psammosarcoma (sam″o-sar-ko′mah) [psammo- + sarcoma] a sarcoma containing a sandy deposit.

psammotherapy (sam″o-ther′ah-pe) [psammo- + Gr. *therapeia* treatment] ammotherapy.

psammous (sam′us) sandy.

psauoscopy (saw-os′ko-pe) [Gr. *psauein* to touch + *skopein* to examine] a method of physical examination by passing the ball of the index finger back and forth lightly over the margin of an abnormal area. Over the pathological area the finger seems to encounter greater resistance and the skin seems more tense and less supple.

pselaphesia (sel-ah-fe′ze-ah) [Gr. *psēlaphēsis* touching] the tactile sense.

psellism (sel′izm) [Gr. *psellisma* stammer] stammering or stuttering; see *stuttering.*

pseudacousis (soo″dah-koo′sis) [pseud- + Gr. *akousis* hearing] pseudacousma.

pseudacousma (soo″dah-kōōz′mah) [pseud- + Gr. *akousma* thing heard] a subjective sensation as if sounds were altered in pitch and quality.

pseudactinomycosis (soo-dak″tĭ-no-mi-ko′sis) pseudoactinomycosis.

pseudagraphia (soo″dah-gra′fe-ah) pseudoagraphia.

pseudalbuminuria (soo″dal-bu″mĭ-nu′re-ah) adventitious proteinuria.

Pseudamphistomum (sood″am-fis′to-mum) [pseud- + amphi- + Gr. *stoma* mouth] a genus of flukes; called also *Metorchis* and *Pseudoamphistomum.* **P. trunca′tum,** a species found in the bile ducts of cats, dogs, seals, and deer, and occasionally in man in Europe and India.

pseudangina (soo″dan-ji′nah) pseudoangina.

pseudankylosis (soo″dang-kĭ-lo′sis) pseudoankylosis.

pseudaphia (soo-da′fe-ah) [pseud- + Gr. *haphē* touch + -ia] defect in the power of perceiving touch.

pseudarthrosis (soo″dar-thro′sis) [pseud- + Gr. *arthrōsis* joint] a pathologic entity characterized by deossification of a weight-bearing long bone, followed by bending and pathologic fracture, with inability to form normal callus leading to existence of the "false joint" that gives the condition its name.

Pseudechis (soo-dek′is) [pseud- + Gr. *echis* viper] a genus of venomous elapid snakes of Australia, including *P. porphyria′cus,* the blacksnake. See table accompanying *snake.*

pseudencephalus (soo″den-sef′ah-lus) [pseud- + Gr. *enkephalos* brain] a monster with a vascular tumor in place of the brain.

pseudesthesia (soo″des-the′ze-ah) [pseud- + Gr. *aisthēsis* perception] any imaginary sensation; a sensation which is felt without any external stimulus, or a sensation which does not correspond to the stimulus that causes it.

pseud(o)- [Gr. *pseudēs* false] combining form signifying false or spurious.

pseudoacanthosis (soo″do-ak″an-tho′sis) [pseudo- + acanthosis] a condition clinically resembling acanthosis. **p. ni′gricans,** a benign form of acanthosis nigricans associated with obesity; the obesity is sometimes associated with endocrine disturbance.

pseudoacephalus (soo″do-a-sef′ah-lus) [pseudo- + acephalus] a placental parasitic twin, apparently headless, but with a rudimentary cranium contained in the autosite.

pseudoactinomycosis (soo″do-ak″tĭ-no-mi-ko′sis) [pseudo- + actinomycosis] a variety of chronic pulmonary disease resembling actinomycosis, usually nocardiosis.

pseudoagglutination (soo″do-ah-gloo″tĭ-na′shun) pseudohemagglutination.

pseudoagraphia (soo″do-ah-graf′e-ah) a condition in which the patient can copy writing, but cannot write except in a meaningless and illegible manner.

pseudoalbuminuria (soo″do-al″bu-mĭ-nu′re-ah) adventitious proteinuria.

pseudoalleles (soo″do-ah-lēlz′) [pseudo- + allele] genes that are seemingly allelic but can eventually be shown to have distinct but closely linked loci.

pseudoallelic (soo″do-ah-lel′ik) pertaining to pseudoalleles; seemingly allelic but located at different sites on homologous chromosomes.

pseudoallelism (soo″do-al′lĕ-lizm) the possession of pseudoalleles.

pseudoalveolar (soo″do-al-ve′o-lar) simulating an alveolar structure.

Pseudoamphistomum (soo″do-am-fis′to-mum) *Pseudamphistomum.*

pseudoanaphylactic (soo″do-an″ah-fi-lak′tik) pertaining to pseudoanaphylaxis.

pseudoanaphylaxis (soo″do-an″ah-fĭ-lak′sis) [*pseudo-* + *anaphylaxis*] a reaction resembling generalized anaphylaxis or anaphylactic shock that is produced by intravenous administration of serum that has been treated with agar, kaolin, or starch; it does not involve antigen-antibody reactions. Called also *anaphylactoid reaction* or *shock*.

pseudoanemia (soo″do-ah-ne′me-ah) [*pseudo-* + *anemia*] marked pallor with no clinical or hematological evidence of anemia. **p. angiospas′tica,** a form due to vasoconstriction.

pseudoaneurysm (soo″do-an′u-rizm) dilatation and tortuosity of a vessel, giving the appearance of an aneurysm.

pseudoangina (soo″do-an-ji′nah) [*pseudo-* + *angina*] false angina; a syndrome occurring in nervous individuals, marked by precordial pain, fatigue, and lassitude, without evidence of organic disease of the heart. See *angina pectoris vasomotoria*.

pseudoankylosis (soo″do-ang″kĭ-lo′sis) a false ankylosis.

pseudoanodontia (soo″do-an″o-don′she-ah) [*pseudo-* + *anodontia*] a condition characterized by the presence of multiple unerupted permanent teeth.

pseudoantagonist (soo″do-an-tag′o-nist) a muscle which by flexing a joint enhances the effect of another muscle crossing that joint to act on a more distant one.

pseudoapoplexy (soo″do-ap′o-plek″se) [*pseudo-* + *apoplexy*] a condition resembling apoplexy, but without cerebral hemorrhage.

pseudoappendicitis (soo″do-ah-pen″dĭ-si′tis) a condition with symptoms simulating appendicitis, sometimes hysterical and sometimes of syphilitic origin, but without affection of the appendix. **p. zooparasit′ica,** a condition in which parasites are present in the vermiform appendix.

pseudoarthrosis (soo″do-ar-thro′sis) pseudarthrosis.

pseudoasthma (soo″do-as′mah) paroxysmal dyspnea.

pseudoathetosis (soo″do-ath″e-to′sis) movements of the fingers elicited when the patient closes his eyes and extends his arms, associated with impairment of joint position sense.

pseudoatrophoderma colli (soo″do-at″ro-fo-der′mah kol′le) a skin disease characterized by papillomatous, depigmented, glossy lesions on the sides of the neck; the depigmented areas resemble vitiligo. It probably differs from confluent reticulated papillomatosis chiefly in its location.

pseudobacillus (soo″do-bah-sil′us) an exceedingly small, rodlike poikilocyte, resembling a microorganism.

pseudobacterium (soo″do-bak-te′re-um) [*pseudo-* + Gr. *baktērion* little rod] a cell that resembles a bacterium.

pseudobasedow (soo″do-baz′ĕ-dow) basedoid.

pseudobronchiectasis (soo″do-brong″ke-ek′tah-sis) a condition in which a bronchiectasis-like pattern appears in the bronchogram of partially atelectatic pulmonary segments when the larger bronchi have become shortened and broadened in outline; these reversible changes do not indicate destruction of the bronchial walls.

pseudobulbar (soo″do-bul′bar) apparently, but not really, due to a bulbar lesion.

Pseudocaedibacter (soo″do-se″dĭ-bak′ter) [*pseudo-* + *caedibacter*] a genus of bacteria of uncertain affiliation that are parasites of paramecia.

pseudocartilage (soo″do-kar′tĭ-lij) chondroid tissue.

pseudocartilaginous (soo″do-kar″tĭ-laj′ĭ-nus) composed of a substance resembling cartilage.

pseudocast (soo′do-kast) a false cast: a form of urinary sediment resembling true casts, but being an accidental formation, taking the shape of casts by adherence to mucous threads, cotton fibers, etc.

pseudocele (soo′do-sēl) cavitas septi pellucidi.

pseudocephalocele (soo″do-sef′ah-lo-sēl) a hernia of the brain not congenital, but due to disease or injury of the skull.

pseudochancre (soo″do-shang′ker) an indurated lesion resembling or simulating chancre. **p. re′dux,** a gummatous recurrence at the site of a primary syphilitic lesion.

pseudocholecystitis (soo″do-ko″le-sis-ti′tis) a syndrome resembling cholecystitis but occurring as an allergic response to eating certain foods.

pseudocholesteatoma (soo″do-ko″les-te-ah-to′mah) a

mass of cornified epithelial cells resembling cholesteatoma in the tympanic cavity in chronic middle ear inflammation.

pseudocholinesterase (soo″do-ko″lin-es′ter-ās) cholinesterase.

pseudochorea (soo″do-ko-re′ah) [*pseudo-* + *chorea*] a condition of complete general incoordination with symptoms like those of chorea.

pseudochromesthesia (soo″do-kro″mes-the′ze-ah) [*pseudo-* + Gr. *chrōma* color + *esthesia*] a synesthesia in which certain sounds induce sensations of color.

pseudochromidrosis (soo″do-kro″mid-ro′sis) [*pseudo-* + *chromidrosis*] the presence of pigment on the skin caused by the action of pigment-producing bacteria.

pseudochromosome (soo″do-kro′mo-sōm) rodlike Golgi bodies of the spermatocytes.

pseudochylous (soo″do-ki′lus) resembling chyle, but containing no fat.

pseudocirrhosis (soo″do-sĭ-ro′sis) [*pseudo-* + *cirrhosis*] an obsolete term used in the phrase *pericardial pseudocirrhosis of the liver* (Pick's disease, def. 2).

pseudoclaudication (soo″do-claw″dĭ-ka′shun) intermittent claudication due to compression of the cauda equina.

pseudoclonus (soo″do-klo′nus) a short-lived clonic response.

pseudocoarctation (soo″do-ko″ark-ta′shun) a substandard term used to refer to a condition roentgenologically resembling coarctation, but without compromise of the lumen of the affected structure; a "kinked aorta," possibly an aortic arch anomaly. **p. of the aorta,** an uncommon congenital anomaly of the arch of the aorta that simulates coarctation roentgenologically but does not produce occlusion of the vessel.

pseudocoele (soo′do-sēl) [*pseudo-* + Gr. *koilia* hollow] cavitas septi pellucidi.

pseudocoelom (soo″do-se′lom) in zoology, a body cavity between the mesoderm and endoderm; a persistent blastocoele.

pseudocoelomate (soo″do-sēl′o-māt) 1. having a pseudocoelom. 2. an animal having a pseudocoelom, as the aschelminths.

pseudocolloid (soo″do-kol′oid) a mucoid substance sometimes found in ovarian cysts.

pseudocoloboma (soo″do-kol″o-bo′mah) a line or scar on the iris giving the appearance of a coloboma.

pseudocopulation (soo″do-kop″u-la′shun) bodily association of male and female associated with liberation of gametes in proximity of space and time but without sexual union.

pseudo-corpus luteum (soo″do-kor′pus loo′te-um) a maturing graafian follicle which does not rupture but retains its ovum and then becomes luteinized.

pseudocowpox (soo″do-kow′poks) paravaccinia.

pseudocoxalgia (soo″do-kok-sal′je-ah) osteochondrosis of the capitular epiphysis of the femur; see under *osteochondrosis*.

pseudocrisis (soo-dok′rĭ-sis) [*pseudo-* + Gr. *krisis* crisis] a false crisis; a sudden but temporary abatement of febrile symptoms.

pseudocroup (soo″do-krōōp′) 1. laryngismus stridulus. 2. thymic asthma.

pseudocyanin (soo″do-si′ah-nin) pseudoisocyanin.

pseudocyesis (soo″do-si-e′sis) [*pseudo-* + Gr. *kyēsis* pregnancy] false pregnancy.

pseudocylindroid (soo″do-sĭ-lin′droid) a shred of mucin in the urine resembling a cylindroid; sometimes of spermatic origin.

pseudocyst (soo′do-sist) [*pseudo-* + *cyst*] 1. an abnormal or dilated cavity resembling a true cyst but not lined with epithelium. Called also *adventitious* or *false cyst*. 2. a cystic collection of fluid and necrotic debris whose walls are formed by the pancreas and other surrounding organs. It occurs as a complication of acute pancreatitis, and may subside spontaneously or become secondarily infected and develop into an abscess. Cf. *phlegmon*, def. 2. 3. a cluster of small, comma-shaped forms of *Toxoplasma gondii* (bradyzoites), perhaps containing thousands of organisms, enclosed by an irregular wall, and representing a resting stage, as opposed to the active, motile stage (*tachyzoite*); pseudocysts are found in the tissues, especially muscles and the brain, in chronic (latent) *toxoplasmosis.* Called also *tissue cyst.* **pancreatic p.,** see *pseudocyst,* def. 2.

pseudodementia (soo″do-de-men′she-ah) 1. a disorder resembling dementia that is not due to organic brain disease and can be reversed by treatment. 2. extreme apathy and indifference to one's surroundings in the absence of a mental disorder. **hysterical p.,** a condition marked by failure of memory, with seeming inability to answer simple questions, and by a psychotic-like state accompanied by bizarre behavior and episodes of excitement or stupor.

pseudodextrocardia (soo″do-deks″tro-kar′de-ah) a condition in which the heart is displaced to the right, but the ventricles are not inverted nor are the great vessels transposed.

pseudodiabetes (soo″do-di″ah-be′tēz) subclinical diabetes.

pseudodiastolic (soo″do-di″ah-stol′ik) apparently but not truly diastolic.

pseudodiphtheria (soo″do-dif-the′re-ah) the presence of a false membrane not due to *Corynbacterium diphtheriae.*

pseudodominant (soo″do-dom′ĭ-nant) quasidominant.

pseudodysentery (soo″do-dis′en-ter″e) a condition marked by the symptoms of dysentery, but due to some local irritation and not to the organisms of dysentery.

pseudoedema (soo″do-ĕ-de′mah) a puffy state resembling edema.

pseudoembryonic (soo″do-em″bre-on′ik) apparently, but not truly, embryonic.

pseudoemphysema (soo″do-em″fĭ-ze′mah) a condition resembling emphysema, but due to temporary blocking of the bronchial tubes.

pseudoencephalomalacia (soo″do-en-sef″ah-lo-mah-la′she-ah) a highly fatal disease of cattle, sheep, and pigs, marked by edema of the brain, with muzzle twitching, opisthotonos, blindness, and inability to stand.

pseudoendometritis (soo″do-en″do-mě-tri′tis) a condition simulating endometritis, in which there are changes in the blood vessels, hyperplasia of the stroma and glands, and atrophy.

pseudoeosinophil (soo″do-e″o-sin′o-fil) neutrophilic leukocytes with granules showing a predilection for acid dyes.

pseudoephedrine (soo″do-ě-fed′rin) chemical name: [S-($R*,R*$)]-α-[1-(methylamino)ethyl]benzenemethanol. One of the stereoisomers of ephedrine, $C_{10}H_{15}NO$, having less pressor action and central stimulant effects than ephedrine. **p. hydrochloride** [USP], the hydrochloride salt of pseudoephedrine, $C_{10}H_{15}NO \cdot HCl$, occurring as fine, white to off-white crystals or as a powder; used as a nasal decongestant, and as a bronchodilator, administered orally.

pseudoepiphysis (soo″do-e-pif′ĭ-sis) an accessory bone at the distal and the proximal end of the second metacarpal bone.

pseudoesthesia (soo″do-es-the′ze-ah) pseudesthesia.

pseudoexfoliation (soo″do-eks″fo-le-a′shun) a condition resembling exfoliation but actually resulting from deposition, as from the deposition of small grayish particles on the capsule of the crystalline lens.

pseudoexophoria (soo″do-ek″so-fo′re-ah) [*pseudo-* + *exophoria*] an outward tendency of the visual axis excited by diminishing the activity of the accommodative centers.

pseudoextrophy (soo″do-ek′stro-fe) a developmental anomaly marked by the characteristic musculoskeletal defects of exstrophy of the bladder but with no major defect of the urinary tract.

pseudofarcy (soo′do-far′se) lymphangitis epizootica.

pseudofluctuation (soo′do-fluk″tu-a′shun) a tremor resembling fluctuation, such as is sometimes seen on tapping lipomas or muscular tissue.

pseudofolliculitis (soo″do-fo-lik″u-li′tis) [*pseudo-* + *folliculitis*] a bacterial disorder, usually caused by *Staphylococcus aureus,* occurring chiefly in the beard of blacks, especially in the submandibular region of the neck, the characteristic lesions being erythematous papules, sometimes pustules, containing buried hairs whose tips can easily be freed up; in contrast to sycosis barbae, which is most often seen in bearded men, pseudofolliculitis affects exclusively those who shave. Called also *barber's itch* and *p. barbae.*

pseudofracture (soo″do-frak′tūr) a condition seen in the roentgenogram of a bone as a thickening of the periosteum and formation of new bone over what looks like an incomplete fracture.

pseudofructose (soo″do-fruk′tōs) a form of fructose, differing from it in the carbon atom configuration.

pseudoganglion (soo″do-gang′gle-on) a thickening of a nerve simulating a ganglion. **Bochdalek's p.,** plexus dentalis superior. **Cloquet's p.,** see under *ganglion.* **Valentin's p.,** intumescentia tympanica.

pseudogene (soo″do-jēn) [*pseudo-* + *gene*] a DNA sequence that is similar to an active gene in base sequence but is not transcribed.

pseudogestation (soo″do-jes-ta′shun) false pregnancy.

pseudogeusesthesia (soo″do-gūs″es-the′ze-ah) [*pseudo-* + Gr. *geusis* taste + *aisthēsis* perception + *-ia*] a false sensation of taste associated with a sensation of another modality.

pseudogeusia (soo″do-gu′ze-ah) [*pseudo-* + Gr. *geusis* taste + *-ia*] a sensation of taste inappropriate to the exciting stimulus or occurring in the absence of a stimulus.

pseudoglanders (soo″do-glan′derz) lymphangitis ulcerosa pseudofarcinosa.

pseudoglioma (soo″do-gli-o′mah) a condition resembling glioma, a membrane being produced behind the lens because of failure of the posterior vascular sheath of the lens to atrophy, or because of its replacement by connective tissue.

pseudoglobulin (soo″do-glob′u-lin) one of a class of globulins characterized by being soluble in water in the absence of neutral salts and thus not a true globulin (euglobulin); see also under *globulin.*

pseudoglottic (soo″do-glot′ik) pertaining to the pseudoglottis.

pseudoglottis (soo″do-glot′is) 1. the aperture between the false vocal cords. 2. neoglottis.

pseudoglucosazone (soo″do-gloo″ko-sa′zōn) a crystalline substance sometimes developed in normal urine in testing for sugar.

pseudogonorrhea (soo″do-gon″o-re′ah) nongonococcal urethritis.

pseudogout (soo′do-gowt) [*pseudo-* + *gout*] an apparently hereditary, arthritic condition marked by attacks of goutlike symptoms, usually affecting a single joint (particularly the knee) and associated with chondrocalcinosis.

pseudographia (soo″do-graf′e-ah) [*pseudo-* + Gr. *graphein* to write + *-ia*] the production of meaningless written symbols.

pseudogynecomastia (soo″do-jin″ě-ko-mas′te-ah) an excess of adipose tissue in the male breast with no increase in glandular tissue.

pseudohallucination (soo″do-hah-loo″sǐ-na′shun) a hallucination brought about by the exercise of memory and imagination; the person experiencing it realizes that it is not real.

pseudohaustration (soo″do-haw-stra′shun) a false appearance of normal sacculation of the wall of the colon, the roentgenographic appearance being produced by edematous islands of mucosa regularly placed between deep areas of ulceration in the muscle layers.

pseudohelminth (soo″do-hel′minth) [*pseudo-* + Gr. *helmins* worm] a structure or object that resembles an endoparasitic worm.

pseudohemagglutination (soo″do-hem″ah-gloo″tǐ-na′shun) a clumping of erythrocytes due to rouleau formation.

pseudohematuria (soo″do-he″mah-tu′re-a) the presence in the urine of pigments that impart to it a pink or red color, but with no detectable hemoglobin or blood cells.

pseudohemophilia (soo″do-he″mo-fil′e-ah) von Willebrand's disease.

pseudohemoptysis (soo″do-he-mop′tǐ-sis) spitting of blood which comes from some source other than the lungs or bronchial tubes.

pseudohereditary (soo″do-hě-red′ĭ-tār″e) occurring in successive generations because of imposition of the same environmental factors and not because of genetic transmission.

pseudohermaphrodism (soo″do-her-maf′ro-dizm) pseudohermaphroditism.

pseudohermaphrodite (soo″do-her-maf′ro-dīt) an individual who has gonadal tissue of one sex and shows one or more contradictions of the morphological criteria of sex. See also *intersex* and *hermaphrodite.* **female p.,** a genetic and gonadal female, with partial masculinization; called also *female intersex.* **male p.,** a genetic and gonadal male with incomplete masculinization; called also *male intersex.*

pseudohermaphroditism (soo″do-her-maf′ro-dīt-izm″) a condition in which the gonads are of one sex but one or more contradictions exist in the morphologic criteria of sex. See also *intersexuality* and *hermaphroditism.* **female p.,** a form in which the affected individual is a genetic and gonadal female with partial masculinization. **male p.,** a form in which the affected individual is a genetic and gonadal male with incomplete masculinization.

pseudohernia (soo″do-her′ne-ah) an inflamed sac or gland simulating strangulated hernia.

pseudoheterotopia (soo″do-het″er-o-to′pe-ah) displacement of gray or white matter of the brain or cord, produced by unskillful manipulation during the autopsy.

pseudohydrocephalus (soo″do-hi″dro-sef′ah-lus) abnormally large appearance of a normal-sized head, due to smallness of the face and body, as in Russell's syndrome.

pseudohydronephrosis (soo″do-hi″dro-ne-fro′sis) a paranephritic cyst.

pseudohyoscyamine (soo″do-hi″o-si′ah-min) norhyoscyamine.

pseudohyperkalemia (soo″do-hi″per-kah-le′me-ah) a laboratory artifact in which serum potassium is elevated when plasma potassium is normal. It occurs in the presence of thrombocytosis or leukocytosis, most commonly in myeloproliferative disorders, because blood clotting causes the release of potassium from platelets and leukocytes.

pseudohypertrichosis (soo″do-hi″per-tri-ko′sis) persistence after birth of the fine hair present during fetal life, owing to inability of the skin to throw it off.

pseudohypertrophic (soo″do-hi″per-trof′ik) characterized by apparent, but not real, hypertrophy.

pseudohypertrophy (soo″do-hi-per′tro-fe) false hypertrophy; increase of size without true hypertrophy. **muscular p.,** an increase in the size of a muscle which is not due to enlargement of muscle fibers but to infiltration of the muscle with other tissue.

pseudohypoaldosteronism (soo″do-hi″po-al-dos′ter-ōn-izm) a hereditary disorder of infancy characterized by severe salt loss by the kidneys despite elevated secretion and urinary excretion of aldosterone; it is thought to be due to unresponsiveness of the distal renal tubule to aldosterone. Affected infants outgrow the need for dietary salt supplements in early childhood. The term is also applied to the endocrine abnormality associated with sodium-losing nephropathy, usually due to chronic pyelonephritis, in adults.

pseudohyponatremia (soo″do-hi″po-nah-tre′me-ah) a decreased serum sodium concentration that does not correspond to a real hypotonic disorder, i.e., the serum osmolality is normal. It occurs when hyperlipemia increases the serum non-water volume or hyperproteinemia increases the serum non-sodium solute.

pseudohypoparathyroidism (soo″do-hi″po-par″ah-thi′-roi-dizm) a hereditary condition clinically resembling hypoparathyroidism, but caused by failure of response to rather than deficiency of parathyroid hormone. It is characterized by hypocalcemia and hyperphosphatemia, and is commonly associated with short stature, obesity, short metacarpals, and ectopic calcification.

pseudohypophosphatasia (soo″do-hi″po-fos″fah-ta′ze-ah) a condition resembling hypophosphatasia, characterized by osteopathy of the skull and long bones, muscular hypotonia, hypercalcemia, and phosphoethanolaminuria. It is distinguished by normal alkaline phosphatase activity.

pseudohypothyroidism (soo″do-hi″po-thi′roi-dizm) the inability to utilize thyroxine in tissue cells, despite normal thyroid function, leading to development of the symptoms and certain stigmata of hypothyroidism.

pseudoicterus (soo″do-ik′ter-us) pseudojaundice.

pseudoinfarction (soo″do-in-fark′shun) the simulation in the electrocardiographic pattern of myocardial infarction, due to other cardiopathies.

pseudoion (soo″do-i′on) one of the electrically charged particles of a colloidal solution.

pseudoisochromatic (soo″do-i″so-kro-mat′ik) seemingly of the same color throughout: applied to solutions for testing color blindness, containing two pigments which will be distinguished by the normal eye, but not by the color blind. Cf. *anisochromatic.*

pseudoisocyanin (soo″do-i″so-si′ah-nin) an orange metachromatic dye, N,N^1-diethyl pseudoisocyanin, used for the selective demonstration of insulin in pancreatic islet beta cells.

pseudojaundice (soo″do-jawn′dis) skin discoloration caused by blood changes and not due to liver disease, as in carotinemia. Called also *pseudoicterus.*

pseudokeratin (soo″do-ker′ah-tin) false keratin, found in the skin and the nervous system.

pseudolamellar (soo″do-lah-mel′ar) resembling lamellae.

pseudoleukemia (soo″do-lu-ke′me-ah) an obsolete term for a group of conditions resembling one another in showing enlargement of the lymph glands and in characteristics which resemble the conditions present in leukemia, but without leukemic blood findings. The term included aleukemic lymphadenosis, aleukemic myelosis, Hodgkin's disease, Kundrat's lymphosarcoma, multiple myeloma, and tuberculosis and syphilis of the lymph glands. See *lymphogranulomatosis,* and *agnogenic myeloid metaplasia,* under *metaplasia.* **p. cu′tis,** pseudoleukemia with the development of skin lesions. **p. gastrointestina′lis,** a condition characterized by extensive lymphocytic infiltration of the gastrointestinal tract, without the typical clinical picture of leukemia. **p. lymphat′ica,** nonsplenic leukemia, a state associated with Hodgkin's disease and also with lymphomatous tumors of the kidneys and intestines in children. **myelogenous p.,** former term for multiple myeloma.

pseudoleukocythemia (soo″do-lu″ko-si-the′me-ah) pseudoleukemia.

pseudolithiasis (soo″do-li-thi′ah-sis) a condition with symptoms of spasm resembling biliary colic.

pseudologia (soo″do-lo′je-ah) [*pseudo-* + Gr. *logos* word + *-ia*] lying; falsehood. **p. fantas′tica,** a tendency to tell extravagant and fantastic falsehoods centered about one's self.

pseudoluxation (soo″do-luk-sa′shun) partial dislocation of a bone.

pseudolymphoma (soo″do-lim-fo′mah) [*pseudo-* + *lymphoma*] a group of disorders having a benign course but exhibiting clinical and histologic features suggestive of malignant lymphoma. Called also *lymphocytoma.* **p. of Spiegler-Fendt,** lymphocytoma cutis.

Pseudolynchia (soo″do-linch′e-a) a genus of parasitic flies of the family Hippoboscidae. **P. canarien′sis, P. mau′rah,** a species of pigeon flies that are vectors of *Haemoproteus columbae;* called also *Lynchia maura.*

pseudomalignancy (soo″do-mah-lig′nan-se) [*pseudo-* + *malignancy*] a group of tumors exhibiting benign clinical behavior but having a distinctly malignant microscopic appearance; the group includes pseudolymphoma, pseudomelanoma, and pseudosarcoma.

pseudomamma (soo″do-mam′ah) a structure resembling a nipple, or even a complete breast, sometimes found on ovarian dermoids.

pseudomania (soo″do-ma′ne-ah) [*pseudo-* + Gr. *mania* madness] 1. false or pretended mental disorder. 2. a mental disorder in which the patient admits to crimes of which he is innocent.

pseudomasturbation (soo″do-mas″tur-ba′shun) peotillomania.

pseudomegacolon (soo″do-meg″ah-ko″lon) dilatation of the colon in adults. Cf. *megacolon.*

pseudomelanoma (soo″do-mel″ah-no′mah) [*pseudo-* + *melanoma*] a benign melanotic lesion resembling a superficial spreading melanoma occurring at the site of an incompletely removed melanocytic nevus.

pseudomelanosis (soo″do-mel″ah-no′sis) a staining of the tissue after death with pigments from the blood.

pseudomelia (soo″do-me′le-ah) [*pseudo-* + Gr. *melos* limb + *-ia*] phantom limb. **p. paraesthet′ica,** the perception of various morbid or perverted sensations as occurring in an absent or paralyzed limb.

pseudomembrane (soo″do-mem′brān) false membrane; see under *membrane.*

pseudomembranelle (soo″do-mem′brah-nel) [*pseudo-* + *membranelle*] 1. a membranelle-like organelle, composed of a group of complex kinetofragments, representing a modified frange in certain ciliate protozoa. Called also *pavé.* 2. loosely, any of various membranelle-like ciliary complexes seen in protozoa.

pseudomembranous (soo″do-mem′brah-nus) marked by or pertaining to a *pseudomembrane.*

pseudomeningitis (soo″do-men″in-ji′tis) pial inflammation with symptoms resembling meningitis.

pseudomenstruation (soo″do-men″stroo-a′shun) uterine discharge unattended with endometrial changes of menstruation, usually occurring in newborn babies.

pseudomethemoglobin (soo″do-met-he″mo-glo′bin) methemalbumin.

pseudomicrocephalus (soo″do-mi″kro-sef′ah-lus) an individual with a small brain due to the atrophy of one hemisphere, probably acquired secondarily.

pseudomonad (su″do-mo′nad) any member of the genus *Pseudomonas.*

Pseudomonadaceae (soo″do-mo″nah-da′se-e) a family of bacteria consisting of gram-negative, aerobic, straight or curved rods that are motile with polar flagella, occurring in soil and fresh and salt water. It contains the genera *Frateuria, Pseudomonas, Xanthomonas,* and *Zoogloea.*

Pseudomonadales (soo″do-mo″nah-da′lēz) an order of bacteria used in some systems of classification to denote those organisms that possess polar flagella; cf. *Eubacteriales.*

Pseudomonadineae (soo″do-mo″nah-di′ne-e) in former systems of classification, a suborder of Pseudomonadales, made up of bacteria containing pigments.

Pseudomonas (soo″do-mo′nas) [*pseudo-* + Gr. *monas* unit, from *monos* single] a genus of gram-negative bacteria of the family Pseudomonadaceae, consisting of straight or curved rods that are motile by polar flagella. The genus comprises several hundred species, including many of uncertain status. Most species are strict aerobes and some produce pigments. The organisms are usually saprophytic, being found in soil, water, and decomposing matter; some are pathogenic for plants and animals. **P. acidov′orans,** a widespread species that is an occasional opportunistic pathogen. **P. aerugino′sa,** the type species of the genus. The organisms produce pyocyanin and fluorescein, which give the color to "blue pus" observed in certain suppurative infections. *P. aeruginosa* is a major agent of nosocomial infection, especially in debilitated patients, causing severe and often fatal infections most commonly involving the urinary tract, wounds, abscesses, or the bloodstream; it may also cause eye infections in those who use contact lenses. It produces a variety of toxins and enzymes. Called also *Bacterium aeruginosum, Bacillus pyocyaneus, P. polycolor,* and *P. pyocyanea.* **P. alcali′genes,** an occasionally opportunistic species found in water reservoirs and recovered from clinical specimens of blood, urine, respiratory tract, and abscesses. It has been associated with empyema and eye infections. **P. cepa′cia,** a widespread species isolated from clinical specimens and hospital equipment and supplies that is an opportunistic pathogen and causes various nosocomial infections. It appears to be an important respiratory pathogen in children with cystic fibrosis. Called also *P. multivorans.* **P. diminu′ta,** a species isolated from waters of streams and ditches and from clinical specimens. **P. eisenber′gii,** *P. putida.* **P. fluores′cens,** a fluorescent species that is an environmental contaminant and occasionally an opportunistic pathogen for humans, causing infections of the urinary tract, wounds, and the bloodstream. It also occurs as a contaminant of blood and blood products used for transfusion, sometimes causing fatal shock. **P. mal′lei,** a nonmotile species that is pathogenic chiefly for horses, causing glanders; it may also infect other animals and humans. Called also *Actinobacillus mallei, Bacillus mallei,* and *Pfeifferella mallei.* **P. maltophil′ia,** a widespread species that is occasionally an opportunistic pathogen, causing infections of the upper respiratory tract, wounds, blood, and urine. **P. mendoci′na,** a nonpathogenic species isolated from soil, water, and urine. **P. multivo′rans,** *P. cepacia.* **P. paucimobil′is,** a species isolated from clinical specimens and environmental sources that may be an opportunistic pathogen. **P. pertucinog′ena,** a species that produces

pertucin. Called also *Bordetella pertussis,* Phase IV. **P. picket′tii,** a species isolated from numerous clinical and environmental sources that is a potential human pathogen. One biovar, a strain formerly called *P. thomasii,* has been isolated from contaminated intravenous fluids and identified as the cause of nosocomial infections of the blood and urinary and respiratory tracts. **P. polyco′lor,** *P. aeruginosa.* **P. pseudoalcali′genes,** a species isolated from water reservoirs and clinical specimens that is sometimes associated with infection. **P. pseudomal′lei,** the species that causes melioidosis, an endemic glanders-like disease of humans and animals, especially in Southeast Asia. It has been isolated from soil and water in tropical regions. Called also *Actinobacillus pseudomallei, Bacillus pseudomallei, Malleomyces pseudomallei,* and *Whitmore's bacillus.* **P. pu′tida,** a fluorescent species that is a common inhabitant of soil, water, and plants. It is frequently isolated from clinical specimens, and is occasionally an opportunistic pathogen. Called also *P. eisenbergii.* **P. putrefa′ciens,** a species of wide distribution that causes spoilage in marine foods, butter, and meats. It has been recovered from clinical specimens, occasionally associated with infection. Called also *Alteromonas putrefaciens.* **P. pyocya′nea,** *P. aeruginosa.* **P. reptiliv′ora,** a species which is pathogenic for lizards. **P. sep′tica,** a species which causes a disease of caterpillars. **P. stani′eri,** *P. stutzeri.* **P. stut′zeri,** a widespread species often recovered from clinical specimens. It is an occasional opportunistic pathogen, particularly in drug addicts. Called also *P. stanieri.* **P. syncya′nea,** a species isolated from blue milk, which produces the blue pigment responsible for its color. **P. testostero′ni,** a widespread species found in soil and isolated from clinical specimens. **P. thoma′sii,** *P. pickettii.* **P. vesicula′ris,** a species isolated from water and clinical specimens. It has been associated with genitourinary tract infections. Called also *Corynebacterium vesiculare.*

Pseudomonilia (soo″do-mo-nil′e-ah) *Candida.*

pseudomorphine (soo″do-mor′fin) a compound, $C_{34}H_{36}N_2O_6 \cdot 3H_2O$, occurring in opium and prepared by the oxidation of morphine; called also *dehydromorphine.*

pseudomotor (soo″do-mo′tor) producing movements which are not normal.

pseudomucin (soo″do-mu′sin) a substance resembling mucin found in ovarian cysts.

pseudomucinous (soo″do-mu′sĭ-nus) pertaining to pseudomucin.

pseudomyiasis (soo″do-mi-i′ah-sis) the presence of fly maggots in the digestive tract due to ingestion; if present in large numbers, they may cause diarrhea and other symptoms.

pseudomyopia (soo″do-mi-o′pe-ah) [*pseudo-* + *myopia*] defective vision resembling myopia, caused by spasm of the ciliary muscle or by failure of relaxation of accommodation.

pseudomyxoma (soo″do-mik-so′mah) a colloid growth developed upon the peritoneum, often secondary to an ovarian dermoid cyst. **p. peritone′i,** the presence in the peritoneal cavity of mucoid matter from a ruptured ovarian cyst or a ruptured mucocele of the appendix; called also *hydrops spurius.*

pseudonarcotic (soo″do-nar-kot′ik) sedative and apparently, but not directly, narcotic.

pseudonarcotism (soo″do-nar′ko-tizm) a hysterical condition simulating narcosis.

pseudoneoplasm (soo″do-ne′o-plazm) [*pseudo-* + *neoplasm*] a temporary formation resembling a tumor.

pseudoneuritis (soo″do-nu-ri′tis) [*pseudo-* + *neuritis*] a hyperemic condition of the optic papilla, occurring as a congenital anomaly.

pseudoneuroma (soo″do-nu-ro′mah) [*pseudo-* + *neuroma*] a tumor on a nerve simulating a neuroma; false neuroma.

pseudoneuronophagia (soo″do-nu-ro″no-fa′je-ah) a false appearance of phagocytosis of nerve cells.

Pseudonocardia (soo″do-no-kar′de-ah) [Gr. *pseudes* false + *nocardia*] in former systems of classification, a genus of bacteria of the family Nocardiaceae, order Actinomycetales, characterized by aerial hyphae that grow by budding. The organisms have now been assigned to other genera.

pseudonucleolus (soo″do-nu-kle′o-lus) [*pseudo-* + *nucleolus*] karyosome.

pseudonystagmus (soo″do-nis-tag′mus) end-position nystagmus.

pseudo-obstruction (soo″do-ob-struk′shun) a condition simulating obstruction. **intestinal p.,** a condition characterized by constipation, colicky pain, and vomiting, but without evidence of organic obstruction apparent at laparotomy.

pseudo-ochronosis (soo″do-o-kro′no-sis) a condition resembling ochronosis, but not caused by a disorder of metabolism.

pseudo-optogram (soo″do-op′to-gram) an optogram in which the rods strip off from the illuminated spot and only the cones remain.

pseudo-osteomalacia (soo″do-os″te-o-mah-la′she-ah) rachitic contraction of the pelvis.

pseudo-ovum (soo″do-o′vum) a large prominent cell, resembling an ovum, seen in granuloma-cell tumor.

pseudopapilledema (soo″do-pap″ĭ-lĕ-de′mah) [pseudo- + papilledema] anomalous elevation of the optic disk.

pseudoparalysis (soo″do-pah-ral′ĭ-sis) false paralysis: apparent loss of muscular power, without true paralysis, marked by defective coordination of movements or by repression of movement on account of pain. **p. ag′itans,** paralysis agitans. **arthritic general p.,** a condition resembling general paralysis, dependent on intracranial atheroma in arthritic persons; called also *Klippel's disease.* **congenital atonic p.,** amyotonia congenita. **Parrot's p., syphilitic p.,** pseudoparalysis of one or more of the extremities in infants caused by syphilitic osteochondritis of an epiphysis.

pseudoparaplegia (soo″do-par″ah-ple′je-ah) spurious paralysis of the lower limbs, as in malingering or hysteria.

pseudoparasite (soo″do-par′ah-sīt) any object resembling or mistaken for a parasite.

pseudoparesis (soo″do-pah-re′sis) a hysterical or other nonorganic condition simulating paresis.

pseudopelade (soo″do-pe′lād) [pseudo- + pelade] an uncommon type of alopecia characterized by the asymptomatic development of a distinctive cicatricial patchy alopecia in adults.

pseudopellagra (soo″do-pĕ-lag′rah) a condition in alcoholics once thought to be similar but not known to be identical to pellagra.

pseudopeptone (soo″do-pep′tōn) ovomucoid.

pseudopericardial (soo″do-per″ĭ-kar′de-al) seemingly, but not actually, arising from the pericardium.

pseudoperitonitis (soo″do-per″ĭ-to-ni′tis) peritonism.

pseudophakia (soo″do-fa′ke-ah) a condition in which the degenerated crystalline lens is replaced by mesodermal tissue. **p. adipo′sa,** a condition in which the crystalline lens is replaced by a mass of fatty tissue. **p. fibro′sa,** replacement of the crystalline lens by a mass of connective tissue that represents hyperplasia of both the anterior and posterior vascular sheaths of the lens.

pseudophotesthesia (soo″do-fo″tes-the′ze-ah) the perception of light on receipt of a stimulus other than light.

pseudophthisis (soo-dof′thi-sis) a wasting disease not of the nature of tuberculosis.

Pseudophyllidea (soo″do-fĭ-lid′e-ah) an order of cestodes in which the scolex typically has two opposing sucking organs. It includes the family Diphyllobothriidae.

pseudophyllidean (soo″do-fil-lid′e-an) pertaining to or caused by tapeworms of the order Pseudophyllidea.

pseudoplasm (soo′do-plazm) a new growth which disappears spontaneously.

pseudoplasmodium (soo″do-plaz-mo′de-um) [pseudo- + plasmodium] a multinucleate plasmodium-like body formed by aggregation of myxamebae without fusion of their protoplasm.

pseudoplegia (soo″do-ple′je-ah) [pseudo- + Gr. plēgē stroke + -ia] hysterical paralysis or pseudoparalysis.

pseudopneumonia (soo″do-nu-mo′ne-ah) a condition marked by the symptoms of pneumonia, but without any lesions in the lungs.

pseudopodia (soo″do-po′de-ah) [L.] plural of pseudopodium.

pseudopodiospore (soo″do-po′de-o-spōr) [pseudopodium + spore] amebula, def. 2.

pseudopodium (soo″do-po′de-um), pl. *pseudopo′dia* [L., from pseudo- + Gr. pous foot] a temporary cytoplasmic extrusion by means of which an ameba or other ameboid organism or cell moves about or engulfs food. Pseudopodia are of four types: axopodia, filopodia, lobopodia, and reticulopodia.

pseudopoliomyelitis (soo″do-po″le-o-mi″ĕ-li′tis) a poliomyelitis-like disease caused by an enterovirus other than poliovirus.

pseudopolycythemia (soo″do-pol′e-si-the′me-ah) 1. stress polycythemia. 2. relative polycythemia.

pseudopolymelia (soo″do-pol′e-me′le-ah) an illusory sensation which may be referred to many extreme portions of the body, including the nose, nipples, and glans penis, as well as the hands and feet. **p. paraesthet′ica,** the perception of various morbid or perverted sensations, referred to various extreme portions of the body.

pseudopolyp (soo″do-pol′ip) a hypertrophied tab of mucous membrane resembling a polyp, but caused by ulceration surrounding and sometimes undermining a portion of intact mucosa; frequently observed in chronic inflammatory diseases, such as ulcerative colitis.

pseudopolyposis (soo″do-pol″ĭ-po′sis) the occurrence of numbers of pseudopolyps in the colon and rectum, as the result of long-standing inflammation.

pseudopregnancy (soo″do-preg′nan-se) 1. false pregnancy. 2. the premenstrual stage of the endometrium; so called because it resembles the endometrium just before implantation of the blastocyst.

pseudoproteinuria (soo″do-pro″te-in-u′re-ah) adventitious proteinuria.

pseudopseudohypoparathyroidism (soo″do-soo″do-hi″po-par″ah-thi′roid-izm) an incomplete form of pseudohypoparathyroidism characterized by the same constitutional features but by normal levels of calcium and phosphorus in the serum.

pseudopsia (soo-dop′se-ah) [pseudo- + Gr. opsis vision + -ia] a visual hallucination or illusion.

pseudopsychosis (soo″do-si-ko′sis) Ganser syndrome.

pseudopterygium (soo″do-ter-ij′e-um) a conjunctival scar attached to the cornea, superficially resembling a true pterygium, but usually not firmly adherent to the underlying tissue.

pseudoptosis (soo″do-to′sis) [pseudo- + ptosis] decrease in the size of the palpebral aperture.

pseudoptyalism (soo″do-ti′al-izm) accumulation and drooling of saliva due to dysphagia.

pseudorabies (soo″do-ra′be-ēz) a highly contagious disease affecting the central nervous system of swine, cattle, dogs, cats, rats, and other animals; in swine the infection usually runs a milder course than in other species. Caused by a herpesvirus, it is characterized by sudden onset, severe pruritus, late paralysis, convulsions, and death within three to four days after onset. Called also *Aujeszky's disease, mad itch,* and *infectious bulbar paralysis.* **bovine p.,** pseudorabies of cattle.

pseudoreaction (soo″do-re-ak′shun) a false or deceptive reaction; a skin reaction in intradermal tests which is not due to the specific protein used in the test but to the protein of the medium employed in producing the toxin.

pseudoreduction (soo″do-re-duk′shun) the apparent halving of the chromosome number by synapsis.

pseudoretinitis pigmentosa (soo″do-ret″in-i′tis pig″-men-to′sah) pigmentary degeneration of the retina mimicking retinitis pigmentosa, but arising from intrauterine viral infections, vascular lesions, and other causes.

pseudorheumatism (soo″do-roo′mah-tizm) a condition resembling rheumatic fever, due to some nonrheumatic disease, as gonorrhea.

pseudorickets (soo″do-rik′ets) renal osteodystrophy.

pseudosarcoma (soo″do-sar-ko′mah) [pseudo- + sarcoma] sarcomatoid transformation of a carcinoma histologically resembling a sarcoma.

pseudoscarlatina (soo″do-skar″lah-ti′nah) a febrile condition with an eruption like that of scarlet fever, but due to septic poisoning.

pseudosclerema (soo″do-skle-re′mah) adiponecrosis subcutanea neonatorum.

pseudosclerosis (soo″do-skle-ro′sis) [pseudo- + Gr. sklērōsis hardening] a condition with the symptoms but without the lesions of multiple sclerosis. **spastic p., p. spas'tica,** Creutzfeldt-Jakob syndrome. **Strümpell-Westphal p.,** Wilson disease. **Westphal-Strümpell p.,** Wilson disease.

pseudoscrotum (soo″do-skro′tum) a solid partition with a median raphe, resembling the scrotum in the male, obliterating the opening into the vagina in female pseudohermaphrodites.

pseudosmia (soo-doz′me-ah) [pseudo- + Gr. osmē odor + -ia] a hallucination of smell.

pseudosolution (soo″do-so-lu′shun) solutions which do not act according to the usual physical laws of solutions; the term is sometimes applied to colloidal solutions.

pseudostoma (soo-dos′to-mah) [pseudo- + Gr. stoma mouth] an apparent communication between silver-stained endothelial cells.

pseudostrabismus (soo″do-strah-bis′mus) apparent strabismus due to an overhanging epicanthus which narrows the visible width of the sclera medial to the iris.

pseudostrophanthin (soo″do-stro-fan′thin) a poisonous glycoside, $C_{40}H_{60}O_{16}\cdot H_2O$, from the African shrub *Strophanthus hispidus* DC. (Apocynaceae).

pseudostructure (soo″do-struk′chur) reticular substance.

pseudotabes (soo″do-ta′bēz) [pseudo- + L. tabes wasting] (obs.) any neuropathy with symptoms like those of tabes dorsalis but not due to syphilis. Called also *Leyden's ataxia.* **pupillotonic p.,** Adie's syndrome.

pseudotetanus (soo″do-tet′ah-nus) persistent muscular contractions resembling tetanus but not associated with the presence of *Clostridium tetani.*

pseudothrill (soo′do-thril) a condition that simulates a true thrill.

pseudotoxin (soo″do-tok′sin) a poisonous extract from belladonna leaves.

pseudotrachoma (soo″do-trah-ko′mah) a disease of the eye and lids resembling trachoma.

pseudotrismus (soo″do-tris′mus) a motor disorder of the mouth with symptoms similar to those of trismus.

pseudotropine (soo-dot′ro-pin) a dark-brown, syrupy, liquid base, a decomposition product of tropine.

pseudotruncus arteriosus (soo″do-trunk′us ar-te″re-o′sus) the most severe form of tetralogy of Fallot.

pseudotubercle (soo″do-tu′ber-k'l) a tubercle resembling that of tuberculosis, but not due to the tubercle bacillus.

pseudotuberculoma (soo″do-tu-ber″ku-lo′mah) a tumor resembling in structure a tuberculoma. **p. silicot′icum,** a pseudotuberculoma due to the presence in the tissue of silica.

pseudotuberculosis (soo″do-too-ber″ku-lo′sis) [pseudo- + tuberculosis] 1. any of various animal diseases caused by pathogens other than the tubercle bacillus, e.g., *Yersinia pseudotuberculosis* in rodents, especially guinea pigs, white rats, and rabbits, in which caseous swellings resembling tubercular nodules (pseudotubercles) form in organs throughout the body. **p. hom′inis streptoth′rica,** a disease of man closely resembling tuberculosis, but due to a streptothrix.

pseudotumor (soo″do-tu′mor) an enlargement that resembles a tumor. **p. cer′ebri,** a condition caused by cerebral edema, marked by raised intracranial pressure with headache, nausea, vomiting, and papilledema, but without neurological signs except occasional sixth-nerve palsy. Called also *benign intracranial hypertension* and *meningeal hydrops.* **orbital p.,** a distinctive, chronic inflammatory reaction in the orbital tissues of the eye, of unknown etiology, that may closely resemble a neoplasm and often becomes bilateral. Symptoms include exophthalmos and congestion of the lids with edema. When limitation of ocular motility also occurs, it is sometimes called *orbital myositis.*

pseudotympanites, pseudotympany (soo″do-tim″pah-ni′tēz, soo″do-tim′pah-ne) (obs.) false tympanites, as in accordion abdomen.

pseudotyphus (soo″do-ti′fus) a disease of Sumatra resembling scrub typhus (tsutsugamushi disease).

pseudouremia (soo″do-u-re′me-ah) uremia-like symptoms occurring in acute glomerulonephritis and in hypertensive vascular disease (hypertensive encephalopathy).

pseudouridine (soo′do-ūr′ĭ-dēn) 5-ribosyluracil, a constituent of transfer-RNA differing from uridine in having the linkage between the 5-carbon of uracil and the 1-carbon of ribose.

pseudovalve (soo′do-valv) a peculiar formation on the parietal endocardium of the left ventricle, seen especially in insufficiency of the aortic valves.

pseudoventricle (soo″do-ven′tre-k'l) cavitas septi pellucidi.

pseudovoice (soo′do-vois) the vocal sounds produced under proper training by a person who has lost his larynx.

pseudovomiting (soo″do-vom′it-ing) regurgitation of matter from the stomach.

pseudoxanthoma elasticum (soo″do-zan-tho′mah e-las′tĭ-kum) [pseudo- + Gr. xanthos yellow + -oma; Gr. elastikos elastic] a rare, progressive inherited disorder usually presenting after puberty, occurring in autosomal recessive and dominant forms, involving the skin, eye, and cardiovascular system, most of the manifestations of which occur as a result of basophilic degeneration of elastic tissue. The chief characteristics include small yellow cutaneous macules and papules that become confluent to form plaques, principally confined to flexural areas; lax, inelastic, and redundant skin; angioid streaks in the retina; arterial insufficiency in the lower extremities, premature calcification of peripheral arteries, reduced arterial pulses, symptoms of coronary insufficiency, hypertension, and mitral valve prolapse; and gastrointestinal and other hemorrhages. Called also *nevus elasticus.*

p.s.i. pounds per square inch.

psicofuranine (si″ko-fer′a-nēn) a nucleoside antibiotic produced by *Streptomyces hygroscopicus* that has antibacterial and antitumor activity.

psilocin (si′lo-sin) a hallucinogenic substance closely related to psilocybin.

psilocybin (si″lo-si′bin) chemical name: 3-[2-(dimethylamino)ethyl]indol-4-ol dihydrogen phosphate ester. A hallucinogenic crystalline compound, $C_{13}H_{18(20)}O_3N_2P_2$, possessing indole characteristics, isolated from the mushroom *Psilocybe mexicana* Heim.

psittacine (sit′ah-sīn) [Gr. psittakos parrot] of or relating to an order of birds including the parrot and related birds (parakeets, macaws, etc.)

psittacosis (sit-ah-ko′sis) [Gr. psittakos parrot + -osis] primarily an acute or chronic respiratory and systemic disease of various wild and domestic birds, originally thought to be seen only in psittacine birds (hence the name), which is caused by *Chlamydia psittaci* and is transmissible to humans and other animals. Human infection, generally acquired by inhalation of dried bird excreta containing the pathogen or rarely by handling feathers or tissues of infected birds or through an open lesion or the bite of an infected bird, may be asymptomatic, or it may be manifested by mild influenza-like symptoms or sometimes by a severe and highly fatal pneumonia. Called also *parrot fever.* See *ornithosis.*

psoas (so′as) see *Table of Musculi.*

psoitis (so-i′tis) [Gr. psoa muscle of the loin + -itis] inflammation of a psoas muscle or of its sheath.

psoralen (sor′ah-len) any of the constituents of certain plants (*Ammi majus, Psoralea corylifolia,* etc.) collectively known as "psoralens"; exposure to substances containing psoralens, such as certain perfumes and drugs (including methoxsalen and trioxsalen) and then to sunlight may produce phototoxic dermatitis (q.v.).

psorenteritis (so″ren-ter-i′tis) [psora + enteritis] a condition of the intestinal mucosa thought to be peculiar to cholera, marked by loss of villi and a granular debris in the surface mucous sheath.

psoriasiform (so″re-as′ĭ-form) resembling psoriasis.

psoriasis (so-ri′ah-sis) [Gr. psōriasis] a common chronic, squamous dermatosis, marked by exacerbations and remissions and having a polygenic inheritance pattern. The most distinctive histological findings in well-developed psoriasis are Munro microabscesses and spongiform pustules. It is characterized clinically by the presence of rounded, circumscribed, erythematous, dry, scaling patches of various sizes, covered by grayish white or silvery white, umbilicated, and lamellar scales, which have a predilection for the extensor surfaces, nails, scalp, genitalia, and lumbosacral region. Central clearing and coalescence of the lesions produce a wide variety of clinical configurations, including annular or circinate, discoid or nummular, figurate, and gyrate arrangements. Called also *p. vulgaris.* **annular p., p. annula′ris, p. annula′ta,** see *psoriasis.* **arthritic p., p. arthropath′ica, p. arthop′ica,** psoriatic arthritis. **Barber's p.,** localized pustular p. **p. bucca′lis,** a rare form of psoriasis affecting the oral mucosa. **circinate p., p. circina′ta,** see *psoriasis.* **discoid p., p. discoi′dea,** see *psoriasis.* **erythrodermic p.,** a severe generalized erythrodermic condition usually developing in chronic forms of psoriasis, e.g., as a reaction to topical therapy or as a result of ultraviolet exposure, or rarely occurring as the initial manifestation of psoriasis, which may be characterized by massive exfoliation of the skin and serious systemic illness associated with abnormalities of temperature and cardiovascular regulation. Called also *erythroderma psoriaticum* and *exfoliative p.* **exfoliative p.,** erythrodermic p. **p. figura′ta, figurate p.,** see *psoriasis.* **flexural p.,** inverse p. **follicular p.,** a form of psoriasis characterized by the presence of prominent follicularly oriented papules, involving mainly the thighs in adults, principally in females, and the trunk in children; in the latter, the lesions extend to form large plaques. Older lesions show nucleated cells in the openings of the hair follicles, along with other epidermal and dermal changes. **p. gutta′ta, guttate p.,** a form of psoriasis seen primarily in children and young adults, especially following streptococcal infections, and characterized by the abrupt appearance of small droplike lesions over much of the skin surface, generally involving the trunk and proximal extremities. **p. gyra′ta, gyrate p.,** see *psoriasis.* **inverse p.,** a seborrheic dermatitis–like form of psoriasis in which the lesions are moist and erythematous with a minimal amount of greasy, soft scales, and occur in a flexural distribution with involvement of the intertriginous folds of the axillae and inguinal region, of the inframammary, intergluteal, and perianal skin, and of the palms, soles, and nails. Called also *flexural p., seborrheic p., seborrhiasis,* and *volar p.* **p. invetera′ta,** a form with confluent lesions and with thickening and hardening of the skin. **p. lin′guae,** a rare form of psoriasis affecting the mucosa of the tongue. **nummular p., p. nummula′ris,** see *psoriasis.* **p. ostra′cea, ostraceous p.,** psoriasis in which the lesions form thick, tough patches covered with scales, giving them a resemblance to the outside of an oyster shell. Called also *p. rupioides.* **palmar p.,** a patchy hyperkeratotic form of psoriasis chiefly involving the contact points of the volar surfaces of the palms and fingers, which is thought to be related to local physical or chemical injury, thus representing the Koebner phenomenon; the same changes are less common on the soles. **p. of palms and soles,** see *inverse p., localized pustular p., palmar p.,* and *localized pustular p.* **pustular p., generalized,** a severe, acute, generalized, sometimes fatal, erythematous pustular eruption in patients with mild to moderate psoriasis or in those with psoriatic arthritis or exfoliative psoriasis, which is accompanied by high fever, leukocytosis, hypocalcemia, arthralgia, malaise, and other systemic symptoms. Called also *von Zumbush's p.* and *Zumbush's p.* **pustular p., localized,** a sterile eruption of pustules superimposed on discrete erythematous plaques involving the volar skin of the hands or feet, or both, usually in the presence of psoriasis at other sites, which may also involve the paronychial skin, and associated with swelling, erythema, and local discomfort. Called also *Barber's p., pustulosis palmaris et plantaris,* and *palmoplantar pustulosis.* Cf. *pustulosis palmaris et plantaris,* def. 2. **p. rupioi′des,** p. ostracea. **seborrheic p.,** inverse p. **volar p.,** 1. inverse p. 2. palmar p. 3. see *localized pustular p.* **von Zumbush's p.,** generalized pustular p. **p. vulga′ris,** psoriasis.

psoriatic (so″re-at′ik) 1. pertaining to, affected with, or of the nature of, psoriasis. 2. a person affected with psoriasis.

Psorophora (so-rof′o-rah) a genus of large, annoying mosquitoes, the larvae of which prey on the larvae of other kinds of mosquitoes. Some species, particularly *P. ferox* and *P. lutzii,* act as carrier hosts of the eggs of *Dermatobia hominis.*

psorophthalmia (so″rof-thal′me-ah) [Gr. *psōrophthalmia*] a form of ulcerative marginal blepharitis.

Psoroptes (so-rop′tēz) a genus of mites. **P. bo′vis,** *P. ovis.* **P. cunic′uli,** a common external parasite of rab-

bits, leading to secondary infections that may extend to the inner ear and involve the central nervous system. **P. e′qui,** a species causing skin lesions (psoroptic mange) in horses, especially in areas covered with long hair. **P. o′vis,** a species which causes the most common type of mange in sheep (sheep scab), cattle (bovine scabies), and horses, with intense itching and sometimes general symptoms.

P.S.P. phenolsulfonphthalein.

PSRO Professional Standards Review Organization: an organization of physicians and in some cases allied health professionals in a designated area, state, or community established to monitor health care services paid for through Medicare, Medicaid, and Maternal and Child Health programs to assure that services provided are medically necessary, meet professional standards, and are provided in the most economic medically appropriate health care agency or institution. The requirement for the establishment of PSRO's was added to the Social Security Amendments of 1972 (Public Law 92-603).

psychalgalia (si″kal-ga′le-ah) psychalgia.

psychalgia (si-kal′je-ah) 1. pain, usually in the head and perceived as being of emotional origin, that may accompany intolerable ideas, obsessions, or hallucinations; called also *algopsychalia* and *psychic pain.* 2. psychogenic pain, pain of hysterical origin perceived as physical pain. See *psychogenic pain disorder,* under *disorder.*

psychalgic (si-kal′jik) pertaining to or characterized by psychalgia.

psychanalysis (si-kah-nal′ĭ-sis) psychoanalysis.

psychanopsia (si-kah-nop′se-ah) [*psych-* + *an* neg. + Gr. *opsis* vision + *-ia*] psychic blindness.

psychasthenia (si″kas-the′ne-ah) [*psych* + Gr. *asthenia* debility] (*obs.*) a term used by Janet to cover all psychoneuroses not classified as hysteria; it mainly included what now would be called phobias and anxiety neuroses.

psychasthenic (si″kas-then′ik) (*obs.*) marked by, or characteristic of psychasthenia.

psychataxia (si″kah-tak′se-ah) a disordered mental condition marked by confusion and inability to concentrate.

psyche (si′ke) [Gr. *psychē* the organ of thought and judgment] the human faculty for thought, judgment, and emotion; the mental life, including both conscious and unconscious processes.

psychedelic (si″kĕ-del′ik) [*psyche* + Gr. *dēlos* manifest, evident] pertaining to or characterized by visual hallucinations, intensified perception, and, sometimes, behavior similar to that seen in psychosis. By extension, a drug that produces such effects.

psychiatric (si″ke-at′rik) pertaining to or within the purview of psychiatry.

psychiatrics (si″ke-at′riks) psychiatry.

psychiatrist (si-ki′ah-trist) a physician who specializes in psychiatry.

psychiatry (si-ki′ah-tre) [*psyche* + Gr. *iatreia* healing] that branch of medicine which deals with the study, treatment, and prevention of mental disorders. **biological p.,** that which emphasizes biochemical, neurological, and pharmacological causes and treatment approaches. **community p.,** the branch of psychiatry concerned with the detection, prevention, and treatment of mental disorders in designated psychosocial, cultural, or geographical areas, with emphasis given to the role of environmental factors. **cross-cultural p.,** the comparative study of mental illness and mental health among different societies, nations, and cultures; called also *transcultural p.* **cultural p.,** the branch of social psychiatry concerned with the mentally ill in relation to their cultural environment. **descriptive p.,** psychiatry based on the study of observable symptoms and behavioral phenomena, rather than underlying psychodynamic processes; cf. *dynamic p.* **dynamic p.,** psychiatry based on the study of the unconscious mechanisms, conflicts, and other emotional processes that motivate and underlie human behavior, rather than the more observable behaviors themselves; cf. *descriptive p.* **existential p.,** that based on the existential philosophy of Kierkegaard, Heidegger, Jaspers, etc., that holds the view that a person takes responsibility for his own existence. **forensic p.,** psychiatry which deals with the legal aspects of mental disorders. **industrial p.,** occupational p. **occupational p.,** that concerned with the diagnosis and prevention of mental illness in industry, with the return of the psychiatric patient to work, and with psychiatric aspects of absenteeism, accident proneness, personnel policies, occupational fatigue, vocational adjustment, retirement, and related phenomena. Called also *industrial p.* **organic p.,** 1. that dealing with the psychological aspects of organic brain disease. 2. biological p. **orthomolecular p.,** psychiatry based on the theory that psychiatric illnesses are due to disturbances in the molecular environment of the brain and can be cured by restoration of optimal concentrations of substances normally present in the body, such as vitamins. **preventive p.,** a broad term referring to the amelioration, control, and limitation of psychiatric disability. It is often categorized as *primary*—measures to prevent a disorder; *secondary*—therapeutic measures to limit a disorder; and *tertiary*—measures and intervention to reduce impairment or disability following a disorder. **social p.,** that concerned with the cultural, ecologic, and sociologic facts that engender, precipitate, intensify, prolong, or otherwise complicate maladaptive patterns of behavior and their treatment. **transcultural p.,** cross-cultural p.

psychic (si′kik) [Gr. *psychikos*] pertaining to the psyche or to the mind; mental.

psychism (si′kizm) a 19th-century theory that there is a fluid diffused through all living beings, animating all alike.

psych(o)- [Gr. *psyche* the organ of thought and reason] a combining form denoting relationship to the psyche, or to the mind.

psychoactive (si″ko-ak′tiv) affecting the mind or behavior, as psychoactive drugs.

psychoanaleptic (si″ko-an″ah-lep′tik) [*psycho-* + Gr. *analepsis* a taking up] exerting a stimulating effect upon the mind.

psychoanalysis (si″ko-ah-nal′ĭ-sis) methods of eliciting from patients their past emotional experiences and their role in influencing their current mental life, in order to discover the conflicts and mechanisms by which their pathologic mental state has been produced, and to furnish hints for psychotherapeutic procedures; the method employs free association, recall and interpretation of dreams, and interpretation of transference and resistance phenomena. Also, a system of theoretical psychology.

psychoanalyst (si″ko-an′ah-list) a practitioner of psychoanalysis.

psychoanalytic (si″ko-an″ah-lit′ik) pertaining to psychoanalysis.

psychoauditory (si″ko-aw′dĭ-to″re) pertaining to the conscious and intelligent perception of sound.

psychobiological (si″ko-bi′o-loj′e-kal) pertaining to psychobiology.

psychobiology (si″ko-bi-ol′o-je) Adolf Meyer's school of psychiatric thought, in which the human being is viewed as an integrated unit, incorporating psychological, social, and biological functions.

psychocatharsis (si″ko-kah-thar′sis) [*psycho-* + Gr. *katharsis* purging] catharsis (def. 2).

psychochemistry (si″ko-kem′is-tre) the science that deals with the relationship between chemistry and psychologic processes.

psychochrome (si′ko-krōm) [*psycho-* + Gr. *chroma* color] a subjective mental association between any bodily sensation and some particular color.

psychochromesthesia (si″ko-krōm″es-the′ze-ah) [*psycho-* + Gr. *chroma* color + *aisthesis* perception + *-ia*] the condition in which auditory or other nonvisual stimuli produce sensations or associated sensations of color.

psychocortical (si″ko-kor′te-kal) pertaining to the mind and to the cortex of the brain as the site of mental functions.

psychocutaneous (si″ko-ku-ta′ne-us) pertaining to the relations between mental or emotional factors and skin disorders.

psychodelic (si″ko-del′ik) psychedelic.

psychodiagnosis (si″ko-di″ag-no′sis) the use of psychological methods of assessment in the diagnosis of psychiatric disorders.

psychodiagnostics (si″ko-di″ag-nos′tiks) psychodiagnosis.

Psychodidae (si-ko′dĭ-de) a family of flies, the owl flies or sandflies, of the order Diptera, characterized by small size, long legs, and abundant hair on both wings and body. It includes the genera *Lutzomyia, Phlebotomas,* and *Psychodopygas.*

psychodometer (si″ko-dom′ĕ-ter) an instrument for measuring the rate of mental processes.

psychodometry (si″ko-dom′ĕ-tre) [*psycho-* + Gr. *hodos* way + *metron* measure] measurement of the rate of mental processes.

Psychodopygus (si″ko-do-pi′gus) [Gr. *psyche* butterfly + *pyge* rump] a genus of sandflies of the family Psychodidae, including *P. wellcomei,* a vector of *Leishmania donovani,* the etiologic agent of visceral leishmaniasis.

psychodrama (si″ko-dram′ah) the psychiatric group-therapy technique of having patients dramatize their own or assigned emotional conflicts.

psychodynamics (si″ko-di-nam′iks) [*psycho-* + Gr. *dynamis* power] the interplay of forces, such as anxiety, conflict, and mechanisms, that give rise to the expression of mental processes.

psychodysleptic (si″ko-dis-lep′tik) [*psycho-* + Gr. *dys-* bad + *lepsis* a taking hold] inducing a dreamlike or delusional state of mind.

psychogalvanometer (si″ko-gal″vah-nom′ĕ-ter) an instrument for determining changes in skin resistance to electric current applied to electrodes on the skin.

psychogenesis (si″ko-jen′ĕ-sis) 1. mental development. 2. production of a symptom or illness by psychic, as opposed to organic, factors.

psychogenic (si″ko-jen′ik) produced or caused by psychic or mental factors rather then organic factors.

psychogeriatrics (si″ko-jer″e-at′riks) management of the psychologic and psychiatric problems of the aged.

psychogogic (si″ko-goj′ik) increasing intrapsychic tensions and acting as a stimulant.

psychogram (si′ko-gram) [*psycho-* + Gr. *gramma* a writing] 1. psychograph. 2. a visual sensation associated with a mental idea, as of a certain number which appears visualized when it is thought of.

psychograph (si′ko-graf) [*psycho-* + Gr. *graphein* to write] 1. a chart for recording graphically the personality traits of an individual. 2. a written description of the mental functioning of an individual.

psychokinesia (si″ko-ki-ne′ze-ah) psychokinesis.

psychokinesis (si″ko-ki-ne′sis) [*psycho-* + Gr. *kinesis* motion] 1. the postulated direct influence of volitional action on a physical object, or the influence of mind on matter without the intermediation of physical force. 2. explosive action due to defective inhibition of primitive instincts.

psycholagny (si′ko-lag″ne) [*psycho-* + Gr. *lagneia* lust] the experiencing of sexual enjoyment from imagining or thinking of sexual acts.

psycholepsy (si′ko-lep″se) [*psycho-* + Gr. *lepsis* a taking hold, a seizure] a sudden, intense lowering of mood level, usually of short duration.

psycholinguistics (si″ko-ling-gwis′tiks) the study of psychological factors involved in the development and use of language.

psychologic, psychological (si″ko-loj′ik; si″ko- loj′e-kal) pertaining to psychology.

psychologist (si-kol′o-jist) a qualified specialist in psychology.

psychology (si-kol′o-je) [*psycho-* + *-logy*] that branch of science which deals with the mind and mental processes, especially in relation to human and animal behavior. **abnormal p.,** the study of mental disorders and behavior disturbances. **analytic p., analytical p.,** the system of psychology founded by Carl Gustav Jung, based on the concepts of the collective unconscious and the complex. **animal p.,** the study of the mental activity of animals. **behavioristic p.,** see *behaviorism.* **child p.,** the study of the development of the mind of the child. **clinical p.,** the use of psychologic knowledge and techniques in the treatment of persons with mental, emotional, behavior, and developmental disorders. **cognitive p.,** that branch of psychology which deals with how the human mind receives and interprets impressions and ideas. **community p.,** the application of psychological principles to the study and support of the mental health of individuals in their social context. **comparative p.,** the study of behavior using a comparison of species as a source of knowledge. **criminal p.,** the study of the mentality, the motivation, and the social behavior of criminals. **depth p.,** the study of unconscious mental processes. **developmental p.,** the study of changes in behavior that occur through the life span. **dynamic p.,** psychology that stresses the causes of and motivations for behavior. **environmental p.,** study of the effects of the physical and social environment on behavior. **experimental p.,** the study of mental operations and behaviors by the employment of controlled laboratory procedures. **gestalt p.,** see *gestaltism*. **individual p.,** Alfred Adler's psychiatric theory that stresses the role of compensation for feelings of inferiority as the source of psychological and interpersonal problems. **physiologic p., physiological p.,** the branch of psychology that studies the relationship between physiologic processes and behavior. **social p.,** psychology that focuses on social interaction, on the ways in which actions of others influence the behavior of an individual.

psychometer (si-kom′ĕ-ter) an instrument used in psychometry.

psychometrician (si″ko-mĕ-trish′an) a person skilled in psychometry.

psychometrics (si″ko-met′riks) psychometry.

psychometry (si-kom′ĕ-tre) [*psycho-* + Gr. *metron* measure] systematic measurement of mental processes and behavioral acts.

psychomotor (si″ko-mo′tor) pertaining to motor effects of cerebral or psychic activity.

psychoneural (si″ko-nu′ral) relating to the totality of neural events initiated by a sensory input and leading to storage, to discrimination, or to an output of any kind.

psychoneurosis (si″ko-nu-ro′sis), pl. *psychoneuroses* [*psycho-* + Gr. *neuron* nerve + *-osis*] 1. (*obs.*) Freud's term for neuroses such as hysteria, obsessions, and phobias originating in childhood experiences; cf. *actual neurosis*, under *neurosis*. 2. neurosis.

psychonomy (si″kon-o′me) [*psycho-* + Gr. *nomos* law] the science of the laws of mental activity.

psychopath (si′ko-path) a person affected with antisocial (psychopathic) personality disorder (see under *personality*).

psychopathic (si″ko-path′ik) 1. pertaining to antisocial behavior or antisocial personality disorder. 2. (*obs.*) pertaining to mental disease.

psychopathology (si″ko-pah-thol′o-je) [*psycho-* + *pathology*] 1. the pathology of mental disorders; the branch of medicine which deals with the causes and nature of mental disease. 2. abnormal, maladaptive behavior or mental activity.

psychopathy (si-kop′ah-the) [*psycho-* + Gr. *pathos* disease] a disorder of the psyche, whether or not associated with subnormal intelligence.

psychopharmacology (si″ko-fahr″mah-kol′o-je) 1. the study of the action of drugs on psychological functions and mental states. 2. the use of drugs to modify psychological functions and mental states.

psychophysical (si″ko-fiz′e-kal) pertaining to the mind and its relation to physical manifestations.

psychophysics (si″ko-fiz′iks) [*psycho-* + Gr. *physikos* natural] the science dealing with the quantitative relationships between the characteristics or patterns of physical stimuli and the resultant sensations.

psychophysiologic (si″ko-fiz″e-o-loj′ik) [*psycho-* + *physiology*] pertaining to psychophysiology; psychosomatic.

psychophysiology (si″ko-fiz″e-ol′o-je) physiologic psychology.

psychoplasm (si′ko-plazm) protyl.

psychoplegia (si″ko-ple′je-ah) [*psycho-* + Gr. *plēgē* stroke + *-ia*] a sudden attack of dementia.

psychoplegic (si″ko-ple′jik) an agent that lessens cerebral activity or excitability.

psychoprophylactic (si″ko-pro″fĭ-lak′tik) pertaining to psychoprophylaxis.

psychosedation (si″ko-sĕ-da′shun) a procedure whereby the patient is rendered free from fear and apprehension through the administration of a psychosedative agent.

psychosedative (si″ko-sed′ah-tiv) an agent that allays apprehension by its action on subcortical centers, while producing minimal motor and sensory impairment because of its limited effect on the cerebral cortex.

psychosensorial (si″ko-sen-so′re-al) psychosensory.

psychosensory (si″ko-sen′so-re) pertaining to the conscious perception of sensory impulses to the mind and to sensation.

psychoses (si-ko′sēz) plural of *psychosis*.

psychosexual (si″ko-seks′u-al) pertaining to the mental or emotional aspects of sex.

psychosin (si-ko′sin) a galactoside, $C_{23}H_{45}N_7O$, resulting from the decomposition of phrenosin. On hydrolysis it yields galactose and sphingosine.

psychosis (si-ko′sis), pl. *psycho′ses* [*psych-* + *-osis*] a mental disorder characterized by gross impairment in reality testing as evidenced by delusions, hallucinations, markedly incoherent speech, or disorganized and agitated behavior without apparent awareness on the part of the patient of the incomprehensibility of his behavior; the term is also used in a more general sense to refer to mental disorders in which mental functioning is sufficiently impaired as to interfere grossly with the patient's capacity to meet the ordinary demands of life. Historically, the term has been applied to many conditions, e.g., manic-depressive psychosis, that were first described in psychotic patients, although many patients with the disorder are not judged psychotic. **affective p.,** mood disorder. **alcoholic p's,** psychoses associated with alcohol use, a category that includes delirium tremens, Korsakoff's syndrome, alcohol hallucinosis, and alcoholic paranoia (concurrent paranoia and alcoholism). **bipolar p.,** see under *disorder*. **brief reactive p.** [DSM III-R], an episode of psychotic symptoms (incoherence, loosening of associations, delusions, hallucinations, disorganized or catatonic behavior) with sudden onset that is a reaction to a recognizable and distressing life event and that lasts less than one month. **circular p.,** obsolete term for bipolar (manic-depressive) disorder with alternating manic and depressive episodes. **depressive p.,** major depression. **drug p.,** any psychosis associated with drug use. **functional p.,** a psychosis in which organic disease or dysfunction does not play a part. **hysterical p.** (*obs.*), a brief reactive psychosis occurring in a person with histrionic (hysterical) personality disorder. **involutional p.,** see under *melancholia*. **Korsakoff's p.,** see under *syndrome*. **manic p.,** bipolar disorder, manic. **manic-depressive p.,** bipolar disorder. **organic p.,** a psychotic organic mental disorder. **postpartum p.,** a psychotic episode occurring in the postpartum period. **prison p.,** any psychosis for which a prison environment has been a precipitating factor. **schizoaffective p.,** see under *disorder*. **senile p.,** senile dementia with depressive or paranoid delusions or hallucinations. **situational p.** (*obs.*), brief reactive p. **symbiotic p., symbiotic infantile p.,** a condition seen in two- to four-year-old children having an abnormal relationship to the mothering figure, characterized by intense separation anxiety, severe regression, giving up of useful speech, and autism; now included in childhood-onset pervasive developmental disorder. **toxic p.,** a psychosis due to the ingestion of toxic agents (e.g., alcohol, opium) into the body, or to the presence of toxins within the body. **unipolar p.,** major depression.

psychosocial (si″ko-so′shal) pertaining to or involving both psychic and social aspects.

psychosomatic (si″ko-so-mat′ik) [*psycho-* + Gr. *sōma* body] pertaining to the mind-body relationship; having bodily symptoms of psychic, emotional, or mental origin; called also *psychophysiologic*. See also under *disorder*.

psychosomimetic (si-ko″so-mi-met′ik) psychotomimetic.

psychostimulant (si″ko-stim′u-lant) 1. producing a transient increase in psychomotor activity. 2. a drug, such as amphetamine, methylphenidate, and caffeine, that produces such effects.

psychosurgery (si″ko-ser′jer-e) brain surgery performed for treatment of psychiatric disorders.

psychotechnics (si″ko-tek′niks) [*psycho-* + Gr. *technē* art] the employment of psychological methods in studying sociological and other problems.

psychotherapeutics (si″ko-ther″ah-pu′tiks) psychotherapy.

psychotherapy (si″ko-ther′ah-pe) [*psycho-* + Gr. *therapeia* treatment] treatment of mental disorders and behavioral disturbances using such psychological techniques as support, suggestion, persuasion, reeducation, reassurance, and insight in order to alter maladaptive patterns of coping and to encourage personality growth. **brief p.,** psychotherapy limited in number of sessions to 10 to 20, usually active and directive, and often oriented toward a specific problem or symptom. **existential p.,** that based on the existential philosophy of Kierkegaard, Heidegger, Jaspers, etc., in which the emphasis is on present interactions and feeling experiences rather than on rational thinking. **group p.,** see under *therapy*. **personologic p.,** a form of therapy designed to focus on the underlying personality of patients rather than their presenting clinical syndrome. **supportive p.,** a technique aimed at reinforcing a patient's defenses and helping suppress disturbing psychological material, while avoiding the probing of emotional conflicts; used when symptoms are insufficient to warrant intensive psychotherapy.

psychotic (si-kot′ik) 1. pertaining to, characterized by, or caused by psychosis. 2. a person exhibiting psychosis.

psychotogenic (si-kot″o-jen′ik) 1. producing a state of psychosis. 2. a drug that produces such effects.

psychotomimetic (si-kot″o-mi-met′ik) [*psychosis* + Gr. *mimētikos* imitative] pertaining to, characterized by, or producing manifestations resembling those of a psychosis, e.g., visual hallucinations, distortion of perception, and schizophrenia-like behavior; applied to a drug that produces these effects.

psychotropic (si″ko-trop′pik) [*psycho-* + Gr. *tropē* a turning] exerting an effect upon the mind; capable of modifying mental activity; usually applied to drugs that affect the mental state.

psychr(o)- [Gr. *psychros* cold] a combining form denoting relationship to cold.

psychroalgia (si″kro-al′je-ah) a painful feeling of cold.

psychroesthesia (si″kro-es-the′ze-ah) [*psychro-* + Gr. *aisthēsis* perception + *-ia*] a state in which a part of the body, though warm, seems cold.

psychrolusia (si″kro-loo′se-ah) [*psychro-* + Gr. *louein* to wash] bathing in cold water.

psychrometer (si-krom′ĕ-ter) [*psychro-* + Gr. *metron* measure] an apparatus for measuring atmospheric moisture by the difference in reading of two thermometers, one with a dry bulb and one with a wet bulb. **sling p.,** an instrument in which the thermometers are swung through the air to facilitate evaporation from the wet bulb.

psychrophile (si′kro-fīl) an organism which grows best at low temperatures.

psychrophilic (si″kro-fil′ik) [*psychro-* + Gr. *philein* to love] fond of cold; said of bacteria that grow in the cold, often growing best between 15° and 20° C. See also *mesophilic* and *thermophilic*.

psychrophore (si′kro-fōr) [*psychro-* + Gr. *pherein* to bear] a double-lumen catheter for applying cold to the urethra.

psychrotherapy (si″kro-ther′ah-pe) [*psychro-* + Gr. *therapeia* treatment] the treatment of disease by the application of cold.

psyllium (sil′e-um) a plant of the genus *Plantago*. *Blond p.* is *P. ovata* Forskal; *Spanish p.* is *P. psyllium* L. See also *plantago (psyllium) seed*, under *seed*.

Pt chemical symbol for *platinum*.

PTA plasma thromboplastin antecedent (blood coagulation Factor XI).

ptarmic (tar′mik) [Gr. *ptarmikos* making to sneeze] relating to or producing spasmodic sneezing.

ptarmus (tar′mus) [Gr. *ptarmos*] spasmodic sneezing.

PTC plasma thromboplastin component (blood coagulation Factor IX); phenylthiocarbamide.

PTEN pentaerythritol tetranitrate.

pteridine (ter′ĭ-dēn) a bicyclic nitrogenous base characteristic of the pterins and folic acids.

pteridophyte (ter′ĭ-do-fīt) one of the Pteridophyta.

pterin (ter′in) [Gr. *pteron* wing] any compound containing pteridine; the pterins are derivatives of 2-amino-4-hydroxypteridine and are constituents of folic acids. They were first

identified in the wings of butterflies. See also *aminopterin, leucopterin, uropterin,* and *xanthopterin*.

pterion (te′re-on) [Gr. *pteron* wing] [NA] a point at the junction of the frontal, parietal, temporal, and great wing of the sphenoid bone; about 3 cm. behind the external angular process of the orbit.

pternalgia (ter-nal′je-ah) [Gr. *pterna* heel + *algos* pain + *-ia*] pain in the heel.

pteroic acid (tĕ-ro′ik) a constituent of folic acid consisting of *p*-aminobenzoic linked to pteridine by a methylene bridge.

pteropterin (ter-op′ter-in) pteroyltriglutamic acid, or folic acid (q.v.), conjugated to two glutamate residues. Called also *fermentation Lactobacillus casei factor*.

pteroylglutamate (ter″o-il-gloo′tah-mate) an anionic form of pteroylglutamic (folic) acid. See *folic acid*.

pteroylglutamic acid (ter″o-il-gloo-tam′ik) folic acid.

pteroyltriglutamic acid (ter″o-il-tri″gloo-tam′ik) pteropterin.

pterygium (tĕ-rij′e-um), pl. *ptery′gia* [Gr. *pterygion* wing] a winglike structure, applied especially to an abnormal triangular fold of membrane, in the interpalpebral fissure, extending from the conjunctiva to the cornea, being immovably united to the cornea at its apex, firmly attached to the sclera throughout its middle portion, and merged with the conjunctiva at its base. **p. col′li,** a congenital condition in which

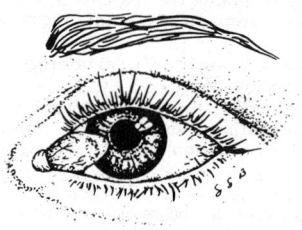

Pterygium.

a thick fold of skin extends from the mastoid region to the acromion on the lateral aspect of the neck; it occurs in association with various genetic syndromes, such as Turner's syndrome and Noonan's syndrome. Called also *webbed neck*. **congenital p.,** epitarsus.

pterygoid (ter′ĭ-goid) [Gr. *pterygōdes* like a wing] shaped like a wing.

pterygomandibular (ter″ĭ-go-man-dib′u-lar) pertaining to the pterygoid process and the mandible.

pterygomaxillary (ter″ĭ-go-mak′sĭ-ler″e) pertaining to a pterygoid process and the upper jaw.

pterygopalatine (ter″ĭ-go-pal′ah-tin) pertaining to a pterygoid process and to the palate bone.

PTFE abbreviation for polytetrafluroethylene; see *polytef*.

PTH parathyroid hormone.

Pthirus (thir′us) *Phthirus*.

ptilosis (ti-lo′sis) [Gr. *ptilōsis*] 1. a falling out or loss of the eyelashes. 2. a form of pneumoconiosis caused by inhaling the dust from ostrich feathers.

ptisan (tiz′an) [L. *ptisana*; Gr. *ptisanē*] (obs.) sweetened barley water, or other similar preparation; a decoction or medicinal tea.

ptomaine (to′mān, to-mān′) [Gr. *ptōma* carcass] a toxic base formed by decarboxylation of an amino acid, often by bacterial action, e.g., cadaverine, muscarine, neurine, ptomatropine, and putrescine. Called also *animal alkaloid, putrefactive alkaloid,* and *cadaveric alkaloid*.

ptomainemia (to″mān-e′me-ah) [*ptomaine* + Gr. *haima* blood + *-ia*] the presence of ptomaines in the blood.

ptomainotoxism (to″mān-o-tok′sizm) poisoning by a ptomaine.

ptomatine (to′mah-tin) ptomaine.

ptomatopsia (to″mah-top′se-ah) [Gr. *ptōma* corpse + *opsis* vision + *-ia*] necropsy.

ptomatopsy (to″mah-top′se) necropsy.

ptomatropine (to-mat′ro-pin) [*ptomaine* + *atropine*] a poison from putrid sausages and the viscera of corpses of those dead from typhoid fever; it has effects somewhat like those of atropine.

ptosed (tōst) affected with ptosis; prolapsed.

ptosis (to′sis) [Gr. *ptōsis* fall] 1. prolapse of an organ or part. 2. drooping of the upper eyelid from paralysis of the third nerve or from sympathetic innervation. **abdominal p.** (*obs.*), splanchnoptosis. **p. adipo′sa, false p.,** an apparent ptosis caused by a fold of skin and fat hanging down below the border of the eyelid. **Horner′s p.,** moderate ptosis of an eye, with retraction of the eyeball, miosis, and flushing of the affected side of the face, due to lesions of the cervical sympathetic; called also *p. sympathetica.* **p. lipomato′sis,** ptosis produced by lipoma of the eyelid. **morning p.,** waking ptosis. **p. sympathe′tica,** Horner′s p. **visceral p.** (*obs.*), splanchnoptosis. **waking p.,** temporary paralysis of the upper lid on awakening from sleep.

-ptosis [Gr. *ptōsis* fall] a word termination indicating downward displacement.

ptotic (tot′ik) pertaining to or affected with ptosis.

PTT partial thromboplastin time; see under *test.*

ptyalagogue (ti-al′ah-gog) [*ptyalo-* + Gr. *agōgos* leading] sialagogue.

ptyalectasis (ti″ah-lek′tah-sis) [*ptyalo-* + Gr. *ektasis* distention] 1. operative dilatation of a salivary duct. 2. dilatation of one of the ducts of the salivary glands.

ptyalin (ti′ah-lin) [Gr. *ptyalon* spittle] α-amylase occurring in saliva.

ptyalism (ti′ah-lizm) [Gr. *ptyalismos*] excessive flow of saliva. Called also *hyperptyalism, hypersalivation, polysialia, ptyalorrhea, salivation, sialism, sialismus,* and *sialorrhea.*

ptyalize (ti′ah-līz) to increase or stimulate the secretion of saliva.

ptyal(o)- [Gr. *ptyalon* saliva] a combining form denoting relationship to saliva. See also words beginning *sial(o)-.*

ptyalocele (ti-al′o-sēl) [*ptyalo-* + Gr. *kēlē* tumor] a cystic tumor containing saliva. **sublingual p.,** ranula.

ptyalogenic (ti″ah-lo-jen′ik) [*ptyalo-* + Gr. *gennan* to produce] formed from or by the action of saliva.

ptyalography (ti″ah-log′rah-fe) [*ptyalo-* + Gr. *graphein* to write] sialography.

ptyalolithiasis (ti″ah-lo-lĭ-thi′ah-sis) [*ptyalo-* + *lith-* + *-iasis*] sialolithiasis.

ptyalolithotomy (ti″ah-lo-lĭ-thot′o-me) sialolithotomy.

ptyaloreaction (ti″ah-lo-re-ak′shun) a reaction occurring in the saliva.

ptyalorrhea (ti″ah-lo-re′ah) [*ptyalo-* + Gr. *rhoia* flow] ptyalism.

ptyalose (ti′ah-lōs) maltose produced by the action of ptyalin on starch.

ptyocrinous (ti-ok′rĭ-nus) [Gr. *ptyon* a winnowing shovel, or fan + *krinein* to separate] elaborating secretion in the form of granules which are eventually extruded; said of unicellular glands, as goblet cells, which secrete in this way. Cf. *diacrinous.*

Pu chemical symbol for *plutonium.*

pubarche (pu-bar′ke) the beginning of growth of the pubic hair.

puberal (pu′ber-al) [L. *puber* of marriageable age] pubertal.

pubertal (pu′ber-tal) pertaining to or characteristic of puberty.

pubertas (pu-ber′tas) [L.] puberty. **p. prae′cox,** precocious puberty.

puberty (pu′ber-te) [L. *pubertas*] the period during which the secondary sex characteristics begin to develop and the capability of sexual reproduction is attained. **precocious p.,** unusually early sexual maturity, either idiopathic or pathological and either isosexual or with development of sex characters of the opposite sex; called also *pubertas praecox.*

pubes (pu′bēz) [L., pl. of *pubis*] 1. pubic hairs; the hairs covering the pubic region. 2. regio pubica.

pubescence (pu-bes′ens) the state of being pubescent.

pubescent (pu-bes′ent) [L. *pubescens* becoming hairy] 1. arriving at the age of puberty. 2. covered with down or lanugo.

pubic (pu′bik) pertaining to or situated near the pubes, the os pubis, or the regio pubica.

pubioplasty (pu′be-o-plas″te) a plastic operation on the pubes.

pubiotomy (pu″be-ot′o-me) [*pubis* + Gr. *tomē* a cutting] surgical separation of the pubic bone lateral to the median line.

pubis (pu′bis), pl. *pu′bes* [L.] NA alternative for *os pubis.* See illustration accompanying *skeleton.*

pubococcygeal (pu″bo-kok-sij′e-al) pertaining to the pubis and coccyx or to the musculus pubococcygeus.

pubofemoral (pu″bo-fem′o-ral) pertaining to the os pubis and femur.

puboprostatic (pu″bo-pros-tat′ik) pertaining to the os pubis and prostate gland.

puborectal (pu″bo-rek′tal) pertaining to the pubis and rectum or to the musculus puborectalis.

pubotibial (pu″bo-tib′e-al) pertaining to the pubes and tibia.

pubovesical (pu″bo-ves′ĭ-kal) pertaining to the pubes and bladder.

pudenda (pu-den′dah) [L.] plural of *pudendum.*

pudendal (pu-den′dal) pertaining to the pudenda.

pudendum (pu-den′dum), pl. *puden′da* [L., from *pudere* to be ashamed.] the external genitalia of humans, especially of the female; see *p. femininum.* **female p.,** p. femininum. **p. femini′num** [NA], female pudendum: that portion of the female genitalia comprising the mons pubis, labia majora, labia minora, vestibule of the vagina, bulb of the vestibule, greater and lesser vestibular glands, and vaginal orifice. Commonly used to denote the entire external female genitalia (partes genitales femininae externae). Called also *p. muliebre* and *vulva.* **p. mulie′bre,** p. femininum.

pudic (pu′dik) [L. *pudicus*] pertaining to the pudenda.

puericulture (pu′er-ĭ-kul″tūr) [L. *puer* child + *cultura* culture] the art of rearing and training children.

puericulturist (pu″er-ĭ-kul′tūr-ist) a specialist in the training of children.

puerile (pu′er-il) [L. *puerilis; puer* child] pertaining to childhood or to children; childish.

puerpera (pu-er′per-ah) [L. *puer* child + *parere* to bring forth, to bear] a woman who has just given birth to an infant.

puerperal (pu-er′per-al) [L. *puerperalis*] pertaining to the puerperium.

puerperalism (pu-er′per-al-izm) a disease condition incident to childbirth.

puerperant (pu-er′per-ant) 1. giving birth. 2. a puerpera.

puerperium (pu″er-pe′re-um) [L.] the period or state of confinement after labor.

puff (puf) [A.S. *pyffan*] 1. a short, blowing, auscultation sound. 2. in genetics, any of the regions of the giant chromosomes of certain flies at which disorganized arrangement and most of RNA synthesis occurs. **chromosome p′s,** active loci of RNA and DNA synthesis in the giant salivary gland chromosomes of insects. **veiled p.,** a faint, muffled pulmonary murmur.

puffing (puf′ing) enlargement in giant polytene chromosomes of fly larval organs; these chromosome puffs are repositories of RNA and DNA synthesis.

pugil, pugillus (pu′jil, pu-jil′us) [L. *pugillus*] a handful.

pukateine (pu-kat′e-in) chemical name: 1,2-methylenedioxy-11-hydroxyaporphine. A crystalline alkaloid, $C_{18}H_{17}NO_3$, from the bark of *Laurelia novaezelandiae* A. Cunn., Lauraceae.

pulegone (pu′le-gōn) chemical name: *p*-menth-4(8)-en-3-one. A volatile oil, a menthene, $(CH_3)_2C:C_6H_7(O)·CH_3$, from pennyroyal oil.

Pulex (pu′leks) [L. "flea"] a genus of fleas which are parasitic on man, dogs, cats, and badgers. **P. cheo′pis,** *Xenopsylla cheopis.* **P. duge′si,** *P. irritans.* **P. ir′ritans,** the common flea or human flea, which is parasitic on the skin of man, its bite producing itching. **P. pen′etrans,** *Tunga penetrans;* see *chigoe.* **P. serrat′iceps,** *Ctenocephalides canis.*

pulex (pu′leks), pl. *pu′lices* [L.] an organism of the genus *Pulex;* a flea.

Pulheems (pul′hēmz) a system of medical classification

for recording the physical and mental status of recruits in the British armed services, representing: P, physical capacity; U, upper limbs; L, lower limbs; H, hearing (acuity); EE, eyesight (visual acuity); M, mental capacity; S, stability (emotional).

pulicicide (pu-lis′ĭ-sīd) [L. *pulex* flea + *caedere* to kill]   an agent destructive to fleas.

Pulicidae (pu-lis′ĭ-de)   a family of the Siphonaptera which includes most of the fleas. Four genera are important to man: *Ctenocephalides, Hoplopsyllus, Pulex,* and *Xenopsylla.*

pull (pul)   1. to strain a muscle.   2. the injury sustained in a muscle strain.

Pullularia (pul″u-la′re-ah)   *Aureobasidium.*   **p. pul′lulans,** *Aureobasidium pullulans.*

pullulate (pul′u-lāt)   to germinate.

pullulation (pul″u-la′shun) [L. *pullulare* to sprout]   the act or process of budding, as in yeast, or of sprouting; germination.

pulmo (pul′mo), gen. *pulmo′nis,* pl. *pulmo′nes* [L.]   the organ of respiration; see *lung.*   **p. dex′ter** [NA], right lung.   **p sinis′ter** [NA], left lung.

pulmo- [L. *pulmo* lung]   a combining form denoting relationship to the lungs; see also words beginning *pulmon(o)-.*

pulmoaortic (pul″mo-a-or′tik)   pertaining to the lungs and the aorta.

pulmogram (pul′mo-gram)   a roentgenogram of the lungs.

pulmolith (pul′mo-lith) [*pulmo-* + Gr. *lithos* stone]   a lung calculus.

pulmometer (pul-mom′ĕ-ter) [*pulmo-* + Gr. *metron* measure]   a form of spirometer for measuring the capacity of the lungs for air.

pulmometry (pul-mom′ĕ-tre)   the measurement of the lung capacity.

pulmonal (pul′mo-nal)   pulmonary.

pulmonary (pul′mo-ner″e) [L. *pulmonarius*]   pertaining to the lungs.

pulmonectomy (pul″mo-nek′to-me)   pneumonectomy.

pulmones (pul-mo′nes) [L.]   1. plural of *pulmo.*   2. [NA] the right and left lungs.

pulmonic (pul-mon′ik)   1. pertaining to the lungs; pulmonary.   2. pertaining to the pulmonary artery.

pulmonitis (pul″mo-ni′tis)   inflammation of the lungs; pneumonia.

pulmon(o)- [L. *pulmo,* gen. *pulmonis* lung]   a combining form denoting relationship to the lungs; see also words beginning *pulmo-.*

pulmonohepatic (pul″mo-no-hĕ-pat′ik)   pertaining to or communicating with the lungs and the liver; hepatopulmonary.

pulmonologist (pul″mo-nol′o-jist)   an individual skilled in pulmonology.

pulmonology (pul″mo-nol′o-je)   the science concerned with the anatomy, physiology, and pathology of the lungs.

pulmonoperitoneal (pul″mo-no-per″ĭ-to-ne′al)   pertaining to or communicating with the lungs and the peritoneum.

pulmotor (pul′mo-tor) [*pulmo-* + L. *motor* mover]   an apparatus for producing artificial respiration by forcing oxygen into the lungs, and, when they are distended, sucking out the air.

pulp (pulp) [L. *pulpa* flesh]   any soft, juicy animal or vegetable tissue, such as that contained within the spleen or the pulp chamber of a tooth (*dental pulp;* see *pulpa dentis* [NA]).   **coronal p.,** pulpa coronalis.   **dead p.,** necrotic p.   **dental p.,** pulpa dentis.   **devitalized p.,** necrotic p.   **digital p.,** the mass of tissue forming the soft cushion on the palmar or plantar surface of the distal phalanx of a finger or toe.   **enamel p.,** stellate reticulum.   **exposed p.,** dental pulp which, through trauma or disease, has become exposed to the external environment.   **mummified p.,** the dry, shriveled pulp seen in dry gangrene.   **necrotic p., nonvital p.,** dental pulp which has been deprived of its blood and nerve supply and is no longer composed of living tissue, with or without bacterial invasion, as evidenced by its insensitivity to stimulation by electricity, heat, cold, or trauma. Called also *dead p.* and *devitalized p.* See also *gangrenous pulp necrosis,* under *necrosis.*   **putrescent p.,** a necrotic pulp which has been invaded by putrefactive microorganisms and is characterized by a particularly foul odor.   **radicular p.,** pulpa radicularis.   **red p., p. of**

spleen, splenic p., pulpa splenica.   **tooth p.,** pulpa dentis.   **vertebral p.,** the soft central portion of an intervertebral disk.   **vital p.,** a dental pulp which is characterized by vascularity and sensation; one that is not necrotic.   **white p.,** folliculi lymphatici splenici.

pulpa (pul′pah), gen. and pl. *pul′pae* [L. "flesh"]   pulp.   **p. corona′le** [NA], coronal pulp; the portion of the dental pulp in the crown portion of the pulp cavity.   **p. den′tis** [NA], dental pulp: the richly vascularized and innervated connective tissue of mesodermal origin contained in the central cavity of a tooth and delimited by the dentin, and having formative, nutritive, sensory, and protective functions. The portion within the tooth chamber proper is the *pulpa coronalis* (coronal pulp); that within the root is the *pulpa radicularis* (radicular pulp). Called also *endodontium* and *tooth p.*   **p. lie′nis,** NA alternative for *p. splenica.*   **p. radicula′ris** [NA], radicular pulp; the portion of the dental pulp in the root canal of a tooth.   **p. sple′nica** [NA], splenic pulp: the dark, reddish-brown substance that fills up the interspaces of the sinuses of the spleen; called also *pulp of spleen, pulpa lienis* [NA alternative] and *red pulp.*

pulpal (pul′pal)   pertaining to the pulp.

pulpalgia (pul-pal′je-ah)   pain in the pulp of a tooth.

pulpectomy (pul-pek′to-me) [*pulp* + Gr. *ektomē* excision]   complete extirpation of the dental pulp from the pulp. Called also *dental pulp extirpation.*

pulpitides (pul-pit′ĭ-dēz)   plural of *pulpitis;* applied to all types of pulp inflammation collectively.

pulpitis (pul-pi′tis), pl. *pulpit′ides* [*pulp* + *-itis*]   inflammation of the dental pulp, usually due to bacterial infection in dental caries, tooth fracture, or other conditions causing exposure of the pulp to bacterial invasion. Chemical irritants, thermal factors, hypremic changes, and other factors may also cause pulpitis.   **anachoretic p.,** that caused by bacteria circulating in the blood stream, which settle at sites of pulpal inflammation resulting from a chemical or mechanical injury.   **closed p.,** that characterized by the absence of a direct communication between the dental pulp and the oral environment.   **hyperplastic p.,** a chronic productive type of pulpitis usually occurring in teeth with large carious lesions; it is characterized by proliferation of the dental pulp tissue, filling the cavity with a pedunculated or sessile, pinkish red, fleshy mass.   **open p.,** that characterized by the presence of a direct communication between the dental pulp and the oral environment.

pulpless (pulp′les)   without pulp; having the pulp removed.

pulpotomy (pul-pot′o-me) [*pulp* + Gr. *tomē* a cutting]   partial excision of the dental pulp. Called also *pulp amputation.*

pulpy (pul′pe)   soft or pulpaceous.

pulque (pul′ke)   a fermented drink made in Mexico and Central America from the juice of *Agave;* it is the source of mescal (def. 2).

pulsate (pul′sāt)   to beat rhythmically, as the heart.

pulsatile (pul′sah-tīl)   characterized by a rhythmical pulsation.

pulsatilla (pul″sah-til′ah)   the dried herb of the ranunculaceous flowering plants *Anemone pulsatilla* L., *A. pratensis* L., or *A. patens* L. Formerly used in a variety of conditions, such as dysmenorrhea, epididymitis, and orchitis, its use has been largely abandoned.

pulsation (pul-sa′shun) [L. *pulsatio*]   a throb or rhythmical beat, as of the heart.   **expansile p.,** a pulsation which is seen or felt to become larger and wider with each impact of the pulse; it reflects an increase in volume of a mass, usually an aneurysm.   **suprasternal p.,** arterial pulsation in the region of the suprasternal notch, due to dilatation and/or elongation of the aortic arch or to aneurysm.

pulsator (pul′sa-tor)   an apparatus for maintaining respiration.   **Bragg-Paul p.,** a pulsator consisting of an air bag placed around the patient's chest and abdomen and rhythmically inflated and deflated by an electric pump.

pulse (puls) [L. *pulsus* stroke]   1. the rhythmic expansion of an artery which may be felt with the finger. The *pulse rate* or number of pulsations of an artery per minute normally varies from 50 to 100. See also *beat.*   2. a brief surge, as of current or voltage.   **abdominal p.,** the pulse over the abdominal aorta.   **abrupt p.,** a pulse which strikes the finger rapidly; a quick or rapidly rising pulse.   **allorhythmic p.,** a pulse marked by irregularities in rhythm.

alternating p., pulsus alternans. **anacrotic p.,** one in which the ascending limb of the tracing shows a transient drop in amplitude, or a notch. **anadicrotic p.,** one in which the ascending limb of the tracing shows two small additional waves or notches. **anatricrotic p.,** one in which the ascending limb of the tracing shows three small additional waves or notches. **atrial liver p.,** a presystolic pulse corresponding to the atrial venous pulse, sometimes occurring in tricuspid stenosis. **atrial venous p., atriovenous p.,** a cervical venous pulse having an accentuated "a" wave during atrial systole, owing to increased force of contraction of the right atrium; a characteristic of tricuspid stenosis. **biferious p., bisferious p.,** pulsus bisferiens. **bigeminal p.,** a pulse in which two beats follow each other in rapid succession, each group of two being separated from the following by a longer interval, usually related to regularly occurring ventricular premature beats. **cannon ball p.,** Corrigan's p. **capillary p.,** Quincke's p. **carotid p.,** the pulse in the carotid artery, tracings of which are used in timing the phases of the cardiac cycle. **catadicrotic p.,** one in which the descending limb of the tracing shows two small additional waves or notches. **catatricrotic p.,** one in which the descending limb of the tracing shows three small additional waves or notches. **centripetal venous p.,** a venous pulse caused by a systolic volume expansion passed from the arteries through the capillaries and venules into the larger veins. **collapsing p.,** Corrigan's p. **Corrigan's p.,** a jerky pulse with a full expansion, followed by a sudden collapse, occurring in aortic regurgitation; called also *water-hammer p.* See also *Corrigan's sign* (def. 2), under *sign*. **coupled p.,** bigeminal p. **dicrotic p.,** a pulse characterized by two peaks, the second peak occurring in diastole and being an exaggeration of the dicrotic wave. **dropped-beat p.,** intermittent p. **elastic p.,** a full pulse which gives an elastic feeling to the finger. **entoptic p.,** the subjective sensation of seeing in the dark a flash of light at each heart beat. **epigastric p.,** abdominal p. **equal p.,** one in which all of the beats are of the same strength. **febrile p.,** a pulse characteristic of fever, often described as full and bounding. **filiform p.,** thready p. **formicant p.,** a small, nearly imperceptible pulse. **frequent p.,** one which is faster in rate than normal. **full p.,** an easily felt pulse; one with a large amplitude of expansion of the vessel palpated. **funic p.,** the arterial tide in the umbilical cord. **gate p.,** an electrical pulse that serves as a control signal for a gate (q.v.). **hard p.,** one which is characterized by very high tension. **hepatic p.,** the pulsations of the liver. **high-tension p.,** one characterized by a gradual impulse, long duration, slow subsidence, and a firm, cordy state of the artery between the beats. **infrequent p.,** one which is slower in rate than normal. **intermittent p.,** one in which various beats are dropped. **irregular p.,** one in which the beats occur at irregular intervals. **jerky p.,** one in which the artery is suddenly and markedly distended. **jugular p.,** a pulsation seen or felt over the jugular vein. **Kussmaul's p.,** paradoxical p. **labile p.,** a pulse which is normal when the patient is resting, but which is increased by sitting, standing, or exercise. **low-tension p.,** a pulse with sudden onset, short duration, and quick decline, and which is easily obliterated by pressure. **Monneret's p.,** a full, slow, and soft pulse said to be characteristic of jaundice. **monocrotic p.,** one in which the tracing shows only one expansion in one beat of the artery. **nail p.,** the pulsation of blood under the nails; sometimes demonstrated by the onychograph. **paradoxical p.,** a pulse that markedly decreases in size during inspiration, as that which often occurs in constrictive pericarditis. **pistol-shot p.,** a form in which the arteries are subject to sudden distention and collapse. **plateau p.,** a pulse which is slowly rising and sustained. **polycrotic p.,** one in which the tracing shows secondary pulse waves. **quadrigeminal p.,** one with a pause after every fourth beat. **quick p.,** 1. one which strikes the finger smartly and leaves it quickly; called also *short p.* 2. one with a faster rate than normal. **Quincke's p.,** alternate blanching and flushing of the skin that may be elicited in several ways, e.g., by observing the nail bed or skin at the root of the nail while pressing on the end of the nail. Caused by pulsation of subpapillary arteriolar and venous plexuses, it is sometimes seen in aortic insufficiency and other disorders, but may occur in normal persons under certain conditions. It was originally thought to be due to pulsation of the capillaries, hence the name *capillary pulse.*

Called also *Quincke's sign.* **radial p.,** that felt over the radial artery. **respiratory p.,** a pulsation observed even in health in the superficial cervical veins after rapid exercise. **retrosternal p.,** a venous pulse perceptible just above the suprasternal notch. **Riegel's p.,** a pulse which is diminished in size during expiration. **running p.,** a pulse with small irregular excursions. **sharp p.,** jerky p. **short p.,** quick p., def. 1. **slow p.,** one with less than the usual number of pulsations per minute. **soft p.,** a pulse of low tension. **strong p.,** a forcible pulse; a pulse of high amplitude. **tense p.,** a pulse that is hard and full, but without wide excursions. **thready p.,** one that is very fine and scarcely perceptible. **trembling p., tremulous p.** (obs.), running p. **tricrotic p.,** one in which the tracing shows three marked expansions in one beat of the artery. **trigeminal p.,** one with a pause after every third beat. **trip-hammer p.,** Corrigan's p. **undulating p.,** a pulse giving the sensation of successive waves. **unequal p.,** a pulse in which some of the beats are strong and others weak. **vagus p.,** a slow pulse. **venous p.,** the pulsation which occurs in a vein, usually observed at the right jugular vein just above the sternoclavicular junction. **vermicular p.,** a small rapid pulse giving to the finger a sensation of wormlike movement. **vibrating p.,** jerky p. **water-hammer p.,** Corrigan's p. **wiry p.,** a small, tense pulse.

pulsimeter (pul-sim′ĕ-ter) [*pulse* + L. *metrum* measure] (*obs.*) an apparatus for measuring the force of the pulse.

pulsion (pul′shun) a pushing forward, or outward or to either side.

pulsus (pul′sus), pl. *pul′sus* [L., from *pellere* to beat] pulse. **p. abdomina′lis,** abdominal pulse. **p. aequa′lis,** equal pulse. **p. alter′nans,** alternating pulse; a pulse in which there is regular alternation of weak and strong beats without changes in cycle length. **p. bifer′iens, p. bisfer′iens,** a pulse characterized by two strong systolic peaks separated by a midsystolic dip, most commonly occurring in pure aortic regurgitation and aortic regurgitation with stenosis. **p. bigem′inus,** bigeminal pulse. **p. ce′ler,** quick pulse. **p. dif′ferens,** inequality of the pulse observable at corresponding sites on either side of the body. **p. filifor′mis,** thready pulse. **p. for′micans,** formicant pulse. **p. for′tis,** a strong pulse. **p. fre′quens,** frequent pulse. **p. irregula′ris perpet′uus,** a pulse which is wholly irregular. **p. mag′nus,** a large, full pulse. **p. mag′nus et ce′ler,** a large, full, and rapid pulse. **p. mol′lis,** soft pulse. **p. monoc′rotus,** monocrotic pulse. **p. oppres′sus,** a pulse which appears to be pushing its way through a contracted artery. **p. parado′xus,** paradoxical pulse. **p. par′vus,** a small pulse. **p. par′vus et tar′dus,** a small hard pulse which rises and falls slowly. **p. ple′nus,** full pulse. **p. tar′dus,** an abnormally slow pulse due to a prolongation of the systole or diastole. **p. trigem′inus,** trigeminal pulse. **p. undulo′sus,** undulating pulse. **p. vac′uus,** an extremely weak pulse. **p. veno′sus,** venous pulse.

pultaceous (pul-ta′shus) [L. *pultaceus*] like a pulp or poultice.

pulv. abbreviation for L. *pulvis* powder.

pulverization (pul″ver-i-za′shun) [L. *pulvis* powder] the reduction of any substance to powder.

pulverulent (pul-ver′u-lent) [L. *pulverulentus*] powdery; dustlike.

pulvinar (pul-vi′nar) [L. "a cushioned seat"] [NA] the prominent, cushion-like mass of nuclei that forms the medial portion of the posterior extremity of the thalamus, which partly overhangs the rostral colliculus and its brachium and is separated inferiorly from the geniculate body by the brachium of the rostral colliculus; it receives fibers from other thalamic nuclei and gives off widespread cortical projections. **p. thal′ami,** nuclei posteriores thalami. **p. tuni′cae inter′nae segmen′ti arteria′lis anastomo′sis arteriove′nae glomerifor′mis** [NA], the wall of the internal coat of the arterial segment of the anastomosis arteriovenosa glomeriformis, consisting of three to six layers of contractile glomus cells. Called also *p. tunicae intimae segmenti arterialis anastomosis arteriovenae glomeriformis* [NA alternative].

pulvinate (pul′vĭ-nāt) [L. *pulvinus* cushion] shaped like a cushion.

pulvis (pul′vis) [L.] powder.

pumex (pu′meks) [L.] pumice.

pumice (pum′is) [USP] a substance of volcanic origin, consisting chiefly of complex silicates of aluminum, potassium, and sodium, occurring as a very light, hard, rough, porous, grayish powder; used in dentistry as an abrasive or polishing agent, the effect achieved depending on the particle size.

pump (pump) 1. an apparatus for drawing or forcing fluids or gases. 2. to draw or force fluids or gases. **air p.**, a pump for exhausting or forcing in air. **Alvegniat's p.**, a mercurial air pump used in measuring the free gaseous constituents of the blood. **blood p.**, a machine used to propel blood through the tubing of extracorporeal circulation devices, especially designed to achieve this without causing damage to the blood constituents, particularly the erythrocytes. **breast p.**, a manual or electric pump for abstracting milk from the breast. **calcium p.**, the mechanism of active transport of calcium (Ca^{++}) across a membrane, as of the sarcoplasmic reticulum of muscle cells, against a concentration gradient; the mechanism is driven by hydrolysis of ATP by the membrane-bound enzyme ATPase. **cardiac balloon p.**, a device for augmenting blood flow to the heart while relieving the cardiac work load. **infusion p.**, a device for injecting a measured amount of fluid during a specific interval of time. **infusion-withdrawal p.**, a pump for the simultaneous injection and withdrawal of fluid at the same rate. **Lindbergh p.**, a perfusion apparatus by means of which an organ removed from the body may be kept alive indefinitely. **Na$^+$-K$^+$ p.**, sodium p. **peristaltic p.**, a pump that moves liquid through tubing by alternate contractions and relaxations on the tubing. **sodium p.**, **sodium-potassium p.**, the mechanism of active transport, involving membrane-bound ATPase, by which sodium (Na$^+$) is extruded from a cell and potassium (K$^+$) is brought in, so as to maintain the low concentration of Na$^+$ and the high concentration of K$^+$ within the cell with respect to the surrounding medium, the high concentration of K$^+$ being necessary for vital processes such as protein biosynthesis, certain enzymes activities, and maintenance of the membrane potential of excitable cells. Called also *Na$^+$-K$^+$ p.* **stomach p.**, a pump for removing the contents from the stomach.

pumpkin (pump′kin) the edible fruit of the plant *Cucurbita pepo* L. (Curcurbitaceae), whose dried, ripe seeds were once used as an anthelmintic.

pump-oxygenator (pump′-ok″sĭ-jĕ-na′tor) an apparatus, usually extracorporeal, comprising an arterial pump and blood oxygenator plus filters and traps, for saturating blood with oxygen and perfusing the body tissue; used for cardiopulmonary bypass during cardiac surgery.

puna (poo′nah) mountain sickness.

punch (punch) an instrument for indenting, perforating, or excising a disk or segment of tissue or material. **kidney p., Murphy's kidney p.**, see *Murphy's test*, under *tests*. **pin p.**, an instrument for perforating a metal backing to receive the pins for fastening artificial teeth. **plate p.**, a punch for cutting out parts of an artificial dental plate. **rubber dam p.**, a hand instrument for punching holes in a rubber dam in order to permit the passage of the dam over the crowns of the teeth.

punchdrunk (punch′drunk) see under *encephalopathy*.

punched-out (puncht′owt) having the appearance of substance or tissue having been removed with a punch.

puncta (punk′tah) [L.] plural of *punctum*.

punctate (punk′tāt) [L. *punctum* point] resembling or marked with points or dots.

punctiform (punk′tĭ-form) [L. *punctum* point + *forma* shape] like a point; located in a point. In bacteriology, said of very minute colonies.

punctograph (punk′to-graf) [L. *punctum* point + Gr. *graphein* to write] an instrument for the roentgenographic localization of foreign bodies in the tissues.

punctum (punk′tum), pl. *punc′ta* [L.] an extremely small spot, or point; used in anatomical nomenclature as a general term to designate an extremely small area, or point of projection. **p. cae′cum**, blind spot; see under *spot*. **punc′ta doloro′sa**, Valleix's points. **p. lacrima′le** [NA], lacrimal point: the opening on the lacrimal papilla of an eyelid, near the medial angle of the eye, into which tears from the lacrimal lake drain to enter the lacrimal canaliculi. **punc′ta lacrima′lia**, see *punctum lacrimale*. **p. lu′-**

teum, macula retinae. **p. nasa′le infe′rius**, the rhinion. **p. ossificatio′nis**, [NA], ossification point: any point at which the process of ossification begins in bones; in a long bone there is a primary point for the diaphysis and one secondary point for epiphysis. Called also *ossification center* and *centrum ossificationis*. **p. ossificatio′nis prima′rium** [NA], primary ossification point: the first point at which bone begins to ossify. Called also *centrum ossificationis primarium* and *primary ossification center*. **p. ossificatio′nis secunda′rium** [NA], secondary ossification point: the point occurring secondary to the primary ossification center that is concerned with progressive ossification toward the end of bones. Called also *centrum ossificationis secundarium* and *secondary ossification center*. **p. prox′imum**, near point. **p. remo′tum**, far point. **punc′ta vasculo′sa**, minute red spots marking the cut surface of the white substance of the brain, produced by blood from divided vessels.

punctumeter (punk-tum′ĕ-ter) [L. *punctum* point + -*meter*] an instrument for measuring the range of accommodation.

punctura (punk-tu′rah) [L.] puncture.

puncture (pungk′chur) [L. *punctura*] 1. the act of piercing or penetrating with a pointed object or instrument. 2. a wound so made. **Bernard's p.**, in experimental medicine, puncture on a definite point of the floor of the fourth ventricle causing glycosuria; called also *diabetic p.* **cisternal p.**, puncture of the cisterna cerebellomedullaris through the occipitoatlantoid ligament for the purpose of withdrawing cerebrospinal fluid. **cranial p.**, cisternal p. **diabetic p.**, Bernard's p. **exploratory p.**, puncture of a cavity or tumor and removal of some portion of the contents for examination. **heat p.**, elevation of the temperature of the animal body produced by puncturing the base of the brain. **intracisternal p.**, cisternal p. **Kronecker's p.**, in experimental medicine, puncture of the inhibitory nerve center of the heart by means of a long fine needle. **lumbar p.**, the tapping of the subarachnoid space in the lumbar region, usually between the third and fourth lumbar vertebrae. **Quincke's p.**, **spinal p.**, lumbar p. **splenic p.**, puncture of the spleen to obtain a specimen of splenic tissue for examination or to measure portal pressure. **sternal p.**, removal of bone marrow from the manubrium of the sternum through an appropriate needle. **suboccipital p.**, cisternal p. **thecal p.**, puncture of the spinal membranes. **transethmoidal p.**, a technique for obtaining postmortem biopsy specimens of the brain, using a tracer inserted through the nostril. **ventricular p.**, puncture of a cerebral ventricle for the purpose of withdrawing fluid.

pungent (pun′jent) [L. *pungens* pricking] sharp or biting; somewhat acrid.

punizin (pu′nĭ-zin) a purple dye formed by the action of light and air on a colorless chromogen found in the secretions of the snails *Murex trunculus* and *Purpura lapillus*.

Punnett square (pun′it) [Reginald Crundall *Punnett*, English geneticist, 20th century] see *checkerboard*.

Puntius (pun′te-us) a genus of fresh-water fish. **P. javan′icus**, a species placed in fresh-water ponds in certain areas of the world, because it eliminates the weeds necessary for the propagation of mosquitoes.

P.U.O. pyrexia of unknown origin.

pupa (pu′pah) [L. "a doll"] the second stage in the development of an insect, between the larva and the imago.

pupal (pu′pal) pertaining to a pupa.

pupil (pu′pil) [L. *pupilla* girl] the opening at the center of the iris of the eye, through which light enters the eye; see *iris*. Called also *pupilla* [NA]. **Adie's p.**, tonic p. **Argyll Robertson p.**, one which is miotic and which responds to accommodation effort, but not to light. **artificial p.**, one made by iridectomy. **Behr's p.**, contralateral dilatation of the pupil in lesions of the optic tract. **bounding p.**, a pupil which shows alternating dilatation and contraction. **Bumke's p.**, dilation of the pupil after a psychic stimulus. **cat's-eye p.**, one with a narrow vertical aperture. **cornpicker's p's**, dilated pupils resulting from exposure to dust from Jimsonweed (which contains stramonium) in the cornfield. **fixed p.**, a pupil which does not react either to light or on convergence, or in accommodation. **Hutchinson's p.**, a condition of the pupils in which one is dilated and the other not. **keyhole p.**, a pupil with a coloboma or a sector iridectomy on one side of the margin.

Marcus Gunn p., an afferent pupillary defect; see *swinging flashlight sign,* under *sign.* **pinhole p.,** one which is extremely contracted. **skew p's,** a condition in which one of the ocular axes deviates upward and the other downward. **stiff p.,** Argyll Robertson p. **tonic p.,** a usually unilateral condition of the eye in which the affected pupil is larger than the other, responds to accommodation and convergence in a slow, delayed fashion, and reacts to light only after prolonged exposure to dark or light. Called also *Adie's pupil* and *papillotonia.* See also *Adie's syndrome,* under *syndrome.*

pupilla (pu-pil′ah) [L. "girl"], pl. *pupil′lae* [NA] the pupil: the opening at the center of the iris of the eye, through which light enters the eye; see *iris.*

pupillary (pu′pĭ-ler-e) pertaining to the pupil.

pupillatonia (pu″pil-ah-to′ne-ah) tonic pupil.

Pupillidae (pu-pil′ĭ-de) a family of small to minute terrestrial gastropods (suborder Stylommatophora, order Pulmonata) that are commonly found in moist wooded regions in North America; the genus *Chondrina* serves as a host of *Dicrocoelium dentriticum.*

pupill(o)- [L. *pupilla* pupil] a combining form denoting relationship to the pupil.

pupillograph (pu-pil′o-graf) [*pupillo-* + *-graph*] an instrument that detects responses of the pupil of the eye.

pupillometer (pu″pĭ-lom′ĕ-ter) [*pupillo-* + *-meter*] an instrument for measuring the width or diameter of the pupil; called also *coreometer.*

pupillometry (pu″pil-lom′ĕ-tre) measurement of the diameter or width of the pupil of the eye; called also *coreometry.*

pupillomotor (pu″pĭ-lo-mo′tor) pertaining to the movement of the pupil.

pupilloplegia (pu″pĭ-lo-ple′je-ah) [*pupillo-* + *-plegia*] tonic pupil.

pupilloscope (pu-pil′o-skōp) 1. an instrument for observing the pupil and its reactions. 2. retinoscope.

pupilloscopy (pu″pĭ-los′ko-pe) [*pupillo-* + *-scopy*] retinoscopy.

pupillostatometer (pu-pil″o-stah-tom′ĕ-ter) [*pupillo-* + Gr. *statos* placed + *-meter*] an instrument for measuring the distance between the pupils.

pupillotonia (pu″pĭ-lo-to′ne-ah) tonic pupil.

Purdy's method, test (per′dēz) [Charles Wesley *Purdy,* American physician, 1846–1901] see under *method* and *tests.*

pure (pūr) [L. *purus*] free from mixture with or contamination by other materials; a reagent is *chemically pure* when it contains no other chemicals that might interfere with its action.

purgation (pur-ga′shun) [L. *purgatio*] catharsis; purging effected by a cathartic medicine.

purgative (pur′gah-tiv) [L. *purgativus*] 1. cathartic (def. 1); causing evacuation of the bowels. 2. a cathartic, particularly one that stimulates peristaltic action.

purge (purj) [L. *purgare* to cleanse, to purify] 1. to relieve of fecal matter. 2. a purgative remedy or dose.

puric (pu′rik) 1. pertaining to pus. 2. pertaining to purine.

puriform (pu′rĭ-form) [L. *pus* pus + *forma* form] resembling pus; the term is applied to the contents of cold abscesses which resemble pus.

purine (pu′rin) [L. *purum* pure + *urine*] a colorless crystalline heterocyclic compound, $C_5H_4N_4$, which is not found free in nature, but is variously substituted to produce a group of compounds known as *purines* or *purine bases* (purine bodies), of which uric acid is a metabolic end product. The purine bases include adenine and guanine, which are constituents of nucleic acids, and hypoxanthine and xanthine. **amino p.,** aminopurine. **methyl p's,** alkaloids formed from purines by substituting methyl groups, usually in positions 1, 3, 7. The principal ones are caffeine, theobromine, and theophylline.

purinemia (pu″rĭ-ne′me-ah) [*purine* + Gr. *haima* blood + *-ia*] the presence of purine bases in the blood.

purinemic (pu″rĭ-ne′mik) pertaining to or characterized by purinemia.

purine-nucleoside phosphorylase (pu′rēn noo″kle-o-sīd fos-for′ĭ-lās) [EC 2.4.2.1] an enzyme of the transferase class that catalyzes the reaction purine nucleoside + ortho-

phosphate = purine + α-D-ribose 1-phosphate. The reaction is a step in the degradation of nucleotides and nucleic acids. Deficiency of the enzyme, an autosomal recessive trait, results in defective T-cell immunity.

purine-5′-nucleotidase (pu′rēn noo″kle-o-ti′dās) 5′ nucleotidase.

Purinethol (pu′rēn-thol) trademark for a preparation of mercaptopurine.

purinolytic (pu″rin-o-lit′ik) [*purine* + Gr. *lytikos* loosing] splitting up purines.

purinometer (pu″rin-om′ĕ-ter) [*purine* + Gr. *metron* measure] an apparatus for estimating the quantity of purine bodies in the urine.

Purkinje's cells, fibers, etc. (pur-kin′jēz) [Johannes Evangelista von *Purkinje,* Bohemian anatomist, physiologist, and microscopist, 1787–1869] see under *cell, fiber, image, layer, network, phenomenon, shift,* and *vesicle.*

Purkinje-Sanson mirror images (pur-kin′je-sah-sō′) [J. E. *Purkinje;* Louis Joseph *Sanson,* French physician, 1790–1841] Purkinje's images; see under *image.*

Purodigin (pu″ro-di′jin) trademark for a preparation of crystalline digitoxin.

purohepatitis (pu″ro-hep″ah-ti′tis) [*pus* + *hepatitis*] hepatic abscess.

puromucous (pu″ro-mu′kus) consisting of or containing pus and mucus; mucopurulent.

puromycin (pūr″o-mi′sin) chemical name: (S)-3′-[(2-amino-3-(4-methoxyphenyl)-1-oxopropyl]amino-3′-deoxy-N,N-dimethyladenosine. An antibiotic produced by *Streptomyces alboniger,* $C_{22}H_{29}N_7O_5$, which has the ability to inhibit protein synthesis and so has been used experimentally as an antineoplastic. It also has trypanosomicidal and amebicidal activity, and was formerly used in the treatment of African trypanosomiasis and amebic dysentery. **p. hydrochloride,** the dihydrochloride salt of puromycin, $C_{22}H_{29}N_7O_5 \cdot 2HCl$, having the same actions as the base.

puron (pu′ron) a compound, $C_5H_8N_4O_2$, obtained by electrolysis of uric acid.

purple (pur′p'l) 1. a color, between blue and red. 2. a substance of this color used as a dye or indicator. **bromcresol p.,** an indicator, dibromorthocresol sulfonphthalein, used in the determination of hydrogen ion concentration; it has a pH range of 5.2 to 6.8, being yellow at 5.2 and purple at 6.8. **royal p.,** tyrian purple. **Stewart's p.,** 1 grain of iodine in 1 oz. of petrolatum. **tyrian p.,** a dye of the ancients which was obtained from the snails *Murex trunculus* and *Purpura lapillus.* **visual p.,** rhodopsin.

Purpura (pur′pu-rah) a genus of marine snails, some species of which furnish a purple dye. See *purpurine.*

purpura (pur′pu-rah) [L. "purple"] 1. a small hemorrhage (up to about 1 cm in diameter) in the skin, mucous membrane, or serosal surface, which may be caused by various factors, including blood disorders, vascular abnormalities, and trauma. Purpuric lesions may be associated with inflammation, in which case they present as papular purpura, or the hemorrhage may not be accompanied by inflammation, in which case they are macular. The term also comprises a group of hemorrhagic diseases characterized by the presence of purpuric lesions, ecchymoses, and a tendency to bruise easily, which may be caused by decreased platelet counts, the presence of abnormal platelets, vascular defects, or reactions to certain drugs. **allergic p., anaphylactoid p.,** Schönlein-Henoch p. **p. annula′ris telangiecto′des,** a rare purpuric eruption, commonly beginning on the lower extremities and becoming generalized, the original punctate erythematous lesions coalescing to form an annular or serpiginous pattern; involution is gradual, sometimes followed by atrophy and loss of hair in the area. Called also *Majocchi's purpura* or *disease.* **brain p.,** cerebral toxic pericapillary hemorrhage. **fibrinolytic p., p. fibrinolyt′ica,** purpura secondary to and accompanied by increased fibrinolytic activity of the blood. **p. ful′minans,** a form of nonthrombocytopenic purpura, observed mainly in children, usually following an infectious disease such as scarlet fever, and characterized by fever, shock, anemia, and sudden and rapidly spreading symmetrical skin hemorrhages of the lower extremities, often associated with extensive intravascular thromboses and gangrene. **p. hemorrha′gica,** thrombocytopenic p., idiopathic. **Henoch's p.,** a variety of Schönlein-Henoch purpura characterized by acute visceral symptoms such as vomiting, diarrhea, abdominal distention, hematuria, and renal colic, and without articular symptoms. Called also *p. nervosa.* **Henoch-Schönlein p.,** Schönlein-Henoch p. **p. hyperglobuline′mica,** originally used to designate prolonged, repetitive episodes of purpura associated with an increase in gamma globulins; no longer considered a specific entity inasmuch as the clinical and laboratory findings are observed in a variety of hematologic conditions. **idiopathic p.,** see *thrombocytopenic p., idiopathic.* **itching p.,** an extremely pruritic, episodically recurring eruptive hemorrhagic dermatosis, tending to occur in males, manifested as erythematous macules containing punctate purpura that are usually localized to the legs, with dissemination to the thighs, trunk, upper extremities, and, in more severe cases, the large flexural areas. It is usually seen in the spring and summer, and it clears spontaneously. Called also *disseminated pruritic angiodermatitis.* **Landouzy′s p.,** a term originally used to designate a form of purpura with grave systemic manifestations. **Majocchi′s p.,** p. annularis telangiectodes. **malignant p.,** epidemic cerebrospinal meningitis. **p. nervo′sa,** Henoch′s p. **p. of newborn,** a form of thrombocytopenia observed soon after birth, presumed in certain instances to be due to the passage of anti-platelet factor(s) across the placenta. **nonthrombocytopenic p.,** purpura without any decrease in the platelet count of the blood. **psychogenic p.,** a psychosomatic condition similar to painful bruising syndrome (q.v.), but without any evidence of sensitivity to erythrocytes, as may be seen in the latter disorder. **p. rheumat′ica,** Schönlein′s p. **Schönlein p.,** Schönlein-Henoch purpura with articular symptoms and without gastrointestinal symptoms. Called also *p. rheumatica, rheumatocelis,* and *Schönlein disease.* **Schönlein-Henoch p.,** a form of nonthrombocytopenic purpura probably due to a vasculitis of unknown cause, most commonly observed in children and associated with a variety of clinical symptoms including urticaria and erythema, arthropathy and arthritis, gastrointestinal symptoms, and renal involvement. Called also *allergic p., anaphylactoid p.,* and *Schönlein-Henoch disease.* **p. seni′lis,** dark purplish red ecchymoses occurring on the forearms and back of the hands in the elderly. See also *steroid p.* **p. sim′plex,** a general designation for nonthrombocytopenic purpura unaccompanied by defined vascular or intravascular abnormalities. **steroid p.,** bizarre-shaped broad hemorrhages beneath the skin of the back of the forearms, hands, or shins caused by attrition of dermal and vascular connective tissue due to long-term treatment with adrenocortical steroid hormones. Identical with purpura senilis in appearance. **thrombocytopenic p.,** any form of purpura in which the platelet count is decreased; it may be either primary (idiopathic) or secondary. **thrombocytopenic p., idiopathic,** thrombocytopenic purpura unassociated with any definable systemic disease but often accompanied by the presence of a serum antiplatelet factor, now characterized as an IgG immunoglobulin. **thrombocytopenic p., secondary,** thrombocytopenic purpura occurring as a consequence of a primary hematologic disease such as leukemia, or an underlying systemic nonhematologic entity. **thrombocytopenic p., thrombotic,** a disease of undefined cause, characterized by thrombocytopenia, hemolytic anemia, bizarre neurological manifestations, azotemia, fever, and thromboses in terminal arterioles and capillaries; called also *microangiopathic hemolytic anemia* and *Moschcowitz′s disease.* **thrombopenic p.,** thrombocytopenic p.

purpureaglycoside (pur-pu″re-ah-gli′ko-sīd) a cardiac glycoside, $C_{47}H_{74}O_{18}$, from the leaves of *Digitalis purpurea* L. (Schrophulariaceae). **p. C.,** see *deslanoside.*

purpuric (pur-pu′rik) of the nature of, pertaining to, or affected with purpura.

purpuric acid (pur-pūr-ik) an imino-condensation product of alloxan, $CO(NH·CO)_2C·NH·C(NH·CO)_2$, found in Weidel′s test for uric acid. See also *murexide,* and *Weidel′s test* (1), under *tests.*

purpuriferous (pur″pu-rif′er-us) [L. *purpura* purple + *ferre* to bear] producing a purple pigment.

purpurin (pur′pu-rin) 1. a glycoside from madder root that has been used as a nuclear stain. It is 1,2,4-trihydroxy-anthraquinone, $C_6H_4(CO)_2C_6H(OH)_3$. 2. uroerythrin. 3. purpurine.

purpurine (pur′pu-rēn) 1. a neurotoxic substance derived from the median zone of the hypobranchial or purple gland

of gastropods of the genus *Purpura,* thought to be an ester or a mixture of esters of choline; the substance is called *murexine* when derived from snails of the genus *Murex.* 2. purpurin.

purpurinuria (pur″pu-rin-u′re-ah) the presence of uroerythrin in the urine.

purpuriparous (pur″pu-rip′ah-rus) [L. *purpura* purple + *parere* to produce] purpuriferous.

purpurogenous (pur″pu-roj′ĕ-nus)[L. *purpura* purple + Gr. *gennan* to produce] producing visual purple (rhodopsin).

purr (pur) a low vibratory murmur, or purring sound.

purring (pur′ing) having a tremulous quality, like the purr of a cat.

purshianin (pur-shi′ah-nin) a brown, oily liquid glycoside mixture from *Rhamnus purshiana* D.C. (Rhamnaceae), having laxative action.

Purtscher′s disease (angiopathic retinopathy) (poor′cherz) [Otmar *Purtscher,* Swiss ophthalmologist, 1852–1927] see under *disease.*

purulence (pu′roo-lens) [L. *purulentia*] the condition or fact of being purulent.

purulency (pu′roo-len″se) purulence.

purulent (pu′roo-lent) [L. *purulentus*] consisting of or containing pus; associated with the formation of or caused by pus.

puruloid (pu′roo-loid) resembling pus; puriform.

pus (pus), pl. *pu′ra,* gen. *pu′ris* [L.] a liquid inflammation product made up of cells (leukocytes) and a thin fluid called liquor puris. **anchovy sauce p.,** the brownish pus seen in amebic abscess of the liver. **blue p.,** pus with a bluish tint, seen in certain suppurative infections, the color occurring as a result of the presence of an antibiotic pigment (pyocyanin) produced by *Pseudomonas aeruginosa.* **p. bo′num et laudab′ile,** laudable pus. **burrowing p.,** pus which is not walled off but may extend between fascial planes for considerable distances. **cheesy p.,** thick, nearly solid pus. **curdy p.,** pus mixed with cheesy flakes. **green p.,** pus having a greenish tint. **ichorous p.,** a thin, acrid pus, often having an ill smell, secreted by unhealthy surfaces. **laudable p., p. laudan′dum,** a term once applied to a creamy yellow, inodorous pus, secreted by a healthy granulating surface, and regarded as indicative of less danger than other varieties. **sanious p.,** bloody pus, often ichorous and ill smelling.

Pusey′s emulsion (pu′sēz) [William Allen *Pusey,* American dermatologist, 1865–1940] see under *emulsion.*

pustula (pus′tu-lah), pl. *pus′tulae* [L.] pustule.

pustular (pus′tu-lar) pertaining to or of the nature of a pustule; consisting of pustules.

pustulation (pus″tu-la′shun) the formation of pustules.

pustule (pus′tūl) [L. *pustula*] a visible collection of pus within or beneath the epidermis, often in a hair follicle or sweat pore. **malignant p.,** see *cutaneous anthrax,* under *anthrax.* **multilocular p.,** a pustule with several compartments, indicating origin from a spongiotic vesicle within the epidermis rather than from infection arising in a follicle or sweat pore, or beneath the epidermis. **simple p.,** unilocular p. **spongiform p., spongiform p. of Kogoj,** a focal subcorneal area of epidermal spongiosis lined with edematous epidermal cells and containing neutrophils in the intercellular spaces, which is a cardinal sign of active psoriasis, and found also in other dermatologic conditions such as seborrheic dermatitis and Reiter′s disease. Cf. *Munro microabscess.* **unilocular p.,** one consisting of a single cavity filled with pus, suggesting origin within a follicle or sweat pore or from beneath the epidermis, rather than within it; called also *simple p.*

pustulosis (pus″tu-lo′sis) a condition marked by an outbreak of pustules. **p. palma′ris et planta′ris, palmoplantar p.,** 1. localized pustular psoriasis. 2. a pustular eruption similar to localized pustular psoriasis except that psoriasis is not present. **p. vaccinifor′mis acu′ta, p. variolifor′mis acu′ta,** Kaposi′s varicelliform eruption.

putamen (pu-ta′men) [L. "shell"] [NA] the larger, darker and more lateral part of the lentiform nucleus, separated from the lateral globus pallidus by the lateral medullary lamina.

Putnam type (put′nam) [James Jackson *Putnam,* Boston

neurologist, 1846–1918] subacute combined degeneration of the spinal cord; see under *degeneration*.

Putnam-Dana syndrome (put′nam-da′nah) [J. J. *Putnam;* Charles Loomis *Dana,* neurologist in New York, 1852–1935] subacute combined degeneration of spinal cord (see under *degeneration*).

putrefaction (pu″trĕ-fak′shun) [L. *putrefactio*] enzymic decomposition, especially of proteins, with the production of foul-smelling compounds, such as hydrogen sulfide, ammonia, and mercaptans. Cf. *fermentation.*

putrefactive (pu″trĕ-fak′tiv) pertaining to or of the nature of putrefaction.

putrefy (pu′trĕ-fi) to decompose, with the production of foul-smelling compounds; a term applied especially to the decomposition of proteins and organic matter.

putrescence (pu-tres′ens) partial or complete rottenness.

putrescent (pu-tres′ent) [L. *putrescens* decaying] rotting; undergoing putrefaction.

putrescine (pu-tres′in) chemical name: tetra-methylene-diamine. A polyamine, $NH_2(CH_2)_4NH_2$, first found in decaying animal tissues but now known to occur in almost all tissues and in cultures of certain bacteria. It is formed by decarboxylation of ornithine and is itself a precursor of spermidine.

putrid (pu′trid) [L. *putridus*] characterized by putrefaction; rotten or corrupt.

putrilage (pu′tri-lij) [L. *putrilago*] putrescent or putrid matter.

putromaine (pu-tro′mān) any poison produced by the decomposition of food within the living body.

Puusepp's reflex (poos′eps) [Lyudvig Martinovich *Puusepp,* Estonian neurosurgeon, 1875–1942] see under *reflex.*

PVP polyvinylpyrrolidone.

PVP-I povidone-iodine.

PWM pokeweed mitogen.

pyarthrosis (pi″ar-thro′sis) [Gr. *pyon* pus + *arthron* joint + *-osis*] acute suppurative arthritis.

Pycnanthemum (pik-nan′the-mum) [Gr. *pyknos* dense + *anthemon* bloom] a genus of American mints, called *mountain basil* and *mountain mint,* aromatic and carminative; resembling pennyroyal and spearmint in taste and smell.

pycn(o)- for words thus beginning, see those beginning *pykn(o)-.*

pyecchysis (pi-ek′ki-sis) [Gr. *pyon* pus + *ek* out + *chein* to pour] the effusion of purulent matter.

pyelectasia (pi″e-lek-ta′ze-ah) pyelectasis.

pyelectasis (pi″ĕ-lek′tah-sis) [*pyel-* + Gr. *ektasis* distention] dilatation of the renal pelvis.

pyelic (pi-el′ik) pertaining to the pelvis of the kidney.

pyelitic (pi″ĕ-lit′ik) pertaining to or affected with pyelitis.

pyelitis (pi″ĕ-li′tis) [*pyel-* + *-itis*] inflammation of the pelvis of the kidney. It is attended by pain and tenderness in the loins, irritability of the bladder, remittent fever, bloody or purulent urine, diarrhea, vomiting, and a peculiar pain on flexion of the thigh. See also *pyelonephritis.* **calculous p.,** that which is caused by calculi. **p. cys′tica,** pyelitis with the formation of multiple submucosal cysts. **defloration p.,** pyelitis in women after the first sexual intercourse, as a result of infection following rupture of the hymen. **encrusted p.,** pyelitis with ulcers which are encrusted with urinary salts. **p. glandula′ris,** pyelitis with conversion of transitional mucosal into cylindrical epithelium, with formation of glandular acini. **p. granulo′sa,** pyelitis marked by the presence of exuberant granulations. **p. gravida′rum,** inflammation of the kidney and ureter occurring in pregnancy. **hematogenous p.,** pyelitis in which the infection comes from the blood. **hemorrhagic p.,** that which is attended with hemorrhage. **suppurative p.,** a form with development of pus which causes abscess of the kidney, or pyonephrosis. **urogenous p.,** pyelitis in which the infection comes from the urine.

pyel(o)- [Gr. *pyelos* pelvis] combining form denoting relationship to the renal pelvis.

pyelocaliectasis (pi″ĕ-lo-kal″e-ek′tah-sis) [*pyelo-* + *calix* + *ektasis* distention] dilatation of the kidney pelvis and calices.

pyelocystitis (pi″ĕ-lo-sis-ti′tis) [*pyelo-* + Gr. *kystis* bladder + *-itis*] inflammation of the renal pelvis and of the bladder.

pyelofluoroscopy (pi″ĕ-lo-floo″o-ros′ko-pe) examination of the renal pelvis by means of the fluoroscope.

pyelogram (pi′ĕ-lo-gram″) [*pyelo-* + Gr. *gramma* mark] a roentgenogram of the kidney and ureter, especially showing the pelvis of the kidney. **dragon p.,** bizarre forms in the pyelogram seen in polycystic kidney.

pyelograph (pi′ĕ-lo-graf) pyelogram.

pyelography (pi″ĕ-log′rah-fe) [*pyelo-* + Gr. *graphein* to draw] roentgenography of the renal pelvis and ureter after the structures have been filled with a contrast solution. **air p.,** pneumopyelography. **antegrade p.,** that in which the contrast medium is introduced by percutaneous needle puncture into the renal pelvis. **ascending p.,** retrograde p. **p. by elimination,** intravenous p. **excretion p.,** intravenous p. **intravenous p.,** pyelography in which an intravenous injection is made of a contrast medium which passes quickly into the urine. **lateral p.,** pyelography in which the patient lies in lateral position with his questionable side next to the film. **respiration p.,** pyelography with a diphasic film showing the kidney under several phases of the respiratory cycle. **retrograde p.,** pyelography in which the contrast fluid is injected into the renal pelvis through the ureter. **wash-out p.,** that in which the roentgenogram is taken after the kidneys have been filled with a contrast solution and then "washed-out" by water diuresis; this procedure increases the contrast between a normal and a malfunctioning kidney.

pyeloileocutaneous (pi″ĕ-lo-il″e-o-ku-ta′ne-us) pertaining to the renal pelvis, ileum, and skin; see under *anastomosis.*

pyelointerstitial (pi″ĕ-lo-in″ter-stish′al) pertaining to the interstitial tissue of the renal pelvis.

pyelolithotomy (pi″ĕ-lo-li-thot′o-me) [*pyelo-* + Gr. *lithos* stone + *tomē* a cutting] the operation of excising a renal calculus from the pelvis of the kidney.

pyelometry (pi″ĕ-lom′e-tre) [*pyelo-* + Gr. *metron* measure] the measurement by tracings of the waves of contraction and relaxation of the renal pelvis, recorded by changes of pressure through a ureteral catheter.

pyelonephritis (pi″ĕ-lo-nĕ-fri′tis) [*pyelo-* + Gr. *nephros* kidney + *-itis*] inflammation of the kidney and its pelvis, beginning in the interstitium and rapidly extending to involve the tubules, glomeruli, and blood vessels; due to bacterial infection. **acute p.,** pyelonephritis of sudden onset characterized by fever, shaking chills, pain in the costovertebral region or flanks, and symptoms of bladder inflammation; it is a self-limited bacterial disease caused most often by gram-negative enteric bacilli. **chronic p.,** pyelonephritis attributed to cicatricial effects of a previous infection or to recurring or progressive infection. Typically, it is of insidious onset, manifested by symptoms of chronic renal insufficiency, with fatigue, headache, loss of appetite, weight loss, excessive thirst, and polyuria. **p. of pregnancy,** a renal infection during pregnancy characterized by dilatation of the renal pelvis and the ureters; some degree of ureteric obstruction may be caused by the gravid uterus.

pyelonephrosis (pi″ĕ-lo-nĕ-fro′sis) [*pyelo-* + Gr. *nephros* kidney + *-osis*] any disease of the kidney and its pelvis.

pyelopathy (pi″ĕ-lop′ah-the) [*pyelo-* + Gr. *pathos* disease] any disease of the renal pelvis.

pyelophlebitis (pi″ĕ-lo-fle-bi′tis) [*pyelo-* + Gr. *phleps* vein + *-itis*] inflammation of the veins of the renal pelvis.

pyeloplasty (pi′ĕ-lo-plas″te) [*pyelo-* + Gr. *plassein* to form] a plastic operation on the pelvis of the kidney.

pyeloscopy (pi″ĕ-los′ko-pe) [*pyelo-* + Gr. *skopein* to examine] observation of the kidney pelvis under the fluoroscope after intravenous or retrograde injection of a contrast medium.

pyelostomy (pi″ĕ-los′to-me) [*pyelo-* + Gr. *stomoun* to provide with an opening, or mouth] the operation of forming an opening into the renal pelvis for the purpose of temporarily diverting the urine from the ureter.

pyelotomy (pi″ĕ-lot′o-me) [*pyelo-* + Gr. *tomē* a cutting] incision of the pelvis of the kidney.

pyeloureterectasis (pi″ĕ-lo-u-re″ter-ek′tah-sis) dilatation of a renal pelvis and a ureter.

pyeloureterography (pi″ĕ-lo-u-re″ter-og′rah-fe) pyelography.

pyeloureterolysis (pi″ĕ-lo-u-re″ter-ol′ĭ-sis) [*pyelo-* + *ureter* + Gr. *lysis* dissolution] the surgical freeing of fibrous bands or adhesions near the junction of the renal pelvis and ureter.

pyeloureteroplasty (pi″ĕ-lo-u-re″ter-o-plas″te) plastic operation on the renal pelvis and ureter.

pyelovenous (pi″ĕ-lo-ve′nus) pertaining to the kidney pelvis and renal veins.

pyemesis (pi-em′ĕ-sis) [Gr. *pyon* pus + *emesis* vomiting] vomiting of purulent matter.

pyemia (pi-e′me-ah) [Gr. *pyon* pus + *haima* blood + *-ia*] a general septicemia in which secondary foci of suppuration occur and multiple abscesses are formed. The condition is marked by fever, chills, sweating, jaundice, and abscess in various parts of the body. Called also *metastatic infection*. **arterial p.,** a form due to the dissemination of septic emboli from the heart. **cryptogenic p.,** that in which the source of infection is in an unidentified tissue. **otogenous p.,** that which originates from inflammation in the ear. **portal p.,** suppurative pylephlebitis; see *pylephlebitis.*

pyemic (pi-e′mik) pertaining to or marked by pyemia.

Pyemotes (pi-ĕ-mo′tez) a genus of parasitic mites; formerly called *Pediculoides*. **P. ventrico′sus,** a predaceous mite which attacks the larvae of a number of insects. Found in the straw of various cereals, it produces a vesiculopapular dermatitis (grain itch) in man. Formerly known as *Pediculoides ventricosus* and *Acarus tritici.*

pyencephalus (pi″en-sef′ah-lus) [Gr. *pyon* pus + *enkephalos* brain] abscess of the brain.

pyesis (pi-e′sis) suppuration.

pygal (pi′gal) [Gr. *pyge* rump] pertaining to the buttocks; natal.

pygalgia (pi-gal′je-ah) [*pygo-* + *-algia*] pain in the buttocks.

pygmalionism (pig-ma′le-on-izm) [*Pygmalion*, a Greek sculptor who fell in love with a statue he had carved] the falling in love with an object made by oneself.

pygmy (pig′me) [Gr. *pygmaios* dwarfish] a small individual; a dwarf.

pyg(o)- [Gr. *pyge* rump] a combining form denoting relationship to the buttocks.

pygoamorphus (pi″go-ah-mor′fus) asymmetrical conjoined twins, in which the parasite, or teratoma, is an amorphous mass attached to the sacral region of the autosite.

pygodidymus (pi″go-did′ĭ-mus) [*pygo-* + Gr. *didymos* twin] a fetus with double hips and pelvis.

pygomelus (pi-gom′ĕ-lus) [*pygo-* + Gr. *melos* limb] a fetus with a supernumerary limb or limbs attached to or near the buttock.

pygopagus (pi-gop′ah-gus) [*pygo-* + Gr. *pagos* thing fixed] a double monster consisting of two nearly complete individuals joined at the sacrum, so the two components are back to back. **p. parasit′icus,** an asymmetrical double monster in which the parasitic component is attached to the sacral region of the autosite.

pygopagy (pi-gop′ah-je) the condition of being a pygopagus.

pyic (pi′ik) of or pertaining to pus.

pyin (pi′in) [Gr. *pyon* pus] an albuminoid mucus-like substance found in pus, and separated from it by adding sodium chloride and filtering.

pyknic (pik′nik) [Gr. *pyknos* thick] having a short, thick, stocky build.

pykn(o)- [Gr. *pyknos* thick, frequent] a combining form meaning thick, compact, or frequent.

pyknocyte (pik″no-sīt) a distorted and contracted, occasionally spiculed erythrocyte normally occurring in small numbers in the full-term infant, but in greater numbers in hemolytic disorders.

pyknocytoma (pik″no-si-to′mah) oxyphilic granular cell adenoma.

pyknocytosis (pik″no-si-to′sis) conspicuous increases in the numbers of pyknocytes.

pyknodysostosis (pik″no-dis″os-to′sis) a symptom complex inherited as an autosomal recessive trait, consisting of dwarfism, osteopetrosis, partial agenesis of the terminal digits of the hands and feet, cranial anomalies, frontal and occipital bossing, and hypoplasia of the angle of the mandible.

pyknoepilepsy (pik″no-ep′ĭ-lep″se) [*pykno-* + Gr. *epilēpsia* seizure] petit mal epilepsy.

pyknolepsy (pik″no-lep′se) [*pykno-* + Gr. *lepsis* seizure] (*obs.*) frequent, brief attacks of unawareness in childhood that terminate by puberty.

pyknometer (pik-nom′ĕ-ter) [*pykno-* + Gr. *metron* measure] an instrument for determining the specific gravity of fluids.

pyknometry (pik-nom′ĕ-tre) measurement by the pyknometer.

pyknomorphic (pik″no-mor′fik) pyknomorphous.

pyknomorphous (pik″no-mor′fus) [*pykno-* + Gr. *morphē* form] having the stainable elements compactly arranged; a term applied to certain nerve cells.

pyknophrasia (pik″no-fra′ze-ah) [*pykno-* + Gr. *phrasis* speech + *-ia*] thickness of speech.

pyknoplasson (pik″no-plas′on) [*pykno-* + *plasson*] the plasson in its unexpanded form. Cf. *chasmatoplasson.*

pyknosis (pik-no′sis) [Gr. *pyknōsis* condensation] a thickening, especially degeneration of a cell in which the nucleus shrinks in size and the chromatin condenses to a solid, structureless mass or masses.

pyknotic (pik-not′ik) [Gr. *pyknōtikos*] 1. serving to close the pores. 2. pertaining to pyknosis.

pyle- [Gr. *pylē* gate] a combining form denoting relationship to the portal vein.

pylephlebectasis (pi″le-fle-bek′tah-sis) [*pyle-* + Gr. *phleps* vein + *ektasis* dilatation] dilatation of the portal vein.

pylephlebitis (pi″le-fle-bi′tis) [*pyle-* + Gr. *phleps* vein + *-itis*] inflammation of the portal vein; it usually results from intestinal disease. Suppurative pylephlebitis, or portal pyemia, is marked by symptoms of pyemia. **adhesive p.,** inflammation of the portal vein producing thrombosis; pylethrombophlebitis.

pylethrombophlebitis (pi″le-throm″bo-fle-bi′tis) [*pyle-* + Gr. *thrombos* clot of blood + *phleps* vein + *-itis*] thrombosis and inflammation of the portal vein.

pylethrombosis (pi″le-throm-bo′sis) thrombosis of the portal vein, as in adhesive pylephlebitis.

pylic (pi′lik) [Gr. *pylē* gate] pertaining to the portal vein.

pylon (pi′lon) a temporary artificial leg.

pyloralgia (pi″lo-ral′je-ah) [*pylorus* + Gr. *algos* pain + *-ia*] pain in the region of the pylorus.

pylorectomy (pi″lo-rek′to-me) [*pylorus* + Gr. *ektomē* excision] excision of the pylorus.

pyloric (pi-lor′ik) pertaining to the pylorus or to the pyloric part of the stomach (pars pylorica ventriculi).

pyloristenosis (pi-lor″e-stĕ-no′sis) [*pylorus* + Gr. *stenōsis* narrowing] stenosis, or narrowing, of the caliber of the pylorus; pyloric stenosis.

pyloritis (pi″lo-ri′tis) inflammation of the pylorus.

pylor(o)- [L. *pylorus*, q.v.] a combining form denoting relationship to the pylorus.

pylorodiosis (pi-lo″ro-di-o′sis) [*pyloro-* + Gr. *diōsis* pushing asunder] dilation of a stricture of the pylorus with the finger.

pyloroduodenitis (pi-lo″ro-du″o-de-ni′tis) inflammation of the pyloric and duodenal mucosa.

pylorogastrectomy (pi-lo″ro-gas-trek′to-me) excision of the pylorus.

pyloromyotomy (pi-lo″ro-mi-ot′o-me) the operation for congenital stenosis of the pylorus, performed by longitudinally incising the thickened serosa and muscularis down to the mucosa; called also *Fredet-Ramstedt operation.*

pyloroplasty (pi-lo′ro-plas″te) [*pyloro-* + Gr. *plassein* to form] incision of the pylorus and reconstruction of the pyloric channel to relieve pyloric obstruction or to accelerate gastric emptying after truncal or selective vagotomy in treatment of duodenal ulcer. **double p.,** posterior pyloromyotomy combined with the Heineke-Mikulicz pyloroplasty. **Finney p.,** reconstruction of the pyloric channel by means of a longitudinal incision through the pylorus and adjacent walls of the stomach and duodenum and the establishment of an inverted U-shaped anastomosis between the stomach and duodenum. **Heineke-Mikulicz p.,** reconstruction of the pyloric channel by incising the pylorus longitudinally and suturing the incision transversely.

pyloroscopy (pi″lo-ros′ko-pe) [*pyloro-* + Gr. *skopein* to examine] inspection of the pylorus with an endoscope.

pylorospasm (pi-lo′ro-spazm) [*pyloro-* + Gr. *spasmos* spasm] spasm of the pylorus or of the pyloric portion of the stomach. **congenital p.,** spasm of the pylorus in infants due to prenatal conditions. **reflex p.,** pylorospasm due to extragastric conditions.

pylorostenosis (pi-lo″ro-stĕ-no′sis) pyloristenosis.

pylorostomy (pi″lo-ros′to-me) [*pyloro-* + Gr. *stomoun* to provide with an opening, or mouth] surgical formation of an opening through the abdominal wall into the stomach near the pylorus.

pylorotomy (pi″lo-rot′o-me) [*pyloro-* + Gr. *tomē* a cutting] surgical incision of the pylorus.

pylorus (pi-lo′rus) [Gr. *pyloros,* from *pylē* gate + *ouros* guard] [NA] the distal aperture of the stomach surrounded by a strong band of circular muscle, and through which the stomach contents are emptied into the duodenum. It is variously used to mean pyloric part of the stomach, pyloric antrum, pyloric canal, pyloric opening, and pyloric sphincter.

py(o)- [Gr. *pyon* pus] a combining form denoting relationship to pus.

pyoarthrosis (pi″o-ar-thro′sis) acute suppurative arthritis.

pyoblennorrhea (pi″o-blen″o-re′ah) suppurative blennorrhea.

pyocalix (pi″o-ka′liks) the presence of pus in a calix of the renal pelvis.

pyocele (pi′o-sēl) [*pyo-* + Gr. *kēlē* hernia] distention of a cavity or tube with pus due to retention; as an accumulation of pus in the scrotum.

pyocelia (pi″o-se′le-ah) [*pyo-* + Gr. *koilia* cavity] pus in the abdominal cavity.

pyocephalus (pi″o-sef′ah-lus) [*pyo-* + Gr. *kephalē* head] the presence of purulent fluid in the cerebral ventricles.

pyochezia (pi″o-ke′ze-ah) [*pyo-* + Gr. *chezein* to defecate + *-ia*] presence of pus in the stools.

pyocin (pi′o-sin) [*pyo-* + *-cin* from L. caedere to kill] a protein bacteriocin produced by certain strains of *Pseudomonas aeruginosa.*

pyococcic (pi″o-kok′sik) pertaining to or produced by pus-forming cocci.

pyococcus (pi″o-kok′us) any pus-forming coccus.

pyocolpocele (pi″o-kol′po-sēl) [*pyo-* + Gr. *kolpos* vagina + *kēlē* tumor] a tumor of the vagina containing pus.

pyocolpos (pi″o-kol′pos) [*pyo-* + Gr. *kolpos* vagina] a collection of pus within the vagina.

pyocyanase (pi″o-si′ah-nās) a preparation from cultures of *Pseudomonas aeruginosa,* formerly used as an antibiotic. It is composed of three fractions, one of which is pyocyanin.

pyocyanic (pi″o-si-an′ik) pertaining to blue pus, or to *Pseudomonas aeruginosa* (*P. pyocyanea*).

pyocyanin (pi″o-si′ah-nin) [*pyo-* + Gr. *kyanos* blue + *-in,* a chemical suffix] a blue-green antibiotic pigment produced by *Pseudomonas aeruginosa;* it gives the color to blue pus.

pyocyanogenic (pi″o-si″ah-no-jen′ik) producing pyocyanin.

pyocyanosis (pi″o-si″ah-no′sis) any disease due to infection with *Pseudomonas aeruginosa* (*P. pyocyanea*).

pyocyst (pi′o-sist) [*pyo-* + *cyst*] a cyst containing pus.

pyocystis (pi″o-sis′tis) pus in the urinary bladder.

pyoderma (pi″o-der′mah) [*pyo-* + Gr. *derma* skin] any purulent skin disease. Called also *pyodermia.* **chancriform p., p. chancrifor′me faci′ei,** an eroded, ulcerated, nodular, solitary lesion with a rolled edge, closely resembling a syphilitic chancre, and generally occurring in association with regional lymphadenopathy. The lesion, which usually involutes and heals with scarring, is most often located on the face, especially near the eyes, although some genital lesions have been reported. **p. facia′le,** an acute, localized skin disease occurring on the face of young women and preadolescent girls, usually in the absence of acne, and characterized by the presence of intense erythema and the development of numerous abscesses and cysts, with the formation of sinus tracts between deep-seated lesions, which may heal with severe scarring if untreated. **p. gangreno′sum,** a rapidly evolving, idiopathic, chronic and severely debilitating skin disease occurring most commonly in association with a systemic disease, especially chronic ulcerative colitis, and characterized by the presence of irregular, boggy, blue-red ulcers with undermined borders surrounding purulent necrotic bases. **malignant p.,** a destructive, progressive ulcerative and suppurative skin disease located predominantly on the head and neck region and trunk, which may develop spontaneously or at the site of trauma and enlarge peripherally, and sometimes associated with neurological disturbances. **p. veg′etans,** see under *dermatitis.*

pyodermia (pi″o-der′me-ah) pyoderma.

pyofecia (pi″o-fe′se-ah) pus in the feces.

pyogenesis (pi″o-jen′ĕ-sis) [*pyo-* + Gr. *genesis* production] the formation of pus; pyopoiesis.

pyogenic (pi″o-jen′ik) producing pus; pyopoietic.

pyogenin (pi-oj′e-nin) a compound, $C_{63}H_{128}N_2O_{19}$, derived from the body of pus cells.

pyogenous (pi-oj′ĕ-nus) caused by pus.

pyohemia (pi″o-he′me-ah) pyemia.

pyohemothorax (pi″o-he″mo-tho′raks) [*pyo-* + Gr. *haima* blood + *thōrax* chest] a collection of pus and blood in the pleural space.

pyohydronephrosis (pi″o-hi″dro-nĕ-fro′sis) the accumulation of pus and urine in the kidney.

pyoid (pi′oid) [*pyo-* + Gr. *eidos* form] 1. resembling pus. 2. a puslike substance from raw or granulating surfaces, but free from bacteria and nontoxic.

pyolabyrinthitis (pi″o-lab″ĭ-rin-thi′tis) inflammation of the labyrinth of the ear, with suppuration.

pyometra (pi″o-me′trah) [*pyo-* + Gr. *mētra* womb] an accumulation of pus within the uterus.

pyometritis (pi″o-mĕ-tri′tis) purulent inflammation of the uterus.

pyometrium (pi″o-me′tre-um) pyometra.

pyomyoma (pi″o-mi-o′mah) a leiomyoma that has undergone suppuration.

pyomyositis (pi″o-mi″o-si′tis) [*pyo-* + *myositis*] an acute bacterial infection of skeletal muscle, usually seen in the tropics, especially in Africa and less often in South America and Asia, which occurs spontaneously without other foci of infection. It is most commonly caused by *Staphylococcus aureus,* and is characterized by suppuration followed by abscess formation within the fascial covering of the affected muscle(s). Called also *spontaneous bacterial myositis* and *tropical p.* **tropical p.,** pyomyositis.

pyonephritis (pi″o-nĕ-fri′tis) purulent inflammation of the kidney.

pyonephrolithiasis (pi″o-nef″ro-lĭ-thi′ah-sis) [*pyo-* + Gr. *nephros* kidney + *lithos* stone + *-iasis*] the presence of stones and pus in the kidney.

pyonephrosis (pi″o-nĕ-fro′sis) [*pyo-* + Gr. *nephros* kidney + *-osis*] suppurative destruction of the parenchyma of the kidney, with total or almost complete loss of renal function.

pyonephrotic (pi″o-nĕ-frot′ik) pertaining to or characterized by pyonephrosis.

pyo-ovarium (pi″o-o-va′re-um) abscess of an ovary.

Pyopen (pi′o-pen) trademark for a preparation of carbenicillin disodium.

pyopericarditis (pi″o-per″ĭ-kar-di′tis) purulent inflammation of the pericardium.

pyopericardium (pi″o-per″ĭ-kar′de-um) the presence of pus in the pericardial cavity.

pyoperitoneum (pi″o-per″ĭ-to-ne′um) [*pyo-* + *peritoneum*] pus in the peritoneal cavity.

pyoperitonitis (pi″o-per″ĭ-to-ni′tis) purulent inflammation of the peritoneum.

pyophagia (pi″o-fa′je-ah) [*pyo-* + Gr. *phagein* to eat] the swallowing of pus.

pyophthalmia (pi″of-thal′me-ah) [*py-* + *ophthalmia*] a suppurative condition of the eye; called also *pyophthalmitis.*

pyophthalmitis (pi″of-thal-mi′tis) pyophthalmia.

pyophylactic (pi″o-fi-lak′tik) [*pyo-* + Gr. *phylaktikos* guarding] serving as a defense against purulent infection.

pyophysometra (pi″o-fi″so-me′trah) [*pyo-* + Gr. *physa* air + *mētra* uterus] a collection of pus and gas in the uterus.

pyoplania (pi″o-pla′ne-ah) [*pyo-* + Gr. *planē* wandering] wandering of pus from one part to another.

pyopneumocholecystitis (pi″o-nu″mo-ko″le-sis-ti′tis) [*pyo-* + Gr. *pneuma* air + *cholecyst* + *-itis*] distention of the gallbladder with pus and gas.

pyopneumocyst (pi″o-nu″mo-sist) [*pyo-* + Gr. *pneuma* air + *cyst*] a cyst containing pus and gas.

pyopneumohepatitis (pi″o-nu″mo-hep″ah-ti′tis) abscess of the liver with pus and gas in the abscess cavity.

pyopneumopericardium (pi″o-nu″mo-per″ĭ-kar′de-um) [*pyo-* + Gr. *pneuma* air + *pericardium*] the presence of pus and gas in the pericardial cavity.

pyopneumoperitoneum (pi″o-nu″mo-per″ĭ-to-ne′um) the presence of pus and gas in the peritoneal cavity.

pyopneumoperitonitis (pi″o-nu″mo-per″ĭ-to-ni′tis) [*pyo-* + Gr. *pneuma* air + *peritonitis*] peritonitis with the presence of pus and gas in the peritoneal cavity.

pyopneumothorax (pi″o-nu″mo-tho′raks) [*pyo-* + Gr. *pneuma* air + *thōrax* chest] a collection of pus and air or gas in the pleural cavity.

pyopoiesis (pi″o-poi-e′sis) [*pyo-* + Gr. *poiein* to make] the formation of pus; pyogenesis.

pyopoietic (pi″o-poi-et′ik) producing pus; pyogenic.

pyoptysis (pi-op′tĭ-sis) [*pyo-* + Gr. *ptysis* spitting] spitting of purulent matter.

pyopyelectasis (pi″o-pi″ĕ-lek′tah-sis) [*pyo-* + Gr. *pyelos* pelvis + *ektasis* dilatation] dilatation of the renal pelvis with purulent fluid.

pyorrhea (pi″o-re′ah) [*pyo-* + Gr. *rhoia* flow] 1. periodontitis (def. 1). 2. marginal periodontitis. **p. alveola′ris,** marginal periodontitis. **Schmutz p.,** marginal periodontitis.

pyorrheal (pi″o-re′al) pertaining to or characterized by periodontitis or marginal periodontitis.

pyorubin (pi″o-roo′bin) a bright-red, water-soluble, non-fluorescent pigment produced by some strains of *Pseudomonas aeruginosa*.

pyosalpingitis (pi″o-sal″pin-ji′tis) [*pyo-* + Gr. *salpinx* tube + *-itis*] purulent salpingitis.

pyosalpingo-oophoritis (pi″o-sal-ping″go-o″of-o-ri′tis) inflammation of the ovary and oviduct, with the formation and accumulation of pus.

pyosalpingo-oothecitis (pi″o-sal-ping″go-o″o-the-si′tis) pyosalpingo-oophoritis.

pyosalpinx (pi″o-sal′pinks) [*pyo-* + Gr. *salpinx* tube] a collection of pus in an oviduct.

pyosapremia (pi″o-sap-re′me-ah) [*pyo-* + Gr. *sapros* rotten + *haima* blood + *-ia*] infection of the blood with purulent matter.

pyosclerosis (pi″o-skle-ro′sis) an inflammatory, purulent sclerosis.

pyosepticemia (pi″o-sep″tĭ-se′me-ah) pyemia combined with septicemia.

pyosin (pi′o-sin) a compound, $C_{57}H_{110}N_2O_{15}$, derived from the plasma of pus cells.

pyospermia (pi″o-sper′me-ah) [*pyo-* + Gr. *sperma* seed + *-ia*] presence of pus in the semen.

pyostatic (pi″o-stat′ik) [*pyo-* + Gr. *statikos* halting] 1. arresting suppuration. 2. an agent that arrests the formation of pus.

pyostomatitis (pi″o-sto″mah-ti′tis) [*pyo-* + *stomatitis*] a suppurative inflammation of the mouth. **p. veg′etans,** a variant of dermatitis vegetans involving the oral mucosa, sometimes occurring in association with ulcerative colitis and other gastrointestinal disturbances. The primary lesions are miliary abscesses with a tendency to form groups and become proliferative, soft, red, folded, and verrucous, sometimes spreading over the entire oral cavity. They may remain confined to the mouth or may coexist with typical dermatitis vegetans.

pyothorax (pi″o-tho′raks) [*pyo-* + Gr. *thōrax* chest] thoracic empyema.

pyotoxinemia (pi″o-tok″sĭ-ne′me-ah) [*pyo-* + *toxin* + Gr. *haima* blood + *-ia*] presence in the blood of the toxins of pus-forming organisms.

pyoumbilicus (pi″o-um-bil′ĭ-kus) infection of the umbilicus.

pyourachus (pi″o-u′rah-kus) the presence of pus in the urachus.

pyoureter (pi″o-u-re′ter) [*pyo-* + *ureter*] an accumulation of pus in a ureter.

pyovesiculosis (pi″o-vĕ-sik″u-lo′sis) an accumulation of pus in the seminal vesicles.

pyoxanthine (pi″o-zan′thin) a brownish red pigment derivable by oxidation from pyocyanin.

pyoxanthose (pi″o-zan′thōs) [*pyo-* + Gr. *xanthos* yellow] a yellow pigment produced by the oxidation of pyocyanin in blue pus when exposed to air.

pyrabrom (pēr′ah-brom) chemical name: 8-bromo-3,7-dihydro-1,3-dimethyl-1*H*-purine-2,6-dione compound with *N*-[(4-methoxyphenyl)methyl]-*N*′,*N*′-dimethyl-*N*-2-pyridinyl-1,2-ethanediamine (1:1); an antihistaminic, $C_{24}H_{30}BrN_7O_3$.

pyracin (pi′rah-sin) a derivative of pyridoxine.

Pyralis (pēr′ah-lis) a genus of widely distributed, small moths. **P. farina′lis,** the grain-infesting meal moth that serves as an intermediate host of helminthic parasites, such as *Hymenolepis*.

pyramid (pēr′ah-mid) [Gr. *pyramis*] a pointed or cone-shaped structure or part; called also *pyramis* [NA]. The term is often used alone to indicate the pyramis medullae oblongatae. **p. of cerebellum,** pyramis vermis. **p. of Ferrein,** pars radiata lobuli corticalis renis. **p′s of kidney,** pyramides renales; see under *pyramis*. **Lalouette's p.,** lobus pyramidalis glandulae thyroideae. **p. of light,** a triangular reflection seen upon the membrana tympani. **Malacarne's p.,** the posterior end of the pyramid of the vermis. **p′s of Malpighi,** pyramides renales; see under *pyramis*. **p. of medulla oblongata,** pyramis medullae oblongatae. **p. of medulla oblongata, anterior** (*obs.*), pyramis medullae oblongatae. **p. of medulla oblongata, posterior** (*obs.*), fasciculus gracilis medullae oblongatae. **olfactory p.** (*obs.*), trigonum olfactorium. **petrous p.,** pars petrosa ossis temporalis. **renal p′s,** pyramides renales; see under *pyramis*. **p. of temporal bone,** pars petrosa ossis temporalis. **p. of temporal bone, of Arnold,** pars mastoidea ossis temporalis. **p. of thyroid,** lobus pyramidalis glandulae thyroideae. **p. of tympanum,** eminentia pyramidalis. **p. of vermis,** pyramis vermis. **p. of vestibule,** pyramis vestibuli. **Wistar's p′s,** see *concha sphenoidalis*.

pyramidal (pĭ-ram′ĭ-dal) [L. *pyramidalis*] shaped like a pyramid; see also under *tract*.

pyramidale (pi-ram″ĭ-da′le) os triquetrum.

pyramidalis (pi-ram″ĭ-da′lis) [L.] pyramidal.

pyramides (pi-ram′ĭ-dēz) [Gr.] plural of *pyramis*.

Pyramidon (pi-ram′ĭ-don) trademark for a preparation of aminopyrine.

pyramidotomy (pēr″am-ĭ-dot′o-me) section of the pyramidal tract.

pyramis (pēr′ah-mis), pl. *pyram′ides* [Gr.] pyramid; [NA] a general term for a part or structure resembling a pyramid. **p. cerebel′li,** p. vermis. **pyram′ides Malpig′hii,** pyramides renales. **p. medul′lae oblonga′tae** [NA], pyramid of medulla oblongata: either of two rounded masses, one on either side of the anterior median fissure of the medulla oblongata, composed of motor fibers (pyramidal tract) from the cerebral cortex to the spinal cord and medulla oblongata. **p. os′sis tempora′lis,** pars petrosa ossis temporalis. **pyram′ides rena′les** [NA], **pyram′ides rena′les [Malpig′hii],** renal pyramids: the conical masses that make up the medullary substance of the kidney; they contain the loops of Henle, the collecting ducts, and the arteriolae rectae renis. **p. ver′mis** [NA], pyramid of vermis: the part of the vermis of the cerebellum between the tuber vermis and the uvula. **p. vestib′uli** [NA], pyramid of vestibule: the triangular-shaped anterior end of the vestibular crest.

pyran (pi′ran) 1. a cyclic compound, C_5H_6O, in which the ring consists of 5 carbon atoms and 1 oxygen atom. 2. (*obs.*) an antineuralgic and antirheumatic preparation of benzoic acid, salicylic acid, and thymol.

pyranisamine maleate (pi″rah-nis′ah-mēn) pyrilamine maleate.

pyranose (pi′rah-nōs) a hexose in which the oxygen ring bridges carbon atoms 1 and 5 in the aldoses or carbon atoms 2 and 6 in the ketoses.

pyrantel (pĭ-ran′tel) chemical name: (*E*)-1,4,5,6-tetrahydro-1-methyl-2-[2-(2-thienyl)vinyl]pyrimidine. A broad-spectrum anthelmintic, $C_{11}H_{14}N_2S$, effective against pinworms (*Enterobius vermicularis*) and roundworms (*Ascaris lumbricoides*). It acts as a depolarizing neuromuscular blocking agent, producing spastic paralysis of the parasite. **p. pamoate** [USP], the pamoate salt of pyrantel, $C_{11}H_{14}N_2S \cdot C_{23}H_{16}O_6$, occurring as a yellow to tan solid; used in the treatment of ascariasis and enterobiasis, administered orally. **p. tartrate,** the tartrate salt of pyrantel, $C_{11}H_{14}N_2S \cdot C_4H_6O_6$, occurring as a white to greenish-yellow, crystalline powder, having the same actions as the pamoate salt.

pyranyl (pi′ran-il) the radical C_5H_5O, of which pyran is the hydride.

pyrathiazine hydrochloride (per″rah-thi′ah-zēn) chemical name: 10-[2-(1-pyrrolidinyl)ethyl]-phenothiazine hydrochloride, $C_{18}H_{20}N_2S_4HCl$; used as an antihistaminic.

pyrazinamide (pi″rah-zin′ah-mīd) [USP] chemical name: pyrazinecarboxamide. An antibacterial derived from nicotinic acid, $C_5H_5N_3O$, occurring as a white to practically white, crystalline powder; used as a tuberculostatic, administered orally.

pyrazine (pi′rah-zēn) a volatile compound, $C_4H_4N_2$, with the odor of heliotrope.

pyrazofurin (per″ah-zo-fūr′in) chemical name: 4-hydroxy-3-β-D-ribofuranosyl-1H-pyrazole-5-carboxamide; an antineoplastic, $C_9H_{13}N_3O_6$.

pyrazolone (pir-āz′o-lōn) any of a class of ketone derivatives of pyrazole having anti-inflammatory, analgesic, and antipyretic effects.

pyrectic (pi-rek′tik) [Gr. *pyrektikos* feverish] 1. pertaining to or of the nature of fever. 2. an agent that induces fever.

pyrene (pi′ren) a polycyclic hydrocarbon, $C_{16}H_{10}$.

pyrenoid (pi′rĕ-noid) [Gr. *pyrēn* fruit stone + *eidos* form] one of the proteinaceous refringent bodies found closely associated with the chloroplasts of most phytoflagellates; involved in the synthesis and storage of polysaccharide.

pyrenolysis (pi″rĕ-nol′ĭ-sis) [Gr. *pyrēn* fruit stone + *lysis* solution] the breaking down of the nucleolus of a cell.

Pyrenomycetes (pi-re″no-mi-se′tēz) a series of ascomycetous fungi of subclass Euascomycetidae, including the orders Clavicipitales and Erysiphales; their fruiting body is a perithecium.

pyretherapy (pi″rĕ-ther′ah-pe) [Gr. *pyr* fever + *therapy*] pyretotherapy.

pyrethron (pi′rĕ-thron) a neutral ester from pyrethrum.

pyrethrum (pi-re′thrum) [Gr. *pyrethron*] see under *flower.*

pyretic (pi-ret′ik) [Gr. *pyretos* fever] pertaining to or of the nature of fever.

pyreticosis (pi-ret″ĭ-ko′sis) any febrile affection.

pyret(o)- [Gr. *pyretos* fever] a combining form denoting relationship to fever.

pyretogen (pi-ret′o-jen) a substance which excites fever.

pyretogenesis (pi″rĕ-to-jen′ĕ-sis) [pyreto- + Gr. *genesis* production] the origin and causation of fever.

pyretogenetic (pi″rĕ-to-jĕ-net′ik) pertaining to pyretogenesis.

pyretogenic (pi″rĕ-to-jen′ik) producing fever.

pyretogenous (pi″rĕ-toj′ĕ-nus) 1. caused by high body temperature. 2. pyrogenic.

pyretography (pi″rĕ-tog′rah-fe) [pyreto- + Gr. *graphein* to write] a description of fever.

pyretology (pi″rĕ-tol′o-je) [pyreto- + -*logy*] the sum of what is known regarding fevers; the science of fevers.

pyretolysis (pi″rĕ-tol′ĭ-sis) [pyreto- + Gr. *lysis* dissolution] 1. reduction of fever. 2. lysis which is hastened by fever.

pyretotherapy (pi″rĕ-to-ther′ah-pe) [pyreto- + Gr. *therapeia* treatment] 1. treatment of a disease by raising the patient's temperature, especially by means of injecting fever-producing vaccines. 2. the treatment of fever.

pyretotyphosis (pi″rĕ-to-ti-fo′sis) [pyreto- + Gr. *typhōsis* delirium] the delirium of fever.

pyrexia (pi-rek′se-ah), pl. *pyrex′iae* [Gr. *pyressein* to be feverish] a fever, or a febrile condition; abnormal elevation of the body temperature. **Pel-Ebstein p.,** see under *fever.*

pyrexial (pi-rek′se-al) pertaining to or characterized by pyrexia.

pyrexiogenic (pi-rek″se-o-jen′ik) pyrogenic.

pyrexy (pi′rek-se) pyrexia.

Pyribenzamine (per″ĭ-ben′zah-mēn) trademark for preparations of tripelennamine.

pyridine (per′ĭ-dēn) 1. a colorless, liquid, basic coal tar derivative, C_5H_5N, derived also from tobacco and various organic matters. 2. any one of a large group of substances homologous with normal pyridine.

Pyridium (pĭ-rid′e-um) trademark for preparations of phenazopyridine hydrochloride.

pyridostigmine bromide (per″ĭ-do-stig′mēn) [USP] chemical name: 3-[[(dimethyl-amino)carbonyl]oxy]-1-methyl pyridinium bromide. A cholinergic, $C_9H_{13}BrN_2O_2$, used in the treatment of myasthenia gravis and as an antidote for nondipolarizing muscle relaxants, such as curariform drugs, administered orally and parenterally.

pyridoxal (per″ĭ-dok′sal) chemical name: 2-methyl-3-hydroxy-4-formyl-5-hydroxymethylpyridine. One of the forms of vitamin B₆; see *Table of Vitamins*, under *vitamin.* **p. phosphate,** a major coenzyme involved in amino acid metabolism.

pyridoxamine (per″ĭ-doks′ah-mēn) one of the three active forms of vitamin B₆. **p. phosphate,** a coenzyme involved in many amino acid reactions.

pyridoxic acid (pir″ĭ-dok′sik) oxidation product of pyridoxal, the principal urinary excretion product of vitamin B₆.

pyridoxine (per″ĭ-dok′sēn) chemical name: 5-hydroxy-6-methyl-3,4-pyridinedimethanol. One of the forms of vitamin B₆; see *Table of Vitamins*, under *vitamin.* **p. hydrochloride** [USP], the hydrochloride salt of pyridoxine, $C_8H_{11}NO_3 \cdot HCl$, occurring as colorless or white crystals or white crystalline powder; used in the prophylaxis and treatment of vitamin B₆ deficiency. It has also been used in neuromuscular and neurological diseases, in dermatoses, and in the management of nausea and vomiting of pregnancy and irradiation sickness. **p. phosphate,** a coenzyme involved in many amino acid reactions.

pyriform (per′ĭ-form) piriform.

pyrilamine maleate (per-il′ah-mēn) [USP] chemical name: N-[(4-methoxyphenyl)methyl]-N′,N′-dimethyl-N-2-pyridinyl-1,2- ethane diamine (Z)-2-butenedioate (1:1). An antihistaminic, $C_{17}H_{23}N_3O \cdot C_4H_4O_4$, occurring as a white, crystalline powder; administered orally. Called also *mepyramine maleate* and *pyranisamine maleate.*

pyrimethamine (per″ĭ-meth′ah-mēn) [USP] chemical name: 5-(4-chlorophenyl)-6-ethyl-2,4-pyrimidinediamine. A folic acid antagonist, $C_{12}H_{13}ClN_4$, occurring as a white crystalline powder; used as an antimalarial, especially for suppressive prophylaxis, and also used concomitantly with a sulfonamide in the treatment of toxoplasmosis, administered orally.

pyrimidine (pi-rim′ĭ-dēn) an organic compound, a metadiazine, $C_4H_4N_2$, which is the fundamental form of the pyrimidine bases. These are mostly oxy or amino derivatives, for example, 2,4-dioxypyrimidine is uracil, 2-oxy-4-aminopyrimidine is cytosine, and 2,4-dioxy-5-methylpyrimidine is thymine. Some of these are constituents of nucleic acid (uracil, thymine, and cytosine). It is also the parent substance of the barbiturates.

pyrinoline (per-in′o-lēn) chemical name: 3-(di-2-pyridylmethylene)-α,α,α-di-2-pyridyl-1,4-cyclopentadiene-1-methanol; an antiarrhythmic cardiac depressant, $C_{27}H_{20}N_4O$.

pyrithiamine (per″ĭ-thi′ah-min) a synthetic compound, $CH_3 \cdot C_4N_2H(NH_2) \cdot CH_2 \cdot CH_2 \cdot SNH_3(CH_3) \cdot CH_2 \cdot CH_2OH$, which by metabolic competition can cause symptoms of thiamine deficiency.

pyr(o)- [Gr. *pyr* fire] a combining form denoting relationship to fire or heat; in chemistry, produced by heating. In inorganic chemistry, it indicates a dimeric acid anhydride, e.g., pyrophosphoric acid.

pyroborate (pi-ro-bo′rāt) any salt of pyroboric acid.

pyroboric acid (pi″ro-bor′ik) a dimer of boric acid, $H_2B_4O_7$, produced by heating boric acid. Called also *tetraboric acid.*

pyrocatechin (pi″ro-kat′ĕ-kin) pyrocatechol.

pyrocatechol (pi″ro-kat′ĕ-kol) chemical name: 1,2-benzenediol. A compound, $C_6H_4(OH)_2$, comprising the aromatic portion in the synthesis of endogenous catecholamines; it is obtained by distilling catechu, etc., or produced synthetically, and has been used as a topical antiseptic and as a reagent. Called also *catechol* and *pyrocatechin.*

pyrodextrin (pi″ro-deks′trin) a brown substance produced by the action of heat upon starch.

pyrogallol (pi″ro-gal′ol) chemical name: 1,2,3-trihydroxybenzene. A poisonous acid, $C_6H_6O_3$, derived from gallic acid, and used externally as an antimicrobial and irritant; it is also used as a reagent. Called also *pyrogallic acid.*

pyrogen (pi′ro-jen) [*pyro-* + Gr. *gennan* to produce] a fever-producing substance. **bacterial p.,** a fever-producing agent of bacterial origin; endotoxin. **endogenous p.,** a low-molecular-weight protein that is produced by phagocytic leukocytes in response to stimulation by exogenous pyrogens and released into the circulation and which induces fever by acting on the preoptic area of the hypothalamus to raise the set-point of the hypothalamic thermostat. The pyrogen produced by monocytes and macrophages is not identical to that produced by neutrophils and eosinophils; the mononuclear phagocytes also produce a greater amount of pyrogen for a longer period of time than do the polymorphonuclear cells. Called also *leukocytic p.* **exogenous p's,** fever producing agents of external origin, e.g., bacterial endotoxins and other microbial products, antigen-antibody complexes, viruses and synthetic polynucleotides, incompatible blood and blood products, and androgen breakdown products such as etiocholanone; the action is mediated by endogenous pyrogen. **leukocytic p.,** endogenous p.

pyrogenetic (pi″ro-jĕ-net′ik) pyrogenic.

pyrogenic (pi″ro-jen′ik) [*pyro-* + Gr. *gennan* to produce] inducing fever.

pyrogenous (pi-roj′ĕ-nus) pyretogenous.

pyroglobulin (pi″ro-glob′u-lin) [*pyro-* + *globulin*] a monoclonal immunoglobulin that precipitates irreversibly upon heating to 56°C (as opposed to Bence Jones proteins, which precipitate but redissolve on cooling).

pyroglobulinemia (pi″ro-glob″u-lĭ-ne′me-ah) the presence of pyroglobulin in the blood, occurring most frequently in multiple myeloma, Waldenström's macroglobulinemia, and other lymphoproliferative disorders but also occasionally without known associated disease.

pyroglutamase (pi″ro-gloo′tah-mās) 5-oxoprolinase (ATP hydrolyzing).

pyroglutamate (pi″ro-gloo′tah-māt) 5-oxoproline.

pyroglutamate hydrolase (pi″ro-gloo′tah-māt hi′dro-lās) 5-oxoprolinase (ATP hydrolyzing).

pyroglutamic acid (pi″ro-gloo-tam′ik) 5-oxoproline.

pyrolagnia (pi″ro-lag′ne-ah) [*pyro-* + Gr. *lagneia* lust] sexual gratification from witnessing or making fires.

pyroligneous (pi″ro-lig′ne-us) [*pyro-* + L. *lignum* wood] pertaining to the destructive distillation of wood.

pyrolusite (pi″ro-lu′sīt) native manganese dioxide, a black powder used in dry-cell batteries.

pyrolysis (pi-rol′ĭ-sis) [*pyro-* + Gr. *lysis* dissolution] decomposition of organic substances under the influence of a rise in temperature.

pyromania (pi″ro-ma′ne-ah) [*pyro-* + Gr. *mania* madness] [DSM III] a compulsion to set fires; an obsessive preoccupation with fire. **erotic p.,** pyrolagnia.

pyrometer (pi-rom′ĕ-ter) [*pyro-* + Gr. *metron* measure] an instrument for measuring the intensity of heat, especially for temperatures which cannot be measured with a mercury thermometer.

pyrone (pi′rōn) a principle, $CO(CH)_4O$, found in opium, from which several other constituents are derived by substitution.

Pyronil (pi′ro-nil) trademark for a preparation of pyrrobutamine.

pyronin (pi′ro-nin) a dye used in histology; the pyronines are methylated diamine xanthines. **p. B,** a basic dye, the tetraethylpyronine chloride, $(C_2H_5)_2N \cdot C_6H_3(O)CH \cdot C_6H_3 \cdot N \cdot (C_3H_5)_2Cl$. **p. G,** a basic dye, the tetramethylpyronine chloride, $(CH_3)_2N \cdot C_6H_3(O)CH \cdot C_6H_3N(CH_3)_2Cl$.

pyroninophilia (pi″ro-nin″o-fil′e-ah) [*pyronine* + Gr. *philein* to love] increased affinity for pyronine, sometimes observed in plasma and reticuloendothelial cells.

pyrophobia (pi″ro-fo′be-ah) [*pyro-* + *phobia*] abnormal dread of fire.

pyrophosphatase (pi″ro-fos′fah-tās) any enzyme that catalyzes the hydrolysis of a pyrophosphate bond, cleaving between the two phosphoric groups. **inorganic p.,** see *inorganic pyrophosphatase.*

pyrophosphate (pi″ro-fos′fāt) any salt of pyrophosphoric acid. **stannous p.,** chemical name: diphosphoric acid ditin (2+) salt; a diagnostic aid (bone imaging), $Sn_2P_2O_7$.

pyrophosphate ribose-P-synthetase (pi″ro fos′fāt ri″bōs-sin′thĕ-tās) ribose-phosphate pyrophosphokinase.

pyrophosphokinase (pi″ro-fos″fo-ki′nās) [EC 2.7.6] one of a sub-subclass of enzymes of the transferase class that catalyze the transfer of a pyrophosphate group from one molecule to another.

pyrophosphoric acid (pi″ro-fos-for′ik) a dimer of phosphoric acid, $H_4P_2O_7$.

pyrophosphotransferase (pi″ro-fos′fo-trans′fer-ās) pyrophosphokinase.

pyroscope (pi′ro-skōp) [*pyro-* + Gr. *skopein* to examine] an instrument for measuring the intensity of heat radiations.

pyrosis (pi-ro′sis) [Gr. *pyrōsis* burning] heartburn.

pyrotic (pi-rot′ik) [Gr. *pyrōtikos*] caustic; burning.

pyrotoxin (pi″ro-tok′sin) [*pyro-* + Gr. *toxikon* poison] a toxin developed during a fever.

pyrovalerone hydrochloride (pēr-o-val′er-ōn) chemical name: 1-(4-methylphenyl)-2-(1-pyrrolidinyl)-1-pentanone hydrochloride; a central nervous system stimulant, $C_{16}H_{23}$-$NO \cdot HCl$.

pyroxamine maleate (pēr-oks′ah-mēn) chemical name: 3-[(*p*- chloro-α-phenylbenzyl)oxy]-1-methylpyrrolidine maleate (1:1); an antihistaminic, $C_{18}H_{20}ClNO \cdot C_4H_4O_4$.

pyroxylin (pi-rok′sĭ-lin) [Gr. *pyr* fire + *xylon* wood] [USP] a product of the action of a mixture of nitric and sulfuric acids on cotton, consisting chiefly of cellulose tetranitrate; a necessary ingredient of collodion. Called also *colloxylin, dinitiocellulose, nitrocellulose,* and *guncotton.*

pyrrobutamine phosphate (pēr″ro-bu′tah-mēn) [USP] chemical name: 1-[4-(4-chlorophenyl)-3-phenyl-2-butenyl] pyrrolidine phosphate (1:2). A long-acting antihistaminic, $C_{20}H_{22}ClN \cdot 2H_3PO_4$, occurring as a white, or almost white, crystalline powder; administered orally.

pyrrocaine (pēr′o-kān) chemical name: N-(2,6-dimethylphenyl)-1-pyrrolidineacetamide; a local anesthetic, $C_{14}H_{20}$-N_2O. **p. hydrochloride** the monohydrochloride salt of pyrrocaine, occurring as a white, crystalline powder; used as a local anesthetic in dentistry to produce infiltration and nerve block anesthesia.

pyrrole (pēr′ol) a liquid, basic, cyclic substance, $(CH)_4NH$, obtained in the destructive distillation of various animal substances. Four pyrrole groups (tetrapyrrole) are formed into a ring in the biosynthesis of the porphyrins.

pyrrolidine (pĭ-rol′ĭ-din) a simple base, tetramethylene imine, $(CH_2)_4NH$, which may be obtained from tobacco or prepared from pyrrole.

pyrroline (pir′o-lin) an oily liquid, C_4H_6NH, formed by the action of acetic acid and zinc dust on pyrrole.

Δ¹-pyrroline-5-carboxylate dehydrogenase (pir′o-lēn kar-bok′sĭ-lāt de-hi′dro-jĕ-nās) [EC 1.5.1.12] an enzyme of the oxidoreductase class that catalyzes the reaction L-pyrroline-5-carboxylate + NAD⁺ + H_2O = L-glutamate + NADH, a step in the degradation of proline. The enzyme also oxidizes 3-hydroxy-1-pyrroline-5-carboxylate to 4-hydroxyglutamate. Deficiency of the enzyme, an autosomal recessive trait, is the cause of hyperprolinemia Type II.

pyrroline-5-carboxylate reductase (pir′o-lēn kar-bok′sĭ-lāt re-duk′tās) [EC 1.5.1.2] an enzyme of the oxidoreductase class that catalyzes the reaction 1-pyrroline-5-carboxylate + NAD(P)H = L-proline + NAD(P)⁺, an irreversible step in the biosynthesis of proline from glutamic acid by way of pyrroline-1-carboxylate. The enzyme also reduces 1-pyrroline-3-hydroxy-5-carboxylate to L-hydroxyproline.

pyrrolnitrin (pēr-ōl-ni′trin) chemical name: 3-chloro-4-(3-chloro-2-nitrophenyl)-1*H*-pyrrole; an antifungal antibiotic isolated from *Pseudomonas pyrrocinia,* $C_{10}H_6Cl_2N_2O_2$, effective against *Trichophyton* species.

pyrroloporphyria (pir″o-lo-por-fir′e-ah) acute intermittent porphyria.

Pyrsonympha (pēr″so-nim′fah) a genus of parasitic flagellate protozoa (order Oxymonadida, class Zoomastigophorea) found in the termite gut.

pyruvate (pi′roo-vāt) a salt, ester, or anionic form of pyruvic acid,

$$CH_3C-C-O^-.$$

In biochemistry, the term is used interchangeably with pyruvic acid, even though pyruvate technically refers to the negatively charged ion. Pyruvate is the end product of glycolysis, and it in turn may be converted to lactate or acetyl CoA or to ethanol (as in yeasts).

pyruvate carboxylase (pi′roo-vāt kar-bok′sĭ-lās) [EC 6.4.1.1] an enzyme of the ligase class that catalyzes the irreversible reaction ATP + pyruvate + HCO_3 = ADP + orthophosphate + oxaloacetate. The enzyme is a biotinyl protein requiring Mg^{2+} or Mn^{2+} and acetyl coenzyme A and occurs in the liver but not in muscle. The reaction is necessary for gluconeogenesis from lactate or amino acids forming pyruvate and also provides four carbon compounds for the tricarboxylic acid cycle. Deficiency of the enzyme, an autosomal recessive trait, causes severe psychomotor retardation and lactic acidosis in infants.

pyruvate carboxylase (PC) deficiency an autosomal recessive disorder involving PC, which catalyzes CO_2 fixation, and characterized by lactic acidosis and profound psychomotor retardation.

pyruvate decarboxylase (pi′roo-vāt de″kar-bok′sĭ-lās) [EC 4.1.1.1] 1. an enzyme of the lyase class that catalyzes the reaction 2-keto acid = an aldehyde + CO_2, part of the anaerobic fermentation pathway that produces ethanol and CO_2 from glucose. The enzyme, a thiamin-diphosphate protein, occurs in yeast. Called also α-carboxylase. 2. Formerly, pyruvate dehydrogenase (lipoamide)

pyruvate dehydrogenase (pi′roo-vāt de-hi′dro-jĕ-nās) a multienzyme complex that catalyzes the overall reaction pyruvate + NAD^+ + CoA-SH = acetyl CoA + CO_2 + NADH. The complex consists of three enzymes: pyruvate dehydrogenase (lipoamide) [EC 1.2.4.1], dihydrolipoamide acetyltransferase [EC 2.3.1.12] and dihydrolipoamide dehydrogenase [EC 1.8.1.4]. It requires five cofactors: thiamine pyrophosphate, lipoic acid, coenzyme A, flavin adenine dinucleotide, and NAD^+. The reaction occurs in the mitochondria and produces acetyl-CoA for fatty acid synthesis, for acetylations, and for oxidation to CO_2 and water by the tricarboxylic acid cycle. Deficiency of any component of the enzyme complex results in ataxia and psychomotor retardation.

pyruvate dehydrogenase complex (PDHC) deficiency an inborn error of metabolism involving the PDHC that catalyzes the oxidation of pyruvate to CO_2 and acetyl CoA. The chief clinical abnormality is in the nervous system, causing ataxic encephalopathy and psychomotor retardation; lactic acidosis is conspicuous in severe, infantile cases.

pyruvate dehydrogenase (lipoamide) (pi′roo-vāt de-hi′dro-jĕ-nās lip-o′ah-mĭd, mid) [EC 1.2.4.1] an enzyme of the oxidoreductase class that catalyzes the reaction pyruvate + lipoamide = S-acetyldihydrolipoamide + CO_2. The enzyme is a component of the multienzyme pyruvate dehydrogenase complex and requires thiamin diphosphate. Formerly also called pyruvate decarboxylase.

pyruvate kinase (PK) (pi′roo-vāt ki′nās) [EC 2.7.1.40] an enzyme of the transferase class that catalyzes the reaction phosphopyruvate + ADP = pyruvate + ATP. The enzyme has three distinct isoenzymes and is a site for regulation of the Embden-Meyerhof pathway. Deficiency of the enzyme, an autosomal recessive trait, results in hemolytic anemia.

pyruvate kinase (PK) deficiency, erythrocyte the most common glycolytic enzyme defect in the Embden-Meyerhof pathway; deficient product (ATP) causes chronic hemolytic anemia of widely variable severity. PK deficiency is an autosomal recessive trait and has no distinguishing clinical features from the other hemolytic disorders.

pyruvemia (pi″roo-ve′me-ah) a condition characterized by an increased amount of pyruvic acid in the blood.

pyruvic acid (pi-roo′vik) α-ketopropionic acid, CH_3 CO-COOH, the end product of the Embden-Meyerhof pathway (q.v.) of glucose metabolism, also produced by the catabolism of several amino acids. Pyruvate can be converted to acetyl coenzyme A, which can enter the tricarboxylic acid cycle (q.v.) for aerobic production of energy or be used for fatty acid synthesis. Energy can be obtained anaerobically by conversion of pyruvate to lactate (which occurs in mammalian muscle tissue) or to ethanol, small organic acids, and many other compounds (microbial fermentations). Pyruvate can also be converted to oxaloacetate, the first step in gluconeogenesis.

pyrvinium pamoate (pir-vin′e-um) [USP] chemical name: 6-(dimethylamino)-2-[2-(2,5-dimethyl-1-phenyl-1H-pyrrol-3-yl)ethenyl]-1-methylquinolinium salt with 4 4′-methylenebis[3-hydroxy-2-naphthalenecarboxylic acid] (2:1). An anthelmintic, $C_{75}N_{70}N_6O_6$; it acts by preventing the uptake of exogenous glucose and is administered orally in the treatment of enterobiasis.

pythogenesis (pi″tho-jen′ĕ-sis) [Gr. pythein to rot + genesis production] 1. the origination of a process of decay or decomposition. 2. generation from filth.

pythogenic (pi″tho-jen′ik) [Gr. pythein to rot + gennan to produce] causing decay or decomposition.

pythogenous (pi-thoj′ĕ-nus) caused by putrefaction or filth.

pyuria (pi-u′re-ah) [Gr. pyon pus + ouron urine + -ia] the presence of pus in the urine. **miliary p.,** the presence in the urine of miliary bodies consisting of pus cells, blood cells, and epithelium.

PZI protamine zinc insulin; see under insulin.

Q, q quantity of electric charge, quantity of heat.

q symbol for the long arm of a chromosome.

q.d. abbreviation for L. qua′que di′e, every day.

Q fever (Q for query) see under fever.

q.h. abbreviation for L. qua′que ho′ra, every hour.

q.i.d. abbreviation for L. qua′ter in di′e, four times a day.

q.l. abbreviation for L. quan′tum li′bet, as much as desired.

Q.N.S. abbreviation for Queen's Nursing Sister (of Queen's Institute of District Nursing).

q.n.s. quantity not sufficient.

q.p. abbreviation for L. quan′tum pla′ceat, as much as desired.

q.q.h. abbreviation for L. qua′que quar′ta ho′ra, every four hours.

Qq.hor. abbreviation for L. qua′que ho′ra, every hour.

q.s. abbreviation for L. quan′tum sa′tis, sufficient quantity.

q-sort (ku′sort) a technique of personality assessment in which the subject (or an observer) indicates the degree to which a standardized set of descriptive statements applies to the subject.

q.suff. abbreviation for L. quan′tum suf′ficit, as much as suffices.

Quaalude (kwa′lood) trademark for a preparation of methaqualone.

quack (kwak) [from quacksalver] one who fraudulently misrepresents his ability and experience in the diagnosis and treatment of disease or the effects to be achieved by the treatment he offers.

quackery (kwak′er-e) the fraudulent misrepresentation of one's ability and experience in the diagnosis and treatment of disease or of the effects to be achieved by the treatment offered.

quacksalver (kwak-sal′ver) [Dutch "salve peddler"] one claiming special merit for treatment with his medications and salves.

Quadramoid (quad′rah-moid) trademark for an oral suspension of trisulfapyrimidines.

quadrangle (kwod′rang-g'l) 1. a figure having four angles, or sides. 2. a dental instrument having four angulations in the shank connecting the handle, or shaft, with the working portion of the instrument, known as the blade, or nib. Cf. *binangle, monangle,* and *triple-angle.*

quadrangular (kwod-rang′gu-lar) [L. *quadri* four + *angulus* angle] having four angles.

quadrant (kwod′rant) [L. *quadrans* quarter] 1. one quarter of a circle; that portion of the circumference of a circle that subtends an angle of 90 degrees. 2. any one of four corresponding parts or quarters, as of the abdominal surface or of the eardrum.

quadrantal (kwod-ran′tal) resembling or affecting a quadrant.

quadrantanopia (kwod″rant-ah-no′pe-ah) [*quadrant* + *an-* neg. + *-opia*] hemianopia in one fourth of the visual field, bounded by a vertical and a horizontal radius. Called also *tetartanopia* and *quadrant hemianopia.*

quadrantanopsia (kwod″rant-ah-nop′se-ah) quadrantanopia.

quadrat (kwod′rat) [L. *quadratus* squared] a rectangular, usually square, sample plot used in ecological studies, especially a plot containing 1 square meter. A sample plot of larger area is often called a *major quadrat.*

quadrate (kwod′rāt) [L. *quadratus* squared] square or squared; four sided.

quadratipronator (kwod-ra″te-pro-na′tor) musculus pronator quadratus.

quadratus (kwod-ra′tus) [L.] squared; four sided.

quadri- [L. *quattuor* four; in combination, *quadri-*] a prefix signifying four, or fourfold.

quadribasic (kwod″rĭ-ba′sik) having four replaceable atoms of hydrogen.

quadriceps (kwod″rĭ-seps) [*quadri-* + L. *caput* head] four headed; possessing four heads. See *Table of Musculi.*

quadricepsplasty (kwod″rĭ-seps′plas-te) plastic repair of a ruptured quadriceps femoris muscle.

quadriceptor (kwod″rĭ-sep′tor) [*quadri-* + L. *ceptor*] an intermediary body having four combining groups.

quadricuspid (kwod″rĭ-kus′pid) [*quadri-* + *cuspid*] 1. having four cusps; said of a tooth, or of a semilunar (aortic or pulmonary) valve with four cusps. 2. a tooth with four cusps.

quadridentate (quod′rĭ-den′tāt) forming four coordinate covalent bonds in a chelate.

quadridigitate (kwod″rĭ-dij′ĭ-tāt) tetradactylous.

quadrigeminal (kwod″rĭ-jem′ĭ-nal) [L. *quadrigeminus*] fourfold, or in four parts; forming a group of four.

quadrigeminus (kwod″rĭ-jem′ĭ-nus) [L.] quadrigeminal.

quadrilateral (kwod″rĭ-lat′er-al) [*quadri-* + L. *latus* side] 1. having four sides. 2. a four-sided figure, or postulate. **Celsus' q.,** "Notae vero inflammationis sunt quattuor, rubor et tumor, cum calore et dolore." There are in fact four signs of inflammation—redness, swelling, heat, and pain.

quadrilocular (kwod″rĭ-lok′u-lar) [*quadri-* + L. *loculus* a small space] having four cells, cavities, or chambers.

quadripara (kwod-rip′ah-rah) [*quadri-* + L. *parere* to bring forth, produce] a woman who has had four pregnancies which resulted in viable offspring; also written *para IV.*

quadripartite (kwod″rĭ-par′tīt) having four parts or divisions.

quadriplegia (kwod″rĭ-ple′je-ah) paralysis of all four limbs; tetraplegia.

quadripolar (kwod″rĭ-po′lar) having four poles, as a cell.

quadrisect (kwod″rĭ-sekt) [*quadri-* + L. *secare* to cut] to cut into four parts.

quadrisection (kwod″rĭ-sek′shun) [*quadri-* + L. *sectio* cut] division into four parts.

quadritubercular (kwod″rĭ-tu-ber′ku-lar) having four tubercles or cusps.

quadrivalent (kwod″rĭ-va′lent) tetravalent.

quadruped (kwod′roo-ped) [*quadri-* + L. *pes* foot] 1. four footed. 2. an animal having four feet.

quadrupl. abbreviation for L. *quadruplica′to,* four times as much.

quadruplet (kwod′rup-let, kwod-roo′plet) [L. *quadrupulus* fourfold] one of four offspring produced in one gestation period.

Quain's degeneration, fatty heart (kwānz) [Sir Richard

Quain, British physician, 1816–1898] see under *degeneration* and *heart.*

quale (kwa′le) the quality of a thing; especially the quality of a sensation or other conscious process.

qualitative, qualitive (kwol′ĭ-ta″tiv) [L. *qualitativus*] pertaining to quality.

quality (kwol′ĭ-te) in radiology, the ability of a particular form or type of ionizing radiation to penetrate matter.

quanta (kwon′tah) [L.] plural of *quantum.*

quantal (kwon′tal) denoting an all-or-none response, one for which partial responses are undetectable or are not measured, or a procedure (a quantal assay) in which such a response is measured.

quantasome (kwon′tah-sōm) [L. *quantum* + Gr. *sōma* body] one of the uniform oblate spheroids of about 100 by 200 Å, which are present within the chloroplasts and are postulated to be the units of photosynthesis, each consisting of 250 molecules of chlorophyll, the minimum amount found necessary for photosynthesis.

quantatrope (kwon′tah-trōp) [L. *quantum* + Gr. *tropos* a turning] the site of the quantasome that is directly involved in the transfer of electrons.

quantile (kwon′tīl) [*quantity* + *-ile* (by analogy with *quartile, percentile,* etc.)] a value that divides the range of an observed or theoretical probability distribution into equal parts; examples are the median, quartiles, percentiles.

quantimeter (kwon-tim′ĕ-ter) [L. *quantus* how much + *metrum* measure] an apparatus for measuring the quantity of roentgen rays generated by a tube.

quantitative (kwon′tĭ-ta-tiv) [L. *quantitativus*] denoting or expressible as quantity; relating to the proportionate quantities or to the amount of the constituents of a compound.

quantity (kwon′tĭ-te) 1. a characteristic, as of energy or mass, susceptible of precise physical measurement. 2. a measurable amount.

quantum (kwon′tum), pl. *quan′ta* [L. "as much as"] a unit of energy under the quantum theory. It is hν, in which h is Planck's constant, 6.55×10^{-27}, and ν is the frequency of vibration with which the energy is associated. See *quantum theory,* under *theory.* **q. of light,** a quantity of light (radiant energy) equivalent to the frequency of the light times 6.55×10^{-27} erg. sec.

quantum libet (kwon′tum li′bet) [L.] as much as desired.

quantum satis (kwon′tum sat′is) a sufficient quantity.

quantum sufficit (kwon′tum suf′fi-sit) [L.] as much as suffices.

quarantine (kwor′an-tēn) [Ital. *quarantina,* from L. *quadraginta* forty] 1. restriction of freedom of movement of apparently well individuals who have been exposed to infectious disease, which is imposed for the usual maximal incubation period of the disease (*quarantine period*). Cf. *insolation* (def. 4) and *surveillance* (def. 2). 2. a period (originally of 40 days' duration) of detention of vessels, vehicles, or travelers coming from infected or suspected ports or places. 3. the place where persons are detained for inspection. 4. to detain or isolate on account of suspected contagion.

quart (kwort) [L. *quartus* fourth] the fourth part of a gallon (946 ml.).

quartan (kwor′tan) [L. *quartanus,* pertaining to the fourth] recurring every 72 hours (fourth day, counting the day of the previous paroxysm). See *malaria.* **double q.,** a fever in which the paroxysms occur on each of two successive days followed by an afebrile day, and continuing in this pattern. **triple q.,** a fever in which the paroxysms occur every day, i.e., quotidian, because of infection with three different groups of quartan parasites.

quarter (kwor′ter) the part of a horse's hoof lying between the heel and the toe. **false q.,** a cleft in the quarter of a horse's hoof from the top to the bottom.

quartile (kwor′tīl) [L. *quartilis* pertaining to a fourth, from *quartus* fourth] any of the three values that divide the range of a probability distribution into four parts of equal probability; i.e., the 1st, 2nd, and 3rd quartiles are the 25th, 50th, and 75th percentiles.

quartipara (kwor-tip′ah-rah) quadripara.

quartisect (kwor′tĭ-sekt) [L. *quartus* fourth + *secare* to cut] to cut into four parts.

quartisternal (kwor″tĭ-ster′nal) [L. *quartus* fourth + *sternum* sternum] pertaining to the fourth sternebra, or the bony segment of the sternum opposite the fourth intercostal space.

quartz (kwarts) a crystalline form of silicon dioxide (silica), SiO_2; called also *rock crystal*.

Quarzan (kwahr′zan) trademark for a preparation of clidinium bromide.

quasi- [L. *quasi* as if, as though] a prefix meaning almost, seemingly, or resembling.

quasidiploid (kwa″si-dip′loid) [*quasi-* + *diploid*] 1. having two sets of chromosomes but with an abnormal distribution. In tissue cell cultures, a chromosome of one pair may be missing and may be replaced by an extra chromosome from another pair. 2. an organism or cell that is quasidiploid.

quasidominance (kwa″zi-dom′ĭ-nans, kwah″zĭ-dom′ĭ-nans) [*quasi-* + *dominance*] the mimicking of dominant inheritance by the direct transmission, generation to generation, of a recessive trait, produced by mating of a recessive homozygote and a heterozygote, the proportion of affected offspring thus resembling that in dominant inheritance.

quasidominant (kwa″zi-dom′ĭ-nant, kwah-zĭ-dom′ĭ-nant) pertaining to or exhibiting quasidominance.

quassation (kwŏ-sa′shun) [L. *quassatio*] the crushing of drugs, or their reduction to small pieces.

Quassia (kwosh′e-ah) [after *Quassi*, a Negro who used it as a remedy] a genus of simaroubaceous tropical trees, the wood of which was first used in the 18th century in the treatment of fevers.

quassia (kwash′e-ah) [after *Quassi*, black slave of Surinam who used it in the treatment of malignant fevers in the 18th century] the dried, intensely bitter heart-wood of the simaroubaceous trees *Picrasma excelsa* (Sw.) Planch. (Jamaica quassia), or *Quassia amara* L. (Surinam quassia); it has been used as an enema for seatworms.

quassin (kwash′in) the major bitter principle, $C_{22}H_{30}O_6$, of quassia.

Quat., quat. abbreviation for L. *quat′tuor*, four.

quater in die (kwah′ter in de′a) [L.] four times a day.

quaternary (kwah′ter-ner″e, kwah-ter′nah-re) [L. *quaternarius*, from *quattuor* four] 1. fourth in order. 2. containing four elements or groups.

Quatrefages' angle (katr′fazh-ez) [Jean Louis Armand de *Quatrefages* de Bréau, French naturalist, 1810–1892] parietal angle.

quazepam (kwah′zĕ-pam) chemical name: 7-chloro-5-(2-fluorophenyl)-1,3-dihydro-1-(2,2,2-trifluoroethyl)-2*H*-1,4-benzodiazepine-2-thione; a sedative and hypnotic, $C_{17}H_{11}Cl-F_4N_2S$.

quazodine (kwa′zo-dēn) chemical name: 4-ethyl-6,7-dimethoxyquinazoline; a cardiotonic and bronchodilator, $C_{12}H_{14}N_2O_2$.

quebrachitol (ka-brah′chĭ-tol) chemical name: 1-methylinositol. A sugar from quebracho bark, which has been suggested as a sugar substitute in diabetes.

Queckenstedt's sign (phenomenon, test) (kwek′enstets″) [Hans Heinrich Georg *Queckenstedt*, German physician, 1876–1918] see under *sign*.

Quelicin (kwel′ĭ-sin) trademark for a preparation of succinylcholine.

quenching (kwench′ing) any type of interference that reduces the intensity of fluorescence, such as deexcitation of the fluorescent molecule by collision with other molecules, absorption of fluorescent emission by the surrounding medium, or a decrease or shift in wavelength of fluorescence due to chemical interaction of the flourescent molecule with other molecules. **fluorescence q.,** a technique for measuring the primary interaction of antigen and antibody by determination of the amount of light absorbed by bound antigen from fluorescent-labeled antibody exposed to ultraviolet light.

Quénu-Muret sign (ka′nu-mü-rĕ′) [Eduard André Victor Alfred *Quénu*, French surgeon, 1852–1933; Paul Louis *Muret*, French surgeon, born 1878] see under *sign*.

quercetin (kwer′sĕ-tin) chemical name: 2-(3,4-dihydroxyphenyl)-3,5,7-trihydroxy-4*H*-1-benzopyran-4-one. The aglycon of rutin and other glycosides, which has been used to reduce abnormal capillary fragility; called also *meletin* and *sophoretin*. **q.-3-rutinoside**, rutin.

Quercus (kwer′kus) [L.] a genus of trees including the oaks, certain species of which (e.g., *Q. infectoria* Oliv., Fagaceae) harbor nutgalls, a source of gallic and tannic acids, which are used in various pharmaceuticals for their astringent properties.

Quervain's disease (kār′vanz) [Fritz de *Quervain*, Swiss surgeon, 1868–1940] see under *disease*.

Questran (kwes′tran) trademark for a preparation of cholestyramine resin.

Quetelet's rule (ket″ĕ-lāz′) [Lambert Adolphe Jacques *Quetelet*, Belgian mathematician, 1796–1874] see under *rule*.

Queyrat's erythroplasia (ka-rahz′) [Auguste *Queyrat*, French dermatologist, born 1872] see under *erythroplasia*.

quick (kwik) 1. rapid. 2. alive. 3. pregnant and able to feel the fetal movements.

Quick test (kwik) [Armand James *Quick*, Milwaukee physician, born 1894] see under *tests*.

quicklime (kwik′līm) calcium oxide.

quickening (kwik′en-ing) the first recognizable movements of the fetus, appearing usually from the sixteenth to the eighteenth week of pregnancy.

quidding (kwid′ing) a condition in horses in which food is taken into the mouth, repeatedly chewed, and then expelled; it may be caused by injuries to the mouth, disorders of the teeth or gums, paralysis of the muscles of mastication, or some other condition causing inability to swallow. Called also *cudding*.

Quide (kwīd) trademark for a preparation of piperacetazine.

quillaia (kwil-la′yah) the dried inner part of the bark of *Quillaja saponaria* Molina (Rosaceae); formerly used in medicine for its local irritant action. Its chief constituent is quillaic acid, and it is used in the manufacture of saponin, in shampoo formulations for its foaming qualities, and as a detergent in the film industry. Called also *soap bark, soap tree bark*, and *quillay bark*.

Quillaja (kwil-la′yah) [Chilian *quillai*] a genus of rosaceous trees. *Q. sapona′ria* Molina, a species native to South America, which was first described in 1782. See also *quillaia*.

quinacrine hydrochloride (kwin′ah-krin) [USP] chemical name: N^4-(6-chloro-2-methoxy-9-acridinyl)-N^1,N^1-diethyl-1,4-pentanediamine dihydrochloride dihydrate. An antimalarial, antiprotozoal, and anthelmintic, $C_{23}H_{30}Cl-N_3\cdot 2HCl\cdot 2H_2O$, occurring as a bright yellow, crystalline powder; used especially for suppressive therapy of malaria and in the treatment of giardiasis and tapeworm infestations, administered orally. Called also *chinacrin hydrochloride* and *mepacrine hydrochloride*.

quinalbarbitone (kwin″al-bar′bĭ-tōn) secobarbital.

quinaldic acid (kwin-al′dik) quinoline-2-carboxylic acid, a catabolite of tryptophan that is excreted in the urine. Called also *quinaldinic acid*.

quinaldinic acid (kwin″al-din′ik) quinaldic acid.

Quincke's disease, edema, meningitis, pulse (sign), puncture (kwink′ez) [Heinrich Irenaeus *Quincke*, physician in Kiel, 1842–1922] see *angioedema*, see *lumbar puncture*, under *puncture*, and see under *meningitis* and *pulse*.

quinestrol (kwin-es′trol) chemical name: 3-(cyclopentyloxy)-19-nor-17α-pregna-1,3,5(10)-trien-20-yn-17-ol; an estrogen, $C_{25}H_{32}O_2$.

quinethazone (kwin-eth′ah-zōn) [USP] chemical name: 7-chloro-2-ethyl-1,2,3,4-tetrahydro-4-oxo-6-quinazolinesulfonamide. An orally effective diuretic, $C_{10}H_{12}ClN_3O_3S$, with the same pharmacologic action as the thiazide diuretics; used in the treatment of edema associated with various conditions and of hypertension.

quinfamide (kwin′fah-mīd) chemical name: 1-(dichloroacetyl)-1,2,3,4-tetrahydro-6-quinolinyl ester 2-furancarboxylic acid; an antiamebic, $C_{16}H_{13}Cl_2NO_4$.

quingestanol acetate (kwin-jes′tah-nōl) chemical name: 3-(cyclopentyloxy)-19-nor-17α-pregna-3,5-dien-20-yn-17-ol acetate; a progestin, $C_{27}H_{38}O_3$.

quingestrone (kwin-jes′trōn) chemical name: 3-(cyclopentyloxy)pregna-3,5-dien-20-one; a progestin, $C_{26}H_{38}O_2$.

quinic acid (kwin′ik) 1,3,4,5-tetrahydroxycyclohexanecarboxylic acid, a compound found in cinchona bark and in many plants. Called also *kinic acid*.

Quinidex (kwin′ĭ-deks) trademark for a preparation of quinidine sulfate.

quinidine (kwin′ĭ-din) chemical name: 6-methoxycinchonan-9-ol. The dextrorotatory isomer of quinine, $C_{20}H_{24}N_2O_2$, obtained from various species of *Cinchona* and their hybrids, and from *Remijia pedunculata*, or prepared from quinine. It has cardiac depressant activity, and is as potent an antimalarial as quinine but is rarely used for the latter effect except in those having an idiosyncrasy to quinine. **q. gluconate** [USP], the gluconate salt of quinidine, $C_{20}H_{24}N_2O_2 \cdot C_6H_{12}O_7$; occurring as a white powder, having the same actions as the base; used in the treatment of certain cardiac arrhythmias, administered intravenously and intramuscularly. **q. polygalacturonate,** a salt of quinidine, $(C_{20}H_{24}N_2O_2 \cdot C_6H_{10}O_7 \cdot H_2O)_x$, having actions and uses the same as the other salts of quinidine; administered orally. **q. sulfate** [USP], the sulfate salt of quinidine, occurring as fine, needle-like crystals or as a fine, white powder, which is odorless, has a bitter taste, and darkens on exposure to light; administered orally for the treatment of cardiac arrhythmias.

quinine (kwin′in, kwin-ēn′, kwi′nīn) [L. *quinina*] an alkaloid of cinchona, $C_{20}H_{24}N_2O_2 \cdot 3H_2O$, occurring as a white microcrystalline powder, which suppresses the asexual erythrocytic forms of all malarial parasites and has a slight effect on the gametocytes of *Plasmodium vivax* and *P. malariae* but none on those of *P. falciparum*. Once widely used to prevent and control malaria, it has been largely replaced by less toxic and more effective synthetic antimalarials, and is now used chiefly (usually in the form of one of its soluble salts) in the treatment of falciparum malaria resistant to other antimalarials. Quinine also has analgesic antipyretic, mild oxytocic, cardiac depressant, and sclerosing properties, and it decreases the excitability of the motor endplate. **q. and urea hydrochloride,** a double salt of quinine and urea hydrochloride, $C_{20}H_{24}N_2O_2 \cdot HCl \cdot CH_4N_2O_2 \cdot HCl \cdot 5H_2O$, occurring as colorless translucent prisms, white granules, or white powder. It has been used to produce sclerosing, thrombosis, and obliteration of internal hemorrhoids and varicose veins, and as a local anesthetic. **q. bismuth iodide,** a compound of quinine and bismuth iodide formerly used in the treatment of syphilis. **q. bisulfate,** a colorless, crystalline cinchona salt, $C_{20}H_{24}O_2N_2 \cdot H_2SO_4 + 7H_2O$. It is much more soluble than the ordinary sulfate, and was formerly used in solution in the treatment of various ophthalmic disorders. **q. dihydrochloride,** the dihydrochloride salt of quinine, $C_{20}H_{24}N_2O_2 \cdot 2HCl$, occurring as a white powder, having the same actions and uses as the base; administered intravenously. **q. ethylcarbonate,** a white crystalline compound, $C_2H_5 \cdot O \cdot CO \cdot C_{20}H_{28}N_2O$, formed by the action of ethyl chlorocarbonate on quinine; it has been used like quinine sulfate. **q. hydrobromide,** a salt, $C_{20}H_{24}O_2N_2 \cdot HBr + H_2O$, formerly used in the treatment of hyperthyroidism and pneumococcal pneumonia. **q. hydrochloride,** a white salt, $C_{20}H_{24}O_2N_2 \cdot HCl + 2H_2O$, resembling the sulfate in taste and uses. **q. salicylate,** a salt, $C_{20}H_{24}N_2O_2 \cdot C_7H_6O_3 + H_2O$, in slender white needles, formerly used as an antipyretic and antirheumatic. **q. sulfate** [USP], the dihydrate sulfate salt of quinine, $(C_{20}H_{24}N_2O_2) \cdot H_2SO_4 \cdot 2H_2O$, occurring as white, fine needle-like crystals, having the same actions and uses as the base, and also used to prevent nocturnal cramps in the legs and feet; administered orally. **q. tannate,** a yellowish powder, containing 33 per cent anhydrous quinine, formerly used in whooping cough and diarrhea.

quininism (kwin′ĭ-nizm) cinchonism.

quinoid (kwin′oid) containing the chromatophoric group:

$$= C \underset{C\quad C}{\overset{C = C}{\diagdown}} C =$$

quinoline (kwin′o-lēn) a tertiary amine or alkaloid, $C_6H_4(CH)_3N$, a yellowish, aromatic liquid derivable from quinine, coal tar, and various other sources, which has antiseptic, antipyretic, and antiperiodic properties.

quinometry (kwĭ-nom′ĕ-tre) the standardization of the alkaloids of quinine.

quinone (kwi-nōn′, kwin′ōn) 1. a substance, $CO(CH \cdot CH)_2 \cdot CO$, in golden-yellow crystals, obtained by oxidizing quinic acid. 2. any benzene derivative in which two hydrogen atoms are replaced by two oxygen atoms.

Quinora (kwin′o-rah) trademark for a preparation of quinidine sulfate.

quinovin (kwin-o′vin) a bitter glycosidal mixture from cinchona.

quinovose (kwin′o-vōs) isorhodeose; 6-deoxy-D-glucose.

quinoxin (kwin-ok′sin) nitrosophenol, $C_6H_4(NO)OH$, a pale yellow, crystalline substance prepared from phenol by the action of nitrous acid.

Quinq. abbreviation for L. *quin'que,* five.

quinquecuspid (kwin″kwe-kus′pid) [L. *quinque* five + *cuspid*] 1. having five cusps. 2. a tooth with five cusps.

quinquetubercular (kwin″kwe-tu-ber′ku-lar) having five tubercles or cusps.

quinquevalent (kwing″kwĕ-va′lent) pentavalent.

quinquina (kin-ke′nah) cinchona.

quinsy (kwin′ze) [Gr. *kynanche* sore throat] peritonsillar abscess. **lingual q.,** suppurative inflammation of the lingual tonsil.

Quint. abbreviation for L. *quin'tus,* fifth.

quintan (kwin′tan) [L. *quintanus* of the fifth] recurring every fifth day, as a fever.

quintessence (kwin-tes′ens) [L. *quintus* fifth + *essentia* essence] the highly concentrated extract of any substance.

quintile (kwin′tīl) [L. *quintilis* pertaining to a fifth, from *quintus* fifth] any of the four values that divide the range of a probability distribution into five parts of equal probability, i.e., the 1st, 2nd, 3rd, and 4th quintiles are the 20th, 40th, 60th, and 80th percentiles.

quintipara (kwin-tip′ah-rah) [L. *quintus* fifth + *parere* to bring forth, produce] a woman who has had five pregnancies which resulted in viable offspring; also written para V.

quintisternal (kwin″tĭ-ster′nal) [L. *quintus* fifth + *sternum*] denoting the fifth bony portion of the sternum, or the part above the xiphoid process and adjacent to the fifth intercostal space.

quintuplet (kwin′tup-let, kwin-tup′let) [L. *quintuplex* five-fold] one of five offspring produced in one gestation period.

quittor (kwit′or) a fistulous sore on the quarters or the coronet of a horse's foot. **simple q.,** local inflammation resulting in a slough, with formation of pus immediately above the hoof. **skin q.,** a very painful ulcer of the skin above the hoof. **subhorny q.,** inflammation beginning at the coronary band and extending beneath the hoof and producing pus formation in the sensitive tissue. **tendinous q.,** a condition in which the inflammation has extended into the tendons of the leg and the ligaments of the joint.

quoad vitam (kwo′ad vi′tam) [L.] so far as life is concerned.

Quotane (kwo′tān) trademark for preparations of dimethisoquin hydrochloride.

Quotid. abbreviation for L. *quotid'ie,* daily.

quotidian (kwo-tid′e-an) [L. *quotidianus* daily] recurring every day; applied to the type of fever caused by certain forms of malarial parasites.

quotient (kwo′shent) a number obtained as the result of division. **achievement q.,** a percentage statement of the extent to which a child has progressed in learning in proportion to his ability. Abbreviated A.Q. **albumin q.,** the amount of albumin in the blood plasma divided by the amount of albumin present in the blood. **Ayala's q.,** a quotient in examination of the cerebrospinal pressure, obtained by dividing the pressure after removal of 10 ml. of cerebrospinal fluid by that registered before such removal, and multiplying by 10. Normal values are 5.5 to 6.5. A result under 5 indicates a small reservoir, as in subarachnoid block; over 7 means a large reservoir, as may be encountered in serous meningitis or hydrocephalus. **caloric q.,** the quotient obtained by dividing the heat evolved (expressed in calories) by the oxygen consumed (expressed in milligrams) in a metabolic process. **D q.,** the ratio of glucose to nitrogen in the urine. **growth q.,** that portion of the entire food energy which is utilized for the purpose of growth. **intelligence q.,** the measure of intelligence obtained by dividing the patient's mental age, as ascertained by the Binet test, by his chronological age and multiplying the result by 100. Abbreviated I.Q. **protein q.,** the number obtained by dividing the quantity of globulin of the blood plasma by the quantity of albumin. **rachidian q.**, Ayala's q. **reaction q.**, for a balanced chemical equation,

$$aA + bB + \ldots \rightleftarrows rR + sS + \ldots,$$

the product of the concentrations of the reaction products, each raised to the power equal to the coefficient of the product in the equation, divided by the concentrations of the reactants, each raised to the power equal to its coefficient:

$$Q = \frac{[R]^r\,[S]^s}{[A]^a\,[B]^b}$$

At equilibrium the reaction quotient equals the equilibrium constant. **respiratory q.**, the ratio of the volume of carbon dioxide given off by the body tissues to the volume of oxygen absorbed by them; usually equal to the corresponding volumes given off and taken up by the lungs. Abbreviated R.Q. **spinal q.**, Ayala's q.

q.v. abbreviation for L. *quan'tum vis*, as much as you please, and for *quod vi'de*, which see.

R

R symbol for *roentgen*; chemical symbol for an *organic radical*.

R symbol for electrical *resistance* and the *gas constant*.

R- [L. *rectus* right] a stereodescriptor used to specify the absolute configuration of compounds having asymmetric carbon atoms. The four different substituents at the asymmetric carbon atom are ranked according to certain sequence rules (described at *E-*); then, looking at the molecule with the lowest ranking substituent pointing directly away from the viewer, if the other three substituents are in clockwise order going from highest to lowest ranked, the configuration is *R*; otherwise S. Example: L-threonine is (2S:3R)-2-amino-3-hydroxybutanoic acid.

℞ symbol for L. *rec'ipe*, take. See *prescription*.

R_f in paper or thin-layer chromatography, the distance moved by a solute spot from the origin expressed as a fraction of the distance moved by the solvent front.

r symbol for *ring chromosome*; former symbol for *roentgen*, officially replaced by capital R.

ρ rho, the seventeenth letter of the Greek alphabet; symbol for *correlation coefficient*, mass *density* and electric charge *density*.

Ra chemical symbol for *radium*.

Raabe's test (rah'bez) [Gustav *Raabe*, German physician, born 1875] see under *tests*.

rabbetting (rab'et-ing) impaction of the denticulated broken surfaces of a fractured bone.

rabbitpox (rab'it-poks) an acute eruptive disease of laboratory rabbits, caused by a virus closely related to the vaccinia virus.

rabelaisin (rab"e-la'i-sin) a poisonous glycoside. from *Rabelaisia philippinensis*, a plant of the Philippine Islands: a heart stimulant.

rabid (rab'id) [L. *rabidus*] affected with rabies; mad.

rabies (ra'bēz, ra'be-ēz) [L. *rabere* to rage] an acute infectious disease of the central nervous system affecting almost all mammals, including humans, caused by a rhabdovirus, and usually spread by contamination with virus-laden saliva of bites inflicted by rabid animals, although aerosol infection via the respiratory route and transmission through transplantation or ingestion of infected tissues can occur. Important animal vectors include the dog, cat, vampire bat, mongoose, skunk, wolf, raccoon, and fox. The incubation period in both humans and animals is highly variable, depending on the size of the inoculum and the site of the bite, being shorter after a bite near the brain than following one farther away. Typical signs exhibited by rabid individuals include paresthesia and a burning sensation or pain at the site of inoculation; periods of hyperexcitability, agitation, delirium, hallucinations, and bizarre behavior, between which the individual is often cooperative and lucid; painful spasms of the pharyngeal and laryngeal muscles, hypersalivation, and fearfulness provoked by attempts to drink or even by the sight of fluids (hydrophobia); convulsions; meningismus; paralysis; and coma. Recovery is extremely rare, with death usually being associated with progressive respiratory depression and cardiorespiratory failure. Formerly called *hydrophobia*, *lyssa*, and *lytta*. **dumb r.**, paralytic r. **furious r.**, a stage or form of rabies in which excessive motor activity is prominent. **paralytic r.**, a stage or form of rabies most often associated with the bite of an infected vampire bat or seen in those inoculated against rabies before exposure, in which the most prominent symptom is ascending paralysis. Called also *dumb r.* and *paralyssa*.

rabiform (ra'bi-form) resembling rabies.

race (rās) 1. an ethnic stock, or division of mankind; in a narrower sense, a national or tribal stock; in a still narrower sense, a genealogic line of descent; a class of persons of a common lineage. In genetics, races are considered as populations having different distributions of gene frequencies. 2. a class or breed of animals; a group of individuals having certain characteristics in common, owing to a common inheritance; a subspecies.

racemase (ra'se-mās) an enzyme that catalyzes the racemization of an optically active substance, such as lactic acid.

racemate (ra'se-māt) an equimolecular mixture of two enantiomorphic isomers, being optically inactive in solution because of the presence of the same number of dextro- and levorotatory molecules. In the solid state it may have the properties of a loosely bound molecular compound. Called also *racemic form*, *racemic mixture*, or *racemic modification*.

raceme (ra-sēm') [L. *racemus* a bunch of grapes] 1. a form of inflorescence in which the individual flowers are borne on stalks which spring from a long central stem. 2. racemate.

racemethionine (rās"e-me-thi'o-nēn) [USP] chemical name: DL-methionine. A compound, $C_5H_{11}NO_2S$, occurring as white, crystalline platelets or powder. It is used as a dietary supplement with lipotropic action.

racemic (ra-se'mik) made up of two enantiomorphic isomers and therefore optically inactive.

racemization (ra"se-mi-za'shun) the transformation of one half of the molecules of an optically active compound into molecules which possess exactly the opposite (mirror-image) configuration, with complete loss of rotatory power because of the statistical balance between equal numbers of dextro- and levorotatory molecules. Cf. *mutarotation*.

racemose (ras'e-mōs) [L. *racemosus*] resembling a bunch of grapes on its stalk.

racephedrine hydrochloride (ra-sef'e-drin) chemical name: dl-α-[1-(methylamino)ethyl]benzyl alcohol hydrochloride. The racemic form of ephedrine hydrochloride, $C_{10}H_{15}$-NO·HCl, occurring as fine, white crystals or as a powder and used as a sympathomimetic.

racephenicol (rās-e-fen'i-kōl) chemical name: (R', R')-(±)-2,2-dichloro-N-[2-hydroxy-1-(hydroxymethyl)-2-[4-methylsulfonyl)phenyl]ethyl]acetamide; an antibacterial, $C_{12}H_{15}Cl_2$-NO_5S.

rachial (ra'ke-al) rachidial.

rachialbuminimeter (ra"ke-al-bu"mi-nim'e-ter) an apparatus for measuring the albumin in a specimen of the cerebrospinal fluid.

rachialbuminimetry (ra"ke-al-bu"mi-nim'e-tre) the measurement of the amount of albumin in the cerebrospinal fluid.

rachialgia (ra"ke-al'je-ah) [*rachi-* + Gr. *algos* pain + *-ia*] pain in the vertebral column.

rachianalgesia (ra"ke-an"al-je'ze-ah) rachianesthesia.

rachianesthesia (ra"ke-an"es-the'ze-ah) spinal anesthesia; anesthesia produced by the injection of the anesthetic into the spinal canal.

rachicentesis (ra"ke-sen-te'sis) [*rachi-* + Gr. *kentēsis* puncture] lumbar puncture.

rachidial (ra-kid'e-al) pertaining to the spine.

rachidian (ra-kid'e-an) pertaining to the spine.

rachigraph (ra'ke-graf) [*rachi-* + Gr. *graphein* to write] an instrument for recording the outlines of the spine and back.

rachilysis (ra-kil′ĭ-sis) [*rachi-* + Gr. *lysis* dissolution] mechanical treatment of a curved vertebral column by combined traction and pressure.

rachi(o)- [Gr. *rhachis* spine] a combining form denoting relation to the spine.

rachiocampsis (ra″ke-o-kamp′sis) [*rachio-* + Gr. *kampsis* curve] curvature of the spinal column.

rachiocentesis (ra″ke-o-sen-te′sis) [*rachio-* + Gr. *kentēsis* puncture] lumbar puncture.

rachiochysis (ra″ke-ok′ĭ-sis) [*rachio-* + Gr. *chysis* a pouring] the effusion of a fluid within the vertebral canal.

rachiocyphosis (ra″ke-o-si-fo′sis) kyphosis.

rachiodynia (ra″ke-o-din′e-ah) [*rachio-* + Gr. *odynē* pain + *-ia*] pain in the spinal column.

rachiokyphosis (ra″ke-o-ki-fo′sis) kyphosis.

rachiometer (ra″ke-om′ĕ-ter) [*rachio-* + Gr. *metron* measure] an instrument for measuring curvatures of the vertebral column.

rachiomyelitis (ra″ke-o-mi″ĕ-li′tis) [*rachio-* + Gr. *myelos* marrow + *-itis*] inflammation of the spinal cord.

rachiopagus (ra″ke-op′ah-gus) [*rachio-* + Gr. *pagos* thing fixed] symmetrical conjoined twins united back to back in the sagittal plane, fusion being limited to the upper trunk and cervical region.

rachiopathy (ra″ke-op′ah-the) [*rachio-* + Gr. *pathos* disease] any disease of the spine.

rachioscoliosis (ra″ke-o-sko″le-o′sis) lateral curvature of the spine.

rachiotome (ra′ke-o-tōm) an instrument for cutting the vertebrae.

rachiotomy (ra″ke-ot′o-me) [*rachio-* + Gr. *tomē* a cutting] incision of a vertebra, or of the vertebral column.

rachipagus (ra-kip′ah-gus) [*rachi-* + Gr. *pagos* thing fixed] a double monster joined at the vertebral column.

rachiresistance (ra″ke-re-zis′tans) a condition in which the injection of a spinal anesthetic produces little or no effect.

rachiresistant (ra″ke-re-zis′tant) abnormally insensitive to spinal anesthetics.

rachis (ra′kis) [Gr. *rhachis* spine] the vertebral column.

rachisagra (ra″kis-ag′rah) [*rachis* + Gr. *agra* seizure] pain or gout in the spine.

rachischisis (ra-kis′kĭ-sis) [*rachi-* + Gr. *schisis* cleft] congenital fissure of the spinal column. **r. partia′lis,** fissure of the spinal column of limited extent; merorachischisis. **r. poste′rior,** spina bifida. **r. tota′lis,** holorachischisis.

rachisensibility (ra″ke-sen″sĭ-bil′ĭ-te) the condition of being abnormally sensitive to spinal anesthetics.

rachisensible (ra″ke-sen′sĭ-b′l) abnormally sensitive to spinal anesthetics.

rachitic (ra-kit′ik) pertaining to or affected with rickets.

rachitis (ra-ki′tis) [Gr. *rachitis*] 1. rickets. 2. inflammatory disease of the vertebral column. **r. feta′lis annula′ris,** the formation before birth of annular thickenings on the long bones. **r. feta′lis micromel′ica,** deficient longitudinal growth of the bones of the fetus. **r. tar′da,** late rickets.

rachitism (rak′ĭ-tizm) a tendency to rickets.

rachitogenic (rah-kit″o-jen′ik) causing rickets.

rachitome (rak″ĭ-tōm) a cutting instrument used in opening the spinal canal.

rachitomy (rah-kit′o-me) [*rachi-* + Gr. *tomē* a cutting] the surgical opening of the vertebral canal.

racial (ra′shal) pertaining to a particular race.

rad [acronym for *r*adiation *a*bsorbed *d*ose] 1. a unit of measurement of the absorbed dose of ionizing radiation; it corresponds to an energy transfer of 100 ergs per gram of any absorbing material (including tissues). The biological effect of 1 rad varies with the kind of radiation the tissue is exposed to. Cf. *gray* (def. 3.). 2. abbreviation for *radian.*

rad. abbreviation for L. *ra′dix,* root.

radarkymography (ra″dar-ki-mog′rah-fe) the recording on a television monitor, by means of a radar tracking instrument, of cardiac motion displayed on a fluoroscope.

radectomy (ra-dek′to-me) [L. *radix* root + Gr. *ektomē* excision] partial or complete excision of a portion of the root of a tooth.

radiability (ra″de-ah-bil′ĭ-te) the property of being radiable.

radiable (ra′de-ah-b′l) capable of being penetrated by radiation, especially by roentgen rays.

radiad (ra′de-ad) toward the radius or radial side.

radial (ra′de-al) [L. *radialis*] 1. pertaining to the radius of the forearm or to the radial (lateral) aspect of the arm as opposed to the ulnar (medial) aspect; pertaining to a radius. 2. radiating; spreading outward from a common center.

radialis (ra″de-a′lis) [L.] radial; [NA] a term designating relationship to the radius.

radian (ra′de-an) [from *radius*] a unit of plane angle equal to the angle subtended at the center of a circle by an arc whose length is equal to the radius of the circle. One radian equals 360°/2π or approximately 57.295°. Abbreviated rad.

radiant (ra′de-ant) [L. *radians*] 1. diverging from a common center. 2. emitting radiation or heat. 3. transmitted by radiation.

radiate (ra′de-āt) [L. *radiare, radiatus*] 1. to diverge or spread from a common point. 2. arranged in a radiating manner.

radiathermy (ra-di″ah-ther′me) short wave diathermy.

radiatio (ra-de-a′she-o), pl. *radiatio′nes* [L., from *radiare* to furnish with spokes] a radiation or radiating structure; used in anatomical nomenclature to designate a collection of nerve fibers connecting different portions of the brain. **r. acus′tica** [NA], acoustic radiation: a fiber tract arising in the medial geniculate nucleus and passing laterally in the sublenticular portion of the internal capsule to terminate in the transverse temporal gyri of the temporal lobe; the radiation provides reciprocal connections and forms part of the caudal peduncle of the thalamus. **r. cor′poris callo′si** [NA], radiation of corpus callosum: the fibers of the corpus callosum radiating to all parts of the neopallium. **r. cor′poris stria′ti,** the extension of fibers from the thalamus and hypothalamus to the corpus striatum. **r. op′tica** [NA], optic radiation: a fiber tract which begins at the lateral geniculate body, passes laterally through the pars retrolentiformis of the internal capsule, and finally projects posteriorly to end in the striate area on the medial surface of the occipital lobe, on either side of the calcarine sulcus; the radiation provides reciprocal connections and forms part of the posterior thalamic peduncle. Called also *geniculocalcarine tract, occipitothalamic radiation,* and *radiation of Gratiolet.* **r. pyramida′lis,** pyramidal radiation: the projection of fibers from the cerebral cortex to the pyramidal tract. **radiatio′nes thala′micae anterio′res** [NA], anterior thalamic radiations: the thalamocortical fibers of the anterior limb of the internal capsule that connect the medial and anterior thalamic nuclei and the cortex of the frontal lobe. **radiatio′nes thala′micae centra′les** [NA], central thalamic radiations: the thalamocortical fibers of the posterior limb of the internal capsule that carry general sensory impulses from the ventral thalamic nuclei to the postcentral gyrus. Called also *superior thalamic radiations.* **radiatio′nes thala′micae posterio′res** [NA], posterior thalamic radiations: the thalamocortical fibers of the retrolentiform part of the internal capsule that connect the cortices of the occipital and parietal lobes and the caudal parts of the thalamus.

radiation (ra-de-a′shun) [L. *radiatio,* q.v.] 1. divergence from a common center. 2. a structure made up of divergent elements, as one of the fiber tracts in the brain; for official names of specific structures, see under *radiatio.* 3. energy transmitted by waves through space or through some medium; usually referring to electromagnetic radiation when used without a modifier. By extension, a stream of particles, such as electrons, neutrons, protons, or alpha particles. **acoustic r.,** radiatio acustica. **adaptive r.,** evolution from a generalized, primitive species to diverse, specialized species, each adapted to a distinct mode of life. **alpha r.,** α-r., see under *ray.* **annihilation r.,** radiation produced by the collision and annihilation of a particle and its antiparticle, especially the two 0.511-MeV gamma ray photons produced by the annihilation of a positron and an electron. **auditory r.,** radiatio acustica. **background r.,** radiation arising from radioactive material other than that directly under consideration or study. Background radiation due to cosmic rays and natural radioactivity in the environment is always present; additional background radiation may be due to the presence of other radioactive material in the vicinity, or radioactive components of building materials, etc. **beta r.**, *β*-**r.**, see under *ray*. **braking r.**, bremsstrahlung. **Cerenkov r.**, visible light emitted by a high-speed charged particle moving through a transparent medium at a speed greater than the speed of light in that medium. **r. of corpus callosum**, radiatio corporis callosi. **corpuscular r's**, radiations consisting of streams of subatomic particles, such as protons, deuterons, electrons, positrons, and neutrons. **electromagnetic r.**, see under *wave*. **gamma r.**, *γ*-**r.**, see under *ray*. **r. of Gratiolet**, radiatio optica. **heterogeneous r.**, radiation consisting of a beam of particles of various energies, or having different frequencies, or containing different types of particles. **homogeneous r.**, radiation consisting of an extremely narrow band of frequencies or a beam of monoenergetic particles of a single type. **Huldshinsky's r.**, a course of three months' treatment with ultraviolet rays from the quartz-mercury vapor lamp. **interstitial r.**, energy emitted by radium or radon inserted directly into the tissue. **ionizing r.**, corpuscular or electromagnetic radiation capable of producing ionization, directly or indirectly, in its passage through matter. **irritative r.**, radiation with ultraviolet rays to the point of erythema. **mitogenetic r.**, **mitogenic r.**, specific energy allegedly given off by a cell undergoing mitosis. **monochromatic r.**, radiation having a single wavelength. **monoenergetic r.**, radiation of a given type, as of alpha, beta, or gamma rays, in which all particles or photons originate with and have the same energy. **occipitothalamic r.**, **optic r.**, radiatio optica. **photochemical r.**, that part of the radiant spectrum which produces chemical changes. **pyramidal r.**, radiatio pyramidalis. **Rollier's r.**, exposure of the tuberculous patient to gradually increasing doses of the ultraviolet rays of the sun. **tegmental r.**, fibers radiating laterally from the red nucleus. **thalamic r.**, fiber tracts that reciprocally connect the thalamus and cerebral cortex by way of the internal capsule; see terms beginning *radiationes thalamicae*. **thalamic r's, anterior**, radiationes thalamicae anteriores. **thalamic r's, central**, radiationes thalamicae centrales. **thalamic r's, posterior**, radiationes thalamicae posteriores. **thalamic r's, superior**, radiationes thalamicae centrales. **thalamotemporal r.**, radiatio acustica. **white r.**, bremsstrahlung, def. 1.

radiationes (ra-de-a″she-o′nēz) [L.] plural of *radiatio*.

radical (rad′ĭ-kal) [L. *radicalis*] 1. directed to the cause; directed to the root or source of a morbid process, as radical surgery. 2. a group of atoms which enters into and goes out of chemical combination without change, and which forms one of the fundamental constituents of a molecule. **acid r.**, 1. the electronegative element which combines with hydrogen to form an acid. 2. all of the acid except the hydroxyl group. **alcohol r.**, all of the alcohol molecule except the hydrogen atom of the –OH group; an alkoxy radical. **color r.**, chromophore. **free r.**, a radical, extremely reactive and having a very short half-life (10^{-5} seconds or less in an aqueous solution), which carries an unpaired electron.

radices (rad′ĭ-sēz) [L.] plural of *radix*.

radiciform (ra-dis′ĭ-form) [L. *radix* root + *forma* shape] shaped like a root; shaped like the root of a tooth.

radicle (rad′ĭ-k′l) [L. *radicula*] 1. any one of the smallest branches of a vessel or nerve. 2. the embryonic, or primary, root that grows out of the hypocotyl of seed plants.

radicotomy (rad″ĭ-kot′o-me) rhizotomy.

radicula (rah-dik′u-lah) [L.] radicle, def. 1.

radicularia (rah-dik″u-lal′je-ah) pain due to disease of the spinal nerve roots.

radicular (rah-dik′u-lar) of or pertaining to a radical or root.

radiculectomy (rah-dik″u-lek′to-me) [L. *radicula* radicle + Gr. *ektomē* excision] excision of a rootlet, especially resection of spinal nerve roots.

radiculitis (rah-dik″u-li′tis) [L. *radicula* radicle + -*itis*] inflammation of the root of a spinal nerve, especially of that portion of the root which lies between the spinal cord and the intervertebral canal.

radiculoganglionitis (rah-dik″u-lo-gang″gle-o-ni′tis) inflammation of the posterior spinal nerve roots and their ganglions.

radiculomedullary (rah-dik″u-lo-med′u-ler″e) pertaining to or affecting the nerve roots and the spinal cord.

radiculomeningomyelitis (rah-dik″u-lo-mě-ning″go-mi″ě-li′tis) inflammation of the nerve roots, the meninges, and the spinal cord.

radiculomyelopathy (rah-dik″u-lo-mi″ě-lop′ah-the) disease of the nerve roots and spinal canal.

radiculoneuritis (rah-dik″u-lo-nu-ri′tis) acute febrile polyneuritis.

radiculoneuropathy (rah-dik″u-lo-nu-rop′ah-the) disease of the nerve roots and nerve.

radiculopathy (rah-dik″u-lop′ah-the) disease of the nerve roots. **spondylotic caudal r.**, compression of the cauda equina due to encroachment upon a congenitally small spinal canal by spondylosis, resulting in pseudoclaudication or more profound neural disorders of the lower limbs.

radiectomy (ra″de-ek′to-me) [L. *radix* root + Gr. *ektomē* excision] root amputation.

radiferous (ra-dif′er-us) containing radium.

radii (ra′de-i) [L.] genitive and plural of *radius*.

radio- [L. *radius*, q.v.] 1. a combining form denoting relationship (*a*) to the radius (def. 2), or (*b*) to radiant energy, rays, or ionizing radiation. 2. in chemistry, a combining form denoting a radioactive isotope of the element to which it is affixed, e.g., radiocarbon, radiogold.

radioactinium (ra″de-o-ak-tin′e-um) a substance formed by the disintegration of actinium.

radioaction (ra″de-o-ak′shun) radioactivity.

radioactive (ra″de-o-ak′tiv) having the property of radioactivity.

radioactivity (ra″de-o-ak-tiv′ĭ-te) the quality of emitting or the emission of corpuscular or electromagnetic radiations consequent to nuclear disintegration, a natural property of all chemical elements of atomic number above 83, and possible of induction in all other known elements. **artificial r.**, **induced r.**, radioactivity produced by bombarding an element with high velocity particles, as the radioactivity of synthetic nuclides.

radioactor (ra″de-o-ak′tor) an apparatus used for collecting and purifying radium emanation.

radioallergosorbent (ra″de-o-al″er-go-sor′bent) denoting a radioimmunoassay technique for the measurement of specific IgE antibody to a variety of allergens; see under *tests*.

radioanaphylaxis (ra″de-o-an″ah-fi-lak′sis) anaphylactic sensitization to the roentgen ray or other form of radiant energy.

radioautogram (ra″de-o-aw′to-gram) autoradiograph.

radioautograph (ra″de-o-aw′to-graf) autoradiograph.

radioautography (ra″de-o-aw-tog′rah-fe) autoradiography.

radiobe (ra′de-ōb) [radio- + Gr. *bios* life] one of the peculiar microscopical condensations of sterilized bouillon produced by radium, discovered by J. B. Burke, which, by their appearance and the way in which they divide, have suggested the similar phenomena of bacteria.

radiobicipital (ra″de-o-bi-sip′ĭ-tal) pertaining to the radius and the biceps muscle of the arm.

radiobiological (ra″de-o-bi″o-loj′ĭ-kal) pertaining to radiobiology: concerning cellular and tissue response to irradiation.

radiobiologist (ra″de-o-bi-ol′o-jist) one who devotes his studies to radiobiology.

radiobiology (ra″de-o-bi-ol′o-je) that branch of science which is concerned with the effect of light and of ultraviolet and ionizing radiations upon living tissue or organisms.

radiocalcium (ra″de-o-kal′se-um) a radioactive isotope of calcium. ^{45}Ca, with a half-life of 180 days, is used as a tracer in the study of calcium metabolism.

radiocarbon (ra″de-o-kar′bon) a radioactive isotope of carbon such as ^{14}C, with a half-life of over 5000 years.

radiocarcinogenesis (ra″de-o-kar″sĭ-no-jen′ě-sis) cancer formation caused by exposure to radiation.

radiocardiogram (ra″de-o-kar′de-o-gram) the graphic record obtained by radiocardiography.

radiocardiography (ra″de-o-kar″de-og′rah-fe) 1. the graphic recording of the variation with time of the concentration, in a selected chamber of the heart, of a radioactive isotope, usually injected intravenously. 2. radioelectrocardiography.

radiocarpal (ra″de-o-kar′pal) pertaining to the radius and carpus.

radiocarpus (ra″de-o-kar′pus) musculus flexor carpi radialis.

radiochemistry (ra″de-o-kem′is-tre) the branch of chemistry which treats of radioactive materials.

radiochemy (ra″de-o-kem′e) the effects produced by radioactive rays.

radiochroism (ra″de-o-kro′izm) [*radio-* + Gr. *chroa* color] the capacity of a substance to absorb certain radioactive and roentgen rays.

radiocinematograph (ra″de-o-sin″ĕ-mat′o-graf) an apparatus combining the moving picture camera and the roentgen ray machine, making possible moving pictures of the internal organs.

radiocolloids (ra″de-o-kol′oids) radioisotopes in pure form in solution, which tend to behave more like colloids than solutes.

radiocurable (ra″de-o-kūr′ah-b'l) curable by radiation therapy.

radiocystitis (ra″de-o-sis-ti′tis) acute or chronic inflammatory tissue changes in the urinary bladder caused by ionizing irradiation.

radiode (ra′de-ōd) an instrument for the therapeutic application of a radioactive source.

radiodense (ra′de-o-dens″) radiopaque.

radiodensity (ra″de-o-den′sĭ-te) radiopacity.

radiodermatitis (ra″de-o-der-mah-ti′tis) a cutaneous inflammatory reaction occurring as a result of exposure to biologically effective levels of ionizing radiation.

radiodiagnosis (ra″de-o-di″ag-no′sis) diagnosis by means of roentgen rays and roentgenograms.

radiodiagnostics (ra″de-o-di″ag-nos′tiks) the art of roentgen-ray diagnosis.

radiodiaphane (ra″de-o-di′ah-fān) an instrument for performing transillumination by means of radium.

radiodigital (ra″de-o-dig′ĭ-tal) pertaining to the radius and to the fingers.

radiodontics (ra″de-o-don′tiks) dental radiology.

radiodontist (ra″de-o-don′tist) dental radiologist.

radioecology (ra″de-o-e-kol′o-je) the science dealing with the effects of radiation on species of plants and animals in natural communities or ecosystems.

radioelectrocardiogram (ra″de-o-e-lek″tro-kar′de-o-gram) the graphic recording obtained by radioelectrocardiography.

radioelectrocardiograph (ra″de-o-e-lek″tro-kar′de-o-graf″) a battery-operated device by means of which cardiographic signals from electrodes attached at desired body sites are transmitted to a recorder close to or at a distance from the subject.

radioelectrocardiography (ra″de-o-e-lek″tro-kar″de-og′-rah-fe) electrocardiography in which impulses are beamed by radio from the subject to a receiver close to or at a distance from the subject.

radioelement (ra″de-o-el′ĕ-ment) any chemical element having radioactive properties.

radioencephalogram (ra″de-o-en-sef′ah-lo-gram″) a curve showing the passage of an injected tracer through the cerebral blood vessels as revealed by an external scintillation counter.

radioencephalography (ra″de-o-en-sef″ah-log′rah-fe) the recording of changes in the electric potential of the brain without direct attachment between the recording apparatus and the subject, the impulses being beamed by radio waves from the subject to the receiver.

radioepidermitis (ra″de-o-ep″ĭ-der-mi′tis) radiodermatitis.

radioepithelitis (ra″de-o-ep″ĭ-the-li′tis) radiodermatitis.

radiogen (ra′de-o-jen) any radioactive substance.

radiogenesis (ra″de-o-jen′ĕ-sis) the production of rays or radioactivity.

radiogenic (ra″de-o-jen′ik) [*radio-* + Gr. *gennan* to produce] produced by irradiation.

radiogold (ra′de-o-gold) a radioactive isotope of gold, viz., ^{195}Au, ^{198}Au, or ^{199}Au. The isotope ^{198}Au is the most commonly used in solid form or in colloidal solution. It has a half-life of 2.7 days and emits gamma (0.411 MeV) as well as beta radiation (E max = 0.96 MeV). The gamma rays contribute from 6 to 10 per cent of the total dose. It is used both as a diagnostic scintiscanning agent and as a therapeutic cancericidal agent.

radiogram (ra′de-o-gram″) radiograph.

radiograph (ra′de-o-graf″) a film produced by radiography. **bite-wing r.,** a type of dental radiograph that reveals the crowns, necks, coronal thirds of the roots of both the upper and lower teeth, and the dental arches, produced on dental x-ray film that has a central protruding tab or wing on which the teeth close to hold the film in position (bite-wing film). **cephalometric r.,** cephalogram. **lateral oblique jaw r.,** a radiograph of the mandible that unilaterally reveals the mandible from symphysis to condyle. **lateral ramus r.,** a radiograph of the mandibular ramus and condyle. **lateral skull r.,** a radiograph of the sinuses and lateral aspects of the skeletal structures of the cranium. **maxillary sinus r.,** a radiograph of the maxillary sinuses and the zygomas that permits direct comparison of the two sides; called also *Waters view r.* **panoramic r.,** a type of extraoral body-section radiograph on which the maxilla and the mandible are depicted on a single film. Called also *Orthopantograph.* **submental vertex r.,** a radiograph that permits visualization of the lateral movements of the condyle, lateral displacement of the condyle and/or the coronoid process, and the contour of the zygomatic arches. **Towne projection r.,** a radiograph of the mandibular condyles and the midfacial skeleton. **Waters view r.,** maxillary sinus r.

radiographic (ra″de-o-graf′ik) pertaining to or produced by radiography.

radiography (ra″de-og′rah-fe) [*radio-* + Gr. *graphein* to write] the making of film records (radiographs) of internal structures of the body by passage of x-rays or gamma rays through the body to act on specially sensitized film. See also *roentgenography.* **body section r.,** a special technique to show in detail images of structures lying in a predetermined plane of tissue, while blurring or eliminating detail in images of structures in other planes. See *tomography.* Various mechanisms and methods for such radiography have been given various names, such as *laminagraphy, laminography, planigraphy, radiotomy, stratigraphy,* and *vertigraphy.* **digital r.,** a technique in which x-ray absorption is quantified by the assignment of a number to the amount of x-rays reaching the detector; the information is entered into a computer and manipulated to produce an optimal image. **double contrast r.,** mucosal relief radiography. **electron r.,** a technique in which a latent electron image is produced on clear plastic by passing x-ray photons through a gas with a high atomic number; this image is then developed into a black-and-white picture. **mass r.,** examination by x-rays of the general population or of large groups of the population. **miniature r., mass,** the use of miniature x-ray film in mass radiography. **mucosal relief r.,** a technique for revealing any abnormality of the intestinal mucosa, involving injection and evacuation of a barium enema, followed by inflation of the intestine with air under light pressure. The light coating of barium on the walls of the inflated intestine in the radiography reveals clearly even small abnormalities. **neutron r.,** that in which a narrow beam of neutrons from a nuclear reactor is passed through tissues, especially useful in visualizing bony tissue. **panoramic r.,** pantomography. **selective r.,** radiography of certain segments of the population, chosen on some specific basis such as symptoms. **serial r.,** the taking of several exposures of a selected area at arbitrary intervals. **spot-film r.,** the making of localized instantaneous radiographs during the course of a fluoroscopic examination.

radiohumeral (ra″de-o-hu′mer-al) pertaining to the radius and humerus.

radioimmunity (ra″de-o-ĭ-mu′nĭ-te) a condition of decreased sensitivity to radiation sometimes produced by repeated irradiation.

radioimmunoassay (ra″de-o-im″u-no-as′a) a highly sensitive and specific assay method that uses the competition between radiolabeled and unlabeled substances in an antigen-antibody reaction to determine the concentration of the unlabeled substance; it can be used to determine antibody concentrations or to determine the concentration of any substance against which specific antibody can be produced. Abbreviated RIA.

radioimmunodiffusion (ra″de-o-im″u-no-dif-fu′zhun) immunodiffusion conducted with radioisotope-labeled antibodies or antigens.

radioimmunoelectrophoresis (ra″de-o-im″u-no-e-lek″tro-fo-re′sis) immunoelectrophoresis in which a radiolabeled antigen or antibody is located within a specific precipitin arc using autoradiography.

radioimmunoprecipitation (ra″de-o-im″u-no-pre-sip″-ĭ-ta′shun) immunoprecipitation conducted with radioisotope- labeled antibody or antigen.

radioimmunosorbent (ra″de-o-im″u-no-sor′bent) denoting a radioimmunoassay technique for measuring IgE in samples of serum; see under *tests*.

radioiodine (ra″de-o-i′o-dīn) a radioactive isotope of iodine; of the nine isotopes, ^{131}I and ^{125}I are the most commonly used in the diagnosis and treatment of both benign and malignant disease of the thyroid gland and in the scintiscanning of such organs as the lung, liver, kidney, etc. ^{131}I has a half-life of 8.04 days and emits both beta and gamma rays. ^{125}I has a half-life of 60 days and emits only gamma radiation.

radioiron (ra″de-o-i′ern) a radioactive isotope of iron. ^{55}Fe has a half-life of about 4 years, ^{59}Fe, a half-life of 47 days. A mixture of these has been used in study of the blood.

radioisotope (ra″de-o-i′so-tōp) an isotope which is radioactive, i.e., one having an unstable nucleus, which gives it the property of decay by one or more of several processes. It may be produced from the stable isotope of the element by irradiation in a cyclotron or nuclear reactor. Radioisotopes have important diagnostic and therapeutic uses in clinical medicine and research. **carrier-free r.,** see *carrier-free*.

radiokymography (ra″de-o-ki-mog′rah-fe) roentgenkymography.

Radiolaria (ra″de-o-la′re-ah) [L. *radiolus* small sunbeam] in former systems of classification, a subclass or an order of rhizopod marine planktonic protozoa, the members of which have been assigned to the classes Phaeodarea and Polycystinea.

radiolarian (ra″de-o-lar′e-an) any protozoan belonging to the Radiolaria (see Phaeodarea and Polycystinea). Traditionally, the term radiolarian has also been used to include acantharians.

radiolead (ra″de-o-led′) a radioactive isotope of lead.

radiolesion (ra″de-o-le′zhun) a lesion caused by exposure to radiation.

radioligand (ra″de-o-li′gand, rad″de-o-lig′and) a radioactive-labeled substance, e.g., an antigen, used in the quantitative measurement of an unlabeled substance by its binding reaction to a specific antibody or other receptor site.

radiologic, radiological (ra″de-o-loj′ik; ra″de-o-loj′ĭ-kal) pertaining to radiology.

radiologist (ra″de-ol′o-jist) a physician who specializes in the use of roentgen rays and other forms of radiation in the diagnosis and treatment of disease. **dental r.,** a dentist who specializes in dental radiology. Called also *radiodontist*.

radiology (ra″de-ol′o-je) [radio- + -logy] that branch of the health sciences dealing with radioactive substances and radiant energy and with the diagnosis and treatment of disease by means of both ionizing (e.g., roentgen rays) and nonionizing (e.g., ultrasound) radiations. **dental r., oral r.,** the branch of radiology dealing primarily with orofacial structures. Called also *radiodontics*.

radiolucency (ra″de-o-loo′sen-se) the property of being radiolucent.

radiolucent (ra-de-o-loo′sent) [radio- + L. *lucēre* to shine] permitting the passage of roentgen rays or other forms of radiant energy with little attenuation; radiolucent areas appear dark on the exposed film.

radiolus (ra-de′o-lus) [L., dim. of *radius* ray] a probe, staff, or sound.

radiometer (ra″de-om′ĕ-ter) an instrument for detecting and measuring radiant energy.

radiomicrometer (ra″de-o-mi-krom′ĕ-ter) [radio- + micro- + -meter] a sensitive radiometer for detecting minute amounts of radiant energy.

radiomimetic (ra″de-o-mi-met′ik) [radio- + Gr. *mimētikos* imitative] exerting effects similar to those of ionizing radiation.

radiomuscular (ra″de-o-mus′ku-lar) going from the radial artery or nerve to the muscles.

radiomutation (ra″de-o-mu-ta′shun) change in the character of cells caused by exposure to radiation.

radion (ra′de-on) one of the radiant particles thrown off by a radioactive substance.

radionecrosis (ra″de-o-ne-kro′sis) destruction of tissue caused by radiant energy.

radioneuritis (ra″de-o-nu-ri′tis) a form of neuritis resulting from exposure to roentgen rays or other radiant energy.

radionitrogen (ra″de-o-ni′tro-jen) a radioactive substance produced by bombarding boron with alpha rays.

radionuclide (ra″de-o-nu′klīd) a radioactive nuclide; one that disintegrates with the emission of corpuscular or electromagnetic radiations.

radio-opacity (ra″de-o-o-pas′ĭ-te) radiopacity.

radiopacity (ra″de-o-pas′ĭ-te) the property of being radiopaque.

radiopaque (ra″de-o-pāk′) [radio- + L. *opacus* dark, obscure] not penetrable by roentgen rays or other forms of radiant energy; radiopaque areas appear light or white on the exposed film.

radioparency (ra″de-o-par′en-se) radiolucency.

radioparent (ra″de-o-par′ent) radiolucent.

radiopathology (ra″de-o-pah-thol′o-je) pathology having to do with the effects of radiation on tissues.

radiopelvimetry (ra″de-o-pel-vim′ĕ-tre) measurement of the pelvis by roentgen-ray examination.

radiopharmaceutical (ra″de-o-fahr″mah-su′tĭ-kal) a radioactive pharmaceutical or chemical (e.g., radioactive iodine, cobalt, etc.) used for diagnostic or therapeutic purposes.

radiopharmacy (ra″de-o-fahr′mah-se) the preparation of radioactive pharmaceuticals and radionuclides.

radiophobia (ra″de-o-fo′be-ah) irrational anxiety about the damaging effects of x-rays and radium.

radiophosphorus (ra″de-o-fos′fo-rus) either of two radioactive isotopes of phosphorus, ^{32}P and ^{33}P. The former, a pure beta emitter, has a half-life of 14.3 days and is used in solution or colloidal form as a diagnostic and therapeutic agent.

radiophotography (ra″de-o-fo-tog′rah-fe) photography of the fluorescent image produced by an x-ray beam.

radiophylaxis (ra″de-o-fi-lak′sis) the modifying effect of a small dose of radiation on the reaction to a large subsequent radiation.

radiophysics (ra″de-o-fiz′iks) the physics of radiology.

radiopotassium (ra″de-o-po-tas′e-um) a radioactive isotope of potassium. ^{42}K, with a half-life of 12.4 hours, is used in tracer studies of potassium interchange in the body.

radiopotentiation (ra″de-o-po-ten″-she-a′shun) the action of a drug in enhancing the effect of irradiation.

radiopraxis (ra″de-o-prak′sis) [radio- + Gr. *praxis* practice] use of rays of light, electricity, etc., in treatment of disease.

radiopulmonography (ra″de-o-pul″mo-nog′rah-fe) a rapid method for estimation of ventilation of localized lung areas, based on measurement of variation in intensity of low-voltage x-rays passed through the lungs during breathing.

radioreaction (ra″de-o-re-ak′shun) a bodily reaction, especially a skin reaction, to radiation.

radioreceptor (ra″de-o-re-sep′tor) a receptor for the stimuli which are excited by radiant energy, such as light or heat.

radioresistance (ra″de-o-re-zis′tans) resistance, as of tissue or cells, to the injurious effects of radiation.

radioresistant (ra″de-o-re-zis′tant) exhibiting the property of radioresistance.

radioscopy (ra″de-os′ko-pe) [radio- + Gr. *skopein* to examine] fluoroscopy.

radiosensibility (ra″de-o-sen″sĭ-bil′ĭ-te) radiosensitivity.

radiosensitive (ra″de-o-sen′sĭ-tiv) sensitive to radiant energy, as roentgen ray or other radiations; said of skin, tumor tissue, etc.

radiosensitiveness (ra″de-o-sen′sĭ-tiv-nes) radiosensitivity.

radiosensitivity (ra″de-o-sen″sĭ-tiv′ĭ-te) sensitivity, as of the skin or other tissue, to radiant energy, such as roentgen-ray or other radiations.

radiosensitizer (ra″de-o-sen′sĭ-ti″zer) a chemotherapeutic agent used to enhance the effect of radiation therapy.

radiosodium (ra″de-o-so′de-um) a radioactive isotope of sodium, ^{24}Na and ^{22}Na are used in the study of blood flow, water balance, and peripheral vascular diseases.

radiostereoscopy (ra″de-o-ster″e-os′ko-pe) [radio- + Gr. stereos solid + skopein to examine] the inspection of the interior organs by means of roentgen rays.

radiostrontium (ra″de-o-stron′she-um) a radioactive isotope of strontium, of which there are four: ^{85}Sr, ^{87}Sr, ^{89}Sr, and ^{90}Sr. The half-lives are, respectively, 65 days, 2.8 hours, 51 days, and 28 years. Their importance in clinical scintiscanning and nuclear fallout is primarily due to their affinity for bone.

radiosulfur (ra″de-o-sul′fur) a radioactive isotope of sulfur.

radiotelemetry (ra″de-o-tel-em′ĕ-tre) the determination of measurement of various factors, the specific data being transmitted by radio waves from the object of measurement to the recording apparatus.

radiotellurium (ra″de-o-tel-lu′re-um) any radioactive isotope of the element tellurium.

radiothanatology (ra″de-o-than″ah-tol′o-je) [radio- + Gr. thanatos death + logos treatise] the study of the effect of radiant energy on dead tissue.

radiotherapeutics (ra″de-o-ther″ah-pu′tiks) 1. the body of knowledge comprising the available information regarding the therapeutic use of ionizing radiation. 2. radiotherapy.

radiotherapist (ra″de-o-ther′ah-pist) a specialist in radiotherapy.

radiotherapy (ra″de-o-ther′ah-pe) [radio- + Gr. therapeia cure] the treatment of disease by ionizing radiation. **interstitial r.,** that administered with the radioactive element contained in devices (e.g., needles or wire) inserted directly into the tissues. **intracavitary r.,** that in which the radioactive element is introduced into a natural body cavity.

radiothermy (ra″de-o-ther′me) [radio- + Gr. thermē heat] 1. therapeutic use of radiant heat or of heat emanating from radioactive substances. 2. short wave diathermy.

radiothorium (ra″de-o-tho′re-um) a radioactive isotope of thorium.

radiotomy (ra″de-ot′o-me) [radio- + Gr. tomē a cutting] see body section roentgenography, under roentgenography.

radiotoxemia (ra″de-o-tok-se′me-ah) toxemia produced by radiation or a radioactive substance.

radiotracer (ra″de-o-tra′ser) a radioactive tracer.

radiotransparency (ra″de-o-trans-par′en-se) radiolucency.

radiotransparent (ra″de-o-trans-par′ent) radiolucent.

radiotropic (ra″de-o-trop′ik) influenced by radiation.

radiotropism (ra″de-ot′ro-pizm) a tropism with regard to radiation.

radioulnar (ra″de-o-ul′nar) pertaining to the radius and ulna.

radisectomy (ra″de-sek′to-me) [L. radix root + Gr. ektome excision] root amputation.

radium (ra′de-um) [so called from its radiant quality] a rare radioactive element in the uranium decay series. It has an atomic weight of 226, an atomic number of 88, and a half-life of 1622 years. It is found mainly in pitchblende and undergoes spontaneous disintegration with formation of a gas called radon (half-life = 3.85 days). In this process it emits alpha particles. Radon (alpha emitter) on deposit in solid form disintegrates into a series of decay products: radium A (half-life = 3 minutes), radium B (half-life = 26.7 minutes), and radium C (half-life = 19.5 minutes). The beta particles and gamma radiations used in clinical therapy originate from radium B and C. With radium in a sealed container and the same number of atoms of each decay product disintegrating per second, radium and its decay products are in equilibrium. In this state, the formation of beta particles and gamma rays reaches its maximum. In clinical gamma-ray therapy, shielding off of the beta particles can be accomplished by a metallic container, e.g., of gold or platinum. A glass wall container permits irradiation with beta particles as well as gamma rays.

radius (ra′de-us), gen. and pl. ra′dii [L. "spoke" (of a wheel)] 1. a line segment from the center to the circumference of a circle or the surface of a sphere; the length of such a segment. 2. [NA] the bone on the outer or thumb side of the forearm, articulating proximally with the humerus and ulna and distally with the ulna and carpus; see Plate accompanying skeleton. **r. cur′vus,** Madelung's deformity. **r. fix′us,** a straight line from the hormion to the inion. **radii of lens, ra′dii len′tis** [NA], imaginary lines extending from the midpoint of the axis of the lens of the eye to the capsule of the lens. **Van der Waals r.,** the distance at which there is a balance between Van der Waals attractive and repulsive forces in the formation of chemical bonds.

radix (ra′diks), gen. rad′icis, pl. rad′ices [L.] the lowermost part, or a structure by which something is firmly attached; [NA] a general term for the lowermost part, or a part by which a structure is anchored, as the portion of a hair, nail, or tooth that is buried in the tissues, or the part of a nerve adjacent to the center to which it is connected. Called also root. **r. ante′rior nervo′rum spina′lium,** NA alternative for r. ventralis nervorum spinalium. **r. ar′cus ver′tebrae,** pediculus arcus vertebrae. **r. bre′vis gan′glii cilia′ris,** r. oculomotoria ganglii ciliaris. **r. clin′ica** [NA], clinical root: that portion of a tooth below the clinical crown, being attached to the gingiva or alveolus. **r. cochlea′ris ner′vi acus′tici,** r. inferior nervi vestibulocochlearis. **rad′ices crania′les ner′vi accesso′rii** [NA], the cranial roots of the accessory nerve. Originating from the nucleus ambiguus and emerging from the side of the medulla oblongata below the roots of the vagus nerve, they unite with the spinal portion in the jugular foramen. Their constituent fibers then form the internal branch, which joins the vagus nerve and is distributed to the soft palate, constrictors of the pharynx, and the larynx. Called also pars vagalis nervi accessorii [NA alternative]. **r. den′tis** [NA], root of tooth: the portion of a tooth which is covered by cementum, proximal to the neck of the tooth and ordinarily embedded in the dental alveolus; called also anatomical root. **r. dorsa′lis nervo′rum spina′lium** [NA], dorsal root of spinal nerves: the sensory division of each spinal nerve, attached centrally to the spinal cord and joining peripherally with the ventral (motor) root to form the nerve before it emerges through the intervertebral foramen: each dorsal root bears a spinal ganglion and conveys sensory fibers to the spinal cord. Called also r. posterior, or sensory, root of spinal nerves, r. posterior nervorum spinalium [NA alternative], and r. sensorialis nervorum spinalium. **r. facia′lis,** nervus

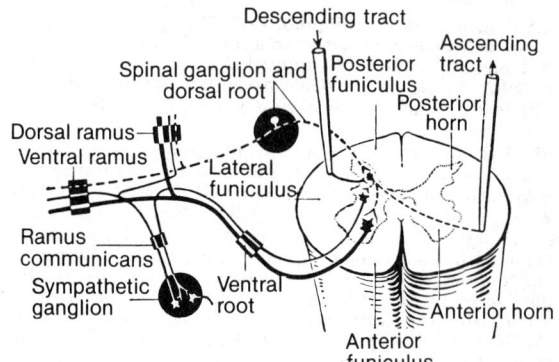

Diagram of a horizontal section of the spinal cord, with dorsal and ventral roots and a spinal nerve.

canalis pterygoidei. **r. infe′rior an′sae cervica′lis** [NA], inferior foot of ansa cervicalis: a strand of filaments connecting the ansa cervicalis with branches of the second and third cervical nerves. **r. infe′rior ner′vi vestibulocochlea′ris** [NA], inferior root of vestibulocochlear nerve: the central continuation of the pars cochlearis nervi octavi from the spiral ganglion, passing dorsal to the inferior cerebellar peduncle to enter the brain; called also r. cochlearis nervi acustici. **r. latera′lis ner′vi media′ni** [NA], lateral root of median nerve: the fibers contributed to the median nerve by the lateral cord of the brachial plexus. **r. latera′lis trac′tus op′tici** [NA], lateral root of optic tract: fibers from the optic tract that enter the lateral geniculate body. **r. lin′guae** [NA], root of tongue: the portion of the tongue posterior to the sulcus terminalis, being attached below to the hyoid bone, and directed backward as well as upward. **r. lon′ga gan′glii cilia′ris,** r. nasociliaris ganglii ciliaris. **r. media′lis ner′vi media′ni** [NA], medial root of median nerve: the fibers contributed to the median nerve by the medial cord of the brachial plexus. **r. media′lis trac′tus op′tici** [NA], medial root of optic tract: fibers from the optic tract that enter the superior colliculus and the pretectal region. **r. mesencephal′ica ner′vi trigem′ini,** tractus mesencephalicus nervi trigemini. **r. mesente′rii** [NA], root of mesentery: the line of attachment of the mesentery to the posterior abdominal wall, extending from the duodenojejunal flexure at the left of the second lumbar vertebra diagonally downward to the upper border of the right sacroiliac articulation. **rad′ices mol′les gan′glii cilia′ris,** see ramus sympathicus ad ganglion ciliare. **r. moto′ria ner′vi trigem′ini** [NA], motor root of trigeminal nerve: the smaller of the two roots by which the trigeminal nerve is attached to the side of the pons; it contains proprioceptive as well as motor fibers, and continues deep to the trigeminal ganglion to join the mandibular nerve. Called also portio minor nervi trigemini. **r. moto′ria nervo′rum spina′lium,** NA alternative for r. ventralis nervorum spinalium. **r. na′si** [NA], root of nose: the upper portion of the nose, which is attached to the frontal bone. **r. nasocilia′ris gan′glii cilia′ris** [NA], nasociliary root of ciliary ganglion: sensory fibers from the cornea, iris, ciliary body, and choroid that pass through the ciliary ganglion to the nasociliary nerve. Called also long or sensory root of ciliary ganglion, r. longa ganglii ciliaris, ramus communicans cum nervo nasociliaris, and ramus nasociliaris ganglii ciliaris [NA alternative]. **r. ner′vi facia′lis,** the root of the facial nerve, consisting of fibers passing from the nucleus of the facial nerve to the facial colliculus, and from there to the ventral surface of the lower portion of the pons. **r. oculomoto′ria gan′glii cilia′ris** [NA], oculomotor root of cilary ganglion: a short collection of fibers passing from the inferior branch of the oculomotor nerve to the posterior inferior portion of the ciliary ganglion; it contains preganglionic parasympathetic fibers for the sphincter pupillae and ciliary muscle. Called also r. brevis ganglii ciliaris, parasympathetic root of ciliary ganglion, r. parasympathetica ganglii ciliaris [NA alternative], r. parasympathica ganglii ciliaris [NA alternative], and short root of ciliary ganglion. **r. parasympathe′tica gan′glii cilia′ris, r. parasympa′thica gan′glii cilia′ris,** NA alternative for r. oculomotoria ganglii ciliaris. **rad′ices parieta′les ve′nae ca′vae inferio′ris,** vessels draining blood from the abdominal wall into the inferior vena cava, including the venae lumbales and vena phrenica inferior. **r. pe′nis** [NA], root of penis: the proximal, attached portion of the penis, consisting of the diverging crura of the corpora cavernosa and the bulb. **r. pi′li** [NA], root of hair: the proximal portion of a hair embedded in the hair follicle. **r. poste′rior, nervo′rum spina′lium,** NA alternative for r. dorsalis nervorum spinalium. **r. pulmo′nis** [NA], root of lung: the attachment of either lung, comprising the structures entering and emerging at the hilum; called also pedicle of lung and pediculus pulmonis [NA alternative]. **r. senso′ria ner′vi trigem′ini** [NA], sensory root of trigeminal nerve: the larger of the two roots by which the trigeminal nerve is attached to the side of the pons. It contains sensory fibers and expands into a large flat ganglion (the trigeminal ganglion) which gives rise to the ophthalmic, maxillary, and mandibular nerves. Called also portio major nervi trigemini. **r. senso′ria nervo′rum spina′lium,** NA alternative for r. dorsalis nervorum spinalium. **r. sensoria′lis nervo′rum spina′lium,** r. dorsalis nervorum spinalium. **rad′ices spina′les ner′vi acces-so′rii** [NA], the spinal roots of the accessory nerve. Originating from the gray matter of the spinal cord and emerging from the side of the cord as far down as a level between the third and seventh cervical nerves, they form a trunk that ascends in the vertebral canal, passes through the foramen magnum, and unites with the cranial portion in the jugular foramen. The constituent fibers then form the external branch, which supplies the sternocleidomastoid and trapezius muscles. Called also pars spinalis nervi accessorii [NA alter-

native]. **r. supe′rior an′sae cervica′lis** [NA], superior root of ansa cervicalis: fibers of the first or second cervical nerve, descending in company with the hypoglossal nerve, connecting it and the ansa cervicalis and helping supply the infrahyoid muscles. Called also ramus descendens nervi hypoglossi. **r. supe′rior ner′vi vestibulocochlea′-ris,** r. vestibularis nervi vestibulocochlearis. **r. sympa-the′tica gan′glii cilia′ris** [NA], **r. sympa′thica gan′-glii cilia′ris** [NA], sympathetic root of ciliary ganglion: postganglionic fibers from the superior cervical ganglion, derived from the internal carotid plexus, to the ciliary ganglion, for distribution by the short ciliary nerves to the dilator muscle of the pupil, orbital muscle and tarsal muscles, and blood vessels of the eyeball. Called also ramus sympathetica ganglii ciliaris [NA alternative] and ramus sympathica ganglii ciliaris [NA alternative]. **r. sympath′ica gan′glii submaxilla′ris,** ramus sympathicus ad ganglion submandibulare. **r. un′guis** [NA], root of nail: the proximal portion of the nail, situated in the sulcus of the matrix of the nail. **r. ventra′lis nervo′rum spina′lium** [NA], ventral root of spinal nerves: the motor division of each spinal nerve, attached centrally to the spinal cord and joining peripherally with the dorsal (sensory) root to form the nerve before it emerges through the intervertebral foramen. It conveys motor fibers to skeletal muscle and contains preganglionic autonomic fibers at thoracolumbar and sacral levels. Called also anterior, or motor, root of spinal nerves, r. anterior nervorum spinalium [NA alternative], and r. motoria nervorum spinalium [NA alternative]. **r. vestibula′ris ner′vi vestibulocochlea′ris** [NA], vestibular root of vestibulocochlear nerve: the central continuation of the vestibular nerve from the vestibular ganglion, entering the brain, just lateral to the intermediate nerve and in front of the inferior cerebellar peduncle. Called also r. superior nervi vestibulocochlearis and superior root of vestibulocochlear nerve. **rad′ices viscera′les ve′nae ca′vae inferio′-ris,** vessels draining blood from the viscera of the abdominal and pelvic cavities to the inferior vena cava, including the venae hepaticae, renales, and suprarenales, the vena spermatica, testicularis, and ovaricus, and the plexus pampiniformis.

radon (ra′don) a heavy, colorless, gaseous, radioactive element, symbol Rn, atomic weight 222, atomic number 86, obtained by the breaking up of radium, and used in radiotherapy. Called also radium emanation (RE). Cf. radium. ^{219}Rn is a radioactive isotope of the actinium radioactive series. ^{220}Rn is a radioactive isotope of the thorium radioactive series.

raffinose (raf′ĭ-nōs) melitose.

rafoxanide (rah-foks′ah-nīd) chemical name: N-3-chloro-4-(4-chlorophenoxy)phenyl-2-hydroxy-3,5-diiodobenzamide; an anthelmintic, $C_{19}H_{11}Cl_2I_2NO_3$.

rage (rāj) a state of violent anger. **sham r.,** an outburst of behavior in a decorticated animal, resembling that manifested in fear and anger; a similar phenomenon may be observed in man in cases of insulin hypoglycemia or carbon monoxide poisoning.

ragocyte (rag′o-sīt) [Ragg (rheumatoid serum agglutinator + -cyte] a polymorphonuclear leukocyte with cytoplasmic inclusions of ingested aggregated IgG, rheumatoid factor, fibrin, and complement, found in the joints in rheumatoid arthritis. Called also RA cell.

Rahnella (rah′nel-ah) [Otto Rahn, German-American microbiologist] a genus of gram-negative, facultatively anaerobic, rod-shaped bacteria of the family Enterobacteriaceae, occurring in fresh water and occasionally isolated from human clinical specimens. The type species is R. aqua′tilis.

raigan (ra′ĭ-gan) a native Chinese name for dried mushrooms, Omphalia lapidescens; anthelmintic.

Raillietina (ri″le-ĕ-ti′nah) a genus of tapeworms of the family Davaineidae, many species of which infect birds, domestic fowl, and mammals. R. madagascarien′sis (Taenia madagascariensis, Madagascar tapeworm), R. asiat′ica, R. formosa′na, R. demararien′sis (Taenia demarariensis), and R. loechesal′avezi have been reported from man.

raillietiniasis (ri″le-ĕ-tĭ-ni′ah-sis) infection with a parasite of the genus Raillietina.

Rainey's tube, tubule (ra′nēz) [George Rainey, English anatomist, 1801–1884] sarcocyst.

rale (rahl) [Fr. râle rattle] an abnormal respiratory sound heard in auscultation, and indicating some pathologic condition. Rales are distinguished as dry or moist, according to the absence or presence of fluid in the air passages, and are classified according to their site of origin as *bronchial, cavernous, laryngeal, pleural, tracheal,* and *vesicular* (*crepitant*). **amphoric r.,** a coarse, musical, and tinkling rale caused by the splashing of fluid in a cavity connected with a bronchus. **atelectatic r.,** a nonpathologic rale which is dissipated by deep breathing or coughing. Such rales are frequently heard in those who breathe feebly and superficially, when on deep inspiration the moist walls of the unexpanded alveoli are suddenly forced apart by the entering air; after a few deep inspirations such rales become lost. These rales are best observed at the margins or borders of the lung and are sometimes known as *marginal* or *border rales.* **border r.,** atelectatic r. **bronchial r.,** a rale produced in a bronchus. **bubbling r.,** a moist rale, finer than a subcrepitant rale, heard in bronchitis, in the resolving stage of croupous pneumonia, and over small cavities. **cavernous r.,** a hollow and metallic rale caused by the alternate expansion and contraction of a pulmonary cavity during respiration. **cellophane r.,** a dry crackling chest sound, as heard in interstitial pulmonary fibrosis. **clicking r.,** a small, sticky sound heard in inspiration, and caused by the passage of air through secretions in the smaller bronchi. **collapse r.,** a fine crepitant rale heard over collapsed lung tissue; also at the base of the healthy lung of a bedridden patient, due to incomplete expansion of the air vesicles. **consonating r.,** a clear, ringing sound produced in bronchial tubes that are surrounded by consolidation tissues. **crackling r.,** subcrepitant r. **crepitant r.,** a very fine rale, resembling the sound produced by rubbing a lock of hair between the fingers or by particles of salt thrown on fire; heard at the end of inspiration. **dry r.,** a rale produced by the presence of viscid secretion in the bronchial tubes or by spastic contraction of the walls of the tubes; it has a whistling, musical, or squeaking quality. Dry rales are heard in asthma and bronchitis. **extrathoracic r.,** a rale produced in the larynx or trachea. **gurgling r.,** a very coarse rale resembling the bursting of large bubbles; in pulmonary edema, heard over large cavities that contain fluid, and in the trachea in the "death rattle." **guttural r.,** a rale produced in the throat. **r. in'dux,** a crepitant rale heard in the stage of beginning consolidation in pneumonia. **laryngeal r.,** a rale produced in the larynx. **marginal r.,** atelectatic r. **metallic r.,** consonating r. **moist r.,** a rale produced by the presence of liquid in the bronchial tubes. **mucous r., r. muqueux,** a modified subcrepitant rale resembling the sound produced by blowing through a pipe into soapy water; it is caused by the bursting of viscid bubbles in the bronchial tubes. **pleural r.,** a pleural friction sound. **r. redux, r. de retour,** an unequal crackling sound produced by air passing through fluid in a bronchial tube; heard in the resolution stage of pneumonia. **sibilant r.,** a hissing sound resembling that produced by suddenly separating two oiled surfaces. It is produced by the presence of a viscid secretion in the bronchial tubes or by thickening of the walls of the tubes; heard in asthma and bronchitis. **sonorous r.,** a fine, moist sound resembling the cooing of a dove, produced by the passage of air through mucus in the capillary bronchial tubes; heard in capillary bronchitis and asthma. **subcrepitant r.,** a fine, moist rale heard in conditions that are associated with liquid in the smaller tubes; called also *crackling r.* **tracheal r.,** a rale produced in the trachea. **vesicular r.,** crepitant r. **whistling r.,** sibilant r.

Ralfe's test (ralfs) [Charles Henry *Ralfe,* English physician, 1842–1896] see under *tests.*

ramal (ra'mal) pertaining to a ramus; branching.

Raman effect (ram'an) [Sir Chandrasekhara Venkata *Raman,* Indian physicist, 1888–1970; winner of the Nobel prize for physics in 1930] see under *effect.*

ramaninjana (ram″an-in-jah'nah) a form of palmus, or jumping disease, prevailing in Madagascar.

R.A.M.C. Royal Army Medical Corps.

rami (ra'mi) [L.] genitive and plural of *ramus.*

Ramibacterium (ra″me-bak-te're-um) [L. *ramus* branch + *bacterium*] in former systems of classification, a genus of bacteria of the family Lactobacillaceae, made up of nonsporulating, anaerobic, gram-positive, rod-shaped organisms. These organisms are now assigned to the genus *Eubacterium.*

ramicotomy (ram″ĭ-kot'o-me) [*ramus* + Gr. *tomē* a cutting] ramisection.

ramification (ram″ĭ-fĭ-ka'shun) [*ramus* + L. *facere* to make] 1. distribution in branches. 2. a branch or set of branches. 3. the manner of branching.

ramify (ram'ĭ-fi) [*ramus* + L. *facere* to make] 1. to branch; to diverge in various directions. 2. to traverse in branches.

ramisection (ram″ĭ-sek'shun) [*ramus* + L. *sectio* a cutting] the operation of cutting the appropriate rami communicantes of the sympathetic nervous system (*sympathetic ramisection*).

ramisectomy (ram″ĭ-sek'to-me) ramisection.

ramitis (ram-i'tis) [*ramus* + *-itis* inflammation] inflammation of a ramus.

Rammstedt (rahm'stet) see *Ramstedt.*

ramollissement (rah″mol-ēs-maw') [Fr.] softening.

Ramon's flocculation, flocculation test [Gaston *Ramon,* French bacteriologist 1886–1963] see under *tests.*

Ramón y Cajal (rah-mōn e ka-hal') Santiago. Spanish physician and histologist, 1852–1934; co-winner, with Camillo Golgi, of the Nobel prize for medicine or physiology in 1906 for describing the terminal branches of neurons, developing a method of staining nerve tissues, and discovering the structure of the nervous system.

Ramond's sign (ram-onz') [Louis *Ramond,* French internist, 1879–1952] see under *sign.*

ramose (ra'mos) [L. *ramus* branch] branching; having many branches.

rampart (ram'part) a broad, encircling embankment. **maxillary r.,** a ridge or mound of epithelial cells seen in that portion of the jaw of the embryo which is to become the alveolar border.

Ramsay Hunt disease, syndrome (ram'se hunt) [James *Ramsay Hunt,* American neurologist, 1872–1937] see *dyssynergia cerebellaris progressiva;* see *juvenile paralysis agitans (of Hunt),* under *paralysis;* and see under *syndrome,* def. 1.

Ramsden's eyepiece (ramz'denz) [Jesse *Ramsden,* English instrument maker and optician, 1735–1800] see under *eyepiece.*

Ramstedt operation (rahm'stet) [Wilhelm Conrad *Ramstedt,* surgeon in Münster, 1867–1963] see *Fredet-Ramstedt operation,* under *operation.*

ramulus (ram'u-lus), pl. *ram'uli* [L., dim. of *ramus*] a small branch or terminal division.

ramus (ra'mus), gen. and pl. *ra'mi* [L.] a branch; [NA] a general term for a smaller structure given off by a larger one, or into which the larger structure, such as a blood vessel or nerve, divides. **r. acetabula'ris arte'riae circumflex'ae fem'oris media'lis** [NA], acetabular branch of medial circumflex femoral artery: a branch of the medial circumflex artery of the thigh, distributed to the head of the femur and to the acetabulum (hip joint); called also *r. acetabuli arteriae circumflexae femoris medialis.* **r. acetabula'ris arte'riae obturato'riae** [NA], acetabular branch of obturator artery: it is distributed to the hip joint; called also *arteria acetabuli.* **r. acetab'uli arte'riae circumflex'ae fem'oris media'lis,** r. acetabularis arteriae circumflexae femoris medialis. **r. acromia'lis arte'riae suprascapula'ris** [NA], acromial branch of suprascapular artery: it is distributed to the acromion process; called also *r. acromialis arteriae transversae scapulae.* **r. acromia'lis arte'riae thoracoacromia'lis** [NA], acromial branch of thoracoacromial artery: it is distributed to the deltoid muscle and acromion process. **r. acromia'lis arte'riae transver'sae scap'ulae,** r. acromialis arteriae suprascapularis. **ra'mi alveola'res superio'res anterio'res ner'vi infraorbita'lis** [NA], anterior superior alveolar branches of infraorbital nerve: branches from the infraorbital nerve that innervate the incisor and canine teeth of the upper jaw, help form the superior dental plexus, and give terminal twigs to the floor of the nose; modality, general sensory. **r. alveola'ris supe'rior me'dius ner'vi infraorbita'lis** [NA], middle superior alveolar branch of infraorbital nerve: a branch from the infraorbital nerve that innervates the premolar teeth of the upper jaw by way of the superior dental plexus; modality, general sensory. **ra'mi alveola'res superio'res posterio'res ner'vi maxilla'ris** [NA], posterior superior alveolar branches of maxillary nerve: they innervate the maxillary sinus, cheek, gums, and molar and premolar teeth of the upper jaw; they form part of the superior dental plexus; modality, general sensory. **r.**

anastomot′icus, a structure connecting one nerve to another; see terms beginning *r. communicans.* **r. anastomo′ticus arte′riae lacrima′lis cum arte′ria menin′gea me′dia** [NA], a branch of the lacrimal artery that anastomoses with the meningeal artery. **r. anastomot′icus arte′riae menin′geae me′diae cum arte′ria lacrima′li** [NA], a branch of the middle meningeal artery that is distributed to the orbit and anastomoses with the recurrent meningeal branch of the lacrimal artery. **r. ante′rior arte′riae obturato′riae** [NA], anterior branch of obturator artery: it passes forward around the medial margin of the obturator foramen, on the obturator membrane, and is distributed to the obturator and adductor muscles. **r. ante′rior arte′riae pancreaticoduodena′lis inferio′ris** [NA], anterior branch of inferior pancreaticoduodenal artery: a branch that passes in front of the head of the pancreas and then ascends to anastomose with the anterior superior pancreaticoduodenal artery; it supplies the head of the pancreas and adjoining parts of the duodenum. **r. ante′rior arte′riae recurren′tis ulna′ris** [NA], anterior branch of ulnar recurrent artery: it helps supply the pronator teres and brachialis muscles and runs to the front of the medial epicondyle, supplying the elbow joint and adjacent structures. **r. ante′rior arte′riae rena′lis** [NA], the anterior branch of the renal artery, supplying the anterior, superior, and inferior segments of the kidney. **r. ante′rior arte′riae thyroi′deae superio′ris** [NA], anterior branch of superior thyroid artery: it helps supply the upper part of the gland, anastomosing with its fellow of the opposite side along the upper border of the isthmus. **r. ante′rior ascen′dens fissu′rae cer′ebri latera′lis [Syl′vii],** r. ascendens sulci lateralis cerebri. **r. ante′rior duc′tus hepat′ici dex′tri** [NA], the anterior branch of the right hepatic duct. **r. ante′rior horizonta′lis fissu′rae cer′ebri latera′lis [Syl′vii],** r. anterior sulci lateralis cerebri. **r. ante′rior ner′vi auricula′ris mag′ni** [NA], anterior branch of great auricular nerve; it is distributed to the skin of the face over the parotid gland; modality, general sensory. **ra′mi anterio′res nervo′rum cervica′lium,** rami ventrales nervorum cervicalium. **r. ante′rior ner′vi coccyg′ei,** r. ventralis nervi coccygei. **r. ante′rior ner′vi cuta′nei antebrach′ii media′lis** [NA], anterior branch of medial cutaneous nerve of forearm; it innervates the skin of the front and medial aspect of the forearm; modality, general sensory; called also *r. volaris nervi cutanei antibrachii medialis.* **r. ante′rior ner′vi laryn′gei inferio′ris,** anterior branch of inferior laryngeal nerve. **ra′mi anterio′res nervo′rum lumba′lium,** rami ventrales nervorum lumbalium. **r. ante′rior ner′vi obturato′rii** [NA], anterior branch of obturator nerve; it supplies the gracilis and the adductor longus and brevis muscles and the pectineus, and occasionally gives off a branch to the skin of the medial side of the thigh and leg; modality, motor and general sensory. **ra′mi anterio′res nervo′rum sacra′lium,** rami ventrales nervorum sacralium. **r. ante′rior nervo′rum spina′lium,** NA alternative for *r. ventralis nervorum spinalium.* **ra′mi anterio′res nervo′rum thoraca′lium,** rami ventrales nervorum thoracicorum. **r. ante′rior ramo′rum cutaneo′rum latera′lium [pectora′lium et abdomina′lium] arterio′rum intercosta′lium,** the anterior branch of the lateral cutaneous branches of the intercostal arteries. **r. ante′rior ramo′rum cutaneo′rum latera′lium [pectora′lium et abdomina′lium] nervo′rum intercosta′lium,** the anterior branch of the lateral cutaneous branches of the intercostal nerve. **r. ante′rior sul′ci latera′lis cer′ebri** [NA], anterior branch of lateral cerebral sulcus; it runs forward a short distance into the inferior frontal gyrus; called also *r. anterior horizontalis fissurae cerebri lateralis [Sylvii].* **ra′mi arterio′si interlobula′res hep′atis,** arteriae interlobulares hepatis. **ra′mi articula′res arte′riae descen′dentis genicula′ris** [NA], articular branches of descending genicular artery: they pass downward in the vastus medialis muscle and help supply the knee joint. Called also *rami articulares arteriae genus descendentis.* **ra′mi articula′res arte′riae ge′nus descenden′tis,** rami articularis arteriae descendentis genicularis. **r. ascen′dens arte′riae circumflex′ae fem′oris latera′lis** [NA], ascending branch of lateral circumflex femoral artery: it runs upward along the trochanteric line of the femur and between the gluteus medius and minimus muscles, and

anastomoses with branches of the superior gluteal artery. It helps supply the upper thigh muscles. **r. ascen′dens arte′riae circumflex′ae fem′oris media′lis** [NA], ascending branch of medial circumflex femoral artery: it ascends in front of the quadratus femoris muscle to the trochanteric fossa, and there anastomoses with gluteal arteries. **r. ascen′dens arte′riae circumflex′ae il′ium profun′dae** [NA], ascending branch of deep circumflex iliac artery: a branch leaving the deep circumflex iliac artery near the anterior superior iliac spine, rising between and distributing to the transversus abdominis and internal oblique muscles. **r. ascen′dens arte′riae transver′sae col′li,** r. superficialis arteriae transversae cervicis. **r. ascen′dens ra′mi superficia′lis arte′riae transver′sae cer′vicis** [NA], the ascending branch of the superficial branch of the transverse cervical artery. **r. ascen′dens sul′ci latera′lis cer′ebri** [NA], ascending branch of lateral cerebral sulcus: it runs superiorly a short distance into the inferior frontal gyrus; called also *r. anterior ascendens fissurae cerebri lateralis [Sylvii].* **r. atria′lis anastomo′ticus arte′riae corona′riae sinis′trae** [NA], a branch of the circumflex branch of the left coronary artery that passes the interatrial septum to anastomose with the right coronary artery; called also *atrial anastomotic artery* and *anastomotic atrial artery.* **ra′mi atria′les arte′riae corona′riae dex′trae** [NA], branches of the right coronary artery, consisting of anterior and lateral branches chiefly distributed to the right atrium, and usually a single posterior branch distributed to the right and left atria. **ra′mi atria′les arte′riae corona′riae sinis′trae** [NA], branches of the left circumflex branch of the left coronary artery, consisting of anterior, lateral, and posterior groups of vessels distributed to the left atrium. **r. atria′lis interme′dius arte′riae corona′riae dex′trae** [NA], a branch of the right coronary artery arising opposite to the marginal branch and ascending to over the right atrium; called also *right intermediate atrial artery.* **r. atria′lis interme′dius ra′mi circumflex′i arte′riae corona′riae sinis′tri** [NA], a branch of the circumflex branch of the left coronary artery that distributes along the left atrium above the coronary sulcus; called also *left intermediate atrial artery.* **ra′mi atrioventricula′res arte′riae corona′riae sinis′trae** [NA], small recurrent branches of the circumflex branch of the left coronary artery distributed to the atria and ventricles. **ra′mi auricula′res anterio′res arte′riae tempora′lis superficia′lis** [NA], anterior auricular branches of superficial temporal artery: they supply the lateral aspect of the pinna and the external acoustic meatus. **r. auricula′ris arte′riae auricula′ris posterio′ris** [NA], auricular branch of posterior auricular artery: a branch supplying the pinna and adjacent skin. **r. auricula′ris arte′riae occipita′lis** [NA], auricular branch of occipital artery: an inconstant branch of the occipital artery that helps supply the medial aspect of the pinna. **r. auricula′ris ner′vi va′gi** [NA], auricular branch of vagus nerve: a branch arising from the superior ganglion of the vagus, innervating the cranial surface of the auricle, the floor of the external acoustic meatus, and the adjacent part of the tympanic membrane; modality, general sensory. **r. basa′lis tento′rii arte′riae caro′tidis inter′nae** [NA], a twig from the cavernous part of the internal carotid artery that supplies the base of the tentorium; called also *r. tentorii basalis arteriae carotidis internae.* **ra′mi bronchia′les anterio′res ner′vi va′gi,** see *rami bronchiales nervi vagi.* **ra′mi bronchia′les aor′tae thora′cicae** [NA], bronchial branches of thoracic aorta: branches arising from the thoracic aorta to supply the bronchi and lower trachea, and passing along the posterior sides of the bronchi to ramify about the respiratory bronchioles; distributed also to adjacent lymph nodes, pulmonary vessels, and pericardium, and to part of the esophagus. Called also *arteriae bronchiales* or *bronchial arteries.* **ra′mi bronchia′les arte′riae mamma′riae inter′nae,** rami bronchiales arteriae thoracicae internae. **ra′mi bronchia′les arte′riae thora′cicae inter′nae** [NA], bronchial branches of internal thoracic artery: small, variable branches of the internal thoracic artery, with distribution to the bronchi and trachea; called also *rami bronchiales arteriae mammariae internae.* **ra′mi bronchia′les bron′chi,** a name applied to the first, extrapulmonary divisions of the main bronchi, the eparterial and hyparterial bronchial rami. **r. bronchia′lis eparteria′lis,** a name given to the superior lobar bronchus on the right, which arises above the level of the pulmonary artery; called also *eparterial bronchus*. **r. bronchia′les hyparteria′les,** a name given to the middle and inferior lobar bronchi on the right and the lobar bronchi on the left, all of which arise below the level of the pulmonary artery; called also *hyparterial bronchi*. **ra′mi bronchia′les ner′vi va′gi** [NA], branches of the vagus that supply the bronchi and the pulmonary vessels, both directly and by way of the anterior and posterior parts of the pulmonary plexus; modality, parasympathetic and visceral afferent. **ra′mi bronchia′les posterio′res ner′vi va′gi,** see *rami bronchiales nervi vagi*. **ra′mi bronchia′les pulmo′nis,** a name given to intrapulmonary bronchial divisions smaller than the main bronchi and larger than the bronchioles; in NA, they are classified as lobar and segmental bronchi, and branches (rami) of the latter. **ra′mi bronchia′les segmento′rum** [NA], intrasegmental bronchial branches: smaller branches arising from the segmental bronchi. **ra′mi bucca′les ner′vi facia′lis** [NA], buccal branches of facial nerve: they innervate the zygomatic, levator labii superioris, buccinator, and orbicularis oris muscles; modality, motor and general sensory. **ra′mi calca′nei latera′les ner′vi sura′lis** [NA], lateral calcaneal branches of sural nerve: they innervate the skin on the back of the leg and the lateral side of the foot and heel; modality, general sensory. **ra′mi calca′nei media′les arte′riae perone′ae,** rami calcanei ramorum malleolarium medialium arteriae tibialis posterioris. **ra′mi calca′nei media′les ner′vi tibia′lis** [NA], medial calcaneal branches of tibial nerve: branches supplying the medial side of the heel and of the posterior part of the sole; modality, general sensory. **ra′mi calca′nei ramo′rum malleola′rium latera′lium arte′riae fibula′ris** [NA], calcaneal branches of lateral malleolar branches of fibular artery: they are distributed to the lateral aspect and back of the heel; called also *rami calcanei ramorum malleolarium lateralium arteriae peroneae* [NA alternative]. **ra′mi calca′nei ramo′rum malleola′rium latera′lium arte′riae perone′ae,** NA alternative for *rami calcanei ramorum malleolarium lateralium arteriae fibularis*. **ra′mi calca′nei ramo′rum malleola′rium media′lium arte′riae tibia′lis posterio′ris** [NA], calcaneal branches of medial malleolar branches of posterior tibial artery: branches that arise from the medial malleolar branches of the posterior tibial artery and are distributed to the medial aspect and back of the heel; called also *rami calcanei mediales arteriae peroneae*. **r. calcari′nus arte′riae occipita′lis media′lis** [NA], a branch of the middle occipital artery that supplies the calcarine fissure. **ra′mi cap′sulae inter′nae** [NA], small branches of the anterior choroidal artery that supply the internal capsule. **ra′mi capsula′res arte′riae re′nis** [NA], capsular branches of renal artery: they supply the renal capsule. **ra′mi cardi′aci cervica′les inferio′res ner′vi va′gi** [NA], inferior cardiac branches of the vagus nerve: branches (sometimes called cervicothoracic) arising from the vagi and from the recurrent laryngeal nerves at the thoracic inlet, and joining cervicothoracic sympathetic cardiac nerves, the combined nerves passing to the cardiac plexus; modality, parasympathetic and visceral afferent. Called also *inferior cardiac branches of recurrent laryngeal nerve*. **ra′mi cardi′aci cervica′les superio′res ner′vi va′gi** [NA], superior cervical cardiac branches of vagus nerve: variable branches arising from the vagus in the cervical region and usually joining the cervical sympathetic cardiac nerves. The conjoined nerves then descend in front of, or behind, the arch of the aorta to the cardiac plexus; modality, parasympathetic and visceral afferent. **ra′mi cardi′aci inferio′res ner′vi recurren′tis,** r. cardiaci cervicales inferiores nervi vagi. **ra′mi cardi′aci thora′cici ner′vi va′gi** [NA], thoracic cardiac branches of the vagus nerve: branches which arise in the thorax from the right and left vagus and left recurrent laryngeal nerves. They go directly to the posterior walls of the atria, to the coronary plexuses, and to the anterior pulmonary plexuses. **ra′mi caroticotympan′ici arte′riae carot′idis inter′nae,** arteriae caroticotympanicae. **r. carpa′lis dorsa′lis arte′riae radia′lis** [NA], **r. car′peus dorsa′lis arte′riae radia′lis,** dorsal carpal branch of radial artery: it runs medially deep to the extensor tendons, and helps form the dorsal carpal rete. **r. carpa′lis dorsa′lis arte′riae ulna′ris** [NA], **r. car′peus dorsa′lis arte′riae ulna′ris,** dorsal carpal branch of ul-

nar artery: a variable branch of the ulnar artery that runs laterally deep to the tendons of the ulnar muscles of the wrist, helping to form the dorsal carpal rete. **r. carpa′lis palma′ris arte′riae radia′lis** [NA], **r. car′peus palma′ris arte′riae radia′lis,** palmar carpal branch of radial artery: a branch that passes medially behind the flexor tendons on the palmar aspect of the wrist and forms a network with a corresponding branch of the ulnar artery. **r. carpa′lis palma′ris arte′riae ulna′ris** [NA], **r. car′peus palma′ris arte′riae ulna′ris,** palmar carpal branch of ulnar artery: a branch that passes laterally behind the flexor tendons on the palmar aspect of the wrist and forms a network with a corresponding branch of the radial artery. **ra′mi cau′dae nuc′lei cauda′ti** [NA], small branches of the anterior choroidal artery that supply the tail of the caudate nucleus. **r. cau′dae nu′clei cauda′ti arte′riae posterio′ris** [NA], a branch of the posterior communicating artery that supplies the tail of the caudate nucleus. **ra′mi cauda′ti** [NA], the caudate branches of the transverse part of the left branch of the portal vein. **ra′mi celi′aci ner′vi va′gi,** rami coeliaci nervi vagi. **ra′mi centra′les anteromedia′les arte′riae cer′ebri anterio′ris,** the anteromedial central branches of the precommunical part of the anterior cerebral artery. **r. chiasma′ticus arte′riae communican′tis posterio′ris** [NA], a branch of the posterior communicating artery that supplies the optic chiasm. **ra′mi choroi′dei media′les arte′riae cer′ebri posterio′ris** [NA], the medial choroid branches of the posterior cerebral artery that supply the choroid plexuses of the third ventricle. **ra′mi choroi′dei posterio′res latera′les arte′riae cer′ebri posterio′ris** [NA], the lateral choroid branches of the posterior cerebral artery that supply the lateral ventricle. **r. cingula′ris arte′riae callosomargina′lis** [NA], the cingular branch of the callosomarginal branch (artery) of the anterior cerebral artery. **r. circumflex′us arte′riae corona′riae sinis′trae** [NA], circumflex branch of left coronary artery: it curves around to the back of the left ventricle in the coronary sulcus, supplying the left ventricle and left atrium. **r. circumflex′us fib′ulae arte′riae tibia′lis posterio′ris,** r. circumflexus fibularis arteriae tibialis posterioris. **r. circumflex′us fibula′ris arte′riae tibia′lis posterio′ris** [NA], fibular circumflex branch of posterior tibial artery: it winds laterally around the neck of the fibula, helping supply the soleus muscle and contributing to the anastomosis around the knee joint; called also *r. circumflexus fibulae arteriae tibialis posterioris*. **r. clavicula′ris arte′riae thoracoacromia′lis** [NA], clavicular branch of thoracoacromial artery: a vessel that passes medially to supply the subclavius muscle. **r. cli′vi** [NA], a twig from the cerebral part of the internal carotid artery that supplies the clivus. **r. coch′leae arte′riae auditi′vae inter′nae,** r. cochleae arteriae labyrinthi. **r. cochlea′ris arte′riae labyrin′thi** [NA], cochlear branch of labyrinthine artery: it supplies the cochlea. **ra′mi coeli′aci ner′vi va′gi** [NA], celiac branches of vagus nerve: branches that arise from both the anterior and posterior vagal trunks and join the celiac plexus; modality, parasympathetic and visceral afferent. Called also *celiac nerves* and *rami celiaci nervi vagi* [NA alternative]. **r. co′licus arte′riae ileoco′licae** [NA], colic branch of ileocolic artery; a branch that passes upward on the ascending colon and anastomoses with the right colic artery; called also *arteria ascendens ileocolica* and *ascending ileocolic artery*. **r. collatera′lis arteria′rum intercosta′lium posterio′rum** [NA], collateral branch of posterior intercostal arteries: a branch helping supply the thoracic wall, arising from the posterior intercostal arteries near the angle of the rib and running forward in the lower part of the corresponding intercostal space. **r. col′li ner′vi facia′lis** [NA], cervical branch of facial nerve: it lies deep to and innervates the platysma muscle; modality, motor. **r. commu′nicans,** 1. [NA] a communicating branch between two nerves. 2. a branch connecting two arteries. **r. commu′nicans al′bus** [NA], any of the whitish, predominantly myelinated preganglionic nerve fibers that run from the sympathetic ganglia to dorsal and ventral roots of a spinal nerve. **r. commu′nicans arte′riae fibula′ris** [NA], communicating branch of fibular artery: a communicating branch between the fibular and the posterior tibial arteries, distributed to the interosseous membrane and supramalleolar region. Called also *r. communicans arteriae peroneae* [NA alternative]. **r. commu′nicans arte′riae perone′ae,**

NA alternative for *r. communicans arteriae fibularis*. **r. commu′nicans co′chlearis** [NA], a branch of the vestibular nerve that unites with the cochlear nerve. **r. commu′nicans fibula′ris ner′vi fibula′ris commu′nis** [NA], communicating branch of common fibular nerve: a small branch arising from the common fibular nerve, either with the lateral cutaneous sural nerve or separately; distally it joins the medial sural cutaneous nerve to form the sural nerve. Called also *r. communicans peroneus nervi peronei communis* [NA alternative]. **r. commu′nicans gan′glii cilia′ris cum ner′vo nasocilia′ri** [NA], communicating branch of ciliary ganglion with nasociliary nerve: a branch or branches carrying sensory fibers from the cornea, iris, ciliary body, and choroid, and passing through the ciliary ganglion to the nasociliary nerve. Called also *sensory root of ciliary ganglion*. **r. commu′nicans gan′glii o′tici cum chor′da tym′pani** [NA], communicating branch of otic ganglion with chorda tympani: a small branch that interconnects the otic ganglion and the chorda tympani. **r. commu′nicans gan′glii o′tici cum ner′vo auriculotempora′li** [NA], communicating branch of otic ganglion with auriculotemporal nerve: a branch carrying postganglionic parasympathetic fibers from the otic ganglion to the auriculotemporal nerve for distribution to the parotid gland. **r. commu′nicans gan′glii o′tici cum ner′vo pterygoi′deo media′li** [NA], communicating branch of otic ganglion with medial pteryoid nerve: a branch of the medial pterygoid nerve that communicates with the otic ganglion. **r. commu′nicans gan′glii o′tici cum ra′mo menin′geo ner′vi mandibula′ris** [NA], communicating branch of otic ganglion with meningeal branch of mandibular nerve: a branch that carries autonomic fibers destined for the meninges from the otic ganglion to the meningeal branch of the mandibular nerve. **ra′mi communican′tes gan′glii submandibula′ris cum ner′vo lingua′li** [NA], communicating branches of submandibular ganglion with lingual nerve: branches which interconnect the lingual nerve and the submandibular ganglion, and by which the ganglion is suspended from the nerve; they carry preganglionic fibers that derive from the chorda tympani and synapse in the submandibular ganglion, and postganglionic fibers. Called also *motor root(s) of submandibular ganglion*. **r. commu′nicans gri′seus** [NA], any of the grayish, predominantly unmyelinated postganglionic nerve fibers that run from the sympathetic ganglia as visceral efferent fibers to supply the blood vessels, sweat glands, and smooth muscles. **ra′mi communican′tes ner′vi auriculotempora′lis cum ner′vo facia′li** [NA], communicating branches of auriculotemporal nerve with facial nerve: branches containing sensory fibers from the auriculotemporal nerve that join the facial nerve within the parotid gland, to be distributed with branches of the latter. **r. commu′nicans ner′vi facia′lis cum ner′vo glossopharyn′geo** [NA], communicating branch of facial nerve with glossopharyngeal nerve: a branch that interconnects the glossopharyngeal nerve and the facial nerve after emergence of the latter from the stylomastoid foramen. **r. commu′nicans ner′vi facia′lis cum plex′u tympan′ico** [NA], communicating branch of facial nerve with tympanic plexus: a branch that interconnects the facial nerve and the tympanic plexus of the glossopharyngeal nerve. **r. commu′nicans ner′vi glossopharyn′gei cum ra′mo auricula′ri ner′vi va′gi** [NA], communicating branch of glossopharyngeal nerve with auricular branch of vagus nerve: a small branch connecting the glossopharyngeal nerve with the auricular branch of the vagus nerve. **r. commu′nicans ner′vi interme′dii cum ner′vo va′go** [NA], a branch of the intermediate nerve that communicates with the vagus nerve. **r. commu′nicans ner′vi interme′dii cum plex′u tympan′ico** [NA], a branch of the intermediate nerve that communicates with the tympanic plexus. **r. commu′nicans ner′vi lacrima′lis cum ner′vo zygomat′ico** [NA], communicating branch of lacrimal nerve with zygomatic nerve: a branch that carries parasympathetic postganglionic fibers originating in the pterygopalatine ganglion and destined for the lacrimal gland. **r. commu′nicans ner′vi laryn′gei inferio′ris cum ra′mo laryn′geo inter′no** [NA], communicating branch of inferior laryngeal nerve with internal laryngeal branch: a small branch interconnecting the inferior laryngeal nerve with the internal branch of the superior laryngeal nerve, behind or in the posterior cricoarytenoid muscle. **r. commu′nicans**

ner′vi laryn′gei superio′ris cum ner′vo laryn′geo inferio′re [NA], communicating branch of superior laryngeal nerve with inferior laryngeal nerve: a small branch interconnecting the internal branch of the superior laryngeal nerve with the inferior laryngeal nerve, behind or in the posterior cricoarytenoid muscle. **r. commu′nicans ner′vi lingua′lis cum chor′da tym′pani** [NA], communicating branch of lingual nerve with chorda tympani: the chorda tympani as it joins the lingual nerve in the infratemporal fossa medial to the lateral pterygoid muscle; modality, parasympathetic and special sensory. **ra′mi communican′tes ner′vi lingua′lis cum ner′vo hypoglos′so** [NA], communicating branches of lingual nerve with hypoglossal nerve: plexiform terminal branches interconnecting the lingual and hypoglossal nerves just in front of the hyoglossus muscle. **r. commu′nicans ner′vi media′ni cum ner′vo ulna′ri** [NA], communicating branch of median nerve with ulnar nerve: a small branch across the flexor digitorum profundus muscle, connecting the median with the ulnar nerve. **r. commu′nicans cum ner′vo nasocilia′ri,** radix nasociliaris ganglii ciliaris. **r. commu′nicans ner′vi nasocilia′ris cum ganglio′ne cilia′ri** [NA], communicating branch of nasociliary nerve with ciliary ganglion: a branch or branches carrying sensory fibers from the cornea, iris, ciliary body, and choroid, and passing through the ciliary ganglion to the nasociliary nerve. **ra′mi communican′tes nervo′rum spina′lium** [NA], communicating branches of spinal nerves: branches connecting spinal nerves with sympathetic ganglia, each spinal nerve receiving a gray communicating ramus, and the thoracic and upper lumbar spinal nerves having in addition a white communicating ramus. **r. commu′nicans ner′vi va′gi cum ner′vo glossopharyn′geo** [NA], communicating branch of vagus nerve with glossopharyngeal nerve: a small branch connecting the auricular branch of the vagus nerve with the glossopharyngeal nerve. **r. commu′nicans pero′neus ner′vi perone′i commu′nis,** r. communicans fibularis nervi fibularis communis. **r. commu′nicans ulna′ris ner′vi radia′lis** [NA], ulnar communicating branch of radial nerve: a small branch in the hand that interconnects the most medial dorsal digital nerve from the superficial branch of the radial nerve with the adjacent most lateral dorsal digital nerve from the dorsal branch of the ulnar nerve. **r. co′ni arterio′si arte′riae corona′riae dex′trae** [NA], the first ventricular branch of the right coronary artery, which supplies the conus arteriosus, and anastomoses with the left conus artery (branch) of the anterior interventricular branch of the left coronary artery; called also *conal* or *conus artery, right conus artery,* and *third coronary artery.* **r. co′ni arterio′si arte′riae corona′riae sinis′trae** [NA], a small branch of the anterior interventricular branch of the left coronary artery, which supplies the conus arteriosus, and anastomoses with the right conus artery (branch) of the right coronary artery; called also *conal* or *conus artery* and *left conus artery.* **ra′mi cor′poris amygdaloi′dei** [NA], small branches of the anterior choroidal artery that supply the amygdaloid body. **r. cor′poris callo′si dorsa′lis arte′riae occipita′lis media′lis** [NA], a branch of the middle occipital artery that supplies the dorsum of the corpus callosum. **ra′mi cor′poris genicula′ti latera′lis** [NA], small branches of the anterior choroidal artery that supply the lateral geniculate body. **r. costa′lis latera′lis arte′riae mamma′riae inter′nae,** r. costalis lateralis arteriae thoracicae internae. **r. costa′lis latera′lis arte′riae thora′cicae inter′nae** [NA], lateral costal branch of internal thoracic artery: an occasional branch passing inferolaterally behind the ribs, supplying ribs and costal cartilages, and anastomosing with the posterior intercostal arteries. **r. cricothyroi′deus arte′riae thyroi′deae superio′ris** [NA], cricothyroid branch of superior thyroid artery: a vessel running medially over the cricothyroid muscle, toward the cricothyroid ligament, and anastomosing with its fellow of the opposite side. **ra′mi cuta′nei anterio′res ner′vi femora′lis** [NA], anterior cutaneous branches of femoral nerve: they innervate the skin on the front and medial aspect of the thigh and patella and contribute to the subsartorial and patellar plexuses; modality, general sensory. **r. cuta′neus ante′rior ner′vi iliohypogas′trici** [NA], anterior cutaneous branch of iliohypogastric nerve: it runs forward between the internal and external oblique muscles and innervates the skin over the pubis; modality, general sensory. **r. cuta′neus an-**

te′rior [pectora′lis/abdomina′lis] nervo′rum intercosta′lium, NA alternative for *r. cutaneus anterior [pectoralis/abdominalis] ramorum ventralium nervorum thoracicorum.* **r. cuta′neus ante′rior [pectora′lis/abdomina′lis] ramo′rum ventra′lium nervo′rum thoracico′rum** [NA], anterior cutaneous branch (pectoral and abdominal) of ventral branches of thoracic nerves: they help innervate the skin in the anteromedial thoracic and abdominal regions, with medial mammary branches given off in the breast region; modality, general sensory. Called also *r. cutaneus anterior [pectoralis/abdominalis] nervorum intercostalium* [NA alternative]. **ra′mi cuta′nei cru′ris media′les ner′vi saphe′ni** [NA], medial crural cutaneous branches of saphenous nerve: branches distributed by the saphenous nerve to the skin of the medial aspect of the leg; modality, general sensory. **r. cuta′neus latera′lis arteria′rum intercosta′lium posterio′rum** [NA], lateral cutaneous branch of posterior intercostal arteries: a branch arising from the posterior intercostal arteries, supplying the anterolateral thoracic wall. The branches of the third through fifth give off small mammary branches. **r. cuta′neus latera′lis ner′vi iliohypogas′trici** [NA], lateral cutaneous branch of iliohypogastric nerve: it is distributed to the skin over the side of the buttock; modality, general sensory. **r. cuta′neus latera′lis [pectora′lis/abdomina′lis] nervo′rum intercosta′lium,** NA alternative for *r. cutaneus lateralis [pectoralis/abdominalis] ramorum ventralium nervorum thoracicorum.* **r. cuta′neus latera′lis [pectora′lis/abdomina′lis] ramo′rum ventra′lium nervo′rum thoracico′rum** [NA], lateral cutaneous branch (pectoral and abdominal) of any of the ventral branches of thoracic nerve (intercostal nerves): the lateral branches divide further into anterior and posterior branches to innervate the skin of the lateral and posterior body wall; modality, general sensory. Those of the fourth through sixth intercostal nerves give off lateral mammary branches. Called also *r. cutaneus lateralis [pectoralis/abdominalis] nervorum intercostalium* [NA alternative]. **r. cuta′neus latera′lis ra′mi dorsa′lis arteria′rum intercosta′lium posterio′rum** [NA], lateral cutaneous branch of dorsal branch of posterior intercostal arteries: it supplies the posterolateral aspect of the thorax. The branches of the third through fifth arteries give off small mammary branches. **r. cuta′neus latera′lis ramo′rum dorsa′lium nervo′rum thoracico′rum** [NA], lateral cutaneous branch of dorsal branches of thoracic nerves: the lateral of the two terminal divisions of the dorsal branch of each thoracic nerve; each supplies first the corresponding levator costae muscle, then the longissimus thoracis and iliocostalis thoracis muscles; the lower ones pierce the latissimus dorsi and supply the skin of the back. Called also *r. cutaneus lateralis ramorum posteriorum nervorum thoracalium.* **r. cuta′neus latera′lis ramo′rum posterio′rum nervo′rum thoraca′lium,** r. cutaneus lateralis ramorum dorsalium nervorum thoracicorum. **r. cuta′neus media′lis ra′mi dorsa′lis arteria′rum intercosta′lium posterio′rum** [NA], medial cutaneous branch of dorsal branch of posterior intercostal arteries: it supplies the skin adjacent to the vertebral column. **r. cuta′neus media′lis ramo′rum dorsa′lium nervo′rum thoracico′rum** [NA], medial cutaneous branch of dorsal branches of thoracic nerves: the medial of the two terminal divisions of the dorsal branch of a thoracic nerve; those of the upper nerves supplying the skin of the back, and those of the lower ones chiefly supplying the erector spinae muscle. Both groups supply adjacent periosteum, ligaments, and joints. Called also *r. cutaneus medialis ramorum posteriorum nervorum thoracalium.* **r. cuta′neus media′lis ramo′rum posterio′rum nervo′rum thoraca′lium,** r. cutaneus medialis ramorum dorsalium nervorum thoracicorum. **r. cuta′neus ner′vi obturato′rii** [NA], cutaneous branch of obturator nerve: a variable branch arising from the anterior branch of the obturator nerve, forming part of the subsartorial plexus, and supplying the skin of the medial aspect of the thigh and leg; modality, general sensory. **r. cuta′neus palma′ris ner′vi ulna′ris,** r. palmaris nervi ulnaris. **r. deltoi′deus arte′riae profun′dae bra′chii** [NA], deltoid branch of deep brachial artery: it is distributed to the brachialis and deltoid muscles and anastomoses with the posterior circumflex humeral artery; called also *deltoid artery.* **r. deltoi′deus arte′riae thoracoacromia′lis** [NA], deltoid branch of thoracoacromial artery: a branch of the thoracoacromial artery descend-

ing with the cephalic vein and helping to supply the deltoid and pectoralis major muscles. **ra′mi denta′les arte′riae alveola′ris inferio′ris** [NA], dental branches of inferior alveolar artery: branches arising from the inferior alveolar artery in the mandibular canal and supplying the inferior teeth. **ra′mi denta′les arteria′rum alveola′rium superio′rum anterio′rum** [NA], dental branches of anterior superior alveolar arteries: they supply the incisor and canine teeth. **ra′mi denta′les arte′riae alveola′ris superio′ris posterio′ris** [NA], dental branches of posterior superior alveolar artery: they supply the molar and premolar teeth. **ra′mi denta′les inferio′res plex′us denta′lis inferio′ris** [NA], inferior dental branches of inferior dental plexus: they supply the lower teeth; modality, general sensory. **ra′mi denta′les superio′res plex′us denta′lis superio′ris** [NA], superior dental branches of superior dental plexus: they innervate the teeth of the upper jaw; modality, general sensory. **r. descen′dens ante′rior arte′riae corona′riae [cor′dis] sinis′trae,** r. interventricularis anterior arteriae coronariae sinistrae. **r. descen′dens arte′riae circumflex′ae fem′oris latera′lis** [NA], descending branch of lateral circumflex femoral artery: a branch passing from the lateral circumflex artery (sometimes directly from the deep femoral) to the knee, and supplying the thigh muscles. **r. descen′dens arte′riae occipita′lis** [NA], descending branch of occipital artery: a branch that arises from the occipital artery on the obliquus capitis superior muscle and divides into superficial and deep branches, supplying the trapezius and deep neck muscles. **r. descen′dens ner′vi hypoglos′si,** radix superior ansae cervicalis. **r. descen′dens poste′rior arte′riae corona′riae [cor′dis] dex′trae,** r. interventricularis posterior arteriae coronariae dextrae. **r. descen′dens ra′mi superficia′lis arte′riae transver′sae cer′vicis** [NA], the descending branch of the superficial branch of the transverse cervical artery. **r. dex′ter arte′riae hepat′icae pro′priae** [NA], right branch of proper hepatic artery: the right of the two branches into which the proper hepatic artery normally divides; it supplies the right lobe of the liver and a branch, the cystic artery, to the gallbladder. **r. dex′ter arte′riae pulmona′lis,** arteria pulmonalis dextra. **r. dex′ter ve′nae por′tae hep′atis** [NA], the right branch of the portal vein of the liver, distributed to the right lobe of the liver. **r. digas′tricus ner′vi facia′lis** [NA], digastric branch of facial nerve: a branch that innervates the posterior belly of the digastric muscle; modality, motor; called also *digastric nerve.* **r. dorsa′lis arteria′rum intercosta′lium posterio′rum** [NA], dorsal branch of posterior intercostal arteries: a branch arising from a posterior intercostal artery, passing backward with the dorsal branch of the corresponding intercostal nerve to supply the posterior thoracic wall; it has a spinal branch and a medial and a lateral cutaneous branch. **ra′mi dorsa′les arte′riae intercosta′lis supre′mae** [NA], dorsal branches of highest intercostal artery: the dorsal branches arising from the first and second posterior intercostal arteries, which stem from the highest intercostal artery. Their distribution is similar to that of the other posterior intercostals; see *ramus dorsalis arteriarum intercostalium posteriorum.* **r. dorsa′lis arteria′rum lumba′lium** [NA], dorsal branch of lumbar arteries: the larger of the two branches into which each lumbar artery (four or five) divides; it supplies lumbar back muscles and gives off a spinal branch. **r. dorsa′lis arte′riae subcosta′lis** [NA], dorsal branch of subcostal artery: a branch supplying back muscles, its distribution being similar to that of the dorsal branches of the lower posterior intercostal arteries. **ra′mi dorsa′les lin′guae arte′riae lingua′lis** [NA], dorsal lingual branches of lingual artery: branches of the lingual artery arising beneath the hyoglossus muscle and supplying the tonsil and the back of the tongue. **r. dorsa′lis ma′nus ner′vi ulna′ris,** r. dorsalis nervi ulnaris. **ra′mi dorsa′les nervo′rum cervica′lium** [NA], the dorsal branches of the eight cervical spinal nerves; called also *rami posteriores nervorum cervicalium.* **r. dorsa′lis ner′vi coccyg′ei** [NA], dorsal branch of coccygeal nerve: the dorsal branch of the last spinal nerve, which helps innervate the skin over the coccyx; called also *r. posterior nervi coccygei.* **ra′mi dorsa′les nervo′rum lumba′lium** [NA], the dorsal branches of the five lumbar spinal nerves; called also *rami posteriores nervorum lumbalium.* **ra′mi dorsa′les nervo′rum sacra′lium** [NA], the dorsal branches of the five sacral spinal nerves, which emerge from the sacrum through the dorsal sacral foramina; called also *rami posteriores nervorum sacralium.* **r. dorsa'lis nervo'rum spina'lium** [NA], dorsal branch of spinal nerves: the smaller of the two chief branches into which each spinal nerve divides almost as soon as it emerges from the intervertebral foramen. The dorsal branches supply the skin, muscles, joints, and bone of the dorsal part of the neck and trunk. Commonly each branch divides into a medial and a lateral portion. Called also *r. posterior nervorum spinalium* [NA alternative]. **ra'mi dorsa'les nervo'rum thoracico'rum** [NA], the dorsal branches of the twelve thoracic spinal nerves; called also *rami posteriores nervorum thoracalium.* **r. dorsa'lis ner'vi ulna'ris** [NA], dorsal branch of ulnar nerve: a large cutaneous branch that arises from the ulnar nerve and passes down the distal portion of the forearm to the medial side of the back of the hand, where it divides usually into three, sometimes four, dorsal digital nerves; modality, general sensory. Called also *r. dorsalis manus nervi ulnaris.* **r. dorsa'lis vena'rum intercosta'lium,** *r.* dorsalis venarum intercostalium posteriorum [IV–XI]. **r. dorsa'lis vena'rum intercosta'lium posterio'rum [IV–XI]** [NA], the dorsal branch of the posterior intercostal veins, corresponding to the dorsal branch of the posterior intercostal arteries. **ra'mi duodena'les arte'riae pancreaticoduodena'lis superio'ris anterio'ris** [NA], duodenal branches of anterior superior pancreaticoduodenal artery; vessels that supply the duodenum. **ra'mi duodena'les arte'riae pancreaticoduodena'lis superio'ris posterio'ris** [NA], duodenal branches of posterior superior pancreaticoduodenal artery; vessels supplying the duodenum. **ra'mi epididyma'les arte'riae testicula'ris** [NA], epididymal branches of testicular artery: they are distributed to the epididymis. **ra'mi epiplo'ici arte'riae gastroepiplo'icae dex'trae,** NA alternative for *rami omentalis arteriae gastro-omentalis dextrae.* **ra'mi epiplo'ici arte'riae gastroepiplo'icae sinis'trae,** NA alternative for *rami omentalis arteriae gastro-omentalis sinistrae.* **ra'mi esopha'gei aor'tae thora'cicae,** NA alternative for *rami oesophagei aortae thoracicae.* **ra'mi esopha'gei arte'riae gas'tricae sinis'trae,** NA alternative for *rami oesophagei arteriae gastricae sinistrae.* **ra'mi esopha'gei arte'riae thyroi'deae inferio'ris,** NA alternative for *r. oesophagei arteriae thyroideae inferioris.* **ra'mi esopha'gei ner'vi laryn'gei recurren'tis,** NA alternative for rami oesophagei nervi laryngei recurrentis. **r. exter'nus ner'vi accesso'rii** [NA], external branch of accessory nerve: the branch of the accessory nerve eleventh cranial that originates from the spinal roots of the nerve; it sends muscular branches to supply the sternocleidomastoid and trapezius muscles. **r. exter'nus ner'vi laryn'gei superio'ris** [NA], external branch of superior laryngeal nerve: the smaller of the two branches into which the superior laryngeal nerve divides, descending under cover of the sternothyroid muscle and innervating the cricothyroid and the inferior constrictor of the pharynx; modality, motor. **ra'mi faucia'les ner'vi lingua'lis,** rami isthmi faucium nervi lingualis. **r. femora'lis ner'vi genitofemora'lis** [NA], femoral branch of genitofemoral nerve: a branch arising by division of the genitofemoral nerve above the inguinal ligament; entering the femoral sheath, it turns forward and supplies the skin of the femoral triangle; modality, general sensory. Called also *nervus lumboinguinalis.* **r. fronta'lis anteromedia'lis arte'riae callosomargina'lis** [NA], the anteromedial frontal branch of the callosomarginal branch (artery) of the anterior cerebral artery. **r. fronta'lis arte'riae menin'geae me'diae** [NA], frontal branch of middle meningeal artery: a branch lodged in grooves on the sphenoid and parietal bones, and supplying the dura mater of the front of the brain. A part of it is sometimes enclosed in a bony canal. **r. fronta'lis arte'riae tempora'lis superficia'lis** [NA], frontal branch of superficial temporal artery: a tortuous terminal branch that supplies the forehead and frontal scalp. **r. fronta'lis ner'vi fronta'lis,** the frontal branch of the frontal nerve. **r. fronta'lis posteromedia'lis arte'riae callosomargina'lis** [NA], the posteromedial frontal branch of the callosomarginal branch (artery) of the anterior cerebral artery. **ra'mi gangliona'res ner'vi lingua'lis** [NA], ganglionic branches of lingual nerve: fibers connecting the lingual nerve to the submandibular ganglion. **ra'mi gangliona'res ner'vi maxilla'ris** [NA], gangli-

onic branches of maxillary nerve: fibers connecting the maxillary nerve to the pterygopalatine ganglion. **r. ganglio'nis trige'mini** [NA], a twig from the cavernous part of the internal carotid artery that supplies the trigeminal ganglion. **ra'mi gas'trici anterio'res ner'vi va'gi** [NA], anterior gastric branches of vagus nerve: branches arising from the anterior trunk of the vagus near the cardiac end of the stomach, innervating the anterior aspect of the lesser curvature and the anterior surface of the stomach almost to the pylorus; modality, parasympathetic and visceral afferent. Called also *plexus gastricus anterior.* **ra'mi gas'trici arte'riae gastroepiplo'icae dex'trae,** NA alternative for *rami gastrici arteriae gastro-omentalis dextrae.* **ra'mi gas'trici arte'riae gastro-omenta'lis dex'trae** [NA], gastric branches of right gastroepiploic artery: vessels that supply both surfaces of the stomach; called also *rami gastrici arteriae gastroepiploicae dextrae* [NA alternative]. **ra'mi gas'trici arte'riae gastro-omenta'lis sinis'trae** [NA], gastric branches of left gastroepiploic artery: vessels that supply both surfaces of the stomach; called also *rami gastrici arteriae gastroepiploicae sinistrae* [NA alternative]. **ra'mi gas'trici ner'vi va'gi,** see *rami gastrici anteriores nervi vagi* and *rami gastrici posteriores nervi vagi.* **ra'mi gas'trici posterio'res ner'vi va'gi** [NA], posterior gastric branches of vagus nerve: branches arising from the posterior vagal trunk near the cardiac end of the stomach, and innervating the cardiac orifice and fundus, the posterior aspect of the lesser curvature, and the posterior surface of the stomach to the pyloric antrum; modality, parasympathetic and visceral afferent. Called also *plexus gastricus posterior.* **r. genita'lis ner'vi genitofemora'lis** [NA], genital branch of genitofemoral nerve: a branch arising from the genitofemoral nerve above the inguinal ligament; entering the inguinal canal through the deep ring, it supplies the cremaster and continues to the skin of the scrotum or of the labium majus, and that of the adjacent area of the thigh; modality, general sensory and motor. Called also *nervus spermaticus externus.* **ra'mi gingiva'les inferio'res plex'us denta'lis inferio'ris** [NA], inferior gingival branches of inferior dental plexus: branches originating from the inferior dental plexus and innervating the gingivae of the lower jaw; modality, general sensory. **ra'mi gingiva'les superio'res plex'us denta'lis superio'ris** [NA], superior gingival branches of superior dental plexus: branches arising from the superior dental plexus and innervating the gingivae of the upper jaw; modality, general sensory. **r. glandula'ris ante'rior arte'riae thyreoi'deae superio'ris** [NA], anterior branch of the superior thyroid artery: principally supplying the anterior surface of the thyroid gland, and anastomosing with the artery of the opposite side. **ra'mi glandula'res arte'riae facia'lis** [NA], **ra'mi glandula'res arte'riae maxilla'ris exter'nae,** glandular branches of facial artery: branches given off to the submandibular gland by the facial artery as it passes over the lateral surface of the gland. **ra'mi glandula'res arte'riae thyreoi'deae inferio'ris,** glandular branches of the inferior thyroid artery. **ra'mi glandula'res arte'riae thyreoi'deae superio'ris,** glandular branches of the superior thyroid artery. **ra'mi glandula'res gan'glii submandibula'ris** [NA], glandular branches of submandibular ganglion: short branches running from the submandibular ganglion to innervate the submandibular gland, bearing postganglionic parasympathetic (secretory) fibers from this ganglion and sympathetic fibers that are postganglionic from the superior cervical ganglion. Called also *rami submaxillares ganglii submaxillaris* and *submaxillary nerves.* **r. glandula'ris latera'lis arte'riae thyreoi'deae superio'ris** [NA], lateral branch of superior thyroid artery: distributed to the lateral surface of the thyroid gland. **r. glandula'ris poste'rior arte'riae thyreoi'deae superio'ris** [NA], posterior glandular branch of the superior thyroid artery; distributed mainly to the medial and lateral surfaces of the thyroid gland; it anastomoses with the inferior thyroid artery. **ra'mi glo'bi pal'lidi** [NA], small branches of the anterior choroidal artery that supply the globus pallidus. **ra'mi helici'ni arte'riae uteri'nae** [NA], helicine branches of uterine artery: the exceedingly tortuous terminal branches of the uterine artery in the uterine muscle. Called also *helicine arteries.* **ra'mi hepat'ici ner'vi va'gi** [NA], hepatic branches of vagus nerve: branches (sometimes only one) arising from the anterior vagal trunk, contributing to the hepatic plexus, and helping innervate the liver, gallbladder, pancreas, pylorus, and duodenum; modality, parasympathetic and visceral afferent. **r. hyoi′deus ar-te′riae lingua′lis,** r. suprahyoideus arteriae lingualis. **r. hyoi′deus arte′riae thyreoi′deae superio′ris,** r. infrahyoideus arteriae thyroideae superioris. **r. hypo-thala′micus arte′riae communican′tis posterio′-ris** [NA], a branch of the posterior communicating artery that supplies the hypothalamus. **r. ilea′lis arte′riae ileoco′licae** [NA], ileal branch of ileocolic artery: a branch that passes upward and to the left of the lower ileum and anastomoses with the end of the superior mesenteric artery. **r. ili′acus arte′riae iliolumba′lis** [NA], iliac branch of iliolumbar artery: one of the two branches into which the iliolumbar artery divides in the iliac fossa; it supplies the iliacus muscle and sends a large nutrient branch to the ilium. **r. infe′rior arte′riae glu′teae superio′ris** [NA], infe-rior branch of superior gluteal artery: the lower division of the deep branch of the superior gluteal artery, accompanied by the superior gluteal artery, accompanied by the superior gluteal nerve and helping supply the gluteus medius, gluteus minimus, and tensor fasciae latae muscles and the hip joint and ilium. **ra′mi inferio′res ner′vi cuta′nei col′li,** rami inferiores nervi transversi colli. **r. infe′rior ner′vi oculomoto′rii** [NA], inferior branch of oculomotor nerve: the branch of the oculomotor nerve that innervates the medial and inferior rectus and inferior oblique muscles of the eyeball and, via the motor root of the ciliary ganglion and then the short ciliary nerves, supplies the sphincter pupillae and ciliary muscles; modality, motor and parasympathetic. **ra′mi inferio′res ner′vi transver′si col′li** [NA], infe-rior branches of transverse nerve of neck: the more inferior of the branches that arise from the transverse cervical nerve near the anterior border of the sternocleidomastoid muscle, innervating skin and subcutaneous tissue in the anterior cervical region; modality, general sensory. Called also *rami inferiores nervi cutanei colli.* **r. infe′rior os′sis is′chii,** r. ossis ischii. **r. infe′rior os′sis pu′bis** [NA], infe-rior r. of pubis, the short flattened bar of bone that projects from the body of the pubic bone in a posteroin-ferolateral direction to meet the ramus of the ischium. **r. infrahyoi′deus arte′riae thyroi′deae superio′ris** [NA], infrahyoid branch of superior thyroid artery: a vessel running along the inferior border of the hyoid bone, supply-ing the infrahyoid region, and anastomosing with its fellow of the opposite side; called also *r. hyoideus arteriae thyreoi-deae superioris.* **r. infrapatella′ris ner′vi saphe′ni** [NA], infrapatellar branch of saphenous nerve: a branch running inferolaterally from the saphenous nerve to the patellar plexus; modality, general sensory. **ra′mi in-guina′les arte′riae femora′lis** [NA], inguinal branches of femoral artery: branches arising from the external puden-dal arteries and supplying the inguinal region. **ra′mi in-tercosta′les anterio′res arte′riae thora′cicae in-ter′nae,** **ra′mi intercosta′les arte′riae mam-ma′riae inter′nae,** anterior intercostal branches of inter-nal thoracic artery: twelve branches, two in each of the upper six intercostal spaces, that supply the intercostal spaces and the pectoralis major muscle. Within each space both branches run laterally, the upper anastomosing with the posterior intercostal artery, the lower with the collateral branch of that artery. **r. interfunicula′ris** (*obs.*), a branch connecting the two trunks of the sympathetic nervous system. **ra′mi intergangliona′res** [NA], interglangli-onic branches: the branches that interconnect the ganglia of the sympathetic trunk. **r. inter′nus ner′vi acces-so′rii** [NA], internal branch of accessory nerve: the branch that continues from the cranial roots of the nerve, carrying motor fibers that are distributed by branches of the vagus to the soft palate, pharyngeal constrictors, and larynx. **r. inter′nus ner′vi laryn′gei superio′ris** [NA], internal branch of superior laryngeal nerve: the larger of the two branches of the superior laryngeal nerve, which innervates the mucosa of the epiglottis, base of the tongue, and larynx; modality, general sensory. Called also *rami fauciales nervi lingualis.* **r. interventricula′ris ante′rior ar-te′riae corona′riae sinis′trae** [NA], anterior interven-tricular branch of left coronary artery: the branch of the left coronary artery that runs to the apex of the heart in the anterior interventricular sulcus, supplying the ventricles and most of the interventricular septum; called also *r. descendens anterior arteriae coronariae* [*cordis*] *sinistrae.* **r. inter-ventricula′ris poste′rior arte′riae corona′riae**

dex′trae [NA], posterior interventricular branch of right coronary artery: a branch running toward the apex of the heart in the posterior interventricular sulcus, supplying the diaphragmatic surface of the ventricles and part of the interventricular septum. Called also *r. descendens posterior arteriae coronariae* [*cordis*] *dextrae.* **ra′mi interven-tricula′res septa′les ra′mi interventricula′ris an-terio′ris arte′riae corona′riae sinis′trae** [NA], inter-ventricular septal branches of anterior interventricular branch of left coronary artery: branches of the anterior interventricular branch of the left coronary artery that supply about the ventral two-thirds of the anterior interven-tricular septum; called also *anterior interventricular septal arteries* and *anterior septal arteries.* **ra′mi interven-tricula′res septa′les ra′mi interventricula′ris posterio′ris arte′riae corona′riae dex′trae** [NA], in-terventricular septal branches of posterior interventricular branch of right coronary artery: numerous, relatively small branches of posterior interventricular branch of the right coronary artery that supply about one-third of the posterior of the interventricular septum. Called also *posterior interven-tricular septal arteries* and *posterior septal arteries.* **r. of ischium,** r. ossis ischii. **ra′mi isth′mi fau′cium ner′vi lingua′lis** [NA], branches from the lingual nerve to the isthmus of the fauces; modality, general sensory. **r. of jaw,** r. mandibulae. **ra′mi labia′les anterio′res ar-te′riae femora′lis** [NA], anterior labial branches of femo-ral artery: branches that arise from the external pudendal arteries and supply the labium majus; called also *arteriae labiales anteriores vulvae.* **ra′mi labia′les inferio′res ner′vi menta′lis** [NA], inferior labial branches of mental nerve: branches of the mental nerve that innervate the lower lip; modality, general sensory. **ra′mi labia′les post-erio′res arte′riae puden′dae inter′nae** [NA], poste-rior labial branches of internal pudendal artery: two branches arising from the internal pudendal artery in the anterior part of the ischiorectal fossa, helping to supply the ischiocavernosus and bulbospongiosus muscles, and supply-ing the labium majus and labium minus. Called also *arteriae labiales posteriores vulvae.* **ra′mi labia′les superi-o′res ner′vi infraorbita′lis** [NA], superior labial branches of infraorbital nerve: branches of the infraorbital nerve that are distributed to mucous membranes of the mouth and skin of the upper lip; modality, general sensory. **ra′mi laryngopharyn′gei gan′glii cervica′lis su-perio′ris** [NA], laryngopharyngeal branches of superior cervical ganglion: branches from the superior cervical gan-glion to the larynx and walls of the pharynx; modality, sympathetic. **ra′mi latera′les arteria′rum cen-tra′lium anterolatera′lium** [NA], the lateral branches of the anterolateral central branches (arteries) of the middle cerebral artery that supply the basal nuclei of the brain and its internal capsule. Called also *lateral striate arteries.* **r. latera′lis duc′tus hepat′ici sinis′tri** [NA], the lat-eral branch of the left hepatic duct. **r. latera′lis inter-ventricula′ris anterio′ris arte′riae corona′riae sinis′trae** [NA], lateral branch of the anterior interventric-ular branch of the left coronary artery. **r. latera′lis na′si arte′riae facia′lis** [NA], lateral nasal branch of the facial artery: a branch supplying the ala and dorsum of the nose. **r. latera′lis ner′vi supraorbita′lis** [NA], lat-eral branch of supraorbital nerve: a branch of the supraor-bital nerve that supplies the frontal sinus, upper eyelid, and skin and subcutaneous tissue of the forehead and scalp laterally as far as the temporal region; modality, general sensory. **r. latera′lis ramo′rum dorsa′lium ner-vo′rum cervica′lium** [NA], lateral branch of dorsal branches of cervical nerves: the lateral branch that arises from the dorsal branch of each of the eight cervical nerves, supplying adjacent muscles; called also *r. lateralis ramorum posteriorum nervorum cervicalium.* **r. latera′lis ramo′-rum dorsa′lium nervo′rum lumba′lium** [NA], lat-eral branch of dorsal branches of lumbar nerves: the branch that runs inferolaterally from the dorsal branch of each lumbar nerve, innervating adjacent muscle; the upper of these branches terminally constitute the superior cluneal nerves, supplying skin of the buttock. Called also *r. lateralis ramorum posteriorum nervorum lumbalium.* **r. latera′lis ramo′rum dorsa′lium nervo′rum sacra′lium** [NA], lateral branch of dorsal branches of sacral nerves: the lateral branch that arises from the dorsal branch of each of the three upper sacral nerves; called also *r. lateralis ramorum posteri-orum nervorum sacralium.* **r. latera′lis ramo′rum**

posterio′rum nervo′rum cervica′lium, r. lateralis ramorum dorsalium nervorum cervicalium. **r. latera′lis ramo′rum posterio′rum nervo′rum lumba′lium,** r. lateralis ramorum dorsalium nervorum lumbalium. **r. latera′lis ramo′rum posterio′rum nervo′rum sacra′lium,** r. lateralis ramorum dorsalium nervorum sacralium. **r. liena′lis arte′riae liena′lis** [NA], NA alternative for *r. splenici arteriae splenicae.* **ra′mi liena′les arte′riae liena′lis,** NA alternative for *rami splenici arteriae splenicae.* **ra′mi liena′les plex′us coeli′aci,** splenic branches of celiac plexus. **r. lingua′lis ner′vi facia′lis** [NA], lingual branch of facial nerve: an inconstant branch of the facial nerve sometimes arising together with the stylohyoid branch, and helping to supply the styloglossal and glossopalatine muscles; modality, motor. **ra′mi lingua′les ner′vi glossopharyn′gei** [NA], lingual branches of glossopharyngeal nerve: branches of the glossopharyngeal nerve that innervate the posterior third of the tongue; modality, general and special sensory. **ra′mi lingua′les ner′vi hypoglos′si** [NA], lingual branches of hypoglossal nerve: branches of the hypoglossal nerve that innervate the intrinsic and extrinsic muscles of the tongue; modality, motor. **ra′mi lingua′les ner′vi lingua′lis** [NA], lingual branches of lingual nerve: branches that innervate the anterior two-thirds of the tongue, adjacent areas of the mouth, and the gums; modality, general and special sensory. **r. lumba′lis arte′riae iliolumba′lis** [NA], lumbar branch of iliolumbar artery: a branch that arises from the iliolumbar artery in the iliac fossa and ascends to supply the psoas and quadratus lumborum muscles, sending a spinal branch through the intervertebral foramen just above the sacrum. **ra′mi malleola′res latera′les arte′riae fibula′ris** [NA], lateral malleolar branches of fibular artery: they supply the lateral aspect of the ankle and give off calcaneal branches to the lateral aspect and back of the heel; called also *rami malleolares laterales peroneae* [NA alternative]. **ra′mi malleola′res latera′les arte′riae perone′ae,** NA alternative for *rami malleolares laterales fibularis.* **ra′mi malleola′res media′les arte′riae tibiales posterioris** [NA], medial malleolar branches of posterior tibial artery: vessels supplying the area of the medial malleolus and giving off calcaneal branches to the medial aspect and back of the heel; called also *arteria malleolaris posterior medialis.* **ra′mi mamma′rii arte′riae mamma′riae inter′nae,** rami mammarii arteriae thoracicae internae. **ra′mi mamma′rii arte′riae thora′cicae inter′nae,** rami mammarii mediales arteriae thoracicae internae. **ra′mi mamma′rii exter′ni arte′riae thoraca′lis latera′lis,** rami mammarii laterales arteriae thoracicae lateralis. **ra′mi mamma′rii latera′les arte′riae thora′cicae latera′lis** [NA], lateral mammary branches of lateral thoracic artery: they supply the mammary gland. **ra′mi mamma′rii latera′les ra′mi cuta′nei latera′lis arte′riarum intercosta′lium posterio′rium** [NA], lateral mammary branches of lateral cutaneous branch of posterior intercostal arteries: they arise from the third, fourth and fifth posterior intercostal arteries. **ra′mi mamma′rii latera′les ra′mi cuta′nei latera′lis nervo′rum intercosta′lium,** NA alternative for *rami mammarii laterales rami cutanei lateralis ramorum ventralium nervorum thoracicorum.* **ra′mi mamma′rii latera′les ra′mi cuta′nei latera′lis ramo′rum ventra′lium nervo′rum thoracico′rum** [NA], the lateral mammary branches of the lateral cutaneous branch of the ventral branches of the thoracic nerves (intercostal nerves): modality, general sensory. Called also *rami mammarii laterales rami cutanei lateralis nervorum intercostalium* [NA alternative]. **ra′mi mamma′rii media′les arte′riae thora′cicae inter′nae** [NA], medial mammary branches of internal thoracic artery; they arise from the second, third, and fourth perforating branches of the internal thoracic artery and help supply the mammary gland. Called also *rami mammarii arteriae thoracicae internae.* **ra′mi mamma′rii media′les ra′mi cuta′nei anterio′ris nervo′rum intercosta′lium** NA alternative for *rami mammarii mediales rami cutanei anterioris ramorum ventralium nervorum thoracicorum.* **ra′mi mamma′rii media′les ra′mi cuta′nei anterio′ris ramo′rum ventra′lium nervo′rum thoracico′rum** [NA], medial mammary branches of anterior cutaneous branch of ventral branches of thoracic nerves (intercostal nerves); modality, general sensory. Called also *rami mammarii medialis rami cutanei*

anterioris nervorum intercostalium thoracicorum [NA alternative]. **ra′mi mamma′rii ra′mi cuta′nei latera′lis arteria′rum intercosta′lium posterio′rum** [NA], mammary branches of lateral cutaneous branch of posterior intercostal arteries: branches arising from the lateral cutaneous branches of the third through fifth posterior intercostal arteries and supplying the mammary region. **r. of mandible, r. mandib′ulae** [NA], a quadrilateral process projecting superiorly from the posterior part of either side of the mandible. **r. margina′lis dex′ter** [NA], a branch of the right coronary artery that passes toward the apex of the heart along the acute margin of the heart and ramifies over the right ventricle; called also *right marginal artery.* **r. margina′lis mandib′ulae ner′vi facia′lis** [NA], marginal mandibular branch of facial nerve: a branch of the facial nerve that runs forward from the front of the parotid gland along the border of the mandible, deep to the platysma and depressor anguli oris muscles, supplying the latter and the risorius, depressor labii inferioris, and mentalis muscles; modality, motor. **r. margina′lis sinis′ter** [NA], a branch of the circumflex branch of left coronary artery that follows the left margin of the heart and supplies the left ventricle; called also *left marginal artery.* **r. margina′lis tento′rii arter′iae caro′tidis inter′nae** [NA], a twig from the cavernous part of the internal carotid artery that supplies the margin of the tentorium; called also *r. tentorii marginalis arteriae carotidis internae.* **ra′mi mastoi′dei arte′riae auricula′ris posterio′ris** [NA], mastoid branches of posterior auricular artery: they supply the mastoid cells. **r. mastoi′deus arte′riae oc′cipita′lis** [NA], mastoid branch of occipital artery: it enters the cranial cavity through the mastoid foramen and supplies the dura mater, diploe, and mastoid cells. **r. mea′tus acus′tici inter′ni arte′riae basila′ris,** NA alternative for *arteria labyrinthi.* **ra′mi media′les arteria′rum centra′lium anterolatera′lium** [NA], the medial branches of the anterolateral central branches (arteries) of the middle cerebral artery that supply anterior lenticular and caudate nuclei and internal capsule; called also *medial striate arteries.* **r. media′lis duc′tus hepat′ici sinis′tri** [NA], the medial branch of the left hepatic duct. **r. media′lis ner′vi supraorbita′lis** [NA], medial branch of supraorbital nerve: it supplies the frontal sinus, upper eyelid, and skin and subcutaneous tissue of the forehead and scalp as far back as the parietal bone; modality, general sensory. **r. media′lis ramo′rum dorsa′lium nervo′rum cervica′lium** [NA], medial branch of dorsal branches of cervical nerves: the medial branch arising from the dorsal branch of each of the eight cervical nerves, supplying muscle, periosteum, ligaments, and joints; also, except for those of the first, and generally the sixth, seventh, and eighth cervical nerves, having an eventual cutaneous distribution. Called also *r. medialis ramorum posteriorum nervorum cervicalium.* **r. media′lis ramo′rum dorsa′lium nervo′rum lumba′lium** [NA], medial branch of dorsal branches of lumbar nerves: the medial branch that arises from the dorsal branch of each lumbar nerve, mainly innervating deep muscle, but also helping supply ligaments, periosteum, and joints; called also *r. medialis ramorum posteriorum nervorum lumbalium.* **r. media′lis ramo′rum dorsa′lium nervo′rum sacra′lium** [NA], medial branch of dorsal branches of sacral nerves: the medial branch that arises from the dorsal branch of each of the upper three sacral nerves; called also *r. medialis ramorum posteriorum nervorum sacralium.* **r. media′lis ramo′rum posterio′rum nervo′rum cervica′lium,** r. medialis ramorum dorsalium nervorum cervicalium. **r. media′lis ramo′rum posterio′rum nervo′rum lumba′lium,** r. medialis ramorum dorsalium nervorum lumbalium. **r. media′lis ramo′rum posterio′rum nervo′rum sacra′lium,** r. medialis ramorum dorsalium nervorum sacralium. **r. media′lis mediastina′les aor′tae thoraca′lis, ra′mi mediastina′les aor′tae thora′cicae** [NA], mediastinal branches of thoracic aorta: small vessels supplying connective tissue and lymph nodes in the posterior mediastinum. **ra′mi mediastina′les arte′riae thora′cicae inter′nae** [NA], mediastinal branches of internal thoracic artery: they supply areolar tissue, pericardium, lymph nodes, and the thymus in the anterior and superior mediastinum; called also *arteriae mediastinales anteriores.* **ra′mi ad medul′lam oblonga′tam arte′riae inferio′ris posterio′ris cerebel′li** [NA], branches of the posterior inferior cerebellar artery that supply the medulla oblongata.

ra′mi medulla′res media′lis et latera′lis arte′riae inferio′ris posterio′ris cerebel′li [NA], lateral and medial medullary branches of posterior inferior cerebellar artery: the lateral branch supplies the undersurface of the hemisphere of the cerebellum and anastomoses with the anterior inferior cerebellar and superior cerebellar branches of the basilar artery; the medial branch ramifies on the cerebellar vermis between the hemispheres. **r. membra′nae tym′pani ner′vi auriculotempora′lis** [NA], branch to tympanic membrane of auriculotemporal nerve: a branch given to the tympanic membrane by the nerve of the external acoustic meatus, a branch of the auriculotemporal nerve; modality, general sensory. **r. menin′geus accesso′rius arte′riae menin′geae me′diae** [NA], accessory meningeal branch of middle meningeal artery: a branch arising from the middle meningeal artery, or directly from the maxillary artery, and entering the middle cranial fossa through the foramen ovale to supply the trigeminal ganglion, walls of the cavernous sinus, and neighboring dura mater. **r. menin′geus ante′rior arte′riae ethmoida′lis anterio′ris,** [NA], anterior meningeal branch of anterior ethmoidal artery; it supplies the dura mater. Called also *arteria meningea anterior* and *anterior meningeal artery.* **r. menin′geus ante′rior arte′riae vertebra′lis,** see *rami meningei arteriae vertebralis.* **r. meninge′us arte′riae caro′tidis inter′nae** [NA] a twig from the cavernous part of the internal carotid artery that supplies the meninges of the anterior cranial fossa. **r. menin′geus arte′riae occipita′lis** [NA], meningeal branch of occipital artery: one or more variable branches of the occipital artery that enter the posterior fossa and supply the dura mater. **ra′mi menin′gei arte′riae vertebra′lis** [NA], meningeal branches of vertebral artery: branches, anterior and posterior, arising from the vertebral artery in the foramen magnum, and ramifying in the posterior cranial fossa to supply the dura mater, including the falx cerebelli and bone. **r. menin′geus me′dius ner′vi maxilla′ris** [NA], middle meningeal branch of maxillary nerve: a branch arising from the maxillary nerve in the middle cranial fossa, accompanying the middle meningeal artery, and supplying the dura mater; modality, general sensory. Called also *meningeal nerve* and *nervus meningeus medius.* **r. menin′geus ner′vi mandibula′ris** [NA], meningeal branch of mandibular nerve: a branch that arises from the trunk of the mandibular nerve, re-enters the cranium through the foramen spinosum, accompanies the middle meningeal artery to supply the dura mater, and also helps innervate the mucous membrane of the mastoid air cells. Called also *nervus spinosus.* **r. menin′geus ner′vi ophthal′mici,** NA alternative for *r. tentorii nervi ophthalmici.* **r. menin′geus nervo′rum spina′lium** [NA], meningeal branch of spinal nerves: the small branch of each spinal nerve that re-enters the intervertebral foramen to supply the dura mater, vertebral column, and associated ligaments. **r. menin′geus ner′vi va′gi** [NA], meningeal branch of vagus nerve: a branch that arises in the jugular foramen from the superior ganglion of the vagus nerve, innervating dura mater of the posterior cranial fossa. **r. menin′geus poste′rior arte′riae vertebra′lis,** see *rami meningei arteriae vertebralis.* **r. menin′geus recur′rens arte′riae lacrima′lis,** recurrent meningeal branch of the lacrimal artery; it anastomoses with a branch of the meningeal artery between the internal and external carotid arteries. **r. menta′lis arte′riae alveola′ris inferio′ris** [NA], mental branch of inferior alveolar artery: a branch arising from the inferior alveolar artery in the mandibular canal, which leaves the canal at the mental foramen, supplies the chin, and anastomoses with its fellow of the opposite side and with the submental and inferior labial arteries. **ra′mi menta′les ner′vi menta′lis** [NA], mental branches of mental nerve: they innervate the skin of the chin; modality, general sensory. **ra′mi muscula′res** [NA], muscular branches: any branches of a peripheral nerve or vessel that supply muscle, many not being more specifically named. **ra′mi muscula′res arte′riae vertebra′lis** [NA], branches of the transverse part of the vertebral artery that supply the deep muscles of the neck and anastomose with the descending branch of the occipital artery and the deep cervical artery. **ra′mi muscula′res ner′vi accesso′rii** [NA], the branches of the external branch of the accessory nerve that supply the sternocleidomastoid and trapezius muscles. **ra′mi muscula′res ner′vi axilla′ris** [NA], muscular branches of

axillary nerve: they innervate the deltoid and teres minor muscles; modality, motor. **ra′mi muscula′res ner′vi femora′lis** [NA], muscular branches of femoral nerve: they innervate the anterior thigh muscles; modality, motor. **ra′mi muscula′res ner′vi fibula′ris profun′di** [NA], muscular branches of deep fibular nerve: they innervate the tibialis anterior, extensor hallucis longus, extensor digitorum longus, and peroneus tertius muscles; modality, motor. Called also *rami musculares nervi peronei profundi* [NA alternative]. **ra′mi muscula′res ner′vi fibula′ris superficia′lis** [NA], muscular branches of superficial fibular nerve: they innervate the peroneus longus and peroneus brevis muscles; modality, motor; called also *rami musculares nervi peronei superficialis* [NA alternative]. **ra′mi muscula′res ner′vi iliohypogas′trici,** muscular branches of iliohypogastric nerve; modality, probably sensory except for an occasional motor twig to the pyramidalis. **ra′mi muscula′res ner′vi ilioinguina′lis,** muscular branches of ilioinguinal nerve, probably sensory in nature. **ra′mi muscula′res nervo′rum intercosta′lium,** muscular branches of the intercostal nerves. **ra′mi muscula′res ner′vi ischiad′ici,** muscular branches of the sciatic nerve. **ra′mi muscula′res ner′vi media′ni** [NA], muscular branches of median nerve: they innervate most of the flexor muscles on the front of the forearm and most of the short muscles of the thumb; modality, motor. **ra′mi muscula′res ner′vi musculocuta′nei** [NA], muscular branches of musculocutaneous nerve: they innervate the coracobrachialis, biceps, and brachialis muscles; modality, motor and general sensory. **ra′mi muscula′res ner′vi obturato′rii** [NA], muscular branches of obturator nerve: branches arising from the anterior and posterior rami of the obturator nerve and innervating the obturator externus, gracilis, and adductor muscles, and sometimes the pectineus; modality, motor. **ra′mi muscula′res ner′vi perone′i profun′di,** NA alternative for *rami musculares nervi fibularis profundi.* **ra′mi muscula′res ner′vi perone′i superficia′lis,** NA alternative for *rami musculares nervi fibularis superficialis.* **ra′mi muscula′res ner′vi radia′lis** [NA], muscular branches of radial nerve: they innervate the triceps, anconeus, brachioradialis, and extensor carpi radialis muscles; a branch to the brachialis muscle is probably sensory; modality, motor and sensory. **ra′mi muscula′res ner′vi tibia′lis** [NA], muscular branches of tibial nerve: they supply muscles of the back of the leg; modality, motor. **ra′mi muscula′res ner′vi ulna′ris** [NA], muscular branches of ulnar nerve: they innervate the flexor carpi ulnaris muscle and the ulnar half of flexor digitorum profundus; modality, motor. **ra′mi muscula′res plex′us lumba′lis,** muscular branches of the lumbar plexus. **r. mus′culi stylopharyn′gei ner′vi glossopharyn′gei** [NA], stylopharyngeal branch of glossopharyngeal nerve: it supplies the stylopharyngeal muscle; modality, motor; called also *r. stylopharyngeus nervi glossopharyngei.* **r. mylohyoi′deus arte′riae alveola′ris inferio′ris** [NA], mylohyoid branch of inferior alveolar nerve: it descends with the mylohyoid nerve in the mylohyoid sulcus to supply the floor of the mouth. **ra′mi nasa′les anterio′res latera′les arte′riae ethmoida′lis anterio′ris** [NA], anterior lateral nasal branches of anterior ethmoidal artery; they supply twigs to the lateral wall and septum of the nose. **ra′mi nasa′les anterio′res ner′vi ethmoida′lis anterio′ris,** rami nasales nervi ethmoidalis anterioris. **r. nasa′lis exter′nus ner′vi ethmoida′lis anterio′ris** [NA], external nasal branch of anterior ethmoidal nerve: essentially a continuation, or terminal branch, of the anterior ethmoidal nerve, it innervates the skin of the dorsal part of the nose; modality, general sensory. **ra′mi nasa′les exter′ni ner′vi infraorbita′lis** [NA], external nasal branches of infraorbital nerve: they innervate the skin of the side of the nose; modality, general sensory. **ra′mi nasa′les inter′ni ner′vi ethmoida′lis anterio′ris** [NA], internal nasal branches of anterior ethmoidal nerve: through medial and lateral branches, they innervate the nasal septum and the mucous membrane of the lateral wall of the nasal cavity; modality, general sensory. **ra′mi nasa′les inter′ni ner′vi infraorbita′lis** [NA], internal nasal branches of infraorbital nerve: they innervate the mobile septum of the nose; modality, general sensory. **ra′mi nasa′les latera′les ner′vi ethmoida′lis anterio′ris** [NA], lateral nasal branches of anterior ethmoidal nerve: branches arising from the internal nasal branches of the anterior ethmoidal nerve and innervating the mucosa of the lateral wall of the nasal cavity; modality, general sensory. **ra′mi nasa′les media′les ner′vi ethmoida′lis anterio′ris** [NA], medial nasal branches of anterior ethmoidal nerve: branches arising from the internal nasal branches of the anterior ethmoidal nerve and supplying the nasal septum; modality, general sensory. **ra′mi nasa′les ner′vi ethmoida′lis anterio′ris** [NA], nasal branches of anterior ethmoidal nerve: the internal and external nasal branches of the anterior ethmoidal nerve, and their subdivisions; called also *rami nasales anteriores nervi ethmoidalis anterioris*. **ra′mi nasa′les posterio′res inferio′res [latera′les] gan′glii pterygopalati′ni** [NA], **ra′mi nasa′les posterio′res inferio′res [latera′les] gan′glii sphenopalati′ni**, [lateral] inferior posterior nasal branches of pterygopalatine ganglion: they are usually branches of the greater palatine nerve and they supply the middle and inferior nasal meatu and inferior conchae; modality, general sensory. **ra′mi nasa′les posteri-o′res inferio′res ner′vi palati′ni** [NA], the posterior inferior branches of the greater palatine nerve. **ra′mi nasa′les posterio′res superio′res latera′les gan′glii pterygopalati′ni** [NA], **ra′mi nasa′les posteri-o′res superio′res latera′les gan′glii sphenopalati′ni**, lateral superior posterior nasal branches of pterygopalatine ganglion: they supply the superior and middle nasal conchae and the posterior ethmoidal sinuses; modality, general sensory. **ra′mi nasa′les posterio′res superio′res media′les gan′glii pterygopalati′ni** [NA], **ra′mi nasa′les posterio′res superio′res media′les gan′glii sphenopalati′ni**, medial superior posterior nasal branches of pterygopalatine ganglion: they are usually branches of the nasopalatine nerve, and they supply the nasal septum; modality, general sensory. **r. nasocilia′ris gan′glii cilia′ris**, NA alternative for *radix nasociliaris ganglii ciliaris*. **r. ner′vi oculomoto′rii arte′riae communican′tis posterio′ris** [NA], a branch of the posterior communicating artery that supplies the oculomotor nerve. **r. no′di atrioven-tricula′ris arte′riae corona′riae dex′trae** [NA], a branch of the right coronary artery usually arising opposite the origin of the posterior interventricular artery and inserting into the atrioventricular node; occasionally, the atrioventricular node is supplied by a branch of the circumflex branch of the left coronary artery (*r. nodi atrioventricula-ris arteriae coronariae sinistrae* [NA]). Called also *atrioven-tricular nodal artery*. **r. no′di sinuatria′lis arte′riae corona′riae dex′trae** [NA], a branch of the right coronary artery that supplies the right atrium, encircles the base of the superior vena cava, and inserts into the sinoatrial node; occasionally, the sinoatrial node is supplied by a branch arising from the circumflex branch of the left coronary artery (*r. nodi sinustrialis arteriae coronariae sinistrae* [NA]). Called also *nodal artery, sinoatrial* or *sinuatrial nodal artery*, and *sinus node artery*. **ra′mi nu′clei ru′bris** [NA], small branches of the anterior choroidal artery that supply the red nucleus. **ra′mi nucleo′rum hypothalamico′rum** [NA], small branches of the anterior choroidal artery that supply the hypothalamic nuclei. **r. obturato′rius ar-te′riae epigas′tricae inferio′ris** [NA], obturator branch of inferior epigastric artery: a vessel connecting the pubic branches of the inferior epigastric and the obturator arteries. The obturator artery is sometimes replaced by an accessory obturator that arises from the inferior epigastric artery by way of this communication. **r. occipita′lis arte′riae auricula′ris posterio′ris** [NA], occipital branch of posterior auricular artery: it is distributed to the epicranius muscle. **ra′mi occipita′les arte′riae oc-cipita′lis** [NA], occipital branches of occipital artery: a medial and a lateral branch of the occipital artery, distributed to the scalp and, through the meningeal branch, to the dura mater. **r. occipita′lis ner′vi auricula′ris posteri-o′ris** [NA], occipital branch of posterior auricular nerve: a branch supplying the occipital belly of the occipitofrontalis muscle; modality, motor. **r. occipitotempora′lis ar-te′riae occipita′lis media′lis** [NA], a branch of the middle occipital artery that supplies the occipital and temporal areas of the cerebral cortex. **ra′mi oesopha′gei aor′-tae thora′cicae** [NA], esophageal branches of thoracic aorta: branches, usually two, that arise from the front of the aorta to supply the esophagus; called also *rami esophagei aortae thoracicae* [NA alternative]. **ra′mi oesopha′gei arte′riae gas′tricae sinis′trae** [NA], esophageal

branches of left gastric artery: they supply the esophagus; called also *rami esophagei arteriae gastricae sinistrae* [NA alternative]. **ra′mi oesopha′gei arte′riae thyroi′-deae inferio′ris** [NA], esophageal branches of inferior thyroid artery: they supply the esophagus; called also *rami esophagei arteriae thyroideae inferioris* [NA alternative]. **ra′mi oesopha′gei ner′vi laryn′gei recurren′tis** [NA], esophageal branches of recurrent laryngeal nerve: they help innervate the esophagus; modality, visceral afferent and general sensory; called also *rami esophagei nervi laryngei recurrentis* [NA alternative]. **ra′mi omenta′les ar-te′riae gastro-omentalis dex′trae** [NA], omental branches of right gastro-omental artery: they supply the greater omentum. Called also *rami epiploici arteriae gastroep-iploicae dextrae* [NA alternative]. **ra′mi omenta′les arte′riae gastro-omentalis sinis′trae** [NA], omental branches of left gastro-mental artery; they supply the stomach and greater omentum. Called also *rami epiploici arteriae gastroepiploicae sinistrae* [NA alternative]. **r. or-bita′lis arte′riae menin′geae me′diae** [NA], the orbi-tal branch of the middle meningeal artery. **ra′mi or-bita′les gan′glii pterygopalati′ni** [NA], **ra′mi or-bita′les gan′glii sphenopalati′ni**, orbital branches of pterygopalatine ganglion: branches passing from the ptery-gopalatine ganglion through the inferior orbital fissure to supply orbital periosteum and the ethmoidal and sphenoidal sinuses; modality, general sensory and parasympathetic. **r. orbitofronta′lis media′lis arte′riae cer′ebri an-terio′ris**, NA alternative for *arteria frontobasalis medialis*. **r. orbitofronta′lis media′lis arte′riae cer′ebri me′-diae**, NA alternative for *arteria frontobasalis lateralis*. **r. os′sis is′chii** [NA], ramus of ischium: the flattened bar of bone that projects from the inferior end of the body of the ischium in an anterosuperomedial direction to meet the inferior ramus of the pubis. It forms part of the border of the obturator foramen. Called also *r. inferior ossis ischii*. **r. os′sis pu′bis**, see *r. inferior ossis pubis* and *r. superior ossis pubis*. **r. ova′ricus arte′riae uteri′nae** [NA], **r. ova′rii arte′riae uteri′nae**, ovarian branch of uterine artery: the terminal branch of the uterine artery, which supplies the ovary and anastomoses with the ovarian artery. **r. palma′ris ner′vi media′ni** [NA], palmar branch of median nerve: a branch arising from the median nerve in the lower part of the forearm and supplying the skin of the outer part of the palm; modality, general sensory. **r. palma′-ris ner′vi ulna′ris** [NA], palmar branch of ulnar nerve: it arises from the ulnar nerve in the lower part of the forearm, supplying the cutaneous structures of the medial part of the palm; modality, general sensory. Called also *r. volaris manus nervi ulnaris*. **r. palma′ris profun′dus arte′riae ul-na′ris** [NA], deep palmar branch of ulnar artery: it accom-panies the deep palmar branch of the ulnar nerve and joins the radial artery to form the deep palmar arch; called also *r. volaris profundus arteriae ulnaris*. **r. palma′ris super-ficia′lis arte′riae radia′lis** [NA], superficial palmar branch of radial artery: a branch arising from the radial artery in the lower part of the forearm and supplying the thenar eminence; called also *r. volaris superficialis arteriae radialis*. **ra′mi palpebra′les inferio′res ner′vi in-fraorbita′lis** [NA], inferior palpebral branches of infraor-bital nerve: they supply the skin and conjunctiva of the lower eyelid; modality, general sensory. **r. palpebra′lis in-fe′rior ner′vi infratrochlea′ris**, see *rami palpebrales nervi infratrochlearis*. **ra′mi palpebra′les ner′vi in-fratrochlea′ris** [NA], palpebral branches of infratrochlear nerve: they help supply the eyelids; modality, general sen-sory. **r. palpebra′lis supe′rior ner′vi infratro-chlea′ris**, see *rami palpebrales nervi infratrochlearis*. **ra′mi pancreat′ici arte′riae liena′lis**, NA alternative for *rami pancreatici arteriae splenicae*. **ra′mi pan-creat′ici arte′riae pancreaticoduodena′lis superi-o′ris anterio′ris** [NA], pancreatic branches of the anterior superior pancreaticoduodenal artery: vessels that supply the pancreas. **ra′mi pancreat′ici arte′riae pan-creaticoduodena′lis superio′ris posterio′ris** [NA], pancreatic branches of posterior superior pancreaticoduode-nal artery: vessels that supply the pancreas. **ra′mi pan-creat′ici arte′riae sple′nicae** [NA], pancreatic branches of splenic artery: branches that supply the pan-creas, arising from the splenic artery during its tortuous course along the superior border of the body of the pancreas. Called also *rami pancreatici arteriae lienalis* [NA alterna-tive]. **ra′mi parieta′les aor′tae abdomina′lis**, parietal branches of the abdominal aorta. **ra'mi parieta'les aor'tae thoraca'lis,** parietal branches of the thoracic aorta. **ra'mi parieta'les arte'riae hypogas'tricae,** parietal branches of the hypogastric artery. **r. parieta'lis arte'riae menin'geae me'diae** [NA], parietal branch of middle meningeal artery: a vessel that arises in the middle cranial fossa, grooves the temporal and parietal bones, and supplies the posterior dura mater. **r. parieta'lis arte'riae occipita'lis media'lis** [NA], the branch of the middle occipital artery that supplies the parietal lobe. **r. parieta'lis arte'riae tempora'lis superficia'lis** [NA], parietal branch of superficial temporal artery: the posterior terminal branch of the superficial temporal artery, supplying the scalp in the parietal region. **r. parieto-occipita'lis arte'riae cer'ebri posterio'ris** [NA], parieto-occipital branch of posterior cerebral artery: a vessel that supplies the cortex of the medial surface of the hemisphere up to the area of the parieto-occipital sulcus. **r. parieto-occipita'lis arte'riae occipita'lis media'lis** [NA], a branch of the middle occipital artery that supplies the cuneus and precuneus. **r. paroti'deus arte'riae auricula'ris posterio'ris** [NA], parotid branch of the posterior auricular artery; a branch supplying the parotid gland. **r. paroti'deus arte'riae tempora'lis superficia'lis** [NA], parotid branch of superificial temporal artery: a branch supplying the parotid gland and the temporomandibular joint. **ra'mi paroti'dei ner'vi auriculotempora'lis** [NA], parotid branches of auriculotemporal nerve: branches that bear postganglionic fibers from the otic ganglion to the parotid gland; modality, parasympathetic. **ra'mi paroti'dei ve'nae facia'lis** [NA], parotid branches of facial vein: small veins from the substance of the parotid gland which follow the parotid duct and open into the facial vein; called also *venae parotideae anteriores*. **ra'mi pectora'les arte'riae thoracoacromia'lis** [NA], pectoral branches of thoracoacromial artery: they descend between the pectoralis major and minor muscles, supplying these muscles and the mammary gland. **rami peduncula'res arte'riae cer'ebri poste'rioris** [NA], the branches of the posterior cerebral artery that supply the cerebral peduncles. **r. per'forans arte'riae fibula'ris** [NA], perforating branch of fibular artery: a branch passing forward from the fibular artery where the interosseous membrane and the tibiofibular syndesmosis are continuous and descending to supply the syndesmosis and the ankle joint. Called also *r. perforans arteriae peroneae* [NA alternative]. **ra'mi perforan'tes arte'riae mamma'riae inter'nae,** rami perforantes arteriae thoracicae internae. **ra'mi perforan'tes arteria'rum metacarpea'rum palma'rium** [NA], **ra'mi perforan'tes arteria'rum metacarpea'rum vola'rium,** perforating branches of palmar metacarpal arteries: vessels connecting the palmar metacarpal arteries and deep palmar arch with the dorsal metacarpal arteries, between the bases of the metacarpal bones and in the interosseous spaces. **ra'mi perforan'tes arteria'rum metatarsea'rum planta'rium** [NA], perforating branches of plantar metatarsal arteries: vessels connecting the plantar metatarsal arteries with the dorsal metatarsal arteries through the interosseous spaces. **r. per'forans arte'riae perone'ae,** NA alternative for *r. perforans arteriae fibularis.* **ra'mi perforan'tes arte'riae thora'cicae inter'nae** [NA], perforating branches of internal thoracic artery: six branches, one in each of the upper six intercostal spaces, supplying the pectoralis major muscle and adjacent skin; the second, third, and fourth branches give off mammary branches. Called also *rami perforantes arteriae mammariae internae.* **ra'mi pericardi'aci aor'tae thoraca'lis,** rami pericardiaci aortae thoracicae. **ra'mi pericardi'aci aor'tae thora'cicae** [NA], pericardiac branches of thoracic aorta: small branches from the aorta distributed to the surface of the pericardium. **r. pericardi'acus ner'vi phren'ici** [NA], pericardiac branch of phrenic nerve: a branch arising from the phrenic or accessory phrenic nerve and supplying the pericardium; modality, general sensory. **ra'mi denta'les arte'riae alveola'ris inferio'ris** [NA], peridental branches of inferior alveolar artery: branches arising from the inferior alveolar artery in the mandibular canal and supplying the roots and pulp of the teeth. **ra'mi peridenta'les arte'riae alveola'ris superio'ris posterio'ris** [NA], peridental branches of posterior superior alveolar artery: branches arising from the posterior superior alveolar artery and supplying the maxillary gingivae.

ra'mi perinea'les ner'vi cuta'nei fem'oris posterio'ris [NA], perineal branches of posterior femoral cutaneous nerve: branches arising from the posterior femoral cutaneous nerve at the lower margin of the gluteus maximus muscle and innervating the skin of the external genitalia; modality, general sensory. **r. petro'sus arte'riae menin'geae me'diae** [NA], **r. petro'sus superficia'lis arte'riae menin'geae me'diae,** petrosal branch of middle meningeal artery: a branch that arises in the region of the petrous part of the temporal bone, entering the hiatus for the greater petrosal nerve and anastomosing with the stylomastoid artery. **ra'mi pharyngea'les ner'vi glossopharyngea'les,** NA alternative for *rami pharyngei nervi glossopharyngeales.* **ra'mi pharyngea'les ner'vi va'gi,** NA alternative for *rami pharyngei nervi vagi.* **r. pharyn'geus arte'riae cana'lis pterygoi'dei** [NA], the pharyngeal branch of artery of the pterygoid canal; it lies medial to the pterygopalatine ganglion. **ra'mi pharyn'gei arte'riae pharyn'geae ascenden'tis** [NA], pharyngeal branches of ascending pharyngeal artery: irregular vessels supplying the pharynx. **ra'mi pharyn'gei arte'riae thyroi'deae inferio'ris** [NA], pharyngeal branches of inferior thyroid artery: vessels that supply the pharynx. **r. pharyn'geus gan'glii pterygopalati'ni** [NA], a nerve branch running from the posterior part of the pterygopalatine ganglion, through the pharyngeal canal with the pharyngeal branch of the maxillary artery, to the mucous membrane of the nasal part of the pharynx posterior to the auditory tube; called also *pharyngeal branch of pterygopalatine ganglion.* **ra'mi pharyn'gei ner'vi glossopharyn'gei** [NA], pharyngeal branches of glossopharyngeal nerve: they innervate the mucous membrane of the oropharynx; modality, general sensory. Called also *rami pharyngeales nervi glossopharyngei* [NA alternative]. **ra'mi pharyn'gei ner'vi va'gi** [NA], pharyngeal branches of vagus nerve: they innervate pharyngeal muscles and mucosa; modality, motor and general sensory. Called also *rami pharyngeales nervi vagi* [NA alternative]. **ra'mi phrenicoabdomina'les ner'vi phren'ici** [NA], phrenicoabdominal branches of phrenic nerve: branches of the phrenic or accessory phrenic nerve that supply the diaphragm and contribute to the celiac plexus; modality, general sensory and motor. **r. planta'ris profun'dus arte'riae dorsa'lis pe'dis,** arteria plantaris profundus. **ra'mi ad pon'tem arte'riae basil'aris,** arteriae pontis. **r. poste'rior arte'riae obtura'to'riae** [NA], posterior branch of obturator artery: it passes backward around the lateral margin of the obturator foramen, on the obturator membrane, supplying muscles around the ischial tuberosity and giving off an acetabular branch. **r. poste'rior arte'riae pancreaticoduodena'lis inferio'ris** [NA], posterior branch of inferior pancreaticoduodenal artery: a branch that ascends behind the head of the pancreas, which it sometimes pierces, and anastomoses with the posterior superior pancreaticoduodenal artery; it supplies the head of the pancreas and adjoining parts of the duodenum. **r. poste'rior arte'riae recurren'tis ulna'ris** [NA], posterior branch of ulnar recurrent artery: it runs to the back of the medial epicondyle, supplying the elbow joint and neighboring muscles. **r. poste'rior arte'riae rena'lis** [NA], the posterior branch of the renal artery, supplying the posterior segment of the kidney. **r. poste'rior arte'riae thyroi'deae superio'ris** [NA], posterior branch of superior thyroid artery: a vessel supplying the posterior part of the thyroid gland. **r. poste'rior duc'tus hepat'ici dex'tri** [NA], the posterior branch of the right hepatic duct. **r. poste'rior fissu'rae cer'ebri latera'lis [Syl'vii],** r. posterior sulci lateralis cerebri. **r. poste'rior ner'vi auricula'ris mag'ni** [NA], posterior branch of great auricular nerve: a branch, formed by division of the great auricular nerve, that innervates the skin over the mastoid process and the back of the external ear; modality, general sensory. **ra'mi posterio'res nervo'rum cervica'lium,** rami dorsales nervorum cervicalium. **r. poste'rior ner'vi coccyg'ei,** r. dorsalis nervi coccygei. **r. poste'rior ner'vi cuta'nei antebra'chii media'lis** [NA], posterior branch of medial antebrachial cutaneous nerve: a branch that innervates the skin of the posteromedial and medial aspects of the forearm; modality, general sensory. Called also *r. ulnaris nervi cutanei antebrachii medialis.* **r. poste'rior ner'vi laryn'gei inferio'ris,** posterior branch of inferior laryngeal nerve. **ra'mi posterio'res**

nervo′rum lumba′lium, rami dorsales nervorum lumbalium. **r. poste′rior ner′vi obturato′rii** [NA], posterior branch of obturator nerve: a branch that descends to innervate the knee joint, giving muscular branches to the obturator externus, adductor magnus, and sometimes the adductor brevis muscle; modality, general sensory and motor. **ra′mi posterio′res nervo′rum sacra′lium,** rami dorsales nervorum sacralium. **r. poste′rior nervo′rum spina′lium,** NA alternative for *r. dorsalis nervorum spinalium.* **ra′mi posterio′res nervo′rum thoraca′lium,** rami dorsales nervorum thoracicorum. **r. poste′rior ramo′rum cutaneo′rum latera′lium [abdomina′lium et pectora′lium] arteria′rum intercosta′lium,** posterior branch of (abdominal and thoracic) lateral cutaneous branches of intercostal arteries. **r. poste′rior ramo′rum cutaneo′rum latera′lium [abdomina′lium et pectora′lium] nervo′rum intercosta′lium,** posterior branch of (abdominal and thoracic) lateral cutaneous branches of intercostal nerves. **r. poste′rior sul′ci latera′lis cer′ebri** [NA], posterior branch of lateral cerebral sulcus: the part of the lateral cerebral sulcus that runs obliquely posteriorly between the temporal and the parietal lobes; called also *r. posterior fissurae cerebri lateralis [Sylvii].* **r. poste′rior ventri′culi sinis′tri** [NA], an interventricular continuation of the circumflex branch of the left coronary artery; it often consists of two or three vessels. Called also *r. ventriculi sinistri posterior.* **r. posterolatera′lis dex′ter,** an inconstant branch of the right coronary artery. **r. profun′dus arte′riae circumflex′ae fem′oris media′lis** [NA], deep branch of medial circumflex femoral artery: a branch ascending toward the trochanteric fossa, and anastomosing with gluteal branches. **r. profun′dus arte′riae glu′teae superio′ris** [NA], deep branch of superior gluteal artery: a branch passing forward between the gluteus medius and minimus muscles, and dividing into superior and inferior branches. **r. profun′dus arte′riae planta′ris media′lis** [NA], deep branch of medial plantar artery: it supplies the anteromedial aspect of the sole, anastomosing with the medial three plantar metatarsal arteries. **r. profun′dus arte′riae transver′sae cer′vicis** [NA], **r. profun′dus arte′riae transver′sae col′li,** deep branch of transverse cervical artery: it descends to supply medial and deep back muscles; sometimes replaced by an artery stemming directly from the subclavian artery (*arteria dorsalis scapularis*). Called also *descending* or *dorsal scapular artery, a. scapularis descendens,* and *a. scapularis dorsalis* [NA alternative]. **r. profun′dus ner′vi planta′ris latera′lis** [NA], deep branch of lateral plantar nerve: it accompanies the lateral plantar artery on its medial side and the plantar arch, innervating the interossei, the second, third, and fourth lumbrical, and the adductor hallucis muscles, and some articulations; modality, general sensory. **r. profun′dus ner′vi radia′lis** [NA], deep branch of radial nerve: a branch arising from the radial nerve and winding laterally around the radius to the back of the forearm, supplying the supinator, extensor digitorum, extensor digiti minimi, and extensor carpi ulnaris muscles, and often the extensor carpi radialis brevis muscle. Its continuation, the posterior interosseous nerve, supplies distal forearm muscles and the carpal and intercarpal joints; modality, motor. **r. profun′dus ner′vi ulna′ris** [NA], deep branch of ulnar nerve: the deep branch that is accompanied by the deep palmar branch of the ulnar artery, rounds the hook of the hamate bone, and follows the deep palmar arch beneath the flexor tendons, supplying the wrist joint, the interossei, third and fourth lumbrical, and adductor pollicis muscles, and usually the deep head of the flexor pollicis brevis muscle; modality, general sensory and motor. **ra′mi prosta′tici arte′riae vesica′lis inferio′ris** [NA], prostatic branches of inferior vesical artery: they supply the prostate and communicate with corresponding vessels on the opposite side. **ra′mi pterygoi′dei arte′riae maxilla′ris** [NA], **ra′mi pterygoi′dei arte′riae maxilla′ris inter′nae,** pterygoid branches of maxillary artery: they supply the pterygoid muscles. **r. pu′bicus arte′riae epigas′tricae inferio′ris** [NA], pubic branch of inferior epigastric artery: it arises from the inferior epigastric artery near the deep inguinal ring and descends on the back of the pubis, anastomosing through an obturator branch with the pubic branch of the obturator artery. **r. pu′bicus arte′riae obturato′riae** [NA], pubic branch of obturator artery: it ascends on the pelvic

surface of the ilium, anastomosing with its fellow of the other side and with the pubic branch of the inferior epigastric artery. **r. of pubis,** see *r. inferior ossis pubis* and *r. superior ossis pubis.* **r. of pubis, ascending,** r. superior ossis pubis. **r. of pubis, descending,** r. inferior ossis pubis. **ra′mi pulmona′les plex′us cardi′aci,** rami pulmonales systematis autonomici. **ra′mi pulmona′les systema′tis autonom′ici** [NA], pulmonary branches of autonomic system: branches from the sympathetic trunks and cardiac plexus, which, via the pulmonary plexuses, accompany the blood vessels and bronchi into the lungs; modality, sympathetic and visceral afferent. **ra′mi radicula′res arte′riae vertebra′lis,** NA alternative for *rami spinales arteriae vertebralis.* **r. rena′lis ner′vi splanch′nici mino′ris** [NA], renal branch of lesser splanchnic nerve: a branch from the lesser splanchnic nerve to the aorticorenal ganglion; modality, sympathetic preganglionic fibers and visceral afferent. **ra′mi rena′les ner′vi va′gi** [NA], **ra′mi rena′les plex′us coeli′aci,** renal branches of vagus nerve: branches passing from the vagal trunks via the celiac plexus to the kidney; modality, parasympathetic and visceral afferent. **ra′mi sacra′les latera′les arte′riae sacra′lis media′nae** [NA], lateral sacral branches of median sacral artery; they anastomose with the lateral sacral arteries laterally. **r. saphe′nus arte′riae descen′dentis genicula′ris** [NA], saphenous branch of descending genicular artery: a vessel that accompanies the saphenous nerve between the sartorius and gracilis muscles on the medial side of the knee, supplying the skin and anastomosing with the medial inferior genicular artery. Called also *r. saphenus arteriae genus descendentis.* **r. saphe′nus arte′riae ge′nus descen′dentis,** r. saphenus arteriae descendentis genicularis. **r. saphe′nus arte′riae ge′nu supre′mae,** r. saphenus arteriae genus descendens. **ra′mi scrota′les anterio′res arte′riae femora′lis** [NA], anterior scrotal branches of femoral artery: branches arising from the external pudendal arteries and supplying the anterior scrotal region in the male; called also *arteriae scrotales anteriores.* **ra′mi scrota′les posterio′res arte′riae puden′dae inter′nae** [NA], posterior scrotal branches of internal pudendal artery; two branches arising from the internal pudendal artery in the anterior part of the ischiorectal fossa, helping to supply the ischiocavernosus and bulbospongiosus muscles, and distributed to the scrotum; called also *arteriae scrotales posteriores.* **ra′mi septa′les anterio′res arte′riae ethmoida′lis anterio′ris** [NA], anterior septal branches of anterior ethmoidal artery: twigs of the posterior lateral nasal branch that supply the lateral wall and septum of the nose. **ra′mi septa′les posterio′res arte′riae sphenopalati′nae** [NA], posterior septal branches of sphenopalatine artery; they anastomose with the ethmoidal arteries. **r. sep′ti na′si arte′riae labia′lis superio′ris** [NA], nasal septum branch of superior labial artery: a branch that ramifies on the lower and front part of the nasal septum. **r. sinis′ter arte′riae hepat′icae pro′priae** [NA], left branch of proper hepatic artery: it supplies the left lobe of the liver. **r. sinis′ter arte′riae pulmona′lis,** arteria pulmonalis sinistra. **r. sinis′ter ve′nae por′tae hep′atis** [NA], the left branch of the portal vein of the liver, distributed to the left lobe of the liver. **r. si′nus carot′ici ner′vi glossopharyn′gei** [NA], branch of glossopharyngeal nerve to carotid sinus: a branch that supplies the pressoreceptors and chemoreceptors of the carotid sinus and carotid body with visceral afferent fibers. **r. si′nus caverno′si** [NA], a twig from the cavernous part of the internal carotid artery that supplies the walls of the cavernous sinus. **ra′mi spina′les arte′riae cervica′lis ascenden′tis** [NA], spinal branches of ascending cervical artery: they help supply the vertebral canal. **r. spina′lis arte′riae iliolumba′lis,** r. spinalis rami lumbalis arteriae iliolumbalis. **ra′mi spina′les arte′riae intercosta′lis supre′mae** [NA], spinal branches of highest intercostal artery: vessels arising from the dorsal branches of the first and second posterior intercostal arteries, entering intervertebral foramina with the corresponding two spinal nerves to help supply the contents of the vertebral canal. **r. spina′lis arteria′rum lumba′lium** [NA], spinal branch of lumbar arteries: a branch arising from the dorsal branch of the lumbar arteries and entering an intervertebral foramen with the spinal nerve to help supply the contents of the vertebral canal. **ra′mi spina′les arteria′rum sacra′lium latera′lium** [NA], spinal branches of lateral sacral arteries:

vessels arising from the two lateral sacral arteries and entering the pelvic sacral foramina to help supply the contents of the vertebral canal. **r. spina′lis arte′riae subcosta′lis** [NA], spinal branch of subcostal artery: a spinal branch corresponding to those arising from the dorsal branches of the posterior intercostal arteries; it enters the vertebral canal to help supply the contents of the canal. **ra′mi spina′les arte′riae vertebra′lis** [NA], branches of the transverse part of the vertebral artery that supply spinal cord and its meninges, the vertebral bodies, and the intervertebral disks; called also *rami radiculares arteriae vertebralis* [NA alternative], *radicular arteries,* and *spinal arteries.* **r. spina′lis ra′mi dorsa′lis arteria′rum intercosta′lium posterio′rum** [NA], spinal branch of dorsal branch of posterior intercostal arteries: one of the two branches into which the dorsal branch of a posterior intercostal artery divides, passing through the intervertebral foramen with the corresponding spinal nerve to help supply the contents of the vertebral canal. **r. spina′lis ra′mi lumba′lis arte′riae iliolumba′lis** [NA], spinal branch of lumbar branch of iliolumbar artery; it passes through the intervertebral foramen between the fifth lumbar vertebra and the sacrum to help supply the contents of the vertebral canal. **r. spina′lis vena′rum intercosta′lium,** r. spinalium venarum intercostalium posteriorum [IV–XI]. **r. spina′lis vena′rum intercosta′lium posterio′rum [IV–XI]** [NA], spinal branch of posterior intercostal veins: a vessel, the vena comitans of the arterial spinal branch, that emerges from the vertebral canal and contributes to the dorsal branch of each posterior intercostal vein. **ra′mi sple′nici arte′riae sple′nicae** [NA], splenic branches of splenic artery: the terminal branches of the splenic artery, which follow the trabeculae; called also *rami lienales arteriae lienales* [NA alternative]. **r. stape′dius arte′riae stylomastoi′deae** [NA], stapedial branch of stylomastoid artery: a variable branch supplying the stapedius muscle and tendon. **ra′mi sterna′les arte′riae mamma′riae inter′nae,** rami sternales arteriae thoracicae internae. **ra′mi sterna′les arte′riae thora′cicae inter′nae** [NA], sternal branches of internal thoracic artery: they supply the sternum and the transversus thoracis muscle. **ra′mi sternocleidomastoi′dei arte′riae occipita′lis** [NA], sternocleidomastoid branches of occipital artery: branches of the occipital artery, usually an upper and a lower, that supply the sternocleidomastoid and adjacent muscles. **r. sternocleidomastoi′deus arte′riae thyroi′deae superio′ris** [NA], sternocleidomastoid branch of superior thyroid artery: a branch that arises from the superior thyroid artery, but sometimes directly from the external carotid artery, passing across the carotid sheath to supply the middle portion of the sternocleidomastoid muscle. **r. stylohyoi′deus ner′vi facia′lis** [NA], stylohyoid branch of facial nerve: a branch that arises from the facial nerve just below the base of the skull to innervate the stylohyoid muscle; modality, motor. **r. stylopharyn′geus ner′vi glossopharyn′gei,** r. musculi stylopharyngei nervi glossopharyngei. **ra′mi subendocardia′les** [NA], the subendocardial ramifications of the conducting system of the heart (Purkinje fibers), which form a plexus in the papillary muscles and ventricles. Called also *Purkinje network* and *subendocardial terminal network.* **ra′mi submaxilla′res gan′glii submaxilla′ris,** rami glandulares ganglii submandibularis. **ra′mi subscapula′res arte′riae axilla′ris** [NA], subscapular branches of axillary artery: they supply the subscapularis muscle. **ra′mi substan′tiae ni′grae** [NA], small branches of the anterior choroidal artery that supply the substantia nigra. **ra′mi substan′tiae perfora′tae anterio′ris** [NA], small branches of the anterior choroidal artery that supply the anterior perforated substance. **r. superficia′lis arte′riae circumflex′ae fem′oris media′lis,** the superficial branch of the medial circumflex femoral artery. **r. superficia′lis arte′riae glu′teae superio′ris** [NA], superficial branch of superior gluteal artery: it ramifies to supply the gluteus maximus muscle. **r. superficia′lis arte′riae planta′ris media′lis** [NA], superficial branch of medial plantar artery: it supplies the medial side of the great toe. **r. superficia′lis arte′riae transver′sae cer′vicis** [NA], **r. superficia′lis arte′riae transver′sae col′li,** superficial branch of transverse cervical artery: a branch that arises from the transverse cervical artery at the anterior border of the levator scapulae muscle, it has ascending and descending

branches that supply the levator scapulae, trapezius, and splenius muscles. Called also *arteria cervicalis superficialis* [NA alternative] and *r. ascendens arteriae transversae colli.* **r. superficia′lis ner′vi planta′ris latera′lis** [NA], superficial branch of lateral plantar nerve: a branch that arises from the lateral plantar nerve at the lateral border of the quadratus plantae muscle and passes forward, dividing into a lateral part that innervates skin of the lateral side of the sole and little toe, joints of the toe, and the flexor digiti minimi brevis muscle, and a medial part, a common plantar digital nerve, that gives two proper plantar digital nerves to the adjacent sides of the fourth and fifth toes; modality, general sensory. **r. superficia′lis ner′vi radia′lis** [NA], superficial branch of radial nerve: the continuation of the radial nerve that accompanies the radial artery in the forearm, winds dorsalward, supplies the lateral side of the back of the hand, and divides into dorsal digital nerves that supply the skin of the dorsal surface and adjacent surfaces of the thumb, index, and middle fingers, and sometimes the radial side of the ring finger; modality, general sensory. **r. superficia′lis ner′vi ulna′ris** [NA], superficial branch of ulnar nerve: the branch of the ulnar nerve in the hand that supplies the palmaris brevis muscle and divides into a proper palmar digital nerve for the medial side of the little finger, a common palmar digital nerve giving off two proper nerves to supply adjacent sides of the little and fourth fingers, and sometimes palmar digital nerves also for the adjacent sides of the third and fourth fingers; modality, general sensory and motor. **r. supe′rior arte′riae glu′teae superio′ris** [NA], superior branch of superior gluteal artery: the upper division of the deep branch of the superior gluteal artery, extending as far as the anterior superior iliac spine and helping supply the gluteus medius, gluteus minimus, and tensor fasciae latae muscles. **ra′mi superio′res ner′vi cuta′nei col′li,** rami superiores nervi transversi colli. **r. supe′rior ner′vi oculomoto′rii** [NA], superior branch of oculomotor nerve: the upper and smaller of the two branches of the oculomotor nerve, which supplies the superior rectus muscle and, terminally, the levator palpebrae superioris; modality, motor. **ra′mi superio′res ner′vi transver′si col′li** [NA], superior branches of transverse cervical nerve: the upper of the branches that arise from the transverse cervical nerve near the anterior border of the sternocleidomastoid muscle, innervating skin and subcutaneous tissue in the anterior cervical region; modality, general sensory. Called also *rami superiores nervi cutanei colli.* **r. supe′rior os′sis is′chii,** a name formerly given to what is now considered the lower part of the body of the ischium (corpus ossis ischii). **r. supe′rior os′sis pu′bis** [NA], **superior r. of pubis,** the bar of bone projecting from the body of the pubic bone in a posterosuperolateral direction to the iliopubic eminence, and forming part of the acetabulum. **r. suprahyoi′deus arte′riae lingua′lis** [NA], suprahyoid branch of lingual artery: it passes along the upper border of the hyoid bone, supplying suprahyoid muscles and anastomosing with its fellow of the other side; called also *r. hyoideus arteriae lingualis.* **ra′mi suprarena′les superio′res arte′riae phren′icae inferio′ris,** see *arteria suprarenalis superior.* **r. sympathet′icus ad gan′glion submandibula′re,** NA alternative for *r. sympathicus ad ganglion submandibulare.* **r. sympathet′icus gan′glii cilia′res, r. sympath′icus gan′glii cilia′ris,** NA alternatives for *radix sympathica ganglii ciliaris.* **r. sympath′icus ad gan′glion submandibula′re** [NA], sympathetic branch to submandibular ganglión: a branch bearing sympathetic fibers, postganglionic from the superior cervical ganglion and derived from a plexus on the facial artery, to the submandibular ganglion, for distribution to the submandibular gland. Called also *r. sympatheticus ad ganglion submandibulare* [NA alternative] and *radix sympathica ganglii submaxillaris.* **ra′mi tempora′les anterio′res arte′riae occipita′lis latera′lis** [NA], the anterior temporal branches of the lateral occipital artery that supply the cortex of the anterior part of the temporal lobe. **ra′mi tempora′les interme′dii media′les arte′riae occipita′lis latera′lis** [NA], the medial intermediate branches of the lateral occipital artery that supply the cortex of the mediate and intermediate part of the temporal lobe. **ra′mi tempora′les ner′vi facia′lis** [NA], temporal branches of facial nerve: terminal branches of the facial nerve that innervate the anterior and superior auricular muscles, the frontal belly of the occipitofrontal muscle, and the orbicularis oculi and corrugator muscles; modality, motor. **r. tempora′les posterio′res arte′riae oc-cipita′lis latera′lis** [NA], the posterior temporal branches of the lateral occipital artery that supply the posterior part of the temporal lobe. **ra′mi tempora′les super-ficia′les ner′vi auriculotempora′lis** [NA], superficial temporal branches of auriculotemporal nerve: branches to the skin of the scalp in the temporal region; modality, general sensory. **r. tento′rii basa′lis arte′riae carot′idis inter′nae** [NA], r. basalis tentorii basalis arteriae carotidis internae. **r. tento′rii margina′lis arte′riae carot′i-dis inter′nae,** r. marginalis tentorii arteriae carotidis internae. **r. tento′rii ner′vi ophthal′mici** [NA], ten-torial branch of ophthalmic nerve: a branch that arises from the ophthalmic nerve close to its origin from the trigeminal ganglion, turning back to innervate the dura mater of the tentorium cerebelli and falx cerebri; modality, general sensory. Called also *r. meningeus nervi ophthalmici* [NA alterna-tive]. **ra′mi thalam′ici arte′riae cer′ebri posteri-o′ris** [NA], branches of the postcommunical part of the pos-terior cerebral artery that supply the thalamus. **r. thalam′icus arte′riae communican′tis posterio′-ris** [NA], a branch of the posterior communicating artery that supplies the thalamus. **ra′mi thy′mici arte′riae thora′cicae inter′nae** [NA], thymic branches of internal thoracic artery: branches distributed to the thymus gland in the anterior mediastinum; called also *arteriae thymicae*. **r. thyreohyoi′deus ner′vi hypoglos′si,** r. thyrohyoi-deus ansae cervicalis. **r. thyrohyoi′deus an′sae cer-vica′lis** [NA], thyrohyoid branch of ansa cervicalis: a branch from the superior root of the ansa cervicalis, innervating the thyrohyoid muscle; modality, motor. **r. tonsil′lae cerebel′li arte′riae inferio′ris posterio′ris cerebel′li** [NA], tonsillar branch of posterior inferior cere-bellar artery: a branch that ascends upward from the posterior inferior cerebellar artery to the tonsil of the cerebellum to supply the dentate nucleus of the cerebellum. **r. tonsilla′ris arte′riae facia′lis** [NA], **r. tonsilla′ris arte′riae maxilla′ris exter′ni,** tonsillar branch of facial artery: a vessel ascending from the facial artery on the pharynx to supply the tonsil and the root of the tongue. **ra′mi tonsilla′res ner′vi glossopharyn′gei** [NA], tonsillar branches of glossopharyngeal nerve: they supply the mucosa over the palatine tonsil and the adjacent portion of the soft palate; modality, general sensory. **ra′mi tra-chea′les arte′riae thora′cicae inter′nae** [NA], the tracheal branches of internal thoracic artery. **ra′mi tra-chea′les arte′riae thyroi′deae inferio′ris** [NA], tracheal branches of inferior thyroid artery: vessels supply-ing the trachea. **ra′mi trachea′les ner′vi laryn′gei recurren′tis** [NA], **ra′mi trachea′les ner′vi recur-ren′tis,** tracheal branches of recurrent laryngeal nerve: they are distributed to the tracheal mucosa; modality, general sensory. **ra′mi trac′tus op′tici** [NA], small branches of the anterior choroid artery that supply the optic tract. **r. transver′sus arte′riae circumflex′ae fem′oris latera′lis** [NA], transverse branch of lateral cir-cumflex femoral artery: a branch that pierces the vastus lateralis muscle, turning around the femur to anastomose with the transverse branch of the medial circumflex femoral artery and with other arteries, deep to the gluteus maximus muscle. **r. transver′sus arte′riae circumflex′ae fem′oris media′lis** [NA], transverse branch of medial cir-cumflex femoral artery: it passes between the quadratus femoris and adductor magnus muscles, supplying them, and then turning around the femur to anastomose with the transverse branch of the lateral circumflex femoral artery and with other arteries, deep to the gluteus maximus muscle. **r. trigemina′les et trochlea′res** [NA], a twig from the cavernous portion of the internal carotid artery that supplies the trigeminal and trochlear nerves. **r. tuba′lis ar-te′riae uteri′nae,** NA alternative for *r. tubarius arteriae uterinae.* **r. tuba′lis plex′us tympan′ici,** NA alter-native for *r. tubarius plexus tympanici.* **ra′mi tuba′rii arte′riae ova′ricae** [NA], tubal branches of ovarian ar-tery: they are distributed to the uterine tubes; called also *rami tubales arteriae ovaricae* [NA alternative]. **r. tuba′rius arte′riae uteri′nae** [NA], tubal branch of uterine artery: it supplies the uterine tube and the round ligament. Called also *r. tubalis arteriae uterina* [NA alterna-tive]. **r. tuba′rius plex′us tympan′ici** [NA], tubal branch of tympanic plexus: a branch given to the auditory tube from the tympanic plexus; modality, general sensory.

Called also *r. tubalis plexus tympanici* [NA alternative]. **ra′mi tu′beris cine′rei** [NA], small branches of the ante-rior choroidal artery that supply the tuber cinereum. **r. ulna′ris ner′vi cuta′nei antebra′chii media′lis,** r. posterior nervi cutanei antebrachii medialis. **ra′mi ureter′ici arte′riae duc′tus deferen′tis** [NA], ure-teral branches of artery of ductus deferens: they supply the lower portion of the ureter. **ra′mi ureter′ici arte′riae ova′ricae** [NA], ureteral branches of ovarian artery: they are distributed to the ureter. **ra′mi ureter′ici ar-te′riae rena′lis** [NA], ureteral branches of renal artery: they supply the upper portion of the ureter. **ra′mi ureter′ici arte′riae testicula′ris** [NA], ureteral branches of testicular artery: they are distributed to the ureter. **ra′mi vagina′les arte′riae recta′lis me′-diae** [NA], a branch of the middle rectal artery that supplies the vagina. **ra′mi vagina′les arte′riae uteri′nae** [NA], vaginal branches of uterine artery: two median longitu-dinal vessels formed by anastomosis of branches of the uterine and vaginal arteries, one of which descends in front of and the other behind the vagina. Called also *arteriae azygoi vaginae* [NA alternative] and *azygous arteries of vagina.* **ra′mi ventra′les nervo′rum cervica′lium** [NA], ven-tral branches of cervical nerves: the upper four form the cervical plexus, and the lower four form most of the brachial plexus; called also *rami anteriores nervorum cervicalium.* **r. ventra′lis ner′vi coccyg′ei** [NA], ventral branch of coccygeal nerve: the ventral branch of the last spinal nerve, which emerges from the sacral hiatus and helps form the coccygeal plexus; called also *r. anterior nervi coccygei.* **ra′mi ventra′les nervo′rum lumba′lium** [NA], ven-tral branches of lumbar nerves: the ventral branches of the five lumbar sacral nerves. The upper four branches form the lumbar plexus, and the fifth and a part of the fourth participate in formation of the sacral plexus. Called also *rami anteriores nervorum lumbalium.* **ra′mi ventra′les ner-vo′rum sacra′lium** [NA], ventral branches of sacral nerves: the ventral branches of the five sacral spinal nerves. The upper four branches emerge from the sacrum through the anterior sacral foramina and help form the sacral plexus; the fifth emerges through the sacral hiatus and, with a communication from the fourth, participates in formation of the coccygeal plexus. Called also *rami anteriores nervorum sacralium.* **r. ventra′lis nervo′rum spina′lium** [NA], ventral branch of spinal nerves: the larger, usually, of the two branches into which each spinal nerve divides almost as soon as it emerges from the intervertebral foramen; the ventral branches supply the ventral and lateral parts of the trunk and all parts of the limbs. Called also *r. anterior nervorum spinalium* [NA alternative]. **ra′mi ventra′les nervo′rum thoracico′rum** [NA], ventral branches of thoracic nerves: the ventral branches of the first eleven thoracic spinal nerves situated between the ribs, the first three of which give branches to the brachial plexus as well as to the thoracic wall; the fourth, fifth, and sixth supply only the thoracic wall; and the seventh to eleventh are thoracoab-dominal in distribution. Called also *intercostal nerves, nervi intercostales* [NA alternative], and *rami anteriores nervorum thoracalium.* The anterior primary division of the twelfth thoracic nerve is subcostal rather than intercostal in position, differing in course and relationships from the other ventral branches, and is known as the subcostal nerve (*nervus subcostales* [NA]). **r. ventri′culi sinis′tri poste′rior,** r. posterior ventriculi sinistri. **ra′mi vestibula′res ar-te′riae audi′ti′vae inter′nae,** rami vestibulares arteriae labyrinthi. **ra′mi vestibula′res arte′riae labyrin′-thi** [NA], vestibular branches of labyrinthine artery: vessels supplying the vestibule of the ear. **ra′mi viscera′les aor′tae abdomina′lis,** visceral branches of the abdomi-nal aorta. **ra′mi viscera′les aor′tae thoraca′lis,** visceral branches of the thoracic aorta. **ra′mi vis-cera′les arte′riae hypogas′tricae,** visceral branches of the hypogastric artery. **r. vola′ris ma′nus ner′vi ulna′ris,** r. palmaris nervi ulnaris. **r. vola′ris ner′vi cuta′nei antibrach′ii media′lis,** r. anterior nervi cuta-nei antebrachii medialis. **r. vola′ris profun′dus ar-te′riae ulna′ris,** r. palmaris profundus arteriae ulnaris. **r. vola′ris superficia′lis arte′riae radia′lis,** r. pal-maris superficialis arteriae radialis. **ra′mi zygomat′ici ner′vi facia′lis** [NA], zygomatic branches of facial nerve: branches that cross the zygomatic bone and innervate the orbicularis oculi muscle; modality, motor. **r. zygomaticofacia′lis ner′vi zygomat′ici** [NA], zygomaticofacial branch of zygomatic nerve: a branch that passes from the lateral wall of the orbit, piercing the zygomatic bone to supply overlying skin; modality, general sensory. **r. zygomaticotempora'lis ner'vi zygomat'ici** [NA], zygomaticotemporal branch of zygomatic nerve: a branch that passes from the lateral wall of the orbit, piercing the zygomatic bone to innervate skin of the anterior temporal region; modality, general sensory.

rancid (ran'sid) [L. *rancidus*] having a musty, rank taste or smell; applied to fats that have undergone decomposition, with the liberation of fatty acids.

rancidify (ran-sid'ĭ-fi) to decompose, with the liberation of fatty acids; a term applied especially to the decomposition of fats.

rancidity (ran-sid'ĭ-te) the quality of being rancid.

Randolph's test (ran'dolfs) [Nathaniel Archer *Randolph*, American physician, 1858–1887] see under tests.

random (ran'dom) [Old French *randon* violence] pertaining to a chance-dependent process, particularly one that occurs according to a known probability distribution.

randomize (ran'do-mīz) to assign experimental subjects to treatment groups according to some known probability distribution.

range (rānj) 1. the difference between the upper and lower limits of a variable or of a series of values. 2. the geographic region in which a given species is found. **r. of accommodation,** the alteration in the refractive state of the eye produced by accommodation. It is the difference in diopters between the refraction by the eye adjusted for its far point and that when adjusted for its near point. Called also *amplitude of accommodation.* **r. of audibility,** see under *limit.* **r. of motion,** the range, measured in degrees of a circle, through which a joint can be extended and flexed. **normal r., r. of normal,** see *reference values,* under *value.*

ranimycin (ran-ĭ-mi'sin) an antibacterial antibiotic derived from a variant of *Streptomyces lincolnensis.*

ranine (ra'nīn) [L. *raninus; rana* frog] pertaining to (*a*) a frog; (*b*) a ranula, or to the lower surface of the tongue; (*c*) the sublingual vein.

rank (rangk) in statistics, the position of a sample observation (or population value) in the sequence of sample values (or population values) arranged in order from lowest to highest.

Ranke's angle (rahn'kēz) [Hans Rudolph *Ranke*, Dutch anatomist, 1849–1887] see under *angle.*

Ranke's complex, formula, stages (rahn'kēz) [Karl Ernst *Ranke*, Munich internist, 1870–1926] see *primary complex,* under *complex,* and see under *formula* and *stage.*

ranula (ran'u-lah) [L., dim. of *rana* frog] a form of retention cyst of the floor of the mouth, usually due to obstruction of the ducts of the submaxillary or sublingual glands, presenting a slowly enlarging painless deep burrowing mucocele of one side of the mouth. Called also *sublingual cyst* and *sublingual ptyalocele.* **pancreatic r.,** a retention cyst of the pancreatic duct.

ranular (ran'u-lar) pertaining to or of the nature of a ranula.

Ranunculus (rah-nung'ku-lus) a genus of plants, the crowfoots and buttercups, certain species of which are poisonous; see also *risus sardonicus.*

Ranvier's crosses, etc. (rahn-ve-āz') [Louis Antoine *Ranvier,* French pathologist, 1835–1922] see under *cross, disk, node,* and *segment.*

Raoult's law (rah-ōlz') [François Marie *Raoult,* French physicist, 1830–1901] see under *law.*

raphania (rah-fa'ne-ah) [L. *raphanus;* Gr. *raphanos* radish] a chronic poisoning ascribed to the seeds of wild radish.

raphe (ra'fe) pl *ra'phae* [Gr. *rhaphē*] a seam; [NA] a general term for the line of union of the halves of various symmetrical parts. **abdominal r.,** linea alba. **amniotic r.,** the line of junction of the amniotic folds in the amnion of those vertebrates in which it is formed by folding. **r. anococcyg'ea, anococcygeal r.,** ligamentum anococcygeum. **r. cor'poris callo'si,** see *stria longitudinalis medialis corpus callosi* and *stria longitudinalis lateralis corporis callosi.* **longitudinal r. of tongue,** sulcus medianus linguae. **median r. of medulla oblongata, media'na medul'lae oblonga'tae,** r. medullae oblongatae. **median r. of neck, posterior,** ligamentum nuchae. **median r. of perineum,** r. perineales. **me-**

dian r. of pons, r. media'na ponti'na, r. pontis. **r. of medulla oblongata, r. medul'lae oblonga'tae** [NA], a median line at the union of the two lateral halves of the medulla oblongata which continues into the dorsal part of the pons; called also *median r. of medulla oblongata* and *r. mediana medullae oblongatae.* **r. pala'ti** [NA], **palatine r.,** a narrow whitish streak in the midline of the palate, extending from the incisive papilla to the tip of the uvula; it may present as a ridge in front and as a groove posteriorly. **palpebral r., lateral, r. palpebra'lis latera'lis** [NA], a thin horizontal band of connective tissue extending from the external angle of the rima palpebralis to the lateral margin of the orbit. **r. pe'nis** [NA], a narrow dark streak or ridge continuous posteriorly with the raphe scroti and extending forward for a variable distance along the midline on the under side of the penis; in the newborn it may extend to the tip of the glans. **perineal r., r. perinea'lis** [NA], **r. perine'i, r. of perineum,** a ridge along the median line of the perineum that runs forward from the anus; in the male, it is continuous with the raphe of the scrotum and raphe of the penis. Called also *median r. of perineum.* **r. pharyn'gis** [NA], **r. of pharynx,** a more or less distinct band of connective tissue extending downward from the base of the skull along the posterior wall of the pharynx in the median plane, and giving attachment to the constrictor muscles of the pharynx. **r. of pons, r. pon'tis** [NA], a median line at the union of the two lateral halves of the pons, which is a continuation of the raphe of the medulla oblongata into the dorsal part of the pons; called also *median r. of pons* and *r. mediana pontina.* **pterygomandibular r., r. pterygomandibula'ris** [NA], a tendinous line between the buccinator and the constrictor pharyngis superior muscles, from which the middle portions of both muscles originate. **scrotal r., r. scrota'lis,** r. scroti. **r. scro'ti** [NA], **r. of scrotum,** a ridge along the surface of the scrotum in the median line, dividing it into nearly equal lateral parts; called also *r. scrotalis* and *scrotal r.*

rapport (rah-por') [Fr.] a relation of harmony and accord between two persons, as between patient and physician.

rarefaction (rār''ĕ-fak'shun) [L. *rarefactio*] the condition of being or becoming less dense; diminution in density and weight, but not in volume.

Ras. abbreviation for L. *rasu'rae,* scrapings or filings.

rash (rash) a temporary eruption on the skin, as in urticaria; a drug eruption or viral exanthem. **brown-tail r.,** see under *dermatitis.* **butterfly r.,** butterfly, def. 3. **caterpillar r.,** see *insect dermatitis,* under *dermatitis.* **diaper r.,** see under *dermatitis.* **drug r.,** drug eruption. **heat r.,** miliaria rubra. **hydatid r.,** an urticarial eruption which sometimes follows tapping or rupture of a hydatid cyst. **wandering r.,** benign migrating glossitis.

rasion (ra'zhun) [L. *rasio*] the grating of drugs with a file.

Rasmussen's aneurysm (ras'mus-ens) [Fritz Waldemar *Rasmussen,* Danish physician, 1834–1877] see under *aneurysm.*

raspatory (ras'pah-to-re) [L. *raspatorium*] a file or rasp for surgical use; a xyster.

RAST radioallergosorbent test; see under *tests.*

rasura (rah-su'rah) [L.] scrapings or filings.

rat (rat) a small, aggressive, and omnivorous rodent of the genus *Rattus* and related genera of the family Muridae, commonly found about human habitations. Rats not only cause great economic loss but are vectors of human disease; they harbor at least eleven different species of intestinal parasites that may be transmitted to man, such as tapeworms, roundworms, and trichinae; they are the reservoirs for the infective agents of plague, typhus, Weil's disease, and rat-bite fever. Albino mutants of *R. norvegicus* are used as laboratory animals. **albino r.,** white r. **BBr.,** a strain that serves as a model of type I diabetes mellitus. **black r.,** *Rattus rattus,* the European black rat and the one most commonly responsible for transmitting plague to man by means of its flea (*Xenopsylla cheopis*). **brown r.,** *Rattus norvegicus;* also called the barn rat, gray rat, Norway rat, sewer rat, and wharf rat. It is larger than the black rat, has a brownish gray color, and short ears and tail. **Egyptian r.,** *Rattus rattus alexandrinus,* a black rat originally found in North Africa, but now distributed worldwide. **Holtzman r.,** a strain of albino rat descended originally from S–D strain which originated from Wistar Institute sometime before 1929. **Long-Evans r.,** a strain of rat, developed at the

University of Rochester, characterized by a brownish to black color of the head and shoulders. **roof r.,** Egyptian r. **Sprague-Dawley r.,** a strain of albino rat developed by the Sprague-Dawley Animal Company, which is widely used in experimental work because of its calmness and ease of handling. **white r.,** an albino form of *Rattus rattus* or of *R. norvegicus* which is much used as a laboratory animal. **Wistar r.,** a strain of albino rat developed at the Wistar Institute but which has spread so widely to other institutions that there is probably marked dilution of the strain. **wood r.,** a rat of the genus *Neotoma;* they are hosts of fleas and ticks. Called also *pack rat, trade rat, mountain rat,* and *brush rat.*

rate (rāt) [L. *rata,* from *ratus* calculated] 1. the amount of change of a physical quantity per unit time. 2. the number of occurrences of an event per unit time. In epidemiology and demography, correctly applied only fractions for which all of the cases contributing to the numerator are also counted in the denominator and for which the denominator is the entire population at risk. Rates are often multiplied by a factor to give the number of events per 1000, 10,000, or 100,000 population. 3. generally, a proportion that does not include a unit of time, e.g., case fatality rate, prevalence rate. **adjusted r.,** a fictitious summary rate statistically adjusted to remove the effect of a demographic variable such as age or sex, thus permitting unbiased comparison between groups with different demographic structure. Called also *standardized r.* Cf. *crude r.* and *specific r.* **attack r.,** an incidence rate, especially one that varies over time, e.g., the incidence rate during an epidemic. **basal metabolic r.,** an expression of the rate at which oxygen is utilized by the body cells, or the calculated equivalent heat production by the body, in a fasting subject at complete rest. Abbreviated B.M.R. See also *basal metabolism,* under *metabolism.* **birth r.,** a rate in which the numerator is the number of live births in a geographic area in one year. The denominator of the *crude birth rate* is the average total population or the midyear population in the area during the year. To obtain the *true birth rate* the average or midyear female population of childbearing age is used as the denominator. **case r.,** attack r. **case fatality r.,** the proportion of persons contracting a disease who die of that disease: the numerator is the number of deaths caused by a disease and the denominator is the number of diagnosed cases of the disease. Called also *case fatality ratio, fatality r.,* and *lethality r.* **circulation r.,** an expression of the amount of blood pumped per minute by the heart through the body. **crude r.,** a summary rate based on the total number of events occurring in an entire population over a period of time: the numerator is the actual number of events in a population and the denominator is the total population. Cf. *adjusted r.* and *specific r.* **death r.,** a rate expressing the number of deaths in a population at risk. The *crude death rate* is the ratio of the number of deaths in a geographic area in one year divided by the average or midyear population in the area during the year. An *age-specific death rate* is the ratio of the number of deaths occurring in a specified age group in one year to the average or midyear population of that group. A *cause-specific death rate* is the ratio of the number of deaths due to a specified cause in one year to the average or midyear total population. Called also *mortality r.* **DEF r.,** an expression of dental caries experience in deciduous teeth: calculated by adding number of decayed primary teeth requiring filling (*D*), decayed primary teeth requiring extraction (*E*), and primary teeth successfully filled (*F*); missing primary teeth are not included in the calculation. **DMF r.,** an expression of the condition of the teeth based on the number of teeth decayed, missing, or indicated for removal and of those filled or bearing restorations: calculated by adding number of carious permanent teeth requiring filling (*D*), carious permanent teeth requiring extraction (*Mr*), permanent teeth previously extracted because of caries (*Mp*), and permanent teeth filled (*F*). Number of DMF teeth per child of a specific age or age group is calculated by the formula:

$$\frac{D \text{ teeth} + Mr \text{ teeth} + Mp \text{ teeth} + F \text{ teeth}}{\text{number of children examined}} = \text{DMF}$$

dose r., the amount of any agent administered per unit of time. **erythrocyte sedimentation r. (ESR),** the rate at which erythrocytes sediment from a well-mixed specimen of venous blood, as measured by the distance that the top of the column of erythrocytes falls in a specified time interval under specified conditions; an increase in ESR is usually due to elevated levels of plasma proteins, especially fibrinogen and immunoglobulins, which decrease the zeta potential on erythrocytes by dielectric shielding and thus promote rouleaux formation; marked elevations are seen in monoclonal gammopathies, hypergammaglobulinemias due to inflammatory disease, and in hyperfibrinogenemias; moderate elevation usually indicates active inflammatory disease; the ESR is also increased in anemia. See *Westergren method* and *Wintrobe method* under *method,* and cf. *zeta sedimentation ratio (ZSR)* under *ratio.* **fatality r.,** case fatality r. **fetal death r.,** the ratio of the number of fetal deaths in one year to the number of live births and fetal deaths in that year. **five-year survival r.,** an expression of the number of survivors with no trace of disease five years after each has been diagnosed or treated for the same disease. **glomerular filtration r. (GFR),** the quantity of glomerular filtrate formed per unit time in all nephrons of both kidneys, equal to the inulin clearance, usually measured clinically by the endogenous creatinine clearance. **growth r.,** an expression of the increase in size of an organic object per unit time, calculations usually being made as to both the absolute and the relative increment. **heart r.,** the number of contractions of the ventricles of the heart per unit of time (usually a minute). It usually corresponds to the pulse rate, but occasionally some of the contractions of the left ventricle fail to produce peripheral pulse waves, so that the rate of the pulse at the wrist is less than that of the heart. **incidence r.,** the number of new cases of disease in a population over a period of time: the numerator of the rate is the number of new cases during a specified time period and the denominator is the population at risk during the period. Cf. *prevalence r.* **infant mortality r.,** the ratio of the number of deaths in one year of children less than one year of age to the number of live births in that year. **lethality r.,** case fatality r. **maternal mortality r.,** a rate in which the numerator is the number of maternal deaths ascribed to puerperal causes in one year; the number of live births in that year is often used as the denominator although to make a true rate the denominator should be the number of live births and fetal deaths. Called also *puerperal mortality r.* **morbidity r.,** a rate in which the numerator is a number of cases of a disease, e.g., an *incidence r.* or *prevalence r.* **mortality r.,** death r. **mutation r.,** the number of mutations at a given locus per gamete per generation. See also *mutant proportion,* under *proportion.* **neonatal mortality r.,** the ratio of the number of deaths in one year of children less than 28 days of age to the number of live births in that year. **oocyst r.,** the percentage of wild female mosquitoes found to contain oocysts in the midgut. **output exposure r.,** in radiology, the exposure to radiation at a specified point per unit of time, usually expressed in roentgens per minute. **parasite r.,** the percentage of persons, in a particular age group or area, in whom parasites, especially malarial parasites, can be found. **perinatal mortality r.,** the ratio of the number of fetal deaths after 28 or more weeks of gestation and deaths of infants less than 7 days of age in one year to the number of live births and fetal deaths after 28 or more weeks of gestation in that year. **prevalence r.,** the number of people in a population who have a disease at a given time: the numerator of the rate is the number of existing cases of disease at a point in time and the denominator is the total population. **puerperal mortality r.,** maternal mortality r. **pulse r.,** the rate of pulsation noted in a peripheral artery per minute, normally from 50 to 100. **respiration r.,** an expression of the number of movements of the chest, indicative of inspiration and expiration, occurring per minute. **secondary attack r.,** the attack rate in a closed exposed group, such as a household. The index case, which brings the group to the attention of the investigator, and also other initial cases occurring too early to be related to the index case are excluded from both the numerator and the denominator. **sedimentation r.,** the rate at which a sediment is deposited in a given volume of solution, especially when subjected to the action of a centrifuge; see also *erythrocyte sedimentation r.* **sickness r.,** morbidity r. **specific r.,** a rate that applies to a specific demographic subgroup, e.g., individuals of a specific age, sex, or race. Cf. *adjusted r.* and *crude r.* **sporozoite r.,** the percentage of wild female mosquitoes found to contain sporozoites in the glands. **standardized r.,** adjusted r. **stillbirth r.,** an expression of the relation of the number of stillbirths to the total number of births.

Rathke's pouch, etc. (rahth′kez) [Martin Heinrich *Rathke*, German anatomist, 1793–1860]   see under *column, cyst, fold, pouch, trabecula,* and *tumor.*

raticide (rat′ĭ-sīd)   an agent destructive to rats.

ratio (ra′she-o) [L.]   an expression of the quantity of one substance or entity in relation to that of another; the relationship between two quantities expressed as the quotient of one divided by the other.   **A-G r., albumin-globulin r.,** the ratio of albumin to globulin in the blood serum, plasma, or the urine in various types of renal disease.   **arm r.,** a figure expressing the relation of the length of the longer arm of a mitotic chromosome to that of the shorter arm.   **birth-death r.,** vital index.   **body-weight r.,** body weight in grams divided by stature in centimeters.   **cardiothoracic r.,** the ratio of the transverse diameter of the heart to the internal diameter of the chest at its widest point just above the level of the dome of the diaphragm, a rough guide to cardiac enlargement, being normally less than 0.5.   **case fatality r.,** case fatality rate.   **cell color r.,** the result obtained by dividing the percentage of red cells by the percentage of hemoglobin.   **concentration r.,** the ratio of the average concentration of a solid in the urine to its concentration in the blood.   **curative r.,** therapeutic r.   **D-N r., dextrose-nitrogen r.,** the ratio between the dextrose and the nitrogen of the urine.   **expiratory exchange r.,** the ratio of carbon dioxide output to oxygen uptake in respiration.   **fetal death r.,** the ratio of fetal deaths in one year to the number of live births in that year.   **G-N r., glucose-nitrogen r.,** D-N r.   **grid r.,** in radiology, the ratio of the height of the lead strips to the width of the interspacing of a grid.   **hand r.,** the ratio of the length of the hand to its width.   **holdaway r.,** a means of expressing the relationship of the pogonion and the lower incisor to the nasion-basion plane; used in roentgenographic cephalometric diagnosis.   **karyoplasmic r.,** nucleocytoplasmic r.   **ketogenic-antiketogenic r.,** the proportion between substances that form glucose in the body and those that form fatty acids.   **lecithin-sphingomyelin r. (L/S r.),** the ratio of lecithin to sphingomyelin concentration in the amniotic fluid, used to predict the degree of pulmonary maturity of the fetus and thus the risk of respiratory difficulties.   **mendelian r.,** an expression of the occurrence of distinctly contrasted mendelian characters in succeeding generations of hybrid offspring.   **nucleocytoplasmic r., nucleoplasmic r.,** the ratio of nuclear to cytoplasmic volume.   **nutritive r.,** the ratio between the digestible protein and the digestible fats and carbohydrates in a ration in stock feeding.   **proportionate mortality r. (PMR),** 1. the ratio of the number of deaths from a particular cause to the total number of deaths in the same time period.   2. in occupational epidemiology, the ratio of observed deaths due to a specific cause in an occupational cohort to the expected deaths due to that cause, as determined by the proportion of deaths from the cause in the general population or comparison population, multiplied by 100. Cf. *standardized mortality r.*   **respiratory exchange r.,** expiratory exchange r.   **sex r.,** an expression of the number of males in a population to the number of females, usually stated as the number of males per 100 females.   **standardized morbidity r. (SMR),** a ratio like a standardized mortality ratio except that cases of disease rather than deaths are the observed data.   **standardized mortality r. (SMR),** the ratio of the number of observed deaths in a study population to the number of expected deaths in that population. The expected deaths are calculated by classifying the study group by demographic variables such as age, sex, or race; computing the expected deaths for each class by multiplying the number of individuals in the study group in that class by the class-specific death rate in a standard reference population; and adding the expected deaths in all classes. Cf. *proportionate mortality r.,* def 2.   **stimulation r. (SR),** see *lymphocyte proliferation test* under *tests.*   **therapeutic r.,** the fraction of the minimal lethal dose of a drug that is therapeutically effective; called also *curative r.*   **urea excretion r.,** the ratio of the number of milligrams of urea in the urine excreted in one hour to the number of milligrams in 100 ml. of blood; the normal ratio is 50.   **zeta sedimentation r. (ZSR),** a measurement comparable to the erythrocyte sedimentation rate (ESR), except that it is unaffected by anemia. Blood specimens are centrifuged in an instrument (the Zetafuge) that produces controlled cycles of compaction and dispersion that allow rouleaux to form and sediment rapidly; the packed cell volume (zetacrit) produced by this procedure divided into the true hematocrit gives the ZSR.

ration (ra′shun) [L. *ratio* proportion]   a fixed allowance of food or drink per day or other unit of time.   **basal r.,** a ration giving the required energy, but lacking in one or more vitamins.

rational (rash′un-al) [L. *rationalis* reasonable]   based upon reason; characterized by possession of one's reason.

rationale (rash″un-al′) [L.]   a rational exposition of principles; the logical basis of a procedure.

rationalization (rash″un-al-i-za′shun)   an unconscious defense mechanism by which one justifies, by an incorrect application of reason, attitudes and behavior that would otherwise be intolerable.

rat-tails (rat′tālz)   a swollen condition of the hair papillae over the flexor tendons of a horse's legs, due to filth and bacteria.

rattlesnake (rat″l-snāk)   any of the New World pit vipers of the genera *Crotalus* and *Sistrurus,* having a series of cornified interlocking segments at the tip of the tail; when disturbed they vibrate the tail to produce the characteristic rattling or buzzing sound. See table accompanying *snake.*

Rattus (rat′us)   a genus of small rodents, the rats (see *rat*).   **R. norve′gicus,** the brown rat.   **R. rat′tus,** the black rat.   **R. rat′tus alexandri′nus,** the Egyptian, or roof, rat.

Rau's apophysis, process (row) [Johann J. *Rau* (Ravius), Dutch anatomist, 1658–1719]   processus anterior mallei.

Rauber's layer (row′berz) [August Antinous Rauber, German anatomist, 1841–1917]   see under *layer.*

Rauchfuss' triangle (rowsh′foos) [Karl Andreyevich *Rauchfuss,* pediatrician in Leningrad, 1835–1915]   see *Grocco's sign* (def. 1), under *sign.*

rauschbrand (rowsh′brahnt) [Ger.]   blackleg.

Rau-Sed (row′sed)   trademark for a preparation of reserpine.

Rauserpa (raw-ser′pah)   trademark for a preparation of rauwolfia serpentina.

Rauwiloid (row′wĭ-loid)   trademark for preparations of alseroxylon.

Rauwolfia (raw-wul′fe-ah)   a genus of apocyanaceous tropical trees and shrubs, including over 100 species, and providing numerous alkaloids, including reserpine, of medical interest. Many species have been used in South America, Africa, and Asia, as a source of several medicines.   **R. serpenti′na,** (L.) Benth. ex Kurz, a small shrub native to India and the Orient, containing many alkaloids, of which reserpine and rescinnamine are the most important therapeutically; the root is used as the whole root or as isolated alkaloids as a hypotensive, tranquilizer, and sedative.

rauwolfia (raw-wol′fe-ah)   any member of the genus *Rauwolfia;* the dried root or an extract of the dried root of *Rauwolfia.*   **r. serpenti′na** [USP], the dried root of *Rauwolfia serpentina,* sometimes with fragments of rhizome and aerial stem bases attached, containing not less than 0.15 per cent of reserpine-rescinnamine group alkaloids, calculated as reserpine; used as an antihypertensive. It is also used as a sedative and tranquilizer.   **r. serpenti′na, powdered** [USP], rauwolfia serpentina reduced to a very fine powder adjusted, if necessary, to contain between 0.15 and 0.20 per cent of reserpine-rescinnamine group alkaloids.

Rauzide (rou′zīd)   trademark for preparations of rauwolfia serpentine with bendroflumethiazide.

RAV   Rous associated virus.

Ravius (ra′ve-us)   see *Rau.*

ray (ra) [L. *radius* spoke]   a line emanating from a center, as (*a*) a more or less distinct portion of radiant energy (light or heat), proceeding in a specific direction (used in the plural as a general term for any form of radiant energy, whether vibratory or particulate), or (*b*) one of the individual elements at the distal end of the limb of an early embryo, foretelling development of the metacarpal or metatarsal bones and the phalanges of the digits.   **actinic r.,** a light ray which produces chemical changes. In general, light rays become more actinic as one passes from the red through the spectrum to the violet and even into the ultraviolet.   **alpha r's, α-r's,** high-speed helium nuclei which have been ejected from radioactive substances. Owing to their high velocity (one tenth that of light) their kinetic energy is so great that a single alpha particle produces a microscopic flash of light when it hits a spinthariscope; when it hits another atom (as of nitrogen) it may cause it to disintegrate. **anode r's,** positive r's. **antirachitic r's,** ultraviolet rays between 2700 and 3020 A.U. **astral r.,** one of the rays of an aster. Called also *polar r.* **Becquerel r's,** former name for rays emitted from uranium and other radioactive substances, and now known as alpha, beta, and gamma rays. **beta r's,** β-r's, electrons ejected from radioactive substances with velocities which may be as high as 0.98 of the velocity of light. **Blondlot r's,** n r's. **caloric r.,** radiant energy which is converted into heat when applied to the body. **canal r's,** positive rays in a vacuum tube; so called from having been first obtained by allowing the discharge from the anode to pass through a perforated (canalized) cathode. **cathode r's,** negative particles of electricity streaming out in a vacuum tube at right angles to the surface of the cathode and away from it irrespective of the position of the anode. They move in a straight line unless deflected by a magnet. By striking on solids they generate roentgen rays. See also *electron stream.* **central r.,** the straight line passing through the center of the radiation source and the center of the final beam-limiting diaphragm. **characteristic r's,** roentgen rays emitted as a result of the rearrangement of electrons in the inner shells of atoms following the ejection of electrons from the inner shells by high-speed bombarding electrons; the wavelengths of the rays produced depend on the element and the energy levels involved. Cf. *characteristic fluorescent r's.* **characteristic fluorescent r's,** secondary rays emitted as a result of the rearrangement of electrons in the inner shells of atoms; identical with characteristic rays (q.v.) except that characteristic rays are caused by the bombardment of the x-ray tube target by electrons, whereas characteristic fluorescent rays are caused by primary ray photon bombardment of an absorbing material. **chemical r.,** actinic r. **convergent r.,** a ray which is approaching a focus; it may be produced by passage through a convex lens or by reflection from a concave mirror. **cosmic r's,** a form of very penetrating radiations which apparently move through interplanetary space in every direction; called also *Millikan rays* and *ultra x-rays.* **delta r's,** δ-r's, secondary beta rays produced in a gas by the passage of alpha particles. **digital r.,** a digit of the hand or foot and the corresponding portion of the metacarpus or metatarsus, considered as a continuous structural unit. **direct r.,** primary r. **divergent r's,** rays coming from a source nearer than infinity, or a pencil or bundle of light rays directed away from a focus after passing through a concave lens or after being reflected from a convex mirror. **Dorno's r's,** the active biological ultraviolet rays, i.e., those below 2890 A.U. **dynamic r's,** rays that are active physically or therapeutically. **erythema-producing r's,** rays that cause erythema, 2050 to 3100 A.U. **Finsen r's,** see under *light.* **fluorescent r's,** characteristic fluorescent r's. **gamma r's,** γ-r's, electromagnetic radiation of short wavelengths emitted by the nucleus of an atom during a nuclear reaction. They consist of high energy photons, have no mass and no electric charge, and travel with the speed of light and are usually associated with beta rays. **glass r's,** the rays formed in a roentgen-ray tube by the cathode rays striking the glass wall of the tube, so called to distinguish them from the roentgen rays originating at the anticathode. **Goldstein's r's,** rays formed when roentgen rays pass through some transparent medium; called also s r's. **grenz r's,** very soft roentgen rays with a wavelength of about 2 A.U., lying between roentgen rays and ultraviolet rays in the electromagnetic spectrum. **H r's,** a stream of hydrogen nuclei. **hard r's,** roentgen rays of short wavelength, high energy, and great penetrative power. **heat r's,** see *radiant heat,* under *heat.* **hertzian r's,** see under *wave.* **incident r.,** see reflection, def. 2., and refraction, def. 2. **indirect r's,** rays formed at the surface of the glass of the cathode ray tube. **infrared r's,** radiations just beyond the red end of the visible spectrum; their wavelengths range between 0.75 and 1000 μm; see *infrared.* **infra roentgen r's,** grenz r's. **intermediate r's,** wavelengths between the ultraviolet and the roentgen rays. **Lenard r's,** cathode rays after they have passed outside the discharge tube. **luminous r's,** the visible rays of the spectrum. **Lyman r's,** electromagnetic vibrations of wavelength between 600 and 12,300 A.U. **medullary r.,** any cortical extension of a bundle of tubules from a malpi-

ghian pyramid of the kidney. **Millikan r's,** cosmic r's. **minin r's,** rays generated by passing incandescent light through dark-blue glass. **n r's,** an alleged form of radiation, the identity of which is not well established. Called also *Blondlot r's.* A variety of n rays (called *n' rays*) differ from other n rays in diminishing the luminosity of light and of faintly luminous surfaces. **necrobiotic r's,** short ultraviolet rays which kill living cells. **Niewenglowski's r's,** luminous rays given out by substances which have been exposed to the sun. **paracathodic r's,** rays formed by the impaction of cathode rays against a body (the anticathode) in their path. **parallel r's,** rays which come from a source at an infinite distance; divergent rays may be made parallel by means of a convex lens or a concave mirror. **pigment-producing r's,** rays that cause pigmentation, with a wavelength of 2500–3000 A.U. **polar r.,** astral r. **positive r's,** streams of positively charged atoms traveling at high speed from the anode of a partially evacuated tube under the influence of an applied voltage. **primary r's,** rays coming directly from a source, such as a radioactive substance or an x-ray tube, without interactions with matter. **reflected r.,** see reflection, def. 3. **refracted r.,** see refraction, def. 2. **roentgen r's,** electromagnetic vibrations of short wavelengths (from 5 A.U. down) or corresponding quanta (wave mechanics) that are produced when electrons moving at high velocity impinge on various substances, especially the heavy metals. They are commonly generated by passing a current of high voltage (from 10,000 volts up) through a Coolidge tube (see under *tube*). They are able to penetrate most substances to some extent, some much more readily than others, and to affect a photographic plate. These qualities make it possible to use them in taking roentgenograms of various parts of the body, thus revealing the presence and position of fractures or foreign bodies or of radiopaque substances that have been purposely introduced. They can also cause certain substances to fluoresce and this makes fluoroscopy possible, by which the size, shape and movements of various organs such as the heart, stomach and intestines can be observed. By reason of the high energy of their quanta, they strongly ionize tissue through which they pass by means of the photoelectrons, both primary and secondary, which they liberate. Because of this effect they are used in treating various pathological conditions. Called also *x-rays.* **s r's,** Goldstein's r's. **Sagnac r's,** secondary beta rays formed when gamma rays are reflected from a metal surface. **scattered r's,** secondary rays whose direction has been changed by interaction with matter in their passage through a substance. See also *scattering.* **Schumann r's,** rays of wavelengths between 1850 and 1220 A.U. **secondary r.,** rays generated by the interaction of primary rays with matter. **soft r's,** roentgen rays of long wavelength, low energy, and little penetrative power. **titanium r.,** the radiation produced between metallic electrodes which consist of a tungsten alloy containing titanium. **ultraviolet r's,** those invisible rays of the spectrum which are beyond the violet rays; their wavelengths range between 4 and 400 nm.; see *ultraviolet.* **ultra x-r.,** Millikan r's. **vital r's,** ultraviolet rays, between 2900 and 3200 A.U., which are the rays that act on the body therapeutically. **W r's,** intermediate r's. **x-r's,** the name given by Röntgen to roentgen rays.

Raymond's apoplexy (ra-mawz′) [Fulgence *Raymond,* French neurologist, 1844–1910] see under *apoplexy.*

Raymond-Cestan (ra-maw′-ses-tan′) [F. *Raymond;* Etienne Jacques Marie Raymond *Cestan,* French surgeon, 1867–1912] see under *syndrome.*

Raynaud's disease (gangrene), phenomenon (ra-nōz′) [Maurice *Raynaud,* French physician, 1834–1881] see under *disease* and *phenomenon.*

Rb chemical symbol for *rubidium.*

R.B.C. red blood cell; red blood [cell] count (see *blood count,* under *count*).

RBC IT red blood cell iron turnover.

RBE relative biological effectiveness; see under *effectiveness.*

R.C.M. Royal College of Midwives.

R.C.N. Royal College of Nursing.

R.C.O.G. Royal College of Obstetricians and Gynaecologists.

R.C.P. Royal College of Physicians.

rcp   reciprocal translocation.

R.C.S.   Royal College of Surgeons.

RCU   red cell utilization.

R.C.V.S.   Royal College of Veterinary Surgeons.

R.D.   reaction of degeneration; see under *reaction*.

rd.   abbreviation for *rutherford*.

RDE   receptor-destroying enzyme.

R.E.   radium emanation (see *radon*); right eye.

Re   chemical symbol for *rhenium*.

re- [L.]   a prefix meaning back or again.

reablement (re-a′b′l-ment)   rehabilitation.

reabsorb (re″ab-sorb′)   to absorb again; to undergo or to subject to reabsorption (q.v.); to resorb.

reabsorption (re″ab-sorp′shun)   1. the act or process of absorbing again, as the selective absorption by the kidneys of substances (glucose, proteins, sodium, etc.) already secreted into the renal tubules, and their return to the circulating blood. 2. resorption.

react (re-akt′)   1. to respond to a stimulus. 2. to enter into chemical action.

reactance (re-ak′tans)   the weakening of an alternating electric current caused by passage through a coil of wire.

reactant (re-ak′tant)   an original substance entering into a chemical reaction. **acute phase r.,** a plasma protein whose concentration increases or decreases in conjunction with inflammatory processes, e.g., haptoglobin, alpha₁-antitrypsin, orosmucoid, C3, ceruloplasmin, fibrinogen, and C-reactive protein.

reaction (re-ak′shun) [re- + L. *agere* to act]   1. opposite action, or counteraction; the response to stimulation. 2. the phenomena caused by the action of chemical agents; a chemical process in which one substance is transformed into another substance or substances. For specially named reactions not defined here, see under *tests*. 3. in psychology, the mental and/or emotional state elicited in response to any particular situation. **accelerated r.,** a reaction or response which occurs in a shorter time than is usual. **acetic acid r.,** Rivalta's r. **acid r.,** 1. a surplus of hydrogen ions in a solution or a pH below 7. 2. any test by which an acid reaction is recognized, such as the reddening of blue litmus. **acrosome r.,** a sequence of structural changes that occur in spermatozoa when in the vicinity of an ovum in the oviduct, and that are believed to facilitate entry of a spermatozoon into the ovum: the outer membrane of the acrosome fuses at multiple points with the overlying plasma membrane of the sperm head, creating openings through which the enzymes of the acrosome are liberated. **acute situational r., acute stress r.,** a transient, self-limiting acute emotional reaction to severe psychological stress; equivalent DSM III categories are *adjustment disorder* (nonpsychotic reactions), *brief reactive psychosis* (psychotic reactions), and *post-traumatic stress disorder* (characteristic symptomatology). Called also *transient situational disturbance.* **adjustment r.,** see under *disorder.* **alarm r.,** the physiologic effects (increased blood pressure and cardiac output, increased blood flow to skeletal muscles, decreased flow to the viscera, increased rate of glycolysis and blood glucose concentration) mediated by sympathetic nervous system discharge and release of adrenal medullary hormones in response to acute stress, fright, or rage. Called also *fight-or-flight r.* and *stress r.* **alkaline r.,** 1. the presence in a solution of more hydroxyl ions than hydrogen ions, i.e., a pH greater than 7. 2. any test by which an alkaline reaction is recognized, such as the bluing of red litmus. **allergic r.,** a local or general reaction characterized by altered reactivity of the animal body to an antigenic substance. **allograft r.,** the rejection of an allogeneic graft by a normal host; called also *homograft r.* **alphanaphthol r.,** Molisch's test, defs. 2 and 3. **anamnestic r.,** see under *response.* **anaphylactic r.,** generalized anaphylaxis, anaphylactic shock; see *anaphylaxis.* **anaphylactoid r.,** pseudoanaphylaxis. **antigen-antibody r.,** the reversible binding of antigen to homologous antibody brought about by the formation of weak bonds between antigenic determinants on antigen molecules and antigen binding sites on immunoglobulin molecules. Certain effects, e.g., precipitation and agglutination reactions and viral neutralization, result from the binding itself; other effects, e.g., complement activation and opsonization, result from conformational changes that occur in immunoglobulin mole-

cules with antigen binding and enable them to interact with complement proteins and Fc receptors on phagocytes. **antiglobulin r.,** the agglutination of particles (usually erythrocytes) that have been (1) sensitized by the adsorption of soluble antigen, (2) treated with antibody to that antigen, and (3) treated with antiserum to the serum globulin of the animal species that produced the antibody. **antitryptic r.,** the reaction produced by the blood upon mixtures of trypsin and casein solutions. Such reaction is modified by various disease conditions, such as cancer and tuberculosis, and by pregnancy. **anxiety r.,** see under *neurosis.* **Arias-Stella r.,** changes in the cells of the endometrial epithelium consisting chiefly of bizarre-shaped hyperchromatic enlarged nuclei associated with a loss of cellular polarity; cytoplasmic vacuolization is occasionally present. The changes are thought to be associated with the presence of chorionic tissue in an intrauterine or extrauterine site, and are seen in some cases of ectopic pregnancy. **Arthus r.,** the development of an inflammatory lesion, characterized by induration, erythema, edema, hemorrhage, and necrosis, a few hours after intradermal injection of antigen into a previously sensitized animal producing precipitating antibody; it is classed as a type III reaction in the Gell and Coombs classification of immune responses. The lesion results from the precipitation of antigen-antibody complexes, which causes complement activation and the release of complement fragments that are chemotactic for neutrophils; large numbers of neutrophils infiltrate the site and cause tissue destruction by release of lysosomal enzymes. Called also *Arthus phenomenon.* **Arthus-type r.,** any pathologic process involving the same mechanism as the Arthus reaction, i.e., deposition of immune complexes and complement activation, as in immune complex disease. **Ascoli's r.,** miostagmin r. **associative r.,** a reaction in which the response is withheld until the idea presented has suggested an associated idea. **axon r., axonal r.,** the series of changes in the ganglion cell (central chromatolysis with displacement of the nucleus) following the severing of its axon. **Bareggi's r.,** the formation in a test tube of an unretracted clot, with but little serum, from the blood of typhoid fever; if the blood is from a patient with tuberculosis, the clot retracts with the separation of much serum. **Bekhterev's r.,** in cases of tetany, the minimum of electric current needed to arouse muscular contraction needs to be diminished at every interruption or change of density in order to prevent tetanic contraction. **Bence Jones r.,** the precipitation of protein by heat followed by its redissolving on boiling and being precipitated again on cooling. **Bittorf's r.,** in renal colic the pain produced by squeezing the testicle or pressing the ovary radiates to the kidney. **biuret r.,** biuret (H_2N—CO—NH—CO—NH_2) forms a chelate having an intense violet-red color with the Cu^{2+} ion in alkaline solution; the same reaction also occurs with tripeptides and polypeptides, but not with dipeptides or amino acids and is used in colorimetric methods for total protein. **Blackman r.,** the fundamental thermochemical dark reaction in which carbon dioxide fixation takes place during photosynthesis. **Bordet and Gengou r.,** complement fixation. **Brieger's cachexia r.,** cachexia r. **cachexia r.,** increase in the antitryptic power of the blood serum seen in malignant disease and other diseases characterized by cachexia. **cadaveric r.,** total loss of electrical response in the affected muscles in familial periodic paralysis. **cancer r.,** see specific reactions, including *antitryptic r., cachexia r., Freund's r., Klein's r., miostagmin r., Penn seroflocculation r., Stammler's r.* See also *cancer test,* under *tests.* **Cannizzaro's r.,** the reaction which aldehydes may undergo in alkali or when brought in contact with animal tissue; one molecule of the aldehyde is reduced to the corresponding alcohol and another molecule is simultaneously oxidized to the corresponding acid. **capsular r.,** the reaction of the capsular substance of bacteria with a homologous antibody. **carbamino r.,** alpha-amino acids unite with CO_2 in the presence of alkalis or alkaline earths to form salts of carbamino-carboxylic acids. This reaction is used in studying the course of protein digestion. See *formol titration,* under *method.* **Casoni's r.,** see *Casoni's intradermal test,* under *tests.* **chain r.,** a nuclear (neutron) reaction which once started will proceed and multiply of its own accord by emitting particles that propagate the reaction in adjacent nuclei. **chromaffin r.,** see *chromaffin.* **cockade r.,** the reaction of a sensitized guinea pig to intradermal injection of tuberculin; it consists of a large papule with a necrotic, hemorrhagic center. **colloidal gold r.,** see under *tests.* **complement fixation r.,** see under *fixation.* **compluetic r.,** Wassermann r. **conglutination r.,** a characteristic agglutination reaction obtained by a mixture of conglutinin, cells (e.g., bacteria or red cells), fresh complement, and a cell-specific immune serum from which the agglutinins have been removed by absorption. See *conglutinin.* **consensual r.,** 1. crossed reflex. 2. an involuntary action that accompanies a voluntary action. **conversion r.,** see under *disorder.* **cross r.,** the interaction of an antibody with antigen that did not specifically stimulate its synthesis; it may be weaker than the reaction of an antibody with its homologous antigen; the interaction of an antigen with an antibody formed against a different antigen with which the first antigen shares identical or closely related antigenic determinants. **cutaneous r.,** a positive reaction indicating immunity or hypersensitivity in a skin test. Called also *cutireaction* and *dermoreaction.* **Dale r.,** an *in vitro* test for anaphylactic sensitization in the guinea pig: a small amount of the antigen, added to a tissue bath in which is immersed the excised uterine horn (smooth muscle) of an anaphylactically sensitized guinea pig, causes contraction of the sensitized uterine muscle. Called also *Schultz-Dale reaction.* Schultz employed intestinal muscle; Dale used uterine muscle from virgin guinea pigs. **dark r.,** in photosynthesis, the series of reactions by which fixation of carbon dioxide into carbohydrate is accomplished; these reactions are driven by the products of the light reaction and do not require the presence of light. **defense r.,** see under *mechanism.* **r. of degeneration,** the reaction to electric stimulation of muscles whose nerves have degenerated. It consists of a loss of response to a faradic stimulus in a muscle, and to galvanic and faradic stimulus in a nerve. Galvanic irritability of the muscle is increased. Abbreviated Ea. R. (Ger. *Entartungs-Reaktion*) and R.D. **r. of degeneration, franklinic,** a form of reaction elicited by static electricity and similar to the reaction produced by the faradic current. **delayed hypersensitivity r., delayed-type hypersensitivity r.,** see under *hypersensitivity.* **depressive r.,** dysthymia. **dermotuberculin r.,** Pirquet's test. **desmoplastic r.,** see *desmoplastic.* **diazo r.,** Ehrlich's diazo r. **Dick r.,** see under *tests.* **digitonin r.,** the formation of a precipitate on treating a sterol, such as cholesterol or ergosterol, with digitonin; employed to define cholesterol esters which do not precipitate in total serum cholesterol determinations. **displacement r.,** a chemical reaction in which a reactant displaces a functional group from a substrate and becomes bound in the position formerly occupied by the leaving group; see also *displacement.* **dissociative r.,** see under *disorder.* **dopa r.,** the reaction by which dopa is changed into melanin under the influence of dopa-oxidase. **downgrading r.,** a lepra reaction, similar in appearance to the reversal ("upgrading") reaction, representing a deterioration in the immune response to *Mycobacterium leprae* with worsening of the clinical symptoms of leprosy and an increased index of *M. leprae* in the tissues; it may be seen during antileprosy treatment in those in whom *M. leprae* has become drug resistant or in those with poor compliance with the chemotherapeutic regimen. **dysergastic r.,** a disorder characterized by disorientation, hallucinations, daydreams and fears, due to impaired cerebral circulation and to the resulting reduced nutrition of the brain. **egg yellow r.,** a yellow foam appearing in Ehrlich's diazo reaction before the addition of ammonia; believed to indicate acute pneumonia. **Ehrlich's diazo r.,** a reaction of a pure pink or red color resulting from the action of diazotized sulfanilic acid and ammonia upon certain aromatic substances, e.g., urobilinogen, found in the urine in some conditions. This reaction has diagnostic value in hepatic disease, typhoid fever, and measles and prognostic value in tuberculosis. **electric r.,** a reaction, such as muscular contraction, caused by the application of electricity to the body. **erythrocyte sedimentation r.,** see under *rate.* **r. of exhaustion,** reaction to electric stimulation seen in conditions of exhaustion. In it the reaction normally produced by a certain current can be reproduced only by an increase in the current. **Felix-Weil r.,** Weil-Felix r. **Fernandez r.,** see *lepromin test,* under *test.* **Feulgen r.,** a specific histochemical reaction for DNA (deoxyribonucleic acid): after acid hydrolysis at 60° C, tissue sections are stained in Schiff's reagent; DNA stains magenta. **fight-or-flight r.,** alarm r. **foreign body r.,** a granulomatous inflammatory reaction evoked by the

presence of an exogenous material in the tissues, a characteristic feature of which is the formation of foreign body giant cells. **fuchsinophil r.,** certain substances when stained with fuchsin retain the stain on being treated with picric acid alcohol. **Gangi's r.,** a test of a liquid to determine whether it is a transudate or exudate, utilizing hydrochloric acid. **Gerhardt's r.,** see under *tests.* **Ghilarducci's r.,** contraction of the muscles of a limb when the active electrode is placed on a part somewhat removed from them. **Gmelin's r.,** see under *tests.* **gold r.,** colloidal gold test. **graft-vs.-host r.,** see under *disease.* **Grignard's r.,** see under *reagent.* **gross stress r.,** post-traumatic stress disorder. **group r.,** see *group agglutination,* under *agglutination.* **Gruber's r., Gruber-Widal r.,** Widal's test. **Gubler's r.,** the formation of a brown color on gradually adding nitrosonitric acid to urine; seen in urobilin jaundice. **Gunning r.,** see under *tests.* **hemagglutination-inhibition r.,** the inhibition by antibodies of viral agglutination of red cells. **hemiopic pupillary r.,** reaction in certain cases of hemianopia in which the stimulus of light thrown upon one side of the retina causes the iris to contract, while light thrown on the other side arouses no response. Called also *Wernicke's r.* **hemoclastic r.,** laking of blood due to hemolysis; see *hemoclastic crisis,* under *crisis.* **Henle's r.,** the medullary cells of the adrenals stain dark brown on treatment with chromium salts. **Henry's melanoflocculation r.,** see under *tests.* **Herxheimer's r.,** Jarisch-Herxheimer r. **Hill r.,** the primary reaction of photosynthesis in which light is absorbed and used by chlorophyll. **homograft r.,** allograft r. **hunting r.,** periods of vasoconstriction alternating with periods of vasodilatation in a finger or other part exposed to temperatures below 15° C. **hyperkinetic r. of childhood,** attention-deficit hyperactivity disorder. **hypersensitivity r.,** see *hypersensitivity.* **id r.,** a localized or generalized, sterile secondary skin eruption occurring in sensitized patients as a result of circulation of allergenic products from a primary site of infection; the morphology and site of the lesion vary. See also *id,* def. 2. **Ide r.,** see under *tests.* **r. of identity,** a reaction pattern seen in double diffusion in two dimensions: the precipitin lines between the antigen wells and the antiserum well stop at their point of intersection, indicating that the antigen samples are identical. See also *r. of nonidentity* and *r. of partial identity.* **immediate hypersensitivity r.,** see under *hypersensitivity.* **immune r.,** see under *response.* **indophenol r.,** see under *tests.* **intracutaneous r.,** the reaction to an intracutaneous injection of antigen in a skin test. **intracuti r.,** see *Frei test,* under *tests.* **intradermal r.,** intracutaneous r. **involutional psychotic r.,** involutional melancholia. **Israelson's r.,** see under *tests.* **Ito-Reenstierna r.,** see under *tests.* **Jaffé r.,** creatinine when treated with picric acid in strongly alkaline solution gives an intense red color. **Jarisch-Herxheimer r.,** a transient, short-term immunologic reaction commonly seen following antibiotic treatment of early and later stages of syphilis and less often in other diseases, such as borreliosis, brucellosis, typhoid fever, and trichinellosis, which is manifested by fever, chills, headache, myalgias, and exacerbation of cutaneous lesions. The reaction has been attributed to liberation of endotoxin-like substances or of antigens from the killed or dying microorganisms, but its exact pathogenesis is unclear. Called also *Herxheimer's r.* **johnin r.,** a skin reaction like the tuberculin reaction, produced by filtrates of cultures of *Mycobacterium paratuberculosis* (johnin); used in the diagnosis of Johne's disease in cattle. **Jolly's r.,** failure of response to faradic stimulation in a muscle, the power of voluntary contraction as well as the response to galvanic stimulation being retained. **Jones-Mote r.,** a weak delayed hypersensitivity reaction that occurs on challenge a few days after priming with a protein antigen in aqueous solution (i.e., not with Freund's complete adjuvant). Called also *cutaneous basophil hypersensitivity.* **Kahn's albumin A r.,** see under *tests,* def. 2. **Keller-Killian r.** (*for 2-desoxy sugars*)*:* dissolve the sugar in glacial acetic acid that contains some ferric chloride, underlay it with concentrated sulfuric acid and the upper layer will take on a deep blue color. **Klein r.,** a modification of Freund's reaction for cancer, using for carcinolysis a cell suspension from an adenocarcinoma of the mouse. **Koch's r.,** see *tuberculin test,* under *tests.* **Koler r.,** Adamkiewicz's test. **Konsuloff's r.,** see under *tests.* **Lange's r.,** 1. colloidal gold test. 2. see under *tests.* **lengthening r.,** the elongation of the extensor muscles which permits flexion of a limb; called also *clasp-knife reflex*. **lentochol r.,** see *Sachs-Georgi test,* under *tests*. **lepra r.,** an acute or subacute hypersensitivity state occurring during the course of antileprosy treatment or in untreated leprosy categories, involving two types of immunological reactions, one a delayed hypersensitivity reaction (see *reversal r's*) and the other an immune complex reaction (see *erythema nodosum leprosum*). **lepromin r.,** see under *tests*. **leukemic r., leukemoid r.,** a peripheral blood picture resembling that of leukemia or indistinguishable from it on the basis of morphologic appearance alone. **Lewis' r.,** the urticaria produced by histamine; see *histamine test,* def. 2, under *tests*. **Lieben's r.,** see under *tests*. **Liebermann-Burchard r.,** a green color is produced when concentrated sulfuric acid in acetic anhydride is added to a mixture of chloroform solution of cholesterol. **light r.,** in photosynthesis, the photochemical process in which a series of reactions driven by light energy results in the generation of ATP and reduced coenzymes (NADH or NADPH); these substances then drive the dark reaction. **lignin r.,** a color reaction given by wood cellulose, consisting of a yellow color with aniline salts and a red color with a solution of phloroglucinol in concentrated hydrochloric acid. **Loeb's decidual r.,** the presence of a glass bead or other irritant causes the formation of a small deciduoma in the uterine mucosa when corpora lutea are developing normally. **Loewi's r.,** see under *tests*. **Lohmann r.,** an easily reversible reaction occurring in muscle, in which the high-energy phosphate bond of ATP is transferred to creatine, forming creatine phosphate; the reaction is catalyzed by creatine kinase. **Machado r., Machado-Guerreiro r.,** see under *tests*. **Malmejde r.,** see under *tests*. **manic-depressive r.,** bipolar disorder. **Mantoux r.,** see under *tests*. **Marchi's r.,** failure of the myelin sheath of a nerve to become discolored when treated with osmic acid. **Meinicke r.,** see under *tests*. **Millon's r.,** see under *tests*. **Mitsuda r.,** see *lepromin test,* under *tests*. **mixed agglutination r.,** agglutination of a mixture of different cell types by antibody directed against an antigenic determinant present on all of the cells. **mixed leukocyte r., mixed lymphocyte r.,** the appearance of blast cells in a culture of leukocytes from two individuals; histocompatibility varies inversely with the number of blast cells. **Molisch's r.,** see under *tests*. **Moloney r.,** see under *tests*. **Montenegro r.,** see *leishmanin test,* under *tests*. **Morelli's r.,** see under *tests*. **Moritz r.,** Rivalta's r. **mouse tail r.,** stiffening of the tail in rats and mice following the administration of a small dose of morphine. **myasthenic r.,** progressively diminished response of a muscle to repeated electric stimuli. **myotonic r.,** failure of muscle to relax immediately upon cessation of voluntary or electrically induced contraction. **Nadi r.,** the production of a blue color when alphanaphthol and dimethyl paraphenylenediamine are injected into animals; see *indophenol test*. **Nagler's r.,** the formation of an opaque zone around colonies of *Clostridium perfringens* on egg yolk agar, produced by the action of a diffusible lecithinase (α toxin). **near-point r.,** constriction of the pupil when the gaze is fixed on a near point. **Neill-Mooser r.,** a reaction in laboratory animals produced by inoculation with rickettsiae of murine typhus. The inflammatory exudate of the scrotal swelling contains large mononuclear cells filled with rickettsiae. **Neisser's r.,** a general reaction sometimes following an initial dose of arsphenamine, characterized by transitory increase of headache in cerebral syphilis and of the lightning pains in tabes. **Neufeld's r.,** when pneumococci and other capsulated microorganisms are mixed with specific immune serum there occurs in addition to agglutination a swelling (quellung) of the capsules of the organisms, owing to the binding of antibody with the capsular polysaccharide; called also *capsular swelling* and *quellung r.* **neurotonic r.,** muscular contraction persisting after the stimulus which produced it has ceased. **neutral r.,** the presence of an equal number of H$^+$ and OH$^-$ ions in a solution, i.e., a pH of 7.0. **ninhydrin r.,** see *triketohydrindene hydrate test,* under *tests*. **nitritoid r.,** see under *crisis*. **r. of nonidentity,** a reaction pattern seen in double diffusion in two dimensions: the precipitin lines between the antigen wells and the antiserum well cross, indicating that the antigen samples have no antigenic determinants in common. See also *r. of identity* and *r. of partial identity*. **Nonne-Apelt r.,** 2 ml. of cerebrospinal fluid is mixed with an equal quantity of a neutral saturated solution of ammonium sulfate and compared after three minutes with another tube containing spinal fluid only; if there is no difference or only a faint opalescence the reaction is said to be *negative*. If there is an opalescence or turbidity the reaction is said to be *positive phase 1,* which indicates an excess of globulin in the fluid and points to nervous disorder. A normal fluid treated with heat and acetic acid only becomes turbid and is called *positive phase 2*. **nucleal r.,** upon the addition of fuchsin-sulfonic acid to any solution containing aldehydes, a bluish-red color is produced. **obsessive-compulsive r.,** see under *disorder*. **Oestreicher's r.,** xanthydrol r. **orbicularis r.,** orbicularis pupillary reflex. **oxidase r.,** the formation of dark-blue granulations in myeloid cells when treated with alphanaphthol and dimethyl paraphenylenediamine. See *indophenol test,* under *tests*. **pain r.,** dilatation of the pupil on a feeling of pain. **Pándy's r.,** see under *tests*. **parallergic r.,** see *parallergy*. **r. of partial identity,** a reaction pattern seen in double diffusion in two dimensions: one of the precipitin lines between the antigen wells and the antiserum well stops at the point of intersection, whereas the other continues past it, indicating that the antigen samples have some, but not all, antigenic determinants in common. See also *r. of identity* and *r. of nonidentity*. **passive cutaneous anaphylaxis r.,** passive cutaneous anaphylaxis. **Pasteur's r.,** see under *effect*. **paternity r.,** Manoiloff's r., def 1. See also *paternity test,* under *tests*. **Paul-Bunnell r.,** see under *tests*. **Penn seroflocculation r.** (*for cancer*) : plasma separated from a small amount of the patient's blood is mixed with a lipoid fraction derived from the liver of a patient who died of cancer. Resulting turbidity constitutes a negative reaction. **periodic acid–Schiff r.,** a tissue section is exposed to periodic acid, which oxidizes hydroxyl groups on adjacent carbon atoms or adjacent hydroxyl groups and amino groups to aldehydes, and then is stained with Schiff's reagent, which forms an additional product with aldehydes to produce a red or magenta reaction product; used to test for glycogen, epithelial mucins, neutral polysaccharides, and glycoproteins; called also *PAS r*. **peroxidase r.,** the appearance of deep-blue granules in leukocytes of marrow origin when stained with Goodpasture's stain, distinguishing them from cells of lymphatic origin. **Petri r.,** see under *tests*. **Petzetaki's r.,** see under *tests*. **Pfeiffer's r.,** see under *phenomenon*. **phobic r.,** phobic disorder or neurosis; see *phobia*. **photochemical r.,** photoreaction. **Piazza's r.,** see under *tests*. **Pirquet r.,** see under *test*. **P-K r.,** Prausnitz-Küstner r. **Porges-Meier r.,** see under *tests*. **Porter-Silber r.,** the reaction of the dihydroxyacetone side chain of 17-hydroxycorticosteroids with phenylhydrazine in acid, which produces a yellow color; an index of adrenocortical function now largely supplanted by immunoassay techniques. **Posner's r.,** see under *tests*. **Prausnitz-Küstner r.,** an immediate hypersensitivity reaction produced in a nonatopic subject by intradermal injection of serum from an atopic subject followed 12 or more hours later by an injection of antigen into the same site; the presence of specific reaginic (IgE) antibody in the transferred serum results in a classic wheal and flare reaction to the antigen. Once the standard method of demonstrating reaginic antibody, this test is no longer used because of the risk of transmitting serum hepatitis and because serum IgE can now be measured by in vitro assays, e.g., RAST and RIST. **precipitin r.,** the formation of an insoluble precipitate by reaction of antigen and antibody; it occurs only with multivalent antigens and is dependent on electrolyte concentration, pH, temperature, and the relative concentrations of antigen and antibody, the amount of precipitate formed increasing to a maximum and then decreasing as the relative antigen concentration is increased. **prozone r.,** see *prozone*. **pseudoallergic r.,** a clinical state exhibiting what appear to be the signs and symptoms of an immediate hypersensitivity reaction, but with no evidence for an immunologic mechanism. **psychotic depressive r.** (*obs*.), major depression with psychotic features and onset associated with an identifiable psychosocial stressor. **quellung r.** [Ger. "swelling"], Neufeld's r. **reversal r.,** a lepra reaction usually occurring during chemotherapy in borderline leprosy representing a delayed-type hypersensitivity reaction with "upgrading" of cell-mediated immunity to *Mycobacterium leprae,* which tends to move the disease toward the tuberculoid pole. It is chiefly characterized by erythema, edema, and tenderness of preexisting quiescent lesions, the appearance of new lesions, neuritis with nerve damage, fever, adenopathy, and elevation of the leukocyte count. See also *downgrading r.* **reverse passive Arthus r.,** the reaction produced when precipitating antibody is inoculated into a skin site in an experimental animal followed in 30 minutes to 2 hours by the intravenous inoculation of the homologous antigen. Thus the usual anatomical locations of precipitating antibody and antigen in an Arthus reaction are reversed. **reversible r.,** a chemical reaction which occurs in either direction, depending on conditions; a reaction in which the products react to re-form the reactants. **Rivalta's r.,** a reaction for distinguishing fluids of transudation and exudation, utilizing acetic acid. **Roger's r.,** the existence of albumin in the sputum, indicating tuberculosis. **Rosenbach's r.,** the formation of a deep-red color when concentrated nitric acid containing a small amount of nitrous acid is gradually added to boiling urine, indicative of an increase in the putrefactive processes of the intestine. **Russo r.,** a reaction of the urine of typhoid patients on adding 4 drops of a solution of methylene blue to 15 ml. of urine. In the first stage of typhoid, the urine becomes light green; at the height of the disease, an emerald color; and during the decline, a bluish color. **Sahli's r.,** desmoid r. **Schardinger's r.,** a reaction of oxidation or reduction made possible by a simultaneous and compensating reaction of reduction or oxidation. Cf. *Cannizzaro's reaction.* This reaction is used to distinguish between fresh milk and milk which has been heated. The milk is treated with aldehyde and methylene blue or indigo blue; if the milk is fresh the dye is reduced to a colorless compound. **Schick r.,** see under *tests.* **schizophrenic r.** (*obs.*), reactive schizophrenia. **Schönbein's r.,** iodine is set free when potassium iodide and iron sulfate are added to a solution of hydrogen peroxide. **Schultz-Charlton r.,** when scarlet fever antitoxin or scarlet fever convalescent serum is injected into an area of the skin showing a bright red rash, a blanching of the skin at the site of the injection occurs. Serum from scarlet fever patients does not produce this reaction. **Schultz-Dale r.,** see *Dale r.* **second-set r.,** see under *phenomenon.* **sedimentation r.,** erythrocyte sedimentation rate. **Selivanoff r., Seliwanow's r.,** see under *tests.* **serological r.,** seroreaction. **serum r.,** seroreaction. **serum sickness–like r.,** see *serum sickness,* under *sickness.* **shortening r.,** the shortening that succeeds the lengthening reaction when a limb is brought back into the extended position. **Shwartzman r., generalized,** a generalized reaction following two intravenous injections of endotoxin separated by 24 hours; it is characterized by widespread hemorrhages, bilateral cortical necrosis of the kidneys, and a marked fall in leukocyte and platelet counts and usually results in death of the animal. **Shwartzman r., localized,** a localized cutaneous reaction consisting of vascular necrosis, petechial hemorrhages, and leukocyte infiltration that occurs at the site of an original subcutaneous injection of endotoxin approximately 24 hours after an intravenous injection of the same or another endotoxin given at a site other than the original injection site. **skin r.,** see *cutaneous r.* **Stammler's r.,** cancer serum when added to a tumor extract clears up the opalescence normal to the extract: normal sera fail to act in this manner. **startle r.,** the various psychophysiological phenomena, including involuntary motor and autonomic reactions, evidenced by an individual in reaction to a sudden, unexpected stimulus, as a loud noise. **stemming r.,** resistance in the leg of a standing animal to forward displacement. **Straus' r.,** when material containing virulent glanders bacilli is inoculated into the peritoneal cavity of male guinea-pigs, scrotal lesions develop; called also *Straus' phenomenon.* **stress r.,** any reaction to physical or psychological stress; see *alarm r.* and *acute stress r.,* and *adjustment disorder* and *post-traumatic stress disorder,* under *disorder.* **sympathetic stress r.,** alarm r. **Szent-Györgyi r.,** a deep violet color develops when a 1 per cent solution of ascorbic acid is mixed with a solution of ferrous sulfate; this color disappears on reduction with sodium hyposulfite. **Tanret's r.,** see under *tests.* **tendon r.,** see under *reflex.* **thyroid function r.,** see specific reactions, including *Goetsch's skin r.* and *Hunt's r.* See also *thyroid function test,* under *tests.* **toxin-antitoxin r.,** the antigen-antibody reaction between a toxin and antitoxin. **trigger r.,** see under *action.* **tryptophan r.,** see under *tests.* **tuberculin r.,** see under *tests.* **Turnbull's blue r.,** blue-black coloration produced when tissue containing chemically active iron is treated with potassium ferrocyanide and

hydrochloric acid. **upgrading r.,** see *reversal r.* **vestibular pupillary r.,** dilatation of the pupils arising from stimulation of the external auditory canal. **Voges-Proskauer r.,** see under *tests.* **von Pirquet's r.,** Pirquet's test. **Weichbrodt's r.,** three parts of a 1 per cent solution of sublimate solution are added to seven parts of cerebrospinal fluid; cloudiness of the mixture indicates pathologic changes in the fluid, especially syphilis. **Weil-Felix r.,** see under *tests.* **Wernicke's r.,** hemiopic pupillary r. **wheal and erythema r., wheal and flare r.,** the characteristic local cutaneous reaction consisting of an elevated, blanched wheal surrounded by a spreading "flare" of erythema that occurs within a few minutes at the site of a minor nonpenetrating skin injury and also in response to administration of allergen to an atopic individual; it is caused by release of histamine from mast cells. Called also the *triple response (of Lewis).* **white-graft r.,** an immune reaction to a tissue graft, e.g., a skin graft, as a result of which the grafted tissue does not become vascularized and is rapidly rejected. **Widal's r.,** see under *tests.* **xanthoproteic r.,** see *Mulder's test,* under *tests.* **xanthydrol r.,** when tissue from a uremic patient is fixed in a solution of xanthydrol in glacial acetic acid, a large deposit of xanthydrol occurs in the tissue. **zed r.,** a reaction which appears in infants in cases of starvation after the starvation is relieved; it consists of a slight gain in weight, elevation of temperature, and the appearance of watery stools containing a large number of cells.

reaction-formation (re-ak′shun for-ma′shun) an unconscious defense mechanism in which a person assumes an attitude that is the reverse of a wish or impulse that he harbors.

reactivate (re-ak′tĭ-vāt) to make active again; especially the restoring of the activity to immune serum that has had its activity destroyed.

reactivation (re-ak″tĭ-va′shun) the restoration of activity to something that has been inactivated. **r. of serum,** restoration of immunological activity to serum by adding fresh complement.

reactivator (re-ak′tĭ-va-tor) an agent that restores activity. **cholinesterase r.,** an agent that restores the activity of acetylcholinesterase that has been inactivated by an organophosphate compound; see *pralidoxime.*

reactivity (re″ak-tiv′ĭ-te) the process or property of reacting.

reactor (re-ak′tor) a person or thing that reacts. **nuclear r.,** a device in which the chain reaction of neutron-induced nuclear fission is sustained in a self-supporting reaction at a controlled rate.

Reactrol (re-ak′trol) trademark for a preparation of clemizole hydrochloride.

Read's formula (rēdz) [Jay Marion *Read,* American physician, born 1889] see under *formula.*

reading (rēd′ing) understanding of written or printed symbols representing words. **lip r., speech r.,** the understanding of speech through observation of the movement of the lips of the speaker.

reagent (re-a′jent) [*re-* + L. *agere* to act] a substance employed to produce a chemical reaction so as to detect, measure, produce, etc., other substances. **acid molybdate r.,** Folin's acid molybdate r. **amino-acid r.,** a 0.5 per cent solution of the sodium salt of beta-naphthaquinone sulfonate acid freshly prepared. **arsenic-sulfuric acid r.,** Rosenthaler's r. **Bial's r.,** orcinol 1.5 gm., fuming hydrochloric acid 500 gm., ferric chloride (10 per cent) 20–30 drops. **biuret r.,** see *Gies' biuret test,* under *tests.* **Black's r.,** 5 gm. of ferric chloride and 0.4 gm. of ferrous chloride dissolved in 100 ml. of water. **Bogg's r.,** dissolve 25 gm. of phosphotungstic acid in 125 ml. of water. Dilute 25 ml. of concentrated HCl to 100 ml. Mix the two solutions. **Bohme's r.,** two reagents for use in testing for indol. **Bonchardat's r.,** a general alkaloidal reagent, consisting of 1 per cent of iodine dissolved in a 1 per cent solution of potassium iodide. **Brücke's r.,** 50 gm. of KI, 120 gm. of HgI_2, water up to 1000 ml.: a modification of Meyer's reagent. **Cramer's 2.5 r.,** 0.4 gm. of mercuric oxide and 6 gm. of potassium iodide dissolved in 100 ml. of water with the reagent so adjusted that 10 ml. will be neutralized to the phenolphthalein end point by 2.5 ml. of N/10 acid. **Cross and Bevan's r.,** two parts of concentrated hydrochloric acid and 1 part of zinc chloride by weight; used for dissolving cellulose. **Denigès' r.**, the reagent used in Denigès' test (def. 2). **diazo r.**, a reagent consisting of two solutions which are mixed just prior to the test in the proportion of 25 ml. of solution *A* to 0.75 ml. of *B*. Solution *A*: sulfanilic acid, 1 gm.; distilled water, 1000 ml. Solution *B*: sodium nitrite, 0.5 gm.: distilled water, 100 ml. **dinitrosalicylic acid r.**, Sumner's r. **Ehrlich's aldehyde r.**, 4 gm. of paradimethylaminobenzaldehyde in a mixture of 80 ml. of concentrated hydrochloric acid and 380 ml. of ethyl alcohol. **Ehrlich's diazo r.**, Solution *A*: dissolve 5 gm. of sodium nitrite in 1 liter of distilled water. Solution *B*: dissolve 5 gm. of sulfanilic acid and 50 ml. of HCl in 1 liter of distilled water. For use mix 1 part of *A* with 50 to 100 parts of *B*. **formalin- sulfuric acid r.**, see *Marquis' test*, under *tests*. **Fröhde's r.**, see under *tests*. **Frohn's r.**, see under *tests*. **general r.**, a reagent that indicates the general class of bodies to which a substance belongs. **Gies' biuret r.**, see under *tests*. **Grignard's r.**, any of several compounds of magnesium with an organic radical and a halogen; these reagents undergo reactions with many substances producing important products. **Hager's r.**, a reagent for detecting sugar in the urine, consisting of iron ferrocyanide and potassium hydroxide. **Hahn oxine r.**, a 5 per cent solution of hydroxyquinoline in alcohol. **Haines' r.**, copper sulfate, 2 parts; potassium hydroxide, 7.5 parts; glycerin, 15 parts; distilled water, 150 parts. **Ilosvay's r.**, a reagent used as a test for nitrites. It is prepared by treating a mixture of 0.5 gm. of sulfanilic acid and 150 ml. of dilute acetic acid with 0.1 gm. of naphthylamine, and then with 20 ml. of boiling water. The sediment produced by this reaction is dissolved in 150 ml. of dilute acetic acid. The suspected substance is heated with this reagent to 80° C., when a red color is formed if nitrites are present. **Izar's r.**, equal parts of linoleic and ricinoleic acid. **Lloyd's r.**, a specially fine preparation of fuller's earth obtained by elutriation; used to absorb alkaloids from solutions. **Mandelin's r.** (*for alkaloids*), 1 part of ammonium vanadate in 200 parts of cold concentrated sulfuric acid. **Marme's r.**, a solution of cadmium iodide and potassium iodide for the precipitation of alkaloids. **Marquis' r.**, see under *tests*. **Mayer's r.**, see under *tests*. **Mecke's r.**, 1 part of selenious acid in 200 parts of concentrated sulfuric acid. **Meyer's r.**, phenolphthalein, 0.032 part; decinormal sodium hydroxide, 21 parts; enough water to make 100 parts; used in testing for blood, which even in minute quantities gives the solution a purple color. **Millon's r.**, see under *tests*. **Mörner's r.**, a solution of 1 volume of formalin, 45 volumes of distilled water, 55 volumes of concentrated sulfuric acid; used as a test for tyrosine. See under *tests*. **Nadi r.**, a mixture of alphanaphthol and dimethyl paraphenylenediamine, which combine to form indophenol blue from cytochrome C under the influence of cytochrome oxidase. See *indophenol test*, under *tests*. **Nakayama r.**, ferric chloride, 0.4 gm., concentrated hydrochloric acid, 1 ml., 95 per cent alcohol, 99 ml. **Nessler's r.**, an aqueous solution of 5 per cent of potassium iodide, 2.5 per cent of mercuric chloride, and 16 per cent of potassium hydroxide; used as a test for ammonia. **Ninhydrin r.**, trademark for a preparation of triketohydrindene hydrate (q.v.). **Noguchi's r.**, butyric acid 10 parts, 0.9 per cent sodium chloride 90 parts. **Obermayer's r.**, a solution of 2 gm. of ferric chloride in 1 liter of hydrochloric acid. **Penzoldt's r.**, see under *tests*. **Porges-Meier r.**, see under *tests*. **Rosenthaler's r.** (*for alkaloids*), 1 part of potassium arsenate in 100 parts of concentrated sulfuric acid. **Sahli's r.**, mix equal parts of a 48 per cent solution of potassium iodide and an 8 per cent solution of potassium iodate. **Schaer's r.** (*for alkaloids*), one volume of 30 per cent pure hydrogen peroxide in 10 volumes of concentrated sulfuric acid. Use while fresh. **Scheibler's r.**, a reagent made by boiling sodium tungstate with half as much phosphoric acid and water, precipitating with barium chloride, dissolving in hot dilute hydrochloric acid, treating with sulfuric acid, and evaporating. **Schiff's r.**, a reagent for testing for the presence of aldehydes, prepared by dissolving 0.25 gm. of fuchsin in 1 liter of water and decolorizing by passing sulfur dioxide into it. In the presence of aldehyde the blue color is restored. **Schweitzer's r.**, a solution of cupric hydroxide, $Cu(OH)_2$, in ammonia water; used as a solvent for cellulose. Called also *cuprammonia*. **Scott-Wilson r.**, (1) mercuric cyanide, 5 gm., (2) sodium hydroxide, 90 gm., (3) silver nitrate, 1.45 gm. Dissolve each separately in water and cool. Add (2) to (1), then add (3) with constant stirring.

selenious-sulfuric acid r., Mecke's r. **Soldaini's r.**, see under *tests*. **Sörensen's r.**, an acetate buffer solution for combining with Pardy's test for albumin: 188 gm. of sodium acetate and 56.5 gm. of glacial acetic acid brought up to 1 liter with distilled water. **Spiegler's r.**, see under *tests*. **splenic r.**, any drug or stimulus which causes the spleen to contract. **Sumner's r.**, to 10 gm. crystallized phenol add 22 ml. of 10 per cent NaOH and dilute to 100 ml. To 6.9 gm. of sodium bisulfite add 69 ml. of the alkaline phenol solution. To this add a solution containing 300 ml. of 4.5 per cent NaOH, 255 gm. $NaKC_4H_4O_6 \cdot 4H_2O$, and 880 ml. of 1 per cent dinitrosalicylic acid; used for the estimation of sugar in normal and diabetic urine. **Takata's r.**, the reagent (a mixture of mercuric chloride solution and basic fuchsin solution) used in Takata-Ara test. **Tanret's r.** (*for albumin in urine, etc.*): mercuric chloride, 1.35 gm.; potassium iodide, 3.32 gm.; acetic acid, 20 ml.; distilled water, to make 80 ml.; it gives a white precipitate with albumin. **Triboulet's r.**, bichloride of mercury, 3.5 gm., acetic acid, 1 ml., water, 100 ml. **Tsuchiya r.**, an acid alcoholic solution of phosphotungstic acid for detecting small amounts of protein in the urine. **Uffelmann's r.**, see under *tests*. **vanadic-sulfuric acid r.**, Mandelin's r. **Wolff's r.**, phosphotungstic acid, 0.3 gm.; concentrated hydrochloric acid, 1 ml.; absolute alcohol, 20 ml.; distilled water, 200 ml.

reagin (re'ah-jin) [*reagent* + *-in*] 1. the antibody that mediates immediate hypersensitivity reactions; in humans reagins are IgE antibodies. 2. (*obs.*) the serum antibody detected by the Wassermann reaction. **atopic r.**, reagin, def. 1.

reaginic (re-ah-jin'ik) pertaining to reagin.

realgar (re'al-gar') [Arabic *rahj al-ghar* powder of the mine] arsenic disulfide, As_2S_2: a pigment.

reamer (re'mer) an engine-driven or hand-operated endodontic instrument for enlarging root canals, consisting of a triangular shaft twisted into a loosely spiraled serrated instrument.

reattachment (re"ah-tach'ment) 1. joining together parts that have been separated. 2. the recementing of a dental crown or other prosthesis. 3. embedding of new periodontal ligament fibers into new cementum and the attachment of gingival epithelium to tooth surface previously denuded by disease.

Réaumur's scale, thermometer (ra"o-merz') [René Antoine Ferschault *Réaumur*, French natural philosopher, 1683–1757] see under *scale* and *thermometer*.

rebase (re-bās') to refit a denture by means of the replacement of the denture base material without changing the occlusal relations of the teeth.

rebound (re'bownd) a reversed response on the withdrawal of a stimulus; see also under *phenomenon* and *tenderness*. **REM r.**, the phenomenon in which a subject deprived of REM (rapid eye movement) sleep for a prolonged period will, on being permitted to sleep undisturbed, compensate by having increased REM sleep.

recalcification (re-kal"sĭ-fi-ka'shun) the restoration of calcium salts to the bodily tissues.

recall 1. (re'kol, rĕ-kol') to remember or recollect. 2. the process of bringing a memory into consciousness.

recapitulation (re"kah-pit"u-la'shun) see under *theory*.

receiver (re-sēv'er) 1. a vessel for collecting a gas or a distillate. 2. the portion of an apparatus by which electric energy is converted into signals which may be seen or heard.

receptaculum (re"sep-tak'u-lum), pl. *receptac'ula* [L., from *recipere* to receive] a receptacle or container; that which serves for receiving or containing something. **r. chy'li,** cisterna chyli. **r. gan'glii petro'si,** fossula petrosa. **r. Pecquet'i,** cisterna chyli.

receptor (re-sep'tor) 1. a molecular structure within a cell or on the surface characterized by (1) selective binding of a specific substance and (2) a specific physiologic effect that accompanies the binding, e.g., cell-surface receptors for peptide hormones, neurotransmitters, antigens, complement fragments, and immunoglobulins and cytoplasmic receptors for steroid hormones. 2. a sensory nerve terminal that responds to stimuli of various kinds; see *exteroceptive, interoceptive,* and *proprioceptive*. **adrenergic r's,** postulated sites on effector organs innervated by postganglionic adrenergic fibers of the sympathetic nervous system, classified as α-adrenergic and β-adrenergic receptors according to their reaction to norepinephrine and epinephrine, respectively, and to certain blocking and stimulating agents. Called also *adrenoceptor* and *adrenoreceptor*. **α-adrenergic r's,** adrenergic receptors that respond to norepinephrine and to such blocking agents as phenoxybenzamine and phentolamine. **β-adrenergic r.,** adrenergic receptors that respond to epinephrine and to such blocking agents as propranolol; they are of two types: β_1 (lipolysis and cardiostimulation) and β_2 (bronchodilation and vasodilation). **B cell antigen r's,** monomeric IgM, IgD, and, (on memory cells only) IgG that is attached to the cell membrane of B lymphocytes and which, in conjunction with T cell help, triggers B cell activation on contact with antigen. **cholinergic r's,** cell-surface receptor molecules that bind the neurotransmitter acetylcholine and mediate its action on postjunctional cells, including parasympathetic autonomic effector cells, sympathetic and parasympathetic autonomic ganglion cells, striated muscle, and certain central neurons. See *muscarinic r's* and *nicotinic r's.* **complement r's,** cell-surface receptors for complement components. **contact r.,** a sense

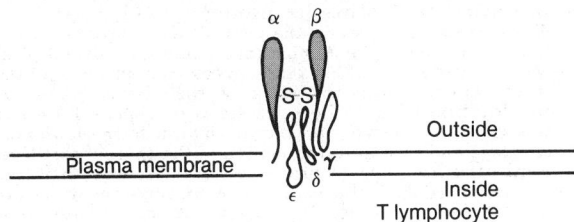

A model of the T cell receptor / T3 complex.

organ which responds to stimuli from objects in contact with the body. **contiguous r.,** a receptor which must be in direct contact with the stimulant, such as touch and taste receptors. **distance r.,** a sense organ which responds to stimuli from objects remote from the body, as a receptor for the stimuli of hearing, vision, or smell. **Fc r's,** specific cell-surface receptors for antigen-antibody complexes or aggregated immunoglobulins that bind a site in the Fc portion of the immunoglobulin molecule and may exhibit specificity for particular immunoglobulin classes. Fc receptors are found on B cells, K cells, macrophages, neutrophils, and eosinophils, and, during some developmental stages, on T cells; those on K cells, macrophages, and neutrophils bind to opsonizing antibodies bound to antigens and trigger phagocytosis of the antigen. **gustatory r.,** a receptor for the sense of taste; a taste bud. **H_1, H_2 r's,** see *histamine.* **IgE r's,** cell-surface receptors for IgE on mast cells and basophils; the IgE molecules are bound by a site in the Fc region leaving their antigen-binding sites exposed; binding of a multivalent antigen that cross-links the receptors triggers release of mediators of immediate hypersensitivity. **insulin r's,** specific receptors for insulin found on the surface of target cells. When insulin binds, the occupied receptors move to coated pits and are endocytosed. The endocytotic vesicles then fuse with lysosomes and insulin is degraded by proteases. Some degradation product released from the lysosome may be the direct intracellular mediator of insulin action. **low-density lipoprotein (LDL) r's,** specific receptors for LDL found in coated pits on the surface of mammalian cells. The coated pits are internalized forming coated vesicles from which LDL receptors are recycled back to the plasma membrane while LDL particles are transferred to lysosomes where they are degraded releasing free cholesterol, phospholipids, and amino acids. Genetic defects in LDL receptors are responsible for familial hypercholesterolemia. **muscarinic r's,** cholinergic receptors that are stimulated by the alkaloid muscarine and blocked by atropine; they are found on autonomic effector cells and on central neurons in the thalamus and cerebral cortex. **N_1-r's,** nicotinic receptors that are preferentially blocked by hexamethonium; they occur on autonomic ganglion cells. **N_2-r's,** nicotinic receptors that are preferentially blocked by decamethonium; they occur on striated muscle. **nicotinic r's,** cholinergic receptors that are stimulated initially and blocked at high doses by the alkaloid nicotine and blocked by tubocurarine;

they are found on autonomic ganglion cells, on striated muscle, and on spinal central neurons. See N_1-*r's* and N_2-*r's.* **pressure r.,** a receptor for stimuli of pressure or touch; a touch corpuscle. **T cell antigen r's,** receptors on T cells that recognize (1) specific foreign antigens and (2) self MHC antigens; both must be seen simultaneously to trigger T cell activation; the T cell receptor has a constant and a variable (antigen-finding) portion; the T cell antigen receptor has α and β chains which carry the idiotype (presumably the antigen binding site) and which are associated with the T3 molecule. **visual r.,** the layer of rods and cones of the retina. **volume r's,** postulated receptors which respond to increased plasma extracellular fluid volume and stimulate corrective measures.

recess (re′ses) a small empty space, hollow, or cavity; called also *recessus.* **accessory r. of elbow,** recessus sacciformis articulationis cubiti. **acetabular r.,** fossa acetabuli. **chiasmatic r.,** recessus opticus. **cochlear r. of vestibule,** recessus cochlearis vestibuli. **conarial r.,** recessus pinealis. **costodiaphragmatic r. of pleura,** recessus costodiaphragmaticus pleurae. **costomediastinal r. of pleura,** recessus costomediastinalis pleurae. **duodenal r., inferior,** recessus duodenalis inferior. **duodenal r., superior, duodenojejunal r.,** recessus duodenalis superior. **elliptical r. of vestibule,** recessus ellipticus vestibuli. **epitympanic r.,** recessus epitympanicus. **r. of fourth ventricle, lateral,** recessus lateralis ventriculi quarti. **hepatorenal r.,** recessus hepatorenalis. **Hyrtl's r.,** recessus epitympanicus. **ileocecal r., inferior,** recessus ileocaecalis inferior. **ileocecal r., superior,** recessus ileocaecalis superior. **infundibular r.,** recessus infundibuli. **infundibuliform r.,** recessus pharyngeus. **r. of infundibulum,** recessus infundibuli. **intersigmoidal r.,** recessus intersigmoideus. **laryngopharyngeal r.,** recessus piriformis. **r. of lesser omental cavity,** recessus lienalis. **r. of nasopharynx, lateral,** recessus pharyngeus. **omental r., inferior,** recessus inferior omentalis. **omental r., superior,** recessus superior omentalis. **optic r.,** recessus opticus. **paracolic r's,** sulci paracolici. **paraduodenal r.,** recessus paraduodenalis. **r. of pelvic mesocolon,** recessus intersigmoideus. **pharyngeal r.,** recessus pharyngeus. **pharyngeal r., middle,** bursa pharyngea. **phrenicohepatic r's,** see *recessus subhepatici, recessus subphrenici,* and *recessus hepatorenalis.* **phrenicomediastinal r.,** recessus phrenicomediastinalis. **phrenicomediastinal r. of pleura,** recessus phrenicomediastinalis pleurae. **pineal r.,** recessus pinealis. **piriform r.,** recessus piriformis. **pleural r's,** recessus pleurales. **Reichert's r.,** recessus cochlearis vestibuli. **retroannular r.,** a deep groove formed by the cell membrane immediately behind the annulus of spermatozoa of some species. **retrocecal r.,** recessus retrocaecalis. **retroduodenal r.,** recessus retroduodenalis. **r. of Rosenmüller,** recessus pharyngeus. **sacciform r. of articulation of elbow,** recessus sacciformis articulationis cubiti. **sacciform r. of distal radioulnar articulation,** recessus sacciformis articulationis radioulnaris distalis. **sphenoethmoidal r.,** recessus sphenoethmoidalis. **spherical r. of vestibule,** r. sphericus vestibuli. **splenic r.,** recessus lienalis. **subhepatic r's,** recessus subhepatici. **subphrenic r's,** recessus subphrenici. **subpopliteal r.,** recessus subpopliteus. **suprapineal r.,** recessus suprapinealis. **supratonsillar r.,** fossa supratonsillaris. **Tarini's r.,** recessus anterior fossae interpeduncularis [Tarini]. **triangular r.,** recessus triangularis. **r's of Tröltsch,** see *recessus membranae tympani anterior* and *recessus membranae tympani posterior.* **r. of tympanic membrane, anterior,** recessus membranae tympani anterior. **r. of tympanic membrane, posterior,** recessus membranae tympani posterior. **r. of tympanic membrane, superior,** recessus membranae tympani superior. **utricular r.,** utriculus, def. 2. **r. of vestibule,** recessus sphericus vestibuli.

recession (re-sesh′un) [L. *recedere* to draw back or away] the act or process of drawing away of a tissue or part from its normal position. **angle r.,** recession of the angle of the anterior chamber of the eye; see also under *glaucoma.* **clitoral r.,** surgical displacement of the clitoris by suturing the corpus back to the ramus; done to reduce its size in clitoral hypertrophy. **gingival r.,** the drawing back of the gingivae from the necks of the teeth with subsequent exposure of root surfaces. **r. of ocular muscle,** surgical displacement of the insertion of an ocular muscle posteriorly; done to weaken the stronger muscle in strabismus.

recessive (re-ses'iv) 1. tending to recede; not exerting a ruling or controlling influence; in genetics, incapable of expression unless the responsible allele is carried by both members of a pair of homologous chromosomes. 2. a recessive allele or trait.

recessus (re-ses'sus), pl. *reces'sus* [L.] a recess; a small empty space, hollow, or cavity; [NA] a general term for such potential spaces. **r. ante'rior fos'sae interpeduncula'ris [Tari'ni],** the portion of the interpeduncular fossa that passes under the corpora mamillaria; called also *Tarini's recess* and *Tarin's space.* **r. chi'asmatis,** r. opticus. **r. cochlea'ris vestib'uli** [NA], cochlear recess of vestibule: a small depressed area on the medial wall of the vestibule of the ear, situated just below the posterior end of the crista vestibuli, and perforated with foramina through which nerve fibers pass to the posterior portion of the ductus cochlearis. Called also *Reichert's recess.* **r. costodia-phragmat'icus pleu'rae** [NA], costodiaphragmatic recess of pleura: the pleural recess situated at the junction of the costal and diaphragmatic pleurae; called also *sinus phrenicocostalis.* **r. costomediastina'lis pleu'rae** [NA], costomediastinal recess of pleura: a wedge-shaped space, not completely filled with lung tissue, along the line at which the costal pleura meets the mediastinal pleura in front; called also *sinus costomediastinalis pleurae.* **r. duodena'lis infe'rior** [NA], inferior duodenal recess: a pocket in the peritoneum on the left side of the ascending portion of the duodenum, bounded by the inferior duodenal fold. **r. duodena'lis supe'rior** [NA], **r. duo-denojejuna'lis,** superior duodenal recess: a peritoneal pocket behind the superior duodenal fold. **r. ellip'ticus vestib'uli** [NA], elliptical recess of the vestibule: an oval depressed area in the roof and medial wall of the vestibule of the inner ear, situated above and behind the crista and pierced by 25 to 30 small foramina through which nerves come from the internal acoustic meatus to the utricle, which occupies the depression. **r. epitympan'icus** [NA], epitympanic recess: the upper portion of the tympanic cavity, extending above the level of the tympanic membrane and containing the greater part of the incus and the upper half of the malleus. **r. hepatorena'lis** [NA], hepatorenal recess: a peritoneal pouch between the liver and the kidney. **r. ileocaeca'lis infe'rior** [NA], inferior ileocecal recess: a peritoneal pocket situated behind the ileocecal fold, above the vermiform appendix below the ileum, and medial to the cecum; called also *r. ileocecalis inferior* [NA alternative]. **r. ileocaeca'lis supe'rior** [NA], superior ileocecal recess: a peritoneal pocket situated behind and below the vascular cecal fold, above the ileum and medial to the lower end of the ascending colon; called also *r. ileocecalis superior* [NA alternative]. **r. infe'rior omenta'lis** [NA], inferior omental recess: the lower portion of the omental bursa, including its extension down into the great omentum. It is bounded in front by the posterior wall of the stomach, and behind by the pancreas, the transverse colon and its mesocolon, the left suprarenal gland, and part of the left kidney. **r. infun-dib'uli** [NA], recess of infundibulum: a funnel-shaped depression in the anterior part of the floor of the third ventricle of the brain, within the infundibulum of the hypophysis. **r. intersigmoi'deus** [NA], intersigmoidal recess: a shallow peritoneal pocket running downward and to the left at the base of the sigmoid mesocolon. **r. latera'lis fos'sae rhomboi'dei,** r. lateralis ventriculi quarti. **r. latera'-lis ventric'uli quar'ti** [NA], lateral recess of fourth ventricle: a narrow, curved prolongation of the cavity of the fourth ventricle of the brain, extending laterally onto the dorsal surface of the inferior cerebellar peduncle; it contains a lateral prolongation of the choroid plexus and provides for the passage of cerebrospinal fluid into the subarachnoid space. **r. liena'lis,** NA alternative for *r. splenicus.* **r. membra'nae tym'pani ante'rior** [NA], anterior recess of tympanic membrane: a pocket in the tympanic membrane formed by the tunica mucosa between the anterior mallear fold and the anterior superior part of the pars tensa of the membrane, ending blindly above. **r. membra'nae tym'pani poste'rior** [NA], posterior recess of tympanic membrane: a pocket in the tympanic membrane formed by

the tunica mucosa between the posterior mallear fold and the posterior superior part of the pars tensa of the membrane, ending blindly above. **r. membra'nae tym'pani supe'rior** [NA], superior recess of tympanic membrane: a recess in the tympanic membrane formed by the tunica mucosa between the neck of the malleus and the pars flaccida of the membrane, and ending blindly below. Called also *Prussak's pouch* or *space.* **r. op'ticus** [NA], optic recess: a depression in the floor of the third ventricle of the brain, between the chiasma behind and the lamina terminalis in front. **r. paracol'ici,** sulci paracolici. **r. paraduodena'lis** [NA], paraduodenal recess: a pocket occasionally found in the peritoneum behind a fold containing a branch of the left colic artery. **r. pharyngea'lis,** NA alternative for *r. pharyngeus.* **r. pharyn'geus** [NA], **r. pharyn'geus [Rosenmül'leri],** pharyngeal recess: a wide, slitlike lateral extension in the wall of the nasopharynx, cranial and dorsal to the pharyngeal orifice of the auditory tube; called also *Rosenmüller's cavity, fossa,* or *cavity.* **r. phrenicohepat'ici,** see *r. subhepatici, r. subphrenici,* and *r. hepatorenalis.* **r. phrenicomedias-tina'lis** [NA], phrenicomediastinal recess: the pleural recess between the diaphragmatic and mediastinal pleurae. **r. phrenicomediastina'lis pleu'rae** [NA], phrenicomediastinal recess of pleura: the pleural recess situated at the line of junction of the diaphragmatic and mediastinal pleurae. **r. pinea'lis** [NA], pineal recess: an extension of the third ventricle into the stalk of the pineal body. **r. pirifor'mis** [NA], piriform recess: a pear-shaped fossa in the wall of the laryngeal pharynx lateral to the arytenoid cartilage and medial to the lamina of the thyroid cartilage. **r. pleura'les** [NA], pleural recesses: the spaces where the different portions of the pleura join at an angle and which are never completely filled by lung tissue; called also *sinus pleurae.* **r. pneumatoenter'icus,** either of the paired embryonic excavations alongside the dorsal mesogastrium, the right one sometimes persisting as the infracardiac bursa. **r. poste'rior fos'sae interpeduncula'ris [Tari'ni],** the portion of the interpeduncular fossa that slightly undermines the anterior margin of the pons. **r. pro utric'-ulo,** r. ellipticus vestibuli. **r. retrocaeca'lis** [NA], retrocecal recess: a peritoneal pocket extending upward behind the cecum and sometimes behind the colon; called also *r. retrocecalis* [NA alternative]. **r. retroduodena'lis** [NA], retroduodenal recess: an occasional peritoneal pocket extending behind the horizontal and ascending parts of the duodenum. **r. saccifor'mis articulatio'nis cu'biti,** sacciform recess of articulation of elbow: the distal bulging of the articular capsule of the elbow joint, situated between the incisura radialis ulnae and the circumferentia articularis radii. **r. saccifor'mis articulatio'nis radioulna'-ris dista'lis** [NA], sacciform recess of distal radioulnar articulation: a bulging of the synovial membrane of the articular capsule of the distal radioulnar joint, which extends proximally between the radius and ulna beyond the point of their articular surfaces. **r. sphenoethmoida'lis** [NA], sphenoethmoidal recess: the most superior and posterior part of the nasal cavity, above the superior nasal concha, into which the sphenoidal sinus opens. **r. spher'icus vestib'uli** [NA], spherical recess of vestibule: a circular depressed area in the anteroinferior portion of the medial wall of the vestibule of the inner ear. It is pierced by 12 to 15 small foramina through which nerves come from the internal acoustic meatus to the saccule, which occupies the depression. **r. sple'nicus** [NA], splenic recess: an extension of the omental bursa to the left behind the gastrosplenic ligament almost to the spleen; called also *r. lienalis* [NA alternative]. **r. subhepat'ici** [NA], subhepatic recesses: peritoneal pockets located beneath the liver. **r. subphren'ici** [NA], subphrenic recesses: peritoneal pockets located beneath the diaphragm. **r. subpopli'teus** [NA], subpopliteal recess: a prolongation of the synovial tendon sheath of the popliteus muscle outside the knee joint into the popliteal space; called also *bursa musculi poplitei.* **r. supe'rior omenta'lis** [NA], superior omental recess: a rather long, narrow peritoneal pocket leading from the vestibule upward toward the liver, between the inferior vena cava on the right, the esophagus on the left, the gastrohepatic ligament in front, and the diaphragm behind. **r. suprapinea'lis** [NA], suprapineal recess: the posterior extension of the third ventricle of the brain above and around the pineal body. **r. triangula'ris,** triangular recess: a small triangular recess on the anterior wall of the third ventricle of the brain, its base below the anterior commissure, and its sides formed by the converging columns of the fornix.

recidivation (re-sid″ĭ-va′shun) recidivism.

recidivism (re-sid′ĭ-vizm) 1. the repetition of an offense or crime. 2. the relapse or recurrence of a disease.

recidivist (re-sid′ĭ-vist) [Fr. *récidiviste*, from L. *recidere* to fall back] one who tends to relapse, especially a person who tends to return to criminal habits after treatment or punishment.

recipe (res′ĭ-pe) 1. [L.] take; used at the head of a physician's prescription, and usually indicated by the symbol ℞. See *prescription*. 2. a formula for the preparation of a specific combination of ingredients.

recipient (re-sip′e-ent) one who receives, as blood in transfusion, or a tissue or organ graft. **universal r.**, a person thought to be able to receive blood of any "type" without agglutination of the donor cells.

recipiomotor (re-sip″e-o-mo′tor) [L. *recipere* to receive + *motor* mover] pertaining to the reception of motor impressions.

reciprocation (re-sip″ro-ka′shun) [L. *reciprocare* to move backward and forward] to give and receive in exchange; the complementary interaction of two distinct entities. In dentistry, the means by which one part of a removable partial denture framework is made to counter the effect created by another part of the framework.

Recklinghausen's canals, disease, disease of bone (rek′ling-how″zenz) [Friedrich Daniel von *Recklinghausen*, German pathologist, 1833–1910] see under *canal*, and see *neurofibromatosis* and *osteitis fibrosa cystica*.

recognin (re-kog′nin) any of a group of protein fragments produced from cancer cells that are capable of recognizing specific cells; they include astrocytin and malignin.

recognition (rek″og-nish′un) 1. the act of recognizing or state of being recognized. 2. antigen recognition; the interaction of immunologically competent cells with antigen that begins with the binding of the antigen to specific antigen receptors on B and T lymphocytes and results in an immune response directed against the antigen.

recombinant (re-kom′bĭ-nant) 1. a cell or an individual with a new combination of genes not found together in either parent; usually applied to linked genes. **r. DNA**, see under *DNA*. **hGH-r.**, growth hormone recombinant.

recombination (re″kom-bĭ-na′shun) the reunion, in the same or a different arrangement, of formerly united elements which have become separated. In genetics, the formation of new combinations of genes as a result of crossing over between homologous chromosomes. **bacterial r.**, in bacterial genetics, the process of producing a new gene by any of several processes, e.g., the sexual union of two parents, molecular crossing over between two DNA chains, or transformation.

recompression (re″kom-presh′un) the restoration of pressure, especially the return to conditions of normal pressure after exposure to greatly diminished atmospheric pressure.

reconstitution (re″kon-stĭ-tu′shun) 1. a type of regeneration in which a new organ forms by the rearrangement of tissues rather than from new formation at an injured surface. 2. The restoration to original form of a substance previously altered for preservation and storage, as the restoration to a liquid state of blood serum or plasma that has been dried and stored.

reconstruction (re″kon-struk′shun) to reassemble or reform from constituent parts. **image r. from projections**, radiography in which two- or three-dimensional images of an object are reconstructed from a set of mathematical projections, as in transverse axial tomography.

recontour (re-kon′toor) to give new shape or contour to. In dentistry, to change the contour of a crown or a complete or partial denture.

record (rek′ord) 1. a permanent or long-lasting account of something (as on film, in writing, etc.). 2. See *registration*. **chew-in r., functional,** 1. a record of the natural chewing movements of the mandible made on the occlusion rim by the teeth or scribing studs. 2. a record of movements of the mandible made on the occluding surface of the opposing occlusion rim by the teeth or scribing studs; produced by simulated chewing movements. 3. a record of lateral and protrusive movements of the mandible made on the occlusal surface of the occlusion rim by the teeth or scribing studs on an opposing rim; produced during simulated movements of bruxism. **face-bow r.**, a registration by means of a face-bow of the position of the hinge axis and/or the condyles; used to orient the maxillary cast to the opening and closing axis of the articulator. **interocclusal r.**, a record of the positional relation of the teeth or jaws to each other, made on occlusal surfaces of occlusion rims or teeth in a plastic material which hardens, such as plaster of Paris, wax, or zinc oxide and eugenol paste. **interocclusal r., centric**, a record of the centric jaw position (relation). **interocclusal r., eccentric**, a record of a jaw relation other than the centric relation. **interocclusal r., lateral**, a record of a lateral eccentric jaw position. **interocclusal r., protrusive**, a record of a protruded eccentric jaw position. **jaw relation r.**, a registration of any positional relationship of the mandible in reference to the maxillae; these records may be of any of the many vertical, horizontal, or orientation relations. **maxillomandibular r.**, a record of the relation of the mandible to the maxillae. Called also *maxillomandibular registration*. **occluding centric relation r.**, a registration of centric relation made at the established occlusal vertical dimension. **problem-oriented r. (POR)**, an approach to patient care record keeping that focuses on those specific health problems of the patient that require immediate attention and on the structuring of a cooperative health care plan designed to cope with the identified problems. The components basic to the POR are: *the data base*, which provides information obtained from the variety of sources required for each patient regardless of diagnosis or presenting problems; *the problem list*, which contains those major problems currently needing attention and serves as the basis of a plan of care; *the plan*, which specifies what is to be done with regard to each problem; *the progress notes*, which document the observations, assessments, nursing care plans, physician's orders, etc., of all health care personnel directly involved in the care of the patient. See also *SOAP*. **profile r.**, a record showing the sagittal outline form or profile of the face. **protrusive r.**, a registration of a forward position of the mandible with reference to the maxillae. **terminal jaw relation r.**, a record of the relationship of the mandible to the maxilla made at the vertical relation of occlusion and at the centric position.

recrement (rek′rĕ-ment) [L. *recrementum*] the saliva or other material which, after secretion, is reabsorbed into the blood.

recrementitious (rek″rĕ-men-tish′us) of the nature of a recrement.

recrudescence (re″kroo-des′ens) [L. *recrudescere* to become sore again] the recurrence of symptoms after a temporary abatement. See *relapse*. The chief distinction between a recrudescence and a relapse is the time interval, a recrudescence occurring after some days or weeks, a relapse after some weeks or months.

recrudescent (re″kroo-des′ent) [L. *recrudescens*] breaking out afresh.

recruitment (re-kroot′ment) 1. the gradual increase to a maximum in a reflex when a stimulus of unaltered intensity is prolonged. 2. in audiology, an abnormally large increase in the loudness of a sound caused by a slight increase in its intensity.

Rect. abbreviation for L. *rectifica′tus*, rectified.

rectal (rek′tal) pertaining to the rectum.

rectalgia (rek-tal′je-ah) [*rectum* + *-algia*] proctalgia.

rectectomy (rek-tek′to-me) [*rectum* + Gr. *ektomē* excision] proctectomy.

rectification (rek″tĭ-fi-ka′shun) [L. *rectificatio*] 1. the act of making straight, pure, or correct. 2. redistillation of a liquid to purify it. 3. conversion of alternating current to direct current. **spontaneous r.**, a transverse lie which rectifies itself before labor begins.

rectified (rek″tĭ-fīd) refined; made straight; converted to direct current (DC).

rectifier (rek′tĭ-fi″er) a device for obtaining a direct (unidirectional) current from an alternating current. **thermionic r.**, a rectifier consisting of an electric valve in which the electrons are supplied by a heated electrode.

rectischiac (rek-tis′ke-ak) pertaining to the rectum and the ischium.

rectitis (rek-ti′tis) proctitis.

rect(o)- [L. *rectum*] a combining form designating relationship to the rectum. See also words beginning *proct(o)*.

rectoabdominal (rek″to-ab-dom′ĭ-nal) pertaining to the rectum and abdomen.

rectocele (rek′to-sēl) [*recto-* + Gr. *kēlē* hernia] hernial protrusion of part of the rectum into the vagina; called also *proctocele*.

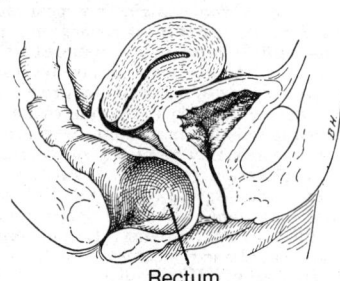

Rectum

Rectocele.

rectoclysis (rek-tok′lĭ-sis) proctoclysis.

rectococcygeal (rek″to-kok-sij′e-al) pertaining to the rectum and the coccyx.

rectococcypexy (rek″to-kok′sĭ-pek-se) proctococcypexy.

rectocolitis (rek″to-ko-li′tis) coloproctitis.

rectocutaneous (rek″to-ku-ta′ne-us) pertaining to the rectum and the skin.

rectocystotomy (rek″to-sis-tot′o-me) proctocystotomy.

rectolabial (rek″to-la′be-al) pertaining to or communicating with the rectum and a labium majus, as a rectolabial fistula.

rectoperineorrhaphy (rek″to-per″ĭ-ne-or′ah-fe) proctoperineorrhaphy.

rectopexy (rek′to-pek″se) proctopexy.

rectoplasty (rek′to-plas″te) proctoplasty.

rectoromanoscope (rek″to-ro-man′o-skōp) an endoscope for examining the rectum and sigmoid.

rectoromanoscopy (rek″to-ro″mah-nos′ko-pe) [*rectum* + L. *romanum* sigmoid + Gr. *skopein* to examine] inspection of the rectum and sigmoid through an endoscope.

rectorrhaphy (rek-tor′ah-fe) [*rectum* + Gr. *rhaphē* suture] proctorrhaphy.

rectoscope (rek′to-skōp) proctoscope.

rectoscopy (rek-tos′ko-pe) proctoscopy.

rectosigmoid (rek″to-sig′moid) the rectum and sigmoid colon.

rectosigmoidectomy (rek″to-sig″moi-dek′to-me) excision of the rectum and sigmoid.

rectostenosis (rek″to-stĕ-no′sis) stenosis, or stricture, of the rectum.

rectostomy (rek-tos′to-me) proctostomy.

rectotome (rek′to-tōm) proctotome.

rectotomy (rek-tot′o-me) proctotomy.

rectourethral (rek″to-u-re′thral) pertaining to or communicating with the rectum and urethra, as a rectourethral fistula.

rectouterine (rek″to-u′ter-in) pertaining to the rectum and uterus.

rectovaginal (rek″to-vaj′ĭ-nal) pertaining to or communicating with the rectum and vagina, as a rectovaginal fistula.

rectovesical (rek″to-ves′ĭ-kal) pertaining to or communicating with the rectum and urinary bladder, as a rectovesical fistula.

rectovestibular (rek″to-ves-tib′u-lar) pertaining to or communicating with the rectum and the vestibule of the vagina, as a rectovestibular fistula.

rectovulvar (rek″to-vul′var) pertaining to or communicating with the rectum and vulva, as a rectovulvar fistula.

Rectules (rek′tūlz) trademark for a preparation of chloral hydrate.

rectum (rek′tum) [L. "straight"] [NA] the distal portion of the large intestine, beginning anterior to the third sacral vertebra as a continuation of the sigmoid and ending at the anal canal; called also *intestinum rectum.*

rectus (rek′tus) [L.] straight; [NA] a general term denoting a straight structure, as a muscle (see entries beginning *musculus rectus*).

recumbent (re-kum′bent) lying down.

recuperation (re-ku″per-a′shun) [L. *recuperatio*] the recovery of health and strength.

recurrence (re-kur′ens) [L. *re-* again + *currere* to run] the return of symptoms after a remission.

recurrent (re-kur′ent) [L. *recurrens* returning] 1. running back, or toward the source. 2. returning after intermissions.

recurvation (re″kur-va′shun) [L. *recurvatio*] a backward bending or curvature.

red (red) [L. *rubrum*] 1. one of the primary colors produced by the longest waves of the visible spectrum. 2. a red dye or stain. **alizarin r.**, the sodium salt of alizarin monosulfonate. **alizarin r. S, alizarin water-soluble r.,** sodium alizarinsulfonate. **aniline r.**, basic fuchsin. **bordeaux r.**, cerasine. **bromphenol r.**, an indicator, dibromphenol-sulfonphthalein, $(CH_2Br_2OH)_2 \cdot C_6H_4 \cdot SO_2 \cdot \cdot ONa$. **carmine r.**, a stain, $C_{11}H_{12}O_7$, derived from carmine. **cerasine r.**, sudan III. **chlorophenol r.**, dichlorosulfonphthalein, a pH indicator with a range of 5.2 (yellow) to 6.8 (red). **cholera r.**, see *cholera red test*, under *tests*. **Congo r.**, chemical name: 3,3′- [4,4′-biphenylene-bis(azo)]bis[4-amino-1-naphthalenesulfonic acid] disodium salt. An odorless dark red or reddish brown powder, $C_{32}H_{22}N_6Na_2O_6S_2$, which decomposes on exposure to acid fumes. It is used as a diagnostic aid in amyloidosis, and has been used as an antihemolytic and detoxicant. See also under *tests*. **cotton r.**, Congo r. **cotton r. 4 B**, benzopurpurine 4 B. **cresol r.**, an indicator, ortho-cresol-sulfonphthalein, $(CH_3 \cdot C_6H_4 \cdot OH)_2C \cdot C_6H_4 \cdot SO_2 \cdot ONa$, used in the determination of the hydrogen ion concentration. It has a pH range of 7.2 to 8.8, being yellow at 7.2 and red at 8.8. **dianil r. 4 C, dianin r. 4 B**, benzopurpurine 4 B. **direct r.**, congo r. **direct r. 4 B**, benzopurpurine 4 B. **fast r.**, amaranth. **fast r. B** or **P**, cerasine. **indigo r., indoxyl r.**, a coloring matter produced by heating an aqueous solution of indoxyl to 130° C. **magdala r.**, a basic dye used for staining connective tissue. It is a mixture of monoamino- and diamino-naphthosafranins. The diamino compound is $NH_2C_{10}H_5 \cdot N_2Cl(C_{10}H_7) \cdot C_{10}H_5 \cdot NH_2$. **methyl r.**, a dye, para-dimethyl-amino-azo-benzene-ortho-carboxylic acid, $(CH_3)_2N \cdot C_6H_4 \cdot N{:}N \cdot C_6H_4 \cdot COOH$, used as an indicator in the determination of hydrogen ion concentration; it has a pH range of 4.4 to 6, being red at 4.4, and yellow at 6. **naphthaline r.**, magdala r. **naphthol r.**, amaranth. **neutral r.**, a dye, amino-dimethylaminotoluphenazonium chloride, $(CH_3)_2N \cdot C_6H_3 \cdot N_2C_6H_2(CH_3) \cdot \cdot NH_2HCl$. As an indicator it has a pH range of 6.8 to 8, being red at 6.8 and yellow at 8. **oil r.**, sudan III. **oil r. IV**, scarlet r. **orange r.**, the red oxide of lead, Pb_3O_4, used as a pigment. **phenol r.**, phenolsulfonphthalein. **provisional r.**, a colored layer obtained from rhodopsin. **scarlet r.**, chemical name: ortho-tolylazo-ortho-tolylazo-beta-naphthol. A fat-soluble azo dye, $C_{24}H_{20}N_4O$, which has some power to stimulate the proliferation of cells, and has been used to enhance wound healing. Called also *oil r. IV, ponceau 3B, rubrum scarlatinum, scarlet R, scharlach R,* and *Sudan IV.* **scarlet r. sulfonate**, the sodium salt of azo-benzene-disulfonic acid azobeta-naphthol; used for the same purpose as scarlet red. **senitol r.**, a dye, $C_2H_5 \cdot NC_9H_6 \cdot (CH)_3 \cdot C_9H_6N(I) \cdot C_2H_5$, with a highly selective germicidal action on staphylococci; it is also used to sensitize photographic plates to red rays of light. **sudan r.**, magdala r. **toluylene r.**, the base, the hydrochloride of which is neutral red. **tony r.**, sudan III. **trypan r.**, an acid azo dye used as a vital stain and which possesses some trypanocidal activity. **vital r.**, chemical name: 3-amino-4-[[4′-[(2-amino-6-sulfo-1-naphthyl)azo]-3,3′-dimethyl-4-biphenylyl]azo]-2,7-naphthalene disulfonic acid trisodium salt. A dye, which is introduced directly into the circulation by venipuncture for the purpose of estimating the volume of the blood in the body by determining the concentration of the dye in the blood plasma. **wool r.,** amaranth.

redecussate (re″de-kus′āt) to form a secondary decussation.

redfoot (red′foot) a fatal condition of unknown etiology affecting newborn lambs, in which the sensitive lamina of the feet become exposed owing to detachment of the overlying horn.

redia (re′de-ah), pl. *re′diae* [named after F. *Redi,* Italian naturalist, 1626–1698] a larval stage of certain trematode parasites, which develops in the body of a snail host and gives rise to daughter rediae, or to the cercariae.

rediae (re′de-e) plural of *redia.*

redifferentiation (re″dif-er-en″she-a′shun) the return of a dedifferentiated tissue or part to its original or another more or less similar condition.

Redig. in pulv. abbreviation for L. *rediga′tur in pul′verem,* let it be reduced to powder.

Red. in pulv. abbreviation for L. *reduc′tus in pul′verem,* reduced to powder.

redintegration (red-in″tě-gra′shun) [L. *redintegratio*] 1. the restoration or repair of a lost or damaged part. 2. that type of psychic process in which a part of a complex stimulus revokes the complete reaction that was previously made to the complex stimulus as a whole.

redislocation (re″dis-lo-ka′shun) dislocation recurring after reduction.

Redisol (red′ĭ-sol) trademark for a preparation of crystalline vitamin B$_{12}$; see *cyanocobalamin.*

Redlich-Obersteiner (red′likh o″ber-sti′ner) see *Obersteiner-Redlich.*

redox (red′oks) oxidation-reduction.

redressement (rĕ-dres-maw′) [Fr.] 1. a second or repeated dressing. 2. correction of a deformity.

red tide (red tīd) see *Gonyaulax.*

reduce (re-dūs′) [re- + L. *ducere* to lead] 1. to restore to the normal place or relation of parts, as to *reduce* a fracture. 2. in chemistry, to submit to reduction. 3. to decrease in weight.

reduced (re-dūst′) 1. returned to the proper place or position, as a *reduced* fracture. 2. restored to a metallic form, as *reduced* iron. 3. altered by a chemical change involving a gain of electrons.

reducible (re-du′sĭ-b'l) permitting of reduction; capable of being reduced.

reductant (re-duk′tant) the electron donor in an oxidation-reduction (redox) reaction.

reductase (re-duk′tās) [EC 1] an enzyme of the oxidoreductase class that catalyzes reactions used physiologically solely for the reduction of metabolites. **5α-r.,** an enzyme that catalyzes the irreversible reduction of testosterone to dihydrotestosterone with NADPH as the hydrogen donor. Deficiency of the enzyme, an autosomal recessive trait, leads to a form of male pseudohermaphroditism.

reduction (re-duk′shun) [L. *reductio*] 1. the correction of a fracture, dislocation, or hernia. 2. in chemistry, the addition of hydrogen to a substance, or more generally, the gain of electrons. **r. of chromosomes,** the passing of the members of a chromosome pair to the daughter cells during meiosis, each daughter cell receiving half the diploid number. **closed r.,** the manipulative reduction of a fracture or dislocation without incision. **r. en masse,** reduction of a strangulated hernia included within its sac, so that the strangulation is not relieved. **open r.,** reduction of a fracture or dislocation after incision into the site. **weight r.,** the lessening of one's body weight by a specific regimen which is especially designed for that purpose.

reductone (re-duk′tōn) glucic acid.

reduplication (re″du-plĭ-ka′shun) [L. *reduplicatio*] 1. a doubling back. 2. the recurrence of paroxysms of a double type. 3. a doubling of parts, connected at some point, the extra part being usually a mirror image of the other.

reduviid (re-du′vĭ-id) belonging to the family Reduviidae.

Reduviidae (re″du-vi′ĭ-de) a family of winged hemipterous insects of the suborder Heteroptera, called cone-nose bugs or kissing bugs; they are also known as assassin bugs because they prey on other insects. They attack man and other mammals; some species transmit Chagas' disease. It includes the genera *Eratyrus, Eutriatoma, Panstrongylus, Reduvius* (type genus), *Rhodnius,* and *Triatoma.*

Reduvius (re-du′ve-us) a genus of hemipterous blood-sucking insects. **R. persona′tus,** a species whose bite may cause nausea, generalized urticaria, or other allergic symptoms.

redwater (red′wah-ter) 1. Texas fever. 2. bacillary hemoglobinuria.

Reed's cells (rēdz) [Dorothy *Reed,* American pathologist, 1874–1964] Reed-Sternberg cells.

reef (rēf) an infolding or tuck of tissue, as a tuck made in plication.

reentry (re-en′tre) in cardiology, a postulated mechanism by which a premature heart beat can be coupled to the normal beat: the normal sinus impulse activates the heart except for an area of diminished responsiveness; by the time this abnormal area is activated, the remainder of the heart has recovered, and the impulse "reenters" the normal zone from the abnormal area, eliciting a premature contraction.

Rees's test (rēs′ez) [George Owen *Rees,* English physician, 1813–1889] see under *tests.*

refect (re-fekt′) to induce refection.

refection (re-fek′shun) [L. *reficere* to restore] recovery; repair: applied specifically to the ability of the flora of the cecum of rats to synthesize vitamins of the B group from deficient diets and supply them to the host animal.

refectious (re-fek′shus) capable of causing, or pertaining to, refection.

refine (re-fīn′) to purify or free from foreign matter.

reflected (re-flekt′ed) turned or bent back; mirrored.

reflection (re-flek′shun) [L. *reflexio*] 1. a turning or bending back; a bending back upon its course. 2. an image produced by reflection. 3. in physics, the turning back of a ray of light, sound, or heat when it strikes against a surface that it does not penetrate. The ray before reflection is known as the *incident ray;* after reflection, it is the *reflected ray.*

reflector (re-flek′tor) a device for reflecting light or sound. **dental r.,** a mouth mirror used to reflect light on the field of action during a dental operation or examination.

reflex (re′fleks) [L. *reflexus*] 1. reflected. 2. a reflected action or movement; the sum total of any particular involuntary activity. See *reflex arc* and *reflex action.* 3. a reflection or a reflected image of an object. **abdominal r's,** contractions of the abdominal muscles on scratching the abdominal wall. **abdominocardiac r.,** any reflex in the heart produced by stimulating the abdominal sympathetic nerves. Cf. *Livierato's sign* and *Prevel's sign,* under *sign.* **Abrams' r.,** reflex contraction of the lung following stimulation of the chest wall. **Abrams' heart r.,** contraction of the myocardium, with reduction in the area of cardiac dullness, which results when the skin of the precordial region is irritated. It is observed with the fluoroscope. **accommodation r.,** the coordinated changes that occur when the eye adapts itself for near vision; they are constriction of the pupil, convergence of the eyes, and increased convexity of the lens. **Achilles tendon r.,** triceps surae jerk. **acoustic r.,** contraction of the stapedius muscle in response to intense sound. Called also *stapedial r.* **acquired r.,** conditioned response. **adductor r.,** on tapping the tendon of the adductor magnus with the thigh in abduction, contraction of the adductors results. **adductor r. of foot,** Hirschberg's sign. **allied r's,** reflexes in which two afferent stimuli use the same common pathway or produce effects on two synergistic muscles. **anal r.,** contraction of the anal sphincter on irritation of the skin of the anus. **ankle r.,** triceps surae jerk. **antagonistic r's,** reflex movements occurring not in the muscle which has been stretched but in its antagonist. **anticus r.,** Piotrowski's sign. **Aschner's r.,** oculocardiac r. **atriopressor r.,** rise in arterial blood pressure (vasoconstriction) attributed to a change of pressure in the right atrium and great veins. **attention r. of pupil,** alteration of size in the pupil when the attention is suddenly fixed; called also *Piltz's r.* **attitudinal r's,** those reflexes having to do with the position of the body. **audito-oculogyric r.,** a turning of both eyes in the direction of a sudden sound. **auditory r.,** any reflex caused by stimulation of the auditory nerve, especially momentary closure of both eyes produced by a sudden sound. **aural r.,** any reflex connected with the auditory apparatus. **auricle r.,** involuntary movement of the ear produced by auditory stimuli. **auriculocervical nerve r.,** Snellen's r. **auriculopalpebral r.,** Kehrer's r. **autonomic r.,** a response of smooth muscle, glands, and conducting tissue of the heart, which alters the functional state of the innervated organ. **axon r.,** a reflex resulting from a stimulus applied to one branch of a nerve which sets up an impulse that moves centrally to the point of division of the nerve where it is reflected down the other branch to the effector organ. **Babinski's r.** (1896), dorsiflexion of the big toe on stimulating the sole of the foot; it occurs in lesions of the pyramidal tract, and indicates organic, as distinguished from hysteric, hemiplegia. Called also *Babinski's sign* or *toe sign.* **Babkin r.,** pressure by the examiner's thumbs on the palms of both hands of the infant results in opening of the infant's mouth; it is elicited in many newborn infants, normal and abnormal, except when lethargic or comatose. **Bainbridge r.,** rise in pressure in, or increased distention of, the large somatic veins or the right atrium, with acceleration of the heart beat. **Barkman's r.,** contraction of the rectus abdominis muscle on the same side after stimulation of the skin just below one of the nipples. **basal joint r.,** finger-thumb r. **behavior r.,** conditioned response. **Bekhterev's r.,** 1. *deep:* passive flexion of the toes and foot in a plantar direction is followed by flexion in a dorsal direction and by flexive movements of the knee and hip. 2. *hypogastric:* contraction of the muscles of the lower abdomen on stroking the skin of the inner surface of the thigh. 3. *pupil:* dilatation of the pupil on exposure to light; sometimes seen in tabes and general paralysis. 4. tickling of the mucosa of the nasal cavity with a feather or piece of paper produces contraction of the facial muscles on the same side of the face; called also *nasal r.* **Bekhterev-Mendel r.,** Mendel-Bekhterev r. **biceps r.,** contractions of the biceps muscle of the arm when its tendon is tapped; this reflex is normal but when greatly increased it indicates the same disease as increased knee jerk. **bladder r.,** any of the reflexes of the bladder necessary for effortless evacuation of urine and subconscious maintenance of continence: vesical contraction following distention of the bladder, vesical contraction evoked by urethral flow, vesical contraction evoked by proximal urethral distention, relaxation of the urethra resulting from running liquid in the urethra, distention of the bladder resulting in relaxation of the external sphincter, relaxation of the proximal urethral smooth muscle by distention of the bladder, and vesical contraction related to running liquid through the urethra. **blink r.,** corneal r. **Brain's r.,** an extension of the hemiplegic flexed arm when the patient assumes the quadrupedal position; called also *quadrupedal extensor reflex.* **bregmocardiac r.,** pressure upon the bregmatic fontanel slows the action of the heart. **Brissaud's r.,** contraction of the tensor muscle of fascia lata on tickling the sole. **Brudzinski's r.,** see under *sign.* **bulbocavernous r.,** a tap on the dorsum of the penis causes retraction of the bulbocavernous portion. **bulbomimic r.,** in coma from apoplexy, pressure on the eyeball causes contraction of the facial muscles on the side opposite to the lesion; in coma from toxic causes, the reflex occurs on both sides. Called also *facial r.* and *Mondonesi's r.* **carotid sinus r.,** pressure on, or in, the carotid artery at the level of its bifurcation causing reflex slowing of the heart rate; this reflex originates in the wall of the sinus of the internal carotid artery. See *carotid sinus syndrome,* under *syndrome.* **cat's eye r.,** see under *amaurosis.* **cerebral cortex r.,** Haab's r. **Chaddock r.,** stimulation below the external malleolus produces extension of the great toe; it occurs in lesions of the pyramidal tract. **chain r.,** a series of reflexes, each serving as a stimulus to the next one, representing a complete activity. **chin r.,** stroking of the chin causes closing of the mouth. **chocked r.,** in skiascopy, absence of movement of the retinal illumination on reaching the point of reversal. **ciliary r.,** the movement of the pupil in accommodation. **ciliospinal r.,** painful stimulation of the skin of the neck dilates the pupil. **clasp-knife r.,** lengthening reaction. **cochleo-orbicular r., cochleopalpebral r.,** contraction of the orbicularis palpebrarum muscle when a sharp, sudden noise is made close to the ear; does not occur in total deafness from labyrinthine disease. **cochleopupillary r.,** a reaction of the iris (contraction of the pupil followed by dilatation) to a loud sound. **cochleostapedial r.,** the reflex contraction of the stapedius muscle from noises. **concealed r.,** one elicited by a stimulus but concealed by a more dominant reflex elicited by the same stimulus. **conditioned r.,**

see under *response.* **conjunctival r.,** closure of the eyelid when the conjunctiva is touched. **consensual r.,** crossed r. **consensual light r.,** stimulation of one eye by light produces a reflex response in the opposite pupil. **convergency r.,** convergence of the visual axes with fixation on a near point. **convulsive r.,** one in which several muscles contract convulsively without coordination. **coordinated r.,** one in which several muscles react so as to produce an orderly and useful movement. **corneal r.,** 1. irritation of the cornea results in reflex closure of the lids; called also *blink r., eyelid closure r.,* and *lid r.* 2. reflection of light from the cornea. **corneomandibular r., corneopterygoid r.,** movement of the lower jaw toward the side opposite the eye whose cornea is lightly touched, the mouth being open. **corneomental r.,** unilateral wrinkling of the muscles of the chin when pressure is applied to the cornea. **coronary r.,** the reflex that controls the caliber of the coronary blood vessels. **cough r.,** the sequence of events initiated by the sensitivity of the lining of the airways of the lung and mediated by the medulla as a consequence of impulses transmitted by the vagus nerve, resulting in coughing, i.e., the clearing of the passageways of foreign matter. **cranial r.,** any reflex whose paths are connected directly with the brain. **cremasteric r.,** stimulation of the skin on the front and inner side of the thigh retracts the testis on the same side. The presence of this reflex indicates integrity of the first lumbar nerve segment of the spinal cord or its root; absence indicates damage of the first lumbar nerve segment or its root or lesion of the corticospinal tract. Cf. *Geigel's r.* **crossed r.,** stimulation of one side of the body often causes also a corresponding response on the other side, especially in the eye. **cuboidodigital r.,** Mendel-Bekhterev r. **cutaneous pupillary r.,** dilatation of the pupil on pinching the skin of the cheek or neck. **dartos r.,** the patient stands with his feet wide apart and the examiner suddenly applies cold to the perineum; the dartos muscle undergoes vermicular contraction. **dazzle r.,** a reflex by which a strong light shining on the eyes causes an immediate closing of the eyelids which lasts as long as the stimulus. **deep r.,** one elicited by a sharp tap on the appropriate tendon or muscle to induce brief stretch of the muscle, followed by contraction. Called also *tendon r.* **defecation r.,** rectal r. **defense r.,** contraction and extension motions in a paralyzed limb produced by plantar flexion of the toes. **delayed r.,** a reflex which occurs some time after the stimulus provoking it has been received. **depressor r.,** a reflex to stimulation resulting in decreased activity of the motor center. **digital r.,** see *Hoffmann's sign,* def. 2, under *sign.* **direct r.,** a contraction on the same side as that of the stimulation. **direct light r.,** when a ray of light is thrown upon the retina through the pupil there is immediate contraction of the sphincter iridis, reducing the size of the pupillary aperture. **diving r.,** a reflex involving cardiovascular and metabolic adaptations to conserve oxygen occurring in animals during diving into water; observed in reptiles, birds, and mammals, including man. **doll's eye r.,** when the premature infant's head is rotated laterally, the eyes are pulled synergistically in the opposite direction, then return to the middle of the palpebral fissure. **dorsal r.,** contraction of the back muscles in response to stimulation of the skin along the erector spinae. **dorsocuboidal r.,** Mendel-Bekhterev r. **elbow r.,** triceps r. **embrace r.,** Moro's r. **emergency light r.,** excessive stimulation of the retina by light produces contraction of the pupils, closure of the eyelids, and lowering of the eyebrows. **enterogastric r.,** inhibition of gastric motility when irritants enter the duodenum. **epigastric r.,** contraction of the abdominal muscles caused by stimulating the skin of the epigastrium or over the fifth and sixth intercostal spaces near the axilla. **Erben's r.,** slowing down of the pulse on bending the head and trunk strongly forward; said to indicate vagal excitability. **erector spinae r.,** contraction of the erector spinae muscle on irritation of the skin along its border. **Escherich's r.,** see under *sign.* **esophagosalivary r.,** Roger's r. **ether r.,** the sudden and increased flow of duodenal secretion following the introduction of ether and certain other substances into the duodenum. **external auditory meatus r.,** Kisch's r. **eyeball compression r., eyeball-heart r.,** oculocardiac r. **eyelid closure r.,** 1. corneal r. (def. 1). 2. conjunctival r. **facial r.,** bulbomimic r. **faucial r.,** reflex vomiting caused by irritation of the fauces. **femoral r.,** Remak's r. **finger-thumb**

r., passive flexion of the metacarpophalangeal joint of one of the fingers causes flexion of the basal joint and extension of the terminal joint of the thumb. **flexion r. of leg,** tapping of the tendons of the semimembranosus and semitendinosus muscles causes flexion of the leg. **flexor r., paradoxical,** dorsiflexion of the great toe or of all the toes when the deep muscles of the calf are pressed upon. **fontanel r.,** Grünfelder's r. **foveolar r.,** the ophthalmoscopic reflex in the form of a dot caused by the foveola. **front-tap r.,** a tap on the skin muscles of the extended leg contracts the gastrocnemius. **fundus r.,** red r. **fusion r.,** the reflex which tends to merge the images on the two retinas into a single impression. **gag r.,** pharyngeal r. **gastrocolic r.,** an increase in intestinal and colonic peristaltic activity following entrance of food into the empty stomach. **gastroileal r.,** an increase in ileal motility and opening of the ileocecal valve when food enters the empty stomach. **gastropancreatic r.,** an increase in pancreatic secretion induced by distention of the corpus of the stomach; it is mediated by the vagus nerve. **Gault's cochleopalpebral r.,** cochleopalpebral r. **Geigel's r.,** a reflex in the female corresponding to the cremasteric reflex in the male; i.e., on stroking of the inner anterior aspect of the upper thigh there is a contraction of the muscular fibers at the upper edge of Poupart's ligament. **genital r.,** any reflex irritability due to disorder of the genital organs. **Gifford's r., Gifford-Galassi r.,** orbicularis pupillary r. **gluteal r.,** a stroke over the skin of the buttock contracts the glutei muscles. **Gordon's r.,** flexor r., paradoxical. **grasp r., grasping r.,** a reflex consisting of a grasping motion of the fingers or of the toes in response to stimulation. **Grünfelder's r.,** dorsal flexion of the great toe with a fan-wise spreading of the other toes elicited by continued pressure at the corner of the posterior lateral fontanel; occurs in the presence of disease of the middle ear in children up to the age of five years. **gustolacrimal r.,** an anomalous reflex by which food taken into the mouth tends to stimulate the secretion not only of saliva but also of tears. **H-r.,** a monosynaptic reflex elicited by stimulating a nerve, particularly the tibial nerve, with an electric shock. **Haab's r.,** bilateral pupillary contraction when the patient sits in a darkened room, and without accommodation or convergence directs his attention to a bright object already within the field of vision. Called also *cerebral cortex r.* **heart r.,** Abrams' heart r. **heel-tap r.,** a reflex occurring in disease of the pyramidal tract and consisting of fanning and plantar flexion of the toes produced by tapping the patient's heel. **hepatojugular r.,** see under *reflux.* **Hering-Breuer r.,** the nervous mechanism which tends to limit the respiratory excursions. Stimuli from the sensory endings in the lungs and perhaps in other parts passing up the vagi tend to limit both inspiration and expiration in ordinary breathing. **Hirschberg's r.,** tickling of the sole at the base of the great toe causes adduction of the foot. **Hoffmann's r.,** see under *sign,* def. 2. **Hughes's r.,** see *virile r.,* def. 2. **hypochondrial r.,** sudden inspiration caused by quick pressure beneath the lower border of the ribs. **ileogastric r.,** inhibition of gastric motility by distension of the ileum. **inborn r.,** unconditioned r. **indirect r.,** crossed r. **infraspinatus r.,** obtained by tapping a certain spot over the shoulder blade, on a line bisecting the angle formed by the spine of the bone and its inner border; outward rotation of the arm occurs, with simultaneous straightening of the elbow. **inguinal r.,** Geigel's r. **interscapular r.,** a stimulus applied between the scapulae contracts the scapular muscles; called also *scapular r.* **intestinointestinal r.,** when a part of the intestine becomes overdistended or its mucosa becomes excessively irritated, activity in other parts of the intestine is inhibited as long as the distention persists. **inverted radial r.,** a flexion of the fingers without movement of the forearm, produced by tapping the lower end of the radius; it indicates disease of the fifth cervical segment of the spinal cord associated with damage of the pyramidal tract below that level. **iris contraction r.,** pupillary r. **ischemic r.,** the elevation of arterial pressure in response to cerebral ischemia. **jaw r., jaw jerk r.,** closure of the mouth caused by a downward blow on the lower jaw while it hangs passively open. It is seen only rarely in health, but is very noticeable in lesions of the corticospinal tract. **Joffroy's r.,** twitching of the gluteal muscles on pressure against the nates in spastic paralysis. **Juster r.,** extension of the fingers instead of flexion on stimulation of the palm. **juvenile r.,** a glistening white reflection from the

smooth surface of the retina in young people. **Kehrer's r., Kisch's r.,** closure of the eye as a result of tactile or thermal stimulation of the deepest part of the external auditory meatus and tympanum. **knee jerk r.,** quadriceps jerk. **Kocher's r.,** contraction of the abdominal muscle on compression of the testicle. **lacrimal r.,** secretion of tears elicited by touching the conjunctiva over the cornea. **Landau r.,** when an infant is held in the prone position, the entire body forms a convex upward arc; gentle pressure on the head or gravity flexes the neck and hip, reversing the arc. **laryngeal r.,** irritation of the fauces and larynx causing cough. **laughter r.,** laughter brought on by tickling. **let-down r.,** the ejection or release of milk from the alveoli of the breast into the ducts, caused by a combination of neurogenic and hormonal reflexes involving the hormone oxytocin and, to a lesser extent, vasopressin; called also *milk ejection* and *milk let-down r.* **lid r.,** corneal r. **Liddell and Sherrington r.,** stretch r. **light r.,** 1. a luminous image reflected from the membrana tympani. 2. a circular spot of light seen reflected from the retina with the retinoscopic mirror. 3. contraction of the pupil when light falls on the eye. **lip r.,** a reflex movement of the lips of sleeping babies which occurs on tapping near the angle of the mouth. **Livierato's r.,** Abrams' heart r. **Lovén r.,** general vasodilatation of an organ when its afferent nerve is stimulated; this secures a maximal supply of blood to the organ, together with a general rise of blood pressure. **lumbar r.,** dorsal r. **Lust's r.,** abduction of the foot with dorsal flexion on percussion of the common peroneal nerve. **McCarthy's r.,** contraction of the orbicularis oculi muscle on tapping the supraorbital nerve. **McCormac's r.,** percussing the patellar tendon produces adduction of the opposite leg. **McDowall r.,** a decrease in systemic blood pressure following vagotomy, due to abolishment of the afferent impulses from the atria, which normally induce vasoconstriction. **Magnus and de Kleijn neck r's,** extension of both ipsilateral limbs, or one, or part of a limb, and increase of tonus on the side to which the chin is turned when the head is rotated to the side, and flexion with loss of tonus on the side to which the occiput points. Essentially it is a sign of *decerebrate rigidity.* **mandibular r.,** jaw r. **Marinesco-Radovici r.,** palm-chin r. **mass r.,** a reflex exhibited by the entire area controlled by the portion of the spinal cord which has been injured. **Mayer's r.,** opposition and adduction of the thumb combined with flexion at the metacarpophalangeal joint and extension at the interphalangeal joint, on downward pressure of the index finger. **Mendel's r., Mendel's dorsal r. of foot,** Mendel-Bekhterev r. **Mendel-Bekhterev r.,** percussion of the dorsum of the foot normally causes dorsal flexion of the second to fifth toes; in certain organic nervous conditions it causes plantar flexion of the toes. Called also *cuboidodigital r., dorsocuboidal r., Mendel-Beckterew r.,* and *tarsophalangeal r.* **milk ejection r., milk let-down r.,** let-down r. **Mondonesi's r.,** bulbomimic r. **Morley's peritoneocutaneous r.,** when any of the cerebrospinal nerve endings in the peritoneum or subperitoneal tissues are irritated, pain will be referred to the corresponding segmental skin area. **Moro's r., Moro embrace r.,** flexion of an infant's thighs and knees, fanning and then clenching of the fingers, with the arms first thrown outward then brought together in an embrace attitude, produced by a sudden stimulus, such as striking the table on either side of the child, or by sudden extension of the neck, as by allowing the head to fall backward or pulling the child up by both hands from the supine position and then letting go. It is seen normally in infants up to 3 to 4 months of age. Called also *embrace r.* and *startle r.* **motor r.,** a reflex brought about by stimulation upon the periphery of the motor mechanism. **muscular r.,** a reflex movement due to the stretching of a muscle. **myenteric r.,** contraction of the intestine above and relaxation below a portion of the intestine that is irritated or distended. **myopic r.,** Weiss's r. **myotatic r.,** stretch r. **nasal r.,** 1. irritation of the schneiderian membrane provokes sneezing. 2. see *Bekhterev's r.,* def. 4. **nasolabial r.,** sudden retroversion of the head, stretching of the back, retroversion of the arms at the shoulder, extension and pronation of the forearms, and extension and adduction of the legs, elicited by a slight vertical sweeping motion touching the tip of the nose; it frequently occurs in healthy infants, and disappears around the fifth month of age. **nasomental r.,** contraction of the mentalis muscle on tapping the side of the nose with a percussion hammer. **neck righting r.,** rotation of the trunk in the direction in which the head of the supine infant is turned; this reflex is absent or decreased in infants with spasticity. **nociceptive r's,** reflexes initiated by painful stimuli. **nostril r.,** reduction of the size of the opening of the naris, said to occur on the affected side in pulmonary disease. **obliquus r.,** stimulation of the skin below Poupart's ligament contracts a part of the external oblique muscle. **oculocardiac r.,** a slowing of the rhythm of the heart following compression of the eyes or pressure on the carotid sinus. A slowing of from 5 to 13 beats per minute is normal; one of from 13 to 50 or more is exaggerated; one of from 1 to 5 is diminished. If ocular compression produces acceleration of the heart, the reflex is called *inverted.* See also *Aschner's phenomenon,* under *phenomenon.* **oculocephalogyric r.,** the reflex by which the movements of the eye, the head, and the body are directed in the interest of visual attention. **oculopharyngeal r.,** rapid deglutition together with spontaneous closing of the eyes. **oculopupillary r.,** trigeminus r. **oculosensory cell r.,** trigeminus r. **oculovagal r.,** pressure on the eyeball induces atrioventricular beats or rhythm. **Oppenheim's r.,** see under *sign.* **opticofacial winking r.,** closure of the lids when an object is brought suddenly into the field of vision. **orbicularis r.,** orbicularis pupillary r. **orbicularis oculi r.,** normal contraction of the orbicularis oculi muscle, with resultant closing of the eye, on percussion at the outer aspect of the supraorbital ridge, over the glabella, or around the margin of the orbit. **orbicularis pupillary r.,** unilateral contraction of the pupil, followed by dilatation after closure or attempted closure of eyelids that are forcibly held apart. Called also *Galassi's pupillary, orbicularis,* and *Westphal-Piltz phenomenon* and *Gifford's, Gifford-Galassi,* and *Westphal's pupillary r.* **orthocardiac r.,** see *Livierato's test,* 2d def. **palatal r., palatine r.,** stimulation of the palate causing swallowing. **palm-chin r.,** twitching of the chin produced by stimulating (scratching) the palm. **palmomental r.,** palm-chin r. **paradoxical pupillary r.,** 1. reversed pupillary r. 2. dilatation of the pupil on exposure to light; sometimes seen in conditions such as tabes dorsalis. Called also *Bekhterev's r.* and *paradoxical pupillary phenomenon.* **patellar r.,** quadriceps jerk. **patelloadductor r.,** crossed adduction of the thigh produced by tapping the quadriceps tendon as in the patellar reflex. **pathologic r.,** one which is not normal, but is the result of a pathologic condition, and may serve as a sign of disease. **pectoral r.,** the subject's arm is placed half way between adduction and abduction and the examiner's finger in the muscle tendon near the humerus: a sharp blow of the finger elicits adduction and slight internal rotation. **penile r., penis r.,** bulbocavernous r. **perianal r.,** anal r. **peritoneointestinal r.,** inhibition of motility of the stomach and intestine resulting from retroperitoneal irritation or hemorrhage. **pharyngeal r.,** contraction of the constrictor muscle of the pharynx elicited by touching the back of the pharynx; called also *gag r.* **phasic r.,** an active and coordinated movement occurring as a response to stimulation. **Philippson's r.,** excitation of the knee extensor in one leg induced by inhibition in the knee extensor of the other leg. **pilomotor r.,** the production of goose flesh on stroking the skin; trichographism. **Piltz's r.,** attention r. of pupil. **placing r.,** flexion followed by extension of the leg when the infant is held erect and the dorsum of the foot is drawn along the under edge of a table top; it is obtainable in the normal infant up to the age of six weeks. **plantar r.,** irritation of the sole contracts the toes. **platysmal r.,** the act of nipping the platysma contracts the pupil. **postural r.,** a reflex which consists of some assumption of posture. **pressor r.,** a reflex to stimulation resulting in increased activity of a motor center. **Preyer's r.,** involuntary movements of the ears produced by auditory stimulation. **proprioceptive r.,** a reflex that is initiated by stimuli arising from some function of the reflex mechanism itself. **psychic r.,** a reflex aroused by a stored-up impression of memory, such as the secretion of saliva at the sight or thought of good-tasting food. **psychocardiac r.,** increase in the pulse rate on recalling an individual emotional experience. **psychogalvanic r.,** galvanic skin response. **pulmonocoronary r.,** reflex vasoconstriction of the coronary arteries, mediated by the vagus nerves. **pupillary r.,** 1. contraction of the pupil on exposure of the retina to light. 2. any reflex involving the iris, resulting in change in the size of the pupil, occurring

in response to various stimuli, e.g., change in illumination or point of fixation, sudden loud noise, emotional stimulation. **Puusepp's r.,** abduction of the little toe on stimulating the posterior external part of the sole of the foot; indicative of lesions of the extrapyramidal and pyramidal tracts. **quadriceps r.,** contraction of the quadriceps and extension of the leg when the quadriceps tendon is tapped between the patella and the tibial tubercle. **quadrupedal extensor r.,** Brain's r. **radial r.,** flexion of the forearm, following tapping on the lower end of the radius; when the fingers flex as well, it indicates hyperreflexia. **rectal r.,** the process by which the accumulation of feces in the rectum excites defecation; called also *defecation r.* **red r.,** a luminous red appearance seen upon the retina; called also *fundus r.* **regional r.,** segmental r. **Remak's r.,** plantar flexion of the first three toes and sometimes of the foot, with extension of the knee on stroking of the upper anterior surface of the thigh. **renointestinal r.,** inhibition of motility of the intestine resulting from renal irritation. **renorenal r.,** a reflex pain or anuria in a sound kidney in cases in which the other kidney is diseased. **resistance r.,** Babinski r. **retrobulbar pupillary r.,** slight dilatation of the pupil which contracts under light stimulation, and then dilates while the light stimulation is still present. **reversed pupillary r.,** any abnormal *pupillary reflex* opposite of that which occurs normally; e.g., stimulation of the retina by light dilates the pupil. Called also *paradoxical pupillary r.* or *phenomenon.* **Riddoch's mass r.,** in severe injury of the spinal cord, stimulation below the level of the lesion produces flexion reflexes of the lower extremity, evacuation of the bowels and bladder, and sweating of the skin below the level of the lesion. **righting r.,** the ability to assume optimal position when there has been a departure from it. **Roger's r.,** salivation on irritation of the esophagus. **rooting r.,** a reflex in the newborn in which stimulation of the side of the cheek or the upper or lower lip causes the infant to turn his mouth and face to the stimulus. **Rossolimo's r.,** on tapping the plantar surface of the toes, plantar flexion of the toes occurs when there are lesions of the pyramidal tract. **Ruggeri's r.,** acceleration of the pulse following strong convergence of the eyeballs toward something very close to the eyes; it indicates sympathetic excitability. **Saenger's r.,** see under *sign.* **scapular r.,** interscapular r. **scapulohumeral r.,** adduction with outward rotation of the humerus produced by percussing along the inner edge of the scapula. **Schäfer's r.,** flexion of the foot and toes on pinching the Achilles tendon at its middle third; seen in organic hemiplegia. **scrotal r.,** a slow, vermicular contraction of the dartos muscle obtained by stroking the perineum or by applying a cold object to it. **segmental r.,** a reflex controlled by a single segment or region of the spinal cord. **senile r.,** a gray reflection from the pupil of aged people due to hardening of the lens. **sexual r.,** the reflex of erection and ejaculation produced by stimulation of the genitals. **shot-silk r.,** see *shot-silk retina,* under *retina.* **simple r.,** a reflex involving a single muscle. **skin r.,** a reflex which occurs on stimulation of the skin. **skin pupillary r.,** dilatation of the pupil produced by irritation of the skin of the neck. **Snellen's r.,** unilateral congestion of the ear upon stimulation of the distal end of the divided auriculocervical nerve. **sole r.,** plantar r. **somatointestinal r.,** inhibition of intestinal motility when the skin over the abdomen is stimulated. **spinal r.,** any reflex whose arc is connected with a center in the spinal cord. **stapedial r.,** acoustic r. **startle r.,** Moro's r. **static r.,** the reflex pose and righting of the body. **statotomic r's,** attitudinal r's. **stepping r.,** 1. movements of progression elicited when the infant is held upright and inclined forward with the soles of the feet touching a flat surface; it is obtainable in the normal infant up to the age of six weeks. 2. extension of the hind leg of a dog on pressing the plantar surface of the foot. **Stookey r.,** with the leg semiflexed at the knee, the tendons of the semimembranosus and the semitendinosus muscles are tapped: flexion of the leg results. **stretch r.,** reflex contraction of a muscle in response to passive longitudinal stretching; called also *Liddell and Sherrington r.* and *myotatic reflex.* **Strümpell's r.,** leg movement with adduction of the foot produced by stroking the thigh or abdomen. **sucking r.,** sucking movements of the mouth elicited by the touching of an object to an infant's lips. **superficial r.,** any withdrawal reflex elicited by noxious or tactile stimulation of the skin, cornea, or mucous membrane, including the corneal reflex, pharyngeal reflex, cremasteric reflex, etc. **supinator longus r.,** tapping on the lower end of the radius produces flexion of the forearm. **supraorbital r.,** McCarthy's r. **suprapatellar r.,** with the subject's leg extended the index finger of the examiner is crooked above the patella and is struck; the result is a kick-back of the patella. **suprapubic r.,** stroking the abdomen above Poupart's ligament causes deviation of the linea alba toward the side that is stroked. **supraumbilical r.,** epigastric reflex. **swallowing r.,** palatal r. **tapetal light r.,** the glowing of eyes in the dark, just as do the eyes of carnivorous animals. **tarsophalangeal r.,** Mendel-Bekhterev r. **tendon r.,** involuntary contraction of a muscle after brief stretching caused by percussion of its tendon; tendon reflexes include the biceps reflex, triceps reflex, quadriceps reflex, etc. Called also *deep r.* and *tendon jerk* or *reaction.* **threat r.,** sudden closure of the eyes at a sign of danger. **Throckmorton's r.,** a variation of the Babinski reflex elicited by percussion of the metatarsophalangeal region in the dorsum of the foot. **tibioadductor r.,** tapping of the tibia on the inner side of the leg results either in homolateral adduction of the leg or crossed adduction from side to side. **toe r.,** strong flexion of the great toe flexes all the muscles of the lower extremity; it is seen in pathologic states in which there is hyperreflexia. **tonic r.,** the passing of an appreciable period of time after the occurrence of a reflex before relaxation; a reflex which maintains the reflex contractions that are the basis of posture and attitude. **tonic neck r.,** a reflex in the newborn consisting of extension of the arm and sometimes of the leg on the side to which the head is forcibly turned, with flexion of the contralateral limbs. **trained r.,** conditioned response. **triceps r.,** contraction of the belly of the triceps muscle and slight extension of the arm when the tendon of the muscle is tapped directly, with the arm flexed and fully supported and relaxed. **triceps surae r.,** plantar flexion of the foot elicited by a tap on the Achilles tendon preferably while the patient kneels on a bed or chair, the feet hanging free over the edge; ankle jerk. **trigeminus r.,** stimulation of the cornea or of the eyelid results in dilatation of the ipsilateral and the contralateral pupil; called also *oculopupillary r.* and *oculosensory cell r.* **ulnar r.,** tapping of the styloid process of the ulna results in pronation of the hand. **unconditioned r.,** see under *response.* **urinary r's,** bladder r. **vagus r.,** abnormal sensitiveness to pressure over the course of the vagus nerve. **vascular r.,** constriction of an artery produced by peripheral irritation. **vasopressor r's,** rise in pressure from reflex vasoconstriction. **vertebra prominens r.,** pressure upon the last cervical vertebra of an animal reduces the tone of all four limbs. **vesical r.,** desire to urinate produced by moderate distention of the bladder. **vesicointestinal r.,** inhibition of intestinal motility due to irritation of the bladder. **vestibular r's,** the reflexes for maintaining the position of the eyes and body in relation to changes in orientation of the head; the neural pathways are complex, traveling from the vestibular nerve to the vestibular nuclei and thence to the involved muscles of the eye and body. **vestibulo-ocular r.,** nystagmus or deviation of the eyes in response to stimulation of the vestibular system by angular acceleration or deceleration or by irrigation of the ears with warm or cool water or air (caloric test). **virile r.,** 1. bulbocavernous reflex. 2. a reflex in the flaccid penis elicited by pulling upward the foreskin or glans penis, when a sudden downward jerk results. Called also *Hughes's r.* **visceral r.,** that in which the stimulus is set up by some state of an internal organ. **viscerocardiac r.,** reflex alteration in cardiac rhythm or contractility caused by visceral excitation. **visceromotor r.,** contraction of abdominal muscles (abdominal rigidity) over a diseased viscus. **viscerosensory r.,** a region of sensitiveness to pressure on some part of the body due to disease of some internal organ. **viscerotrophic r.,** degeneration of any peripheral tissue as a result of chronic inflammation of any of the viscera. **von Mering r.,** relaxation of overlying abdominal muscles following ingestion of food. **water-silk r.,** see *shot-silk retina,* under *retina.* **Weiss's r.,** a curved reflection seen with the ophthalmoscope on the fundus of the eye to the nasal side of the disk; believed to be indicative of myopia. **Westphal's pupillary r., Westphal-Piltz r.,** orbicularis pupillary r. **zygomatic r.,** lateral motion of the lower jaw to the percussed side on percussion over the zygoma.

reflexogenic (re-flek″so-jen′ik) [*reflex* + Gr. *gennan* to produce] producing or increasing reflex action.

reflexogenous (re″fleks-oj′ĕ-nus) reflexogenic.

reflexograph (re-flek′so-graf) [*reflex* + Gr. *graphein* to write] an instrument for graphically recording a reflex.

reflexology (re″flek-sol′o-je) the science or study of reflexes.

reflexometer (re″flek-som′ĕ-ter) [*reflex* + L. *metrum* measure] an instrument for measuring the force necessary to produce myotatic contraction.

reflexophil (re-flek′so-fil) [*reflex* + Gr. *philein* to love] characterized by activity of reflexes.

reflexotherapy (re-flek″so-ther′ah-pe) reflex therapy.

reflux (re′fluks) [*re-* + L. *fluxus* flow] a backward or return flow. **gastroesophageal r.,** reflux of the stomach and duodenal contents into the esophagus, which may sometimes occur normally, particularly in the distended stomach postprandially, or as a chronic pathological condition (see *reflux esophagitis,* under *esophagitis*). Called also *esophageal r.* **hepatojugular r.,** distention of the jugular vein induced by pressure over the liver; it suggests insufficiency of the right heart; formerly called *hepatojugular reflex.* **intrarenal r.,** reflux of urine into the renal parenchymal tissue. **urethrovesiculo-differential r.,** the passage of a liquid, sperm, or injected substance from the posterior urethra into the genital system. **vesicoureteral r., vesicoureteric r.,** the passage of urine from the bladder back into a ureter; called also *vesicoureteral regurgitation.*

refract (re-frakt′) [L. *refringere* to break apart] 1. to cause to deviate. 2. to ascertain errors of ocular refraction.

refracta dosi (re-frak′tah do′si) [L.] in repeated and divided doses.

refractile (re-frak′til) capable of refracting.

refraction (re-frak′shun) 1. the act or process of refracting; specifically the determination of the refractive errors of the eye and their correction by glasses. 2. the deviation of light in passing obliquely from one medium to another of different density. The deviation occurs at the surface of junction of the two mediums, which is known as the refracting surface. The ray before refraction is called the *incident ray;* after refraction it is the *refracted ray.* The point of junction of the incident and the refracted ray is known as the *point of incidence.* The angle between the incident ray and a line perpendicular to the refracting surface at the point of incidence is known as the *angle of incidence;* that between the refracted ray and this perpendicular is called the *angle of refraction.* The sine of the angle of incidence divided by the sine of the angle of refraction gives the *relative index of refraction.* **double r.,** that in which the incident ray is

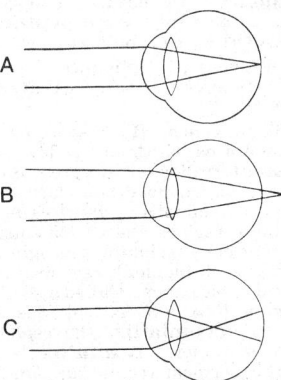

Refraction by the eye in (*A*) emmetropia; (*B*) hyperopia; and (*C*) myopia.

divided into two refracted rays, so as to produce a double image. Double refraction is produced by Iceland spar. See *Nicol prism,* under *prism.* **dynamic r.,** the normal accommodation of the eye which is being continually exerted without conscious effort. **ocular r.,** the refraction of light produced by the mediums of the normal eye and resulting in the focusing of images upon the retina. **static r.,** the refraction of the eye when its accommodation is paralyzed.

refractionist (re-frak'shun-ist) one skilled in determining the refracting power of the eyes and correcting refractive defects.

refractive (re-frak'tiv) pertaining to or subserving a process of refraction; having the power to refract.

refractivity (re″frak-tiv'ĭ-te) the quality of being refractive; the power or ability to refract.

refractometer (re″frak-tom'ĕ-ter) [*refraction* + Gr. *metron* measure] 1. an instrument for measuring the refractive power of the eye. 2. an instrument for determining the indexes of refraction of various substances, particularly for determining the strength of lenses of spectacles.

refractometry (re″frak-tom'ĕ-tre) the measurement of refractive power with the refractometer.

refractor (re-frakt'or) a device for retinoscopic examination of the eye to determine its refractive power.

refractory (re-frak'to-re) [L. *refractorius*] not readily yielding to treatment.

refracture (re-frak'chur) the operation of breaking over again a bone which has been fractured and has united with a deformity; called also *anaclasis.*

refrangibility (re-fran″jĭ-bil'ĭ-te) susceptibility of being refracted; the quality of being refrangible.

refrangible (re-fran'jĭ-b'l) susceptible of being refracted.

refresh (re-fresh') to freshen; to denude a wound of epithelium to enhance tissue repair.

refrigerant (re-frij'er-ant) [L. *refrigerans*] 1. relieving fever and thirst. 2. a cooling remedy. The refrigerants consist of cooling, acidulous drinks and evaporating lotions. Called also *algefacient.*

refrigeration (re-frij″er-a'shun) [L. *refrigeratio*] the therapeutic application of or exposure to low temperatures.

refringent (re-frin'jent) refractive.

Refsum's disease (syndrome) (ref'soomz) [Sigvald *Refsum,* Norwegian physician] see under *disease.*

refusion (re-fu'zhun) [L. *refusio*] the return of blood to the circulation after temporary removal or stoppage of flow.

R.E.G. radioencephalogram.

regainer (re-gān'er) space regainer; a space maintainer that pushes back teeth that have crowded the edentulous area. See also under *maintainer* and *retainer.* **space r.,** regainer.

regainer-maintainer (re-gān'er-mān-tān'er) an orthodontic appliance combining the characteristics of a space regainer and a maintainer.

regeneration (re-jen″er-a'shun) [*re-* + L. *generare* to produce, bring to life] the natural renewal of a structure, as of a lost tissue or part. **epimorphic r.,** epimorphosis. **morphallactic r.,** morphallaxis.

regimen (rej'ĭ-men) [L. "guidance"] a strictly regulated scheme of diet, exercise, or other activity designed to achieve certain ends.

regio (re'je-o), pl. *regio'nes* [L. "a space enclosed by lines"] a region: a plane area with more or less definite boundaries; [NA] a general term for certain areas on the surface of the body within certain defined boundaries. **r. abdomina'lis,** cavitas abdominalis. **regio'nes abdomina'les** [NA], abdominal regions: the various anatomical regions of the abdomen or belly including the right and left hypochondriac, lateral, and inguinal regions, and the epigastric, umbilical, and pubic regions. Called also *abdominal zones* and *hypochondrium* [NA alternative]. See illustration under *abdomen.* **r. acromia'lis,** the region of the shoulder overlying the acromion. **r. ana'lis** [NA], anal region: the portion of the perineal region surrounding the anus. **r. antebrachia'lis ante'rior** [NA], anterior antebrachial region: the anterior, or palmar, region of the forearm; called also *anterior antebrachial facies, facies antebrachialis anterior* [NA alternative], *r. antibrachii volaris,* and *volar antebrachial r.* **r. antebrachia'lis poste'rior** [NA], posterior antebrachial region: the posterior, or dorsal, region of the forearm; called also *facies antebrachialis posterior* [NA alternative] and *posterior antebrachial facies.* **r. antibra'chii radia'lis,** radial antebrachial region: the radial aspect of the forearm. **r. antibra'chii ulna'ris,** ulnar

antebrachial region: the ulnar aspect of the forearm. **r. antibra'chii vola'ris,** r. antebrachialis anterior. **r. auricula'ris,** auricular region: the region of the head on either side, about the ear. **r. axilla'ris** [NA], axillary region: the region of the chest about the fossa axillaris. **r. brachia'lis ante'rior** [NA], anterior brachial region: the anterior region of the arm; called also *anterior brachial facies* and *facies brachialis anterior* [NA alternative]. **r. brachia'lis poste'rior** [NA], posterior brachial region: the posterior region of the arm; called also *facies brachialis posterior* [NA alternative] and *posterior brachial facies.* **r. bucca'lis** [NA], buccal region: the region of the cheek. **r. calca'nea** [NA], the hindmost projection of the foot; called also *calx* [NA alternative] and *heel*). **regio'nes cap'itis** [NA], the various anatomical regions of the head, including the frontal, parietal, occipital, and infratemporal regions. **r. carpa'lis ante'rior** [NA], anterior carpal region: the anterior aspect of the wrist. **r. carpa'lis poste'rior** [NA], posterior carpal region: the posterior aspect of the wrist. **regio'nes cervica'les** [NA], cervical regions: the various anatomical regions of the neck, including the anterior, sternocleidomastoid, lateral, and posterior regions; called also *regiones colli.* **r. cervica'lis ante'rior** [NA], anterior cervical region: the anterior region of the neck, subdivided into the submandibular, carotid, muscular, and submental triangles; called also *r. colli anterior* and *trigonum cervicale anterius* [NA alternative]. **r. cervica'lis latera'lis** [NA], lateral cervical region: the region of the neck lateral to the regio sternocleidomastoidea; called also *r. colli lateralis, lateral region of neck, trigonum cervicale posterius* [NA alternative], and *trigonum colli laterale.* **r. cervica'lis poste'rior** [NA], posterior cervical region: the region of the neck adjoining the regio cervicalis lateralis; the back of the neck. Called also *r. nuchalis* [NA alternative], *nuchal region, posterior cervical region,* and *posterior region of neck.* **r. clavicula'ris,** clavicular region: the region of the front of the chest, overlying the clavicle. **regio'nes col'li** [NA], regiones cervicales. **r. col'li ante'rior,** r. cervicalis anterior. **r. col'li latera'lis,** r. cervicalis lateralis. **r. col'li poste'rior,** r. cervicalis posterior. **regio'nes cor'poris, regio'nes cor'poris huma'ni,** see *regiones et partes corporis.* **r. costa'lis latera'lis,** the lateral region of the thorax, or chest, overlying the ribs. **r. cox'ae,** the region of the hip. **r. crura'lis ante'rior** [NA], anterior crural region: the anterior region of the leg; called also *facies cruralis anterior* [NA alternative]. **r. crura'lis poste'rior** [NA], posterior crural region: the posterior region of the leg; called also *facies cruralis posterior* [NA alternative]. **r. cubita'lis ante'rior** [NA], anterior cubital region: the anterior region about the elbow; called also *anterior cubital facies* and *facies cubitalis anterior* [NA alternative]. **r. cubita'lis poste'rior,** [NA], posterior cubital region: the posterior or dorsal region about the elbow. Called also *facies cubitalis posterior* [NA alternative] and *posterior cubital facies.* **r. deltoi'dea** [NA], deltoid region: the region overlying the deltoid muscle. **r. dorsa'lis ma'nus,** dorsum manus. **r. dorsa'lis pe'dis,** NA alternative for *dorsum pedis.* **regio'nes dorsa'les** [NA], dorsal regions: the various anatomical regions of the back, including the vertebral, sacral, scapular, infrascapular, and lumbar regions. **r. epigas'trica** [NA], epigastric region: the upper middle region of the abdomen, located within the sternal angle; called also *antecardium* and *epigastrium* [NA alternative]. **regio'nes extremita'tis inferio'ris,** regiones membri inferioris. **regio'nes extremita'tis superio'ris,** regiones membri superioris. **regio'nes facia'les** [NA], the various anatomical regions of the face, including the orbital, nasal, oral, mental, infraorbital, buccal, and zygomatic regions. **r. femora'lis ante'rior** [NA], the anterior region of the thigh; called also *facies femoralis anterior* [NA alternative]. **r. femora'lis poste'rior** [NA], the posterior region of the thigh; called also *facies femoralis posterior* [NA alternative]. **r. fronta'lis** [NA], frontal region: the region of the head overlying the frontal bone; the forehead. **r. genua'lis ante'rior,** NA alternative for r. genus anterior. **r. genua'lis poste'rior,** NA alternative for r. genus posterior. **r. ge'nus ante'rior** [NA], the anterior region about the knee; called also *r. genualis anterior* [NA alternative]. **r. ge'nus poste'rior,** [NA], the posterior region about the knee; called also *r. genualis posterior* [NA alternative]. **r. glutea'lis** [NA], gluteal region: the region overlying the gluteal muscles. **r. hyoi'dea,** hyoid region: the part of the anterior region of the neck about the hyoid bone. **r. hypochondri'aca [dex'tra et sinis'tra]** [NA], hypochondriac region (right and left): the upper lateral region of the abdomen, about the costal cartilages, on either side of the epigastric region. **r. hypogas'trica,** r. pubica. **r. hypothala'mica ante'rior** [NA], anterior hypothalamic region: the most anterior part of the hypothalamus, lying adjacent to the lamina terminalis and superior to the optic chiasm, and comprising the lateral and medial preoptic nuclei, the supraoptic and paraventricular nuclei; and the anterior hypothalamic nucleus; called also *preoptic area* or *region.* **r. hypothala'mica dorsa'lis** [NA], dorsal hypothalamic region: the most dorsal part of the hypothalamus, comprising the entopeduncular nucleus, nucleus of the ansa lenticularis, anterior hypothalamic region, medial and lateral preoptic nuclei, and supraoptic, paraventricular, and anterior hypothalamic nuclei. Called also *area hypothalamica dorsalis* [NA alternative] and *dorsal hypothalamic area.* **r. hypothala'mica interme'dia** [NA], intermediate hypothalamic nucleus: the part of the hypothalamus comprising the arcuate and tuberal nuclei, the lateral hypothalamic area, the ventromedial, dorsomedial, and dorsal hypothalamic nuclei, and the posterior periventricular and the infundibular nuclei. **r. hypothala'mica poste'rior** [NA], posterior hypothalamic region: the most posterior part of the hypothalamus, consisting of the lateral and medial nuclei of the mamillary body and the posterior hypothalamic nucleus. **r. infraclavicula'ris,** fossa infraclavicularis. **r. inframamma'ria** [NA], inframammary region: the region of the front of the chest situated below either mamma and above the lower border of the twelfth rib. **r. infraorbita'lis** [NA], infraorbital region: the region beneath the eye, adjacent to the regio nasalis. **r. infrascapula'ris** [NA], infrascapular region: the region of the back below the scapula and lateral to the lower thoracic vertebrae. **r. infratempora'lis,** fossa infratemporalis. **r. inguina'lis [dex'tra et sinis'tra]** [NA], inguinal region (right and left): the region of the abdomen on either side, lateral to the pubic region and about the inguinal canal. Called also *iliac region.* **r. interscapula'ris,** interscapular region: the region of the back between the scapulae. **r. labia'lis infe'rior,** inferior labial region: the region of the face about the lower lip. **r. labia'lis supe'rior,** superior labial region: the region of the face about the upper lip. **r. laryn'gea,** laryngeal region: the part of the anterior region of the neck overlying the larynx. **r. latera'lis [dex'tra/sinis'tra]** [NA] lateral region (right and left): the region of the abdomen on either side of the umbilical region; called also *external region* and *lumbar region.* **r. lumba'lis** [NA], lumbar region: the region of the back lying lateral to the lumbar vertebrae; called also *r. lumbaris* [NA alternative]. **r. lumba'ris,** NA alternative for *r. lumbalis.* **r. malleola'ris latera'lis,** the region overlying the lateral malleolus. **r. malleola'ris media'lis,** the region overlying the medial malleolus. **r. mamma'ria** [NA], mammary region: the region of the front of the chest, about the mammary gland. **r. mastoi'dea,** mastoid region: the region of the head on either side, about the mastoid process of the temporal bone. **r. media'na dor'si,** r. vertebralis. **regio'nes mem'bri inferio'ris** [NA], the various anatomical regions of the lower limb; called also *regiones extremitatis inferioris.* **regio'nes mem'bri superio'ris** [NA], the various anatomical regions of the upper limb; including the regio deltoidea, brachium (arm), cubitus (elbow), antebrachium (forearm), carpus (wrist), and manus (hand); called also *regiones extremitatis superioris.* **r. menta'lis** [NA], mental region: the region of the chin. **r. nasa'lis** [NA], nasal region: the region of the face about the nose. **r. nucha'lis,** NA alternative for *r. cervicalis posterior.* **r. occipita'lis** [NA], occipital region: the region of the head overlying the occipital bone. **r. olec'rani,** olecranal region: the region of the elbow overlying the olecranon. **r. olfacto'ria** [NA], olfactory region: the upper part of the nasal cavity, the mucosa of which contains most of the receptors for the sense of smell. **r. ora'lis** [NA], oral region: the region of the face about the mouth. **r. orbita'lis** [NA], orbital region: the region of the face about the eye; called also *ocular region.* **r. palpebra'lis infe'rior,** inferior palpebral region: the region of the lower eyelid. **r. palpebra'lis supe'rior,** superior palpebral region: the region of the upper eyelid. **r. parieta'lis** [NA], parietal region: the region of the head on either side, about the parietal bone. **r. parotideomas-**

seter'ica, parotideomasseteric region: the region of the face on either side, about the parotid gland and masseter muscle. **regio'nes et par'tes cor'poris** [NA], regions and parts of the body: the category in anatomical nomenclature embracing the names of all of the regions and parts of the human body. **r. patella'ris,** the region of the knee overlying the patella. **r. pectora'lis** [NA], the aspect of the thorax, or chest, bounded by the pectoralis major muscle. **regio'nes pectora'les** [NA], pectoral regions: the various regions of the chest, including the presternal, infraclavicular, pectoralis, mammary, inframammary, and axillary regions, infraclavicular fossa, and clavipectoral trigone. **r. perinea'lis** [NA], perineal region: the region overlying the pelvic outlet, including the anal and urogenital regions. **regio'nes planta'res digito'rum pe'dis,** the plantar aspect of the several toes. **r. planta'ris pe'dis,** NA alternative for *planta pedis.* **regio'nes pleuropulmona'les** [NA], pleuropulmonary regions: one-half of the thoracic cavity excluding the mediastinum. **r. presterna'lis** [NA], presternal region: the region of the chest superficial to the sternum. **r. pu'bica** [NA], pubic region: the middle portion of the most inferior region of the abdomen, located below the umbilical region and between the inguinal regions. Called also *r. hypogastrica, hypogastric region,* and *hypogastrium* [NA alternative]. **r. pudenda'lis,** the region of the external genital organs (scrotum or vulva). **r. respirato'ria** [NA], respiratory region: the part of the nasal cavity below the olfactory region. **r. retromalleola'ris latera'lis,** the region back of the lateral malleolus. **r. retromalleola'ris media'lis,** the region back of the medial malleolus. **r. sacra'lis** [NA], sacral region: the region of the back overlying the sacrum. **r. scapula'ris** [NA], scapular region: the region of the back overlying the scapula. **r. sterna'lis,** the region of the front of the chest overlying the sternum. **r. sternocleidomastoi'dea** [NA], sternocleidomastoid region: the region of the neck overlying the sternocleidomastoid muscle. **r. subhyoi'dea,** subhyoid region: the part of the anterior region of the neck below the hyoid bone. **r. submaxilla'ris,** trigonum submandibulare. **r. supraorbita'lis,** supraorbital region: the region of the head immediately above the orbit. **r. suprascapula'ris,** suprascapular region: the region of the back above the scapula. **r. suprasterna'lis,** suprasternal region: the part of the anterior region of the neck above the sternum. **r. sura'lis,** NA alternative for *sura.* **regio'nes talocrura'les ante'rior et poste'rior** [NA], the regions of the leg, anterior and posterior, between the ankle and the foot. **r. tempora'lis** [NA], temporal region: the region of the head on either side, about the temporal bone. **r. thyreoi'dea,** thyroid region: the part of the anterior region of the neck about the thyroid gland. **r. trochanter'ica,** the portion of the lateral region of the thigh overlying the greater trochanter. **r. umbilica'lis** [NA], umbilical region: the region of the abdomen about the umbilicus. **regio'nes unguicula'res digito'rum ma'nus,** the region of the several fingers about the nails. **regio'nes unguicula'res digito'rum pe'dis,** the region of the several toes about the nails. **r. urogenita'lis** [NA], urogenital region: the portion of the perineal region surrounding the urogenital organs. **r. vertebra'lis** [NA], vertebral region: the middle region of the back, overlying the vertebral column; called also *r. mediana dorsi.* **regio'nes vola'res digito'rum ma'nus,** volar region of fingers: the palmar aspect of the several fingers. **r. vola'ris ma'nus,** palma manus. **r. zygomati'ca** [NA], zygomatic region: the region of the face on either side, about the zygomatic bone.

region (re'jun) a plane area with more or less definite boundaries; see also *regio.* **abdominal r.,** cavitas abdominalis. **abdominal r's,** the various anatomical regions of the abdomen; see *regiones abdominis* [NA], and illustration under *abdomen.* **r. of accommodation,** the space including all points to which the eye can be adjusted by accommodation. **anal r.,** regio analis. **antebrachial r., anterior,** regio antebrachialis anterior. **antebrachial r., posterior,** regio antebrachialis posterior. **antebrachial r., radial,** regio antibrachii radialis. **antebrachial r., ulnar,** regio antibrachii ulnaris. **antebrachial r., volar,** regio antebrachialis anterior. **anterior r. of neck,** regio cervicalis anterior. **auricular r.,** regio auricularis. **axillary r.,** regio axillaris. **basilar r.,** the base of the skull. **brachial r., anterior,** regio brachialis anterior. **brachial r., posterior,** regio brachialis posterior. **Broca's r.,** see under *convolution*. **buccal r.,** regio buccalis. **calcaneal r.,** regio calcanea. **carpal r., anterior,** regio carpalis anterior. **carpal r., posterior,** regio carpalis posterior. **cervical r's,** regiones cervicales. **cervical r., anterior,** regio cervicalis anterior. **cervical r., lateral,** regio cervicalis lateralis. **cervical r., posterior,** regio cervicalis posterior. **ciliary r.,** the part of the eye occupied by the ciliary body and its adjuncts. **clavicular r.,** regio clavicularis. **constant (C) r.,** the C-terminal portion of an immunoglobulin heavy (C_H) or light (C_L) chain, comprising one homology region in light chains and three or four in heavy chains, that has a constant amino acid sequence for chains of a single type produced by one individual. Constant regions vary among the heavy chain classes and subclasses (isotypic variation) and among individuals (allotypic variation). **crural r., anterior,** regio cruralis anterior. **crural r., posterior,** regio cruralis posterior. **cubital r., anterior,** regio cubitalis anterior. **cubital r., posterior,** regio cubitalis posterior. **deltoid r.,** regio deltoidea. **dorsal r's,** regiones dorsales. **dorsal hypothalamic r.,** regio hypothalamica dorsalis. **dorsal lip r.,** the mesodermal tissue around the dorsal lip of the blastopore; it is the organizer which by induction initiates and controls the early development of the embryo. **encephalic r.,** lamina alaris. **epigastric r.,** regio epigastrica. **external r.,** see *regio lateralis [dextra et sinistra]*. **extrapolar r.,** that region of the body which lies outside the influence of the poles in electrotherapy. **facial r's,** regiones faciales. **frontal r.,** regio frontalis. **genitourinary r.,** regio urogenitalis. **gluteal r.,** regio glutealis. **hinge r.,** a short flexible region between the C_H1 and C_H2 domains of immunoglobulin heavy chains which allows each of the Fab regions (the "arms" of the Y-shaped immunoglobulin molecule) to move independently as necessary to bind to antigens. **homology r's,** regions of immunoglobulin heavy and light chains containing about 110 amino acid residues and forming compact globular domains stabilized by one intrachain disulfide bond; they have a high degree of sequence homology and similar three-dimensional structure. Each variable region (V_H and V_L) of heavy and light chains and the light chain constant region (C_L) are coextensive with a single homology region. Heavy chain constant regions are composed of three (in γ, δ, and α chains) or four (in μ and ϵ chains) homology regions, C_H1, C_H2, C_H3, and C_H4, and a hinge region separating C_H1 and C_H2. **hyoid r.,** regio hyoidea. **hypervariable r's,** regions a few amino acids in length within immunoglobulin heavy and light chain variable regions at which the amino acid sequence is extremely variable; there are three in light chains and four in heavy chains. They contain most of the amino acid residues forming the antigen binding site. **hypochondriac r.,** see *regio hypochondriaca [dextra et sinistra]*. **hypogastric r.,** regio pubica. **hypothalamic r., anterior,** regio hypothalamica anterior. **hypothalamic r., intermediate,** regio hypothalamica intermedia. **hypothalamic r., posterior,** regio hypothalamica posterior. **I r.,** that part of the mouse major histocompatibility complex (H-2 complex) containing the immune response genes. **iliac r.,** regio inguinalis. **infraclavicular r.,** fossa infraclavicularis. **inframammary r.,** regio inframammaria. **infraorbital r.,** regio infraorbitalis. **infrascapular r.,** regio infrascapularis. **infratemporal r.,** fossa infratemporalis. **inguinal r.,** see *regio inguinalis [dextra et sinistra]*. **interscapular r.,** regio interscapularis. **labial r., inferior,** regio labialis inferior. **labial r., superior,** regio labialis superior. **laryngeal r.,** regio laryngea. **lateral r.,** see *regio lateralis [dextra et sinistra]*. **lateral r. of neck,** regio cervicalis lateralis. **r's of leg, anterior and posterior,** regiones talocrurales anterior et posterior. **lumbar r.,** 1. regio lumbalis. 2. See *regio lateralis [dextra et sinistra]*. **mammary r.,** regio mammaria. **mastoid r.,** regio mastoidea. **mental r.,** regio mentalis. **motor r.,** the ascending frontal and parietal convolutions of the cerebrum; called also *rolandic r.* **mylohyoid r.,** the region on the lingual surface of the mandible to which the mylohyoid muscle is attached. **r. of nape,** regio nuchae. **nasal r.,** regio nasalis. **nuchal r.,** regio cervicalis posterior. **occipital r.,** regio occipitalis. **ocular r.,** regio orbitalis. **olecranal r.,** regio olecrani. **olfactory r.,** regio olfactoria. **opticostriate r.,** the basal ganglia and the capsule. **oral r.,** regio oralis. **orbital r.,** regio orbitalis.

palpebral r., inferior, regio palpebralis inferior. **palpebral r., superior,** regio palpebralis superior. **parietal r.,** regio parietalis. **parietotemporal r.,** sensory r. **parotideomasseteric r.,** regio parotideomasseterica. **pectoral r's,** regiones pectorales. **perineal r.,** regio perinealis. **plantar r's of toes,** regiones plantares digitorum pedis. **pleuropulmonary r's,** regiones pleuropulmonales. **posterior r. of neck,** regio cervicalis posterior. **precordial r.,** a part of the anterior surface of the body covering the heart and the pit of the stomach. **prefrontal r.,** the part of the frontal lobe of the cerebrum in front of the precentral fissures. **preoptic r.,** regio hypothalamica anterior. **presternal r.,** regio presternalis. **presumptive r.,** an area of the blastula which has been proved under normal conditions to develop into a specific organ or type of tissue. **pretectal r.,** area pretectalis. **pterygomaxillary r.,** the region of the face about the zygoma and the prominences of the lower jaw. **pubic r.,** regio pubica. **respiratory r.,** regio respiratoria. **rolandic r.,** motor r. **sacral r.,** regio sacralis. **scapular r.,** regio scapularis. **sensory r.,** a part of the cerebral cortex located in part behind the central sulcus; called also *parietotemporal r.* **sternocleidomastoid r.,** regio sternocleidomastoidea. **subauricular r.,** fossa retromandibularis. **subhyoid r.,** regio subhyoidea. **submaxillary r.,** trigonum submandibulare. **supraclavicular r.,** the region above the clavicle. **supraorbital r.,** regio supraorbitalis. **suprasternal r.,** regio suprasternalis. **temporal r.,** regio temporalis. **thyroid r.,** regio thyreoidea. **trabecular r.,** the region of the embryonic skull from which the sphenoid bone is developed. **umbilical r.,** regio umbilicalis. **urogenital r.,** regio urogenitalis. **variable (V) r.,** the N-terminal portion, composing one homology region, of an immunoglobulin heavy (V_H) or light (V_L) chain that varies in amino acid sequence among chains of a single type. The antigen binding sites of immunoglobulin molecules are formed by parts of the V_H and V_L regions; thus the V_H and V_L amino acid sequences determine the antigenic specificity of the antibody molecule. Although variable regions vary among antibodies of different specificity (idiotype variation), all of the immunoglobulins produced by a single clone of plasma cells (a clonotype) have the same variable regions but may have different constant regions. **vertebral r.,** regio vertebralis. **vestibular r.,** the lowest and the movable portion of the nose; it is lined with stratified squamous cell epithelium and possesses hairs and sebaceous glands. **volar r's of fingers,** regiones volares digitorum manus. **volar r. of hand,** palma manus. **zygomatic r.,** regio zygomatica.

regional (re′jun-al) pertaining to, limited to, or affecting a certain region or regions.

regiones (re″je-o′nēz) [L.] plural of *regio*.

registrant (rej′is-trant) a nurse who is listed on the books of a registry as available for duty.

registrar (rej′is-trar) 1. an official keeper of records. 2. in British hospitals, a resident specialist who acts as assistant to the chief or attending specialist.

registration (rej″is-tra′shun) the act of recording. In dentistry, the making of a record of the jaw relations present, or of those desired, in order to transfer them to an articulator to facilitate proper construction of a dental prosthesis. **maxillomandibular r.,** see under *record*.

registry (rej′is-tre) 1. an office where a nurse may have his or her name listed as being available for duty. 2. a central agency for the collection of pathologic material and related clinical, laboratory, x-ray, and other data in a specified field of pathology, so organized that the data can be properly processed and made available for study.

Regitine (rej′ĭ-tēn) trademark for a preparation of phentolamine.

Regonol (reg′o-nōl) trademark for preparations of pyridostigmine bromide.

regression (re-gresh′un) [L. *regressio* a return] 1. a return to a former or earlier state. 2. a subsidence of symptoms or of a disease process. 3. in biology, the tendency in successive generations toward the mean; see *Galton's law of regression*, under *law*. 4. a return to earlier, especially to infantile, patterns of thought or behavior, a characteristic of many mental disorders also exhibited by normal persons in many situations, e.g., feelings of helplessness and dependency in a patient with a serious physical illness. 5. a functional relationship between a random variable (the dependent variable) and one or more variables fixed by the experimenter (the independent variables), usually the conditional mean of the dependent variable, e.g., the regression (or *regression curve*) of *Y* on *X* is the graph of the average value of *Y* associated with each value of *X;* so called because Galton's law of regression involves the determination of such relationships. **linear r.,** the statistical procedure for fitting a straight regression line to observed data, usually by minimizing the sum of the squared deviations of the observed values of the dependent variable from the regression line (*least-squares regression*).

regressive (re-gres'iv) going back; subsiding; characterized by regression.

Regroton (reg'ro-ton) trademark for preparations of chlorthalidone and reserpine.

regular (reg'u-lar) [L. *regularis; regula* rule] normal or conforming to rule; occurring at proper or fixed intervals.

regulation (reg"u-la'shun) [L. *regula* rule] 1. the act of adjusting or state of being adjusted to a certain standard. 2. in biology, the adaptation of form or behavior of an organism to changed conditions. 3. the power of a pregastrula stage to form a whole embryo from a part. **menstrual r.,** removal of the uterine contents, without dilatation, by application of a vacuum through a cannula introduced into the uterus.

Reg. umb. abbreviation for L. *re'gio umbili'ci,* umbilical region.

regurgitant (re-gur'ji-tant) [re- + L. *gurgitare* to flood] flowing back or in the opposite direction from normal.

regurgitation (re-gur"ji-ta'shun) [re- + L. *gurgitare* to flood] a backward flowing, as the casting up of undigested food, or the backward flowing of blood into the heart, or between the chambers of the heart when a valve is incompetent. **aortic r.,** the backflow of blood from the aorta into the left ventricle, owing to imperfect functioning (insufficiency or incompetence) of the aortic semilunar valve. **mitral r.,** the backflow of blood from the left ventricle into the left atrium, owing to inadequate functioning (insufficiency) of the mitral valve. **pulmonic r.,** the backflow of blood from the pulmonary artery into the right ventricle, owing to inadequate functioning (insufficiency) of the pulmonic semilunar valve. **tricuspid r.,** the backflow of blood from the right ventricle into the right atrium, owing to imperfect functioning (insufficiency) of the tricuspid valve. **valvular r.,** regurgitation of the blood through the orifices of the heart valves owing to imperfect closing (insufficiency or incompetence) of the valves; named, according to the valve affected, *aortic, mitral, pulmonic,* or *tricuspid r.* **vesico-ureteral r.,** see under *reflux.*

rehabilitation (re"hah-bil"i-ta'shun) 1. the restoration of normal form and function after injury or illness. 2. the restoration of an ill or injured patient to self-sufficiency or to gainful employment at his highest attainable skill in the shortest possible time.

rehabilitee (re"hah-bil'i-te") the subject of rehabilitation.

rehalation (re"hah-la'shun) [re- + L. *halare* to breathe] rebreathing.

Rehfuss' test (method), tube (ra'fus) [Martin Emil *Rehfuss,* American physician, 1887–1964] see under *tests* and *tube.*

rehydration (re"hi-dra'shun) the restoration of water or of fluid content to a body or to substance which has become dehydrated.

Reichel's cloacal duct (ri'kelz) [Friedrich Paul *Reichel,* German obstetrician, 1858–1934] see under *duct.*

Reichert's canal, etc. [Karl Bogislaus *Reichert,* German anatomist, 1811–1883] see under *canal, cartilage, membrane, recess, scar,* and *substance.*

Reichmann's disease (syndrome) (rik'manz) [Nikolas *Reichmann,* Warsaw physician, 1851–1918] gastrosuccorrhea.

Reichstein (rik'shtin), Tadeus. Polish-born Swiss organic chemist, born 1897; co-winner, with Edward Calvin Kendall and Philip Showalter Hench, of the Nobel prize for medicine or physiology in 1950 for his research on the structure and biological effects of the hormones of the adrenal cortex.

Reid's base line (redz) [Robert William *Reid,* Scottish anatomist, 1851–1939] see *base line,* under *line.*

Reil's insula, etc. (rilz) [Johann Christian *Reil,* German anatomist, 1759–1813] see under *insula, ribbon, sulcus,* and *trigone.*

reimplantation (re"im-plan-ta'shun) replantation of tissue or a structure, such as a tooth, in the site from which it was previously lost or removed.

reinfection (re"in-fek'shun) a second infection by the same pathogenic agent, or a second infection of an organ such as the kidney by a different pathogenic agent.

reinforcement (re"in-fors'ment) the increasing of force or strength. In behavioral science, the presentation of a stimulus that serves to strengthen responses preceding its occurrence. **r. of reflex,** the increasing of a reflex response by causing the patient to perform some mental or physical concentration while the reflex is being elicited.

reinforcer (re"in-fors'er) anything that produces reinforcement; a reinforcing stimulus.

reinfusate (re'in-fu"sat) fluid for reinfusion into the body, usually after being subjected to a treatment process.

reinfusion (re"in-fu'zhun) infusion of body fluid that has previously been withdrawn from the same individual, e.g., reinfusion of ascitic fluid after ultrafiltration.

Reinke's crystalloids (crystals) (rin'kez) [Friedrich Berthold *Reinke,* German anatomist, 1862–1919] see under *crystalloids.*

reinnervation (re"in-er-va'shun) restoration of nerve function to a part from which it was lost; it may occur spontaneously or be achieved by nerve grafting.

reinoculation (re"in-ok"u-la'shun) an inoculation that follows a previous one with the same virus.

reintegration (re"in-te-gra'shun) 1. biological integration after a state of disruption. 2. restoration of harmonious mental function after disintegration of the personality in mental illness.

reintubation (re"in-tu-ba'shun) intubation performed after extubation.

reinversion (re"in-ver'zhun) restoration to its normal place of an inverted organ, especially restoration of an inverted uterus.

reinvocation (re"in-vo-ka'shun) reactivation.

Reisseisen's muscles (ris'i-senz) [Franz Daniel *Reisseisen,* German anatomist, 1773–1828] see under *muscle.*

Reissner's fiber, membrane (ris'nerz) [Ernst *Reissner,* German anatomist, 1824–1878] see under *fiber,* and see *paries vestibularis ductus cochlearis.*

Reiter's syndrome (disease) (ri'terz) [Hans *Reiter,* German physician, 1881–1969] see under *syndrome.*

reiterature (re-it"er-a-tu're) [L.] repeat or renew, as a prescription.

rejection (re-jek'shun) graft rejection; an immune response against grafted tissue that results in failure of the graft to survive. **acute r., acute cellular r.,** the classic type of graft rejection, occurring 1 to 3 weeks after transplantation or following a cessation of immunosuppressive therapy and resulting primarily from the cell-mediated immune response of the recipient against incompatible HLA antigens; it is manifested histologically as extensive infiltration by mononuclear cells, primarily small lymphocytes, accompanied by edema and interstitial hemorrhage. **cellular r.,** acute r. **chronic r.,** a gradual progressive loss of function of the transplanted organ occurring months or years after transplantation. **first-set r.,** see under *phenomenon.* **hyperacute r.,** graft rejection occurring immediately after transplantation and resulting from the presence of preformed, circulating cytotoxic antibodies against antigens (often non-HLA antigens) on the graft. Antigen-antibody complexes on vascular endothelium initiate an Arthus-type (type III) reaction in which complement activation results in infiltration by neutrophils, endothelial injury, and occlusion of capillaries with fibrin-platelet thrombi; adequate blood flow to the graft is never established. **second-set r.,** see under *phenomenon.*

rejuvenescence (re-ju"ve-nes'ens) [re- + L. *juvenescere* to become young] a renewal of youth or of strength and vigor.

relapse (re-laps') [L. *relapsus*] the return of a disease after its apparent cessation. Cf. *recrudescence.* **intercurrent r.,** a relapse occurring before the temperature has reached a normal level. **rebound r.,** return of some of the symptoms of a disease on cessation of treatment, applied especially to the relapse of patients with rheumatoid arthritis on withdrawal of cortisone or ACTH (Hench).

relation (re-la'shun) [L. *relatio* a carrying back] the condition or state of one object or entity when considered in connection with another. **acentric r.**, eccentric jaw r. **buccolingual r.**, the position of a tooth or space in the dental arch in relation to the tongue and the cheek. **centric r., centric jaw r.**, the position of the mandible, obtained principally by operator guidance, in which the condyles are in the rearmost uppermost position in the fossae of the temporomandibular joint. Called also *median retruded r., terminal hinge position,* and *true centric.* **dynamic r's,** those existing between two objects or entities when one or both of them are moving or constantly changing, as the relation between the mandible and the maxilla. **eccentric r., eccentric jaw r.**, any relation of the mandible to the maxillae other than the centric relation; called also *acentric r.* and *eccentric position.* **eccentric jaw r., acquired,** an eccentric relation of the mandible to the maxilla that is assumed in order to bring the teeth into centric occlusion. **jaw r.**, any relation of the mandible to the maxilla, variously designated as centric, eccentric, median, occlusal, protrusive, and the like. Called also *maxillomandibular r.* **lateral occlusal r.**, the relation of the mandible to the maxilla when the lower jaw is in a position to either side of centric relation. **maxillomandibular r.**, jaw r. **median jaw r.**, the relation between the maxilla and the mandible when the lower jaw is in the median sagittal plane, without being displaced to either side; ideally, median and centric relations should coincide. **median retruded jaw r.**, centric r. **object r.**, the emotional bond formed between one person and another, as contrasted with interest in and love for oneself. **occlusal r.**, see under *position.* **posterior border jaw r.**, see under *position.* **protrusive jaw r.**, an occlusal position in which the mandible is protruded. See also *prognathism.* **rest jaw r.**, rest position. **ridge r.**, the positional relation of the mandibular ridge to the maxillary ridge. **static r's**, those existing between two objects or entities when neither one of them is moving or changing in any way. **unstrained jaw r.**, that maintained when a state of balanced tonus exists among all the muscles involved, being achieved without undue or unnatural force and causing no distortion of the tissues of the temporomandibular joints.

relaxant (re-lak'sant) [L. *relaxare* to loosen] 1. lessening or reducing tension. 2. an agent that lessens tension. **muscle r.**, an agent that specifically aids in reducing muscle tension, as those acting at the polysynaptic neurons of motor nerves (e.g., meprobamate) or at the myoneural junction (curare and related compounds).

relaxation (re″lak-sa'shun) 1. a lessening of tension. 2. a mitigation of pain. **isometric r.**, relaxation of a muscle without shortening.

relaxin (re-lak'sin) a water-soluble polypeptide (molecular weight approx. 8000) extracted from the corpus luteum during pregnancy; it produces relaxation of the pubic symphysis and dilation of the uterine cervix in certain animal species. Its role in the human pregnant female is unknown. A pharmaceutical preparation, extracted from the ovaries of pregnant sows, has been used in treatment of dysmenorrhea and premature labor, and to facilitate labor at term.

reliability (re-li″ah-bil'ĭ-te) the extent to which a statistically derived measure (mean, median, standard deviation, etc.) from a simple gives the same results upon repeated sampling under identical conditions.

relief (re-lēf') [L. *relevatio*] 1. the mitigation or removal of pain or distress. 2. the projection of a figure, part, or structure above the ground on which it is formed. 3. the reduction or elimination of undesirable pressure or force from a specific area under a denture base. See also under *chamber,* and *space.* 4. a thin lining of adhesive or hard baseplate wax in the master cast beneath lingual bar connectors or bar portions of the lingual plates, areas where major connectors will contact thin tissue, and beneath framework extension onto bridge areas for attachment of resin bases, which correspond accurately to the tissue topography. See also *blockout.*

relieve (re-lēv') [L. *relevare* to lighten] to mitigate or remove pain or distress.

reline (re-līn') to resurface the tissue side of a denture

with new base material in order to achieve a more accurate fit.

reluxation (re″luk-sa'shun) redislocation.

REM rapid eye movements (see under *sleep*).

rem (rem) [*r*oentgen-equivalent–*m*an] the quantity of any ionizing radiation which has the same biological effectiveness as 1 rad of x-rays; 1 rem = 1 rad × RBE (relative biological effectiveness).

Remak's band, fibers, ganglion, plexus, etc. (ra'maks) [Robert *Remak,* German neurologist, 1815–1865] see *axon;* see *gray fibers,* under *fiber;* see under *ganglion;* and see *plexus submucosus.*

Remak's paralysis (type), reflex, symptom (sign) (ra'maks) [Ernst Julius *Remak,* German neurologist, 1848–1911] see under *paralysis, reflex,* and *symptom.*

remedial (re-me'de-al) [L. *remedialis*] curative, acting as a remedy.

remedy (rem'ĕ-de) [L. *remedium*] anything that cures, palliates, or prevents disease. **concordant r's**, a homeopathic term for remedies of similar action, but of dissimilar origin. **Ehrlich-Hata r.**, arsphenamine. **inimic r's**, a homeopathic term for remedies whose actions are antagonistic. **tissue r's**, the twelve remedies which, according to the biochemical school of homeopathy, form the mineral bases of the body.

Remijia (re-mij'e-ah) a genus of rubiaceous shrubs. *R. peduncula'ta* Flueck. furnishes cuprea bark, a source of hydroxycinchonidine.

remineralization (re-min″er-al-i-za'shun) the restoration of mineral elements, as to the human body.

remission (re-mish'un) [L. *remissio*] a diminution or abatement of the symptoms of a disease; also the period during which such diminution occurs.

remittence (re-mit'ens) temporary abatement, without actual cessation, of symptoms.

remittent (re-mit'ent) [L. *remittere* to send back] having periods of abatement and of exacerbation.

remnant (rem'nant) something remaining; a residue; a vestige. **acroblastic r.**, the peripheral part of the acroblast which recedes into the protoplasm of the spermatid and later disintegrates.

remotivation (re-mo″tĭ-va'shun) in psychiatry, a group therapy technique administered by the nursing staff in a mental hospital, which is used to stimulate the communication skills and an interest in the environment of long-term, withdrawn patients.

ren (ren), pl. *re'nes*, gen. *re'nis* [L.] [NA] either of the two organs (i.e., the kidneys) in the lumbar region that excrete the urine; see *kidney.* **r. mo'bilis**, hypermobile kidney. **r. ungulifor'mis**, horseshoe kidney.

Renacidin (re-nas'ĭ-din) trademark for a preparation of hemiacidrin.

renal (re'nal) [L. *renalis*] pertaining to the kidney; nephric.

Renaut's bodies (ren-ōz') [Joseph Louis *Renaut,* French physician, 1844–1917] see under *body.*

renculi (ren'ku-li) [L.] plural of *renculus.*

renculus (ren'ku-lus), pl. *ren'culi* [L.] reniculus.

Rendu-Osler-Weber disease, syndrome (ron-duh'-ōs'ler-web'er) [Henri Jules Louis Marie *Rendu,* French physician, 1844–1902; Sir William *Osler,* Canadian-born physician; 1849–1919; Frederick Parkes *Weber,* British physician, 1863–1962] hereditary hemorrhagic telangiectasia.

renes (re'nēz) [L.] plural of *ren.*

Renese (rēn'ēs) trademark for preparations of polythiazide (Renese-R also contains reserpine).

renicapsule (ren'ĭ-kap″sūl) [*ren* + L. *capsula* capsule] an adrenal gland.

reniculi (rĕ-nik'u-li) [L.] plural of *reniculus.*

reniculus (rĕ-nik'u-lus), pl. *renic'uli* [L.] one of the lobules composing the kidney, and consisting of a pyramid and its enclosing cortical substance.

reniform (ren'ĭ-form) [*ren* + L. *forma* form] shaped like a kidney.

renin (re'nin) [EC 3.4.23.15] an enzyme of the hydrolase class that catalyzes cleavage of the leucine-leucine bond in angiotensin to generate angiotensin 1. The enzyme is synthesized as inactive prorenin in the kidney and released into the blood in the active form in response to various metabolic stimuli. Not to be confused with *rennin* (chymosin). **big r.**, prorenin.

reninism (re′nin-izm) a condition marked by overproduction of renin. **primary r.**, a syndrome of hypertension, hypokalemia, hyperaldosteronism, and elevated plasma renin activity, due to proliferation of juxtaglomerular cells.

renipelvic (ren″ĭ-pel′vik) pertaining to the pelvis of the kidney.

reniportal (ren″ĭ-pōr′tal) [ren + L. *porta* gate] pertaining to the portal system of the kidneys.

rennet (ren′et) chymosin.

rennin (ren′in) chymosin.

ren(o)- [L. *ren*, q.v.] a combining form denoting relationship to a kidney.

renocortical (re″no-kor′tĭ-kal) pertaining to the cortex of a kidney.

renocutaneous (re″no-ku-ta′ne-us) pertaining to the kidneys and skin.

renocystogram (re″no-sis′to-gram) renogram.

renogastric (re″no-gas′trik) pertaining to the kidney and stomach; nephrogastric.

Renografin (re″no-graf′in) trademark for preparations of diatrizoate sodium and diatrizoate meglumine.

renogram (re′no-gram) a graphic record of kidney function produced by externally monitoring the level of radioactivity in the bladder as a radiopharmaceutical agent enters it from the kidney via the ureters; called also *renocystogram.*

renography (re-nog′rah-fe) [ren + Gr. *graphein* to write] radiography of the kidney.

renointestinal (re″no-in-tes′tĭ-nal) pertaining to the kidney and intestine.

renopathy (re-nop′ah-the) [ren + Gr. *pathos* disease] nephropathy.

renoprival (re″no-pri′val) pertaining to, characterized by, or resulting from deprivation of kidney function.

Renoquid (re′no-kwid) trademark for a preparation of sulfacytine.

renotrophic (re″no-trof′ik) having the ability to increase kidney size.

renotropic (re″no-trop′ik) having a special affinity for kidney tissue.

Renovist (re″no-vist′) trademark for preparations of diatrizoate sodium and diatrizoate meglumine.

renule (ren′ūl) an area of the kidney supplied by a branch of the renal artery, usually consisting of three or four medullary pyramids and their corresponding cortical substance.

renunculus (re-nung′ku-lus) reniculus.

reovirus (re″o-vi′rus) [respiratory and *enteric orphan* + *virus*] a group of ether-resistant RNA viruses, formerly classified as a subgroup of the echoviruses. Reoviruses are separable into three serotypes, and have been isolated from healthy children, children with febrile and afebrile upper respiratory disease, children with diarrhea, and many animals.

reoxidation (re-ok″sĭ-da′shun) the act of taking up oxygen again, as by hemoglobin.

reoxygenation (re-ok″sĭ-jen-a′shun) in radiobiology, the phenomenon in which hypoxic (and thus radioresistant) tumor cells become more exposed to oxygen (and thus more radiosensitive) by coming into closer proximity to capillaries after death and loss of other tumor cells due to previous irradiation.

Rep. abbreviation for L. *repeta′tur*, let it be repeated.

rep (rep) [*r*oentgen *e*quivalent *p*hysical] an unofficial unit of amount of radiation of any kind which yields an amount of energy transferred to the tissue equal to that transferred by 1 roentgen of hard x- or γ-radiation (200 kv. or greater). This amount of energy turns out to be about 93 ergs per gram of water or soft tissue.

repair (re-pār′) the physical or mechanical restoration of damaged or diseased tissues by the growth of healthy new cells or by surgical apposition.

repatency (re-pa′ten-se) [re- + L. *patens* open] reestablishment of the opening in a part or vessel which has been closed.

repellent (re-pel′ent) [L. *repellere* to drive back] 1. able to repel or drive off; also an agent so acting, as *insect repellent.* 2. (*obs.*) capable of dispersing a swelling; also an agent or remedy which causes a swelling to disappear.

repeller (re-pel′er) an instrument used in labor of animals to push back the fetus until the head and limbs can be properly placed for normal delivery.

repercolation (re″per-ko-la′shun) [L. *re-* again + *percolare* to filter] a second or repeated percolation with the same materials.

repercussion (re″per-kush′un) [L. *repercussio* rebound] 1. the driving in of an eruption or the scattering of a swelling. 2. ballottement.

repercussive (re″per-kus′iv) 1. causing or pertaining to repercussion. 2. an agent causing repercussion; a repellent.

repetatur (re″pe-ta-tūr′) [L.] let it be repeated.

replantation (re″plan-ta′shun) the replacement of an organ or other structure, such as a digit, limb, or tooth, to the site from which it was previously lost or removed; called also reimplantation.

replenisher (re-plen′ish-er) an agent that restores what has been lost, used up, or is lacking.

repletion (re-ple′shun) [L. *repletio*] the condition of being full.

replication (rep″lĭ-ka′shun) [L. *replicatio* a fold backwards] 1. a turning back of a part so as to form a duplication. 2. repetition of an experiment to ensure accuracy. 3. the process of duplicating or reproducing, as the replication of an exact copy of a polynucleotide strand of DNA or RNA. **DNA r.**, the production of multiple identical copies of a DNA molecule by unwinding the two strands of the double helix and forming new complementary strands thereto. **semiconservative r.**, a term used to characterize the mode in which DNA is replicated, to wit, each daughter molecule has one newly synthesized strand and one strand from the parent molecule.

replicon (rep′lĭ-kon) a unit of DNA that contains an initiation point and a termination point and is capable of self-replication. A bacterial chromosome or plasmid consists of a single replicon, while a mammalian chromosome may contain 30,000 to 40,000 replicon units.

Repoise (re-pōz′) trademark for preparations of butaperazine.

repolarization (re-po″lar-ĭ-za′shun) the reestablishment of polarity, especially the return of cell membrane potential to resting potential after depolarization.

repositioning (re″po-zish′un-ing) the replacing of a structure or part to its normal site. **jaw r.**, the changing of any relative position of the mandible to the maxilla, usually by altering the occlusion of the natural or artificial teeth. **muscle r.**, surgical replacement of a muscle attachment into a more acceptable functional position.

repositor (re-poz′ĭ-tor) an instrument used in returning a displaced organ, especially the uterus, to the normal position.

repository (re-poz′ĭ-to-re) a place where something is stored; used in pharmacology to refer to the injection, usually intramuscularly, of a long-acting drug, which is slowly absorbed and is therefore prolonged in its action.

repression (re-presh′un) 1. the act of restraining, inhibiting, or suppressing. 2. in psychiatry, an unconscious defense mechanism in which unacceptable ideas and impulses are thrust out or kept out of consciousness. 3. in genetic theory, inhibition or gene transcription by a repressor; called also *gene r.* Cf. *derepression*, def. 2. **coordinate r.**, parallel diminution of the concentrations of the several enzymes of a metabolic pathway, resulting from increases in the level of repressor. **endproduct r.**, enzyme r. **enzyme r.**, interference, usually by the endproduct of a pathway, with synthesis of the enzymes of that pathway. **gene r.**, see *repression.*

repressor (re-pres′or) [L. "a restrainer"] in genetics, a substance produced by a regulator gene which acts through the cytoplasm to prevent initiation by the operator gene of protein synthesis by the operon.

reproduction (re″pro-duk′shun) [L. *re-* again + *productio* production] 1. the production of offspring by organized bodies. 2. the creation of a similar object or situation; duplication; replication. **asexual r.**, reproduction without the fusion of sexual cells, as by fission or budding. **bisex-**

ual r., see *sexual r.* **cytogenic r.,** reproduction in which the new individual proceeds from a single germ cell or zygote. **sexual r.,** reproduction by the fusion of a female sexual cell with a male sexual cell (*bisexual r., amphigony, gamogenesis, syngamy*) or by the development of an unfertilized egg (*unisexual r., parthenogenesis*). **somatic r.,** reproduction in which the new individual proceeds from a multicellular fragment produced by fission or budding. **unisexual r.,** see *sexual r.*

reproductive (re″pro-duk′tiv) subserving or pertaining to the production of offspring.

repromicin (rep″ro-mi′cin) chemical name: 12,13-deepoxy-12,13-didehydro-4′-deoxycirramycin A₁; an antibiotic, $C_{31}H_{51}NO_8$.

reproterol hydrochloride (re″pro-ter′ol) chemical name: 7-[3-[[2-(3,5-dihydroxyphenyl)-2-hydroxy ethyl]amino]propyl]-3,7-dihydro-1,3-dimethyl-1*H*-purine-2,6-dione monohydrochloride; a bronchodilator, $C_{18}H_{23}N_5O_5 \cdot HCl$.

reptilase (rep′til-ās) an enzyme from Russell's viper venom used in determining blood clotting time.

reptile (rep′til) any member of the class Reptilia.

Reptilia (rep-til′e-ah) a class of aquatic or terrestrial, cold-blooded vertebrates, including snakes, lizards, turtles, alligators, and crocodiles, as well as the extinct dinosaurs, which have bodies covered with horny scales or plates and breathe by means of lungs; most lay eggs outside of the body.

repullulation (re-pul″u-la′shun) [L. *re-* back + *pullulare* to sprout out] renewed growth by sprouting.

repulsion (re-pul′shun) [L. *re-* back + *pellere* to drive] the act of driving apart or away; a force which tends to drive two bodies apart. It is the opposite of attraction. In genetics, occurrence on opposite chromosomes in a double heterozygote of the two mutant alleles of interest. Cf. *coupling.*

RES reticuloendothelial system.

resazurin (re-sa′zu-rin) a quinone-imine compound used as a pH indicator with a pH range of 3.8 (orange) to 6.5 (violet). It is also used as an indicator of redox potential, turning from blue (oxidized) to pink (partially reduced) to colorless (fully reduced).

rescinnamine (re-sin′ah-min) an alkaloid, the 3,4,5-trimethoxycinnamic acid ester of methyl reserpate, obtained from *Rauwolfia serpentina* and other species of *Rauwolfia*. It occurs as a white or pale buff to cream colored crystalline powder, $C_{35}H_{42}N_2O_9$; used as an antihypertensive and also as a tranquilizer.

resect (re-sekt′) to remove part or all of an organ or tissue.

resectable (re-sek′tah-b'l) capable of being resected; lending itself to resection.

resection (re-sek′shun) [L. *resectio*] excision of a portion or all of an organ or other structure. **gastric r.,** partial gastrectomy; see *gastrectomy.* **root r.,** apicoectomy. **submucous r.,** excision of a portion of a deviated nasal septum after first laying back a flap of mucous membrane, which is replaced, or repositioned, after the operation. **transurethral prostatic r. (TURP),** resection of the prostate by means of a cystoscope passed through the urethra. **wedge r.,** removal of a triangular-shaped segment of tissue.

resectoscope (re-sek′to-skōp) an instrument with a wide-angle telescope and an electrically activated wire loop for transurethral removal or biopsy of lesions of the bladder, prostate, or urethra.

resectoscopy (re″sek-tos′ko-pe) resection or biopsy of lesions by means of the resectoscope.

resene (res′ēn) any one of a class of resin derivatives.

reserpine (res′er-pēn, rĕ-ser′pin) [USP] chemical name: 11,17β-dimethoxy-18β-[(3,4,5-trimethoxybenzoyl)oxy]-3β-20-α-yohimban-16β-carboxylic acid methyl ester. An alkaloid, $C_{33}H_{40}N_2O_9$, isolated from the root of *Rauwolfia serpentina* (L.) Benth. ex Kurz (Apocyanaceae) and other species of *Rauwolfia*, and occurring as a white or pale buff to slightly yellowish crystalline powder; used as an antihypertensive, and also as a sedative, administered orally and intramuscularly.

Reserpoid (res′er-poid) trademark for a preparation of reserpine.

reserve (re-zerv′) 1. to hold back for future use. 2. a supply, beyond that ordinarily used, which may be utilized in an emergency. **alkali r., alkaline r.,** the amount of conjugate base components of the blood buffers; since bicarbonate

is the most important of these conjugate bases, the term blood bicarbonate is often preferred to alkali reserve. **cardiac r.,** the potential ability of the heart to perform a wide range of work beyond that required under basal conditions, depending on changing demands of various physiological or pathological states.

reservoir (rez′er-vwar) [Fr. *réservoir*, from *réserver* to reserve] 1. a place or cavity for storage; for anatomical structures serving as a storage space for fluids; see *cisterna.* 2. reservoir host or reservoir of infection; an alternate or passive host or carrier that harbors pathogenic organisms, without injury to itself, and serves as a source from which other individuals can be infected. **chromatin r.,** karyosome. **r. of infection,** see *reservoir,* def. 2. **Ommaya r.,** a device implanted beneath the galea aponeurotica for instillation of medication or removal of fluid through a catheter positioned in a lateral ventricle of the brain. **Pecquet's r.,** cisterna chyli.

reshaping (re-shāp′ing) a restoration or change of shape, as of a crown, bridge, or denture.

resident (rez′i-dent) a graduate and licensed physician receiving training in a specialty in a hospital.

residua (re-zid′u-ah) [L.] plural of *residuum.*

residual (re-zid′u-al) [L. *residuus*] remaining or left behind.

residue (rez′i-du) [L. *residuum*, from *re-* back + *sidere* to sit] 1. a remainder; that which remains after the removal of other substances. In biochemistry, the portion of a molecule that remains after it has lost some of its components, as an amino acid residue, which loses a water molecule when it is joined to another amino acid. 2. see *Vaughn's split products,* under *product.* **day r.,** any element of a dream that is derived from an occurrence of the preceding day.

residuum (re-zid′u-um), pl. *resid′ua* [L.] 1. a residue or remainder. 2. in coccidian protozoa, the material remaining after completion of different stages in the life cycle of the parasite. Called also *residual body.* **gastric r.,** the contents of the stomach during the interdigestive period, as in the morning before eating.

resilience (re-zil′e-ens) [L. *resilire* to leap back] 1. the property of being able to return to the original form after distortion, as by bending, compressing, or stretching. 2. the ability to recover readily from an illness. 3. resiliency, def. 2.

resiliency (re-zil′yen-se) 1. resilience. 2. a measure of the energy required to stress an object to the limit above which permanent deformation will occur (proportional limit).

resilient (re-zil′e-ent) [L. *resiliens*] elastic; returning to its former shape or size after distortion.

resilin (rĕ-zil′in) an elastic protein present in the wing-hinge of dragonflies, locusts, and fleas, which stores and releases energy with extremely high efficiency.

resin (rez′in) [L. *resina*] a mixture of carboxylic acids, essential oils, and terpenes, occurring as exudations on various trees and shrubs, or produced synthetically. Resins are highly combustible semisolids or amorphous solids that are insoluble in water, while some are soluble in ethanol and others in carbon tetrachloride, ether, and volatile oils. Most are soft and sticky, but harden after exposure to cold. **acrylic r's,** a class of thermoplastic resins, ethylene derivatives containing a vinyl group, produced by polymerization of acrylic or methacrylic acid or their derivatives; used in the fabrication of medical prostheses and dental restorations and appliances. **activated r.,** self-curing r. **anion-exchange r.,** see *ion-exchange r.* **autopolymer r.,** self-curing r. **azure A carbacrylic r.,** azuresin. **carbacrylamine r's,** a mixture of 87.5 per cent of cation exchangers, carbacrylic resin, and potassium carbacrylic resin, with 12.5 per cent of the anion exchanger, polyamine-methylene resin; used to increase fecal excretion of sodium in the treatment of edema. **cation-exchange r.,** see *ion-exchange r.* **cholestyramine r.** [USP], a strongly basic anion exchange resin in the chloride form, consisting of styrene-divinylbenzene copolymer with quaternary ammonium functional groups, having an affinity for bile acids, which it binds into an insoluble complex that is excreted in the feces, resulting in elimination of bile acids from the enterohepatic circulation and in increased oxidation of cholesterol to bile acids; administered orally for the relief of pruritus associated with cholestasis occurring in partial biliary obstruction and as adjunctive therapy to diet in the management of patients with elevated cholesterol due to primary type II hyperlipoproteinemia (patients with pure hypercholesterolemia). **cold-curing r.,** self-curing r. **composite r.,** a synthetic resin, usually acrylic based, to which a high percentage (about 75 to 80 per cent) of an inert filler has been added; glass beads or rods, borosilicate glass powder, and natural silica are the most commonly used fillers. Filler particles are coated with a coupling agent that binds the particles to the resin matrix. Used chiefly in dental restorative procedures. **copolymer r.,** one that is produced by the concurrent and joint polymerization of two or more different monomers or polymers. **direct filling r.,** a resin or a composite, usually an acrylic, that is inserted directly into the prepared cavity and allowed to polymerize at mouth temperature. **epoxy r.,** a thermosetting resin based on reactivity of the epoxide group, which is characterized by toughness, adhesibility, chemical resistance, dielectric properties, and dimensional stability; several modified types are used as denture base material. **heat-curing r.,** one that requires the use of heat to effect its polymerization. **ion exchange r.,** a high molecular weight, insoluble polymer of simple organic compounds with the ability to exchange its attached ions for other ions in the surrounding solution. They are classified as (a) *cation* or *anion exchange resins,* depending on which ions the resin exchanges, and (b) carboxylic, sulfonic, etc., depending on the nature of the active groups. *Cation exchange resins* are used to restrict intestinal sodium absorption in edematous states; *anion exchange resins* are used as antacids in the treatment of ulcers. **podophyllum r.** [USP], a powdered mixture of resins removed from podophyllum by percolation with alcohol and subsequent precipitation upon addition of acidified water; used as a topical caustic in the treatment of certain papillomas as a 25 per cent dispersion in compound benzoin tincture, or as a solution in alcohol. Formerly used as a cathartic. Called also *podophyllin.* **polyamine-methylene r.,** a polyethylene polyamine methylene substituted resin of diphenylol dimethylmethane and formaldehyde in basic form; because of its exchange-resin action it has been used as a gastric antacid. **quick-cure r.,** self-curing r. **self-curing r.,** any resin which can be polymerized by the addition of an activator and a catalyst without the use of external heat. **styrene r.,** polystyrene. **synthetic r.,** an amorphous, organic, semisolid or solid material produced from simpler compounds by polymerization or condensation. **vinyl r.,** a thermoplastic resin, an ethylene derivative containing the vinyl radical, CH_2:CH—.

resina (re-zi′nah) [L.] resin.

Resinat (rez′ĭ-nat) trademark for preparations of polyamine-methylene resin.

resinoid (rez′ĭ-noid) 1. resembling a resin. 2. a substance resembling a resin. 3. a dry therapeutic precipitate prepared from a vegetable tincture.

resinotannol (rez″ĭ-no-tan′ol) any resin alcohol which gives a tannin reaction.

resinous (rez′ĭ-nus) [L. *resinosus*] of the nature of a resin.

resistance (re-zis′tans) [L. *resistentia*] 1. opposition, or counteracting force. 2. in psychiatry, conscious or unconscious defenses that prevent repressed material from coming into awareness and being subject to treatment efforts. 3. the natural ability of an organism to resist microorganisms or toxins produced in disease. 4. electrical resistance, the opposition of the flow of electrical current between two points of a circuit: the voltage drop between the two points divided by the current flow, expressed in ohms. 5. vascular resistance, the opposition to blood flow in a vascular bed: the pressure drop across the bed divided by the blood flow, conventionally expressed in peripheral resistance units. 6. airway resistance, the opposition of the tracheobronchial tree to air flow: the mouth-to-alveoli pressure difference divided by the air flow. **airway r.,** resistance, def. 6. **drug r.,** the ability of a microorganism to withstand the effects of a drug that are lethal to most members of its species. Primary drug resistance refers to initial infection by a resistant organism; secondary drug resistance to resistance that develops during the course of therapy. **electrical r.,** resistance, def. 4. **environmental r.,** the sum of the physical and biologic factors that prevent a species from reproducing at its maximum rate. **internal r.,** the electrical resistance within a voltage source, e.g., a battery, power supply, or generator. **total peripheral r.,** the vascular resis-

tance of the systemic circulation: the difference between the mean arterial pressure and central venous pressure divided by the cardiac output. **total pulmonary r.,** the vascular resistance of the pulmonary circulation: the difference between the mean pulmonary arterial pressure and the left atrial filling pressure divided by the cardiac output. **vascular r.,** resistance, def. 5.

resite (res′it) an insoluble, infusible compound formed by further reaction of resole under heat.

resole (res′ōl) a condensation polymer of an alcohol formed by interaction of phenol and formaldehyde, which is of relatively low molecular weight, thermoplastic, and alcohol soluble.

resolution (rez″o-lu′shun) [L. *resolutum,* from *resolvere* to unbind] 1. the subsidence of a pathologic state, as the subsidence of an inflammation, or the softening and disappearance of a swelling. 2. the perception as separate of two adjacent objects or points. In microscopy, it is the minimal distance at which two adjacent objects can be distinguished as separate. The resolving power of an instrument depends on the wavelength of the radiation used and the numerical aperture of the system; it is expressed in microns distance or lines per millimeter.

resolve (re-zolv′) [L. *resolvere*] 1. to restore to the normal state after some pathologic process. 2. to separate a thing into its component parts.

resolvent (re-zol′vent) [L. *resolvens* dissolving] 1. promoting resolution or the dissipation of a pathologic growth. 2. an agent that promotes resolution.

resonance (rez′o-nans) [L. *resonantia*] 1. the prolongation and intensification of sound produced by the transmission of its vibrations to a cavity, especially a sound elicited by percussion. Decrease of resonance is called *dullness;* absence of resonance, *flatness.* 2. a vocal sound as heard in auscultation. 3. mesomerism. **amphoric r.,** a sound resembling that produced by blowing over the mouth of an empty bottle. **bandbox r.,** the extremely resonant sound elicited by percussion in cases of emphysema of the lungs. **bell-metal r.,** a peculiar sound heard in pneumothorax when a coin placed on the chest wall is struck by another coin. **cough r.,** a peculiar auscultatory sound elicited by coughing. **cracked-pot r.,** a peculiar sound elicited by percussion over a pulmonary cavity that communicates with a bronchus. **electron spin r.,** in spectrometry, a measure of electron spin as an indication of the extent of activity of free radicals in an organic reaction. **hydatid r.,** a peculiar sound heard in the combined auscultation and percussion of a hydatid cyst. **nuclear magnetic r.,** a measure, by means of applying an external magnetic field to a solution in a constant radio frequency field, of the magnetic moment of atomic nuclei to determine the structure of organic compounds. An application of this technique, called magnetic resonance imaging, permits imaging of soft tissues of the body by distinguishing between hydrogen atoms in different environments. **osteal r.,** the sound elicited by percussion over a bony structure. **shoulder-strap r.,** pulmonary resonance in the apex of the lung above the clavicle. **skodaic r.,** increased percussion resonance at the upper part of the chest, with flatness below it. **tympanic r.,** the drumlike reverberation of a cavity full of air. **tympanitic r.,** the peculiar sound elicited by percussing a tympanitic abdomen. **vesicular r.,** the normal pulmonary resonance. **vesiculotympanic r.,** a resonance partly vesicular and partly tympanic. **vocal r.,** the sound of ordinary speech as heard through the chest wall. **whispering r.,** the auscultatory sound of whispered words heard through the chest wall. **wooden r.,** vesiculotympanic r.

resonant (rez′o-nant) giving a vibrant sound on percussion.

resonator (rez′o-na″ter) an instrument used to intensify sounds. In electricity, an electrical circuit in which oscillations of a certain frequency are set up by oscillations of the same frequency in another circuit. **Oudin r.,** a coil of wire of adjustable number of turns which is designed to be connected to a source of high-frequency current, such as a spark gap and induction coil, for the purpose of applying an effluve to a patient.

resorb (re-sorb′, re-zorb′) to take up or absorb again; to undergo resorption.

resorcin (rĕ-zor′sin) resorcinol.

resorcinism (rĕ-zor′sĭ-nizm) chronic poisoning by resorcinol, resulting in methemoglobinemia, paralysis, and damage to the capillaries, kidneys, heart, and nervous system.

resorcinol (rĕ-zor′sĭ-nol) [USP] chemical name: 1,3-benzenediol. A bactericidal, fungicidal, keratolytic, exfoliative, and antipruritic agent, $C_6H_6O_2$, occurring as white, or nearly white, needle-shaped crystals or powder; used especially as a topical keratolytic in the treatment of acne and other dermatoses, such as seborrheic dermatitis. Called also *resorcin*. **r. monoacetate** [USP], the monoacetate salt of resorcinol, $C_8H_8O_3$, occurring as a viscous, pale yellow or amber liquid; used topically as an antiseborrheic and keratolytic.

resorcinolphthalein (re-zor″sĭ-nol-thal′e-in) fluorescein.

resorcinum (re″zor-si′num) resorcinol.

resorption (re-sorp′shun) [L. *resorbere* to swallow again] the loss of substance through physiologic or pathologic means, such as loss of dentin and cementum of a tooth, or of the alveolar process of the mandible or maxilla. **bone r.,** a type of bone loss (resorption) due to osteoclastic activity. **idiopathic r.,** resorption of calcified tissues without apparent cause. **root r.,** resorption in which cementum or dentin is lost from the root of a tooth owing to cementoclastic or osteoclastic activity in conditions such as trauma of occlusion or neoplasms. **tooth r., external,** resorption of calcified dental tissue, beginning on the external surface of the root and extending to the cementum, dentin, and eventually into the root canal. See also *internal tooth r.,* def. 1. **tooth r., internal,** 1. an unusual form of tooth resorption beginning centrally in a tooth, and apparently initiated by inflammatory hyperplasia of the pulp, characterized by a pink hued area on the crown showing the hyperplastic vascular pulp tissue filling the resorbed area. Called also *chronic perforating hyperplasia* and *pink tooth of Mummery.* 2. external tooth resorption that ramifies into the dentin. **tubular r.,** resorption by renal tubular cells of elements of the fluid filtered at the glomerulus.

respirable (rĕ-spīr′ah-b'l) suitable for respiration, or able to be respired.

respiration (res″pĭ-ra′shun) [L. *respiratio*] 1. the exchange of oxygen and carbon dioxide between the atmosphere and the cells of the body. The process includes ventilation (inspiration and expiration), the diffusion of oxygen from pulmonary alveoli to the blood and of carbon dioxide from the blood to the alveoli, and the transport of oxygen to and carbon dioxide from the body cells. 2. the exergonic metabolic processes in living cells by which molecular oxygen is taken in, organic substances are oxidized, free energy is released, and carbon dioxide, water, and other oxidized products are given off by the cell; called also *cell r.* **abdominal r.,** respiration maintained by contribution of the diaphragm and respiratory muscles. Cf. *thoracic r.* **absent r.,** that in which the respiratory sounds are suppressed. **accelerated r.,** respiration at a faster than normal frequency. **aerobic r.,** the oxidative transformation of certain substrates into secretory products, the released energy being used in the process of assimilation. **amphoric r.,** that which is characterized by amphoric resonance, or a quality like that of the sound produced by blowing over the mouth of an empty jar. It is heard over tuberculous or bronchiectatic cavities, in pneumothorax, in compression of lung from effusion. **anaerobic r.,** a form of respiration in which energy is released from chemical reactions in which free oxygen takes no part. **artificial r.,** that which is maintained by artificial means. Among the various methods of artificial respiration are the following: *Buist's method* is employed in asphyxiation of the newborn, and consists of holding the infant alternately on the stomach and back. *Eve's method:* ". . . the victim is laid face downward on a stretcher and is well wrapped with blankets. His wrists and ankles are lashed to the handles. Then he is hoisted on a trestle or sling and rocking is begun. The first tilt should be head down and steep (50 degrees) and should produce full expiration by the weight of the abdominal contents pressing on the diaphragm. It will also force aortic blood through the coronaries and empty the stomach and lungs of water. Then full inspiration is produced by tilting the foot end down to 50 degrees. The rocking is done a dozen times a minute through an angle of 45 degrees each way." (J.A.M.A.) *Method of Marshall Hall:* Put the body prone, gently press on the back, then removing the back pressure, turn the body on its side and press a little more, repeating this formula sixteen times every minute. It is known as the method of *prone* or *postural respiration,* or

"ready method." *Howard method:* Place the body supine, with a cushion under the back, so that the head is lower than the abdomen; the arms are held over the head, forcible pressure is made with both hands inward and upward, over the lower ribs, about sixteen times per minute. *Mouth-to-mouth method:* The rescuer applies his mouth directly to the mouth of the patient and regularly inflates the patient's lungs with his own expired air. *Schafer's method:* Patient prone with forehead on one of his arms: straddle across patient with knees on either side of his hips, and press with both hands firmly upon the back over the lower ribs; then raise your body slowly, at the same time relaxing the pressure with your hands. Repeat this forward and backward movement about every five seconds. *Silvester's method:* Patient supine. The arms are pulled firmly over the head to raise the ribs, and kept there until air ceases to enter the chest. The arms are brought down to the chest, and are pressed against it for a second or so after air ceases to escape. This formula is repeated sixteen times per minute. See also *respirator.* **asthmoid r.,** respiration in which expiration is accompanied by a wheezing sound like that of bronchial asthma. **Austin Flint r.,** cavernous r. **Biot's r.,** breathing characterized by irregular periods of apnea alternating with periods in which four or five breaths of identical depth are taken; seen in patients with increased intracranial pressure. **Bouchut's r.,** respiration in which the inspiratory phase is shorter than the expiratory phase; seen in children with bronchopneumonia. **bronchial r.,** tubular r. **bronchocavernous r.,** that which is intermediate in character between bronchial and cavernous; it is heard over a lung cavity with solidified lung tissue adjacent to it. **bronchovesicular r.,** a variety intermediate between the bronchial and vesicular forms. **cavernous r.,** a respiration marked by a peculiar prolonged hollow resonance, usually due to a cavity in the lung; it is heard in the same conditions as amphoric respiration. **cell r.,** respiration, def. 2. **cerebral r.,** Corrigan's r. **Cheyne-Stokes r.,** breathing characterized by rhythmic waxing and waning of the depth of respiration, with regularly recurring periods of apnea; seen especially in coma resulting from affection of the nervous centers. **cogwheel r.,** a form with a peculiar jerky inspiration; breathing in which the expiratory and inspiratory sounds are not continuous, but are split into two or more separate sounds. Called also *interrupted r.* **collateral r.,** the entrance of air into alveoli through pulmonary alveolar pores and other pathways so that a lobule may remain aerated even though its bronchiole is obstructed. **controlled diaphragmatic r.,** the intentional use of abdominal respiration for the purpose of limiting the motion of the apices of the lung. **Corrigan's r.,** a shallow and frequent blowing respiration in a low fever. **costal r.,** that which is performed mainly by the rib muscles. **diaphragmatic r.,** that which is mainly performed by the diaphragm. **divided r.,** respiration marked by a pause between the inspiratory and expiratory sounds. **electrophrenic r.,** artificial respiration induced by electric stimulation of the phrenic nerve. Abbreviated EPR. **external r.,** the exchange of gases between the lungs and the blood. **fetal r.,** gaseous interchange through the placenta. **forced r.,** deliberate hyperventilation. **granular r.,** a vesicular respiration, giving a sound as if the air were passing through a tube with an uneven surface. **harsh r.,** bronchovesicular r. **indefinite r.,** a respiratory sound so feeble or so confused that it is difficult to assign to it a definite character. **internal r.,** the exchange of gases between the body cells and the blood; called also *tissue r.* **interrupted r.,** cogwheel r. **jerky r.,** cogwheel r. **Kussmaul's r., Kussmaul-Kien r.,** air hunger; see under *hunger.* **labored r.,** that which is performed with difficulty. **meningitic r.,** short and rapid breathing interrupted by pauses of ten to thirty seconds; occurring in healthy persons during sleep it has no important significance, but in meningitis it is regarded as an unfavorable sign. **metamorphosing r.,** bronchocavernous r. **nervous r.,** Corrigan's r. **paradoxical r.,** respiration in which a lung, or a portion thereof, is deflated during inspiration and inflated during expiration. **periodic r.,** Cheyne-Stokes r. **puerile r.,** that in which the breathing sounds are more intense than those of normal adult respiration and resemble those of childhood. **rude r.,** bronchovesicular r. **Seitz's metamorphosing r.,** a variety of bronchial respiration consisting of an inspiratory murmur, beginning as a tubular bronchial sound and ending as either a cavernous or an

Place one hand under the patient's chin and the other on top of his head. Lift up on the chin and push down on the top of the head to tilt the head backwards.

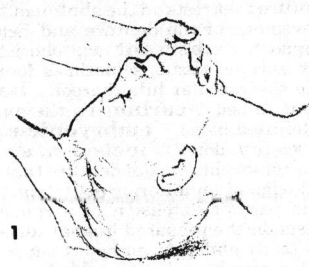

1

Put the thumb of the hand under the jaw into the patient's mouth; grasp the jaw and pull it forward.

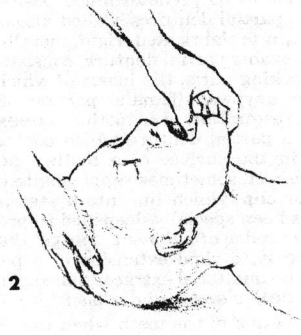

2

While holding the jaw forward pinch the nostrils closed with the other hand to prevent leakage of air through the nose.

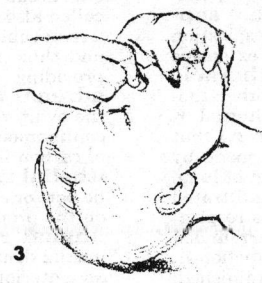

3

Take a deep breath; place your mouth tightly over the patient's and blow forcefully into his lungs.

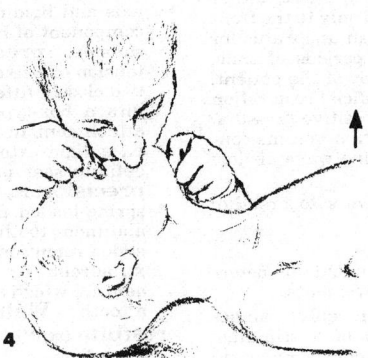

4

Blowing into the lungs causes the chest to expand. When the chest has expanded adequately remove your mouth from the patient's so that he can exhale.

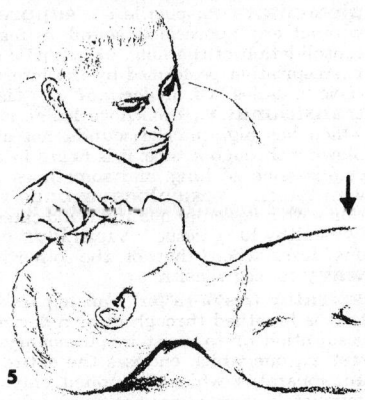

5

Repeat this sequence of maneuvers every 3 to 4 seconds until other means of ventilation are available.

If you cannot open his mouth blow through his nose. In infants cover both mouth and nose with your mouth. Blow gently into a child's mouth, and in infants use only small puffs from your cheeks.

The patient is placed in a supine position on a rigid support so that there is no give under the patient as pressure is applied. The individual applying the pressure stands or kneels at right angles to the patient. He places the heel of one hand with the heel of the other on top of it on the sternum, just cephalad to the xiphoid process.

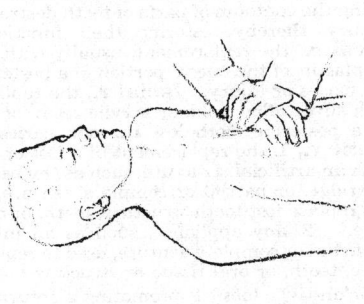

Firm pressure is applied vertically downward about 60 times a minute. At the end of each pressure stroke the hands are relaxed to permit full expansion of the chest. The position of the operator should be such that he can use his body weight while applying the pressure. Sufficient pressure should be exerted to move the sternum 3 or 4 cm. toward the vertebral column.

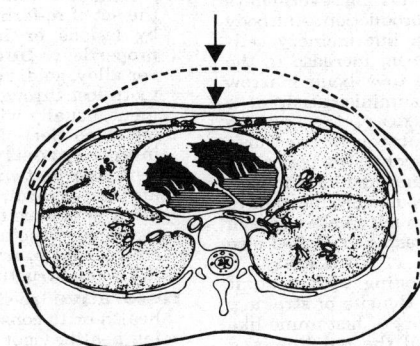

Children up to 10 years of age require the force of only one hand.

Only moderate pressure by the finger tips on the middle third of the sternum should be used on infants.

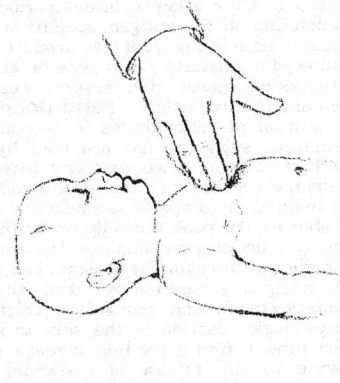

PLATE 41 — TECHNIQUE OF RESUSCITATION BY CLOSED CARDIAC MASSAGE

amphoric tone. **slow r.,** that in which there are less than twelve respirations in each minute. **stertorous r.,** that which is accompanied by abnormal snoring sounds. **supplementary r.,** puerile r. **suppressed r.,** respiration without any appreciable sound, as may occur in extensive consolidation of the lung, or pleuritic effusion. **thoracic r.,** respiration performed by the intercostal and other thoracic muscles. Cf. *abdominal r.* **tissue r.,** internal r. **transitional r.,** bronchovesicular r. **tubular r.,** that which has high-pitched sounds, not unlike those made by blowing through a tube; it is heard in consolidation of lung, compression of lung, and sometimes over lung infiltrated with tumor. **vesiculocavernous r.,** cavernous respiration with a vesicular quality; it indicates a cavity surrounded by healthy lung tissue. **vicarious r.,** increased action in one lung when that of the other lung is diminished. **wavy r.,** cogwheel r.

respirator (res'pĭ-ra″tor) an apparatus to qualify the air that is breathed through it, or a device for giving artificial respiration or to assist in pulmonary ventilation. **cabinet r.,** one which encloses the entire body. **cuirass r.,** an apparatus which is applied only to the chest, either completely surrounding the trunk or applied only to the front of the chest and abdomen. **Drinker r.,** an apparatus for producing artificial respiration over long periods of time, consisting of a metal tank, enclosing the body of the patient, with his head outside, and within which artificial respiration is maintained by alternating negative and positive pressure. Popularly called *iron lung.* **Engström r.,** a volume-controlled, piston-operated respirator with a sine wave airflow pattern.

respiratory (re-spi'rah-to″re) [re- + L. *spirare* to breathe] pertaining to respiration.

respiratory system see under *system.*

respirometer (res″pĭ-rom'ĕ-ter) an instrument for determining the character of the respiratory movements.

response (re-spons') [L. *respondere* to answer, reply] an action or movement due to the application of a stimulus. **anamnestic r.,** the manifestation of immunologic memory; the larger, more rapid immune response that occurs on the second exposure to an antigen. See *secondary immune r.* **autoimmune r.,** an immune response against an autoantigen. **booster r.,** anamnestic r. **conditioned r.,** a response evoked by a conditioned stimulus; one occurring to a stimulus that was incapable of evoking it before conditioning. **galvanic skin r.,** the alteration in electrical resistance of the skin associated with sympathetic nerve discharge. **immune r.,** any response of the immune system to an antigenic stimulus, including antibody production, cell-mediated immunity, and immunological tolerance. The responses causing tissue injury have been divided into four types: *type I,* immediate hypersensitivity; *type II,* cytotoxicity, mediated by antibody and complement; *type III,* serum sickness and immune complex diseases, and *type IV,* delayed hypersensitivity, or cell-mediated immunity; see *Gell and Coombs classification,* under *classification.* **primary immune r.,** the immune response occurring on the first exposure to an antigen. After a lag or latent period of from 3 to 14 days depending on the antigen, specific antibodies appear in the blood. There is a peak of IgM production lasting several days followed immediately by a peak of IgG production. Antibody production ceases after several weeks, but memory cells remain in circulation. **reticulocyte r.,** increase in the formation of reticulocytes in response to a bone marrow stimulus, such as that provided by administration of a hematinic agent. **secondary immune r.,** the immune response occurring on the second and subsequent exposures to an antigen; compared to a primary response, the lag period is shorter, the peak antibody titer is higher and lasts longer, IgG production predominates, the antibodies produced have a higher affinity for the antigen, and a much smaller dose of the antigen is required to initiate the response. Called also *anamnestic h.* and *booster r.* **triple r. (of Lewis),** a physiologic reaction of the skin to stroking with a blunt instrument: first a red line develops at the site of stroking, owing to the release of histamine or a histamine-like substance, then a flare develops around the red line, and lastly a wheal is formed as a result of local edema. **unconditioned r.,** a response elicited by an unconditioned stimulus; an unlearned response, i.e., one that occurs naturally.

rest (rest) 1. repose after exertion. 2. a fragment of embryonic tissue that has been retained within the adult organism; called also *embryonic, epithelial,* and *fetal r.* 3. that part of a removable partial denture that rests on the abutment tooth, and thus prevents movement of the denture and helps in providing occlusal support. **aberrant r.,** choristoma. **adrenal r.,** accessory adrenal tissue, sometimes found in the ovary or testis or in the vascular hila thereof. **bed r.,** confinement of a patient to bed. **carbon r.,** the amount of carbon in the deproteinized blood. **embryonic r., epithelial r., fetal r.,** see *rest,* def. 2. **incisal r.,** a metallic part or extension of a removable partial denture that rests on the prepared incisal edge of an anterior abutment tooth. **lingual r.,** a metallic part or extension of a removable partial denture that rests on the prepared lingual surface of an anterior abutment tooth and thus provides support or indirect retention. Called also *cingulum r.* **Malassez r.,** the remaining cells of the root sheath in the periodontal ligament, which persist and sometimes form an epithelial network and occasionally develop into a dental cyst. **occlusal r.,** a rest placed on the occlusal surface of a posterior tooth for transmitting occlusal stresses parallel to its long axis and holding the clasp in its predetermined position; a component of removable partial dentures. Called also *occlusal stop.* **precision r.,** a prefabricated, rigid, metallic extension of a fixed or removable partial denture, consisting of two closely fitted interlocking parts, the insert of which fits into a box-type rest or keyway (female) portion of the attachment in the cast restoration of a tooth. **recessed r.,** a rigid extension of a partial denture which contacts a definite seat prepared in the surface of a tooth. **semiprecision r.,** a denture rest, sometimes supplemented by a spring-loaded plunger or clip, which fits into a seat in an abutment tooth that has been specially deepened to provide added retention. See also under *attachment.* **suprarenal r.,** adrenal r. **surface r.,** a rigid extension of a partial denture which contacts the unaltered extracoronal surface of a tooth. **Walthard's cell r's,** see under *islet.*

restbite (rest'bīt) the relation of the teeth when the jaw is at rest.

restenosis (re″stĕ-no'sis) recurrent stenosis, especially of a valve of the heart, after surgical correction of the primary condition. **false r.,** stenosis recurring after failure to divide either commissure of the cardiac valve beyond the area of incision of the papillary muscles. **true r.,** restenosis occurring after complete opening of one or both of the commissures of the cardiac valve involved.

restiform (res'tĭ-form) [L. *restis* rope + *forma* form] shaped like a rope.

restitutio (res″tĭ-tu'she-o) [L.] restitution. **r. in'tegrum,** complete return to health.

restitution (res″tĭ-tu'shun) [L. *restitutio*] 1. an active process of restoration. 2. the spontaneous realignment of the fetal head with the fetal body, after delivery of the head.

restoration (res″to-ra'shun) [L. *restaurare* to review, rebuild] 1. the act of renewing, rebuilding, or reconstructing. 2. the return to a previous state or condition, as of health. 3. the process of replacing by artificial means a missing, damaged, or diseased tooth or teeth or any part thereof. See also *prosthetic r.* and *restorative dentistry,* under *dentistry.* 4. the act of re-forming the contours of parts of teeth destroyed by lesions or injury, thereby restoring their functional properties. **buccal r.,** the replacement, usually with silver alloy, gold, or plastic, of the buccal portion of a posterior tooth lost through caries or injury. **facial r.,** the replacement, usually with silver alloy, gold, or acrylic resin, of the facial portion of a posterior tooth lost through caries or injury. **prosthetic r.,** 1. the replacement of a lost or absent body part with an artificial structure, such as the use of an inlay, crown, bridge, or partial or complete denture, or other appliance to replace lost tooth structure, teeth, or oral tissue or structure. 2. any appliance, such as an inlay, crown, bridge, or partial or complete denture, used to replace lost tooth structure, teeth, or oral tissue or structure.

restorative (re-stōr'ah-tiv) *(obs.)* 1. promoting a return to health or to consciousness. 2. a remedy that aids in restoring health, vigor, or consciousness; called also *anastatic.*

restraint (re-strānt') the forcible confinement of a violently psychotic or irrational person.

restriction (re-strik'shun) anything that limits; also, a limitation. **MHC r.,** the phenomenon of certain cell-cell interactions in the immune response occurring only between MHC haploidentical cells. Helper T cells are activated by antigen only when the antigen is "seen" in conjunction with self class II MHC antigens (Ia antigens in mice, HLA-DR antigens in humans) as is the case when antigen is presented by macrophages. Cytotoxic T cells are activated by and kill only cells displaying foreign antigens (e.g., viral antigens or tumor antigens) plus self class I MHC antigens (K or D antigens in mice, HLA-A, -B, or -C antigens in humans).

resublimed (re″sub-līmd′) subjected to repeated processes of sublimation.

resultant (re-zul′tant) any of the products of a chemical reaction.

resupination (re″su-pĭ-na′shun) [L. *resupinare* to turn on the back] 1. the act of turning upon the back or dorsum. 2. the position of one lying upon the back.

resuscitation (re-sus″ĭ-ta′shun) [L. *resuscitare* to revive] the restoration to life or consciousness of one apparently dead; it includes such measures as artificial respiration and cardiac massage. **cardiopulmonary r. (CPR),** the artificial substitution of heart and lung action as indicated for cardiac arrest or apparent sudden death resulting from electric shock, drowning, respiratory arrest, and other causes. The two major components of CPR are artificial ventilation and closed chest cardiac massage; see illustration accompanying *respiration.* **r. of the heart,** restoration of spontaneous cardiac contractions. See illustration accompanying *respiration.*

resuscitator (re-sus′ĭ-ta″tor) an apparatus for initiating respiration in cases of asphyxia. **cardiopulmonary r.,** an apparatus that simultaneously assists the patient's breathing and applies external cardiac massage.

resuture (re-soo′tūr) secondary suture.

retainer (re-ta′ner) 1. a device for retaining or keeping something in position. 2. the part of a denture that unites the abutment tooth with the suspended portion of the bridge, such as an inlay, partial crown, or complete crown. 3. an orthodontic device for maintaining in position the teeth and jaws. 4. any form of clasp, attachment, or other device used for the fixation or stabilization of a prosthetic appliance. 5. the portion of a fixed prosthesis attaching a pontic to the abutment teeth. **continuous bar r.,** continuous clasp. **direct r.,** a clasp or attachment applied to an abutment tooth, by which a removable partial denture is maintained in position. **Hawley r.,** an orthodontic appliance consisting of a removable palatal wire and an acrylic biteplate resting against the palate, used to stabilize teeth after their movement or as a basis for tooth movement by providing anchorage for other attachments. Called also *Hawley appliance.* **indirect r.,** a part of a removable partial denture that assists the direct retainers in preventing displacement of distal-extension denture bases by functioning through lever action on the opposite side of the fulcrum line. **matrix r.,** a mechanical device designed to engage the ends of a matrix band or strip and to tighten the matrix around the tooth. **space r.,** an orthodontic appliance that retains the space created by premature loss of a tooth or the space to be filled by an erupting tooth. See also under *maintainer* and *regainer.*

retamine (ret′ah-min) an alkaloid, $C_{15}H_{26}N_2O$, from the young branches and bark of *Genista sphaerocarpa* Lam. (Leguminosae).

retardate (re-tar′dāt) a mentally retarded person.

retardation (re″tar-da′shun) [L. *retardare* to slow down, impede] delay; hindrance; delayed development. **mental r.,** [DSM III-R], a mental disorder characterized by significantly subaverage general intellectual functioning associated with impairments in adaptive behavior and manifested during the developmental period; classified as *mild* (IQ 50–70)—can develop social and communication skills during the preschool period, have minimal sensorimotor impairment, can by their late teens learn academic skills up to the sixth grade level, and usually achieve social and vocational skills adequate for minimal self-support; *moderate* (IQ 35–50)—can talk or learn to communicate but have poor social awareness and only fair motor development, are unlikely to progress to the second grade level in academic skills but can profit from vocational training, and can take care of themselves under supervision; *severe* (IQ 20–35)—have poor motor development and minimal speech in the preschool period, may learn to talk by their late teens and

can be trained in elementary hygiene skills, and as adults may learn to perform simple work under close supervision; *profound* (IQ below 20)—have limited sensorimotor development, may achieve very limited self-care, and require a highly structured environment and constant supervision. *Borderline* mental retardation (IQ 70–85), now called borderline intellectual functioning, is used to refer to very mild forms with only slight impairments in adaptive behavior. Called also *mental deficiency* or *subnormality.* **psychomotor r.,** generalized slowing of mental and physical activity; seen in depression.

retching (rech′ing) a strong involuntary effort to vomit.

rete (re′to), pl. *re′tia* [L. "net"] a net or meshwork; used in anatomical nomenclature as a general term to designate a network, especially of arteries or veins. **acromial r., r. acromia′le** [NA], a network formed by ramification of the acromial branch of the thoracoacromial artery on the acromion process. **r. arterio′sum** [NA], an anastomotic network formed by arteries just before they become arterioles or capillaries. **articular r.,** r. vasculosum articulare. **articular cubital r., articular r. of elbow,** r. articulare cubiti. **articular r. of knee,** r. articulare genus. **r. articula′re cu′biti** [NA], articular rete of elbow: an arterial network formed on the posterior aspect of the elbow by the posterior ulnar recurrent, inferior and superior ulnar collateral, and interosseous recurrent arteries. **r. articula′re ge′nu,** r. articulare genus. **r. articula′re ge′nus** [NA], articular rete of knee: an extensive arterial rete on the capsule of the knee joint, supplying branches to the contiguous bones and joints. It is formed by the genicular arteries, the termination of the deep femoral artery, the descending branch of the lateral circumflex artery, and the tibial recurrent artery. **calcaneal r., r. calca′neum** [NA], an arterial rete on the posterior and lower surfaces of the calcaneus, receiving branches from the calcaneal branches of the fibular artery and the lateral malleolar branches of the fibular artery. **r. cana′lis hypoglos′si,** plexus venosus canalis hypoglossi. **carpal r., dorsal,** r. carpale dorsale. **r. carpa′le dorsa′le** [NA], **r. car′pi dorsa′le,** dorsal carpal rete: an arterial rete formed by the dorsal radial carpal and dorsal ulnar carpal arteries and giving off the second, third, and fourth dorsal metacarpal arteries to the dorsum of the hand and the second, third, and fourth fingers. **r. cuta′neum,** the network of arteries at the boundary between the corium and the tela subcutanea. **dorsal venous r. of foot,** r. venosum dorsale pedis. **dorsal venous r. of hand,** r. venosum dorsale manus. **r. dorsa′le pe′dis,** an arterial rete on the dorsum of the foot. **r. foram′inis ova′lis,** plexus venosus foraminis ovalis. **r. of Haller, r. Halle′ri,** r. testis. **r. lymphocapilla′re** [NA], any of the closed, freely communicating networks formed by the lymphocapillary vessels. **malleolar r., lateral,** r. malleolare laterale. **malleolar r., medial,** r. malleolare mediale. **r. malleola′re latera′le** [NA], lateral malleolar rete: a small arterial rete on the lateral malleolus, formed by the lateral anterior malleolar artery, the perforating branch of the peroneal artery, and the lateral tarsal artery. **r. malleola′re media′le** [NA], medial malleolar rete: a small arterial rete on the medial malleolus, formed by the medial anterior malleolar artery and branches from the posterior tibial artery. **malpighian r.,** stratum germinativum. **r. mira′bile,** 1. [NA] a vascular network formed by division of an artery or a vein into a large number of smaller vessels that subsequently reunite into a single vessel; in the human this occurs only in the arterioles that supply the glomeruli of the kidney. 2. arterial anastomosis of the brain occurring between the external and internal carotid arteries as a result of longstanding thrombosis of the internal carotid arteries. **r. na′si,** a venous plexus in the inferior nasal concha. **r. olec′rani,** r. articulare cubiti. **r. ova′rii,** a homologue of the rete testis, developed in the early female fetus, but vestigial in the adult. **r. of patella, r. patel′lae** [NA], a network of arterial branches surrounding the patella, and derived from the various arteries of the knee. Called also *r. patellare.* **r. patella′re,** r. patellae. **plantar r., plantar venous r.,** r. venosum plantare. **r. subpapilla′re,** the network of arteries at the boundary between the papillary and reticular layers of the corium. **r. test′is** [NA], **r. test′is [Halle′ri],** a network of channels, formed by the straight seminiferous tubules, traversing the mediastinum testis and drain-

ing into the efferent ductules; called also *rete of Haller.*
r. vasculo′sum articula′re [NA], a anastomotic network of blood vessels in or around a joint; called also *articular r.*
r. veno′sum [NA], venous network: an anastomotic network of small veins. **r. veno′sum dorsa′le ma′nus** [NA], dorsal venous rete of hand: a venous network on the back of the hand, formed by the dorsal metacarpal veins. **r. veno′sum dor′sale pe′dis** [NA], dorsal venous rete of foot: a superficial network of anastomosing veins on the dorsum of the foot proximal to the transverse venous arch, draining into the great and the small saphenous veins. **r. veno′sum planta′re** [NA], plantar venous rete: a thick venous rete in the subcutaneous tissue of the sole of the foot. **re′tia veno′sa vertebra′rum,** networks of veins inside the vertebral canal.

retention (re-ten′shun) [L. *rententio,* from *retentare* to hold firmly back] 1. the act or process of keeping in possession, or of holding in place or position. 2. the persistent keeping within the body of matters normally excreted. 3. in cavity preparation, the prevention of displacement of a restoration. 4. in orthodontic therapy, the period during which the patient is wearing an appliance(s) to maintain and stabilize the teeth in the position into which they were moved. **denture r.,** the holding in proper position in the mouth of a removable denture. See *direct r.* and *indirect r.* **direct r.,** denture retention through the use of attachments or clasps that resist removal from the abutment teeth. See under *retainer.* **indirect r.,** retention in the mouth of a removable partial denture by means of an indirect retainer. **surgical r.,** retention in the mouth of a dental prosthesis by means of attachments embedded in the oral tissues. **r. of urine,** accumulation of urine within the bladder because of inability to urinate.

retethelioma (re″te-the-le-o′mah) malignant lymphoma.

retia (re′te-ah) [L.] plural of *rete.*

retial (re′te-al) pertaining to or of the nature of a rete.

reticula (rĕ-tik′u-lah) [L.] plural of *reticulum.*

reticular (rĕ-tik′u-lar) [L. *reticularis*] pertaining to or resembling a net.

reticulated (rĕ-tik′u-lāt″ed) reticular.

reticulation (rĕ-tik″u-la′shun) [L. *reticulum* a net] in radiology, a network of wrinkles or corrugations in the emulsion of an x-ray film resulting from sharp temperature differences between processing solutions. **dust r.,** an early stage of pneumoconiosis, seen especially in coal miners, which may go on to an anthracosilicosis.

reticulin (rĕ-tik′u-lin) a scleroprotein from the connective fibers of reticular tissue. **r. M,** an internal secretion produced by the reticuloendothelial system.

reticulitis (rĕ-tik″u-li′tis) [*reticul-* + *-itis*] inflammation of the reticulum of a ruminant animal.

reticul(o)- [L. *reticulum* dim. of *rete* net] 1. a combining form denoting a relationship to a reticulum or to a reticular structure.

reticulocyte (rĕ-tik′u-lo-sīt″) [*reticulo-* + *-cyte*] a young red blood cell showing a basophilic reticulum under vital staining.

reticulocytogenic (rĕ-tik″u-lo-si″to-jen′ik) causing the formation of reticulocytes.

reticulocytopenia (rĕ-tik″u-lo-si″to-pe′ne-ah) [*reticulocyte* + Gr. *penia* poverty] a decrease in the number of reticulocytes of the blood.

reticulocytosis (rĕ-tik″u-lo-si-to′sis) [*reticulocyte* + *-osis*] an increase in the number of reticulocytes in the peripheral blood.

reticuloendothelial (rĕ-tik″u-lo-en″do-the′le-al) pertaining to tissues having both reticular and endothelial attributes; see under *system.*

reticuloendothelioma (rĕ-tik″u-lo-en″do-the-le-o′mah) [*reticuloendothelium* + *-oma*] malignant lymphoma.

reticuloendotheliosis (rĕ-tik″u-lo-en″do-the-le-o′sis) [*reticuloendothelium* + *-osis*] hyperplasia of reticuloendothelial tissue. **leukemic r.,** hairy-cell leukemia.

reticuloendothelium (rĕ-tik″u-lo-en″do-the′le-um) the tissue of the reticuloendothelial system.

reticulohistiocytary (re-tik″u-lo-his″te-o-si′ter-e) pertaining to or composed of histiocytes of the reticuloendothelial system.

reticulohistiocytoma (re-tik″u-lo-his″te-o-si-to′mah) [*reticulo-* + *histiocytoma*] 1. a granulomatous proliferation of lipid-laden histiocytes and multinucleated giant cells with pale eosinophilic cytoplasm having a ground-glass appearance. Called also *reticulohistiocytic granuloma.* 2. multicentric reticulohistiocytosis.

reticulohistiocytosis (re-tik″u-lo-his″te-o-si-to′sis) [*reticulo-* + *histiocytosis*] the formation of multiple reticulohistiocytomas. **multicentric r.,** a rare systemic disease, predominantly occurring in women, characterized by polyarthritis of the hands and large joints and the development of nodular reticulohistiocytomas in the skin, bone, and mucous and synovial membranes, and sometimes associated with the presence of soft, cystic ganglia-like swellings over the extensor and flexor surfaces of the wrists and with evidence of internal malignancy. The disease may become quiescent, with crippling arthropathy and disfigured skin as sequelae, or it may progress to polyvisceral involvement and eventual death. Called also *lipid* or *lipoid dermatoarthritis,* *reticulohistiocytic granuloma,* and *reticulohistiocytoma.* Cf. *reticulohistiocytic granuloma,* def. 2.

reticuloid (rĕ-tik′u-loid) 1. resembling reticulosis. 2. a condition resembling reticulosis. **actinic r.,** dermatosis aggravated by exposure to light, usually affecting the elderly, characterized by a chronic eczematous eruption predominantly on the exposed skin of the face, hands, and forearms, and extending to contiguous unexposed areas. Often there are episodes of almost universal erythroderma. In severe cases, edematous plaques produce gross furrowing and distortion of features. The eruption clears slowly on avoidance of light.

reticuloma (rĕ-tik″u-lo′mah) [*reticul-* + *-oma*] histiocytic malignant lymphoma.

reticulopenia (rĕ-tik″u-lo-pe′ne-ah) [*reticulo-* + *-penia*] reticulocytopenia.

reticuloperithelium (rĕ-tik″u-lo-per″ĭ-the′le-um) [*reticulo-* + *peri-* + Gr. *thēlē* papilla] retoperithelium.

reticulopituicyte (rĕ-tik″u-lo-pĭ-tu′ĭ-sīt) see *pituicyte.*

reticulopodia (rĕ-tik″u-lo-po′de-ah) plural of *reticulopodium.*

reticulopodium (rĕ-tik″u-lo-po′de-um) [*reticulo-* + Gr. *pous* foot] a filamentous pseudopodium with interconnected branches. Called also *rhizopodium.* Cf. *axopodium, filopodium,* and *lobopodium.*

reticulosis (rĕ-tik″u-lo′sis) [*reticul-* + *-osis*] an abnormal increase in cells derived from or related to reticuloendothelial cells. **familial hemophagocytic r.,** histiocytic medullary r. **familial histiocytic r.,** histiocytic medullary r. **histiocytic medullary r.,** a fatal hereditary disorder transmitted as an autosomal recessive trait, characterized by anemia, granulocytopenia, thrombocytopenia, intense phagocytosis of red blood cells, diffuse proliferation of histiocytes of various organs, and enlargement of the liver, spleen, and lymph nodes; called also *familial hemophagocytic r.* and *familial histiocytic r.* **lipomelanic r.,** dermatopathic lymphadenopathy. **pagetoid r.,** a solitary skin lesion of long duration and slow growth characterized histologically by large numbers of abnormal mononuclear cells infiltrating the epidermis with an underlying reactive mixed dermal infiltrate, which is considered by some authorities to represent an indolent, epidermotropic form of cutaneous T cell lymphoma, although some studies suggest that the characteristic cells are not T cells but are of the monocyte-macrophage series or are Merkel cells. Called also *Woringer-Kolopp disease* or *syndrome.*

reticulothelium (rĕ-tik″u-lo-the′le-um) the retothelium.

reticulum (rĕ-tik′u-lum), pl. *retic′ula* [L., dim. of *rete* net] 1. a network, especially a protoplasmic network in cells, as the flattened double membrane sheets of the endoplasmic reticulum. 2. reticular tissue. 3. the second division of the stomach of a ruminant animal. **agranular r.,** see *endoplasmic r.* **Chiari's r.,** Chiari's network. **Ebner's r.,** a network of cells in the seminiferous tubules. **endoplasmic r.,** an ultramicroscopic organelle of nearly all cells of higher plants and animals, consisting of a more or less continuous system of membrane-bound cavities that ramify throughout the cytoplasm of a cell. Two forms have been distinguished: *granular reticulum* (chromidial substance, ergastoplasm), which bears large numbers of ribosomes on the outer surface of its membrane and is basophilic, and *agranular reticulum,* which contains no ribosomes and has no distinctive staining properties. Called also *superior protoplasm*. **granular r.,** see *endoplasmic r.* **retic′ula lie′nis,** trabeculae splenicae. **sarcoplasmic r.,** a special form of agranular reticulum found in the sarcoplasm of striated muscle and comprising a system of smooth-surfaced tubules forming a plexus around each myofibril. **stellate r.,** the soft, middle part of the enamel organ of a developing tooth, the cells being separated by an increase in the gelatinous intercellular substance which forces the cells apart without breaking the intercellular connections, giving them a stellate appearance and providing protection later for the enamel-forming cells. **r. trabecula′re an′guli iridocornea′lis** [NA], a trabeculum of loose fibers found at the iridocorneal angle between the anterior chamber of the eye and the venous sinus of the sclera; the aqueous humor filters through the spaces between the fibers into the sinus and passes into the bloodstream. The reticulum is divided into a corneoscleral part and a uveal part. Called also *Hueck's ligament, ligamentum pectinatum iridis, ligamentum pectinatum anguli iridocornealis* [NA alternative], *pectinate ligament of iridocorneal angle,* and *pectinate ligament of iris.*

retiform (re′tĭ-form, ret′ĭ-form) [L. *rete* net + *forma* form] resembling a network.

retina (ret′ĭ-nah) [L.] [NA] the innermost of the three tunics of the eyeball, surrounding the vitreous body and continuous posteriorly with the optic nerve. It is divided into the *pars optica,* which rests upon the choroid, the *pars ciliaris,* which rests upon the ciliary body, and the *pars iridica,* which rests upon the posterior surface of the iris. Grossly, the retina is composed of an outer, pigmented layer (*pars pigmentosa*) and an inner, transparent layer (*pars nervosa*), which make up the *pars optica.* The latter comprises nine layers, named from within outward, as follows (see illustration): (1) the internal limiting membrane; (2) the nerve fiber layer; (3) the layer of ganglion cells; (4) the inner plexiform layer; (5) the inner nuclear layer; (6) the outer plexiform layer; (7) the outer nuclear layer; (8) the external limiting membrane; (9) the layer of rods and cones. The pigmented part overlies the optic part and continues forward over the inner surface of the ciliary body, constituting the *pars ciliaris retinae.* The various layers are connected transversely by fibers of connective tissue (*fibers of Müller*). The layer of rods and cones forms the percipient element of the retina (i.e., the element that responds to visual stimuli by a photochemical reaction) and is connected with the nerve fiber layer by nerve fibers which join to form the optic nerve. In the center of the posterior part of the retina is the *macula lutea,* the most sensitive portion of the retina; and in the center of the macula lutea is a depression, the *fovea centralis,* from which the rods are absent. About 0.25 cm. inside the fovea is the point of entrance of the optic nerve and its central artery (*central artery of the retina*). At this point the retina is incomplete and forms the blind spot. **coarctate r.,** a funnel-shaped con-

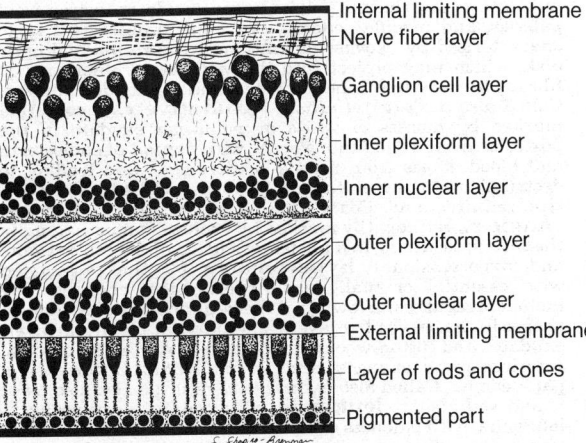

Internal limiting membrane
Nerve fiber layer
Ganglion cell layer
Inner plexiform layer
Inner nuclear layer
Outer plexiform layer
Outer nuclear layer
External limiting membrane
Layer of rods and cones
Pigmented part

Schematic representation of the optic part of the retina.

dition of the retina caused by a fluid exudation between the retina and the choroid. **detached r., detachment of**

r., separation of the inner layers of the retina (neural retina) from the pigment epithelium; called also *ablatio retinae* and *amotio retinae.* **shot-silk r.,** an opalescent effect, as of changeable silk, sometimes seen in the retinas of young persons. **tigroid r.,** see under *fundus.* **watered-silk r.,** shot-silk retina.

Retin-A (ret′in-a) trademark for preparations of tretinoin.

retinaculum (ret″ĭ-nak′u-lum), pl. *retinac′ula* [L. "a rope, cable"] 1. a structure which retains an organ or tissue in place; [NA] a general term for such a structure. 2. an instrument or device for retracting tissues during surgery. See *tenaculum.* **r. of arcuate ligament,** r. ligamenti arcuati. **r. cap′sulae articula′ris cox′ae,** one of the longitudinal folds of the cervical portion of the articular capsule of the hip. **caudal r., r. cauda′le** [NA], a fibrous band that extends from the tip of the coccyx to the adjacent skin and thus forms the foveola coccygea; called also *ligamentum caudale integumenti communis.* **r. cos′tae ul′timae,** ligamentum lumbocostale. **retinac′ula cu′tis** [NA], bands of connective tissue attaching the corium to the subcutaneous tissue. **extensor r. of foot, inferior,** r. musculorum extensorum pedis inferioris. **extensor r. of foot, superior,** r. musculorum extensorum pedis superius. **extensor r. of hand,** r. extensorum manus. **r. extenso′rum ma′nus** [NA], extensor retinaculum of hand: the distal part of the antebrachial fascia, overlying the extensor tendons; called also *ligamentum carpi dorsale.* **flexor r. of foot,** r. musculorum flexorum pedis. **flexor r. of hand,** r. flexorum manus. **r. flexo′rum ma′nus** [NA], flexor retinaculum of hand: a heavy fibrous band continuous with the distal part of the antebrachial fascia, completing the carpal canal through which pass the tendons of the flexor muscles of the hand and fingers; called also *ligamentum carpi transversum.* **r. ligamen′ti arcua′ti,** retinaculum of arcuate ligament: a band of converging fibers passing from the convex lower margin of the arcuate popliteal ligament to the head of the fibula. **r. musculo′rum extenso′rum pe′dis infe′rius** [NA], inferior extensor of foot: a thickened band of the fascia cruris passing from each malleolus across the front of the ankle joint, there crossing the other and passing onto the dorsum of the foot; called also *ligamentum cruciatum cruris.* **r. musculo′rum extenso′rum pe′dis supe′rius** [NA], superior extensor retinaculum of foot: the thickened lower portion of the fascia on the front of the leg, attached to the tibia on one side and the fibula on the other, and serving to hold in place the extensor tendons that pass beneath it; called also *ligamentum transversum cruris.* **r. musculo′rum fibula′rium infe′rius,** NA alternative for *r. musculorum peroneorum inferius.* **r. musculo′rum fibula′rium supe′rius,** NA alternative for *r. musculorum peroneorum superius.* **r. musculo′rum flexo′rum pe′dis** [NA], a strong band of fascia that extends from the medial malleolus down onto the calcaneus. It holds in place the tendons of the tibialis posterior, flexor digitorum, and flexor hallucis muscles as they pass to the sole of the foot, and gives protection to the posterior tibial vessels and tibial nerve. Called also *ligamentum laciniatum* and *flexor r. of foot.* **r. musculo′rum peronaeo′rum infe′rius,** r. musculorum peroneorum inferius. **r. musculo′rum peronaeo′rum supe′rius,** r. musculorum peroneorum superius. **r. musculo′rum peroneo′rum infe′rius** [NA], a fibrous band that arches over the tendons of the peroneal muscles and holds them in position on the lateral side of the calcaneus; called also *inferior peroneal r.* **r. musculo′rum peroneo′rum supe′rius** [NA], a fibrous band that arches over the peroneal tendons and helps to hold them in place below and behind the lateral malleolus; it extends from the malleolus downward and backward to the calcaneus. Called also *superior peroneal r.* **r. patel′lae latera′le** [NA], lateral patellar retinaculum: a fibrous membrane from the tendon of the vastus lateralis muscle, attached to the lateral margin of the patella and then along the side of the patellar ligament, and inserted into the tibia as far distal as the fibular collateral ligament; it also blends with the iliotibial tract of the fascia lata. Called also *lateral patellar ligament.* **r. patel′lae media′le** [NA], medial patellar retinaculum: a fibrous membrane from the tendon of the vastus medialis muscle, attached to the medial margin of the patella and then along the side of the patellar ligament, and inserted into the tibia as far distal as the tibial collateral ligament. **patellar r., lateral,** r. patellae laterale. **patellar r., medial,** r. patellae mediale. **peroneal r.,**

inferior, r. musculorum peroneorum inferius. **peroneal r., superior,** r. musculorum peroneorum superius. **r. ten′dinum,** a tendinous restraining structure, such as an annular ligament. **r. ten′dinum musculo′rum extenso′rum,** r. extensorum manus. **r. ten′dinum musculo′rum extenso′rum infe′rius,** r. musculorum extensorum pedis inferius. **r. ten′dinum musculo′rum extenso′rum supe′rius,** r. musculorum extensorum pedis superius. **r. ten′dinum musculo′rum flexo′rum,** r. flexorum manus. **retinac′ula un′guis** [NA], structures homologous to the retinacula cutis, attaching the nail to underlying tissue. **Weitbrecht′s r.,** retinacular fibers attached to the neck of the femur.

retinal (ret′ĭ-nal) 1. pertaining to the retina. 2. the aldehyde of retinol, derived by the oxidative enzymatic splitting of absorbed dietary carotene, and having vitamin A activity. In the retina, retinal combines with opsins to form visual pigments. One isomer, 11-*cis* retinal combines with opsin in the rods (scotopsin) to form rhodopsin, or visual purple. Another, all-*trans* retinal (*trans*-r.; visual yellow; xanthopsin), results from the bleaching of rhodopsin by light, in which the 11-*cis* form is converted to the all-*trans* form. Retinal also combines with opsins in the cones (photopsins) to form the three pigments responsible for color vision. Called also *retinal₁* and *retinene₁*.

retinal₁ (ret′ĭ-nal) retinal.

retinal₂ (ret′ĭ-nal) dehydroretinal.

retinal isomerase (ret′ĭ-nal i-som′er ās) [EC 5.2.1.3] an enzyme of the isomerase class that catalyzes the reaction all-*trans*-retinal = 11-*cis*-retinal. The reaction is important in the visual cycle.

retine (ret′ēn) a substance stated to be widely distributed in animal cells, which is characterized by its ability to retard cell division and growth. Cf. *promine*.

retinene (ret′ĭ-nēn) the aldehyde of vitamin A, occurring in two forms: *retinene₁* is the aldehyde of retinol (see *retinal*, def. 2), and *retinene₂* is the aldehyde of dehydroretinol.

retinitis (ret′ĭ-ni′tis) inflammation of the retina; used in the older ophthalmological literature to denote impairment of sight, perversion of vision, edema, and exudation into the retina, and occasionally by hemorrhages into the retina. **actinic r.,** retinitis due to exposure to actinic light rays. **r. albuminu′rica,** that which is associated with kidney disease. Cf. *arteriosclerotic retinopathy* and *hypertensive retinopathy*. **apoplectic r.,** that which is characterized by extravasations of blood within the retina. **azotemic r.,** retinitis due to nitrogenous waste products in renal disease. **central angiospastic r.,** central serous retinopathy. **r. circina′ta, circinate r.,** circinate retinopathy. **Coats′ r.,** exudative retinopathy. **diabetic r.,** see under *retinopathy*. **disciform r.,** disciform macular degeneration. **exudative r.,** see under *retinopathy*. **gravidic r.,** inflammation of the retina occurring along with the albuminuria of pregnancy. **hypertensive r.,** see under *retinopathy*. **Jacobson′s r.,** syphilitic r. **Jensen′s r.,** retinochoroiditis juxtapapillaris. **leukemic r.,** see under *retinopathy*. **metastatic r.,** retinitis caused by the location of septic emboli in the retinal vessels. **nephritic r.,** renal retinopathy. **r. pigmento′sa,** a group of diseases, frequently hereditary, marked by progressive loss of retinal response (as elicited by the electroretinogram), retinal atrophy, attenuation of the retinal vessels, and clumping of the pigment, with contraction of the field of vision. It may be transmitted as a dominant, recessive, or X-linked trait and is sometimes associated with other genetic defects. **r. pigmento′sa si′ne pigmen′to,** retinitis pigmentosa without clumping of pigment. **r. prolif′erans, proliferating r.,** a condition sometimes resulting from intraocular hemorrhage, with neovascularization and the formation of fibrous tissue bands extending into the vitreous from the surface of the retina; retinal detachment is sometimes a sequel. **r. puncta′ta albes′cens,** a type of retinal disorder in which there is a diffusion of white spots on the retina. **renal r.,** see under *retinopathy*. **r. sclopeta′ria,** a severe traumatic retinal lesion, as from the impact of a bullet. **serous r.,** simple inflammation of the superficial layers of the retina; called also *simple r.* **solar r.,** retinitis due to excessive exposure to sunlight. **r. stella′ta,** stellate retinopathy. **striate r.,** a form marked by the presence of gray or yellowish streaks just behind the retinal vessels. **suppurative r.,** retinitis due to pyemic infection. **syphi-**

litic r., r. syphilit′ica, retinitis complicating syphilitic iritis. **uremic r.,** retinitis occurring in uremia.

retinoblastoma (ret′′ĭ-no-blas-to′mah) [retina + blastoma] a malignant congenital hereditary blastoma composed of tumor cells arising from the retinoblasts, appearing in one or both eyes in children under 5 years of age, and usually diagnosed initially by a bright white or yellow pupillary reflex (leukokoria).

retinochoroid (ret′′ĭ-no-ko′roid) pertaining to the retina and the choroid.

retinochoroiditis (ret′′ĭ-no-ko-roi-di′tis) chorioretinitis. **r. juxtapapilla′ris,** a condition seen in young healthy subjects marked by a small inflammatory area on the fundus close to the papilla; called also *Jensen′s retinitis* or *retinochoroiditis*. **toxoplasmic r.,** see under *chorioretinitis*.

retinodialysis (ret′′ĭ-no-di-al′ĭ-sis) [retina + dialysis] disinsertion of the retina; detachment of the retina at its peripheral insertion.

retinograph (ret′ĭ-no-graf) a photograph of the retina.

retinography (ret′′ĭ-nog′rah-fe) photography of the retina.

retinoic acid (ret′in-o′ik) tretinoin.

retinoid (ret′ĭ-noid) 1. resembling the retina. 2. any derivative of retinal, whether naturally occurring or synthetic. 3. [Gr. *rhētīnē* resin + *eidos* form] resembling a resin.

retinol (ret′ĭ-nol) vitamin A₁, the form of vitamin A found in mammals; it is a 20-carbon alcohol, C₂₀H₃₀O, that is reversibly dehydrogenated by enzymatic action into its aldehyde (q.v.). Called also *retinol₁*.

retinol₁ (ret′ĭ-nol) retinol.

retinol₂ (ret′ĭ-nol) dehydroretinol.

retinomalacia (ret′′ĭ-no-mah-la′she-ah) [retina + malacia] softening of the retina.

retinopapillitis (ret′′ĭ-no-pap′′ĭ-li′tis) inflammation of the retina and the optic papilla.

retinopathy (ret′′ĭ-nop′ah-the) [retina + -pathy] 1. retinitis. 2. retinosis. **arteriosclerotic r.,** sclerosis of retinal arterioles marked by increased tortuosity, attenuation, copper-wire appearance, perivascular sheathing, nipping at arteriovenous crossings, small, scattered hemorrhaging, and small, white, well defined exudates with no surrounding edema. **central angiospastic r.,** central serous r. **central disk-shaped r.,** disciform macular degeneration. **central serous r.,** a usually self-limiting condition marked by acute localized detachment of the neural retina or retinal pigment epithelium in the region of the macula, with hypermetropia; called also *central angiospastic retinitis* and *retinopathy*. **circinate r.,** a condition marked by a circle of white spots enclosing the macular area, leading to complete foveal blindness; called also *retinitis circinata* or *circinate retinitis*. **diabetic r.,** retinopathy associated with diabetes mellitus, which may be of the background type, progressively characterized by microaneurysms, intraretinal punctate hemorrhages, yellow, waxy exudates, cotton-wool patches, and macular edema, or of the proliferative type, characterized by neovascularization of the retina and optic disk, which may project into the vitreous, proliferation of fibrous tissue, vitreous hemorrhage, and retinal detachment. Called also *diabetic retinitis*. **exudative r.,** a condition marked by masses of white or yellowish exudate in the posterior part of the fundus oculi, with deposit of cholesterin and blood debris from retinal hemorrhage, and leading to destruction of the macula and blindness. Called also *exudative retinitis*, and *Coats′ disease* or *retinitis*. **hemorrhagic r.,** retinopathy marked by profuse hemorrhaging in the retina, occurring in diabetes, occlusion of the central vein, and hypertension. **hypertensive r.,** that associated with essential or malignant hypertension; changes may include irregular narrowing of the retinal arterioles, hemorrhages in the nerve fiber layers and the outer plexiform layer, exudates and cotton-wool patches, a lipid star in the macula, arteriosclerotic changes, and, in malignant hypertension, papilledema. Called also *hypertensive retinitis*. See also *renal r.* and *stellate r.* **leukemic r.,** a condition occurring in leukemia, with paleness of the fundus resulting from infiltration of the retina and choroid with leukocytes, and swelling of the disk with blurring of its margin. **r. of prematurity,** retrolental fibroplasia. **pigmentary r.,** see *retinitis pigmentosa*. **proliferative r.,** the proliferative type of diabetic retinopathy (q.v.). **Purtscher′s angio-**

pathic r., Purtscher's disease. **renal r.,** a retinopathy associated with renal and hypertensive disorders, and presenting the same symptoms as hypertensive retinopathy; called also *renal retinitis.* See also *stellate r.* **stellate r.,** a retinopathy not associated with hypertensive, renal, or arteriosclerotic disorders, but presenting the same symptoms as hypertensive retinopathy; called also *stellate retinitis.* See also *renal r.*

retinoschisis (ret″ĭ-nos′kĭ-sis) [*retina* + Gr. *schisis* division] splitting of the retina: in the *juvenile form* the splitting occurs in the nerve fiber layer, and in the *adult form* in the external plexiform layer. The disorder is usually more benign and slowly progressive than retinal detachment.

retinoscope (ret′ĭ-no-skōp″) an instrument for performing retinoscopy; called also *skiascope.*

retinoscopy (ret″ĭ-nos′ko-pe) [*retina* + *-scopy*] an objective method for investigating, diagnosing, and evaluating refractive errors of the eye, by projection of a beam of light into the eye and observation of the movement of the illuminated area on the retina surface and of the refraction by the eye of the emergent rays. Called also *pupilloscopy, skiascopy, skiametry, shadow test,* and *umbrascopy.*

retinosis (ret″ĭ-no′sis) [*retina* + *-osis*] a general term for degenerative, noninflammatory conditions of the retina.

retinotopic (ret″ĭ-no-top′ik) relating to the organization of the visual pathways and visual area of the brain.

retinotoxic (ret″ĭ-no-tok′sik) exerting a toxic or deleterious effect upon the retina.

retisolution (ret″ĭ-so-lu′shun) [L. *rete* net + *solution*] dissolution of the Golgi apparatus.

retispersion (ret″ĭ-sper′shun) [L. *rete* net + *spargere* to throw about] migration of the Golgi apparatus from its normal position to the periphery of the cell.

retoperithelium (re″to-per″ĭ-the′le-um) [L. *rete* net + Gr. *peri* around + *thēlē* papilla] the layer of cells covering a reticular framework.

retort (re-tort′) [L. *retorta* bent back] a long-necked globular vessel formerly used in distillation.

Retortamonadida (re-tor″tah-mo-nad′ĭ-dah) an order of parasitic intestinal flagellate protozoa (class Zoomastigophorea, subphylum Mastigophora), characterized by the presence of two to four flagella, one of which is turned posteriorly and associated with a ventral cytosomal region; Golgi apparatus and mitochondria are absent. Representative genera include *Chilomastix* and *Retortamonas.*

Retortamonas (re″tor-tam′o-nas) [L. *retortus* bent back + Gr. *monas* unit, from *monos* single] a genus of biflagellate nonpathogenic parasitic intestinal protozoa (order Retortamonadida, class Zoomastigophorea), found in various insects, amphibians, reptiles, and mammals, and characterized by the presence of two anterior flagella, one of which extends posteriorly and trails from the body.

retothel (re′to-thel) reticuloendothelial.

retothelial (re″to-the′le-al) pertaining to the retothelium; containing reticulum cells.

retothelium (re″to-the′le-um) [L. *rete* net + Gr. *thēlē* papilla] the layer of cells covering a reticular tissue.

retractile (re-trak′til) [L. *retractilis*] susceptible of being drawn back.

retraction (re-trak′shun) [L. *retrahere* to draw back] 1. the act of drawing back; the condition of being drawn back. 2. distal movement of teeth, usually accomplished with an orthodontic appliance. **clot r.,** the drawing away of a blood clot from the wall of a vessel; it is a function of blood platelets. **gingival r.,** the displacement of the marginal gingiva away from a tooth. **mandibular r.,** 1. drawing back or retracting the mandible, accomplished by contraction of the middle and posterior parts of the temporal muscles and the suprahyoid muscle. 2. the condition of the mandible in which it lies posterior to the orbital plane. Cf. *mandibular protraction.*

retractor (re-trak′tor) 1. an instrument for maintaining operative exposure by separating the edges of a wound and holding back underlying organs and tissues; many shapes, sizes, and styles are available. 2. any retractile muscle. **Emmet's r.,** a self-retaining vaginal speculum. **Moorehead's r.,** one for retracting the lips, cheeks, or margins of a surgical wound. It fits over the crown of the head and is

provided with metal buttons, to which shields (or retractors) of desired shapes or sizes may be attached.

retrad (re′trad) [L. *retro* backward] toward a posterior or dorsal part.

retrieval (re-tre′val) in psychology, the process of obtaining memory information from wherever it has been stored.

retr(o)- [L. *retro* backward] a prefix meaning backward, or located behind.

retroaction (ret″ro-ak′shun) action in a reversed direction; reaction.

retrobuccal (ret″ro-buk′al) pertaining to the back part of the mouth near the cheek.

retrobulbar (ret″ro-bul′bar) [*retro-* + L. *bulbus* bulb] 1. behind the pons. 2. behind the eyeball.

retrocalcaneobursitis (ret″ro-kal-ka″ne-o-bur-si′tis) achillobursitis.

retrocervical (ret″ro-ser′ve-kal) behind the cervix uteri.

retrocession (ret″ro-sesh′un) [L. *retrocessio*] a going backward; backward displacement; specifically a dropping backward of the entire uterus.

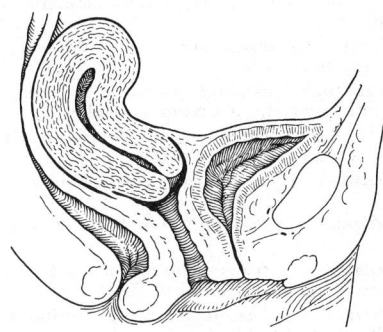

Retrocession of uterus.

retrocochlear (ret″ro-kok′le-ar) 1. behind the cochlea. 2. denoting the eighth cranial nerve and cerebellopontine angle as opposed to the cochlea.

retrocollic (ret″ro-kol′ik) pertaining to the back of the neck; nuchal.

retrocollis (ret″ro-kol′is) [*retro-* + L. *collum* neck] spasmodic wryneck in which the head is drawn directly backward.

retrocrural (re″tro-kru′ral) situated at the back of the leg, or crus.

retrocursive (re″tro-kur′siv) [*retro-* + L. *currere* to run] marked by stepping backward.

retrodeviation (re″tro-de″ve-a′shun) a general term inclusive of retroversion, retroflexion, retroposition, etc.

retrodisplacement (re″tro-dis-plās′ment) backward or posterior displacement.

retrofilling (ret″ro-fil′ing) a method of filling the root canal of a tooth from the apex of a root which has been surgically exposed; zinc-free silver alloy is the most commonly used filling material. Called also *reverse filling* and *root-end filling.*

retroflexed (ret′ro-flekst) [*retro-* + L. *flexus* bent] bent backward; in a state of retroflexion.

retroflexion (ret″ro-flek′shun) [L. *retroflexio*] the bending of an organ so that its top is turned backward; specifically, the bending backward of the body of the uterus toward the cervix, resulting in a sharp angle at the point of bending.

retrogasserian (ret″ro-gas-se′re-an) pertaining to the sensory (posterior) root of the trigeminal (gasserian) ganglion.

retrognathia (ret″ro-nath′e-ah) [*retro-* + Gr. *gnath-* + *-ia*] retrusion of the mandible.

retrognathic (ret″ro-nath′ik) pertaining to or characterized by retrognathia.

retrognathism (ret″ro-nath′ism) retrognathia.

retrograde (ret′ro-grād) [*retro-* + L. *gradi* to step] 1. moving backward or against the usual direction of flow. 2. degenerating, deteriorating, or catabolic.

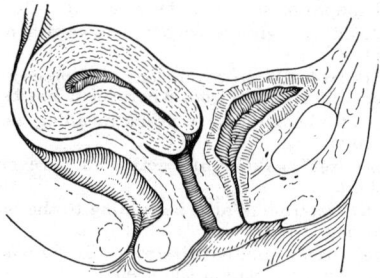

Retroflexion of uterus.

retrography (re-trog′rah-fe) [retro- + Gr. *graphein* to write] mirror writing.

retrogression (ret″ro-gresh′un) [retro- + L. *gressus* course] degeneration; deterioration; regression; return to an earlier, less complex condition.

retroinfection (re″tro-in-fek′shun) infection of the mother by the fetus.

retrojection (re″ro-jek′shun) [retro- + L. *jacere* to throw] irrigation of a cavity by injection of fluid.

retromorphosis (re″tro-mor-fo′sis) [retro- + Gr. *morphē* form] retrograde metamorphosis.

retroperitoneal (re″tro-per″ĭ-to-ne′al) behind the peritoneum.

retroperitoneum (re″tro-per″ĭ-to-ne′um) the retroperitoneal space.

retroperitonitis (re″tro-per″ĭ-to-ni′tis) inflammation in the retroperitoneal space.

retropharyngitis (re″tro-far″in-ji′tis) inflammation of the posterior part of the pharynx.

retropharynx (re″tro-far′inks) the posterior part of the pharynx.

retroplacental (re″tro-plah-sen′tal) behind the placenta.

retroplasia (ret″ro-pla′se-ah) [retro- + Gr. *plasis* formation + -ia] retrograde metaplasia; degeneration of a tissue or cell into a more primitive type.

retroposed (re′tro-pōzd) [retro- + L. *positus* placed] displaced backward or posteriorly.

retroposition (re″tro-po-zish′un) backward displacement.

retropulsion (re″tro-pul′shun) [retro- + L. *pellere* to drive] 1. a driving back, as of the fetal head in labor. 2. a tendency to walk backward, as in some cases of tabes dorsalis; opisthoporeia. 3. an abnormal gait in which the body is bent backward.

retrorsine (ret′ror-sin) a poisonous alkaloid, $C_{18}H_{25}O_6N$, from *Senecio retrorsus*, which may cause a fatal cirrhosis of the liver in horses and cattle that eat the plant.

retrosinus (ret″ro-si′nus) the air cells behind the sigmoid sinus in the mastoid process of the temporal bone.

retrospondylolisthesis (ret″ro-spon″dĭ-lo-lis-the′sis) posterior displacement of one vertebral body on the subjacent body.

retrostalsis (re″tro-stal′sis) reversed or backward peristaltic action.

retrosternal (re″tro-ster′nal) [retro- + *sternum*] situated or occurring behind the sternum.

retrosymphysial (re″tro-sim-fiz′e-al) behind the symphysis pubis.

retrouterine (re″tro-u′ter-in) [retro- + *uterus*] behind the uterus.

retroversioflexion (re″tro-ver″se-o-flek′shun) retroversion combined with retroflexion.

retroversion (ret″ro-ver′zhun) [L. *retroversio; retro* back + *versio* turning] the tipping of an entire organ backward. **r. of uterus,** the turning backward of the entire uterus in relation to the pelvic axis.

retroverted (ret″ro-vert′ed) in a condition of retroversion.

retrovesical (re″tro-ves′ĭ-kal) behind the urinary bladder.

retrovirus (re″tro-vi′rus, ret″ro-vi′rus) a large group of

RNA viruses that includes the leukoviruses and lentiviruses; so called because they carry reverse transcriptase.

retrusion (re-troo′zhun) [L. *re*-back + *trudere* to shove] 1. the state of being located posterior to the normal position, as malposition of a tooth posteriorly in the line of occlusion. 2. the backward movement or position of the mandible. 3. the act or process of pressing the teeth backward.

Rett syndrome (ret) [A. *Rett*, Austrian physician, 20th century] see under *syndrome*.

Retzius' fibers, space (cavity), veins (ret′ze-us) [Anders Adolf *Retzius*, Swedish anatomist, 1796–1860] see under *fiber* and *vein*, and see *spatium retropubicum*.

Retzius' foramen, lines (striae, stripes) (ret′ze-us) [Magnus Gustav *Retzius*, Swedish anatomist, 1842–1919] see *apertura lateralis ventriculi*, and see *incremental lines*, under *line*.

Reuss's color charts (tables) (rois′ez) [August Ritter von *Reuss*, Vienna ophthalmologist, 1841–1924] see under *chart*.

revaccination (re″vak-sĭ-na′shun) a second vaccination.

revascularization (re-vas″ku-lar-ĭ-za′shun) 1. the restoration of blood supply, as after a wound. 2. the restoration of an adequate blood supply to a part, as by means of a vascular graft or prosthesis.

revellent (re-vel′ent) [L. *re*- back + *vellere* to draw] causing revulsion; revulsive.

Reverdin's graft, needle (ra-ver-danz′) [Jacques Louis Reverdin, surgeon at Geneva, 1842–1929] see *epidermic graft*, under *graft*, and see under *needle*.

reversal (re-ver′sal) a turning or change in the opposite direction. **r. of gradient,** a changing of direction of the fecal stream due to an area of irritation causing local spasticity of the intestine with higher tonus than that of the proximal area.

reverse transcriptase RNA-directed DNA polymerase.

reversible (re-ver′sĭ-b′l) capable of going through a series of changes in either direction, forward or backward, as a reversible chemical reaction. **antigenic r.,** a change in the antigenic structure of adult cells to that of immature cells, as in certain tumors.

Revilliod's sign (ra-ve-yōz′) [Jean Léonard Adolphe Revilliod, Swiss physician, 1835–1918] see under *sign*.

revivescence (re″vi-ves′ens) [L. *revivescere* to revive] the renewal of vital activities.

revivification (re-viv″ĭ-fĭ-ka′shun) [L. *re*- again + *vivus* alive + *facere* to make] 1. restoration to life or consciousness. 2. refreshing of diseased surfaces to promote their union.

revolute (rev′o-lūt) turned back or curled back.

revulsant (re-vul′sant) [L. *revulsans*] revulsive.

revulsion (re-vul′shun) [L. *revulsio;* from *re*- back + *vellere* to draw] the drawing of blood from one part to another, as occurs in counterirritation.

revulsive (re-vul′siv) [L. *re*- back + *vellere* to draw] 1. effecting revulsion. 2. an agent causing revulsion; a counterirritant.

Reynals see *Duran-Reynals*.

Reynold's test (ren′oldz) [James Emerson *Reynold*, Scottish physician, 1844–1920] see under *tests*.

Rezipas (rez′ĭ-pas) trademark for a preparation of para-aminosalicylic acid.

RF rheumatoid factor.

Rf symbol for *rutherfordium*.

R.F.A. right frontoanterior (position of the fetus).

RFLP restriction fragment length polymorphism; see under *polymorphism*.

R.F.P. right frontoposterior (position of the fetus).

R.F.P.S.(Glasgow) Royal Faculty of Physicians and Surgeons of Glasgow.

R.F.T. right frontotransverse (position of the fetus).

R.G.N. Registered General Nurse (Scotland).

Rh 1. chemical symbol for *rhodium*. 2. symbol for *rhesus factor* (see under *factor*).

Rh$_{null}$ symbol for a rare blood type in which all Rh factors are lacking; see also under *syndrome*.

Rhabdiasoidea (rab″dĭ-ah-soi′de-ah) in some classifications, a superfamily of phasmids, including the genus *Strongyloides*.

rhabditic (rab-dit′ik)   pertaining or belonging to *Rhabditis*, or to the Rhabditoidea.

rhabditiform (rab-dit′ĭ-form)   rhabdoid.

Rhabditis (rab-di′tis) [Gr. *rhabdos* rod]   a genus of minute phasmid nematodes of the superfamily Rhabditoidea, living mostly in damp earth, and as an accidental parasite in man. *R. hominis* and *R. intestinalis* have been found in the stools. *R. niellyi* is found in the skin. *R. pellio* (*R. genitalis, Leptodera pellio*) is sometimes found in the genitourinary organs.

rhabditoid (rab′dĭ-toid)   rhabdoid.

Rhabditoidea (rab″dĭ-toi′de-ah)   a superfamily of phasmids, some members of which are free-living and others are parasites of plants and animals; it includes the genera *Rhabditis* and *Strongyloides*.

rhabdium (rab′de-um) [Gr. *rhabdion* a little rod]   a voluntary muscle fiber.

rhabd(o)- [Gr. *rhabdos* rod]   a combining form meaning rod-shaped or denoting relationship to a rod.

rhabdocyte (rab′do-sīt) [*rhabdo-* + *-cyte*]   (*obs.*) metamyelocyte.

rhabdoid (rab′doid) [Gr. *rhabdo-eides* like a rod, striped looking]   resembling a rod; rod-shaped.

Rhabdomonadina (rab″do-mo″nah-di′nah)   a suborder of colorless, plantlike, biflagellate protozoa (order Euglenida, class phytomastigophorea). *Rhabdomonas* is a representative genus.

Rhabdomonas (rab″do-mo′nas) [*rhabdo-* + Gr. *monas* unit, from *monos* single]   1. a genus of plantlike flagellate protozoa, suborder Rhabdomonadina, order Euglenida. 2. in former systems of classification, a genus of bacteria, species of which are now assigned to the genus *Chromatium*.

rhabdomyoblastoma (rab″do-mi″o-blas-to′mah) [*rhabdo-* + Gr. *mys* muscle + *blastos* germ + *-oma*]   rhabdomyosarcoma.

rhabdomyochondroma (rab″do-mi″o-kon-dro′mah)   benign mesenchymoma.

rhabdomyolysis (rab″do-mi-ol′ĭ-sis) [*rhabdo-* + Gr. *mys* muscle + *lysis* dissolution]   disintegration or dissolution of muscle, associated with excretion of myoglobin in the urine. **exertional r.,** that due to intense, prolonged physical exertion, with symptoms often resembling those elicited by exercise in persons with occlusive arterial disease.

rhabdomyoma (rab″do-mi-o′mah)   a benign tumor derived from striated muscle; called also *myoma striocellulare*.

rhabdomyomyxoma (rab″do-mi″o-mik-so′mah)   benign mesenchymoma.

rhabdomyosarcoma (rab″do-mi″o-sar-ko′mah)   a highly malignant tumor of striated muscle derived from primitive mesenchymal cells and exhibiting differentiation along rhabdomyoblastic lines, including but not limited to the presence of cells with recognizable cross striations. It occurs in three forms: the *pleomorphic* form affects predominantly the extremities of adults; the *alveolar* form, occurring mainly in adolescents and young adults, affects muscles of the extremities, trunk, orbital region, etc.; the *embryonal* form, occurring predominantly in infants and children, affects the head and neck, lower genitourinary tract, pelvis, and extremities.

Rhabdonema (rab″do-ne′mah)   *Rhabditis*.

rhabdos (rab′dos) [Gr. "rod"]   a straight cytopharyngeal apparatus with walls supported by nematodesmata and sometimes containing toxicysts; it is characteristic of the lower ciliate protozoa. Cf. *cyrtos*.

rhabdosarcoma (rab″do-sar-ko′mah)   rhabdomyosarcoma.

rhabdovirus (rab″do-vi′rus) [*rhabdo-* + *virus*]   any of a group of morphologically similar, bullet-shaped or bacilliform RNA viruses, including the viruses of vesicular stomatitis and rabies.

rhachi-   for words beginning thus, see those beginning *rachi-*.

rhacoma (ra-ko′mah) [Gr. *rhakōma* rags]   a pendulous scrotum.

rhaebocrania (re″bo-kra′ne-ah) [Gr. *rhaibos* crooked + *kranion* skull + *-ia*]   torticollis, or wryneck.

rhaeboscelia (re″bo-se′le-ah) [Gr. *rhaibos* crooked + *skelos*

leg + *-ia*]   genu varum (bowleg), or genu valgum (knock knee).

rhaebosis (re-bo′sis) [Gr. *rhaibos* crooked + *-osis*]   crookedness of the legs or of any normally straight part.

rhagades (rag′ah-dēz) [pl. of Gr. *rhagas* rent]   fissures, cracks, or fine linear scars in the skin, especially such lesions around the mouth or other regions subjected to frequent movement.

rhagadiform (ra-gad′ĭ-form) [Gr. *rhagas* rent + L. *forma* shape]   resembling rhagades.

rhagiocrine (raj′e-o-krīn) [Gr. *rhax* grape + *krinein* to separate]   denoting colloid vacuoles in the cytoplasm of gland cells that represent a stage in the development of secretory granules.

rhagionid (raj″e-on′id)   a fly of the family Rhagionidae.

Rhagionidae (raj″e-on′ĭ-de)   a family of biting flies, the snipe flies, of the order Diptera; the genera, *Spaniopsis, Suragina,* and *Symphoromyia,* contain species that are vicious biters.

rhamninose (ram′nĭ-nōs)   a trisaccharide which occurs in the glycosides rutin and xanthorhamnin.

rhamnose (ram′nōs)   6-deoxy-L-mannose, $C_6H_{12}O_5$.

rhamnoside (ram′no-sīd)   a glycoside which on hydrolysis yields rhamnose.

Rhamnus (ram′nus) [L.; Gr. *rhamnos* a kind of prickly shrub]   a genus of rhamnaceous trees and shrubs, often with a purgative bark and fruit. Among them are *R. cathar′tica* L., or buckthorn, *R. purshia′na* D.C. (the source of cascara sagrada), and *R. fran′gula* L. *R. califor′nica* L., California buckthorn or coffee tree, has been used in rheumatism. *R. cro′ceus* Nutt. is a species of buckthorn with edible red fruit, the excessive use of which tinges the skin red.

rhaphania (rah-fa′ne-ah)   raphania.

rhaphe (ra′fe) [Gr. *rhaphē*]   raphe.

rhatany (rat′ah-ne) [Port. *ratanhia*]   *Krameria*. **Brazilian r.,** *Krameria argentea* Mart. (Leguminosae). **Peruvian r.,** *Krameria triandra* R. et P. (Leguminosae).

Rhazes (ra′zes) [Ar. Abu Bakr Mohammad Ibn Zakariya *Razi*, c. 845 to c. 930]   a Persian physician distinguished for his clinical practice and scholarship. He published the first known monograph distinguishing smallpox and measles (*Liber de variolis et morbillis*); and his students made a posthumous compilation of his medicine and surgery (*Liber continens, The Comprehensive Book*), which was a standard textbook in western Europe for more than 600 years.

rhe (re) [Gr. *rheos* current]   the unit of fluidity, being the reciprocal of the unit of velocity or centipoise.

rhegma (reg′mah) [Gr. *rhēgma* rent]   a rupture, rent, or fracture.

rhegmatogenous (reg″mah-toj′ĕ-nus)   arising from a rhegma, as rhegmatogenous detachment of the retina.

rhenium (re′ne-um)   a chemical element, atomic number 75, atomic weight 186.2, symbol Re.

rheo- [Gr. *rheos* current]   a combining form denoting relationship to an electric current, or to a flow, as of fluids.

rheocord (re′o-kord) [*rheo-* + Gr. *chordē* chord]   rheostat.

rheology (re-ol′o-je)   the science of the deformation and flow of matter, such as the flow of blood through the heart and blood vessels.

Rheomacrodex (re″o-mak′ro-deks)   trademark for a preparation of dextran 40.

rheometer (re-om′ĕ-ter) [*rheo-* + Gr. *metron* measure]   galvanometer.

rheonome (re′o-nōm) [*rheo-* + Gr. *nemein* to distribute]   an apparatus for determining the effect of irritation on a nerve.

rheophore (re′o-fōr) [*rheo-* + Gr. *phoros* carrying]   an electrode.

rheoscope (re′o-skōp) [*rheo-* + Gr. *skopein* to examine]   an instrument for detecting the presence of an electric current.

rheostat (re′o-stat) [*rheo-* + Gr. *histanai* to place]   an appliance for regulating the resistance and thus controlling the amount of current entering an electric circuit.

rheostosis (re″os-to′sis) [*rheo-* + *ostosis*]   a condition of hyperostosis marked by the presence of streaks in the bones; see also *melorheostosis*.

rheotachygraphy (re″o-tah-kig′rah-fe) [*rheo-* + Gr. *tachys* swift + *graphein* to write] the photographic record of the curve of variation in experiments upon the electromotive action of muscles.

rheotaxis (re″o-tak′sis) [*rheo-* + Gr. *taxis* arrangement] the orientation of an organism in a stream of liquid, with its long axis parallel with the direction of fluid flow. **negative r.,** rheotaxis with movement of the organism in the same direction as that of the liquid. **positive r.,** rheotaxis with movement of the organism in the opposite direction to that of the liquid.

rheotome (re′o-tōm) [*rheo-* + Gr. *tomē* a cutting] a device in a faradic battery for interrupting the current with an adjustable speed control.

rheotrope (re′o-trōp) [Gr. *rheos* current + *trepein* to turn] an instrument for reversing an electric current.

rheotropism (re-ot′ro-pizm) rheotaxis.

rhestocythemia (res″to-si-the′me-ah) [Gr. *rhaiein* to break, ruin + *-cyte* + *haima* blood + *-ia*] (obs.) the occurrence of broken-down erythrocytes in the blood.

Rheum (re′um) a genus of cathartic polygonaceous plants; see *rhubarb.*

rheum, rheuma (rōōm, roo′mah) [Gr. *rheuma* flux] any watery or catarrhal discharge.

rheumapyra (roo″mah-pi′rah) [Gr. *rheuma* flux + *pyr* fire] acute rheumatism; rheumatic fever.

rheumarthritis (roo″mar-thri′tis) rheumatoid arthritis.

rheumatalgia (roo″mah-tal′je-ah) chronic rheumatic pain.

rheumatic (roo-mat′ik) [Gr. *rheumatikos*] pertaining to or affected with rheumatism.

rheumaticosis (roo-mat″ĭ-ko′sis) a term suggested to express the general condition seen in the rheumatism of childhood.

rheumatid (roo′mah-tid) any skin lesion or eruption etiologically associated with rheumatism.

rheumatism (roo′mah-tizm) [L. *rheumatismus;* Gr. *rheumatismos*] any of a variety of disorders marked by inflammation, degeneration, or metabolic derangement of the connective tissue structures of the body, especially the joints and related structures, including muscles, bursae, tendons and fibrous tissue. It is attended by pain, stiffness, or limitation of motion of these parts. Rheumatism confined to the joints is classified as arthritis. **apoplectic r.,** rheumatism associated with brain hemorrhage. **articular r., acute,** rheumatic fever. **articular r., chronic,** see *rheumatoid arthritis,* under *arthritis,* and *osteoarthritis.* **Besnier's r.,** chronic arthrosynovitis. **cerebral r.,** acute rheumatic fever marked by chorea, delirium, convulsions, and coma. **desert r.,** the primary stage of coccidioidomycosis. **gonorrheal r.,** acute articular rheumatism associated with gonorrheal urethritis, and frequently producing ankylosis of the joints. **r. of the heart,** involvement of the heart by the rheumatic fever process. **Heberden's r.,** rheumatism of the finger joint, marked by the formation of nodosities. **inflammatory r.,** rheumatic fever. **lumbar r.,** lumbago. **MacLeod's capsular r.,** a rheumatoid arthritis with effusion into the synovial capsules, bursae, and sheaths. **muscular r.,** fibrositis. **nodose r.,** 1. articular rheumatism with the formation of nodules in the region of the joints. 2. rheumatoid arthritis. **osseous r.,** rheumatoid arthritis. **palindromic r.,** a condition in which there are repeated episodes of arthritis and periarthritis without fever and without producing irreversible changes in the joints. **Poncet's r.,** tuberculous rheumatism. **subacute r.,** a mild but protracted form of rheumatism. **tuberculous r.,** see under *arthritis.* **visceral r.,** that which involves a viscus, more commonly the heart or pericardium.

rheumatismal (roo″mah-tiz′mal) pertaining to or of the nature of rheumatism.

rheumatogenic (roo″mah-to-jen′ik) [*rheumatism* + Gr. *gennan* to produce] producing or causing rheumatism.

rheumatoid (roo′mah-toid) [Gr. *rheuma* flux + *eidos* form] resembling rheumatism.

rheumatologist (roo″mah-tol′o-jist) a specialist in rheumatic conditions.

rheumatology (roo″mah-tol′o-je) the branch of medicine dealing with rheumatic disorders, their causes, pathology, diagnosis, treatment, etc.

rheumatopyra (roo″mah-to-pi′rah) rheumapyra.

rheumatosis (roo″mah-to′sis) any disorder attributed to rheumatic origin.

rheumic (roo′mik) pertaining to a rheum or flux.

rhexis (rek′sis) [Gr. *rhēxis* a breaking forth, bursting] the rupture of an organ or vessel.

Rh factor see under *factor.*

rhigosis (rĭ-go′sis) [Gr. *rhigōsis* a shivering] the cold sense; the perception of cold.

rhigotic (rĭ-got′ik) pertaining to rhigosis.

rhinal (ri′nal) [Gr. *rhis* nose] pertaining to the nose.

rhinalgia (ri-nal′je-ah) [*rhin-* + *-algia*] pain in the nose.

rhinallergosis (rin″al-er-go′sis) [*rhin-* + *allergy* + *-osis*] allergic rhinitis.

rhinedema (ri″nĕ-de′mah) [*rhin-* + *edema*] edema of the nose.

rhinencephalia (ri″nen-sĕ-fa′le-ah) rhinocephaly.

rhinencephalon (ri″nen-sef′ah-lon) [*rhin-* + Gr. *enkephalos* brain] 1. a term generally applied to certain parts of the brain previously thought to be concerned entirely with olfactory mechanisms, including the olfactory nerves, bulbs, tracts, and subsequent connections (all olfactory in function) and the limbic system (not primarily olfactory in function); it is homologous with the olfactory portions of the brain in lower animals. Called also *olfactory brain* and *smell brain.* 2. [NA] the area of the brain comprising the substantia perforata, rostralis, bandaletta diagonalis (Broca), area subcallosa, and gyrus paraterminalis. 3. one of the portions of the telencephalon in the embryo.

rhinencephalus (ri″nen-sef′ah-lus) rhinocephalus.

rhinenchysis (ri-nen′kĭ-sis) [*rhin-* + Gr. *enchein* to pour in] injection of a medicinal fluid into the nose.

rhinesthesia (ri″nes-the′ze-ah) [*rhin-* + Gr. *aisthēsis* perception] the sense of smell.

rhineurynter (rin″u-rin′ter) [*rhin-* + Gr. *eurynein* to widen] a dilatable rubber bag for distending a nostril.

rhinion (rin′e-on) [Gr., dim. of *rhis*] the lower end of the suture between the nasal bones.

rhinism (ri′nizm) a nasal quality of voice.

rhinitis (ri-ni′tis) [*rhin-* + *-itis*] inflammation of the mucous membrane of the nose. **acute catarrhal r.,** coryza, or cold in the head; an acute congestion of the mucous membrane of the nose, marked by dryness, followed by increased mucous secretion from the membrane, impeded respiration through the nose, and some pain. **allergic r., anaphylactic r.,** a general term used to denote any allergic reaction of the nasal mucosa; it may occur perennially (*nonseasonal allergic rhinitis*) or seasonally (*hay fever*). **atopic r.,** nonseasonal allergic r. **atrophic r.,** a chronic form marked by wasting of the mucous membrane and the glands. **atrophic r. of swine,** a disease of very young swine that may result in marked displacement or atrophy of the turbinate bones in severe cases, due to severe persistent inflammation of the nasal mucosa; the primary inflammatory reaction may be caused by a variety of agents, including a virus (see *inclusion-body r.*). **r. caseo′sa,** rhinitis with a caseous, gelatinous, and fetid discharge. **chronic catarrhal r.,** a form characterized by hypertrophy and later by atrophy of the mucous and submucous tissues. **croupous r., fibrinous r. dyscrinic r.,** rhinitis associated with and dependent on endocrine imbalance. **fibrinous r.,** a form characterized by the development of a false membrane; called also *croupous r.* **gangrenous r.,** a gangrene-like inflammation of the nasal mucosa. **hypertrophic r.,** a form in which the mucous membrane thickens and swells. **inclusion-body r.,** atrophic rhinitis of swine due to a viral infection, frequently marked by atrophy of the turbinate bones and distortion of the snout, sneezing, stunting of growth, and, histologically, by the presence of inclusion bodies in scrapings of the nasal mucous membranes. **membranous r.,** chronic rhinitis with the formation of a membranous exudate. **nonseasonal allergic r.,** allergic rhinitis that may occur continuously or intermittently all year round; it is caused by an allergen to which the individual is more or less always exposed, such as house dust, danders, and food, and is characterized by sudden attacks of sneezing, swelling of the nasal mucosa with a profuse watery discharge, itching of the eyes, and lacrimation. Called also *atopic* or *perennial r.* Cf. *hay fever.* **pe-**

rennial r., nonseasonal allergic r. **porcine inclusion body r.,** a severe mucopurulent rhinitis and sinusitis of young pigs, often with turbinate bone atrophy and hemorrhage of the parenchymatous organs. It is caused by a type B herpesvirus. **pseudomembranous r.,** a form in which the inflamed region is covered with an opaque exudation. **purulent r.,** chronic rhinitis with the formation of pus. **scrofulous r.,** tuberculous rhinitis. **r. sic′ca,** a variety of atrophic rhinitis in which the secretion is entirely absent. **syphilitic r.,** a variety caused by syphilis, and marked by ulceration, caries of the nasal bone, and a fetid discharge. **tuberculous r.,** a variety due to tuberculosis, and attended with ulceration, caries of the nasal bone, and ozena. **vasomotor r.,** 1. a form of nonallergic rhinitis in which transient changes in vascular tone and permeability, with the same symptoms as in allergic rhinitis, are brought on by such stimuli as mild chilling, fatigue, anger, and anxiety. 2. any condition of allergic or nonallergic rhinitis, as opposed to infectious rhinitis.

rhin(o)- [Gr. *rhis,* gen. *rhinos* nose] a combining form denoting relationship to the nose, or a noselike structure.

rhinoanemometer (ri″no-an″ĕ-mom′ĕ-ter) [*rhino-* + *anemometer*] an apparatus for measuring the air passing through the nose during respiration.

rhinoantritis (ri″no-an-tri′tis) [*rhino-* + *antrum* + *-itis*] inflammation of the nasal cavity and the antrum of Highmore.

rhinobyon (ri-no′be-on) [*rhino-* + Gr. *byein* to plug] a nasal tampon.

rhinocanthectomy (ri″no-kan-thek′to-me) rhinommectomy.

rhinocele (ri′no-sēl) rhinocoele.

Rhinocephalus annulatus (ri″no-sef′ah-lus an″u-la′tus) *Boophilus annulatus.*

rhinocephalus (ri″no-sef′ah-lus) a fetus exhibiting rhinocephaly.

rhinocephaly (ri″no-sef′ah-le) [*rhino-* + Gr. *kephalē* head + *-ia*] a developmental anomaly characterized by the presence of a proboscis-like nose above eyes partially or completely fused into one.

rhinocheiloplasty (ri″no-ki′lo-plas″te) [*rhino-* + Gr. *cheilos* lip + *plassein* to form] plastic surgery of the nose and lip.

rhinocleisis (ri″no-kli′sis) [*rhino-* + Gr. *kleisis* closure] obstruction of the nasal passages.

rhinocoele (ri′no-sēl) [*rhino-* + Gr. *koilia* hollow] the ventricle of the olfactory lobe of the brain.

rhinodacryolith (ri″no-dak′re-o-lith″) [*rhino-* + Gr. *dakryon* tear + *lithos* stone] a lacrimal concretion in the nasal duct.

rhinodynia (ri″no-din′e-ah) [*rhino-* + Gr. *odynē* pain + *-ia*] pain in the nose.

rhinoentomophthoromycosis (ri″no-en″to-mof″tho-ro-mi-ko′sis) rhinophycomycosis.

Rhinoestrus (rīn-es′trus) a genus of flies of the family Oestridae whose larvae occur in the nasal passages of horses in Europe, Asia and Africa; they may deposit larvae in the human eye.

rhinogenous (ri-noj′ĕ-nus) [*rhino-* + Gr. *gennan* to produce] arising in the nose.

rhinokyphosis (ri″no-ki-fo′sis) [*rhino-* + Gr. *kyphos* hump] the presence of an abnormal hump in the ridge of the nose.

rhinolalia (ri″no-la′le-ah) [*rhino-* + Gr. *lalia* speech] a nasal quality of voice due to some disease or defect of the nasal passages. **r. aper′ta,** that which is caused by undue patency of the posterior nares. **r. clau′sa,** that which is due to undue closure of the nasal passages. **open r.,** r. aperta.

rhinolaryngitis (ri″no-lar″in-ji′tis) inflammation of the mucous membrane of the nose and larynx.

rhinolaryngology (ri″no-lar″in-gol′o-je) [*rhino-* + Gr. *larynx* larynx + *-logy*] the sum of knowledge concerning the nose and larynx and their diseases.

rhinolith (ri′no-lith) [*rhino-* + Gr. *lithos* stone] a nasal stone or concretion.

rhinolithiasis (ri″no-li-thi′ah-sis) a condition associated with the formation of rhinoliths.

rhinologist (ri-nol′o-jist) a specialist in rhinology.

rhinology (ri-nol′o-je) [*rhino-* + *-logy*] the sum of knowledge regarding the nose and its diseases.

rhinomanometer (ri″no-mah-nom′ĕ-ter) [*rhino-* + *manometer*] a manometer used in rhinomanometry.

rhinomanometry (ri″no-mah-nom′ĕ-tre) measurement of the airflow and pressure within the nose during respiration; nasal resistance or obstruction can be calculated from the data obtained.

rhinometer (ri-nom′ĕ-ter) [*rhino-* + Gr. *metron* measure] an instrument for measuring the nose or its cavities.

rhinommectomy (ri″nom-mek′to-me) [*rhin-* + Gr. *omma* eye + *ectomy*] excision of the inner canthus of the eye.

rhinomycosis (ri″no-mi-ko′sis) fungal infection of the nasal mucosa.

rhinonecrosis (ri″no-nĕ-kro′sis) necrosis of the nasal bones.

rhinonemmeter (ri″no-nem′ĕ-ter) a device for measuring nasal air flow rates.

rhinoneurosis (ri″no-nu-ro′sis) a neurosis or functional disease of the nose.

rhinopathia (ri″no-path′e-ah) rhinopathy. **r. vasomoto′ria,** vasomotor rhinitis.

rhinopathy (ri-nop′ah-the) [*rhino-* + Gr. *pathos* disease] any disease of the nose.

rhinopharyngeal (ri″no-fah-rin′je-al) nasopharyngeal.

rhinopharyngitis (ri″no-far″in-ji′tis) inflammation of the nasopharynx. **r. mu′tilans,** gangosa.

rhinopharyngocele (ri″no-fah-ring′go-sēl) a tumor, usually an aerocele, of the nasopharynx.

rhinopharyngolith (ri″no-fah-ring′go-lith) [*rhino-* + Gr. *pharynx* pharynx + *lithos* stone] calculus of the nasal pharynx.

rhinopharynx (ri″no-far′inks) nasopharynx (pars nasalis pharyngis [NA]).

rhinophonia (ri″no-fo′ne-ah) [*rhino-* + Gr. *phōnē* voice] a nasal twang or quality of voice.

rhinophycomycosis (ri″no-fi″ko-mi-ko′sis) a fungal infection caused by *Entomophthora coronata,* marked by development of large polyps in the subcutaneous tissues of the nose and paranasal sinuses; orbital involvement with unilateral blindness may follow. It usually leads to cerebral involvement. Called also *phycomycosis entomophthorae* and *rhinoentomophthoromycosis.*

rhinophyma (ri″no-fi′mah) [*rhino-* + Gr. *phyma* growth] a manifestation of severe rosacea involving the lower half of the nose and sometimes spreading to adjacent cheek areas, usually seen in men, and characterized by thickened, lobulated overgrowth of the sebaceous glands and epithelial connective tissue.

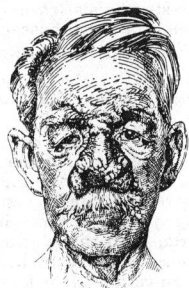

Rhinophyma.

rhinoplastic (ri″no-plas′tik) pertaining to rhinoplasty.

rhinoplasty (ri′no-plas″te) [*rhino-* + Gr. *plassein* to form] a plastic surgical operation on the nose, either reconstructive, restorative, or cosmetic. **Carpue's r.,** Indian r. **English r.,** that in which a nose is formed out of flaps from the cheeks. **Indian r.,** the reconstruction of a nose by a flap of skin taken from the forehead, with its pedicle at the root of the nose; called also *Carpue's operation.* **Joseph r.,** an operation for modification of the shape of the nose by resection of the dorsal osteocartilaginous hump with a saw. **Italian r.,** tagliacotian r. **tagliacotian r.,** the reconstruction of a nose by a flap of skin taken from the arm, the flap remaining attached to the arm until union has taken place; called also *Italian* or *tagliacotian operation.*

rhinopneumonitis (ri″no-nu″mo-ni′tis) [*rhino-* + Gr. *pneumōn* lung + *-itis*] inflammation of the nasal and pulmonary mucous membranes. **equine viral r.,** a highly contagious disease of horses caused by a herpesvirus, which is marked by a mild respiratory infection in young animals and abortion in young mares exposed to the infection for the first time; in the latter instance, it is called *equine virus abortion.*

rhinopolypus (ri″no-pol′ĭ-pus) a nasal polyp.

rhinorrhagia (ri″no-ra′je-ah) [*rhino-* + Gr. *rhēgnynai* to burst forth] nosebleed; epistaxis.

rhinorrhaphy (ri-nor′ah-fe) [*rhino-* + Gr. *rhaphē* suture] an operation for epicanthus performed by excising a fold of skin from the nose and closing the opening with sutures.

rhinorrhea (ri″no-re′ah) [*rhino-* + Gr. *rhoia* flow] the free discharge of a thin nasal mucus. **cerebrospinal r.,** discharge of cerebrospinal fluid through the nose.

rhinosalpingitis (ri″no-sal-pin-ji′tis) [*rhino-* + Gr. *salpinx* tube + *-itis*] inflammation of the nasal mucosa and the eustachian tube.

rhinoscleroma (ri″no-skle-ro′mah) [*rhino-* + Gr. *sklērōma* a hard swelling] a granulomatous disease involving the nose and nasopharynx. The growth forms hard patches or nodules, which tend to increase in size and are painful on pressure. The disease occurs in Egypt, Eastern Europe, and Central and South America and is ascribed to the presence of the *Klebsiella rhinoscleromatis.*

rhinoscope (ri′no-skōp) [*rhino-* + Gr. *skopein* to examine] a speculum for use in nasal examinations.

rhinoscopic (ri″no-skop′ik) pertaining to rhinoscopy.

rhinoscopy (ri-nos′ko-pe) the examination of the nasal passages, either through the anterior nares (*anterior r.*) or through the nasopharynx (*posterior r.*). **median r.,** examination of the nasal cavity and the openings of the ethmoid cells, etc., by means of a long nasal speculum.

rhinosporidiosis (ri″no-spo-rid″e-o′sis) [*rhino-* + Gr. *sporidion* dim. of *sporos* seed] a chronic, localized granulomatous fungal infection of the mucocutaneous tissues, especially of the nose, caused by *Rhinosporidium seeberi,* usually found in India and Sri Lanka but also seen in many temperate and tropical regions worldwide, characterized by the development of polyps, tumors, papillomas, or wartlike lesions; other areas of infection may involve the conjunctiva and rarely the anus, penis, vagina, ears, pharynx, and larynx. The infection has also been described in various wild and domestic animals.

Rhinosporidium seeberi (ri″no-spo-rid′e-um se′ber-i) an as yet unisolated fungus that causes rhinosporidiosis.

rhinostegnosis (ri″no-steg-no′sis) [*rhino-* + Gr. *stegnōsis* obstruction] obstruction of a nasal passage.

rhinostenosis (ri″no-stĕ-no′sis) narrowing of a nasal passage.

rhinotomy (ri-not′o-me) [*rhino-* + Gr. *tomē* a cutting] incision into the nose.

rhinotracheitis (ri″no-tra″ke-i′tis) [*rhino-* + L. *trachea* + *-itis*] inflammation of the nasal mucous membranes and trachea. **feline r., feline viral r.,** an acute, febrile, herpesvirus infection of the upper respiratory tract and conjunctivae affecting young kittens; it is marked by a mucopurulent discharge from the eyes and nose, photophobia, coughing, and sneezing. **infectious r., infectious bovine r.,** an acute, infectious, febrile, herpesvirus disease of cattle, marked by inflammation and ulceration of the upper respiratory tract, which may be followed by pneumonia, coughing, profuse discharge from the eyes and nose, excessive salivation, anorexia, and, in pregnant cows, abortion.

rhinoviral (ri″no-vi′ral) pertaining to or caused by rhinoviruses.

rhinovirus (ri″no-vi′rus) any of a subgroup of the picornaviruses considered to be etiologically associated with the common cold and certain other upper respiratory ailments; over 90 antigenically distinct strains are known to cause the common cold. Called also *coryzavirus.*

rhiotin (ri′o-tin) a biotin vitamin which is active for *Rhizobium* but not for yeast, is avidin-combinable, and stable to acid or neutral autoclaving.

Rhipicentor (ri″pĭ-sen′tor) [Gr. *rhipis* fan + *kentein* to prick or stab] a genus of ticks. The bite of *R. bicor′nis* (*Ixodes bicornis*), a Mexican tick that infests the cougar, may cause a high fever in the human adult and may kill a child.

Rhipicephalus (ri″pĭ-sef′ah-lus) [Gr. *rhipis* fan + *kephalē* head] a genus of cattle ticks, species of which are the agents in transmitting *Babesia* of cattle fever, and other diseases. **R. appendicula′tus,** the brown tick; it transmits *Theileria parva,* the cause of East Coast fever in African cattle. **R. bur′sa,** a species that transmits *Babesia ovis,* which causes icterohematuria and carceag of sheep. **R. capen′sis,** an African species found on cattle and horses, which may transmit *Theileria parva,* the cause of East Coast fever. **R. decolora′tus,** a species regarded as the transmitter of *Borrelia theileri,* the cause of tickborne relapsing fever, of *Rickettsia conorii,* causing tickborne typhus, and of bovine anaplasmosis in some parts of Africa. **R. ever′t′si,** an African species found on horses and cattle; it may transmit *Theileria parva* and *Rickettsia conorii.* **R. sanguin′eus,** the brown dog tick, a species found on many domestic animals; it transmits *Rickettsia rickettsii,* the cause of Rocky Mountain spotted fever, *R. conorii,* the cause of tickborne typhus and Boutonneuse fever in humans, and various species of *Babesia.* **R. si′mus,** the black pitted tick, a species which transmits *Theileria parva,* the cause of East Coast fever.

rhitid- for words beginning thus, see those beginning *rhytid-.*

rhizanesthesia (ri-zan″es-the′ze-ah) anesthesia produced by injecting a local anesthetic into the spinal arachnoid space.

rhiz(o)- [Gr. *rhiza* root] a combining form denoting relationship to a root.

Rhizobiaceae (ri-zo″be-a′se-e) a family of gram-negative, aerobic, rod-shaped bacteria without endospores, found on plant roots; it consists of the genera *Agrobacterium, Bradyrhizobium, Phyllobacterium,* and *Rhizobium.*

Rhizobium (ri-zo′be-um) [Gr. *rhiza* root + *bios* life] a genus of gram-negative, aerobic, rod-shaped bacteria of the family Rhizobiaceae. The organisms produce nodules on the roots of leguminous plants and fix free nitrogen symbiotically.

rhizoblast (ri′zo-blast) [*rhizo-* + Gr. *blastos* germ] flagellar rootlet.

rhizodontropy (ri″zo-don′tro-pe) [*rhizo-* + *odont-* + *tropos* a turning] 1. the act of rotating a tooth root. 2. the act of attaching an artificial crown to a tooth root by means of a pivot.

rhizodontrypy (ri″zo-don′trĭ-pe) [*rhizo-* + *odont-* + Gr. trephination] surgical perforation of a tooth root to provide a channel of egress for a confined fluid.

Rhizoglyphus (ri-zog′lĭ-fus) a genus of mites. **R. parasit′icus,** the coolie-itch mite, which lives on the ground in India and is reported to cause sore feet in the tea plantation workers.

rhizoid (ri′zoid) [*rhizo-* + Gr. *eidos* form] rootlike; resembling a root.

rhizoidal (ri-zoi′dal) rhizoid.

rhizolysis (ri-zol′ĭ-sis) radiofrequency neurotomy.

Rhizomastigida (ri″zo-mas-tij′ĭ-dah) [*rhizo-* + Gr. *mastix* whip] in former systems of classification, an order of zooflagellates characterized by the presence of one to many flagella and pseudopodia occurring simultaneously or at different times in the trophozoite.

rhizome (ri′zōm) [Gr. *rhizōma* root stem] the subterraneous root stock of a plant.

rhizomelic (ri-zo-mel′ik) [*rhizo-* + Gr. *melos* limb] pertaining to or involving the hip joint and shoulder joint.

rhizomeningomyelitis (ri″zo-mě-nin″go-mi″ě-li′tis) radiculomeningomyelitis.

rhizoneure (ri′zo-nūr) [*rhizo-* + Gr. *neuron* nerve] a nerve cell which forms a nerve root.

rhizoplast (ri′zo-plast) [*rhizo-* + Gr. *plastos* formed] flagellar rootlet.

Rhizopoda (ri-zop′o-dah) [*rhizo-* + Gr. *pous* foot] 1. a superclass of protozoa (subphylum Sarcodina, phylum Sarcomastigophora), comprising the amebae, which move about and acquire food by means of filopodia, lobopodia, or reticulopodia, or by protoplasmic flow without production of discrete pseudopodia. The majority are free-living in soil and water, but some are parasitic and pathogenic in humans. It comprises eight classes: Lobosea, Acarpomyxea, Acrasea, Eumycetozoea, Plasmodiophorea, Filosea, Granuloreticulosa, and Xenophyophorea. 2. Sarcodina.

rhizopodium (ri″zo-po′dĭ-um), pl. *rhizopo′dia* [*rhizo-* + Gr. *pous* foot] reticulopodium.

Rhizopus (ri-zo′pus) a genus of fungi of the family Mucoraceae, order Mucorales; see *mucormycosis. R. arrhizus* and *R. oryzae* have been isolated from uncontrolled acidotic diabetics demonstrating cerebral infections, and *R. rhizopodoformis* has been isolated from cutaneous lesions of diabetics and severely burned patients.

rhizotomy (ri-zot′o-me) [*rhizo-* + Gr. *tomē* a cutting] interruption of the roots of spinal nerves within the spinal canal. **anterior r.,** division of the anterior or motor spinal nerve roots. **dorsal r., posterior r.,** division of the posterior or sensory spinal nerve roots; done for relief of intractable pain. **retrogasserian r.,** transection of the sensory root fibers of the trigeminal nerve for the permanent relief of trigeminal neuralgia; called also *retrogasserian neurotomy.*

rho (ro) [P, ρ] the seventeenth letter of the Greek alphabet.

rhodamine (ro-dah′min) [Gr. *rhodon* rose + *amine*] a red fluorescent dye.

rhodanate (ro′dah-nāt) a salt of rhodanic acid.

rhodanic acid (ro-dan′ik) 1. thiocyanic acid. 2. rhodanine.

rhodanine (ro′dah-nēn) 2-thio-4-oxothiazolidine, a reagent that gives colored products with aldehydes and ketones.

rhodium (ro′de-um) [Gr. *rhodon* rose] a hard and rare metal of the platinum group; atomic number, 45; atomic weight, 102.905; symbol, Rh.

Rhodnius prolixus (rod′ne-us pro-lik′sus) a reduviid bug of South America capable of transmitting *Trypanosoma cruzi,* the etiologic agent of Chagas' disease.

rhod(o)- [Gr. *rhodon* rose] a combining form meaning red.

rhodogenesis (ro″do-jen′ĕ-sis) [*rhodo-* + Gr. *genesis* production] the restoration of the purple tint to rhodopsin after it has become bleached by the action of light.

Rhodomicrobium (ro″do-mi-kro′be-um) [*rhodo-* + *microbe*] a genus of photosynthetic aquatic bacteria of the family Rhodospirillaceae, order Rhodospirillales, consisting of ovoid, gram-negative cells connected by filaments that produce pink to reddish brown pigments. The type species is *R. vanniel′ii.*

rhodophane (ro′do-fān) [*rhodo-* + Gr. *phainein* to show] a red pigment, or chromophane, from the retinal cones of birds and fishes.

rhodophylactic (ro″do-fi-lak′tik) tending to preserve or restore rhodopsin; pertaining to rhodophylaxis.

rhodophylaxis (ro″do-fi-lak′sis) [*rhodo-* + *phylaxis*] the ability of the retinal epithelium to regenerate rhodopsin.

Rhodopseudomonas (ro″do-soo″do-mo′nas) [*rhodo-* + *pseudo-* + Gr. *monas* unit, from *monos* single] a genus of photosynthetic aquatic bacteria of the family Rhodospirillaceae, order Rhodospirillales, consisting of rod-shaped, ovoid or spherical, gram-negative cells that produce yellow-green to brown and red pigments. The type species is *R. palus′tris.*

rhodopsin (ro-dop′sin) [*rhodo-* + Gr. *opsis* vision] visual purple: a photosensitive purple-red chromoprotein in the retinal rods which is bleached to visual yellow (all-*trans* retinal) by light, thereby producing stimulation of the retinal sensory endings. It is a conjugated protein, the prosthetic group of which is 11-*cis* retinal.

Rhodospirillaceae (ro″do-spi″ril-la′se-e) a family of photosynthetic aquatic bacteria of the order Rhodospirillales, comprising the purple nonsulfur bacteria. It consists of motile, anaerobic cells that produce purple, red, and brown pigments, and that do not utilize sulfur as an electron donor. It contains the genera *Rhodomicrobium, Rhodopseudomonas,* and *Rhodospirillum.* Called also *Athiorhodaceae.*

Rhodospirillales (ro″do-spi″ril-la′lēz) an order of phototrophic bacteria, composed of gram-negative cells that are primarily aquatic and contain bacteriochlorophylls and carotenoids. Photosynthesis occurs anaerobically. It contains the families *Rhodospirillaceae, Chromatiaceae,* and *Chlorobiaceae.*

Rhodospirillum (ro″do-spi-ril′um) [*rhodo-* + *spirillum*] a genus of photosynthetic aquatic bacteria of the family Rhodospirillaceae, order Rhodospirillales, consisting of spiral, gram-negative cells that multiply by binary fission and produce red to brown pigments. The type species is *R. ru′brum.*

Rhodothece (ro′do-the′se) in former systems of classification, a genus of bacteria, species of which are now assigned to the genus *Amoebobacter.*

Rhodotorula (ro″do-tor′u-lah) a genus of imperfect yeasts. **R. glu′tinis,** a nonpathogenic species from air, potatoes, and the skin in seborrhea; its cells are cylindrical, oval, or spherical and it forms a rosy pigment. Called also *Saccharomyces glutinis.* **R. ru′bra,** a skin contaminant which rarely causes opportunistic infections in man.

rhodotoxin (ro″do-tok′sin) a poisonous compound from the flowers and leaves of various shrubs and trees, such as *Rhododendron;* it is also found in honey from *Rhododendron* flowers.

RhoGAM (ro′gam) trademark for a preparation of Rh₀ (D) immune globulin.

rhombencephalon (rom″ben-sef′ah-lon) [Gr. *rhombos* rhomb + *enkephalos* brain] 1. the part of the brain developed from the posterior of the three primary brain vesicles of the embryonic neural tube; it comprises the metencephalon (cerebellum and pons) and myelencephalon (medulla oblongata). In official anatomical nomenclature [NA], the rhombencephalon comprises only the medulla oblongata and pons. 2. the most caudal of the three primary brain vesicles in the embryo, later dividing into the metencephalon and myelencephalon. Called also *hindbrain.*

rhombocoele (rom′bo-sēl) [Gr. *rhombos* rhomb + *koilia* cavity] the terminal distention of the canal of the spinal cord.

rhomboid (rom′boid) [Gr. *rhombos* rhomb + *eidos* form] having a shape similar to a rectangle that has been skewed to one side so that the angles are oblique. **Michaelis's r.,** a diamond-shaped area over the posterior aspect of the pelvis formed by the dimples of the posterior-superior spines of the ilia, the lines formed by the gluteal muscles, and the groove at the end of the spine.

rhombomere (rom′bo-mēr) neuromere, def. 1.

rhonchal, rhonchial (rong′kal, rong′ke-al) pertaining to, or of the nature of, a rhonchus.

rhonchus (rong′kus), pl. *rhon′chi* [L.; Gr. *rhonchos* a snoring sound] a rattling in the throat; also a dry, coarse rale in the bronchial tubes, due to a partial obstruction. See *rale.*

Rhopalopsyllus cavicola (ro″pah-lo-sil′us kah-vik′o-lah) the South American cavy flea, which transmits *Pasteurella pestis.*

rhoptry (rōp′tre) [Gr. *rhopalon* club] either of the electron-dense, paired, tubular, saccular, or club-shaped organelles arising anteriorly and extending toward the posterior end of the body of apicocomplexan, forming part of the apical complex. Called also *toxoneme.*

rhubarb (roo′barb) the dried rhizome and root of *Rheum officinale* Baill., used in fluidextract or aromatic tincture as a cathartic. The common garden rhubarb, *R. rhaponticum* L., is edible and devoid of cathartic principles.

Rhus (rus) [L., gen. *rhois*] a genus of anacardiaceous vines and shrubs, many of them poisonous. Some species contain a highly allergenic oleoresin mixture known as *urushiol;* contact with these species produces a severe dermatitis in sensitive persons (see *rhus dermatitis,* under *dermatitis*). The most important toxic species are *R. radicans* L. (poison ivy), *R. diversiloba* L. (poison oak or western poison oak), and *R. vernix* L. (poison sumac). Extracts of the leaves and twigs of these plants (poison ivy extract, poison oak extract) have been used in the prophylaxis and treatment of dermatitis associated with these species. Called also *Toxicodendron.*

Rhynchocoela (rin-ko-sēl′ah) [Gr. *rhynchos* snout, bill, beak + *-coele*] the ribbon worms, a phylum of slender, flat, soft, often brightly colored, acoelmate worms which have unsegmented bodies and an eversible proboscis that lies in a special cavity in front of the mouth; most species are marine inhabitants. Called also *Nemertea* and *Nemertina.*

rhynchocoelan (rin-ko-sēl′an) a ribbon worm; any individual of the Rhynchocoela; called also *nemertean.*

Rhynchodea (rin-ko′de-ah) [Gr. *rhynchos* snout] a superorder of commensal or pathogenic ciliate protozoa (subclass

Hypostomatia, class Kinetofragminophorea), most commonly parasitic on the gills of marine bivalves, and characterized by the presence of a suctorial tentacle and toxicysts; the somatic ciliature may be limited to a thigmotactic field, or the body of the mature stage may be naked. It comprises one order: Rhynchodida.

Rhynchodida (rīn-ko′dĭ-dah) an order of ciliate protozoa (superorder Rhynchodea, subclass Hypostomatia) having the characters of the superorder.

rhythm (rith′m) [L. *rhythmus;* Gr. *rhythmos*] a measured movement; the recurrence of an action or function at regular intervals. **alpha r.,** a uniform rhythm of waves in the normal electroencephalogram, showing an average frequency of 10 per second; called also *Berger r.* See under *wave.* **atrioventricular r.,** nodal r. **Berger r.,** alpha r. **beta r.,** a rhythm in the electroencephalogram consisting of waves smaller than those of the alpha rhythm, having an average frequency of 25 per second; see under *wave.* **biological r.,** the established regularity with which certain phenomena recur in living organisms. **cantering r.,** gallop r. **circadian r.,** the regular recurrence in cycles of approximately 24 hours from one stated point to another, as certain biological activities which occur at that interval, regardless of constant darkness or other conditions of illumination. **circus r.,** circus movement or contraction; a movement travelling in circular fashion around a ring of muscle. **coupled r.,** heart beats occurring in pairs, the second beat of the pair usually being a ventricular premature beat; see also *bigeminal pulse* and *bigeminy.* **delta r.,** see under *wave.* **ectopic r.,** a heart rhythm initiated by a focus outside the sinoatrial node. **escape r.,** a heart rhythm initiated by lower centers when the sinoatrial node fails to initiate impulses, its rhythmicity is depressed, or its impulses are completely blocked. **fetal r.,** embryocardia. **gallop r.,** an auscultatory finding of three (*triple r.*) or four heart sounds, the extra sound(s) by convention being in diastole and related either to atrial contraction (*fourth sound, presystolic gallop*), to early rapid filling of a ventricle with an altered ventricular compliance (*protodiastolic gallop*), or to concurrence of atrial contraction and ventricular early rapid filling (*summation gallop*). **gallop r., systolic,** systolic gallop. **gamma r.,** a rhythm of waves in the electroencephalogram having a frequency of 50 per second. **idioventricular r.,** a cardiac rhythm wherein the ventricle follows an intrinsic pacemaker different from that of the atrium; see *atrioventricular dissociation,* under *dissociation.* **infradian r.,** the regular recurrence in cycles of more than 24 hours from one stated point to another, as certain biological activities which occur at such intervals, regardless of conditions of illumination. **isochronal r.,** see *cilium* (def. 3). **metachronal r.,** see *cilium* (def. 3). **nodal r.,** heart rhythm initiated in the specialized junctional tissue, i.e., the atrioventricular node and the main (His) bundle. Called also *nodal arrhythmia.* **nyctohemeral r.,** a day and night rhythm. **pendulum r.,** alternation in the rhythm of the heart sounds in which the diastolic sound is equal in time, character, and loudness to the systolic sound, the beat of the heart resembling the tick of a watch. **reciprocal r.,** a heart rhythm produced with the occurrence of many reciprocal beats. **sinus r.,** normal heart rhythm originating in the sinoatrial node. **theta r.,** see under *wave.* **triple r.,** the cadence produced when three heart sounds recur in successive cardiac cycles; see also *gallop r.* **ultradian r.,** the regular recurrence in cycles of less than 24 hours from one stated point to another, as certain biological activities which occur at such intervals, regardless of conditions of illumination. **ventricular r.,** the ventricular contractions which occur in cases of complete heart block.

rhythmeur (rith-mer′) a device for making rhythmic interruptions of the current in an x-ray machine.

rhythmical (rith′me-kal) characterized by rhythm.

rhythmicity (rith-mis′ĭ-te) in cardiology, the ability to beat, or the state of beating, rhythmically without external stimuli.

rhytidectomy (rit″ĭ-dek′to-me) [Gr. *rhytis* wrinkle + *ektomē* excision] excision of skin for the elimination of wrinkles.

rhytidoplasty (rit′ĭ-do-plas″te) plastic surgery for the elimination of wrinkles from the skin.

rhytidosis (rit″ĭ-do′sis) [Gr. *rhytidōsis; rhytis* wrinkle] a wrinkling of the cornea.

rib (rib) any one of the paired elastic arches of bone, twelve on either side, that extend from the thoracic vertebrae toward the median line on the ventral aspect of the trunk, forming the major part of the thoracic skeleton. The upper seven (true ribs) are connected ventrally with the sternum. The lower five (false ribs) are not. Collectively called *costae* [NA]. **abdominal r's, asternal r's,** false r's. **bicipital r.,** an anomalous rib resulting from fusion of the anterior part of the seventh cervical vertebra with the first thoracic rib. **cervical r.,** costa cervicalis. **false r's,** costae spuriae. **floating r's,** costae fluitantes. **slipping r.,** a rib whose attaching cartilage is repeatedly dislocated. **spurious r's,** costae spuriae. **sternal r's,** costae verae. **Stiller's r.,** an abnormally movable tenth rib. **true r's,** costae verae. **vertebral r's,** costae fluitantes. **vertebrocostal r's,** the upper three false ribs of either side, articulating with the vertebrae and connected by cartilage to the costal cartilage of the ipsilateral seventh rib. **vertebrosternal r's,** costae verae. **Zahn's r's,** see under *line.*

ribaminol (ri-bah′mĭ-nōl) chemical name: ribonucleic acid compound with 2-(diethylamino)ethanol; a memory adjuvant.

ribavirin (ri″bah-vi′rin) chemical name: 1β-D-ribofuranosyl-1*H*-1,2,4-triazole-3-carboxamide; a synthetic nucleoside resembling guanosine and used as an antiviral, $C_8H_{12}N_4O_5$.

Ribbert's theory (rib′erts) [Moritz Wilhelm Hugo *Ribbert,* German pathologist, 1855–1920] see under *theory.*

ribbon (rib′un) a band-like structure. **r. of Reil,** the rostral part of the lemniscus medialis. **synaptic r.,** 1. a dense lamella surrounded by a halo of synaptic vesicles, found at a right angle to the apex of the synaptic ridge in the outer plexiform layer of the retina. 2. a similar structure found in varying numbers in the cytoplasm of the hair cells of the ear.

Ribes's ganglion (rēbz) [François *Ribes,* French surgeon, 1800–1864] see under *ganglion.*

ribitol (ri′bĭ-tol) an alcohol corresponding to the sugar ribose; it is a constituent of a class of teichoic acids.

ribodesose (ri-bo′des-ōs) D-2-deoxyribose.

riboflavin (ri″bo-fla′vin) the heat-stable factor of the vitamin B complex, 6,7-dimethyl-9-[1′-D-ribityl]-isoalloxazin, $C_{17}H_{20}N_4O_6$; called also *lactoflavin* and *vitamin B₂.* A water-soluble vitamin, it serves as a component of two coenzymes or prosthetic groups (FAD and FMN) of flavoproteins, which function as hydrogen carriers in oxidation-reduction processes. It occurs in milk, muscle, liver, kidney, eggs, grass, malt, leafy young vegetables, and various algae, and is an essential nutrient for man, the requirement being related to body size, metabolic rate, and growth rate. Deficiency of the vitamin is known as *ariboflavinosis* (q.v.). A standardized preparation [USP], occurring as a yellow to orange-yellow, crystalline powder, containing 98 to 102 per cent of riboflavin, calculated on the dried basis, is used in the treatment and prophylaxis of riboflavin deficiency, administered orally and parenterally. **r.-5¹-phosphate,** flavin mononucleotide.

riboflavin kinase (ri″bo-fla′vin ki′nās) [EC 2.7.1.26] an enzyme of the transferase class that catalyzes the reaction ATP + riboflavin = ADP + flavin mononucleotide. The reaction produces riboflavin-5′-phosphate (FMN), a cofactor for electron transfer reactions.

ribonuclease (ri″bo-nu′kle-ās) [EC 3.1] one of a group of enzymes of the hydrolase class that catalyze the hydrolysis of phosphate ester linkages in ribonucleic acids. **r. I** [EC 3.1.27.5], pancreatic ribonuclease; an enzyme of the hydrolase class that catalyzes the endonucleolytic cleavage of ribonucleic acids to form 3′-phosphomononucleotides and 3′ phosphooligonucleotides. The enzyme, found in the pancreas of ruminants, has been used extensively in studies of enzyme mechanics. Called also *RNase.*

ribonucleic acid (ri″bo-nu-kle′ik) RNA; the nucleic acid composed of ribonucleotide monomers, each containing ribose (a five-carbon sugar), a phosphate group, and a nitrogenous base. It is a linear polymer with a backbone composed of alternating phosphate and sugar moieties; the bases are attached to the sugars as side chains. The base sequence of an RNA is specified by the base sequence of a section of DNA (a gene) which is used as a template for RNA synthesis (transcription). The bases adenine (A), uracil (U), cytosine (C), and guanosine (G) are incorporated into the growing RNA chain, when thymine (T), A, G, and C, respectively are encountered in the DNA template. The RNA transcript is complementary to the DNA template. Many RNAs contain modified bases produced by posttranscriptional processing (methylation, deamination, and isomerization). Some RNAs contain self-complementary sequences; the chain folds back on itself forming short sections of double helix, like DNA, which stabilize the RNA in its native conformation. See also *deoxyribonucleic acid.* **heterogenous nuclear RNA (hnRNA),** a group of RNAs of diverse sizes, some much larger than other RNAs. Most of the hnRNA consists of primary transcripts that are processed by excision of intervening sequences, to form mature mRNA which then moves from the nucleus to the cytoplasm. However, much of the hnRNA is degraded in the nucleus shortly after synthesis, and it may contain fractions having other functions. **messenger RNA (mRNA),** RNA sequences, usually 400-3000 bases long, that serve as templates for protein synthesis; in eukaryotes they have characteristic structures, the 5'-cap and polyA tail, which are added during posttranscriptional processing. The amino acid sequence of a polypeptide is completely specified by the base sequence of a mRNA gene transcript. See *translation.* **ribosomal RNA (rRNA),** four RNA chains conventionally designated by their sedimentation coefficients (28S, 18S, 5.8S, and 5S in eukaryotic ribosomes). The 28S, 18S, and 5.8S mRNAs are cleaved from a 45S primary transcript in posttranscriptional processing. The 18S mRNA is part of the ribosome small subunit; the other three are part of the large subunit, rRNA makes up about 50 per cent of the ribosome, the rest is made up of about 70 different proteins. In addition to a structural role, mRNA is involved in the binding of mRNA and tRNAs to the ribosome. **transfer RNA (tRNA),** small RNA molecules (75–93 nucleotides) that match specific amino acids to mRNA codons (see *translation*). All have a similar "cloverleaf" structure with three hairpin turns. In the native conformation, the CCA acceptor stem where the amino acid is attached is at one end and the anticodon, a three base sequence that bonds to one or more specific codons, is at the other end. The attachment of a tRNA to its specific amino acid is catalyzed by an aminoacyl-tRNA synthetase, which recognizes a binding site on the tRNA. There is also a binding site for attachment to ribosomes found on all tRNAs. Specific tRNAs are designated by the amino acid they carry and the codon(s) they recognize, e.g.,

$$\text{tRNA} \begin{array}{c} \text{Gly I} \\ \text{CCC} \end{array} \quad \text{and} \quad \text{tRNA} \begin{array}{c} \text{Gly II} \\ \text{CCA/C} \end{array}$$

ribonucleoprotein (ri″bo-nu″kle-o-pro′te-in) a substance composed of both protein and ribonucleic acid.

ribonucleoside (ri″bo-nu′kle-o-sīd) a nucleoside in which the purine or pyrimidine base is combined with ribose.

ribonucleoside diphosphate reductase (ri″bo-noo′-kle-o-sīd di-fos′fāt re-duk′tās) [EC 1.17.4.1] an enzyme of the oxidoreductase class that catalyzes the formation of 2′-deoxyribonucleotides from the corresponding ribonucleotides using NADPH as the ultimate electron donor. The deoxyribonucleoside diphosphates are used in DNA synthesis. Called also *ribonucleotide reductase.*

ribonucleotide (ri″bo-nu′kle-o-tīd) a nucleotide in which the purine or pyrimidine base is combined with ribose.

ribonucleotide reductase (ri″bo-noo′kle-o-tīd re-duk′tās) ribonucleoside diphosphate reductase.

riboprine (ri′bo-prēn) chemical name: *N*-(3-methyl-2-butenyl)adenosine; an antineoplastic, $C_{43}H_{58}N_2O_{13}$.

ribopyranose (ri″bo-pi′rah-nōs) ribose in cyclic hemiacetal form.

ribose (ri′bōs) an aldopentose, $CH_2OH(CHOH)_3CHO$, found in ribonucleic acid (RNA) and in adenosine triphosphate (ATP).

ribose nucleic acid (ri′bōs noo-kle′ik) ribonucleic acid.

ribose-5-phosphate isomerase (ri′bōs fos′fāt i-som′er-ās) [EC 5.3.1.6] an enzyme of the isomerase class that catalyzes the reaction D-ribose 5-phosphate = D-ribulose 5-phosphate. The reaction is part of the overall pentose phosphate pathway and is important in ribose metabolism. Called also *phosphoriboisomerase.*

ribose-phosphate pyrophosphokinase (ri-bōs-fos′fāt pi′ro-fos″fo ki′nās) [EC 2.7.6.1] an enzyme of the transferase class that catalyzes the reaction ATP + D-ribose 5-phosphate = AMP + 5-phospho-α-D ribose 1-diphosphate. The reaction requires Mg^{2+}. The product, phosphoribosyl pyro-

phosphate, is the initial reactant in purine and pyrimidine nucleotide biosynthesis. Increased production of the enzyme, an X-linked recessive trait, leads to increased purine synthesis and causes primary gout. Called also *phosphoribosylpyrophosphate synthetase.*

ribosome (ri′bo-sōm) a large molecular structure having two dissociable subunits that is the site of protein synthesis (see *translation*). The two subunits together contain 4 different ribosomal RNA (rRNA) chains and about 70 different proteins. Ribosomes found in the cytosol of eukaryotes have a molecular weight of 4.5 million and a sedimentation coefficient of 80S; the subunits have coefficients of 60S and 40S. Ribosomes found in prokaryotes and mitochondria are smaller (70S) and also differ from eukaryotic ribosomes in their sensitivity to certain antibiotics.

ribosyl (ri′bo-sil) a glycosyl radical, $C_5H_9O_4$, formed from ribose.

5-ribosyluridine (ri″bo-sil-u′rĭ-dēn) pseudouridine.

ribothymidine (ri″bo-thi″mĭ-dēn) the ribosyl analogue of thymidine, a rare base found in small amounts in transfer-RNA.

ribulose (ri′bu-lōs) the 2-ketose isomer of ribose.

ribulose-phosphate 3-epimerase (ri′bu-lōs fos′fāt ĕ-pim′er-ās) [EC 5.1.3.1] an enzyme of the isomerase class that catalyzes the reaction D-ribulose-5-phosphate = D-xylulose 5-phosphate. The reaction is a part of the pentose phosphate pathway.

R.I.C. Royal Institute of Chemistry.

rice (rīs) the cereal plant, *Oryza sativa;* also its seed or grain. The grain consists mainly of starch, and is used as a food and as a dusting powder. **r. polishings,** fine yellowish powder from the pericarp and germ of rice; used in vitamin B deficiency. **white r.,** rice from which the outer brown coats have been removed; a diet composed too exclusively of white rice is apt to produce beriberi.

Richards (rich′ardz), Dickinson Woodruff, Jr. American physician, 1895–1973; co-winner, with Werner Theodor Otto Forssmann and André Frédéric Cournand, of the Nobel prize for medicine or physiology in 1956 for research on pathological changes in the circulatory system and for developing cardiac catheterization.

Richardson's sign (rich′ard-sunz) [Sir Benjamin Ward *Richardson,* London physician, 1828–1896] see under *sign.*

Richet (re-sha′), Charles Robert. French physiologist, 1850–1935; winner of the Nobel prize for medicine or physiology in 1913 for his research on anaphylaxis.

Richet's aneurysm (re-shāz′) [Didier Dominique Alfred *Richet,* French surgeon, 1816–1891] a fusiform aneurysm.

Richter's hernia (rik′terz) [August Gottlieb *Richter,* surgeon in Göttingen, 1742–1812] see under *hernia.*

Richter's syndrome (rik′terz) [Maurice N. *Richter,* American pathologist, born 1897] see under *syndrome.*

Richter-Monro line (rik′ter mon-ro′) see *Monro-Richter,* and under *line.*

ricin (ri′sin) a poisonous substance (phytotoxin) found in the seeds of the castor oil plant (*Ricinus communis*).

ricinism (ri′sĭ-nizm) intoxication caused by inhalation or ingestion of a poisonous principle of castor bean, producing superficial inflammation of the respiratory mucosa with hemorrhages into the lungs, or edema of the gastrointestinal tract with hemorrhages.

ricinoleic acid (ri″sin-o-le′ik) *d*-12-hydroxyoleic acid, a hydroxylated unsaturated fatty acid occurring in castor oil.

Ricinus (ris′ĭ-nus) [L.] the name of a genus of euphorbiaceous plants. The seeds of *R. commu′nis,* or castor oil plant, are highly poisonous but afford castor oil. The leaves of the castor oil plant are galactagogic.

rickets (rik′ets) [thought to be a corruption of Gr. *rhachitis* a spinal complaint] a condition caused by deficiency of vitamin D, especially in infancy and childhood, with disturbance of normal ossification. The disease is marked by bending and distortion of the bones under muscular action, by the formation of nodular enlargements on the ends and sides of the bones, by delayed closure of the fontanels, pain in the muscles, and sweating of the head. Vitamin D and sunlight together with an adequate diet are curative, provided that the parathyroid glands are functioning properly. **acute r.,** infantile scurvy. **adult r.,** osteomalacia. **beryllium r.,** a form of rickets produced by adding beryllium to an otherwise normal diet. **fat r.**, a form in which the infant is plump and seems well nourished. **fetal r.**, achondroplasia. **glissonian r.**, rickets as described by Glisson. **hemorrhagic r.**, infantile scurvy. **hepatic r.**, a rickets-like condition with cirrhosis of the liver. **late r.**, rickets occurring in older children. **lean r.**, rickets with wasting and progressive emaciation. **pseudodeficiency r.**, vitamin D–resistant r. **refractory r.**, vitamin D–resistant r. **renal r.**, a condition characterized by rachitic changes in the skeleton and resulting from dysfunction of the kidneys; see *renal osteodystrophy*, under *osteodystrophy*. **scurvy r.**, rachitic changes in the skeleton associated with infantile scurvy. **tardy r.**, late r. **vitamin D–refractory r.**, vitamin D–resistant r. **vitamin D–resistant r.**, a condition almost indistinguishable from ordinary rickets clinically but resistant to unusually large doses of vitamin D; it is often familial but may occur sporadically. In *hypophosphatemic vitamin D–resistant rickets*, hypophosphatemia is the main characteristic, while in *hypocalcemic vitamin D–resistant rickets*, the serum concentration of phosphate is within normal limits or nearly so, and the concentration of calcium is abnormally low. Called also *pseudodeficiency r.* and *vitamin D–refractory r.*

rickettsemia (rik″et-se′me-ah) the presence of rickettsiae in the blood.

Rickettsia (rĭ-ket′se-ah) [Howard Taylor *Ricketts*, American pathologist, 1871–1910] a genus of bacteria of the tribe Rickettsieae, family Rickettsiaceae, order Rickettsiales, made up of small rod-shaped to coccoid, often pleomorphic microorganisms. The cells have typical cell walls, possess no flagella, are gram-negative, and multiply only inside host cells. They occur intracytoplasmically or free in the lumen of the gut in lice, fleas, ticks, and mites, by which they are transmitted to man and other animals. The various species contain the organisms causing typhus fevers, spotted fevers and scrub typhus (tsutsugamushi disease). **R. akamu′shi**, *R. tsutsugamushi*. **R. ak′ari**, the etiologic agent of rickettsialpox, transmitted by the mite *Allodermanyssus sanguineus* from the reservoir of infection in house mice. **R. austra′lis**, the etiologic agent of North Queensland tick typhus, transmitted from infected marsupials by Ixodes ticks. **R. burnet′ii**, *Coxiella burnetii*. **R. ca′nis**, *Ehrlichia canis*. **R. cono′rii**, the etiologic agent of boutonneuse fever, transmitted by the bites of various species of ixodid ticks, including those of the genera *Rhipicephalus, Amblyomma, Haemaphysalis,* and *Hyalomma*. The principal animal reservoirs are dogs and rodents. **R. diapor′ica**, *Coxiella burnetii*. **R. moo′seri**, *R. typhi*. **R. murico′la**, *R. typhi*. **R. nippon′ica, R. orienta′lis**, *R. tsutsugamushi*. **R. pedic′uli**, *Rochalimaea quintana*. **R. prowaze′kii**, the etiologic agent of epidemic typhus and the recrudescent infection Brill-Zinsser disease. The organisms are transmitted from man to man via the louse *Pediculus humanus* var. *corporis* and from flying squirrels to man by fleas and lice. **R. quinta′na**, *Rochalimaea quintana*. **R. rickett′sii**, the etiologic agent of Rocky Mountain spotted fever, transmitted by *Dermacentor, Rhipicephalus, Haemaphysalis, Amblyomma* and *Ixodes* ticks from a natural reservoir in rodents, dogs, and foxes. Called also *Dermacentroxenus rickettsii*. **R. sennet′su**, *Ehrlichia sennetsu*. **R. sibi′rica**, the etiologic agent of Siberian tick typhus, which is transmitted from infected rodents by *Ixodes* ticks. **R. tsutsugamu′shi**, the etiologic agent of scrub typhus, transmitted by larval mites of the genus *Trombicula*, including *T. akamushi* and *T. deliensis*, from rodent reservoirs of infection. Called also *R. akamushi, R. nipponica,* and *R. orientalis*. **R. ty′phi**, the etiologic agent of murine typhus, transmitted from infected rats to humans chiefly by rat fleas. Called also *Dermacentroxenus typhi, R. mooseri, R. muricola,* and *R. typhi (mooseri)*. **R. ty′phi (moo′seri)**, *R. typhi*. **R. wolhyn′ica**, *Rochalimaea quintana*.

rickettsia (rĭ-ket′se-ah), pl. *rickett′siae*. any scotobacterium of the order Rickettsiales.

Rickettsiaceae (rĭ-ket″se-a′se-e) a family of bacteria of the order Rickettsiales, made up of small rod-shaped, ellipsoidal, coccoid, or diplococcus-shaped, often pleomorphic microorganisms often occurring intracellularly in arthropods, by which they are transmitted to man and other animals, causing disease. It includes three tribes, Ehrlichieae, Rickettsieae, and Wolbachieae.

Rickettsiae (rĭ-ket′se-e) Rickettsieae.

rickettsiae (rĭ-ket′se-e) plural of *rickettsia*.

rickettsial (rĭ-ket′se-al) caused by rickettsiae.

Rickettsiales (rĭ-ket″se-a′lēz) an order of bacteria, class Scotobacteria, division Gracilicules, kingdom Procaryotae, comprising small, gram-negative, rod-shaped or coccoid, often pleomorphic microorganisms occurring as elementary bodies that typically multiply only inside the cells of the host. Found as parasites in both vertebrates and invertebrates, which may serve as vectors, they may be pathogenic for both man and other animals. The order includes the families Anaplasmataceae, Bartonellaceae, and Rickettsiaceae.

rickettsialpox (rĭ-ket′se-al-poks″) a mild self-limited febrile disease caused by *Rickettsia akari*, transmitted by the mite *Allodermanyssus sanguineus*, an ectoparasite of the house mouse, and characterized principally by the presence of an eschar-like primary cutaneous lesion, generalized papulovesicular rash, headache, and backache. Called also *Kew Gardens fever*.

rickettsicidal (rĭ-ket″sĭ-si′dal) destructive to rickettsiae.

Rickettsieae (rik″et-si′e-e) a tribe of bacteria of the family Rickettsiaceae, order Rickettsiales, made up of small pleomorphic, most intracellular organisms, which are classified in three genera, *Coxiella, Rickettsia,* and *Rochalimaea*. They occur as parasites in arthropods and cause disease in vertebrate hosts. Pathogenic species fall generally into four groups, based upon immunologic characterization (Weil-Felix reaction): I, classic typhus (epidemic typhus, Brill-Zinsser disease, murine typhus); II, spotted fever (Rocky Mountain spotted fever, boutonneuse fever, rickettsialpox, Siberian tick typhus, Queensland tick typhus); III, scrub typhus (tsutsugamushi disease); and IV, miscellaneous organisms (Q fever and trench fever). Called also *Rickettsiae*. See also *typhus*.

Rickettsiella (rĭ-ket″se-el′ah) [*rickettsia* + *-ella* diminutive ending] a genus of bacteria of the tribe Wolbachieae, family Rickettsiaceae, order Rickettsiales, made up of minute intracellular rickettsia-like organisms, parasitic on the Japanese beetle (*Popillia japonica*) and many other species of insects. It is not pathogenic for mammals. The type species is *R. popil′liae*.

rickettsiosis (rĭ-ket″se-o′sis) infection with rickettsiae. **canine r.**, an often fatal febrile disease of dogs in Africa, the Mediterranean area, and India, caused by *Rickettsia canis*, which is transmitted by the brown dog tick (*Rhipicephalus sanguineus*). It is characterized by high fever, mucopurulent discharge from the nose and eyes, gastritis, thirst, anorexia, emaciation, fetid breath, enlargement of lymph and spleen, erythematous pustules on the axilla and groin, hysteria, convulsions, meningoencephalitis, and paralysis; dogs that recover may become carriers.

rickettsiostatic (rĭ-ket″se-o-stat′ik) inhibiting the growth and activity of rickettsiae.

Ricolesia (ri″ko-le′ze-ah) [*Ricketts* + J. D. W. A. *Coles*] a genus of bacteria of uncertain status of the order Chlamydiales, reported to be the cause of keratoconjunctivitis in cattle, goats, fowl, and swine.

rictal (rik′tal) pertaining to a fissure.

rictus (rik′tus) [L.] 1. a fissure or cleft. 2. a gaping, as of the mouth.

RID radial immunodiffusion; see *single radial diffusion*, under *diffusion*.

Riddoch's reflex (rid′oks) [George *Riddoch*, British neurologist, 1888–1947] see under *reflex*.

Rideal-Walker coefficient (rid′e-al-waw′ker) [Samuel *Rideal*, English chemist, 1863–1929; J. F. Ainslie *Walker*, English chemist, 1868–1930] phenol coefficient.

ridge (rij) a projection or projecting structure; see also *crest* and *crista*. **alveolar r.**, the bony ridge of the maxilla or mandible which contains the alveoli. **alveolar r., residual**, the bony ridge remaining after disappearance of the alveoli from the alveolar process following removal or loss of the teeth. Called also *edentulous r.* and *residual r.* **basal r.**, cingulum (def. 3). **bicipital r., anterior**, crista tuberculi minoris. **bicipital r., external**, crista tuberculi majoris. **bicipital r., internal**, crista tuberculi minoris. **bicipital r., outer, bicipital r., posterior**, crista tuberculi majoris. **buccocervical r., buccogingival r.**, a ridge or prominence on the buccal surface above the cementoenamel junction of posterior teeth. **bulbar r's**, spiral endocardial thickenings in the bulbus cordis that fuse and form the bulbar septum, separating the bulbus cordis into aortic and pulmonary trunks. **cerebral r's of cranial bones,** juga cerebralia ossium cranii. **deltoid r.,** tuberositas deltoidea humeri. **dental r.,** any linear elevation on the crown of a tooth named according to the surface on which it is located, such as buccal or lingual, or in recognition of some other characteristic. **dermal r's,** cristae cutis. **edentulous r.,** alveolar r., residual. **epicondylic r., lateral,** supracondylar r., lateral. **epicondylic r., medial,** supracondylar r., medial. **epipericardial r.,** a ventral ridge separating the ventral ends of the branchial arches in the embryo from the pericardial swelling. **gastrocnemial r.,** a ridge on the posterior surface of the femur, giving attachment to the gastrocnemius muscle. **genital r.,** the more medial portion of the urogenital ridge, which gives rise to the gonad. **germ r.,** genital r. **gluteal r. of femur,** tuberositas glutea femoris. **healing r.,** an indurated ridge that normally forms deep to the skin along the length of a healing wound and extends about 1 cm. on each side of the wound. **r. of humerus,** tuberositas deltoidea humeri. **incisal r.,** that portion of the crown of an anterior tooth which makes up the actual incisal portion. **interarticular r. of head of rib,** crista capitis costae. **interosseous r. of fibula,** margo interosseus fibulae. **interosseous r. of radius,** margo interosseus radii. **interosseous r. of tibia,** margo interosseus tibiae. **interosseous r. of ulna,** margo interosseus ulnae. **intertrochanteric r.,** crista intertrochanterica. **interureteric r.,** a smooth ridge extending across the bladder from one ureteral opening to the other, produced by a transverse bundle of muscle fibers; called also *plica interureterica* [NA], and *plica ureterica.* **linguocervical r., linguogingival r.,** cingulum (def. 3). **longitudinal r. of hard palate,** raphe palati. **Mall's r.,** pulmonary r. **mammary r.,** milk line. **r. of mandibular neck,** a blunt, smooth ridge passing obliquely downward and forward from the mandibular condyle on the medial surface of the mandibular neck and ramus, serving as their buttress. **marginal r.,** crista marginalis. **mesonephric r.,** the more lateral portion of the urogenital ridge, which gives rise to the mesonephros. **middle r. of femur,** linea pectinea femoris. **milk r.,** see under *line.* **mylohyoid r.,** linea mylohyoidea mandibulae. **r. of neck of rib,** crista colli costae. **r. of nose,** agger nasi. **oblique r.,** 1. an elevated crest of variable prominence, comprised jointly of the triangular ridge of the distobuccal cusp and the distal ridge of the mesiolingual cusp, coursing obliquely across the occlusal surface of the maxillary molars to link the apices of the distobuccal and the mesiolingual cusps. 2. tuberositas masseterica. **oblique r's of scapula,** lineae musculares scapulae. **palatine r's, transverse,** plicae palatinae transversae. **Passavant's r.,** see under *bar.* **pectoral r.,** crista tuberculi majoris. **pharyngeal r.,** Passavant's bar. **pterygoid r.,** crista infratemporalis. **pulmonary r.,** a ridge along the common cardinal vein in the embryo, which develops into the pleuropericardial membrane. **radial r. of wrist,** eminentia carpi radialis. **residual r.,** alveolar r., residual. **rough r. of femur,** linea aspera femoris. **semicircular r. of parietal bone, inferior,** linea temporalis inferior ossis parietalis. **semicircular r. of parietal bone, superior,** linea temporalis superior ossis parietalis. **skin r's,** cristae cutis. **sublingual r.,** frenulum linguae. **superciliary r.,** arcus superciliaris. **supinator r.,** crista musculi supinatoris. **supplemental r.,** an abnormal ridge on the surface of a tooth. **supracondylar r., of humerus, lateral,** crista supracondylaris lateralis humeri. **supracondylar r., of humerus, medial,** crista supracondylaris medialis humeri. **supraorbital r.,** arcus superciliaris. **suprarenal r.,** a caudal projection of the dorsal portion of the pleuroperitoneal membrane of the embryo, in which the adrenal cortex develops. **synaptic r.,** a wedge-shaped projection in the retina of a cone pedicle or of a rod spherule, on either side of which lie the horizontal cells whose dendrites are inserted into the ridge. **taste r's,** papillae foliatae. **tentorial r.,** a ridge on the inner surface of the cranium just above the groove for the transverse sinus, to which the tentorium is attached. **transverse r.,** crista transversalis. **transverse r's of sacrum,** lineae transversae ossis sacri. **transverse r's of vaginal wall,** rugae vaginales. **trapezoid r.,** linea trapezoidea. **triangular r.,** crista triangularis. **tuber-**

cular r. of sacrum, crista sacralis mediana. **ulnar r. of wrist,** eminentia carpi ulnaris. **urethral r.,** carina urethralis vaginae. **urogenital r.,** a longitudinal ridge or fold in the embryo, lateral to the root of the mesentery, which later subdivides longitudinally into the mesonephric and the genital ridge. **wolffian r.,** mesonephric r.

ridgel (rid′jel) ridgling.

ridging (rij′ing) in plastic surgery, a visible line or ridge at the margin of an area that has been surgically planed; occasionally encountered when beveling at the junction of treated and untreated areas has not been performed.

ridgling (rij′ling) an animal, especially a horse, with one or both testes undescended.

Ridley's sinus (rid′lēz) [Humphrey *Ridley,* English anatomist, 1653–1708] sinus circularis.

Riedel's lobe, thyroiditis (disease, struma) (re′delz) [Bernhard Moritz Carl Ludwig *Riedel,* surgeon in Jena, 1846–1916] see under *lobe* and *thyroiditis.*

Rieder's cell, cell leukemia, lymphocyte (re′derz) [Hermann *Rieder,* German roentgenologist, 1858–1932] see under *cell, leukemia,* and *lymphocyte.*

Riegel's pulse (re′-gelz) [Franz *Riegel,* German physician, 1843–1904] see under *pulse.*

Rieger's anomaly, syndrome (re′gerz) [Herwigh *Rieger,* German ophthalmologist, born 1898] see under *anomaly* and *syndrome.*

Riegler's test (rēg′lerz) [Emanuel *Riegler,* German chemist, 1854–1929] see under *tests.*

Riehl's melanosis (rēlz) [Gustav *Riehl,* Vienna dermatologist, 1855–1943] see under *melanosis.*

Riesman's pneumonia, sign (rēs′manz) [David *Riesman,* American physician, 1867–1940] see under *pneumonia* and *sign.*

Rieux's hernia (re-uhz′) [Léon *Rieux,* French surgeon] retrocecal hernia.

R.I.F. right iliac fossa.

Rifadin (rif′ah-din) trademark for a preparation of rifampin.

rifamide (rif′ah-mīd) chemical name: 4-*O*-[2-(diethylamino)-2-oxoethyl]rifamycin. A semisynthetic antibacterial antibiotic, $C_{43}H_{58}N_2O_{13}$, derived from rifamycin B, having the actions of the other rifamycins; it has been used in the treatment of respiratory infections due to gram-positive cocci and in biliary tract infections due to gram-negative and gram-positive organisms. See also *rifamycin.*

rifampicin (rif′am-pĭ-sin) the international nonproprietary name for rifampin.

rifampin (rif′am-pin) [USP] chemical name: 3-[[(4-methyl-1-piperazinyl)imino]methyl]rifamycin. A semisynthetic derivative of rifamycin SV, $C_{43}H_{58}N_4O_{12}$, occurring as a red-brown, crystalline powder, having the antibacterial actions of the rifamycin (q.v.) group of antibiotics; administered orally. Called also *rifampicin.*

rifamycin (rif″ah-mi′sin) any of a family of antibiotics biosynthesized by a strain of *Streptomyces mediterranei,* effective against a broad spectrum of bacteria, including gram-positive cocci, some gram-negative bacilli, and *Mycobacterium tuberculosis* and certain other mycobacteria. The five components are designated A, B, C, D, and E; rifamycins O, S, and SV are derivatives of the B component, and AG and X are derivatives of the O component. In the United States the rifamycins are used only for the initial treatment and re-treatment of pulmonary tuberculosis and for treatment of asymptomatic nasopharyngeal carriers of *Neisseria meningitidis;* they have been used in other countries to treat various infectious diseases due to susceptible organisms, such as leprosy, gonorrhea, and biliary tract and respiratory infections. Formerly called *rifomycin.*

rifomycin (rif″o-mi′sin) former name for rifamycin.

Riga-Fede disease [Antonio *Riga,* 1832–1919; Francesco *Fede,* 1832–1913] see under *disease.*

Riggs' disease (rigz) [John M. *Riggs,* American dentist, 1811–1885] marginal periodontitis.

right-handed (rīt-han′ded) using the right hand preferentially, or more skillfully than the left, in voluntary motor acts. See also *laterality.*

rigidity (rĭ-jid′ĭ-te) [L. *rigiditas; rigidus* stiff] stiffness or inflexibility, chiefly that which is abnormal or morbid; rigor.

anatomical r., rigidity of the cervix uteri in labor so that it dilates to only a limited extent, beyond which uterine contractions are of no avail. **cadaveric r.,** rigor mortis. **clasp-knife r.,** increased resistance of the extensors (induced by passive flexion of a joint), which suddenly gives way on exertion of further pressure. **cogwheel r.,** rigidity of a muscle which gives way in a series of little jerks when the muscle is passively stretched. **decerebrate r.,** the posture produced in an experimental animal by decerebration (q.v.), marked by rigid extension of the legs. It occurs in man as a result of lesions of the upper part of the brain stem and is manifested as follows: the patient lies in rigid extension with his arms internally rotated at the shoulder, extended at the elbow, and pronated, his fingers flexed at the interphalangeal joints and extended at the metacarpophalangeal joints, and his legs extended at the hips and knees, with the ankles and toes flexed. **hemiplegic r.,** rigidity of the paralyzed limbs in hemiplegia. **lead-pipe r.,** the diffuse muscular rigidity seen in parkinsonism. **mydriatic r.,** Westphal's pupillary reflex. **paratonic r.,** an intermittent abnormal increase in resistance to passive movement in a comatose patient. **pathologic r.,** rigidity of the cervix uteri in labor from some disease. **postmortem r.,** rigor mortis. **spasmodic r.,** rigidity of the cervix uteri due to spasmodic contraction.

rigor (rig′or, ri′gor) [L.] 1. a chill. 2. rigidity. **acid r.,** coagulation of the protein of muscle produced by acids. **calcium r.,** systolic cardiac arrest caused by an excess of calcium. **heat r.,** rigidity of muscles induced by heat. **r. mor′tis,** the stiffening of a dead body, accompanying the depletion of adenosine triphosphate in the muscle fibers. **r. tre′mens,** parkinsonism. **water r.,** a condition of rigor in a muscle caused by immersing it in water.

Riley-Day syndrome (ri′le da) [Conrad Milton *Riley*, American pediatrician, born 1913; Richard Lawrence *Day*, American pediatrician, born 1905] dysautonomia.

Riley-Smith syndrome (ri′le smith) [H. D. *Riley*, Jr., W. R. *Smith*] see under *syndrome*.

rim (rim) a border, or edge. **bite r.,** occlusion r. **occlusion r., record r.,** a border constructed on temporary or permanent denture bases for the purpose of recording the maxillomandibular relation and for positioning the teeth. Called also *bite-block, bitelock,,* and *bite r.*

rima (ri′mah), pl. *ri′mae* [L.] a cleft or crack; [NA] a general term for such an opening. **r. glot′tidis** [NA], the elongated opening between the true vocal cords and between the arytenoid cartilages; called also *fissure of glottis.* **r. glot′tidis cartilagin′ea,** pars intercartilaginea rimae glottidis. **r. glot′tidis membrana′cea,** pars intermembranacea rimae glottidis. **intercartilaginous r.,** pars intercartilaginea rimae glottidis. **intermembranous r.,** pars intermembranacea rimae glottidis. **r. o′ris** [NA], the longitudinal opening of the mouth, between the lips; called also *oral fissure.* **r. palpebra′rum** [NA], the longitudinal opening between the eyelids; called also *palpebral fissure.* **r. puden′di** [NA], the cleft between the labia majora in which the urethra and vagina open; called also *pudendal fissure.* **r. respirato′ria,** pars intercartilaginea rimae glottidis. **r. vestib′uli** [NA], the space between the right and left vestibular folds of the larynx; called also *fissure of vestibule.* **r. voca′lis,** pars intermembranacea rimae glottidis. **r. vul′vae,** r. pudendi.

Rimactane (rim-ak′tān) trademark for a preparation of rifampin.

rimae (ri′me) [L.] plural of *rima.*

rimal (ri′mal) pertaining to a rima.

rimantadine hydrochloride (ri-man′tah-dēn) chemical name: α-methyltricyclo[3.3.1³,⁷]-decane-1-methanamine hydrochloride. An antiviral agent, $C_{12}H_{21}N \cdot HCl$, which has been used in the prophylaxis of influenza type A.

Rimifon (rim′ĭ-fon) trademark for a preparation of isoniazid.

rimiterol hydrobromide (rim″ĭ-ter′ŏl) chemical name: (R^*,S^*)-α-(3,4-dihydroxyphenyl)-2-piperidinemethanol hydrobromide. An adrenergic, $C_{12}H_{17}NO_3 \cdot HBr$, used as a bronchodilator.

rimose (rim′ōs) [L. *rima* crack] marked by cracks and fissures.

rimula (rim′u-lah), pl. *rim′ulae* [L.] a minute fissure, especially of the spinal cord or brain.

rinderpest (rind′er-pest) [Ger. *Rinder* cattle + *pest* plague] cattle plague.

Rindfleisch's cells, folds (rint′flish-ez) [Georg Eduard *Rindfleisch*, German physician, 1836–1908] see *eosinophil,* and under *fold.*

ring (ring) [L. *annulus, circulus, orbiculus*] 1. any annular or circular organ or area; for names of specific anatomical structures, see under *annulus.* See also *circle* and *circulus.* 2. in chemistry, a collection of atoms united in a continuous or closed chain. **abdominal r., deep,** annulus inguinalis profundus. **abdominal r., external,** annulus inguinalis superficialis. **abdominal r., internal,** annulus inguinalis profundus. **abdominal r., superficial,** annulus inguinalis superficialis. **Albl's r.,** a ring-shaped shadow observed in a roentgenogram of the skull, caused by an aneurysm of a cerebral artery. **amnion r.,** the attached margin of the amnion about the umbilicus of the fetus. **annular r's,** round or oval opacities surrounding a translucent area in the roentgenogram, indicative of cavitation of the lung in tuberculosis; called also *pleural rings.* **apical r.,** polar r. **atrial r.,** the ring surrounding the opening between the atrium and ventricle of the primitive vertebrate heart; represented in the mammalian heart by the atrioventricular node. **Balbiani's r's,** a series of loops of the chromonemata of polytene chromosomes, similar in nature to chromosome puffs and in appearance to lampbrush chromosomes. **Bandl's r.,** pathologic retraction r.; see *retraction r.* **benzene r.,** the closed hexagon of carbon atoms in benzene (C_6H_6), from which the different benzene compounds are derived by replacement of the hydrogen atoms. **Bickel's r.,** Waldeyer's tonsillar ring. **Braun's r.,** pathologic retraction r.; see *retraction r.* **Cabot's r's,** see *Cabot's ring bodies,* under *body.* **Cannon's r.,** in the roentgenogram after a barium meal, a narrow area or focal contraction at the mid-third of the transverse colon, representing the junction of the primitive midgut and hindgut and marking an area of overlap between the superior and inferior nerve plexuses. **carbocyclic r.,** a chemical ring which includes only carbon atoms. **cardiac lymphatic r.,** annulus lymphaticus cardiae. **casting r.,** 1. a cylinder used as a container for the investment and mold during the process of casting. 2. refractory flask. **ciliary r.,** orbiculus ciliaris. **closing r. of Winkler-Waldeyer,** a slight thickening at the edge of the placenta, due to piling up of fetal and maternal tissues. **conjunctival r.,** annulus conjunctivae. **constriction r.,** a contracted area of the uterus, allegedly possible at any level, occurring where the resistance of the uterine contents is slight, as over a depression in the contour of the fetal body, or below the presenting part. Cf. *retraction r.* **contact r.,** the wound inflicted at the site of entrance of a bullet on the surface of the body. **contraction r.,** see *constriction r.* and *retraction r.* **coronary r.,** see under *band.* **crural r.,** annulus femoralis. **Döllinger's tendinous r.,** thickening of Descemet's membrane, forming an elastic ring around the limbus. **esophageal r.,** an annular constriction of the lower esophagus, usually at the junction of the esophageal and gastric mucosa. The term is sometimes used interchangeably with *esophageal web.* Called also *Schatzki's r.* **femoral r.,** annulus femoralis. **fibrocartilaginous r. of tympanic membrane,** annulus fibrocartilagineus membranae tympani. **fibrous r., interpubic,** discus interpubicus. **fibrous r's of heart,** annuli fibrosi cordis. **fibrous r. of intervertebral disk,** anulus fibrosus disci intervertebralis. **Fleischer r.,** an incomplete annular pigmented line at the base of the cone in keratoconus. **Fleischer-Strümpell r.,** Kayser-Fleischer r. **furan r.,** a ring containing four atoms of carbon and one of oxygen. **germ r.,** the proliferating marginal zone of the early blastoderm that is about to become the lips of the blastopore. **glaucomatous r.,** a light yellowish ring around the optic disk in glaucoma, indicating atrophy of the choroid. **r. of iris, greater,** annulus iridis major. **heterocyclic r.,** a chemical ring which includes atoms of different elements. **homocyclic r.,** a chemical ring in which all the members are atoms of the same element. **inguinal r., deep,** annulus inguinalis profundus. **inguinal r., external,** annulus inguinalis superficialis. **inguinal r., internal,** annulus inguinalis profundus. **inguinal r., superficial,** annulus inguinalis superficialis. **isocyclic r.,** homocyclic r. **Kayser-Fleischer r.,** a golden brown or green discoloration at the level of Descemet's membrane in the limbic region of the cornea seen in Wilson's disease and other liver disorders. **r. of iris, lesser,** annulus iridis minor. **Liesegang r's,** see under *phenomenon.* **Löwe's r.,** a ring in the visual field caused by the macula lutea. **Lower's r's,** annuli fibrosi cordis. **lymphoid r.,** Waldeyer's tonsillar ring. **Maxwell's r.,** a ring resembling Löwe's, but smaller and fainter. **neonatal r.,** see *neonatal line,* under *line.* **Newton's r's,** colored rings seen on the surface of thin, transparent membranes, as soap-bubbles, due to light wave interference. **Ochsner's r.,** a circular mucosal thickening at the opening of the pancreatic duct into the common bile duct. **periosteal bone r.,** see under *collar.* **pleural r's,** annular r's. **polar r.,** an electron-dense, annular, anterior thickening of the pellicle of apicomplexan protozoa, occurring at some stage in the life cycle, and forming part of the apical complex. Called also *apical r.* **pyran r.,** a ring containing five atoms of carbon and one of oxygen. **retraction r.,** a ringlike thickening and indentation occurring in normal labor at the junction of the isthmus and corpus uteri, delineating the upper contracting portion and the lower dilating portion (*physiologic retraction r.*), or a persistent retraction ring in abnormal or prolonged labor that obstructs expulsion of the fetus (*pathologic retraction r.*). Cf. *constriction r.* **Schatzki's r.,** esophageal r. **Schwalbe's r., Schwalbe's anterior border r.,** a circular ridge composed of collagenous fibers surrounding the outer margin of Descemet's membrane (lamina limitans posterior corneae). **signet r.,** ring form. **Soemmering's r.,** 1. a doughnut-shaped remnant of lens behind the pupil, occurring after cataract surgery or secondary to trauma as a result of contact between the anterior capsule and the posterior capsule, which traps varying amounts of lens substance peripherally; called also *Soemmering's ring cataract.* 2. a developmental cataract in which the primary lens cells fail to develop or are absorbed during intrauterine disease. Later developing subcapsular cells, having no fetal nucleus around which to grow, form doughnut-shaped ring cataracts. **tendinous r., common,** annulus tendineus communis. **tracheal r's,** cartilagines tracheales. **tympanic r.,** annulus tympanicus. **umbilical r.,** annulus umbilicalis. **vascular r.,** a developmental anomaly of the aortic arches wherein the trachea and esophagus are encircled by vascular structures, many variations being possible. **r. of Vieussens,** limbus fossae ovalis. **Vossius' r.,** a ring of pigment on the lens caused by pressure of the pupillary margin against the lens following a contusion. **Waldeyer's tonsillar r.,** the circular series of lymphoid tissue formed by the lingual, pharyngeal, and faucial tonsils. **Zinn's r.,** annulus tendineus communis.

ring-bone (ring'bōn) exostosis involving the first or second phalanx of the horse, resulting in lameness if the articular surfaces are affected. **low r.,** buttress foot.

Ringer's injection, irrigation (mixture, solution) (ring'erz) [Sydney *Ringer,* English physiologist, 1835–1910] see under *injection* and *irrigation.*

ringworm (ring'werm) popular name for tinea; so called because of the ring-shaped configuration of the lesions. **r. of the beard,** tinea barbae. **black-dot r.,** tinea capitis usually due to *Trichophyton tonsurans* and occasionally to *T. violaceum,* manifested as multiple areas of alopecia studded with black dots representing infected hairs broken off at or below the surfaces of the scalp. **r. of the body,** tinea corporis. **r. of the face,** tinea faciale. **r. of the feet,** tinea pedis. **gray-patch r.,** the classic form of tinea capitis, most often caused by *Microsporum audouinii* but also by *M. canis, M. ferrungineum,* and *M. gypseum,* and manifested by multiple gray scaly lesions, stubs of broken hairs, and minimal inflammatory response; it is benign and resolves spontaneously. **r. of the groin,** tinea cruris. **r. of the hand,** tinea manus. **honeycomb r.,** favus. **r. of the nails,** tinea unguium. **r. of the scalp,** tinea capitis.

Rinne's test (rin'nez) [Heinrich Adolf *Rinne,* German otologist, 1819–1868] see under *tests.*

Riolan's anastomosis, arch, etc. (re''o-lanz') [Jean *Riolan,* French physician and physiologist, 1580–1657] see under *anastomosis, arch, bone, muscle, nosegay,* and *ossicle.*

Riopan (ri'o-pan) trademark for preparations of magaldrate.

Ripault's sign (re-pōz') [Louis Henry Antoine *Ripault,* French physician, 1807–1856] see under *sign.*

ripazepam (rĭ-pah'zĕ-pam) chemical name: 1-ethyl-4,6-d hydro -3- methyl -8-phenypyrazolo[4,3-*e*][1,4]diazepin -5(1*H* one; a minor tranquilizer, $C_{15}H_{16}N_4O.$

R.I.P.H.H. Royal Institute of Public Health and Hygiene

risk (risk) [Fr. *risque,* from L. *rescare* to cut off] a dange or hazard, the probability of suffering harm. **attributa ble r.,** the arithmetic difference between the incidence rat of a disease among individuals exposed to a risk factor and th incidence rate among unexposed individuals. **empiric r.** the probability that a trait will occur or recur in a family based solely on experience rather than on knowledge of th causative mechanism. See also *genetic r.* **genetic r.,** th probability that a trait will occur or recur in a family, based on knowledge of its pattern of genetic transmission. See als *empiric r.* **relative r.,** the ratio of the incidence rate of ɛ disease among individuals exposed to a particular risk facto to the incidence rate among unexposed individuals.

Risley's prism (riz'lēz) [Samuel Doty *Risley,* American ophthalmologist, 1845–1920] see under *prism.*

risocaine (riz'o-kān) chemical name: 4-aminobenzoic acid propyl ester; a local anesthetic and antipruritic, $C_{10}H_{13}NO_2.$

RIST radioimmunosorbent test; see under *tests.*

Ristella melaninogenica (ris-tel'ah mel''ah-nin-o-jen'ĭ-kah) *Bacteroides melaninogenicus.*

ristocetin (ris''to-se'tin) an antibiotic substance produced by the fermentation of *Nocardia lurida;* formerly used in treatment of severe staphylococcal infections resistant to other antibiotics.

risus (ri'sus) [L.] laughter. **r. cani'nus,** r. sardonicus. **r. sardon'icus,** a grinning expression produced by spasm of the facial muscles; see *sardonic.*

Ritalin (rit'ah-lin) trademark for preparations of methylphenidate hydrochloride.

Ritgen maneuver (method) (rit'gen) [Ferdinand August Marie Franz von *Ritgen,* German gynecologist, 1787–1867] see under *maneuver.*

ritodrine (rit'o-drēn) chemical name: (*R**,*S**)-4-hydroxy-α-[1-[[2-(4-hydroxyphenyl)ethyl]amino]ethyl]benzene methanol. A beta$_2$-adrenergic agent, $C_{17}H_{21}O_3,$ used as a smooth muscle (uterine muscle) relaxant to delay uncomplicated premature labor.

Ritter's disease (rit'erz) [Gottfried *Ritter* von Rittershain, German physician, 1820–1883] staphylococcal scalded skin syndrome.

Ritter-Rollet phenomenon (sign) (rit'er-ro-la') [J. W. *Ritter*] see under *phenomenon.*

Ritter-Valli law [J. W. *Ritter;* Eusebio *Valli,* Italian physician, 1755–1816] see under *law.*

ritual (rich'u-al) in psychiatry, a series of repetitive acts performed compulsively to relieve anxiety, as in obsessive-compulsive neurosis.

rivalry (ri'val-re) a state of competition or antagonism. **binocular r., retinal r.,** the apparent alternate displacement of two figures when viewed together, there being no fusion into a continuous picture of the images of the two eyes. **sibling r.,** competition between siblings for the love, affection, and attention of one or both parents or for other recognition or gain.

Rivalta's reaction (test) (re-val'tahz) [Fabio *Rivalta,* pathologist in Bologna, born 1863] see under *reaction.*

Riva-Rocci sphygmomanometer (re''vah-ro'che) [Scipione *Riva-Rocci,* Italian physician, 1863–1937] see under *sphygmomanometer.*

Riverius' draft (re-ve're-us) Rivière's potion.

Rivière's potion (re''ve-ārz') [Lazare *Rivière,* French physician, 1589–1655] see under *potion.*

Riviere's sign (riv-ērz') [Clive *Riviere,* British physician, 1873–1929] see under *sign.*

Rivinus's ducts (canals), gland, incisure (foramen, notch, segment) (re-ve'nus) [Augustus Quirinus *Rivinus,* anatomist and botanist in Leipzig, 1652–1723] see *ductus sublinguales minores, glandula sublinguales,* and *incisura tympanica* [*Rivini*].

rivus (ri'vus), pl. *ri'vi* [L.] a brook, or little stream. **r. lacrima'lis** [NA], the pathway by which the tears reach the lacrimal lake from the excretory ductules of the lacrimal gland.

riziform (riz'ĭ-form) resembling grains of rice.

RKY   roentgenkymography.

R.L.L.   right lower lobe (of lungs).

R.M.A.   right mentoanterior (position of the fetus).

R.M.L.   right middle lobe (of lungs).

R.M.P.   right mentoposterior (position of the fetus).

R.M.T.   right mentotransverse (position of the fetus).

R.N.   Registered Nurse.

Rn   chemical symbol for *radon*.

RNA (ar′en-a)   ribonucleic acid. **messenger RNA, ribosomal RNA, soluble RNA, transfer RNA,** see definitions on *ribonucleic acid.*

RNase   ribonuclease I.

RNA-directed DNA polymerase (pol-im′er-ās) [EC 2.7.7.49]   an enzyme of the transferase class that catalyzes the reaction n deoxynucleoside triphosphate = n pyrophosphate + DNA$_n$. The enzyme occurs in oncogenic viruses of eukaryotic cells in the leukoviruses and in HIV viruses such as the AIDS virus. The reaction uses RNA as a template for the synthesis of single stranded DNA. Called also *reverse transcriptase.*

RNA directed RNA polymerase (pol-im′er-ās) [EC 2.7.7.48]   an enzyme of the transferase class that catalyzes the reaction n nucleoside triphosphate = n pyrophosphate + RNA$_n$. The enzyme uses RNA as a template for the synthesis of ribonucleic acids. It occurs in RNA viruses.

RNA nucleotidyltransferase (noo″kle-o-tīd′il-trans′-fer-ās)   DNA-directed RNA nucleotidyltransferase.

RNA polymerase (pol-im′er-ās)   see *DNA-directed RNA polymerase* and *RNA directed RNA polymerase.*

R.O.A.   right occipitoanterior (position of the fetus).

roach (rōch)   see *Blatta.*

roaring (rōr′ing)   a condition in the horse marked by a rough sound on inspiration and sometimes on expiration, due to some obstruction in the respiratory tract or to paralysis of the vocal cords.

Robalate (ro′bah-lāt)   trademark for preparations of dihydroxyaluminum aminoacetate.

Robaxin (ro-bak′sin)   trademark for preparations of methocarbamol.

Robbins (rob′inz), **Frederick Chapman.**   American pediatrician, born 1916; co-winner, with John Franklin Enders and Thomas Huckle Weller, of the Nobel prize in medicine or physiology for 1954 for the discovery that viruses (specifically, poliomyelitis viruses) can be grown in tissue culture and thereby be isolated and studied, making possible the production of vaccines.

robenidine hydrochloride (ro-ben′ĭ-den)   chemical name: bis[(4-chlorophenyl)methylene]carbonimidic dihydrazide monohydrochloride; a coccidiostat for poultry $C_{15}H_{13}$-Cl_2N·$_5HCl$.

Robert's ligament (ro-bārz′) [Cesar Alphonse *Robert,* French surgeon, 1801–1862]   see under *ligament.*

Robert's pelvis (ro′bārts) [Heinrich Ludwig Ferdinand *Robert,* German gynecologist, 1814–1874]   see under *pelvis.*

Roberts' test (rob′erts) [Sir William *Roberts,* English physician, 1830–1899]   see under *tests.*

Robertson's pupil (rob′ert-sunz)   see *Argyll Robertson,* and under *pupil.*

Robertson's sign (rob′ert-sunz) [William Egbert *Robertson,* American physician, 1869–1956]   see under *sign.*

robin (ro′bin)   a poisonous substance (phytotoxin) found in the bark of the North American locust tree (*Robinia pseudacacia*).

Robin's anomalad, syndrome (ro-baz′) [Pierre *Robin,* French pediatrician, 1867–1950]   Pierre Robin syndrome.

Robinson's circle (rob′in-sunz) [Frederick Byron *Robinson,* American anatomist, 1857–1910]   see under *circle.*

Robinul (ro′bĭ-nul)   trademark for preparations of glycopyrrolate.

Robison ester, ester dehydrogenase (ro′bĭ-sun) [Robert *Robison,* British chemist, 1884–1941]   see *glucose-6-phosphate,* and see under *dehydrogenase.*

Robitussin (ro″bĭ-tus′in)   trademark for preparations of guaifenesin.

roborant (rob′o-rant) [L. *roborans* strengthening]   conferring strength; strengthening.

Robson's line, point, position (rōb′sonz) [Sir Arthur William Mayo *Robson,* London surgeon, 1853–1933]   see under *line, point,* and *position.*

robust (ro-bust′)   in statistics, a somewhat imprecise term that is applied to a procedure that is relatively insensitive to violations of the assumptions on which it is based or to procedures that are based on weaker (more easily satisfied) assumptions, e.g., nonparametric tests.

Rocephin (ro-sef′in)   trademark for a preparation of ceftriaxone sodium.

Rochalimaea (ro″kah-li-me′ah) [H. da *Rocha-Lima*]   a genus of bacteria of the tribe Rickettsieae, family Rickettsiaceae, order Rickettsiales, resembling the genus *Rickettsia,* but usually found extracellularly in the arthropod host, and capable of growth in a cell-free medium. **R. quinta′na,** the etiologic agent of trench fever, transmitted by the body louse *Pediculus humanus.* Called also *Rickettsia quintana* and *Rickettsia wolhynica.*

rod (rod)   a straight, slim mass of substance; specifically, one of the rodlike bodies of the retina. See *retinal r's.* **Corti's r's,** *pillar cells;* see under *cell.* **enamel r's,** the approximately parallel rods or prisms forming the enamel of teeth. They are enclosed in a sheath of organic matter (the enamel rod sheath, or prism sheath) and are embedded in the interprismatic or cement substance. **r's of Heidenhain,** the rodlike cells of the renal tubules. **König's r's,** a series of steel bars each of which gives a note of certain pitch when struck. **Maddox r's,** a set of parallel cylindrical glass rods used in testing for heterophoria. The rods, placed before the eye, distort the image of a point source of light into a long streak perpendicular to the axis of the rods, interfere with fusion, and break up binocular vision. **Meckel's r.,** Meckel's cartilage. **muscle r.,** myofibril. **olfactory r.,** the slender apical portion of an olfactory bipolar neuron, a modified dendrite, extending as a cylindrical process from the nucleus to surface of the epithelium. **Reichmann's r.,** a short ivory rod with circular grooves and intervening projections, used in auscultatory percussion of the stomach. **retinal r.,** a visual cell that serves night vision and detection of motion. The synaptic terminal is a rounded spherule; the dendritic inner and outer segments are long and cylindrical; the membranous disks contain rhodopsin and are free saccules completely enclosed by the outer cell membrane. There are about 120 million rods in the retina—none in the foveola, the greatest concentration about 20 degrees away from the fovea, and a gradually decreasing density approaching the retinal periphery. Called also *rod* and *rod cell.* See also *retinal cone,* under *cone,* and *visual cell,* under *cell.*

rodenticide (ro-den′tĭ-sīd)   1. destructive to rodents.   2. any agent for destroying rodents.

rodentine (ro-den′tīn)   pertaining to a rodent.

rodocaine (ro′do-kān)   chemical name: *trans*-(2-chloro-6-methylphenyl)octahydropyrindine-1-propanamide; a local anesthetic, $C_{18}H_{25}ClN_2O$.

roentgen (rent′gen) [for Wilhelm Conrad *Röntgen,* German physicist, 1845–1923, who discovered roentgen rays in 1895; winner of the Nobel prize in physics for 1901]   the international unit of x- or γ-radiation. It is the quantity of x- or γ-radiation such that the associated corpuscular emission per 0.001293 gram of dry air (1 cm³ at 0° C and 760 mm Hg) produces in air ions carrying 1 electrostatic unit of electrical charge of either sign. Abbreviated R.

roentgenkymograph (rent″gen-ki′mo-graf)   the apparatus used in radiokymography.

roentgenkymography (rent″gen-ki-mog′rah-fe)   a technique of graphically recording the movements of an organ or structure on a single x-ray film; abbreviated RKY.

roentgenocardiogram (rent″gen-o-kar′de-o-gram)   a polygraphic tracing of cardiac pulsation made by roentgen rays.

roentgenocinematography (rent″gen-o-sin″ĕ-mah-tog′-rah-fe)   radiocinematography.

roentgenogram (rent-gen′o-gram″)   a film produced by roentgenography; radiograph.

roentgenograph (rent′gen-o-graf″)   radiograph.

roentgenographic (rent″gen-o-graf′ik)   radiographic.

roentgenography (rent″gen-og′rah-fe) [*roentgen* + Gr. *graphein* to write]   the making of a record (roentgenogram) of internal structures of the body by passage of x-rays through the body to act on specially sensitized film. See also *radiography*.

roentgenokymograph (rent″gen-o-ki′mo-graf)   roentgenkymograph.

roentgenologist (rent″gĕ-nol′o-jist)   a physician who specializes in diagnosis and treatment by roentgen rays; radiologist.

roentgenology (rent″gĕ-nol′o-je) [*roentgen rays* + *-logy*]   the branch of radiology which deals with the diagnostic and therapeutic use of roentgen rays. Cf. *radiology*.

roentgenolucent (rent″gen-o-lu′sent)   radiolucent.

roentgenometer (rent″gĕ-nom′ĕ-ter)   an instrument for measuring the intensity of roentgen rays.

roentgenometry (rent″gĕ-nom′ĕ-tre)   1. measurement of the intensity of x-rays. 2. the direct measurement of structures shown in the roentgenogram with or without the necessity of correcting for magnification.

roentgenopaque (rent″gen-o-pāk′)   radiopaque.

roentgenoparent (rent″gen-o-par′ent)   radioparent.

roentgenoscope (rent-gen′o-skōp)   a fluoroscope; an apparatus for examining the body by means of the fluorescent screen excited by the roentgen rays.

roentgenoscopy (rent″gĕ-nos′ko-pe) [*roentgen rays* + Gr. *skopein* to examine]   examination by means of roentgen rays; fluoroscopy.

roentgenotherapy (rent″gen-o-ther′ah-pe) [*roentgen rays* + Gr. *therapeia* treatment]   therapeutic use of roentgen rays.

roeteln (ret′eln) [Ger.]   rubella.

Roger's disease, reaction, symptom (ro-zhāz′) [Henri Louis *Roger*, French physician, 1809–1891]   see under *disease*, *reaction*, and *symptom*.

Roger-Josué test (ro-zha′ zho-zu-a′) [H. L. *Roger*; Otto *Josué*, French physician, 1869–1923]   see *blister test*, under *tests*.

Rogers' sphygmomanometer (roj′erz) [Oscar H. *Rogers*, American physician, born 1857]   see under *sphygmomanometer*.

Röhl's marginal corpuscles (rālz) [Wilhelm *Röhl*, German physician, 1881–1929]   see under *corpuscle*.

roka (ro′kah)   a tree of Arabia and Africa, *Trichilia emetica* Vahl.; it affords various remedial products.

Rokitansky's disease, diverticulum, pelvis (ro″kĭ-tan′skēz) [Karl Freiherr von *Rokitansky*, pathologist in Vienna, 1804–1878]   see *massive hepatic necrosis*, under *necrosis*, see *spondylolisthetic pelvis*, under *pelvis*, and see under *diverticulum*.

rolandic (ro-lan′dik)   described by or named in honor of Luigi *Rolando*.

Rolando (ro-lan′do), Luigi.   An Italian anatomist (1773–1831), known for his studies on the brain and spinal cord, who had a number of anatomical structures named in his honor. See under *angle*, *area*, *cell*, *fissure*, *line*, *point*, *substance*, *tubercle*, and *zone*.

rolandometer (ro″lan-dom′ĕ-ter)   an instrument for determining the positions of the various fissures of the surface of the brain.

role (rōl)   the behavior pattern that an individual presents to others.   **gender r.,** the image projected by a person that identifies him or her as being boy or girl, man or woman. It is the public expression of gender identity. Cf. *gender identity*, under *identity*.

roletamide (ro-let′ah-mīd)   chemical name: 3-(2,5-dihydro-1*H*-pyrrol-1-yl)-1-(3,4,5-trimethoxyphenyl)-2-propen-1-one; a hypnotic, $C_{16}H_{19}NO_4$.

rolitetracycline (ro-le-tet″rah-si′klen) [USP]   chemical name: [4S-(4α,4aα,5aα,6β,12aα)]-4-(dimethylamino)-1,4,4a,5,5a,6,11,12a-octahydro-3,6,10,12,12a-pentahydroxy-6-methyl-1,11,dioxo-*N*-(1-pyrrolidinylmethyl)-2-naphthacenecarboxamide. A semisynthetic broad-spectrum antibiotic of the tetracycline group, $C_{27}H_{33}N_3O_8$, occurring as a yellow, crystalline powder; used as an antibacterial, administered intravenously or intramuscularly.   **r. nitrate,** a salt of rotitetracycline, having the same actions and uses as the base.

roll (rōl)   a cylindrical structure.   **iliac r.,** a mass shaped like a sausage, located in the left iliac fossa and produced by a collection of feces or by induration of the walls of the

sigmoid fossa; called also *sigmoid sausage*.   **jelly r.,** see under *hypothesis*.   **scleral r.,** see under *spur*.

roller (rōl′er)   a small cylinder of rolled cotton, linen, or flannel for surgical use.

Roller's nucleus (rol′erz) [Christian Friedrich Wilhelm *Roller*, German neurologist, 1802–1878]   sublingual nucleus.

Rolleston's rule (rol′es-tonz) [Sir Humphrey Davy *Rolleston*, London physician, 1862–1944]   see under *rule*.

Rollet's stroma (rol′ets) [Alexander *Rollet*, Austrian physiologist, 1834–1903]   see under *stroma*.

Rollier's radiation, treatment (rol-yāz′) [Auguste *Rollier*, Swiss physician, 1874–1954]   see under *radiation* and *treatment*.

Romaña's sign (ro-mahn′yahz) [Cecilio *Romaña*, Brazilian physician]   see under *sign*.

romanoscope (ro-man′o-skōp) [L. *romanum* the sigmoid + Gr. *skopein* to examine]   sigmoidoscope.

Romanovsky's (Romanowsky's) stain (method) (ro″man-of′skēz) [Dimitri Leonidovich *Romanovsky*, Russian physician, 1861–1921]   see Table of Stains.

Romberg's disease (trophoneurosis), sign, spasm, station (rom′bergz) [Moritz Heinrich *Romberg*, physician in Berlin, 1795–1873]   see *facial hemiatrophy*, under *hemiatrophy*, and see under *sign*, *spasm*, and *station*.

rombergism (rom′berg-izm)   the tendency of a patient to fall when he closes his eyes while standing still with his feet close together (Romberg's sign), due to loss of joint position sensation, as in tabes dorsalis.

Romilar (ro′mil-ar)   trademark for preparations of dextromethorphan hydrobromide.

Rommelaere's sign (rom″el-a-erz′) [Guillaume *Rommelaere*, Belgian physician, 1836–1916]   see under *sign*.

Rondomycin (ron″do-mi′sin)   trademark for a preparation of methacycline hydrochloride.

rongeur (raw-zhur′) [Fr. "gnawing, biting"]   an instrument for cutting tough tissue, particularly bone.

Roniacol (ro-ni′ah-kol)   trademark for preparations of nicotinyl alcohol.

ronidazole (ro-nid′ah-zōl)   chemical name: 1-methyl-5-nitro-1*H*-imidazole-2-methanol carbamate (ester); a veterinary antiprotozoal, $C_6H_8N_4O_4$.

Rönne's nasal step (ren′ēz)   see under *step*.

ronnel (ron′el)   chemical name: phosphorothioic acid, *O,O*-dimethyl *O*-(2,4,5-trichlorophenyl) ester; a cholinesterase inhibitor, $C_8H_8Cl_3O_3PS$, used as an insecticide, effective against flies, roaches, screw worms, and cattle grub.

röntgenography (rent″gen-og′rah-fe)   roentgenography.

roof (roof)   a covering structure.   **r. of orbit,** paries superior orbitae.   **r. of skull,** calvaria.   **r. of tympanum,** tegmen tympani, def. 1.

room (rōōm)   a place in a building enclosed and set apart for occupancy or for performance of certain procedures.   **anechoic r.,** an echo-free room used for acoustical testing.   **delivery r.,** a hospital room to which an obstetrical patient is taken for delivery.   **intensive therapy r.,** intensive care unit.   **labor r.,** predelivery room.   **operating r.,** a room in a hospital equipped and used for surgical operations.   **postdelivery r.,** a recovery room for the care of obstetrical patients immediately after delivery.   **predelivery r.,** a hospital room where an obstetrical patient remains during the first stage of labor, i.e., from the time the pains begin until she is ready for delivery; called also *labor r*.   **recovery r.,** a hospital unit adjoining operating or delivery rooms, with special equipment and personnel for the care of postoperative or postpartum patients until they may safely be returned to general nursing care in their own rooms or wards.

rooming-in (rōōm′ing-in)   the practice of keeping a newly born infant in a crib near the mother's bed, instead of in a nursery, during the hospital stay.

root (root)   the lowermost part, or a structure by which something is firmly attached. For official names of various anatomical structures, see under *radix*.   **anatomical r.,** the portion of a tooth that is covered by cementum; see *radix dentis* [NA].   **r. of ansa cervicalis, inferior,** radix inferior ansae cervicalis.   **r. of ansa cervicalis, superior,** radix superior ansae cervicalis.   **r. of arch of vertebra,** pediculus arcus vertebrae.   **belladonna r.,** the dried root of *Atropa belladonna*, which contains various anticholinergic alkaloids; called also *deadly nightshade root.* See *belladonna.* **bitter r.,** gentian. **clinical r.,** radix clinica. **r. of clitoris,** crus clitoridis. **cochlear r. of vestibulocochlear nerve,** radix cochlearis nervi vestibulocochlearis. **cranial r's of accessory nerve,** radices craniales nervi accessorii. **dandelion r.,** taraxacum. **deadly nightshade r.,** belladonna r. **facial r.,** radix nervi facialis. **r. of hair,** radix pili. **insane r.,** hyoscyamus. **intermediate r. of olfactory trigone,** stria intermedia trigoni olfactorii. **licorice r.,** glycyrrhiza. **lingual r.,** that root of a posterior tooth, especially a maxillary molar, which is situated nearest the tongue. **long r. of ciliary ganglion,** radix nasociliaris ganglii ciliaris. **r. of lung,** radix pulmonis. **mandrake r.,** podophyllum. **r. of median nerve, lateral,** radix lateralis nervi mediani. **r. of median nerve, medial,** radix medialis nervi mediani. **r. of mesentery,** radix mesenterii. **motor r. of ciliary ganglion,** radix oculomotoria ganglii ciliaris. **motor r's of submandibular ganglion,** rami communicantes ganglii submandibularis cum nervo linguali. **motor r. of trigeminal nerve,** radix motoria nervi trigemini. **r. of nail,** radix unguis. **nasociliary r. of ciliary ganglion,** radix nasociliaris ganglii ciliaris. **nerve r's,** the series of paired bundles of nerve fibers which emerge at each side of the spinal cord, termed dorsal or posterior (see *radix dorsalis*), or ventral or anterior (see *radix ventralis*) according to their position. There are 31 pairs (8 cervical, 12 thoracic, 5 lumbar, 5 sacral, and 1 coccygeal), each corresponding dorsal and ventral root joining to form a spinal nerve. Called also *spinal r's.* Certain cranial nerves, e.g., the trigeminal, also have nerve roots. **r. of nose,** radix nasi. **oculomotor r. of ciliary ganglion,** radix oculomotoria ganglii ciliaris. **olfactory r., internal,** stria medialis trigoni olfactorii. **r. of optic tract, lateral,** radix lateralis tractus optici. **r. of optic tract, medial,** radix medialis tractus optici. **orizaba jalap r.,** ipomea. **orris r.,** orris. **palatine r.,** that root of a maxillary molar tooth which is situated nearest the palate; lingual root. **parasympathetic r. of ciliary ganglion,** radix oculomotoria ganglii ciliaris. **r. of penis,** radix penis. **physiological r.,** the portion of a tooth proximal to the gingival crevice, or embedded in the dental alveolus. **puccoon r., red r.,** sanguinaria. **retained r.,** 1. a tooth root, or part of a root, remaining in the soft tissue or in bone following trauma, extensive tooth decay, or incomplete extraction. 2. a tooth root intentionally retained to prevent resorption of the alveolar process. **sensory r. of ciliary ganglion,** radix nasociliaris ganglii ciliaris. **sensory r. of trigeminal nerve,** radix sensoria nervi trigemini. **short r. of ciliary ganglion,** radix oculomotoria ganglii ciliaris. **spinal r's,** nerve r's. **spinal r's of accessory nerve,** radices spinales nervi accessorii. **r. of spinal nerves, anterior,** radix ventralis nervorum spinalium. **r. of spinal nerves, dorsal,** radix dorsalis nervorum spinalium. **r. of spinal nerves, motor,** radix ventralis nervorum spinalium. **r. of spinal nerves, posterior,** radix dorsalis nervorum spinalium. **r. of spinal nerves, sensory,** radix dorsalis nervorum spinalium. **r. of spinal nerves, ventral,** radix ventralis nervorum spinalium. **sweet r.,** glycyrrhiza. **sympathetic r. of ciliary ganglion,** radix sympathica ganglii ciliaris. **r. of tongue,** radix linguae. **r. of tooth,** radix dentis. **vestibular r. of vestibulocochlear nerve,** radix vestibularis nervi vestibulocochlearis. **r. of vestibulocochlear nerve, inferior,** radix cochlearis nervi vestibulocochlearis. **r. of vestibulocochlear nerve, superior,** radix vestibularis nervi vestibulocochlearis.

rootlet (root'let) a small root or rootlike structure or a division of such a structure. **flagellar r.,** one of the delicate striated fibrils of the flagellar root system that arise from the basal body and run deep into the cytoplasm, perhaps serving as anchoring organelles or having a skeletal function. They occur most commonly in phytoflagellate protozoa, and were formerly thought to connect the basal body to the nucleus of the cell. Called also *rhizoblast* and *rhizoplast.*

R.O.P. right occipitoposterior (position of the fetus).

ropizine (ro'pĭ-zēn) chemical name: 4-(diphenylmethyl)-*N*-[(6-methyl-2-pyridinyl)methylene]-1-piperazinamine; an anticonvulsant, $C_{24}H_{26}N_4$.

Rorschach test (ror'shahk) [Hermann *Rorschach,* Swiss psychiatrist, 1884–1922] see under *tests.*

rosacea (ro-za'she-ah) a chronic hyperemic disease of the skin, usually involving the middle third of the face, characterized by persistent erythema and often by telangiectasia with acute episodes of edema, papules, and pustules, and usually affecting both men and women, although the most severe cases (see *rhinophyma,* and rosacea keratitis, under *keratitis*) are usually seen in men. Called also *acne rosacea.* **granulomatous r.,** rosacea in which discrete papules occur on the medial and lateral facial areas of the face as well as periorally; on diascopy the lesions appear as yellowish brown nodules, and as noncaseating epithelioid cell granulomas histologically. Called also *granulomatous r., lupoid r.,* and *micronodular* or *rosacea-like tuberculid.* **lupoid r.,** granulomatous r. **papular r.,** granulomatous r.

rosacic acid (ro-zas'ik) purpurin (def. 2).

rosamicin (ro"zah-mi'sin) a macrolide antibiotic, $C_{31}H_{51}NO_9$, derived from *Micromonospora rosaria,* having a broad spectrum of antibacterial activity against gram-positive bacteria and some activity against gram-negative bacteria; the butyrate, propionate, sodium phosphate, and stearate salts have antibacterial activity similar to that of the base.

rosaniline (ro-zan'ĭ-lin) a basic dye derived from triphenylmethane, $C_{20}H_{21}N_3O$, occurring as reddish brown crystals, which is soluble in acids and alcohol and slightly soluble in water. It is used, usually as the hydrochloride, in the preparation of other dyes and as a component of basic fuchsin.

rosary (ro'zah-re) a structure resembling a string of beads. **rachitic r.,** rachitic beads; see under *bead.*

rose (rōz) [L. *rosa*] any plant or species of the genus *Rosa.* The flowers of *R. gallica* L., *R. damascena* Mill., *R. alba* L., *R. centifolia* L., and varieties of these species afford rose oil. **r. bengal,** a dye, the dichlor- or the tetrachlorerythrosin, $NaO \cdot (C_6HI_2 \cdot O)_2C \cdot C_6H_2Cl_2 \cdot COONa$.

Rose's position (ro'zez) [Frank Atcherly *Rose,* British surgeon] see under *position.*

Rose's test (ro'zez) [Joseph Constantin *Rose,* German physician, 1826–1893] see under *tests.*

rosein (ro'ze-in) fuchsin.

Rosenbach's sign, syndrome (ro'zen-bahks) [Ottomar *Rosenbach,* physician in Berlin, 1851–1907] see under *sign* and *syndrome.*

Rosenmüller's body (organ), gland (node), valve, recess (cavity, fossa) (ro'zen-mil"erz) [Johann Christian *Rosenmüller,* German anatomist, 1771–1820] see *epoöphoron, nodi lymphatici inguinalis profundi, plica lacrimalis,* and *recessus pharyngeus.*

Rosenthal's canal (ro'zen-tahlz) [Isidor *Rosenthal,* German physiologist, 1836–1915] canalis spiralis modioli.

Rosenthal's test (ro'zen-thahlz) [Sanford Morris *Rosenthal,* American physician, born 1897] see under *tests.*

Rosenthal's vein (ro'zen-tahlz) [Friedrich Christian *Rosenthal,* German anatomist, 1779–1829] vena basalis.

roseola (ro-ze'o-lah, ro"ze-o'lah) [L.] 1. a rose-colored rash, as may be seen in measles, syphilis, and certain other exanthematous diseases. 2. exanthem subitum. **r. infan'tum,** exanthema subitum. **syphilitic r.,** an eruption of macular, rose-colored syphilids which is the earliest cutaneous manifestation of secondary syphilis.

Roser's sign (ro'zerz) [Wilhelm *Roser,* German surgeon, 1817–1888] see under *sign.*

roset (ro-zet') rosette.

rosette (ro-zet') [Fr. "little rose"] a structure, formation, or part occurring in a loosely attached cluster somewhat resembling a rose, such as (*a*) the clusters of polymorphonuclear leukocytes around a globule of lysed nuclear material, as observed in the test for disseminated lupus erythematosus; (*b*) a figure formed by the chromosomes in an early stage of mitosis; (*c*) a unique glandular complex present near the oral area of certain ciliate protozoa, the function of which is unclear; or (*d*) the symmetrical segmenter stage of certain malarial plasmodia, especially *Plasmodium malariae.* **E r.,** see under *assay.* **EAC r.,** see under *assay.*

rosin (roz'in) [L. *resina*] [NF] the solid resin obtained from *Pinus palustris* Mill. (Pinaceae) and other species of pine, occurring as sharply angular, translucent, amber-colored fragments, frequently covered with yellow dust. It contains about 90 per cent resin and 10 per cent neutral matter. Most of the resin acids are isomeric with abietic acid, $C_{44}H_{62}O_4$. It is used as a stiffening agent in the preparation of plasters and ointments. Formerly called *colophony*.

Rosin's test (ro′zenz) [Heinrich *Rosin*, German physician, born 1863] see under *tests*.

Rosmarinus (ros″mah-ri′nus) [L. "sea-dew"] a genus of labiate plants. *R. officina′lis*, L., or common rosemary, affords the fragrant volatile oil of rosemary.

rosoxacin (ro-soks′ah-sin) chemical name: 1-ethyl-1,4-dihydro-4-oxo-7-(4-pyridinyl)-3-quinolinecarboxylic acid; an antibacterial, $C_{17}H_{14}N_2O_3$.

Ross (ros) Sir Ronald. British physician and protozoologist, 1857–1932; winner of the Nobel prize for medicine or physiology in 1902 for his demonstration of the life history of the malarial parasite *Plasmodium* in the stomach of the *Anopheles* mosquito and its transmission by the bite of the female anopheline mosquito.

Ross' black spores (ros′ez) [Sir Ronald *Ross*] see under *spore*.

Ross' bodies (ros′ez) [Edward Halford *Ross*, English pathologist, 1875–1928] see under *body*.

Rossbach's disease (ros′bahks) [Michael Josef *Rossbach*, German physician, 1842–1894] hyperchlorhydria.

Rossolimo's reflex (sign) (ros″o-le′mōz) [Gregorij Ivanovich *Rossolimo*, Russian neurologist, 1860–1928] see under *reflex*.

Rostan's asthma (ros-tahz′) [Louis Léon *Rostan*, Paris physician, 1790–1866] cardiac asthma.

rostellum (ros-tel′um), pl. *rostel′la* [L. "little beak"] a small protuberance or beak, especially the fleshy protuberance of the scolex of a tapeworm, which may or may not bear hooks.

rostrad (ros′trad) 1. toward a rostrum; situated nearer the rostrum in relation to a specific point of reference. 2. cephalad.

rostral (ros′tral) [L. *rostralis*, from *rostrum* beak] 1. pertaining to or resembling a rostrum; having a rostrum or beak. 2. situated toward a rostrum or toward the beak (oral and nasal region), which may mean superior (in relationships of areas of the spinal cord) or anterior or ventral (in relationships of brain areas).

rostralis (ros-tra′lis) [L.] rostral.

rostrate (ros′trāt) [L. *rostratus* beaked] having a beaklike process.

rostriform (ros′tri-form) [L. *rostrum* beak + *forma* form] shaped like a beak.

rostrum (ros′trum), pl. *ros′trums* or *ros′tra* [L. "beak"] a beaklike appendage or part; [NA] a general term for such a structure. **r. cor′poris callo′si** [NA], **r. of corpus callosum,** the anterior and lower end of the corpus callosum. **sphenoidal r., r. sphenoida′le** [NA], the prominent ridge on the inferior surface of the sphenoid bone that articulates with a deep depression between the wings of the vomer.

R.O.T. right occipitotransverse (position of the fetus).

Rot see *Roth*.

rot (rot) 1. decay. 2. a disease of sheep, and sometimes of man, caused by *Fasciola hepatica*. **Barcoo r.,** desert sore. **black r.,** a condition sometimes seen in storage eggs, even when kept in a refrigerator; it is caused by *Proteus melanovogenes*. **foot r.,** a disease of the feet of cattle and sheep, marked by decay of the hoof and an offensive discharge; it is caused by *Fusobacterium necrophorum* in cattle and *Bacteroides nodosus* in sheep, especially on soft, wet pasture. Called also *leg ill*. **liver r.,** a disease of sheep and cattle caused by the liver fluke, *Fasciola hepatica*. **pizzle r.,** enzootic balanoposthitis. **sheath r.,** enzootic balanoposthitis.

Rotaliina (ro″tah-li′i̇-nah) [L. *rotalis* wheel] a suborder of protozoa (order Foraminiferida, class Granuloreticulosea) having a calcareous, hyaline test. Fossil and recent species are known.

rotameter (ro-tam′ĕ-ter) a flow-rate meter of variable area with a rotating float in a tapered tube, used for measuring the gases in administering an anesthetic.

rotary (ro′ter-e) marked by or produced by rotation.

rotate (ro′tāt) to turn around an axis; to twist.

rotation (ro-ta′shun) [L. *rotare* to turn] 1. the process of turning around an axis; movement of a body about its axis, called the *axis of rotation*. 2. the turning of the fetal head through 90 degrees during labor so that the long diameter of the head corresponds with the long diameter of the pelvic outlet. It should occur naturally, but if it does not the rotation must be accomplished manually or instrumentally by the obstetrician. See also *maneuver*. 3. a turning around a central axis without undergoing any displacement from the axis. See also *hinge movement*, under *movement*. 4. a procedure whereby a malturned tooth is turned into its normal position. 5. malposition due to an abnormal turning of a tooth around its longitudinal axis. **molecular r.,** the figure obtained by multiplying the specific rotation by the molecular weight and dividing by 100. **optical r.,** the quality of certain optically active substances whereby the plane of polarized light is changed, so that it is rotated in an arc the length of which is characteristic of the substance. **specific r.,** the arc through which a substance rotates the plane of polarization as observed in a polarimeter. **van Ness r.,** fusion of the knee joint and rotation of the ankle to function as the knee; done to correct a congenitally missing femur.

rotatory (ro′tah-to′re) occurring in or caused by rotation.

rotavirus (ro′tah-vi″rus) [L. *rota* wheel + *virus*] a group of doubled-stranded RNA viruses having a wheel-like appearance and responsible for acute infantile gastroenteritis and for diarrhea in several animal species and in young children.

Rotch's sign (roch′es) [Thomas Morgan *Rotch*, physician in Boston, 1849–1914] see under *sign*.

röteln (ret′eln) [Ger.] rubella.

rotenone (ro′tĕ-nōn) a poisonous compound, $C_{23}H_{22}O_6$, from derris root and other roots; used as an insecticide and as a scabicide.

rotexed (ro′tekst) rotated and bent to one side.

rotexion (ro-tek′shun) act of rotating and flexing; also the state of being rotated and flexed.

Roth's (Rot's) disease, syndrome (rōts) [Vladimir Karlovich *Roth*, Russian neurologist, 1848–1916] meralgia paraesthetica.

Roth's spots, vas aberrans (rōts) [Moritz *Roth*, Swiss physician, 1839–1915] see under *spot*, and see *ductuli aberrantes*.

Roth-Bernhardt disease, syndrome (rōt-bern′hart) [Vladimir K. *Roth*, Russian neurologist, 1848–1916; Martin *Bernhardt*, neurologist in Berlin, 1844–1915] meralgia paraesthetica.

Rothia (roth′e-ah) [Genevieve D. *Roth*] a genus of bacteria of the family Actinomycetaceae, order Actinomycetales, made up of aerobic, gram-positive, nonacid-fast, nonspore-forming organisms occurring in coccoid, diphtheroid, and branched filament forms. **R. dentocario′sus,** a species found in the oral cavity of man and other primates, particularly in plaque and calculus deposits on the teeth and in carious material. Called also *Actinomyces dentocariosus*.

Rothman-Makai syndrome (rōt′mahn maw′koi) [Max *Rothman*, German pathologist, 1868–1915; Endre *Makai*, Hungarian surgeon, 20th century] see under *syndrome*.

Rothmund-Thomson syndrome (rōt′mund tom′son) [August von *Rothmund*, Jr., German physician, 1830–1906; Mathew Sidney *Thomson*, English dermatologist, 1894–1969] see under *syndrome*.

rotifer (ro′ti-fer) any individual of the class Rotifera.

Rotifera (ro-tif′er-ah) [L. *rota* wheel + *ferre* to bear] a class of small, usually transparent, mostly free-living animals of the phylum Aschelminthes, the rotifers, which characteristically possess a corona of cilia around the anterior end, a cleft foot at the posterior end, and internal jaws. In some systems of classification, they are considered to be a separate phylum.

rotlauf (rot′lowf) [Ger.] swine erysipelas.

rotoxamine (ro-toks′ah-mēn) chemical name: (-)-2-[(4-chlorophenyl)(2-pyridinyl)methoxy]-*N*,*N*-dimethylethanamine. The *l*-isomer of carbinoxamine, $C_{16}H_{19}ClN_2O$, having antihistaminic potency about twice that of the racemic form. **r. tartrate,** the tartrate salt of rotoxamine, $C_{16}H_{19}ClN_2O\cdot C_4H_6O_4$, occurring as a white to creamy white, crystalline powder, having the same actions as the base; used in the treatment of allergic disorders, administered orally.

Rotter's test (rot′erz) [H. *Rotter*, physician in Budapest] see under *tests*.

rottlera (rot′ler-ah) kamala.

rottlerin (rot′ler-in) a powerful and toxic chromene derivative, $C_{30}H_{28}O_8$, obtained from *Kamala* or *Mallotus philippinensis* (Lam.) Muell.-Arg. (Euphorbiaceae); called also *mallotoxin*.

rotz (rōts) [Ger.] glanders in horses.

rouge (roozh) a fine red powder composed of iron oxide (Fe_2O_3), usually in cake form but sometimes impregnated on paper or cloth; used in dentistry as a polishing agent for restorations of gold and precious metal alloys.

rouget du porc (roo-zha′ du pork′) [Fr.] the urticarial form of swine erysipelas.

Rouget's bulb (roo-zhāz′) [Antoine D. *Rouget*, French physiologist] bulb of the ovary.

Rouget's cells, muscle (roo-zhāz′) [Charles Marie Benjamin *Rouget*, French physiologist and anatomist, 1824–1904] see *pericyte*, and see under *cell*.

rough (ruf) not smooth; having an irregular, roughened surface.

roughage (ruf′ij) indigestible material such as fibers, cellulose, etc., in the diet.

Rougnon-Heberden disease (roon-yaw′-heb′er-den) [Nicholas François *Rougnon* de Magny, French physician, 1727–1799; William *Heberden*, Sr., English physician, 1710–1801] angina pectoris.

rouleau (roo-lo′), pl. *rouleaux′* [Fr. "roll"] a roll of red blood corpuscles like a pile of coins.

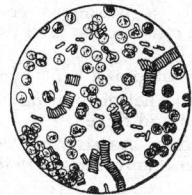

Human red blood cells arranged in rouleaux.

rouleaux (roo-lo′) [Fr.] plural of *rouleau*.

roundworm (rownd′wurm) any worm of the class Nematoda; a nematode.

Rous (rows) Francis Peyton. American pathologist, 1879–1970; co-winner, with Charles Brenton Huggins, of the Nobel prize for medicine or physiology in 1966 for his discovery of tumor-inducing viruses in 1910.

Rous sarcoma, test (rows) [Francis Peyton *Rous*] see under *sarcoma* and *tests*.

Roussy-Dejerine syndrome (roo-se′-deh″zher-ēn′) [Gustave *Roussy*, French pathologist, 1874–1948; Joseph Jules *Dejerine*, French neurologist, 1849–1917] thalamic syndrome.

Roussy-Lévy syndrome (disease, hereditary ataxic dystasia) (roo-se′ la′ve) [Gustave *Roussy*; Gabrielle *Lévy*, French neurologist, 1886–1935] see under *syndrome*.

Roux's anastomosis (rooz) [César *Roux*, Swiss surgeon, 1857–1926] see *Roux-en-Y anastomosis*.

Roux-en-Y see under *anastomosis*.

Rovighi's sign (ro-vig′ēz) [Alberto *Rovighi*, Bologna physician, 1856–1919] see under *sign*.

Rowntree-Geraghty test (roun′tre-ger′ah-te) [Leonard George *Rowntree*, American physician, born 1883; John Timothy *Geraghty*, Baltimore physician, 1876–1924] the phenolsulfonphthalein test.

RPF renal plasma flow.

R. Ph. abbreviation for Registered Pharmacist.

rpm revolutions per minute.

RPS renal pressor substance.

R.Q. respiratory quotient.

-rrhage, -rrhagia [Gr. *rhegnynai* to burst forth] word terminations denoting abnormal or excessive flow.

-rrhaphy [Gr. *rhaphē* suture] a word termination denoting suture or operative repair.

-rrhea [Gr. *rhoia* flow] a word termination denoting flow or discharge.

R.R.L. Registered Record Librarian.

rRNA ribosomal RNA; see *ribonucleic acid*.

R.S.A. right sacroanterior (position of the fetus).

R.Sc.A. right scapuloanterior (position of the fetus).

R.S.C.N. Registered Sick Children's Nurse.

R.Sc.P. right scapuloposterior (position of the fetus).

R.S.M. Royal Society of Medicine.

R.S.N.A. Radiological Society of North America.

R.S.P. right sacroposterior (position of the fetus).

R.S.T. right sacrotransverse (position of the fetus).

R.S.T.M.H. Royal Society of Tropical Medicine and Hygiene.

RSV Rous sarcoma virus.

RTF resistance transfer factor.

R.U. rat unit.

Ru chemical symbol for *ruthenium*.

rub (rub) an auscultatory sound caused by the rubbing together of two serous surfaces, as in pericardial rub; called also *friction r*. **friction r.,** see *rub*. **pericardial r.,** a scraping or grating noise heard with the heart beat, usually a to-and-fro sound, associated with an inflamed pericardium. **pleural r., pleuritic r.,** a rub produced by friction between the visceral and costal pleurae.

rubber dam (rub′er-dam) see under *dam*.

rubefacient (roo″bĕ-fa′shent) [L. *ruber* red + *facere* to make] 1. reddening the skin. 2. an agent that reddens the skin by producing active or passive hyperemia.

rubella (roo-bel′ah) [L. from *rubellus* reddish, from *ruber* red] an acute, usually benign, infectious disease caused by a togavirus and most often affecting children and nonimmune young adults, in which the virus enters the respiratory tract via droplet nuclei and spreads to the lymphatic system. It is characterized by a slight cold, sore throat, and fever, followed by enlargement of the postauricular, suboccipital, and cervical lymph nodes, and the appearance of a fine pink rash that begins on the head and spreads to become generalized. Transplacental infection of the fetus as a result of maternal infection in the first trimester can cause death of the conceptus or severe developmental abnormalities in the newborn infant (see *congenital rubella syndrome*, under *syndrome*). Called also *German measles, roeteln, röteln,* and *three-day measles,* and *rubeola* in French and Spanish.

rubeola (roo-be′o-lah, roo-be-o′lah) [dim. of h. *rubeus* red] 1. measles. 2. in French and Spanish, rubella.

rubeosis (roo″be-o′sis) redness. **r. i′ridis,** a condition characterized by a new formation of vessels and connective tissue on the surface of the iris, frequently seen in diabetics (*r. i′ridis diabe′tica*) and following occlusion of the central retinal vein or artery. It gives rise to severe intractable glaucoma. **r. re′tinae,** a name proposed for a condition characterized by formation of new vessels in front of the optic papilla in retinitis proliferans, seen in nondiabetics, as well as in diabetics (*r. re′tinae diabe′tica*), and usually leading to retinal detachment.

ruber (roo′ber) [L.] red.

rubescent (roo-bes′ent) [L. *rubescere* to become red] reddish; becoming red.

rubidiol (roo-bid′e-ol) a solution in oil of rubidium and potassium mercuric iodide, used externally as a resolvent.

rubidium (roo-bid′e-um) [L. *rubidus* red] a rare metallic alkaline element; atomic number, 37; atomic weight, 85.47; symbol, Rb. **r. and ammonium bromide,** a substance, $RbBr + 3NH_4Br$, used like potassium bromide.

rubidomycin (roo-bid′o-mi″sin) daunorubicin.

rubiginous, rubiginose (roo-bij′ĭ-nus; roo-bij′ĭ-nōs) [L. *rubigo* rust] having a rusty, brownish color; said of sputum.

rubin (roo′bin) fuchsin.

Rubin's test (roo′binz) [Isidor Clinton *Rubin*, New York physician, 1883–1958] see under *tests*.

Rubner's law, test (roob′nerz) [Max *Rubner*, German physiologist, 1854–1932] see under *law* and *tests*.

rubor (roo′bor) [L.] redness, one of the cardinal signs of inflammation.

rubriblast (roo′brĭ-blast) pronormoblast.

rubric (roo′bric) red; specifically, pertaining to the red nucleus.

rubricyte (roo′brĭ-sīt) [L. *rubrum* red + Gr. *kytos* cell] polychromatic normoblast.

rubrospinal (roo″bro-spi′nal) pertaining to the red nucleus and the spinal cord.

rubrothalamic (roo″bro-thah-lam′ik) pertaining to the red nucleus and the thalamus.

rubrum (roo′brum) [L.] red. **r. Con′go,** Congo red. **r. scarlati′num,** scarlet red.

Rubus (roo′bus) [L.] a genus of rosaceous plants, including the blackberries, raspberries, brambles, dewberries, and cloudberries. The root barks of several species of blackberry are tonic and astringent, and have been used in diarrhea. The fruits of R. *idae′us* L. and R. *strigo′sus* Michx. (Rosaceae), red raspberries, are used in pharmacy as vehicles for syrups, etc. See *raspberry juice,* under *juice.*

ructus (ruk′tus) [L.] the belching of wind; eructation.

Rudbeckia (rud-bek′e-ah) [O. *Rudbeck,* 1630–1702, and O. *Rudbeck,* Jr., 1660–1740] a genus of composite-flowered herbs of North America; the cone flower, R. *lacinia′ta,* thimble weed, is diuretic and tonic.

rudiment (roo′dĭ-ment) 1. primordium; the first indication of a structure in the course of its development. 2. a structure that has remained undeveloped, or one with little or no function at present but which was functionally developed earlier either in the individual or in its phylogenetic ancestors. **lens r.,** a thickening of the ectoderm of the sides of the embryonic head, from which the crystalline lens develops. **r. of vaginal process,** vestigium processus vaginalis.

rudimentary (roo″dĭ-men′tah-re) 1. imperfectly developed. 2. vestigial.

rudimentum (roo″dĭ-men′tum), pl. *rudimen′ta* [L. "a first beginning"] 1. [NA] the first indication of a structure in the course of its development; a primordium. 2. a vestigial structure. **r. processus vaginalis,** vestigium processus vaginalis.

Rudimicrosporea (roo″dĭ-mi″kro-spor′e-ah) [*rudiment* + *micro-* + *spore*] a class of protozoa (phylum Microspora) found as hyperparasites of gregarines in annelids, the spores of which have a simple extrusion apparatus consisting of a polar cap and a thick polar tube extending backward from the cap, bending laterally and terminating in an infundibulum; a polaroplast and posterior vacuole are absent. It comprises one order: Metchnikovellida.

rue (roo) [L. *Ruta*] the rutaceous herb, *Ruta graveolens;* the volatile oil (*oleum rutae*) from the leaves is an irritant poison.

Rufen (roo′fen) trademark for preparations of ibuprofen.

rufescine (roo′fĕ-sin) a substance obtained from a mollusk, *Haliotis rufescens,* which corresponds to the bile pigments in man.

Ruffini's brushes (organ), corpuscles (cylinders) (roo-fe′nēz) [Angelo *Ruffini,* Italian anatomist, 1864–1929] see under *brush* and *corpuscle.*

rufiopin (roo″fe-o′pin) a reddish yellow, crystalline substance, $C_{14}H_8O_4$, derivable from opianic acid, and isomeric with rufigallic acid.

rufous (roo′fus) [L. *rufus* red] erythristic.

ruga (roo′gah), pl. *ru′gae* [L.] a ridge, wrinkle, or fold, as of mucous membrane. **rugae gas′tricae,** rugae of stomach. **ru′gae palati′nae, palatine rugae,** plicae palatinae transversae. **rugae of stomach,** large folds of the mucous membrane of the stomach, occurring especially in the corpus, which are seen when the stomach is empty or undistended. **rugae of vagina, ru′gae vagina′les** [NA], small transverse folds of the mucous membrane of the vagina extending outward from the columns.

rugae (roo′je) [L.] plural of *ruga.*

rugine (roo-zhēn′) a raspatory.

rugitus (roo′jĭ-tus) [L. "roaring"] rumbling in the intestines caused by movement of flatus; see *borborygmus.*

rugose, rugous (roo′gōs, roo′gus) [L. *rugosus*] characterized by wrinkles.

rugosity (roo-gos′ĭ-te) [L. *rugositas*] 1. the condition of being wrinkled. 2. a fold, wrinkle, or ruga.

R.U.L. right upper lobe (of a lung).

rule (rōōl) [L. *regula*] a statement of conditions commonly observed in a given situation, or a statement of a prescribed course of action to obtain a result. **Abegg's r.** (obs.), all atoms have the same number of valences. **Allen's r.,** the

extended body parts of warm-blooded species (tail, ears, and limbs) are relatively shorter in the colder regions of a species range than in the warmer. **Arey's r.,** the total length of an embryo or fetus in inches, for the first five months, equals the numerical sum of the number of the previous lunar months since conception; for the last five lunar months, it equals the product of the number of the month multiplied by 2. **Bartholomews' r. of fourths,** if the uterine fundus is one-fourth of the way from the pubic symphysis to the umbilicus, the pregnancy is of two months duration; one-half of the way, three months duration; three-quarters of the way, four months duration; at the umbilicus, five months duration. The fundus then rises one-quarter of the way to the ensiform process each month until the ninth, when it sinks to the level it occupied at eight months. **Bastedo's r.,** the dose of a drug for a child is obtained by multiplying the adult dose by the child's age in years, adding 3 to the product, and dividing the sum by 30. **Bergmann's r.,** the body size of geographical races of warm-blooded species is smaller in the warmer parts of the species range than in the colder parts of the range. **Budin's r.,** a bottle-fed baby should not take more than $\frac{1}{10}$ of its own weight of cow's milk per day. **Clark's r.,** the dose of a drug for a child is obtained by multiplying the adult dose by the weight of the child in pounds and dividing the result by 150. **Cowling's r.,** the dose of a drug for a child is obtained by multiplying the adult dose by the age of the child at his next birthday and dividing by 24. **delivery date r.,** Nägele's r. **dermatomal r.,** visceral pain is referred to the dermatomes supplied by the posterior roots through which the visceral afferent impulses reach the spinal cord. **Durham r.,** a definition of criminal responsibility from a 1954 federal court of appeals case, Durham vs. United States; the court held that "an accused is not criminally responsible if his unlawful act was the product of mental disease or mental defect." In 1972 the same court reversed itself and adopted the American Law Institute formulation (see under *formulation*). **Fried's r.,** the dose of a drug for an infant less than 2 years old is obtained by multiplying the child's age in months by the adult dose and dividing the result by 150. **Gibson's r.,** in pneumonia, if the pulse pressure in millimeters of mercury does not fall below the pulse rate, the prognosis is good; if it does, prognosis is bad. **Haase's r.,** the total length of an embryo or fetus in centimeters, for the first five months, equals the square of the number of lunar months since conception; for the last five months it equals the product of the number of the month multiplied by 5. **Hardy-Weinberg r.,** see under *law.* **Hudson's lactone r.,** molecular optical rotation of a carbohydrate or its derivatives is given as the sum of the rotation contributions at each asymmetric center. Certain other empirical conclusions may also be drawn from existing data. **Jackson's r.,** after epileptic attacks, simple nervous processes are more quickly recovered from than complex ones. **Liebermeister's r.,** in febrile tachycardia, the pulse beats increase at the rate of about eight to every degree centigrade of temperature. **Lossen's r.,** in hemophilia, only women transmit the condition, only men inherit it. **McDonald's r.,** the length in centimeters of the abdominal contour from the upper margin of the pubic symphysis to the fundus divided by 3.5 gives the duration of pregnancy in lunar months. **M'Naghten r.,** a definition of criminal responsibility formulated in 1843 by English judges questioned by the House of Lords as a result of the acquittal of Daniel M'Naghten on grounds of insanity. It holds that "to establish a defense on the ground of insanity, it must be clearly proved that, at the time of committing the act, the party accused was laboring under such a defect of reason, from disease of the mind, as not to know the nature and quality of the act he was doing, or, if he did know it, he did not know he was doing what was wrong" and further that a defendant who "labors under partial delusions only and is not in other respects insane ... must be considered in the same situation as to responsibility as if the facts with respect to which the delusion exists were real." These rules are still used in many American jurisdictions. **Nägele's r.** (for predicting day of labor), subtract three months from the first day of the last menstruation and add seven days. **octet r.,** when atoms combine to form molecules, they tend to share or transfer electrons until eight (four pairs) are in the valence shell of each atom. **phase r.,** a homogeneous chemical substance of n components is capable of $n + 1$ modifications of phase; e.g., the phases of H_2O are ice, water, and steam. A heterogeneous chemical system of p coexistent phases and c variable components has

$p + 2 - c$ degrees of freedom or variations of phase, i.e., the sum of its coexistent phases and its possible changes of phase exceeds the number of its components by 2. **Quetelet's r.,** the body weight of an adult ought to be as many kilograms as his body length in centimeters exceeds 100. **Rolleston's r.,** the ideal systolic pressure for an adult is the figure represented by 100 plus half the age in years. **van't Hoff's r.,** the velocity of chemical reactions is increased twofold or more for each rise of 10° C. in temperature; called also *van't Hoff's law.* Cf. *temperature coefficient,* under *coefficient.* **Weinberg's r.,** the total number of dizygotic twins in any population is twice the number of twins of different sex, and the sum of these subtracted from the total number of all twins gives the number of monozygotic twins. **Young's r.,** the dose of a drug for a child is obtained by multiplying the adult dose by the age in years and dividing the result by the sum of the child's age plus 12.

rumbatron (rum′bah-tron) a high efficiency radio oscillator in which atoms are shattered and which employs electrons as the bombarding particles.

rumen (roo′men) the first stomach of a ruminant, or cud-chewing animal; also called *paunch.*

rumenitis (roo″mĕ-ni′tis) inflammation of the rumen.

rumenotomy (roo″mĕ-not′o-me) [*rumen* + Gr. *tomē* a cutting] the operation of cutting into the rumen of an animal for the purpose of removing foreign bodies or impacted food or for evacuating gases.

ruminant (roo′mĭ-nant) 1. chewing the cud. 2. one of the order of animals which have a stomach with four complete cavities (1, rumen; 2, reticulum; 3, omasum; 4, abomasum), through which the food passes in digestion. The division includes oxen, sheep, goats, deer, and antelopes.

rumination (roo″mĭ-na′shun) [L. *ruminatio*] 1. the casting up of the food to be chewed a second time, as in cattle. In man, the regurgitation of food after almost every meal, part of it being vomited and the rest swallowed: a condition seen in infants. 2. meditation. **obsessive r.,** the constant preoccupation with certain thoughts, with inability to dismiss them from the mind.

ruminative (roo″mĭ-na′tiv) characterized by rumination; constantly dwelling on certain topics or ideas.

Ruminococcus (ru″mĭ-no-kok′us) [L. *ruminalis* of the urine + Gr. *kokkos* berry] a genus of anaerobic, gram-positive bacteria of the family Peptococcaceae, occurring as spherical to elongated cocci, which are involved in the fermentation of cellulose in the rumens of cattle and sheep.

rump (rump) the buttock or gluteal region.

Rumpel-Leede phenomenon (sign, test) (room′pel-la′dĕ) [Theodor *Rumpel*, German physician, 1862–1923; Carl Stockbridge *Leede*, American physician, born 1882] see under *phenomenon.*

Runeberg's anemia (disease, type) formula (roo′nĕ-bergs) [Johan Wilhelm *Runeberg*, Finnish physician, 1843–1918] see under *anemia* and *formula.*

Runella (roo-nel′ah) a genus of nonmotile, gram-negative, straight to curved, rod-shaped bacteria of the family Spirosomaceae; they have been isolated from eutrophic fresh waters. The type species is *R. slithyfor′mis.*

rupia (roo′pe-ah) [Gr. *rhypos* filth] thick, dark, raised, lamellated, adherent crusts on the skin somewhat resembling oyster shells, as in late recurrent secondary syphilis.

rupial (roo′pe-al) pertaining to or resembling rupia.

rupioid (roo′pe-oid) resembling rupia.

rupture (rup′chur) 1. forcible tearing or disruption of tissue. 2. a hernia. **defense r.,** a breaking down of the body's defense against infection, such as is seen when silica particles inhaled by a worker break down the resistance against tuberculosis.

Rusconi's anus (roos-ko′nēz) [Mauro *Rusconi*, Italian biologist, 1776–1849] the blastopore.

Rush (rush) Benjamin (1745–1813) American physician and statesman, born in Philadelphia; he was the first

professor of chemistry at the College of Philadelphia and wrote the first American book on chemistry; he was a Surgeon General in the Continental Army and physician to Pennsylvania Hospital, where he introduced clinical instruction; he was the founder of the Philadelphia Dispensary (the first in America), founder of the Philadelphia College of Physicians, and professor of the Institutes of Medicine (i.e., physiology and pathology) and Clinical Medicine at the University of Pennsylvania. Rush was the first American to investigate mental illness, to write on cholera infantum, and to notice focal infection in teeth; he was a founder of experimental physiology; and he also wrote on alcoholism, personal hygiene, and public health and on the great yellow fever epidemic in Philadelphia (1793). Rush's views on that epidemic (that it originated locally and was not imported) and his treatment of the sufferers (excessive purging and blood letting) caused controversy and lawsuits.

rush (rush) a powerful wave of contractile activity which travels extremely long distances down the small intestine; it is caused by intense irritation or unusual distention. Called also *peristaltic r.*

Russell's bodies (rus′elz) [William *Russell*, physician in Edinburgh, 1852–1940] see under *body.*

Russell effect (rus′el) [W. J. *Russell*, British physicist] see under *effect.*

Russell's viper, viper venom (rus′elz) [Patrick *Russell*, Aleppo physician, 1727–1805] see under *viper* and *venom.*

Russo's reaction (test) (roo′sōz) [Mario *Russo*, Italian physician, born 1866] see under *reaction.*

rust (rust) 1. iron oxide or hydroxide, forming a reddish deposit on metallic iron where the latter has been exposed to moisture; also a similar deposit on other metals that have been exposed to dampness. 2. a fungal disease of plants characterized by the formation of rust-like spots on them.

Rust's disease, phenomenon (sign), syndrome (roosts) [Johann Nepomuk *Rust*, German surgeon, 1775–1840] see under *disease, phenomenon,* and *syndrome.*

rut (rut) [L. *rugitus* roaring] 1. the period or season of heightened sexual activity in some male mammals that coincides with the season of estrus in the females. 2. estrus.

rutaecarpine (roo″te-kar′pin) a crystalline alkaloid, $C_{18}H_{13}ON_3$, from *Evodia rutaecarpa* Hook and Thoms. (Rutaceae), a small Asiatic shrub or tree.

ruthenium (roo-the′ne-um) a rare, very hard metallic element; symbol, Ru; atomic weight, 101.07; atomic number, 44.

rutherford (ruth′er-ford) [Ernest *Rutherford*, British physicist, 1871–1937] the unit representing one million disintegrations of radioactive matter per second. Abbreviated rd.

rutherfordium (ruth″er-ford′e-um) [named for Sir Ernest *Rutherford*, British physicist, 1871–1937] a transuranic element, atomic number 104, atomic weight 261, symbol Rf, produced by an induced nuclear reaction.

rutidosis (roo″tĭ-do′sis) rhytidosis.

rutin (roo′tin) chemical name: 3-[[6-O-(6-deoxy-α-L-mannopyranosyl)-β-D-glucopyranosyl]oxy]-2-(3,4-dihydroxyphenyl)-5,7-dihydroxy-4*H*-1-benzopyran-4-one. A bioflavonoid, $C_{27}H_{30}O_{16}$, obtained from buckwheat or other sources; it has been reported to reduce capillary fragility.

rutinose (roo′tĭ-nōs) rhamnosidoglucose, a disaccharide occurring in rutin.

rutoside (roo′to-sīd) rutin.

Ruysch's glomeruli, membrane (tunic), muscle, tube, veins (roish′ez) [Frederic *Ruysch*, Dutch anatomist, 1638–1731] see *glomeruli renis, lamina choriocapillaris,* and *venae vorticosae,* and see under *muscle* and *tube.*

RV residual volume.

R.V.H. right ventricular hypertrophy.

rye (ri) the cereal plant, *Secale cereale* L. (Gramineae), and its nutritious seed. **spurred r.,** see *ergot,* def. 1.

Ryle tube (rīl) [G. A. *Ryle*, British physician] see under *tube.*

S chemical symbol for *sulfur*; symbol for *siemens* and *Svedberg unit* (S_f Svedberg flotation unit).

S symbol for *entropy*.

S- [L. *sinister* left] a stereodescriptor used to specify the absolute configuration of compounds having asymmetric carbon atoms. See *R-*.

s SI symbol for *second*.

Σ the Greek capital letter sigma; used in mathematics to indicate a sum; $\Sigma_{i=1}^{n}$ $x_i = x_1 + x_2 + x_3 + \ldots + {}^{i} x_n$.

σ sigma, the eighteenth letter of the Greek alphabet; symbol for standard deviation.

S.A. abbreviation for L. *secun'dum ar'tem*, according to art.

Saathoff's test (saht'ofs) [Lübhard *Saathoff*, German physician, 1877–1929] see under *tests*.

saber-legged (sa'ber-legd) having the angle of the hock more acute than normal, so that the hind feet stand well under the body; said of horses.

Sabin's vaccine (sa'binz) [Albert Bruce *Sabin*, American virologist, born 1906] live oral poliovirus vaccine; see under *vaccine*.

sabinism (sab'ĭ-nizm) poisoning by savin.

sabinol (sab'ĭ-nol) a terpene alcohol, $(CH_3)_2CH \cdot C_6H_8$-$(OH){:}CH_2$, from the evergreen shrub, *Juniperus sabina* L., which is the chief constituent of savin oil; see *savin*.

Sabouraud's dextrose agar (sab'oo-rōz) [Raymond Jacques Adrien *Sabouraud*, French dermatologist, 1864–1938] see under *culture medium*.

Sabouraudia (sab"oo-ro'de-ah) Trichophyton.

Sabouraudites (sab"oo-ro-di'tēz) Microsporum.

sabulous (sab'u-lus) [L. *sabulosus; sabulum* sand] gritty or sandy.

saburra (sah-bur'ah) [L.] foulness of the stomach, mouth, or teeth.

saburral (sah-bur'al) [L. *saburra* sand] pertaining to or of the nature of sordes, or of foulness of the stomach.

sac (sak) [L. *saccus;* Gr. *sakkos*] a pouch; a baglike organ or structure. **abdominal s.,** a serous sac in the embryo which develops into the abdominal cavity. **air s.,** in birds, one of the air-filled cavities connected with the air passages of the lungs and, usually, with cavities in the bones; they assist in respiration and lower the body's specific gravity; they include cervicocephalic, tracheal, pulmonary, thoracic, and abdominal air sacs. **air s's,** alveoli pulmonis. **allantoic s.,** the dilated portion of the allantois which becomes a part of the placenta in many mammals. **alveolar s's,** sacculi alveolares. **amniotic s.,** amnion. **aneurysmal s.,** the chamber of a sacculated aneurysm. **aortic s.,** the homologue in mammalian embryos of the ventral aorta, from which arise the series of aortic arches. **chorionic s.,** the mammalian chorion. **conjunctival s.,** saccus conjunctivalis. **dental s.,** a concentric layer of connective tissue in which the enamel organ and dental papilla are embedded, which completely surrounds the developing tooth after the epithelial attachment that connects the enamel organ with the dental lamina disentegrates. Called also *sacculus dentis*. **dural s.,** the continuation of the dura mater below the caudal end of the spinal cord. **embryonic s.,** the blastocyst. **enamel s.,** the enamel organ during the stage in which its outer layer forms a sac enclosing the whole dental germ. **endolymphatic s.,** saccus endolymphaticus. **epiploic s.,** omental bursa. **gestation s.,** the extraembryonic membranes that envelop the embryo or fetus; in man, the fused amnion and chorion. **greater s. of peritoneum,** the peritoneum of the peritoneal cavity proper. **heart s.,** the pericardium. **hernial s.,** the pouch of peritoneum enclosing a hernia. **Hilton's s.,** sacculus laryngis. **lacrimal s.,** saccus lacrimalis. **laryngeal s.,** ventriculus laryngis. **lesser s. of peritoneal cavity,** omental bursa. **Lower's s's,** sacculated portions of the jugular vein at exit of the vein from the skull. **omental s.,** omental bursa. **pericardial s.,** pericardium. **pleural s.,** cavum pleurae. **serous s.,** the sac made up of the pleura, pericardium, and peritoneum. **splenic s.,** recessus splenicus. **tear s.,** saccus lacrimalis. **vitelline s.,** yolk s. **yolk s.,** the extraembryonic membrane that connects with the midgut; at the end of the fourth week of development it expands into a pear-shaped vesicle (*umbilical vesicle*) connected to the body of the embryo by a long narrow tube (*yolk stalk*). In marsupial and placental mammals, it produces a complete vitelline circulation in the early embryo and then undergoes regression; in oviparous vertebrates, it encloses the yolk mass, breaks down yolk, and makes it available to the developing organism.

sacbrood (sak'brood) an infectious disease of the larvae of bees, caused by a virus.

saccade (sah-kād') [Fr. "jerking"] the series of involuntary, abrupt, rapid, small movements or jerks of both eyes simultaneously in changing the point of fixation.

saccadic (sah-kad'ik) denoting the rapid involuntary small movements of both eyes simultaneously in changing the point of fixation on a visualized object, such as the series of jumps the eyes make in scanning a line of print.

saccate (sak'āt) [L. *saccatus*] 1. shaped like a sac. 2. contained in a sac.

saccharascope (sak'ah-rah-skōp) [Gr. *sakcharon* sugar + *skopein* to examine] a fermentation saccharimeter; see *saccharimeter*.

saccharate (sak'ah-rāt) a salt of saccharic acid.

saccharated (sak'ah-rāt"ed) [L. *saccharatus*, from *saccharum* sugar] charged with or containing sugar.

saccharephidrosis (sak"ar-ef"ĭ-dro'sis) [Gr. *sakcharon* sugar + *ephidrōsis* sweating] the discharge of sugar in the sweat.

saccharic acid (sak-kar'ik) 1. glucaric acid. 2. any dicarboxylic sugar acid.

saccharide (sak'ah-rid) one of a series of carbohydrates, including the sugars. The saccharides are divided into monosaccharides, disaccharides, trisaccharides, etc., or into oligosaccharides and polysaccharides, according to the number of saccharide groups ($C_nH_{2n}O_{n-1}$) composing them.

sacchariferous (sak"ah-rif'er-us) [L. *saccharum* sugar + *ferre* to bear] containing or yielding sugar.

saccharification (sak"ar-ĭ-fi-ka'shun) [L. *saccharum* sugar + *facere* to make] conversion into sugar.

saccharimeter (sak"ah-rim'ĕ-ter) [L. *saccharum* sugar + *metrum* measure] a device for estimating the proportion of sugar in a solution. It is either a polarimeter, indicating the proportion of sugar by the number of degrees through which it rotates the plane of polarization, or a hydrometer, indicating the proportion of sugar by the specific gravity of the solution. **Einhorn's s.,** a form of fermentation saccharimeter. **fermentation s.,** a saccharimeter in the form of a bent graduated tube and closed at one end. The amount of sugar in the urine is indicated by the gas which collects at the closed end when yeast is added to the urine. **Lohnstein's s.,** an instrument for performing a quantitative fermentation test of sugar in the urine.

saccharin (sak'ah-rin) [NF] chemical name: 1,2-benzisothiazolin-3-(2*H*)-one-1,1-dioxide. A white crystalline compound, $C_7H_5NO_3S$, several hundred times sweeter than sucrose; used as a sweetening agent in pharmaceutical preparations. **s. calcium** [USP], a salt, $C_{14}H_8CaN_2O_2 \cdot 3\frac{1}{2}H_2O$, used as a non-nutritive sweetener when sugar is contraindicated. **s. sodium** [USP], a salt, $C_7H_4NNaO_3$-$S \cdot 2H_2O$, used like the calcium salt.

saccharine (sak'ah-rīn) [L. *saccharinus*] sugary; having a sweet taste.

saccharinol (sah-kar'ĭ-nol) saccharin.

saccharinum (sak"ah-ri'num) saccharin.

racchar(o)- [L. *saccharum*, from Gr. *sakcharon* sugar] a combining form denoting relationship to sugar.

saccharobiose (sak"ah-ro-bi'ōs) a disaccharide.

saccharocoria (sak"ah-ro-ko're-ah) abhorrence of sugar.

saccharogalactorrhea (sak"ah-ro-gah-lak"to-re'ah) [*saccharo-* + Gr. *gala* milk + *rhoia* flow] the secretion of milk containing an excess of sugar.

saccharolytic (sak"ah-ro-lit'ik) [*saccharo-* + Gr. *lysis* dissolution] capable of chemically splitting up sugar.

saccharometabolic (sak″ah-ro-met″ah-bol′ik) pertaining to the metabolism of sugar.

saccharometabolism (sak″ah-ro-mĕ-tab′o-lizm) the metabolism of sugar.

saccharometer (sak″ah-rom′ĕ-ter) saccharimeter.

Saccharomyces (sak″ah-ro-mi′sēz) [*saccharo-* + Gr. *mykēs* fungus] a genus of ascomycetous fungi of the family Saccharomycetaceae, the yeasts. **S. al′bicans,** *Candida albicans.* **S. an′ginae,** *Candida albicans.* **S. apicula′tus,** *Kloekera apiculatus.* **S. baya′nus,** a species from fermenting wine and beer; called also *S. pastorianus.* **S. cant′liei,** a species reported from a tropical blastomycosis; it is now known to be *Pityrosporon ovale.* **S. capillit′ii,** a species from the scalp, with spherical cells, said to cause alopecia seborrheica; it is now known to be *Pityrosporon ovale.* **S. carlsbergen′sis,** a species used in microbiological assay in measuring vitamin B₆ in the urine, and in the brewing of beer. **S. cerevis′iae,** a species with oval or spherical cells, known as *brewers'* or *bakers' yeast;* it causes alcoholic fermentation, and is a very rare cause of lung disease. **S. dairen′sis,** a species with oval or elliptical cells that produces a fermentation in milk; called also *S. galacticolus.* **S. ellipsoi′deus,** a form from wine yeast, forming elliptical cells, solitary or in branching chains; it causes alcoholic fermentation in wines. **S. exig′uus,** a form in beer yeast, whose cells are elliptical and solitary, or in branching chains; it causes late fermentation in beer. **S. galactic′olus,** *S. dairensis.* **S. glu′tinis,** *Rhodotorula glutinis.* **S. granulomato′sus,** *Cryptococcus neoformans.* **S. guttula′tus,** *Saccharomycopsis guttulatus.* **S. hansen′ii,** *Debaryomyces hansenii.* **S. hom′inis,** a species once isolated in chronic infectious pyemia; it is now known to be *Bacillus megatherium.* **S. lemonnie′ri,** a pathogenic fungus found in bronchitis; it was probably *Candida albicans.* **S. litho′genes,** a species from the lymph glands of an ox suffering from carcinoma of the liver; it is pathogenic to animals. It is now known to be *Cryptococcus neoformans.* **S. mesenter′icus,** *Candida mesenterica.* **S. mycoder′ma,** *Candida vini.* **S. neofor′mans,** *Cryptococcus neoformans.* **S. pastoria′nus,** *S. bayanus.* **S. ru′brum,** a Brazilian species reported to cause a parapsoriasic affection; it was probably the skin contaminant *Rhodotorula rubra.* **S. subcuta′neus tumefa′ciens,** a species, which is probably the same as *Cryptococcus neoformans,* once found in a myxoma of the thigh; it is pathogenic for animals. **S. tumefa′ciens al′bus,** a species discovered in certain cases of pharyngitis, pathogenic for mice, guinea pigs, and rabbits; it is now known to be *Candida albicans.*

saccharomyces (sak″ah-ro-mi′sēz), pl. *saccharomyce′tes.* An organism of the genus *Saccharomyces.* **Busse's s.,** *Cryptococcus neoformans.*

Saccharomycetacea (sak″ah-ro-mi-sĕ-ta′se-e) a family of ascomycetous fungi of the order Endomycetales, subclass Hemiascomycetidae, the members of which are usually unicellular yeasts and reproduce sexually by formation of ascospores; it includes the genus *Saccharomyces.*

saccharomycetes (sak″ah-ro-mi-se′tēz) plural of *saccharomyces.*

saccharomycetic (sak″ah-ro-mi-set′ik) pertaining to or due to the presence of yeastlike fungi.

saccharomycetolysis (sak″ah-ro-mi″sĕ-tol′ĭ-sis) [*saccharomyces* + Gr. *lysis* dissolution] the splitting up of saccharomyces.

Saccharomycopsis (sak″ah-ro-mi-kop′sis) a genus of perfect yeasts of the family Saccharomycetaceae. **S. guttula′tus,** a species found in the intestinal tract of herbivorous animals; formerly called *Saccharomyces guttulatus.*

saccharopine (sak′ah-ro-pēn″) *N⁶*-(L-1,3-dicarboxypropyl)-L-lysine, an intermediate in the metabolism of lysine.

saccharopine dehydrogenase (NADP⁺, L-lysine forming) (sak′ah-ro-pēn de-hi′dro-jĕ-nās) [EC 1.5.1.8] an enzyme of the oxidoreductase class that catalyzes the reaction L-lysine + 2-ketoglutarate + NADPH = saccharopine + NADP⁺ + H₂O, the initial step in the major route of lysine metabolism. Deficient enzyme activity, an autosomal recessive trait, causes persistent hyperlysinemia. Called also *lysine ketoglutarate reductase.*

saccharorrhea (sak″ah-ro-re′ah) [*saccharo-* + Gr. *rhoia* flow] glycosuria.

saccharosan (sak′ah-ro-san) a form of anhydrosugar.

saccharose (sak′ah-rōs) [*saccharo-* + *-ose*] sucrose.

saccharosuria (sak″ah-ro-su′re-ah) [*saccharose* + Gr. *ouron* urine + *-ia*] sucrosuria.

Saccharum (sak′ah-rum) a genus of graminaceous plants. *S. officina′rum* L., sugar cane, affords a large part of the commercial supply of sugar.

saccharum (sak′ah-rum) [L.; Gr. *sakcharon*] sugar, especially cane sugar, or sucrose. **s. acer′num, s. canaden′se,** maple sugar. **s. lac′tis,** sugar of milk; lactose. **s. us′tum,** caramel.

saccharuria (sak″ah-roo′re-ah) [*saccharo-* + Gr. *ouron* urine + *-ia*] glycosuria.

sacciform (sak′sĭ-form) [L. *saccus* sac + *forma* form] shaped like a sac or bag.

saccular (sak′u-lar) shaped like a sac.

sacculated (sak′u-lāt″ed) [L. *sacculatus*] characterized by sacculation or by the presence of saccules.

sacculation (sak″u-la′shun) 1. a sacculus, or pouch. 2. the quality of being sacculated, or pursed out with little pouches. **s's of colon,** haustra coli.

saccule (sak′ūl) [L. *sacculus*] 1. a little bag or sac. 2. see *sacculus.* **air s's, alveolar s's,** sacculi alveolares. **laryngeal s., s. of larynx,** sacculus laryngis.

sacculi (sak′u-li) [L.] genitive and plural of *sacculus.*

sacculocochlear (sak″u-lo-kok′le-ar) pertaining to the sacculus and cochlea.

sacculus (sak′u-lus), gen. and pl. *sac′culi* [L., dim. of *saccus*] a little bag or sac; applied in official anatomical nomenclature specifically to the smaller of the two divisions of the membranous labyrinth of the vestibule, which communicates with the cochlear duct by way of the ductus reuniens. Called also *s. proprius, s. rotundus, s. sphaericus, s. vestibularis,* and *saccule.* **sac′culi alveola′res** [NA], alveolar saccules: the spaces into which the alveolar ducts open distally, and with which the alveoli communicate; called also *alveolar sacs.* **s. commu′nis,** utriculus. **s. den′tis,** dental sac. **s. endolymphat′icus,** saccus endolymphaticus. **s. lacrima′lis,** saccus lacrimalis. **s. laryn′gis** [NA], laryngeal saccule: a diverticulum extending upward from the front of the laryngeal ventricle, between the vestibular fold medially and the thyroarytenoid muscle and thyroid cartilage laterally; called also *appendix ventriculi laryngis.* **s. Morgag′nii,** ventriculus laryngis. **s. pro′prius, s. rotun′dus, s. sphae′ricus,** see *sacculus.* **s. ventricula′ris,** s. laryngis. **s. vestibula′ris,** see *sacculus.*

saccus (sak′kus), pl. *sac′ci* [L.; Gr. *sakkos*] a sac or pouch; [NA] a general term for a saclike structure. **s. conjunctiva′lis** [NA], conjunctival sac: the potential space, lined by conjunctiva, between the eyelids and the eyeball. **s. endolymphat′icus** [NA], endolymphatic sac: the blind, flattened cerebral end of the endolymphatic duct. **s. lacrima′lis** [NA], lacrimal sac: the dilated upper end of the nasolacrimal duct.

Sachs' disease [Bernard (Barney) *Sachs,* New York neurologist, 1858–1944] see *Tay-Sachs disease,* under *disease.*

Sachsse's test (zahk′sez) [Georg Robert *Sachsse,* German chemist, 1840–1895] see under *tests.*

sacrad (sa′krad) toward the sacrum, or sacral aspect.

sacral (sa′kral) [L. *sacralis*] pertaining to or situated near the sacrum.

sacralgia (sa-kral′je-ah) [*sacrum* + *-algia*] pain in the sacrum.

sacralization (sa″kral-i-za′shun) anomalous fusion of the fifth lumbar vertebra to the first segment of the sacrum, so that the sacrum consists of six segments.

sacrarthrogenic (sa″krar-thro-jen′ik) [*sacrum* + Gr. *arthron* joint + *gennan* to produce] resulting from disease of a sacral joint.

sacrectomy (sa-krek′to-me) [*sacrum* + Gr. *ektomē* excision] excision or resection of the sacrum.

sacrifice (sak′rĭ-fīs) to kill an experimental animal.

sacr(o)- [L. *sacrum,* q.v.] a combining form denoting relationship to the sacrum.

sacroanterior (sa″kro-an-te′re-or) having the sacrum directed forward; see under *position.*

sacrococcygeal (sa″kro-kok-sij′e-al) pertaining to or located in the region of the sacrum and coccyx.

sacrococcyx (sa″kro-kok′siks) the sacrum and coccyx together.

sacrocoxalgia (sa″kro-kok-sal′je-ah) pain in the sacroiliac joint.

sacrocoxitis (sa″kro-kok-si′tis) [sacro- + L. coxa hip + -itis] inflammation of the sacroiliac joint.

sacrodynia (sa″kro-din′e-ah) [sacro- + Gr. odynē pain] pain in the sacral region.

sacroiliac (sa″kro-il′e-ak) pertaining to the sacrum and ilium; denoting the joint or articulation between the sacrum and ilium and the ligaments associated therewith.

sacroiliitis (sa″kro-il″e-i′tis) inflammation in the sacroiliac joint.

sacrolisthesis (sa″kro-lis-the′sis) the condition in which the sacrum lies anterior to the fifth lumbar vertebra.

sacrolumbar (sa″kro-lum′bar) [sacro- + L. lumbus loin] pertaining to the sacrum and the loin.

sacroperineal (sa″kro-per″ĭ-ne′al) pertaining to the sacrum and the perineum.

sacroposterior (sa″kro-pos-te′re-or) having the sacrum directed backward; see under position.

sacropromontory (sa″kro-prom′on-to-re) the promontory of the sacrum.

sacrosciatic (sa″kro-si-at′ik) pertaining to the sacrum and the ischium.

sacrospinal (sa″kro-spi′nal) [sacro- + L. spina spine] pertaining to the sacrum and the spine, or vertebral column.

sacrotomy (sa-krot′o-me) [sacro- + Gr. temnein to cut] the operation of cutting into the lower end of the sacrum.

sacrotransverse (sa″kro-trans-vers′) relating to the direction of the fetal sacrum in breech presentation; see under position.

sacrouterine (sa″kro-u′ter-in) pertaining to the sacrum and the uterus.

sacrovertebral (sa″kro-ver′tĕ-bral) pertaining to the sacrum and the vertebral column.

sacrum (sa′krum) [L. "sacred"] the triangular bone just below the lumbar vertebrae, formed usually by five fused vertebrae (sacral vertebrae) that are wedged dorsally between the two hip bones; called also os sacrum [NA]. See Plate accompanying skeleton. **assimilation s.,** see assimilation pelvis, under pelvis. **tilted s.,** a condition marked by separation of the sacroiliac joint and forward displacement of the sacrum.

sactosalpinx (sak″to-sal′pinks) [Gr. saktos stuffed + salpinx tube] dilatation of the inflamed uterine tube by retained secretions.

saddle (sad′'l) 1. a support whose shape fits the contour of the object resting upon it. 2. a saddle-shaped structure or part. 3. denture base s. **denture base s.,** that part of a complete or partial denture which rests upon the basal seat and to which the teeth are attached. Called also saddle. See also denture base, under base.

sadism (sad′izm) [Marquis de Sade, 1740–1814] a paraphilia in which sexual gratification is derived from humiliating or hurting another. Called sexual sadism in DSM III. **anal s.,** in Freudian theory, the sadistic manifestations of anal erotism, such as aggressiveness, selfishness, and stinginess. **oral s.,** in Freudian theory, a sadistic form of oral erotism manifested by fantasies of chewing, biting, etc.

sadist (sad′ist) a practicer of sadism.

sadistic (să-dis′tik) pertaining to or characterized by sadism.

sadomasochism (sad″o-mas′o-kizm) a state characterized by both sadistic and masochistic tendencies.

sadomasochistic (sad″o-mas″o-kis′tik) characterized by both sadism and masochism.

Saemisch's operation (section), ulcer (sa′mish-ez) [Edwin Theodor Saemisch, ophthalmologist in Bonn, 1833–1909] see under operation, and see ulcus serpens corneae.

Saenger's macula (zeng′erz) [Max Saenger, gynecologist in Prague, 1853–1903] see macula gonorrhoeica.

Saenger's sign (reflex) (zeng′erz) [Alfred Saenger, German neurologist, 1861–1921] see under sign.

Saff (saf) trademark for a preparation of safflower oil.

Safflor (saf′flor) trademark for a preparation of safflower oil.

safrene (saf′rēn) a hydrocarbon, $C_{10}H_{16}$, obtained from sassafras oil.

safrol (saf′rol) an oily, volatile (melting point, 11° C.) substance, the methylene ether of 3,4-dihydroxyallylbenzene from sassafras oil; has been used as anodyne.

safrosin (saf′ro-sin) bluish eosin.

sagittal (saj′ĭ-tal) [L. sagittalis; sagitta arrow] 1. shaped like or resembling an arrow; straight. 2. situated in the plane of the sagittal suture or parallel to it; said of an anteroposterior plane or section parallel to the median plane of the body.

sagittalis (saj″ĭ-ta′lis) sagittal; [NA] a general term denoting a structure situated in the plane of the sagittal suture.

sago (sa′go) a starch mainly derived from the pith of various species of palm, chiefly of the genus Sagus.

Sahli's reaction, method, test (sah′lēz) [Herman Sahli, physician in Bern, 1856–1933] see desmoid reaction, under reaction, and see under method and tests.

S.A.L. abbreviation for L. secun′dum ar′tis le′ges, according to the rules of art.

sal (sal) [L.] salt. **s. ammoniac,** ammonium chloride. **s. diuret′icum,** potassium acetate. **s. so′da,** sodium carbonate. **s. volat′ile, volat′ilis,** ammonium carbonate.

Sala's cells (sal′ahz) [Luigi Sala, Italian zoologist, 1863–1930] see under cell.

salamander (sal″ah-man′der) [Gr. salamandra a kind of lizard] a tailed amphibian, many species of which are used in various types of experiments.

salamanderin (sal″ah-man′der-in) a poisonous base from the skin of a species of salamander.

salantel (sal′an-tel) chemical name: N-[3-chloro-4-(4-chlorobenzoyl)phenyl]-2-hydroxy-3,5-diiodobenzamide; a veterinary anthelmintic, $C_{20}H_{11}Cl_2I_2NO_3$.

salazosulfapyridine (sal″ah-zo-sul″fah-pir′ĭ-den) sulfasalazine.

salbutamol (sal-bu′tah-mol) albuterol.

salcolex (sal′ko-leks) chemical name: 2-hydroxy-N,N,Ntrimethylethanaminium 2-hydroxybenzoate(salt) compounded with tetrahydrate magnesium sulfate (2:1); an analgesic, anti-inflammatory, and antipyretic, $[C_{12}H_{19}NO_4]_2$ · $MgSO_4$ · $4H_2O$.

salethamide maleate (sal-eth′ah-mīd) chemical name: N-[2-(diethylamino)ethyl]-2-hydroxybenzamide (Z)-2-butenedioate (1:1) (salt); an analgesic, $C_{13}H_{20}N_2$ · $O_2C_4H_4O_4$.

salicylaldehyde (sal″ĭ-sil-al′dĕ-hīd) salicylic aldehyde.

salicylamide (sal″ĭ-sil-am′īd) chemical name: 2-hydroxybenzamide. An amide of salicylic acid, $C_7H_7NO_2$, occurring as a white, crystalline powder; used as an analgesic and antipyretic, administered orally.

salicylanilide (sal″ĭ-sil-an′ĭ-lid) chemical name: 2-hydroxy-N-phenylbenzamide. A compound usually prepared by the interaction of salicylic acid and aniline, $C_{13}H_{11}NO_2$, occurring as white or slightly pink crystals; used as a topical antifungal in the treatment of tinea capitis.

salicylate (sal′ĭ-sil″āt, sah-lis′ĭ-lāt) a salt, ester of salicylic acid (e.g., methyl salicylate), or salicylate ester of an organic acid (e.g., aspirin, acetylsalicylic acid); such compounds have analgesic, antipyretic, and anti-inflammatory activity; they act by inhibiting prostaglandin synthesis. **s. meglumine,** chemical name: 2-hydroxybenzoic acid compound with 1-deoxy-1-(methylamino)-D-glucitol; an antirheumatic and analgesic, $C_7H_{17}NO_5 \cdot C_7H_6O_3$.

salicylated (sal′ĭ-sil″āt-ed) containing or impregnated with salicylic acid.

salicylazosulfapyridine (sal″ĭ-sil″ah-zo-sul″fah-pir′ĭ-den) sulfasalazine.

salicylemia (sal″ĭ-sil-e′me-ah) [salicylate + Gr. haima blood + -ia] the presence of salicylate in the blood.

salicylic (sal″ĭ-sil′ik) pertaining to the radical salicyl; see under acid.

salicylic acid (sal′ĭ-sil′ik) [USP] orthohydroxybenzoic acid, obtained from the bark of the white willow and wintergreen leaves, and also prepared synthetically; it has bacteriostatic, fungicidal, and keratolytic actions; its salts, the salicylates, are used as analgesics.

salicylism (sal″ĭ-sil″izm) a group of commonly occurring toxic effects of excessive dosage with salicylic acid or its salts, usually marked by tinnitus, nausea, and vomiting.

salicylsalicylic acid (sal-is″il-sal″is-il′ik) salsalate.

salicylsulfonic acid (sal″ĭ-sil-sul-fon′ik) sulfosalicylic acid.

salicyluric acid (sal″ĭ-sil-ūr′ik) the glycine conjugate of salicylic acid, a form in which salicylates are excreted in the urine.

salifiable (sal′ĭ-fi″ah-b'l) [L. *sal* salt + *fieri* to become] capable of combining with acids so as to form salts.

salify (sal′ĭ-fi) to convert into a salt.

salimeter (sah-lim′ĕ-ter) [L. *sal* salt + *metrum* measure] a hydrometer for ascertaining the concentration of saline solutions.

saline (sa′lēn, sa′līn) [L. *salinus; sal* salt] salty; of the nature of a salt; containing a salt or salts. **physiological s.,** an isotonic aqueous solution of NaCl for temporarily maintaining living cells.

salinigrin (sal″ĭ-ni′grin) a glycoside, $C_{13}H_{16}O_7$, from the bark of several species of *Salix* (willow) of the family Salicaceae, and from the needles and sprouts of certain coniferous trees.

salinometer (sal″ĭ-nom′ĕ-ter) an instrument (hydrometer) for direct reading of the salt content of a liquid.

saliva (sah-li′vah) [L.] the clear, alkaline, somewhat viscid secretion from the parotid, submaxillary, sublingual, and smaller mucous glands of the mouth. It serves to moisten and soften the food, keeps the mouth moist, and contains α-amylase, a digestive enzyme which converts starch into maltose. The saliva also contains mucin, serum albumin, globulin, leukocytes, epithelial debris, and potassium thiocyanate. Certain toxins frequently occur in it. **chorda s.,** submaxillary saliva produced in response to stimulation of the chorda tympani nerve, less viscid and turbid than that of the unstimulated gland. **ganglionic s.,** saliva obtained by irritating the submaxillary gland. **lingual s.,** the secretion of Ebner's glands and other serous glands of the tongue. **parotid s.,** saliva produced by the parotid gland; thinner and less viscid than the other varieties. **ropy s.,** saliva which is highly viscid. **sublingual s.,** that produced by the sublingual gland, the most viscid of all. **submaxillary s.,** that produced by the submaxillary gland. **sympathetic s.,** submaxillary saliva produced in response to stimulation of its sympathetic nerve supply; more viscid and turbid than that of the unstimulated gland.

salivant (sal′ĭ-vant) provoking a flow of saliva.

salivaria (sal″ĭ-va′re-ah) in some systems of classification, a group or section comprising those trypanosomes in which the developmental cycle is completed in the salivary glands (anterior station) of the vector and transmission is usually by inoculation through the hypopharynx. The group includes the subgenera *Duttonella, Nannomonas,* and *Trypanozoon.* Cf. *stercoraria.*

salivarian (sal″ĭ-va′re-an) pertaining to or caused by trypanosomes of the salivaria group or section.

salivary (sal′ĭ-ver-e) [L. *salivarius*] pertaining to the saliva.

salivate (sal′ĭ-vāt) to produce an excessive flow of saliva.

salivation (sal″ĭ-va′shun) [L. *salivatio*] 1. the secretion of saliva. 2. ptyalism.

salivator (sal′ĭ-va″tor) an agent that causes salivation.

salivatory (sal′ĭ-vah-to″re) causing salivation.

Salk vaccine (sahlk) [Jonas Edward *Salk,* American physician and virologist, born 1914] see under *vaccine.*

Salkowski's method, test (sal-kow′skēz) [Ernst Leopold *Salkowski,* physiologic chemist in Berlin, 1844–1923] see under *method* and *tests.*

salmiac (sal′me-ak) ammonium chloride.

salmin (sal′min) a toxic substance derived from the milt of salmon.

Salmonella (sal″mo-nel′ah) [Daniel Elmer *Salmon,* American pathologist, 1850–1914] a genus of gram-negative, facultatively anaerobic bacteria of the family Enterobacteriaceae, made up of nonspore-forming rods, usually motile with peritrichous flagella. They utilize citrate as a sole carbon source and generally ferment glucose but not sucrose or lactose. The genus is separated into species or serotypes on

the basis of O (somatic), Vi (capsular), and H (flagellar) antigens (Kauffman-White scheme). The somatic antigen is the basis for separation into serogroups not contained in another group. Agglutination tests with pooled (polyvalent) antisera for groups A through E and Vi antigen can detect 95 per cent of the serotypes isolated from humans and lower animals. The H antigen of *Salmonella* is biphasic, designated as phase 1 (specific) or phase 2 (nonspecific). Serotypes (more than 1500 have been described) are identified by antigenic formulae, taking the general form O antigen: phase 1 ⇄ phase 2, in which the O antigens are designated by numerals, the phase 1 antigens by lowercase letters, and the phase 2 antigens by numerals. Clinical laboratories frequently report salmonellae as one of three species, differentiated on the basis of serologic and biochemical reactions: *S. typhi, S. choleraesuis,* and *S. enteritidis;* the last contains all serotypes except the first two (Ewing scheme). Numerous strains familiarly named as species are thus designated as serotypes of *S. enteritidis.* For taxonomic purposes the salmonellae are grouped in five subgenera on the basis of biochemical characteristics and are separated into species on the basis of antigenic reactions. The subgenera and selected representative serovars are: subgenus I (containing most serotypes), *S. choleraesuis, S. hirschfeldii, S. typhi, S. paratyphi-A, S. schottmuelleri, S. typhimurium, S. enteritidis,* and *S. gallinarum;* subgenus II, *S. salamae;* subgenus III, *S. ariyonae;* subgenus IV, *S. houtenae;* and subgenus V, *S. bongor.* The genus contains pathogenic species causing enteric fevers (typhoid and paratyphoid), septicemias, and gastroenteritis. The most frequent clinical manifestation is food poisoning. *Salmonella* species are widely distributed in lower animals, frequently producing disease. **S. abor′tus e′qui,** *S. enteritidis* serotype *abortus equi.* **S. abor′tus o′vis,** *S. enteritidis* serotype *abortus ovis.* **S. ago′na,** *S. enteritidis* serotype *agona.* **S. arizo′nae,** a species originally found in reptiles, which also occurs in fowl and other domestic animals, and has been isolated from dried egg powder and other food sources. Ingestion of contaminated food produces gastroenteritis and enteric fever (salmonellosis); the organisms can also cause bacteremias and local infections. The organisms may ferment lactose rapidly. The members of this species are frequently classified in a separate genus, *Arizona.* **S. bon′gor,** the type species of subgenus V. **S. choleraesu′is,** a group C species, pathogenic for man and animals. It is found as a secondary invader in hog cholera and has been associated with paratyphoid, gastroenteritis, and septicemia in humans. Called also *Bacterium choleraesuis* and *S. suipestifer.* See also *suipestifer.* **S. chol′eraesu′is** var. **ku′zendorf,** a strain associated with paratyphoid gastroenteritis; seen with increasing frequency in the United States. **S. chol′eraesu′is** var. **typhisu′is,** a strain pathogenic for pigs that may infect humans. **S. enterit′idis,** a species containing group A, B, C, and D serotypes, occurring frequently in humans and animals. It comprises more than 1500 different serotypes, known also by their individual names, which may produce paratyphoid fever, septicemia, and gastroenteritis. Called also *Gärtner bacillus.* **S. enterit′idis** serotype **abor′tus e′qui,** a group B serotype causing infectious abortion in mares; not found in other animals. Called also *S. abortus equi.* **S. enterit′idis** serotype **abor′tus o′vis,** a group B serotype causing abortion in sheep. **S. enterit′idis** serotype **ago′na,** a group B serotype sometimes isolated in the United States. Called also *S. agona.* **S. enterit′idis** serotype **gallina′rum,** a group D_1 serotype, the causative agent of fowl typhoid; it has little or no pathogenicity for humans. It is nonmotile and contains somatic O antigen but no H antigen. Called also *S. gallinarum.* **S. enterit′idis** serotype **hei′delberg,** a group B serotype frequently isolated in the United States. Called also *S. heidelberg.* **S. enterit′idis** serotype **hirschfel′dii,** a group C serotype, closely related to strains of *S. choleraesuis;* it is the etiologic agent of human paratyphoid fever in parts of Asia, Africa, and northeastern Europe and is reported as an important cause of illness and death in British Guiana. Called also *S. hirschfeldii* and *S. paratyphi* C. **S. enterit′idis** serotype **infan′tis,** a group C serotype sometimes isolated in the United States. Called also *S. infantis.* **S. enterit′idis** serotype **new′port,** a group C serotype, one of the most common types isolated in the United States. Called also *S. newport.* **S. enterit′idis** serotype **paraty′phi A,** a group A serotype causing mild paratyphoid fever in humans; it is one of the most frequent causes of the disease in India.

Called also *S. paratyphi* and *S. paratyphi A*. **S. enterit′i-dis** serotype **pullo′rum**, the causative agent of bacillary white diarrhea of chicks; serologically identical with *S. enteritidis* serotype *gallinarum*. Called also *S. pullorum*. **S. enterit′idis** serotype **schottmuel′leri**, a group B serotype, the most common cause of paratyphoid fever in the northern United States and northern Europe. Some strains also infect animals. Called also *S. paratyphi B* and *S. schottmuelleri*. **S. enterit′idis** serotype **sen′dai**, a group D serotype found in Japan and the Far East. **S. enterit′idis** serotype **typhimu′rium**, a group B serotype, a parasite of rats and mice, which is the serotype most frequently isolated in the United States and the most frequent agent of food poisoning; it also causes paratyphoid fever. Called also *S. typhimurium*. **S. gallina′rum**, *S. enteritidis* serotype *gallinarum*. **S. hei′delberg**, *S. enteritidis* serotype *heidelberg*. **S. hirschfel′dii**, *S. enteritidis* serotype *hirschfeldii*. **S. hou′tenae**, the type species of subgenus IV. **S. infan′tis**, *S. enteritidis* serotype *infantis*. **S. morga′ni**, *Morganella morganii*. **S. new′port**, *S. enteritidis* serotype *newport*. **S. paraty′phi**, *S. enteritidis* serotype *paratyphi A*. **S. paraty′phi A**, *S. enteritidis* serotype *paratyphi A*. **S. paraty′phi B**, *S. enteritidis* serotype *schottmuelleri*. **S. paraty′phi C**, *S. enteritidis* serotype *hirschfeldii*. **S. pullo′rum**, *S. enteritidis* serotype *pullorum*. **S. sala′mae**, the type species of subgenus II, a group D serotype originally isolated in Dar-es-Salaam, Tanzania. Called also *Dar es Salaam bacterium*. **S. schottmuel′leri**, *S. enteritidis* serotype *schottmuelleri*. **S. sen′dai**, *S. enteritidis* serotype *sendai*. **S. suipes′tifer**, *S. choleraesuis*. **S. ty′phi**, a group D serotype, a strict parasite of humans and the cause of typhoid fever. Strains containing the Vi (virulence) antigen are designated V strains; those that have partially lost Vi antigen, V-W strains; and those that do not contain Vi antigen, W strains. The species is also subdivided into phage types on the basis of susceptibility to empirically numbered bacteriophages. The organism is transmitted by water or food contaminated by human excreta. Called also *typhoid bacillus*. Formerly called *Bacillus typhi*, *Bacillus typhosus*, *Eberthella typhi*, and *S. typhosa*. **S. typhimu′rium**, *S. enteritidis* serotype *typhimurium*. **S. typhisu′is**, *S. choleraesuis var. typhisuis*. **S. typho′sa**, *S. typhi*.

salmonella (sal″mo-nel′ah), pl. *salmonel′lae*. a bacterium of the genus *Salmonella*.

salmonellae (sal″mo-nel′e) plural of *salmonella*.

salmonellal (sal-mo-nel′al) caused by salmonellae.

Salmonelleae (sal″mo-nel′e-e) in some systems of classification, a tribe of gram-negative, facultatively anaerobic, rod-shaped bacteria of the family Enterobacteriaceae, made up of the genera *Arizona*, *Citrobacter*, and *Salmonella*.

salmonellosis (sal″mo-nel-o′sis) any disease caused by a salmonellal infection, which may be manifested as food poisoning with acute gastroenteritis, vomiting, diarrhea, and rarely septicemia, or as typhoid or paratyphoid fever.

salocoll (sal′o-kol) phenocoll salicylate, $C_2H_5O \cdot C_6H_4 \cdot NH \cdot CO \cdot CH_2 \cdot NH_2 \cdot C_6H_4(OH)CO_2H$, a crystalline salt used as an antirheumatic.

salol (sa′lol) phenyl salicylate.

Salomon's test (sal′o-monz) [Hugo *Salomon*, German physician in Buenos Aires, 1872–1954] see under *tests*.

salpingectomy (sal″pin-jek′to-me) [*salpingo-* + Gr. *ektomē* excision] surgical removal of the uterine tube.

salpingemphraxis (sal″pin-jem-frak′sis) [*salpingo-* + Gr. *emphraxis* stoppage] obstruction of the auditory tube.

salpingian (sal-pin′je-an) pertaining to the auditory or to the uterine tube.

salpingion (sal-pin′je-on) a point at the apex of the petrous bone on its lower surface.

salpingitic (sal″pin-jit′ik) pertaining to or characterized by salpingitis.

salpingitis (sal″pin-ji′tis) [*salpingo-* + *-itis* inflammation] 1. inflammation of the uterine tube.   2. inflammation of the auditory tube. **chronic interstitial s.,** inflammation of the uterine tube associated with infiltration of connective tissue and muscle with lymphocytes and plasma cells. **chronic vegetating s.,** inflammation of the uterine tube, with marked hypertrophy of the mucosa. **eustachian s.,** inflammation of the auditory tube. **hemorrhagic s.,** inflammation of the uterine tube associated with rupture of a blood vessel and effusion of blood. **hypertrophic s.,** pachysalpingitis.   **s. isth′mica nodo′sa,** a condition marked by nodular thickening of parts of both uterine tubes, most characteristically of the isthmic portion, pathogenically related to adenomyosis of the uterus. **mural s.,** pachysalpingitis.   **nodular s.,** inflammation attended with formation of nodules in the wall and mucous lining of the uterine tube. **parenchymatous s.,** pachysalpingitis.   **s. prof′luens,** inflammation of the uterine tube, with accumulation in its lumen of fluid that ultimately escapes. **pseudofollicular s.,** inflammation of the uterine tube characterized by agglutination of its walls, causing a formation of cacculoo. **purulent s.,** inflammation of the uterine tube attended with suppuration; called also *pyosalpingitis*. **tuberculous s.,** infection of the uterine tube by the tubercle bacillus, *Mycobacterium tuberculosis*.

salping(o)- [Gr. *salpinx* tube] a combining form denoting relationship to a tube, specifically to the uterine or to the auditory tube.

salpingocele (sal-ping′go-sēl) [*salpingo-* + Gr. *kēlē* hernia] hernial protrusion of a uterine tube.

salpingography (sal″ping-gog′rah-fe) [*salpingo-* + Gr. *graphein* to write] roentgenography of the uterine tubes after the injection of an opaque medium.

salpingolithiasis (sal-ping″go-lĭ-thi′ah-sis) the presence of calcareous deposits in the wall of the uterine tubes.

salpingolysis (sal″ping-gol′ĭ-sis) surgical lysis of adhesions involving the uterine tubes.

salpingo-oophorectomy (sal-ping″go-o″of-o-rek′to-me) surgical removal of a uterine tube and ovary.

salpingo-oophoritis (sal-ping″go-o″of-o-ri′tis) inflammation of a uterine tube and ovary.

salpingo-oophorocele (sal-ping″go-o-of′or-o-sēl) hernia containing a uterine tube and ovary.

salpingo-oothecitis (sal-ping″go-o″o-the-si′tis) [*salpingo-* + Gr. *ōon* egg + *thēkē* case + *-itis*] salpingo-oophoritis.

salpingo-oothecocele (sal-ping″go-o″o-the′ko-sēl) [*salpingo-* + Gr. *ōon* egg + *thēkē* case + *kēlē* hernia] salpingo-oophorocele.

salpingo-ovariectomy (sal-ping″go-o-va″re-ek′to-me) salpingo-oophorectomy.

salpingo-ovariotomy (sal-ping″go-o-va″re-ot′o-me) salpingo-oophorectomy.

salpingoperitonitis (sal-ping″go-per″ĭ-to-ni′tis) inflammation of the peritoneum covering the uterine tube.

salpingopexy (sal-ping′go-pek″se) [*salpingo-* + Gr. *pēxis* fixation] operative fixation of the uterine tube.

salpingopharyngeal (sal-ping″go-fah-rin′je-al) pertaining to the auditory tube and the pharynx.

salpingoplasty (sal-ping′go-plas″te) [*salpingo-* + Gr. *plassein* to form] plastic repair of the uterine tube; called also *tuboplasty*.

salpingorrhaphy (sal″ping-gor′ah-fe) [*salpingo-* + *-rrhaphy*] suture of the fallopian tube.

salpingoscopy (sal″ping-gos′ko-pe) inspection of the auditory tube.

salpingostaphyline (sal-ping″go-staf′ĭ-lin) pertaining to the auditory tube and the uvula.

salpingostomatomy (sal-ping″go-sto-mat′o-me) [*salpingo-* + Gr. *stoma* mouth + *tomē* a cutting] surgical resection of a portion of the uterine tube, with creation of a new abdominal ostium.

salpingostomatoplasty (sal-ping″go-sto-mat′o-plas″te) salpingostomatomy.

salpingostomy (sal″ping-gos′to-me) [*salpingo-* + Gr. *stomoun* to provide with an opening or mouth] 1. formation of an opening or fistula into a uterine tube for the purpose of drainage.   2. surgical restoration of the patency of a uterine tube.

salpingotomy (sal″ping-got′o-me) [*salpingo-* + Gr. *tomē* a cutting] surgical incision of a uterine tube.

salpinx (sal′pinks) [Gr.] a tube. **s. auditi′va,** tuba auditiva. **s. uteri′na,** [NA] alternative for *tuba uterina*.

salsalate (sal′sah-lāt) the salicylate ester of salicylic acid, which hydrolyzes in vivo to form salicylate; used for treatment of osteoarthritis and rheumatoid arthritis. Formerly called *salicylsalicylic acid*.

salt (sawlt) [L. *sal;* Gr. *hals*] 1. sodium chloride, or common salt. 2. any compound of a base and an acid; any compound of an acid some of whose replaceable hydrogen atoms have been substituted. 3. [pl.] a saline purgative. See *magnesium sulfate* (Epsom s.), *sodium sulfate* (Glauber's s.), and *potassium sodium tartrate* (Preston's, Rochelle, or Seignette's s.). **acid s.,** any salt in which the combining power of the acid is not completely exhausted. **baker's s.,** ammonium carbonate; sometimes used in leavening cakes. **basic s.,** any salt with more than the normal proportion of the basic elements. **bile s's,** glycine or taurine conjugates of bile acids that are formed in the liver and excreated in the bile; they are powerful detergents that disperse fat globules in the intestine, enabling fats to be digested and absorbed. **bone s's,** the crystalline salts deposited in the organic matrix (principally collagen fibers) of bone, composed chiefly of calcium and phosphate. **buffer s.,** a salt, such as sodium bicarbonate and sodium phosphate, the anion of which functions as a conjugate base in a buffer system. **Carlsbad s.,** a mixture of sodium sulfate, potassium sulfate, sodium chloride, and sodium bicarbonate, used as a purgative. **common s.,** sodium chloride, NaCl. **diuretic s.,** potassium acetate. **double s.,** any salt in which the two hydrogen atoms of a dibasic acid have been replaced by two separate metals or basic radicals, as in potassium ammonium tartrate. **Epsom s.,** magnesium sulfate. **Everitt's s.,** potassium ferrous ferrocyanide, $K_2Fe[Fe(CN)_6]$. **Glauber's s.,** sodium sulfate. **halide s., haloid s.,** any binary compound of a metal or basic radical with a halogen—i.e., chlorine, iodine, bromine, fluorine. **Kissingen s's,** an aperient salt from the waters of a spring at Kissingen, Bavaria. **Monsel's s.,** iron subsulfate. **neutral s., normal s.,** any salt which is neither acidic nor basic in reaction. **pancreatic s.,** a mixture of the pancreatic ferments with common salt, used as a digestant. **peptic s.,** common salt mixed with pepsin, used as a digestant. **Plimmer's s.,** sodium antimony tartrate. **Preston's s., Rochelle s., Seignette's s.,** potassium sodium tartrate. **smelling s's,** aromatized ammonium carbonate: stimulant and restorative. **table s.,** sodium chloride, NaCl. **Wurster's s's,** the univalent oxidation products of the aromatic *p*-diamines. They are free radicals which may polymerize in a sufficiently concentrated solution and at low temperatures or in the solid state.

saltation (sal-ta′shun) [L. *saltatio* from *saltare* to jump] the action of leaping, especially (1) chorea, or the dancing which sometimes accompanies it; (2) conduction along myelinated nerves; (3) in genetics, an abrupt variation in species; a mutation.

saltatorial, saltatoric (sal″tah-to′re-al; sal″tah-to′rik) saltatory.

saltatory (sal′tah-to″re) pertaining to or characterized by saltation; see also under *evolution* and *spasm*.

Salter's line (sawl′terz) [Sir James A. *Salter*, English dentist, 1825–1897] see under *line.*

salting in (sawl′ting in) dissolving proteins by raising the salt concentration; certain proteins that are insoluble in pure water dissolve when small amounts of neutral salt are added.

salting out (sawl′ting out) precipitation of proteins by raising the salt concentration; any soluble protein will precipitate out of solution if enough neutral salt is added.

saltpeter (sawlt-pe′ter) [L. *salpetra* or *sal petrae*] potassium nitrate, KNO_3. **Chile s.,** sodium nitrate.

salubrious (sah-lu′bre-us) [L. *salubris*] conducive to health; wholesome.

saluresis (sal″u-re′sis) [L. *sal* salt + Gr. *ourēsis* a making water] the excretion of sodium and chloride ions in the urine.

saluretic (sal″u-ret′ik) 1. pertaining to, characterized by, or promoting saluresis. 2. an agent that promotes saluresis.

Saluron (sal′u-ron) trademark for a preparation of hydroflumethiazide.

salutary (sal′u-ta″re) [L. *salutaris*] favorable to the preservation or restoration of health.

Salutensin, Salutensin-Demi (sal″u-ten′sin) trademarks for preparations of hydroflumethiazide with reserpine, an antihypertensive.

salvarsan (sal′var-san) see *arsphenamine.* **s. copper,** a yellowish-red powder, a combination of arsphenamine and copper, suggested by Ehrlich for use in protozoan infections. **silver s.,** silver arsphenamine. **sulfoxylate s.,** a modified arsphenamine.

salve (sav) a thick ointment or cerate; see *ointment.* **Dreuw's s.,** salicylic acid 10, chrysarobin 20, birch tar 20, green soap 25, petrolatum 25. **fetron s.,** a salve composed of from 3 to 5 per cent of the anilide of stearic acid with petrolatum. **scarlet s.,** a synthetic cell proliferant, toluylazo-toluyl-azo-beta-naphthol.

Salvia (sal′ve-ah) [L.] a genus of labiate plants. The leaves of *S. officinalis* L., sage, contain a volatile oil, and are sudorific, carminative, and astringent. The dried leaves are used as an antisecretory agent in hyperhidrosis, sialorrhea, pharyngitis, and bronchitis, and have been used to check excessive milk secretion. *S. reflexa* L., mint weed, sometimes causes poisoning in stock.

Salyrgan (sal′er-gan) trademark for a preparation of mersalyl.

Salzmann's nodular corneal dystrophy (salz′manz) [Maximilian *Salzmann*, German ophthalmologist, 1862–1954] see under *dystrophy.*

samaderin (sah-mad′er-in) a light-yellow, bitter, crystalline principle from the fruit and bark of *Samadera indica,* a tree of India, Ceylon, and Java; a decoction of the leaf is used as an emetic and purgative.

samandaridine (sam″an-dar′ĭ-din) an alkaloid, $C_{21}H_{31}$-O_3N, from the skin of various salamanders; less poisonous than samandarine.

samandarine (sah-man′dah-rin) a poisonous alkaloid, $C_{19}H_{31}O_2N$, from the skin of various salamanders.

samarium (sah-ma′re-um) a very rare metallic element; symbol, Sm; atomic number, 62; atomic weight, 150.35.

Sambucus (sam-bu′kus) [L. "the elder-tree"] a genus of caprifoliaceous trees and shrubs; elder. The dried flowers have been used as a carminative, stimulant, and diuretic; the berries (elder berries) were thought to possess some laxative principles.

sample (sam′p'l) [L. *exemplum* example] a representative part taken to typify the whole. **random s.,** a sample chosen from a population in such a way that each choice is independent of the other choices and every member of the population has a fixed and determinate probability of being chosen (usually an equal probability).

sampling (sam′pling) the selection or making of a sample. **chorionic villus s. (CVS),** a procedure used for prenatal diagnosis at nine to 12 weeks' gestation. Fetal tissue for analysis is aspirated by catheter through the cervix from the villous area of the chorion (chorion frondosum), under ultrasonic guidance. Spelled also *chorionic villous sampling.* Called also *chorionic villus biopsy.*

Sampson's cyst (samp′sunz) [John Albertson *Sampson,* American gynecologist, 1873–1946] chocolate cyst.

Samuelsson (sam′u-el-son), Bengt Ingemar. Swedish biochemist, born 1934; co-winner, with Sune Bergström and John Robert Vane, of the Nobel prize for medicine or physiology in 1982 for their discovery of prostaglandins and related substances.

sanative (san′ah-tiv) [L. *sanare* to heal] having a tendency to heal; curative.

sanatorium (san″ah-to′re-um) [L. *sanatorius* conferring health, from *sanare* to cure] 1. an establishment for the treatment of sick persons, especially a private hospital for convalescents or those who are not extremely ill. The term is now applied particularly to an establishment for the open-air treatment of tuberculous patients. 2. a health station; a health resort in a hot region.

sanatory (san′ah-to″re) [L. *sanatorius*] conducive to health; salubrious.

Sanctorius (sank-to′re-us) [It. Santorio Santorio, 1561–1636] an Italian physician, professor of medicine at Padua, who devised several instruments of precision (e.g., a clinical thermometer and a pulse clock), and made quantitative experiments on basal metabolism or "insensible perspiration."

sand (sand) material occurring in small, gritty particles. **brain s.,** acervulus. **intestinal s.,** small gritty particles made up of oxides of calcium and phosphorus, bacteria, bile pigment, etc., formed in the intestine.

sandalwood (san′dal-wood) [L. *santalum*] 1. the fragrant wood of *Santalum album*, L. (Santalaceae), white or yellow sandal, and of other trees of the genera *Santalum* and *Fusanus*. See also *santal oil*, under *oil*. 2. the dried heart wood of the leguminous tree *Pterocarpus santalinus*, red sandal or santalum rubrum, used as a coloring agent.

sand crack (sand krak) a crack starting at the bearing surface of a horse's hoof; it rarely causes lameness.

Sanders' disease [Murray *Sanders*, New York bacteriologist, born 1910] epidemic keratoconjunctivitis.

sandfly (sand′fli) a name applied to various two-winged flies of the families Heleidae, Simuliidae, and Psychodidae, but especially to flies of the latter family (of the genus *Phlebotomus*).

Sandril (san′dril) trademark for preparations of reserpine.

Sandström's bodies, glands (zant-strämz) [Ivar Victor *Sandström*, Swedish anatomist, 1852–1889] see *parathyroid glands*, under *gland*, and see *glandulae thyroideae accessoriae*.

Sandwith's bald tongue (sand′withs) [Fleming Mant *Sandwith*, British physician, 1853–1918] see under *tongue*.

sane (sān) [L. *sanus*] of sound mind; compos mentis.

Sänger see *Saenger*.

Sanger (Sang′er), Frederick. British biochemist, born 1918; winner of the Nobel prize for chemistry in 1958 for isolating and identifying the amino acid components of the insulin molecule and creating a method to identify the order of amino acids in more complicated protein molecules.

sangui- [L. *sanguis* blood] a combining form denoting relationship to blood.

sanguicolous (sang-gwik′o-lus) [*sangui-* + L. *colere* to dwell] inhabiting or living in the blood.

sanguifacient (sang″gwĭ-fa′shent) [*sangui-* + L. *facere* to make] hematopoietic.

sanguiferous (sang-gwif′er-us) [*sangui-* + L. *ferre* to bear] conveying or containing blood.

sanguification (sang″gwĭ-fi-ka′shun) [*sangui-* + L. *facere* to make] hematopoiesis.

sanguimotor, sanguimotory (sang″gwĭ-mo′tor; sang″wĭ-mo′tor-e) [*sangui-* + L. *motor* mover] pertaining to blood circulation.

sanguinaria (sang″gwĭ-na′re-ah) the dried rhizome and root of the bloodroot, *Sanguinaria canadensis*, a perennial herb, used as an ingredient of compound white pine syrup. It was formerly used as an expectorant and externally in the treatment of chronic eczema and cancer of the skin. It contains several alkaloids, e.g., sanguinarine.

sanguinarine (sang″gwĭ-na′rēn) an alkaloid obtained from sanguinaria and other species of the same family, including the prickly poppy (*Argemona Mexicana*), the cause of epidemic dropsy.

sanguine (sang′gwin) [L. *sanguineus; sanguis* blood] 1. abounding in blood. 2. ardent; hopeful.

sanguineous (sang-gwin′e-us) abounding in blood; pertaining to the blood.

sanguinolent (sang-gwin′o-lent) [L. *sanguinolentus*] of a bloody tinge.

sanguinopoietic (sang″gwĭ-no-poi-et′ik) hematopoietic.

sanguinopurulent (sang″gwĭ-no-pu′ru-lent) containing both blood and pus.

sanguinous (sang′gwĭ-nus) sanguineous.

sanguirenal (sang″gwĭ-re′nal) [*sangui-* + L. *ren* kidney] pertaining to the blood and the kidneys.

sanguis (sang′gwis) [L.] blood.

sanguivorous (sang-gwiv′o-rus) [*sangui-* + L. *vorare* to eat] blood-eating; said of female mosquitoes, which prefer blood to other nutrients.

sanies (sa′ne-ēz) [L.] a fetid, ichorous discharge from a wound or ulcer, containing serum, pus, and blood.

saniopurulent (sa″ne-o-pu′roo-lent) partly sanious and partly purulent.

sanioserous (sa″ne-o-se′rous) partly sanious and partly serous.

sanious (sa′ne-us) [L. *saniosus*] of the nature of sanies.

sanitarian (san″ĭ-ta′re-an) a person who is expert in matters of sanitation and public health.

sanitarium (san″ĭ-ta′re-um) [L.] an institution for the promotion of health. The word was originally coined to designate the institution established by the Seventh Day Adventists at Battle Creek, Michigan, to distinguish it from institutions providing care for mental or tuberculous patients.

sanitary (san′ĭ-ta″re) [L. *sanitarius*] pertaining to health or promoting or conducive to health; usually used in reference to an environment that is clean, i.e., without an agent that is deleterious to health.

sanitation (san″ĭ-ta′shun) [L. *sanitas* health] the establishment of environmental conditions favorable to health.

sanitization (san″ĭ-ti-za′shun) the process of making or the quality of being made sanitary; see *sanitize*.

sanitize (san′ĭ-tīz) to clean and sterilize, as eating or drinking utensils.

sanity (san′ĭ-te) [L. *sanitas* soundness] soundness, especially soundness of mind.

Sanorex (san′o-reks) trademark for a preparation of mazindol.

Sansert (san′sert) trademark for a preparation of methysergide maleate.

Sansom's sign (san′somz) [Arthur Ernest *Sansom*, English physician, 1838–1907] see under *sign*.

Sanson's images (san′sonz) [Louis Joseph *Sanson*, French physician, 1790–1841] *Purkinje's images*; see under *image*.

santalum (san′tah-lum) sandalwood. **s. ru′brum,** the dried heart wood of *Pterocarpus santalinus*; used as a coloring agent.

santonica (san-ton′ĭ-kah) [L.] the dried unexpanded flower heads of *Artemisia maritima*, formerly used as an anthelmintic and stomachic; called also *semen contra*.

santonin (san′to-nin) a lactone, $C_{15}H_{18}O_3$, which may be obtained from the unexpanded flower heads of *Artemisia maritima* L. (Compositae), santonica, or other species of *Artemisia*; used as an anthelmintic against *Ascaris lumbricoides*.

Santorini's cartilages, etc. (sahn″to-re′nēz) [Giovanni Domenico *Santorini*, Italian anatomist, 1681–1737] see under *cartilage, duct, fissure, ligament, muscle, papilla, plexus,* and *tubercle*.

sap (sap) the natural juice of a living organism or tissue. **cell s.,** hyaloplasm, def. 1. **nuclear s.,** karyolymph.

saphena (sah-fe′nah) [L.; Gr. *saphēnēs* manifest] either of two large superficial veins of the leg; see *vena saphena*.

saphenectomy (saf″ĕ-nek′to-me) [*saphena* + Gr. *ektomē* excision] excision of a saphenous vein.

saphenous (sah-fe′nus) pertaining to or associated with a saphena; applied to certain arteries, nerves, veins, etc.

sapid (sap′id) [L. *sapidus*] having or imparting an agreeable taste.

sapin (sa′pin) a nontoxic ptomaine, $C_5H_{14}N_2$, isomeric with cadaverine and neuridine.

sapo (sa′po) [L. "soap"] 1. soap; a compound of a fatty acid with a suitable base. 2. white castile soap made of soda and olive oil, used in pills, suppositories, plasters, and liniments: detergent. **s. anima′lis,** s. domesticus. **s. cine′reus,** gray soap, or mercurial salve soap, a soap containing 50 per cent, by weight, of mercury and 5 per cent of benzoinated fat. **s. domes′ticus,** a preparation of a soft soap made of animal fat and potash. **s. du′rus,** soda soap. **s. mol′lis,** soft soap. **s. mol′lis medicina′lis,** green soap. **s. vir′idis,** green soap.

sapogenin (sah-poj′ĕ-nin) a compound resulting from the decomposition of saponin, $C_{14}H_{22}O_2$.

saponaceous (sa″po-na′shus) [L. *sapo* soap] of a soapy quality or nature.

Saponaria (sa″po-na′re-ah) a genus of plants. The root of *S. officinalis*, or soapwort, has alterative properties and was formerly used in skin diseases. It contains saponin, saponarin, and sapotoxin.

saponarin (sa″po-na′rin) a glycoside, $C_{27}H_{30}O_{16}$, from *Saponaria officinalis* L. (Caryophyllaceae).

saponatus (sa″po-na′tus) [L., from *sapo* soap] charged or mixed with soap.

saponification (sah-pon″ĭ-fi-ka′shun) [L. *sapo* soap + *facere* to make] the act or process of converting fats into soaps and glycerol by heating with alkalis. In chemistry, the term now denotes hydrolysis of an ester by an alkali, resulting in the production of a free alcohol and an alkali salt of the ester acid.

saponin (sap'o-nin) a group of glycosides, widely distributed in plants, such as *Quillaja saponaria* Molina (Rosaceae) and *Saponaria officinalis* L. (Caryophyllaceae), and characterized (1) by their property of forming a durable foam when their watery solutions are shaken, (2) by their ability to dissolve red blood cells even in high dilutions, and (3) by their having sapogenin as their aglycones. **cholan s's,** a group of saponins that on hydrolysis yield sterol-like compounds. **triterpenoid s's,** a group of saponins that on hydrolysis yield 1,2,7-trimethyl naphthalene.

sapophore (sap'o-for) [L. *sapor* taste + Gr. *phoros* bearing] the group of atoms in the molecule of a compound that gives the substance its characteristic taste.

sapotalene (sap'o-tal''ēn) a hydrocarbon, 1,2,7-trimethyl-naphthalene, formed by the reduction of sapogenin.

sapotoxin (sa''po-tok'sin) any of various toxic saponins found in such plants as *Quillaja saponaria* Molina (Rosaceae) and *Saponaria officinalis* L. (Caryophyllaceae).

Sappey's fibers, ligament, nucleus, veins (sahp-pāz') [Marie Philibert Constant *Sappey*, French anatomist, 1810–1896] see under *fiber* and *ligament*, and see *venae paraumbicales* and *nucleus ruber*.

sapphism (saf'izm) [*Sappho*, Greek poetess, about 600 B.C.] homosexuality between women; lesbianism.

saprin (sa'prin) [Gr. *sapros* rotten] a ptomaine, $C_5H_{14}N_2$, from decaying visceral substances; not poisonous.

sapr(o)- [Gr. *sapros* rotten] a combining form meaning rotten or putrid, or designating relationship to decay or to decaying material.

saprobe (sah'prōb) [*sapro-* + Gr. *bios* life] an organism that feeds on dead or decaying organic matter.

saprobic (sah-prōb-ik) of the nature of, or being a saprobe.

Saprolegnia (sap''ro-leg'ne-ah) [*sapro-* + Gr. *legnon* border] a genus of partially saprophytic, phycomycetous water molds of the order Saprolegniales, subclass Oomycetes. *S. fe'rax* is destructive to salmon and to various water animals.

Saprolegniales (sap''ro-leg''ne-a'lēz) an order of mostly saprophytic molds of the subclass Oomycetes, class Phycomycetes, which have an extensive mycelial thallus that has no cross walls, including the genera *Saprolegnia* and *Achlya*. These fungi are commonly called "water molds," although some inhabit soil.

sapronosis (sap''ro-no'sis) a disease caused by organisms of the environment.

saprophilous (sah-prof'ĭ-lus) [*sapro-* + Gr. *philein* to love] saprophytic.

saprophyte (sap'ro-fīt) [*sapro-* + Gr. *phyton* plant] a saprophytic organism. Cf. *autophyte*.

saprophytic (sap''ro-fit'ik) 1. having a type of nutrition involving uptake of organic materials in dissolved form obtained for dead or decaying plant or animal matter; said of plants or so-called plantlike organisms (e.g., certain protozoa, bacteria, or fungi). Cf. *saprozoic*. 2. saprozoic.

Saprospira (sap''ro-spi'rah) [*sapro-* + Gr. *speira* coil] a genus of gliding bacteria of the family Cytophagaceae, found free-living in fresh and salt water, made up of helical filament cells. The type species is *S. gran'dis*.

saprozoic (sap''ro-zo'ik) [*sapro-* + Gr. *zōon* animal] having a type of nutrition involving uptake of organic materials in dissolved form obtained from dead or decaying plant or animal matter; said of animals or so-called animal-like organisms (e.g., certain protozoa). Called also *saprophytic*. Cf. *holozoic* and *saprophytic*.

saralasin acetate (sar-al'ah-sin) chemical name: 1-(*N*-methylglycine)-5-L-valine-8-L-alaninangiotensin II acetate (salt) hydrate. An angiotensin-II antagonist, $C_{42}H_{65}N_{13}O_{10}$·-$xC_2H_4O_2$·xH_2O, used as an antihypertensive in the treatment of severe hypertension and in the diagnosis of renin-dependent hypertension.

Sarbó's sign (sar'bōz) [Arthur von *Sarbó*, Budapest neurologist, born 1867] see under *sign*.

Sarcina (sar'sĭ-nah) [L. "package," "bundle"] a genus of spherical, gram-positive bacteria of the family Micrococcaceae, occurring in cubical packets of eight or more cells. They are strict anaerobes found in soil and on grains and occasionally in clinical specimens.

sarcina (sar'sĭ-nah), pl. *sar'cinae*. 1. a spherical bacterium occurring predominantly in cubical packets of eight cells as a consequence of failure of daughter cells to separate following cell division in three planes. 2. an organism of the genus *Sarcina*.

sarcinae (sar'sĭ-ne) [L.] plural of *sarcina*.

sarc(o)- [Gr. *sarx, sarkos* flesh] a combining form denoting relationship to flesh.

sarcoblast (sar'ko-blast) [*sarco-* + Gr. *blastos* germ] the primitive cell which develops into a muscle cell.

sarcocarcinoma (sar''ko-kar''sĭ-no'mah) sarcoma and carcinoma combined.

sarcocele (sar'ko-sēl) [*sarco-* + Gr. *kēlē* tumor] any fleshy swelling or tumor of the testis.

sarcocyst (sar'ko-sist) [*sarco-* + *cyst*] 1. a protozoan of the genus *Sarcocystis*. 2. one of the elongated, fusiform, cylindrical, membrane-bound hyaline bodies containing the numerous crescentic or banana-shaped, uninucleate trophozoites (Rainey's corpuscles) of the protozoan *Sarcocystis*, found in the muscles of those with sarcocystosis. Called also *Miescher tube* or *tubule*, *Rainey's tube* or *tubule*, and *sarcosporidian cyst*.

sarcocystin (sar''ko-sis'tin) a toxin obtained from species of *Sarcocystis*.

Sarcocystis (sar''ko-sis'tis) [*sarco-* + Gr. *kystis* bladder] a genus of coccidian protozoa (suborder Eimeriina, order Eucoccidiida) parasitic in birds, reptiles, and mammals, including humans, cattle, horses, sheep, swine, rabbits, and rodents, occurring as elogated cylindrical bodies (sarcocysts) in the host's muscles. They have an obligatory two-host life cycle, involving sexual reproduction in the definitive host (a carnivore), and asexual reproduction, including schizogony and sarcocyst formation, occurs in the intermediate host. Infection is transmitted by ingestion of the sporocysts in the feces passed by infected animals (see *sarcocystosis*). **S. bovihom'inis,** a species for which cattle are the specific intermediate hosts and humans the definitive hosts; it causes intestinal sarcocystosis in the latter. Together with *S. suihominis*, formerly considered to be a single species, *S. hominis* (*Isospora hominis*). **S. hom'inis,** see *S. bovihominis* and *S. suihominis*. **S. lindeman'ni,** a species causing human infection, most cases of which are asymptomatic, although it may cause polymyositis sometimes associated with eosinophilia. **S. suihom'inis,** a species for which swine are the specific intermediate hosts and humans the definitive hosts; it causes intestinal sarcocystosis in the latter. Together with *S. bovihominis*, formerly considered to be a single genus, *S. hominis* (*Isospora hominis*).

sarcocystosis (sar''ko-sis-to'sis) infection with protozoa of the genus *Sarcocystis*, which in humans is usually asymptomatic or manifested either by muscle cysts associated with myositis or myocarditis or by intestinal infection. It is usually transmitted by the eating of raw or undercooked beef or pork containing sporocysts of the parasites or by ingestion of sporocysts from the feces of an infected animal, usually in contaminated soil. Heavy infections in cattle and other animals may be associated with anorexia, emaciation, fever, nervousness, lameness, hypersalivation, anemia, and abortion. Called also *sarcosporidiasis* and *sarcosporidiosis*.

Sarcodina (sar''ko-di'nah) [Gr. *sarkōdēs* fleshlike] a subphylum of protozoa (phylum Sarcomastigophora), the organisms of which alter their body shape and move about and acquire food by extension of cytoplasmic organelles (pseudopodia) of various types, or by protoplasmic flow without producing discrete pseudopodia. Some have flagella during developmental or other temporary stages. The body of some sarcodines is naked, while in others an external or internal test or skeleton is present. It comprises two superclasses: Actinopoda and Rhizopoda; the latter has been used as a synonym of Sarcodina.

sarcodine (sar'ko-dīn) 1. pertaining to the subphylum Sarcodina. 2. any individual protozoan of the subphylum Sarcodina. Called also *sarcodinian*.

sarcodinian (sar''ko-din'e-an) sarcodine.

sarcoenchondroma (sar''ko-en''kon-dro'mah) chondrosarcoma.

sarcogenic (sar''ko-jen'ik) [*sarco-* + Gr. *gennan* to produce] forming flesh.

sarcoglia (sar-kog'le-ah) [*sarco-* + Gr. *glia* glue] the substance which composes Doyére's eminence at the entrance of nerve filament into a muscle fiber.

sarcohydrocele (sar″ko-hi′dro-sēl)   sarcocele combined with hydrocele.

sarcoid (sar′koid) [sarc- + -oid]   1. sarcoidosis. 2. a sarcoma-like tumor. 3. fleshlike. **Boeck's s., s. of Boeck,** sarcoidosis. **Darier-Roussy s.,** a form of sarcoidosis characterized by the large size of the nodules and their subcutaneous location. **Schaumann's s.,** sarcoidosis. **Spiegler-Fendt s.,** lymphocytoma cutis.

sarcoidosis (sar″koi-do′sis) [sarcoid + -osis]   a chronic, progressive, systemic granulomatous reticulosis of unknown etiology, involving almost any organ or tissue, including the skin, lungs, lymph nodes, liver, spleen, eyes, and small bones of the hands and feet. It is characterized histologically by the presence in all affected organs or tissues of noncaseating epithelioid cell tubercles (naked or hard tubercles). Laboratory findings may include hypercalcemia and hypergammaglobinemia; there is usually diminished or absent reactivity to tuberculin and in most active cases, a positive Kveim reaction. The acute form has an abrupt onset and a high spontaneous remission rate, whereas the chronic form, insidious in onset, is progressive. Called also Besnier-Boeck or Boeck's disease, sarcoid, sarcoid of Boeck, and Schaumann's disease, sarcoid, and syndrome. **s. cor′dis,** involvement of the heart in sarcoidosis, with lesions ranging from a few asymptomatic, microscopic granulomas to widespread infiltration of the myocardium by large masses of sarcoid tissue. **muscular s.,** sarcoidosis involving the skeletal muscles, with sarcoid tubercles, interstitial inflammation with fibrosis, and disruption and atrophy of the muscle fibers.

sarcolactic acid (sar″ko-lak′tik)   an old term for L-lactic acid; so-called because it is produced in muscle during anaerobic exercise.

sarcolemma (sar″ko-lem′ah) [sarco- + Gr. lemma husk]   the delicate plasma membrane which invests every striated muscle fiber.

sarcolemmic (sar″ko-lem′ik)   pertaining to or of the nature of sarcolemma.

sarcolemmous (sar″ko-lem′us)   sarcolemmic.

L-sarcolysin (sar″ko-li′sin)   melphalan.

sarcoma (sar-ko′mah), pl. sarcomas or sarco′mata [sarco- + -oma]   a tumor made up of a substance like the embryonic connective tissue; tissue composed of closely packed cells embedded in a fibrillar or homogeneous substance. Sarcomas are often highly malignant. See also chondrosarcoma, fibrosarcoma, lymphosarcoma, melanosarcoma, myxosarcoma, osteosarcoma, etc. **Abernethy's s.,** a variety of fatty tumor found principally on the trunk. **adipose s.,** liposarcoma. **alveolar soft part s.,** a variety having a reticulated fibrous stoma enclosing groups of sarcoma cells, which resemble epithelial cells and are enclosed in alveoli walled with connective tissue. **ameloblastic s.,** the malignant counterpart of ameloblastic fibroma. **botryoid s., s. botryoi′des,** a variety of embryonal rhabdomyosarcoma, arising in submucosal tissue, presenting grossly as a polypoid grapelike structure, and found most often in young children or infants in the upper vagina, cervix uteri, or neck of the urinary bladder. **chicken s.,** a sarcoma of chickens which may be of several various cell types. **chloromatous s.,** chloroma. **chondroblastic s.,** see osteogenic s. **s. col′li u′teri hydro′picum papilla′re,** botryoid s. **deciduocellular s.,** choriocarcinoma. **embryonal s.,** Wilms' tumor. **endometrial stromal s.,** a pale, polypoid, fleshy, malignant tumor of the endometrial stroma, usually arising from the uterine fundus. **Ewing's s.,** see under tumor. **fascial s.,** a sarcoma arising in the fasciae about the joints, especially in the lower extremities. **fibroblastic s.,** see osteogenic s. **fowl s.,** chicken s. **giant cell s.,** a malignant form of giant cell tumor of bone; see under tumor. **granulocytic s.,** chloroma. **Hodgkin's s.,** Hodgkin's disease of the lymphocytic depletion type. **idiopathic multiple pigmented hemorrhagic s.,** Kaposi's s. **immunoblastic s. of B cells,** an aggressive B-cell lymphoma believed to arise from transformed interfollicular B lymphocytes, which in many cases is associated with a preexisting immunologic disorder, e.g., Sjögren's syndrome, systemic lupus erythematosus, or Hashimoto's thyroiditis, or with an immunosuppressed state. **immunoblastic s. of T cells,** a group of T-cell lymphomas comprising tumors derived from T lymphocytes in the

paracortical area arising from a mixture of small lymphocytes and many large transformed cells; the latter are characterized by one or more small but distinctly eosinophilic nucleoli. **Jensen's s.,** a malignant tumor in mice transmissible to healthy mice by transplanting a small portion of the tumor. **Kaposi's s.,** a multicentric, malignant neoplastic vascular proliferation characterized by the development of bluish-red cutaneous nodules, usually on the lower extremities, most often on the toes or feet, and slowly increasing in size and number and spreading to more proximal sites. The tumors have endothelium-lined channels and vascular spaces admixed with variably sized aggregates of spindle-shaped cells, and often remain confined to skin and subcutaneous tissue, but widespread visceral involvement may occur. Kaposi's sarcoma occurs endemically in certain parts of Central Africa and Central and Eastern Europe, and a particularly virulent and disseminated form occurs in immunocompromised patients, e.g., transplant recipients and those with acquired immunodeficiency syndrome. Called also multiple idiopathic hemorrhagic s. and idiopathic multiple pigmented hemorrhagic s. **Kupffer cell s.,** angiosarcoma of the liver in adults. **leukocytic s.,** leukosarcoma. **lymphatic s.,** diffuse lymphoma. **melanotic s.,** malignant melanoma. **mixed cell s.,** malignant mesenchymoma. **multiple idiopathic hemorrhagic s.,** Kaposi's s. **osteoblastic s.,** see osteogenic s. **osteogenic s.,** a malignant primary tumor of bone composed of a malignant connective tissue stroma with evidence of malignant osteoid, bone, and/or cartilage formation. Depending on which component is dominant, three major subtypes are recognized: osteoblastic, fibroblastic, and chondroblastic. Called also osteosarcoma, osteoid s., and osteolytic s. **osteoid s.,** osteogenic s. **osteolytic s.,** osteogenic s. **parosteal s.,** a sarcoma situated close to the outer surface of a bone. **polymorphous s.,** malignant mesenchymoma. **pseudo-Kaposi s.,** unilateral subacute to chronic dermatitis, often with postinflammatory hyperpigmentation, occurring in association with underlying arteriovenous fistula, which closely resembles Kaposi's sarcoma both clinically and histologically. **reticulocytic s., reticuloendothelial s.,** reticulum cell s. **reticulum cell s.,** histiocytic lymphoma. **retothelial s.,** reticulum cell s. **Rous s.,** a peculiar sarcoma-like growth found in some fowls; from it can be obtained a filterable virus, the first known to cause tumors, which on inoculation into other fowls produces similar growths. **serocystic s.,** a proliferous cyst with intracystic growths. **synovial s.,** synoviosarcoma. **telangiectatic s.,** a sarcoma which develops such a rich vascular network that the endothelial cells are mistaken for the neoplastic element.

sarcomagenic (sar″ko-mah-jen′ik)   causing sarcoma.

Sarcomastigophora (sar″ko-mas″tĭ-gof′o-rah) [sarco- + Gr. mastix whip + phoros bearing]   a phylum comprising protozoa that typically possess an endosome nucleus characterized by a ring of nuclear chromatin around a central chromatin-free region, and are motile by means of flagella, pseudopodia, or both types of locomotor organs. The phylum includes the subphyla Mastigophora (flagellates), Sarcodina (amebae), and Opalinata (opalinids).

sarcomata (sar-ko′mah-tah)   plural of sarcoma.

sarcomatoid (sar-ko′mah-toid)   resembling sarcoma.

sarcomatosis (sar″ko-mah-to′sis)   a condition characterized by the formation of sarcomas. **s. cu′tis,** the development of sarcomatous growths on the skin. **general s.,** the occurrence of sarcomas in several parts of the body at the same time.

sarcomatous (sar-ko′mah-tus)   pertaining to or of the nature of sarcoma.

sarcomere (sar′ko-mēr) [sarco- + Gr. meros part]   the contractile unit of myofibrils; sarcomeres are repeating units, delimited by the Z bands along the length of the myofibril.

sarcomphalocele (sar″kom-fal′o-sēl) [sarco- + Gr. omphalos navel + kēlē tumor]   a fleshy tumor of the umbilicus.

sarconeme (sar′ko-nēm) [sarco- + Gr. nēma thread]   microneme.

Sarcophaga (sar-kof′ah-gah) [sarco- + Gr. phagein to eat]   a genus of flies of the family Sarcophagidae. The larvae of several species have been found in wounds, ulcers, the nasal passages, and sinuses. The most important species is S. haemorrhoida′lis. Other species are S. carna′ria, S. fuscicau′da, S. dux, S. nificor′nis, and S. rubicor′nis.

Sarcophagidae (sar″ko-faj′ĭ-de) a family of flies of the order Diptera, including the flesh flies; two genera *Sarcophaga* (type genus) and *Wohlfahrtia* produce myiasis in man and domestic animals.

sarcoplasm (sar′ko-plazm) [*sarco-* + Gr. *plasma* anything formed or molded] the interfibrillary matter of the striated muscles; the substance in which the fibrillae of the muscle fiber are embedded.

sarcoplasmic (sar″ko-plaz′mik) composed of or containing sarcoplasm; see also under *reticulum*.

sarcoplast (sar′ko-plast) [*sarco-* + Gr. *plastos* formed] an interstitial cell of a muscle, itself capable of being transformed into a muscle.

sarcopoietic (sar″ko-poi-et′ik) [*sarco-* + Gr. *poiein* to make] producing flesh or muscle.

Sarcopsylla (sar″kop-sil′ah) *Tunga*. **S. pen′etrans,** *Tunga penetrans*.

Sarcoptes (sar-kop′tēz) [*sarco-* + Gr. *koptein* to cut] a genus of acarids, including *S. scabie′i* (*Acarus scabiei*), the itch mite of humans, which produces scabies (q.v.). Varieties of *S. scabiei* cause mange of domestic animals, including pigs, horses, cows, and dogs.

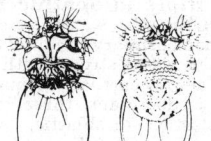

Sarcoptes scabiei, male and female.

sarcoptic (sar-kop′tic) of, relating to, or caused by *Sarcoptes*.

sarcoptidosis (sar-kop″tĭ-do′sis) infestation with *Sarcoptes*.

sarcosine (sar′ko-sēn) chemical name: *N*-methylglycine. An amino acid intermediate between glycine and dimethyl glycine in the one-carbon cycle, $C_3H_7NO_2$, found in shellfish, peanut protein, actinomycins, and, in low levels, in normal human blood.

sarcosine dehydrogenase (sar′ko-sēn de-hi′dro-jĕ-nās) [EC 1.5.99.1] an enzyme of the oxidoreductase class that catalyzes the reaction sarcosine + ubiquinone + H_2O = glycine + formaldehyde + ubiquinol in choline catabolism. The enzyme is a flavoprotein found in mitochondrial inner membrane; deficiency in it, an autosomal recessive trait, results in hypersarcosinemia.

sarcosis (sar-ko′sis) [*sarco-* + *-osis*] abnormal increase of flesh.

sarcosome (sar′ko-sōm) [*sarco-* + Gr. *sōma* body] former name for one of the mitochondria of a myofibril.

Sarcosporidia (sar″ko-spo-rid′e-ah) in former systems of classification, an order of sporozoan protozoa that included the genus *Sarcocystis*.

sarcosporidiasis (sar″ko-spo″rĭ-di′ah-sis) sarcocystosis.

sarcosporidiosis (sar″ko-spo-rid″e-o′sis) sarcocystosis.

sarcostosis (sar″kos-to′sis) [*sarco-* + Gr. *osteon* bone] ossification of fleshy tissues.

sarcostyle (sar′ko-stīl) [*sarco-* + Gr. *stylos* column] 1. a myofibril. 2. a bundle of myofibrils; called also *column of Kolliker* and *muscle column*.

sarcotherapeutics (sar″ko-ther″ah-pu′tiks) treatment of disease by the use of animal extracts.

sarcotherapy (sar″ko-ther′ah-pe) sarcotherapeutics.

sarcotic (sar-kot′ik) [Gr. *sarkōtikos*] promoting the growth of flesh.

sarcotubules (sar″ko-tu′būlz) membrane-limited structures that extend throughout the sarcoplasm and form a closely meshed canalicular network around each myofibril.

sarcous (sar′kus) pertaining to flesh or to muscular tissues.

sardonic (sar-don′ik) [L. *sardonicus, sardonius;* from Gr. *sardonios* Sardinian; an alteration (influenced by *sardonion*, a poisonous Sardinian herb that supposedly distorted the eater's face) of *sardanios* scornful, bitter] denoting a kind

of spasmodic or tetanic grin or involuntary smile, as *risus sardonicus*.

sarmentocymarin (sar-men″to-si′mah-rin) a cardiac glycoside, $C_{30}H_{46}O_8$, from the seeds of *Strophanthus sarmentosus* DC. var. *senegambiae* (A. DC.). On hydrolysis, it yields sarmentogenin and sarmentose.

sarmentogenin (sar″men-toj′ĕ-nin) an aglycone, $C_{23}H_{34}$-O_5, from sarmentocymarin; it has been studied as a possible source of cortisone.

sarmentose (sar′men-tōs) a methyl ether of a 2-desoxyhexomethyl sugar from sarmentocymarin.

Sarothamnus (sa″ro-tham′nus) [Gr. *saron* broom + *thamnos* shrub] *Cytisus*.

sarpicillin (sar″pĭ-sil′in) chemical name: 6-(2,2-dimethyl-5- oxo-4- phenyl -1-imidazolidinyl) -3,3- dimethyl -7- oxo -4-thia-1-azabicyclo[3.2.0]heptane-2-carboxylic acid; an antibacterial, $C_{21}H_{27}N_3O_5S$.

Sarracenia (sar″ah-se′ne-ah) [Michel *Sarrazin*, Quebec physician and naturalist, 1659–1734] a genus of polypetalous plants, known as *side-saddle flower* and *pitcher plant*, type of the order Sarraceniaceae. *S. purpu′rea* L. (Sarraceniaceae) is the commonest of the pitcher plants of North America. The secretion of the pitcher of this plant is said to contain digestant enzymes. It is a stimulant, diuretic, and aperient.

sarsa (sar′sah), gen. *sar′sae* [L.; Sp. *sarça* briar] sarsaparilla.

sarsaparilla (sar″sap-ah-ril′ah) [L.; Sp. ''briar vine''] the dried root of *Smilax aristolochiaefolia* Mill. (Liliaceae) and other related species; used as a flavoring agent in beverages, and in the treatment of psoriasis. It contains sarsasapogenin, a precursor in the manufacture of compounds in the pregnane series. Called also *sarsa*.

sarsasapogenin (sar″sah-sap″o-jen′in) a steroid sapogenin from sarsaparilla, used in the synthesis of hormones of the pregnane series.

Sassafras (sas′ah-fras) [L.] a genus of lauraceous trees. The root bark of *S. albi′dum* Nutt. (Lauraceae) (*S. variifo′lia, S. officina′le*), or sassafras, a tree of North America, is used as an aromatic and flavoring agent, and was formerly used as a sudorific. The volatile oil contains safrene and safrol. It is the source of the popular American beverage, root beer.

satellite (sat′ĕ-līt) [L. *satelles* companion] 1. a vein that closely accompanies an artery, such as the brachial. 2. a minor, or attendant, lesion situated near a larger one. 3. a globoid mass of chromatin attached at the secondary constriction to the ends of the short arms of acrocentric autosomes. 4. exhibiting satellitism. 5. the posterior of a pair of gregarines undergoing syzygy. Cf. *primite*. **bacterial s.,** satellite colony. **centriolar s.,** one of the small dense, amorphous bodies associated with the centrioles, which serve as nucleatin sites for polymerization of tubulin to form microtubules. **chromosomal s.,** see *satellite*. **nucleolar s.,** a small mass of chromatin found next to the nucleolar membrane in most nerve cells of the female; sex chromatin.

satellitism (sat′ĕ-li-tizm) the phenomenon in which certain bacterial species grow more vigorously in the immediate vicinity of colonies of other unrelated species (e.g., *Haemophilus influenzae* near a colony of staphylococci), owing to the production of an essential metabolite by the latter species.

satellitosis (sat″ĕ-li-to′sis) accumulation of neuroglial cells about neurons; seen whenever neurons are damaged.

satiety (sah-ti′e-ty) [L. *satis* sufficient + *-ety* state or condition of] sufficiency, or satisfaction, as full gratification of appetite or thirst, with abolition of the desire to ingest food or liquids.

Satterthwaite's method (sat′er-thwāts) [Thomas Edward *Satterthwaite*, New York physician, 1843–1934] see under *method*.

Sattler's layer (sat′lerz) [Hubert *Sattler*, Austrian ophthalmologist, 1844–1928] see under *layer*.

saturated (sach′ĕ-rāt″ed) 1. having all the chemical affinities satisfied. 2. unable to hold in solution any more of a given substance. 3. denoting a fatty acid having only single bonds in its carbon chain.

saturation (sach′ĕ-ra′shun) [L. *saturatio*] 1. the act of saturating or condition of being saturated. 2. in radiotherapy, the delivery of a maximum tolerable tissue dose within a short time period and then maintenance of this biologic effect for an extended period of time by additional smaller fractional doses. 3. an effervescing draft or potion. **oxygen s.,** a measure of the degree to which oxygen is bound to hemoglobin, given as a percentage calculated by dividing the maximum oxygen capacity into the actual oxygen content and multiplying by 100.

saturnine (sat′ur-nīn) [L. *saturninus; saturnus* lead] pertaining to or produced by lead; having the dull, heavy properties associated with lead.

saturnism (sat′ur-nizm) [L. *saturnus* lead] lead poisoning.

satyriasis (sat″ĭ-ri′ah-sis) [Gr. *satyros* satyr] abnormal, excessive, insatiable sexual desire in the male. Cf. *nymphomania*.

satyromania (sat″ĭ-ro-ma′ne-ah) [Gr. *satyros* satyr + *mania* madness] satyriasis.

saucer (saw′ser) a rounded, shallow depression. **auditory s.,** see under *placode*.

saucerization (saw″ser-i-za′shun) 1. the excavation of tissue to form a shallow shelving depression usually performed to facilitate drainage from infected areas of bone. 2. the shallow, saucer-like depression on the upper surface of a vertebra which has suffered a compression fracture.

Sauerbruch's cabinet, prosthesis (sow′er-brooks) [Ernst Ferdinand *Sauerbruch*, surgeon in Berlin, 1875–1951] see under *cabinet* and *prosthesis*.

Saundby's test (sawnd′bēz) [Robert *Saundby*, English physician, 1849–1918] see under *tests*.

Saunders' disease, sign (sawn′derz) [Edward Watt *Saunders*, physician in St. Louis, 1854–1927] see under *disease* and *sign*.

sauroid (saw′roid) [Gr. *sauros* lizard + *eidos* form] resembling a reptile.

Saussure's hygrometer (so-sürz′) [Horace Bénédict de *Saussure*, Swiss physicist, 1740–1779] see under *hygrometer*.

savin (sav′in) [L. *sabina*] the evergreen shrub, *Juniperus sabina* L. Cupressaceae. The fresh tops afford an acrid volatile oil which has been used in folk medicine for its emmenagogic, antirheumatic, and anthelmintic properties, and is used in perfumery. A preparation of the young twigs was formerly used as a diuretic.

saw (saw) a cutting instrument with a cutting or serrated edge. **Adams' s.,** a small straight saw with a long handle, for osteotomy. **amputating s.,** one for use in performing amputations. **bayonet s.,** a surgical bone saw used for the excision of the nasal dorsal hump. **Butcher's s.,** an amputating saw with a blade that can be set at various angles. **chain s.,** one in which the teeth are set on links, the saw being moved by pulling one or the other handle. **crown s.,** a form of trephine. **Farabeuf's s.,** a saw the blade of which can be set at any desired angle. **Gigli's wire s.,** a flexible wire with saw teeth. **Hey's s.,** a small saw for enlarging orifices in bones. **hole s.,** a trephine. **separating s.,** a saw for separating teeth. **Shrady's s., subcutaneous s.,** a saw for bone work operated through a fenestrated cannula which has been introduced alongside the bone by a trocar.

saxitoxin (sak″sĭ-tok′sin) a powerful, heat-stable, low molecular weight neurotoxin synthesized and secreted by certain dinoflagellates, such as species of *Gonyaulax*, which accumulates in the tissues of bivalve mollusks feeding on the dinoflagellates, and may cause a severe toxic reaction in those who ingest contaminated shellfish. See also *shellfish poisoning*, under *poisoning*.

Sayre's apparatus (sa′erz) [Lewis Albert *Sayre*, American surgeon, 1820–1900] see under *apparatus*.

Sb chemical symbol for *antimony* (L. *stibium*).

SbCl₃ antimony trichloride.

Sb₂O₃ antimony trioxide.

Sb₂O₅ antimony pentoxide.

Sb₄O₆ antimony trioxide.

SC secretory component.

S.C. closure of the semilunar valves.

Sc chemical symbol for *scandium*.

SCAB a regimen of streptozocin, CCNU (lomustine), Adriamycin (doxorubicin), and bleomycin, used in cancer chemotherapy.

scab (skab) 1. crust. 2. to become covered with a crust or scab. **foot s.,** sheep scab. **head s.,** any acariasis of the

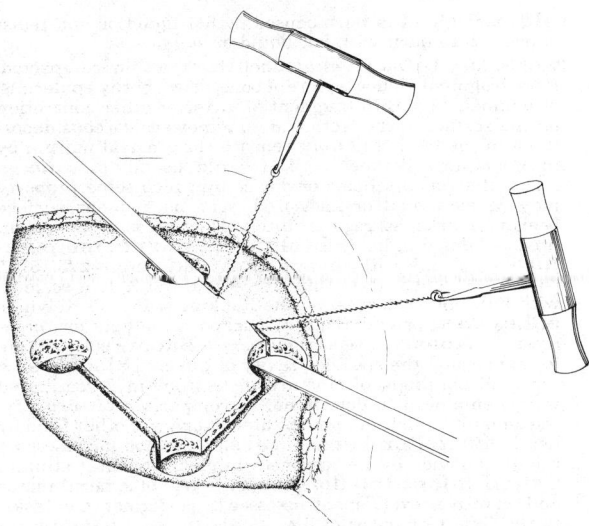

Gigli's wire saw as used in removing segment of the skull.

head, especially the sarcoptic scab of the head of sheep. **sheep s.,** a disease of sheep caused by the mite *Psoroptes ovis*, which infests the skin at the base of the hairs. A scab is formed which comes off, bringing the wool along with it.

scabetic (skah-bet′ik) scabietic.

scabicide (ska′bĭ-sīd) 1. destructive to *Sarcoptes scabiei*; used in the treatment of scabies. 2. an agent for destroying *Sarcoptes scabiei*.

scabies (ska′bēz) [L., from *scabere* scratch] a contagious dermatitis of humans and various wild and domestic animals (see *mange*) caused by the itch mite, *Sarcoptes scabiei*, transmitted by close contact, and characterized by a papular eruption over tiny, raised sinuous burrows (cuniculi) produced by digging into the upper layer of the epidermis by the egg-laying female mite, which is accompanied by intense pruritus and sometimes associated with eczema from scratching and secondary bacterial infection. Called also the *itch* and *seven-year itch*. **crusted s.,** Norwegian s. **Norwegian s.,** a rare, severe form of scabies associated with an extremely heavy infestation of *Sarcoptes scabiei*, which is seen especially in the senile and mentally retarded, in patients with poor sensation or severe systemic disease, and in immunosuppressed patients, and presumably representing an abnormal host immune response to the etiologic agent. It is characterized by a marked crusting dermatitis of the hands and feet with subungual horny debris, erythematous scaling plaques on the neck, scalp, and trunk that may become generalized, and usually lymphadenopathy and eosinophilia. Called also *crusted s.*

scabietic (ska″be-et′ik) pertaining to or affected with scabies.

scala (ska′lah), pl. *sca′lae* [L. "staircase"] a stairlike structure; applied especially to various passages of the cochlea. **s. me′dia, s. of Löwenberg,** ductus cochlearis. **s. tym′pani** [NA], the perilymph-filled part of the cochlea that is continuous with the scala vestibuli at the helicotrema, is separated from other cochlear structures by the spiral lamina and the cochlear duct, and ends blindly near the fenestra cochleae. Called also *tympanic canal of cochlea*. **s. vestib′uli** [NA], the perilymph-filled part of the cochlea that begins in the vestibule, is separated from other cochlear structures by the spiral lamina and the cochlear duct, and becomes continuous with the scala tympani at the helicotrema. Called also *vestibular canal*.

scalar (ska′lar) [L. *scalaris* pertaining to a ladder or staircase] 1. a quantity that has magnitude only, such as mass or temperature. Cf. *vector*. 2. pertaining to a scalar.

scalariform (skah-lar′ĭ-form) [L. *scalaris* like a ladder + *forma* shape] resembling the rungs of a ladder.

scald (skawld) 1. a burn caused by hot liquid or hot, moist vapor. 2. to burn with hot liquid or steam.

scale (skāl) 1. [Old Fr. *escale* shell, husk] a thin, compacted, flaky fragment; delicate plate of bone; dried, horny epidermis; or enamel. 2. a thin fragment of tartar or other concretion on the surface of the teeth. 3. to remove calcareous deposits from the teeth and from beneath the gingival margin by means of an instrument. 4. [L. *scala*, usually pl. *scalae*, a series of steps] a scheme or device by which some property may be evaluated or measured, such as a linear surface bearing marks at regular intervals, representing certain predetermined units. **absolute s., absolute temperature s.**, 1. one with its zero at absolute zero (−273.15° C, −459.67° F) and with Celsius degrees on the Kelvin scale or with Fahrenheit degrees on the Rankine scale. 2. Kelvin s. **adhesive s.**, one not readily sloughed, as in lupus erythematosus. **Apgar s.**, see under *score*. **Baumé's s.**, a scale for expressing the specific gravity of fluids. **Bloch's s.**, a series of solutions of tincture of benzoin in glycerinated water, employed to determine, by comparison of turbidity, the amount of albumin precipitated in urine or other fluid by heat. **Brazelton behavioral s.**, a method for assessing infant behavior by its responses to environmental stimuli. **Cattell Infant Intelligence S.**, a test of general motor and cognitive development, assessed by performance of tasks, in the first 18 months of life. **Celsius s.**, a temperature scale on which 0 is officially 273.15 kelvins and 100° is 373.15 kelvins; abbreviated C or Cel. Before 1948 (and still, unofficially) the degree Celsius (°C) was called the degree centigrade (symbol ° C) with 0° at the freezing point of fresh water and 100° at the boiling point, at normal atmospheric pressure (760 mm Hg). See also *kelvin* and Appendix 1 for Celsius-Fahrenheit, Fahrenheit-Celsius equivalents. **centigrade s.**, 1. one in which the interval between two fixed points is divided into 100 equal units. 2. Celsius s. **Charrière s.**, French s. **Clark's s.**, a scale used in denoting the hardness of water, based on the number of grains of calcium carbonate per imperial gallon. **Columbia Mental Maturity S.**, a test of specific kinds of mental function and general abilities, suitable for children (ages 3 to 12) with no speech or with limited physical capabilities, such as those with cerebral palsy. **dichotomous s.**, a nominal scale (q.v.) with two categories. **Dunfermline s.**, a scheme used in denoting the nutritional status of children: 1, superior condition; 2, passable condition; 3, requiring supervision; 4, requiring medical treatment. **Fahrenheit s.**, a temperature scale, obsolescent but still commonly, unofficially used in the United States, in which the interval between Fahrenheit's two original fixed points, which are the lowest temperature attainable by a freezing mixture of ice and salt (0) and the normal temperature of the human body (96° originally), is divided into 96 degrees (96 having 10 factors besides itself and 1); fresh water freezes at about 32° and boils at about 212° under average atmospheric pressure. Abbreviated *F.* and *Fahr.* See *Celsius s.* and *Appendix 1* for Celsius-Fahrenheit, Fahrenheit-Celsius equivalents. **French s.**, a scale used for denoting the size of catheters, sounds, and other tubular instruments, each unit being roughly equivalent to 0.33 mm. in diameter, i.e., 18 French indicates a diameter of 6 mm. **Gaffky s.**, a scale used in denoting the prognosis in tuberculosis, based on the number of tubercle bacilli in the sputum. **gray s.**, see under *ultrasonography*. **homigrade s.**, a temperature scale in which 0 represents the melting point of ice (0 C, 32° F), 100°, normal human temperature (37° C, 98.6° F), and 270° the boiling point of water. **hydrometer s.**, a scale used for expressing the specific gravity of liquids. **interval s.**, an ordinal scale (q.v.) with a distance measure; the sample points are numerical, but the zero is arbitrary (as in the Celsius and Fahrenheit temperature scales). **Kelvin s.**, an absolute temperature scale whose unit of measurement, the kelvin, is equivalent to the degree Celsius, the ice point therefore being at 273.15 degrees Celsius (273.15 kelvins). **nominal s.**, the weakest qualitative, not quantitative, classification of the samples into separate categories so that each possible result belongs to only one category, e.g., one dealing with eye, hair, or skin color and not size, weight, or temperature. See *ordinal s.* **nonlinear s.**, one in which the divisions corresponding to the steps are unequal, e.g., a scale with divisions showing logarithmic or exponential growth or change. **ordinal s.**, an ordered nominal scale (q.v.) in which the sample points are numbers, of which only the relative sizes (larger than, smaller than) are important, e.g., a classification of disease symptoms as mild (1), moderate

(2), or severe (3). **Rankine s.**, an absolute scale on which the unit of measurement corresponds with that of the Fahrenheit scale, but the ice point is at 491.67 degrees (491.67° R). **ratio s.**, an interval scale (q.v.) with a meaningful zero point, e.g., mass or length; thus products involving the data points, like volume or density, demonstrate the relations between the data points. Used in the psychophysical measurement of sensations. **Réaumur s.**, a temperature scale with the ice point at 0 and the normal boiling point of water at 80 degrees (80° R). **Tallqvist's s.**, a series of lithographed colors formerly used to quantitate hemoglobin. **temperature s.**, a scale used for expressing the degree of heat, based on absolute zero as a reference point (absolute scale), or with a certain value arbitrarily assigned to such temperatures as the ice point and boiling point of water under certain stipulated conditions, the range between and beyond them being divided into a designated number of identical units. **Wechsler Adult Intelligence s. (WAIS)**, a group of tests for assessment of intellectual functioning in adults. **Wechsler Intelligence S. for Children (WISC)**, a group of tests for assessment of intellectual functioning in children ages 5 to 15.

scalene (ska'lēn) [Gr. *skalēnos* uneven] 1. unequally three-sided. 2. pertaining to one of the scalene muscles.

scalenectomy (ska″lĕ-nek′to-me) [*scalenus* + Gr. *ektomē* excision] the operation of resecting a scalenus muscle.

scalenotomy (ska″lĕ-not′o-me) [*scalenus* + *-tomy*] sectioning of the scaleni muscles to restrict respiratory activity of the upper thorax and thus induce apical rest; formerly used in treatment of pulmonary tuberculosis.

scalenus (ska-le′nus) [L.; Gr. *skalēnos*] uneven; a name given to various muscles of the neck. See *Table of Musculi*.

scaler (ska′ler) 1. a dental instrument used in removing calculus from tooth surfaces. See also *scaling*. 2. an electronic instrument for rapid counting of radiation-induced pulses emitted from a Geiger counter or other radiation detectors. **chisel s.**, periodontal chisel. **deep s.**, one of several types of scalers designed for removal of subgingival deposits from the teeth. **double-ended s.**, one with blades on both sides of the handle, one blade for the right side, the other for the left. **hoe s.**, one made with different angular relationships of shank and handle, but with the blade bent at a 99° angle, and the flattened termination surface beveled at an angle of 45°, used for planing and smoothing root surfaces. **sickle s.**, a scaler for removing tenacious supragingival or subgingival deposits from the teeth, having a sickle-like blade with flattened sides and a trapezoidal cross section. **superficial s.**, one of several types of scalers designed for removal of supragingival deposits from the teeth. **ultrasonic s.**, an ultrasonic instrument with a tip for supplying high-frequency vibrations, used to remove adherent deposits from the teeth and bits of inflamed tissue from the walls of the gingival crevice.

scaling (skāl′ing) removal of plaque and calculus from the surface of a tooth by means of a scaler. **deep s.**, removal of plaque and calculus from the surface of a tooth apical to the gingival margin, usually accumulated in periodontal pockets. Called also *subgingival s., root s.* **root s.**, deep s. **subgingival s.**, deep s. **ultrasonic s.**, removal of debris, plaque, and calculus from the surface of the teeth with an ultrasonic scaler.

scall (skawl) (*obs.*) 1. any scaly, or scabby, disease of the skin. 2. favus of animals. **honeycomb s.** (*obs.*), an eruption consisting of small ulcers separated by raised edges. **milk s.**, crusta lactea.

scalp (skalp) that part of the skin of the head, exclusive of the face and ears, which normally is covered with hair. **gyrate s.**, cutis verticis gyrata.

scalpel (skal′pel) [L. *scalpellum*] a small surgical knife with a straight handle and, usually, a blade with a convex edge.

scalpriform (skal′prĭ-form) shaped like a chisel.

scaly (ska′le) [L. *squamosus*] 1. scalelike. 2. characterized by scales.

scammonia (skah-mo′ne-ah) scammony.

scammony (skam′o-ne) [L. *scammonium, scammonia*] the plant *Convolvulus scammonia* L. (Convolvulaceae), of Asia Minor and Syria; the root affords a gummy and resinous exudate, which has anthelmintic and cathartic properties. **Mexican s.**, ipomea.

scan (skan) 1. shortened form of *scintiscan*, q.v.; variously designated, according to the organ under examination, as *brain scan*, *kidney scan*, *thyroid scan*, etc. 2. a visual display of ultrasonographic echoes. An *A-scan* is a display on a cathode ray tube in which one axis represents the time required for return of the echo and the other corresponds to the strength of the echo. In *B-scan*, the position of a bright dot on the tube corresponds to the time elapsed, and the brightness of the spot to the strength of the echo; movement of the transducer across the skin surface yields a two-dimensional cross-sectional display. **CAT s.,** computerized axial tomography; see under *tomography*. **Meckel s.,** a technetium-99m pertechnetate gastrio-mucosa scan used to demonstrate ectopic gastric mucosa, particularly in Meckel diverticulum.

scandium (skan′de-um) a very rare metallic element; symbol, Sc; atomic number, 21; atomic weight, 44.956.

scanner (skan′er) something that scans; a scintiscanner. **EMI s.,** an instrument for reconstructing tomographic images for display on a cathode ray tube; see *computerized axial tomography*, under *tomography*. **scintillation s.,** scintiscanner.

scanning (skan′ning) 1. the act of examining visually, as a small area or different isolated areas, in detail. 2. a manner of utterance characterized by somewhat regularly recurring pauses. **radioisotope s.,** the production of a two-dimensional picture (scintiscan, or scan) representing the gamma rays emitted by a radioactive isotope concentrated in a specific tissue of the body, such as the brain or thyroid gland.

scanography (skan-og′rah-fe) a method of making radiographs by the use of a narrow slit beneath the tube in such a manner that only a line or sheet of x-rays is employed and the x-ray tube moves over the object so that all the rays of the central beam pass through the part being radiographed at the same angle.

scansion (skan′shun) scanning.

Scanzoni's maneuver (operation) (skan-tso′nēz) [Friedrich Wilhelm *Scanzoni*, German obstetrician, 1821–1891] see under *operation*.

scapha (ska′fah) [L. "a skiff"] [NA] the long curved depression which separates the helix from the anthelix; called also *scaphoid fossa* and *fossa helicis*.

scaphion (ska′fe-on) [Gr. *skaphion* a small bowl or basin] basis cranii externa.

scaph(o)- [Gr. *skaphē* skiff or light boat] a combining form meaning boat-shaped.

scaphocephalia (skaf″o-sě-fa′le-ah) scaphocephaly.

scaphocephalic (skaf″o-sě-fal′ik) pertaining to or characterized by scaphocephaly.

scaphocephalism (skaf″o-sef′ah-lizm) scaphocephaly.

scaphocephalous (skaf″o-sef′ah-lus) scaphocephalic.

scaphocephaly (skaf″o-sef′ah-le) [Gr. *skaphē* skiff + *kephalē* head] a condition in which the skull is abnormally long and narrow, as a result of premature closure of the sagittal suture, with heavy centers of ossification in the line of the suture, usually accompanied by inflammation and atrophy of the optic papillae and by mental retardation. Called also *sagittal synostosis*.

scaphohydrocephalus (skaf″o-hi″dro-sef′ah-lus) hydrocephalus in which the head assumes a boatlike shape.

scaphohydrocephaly (skaf″o-hi″dro-sef′ah-le) scaphohydrocephalus.

scaphoid (skaf′oid) [Gr. *skaphē* skiff + *eidos* form] shaped like a boat; navicular. Used especially in reference to the most lateral bone in the proximal row of carpal bones (os scaphoideum [NA]). See also os *naviculare*.

scaphoiditis (skaf″oi-di′tis) inflammation of the scaphoid bone. **tarsal s.,** inflammation involving the navicular (scaphoid) bone of the tarsus. See also *Köhler's bone disease* (def. 1), under *disease*.

Scaptocosa (skap″to-co′sah) a genus of wolf spiders. **S. rapto′ria,** a species of Brazil that has a powerful hemolytic venom that has been shown to cause necrotic arachnidism.

scapula (skap′u-lah), pl. *scap′ulae* [L.] [NA] the flat, triangular bone in the back of the shoulder; the shoulder blade. See illustration. **alar s., s. ala′ta,** winged s. **elevated s.,** Sprengel's deformity. **Graves′ s.,** scaphoid s.

scaphoid s., a scapula in which the vertebral border is more or less concave. **winged s.,** a scapula having a prominent vertebral border.

scapulalgia (skap″u-lal′je-ah) pain in the scapular region.

scapular (skap′u-lar) of or pertaining to the scapula.

scapulary (skap′u-la′re) a shoulder bandage, with the appearance of a pair of suspenders or braces, to hold in place a body bandage or girdle.

scapulectomy (skap″u-lek′to-me) [*scapula* + Gr. *ektomē* excision] surgical removal or resection of the scapula.

scapuloanterior (skap″u-lo-an-te′re-or) denoting a position of the fetus in transverse lie, with the scapula directed anteriorly.

scapuloclavicular (skap″u-lo-klah-vik′u-lar) pertaining to the scapula and the clavicle.

scapulodynia (skap″u-lo-din′e-ah) [*scapula* + Gr. *odynē* pain + *-ia*] pain in the region of the shoulder.

scapulohumeral (skap″u-lo-hu′mer-al) pertaining to the scapula and the humerus.

scapulopexy (skap′u-lo-pek″se) [*scapula* + Gr. *pēxis* fixation] surgical fixation of the scapula.

scapuloposterior (skap″u-lo-pos-te′re-or) denoting a position of the fetus in transverse lie, with the scapula directed posteriorly.

scapus (ska′pus), pl. *sca′pi* [L.] shaft; [NA] a general term for a shaftlike structure. **s. pe′nis,** corpus penis. **s. pi′li** [NA], hair shaft: the major portion of a hair, designating especially the portion that extends beyond the surface of the skin.

scar (skahr) [Gr. *eschara* the scab or eschar on a wound caused by burning] a mark remaining after the healing of a wound or other morbid process; a cicatrix. By extension applied to other visible manifestations of an earlier event. **hypertrophic s.,** one formed by exuberant cicatrization, giving it the appearance of a keloid but without the latter's tendency to progressive extension or to recurrence after excision. **Reichert's s.,** an area over the implanting blastocyst of some species, consisting of a fibrinous membrane in place of the decidual tissue. **white s. of ovary,** corpus albicans, def. 1.

scarification (skar″ĭ-fĭ-ka′shun) [L. *scarificatio*, Gr. *skariphismos* a scratching up] production in the skin of many small, superficial scratches or punctures, as for the introduction of smallpox vaccine. The term is sometimes used erroneously for scarring.

scarificator (skar′ĭ-fi-ka″tor) scarifier.

scarifier (skar′ĭ-fi′er) an instrument bearing many sharp points, used in scarification.

scarlatina (skahr″lah-te′nah) [L. "scarlet"] scarlet fever; see under *fever*. **s. angino′sa,** scarlet fever associated with painful pharyngitis, with tonsillar enlargement or peritonsillar abscess. Called also *Fothergill's disease* and *Fothergill's sore throat*. **s. haemorrha′gica,** (obs.), scarlet fever in which there is extravasation of the blood into skin and mucous membranes. **puerperal s.,** a scarlet rash sometimes seen in puerperal fever.

scarlatinal (skahr-lat′ĭ-nal) pertaining to or due to scarlatina (scarlet fever).

scarlatinella (skahr-lat″ĭ-nel′ah) Duke's disease.

scarlatiniform (skahr″lah-tin′ĭ-form) resembling scarlet fever, especially the skin eruption of scarlet fever; scarlatinoid.

scarlatinoid (skahr-lat′ĭ-noid) scarlatiniform.

scarlet (skar′let) 1. bright red tinged with orange or yellow. 2. a scarlet dye. **Biebrich s., water-soluble,** an azo dye used as a plasma stain, $C_6H_2 2 \cdot ONa) \cdot N{:}N \cdot C_6H_2{-} (SO_2 \cdot ONa) \cdot N{:}N \cdot C_{10}H_3 \cdot OH$. **s. G,** sudan III. **s. R,** scarlet red.

Scarpa's fascia, etc. (skar′pahz) [Anthony *Scarpa*, Italian anatomist and surgeon, 1747–1832] see under *fascia, fluid, foramen, ganglion, ligament, membrane, nerve, sheath, staphyloma,* and *triangle*.

SCAT sheep cell agglutination test.

scatemia (skah-te′me-ah) [*scato*- + Gr. *haima* blood + *-ia*] alimentary toxemia in which the chemical poisons are absorbed through the intestine.

scat(o)- [Gr. *skōr, skatos* dung] a combining form denoting relation to dung, or fecal matter; see also words beginning *skat(o)-*.

scatol (ska′tōl) skatole.

scatologic (skat″o-loj′ik) pertaining to fecal matter, or to scatology.

scatology (skah-tol′o-je) [*scato- + -logy*] 1. the study of the feces. 2. a preoccupation with feces and filth.

scatoma (skah-to′mah) [*scato- + -oma*] stercoroma.

scatophagy (skah-tof′ah-je) [*scato- +* Gr. *phagein to eat*] the eating of excrement.

scatoscopy (skah-tos′ko-pe) [*scato- +* Gr. *skopein to examine*] inspection of the feces.

scatter (skat′er) the diffusion or deviation of roentgen rays produced by a medium through which the rays pass. See also *backscatter*.

scattergram (skat′er-gram) scatterplot.

scattering (skat′er-ing) a change in direction of a photon or subatomic particle as the result of a collision or interaction. **Compton s.,** modified scattering; the deflection of an incident photon by interaction with a free electron or an orbital electron of much lower energy than the photon; the photon is deflected from its original path and gives up part of its energy to displace the electron. **Thomson s.,** unmodified scattering; deflection of a photon by interaction with an atom with no loss of energy by the photon.

scatterplot (skat′er-plot) a plot in rectangular coordinates of paired observations of two random variables, each observation plotted as one point on the graph; the scatter or clustering of points provides an indication of the relationship between the two variables. Called also *scatterdiagram* or *scattergram*.

scatula (skat′u-lah) [L. "parallelepiped"] an oblong paper box for powders or pills.

scavenger (skav′en-jer) a substance that influences the course of a chemical reaction by ready combination with free radicals, e.g., diphenylpicrylhydrazyl.

Sc.D. Doctor of Science.

Sc.D.A. abbreviation for L. *scapulodextra anterior* (right scapuloanterior; a presentation of the fetus).

Sc.D.P. abbreviation for L. *scapulodextra posterior* (right scapuloposterior; a presentation of the fetus).

Scedosporium (se-do-spo′re-um) *Monosporium.*

scelalgia (ske-lal′je-ah) [Gr. *skelos* leg + *algos* pain + *-ia*] pain in the leg.

scelotyrbe (sel-o-ter′be) [Gr. *skelos* leg + *tyrbē* disorder] spastic paralysis of the legs.

Schacher's ganglion (shah′kerz) [Polycarp Gottlieb *Schacher*, German physician, 1674–1737] the ciliary ganglion.

Schachowa's spiral tubes (shah′ko-vahz) [Seraphina *Schachowa*, Russian histologist in Bern, born 1854] tubuli renales.

Schafer's method (sha′ferz) [Sir Edward Albert Sharpey-*Schafer*, English physiologist, 1850–1935] see under *respiration, artificial.*

Schäffer's reflex (shef′erz) [Max *Schäffer*, German neurologist, 1852–1923] see under *reflex.*

Schally (shal′e), Andrew Victor. Lithuanian-born American biochemist, born 1926; co-winner, with Roger Charles Louis Guillemin and Rosalyn Sussman Yalow, of the Nobel prize for medicine or physiology in 1977 for the discovery of releasing factors, low-molecular-weight polypeptides secreted by the hypothalamus that regulate the release of hormones by the pituitary gland.

Schamberg's disease (dermatosis, progressive pigmented purpuric dermatosis) (sham′bergz) [Jay Frank *Schamberg*, Philadelphia dermatologist, 1870–1934] see under *disease.*

Schanz's disease, syndrome (shants′ez) [Alfred *Schanz*, German orthopedist, 1868–1931] see under *disease* and *syndrome.*

Schardinger's enzyme, reaction (shar′ding-er) [Franz *Schardinger*, Austrian chemist, 19th century] see under *enzyme* and *reaction.*

scharlach R (shar′lak) scarlet red.

Schaudinn's fluid (shaw-dinz′) [Fritz Richard *Schaudinn*, German bacteriologist, 1871–1906] see under *fluid.*

Schaumann's bodies, disease, sarcoid, syndrome (shaw′manz) [Jörgen *Schaumann*, Swedish dermatologist, 1879–1953] see under *body*, and see *sarcoidosis.*

Schauta's operation (shaw′tahz) [Friedrich *Schauta*, Vienna gynecologist, 1849–1919] see under *operation.*

schedule (sked′ūl) a formal list, plan of procedure, or timetable. **Gesell developmental s.,** a test of the developmental status of infants that includes assessment of motor development, adaptive behavior, language development, and personal-social behavior.

Scheiner's experiment (shi′nerz) [Christoph *Scheiner*, German mathematician, 1575–1650] see under *experiment.*

schema (ske′mah) [Gr. *schēma* form, shape] a plan, outline, or arrangement. **Hamberger's s.,** the external intercostal and the intercartilaginous muscles are inspiratory muscles, the internal intercostal muscles are expiratory.

schematic (ske-mat′ik) serving as a diagram or model.

Scherer's test (shār′erz) [Johann Joseph von *Scherer*, German physician, 1814–1869] see under *tests.*

scheroma (ske-ro′mah) xerophthalmia.

Scheuermann's disease, kyphosis (shoi′er-manz) [Holger Werfel *Scheuermann*, Danish surgeon, 1877–1960] osteochondrosis of the vertebrae; see *osteochondrosis.*

Schick's sign, test (reaction) (shiks) [Béla *Schick*, Hungarian pediatrician in the United States, 1877–1967] see under *sign* and *tests.*

Schiefferdecker's disk, theory (she-fer-dek′erz) [Paul *Schiefferdecker*, Bonn anatomist, 1849–1931] see under *disk*, and *theory.*

Schiff's biliary cycle (shifs) [Moritz *Schiff*, German physiologist, 1823–1896] see under *cycle.*

Schiff's reagent, test (shifs) [Hugo (Ugo) *Schiff*, German chemist in Florence, 1834–1915] see under *reagent* and *tests.*

Schilder's disease (encephalitis) (shil′derz) [Paul Ferdinand *Schilder*, Austrian neurologist in the United States, 1886–1940] see under *disease.*

Schiller's test (shil′erz) [Walter *Schiller*, Austrian pathologist in the United States, 1887–1960] see under *tests.*

Schilling blood count (shil′ing) [Victor *Schilling*, German hematologist, 1883–1960] see under *count.*

Schilling test (shil′ing) [Robert Frederick *Schilling*, American hematologist, born 1919] see under *tests.*

Schimmelbusch's disease (shim′el-boosh″ez) [Curt *Schimmelbusch*, German surgeon, 1860–1895] cystic disease of the breast; see under *disease.*

schindylesis (skin″dĭ-le′sis) [Gr. *schindylēsis* a splintering] a form of articulation in which a thin plate of one bone is received into a cleft in another, as in the articulation of the perpendicular plate of the ethmoid bone with the vomer.

Schinus (ski′nus) [Gr. *schinos* mastic] a genus of anacardiaceous trees of warm regions. *S. mol′le,* L., of tropical America (pepper tree), affords a kind of American mastic, and is a mild purgative and aromatic.

Schiotz's tonometer (she-ets′) [Hjalmar *Schiotz*, Norwegian physician, 1850–1927] see under *tonometer.*

schistasis (skis′tah-sis) a splitting; specifically, a congenital defect consisting of a cleft or fissure of the body, as schistocormia, schistomelia, schistosomia.

schist(o)- [Gr. *schistos* split] a combining form meaning split or cleft.

schistocelia (shis″, skiz″to-se′le-ah) schistocoelia.

schistocephalus (shis″, skis″to-sef′ah-lus) [*schisto- +* Gr. *kephalē* head] a fetus born with a cleft head.

schistocoelia (shis″, skiz″to-se′le-ah) [*schisto- +* Gr. *koilia* belly] congenital fissure of the abdomen.

schistocormia (shis″, skiz″to-kor′me-ah) [*schisto- +* Gr. *kormos* trunk + *-ia*] a developmental anomaly characterized by a cleft condition of the trunk.

schistocormus (shis″, skiz″to-kor′mus) a fetus exhibiting schistocormia.

schistocystis (shis″to-sis′tis) [*schisto- +* Gr. *kystis* bladder] fissure of the bladder.

schistocyte (shis′, skis′to-sīt) a fragment of a red blood corpuscle, commonly observed in the blood in hemolytic anemias; called also *helmet cell.*

schistocytosis (shis″, skis″to-si-to′sis)　the accumulation of schistocytes in the blood.

schistomelia (shis″, skis″to-me′le-ah) [*schisto-* + Gr. *melos* limb + *-ia*] a developmental anomaly characterized by a cleft condition of a limb.

schistomelus (shis-, skis-tom′e-lus)　a fetus exhibiting schistomelia.

schistoprosopia (shis″, skis″to-pro-so′pe-ah) [*schisto-* + Gr. *prosōpon* face + *-ia*] a developmental anomaly characterized by fissure of the face; schizoprosopia.

schistoprosopus (shis″, skis″to-pros′o-pus)　a fetus exhibiting schistoprosopia.

schistorachis (shis-, skis-tor′ah-kis) [*schisto-* + Gr. *rachis* spine] rachischisis.

schistosis (shis-, skis-to′sis) [*Schist* a form of slate + *-osis*] pneumoconiosis in slate workers.

Schistosoma (shis″, skis″to-so′mah) [*schisto-* + Gr. *sōma* body] a genus of trematode parasites or flukes; the blood flukes; sometimes called also *Bilharzia*. **S. bo′vis,** a species found in the portal system of sheep and oxen in Africa, Mesopotamia, Corsica, Sardinia, and Sicily. **S. haemato′bium,** a common parasite of Africa, especially Egypt, the Mediterranean littoral, and the Arabian peninsula. The adult worms are found in the veins, especially those of the vesical plexus, producing irritability of the bladder, hematuria, and dysentery. The parasites enter the body through the skin of persons coming in contact with infested waters, the invertebrate hosts being small snails of the genus

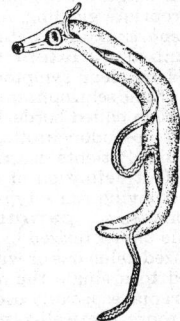

Schistosoma haematobium, male carrying female in gynecophoral canal (×6).

Bulinus, including the subgenus *Physopsis.* Called also *Bilharzia haematobia* and, formerly, *Distoma haematobium* and *D. capense.* **S. in′dicum,** a species occurring in cattle, sheep, goats, etc., in India and Rhodesia. **S. intercala′tum,** a species found in West Central Africa, which causes schistosomiasis intercalatum by penetrating the skin of persons coming in contact with infested water; the proven transmitting hosts are certain snails of the genus *Bulinus.* **S. japon′icum,** a species found in Japan, China, the Philippines, Taiwan, and the Celebes, which causes schistosomiasis japonica by penetrating the skin of persons coming in contact with infested waters; the usual transmitting hosts are small snails of the genus *Oncomelania.* **S. manso′ni,** a species found in Egypt and elsewhere in Africa as well as in South America and the West Indies, including Puerto Rico, which causes schistosomiasis mansoni by penetrating the skin of persons coming in contact with infested waters; the transmitting hosts are planorbid snails, especially those of the genus *Biomphalaria.* **S. mat′thei,** a species found in the portal mesenteric vein of sheep, goats, game animals, monkeys, and rarely man in South Africa. **S. mekon′gi,** a species found in Laos and Cambodia that differs from *S. japonicum* chiefly in requiring a different intermediate host. **S. spinda′le,** a species parasitic in water buffalo, cattle, sheep, and goats in India, Malaya, Sumatra, Northern Rhodesia, and South Africa.

schistosomacidal (shis″, skis″to-so″mah-si′dal)　schistosomicidal.

schistosomacide (shis″, skis″to-so′mah-sīd)　schistosomicide.

schistosomal (shis″, skis″to-so′mal)　pertaining to or caused by *Schistosoma.*

Schistosomatium (shis″, skis″to-so-ma′she-um)　a genus

of blood flukes allied to *Schistosoma. S. douthitti* is found in the hepatic portal veins of the meadow mouse.

schistosome (shis′, skis′to-sōm)　an individual of the genus *Schistosoma.*

schistosomia (shis″, skis″to-so′me-ah) [*schisto-* + Gr. *soma* body + *-ia*] a developmental anomaly characterized by a fissure of the abdomen, with lower extremities rudimentary or lacking.

schistosomiasis (shis″, skis″to-so-mi′ah-sis)　the state of being infected with flukes of the genus *Schistosoma;* sometimes called *bilharziasis.* **cutaneous s.,** cercarial dermatitis. **eastern s.,** s. japonica. **s. haemato′bia,** urinary s. **hepatic s.,** the chronic form of schistosomiasis mansoni and japonica in which the liver is involved. Ova of the parasites lodge in the hepatic portal venules, stimulating an inflammatory reaction with fibrosis; portal venous destruction leads to portal hypertension. **s. intercala′tum,** an endemic intestinal disease of West Central Africa due to infection by flukes of the species *Schistosoma intercalatum,* with abdominal pain, diarrhea in which the stools may contain blood and mucus, hyperplasia of the mucosa of the rectal valves, inflammation of the rectal walls, and sometimes polyposis. **intestinal s.,** the chronic form of schistosomiasis mansoni and japonica in which the intestinal tract is involved. Most of those infected are asymptomatic but some have intermittent diarrhea and blood and mucus in the stools. **s. japon′ica,** infection by flukes of the species *Schistosoma japonicum.* The acute infection in its early stages produces a serum sickness–like illness (see *Katayama fever,* under *fever*). Chronic effects of infection, which may be very severe, are caused by fibrosis around the eggs deposited by the parasite in the liver, lungs, and central nervous system. **Manson's s., s. manso′ni,** infection with flukes of the species *Schistosoma mansoni,* living principally in the inferior and superior mesenteric veins but migrating to deposit their eggs in venules, primarily of the large intestine. Eggs lodging in the liver may lead to peripheral fibrosis, hepatosplenomegaly, and ascites. Called also *intestinal bilharziasis* and *Manson's disease.* **Oriental s.,** s. japonica. **pulmonary s.,** schistosomiasis in which migrating cercariae cause a type of pneumonia, and the ova, and sometimes the adult worms, cause embolization of pulmonary arterioles. Allergic pneumonia, allergic asthma, and emphysema may occur. **urinary s., vesical s.,** infection with *Schistosoma haematobium,* involving the urinary tract and causing cystitis and hematuria; called also *endemic hematuria, genitourinary schistosomiasis,* and *schistosomiasis haematobia.* **visceral s.,** infection with *Schistosoma mansoni* or *S. japonicum,* in contradistinction to urinary schistosomiasis caused by *S. haematobium.*

schistosomicidal (shis″, skis″to-so″mĭ-si′dal)　destructive to schistosomes.

schistosomicide (shis″, skis″to-so′mĭ-sīd)　an agent which destroys schistosomes.

Schistosomum (shis″, skis″to-so′mum)　*Schistosoma.*

schistosomus (shis″, skis″to-so′mus)　a monster exhibiting schistosomia.

schistosternia (shis″, skis″to-ster′ne-ah) [*schisto-* + *sternum*] schistothorax.

schistothorax (shis″, skis″to-tho′raks) [*schisto-* + Gr. *thōrax* chest] a developmental anomaly characterized by fissure of the chest.

schistotrachelus (shis″, skis″to-trah-ke′lus) [*schisto-* + *trachēlos* neck] a fetus with fissure of the neck.

schizamnion (skiz-am′ne-on) [Gr. *schizein* to divide + *amnion*] an amnion formed by cavitation over or in the inner cell mass, as occurs in human development.

schizaxon (skiz-ak′sōn)　an axon which is divided into two equal, or nearly equal, branches.

schizencephalic (skiz″en-sĕ-fal′ik)　having abnormal clefts in the brain substance; see under *porencephaly,* def. 2.

schizencephaly (skiz″en-sef′ah-le) [Gr. *schizein* to divide + *enkephalos* brain] schizencephalic porencephaly.

schiz(o)- [Gr. *schizein* to divide]　a combining form meaning divided, or denoting relationship to division.

schizoaffective (skiz″o-ah-fek′tiv, skit″so-ah-fek′tiv)　pertaining to or exhibiting features of both schizophrenic and mood disorders (mania and depression).

Schizoblastosporion (skiz″o-blas″to-spo′re-on) *Geotrichum.*

schizocephalia (skiz″o-sĕ-fa′le-ah) a developmental anomaly characterized by a longitudinal fissure of the head.

schizocyte (skiz′o-sīt) schistocyte.

schizocytosis (skiz″o-si-to′sis) schistocytosis.

schizogenesis (skiz″o-jen′ĕ-sis) [*schizo-* + Gr. *genesis* production] reproduction by fission.

schizogenous (skĭ-zoj′ĕ-nus) reproducing by fission.

schizogony (skĭ-zog′o-ne) [*schizo-* + Gr. *gonē* seed] a form of asexual reproduction characteristic of certain sarcodines and sporozoa in which daughter cells are produced by multiple fission of the nucleus of the parasite (schizont) followed by segmentation of the cytoplasm to form separate masses around each smaller nucleus. Called also *agametogeny* and *agamogenesis.* See also *gametogony, merogony,* and *sporogony.*

schizogyria (skiz″o-ji′re-ah) a condition in which the cerebral convolutions are marked by wedge-shaped cracks.

schizoid (skiz′oid, skit′soid) 1. the traits of shyness, sensitivity, social withdrawal, and introversion that characterize the schizoid personality. 2. schizophrenia-like traits that are held by some to indicate a predisposition to schizophrenia, not only the shyness and aloofness of schizoid personality disorder but also the eccentricity and illogical or magical thinking of schizotypal personality disorder.

schizoidism (skiz′oi-dizm) (*obs.*) the state characterized by the presence of schizoid personality traits.

schizokinesis (skiz″o-ki-ne′sis) the condition in which, when an overt specific conditioned response has been extinguished, concomitant nonspecific responses continue to be elicited by the stimulus.

schizomycete (skiz″o-mi-sēt′) any organism or species belonging to the Schizomycetes; a bacterium.

Schizomycetes (skiz″o-mi-se′tēz) [*schizo-* + Gr. *mykēs* fungus] a former taxonomic class comprising the bacteria, consisting of unicellular organisms that commonly multiply by cell division. As originally proposed, it included eight orders, Actinomycetales, Chlamydiales, Cytophagales, Mycoplasmatales, Myxobacteriales, Rhodospirillales, Rickettsiales, and Spirochaetales.

schizont (skiz′ont) [*schizo-* + Gr. *ōn, ontos* being] the multinucleate stage or form in the development of certain sarcodines and sporozoa during schizogony. See also *meront* and *segmenter.*

schizonticide (skĭ-zon′tĭ-sīd) an agent that destroys schizonts.

schizonychia (skiz″o-nik′e-ah) [*schizo-* + Gr. *onyx* nail + *-ia*] splitting of the nails.

schizophasia (skiz″o-fa′ze-ah) the incomprehensible, disordered speech characteristic of schizophrenia.

schizophrenia (skiz″o-fre′ne-ah, skit″so-fre′ne-ah) [*schizo-* + Gr. *phrēn* mind + *-ia*] [DSM III-R] a mental disorder or heterogeneous group of disorders (the schizophrenias or schizophrenic disorders) comprising most major psychotic disorders and characterized by disturbances in form and content of thought (loosening of associations, delusions, and hallucinations), mood (blunted, flattened, or inappropriate affect), sense of self and relationship to the external world (loss of ego boundaries, dereistic thinking, and autistic withdrawal), and behavior (bizarre, apparently purposeless, and sterotyped activity or inactivity). The definition and clinical application of the concept of schizophrenia have varied greatly. The DSM III-R criteria emphasize marked disorder of thought (delusions, hallucinations, or other thought disorder accompanied by disordered affect or behavior), deterioration from a previous level of functioning, and chronicity (duration of more than 6 months), thus excluding from this classification conditions referred to by others as acute, borderline, simple, or latent schizophrenia. Originally called *dementia praecox* and characterized as a psychosis with adolescent onset and a chronic course ending in deterioration. The term schizophrenia was introduced by Bleuler because neither early onset nor terminal deterioration is an essential feature; he emphasized the splitting and lack of personality integration seen in the disorder. **acute s.,** acute schizophrenic episode; a condition characterized by acute onset of schizophrenic symptoms; since DSM III-R defines schizophrenia as a chronic disorder, such conditions must now be classified in another psychotic syndrome, such as schizophreniform disorder, brief reactive psychosis, or schizoaffective disorder. **ambulatory s.,** mild schizophrenia sufficiently well compensated so that the patient can maintain himself in the community without hospitalization. **borderline s.,** latent s. **catatonic s.** [DSM III-R], a type of schizophrenia characterized by marked psychomotor disturbance: *catatonic stupor* (marked decrease in reactivity to the environment and in spontaneous activity) or *mutism, catatonic negativism* (resistance to all instructions or attempts to be moved), *catatonic rigidity* (maintenance of a rigid posture), *catatonic excitement* (excited, uncontrollable, and apparently purposeless motor activity), or *catatonic posturing* (assumption of bizarre fixed postures); associated features are stereotyped behaviors, mannerisms, and waxy flexibility. Called also *catatonia.* **childhood s.,** schizophrenia with onset before puberty, characterized by autistic, withdrawn behavior, failure to develop an identity separate from the mother's, and gross developmental immaturity, a category that formerly included all types of childhood "psychosis" including symbiotic psychosis and infantile autism. DSM III-R, taking the position that there is no clear relationship between these disorders and adolescent and adult schizophrenia and other psychotic disorders, has renamed them pervasive developmental disorders. **disorganized s.** [DSM III-R], a type of schizophrenia characterized by frequent incoherence; marked loosening of associations, or grossly disorganized behavior and flat or grossly inappropriate affect that does not meet the criteria for the catatonic type; associated features include extreme social withdrawal, grimacing, mannerisms, mirror gazing, inappropriate giggling, and other odd behavior. Called also *hebephrenia* and *hebephrenic s.* **hebephrenic s.,** disorganized s. **latent s.,** a type of schizophrenia characterized by clear symptoms of schizophrenia but no history of a psychotic schizophrenic episode; it includes conditions that have been called borderline, incipient, prepsychotic, prodromal, pseudoneurotic, and pseudopsychopathic schizophrenia. Patients described by these terms do not fit the DSM III-R definition of schizophrenia; most would be classified as having schizotypal personality disorder. **nuclear s.,** process s. **paranoid s.,** [DSM III-R], a type of schizophrenia characterized by preoccupation with one or more systematized delusions or with frequent auditory hallucinations related to a single theme. **paraphrenic s.,** paranoid schizophrenia, especially used to refer to chronic conditions in which there are well-systematized grandiose delusions. **prepsychotic s.,** latent s. **process s.,** a subset of schizophrenias assumed (like the original concept of dementia praecox) to have endogenous origin and poor prognosis as compared to other cases, termed reactive schizophrenia or schizophrenic reaction, that are assumed to be caused by predisposing or precipitating environmental factors and to have a better prognosis; called also *schizophrenic process* and *nuclear schizophrenia.* **pseudoneurotic s.,** a term applied to patients who fit the diagnostic criteria for a neurotic disorder but have abnormalities of thought and emotion resembling those seen in schizophrenia; there is pananxiety (diffuse, all-pervading anxiety) and panneurosis (symptoms of many neurotic syndromes). **pseudopsychopathic s.,** a term applied to patients who fit the diagnostic criteria of antisocial (psychopathic) personality disorder but have abnormalities of thought and emotion resembling those seen in schizophrenia. **reactive s.,** a subset of schizophrenias assumed to be caused by predisposing or precipitating environmental factors and to have a more favorable prognosis than process schizophrenia. **residual s.,** [DSM III-R], a type of schizophrenia characterized by a history of one or more episodes of schizophrenia with prominent psychotic symptoms, current lack of such symptoms, but continuing presence of other schizophrenic symptoms, such as blunted or inappropriate affect, social withdrawal, eccentric behavior, illogical thinking, or loosening of associations. **schizo-affective s.,** see under *disorder.* **simple s.,** schizophrenia without prominent psychotic features; schizotypal personality disorder (see under *personality*). **undifferentiated s.** [DSM III-R], a type of schizophrenia characterized by the presence of prominent psychotic symptoms but not classifiable as catatonic, disorganized, or paranoid.

schizophrenic (skiz″o-fren′ik) 1. pertaining to or characterized by schizophrenia. 2. a person affected with schizophrenia.

schizophreniform (skiz″o-fren′ĭ-form) resembling schizophrenia.

Schizophyceae (skiz″o-fi′se-e) [schizo- + Gr. *phykos* seaweed] Cyanophyceae.

schizoprosopia (skiz″o-pro-so′pe-ah) ununited fissure of the face, as in harelip, cleft palate, etc.; schistoprosopia.

Schizopyrenida (shiz″o-pĭ-ren′ĭ-dah) [schizo- + Gr. *pyrēn* fruit stone] an order of cylindrical, monopodial, typically uninucleate ameboid protozoa (subclass Gymnamoebia, class Lobosea), some species of which exhibit temporary flagellate stages during their life cycle. Representative genera include *Naegleria* and *Vahlkampfia.*

Schizosaccharomyces hominis (skiz″o-sak″ah-ro-mi′sēz hom′ĭ-nis) *Saccharomyces hominis.*

schizothorax (skiz″o-tho′raks) a fetus with a fissure of the chest wall.

schizotonia (skiz″o-to′ne-ah) [schizo- + Gr. *tonos* tension + *-ia*] division of the influx of tone to the muscles, so that, for instance, the flexor groups of the arm become hypertonic, while in the leg the extensors become hypertonic.

schizotrichia (skiz″o-trik′e-ah) [schizo- + Gr. *thrix* hair] splitting of the hairs at the ends.

schizotrypanosomiasis (skiz″o-trip″ah-no-so-mi′ah-sis) Chagas' disease.

Schizotrypanum (skiz″o-trip′ah-num) [schizo- + Gr. *trypanon* borer] 1. in some systems of classification: (*a*) a subgenus of stercorarian trypanosomes comprising *Trypanosoma cruzi;* and (*b*) a genus of trypanosomes comprising the etiologic agent of Chagas' disease when it is considered genically distinct from *Trypanosoma,* in which case the agent is known as *S. cruzi.*

schizozoite (skiz″o-zo′īt) [schizo- + Gr. *zōon* animal] merozoite.

schlammfieber (shlahm′fe-ber) [Ger. "slime fever"] a disease resembling leptospiral jaundice, due to *Leptospira grippotyphosa,* which prevailed among young persons who worked in the flooded districts near Breslau in the summer of 1891.

Schlatter's disease (sprain) (shlat′erz) [Carl *Schlatter,* surgeon in Zurich, 1864–1934] see *Osgood-Schlatter disease,* under *disease.*

Schlatter-Osgood disease (shlat′er-oz′good) [Carl *Schlatter;* Robert Bayley *Osgood,* Boston orthopedist, 1873–1956] Osgood-Schlatter disease.

Schlemm's canal, ligaments (shlemz) [Friedrich S. *Schlemm,* German anatomist, 1795–1858] see *sinus venosus sclerae,* and under *ligament.*

Schlepper (shlep′er) [Ger. *Schlepper,* hauler, tractor, tugboat] carrier (def. 7).

Schlesinger's sign (phenomenon) (shla′zing-erz) [Hermann *Schlesinger,* Austrian physician, 1866–1934] see under *sign.*

Schlichter test (shlik′ter) [Jakub G. Schlichter, American internist, born 1912] see *serum bactericidal activity test,* under *test.*

Schlösser's treatment (shles′erz) [Carl *Schlösser,* German ophthalmologist, 1857–1925] see under *treatment.*

Schlusskoagulum (shluss″ko-ag′u-lum) [Ger.] the clot that closes the gap made in the uterine lining by the implanting blastocyst; called also *closing coagulum.*

Schmidt's diet, syndrome, test (shmits) [Adolf *Schmidt,* physician in Bonn, 1865–1918] see under *diet, syndrome,* and *tests.*

Schmidt's syndrome (shmits) [Martin Benno *Schmidt,* German pathologist, 1863–1949] see under *syndrome.*

Schmidt-Lanterman incisures (clefts), segment (shmit′lahn″ter-mahn′) [Henry D. *Schmidt,* American anatomist, 1823–1888; A. J. *Lantermann,* American anatomist at Strassburg, 19th century] see *incisures of Lanterman,* under *incisure,* and *medullary segment,* under *segment.*

Schmincke tumor (shmin′kĕ) [Alexander *Schmincke,* German pathologist, 1877–1953] lymphoepithelioma.

Schmitz bacillus (shmits) [Karl Eitel Friedrich *Schmitz,* German physician, born 1889] *Shigella dysenteriae* type 2.

Schmorl's body, disease, nodule (shmorlz) [Christian Georg *Schmorl,* German pathologist, 1861–1932] see under *body, disease,* and *nodule.*

Schnabel's caverns (shnab′elz) [Isidor *Schnabel,* Vienna ophthalmologist, 1842–1908] see under *cavern.*

schnauzkrampf (shnowts′krampf) [Ger.] a facial grimace resembling pouting.

Schneider's carmine (shni′derz) [Franz Coelestin Schneider, German chemist, 1813–1897] see under *carmine.*

schneiderian membrane (shni-de′re-an) [Conrad Victor *Schneider,* German physician, 1614–1680] see under *membrane.*

Schoemaker's line (she′mah-kerz) [Jan *Schoemaker,* Dutch surgeon, 1871–1940] see under *line.*

Scholz's disease (shōlts′ez) [Willibald Oscar *Scholz,* German neurologist, born 1889] see under *disease.*

Schön's theory (shānz) [Wilhelm *Schön,* German ophthalmologist, 1848–1917] see under *theory.*

Schönbein's reaction, test (shān′bīnz) [Christian Friedrich *Schönbein,* German chemist, 1799–1868] see under *reaction* and *tests.*

Schönlein's purpura (disease) (shān′līnz) [Johann Lukas *Schönlein,* German physician, 1793–1864] purpura rheumatica.

Schönlein-Henoch purpura (disease, syndrome) (shān′lĭn-hen′ōk) [J. L. *Schönlein;* Edouard Heinrich *Henoch,* German pediatrician, 1820–1910] see under *purpura.*

Schott's treatment (bath) (shots) [Theodor *Schott,* physician in Nauheim, 1850–1921] see under *treatment.*

Schottmüller's disease (shot′mil-erz) [Hugo *Schottmüller,* physician in Hamburg, 1867–1936] paratyphoid.

schradan (schra′dan) octamethyl pyrophosphoramide.

Schreger's lines (band, striae, zones) (shra′gerz) [Bernhard Gottlob *Schreger,* German anatomist, 1766–1825] lines of Schrager.

Schreiber's maneuver (shri′berz) [Julius *Schreiber,* German physician, 1849–1932] see under *maneuver.*

Schroeder's disease (shra′derz) [Robert *Schroeder,* German gynecologist, 1884–1959] see under *disease.*

Schroeder's test (shra′derz) [Woldemar von *Schroeder,* German physician, 1850–1898] see under *tests.*

Schroetter see *Schrötter.*

Schrön's granule (shrānz) [Otto von *Schrön,* German pathologist in Naples, 1837–1917] see under *granule.*

Schrön-Much granules (shrān-mook) [Otto von *Schrön;* Hans Christian *Much,* German physician, 1880–1932] Much's granules.

Schroth's treatment (shrōts) [Johann *Schroth,* German physician, 1800–1856] see under *treatment.*

Schrötter's chorea (shret′erz) [Leopold *Schrötter* von Kristelli, Viennese laryngologist, 1837–1908] see *diaphragmatic chorea,* under *chorea.*

Schuchardt's incision (shoo′karts) [Karl August *Schuchardt,* German surgeon, 1856–1901] paravaginal incision.

Schüffner's dots (granules, punctuation, stippling) (shif′nerz) [Wilhelm August Paul *Schüffner,* German pathologist, 1867–1949] see under *dot.*

Schüller's disease (syndrome), phenomenon (shil′erz) [Artur *Schüller,* Vienna neurologist, born 1874] see *Hand-Schüller-Christian disease,* under *disease,* see *osteoporosis circumscripta cranii,* and see under *phenomenon.*

Schüller's method (shil′erz) [Karl Heinrich Anton Ludwig Max *Schüller,* surgeon in Berlin, 1843–1907] see under *method.*

Schüller-Christian disease (syndrome) (shil′er-kris′chan) [Artur *Schüller;* Henry A. *Christian,* American physician, 1876–1951] Hand-Schüller-Christian disease.

Schultz's angina (disease, syndrome) (shoolt′sez) [Werner *Schultz,* German internist, 1878–1947] agranulocytosis.

Schultz-Charlton reaction (phenomenon, test) (shoolts-charl′ton) [Werner *Schultz;* Willy *Charlton,* Berlin physician, born 1889] see under *reaction.*

Schultz-Dale reaction (shoolts-dāl) [Werner *Schultz,* German internist, 1878–1947; Sir Henry Hallett *Dale,* British physiologist and pharmacologist, 1875–1968] see under *reaction.*

Schultze's bundle (tract), cells (shoolt′sez) [Max Johann Sigismund *Schultze,* German biologist, 1825–1874] see *in-*

terfascicular fasciculus, under *fasciculus,* and *olfactory cells,* under *cell.*

Schultze's fold (shoolt′sez) [Bernhard Sigismund *Schultze,* German gynecologist, 1827–1919] see under *fold.*

Schultze's sign, type (shoolt′sez) [Friedrich *Schultze,* German physician, 1848–1934] see *Chvostek's sign,* under *sign, tongue phenomenon,* under *phenomenon,* and see (for type) under *acroparesthesia.*

Schultze's test (shoolt′sez) [Ernst *Schultze,* Swiss chemist, 1860–1912] see under *tests.*

Schultze-Chvostek's sign (shoolt′se-vos′tek) [Friedrich *Schultze;* Franz *Chvostek,* Austrian surgeon, 1835–1884] Chvostek's sign.

Schumm's test (shoomz) [Otto *Schumm,* German chemist, born 1874] see under *tests.*

Schütz's micrococcus (shitz′ez) [Johann Wilhelm *Schütz,* German veterinarian, 1839–1920] *Streptococcus equi.*

Schwabach's test (shvah′baks) [Dagobert *Schwabach,* otologist in Berlin, 1846–1920] see under *tests.*

Schwalbe's corpuscles, etc. (shvahl′bez) [Gustav Albert *Schwalbe,* German anatomist, 1844–1917] see under *corpuscle, foramen, fissure, nucleus, ring, sheath,* and *space.*

Schwann's cell, membrane (sheath), nucleus, substance (shvonz) [Theodor *Schwann,* German anatomist and physiologist, 1810–1882; professor of anatomy at Louvain, and the founder of the cell theory] see under *cell* and *nucleus,* and see *myelin* and *neurilemma.*

schwannitis (shwon-ni′tis) schwannosis.

schwannoglioma (shwon″o-gli-o′mah) schwannoma.

schwannoma (shwon-no′mah) a neoplasm originating from Schwann cells (of the myelin sheath) of neurons; schwannomas include neurofibromas and neurilemomas. **granular cell s.,** see under *tumor.*

schwannosis (shwon-no′sis) hypertrophy of the sheaths of Schwann.

Schwarz activator, appliance (shvarts) [A. Martin *Schwarz,* Austrian orthodontist] see *bow activator,* under *activator,* and see under *appliance.*

Schwediauer (shva′de-ow″er) see *Swediaur.*

Schweigger-Seidel sheath (shvi′ger-si′del) [Franz *Schweigger-Seidel,* Leipzig physiologist, 1834–1871] see under *sheath.*

schweinerotlauf (shvi″ně-rot′lowf) [Ger.] swine erysipelas.

schweineseuche (shvi″ně-zoi′ke) [Ger.] hemorrhagic septicemia of swine.

Schweitzer's reagent (shvīt′serz) [Matthias Eduard *Schweitzer,* German chemist, 1818–1860] see under *reagent.*

Schweninger's method (shven′in-gerz) [Ernst *Schweninger,* German physician, 1850–1924] see under *method.*

Schweninger-Buzzi anetoderma (shven′in-ger boots′e) [Ernst *Schweninger;* Fausto *Buzzi*] see under *anetoderma.*

scia- for other words beginning thus, see also those beginning *skia-.*

sciage (se-azh′) [Fr.] a sawing movement in massage.

sciatic (si-at′ik) [L. *sciaticus;* Gr. *ischiadikos*] 1. pertaining to or located near the sciatic nerve or vein; ischiadic; ischiatic. 2. ischial.

sciatica (si-at′ĭ-kah) [L.] a syndrome characterized by pain radiating from the back into the buttock and into the lower extremity along its posterior or lateral aspect, and most commonly caused by prolapse of the intervertebral disk; the term is also used to refer to pain anywhere along the course of the sciatic nerve.

SCID severe combined immunodeficiency.

science (si′ens) [L. *scientia* knowledge] 1. the systematic observation of natural phenomena for the purpose of discovering laws governing those phenomena. 2. the body of knowledge accumulated by such means. **applied s.,** that concerned with the application of discovered laws to the matters of everyday living. **behavioral s.,** the interdisciplinary study of the behavior of man and lower animals for the purpose of understanding man as an individual and social being; it involves principally psychology, sociology, and anthropology, but also political science and other social sciences. **pure s.,** that concerned solely with the discovery of unknown laws relating to particular facts.

scientist (si′en-tist) one learned in science, especially one active in some particular field of investigation.

scieropia (si-er-o′pe-ah) [Gr. *skieros* shady + *-opia*] visual defect in which objects appear in a shadow.

scilla (sil′ah) [L.] squill.

scillabiose (sil″ah-bi-ōs) glucosidorhamnose, $C_{12}H_{22}O_{10}$, obtained by acid hydrolysis of scillaren A.

scillaren (sil′ah-ren) a mixture of cardioactive glycosides, scillaren A and B, from fresh squill.

scilliroside (sil′ir-o-sīd) a cardioactive glycoside from red squill that is poisonous to rodents.

scillism (sil′izm) poisoning from squill.

scillitic (sil′it-ik) pertaining to squill.

scintigram (sin′tĭ-gram) scintiscan.

scintigraphic (sin″tĭ-graf′ik) pertaining to scintigraphy.

scintigraphy (sin-tig′rah-fe) the production of two-dimensional images of the distribution of radioactivity in tissues after the internal administration of radionuclide, the images being obtained by a scintillation camera. **thyroidal lymph node s.,** radioisotopic thyroidolymphography.

scintillascope (sin-til′ah-skōp) [L. *scintilla* spark + Gr. *skopein* to examine] spinthariscope.

scintillation (sin″tĭ-la′shun) [L. *scintillatio*] 1. an emission of sparks. 2. a subjective visual sensation, as of seeing sparks. 3. a particle emitted in disintegration of a radioactive element; see also under *counter.*

scintiphotograph (sin″tĭ-fo′to-graf) a photograph made with a camera using scintillation energy sources.

scintiphotography (sin″tĭ-fo-tog′rah-fe) photography of the pattern of radioactivity of tissues after administration of radionuclides.

scintiscan (sin′tĭ-skan) a two-dimensional representation (map) of the gamma rays emitted by a radioisotope, revealing its varying concentration in a specific tissue of the body, such as the brain, kidney, or thyroid gland.

scintiscanner (sin″tĭ-skan′er) the system of equipment used in the making of a scintiscan.

sciopody (ski-op′o-de) unusually large feet, especially in children.

scirrh(o)- [Gr. *skirrhos* hard] a combining form meaning hard, or denoting relationship to a hard cancer or scirrhous carcinoma.

scirrhoid (skir′oid) [*scirrho-* + Gr. *eidos* form] resembling scirrhous carcinoma.

scirrhoma (skir-ro′mah) [*scirrho-* + *-oma*] scirrhous carcinoma. **s. caminiano′rum,** chimney-sweeper's cancer, or soot cancer.

scirrhophthalmia (skir″of-thal′me-ah) [*scirrho-* + Gr. *ophthalmos* eye + *-ia*] scirrhous carcinoma of the eye.

scirrhous (skir′us) [L. *scirrhosus*] pertaining to or of the nature of a hard cancer; see also under *carcinoma.*

scirrhus (skir′us) [Gr. *skirrhos*] scirrhous carcinoma.

scission (sizh′un) [L. *scindere* to split] fission; splitting. In chemistry, the splitting of a molecule into two or more simpler molecules.

scissors (siz′erz) a cutting instrument with two opposed shearing blades. **canalicular s.,** delicate scissors with one of the blades probe pointed; used in slitting the lacrimal canal. **cannula s.,** scissors used in slitting a canal lengthwise. **craniotomy s.,** strong *f*-shaped shears for use in opening the fetal head. **Fox s.,** delicate, fine-pointed scissors designed to gain access to interproximal areas for the removal of small tissue tabs or slight soft tissue deformities during gingivoplasty or gingivectomy. **Liston's s.,** scissors for cutting plaster-of-Paris bandages. **Smellie's s.,** short, strong-bladed scissors with external cutting edges, used in craniotomy.

scissors-bite (siz′erz-bīt′) see under *bite.*

scissura (sĭ-su′rah), pl. *scissu′rae* [L.] an incisure; a splitting.

Sc.L.A. abbreviation for L. *scapulolaeva anterior* (left scapulo-anterior; a presentation of the fetus).

sclera (skle′rah), gen. and pl. *scle′rae* [L.; Gr. *skleros* hard] [NA] the tough white outer coat of the eyeball, covering approximately the posterior five-sixths of its surface, and continuous anteriorly with the cornea and posteriorly with the external sheath of the optic nerve. **blue s.,** a condition of unusual blueness of the sclera; it is normal in infants, but is also a prominent feature of osteogenesis imperfecta, and is seen in certain other abnormalities.

scleradenitis (skle″rad-ĕ-ni′tis) [*sclero-* + Gr. *adēn* gland + *-itis*] inflammation and hardening of a gland.

scleral (skle′ral) pertaining to the sclera.

scleratitis (skle″rah-ti′tis) scleritis.

scleratogenous (skle″rah-toj′ĕ-nus) sclerogenous.

sclerectasia (skle″rek-ta′ze-ah) [*scler-* + *ectasia*] a bulging out of the sclera.

sclerectasis (skle-rek′tah-sis) sclerectasia.

sclerectoiridectomy (skle-rek″to-ir″ĭ-dek′to-me) [*sclerectomy* + *iridectomy*] the operation of excision of a portion of the sclera and of the iris for glaucoma; called also *Lagrange's operation.*

sclerectoiridodialysis (skle-rek″to-ir″ĭ-do-di-al′ĭ-sis) sclerectomy and iridodialysis.

sclerectome (skle-rek′tōm) an instrument for performing sclerectomy.

sclerectomy (skle-rek′to-me) [*sclero-* + *ectomy*] excision of the sclera by scissors (Lagrange's operation), by punch (Holth's operation), or by trephining (Elliot's operation).

scleredema (skle″rĕ-de′mah) [*scler-* + *edema*] diffuse, symmetrical, wooden-like, nonpitting induration of the skin of unknown etiology, typically beginning on the face, head, or neck and spreading progressively to involve the shoulders, arms, thorax, and sometimes extracutaneous sites, and usually preceded by any of various infectious processes, especially a staphylococcal infection. It occurs in association with diabetes mellitus in most cases, predominantly in females, and usually resolves spontaneously in 6 months to 2 years. Called also *Buschke's s.,* and although the disorder is not restricted to adults, it is called also *s. adultorum,* and sometimes, erroneously, *sclerema adultorum.* **s. adulto′rum, Buschke's s.,** scleredema. **s. neonato′rum,** sclerema.

sclerema (skle-re′mah) [*scler-* + (ed)*ema*] a severe, sometimes fatal, disorder of adipose tissue occurring chiefly in preterm, sick, or debilitated infants suffering from a serious underlying illness, manifested by diffuse, rapidly progressive, nonpitting induration of the involved tissue, causing the skin to become cold, yellowish white, mottled, boardlike, and inflexible. Called also *s. adiposum, s. neonatorum, Underwood's disease,* and sometimes, erroneously, *scleredema neonatorum.* **s. adipo′sum,** sclerema. **s. adulto′rum,** scleredema. **s. neonato′rum,** sclerema.

sclerencephalia (skle″ren-sĕ-fa′le-ah) sclerencephaly.

sclerencephaly (skle″ren-sef′ah-le) [*sclero* + Gr. *enkephalos*] sclerosis of the brain.

sclerenchyma (skle-reng′kĭ-mah) [Gr. *sklēros* hard + *enchyma* infustion] supportive tissue occurring in many plant stems and roots, composed of thick-walled, usually dead cells impregnated with lignin. Cf. *collenchyma*

sclerenchymatous (skle″reng-kim′ah-tus) of the nature of sclerenchyma.

sclererythrin (skle-rer′ĭ-thrin) [*sclerotium* + Gr. *erythros* red] a red coloring matter from ergot.

scleriasis (skle-ri′ah-sis) [Gr. *sklēriasis*] a hardened state of an eyelid.

scleriritomy (skle″rĭ-rit′o-me) [*sclera* + *iris* + *-tomy*] incision of the sclera and iris in anterior staphyloma.

scleritis (skle-ri′tis) [*sclera* + *-itis*] inflammation of the sclera; it may be superficial (*episcleritis*) or deep, the latter form causing bulging and thinning of the sclera. It may occur alone or with keratitis or uveitis. **annular s.,** scleritis occurring in a ring around the limbus of the cornea. **anterior s.,** inflammation of the sclera adjoining the limbus of the cornea. **brawny s.,** a virulent, usually bilateral scleritis involving a thickening of the periphery of the cornea; called also *gelatinous s.* **s. necro′ticans, necrotizing s.,** scleromalacia. **nodular s.,** that marked by localized dark blue patches in the anterior portion of the sclera, resulting from the choroid being visible through a translucent sclera. **posterior s.,** scleritis involving the posterior sclera, the vagina bulbi, and the underyling retina and choroid.

scler(o)- [Gr. *sklēros* hard] a combining form meaning hard, often used especially to denote relationship to the sclera.

scleroadipose (skle″ro-ad′ĭ-pōs) composed of fibrous and fatty tissue.

scleroblastema (skle″ro-blas-te′mah) [*sclero-* + *blastema*] the embryonic tissue which takes part in the formation of bone.

scleroblastemic (skle″ro-blas-tem′ik) pertaining to the scleroblastema.

sclerochoroiditis (skle″ro-ko″roi-di′tis) inflammation of the sclera and the choroid coat, resulting in atrophy of both coats and protrusion of the former. **s. ante′rior,** a form involving the anterior portions of the sclera and causing anterior staphyloma. **s. poste′rior,** a condition seen in progressive myopia in which posterior staphyloma occurs in the region of the optic disk.

scleroconjunctival (skle″ro-kon″junk-ti′val) pertaining to the sclera and conjunctiva.

scleroconjunctivitis (skle″ro-kon-junk″tĭ-vi′tis) inflammation of the sclera and the conjunctiva.

sclerocornea (skle″ro-kor′ne-ah) the sclera and the cornea considered as forming a single coat or layer.

sclerocorneal (skle″ro-kor′ne-al) pertaining to the sclera and the cornea.

sclerodactylia (skle″ro-dak-til′e-ah) sclerodactyly.

sclerodactyly (skle″ro-dak′tĭ-le) [*sclero-* + Gr. *daktylos* finger] localized scleroderma of the digits, as in acrosclerosis.

scleroderma (skle″ro-der′mah) [*sclero-* + *derma*] chronic hardening and thickening of the skin, which may be a finding in several different diseases, occurring in a localized or focal form and as a systemic disease. Called also *dermatosclerosis.* **circumscribed s.,** 1. localized s. 2. morphea. **diffuse s.,** see *systemic s.* **generalized s.,** see *systemic s.* **linear s.,** a form of localized scleroderma characterized by bandlike lesions of induration with hyper- and hypopigmentation and atrophy of the skin, underlying subcutaneous tissue, muscle, and bone. When it involves the frontal or frontoparietal area of the forehead and a scalp the lesion is known as *en coup de sabre.* Called also *linear morphea.* **localized s.,** 1. scleroderma confined to the skin and subcutaneous tissue or secondarily involving the musculoskeletal system. It occurs in three forms: morphea, linear scleroderma, and en coup de sabre. Called also *circumscribed s.* Cf. *systemic s.* 2. morphea. **systemic s.,** a systemic disorder of the connective tissue characterized by induration and thickening of the skin, by abnormalities involving both the microvasculature (*telangiectasia*) and larger vessels (*Raynaud's phenomenon*), and by fibrotic degenerative changes in various body organs, including the heart, lungs, kidneys, and gastrointestinal tract. The disease may remain confined to the face and hands for long periods or may be progressive and spread diffusely and become generalized. Called also *systemic sclerosis.* See also *CREST syndrome,* under *syndrome.*

sclerodermatous (skle″ro-der′mah-tous) pertaining to or characterized by scleroderma.

sclerodesmia (skle″ro-des′me-ah) [*sclero-* + Gr. *desmos* ligament + *-ia*] hardening of ligaments.

sclerogenic (skle″ro-jen′ik) sclerogenous.

sclerogenous (skle-roj′ĕ-nus) [*sclero-* + Gr. *gennan* to produce] producing sclerosis or sclerous tissue.

sclerogummatous (skle″ro-gum′ah-tus) composed of fibrous and gummatous tissue.

scleroid (skle′roid) [*sclero-* + Gr. *eidos* form] having a hard texture.

scleroiritis (skle″ro-i-ri′tis) inflammation of the sclera and of the iris.

sclerokeratitis (skle″ro-ker″ah-ti′tis) inflammation of the sclera and of the cornea.

sclerokeratoiritis (skle″ro-ker″ah-to-i-ri′tis) inflammation of the sclera, cornea, and iris.

sclerokeratosis (skle″ro-ker″ah-to′sis) sclerokeratitis.

scleroma (skle-ro′mah) [Gr. *sklērōma* induration] a hardened patch or induration, especially of the nasal or laryngeal tissues. **s. respirato′rium,** rhinoscleroma.

scleromalacia (skle″ro-mah-la′she-ah) [*sclero-* + *malacia*] degeneration and thinning (softening) of the sclera, occurring in patients with rheumatoid arthritis; called also s. *eromalacia perforans.*

scleromeninx (skle″ro-me′ninks) [*sclero-* + Gr. *mēninx* membrane] the dura mater.

scleromere (skle′ro-mēr) [*sclero-* + Gr. *meros* part] 1. any segment or metamere of the skeletal system. 2. the caudal half of a sclerotome (def. 3).

sclerometer (skle-rom′ĕ-ter) [*sclero-* + Gr. *metron* measure] an instrument for determining the hardness of substances.

scleromucin (skle″ro-mu′sin) a slimy, active principle from ergot.

scleromyxedema (skle″ro-mik″sĕ-de′mah) [*sclero-* + *myxedema*] 1. lichen myxedematosus. 2. a term sometimes used to refer to lichen myxedematosus associated with scleroderma, producing, especially on the face, exaggerated furrowing of the skin.

scleronychia (skle″ro-nik′e-ah) [*sclero-* + Gr. *onyx* nail + *-ia*] a simultaneous thickening and dryness of the nails.

scleronyxis (skle″ro-nik′sis) [*sclero-* + *nyxis*] surgical puncture of the sclera.

sclero-oophoritis (skle″ro-o-of″o-ri′tis) sclerosing inflammation of an ovary.

sclero-oothecitis (skle″ro-o″o-the-si′tis) sclero-oophoritis.

sclerophthalmia (skle″rof-thal′me-ah) [*sclero-* + *-ophthalmia*] the condition in which, from imperfect differentiation of the sclera and cornea, the periphery of the cornea is opaque and only the central part remains clear.

scleroprotein (skle″ro-pro′te-in) [*sclero-* + *protein*] a simple protein which is characterized by its insolubility and fibrous structure, and which usually serves a supportive or protective function in the body; called also *albuminoid.*

sclerosal (skle-ro′sal) sclerous.

sclerosant (skle-ro′sant) a chemical irritant injected into a vein to produce inflammation and eventual fibrosis and obliteration of the lumen, used in the treatment of varicose veins.

sclerosarcoma (skle″ro-sar-ko′mah) [*sclero-* + Gr. *sarkōma*] a fleshy excrescence] a fibrosing sarcoma.

scleroscope (skle″ro-skōp′) [*sclero-* + *-scope*] an instrument for determining the hardness of materials. See under *test.*

sclerose (skle-rōs′) to become sclerotic; to harden.

sclerosed (skle-rōst′) affected with sclerosis.

sclérose en plaques (skla-rōz″ aw-plak′) [Fr.] multiple sclerosis.

sclerosing (skle-rōs′ing) causing or undergoing sclerosis.

sclerosis (skle-ro′sis) [Gr. *sklērōsis* hardness] an induration, or hardening; especially hardening of a part from inflammation and in diseases of the interstitial substance. The term is used chiefly for such a hardening of the nervous system due to hyperplasia of the connective tissue or to designate hardening of the blood vessels. **amyotrophic lateral s.,** a disease marked by progressive degeneration of the neurons that give rise to the corticospinal tract and of the motor cells of the brain stem and spinal cord, and resulting in a deficit of upper and lower motor neurons; it usually ends fatally within two to three years. Called also *Charcot syndrome, Dejerine type,* and *Lou Gehrig disease.* **annular s.,** sclerosis of the spinal cord, forming a band around it. **anterolateral s.,** sclerosis of the ventral and lateral columns of the spinal cord, leading to spastic paraplegia; called also *ventrolateral s.* **arterial s., arteriocapillary s.,** arteriosclerosis. **arteriolar s.,** arteriolosclerosis. **bone s.,** eburnation. **combined s.,** subacute combined degeneration of the spinal cord; see under *degeneration.* **dentinal s.,** regressive alteration in tooth substance with calcification of the dentinal tubules, usually caused by trauma, abrasion, or normal aging processes, and producing translucent zones (transparent dentin). **diaphyseal s.,** diaphyseal dysplasia. **diffuse s.,** a form affecting large areas of the brain and spinal cord. **diffuse systemic s.,** see *systemic scleroderma,* under *scleroderma.* **disseminated s.,** multiple sclerosis. **endocardial s.,** see under *fibroelastosis.* **Erb's s.,** primary lateral spinal sclerosis; see under *lateral s.* **familial centrolobar s.,** Pelizaeus-Merzbacher disease. **focal s.,** multiple s. **focal glomerular s.,** the occurrence of focal sclerosing lesions of the renal glomeruli, marked by proteinuria, hematuria, hypertension, and the nephrotic syndrome; it may be idio-

pathic or secondary to other diseases, including heroin-abuse nephropathy, chronic interstitial nephritis, and malignancies. Exacerbations and remissions may occur, most often in children; progression to renal failure occurs at a variable and unpredictable rate. **gastric s.,** linitis plastica. **hyperplastic s.,** a form of arteriosclerosis seen in small arteries and arterioles as a subintimal thickening of the wall of the vessel. **insular s.,** multiple s. **lateral s.,** a degeneration of the lateral columns of the spinal cord. It may occur as a *primary* affection, resulting in spastic paraplegia, attended with rigidity of the limbs, increase of the tendon reflexes, and absence of nutritive and sensory disturbance; called also *Erb's sclerosis.* Or it may be *secondary* to myelitis, in which there is spastic paraplegia, with sensory and other disturbances; called also *spastic spinal paralysis.* **lobar s.,** presence of narrow, scar-distorted convolutions over a large area (lobe) of the surface of the cerebral hemispheres; seen frequently in cerebral palsy. **Marie's s.,** hereditary cerebellar ataxia. **miliary s.,** sclerosis occurring in minute spots. **Mönckeberg's s.,** see under *arteriosclerosis.* **multiple s.,** a disease in which there are patches of demyelination throughout the white matter of the central nervous system, sometimes extending into the gray matter. Typically, the symptoms of lesions of the white matter are weakness, incoordination, paresthesias, speech disturbances, and visual complaints. The course of the disease is usually prolonged, with remissions and relapses over a period of many years. The etiology is unknown. Called also *disseminated s.* and *insular s.* **Pelizaeus-Merzbacher s.,** familial centrolobar s. **posterior s., posterior spinal s.,** tabes dorsalis. **posterolateral s.,** subacute combined degeneration of spinal cord; see under *degeneration.* **progressive systemic s.,** see *systemic scleroderma,* under *scleroderma.* **renal arteriolar s.,** arteriosclerosis involving chiefly the renal arterioles, resulting in contracted kidney. **subendocardial s.,** endocardial fibroelastosis. **systemic s.,** see under *scleroderma.* **tuberous s.,** an autosomal dominant disease characterized principally by the presence of hamartomas of the brain (tubers), retina (phakomas), and viscera, mental retardation, seizures, and adenoma sebaceum, and often associated with other skin lesions, including subungual fibromas, vitiliginous patches, shagreen patches, and café-au-lait spots. Called also *Bourneville's disease* and *epiloia.* **unicellular s.,** the development of bands of fibrous material between the cells of a gland. **vascular s.,** arteriosclerosis. **valvular s.,** fibrous thickening of a cardiac valve, especially the mitral valve. **venous s.,** phlebosclerosis. **ventrolateral s.,** anterolateral s.

scleroskeleton (skle″ro-skel′ĕ-ton) [*sclero-* + *skeleton*] those parts of the bony skeleton that are formed by the ossification of ligaments, tendons, or fasciae.

sclerostenosis (skle″ro-stĕ-no′sis) [Gr. *sklērōs* hard + *stenōsis* narrowing] induration or hardening combined with contraction.

Sclerostoma (skle-ros′to-mah) *Strongylus.* **S. duodena′le,** *Ancylostoma duodenale.* **S. syn′gamus,** *Syngamus trachea.*

sclerostomy (skle-ros′to-me) [*sclero-* + *-stomy*] the surgical creation of an opening through the sclera; it is usually performed in the treatment of glaucoma.

sclerotherapy (skle″ro-ther′ah-pe) the injection of sclerosing solutions in the treatment of hemorrhoids, varicose veins, or esophageal varices.

sclerotia (skle-ro′she-ah) plural of *sclerotium.*

sclerotic (skle-rot′ik) 1. hard, or hardening; affected with sclerosis. 2. sclera.

sclerotica (skle-rot′ĭ-kah) [L. *scleroticus;* Gr. *sklēros* hard] sclera.

sclerotic acid (skle-rot′ik) an acid found in ergot, of which it is one of the active principles.

scleroticochoroiditis (skle-rot″ĭ-ko-ko″roid-i′tis) sclerochoroiditis.

Sclerotinia (skle″ro-tin′ĭ-ah) a genus of ascomycetous fungi of the order Helotiales, family Sclerotiniaceae, which includes many pathogens of plants. Its imperfect (sexual) stage is *Monilia.*

Sclerotiniaceae (skle″ro-tin-i-a′she-e) a family of ascomycetes of the order Heleotiales, series Pyrenomycetes, including the genus *Sclerotina.*

sclerotinic acid (skle″ro-tin′ik) sclerotic acid.

sclerotitis (skle″ro-ti′tis) scleritis.

sclerotium (skle-ro′she-um) [L. *sclerotica* hard] 1. in fungi, a hard mass of intertwined mycelia, usually with pigmented walls resistant to adverse environmental conditions; it will germinate to produce new hyphae under favorable conditions or in response to a chemical stimulus from a prospective host. 2. in certain protoza, a multinucleate hard cyst into which the plasmodium divides in response to adverse environmental conditions, such as desiccation; sclerotia will germinate and fuse together to produce a new plasmodium under favorable conditions.

sclerotome (skle′ro-tōm) [*sclero-* + *-tome*] 1. an instrument used in the incision of the sclera. 2. the area of a bone innervated from a single spinal segment. 3. one of the paired masses of mesenchymal tissue, separated from the ventromedial part of a somite, which develop into vertebrae and ribs.

sclerotomy (skle-rot′o-me) [*sclero-* + *-tomy*] surgical incision of the sclera. **anterior s.,** the surgical opening of the anterior chamber of the eye, chiefly done for the relief of glaucoma. **posterior s.,** an opening made into the vitreous through the sclera, as for detached retina or the removal of a foreign body.

sclerous (skle′rus) hard; indurated.

sclerozone (skle′ro-zōn) [*sclero-* + Gr. *zōnē* zone] any surface on a bone giving attachment to the muscles from a given myotome.

Sc.L.P. abbreviation for *L. scapulolaeva posterior* (left scapuloposterior; a presentation of the fetus).

S.C.M. State Certified Midwife.

scoleces (sko′lĕ-sēz) [L.] plural of *scolex*.

scoleciasis (sko-lĕ-si′ah-sis) [*scoleco-* + *-iasis*] the condition caused by the presence of larvae of moths or butterflies in the body.

scoleciform (sko-les′ĭ-form) resembling a scolex.

scoleco- [Gr. *skōlĕx* worm] a combining form denoting relationship to a worm.

scolecoid (sko′lĕ-koid) [Gr. *skōlekoeidēs* vermiform] 1. resembling a worm. 2. resembling a scolex; hydatid.

scolecology (sko″lĕ-kol′o-je) [*scoleco-* + *-logy*] helminthology.

scolex (sko′leks), pl. *sco′leces* [Gr. *skōlĕx* worm] the attachment (or holdfast) organ, of a tapeworm, generally considered the anterior, or cephalic end.

scolio- [Gr. *skolios* twisted] a combining form meaning twisted or crooked.

scoliokyphosis (sko″le-o-ki-fo′sis) [*scolio-* + *kyphosis*] combined lateral (scoliosis) and posterior (kyphosis) curvature of the spine.

scoliorachitic (sko″le-o-rah-kit′ik) affected with scoliosis and rickets.

scoliosiometry (sko″le-o-se-om′ĕ-tre) [*scoliosis* + Gr. *metron* measure] measurement of curvatures, especially those of the vertebral column.

scoliosis (sko″le-o′sis) [Gr. *skoliōsis* curvation] an appreciable lateral deviation in the normally straight vertical line of the spine. Cf. *kyphosis* and *lordosis*. **Brissaud's s.,** sciatic s. **cicatricial s.,** that which is due to a cicatricial contraction following caries or necrosis. **coxitic s.,** scoliosis in the lumbar region caused by hip disease. **empyematic s.,** that which is caused by empyema. **habit s.,** scoliosis due to improper posture. **inflammatory s.,** that which is due to vertebral disease. **ischiatic s.,** that which is due to hip disease. **myopathic s.,** paralytic s. **ocular s., ophthalmic s.,** scoliosis attributed to tilting of the head on account of astigmatism or muscle imbalance. **osteopathic s.,** that which is caused by disease of the vertebrae. **paralytic s.,** lateral curvature of the spinal column due to muscle paralysis; called also *myopathic s.* **rachitic s.,** spinal curvature due to rickets. **rheumatic s.,** that which is due to rheumatism of the dorsal muscles. **sciatic s.,** a list of the lumbar part of the spine away from the affected side in sciatica; called also *Brissaud's s.* **static s.,** that which is due to difference in the length of the legs.

scoliosometer (sko″le-o-som′ĕ-ter) an apparatus for measuring curves, especially those of the spinal column.

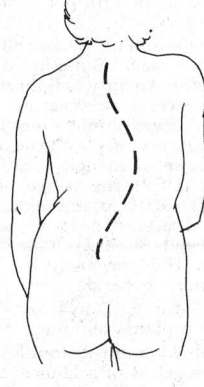

Scoliosis.

scoliotic (sko″le-ot′ik) [Gr. *skoliōtos* looking askew] pertaining to or characterized by scoliosis.

scoliotone (sko′le-o-tōn) an apparatus for the forcible correction of scoliosis.

Scolopendra (sko″lo-pen′drah) [Gr. *skolops* anything pointed] a genus of venomous centipedes of the class Chilopoda. The bite of some large species may produce a severe local inflammation attended with pain, glandular enlargement, vomiting, headache, vertigo, and fever. *S. he′ros* and *S. mor′sitans* are American species; *S. gigan′tea* is a tropical species.

scolopsia (sko-lop′se-ah) [Gr. *skolops* anything pointed] a suture between two bones that allows motion of one on the other.

scombrine (skom′brin) a protamine found in mackerel sperm.

scombroid (skom′broid) 1. of or pertaining to the suborder Scombroidea. 2. a fish of the suborder Scombroidea. See also under *poisoning.*

Scombroidea (skom-broi′de-ah) a suborder of larger, bony, marine fish having oily flesh, including tunas, bonitos, mackerels, albacores, and skipjacks. The flesh of these fish may contain a toxic histamine-like substance and, if ingested, can cause a condition known as *scombroid poisoning* (q.v.).

scombrone (skom′bron) a histone from spermatozoa of mackerel.

scombrotoxic (skom″bro-toks′ik) pertaining to or caused by the histamine-like toxin of scombroid fish; see *scombroid poisoning,* under *poisoning.*

scombrotoxin (skom″bro-toks′in) the histamine-like toxin formed in scombroid fish by bacterial action; it causes scombroid poisoning.

scoop (skōōp) a spoonlike instrument for evacuating cavities. **Mules's s.,** a form of curet used in eye operations.

scopafungin (sko-pah-fun′jin) an antibacterial and antifungal antibiotic derived from a variant of *Streptomyces hygroscopicus.*

scoparin (sko-pa′rin) chemical name: 8-glycosyl-4′,5,7-trihydroxy-3′-methoxyflavone. A yellowish, crystalline diuretic principle, $C_{22}H_{22}O_{11}$, from scoparius, the tops of *Cytisus scoparius* (L.) Link. (Leguminosae).

scoparius (sko-pa′re-us) the tops of *Cytisus scoparius,* (L.) Link. (Leguminosae), or broom, a leguminous shrub; they contain the alkaloid sparteine and the principle scoparin, and are diuretic, purgative, and emetic. Scoparius is also abused by being smoked for its euphoric properties.

-scope [Gr. *skopein* to view, examine] a word termination denoting an instrument for examining or observing.

scopin (sko′pin) a substance formed by the gentle hydrolysis of scopolamine. It is $OH \cdot C_6H_8O \cdot N \cdot CH_3$, and readily changes into oscine.

scopola (sko-po′lah) the dried rhizome and larger roots of *Scopolia carniolica* Jacq. (Solanaceae). It contains the same constituents as belladonna, is used as an anticholinergic, and is a source of scopoletin.

scopolagnia (sko″po-lag′ne-ah) [Gr. *skopein* to view + *lagneia* lust]　scopophilia.

scopolamine (sko-pol′ah-mēn)　chemical name: α-(hydroxymethyl)benzeneacetic acid 9-methyl-3-oxa-9-azatricyclo-[3.3.1.0²,⁴] non-7-yl ester. An anticholinergic alkaloid, $C_{17}H_{21}NO_4$, derived from several solanaceous plants, including *Atropa belladonna* L., *Hyoscyamus niger* L., *Datura* species, and *Scopolia* species. It has effects on the autonomic nervous system similar to those of atropine. Called also *hyoscine*. **s. hydrobromide** [USP], the trihydrate salt of scopolamine, $C_{17}H_{21}NO_4 \cdot HBr \cdot 3H_2O$, occurring as colorless or white crystals. It is used as a cerebral sedative, administered orally or subcutaneously, and as a cycloplegic and mydriatic, applied topically to the conjunctiva. **s. methylbromide,** methscopolamine bromide.

scopoletin (sko-pol′ĕ-tin)　7 - hydroxy - 5 - methoxycoumarin, a growth factor in plants obtained from scopola.

Scopolia (sko-po′le-ah) [Johann-Antoni *Scopoli*, physician in Pavia, 1723–1788]　a genus of solanaceous plants. *S. carniolica atropoi′des* Jacq. (solanaceae), of Europe, and *S. japon′ica* and *S. lu′rida*, of Asia, have properties like those of hyoscyamus and belladonna.

scopometer (sko-pom′ĕ-ter) [Gr. *skopein* to examine + *metron* measure]　an instrument for measuring the turbidity of solutions, i.e., the density of a precipitate.

scopometry (sko-pom′ĕ-tre)　measurement of the optical density of a precipitate to determine the amount of a substance in suspension.

scopophilia (sko-po-fil′e-ah) [Gr. *skopein* to view + *philein* to love]　1. voyeurism; the derivation of sexual pleasure from looking at another's genital organs (*active* s.).　2. exhibitionism; the desire to be looked at by others (*passive* s.).

scopophobia (sko″po-fo′be-ah) [Gr. *skopein* to view + *phobia*]　irrational fear of being seen.

scoptophilia (skop″to-fil′e-ah)　scopophilia.

scoptophobia (skop″to-fo′be-ah)　scopophobia.

scopula (skop′u-lah) [L. "small brush"]　an aboral organelle of peritrichous protozoa comprising a field of kinetosomes and immobile cilia, which may function as a holdfast organ or may be the origin of the stalk.

Scopulariopsis (skop″u-la″re-op′sis)　a genus of imperfect fungi of the family Moniliaceae, order Moniliales. *S. brevicaulis* sometimes causes onychomycosis. Formerly called *Acaulium*.

scopulariopsosis (skop″u-la″re-op-so′sis)　infection with a fungus of the genus *Scopulariopsis*.

-scopy [Gr. *skopein* to examine]　word termination denoting the act of examining.

scorbutic (skōr-bu′tik) [L. *scorbuticus*]　pertaining to or affected with scurvy.

scorbutigenic (skōr-bu″tĭ-jen′ik)　causing scurvy.

scorbutus (skōr-bu′tus) [L.]　scurvy.

scordinema (skōr″dĭ-ne′mah) [Gr. *skordinēma*]　yawning and stretching with a feeling of lassitude, occurring as a preliminary symptom of some infectious disease.

score (skōr)　a rating, usually expressed numerically, based on achievement or the degree to which certain qualities are present.　**Apgar s.,** a numerical expression of the condition of a newborn infant, usually determined at 60 seconds after birth, being the sum of points gained on assessment of the heart rate, respiratory effort, muscle tone, reflex irritability, and color. Cf. *recovery s.*　**Bishop s.,** a score for estimating the prospects of induction of labor, arrived at by evaluating the extent of cervical dilatation, effacement, the station of the fetal head, consistency of the cervix, and the cervical position in relation to the vaginal axis.　**lod s.,** "logarithm of the *odds*" score, which measures the likelihood of two genes being within measurable distance of each other.　**recovery s.,** a number expressing the condition of an infant at various intervals, which should be stipulated, greater than 1 minute after birth, based on the same features assessed by the Apgar score at 60 seconds after birth.

scorings (skōr′ingz)　small transverse lines caused by increased density of bone, seen in roentgenograms at the metaphysis of growing bones, and due to temporary cessation of growth.

scorpion (skōr′pe-on)　an arthropod of warm countries, having a venomous sting. More important species are *Buthus quinquestriatus* of Egypt, *Centruroides suffusus* of Mexico,

Euscorpius italicus, or black scorpion, of Europe and North Africa, and *Tityus serrulatus* of Brazil.

scorpionism (skōr′pe-un-izm)　poisoning by scorpion stings.

scot(o)- [Gr. *skotos* darkness]　a combining form denoting relationship to darkness.

Scotobacteria (sko″to-bak-te′re-ah) [scoto- + *bacteria*]　a class of bacteria of the division Gracilicutes, kingdom Procaryotae, made up of gram-negative organisms that do not derive energy from light (nonphototrophic metabolism). It contains aerobic and anaerobic rods and cocci, including the medically important families Spirochaetaceae, Spirosomaceae, Pseudomonadaceae, Enterobacteriaceae, Vibrionaceae, Bacteroidaceae, Neisseriaceae, Legionellaceae, Pasteurellaceae, and Veillonellaceae and the orders Rickettsiales and Chlamydiales.

scotobacterium (sko″to-bak-te′re-um)　1. an individual organism of the class Scotobacteria.　2. a bacterium capable of growing in the dark.

scotochromogen (sko″to-kro′mo-jen) [scoto- + Gr. *chrōma* color + *gennan* to produce]　a microorganism whose pigmentation develops in the dark as well as in the light; specifically, a member of Runyon Group II of the nontuberculous mycobacteria, but applicable also to many other organisms. See also *nontuberculous mycobacteria*, under *mycobacterium*.

scotochromogenic (sko″to-kro″mo-jen′ik)　pertaining to or characterized by scotochromogenicity.

scotochromogenicity (sko″to-kro″mo-jĕ-nis′ĭ-te)　the property of forming pigment in the dark, the coloration occurring irrespective of exposure to light.

scotodinia (sko″to-din′e-ah) [Gr. *skotos* darkness + *dinos* whirl]　dizziness with blurring of vision and headache.

scotogram, scotograph (sko′to-gram; sko′to-graf) [Gr. *skotos* darkness + *graphein* to write]　1. roentgenogram.　2. the effect produced upon a photographic plate in the dark by certain substances.

scotographic (sko″to-graf′ik)　affecting a photographic plate in the dark.

scotography (sko-tog′rah-fe)　roentgenography.

scotoma (sko-to′mah), pl. *scoto′mata* [Gr. *skotōma*]　1. an area of lost or depressed vision within the visual field, surrounded by an area of less depressed or of normal vision.　2. mental s.　**absolute s.,** an area within the visual field in which perception of light is entirely lost.　**annular s.,** a circular area of depressed vision in the visual field, surrounding the point of fixation.　**arcuate s.,** a scotoma arising at or near the blind spot and arching inferiorly or superiorly toward the nasal field, following the paths of the retinal nerve fibers.　**aural s., s. au′ris,** loss of ability to perceive auditory stimuli coming from a certain direction.　**Bjerrum's s.,** a further development of Seidel's scotoma, the sickle-shaped defect contiguous to the blind spot extending above and below the fixation point and encircling it more or less completely.　**cecocentral s.,** centrocecal s.　**central s.,** an area of depressed vision corresponding with the point of fixation and either surrounding or entirely abolishing central vision.　**centrocecal s.,** a horizontal oval defect in the field of vision situated between and embracing both the point of fixation and the blind spot.　**color s.,** an isolated area of depressed or defective vision for color in the visual field.　**flittering s.,** teichopsia.　**hemianopic s.,** depressed or lost vision affecting half of the central visual field. Cf. *hemianopia*.　**mental s.,** in psychiatry, a figurative blind spot in a person's psychological awareness, the patient being unable to gain insight into and to understand his mental problems; lack of insight. See also *scotomization*.　**motile s's,** floating opacities, not true scotomata, occurring in the vitreous, muscae volitantes being an example of such a defect.　**negative s.,** a scotoma appearing as a blank spot in the visual field; the patient is unaware of it, and it is detected only by examination.　**paracentral s.,** an area of depressed vision situated near the point of fixation.　**peripapillary s.,** an area of depressed vision in the visual field near that corresponding with the optic disk.　**peripheral s.,** an area of depressed vision distant from the point of fixation, toward the periphery of the visual field.　**physiologic s.,** that area of the visual field corresponding with the optic disk, in which the photosensitive receptors are absent.　**positive s.,** a scotoma subjectively perceived as a black spot in the visual field, and of which the patient is aware. **relative s.,** an area of the visual field in which perception of light is only diminished, or the loss is restricted to light of certain wavelengths. **ring s.,** annular s. **scintillating s.,** teichopsia. **Seidel's s.,** a further development of an arcuate scotoma, which extends at either or both ends, the concavity of the prolongation always being directed toward the fixation point.

scotomagraph (sko-to′mah-graf) [scotoma + -graph] an instrument for recording a scotoma.

scotomata (sko-to′mah-tah) plural of scotoma.

scotomatous (sko-tom′ah-tus) pertaining to or affected with scotoma.

scotometer (sko-tom′ĕ-ter) [scotoma + -meter] an instrument for diagnosing and measuring scotomata. **Bjerrum's s.,** campimeter.

scotometry (sko-tom′ĕ-tre) the measurement of isolated areas of depressed vision (scotomata) within the visual field.

scotomization (sko″to-mi-za′shun) [scotoma + -izein to make into] the development of scotomata, or blind spots, especially the development of mental scotomata (mental "blind spots"), the patient attempting to deny existence of everything which conflicts with his ego.

scotophilia (sko″to-fil′e-ah) [scoto- + Gr. philein to love] preference for night.

scotophobia (sko″to-fo′be-ah) [scoto- + phobia] irrational fear of darkness.

scotophobin (sko″to-fo′bin) [scoto- + Gr. phobein to be affrighted by] a peptide composed of 15 amino acids that has been isolated from the brain tissue of rats and mice conditioned to fear the dark; on injection into normal rodents, it is said to induce fear of dark.

scotopia (sko-to′pe-ah) [scot- + -opia] night vision; see also dark adaptation.

scotopic (sko-top′ik) pertaining to scotopia.

scotopsin (sko-top′sin) the protein moiety in the rods of the retina that combines with retinal (11-cis retinal) to form rhodopsin.

scotoscopy (sko-tos′ko-pe) [scoto- + Gr. skopein to examine] skiascopy.

scototherapy (sko″to-ther′ah-pe) [scoto- + Gr. therapeia treatment] treatment of disease by the complete exclusion of light rays.

scours (skowrz) diarrhea or dysentery, especially in newborn animals; see white s. **black s.,** acute dysentery in cattle, accompanied by intestinal hemorrhage producing a dark color of the feces; the etiology is unknown. **bloody s.,** black scours in swine. **calf s.,** white scours in calves. **peat s.,** molybdenum poisoning in grazing cattle. **white s.,** an acute infectious disease of calves, lambs, and foals during the first few days after birth, caused by enteropathogenic strains of Escherichia coli and marked by fever, dehydration, depression, and diarrhea, with fetid feces that are light in color but may be blood-stained late in the disease. **winter s.,** black scours occurring in cattle when stabled for the winter.

scr. scruple.

scrapie (skra′pe) one of the transmissible spongiform encephalopathies occurring in sheep and goats, characterized by severe pruritus, debility, and muscular incoordination, and invariably ending fatally.

scratches (skrach′ez) eczematous inflammation of the feet of a horse.

screen (skrēn) 1. a structure resembling a curtain or partition, used as a protection or shield; such a structure used in fluoroscopy; or such a structure on which light rays are projected. 2. to examine by fluoroscopy (Great Britain). 3. an agent that affords defense against a deleterious influence, such as a substance applied to the skin (skin s.) to protect against the effects of the sun's rays (solar s.) or other noxious influences; called also protectant and protective. 4. to separate well individuals in a population from those who have an undiagnosed disease, defect, or other pathologic condition or who are at high risk, by means of tests, examinations, or other procedures. See also screening. **Bjerrum s.,** tangent s. **fluorescent s.,** 1. a sheet of cardboard, paper, or glass coated with suitable material, which fluoresces visibly, as calcium tungstate, used as an intensifying screen in roentgenography; as the chief part of a fluoroscope; as a

substitute for a fluoroscope in a darkened room. 2. a sheet of cardboard, paper, or glass coated with anthracene or other fluorescing materials to observe the ultraviolet radiations. **intensifying s.,** a thin sheet of celluloid or other substance coated with a finely divided substance which fluoresces under the influence of roentgen rays and intended to be used in close contact with the emulsion of a photographic plate or film for the purpose of reinforcing the image. **oral s.,** vestibular s. **tangent s.,** a large square of black cloth, stretched on a frame, hung from a roller, and having a central mark for fixation; used with a campimeter to map the field of vision. Called also Bjerrum screen. **vestibular s.,** an acrylic resin removable orthodontic appliance that covers the labial or buccal surface of one or both dental arches, fitting between the oral mucosa and the teeth; used to treat oral habits and to stimulate tooth movement. Called also oral s. and oral shield.

screening (skrēn′ing) 1. examination or testing of a group of individuals to separate those who are well from those who have an undiagnosed disease or defect or who are at high risk. 2. fluoroscopy (Great Britain). **mass s.,** that performed on or made available to an entire population. **multiphasic s., multiple s.,** that in which various diagnostic procedures are employed during the same screening program. **prescriptive s.,** that performed for the early detection of disease or disease precursors in apparently well individuals so that health care can be provided early in the course of the disease or before the disease becomes manifest.

screwworm (skru′werm) the larva of Cochliomyia hominivorax.

scribomania (skrib″o-ma′ne-ah) graphorrhea.

scrobiculate (skro-bik′u-lāt) [L. scrobiculatus] marked with pits or cavities.

scrobiculus (skro-bik′u-lus) [L. "little trench," "pit"] a small hollow, pit, or cavity. **s. cor′dis,** fossa epigastrica.

scrofula (skrof′u-lah) [L. "brood sow"] former name for tuberculous cervical lymphadenitis. See also scrofuloderma.

scrofuloderma (skrof″u-lo-der′mah) [scrofula + Gr. derma skin] a tuberculous or nontuberculous mycobacterial infection affecting children and young adults, representing direct extension of tuberculosis into the skin from underlying structures such as lymph nodes (especially the cervical), bone or lung or by contact exposure to tuberculosis. It is manifested by the development of painless subcutaneous swelling that evolve into cold abscesses, multiple ulcers, and draining sinus tracts. Called also t. colliquativa and tuberculosis cutis colliquativa. Cf. tuberculous gumma.

scrofulous (skrof′u-lus) pertaining or relating to, characterized by, or affected with scrofula.

scrotal (skro′tal) pertaining to the scrotum.

scrotectomy (skro-tek′to-me) [scrotum + Gr. ektomē excision] partial or complete excision of the scrotum.

scrotitis (skro-ti′tis) inflammation of the scrotum.

scrotocele (skro′to-sēl) [scrotum + Gr. kēlē hernia] scrotal hernia.

scrotoplasty (skro′to-plas″te) [scrotum + Gr. plassein to form] plastic operation on the scrotum.

scrotum (skro′tum) [L. "bag"] [NA] the pouch which contains the testes and their accessory organs. It is composed of skin, the dartos, the spermatic, cremasteric, and infundibuliform fasciae, and the tunica vaginalis. **s. lapillo′sum,** calcareous atheroma of the scrotum. **lymph s.,** elephantiasis scroti. **watering-can s.,** a condition in which the undersurface of the scrotum and the perineum are marked by multiple sinuses discharging urine; due to neglected stricture of the perineal urethra.

scruple (skroo′p'l) [L. scrupulus, dim. of scrupus a sharp stone, a worry or anxiety] 1. a fear of transgression. 2. a unit of mass (weight) of the apothecaries' system, being 20 grains, or the equivalent of 1.296 gm. Abbreviated scr.; symbol ℈.

scrupulosity (skroo″pu-los′ĭ-te) excessive meticulousness or punctiliousness, usually related to moral or religious questions.

scultetus (skul-te′tus) [named for Johann Schultes (Scultetus), German surgeon, 1595–1645] scultetus bandage, a many-tailed binder; see under bandage.

scurvy (skur′ve) [L. scorbutus] a condition due to deficiency of ascorbic acid (vitamin C) in the diet and marked by weakness, anemia, spongy gums, a tendency to mucocutaneous hemorrhages and a brawny induration of the muscles of the calves and legs. **hemorrhagic s.,** infantile scurvy. **infantile s.,** a nutritional disease of infants characterized by the same symptoms as scurvy in adults; called also *Barlow's disease.* **sea s.,** true scurvy; so called because it was most often seen in mariners.

scute (skūt) [L. *scutum* shield] 1. any squama or scalelike structure. 2. the tympanic scute. **tympanic s.,** the bony plate which divides the upper part of the tympanic cavity from the mastoid cells.

scutica (sku′tĭ-kah), pl. *scu′ticae* [L. "whip," "lash"] a transient multikinetosomal structure seen in certain ciliate protozoa during the process of stomatogenesis, typically having a hooklike or whiplike shape.

Scuticociliatida (sku″te-ko-sil″e-a′tĭ-dah) [L. *scutum* shield + *ciliate*] an order of large, uniformly or sparsely ciliated protozoa (subclass Hymenostomatia, class Oligohymenophorea), characterized by the presence of buccal ciliature often dominated by a tripartite (anterior, middle, posterior) paroral membrane; the appearance of a scutica during morphogenesis; mucocysts; and long mitochondria, sometimes fused to form a large chondriome. They are found chiefly in marine habitats, free-living or symbiotic with mostly invertebrates, such as echinoids, mollusks, and annelids. It comprises three suborders: Philasterina, Pleuronematina, and Thigmotrichina.

scutiform (sku′tĭ-form) [L. *scutum* shield + *forma* form] shaped like a shield; thyroid.

scutular (sku′tu-lar) marked by scutula, or small, saucer-shaped crusts.

scutulum (sku′tu-lum), pl. *scu′tula* [L.] one of the disklike or saucer-like crusts characteristic of favus.

scutum (sku′tum) [L. "shield"] 1. the tympanic scute. 2. the thyroid cartilage. 3. a hard chitinous plate on the anterior portion of the dorsal surface of the Ixodidae, or hard-bodied ticks. **s. pec′toris,** the sternum.

scybala (sib′ah-lah) [Gr.] plural of *scybalum.*

scybalous (sib′ah-lus) of the nature of or composed of scybala.

scybalum (sib′ah-lum), pl. *scyb′ala* [Gr. *skybalon*] a dry, hard mass of fecal matter in the intestine.

scyllite (sil′īt) a hexose from the liver and kidneys of sharks, skates, etc.

scyllitol (sil′ĭ-tol) the 2-isomer of inositol isolated from the dog fish, *Scyllum canicula,* as well as from sharks and rays.

scymnol (sim′nol) a bile alcohol, $C_{27}H_{48}O_5$, with a 24:26-epoxy group, and a ring-system similar to that of cholic acid; found in the bile of *Scymnus borealis,* a marine fish of the shark family, and in other elasmobranchi.

scyphoid (si′foid) [Gr. *skyphos* cup + *-oid*] shaped like a cup.

scythropasmus (si″thro-paz′mus) [Gr. *skythrōpasmos; skythōpazein* to look sullen] a dull, fatigued expression, regarded as a grave symptom in serious disease.

scytoblastema (si″to-blas-te′mah) [Gr. *skytos* skin + *blastēma* sprout] the rudimentary skin of the embryo.

Scytonema (si″to-ne′mah) [Gr. *skytos* skin + *nēma* thread] a genus of blue-green algae with cylindrical branching filaments.

S.D. skin dose; standard deviation.

S.D.A. abbreviation for L. *sacrodex′tra ante′rior* (right sacroanterior; a presentation of the fetus), and specific dynamic action.

S.D.E. specific dynamic effect (or action); see under *action.*

S.D.P. abbreviation for L. *sacrodex′tra poste′rior* (right sacroposterior; a presentation of the fetus).

S.D.T. abbreviation for L. *sacrodex′tra transver′sa* (right sacrotransverse; a presentation of the fetus).

S.E. standard error.

SE sphenoethmoidal suture, def. 2.

Se chemical symbol for *selenium.*

seal (sēl) 1. something that effects a firm closure. 2. to secure or close tightly. 3. in dentistry, a material, usually a plastic, that hardens in the mouth; used to close the coronal opening in a tooth during endodontic treatment. See also *sealant.* **border s.,** the contact of the denture border with the underlying or adjacent tissues to prevent the passage of air or other substances. **double s.,** a seal con-

sisting of gutta-percha underneath another material (e.g., temporary cement); used to close the coronal opening in a tooth during endodontic treatment. **posterior palatal s.,** the seal at the posterior border of a denture produced by displacing some of the soft tissue covering the palate by extra pressure developed in the impression or by scraping a depression in the cast. **velopharyngeal s.,** closure between the oral and nasopharyngeal cavities, accomplished by the action of the muscles of the soft palate and the superior constrictor muscle.

sealant (se′lant) an agent that protects against access from the outside or leakage from the inside; sealer. **dental s.,** a sealant resin capable of mechanically bonding to the surface of a tooth and offering protection against outside chemical or physical agents. Called also *dental adhesive.* **fissure s.,** see *pit and fissure s.* **pit and fissure s.,** a dental sealant used to occlude noncarious pits and fissures, thereby preventing caries-producing microorganisms and debris from entering.

sealer (se′ler) an agent that protects against access from the outside or leakage from the inside; sealant. **endodontic s.,** root canal s. **root canal s.,** a substance used for cementing silver and gutta-percha cones to the tooth structure in root canal therapy. Called also *endodontic s.* and *root canal cement.*

seam (sēm) a line of union. **pigment s.,** the portion of the pigmented epithelium of the iris which bends forward around the pupillary border.

searcher (surch′er) a sound used in searching for calculi in the bladder.

seat (sēt) a part on which the base of something rests or sits. **basal s.,** oral tissues which support a complete or partial denture. **rest s.,** see under *area.*

seatworm (sēt′werm) any oxyurid, especially *Enterobius vermicularis.*

seaweed (se′wēd) a plant growing in the sea, especially one of the algae.

sebaceous (sĕ-ba′shus) [L. *sebaceus*] 1. pertaining to sebum. 2. secreting a greasy lubricating substance, sebum. See under *gland.*

sebiferous (sĕ-bif′er-us) [L. *sebiferus,* from *sebum* suet + *ferre* to bear] sebiparous.

Sebileau's bands, hollow (seb″ĭ-lōz′) [Pierre Sebileau, French surgeon, 1860–1953] see under *band* and *hollow.*

sebiparous (sĕ-bip′ah-rus) [L. *sebiparus; sebum* suet + *parere* to produce] producing a fatty secretion.

sebolith (seb′o-lith) [*sebum* + Gr. *lithos* stone] a concretion formed in a sebaceous gland.

seborrhea (seb″o-re′ah) [L. *sebum* suet + Gr. *rhoia* flow] 1. excessive secretion of sebum; called also *hypersteatosis.* 2. seborrheic dermatitis. **s. adipo′sa,** that in which the secretion is oily, especially occurring about the nose and forehead; called also *s. oleo′sa.* **s. oleo′sa,** seborrhea adiposa. **s. sic′ca,** dry, scaly seborrheic dermatitis.

seborrheal (seb″o-re′al) characterized by or pertaining to seborrhea.

seborrheic (seb″o-re′ik) 1. affected with or of the nature of seborrhea. 2. pertaining to those areas of the body in which sebaceous glands are abundant; i.e., the scalp, face, chest, back, axilla, and groin.

seborrhiasis (seb″o-ri′ah-sis) inverse psoriasis.

sebotropic (seb″o-trop′ik) having an affinity for or a stimulating effect on sebaceous glands; promoting the excretion of sebum.

sebum (se′bum) [L.] 1. suet. 2. the secretion of the sebaceous glands; a thick, semifluid substance composed of fat and epithelial debris from the cells of the malpighian layer. **cutaneous s., s. cuta′neum,** the fatty secretion of the sebaceous glands. **s. palpebra′le,** the secretion of the tarsal glands; called also *lema.*

Secale (se-ka′le) [L. "rye"] a genus of graminaceous plants, including *S. cereále* L. (Gramineae), the common rye.

secale cornutum (se-ka′le kor-nu′tum) the name under which ergot was adopted in the first edition of the U.S.P.

secalin (sek′ah-lin) one of the active principles of ergot; said to be identical with trimethylamine, $N(CH_3)_3$.

secalintoxin (sek″ah-lin-tok′sin) a principle obtainable from ergot.

secalose (sek′ah-lōs) a carbohydrate obtainable from rye; when dried, it forms a white, hygroscopic powder, convertible by inversion into levulose.

Sechenoff's center (setsh′en-ofs) see *Setschenow.*

seclazone (sek′lah-zōn) chemical name: 7-chloro-3,3a-dihydro-2*H*,9*H*-isorazolo[3,2-*b*][1,3]benzoxazin-9-one; an anti-inflammatory with uricosuric properties, $C_{10}H_8ClNO_3$.

secobarbital (se″ko-bar′bĭ-tal) [USP] chemical name: 5-(1-methylbutyl)-5-(2-propenyl)-2,4,6(1*H*,3*H*,5*H*)pyrimidinetrione. A short-acting barbiturate, $C_{12}H_{18}N_2O_3$, occurring as a white, amorphous or crystalline powder; used as a hypnotic and sedative, administered orally. Called also *quinalbarbitone.* **s. sodium** [USP], the monosodium salt of secobarbital, $C_{12}H_{17}N_2NaO_3$, occurring as a white powder, having the actions and uses of the base; administered orally, intravenously, and intramuscularly.

secodont (se′ko-dont) [L. *secare* to cut + Gr. *odous* tooth] having teeth in which the tubercles of the molars are provided with cutting edges, as in many carnivorous mammals.

Seconal (sek′ŏ-nol) trademark for preparations of secobarbital.

second (sek′und) the unit of time equal to $\frac{1}{60}$ of a minute. **milliampere s's,** in radiographic exposure technique, the product of the milliamperes and the time in seconds.

secondary (sek′un-der″e) [L. *secundarius; secundus* second] second or inferior in order of time, place, or importance; derived from or consequent to a primary event or thing.

second intention (sek′und in-ten′shun) see under *healing.*

secreta (se-kre′tah) [L. pl.] secretion products.

secretagogue (se-krēt′ah-gog) [*secretion* + Gr. *agōgos* drawing] 1. stimulating secretion. 2. an agent that stimulates secretion.

secrete (se-krēt′) [L. *secernere, secretum* to separate] to separate or elaborate cell products.

secretin (se-kre′tin) a strongly basic polypeptide hormone secreted by the mucosa of the duodenum and upper jejunum when acid chyme enters the intestine. It stimulates the pancreatic acinar cells to release bicarbonate and water, which are excreted into the duodenum and change pH from acid to alkaline, thereby facilitating the action of digestive enzymes. It has a lesser stimulatory effect on bile and intestinal secretion. Secretin is used as a diagnostic test for gastrinoma and as a test of pancreatic acinar function. **gastric s.,** former term for gastrin.

secretion (se-kre′shun) [L. *secretio,* from *secernere* to secrete] 1. the process of elaborating a specific product as a result of the activity of a gland; this activity may range from separating a specific substance of the blood to the elaboration of a new chemical substance. 2. any substance produced by secretion. **antilytic s.,** saliva secreted by the submaxillary gland with nerves intact, as distinguished from that secreted when the nerve is divided. **external s.,** one that is discharged upon an external or internal surface of the body; the glands of external secretion are the exocrine glands (q.v.). Cf. *internal s.* **internal s.,** any of the specific substances (hormones) that are not discharged by a duct from the body, but are given off into the blood and lymph, and effect a response distant from the site of origin. Such substances are secreted by the organs and structures of the endocrine system (q.v.). Cf. *external s.* **paralytic s.,** secretion from a gland after paralysis or division of its nerve.

secretogogue (se-kre′to-gog) secretagogue.

secretoinhibitory (se-kre″to-in-hib′ĭ-to″re) inhibiting secretion; antisecretory.

secretomotor (se-kre″to-mo′tor) exciting or stimulating secretion; said of nerves.

secretomotory (se-kre″to-mo′tor-e) secretomotor.

secretor (se-kre′tor) in genetics, an individual who secretes the ABH antigens of the ABO blood group in the saliva and other body fluids. Also, the autosomal dominant gene that determines this trait.

secretory (se-kre′to-re) pertaining to secretion or affecting the secretions.

sectile (sek′tīl) [L. *sectilis,* from *secare* to cut] 1. susceptible of being cut. 2. one of several parts into which a whole is divided.

sectio (sek′she-o) pl. *sectio′nes* [L., from *secare* to cut] 1. an act of cutting. 2. a section; [NA] a general term for a segment or subdivision of an organ. **sectio′nes cerebel′li** [NA], the various internal anatomical subdivisions of the cerebellum. **sectio′nes corpo′rum quadrigemino′rum,** the anatomical divisions of the corpora quadrigemina. **sectio′nes hypothal′ami** [NA], the various internal anatomical subdivisions of the hypothalamus. **sectio′nes isth′mi,** see *sectiones mesencephali.* **sectio′nes medul′lae oblonga′tae** [NA], the various internal anatomical subdivisions of the medulla oblongata. **sectio′nes medul′lae spina′lis** [NA], the various internal anatomical subdivisions of the spinal cord. **sectio′nes mesencephal′icae, sectio′nes mesence′phali** [NA], the various internal anatomical subdivisions of the mesencephalon. **sectio′nes pedun′culi cer′ebri,** sectiones mesencephali. **sectio′nes pon′tis** [NA], the various internal anatomical subdivisions of the pons. **sectio′nes telence′phali** [NA], the various internal anatomical subdivisions of the telencephalon. **sectio′nes thalamence′phali,** the various internal anatomical subdivisions of the thalamencephalon. **sectio′nes thal′ami et metathal′ami** [NA], the various internal anatomical subdivisions of the thalamus and metathalamus.

section (sek′shun) [L. *sectio*] 1. an act of cutting. 2. a cut surface. 3. a segment or subdivision of an organ; called also *sectio* [NA]. **abdominal s.,** laparotomy. **celloidin s.,** a section cut by a microtome from tissue that has been embedded in celloidin. **cesarean s.,** incision through the abdominal and uterine walls for delivery of a fetus. **cesarean s., cervical,** cesarean s., lower segment. **cesarean s., classic, cesarean s., corporeal,** cesarean section in which the upper segment, or corpus, of the uterus is incised. **cesarean s., extraperitoneal,** cesarean section performed without incision of the peritoneum, the peritoneal fold being displaced upward and the bladder being displaced downward or to the midline, the uterus then being opened by an incision in its lower segment. **cesarean s., Latzko's,** extraperitoneal cesarean section with the uterine incision made through one side of the lower segment of the uterus. **cesarean s., lower segment,** cesarean section in which the lower uterine segment is incised, either transperitoneally or extraperitoneally. **cesarean s., Munro Kerr,** cesarean section in which the lower uterine segment is opened transversely through the uterovesical fold, without displacement of the bladder. **cesarean s., Porro,** cesarean section with extirpation of the uterine corpus and ovaries; of historical interest. **cesarean s., transperitoneal,** cesarean section performed with an incision through the uterovesical fold of peritoneum. **coronal s., frontal s.,** a longitudinal section parallel with the long axis of the body and at right angles to a sagittal section; it divides the body into a dorsal and ventral part. Called also *coronal s.* **frozen s.,** a section cut by a microtome from tissue that has been frozen. **paraffin s.,** a section cut by a microtome from tissue which has been embedded in paraffin. **perineal s.,** external urethrotomy. **Pitres' s's,** a series of six coronal sections through the brain: a *prefrontal* section, through the prefrontal part of the frontal lobe; two *frontal* sections, the first being 2 cm. in front of the central sulcus (*pediculofrontal s.*), and the second being through the precentral gyrus; two *parietal* sections, one through the postcentral gyrus, and the other (*pediculoparietal s.*) 3 cm. behind the central sulcus; and an *occipital* section, through the middle of the occipital lobe. **Saemisch's s.,** Saemisch's operation. **sagittal s.,** a longitudinal section that follows the sagittal suture and runs the entire length of the body, thus dividing the latter into more or less equal right and left halves, or a section parallel to it. **serial s.,** histologic section made in a consecutive order and so arranged for the purpose of microscopical examination. **transverse s.,** one made at right angles to the long axis of a body or structure.

sectiones (sek″she-o′nēz) [L.] plural of *sectio.*

sector (sek′tor) [L. "cutter"] 1. the area of a circle included between an arc and the radii bounding it. 2. an area, zone, or part of something. 3. to divide into sectors.

sectorial (sek-to′re-al) [L. *sector* cutter] 1. pertaining or relating to a sector. 2. in genetics, pertaining to the presence of a sector of tissue which carries a somatic mutation and which is therefore different phenotypically from the tissues of the rest of the body; also, an individual having such a sector of tissue (a mosaic). 3. cutting or adapted for cutting, as the molar teeth of carnivores.

secundigravida (se-kun″dĭ-grav′ĭ-dah) [L. *secundus* second + *gravida* pregnant] a woman pregnant for the second time; written gravida II.

secundina (se″kun-di′nah), pl. *secundi′nae* [L., from *secundus* following] that which follows; see *secundines*. **s. u′teri,** the chorion.

secundinae (se″kun-di′ne) [L.] plural of *secundina*; secundines.

secundines (se-kun′dinz, se-kun-denz) [L. *secundinae*] the placenta and membranes expelled after childbirth; the afterbirth.

secundipara (se″kun-dip′ah-rah) [L. *secundus* second + *parere* to bring forth, produce] a woman who has had two pregnancies which resulted in viable offspring; written para II or II-para.

secundiparity (se-kun″dĭ-par′ĭ-te) the condition of being a secundipara.

secundiparous (se″kun-dip′ah-rus) having borne viable offspring in two separate pregnancies.

secundum artem (se-kun′dum ar′tem) [L. "according to the art"] in an approved or professional manner.

securinine (se-ku′rĭ-nen) an alkaloid, $C_{13}H_{15}NO_2$, obtained from the leaves and roots of *Securinega suffruticosa* Rehder (Euphorbiaceae); its nitrate salt is used in neurasthenic states and cardiac insufficiency, and in the treatment of impotence.

S.E.D. skin erythema dose.

sedation (se-da′shun) [L. *sedatio*] the production of a sedative effect; the act or process of calming.

sedative (sed′ah-tiv) [L. *sedativus*] 1. allaying activity and excitement. 2. an agent that allays excitement. **Battley's s.,** a solution made up of extract of opium, boiling water, alcohol, and cold water. **cardiac s.,** one that abates the force of the heart's action. **cerebral s.,** one which principally affects the brain. **gastric s.,** one which soothes or lessens irritability of the stomach. **general s.,** one which affects all the organs and functions. **intestinal s.,** one which diminishes intestinal irritation; in general, they are also gastric sedatives. **nerve trunk s.,** one which acts upon the trunks of the nerves. **nervous s.,** a sedative which acts upon and through the nervous system; the cerebral, spinal, and nerve trunk sedatives belong to this class. **respiratory s.,** one which affects especially the respiratory centers and organs. **spinal s.,** any drug which abates the functional or abnormal activity of the spinal cord. **vascular s.,** one which affects the vasomotor activities.

sedentary (sed′en-ter″e) [L. *sedentarius*] 1. sitting habitually; of inactive habits. 2. pertaining to a sitting posture.

Sédillot's operation (sa-de-yoz′) [Charles Emmanuel *Sédillot*, French surgeon, 1804–1883] see under *operation*.

sediment (sed′ĭ-ment) [L. *sedimentum*] a precipitate, especially one that is formed spontaneously. **urinary s.,** the deposit of solid matter left after the urine has been allowed to stand for some time.

sedimentable (sed″ĭ-ment′ah-b'l) in microbiology, capable of forming sediment.

sedimentation (sed″ĭ-men-ta′shun) the act of causing the deposit of sediment, especially by the use of a centrifugal machine. **erythrocyte s.,** the sinking of red cells in a volume of drawn blood; see *erythrocyte sedimentation rate*, under *rate*. **formalin-ether s. (Ritchie),** a technique for detecting parasites in the feces, involving the centrifugation of diluted feces, the addition of formalin and ether to the sample, recentrifugation, and examining the final sediment as a wet mount.

sedimentator (sed″ĭ-men-ta′tor) a centrifugal machine for separating sediments from the urine.

sedopeptose (se″do-pep′tos) a monosaccharide occurring in herbs of the genus *Sedum*.

seed (sed) 1. the mature ovule of a flowering plant. 2. semen. 3. a small cylindrical shell of gold or other suitable material, used in application of radiation therapy. 4. to inoculate a culture medium with microorganisms. **cardamom s.** [NF], the dried ripe seed of *Elettaria cardamomum*, a perennial herb of the ginger family of tropical Asia; used as a flavoring agent. **celery s.,** see *Apium*. **larkspur s.,**

see *Delphinium*. **plantago s.** [USP], **psyllium s.,** the cleaned dried, ripe seed of *Plantago psyllium, P. indica,* or *P. ovata,* used as a fecal softener. The mucilaginous portion of the seeds of *P. ovata* is used in preparing psyllium hydrophilic mucilloid. **radiogold** (^{198}Au) **s.,** a solid piece of radioactive gold wire about 2.5 mm. long and 0.8 mm. thick, used as a permanent interstitial radioactive implant in the treatment of cancer. **radon s.,** a small sealed container or tube for carrying radon, made of gold or glass, for insertion into tissues for the treatment of certain malignant diseases; it is visible roentgenographically.

Seeligmüller's sign (za′lik-mil″erz) [Otto Ludovicus G. A. *Seeligmüller,* German neurologist, 1837–1912] see under *sign*.

Seessel's pouch (pocket) (za′selz) [Albert *Seessel,* American embryologist and neurologist, 1850–1910] see under *pouch*.

Séglas type (sa-glahz′) [Jules Ernest *Séglas,* French psychiatrist, 1856–1939] see under *type*.

segment (seg′ment) [L. *segmentum* a piece cut off] a portion of a larger body or structure, set off by natural or arbitrarily established boundaries. **arterial s. of glomeriform arteriovenous anastomosis,** segmentum arteriale anastomosis arteriovenae glomeriformis. **bronchopulmonary s.,** one of the smaller subdivisions of the lobes of the lungs; see *segmenta bronchopulmonalia*. **cranial s's,** three segments into which the bones of the cranium may be divided; they are distinguished as the occipital, the parietal, and the frontal. **frontal s.,** the anterior of the three cranial segments. **hepatic s's,** segmenta hepatis. **interannular s.,** the portion of a nerve fiber between two consecutive nodes of Ranvier. **s's of kidney,** segmenta renalia. **medullary s.,** a division of the medullary sheath of a nerve fiber between two incisures of Lanterman. Called also *Schmidt-Lanterman s.* **mesoblastic s., mesodermal s.,** a somite. **neural s.,** neuromere (def. 2). **occipital s.,** the posterior of the three cranial segments. **parietal s.,** the central of the three cranial segments. **primitive s., protovertebral s.,** somite. **pubic s. of the pelvis,** that portion of the floor of the pelvis which is between the symphysis pubis and the anterior wall of the vagina, which latter it includes. **Ranvier's s's,** the portions of the medullary substance of a nerve fiber between the nodes of Ranvier. **renal s's,** segmenta renalia. **rivinian s., s. of Rivinus,** an irregular notch at the upper border of the tympanic sulcus; called also *incisura tympanica* [*Rivini*]. **sacral s.,** that portion of the floor of the pelvis which lies between the sacrum and the posterior vaginal wall. **Schmidt-Lanterman s.,** medullary s. **spinal s.,** segmenta medullae spinalis. **s's of spinal cord,** segmenta medullae spinalis. **uterine s.,** either of the portions into which the uterus becomes differentiated early in labor: the upper contractile portion (corpus uteri) becomes thicker as labor advances, and the lower noncontractile portion is thin-walled and passive in character. **venous s. of glomeriform arteriovenous anastomosis,** segmentum venosum anastomosis arteriovenae glomeriformis.

segmenta (seg-men′tah) [L.] plural of *segmentum*.

segmental (seg-men′tal) pertaining to or forming a segment or a product of division, especially into serially arranged or nearly equal parts; undergoing segmentation.

segmentation (seg″men-ta′shun) 1. division into parts more or less similar, such as somites or metameres. 2. cleavage. **haustral s.,** the formation of pouches in the wall of the large intestine, by alternating contraction and relaxation of circular muscle fibers. It keeps the intestinal contents plastic and assists in propelling them toward the rectum.

segmenter (seg′men-ter) a late meront or schizont; applied to that stage during schizogony when the cytoplasm segments into daughter cells.

Segmentina (seg″men-ti′nah) a genus of fresh-water snails of the Orient; *S. hemisphaerula, S. trochoideus,* and *S. largillierti* are first intermediate hosts of the intestinal fluke *Fasciolopsis buski*.

segmentum (seg-men′tum), pl. *segmen′ta* [L.] a portion of a larger body or structure; [NA] a general term for a part of an organ or other structure set off by natural or arbitrarily established boundaries. **s. arteria′le anastomo′sis arteriove′nae glomerifor′mis** [NA], the arterial segment of the anastomosis arteriovenosa glomeriformis, which has a narrow lumen and a thick wall consisting of three to six layers of contractile glomus cells (*pulvinar tunicae internae*). Called also *Sucquet-Hoyer anastomosis* or *canal*. **seg-men'ta bronchopulmona'lia** [NA], bronchopulmonary segments: the smaller subdivisions of the lobes of the lungs, separated by connective tissue septa and supplied by branches of the respective lobar bronchi; called also *lobuli pulmonum*. Roman numerals are used to designate the bronchopulmonary segments. The *lobus superior pulmonis dextri* has three segments: *s. apicale* (s. I) *s. posterius* (s. II), and *s. anterius* (s. III); the *lobus medius pulmonis dextri* has two segments: *s. laterale* (s. IV) and *s. mediale* (s. V); the *lobus inferior pulmonis dextri* has five segments: *s. apicale* (s. VI) [alternative *s. superius*], *s. basale mediale* (s. VII) [alternative *s. cardiacum*], *s. basale anterius* (s. VIII), *s. basale laterale* (s. IX), and *s. basale posterius* (s. X); the *lobus superior pulmonis sinistri* has four segments: *s. apicoposterius* (s. I + II), *s. anterius* (s. III), *s. lingulare superius* (s. IV), and *s. lingulare inferius* (s. V); the *lobus inferior pulmonis sinistri* has five segments: *s. apicale* (s. VI) [alternative *s. superius*], *s. basale mediale* (s. VIII) [alternative *s. cardiacum*], *s. basale anterius* (s. VIII), *s. basale laterale* (s. IX), and *s. basale posterius* (s. X). See also *bronchi segmentales*. See the Plate of Pulmonary Segments. **segmen'ta hep'atis** [NA], hepatic segments: subdivisions of the hepatic lobes based on arterial and biliary supply and venous drainage; they are the *segmentum anterius* and *s. posterius* of the right lobe, and the *s. mediale* and *s. laterale* of the left lobe. **segmen'ta medul'lae spina'lis** [NA], segments of spinal cord: the regions of the spinal cord to each of which is attached a pair of dorsal and a pair of ventral roots of the spinal nerves. The spinal cord gives rise to thirty-three pairs of spinal nerves: eight cervical (**cervica'lia [1–8]**—see *pars cervicalis medullae spinalis*), twelve thoracic (**thora'cica [1–12]**—see *pars thoracica medullae spinalis*), five lumbar (**lumba'lia [1–5]**—see *pars lumbalis medullae spinalis*), five sacral (**sacra'lia [1–5]**—see *pars sacralis medullae spinalis*), and three coccygeal (**coccyg'ea [1–3]**—see *pars coccygea medullae spinalis*). **segmen'ta rena'lia** [NA], renal segments: subdivisions of the kidney that have independent blood supply from branches of the renal artery; they are: *segmentum superius, s. anterius superius, s. anterius inferius, s. inferius*, and *s. posterius*. **s. veno'sum anastomo'sis arteriove'nae glomerifor'mis** [NA], the thin-walled venous segment of the anastomosis arteriovenosa glomeriformis, which has a wide lumen that drains into a subpapillary vein.

segregation (seg"re-ga'shun) [L. *segregatio* separation] 1. in genetics the separation of allelic genes during meiosis as homologous chromosomes begin to migrate toward the poles of the cell, so that eventually the members of each pair of allelic genes go to separate gametes. 2. the separation of different elements of a population. 3. the progressive restriction of potencies in the zygote to the various regions of the forming embryo.

segregator (seg're-ga"tor) an instrument for securing the urine from each kidney separately.

Séguin's signal symptom (sign) (sa-ganz') [Edouard *Séguin*, French alienist, 1812–1880] see under *symptom*.

Sehrt's clamp (compressor) (sārts) [Ernst *Sehrt*, German surgeon, born 1879] see under *clamp*.

Seidel's scotoma (sign) (si'delz) [Erich *Seidel*, German ophthalmologist, 1882–1948] see under *scotoma*.

Seidelin bodies (si'dĕ-lin) [Harold *Seidelin*, British physician] see under *body*.

Seidlitz powder, powder test (sīd'litz) [named from a mineral spring in Bohemia] see under *powder* and *tests*.

Seignette's salt (sīn-yets') [Pierre *Seignette*, apothecary in Rochelle, 1660–1719] potassium sodium tartrate.

seisesthesia (sīs"es-the'ze-ah) seismesthesia.

seismesthesia (sīs"mes-the'ze-ah) [Gr. *seismos* a shaking + *aisthēsis* perception + *-ia*] tactile perception of vibrations in a liquid or aerial medium.

seismocardiogram (sīz"mo-kar'de-o-gram") the graphic record obtained by seismocardiography.

seismocardiography (sīz"mo-kar"de-og'rah-fe) [Gr. *seismos* a shaking, shock + *kardia* heart + *graphē* representation by means of lines] the selective recording of cardiac vibrations.

seismotherapy (sīz"mo-ther'ah-pe) [Gr. *seismos* a shaking + *therapy*] the treatment of disease by mechanical vibration.

seizure (se'zhur) 1. the sudden attack or recurrence of a disease. 2. an attack of epilepsy. See also *ictus*. **absence s.**, an epileptic seizure marked by a momentary break in the stream of thought and activity, accompanied by a symmetrical 3-c.p.s. spike and wave activity on the electroencephalogram; called also *petit mal epilepsy*. **audiogenic s.**, an epileptic seizure brought on by sound. **cerebral s.**, an attack of epilepsy. **febrile s.**, convulsions associated with high fever, occurring in infants and children. **jackknife s.**, a severe myoclonus appearing in the first 18 months of life and associated with general cerebral deterioration; it is marked by severe flexion spasms of the head, neck, and trunk and extension of the arms and legs. Called also *infantile massive spasms*. **photogenic s.**, an epileptic seizure brought on by light. **psychomotor s.**, psychomotor epilepsy. **uncinate s.**, see under *epilepsy*.

sejunction (se-junk'shun) an interruption of the continuity of association complexes which leads to a breaking up of the personality.

sekisanine (sek-is'ah-nin) an alkaloid, $C_{16}H_{19}O_4N$, from *Lycoris radiata* Herb. (Amaryllidaceae).

selachian (sĕ-la'ke-an) one of a class of vertebrates which includes the sharks and rays.

Selacryn (sel'ah-krin) trademark for a preparation of ticrynafen (withdrawn).

selection (sĕ-lek'shun) [L. *selectio* choice] the play of forces that determines the relative reproductive performance of the various genotypes in a population. **artificial s.**, the interference by man in the selection of the genotypes to produce succeeding generations of a given organism. **directional s.**, selection favoring individuals at one extreme of the distribution. **disruptive s., diversifying s.**, selection favoring the two extremes rather than the intermediate. **natural s.**, the survival in nature of those individuals and their progeny best equipped to adapt to environmental conditions. **progeny s.**, a breeding program in which the genotype is determined by making test matings and observing the offspring. **sexual s.**, natural selection in which certain characteristics attract male or female members of a species, thus ensuring survival of those characteristics. **stabilizing s.**, selection favoring intermediate phenotypes rather than those at one or both extremes. **truncate s.**, in medical genetics, the selection of families for a genetic study in such a way that one or more kinds of sibships are not ascertained, usually those sibships in which no member is affected with the trait under study. See also *ascertainment* and *truncate ascertainment*.

selective (sĕ-lek'tiv) having a high degree of selectivity.

selectivity (sĕ-lek-tiv'ĭ-te) in pharmacology, the degree to which a dose of a drug produces the desired effect in relation to adverse effects.

selene (sĕ-le'ne) [L.; Gr. *selēnē* moon] a moon-shaped object or structure. **s. un'guium** ["moon of the nails"], lunula unguis.

selenide (sel'ĕ-nīd) a compound of selenium with another element or radical.

Selenidium (sel"ĕ-nid'ĭ-um) [Gr. *selēnē* moon, crescent-shaped] a genus of parasitic gregarine protozoa (suborder Aseptina, order Eugregarinida) found in the gut of annelids.

selenium (sĕ-le'ne-um) [Gr. *selēnē* moon] a nonmetallic element resembling sulfur; symbol, Se; atomic number, 34; atomic weight, 78.96. It is an essential mineral, being a constituent of the enzyme glutathione peroxidase, and believed to be closely associated with vitamin E in its functions, but it occurs in toxic levels in several kinds of plants growing in soil with high levels, causing disease in grazing animals (see *selenium poisoning*, under *poisoning*). Dietary deficiency, occurring where the soil has a low sodium content, results in cardiomyopathy (see *Kashan disease*, under *disease*). **s. sulfide** [USP], the sulfide salt of selenium, SeS_2, occurring as a reddish brown to bright orange powder; used as a topical antifungal in the treatment of tinea versicolor, as a topical keratolytic, and applied topically to the scalp to control seborrheic dermatitis and dandruff.

selenodont (sĕ-le'no-dont) [Gr. *selēnē* moon + *odous* tooth] having posterior teeth on which the individual cusps assume a crescentic outline, as in many herbivorous mammals.

selenomethionine (sel"en-o-mĕ-thi'o-nēn) methionine in

which selenium replaces the sulfur atom; the radioactive form (^{75}Se) is used in tests of tissue uptake of methionine.

Selenomonas (se″le-no-mo′nas) [Gr. *selēnē* moon + *monas* unit, from *monos* single] a genus of gram-negative, anaerobic bacteria of the family Bacteroidaceae, found in the gastrointestinal tract of mammals and in contaminated river water, made up of motile, kidney- to crescent-shaped cells occurring singly and in chains. It includes the species *S. sputigena*, found in the human oral cavity, and *S. ruminantium*, found in the rumen contents of animals.

selenosis (se″le-no′sis) selenium poisoning; see under *poisoning*.

self (self) pertaining to an individual's own tissue constituents (self antigens or autoantigens). Normal animals exhibit self tolerance, lack of immune response to autoantigens, acquired during fetal life by a process of "self recognition."

self-antigen (self′an″tĭ-gen) autoantigen.

self-differentiation (self″dif-er-en″she-a′shun) perseverance in a course of development by a part independently of outside influences or changed surroundings.

self-digestion (self″di-jes′chun) autodigestion; autolysis (def. 1).

self-fermentation (self″fer-men-ta′shun) autolysis; (def. 1); autodigestion.

self-fertilization (self″fer-tĭ-lĭ-za′shun) the fusion of male and female gametes from the same individual.

self-hypnosis (self″hip-no′sis) the act or process of hypnotizing oneself.

self-inductance (self″in-duk′tans) the property of an electric circuit which determines, for a given rate of change of current in the circuit, the electromotive force induced in the circuit itself.

self-infection (self″in-fek′shun) autoinfection.

selfing (self′ing) continuous cross-fertilization between different proglottids of the same tapeworm.

self-limited (self-lim′it-ed) limited by its own peculiarities, and not by outside influence; said of a disease that runs a definite limited course.

self-suspension (self″sus-pen′shun) the suspension of the body by the head and axillae (*axillocephalic s.*) or by the head (*cephalic s.*) for the purpose of stretching the vertebral column.

self-tolerance (self-tol′er-ans) see under *tolerance*.

selfwise (self′wīz) developing in a previously determined manner despite transplantation to a new and strange location; said of embryonic cells or tissue. Cf. *neighborwise*.

Seliberia (se″lĭ-be′re-ah) [G.L. *Seliber*, Russian microbiologist] a genus of budding bacteria found in soil, made up of rod-shaped twisted cells attached in star or rosette formations. The type species is *S. stella′ta*.

Selivanoff's (Seliwanow's) test (reaction) [Feodor Fedorowich *Selivanoff*, Russian chemist, born 1859] see under *tests*.

sella (sel′ah), gen. and pl. *sel′lae* [L.] a saddle-shaped depression. **s. tur′cica** [NA], a transverse depression crossing the midline on the superior surface of the body of the sphenoid bone, and containing the hypophysis.

sellae (sel′e) [L.] genitive and plural of *sella*.

sellanders (sel′an-derz) malanders.

sellar (sel′ar) pertaining to the sella turcica.

Sellick maneuver (sel′ik) [Brian A. *Sellick*, British anesthetist, of the 20th century] see under *maneuver*.

Selsun (sel′sun) trademark for a preparation of selenium sulfide. **S. Blue,** trademark for a preparation of selenium sulfide.

Selter's disease (sel′terz) [Paul *Selter*, German pediatrician, 1866–1941] acrodynia.

Selye syndrome (sel′yeh) [Hans *Selye*, Canadian biochemist, born 1907] see under *syndrome*.

semantic (se-man′tik) pertaining to or affecting the meanings or significance of words.

semantics (se-man′tiks) [Gr. *sēmantikos* significant, from *sēma* a sign] the study of the meanings of words and the rules of their use; the study of the relationship between language and significance.

semasiology (se-ma″se-ol′o-je) semantics.

semeiography (se″mi-og′rah-fe) [Gr. *sēmeion* sign + gra-

phein to write] a description of the signs or symptoms of disease.

semeiology (se″mi-ol′o-je) [Gr. *sēmeion* sign + -*logy*] symptomatology.

semeiotic (se″mi-ot′ik) [Gr. *semeiōtikos*] 1. pertaining to the signs or symptoms of disease. 2. pathognomonic.

semeiotics (se″mi-ot′iks) symptomatology.

semelincident (sem″el-in′sĭ-dent) [L. *semel* once + *incidens* falling upon] attacking only once, as an infectious disease which induces immunity thereafter.

semel in d. abbreviation for L. *sem′el in di′e*, once a day; written also *s.i.d.*

semelparity (sem″el-par′ĭ-te) [L. *semel* once + *parere* to bear] the state, in an individual organism, of reproducing only once in a lifetime.

semelparous (sem-el′pah-rus) pertaining to or characterized by semelparity.

semen (se′men), gen. *sem′inis* [L. "seed"] 1. any seed or seedlike fruit. 2. the thick, whitish secretion of the reproductive organs in the male; composed of spermatozoa in their nutrient plasma, secretions from the prostate, seminal vesicles, and various other glands, epithelial cells, and minor constituents. **s. con′tra,** santonica.

semenologist (se″mĕ-nol′o-jist) seminologist.

semenology (se″mĕ-nol′o-je) seminology.

semenuria (se″mĕ-nu′re-ah) seminuria.

semi- [L. *semis* half] a prefix signifying one half, or partly.

semiapochromat (sem″e-ap″o-kro′mat) [*semi-* + *apo-* + *chromatic* aberration] semiapochromatic objective.

semiapochromatic (sem″e-ap″o-kro-mat′ik) see under *objective*.

semicanal (sem″e-kah-nal′) a channel which is open on one side; called also *semicanalis*. **s. of auditory tube,** semicanalis tubae auditivae. **s. of humerus,** sulcus intertubercularis humeri. **s. of tensor tympani muscle,** semicanalis musculi tensoris tympani.

semicanales (sem″e-kah-na′lēz) [L.] plural of *semicanalis*.

semicanalis (sem″e-kah-na′lis), pl. *semicana′les* [L.] semicanal: a channel which is open on one side. **s. mus′culi tenso′ris tym′pani** [NA], semicanal of tensor tympani muscle: a small canal hidden in the temporal bone, constituting the superior part of the musculotubal canal, and lodging the tensor tympani muscle. **s. tu′bae auditi′vae** [NA], semicanal of auditory tube: a small canal in the temporal bone, opening on the inferior surface of the skull just posterior and superior to the foramen spinosum. It constitutes the inferior part of the musculotubal canal and lodges the auditory tube.

semicartilaginous (sem″e-kar″tĭ-laj′ĭ-nus) partially cartilaginous.

semicoma (sem″e-ko′mah) a stupor from which the patient may be aroused.

semicomatose (sem″e-ko′mah-tōs) in a condition of semicoma.

semicrista (sem″e-kris′tah), pl. *semicris′tae* [L.] a small or rudimentary crest. **s. incisi′va,** crista nasalis maxilla.

semidecussation (sem″e-de″kus-sa′shun) 1. an incomplete crossing of nerve fibers. 2. decussatio pyramidum.

semidiagrammatic (sem″e-di″ah-grah-mat″ik) partly diagrammatic; modified so as to illustrate a principle, rather than to serve as an exact copy of nature.

semiflexion (sem″e-flek′shun) 1. the position of a limb midway between flexion and extension. 2. the act of bringing to such a position.

semifluctuating (sem″e-fluk′chu-āt″ing) giving a somewhat fluctuating sensation on palpation.

semiglutin (sem″e-gloo′tin) a substance, $C_{55}H_{85}N_{17}O_{22}$, derived from gelatin and resembling a peptone.

Semih. abbreviation for L. *semiho′ra*, half an hour.

Semikon (sem′ĭ-kon) trademark for preparations of methapyrilene.

semilunar (sem″e-lu′nar) [L. *semilunaris*; *semi-* half + *luna* moon] resembling a crescent, or half-moon.

semilunare (sem″e-lu-na′re) [L.] the second bone of the first row of carpal bones, counting from the thumb side (os lunatum [NA]).

semiluxation (sem″e-luk-sa′shun) subluxation.

semimembranous (sem″e-mem′brah-nus) made up in part of membrane or fascia.

seminal (sem′ĭ-nal) [L. *seminalis*] pertaining to seed or to the semen.

seminarcosis (sem″e-nar-ko′sis) twilight sleep.

semination (sem″ĭ-na′shun) [L. *seminatio*] insemination.

seminiferous (se″mĭ-nif′er-us) [L. *semen* seed + *ferre* to bear] producing or conveying semen.

seminologist (se″mĭ-nol′o-jist) a specialist in the study of semen and spermatozoa.

seminology (se″mĭ-nol′o-je) the scientific study of the semen, in relation to the possible causes of infertility in the male.

seminoma (se″mĭ-no′mah) [*semen* + *-oma*] a radiosensitive, malignant neoplasm of the testis, thought to be derived from primordial germ cells of the sexually undifferentiated embryonic gonad, and occurring as a gray to yellow-white nodule or mass; three histologic variants are recognized: *classical* (typical), the most common type; *anaplastic;* and *spermatocytic.* The classical tumor is composed of fairly well differentiated sheets or cords of uniform polygonal or round cells (seminoma cells), each cell having abundant clear cytoplasm, distinct cell membranes, a centrally placed round nucleus, and one or more nucleoli. In the female, a grossly and histologically identical neoplasm, known as *dysgerminoma,* occurs. **ovarian s.,** a dysgerminoma of an ovary.

seminormal (sem″e-nor′mal) of one-half the normal or standard strength.

seminose (sem′ĭ-nōs) mannose.

seminuria (se″mĭ-nu′re-ah) [L. *semen* seed + Gr. *ouron* urine + *-ia*] the presence of semen in the urine.

semiography (se″me-og′rah-fe) semeiography.

semiology (se″me-ol′o-je) symptomatology.

semiorbicular (sem″e-or-bik′u-lar) semicircular.

semiotic (se″mi-ot′ik) semeiotic.

semiparasite (sem″e-par′ah-sīt) an organism having potential pathogenicity, occurring both as a saprophyte and as a parasite.

semipenniform (sem″e-pen′ĭ-form) penniform on one side; said of a muscle the fibers of which are attached to one side of the tendon.

semipermeable (sem″e-per′me-ah-b′l) permitting the passage of certain molecules and hindering that of others; see under *membrane.*

semiplacenta (sem″e-plah-sen′tah) Strähl's term for a placenta in certain animals in which the fetal and maternal sections of the organ can be separated without tearing.

semiplegia (sem″e-ple′je-ah) hemiplegia.

semipronation (sem″e-pro-na′shun) 1. the act of bringing to a semiprone position from a position of supination. 2. a semiprone position.

semiprone (sem″e-prōn′) [L. *semis* half + *pronus* prone] partly prone; see *Sims's position,* under *position.*

semiquantitative (sem″ĭ-kwon′tĭ-ta′tiv) denoting a test that is more specific than a qualitative test (a positive or negative result) but less so than a quantitative test (a numerical result), usually referring to a test in which results are scored on an arbitrary scale, e.g., 0 to $+ + + +$.

semiquinone (sem″e-kwin′ōn) a free radical derived from quinones or quinone imines by the addition of a single H atom to a molecule.

semirecumbent (sem″e-re-kum′bent) reclining but not completely recumbent.

semis (se′mis) [L.] half; abbreviated *ss.*

semisideratio (sem″e-sid′er-a′she-o) hemiplegia.

semisomnus (sem″e-som′nus) semicoma.

semisopor (sem″e-so′por) semicoma.

semisulcus (sem″e-sul′kus) [L. *semis* half + *sulcus* furrow] a slight channel on the edge of a bone or other structure, which unites with a similar channel on a corresponding adjoining structure to form a complete sulcus.

semisupination (sem″e-su″pĭ-na′shun) 1. a position of partial or incomplete supination. 2. the act of bringing to such a position.

semisupine (sem″e-su′pīn) partly but not completely supine.

semisynthetic (sem″e-sin-thet′ik) produced by chemical manipulation of naturally occurring substances.

Semitard (sem′ĭ-tard) trademark for preparations of prompt insulin zinc suspension.

semitendinous (sem″e-ten′dĭ-nus) in part having a tendinous structure.

semivalent (sem-iv′ah-lent) (*obs.*) having one-half the power which is normal.

Semmelweis (zem′el-vīs), Ignaz Philipp (1818–1865). A Hungarian physician, who in Vienna (1847–1849) proved that puerperal fever is a form of septicemia, thus becoming the pioneer of antisepsis in obstetrics. Semmelweis's methods were not fully recognized till about 1890 even though the contagiousness of puerperal fever had been affirmed by Oliver Wendell Holmes of Boston in 1843, and important observations had been made even earlier by Alexander Gordon of Aberdeen and Charles White of Manchester.

Semon's law, sign (se′monz) [Sir Felix *Semon,* German laryngologist in London, 1849–1921] see under *law* and *sign.*

Semon-Hering hypothesis, theory (za′mon-ha′ring) [Richard Wolfgang *Semon,* German naturalist, 1859–1918; Ewald *Hering,* German physiologist, 1834–1918] see *mnemic theory,* under *theory.*

Semoxydrine (sem-ok′sĭ-drin) trademark for a preparation of methamphetamine hydrochloride.

Semple's vaccine (sem′p'lz) [Sir David *Semple,* British physician, 1856–1937] see under *vaccine.*

semustine (sĕ-mus′tēn) methyl CCNU; MeCCNU: the methyl analog of lomustine, a cytotoxic alkylating agent of the nitrosourea (q.v.) group, used as an antineoplastic, primarily for treatment of brain tumors, colorectal carcinoma, gastric carcinoma, Hodgkin's disease, and malignant melanoma.

Senear-Usher syndrome (se-nēr′ush′er) [Francis Eugene *Senear,* Chicago dermatologist, 1889–1958; Barney *Usher,* Canadian dermatologist, born 1899] pemphigus erythematosus.

senecifolin (sen″ĕ-sif′o-lin) a poisonous alkaloid, $C_{18}H_{27}$-O_8N, of *Senecio,* found in the vascular bundles of the young plant before flowering.

Senecio (sĕ-ne′she-o) [L. "old man"] a genus of composite-flowered plants. *S. aureus* L. (golden ragwort) and related species were once used as emmenagogues, but are now listed as poisonous to livestock; they contain senecine, senecifoline, and similar alkaloids. **S. jaco′bae** L. (Compositae), a species causing Pictou's disease in horses and cattle in Nova Scotia; also known as *Tansy ragwort.*

senega (sen′e-gah) [L.] the dried root of *Polygala senega* L. (Polygalaceae), seneca or senega snakeroot, a plant of North America, the main constituents of which are polygalic acid and senegenin; expectorant and emetic. It has been used in veterinary medicine as an expectorant.

senegenin (sen″ĕ-jen′in) a bitter saponin, $C_{30}H_{45}ClO_6$, which is an active principle of senega; called also *polygalin.*

senescence (se-nes′ens) [L. *senescere* to grow old] the process or condition of growing old, especially the condition resulting from the transitions and accumulations of the deleterious aging processes. Cf. *aging.* **dental s.,** deterioration of the teeth and other oral structures as a consequence of advancing age or of premature aging processes.

senescent (se-nes′ent) exhibiting senescence.

Sengstaken-Blakemore tube (sengz′ta-ken-blāk′mōre) [Robert William *Sengstaken,* American neurosurgeon, born 1923; Arthur H. *Blakemore,* American surgeon, born 1897] see under *tube.*

senile (se′nīl) [L. *senilis*] pertaining to or characteristic of old age; manifesting senility.

senilism (se′nil-izm) premature old age.

senility (sĕ-nil′ĭ-te) [L. *senilitas*] old age; the physical and mental deterioration associated with old age.

senium (se′ne-um) [L. "the weakness of old age"] old age; the period of life marked by the weaknesses and deterioration that may accompany advanced years.

senna (sen′ah) [USP], the dried leaflets of *Cassia senna* L. (Alexandria senna) or of *C. angustifolia* Vahl. (India or

Tinnevelly senna) (Leguminosae). They contain sennoside A and B, glycosides of rhein, and chrysophanic acid. Used chiefly as a cathartic.

sennoside (sen′o-sid) either of two anthraquinone glucosides, sennoside A and B, found in senna. A mixture of *sennosides A and B* [USP] is used as a cathartic, administered orally.

senograph (se′no-graf) the apparatus used in senography; also, the resultant film.

senography (se-nog′rah-fe) a low voltage, constant-potential x-ray technique designed especially for mammography.

Senokot (sen′ŏh-kot) trademark for preparations of senna.

senopia (se-no′pe-ah) [L. *senex* old man + *opia*] an apparent decrease in presbyopia in the elderly, which is related to the development of nuclear sclerosis and resultant myopia.

sensation (sen-sa′shun) [L. *sensatio*] an impression conveyed by an afferent nerve to the sensorium. **articular s.,** the sensation produced by the contact of moving joint surfaces. **cincture s.,** zonesthesia. **common s.** (Gemeingefühl), the general feeling superinduced by the summation of all the bodily sensation (E. H. Weber, 1846). **concomitant s.,** a secondary sensation, developed, without special stimulation, along with a primary sensation. **cutaneous s.,** dermal s. **delayed s.,** a sensation which is not perceived until some time after the application of the stimulation. **dermal s.,** a sensation that arises from a receptor situated in the skin. **epigastric s.,** a peculiar, weak, sinking or anxious feeling localized in the stomach; a visceral sensation of undefined nature. **external s.,** the effect produced upon the mind by an external object through the medium of the senses. **general s.,** a sensation felt throughout the body. **girdle s.,** zonesthesia. **gnostic s′s,** sensations that are perceived by the more recently developed senses, such as those of light touch and the epicritic sensibility to muscle, joint, and tendon vibrations; called also *new sensations.* **internal s.,** a sensation perceptible only to the subject himself, and not connected with any object external to his body. **joint s.,** articular s. **light s.,** the sensation produced when radiant energy of wavelength from 400 to 760 mμ enters a normal eye. **negative s.,** the condition produced by a stimulation below the threshold. **new s′s,** gnostic s′s. **objective s.,** external s. **palmesthetic s.,** pallesthesia. **primary s.,** a sensation which is the direct result of the reception of a stimulus. **referred s., reflex s.,** a sensation felt at a place other than the point of application of the stimulus. **skin s.,** dermal s. **strain s.,** a sensation as of a strain or straining. **subjective s.,** internal s. **transferred s.,** referred s. **vascular s.,** the sensation felt when there is a change in vascular tone, as in blushing. **s. of warmth,** the comfortable sensation experienced when the environment is not too cold, also the sensation felt when moderate heat is imparted to the body by radiation or contact.

sense (sens) [L. *sensus,* from *sentire* to perceive, feel] 1. a faculty by which the conditions or properties of things are perceived. Hunger, thirst, malaise, and pain are varieties of sense; a sense of equilibrium, of well being (euphoria), and other senses are also distinguished. 2. in molecular genetics, referring to the strand of a double-stranded DNA that is transcribed and specifies a product (RNA or protein). Cf. *antisense.* **chemical s.,** a general sense which causes avoidance reactions in water creatures and residual reactions in man to various irritants, such as onion, pepper, snuff, ammonia, and war gases. **color s.,** the faculty by which various colors are perceived and distinguished. **equilibrium s.,** static s. **form s.,** the ability of the eye to recognize objects as solid. **internal s.,** any sense that is normally stimulated from within the body. **kinesthetic s.,** muscle s. **labyrinthine s.,** static s. **light s.,** the faculty by which different degrees of brilliancy are distinguished. **muscle s., muscular s.,** the faculty by which muscular movements are perceived. **pain s.,** the sense by which pain is perceived. **posture s.,** a variety of muscular sense by which the position or attitudes of the body or its parts are perceived. **pressure s.,** the faculty by which pressure upon the surface of the body is perceived; called also *baresthesia.* **proprioceptive s.,** proprioceptive sensibility. **seventh s.,** visceral s. **sixth s.,** the general feeling of consciousness of the entire body; cenesthesia. **space s.,** that combination of the senses (chiefly of sight and touch) which gives information as to the relative positions

and relations of objects in space. **special s.,** any one of the five senses of seeing, feeling, hearing, taste, and smell. **static s.,** the sense that enables man to maintain an upright position. **stereognostic s.,** the sense by which form and solidity are perceived. **temperature s.,** the faculty by which a person is able to appreciate differences of temperature. **time s.,** the ability to appreciate time intervals, especially in sound and in music. **tone s.,** the power of distinguishing one tone from another. **visceral s.,** the internal and subjective sensations supposed to appertain to the ganglionic portion of the nervous system.

Sensibamine (sen-sib′ah-mīn) trademark for an equimolar mixture of ergotamine and ergotaminine.

sensibility (sen″sĭ-bil′ĭ-te) [L. *sensibilitas*] susceptibility of feeling; ability to feel or perceive. **bone s.,** pallesthesia. **common s.,** cenesthesia. **cortical s.,** the sensibility controlled by the cerebral cortex which is concerned with the recognition and discrimination of sensory impressions. **deep s.,** the sensibility to pressure and movement which exists after the skin area is made completely anesthetic. **electromuscular s.,** sensibility of muscles to electric stimulation. **epicritic s.,** the sensibility to gentle stimulations which furnishes the means for making fine discriminations of touch and temperature; this sensibility exists in the skin only. **joint s.,** arthresthesia. **mesoblastic s.,** deep s. **pallesthetic s., palmesthetic s.,** pallesthesia. **proprioceptive s.,** the largely ignored and unconscious sense that gives us knowledge of the position and state of muscles, joints, limbs, and other parts; see *proprioceptor.* **protopathic s.,** the sensibility to stimulations of pain and temperature which is low in degree and poorly localized. Such sensibility exists in the skin and in the viscera, and acts as a defensive agency against pathologic changes in the tissues. **recurrent s.,** sensibility exhibited in the anterior root of a spinal nerve when the distal portion is stimulated after division. **somesthetic s.,** proprioceptive s. **splanchnesthetic s.,** the consciousness or sensibility dependent on the splanchnic receptors. **vibratory s.,** pallesthesia.

sensibilization (sen″sĭ-bil-i-za′shun) 1. the act of making more sensitive. 2. sensitization.

sensibilizer (sen′sĭ-bil-īz″er) obsolete term for antibody.

sensible (sen′sĭ-b′l) [L. *sensibilis*] capable of sensation; perceptible to the senses.

sensiferous (sen-sif′er-us) [L. *sensus* sense + *ferre* to carry] transmitting sensations.

sensigenous (sen-sij′ĕ-nus) [L. *sensus* sense + Gr. *gennan* to produce] producing sensory impulses.

sensimeter (sen-sim′ĕ-ter) an instrument for measuring the degree of sensitiveness of anesthetic and hyperesthetic areas on the body.

sensitive (sen′sĭ-tiv) [L. *sensitivus*] able to receive or respond to stimuli; often used to mean abnormally responsive to stimulation, or responding quickly and acutely.

sensitivity (sen″sĭ-tiv′ĭ-te) 1. the state or quality of being sensitive; often used to denote a state of abnormal responsiveness to stimulation, or of responding quickly and acutely. 2. analytical sensitivity, the smallest concentration of a substance that can be reliably measured by a particular analytical method. 3. diagnostic sensitivity; the conditional probability that a person having a disease will be correctly identified by a clinical test, i.e., the number of true positive results divided by the number of true positive and false negative results. Cf. *specificity* and *predictive value.* **proportional s.,** the relationship in which a response bears some quantitative algebraic relationship to the intensity of the stimulus.

sensitization (sen″sĭ-tĭ-za′shun) 1. administration of antigen to induce a primary immune response; priming; immunization. 2. exposure to allergen that results in the development of hypersensitivity. 3. the coating of erythrocytes with antibody so that they are subject to lysis by complement in the presence of homologous antigen, the first stage of a complement fixation test. **autoerythrocyte s.,** see under *syndrome.* **photodynamic s.,** the increased lethal effects of light on microorganisms when certain dyes are present in the solution. **Rh s.,** see under *isoimmunization.*

sensitized (sen′sĭ-tīzd) rendered sensitive.

sensitizer (sen′sĭ-ti″zer) an allergen or irritant that, after an initial sensitizing exposure, produces atopic or contact dermatitis in secondary exposures.

sensomobile (sen″so-mo′bil) moving in response to a stimulus.

sensomobility (sen″so-mo-bil′ĭ-te) the capacity of man or animals for movement in response to a sensory stimulus.

sensomotor (sen″so-mo′tor) sensorimotor.

sensor (sen′sor) something that senses; a device specifically designed to respond to a physical stimulus (light, heat, pressure, etc.) by generating an impulse that can be measured or otherwise interpreted, or used as a control.

sensorial (sen-so′re-al) [L. *sensorialis*] pertaining to the sensorium.

sensoriglandular (sen″so-re-glan′du-lar) producing glandular activity as one of the consequences of stimulation of the sensory nerves.

sensorimetabolism (sen″so-re-mĕ-tab′o-lizm) the production of some metabolic action as a result of stimulation of the sensory nerves.

sensorimotor (sen″so-re-mo′tor) both sensory and motor.

sensorimuscular (sen″so-re-mus′ku-lar) producing reflex muscular action in response to a sensory impression.

sensorineural (sen″so-re-nu′ral) of or pertaining to a sensory nerve; pertaining to or affecting a sensory mechanism and/or a sensory nerve (see under *deafness* and *hearing loss*).

sensorium (sen-so′re-um) [L. *sentire* to experience, to feel the force of] 1. a sensory nerve center. 2. the seat of sensation, located in the brain (s. *commu′ne*); the term is often used to designate the condition of a subject relative to his consciousness or mental clarity.

sensorivascular (sen″so-re-vas′ku-lar) producing vascular changes as a result of stimulation applied through the sensory nerves.

sensorivasomotor (sen″so-re-vas″o-mo′tor) sensorivascular.

sensory (sen′so-re) [L. *sensorius*] pertaining to or subserving sensation.

sensualism (sen′shu-al-izm) [L. *sensus* sense] the condition of being dominated by bodily passions.

sentient (sen′she-ent) [L. *sentiens*] able to feel; sensitive; having sensation or feeling.

sepal (se′pal) one of the divisions of leaves of the calyx of a flower.

sepaloid (sep′ah-loid) resembling or shaped like a sepal.

separation (sep″ah-ra′shun) the forcing apart of adjacent teeth having tight contact, as with a separating wire prior to banding in orthodontic therapy.

separator (sep′ah-ra″tor) 1. a device for separating one thing from another. 2. a device or instrument for wedging teeth apart, especially proximal teeth having a tight contact, as for the examination of proximal surfaces, finishing a restoration, or before banding in orthodontic therapy. Called also *space maintainer*.

sepazonium chloride (sep″ah-zo′ne-um) chemical name: 1-[2-(2,4-dichlorophenyl)-2-[2,4-dichlorophenyl)methoxy]ethyl]-3-(2-phenylethyl)-1*H*-imidazolium chloride; a topical anti-infective, $C_{26}H_{23}Cl_5N_2O$.

sepedogenesis (sep″ĕ-do-jen′ĕ-sis) sepedonogenesis.

sepedon (sep′ĕ-don′) [Gr. *sēpedōn* rottenness, putrefaction] a septic condition; putridity.

sepedonogenesis (sep″ĕ-do″no-jen′ĕ-sis) [*sepedon* + Gr. *genesis* production] the production of septic conditions.

seperidol hydrochloride (sĕ-per′ĭ-dōl) chemical name: 4-[4-[4-chloro-3-(trifluoromethyl)phenyl]-4-hydroxy-1-piperidinyl]-1-(4-fluorophenyl)-1-butanone; a tranquilizer, $C_{22}H_{22}ClF_4NO_2 \cdot HCl$.

Sephadex (sef′ah-deks) trademark cross-linked dextran beads, a medium for molecular sieve chromatography.

sepia (se′pe-ah) [L.; Gr. *sēpia* cuttlefish] a dark brown, inspissated inky juice secreted by cuttlefish (*Sepia*), squidlike cephalopod marine mollusks; also, the dark brown colored pigment originally prepared from the juice.

sepiapterin reductase (sēp-e-ap′ter-in re-duk′tās) [EC 1.1.1.153] an enzyme that catalyzes the reaction sepiapterin + NADPH = dihydrobiopterin + NADP$^+$, a step in the synthesis of the coenzyme tetrahydrobiopterin.

sepium (se′pe-um) [L.; Gr. *sēpia* cuttlefish] the bone or internal shell of the cuttlefish; cuttlebone. It is used in preparing polishing agents and tooth powder, and is hung in bird cages for the purpose of supplying supplementary lime.

sepsin (sep′sin) [Gr. *sēpsis* decay] a poisonous crystallizable substance from decaying yeast and from animal matter.

sepsis (sep′sis) [Gr. *sēpsis* decay] the presence in the blood or other tissues of pathogenic microorganisms or their toxins; the condition associated with such presence. **s. agranulocyt′ica,** agranulocytosis. **catheter s.,** sepsis occurring as a complication of intravenous catheterization. **incarcerated s.,** an infection which is latent after the primary lesion has apparently healed, but which may be stirred into activity by a slight trauma. **s. intestina′lis,** poisoning from the eating of contaminated food, such as canned meats, ice cream, sausages, or cheese. **s. len′ta,** a condition produced by infection with α-hemolytic streptococci, characterized by a febrile illness with endocarditis. **mouse s., murine s.,** see under *septicemia*. **oral s.,** a disease condition in the mouth or adjacent parts which may affect the general health through the dissemination of toxins. **puerperal s.,** sepsis occurring after childbirth, due to matter absorbed from the parturient canal.

Sepsis violacea (sep′sis vi″o-la′se-ah) the common dung fly, which may be found in houses.

Sept. abbreviation for L. *sep′tem,* seven.

septa (sep′tah) [L.] plural of *septum.*

septal (sep′tal) pertaining to a septum; see also under *area.*

septan (sep′tan) [L. *septem* seven] recurring every seventh (sixth) day, as a fever.

septanose (sep′tah-nōs) a monosaccharide having a seven-numbered ring structure.

septate (sep′tāt) divided by a septum or septa.

Septatina (sep″tah-ti′nah) [L. *septum* dividing wall or partition] a suborder of parasitic protozoa (order Eugregarinida, subclass Gregarinia), in which gametocytes are present and the gamont is compartmentalized into a protomerite and deutomerite by an ectoplasmic septum; an epimerite is present. They are found in the alimentary canal of invertebrates, especially arthropods. Representative genera include *Actinocephalus* and *Gregarina*. Called also *Cephalina*.

septation (sep-ta′shun) division into parts by a septum or septa.

septatome (sep′tah-tōm) septotome.

septectomy (sep-tek′to-me) [*septum* + Gr. *ektomē* excision] excision of a portion of the nasal septum.

septemia (sep-te′me-ah) septicemia.

septic (sep′tik) [L. *septicus;* Gr. *sēptikos*] produced by or due to decomposition by microorganisms; putrefactive.

septicemia (sep″tĭ-se′me-ah) [*septic* + Gr. *haima* blood + *-ia*] systemic disease associated with the presence and persistence of pathogenic microorganisms or their toxins in the blood. Called also *blood poisoning.* **bronchopulmonary s.,** septicemia resulting from the aspiration of infected wound secretions into the trachea in operations on the larynx. **cryptogenic s.,** septicemia in which the focus of infection is not evident during life. **fowl s.,** a disease of fowls resembling fowl cholera caused by *Vibrio metschnikovii,* marked by diarrhea, hyperemia of the alimentary canal, and the presence of a blood-tinged yellowish liquid in the small intestine. **hemorrhagic s., s. hemorrhagica,** any of a group of animal diseases caused by *Pasteurella multocida,* marked by the presence of pneumonia and some hemorrhagic areas in the subcutaneous tissues, serous membranes, muscles, lymph glands, and throughout the internal organs. It includes fowl cholera, swine plague, and bovine and swine pneumonias. **s. hemorrhag′ica bo′vum,** hemorrhagic septicemia of cattle. **s. hemorrhag′ica bubalo′rum,** pasteurellosis in the buffalo. **s. hemorrhag′ica o′vum,** hemorrhagic septicemia of sheep. **lymphovenous s.,** infection of the deep cellular planes of the body. **metastasizing s.,** pyemia. **morphine injector's s.,** melioidosis in man. **mouse s.,** an infectious disease of mice, due to *Erysipelothrix insidiosa.* **phlebitic s.,** pyemia. **plague s.,** septicemic plague. **s. plurifor′mis,** hemorrhagic septicemia of sheep. **puerperal s.,** see under *fever.* **rabbit s.,** pasteurellosis in rabbits. **sputum s.,** a form produced by inoculation of certain of the microorganisms of the sputum.

septicemic (sep″tĭ-se′mik)   pertaining to, or of the nature of, septicemia.

septicine (sep′tĭ-sin)   a ptomaine, or compound of hexylamine and amylamine, from putrid flesh.

septicopyemia (sep″tĭ-ko-pi-e′me-ah)   septicemia and pyemia combined.   **cryptogenic s.,** spontaneous septicopyemia.   **metastatic s.,** a form marked by septic deposits in the lungs caused by embolism from putrid thrombi. **spontaneous s.,** a variety developing without obvious cause or from a slight wound of the skin; called also *cryptogenic s.*

septicopyemic (sep″tĭ-ko-pi-e′mik)   pertaining to septicopyemia.

septigravida (sep″tĭ-grav′ĭ-dah) [L. *septem* seven + *gravida* pregnant]   a woman pregnant for the seventh time; also written gravida VII.

septile (sep′tīl)   of or pertaining to a septum.

septimetritis (sep″tĭ-mĕ-tri′tis) [*septic* + *metritis*]   septic inflammation of the uterus.

septineuritis (sep″te-noo-ri′tis)   neuritis due to sepsis. **Nicolau's s.,** a generalized, diffuse neuritis of the entire nervous system due to the multiplication and migration of viruses in nervous tissue, as occurs in rabies.

septipara (sep-tip′ah-rah) [L. *septem* seven + *parere* to bring forth, produce]   a woman who has had seven pregnancies which resulted in viable offspring; also written para VII or VII-para.

septivalent (sep″tĭ-va′lent) [L. *septem* seven + *valens* able]   able to combine with or to replace seven hydrogen atoms.

sept(o)- [L. *septum*, q.v.]   a combining form denoting relationship to a septum.

septomarginal (sep″to-mar′ji-nal)   pertaining to the margin of a septum.

septonasal (sep-to-na′zal)   pertaining to the nasal septum.

septoplasty (sep″to-plas′te) [*septum* + Gr. *plassein* to form or mold]   surgical reconstruction of the nasal septum.

septostomy (sep-tos′to-me) [*septum* + Gr. *stomoun* to provide with an opening]   surgical creation of an opening in a septum.   **balloon atrial s.,** surgical creation of an opening in the interatrial septum of the heart by passage of a balloon catheter from the right atrium through the septum to the left atrium, at which point the balloon is inflated and the catheter is then withdrawn to create an interatrial septal defect; performed in transposition of the great vessels with an intact septum.

septotome (sep′to-tōm)   an instrument for operating on the nasal septum.

septotomy (sep-tot′o-me) [*septum* + Gr. *tomē* a cutting]   incision of the nasal septum.

septula (sep′tu-lah) [L.]   plural of *septulum.*

septulum (sep′tu-lum), pl. *sep′tula* [L., dim. of *septum*]   a small separating wall or partition; used in anatomical nomenclature as a general term to designate such a structure.   **sep′tula tes′tis** [NA], septa of testis: connective tissue lamellae from the inner surface of the tunica albuginea, which unite to form the mediastinum testis.

septum (sep′tum), pl. *sep′ta* [L.]   a dividing wall or partition; [NA] a general term for such a structure. The term is often used alone to refer to the septal area (see under *area*) or to the septum pellucidum.   **s. alve′oli,** see *interalveolar s.* and *interradicular s.*   **s. atrio′rum cor′dis,** s. interatriale cordis.   **atrioventricular s. of heart, s. atrioventricula′re cor′dis** [NA], the portion of the membranous part of the interventricular septum between the right atrium and left ventricle.   **s. of auditory tube,** s. canalis musculotubarii.   **s. auricula′rum,** s. interatriale cordis.   **Bigelow's s.,** a layer of hard, bony tissue in the neck of the femur.   **bony s. of eustachian canal,** s. canalis musculotubarii.   **bony s. of nose,** s. nasi osseum.   **bronchial s., s. bronchia′le,** carina tracheae.   **bulbar s.,** a septum, formed by fusion of the bulbar ridges, that divides the bulbus cordis into aortic and pulmonary trunks.   **s. bul′bi ure′thrae,** the fibrous septum dividing the interior of the bulb of the urethra into two approximately equal parts.   **s. cana′lis musculotuba′rii** [NA], septum of musculotubal canal: the thin lamella of bone that divides the musculotubal canal into the semicanals for the tensor tympani muscle and the auditory tube.   **s. cartilagin′eum na′si,** pars cartilaginea septi

nasi.   **cervical s., intermediate, s. cervica′le interme′dium** [NA], a glial–pia mater septum which dips into the dorsal intermediate sulcus of the dorsal funiculus of the cervical and upper lumbar parts of the spinal cord; it separates the fasciculus gracilis and fasciculus cuneatus. **cloacal s.,** urorectal s.   **s. of Cloquet,** s. femorale. **s. corpo′rum cavernoso′rum clitor′idis** [NA], an incomplete fibrous septum between the two lateral halves of the clitoris.   **crural s.,** s. femorale.   **Douglas' s.,** the septum formed by the union of Rathke's folds, forming the rectum of the fetus.   **enamel s.,** enamel cord.   **femoral s., s. femora′le** [NA], **s. femora′le [Cloque′ti],** the thin fibrous membrane that helps to close the anulus femoralis; it is derived from the fascia transversalis, is perforated for the passage of lymphatic vessels, and is embedded in fat.   **s. of frontal sinuses,** s. sinuum frontalium.   **gingival s.,** the part of the gingiva interposed between adjoining teeth. **s. glan′dis pe′nis** [NA], **s. of glans penis,** an incomplete fibrous septum in the median plane of the glans penis, especially below the urethra.   **gum s.,** gingival s.   **hemal s.,** a structure of lower animals which in man is represented by the linea alba and the transversalis, iliac, and rectovesical fasciae.   **interalveolar s.,** 1. one of the partitions of bone separating the alveoli of different teeth (*septa interalveolaria mandibulae* [NA] and *septa interalveolaria maxillae* [NA]). 2. one of the thin septa that separate adjacent pulmonary alveoli, containing connective tissue constituents of the respiratory tissue and the capillary network of the blood supply of the lung.   **sep′ta interalveola′ria mandib′ulae** [NA], interalveolar septa of mandible: the partitions between the tooth sockets in the alveolar part of the mandible.   **sep′ta interalveola′ria maxil′lae** [NA], interalveolar septa of maxilla: the partitions between the tooth sockets in the alveolar process of the maxilla. **interatrial s. of heart, s. interatria′le cor′dis** [NA], **interauricular s.,** the wall that separates the atria of the heart; called also *s. atriorum cordis*.   **interdental s.,** interalveolar s.   **intermuscular s. of arm, external,** s. intermusculare brachii laterale.   **intermuscular s. of arm, internal,** s. intermusculare brachii mediale.   **intermuscular s. of arm, lateral,** s. intermusculare brachii laterale.   **intermuscular s. of arm, medial,** s. intermusculare brachii mediale.   **intermuscular s., crural, anterior,** s. intermusculare cruris anterius.   **intermuscular s., crural, posterior,** s. intermusculare cruris posterius.   **intermuscular s. of leg, anterior,** s. intermusculare cruris anterius.   **intermuscular s. of leg, posterior,** s. intermusculare cruris posterius.   **intermuscular s. of thigh, external,** s. intermusculare femoris laterale.   **intermuscular s. of thigh, lateral,** s. intermusculare femoris laterale.   **intermuscular s. of thigh, medial,** s. intermusculare femoris mediale.   **s. intermuscula′re cru′ris anterius,** s. intermusculare cruris anterius.   **s. intermuscula′re bra′chii latera′le** [NA], lateral intermuscular septum of arm: the fascial sheet extending from the lateral border of the humerus to the under surface of the fascia investing the arm; called also *s. intermusculare humeri laterale*.   **s. intermuscula′re bra′chii media′le** [NA], medial intermuscular septum of arm: the fascial sheet extending from the medial border of the humerus to the under surface of the fascia investing the arm; called also *s. intermusculare humeri mediale*.   **s. intermuscula′re cru′ris ante′rius** [NA], anterior crural intermuscular septum: a fascial sheet extending between the extensor digitorum longus and the peroneal muscles to the anterior fibular crest. Called also *anterior intermuscular s. of leg* and *s. intermusculare anterius cruris*.   **s. intermuscula′re cru′ris poste′rius** [NA], posterior crural intermuscular septum: the fascial sheet extending between the peroneal muscles and soleus to the lateral fibular crest. Called also *posterior intermuscular s. of leg* and *s. intermusculare posterius cruris*.   **s. intermuscula′re fem′oris latera′le** [NA], lateral intermuscular septum of thigh: the fascial sheet in the thigh separating the vastus lateralis muscle from the biceps femoris.   **s. intermuscula′re fem′oris media′le** [NA], medial intermuscular septum of thigh: the fascial sheet in the thigh separating the vastus medialis from the adductor and the pectineus muscles. **s. intermuscula′re hu′meri latera′le,** s. intermusculare brachii laterale.   **s. intermuscula′re hu′meri media′le,** s. intermusculare brachii mediale.   **s. intermuscula′re poste′rius cru′ris,** s. intermusculare cruris posterius.   **interradicular s., s. interradicula′re,** one of the thin bony partitions separating the crypts of a dental alveolus occupied by the separate roots of a multi-rooted tooth. **interventricular s. of heart, s. interventricula′re cor′dis** [NA], the partition that separates the left ventricle from the right ventricle, consisting of a muscular and a membranous part; called also *s. ventriculorum cordis*. **s. intra-alveola′rium,** interradicular s. **Körner's s.,** petrosquamosal lamina. **s. lin′guae** [NA], lingual s., the median vertical fibrous part of the tongue. **s. lu′cidum,** septum pellucidum. **median s., dorsal, median s., posterior,** s. medianum dorsale. **s. media′num dorsa′le** [NA], dorsal median septum: a neuroglial septum, which is a continuation of the dorsal median sulcus of the spinal cord, that penetrates the substance of the cord and extends almost to the central canal. Called also *posterior median s.* and *s. media′num posterius* [NA alternative]. **s. media′num poste′rius** NA alternative for *s. medianum dorsale.* **mediastinal s., s. mediastina′le,** mediastinum, def. 2. **s. membrana′ceum na′si,** pars membranacea septi nasi. **s. membrana′ceum ventriculo′rum cor′dis,** pars membranacea septi interventricularis cordis. **membranous s. of nose,** pars membranacea septi nasi. **s. mo′bile na′si, mobile s. of nose,** pars mobilis septi nasi. **s. muscula′re ventriculo′rum cor′dis,** pars muscularis septi interventricularis cordis. **s. of musculotubal canal,** s. canalis musculotubarii. **nasal s., s. na′si** [NA], the partition separating the two nasal cavities in the midplane, composed of cartilaginous, membranous, and bony parts. **s. na′si os′seum** [NA], osseous septum of nose: the bone of the skull interposed between the openings of the nose, consisting primarily of the vomer below and the perpendicular plate of the ethmoid bone above. Called also *bony s. of nose.* **neural s.,** a prolongation, chiefly in the lower vertebrates, of the general investing fascia, extending medially from the surface toward the skeleton; represented in man by the ligamentum nuchae and the supraspinous and interspinous ligaments. **orbital s., s. orbita′le** [NA], a fibrous membrane anchored to the periorbita along the entire margin of the orbit, extending to the levator palpebrae superioris muscle in the upper lid and to the tarsal plate in the lower lid; called also *tarsal membrane.* **osseous s. of nose,** s. nasi osseum. **parietal s.,** cuspis posterior valvae atrioventricularis sinistrae. **s. pectinifor′me,** s. penis. **pellucid s., s. pellu′cidum** [NA], a triangular double membrane separating the anterior horns of the lateral ventricles of the brain; situated in the median plane, it is bounded by the corpus callosum and the body and columns of the fornix. Called also *s. lucidum.* **s. pe′nis** [NA], the fibrous sheet between the two corpora cavernosa of the penis, formed by union of the tunicae albugineae of the two sides. **pharyngeal s.,** the transitory partition which separates the mouth cavity from the pharynx in the embryo; called also *buccopharyngeal membrane.* **placental s.,** tissue that divides the placenta into cotyledons. **s. pon′tis,** raphe pontis. **precommissural s., s. precommissura′le** [NA], a septum situated anterior to the rostral commissure of the cerebrum, corresponding in part to the paraterminal gyrus, which consists of dorsal, ventral, medial, and caudal nuclear groups; called also *s. verum.* **s. pri′mum,** a septum in the embryonic heart, dividing the primitive atrium into right and left chambers. **rectovaginal s., s. rectovagina′le** [NA], the membranous partition between the rectum and the vagina. **rectovesical s., s. rectovesica′le** [NA], a membranous partition separating the rectum from the prostate and urinary bladder. **s. re′nis,** see *columnae renales.* **scrotal s., s. scrota′le,** s. scroti. **s. scro′ti** [NA], **s. of scrotum,** a fibromuscular partition in the median plane, dividing the scrotum into two nearly equal parts; called also *s. scrotale* and *scrotal s.* **s. secun′dum,** a septum in the embryonic heart to the right of the septum primum; after birth it fuses with the septum primum to close the foramen ovale. **s. si′nuum fronta′lium** [NA], septum of frontal sinuses: a thin lamina of bone, in the lower front part of the frontal bone, that lies more or less in the median plane and separates the frontal sinuses. **s. si′nuum sphenoida′lium** [NA], **sphenoidal s., s. of sphenoidal sinuses,** a thin lamina of bone in the body of the sphenoid bone, lying more or less in the median plane and separating the sphenoidal sinuses. **spurious s., s. spu′rium,** a structure formed by union of the two folds, one on either side, guarding the opening of the sinus venosus into the dorsal wall of the right atrium of the heart in the early

embryo. **subarachnoidal s.,** an incomplete fibrous sheath which lies in the median plane and which connects the arachnoid to the pia mater along the posterior median sulcus of the cervical and upper thoracic parts of the spinal cord. **septa of testis,** septula testis. **s. of tongue,** s. linguae. **tracheoesophageal s.,** the septum that, during the fourth week of embryonic development, separates the trachea from the ventral surface of the foregut. **transverse s. of ampulla,** crista ampullaris. **s. tu′bae,** processus cochleariformis. **urorectal s.,** the caudally and outwardly growing wedge of endoderm-covered mesoderm that divides the cloaca into urogenital sinus and rectum; called also *cloacal s.* **s. of ventricles of heart, s. ventriculo′rum cor′dis,** s. interventriculare cordis. **s. ve′rum,** s. precommissurale.

septuplet (sep′tu-plet, sep-tup′let, sep-too′plet) [L. *septuplum* a group of seven] one of seven offspring produced in one gestation period.

seq. luce. abbreviation for L. *sequen′ti lu′ce,* the following day.

sequel (se′kwel) sequela.

sequela (se-kwe′lah), pl. *seque′lae* [L.] any lesion or affection following or caused by an attack of disease.

sequelae (se-kwe′le) [L.] plural of *sequela.*

sequence (se′kwens) [L. *sequi* to follow] 1. a connected series of events or things. 2. in dysmorphology, a pattern of multiple anomalies derived from a single known or presumed prior anomaly or mechanical factor. Sometimes called *anomalad* or *complex.* **flanking s.,** a region of a gene preceding or following the transcribed region. **intervening s.,** intron. **nearest neighbor s.,** in biochemistry, the relative frequency with which pairs of the four nucleotide bases occur next to one another.

sequester (se-kwes′ter) [L.; Fr. *sequestrer* to shut up illegally] to detach or separate abnormally a small portion from the whole; see *sequestration* and *sequestrum.*

sequestra (se-kwes′trah) [L.] plural of *sequestrum.*

sequestral (se-kwes′tral) pertaining to or of the nature of a sequestrum.

sequestrant (se-kwes′trant) a sequestering agent, as, for example, cholestyramine resin, which binds bile acids in the intestine, thus preventing their absorption.

sequestration (se″kwes-tra′shun) [L. *sequestratio*] 1. the formation of a sequestrum. 2. the isolation of a patient. 3. a net increase in the quantity of blood within a limited vascular area, occurring physiologically, with or without forward flow persisting, or produced artificially by the application of tourniquets. **pulmonary s.,** loss of connection of lung tissue with the bronchial tree and with the pulmonary veins, the tissue receiving its arterial supply from the systemic circulation. The mass may be completely separated anatomically and physiologically from normally connected lung (*extralobar pulmonary s.*) or be in anatomical contiguity with and partly surrounded by normal lung (*intralobar pulmonary s.*).

sequestrectomy (se″kwes-trek′to-me) [*sequestrum* + Gr. *ektomē* excision] the surgical removal of a sequestrum.

sequestrotomy (se″kwes-trot′o-me) [*sequestrum* + Gr. *tomē* a cutting] sequestrectomy.

sequestrum (se-kwes′trum), pl. *seques′tra* [L.] a piece of dead bone that has become separated during the process of necrosis from the sound bone. **primary s.,** a sequestrum

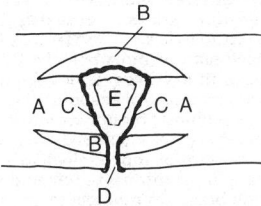

Formation of a sequestrum: *A, A,* Sound bone; *B, B,* new bone; *C, C,* granulations lining involucrum; *D,* cloaca; *E,* sequestrum.

that is entirely detached. **secondary s.,** a sequestrum that is partially detached and may be pushed into place.

tertiary s., a sequestrum that is separated by only a slight dividing line and remains in its place.

sequoiosis (se″kwoi-o′sis) a form of allergic alveolitis due to inhalation of and tissue reaction to dust from moldy redwood bark; species of *Graphium* provide the offending antigen.

Ser serine.

sera (se′rah) [L.] plural of *serum.*

seractide acetate (ser-ak′tīd) chemical name: 25-L-aspartic acid-26-L-alanine-27-glycine-30-L-glutamine-31-L-serine-α^{1-39}-corticotropin (pig); a synthetic adrenocorticotropic hormone, $C_{207}H_{308}N_{56}O_{58}S \cdot (C_2H_4O_2)_x \cdot xH_2O$.

seral (sēr′al) of or pertaining or relating to a sere, as a seral stage.

seralbumin (se″ral-bu′min) serum albumin.

serangitis (se″ran-ji′tis) [Gr. *sēranx* cavern + *-itis*] cavernitis.

Ser-Ap-Es (ser-ap-es) trademark for preparations of reserpine with hydralazine hydrochloride and hydrochlorothiazide.

Serapion (sĕ-ra′pe-on) **of Alexandria** (c. 280 B.C.) a Greek physician who is believed to have been one of the founders of the Empiric school of medicine.

Serax (ser′aks) trademark for a preparation of oxazepam.

sere (sēr) the entire sequence of ecological communities that successively occupy a given area, the transitory communities of which are called *seral stages,* or seral communities. The series finally lead to a stable, mature climax community.

serendipity (ser″en-dip′ĭ-te) the discovery of some important scientific fact, by accident or sagacity, which was not the original objective of the quest.

Serenium (sĕ-re′ne-um) trademark for a preparation of ethoxazene hydrochloride.

Serenoa (ser″e-no′ah) [*Sereno* Watson] a genus of palms. S. *serrula′ta* (Michx.) Hook f. (Palmaceae) is the saw palmetto or sabal of the southern United States. A fluid extract of the berries is diuretic, expectorant, and aphrodisiac, and has been used in diseases of the prostate and bladder.

Serentil (sĕ-ren′til) trademark for preparations of mesoridazine besylate.

seretin (ser′e-tin) carbon tetrachloride.

Serfin (ser′fin) trademark for a preparation of reserpine.

Sergent's white adrenal line (sār-zhawz′) [Emile *Sergent,* French physician, 1867–1943] see under *line.*

serial (se′re-al) arranged in or forming a series.

serialograph (se″re-al′o-graf) an apparatus for making series of x-ray pictures.

sericin (ser′ĭ-sin) silk glue or silk gelatin; a protein, $C_{15}H_{25}N_5O_3$, derivable from silk.

sericite (se′rĭ-sīt) a form of mica or muscovite, a complex silicate, causing pneumoconiosis.

Sericopelma (ser″ĭ-ko-pel′mah) a genus of huge hairy spiders of the family Theraphosidae. **S. commu′nis,** a large black species found in the Canal Zone whose venom is harmful to man.

series (sēr′ēz) [L. "row"] 1. a group or succession of objects or substances arranged in regular order or forming a kind of chain. 2. pertaining to electric circuit components connected "in series" so that the current flow goes through each component without branching; applied by extension to any similar series circuit, e.g., the pulmonary and systemic circulations. Cf. *parallel.* 3. a taxonomic category assigned different ranks by different authors. **basophil s., basophilic s.,** see *granulocytic s.* **eosinophil s., eosinophilic s.,** see *granulocytic s.* **erythrocyte s., erythrocytic s.,** the succession of morphologically distinguishable cells that are stages in erythrocyte development: in order of maturity, the pronormoblast, basophilic normoblast, polychromatophilic normoblast, orthochromatic normoblast, reticulocyte, and erythrocyte. **granulocyte s., granulocytic s.,** the succession of morphologically distinguishable cells that are stages in granulocyte development: in order of maturity, the myeloblast, promyelocyte, myelocyte, metamyelocyte, the band or stab cell, which is the least mature form normally found in the peripheral blood, and the mature segmented (polymorphonuclear) granulocyte. Commitment to one of the granulocyte lines occurs in stem cells before the myeloblast stage is reached; thus there are distinct neutro-

phil, eosinophil, and basophil series; however, the morphologic stages are the same. Formerly called the *myeloid, myelocytic,* or *leukocytic s.* **Hofmeister s.,** the sequence of ions arranged with respect to their effects on the solubility of proteins, e.g., on their salting-out effects; called also *lyotropic s.* **homologous s.,** a series of compounds each member of which differs from the one preceding it by having one more methylene (CH_2) group. **leukocytic s.,** granulocytic s. **lymphocyte s., lymphocytic s.,** a series of morphologically distinguishable cells once thought to represent stages in lymphocyte development: in order of maturity, the lymphoblast, "prolymphocyte," and lymphocyte. It is now known that lymphocyte precursors are morphologically indistinguishable from small lymphocytes and that lymphoblasts are not precursors but activated lymphocytes that have been transformed in response to antigenic stimulation. **lyotropic s.,** Hofmeister s. **monocyte s., monocytic s.,** the succession of developing cells that ultimately culminates in the monocyte; it begins with the monoblast, which matures to form sequentially the promonocyte and the mature cell. **myeloid s., myelocytic s.,** granulocytic s. **neutrophil s., neutrophilic s.,** see *granulocytic s.* **plasmacyte s., plasmacytic s.,** a series of morphologically distinguishable cells that are stages in plasma cell development: in order of maturity, the plasmablast (an activated B cell usually referred to as a large lymphocyte or lymphoblast), proplasmacyte, and plasmacyte. **thrombocyte s., thrombocytic s.,** the succession of morphologically distinguishable cells that are stages in platelet (thrombocyte) development: in order of maturity, the megakaryoblast, promegakaryocyte, and megakaryocyte, which fragments to form platelets.

seriflux (ser′ĭ-fluks) [L. *serum* whey + *fluxus* flow] a thin, watery discharge.

serine (ser′ēn) chemical name: 2-amino-3-hydroxypropionic acid. A naturally occurring, nonessential amino acid, $C_3H_7NO_3$. It may be synthesized from glycine, and is used as a dietary supplement and feed additive, in biological studies and tests, and in culture media.

serine carboxypeptidase (ser′ēn kar-bok″se-pep′tĭ-dās) 1. [EC 3.4.16] one of a sub-subclass of enzymes of the hydrolase class consisting of peptidases that hydrolyze single amino acid residues from the C-terminus of peptide chains, and contain a diisopropyl fluorophosphate-sensitive serine in their catalytic site; they have optimum activity at acid pH. 2. [EC 3.4.16.1] one of the lysosomal serine carboxypeptidases of broad specificity that catalyzes the reaction peptidyl-L-amino acid + H_2O = peptide + L-amino acid. Formerly called *cathepsin A* and *cathepsin B_2.*

serine proteinase (ser′ēn pro′te-ĭ-nās) [EC 3.4.21] a sub-subclass of enzymes of the hydrolase class that hydrolyze proteins and have a serine and histidine involved at the active site of catalysis. They include enzymes active in digestion, blood coagulation, immune reactions, and fertilization of the ovum.

serioscopy (se″re-os′ko-pe) roentgenographic visualization of the body in a series of parallel planes by means of multiple exposures. Two or more roentgenograms are taken from different directions. They are laid on each other and moved until the projections of the various planes of the object coincide consecutively.

seriscission (ser″ĭ-sizh′un) [L. *sericum* silk + *scindere* to cut] the division of soft tissues by an encircling silk ligature pulled tightly.

seroalbuminous (se″ro-al-bu′mĭ-nus) containing serum and albumin; containing serum albumin.

seroalbuminuria (se″ro-al-bu″mĭ-nu′re-ah) the presence in the urine of serum albumin.

serochrome (se′ro-krōm) [*serum* + Gr. *chrōma* color] (obs.) the coloring matter of normal serum.

serocolitis (se″ro-ko-li′tis) inflammation of the serous surface of the colon.

seroconversion (se″ro-kon-ver′shun) the change of a serologic test from negative to positive, indicating the development of antibodies in response to infection or immunization.

seroconvert (se″ro-kon-vert′) to undergo seroconversion.

seroculture (se′ro-kul-tūr) a bacterial culture on blood serum.

serocystic (se″ro-sis′tik) made up of serous cysts.

serodiagnosis (se″ro-di″ag-no′sis) diagnosis made by using serologic tests.

serodiagnostic (se″ro-di″ag-nos′tik) pertaining to serodiagnosis.

seroenteritis (se″ro-en″tĕ-ri′tis) inflammation of the serous coat of the intestine.

sero-fast (se′ro-fast′) serum-fast.

serofibrinous (se″ro-fib′rin-us) both serous and fibrinous.

serofibrous (se″ro-fi′brus) pertaining to serous and fibrous surfaces; as, *serofibrous* apposition.

seroflocculation (se″ro-flok″u-la′shun) flocculation produced in blood serum by an antigen. Cf. *Henry test*, under tests.

serofluid (se″ro-floo′id) a serous fluid.

seroglobulin (se″ro-glob′u-lin) serum globulin; the globulin of the blood serum.

serogroup (se′ro-groop) a group of bacteria containing a common antigen, possibly including more than one serotype (q.v.), species, or genus. A serogroup is a tentative and unofficial designation, used in the classification of certain genera of bacteria, e.g., *Leptospira, Salmonella, Shigella,* and *Streptococcus.*

serologic, serological (se″ro-loj′ik; se″ro-loj′ĕ-kal) pertaining to serology.

serologist (se-rol′o-jist) one who is an expert in serology.

serology (se-rol′o-je) [*serum* + *-logy*] originally, the study of the in vitro reactions of immune sera, e.g., precipitin, agglutination, and complement fixation reactions. The term is now used to refer to the use of such reactions to measure serum antibody titers in infectious disease (serologic tests), to the clinical correlations of the antibody titer (the "serology" of a disease), and to the use of serologic reactions to detect antigens (e.g., "serologically defined" HLA antigens). **diagnostic s.,** serodiagnosis.

serolysin (se-rol′ĭ-sin) a lysin present in the blood serum.

seroma (sēr-o′mah) a tumor-like collection of serum in the tissues.

seromembranous (se″ro-mem′brah-nus) both serous and membranous; composed of serous membrane.

seromucoid (se″ro-mu′koid) seromucous.

seromucous (se″ro-mu′kus) partly serous and partly mucous.

seromucus (se″ro-mu′kus) a secretion which is part serum and part mucus.

seromuscular (se″ro-mus′ku-lar) pertaining to the serous and muscular coats of the intestine.

Seromycin (ser′o-mi″sin) trademark for preparations of cycloserine.

seronegative (se″ro-neg′ah-tiv) serologically negative; showing negative results on serological examination; showing a lack of antibody.

seronegativity (se″ro-neg″ah-tiv′ĭ-te) the state of being seronegative, or of showing negative results on serological examination.

seroperitoneum (se″ro-per″ĭ-to-ne′um) the presence of free fluid in the peritoneum; ascites.

serophilic (se″ro-fil′ik) a term used to describe a bacterium whose growth is enhanced in the presence of serum.

seroplastic (se″ro-plas′tik) serofibrinous.

seropneumothorax (se″ro-nu″mo-tho′raks) pneumothorax with a serous effusion in the pleural cavity.

seropositive (se″ro-poz′ĭ-tiv) serologically positive; showing positive results on serological examination; showing a high level of antibody.

seropositivity (se″ro-poz″ĭ-tiv′ĭ-te) the state of being seropositive, or of showing positive results on serological examination.

seroprognosis (se″ro-prog-no′sis) the prognosis of a disease based on the results of serologic tests.

seropurulent (se″ro-pu″roo-lent) both serous and purulent.

seropus (se″ro-pus′) serum mingled with pus.

seroreaction (se″ro-re-ak′shun) serological reaction; a reaction demonstrating a specific antibody or antigen in serum.

serorelapse (se″ro-re-laps′) a definite rise in serological titer occurring after treatment.

seroresistant (se″ro-re-zis′tant) pertaining to seroresistance; showing a seropositive reaction to a pathogen after treatment.

seroresistance (se″ro-re-zis′tans) failure of the serological titer to fall satisfactorily after treatment.

seroreversal (se″ro-re-vers′al) a fall in serological titer after treatment.

serosa (se-ro′sah; se-ro′zah) 1. any serous membrane (tunica mucosa). 2. the tunica serosa. 3. the chorion.

serosal (se-ro′sal) pertaining to or composed of serosa.

serosamucin (se-ro″sah-mu′sin) a protein resembling mucin, found in inflammatory ascitic exudates.

serosanguineous (se″ro-sang-gwin′e-us) pertaining to or containing both serum and blood.

serose (se′rōs) an albumose obtained from serum albumin.

seroserous (se″ro-se′rus) pertaining to two or more serous membranes.

serositis (se″ro-si′tis), pl. *serositides* [*serous membrane* + *-itis*] inflammation of a serous membrane. **infectious avian s.,** a septicemic disease of ducklings and geese, characterized by fibrinous peritonitis, pericarditis, and airsacculitis, and caused by *Pasteurella anatipestifer.* Called also *new duck disease* in ducklings and *goose influenza* in geese. **multiple s.,** polyserositis.

serosity (se-ros′ĭ-te) the quality possessed by serous fluids.

serosurvey (se″ro-sur′va) a population survey using a serologic test to screen for exposure and immunity to an infectious disease.

serosynovial (se″ro-sĭ-no′ve-al) both serous and synovial.

serosynovitis (se″ro-sin″o-vi′tis) synovitis with effusion of serum.

serotherapy (se″ro-ther′ah-pe) [*serum* + Gr. *therapy*] the treatment of disease by the injection of immune serum or antitoxin.

serothorax (se″ro-tho′raks) hydrothorax.

serotonergic (se″ro-tōn-er′jik) serotoninergic.

serotonin (ser″o-to′nin) chemical name: 3-(2-aminoethyl)-5-indolol. A vasoconstrictor, $C_{10}H_{12}N_2O$, found in various animals from coelenterates to vertebrates, in bacteria, and in many plants. In humans, it is synthesized in the intestinal chromaffin cells or in central or peripheral neurons and is found in high concentrations in many body tissues, including the intestinal mucosa, pineal body, and central nervous system. Produced enzymatically from tryptophan by hydroxylation and decarboxylation, serotonin has many physiologic properties; e.g., it inhibits gastric secretion, stimulates smooth muscle, serves as a central neurotransmitter, and is a precursor of melatonin. Called also *enteramine, thrombocytin, thrombotonin, 5-hydroxytryptamine,* and *5-HT.*

serotoninergic (ser″o-to″nin-er′gik) 1. containing or activated by serotonin, as the neurons of the raphe nuclei of the brain stem. 2. of or pertaining to neurons that secrete serotonin, which, in turn, stimulates release of pituitary hormones. Called also *serotonergic.*

serotoxin (se″ro-tok′sin) (*obs.*) anaphylatoxin.

serotype (se′ro-tīp) 1. the type of a microorganism as determined by the kinds and combinations of constituent antigens present in the cell. 2. to distinguish organisms on the basis of their constituent antigens. 3. a taxonomic subdivision of bacteria based on the kinds and combinations of constituent antigens present in the cell, or a formula expressing the antigenic analysis on which such a subdivision is based. Called also *serovar.* See also *serogroup.* **heterologous s.,** a related but not identical serotype. **homologous s.,** an identical serotype.

serous (se′rus) [L. *serosus*] 1. pertaining to or resembling serum. 2. producing or containing serum, as a serous gland or cyst.

serovaccination (se″ro-vak″sĭ-na′shun) injection of serum combined with bacterial vaccination to produce passive immunity by the former and active immunity by the latter.

serovar (se′ro-var) serotype.

serozyme (se′ro-zīm) [L. *serum* + Gr. *zymē* yeast] (*obs.*) Bordet's name for the prothrombin present in the blood serum.

Serpasil (ser′pah-sil) trademark for preparations of reserpine.

Serpens (ser′pens) [L. *serpens* snake] a genus of gram-negative, aerobic, rod-shaped bacteria of uncertain affiliation, made up of motile flagellated organisms found in sediments of freshwater ponds. The type species is *S. flexi′bilis.*

serpentaria (ser″pen-ta′re-ah) [L. *serpens* snake] the dried rhizome and roots of *Aristolochia serpentaria,* Virginia snakeroot, and *A. reticulata,* or Texas snakeroot, herbs of North America. Serpentaria is an astringent bitter, the major bitter principle of which is aristolochic acid. Formerly used as an analgesic and in the treatment of snakebite.

Serpentes (ser′pen-tēz) *Ophidia.*

serpiginous (ser-pij′ĭ-nus) [L. *serpere* to creep] having a wavy or much indented margin, as a lesion in noduloulcerative cutaneous syphilis.

serrated (ser′āt-ed) [L. *serratus,* from *serra* saw] having a sawlike edge.

Serratia (sĕ-ra′she-ah) [Serafino *Serrati,* Italian physicist of the 18th century] a genus of gram-negative, facultatively anaerobic bacteria of the family Enterobacteriaceae, consisting of motile, peritrichously flagellated rods, sometimes capsulated. Most strains produce white, pink, or red pigments. The organisms occur on plants, in soil, and in water. Many species are opportunistic pathogens, causing infections of the endocardium, blood, wounds, and urinary and respiratory tracts in immunocompromised patients. **S. fica′ria,** a nonpigmented species, isolated from fig trees, that is ornithine decarboxylase negative. **S. liquefa′ciens,** a nonpigmented species sometimes found in clinical specimens as an opportunistic pathogen; it is ornithine decarboxylase positive. Called also *S. proteamaculans.* **S. marces′-cens,** the most frequently isolated species, with red-pigmented varieties, occurring in water, soil, and food and in clinical specimens. It is an opportunistic pathogen, causing nosocomial bacteremia, endocarditis, and pneumonia in immunocompromised patients. It is ornithine decarboxylase positive. **S. odori′fera,** a species with a characteristic musty, potato-like odor, occasionally isolated from plants or food and rarely found as an opportunistic pathogen. **S. plymuth′ica,** a species with pigmented strains that is lysine decarboxylase negative and ornithine decarboxylase negative, reported in human sputum. **S. proteama′culans,** *S. liquefaciens.* **S. rubida′ea,** a species with pigmented strains that is ornithine decarboxylase negative, found in ripe coconuts.

serration (sĕ-ra′shun) [L. *serratio*] a structure or formation with teeth like those of a saw; the condition of being serrated.

serratus (sĕ-ra′tus) [L.] serrated.

serrefine (sār-fēn′) [Fr.] a small spring forceps for compressing bleeding vessels.

Serres' angle, glands (sārz) [Antoine Etienne Reynaud Augustin *Serres,* French physiologist, 1786–1868] see *metafacial angle,* under *angle,* and see under *gland.*

serrulate (ser′u-lāt) [L. *serrulatus*] marked or bordered with small serrations or projections.

Sertoli's cell, column (ser-to′lēz) [Enrico *Sertoli,* Italian histologist, 1842–1910] see under *cell* and *column.*

serum (se′rum), pl. *serums* or *se′ra* [L. "whey"] 1. the clear portion of any body fluid; the clear fluid moistening serous membranes. 2. blood serum; the clear liquid that separates from blood on clotting; see *blood serum,* under *blood.* 3. immune serum; blood serum from an immunized animal used for passive immunization; an antiserum, antitoxin, or antivenin. **active s.,** a serum that contains complement. **anticomplementary s.,** a serum which interferes with or destroys the activity of complement. **antilymphocyte s. (ALS),** equine antiserum against human lymphocytes, a powerful nonspecific immunosuppressive agent that causes destruction of circulating lymphocytes. **antipneumococcus s.,** type-specific horse or rabbit antiserum used effectively to treat pneumococcal pneumonia before the advent of antibiotics. **antirabies s.** [USP], antiserum obtained from horses immunized with rabies vaccine, used concurrently with rabies vaccine for postexposure prophylaxis against rabies; rabies immune globulin is used instead, if available. **antireticular cytotoxic s.,** (*obs.*) an antiserum produced by immunizing horses with human spleen and bone marrow cells; said to have a stimulating effect on the reticuloendothelial system in small doses and a cytotoxic effect in large doses. Called also *ACS s.* **antitetanic s.**

(A.T.S.), tetanus antitoxin. **antitoxic s.,** antitoxin. **articular s.,** synovia. **bacteriolytic s.,** serum containing a bacteriolysin capable of inducing complement-dependent lysis of a bacterium. **blood s.,** see *blood serum,* under B. **blood grouping s's** [USP], preparations containing particular antibodies against red cell antigens, used for blood typing. Those most commonly used are the anti-A and anti-B blood grouping serums, used to determine ABO blood types, and the anti-Rh blood grouping serums (anti-D, anti-C, anti-E, anti-c, and anti-e), used to determine Rh blood types. **convalescence s., convalescent s., convalescents' s.,** blood serum from a patient who is convalescent from an infectious disease; such a serum was once used as a prophylactic injection in such diseases as measles, scarlet fever, whooping cough, etc. **despeciated s.,** a heterologous antiserum treated to remove some of the species-specific proteins so that it is less likely to cause anaphylaxis. **foreign s.,** heterologous s., def. 1. **heterologous s.,** 1. serum obtained from an animal belonging to a species different from that of the recipient. 2. serum prepared from an animal immunized by an organism differing from that against which it is to be used. **homologous s.,** 1. serum obtained from an animal belonging to the same species as the recipient. 2. serum prepared from an animal immunized by the same organism against which it is to be used. **hyperimmune s.,** antiserum with an especially high antibody titer produced by repeated antigen injections. **immune s.,** antiserum. **inactivated s.,** serum which has been heated, usually at 56° C. for 30 minutes, to destroy the lytic activity of contained complement components. **Löffler's s.,** see *Löffler's coagulated serum medium* in *Table of Culture Media,* under *culture medium.* **lymphatolytic s.,** serum which destroys lymphatic tissues, such as the spleen and lymph glands. **monovalent s.,** antiserum containing antibodies against only one of several strains or species of microorganisms or only one of a group of antigens. **muscle s.,** muscle plasma deprived of its myosin. **normal s.,** serum from a normal untreated animal. **pericardial s.,** liquor pericardii. **polyvalent s.,** antiserum containing antibodies to a group of two or more strains or species of microorganism or to a group of two or more antigens. **pooled s.,** the mixed serum from a number of individuals. **pregnancy s.,** blood serum taken from pregnant women. **Sclavo's s.,** a specific anti-anthrax serum that may be used against human anthrax. **specific s.,** monovalent s. **truth s.,** a misnomer for the drugs sometimes employed in narcoanalysis, especially sodium amobarbital and sodium thiopental; the agent used is not a serum and its use does not guarantee truthfulness.

serumal (se-roo′mal) pertaining to or formed from serum.

serum-fast (se′rum-fast) resistant to the destructive effect of serum; said of bacteria.

serumuria (se″rum-u′re-ah) albuminuria.

Serv. abbreviation for L. *ser′va,* keep, preserve.

Servetus (ser-ve′tus), Michael (1511–1553). A Spanish theologian who also wrote, among other subjects, on geography, astrology, and medicine. His *Christianismi restitutio* (1553) contains the first printed description of the lesser circulation; Servetus was burned at the stake for heresy the same year, and only three copies of the book have survived.

servomechanism (ser″vo-mek′ah-nizm) a control system in which feedback is used to control errors in another system. The term is also applied to biological systems, such as the mechanism that controls the diameter of the pupil of the eye according to the amount of incident light.

seryl (sēr′il, ser′il) the acyl radical of serine.

sesame (ses′ah-me) [L. *sesamum;* Gr. *sēsamon*] the plant *Sesamum indicum* L.; also its oil-bearing seeds. The oil, called oil of benne, is used like olive oil. The seeds are demulcent, and are used as a laxative. Currently also used in topical skin lotions, as an emollient, and as a parenteral vehicle for intramuscular injections.

sesamoid (ses′ah-moid) [L. *sesamoides;* Gr. *sēsamon* sesame + *eidos* form] 1. denoting a small nodular bone embedded in a tendon or joint capsule. 2. a sesamoid bone. See under *bone.*

sesamoiditis (ses″-moi-di′tis) inflammation of the sesamoid bones and surrounding structures of a horse's foot.

sesqui- [L. *sesqui* a half more] a prefix meaning one and a half.

sesquih. abbreviation for L. *sesquiho′ra,* an hour and a half.

sesquihora (ses″kwe-ho′rah) [L.] an hour and a half.

sesquioxide (ses″kwe-ok′sid) a compound of three parts of oxygen with two of another element.

sesquisulfate (ses″kwe-sul′fāt) a sulfate containing three parts of sulfuric acid united with two of another element.

sesquisulfide (ses″kwe-sul′fid) a sulfide containing three parts of sulfur united with two of another element.

sessile (ses′il) [L. *sessilis*] attached by a base; not pedunculated or stalked.

Sessilina (ses″sĭ-li′nah) [L. *sessilis* sessile] a suborder of usually bell- or goblet-shaped protozoa (order Peritrichida, subclass Peritrichia) comprising sedentary and sessile forms with a stalk at the tapered end of the body. Most are free-living and are found attached to various substrates in a wide range of habitats. *Vorticilla* is a representative genus.

Sessinia (ses-sin′e-ah) a genus of blistering beetles, coconut beetles, of certain Pacific islands.

sesunc. abbreviation for L. *sesun′cia,* an ounce and a half.

set (set) 1. to align bones or bone fragments, as in reducing a fracture. 2. in psychology, a readiness to perceive or respond in a certain way because of past experience, requirements of a task, etc. **phalangeal s.,** a surgical office procedure for correction of deformities of the lesser toes, involving incision to reach the bony joint and manipulation for proper positioning.

seta (se′tah), pl. *se′tae* [L.] 1. bristle. 2. any bristle-like structure, such as the multicellular stalk of certain plants.

setaceous (se-ta′shus) [L. *setaceus; seta* bristle] slender and rigid, like a bristle.

Setaria (se-ta′re-ah) a genus of filarial nematodes. **S. cer′vi, S. cervi′na,** S. *labiatopapillosa.* **S. equi′na,** a species found in the abdominal cavity of the horse and related species, buffalo, cattle, and sometimes man. **S. labiatopapillo′sa,** a species found in the peritoneal cavity of cattle and various game animals in Africa.

Setchenow's centers (nuclei) (sech′ĕ-nofs) [Ivan Mikhailovich *Setchenow,* Russian neurologist, 1829– 1905, the father of Russian physiology and neurology] see under *center.*

setiferous (se-tif′er-us) [L. *seta* bristle + *ferre* to bear] bearing bristles; covered with bristles.

setigerous (se-tij′er-us) [L. *seta* bristle + *gerere* to carry] setiferous.

seton (se′ton) [Fr. *seton;* L. *seta* bristle] a thread of silk, linen, or other finely drawn material for passage through a sinus, fistula, or epithelial tract, often to serve as a guide for subsequent dilatation with instruments of larger diameter.

set-point (set′point) the target value of the controlled variable that is maintained by an automatic control system, e.g., the point at which body temperature is controlled by the hypothalamic thermostat. Written also *set point.*

setup (set′up) 1. organization or arrangement. 2. the arrangement of teeth on a trial denture base. **diagnostic s.,** a procedure involving dissection of teeth from a plaster model and repositioning of the teeth in desired positions to aid in case analysis preliminary to constructing an orthodontic appliance.

Seutin's bandage (su-tanz′) [Louis Joseph *Seutin,* Brussels surgeon, 1793–1862] see under *bandage.*

Sever's disease (se′verz) [James Warren *Sever,* Boston orthopedic surgeon, born 1878] see under *disease.*

sevoflurane (se″vo-floo′rān) chemical name: 1,1,1,3,3,3-hexafluoro-2-(fluoromethoxy)propane; an inhalation anesthetic, $C_4H_3F_7O$.

sewage (soo′ij) the used water supply of a community, consisting of an aqueous suspension of human and animal excreta and other waste materials from structures inhabited by humans; the contents of sewers. **activated s.,** sewage mixed with activated sludge. **domestic s.,** sewage from dwellings, business buildings, factories, or institutions. **septic s.,** sewage undergoing anaerobic bacterial decomposition.

sex (seks) [L. *sexus*] 1. the fundamental distinction, found in most species of animals and plants, based on the type of gametes produced by the individual or the category into which the individual fits on the basis of that criterion; ova, or macrogametes, are produced by the female, and spermatozoa, or microgametes, are produced by the male, the union of these distinctive germ cells being the natural prerequisite for the production of a new individual in sexual reproduction. 2. to determine the sex of an organism. **chromosomal s.,** sex as determined by the presence of the XX (female) or the XY (male) genotype in somatic cells, and without regard to phenotypic manifestations; called also *genetic s.* **endocrinologic s.,** the phenotypic manifestations of sex determined by endocrine influences, such as breast development in the female, phallic enlargement in the male. **genetic s.,** chromosomal s. **gonadal s.,** the sex as determined on the basis of the gonadal tissue present, whether ovarian or testicular. **morphological s.,** sex determined on the basis of the morphology of the external genitals. **nuclear s.,** the sex as determined on the basis of the presence or absence of sex chromatin in somatic cells, its presence normally indicating the XX (female) genotype, and its absence the XY (male) genotype. **psychological s.,** the self-image of the gender role of an individual. **social s.,** the complex of attitudes, expectations, etc., that a society attaches to the male and female roles.

sex-conditioned (seks″kon-dish′und) see under *gene.*

sexdigitate (seks-dij′ĭ-tāt) [L. *sex* six + *digitus* digit] having six fingers on the hand or six toes on the foot.

sexduction (seks-duk′shun) F-duction.

sex-influenced (seks-in′floo-enst) see under *gene.*

sexivalent (sek-siv′ah-lent) hexivalent.

sex-limited (seks-lim′it-ed) see under *gene.*

sex-linked (seks′linkt) see under *gene.*

sexology (seks-ol′o-je) the study of sex and sexual relations and their evolutionary, physiological, developmental, and sociological aspects.

sexopathy (seks-op′ah-the) abnormality or perversion of sexual expression.

sextan (seks′tan) [L. *sextanus* of the sixth] recurring every sixth day; said of fevers.

sextigravida (seks″tĭ-grav′ĭ-dah) [L. *sextus* sixth + *gravida* pregnant] a woman pregnant for the sixth time; also written gravida VI.

sextipara (seks-tip′ah-rah) [L. *sextus* sixth + *parere* to bring forth, produce] a woman who has had six pregnancies which resulted in viable offspring; also written para VI or VI-para.

sextuplet (seks′tu-plet, seks-tup′let) [L. *sextus* sixth] one of six offspring produced in one gestation period.

sexual (seks′u-al) [L. *sexualis*] 1. pertaining to sex. 2. a person considered in his sexual relations.

sexuality (seks″u-al′ĭ-te) 1. the characteristic quality of the male and female reproductive elements. 2. the constitution of an individual in relation to sexual attitudes or activity. **infantile s.,** in freudian theory, the erotic life of infants and children, encompassing the oral, anal, and phallic phases of psychosexual development.

Seyderhelm's solution (si′der-helmz) [Richard *Seyderhelm,* Göttingen physician, 1888–1940] see under *solution.*

Sézary cell, syndrome (erythroderma) (sa′zah-re) [Albert *Sézary,* French dermatologist, 1880–1956] see under *cell* and *syndrome.*

SGOT serum glutamic-oxaloacetic transaminase; see *aspartate aminotransferase.*

SGPT serum glutamate pyruvate transaminase; see *alanine aminotransferase.*

SH serum hepatitis.

shadow (shad′o) 1. an attenuated image of an actual object, as a faded or colorless erythrocyte. 2. a figure or image created by the interruption of light or other rays, such as the representation on a roentgenogram of radiopaque structures. **bat's wing s.,** a roentgenographic shadow that radiates through both lungs from the hilar region toward the periphery, leaving a clear zone at the apices, periphery, and bases. **heart s.,** the shadow of the heart on a roentgenogram. **Purkinje's s's,** see under *image.*

shadow-casting (shad″o-kast′ing) a technique for increasing the visibility of ultramicroscopic specimens under the microscope by applying a coating of chromium, gold, or other metal.

shadowgram, shadowgraph (shad′o-gram, shad′o-graf) roentgenogram.

shadowgraphy (shad′o-graf″e) roentgenography.

Shaffer's method (sha′ferz) [Philip Anderson *Shaffer*, American biochemist, 1881–1960] see under *method*.

shaft (shaft) a long slender part, such as the portion of a long bone between the wider ends or extremities; see also *diaphysis* [NA]. **s. of femur,** corpus femoris. **s. of fibula,** corpus fibulae. **hair s.,** scapus pili. **s. of humerus,** corpus humeri. **s. of metacarpal bone,** corpus ossis metacarpalis. **s. of metatarsal bone,** corpus ossis metatarsalis. **s. of penis,** corpus penis. **s. of phalanx of fingers,** corpus phalangis digitorum manus. **s. of phalanx of toes,** corpus phalangis digitorum pedis. **s. of radius,** corpus radii. **s. of rib,** corpus costae. **s. of tibia,** corpus tibiae. **s. of ulna,** corpus ulnae.

shakes (shāks) a vernacular term for the cold paroxysm of intermittent fever. **hatter's s.,** mercury poisoning among fur hat workers. **kwaski s.,** a condition seen in children who, having been severely malnourished, suffer rhythmic twitches and shaking a week or two after introduction of a better diet. The "shakes" gradually disappear over a period of a few weeks. **spelter s.,** metal fume fever seen among brass-founders. **Teflon s.,** polymer fume fever.

sham-feeding (sham-fēd′ing) sham feeding; see under *feeding.*

shank (shangk) a leg, or leglike part.

shaping (shāp′ing) an operant conditioning technique used in behavior therapy in which new behavior is produced by providing reinforcement for progressively closer approximations of the final desired behavior. Called also *successive approximation.*

Sharpey's fibers (shar′pēz) [William *Sharpey,* English anatomist and physiologist, 1802–1880] see under *fiber.*

shear (shēr) an applied force that tends to cause an opposite but parallel sliding motion of the planes of an object. Also, the strain resulting from such force.

Shear's test (sherz) [Murray Jacob *Shear,* American chemist, born 1899] see under *tests.*

sheath (shēth) [L. *vagina;* Gr. *thēkē*] a tubular structure enclosing or surrounding some organ or part. **arachnoid s.,** the delicate membrane between the pial and dural sheaths of the optic nerve. **bulbar s.,** vagina bulbi. **carotid s.,** a portion of the cervical fascia enclosing the carotid artery, the internal jugular vein, and the vagus nerve. **caudal s.,** a tubular cytoplasmic structure at the base of the nucleus in the early spermatid. **chordal s.,** notochordal s. **common s. of tendons of peroneal muscles,** vagina synovialis musculorum peroneorum communis. **common s. of testis and spermatic cord,** fascia spermatica interna. **connective tissue s. of Key and Retzius,** endoneurium, especially the delicate continuation around terminal branches of nerve fibers. **crural s.,** femoral s. **dentinal s.,** Neumann s. **dural s.,** the external investment of the optic nerve, overlying the arachnoid sheath. **enamel prism s., enamel rod s.,** a sheath of organic tissue completely or partially surrounding each enamel prism. Called also *prism s.* and *rod s.* **s. of eyeball,** vagina bulbi. **fascial s. of prostate,** the sheath, derived from the rectovesical fascia, which surrounds the prostate. **female s.,** vagina (def. 2). **femoral s.,** the fascial covering of the proximal portion of the femoral vessels, derived from the intra-abdominal fascia; the most medial portion of the sheath, separated by a septum, forms the canalis femoralis. Called also *crural s.* **fibrous s's of fingers,** vaginae fibrosae digitorum manus. **fibrous s. of optic nerve,** vagina externa nervi optici. **fibrous s. of spermatozoon,** the fibrous sheath surrounding the principal piece of the tail of a spermatozoon. **fibrous s. of tendon,** vagina fibrosa tendinis. **fibrous s's of toes,** vaginae fibrosae digitorum pedis. **s. of Henle,** connective tissue s. of Key and Retzius. **Hertwig s., s. of Hertwig,** root s., def. 1. **s. of Key and Retzius,** connective tissue s. of Key and Retzius. **lamellar s.,** perineurium. **masculine s.,** utriculus prostaticus. **Mauthner's s.,** axolemma. **medullary s.,** myelin s. **mitochondrial s.,** the sheath of circumferentially oriented mitochondria arranged end to end, which surrounds the middle piece of a spermatozoon and is thought to control the movements of the tail. **mucous s's,** bursa synovialis

and vaginal synoviales. **mucous s., intertubercular,** septum intermusculare anterius cruris. **mucous s. of tendon,** vagina synovialis tendinis. **mucous s's of tendons of fingers,** vaginae synoviales digitorum manus. **mucous s's of tendons of toes,** vaginae synoviales digitorum pedis. **myelin s.,** the sheath surrounding the axon of some (the myelinated) nerve cells, consisting of concentric layers of myelin, formed in the peripheral nervous system by the plasma membrane of Schwann cells, and in the central nervous system by oligodendrocytes. It is interrupted at intervals along the length of the axon by gaps known as nodes of Ranvier. Myelin is an electrical insulator that serves to speed the conduction of nerve impulses. **Neumann s., s. of Neumann,** an area of interface between peri- and intertubular dental structures. Called also *dentinal s.* **neurilemmal s.,** neurilemma. **notochordal s.,** an elastic sheath surrounding the notochord. **nucleated s.,** neurilemma. **s's of optic nerve,** vaginae nervi optici. **s. of optic nerve, external,** vagina externa nervi optici. **s. of optic nerve, internal,** vagina interna nervi optici. **perinephric s.,** the sheath of fascia investing the kidney. **perivascular s.,** a pia glial membrane which accompanies blood vessels into the brain. **pial s.,** the innermost of the three sheaths of the optic nerve, underlying the arachnoid sheath. **s. of plantar tendon of long peroneal muscle,** vagina tendinis musculi peronei longi plantaris. **periarterial lymphatic s., periarterial lymphoid s. (PALS),** any of the sheaths of lymphatic tissue that make up the white pulp of the spleen. **primitive s.,** neurilemma. **prism s.,** enamel prism s. **s. of rectus abdominis muscle,** vagina musculi recti abdominis. **rod s.,** enamel prism s. **root s.,** 1. an epithelial extension of the cervical loop of the enamel organ, consisting of the inner and outer enamel epithelium, and directing the number and morphological growth of the roots. It is bordered externally by the dental sac and internally by developing cementum and root dentin, and ultimately becomes the epithelial diaphragm. Called also *Hertwig's s.* and *s. of Hertwig.* 2. the epithelial portion of the hair follicle, divided into the inner root sheath and the outer root sheath, which gives rise to the sebaceous glands. **Scarpa's s.,** fascia cremasterica. **Schwalbe's s.,** the thin envelope of an elastic fiber. **s. of Schwann,** neurilemma. **Schweigger-Seidel s.,** a spindle-shaped thickening in the walls of the second portion of the arterial branches forming the penicilli in the spleen. See *sheathed artery,* under *artery.* **spiral s.,** a heavily staining filament winding around the axial filament of the middle piece of a spermatozoon. **s. of styloid process,** vagina processus styloidei. **synovial s. of bicipital groove,** vagina synovialis intertubercularis. **synovial s. of intertubercular groove,** vagina synovialis intertubercularis. **synovial s. of tendon,** vagina synovialis tendinis. **synovial s. of tendons of foot,** vaginae synoviales digitales pedis. **tendinous s's of flexor muscles of fingers,** vaginae fibrosae digitorum manus. **tendinous s's of flexor muscles of toes,** vaginae fibrosae digitorum pedis. **tendinous s. of leg,** fascia cruris. **tendinous s. of long peroneal muscle, plantar,** vagina tendinis musculi peronei longi plantaris. **tendon s. of anterior tibial muscle,** vagina tendinis musculi tibialis anterioris. **tendon s's of long extensor muscles of toes,** vaginae tendinum musculi extensoris digitorum pedis longi. **tendon s's of long flexor muscles of toes,** vaginae tendinum musculi flexoris digitorum pedis longi. **tendon s. of posterior tibial muscle,** vagina tendinis musculi tibialis posterioris.

sheep-pox (shēp-poks) a contagious, often fatal, disease of sheep caused by a poxvirus, which is characterized by fever, systemic disturbances, and widespread skin lesions on non-wool-bearing areas or where the hair is not long. Called also *ovinia, ovine smallpox,* and *variola ovina.*

sheet (shēt) a rectangular piece of cotton, linen, etc., for a bed covering. *β*-s., **beta s.,** *β*-pleated s., **beta pleated s.,** pleated s. **draw s.,** a folded sheet placed under a patient in bed so that it may be withdrawn without lifting the patient. **drip s.,** a wet sheet from which the water is wrung out and which is then wrapped around a patient standing in a tub of water. **pleated s.,** a secondary structure occurring in many proteins, consisting of several polypeptide chains running in the same direction (a parallel pleated sheet) or in alternating directions (an antiparallel pleated sheet) and joined by hydrogen bonds between the imino hydrogen of each peptide bond and the carbonyl oxygen of a peptide bond in the next chain over. Called also *β-structure*, *β-sheet*, and *β-pleated sheet*. **secretory s.**, the simplest form of multicellular gland, consisting of secreting cells alone, e.g., the surface epithelium of the mammalian gastric mucosa.

shelf (shelf) a shelflike structure, normal or abnormal, in the body. **buccal s.**, the surface of the mandible from the residual alveolar ridge or the alveolar ridge to the external oblique line in the region of the lower buccal vestibule; it is covered with cortical bone. **dental s.**, the shelflike epithelial invagination formed by the dental ridge, beneath which the dental papillae are formed. **mesocolic s.**, the transverse mesocolon and the great omentum taken together. **palatine s.**, see *lateral palatine process* and *median palatine process*, under *process*.

shell (shel) a covering or encasement, such as the calcareous, horny, or chitinous covering of an animal. **egg s.**, the thin, hard, brittle, outer covering of an egg; called also *testa ovi*.

shellac (shĕ-lak′) a product of lac from India, produced on various plants by an insect, *Laccifer lacca* Kerr (Coccidae); sometimes used in dentistry and surgery, and in coating confections and medicinal tablets.

Shenton's line (arch) (shen′tonz) [Thomas *Shenton*, English radiologist] see under *line*.

Shepherd's fracture (shep′ards) [Francis John *Shepherd*, Canadian surgeon, 1851–1929] see under *fracture*.

Sherman unit (shur′man) [Henry Clapp *Sherman*, American biochemist, 1875–1955] Sherman-Munsell unit.

Sherman-Bourquin unit (shur′man boor′kwin) [Henry C. *Sherman*; Ann *Bourquin*, American nutritionist, born 1897] see under *unit*.

Sherman-Munsell unit (shur′man-mun′sel) [Henry C. *Sherman*; Hazel E. *Munsell*, American nutritionist, born 1891] see under *unit*.

Sherrington (sher′ing-ton) Sir Charles Scott. English physiologist, 1857–1952; co-winner, with Baron Adrian of Cambridge, of the Nobel prize for medicine or physiology in 1932 for their work on the function of the neuron and particularly for his studies of reflex action and neurophysiology.

Sherrington's law (sher′ing-tonz) [Sir Charles Scott *Sherrington*] see under *law*.

shield (shēld) any protecting structure. **Buller's s.**, a watch glass fitted over the unaffected eye to guard it from infection from the affected eye. **embryonic s.**, the double-layered disk from which the embryo proper develops. **eye s.**, a covering for the eyes to protect them from light or injury. **lead s.**, in radiology, a lead barrier for protecting personnel from radiation. **nipple s.**, a cover to protect the nipple of a nursing woman. **oral s.**, see under *screen*.

shift (shift) a change, as of position, status, etc. **chloride s.**, the exchange of chloride (Cl) and bicarbonate (HCO₃⁻) between the plasma and the red blood cells which takes place whenever HCO₃⁻ is generated or decomposed within the red cells. Called also *Hamburger's phenomenon*. **Doppler s.**, the magnitude of the change in frequency caused by the Doppler effect. **s. to the left**, an increase in the percentage of neutrophils having only one or a few lobes; see *Arneth count*, under *count*. **Purkinje s.**, see under *phenomenon*. **regenerative blood s.**, the rapid outpouring of leukocytes of the juvenile and myelocyte type, occurring as the result of an acute stimulus to the bone marrow. **s. to the right**, an increase in the percentage of multisegmented neutrophils; see *Arneth count*, under *count*.

Shiga's bacillus, toxin (she′gahz) [Kiyoshi *Shiga*, Japanese physician, 1870–1957] see *Shigella dysenteriae* type 1, and see under *toxin*.

Shigella (shĭ-gel′ah) [Kiyoshi *Shiga*, Japanese physician, 1870–1957] a genus of gram-negative, facultatively anaerobic, rod-shaped bacteria of the family Enterobacteriaceae, made up of nonmotile bacilli that cannot utilize citrate as a sole carbon source and that ferment carbohydrates with acid but no gas production. The genus consists of four species, differentiated by biochemical reactions: *S. dysenteriae* (subgroup A), *S. flexneri* (subgroup C), *S. boydii* (subgroup C), and *S. sonnei* (subgroup D). Their normal habitat is the intestinal tract of humans and higher monkeys; all species cause dysentery. **S. alkales′cens**, *Escherichia coli*. **S. am-**

big′ua, *S. dysenteriae* type 2. **S. arabinotar′da type A**, *S. dysenteriae* type 3. **S. arabinotar′da type B**, *S. dysenteriae* type 4. **S. boy′dii**, a species that causes acute diarrheal disease in humans, especially in tropical regions. It has 15 serological types; all ferment mannitol but not lactose. **S. ceylonen′sis**, *S. sonnei*. **S. dispar**, *Escherichia coli*. **S. dysente′riae**, a highly pathogenic species that causes severe dysentery, separable into 10 serologic types; it does not ferment lactose or mannitol. *S. dysenteriae* type 1, the classic Shiga bacillus, produces a potent neurotoxin and causes epidemic dysentery, which can be fatal in children. *S. dysenteriae* type 2, the Schmitz bacillus, is serologically related to *Escherichia coli* type 0112; it is the cause of occasional epidemic diarrheal disease in humans and among captive chimpanzees. The other numbered types of dysentery bacilli include the parashiga, the Large-Sachs, and the arabinotarda groups. Formerly called *Bacillus dysenteriae* and *Bacterium dysenteriae*. **S. etou′sae**, *S. boydii* type 7. **S. flexne′ri**, a species that causes severe dysentery. It has six serotypes and two variants (X and Y); type 2 produces an enterotoxin. The organisms ferment mannitol but not lactose. Called also *S. paradysenteriae* and *Flerner's bacillus*. **S. madampen′sis**, *Escherichia coli*. **S. new′castle**, *S. flexneri* type 6. **S. paradysente′riae**, *S. flexneri*. **S. parashi′gae**, a name formerly given to a group of non-mannitol-fermenting dysentery bacilli serologically differentiable from the Shiga bacillus (now *S. dysenteriae* type 1); also known as the Large-Sachs group of parashiga bacilli, they are now known as *S. dysenteriae*, types 3 to 7, inclusive. **S. schmit′zii**, *S. dysenteriae* type 2. **S. shi′gae**, *S. dysenteriae* type 1. **S. son′nei**, the least pathogenic species, causing a milder but frequently encountered form of bacillary dysentery. The organisms ferment mannitol; lactose is fermented slowly (5 to 14 days). The genus is serologically homogeneous, but two antigens, designated I and II, occur in varying proportions. Called also *Sonne-Duval bacillus* and, formerly, *Bacterium sonnei*.

shigella (shĭ-gel′ah), pl. *shigel′lae*. a bacterium of the genus *Shigella*.

shigellae (shĭ-gel′e) plural of *shigella*.

shigellosis (shĭ″gel-lo′sis) the condition produced by infection with organisms of the genus *Shigella*. See individual species under *Shigella*, and *bacillary dysentery*, under *dysentery*.

shikimene (shik′ĭ-mēn) sikimin.

shikimic acid (shĭ-kim′ik) 3,4,5-trihydroxy-1-cyclohexene-1-carboxylic acid, a metabolic intermediate in the synthesis of phenylalanine and tyrosine in plants and bacteria.

shin (shin) 1. the crest or anterior edge of the tibia. 2. the anterior aspect of the leg below the knee. **bucked s′s**, sore s′s. **cucumber s.**, a tibia which is curved with the concavity forward. **saber s.**, a tibia with a marked anterior convexity as seen in congenital syphilis, yaws, and osteitis deformans. **sore s′s**, periostitis of the large metacarpal or metatarsal bone of the horse.

shingles (shing′g'lz) [L. *cingulus*] herpes zoster.

shiver (shiv′er) 1. a slight chill or tremor. 2. to tremble, as from a chill.

shivering (shiv′er-ing) 1. involuntary trembling or quivering of the body caused by contraction or twitching of the muscles, a physiologic method of heat production in man and other mammals. 2. a disease of horses characterized by trembling or quivering of various muscles.

shock (shok) 1. a sudden disturbance of mental equilibrium. 2. a condition of profound hemodynamic and metabolic disturbance characterized by failure of the circulatory system to maintain adequate perfusion of vital organs; it may result from inadequate blood volume (hypovolemic shock); inadequate cardiac function (cardiogenic shock), or inadequate vasomotor tone (neurogenic shock, septic shock). The clinical manifestations of hypovolemic or cardiogenic shock include hypotension, hyperventilation, cold, clammy, cyanotic skin, a weak and rapid pulse, oliguria, and mental confusion, combativeness, or anxiety. Septic shock is initially manifested by chills and fever, warm flushed skin, a lesser degree of hypotension, and an increase in cardiac output; if unresponsive to therapy it progresses to the clinical picture associated with hypovolemic or cardiogenic shock. **anaphylactic s.**, see *anaphylaxis*. **anaphylactoid s.**, pseudoanaphylaxis. **anesthesia s.**, a shocklike condition caused by an overdose of anesthetic. **burn s.,** shock resulting from the loss of plasma into a burn wound. **cardiac s.,** cardiogenic s. **cardiogenic s.,** shock resulting from primary failure of the heart in its pumping function, as in myocardial infarction, severe cardiomyopathy, or mechanical obstruction or compression of the heart. **colloidoclastic s.,** see *colloidoclasia*. **deferred s., delayed s.,** shock occurring a considerable time after the injury is received. **diastolic s.,** the cardiac impulse which strikes the palpating hand in early diastole. **electric s.,** the immediate effects produced by the passage of an electric current through any part of the body, e.g., painful stimulation of nerves or tetanic contractions of muscles. **endotoxic s., endotoxin s.,** septic shock due to release of endotoxins by gram-negative bacteria. **hematogenic s.,** hypovolemic s. **hemorrhagic s.,** hypovolemic shock resulting from hemorrhage. **histamine s.,** a reaction resembling anaphylactic shock produced in experimental animals by histamine injection. **hypoglycemic s.,** insulin s. **hypovolemic s.,** shock resulting from insufficient blood volume for the maintenance of adequate cardiac output, blood pressure and tissue perfusion. Without modification the term refers to absolute hypovolemic shock caused by acute hemorrhage or excessive fluid loss. Relative hypovolemic shock refers to a situation in which the blood volume is normal but insufficient because of widespread vasodilation as in neurogenic shock or septic shock. Called also *hematogenic* or *oligemic s.* **insulin s.,** a hypoglycemic reaction to overdosage of insulin, a skipped meal, or strenuous exercise in an insulin-dependent diabetic; early symptoms are tremor, irritability, dizziness, cool moist skin, hunger, and tachycardia; if untreated it may progress to coma and convulsions. **irreversible s.,** a condition in which the changes produced cannot be corrected by treatment, and death is inevitable. **neurogenic s.,** shock resulting from neurogenic vasodilation, which can be produced by cerebral trauma or hemorrhage, spinal cord injury, deep general or spinal anesthesia, or toxic central nervous system depression. **oligemic s.,** hypovolemic s. **osmotic s.,** exposure of cells to an extremely hypotonic environment, which results in rupture of the plasma membrane and loss of cell contents, except for cells that have a rigid cell wall, which prevents rupture of the plasma membrane. **pleural s.,** a hypotensive condition sometimes following thoracentesis, characterized by cyanosis, pallor, dilated pupils, and disturbance of pulse and respiration. **postoperative s.,** a state of shock following a surgical operation. **secondary s.,** shock appearing one or more hours after injury; delayed shock. **septic s.,** shock associated with overwhelming infection, most commonly infection with gram-negative bacteria, although it may be produced by other bacteria, viruses, fungi, and protozoa. It is thought to result from the action of endotoxins or other products of the infectious agent on the vascular system causing large volumes of blood to be sequestered in the capillaries and veins; activation of the complement and kinin systems and the release of histamine, prostaglandins and other mediators may be involved. **serum s.,** anaphylactic shock resulting from administration of foreign serum to a sensitized individual. **shell s.,** a term used during World War I to refer to a wide variety of mental disorders associated with combat experience, so called because it was attributed to concussion from shelling. **spinal s.,** the loss of spinal reflexes after injury of the spinal cord, which affects the muscles innervated by the cord segments situated below the site of the lesion. **surgical s.,** shock that occurs during or after surgical operation. **testicular s.,** the effect of a sharp blow upon the testes. **traumatic s.,** any shock produced by trauma. **vasogenic s.,** shock caused by marked vasodilation.

shoe (shoo) a covering or appliance for the foot. **Charlier's s.,** a horse's shoe which allows the sole and the frog to come to the ground exactly as in the unshod foot. **Scarpa's s.,** a metal brace used in treating talipes equinus by preventing plantar extension of the foot beyond a right angle.

Shope papilloma (shōp) [Richard Edwin *Shope*, American pathologist, 1902–1966] rabbit papilloma.

shortsightedness (short-sīt′ed-nes) myopia.

shot-compressor (shot′kom-pres″or) see under *compressor*.

shotty (shot′e) like shot; resembling the lead pellets used in shotgun cartridges.

shoulder (shōl′der) the junction of the arm and trunk; also that part of the trunk which is bounded at the back by the scapula. **bull's-eye s.,** a horse's shoulder having on it a loose flabby disk of hyperplastic skin with a central denuded surface. **drop s.,** depression of one shoulder below the level of the other. **frozen s.,** adhesive capsulitis. **knocked-down s.,** separation or dislocation of the shoulder at the acromioclavicular joint occurring in athletes. Called also *shoulder separation*. **loose s.,** a condition seen in progressive muscular atrophy in which, when attempts to lift the patient by grasping the upper arms at their sides are made, the arms move up but the trunk remains behind. **stubbed s.,** sprain of the shoulder joint occurring in athletes.

shoulder-blade (shōl′der-blād) the scapula.

shoulder slip (shōl′der slip) inflammation and atrophy of the shoulder muscles and tendons in the horse; called also *sweeny*.

show (sho) the appearance of blood as a forerunner of labor or menstruation.

shower (show′er) a sudden emission or appearance. **uric acid s.,** temporary increase in the uric acid content of the urine; occurring in the course of a gouty attack.

Shrady's saw (shra′dēz) [George Frederick *Shrady*, New York surgeon, 1837–1907] see under *saw*.

Shrapnell's membrane (shrap′nelz) [Henry Jones *Shrapnell*, English anatomist and Army surgeon, 1761–1841] pars flaccida membranae tympani.

shunt (shunt) 1. to turn to one side; to divert; to bypass. 2. a passage or anastomosis between two natural channels, especially between blood vessels. Such structures may be formed physiologically (e.g., to bypass a thrombosis), or they may be structural anomalies (see *cardiovascular s.*). 3. a surgically created anastomosis; also, the operation of forming a shunt. **arteriovenous (A-V) s.,** direct passage of

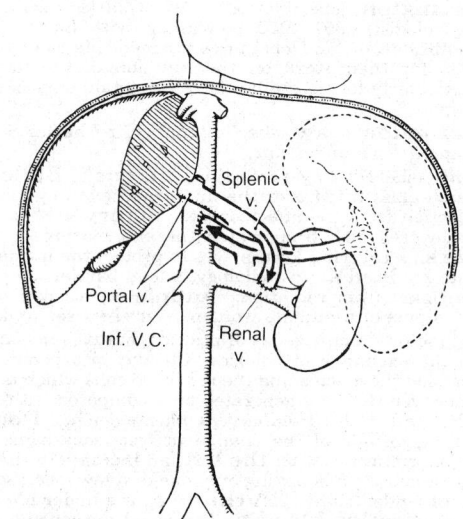

Portal shunts, showing two types of portal to systemic venous shunt.

blood from an artery to a vein. Also a U-shaped plastic tube inserted between an artery and a vein (usually between the radial artery and cephalic vein), bypassing the capillary network; commonly done to allow repeated access to the arterial system for the purpose of hemodialysis. **cardiovascular s.,** an abnormality of blood flow between the sides of the heart or between the systemic and pulmonary circulation; see *left-to-right s.* and *right-to-left s.* **Glenn s.,** see under *operation*. **hexose monophosphate s.,** pentose phosphate pathway. **left-to-right s.,** diversion of blood from the left side of the heart to the right side or from the systemic to the pulmonary circulation through an anomalous opening such as a septal defect or patent ductus arteriosus. **LeVeen peritoneovenous s.,** continuous shunting of ascites fluid from the peritoneal cavity to the jugular vein by means of a surgically implanted subcutaneous plastic tube; a pressure-activated valve buried in the abdominal wall ensures one-way flow. **pentose s.,** pentose phosphate pathway. **peritoneovenous s.,** LeVeen peritoneovenous s. **portacaval s., postcaval s.,** surgical creation of an anastomosis between the portal vein and vena cava. **reversed s.,** right-to-left s. **right-to-left s.,** diversion of blood from the right side of the heart to the left side or from the pulmonary to the systemic circulation through an anomalous opening such as a septal defect or patent ductus arteriosus; called also *reversed s.* **ventriculoatrial s.,** the surgical creation of a communication between a cerebral ventricle and a cardiac atrium by means of a plastic tube, to permit drainage of cerebrospinal fluid for relief of hydrocephalus. **ventriculoperitoneal s.,** a communication between a cerebral ventricle and the peritoneum by means of plastic tubing; done for the relief of hydrocephalus. **ventriculovenous s.,** creation of a communication between a cerebral ventricle and the internal jugular vein by means of a plastic tube, to permit drainage of cerebrospinal fluid for relief of hydrocephalus.

shuttle (shut′el) [A.S. *scytel* a dart] in biochemistry, a mechanism for the transport of electrons or an organic group, or both, across a membrane. **glycerol phosphate s.,** transfer of electrons from cytosolic NADH to oxygen in mitochondria, involving glycerol-3-phosphate dehydrogenase (NAD⁺) in the cytosol and membrane-bound glycerol-3-phosphate dehydrogenase in the mitochondria, occurring primarily in white fibers of striated muscle and nervous tissue. **malate-aspartate s.,** the transfer of electrons into mitochondria from the cytosol of red fibers of skeletal, muscle, heart, and the brain, involving the enzymes malate dehydrogenase and aspartate aminotransferase.

Shwachman syndrome (shwok′man) [Harry *Shwachman*, man, American pediatrician, 1910–1986] see under *syndrome.*

Shwachman-Diamond syndrome (shwak′man di′ah-mond) [Harry *Shwachman;* Louis Klein *Diamond*, American pediatrician, born 1902] see under *syndrome.*

Shwartzman reaction (phenomenon) (shwarts′man) [Gregory *Shwartzman*, Russian bacteriologist in the United States, 1896–1965] see under *reaction.*

SI 1. Système International d'Unites, or International System of Units. See *SI unit,* under *unit.* 2. stimulation index; see *lymphocyte proliferation test,* under *tests.*

Si chemical symbol for *silicon.*

SIADH syndrome of inappropriate antidiuretic hormone.

sialaden (si-al′ah-den) [Gr. *sial-* + Gr. *adēn* gland] a salivary gland.

sialadenectomy (si″al-ad″ĕ-nek′to-me) sialoadenectomy.

sialadenitis (si″al-ad″ĕ-ni′tis) inflammation of a salivary gland. **chronic nonspecific s.,** an inflammatory disease of the major salivary glands, characterized by intermittent swelling that may lead to fibrous degeneration, resulting from obstruction of the salivary ducts by calculi, foreign bodies, tumors, or scar formation, with subsequent bacterial invasion.

sialadenography (si″al-ad″ĕ-nog′rah-fe) radiography of the salivary glands and ducts.

sialadenosis (si″al-ad″ĕ-no′sis) [*sial-* + *adenosis*] a disease of a salivary gland. Called also *sialoadenitis.*

sialadenotomy (si″al-ad″ĕ-not′o-me) sialoadenotomy.

sialagogic (si″ah-lah-goj′ik) promoting the flow of saliva.

sialagogue (si-al′ah-gog) [*sial-* + Gr. *agōgos* leading] an agent that promotes the flow of saliva. Called also *ptyalagogue.*

sialate (si′ah-lāt) any salt of a sialic acid.

sialectasia (si″al-ek-ta′se-ah) dilatation of a salivary duct.

sialemesis (si″al-em′ĕ-sis) [Gr. *sial-* + Gr. *emesis* vomiting] vomiting of saliva.

sialic (si-al′ik) [Gr. *sialikos*] 1. pertaining to the saliva. 2. pertaining to sialic acid.

sialic acid (si-al′ik) an *N*-acyl derivative of neuraminic acid, e.g., *N*-acetylneuraminic acid; sialic acids occur in many polysaccharides, glycoproteins, and glycolipids in animals and bacteria.

sialidase (si-al′ĭ-dās) [EC 3.2.1.18] an enzyme of the hydrolase class that catalyzes the hydrolysis of glucosidic linkages between a sialic acid residue and a hexose or hexosamine residue at the nonreducing terminal of oligosaccharides in glycoproteins, glycolipids, and proteoglycans. The enzyme is a major antigen of myxoviruses. Deficiency of the enzyme, an autosomal recessive trait, causes sialidosis. Called also *neuraminidase.*

sialine (si′ah-lin) [L. *sialinus*] pertaining to the saliva.

sialism, sialismus (si′al-izm; si″al-iz′mus) [Gr. *sialismos*] ptyalism.

sialitis (si″ah-li′tis) inflammation of a salivary gland or duct.

sial(o)- [Gr. *sialon* saliva] combining form denoting relationship to (*a*) saliva or to the salivary glands or (*b*) sialic acid.

sialoadenectomy (si″ah-lo-ad″ĕ-nek′to-me) [*sialo-* + Gr. *adēn* gland + *ektomē* excision] excision of a salivary gland.

sialoadenitis (si″ah-lo-ad″ĕ-ni′tis) sialadenitis.

sialoadenotomy (si″ah-lo-ad″ĕ-not′o-me) [*sialo-* + Gr. *adēn* gland + *tomē* a cutting] incision and drainage of a salivary gland.

sialoaerophagia (si″ah-lo-a″er-o-fa′je-ah) [*sialo-* + Gr. *aēr* air + *phagein* to eat + *-ia*] excessive swallowing of saliva and air.

sialoangiectasis (si″ah-lo-an″je-ek′tah-sis) [*sialo-* + Gr. *angeion* vessel + *ektasis* distention] dilatation of the salivary ducts.

sialoangiitis (si″ah-lo-an″je-i′tis) inflammation of the salivary ducts.

sialoangiography (si″ah-lo-an″je-og′rah-fe) radiography of the ducts of the salivary glands after injection of radiopaque material.

sialoangitis (si″ah-lo-an-ji′tis) sialoangiitis.

sialocele (si′ah-lo-sēl″) [*sialo-* + Gr. *kēlē* tumor] a salivary cyst or tumor.

sialodochitis (si″ah-lo-do-ki′tis) [*sialo-* + Gr. *dochos* receptacle + *-itis*] inflammation of the salivary ducts.

sialodochoplasty (si″ah-lo-do′ko-plas″te) [*sialo-* + Gr. *dochos* receptacle + *plassein* to form] plastic operation on the salivary ducts.

sialoductitis (si″ah-lo-duk-ti′tis) sialoangiitis.

sialogastrone (si″ah-lo-gas′trōn) a substance in saliva reputed to inhibit gastric secretion and motility.

sialogenous (si″ah-loj′ĕ-nus) [*sialo-* + Gr. *gennan* to produce] producing saliva.

sialogogic (si″ah-lo-goj′ik) sialagogic.

sialogogue (si-al′o-gog) sialagogue.

sialogram (si-al′o-gram) [*sialo-* + Gr. *gramma* a mark] a radiograph produced by sialography.

sialograph (si-al′o-graf) sialogram.

sialography (si″ah-log′rah-fe) [*sialo-* + Gr. *graphein* to write] radiographic demonstration of the salivary ducts by means of the injection of substances opaque to x-radiation.

sialolith (si-al′o-lith) [*sialo-* + Gr. *lithos* stone] a calcareous concretion or calculus in the salivary ducts or glands, involving most commonly the submaxillary gland and its duct, less frequently the parotid and sublingual glands and their ducts, and seldom the minor salivary glands. Called also *salivary calculus* and *salivary stone.*

sialolithiasis (si″ah-lo-lĭ-thi′ah-sis) [*sialo-* + Gr. *lithiasis*] a condition characterized by the presence of sialoliths. Called also *ptyalolithiasis.*

sialolithotomy (si″ah-lo-lĭ-thot′o-me) [*sialolith* + Gr. *tomē* a cutting] incision of a salivary gland or duct for the removal of a calculus.

sialoma (si″ah-lo′mah) a salivary tumor.

sialometaplasia (si″ah-lo-met″ah-pla′ze-ah) metaplasia of the salivary glands. **necrotizing s.,** a benign inflammatory condition of the minor salivary glands, simulating mucoepidermoid and squamous cell carcinoma. Histological findings usually show lobular necrosis and ductal and glandular metaplasia.

sialomucin (si″ah-lo-mu′sin) a component of the airway secretions of the lungs.

sialophagia (si″ah-lo-fa′je-ah) [*sialo-* + Gr. *phagein* to eat] excessive swallowing of saliva.

sialorrhea (si″ah-lo-re′ah) [*sialo-* + Gr. *rhoia* flow] ptyalism.

sialoschesis (si″ah-los′kĕ-sis) [sialo- + Gr. *schesis* suppression] suppression of the salivary secretion.

sialosemeiology (si″ah-lo-se″mi-ol′o-je) [sialo- + *semeiology*] analysis of the saliva as a means of determining the physiologic status of the patient, especially in regard to metabolic processes.

sialosis (si″ah-lo′sis) [sial- + -osis] 1. the flow of saliva. 2. ptyalism.

sialostenosis (si″ah-lo-stĕ-no′sis) [sialo- + Gr. *stenos* narrow] stenosis, or narrowing, of a salivary duct.

sialosyrinx (si″ah-lo-si′rinks) [sialo- + Gr. *syrinx* pipe] 1. a salivary fistula. 2. a syringe for washing out the salivary ducts, or a drainage tube for the salivary ducts.

sib (sib) [Anglo-Saxon *sib* kin] 1. a blood relative; one of a group of persons, all of whom are descendants of a common ancestor. 2. sibling.

sibilant (sib′ĭ-lant) [L. *sibilans* hissing] of a shrill, hissing, or whistling character.

sibilus (sib′ĭ-lus) [L.] a whistling or sibilant rale.

sibling (sib′ling) [Anglo-Saxon *sib* kin + *ling* a diminutive] any of two or more offspring of the same parents; a brother or sister. Called also *sib*.

sibship (sib′ship) 1. relationship by blood. 2. a group of persons, all of whom are descendants of a common ancestor, commonly used as the basis of study to determine genetic influences. 3. a group of siblings.

Sibson's aponeurosis (fascia), furrow, groove, notch, vestibule (sib′sunz) [Francis *Sibson*, English physician, 1814–1876] see under *furrow, groove*, and *notch*, and see *membrana suprapleuralis* and *vestibule of aorta*.

Sicard's syndrome (se-karz′) [Jean Athanase *Sicard*, Paris neurologist, 1872–1929] Collet's syndrome.

siccative (sik′ah-tiv) [L. *siccus* dry] drying; removing moisture from surrounding objects; xeransis.

sicchasia (sĭ-ka′ze-ah) [Gr. *sikchasia*] nausea.

siccolabile (sik″o-la′bĭl) altered or destroyed by drying.

siccostabile (sik″o-sta′bĭl) not altered by drying.

siccus (sik′us) [L.] dry.

sick (sik) 1. not in good health; afflicted with disease; ill. 2. affected with nausea.

sick bay (sik′ba) hospital and dispensary quarters on a naval vessel or station.

sicklemia (sik-le′me-ah) sickle cell anemia; see under *anemia*.

sicklemic (sik-le′mik) pertaining to or characterized by sicklemia.

sickling (sik′ling) the development of sickle cells in the blood, as in sickle cell anemia.

sickness (sik′nes) any condition or episode marked by pronounced deviation from the normal healthy state; illness. **aerial s.,** air s. **African horse s.,** an infectious pulmonary disease of horses and mules in South Africa, caused by a virus and marked by serous exudations. Called also *pestis equorum* and *equine plague*. **African sleeping s.,** see under *trypanosomiasis*. **air s.,** sickness due to change in air pressure and to the movements experienced in an airplane, marked by nausea, salivation, and cold sweats. **altitude s.,** high-altitude s. **athletes' s.,** weakness, blurred vision, nausea, and headache, following a short period of intense physical exercise. **aviation s.,** air s. **balloon s.,** a condition similar to mountain sickness occurring during balloon ascents. **bay s.,** Haff disease. **Borna s.,** Borna disease. **bush s.,** a disease similar to enzootic marasmus, occurring in New Zealand. **caisson s.,** decompression s. **car s.,** nausea and malaise produced by the motion of trains or automobiles or other vehicles. **cave s.,** a febrile disease of the lungs occurring in persons who were engaged in excavating in an abandoned mine, due to infection with *Histoplasma capsulatum* (histoplasmosis). **compressed-air s.,** decompression s. **decompression s.,** a disorder characterized by joint pains, respiratory manifestations, skin lesions, and neurologic signs, occurring in aviators flying at high altitudes and following rapid reduction of air pressure in persons who have been breathing compressed air in caissons and diving apparatus. **falling s.,** epilepsy. **gall s.,** see *gallsickness*. **Gambian horse s.,** a fatal infection of horses throughout central Africa caused by *Trypanosoma congolense*. See also *nagana*.

Gambian sleeping s., see under *trypanosomiasis*. **green s.,** chlorosis. **green tobacco s.,** a transient, recurrent occupational illness of tobacco harvesters, marked by headache, dizziness, vomiting, and prostration. **high-altitude s.,** the condition resulting from difficulty in adjusting to diminished oxygen pressure at high altitudes. It may take the form of mountain sickness (q.v.), high-altitude pulmonary edema, or cerebral edema. **Jamaican vomiting s.,** a disease occurring in Jamaica, marked by severe vomiting of acute onset, usually followed by convulsions, coma, and death, due to ingestion of damaged or unripe fruit of akee (*Blighia sapida*). Called also *akee poisoning*. **lambing s.,** a condition of ewes almost identical with milk fever of cows. **laughing s.,** pseudobulbar paralysis. **milk s.,** 1. an acute, often fatal disease caused by the ingestion of milk, milk products, or the flesh of cattle or sheep which have a disease known as trembles. It is marked by weakness, anorexia, vomiting, constipation, and sometimes muscular tremors. 2. trembles. **morning s.,** the nausea of early pregnancy. **motion s.,** sickness caused by motion experienced in any kind of travel, such as sea sickness, train sickness, car sickness, and air sickness. **mountain s.,** a syndrome caused by exposure to altitude high enough to cause hypoxia, occurring as a result of decreased atmospheric pressure with consequent lowering of arterial oxygen content. The *acute* form (Acosta's disease) may appear a few hours after exposure to high altitude, with manifestations that include fatigue, dizziness, breathlessness, headache, nausea, vomiting, insomnia, impairment of mental capacity and judgment, and prostration. The *chronic* form (Andes disease, Monge's disease) is characterized by loss of tolerance to hypoxia in a previously acclimatized person, and by secondary polycythemia. It occurs in two types: an *emphysematasus* type, in which dyspnea is the dominant symptom and bronchitis and laryngitis are common, and cyanosis is present; and in an *erythremic* type, in which the prominent symptoms include an erythremic color that turns to cyanosis on mild exertion, fatigue, headache, episodic stupor, paresthesias, anorexia, nausea, vomiting, and diminution of visual acuity. The *subacute* form is milder than the chronic form and resembles the acute form clinically, but is persistent. Both the chronic and subacute forms can be cured by descent to a lower altitude or to sea level. **radiation s.,** a condition resulting from exposure to a whole-body dose of over 1 gray of ionizing radiation and characterized by the symptoms of the acute radiation syndrome (q.v.). Its severity varies with the dose level. **railroad s.,** transit tetany. **Rhodesian sleeping s.,** see under *trypanosomiasis*. **salt s.,** a disease similar to enzootic marasmus, occurring in Florida. **sea s.,** nausea and malaise caused by the motion of a ship. **serum s.,** a hypersensitivity reaction to the administration of foreign serum or serum proteins characterized by fever, urticaria, arthralgia, edema, and lymphadenopathy. It is caused by the formation of circulating antigen-antibody complexes that are deposited in tissues and trigger tissue injury mediated by complement and polymorphonuclear leukocytes. Serum sickness is classed with the Arthur's reaction and immune complex diseases as Type III in the Gell and Coombs classification of immune reactions. Although serum sickness is now rare because of the replacement of most animal-derived antisera with human immune globulins, an identical illness (*serum sickness–like reaction* or *syndrome*) can be produced by hypersensitivity reactions to penicillin and other drugs. **sleeping s.,** a disease characterized by increasing drowsiness and lethargy, caused by a protozoal infection, such as African trypanosomiasis, or by a viral infection, such as lethargic encephalitis, St. Louis encephalitis, or eastern or western encephalomyelitis. **space s.,** space adaptation syndrome. **stiff s.,** ephemeral fever of cattle. **sweating s.,** a febrile, tickborne illness affecting African cattle, especially calves, due to a toxin produced by *Hyalomma truncatum*, and characterized by the presence of moist eczematous lesions of the mucous membranes. **talking s.,** epidemic encephalitis marked by extreme excitement, muscular twitching, and talkativeness. **three-day s.,** ephemeral fever of cattle. **veld s., veldt s.,** heartwater. **vomiting s.,** Jamaican vomiting s. **x-ray s.,** radiation s.

s.i.d. abbreviation for L. *sem′el in di′e*, once a day; written also *semel in d*.

side (sīd) the lateral (right or left) portion or aspect of the body or a structure. **balancing s.,** the segment of a denture or dental arch on the side opposite to that toward which the mandible is moved. The term pertains to occlusion and bears no relation to masticatory activity. Called also *nonfunctioning s.* **functioning s.,** working s. **nonfunctioning s.,** balancing s. **working s.,** the segment of a denture or dental arch on the same side as that toward which the mandible is moved. The term pertains to occlusion and bears no relation to masticatory activity. Called also *functioning s.*

side-bone (sīd′bōn) a condition of horses marked by ossification of the lateral cartilages of the third phalanx of the foot.

side effect (sīd′ef-fekt″) a consequence other than the one(s) for which an agent or measure is used, as the adverse effects produced by a drug, especially on a tissue or organ system other than the one sought to be benefited by its administration.

siderinuria (sid″er-ĭ-nu′re-ah) [Gr. *sidēros* iron + *ouron* urine + *-ia*] excretion of iron in the urine.

siderism (sid′er-izm) metallotherapy.

sider(o)- [Gr. *sidēros* iron] a combining form denoting relationship to iron.

Siderobacter (sid′er-o-bak′ter) [*sidero-* + Gr. *bactron* a rod] a genus of gram-negative chemolithotrophic bacteria of uncertain status, affiliated with the family Siderocapsaceae.

sideroblast (sid′er-o-blast″) a nucleated red blood cell containing granules of iron in its cytoplasm.

Siderocapsa (sid″er-o-kap′sah) [*sidero-* + L. *capsa* box] a genus of gram-negative chemolithotrophic bacteria of the family Siderocapsaceae, occurring as one to many ellipsoidal cells encased in a common capsule that is crusted with iron compounds or manganese compounds or both. They are found in fresh water, free or attached to a substrate. The type species is S. *treu′bii.*

Siderocapsaceae (sid″er-o-kap-sa′se-e) a family of gram-negative chemolithotrophic bacteria made up of organisms that deposit iron or manganese oxides. It contains the genera *Naumanniella, Ochrobium, Siderocapsa,* and *Siderococcus.*

Siderococcus (sid″er-o-kok′us) [*sidero-* + Gr. *kokkos* berry] a genus of gram-negative chemolithotrophic bacteria of the family Siderocapsaceae, occurring as small, unencapsulated coccoid cells. Colonies may be covered with orange-yellow deposits of ferric hydroxide. They are found in fresh water and bottom muds. The type species is S. *limoni′ticus.*

siderocyte (sid′er-o-sīt″) an erythrocyte containing nonhemoglobin iron.

sideroderma (sid″er-o-der′mah) bronzed coloration of the skin from disorder of the metabolism of the iron from degenerated hemoglobin.

siderofibrosis (sid″er-o-fi-bro′sis) fibrosis of the spleen marked by iron-containing deposits.

siderogenous (sid″er-oj′ĕ-nus) [*sidero-* + Gr. *gennan* to produce] (*obs.*) producing or forming iron.

Sideromonas (sid″er-o-mo′nas) [*sidero-* + Gr. *monas* unit, from *monos* single] a genus of gram-negative chemolithotrophic bacteria of uncertain status, affiliated with the family Siderocapsaceae.

sideromycin (sid″er-o-mi′sin) any of a class of antibiotics structurally related to hydroxamic acid that inhibit bacterial growth by interfering with iron uptake. Sideromycins are synthesized by certain species of actinomycetes.

Sideronema (sid″er-o-ne′mah) [*sidero-* + Gr. *nēma* thread] a genus of gram-negative chemolithotrophic bacteria of uncertain status, affiliated with the family Siderocapsaceae.

sideropenia (sid″er-o-pe′ne-ah) [*sidero-* + Gr. *penia* poverty] iron deficiency; deficiency of iron in the body.

sideropenic (sid″er-o-pe′nik) pertaining to or characterized by deficiency of iron.

Siderophacus (sid″er-o′fah-kus) [*sidero-* + Gr. *phakos* lentil] in former systems of classification, a genus of appendaged bacteria. They appear to belong to the genera *Gallionella* and *Planctomyces.*

siderophage (sid′er-o-fāj″) a histiocyte laden with phagocytosed particles.

siderophil (sid′er-o-fil) 1. siderophilous. 2. a siderophilous tissue or structure.

siderophilin (si″der-of′ĭ-lin) transferrin.

siderophilous (sid″er-of′ĭ-lus) [*sidero-* + Gr. *philein* to love] having a tendency to absorb iron.

siderophone (sid′er-o-fōn) [*sidero-* + Gr. *phonē* voice] an instrument for detecting, by a telephone-like arrangement, the presence of iron splinters in the eyeball.

siderophore (sid′er-o-fōr″) [*sidero-* + Gr. *phoros* bearing] 1. a substance that binds iron. 2. a macrophage containing hemosiderin. 3. a compound produced by certain species of mycobacteria and enterobacteria that chelates iron and facilitates its uptake by the cell.

sideroscope (sid′er-o-skōp) [*sidero-* + *-scope*] a magnet or other appliance for determining the presence of metallic iron as a foreign body in the eye.

siderosilicosis (sid″er-o-sil″ĭ-ko′sis) pneumoconiosis due to the inhalation of iron-ore dust containing silica.

siderosis (sid″er-o′sis) 1. pneumoconiosis due to the inhalation of iron particles. 2. excess of iron in the blood. 3. the deposit of iron in a tissue. **s. bul′bi,** the deposit of an iron pigment within the eyeball. **s. conjuncti′vae,** a rust brown or yellowish discoloration of the conjunctiva due to the presence of an iron foreign body; the condition may also be seen in hemochromatosis. **hepatic s.,** the deposit of an abnormal quantity of iron in the liver; see also under *hemosiderosis.* **nutritional s.,** excessive iron in the blood due to a diet very high in iron and low in protein and calories. **pulmonary s.,** siderosis (def. 1). **urinary s.,** presence of hemosiderin granules in the urine.

Siderosphaera (sid″er-o-sfe′rah) [*sidero-* + Gr. *sphaira* sphere] a genus of gram-negative chemolithotrophic bacteria of uncertain status, affiliated with the family Siderocapsaceae.

siderotic (sid″er-ot′ik) pertaining to or characterized by siderosis.

siderous (sid′er-us) containing iron.

SIDS sudden infant death syndrome; see under *syndrome.*

Siegert's sign (se′gertz) [Ferdinand *Siegert,* German pediatrician, 1865–1946] see under *sign.*

Siegle's otoscope (ze′gelz) [Emil *Siegle,* French aurist in Stuttgart, 1833–1900] see under *otoscope.*

siemens (se′menz) the SI unit of conductivity, measured by the quantity of electricity transferred across the unit area, per unit potential gradient per unit time. Called also *mho.* Abbreviated S.

Siemerling's nucleus (se′mer-lingz) [Ernst *Siemerling,* German neurologist and psychiatrist, 1857–1931] see under *nucleus.*

Sieur's test (sign) (se-erz′) [Célestin *Sieur,* French surgeon, 1860–1955] see *coin test,* under *tests.*

sieve (siv) a device having pores or perforations of uniform size used for separating objects or particles of different sizes. **molecular s.,** a crystalline substance having uniform pores of molecular size that adsorbs smaller but not larger molecules; used in chemical separation.

sievert (se′vert) the SI unit of radiation absorbed dose equivalent, defined as that producing the same biologic effect in a specified tissue as 1 gray of high-energy x-rays; 1 sievert equals 100 rem. Abbreviated Sv.

Sig. abbreviation for L. *signe′tur,* let it be labeled.

sigh (si) [L. *suspirium*] an audible and prolonged inspiration, followed by an audible expiration.

sight (sīt) [A.S. *sihth*] 1. the act or faculty of vision. 2. a thing seen. **day s.,** nyctalopia, or night blindness. **far s., long s.,** hyperopia. **near s.,** myopia. **night s.,** hemeralopia, or day blindness. **old s.,** presbyopia. **second s.,** senopia. **short s.,** myopia.

sigmasism (sig′mah-sizm) sigmatism.

sigmatism (sig′mah-tizm) the incorrect, difficult, or too frequent use of the *s* sound.

sigmoid (sig′moid) [Gr. *sigmoeidēs,* from the letter *sigma* + *eidos* form] 1. shaped like the letter S or the letter C. 2. the sigmoid colon.

sigmoidectomy (sig″moi-dek′to-me) excision of the sigmoid colon.

sigmoiditis (sig″moi-di′tis) inflammation of the sigmoid colon.

sigmoidopexy (sig-moi′do-pek″se) [*sigmoid* + Gr. *pēxis* fixation] suspension of the sigmoid colon, usually performed for treatment of rectal prolapse.

sigmoidoproctostomy (sig-moi″do-prok-tos′to-me) the

creation of an artificial opening between the sigmoid colon and the rectum; also, the opening so created.

sigmoidorectostomy (sig-moi″do-rek-tos′to-me) sigmoidoproctostomy.

sigmoidoscope (sig-moi′do-skōp) [*sigmoid* + Gr. *skopein* to examine] a rigid or flexible endoscope with appropriate illumination for examining the sigmoid colon.

sigmoidoscopy (sig″moi-dos′ko-pe) inspection of the sigmoid colon through a sigmoidoscope.

sigmoidosigmoidostomy (sig-moi″do-sig-moi-dos′to-me) the operative formation of an anastomosis between two portions of the sigmoid colon; also, the opening so created.

sigmoidostomy (sig″moi-dos′to-me) [*sigmoid* + Gr. *stomoun* to provide with a mouth, or opening] the formation of an artificial opening from the surface of the body into the sigmoid colon; also, the opening so produced.

sigmoidotomy (sig″moi-dot′o-me) operative incision into the sigmoid colon.

sigmoidovesical (sig-moi″do-ves′ĭ-kal) pertaining to or communicating with the sigmoid colon and the urinary bladder, as a sigmoidovesical fistula.

Sigmund's glands (zig′moonts) [Karl Ludwig *Sigmund*, Austrian physician, 1810–1883] see under *gland*.

sign (sīn) [L. *signum*] an indication of the existence of something; any objective evidence of a disease, i.e., such evidence as is perceptible to the examining physician, as opposed to the subjective sensations (symptoms) of the patient. **Aaron's s.,** a sensation of pain or distress in the epigastric or precordial region on pressure over McBurney's point in appendicitis. **Abadie's s.,** 1. spasm of the levator palpebrae superioris muscle; a sign of Graves' disease. 2. insensibility of the Achilles tendon to pressure; seen in tabes dorsalis. **Abrahams' s.,** 1. a sound between dull and flat obtained on percussion over the acromion process in early tuberculosis of the apex of the lung. 2. acute pain produced in vesical lithiasis when pressure is applied midway between the umbilicus and the ninth right costal cartilage. **accessory s.,** any nonpathognomonic sign of disease. **air-cushion s.,** Klemm's s. **Allis' s.,** relaxation of the fascia between the crest of the ilium and the greater trochanter: a sign of fracture of the neck of the femur. **Amoss' s.,** in painful flexure of the spine, the patient, when rising to a sitting posture from lying in bed, does so by supporting himself with his hands placed far behind him in the bed. **Andral's s.,** see under *decubitus*. **André-Thomas s.,** if during the finger to nose test, the patient is directed to raise his arm over his head and is then suddenly ordered to let it fall to his head, the arm will rebound; seen in disease of the cerebellum. **Anghelescu's s.,** inability to bend the spine while lying on the back so as to rest on the head and heels alone, seen in tuberculosis of the vertebrae. **antecedent s.,** any precursory indication of an attack of disease. **anterior tibial s.,** involuntary contraction of the tibialis anterior muscle when the thigh is forcibly flexed on the abdomen; seen in spastic paraplegia. **anticus s.,** Piotrowski's s. **Argyll Robertson pupil s.,** see under *pupil*. **Arroyo's s.,** asthenocoria. **Aschner's s.,** oculocardiac reflex. **assident s.,** accessory s. **Auenbrugger's s.,** a bulging of the epigastrium, due to extensive pericardial effusion. **Aufrecht's s.,** noisy breathing heard just above the suprasternal notch, indicative of tracheal stenosis. **Babinski's s's,** 1. loss or lessening of the Achilles tendon reflex in sciatica: this distinguishes it from hysteric sciatica. 2. Babinski's reflex. 3. in hemiplegia, the contraction of the platysma muscle in the healthy side is more vigorous than on the affected side, as seen in opening the mouth, whistling, blowing, etc. 4. the patient lies supine on the floor, with arms crossed upon his chest, and then makes an effort to rise to the sitting posture. On the paralyzed side, the thigh is flexed upon the pelvis and the heel is lifted from the ground, while on the healthy side the limb does not move. This phenomenon is repeated when the patient resumes the lying posture. It is seen in organic hemiplegia, but not in hysterical hemiplegia. 5. when the paralyzed forearm is placed in supination, it turns over to pronation: seen in organic paralysis. Called also *pronation sign*. **Babinski's toe s.,** Babinski's reflex. **Baccelli's s.,** whisper heard over the chest in pleural effusion. **Baillarger's s.,** inequality of the pupils in paralytic dementia. **Ballance's s.,** resonance of right flank when the patient lies on the left side; said to be present in splenic rupture.

Ballet's s., external ophthalmoplegia, with loss of all voluntary eye movements, the pupillary movements and reflex eye movements persisting; seen in Graves' disease and hysteria. **Bamberger's s.,** 1. allochiria. 2. presence of signs of consolidation at the angle of the scapula, which disappear when the patient leans forward; a sign of pericardial effusion. **Bárány's s.,** see *caloric test*, under *test*. **Bard's s.,** in organic nystagmus the oscillations of the eye increase as the patient's attention follows the finger moved alternately from one side to the other; but in congenital nystagmus the oscillations disappear in like condition. **Barré's s.,** contraction of the iris is retarded in mental deterioration. **Barré's pyramidal s.,** the patient lies face down and the legs are flexed at the knee; he is unable to hold the legs in this vertical position if there is disease of the pyramidal tracts. **Baruch's s.,** resistance of the temperature in the rectum to a bath of 75° F. for fifteen minutes; a sign of typhoid fever. **Bastian-Bruns' s.,** see under *law*. **Battle's s.,** discoloration in the line of the posterior auricular artery, the ecchymosis first appearing near the tip of the mastoid process; seen in fracture of the base of the skull. **Becker's s.,** see under *phenomenon*. **Béclard's s.,** a sign of the maturity of the fetus consisting of a center of ossification in the lower epiphysis of the femur. **Beevor's s.,** 1. a sign of functional paralysis consisting in inability of the patient to inhibit the antagonistic muscles. 2. upward deviation of the umbilicus on attempting to lift the head, a sign of weakness of the lower abdominal muscles. **Béhier-Hardy s.,** aphonia in the early stages of pulmonary gangrene. **Bekhterev's s.,** 1. in tabes dorsalis, anesthesia of the popliteal space. 2. Bekhterev's reflex. **Bell's s.,** see under *phenomenon*. **Berger's s.,** an irregularly shaped or elliptical pupil in the early stages of tabes dorsalis, paralytic dementia, and certain paralyses. **Bergman's s.,** in urologic radiography, (*a*) the ureter is dilated immediately below a neoplasm, rather than collapsed as below an obstructing stone and (*b*) the ureteral catheter tends to coil in this dilated portion of the ureter. **Bethea's s.,** when the examiner, standing in back of the patient, places his fingers so that the tips rest on the upper surfaces of corresponding ribs high up in the patient's axillae, unilateral impairment of chest expansion is indicated by the lessened degree of respiratory movement of the ribs on the side affected. **Bezold's s.,** an inflammatory swelling below the apex of the mastoid process; evidence of mastoiditis. **Biederman's s.,** a dark red color (instead of the normal pink) of the anterior pillars of the throat, seen in some patients with syphilis. **Biermer's s.,** the metallic resonance over hydropneumothorax varies in pitch with change of position of the patient; seen in pneumothorax. Called also *change of sound* and *Gerhardt's sign*. **Biernacki's s.,** analgesia of the ulnar nerve in paralytic dementia and tabes dorsalis. **Binda's s.,** a sudden movement of the shoulder when the head is passively and sharply turned toward the other side, an early sign of tuberculous meningitis. **Biot's s.,** see under *respiration*. **Bird's s.,** a definite zone of dullness with absence of the respiratory sounds in hydatid disease of the lung. **Bjerrum's s.,** see under *scotoma*. **Blatin's s.,** hydatid thrill. **Blumberg's s.,** pain on abrupt release of steady pressure (rebound tenderness) over the site of a suspected abdominal lesion; seen in peritonitis. **Bonnet's s.,** pain on thigh adduction in sciatica. **Bordier-Fränkel s.,** an outward and upward rolling of the eye in peripheral facial paralysis. **Borsieri's s.,** when the fingernail is drawn along the skin in early stages of scarlet fever, a white line is left which quickly turns red; called also *Borsieri's line*. **Boston's s.,** in Graves' disease, when the eyeball is turned downward there is arrest of descent of the lid, spasm, and continued descent. **Bouchard's s.,** a few drops of Fehling's solution are added to the urine and the mixture is shaken; if pus from the kidney is present, fine bubbles will form, which push to the surface the coagulum formed by heating. **Bouillaud's s.,** permanent retraction of the chest in the precordial region; a sign of adherent pericardium. **Boyce's s.,** a gurgling sound heard on pressure by the hand on the side of the neck, in diverticulum of the esophagus. **Bozzolo's s.,** a visible pulsation of the arteries within the nostrils; said to indicate aneurysm of the thoracic aorta. **Bragard's s.,** with the knee stiff, the lower extremity is flexed at the hip until the patient experiences pain; the foot is then dorsiflexed. Increase of pain points to disease of the nerve root. **Branham's s.,** bradycardia produced by digital closure of an artery proximal to an arteriovenous fistula. **Braunwald s.,** occurrence of a weak pulse instead of a strong one immediately after a premature ventricular contraction. **Braxton Hicks' s.,** see under *contraction*. **Brickner's s.,** diminished oculoauricular associated movements seen in impairment of function of the facial nerve. **Broadbent's s.,** a retraction seen on the left side of the back, near the eleventh and twelfth ribs, related to pericardial adhesion. **Broadbent's inverted s.,** pulsations synchronizing with ventricular systole on the posterior lateral wall of the chest in gross dilatation of the left atrium. **Brockenbrough's s.,** occurrence of a weak pulse instead of a strong one immediately after a premature ventricular contraction. **Brodie's s.,** 1. a black spot on the glans penis: a sign of urinary extravasation into the spongiosum. 2. Brodie's pain. **Brown-Séquard's s.,** see under *syndrome*. **Brudzinski's s.,** 1. in meningitis, flexion of the neck usually results in flexion of the hip and knee. 2. in meningitis, when passive flexion of the lower limb on one side is made, a similar movement will be seen in the opposite limb; called also *contralateral sign*. **Brunati's s.,** the appearance of opacities in the cornea during the course of pneumonia or typhoid fever. **Bruns' s.,** see under *syndrome*. **Bryant's s.,** lowering of the axillary folds in dislocation of the shoulder. **Burger's s.,** Heryng's s. **Burghart's s.,** see under *symptom*. **Burton's s.,** lead line. **Cantelli's s.,** dissociation between the movements of the head and eyes: as the head is raised the eyes are lowered, and vice versa. Called also *doll's eye s.* **Capps' s.,** see under *reflex*. **Carabelli's s.,** see under *cusp*. **Cardarelli's s.,** transverse pulsation of the laryngotracheal tube in aneurysms and in dilatation of the arch of the aorta. **cardinal s's** (of inflammation), dolor, calor, rubor, tumor, and functio laesa; see *inflammation*. **cardiorespiratory s.,** a change in the normal pulse-respiration ratio from 4 : 1 to 2 : 1; seen in infantile scurvy. **Carman's s.,** meniscus s. **Carnett's s.,** the test for demonstrating parietal tenderness consists of palpation during a period in which the patient holds his anterior abdominal muscles as tense as possible. The tense abdominal muscles prevent the examiner's fingers from coming in contact with the underlying viscera and any tenderness that is elicited over them will be parietal in location. Tenderness elicited over relaxed muscles may be either parietal or intra-abdominal in origin. Tenderness present with relaxed muscles and absent with tense muscles is due to a subparietal lesion and its cause should be sought inside of the abdomen. Tenderness found both when the muscles are relaxed and when voluntarily tensed is due to an anterior parietal lesion and its cause should be sought outside the abdominal cavity. **Carvallo s.,** in tricuspid regurgitation, augmentation of the pansystolic murmur by inspiration. **Castellino's s.,** Cardarelli's s. **Cegka's s.,** invariability of the cardiac dullness during the different phases of respiration; a sign of adherent pericardium. **Chaddock's s.,** see under *reflex*. **Charcot's s.,** 1. the raising of the eyebrow in peripheral facial paralysis, and the lowering of the same part in facial contraction. 2. intermittent limping in arteriosclerosis of the legs and feet. **Cheyne-Stokes s.,** see under *respiration*. **Chilaiditi s.,** hepatoptosis (def. 2). **chin-retraction s.,** a sign of the third stage of anesthesia: the chin and larynx move downward during inspiration. **Chvostek's s., Chvostek-Weiss s.,** spasm of the facial muscles elicited by tapping the facial nerve in the region of the parotid gland; seen in tetany. **Claude's hyperkinesis s.,** reflex movements of paretic muscles elicited by painful stimuli. **clavicular s.,** a tumefaction at the inner third of the right clavicle; seen in congenital syphilis. Called also *Higouménakis's* s. **Cleeman's s.,** creasing of the skin just above the patella, indicative of fracture of the femur with overriding of fragments. **Cloquet's needle s.,** a clean needle is plunged into the biceps muscle; if life is not extinct, the needle oxidizes in 20–60 minutes. **Codman's s.,** in rupture of the supraspinatus tendon, the arm can be passively abducted without pain, but when support of the arm is removed and the deltoid contracts suddenly, pain occurs again. **cogwheel s.,** see under *phenomenon*. **coin s.,** see under *tests*. **Cole's s.,** deformity of the duodenal contour as seen in the roentgenogram, a sign of the presence of duodenal ulcer. **commemorative s.,** any sign of a previous disease. **Comolli's s.,** a sign of scapular fracture consisting in the appearance in the scapular region, shortly after the accident, of a triangular swelling reproducing the shape of the body of the scapula. **complementary op-**

position s., Grasset-Gaussel-Hoover s. **contralateral s.,** Brudzinski's s., def. 2. **Coopernail s.,** ecchymosis on the perineum and scrotum or labia: a sign of fracture of the pelvis. **Cope's s.,** psoas s. **Corrigan's s.,** 1. a purple line at the junction of the teeth and gum in chronic copper poisoning. 2. a peculiar expanding pulsation indicative of aneurysm of the abdominal aorta; see also *Corrigan's pulse*, under *pulse*. 3. see under *respiration*. **coughing s.,** Huntington's s. **Courvoisier's s.,** see under *law*. **Cowen's s.,** jerky constriction of the contralateral pupil when light is shown into the pupil, a sign of Graves' disease. **Crichton-Browne's s.,** tremor of the outer angles of the eyes and of the labial commissures in the earlier stages of paralytic dementia. **Cruveilhier's s.,** a swelling in the groin is palpated when the patient coughs: in saphenous varix there is felt a tremor as of a jet of water entering and filling the pouch. **Cullen's s.,** a bluish discoloration of the skin around the umbilicus sometimes associated with intraperitoneal hemorrhage, especially following rupture of the uterine tube in ectopic pregnancy. A similar discoloration is seen in acute hemorrhagic pancreatitis. **Dalrymple's s.,** abnormal wideness of the palpebral opening in Graves' disease. **D'Amato's s.,** in pleural effusion, the location of dullness is altered from the vertebral area in the sitting position to the heart region when the patient assumes a lateral position on the side opposite the effusion. **Damoiseau's s.,** Ellis' line. **Darier's s.,** urtication and itching occurring on rubbing the lesions of urticaria pigmentosa. **Davidsohn's s.,** decrease of illumination of the pupil on transillumination with an electric light placed in the mouth; indicates tumor or fluid in the maxillary antrum. **Davis' s.,** an empty state and a yellowish or pale tint of the pulseless arteries; a sign of death. **Dawbarn's s.,** in acute subacromial bursitis, when the arm hangs by the side palpation over the bursa causes pain, but when the arm is abducted this pain disappears. **Dejerine's s.,** aggravation of symptoms of radiculitis produced by coughing, sneezing, and straining at stool. **de la Camp's s.,** relative dullness over and at each side of the fifth and sixth vertebrae in tuberculosis of the bronchial lymph nodes. **Delbet's s.,** in aneurysm of the main artery of a limb, if the nutrition of the part distal to the aneurysm is maintained, although the pulse may have disappeared, the collateral circulation is sufficient. **Delmege's s.,** deltoid flattening; said to be an early sign of tuberculosis. **Demarquay's s.,** fixation or lowering of the larynx during phonation and deglutition; a sign of syphilis of the trachea. **Demianoff's s.,** a sign that permits the differentiation of pain originating in the sacrolumbalis muscles from lumbar pain of any other origin. The sign is obtained by placing the patient in dorsal decubitus and lifting his extended leg. In the presence of lumbago this produces a pain in the lumbar region which prevents raising the leg high enough to form an angle of 10 degrees, or even less, with the table or bed on which the patient reposes. The pain is due to the stretching of the sacrolumbalis. **de Musset's s.,** Musset's s. **de Mussy's s.,** see under *point*. **Dennie's s.,** Morgan's line. **Desault's s.,** a sign of intracapsular fracture of the femur, consisting of alteration of the arc described by rotation of the great trochanter, which normally describes the segment of a circle, but in this fracture rotates only as the apex of the femur as it rotates about its own axis. **d'Espine's s.,** in the normal person, on auscultation over the spinous processes, pectoriloquy ceases at the bifurcation of the trachea, and in infants opposite the seventh cervical vertebra. If pectoriloquy is heard lower than this, it indicates enlargement of the bronchial lymph nodes. **Dew's s.,** in diaphragmatic hydatid abscess beneath the right cupola, the area of resonance moves caudally with the patient on hands and knees. **Dixon Mann's s.,** Mann's s. **doll's eye s.,** Cantelli's s. **Dorendorf's s.,** fullness of the supraclavicular groove on one side in aneurysm of the aortic arch. **Drummond's s.,** a whiff heard at the open mouth during respiration in cases of aortic aneurysm. **D.T.P. s.** (*distal tingling on percussion*), Tinel's s. **Du Bois' s.,** shortness of the little finger in congenital syphilis. **Duchenne's s.,** the sinking in of the epigastrium on inspiration in paralysis of the diaphragm or in certain cases of hydropericardium. **Duckworth's s.,** see under *phenomenon*. **Dugas' s.,** see under *tests*. **Duncan-Bird s.,** Bird's s. **Dupuytren's s.,** 1. a crackling sensation on pressure over a sarcomatous bone. 2. in congenital dislocation of the head of the femur, there is a free up-and-down movement of the head of the bone. **Duroziez's s.,** see under *murmur.* **echo s.,** 1. a percussion sound resembling an echo which is heard over a hydatid cyst. 2. the repetition of the last word or clause of a sentence, seen in certain brain diseases; echolalia. **Elliot's s.,** 1. induration of the edge of a syphilitic skin lesion. 2. a scotoma extending from the blind spot and made up of numerous points or spots. **Ellis' s.,** the peculiar curved line of dullness discoverable during resorption of a pleuritic exudate. **Ely's s.,** see under *tests.* **Enroth's s.,** abnormal fullness of the eyelids in Graves' disease. **Erb's s.,** 1. increased electric irritability of motor nerves in cases of tetany. 2. dullness in percussion over the manubrium of the sternum in acromegaly. **Erben's s.,** see under *reflex.* **Erichsen's s.,** when the iliac bones are sharply pressed toward each other pain is felt in sacroiliac disease but not in hip disease. **Erni's s.,** the cavernous tympany developed over an apical cavity that has previously been filled with fluid. Sometimes gently rapping over such a filled cavity with a hard instrument will excite coughing, which will expel the secretion, and thus the cavernous signs are developed. **Escherich's s.,** in tetany, percussion of the inner surface of the lips or tongue produces contraction of the lips, tongue, and masseter muscles. **ether s.,** a sign of death: 1 or 2 ml. of ether is injected subcutaneously. If the ether spurts back when the needle is withdrawn, death has occurred. Its absorption indicates that life still persists. **Eustace Smith's s.,** Smith's s. **Ewart's s.,** 1. undue prominence of the sternal end of the first rib in certain cases of pericardial effusion. 2. bronchial breathing and dullness on percussion at the lower angle of the left scapula in pericardial effusion. **Ewing s.,** tenderness at the upper inner angle of the orbit: a sign of obstruction of the frontal sinus. **external malleolar s.,** Chaddock's reflex. **fabere s.,** see *Patrick's test,* under *tests.* **facial s.,** Chvostek's s. **Fajersztajn's crossed sciatic s.,** in sciatica, when the leg is flexed, the hip can also be flexed, but not when the leg is held straight; flexing the sound thigh with the leg held straight causes pain on the affected side. **fan s.,** spreading apart of the toes following the stroking of the sole of the foot; it forms part of the Babinski reflex. **Federici's s.,** on auscultation of the abdomen, the cardiac sounds can be heard in cases of intestinal perforation with gas in the peritoneal cavity. **Filipovitch's s.,** the yellow discoloration of prominent parts of the palms and soles in typhoid fever; called also *palmoplantar s.* **Fischer's s.,** 1. on auscultation over the manubrium with the patient's head bent backward, there is sometimes heard, in tuberculosis of the bronchial glands, a murmur due to pressure of the glands on the innominate veins. 2. a presystolic murmur in certain cases of adherent pericardium. **flag s.,** dyspigmentation of the hair occurring as a band of light hair, seen in children who have recovered from kwashiorkor. **flushtank s.,** the passage of a large amount of urine and the coincident temporary disappearance of a lumbar swelling; a sign of hydronephrosis. **forearm s.,** Leri's s. **formication s.,** Tinel's s. **Fränkel's s.,** excessive range of passive movement of the hip joint, indicating diminished tone of the surrounding musculature in tabes dorsalis. **Friedreich's s.,** 1. diastolic collapse of the cervical veins due to adherent pericardium. 2. lowering of the pitch of the percussion note over an area of cavitation during forced inspiration; called also *Friedreich's change of note.* **Froment's paper s.,** flexion of the distal phalanx of the thumb when a sheet of paper is held between the thumb and index finger; seen in affections of the ulnar nerve. **Fürbringer's s.,** in cases of subphrenic abscess, the respiratory movements will be transmitted to a needle inserted into the abscess, which is thus distinguished from abscess above the diaphragm. **Gaenslen's s.,** with the patient on his back on the operating table, the knee and hip of one leg are held in flexed position by the patient, while the other leg, hanging over the edge of the table, is pressed down by the examiner to produce hyperextension of the hip: pain occurs on the affected side in lumbosacral disease. **Galeazzi s.,** in congenital dislocation of the hip, apparent shortening of the femur, as shown by the difference of knee levels with the knees and hips flexed at right angles with the patient lying on a flat table. **Garel's s.,** Heryng's s. **Gerhardt's s.,** Biermer's s. **Gianelli's s.,** Tournay's s. **Gifford's s.,** inability to evert the upper lid; seen in Graves' disease. **Gilbert's s.,** opsiuria indicative of hepatic cirrhosis. **Glasgow's s.,** a systolic sound in the brachial artery in

latent aneurysm of the aorta. **Goggia's s.,** in health, the fibrillary contraction produced by striking and then pinching the brachial biceps extends throughout the whole muscle: in debilitating disease, such as typhoid fever, the contraction is local. **Goldstein's s.,** wide space of distance between the great toe and the adjoining toe seen in cretinism and Down's syndrome. **Goldthwait's s.,** the patient lying supine, his leg is raised by the examiner with one hand, the other hand being placed under the patient's lower back; leverage is then applied to the side of the pelvis. If pain is felt by the patient before the lumbar spine is moved, the lesion is a sprain of the sacroiliac joint. If pain does not appear until after the lumbar spine moves, the lesion is in the sacroiliac or lumbosacral articulation. **Golonbov's s.,** tenderness on percussion over the tibia in chlorosis. **Goodell's s.,** if the woman's cervix uteri is soft she is pregnant; if it is hard she is not. **Gordon's s.,** finger phenomenon (def. 1). **Gottron's s.,** 1. a cutaneous sign pathognomonic of dermatomyositis, consisting of symmetrical macular violaceous erythema, with or without edema, overlying the dorsal aspect of the interphalangeal joints of the hands, olecranon processes, patellas, and medial malleoli. 2. see under *papule.* **Gowers' s.,** 1. abrupt intermittent oscillation of the iris under the influence of light; seen in certain stages of tabes dorsalis. 2. a sign of pseudohypertrophic muscular dystrophy; to stand from the supine position, the patient rolls to the prone position, kneels, and raises himself to a standing position by pushing with his hands against shins, knees, and thighs. Called also *Gower's maneuver* and *Gower's phenomenon.* **Graefe's s.,** failure of the upper lid to move downward promptly and evenly with the eyeball in looking downward, instead it moves tardily and jerkingly; seen in Graves' disease. **Grancher's s.,** equality of pitch between expiratory and inspiratory murmurs; a sign of obstruction to expiration. **Granger's s.,** if in the radiograph of an infant two years old or less, the anterior wall of the lateral sinus is visible, extensive destruction of the mastoid is indicated. **Grasset's s., Grasset-Bychowski s.,** Grasset's phenomenon. **Grasset-Gaussel-Hoover s.,** when the patient in a recumbent position attempts to lift the paretic limb, there is greater downward pressure on the examiner's hand with the sound limb than is observed in the test with a normal person. **Greene's s.,** outward displacement of the free cardiac border by the expiratory movement in pleuritic effusion; it is detected by percussion. **Grey Turner's s.,** Turner's s. **Griesinger's s.,** edematous swelling behind the mastoid process; seen in thrombosis of the transverse sinus. **Griffith's s.,** lower lid lag on upward gaze, a sign of Graves' disease. **Grisolle's s.,** the papule of smallpox can be felt beneath the skin when the skin over the lesion is stretched; to the contrary, if the papule becomes impalpable, it is a lesion of measles. **Grocco's s.,** 1. a sign of pleural effusion consisting of the presence of a triangular area of dullness (*Grocco's, Korányi-Grocco, paravertebral,* or *Rauchfuss' triangle*) on the back, on the side opposite to that on which the effusion is present. Called also *Grocco's triangular dullness.* 2. extension of the liver dullness to the left of the midspinal line, indicating enlargement of the organ. **Grossman's s.,** dilatation of the heart as a sign of pulmonary tuberculosis. **Gubler's s.,** see under *tumor.* **Guilland's s.,** brisk flexion at the hip and knee joint when the contralateral quadriceps muscle is pinched; a sign of meningeal irritation. **Gunn's s.,** a raising of a ptosed eyelid on opening the mouth and moving the jaw toward the opposite side in the Gunn syndrome. **Gunn's crossing s.,** a crossing of an artery over a vein in the fundus of the eye, indicative of essential hypertension. **Gunn's pupillary s.,** swinging flashlight s. **Guyon's s.,** the ballottement and palpation of a floating kidney. **Hahn's s.,** persistent rotation of the head from side to side in cerebellar disease of childhood. **Hall's s.,** a tracheal diastolic shock felt in aneurysm of the aorta. **halo s.,** a halo effect produced in the roentgenogram of the fetal head between the subcutaneous fat and the cranium; said to be indicative of intrauterine death of the fetus. **Hamman's s.,** a precordial crunching, clicking, or knocking sound, synchronous with each heart beat, heard on ausculation in such conditions as acute mediastinitis, pneumomediastinum, and pneumothorax. **harlequin s.,** reddening of the lower half of the laterally recumbent body and blanching of the upper half, due to temporary vasomotor disturbance in newborn infants. **Hatchcock's s.,** tenderness on running the finger toward the angle of the jaw in mumps. **Haudek's s.,** a projecting shadow in radiographs of penetrating gastric ulcer, due to settlement of bismuth in pathologic niches of the stomach wall; called also *Haudek's niche.* **Heberden's s's,** see under *node.* **Hefke-Turner s.,** a widening and change in contour of the normal obturator x-ray shadow, indicative of pathologic condition of the hip joint; called also *obturator s.* **Hegar's s.,** softening of the lower segment of the uterus, an indication of pregnancy. **Heilbronner's s.,** see under *thigh.* **Heim-Kreysig s.,** a depression of the intercostal spaces occurring along with the cardiac systole in adherent pericarditis. **Helbing's s.,** medialward curving of the Achilles tendon as viewed from behind; seen in flatfoot. **Hellat's s.** (*obs.*), in mastoid suppuration, a tuning fork placed on the diseased area is heard for a shorter time than when placed on any other part. **Hellendall's s.,** Cullen's s. **Hennebert's s.,** in the labyrinthitis of congenital syphilis, compression of the air in the external auditory canal produces a rotatory nystagmus to the diseased side; rarefaction of the air in the canal produces a nystagmus to the opposite side. Called also *pneumatic s.* or *test.* **Henning's s.,** an angular deformity of the angulus of the stomach, in which it assumes a Gothic arch shape; a sign of chronic gastric ulcer. Called also *Gothic arch formation.* **Heryng's s.,** an infraorbital shadow produced by fluid or by a hypertrophied, hyperplastic, or neoplastic membrane in the maxillary antrum and observable by electric illumination of the buccal cavity; seen in diseases of the antrum of Highmore (maxillary sinus). **Hicks' s.,** see *Braxton Hicks contractions,* under contraction. **Higouménakis' s.,** clavicular s. **Hill's s.,** disproportionate femoral systolic hypertension. **Hirschberg's s.,** adduction, inversion, and slight plantar flexion of the foot on stroking the inner aspect (not the sole) of the foot from the great toe to the heel; called also *adductor reflex of foot.* **Hochsinger's s.,** 1. indicanuria in the tuberculosis of childhood. 2. see under *phenomenon.* **Hoehne's s.,** absence of uterine contractions during delivery despite repeated injections of oxytocics, regarded as a sign of rupture of the uterus. **Hoffmann's s.,** 1. increased mechanical irritability of the sensory nerves in tetany; the ulnar nerve is usually tested. 2. a sudden nipping of the nail of the index, middle, or ring finger produces flexion of the terminal phalanx of the thumb and of the second and third phalanx of some other finger; called also *digital reflex, Hoffmann's reflex,* and *Trömmer's* s. **Holmes' s.,** rebound phenomenon. **Homans' s.,** pain on passive dorsiflexion of the foot; a sign of thrombosis of deep calf veins. **Hoover's s.,** 1. in the normal state or in genuine paralysis, if the patient, lying on a couch, is directed to press the leg against the couch, there will be a lifting movement seen in the other leg; this phenomenon is absent in hysteria and malingering. 2. movement of the costal margins toward the midline in inspiration, occurring bilaterally in pulmonary emphysema and unilaterally in conditions causing flattening of the diaphragm, such as pleural effusion and pneumothorax. **Hope's s.,** double heart beat in aortic aneurysm. **Horn's s.,** pain produced by traction on the right spermatic cord in acute appendicitis. **Horner's s.,** Spalding's s. **Horsley's s.,** if there is a difference in the temperature in the two axillae, the higher temperature will be on the paralyzed side. **Howship-Romberg s.,** pain passing down the inner side of the thigh to the knee due to pressure on the obturator nerve by an obturator hernia. **Hoyne's s.,** a sign elicited in paralytic or nonparalytic poliomyelitis: with the patient in the supine position, his head falls back when his shoulders are elevated. **Huchard's s.,** paradoxic percussion resonance in pulmonary edema. **Hueter's s.,** the absence of the transmission of osseous vibration in cases of fracture with fibrous material interposed between the fragments. **Human's s.,** chin-retraction s. **Huntington's s.,** the patient is recumbent, with his legs hanging over the edge of a table, and is told to cough. If the coughing produces flexion of the thigh and extension of the leg in the paralyzed limb, it indicates that the paralysis is due to an upper motor neuron lesion. **Hutchinson's s.,** 1. interstitial keratitis and a dull-red discoloration of the cornea in inherited syphilis. 2. see under *tooth.* 3. see under *triad.* **hyperkinesis s.,** see *Claude's hyperkinesis s.* **interossei s.,** Souques's phenomenon. **Itard-Cholewa s.,** anesthesia of the tympanic membrane in otosclerosis. **Jaccoud's s.,** prominence of the aorta in the suprasternal notch. **Jackson's s.,** 1. [Chevalier *Jackson*] see *asthmatoid wheeze,* under *wheeze.* 2. [James *Jackson,* Jr.] prolongation of the expiratory sound over the affected area in

pulmonary tuberculosis. **Jellinek's s.,** the pigmentation, usually brownish, occurring on the lid margins in many cases of hyperparathyroidism; called also *Rasin's s.* **Jendrassik's s.,** paralysis of the extraocular muscles in Graves' disease. **Joffroy's s.,** absence of forehead wrinkling in Graves' disease when the patient suddenly turns his eye upward. **jugular s.,** Queckenstedt's s. **Jürgensen's s.,** delicate crepitation sometimes heard in auscultation in acute pulmonary tuberculosis. **Kanavel's s.,** a point of maximum tenderness in the palm 1 inch proximal to the base of the little finger in infection of tendon sheath. **Kantor's s.,** a thin stringlike shadow in the roentgenogram of the colon through the filling defect; seen in colitis and regional ileitis. **Karplus' s.,** a modification of the vocal resonance, in which, on auscultation over a pleural effusion, the vowel *u* spoken by the patient is heard as *a.* **Kashida's s.,** spasm of muscles and hyperesthesia produced by applying heat or cold; seen in tetany. **Keen's s.,** increased diameter of the leg at the malleoli in Pott's fracture of the fibula. **Kehr's s.,** severe pain in the left shoulder in some cases of rupture of the spleen. **Kellock's s.,** increase of the vibration of the ribs on sharp percussion with the right hand, the left hand being placed firmly on the thorax under the nipple; a sign of pleural effusion. **Kelly's s.,** if the ureter is teased with an artery forceps, it will contract like a snake or worm. **Kerandel's s.,** deep hyperesthesia accompanied by pain, often retarded, after some slight blow upon a bony projection of the body; seen in African trypanosomiasis. Called also *Kerandel's symptom.* **Kergaradec's s.,** uterine souffle. **Kernig's s.,** in dorsal decubitus, the patient can easily and completely extend the leg; in the sitting posture or when lying with the thigh flexed upon the abdomen, the leg cannot be completely extended; it is a sign of meningitis. **Kerr's s.,** alteration of the texture of the skin below the somatic level in lesions of the spinal cord. **Kestenbaum's s.,** a decrease in number of arterioles traversing the optic disk margin as a criterion for optic atrophy. **Kleist's s.,** the fingers of the patient when gently elevated by the fingers of the examiner will hook into the examiner's fingers; indicative of frontal and thalamic lesions. **Klemm's s.,** in the roentgenogram in chronic appendicitis, there is often an indication of tympanites in the right lower quadrant. **Klippel-Feil s.,** flexion and adduction of the thumb when the patient's flexed fingers are quickly extended by the examiner; indicative of pyramidal tract disease. **Knie's s.,** unequal dilatation of the pupils in Graves' disease. **Kocher's s.,** a sign of Graves' disease: the examiner places his hand on a level with the patient's eyes and then lifts it higher; the patient's upper lid springs up more quickly than does his eyeball. **Koplik's s.,** see under *spot.* **Korányi's s.,** increase of resonance over the dorsal segment on percussion of the spinal processes of the thoracic vertebrae; a sign of pleural effusion. **Kreysig's s.,** Heim-Kreysig s. **Krisovski's (Krisowski's) s.,** cicatricial lines which radiate from the mouth in congenital syphilis. **Kussmaul's s.,** 1. distention of the jugular veins on inspiration, seen in constrictive pericarditis and mediastinal tumor. 2. convulsions and coma in gastric disease as a result of toxin absorption. 3. paradoxical pulse. **Küstner's s.,** a cystic tumor on the median line anterior to the uterus in cases of ovarian dermoids. **Laborde's s.,** Cloquet's needle s. **Ladin's s.,** a sign of pregnancy, consisting of a circular elastic area, which offers a sensation of fluctuation to the examining finger, situated in the median line of the anterior surface of the body of the uterus just above the junction of the body and the cervix. This area increases in size as pregnancy advances. **Laënnec's s.,** the occurrence of rounded, gelatinous masses (Laënnec's pearls) in the sputum of bronchial asthma. **Lafora's s.,** picking of the nose regarded as an early sign of cerebrospinal meningitis. **Langoria's s.,** relaxation of the extensor muscles of the thigh; a symptom of intracapsular fracture of the femur. **Larcher's s.,** grayish, cloudy discolorations of the conjunctivae that are speedily blackened; a sign of death. **Lasègue's s.,** in sciatica, flexion of the hip is painful when the knee is extended, but painless when the knee is flexed. This distinguishes the disorder from disease of the hip joint. **Laugier's s.,** a condition in which the styloid process of the radius and of the ulna are on the same level; seen in fracture of the lower part of the radius. **leg s.,** 1. Schlesinger's s. 2. Neri's s. **Leichtenstern's s.,** in cerebrospinal meningitis, tapping lightly any bone of the extremities causes the patient to wince suddenly. **Lenn-**

hoff's s., a furrow appearing on deep inspiration below the lowest rib and above an echinococcus cyst of the liver. **Leri's s.,** passive flexion of the hand and wrist of the affected side in hemiplegia shows no normal flexion at the elbow. **Leser-Trélat s.,** the sudden appearance and rapid increase in size and number of seborrheic keratoses may be a sign of internal malignancy, especially of the gastrointestinal tract. **Leudet's s.,** see under *tinnitus*. **Levasseur's s.,** the failure of the scarificator and cupping-glass to draw blood; a sign of death. **Lhermitte's s.,** the development of sudden, transient, electric-like shocks spreading down the body when the patient flexes the head forward; seen mainly in multiple sclerosis but also in compression and other disorders of the cervical cord. **Libman's s.,** extreme tenderness, but without pain on pressure, of the tips of the mastoid bones. **Lichtheim's s.,** in subcortical aphasia, although the patient cannot speak, he is able to indicate with his fingers the number of syllables in the word he is thinking of. **ligature s.,** in hematuria, the development of ecchymoses in the distal part of a limb to which a ligature has been applied. **Linder's s.,** with the patient recumbent or sitting with outstretched legs, passive flexion of the head will cause pain in the leg or the lumbar region in sciatica. **Litten's s.,** see under *phenomenon*. **Livierato's s.,** vasoconstriction when the abdominal sympathetic nerve is irritated by striking the anterior abdomen along the xiphoumbilical line. **Lloyd's s.,** a symptom of renal calculus, consisting of pain in the loin on deep percussion over the kidney, even when pressure causes no pain. **Lombardi's s.,** the appearance of venous varicosities in the region of the spinous processes of the seventh cervical and first three thoracic vertebrae; seen in early pulmonary tuberculosis. **Lucas' s.,** distention of the abdomen in the early stages of rickets. **Ludloff's s.,** swelling and ecchymosis at the base of Scarpa's triangle together with inability to raise the thigh when in a sitting posture, a sign of traumatic separation of the epiphysis of the greater trochanter. **Lust's s.,** see under *phenomenon*. **McBurney's s.,** tenderness at a point two-thirds the distance from the umbilicus to the anterior superior spine of the ilium; indicative of appendicitis. See also under *point*. **Macewen's s.,** on percussion of the skull behind the junction of the frontal, temporal, and parietal bones, there is a more resonant note than normal in internal hydrocephalus and cerebral abscess. **McGinn-White s.,** a Q wave and late inversion of the T wave in lead III, low S-T intervals and T waves in lead II, and inverted T waves in chest leads V_2 and V_3, the electrocardiographic evidence of right ventricular dilatation due to massive pulmonary embolism, plus the clinical signs of acute cor pulmonale. **McMurray s.,** occurrence of a cartilage click during manipulation of the knee; indicative of meniscal injury. **Magendie's s., Magendie-Hertwig s.,** skew deviation. **Magnan's s.,** see under *symptom*. **Mangus' s.,** after death, light ligation of a finger causes no visible change in its distal portion. **Mahler's s.,** a steady increase of pulse rate without corresponding elevation of temperature; seen in thrombosis. **Maisonneuve's s.,** marked hyperextensibility of the hand; a symptom of Colles' fracture. **Mann's s.,** 1. in Graves' disease the two eyes appear not to be on the same level. 2. lessened resistance of the scalp to a constant electric current; seen in certain traumatic neuroses. Called also *Dixon Mann's s.* **Mannkopf's s.,** increase in the frequency of the pulse on pressure over a painful spot; not present in simulated pain. **Marcus Gunn's pupillary s.,** swinging flashlight s. **Marfan's s.,** a red triangle at the tip of a coated tongue indicates typhoid fever; a rarely observed phenomenon. **Marie's s.,** tremor of the body or extremities in Graves' disease. **Marie-Foix s.,** withdrawal of lower leg on transverse pressure of tarsus or forced flexion of toes, even when the leg is incapable of voluntary movement. **Marinesco's s.,** Marinesco's succulent hand; see under *hand*. **Mayo's s.,** relaxation of the muscles controlling the lower jaw, indicative of profound anesthesia. **Means' s.,** lag of the eyeball on upward gaze in Graves' disease. **Meltzer's s.,** loss of the normal second sound, heard on auscultation of the heart after swallowing; symptomatic of occlusion or contraction of the lower part of the esophagus. **Mendel-Bekhterev s.,** see under *reflex*. **meniscus s.,** the radioscopic appearance of a crescentic shadow made by the crater of a gastric ulcer: when the convexity of the crescent points outward the ulcer is on the lesser curvature; when the convexity points downward the ulcer is distal to the angular incisure. **Mennell's s.,** an examining thumb is placed over the posterosuperior spine of the sacrum and then made to slide, first outward and then inward. If on pressure over the former point tenderness is detected, it is due to a sensitive deposit in the structures of the gluteal aspect of the posterosuperior spine. If the tenderness is over the inner point, it is probable that the superior ligaments of the sacroiliac joint are strained and sensitive. If the tenderness is increased by pressure backward on the anterosuperior aspect of the ilium and decreased by pulling forward the crest from behind, this is positive proof that it is caused by the sensitive ligaments. **Minor's s.,** the method of rising from a sitting position characteristic of the patient with sciatica; he supports himself on the healthy side, placing one hand on the back, bending the affected leg and balancing on the healthy leg. **Mirchamp's s.,** when a sapid substance, such as vinegar, is applied to the mucous membrane of the tongue, a painful reflex secretion of saliva in the gland about to be affected is indicative of sialadenitis, e.g., mumps. **Möbius' s.,** inability to keep the eyeballs converged in Graves' disease; due to insufficiency of the internal recti muscles. **Moebius' s.,** Möbius' s. **Monteverde's s.,** failure of any response to the subcutaneous injection of ammonia; a sign of death. **Morquio's s.,** the patient lying supine resists all attempts to raise the trunk to a sitting posture until the legs are passively flexed; noticed in epidemic poliomyelitis. **Moschcowitz's s.,** see under *tests*. **Mosler's s.,** sternal tenderness in acute myeloblastic anemia. **moulage s.,** a waxy cast appearance of bowel segments, a roentgenographic sign of celiac disease. **Müller's s.,** a sign of aortic insufficiency consisting of pulsation of the uvula and redness of the tonsils and velum palati, occurring synchronously with the action of the heart. **Munson's s.,** abnormal bulging of the lower lid when the patient rolls his eyes downward, caused by abnormal curvature of the cornea (keratoconus). **Murat's s.,** in the tuberculous patient there is vibration of the affected side of the chest with a feeling of discomfort when speaking. **Murphy's s.,** a sign of gallbladder disease consisting of interruption of the patient's deep inspiration when the physician's fingers are pressed deeply beneath the right costal arch, below the hepatic margin. **Musset's s.,** rhythmical jerking movement of the head; seen in cases of aortic aneurysm and aortic insufficiency. **Myerson's s.,** ready induction of blepharospasm when the frontalis muscle is tapped, a sign of Parkinson's disease. **neck s.,** Brudzinski's s., def. 1. **Negro s.,** cogwheel phenomenon. **Neri's s.,** 1. a sign of organic hemiplegia, consisting in the spontaneous bending of the knee of the affected side as the leg is passively lifted, the patient being in the dorsal position. 2. with the patient standing, forward bending of the trunk will cause flexion of the knee on the affected side in lumbosacral and iliosacral lesions. **niche s.,** Haudek's s. **Nicoladoni's s.,** Branham's s. **Nikolsky's s.,** ready separation of the outer layer of the epidermis from the basal layer with sloughing of the skin produced by minor trauma, such as by exerting a sliding or rubbing pressure on the area involved, which may occur in pemphigus and in other conditions such as certain hereditary blistering skin diseases, scalded skin syndrome, adult toxic epidermal necrolysis, and thermal burns. **Ober's s.,** see under *tests*. **objective s.,** one that can be seen, heard, or felt by the diagnostician; called also *physical s.* **obturator s.,** 1. hypogastric or adductor pain elicited by passive internal rotation of the flexed thigh, due to contact between an inflammatory process and the internal obturator muscle; a sign of appendicitis. 2. see *Hefke-Turner s.* **Oliver's s.,** tracheal tugging; see under *tugging*. **ophthalmoscopic s.,** as death approaches, the blood in the retinal vessels gradually ceases to move and the column of blood splits into fragments. **Oppenheim's s.,** dorsiflexion of the big toe on stroking downward the medial side of the tibia; seen in pyramidal tract disease. **orbicularis s.,** in hemiplegia, inability to close the eye on the paralyzed side without closing the other. **Ortolani's s.,** the presence of a palpable click in and out as the hip is reduced by abduction and dislocated by adduction in congenital dislocation of the hip; called also *Ortolani's click.* **Osler's s.,** small, painful, erythematous swellings in the skin of the hands and feet in malignant endocarditis; Osler's nodes. **palmoplantar s.,** Filipovitch's s. **Parkinson's s.,** see under *facies*. **Parrot's s.,** 1. dilatation of the pupil on pinching the skin of the neck; seen in meningitis. 2. bony nodes on the outer table of the skull of infants with congenital syphilis, giving it a buttock shape; called also *Parrot's* nodes. **Pastia's s.,** see under *line.* **patent bronchus s.,** the radiologic finding of an unobstructed bronchus supplying a collapsed lung, lobe, or segment. **Patrick's s.,** see under *tests.* **Pende's s.,** André-Thomas s. **Perez's s.,** a friction sound heard over the sternum when the patient raises and drops his arms; a sign of mediastinal tumor or of aneurysm of the arch of the aorta. **peroneal s.,** dorsal flexion and abduction of the foot, a sign of latent tetany elicited by tapping the peroneal nerve just below the head of the fibula, while the knee is relaxed and slightly flexed. **Pfuhl's s.,** inspiration increases the force of flow in paracentesis in the case of subphrenic abscess, but lessens it in the case of pyopneumothorax. This distinction is lost when the diaphragm is paralyzed. **Pfuhl-Jaffé s.,** in pyopneumothorax, the liquid issues from the exploratory puncture or incision with considerable force during inspiration; in true pneumothorax, during expiration. **physical s.,** objective s. **Piltz's s.,** 1. attention reflex of pupil; see under *reflex.* 2. orbicularis pupillary reflex. **Pins' s.,** Ewart's s., def. 2. **Piotrowski's s.,** percussion of the anterior tibialis muscle produces dorsal flexion and supination of the foot. When this reflex is excessive it indicates organic disease of the central nervous system. Called also *anticus s.* or *reflex.* **Piskacek's s.,** asymmetrical enlargement of the corpus uteri, a sign of pregnancy. **Pitres' s.,** 1. hyperesthesia of the scrotum and testes in tabes dorsalis. 2. anterior deviation of the sternum in pleuritic effusion. **placental s.,** implantation bleeding. **plumb-line s.,** the estimation in sternal displacement by a plumb-line in the diagnosis of pleuritic effusion. **Plummer's s.,** inability to step up onto a chair or to walk up steps, in Graves' disease. **pneumatic s.,** Hennebert's s. **Pool-Schlesinger s.,** Schlesinger's s. **Porter's s.,** tracheal tugging; see under *tugging.* **Potain's s.,** 1. extension of percussion dullness over the arch of the aorta, in dilatation of the aorta, from the manubrium to the third costal cartilage on the right-hand side. 2. timbre métallique. **Pottenger's s.,** 1. intercostal muscle rigidity on palpation in pulmonary and pleural inflammatory conditions. 2. different degrees of resistance on light touch palpation, noted (1) over solid organs when compared with hollow organs; (2) over foci of disease in the lungs and pleura when compared with that over normal organs. **Prehn's s.,** elevation and support of the scrotum will relieve the pain in epididymo-orchitis, but not in torsion of the testicle. **Prévost's s.,** conjugate deviation of the head and eyes, the eyes looking toward the affected hemisphere and away from the palsied extremities; seen in hemiplegia. **pronation s.,** 1. Babinski's s. (def. 5). 2. Strümpell's s. (def. 3). **pseudo-Babinski's s.,** in poliomyelitis the Babinski reflex is modified so that only the big toe is extended, because all the foot muscles except the dorsiflexors of the big toe are paralyzed. **pseudo-Graefe's s.,** slow descent of the upper lid on looking down, and quick ascent on looking up; seen in conditions other than Graves' disease. **psoas s.,** flexion of or pain on hyperextension of the hip due to contact between an inflammatory process and the psoas muscle; a sign often seen in appendicitis. Called also *Cope's s.* **puddle s.,** in examination for ascites, a method for detecting free fluid in the abdominal cavity. The patient lies prone for five minutes, then rises to his hands and knees. While the examiner lightly flicks a finger against one flank, a Bowles stethoscope is moved slowly from the most dependent part of the abdomen to the flank. That part of the ventral abdomen containing the fluid "puddle" shows a loss of high-frequency vibration, which will be detected as soon as the edge of the fluid is reached, indicating the amount of fluid. **pyramid s., pyramidal s.,** any sign pointing to disease of the pyramidal tract. **Quant's s.,** a T-shaped depression in the occipital bone, sometimes seen in rickets. **Queckenstedt's s.,** when the veins in the neck are compressed on one or both sides, there is a rapid rise in the pressure of the cerebrospinal fluid of healthy persons, and this rise quickly disappears when pressure is taken off the neck. But when there is a block in the vertebral canal the pressure of the cerebrospinal fluid is little or not at all affected by this maneuver. **Quénu-Muret s.,** in aneurysm, the main artery of the limb is compressed and then a puncture is made at the periphery; if blood flows, the collateral circulation is probably established. **Quincke's s.,** see under *pulse.* **radialis s.,** Strumpell's s., def. 2. **Radovici's s.,** palm-chin reflex. **Raimiste's s.,** the patient's hand and arm are held upright by the exam-

iner: if the hand is sound, it remains upright on being released; if paretic the hand flexes abruptly at the wrist. **Ramond's s.,** rigidity of the erector spinae muscle indicative of pleurisy with effusion; the rigidity relaxes when the effusion becomes purulent. **Rasin's s.,** Jellinek's s. **Raynaud's s.,** acrocyanosis. **Remak's s.,** see under *symptom.* **Revilliod's s.,** orbicularis s. **Richardson's s.,** the application of a tight fillet to the arm as a test of death: if life is present, the veins on the distal side of the fillet become more or less distended. **Riesman's s.,** 1. a bruit heard with the stethoscope over the closed eye in Graves' disease. 2. softening of the eyeball in diabetic coma. **Ripault's s.,** external pressure upon the eye during life causes only a temporary change in the normal roundness of the pupil; but after death the change so caused may be permanent. **Ritter-Rollet s.,** see under *phenomenon.* **Riviere's s.,** an area of change in percussion note denoting a band of increased density across the back at the plane of the spinous processes of the fifth, sixth, and seventh dorsal vertebrae: a sign of pulmonary tuberculosis. **Robertson's s.,** 1. fibrillary contraction of the pectoralis muscle over the cardiac area in approaching death from heart disease. 2. absence of pupillary dilatation on pressure over alleged painful areas in malingering. 3. in ascites, fullness and tension in the patient's flanks, felt by the examiner with the patient supine. **Roche's s.,** in torsion of the testis, the epididymis cannot be distinguished from the body of the testis, whereas in epididymitis the body of the testis can be felt in the enlarged crescent of the epididymis. **Romaña's s.,** unilateral ophthalmia with palpebral edema, conjunctivitis, and swelling of regional lymph glands as a sign of Chagas' disease. **Romberg's s.,** swaying of the body or falling when standing with the feet close together and the eyes closed; observed in tabes dorsalis. **Rommelaere's s.,** an abnormally small proportion of normal phosphates and of sodium chloride in the urine in cancerous cachexia. **rope s.,** acute angulation between chin and larynx, due to weakness of hyoid muscles, noted in bulbar poliomyelitis. **Rosenbach's s.,** 1. absence of the abdominal skin reflex in inflammatory disease of the intestines. 2. absence of the abdominal skin reflex in pinching the skin of the abdomen on the paralyzed side in hemiplegia. 3. a fine rapid tremor of the closed eyelids in Graves' disease. **Roser's s., Roser-Braun s.,** absence of dural pulsation, a sign of cerebral tumor or abscess. **Rossolimo's s.,** see under *reflex.* **Rotch's s.,** dullness on percussion of the right fifth intercostal space, a sign of pericardial effusion. **Rothschild's s.,** 1. preternatural flattening and mobility of the sternal angle; seen in tuberculosis. 2. loss of hair from the outer third of the eyebrows in hypothyroidism. **Rovighi's s.,** a fremitus felt on percussion and palpation of a superficial hepatic hydatid cyst. **Rovsing's s.,** pressure on the left side over the point corresponding to McBurney's point will elicit the typical pain at McBurney's point in appendicitis. **Ruggeri's s.,** see under *reflex.* **Rumpel-Leede s.,** see under *phenomenon.* **Rust's s.,** see under *phenomenon.* **Saenger's s.,** a light reflex of the pupil that has ceased returns after a short stay in the dark; observed in cerebral syphilis but not in tabes dorsalis. **Salisbury and Melvin's s.,** ophthalmoscopic s. **Sansom's s.,** 1. marked increase of the area of dullness in the second and third intercostal spaces, due to pericardial effusion. 2. a rhythmical murmur heard with a stethoscope applied to the lips in aneurysm of the thoracic aorta. **Sarbó's s.,** analgesia of the peroneal nerve; sometimes noticed in tabes dorsalis. **Saunders' s.,** on wide opening of the mouth there take place in children associated movements of the hand consisting of opening of the hand and extension and separation of the fingers; called also *mouth- and-hand synkinesia.* **Schepelmann's s.,** in dry pleurisy, the pain is increased when the patient bends his body toward the normal side, whereas in intercostal neuralgia it is increased by bending toward the affected side. **Schick's s.,** stridor heard on expiration in an infant with tuberculosis of the bronchial glands. **Schlesinger's s.,** in tetany, if the patient's leg is held at the knee joint and flexed strongly at the hip joint, there will follow within a short time an extensor spasm at the knee joint, with extreme supination of the foot. Called also *Pool's phenomenon.* **Schultze's s.,** 1. Chvostek's sign. 2. tongue phenomenon. **Schultze-Chvostek s.,** Chvostek's s. **Seeligmüller's s.,** mydriasis on the side of the face affected with neuralgia. **Séguin's s.,** see *Séguin's signal symptom,* under *symptom.* **Seidel s.,** see under *scotoma.* **Seitz's s.,** bronchial inspiration which begins harshly and then becomes faint; indicative of a cavity in the lung. **Semon's s.,** impairment of the mobility of the vocal cords in malignant disease of the larynx. **setting-sun s.,** downward deviation of the eyes, so that each iris appears to "set" beneath the lower lid, with white sclera exposed between it and the upper lid; indicative of intracranial pressure (hemorrhage or meningoependymitis) or irritation of the brain stem (as in kernicterus). **Shibley's s.,** in the presence of consolidation of the lung or a collection of fluid in the pleural cavity, all spoken vowels are heard through the stethoscope as "ah." **Sicar's s.,** a metallic resonance on percussion with two coins on the front of the chest and auscultation at the back; observed in some cases of effusion within the pleura. **Siegert's s.,** in Down's syndrome, the little fingers are short and curved inward. **Sieur's s.,** see *coin test,* under *tests.* **Signorelli's s.,** extreme tenderness on pressure on the retromandibular point in meningitis. **Silex's s.,** furrows radiating from the mouth in congenital syphilis. **Simon's s.,** 1. [C. E. *Simon*] retraction or fixation of the umbilicus during inspiration. 2. [J. *Simon*] absence of the usual correlation between the movements of the diaphragm and thorax; seen in beginning meningitis. **Sisto's s.,** constant crying as a sign of congenital syphilis in infancy. **Skoda's s.,** a tympanitic sound heard on percussing the chest above a large pleural effusion or above a consolidation in pneumonia. **Smith's s.,** a murmur heard in cases of enlarged bronchial glands on auscultation over the manubrium with the patient's head thrown back. **Snellen's s.,** the bruit heard with a stethoscope over the closed eye in Graves' disease. **Soto-Hall s.,** with the patient flat on his back, on flexion of the spine beginning at the neck and going downward, pain will be felt at the site of the lesion in back abnormalities. **Souques' s.,** 1. when the patient seated in a chair is suddenly thrown back, the lower extremities do not extend normally or otherwise attempt to counteract the loss of balance; it indicates advanced striatal disease. 2. Souques' phenomenon. **Spalding's s.,** in the x-ray film of the fetus in utero, overriding of the bones of the vault of the skull indicates death of the fetus. **spinal s.,** tonic contraction of the spinal muscles on the diseased side in pleurisy. **spine s.,** disinclination to flex the spine anteriorly on account of pain; seen in poliomyelitis. **Squire's s.,** alternate contraction and dilatation of the pupil, indicative of basilar meningitis. **stairs s.,** difficulty in descending a stairway in tabes dorsalis. **Stellwag's s.,** retraction of the upper eyelids producing apparent widening of the palpebral opening with which is associated infrequent and incomplete blinking; seen in Graves' disease. **Sterles' s.,** increased pulsation over the cardiac region in intrathoracic tumors. **Sternberg's s.,** sensitiveness to palpation of the muscles of the shoulder girdle in pleurisy. **Stewart-Holmes s.,** rebound phenomenon. **Stierlin's s.,** see under *symptom.* **Stocker's s.,** in typhoid fever, if the bed clothes are pulled down, the patient takes no notice; but in tuberculous meningitis the patient resents the interference and immediately draws the clothes up again. **Strauss' s.,** increase of fat following the use of fatty foods in chylous ascites. **string s.,** 1. Kantor's s. 2. the stringing out of tubules, observed on pulling the tissues of an intact testis or one in which there is active spermatogenesis, a phenomenon which is prevented by the fibrosis and hyalinization about the tubules when the testis is atrophic. **Strümpell's s.,** 1. dorsal flexion of the foot when the thigh is drawn up toward the body; seen in spastic paralysis of the lower limb. Called also *tibialis s.* 2. inability to close the fist without marked dorsal extension of the wrist; called also *radialis s.* 3. pronation sign: passive flexion of the forearm caused by pronation; seen in hemiplegia. **Strunsky's s.,** a sign for detecting lesions of the anterior arch of the foot. The examiner grasps the toes and flexes them suddenly. This procedure is painless in the normal foot, but causes pain if there is inflammation of the anterior arch. **Suker's s.,** deficient complementary fixation in lateral eye rotation; seen in Graves' disease. **Sumner's s.,** on gentle palpation of the iliac fossa, a slight increase in tonus of the abdominal muscles may indicate appendicitis, stone in the ureter or kidney, or a twisted pedicle of an ovarian cyst. **swinging flashlight s.,** with the patient's eyes fixed at a distance and a strong light shining before the intact eye, a crisp bilateral contraction of the pupil is noted. On moving the light to the affected eye, both pupils dilate for a short period. Then on

return of the light to the intact eye, both pupils contract promptly and remain contracted. Indicative of minimal damage to the optic nerve. Called also *Marcus Gunn pupillary phenomenon* or *sign.* **Tay's s.,** see *cherry-red spot,* under *spot.* **Testivin's s.,** the formation of a collodion-like pellicle on the urine after removing the albumin and treating with acid and then with one third of its volume of ether; said to occur during the incubation of infectious diseases. **Theimich's lip s.,** a protrusion or pouting of the lips elicited by tapping the orbicularis oris muscle. **thermic s.,** Kashida's s. **Thomas' s.,** 1. flexion of the hip joint can be compensated by lordosis. 2. pinching of the trapezius muscle causes goose flesh above the level of a spinal cord lesion. **Thomson's s.,** Pastia's s. **Thornton's s.,** severe pain in the region of the flanks in nephrolithiasis. **tibialis s.,** Strümpell's s., def. 1. **Tinel's s.,** a tingling sensation in the distal end of a limb when percussion is made over the site of a divided nerve. It indicates a partial lesion or the beginning regeneration of the nerve. Called also *formication s.* and *distal tingling on percussion.* **toe s.,** Babinski's reflex. **Tournay's s.,** unilateral dilatation of the pupil of the abducting eye on extreme lateral fixation. **Traube's s.,** a loud "pistol-shot" sound heard in auscultation over the femoral arteries in aortic regurgitation. Called also *pistol-shot sound.* **Trendelenburg's s.,** see under *tests.* **trepidation s.,** patellar clonus. **Tresilian's s.,** a reddish appearance in Stensen's duct in mumps. **Trimadeau's s.,** if the dilatation above an esophageal stricture is conic, the stricture is fibrous; if cup shaped, the stricture is malignant. **Troisier's s.,** enlargement of the lymph nodes above the clavicle; a sign of intra-abdominal malignant disease or of retrosternal tumor. **Trömner's s.,** Hoffmann's s., def. 2. **Trousseau's s.,** 1. see under *phenomenon.* 2. tache cérébrale. **Turner's s.,** discoloration (bruising) of the skin of the loin in acute hemorrhagic pancreatitis. **Turyn's s.,** in sciatica, if the patient's great toe is bent dorsally, pain will be felt in the gluteal region. **Uhthoff's s.,** nystagmus occurring in multiple cerebrospinal sclerosis. **Unschuld's s.,** a tendency to cramp in the calves of the legs; a nonspecific early indication of diabetes. **Vanzetti's s.,** in sciatica the pelvis is always horizontal in spite of scoliosis, but in other lesions with scoliosis the pelvis is inclined. **Vedder's s's** (*of beriberi*), slight pressure on muscles of calf causes pain; ascertain the presence of anesthesia with a pin over anterior surface of leg; note any changes in patellar reflexes; when patient squats upon heels, note the inability to rise without use of hands. **vein s.,** a bluish cord along the midaxillary line formed by the swollen junction of the thoracic and superficial epigastric vein; seen in tuberculosis of the bronchial glands and in superior vena cava obstruction. **vital s's,** the pulse, respiration, and temperature. **Voltolini's s.,** Heryng's s. **von Graefe's s.,** Graefe's s. **Wartenberg's s.,** 1. a sign of ulnar palsy, consisting of a position of abduction assumed by the little finger. 2. reduction or absence of the pendulum movements of the arm in walking; seen in patients with cerebellar disease. **Weber's s.,** paralysis of the oculomotor nerve of one side and hemiplegia of the opposite side. See *syndrome of Weber.* **Wegner's s.,** a broadened, discolored appearance of the epiphyseal line in infants dying from hereditary syphilis. **Weill's s.,** absence of expansion in the subclavicular region of the affected side in infantile pneumonia. **Weiss's s.,** Chvostek's s. **Wernicke's s.,** hemiopic pupillary reaction. **Westermark's s.,** transient clearing (avascularity) of the normal radiologic shadow of pulmonary tissue distal to a pulmonary embolism. **Westphal's s.,** loss of the knee jerk in tabes dorsalis. **Widowitz's s.,** protrusion of the eyeballs and sluggish movements of the eyeballs and eyelids seen in diphtheritic paralysis. **Wilder's s.,** an early sign of Graves' disease consisting in a slight twitch of the eyeball when it changes its movement from adduction to abduction or vice versa. **Williams' s.,** a dull tympanitic resonance heard in the second intercostal space in severe pleural effusion. **Williamson's s.,** markedly diminished blood pressure in the leg as compared with that in the arm on the same side; seen in pneumothorax and pleural effusion. **Winterbottom's s.,** enlargement of posterior cervical lymph nodes in African trypanosomiasis. **Wintrich's s.,** a change in the pitch of the percussion note when the mouth is opened and closed; it indicates a cavity in the lung. **Wood's s.,** relaxation of the orbicularis muscle, fixation of the eyeball, and divergent strabismus, indicative of profound anesthesia.

Wreden's s., presence of a gelatinous matter in the external auditory meatus in children who are born dead. **Zaufal's s.,** saddle nose.

signa (sig′nah) [L.] mark, or write; abbreviated S. or sig. on prescriptions. See *prescription*.

signature (sig′nah-chur) [L. *signatura*] 1. that part of a prescription which gives directions to the patient for taking of medicine; abbreviated S. or sig. See *prescription*. 2. any characteristic feature of a substance formerly regarded as an indication of its medicinal virtues: thus, the eyelike mark on the flower of the euphrasia was supposed to show its usefulness in eye diseases; the liver-like shape of the leaf of liverwort pointed to its use in hepatic diseases; the yellow color of saffron indicated its use in jaundice.

signe (sēn) [Fr.] sign.

significant (sig-nif′ĭ-kant) in statistics, probably resulting from something other than chance.

Signorelli's sign (sēn-yor-el′ēz) [Angelo *Signorelli*, Italian physician, 1876–1952] see under *sign*.

Sig. n. pro. abbreviation for L. *sig′na nom′ine pro′prio*, label with the proper name.

siguatera (sig″wah-ta′rah) [Sp.] ciguatera.

sikimi (sik′ĭ-me) [Japanese] the plant *Illicium religiosum*.

sikimin (sik′ĭ-min) a poisonous hydrocarbon, $C_{10}H_{16}$, found in the leaves of *Illicium religiosum*.

sikimitoxin (sik-im″ĭ-tok′sin) a poisonous substance extracted from sikimi.

silafilcon A (sil″ah-fil′kon) chemical name: poly (dimethyl diphenyl methylvinyl phenyl hydrodimethyl siloxane); a hydrophilic contact lens material.

silafocon A (sil″ah-fo′kon) a hydrophobic contact lens material.

Silain (si′lān) trademark for preparations of simethicone.

silandrone (sĭ-lan′drōn) chemical name: 17β-(trimethylsiloxy)androst-4-en-3-one; an androgenic steroid, $C_{22}H_{36}O_2Si$.

Silastic (sĭ-las′tik) trademark for polymeric silicone substances having the properties of rubber; it is biologically inert and used in surgical prostheses.

silent (si′lent) producing no detectable signs or symptoms; noiseless.

silex (si′leks) [L. "flint"] a refined form of silica powder, which may be mixed with water or a mouthwash solution to form a fine abrasive paste for polishing metal castings.

Silex's sign (se′leks-ez) [Paul *Silex*, German ophthalmologist, 1858–1929] see under *sign*.

silica (sil′ĭ-kah) [L. *silex* flint] silicon dioxide, SiO_2, or silicic anhydride, occurring in nature as agate, amethyst, sand, quartz, chalcedony, cristobalite, and flint. It is one of the major constituents of dental porcelain, and in granular form serves as a dental abrasive and polishing agent.

silicate (sil′ĭ-kāt) [L. *silicus*] a salt of any of the silicic acids.

silicatosis (sil′ĭ-kah-to′sis) pneumoconiosis caused by the inhalation of the dust of silicates.

silicea (sĭ-lis′e-ah) a homeopathic preparation of silica.

siliceous, silicious (sĭ-lish′us) containing silica or a compound of silicon.

silicic acid (sĭ-lik′ik) the molecular species $Si(OH)_4$ occurring in hydrated forms of silica, e.g., silica gel.

silicoanthracosis (sil″ĭ-ko-an″thrah-ko′sis) silicosis combined with pneumoconiosis of coal workers.

Silicoflagellida (sil″ĭ-ko-flah-jel′lĭ-dah) [*silicon* + Gr. *flagellum* whip] an order of plantlike flagellate marine protozoa (class Phytomastigophorea, subphylum Mastigophora) having one flagellum, golden-brown or green-brown chloroplasts, and a star-shaped siliceous skeleton that envelops the body. *Dictyocha* is a representative genus.

silicofluoride (sil″ĭ-ko-floo′o-rīd) fluorosilicate.

silicol (sil′ĭ-kol) an organic silica compound, silicic oxide casein metaphosphate; used in the treatment of tuberculosis.

silicon (sil′ĭ-kon) [L. *silex* flint] a nonmetallic element occurring in nature as silica (s. *dioxide*); symbol, Si; atomic number, 14; atomic weight, 28.086. **s. carbide,** a compound produced by the reaction of silicon and carbon at extremely high temperature, used in dentistry as an abrasive agent. Trade names include Carborundum, Crystolon, and Carbolon. **s. dioxide,** silica. **s. dioxide, colloidal**

[NF], a submicroscopic fumed silica prepared by the vapor-phase hydrolysis of a silicon compound; used as a tablet diluent and as a suspending and thickening agent. **s. fluoride,** SiF_4, a colorless gas sometimes fatal to workers in superphosphate factories.

silicone (sil′ĭ-kōn) any organic compound in which all or part of the carbon has been replaced by silicon.

silicosiderosis (sil″ĭ-ko-sid″er-o′sis) pneumoconiosis in which the inhaled dust is that of silica and iron.

silicosis (sil″ĭ-ko′sis) [L. *silex* flint] pneumoconiosis due to the inhalation of the dust of stone, sand, or flint containing silicon dioxide, with formation of generalized nodular fibrotic changes in both lungs. Called also *grinders' disease*. **infective s.,** silicotuberculosis.

Silicote (sil′ĭ-kōt) trademark for preparations of dimethicone.

silicotic (sil″ĭ-kot′ik) pertaining to or characterized by silicosis.

silicotuberculosis (sil″ĭ-ko-tu-ber″ku-lo′sis) tuberculous infection of the silicotic lung; infective silicosis.

siliqua (sil′ĭ-kwah) [L.] pod, or husk. **s. oli′vae** ["husk of the olive"], the fibers which appear to encircle superficially the inferior olive of the brain; their outer and inner portions are termed *funiculus lateralis medullae oblongatae*. Called also *amiculum olivae*.

siliquose (sil′ĭ-kwōs) pertaining to or resembling a pod or husk; see under *cataract*.

sillonneur (se-yon-nur′) [Fr.] (*obs.*) a three-bladed scalpel for operations on the eye.

Silvadene (sil′vah-dēn) trademark for a preparation of silver sulfadiazine.

silvatic (sil-vat′ik) [L. *silva* a wood or woods] pertaining to or occurring in the woods; as *silvatic plague*.

silver (sil′ver) [L. *argentum*] a white, soft, malleable, and ductile metal; symbol, Ag; atomic number, 47; atomic weight, 107.870. Its compounds are extensively used in medicine, and metallic silver is employed in surgery and in the manufacture of instruments. In dentistry, it is used chiefly in prostheses, in alloys, in soldering, to neutralize the color imparted by copper in alloys, and as points to obliterate the root canal. **s. arsphenamine,** see under *arsphenamine*. **s. chloride,** an insoluble white salt, AgCl, that darkens in light; called *horn silver* in mineral form. **colloidal s.,** a silver preparation in which the silver exists as free ions to only a small extent. See *protein s., mild,* and *protein s., strong.* **s. cyanide,** a soluble salt, AgCN. **s. iodide,** an insoluble, light-yellowish, binary, powdery compound, AgI, that turns black in the light; used in treatment of syphilis, nervous diseases, and conjunctivitis. **s. iodide, colloidal,** silver iodide in solution rendered stable by gelatin, an antiseptic for treating inflammations of mucous membranes. **s. nitrate** [USP], a powerful germicide, $AgNO_3$, occurring as colorless or white crystals; used as an antiseptic, applied topically to the conjunctiva as a prophylactic against ophthalmia neonatorum, and also used as an antiseptic and astringent, especially in infections of the skin and mucous membranes. It has also been used to purify drinking water. **s. nitrate, toughened** [USP], a compound prepared by fusing silver nitrate with hydrochloric acid, sodium chloride, or potassium nitrate, occurring as white crystalline masses molded into pencils or cones, and containing 94.5 per cent of silver nitrate; used as a caustic and applied topically after being dipped in water. Called also *lunar caustic, fused silver nitrate,* and *molded silver nitrate.* **s. orthophosphate,** an insoluble yellow powder, Ag_3PO_4. **s. oxide,** a heavy brownish-black powder, Ag_2O. **s. picrate,** yellow crystals, $C_6H_2(NO_2)_3OAg·H_2O$, used as a topical anti-infective, especially in infections of the skin and mucous membranes; it has been used in the treatment of vaginal trichomoniasis and candidiasis, administered by insufflation or in pessaries. **s. protein, mild,** a preparation containing 19–23 per cent of silver, rendered colloidal by the presence of, or combination with, protein; it occurs as dark brown or almost black scales or granules and is used as a topical anti-infective in various rectal, ocular, vaginal, urethral, otic, nasal, and pharyngeal infections. **s. protein, strong,** a pale yellowish orange to brownish black powdered compound of silver and protein containing 7.5–8.5 per cent of silver, an active germicide with a local irritant and astringent effect. It may cause argyria. **s. sulfadiazine,** the silver derivative of sulfadiazine, $C_{10}H_9Ag\ N_4O_2S$, having bactericidal activity against many gram-positive and gram-negative organisms, as well as being effective against yeasts; used as a topical anti-infective for the prevention and treatment of wound sepsis in patients with second and third degree burns. **s. sulfate,** a moderately soluble colorless salt, Ag_2SO_4. **s. sulfide,** a black insoluble powder, Ag_2S.

Silverman's needle (sil′ver-manz) [Irving *Silverman,* Brooklyn surgeon, born 1904] see under *needle.*

silverskin (sil′ver-skin) the pericarp and germ of grains which are removed in processing, as in polished rice, but which contain the thiamine.

Silvester's method (sil-ves′terz) [Henry Robert *Silvester,* English physician, 1828–1908] see under *respiration, artificial.*

silvestrene (sil-ves′trēn) a hydrocarbon, $C_{10}H_{16}$, obtainable from European oil of turpentine.

Silvius (sil′ve-us) a genus of tabanid flies found abundantly in Australia.

Simaruba (sim′ah-roo′bah) a genus of tropical American trees, several species of which are medicinal. The root bark of *S. ama′ra* Aubl. (Simarubaceae) is a bitter tonic and astringent, and has been used in amebiasis. The active principle is simarubidin.

simarubidin (sim″ah-roo′-bĭ-din) the active principle, $C_{22}H_{32}O_9$, of the bark and wood of *Simaruba amara;* used experimentally in canine amebiasis.

simesthesia (sim″es-the′ze-ah) osseous sensibility.

simethicone (sĭ-meth′ĭ-kōn) [USP] a mixture of dimethicones and silicon dioxide, with a molecular weight between 14,000 and 21,000, occurring as a translucent, gray, viscous fluid. It is administered orally as an antifoaming agent in gastroscopy, and is also used as an antiflatulent and as a releasing agent in pharmaceutical preparations. Called also *dimethicone* or *activated dimethicone.* It is used in veterinary medicine in the treatment and prevention of bloat in cattle.

similia similibus curantur (sĭ-mil′e-ah sĭ-mil′ĭ-bus ku-ran′tur) [L. "likes are cured by likes"] the doctrine, or the brocard expressing it, which lies at the foundation of homeopathy; namely, that a disease is cured by those remedies which produce effects resembling the disease itself.

simillimum (sĭ-mil′ĭ-mum) [L. "likest"] the homeopathic remedy which most exactly reproduces the symptoms of any disease.

Simmonds' disease (syndrome) (sim′ondz) [Morris *Simmonds,* physician in Hamburg, 1855–1925] see *panhypopituitarism.*

Simon's septic factor, sign (si′monz) [Charles Edmund *Simon,* Baltimore physician, 1866–1927] see under *factor* and *sign,* def. 1.

Simon's sign (si′monz) [John *Simon,* English surgeon, 1824–1876] see under *sign.*

Simonart's thread (band) (se″mo-narz′) [Pierre Joseph Cécilien *Simonart,* Belgian obstetrician, 1817–1847] see under *thread.*

Simonea folliculorum (sĭ-mo′ne-ah fŏ-lik″u-lo′rum) *Demodex folliculorum.*

Simonelli's test (si″mo-nel′ēz) [F. *Simonelli,* Italian physician] see under *tests.*

Simons' disease (si′monz) [Arthur *Simons,* Berlin physician, born 1877] partial lipodystrophy.

Simonsiella (si-mon″se-el′ah) [Hellmuth *Simons*] a genus of gliding bacteria of the family Simonsiellaceae, order Cytophagales, found in the oral flora of humans and animals, made up of cells forming flat filaments with rounded ends. It contains the species *S. cras′sa* and *S. muel′leri.*

Simonsiellaceae (si″mon-se″el-a′se-e) a family of gliding bacteria of the order Cytophagales, made up of cells in flat filaments. It contains the genera *Alysiella* and *Simonsiella.*

simple (sim′p'l) [L. *simplex*] 1. neither compound nor complex; single. 2. an old term for any herb with real or supposed medicinal virtues.

Simpson's forceps (simp′sunz) [Sir James Young *Simpson,* Scottish obstetrician, 1811–1870] see under *forceps.*

Simpson light (lamp) (simp′sun) [William Speirs *Simpson,* British civil engineer, died 1917] see under *light.*

Sims' position, etc. (simz) [James Marion *Sims,* New York gynecologist, 1813–1883] see under *depressor, position,* and *speculum.*

simul (sim′ul) [L.] at the same time as.

simulation (sim″u-la′shun) [L. *simulatio*] 1. the act of counterfeiting a disease; malingering. 2. the mimicking of one disease by another.

simulator (sim″u-la′tor) something that simulates, such as an apparatus that simulates conditions that will be encountered in real life. **electrocardiographic s.,** a device that produces simulations of electrocardiographic wave forms.

Simuliidae (si″mu-le′ĭ-de) a family of flies of the suborder Nematocera, order Diptera, characterized by small size, a humped back, and short stubbed antennae of 10 or 11 segments. It contains approximately 600 species, known variously as black flies, buffalo gnats, or turkey gnats. The females of several species are vicious biters.

Simulium (si-mu′le-um) a genus of flies of the family Simuliidae. They are widely distributed and a great pest at times. *S. amazon′icum* is a vector of *Mansonella ozzardi* in Brazil and Guyana. *S. arc′ticum* occurs in Alaska. *S. columbaczen′se,* a species in southern Europe which has been known to kill animals. *S. damno′sum* is an intermediate host of *Onchocerca volvulus* in Africa. *S. metal′licum* and *S. ochra′ceum* transmit *Onchocerca volvulus* in Mexico. *S. pecua′rium,* the buffalo gnat, a terrible scourge to horses and cattle. *S. venus′tum,* a species widely distributed in North America and Denmark.

simultagnosia (si″mul-tag-no′se-ah) simultanagnosia.

simultanagnosia (si″mul-tān″ag-no′se-ah) the inability to comprehend more than one element of a visual scene at the same time or to integrate the parts as a whole.

SIMV synchronized intermittent mandatory ventilation; see under *ventilation.*

sinal (si′nal) pertaining to a sinus; sinusal.

Sinaxar (sin′aks-ar) trademark for a preparation of styramate.

sincalide (sin′kah-līd) chemical name: 1-de(5-oxo-L-proline)-2-de-L-glutamide-5-L-methioninecaerulin; a choleretic, $C_{49}H_{62}N_{10}O_{16}S_3$.

sincipital (sin-sip′ĭ-tal) pertaining to the sinciput.

sinciput (sin′sĭ-put) [L.] [NA] the anterior and upper part of the head.

sinefungin (sin″ĕ-fun′jin) chemical name: 6,9-diamino-1-(6-amino-9H-purin-9-yl)-1,5,6,7,8,9-hexadeoxy-β-D-*ribo*-decofuranuronic acid; an antifungal antibiotic derived from *Streptomyces griseolus,* $C_{15}H_{23}N_7O_5$.

Sinequan (sin′ĕ-kwan) trademark for a preparation of doxepin hydrochloride.

sinew (sin′u) the tendon of a muscle. **back s.,** the large flexor tendon at the back of the cannon bone of quadrupeds. **weeping s.,** an encysted ganglion, chiefly on the back of the hand, containing synovial fluid.

sing. abbreviation of L. *singulo′rum,* of each.

single blind (sing′g'l blind) pertaining to a clinical trial or other experiment in which subjects do not know which treatment they are receiving.

Singoserp (sing′go-serp) trademark for preparations of syrosingopine.

singultation (sing″gul-ta′shun) a hiccup.

singultous (sing-gul′tus) affected with hiccup.

singultus (sing-gul′tus) [L.] hiccup. **s. gas′tricus nervo′sus,** hiccup due to a nervous condition of the stomach.

sinigrin (sin′ĭ-grin) potassium myronate, $CH_2{:}CH{\cdot}CH_2(S{\cdot}C_6H_{11}O_5)N{\cdot}CO{\cdot}SO_2{\cdot}OK$, a glycoside found in black mustard seed (*Brassica nigra* Koch, Cruciferae) and horseradish root (*Alliaria officinalis* Andrz.).

sinister (sin-is′ter) [L.] left; [NA] a term denoting the left-hand one of two similar structures, or the one situated on the left side of the body.

sinistrad (sin-is′trad) to or toward the left.

sinistral (sin-is′tral) [L. *sinistralis*] 1. pertaining to the left side; 2. a left-handed person.

sinistrality (sin″is-tral′ĭ-te) the preferential use, in voluntary motor acts, of the left member of the major paired organs of the body, as the left ear, eye, hand, and foot.

sinistraural (sin″is-traw′ral) [L. *sinister* + *auris* ear] hearing better with the left ear.

sinistr(o)- [L. *sinister* left] a combining form meaning left, or denoting relationship to the left side.

sinistrocardia (sin″is-tro-kar′de-ah) [*sinistro-* + Gr. *kardia* heart] location of the heart in left side of the thorax; levocardia.

sinistrocerebral (sin″is-tro-ser′ĕ-bral) pertaining to or situated in the left cerebral hemisphere.

sinistrocular (sin″is-trok′u-lar) [*sinistro-* + L. *oculus* eye] left eyed; having the left eye the dominant eye.

sinistrocularity (sin″is-trok″u-lar′ĭ-te) the state of having the left eye the dominant eye.

sinistrogyration (sin″is-tro-ji-ra′shun) [*sinistro-* + *gyration*] a turning to the left, as a movement of the eye or the plane of polarization.

sinistromanual (sin″is-tro-man′u-al) [*sinistro-* + L. *manus* hand] left-handed.

sinistropedal (sin″is-trop′ĕ-dal) [*sinistro-* + L. *pes* foot] using the left foot in preference to the right.

sinistrorse (sin′is-trors) turned to the left.

sinistrose (sin′is-trōs) a levorotatory sugar sometimes found in the urine.

sinistrotorsion (sin″is-tro-tor′shun) [*sinistro-* + *torsion*] a twisting toward the left; said mainly of the eye.

sinkaline (sing′kah-lin) choline.

Sinkler's phenomenon (singk′lerz) [Wharton *Sinkler,* Philadelphia neurologist, 1847–1910] see under *phenomenon.*

sinoatrial (si″no-a′tre-al) pertaining to the sinus venosus and the atrium of the heart; see also under *node.*

sinoauricular (si″no-aw-rik′u-lar) sinoatrial.

sinobronchitis (si″no-brong-ki′tis) [*sino-* + Gr. *bronchos* bronchus + *-itis*] chronic paranasal sinusitis with recurrent episodes of bronchitis.

Sinografin (si″no-graf′in) trademark for preparations of diatrizoate meglumine.

sinography (si-nog′rah-fe) [*sinus* + Gr. *graphein* to write] roentgenography of the sinuses.

sinomenine (si-nom′ē-nin) a crystalline alkaloid, $C_{19}H_{23}NO_4$, from the root of *Sinomenium acutum* (Thumb.) Rehd. Wils. (Menispermaciae), a plant of eastern Asia. Called also *coculine* and *cucoline.*

Si non val. abbreviation for L. *si non va′leat,* if it is not enough.

sinopulmonary (si″no-pul′mo-ner″e) involving the paranasal sinuses and the lungs.

sinospiral (si″no-spi′ral) pertaining to the sinus venosus and having a spiral course; said of certain muscle fibers of the heart.

sinoventricular (si″no-ven-trik′u-lar) pertaining to the sinus venosus and the ventricle of the heart.

sinter (sin′ter) 1. the calcareous or silicious matter deposited by mineral springs. 2. [Ger.] to transform into a solid mass by heating without melting.

sintoc (sin′tok) the bark of *Cinnamomum sintoc* Blume (Lauraceae), of the East Indies; it resembles cinnamon. Used in Indonesia for diarrhea and as a vermifuge.

Sintrom (sin′trom) trademark for a preparation of acenocoumarol.

sinuate (sin″u-āt) having a wavy margin.

sinuatrial (sin″u-a′tre-al) sinoatrial.

sinuauricular (sin″u-aw-rik′u-lar) sinoatrial.

sinuous (sin′u-us) [L. *sinuosus*] bending in and out; winding.

sinus (si′nus), pl. *si′nus* or *sinuses* [L. "a hollow"] 1. a cavity, or channel; [NA] a general term for such spaces as the dilated channels for venous blood in the cranium or liver, or the air cavities in the cranial bones. 2. an abnormal channel or fistula permitting the escape of pus. **accessory s′s of the nose,** s. paranasales. **air s.,** an air-containing space within the substance of a bone. **s. a′lae par′vae,** old term for s. sphenoparietalis. **anal s′s, s. ana′les** [NA], furrows, with pouchlike recesses at the lower end, separating the rectal columns; called also *s. rectales* and *crypts of Morgagni.* **anterior s′s, s. anterior′res** [NA], the anterior air cells that together with the middle and

posterior air cells form the ethmoidal sinus; called also *cellulae anteriores.* **s. of anterior chamber,** the narrow space at the edge of the anterior chamber of the eye, between the border of the cornea and the root of the iris. **s. aor′tae** [NA], **s. aor′tae [Valsal′vae], aortic s.,** a dilatation between the aortic wall and each of the semilunar cusps of the aortic valve; from two of these sinuses the coronary arteries take origin. Called also *Petit's s., s. of Morgagni,* and *s. of Valsalva.* **Arlt's s.,** s. of Maier. **s. arte′riae pulmona′lis,** s. trunci pulmonalis. **articular s. of atlas,** fovea dentis atlantis. **articular s. of atlas, superior,** fovea articularis superior atlantis. **articular s. of axis, anterior,** facies articularis anterior axis. **articular s. of vertebrae, inferior,** see *facies articulares inferiores vertebrarum.* **s. of atlas, anterior,** fovea dentis atlantis. **basilar s.,** plexus basilaris. **s. of Bochdalek,** hiatus pleuroperitonealis. **branchial s.,** an abnormal opening between a branchial groove and its corresponding pharyngeal pouch, homologous with an ancestral gill slit. **Breschet's s.,** s. sphenoparietalis. **s. carot′icus** [NA], **carotid s.,** the dilated portion of the internal carotid artery, situated above the division of the common carotid artery into its two main branches, or sometimes on the terminal portion of the common carotid artery, containing in its wall pressoreceptors that are stimulated by changes in blood pressure. Called also *bulbus caroticus.* **s. caverno′sus** [NA], **cavernous s.,** an irregularly shaped venous space in the dura mater at either side of the body of the sphenoid bone, extending from the medial end of the superior orbital fissure in front to the apex of the petrous temporal bone behind. It receives the superior ophthalmic vein, the superficial middle cerebral vein, and the sphenoparietal sinus, and communicates with the opposite cavernous sinus and with the transverse sinus and internal jugular vein by way of the petrosal sinuses. Commonly comprising one or more main venous channels, it contains the internal carotid artery and abducent nerve. **cerebral s.,** any of the ventricles of the brain. **cervical s.,** a temporary depression caudal to the embryonic hyoid arch, containing the succeeding branchial arches; it is overgrown by the hyoid arch and closes off as the cervical vesicle. **circular s., s. circula′ris,** the venous ring around the hypophysis formed by the two cavernous and the anterior and posterior intercavernous sinuses; called also *Ridley's s.* **s. circula′ris i′ridis,** s. venosus sclerae. **coccygeal s.,** a sinus or fistula situated just over or close to the tip of the coccyx, being the remains of the end of the neurenteric canal; see also *pilonidal s.* **s. coch′leae,** vena canaliculi cochleae. **s. condylo′rum fem′oris,** fossa intercondylaris femoris. **s. corona′rius** [NA], **coronary s.,** the terminal portion of the great cardiac vein, which lies in the coronary sulcus between the left atrium and ventricle, and empties into the right atrium. **cortical s′s,** lymph sinuses in the cortex of a lymph node, which arise from the marginal sinuses and continue into the medullary sinuses; called also *intermediate s′s.* **costal s′s of sternum,** incisurae costales sterni. **costodiaphragmatic s.,** recessus costodiaphragmaticus pleurae. **costomediastinal s. of pleura, s. costomediastina′lis pleu′rae,** recessus costomediastinalis pleurae. **costophrenic s.,** recessus costodiaphragmaticus pleurae. **cranial s′s,** s. durae matris. **Cuvier's s′s,** see under *duct.* **dermal s.,** a congenital sinus tract extending from the surface of the body, between the bodies of two adjacent lumbar vertebrae, to the spinal canal. **s′s of dura mater, s. du′rae ma′tris** [NA], large venous channels forming an anastomosing system between the layers of the dura mater encephali. They are devoid of valves, do not collapse when drained, and in some parts contain numerous trabeculae. They drain the cerebral veins and some diploic and meningeal veins into the veins of the neck. Those at the base of the skull also drain most of the blood from the orbit. In some places they communicate with superficial veins by small emissary vessels. Called also *cranial s′s, s. venosi durales,* and *venous s′s of dura mater.* **s. epididym′idis** [NA], **s. of epididymis,** a long, slitlike serous pocket between the upper part of the testis and the overlying epididymis. **Eternod's s.,** a loop of vessels connecting the vessels of the chorion with those in the underside of the yolk sac. **ethmoidal s., s. ethmoida′lis** [NA], one of the paranasal sinuses, located in the ethmoid bone, consisting of air-containing spaces (*sinus anteriores, medii,* and *posteriores,* collectively *cellulae ethmoidalis*), and communicating with the ethmoidal infundibulum and bulla and with the superior and highest meatuses of the nasal cavity. **falcial s., falciform s.,** old term for s. sagittalis inferior. **Forssell's s.,** a smooth space in the wall of the stomach surrounded by folds of the mucosa; seen on roentgen-ray examination. **frontal s.,** s. frontalis. **frontal s., bony,** s. frontalis osseus. **s. fronta′lis** [NA], frontal sinus: one of the paired paranasal sinuses located in the frontal bone, and communicating by way of the nasofrontal duct with the middle meatus of the nasal cavity on the same side. See also *s. frontalis osseus.* **s. fronta′lis os′seus** [NA], bony frontal sinus: an irregular air cavity situated in the frontal bone on either side, deep to the superciliary arch; separated from its fellow of the opposite side by a bony septum, and communicating with the middle meatus of the bony nasal cavity on the same side. **Guérin's s.,** a diverticulum behind Guérin's fold. **Huguier's s.,** a depression in the tympanum between the fenestra ovalis and the fenestra rotunda. **s. interarcua′lis,** fossa tonsillaris. **s. intercaverno′si** [NA], intercavernous sinuses: two venous channels that connect the two cavernous sinuses, one passing anterior and the other posterior to the infundibulum of the hypophysis. **s. intercaverno′sus ante′rior,** the anterior of the two spaces connecting the cavernous sinuses; see *s. intercavernosi.* **s. intercaverno′sus poste′rior,** the posterior of the two spaces connecting the cavernous sinuses; see *s. intercavernosi.* **intercavernous s′s,** s. intercavernosi. **intermediate s′s,** cortical s′s. **s. of internal jugular vein, inferior,** bulbus venae jugularis inferior. **s. of internal jugular vein, superior,** bulbus venae jugularis superior. **s. of kidney,** s. renalis. **lacteal s′s, s. lacteus, s. lactif′eri** [NA], **lactiferous s′s,** enlargements in the lactiferous ducts just before they open onto the mammary papilla. **laryngeal s., s. of larynx,** ventriculus laryngis. **lateral s.,** s. transversus durae matris. **s. lie′nis** NA alternative for *s. splenicus.* **longitudinal s., inferior,** s. sagittalis inferior. **longitudinal s., superior,** s. sagittalis superior. **lunate s. of radius,** incisura ulnaris radii. **lunate s. of ulna,** incisura radialis ulnae. **lymph s′s, lymphatic s′s,** irregular tortuous spaces within lymphoid tissue (nodes) through which a continuous stream of lymph passes, to enter the efferent lymphatic vessels. See also *cortical s′s, marginal s′s,* and *medullary s′s.* **s. of Maier,** a slight diverticulum from the upper part of the lacrimal sac, into which the lacrimal canaliculi open, either together or separately; called also *Arlt's sinus.* **marginal s′s,** 1. marginal lakes; see under *lake.* 2. bow-shaped lymph sinuses separating the capsule from the cortical parenchyma of a lymph mode, and from which lymph flows into the cortical sinuses; called also *subcapsular s′s.* **mastoid s.,** see *cellulae mastoideae.* **s. maxilla′ris** [NA], **s. maxilla′ris [Highmo′ri],** maxillary sinus: one of the paired paranasal sinuses, located in the body of the maxilla on either side and communicating with the middle meatus of the nasal cavity on the same side. Called also *antrum of Highmore.* (See also *s. maxillaris osseus.*) **s. maxilla′ris os′seus** [NA], bony maxillary sinus: an air cavity of variable size and shape located in the body of each maxilla, communicating with the middle meatus of the bony nasal cavity on the same side. **maxillary s.,** s. maxillaris. **maxillary s., bony,** s. maxillaris osseus. **s. me′diae, s. me′dii** [NA], middle sinuses: the middle air cells that together with the anterior and posterior air cells form the ethmoidal sinus; called also *s. mediae* and *cellulae mediae.* **medullary s′s,** lymph sinuses in the medulla of a lymph node, which divide the lymphoid tissue into a number of medullary cords. **Meyer's s., s. Mey′eri,** a small depression in the floor of the external auditory canal just in front of the tympanic membrane. **middle s′s,** s. medii. **middle s. of atlas,** fovea dentis atlantis. **s. of Morgagni,** 1. see *sinus anales.* 2. sinus aortae. 3. ventriculus laryngis. **mucous s′s of male urethra,** lacunae urethrales. **oblique s. of pericardium, s. obli′quus pericar′dii** [NA], a recess of serous pericardium that passes upward behind the left atrium and between the left and right pulmonary veins. **occipital s., s. occipita′lis** [NA], a single venous sinus of the dura mater that begins in right and left branches, the marginal sinuses, and passes upward along the attached margin of the cerebellar falx to end in the confluence of the sinuses. **oral s.,** stomodeum. **paranasal s′s, s. paranasa′les** [NA], the mucosa-lined air cavities in the cranial bones which communicate with the nasal cavity, including the ethmoidal, frontal, maxillary, and sphenoidal sinuses. **parasinoi-**

dal s., any one of several spaces in the dura mater opening into one of the dural sinuses; called also *lacuna lateralis* or *lacus lateralis.* **pericardial s.,** an enlarged blood-filled portion of the hemocoelom surrounding the heart in many invertebrates with open circulatory systems, such as arthropods. Called also *pericardium.* **s. pericar′dii,** s. transversus pericardii. **s. pericra′nii,** a soft fluctuating vascular tumor of the scalp which communicates directly with an intracranial sinus through a defect in the skull. **peroneal s. of tibia,** incisura fibularis tibiae. **Petit's s.,** s. aortae. **petrosal s., inferior,** s. petrosus inferior. **petrosal s., superior,** s. petrosus superior. **s. petro′sus infe′rior** [NA], inferior petrosal sinus: a venous sinus arising from the cavernous sinus and running along the line of the petrooccipital synchondrosis to the superior bulb of the internal jugular vein. **s. petro′sus supe′rior** [NA], superior petrosal sinus: a sinus arising at the cavernous sinus, passing along the attached margin of the cerebellar tentorium, and draining into the transverse sinus. **phrenicocostal s., s. phrenicocosta′lis,** recessus costodiaphragmaticus pleurae. **pilonidal s.,** a suppurating sinus containing a tuft of hair, occurring chiefly in the coccygeal region, but also in other regions of the body. See also *coccygeal s.* **piriform s.,** recessus piriformis. **s. pleu′rae, pleural s.,** recessus pleurales. **pleuroperitoneal s.,** hiatus pleuroperitonealis. **s. pocula′ris,** utriculus prostaticus. **s. poste′rior ca′vi tym′pani** [NA], posterior sinus of tympanic cavity: a groove in the posterior wall of the tympanic cavity above the pyramidal eminence. **posterior s′s, s. posterio′res** [NA], the posterior air cells that together with the anterior and middle air cells form the ethmoidal sinus; called also *cellulae posteriores.* **s. precervica′lis,** the depression at the side of the neck, produced in the developing embryo by the growth of the branchial arches. **prostatic s., s. prostat′icus** [NA], the posterolateral recess between the seminal colliculus and the wall of the urethra. **s′s of pulmonary trunk,** s. trunci pulmonalis. **pyriform s.,** recessus piriformis. **rectal s′s, s. recta′les,** s. anales. **s. rec′tus** [NA], a venous sinus of the dura mater situated in the line of union of the cerebral falx and the cerebellar tentorium, formed by the junction of the great cerebral vein and the inferior sagittal sinus, and commonly ending in the opposite transverse sinus at the confluence of the sinuses. Called also *straight s.* **renal s., s. rena′lis** [NA], a cavity within the substance of the kidney, occupied by the renal pelvis, calices, vessels, nerves, and fat. **s. reu′niens,** the sinus venosus of the embryonic heart into which empty all the veins that go to the heart. **rhomboid s.,** fossa rhomboidea. **rhomboid s. of Henle,** ventriculus terminalis medullae spinalis. **Ridley's s.,** s. circularis. **Rokitansky-Aschoff s′s,** small outpouchings of the mucosa of the gallbladder extending through the lamina propria and the muscular layer. **sacrococcygeal s.,** pilonidal s. **sagittal s., inferior,** s. sagittalis inferior. **sagittal s., superior,** s. sagittalis superior. **s. sagitta′lis infe′rior** [NA], inferior sagittal sinus: a small venous sinus of the dura mater, situated in the posterior half of the lower concave border of the cerebral falx and opening into the upper end of the straight sinus. **s. sagitta′lis supe′rior** [NA], superior sagittal sinus: a single venous sinus of the dura mater which begins in front of the crista galli and extends backward in the convex border of the falx cerebri. Near the internal occipital protuberance it ends in a variable way in the confluence of the sinuses. It receives the superior cerebral veins, communicates with the lateral lacunae of adjacent dura mater, and is partially invaginated by arachnoidal granulations. **semilunar s. of tibia,** incisura fibularis tibiae. **sigmoid s., s. sigmoi′deus** [NA], either of two venous sinuses within the dura mater that are continuations of the transverse sinuses; each curves downward from the tentorium cerebelli to become continuous with the superior bulb of the internal jugular vein. **sphenoidal s.,** s. sphenoidalis. **sphenoidal s., bony,** s. sphenoidalis osseus. **s. sphenoida′lis** [NA], sphenoidal sinus: one of the paired paranasal sinuses, located in the anterior part of the body of the sphenoid bone and communicating with the highest meatus of the nasal cavity on the same side. See also *s. sphenoidalis osseus.* **s. sphenoida′lis os′seus** [NA], bony sphenoidal sinus: an air cavity of variable size and shape situated in the anterior part of the body of the sphenoid bone; separated from its fellow of the opposite side by a septum, and opening into the nasal cavity above the superior nasal concha on the same side. **sphenoparietal s., s. sphenoparieta′lis** [NA], a dural venous sinus which begins at a meningeal vein next to the apex of the small wing of the sphenoid bone and which drains into the anterior part of the cavernous sinus. Called also *Breschet's s.* **s. of spleen, splenic s., s. sple′nicus** [NA], splenic sinus: a dilated venous sinus not lined by ordinary endothelial cells, found in the splenic pulp; called also *s. lienis* [NA alternative] and *s. of spleen.* **straight s.,** s. rectus. **subarachnoidal s′s,** cisternae subarachnoideales. **subcapsular s′s,** marginal s′s (def. 2.) **subpetrosal s.,** s. petrosus inferior. **superpetrosal s.,** s. petrosus superior. **tarsal s., s. tar′si** [NA], the space between the calcaneus and talus, containing the interosseous ligament; called also *tarsal canal.* **tentorial s.,** s. rectus. **terminal s.,** a vein which encircles the vascular area in the blastoderm. **tonsillar s., s. tonsilla′ris,** fossa tonsillaris. **transverse s. of dura mater,** s. transversus durae matris. **transverse s. of pericardium,** s. transversus pericardii. **s. transver′sus du′rae ma′tris** [NA], transverse sinus of dura mater: either of two large venous sinuses of the dura mater that begin in a variable fashion at the confluence of the sinuses near the internal occipital protuberance. Each follows the attached margin of the tentorium cerebelli to the petrous temporal bone, where it becomes the sigmoid sinus. At their origin in the confluence, the right and left sinuses communicate with each other, and with the superior sagittal sinus and the straight sinus. **s. transver′sus pericar′dii** [NA], transverse sinus of pericardium: a passage behind the aorta and pulmonary trunk and in front of the atria; it is lined by serous pericardium. **traumatic s.,** a sinus due to trauma. **s. trun′ci pulmona′lis** [NA], sinuses of pulmonary trunk: slight dilatations in the wall of the pulmonary trunk immediately above the pulmonary valve. **s. tym′pani** [NA], **tympanic s.,** a deep fossa in the posterior part of the tympanic cavity; it is bounded superiorly by the eminentia pyramidalis, inferiorly by the subiculum promontorii, and it opens anteriorly into the fossula fenestrae cochleae. **s. of tympanic cavity, posterior,** s. posterior cavi tympani. **s. un′guis** [NA], the space underlying the advancing free edge of the fingernail or toenail. **urogenital s., s. urogenita′lis** [NA], an elongated sac formed by division of the cloaca in the early embryo, communicating with the mesonephric ducts and bladder, and forming the vestibule, urethra, and vagina in the female and some of the urethra in the male. **uterine s′s,** venous channels in the wall of the uterus in pregnancy. **s. of Valsalva,** s. aortae. **s. of venae cavae, s. vena′rum cava′rum** [NA], the portion of the right atrium bounded medially by the interatrial septum and laterally by the crista terminalis, and into which the superior and inferior venae cavae empty; it is often called the sinus venosus because it develops from that embryonic structure. **s. veno′si dura′les,** s. durae matris. **s. veno′sus,** 1. [NA] the common venous receptacle in the embryo midheart, attached to the posterior wall of the primitive atrium; it receives the umbilical and vitelline veins and the ducts of Cuvier. 2. s. venarum cavarum. **s. veno′sus scle′rae** [NA], venous sinus of sclera: a circular channel at the junction of the sclera and cornea, which is the main pathway for elimination of aqueous humor from the eye. Called also *Schlemm's canal.* **venous s.,** 1. a large vein or channel for the circulation of venous blood. 2. sinus venosus. **venous s′s of dura mater,** s. durae matris. **venous s. of sclera,** s. venosus sclerae. **s. ventric′uli,** Forssell's s. **s. vertebra′les longitudina′les,** old term for internal vertebral venous plexus.

sinusal (si′nus-al) pertaining to a sinus.

sinusitis (si″nŭ-si′tis) inflammation of a sinus. The condition may be purulent or nonpurulent, acute or chronic. Depending on the site of involvement it is known as ethmoid, frontal, maxillary, or sphenoid sinusitis. **infectious s. of turkeys,** a common, sometimes highly fatal respiratory disease of turkeys and game birds, caused by organisms of the pleuropneumonia-like group and marked by swelling below the eyes and sneezing; called also *airsac disease.*

sinusoid (si′nŭ-soid) [*sinus* + Gr. *eidos* form] 1. resembling a sinus. 2. a form of terminal blood channel consisting of a large, irregular anastomosing vessel, having a lining of reticuloendothelium but little or no adventitia. Sinusoids are found in the liver, suprarenals, heart, parathyroid, carotid gland, spleen, hemolymph glands, and pancreas; sinusoids in the anterior pituitary gland, adrenal cortex, and

islets of Langerhans have a continuous basal lamina and a thin endothelium penetrated by pores closed by thin diaphragms (*fenestrated s′s*), and in many mammals the endothelial cells lining those of the liver meet and overlap in some areas, while there are gaps between the cells in other areas (*discontinuous s′s*). Called also *sinusoidal capillaries.* **myocardial s′s,** blood sinusoids that lie between the myocardial bundles or fibers.

sinusoidalization (si″nŭ-soi″dal-i-za′shun) the application of a sinusoidal current.

sinusotomy (si″nŭ-sot′o-me) [*sinus* + Gr. *tomē* a cutting] incision into a sinus.

sinuventricular (si″nu-ven-trik′u-lar) sinoventricular.

SiO₂ silicon dioxide (silica).

Si op. sit abbreviation for L. *si o′pus sit,* if it is necessary.

siphon (si′fun) [Gr. *siphōn* tube] a bent tube with two arms of unequal length, used to transfer liquids from a higher to a lower level by the force of atmospheric pressure.

siphonage (si′fun-ij) the use of the siphon, as in gastric lavage or in draining the bladder.

Siphona irritans (si-fon′ah ir′ĭ-tans) *Haematobia irritans.*

Siphonaptera (si″fo-nap′ter-ah) [Gr. *siphon* tube + *apteros* wingless] an order of laterally compressed, highly chitinized and sclerotized small wingless blood-sucking ectoparasites of mammals and birds, commonly known as fleas. More than 800 species have been described, grouped in six or more families.

Siphunculata (si-fun″ku-la′tah) an order of insects including the lice.

Siphunculina (si-fun″ku-li′nah) a genus of dipterous insects of the family Chloropidae. **S. funic′ola,** the common "eye-fly" of India, where it spreads conjunctivitis; trachoma may also be transmitted by it.

Sippy diet, treatment (method) (sip′e) [Bertram Welton *Sippy,* American physician, 1866–1924] see under *diet* and *treatment.*

siqua (si′kwah) [coined from L. *sidentis altitudinis quadratio,* the square of the sitting height] Pirquet's unit for calculating the area of the absorptive surface of the intestine; it is the square of the sitting height (in centimeters).

sirenomelus (si″ren-om′ĕ-lus) [Gr. *seirēn* siren + *melos* limb] a fetus with fused legs and no feet. Cf. *sympus.*

siriasis (sir-i′ah-sis) [Gr. *seiriasis* a disease produced by the heat of the sun] sunstroke.

sirikaya (sir″ĭ-ka′yah) the tree *Annona squamosa,* L. (Annonaceae), sugar apple or custard apple, whose fruit is edible and whose leaves are sudorific and bark purgative.

sirup (sir′up) syrup.

-sis [Gr. suffix of action] a word termination denoting an action, process, or condition. Appears most commonly in the suffixes *-asis, -esis, -iasis,* and *-osis.*

SISI short increment sensitivity index; see under *index.*

sismotherapy (sis″mo-ther′ah-pe) seismotherapy.

sisomicin (sis″o-mi′sin) chemical name: (2S-*cis*)-4-*O*-[3-amino-6-(aminomethyl)-3, 4-dihydro-2*H*-pyran-2-yl]-2-deoxy-6-*O*[3-deoxy-4-*O*-methyl-3-(methylamino)-β-L-arabinopyranosyl-D-streptamine. An aminoglycoside antibiotic derived from *Micromonospora inyoensis,* $C_{19}H_{37}N_5O_7$, closely related to C_{1a} component of the gentamicin complex; it is bactericidal for many gram-negative and some gram-positive organisms. **s. sulfate,** the sulfate salt of sisomicin, $(C_{19}H_{37}N_5O_7)_2 \cdot 5H_2SO_4$, having the antibacterial properties of the base.

sissorexia (sis″o-rek′se-ah) a tendency of the spleen to accumulate blood corpuscles.

sister (sis′ter) the nurse in charge of a hospital ward (Great Britain).

Sisto's sign (sēs′tōz) [Genero *Sisto,* Chilean pediatrician, died 1923] see under *sign.*

Sistrurus (sis-troo′rus) a genus of small rattlesnakes, the ground rattlesnakes, widely distributed throughout the United States, which have symmetrical plates covering the head. See table accompanying *snake.*

Sisyrinchium galaxioides (sis″ĭ-rin′ke-um gah-lak″se-oi′dēz) a South American iridaceous plant; its bulbs are purgative and diuretic.

site (sīt) a place, position, or locus. **active s.,** that portion of an enzyme molecule containing chemical groups on amino acids in a particular geometric conformation that so bond with the substrate molecule as to facilitate the conversion of the substrate into a reaction product; called also *catalytic s.* **allosteric s.,** that subunit of an enzyme molecule which binds with a nonsubstrate molecule, inducing a conformational change that changes the affinity of the enzyme for its substrate. **antigen-binding s., antigen-combining s.,** the region of the immunoglobulin molecule that binds to antigens; there is one such site on each of the two Fab regions of each immunoglobulin monomer. **binding s's,** those portions of an enzyme molecule that contain chemical groups on amino acid residues in a geometric configuration bonding particular compounds with relatively high affinity. Substrate binding sites so bond the substrate that it becomes susceptible to change by the *active s.* Effector binding sites so bond regulating compounds as to alter the conformation of the enzyme and change its activity. **catalytic s.,** active s. **combining s.,** antigen-binding s. **immunologically privileged s's,** regions of the body that are not normally accessible to effector cells of the immune system and thus sites where allograft rejection does not occur and tumors escape immune surveillance, e.g., the meninges of the brain and the anterior chamber of the eye. **operator s.,** a site adjacent to the structural genes in the operon, believed to be the site on the DNA to which repressor molecules are bound, thereby inhibiting the synthesis of mRNA by the genes in the adjacent operon. **restriction s.,** a base sequence in a DNA segment recognized by a particular restriction endonuclease.

sitfast (sit′fast) an inverted conical area of dry gangrene involving the skin and superficial fasciae of the neck in draft animals, caused by arrest of blood supply from pressure.

sitiology (sit″e-ol′o-je) sitology.

sitiomania (sit″e-o-ma′ne-ah) sitomania.

sit(o)- [Gr. *sitos* food] a combining form denoting relationship to food.

sitology (si-tol′o-je) the sum of knowledge regarding food, diet, and nutrition.

sitomania (si″to-ma′ne-ah) [sito- + Gr. *mania* madness] 1. excessive hunger, or morbid craving for food. 2. periodic bulimia.

sitophobia (si″to-fo′be-ah) [sito- + *phobia*] irrational fear of eating or of food.

sitosterol (si-tos′ter-ol) a generic term for a group of closely related natural plant sterols, the individual compounds being designated by Greek letters, and sometimes subscript numerals, as α_1, α_2, α_3, β, and γ, on the basis of differing characteristics. A pharmaceutical preparation, called *sitosterols,* consisting of β-sitosterol and related sterols of plant origin, and containing not less than 95 per cent of total sterols and not less than 85 per cent of unsaturated sterols, calculated on the dried basis as β-sitosterol, is used as an oral anticholesterolemic agent.

β-sitosterolemia (si-tos″ter-ol-e′me-ah) the presence of excessive levels of plant sterols, especially β-sitosterol, in the blood. A rare form is associated with xanthomatosis, with tuberous and tendon xanthomas appearing in childhood.

sitotaxis (si″to-tak′sis) sitotropism.

sitotherapy (si″to-ther′ah-pe) [sito- + Gr. *therapeia* treatment] dietetic treatment.

sitotoxin (si″to-tok′sin) any basic food poison, especially that generated in a cereal food by a plant microorganism.

sitotoxism (si″to-tok′sizm) [sito- + Gr. *toxikon* poison] poisoning from ingested foods; food poisoning; alimentary toxicosis.

sitotropism (si-tot′ro-pizm) [sito- + Gr. *tropos* a turning] response of living cells to the presence of nutritive elements.

situation (sit″u-a′shun) the combination of factors with which an individual is confronted. In psychology, the total sum of physical, psychological, and sociocultural factors that act on a person and influence his behavior.

situs (si′tus), pl. *si′tus* [L.] site, or position. **s. inver′sus vis′cerum,** lateral transposition of the viscera of the thorax and abdomen; a familial pattern and consanguineous parents have been reported. Complete transposition of the viscera in the absence of other defects is structurally sound, but see *dextrocardia, levocardia,* and *Kartagener's syndrome.* **s. perver′sus,** dislocation of any viscus. **s. sol′itus,** the

normal position of the viscera. **s. transver′sus,** s. inversus viscerum.

Si vir. perm. abbreviation for L. *si vi′res permit′tant,* if the strength will permit.

606 (siks-o-siks) arsphenamine.

Sjögren's syndrome (disease) (sho′grenz) [Henrik Samuel Conrad *Sjögren,* Swedish ophthalmologist, born 1899] see under *syndrome.*

Sjöqvist's method (sho′kwistz) [John August *Sjöqvist,* Swedish physician, 1863–1934] see under *method.*

skatole (skat′ōl) [Gr. *skōr, skatos* dung] chemical name: β-methylindole. A crystalline amine, with a strong characteristic odor,

$$C_6H_4 \cdot C(CH_3):CH \cdot NH,$$

from human feces. It is produced by the decomposition of proteins in the intestine and directly from the amino acid tryptophan by decarboxylation.

skatosin (skah-to′sin) a base, $C_{10}H_{16}N_2O_2$, derived from certain proteins.

skatoxyl (skah-tok′sil) an oxidation product of skatole, $CH_3 \cdot C_8H_6NO$, found in the urine in certain cases of disease of the large intestine.

skein (skān) spireme. **Holmgren's s's, test s's,** skeins of colored worsted used in Holmgren's test of color perception.

skelalgia (ske-lal′je-ah) [Gr. *skelos* leg + *algos* pain + -*ia*] pain in the leg.

skelasthenia (ske″las-the′ne-ah) [Gr. *skelos* leg + *a* neg. + *sthenos* strength + -*ia*] weakness of the legs.

Skelaxin (skĕ-laks′in) trademark for a preparation of metaxalone.

skeletal (skel′ĕ-tal) pertaining to the skeleton.

skeletin (skel′ĕ-tin) any of a number of gelatinous substances occurring in invertebrate tissue, and including chitin, sericin, spongin, etc.

skeletization (skel″ĕ-ti-za′shun) 1. extreme emaciation. 2. the removal of the soft parts from the skeleton.

skeletogenous (skel″ĕ-toj′ĕ-nus) producing skeletal or bony structures.

skeletogeny (skel″ĕ-toj′ĕ-ne) the formation of the skeleton; the origin and development of the skeleton.

skeletography (skel″ĕ-tog′rah-fe) [skeleton + Gr. *graphein* to write] a description of the skeleton.

skeletology (skel″ĕ-tol′o-je) [skeleton + -*logy*] the sum of what is known regarding the skeleton.

skeleton (skel′ĕ-ton) [Gr. "a dried body, mummy"] the hard framework of the animal body, especially the bony framework of the body of higher vertebrate animals; the bones of the body collectively. See *endoskeleton, exoskeleton,* and *splanchnoskeleton.* **appendicular s., s. appendicula′re** [NA], the bones of the upper and lower limbs. **axial s., s. axia′le,** the bones of the cranium, vertebral column, ribs, and sternum. **cardiac s.,** the fibrous or fibrocartilaginous framework that supports and gives attachment to the cardiac musculature, which consists of fibrous rings that send thin sheetlike extensions to the heart valves; it is continuous with the pulmonary trunk and the membranous part of the interventricular septum. Called also *fibrous s. of heart.* **fibrous s. of heart,** cardiac s. **s. of heart,** cardiac s. **s. mem′bri inferio′ris li′beri** pars libera membri superioris. **s. mem′bri superio′ris li′beri** pars libera membri superioris. **thoracic s., s. of thorax,** compages thoracis. **visceral s.,** that portion of the skeleton which protects the viscera, as the sternum, ribs, and os coxae.

skeletopia, skeletopy (skel″ĕ-to′pe-ah; skel′ĕ-to″pe) [skeleton + Gr. *topos* place] the position of an organ in relation to the skeleton.

Skene's glands (ducts, tubules) (skēnz) [Alexander Johnston Chalmers *Skene,* American gynecologist, 1838–1900] see *ductus paraurethrales.*

skenitis (ske-ni′tis) inflammation of the ductus paraurethrales (Skene's glands).

skenoscope (ske′no-skōp) [Skene's glands + Gr. *skopein* to examine] an endoscope for examining Skene's glands.

skeocytosis (ske″o-si-to′sis) [Gr. *skaios* left + *kytos* hollow vessel + -*osis*] (*obs.*) presence of immature forms of white cells (neutrophils) in the blood; called also *shift to the left.*

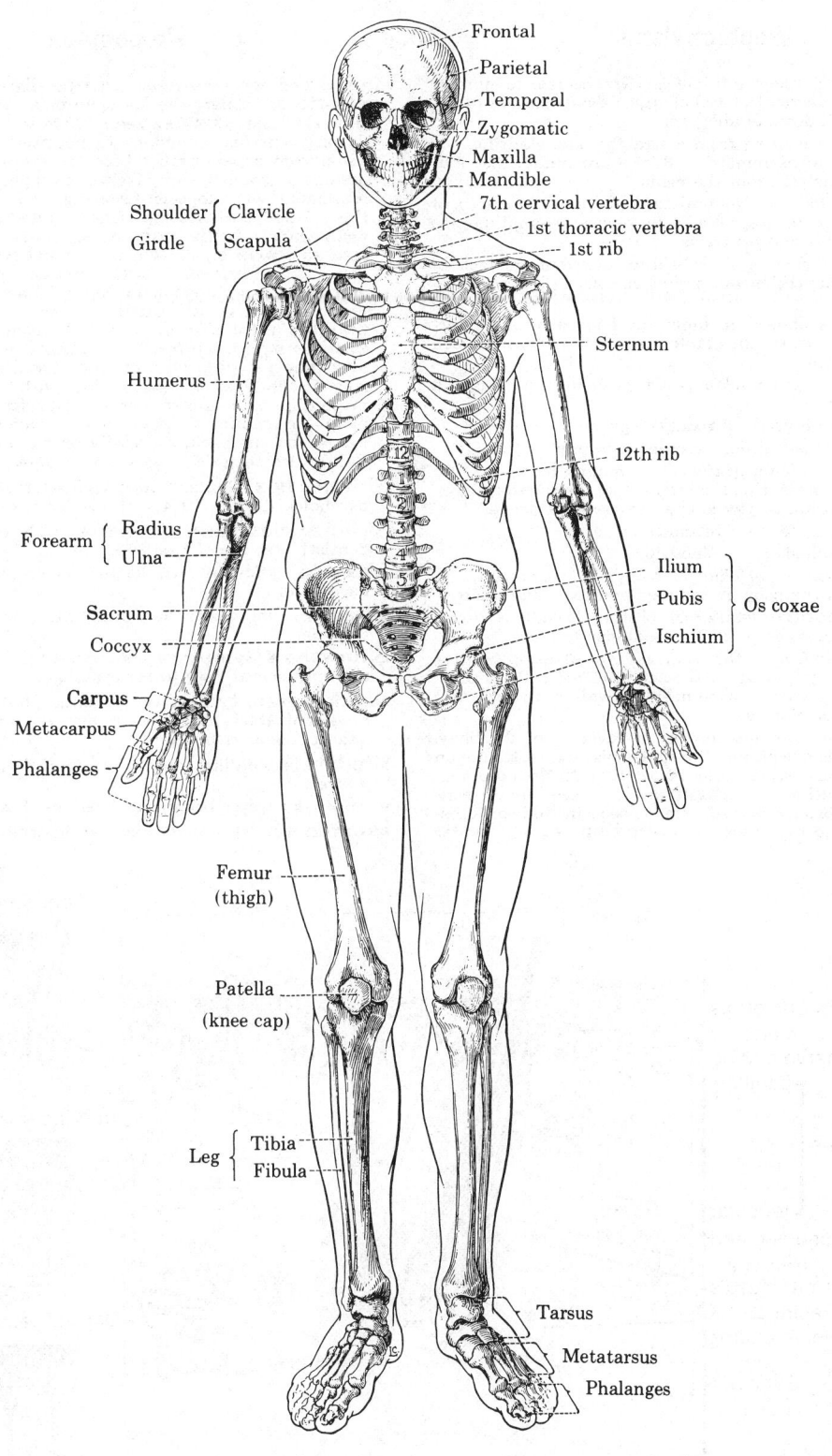

Frontal
Parietal
Temporal
Zygomatic
Maxilla
Mandible
7th cervical vertebra
1st thoracic vertebra
1st rib

Shoulder { Clavicle
Girdle { Scapula

Humerus

Sternum

12th rib

Forearm { Radius
        { Ulna

Ilium
Pubis   } Os coxae
Ischium

Sacrum
Coccyx

Carpus
Metacarpus
Phalanges

Femur
(thigh)

Patella
(knee cap)

Leg { Tibia
    { Fibula

Tarsus
Metatarsus
Phalanges

PLATE 42 — ANTERIOR VIEW OF THE HUMAN SKELETON

1533

skeptophylaxis (skep″to-fi-lak′sis) [Gr. *skēptein* to support + *phylaxis* protection] (*obs.*) allergic desensitization by injection of small doses of allergen.

skew (sku) 1. deviating from a straight line; slanting. 2. asymmetric or antisymmetric. 3. of a probability distribution, not symmetric about the mean.

skewfoot (sku′foot) a general term for any deformity of the foot in which its forepart deviates toward the midline; see *metatarsus varus* and *pes varus*.

skewness (sku′nes) of a probability distribution, lack of symmetry about the mean, or any measure of the lack of symmetry.

skia- [Gr. *skia* shadow] a combining form denoting reference to shadows, especially of internal structures as produced by roentgen rays.

skiagram (ski′ah-gram) [*skia-* + Gr. *gramma* a writing] a roentgenogram.

skiagraph (ski′ah-graf) a roentgenogram.

skiagraphy (ski-ag′rah-fe) roentgenography.

skiameter (ski-am′ĕ-ter) [*skia-* + Gr. *metron* measure] an instrument for measuring the intensity of the roentgen rays, and thus determining how long an exposure is needed.

skiametry (ski-am′ĕ-tre) retinoscopy.

skiascope (ski′ah-skōp) retinoscope.

skiascopy (ski-as′ko-pe) [*skia-* + *-scopy*] 1. retinoscopy. 2. examination of the body by the roentgen ray; fluoroscopy.

Skillern's fracture (skil′ernz) [Penn Gaskell *Skillern*, American surgeon, born 1882] see under *fracture*.

skimming (skim′ing) the removing of floating matter from a liquid. **plasma s.,** the action of red cells in flowing blood which leaves a zone near the wall of a vessel that is relatively free of cells.

skin (skin) the outer integument or covering of the body, consisting of the dermis and the epidermis, and resting upon the subcutaneous tissues; called also *cutis* [NA]. See accompanying illustration. **alligator s.,** see *ichthyosis*. **bronzed s.,** bronze-colored skin, as seen in Addison's disease and hemochromatosis. **collodion s.,** see under baby, and see *ichthyosis*. **crocodile s.,** see *ichthyosis*. **elastic s.,** Ehlers-Danlos syndrome. **farmers' s.,** actinic elastosis. **fish s.,** see *ichthyosis*. **glossy s.,** a condition occurring secondary to neuritis in which the skin, usually on an extremity, becomes erythematous and then assumes a grayish, shiny ivory-like appearance, and may be associated with alopecia, fissuring, and ulceration; nails on the affected part become ridged. Called also *atrophoderma neuriticum*. **India rubber s.,** Ehlers-Danlos syndrome. **lax s., loose s.,** cutis laxa. **marble s.,** cutis marmorata. **parchment s.,** a dry condition of the skin of cattle and sheep, especially such a condition accompanying verminous bronchitis. **piebald s.,** a term applied to the appearance of the skin in partial albinism or vitiligo. **porcupine s.,** see *ichthyosis*. **sailors' s.,** actinic elastosis. **shagreen s.,** a large connective tissue nevus often occurring in children in association with tuberous sclerosis, presenting as a skin-colored or yellowish, elevated, knobby plaque resembling shark or pig skin, which is predominantly located on the back, especially on the lumbosacral region. Called also *peau de chagrin* and *shagreen patch*.

Skinner box (skin′er) [Burrhus Frederic *Skinner*, American psychologist, born 1904] see under *box*.

Skinner classification (skin′er) [C.N. *Skinner*, American dentist] see under *classification*.

Skiodan (ski′o-dan) trademark for preparations of methiodal sodium.

skler(o)- for words beginning thus, see those beginning *scler(o)-*.

Sklowsky's symptom (sklow′skēz) [E. L. *Sklowsky*, German physician] see under *symptom*.

Skoda's sign, tympany (sko′dahz) [Josef *Skoda*, Austrian physician, 1805–1881] see under *sign*, and see *skodaic resonance*, under *resonance*.

skodaic (sko-da′ik) named for Josef *Skoda*; see under *resonance*.

skole- for words beginning thus, see those beginning *scole-*.

skopometer (sko-pom′ĕ-ter) an instrument for measuring

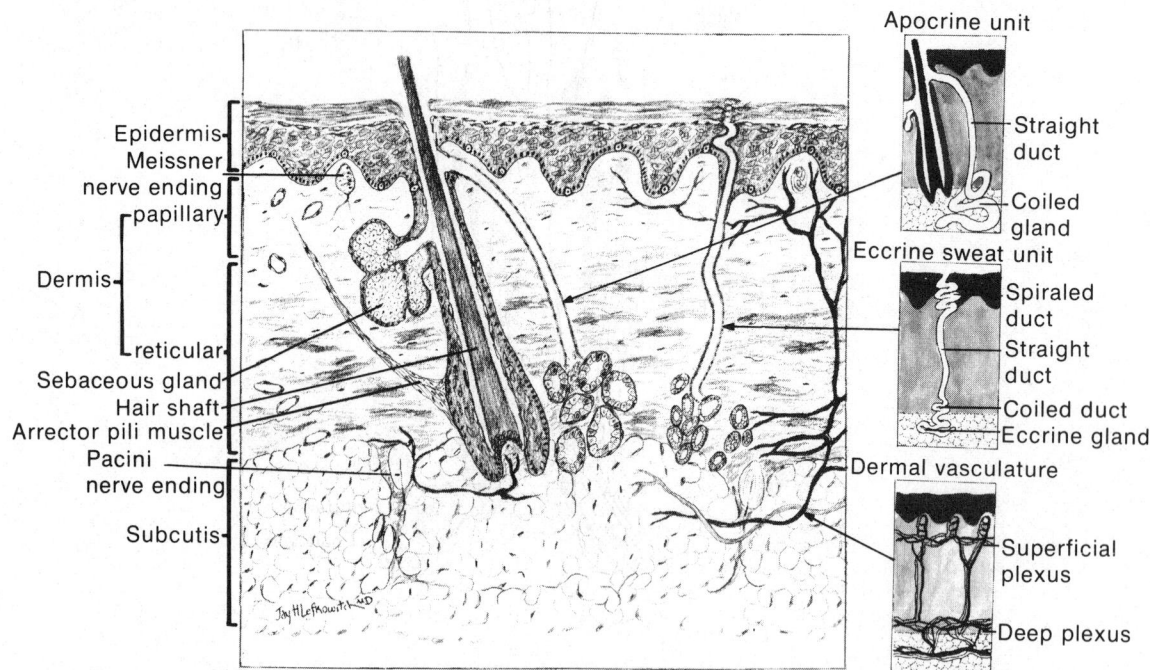

Cross section of the skin.

color, cloudiness, and other optical phenomena of liquids without using standards for comparison.

skot(o)- for words beginning thus, see those beginning *scot(o)-*.

SKSD streptokinase-streptodornase.

skull (skul) the bony framework of the head, composed of the cranial bones and the bones of the face. It includes the ethmoid, frontal, hyoid, lacrimal, nasal, occipital, palatine, parietal, sphenoid, temporal, and zygomatic bones, and the inferior nasal conchae, mandible, maxillae, and vomer. Called also *cranium*. **cloverleaf s.,** kleeblattschädel. **hot cross bun s.,** see *Parrot's sign,* def. 2. **lacuna s.,** craniolacunia. **maplike s.,** a skull marked by irregular tracings resembling outlines on a map; seen in x-ray films of the cranial bones in Hand-Schüller-Christian disease. **natiform s.,** see *Parrot's sign,* def. 2. **steeple s., tower s.,** oxycephaly. **West's lacuna s., West-Engstler's s.,** a honeycomb appearance of the skull in roentgenograms, associated with spina bifida or meningocele and occasionally with encephalocele.

S.L.A. abbreviation for L. *sacrolaeva anterior* (left sacroanterior, a presentation of the fetus).

slant (slant) 1. a sloping surface of agar in a test tube. 2. a slant culture.

SLE systemic lupus erythematosus.

sleep (slēp) a period of rest for the body and mind, during which volition and consciousness are in partial or complete abeyance and the bodily functions partially suspended. Sleep has also been described as a behavioral state marked by a characteristic immobile posture and diminished but readily reversible sensitivity to external stimuli. Sleep is divisible into two stages: *NREM* (non-rapid eye movement) *sleep* and *REM* (rapid eye movement) *sleep*. **active s.,** REM s. **D s.,** REM s. **deep s.,** NREM s. **desynchronized s.,** REM s. **dreaming s.,** REM s. **electric s.,** loss of voluntary movement and presence of general anesthesia induced by the application to the head of a rapidly interrupted electric current. **electrotherapeutic s.,** cerebral electrotherapy. **fast wave s.,** REM s. **non-rapid eye movement s.,** NREM s. **NREM s.,** the dreamless period of sleep, consisting of four stages of succeeding depth, during which the brain waves are slow and of high voltage, and autonomic activities, such as heart rate and blood pressure, are low and regular. Brief episodes of REM sleep occur at intervals during this type of sleep; in adults, about 80 per cent of sleep is NREM sleep. Called also *non-rapid eye movement s., orthodox s., slow wave s.,* and *synchronized s.* **orthodox s.,** NREM s. **paradoxical s.,** REM s. **paroxysmal s.,** narcolepsy. **prolonged s.,** treatment of mental disorders by sustained and continuous sleep for several days under profound drug narcosis. **quiet s.,** NREM s. **rapid eye movement s.,** REM s. **REM s.,** the period of sleep during which the brain waves are fast and of low voltage, and autonomic activities, such as heart rate and respiration, are irregular. This type of sleep is associated with dreaming, mild involuntary muscle jerks, and rapid eye movements (REM). It usually occurs three to four times each night at intervals of 80 to 120 minutes, each occurrence lasting from 5 minutes to more than an hour. In adults, about 20 per cent of sleep is REM sleep and 80 per cent is NREM (non-rapid eye movement) sleep. Called also *desynchronized s., paradoxical s.,* and *rapid eye movement s.* See also *REM rebound,* under *rebound.* **S s.,** NREM s. **slow wave s.,** NREM s. **synchronized s.,** NREM s. **temple s.,** incubation, def. 3. **twilight s.,** a condition of analgesia and amnesia, produced by hypodermic administration of morphine and scopolamine. In this state the patient, although responding to pain, does not retain it in her memory. Formerly widely used in obstetrics. Called also *twilight anesthesia, Freiburg method,* and *seminarcosis.*

sleeptalking (slēp′tok-ing) talking during sleep; called also *somniloquism.*

sleepwalking (slēp′wok-ing) somnambulism.

slide (slīd) a glass plate on which objects are placed for microscopic examination.

sling (sling) a bandage or suspensory for supporting all or a particular part of the body. **Glisson's s.,** a leather collar applied around the neck and under the chin to which is attached an extension apparatus over a pulley at the head of the patient's bed: for applying extension to the vertebral column.

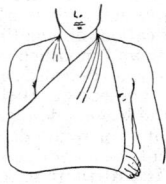

Sling.

slit (slit) 1. a long narrow opening or incision. 2. to make a long narrow opening or incision. **filtration s's,** slit pores. **gill s.,** a long narrow opening from the pharynx to the exterior of the body of many aquatic animals, such as fishes and salamanders, through which water is drawn to bathe the gills.

slope (slōp) 1. an inclined plane; a surface which is neither horizontal nor vertical. 2. to deviate from the horizontal and from the vertical plane; said of a surface intersecting the horizontal at an angle between 1 and 90 degrees. **lower ridge s.,** the slope of the crest of the mandibular residual ridge from the third molar region to its most anterior aspect in relation to the lower border of the mandible as viewed in profile. **mandibular anteroposterior ridge s.,** the slope of the crest of the mandibular residual ridge from the third molar region to its most anterior aspect in relation to the lower border of the mandible as viewed in profile.

slough (sluf) 1. necrotic tissue in the process of separating from viable portions of the body. 2. to shed or cast off.

sloughing (sluf′ing) the formation or separation of a slough.

slows (slōz) trembles.

S.L.P. abbreviation for L. *sacrolaeva posterior* (left sacroposterior, a presentation of the fetus).

S.L.T. abbreviation for L. *sacrolaeva transversa* (left sacrotransverse, a presentation of the fetus).

Sluder's method, neuralgia (syndrome) (slu′derz) [Greenfield *Sluder,* American laryngologist, 1865–1928] see under *method* and *neuralgia.*

sludge (sluj) a suspension of solid or semisolid particles in a fluid which itself may or may not be a truly viscous fluid. **activated s.,** sludge from aerated sewage, consisting mainly of aerobic bacteria (e.g., *Sphaerotilus, Zoogloea*), protozoa (e.g., *Opercularia, Vorticella*), yeasts, and molds. Further treatment consists of anaerobic digestion. A portion serves as inoculum for a succeeding batch of screened and sedimented raw sewage.

sludging (sluj′ing) the settling out of solid particles from solution. **s. of blood,** see *intravascular agglutination,* under *agglutination.*

slug (slug) a large group of terrestrial gastropods closely related to the snails but having a rudimentary or absent shell.

slurry (slur′e) a watery mixture or suspension of insoluble matter.

slyke (slīk) a unit of buffer value, named after D. D. Van Slyke, a pioneer in buffering analysis; abbreviated sl.

Sm chemical symbol for *samarium.*

SMA 6/60 [Sequential Multiple Analyzer] trademark for an automated chemistry system that determines the concentrations of six substances in serum in 60 minutes and reports the results in a fixed sequence; the substances measured are creatinine or glucose, urea nitrogen, chloride, carbon dioxide, sodium, and potassium.

SMA 12/60 [Sequential Multiple Analyzer] trademark for an automated chemistry system that determines the concentrations of 12 substances in serum in 60 minutes and reports the results in a fixed sequence; the substances measured are calcium, inorganic phosphorus, glucose, urea nitrogen, uric acid, cholesterol, total protein, albumin, total bilirubin, alkaline phosphatase, lactate dehydrogenase, and aspartate aminotransferase.

SMAF specific macrophage arming factor.

smallpox (smawl′poks) [compared to "great pox" (syphilis)] variola: an acute, highly contagious, often fatal infectious disease caused by an orthopoxvirus characterized by a biphasic febrile course and distinctive progressive skin eruptions. Vaccination has succeeded in eradicating smallpox worldwide; therefore, since there are no animal vectors of the disease, the only source of the virus is in medical laboratories. One clinical classification of smallpox comprised hemorrhagic, flat, ordinary, and modified varieties, each of which were subdivided into types. See also *variola major* and *variola minor*. **equine s.,** horsepox. **flat s.,** a severe variety of smallpox in which the lesions do not project above the skin surface, and depending upon the density of the rash are of three types: confluent, semiconfluent, and discrete. Called also *malignant s*. **fulminant s.,** hemorrhagic s. **hemorrhagic s.,** a severe and highly fatal variety of smallpox in which hemorrhages occur in the skin and mucous membranes before the onset of the rash (early type) or after the rash appears (late type). Called also *fulminant s*. **malignant s.,** flat s. **modified s.,** a variety of smallpox occurring in previously vaccinated, partially immune individuals in which all signs and symptoms are less severe than in other varieties of smallpox; depending on whether the rash is present and its density, this variety is divided into four types: that in which no rash occurs (variola sine eruptione), and confluent, discrete, and semiconfluent. Called also *varioloid*. **ordinary s.,** the most common variety of smallpox, in which after an incubation period and a prodrome of high fever, chills, myalgia, and malaise, petechial reddish spots appear on the oral mucosa followed by a raised macular cutaneous rash that usually starts on the forehead and spreads to become generalized. The lesions evolve to become papules and vesicles, umbilicate, crust, and scab, leaving small depressed, depigmented scars (pock marks); depending upon the density of the rash, the lesions are of three types: confluent, discrete, and semiconfluent. **ovine s.,** sheeppox.

smear (smēr) a specimen for microscopic study prepared by spreading the material across the glass slide. **Pap s., Papanicolaou s.,** see under *tests*.

smegma (smeg′mah) [Gr. *smēgma* soap] the secretion of sebaceous glands, especially the cheesy secretion, consisting principally of desquamated epithelial cells, found chiefly beneath the prepuce. **s. embryo′num,** vernix caseosa.

smegmatic (smeg-mat′ik) pertaining to or composed of smegma.

smegmalith (smeg′mah-lith) [*smegma* + *-lith*] a calcareous concretion in the smegma.

smell-brain (smel′brān) rhinencephalon, def. 1.

Smellie's method, scissors (smel′ēz) [William *Smellie*, British obstetrician, 1697–1763] see under *method* and *scissors*.

smilacin (smi′lah-sin) [Gr. *smilakinos* pertaining to smilax] a poisonous glycoside, $C_{18}H_{36}O_6$, from sarsaparilla.

smilagenin (smi″lah-jen′in) a steroid precursor, $C_{27}H_{44}O_3$, from several species of *Smilax*; used in the manufacture of compounds of the pregnane series.

Smilax (smi′laks) [L., Gr. "bindweed"] a genus of climbing smilacaceous plants, which are the source of sarsaparilla; the starchy root of several species was used as food by the Indians. Several species yield a steroid precursor, smilagenin. **S. aristolochiaefo′lia,** Mexican sarsaparilla, a species used as a beverage flavor and for digestive disorders, kidney ailments, skin diseases, and rheumatism in several tropical countries and Mexico.

Smith (smith) Hamilton Othanel. American microbiologist, born 1931; co-winner, with Werner Arber and Daniel Nathans, of the Nobel prize for medicine or physiology in 1978 for his work on restriction enzymes.

Smith's disease, sign [Eustace *Smith*, London physician, 1835–1914] see *mucous colitis*, under *colitis*, and see under *sign*.

Smith's dislocation, fracture [Robert William *Smith*, Irish surgeon, 1807–1873] see under *dislocation* and *fracture*.

Smith's operation [Henry *Smith*, English surgeon in India, 1862–1948] see under *operation*.

Smith's test [Walter George *Smith*, Irish physician, 1844–1932] see under *tests*.

Smith-Petersen nail [Marius Nygaard *Smith-Petersen*, American orthopedic surgeon, 1886–1953] see under *nail*.

smog (smog) a mixture of smoke and fog; a colloid system in which the disperse phase consists of a mixture of gas and moisture and the dispersion medium is air.

smoke (smōk) a colloid system in which one or more solids is dispersed in a gas or vapor.

SMR standard mortality (or morbidity) ratio.

smudging (smuj′ing) a defect of speech in which the difficult consonants are omitted.

smut (smut) a disease of cereal grasses (wheat, oats, rye, Indian corn) caused by basidiomycetous fungi of the genera *Tilletia, Ustilago,* and *Urocystis*. See *Tilletia, Ustilago,* and *Urocystis*. **corn s.,** a smut of maize which is caused by *Ustilago maydis*; ingestion of the infected seeds cause ustilaginism, a condition similar to ergotism. **rye s.,** ergot formed by the ascomycete *Claviceps purpurea*.

Sn chemical symbol for *tin* [L. *stannum*].

S.N. abbreviation for L. *secun′dum natu′ram*, according to nature.

sn- [for stereospecific numbering] a chemical prefix used to indicate stereoisomers of glycerol derivatives: the glycerol chain is numbered as if it were derived from L-glyceraldehyde. This provides an unambiguous numbering. The enantiomer is obtained by reversing the numbering. For example sn-glycerol 1-phosphate is the same as L-glycerol 1-phosphate; the enantiomer D-glycerol 1-phosphate is the same as L-glycerol 3-phosphate or sn-glycerol 3-phosphate. See D-.

snail (snāl) a gastropod mollusk with a spiral shell. Certain fresh-water snails in tropical countries are intermediate hosts of parasitic trematodes; the miracidium of the fluke developing into a cercaria in the body of the snail.

snake (snāk) a limbless reptile of the suborder Ophidia, some of which are poisonous. See also *viper*. See table. **brown s.,** a venomous elapid snake of Australia and New Guinea belonging to the genus *Demansia*. **cabbage s.,** see *Mermithidae*. **colubrid s.,** a snake of the family Colubridae, most of which are inoffensive, but the boomslang is venomous. **coral s.,** a venomous elapid snake, *Micrurus fulvius*, found in the southern United States and tropical America, whose body is marked with bright red, yellow, and black bands. **crotalid s.,** a snake of the family Crotalidae, a pit viper. **elapid s.,** any snake of the family Elapidae, including cobras, kraits, mambas, blacksnakes, brown snakes, copperheads, tiger snakes, death adder, and coral snakes. **hair s.,** see *Gordius*. **harlequin s.,** coral s. **poisonous s.,** any snake that contains a poison, either in venom glands or in other organs or tissues; commonly, a venomous snake. **sea s.,** a snake of the family Hydrophidae. **tiger s.,** a very venomous elapid snake, *Notechis scutatus*, of Australia, whose body is chiefly brown with dark bands. **venomous s.,** any snake that secretes substances (venoms) capable of producing a deleterious effect on the blood (hematoxins) or nervous system (neurotoxins), the venom being injected into the body of the victim by the snake's bite. Collectively, they are called the *thanatophidia* or *toxicophidia*. **viperine s.,** any snake of the family Viperidae, the true vipers, including European vipers, Russell's viper, sand vipers, puff adders, Gaboon vipers, and rhinoceros vipers.

snap (snap) a short sharp sound. **opening s.,** a short sharp sound in early diastole caused by the movement of the mitral leaflet into the ventricle at the beginning of ventricular filling.

snare (snār) a wire loop or noose for removing polyps and tumors by encircling them at the base and closing the loop.

Sneddon-Wilkinson disease (sne′den wil′kin-son) [Lan Bruce *Sneddon*, English dermatologist, born 1915; Darrell Sheldon *Wilkinson*, English dermatologist, 20th century] subcorneal pustular dermatosis.

sneeze (snēz) 1. to expel air forcibly and spasmodically through the nose and mouth. 2. an involuntary, sudden, violent, and audible expulsion of air through the mouth and nose.

Snell (snel) George Davis. American geneticist, born 1903; co-winner, with Jean Baptiste Gabriel Dausset and Baruj Benacerraf, of the Nobel prize for medicine or physiology in 1980 for their work on the major histocompatibility complex and the genetic control of immune responses.

Snell's law (snelz) [Willebrord van Roijen Snell, Dutch astronomer and mathematician, 1591–1626] see under *law*.

Snellen's chart, etc. (snel′enz) [Hermann *Snellen*, ophthalmologist in Utrecht, 1834–1908] see under *chart, eye, tests,* and *test type*.

IMPORTANT VENOMOUS SNAKES OF THE WORLD

FAMILY AND TYPE OF FANGS	COMMON NAMES	TYPE OF VENOM	DISTRIBUTION	REMARKS
COLUBRIDAE; rear, immovable, grooved	Colubrids	Mostly mild	Warm parts of both hemispheres	Over 1000 species, the few poisonous ones not dangerous
Example:	Boomslang	Hemorrhagin	South Africa	Arboreal, timid
ELAPIDAE; front, immovable, grooved	Elapids	Predominantly neurotoxin	Mostly in Old World	Over 150 species, very poisonous
Examples:	Cobras	Mostly neurotoxin	Africa, India, Asia, Philippines, Celebes	Spitting cobra in Africa aims at eyes
	Kraits	Strong neurotoxin	India, S.E. Asia, Indonesia	Sluggish, often buried in dust
	Mambas	Neurotoxin	Tropical W. Africa	Arboreal
	Blacksnake	Neurotoxin	Australia	Large snake, wet terrain
	Copperhead	Neurotoxin	Australia, Tasmania, Solomons	Damp environment
	Brown snake	Neurotoxin	Australia, New Guinea	Slender
	Tiger snake	Strong neurotoxin	Australia	Dry environment; aggressive; very dangerous
	Death adder	Neurotoxin	Australia, New Guinea	Sandy terrain
	Coral snakes	Neurotoxin	United States, tropical America	About 26 species, 2 in southern U. S. A.
HYDROPHIDAE; front, immovable, hollow	Sea snakes	Some mild; others very toxic	Tropical, Indian and Pacific Oceans	Gentle. Rudder-like tail. Over 50 species
VIPERIDAE; front, movable, hollow	True vipers; viperines; viperids	Predominantly hematoxin	Entirely in Old World	About 50 species
Examples:	European viper	Hematoxin	Europe (rare), N. Africa, Near East	Dry rocky country
	Russell's viper	Hematoxin	S.E. Asia, Java, Sumatra	Mostly open terrain; deadly
	Sand vipers	Hematoxin	N. Sahara	Buried in sand
	Puff adder	Hematoxin	Arabia, Africa	Open terrain; sluggish
	Gaboon viper	Neurotoxin and hematoxin	Tropical W. Africa	Forests; deadly
	Rhinoceros viper	Hematoxin	Tropical Africa	Wet forests
CROTALIDAE; front, movable, hollow	Pit vipers; crotalids; crotalines	Predominantly hematoxin	Old and New Worlds; none in Africa	Over 80 species; pit between eye and nostril
Examples:	Habu viper	Neurotoxin	Warmer parts of E. Asia; Ryukyu Islands	Caves and dry rocky country
	Rattlesnakes†	Predominantly hematoxin	N., Central and S. America	South American form neurotoxic
	Bushmaster	Hematoxin	Central and S. America	Large. In wet forests
	Fer-de-lance	Hematoxin	Central America, N. South America, few West Indies	Common on plantations
	Palm vipers	Hematoxin(?)	S. Mexico, Central and South America	Arboreal; small, greenish. Bite face
	Copperhead	Hematoxin	United States	Dry stony terrain
	Water moccasin	Hematoxin	Southeast U. S. A. to Texas	Swamps
	Asiatic pit vipers	Hematoxin	Southeast Asia, Taiwan	Most arboreal

†All rattlesnakes are venomous.

1537

Snider match test (sni'der) [Thomas H. *Snider,* American physician, born 1925] see under *test.*

S.N.M. Society of Nuclear Medicine.

snore (snor) 1. rough, noisy breathing during sleep, due to vibration of the uvula and soft palate; called also *stertor.* 2. to produce such sounds during sleep.

snow (sno) a freezing or frozen mixture consisting of discrete particles or crystals. **carbon dioxide s.,** Dry Ice: solid carbon dioxide, formed by rapid evaporation of liquid carbon dioxide; it gives a temperature of about 110 degrees below zero Fahrenheit (−79° C.); it has been used in cryotherapy to freeze the skin, thus producing local anesthesia and arrest of blood flow, and, in the form of a slush, as an escharotic to destroy certain skin lesions, such as warts, moles, etc.

snowblindness (sno'blīnd-nes) temporary loss of sight due to injury to superficial cells of the cornea caused by ultraviolet rays of the sun reinforced by those reflected by snow.

SNS sympathetic nervous system.

snuff (snuf) a medicinal or errhine powder to be inhaled through the nose. **anatomical s.-box,** see under *box.*

snuffles (snuf'f'lz) a catarrhal discharge from the nasal mucous membrane in infants, generally in congenital syphilis.

SO the spheno-occipital synchondrosis, a cephalometric landmark designating the most superior point at the junction of the sphenoid and occipital bones.

SO₂ sulfur dioxide.

SOAP a device for conceptualizing the process of recording the progress notes in the *problem-oriented record* (see under *record*): S indicates subjective data obtained from the patient and others close to him; O designates objective data obtained by observation, physical examination, diagnostic studies, etc.; A refers to assessment of the patient's status through analysis of the problem, possible interaction of the problems, and changes in the status of the problems; P designates the plan for patient care.

soap (sōp) [L. *sapo*] any compound of one or more fatty acids, or their equivalents, with an alkali. Soap is detergent and is much employed in liniments, enemas, and in making pills. It is also a mild aperient, antacid, and antiseptic. **animal s.,** sapo domesticus. **carbolic s.,** a disinfectant soap containing 10 per cent of phenol. **castile s.,** a hard soap, either white or mottled, prepared from olive oil and soda. See *sapo,* def. 2. **curd s.,** sapo domesticus. **green s.** [USP], a potassium soap made by the saponification of vegetable oils, excluding coconut oil and palm kernel oil, without the removal of glycerin. It is the chief ingredient of green soap tincture (q.v.). Called also *medicinal soft s., sapo mollis medicinalis,* and *soft s.* **hexachlorophene liquid s.** [USP], a solution of hexachlorophene in a 10 to 13 per cent solution of potassium soap, containing in each 100 gm., 225 to 260 mg. of hexachlorophene; used as a topical anti-infective and detergent. **guaiac s.,** a resin of guaiacum saponified with liquor potassae. **hard s.,** soda s. **McClintock's s.,** a disinfectant soap containing an active mercury salt. **medicinal soft s.,** green s. **potash s.,** green s. **soda s.,** soap made from soda and olive oil; called also *hard s.* **soft s.,** 1. a liquid soap made from potash and some oil; called also *potash s.* and *sapo mollis.* 2. green s. **Starkey's s.,** a soap made of potassium carbonate, turpentine oil, and Venice turpentine in equal parts. **superfatted s.,** a soap having an excess of fat over that necessary to neutralize all the alkali. **zinc s.,** a soap containing zinc oxide or zinc sulfate; for use as an ointment or plaster.

socaloin (so-kal'o-in) a variety of aloin, $C_{15}H_{16}O_7$, from Socotrine aloes.

socia (so'she-ah) [L. "a comrade, associate"] a detached part or exclave of an organ. **s. parot'idis,** accessory parotid gland.

socialization (so″shă-lĭ-za'shun) the process by which society integrates the individual, and the individual learns to behave in socially acceptable ways.

socioacusis (so″se-o-ah-ku'sis) the acceleration of the normal hearing loss associated with aging, which results from the noise encountered in modern civilization.

sociobiologic, sociobiological (so″se-o-bi″o-loj'ik; so″se-o-bi″o-loj'ĭ-kal) pertaining to sociobiology.

sociobiologist (so″se-o-bi-ol′o-jist) an individual trained in sociobiology.

sociobiology (so″se-o-bi-ol′o-je) the branch of theoretical biology which proposes that all animal (including human) behavior has a biological basis, which is controlled by the genes; the study of the biological basis of behavior.

sociogenic (so″se-o-jen'ik) arising from or imposed by society.

sociologist (so″se-ol′o-jist) an individual trained in sociology.

sociology (so″se-ol′o-je) [L. *socius* fellow + *-logy*] the science dealing with social relations and phenomena.

sociometry (so″se-om′ĕ-tre) [L. *socius* fellow + *metrum* a measure] the branch of sociology concerned with the measurement of human social behavior.

sociopath (so′se-o-path″) a previously used term for a person exhibiting antisocial personality disorder.

sociopathic (so″se-o-path′ik) pertaining to antisocial behavior or to antisocial personality disorder.

sociopathy (so″se-op′ah-the) antisocial personality disorder (see under *personality*).

sociotherapy (so″se-o-ther′ah-pe) any treatment emphasizing socioenvironmental and interpersonal rather than intrapsychic factors.

socket (sok′et) a hollow or depression, into which a corresponding part fits. **dry s.,** a condition sometimes occurring after tooth extraction, particularly after traumatic extraction, resulting in a dry appearance of the exposed bone in the socket, due to disintegration or loss of the blood clot. It is basically a focal osteomyelitis without suppuration and is accompanied by severe pain (alveolalgia) and foul odor. Called also *alveolar osteitis* and *alveolitis sicca dolorosa.* **tooth s's,** dental alveoli.

soda (so'dah) a term loosely applied to sodium bicarbonate (baking s.), sodium hydroxide (caustic s.), or sodium carbonate (washing s.). **baking s.,** sodium bicarbonate. **bicarbonate of s.,** sodium bicarbonate. **caustic s.,** sodium hydroxide. **chlorinated s.,** a mixture of sodium chloride and sodium hypochlorite. **s. cum cal′ce,** an escharotic preparation of equal parts of sodium hydroxide and lime. **s. lime,** [NF], hydroxide with sodium or potassium hydroxide, or both; used as adsorbent of carbon dioxide in equipment for metabolism tests, inhalant anesthesia, or oxygen therapy. **washing s.,** sodium carbonate.

sodiarsphenamine (so″di-ars-fen′ah-min) sodium arsphenamine; see under *arsphenamine.*

sodii (so'de-i) [L.] genitive of *sodium.*

sodiocitrate (so″de-o-sit′rāt) a compound containing sodium and a salt of citric acid.

sodiotartrate (so″de-o-tar′trāt) a compound containing sodium and a salt of tartaric acid.

sodium (so'de-um), gen. *so'dii* [L. *na'trium,* gen. *na'trii*] a soft, silver white, alkaline metallic element; symbol, Na; atomic number, 11; atomic weight, 22.990; specific gravity, 0.971. With a valence of 1, it has a strong affinity for oxygen and other nonmetallic elements. Sodium provides the chief cation of the extracellular body fluids. See also *sodium pump,* under *pump.* The salts of sodium are the most widely used salts in medicine. (NOTE: For sodium salts not listed below, see the name of the active ingredient.) **s. acetate** [USP], the trihydrate sodium salt of acetic acid, $C_2H_3NaO_2 \cdot 3H_2O$, occurring as colorless, transparent crystals, or white, granular crystalline powder, or white flakes; used as a source of sodium ions in solutions for hemodialysis and peritoneal dialysis. It has also been used as a systemic and urinary alkalizer, diuretic, and expectorant. **s. acid phosphate,** s. biphosphate, NaH_2PO_4. **s. alginate** [NF], a purified carbohydrate product extracted from brown seaweeds with dilute alkali; used as a suspending agent. It is also used for its emulsifying, stabilizing, thickening, and water-binding qualities in foods, medicines, and cosmetics. **s. alizarinsulfonate,** chemical name: 9,10-dihydro-3,4-dihydroxy-9,10-dioxo-2-anthracenesulfonic acid sodium salt. A dye, $C_{14}H_5O_2(OH)_2SO_3Na \cdot H_2O$, occurring as a yellow-brown or orange-yellow powder; used as a stain in microscopy, as a reagent for aluminum, as an acid-base indicator, and in the determination of fluorine. Called also *alizarin red S* and *alizarin water-soluble red.* **s. antimony gluconate,** antimony sodium gluconate. **s. antimonylthioglycollate,** antimony sodium thioglycollate. **s. arsenate,** Na₂-

$HAsO_4$, an odorless, amorphous white powder used when effects of arsenic are desired. **s. ascorbate** [USP], the monosodium salt of ascorbic acid, $C_6H_7NaO_6$, occurring as white or very faintly yellow crystals or crystalline powder; used in the preparation of parenteral dosage forms of ascorbic acid. **s. aurothiomalate**, gold sodium thiomalate; see under *gold*. **s. aurothiosulfate**, gold sodium thiosulfate; see under *gold*. **s. benzoate** [NF], the sodium salt of benzoic acid, $C_7H_5NaO_2$, occurring as a white, granular or crystalline powder; used as an antifungal preservative in pharmaceutical preparations and foods. It may also be used as a test for liver function, administered orally or intravenously. **s. bicarbonate** [USP], the monosodium salt of carbonic acid, $NaHCO_3$, occurring as a white, crystalline powder; used as an electrolyte replenisher and systemic alkalizer, administered by intravenous injection or infusion. It is also administered orally as a gastric antacid and urinary alkalizer, and is applied topically in solution to wash the nose, mouth, or vagina, and as a cleansing enema; sometimes used in solution as a dressing for minor burns. Called also *baking soda* and *bicarbonate of soda*. **s. biphosphate** [USP], the monohydrate monosodium salt of phosphoric acid, $NaH_2PO_4 \cdot H_2O$, occurring as colorless crystals or white, crystalline powder. It is given orally with sodium phosphate as an antihypercalcemic; orally and rectally with sodium phosphate as a cathartic; and orally as a urinary acidifier. **s. bisulfite** [NF], the monosodium salt of sulfurous acid, $HNaO_3S$, occurring as white or yellowish white crystals or granular powder; used as an antioxidant in pharmaceutical preparations. **s. borate** [NF], the sodium salt of boric acid, $Na_2B_4O_7$, occurring as a white, crystalline powder, or as colorless transparent crystals; used as an alkalizing agent in pharmaceutical preparations. It has also been used for its weak antibacterial and mild astringent properties in lotions, gargles, and mouthwashes. Called also *borax, sodium pyroborate*, and *s. tetraborate*. **s. bromide**, a sedative, $NaBr$, occurring in white or colorless crystals; used occasionally in the management of grand mal seizures. See also *bromide* and *brominism*. **s. cacodylate**, an arsenical remedy, $(CH_3)_2AsO \cdot ONa \cdot 3H_2O$, in the form of white crystals, or a white, granular powder, soluble in water; formerly used in tuberculosis, anemia, malaria, psoriasis, etc. **s. calcium edetate**, **s. calciumedetate**, edetate calcium disodium. **s. caprylate**, the sodium salt of caprylic acid, $C_8H_{15}NaO_2$; used as a topical antifungal in the treatment of cutaneous mycotic infections. **s. carbonate** [NF], the disodium salt of carbonic acid, Na_2CO_3, occurring as colorless crystals, or white, crystalline powder or granules; used as an alkalizing agent in pharmaceutical preparations. Called also *sal soda* and *washing soda*. **s. caseinate** casein-sodium. **s. cellulose phosphate**, an ion exchange resin used in the treatment of recurrent calcium phosphate renal calculi. **s. chlorate**, a salt, $NaClO_3$, with properties similar to those of potassium chlorate, and occurring in colorless or white crystals or granules. It has been used as an antiseptic wash. **s. chloride**, common salt or table salt: a mineral, $NaCl$, soluble in water and occurring as colorless, cubic crystals or a white, crystalline powder, found widely distributed over the earth, in sea water, etc., which is a necessary constituent of the body and consequently of the diet. It makes up over 90 per cent of the inorganic constituents of the blood serum and is the principal salt involved in maintaining osmotic tension of blood and tissues. It is used in medicine [USP] for many purposes, as in the preparation of isotonic and physiologic saline solutions; as a fluid and electrolyte replenisher, an isotonic vehicle for drugs, an antihypercalcemic, and an antidote to silver nitrate poisoning, administered by intravenous infusion; as a topical anti-inflammatory; to irrigate wounds and body cavities; as an enema to flush the colon and promote evacuation; as a mucolytic, administered by inhalation; and as a topical osmotic agent in ophthalmology. Also used widely as a food preservative and seasoning. **s. citrate** [USP], the trisodium salt of citric acid, $C_6H_5Na_3O_7$, occurring as colorless crystals, or white, crystalline powder; used as an anticoagulant for blood or plasma that is to be fractionated or for blood that is to be stored. It is also administered orally as a urinary alkalizer. **s. dimethylarsenate**, s. cacodylate. **s. fluoride** [USP], a dental caries prophylactic, NaF, occurring as a white powder; used in the fluoridation of water and applied topically to the teeth. **s. fluosilicate**, s. silicofluoride. **s. folate**, chemical name: sodium N-[4-{[(2-amino-4-hydroxy-6-pteridyl)methyl]amino}benzoyl]glutamate. A water-soluble compound, C_{19}-

$H_{18}N_7NaO_6$, used in various anemias and in sprue. **s. glutamate**, the monosodium salt of L-glutamic acid, $COOH \cdot CHNH_2 \cdot CH_2 \cdot CH_2 \cdot COONa$, occurring as a white or nearly white crystalline powder; used in treatment of encephalopathies associated with hepatic disease. It is also used to enhance the flavor of foods and tobacco. See also *Chinese restaurant syndrome*, under *syndrome*. **s. glycerophosphate**, a compound, $C_3H_5(OH)_2PO_4Na_2$, formerly thought useful in various conditions of disordered metabolism. **s. glycocholate**, a yellowish white, bitter salt, $NaC_{26}H_{42}O_6N$, with a pH of 6.6; used as a laboratory reagent. **s. gold thiosulfate**, gold sodium thiosulfate; see under *gold*. **s. hydrate**, s. hydroxide. **s. hydroxide** [NF], a caustic alkali, $NaOH$, occurring as white, or nearly white, fused masses, in small pellets, flakes, sticks, and other forms; used as an alkalizing agent in pharmaceutical preparations. Called also *caustic soda* and *s. hydrate*. **s. hypochlorite**, the sodium salt of hypochlorous acid, $NaClO$, having germicidal and disinfectant properties. **s. hypophosphite**, a salt, $NaPH_2O_2 \cdot H_2O$, occurring in colorless, rectangular plates, or as a white, granular powder. **s. hyposulfite**, s. thiosulfate. **s. iodate**, a white crystalline powder, $NaIO_3$, which has been used as an antiseptic in diseases of the mucous membranes. **s. iodide** [USP], a binary haloid, NaI, occurring in colorless crystals or white crystalline powder, used in various conditions as a source of iodine. It is also used as an expectorant. **s. ipodate** [NF], chemical name: sodium 3- [[(dimethylamino)methylene]amino]-2,4,6-triiodohydrocinnamate. A white to off-white, odorless, fine crystalline powder, $C_{12}H_{12}I_3N_2NaO_2$, used as a radiopaque medium in cholecystography. **s. lactate** [USP], the sodium salt of racemic or inactive lactic acid, $C_3H_5NaO_3$, used intravenously in one-sixth molar solution as a fluid and electrolyte replenisher to combat acidosis. **s. lauryl sulfate** [NF], an anionic surfactant, $CH_3(CH_2)_{10}CH_2OSO_3Na$, occurring in white or light yellow crystals; used as a wetting agent, emulsifying aid, and detergent in various cosmetic and dermatologic preparations, and as an ingredient of toothpastes. Called also *irium*. **s. metabisulfite** [NF], chemical name: disulfurous acid disodium salt. An antioxidant, $Na_2S_2O_5$, occurring as white crystals or as a white to yellowish crystalline powder; used in pharmaceutical preparations. **s. methylarsonate**, a crystalline powder, $CH_3AsO(ONa)_2 \cdot 5H_2O$, easily soluble in water and less soluble in alcohol, sometimes employed for its arsenical effects. **s. monofluorophosphate** [USP], chemical name: phosphorofluoridic acid disodium salt. A dental caries prophylactic, Na_2PFO_3, occurring as a white to slightly gray powder; applied topically to the teeth. **s. nitrate**, a compound, $NaNO_3$, occurring as colorless crystals or in white granules or powder; formerly used as a diuretic and in treatment of dysentery, but now used as a reagent and in certain industrial processes; called also *Chile saltpeter*. **s. nitrite** [USP], a compound, $NaNO_2$, occurring as a white to slightly yellow, granular powder or as white or nearly white, opaque fused masses or sticks, used as an antidote for cyanide poisoning. It is also used in the relief of the pain of angina pectoris, Raynaud's disease, asthma, and such conditions as lead colic and spastic colitis. **s. nitroferricyanide**, s. nitroprusside. **s. nitroprusside**, chemical name: $(OC\text{-}6\text{-}22)$- pentakis(cyano- C)nitrosylferrate(2–) disodium dihydrate. An antihypertensive, $Na_2[Fe(CN)_5NO] \cdot 2H_2O$, occurring as reddish brown crystals or powder; used in the treatment of hypertensive crisis and to produce controlled hypotension during surgery, administered by intravenous infusion. Sterile sodium nitroprusside conforms to USP specifications. It is also used as a reagent and testing solution. Called also *s. nitroferricyanide*. **s. oleate**, the sodium salt of oleic acid, $C_{17}H_{33}COONa$, formerly considered useful in treatment of gallstones. **s. oxybate**, chemical name: 4-hydroxybutanoic acid sodium salt; a hypnotic agent, $C_4H_7NaO_3$, used as an adjunct in anesthesia. **s. para-aminosalicylate**, s. aminosalicylate. **s. perborate**, a compound, $NaBO_3 \cdot 4H_2O$, prepared by interaction of boric acid or sodium borate with sodium or hydrogen peroxide. It is an antiseptic compound, used in 2 per cent solution as a mouthwash and in a 10–20 per cent powder in dentrifices. **s. peroxide**, a white powder, Na_2O_2, soluble in water in which it liberates oxygen, which has been used externally in acne, and as a dental bleach. **s. phenolsulfonate**, chemical name: hydroxybenzenesulfonic acid sodium salt. An odorless, saline compound, $NaC_6H_5OSO_3 \cdot 2H_2O$, in colorless transparent prisms or crystalline granules; formerly used as an intestinal antiseptic. **s. phosphate** [USP], the heptahydrate monosodium salt of phosphoric acid, $Na_2HPO_4 \cdot 7H_2O$, occurring as a colorless or white, granular salt. It is given orally as a cathartic; orally and rectally with sodium biphosphate as a cathartic; and orally with sodium biphosphate as an antihypercalcemic. **s. phosphate, dried** [USP], the anhydrous salt, $NaHPO_4 \cdot xH_2O$, dried at 105° C. for four hours; used as an oral cathartic. **s. phosphate, effervescent** [USP], a dry granular mixture of citric acid, dried sodium phosphate, tartaric acid, and sodium bicarbonate; used as an oral cathartic. **s. phosphate, exsiccated,** dried s. phosphate. **s. phytate,** the sodium salt of phytic acid, $C_6H_9Na_9O_{24}P_6$; a calcium chelating agent. **s. polyphosphate,** disodium salt of polyphosphoric acid; a pharmaceutic aid, $(NaPO_3)_n$. **s. polystyrene sulfonate** [USP], a cation-exchange resin prepared in the sodium form, each gram of which exchanges 110–135 mg. of potassium, calculated on the anhydrous basis; used as an antihyperkalemic, administered orally and rectally. **potassium s. tartrate,** see under *potassium.* **s. propionate** [NF], the sodium salt of propionic acid, CH_3CH_2COONa, occurring as colorless, transparent crystals or as a granular, crystalline powder, having antifungal properties; used alone or in combination with calcium propionate or other agents as a preservative to inhibit mold production in bakery and dairy products and other foods and in pharmaceuticals. It is also used as a topical antifungal in the treatment of various mycoses. **s. psylliate,** the sodium salt of the liquid fatty acids obtained by hydrolysis of the fixed oil of the seeds of *Plantago ovata;* used as a sclerosing agent. **s. pyroborate,** s. borate. **s. pyrophosphate,** a compound, $Na_4P_2O_7$, produced by heating sodium phosphate at a red heat; used in detergents. **radioactive s.,** radiosodium. **s. salicylate** [USP], the monosodium salt of salicylic acid, $C_7H_5NaO_3$, occurring as an amorphous or microcrystalline powder or as scales; used as an analgesic, antipyretic, and antirheumatic, administered orally. **s. silicate,** a compound of sodium, silicon, and oxygen in various ratios, formerly used as an antiseptic, and in tuberculosis, bronchial asthma, and arteriosclerosis. **s. silicofluoride,** a white, granular powder, Na_2SiF_6, which is toxic in high concentrations. It is sometimes added to water to produce 0.7 to 1 part per million of fluorine, to prevent dental caries and is sometimes used in insecticides. Called also s. *fluosilicate.* **s. stearate** [NF], a mixture of sodium stearate, sodium palmitate, and small amounts of the sodium salts of other fatty acids; used as a stiffening and emulsifying agent in pharmaceutical preparations. **s. stibocaptate** [INN], stibocaptate. **s. stibogluconate,** antimony sodium gluconate. **s. succinate,** chemical name: succinic acid sodium salt, $C_4H_4Na_2O_4$; used as a respiratory stimulant, analeptic, urinary alkalizer, diuretic, and laxative. **s. sulfate** [USP], the decahydrate disodium salt of sulfuric acid, $Na_2SO_4 \cdot 10H_2O$, occurring as large, colorless, transparent crystals, or a granular powder; used as an antihypercalcemic and antidote to barium poisoning, administered by intravenous infusion. It is also used orally as a cathartic or laxative and has been applied topically as a lymphagogue for infected wounds. Called also *Glauber's salt.* **s. sulfite,** a compound, $Na_2SO_3 \cdot 7H_2O$, occurring as colorless, efflorescent crystals; formerly used in treatment of dyspepsia, and externally in parasitic infections. **s. sulfite, anhydrous,** a fairly stable compound, Na_2SO_3, occurring as small white crystals or powder; used as a reagent. **s. sulfite, exsiccated,** s. sulfite, anhydrous. **s. sulfocarbolate,** s. phenolsulfonate. **s. tetraborate,** s. borate. **s. tetradecyl sulfate,** an anionic surfactant with sclerosing properties, $C_{14}H_{29}NaSO_4$, occurring as a white, waxy solid; used as a wetting agent and in the treatment of varicose veins and hemorrhoids. **s. thiamylal,** chemical name: sodium 5-allyl-5-(1-methylbutyl)-2-thiobarbiturate; an ultrashort-acting barbiturate, $C_{12}H_{17}N_2NaO_2S$. A sterile mixture of sodium thiamylal with anhydrous sodium carbonate (s. *thiamylal for injection* [NF]) is used intravenously as the sole anesthetic in relatively short surgical procedures, as a supplement to local anesthetics during regional and spinal anesthesia, and for induction prior to general anesthesia in prolonged surgical procedures. **s. thiosulfate** [USP], a compound, $Na_2S_2O_3 \cdot 5H_2O$, occurring as large colorless crystals or as a coarse crystalline powder, used intravenously as an antidote to cyanide poisoning. It is also used in solution as a foot bath to prevent ringworm infection at swimming pools and public shower-baths, topically in tinea versicolor, and in measuring

the volume of extracellular body fluid and the renal glomerular filtration rate. It was formerly used in the treatment of arsenic poisoning. **s. trimetaphosphate,** the trisodium salt of metaphosphoric acid; a pharmaceutic aid, $Na_3P_3O_9$.

sodium-potassium adenosinetriphosphatase (ah-den″o-sin-tri-fos′fah-tās) a complex in the plasma membrane catalyzing the approximate reaction $3 \, NA^+$ (inside) + $2K^+$ (outside) + ATP + H_2O = $3 \, NA^+$ (outside) + $2k^+$ (inside) + ADP + P_i. Called also ($NA^+ + K^+$)-*ATPase* and NA^+ , K^+ *ATPase.*

sodoku (so′do-koo) [Japanese so rat + *doku* poison] the spirillary form of rat-bite fever (see under *fever*), caused by *Spirillum minus.*

sodomist (sod′o-mist) one who practices sodomy.

sodomite (sod′o-mīt) sodomist.

sodomy (sod′o-me) [after the city of *Sodom*] a form of paraphilia, variously defined by law to include sexual contact between humans and animals of other species, and mouth-genital or anal contact between humans; in medical usage, it is restricted to human-animal sexual contact and anal intercourse.

sodophthalyl (so″do-thal′il) disodoquinone phenolphthalein; used as a laxative.

Soemmering's foramen, gray substance, spot (sem′er-ingz) [Samuel Thomas *Soemmering,* German anatomist, 1755–1830] see *fovea centralis retinae, macula retinae,* and *substantia nigra.*

softening (sof′en-ing) [Gr. *malakia*] the process of becoming soft; any morbid process of becoming soft, as of the brain or spinal cord, or of the vascular coats. **anemic s.,** disintegration of brain matter from deficient blood supply. **s. of the brain,** 1. a popular designation for paralytic dementia. 2. true softening of the brain substance; encephalomalacia. **colliquative s.,** softening in which the tissues become liquefied. **gray s.,** a stage in which the fat produced by degeneration has been more or less absorbed. **green s.,** a stage in which there is green pus present in the degenerated spot. **hemorrhagic s.,** softening of a part due to hemorrhage into it. **inflammatory s.,** a form of red softening due to inflammation. **mucoid s.,** myxomatous degeneration. **pyriform s.,** yellow s. **red s.,** softening of a patch or of patches of brain substance, with local redness due to congestion. **s. of the stomach,** gastromalacia; softening of the stomach walls due to an extremely acidic condition of its contents, a condition usually seen after death. **white s.,** the stage next following yellow softening, in which the spot has become white from the presence of fatty deposit. **yellow s.,** the second of the three stages of the myelic process, characterized by fatty degeneration; the stage following red softening, in which the patch has become yellow as a result of degenerative changes in the brain substance.

soja bean (so′yah) soy bean.

Sol. solution.

sol (sol) 1. a colloid system in which the dispersion medium is liquid. 2. a contraction of *solution.* **metal s.,** a colloidal dispersion of a metal in a liquid. Such dispersions often have catalytic properties similar to those of enzymes, and are therefore sometimes called inorganic enzymes. **solid s.,** a colloidal system in which both the dispersed phase and the dispersion medium are solids.

Solanaceae (sōl″ah-na′se-e) a large family of widely distributed herbs, shrubs, and trees, having great economic importance, and including many poisonous species and numerous species that have medicinal properties. *Atropa, Capsicum, Datura, Duboisia, Hyoscyamus, Nicotiana, Scopolia,* and *Solanum* are some of the important genera.

solanaceous (sōl″ah-na′shus) of or pertaining to the family Solanaceae.

solandrine (so-lan′drin) pseudohyoscyamine.

solanine (so′lah-nēn) solatunine; a steroidal glycoalkaloid, $C_{45}H_{73}NO_{15}$, found in several species of *Solanum;* formerly used in bronchitis, epilepsy, and asthma. On hydrolysis, it yields solanidine and three sugars. Its aglycone portion is considered most toxic.

solanoid (so′lah-noid) [L. *solanum* potato + Gr. *eidos* form] resembling a raw potato in texture.

solanoma (so″lah-no′mah) (*obs.*) scirrhous carcinoma.

Solanum (so-la′num) [L. "nightshade"] a genus of solanaceous plants, including the potato, tomato, eggplant, several of the nightshades, and many poisonous and medicinal species. **S. carolinen′se** L., plant of the United States. The fluid extracts of the root and berries were formerly used as anticonvulsive and sedative agents in epilepsy. The fruit is listed as poisonous to both animals and humans. Also known as *bull nettle, sand-briar, radical weed,* and *horse nettle.* **S. tubero′sum** L., the common potato.

solapsone (so-lap′sōn) chemical name: 1,1′-[sulfonylbis(*p*-phenyleneimino)]bis[3-phenyl-1,3-propanedisulfonic acid] tetrasodium salt. An antibacterial derivative of dapsone, $C_{30}H_{28}N_2Na_4O_{14}S_5$, having actions similar to those of the parent compound but less toxic; used as a leprostatic, administered orally and intramuscularly. Called also *solasulfone.*

solar (so′lar) [L. *solaris*] 1. pertaining to the sun. 2. denoting the great sympathetic plexus and its principal ganglia (especially the celiac); so called because of their radiating nerves.

solarium (so-la′re-um) [L.] a room especially designed to allow exposure to light of the sun or to artificial light.

solasulfone (so‴lah-sul′fōn) solapsone.

solation (sol-a′shun) the conversion of a gel into a sol.

Soldaini's test (reagent) (sol″dah-e′nēz) [Arturo *Soldaini,* Italian chemist] see under *tests.*

solder (sod′er) [L. *solidatio* making solid, fastening] 1. a fusible metal or alloy of metals used to unite pieces of less fusible metals. 2. to fasten together pieces of metal through the use of fusible metals or alloys of metal.

sole (sōl) [L. *solea; planta*] the bottom of the foot; called also *planta pedis* [NA]. **convex s., dropped s.,** pumiced foot.

solen(o)- [Gr. *sōlēn* a channel, gutter, pipe] a combining form denoting relationship to a pipe or gutter; tubular or grooved.

Solenoglypha (so″lĕ-nog′lĭ-fah) [*soleno-* + Gr. *glyphein* to cut out with a knife] a group of venomous snakes with fangs that are hollow like a hypodermic needle and that normally fold back against the roof of the mouth but can be erected for striking and piercing. Examples are the massasauga and the rattlesnakes.

solenoid (so′lĕ-noid) [Gr. *sōlēnoeidēs* pipe-shaped, from *sōlēn* pipe] 1. a coil of insulated wire in which a magnetic field is produced by a flow of electric current. 2. a coil surrounding a movable iron core that is pulled in when the coil is energized. It can be used to perform some mechanical work, such as opening a valve, or as a switch.

solenoma (so″lĕ-no′mah) (*obs.*) endometrial carcinoma.

solenonychia (so″lĕ-no-nik′e-ah) [*soleno-* + Gr. *onyx, onychos* nail + *-ia*] dystrophia unguis mediana canaliformis.

Solenopotes (so″lĕ-no-po′tēz) [*soleno-* + Gr. *potēs* a drinker] a genus of lice of the order Anoplura. **S. capilla′tus,** a species of sucking lice occasionally found parasitic on cattle.

Solenopsis (so″lĕ-nop′sis) a genus of stinging ants, including the fire ants that attack man and inflict painful burning stings and may cause severe local and systemic reactions; *S. geminata* is indigenous to the United States; *S. saevissima richteri* is a viciously aggressive South American species that has been imported into the United States and gained a strong foothold.

sole plate, sole-plate (sōl plāt) a specialized region of the surface of a skeletal muscle fiber where a motor nerve terminates. See *neuromuscular junction,* under *junction.*

solferino (sol″fer-e′no) fuchsin.

Solganal (sol′gah-nal) trademark for a preparation of aurothioglucose.

solid (sol′id) [L. *solidus*] 1. not fluid or gaseous; not hollow. 2. a substance or tissue not fluid or gaseous. **color s.,** a three-dimensional geometrical body, devised to show the relation of all hues and brightnesses, including black, white, and grays, in their various modes.

Solidago (sol″ĭ-da′go) [L.] a genus of composite-flowered plants: the golden-rods. *S. virgau′rea* L., of Europe and North America, is aromatic and diuretic. Some species are considered to be toxic to livestock.

solidism (sol′ĭ-dizm) the fundamental theory of Asclepiades and Themison, opposed to humoralism and pneumatism. Solidism is a development of atomism that made possible a new classification for disease: either the atoms were too

distant and the bodily pores too lax, or the atoms too close and the pores too tight.

solipsism (sōl′ip-sizm) [L. *solus* alone + *ipse* one's self] the belief that the world exists only in the mind of the individual, or that it consists solely of the individual himself and his own experiences.

solipsistic (sōl″ip-sis′tik) pertaining to or characterized by solipsism.

solitary (sol′ĭ-ter″e) [L. *solitarius*] placed alone; not grouped with others.

sol-lunar (sol-lu′nar) [L. *sol* sun + *luna* moon] pertaining to or caused by the sun and moon.

solpugid (sol-pu′jid) an individual of the order Solpugida.

Solpugida (sol″pu-jid′ah) the solpugids, a family of hairy, jointed spiders (class Arachnida) that are differentiated from true spiders by having a segmented abdomen, which is more broadly joined to the cephalothorax; solpugids are capable of inflicting deep painful bites and are found mainly in desert, tropical, and subtropical areas.

solubility (sol″u-bil′ĭ-te) the quality or fact of being soluble; susceptibility of being dissolved.

soluble (sol′u-b'l) [L. *solubilis*] susceptible of being dissolved.

Solu-Cortef (sol″u-kor′tef) trademark for a preparation of hydrocortisone sodium succinate.

solum (so′lum), pl. *so′la* [L.] [NA] the bottom or lowest part. **s. tym′pani,** paries jugularis cavi tympani.

solute (so′lūt) a substance dissolved in a solvent; a solution consists of a solute and a solvent.

solutio (so-lu′she-o) [L., from *solvēre* to dissolve] solution.

solution (so-lu′shun) [L. *solutio*] 1. a homogeneous mixture of one or more substances (solutes) dispersed molecularly in a sufficient quantity of dissolving medium (solvent). The solute may be gas, liquid, or solid; the solvent is usually liquid, but may be solid, as in a solid solution of copper in silver (sterling silver). In pharmacology, a liquid preparation containing one or several soluble chemical substances usually dissolved in water and not, for various reasons, falling into another category. 2. the process of dissolving. 3. a loosening or separation. **acetylcysteine s.** [USP], a sterile solution of acetylcysteine in water, prepared with the aid of sodium hydroxide, containing 95 to 105 per cent of the labeled amount of acetylcysteine; administered by nebulization or installation for adjunct therapy in bronchopulmonary disorders when mucolysis is desired. **Albright's s.,** one consisting of 75 gm. of sodium citrate, 25 gm. of potassium citrate, 140 gm. of citric acid, and 1000 ml. of water; used in the treatment of renal tubular acidosis. **alcoholic s.,** a solution in which alcohol is used as the solvent. **aluminum acetate topical s.** [USP], a preparation of aluminum subacetate solution, glacial acetic acid, and water, containing, in each 100 ml., 4.8–5.8 gm. of aluminum acetate, and used topically on the skin and mucous membranes, diluted with 10 to 40 parts of water, as an astringent. Called also *Burow's s.* **aluminum subacetate topical s.** [USP], a solution containing aluminum sulfate, acetic acid, precipitated calcium carbonate, and water, yielding, from each 100 ml., 2.3–2.6 gm. aluminum oxide and 5.43–6.13 gm. acetic acid, and used topically on the skin and mucous membranes as an astringent. It is also used as a topical antiseptic and as a wet dressing in various skin diseases. **amaranth s.,** [USP] a clear, vivid red solution of amaranth in purified water containing, in each 100 ml., 0.9–1.1 gm. of amaranth; used as a coloring agent in pharmaceutical preparations. **amaranth s., compound,** [NF] a solution composed of amaranth solution, caramel, alcohol, and purified water; used as a coloring agent in pharmaceutical preparations. **aminoacetic acid sterile s.,** a sterile, aqueous solution containing 95 to 105 per cent of the labeled amount of aminoacetic acid; used as a nutrient. **aminobenzoic acid s.** [USP], a straw-colored solution containing 5 per cent aminobenzoic acid; applied topically to the skin as a sunscreening agent. **ammonia s., diluted,** a colorless, transparent liquid of alkaline reaction, containing, in each 100 ml., 9–10 gm. of ammonia; used as a pharmaceutic necessity. Called also *ammonia water* or *diluted ammonium hydroxide solution.* **ammonia s., strong** [NF], a colorless, transparent liquid, strongly alkaline in reaction, containing 27–30 per cent of ammonia; used as a solvent and as a source of ammonia in pharmaceutical preparations.

ammonium acetate s., a clear, colorless liquid, containing ammonium acetate, which has been used as a diaphoretic and diuretic. Called also *spirit of Mindererus.* **ammonium citrate s., alkaline,** a preparation of dibasic ammonium citrate and strong ammonia solution; used in tests for zinc. **ammonium hydroxide s., diluted,** ammonia s., diluted. **ammonium hydroxide s., stronger,** ammonia s., strong. **anisotonic s.,** a solution having tonicity differing from that of the standard of reference. **antazoline phosphate ophthalmic s.,** a sterile, aqueous solution, containing 90 to 100 per cent of the labeled amount of antazoline phosphate; used topically in the eye as an antihistaminic. **antipyrine and benzocaine s.** [NF], a solution of antipyrine and benzocaine in glycerin, containing 90 to 110 per cent of the labeled amount of antipyrine and benzocaine; instilled in the ear as a local anesthetic. **antiseptic s.,** a clear, colorless liquid, containing boric acid, thymol, chlorothymol, menthol, eucalyptol, methyl salicylate, thyme oil, alcohol, and purified water, used as an antibacterial for external and oral use. **aqueous s.,** a solution in which water is used as the solvent. **arsenic chloride s.,** a partly hydrolyzed solution of antimony trichloride in water. **arsenical s.,** potassium arsenite s. **arsenious acid s.,** a clear, colorless, odorless liquid, with an acid reaction, containing arsenic trioxide. **atropine sulfate ophthalmic s.** [USP], a sterile, aqueous solution containing 93 to 107 per cent of the labeled amount of atropine sulfate; applied topically to the conjunctiva as an anticholinergic to produce mydriasis or cycloplegia. **Benedict's s.,** sodium citrate, sodium carbonate, and copper sulfate water solution. Its normal blue color changes to yellow, orange, or red in the presence of a reducing sugar such as glucose. It is used in urinalysis. **benzalkonium chloride s.** [USP], a clear, colorless, aqueous solution, with an aromatic odor and a slightly bitter taste, which contains 95–105 per cent of the labeled amount of benzalkonium chloride in concentrations of 1 per cent or more, and 93–107 per cent of the labeled amount in concentrations of less than 1 per cent; used as a topical antiseptic, effective against gram-positive and gram-negative bacteria and certain viruses, fungi, yeasts and protozoa. It is also used as an antimicrobial preservative in ophthalmic solutions. **benzethonium chloride topical s.** [USP], a clear, colorless liquid, without odor and with a slightly bitter taste, which contains 95–105 per cent of the labeled amount of benzethonium chloride; used as a local anti-infective, applied topically to the skin and nasal mucosa, and as a preservative in pharmaceutical preparations. **Bonain's s.,** an anesthetic and antiseptic solution used in operations on the tympanic membrane, consisting of equal parts of menthol, phenol, and cocaine hydrochloride. **boric acid s.,** a clear, colorless, odorless liquid, each 100 ml. of which contains at least 4.25 gm. of boric acid; used as an external anti-bacterial. **Bouin's s.,** see under *fluid.* **buffer s.,** a solution which resists appreciable change in its hydrogen ion concentration when acid or alkali is added to it. **Burnett's s.,** see under *fluid.* **Burow's s.,** aluminum acetate s. **butacaine sulfate s.** [USP], a sterile solution containing 95–105 per cent of the labeled amount of butacaine sulfate in water; used to produce topical anesthesia of the eye. **calciferol s.,** ergocalciferol s. **calcium cyclamate and calcium saccharin s.,** a clear, colorless solution containing 90 to 110 per cent of the labeled amounts of calcium cyclamate and calcium saccharin; used as a non-nutritive sweetener. **calcium hydroxide topical s.** [USP], a clear, colorless liquid with an alkaline reaction, each 100 ml., at 25° C. (77° F.), containing not less than 140 mg. of calcium hydroxide; used in preparing various astringent formulations for topical application to the skin and mucous membranes. It has also been used internally as an antacid and has been added to infant formulas to decrease the curd size formed from cow's milk. Called also *aqua calcis* and *lime water.* **carbachol ophthalmic s.** [USP], a sterile solution of carbol in an isotonic, aqueous medium, containing 95 to 105 per cent of the labeled amount of carbol; used as a cholinergic applied topically to the conjunctiva in the treatment of glaucoma. **carbol-fuchsin topical s.** [USP], a dark purple solution containing, in each 1000 ml., basic fuchsin (3 gm.), phenol (45 gm.), resorcinol (100 gm.), acetone (50 ml.), alcohol (100 ml.), and purified water; used as a local antifungal in the treatment of dermatophytosis, tinea, and other skin infections. Called also *Castellani's paint.* **carmine s.,** a deep red, rather viscous liquid, compounded of carmine, diluted

ammonia solution, glycerin, and water; used as a coloring agent. **Carnoy's s.,** an acid fixative used for studying the cell nucleus and chromosomes, composed of: 3 parts absolute ethanol, 1 part glacial acetic acid (or Bowin's fluid), 5 parts saturated picric acid, 5 parts 40 per cent formaldehyde (formalin), and 1 part glacial acetic acid. **carphenazine maleate s.** [USP], a solution containing 95–110 per cent of the labeled amount of carphenazine maleate; used as an antipsychotic in the treatment of acute and chronic schizophrenic reactions in hospitalized patients. **centinormal s.,** hundredth-normal s. **cetylpyridinium chloride s.** [USP], a clear solution containing 95 to 105 per cent of the labeled amount of cetylpyridinium chloride; used as a local anti-infective applied topically to the skin and mucous membranes, and as a preservative in pharmaceutical preparations. **chloramphenicol ophthalmic s.** [USP], a sterile, buffered solution, containing 90–130 per cent of the labeled amount of chloramphenicol; used as an antibacterial, applied topically to the conjunctiva. **chloramphenicol for ophthalmic s.** [USP], a sterile, dry mixture of chloramphenicol and suitable buffers, containing 90–120 per cent of the labeled amount of chloramphenicol; used as an antibacterial, applied topically to the conjunctiva. **chymotrypsin for ophthalmic s.** [USP], a sterile preparation containing 80–120 per cent of the labeled potency of chymotrypsin; used for enzymatic zonulolysis for intracapsular lens extraction, applied by irrigation to the posterior chamber of the eye, under the iris. **clindamycin palmitate hydrochloride for oral s.** [USP], a dry mixture containing clindamycin palmitate hydrochloride equivalent to 90–120 per cent of the labeled amount of clindamycin; used as an antibacterial, primarily in the treatment of penicillin-resistant gram-positive infections and in patients allergic to penicillin. **cloxacillin sodium for oral s.** [USP], a preparation containing 90–120 per cent of the labeled amount of cloxacillin; used as an oral antibacterial, primarily in the treatment of infections due to penicillinase-resistant staphylococci. **coal tar topical s.** [USP], a solution of coal tar and polysorbate 80 in alcohol, used, diluted, as a local antieczematic. **cochineal s.,** a dark, purplish red fluid with a slightly aromatic odor, compounded of cochineal, potassium carbonate, alum, potassium bitartrate, glycerin, and water; used as a coloring agent. **Cohn's s.,** a synthetic medium for growing yeast and molds, containing monopotassium acid phosphate, calcium phosphate, magnesium sulfate, and ammonium tartrate, in water. **colloid s., colloidal s.,** a preparation consisting of minute particles of matter suspended in a solvent, the solvent being called the continuous phase, and the suspended matter, the disperse phase. Called also *disperse system.* See *dispersoid* and *emulsoid.* **contrast s.,** a solution of a substance opaque to the roentgen ray, used to facilitate roentgen visualization of some organ or structure in the body. **cresol s., compound,** cresol s., saponated. **cresol s., saponated,** a mixture of cresol, vegetable oil, potassium hydroxide, alcohol, and water, and containing, in each 100 ml., 46–52 ml. of cresol; used as a disinfectant, chiefly to sterilize instruments, dishes, utensils, and other inanimate objects. Called also *compound cresol s.* **crystal violet s.,** methylrosaniline chloride s. **cyanocobalamin Co 57 s.** [USP], a clear colorless to pink solution, suitable for oral administration, containing cyanocobalamin in which a portion of the molecules contain radioactive cobalt (^{57}Co); used as a diagnostic aid in pernicious anemia. **cyanocobalamin Co 60 s.** [USP], a clear colorless to pink solution suitable for oral administration, containing cyanocobalamin in which a portion of the molecules contain radioactive cobalt (^{60}Co); used as a diagnostic aid in pernicious anemia. Formerly called *radiocyanocobalamin s.* **cyclopentamine hydrochloride s.** [USP], a solution of cyclopentamine hydrochloride in a suitable isotonic vehicle, containing 95 to 105 per cent of the labeled amount of cyclopentamine hydrochloride; applied intranasally as a vasoconstrictor to reduce nasal congestion. **cyclopentolate hydrochloride ophthalmic s.** [USP], a sterile solution of cyclopentolate hydrochloride in a buffer, isotonic, aqueous medium, containing 95 to 105 per cent of the labeled amount of cyclopentolate hydrochloride; applied topically to the conjunctiva as an anticholinergic. **Czapek-Dox s.,** a solution used for growing molds, containing glucose, sodium nitrate, monopotassium phosphate, potassium chloride, magnesium sulfate, iron sulfate, and water. **Dakin's s., Dakin's s., modified,** sodium hypochlorite s., diluted. **decimolar s.,** a solution having one-tenth the concentration of a molar solution. **decinormal s.,** tenth-normal s. **demecarium bromide ophthalmic s.** [USP], a sterile, aqueous solution containing 92 to 108 per cent of the labeled amount of demecarium bromide; applied topically to the conjunctiva as a cholinergic in treatment of glaucoma and convergent strabismus. **dexamethasone sodium phosphate ophthalmic s.** [NF], a sterile, aqueous solution containing 90 to 115 per cent of the labeled amount of dexamethasone phosphate; applied topically to the eye as an anti-inflammatory glucocorticoid. **diatrizoate sodium s.** [USP], a solution of diatrizoate sodium in purified water, or a solution of diatrizoic acid in purified water prepared with the aid of sodium hydroxide; used orally as a diagnostic radiopaque medium in radiography of the gastrointestinal tract. **diethyltoluamide topical s.** [USP], a solution of diethyltoluamide in alcohol or isopropyl alcohol, containing 92 to 108 per cent of the labeled amount of diethyltoluamide; applied to the skin and clothing to repel arthropods. **dioctyl calcium sulfosuccinate s.,** a clear solution containing 95 to 105 per cent of the labeled amount of dioctyl calcium sulfosuccinate; used as a wetting agent and as a nonlaxative fecal matter softener. **dioctyl sodium sulfosuccinate s.** docusate sodium s. **diphenoxylate hydrochloride and atropine sulfate oral s.** [USP], a solution containing 93 to 107 per cent of the labeled amount of diphenoxylate hydrochloride and 80 to 120 per cent of the labeled amount of atropine sulfate; used as an antiperistaltic in treatment of diarrhea. **disclosing s.,** a solution which is used for the purpose of making something apparent, such as one to be painted on the surface of a tooth in order to stain, and thus render visible, foreign matter or bacterial plaques. **docusate sodium s.** [USP], a solution containing 95 to 105 per cent of the labeled amount of docusate sodium; used as a fecal softener, administered rectally. Called also *dioctyl sodium sulfosuccinate s.* **double-normal s.,** a solution having double the strength of a normal solution: designated 2 N. **Drabkin's s.,** an aqueous solution containing 1.0 g sodium bicarbonate, 0.05 g potassium cyanide, and 0.20 g potassium ferricyanide per liter; used to lyse red cells and convert hemoglobin to cyanmethemoglobin in hemoglobinimetry. **dyclonine hydrochloride topical s.** [USP], a sterile, aqueous solution containing 92 to 108 per cent of the labeled amount of dyclonine hydrochloride; used as a local anesthetic, applied topically to the skin and mucous membranes. **echothiophate iodide for ophthalmic s.** [USP], a preparation containing 95-115 per cent of the labeled amount of echothiophate iodide; a cholinergic used as a miotic in the treatment of certain forms of glaucoma, applied topically to the conjunctiva. **dl-ephedrine hydrochloride s.,** racephedrine hydrochloride s. **ephedrine sulfate nasal s.** [USP], a solution containing 93-107 per cent of the labeled amount of ephedrine sulfate; applied intranasally to decongest the nasal mucous membranes. **epinephrine s.** [USP], a nearly colorless, slightly acid solution of epinephrine in purified water, prepared with the aid of hydrochloric acid, each 100 ml. containing 90-115 mg. of epinephrine; used as a vasoconstrictor. **epinephrine bitartrate ophthalmic s.** [USP], a buffered, aqueous solution, containing 90-115 per cent of the labeled amount of epinephrine bitartrate; used to reduce intraocular pressure in the management of simple chronic (open-angle) glaucoma, applied topically to the conjunctiva. **epinephrine nasal s.** [USP], a solution of epinephrine in purified water prepared with the aid of hydrochloric acid, each ml. containing 90-115 mg. of the labeled amount of epinephrine; applied intranasally to decongest the nasal mucous membranes. **epinephryl borate ophthalmic s.** [USP], a sterile solution containing epinephryl borate equivalent to 90-115 per cent of the labeled amount of epinephrine; used as an adrenergic in ophthalmology, administered by instillation into the eye. **ergocalciferol oral s.** [USP], a solution of ergocalciferol in an edible vegetable oil, in polysorbate 80, or in propylene glycol, containing, in each gram, not less than 0.25 mg. of ergocalciferol; used in the prophylaxis and treatment of vitamin D deficiency. Called also *calciferol s.* **erythrosine sodium topical s.** [USP], a preparation containing 90-110 per cent of the labeled amount of erythrosine sodium in purified water; applied topically to the teeth to disclose plaque. **ethereal s.,** a solution in which ether is used as the solvent. **Farrant's s.,** a mounting preparation used in bacteriological work, containing glycerin, water, arsenious acid solution, and gum arabic. **Fehling's s.,** dissolve

34.66 gm. of copper sulfate in water to make 500 ml.; dissolve 173 gm. of crystallized potassium sodium tartrate and 50 gm. of sodium hydroxide in water to make 500 ml. Keep the two solutions in small well-stoppered bottles; for use, mix equal parts of the two solutions. **ferric chloride s.,** a yellowish orange liquid with a faint odor of hydrochloric acid and an acid reaction, containing 37.2-42.7 gm. of ferric chloride and 3.85-6.6 gm. of hydrochloric acid in each 100 ml.; formerly used as a hematinic in the treatment of iron deficiency anemias. **ferric subsulfate s.,** a reddishbrown, almost odorless, aqueous solution of basic ferric sulfate, used as an astringent. **ferrous sulfate oral s.** [USP], a solution containing 94-106 per cent of the labeled amount of ferrous sulfate; used as a hematinic in the treatment of iron deficiency anemia. **fiftieth-normal s.,** a solution having one-fiftieth the strength of a normal solution: designated N/50 or 0.02 N. **fixative s.,** see *fixative.* **Flemming's s.,** a solution for hardening histological specimens, consisting of chromium trioxide, osmium tetroxide, glacial acetic acid, and water. **fluocinolone acetonide topical s.** [USP], a solution containing 90-110 per cent of the labeled amount of fluocinolone acetonide; used as an anti-inflammatory in glucocorticoid-responsive dermatoses. **fluorouracil topical s.** [USP], a preparation containing 90-110 per cent of the labeled amount of fluorouracil; used as an antineoplastic in the treatment of actinic keratoses. **Fonio's s.,** a solution of magnesium sulfate in water, used as a diluent for blood platelets. **formaldehyde s.** [USP], a solution of formaldehyde in water, containing not less than 37 per cent of formaldehyde; used as a disinfectant. Called also *formalin* and *formol.* **formol-Zenker s.,** a fixing solution consisting of Zenker's solution and formaldehyde solution. **Fowler's s.,** potassium arsenite s. **gelatin s., special intravenous,** a 5 or 6 per cent sterile, pyrogen-free solution of gelatin in isotonic sodium chloride solution; used as a plasma volume expander. **gentian violet topical s.** [USP], a purple liquid with a slight odor of alcohol, containing gentian violet, alcohol, and purified water, each 100 ml. containing 0.95-1.05 gm. of gentian violet, applied topically to the skin and mucous membranes in infections associated with gram-positive bacteria and molds. Called also *crystal violet s.* and *methylrosaniline chloride s.* **Gilson's s.,** a fixative solution consisting of mercuric chloride, nitric acid, glacial acetic acid, 70 per cent alcohol, and water. **glycerin oral s.** [USP], a preparation containing 95-105 per cent of the labeled amount of glycerin; used as a diuretic to reduce intraocular pressure in glaucoma and before cataract surgery. **gold s.,** any of a variety of gold compounds available for medicinal purposes with differences in their physical properties and clinical effectiveness, e.g., aurothioglucose, aurothioglycanide, gold sodium thiomalate, and gold sodium thiosulfate. See also *gold 198Au s.* **gold 198Au s.,** a sterile, pyrogen-free, cherry-red, colloidal solution of radiogold (198Au) stabilized by the addition of gelatin and suitable reducing agents, used by intracavitary or interstitial injection in the treatment of certain types of cancer. Called also *radiogold s.* **Gowers' s.,** a solution of sodium sulfate, glacial acetic acid, and water, used for the dilution of blood prior to enumerating red blood cells microscopically with a hemocytometer. **Gram's s.,** see *Table of Stains and Staining Methods,* under *stain.* **gram molecular s.,** molar s. **half-normal s.,** a solution having half the strength of a normal solution; designated N/2. **haloperidol oral s.** [USP], a solution containing 90 to 110 per cent of the labeled amount of haloperidol; used as a tranquilizer, especially in the management of psychoses and for control of the manifestations of Gilles de la Tourette's syndrome. **Hamdi's s.,** a solution for preserving histological specimens, consisting of sodium sulfate, salt, glycerin, and water. **Harrington's s.,** a solution for hand disinfection, consisting of alcohol, hydrochloric acid, water, and corrosive mercuric chloride. **Hayem's s.,** a solution used in diluting blood prior to enumerating red blood cells microscopically with a hemocytometer, and consisting of mercury bichloride, sodium chloride, sodium sulfate, and water. **hexylcaine hydrochloride topical s.** [NF], a clear, colorless, aqueous solution containing 93 to 107 per cent of the labeled amount of hexylcaine hydrochloride; applied topically as a local anesthetic. **homatropine hydrobromide ophthalmic s.** [USP], a sterile, buffered, aqueous solution containing 95 to 105 per cent of the labeled amount of homatropine hydrobromide; applied topically to the conjunctiva to produce cycloplegia and mydriasis.

hundredth-normal s., a solution having one-hundredth the strength of a normal solution; designated N/100 or 0.01 N. **hydrogen dioxide s.,** hydrogen peroxide s. **hydrogen peroxide topical s.** [USP], a solution containing 2.5–3.5 gm. of hydrogen peroxide per 100 ml.; used as a topical anti-infective to the skin and mucous membranes. Called also *hydrogen dioxide solution.* **hydroxyamphetamine hydrobromide ophthalmic s.** [USP], a sterile, buffered, aqueous solution containing 0.95 to 1.05 per cent of hydroxyamphetamine hydrobromide; applied topically to the conjunctiva as a mydriatic. **hydroxypropyl methylcellulose ophthalmic s.** [USP], a sterile solution containing 85–115 per cent hydroxypropyl methylcellulose; applied topically to the conjunctiva to protect the cornea during certain ophthalmic procedures and to lubricate the cornea. **hyperbaric s.,** a solution having a greater specific gravity than a standard of reference, such as one used for spinal anesthesia having a specific gravity greater than that of the spinal fluid, causing it to migrate downward and produce anesthesia below the level of injection. **hypertonic s.,** see *hypertonic.* **hypobaric s.,** a solution having a specific gravity less than that of a standard of reference, such as one used for spinal anesthesia having a specific gravity less than that of the spinal fluid, causing it to migrate upward and produce anesthesia above the level of injection. **hypotonic s.,** see *hypotonic.* **idoxuridine ophthalmic s.,** [USP], a sterile, aqueous solution containing 0.09 to 0.11 per cent of idoxuridine; used as an antiviral agent in the treatment of herpes virus keratitis, applied topically to the conjunctiva. **iodine topical s.** [USP], a transparent, reddish brown liquid, with the odor of iodine, consisting of iodine and sodium iodide in purified water, each 100 ml. of which contains 1.8–2.2 gm. of iodine and 2.1–2.6 gm. of sodium iodide; used as a topical anti-infective. **iodine s., compound,** iodine s. strong. **iodine s., strong** [USP], a transparent, deep brown liquid, with the odor of iodine, consisting of iodine and potassium iodide in purified water, each 100 ml. containing 4.5–5.5 gm. of iodine and 9.5–10.5 gm. of potassium iodide. It is used as a source of iodine in preparation for thyroid surgery; administered orally. Called also *compound iodine s.* and *Lugol's s.* **iron and ammonium acetate s.,** a clear, reddish brown liquid, with an aromatic odor, compounded of ferric chloride tincture, diluted acetic acid, ammonium acetate solution, aromatic elixir, glycerin, and distilled water. Formerly used as a hematinic and as a diuretic. Called also *Basham's mixture.* **isobaric s.,** a solution having the same specific gravity as a standard of reference, such as one used for spinal anesthesia having a specific gravity the same as that of the spinal fluid, causing it to remain and produce anesthesia at the level of injection. **isoflurophate ophthalmic s.,** a sterile solution containing 0.09–0.11 per cent of isoflurophate in a suitable vegetable oil; used as a cholinergic in the treatment of glaucoma, applied topically to the conjunctiva. **isotonic s.,** see *isotonic.* **Kaiserling s.,** 1. for *fixation:* formalin 400 ml., water 2,000 ml., potassium nitrate 30 gm., potassium acetate 60 gm. 2. *for restoring color:* alcohol 80 per cent. 3. *for preservation:* potassium acetate 200 gm., glycerol 400 ml., sodium arsenate 100 gm., water 2,000 ml. **Labarraque's s.** [NF], sodium hypochlorite solution, diluted with an equal volume of water. **Lang's s.,** see under *fluid.* **Lange's s.,** a solution of colloidal gold. **lead subacetate s.,** an aqueous solution of lead acetate and lead monoxide; used as an astringent and as a local sedative. **lead subacetate s., diluted,** a colorless, slightly turbid liquid, with a sweet, astringent taste, prepared by diluting lead subacetate solution with water. **lime s., sulfurated,** a solution of lime and sublimed sulfur in water; formerly much used as a keratolytic in acne vulgaris and seborrhea. **liver s.,** a brownish liquid prepared from mammalian livers and containing the soluble thermostable fraction which stimulates hematopoiesis in patients with pernicious anemia. Called also *liquid liver extract.* **Locke's s.,** a solution of sodium chloride, calcium chloride, potassium chloride, sodium bicarbonate, and dextrose; used in physiological experiments to keep the mammalian heart beating. **Locke's s., citrated,** a solution of sodium chloride, potassium chloride, calcium chloride, and sodium citrate in distilled water, with pH adjusted to 7.4. **Locke-Ringer's s.,** a test solution containing sodium chloride, potassium chloride, calcium chloride, magnesium chloride, sodium bicarbonate, dextrose, and water. **Lugol's s.,** iodine s., strong. **Magendie's s.,** a solution for par-

enteral use containing morphine sulfate. **magnesium citrate oral s.** [USP], a colorless to slightly yellow, clear, effervescent liquid, with a sweet, aciduous taste and a lemon flavor, which consists of magnesium carbonate, anhydrous citric acid, syrup, talc, lemon oil, potassium bicarbonate, and purified water, each 100 ml. containing an amount of magnesium citrate equal to 1.55–1.9 gm. magnesium oxide. It is used as a cathartic. **Massier's s.,** a solution used as a spray in laryngitis, consisting of resorcinol (1.5 gm.), menthol (0.1 gm.), 3.0 strong tincture of iodine, and glycerin (30 ml.). **merbromin s.,** a clear, red liquid with a yellow-green fluorescence, compounded of merbromin and water, each 100 ml. of which contains 1.8–2.2 gm. of merbromin; used as an antibacterial. **merbromin s., surgical,** a clear, red liquid with a yellow-green fluorescence, compounded of merbromin, water, acetone, and neutralized alcohol, the merbromin containing 24–26.7 per cent of mercury, and 18–21.3 per cent of bromine; used as an antibacterial. **methoxsalen topical s.** [USP], a preparation containing 9.2–10.8 mg. of methoxsalen per milliliter; used in conjunction with exposure to ultraviolet light to facilitate repigmentation in idiopathic vitiligo, and also as a suntan accelerator and sun protectant. **methylcellulose ophthalmic s.** [USP], a sterile solution containing 85–115 per cent of the labeled amount of methylcellulose; applied topically to protect the cornea during certain ophthalmic procedures and to lubricate the cornea. **methylrosaniline chloride s.,** gentian violet s. **molal s.,** a solution containing 1 mole of solute dissolved in 1,000 gm. of solvent. **molar s.,** a solution each liter of which contains 1 gram-molecule of the dissolved substance: designated M/1 or 1 M. The concentration of other solutions may be expressed in relation to that of molar solutions as tenth-molar (M/10 or 0.1 M), etc. **molecular disperse s.,** a solution in which the dispersed particles have a diameter of about 0.1 micromicron. **Monsel's s.,** ferric subsulfate s. **nafcillin sodium for oral s.** [USP], a preparation containing nafcillin sodium equivalent to 90–120 per cent of the labeled amount of nafcillin; used as an antibacterial, chiefly in the treatment of resistant staphylococcal infections. **naphazoline hydrochloride nasal s.** [USP], a solution containing 90–110 per cent of the labeled amount of naphazoline hydrochloride in water; used as a vasoconstrictor, applied topically to the nasal mucosa. **naphazoline hydrochloride ophthalmic s.** [USP], a solution containing 90–110 per cent of the labeled amount of naphazoline hydrochloride in water; used as a vasoconstrictor, applied topically to the conjunctiva. **neomycin and polymyxin B sulfates and gramicidin ophthalmic s.** [USP], a sterile isotonic solution containing 90 to 130 per cent of the labeled amounts of neomycin base, polymyxin B sulfate, and gramicidin; applied topically to the eye as a local anti-infective. **neomycin and polymyxin B sulfates and hydrocortisone otic s.** [USP], a sterile solution containing the equivalent of not less than 90 and not more than 130 per cent of the labeled amounts of neomycin and of polymyxin B and also containing 10 mg. of hydrocortisone per 100 ml. **neomycin sulfate oral s.** [USP], a solution containing, in each 5 ml. of solution, an amount of neomycin sulfate equivalent to 90 to 125 per cent of the equivalent of 87.5 mg. of neomycin base; used as an antibacterial. **Nessler's s.,** see under *reagent.* **nitrofurazone topical s.** [USP], a solution containing 95–105 per cent of the labeled amount of nitrofurazone; used as a local anti-infective against a wide variety of gram-negative and gram-positive bacteria in the treatment of many skin lesions, especially second and third degree burns and to aid healing and prevent infection of skin grafts, applied topically. **nitromersol topical s.** [USP], a clear, reddish orange liquid, compounded of nitromersol, sodium hydroxide, monohydrated sodium carbonate, and purified water, each 100 ml. of which yields 180–220 mg. of nitromersol; used as a topical anti-infective. **normal s.,** a solution each liter of which contains 1 gram equivalent weight of the dissolved substance: designated N/1 or 1 N. **normal saline s., normal salt s.,** physiological salt s. **normobaric s.,** isobaric s. **nortriptyline s.** [NF], a preparation containing nortriptyline hydrochloride equivalent to 90–110 per cent of the labeled amount of nortriptyline; used as an antidepressant, administered orally. **ophthalmic s.,** a sterile solution, essentially free from foreign particles and suitably compounded and dispensed, for instillation into the eye. **Orth's s.,** a solution for fixing histological specimens, consisting of Müller's fluid and formaldehyde solution.

oxacillin sodium for oral s. [USP], a preparation containing 90–120 per cent of the labeled amount of oxacillin; used as an antibacterial, primarily in the treatment of infections due to penicillinase-resistant staphylococci. **oxymetazoline hydrochloride nasal s.** [USP], a solution of oxymetazoline hydrochloride in water adjusted to a suitable pH and tonicity, containing 95 to 115 per cent of the labeled amount of oxymetazoline hydrochloride; instilled into the nostrils as a vasoconstrictor. **paramethadione oral s.** [USP], a solution of paramethadione in dilute alcohol, containing, in each milliliter, 282 to 318 mg. of paramethadione; used as an anticonvulsant, especially in petit mal epilepsy. **parathyroid s.,** parathyroid injection. **Perenyi's s.,** an embryological fixing solution, consisting of 10 per cent solution of nitric acid, alcohol, and 0.5 per cent solution of chromic acid. **phenylephrine hydrochloride nasal s.** [USP], a clear, colorless, or slightly yellow liquid, which contains 95–105 per cent of the labeled amount of phenylephrine hydrochloride; used as a nasal vasoconstrictor and decongestant, applied topically. **phenylephrine hydrochloride ophthalmic s.** [USP], a sterile, buffered, aqueous solution containing 90 to 115 per cent of the labeled amount of phenylephrine hydrochloride; applied topically to the conjunctiva as a vasoconstrictor to produce mydriasis without cycloplegia. **physiological salt s., physiological sodium chloride s.,** an aqueous solution of sodium chloride having an osmolality similar to that of blood serum. **physostigmine salicylate ophthalmic s.** [USP], a sterile, aqueous solution containing 90–110 per cent of the labeled amount of physostigmine salicylate; used as a cholinergic to produce miosis and to decrease intraocular pressure in the treatment of glaucoma, applied topically to the conjunctiva. **pilocarpine hydrochloride ophthalmic s.** [USP], a sterile, buffered, aqueous solution containing 90 to 110 per cent of the labeled amount of pilocarpine hydrochloride; applied topically to the conjunctiva as a cholinergic to produce miosis and to decrease intraocular pressure in the treatment of glaucoma. **pilocarpine nitrate ophthalmic s.** [USP], a sterile, buffered, aqueous solution containing 90 to 110 per cent of the labeled amount of pilocarpine nitrate; applied topically to the conjunctiva as a cholinergic to produce miosis and to decrease intraocular pressure in the treatment of glaucoma, applied topically to the conjunctiva. **Pitkin's s.,** a solution of procaine in a solvent having a specific gravity lower than that of the spinal fluid; used as a spinal anesthetic. **pituitary s., pituitary s., posterior,** posterior pituitary injection. **potassium arsenite s.,** a solution of arsenic trioxide, potassium bicarbonate, and alcohol in water. It has been used in the treatment of chronic myelogenous leukemia and chronic dermatitides. In veterinary medicine, it is used in the treatment of pulmonary emphysema, chronic nonparasitic dermatitides, chronic coughs, and general debility. Called also *arsenical s., Fowler's solution,* and *kali arsenicosum.* **potassium citrate oral s.** [USP], a solution containing 95–105 per cent of the labeled amount of potassium chloride; also used as an electrolyte replenisher. **potassium iodide oral s.** [USP], a solution containing 97–103 gm. of potassium iodide in each ml.; used as an expectorant, as a source of iodine in thyrotoxic crises and in the preparation of thyrotoxic patients for thyroidectomy, and as an antifungal in the treatment of lymphocutaneous sporotrichosis, administered orally. **potassium phenethicillin for oral s.** [NF], a dry mixture of potassium phenethicillin with or without one or more suitable coloring or flavoring agents, which may contain one or more suitable buffers and preservatives; used as an antibacterial. **povidone-iodine topical s.** [USP], a reddish brown, transparent solution of povidone-iodine and water, containing 85 to 120 per cent of the labeled amount of iodine; applied topically as an anti-infective. **prednisolone sodium phosphate ophthalmic s.** [USP], a sterile solution of prednisolone sodium phosphate in a buffered, aqueous medium, containing 90 to 115 per cent of the labeled amount of prednisolone phosphate, present as the disodium salt; used as an anti-inflammatory adrenocortical steroid. **prochlorperazine edisylate oral s.** [USP], a solution containing 92–108 per cent of the labeled amount of prochlorperazine; used as an antiemetic and tranquilizer, administered orally. **promazine hydrochloride oral s.** [USP], a solution containing 95–110 per cent of the labeled amount of promazine hydrochloride; used mainly as an antipsychotic agent, administered orally. **proparacaine hydrochloride ophthalmic s.** [USP], a sterile, aqueous solution containing 95 to 110 per cent of the labeled amount of proparacaine hydrochloride; applied topically to the conjunctiva as an anesthetic. **racephedrine hydrochloride s.,** a clear, colorless solution with a camphoraceous odor and taste, compounded of racephedrine hydrochloride, chlorobutanol, and Ringer's solution, each 100 ml. of which contains between 930 mg. and 1.07 gm. of racephedrine; used as an adrenergic. Called also *dl-ephedrine hydrochloride s.* **radiocyanocobalamin s.,** radioactive cyanocobalamin. **radiogold s.,** gold [198]Au s. **Randall's s.,** a solution consisting of the acetate, bicarbonate, and citrate salts of potassium; used especially in the treatment of potassium deficiency, administered orally. **Rees-Ecker s.,** see under *fluid.* **Ringer's s.,** see under irrigation. **Ruge's s.,** a solution of glacial acetic acid, 40 per cent formalin, and water; used as a stain. **saline s., salt s.,** a solution of sodium chloride, or common salt, in purified water. **saturated s.,** a solution in which the solvent has taken up all of the dissolved substance that it can hold in solution. **Schällibaum's s.,** a solution of celloidin and oil of cloves used in histological work to attach paraffin sections to slides. **sclerosing s.,** a solution of an irritant substance for injection into a vein to produce obliteration of the vein, or into a hernia to induce fibrous formation and obliteration of the sac. **scopolamine hydrobromide ophthalmic s.** [USP], a sterile, buffered, aqueous solution, containing 90 to 110 per cent of the labeled amount of scopolamine hydrobromide; used as a mydriatic and cycloplegic, applied topically to the conjunctiva. **seminormal s.,** half-normal s. **Seyderhelm's s.,** a colloidal mixture of Congo red and trypan blue, for staining urinary sediment. **Shohl's s.,** a solution containing 140 gm. citric acid and 98 gm. hydrated crystalline salt of sodium citrate in distilled water to make 1000 ml.; used to correct electrolyte imbalance in the treatment of renal tubular acidosis. **silver nitrate s., ammoniacal,** an ammonium compound of silver nitrate; used as an antiseptic and in the detection and prevention of dental caries. Because of inflammatory and necrotic tissue reaction, its use has now declined. **silver nitrate ophthalmic s.** [USP], a solution of silver nitrate in a buffered water medium, containing 0.95–1.05 per cent of $AgNO_3$; used as a local anti-infective applied topically to the conjunctiva as a prophylactic against ophthalmia neonatorum. **sodium chloride s.,** see under *irrigation.* **sodium citrate and citric acid s.** [USP], a solution containing, in each ml., 95–105 mg. of sodium citrate dihydrate and 57–63 mg. of anhydrous citric acid in purified water; used as a systemic alkalizer. **sodium cyclamate and sodium saccharin s.,** a clear, colorless solution containing 90 to 110 per cent of the labeled amounts of sodium cyclamate and sodium saccharin; used as a non-nutritive sweetener. **sodium fluorescein ophthalmic s.** [USP], a sterile buffered solution containing, in each 100 ml., 1.86 to 2.10 gm. of sodium fluorescein, and a suitable antimicrobial agent; applied topically to the conjunctiva as a corneal trauma indicator. **sodium fluoride oral s.** [USP], a solution containing 95–105 per cent of the labeled amount of sodium fluoride; used as a dental caries prophylactic, used in the fluoridation of water, and applied topically to the teeth. **sodium fluoride and orthophosphoric acid s.** [NF], a solution containing 90–110 per cent of the labeled amount of fluoride ion; used as a dental caries prophylactic, applied topically to the teeth. **sodium hypochlorite s.** [USP], a clear, pale, greenish yellow liquid with the odor of chlorine, containing 4–6 per cent of sodium hypochlorite; used as a disinfectant for utensils, etc., but not suitable for application to wounds. It has also been used as a deodorant and bleaching agent. **sodium hypochlorite s., diluted,** a colorless to light yellow liquid with a faint odor of chlorine, compounded of sodium hypochlorite solution, sodium bicarbonate, and water, each 100 ml. containing 450–500 mg. of sodium hypochlorite; used as a topical anti-infective. It is also used for wound irrigation, and has been used to irrigate the urinary bladder. Called also *Dakin's antiseptic, Dakin's fluid, Dakin's s., Dakin's modified s.,* and *surgical s. of chlorinated soda.* See also *Carrel's treatment,* under *treatment.* **sodium iodide I 125 s.** [USP], a solution suitable for either oral or intravenous administration, containing radioiodine (^{125}I) as sodium iodide; used in the determination of thyroid function. **sodium iodide I 131 s.** [USP], a solution suitable for either oral or intravenous use, containing radioiodine (^{131}I) as sodium iodide; used for thryoid function determination and thyroid scans, as a thyroid inhibitor in the treatment of hyperthyroidism and cardiac diseases associated with hyperthyroidism, and for the palliation of thyroid cancer. **sodium pertechnetate Tc 99m s.**, see under *injection*. **sodium phosphate s.**, a clear colorless liquid without odor and with a salty taste, the consistency of thick syrup, each 100 ml. of which contains the equivalent of 71–79 gm. of sodium phosphate; used as a mild saline cathartic. It was formerly administered orally or intravenously in the treatment of lead poisoning. **sodium phosphate P 32 s.** [USP], a solution suitable for either oral or intravenous administration, containing radiophosphorus (^{32}P) as sodium phosphate; used especially as an antipolycythemic and as a diagnostic aid for localization of tumors, e.g., intraocular and brain lesions, and has been used in the treatment of certain leukemias. Formerly called *sodium radiophosphate s.* **sodium phosphate and biphosphate oral s.** [USP], a solution of sodium phosphate and sodium biphosphate, or sodium phosphate and phosphoric acid, in purified water, containing in each 100 ml. 17.1–18.9 gm. of sodium phosphate and 45.6–50.4 gm of sodium biphosphate; used as a cathartic. **sodium radioiodide s.**, sodium iodide I 131 s. **sodium radiophosphate s.**, sodium phosphate P 32 s. **sorbitol s.** [USP], a clear, colorless, syrupy liquid with a sweet taste, containing in each 100 ml. 69–71 gm. of total solids consisting essentially of D-sorbitol with a small quantity of mannitol and other isomeric polyhydric alcohols; used as a flavored humectant in pharmaceutic preparations. **standard s.**, one which contains in each liter a definitely stated amount of reagent; usually expressed in terms of normality (equivalent weights of solute per liter of solution) or molarity (g.mol.wts. of solute per liter of solution). **sulfacetamide sodium ophthalmic s.** [USP], a sterile solution containing 95–105 per cent of the labeled amount of sulfacetamide sodium; used as an antibacterial in sulfonamide-responsive eye infections, applied topically to the conjunctiva. **sulfisoxazole diolamine ophthalmic s.**, [USP], a sterile solution containing sulfisoxazole diolamine equivalent to 90–115 per cent of the labeled amount of sulfisoxazole; used as an antibacterial in the treatment of sulfonamide-responsive eye infections. **supersaturated s.**, an unstable solution that contains more of the solute than it can permanently hold. **surgical s. of chlorinated soda**, see *sodium hypochlorite s., diluted*. **susa s.**, a decalcifying solution composed of corrosive sublimate, sodium chloride, trichloracetic acid, glacial acetic acid, formalin, and water. **tenth-normal s.**, one having one-tenth the strength of a normal solution: designated N/10 or 0.1 N. **test s's,** standard solutions (in purity and concentration) of specified chemical substances used in performing certain test procedures. **tetracaine hydrochloride ophthalmic s.** [USP], a sterile aqueous solution containing 90–110 per cent of the labeled amount of tetracaine hydrochloride; used as a topical anesthetic, applied to the conjunctiva. **tetracaine hydrochloride topical s.** [USP], an aqueous solution containing 95–105 per cent of tetracaine hydrochloride; used as a topical anesthetic, applied to the mucous membranes of the nose and throat. **tetrahydrozoline hydrochloride nasal s.** [USP], a solution of tetrahydrozoline hydrochloride in water adjusted to a suitable tonicity, containing 90 to 110 per cent of the labeled amount of tetrahydrozoline hydrochloride; a vasoconstrictor applied in 0.05 or 0.1 per cent solution as nasal drops or spray, or in 0.05 solution to the eye. **tetrahydrozoline hydrochloride ophthalmic s.** [USP], a sterile, aqueous solution containing 90 to 110 per cent of the labeled amount of tetrahydrozoline hydrochloride; a vasoconstrictor applied to the eye in 0.05 per cent solution. **thimerosal topical s.** [USP], a clear solution having a characteristic odor, compounded of thimerosal, ethylenediamine, monoethanolamine, sodium chloride, sodium borate, and purified water, each 100 ml. containing 95 to 105 mg. of thimerosal; applied topically as an anti-infective. **thioridazine hydrochloride oral s.** [USP], a solution containing, in each 100 ml., 2.70 to 3.30 gm. of thioridazine hydrochloride; used as a tranquilizer. **thousandth-normal s.**, a solution having one-thousandth the strength of a normal solution: designated N/1000 or 0.001 N. **Toison's s.**, a fluid used in diluting blood for the counting of the erythrocytes, consisting of crystal violet, sodium chloride, sodium sulfate, glycerin, and water. **tolnaftate topical s.** [USP], a solution containing 90 to 115 per cent of the labeled amount of tolnaftate; used as a topical antifungal. **tribromoethanol s.**, tribromethyl alcohol s., a preparation containing in each 100 ml. 95–105 gm. of tribromoethanol in amylene hydrate; used as a rectally administered basal anesthetic, and has been used as an anticonvulsive. Called also *bromethol*. **tribromoethyl alcohol s.**, tribromoethanol s. **trimethadione s.** [USP], a solution containing 94 to 106 per cent of the labeled amount of trimethadione; used as an oral anticonvulsant for control of petit mal seizures. **tropicamide ophthalmic s.** [USP], a sterile solution of tropicamide in a suitable buffered, aqueous medium, containing 95 to 105 per cent of tropicamide; applied topically to the conjunctiva as an anticholinergic to produce mydriasis and cycloplegia. **tuaminoheptane sulfate nasal s.** [USP], a solution of tuaminoheptane sulfate, sodium hydroxide, phenylmercuric nitrate, monobasic potassium nitrate, sodium chloride, and purified water; used as an adrenergic applied topically to the nasal mucosa to relieve congestion. **Tyrode's s.**, a modified Locke's solution containing magnesium. **Vleminckx's s.**, lime s., sulfurated. **volumetric s.**, one which contains a specific quantity of solute per stated unit of volume; see also *standard s.* **xylometazoline hydrochloride nasal s.** [USP], a solution of xylometazoline hydrochloride in water adjusted to a suitable pH and tonicity, containing 90 to 110 per cent of the labeled amount of $C_{16}H_{24}N_2 \cdot HCl$; applied topically as a vasoconstrictor in nasal congestion. **Zenker's s.**, a fixative solution consisting of mercury bichloride, potassium dichromate, glacial acetic acid, and water. **Ziehl's s.**, see *Table of Stains and Staining Methods*. **zinc sulfate ophthalmic s.** [USP], a sterile solution of zinc sulfate in water rendered isotonic by the addition of suitable salts, containing 95 to 105 per cent of the labeled amount of zinc sulfate; applied topically to the conjunctiva as an astringent. Considered specific for conjunctivitis due to *Haemophilus duplex*.

solv. abbreviation for L. *sol've*, dissolve.

solvable (sol′vah-b'l) soluble.

solvate (sol′vāt) a compound of one or more molecules of a solvent with the ions or with the molecules of a dissolved substance.

solvation (sol-va′shun) chemical combination of a solvent with the solute.

solvent (sol′vent) [L. *solvens*] 1. dissolving; effecting a solution. 2. a liquid that dissolves or that is capable of dissolving; the component of a solution that is present in greater amount. Cf. *solute*.

solvolysis (sol-vol′ĭ-sis) a general term for double decomposition reactions of the type of hydrolysis, ammonolysis, and sulfolysis.

Soma (so′mah) trademark for preparations of carisoprodol.

soma (so′mah) [Gr. *sōma* body] 1. the body as distinguished from the mind. 2. the body tissue as distinguished from the germ cells. 3. the cell body.

somal (so′mal) somatic.

somalin (som′ah-lin) a cardioactive glycoside from plants of the genus *Adenium*.

somaplasm (so′mah-plazm) somatoplasm.

somasthenia (sōm″as-the′ne-ah) [*soma* + *a* neg. + Gr. *sthenos* strength + *-ia*] a condition of bodily weakness, poor appetite and sleep, and inability to maintain a normal active life without easy exhaustion.

somatalgia (so″mah-tal′je-ah) [*somato-* + Gr. *algos* pain + *-ia*] bodily pain.

somatasthenia (so″mat-as-the′ne-ah) somasthenia.

somatesthesia (so″mat-es-the′ze-ah) [*somato-* + Gr. *aisthēsis* perception + *-ia*] the consciousness of having a body.

somatesthetic (so″mat-es-thet′ik) pertaining to somatesthesia.

somatic (so-mat′ik) [Gr. *sōmatikos*] 1. pertaining to or characteristic of the soma or body. 2. pertaining to the body wall in contrast to the viscera.

somaticosplanchnic (so-mat″ĭ-ko-splank′nik) somaticovisceral.

somaticovisceral (so-mat″ĭ-ko-vis′er-al) pertaining to the body proper and viscera.

somatist (so′mah-tist) one who believes that neuroses and psychoses are of physical origin and are based on bodily lesions.

somatization (so″mah-ti-za′shun) in psychiatry, the conversion of mental experiences or states into bodily symptoms.

somat(o)- [Gr. *sōma*, gen. *sōmatos* body] a combining form denoting relationship to the body.

somatoceptor (so-mat′o-sep″tor) a receptor concerned in receiving stimuli of the skeletal and somatic musculature.

somatochrome (so-mat′o-krōm) [*somato-* + Gr. *chrōma* color] any nerve cell which has a well marked cell body completely surrounding the nucleus, its colorable protoplasm having a distinct contour; used also adjectively.

somatoderm (so-mat′o-derm) [*somato-* + Gr. *derma* skin] the somatic layer of mesoderm.

somatodidymus (so″mah-to-did′ĭ-mus) a double fetus exhibiting somatodymia.

somatodymia (so″mah-to-dim′e-ah) [*somato-* + Gr. *didymos* twin + *-ia*] a developmental anomaly resulting in the production of conjoined twins whose trunks are fused into one.

somatoform (so-mat′o-form) denoting psychogenic symptoms resembling those of physical disease.

somatogenesis (so″mah-to-jen′ĕ-sis) [*somato-* + Gr. *genesis* production] the formation or emergence of bodily structure out of hereditary sources; the formation of somatoplasm out of germ plasm.

somatogenetic (so-mat″o-jĕ-net′ik) 1. pertaining to somatogenesis. 2. somatogenic.

somatogenic (so″mah-to-jen′ik) [*somato-* + Gr. *gennan* to produce] originating in the cells of the body, as a disease process; opposed to psychogenic.

somatogram (so-mat′o-gram) [*somato-* + Gr. *gramma* a writing] a roentgenogram of the body.

somatology (so″mah-tol′o-je) [*somato-* + *-logy*] the sum of what is known regarding the body; the study of the anatomy and physiology of the body.

somatomammotropin (so″mah-to-mam″o-tro′pin) a family of three hormones, growth hormone and prolactin, produced by the anterior pituitary, and placental lactogen, of similar structure. **chorionic s.,** human placental lactogen.

somatomedin (so″mah-to-me′din) any of a group of peptides formed in the liver and other tissues (molecular weight, approximately 8000) and found in plasma which mediate the effect of growth hormone (somatotropin) on cartilage; they are responsible for uptake of sulfate and increased synthesis of collagen and other proteins by cartilage. Somatomedins also have insulin-like biological actions and increase ribonucleic acid (RNA) synthesis and promote deoxyribonucleic acid (DNA) synthesis, and thus act as growth factors. Postulated as a "second messenger" in the somatotropic actions of growth hormone. Called also *sulfation factor*.

somatomegaly (so″mah-to-meg′ah-le) [*somato-* + Gr. *megaleios* stately + *-ia*] abnormal size of body; gigantism.

somatometry (so-mah-tom′ĕ-tre) [*somato-* + Gr. *metron* measure] measurement of the body.

somatopagus (so″mah-top′ah-gus) [*somato-* + Gr. *pagos* thing fixed] a double fetus with trunks more or less merged.

somatopathic (so″mah-to-path′ik) [*somato-* + Gr. *pathos* disease] pertaining to or characterized by somatopathy.

somatopathy (so″mah-top′ah-the) a bodily disorder as distinguished from a mental one.

somatophrenia (so″mah-to-fre′ne-ah) [*somato-* + Gr. *phrēn* mind + *-ia*] exaggeration or imagination of bodily ills.

somatoplasm (so-mat′o-plazm) [*somato-* + Gr. *plasma* anything formed or molded] the protoplasm of the body cells as distinguished from that of the germ cells. Cf. *germ plasm.*

somatopleural (so″mah-to-ploor′al) pertaining to the somatopleure.

somatopleure (so-mat′o-ploor) [*somato-* + Gr. *pleura* side] the embryonic body wall, formed by ectoderm and somatic mesoderm.

somatopsychic (so″mah-to-si′kik) [*somato-* + Gr. *psychē* soul] pertaining to both body and mind; denoting a physical disorder that produces mental symptoms.

somatopsychosis (so″mah-to-si-ko′sis) [*somato-* + *psychosis*] a mental disorder associated with a physical disease.

somatoschisis (so″mah-tos′kĭ-sis) [*somato-* + Gr. *schisis* fissure] a developmental anomaly characterized by a fissure of the trunk.

somatoscopy (so″mah-tos′ko-pe) [*somato-* + Gr. *skopein* to examine] viewing or examination of the body.

somatosexual (so″mah-to-seks′u-al) [*somato-* + L. *sexus* sex] pertaining to both physical and sex characteristics; pertaining to the physical manifestations of sexual development.

somatosplanchnopleuric (so″mah-to-splank″no-ploor′ik) pertaining to the somatopleure and the splanchnopleure.

somatostatin (so″mah-to-stat′in) a cyclic tetradecapeptide elaborated primarily by the median eminence of the hypothalamus and by the delta cells of the pancreatic islets; it inhibits release of growth hormone (somatotropin), thyrotropin, and corticotropin by the adenohypophysis, of insulin and glucagon by the pancreas, of gastrin by the gastric mucosa, of secretin by the intestinal mucosa, and of renin by the kidney.

somatostatinoma (so″mah-to-stat″ĭ-no′mah) a rare somatostatin-secreting pancreatic islet-cell tumor, associated with diabetes mellitus or abnormal glucose tolerance.

somatotherapy (so″mah-to-ther′ah-pe) [*somato-* + Gr. *therapeia* treatment] biological treatment of mental disorders.

somatotonia (so″mah-to-to′ne-ah) [*somato-* + *ton-* + *-ia*] a temperament type characterized by love of physical adventure, boundless energy, boldness, aggressiveness, and need for exercise and activity; the behavioral counterpart of mesomorphy.

somatotopic (so″mah-to-top′ik) related to particular areas of the body; describing the organization of the motor area of the brain, control of the movement of different parts of the body being centered in specific regions of the cortex.

somatotridymus (so″mah-to-trid′ĭ-mus) [*somato-* + Gr. *tri-* three + *didymos* twin] a monster with three trunks.

somatotrope (so-mat′o-trōp) somatotroph.

somatotroph (so-mat′o trōf) any of the acidophils (alpha cells) of the adenohypophysis that stain preferentially with orange G, and are thought to be responsible for the secretion of growth hormone. Called also *somatotroph cell.*

somatotrophic (so″mah-to-trōf′ik) [*somato-* + Gr. *trophē* nourishment] somatotropic.

somatotrophin (so″mah-to-tro′fin) somatotropin.

somatotropic (so″mah-to-trop′ik) [*somato-* + Gr. *tropos* a turning] 1. having an affinity for or attacking the body or the body cells; also having an influence on the body. 2. having a stimulating effect on body nutrition and growth. 3. having the properties of somatotropin.

somatotropin (so″mah-to-tro′pin) growth hormone; see under *hormone.*

somatotype (so-mat′o-tīp) [*somato-* + *type*] a particular category of body build, determined on the basis of certain physical characteristics. See *ectomorph*, *endomorph*, and *mesomorph.*

somatotyping (so-mat′o-tīp″ing) a method of studying objectively the physical types of individuals.

somatotypy (so-mat′o-ti″pe) the determination of the type of body build.

somatropin (so-mat′ro-pin) somatotropin.

Sombulex (som′bu-leks) trademark for a preparation of hexobarbital.

-some [Gr. *soma* body] a word termination denoting a body.

somesthesia (so″mes-the′ze-ah) somatesthesia.

somesthetic (so″mes-thet′ik) somatesthetic.

somite (so′mīt) one of the paired, blocklike masses of mesoderm, arranged segmentally alongside the neural tube of the embryo, forming the vertebral column and segmental musculature; called also *mesoblastic* or *mesodermal segment.*

somnambulance (som-nam′bu-lans) somnambulism.

somnambulation (som-nam″bu-la′shun) somnambulism.

somnambulism (som-nam′bu-lizm) [L. *somnus* sleep + *ambulare* to walk] sleepwalking; rising out of bed and walking about during an apparent state of sleep, usually occurring in the first third of the night and lasting a few minutes to a half hour.

somnambulist (som-nam′bu-list) a person who walks in his sleep.

somni- [L. *somnus* sleep] a combining form denoting relationship to sleep.

somnifacient (som″nĭ-fa′shent) [somni- + L. facere to make] 1. causing sleep; hypnotic. 2. an agent that induces sleep.

somniferous (som-nif′er-us) [somni- + L. ferre to bring] inducing or causing sleep.

somnific (som-nif′ik) somniferous.

somniloquence (som-nil′o-kwens) somniloquism.

somniloquism (som-nil′o-kwizm) [somni- + L. loqui to speak] talking during sleep.

somniloquist (som-nil′o-kwist) one who talks in his sleep.

somniloquy (som-nil′o-kwe) somniloquism.

somnocinematograph (som″no-sin″e-mat′o-graf) [somnus + cinematograph] an apparatus for recording movements made during sleep.

somnolence (som′no-lens) [L. somnolentia sleepiness] sleepiness; also unnatural drowsiness.

somnolent (som′no-lent) [L. somnolentus] affected with somnolence; sleepy.

somnolentia (som″no-len′she-ah) [L.] 1. drowsiness, or somnolence. 2. sleep drunkenness; a condition of incomplete sleep marked by loss of orientation and by excited or violent behavior.

Somnos (som′nos) trademark for preparations of chloral hydrate.

somnus (som′nus) [L.] sleep.

Somogyi effect (phenomenon), unit (so′mo-je) [Michael Somogyi, American biochemist, 1883–1971] see under effect and unit.

somosphere (so′mo-sfēr) [Gr. sōma body + sphaira sphere] one of the elements of the archiplasm.

sonarography (so″nar-og′rah-fe) ultrasonic scanning that provides a two-dimensional image corresponding to clear sections of acoustic interfaces in tissues.

sonde (sond) [Fr.] sound. **s. coudé** (sond koo-da′) [Fr. "bent sound"], a catheter with an elbow, or sharp, beaklike bend, near the end.

sone (sōn) a unit of loudness, being the loudness of a simple tone of 1,000 cycles per second, 40 decibels above a listener's threshold.

sonicate (son′ĭ-kāt) 1. to expose to sound waves; to disrupt bacteria by exposure to high-frequency sound waves. 2. the products of such disruption.

sonication (son″ĭ-ka′shun) exposure to sound waves; disruption of bacteria by exposure to high-frequency sound waves.

Sonilyn (son′ĭ-lin) trademark for a preparation of sulfachlorpyridazine.

sonitus (son′ĭ-tus) [L. "sound"] a sounding or tinkling in the ears; tinnitus aurium.

Sonne dysentery (son′e) [Carl Olaf Sonne, Danish bacteriologist, 1882–1948] see under dysentery.

sonogram (so′no-gram) a record or display obtained by ultrasonic scanning.

sonographic (so″no-graf′ik) ultrasonographic.

sonography (so-nog′rah-fe) ultrasonography.

sonolucency (so″no-loo′sen-se) the property of being sonolucent.

sonolucent (so′no-loo′sent) in ultrasonography, permitting the passage of ultrasound waves without reflecting them back to their source (without giving off echoes).

sonorous (so-no′rus) [L. sonorus] resonant; sounding.

sophistication (so-fis″tĭ-ka′shun) [Gr. sophistikos deceitful] the adulteration of food or medicine.

sophomania (sof″o-ma′ne-ah) [Gr. sophos wise + mania madness] an irrational belief in one's own great wisdom.

Sophora (so-fo′ra) [Arabic sofara] a genus of leguminous trees and shrubs. The root and seed of S. tomentosa are used in India to arrest choleraic vomiting. Some species are poisonous; see loco.

sophoretin (sof″o-re′tin) quercetin.

sophorin (sof′o-rin) rutin.

sophorine (sof′o-rēn) cytisine.

sopor (so′por) [L.] unnaturally deep or profound sleep.

soporiferous (so″po-rif′er-us) [L. sopor deep sleep + ferre to bring] inducing deep or profound slumber.

soporific (sop″o-rif′ik, so″po-rif′ik) [L. soporificus] 1. causing or inducing profound sleep. 2. a drug or other agent which induces sleep.

soporous (so′por-us) [L. soporus] associated or affected with coma or profound slumber.

S. op. s. abbreviation for L. si o′pus sit, if it is necessary.

Sorangiaceae (so-ran″je-a′se-e) in former systems of classification, a family of bacteria made up of organisms now included in the family Polyangiaceae.

Sorangium (so-ran′je-um) in former systems of classification, a genus of bacteria made up of organisms now included in the genus Polyangium.

Soranus (so-ran′us) **of Ephesus** (2nd century A.D.) a Greek physician of the Methodist school; he studied in Alexandria and practiced in Rome. His writings on obstetrics, gynecology, and pediatrics survive.

sorb (sorb) to attract and retain substances by absorption or adsorption.

sorbefacient (sor″bĕ-fa′shent) [L. sorbere to suck + facere to make] 1. promoting absorption. 2. an agent that promotes absorption.

sorbent (sor′bent) an agent that sorbs.

sorbic acid (sor′bik) 2,4-hexadecenoic acid, a compound found in berries of the mountain ash Sorbus aucuparia and in many other plants; it inhibits the growth of yeasts and molds and is used as an antimicrobial preservative.

sorbin (sor′bin) sorbose.

sorbinose (sor′bĭ-nōs) sorbose.

sorbitan (sor′bĭ-tan) a generic name for an anhydride of sorbitol, $C_6H_8O(OH)_4$, the fatty acids of which (s. monolaurate [NF], s. monooleate, s. monopalmitate [NF], s. monostearate [NF], s. sesquioleate, s. trioleate, s. tristearate) are surfactants; called also sorbitol anhydride. See also polysorbate.

sorbite (sor′bīt) sorbitol.

sorbitol (sor′bĭ-tol) a crystalline, hexahydric alcohol, $CH_2-OH\cdot(CHOH)_4CH_2OH$, first found in ripe berries of the tree Sorbus aucuparia, and occurring in small quantities in other berries, cherries, plums, pears, etc. It is formed in mammals from glucose and is then converted to fructose; this process is responsible for fructose found in seminal plasma. It is also found in lens deposits in diabetes mellitus. A pharmaceutical preparation [NF] is obtained by catalytic hydrogenation of glucose and certain other sugars; it contains between 91 and 100.6 per cent sorbitol, calculated on the anhydrous basis; used as a sweetening agent and tablet excipient in pharmaceutical preparations and, in a 50 per cent solution, as an intravenous osmotic diuretic.

sorbitol dehydrogenase (sor′bĭ-tol de-hi′dro-jĕ-nās) L-iditol dehydrogenase.

Sorbitrate (sor′bĭ-trāt) trademark for a preparation of isosorbide dinitrate.

sorbose (sor′bōs) a ketohexose, $CH_2OH(CHOH)_3CO\cdot CH_2-OH$, resembling levulose in its properties.

Sordariaceae (sor″dah-re-a′se-e) a family of fungi of the order Sphaeriales, series Pyrenomycetes, including the genus Neurospora.

sordes (sor′dēz) [L. "filth"] dirt; debris; especially the encrustations and accumulations of food, epithelial matter, and bacteria collected on the teeth and lips during a prolonged fever. **s. gas′tricae,** undigested food, mucus, etc., in the stomach.

sore (sōr) 1. a popular term for almost any lesion of the skin or mucous membranes. 2. painful. **bed s.,** decubitus ulcer. **canker s.,** recurrent aphthous stomatitis. **chrome s.,** chrome ulcer. **cold s.,** herpes febrilis. **Delhi s.,** the Old World form of cutaneous leishmaniasis. **desert s.,** a phagedenic ulcer occurring in South Africa and Australia characterized initially by the development of papulovesicular lesions on the extremities, especially on the backs of the hands, forearms, knees, and shins that rupture and form painful, crusted purulent ulcers. The condition probably represents an infected ulcer from some secondarily antecedent neglected lesion. Called also Barcoo rot and veldt s., and also known by various native names and by names having only geographical significance. **hard s.,** chancre, def 1. **Kandahar s., Lahore s.,** the Old World form of cutaneous leishmaniasis. **mixed s.,** see under chancre. **Naga s.,** tropical phagedenic ulcer. **Natal s., oriental s., Penjdeh s.,** the Old World form of cutaneous leishmaniasis. **pressure s.,** decubitus ulcer. **soft s.,** chancroid.

veldt s., desert s. **venereal s.,** any sore that accompanies or manifests a venereal disease, especially a chancroid.

Sörensen's reagent (sor′en-senz) [Sören Peer Lauritz *Sörensen,* Danish biochemist, 1868–1939] see under *reagent.*

sore throat (sōr thrōt) see *laryngitis, pharyngitis,* and *tonsillitis.* **clergyman's s. t.,** dysphonia clericorum. **epidemic streptococcal s. t.,** septic s. t. **Fothergill's s. t.,** (*obs.*), scarlatina angiosa. **hospital s. t.,** septic inflammation of the pharynx and fauces sometimes affecting nurses and interns in hospitals. **putrid s. t.,** gangrenous pharyngitis. **septic s. t.,** a severe type of sore throat occurring in epidemics, marked by intense local hyperemia with or without a grayish exudate and enlargement of the cervical lymph glands. It is usually caused by *Streptococcus pyogenes* and sometimes by *S. equisimilis.* The infection is probably largely spread by droplets or in air, but is also transmitted by direct contact and by food and milk. Called also *streptococcal sore throat* and *streptococcal tonsillitis.* **spotted s. t.,** follicular tonsillitis. **streptococcal s. t.,** septic s. t. **ulcerated s. t.,** gangrenous pharyngitis.

Soret band, effect (phenomenon) (so-ra′) [C. *Soret,* French physicist, died 1931] see under *band* and *effect.*

sori (so′ri) plural of *sorus.*

Sorosphaera (sor″o-sfe′rah) [Gr. *sōros* heap + *sphere*] a genus of ameboid protozoa (order Plasmodiophorida, class Plasmodiophorea) parasitic on plants of the genus *Veronica.*

sorption (sorp′shun) [L. *sorbere* to suck in] the process or state of being sorbed; absorption or adsorption.

sorter (sor′ter) a device for sorting. **fluorescence-activated cell s. (FACS),** an automated instrument that separates cell populations labeled with fluorescent antibodies or other fluorescent labels. The sample stream is broken up into droplets which are electrostatically charged and deflected into different collecting tubes depending on the measured fluorescence of the droplets.

sorus (so′rus), pl. *so′ri* [Gr. *sōros* heap] a mass, group, or cluster of spores, sporangia, or reproductive bodies occurring in certain plants, fungi, and protozoa.

S.O.S. abbreviation for L. *si o′pus sit,* if it is necessary.

sotalol hydrochloride (so′tah-lōl) chemical name: *N*-[4-[1-hydroxy-2-[(1-methylethyl)amino]ethyl]phenyl]methanesulfonamide monohydrochloride; a beta-adrenergic blocking agent, $C_{12}H_{20}N_2O_4 \cdot HCl$, having the same actions as propranolol (q.v.).

soterenol hydrochloride (so-ter′ĕ-nōl) chemical name: *N*-[2-hydroxy-5-[1-hydroxy-2-[(1-methylethyl)amino]ethyl]phenyl]methanesulfonamide monohydrochloride; an adrenergic with bronchodilator properties, $C_{12}H_{20}N_2O_4 \cdot HCl$.

Soto-Hall sign (so′to-hawl) [Ralph *Soto-Hall,* San Francisco surgeon, born 1899] see under *sign.*

Sottas disease (sot′tahz) [Jules *Sottas,* French neurologist, 1866–1943] progressive hypertrophic interstitial neuropathy.

soudan (soo-dan′) Sudan.

souffle (soo′f'l) [Fr. "a puff"; L. *sufflare* to blow] a soft, blowing, auscultatory sound; called also *bruit de soufflet* and *bellows murmur.* **cardiac s.,** any cardiac or vascular murmur of a blowing quality. **fetal s.,** a blowing sound sometimes heard in pregnancy; supposed to be due to compression of the umbilical vessels. **funic s., funicular s.,** a hissing souffle synchronous with the fetal heart sounds, and supposed to be produced in the umbilical cord. **placental s.,** a souffle supposed to be produced by the blood current in the placenta. **splenic s.,** a sound said to be sometimes audible over a diseased spleen. **umbilical s.,** funic s. **uterine s.,** a sound made by the blood within the arteries of the gravid uterus.

sound (sownd) [L. *sonus*] 1. the effect produced on the organ of hearing and its central connections by the vibrations of the air or other medium. 2. mechanical radiant energy, the motion of particles of the material medium through which it travels (air, water, or solids) being along the line of transmission (longitudinal); such energy, of frequency between 8 and 20,000 cycles per second, provides the stimulus for the subjective sensation of hearing. 3. an instrument to be introduced into a cavity to detect a foreign body or to dilate a stricture. 4. a noise, normal or abnormal, heard within the body; for other sounds see under *bruit, fremitus, murmur,* and *rale.* **auscultatory s.,** any sound heard on auscultation. **bandbox s.,** a highly resonant sound elicited by percussion over the chest in cases of emphysema of the lung. **Beatty-Bright friction s.,** the friction sound of pleurisy. **bell s.,** bruit d'airain. **bellows s.,** a double murmur (systolic and diastolic) resembling the sound made by a bellows. **Béniqué's s.,** a lead or tin sound, having a wide curve, for dilating urethral strictures. **bottle s.,** amphoric rale. **cardiac s's,** heart s's. **coin s.,** bruit d'airain. **cracked-pot s.,** a percussion sound indicative of a pulmonary cavity into which the breath may pass. **cracked-pot s., cranial,** a peculiar sound due to the separation of the cranial sutures; seen in children with raised intracranial pressure. **ejection s's,** high-pitched clicking sounds occurring very shortly after the first heart sound, attributed to sudden distention of a dilated pulmonary artery or aorta or to forceful opening of the pulmonic or aortic cusps; most often heard in septal defects or patent ductus associated with high pulmonary resistance and hypertension. Called also *ejection clicks.* **entotic s's,** sounds that originate within the ear, such as tinnitus. **esophageal s.,** a long, flexible sound for exploring the esophagus. **first s.,** see *heart s's.* **flapping s.,** the peculiar sound made by the closure of the heart valves. **fourth s.,** see *gallop rhythm,* under *rhythm.* **friction s.,** any sound produced by the rubbing of one surface over another. **heart s's,** the sounds heard over the cardiac region, which are produced by the functioning of the heart. The *first,* occurring at the beginning of ventricular systole, is dull, firm, and prolonged, and is heard as a "lubb" sound; the *second,* produced essentially by closure of the semilunar valves, is shorter and sharper than the first, and is heard as a "dupp" sound; the *third,* produced by vibrations of the ventricular walls when they are suddenly distended by the rush of blood from the atria, is weak, low-pitched, and dull, and is usually audible only in children and young adults; and the *fourth,* produced by atrial contraction and ventricular filling, is low-pitched and short, and is rarely audible in the normal heart. Called also *cardiac s's.* **hippocratic s.,** the succussion sound heard in pyopneumothorax or seropneumothorax. **Korotkoff s's,** sounds heard during auscultatory determination of blood pressure, produced by sudden distention of the artery, the walls of which were previously relaxed because of the proximally placed pneumatic cuff. **lacrimal s.,** a sound of small caliber for use in the lacrimal canal. **Le-Fort s.,** a sound with a screw tip for attachment of a filiform, used to pass through tight urethral strictures. **metallic s.,** a sound having a metallic quality heard especially over cavities in the chest. **muscle s.,** the sound heard over a muscle when in a condition of contraction. **peacock s.,** a quality of voice due to various defects and lesions of the air passages. **percussion s.,** any sound obtained by percussion. **physiological s's,** sounds heard when the auditory canals are plugged, caused by the rush of blood through blood vessels in or near the inner ear and by adjacent muscles in continuous low frequency vibration. **pistol-shot s.,** Traube's sign. **respiratory s.,** any sound heard on auscultation over any portion of the respiratory tract. **second s.,** see *heart s's.* **second s., pulmonic,** the audible vibrations related to the closure of the pulmonary semilunar valve; abbreviated P₂. **shaking s.,** succussion s. **subjective s.,** 1. phonism. 2. the sound sometimes produced by the blood current in the examiner's ears during auscultation. **succussion s's,** splashing sounds heard on succussion over a distended stomach and in hydropneumothorax. **third s.,** see *heart s's.* **tick-tack s's,** heart sounds in which there is little or no difference in the quality of the first and second sounds. **to-and-fro s.,** a friction sound or murmur heard with both systole and diastole. **urethral s.,** a long, slim, slightly conical instrument of steel for exploring and dilating the urethra. **vesicular breath s's,** sounds heard on auscultation over the normal lung during respiration. **water-wheel s.,** bruit de moulin. **white s.,** that produced by a mixture of all frequencies of mechanical vibration perceptible as sound. **Winternitz's s.,** a double-current catheter. **xiphisternal crunching s.,** a peculiar sound, of unknown origin, frequently heard (20 per cent of healthy men) over the lower sternum and xiphoid process.

Souques's phenomenon, sign (soo′kez) [Alexandre Achille *Souques,* French neurologist, 1860–1944] see under *phenomenon* and *sign.*

Souttar's tube (sow′terz) [Henry Sessions *Souttar,* London surgeon, 1875–1964] see under *tube.*

sowdah (sow′dah) [Ar. "black"] the typical cutaneous manifestation of onchocerciasis in Yemen and Saudi Arabia, usually limited to one or both lower limbs, characterized by black pigmentation, thickening, and roughness of the skin, edema, intense pruritus, papules, and regional lymphadenopathy. Similar cases have been reported from the Sudan and West Africa.

Soxhlet's apparatus (soks′lets) [Franz Ritter von Soxhlet, German chemist, 1848–1926] see under *apparatus*.

soya (soi′ah) see *soy bean*.

soybean (soi′bēn) the bean of the leguminous plant, *Soja hispida* (*Glycine soja*) or Chinese bean. It contains little starch and is rich in protein. From it is prepared a meal which is used as a protein supplement. It also furnishes an enzyme, urease. See *urease*.

Soymida febrifuga Juss. (soi′mĭ-dah feb-rif′u-gah) a tree of southern Asia, known as Indian red wood; the bark is bitter, astringent, and aromatic.

sp. abbreviation for L. *spir′itus*, spirit.

space (spās) 1. a delimited area. 2. an actual or potential cavity of the body; called also *spatium* [NA]. 3. the expanse of the universe beyond the earth and its atmosphere. **anatomical dead s.,** see *dead s*. **apical s.,** the region between the wall of the alveolus and the apex of the root of a tooth. **arachnoid s.,** see *cavum subarachnoideale* and *cavum subdurale*. **axillary s.,** fossa axillaris. **Blessig's s's,** see under *cyst*. **Bogros's s.,** a region bounded by the peritoneum above and the fascia transversalis below, in which the lower part of the external iliac artery can be found without cutting the peritoneum; called also *retroinguinal s*. **Bowman's s.,** capsular s. **bregmatic s.,** the anterior fontanel (fonticulus frontalis). **Burns' s.,** fossa jugularis, def. 1. **capsular s.,** a narrow chalice-shaped cavity between the glomerular and the capsular epithelium of the glomerular capsule of the kidney; called also *Bowman's space*. **cartilage s's,** the spaces in hyaline cartilage which contain the cartilage cells. **cathodal dark s.,** Crookes s. **cell s's,** the spaces in the ground substance of connective tissue enclosing the connective tissue corpuscles. **chyle s's,** the central lymphatic spaces of the villi of the intestine. **circumlental s.,** see *spatia zonularia*, under *spatium*. **Colles' s.,** a space under the perineal fascia containing the transversus perinei, ischiocavernosus, and bulbocavernosus muscles, the posterior scrotal or labial vessels and nerves, and the bulbous portion of the urethra. **complemental s.,** portions of the pleural cavity that are not occupied by lung tissue, such as the triangular spaces below the lower borders of the lungs and irregular spaces about the heart. **corneal s's,** the spaces between the lamellae of the substantia propria of the cornea which contain corneal cells and tissue fluid; called also *interlamellar s's*. **Cotunnius' s.,** the space within the membranous labyrinth. **Crookes s.,** a dark space at the cathode of a nearly exhausted roentgen-ray tube through which a current is being passed; called also *cathodal dark s*. **cupular s.,** pars cupularis recessus epitympanici. **Czermak's s's,** spatia interglobularia; see under *spatium*. **dead s.,** 1. space remaining after closure of surgical or other wounds, permitting the accumulation of blood or serum and resultant delay in healing. 2. in the respiratory tract: (a) *anatomical dead space*, those portions, from the nose and mouth to the terminal bronchioles, in which exchange of oxygen and carbon dioxide does not occur, and (b) *physiologic dead space*, which reflects nonuniformity of ventilation and perfusion in the lung, is the anatomical dead space plus the space in alveoli occupied by air that does not participate in oxygen–carbon dioxide exchange. **s's in dentin,** spatia interglobularia. **Disse's s's,** small spaces which separate the sinusoids of the liver from the liver cells and which carry the lymph of the liver. **Douglas' s.,** excavatio rectouterina. **epicerebral s.,** the potential space between the brain and the pia mater. **epidural s.,** cavitas epiduralis. **episcleral s.,** spatium episclerale. **epispinal s.,** the potential space between the substance of the spinal cord and the pia mater. **epitympanic s.,** recessus epitympanicus. **escapement s's,** spaces which permit the escape of material being comminuted between the occlusal surfaces of the teeth, provided by the cusps and ridges, sulci and developmental ridges of the teeth, and the embrasures between the teeth. **extraperitoneal s.,** spatium extraperitoneale. **Faraday's dark s.,** the dark region separating the negative glow from the positive column in a Crookes tube. **s's**

of Fontana, see *spatia anguli iridis* [*Fontanae*], under *spatium*. **freeway s.,** interocclusal distance. **globular s's of Czermak,** spatia interglobularia. **H. s.,** Holzknecht's s. **haversian s.,** haversian canal (canalis nutricius ossis [NA]). **Henke's s.,** a space containing connective tissue between the spinal column and the pharynx and esophagus. **His's perivascular s.,** the space between the adventitia of the blood vessels of the brain and spinal cord and the perivascular limiting membrane of glia tissue. **Holzknecht's s.,** the middle one of the three clear lung fields in the roentgenogram of the chest in oblique projection when the rays pass from the left posteriorly to the right anteriorly; called also *H. s.*, *prevertebral s.*, and *retrocardiac s*. **iliocostal s.,** the area between the twelfth rib and the crest of the ilium. **interarytenoid s.,** pars intercartilaginea rimae glottidis. **intercostal s.,** spatium intercostale. **intercristal s.,** 1. all of the area within the inner membrane of a mitochondrion. 2. the clefts between the inward extensions of the mitochondrial membrane space. **intercrural s.,** a triangular space between the crura cerebri. **interdental s.,** interproximal s. **interfascial s.,** spatium intervaginale. **interglobular s's (of Owen),** spatia interglobularia. **interlamellar s's,** corneal s's. **interocclusal s.,** interocclusal distance (clearance). **interosseous s's of metacarpus,** spatia interossea metacarpi. **interosseous s's of metatarsus,** spatia interossea metatarsi. **interpeduncular s.,** fossa interpeduncularis. **interpleural s.,** mediastinum, def. 2. **interproximal s., interproximate s.,** the space between the proximal surfaces of adjoining teeth; sometimes used to designate especially the space between the proximal surfaces of adjoining teeth that is gingival to the area of contact (*septal s.*). Cf. *embrasure*. **interradicular s.,** the space between roots; in dentistry, the entire extent of the space between the roots of a tooth, from apex to base. **interseptal s.,** a space between the two folds uniting to form the spurious septum in the heart of the early embryo. **intervaginal s.,** spatium episclerale. **intervaginal s's of optic nerve,** spatia intervaginalia nervi optici. **intervillous s.,** the space of the placenta into which the chorionic villi project and through which maternal blood circulates. **s's of iridocorneal angle,** spatia anguli iridocornealis. **Kiernan's s's,** the triangular spaces bounded by invaginated Glisson's capsule between the liver lobules, containing the larger interlobular branches of the portal vein, hepatic artery, and hepatic duct. **Kiesselbach's s.,** see under *area*. **Kretschmann's s.,** a depressed area in the recessus epitympanicus, below Prussak's space. **Larrey's s's,** intervals between those parts of the diaphragm which are attached to the ribs and that which is attached to the sternum. **leeway s.,** see *Nance's leeway s*. **Lesgaft's s.,** a rhombus which in some persons exists between the external oblique muscle in front, the latissimus dorsi behind, the serratus posticus above, and the internal oblique below; frequently the site of pointing of an abscess, or occurrence of a hernia. Called also *Lesgaft's triangle* and *Grynfeltt's triangle*. **lymph s.,** any space in tissue occupied by lymph. **Magendie's s's,** subarachnoid spaces between the pia and arachnoid, corresponding to the principal sulci of the brain. **Malacarne's s.,** substantia perforata posterior. **Marie's quadrilateral s.,** see *quadrilateral s. of Marie*. **marrow s.,** cavum medullare ossium. **Meckel's s.,** cavum trigeminale. **mediastinal s.,** mediastinum, def. 2. **medullary s.,** cavitas medullaris. **midpalmar s.,** the palmar space lying between the middle metacarpal bone and the radial side of the hypothenar eminence. **mitochondrial membrane s.,** a narrow space between the inner and outer membranes of a mitochondrion, including its inward projections between the cristae. **Mohrenheim's s.,** a groove on the deltoid muscle for the cephalic vein and a branch of the acromiothoracic artery. **Nance's leeway s.,** the amount by which the space occupied by the deciduous canine and first and second deciduous molars exceeds that occupied by the canine and premolar teeth of the permanent dentition, usually averaging 1.7 mm on each side of the dental arch. **Nuel's s's,** fluid-filled spaces in the organ of Corti between the outer hair cells, communicating with the inner tunnel through the spaces between the pillar cells. Called also *outer tunnel*. **Obersteiner-Redlich s.,** see under *area*. **palmar s.,** a large fascial space in the hand, divided by a fibrous septum into the midpalmar space and the thenar space. **parapharyngeal s.,** pharyngomaxillary s. **parasinoidal**

s's, lateral lacunae in the dura mater, along the superior sagittal sinus, which receive meningeal and diploic veins. **Parona's s.,** a space between the pronator quadratus muscle and the deep flexor tendons in the forearm, about 5 cm. above the wrist, in direct continuity with the tendon sheaths and the midpalmar space. **perforated s., anterior,** substantia perforata anterior. **perforated s., posterior,** substantia perforata posterior. **periaxial s.,** a fluid-filled cavity surrounding the nuclear bag and myotubule regions of a muscle spindle. **perichorioidal s., perichoroidal s.,** spatium perichoroideale. **perilymphatic s.,** spatium perilymphaticum. **perineal s., deep,** spatium perinei profundum **perineal s., superficial,** spatium perinei superficiale. **perineuronal s.,** the extracellular compartment surrounding nerve cells of the central nervous system; its histologic appearance as a space is an artefact. **perinuclear s.,** see under *cisterna*. **peripharyngeal s.,** retropharyngeal s. **periplasmic s.,** a zone between the plasma membrane and the outer membrane of the cell wall of gram-negative bacteria. **perisinusoidal s's,** Disse's s's. **perivascular s.,** a lymph space occurring within the walls of an artery. **perivitelline s.,** a space between the ovum and the zona pellucida; in the ovum of some animals, a fluid-filled space separating the fertilization membrane from the surface of the egg. **pharyngomaxillary s.,** the space included between the lateral wall of the pharynx, the internal pterygoid muscle, and the cervical vertebrae. **phrenocostal s.,** the space between the outer edge of the diaphragm and the costal surface. **physiologic dead s.,** see *dead* s. **pneumatic s.,** a portion of bone occupied by air-containing cells; applied especially to spaces in the bones of the head constituting the paranasal sinuses. **Poiseuille's s.,** that part of the lumen of a tube where no flow of liquid occurs, as next to the wall of a blood vessel, where the red cells are virtually motionless and constitute a layer over which the inner layers of liquid slide. **popliteal s.,** fossa poplitea. **postperforated s.,** substantia perforata posterior. **preperitoneal s.,** spatium retropubicum. **preputial s.,** the space between the prepuce and the glans penis. **prevertebral s.,** Holzknecht's s. **prevesical s.,** spatium retropubicum. **prezonular s.,** portion of the eyeball anterior to the zonula ciliaris, occupied by the aqueous humor. **proximal s., proximate s.,** interproximal s. **Prussak's s.,** recessus membranae tympani superior. **quadrilateral s. of Marie,** a space in the cerebral hemisphere bounded externally by the cortex, medially by the internal capsule, and anteriorly and posteriorly by the insula. **relief s.,** the space between the slightly elevated lingual bar type of major connector and the underlying soft tissue that allows for a minor degree of settling of a removable partial denture, without impinging on the structure over which the bar passes. **retrobulbar s.,** the space lying behind the fascia of the bulb of the eye, containing the eye muscles and the ocular vessels and nerves. **retrocardiac s.,** Holzknecht's s. **retroinguinal s.,** Bogros' s. **retromylohyoid s.,** the part of the alveolingual sulcus just lingual to the retromolar pad, bounded anteriorly by the lingual tuberosity, posteriorly by the retromylohyoid curtain, inferiorly by the floor of the alveolingual sulcus, and lingually by the anterior tonsillar pillar. **retro-ocular s.,** retrobulbar s. **retroperitoneal s.,** spatium retroperitoneale. **retropharyngeal s.,** the space behind the pharynx, containing areolar tissue. **retropubic s., Retzius s.,** spatium retropubicum. **Robin's s's,** minute lymph spaces in the external coat of an artery communicating with lymphatic vessels. **Schwalbe's s's,** spatia intervaginalia nervi optici. **semilunar s.,** see *Traube's semilunar s.* **septal s.,** that portion of the interproximal space gingival to the contact area of adjacent teeth in a dental arch. **subarachnoid s.,** cavitas subarachnoidealis. **subchorial s.,** see under *lake*. **subdural s.,** spatium subdurale. **subepicranial s.,** the potential space between the epicranius muscle and the pericranium; it is traversed by small arteries which supply the pericranium and by the emissary veins connecting the intracranial venous sinuses with the superficial veins of the scalp. **subgingival s.,** gingival crevice. **submaxillary s.,** trigonum submandibulare. **subphrenic s.,** the space between the diaphragm and subjacent organs. **subumbilical s.,** the somewhat triangular space within the body cavity just below the umbilicus. **suprasternal s.,** fossa jugularis, def. 1. **Tarin's s.,** recessus anterior fossae interpeduncularis [Tarini]. **Ten-**

on's s., spatium episclerale. **thenar s.,** the palmar space lying between the middle metacarpal bone and the tendon of the flexor pollicis longus. **thiocyanate s.,** a quantitative expression of the space occupied by the extracellular fluid in the body, computed after intravenous injection of sodium thiocyanate. **thyrohyal s.,** the depressed space between the thyroid cartilage and hyoid bone in front. **Traube's semilunar s.,** an area on the left side and front of the lower part of the chest, over which the air in the stomach produces a vesiculotympanitic sound. **Tröltsch's s's,** see *recessus membranae tympani anterior* and *recessus membranae tympani posterior.* **urogenital s.,** rima pudendi **Virchow-Robin s's,** potential spaces surrounding blood vessels for a short distance as they enter the brain, the inner wall being formed by a prolongation of a membrane like the arachnoid, and the outer wall by a continuation of the pia; the intervening channel communicates with the subarachnoid space. **Westberg's s.,** the space between the pericardium and the beginning of the aorta. **yolk s.,** the space formed by retraction of the vitellus of the ovum from the zona pellucida. **Zang's s.,** fossa supraclavicularis minor. **zonular s's,** spatia zonularia.

spadic (spa′dik) the native name in western South America for the leaves of the coca plant, used for chewing.

spagyric (spah-jir′ik) iatrochemical.

Spallanzani's law (spal″an-zan′ēz) [Lazaro *Spallanzani*, eminent Italian anatomist, 1729–1799] see under *law.*

spallation (spawl-la′shun) splintering; the process of breaking into small bits; see *spallation products,* under *product.*

span (span) 1. a measurement of reach or extent. 2. the distance in a fully extended hand between the tips of the thumb and little finger. 3. the distance between the tips of the fingers when the arms are extended.

Spaniopsis (span″ĭ-op′sis) a genus of blood-sucking flies of the family Rhagionidae found in Australia.

Spanish windlass (span′ish wind′las) see *windlass.*

span(o)- [Gr. *spanos* scarce] a combining form meaning scanty or scarce.

spar (spar) a nonmetallic, rather lustrous mineral. **Iceland s.,** a crystalline form of calcium carbonate, usually found in Iceland, and used in making Nicol prisms.

sparganosis (spar″gah-no′sis) infection with the migrating larvae (spargana) of any of several species of pseudophyllidean tapeworms, which invade the subcutaneous tissues, causing inflammation and fibrosis suggestive of cellulitis.

sparganum (spar-ga′num), pl. *sparga′na* [Gr. *sparganon* swaddling clothes] the larval stage (plerocercoid) of various pseudophyllidean cestodes, especially of the genera *Diphyllobothrium* and *Spirometra,* which may migrate in the subcutaneous tissues of man and other animals (see *sparganosis*). Also, a genus name applied to such larvae, usually when the adult stage is not known.

Sparine (spar′ēn) trademark for preparations of promazine hydrochloride.

spark (spark) a flash of light attended with a crackling sound, made by a discharge of electricity. **direct s.,** an electric spark which passes through the body from electrodes without the use of a Leyden jar.

sparteine (spar′te-in) [L. *spartium* broom] chemical name: dodecahydro-7,14-methano-$2H,6H$-dipyrido[1,2-*a*:1′,2′-*e*][1,5]-diazocine. An alkaloid $C_{15}H_{26}N_2$, obtained from the legumes *Cystisus scoparius* (L.) Link. (broom), *Lupinus luteus* L. (yellow lupin bean), *L. niger* Hort. (black lupin bean), and *Anagyris foetida* L. (Mediterranean stinkbush). It is poisonous, and acts like digitalis. **s. sulfate,** the pentahydrate sulfate salt of sparteine, $C_{15}H_{26}N_2 \cdot H_2SO_4 \cdot 5H_2$, used as an oxytocic for the induction of labor and stimulation of hypotonic or subnormal uterine contractions. Formerly used as a substitute for digitalis.

spartium (spar′she-um) [Gr. *sparton*] scoparius.

spasm (spazm) [L. *spasmus;* Gr. *spasmos*] 1. a sudden, violent, involuntary contraction of a muscle or a group of muscles, attended with pain and interference with function, producing involuntary movement and distortion. 2. a sudden but transitory constriction of a passage, canal, or orifice. **s. of accommodation,** spasm of the ciliary muscles, producing excess of accommodation for near objects. **athetoid s.,** a spasm in which the affected member makes movements like those of athetosis. **Bell's s.,** convulsive tic. **bronchial s.,** spasmodic contraction of the muscular coat of the bronchial tubes, such as occurs in asthma. **cadaveric s.,** rigor mortis causing movements of the limbs. **canine s.,** risus sardonicus. **carpopedal s.,** spasm of the hand or foot, or of the thumbs and great toes, seen in tetany. **cerebral s.,** spasm due to a cerebral lesion. **clonic s.,** a spasm in which rigidity of the muscles is followed immediately by relaxation. **cynic s.,** risus sardonicus. **dancing s.,** saltatory s. **diffuse esophageal s.,** strong, incoordinated, nonpropulsive contractions of the esophagus evoked by deglutition, especially in the elderly; on barium radiography, the esophageal lumen appears as an irregular series of concentric narrowings, or a spiral coil (curling). Called also *esophageal dysrhythmia.* **esophageal s.,** diffuse esophageal s. **facial s.,** tonic spasm of the muscles supplied by the facial nerve, either involving the entire side of the face or confined to a limited region around the eye. **fixed s.,** permanent rigidity of a muscle or set of muscles. **glottic s.,** laryngospasm. **habit s.,** tic. **histrionic s.,** convulsion of the facial muscles analogous to writers' cramp. **infantile massive s's,** jackknife seizure. **inspiratory s.,** spasmodic contraction of the muscles of inspiration. **intention s.,** muscular spasm occurring on attempting voluntary movement. **lock s.,** a firm tonic spasm that seems to lock the fingers together, as in writers' cramp and in similar affections. **malleatory s.,** malleation. **massive s.,** a seizure characterized by contraction of most of the body musculature. **mixed s.,** a spasm in which there are both extensor and flexor movements. **mobile s.,** athetosis. **myopathic s.,** that which accompanies a disease of the muscles. **nictitating s.,** winking s. **nodding s.,** clonic spasm of the sternomastoid muscles, producing bowing motions; called also *salaam convulsions.* **perineal s.,** perineal vaginismus. **phonatory s.,** spasm of the tensors of the vocal bands. **progressive torsion s.,** dystonia musculorum deformans. **respiratory s.,** spasm of the muscles of respiration. **retrocollic s.,** spasmodic retroflexion of the head. **Romberg's s.,** masticatory spasm of the muscles supplied by the fifth nerve. **rotatory s.,** intermittent spasm of the splenius muscle causing rotation of the head. **salaam s.,** nodding s. **saltatory s.,** clonic spasm of the muscles of the legs, producing a peculiar jumping or springing motion whenever the patient stands. Called also *Bamberger's disease, palmus,* and *saltatory tic.* **synclonic s.,** clonic spasm of more than one muscle. **tetanic s., tonic s.,** tetanus, def. 2. **tonoclonic s.,** a convulsive twitching of the muscles. **torsion s.,** spasm marked by a twisting or turning of the body, especially of the pelvis, as in dystonia musculorum deformans. **toxic s.,** that which is due to a poison. **winking s.,** spasmodic twitching of the orbicularis palpebrarum muscle and of the eyelid. **writers' s.,** writers' cramp.

spasm(o)- [Gr. *spasmos* spasm] a combining form denoting relationship to a spasm.

spasmodic (spaz-mod′ik) [Gr. *spasmōdēs*] of the nature of a spasm.

spasmogen (spaz′mo-jen) [*spasmo-* + Gr. *gennan* to produce] a substance that produces or causes spasms.

spasmogenic (spaz″mo-jen′ik) relating to the production of or causing spasms.

spasmology (spaz-mol′o-je) [*spasmo-* + *-logy*] the sum of what is known regarding spasms.

spasmolygmus (spaz″mo-lig′mus) [*spasmo-* + Gr. *lygmos* hiccup] hiccup.

spasmolysant (spaz-mol′ĭ-zant) 1. relieving or relaxing spasms. 2. an agent that relieves spasm.

spasmolysis (spaz-mol′ĭ-sis) the elimination or checking of spasm.

spasmolytic (spaz″mo-lit′ik) checking spasms; antispasmodic.

spasmophile (spaz′mo-fīl) spasmophilic.

spasmophilia (spaz″mo-fil′e-ah) [*spasmo-* + Gr. *philein* to love] spasmophilic diathesis; a condition in which the motor nerves show abnormal sensitiveness to mechanical or electric stimulation, and the patient shows a tendency to spasm, tetany, and convulsions.

spasmophilic (spaz″mo-fil′ik) marked by a tendency to spasms.

spasmotin (spaz′mo-tin) a poisonous ecbolic and acid principle, $C_{20}H_{21}O_9$, from ergot, which has oxytocic but not hallucinogenic properties.

spasmus (spaz′mus) [L.] spasm. **s. nu′tans,** nodding spasm.

spastic (spas′tik) [Gr. *spastikos*] 1. of the nature of or characterized by spasms. 2. hypertonic, so that the muscles are stiff and the movements awkward; see *cerebral palsy,* under *palsy.* 3. a person exhibiting spasticity, such as occurs in spastic paralysis or in cerebral palsy.

spasticity (spas-tis′ĭ-te) a state of hypertonicity, or increase over the normal tone of a muscle, with heightened deep tendon reflexes. **clasp-knife s.,** the phenomenon occurring when a hypertonic muscle is passively stretched: after initial increased resistance there is a sudden relaxation.

spatia (spa′she-ah) [L.] plural of *spatium.*

spatial (spa′shal) pertaining to space.

spatium (spa′she-um), pl. *spa′tia* [L.] a space or delimited area; [NA] a general term for an actual or potential open region. **spa′tia an′guli i′ridis** [Fonta′nae], **spa′tia an′guli iridocornea′lis** [NA], spaces of the iridocorneal angle: the spaces between the fibers of the pectinate ligament through which communication is effected between the anterior chamber and the canal of Schlemm. See also *Fontana's spaces,* under *space.* **s. episclera′le** [NA], episcleral space: the space between the bulbar fascia and the eyeball; called also *s. intervaginale, s. interfasciale* [Tenoni], *intervaginal space,* and *Tenon's space.* **s. extraperitonea′le** [NA], extraperitoneal space: the thin space between the abdominal walls and the transverse fascia occupied by the extraperitoneal fascia. **s. intercosta′le** [NA], intercostal space: the space intervening between two adjacent ribs. **spa′tia intercosta′lia,** see *spatium intercostale.* **s. interfascia′le** [Teno′ni], s. episclerale. **spa′tia interglobula′ria** [NA], interglobular spaces: numerous small irregular spaces on the outer surface of the dentin in the root of a tooth. Called also *Czermak's spaces, globular spaces of Czermak,* and *interglobular spaces (of Owen).* **spa′tia interos′sea metacar′pi** [NA], interosseous spaces of the metacarpus: the four spaces between the metacarpal bones. **spa′tia interos′sea metatar′si** [NA], interosseous spaces of metatarsus: the four spaces between the metatarsal bones. **s. intervagina′le,** former NA term for s. episclerale. **spa′tia intervagina′lia ner′vi op′tici** [NA], intervaginal spaces of optic nerve: the subdural and subarachnoid spaces between the internal and external sheaths of the optic nerve; called also *Schwalbe's spaces.* **s. perichorioidea′le, s. perichoroidea′le** [NA], perichoroidal space: any of the spaces between the laminae of the nonvascular layer of the choroid nearest the sclera. **s. perilymphat′icum** [NA], perilymphatic space: the fluid-filled space separating the membranous from the osseous labyrinth; called also *Retzius space.* **s. perine′i profun′dum** [NA], deep perineal space: the region superior (deep) to the perineal membrane; called also *deep perineal pouch.* **s. perine′i superficia′le** [NA], superficial perineal space: the region between the perineal membrane and the superficial perineal fascia; called also *superficial perineal pouch.* **s. retroperitonea′le** [NA], extraperitoneal space: the space between the posterior parietal peritoneum and the posterior abdominal wall, containing the kidneys, suprarenal glands, ureters, duodenum, ascending and descending colon, pancreas, and the large vessels and nerves. **s. retropu′bicum** [NA], retropubic space: the extraperitoneal space between the inferior aspect of the apex of the bladder, and the transversalis fascia and the posterosuperior aspect of the pubic symphysis, extending along the sides of the bladder to the lateral ligaments and limited below by the puboprostatic ligaments. **spa′tia zonula′ria** [NA], zonular spaces: the lymph-filled interstices between the fibers of the zonula ciliaris, communicating with the posterior chamber of the eye; called also *Petit's canal.* **s. subdura′le** [NA], subdural space: a narrow fluid-containing space, often only a potential space, between the dura mater and the arachnoid; called also *cavum subdurale* and *subdural cavity.*

spatula (spach′u-lah) [L.] a flat, blunt, usually flexible instrument, used for spreading plasters and for mixing ointments and masses; a spatulate structure. **s. mal′lei,** the flat end of the handle of the malleus, attached to the membrana tympani.

spatular (spach′u-lar) spatulate.

spatulate (spach′ŭ-lāt) 1. having a flat blunt end. 2. to mix or manipulate with a spatula.

spatulation (spach″u-la′shun) the mixing of combined materials to a homogeneous mass by repeatedly scraping them up and smoothing out the mass on a flat surface with a spatula.

spavin (spav′in) in general, an exostosis, usually medial, of the tarsus of equines, distal to the tibiotarsal articulation and often involving the metatarsals. **blood s.,** a dilatation of either or both of the medial metatarsal or of the saphenous veins, forming a soft enlargement on the dorsomedial surface of the tarsus in equines. **bog s.,** a distention of the synovial capsule of the tibiotarsal joint in equines. **bone s.,** osteoperiostitis or arthritis of the intertarsal or tarsometatarsal articulations in equines, commonly followed by exostosis and ankylosis. Classified as visible, occult, anterior, posterior and high. **Jack s.,** a very large exostotic spavin.

spavined (spav′ind) affected with spavin.

spay (spa) to castrate a female animal, usually by oophorohysterectomy.

SPCA serum prothrombin conversion accelerator (blood coagulation factor VII).

Spearman's rank correlation coefficient (rho) (spēr-manz) [Charles Edward *Spearman*, British psychologist, 1863–1945] see under *coefficient.*

spearmint (spēr′mint) [NF] the dried leaf and flowering top of *Mentha spicata* L. (Labiatae) (*M. viridis* L.), common spearmint, or of *Mentha caridiaca* L., Scotch spearmint; used as a flavoring agent.

specialism (spesh′al-izm) limitation of practice or study to a particular branch of medicine or surgery.

specialist (spesh′al-ist) a physician whose practice is limited to a particular branch of medicine or surgery, especially one who, by virtue of advanced training, is certified by a specialty board as being qualified to so limit his practice. **clinical nurse s., nurse s.,** see under *nurse.*

specialization (spesh″al-i-za′shun) in medicine, medical practice limited to some special department of medicine or surgery.

specialty (spesh′al-te) the field of practice of a specialist.

speciation (spe″se-a′shun) the evolutionary formation of new species, or the process of such formation.

species (spe′shēz, spe′sēz) [L.] 1. a taxonomic category subordinate to a genus (or subgenus), and superior to a subspecies or variety, composed of individuals possessing common characters distinguishing them from other categories of individuals of the same taxonomic level. In taxonomic nomenclature, species are designated by the genus name followed by a Latin or latinized adjective or noun. 2. (*obs.*) a mixture of dried herbs, seeds, or barks, used chiefly as a decoction. **diovulatory s.,** a species of animal, the females of which ordinarily discharge two ova in one ovulatory cycle. **fugative s.,** a species of plant or animal that inhabits or grows in a region for only a short period of time. **monovulatory s.,** a species of animal, the females of which usually discharge only one ovum in any one ovulatory cycle. **polyovulatory s.,** a species of animal, the females of which normally discharge several (3–16) ova at each ovulatory cycle. **type s.,** in bacteriology, the species that characterizes a genus, usually the first species validly described in the genus, but it may be one arbitrarily designated as such for classification purposes.

species-specific (spe′sēz-spĕ-sif′ik) characteristic of a particular species; having a characteristic effect on, or interaction with, cells or tissues of members of a particular species; said of an antigen, drug, or infective agent.

specific (spĕ-sif′ik) [L. *specificus*] 1. pertaining to a species. 2. produced by a single kind of microorganism. 3. restricted in application, effect, etc., to a particular structure, function, etc. 4. a remedy specially indicated for any particular disease. 5. in immunology, pertaining to the special affinity of antigen for the corresponding antibody.

specificity (spes″ĭ-fis′ĭ-te) 1. the quality or state of being specific. 2. diagnostic specificity; the conditional probability that a person not having a disease will be correctly identified by a clinical test, i.e., the number of true negative results divided by the number of true negative and false positive results. Cf. *sensitivity* and *predictive value.* **neuronal s.,** the invariance of the locations, trajectories, and spatial arrangement of neurons in all members of the same species. **organ s.,** the state of being organ-specific. **species s.,** the state of being species-specific.

specificness (spe-sif′ik-nes) specificity.

specimen (spes′ĭ-men) 1. a sample or part of a thing, or of several things, taken to show or to determine the character of the whole, as a specimen of urine. 2. a preparation of tissue for pathological examination or of a normal tissue, organ, or organism for study of its structure. **corrosion s.,** a preparation of an organ, such as the liver, by injection of certain of its structures, as the arteries and veins, and chemical digestion of surrounding substance.

spectacles (spek′tah-k'lz) [L. *spectacula; spectare* to see] a pair of lenses in a frame to assist vision; see also *glasses* and *lens.* **compound s.,** spectacles fitted with extra colored glasses, or extra lenses, to be used as occasion requires. **decentered s.,** spectacles with lenses formed from eccentric portions of two convex lenses. **divided s.,** bifocal glasses. **industrial s.,** protective s. **Masselon's s.,** spectacles with an attachment for keeping the upper lid raised in cases of paralytic ptosis. **mica s.,** spectacles of sheet mica used to protect the eye from foreign bodies. **pantoscopic s.,** bifocal glasses. **periscopic s.,** spectacles with either menisci or concavoconvex lenses, with the concave surfaces toward the eyes; they allow the eyes considerable latitude of motion. **prismatic s.,** spectacles with prismatic lenses for correcting muscular defects. **protective s.,** spectacles designed to protect the eyes rather than to correct defective vision; the spectacles may have side shields, plastic or hardened lenses, or lenses that protect against ultraviolet or infrared rays. **pulpit s.,** spectacles containing the lenses in the lower segments of the glasses only. **safety s.,** protective s. **stenopeic s.,** spectacles fitted with metal plates, having each a small central aperture. **tinted s.,** spectacles of a glass so colored as to protect the eyes from the effects of too bright light. **wire frame s.,** a kind of spectacles of wire gauze worn to protect the eye from the entrance of foreign bodies.

spectinomycin (spek″tĭ-no-mi′sin) chemical name: decahydro -4α,7,9- trihydroxy -2- methyl -6,8- bis(methylamino)- 4 *H*-pyrano[2,3-*b*][1,4]-benzodioxin-4-one. An antibiotic, $C_{14}H_{24}N_2O_7$, derived from *Streptomyces spectabilis,* that has moderate antibacterial activity against many gram-positive and gram-negative organisms, but is especially effective against *Neisseria gonorrhoeae.* It is also used in veterinary medicine in bacterial enteritis and coccidiosis of dogs. **s. hydrochloride,** the pentahydrate dehydrochloride salt of spectinomycin, $C_{14}H_{24}N_2O_7 \cdot 2HCl \cdot 5H_2O$, having the same actions as the base. A preparation suitable for intramuscular administration [USP] is used in the treatment of acute gonorrheal urethritis and proctitis in the male and acute gonorrheal cervicitis and proctitis in the female when due to susceptible strains of *Neisseria gonorrhoeae.*

spectra (spek′trah) plural of *spectrum.*

spectral (spek′tral) pertaining to a spectrum; performed by means of a spectrum.

spectrin (spek′trin) a contractile protein attached to glycophorin at the cytoplasmic surface of the cell membrane of erythrocytes, considered to be important in the determination of red-cell shape.

spectrochrome (spek′tro-krōm) [L. *spectrum* + Gr. *chrōma* color] a term applied to a method of treatment consisting of exposure of the part to be treated to light of various colors.

spectrocolorimeter (spek″tro-kul″or-im′ĕ-ter) [*spectrum* + *colorimeter*] an ophthalmospectroscope using a source of light from a selected wavelength of the spectrum to detect color blindness for one or more color.

spectrofluorometer (spek″tro-floo″or-om′ĕ-ter) an optical instrument for analysis of fluorescence spectra.

spectrograph (spek′tro-graf) an instrument for photographing spectra on a sensitive photographic plate. **mass s.,** mass spectrometer.

spectrometer (spek-trom′ĕ-ter) [*spectrum* + *-meter*] 1. an instrument for measuring the index of refraction by measuring the external angle of a prism of the substance. 2. a spectroscope for measuring the wavelengths of rays of a spectrum. **mass s.,** an analytical instrument which identifies a substance by sorting a stream of electrified particles (ions) according to their mass; the sorting is most commonly done as follows: when the stream of charged particles enters a magnetic field, it is deflected into a semicircular path, ultimately striking a photographic plate or photomultiplier tube sensor. Called also *mass spectrograph*. **Mossbauer s.,** an instrument that detects small changes in interaction between an atomic nucleus and its environment caused by changes in temperature, pressure, and chemical state; used in chemical-physical research with applications in medicine.

spectrometry (spek-trom′ĕ-tre) the determination of the places of the lines in a spectrum.

spectrophotofluorometer (spek″tro-fo″to-floo″or-om′ĕ-ter) an analytical instrument combining the techniques of spectrophotometry and fluorescence analysis.

spectrophotometer (spek″tro-fo-tom′ĕ-ter) [*spectrum* + *photometer*] an apparatus for estimating the quantity of coloring matter in solution by the quantity of light absorbed (as indicated by the spectrum) in passing through the solution. **absorption s.,** an analytical instrument for comparing the absorption of radiation of a given wavelength against a standard to identify a sample material.

spectrophotometry (spek″tro-fo-tom′ĕ-tre) the use of the spectrophotometer.

spectropolarimeter (spek″tro-po″lar-im′ĕ-ter) a combined spectroscope and polariscope for determining optical rotation.

spectropyrheliometer (spek″tro-pir-he″le-om′ĕ-ter) [*spectrum* + Gr. *pyr* fire + *hēlios* sun + *metrum* measure] an instrument for measuring the radiation from the sun.

spectroscope (spek′tro-skōp) [*spectrum* + Gr. *skopein* to examine] an instrument for developing and analyzing spectra.

spectroscopic (spek″tro-skop′ik) of, pertaining to, or performed by, the spectroscope.

spectroscopy (spek-tros′ko-pe) the propagation and analysis of spectra; examination by means of a spectroscope.

spectrum (spek′trum), pl. *spec′tra* [L. "image"] a charted band of wavelengths of electromagnetic vibrations obtained by refraction and diffraction. See *invisible s.* and *visible s.* By extension, a measurable range of activity, such as the range of bacteria affected by an antibiotic (antibacterial s.) or the complete range of manifestations of a disease. **absorption s.,** the spectrum afforded by light which has passed through various gaseous media, each gas absorbing those rays of which its own spectrum is composed. **action s.,** the range of wavelength of incident light producing a response in the material under study (e.g., the inactivation of an enzyme); also, a graph plotting the magnitude of the response as a function of the wavelength of the incident light. **broad-s.,** effective against a wide range of microorganisms; said of an antibiotic. **chemical s.,** that part of the spectrum which includes the ultraviolet or actinic rays. **chro-**

matic s., that portion of the range of wavelengths of electromagnetic vibrations (from 7700 to 3900 A.U.) which gives rise to the sensation of color (red to violet) to the normally perceptive eye; coincident with the visible spectrum. **color s.,** chromatic s. **continuous s.,** one in which Fraunhofer's lines are not developed. **continuous x-ray s.,** bremsstrahlung, def. 1. **diffraction s.,** a spectrum formed by the passage of light through a diffraction grating. **electromagnetic s.,** the continuous range of electromagnetic energy from cosmic rays to electric waves, including gamma, x-, and ultraviolet rays, visible light, infrared waves, and radio waves. **fortification s.,** teichopsia. **gaseous s.,** one which is afforded by an incandescent gas. **invisible s.,** that made up of vibrations of wavelengths less than 3900 A.U. (ultraviolet, grenz rays, x-rays, and gamma rays) and between 7700 and 120,000 A.U. (infrared). **ocular s.,** after-image. **prismatic s.,** one produced by the passage of light through a prism. **solar s.,** that portion of the range of wavelengths of electromagnetic vibrations emanating from the sun, including the visible (chromatic, or color) spectrum and small portions of the infrared and ultraviolet radiations at either extreme. **thermal s.,** that portion of the range of wavelengths of electromagnetic vibrations (> 7700 A.U.) containing the infrared or heat rays. **visible s.,** that portion of the range of wavelengths of electromagnetic vibrations (from 7700 to 3900 A.U.) which is capable of stimulating specialized sense organs and is perceptible as light. **x-ray s.,** the spectrum of a heterogeneous beam of roentgen rays produced by a suitable grating, generally a crystal.

speculum (spek′u-lum), pl. *spec′ula* [L. "mirror"] 1. an instrument that exposes the interior of a passage or cavity of the body by enlarging the opening. 2. the septum pellucidum. **Bozeman's s.,** a bivalve speculum the blades of which remain parallel when separated. **Brinkerhoff's s.,** a rectal speculum consisting of a conical tube having a closed extremity, but provided with a sliding bar on the side which provides an opening. **Cook's s.,** a three-pronged rectal speculum. **duck-billed s.,** a form of two-valved vaginal speculum. **eye s.,** an appliance for keeping the eyelids apart. **Fergusson's s.,** a cylindrical vaginal speculum made of silvered glass. **Fränkel's s.,** a form of nasal speculum. **Gruber's s.,** a form of ear speculum. **Hartmann's s.,** a form of nasal speculum. **s. Helmon′tii,** centrum tendineum. **Kelly's s.,** a rectal speculum tubular in shape and fitted with an obturator; called also *Kelly's sphincteroscope*. **Martin's s.,** Martin and Davy s., a rectal speculum consisting of a conical cylinder with an obturator. **Mathews' s.,** a four-pronged rectal speculum. **Politzer's s.,** a form of ear speculum. **Sims' s.,** a double duck-billed vaginal speculum. **stop s.,**

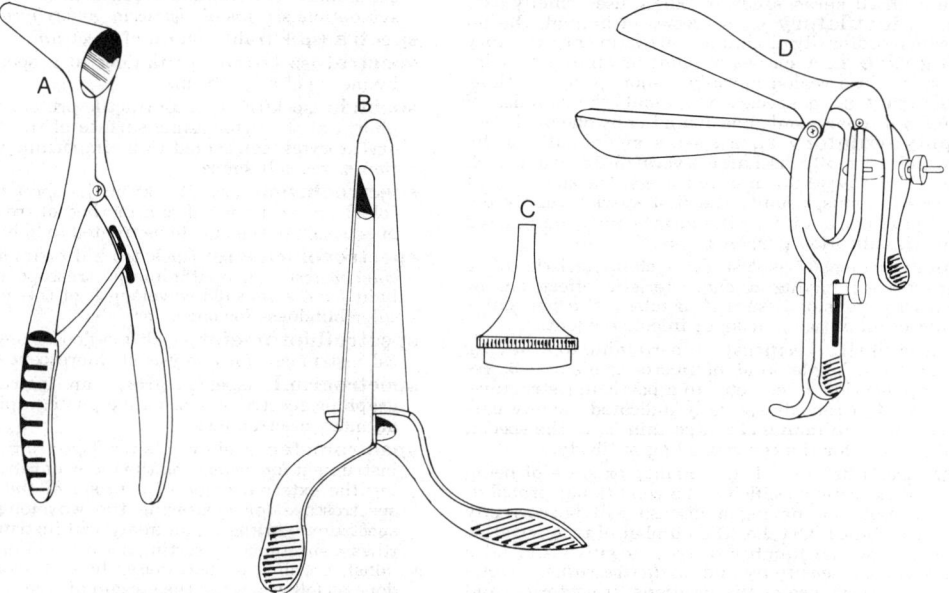

Specula: *A,* Vienna nasal speculum; *B,* Brinckerhoff rectal speculum; *C,* speculum for otoscope; *D,* Graves vaginal speculum.

an eye speculum with an appliance for controlling the degree to which its branches spread. **wire bivalve s.,** a two-valved vaginal speculum made of heavy wire.

Spee's curve (curvature) (spāz) [Ferdinand Graf von *Spee*, German embryologist, 1855–1937] see under *curve.*

speech (spēch)   the utterance of vocal sounds conveying ideas. **alaryngeal s.,** esophageal s. **clipped s.,** speech in which the words are slurred over and uncompleted; sometimes one of the features of dementia paralytica. **echo s.,** echolalia. **esophageal s.,** a method of speech used after laryngectomy, with sound produced by vibration of the column of air in the esophagus against the contracting cricopharyngeal sphincter. **explosive s.,** loud, sudden enunciation, seen in certain brain diseases. **incoherent s.,** speech in which the consecutive ideas expressed are not related; due to disturbance of the train of thought. **jumbled s.,** anarthria. **mirror s.,** a speech abnormality in which the order of syllables in a sentence is reversed. **plateau s.,** speech which is characterized by a level, monotonous, unvaried pitch. **pressured s.,** a rapid, accelerated, frenzied speech, which may exceed the ability of the vocal musculature to articulate or may be incoherent to the listener. **scamping s.,** clipped s. **scanning s.,** speech in which the syllables are separated by pauses. **slurred s.,** clipped s. **staccato s.,** speech in which each syllable is uttered separately; seen in multiple sclerosis.

Spemann (shpa′mahn)   Hans. German zoologist, 1869–1941; winner of the Nobel prize for medicine or physiology in 1935 for investigating the organizer effect in embryonic development.

Spemann's induction (shpa′mahnz) [Hans *Spemann*] see under *induction.*

Spencer Wells facies   see *Wells.*

Spengler's fragments (speng′lerz) [Carl *Spengler,* Swiss physician, 1860–1937] see under *fragment.*

Spens' syndrome (spenz) [Thomas *Spens,* Scottish physician, 1764–1842]   Adams-Stokes disease.

sperm (sperm) [Gr. *sperma* seed]   1. the semen or testicular secretion.   2. one of the mature germ cells of a male animal; see *spermatozoon.* **muzzled s.,** spermatozoa which are unable to adhere to the ovum.

sperma (sper′mah)   semen.

spermaceti (sper″mah-set′e) [Gr. *sperma* seed + *kētos* whale] a waxy substance obtained from the head of the sperm whale, *Physeter macrocephalus,* occurring as white, somewhat translucent, slightly unctuous masses, having a crystalline fracture and a pearly luster; used in the preparation of ointment bases, such as cold cream and rose water ointment. **synthetic s.,** cetyl esters wax.

spermacrasia (sper″mah-kra′zhe-ah) [Gr. *sperma* seed + *akrasia* ill mixture]   deficiency of spermatozoa in the semen.

spermagglutination (sperm″ah-gloo″tĭ-na′shun)   the agglutination of spermatozoa.

spermalist (sper′mah-list)   animalculist.

spermateliosis (sper″mah-te″le-o′sis)   spermiogenesis.

spermatemphraxis (sper″mat-em-frak′sis) [Gr. *sperma* seed + *emphraxis* stoppage]   obstruction to the discharge of semen.

spermatic (sper-mat′ik) [L. *spermaticus;* Gr. *spermatikos*] pertaining to the semen; seminal.

spermaticide (sper-mat′ĭ-sīd)   spermicide.

spermatid (sper′mah-tid)   a cell derived from a secondary spermatocyte by fission, and developing into a spermatozoon; called also *spermatoblast.*

spermatin (sper′mah-tin)   an albuminoid substance derived from the semen; it is related to mucin and to nucleoalbumin.

spermatism (sper′mah-tizm) [Gr. *spermatismos*]   the production or discharge of semen.

spermatitis (sper″mah-ti′tis)   inflammation of a vas deferens; deferentitis or funiculitis.

spermat(o)-, sperm(o)- [Gr. *sperma,* gen. *spermatos* seed] combining forms denoting relationship to seed, specifically to the male generative element.

spermatoblast (sper′mah-to-blast″) [*spermato-* + Gr. *blastos* germ]   a term originally applied to the supporting cells of Sertoli, but now used with the same meaning as *spermatid.*

spermatocele (sper′mah-to-sēl″) [*spermato-* + Gr. *kēlē* tu-

mor]   a cystic distention of the epididymis or the rete testis containing spermatozoa.

spermatocelectomy (sper-mat″o-se-lek′to-me) [*spermatocele* + Gr. *ektomē* excision]   excision of a spermatocele.

spermatocidal (sper″mah-to-si′dal)   spermicidal.

spermatocyst (sper′mah-to-sist″) [*spermato-* + Gr. *kystis* sac, bladder]   1. a seminal vesicle.   2. a spermatocele.

spermatocystectomy (sper″mah-to-sis-tek′to-me) [*spermatocyst* + Gr. *ektomē* excision]   excision of the seminal vesicles.

spermatocystitis (sper″mah-to-sis-ti′tis)   seminal vesiculitis.

spermatocystotomy (sper″mah-to-sis-tot′o-me) [*spermatocyst* + Gr. *tomē* a cutting]   incision of the seminal vesicles.

spermatocytal (sper″mah-to-si′tal)   pertaining to a spermatocyte.

spermatocyte (sper′mah-to-sīt″) [*spermato-* + *-cyte*]   the parent cell of a spermatid. **primary s.,** a cell derived from a spermatogonium and dividing into two secondary spermatocytes; called also *spermiocyte.* **secondary s.,** one of the two cells into which a primary spermatocyte divides, and which in turn gives origin to spermatids; called also *prespermatid.*

spermatocytogenesis (sper″mah-to-si″to-jen′ĕ-sis)   the first stage of formation of spermatozoa in which the spermatogonia develop into spermatocytes and then into spermatids.

spermatocytoma (sper″mah-to-si-to′mah)   seminoma.

spermatogenesis (sper″mah-to-jen′ĕ-sis) [*spermato-* + Gr. *genesis* production]   the process of formation of spermatozoa, including spermatocytogenesis and spermiogenesis.

spermatogenic (sper″mah-to-jen′ik) [*spermato-* + Gr. *gennan* to produce]   producing semen or spermatozoa.

spermatogenous (sper″mah-toj′ĕ-nus)   spermatogenic.

spermatogeny (sper″mah-toj′ĕ-ne)   spermatogenesis.

spermatogone (sper′mah-to-gōn″)   spermatogonium.

spermatogonia (sper″mah-to-go′ne-ah)   plural of *spermatogonium.*

spermatogonium (sper″mah-to-go′ne-um), pl. *spermatogo′nia* [*spermato-* + Gr. *gonē* generation]   an undifferentiated germ cell of a male, originating in a seminiferous tubule and dividing into two primary spermatocytes; called also *spermatophore, spermatospore,* and *spermospore.*

spermatoid (sper′mah-toid) [*spermato-* + Gr. *eidos* form] resembling semen.

spermatology (sper″mah-tol′o-je) [*spermato-* + *-logy*]   the sum of what is known regarding the semen.

spermatolysin (sper″mah-tol′ĭ-sin)   a specific lysin produced by injecting an animal with spermatozoa; spermatotoxin.

spermatolysis (sper″mah-tol′ĭ-sis) [*spermato-* + Gr. *lysis* dissolution]   destruction or solution of spermatozoa.

spermatolytic (sper″mah-to-lit′ik)   pertaining to, characterized by, or causing spermatolysis.

spermatomere (sper′mah-to-mēr″)   spermatomerite.

spermatomerite (sper′mah-to-me′rīt) [*spermato-* + Gr. *meros* part]   one of the chromosomes into which the sperm nucleus resolves during fertilization of the ovum.

spermatomicron (sper″mah-to-mi′kron)   a minute particle found in the semen of various animals; seen best with a dark-field microscope, when they show brownian motion.

spermatopathia (sper″mah-to-path′e-ah) [*spermato-* + Gr. *pathos* affection]   a morbid condition of the semen.

spermatopathy (sper″mah-top′ah-the)   spermatopathia.

spermatophore (sper′mah-to-fōr″) [*spermato-* + Gr. *phorein* to carry]   1. a capsule, containing several spermatozoa, extruded by some of the lower animals.   2. spermatogonium.

spermatopoietic (sper″mah-to-poi-et′ik) [*spermato-* + Gr. *poiētikos* creative, productive]   subserving or promoting the secretion of semen.

spermatorrhea (sper″mah-to-re′ah) [*spermato-* + Gr. *rhoia* flow]   involuntary, too frequent, and excessive discharge of semen without copulation.

spermatoschesis (sper″mah-tos′kĕ-sis) [*spermato-* + Gr. *schesis* check]   suppression of the secretion of semen.

spermatosome (sper-mat′o-sōm)   spermatozoon.

spermatospore (sper-mat′o-spōr) [*spermato-* + Gr. *sporos* spore] a spermatogonium.

spermatotoxin (sper″mah-to-tok′sin) a toxin destructive to spermatozoa; especially a cytotoxic antibody produced by injecting an animal with spermatozoa.

spermatovum (sper″mat-o′vum) [*spermato-* + L. *ovum* egg] a fertilized ovum.

spermatoxin (sper″mah-tok′sin) spermatotoxin.

spermatozoa (sper″mah-to-zo′ah) [Gr.] plural of *spermatozoon*.

spermatozoal (sper″mah-to-zo′al) pertaining to spermatozoa.

spermatozoicide (sper″mah-to-zo′ĭ-sīd) spermicide.

spermatozoid (sper′mah-to-zoid) [*spermatozoon* + Gr. *eidos* form] 1. spermatozoon. 2. the male germ cell in plants.

spermatozoon (sper″mah-to-zo′on), pl. *spermatozo′a* [*spermato-* + Gr. *zōon* animal] a mature male germ cell, the specific output of the testes. It is the generative element of the semen which serves to fertilize the ovum. It consists of a head (or nucleus), a neck, a middle piece, and a tail with an end piece. Spermatozoa, formed in the seminiferous tubules, are derived from spermatogonia, which first develop into spermatocytes, which, in turn, undergo meiosis to produce spermatids; the spermatids then differentiate into spermatozoa.

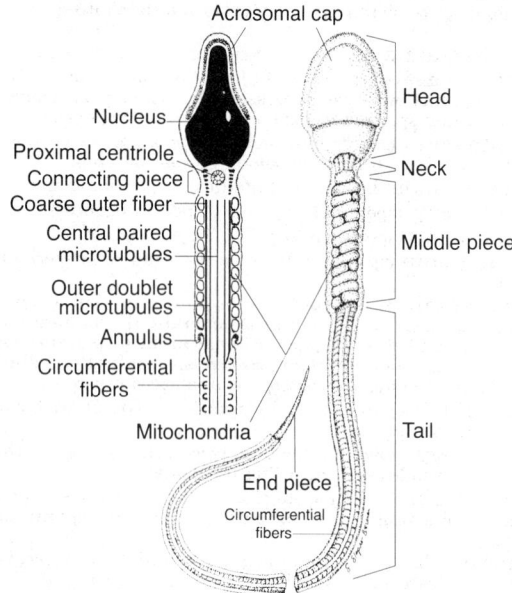

Human spermatozoon: side view (in cross section) and flat view.

spermaturia (sper″mah-tu′re-ah) [*spermato-* + Gr. *ouron* urine + *-ia*] seminuria.

spermectomy (sper-mek′to-me) excision of a portion of the spermatic cord.

spermia (sper′me-ah) [L.] plural of *spermium*.

spermiation (sper″me-a′shun) the freeing of mature spermatozoa from the Sertoli cells.

spermicidal (sper″mĭ-si′dal) [*sperm* + L. *caedere* to kill] destructive to spermatozoa.

spermicide (sper′mĭ-sīd) an agent that is destructive to spermatozoa.

spermid (sper′mid) spermatid.

spermidine (sper′mĭ-din) a polyamine, NH$_2$(CH$_2$)$_3$NH-(CH$_2$)$_4$NH$_2$, first found in human semen but now known to occur in almost all tissues, in association with nucleic acids; it is formed from putrescine and is itself a precursor of spermine.

spermiduct (sper′mĭ-dukt) [*sperm* + L. *ductus* duct] the ejaculatory duct and vas deferens together.

spermine (sper′min) a polyamine, NH$_2$(CH$_2$)$_3$NH(CH$_2$)$_4$-NH(CH$_2$)$_3$NH$_2$, first found in human semen but now known

to occur in almost all tissues in association with nucleic acids, being formed from spermidine. **s. phosphate,** the substance, (C$_2$H$_5$N)$_4$H$_4$Ca(PO$_4$)$_2$, of which the Charcot-Neumann crystals are composed; found also in various organs and secretions in leukemia, asthma, and emphysema.

spermiocyte (sper′me-o-sīt″) [*spermia* + *-cyte*] a primary spermatocyte.

spermiogenesis (sper″me-o-jen′ĕ-sis) the second stage in the formation of spermatozoa in which the spermatids transform into spermatozoa.

spermiogonium (sper″me-o-go′ne-um) spermatogonium.

spermiogram (sper′me-o-gram) a diagram of the various cells formed during the development of the sperm.

spermioteleosis (sper″me-o-te″le-o′sis) [*spermio-* + Gr. *teleiōsis* perfection, completion] the progressive development of the spermatogonium through the successive changes necessary for becoming a mature spermatozoon.

spermioteleotic (sper″me-o-te″le-ot′ik) [*spermio-* + Gr. *teleiōtikos* perfective] pertaining to or characteristic of spermioteleosis.

spermist (sper′mist) animalculist.

spermium (sper′me-um), pl. *sper′mia*. The mature spermatozoon.

sperm(o)- see *spermat(o)-*.

spermoblast (sper′mo-blast) [*spermo-* + Gr. *blastos* germ] a spermatid.

spermocytoma (sper″mo-si-to′mah) seminoma.

spermolith (sper′mo-lith) [*spermo-* + Gr. *lithos* stone] a calculus in the spermiduct.

spermolysin (sper-mol′ĭ-sin) spermatolysin.

spermolysis (sper-mol′ĭ-sis) spermatolysis.

spermolytic (sper″mo-lit′ik) spermatolytic.

spermoneuralgia (sper″mo-nu-ral′je-ah) [*spermo-* + Gr. *neuron* nerve + *-algia*] neuralgic pain in the spermatic cord.

Spermophilus (sper-mof′ĭ-lus) a genus of rodents that harbor organisms transmissible to man. *S. beech′eyi*, the ground squirrel of California, is extensively infected with plague, and, along with *S. mol′lis*, the ground squirrel of Utah, and *S. orego′nus* of Oregon, is a natural reservoir of *Francisella tularensis*.

spermophlebectasia (sper″mo-fle″bek-ta′ze-ah) [*spermo-* + Gr. *phelps* vein + *ektasis* distention + *-ia*] varicosity of the spermatic veins.

spermoplasm (sper′mo-plazm) [*spermo-* + Gr. *plasma* plasm] the protoplasm of the spermatids.

spermosphere (sper′mo-sfēr) [*spermo-* + Gr. *sphaira* sphere] a group or mass of spermatids formed by the segmentation of a secondary spermatocyte.

spermospore (sper′mo-spōr) spermatogonium.

spermotoxic (sper″mo-tok′sik) destructive to spermatozoa.

spermotoxin (sper″mo-tok′sin) spermatotoxin.

Sperry (sper′e) Roger Wolcott. American psychobiologist, born 1913; co-winner, with David Hunter Hubel and Tolsten Nils Wiesel, of the Nobel prize for medicine or physiology in 1981 for his studies of functional specialization of the cerebral hemispheres.

spes (spēs) [L.] hope. **s. phthis′ica** (*obs.*), feeling of hopefulness of recovery frequently characteristic of patients with tuberculosis.

SPF specific-pathogen free, a term applied to animals reared for use in laboratory experiments, and known to be free of specific pathogenic microorganisms.

sp. gr. specific gravity.

sph. spherical or spherical lens.

sphacelate (sfas′ĕ-lāt) to become gangrenous.

sphacelation (sfas″ĕ-la′shun) the formation of a sphacelus; mortification.

sphacelinic acid (sfas‴l-in′ik) a poisonous substance from ergot.

sphacelism (sfas′ĕ-lizm) [Gr. *sphakelismos*] sphacelation or necrosis; sloughing.

sphaceloderma (sfas″ĕ-lo-der′mah) [*sphacelus* + Gr. *derma* skin] gangrene of the skin, or an ulcer resulting from it.

sphacelotoxin (sfas″ĕ-lo-tok′sin) [*sphacelus* + Gr. *toxikon* poison] 1. spasmotin. 2. a poisonous, yellow resin obtainable from ergot.

sphacelous (sfas′ĕ-lus) affected with gangrene; sloughing.

sphacelus (sfas′ĕ-lus) [L.; Gr. *sphakelos*] a slough or mass of gangrenous tissue; mortification.

Sphaenacanthina (sfēn″ah-kan-thi′nah) [Gr. *sphēn* wedge + *akantha* thorn, prickle] a suborder of marine protozoa (order Arthracanthida, class Acantharea), usually characterized by the presence of 20 radial spines joined at the cell center by apposition; the bases of the spines have no lateral wings.

Sphaeranthus (sfe-ran′thus) a genus of herbaceous plants of Asia. *S. indicus* L. furnishes a purported aphrodisiac oil. It is also used in India as an anthelmintic.

Sphaerellarina (sfe″rel-ah-ri′nah) a suborder of marine planktonic protozoa (order Spumellarida, class Polycystinea) occurring as small, solitary cells with a skeleton made up of one latticed piece, consisting of one shell, sometimes two or more concentric ones, more or less complete, with or without radial spines.

Sphaeria (sfe′re-ah) a former genus of fungi, the species of which are now included in various genera. **S. sinen′sis,** *Cordyceps sinensis.*

Sphaeriales (sfe′re-a′lēz) an order of ascomycetes of the series Pyrenomycetes, including the family Sordariaceae.

sphaer(o)- for words beginning thus, see also those beginning *spher(o)-.*

Sphaerocollina (sfe″ro-ko-li′nah) a suborder of marine planktonic protozoa (or Spumellarida, class Polycystinea) occurring as large, solitary cells or cell colonies that have no skeleton or one consisting of one or more isolated spicules or usually of a single, perforated shell.

Sphaeroides maculatus (sfe′roi-dēz mak″u-la′tus) the Atlantic Coast puffer fish that contains a potent toxin concentrated in the gonads and viscera, which when eaten without special cooking preparation causes generalized paralysis and, in severe cases, unconsciousness and death.

Sphaeromyxa (sfēr″o-mik′sah) [*sphero-* + Gr. *myxa* mucus] a genus of parasitic protozoa (suborder Bipolarina, order Bivalvulida) found in marine fish.

Sphaerophorus (sfe-ro′fo-rus) in former systems of classification, a genus of gram-negative anaerobic bacteria the organisms of which have been assigned to *Bacteroides* and *Fusobacterium.* **S. necroph′orus,** *Fusobacterium necrophorum.*

Sphaerotilus (sfe-ro′tĭ-lus) [Gr. *sphaira* sphere + *tilos* anything shredded] a genus of sheathed bacteria found in polluted fresh waters and in sludge, made up of straight rods occurring singly or in chains in a thin sheath and frequently attached to a substrate. The type species is *S. na′tans.*

sphagiasmus (sfa″je-az′mus) [Gr. *sphagiasmos* a slaying, sacrificing] 1. contraction of the neck muscles in an epileptic attack. 2. petit mal; see *epilepsy.*

sphagitides (sfah-jit′ĭ-dēz) [Gr. *sphagitis* jugular; *sphagē* throat] an old name for the so-called jugular vessels.

sphagitis (sfa-ji′tis) [Gr. *sphagē* throat + *-itis*] any throat inflammation.

sphenethmoid (sfen-eth′moid) sphenoethmoid.

sphenion (sfe′ne-on), pl. *sphe′nia* [Gr. *sphēn* wedge + *on* neuter ending] the cranial point at the sphenoid angle of the parietal bone.

sphen(o)- [Gr. *sphēn* wedge] a combining form denoting relationship to the sphenoid bone or to a wedge, or meaning wedge-shaped.

sphenobasilar (sfe′no-bas′ĭ-lar) pertaining to the sphenoid bone and the basilar part of the occipital bone.

sphenoccipital (sfe″nok-sip′ĭ-tal) spheno-occipital.

sphenocephalus (sfe″no-sef′ah-lus) a fetus exhibiting sphenocephaly.

sphenocephaly (sfe″no-sef′ah-le) [*spheno-* + Gr. *kephalē* head] a developmental anomaly characterized by a wedge-shaped appearance of the head.

sphenoethmoid (sfe″no-eth′moid) denoting the curved plate of bone in front of the lesser wing of the sphenoid bone.

sphenofrontal (sfe″no-frun′tal) pertaining to the sphenoid and frontal bones.

sphenoid (sfe′noid) [*spheno-* + Gr. *eidos* form] wedge-shaped; designating especially a very irregular wedge-shaped

bone at the base of the skull (os sphenoidale, or sphenoid bone).

sphenoidal (sfe-noi′dal) pertaining to the sphenoid bone.

sphenoiditis (sfe″noi-di′tis) inflammation of the sphenoidal sinus.

sphenoidostomy (sfe″noi-dos′to-me) [*sphenoid* + Gr. *stomoun* to provide with an opening, or mouth] operative removal of the anterior wall of the sphenoidal sinus.

sphenoidotomy (sfe″noi-dot′o-me) incision into the sphenoidal sinus.

sphenomalar (sfe″no-ma′lar) sphenozygomatic.

sphenomaxillary (sfe″no mak′sĭ ler″e) pertaining to the sphenoid bone and the maxilla.

Sphenomonadina (sfe″no-mo″nah-di′nah) a suborder of colorless, plantlike biflagellate protozoa (order Euglenida, class Phytomastigophora). *Sphenomonas* is a representative genus.

Sphenomonas (sfe″no-mo′nas) [*spheno-* + Gr. *monas* unit] a genus of plantlike biflagellate protozoa (suborder Sphenomonadina, order Euglenida) having one immobile flagellum always directed anteriorly.

spheno-occipital (sfe″no-ok-sip′ĭ-tal) pertaining to the sphenoid and occipital bones.

sphenopagus (sfe″nop′ah-gus) [*spheno-* + Gr. *pagos* a thing fixed] symmetrical twins conjoined at the sphenoid bone at the base of the skull.

sphenopalatine (sfe″no-pal′ah-tin) pertaining to or in relation with the sphenoid and palatine bones.

sphenoparietal (sfe″no-pah-ri′ĕ-tal) pertaining to the sphenoid and parietal bones.

sphenopetrosal (sfe″no-pe-tro′sal) pertaining to the sphenoid bone and the petrosa.

sphenorbital (sfe-nor′bĭ-tal) pertaining to the sphenoid bone and the orbits.

sphenosquamosal (sfe″no-skwa-mo′sal) pertaining to the sphenoid bone and the squamous portion of the temporal bone.

sphenotemporal (sfe″no-tem′po-ral) pertaining to the sphenoid and temporal bones.

sphenotic (sfe-not′ik) [*spheno-* + Gr. *ous* ear] denoting a fetal bone which becomes that part of the sphenoid which is adjacent to the carotid groove.

sphenoturbinal (sfe″no-tur′bĭ-nal) denoting a thin, curved bone in front of each of the lesser wings of the sphenoid, with which bone it becomes fused.

sphenovomerine (sfe″no-vo′mer-in) pertaining to the sphenoid and to the vomer.

sphenozygomatic (sfe″no-zi″go-mat′ik) pertaining to the sphenoid and zygomatic bones.

sphere (sfēr) [Gr. *sphaira* sphere] a ball, globe, or orb. **attraction s.,** centrosome. **embryotic s.,** the morula. **segmentation s.,** 1. the morula. 2. a blastomere. **vitelline s.,** yolk s., the morula.

spheresthesia (sfe″res-the′ze-ah) [Gr. *sphaira* sphere + *aisthēsis* perception + *-ia*] globus hystericus.

spherical (sfer′ĭ-kal) [Gr. *sphairikos*] pertaining to a sphere; sphere-shaped.

spher(o)- [Gr. *sphaira* a ball or globe] a combining form meaning round, or denoting relationship to a sphere.

spherocylinder (sfe″ro-sil′in-der) a combined spherical and cylindrical lens.

spherocyte (sfe′ro-sit) [*sphero-* + Gr. *kytos* cell] a small, globular, completely hemoglobinated erythrocyte without the usual central pallor, found characteristically in hereditary spherocytosis but also observed in acquired hemolytic anemia.

spherocytic (sfe″ro-sit′ik) characterized by the presence of spherocytes.

spherocytosis (sfe″ro-si-to′sis) the presence of spherocytes in the blood. **hereditary s.,** a congenital, familial form of hemolytic anemia characterized by spherocytosis, abnormal fragility of erythrocytes, jaundice, and splenomegaly. Called also *globe cell anemia, congenital hemolytic icterus, constitutional hemolytic anemia, chronic familial icterus, chronic acholuric jaundice,* and *acholuric jaundice.*

spheroid (sfe′roid) [*sphero-* + Gr. *eidos* form] a globular body, or one resembling a sphere.

spheroidal (sfe-roi'dal) having the form or shape of a sphere.

spheroidin (sfe-roi'din) [*Sphaeroides* (Gr. *sphaira* sphere) a puffer fish + -*in*, suffix denoting a chemical compound] a toxic fraction from tetrodotoxin, believed to have the empirical formula $C_{12}H_{17}O_{13}N_3$.

spherolith (sfe'ro-lith) [*sphero-* + Gr. *lithos* stone] any of the minute spherical deposits found in the kidney tissue of the newborn; they are probably uratic deposits.

spheroma (sfe-ro'mah) a globular tumor.

spherometer (sfe-rom'ĕ-ter) [*sphero-* + Gr. *metron* measure] an instrument for measuring the curvature of a surface.

spherophakia (sfe"ro-fa'ke-ah) [*sphero* + *phak-* + *ia*] a developmental defect in which a smaller, more spherical optic lens than normal is formed, with partial or complete aplasia of the zonule.

Spherophorous (sfer-of'o-rus) *Sphaerophorus.*

spheroplast (sfēr'o-plast) a bacterial, yeast, or fungal cell that results after partial removal of the rigid cell wall, which forms a membrane-bound cell with a spherical shape that is dependent for its integrity on an isotonic or hypertonic medium. Cf. *protoplast*, def. 3.

spherospermia (sfe-ro-sper'me-ah) [*sphero-* + Gr. *sperma* seed] a round, tailless spermatozoon.

spherule (sfer'ūl) [L. *sphaerula* little ball] 1. a small sphere. 2. a spherical multinucleate cell of the parasitic stage of *Coccidioides immitis,* in which endospores are developed. **s's of Fulci,** numerous spherical red bodies seen in the spinal cord in inflammatory conditions of the cord. **rod s.,** the pear-shaped ending of a retinal rod cell, which synapses with the bipolar and horizontal cells in the outer plexiform layer.

spherulin (sfēr'u-lin) a skin test antigen prepared from spherule-endospore phase *Coccidioides immitis* organisms, which detects almost all persons who are coccidioidin-positive, as well as a group of coccidioidin-negative persons with previous *C. immitis* exposure. Cf. *coccidioidin.*

sphincter (sfingk'ter) [L.; Gr. *sphinktēr* that which binds tight] a ringlike band of muscle fibers that constricts a passage or closes a natural orifice; called also *musculus sphincter* [NA]. **s. a'ni,** see *musculus sphincter ani externus* and *musculus sphincter ani internus.* **s. of Boyden,** a superior choledochal sphincter encircling the common bile duct just proximal to the duodenum. **cardiac s., cardioesophageal s.,** muscle fibers about the opening of the esophagus into the stomach. **cornual s.,** tubal s. **gastroesophageal s.,** the terminal few centimeters of the esophagus, which prevents reflux of gastric contents into the esophagus. **Giordano's s.,** musculus sphincter ductus choledochi. **Henle's s.,** muscle fibers surrounding the prostatic urethra. **hepatic s.,** a thickened portion of the muscular coat of the hepatic veins near their entrance into the inferior vena cava. **s. of hepatopancreatic ampulla,** musculus sphincter ampullae hepatopancreaticae. **Hyrtl's s.,** an incomplete band or thickening of the muscle fibers in the rectum a few inches above the anus in the upper part of the rectal ampulla; called also *rectal s.* **inguinal s.,** a ring of muscle fibers around the spermatic cord at the internal opening of the inguinal canal. **s. i'ridis,** musculus sphincter pupillae. **Lütkens' s.,** a thickening of the muscle fibers in the neck of the gallbladder. **Nélaton's s.,** an occasional and often incomplete band of muscle fibers about the rectum at the level of the prostate. **O'Beirne's s.,** circular muscle fibers in the wall of the large intestine at the junction of the sigmoid colon and rectum. **s. o'culi,** musculus orbicularis oculi. **Oddi's s.,** the sheath of muscle fibers investing the associated bile and pancreatic passages as they traverse the wall of the duodenum; called also *musculus sphincter ampullae hepatopancreaticae* [NA] and *Oddi's muscle.* **s. o'ris,** musculus orbicularis oris. **palatopharyngeal s.,** a transverse band of muscle fibers in the posterior wall of the pharynx, derived from the superior constrictor or palatopharyngeal muscle, which contracts during swallowing to form Passavant's bar; it also contracts during speech in persons with cleft palate. **pharyngoesophageal s.,** a region of higher muscular tone at the junction of the pharynx and esophagus, which is involved in movements of swallowing. **precapillary s.,** a smooth muscle fiber encircling a true capillary where it originates from the arterial capillary, which can open and close the capillary entrance. **prepyloric s.,** a band of muscle fi-

bers in the wall of the stomach proximal to the pyloric sphincter. **s. pupil'lae,** musculus sphincter pupillae. **pyloric s.,** a thickening of the circular muscle of the stomach around its opening into the duodenum; called also *musculus sphincter pyloricus* [NA]. **rectal s.,** Hyrtl's s. **tubal s.,** an encircling band of muscle fibers at the junction of the uterine tube and the uterus. **s. ure'thrae,** musculus sphincter urethrae. **s. vagi'nae,** the musculus bulbospongiosus in the female. **s. vesi'cae,** musculus sphincter vesicae urinariae.

sphincteral (sfingk'ter-al) pertaining to a sphincter.

sphincteralgia (sfingk"ter-al'je-ah) [*sphincter* + Gr. *algos* pain + -*ia*] pain in a sphincter muscle, as of the anus.

sphincterectomy (sfingk"ter-ek'to-me) [*sphincter* + Gr. *ektomē* excision] excision of any sphincter, such as the sphincter iridis.

sphincteric (sfingk-ter'ik) pertaining to a sphincter.

sphincterismus (sfingk"ter-iz'mus) spasm of the sphincter ani.

sphincteritis (sfingk"ter-i'tis) inflammation of a sphincter, particularly of the sphincter of Oddi.

sphincterolysis (sfingk"ter-ol'ĭ-sis) [*sphincter* + *lysis*] the operation of separating the iris from the cornea in anterior synechia.

sphincteroplasty (sfingk'ter-o-plas"te) [*sphincter* + Gr. *plassein* to mold] surgical repair of a defective sphincter.

sphincteroscope (sfingk'ter-o-skōp") [*sphincter* + Gr. *skopein* to examine] a speculum for inspecting the anal sphincter. **Kelly's s.,** see under *speculum.*

sphincteroscopy (sfingk"ter-os'ko-pe) inspection of a sphincter.

sphincterotome (sfingk'ter-o-tōm") an instrument for cutting a sphincter.

sphincterotomy (sfingk"ter-ot'o-me) [*sphincter* + Gr. *tomē* a cutting] division of a sphincter. **internal s.,** incision of the internal sphincter of the anus.

sphingo- [Gr. *sphingein* to bind fast] a combining form denoting relationship to sphingosine or a sphingolipid.

sphingogalactoside (sfing"go-gah-lak'to-sīd) a substance composing part of the material characteristic of the spleen in Gaucher's disease.

sphingoglycolipid (sfing"go-gli"ko-lip'id) any glycolipid that contains sphingosine, including the cerebrosides, globosides, hematosides, and gangliosides.

sphingoin (sfing'go-in) a leukomaine, $C_{17}H_{35}NO_2$, from the substance of the brain.

sphingol (sfing'gol) an alcohol, $C_9H_{18}O$, obtained from sphingomyelinic acid by hydrolysis.

sphingolipid (sfing"go-lip'id) [Gr. *sphingein* to bind tight + *lipid*] a lipid containing sphingosine; a fatty acid is attached to the nitrogen atom, and these N-acylsphingosines are called ceramides. Sphingolipids are combinations of different compounds with the hydroxyl group of ceramides, e.g., sphingomyelins (with phosphoryl choline), gangliosides (with branched-chain oligosaccharides), and cerebrosides (with glucose or galactose). They occur in membranes and in particularly high concentrations in brain and nerve tissue.

sphingolipidoses (sfing"go-lip"ĭ-do'sēz) [Gr.] plural of *sphingolipidosis.*

sphingolipidosis (sfing"go-lip"ĭ-do'sis) [*sphingolipid* + -*osis*] 1. any lysosomal storage disease characterized by abnormal storage of sphingolipids. 2. Niemann-Pick disease. Called also *sphingolipodystrophy.* **cerebral s.,** a group of hereditary disorders transmitted as an autosomal recessive trait and due to an inborn defect of lipid metabolism in which spingolipids accumulate in the brain. They are characterized by cerebromacular degeneration, progressive dementia, progressive loss of vision resulting in blindness, paralysis, and death, and are classified according to age of onset. The *infantile form* usually occurs between 4 and 6 months of age, chiefly affecting childred of Jewish ancestry, and marked by a cherry-red spot with a gray-white border on both retinas; called also *Sachs'* or *Tay-Sachs disease.* The *late infantile form* occurs between 3 and 4 years of age, shows no racial predilection, and progresses more slowly than the infantile form. The cherry-red spot seen in the infantile form is frequently absent, but there are pigmentary changes of the retina. Called also *Bielschosky's* or *Bielschowsky-Jansky disease.* The *juvenile form* shows no racial predilection, occurs between 5 and 10 years of age, and is marked by "salt and pepper" pigmentation of the retina; called also *Batten-Mayou*, *Spielmeyer-Vogt*, and *Vogt-Spielmeyer disease*. The *late juvenile*, or *adult*, *form* occurs between the ages of 15 and 26, and shows no racial predilection or ocular lesions; clinical findings are those of cerebellar or basal ganglia disorders. Called also *Kufs' disease*.

sphingolipodystrophy (sfing"go-lip"o-dis'tro-fe) sphingolipidosis.

sphingomyelin (sfing"go-mi'ĕ-lin) a general designation of a group of phospholipids which on hydrolysis yield phosphoric acid, choline, sphingosine, and a fatty acid. They occur primarily in nervous tissue and generally in membranes.

sphingomyelin phosphodiesterase (sfing"go-mi'e-lin fos"fo-di-es'ter-ās) [EC 3.1.4.12] an enzyme of the hydrolase class that catalyzes the reaction sphingomyelin + H_2O = N-acylsphingosine + choline phosphate. Deficiency of the enzyme, an autosomal recessive trait, causes Niemann-Pick disease. Called also *sphingomyelinase*.

sphingomyelinase (sfing"go-mi'el-in-ās) sphingomyelin phosphodiesterase.

sphingomyelinase deficiency Niemann-Pick disease.

sphingomyelinosis (sfing"go-mi"ĕ-lin-o'sis) Niemann-Pick disease.

sphingophospholipid (sfing"go-fos"fo-lip'id) a sphingolipid containing sphingosine or a related base and phosphorylcholine.

sphingosine (sfing'go-sin) a long-chain, mono-unsaturated aliphatic amino alcohol, $C_{18}H_{37}O_2N$, usually present in sphingomyelin.

sphygmic (sfig'mik) [Gr. *sphygmikos*] pertaining to the pulse; see *sphygmic period*, under *period*.

sphygm(o)- [Gr. *sphygmos* pulse] a combining form denoting relationship to the pulse.

sphygmobologram (sfig"mo-bo'lo-gram) a tracing made by the sphygmobolometer.

sphygmobolometer (sfig"mo-bo-lom'ĕ-ter) [*sphygmo-* + Gr. *bŏlos* mass + *metron* measure] an instrument for measuring and recording the energy of the pulse wave, and so, indirectly, the strength of the systole.

sphygmobolometry (sfig"mo-bo-lom'ĕ-tre) the use of the sphygmobolometer.

sphygmocardiogram (sfig"mo-kar'de-o-gram) the tracing made by a sphygmocardiograph.

sphygmocardiograph (sfig"mo-kar'de-o-graf) [*sphygmo-* + Gr. *kardia* heart + *graphein* to write] an instrument for recording the pulse waves and heart beat at the same operation.

sphygmocardioscope (sfig"mo-kar'de-o-skōp) [*sphygmo-* + Gr. *kardia* heart + *skopein* to examine] an apparatus that records or displays the behavior of the pulse, heart action, and sounds.

sphygmochronograph (sfig"mo-kro'no-graf) [*sphygmo-* + Gr. *chronos* time + *graphein* to write] a form of self-registering sphygmograph.

sphygmodynamometer (sfig"mo-di"nah-mom'ĕ-ter) [*sphygmo-* + Gr. *dynamis* power + *metron* measure] an instrument for determining the force of the pulse.

sphygmogram (sfig'mo-gram) [*sphygmo-* + Gr. *gramma* a writing] a sphygmographic tracing; the record or tracing made by a sphygmograph. It consists of a curve having a sudden rise (*primary elevation*), followed by a sudden fall, after which there is a gradual descent marked by a number of secondary elevations.

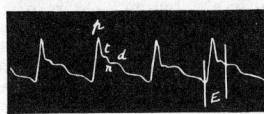

Radial sphygmogram from a healthy person: *p*, percussion wave; *t*, tidal or predicrotic wave; *n*, dicrotic or aortic notch; *d*, dicrotic wave; *E*, the sphygmic period during which the semilunar valves are open.

sphygmograph (sfig'mo-graf) [*sphygmo-* + Gr. *graphein* to write] an instrument for registering the movements, form, and force of the arterial pulse. Vierordt's sphygmograph

(1835) and Marey's (1860) were the earliest. The latter, variously modified, is the kind principally used.

sphygmographic (sfig"mo-graf'ik) pertaining to the sphygmograph.

sphygmography (sfig-mog'rah-fe) the production of pulse tracings with the sphygmograph.

sphygmoid (sfig'moid) [*sphygmo-* + Gr. *eidos* form] resembling the pulse.

sphygmology (sfig-mol'o-je) [*sphygmo-* + *-logy*] the sum of what is known regarding the pulse.

sphygmomanometer (sfig"mo-mah-nom'ĕ-ter) an instrument for measuring the blood pressure in the arteries. There are many forms of the instrument, each named for the person who devised it, as *Riva-Rocci s.*, *Faught's s.*, *Erlanger's s.*, *Janeway's s.*, *Mosso's s.*, *Rogers' s.*, *Stanton's s.*, *Tychos s.*

sphygmometer (sfig-mom'ĕ-ter) [*sphygmo-* + Gr. *metron* measure] an instrument for measuring the force and frequency of the pulse.

sphygmometrograph (sfig"mo-met'ro-graf) an apparatus for recording the maximal and minimal arterial pressures.

sphygmometroscope (sfig"mo-met'ro-skōp) an instrument for taking the blood pressure by the auscultatory method.

sphygmo-oscillometer (sfig"mo-os"ĭ-lom'ĕ-ter) a form of sphygmomanometer in which the disappearance and reappearance of the pulse are indicated by an oscillating needle.

sphygmopalpation (sfig"mo-pal-pa'shun) the act of palpating or feeling the pulse.

sphygmophone (sfig'mo-fōn) [*sphygmo-* + Gr. *phōnē* sound] an apparatus for rendering audible the vibrations of the pulse.

sphygmoplethysmograph (sfig"mo-plĕ-thiz'mo-graf) a plethysmograph which traces a record of the pulse, together with the curve of fluctuation of volume.

sphygmoscope (sfig'mo-skōp) [*sphygmo-* + Gr. *skopein* to examine] a device for rendering the pulse beat visible. **Bishop's s.,** an apparatus for measuring the blood pressure, especially the diastolic pressure.

sphygmoscopy (sfig-mos'ko-pe) examination of the pulse.

sphygmosystole (sfig"mo-sis'to-le) [*sphygmo-* + *systole*] that part of the sphygmogram that corresponds to the systole of the heart.

sphygmotonogram (sfig"mo-to'no-gram) (*obs.*) the graphic record produced by the sphygmotonograph.

sphygmotonograph (sfig"mo-to'no-graf) [*sphygmo-* + Gr. *tonos* tension + *graphein* to write] (*obs.*) an instrument for recording simultaneously the blood pressure, the carotid or jugular pulse, the brachial pulse, and the time in fifths of a second.

sphygmotonometer (sfig"mo-to-nom'ĕ-ter) [*sphygmo-* + Gr. *tonos* tension + *metron* measure] an instrument for measuring the elasticity of the arterial walls.

sphygmoviscosimetry (sfig"mo-vis"ko-sim'ĕ-tre) [*sphygmo-* + *viscosity* + Gr. *metron* measure] measurement of the blood pressure and the viscosity of the blood.

sphyrectomy (sfi-rek'to-me) [Gr. *sphyra* malleus + *ektomē* excision] surgical removal of the malleus.

sphyrotomy (sfi-rot'o-me) [Gr. *sphyra* malleus + *tomē* a cutting] surgical removal of a portion of the malleus.

spica (spi'kah) [L. "ear of wheat"] a figure-of-8 bandage with turns that cross one another usually at the shoulder or hip; see under *bandage*.

spicular (spik'u-lar) pertaining to a spicule.

spicule (spik'ūl) [L. *spiculum*] a sharp, needle-like body.

spiculum (spik'u-lum), pl. *spic'ula* [L.] spicule.

spider (spi'der) 1. an arthropod of the class Arachnida, some species of which have venomous bites. Cf. *arachnidism*. 2. a spider-like nevus; see *vascular s.* **arterial s.,** vascular s. **banana s.,** *Heteropoda venatoria*. **black widow s.,** see *Latrodectus*. **brown recluse s.,** *Loxosceles reclusa*. **cat-headed s.,** *Mastophora gasteracanthoides*. **comb-footed s.,** see *Theridiidae*. **European wolf s.,** European tarantula. **funnel-web s.,** see *Atrax*. **jointed s.,** see *Solpugida*. **lynx s.,** *Peucetia viridans*. **tree funnel-web s.,** *Atrax formidabilis*. **vascular s.,** a telangiectasis due to dilatation and ramification of superficial cutaneous arteries, which presents as a bright red central portion with branching radiations, the whole somewhat resembling the configuration of a spider. The lesions may occur singly or in large numbers, and may be nevoid or acquired, being commonly associated with pregnancy and liver disease. Called also *arterial s.*, *nevus araneus*, and *spider angioma*, *nevus*, or *telangiectasia*. See also under *vascular nevus*, under *nevus*. **wandering s.**, *Ctenus ferus*.

spider burst (spi′der burst) radiating lines of capillaries on the leg caused by venous dilatation but without distinct varicosity.

Spieghel's line (spig′elz) [Adriaan van der *Spieghel* (*L. Spigelius*), Flemish anatomist, 1578–1625] linea semilunaris.

Spiegler's test (reagent) (spe′glerz) [Eduard *Spiegler*, Austrian dermatologist, 1860–1908] see under *tests*.

Spiegler-Fendt sarcoid (spe′gler fent) [Edward *Spiegler*; Heinrich *Fendt*, German physician, 20th century] lymphocytoma cutis.

Spigelia (spi-je′le-ah) [Adriaan van der *Spieghel*, 1578–1625] a genus of loganiaceous plants; the rhizome and roots of *S. marilan′dica* L. (pinkroot) have been used as an anthelmintic.

spigelian (spi-je′le-an) named for Adriaan van der *Spieghel* (*L. Spigelius*), Flemish anatomist, 1578–1625, as *spigelian* line (linea semilunaris) or *spigelian* lobe (lobus caudatus).

spigeline (spi-je′lēn) an alkaloid resembling coniine and nicotine occurring in *Spigelia marilandica* L., a perennial herb of Eastern North America.

spignet (spig′net) *Aralia*.

spike (spīk) a sharp upward deflection in a curve, such as the main deflection of the oscillographic tracing of the action potential wave, the following smaller wave being called the *after-potential*. See also under *potential*.

spikenard (spīk′nard) [L. *nardus*, or *spica nardi*] the plant *Nardostachys jatamansi* DC. (Valerianaceae) and various fragrant valerianaceous and other plants; now chiefly used in oriental medicine for nervous disorders. **American s.**, *Aralia*. **false s.**, *Andropogon nardus*, an aromatic and stimulant East Indian grass; also *Smilacina racemosa*, a North American plant.

Spilanthes (spi-lan′thēz) [Gr. *spilos* spot + Gr. *anthos* flower] a genus of composite-flowered plants. *S. acmella* Murr., the Para cress of tropical America and Asia, was formerly used as a remedy for toothache. It is also a powerful mosquito larvicide.

spillway (spil′wa) embrasure.

spina (spi′nah), pl. *spi′nae* [L.] a spine: a thornlike process or projection; [NA] a general term for such a process. **s. angula′ris**, s. ossis sphenoidalis. **s. bif′ida**, a developmental anomaly characterized by defective closure of the bony encasement of the spinal cord, through which the cord and meninges may (s. bifida cystica) or may not (s. bifida occulta) protrude. **s. bif′ida ante′rior**, a defect of closure on the anterior surface of the bony spinal canal, often associated with defective development of the abdominal and thoracic viscera. **s. bif′ida aper′ta**, s. bifida cystica. **s. bif′ida cys′tica**, spina bifida in which there is protrusion through the defect of a cystic swelling involving the meninges (meningocele), spinal cord (myelocele), or both (meningomyelocele). **s. bif′ida manifes′ta**, s. bifida cystica. **s. bif′ida occul′ta**, spina bifida in which there is a defect of the bony spinal canal without protrusion of the cord or meninges. **s. bif′ida poste′rior**, a defect of closure on the posterior surface of the bony spinal canal. **s. fronta′lis**, s. nasalis ossis frontalis. **s. hel′icis** [NA], spine of helix: a small, forward-projecting cartilaginous process on the anterior portion of the helix at about the junction of the helix and its crus, just above the tragus. **s. ili′aca ante′rior infe′rior** [NA], anterior inferior iliac spine: a blunt bony process projecting forward from the lower part of the anterior margin of the ilium, just above the acetabulum. **s. ili′aca ante′rior supe′rior** [NA], anterior superior iliac spine: a blunt bony projection on the anterior border of the ilium, forming the anterior end of the iliac crest. **s. ili′aca poste′rior infe′rior** [NA], posterior inferior iliac spine: a blunt bony projection from the posterior border of the ilium, corresponding to the posterior lower extremity of the facies auricularis and the posterior upper extremity of the incisura ischiadica major. **s.**

ili′aca poste′rior supe′rior [NA], posterior superior iliac spine: a blunt bony projection on the posterior border of the ilium, forming the posterior end of the iliac crest. **s. intercondyloi′dea**, eminentia intercondylaris. **s. ischiad′ica** [NA], spine of ischium: a strong process of bone projecting backward and medialward from the posterior border of the ischium, on a level with the lower border of the acetabulum and serving to separate the major and minor ischiadic notches. Called also *ischial spine* and *spina ischialis* [NA alternative] **s. ischia′lis**, NA alternative for *s. ischiadica*. **s. mea′tus**, s. suprameatum. **s. menta′lis** [NA], mental spine: any of the small bony projections (usually four in number) located on the internal surface of the mandible, near the lower end of the midline, serving for attachment of the genioglossal and geniohyoid muscles. Called also *genial apophysis*. **s. nasa′lis ante′rior maxil′lae** [NA], anterior nasal spine of maxilla: the sharp anterosuperior projection at the anterior extremity of the nasal crest of the maxilla. **s. nasa′lis os′sis fronta′lis** [NA], nasal spine of frontal bone: a rough and somewhat irregular process of bone projecting downward and forward from the front part of the inferior surface of the pars nasalis of the frontal bone and fitting between the nasal bones and the ethmoid bone; called also *spina frontalis*. **s. nasa′lis os′sis palati′ni** [NA], **s. nasa′lis poste′rior os′sis palati′ni**, nasal spine of palatine bone: a small, sharp, backward-projecting bony spine forming the medial posterior angle of the horizontal portion of the palatine bone; called also *posterior nasal spine*. **s. os′sis sphenoida′lis** [NA], spine of sphenoid bone: a small bony process projecting downward from the inferior aspect of the great wing of the sphenoid bone where the wing projects into the angle between the petrous and squamous portions of the temporal bone; it is just posterior to the foramen spinosum and serves for attachment of the sphenomandibular and pterygospinous ligaments. Called also *s. angularis*. **spi′nae palati′nae** [NA], palatine spines: ridges which are laterally placed on the inferior surface of the maxillary part of the hard palate, separating the palatine sulci. **s. scap′ulae** [NA], spine of scapula: a triangular plate of bone attached by one edge to the back of the scapula, its tip being at the vertebral border of the scapula; it passes laterally toward the shoulder joint and at its base bears the acromion. **s. suprameata′lis**, NA alternative for *s. suprameatica*. **s. su′pramea′tica** [NA], suprameatal spine: a pointed process that sometimes projects from the temporal bone, just above and at the back of the external acoustic meatus. Called also *s. suprameatalis* [NA alternative]. **s. tib′iae**, tuberositas tibiae. **s. trochlea′ris** [NA], trochlear spine: a spicule of bone on the anteromedial part of the orbital surface of the frontal bone for attachment of the trochlea of the superior oblique muscle; when absent, it is represented by the trochlear fovea. **s. tympan′ica ma′jor** [NA], greater tympanic spine: a spine of the temporal bone forming the anterior edge of the tympanic notch (deficient part of tympanic sulcus). **s. tympan′ica mi′nor** [NA], lesser tympanic spine: a spine of the temporal bone forming the posterior edge of the tympanic notch. **s. vento′sa**, a true dactylitis occurring mostly in infants and young children, characterized by enlargement of the fingers or toes, with caseation, sequestration, and sinus formation.

spinacin (spi′nah-sin) a protein obtained from the cytoplasm of the cells of spinach leaves. It is insoluble in water and in salt solutions, but soluble in very slight excess of either acid or alkali.

spinae (spi′ne) [L.] plural of *spina*.

spinal (spi′nal) [L. *spinalis*] pertaining to a spine or to the vertebral column. See also under *animal*.

spinalgia (spi-nal′je-ah) [*spine* + Gr. *algos* pain + *-ia*] pain in the spinal region. **Petruschky's s.**, tenderness in the interscapular region in tuberculosis of the bronchial lymph nodes.

spinalis (spi-na′lis) [L.] spinal.

spinant (spi′nant) any agent that acts directly upon the spinal cord, increasing its reflex activity.

spinate (spi′nāt) [L. *spinatus*] having thorns; shaped like a thorn.

spindle (spin′d′l) 1. the fusiform figure occurring in the cell nucleus during the metaphase of mitosis, composed of microtubules radiating from the centrioles and connecting the chromosomes at their centromeres. Called also *achro-*

matic s., mitotic s., and *nuclear s.* 2. see *brain waves,* under *wave.* 3. **muscle s. aortic s.,** the dilated part of the aorta just below the isthmus. **Axenfeld-Krukenberg s.,** Krukenberg's s. **Bütschli's nuclear s.,** spindle, def. 1. **central s.,** the bundle of fibers in the axial part of the spindle of an amphiaster. **cleavage s.,** any spindle formed during cleavage of the ovum. **enamel s's,** club-like structures in the inner third of the dental enamel, believed to be terminals of protoplasmic processes of the odontoblasts that have passed across the dentinoenamel junction. **His' s.,** aortic s. **Krukenberg's s.,** a vertical spindle-shaped, brownish-red opacity on the posterior surface of the cornea. **Kühno's s.,** muscle s. **mitotic s.,** spindle, def. 1. **muscle s.,** a mechanoreceptor found between skeletal muscle fibers; the muscle spindles are arranged in parallel with muscle fibers, and respond to passive stretch of the muscle but cease to discharge if the muscle contracts isotonically, thus signaling muscle length. The muscle spindle is the receptor responsible for the stretch or myotatic reflex. **neuromuscular s.,** muscle s. **neurotendinal s.,** Golgi tendon organ. **nuclear s.,** see *spindle,* def. 1. **tendon s.,** Golgi tendon organ. **tigroid s's,** Nissl bodies. **urine s's,** spindle-shaped, urine-filled segments of the ureter due to incomplete occlusion of the ureter during peristalsis.

spine (spīn) 1. a thornlike process or projection; called also *spina* [NA]. 2. the spinal column (columna vertebralis [NA]). 3. the central ridge on the internal surface of a horse's hoof, between the branches of the frog; called also *frog stay.* **alar s., angular s.,** spina ossis sphenoidalis. **bamboo s.,** the ankylosed spine produced by rheumatoid spondylitis; so called because of the roentgenographic appearance caused by lipping of the vertebral margins. **basilar s.,** tuberculum pharyngeum. **Civinini's s.,** processus pterygospinosus. **cleft s.,** see *spina bifida.* **dendritic s.,** gemmule, def. 2. **dorsal s.,** columna vertebralis. **Erichsen's s.,** an obscure condition occurring as the result of alleged accidental injury to the vertebral column. **ethmoidal s. of Macalister,** crista sphenoidalis. **frontal s., external,** spina nasalis ossis frontalis. **s. of greater tubercle of humerus,** crista tuberculi majoris. **s. of helix,** spina helicis. **hemal s.,** a ventral projection from the hemal arch, which is attached to the underside of certain vertebral centra in lower vertebrates. **s. of Henle,** spina suprameatica. **iliac s., anterior inferior,** spina iliaca anterior inferior. **iliac s., anterior superior,** spina iliaca anterior superior. **iliac s., posterior inferior,** spina iliaca posterior inferior. **iliac s., posterior superior,** spina iliaca posterior superior. **iliopectineal s.,** eminentia iliopubica. **intercondyloid s.,** eminentia intercondylaris. **ischial s., s. of ischium,** spina ischiadica. **jugular s.,** processus jugularis ossis occipitalis. **kissing s's,** a condition in which the spinous processes of adjacent vertebra are in contact; called also *Baastrup's disease* or *syndrome.* **s. of lesser tubercle of humerus,** crista tuberculi minoris. **s. of maxilla,** spina nasalis anterior maxillae. **meatal s.,** spina suprameatum. **mental s.,** spina mentalis. **mental s., external,** protuberantia mentalis. **nasal s., anterior,** spina nasalis anterior maxillae. **nasal s., posterior,** spina nasalis ossis palatini. **nasal s. of frontal bone,** spina nasalis ossis frontalis. **nasal s. of maxilla, anterior,** spina nasalis anterior maxillae. **nasal s. of palatine bone,** spina nasalis ossis palatini. **neural s.,** processus spinosus vertebrarum. **obturator s.,** crista obturatoria. **occipital s., external,** protuberantia occipitalis externa. **occipital s., internal,** protuberantia occipitalis interna. **palatine s's,** spinae palatinae. **peroneal s. of os calcis,** trochlea peronealis calcanei. **pharyngeal s.,** tuberculum pharyngeum. **poker s.,** the ankylosed spine produced by rheumatoid spondylitis; so called because of its rigidity. **s. of pubic bone, s. of pubis,** tuberculum pubicum ossis pubis. **railway s.,** traumatic neurosis following spinal injury. **rigid s.,** poker s. **s. of scapula,** spina scapulae. **sciatic s.,** spina ischiadica. **s. of sphenoid bone, sphenoidal s.,** spina ossis sphenoidalis. **suprameatal s.,** spina suprameatica. **s. of tibia, tibial s.,** tuberositas tibiae. **trochanteric s., greater,** labium laterale lineae asperae femoris. **trochanteric s., lesser,** labium mediale lineae asperae femoris. **trochlear s.,** spina trochlearis. **tympanic s., anterior, tympanic s., greater,** spina tympanica major. **tympanic s., lesser, tympanic s.,**

posterior, spina tympanica minor. **typhoid s.,** a painful condition of the spine due to osteomyelitis of the vertebrae following typhoid fever. **s. of vertebra,** processus spinosus vertebrarum.

Spinelli's operation (spe-nel'ēz) [Pier Giuseppe *Spinelli,* Italian gynecologist, 1862–1929] see under *operation.*

spinifugal (spi-nif'u-gal) [L. *spina* spine + *fugere* to flee] going, conducting, or moving away from the spinal cord.

spinipetal (spi-nip'e-tal) [L. *spina* spine + *petere* to seek] tending, conducting, or moving toward the spinal cord.

Spinitectus gracilis (spi''ne-tek'tus gras'ĭ-lis) a parasitic nematode in the intestines of fishes in the United States.

spinnbarkeit (spin'bahr-kīt) [Ger.] the formation of a thread by mucus from the cervix uteri when spread onto a glass slide and drawn out by a coverglass; the time at which it can be drawn to the maximum length usually precedes or coincides with the time of ovulation.

spinobulbar (spi''no-bul'bar) pertaining to the spinal cord and the medulla oblongata.

spinocellular (spi''no-sel'u-lar) containing, made up of, or marked by prickle cells.

spinocerebellar (spi''no-ser''e-bel'ar) pertaining to the spinal cord and the cerebellum.

spinocerebellum (spi''no-ser''ĕ-bel'lum) [spino- + *cerebellum*] paleocerebellum.

spinocortical (spi''no-kor'tĭ-kal) corticospinal.

spinocostalis (spi''no-kos-ta'lis) the serratus posterior superior and inferior muscles together.

spinogalvanization (spi''no-gal''vah-ni-za'shun) galvanization of the spinal cord, performed by moving the anode slowly up and down the spine.

spinoglenoid (spi''no-gle'noid) pertaining to the spine of the scapula and the glenoid cavity.

spinogram (spi'no-gram) a roentgenogram of the spine or of the spinal cord.

spinopetal (spi-nop'e-tal) spinipetal.

spinose (spi'nōs) spinous.

spinotectal (spi''no-tek'tal) tectospinal.

spinous (spi'nus) [L. *spinosus*] 1. like a spine; acanthoid. 2. pertaining to a spine or to a spinelike process.

spinthariscope (spin-thar'ĭ-skōp) [Gr. *spintharis* spark + *skopein* to examine] an instrument for viewing the emanations of radium.

spintherism (spin'ther-izm) [Gr. *spinthērizein* to emit sparks] synchysis scintillans.

spintherometer (spin''ther-om'ĕ-ter) [Gr. *spinthēr* spark + *metron* measure] an apparatus for measuring the changes which occur in the vacuum of the roentgen-ray tube, and hence the penetrating power of the rays.

spintheropia (spin''ther-o'pe-ah) [Gr. *spinthēr* spark + *ōpē* sight + *-ia*] synchysis scintillans.

spintometer (spin-tom'ĕ-ter) spintherometer.

spiperone (spip'ĕ-rōn) chemical name: 8-[4-(4-fluorophenyl)-4- oxobutyl-1-phenyl-1,3,8-triazaspirol[4.5]-decan-4-one; a tranquilizer, $C_{23}H_{26}FN_3O_2$, used in treatment of schizophrenia.

spir. abbreviation for L. *spir'itus,* spirit.

spiracle (spir'ah-k'l) [L. *spirare* to breathe] a breathing orifice of arthropods; an accessory respiratory orifice for the intake of water in the respiratory system of cartilaginous fish.

spiradenoma (spi''rad-ĕ-no'mah) [Gr. *speira* coil + *adenoma*] adenoma sudoriparum. **cylindromatous s.,** cylindroma, def. 2. **eccrine s.,** a benign, solitary, deep-seated nodule arising from the coil portion of an eccrine gland; it is covered by normal appearing skin and may be accompanied by paroxysmal pain.

spiral (spi'ral) [L. *spiralis* from *spira;* Gr. *speira*] 1. winding about a center like a coil or the thread of a screw. 2. anything coiled or winding about a center. **Curschmann's s's,** coiled mucinous fibrils sometimes found in the sputum of bronchial asthma. **Golgi-Rezzonico s.,** see under *thread.* **Herxheimer's s's,** see under *fiber.* **Perroncito's s's,** see under *apparatus.* **tendon s.,** a spiral receptor connected with a tendon.

spiramycin (spēr-ah-mi'sin) an antibiotic produced by *Streptomyces ambofaciens;* administered orally.

Spiranthes (spi-ran'thēz) [Gr. *speira* coil + *anthos* flower] a genus of orchidaceous plants. **S. autumna′lis,** a species reputed to be aphrodisiac. **S. diuret′ica,** a species of Chile, said to be a valuable diuretic.

spireme (spi′rēm) [Gr. *speirēma* coil] the threadlike, continuous or segmented figure formed by the chromosome material during the prophase of mitosis or meiosis. Called also *skein.*

spirilla (spi-ril′ah) [L.] plural of *spirillum.*

Spirillaceae (spi″ril-la′se-e) in former systems of classification, a family of spiral and curved bacteria that included the genera *Spirillum* and *Campylobacter.*

spirillemia (spi″ril-e′me-ah) [*spirilla* + Gr. *haima* blood + *-ia*] the presence of spirilla in the blood.

spirillicidal (spi-ril″ĭ-si′dal) destroying spirilla.

spirillicide (spi-ril′ĭ-sīd) [*spirilla* + L. *caedere* to kill] 1. destroying spirilla. 2. an agent that destroys spirilla.

spirillolysis (spi″rĭ-lol′ĭ-sis) [*spirilla* + Gr. *lysis* dissolution] the breaking up or destruction of spirilla.

spirillosis (spi″rĭ-lo′sis) any disease condition attended or marked by the presence of spirilla in the body.

Spirillospora (spi″rĭ-lo-spo′ra) [*spirilla* + Gr. *spora* seed] a genus of soil bacteria of the family Actinoplanaceae, order Actinomycetales, made up of cells bearing spiral sporangia. The type species is *S. al′bida.*

spirillotropic (spi″rĭ-lo-trop′ik) having an affinity for spirilla.

spirillotropism (spi″rĭ-lot′ro-pizm) [*spirilla* + Gr. *tropos* turning] the property of having an affinity for spirilla.

Spirillum (spi-ril′um) [Gr. *speira* spiral] a genus of spiral and curved bacteria of the family Spirillaceae, consisting of short, rigid, helical cells with bipolar flagella. The organisms are motile and microaerophilic or aerobic; they are found in fresh and salt waters that contain organic matter. **S. mi′nus,** a species of uncertain status that is a normal parasite of the nasopharynx of rats and mice; it is the etiologic agent of the spirillary form of rat-bite fever.

spirillum (spi-ril′um), pl. *spiril′la* [L., dim. of *spira* coil] any organism of the genus *Spirillum.* **s. of Finkler and Prior,** *Vibrio cholerae* biotype *proteus.* **s. of Vincent,** *Treponema vincentii.*

spirit (spir′it) [L. *spiritus*] 1. any volatile or distilled liquid. 2. a solution of a volatile material in alcohol. **ammonia s.,** aromatic ammonia s. **ammonia s., aromatic** [USP], **s. of ammonia, aromatic,** a preparation compounded of ammonia, ammonium carbonate, strong ammonia solution, lemon oil, lavender oil, myristica oil, alcohol, and purified oil, and containing, in each 100 ml., 1.7–2.1 gm. ammonia and 3.5–4.5 gm. ammonium carbonate; used as a respiratory stimulant in syncope, weakness, or threatened faint. In veterinary medicine, it is used as a respiratory and circulatory stimulant, and sometimes as a carminative and antacid. Called also *ammonia s.* **anise s.,** a mixture of anise oil and alcohol; used as a carminative. **benzaldehyde s.,** a mixture of benzaldehyde, alcohol, and distilled water; used as a flavoring agent. **camphor s.** [USP], a solution of camphor and alcohol, each 100 ml. of which contains 9–11 gm. of camphor; used topically as a local irritant. It was formerly used for the treatment of diarrhea, and in hysteria and nervous excitement. **cardamom s., compound,** a preparation of cardamom oil, orange oil, cinnamon oil, clove oil, anethole, caraway oil, and alcohol, used as a flavoring vehicle. **cinnamon s.,** an alcoholic solution of cinnamon oil, each 100 ml. of which contains 9–11 ml. of the oil; used as a flavoring agent. **ether s.,** a transparent, colorless liquid with a burning sweetish taste and an ether odor, consisting of ethyl oxide and alcohol; formerly used as a carminative. Called also *Hoffmann's drops.* **ether s., compound,** a mixture of ethyl oxide, alcohol, and ethereal oil, which has been used as a carminative. In veterinary medicine, it is used as a stomachic and carminative. **ethyl nitrite s.,** an alcoholic solution containing 3.5–4.5 per cent of ethyl nitrite, which has been used as a diaphoretic and diuretic. Called also *s. of nitrous ether* and *sweet s. of nitre.* **glyceryl trinitrate s.,** nitroglycerin s. **lavender s.,** an alcoholic solution of lavender oil, each 100 ml. of which contains 4–6 ml. of lavender oil; used as a flavoring agent. **methylated s.,** denatured alcohol. **s. of Mindererus,** ammonium acetate solution. **nitroglycerin s.,** a clear, colorless liquid with the odor of alcohol, compounded of nitroglycerin 1–1.1 per cent in alcohol; used as a

coronary vasodilator. Called also *glyceryl trinitrate s.* **s. of nitrous ether,** ethyl nitrite s. **orange s., compound** [USP], an alcoholic preparation containing orange, lemon, coriander, and anise oils; used as a flavoring agent. **peppermint s.** [USP], a preparation of peppermint, peppermint oil, and alcohol, used as a digestive aid and flavor. Called also *essence of peppermint.* **perfumed s.,** an aqueous solution of various fragrant oils, such as bergamot, lavender, lemon, orange flower, and rosemary, with alcohol, to which ethyl acetate has been added. **proof s.,** a product containing 50 per cent by volume of C_2H_5OH. **rectified s.,** alcohol. **spearmint s.,** an alcoholic solution of spearmint oil and powdered spearmint, each 100 ml. of which contains 9–11 ml. of spearmint oil. It has been used as a carminative. **sweet s. of nitre,** ethyl nitrite s. **s. of turpentine,** turpentine oil. **vanillin s., compound,** a preparation of vanillin and cardamom, cinnamon, and orange oils in alcohol; used as a flavoring agent. **s. of wine,** alcohol.

spirituous (spir′it-u-us) [L. *spirituosus*] alcoholic; containing a considerable proportion of alcohol.

spir(o)- 1. [Gr. *speira* coil] a combining form denoting relationship to a coil or spiral. 2. [L. *spirare* to breathe] a combining form denoting relationship to the breath or to breathing.

Spiro's test (spe′ro) [Karl *Spiro,* German chemist, 1867–1932] see under *tests.*

Spirocerca sanguinolenta (spi″ro-ser′kah sang″gwĭ-no-len′tah) a nematode of the family Spiruroidea, found in the walls of the aorta, esophagus, and stomach of dogs.

Spirochaeta (spi″ro-ke′tah) [Gr. *speira* coil + *chaitē* hair] a genus of microorganisms of the family Spirochaetaceae, order Spirochaetales, made up of characteristically large (up to 500 μm in length) free-living organisms, found in hydrogen sulfide–containing mud, sewage, and polluted water. Most of the organisms formerly in this genus have been assigned to other genera. The type species, is *S. plica′tilis.* **S. pseudoicterog′enes,** the name used in Germany to designate *Leptospira biflexa.*

Spirochaetaceae (spi″ro-ke-ta′se-e) a family of bacteria of the order Spirochaetales consisting of slender, undulating, motile organisms, 6 to 500 μ in length, occurring in the form of spirals with one or more complete turns in the helix. It contains the genera *Borrelia, Cristispira, Spirochaeta,* and *Treponema.*

Spirochaetales (spi″ro-ke-ta′lēz) an order of bacteria comprising the families Spirochaetaceae and Leptospiraceae, the members of which are free-living, commensal, or parasitic, with some species being pathogenic.

spirochetal (spi″ro-ke′tal) pertaining to or caused by spirochetes.

spirochete (spi′ro-kēt) [*spiro-(1)* + Gr. *chaitē* hair] 1. a spiral bacterium; a general term for any microorganism of the order Spirochaetales. 2. an organism of the genus *Spirochaeta.* **Dutton's s.,** *Borrelia duttonii.*

spirochetemia (spi″ro-ke-te′me-ah) [*spirochete* + Gr. *haima* blood + *-ia*] the presence of spirochetes in the blood.

spirocheticidal (spi″ro-ke″tĭ-si′dal) [*spirochete* + L. *caedere* to kill] destructive to spirochetes.

spirocheticide (spi″ro-ke″tĭ-sīd) an agent that causes the destruction of spirochetes.

spirochetogenous (spi″ro-ke-toj′ĕ-nus) caused by spirochetes.

spirochetolysin (spi″ro-ke-tol′ĭ-sin) a substance which causes lysis of spirochetes.

spirochetolysis (spi″ro-ke-tol′ĭ-sis) [*spirochete* + Gr. *lysis* dissolution] the destruction of spirochetes by lysis.

spirochetolytic (spi″ro-ke″to-lit′ik) pertaining to, characterized by, or causing spirochetolysis.

spirochetosis (spi″ro-ke-to′sis) infection with spirochetes. **s. arthrit′ica,** spirochetosis in which there is rheumatoid involvement of the joints. **bronchopulmonary s.,** bronchospirochetosis. **fowl s.,** a septicemic disease of fowls caused by the spirochete *Borrelia anserina,* and spread by the fowl tick *Argas persicus.*

spirocheturia (spi″ro-ke-tu′re-ah) [*spirochete* + Gr. *ouron* urine + *-ia*] the presence of spirochetes in the urine.

spirofibrilla (spi″ro-fi-bril′lah), pl. *spirofibril′lae* [*spiro-(1)* + L. *fibrilla*] Fayod's name for one of the hypothetical hollow, twisted fibrils forming the spirospartae.

spirogram (spi'ro-gram) [L. *spirare* to breathe + Gr. *gramma* a writing] a tracing or graph of respiratory movements.

spirograph (spi'ro-graf) [L. *spirare* to breathe + Gr. *graphein* to write] an instrument for registering the respiratory movements.

spirographidin (spi"ro-graf'ĭ-din) (*obs.*) a hyalin derived from spirographin.

spirographin (spi-rog'rah-fin) a hyalogen derivable from the cartilage and skeletal structures of *Spirographis*, a marine worm.

spirography (spi-rog'rah-fe) the graphic measurement of breathing, including breathing movements and breathing capacity.

Spirogyra (spi"ro-ji'rah) a genus of fresh-water green algae having spiral chlorophyll bands and forming slimy masses in still waters and slow streams.

spiroid (spi'roid) resembling a spiral.

spiro-index (spi"ro-in'deks) [L. *spirare* to breathe + *index*] the value obtained by dividing the vital capacity by the height of the individual.

spirolactone (spi"ro-lak'tōn) a group of compounds bearing 17α-propionic acid as gamma-lactone with 17β-hydroxyl, capable of opposing the action of sodium-retaining steroids on renal transport of sodium and potassium. Three such compounds have been studied. The first contains angular methyl at C_{13} and C_{10}, and is 3-(3-keto-17β-hydroxy-4-androsten-17α-yl)-propionic acid-γ-lactone; the second, without angular methyl at C_{10}, is more potent; and the third (spironolactone), with a thioacetyl group at C_7, is highly active orally.

spiroma (spi-ro'mah) adenoma sudoriparum.

spirometer (spi-rom'ě-ter) [L. *spirare* to breathe + *metrum* measure] an instrument for measuring the air taken into and exhaled from the lungs.

Spirometra (spi"ro-met'rah) [*spiro-* (1) + Gr. *metra* womb, uterus] a genus of tapeworms of the family Diphyllobothriidae, order Pseudophyllidea, which are parasites of fish-eating cats, dogs, and birds. Infection in man is caused by eating inadequately cooked fish. **S. erinaceieuropa'ei**, a species parasitic in man, dogs, and cats. **S. mansonoi'des**, a species parasitic in dogs and cats, especially bobcats, which may cause diarrhea and anemia; infection with the larvae may cause sparganosis in man.

spirometric (spi"ro-met'rik) pertaining to spirometry or the spirometer.

spirometry (spi-rom'ě-tre) the measurement of the breathing capacity of the lungs. **bronchoscopic s.,** bronchospirometry.

Spironema (spi"ro-ne'mah) [Gr. *speira* coil + *nēma* thread] in former systems of classification, a genus of bacteria made up of organisms now assigned to the genus *Treponema*.

spironolactone (spēr"o-no-lak'tōn) [USP] a synthetic 17-spirolactone steroid that is a competitive antagonist of aldosterone, which blocks the aldosterone-dependent exchange of sodium and potassium in the distal tubule, thus increasing the excretion of sodium and water and decreasing the excretion of potassium; used in the treatment of edema due to congestive heart failure or hepatic or renal disease, in the treatment of hypokalemia, in the management of primary hyperaldosteronism, and, usually in combination with other drugs, in the treatment of hypertension.

spirophore (spi'ro-fōr) [L. *spirare* to breathe + Gr. *phorein* to bear] an apparatus to effect artificial respiration.

Spiroplasma (spi"ro-plaz'mah) [*spiro-* + *plasma*] a genus of microorganisms of the family Spiroplasmataceae, order Mycoplasmatales, class Mollicutes, made up of helical organisms bounded by a membrane but lacking a true cell wall. The organisms are pathogens of plants and insects.

Spiroplasmataceae (spi"ro-plaz"ma-ta'se-e) a family of bacteria of the order Mycoplasmatales, class Mollicutes, made up of motile helical organisms that require sterol for growth. It contains the genus *Spiroplasma*.

Spiroptera neoplastica (spi-rop'ter-ah ne"o-plas'tĭ-kah) a nematode which produces gastric carcinoma in certain species of rats.

Spiroschaudinnia (spi"ro-shaw-din'e-ah) in former systems of classification, a genus of bacteria made up of organisms now assigned to the genera *Borrelia* and *Treponema*.

spiroscope (spi'ro-skōp) [L. *spirare* to breathe + Gr. *skopein* to examine] an apparatus for respiration exercises by which the patient can see the amount of water displaced in a given time and thus gauge his respiratory capacity.

spiroscopy (spi-ros'ko-pe) the use of the spiroscope.

Spirosoma (spi"ro-so'ma) [*spiro-*(1) + *soma*] a genus of nonmotile, gram-negative, straight to curved, rod-shaped bacteria of the family Spirosomaceae, occurring as helices or long coiled filaments; they are nonpathogens found in soil and fresh water. The type species is *S. lingua'le*.

Spirosomaceae (spi"ro-so-ma'se-e) a family of nonmotile or rarely motile, gram-negative, curved bacteria comprising the genera *Flectobacillus*, *Runella*, and *Spirosoma*.

spirosparta (spi"ro-spar'tah), pl. *spirospar'tae* [Gr. *speira* coil + *spartē* a rope] Fayod's name for one of the ropelike structures, formed by spirofibrillae, which constitute the protoplasm and nuclei of vegetable cells.

Spirotrichia (spi"ro-trik'e-ah) [*spiro-* + Gr. *thrix* hair] a subclass of ciliate protozoa (class Polyhymenophorea, phylum Ciliophora) having characters of the class. It comprises four orders: Heterotrichida, Odontostomatida, Oligotrichida, and Hypotrichida.

Spirotrichonympha (spi"ro-trik"o-nim'fah) [*spiro-* + *tricho-* + *nymph*] a genus of multiflagellated cellulose-digesting, parasitic protozoa (suborder Trichonymphina, order Hypermastigida) found in the termite gut, and characterized by the presence of flagella arranged in 12 to 40 spiral rows on the anterior end of the body.

Spiruroidea (spi"roo-roi'de-ah) a superfamily of phasmid nematodes, including the genera *Gnathostoma*, *Gongylonema*, *Habronema*, *Physaloptera*, *Physocephalus*, *Spirocerca*, and *Thelazia*.

spissated (spis'āt-ed) [L. *spissatus*] inspissated: thickened by evaporation.

spissitude (spis'ĭ-tūd) [L. *spissitudo*] the state or quality of being inspissated.

Spitzka's nucleus, tract (spits'kahz) [Edward Charles Spitzka, New York neurologist, 1852–1914] see *Perlia's nucleus*, under *nucleus*, and see *tractus dorsolateralis*.

Spitzka-Lissauer tract (column) (spits'kah lis'ow-er) [E. C. *Spitzka*; Heinrich *Lissauer*, German neurologist, 1861–1891] tractus dorsolateralis.

splanchnapophyseal (splank"nap-o-fiz'e-al) pertaining to a splanchnapophysis.

splanchnapophysis (splank"nah-pof'ĭ-sis) [*splanchno-* + *apophysis*] a skeletal element, like the lower jaw, connected with the alimentary canal.

splanchnectopia (splank"nek-to'pe-ah) [*splanchno-* + Gr. *ektopos* out of place + *-ia*] displacement of a viscus.

splanchnesthesia (splank"nes-the'ze-ah) [*splanchno-* + Gr. *aisthēsis* perception + *-ia*] visceral sensation.

splanchnesthetic (splank"nes-thet'ik) pertaining to splanchnesthesia.

splanchnic (splank'nik) [Gr. *splanchnikos*; L. *splanchnicus*] pertaining to the viscera.

splanchnicectomy (splank"ne-sek'to-me) [*splanchnic* + Gr. *ektomē* excision] excision of a section (resection) of the greater splanchnic nerve; splanchnic neurectomy.

splanchnicotomy (splank"ne-kot'o-me) [*splanchnic* + Gr. *tomē* a cutting] division of a splanchnic nerve.

splanchn(o)- [Gr. *splanchnos* viscus] a combining form denoting relationship to a viscus, or to the splanchnic nerve.

splanchnoblast (splank'no-blast) [*splanchno-* + Gr. *blastos* germ] the rudiment or anlage of any viscus.

splanchnocele (splank'no-sēl) [*splanchno-* + Gr. *kēlē* hernia] hernial protrusion of a viscus.

splanchnocoele (splank'no-sēl) [*splanchno-* + Gr. *koilos* hollow] that portion of the embryonic body cavity, or coelom, from which are developed the abdominal, pericardial, and pleural cavities; called also *pleuroperitoneal cavity*.

splanchnocranium (splank"no-kra'ne-um) [*splanchno-* + *cranium*] those parts of the skull that are of branchial arch origin.

splanchnoderm (splank'no-derm) splanchnopleure.

splanchnodiastasis (splank"no-di-as'tah-sis) [*splanchno-* + Gr. *diastasis* separation] separation of a viscus; displacement of a viscus.

splanchnography (splank-nog′rah-fe) [*splanchno-* + Gr. *graphein* to write] the descriptive anatomy of the viscera.

splanchnolith (splank′no-lith) [*splanchno-* + Gr. *lithos* stone] an intestinal calculus or concretion.

splanchnologia (splank″no-lo′je-ah) splanchnology; in NA terminology *splanchnologia* encompasses the nomenclature relating to the viscera.

splanchnology (splank-nol′o-je) [*splanchno-* + Gr. *logos* treatise] the scientific study of the viscera of the body; applied also to the body of knowledge relating thereto.

splanchnomegalia (splank″no-mĕ-ga′le-ah) splanchnomegaly.

splanchnomegaly (splank″no-meg′ah-le) [*splanchno-* + Gr. *megas* large] enlargement of the viscera; visceromegaly.

splanchnomicria (splank″no-mik′re-ah) [*splanchno-* + Gr. *mikros* small] abnormal smallness of the viscera.

splanchnopathy (splank-nop′ah-the) [*splanchno-* + Gr. *pathos* disease] disease of the abdominal viscera.

splanchnopleural (splank″no-ploor′al) pertaining to the splanchnopleure.

splanchnopleure (splank′no-ploor) [*splanchno-* + Gr. *pleura* side] the layer formed by the union of the splanchnic mesoderm with entoderm; from it are developed the muscles and the connective tissue of the digestive tube.

splanchnoptosis (splank″no-to′sis) [*splanchno-* + Gr. *ptosis* falling] the prolapse, or downward displacement, of the viscera; called also *visceroptosis*.

splanchnosclerosis (splank″no-skle-ro′sis) [*splanchno-* + Gr. *sklērōsis* hardening] induration of the viscera.

splanchnoscopy (splank-nos′ko-pe) [*splanchno-* + Gr. *skopein* to examine] inspection of the viscera by endoscopy.

splanchnoskeleton (splank″no-skel′e-ton) [*splanchno-* + Gr. *skeleton* a dried body, mummy] the totality of the skeletal structures connected with the viscera, especially the bony structure that forms within certain organs of animals, as in the gills, tongue, eye, penis, etc.

splanchnosomatic (splank″no-so-mat′ik) [*splanchno-* + Gr. *sōmatikos* of or for the body] pertaining to the viscera and the body proper.

splanchnotomy (splank-not′o-me) [*splanchno-* + Gr. *tomē* a cutting] the anatomy or dissection of the viscera.

splanchnotribe (splank′no-trīb) [*splanchno-* + Gr. *tribein* to crush] an instrument for crushing the intestine and so closing its lumen.

S-plasty in plastic surgery, a technique for distributing the contractile forces of wound healing in more than one direction by making an S-shaped incision, instead of a straight line, in areas where skin is loose.

splayfoot (spla′foot) flatfoot; talipes valgus.

spleen (splēn) [Gr. *splēn*; L. *splen*] a large glandlike but ductless organ situated in the upper part of the abdominal cavity on the left side and lateral to the cardiac end of the stomach. Called also *splen* [NA] and *lien* [NA alternative]. It is of a flattened oblong shape and about 125 mm. long, the largest structure in the lymphoid system; it has a purple color and a pliable consistency, and is distinguished by two types of tissue: red pulp and white pulp (see under *pulp*). It disintegrates the red blood cells and sets free the hemoglobin, which the liver converts into bilirubin; gives rise to new red blood cells during fetal life and in the newborn; serves as a reservoir of blood, produces lymphocytes and plasma cells, and has other important functions, the full scope of which is not entirely determined. **accessory s.**, splen accessorius. **bacon s.**, a spleen with areas of amyloid degeneration, giving its cut surfaces the appearance of fried bacon. **cyanotic s.**, a contracted form of spleen due to passive congestion. **diffuse waxy s.**, amyloid degeneration of the spleen involving especially the coats of the venous sinuses and the reticulum of the organ. **enlarged s.**, splenomegaly. **flecked s. of Feitis**, multiple necroses of the spleen, characterized by nonembolic multiple areas of anemic necrosis. **floating s.**, a spleen displaced and preternaturally movable; called also *wandering s.* **Gandy-Gamna s.**, siderotic splenomegaly. **hard-baked s.**, a condition of the spleen in Hodgkin's disease, marked by the presence of grayish areas resembling the diseased lymph nodes in structure. **lardaceous s.**, waxy s. **movable s.**, floating s. **porphyry s.**, a spleen which is the seat of nodular infiltration. **sago s.**, a spleen having on its cut surface

the appearance of grains of sago; due to amyloid infiltration. **speckled s.**, flecked s. of Feitis. **wandering s.**, floating s. **waxy s.**, a spleen affected with amyloid degeneration; called also *lardaceous s.*

splen (splen) [Gr. *splēn*] a large glandlike but ductless organ situated in the upper part of the abdominal cavity; see *spleen*. Called also *lien* [NA alternative]. **s. accesso′rius** [NA], accessory spleen: a connected or detached outlying portion, or exclave, of the spleen; called also *lien accessorius* [NA alternative].

splenadenoma (splēn″ad-ĕ-no′mah) [*splen-* + Gr. *adēn* gland + *-oma*] hyperplasia of the spleen pulp.

splenalgia (sple-nal′je-ah) [*splen-* + Gr. *algos* pain + *-ia*] neuralgic pain in the spleen.

splenatrophy (splen-at′ro-fe) atrophy of the spleen.

splenauxe (sple-nawk′se) [*splen-* + Gr. *auxē* increase] splenomegaly.

splenceratosis (splen″ser-ah-to′sis) splenokeratosis.

splenculus (spleng′ku-lus) [L. "little spleen"] an accessory spleen, or splenic exclave.

splenectasis (sple-nek′tah-sis) [*splen-* + Gr. *ektasis* enlargement] splenomegaly.

splenectomize (sple-nek′to-mīz) to remove the spleen.

splenectomy (sple-nek′to-me) [*splen-* + Gr. *ektomē* excision] excision or extirpation of the spleen.

splenectopia (sple-nek-to′pe-ah) [*splen-* + Gr. *ek* out + *topos* place + *-ia*] displacement of the spleen; wandering or floating spleen.

splenectopy (sple-nek′to-pe) splenectopia.

splenelcosis (sple″nel-ko′sis) [*splen-* + Gr. *helkōsis* ulceration] ulceration of the spleen.

splenemia (sple-ne′me-ah) [*splen-* + Gr. *haima* blood + *-ia*] congestion of the spleen with blood.

splenemphraxis (sple″nem-frak′sis) [*splen-* + Gr. *emphraxis* stoppage] congestion of the spleen.

spleneolus (sple-ne′o-lus) accessory spleen.

splenetic (sple-net′ik) affected with splenic disorder; ill humored.

splenial (sple′ne-al) pertaining to the splenium or to the splenius muscle.

splenic (splen′ik) [Gr. *splēnikos*; L. *splenicus*] pertaining to the spleen; lienal.

splenicterus (splen-ik′ter-us) [*splen-* + Gr. *ikteros* jaundice] inflammation of the spleen associated with jaundice.

splenification (splen″i-fi-ka′shun) splenization.

spleniform (splen′i-form) resembling the spleen.

spleniserrate (splen″i-ser′āt) pertaining to the splenius and the serratus muscles.

splenitis (sple-ni′tis) [*splen-* + *-itis*] inflammation of the spleen, a condition usually produced by pyemia. It is attended by enlargement of the organ with pus, and is marked by much local pain. **spodogenous s.**, that due to accumulation of foreign particles in the spleen.

splenium (sple′ne-um) [L.; Gr. *splēnion*] a bandlike structure; a bandage or compress. **s. cor′ poris callo′si** [NA], the posterior rounded end of the corpus callosum.

splenization (splen″i-za′shun) that condition of a part, especially the lung, in which it has the appearance of the tissue of the spleen, owing to engorgement and condensation. **hypostatic s.**, splenization produced by hypostatic pneumonia.

splen(o)- [Gr. *splēn* spleen] a combining form denoting relationship to the spleen.

splenoblast (sple′no-blast) the cell from which a splenocyte develops.

splenocele (sple′no-sēl) [*spleno-* + Gr. *kēlē* hernia] hernia of the spleen.

splenoceratosis (sple″no-ser″ah-to′sis) splenokeratosis.

splenocleisis (sple″no-kli′sis) [*spleno-* + Gr. *kleisis* closure] irritation of the surface of the spleen to induce the development of new fibrous tissue.

splenocolic (sple″no-kol′ik) [*spleno-* + Gr. *kolon* colon] pertaining to the spleen and colon.

splenocyte (splen′o-sīt) the monocyte characteristic of the spleen.

splenodynia (sple″no-din′e-ah) [*spleno-* + Gr. *odynē* pain + *-ia*] pain in the spleen.

splenogenous (sple-noj′ĕ-nus) arising in or formed by the spleen.

splenogram (sple′no-gram) 1. a roentgenogram of the spleen. 2. a differential count of the cells found in a stained preparation of material obtained by splenic puncture.

splenography (sple-nog′rah-fe) [*spleno-* + Gr. *graphein* to write] 1. roentgenography of the spleen. 2. a description of the spleen.

splenohepatomegalia (sple″no-hep″ah-to-me-ga′le-ah) splenohepatomegaly.

splenohepatomegaly (sple″no-hep″ah-to-meg′ah-le) [*spleno-* + Gr. *hēpar* liver + *megas* large] enlargement of the spleen and liver.

splenoid (sple′noid) [*spleno-* + Gr. *eidos* form] resembling the spleen.

splenokeratosis (sple″no-ker″ah-to′sis) [*spleno-* + Gr. *keras* horn + *-osis*] hardening of the spleen.

splenolaparotomy (sple″no-lap″ah-rot′o-me) laparosplenotomy.

splenology (sple-nol′o-je) [*spleno-* + *-logy*] the sum of knowledge regarding the spleen, its functions and diseases.

splenolymphatic (sple″no-lim-fat′ik) pertaining to the spleen and lymph nodes.

splenolysin (sple-nol′ĭ-sin) [*spleno-* + Gr. *lyein* to dissolve] a lysin destructive to splenic tissue.

splenolysis (sple-nol′ĭ-sis) destruction of spleen tissue.

splenoma (sple-no′mah), pl. *splenomas* or *spleno′mata* [*spleno-* + *-oma*] a tumor of the spleen.

splenomalacia (sple″no-mah-la′she-ah) [*spleno-* + Gr. *malakia* softness] abnormal softness of the spleen; softening of the spleen.

splenomedullary (sple″no-med′u-ler″e) of or pertaining to the spleen and bone marrow.

splenomegalia (sple″no-me-ga′le-ah) splenomegaly.

splenomegaly (sple″no-meg′ah-le) [*spleno-* + Gr. *megas* large] enlargement of the spleen. **congestive s.,** enlargement of the spleen occurring secondary to portal hypertension, with ascites, anemia, thrombocytopenia, leukopenia, and episodic hemorrhage from the gastrointestinal tract. Called also *Banti's syndrome.* See also *Banti's disease,* under *disease.* **Egyptian s.,** that caused by *Schistosoma mansoni.* **Gaucher's s.,** see under *disease.* **hemolytic s.,** hemolytic anemia. **infective s., infectious s.,** splenomegaly associated with an infection. **myelophthisic s.,** enlargement of the spleen marked by decrease in myeloid tissue and by fibrosis. **siderotic s.,** splenomegaly characterized by marked fibrosis with deposit of iron and calcium (Gamna nodules); called also *Gandy-Gamna disease.* **spodogenous s.,** enlargement of the spleen attributed to accumulation of erythrocytes in the organ. **thrombophlebitic s.,** Opitz's disease. **tropical s.,** the classic form of visceral leishmaniasis. Cf. *tropical splenomegaly syndrome,* under *syndrome.*

splenometry (sple-nom′ĕ-tre) determination of the size of the spleen.

splenomyelogenous (sple″no-mi″ĕ-loj′ĕ-nus) formed in the spleen and bone marrow; splenomedullary.

splenomyelomalacia (sple″no-mi″ĕ-lo-mah-la′she-ah) [*spleno-* + Gr. *myelos* marrow + *malakia* softening] softening of the spleen and bone marrow.

splenoncus (sple-nong′kus) [*spleno-* + Gr. *onkos* bulk, mass] tumor of the spleen.

splenonephric (sple″no-nef′rik) pertaining to the spleen and the kidney.

splenonephroptosis (sple″no-nef′rop-to′sis) [*spleno-* + Gr. *nephros* kidney + *ptōsis* falling] downward displacement of the spleen and kidney on the same side.

splenopancreatic (sple″no-pan″kre-at′ik) pertaining to the spleen and the pancreas.

splenoparectasis (sple″no-pah-rek′tah-sis) [*spleno-* + Gr. *parektasis* extension] excessive enlargement of the spleen.

splenopathy (sple-nop′ah-the) [*spleno-* + Gr. *pathos* disease] any disease of the spleen.

splenopexy (sple′no-pek″se) [*spleno-* + Gr. *pexis* fixation] surgical fixation of a mobile spleen.

splenophrenic (splen-o-fren′ik) [*spleno-* + Gr. *phrēn* diaphragm] pertaining to the spleen and diaphragm.

splenopneumonia (splen″o-nu-mo′ne-ah) pneumonia attended with splenization of the lung.

splenoportography (sple″no-por-tog′rah-fe) splenic portography.

splenoptosia (sple″nop-to′se-ah) splenoptosis.

splenoptosis (sple″nop-to′sis) [*spleno-* + Gr. *ptōsis* falling] prolapse or downward displacement of the spleen.

splenorenal (sple″no-re′nal) pertaining to the spleen and kidney, or to splenic and renal veins.

splenorrhagia (sple″no-ra′je-ah) [*spleno-* + Gr. *rhegnynai* to burst forth] hemorrhage from the spleen.

splenorrhaphy (sple-nor′ah-fe) [*spleno-* + Gr. *rhaphē* suture] surgical repair of the spleen.

splenosis (sple-no′sis) a condition in which multiple implants of splenic tissue are present throughout the peritoneal cavity.

splenotomy (sple-not′o-me) [*spleno-* + Gr. *tomē* a cutting] surgical incision of the spleen.

splenotoxin (sple″no-tok′sin) a toxin produced by or acting on the spleen.

splenulus (splen′u-lus), pl. *sple′nuli* [L.] little spleen; an accessory spleen.

splenunculus (sple-nung′ku-lus) lienunculus.

splicing (spli′sing) [Middle Dutch *splissen*] in genetics, the removal (splicing out) of introns and joining (splicing together) of exons during transcription of a gene.

splint (splint) 1. a rigid or flexible appliance used to maintain in position a displaced or movable part or to keep in place and protect an injured part. 2. the act of fastening or confining with a splint a displaced or movable part, or the support or bracing of such a part. **abutment s.,** adja-

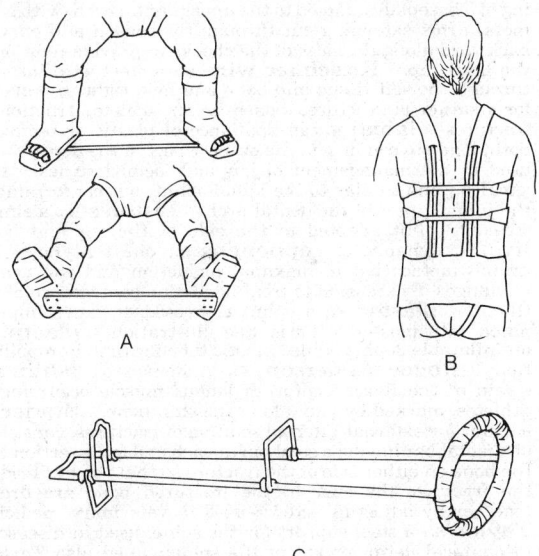

Splints: *A,* Denis Browne splint; *B,* Taylor splint; *C,* Thomas knee splint.

cent tooth restorations that have been rigidly united at their proximal contact areas to form a single abutment with multiple roots. **airplane s.,** one which holds the arm in abduction. **anchor s.,** a splint for fracture of the jaw, with metal loops fitting over the teeth and held together by a rod. **Anderson s.,** a splint for external internal fixation of fractures: two or more long screws, Kirschner wire, or nails are inserted through the tissues into the bone above and below the fracture; each group of screws, wires or nails is attached to an external plate and the plates are joined by an adjustable screw. **Angle's s.,** a splint for fracture of the mandible; see illustration. **Asch s.,** a splint used in operations on the nose. **Balkan s.,** see under *frame.* **banjo traction s.,** a splint for the fingers constructed from a steel rod shaped like a banjo. **cap s.,** a plastic or metallic fracture or stabilization appliance designed to cover the crowns of the teeth and usually cemented in place. **Chatfield-Girdleston s.,** an apparatus for enabling a paralyzed poliomyelitis patient with bilateral deltoid paralysis to walk with crutches. **coaptation s's,** small splints adjusted about a fractured limb for the purpose of producing coaptation of fragments. **Cramer's s.,** a flexible wire splint consisting of parallel stout wires between which smaller wires are stretched like the rungs of a ladder. **Denis Browne s.,** a splint consisting of a pair of metal foot splints joined by a cross bar; used in talipes equinovarus. See illustration. **dynamic s.,** a support or protective apparatus for the hand or any other part of the body which also aids in initiating and performing motion of that part or adjacent parts and assists in dealing with the forces resulting from the action, thus assisting in those motions necessary to perform the activities of daily living. **Essig-type s.,** a stainless steel wire passed labially and lingually around a segment of the dental arch and held in position by individual ligature wires around the contact areas of the teeth; used to stabilize fractured or repositioned teeth. **fracture s.,** 1. a device fabricated of metal or plastic and used to fix segments in the treatment of fractures or facial deformities. 2. a plastic material contoured to the lingual and buccal-labial aspects of the teeth and fixed with wire or cement. **Frejka pillow s.,** one used for maintaining abduction and flexion of the femurs in congenital dislocation of the hip. **functional s.,** dynamic s. **Gilmer's s.,** a stainless steel wire fastening for holding the lower teeth to the upper ones in fracture of the mandible. **Gunning's s.,** an interdental splint used in treating fractured mandible or maxilla. **Hodgen s.,** one similar to the Thomas splint with only half a ring; used for fracture of the femur below the upper third. **interdental s.,** one for fracture of the jaws, held in place by wires passed around the teeth. **Keller-Blake s.,** a hinged half-ring modification of the Thomas splint for fracture of the femur. **Kingsley s.,** one used for jaw fractures, consisting of a baseplate adapted to the upper dental arch, with stout metal arms extending out through the mouth and curving backward along the sides of the cheeks to provide fixation to the head cap. **Kirschner wire s.,** a steel wire inserted through the soft tissue into bone and held tight in a clamp; for fixation of fractured bones or for skeletal traction in fractures. **labial s.,** an appliance of plastic or metal, or both, made to conform to the outer aspect of the dental arch; used in the management of jaw and facial injuries. **lingual s.,** one similar to the labial splint, but conforming to the inner aspect of the dental arch. **Liston's s.,** a simple straight splint adapted to the side of the leg and body. **live s.,** dynamic s. **opponens s.,** one that holds the thumb metacarpal in maximal abduction and the thumb phalanges in extension to treat adduction contracture of the thumb. **plaster s.,** a splint composed of gauze impregnated with plaster of Paris. See illustration. **plastic s.,** an inflatable double-walled plastic tube for limb immobilization. **Roger Anderson s.,** Anderson s. **shin s's,** strain of the flexor digitorum longus muscle occurring in athletes, marked by pain along the shin bone. **Stader s.,** a splint for external-internal fixation of fractures, consisting of a metal bar having a steel pin at each end for insertion into the bone on either side of the fracture so that the bar bridges the fracture; the ends of the fractured bone are drawn together by adjusting screws; used in veterinary medicine. **Taylor s.,** a steel support for the spine, used in disease or mechanical derangement of the spine; called also *Taylor's apparatus* and *Taylor brace.* See illustration. **therapeutic s.,** dynamic s. **Thomas s.,** a leg splint consisting of two rigid rods attached to an ovoid ring that fits around the thigh; it can be combined with other apparatus to provide traction. See illustration. **Tobruk s.,** an immobilizing split plaster cast applied from the foot to the groin, with skin traction tapes through openings in the plaster and connected with a Thomas splint. It was used in the North African campaign of World War II. **Toronto s.,** 1. a splint for poliomyelitis cases in which adjustable splints for the arms and legs are used with and attached to a Bradford frame. 2. a splinting catheter for use in the ureter after plastic operation.

splinter (splin′ter) 1. a small slender fragment, as a piece of fractured bone. 2. to break into small fragments.

splinting (splint′ing) 1. application of a splint, or treatment by use of a splint. 2. in dentistry, the application of a fixed restoration to join two or more teeth into a single rigid unit. 3. rigidity of muscles occurring as a means of avoiding pain caused by movement of a part.

splints (splintz) a condition characterized by the development of exostoses on the rudimentary second or fourth metacarpal or metarsal bone in the horse.

splitting (split′ing) 1. the division of a single object into two or more objects or parts. 2. in psychoanalytic theory, a primitive defense mechanism, characteristic of very young children and of patients with psychotic or borderline personalities, in which "objects" (persons) possessing a natural mix of positive and negative attributes are perceived as being either "all good" or "all bad." **s. of heart sounds,** the presence of two components in the first or second heart sound complexes; used chiefly to denote the separation of the elements of the second sound, which is related to closure of the aortic and pulmonary semilunar valves. **sagittal s. of mandible,** intraoral osteotomy of the ascending mandibular ramus and posterior body of the mandible in the sagittal plane for correction of prognathism, retrognathism, or open bite; an alternative procedure confines the split to the body of the mandible.

spodiomyelitis (spo″de-o-mi″ĕ-li′tis) [Gr. *spodios* ash colored + *myelos* marrow + *-itis*] acute anterior poliomyelitis.

spod(o)- [Gr. *spodos* ashes] a combining form denoting relation to waste materials.

spodogenous (spo-doj′ĕ-nus) [*spodo-* + Gr. *gennan* to produce] pertaining to or caused by waste materials in an organ.

spodogram (spod′o-gram) [*spodo-* + Gr. *gramma* a mark] the pattern created by the ash after incineration of a minute amount of tissue or other material; called also *ash picture.*

spodography (spo-dog′rah-fe) [*spodo-* + Gr. *graphein* to write] the incineration of a minute quantity of tissue and observation of the ashes (spodogram) under a dark-field microscope, as a means of studying the mineral constituents of the cells.

spondee (spon′de) any word (e.g., pancake) of two syllables having equal stress on each syllable; used in tests of speech reception threshold.

spondylalgia (spon″dĭ-lal′je-ah) pain in a vertebra.

spondylarthritis (spon″dil-ar-thri′tis) [*spondyl-* + Gr. *arthron* joint + *-itis*] arthritis of the spine. **s. ankylopoiet′ica,** rheumatoid s.

spondylarthrocace (spon″dil-ar-throk′ah-se) [*spondyl-* + Gr. *arthron* joint + *kakē* badness] tuberculosis of the vertebrae.

spondylexarthrosis (spon″dil-eks″ar-thro′sis) [*spondyl-* + Gr. *exarthrōsis* dislocation] dislocation of a vertebra.

spondylitic (spon″dĭ-lit′ik) pertaining to or characterized by spondylitis.

spondylitis (spon″dĭ-li′tis) inflammation of the vertebrae. **s. ankylopoiet′ica, s. ankylo′sans, ankylosing s.,** rheumatoid s. **Bekhterev's s.,** rheumatoid s. **s. defor′mans,** rheumatoid s. **hypertrophic s.,** spondylitis with evidences of hypertrophic changes in the vertebrae. **s. infectio′sa,** inflammation of the vertebrae caused by a specific pathogen. **Kümmell's s.,** see under *disease.* **Marie-Strümpell s.,** rheumatoid s. **muscular s.,** a morbid condition of the spine resulting from muscular weakness and not a true inflammation. **post-traumatic s.,** Kümmell's disease. **rheumatoid s.,** the form of rheumatoid arthritis that affects the spine. It is a systemic illness of unknown etiology, affecting young males predominantly, and producing pain and stiffness as a result of inflammation of the sacroiliac, intervertebral, and costovertebral joints; paraspinal calcification, with ossification and ankylosis of the spinal joints, may cause complete rigidity of the spine and thorax. Called also *Bekhterev's disease* and *Marie-Strümpell disease.* **rhizomelic s., s. rhizome′lica, s. rhizomélique′,** rheumatoid s. **traumatic s.,** spondylitis occurring as a result of injury to the vertebrae. **s. tuberculo′sa, tuberculous s.,** tuberculosis of the spine. **s. typho′sa,** inflammation of the vertebrae following typhoid fever.

spondylizema (spon″dĭ-li-ze′mah) [*spondyl-* + Gr. *izēmia* depression] downward displacement of a vertebra in consequence of the destruction or softening of the one below it.

spondyl(o)- [Gr. *spondylos* vertebra] combining form denoting relationship to a vertebra, or to the spinal column.

spondyloarthropathy (spon″dĭ-lo-ar-throp′ah-the) disease of the joints of the spine.

spondylocace (spon″dĭ-lok′ah-se) [*spondylo-* + Gr. *kakē* badness] tuberculosis of the vertebrae.

spondylodidymia (spon″dĭ-lo-di-dim′e-ah) [*spondylo-* + Gr. *didymos* twin + *-ia*] teratic union of twins by the vertebrae.

spondylodymus (spon″dĭ-lod′ĭ-mus) twin fetuses united by the vertebrae.

spondylodynia (spon″dĭ-lo-din′e-ah) [*spondyl-* + Gr. *odynē* pain + *-ia*] pain in a vertebra.

spondylolisthesis (spon″dĭ-lo-lis′the-sis) [*spondyl-* + Gr. *olisthanein* to slip] forward displacement of one vertebra over another, usually of the fifth lumbar over the body of the sacrum, or of the fourth lumbar over the fifth, usually due to a developmental defect in the pars interarticularis.

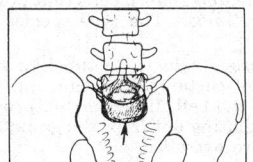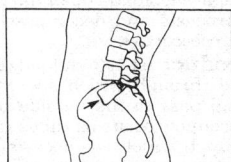

Spondylolisthesis of the fifth lumbar vertebra over the sacrum.

spondylolisthetic (spon″dĭ-lo-lis-thet′ik) pertaining to or caused by spondylolisthesis.

spondylolysis (spon″dĭ-lol′ĭ-sis) [*spondylo-* + Gr. *lysis* dissolution] dissolution of a vertebra; a condition marked by platyspondylia, aplasia of the vertebral arch, and separation of the pars interarticularis.

spondylomalacia (spon″dĭ-lo-mah-la′she-ah) softening of vertebrae. **s. traumat′ica,** Kümmell's disease.

spondylopathy (spon″dĭ-lop′ah-the) [*spondylo-* + Gr. *pathos* disease] any disorder of the vertebrae. **traumatic s.,** Kümmell's disease.

spondyloptosis (spon″dĭ-lo-to′sis) spondylolisthesis.

spondylopyosis (spon″dĭ-lo-pi-o′sis) [*spondylo-* + Gr. *pyōsis* suppuration] suppuration of a vertebra or of vertebrae.

spondyloschisis (spon″dĭ-los′kĭ-sis) [*spondylo-* + Gr. *schisis* fissure] congenital fissure of a vertebral arch.

spondylosis (spon″dĭ-lo′sis) ankylosis of a vertebral joint; also, a general term for degenerative changes due to osteoarthritis. **cervical s.,** degenerative joint disease affecting the cervical vertebrae, intervertebral disks, and surrounding ligaments and connective tissue, sometimes with pain or paresthesia radiating down the arms as a result of pressure on the nerve roots. **s. chron′ica ankylopoiet′ica, rhizomelic s.,** rheumatoid spondylitis. **lumbar s.,** degenerative joint disease affecting the lumbar vertebrae and intervertebral disks, causing pain and stiffness, sometimes with sciatic radiation due to nerve root pressure by associated protruding disks or osteophytes. **s. uncovertebra′lis,** cervical spondylosis affecting the uncinate process of a vertebra.

spondylosyndesis (spon″dĭ-lo-sin′de-sis) [*spondylo-* + Gr. *syndesis* a binding together] spinal fusion.

spondylotherapy (spon″dĭ-lo-ther′ah-pe) [*spondylo-* + Gr. *therapeia* treatment] treatment by physical methods applied to the spinal region; spinal therapeutics.

spondylotic (spon″dĭ-lot′ik) pertaining to or due to spondylosis.

spondylotomy (spon″dĭ-lot′o-me) [*spondylo-* + Gr. *temnein* to cut] rachitomy.

spondylous (spon′dĭ-lus) pertaining to a vertebra; vertebral.

sponge (spunj) [L., Gr. *spongia*] 1. the elastic fibrous skeleton of certain marine animals; used mainly as an absorbent. 2. an absorbent pad of folded gauze or cotton. **Bernays' s.,** compressed disks of cotton which expand under moisture; used in checking epistaxis. **fibrin s.,** a spongy form of fibrin, used as a hemostatic. **gelatin s.,** a spongy form of denatured gelatin used as a hemostatic, especially when wet with thrombin. **gelatin s., absorbable** [USP], a ster-

ile, absorbable, water-insoluble gelatin-base sponge; used as a local hemostatic.

spongeitis (spon″je-i′tis) spongiitis.

spongia (spon′je-ah) [L., from Gr.] sponge.

spongiform (spon′jĭ-form) [L. *spongia* sponge + *forma* shape] resembling a sponge.

spongiitis (spon″je-i′tis) inflammation of the corpus spongiosum of the penis; periurethritis.

spongin (spon′jin) a horny, albuminoid material forming the basis of sponge.

spongi(o)- [L., *spongia* sponge] a combining form meaning like a sponge, or denoting relationship to a sponge.

spongioblast (spun′je-o-blast″) [*spongio-* + *blast* (def. 1)] 1. any of the embryonic epithelial cells, developed about the neural tube, which become transformed, some into neuroglial and some into ependymal cells. 2. amacrine cell; see under *cell*.

spongioblastoma (spun″je-o-blas-to′mah) a tumor containing spongioblasts; gliosarcoma or glioblastoma. **s. multifor′me,** one in which the cells are of various forms of arrangements; called also *glioma multiforme*. **s. unipola′re,** one in which the spongioblasts are mostly unipolar.

spongiocyte (spun′je-o-sīt″) 1. a neuroglial cell. 2. one of the cells with spongy vacuolated protoplasm in the cortex of the suprarenal gland.

spongiocytoma (spun″je-o-si-to′mah) spongioblastoma.

spongioid (spun′je-oid) [*spongio-* + Gr. *eidos* form] resembling a sponge in structure or appearance.

spongioplasm (spun′je-o-plazm) [*spongio-* + Gr. *plasma* anything formed or molded] 1. a substance which forms the network of fibrils pervading the cell substance and forming the reticulum of the fixed cell. 2. the granular material of an axon.

spongiosa (spon″je-o′sah) [L.] spongy; sometimes used alone to mean the substantia spongiosa ossium.

spongiosaplasty (spon″je-o″sah-plas′te) autoplasty of the substantia spongiosa ossium to potentiate formation of new bone or to cover bone defects.

spongiosis (spun″je-o′sis) intercellular edema of the spongy layer (malpighian layer) of the skin.

spongiositis (spun″je-o-si′tis) inflammation of the corpus spongiosum of the penis.

spongiotic (spon″je-ot′ik) pertaining to or characterized by spongiosis.

spongosterol (spon-gos′ter-ol) a mono-unsaturated sterol, 24α-methyl-22-cholestene-3β-ol, found in certain sponges.

spongy (spun′je) of a spongelike appearance or texture.

spontaneous (spon-ta′ne-us) [L. *spontaneus*] 1. voluntary; instinctive. 2. occurring without external influence.

Spontin (spon′tin) trademark for a lyophilized preparation of ristocetins A and B.

spool (spool) a tubular surgical instrument around which suture material is usually wound.

spoon (spoon) 1. a metallic instrument with an oval bowl to which a handle is attached. 2. spoon excavator. **Daviel's s.,** an instrument used in removing the crystalline lens from the eye. **excavator s.,** a spoon-shaped dental excavator. **sharp s.,** a surgical instrument consisting of a spoon with sharp edges for scraping away granulations. **test s.,** a small spoon with a spatula-like handle for taking up small quantities of a powder, etc., in chemical experiments. **Volkmann's s.,** sharp s.

sporadic (spo-rad′ik) [Gr. *sporadikos* scattered; L. *sporadicus*] neither endemic nor epidemic; occurring occasionally in a random or isolated manner.

sporadin (spor′ah-din) 1. a gregarine gamont without an epimerite or mucron that is free-living in the host's gut. 2. a mature trophozoite.

sporadoneure (spo-rad′o-nūr) [Gr. *sporadikos* sporadic + *neuron* nerve] an isolated nerve cell occurring in any of the tissues.

Sporadotrichina (spo″rah-do-trī-ki′nah) [Gr. *sporas* scattered + *thrix* hair] a suborder of mostly free-living ciliate protozoa (order Hypotrichida, subclass Spirotricha) having a body that is often ovoid to elliptical, and nonaligned cirri that are typically heavy and conspicuous and occur in isolated groups in specific regions on the ventral surface.

sporangia (spo-ran′je-ah) plural of *sporangium*.

sporangial (spo-ran′je-al) pertaining to a sporangium.

sporangiophore (spo-ran′je-o-fōr) [*sporangium* + Gr. *phoros* bearing] a specialized hypha that gives rise to a sporangium.

sporangiospore (spo-ran′je-o-spōr) a spore contained in a sporangium.

sporangium (spo-ran′je-um), pl. *sporan′gia* [*spore* + Gr. *angeion* vessel] a fungal or protozoal cell that produces spores internally by a series of progressive cleavages.

sporation (spo-ra′shun) sporulation.

spore (spōr) [L. *spora*, Gr. *spora* seed] 1. a refractile, oval body formed within bacteria, especially genera of the family Bacillaceae (*Bacillus, Clostridium, Desulfotomaculum, Sporolactobacillus, Sporosarcina*), which is regarded as a resting stage during the life history of the cell, and is characterized by its resistance to environmental changes. Called also *bacterial s.* 2. the reproductive element, produced sexually or asexually, of one of the lower organisms, such as protozoa, fungi, algae, etc. Spores arising as a result of a nonsexual process include: *conidia*, which are deciduous and develop from the hyphae by budding; *aleuriospores*, which are nondeciduous and also develop from the hyphae by budding; *endospores*, which are formed in the interior of special spore cases called *sporangia*; *zoospores*, which are flagellated motile spores formed in cases known as *zoosporangia*; and *chlamydospores*, which are resting spores, with thick walls, produced by enlargement of special cells. Those arising as a result of a sexual process include: *ascospores*, which are contained in special spore cases called *asci*; *basidiospores*, which are formed at the ends of club-shaped structures called *basidia*; *zygospores*, which are formed by conjugation between two morphologically identical cells, or from the fusion of like gametangia; and *oospores*, which are formed by heterogamous fertilization. See also *sporulation*. **asexual s.,** a spore produced by various

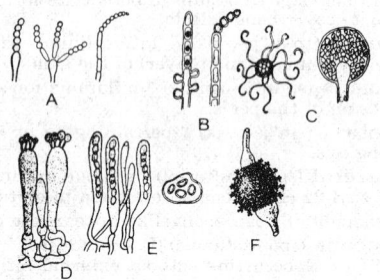

Various types of spores in fungi: *A*, conidiospores; *B*, chlamydospores; *C*, sporangiospores; *D*, basidiospores; *E*, ascospores; *F*, zygospores.

methods, but not involving a sexual process. **bacterial s.,** see *spore*, def. 1. **black s's of Ross,** pigmented malarial oocysts in the stomach wall of a mosquito. **swarm s.,** a spore made up of numerous active motile individuals; a zoospore.

sporetia (spo-re′she-ah) that part of the extranuclear chromatin of a cell that is concerned in the reproductive function of the cell.

Sporichthya (spo-rik′the-ah) [*sporo-* + Gr. *ichthys* fish] a genus of bacteria of the family Streptomycetaceae, order Actinomycetales, consisting of soil organisms forming an aerial mycelium and producing spores that become motile in water. The type species is *S. polymor′pha*.

sporicidal (spo″rĭ-si′dal) [*spore* + L. *caedere* to kill] destroying spores.

sporicide (spo′rĭ-sīd) an agent that destroys spores.

sporidesmin (spōr″ĭ-des′min) a poisonous substance isolated from the fungus *Pithomyces chartarum* (class Deuteromycetes), which causes facial eczema and liver damage in sheep and cattle in New Zealand and Australia.

sporiferous (spo-rif′er-us) [*spore* + L. *ferre* to bear] producing or bearing spores.

sporiparous (spo-rip′ah-rus) [*spore* + L. *parere* to produce] producing spores.

spor(o)- [Gr. *sporos* seed] a combining form denoting relationship to a spore.

sporoagglutination (spo″ro-ah-gloo″tĭ-na′shun) agglutination of spores in the diagnosis of sporotrichosis.

sporoblast (spor′o-blast) [*sporo-* + Gr. *blastos* germ] 1. an immature coccidian sporozoit. 2. a mass of spore-forming cells within a pansporoblastic membrane.

sporocyst (spor′o-sist) [*sporo-* + *cyst*] 1. any cyst, envelope, or sac containing spores or reproductive cells. 2. a germinal saclike stage in the life cycle of digenetic trematodes produced by metamorphosis of a miracidium and giving rise to rediae. 3. a stage in the life cycle of certain coccidian protozoa contained within an oocyst, produced by a sporoblast, and giving rise to sporozoites.

Sporocytophaga (spo″ro-si-to′fah-gah) [*sporo-* + Gr. *phagein* to eat] a genus of gliding bacteria of the family Cytophagaceae, made up of flexible, rod-shaped cells that produce microcysts and decompose cellulose. The type species is *S. myxococcoi′des.*

sporoduct (spor′o-dukt) [*sporo-* + *duct*] a tubelike structure through which spores of certain sporozoan and some fungi pass to the outside of the cell. In gregarine protozoa sporoducts occur as tubes radiating out from the gametocyst through which the oocysts are extruded.

sporogenesis (spor′o-jen′ĕ-sis) [*sporo-* + Gr. *genesis* production] the formation of or reproduction by spores; sporulation.

sporogenic (spo″ro-jen′ik) capable of developing into or producing spores.

sporogenous (spo-roj′ĕ-nus) [*sporo-* + Gr. *gennan* to produce] reproduced by spores.

sporogeny (spo-roj′ĕ-ne) [*sporo-* + Gr. *gennan* to produce] the development of spores.

sporogony (spo-rog′o-ne) [*sporo-* + Gr. *goneia* generation] sporulation involving multiple fission of a sporont (schizogony), resulting in the production of sporocysts (if present in the life cycle) and sporozoites. See also *sporulation*.

Sporolactobacillus (spo″ro-lak″to-bah-sil′us) [*sporo-* + L. *lac* milk + *bacillus* small rod] a genus of endospore-forming, rod-shaped bacteria of the family Bacillaceae, occurring as microaerophilic, gram-positive organisms that do not contain heme compounds. The type species is *S. inuli′nus.*

sporont (spo′ront) [*sporo-* + Gr. *ōn, ontos* being] a zygote of coccidian protozoa enclosed within an oocyst, which undergoes sporogony to produce sporoblasts, each of which forms a sporocyst containing sporozoites.

sporophore (spo′ro-fōr) [*sporo-* + Gr. *phorein* to bear] that part of an organism that supports the spores.

sporophyte (spo′ro-fīt) [*sporo-* + Gr. *phyton* plant] the diploid or asexual stage in the antithetic alternation of generation.

sporoplasm (spo′ro-plazm) [*sporo-* + Gr. *plasma* anything formed or molded] 1. the protoplasm of spores. 2. the central dinucleate mass of cytoplasm of certain protozoa that leaves the spore through the polar tube as an amebula to infect the host.

sporoplasmic (spo″ro-plaz′mik) pertaining to or of the nature of sporoplasm.

Sporosarcina (spo″ro-sar-si′nah) [*sporo-* + L. *sarcina* bundle] a genus of endospore-forming coccoid bacteria of the family Bacillaceae, made up of gram-positive aerobic cells occurring in tetrads and packets. The type species is *S. u′reae.*

Sporothrix (spo′ro-thriks) a genus of imperfect fungi of the family Moniliaceae, order Moniliales. *S. schenck′ii* (formerly called *Sporotrichum schenckii*) causes sporotrichosis, and many species, including *S. car′nis*, cause the formation of white mold on meat in cold storage.

sporotrichin (spo-rot′rĭ-kin) a derivative of *Sporothrix schenkii* used as a skin test in the diagnosis of sporotrichosis.

sporotrichosis (spo″ro-tri-ko′sis) [*sporo-* + Gr. *thrix* hair + *-osis*] a chronic fungal infection due to *Sporothrix schenchii*, most commonly characterized by nodular lesions of the cutaneous and subcutaneous tissues and adjacent lymphatics that suppurate, ulcerate, and drain, and acquired by implantation into the skin, traumatic or through an abrasion, or by inhalation into the lungs of *S. schenchii*. The infection may remain localized or it may be disseminated by the bloodstream to involve the osteoarticular and musculoskeletal tissues, viscera, mucous membranes, central nervous system, eye, and genitourinary system.

sporotrichotic (spo″ro-tri-kot′ik) 1. pertaining to or caused by fungi of the genus *Sporothrix*. 2. pertaining to sporotrichosis.

Sporotrichum (spo-rot′rĭ-kum) [*sporo-* + Gr. *thrix* hair] a genus of soil-inhabiting imperfect fungi of the family Moniliaceae, order Moniliales, which formerly included the etiologic agent of sporotrichosis. See *Sporothrix*.

Sporozoa (spo″ro-zo′ah) [*sporo-* + Gr. *zōon* animal] 1. Sporozoea. 2. in some former systems of classification, a subphylum and in others a class of protozoa, the members of which have been assigned to four phyla: Apicocomplexa, Acetospora, Microspora, and Myxozoa. The organisms in the last three phyla form spores; many of the Apicocomplexa do not. 3. Apicocomplexa.

sporozoa (spo″ro-zo′ah) plural of *sporozoon*.

sporozoan (spo″ro-zo′an) [*sporo-* + Gr. *zōon* animal] 1. any protozoan of the phyla Apicocomplexa (especially those of the class Sporozoea), Ascetospora, Microspora, and Myxozoa. Called also *sporozoon*. 2. pertaining or relating to protozoa of the phyla Apicocomplexa, Ascetospora, Microspora, and Myxozoa.

Sporozoea (spo″ro-zo′e-ah) a class of homoxenous or heteroxenous parasitic protozoa (phylum Apicocomplexa) having a conoid (if present) forming a complete cone; both sexual and asexual phases; oocysts generally containing infective sporozoites that result from sporogeny; flagella in microgametes of some groups; and pseudopods (if present) used for feeding only. Locomotion of mature organisms is by means of body flexion, gliding, or undulation of longitudinal ridges on the body surface. It comprises three subclasses: Gregarinia, Coccidia, and Piroplasmia. Called also *Sporozoa*.

sporozoite (spo″ro-zo′īt) [*sporo-* + Gr. *zōon* animal] the elongate, nucleated, motile infective stage resulting from sporogony in gregarine and coccidian protozoa. In malaria, the sporozoites of *Plasmodium* spp. are liberated from the oocysts in the mosquito, accumulate in the vector's salivary glands, and are transferred to the definitive host by the bite of the infected mosquito.

sporozoon (spo″ro-zo′on), pl. *sporozo′a* [*sporo-* + Gr. *zōon* animal] sporozoan, def. 1.

sporozoosis (spo″ro-zo-o′sis) infection with sporozoa.

sport (spōrt) a mutation; lusus naturae.

sporular (spōr′u-lar) pertaining to a spore.

sporulation (spor″u-la′shun) the formation or liberation of spores; sporogony; sporogenesis.

sporule (spor′ūl) a small spore.

spot (spot) a circumscribed area or place distinguished by its color; a loculus or macula; see also *tache*. **acoustic s's,** the maculae sacculi and maculae utriculi. **Bitot's s's,** superficial, foamy gray, triangular spots on the conjunctiva, consisting of keratinized epithelium; they are associated with vitamin A deficiency. See also *xerosis conjunctivae*. **blind s.,** discus nervi optici. **blind s., mental,** mental scotoma. **blue s.,** 1. [pl.] maculae caeruleae. 2. mongolian spot. **Brushfield's s's,** small white spots on the periphery of the iris, usually crescentic, with the concavity outward, frequently but not exclusively seen in children with Down's syndrome. **café au lait s's** (kah-fa′o-la′) [Fr.], pigmented macules of a distinctive light brown color, like coffee with milk, as in neurofibromatosis and Albright's syndrome. **Carleton's s's,** sclerosed spots in the bones in gonorrheal disease. **Cayenne pepper s's,** red angiomatous puncta within or on the border of the lesions of Schamberg's disease. **cherry-red s.,** a red circular area (the choroid) surrounded by gray-white retina, seen through the fovea centralis of the eye in the infantile and sometimes in the late infantile form of amaurotic familial idiocy; called also *Tay's sign* or *spot*. **Christopher's s's,** Maurer's dots; see under *dot*. **chromatin s.,** sex chromatin. **cold s.,** see *temperature s's*. **cotton-wool s's,** white or gray soft-edged opacities in the retina composed of cytoid bodies; seen in hypertensive retinopathy, lupus erythematosus, and numerous other conditions. Called also *cotton-wool exudates* or *patches*. **cribriform s's,** maculae cribrosae. **deaf s.,** deaf point. **De Morgan's s's,** cherry angiomas. **embryonic s.,** see under *disk*. **epigastric s.,** a point of tenderness exactly over the xiphoid process. **eye s.,** 1. the rudiment of an eye in the embryo. 2. eyespot. 3.

stigma (def. 5). **flame s's,** flame-shaped hemorrhages. **focal s.,** the part of the target of an x-ray tube which is bombarded by the focused electron stream when the tube is energized. **Fordyce's s's,** see under *granule*. **Forschheimer's s's,** a fleeting exanthem consisting of discrete rose spots on the soft palate, which may coalesce into a red blush and may extend over the fauces; sometimes seen in rubella just prior to the onset of the skin rash. **germinal s.,** the nucleolus of an ovum. **Graefe's s's,** spots over the vertebrae, pressure on which produces relaxation of blepharofacial spasm. **hot s.,** 1. see *temperature s's*. 2. the sensitive area of a neuroma. 3. an area of increased density on an x-ray or thermographic film. **hypnogenetic s.,** any superficial area the stimulation of which will bring on sleep. **Koplik's s's,** small, irregular, bright red spots on the buccal and lingual mucosa, with a minute bluish white speck in the center of each; seen in the prodromal stage of measles. Called also *Koplik's sign*. **light s.,** cone of light; see under *cone*. **liver s.,** senile lentigo. **Mariotte's s.,** blind s. **Maurer's s's,** see under *dot*. **Maxwell's s.,** macula retinae. **milk s's,** 1. whitish spots of fibrous thickening seen on the visceral layer of the pericardium in postmortem examination. 2. dense masses of macrophages in the omentum. **milky s's,** aggregations of macrophages in the subserous connective tissue of the pleura and peritoneum. **mongolian s.,** a congenital melanocytic nevus manifested by a flat, smooth, bluish gray to gray-brown macular patch(es), most often located on the central lumbosacral area, occurring especially in Orientals and dark-skinned races, and usually disappearing before 5 years of age. Called also *blue* or *sacral s.* and *mongolian macula*. See also *nevus of Ito* and *nevus of Ota*. **pain s's,** spots on the skin where alone the sense of pain can be produced by a stimulus. **pelvic s's,** round or oval shadows often seen on fluoroscopic examination in the region of the inferior spine of the ilium and the horizontal ramus of the pubic bone. **rose s's,** an eruption of rose-colored macules developing especially on the skin of the abdomen and thighs in the early stage of typhoid fever. Called also *typhoid s's*. **Roth's s's,** round or oval white spots consisting of coagulated fibrin seen in the retina in a number of diseases in which a vascular insult resulting in hemorrhage is followed by healing. **sacral s.,** mongolian s. **shin s's,** diabetic dermopathy. **Soemmering's s.,** macula retinae. **soldier's s's,** milk s's, def. 1. **spongy s.,** zona vasculosa. **Stephen's s's,** Maurer's dots. **Tardieu's s's,** spots of ecchymosis under the pleura following death by suffocation. **Tay's s.,** cherry-red s. **temperature s's,** hot and cold spots: spots on the skin normally anesthetic to pain and pressure and sensitive respectively to heat and cold; they are arranged in lines, often somewhat curved, and show the peculiar arrangement of the end-organ with respect to the temperature sense. **tendinous s's,** maculae albidae. **Trousseau's s.,** tache cérébrale. **typhoid s's,** rose s's. **vital s.,** a name sometimes given to any of the major autonomic centers in the pons and medulla oblongata which are indispensable to life. **Wagner's s.,** the nucleolus of the human ovum. **warm s's,** minute areas in the skin that are peculiarly sensitive to temperatures above body temperature; see *temperature s's*. **yellow s.,** macula retinae.

sprain (sprān) a joint injury in which some of the fibers of a supporting ligament are ruptured but the continuity of the ligament remains intact. **rider's s.,** sprain of the adductor longus muscle of the thigh, resulting from strain in riding horseback. **Schlatter's s.,** Osgood-Schlatter disease.

spray (spra) a liquid minutely divided or nebulized as by a jet of air or steam. **ether s.,** ether applied in a nebulized form to produce local anesthesia by chilling the part. **needle s.,** a water spray administered through a device having needle-sized jets. **Peet-Schultz s.** (*obs.*), a nasal spray for preventive application against poliomyelitis. **Tucker's s.** (*obs.*), a nasal spray for asthma containing 1 per cent cocaine and 5 per cent potassium nitrate. **tyrothricin s.,** a solution of tyrothricin and water, made with suitable, harmless, solubilizing and wetting agents; it may contain a small proportion of alcohol and a suitable vasoconstrictor. It is used as a topical antibiotic.

spreader (spred′er) an instrument for distributing something over a broader area. **root canal filling s.,** a hand-operated, smooth, pointed, and tapered metal endodontic instrument; used to compress filling material laterally against the walls of the root canal to make room for insertion of additional cones in root canal therapy.

Sprengel's deformity (spreng'elz) [Otto Gerhard Karl *Sprengel*, German surgeon, 1852–1915]   see under *deformity.*

sprew (sproo) sprue.

spring (spring)   1. a piece of resilient metal, such as a hardened coiled steel wire, that will return to its original shape after bending.   2. a resilient wire attached to a denture or other appliance.   **auxiliary s.,** a short piece of wire attached to an orthodontic appliance to serve as a lever to apply force to a tooth or teeth.   **bow s.,** a loop spring with the shape of a labial bow; used in a removable orthodontic appliance to move teeth.   **closed s.,** one having both ends attached.   **coil s.,** a spiral winding of fine resilient wire; attached to orthodontic appliances to open or to close spaces between teeth.   **finger s.,** a finger-shaped stainless steel wire spring; used interproximally as an open spring in removable orthodontic appliances.   **Kesling s.,** a tooth-spacing spring used to gain separation between the teeth to facilitate band placement in fitting orthodontic appliances.   **loop s.,** a closed orthodontic spring having a variety of different shapes, from that of a hairpin to that of a bow.   **open s.,** one having free ends; in orthodontic appliances, one having only one end anchored in the active plate.   **paddle s.,** a paddle-shaped wire spring used in removable orthodontic appliances; it is activated by bending it toward the tooth.   **separating s.,** one placed between the teeth to obtain separation.   **uprighting s.,** a coiled spring used for uprighting teeth in orthodontic therapy.   **Z s.,** a spring bent in the form of a Z with a coil loop at each end, used to move an individual tooth or groups of teeth buccally or labially.

sprue (sproo)   1. a chronic form of malabsorption syndrome occurring in both tropical and nontropical forms; called also *catarrhal dysentery.*   2. in a dental casting, an opening in the investment through which the molten alloy or metal can reach the mold after the wax has been eliminated.   **nontropical s.,** a malabsorption syndrome affecting both children and adults, precipitated by the ingestion of gluten-containing foods; its etiology is unknown, but a hereditary factor has been implicated. Pathologically, the proximal intestinal mucosa loses its villous structure, surface epithelial cells exhibit degenerative changes, and their absorptive function is severely impaired. It is characterized by diarrhea in which the stools are bulky, frothy, fatty (steatorrhea), and fetid (occasionally, malabsorption may be associated with the passage of a single bulky stool without diarrhea), and by abdominal distention, flatulence, weight loss, asthenia, deficiency of vitamins B, D, and K, and electrolyte depletion. Called also *celiac disease* and *gluten enteropathy.* In the *infantile form* the onset is insidious, and is marked by irritability, loss of appetite, weakness, extreme wasting, growth retardation, and celiac crisis; called also *infantile celiac disease.* The *adult form* is marked by extreme lassitude, fatigue, difficulty in breathing, clubbing of the fingers, bone pain, cramping of the muscles, tetany, abdominal distention during the day, megacolon, tympanitis, and skin pigmentation; called also *adult celiac disease.*   **tropical s.,** a malabsorption syndrome occurring in the tropics and subtropics. Protein malnutrition is usually precipitated by the malabsorption, and anemia due to folic acid deficiency is particularly common. Administration of antibiotics (especially tetracycline) and folic acid usually results in remission. Called also *Ceylon sore mouth, Cochin-China diarrhea, psilosis stomatitis intertropica,* and *stomatitis tropica.*

Spt.   abbreviation for L. *spir'itus,* spirit.

Spumellarida (spu″mel-lār'ĭ-dah) [L. *spuma* foam]   an order of marine planktonic protozoa (class Polycystinea, superclass Actinopoda), characterized by the presence of a capsular membrane with uniformly distributed pores. It comprises two suborders: Sphaerocollina and Sphaerellarina.

spur (sper)   1. a projecting body, as from a bone.   2. in dentistry, a piece of metal projecting from a plate, band, or other dental appliance.   **calcaneal s.,** a bone excrescence on the lower surface of the calcaneus which frequently causes pain on walking.   **Morand's s.,** calcar avis.   **occipital s.,** an abnormal process of bone on the occipital bone behind the posterior process of the atlas.   **olecranon s.,** an abnormal process of bone at the insertion of the triceps muscle.   **scleral s.,** the posterior lip of the venous sinus of the sclera

to which most of the fibers of the trabecular reticulum of the iridocorneal angle and the meridional fibers of the ciliary muscle are attached; called also *scleral roll.*

spurious (spu're-us) [L. *spurius*]   simulated; not genuine; false.

sputamentum (spu″tah-men'tum) [L.]   sputum.

sputum (spu'tum) [L.]   matter ejected from the lungs, bronchi, and trachea, through the mouth.   **s. aerogino'sum,** green s.   **albuminoid s.,** a yellowish, frothy sputum of persons from whom large amounts of pleural fluid have been withdrawn; believed to be due to pulmonary edema.   **s. coc'tum,** the opaque mucopus of the later stages of bronchitis and laryngitis.   **s. cru'dum,** the clear, tenacious mucus of the early stages of laryngitis and bronchitis.   **s. cruen'tum,** bloody sputum.   **globular s.,** sputum in yellow spherical lumps; said to be characteristic of the late stages of tuberculosis.   **green s.,** sputum stained with a green pigment, as in certain cases of jaundice.   **icteric s.,** sputum stained with a greenish or yellow tint by bile pigments, as in jaundice.   **moss-agate s.,** a grayish, opalescent, gelatinous mottled sputum, usually projected from the mouth in a more or less globular form during coughing; characteristic of diseases of the trachea (Chevalier Jackson).   **nummular s.,** sputum in rounded disks, shaped somewhat like coins.   **prune juice s.,** dark, reddish brown, bloody sputum of certain forms of pneumonia, cancer of the lung, gangrene, etc.   **rusty s.,** sputum stained with blood or blood pigments; seen in pneumonia, etc.

SQ   abbreviation (symbol) for *subcutaneous.*

squalene (skwal'ēn)   an unsaturated terpene hydrocarbon, $[(CH_3)_2C:CH(CH_2)_2C(CH_3):CH(CH_2)_2C(CH_3):CH·CH_2]_2$, from the liver oil of sharks and certain other elasmobranch fishes; it is an intermediate in cholesterol biosynthesis (by way of lanosterol) in all animals examined. It is found in small amounts in human blood plasma and in increased amounts in viral influenza. A preparation [NF] is used as an oleaginous vehicle in pharmaceuticals.

squama (skwa'mah), pl. *squa'mae* [L.]   a scale or platelike structure; [NA] a general term for such a structure.   **s. alveola'ris,** a thin plate covering the bare areas of pulmonary alveoli.   **frontal s., s. of frontal bone, s. fronta'lis** [NA], the broad, curved portion of the frontal bone, situated above the supraorbital margin and forming the forehead.   **mental s., external,** protuberantia mentalis.   **occipital s., s. occipitalis.**   **occipital s., superior,** os interparietale.   **s. occipita'lis** [NA], occipital squama: the largest of the four parts of the occipital bone, extending from the posterior edge of the foramen magnum to the lambdoid suture, its external surface bearing the external occipital protuberance and nuchal lines.   **perpendicular s.,** s. frontalis.   **temporal s., s. of temporal bone, s. tempora'lis,** pars squamosa ossis temporalis.

squamae (skwa'me) [L.]   plural of *squama.*

squamate (skwa'māt) [L. *squamatus,* from *squama* scale]   scaly; having or resembling scales.

squamatization (skwa″mah-ti-za'shun)   the transformation of cells of other types into squamous cells; squamous metaplasia.

squame (skwām) [L. *squama*]   a scale or scalelike substance.

squamocellular (skwa″mo-sel'u-lar) [L. *squama* scale + *cellula* cell]   having squamous cells.

squamofrontal (skwa″mo-fron'tal)   pertaining to the squama frontalis.

squamomastoid (skwa″mo-mas'toid)   pertaining to the squamous and mastoid portions of the temporal bone.

squamo-occipital (skwa″mo-ok-sip'ĭ-tal)   pertaining to the squama occipitalis.

squamoparietal (skwa″mo-pah-ri'ĕ-tal)   pertaining to the pars squamosa ossis temporalis and the parietal bone.

squamopetrosal (skwa″mo-pe-tro'sal)   pertaining to the squamous and petrous portions of the temporal bone.

squamosa (skwa-mo'sah) [L.]   scaly, or platelike; see *pars squamosa.*

squamosal (skwa-mo'sal)   squamous.

squamosoparietal (skwa-mo″so-pah-ri'ĕ-tal)   squamoparietal.

squamosphenoid (skwa″mo-sfe'noid)   pertaining to the

squamous portion of the temporal bone and to the sphenoid bone.

squamotemporal (skwa″mo-tem′po-ral)   pertaining to the squamous portion of the temporal bone.

squamous (skwa′mus) [L. *squamosus* scaly]   scaly, or plate-like.

squamozygomatic (skwa″mo-zi″go-mat′ik)   pertaining to the squamous portions of the temporal bone and the zygomatic bone.

squatting (skwot′ing)   a position of flexion of the knees and hips, the buttocks being lowered to the level of the heels. It is sometimes adopted by the parturient at delivery. Children with certain types of cyanotic cardiac defects, particularly those with tetralogy of Fallot, frequently adopt the position.

squeeze (skwēz)   subjection to pressure; compression. **tussive s.,** the compression of the lung in coughing, which is said to force material from the alveoli and smaller air passages into the bronchi.

squill (skwil) [L. *scilla;* Gr. *skilla*]   the fleshy inner scales of the bulb of the white variety of *Urginea maritima* (L.) Baker (a liliaceous plant). It contains glucoscillaren A, scillaren A, proscillaridin A, other related cardioactive glycosides, and several other principles, and has been used as a diuretic, emetic, expectorant, and cardiotonic. The red variety is used as a rat poison. Called also *scilla*.

squillitic (skwil-lit′ik) [L. *scilliticus;* Gr. *skillitikos*]   pertaining to or containing squill.

squint (skwint)   strabismus; for types of squint not entered here, see under *strabismus.* **accommodative s.,** esotropia. **comitant s., concomitant s.,** concomitant strabismus. **convergent s.,** esotropia. **divergent s.,** exotropia. **upward and downward s.,** hypertropia.

SR   stimulation ratio; see *lymphocyte proliferation test* under *tests.*

Sr   chemical symbol for *strontium.*

sr   abbreviation for *steradian.*

SRBC   sheep red blood cell.

SRF   1. somatotropin releasing factor; see *growth hormone releasing hormone,* under *hormone.* 2. skin reactive factor.

SRH   somatotropin releasing hormone; see *growth hormone releasing hormone,* under *hormone.*

SRIF   somatostatin.

S.R.N.   State Registered Nurse (England and Wales).

sRNA   soluble ribonucleic acid; see *ribonucleic acid.*

SRS-A   slow reacting substance of anaphylaxis.

SS   somatostatin.

ss.   abbreviation for L. *se′mis,* one half.

Ssabanejew-Frank operation (sah-ban′ĕ-jef-frank) [Ivan *Ssabanejew,* Russian surgeon, born 1856; Rudolf *Frank,* Vienna surgeon, 1862–1913]   see under *operation.*

S.S.D.   source-skin distance.

ssDNA   single-stranded DNA.

ssRNA   single-stranded RNA.

SSS   specific soluble substance.

s.s.s.   abbreviation for L. *stra′tum su′per stra′tum,* layer upon layer.

S.S.V.   abbreviation for L. *sub sig′no vene′ni,* under a poison label.

St.   abbreviation for L. *stet,* let it stand; or *stent,* let them stand.

S. T. 37   trademark for a solution of hexylresorcinol.

stab (stab)   see under *culture,* and see *band cell,* under *cell.*

stabilarsan (sta-bil′ar-san)   a double glycoside of arsphenamine, $C_6H_{11}O_5 \cdot NH(OH)C_6H_3As.$

stabilate (sta′bĭ-lāt)   a population of microorganisms preserved in a genetically stable and viable condition (as by freeze-drying or low temperature); distinguished from a strain that may be maintained by subculture.

stabile (sta′bil, sta′bīl) [L. *stabilis* stable, abiding]   not moving; stationary; resistant to chemical change; opposed to *labile.* **heat s.,** thermostabile.

stability (stah-bil′ĭ-te)   the quality of maintaining a constant character in the presence of forces which threaten to disturb it; resistance to change. **dimensional s.,** the re-

sistance of a material to change in its shape or measurements.

stabilization (sta″bil-i-za′shun)   the creation of a stable state.

stable (sta′b'l)   not moving, fixed, firm; resistant to change.

staccato (stah-kah′to) [Ital. "detached"]   denoting a manner of utterance in which the speech is delivered in a quick, jerky manner, with an interval between each two syllables.

stachydrine (stah-kid′rin)   chemical name: *N*-methylproline-methylbetaine. An alkaloid, $C_7H_{13}NO_2,$ found in various plants, such as alfalfa, chrysanthemum, citrus, and species of hedge nettles.

stachyose (stak′e-ōs)   an indigestible tetrasaccharide, $C_{24}H_{42}O_{21},$ from the tubers of the hedge nettle, *Stachys tubifera,* the seeds of various leguminous plants, and the roots and rhizomes of various labiate plants.

Stacke's operation (stak′ez) [Ludwig *Stacke,* German otologist, 1859–1918]   see under *operation.*

stactometer (stak-tom′ĕ-ter) [Gr. *staktos* oozing out in drops + *metron* measure]   an instrument for measuring drops.

Stader splint (sta′der) [Otto *Stader,* American veterinary surgeon]   see under *splint.*

Staderini's nucleus (stad″er-e′nēz) [Rutilio *Staderini,* Italian anatomist]   nucleus intercalatus.

stadium (sta′de-um), pl. **sta′dia** [L.; Gr. *stadion* course]   a stage or period in a disease. See *stage,* def. 1. **s. ac′mes,** the height of a disease. **s. augmen′ti,** s. incrementi. **s. calo′ris,** the hot stage of a fever or disease. **s. decremen′ti,** the period of decrease of severity in a disease; the defervescence of fever. **s. defervescen′tiae,** s. decrementi. **s. fluorescen′tiae,** eruptive stage (of an exanthem). **s. frig′oris,** the cold stage of an intermittent fever. **s. incremen′ti,** the period of increase in the intensity of a disease; the stage of development of fever. **s. invasio′nis,** the incubative stage. **s. sudo′ris,** the sweating stage.

staff (staf)   1. a wooden rod or rodlike structure.   2. a grooved director used as a guide for the knife in lithotomy. 3. the professional personnel of a hospital.   4. see under *cell.* **s. of Aesculapius,** a rod or staff with a snake entwined around it, commonly appearing in the ancient representations of Aesculapius, the god of medicine. It is the symbol of medicine and is the official emblem of the American Medical Association.   **attending s.,** the corps of attending physi-

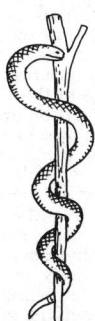

Staff of Aesculapius.

cians and surgeons of a hospital.   **consulting s.,** the corps of physicians and surgeons attached to a hospital who do not visit regularly, but may be consulted by members of the attending staff.   **house s.,** the resident physicians and surgeons of a hospital.   **s. of Wrisberg,** a slight mounding up of the mucosa over Wrisberg's cartilage (cartilago cuneiformis) seen in the normal larynx during examination with the laryngoscope.

stage (stāj)   1. a period or distinct phase in the course of a disease, the life history of an organism, or any biological process. See also *staging.* 2. the platform of a microscope on which a slide is placed for viewing of the specimen. **algid s.,** a condition characterized by a flickering pulse, subnormal temperature, and varied nervous symptoms. **amphibolic s.,** the stage of an infectious disease between the acme and the decline in which the diagnosis is uncertain. **anal s.,** in psychoanalytic theory, the second stage of psychosexual development, occurring between the ages of 1 and 3 years, during which the infant's activities, interests, and concerns are on the anal zone; it is preceded by the oral stage and followed by the phallic stage. **cold s.,** the chill or rigor of a malarial attack. **defervescent s.,** stadium decrementi. **eruptive s.,** that period during the course of an eruptive fever or exanthem when the rash is present. Called also *stadium fluorescentiae.* **expulsive s.,** the stage of labor during which the child is being expelled from the uterus; the second stage of labor. **s. of fervescence,** pyrogenetic s. **first s.** (of labor), the earliest stage of labor, ending with dilatation of the os uteri. **fourth s.** (of labor), a name sometimes applied to the immediate postpartum period. **genital s.,** in psychoanalytic theory, the last stage in psychosexual development, occurring during puberty, during which the person can achieve sexual gratification from genital-to-genital contact and is capable of a mature relationship with a person of the opposite sex; it follows the latency stage. **hot s.,** the period of pyrexia in a malarial paroxysm. **incubative s.,** incubation period. **knäuel s.,** skein. **latency s.,** 1. the incubation period of any infectious disorder. 2. the quiescent period following an active period in certain infectious diseases, during which the pathogen remains dormant for a variable length of time before again initiating signs of active disease. 3. in psychoanalytic theory, the period of relative quiescence in psychosexual development, lasting from age 5 or 6 years to adolescence, during which interest in persons of the opposite sex ceases and the child tends to associate mainly with persons of his own sex; it is preceded by the phallic stage and followed by the genital stage. **mechanical s.,** a platform of a microscope by which the specimen being viewed can be moved in either of two mutually perpendicular directions. **oral s.,** in psychoanalytic theory, the earliest stage of psychosexual development, lasting from birth to about 18 months, during which the oral zone is the center of the infant's needs, expression, and pleasurable erotic experiences; it is followed by the anal stage. **phallic s.,** in psychoanalytic theory, the third stage is psychosexual development, lasting from age 2 or 3 years to 5 or 6 years, during which sexual interest, curiosity, and pleasurable experiences are centered on the penis in boys and the clitoris in girls; it is preceded by the anal stage and followed by the latency stage. **placental s.,** third s. **preeruptive s.,** 1. the stage after infection and before eruption. 2. the period of tooth development, before tooth eruption, characterized by growth of the coronal portion of the tooth, prior to the beginning of the growth of the root. **premenstrual s.,** the condition of the uterine mucosa after ovulation and the formation of a corpus luteum. **prodromal s.,** the period of early symptoms of a disease occurring after the incubation period and just before the appearance of the characteristic symptoms of the disease; called also *prodromal period.* **progestational s.,** the secretory stage of the endometrial cycle immediately preceding menstruation or implantation of the ovum. **proliferative s.,** the phase of the uterine mucosa following the first stage of rest: the mucosa shows hypertrophy of the glands and increase of the lining epithelium. **pyretogenic s., pyrogenic s.,** the stage of invasion of a febrile attack. **Ranke's s's,** the hypothesis that tuberculosis of the lungs develops in three stages: (1) the primary focus, (2) generalized spread of the tubercle bacillus, and (3) isolated organ tuberculosis, chiefly of the lungs. **rest s.,** the stage of the uterine mucosa immediately following the completion of menstruation. **resting s.,** the stage of a cell or its nucleus when no mitotic changes are going on; interphase. **ring s.,** see under *form.* **second s.** (of labor), period during which the infant is expelled from the uterus and vagina. **seral s.,** any of the individual transitional series of communities of an ecological sere, which finally leads to a stable, mature *climax community.* Called also *seral community.* **stepladder s.,** an early stage of enteric fever; so called from the peculiar form of the temperature curve. **sweating s.,** the final stage of a malarial paroxysm, marked by sweating. **third s.** (of labor), the period following expulsion of the infant and ending with expulsion of the placenta and membranes from the uterus. **transitional pulp s.,** a condition of the dental pulp in which chronic inflammatory cells are present but not in sufficient quantities to constitute a typical inflammatory exudate, usually resulting from abrasion, attrition, caries, periodontal disease, or a reaction to a restorative procedure. **ugly duckling s.,** a development stage in the mixed dentition when the upper central and lateral incisors may be flared, with the crowns distally and with diastema present

before the maxillary canine teeth erupt. **vegetative s.,** resting s.

staggers (stag′erz) 1. gid. 2. a form of vertigo occurring in decompression sickness. **blind s.,** 1. gid. 2. an acute form of selenium poisoning in animals. **grass s.,** locoism. **sleepy s., stomach s.,** a disease of horses, of unknown causation, but usually associated with the eating of moldy hay and grain; called also *forage poisoning.*

staging (sta′jing) 1. the determination of distinct phases or periods in the course of a disease, the life history of an organism, or any biological process. 2. the classification of neoplasms according to the extent of the tumor; see *TNM s.* **TNM s.,** staging of tumors according to three basic components: primary tumor (T), regional nodes (N), and metastasis (M). Adscripts are used to denote size and degree of involvement; for example, 0 indicates undetectable, and 1, 2, 3, and 4 a progressive increase in size or involvement. Thus a tumor may be described as T1, N2, M0.

Stahr's gland (stahrz) [Hermann *Stahr,* German anatomist and pathologist, born 1868] see under *gland.*

stain (stān) 1. any dye, reagent, or other material used in producing coloration, such as a substance used in coloring tissues or microorganisms for microscopical study. See *Table of Stains and Staining Methods* and names of specific compounds. 2. a superficial discoloration, or an artificially colored spot in the skin. **acid s.,** a stain which is acid in reaction and more readily colors the protoplasm of cells. **after s.,** see *after-stain.* **basic s.,** a stain which is basic in reaction and shows an affinity for the nuclei of cells. **contrast s.,** material used to color an unstained portion of a tissue after another portion has been stained with another dye. **counter s.,** see *counterstain.* **differential s.,** one which facilitates differentiation of various elements in a specimen. **electron s's,** substances containing heavy atoms, such as osmic tetroxide, uranyl, and lead ions, which, under certain conditions, act as "electron stains," comparable to histologic stains, by combining selectively with certain regions of the specimen; used in the visualization of the ultrastructure. **heavy-metal s.,** any of the elements of high atomic weight often used as stains in electron microscopy. **lipoid s.,** a stain made from any fatlike, or lipid, substance, e.g., Sudan III. **metachromatic s.,** a stain that colors certain cell constituents a color different from that of the stain itself. **neutral s.,** a combination of an acid and a basic stain for staining neutrophil tissues. **nuclear s.,** a stain which has a special affinity for the nuclei of cells. **plasmatic s., plasmic s.,** a stain which colors the tissue uniformly throughout. **port-wine s.,** a persistent dark red to purple nevus flammeus that grows proportionately with the affected child and is usually found on the face. Initially it is macular, but the surface may develop angiomatous overgrowths with time. Port-wine stains occur in association with other congenital abnormalities, such as the Klippel-Trenaunay and Sturge-Weber syndromes. Called also *port-wine mark* or *nevus.* **protoplasmic s.,** a stain which has a special affinity for the protoplasm of cells. **selective s.,** a stain which has a special affinity for a certain tissue element, staining it more vividly than, or to the exclusion of, other elements of the same specimen. **tumor s.,** an area of increased density in a radiograph due to collection of contrast material in distorted and abnormal vessels, prominent in the capillary and venous phase of arteriography, and presumed to indicate neoplasm.

staining (stān′ing) 1. the artificial coloration of a substance, such as the introduction or application of material to facilitate examination of tissues, microorganisms, or other cells under the microscope. For various methods, see *Table of Stains and Staining Methods.* 2. modification of the color of the teeth or denture base to achieve a more lifelike appearance. **bipolar s.,** staining at the two poles only, or staining differently at the two poles. **differential s.,** staining with a substance for which different bacteria or different elements of the bacteria or specimen being stained show varying affinities, resulting in their differentiation. **double s.,** staining with two different dyes which have an affinity for different tissue elements. **fluorescent s.,** the coloration of tissues with a fluorescent dye. **intravital s.,** vital s. **multiple s.,** staining with several different dyes to facilitate identification of different tissue elements. **negative s.,** staining of the background and not the organism, to facilitate the microscopical study of bacteria. **polar s.,** staining in which the ends of the rod stain deeply while the central portion of the organism is nearly or quite unstained, as in the pasteurellas. **postvital s.**, staining that occurs after death of a tissue which has been previously stained by vital methods. **preagonal s.**, vital s. **relief s.**, a method of staining that colors the background and leaves the cells uncolored. **simple s.**, staining with a single substance, such as the staining of microorganisms with a single dye. **substantive s.**, the coloration of tissues by direct absorption of dyes in which they are immersed. **supravital s.**, staining of living tissue removed from the body, but before cessation of the chemical life of the cells.

telomeric s., terminal s., differential staining of chromosomes to stain chromosome telomeric regions, consisting of pretreatment with a heated salt solution before treatment with buffered Giemsa stain or acridine orange; only the telomeric regions of the chromosomes retain the stain. **triple s.**, staining with three different dyes to facilitate identification of the different elements. **vital s.**, staining of a tissue by a dye which is introduced into a living organism and which, by virtue of affinity for certain tissues, will stain those tissues; called also *intravital staining*.

TABLE OF STAINS AND STAINING METHODS

Listing some of the preparations and methods commonly employed in histologic and pathologic technique (*arranged alphabetically*). For other stains, see under *blue, red,* etc.

Achucárro's s., a silver-tannin stain for impregnating connective tissue.

acid-fast s., a staining procedure for demonstrating acid-fast microorganisms. See *Kinyoun carbolfuchsin S.* and *Ziehl-Neelsen S.*

acid fuchsin s., a diffuse stain containing acid fuchsin and diluted hydrochloric acid in purified water, for demonstrating axons.

Albert's diphtheria s., a stain containing toluidine blue and methyl (or malachite) green. Following treatment with iodine solution, the metachromatic granules appear black, the bars dark green to black, and the remainder of the diphtheria bacillus a light green.

alum-carmine s., a preparation of ordinary alum and carmine.

Alzheimer s., a methylene blue and eosin polychrome stain for demonstrating Negri bodies.

Anthony capsule s., a method of demonstrating the capsules of bacteria. A smear of a milk culture is air dried, or a smear is mixed with milk and dried. The slide is stained with crystal violet and washed with copper sulfate. The capsule appears unstained against a purple background; the cells are deeply stained.

auramine-rhodamine s., Truant auramine-rhodamine s.

azan s., Heidenhain's modification of Mallory's triple stain.

basic fuchsin s., a stain containing basic fuchsin in distilled water.

Benda's s., a method for demonstrating nerve tissue.

Bensley's neutral gentian orange G s., a preparation used for demonstrating secretion granules.

Best's carmine s., a stain for demonstrating glycogen.

Bethe's method, a method of fixing methylene blue stains of nerve fibers.

Bielschowsky's s., an ammoniacal silver stain for demonstrating axons and neurofibrils.

Bodian method, a method of staining nerve fibers and nerve endings with colloidal silver.

Bowie s., a stain used to demonstrate the slightly basophilic cytoplasm and the specific granules of juxtaglomerular cells.

Cajal method, a method of staining astrocytes by a gold chloride–mercuric chloride compound.

Cajal's double method, a method of demonstrating ganglion cells.

carbolfuchsin s., a stain for microorganisms containing basic fuchsin with dilute phenol as a mordant. It is also used as a counterstain for *Legionella pneumophilia* following other routine stains. Stained cells appear pink to red.

carbol-gentian violet s., a solution containing gentian violet and carbolic acid.

Castaneda's s., a method of demonstrating rickettsiae. A smear is air dried and treated with methylene blue, then counterstained with safranin O, washed, and air dried. Rickettsiae appear blue against red cellular elements.

Ciaccio's s., a stain for demonstrating lipoids.

Cox's modification of Golgi's corrosive sublimate method, a method for staining ganglion cells.

Davenport's s., a stain for demonstrating various elements of nerve tissue, dependent upon the special affinity of nerve cells and their processes for silver.

Delafield's hematoxylin [USP], a preparation of hematoxylin, alcohol, ammonia alum, water, glycerin, and methanol, used as a nuclear stain.

Dieterle's s., a silver impregnation method for staining *Legionella* and other organisms. Slides are sensitized in uranyl nitrate, treated with gum mastic, incubated in silver nitrate, and developed in a solution of hydroquinone, sodium sulfite, acetone, formaldehyde, pyridine, and gum mastic. Cells stain black on a yellow-tan background.

Ehrlich's acid hematoxylin, a preparation of hematoxylin, used as a nuclear stain.

Ehrlich's neutral s., a mixture of methylene blue and acid fuchsin, used to stain blood corpuscles.

Ehrlich's triacid s., a stain containing acid fuchsin, orange G, and methyl green; used for demonstrating various formed elements in the blood.

F method, F-staining method, chromosomes are treated with phosphate buffer, rinsed and stored for 60–72 hours in saline citrate solution, then fixed in methanol-acetic acid, and stained by the Feulgen method.

Feulgen method, a method of demonstrating chromatin and deoxyribonucleic acid (DNA).

Fontana's s., a method of staining spirochetes by silver impregnation, using ammoniacal silver nitrate solution.

Giemsa s., a solution containing azure II-eosin, azure II, glycerin, and methanol; used for staining protozoan parasites such as *Plasmodium* and *Trypanosoma*, for *Chlamydia*, for differential staining of blood smears, and for viral inclusion bodies. Stained elements appear pink to purple to blue.

Gimenez s., a method for staining *Chlamydia* and other rickettsiae and *Legionella*. Smears are stained with carbol–basic fuchsin solution, washed, and counterstained with malachite green. Cells appear red against a greenish background.

Golgi's mixed method, a method of staining nerve cells and all of their processes; historically of very great importance.

Gomori's s's, stains used for histological demonstration of enzymes, especially phosphatases and lipases in sections; also methods for demonstration of connective tissue fibers and secretion granules. Called also *Gomori-Takamatsu s's*.

Gomori-Takamatsu s's, Gomori's s's.

Gomori-Wheatley s., trichrome s.

Goodpasture's s., a method for demonstrating the peroxidase reaction.

Gram's method, Gram's s., an empirical staining procedure devised by Gram in which microorganisms are stained with crystal violet, treated with 1:15 dilution of Lugol's iodine, decolorized with ethanol or ethanol-acetone, and counterstained with a contrasting dye, usually safranin. Those microorganisms that retain the crystal violet stain are said to be gram-positive, and those that lose the crystal violet stain by decolorization but stain with the counterstain are said to be gram-negative.

Grocott-Gomori methenamine-silver nitrate s., a method for demonstrating actinomycetes and fungi in tissue. Sections are treated with chromic acid, stained with methenamine-silver nitrite solution, and counterstained with light green solution. Cells appear brown against a green background.

Hale's iron s., a stain used on substances with a high acid polysaccharide content because of the ability of polyanionic polysaccharides to bind polyvalent cations. Its main component is colloidal iron (Fe^{+++}).

Harris' hematoxylin, a nuclear stain.

Harris' method, a method for demonstrating Negri bodies.

Heidenhain's iron hematoxylin s., an important cytological method for the demonstration of most cellular structures: nuclei, chromosomes, centrioles, fibrils, mitochondria, cilia, etc.

hemalum s., a nuclear stain containing hematoxylin and alum, widely used, especially in combination with eosin.

hematoxylin-eosin s., a mixture of hematoxylin in distilled water and aqueous eosin solution, employed also universally for routine examination of tissues; numerous variations are employed in execution of the stain.

hematoxylin-eosin-azure II, Maximow's method for the staining of blood-forming organs.

Hiss capsule s., a method of demonstrating bacterial capsules. Smears are treated with crystal violet, heated, and rinsed with copper sulfate solution. Capsules appear as pale blue halos around deep blue to purple cells.

Hortega method, a method of demonstrating microglia, employing ammoniacal silver carbonate.

India ink capsule s., a method of demonstrating cell capsules, especially of *Cryptococcus neoformans.* The smear is mixed with India ink, covered with a coverglass, and examined microscopically. Capsules appear as a clear halo around the cells against a black background.

iron hematoxylin method, a staining procedure in which the sections are treated with an iron salt, stained with hematoxylin, and differentiated with the same iron salt.

Janus green B, a stain used supravitally for the demonstration of mitochondria.

Jenner's method, a method for demonstrating blood corpuscles.

Kinyoun carbolfuchsin s., a stain for acid-fast organisms. A heat-fixed smear is treated with carbolfuchsin solution. The slide is washed with water, decolorized with acid alcohol, and counterstained with methylene blue. Acid-fast organisms appear red against a blue background.

Leifson flagella s., a method for demonstrating bacterial flagella. Smears are air dried, treated with alcoholic pararosaniline–tannic acid solution, and washed. Flagella are visible against a clear background.

Leishman's s., a mixture of methylene blue and eosin for staining blood cells and certain parasites.

Levaditi's method, a method for demonstrating *Treponema pallidum* in sections, employing reduced silver.

lithium-carmine s., a diffuse stain used intravitally for the demonstration of macrophages.

Löffler's alkaline methylene, blue s., a simple stain used especially for demonstrating granules in *Corynebacterium diphtheriae.* Methylene blue made alkaline with potassium hydroxide is applied to a smear briefly and the slide washed. Granules appear deep blue in lighter blue cells.

Lorrain Smith s., Nile blue sulfate staining fatty acids blue and neutral fat pink.

Macchiavellos s., a rickettsial stain, used especially for *Chlamydia.* The heat-fixed smear is stained with basic fuchsin, decolorized in citric acid, and counterstained with methylene blue. Rickettsiae stain red against a blue background.

Mallory's acid fuchsin, orange G, and aniline blue s., a stain for demonstrating connective tissue and secretion granules. Called also *Mallory's triple stain.*

Mallory's phosphotungstic acid–hematoxylin s., a stain used for demonstrating nuclear and cytoplasmic detail and connective tissue fibers.

Mallory's triple s., Mallory's acid fuchsin, orange G, and aniline blue s.

Marchi's method, a method of demonstrating degenerated nerve fibers, the tissue first being fixed in a solution containing potassium bichromate, which prevents the normal myelinated fibers from staining with osmic acid.

Masson s., a trichrome stain for connective tissue.

Maximow's method, hematoxylin-eosin-azure II.

May's spore s., a method of staining the spores of bacteria in which they are treated with 5 per cent chromic acid, then with ammonia, stained with hot carbol-fuchsin, decolorized with dilute sulfuric acid, and counterstained with methylene blue. The spores appear red, the vegetative cells blue.

May-Grünwald s., an alcoholic neutral mixture of methylene blue and eosin.

Mayer's hemalum, an aqueous solution of hematein, alum, thymol, and 90 per cent alcohol.

Mayer's muchematein, a specific stain for mucus.

methyl green-pyronine s., Unna-Pappenheim s.

methyl violet s., an aniline dye used as a bacteriological stain.

methylene blue, an aniline dye much used as a staining agent; prepared in a saturated solution (7 per cent) in absolute alcohol, which is diluted for use.

Michaelis' s., a mixture of alcoholic solution of methylene blue and a solution of eosin in acetone; used for demonstrating blood corpuscles.

Milligan's trichrome s., a differential stain for connective tissue and smooth muscle. Nuclei and muscle appear magenta; collagen appears green or blue, depending on whether fast green or aniline blue is used as a counterstain; and red blood cells appear orange to orange red.

neutral red, an important supravital stain for the demonstration of vacuoles in cells, and especially of the vacuome.

Nissl's method, a method employed in the study of nerve cell bodies.

Pal's modification of Weigert's myelin sheath s., a method for the study of myelinated nerves, the specimen being treated for several weeks in a solution containing potassium bichromate.

Papanicolaou's s., a method of staining smears of various body secretions, from the respiratory, digestive or genitourinary tract, for the examination of exfoliated cells, to detect the presence of a malignant process.

Pappenheim's s., a method for differentiating basophilic granules of erythrocytes and nuclear fragments.

PAS s., periodic acid–Schiff s.

Perdrau's method, a modification of Bielschowsky's method for staining collagen and reticulin.

periodic acid–Schiff (PAS) s., see under *reaction.*

Perls' s., see under *tests.*

peroxidase s., see Goodpasture's s.

phosphotungstic acid–hematoxylin s., see *Mallory's phosphotungstic acid–hematoxylin s.*

polychrome methylene blue, a stain for demonstrating plasma cells and mast cells, employing potassium carbonate and methylene blue.

quinacrine fluorescent method, chromosomes are exposed to quinacrine derivatives, after which they fluoresce, the degree of fluorescence varying from one chromosome segment to another; the resultant fluorescent patterns (Q bands) are characteristic for each chromosome. Called also *Q method.*

Ranson's pyridine silver s., a stain used for demonstrating nerve cells and their processes.

reverse Giemsa method, a method in which the reciprocal (R-bands) of the banding pattern seen in the Giemsa method for chromosomes is obtained; called also *R method.*

Romanovsky's (Romanowsky's) s., the prototype of the many eosin-methylene blue stains for blood smears and malarial parasites, including Giemsa stain, Leishman's stain, and Wright's stain.

Seller's s., a combination of alcoholic solutions of methylene blue and basic fuchsin which stains Negri bodies a bright red against a purplish-pink background; used in rapid diagnosis of rabies.

Sternheimer-Malbin s., a stain used in urinalysis which has ready affinity for hyaline casts, epithelial casts, red cells, bladder epithelial nuclei, nuclei of vaginal epithelium, and trichomonads, staining each a different color.

Sudan black B fat s., a stain used to demonstrate *Legionella* and fat vacuoles in bacterial cells. A heat-fixed smear is treated with Sudan black B, cleared with xylol, and counterstained with safranin. Fat vacuoles stain blue-black; bacterial cells stain pink.

T method, T-staining method, a method for staining only the terminal ends of chromosomes by means of either Giemsa stain or acridine orange; it results in bands (T bands) of dark violet (Giemsa) or fiery orange (acridine orange).

tetrachrome s., a stain combining eosin Y, methylene blue, azur A, and methylene violet, in methyl alcohol.

trichrome s., a rapid staining method which adequately demonstrates structural details of the various intestinal protozoa. The solution is as follows: chromotrope 2R 0.6 gm., light green SF 0.3 gm., phosphotungstic acid 0.7 gm., acetic acid 1.00 ml., and distilled water 100.00 ml. Called also *Gomori-Wheatley s.*

Truant auramine-rhodamine s., a method for demonstrating mycobacteria. A smear is heat fixed, stained with auramine-rhodamine solution, decolorized, counterstained with potassium permanganate, and examined under ultraviolet light; acid-fast organisms glow with a yellow-orange color.

Unna's alkaline methylene blue, a strongly alkaline solution of methylene blue which is valuable for staining plasma cells.

Unna-Pappenheim s., a stain for plasma cells, employing methyl green and pyronine; also widely used for demonstrating nucleoproteins.

van Gieson's solution of trinitrophenol and acid fuchsin, a stain for connective tissue, consisting of acid fuchsin and aqueous solution of trinitrophenol.

Verhoeff's s., a stain for demonstrating elastic tissue.

von Kossa's s., a silver nitrate stain for bone mineral.

Wayson s., a method used to demonstrate polar staining. A smear is treated with a mixture of basic fuchsin and methylene blue with phenol, washed with water, and dried. It is used especially to demonstrate *Yersinia pestis* in specimens from tissues and lymph nodes.

Weigert's fibrin s., a method, many variations of which have been used in both fixation and staining; stains gram-positive bacteria as well as fibrin.

Weigert's iron hematoxylin s., a simple method for staining most nuclear and cytoplasmic constituents.

Weigert's myelin sheath m., a method of demonstrating the myelin sheath of nerve cell processes.

Weigert's neuroglia fiber s., a complicated method for demonstrating fibrous glia, which works best on human material.

Weigert's resorcin-fuchsin s., a method for the demonstration of elastic fibers.

Weil's s., a method for staining myelin sheaths.

Wirtz-Conklin spore s., a smear is heated with malachite green, rinsed, then counterstained with safranin. Spores appear green in red-stained cells.

Wright's s., a mixture of eosin and methylene blue, used for demonstrating blood corpuscles and malarial parasites.

Ziehl-Neelsen s., a stain for acid-fast organisms. A heat-fixed smear is flooded with carbolfuchsin, heated for 5 minutes, cooled, and washed. The slide is decolorized with acid alcohol, washed, and counterstained with methylene blue. Acid-fast organisms appear red against a blue background.

Ziehl-Neelsen carbolfuchsin, a mixture of basic fuchsin, alcohol, liquefied phenol, and purified water.

---

stalagmometer (stal″ag-mom′ĕ-ter) [Gr. *stalagmos* dropping + *meter*] an instrument for measuring surface tension by determining the exact number of drops in a given quantity of a liquid.

stalagmon (stah-lag′mon) a colloidal substance that changes the surface tension of a liquid containing it.

staling (stāl′ing) urination in cattle and horses.

stalk (stawk) an elongated, more or less slender anatomical structure resembling the stalk of a plant. **abdominal s.,** the umbilical cord. **allantoic s.,** the more slender tube interposed in most mammals between the urogenital sinus and the allantoic sac. It is the precursor of the umbilical cord. Called also *connecting s.* **belly s.,** the umbilical cord. **body s.,** a bridge of mesoderm connecting the caudal end of the young embryo with the chorion and eventually giving passage to the allantois with its important accompanying blood vessels; it is the precursor of the allantoic stalk. **cerebellar s.,** any of the cerebellar peduncles. **connecting s.,** allantoic s. **hypophysial s.,** 1. infundibulum hypothalami. 2. pars tuberalis adenohypophyseos. **infundibular s.,** 1. infundibulum hypothalami. 2. see under *stem* (def. 1). **neural s.,** infundibulum hypothalami. **optic s.,** a slender structure attaching the optic vesicle to the brain wall in the early embryo. **pituitary s.,** 1. infundibulum hypothalami. 2. pars tuberalis adenohypophyseos. **s's of thalamus,** see under *peduncle.* **yolk s.,** the narrow tube connecting the yolk sac (umbilical vesicle) with the midgut of the early embryo, which becomes incorporated into the embryo and usually undergoes complete obliteration, but occasionally persists in the embryo, and, rarely, is found in the adult as a diverticulum from the small intestine (*Meckel's diverticulum*). Called also *oomphalomesenteric duct, umbilical duct,* and *vitelline duct.*

stallimycin hydrochloride (stal″ĭ-mi′sin) chemical name: *N*-[5-[[[(3-amino-3-iminopropyl)amino]carbonyl]-1-methy-1*H*-pyr rol-3-yl]-4-[[[4-(formylamino)-1-methyl-1*H*-pyrrol-2-yl]carbonyl]amino]-1-methyl-1*H*-pyrrole-2-carboxamide monohydrochloride; an antibacterial, $C_{22}H_{27}N_9O_4$·HCl.

stamen (sta′men) the structure of a flower which bears the male gamete, or pollen.

stamina (stam′ĭ-nah) [L.] vigor or endurance.

stammering (stam′er-ing) a disorder of speech behavior marked by involuntary pauses in speech; sometimes used synonymously with stuttering, especially in Great Britain.

Stamnosoma (stam″no-so′mah) [Gr. *stamnos* jar + *sōma* body] a genus of flukes. *S. arma′tum* and *S. formosa′num* are parasites of birds, but experimental human infections have been reported.

standard (stan′dard) something established as a measure or model to which other similar things should conform. **Pignet's s.,** see *Pignet's formula,* under *formula.*

standardization (stan″dard-i-za′shun) 1. the bringing of any preparation to a specified standard as to quality or ingredients. 2. the formulation of standards for a substance or for a procedure.

standardize (stan′dard-īz) to compare with or conform to a standard; to establish standards.

standstill (stand′stil) a quiet state resulting from the suspension of activity or movement, as cardiac standstill. **atrial s.,** cardiac arrhythmia in which there is a pause in atrial contraction secondary to sinus arrest or sinoatrial block, the ventricle continuing to respond to its own pacemaker. **auricular s.,** atrial s. **cardiac s.,** cessation of contraction of the myocardium; see also *cardioplegia.* **respiratory s.,** suspension of the movements of respiration; termed *expiratory s.* when it occurs at the end of an expiration, and *inspiratory s.* when it occurs at the end of an inspiration. **sinus s.,** see under *arrest.* **ventricular s.,** cardiac arrhythmia in which there is an absence of ventricular contraction.

Stanley (stan′le), Wendell Meredith. American biochemist, 1904–1971; co-winner, with James Batcheller Sumner and John Howard Northrop, of the Nobel prize for chemistry in 1946 for isolating virus crystals and for isolating nucleic acid from crystallized virus.

Stanley bacillus (stan′le) [*Stanley,* England] see under *bacillus.*

Stanley Kent see *Kent.*

stannate (stan′āt) any salt of stannic acid.

stannic (stan′ik) containing tin as a quadrivalent element. **s. chloride,** an irritant war smoke, $SnCl_4$.

stanniferous (stan-nif′er-us) [L. *stannum* tin + *ferre* to bear] containing tin.

Stannomida (stah-nom′ĭ-dah) an order of testaceous ameboid protozoa (order Xenophyophorea, superclass Rhizopoda) having a flexible body.

stannosis (stan-o′sis) benign pneumoconiosis due to the inhalation of tin oxide; it is symptomless unless accompanied by silicosis.

stannous (stan′us) containing tin as a bivalent element. For stannous compounds, see under the salt, e.g., *chloride* and *fluoride.*

stannum (stan′um) [L.] tin (symbol Sn).

stanolone (stan′o-lōn) chemical name: 17β-hydroxy-5α-androstan-3-one. A semisynthetic androgen (dihydrotestosterone), $C_{19}H_{30}O_2$, occurring as a white crystalline powder, and having the same actions and uses as testosterone. It is used for its anabolic and antineoplastic actions in inoperable breast cancer and in postoperative metastatic breast cancer.

stanozolol (stan′o-zo-lol″) [USP] chemical name: 17-methyl-2′*H*-5α-androst-2-eno[3,2-c]-pyrazol-17β-ol. An androgenic anabolic steroid, $C_{21}H_{32}N_2O$, occurring as a white, crystalline powder; used orally, especially to increase hemoglobin levels in some patients with aplastic (congenital and idiopathic) anemia.

stapedectomy (sta″pĕ-dek′to-me) [L. *stapes* stirrup + Gr. *ektomē* excision] excision of the stapes.

stapedial (stah-pe′de-al) pertaining to the stapes.

stapediolysis (stah-pe″de-ol′ĭ-sis) mobilization of the stapes in the surgical treatment of otosclerosis.

stapedioplasty (stah-pe″de-o-plas′te) replacement of the stapes with other material (wire, bone, plastic) in correction of defective hearing resulting from otosclerosis, the prosthesis serving to conduct the sound waves from the incus to the oval window (fenestra vestibuli).

stapediotenotomy (stah-pe″de-o-tĕ-not′o-me)   the cutting of the tendon of the stapedius muscle.

stapediovestibular (stah-pe″de-o-ves-tib′u-lar)   pertaining to the stapes and vestibule.

stapes (sta′pēz) [L. "stirrup"] [NA]   the innermost of the auditory ossicles, shaped somewhat like a stirrup; it articulates by its head with the incus, and its base is inserted into the fenestra vestibuli. Called also *stirrup*.

Staphcillin (staf-sil′in)   trademark for preparations of sodium methicillin.

staphisagria (staf″ĭ-sa′gre-ah) [Gr. *staphis* raisin + *agrios* wild]   the poisonous seeds of *Delphinium staphisagria*, stavesacre, or lousewort. The plant and its seeds are poisonous and narcotic. The ripe seeds were formerly used externally as a parasiticide.

staphisagrine (staf″ĭ-sa′grin)   a poisonous alkaloid, $C_{22}H_{33}NO_5$, from staphisagria.

staphylagra (staf″ĭ-la′grah) [*staphyl-* + Gr. *agra* a way of catching]   a forceps for holding the uvula.

staphyledema (staf″il-ĕ-de′mah) [*staphyl-* + Gr. *oidēma* swelling]   an enlargement or swollen state of the uvula.

staphylematoma (staf″il-em″ah-to′mah)   hemorrhage from the uvula (Pauli).

staphyline (staf″ĭ-lin)   1. shaped like a bunch of grapes. 2. pertaining to the uvula; uvular.

staphylinid (staf-ĭ-lin′id)   1. pertaining to or due to beetles of the family Staphylinidae. 2. a beetle of the family Staphylinidae.

Staphylinidae (staf″ĭ-lin′ĭ-de)   a family of beetles (order Coleoptera), some members of which produce an irritating substance that causes blistering one or two days after contact.

staphylinus (staf″ĭ-li′nus) [L.]   pertaining to the uvula.

staphylion (stah-fil′e-on) [Gr. "little grape"]   1. an encephalometric landmark on the posterior edge of the hard palate at the median line. 2. the uvula. 3. a nipple or teat.

staphylitis (staf″ĭ-li′tis)   inflammation of the uvula; uvulitis.

staphyl(o)- [Gr. *staphylē* a bunch of grapes]   a combining form denoting resemblance to a bunch of grapes, used especially to denote relationship to the uvula or to staphylococci.

staphyloangina (staf″ĭ-lo-an′jĭ-nah)   a mild form of sore throat, marked by a pseudomembranous deposit in the throat due to a staphylococcus.

staphylococcal (staf″ĭ-lo-kok′al)   pertaining to or caused by staphylococci.

staphylococcemia (staf″ĭ-lo-kok-se′me-ah) [*staphylococcus* + Gr. *haima* blood + *-ia*]   a condition in which staphylococci are present in the blood; septicemia caused by staphylococci.

staphylococci (staf″ĭ-lo-kok′si)   plural of *staphylococcus*.

staphylococcic (staf″ĭ-lo-kok′sik)   pertaining to or caused by staphylococci.

staphylococcin (staf″ĭ-lo-kok′sin)   a bacteriocin produced by certain strains of *Staphylococcus aureus*.

staphylococcosis (staf″ĭ-lo-kok-o′sis)   infection caused by staphylococci.

Staphylococcus (staf″ĭ-lo-kok′us) [Gr. *staphylē* bunch of grapes + *kokkos* berry]   a genus of gram-positive, facultatively anaerobic bacteria of the family Micrococcaceae, order Eubacteriales, consisting of cocci, usually unencapsulated, 0.5 to 1.5 μ in diameter. The organisms occur singly, in pairs, and in irregular clusters, and are nonsporogenous and nonmotile. They are potential pathogens, causing local lesions and serious opportunistic infections. **S. al′bus,** S. aureus. **S. au′reus,** a species comprising the yellow-pigmented, coagulase-positive pathogenic forms of the genus, causing serious suppurative infections and systemic disease; they produce toxins that cause food poisoning and toxic shock syndrome. Called also *S. pyogenes*. **S. epider′midis,** a coagulase-negative species that ferments glucose and produces colonies that are usually white. They are commonly found on normal skin. Many strains are pathogens or secondary invaders in various diseases, such as abscess, infected wounds, and subacute bacterial endocarditis. **S. haemolyt′icus,** S. simulans. **S. hom′inis,** S. simu-

lans. **S. pyog′enes,** S. aureus. **S. saprophyt′icus,** a coagulase-negative species that ferments glucose weakly; they are usually harmless commensals but are occasionally pathogenic, causing urinary tract infections. **S. sim′ulans,** a coagulase-negative species isolated from certain human infections; called also *S. haemolyticus* and *S. hominis*.

staphylococcus (staf″ĭ-lo-kok′us), pl. *staphylococ′ci*.   an organism of the genus *Staphylococcus*.

staphyloderma (staf″ĭ-lo-der′ma)   cutaneous pyogenic infection by staphylococci.

staphylodialysis (staf″ĭ-lo-di-al′ĭ-sis) [*staphylo-* + Gr. *dialysis* loosing]   relaxation of the uvula.

staphyloedema (staf″ĭ-lo-ĕ-de′mah)   staphyledema.

staphylokinase (staf″ĭ-lo-ki′nās)   a bacterial kinase produced by certain strains of staphylococci, which is capable of activating plasminogen in the blood of various species of animals; see also *kinase* (def. 2).

staphylolysin (staf″ĭ-lol′ĭ-sin)   a principle with hemolytic activity produced by staphylococci. **α s., alpha s.,** a hemolysin produced by pathogenic staphylococci which lyses both sheep and rabbit erythrocytes at 37° C. and has leukocidin activity. **β s., beta s.,** a hot-cold hemolysin produced by staphylococci which lyses sheep but not rabbit erythrocytes in the cold following preliminary incubation at 37° C. **δ s., delta s.,** a hemolysin produced by pyogenic staphylococci which lyses red cells from man and several other species; it differs immunologically from the α and β staphylolysins, and is both dermonecrotic and lethal. **ε s., epsilon s.,** a hemolysin formed almost exclusively by nonpathogenic, coagulase-negative strains of staphylococci. **γ s., gamma s.,** a hemolysin produced by staphylococci which is similar to, but serologically distinguishable from, the α staphylolysin.

staphyloma (staf″ĭ-lo′mah) [Gr. *staphylōma* a defect in the eye inside the cornea]   protrusion of the cornea or sclera lined with uveal tissue, resulting from inflammation. **annular s.,** staphyloma of the sclera in the ciliary region, extending around the margin of the cornea. **anterior s.,** scleral or corneal staphyloma in the anterior part of the eye. **ciliary s.,** scleral staphyloma in the part covered by the ciliary body. **s. cor′neae, corneal s.,** 1. ectasia of the cornea with adherent uveal tissue; called also *prolapsus corneae* and *projecting staphyloma*. 2. staphyloma formed by an iris which has protruded through a wound in the cornea. **s. cor′neae racemo′sum,** staphyloma corneae (def. 2) in which there are a number of perforations from which small portions of iris protrude. **equatorial s.,** scleral staphyloma occurring in the equatorial region of the eye. **intercalary s.,** that which occurs in the rim of sclera anterior to the insertion of the ciliary body. **posterior s., s. posti′cum,** backward bulging of the sclera at the posterior pole of the eye; called also *Scarpa's s.* **projecting s.,** s. corneae. **retinal s.,** a forward bulging of the retina. **Scarpa's s.,** posterior s. **scleral s.,** protrusion of the contents of the eyeball at a point where the sclera has become too thin. **uveal s.,** protrusion of the uvea through a ruptured sclera.

staphylomatous (staf″ĭ-lom′ah-tus)   pertaining to or resembling staphyloma.

staphyloncus (staf″ĭ-long′kus) [*staphylo-* + Gr. *onkos* mass]   a tumor or swelling of the uvula.

staphylopharyngorrhaphy (staf″ĭ-lo-far″in-gor′ah-fe) [*staphylo-* + Gr. *pharynx* the throat + *rhaphē* suture]   the stitching of the halves of the velum palatini to the posterior wall of the pharynx.

staphyloplasty (staf″ĭ-lo-plas″te) [*staphylo-* + Gr. *plassein* to mold]   plastic repair of the soft palate and uvula.

staphyloptosia (staf″ĭ-lop-to′se-ah) [*staphylo-* + Gr. *ptōsis* falling + *-ia*]   elongation of the uvula.

staphyloptosis (staf″ĭ-lop-to′sis)   staphyloptosia; uvuloptosis.

staphylorrhaphy (staf″ĭ-lor′ah-fe) [*staphylo-* + Gr. *rhaphē* suture]   surgical correction of a midline cleft in the uvula and soft palate; cionorrhaphy. Cf. *palatorrhaphy*.

staphyloschisis (staf″ĭ-los′kĭ-sis) [*staphylo-* + Gr. *schisis* splitting]   fissure of the uvula and soft palate; a form of cleft palate.

staphylotome (staf′ĭ-lo-tōm) [Gr. *staphylotomon*]   a knife for cutting the uvula; uvulotome.

staphylotomy (staf″ĭ-lot′o-me) [*staphylo-* + *-tomy*] 1. incision of the uvula; uvulotomy. 2. the removal of a staphyloma by cutting.

staphylotoxin (staf″ĭ-lo-tok′sin) any of the several toxins produced by *Staphylococcus aureus*; see *staphylococcal toxin*, under *toxin*.

stapling (sta′pling) the act or process of fastening with staples. **gastric s.**, gastric partitioning.

star (star) any structure with an appearance like that of a star. **daughter s.**, amphiaster. **dental s.**, a marking on the incisor teeth of horses, first appearing in the lower central incisors at about the age of eight years; used in judging a horse's age. **lens s's,** starlike lines formed within the lens of the eye by fibers which pass from the anterior to the posterior surface. **mother s.**, monaster. **polar s's,** the starlike figures of the amphiaster. **s's of Verheyen,** venulae stellatae renis. **Winslow's s's,** whorls of capillary vessels from which arise the vorticose veins of the choroid coat of the eye.

starch (starch) [L. *amylum*] 1. any of a group of polysaccharides of the general formula $(C_6H_{10}O_5)_n$, composed of a long-chain polymer of glucose in the form of amylose and amylopectin; it is the chief storage form of energy reserve (carbohydrates) in plants. 2. [NF] a preparation consisting of the granules separated from the mature grain of corn or wheat, or from potato tubers, occurring as irregular, angular, white masses or fine powder; used as a dusting powder and as a filler, binder, and disintegrant in pharmaceutical preparations. **animal s.**, glycogen. **cassava s.**, the starch from the roots of cassava (*Manihot utilissima* and *M. aipi*) which is the source of tapioca. **corn s.**, a starch from maize. **s. glycerite** [NF], a preparation of starch, benzoic acid, purified water, and glycerin; used as an emollient in pharmaceutical preparations intended for external use. **hydroxyethyl s.**, a starch product which has been suggested as a plasma substitute in man. **lichen s.**, **moss s.**, lichenin. **pregelatinized s.**, [NF], starch chemically or mechanically processed to rupture all or part of the granules in the presence of water, and subsequently dried; it occurs as a moderately coarse to fine, white to off-white powder and is used as a tablet excipient in pharmaceutical preparations. **sago s.**, starch from the sago palm. **soluble s.**, amidulin.

stare (stār) [A.S. *starian*] a fixed, unblinking gaze. **postbasic s.**, a peculiar expression of the eyes in posterior basic meningitis due to downward rolling of the eyeball and retraction of the upper lid.

Starling's hypothesis, law (star′lingz) [Ernest Henry *Starling*, English physiologist, 1866–1927] see under *hypothesis* and *law*.

starter (star′ter) a culture of microorganisms used to initiate fermentation, as in dairy products.

stasimorphia (stas″ĭ-mor′fe-ah) stasimorphy.

stasimorphy (stas″ĭ-mor′fe) [Gr. *stasis* standing + *morphē* form] deformity or abnormality of shape in any organ, due to arrest of development.

stasis (sta′sis) [Gr. "a standing still"] 1. a stoppage or diminution of the flow of blood or other body fluid in any part. 2. a state of equilibrium among opposing forces. **ileal s.**, abnormal delay in the passage of the intestinal contents through the ileum; it is usually associated with dilatation of the ileum. **intestinal s.**, any condition in which normal passage of intestinal content is impaired; it may be due to mechanical obstruction or impaired intestinal motility. **papillary s.**, papilledema. **pressure s.**, stoppage of the circulation caused by undue pressure on a part. **urinary s.**, stoppage of the flow or discharge of urine, which may occur at any level of the urinary tract. **venous s.**, cessation or impairment of venous flow.

-stasis [Gr. "a standing still"] a word termination indicating the maintenance of (or maintaining) a constant level; preventing increase or multiplication.

Stas-Otto method (stahs-ot′o) [Jean Servais *Stas*, a Belgian chemist, 1813–1891] see under *method*.

stat. abbreviation for L. *sta′tim*, immediately.

-stat [Gr. *-states* one who causes to stand, from *histanai* to cause to stand] a word termination denoting an agent that inhibits growth without killing, or a device that maintains something in a steady state.

state (stāt) [L. *status*] 1. condition or situation; status. 2. the crisis, or the turning point of an attack of disease. **acute confusional s.**, delirium. **alpha s.**, the state of relaxation and peaceful awakefulness, associated with prominent alpha brain wave activity. **anelectrotonic s.**, the condition which obtains in a nerve near the anode during the passage of a continuous current. **anxiety s.**, see under *neurosis*. **anxiety tension s. (A.T.S.),** neuromuscular hypertension. **borderline s.**, a diagnostic term used when it is difficult to determine whether symptoms are predominantly neurotic or psychotic. **carrier s.**, see carrier, def. 1. **catelectrotonic s.**, the condition of a nerve near the cathode during the passage of an electric current. **central excitatory s.**, a condition in which there is stored up in a reflex center of the spinal cord a number of stimuli which do not reveal themselves in reflex response. **correlated s.**, dynamic equilibrium. **dreamy s.**, a state of altered consciousness lasting for a few minutes and accompanied by hallucinations; associated with temporal lobe lesions. **epileptic s.**, status epilepticus. **excited s.**, the condition of a nucleus, atom, or molecule produced by the addition of energy to the system as the result of absorption of photons or of inelastic collisions with other particles or systems. **ground s.**, the condition of lowest energy of a nucleus, atom, or molecule, as opposed to the excited state. **hypnagogic s.**, that state of semiconsciousness which immediately precedes falling asleep. **hypnoid s.**, in Freudian theory, an alteration of consciousness, characterized by heightened suggestibility, that occurs in hysteria during emotional stress and provides the basis for hysterical somatic symptom formation. **hypnopompic s.**, that state of semiconsciousness which immediately precedes complete awakening from sleep. **local excitatory s.**, the condition of a nerve produced by an ineffectual stimulus. **marble s.**, status marmoratus. **metastable s.**, the condition of a system (nucleus, atom, or molecule) capable of undergoing quantum transition to a state of lower energy. **oxidation s.**, see under *number*. **persistent vegetative s.**, a condition of profound nonresponsiveness in the wakeful state caused by brain damage at whatever level and characterized by a nonfunctioning cerebral cortex, the absence of any discernible adaptive response to the external environment, akinesia, mutism, and inability to signal; the electroencephalogram may be isoelectric or show abnormal activity. **plastic s.**, **pluripotent s.**, the state of parts of the zygote or early embryo in which they may develop into any adult tissue or part. **refractory s.**, a condition of subnormal excitability of muscle and nerve following excitation. **resting s.**, the physiological condition achieved by complete bed rest for a period of at least one hour, a condition required in a number of different tests of various body functions. **steady s.**, dynamic equilibrium. **triplet s.**, the state resulting when an electron is activated by absorbing a photon, moves to an outer orbital of higher energy, and pairs with an electron of like spin. **twilight s.**, a temporary absence of consciousness in which the patient may perform certain acts involuntarily and without remembrance of them afterward.

stathmokinesis (stath″mo-ki-ne′sis) a state of arrested mitosis, or pseudometaphase, as that induced by subjecting cells to the action of an agent such as colchicine, which destroys the fibrillar structure of cell spindles and thus permits the calculation of mitosis time.

static (stat′ik) [Gr. *statikos* causing to stand, from *histanai* to cause to stand] 1. at rest; in equilibrium; not in motion. 2. not dynamic. 3. a word termination meaning inhibiting, or denoting an agent that inhibits.

statics (stat′iks) that phase of mechanics which deals with the action of forces and systems of forces on bodies at rest.

statim (sta′tim) [L.] immediately, at once. Abbreviated *stat.*

station (sta′shun) [L. *statio*, from *stare* to stand still] 1. the position assumed in standing; the manner of standing; in ataxic conditions it is sometimes pathognomonic. See *attitude*. 2. the location of the presenting part of the fetus in the birth canal, designated as −5 to −1 according to the number of centimeters the part is above an imaginary plane passing through the ischial spines, 0 when at the plane, and +1 to +5 according to the number of centimeters the part is below the plane. 3. a specified site to which the sick and wounded are brought. **anterior s.**, see *salivaria*. **posterior s.**, see *stercoraria*. **Romberg s.**, the position assumed by the patient when the Romberg sign is being sought, i.e., standing upright with the feet close together.

stationary (sta′shun-er″e) [L. *stationarius*] not subject to variations or to changes of place.

statistic (stah-tis′tik) [back formation from *statistics*] any function computed from the values of a random sample, such as the sample mean or median, when considered as a random variable with a known probability distribution.

statistics (stah-tis′tiks) [Ger. *Statistik* originally "political science of state affairs," from L. *status* state] 1. a collection of numerical data. 2. a distinct scientific method that aims at solving real life problems by the use of the theory of probability; it usually deals with the collection, analysis, and interpretation of numerical data, especially with methods for drawing inferences about characteristics of a population from examination of a random sample. **bayesian s.,** a somewhat controversial statistical methodology that, unlike conventional statistics, which treats population parameters as fixed (though unknown) values, treats parameters as random variables with a specified probability distribution, termed the prior (or *a priori*) distribution. Bayes' theorem is then used to convert the probability distribution of an observable statistic (treated as a conditional probability for a given parameter value) to a conditional probability distribution of the parameter values for a given value of the observable statistic. This distribution is termed the posterior (or *a posteriori*) distribution because it assigns a probability to each parameter value that depends on the observed data. The controversial point is the prior distribution, which represents a subjective opinion of the experimenter as to the *a priori* credibility of the various parameter values; for example, in estimating the probability of the presence of a particular disease given a positive test result, the prior distribution represents the experimenter's judgement of the prevalence of the disease in the population under study. **nonparametric s.,** see *nonparametric*. **vital s.,** the data collected by governmental bodies by registration of all births, deaths, fetal deaths, marriages, and divorces.

statoacoustic (stat″o-ah-koo′stik) pertaining to balance and hearing.

statoconia (stat″o-ko′ne-ah), pl. of *statoconium* [Gr. *statos* standing + *konos* dust] [NA] minute calciferous granules within the gelatinous statoconic membrane surmounting the acoustic maculae; called also *otoconia*.

statoconium (stat″o-ko′ne-um) singular of *statoconia*; called also *otoconium* and *otoconite*.

statocyst (stat′o-sist) [Gr. *statos* standing + *kystis* sac, bladder] one of the sacs of the labyrinth of the ear to which is attributed an influence in the maintenance of static equilibrium.

statolith (stat′o-lith) 1. one of the granules constituting the statoconia; called also *ear crystal, otolith, otolite,* and *otosteon.* 2. a solid or semisolid body occurring in the statocyst of animals.

statolon (stat′o-lon) an antiviral agent derived from *Penicillium stoloniferum,* which inhibits the multiplication of certain picornaviruses and arboviruses.

statometer (stah-tom′ĕ-ter) exophthalmometer.

statosphere (stat′o-sfēr) centrosome.

statural (stat′u-ral) pertaining to stature.

stature (stat′ūr) [L. *statura*] the height or tallness of a person standing.

status (sta′tus) [L.] state or condition. **absence s.,** sustained clouding of consciousness for several hours, with no interval of normal mental activity, and with few stereotyped movements or no abnormal motor activity. **s. anginosus,** angina which occurs at rest and is refractory to treatment; called also *preinfarction angina.* **s. arthriticus,** gouty diathesis; predisposition to gout. **s. asthmaticus,** a particularly severe episode of asthma, usually requiring hospitalization, that does not respond adequately to ordinary therapeutic measures. **s. calcifames,** calcium hunger. **s. choreicus,** a severe and persistent form of chorea. **s. convulsivus,** epilepticus. **s. cribalis, s. cribrosus,** a sievelike condition of the brain due to dilatation of the perivascular lymph spaces. **s. criticus,** a severe and persistent form of tabetic crises. **s. dysgraphicus,** dysgraphia. **s. dysmyelinatus, s. dysmyelinisatus,** Hallervorden-Spatz syndrome. **s. dysraphicus,** faulty closure of the embryonic neural tube resulting in faulty formation of midline adult structures, such as the spine, sternum, breasts, and palate; called also

arrhaphia. **s. epilepticus,** a series of rapidly repeated epileptic convulsions without any periods of consciousness between them. **s. hemicranicus,** a state marked by constantly recurring attacks of migraine. **s. lacunaris, s. lacunosus,** a condition of the brain marked by numerous small infarcts or losses of substance. **s. lymphaticus,** hyperplasia of lymphoid tissue and the thymus, formerly thought to be an important cause of sudden death (by airway obstruction) in infants; called also *status thymicolymphaticus,* and *status thymicus.* **s. marmoratus,** a condition marked by excessive myelinization of the nerve fibers of the corpus striatum, as in Vogt's syndrome; called also *état marbré* and *marble state.* **petit mal s.,** a state of mental confusion lasting for minutes or hours, and accompanied by nearly continuous 3-cps spike and wave discharges in the electroencephalogram. **s. praesens,** the condition of a patient at the time of observation. **s. raptus,** a condition of ecstasy. **s. spongiosus,** extensive vacuolization of the cerebral cortex; called also *spongiform encephalopathy.* **s. thymicolymphaticus,** s. lymphaticus. **s. thymicus,** s. lymphaticus. **s. verrucosus,** a wartlike appearance of the cerebral cortex, produced by disorderly arrangement of the neuroblasts so that the formation of fissures and sulci is irregular and unpredictable. **s. vertiginosus,** prolonged vertigo.

statuvolence (stat-u′vo-lens) [L. *status* state + *volens* willing] (*obs.*) a voluntary, self-induced state of hypnotism.

statuvolent (stat-u′vo-lent) (*obs.*) affected with or able to enter a condition of statuvolence.

Staub-Traugott effect (test) (stawb-traw′got) [Hans *Staub,* Swiss (Basel) internist, born 1890; Carl *Traugott,* Frankfort internist, born 1885] see under *effect.*

staurion (staw′re-on) [Gr., dim. of *stauros* cross] a point at the crossing of the median and transverse palatine sutures.

stauroplegia (staw″ro-ple′je-ah) [Gr. *stauros* cross + *plēgē* stroke] alternate hemiplegia.

stavesacre (stāvz′a-ker) staphisagria.

staxis (stak′sis) [Gr. "a dripping"] hemorrhage.

stay (sta) a narrow structure that gives support, such as the bar of a horse's hoof. **s. of white line,** adminiculum lineae albae.

STD sexually transmitted disease.

steal (stēl) the diversion, as of blood flow, from its normal course, as in occlusive arterial disease. **subclavian s.,** in occlusive disease of the subclavian artery, a reversal of blood flow in the ipsilateral vertebral artery (which may deprive the brain of blood) from the basilar artery to the subclavian artery beyond the point of occlusion.

stearaldehyde (ste″ah-ral′dĕ-hīd) a long-chain, aliphatic aldehyde of the class of free aldehydes with the formula $CH_3(CH_2)_{16}CHO$; it is found in plasmalogens, which give the so-called plasmal reaction upon direct treatment of the tissue with Schiff's reagent.

stearate (ste-ah-rāt, stēr′āt) any salt (soap), ester, or anionic form of stearic acid.

stearic acid (ste-ah′rik, stēr′ik) [Gr. *stear* fat + *-ic*] trivial name for octadecanoic acid, the 18-carbon straight-chain fatty acid. Stearic and palmitic acids are the two most common unsaturated fatty acids in body fluids.

steariform (ste-ar′ĭ-form) fatlike.

stearin (ste′ah-rin) tristearin.

stear(o)-, steat(o)- [Gr. *stear,* gen. *steatos* fat] combining forms denoting relationship to fat.

stearopten (ste″ah-rop′ten) [*stearo-* + Gr. *ptēnos* volatile] a camphor; the more solid substance which, combined with an eleopten, constitutes a typical volatile oil.

stearoyl-CoA desaturase (stēr′o-il de-satch′ū-rās) acyl-CoA desaturase.

stearrhea (ste″ah-re′ah) [*stearo-* + Gr. *rhoia* flow] steatorrhea.

steatite (ste′ah-tīt) talc.

steatitis (ste″ah-ti′tis) [*steato-* + *-itis*] inflammation of adipose tissue.

steat(o)- see *stear(o)-.*

steatocele (ste-at′o-sēl) [*steato-* + Gr. *kēlē* tumor] a fatty mass formed within the scrotum.

steatocystoma (ste″ah-to-sis-to′mah) an epithelial cyst. **s. multiplex,** an autosomal dominant disorder chiefly affecting males at birth or presenting about the time of puberty, characterized by the development of numerous flesh-colored to yellow epidermal cysts, especially involving the skin of the sternum, the proximal extremities, and the scrotum in males. The cysts typically have an intricately infolded thin epidermal lining, without a granular layer, incorporating abortive hair follicles and at times sebaceous, eccrine, or apocrine structures, and contain lanugo hair and an oily material.

steatogenous (ste″ah-toj′ĕ-nus) [steato- + Gr. gennan to produce] lipogenic.

steatolysis (ste″ah-tol′ĭ-sis) [steato- + Gr. lysis dissolution] the emulsifying process fats undergo preparatory to absorption.

steatolytic (ste″ah-to-lit′ik) pertaining to, characterized by, or promoting steatolysis.

steatoma (ste″ah-to′mah), pl. steato′mata or steatomas. 1. a lipoma. 2. a fatty mass retained within a sebaceous gland.

steatomatosis (ste″ah-to-mah-to′sis) 1. the presence of numerous steatomas. 2. steatocystoma multiplex.

steatomery (ste″ah-tom′er-e) [steato- + Gr. meros thigh] a deposit of fat on the outer aspect of the thighs and buttocks.

steatonecrosis (ste″ah-to-nĕ-kro′sis) fat necrosis.

steatopygia (ste″ah-to-pij′e-ah) [steato- + Gr. pygē buttock + -ia] excessive fatness of the buttocks, usually seen in women. Sometimes called Hottentot bustle because it is commonly seen in the Hottentot people of southern Africa.

steatopygous (ste″ah-top′ĭ-gus) pertaining to or characterized by steatopygia.

steatorrhea (ste″ah-to-re′ah) [steato- + Gr. rhoia a flow] excessive amounts of fats in the feces, as in malabsorption syndromes. **idiopathic s.,** nontropical sprue.

steatosis (ste″ah-to′sis) fatty degeneration. **s. cardi′aca,** cardiomyoliposis.

stechiology (stek″e-ol′o-je) stoichiology.

stechiometry (stek″e-om′ĕ-tre) stoichiometry.

Steclin (stek′lin) trademark for preparations of tetracycline.

Steell's murmur (stēlz) [Graham Steell, English physician, 1851–1942] Graham Steell's murmur; see under murmur.

Steenbock unit (stēn′bok) [Harry Steenbock, American biochemist, 1886–1967] see under unit.

steffimycin (stef-ĭ-mi′sin) an antibacterial with antiviral properties, produced by Streptomyces steffisburgensis var. steffisburgensis.

stege (ste′je) [Gr. stegos roof] the internal layer of the rods of Corti.

stegnosis (steg-no′sis) [Gr. stegnōsis obstruction] constriction; stenosis.

stegnotic (steg-not′ik) pertaining to, characterized by, or promoting stegnosis; astringent.

Stegomyia (steg″o-mi′yah) [Gr. stegos roof + myia fly] a subgenus of mosquitoes. S. argen′teus, S. cal′opus and S. fascia′tus are old names for Aedes aegypti.

Stein's test (stīnz) [Stanislav Aleksandr Fyodorovich von Stein, Russian otologist, born 1855] see under tests.

Stein-Leventhal syndrome (stīn-lev′en-thal) [Irving F. Stein, Sr., American gynecologist, born 1887; Michael Leo Leventhal, American obstetrician and gynecologist, 1901–1971] see under syndrome.

Steiner's tumors (sti′nerz) [Gabriel Steiner, German neurologist, born 1883] Jeanselme's nodules.

Steinmann's pin (stīn′manz) [Fritz Steinmann, Bern surgeon, 1872–1932] see under pin.

Stelangium (ste-lan′je-um) a genus of bacteria of uncertain status, made up of organisms producing fruiting bodies that contain myxospores.

Stelazine (stel′ah-zēn) trademark for preparations of trifluoperazine hydrochloride.

stele (stēl) [Gr. stechelo stem] the cylindrical central core of vascular tissue of a plant, consisting of the pericycle and the tissues within it—xylem, phloem, and parenchyma.

stella (stel′ah), pl. stel′lae [L.] star. **s. len′tis hyaloi′dea,** the posterior pole of the crystalline lens. **s. len′tis iri′dica,** the anterior pole of the crystalline lens.

Stellaria (stel-la′re-ah) a genus of caryophyllaceous plants, the chickweeds. S. holos′tea and S. me′dia L. were formerly used as demulcent medicines.

stellate (stel′āt) [L. stellatus] shaped like a star; arranged in a roset, or in rosets.

Stellatosporea (stel″ah-to-spor′e-ah) [stellate + spore] a class of parasitic protozoa (phylum Ascetospora), characterized by the presence of haplosporosomes and spores with one or more sporoplasms. It comprises two orders: Occlusosporida and Balanosporida.

stellectomy (stel-lek′to-me) removal of the stellate ganglion; done for the relief of pain.

Stellite (stel′it; stel′līt) trademark for any of a group of nonferrous, very hard, noncorrosive alloys composed chiefly of cobalt and chromium, with or without small amounts of other metals added. Used especially in the manufacture of cutting tools such as surgical instruments.

stellreflexe (stel″re-flek′sĕ) [Ger.] a postural reflex.

stellula (stel′u-lah), pl. stel′lulae [L., dim. of stella] little star. **stel′lulae vasculo′sae winslow′ii,** Winslow's stars. **stellulae of Verheyen,** venulae stellatae renis. **stel′lulae verhey′enii,** venulae stellatae renis.

stellulae (stel′u-le) [L.] plural of stellula.

Stellwag's sign (symptom) (stel′vagz) [Carl Stellwag von Carion, Austrian ophthalmologist, 1823–1904] see under sign.

stem (stem) a supporting structure comparable to the stalk or stem of a plant. **brain s.,** see under B. **infundibular s.,** 1. the inferior part of the infundibulum hypothalami, which contains the neural connections of the pituitary gland and is continuous with the tuber cinereum; called also infundibular stalk. 2. infundibulum hypothalami.

Stemonitida (ste″mo-ni′tĭ-dah) [Gr. stēmōn warp, thread] an order of ameboid protozoa (subclass Myxogastria, class Eumycetozoa), the organisms of which have a spore mass that is usually dark colored. Stemonitis is a representative genus.

Stemonitis (ste″mo-ni′tis) a genus of ameboid protozoa (order Stemonitida, subclass Myxogastria), the organisms of which have evanescent sporangium and a capillitium that ramifies from the columella.

Stender dish (sten′der) [Wilhelm P. Stender, manufacturer in Leipzig] see under dish.

Stenediol (sten′di-ol) trademark for preparations of methandriol.

stenion (sten′e-on), pl. sten′ia [Gr. stenos narrow + -on neuter ending] an encephalometric landmark, the craniometrical point situated at each end of the smallest transverse diameter of the head in the temporal region.

Steno (ste′no) see Stensen.

sten(o)- [Gr. stenos narrow] a combining form meaning contracted or narrow.

stenobregmatic (sten″o-breg-mat′ik) [steno- + Gr. bregma the front part of the head] having the upper and anterior portion of the head narrowed.

stenocardia (sten″o-kar′de-ah) angina pectoris.

stenocephalia (sten″o-sĕ-fa′le-ah) stenocephaly.

stenocephalous (sten″o-sef′ah-lus) having a narrow head.

stenocephaly (sten″o-sef′ah-le) [steno- + Gr. kephalē head] excessive narrowness of the head.

stenochoria (sten″o-ko′re-ah) [steno- + Gr. chōros space] stenosis, or narrowing.

stenocoriasis (sten″o-ko-ri′ah-sis) [steno- + Gr. korē pupil] contraction of the pupil of the eye.

stenocrotaphia (sten″o-kro-ta′fe-ah) [steno- + Gr. krotaphos temple + -ia] narrowness of the temporal region.

stenocrotaphy (sten″o-krot′ah-fe) stenocrotaphia.

stenopeic (sten″o-pe′ik) [sten- + Gr. opē opening] having a narrow slit or opening, as stenopeic spectacles.

stenosal (ste-no′sal) stenotic.

stenosed (stĕ-nōst′, stĕ-nōzd′) narrowed or constricted.

stenosis (stĕ-no′sis) [Gr. stenōsis] narrowing or stricture of a duct or canal. **aortic s.,** a narrowing of the aortic orifice of the heart or of the aorta itself. **buttonhole mitral s.,** mitral stenosis in which adhesion and shortening of the mitral cusps produces a diaphragmatic slit resembling a buttonhole; called also buttonhole deformity and fishmouth mitral s. **caroticovertebral s.,** atherosclerotic stenosis of the cervical portions of the vertebral arteries, resulting in cerebral ischemia. **cicatricial s.,** stenosis caused by the contraction of a cicatrix. **fishmouth mitral s.,** buttonhole mitral s. **granulation s.,** stenosis or narrowing caused by the deposit of granulations or by their contraction. **idiopathic hypertrophic subaortic s.,** a cardiomyopathy of unknown cause, in which the left ventricle is hypertrophied (commonly with disproportionate involvement of the interventricular septum) and the cavity is small; it is marked by obstruction to left ventricular outflow. Called also *muscular subaortic s.* **infundibular s.,** stenosis below the pulmonary valve, within the infundibulum (conus arteriosus) of the right ventricle of the heart. **mitral s.,** a narrowing of the left atrioventricular orifice (mitral orifice). **muscular subaortic s.,** idiopathic hypertrophic subaortic s. **myocardial infundibular s.,** infundibular stenosis due to hypertrophy of the surrounding myocardium, resulting in a long narrow channel. **postdiphtheritic s.,** stenosis of the larynx or trachea following diphtheria. **pulmonary s.,** narrowing of the opening between the pulmonary artery and the right ventricle. **pyloric s.,** obstruction of the pyloric orifice of the stomach; it may be congenital as in hypertrophic pyloric stenosis, or acquired due to peptic ulceration or prepyloric carcinoma. **subaortic s., subvalvular aortic s.,** aortic stenosis due to an obstructive lesion in the left ventricle below the aortic valve, causing a pressure gradient across the obstruction within the ventricle. **supravalvular s.,** a rare form of aortic stenosis occurring above the aortic valve, usually caused by a complete circumferential fibrous ring of constricting tissue at the level of the sinus of Valsalva. **tricuspid s.,** narrowing or stricture of the tricuspid orifice of the heart. **valvular s.,** stenosis affecting any of the valves of the heart; see *aortic s., mitral s., pulmonary s.,* and *tricuspid s.*

stenothermal (sten″o-ther′mal) stenothermic.

stenothermic (sten″o-ther′mik) [steno- + Gr. *thermē* heat] capable of development only within a narrow range of temperature, e.g., a bacterial culture.

stenothorax (sten″o-tho′raks) [steno- + Gr. *thōrax* chest] abnormal narrowness of the chest.

stenotic (stĕ-not′ik) [Gr. *stenotēs* narrowness] pertaining to or characterized by stenosis; abnormally narrowed.

Stensen's canal, duct, experiment, foramen, plexus (sten′senz) [Niels *Stensen,* Danish priest-physician, anatomist, physiologist, and theologian, 1638–1686] see under *experiment* and *plexus,* and see *canalis incisivum, ductus parotideus,* and *foramen incisivum.*

stent (stent) [from Charles R. *Stent* English dentist, died 1901] a mold for keeping a skin graft in place, made of Stent's mass or some acrylic or dental compound. By extension, used to designate a device or mold of a suitable material, used to hold a skin graft in place or to provide support for tubular structures that are being anastomosed.

step (step) one of a series of footrests on different levels, or a structure resembling it. **Rönne's nasal s.,** a steplike defect in the nasal side of the visual field; seen in glaucoma.

stephanial (ste-fa′ne-al) pertaining to the stephanion.

stephanion (stĕ-fa′ne-on) [Gr. *stephanos* crown + -*on* neuter ending] the point on the side of the cranium at which the coronal suture meets the superior temporal line.

Stephanofilaria (stef″ah-no-fĭ-la′re-ah) a genus of filarial nematodes. **S. stile′si,** a species causing dermatitis in cattle in the United States.

stephanofilariasis (stef″ah-no-fil″ah-ri′ah-sis) a chronic skin disease of cattle in certain parts of the United States, due to infestation with the nematode *Stephanofilaria stilesi;* called also *verminous dermatitis.*

Stephanurus (stef″ah-nu′rus) a genus of nematode parasites of the family Syngamidae. **S. denta′tus,** a species parasitic in the urinary tract and occasionally in other tissues of swine.

steradian (ste-ra′de-an) [Gr. *ster-* solid + *radian*] the unit of measurement of solid angles, equivalent to the angle subtended at the center of a sphere by an area on its surface equal to the square of its radius. A full sphere subtends 4π steradians.

Sterane (ster′ān) trademark for preparations of prednisolone.

sterc(o)- [L. *stercus* dung] a combining form denoting relationship to feces.

stercobilin (ster″ko-bi′lin) [*sterco-* + *bilin*] a bile pigment derivative, $C_{33}H_{46}N_4O_6$, formed by air oxidation of stercobilinogen, which is in turn derived by reduction of bilirubin; it is a brown-orange-red pigmentation contributing to the color of feces and urine.

stercobilinogen (ster″ko-bi-lin′o-jen) a bilirubin metabolite and precursor of stercobilin, formed by reduction of urobilinogen.

stercolith (ster′ko-lith) [*sterco-* + Gr. *lithos* stone] a fecal concretion.

stercoraceous (ster″ko-ra′shus) [L. *stercoraceus*] consisting of or containing feces; fecal.

stercoral (ster′ko-ral) stercoraceous.

stercoraria (ster″ko-ra′re-ah) in some systems of classification, a group or section comprising those trypanosomes in which the developmental cycle is completed in the hindgut (posterior station) of the vector and transmission is by fecal contamination during biting of the host by the vector. The group includes the subgenera *Megatrypanum, Herpetosoma,* and *Schizotrypanum.* Cf. *salivaria.*

stercorarian (ster″ko-ra′re-an) pertaining to or caused by trypanosomes of the stercoraria group or section.

stercorin (ster′ko-rin) coprostanol.

stercorolith (ster′ko-ro-lith) stercolith.

stercoroma (ster″ko-ro′mah) a large accumulation of fecal matter forming a tumor-like mass in the rectum.

stercorous (ster′ko-rus) [L. *stercorosus*] of the nature of excrement.

Sterculia (ster-ku′le-ah) a genus of trees and shrubs, including many species, mostly tropical; some have edible seeds and others are medicinal, while still others afford a gummy exudation with cathartic and adhesive properties (see *karaya gum,* under *gum*). The hairs of *S. apetala* of Panama may be very irritating.

stercus (ster′kus), pl. *ster′cora* [L.] dung, or feces.

stere (stēr) [Gr. *stereos* solid] a cubic meter.

stereo- [Gr. *stereos* solid] a combining form meaning solid, having three dimensions, or firmly established.

stereoagnosis (ste″re-o-ag-no′sis) astereognosis.

stereoanesthesia (ste″re-o-an″es-the′ze-ah) reduced tactile ability to identify the form, size, weight, and texture of objects.

stereoarthrolysis (ste″re-o-ar-throl′ĭ-sis) [*stereo-* + Gr. *arthron* joint + *lysis* dissolution] operative formation of a movable new joint in cases of bony ankylosis.

stereoauscultation (ste″re-o-aws″kul-ta′shun) auscultation by means of two phonendoscopes each on different parts of the chest. One tube of each instrument is placed in the ears, the other tube of each being closed with the fingers.

stereoblastula (ste″re-o-blas′tu-lah) a solid blastula, all of whose cells reach the external surface.

stereocampimeter (ste″re-o-kam-pim′ĕ-ter) [*stereo-* + *campimeter*] an instrument for studying unilateral central scotomas and defects in the central retinal area.

stereochemical (ste″re-o-kem′e-kal) pertaining to stereochemistry, or to the space relations of the atoms of a molecule.

stereochemistry (ste″re-o-kem′is-tre) that chemical theory which supposes an arrangement of the atoms of certain molecules in three-dimensional spaces; that branch of chemistry which treats of the space relations between atoms.

stereocilia (ste″re-o-sil′e-ah) [L.] plural of *stereocilium.*

stereocilium (ste″re-o-sil′e-um), pl. *stereocil′ia.* A nonmotile protoplasmic filament on the free surface of a cell. Cf. *kinocilium.*

stereocinefluorography (ste″re-o-sin″ĕ-floo″or-og′rah-fe) photographic recording by motion picture camera of x-ray images produced by stereofluoroscopy, affording three-dimensional visualization.

stereocognosy (ste″re-o-kog′no-se) stereognosis.

stereoencephalotome (ster″e-o-en-sef′ah-lo-tōm″) a guiding instrument used in stereoencephalotomy.

stereoencephalotomy (ster″e-o-en-sef″ah-lot′o-me) [*stereo-* + Gr. *enkephalos* brain + *tomē* a cutting] stereotaxic surgery.

stereofluoroscopy (ste″re-o-floo″o-ros′ko-pe) stereoscopic fluoroscopy.

stereognosis (ste″re-og-no′sis) [*stereo-* + Gr. *gnōsis* knowledge] 1. the faculty of perceiving and understanding the form and nature of objects by the sense of touch. 2. perception by the senses of the solidity of objects.

stereognostic (ste″re-og-nos′tik) pertaining to stereognosis.

stereogram (ste′re-o-gram) 1. a stereoscopic roentgenogram. 2. a stereoscopic drawing.

stereograph (ste′re-o-graf) stereogram.

stereoisomer (ste″re-o-i′so-mer) one of a group of compounds having a stereoisomeric relationship.

stereoisomeric (ster″e-o-i″so-mer′ik) pertaining to or exhibiting stereoisomerism.

stereoisomerism (ster″e-o-i-som′er-izm) [*stereo-* + *isomerism*] the relationship between two or more isomers that have the same structure (the same linkages between atoms) but different configurations (spatial arrangements) in contrast to structural isomerism in which the isomers have different structures. Stereoisomers are further classified into *enantiomers*, those having molecules that are mirror images of each other, and *diastereomers*, those that do not. An older classification used the subdivisions optical and geometric isomerism (q.v.), which did not include all forms of stereoisomerism. Called also *configurational*, *stereochemical*, or *spatial isomerism*.

stereology (ste″re-ol′o-je) the study of the three-dimensional properties of objects usually seen in two dimensions.

stereometer (ste″re-om′ĕ-ter) [*stereo-* + Gr. *metron* measure] an instrument for performing stereometry.

stereometry (ste″re-om′ĕ-tre) the measurement of the cubic or solid contents of a solid body, or of the capacity of a hollow space.

Stereomyxida (ster″e-o-mik′sĭ-dah) an order of ameboid protozoa (class Acarpomyxea, superclass Rhizopoda) comprising marine organisms with more or less branched pseudopodia, producing only very slow motion or serving as flotation organelles.

stereo-ophthalmoscope (ste″re-o-of-thal′mo-skōp) binocular ophthalmoscope.

Stereo-orthopter (ste″re-o-thop′ter) trademark for a mirror-reflecting instrument used to correct strabismus.

stereophorometer (ste″re-o-fo-rom′ĕ-ter) [*stereo-* + *phorometer*] a phorometer with a stereoscopic attachment.

stereophoroscope (ste″re-o-for′o-skōp) [*stereo-* + Gr. *phoros* movement, range + *-scope*] a form of zoetrope, employed in the study of visual perception.

stereophotomicrograph (ste″re-o-fo-to-mi′kro-graf) a stereoscopic photograph of a microscopical subject.

stereoplasm (ste′re-o-plazm″) [*stereo-* + Gr. *plasma* anything formed or molded] the more solid portions of protoplasm.

stereopsis (ste″re-op′sis) [*stereo-* + Gr. *opsis* vision] stereoscopic vision.

stereoradiography (ste″re-o-ra″de-og′rah-fe) stereoroentgenography.

stereoroentgenography (ste″re-o-rent″gen-og′rah-fe) the making of a roentgenogram giving an impression of depth as well as of width and height.

stereoroentgenometry (ste″re-o-rent″gen-om′ĕ-tre) measurement of the solid dimensions of a radiopaque object from its stereoscopic roentgenograms.

stereosalpingography (ste″re-o-sal″ping-gog′rah-fe) salpingography in which an impression of depth is achieved.

stereoscope (ste′re-o-skōp″) [*stereo-* + *-scope*] an instrument for producing the appearance of solidity and relief by combining the images of two pictures of an object seen from slightly dissimilar viewpoints.

stereoscopic (ste″re-o-skop′ik) having the effect of a stereoscope; giving to objects seen a solid or three-dimensional appearance.

stereoskiagraphy (ste″re-o-ski-ag′rah-fe) stereoroentgenography.

stereospecific (ster″e-o-spĭ-sif′ik) exhibiting marked specificity for one of several stereoisomers of a substrate or reactant; said of enzymes or of synthetic organic reactions.

stereotactic (ste″re-o-tak′tik) 1. stereotaxic (def. 1). 2. thigmotactic.

stereotaxic (ste″re-o-tak′sik) 1. pertaining to or characterized by precise positioning in space; said especially of discrete areas of the brain that control specific functions. Called also *stereotactic*. See also under *surgery*. 2. thigmotactic.

stereotaxis (ste″re-o-tak′sis) thigmotaxis.

stereotaxy (ste″re-o-tak′se) stereotaxic surgery.

stereotropic (ste″re-o-trop′ik) thigmotropic.

stereotropism (ste″re-ot′ro-pizm) [*stereo-* + Gr. *tropos* a turning] thigmotropism.

stereotypy (ste′re-o-ti″pe) [*stereo-* + Gr. *typos* type] the persistent repetition of senseless acts or words. It may be a persistent maintaining of a bodily attitude (s. *of attitude*), repetition of senseless movements (s. *of movement*, echopraxia), or constant repetition of certain words or phrases (s. *of speech*, echolalia, verbigeration).

Stereum (ste′re-um) a genus of basidiomycetous fungi of the order Polyporales, series Hymenomycetes, composed of the bracket fungi, and including some species causing tree and wood rot. *S. hirsu′tum* is the source of hirsutic acid.

steric (ste′rik) pertaining to the arrangement of atoms in space; pertaining to stereochemistry.

sterigma (ste-rig′mah), pl. *sterig′mata* [Gr. *stērigma* support] any of the flask-shaped structures projecting radially from the vesicle of fungi of the genus *Aspergillus*, from the tips of which conidia bud off consecutively; also any of the similar structures in *Penicillium* and other conidia-producing fungi.

Sterigmatocystis (ste-rig″mah-to-sis′tis) *Aspergillus*.

Sterigmocystis (ste-rig″mo-sis′tis) *Aspergillus*.

sterilant (ster′ĭ-lant) a sterilizing agent, i.e., an agent that destroys microorganisms.

sterile (ster′il) [L. *sterilis*] 1. unable to produce offspring; barren. 2. aseptic; free from living microorganisms.

sterility (stĕ-ril′ĭ-te) [L. *sterilitas*] 1. the inability to produce offspring, i.e., the inability to conceive (*female s.*) or to induce conception (*male s.*). Cf. *infertility*. 2. the state of being aseptic, or free from microorganisms. **absolute s.**, complete and irremediable inability to produce offspring. **female s.**, inability of the female to conceive as a result of a structural or functional defect in the reproductive organs. **male s.**, inability of the male to fertilize the ovum as a result of failure to produce living spermatozoa (*aspermatogenic s.*), an abnormality in spermatozoa production (*dysspermatogenic s.*), or some cause other than inability to produce live, normal spermatozoa (*normospermatogenic s.*). **one-child s.**, inability to produce further offspring after having produced one. **primary s.**, 1. inability to produce offspring because of the absence of some factor essential for reproduction. 2. sterility in which no offspring has ever been produced. **relative s.**, infertility. **secondary s.**, 1. inability to produce further offspring after having conceived or induced conception. See *one-child s.* and *two-child s.* 2. inability to produce offspring resulting from a noncongenital defect. **two-child s.**, inability to produce further offspring after having produced two.

sterilization (ster″ĭ-lĭ-za′shun) 1. the complete destruction or elimination of all living microorganisms, accomplished by physical methods (dry or moist heat), chemical agents (ethylene oxide, formaldehyde, alcohol), radiation (ultraviolet, cathode), or mechanical methods (filtration). 2. any procedure by which an individual is made incapable of reproduction, as by castration, vasectomy, or salpingectomy. **eugenic s.**, the process of rendering a person incapable of reproduction because the offspring would probably be undesirable types or because the parent is incapable of rearing the child responsibly. **fractional s., intermittent s.**, destruction of microbial viability by successive application of the procedure at intervals, to allow spores to develop into vegetative forms, which are more easily destroyed.

sterilize (ster′ĭ-līz) 1. to render sterile; to free from microorganisms. 2. to render incapable of reproduction.

sterilizer (ster′ĭ-līz″er) an apparatus used for the destruction of microorganisms; see *sterilization*.

Sterisil (ster′ĭ-sil) trademark for a preparation of hexetidine.

Stern's position (sternz) [Heinrich *Stern*, American physician, 1868–1918] see under *position*.

sternad (ster′nad)   toward the sternum, or sternal aspect.

sternal (ster′nal) [L. *sternalis*]   pertaining to the sternum.

sternalgia (ster-nal′je-ah) [Gr. *sternon* sternum + *algos* pain + *-ia*]   1. pain in the sternum.   2. angina pectoris.

Sternberg's disease, giant cells (stern′bergz) [Carl *Sternberg*, Austrian pathologist, 1872–1935]   see *Hodgkin's disease,* under *disease,* and *Reed-Sternberg cells,* under *cell.*

Sternberg-Reed cells (stern′berg-rēd) [Carl *Sternberg;* Dorothy *Reed,* American pathologist, 1874–1964]   see *Reed-Sternberg cells,* under *cell.*

sternebra (ster′ne-brah), pl. *ster′nebrae* [*sternum* + *vertebrae*]   any of the segments of the sternum in early life, which later fuse to form the corpus sterni.

Sterneedle (stern′ne-d′l)   trademark for a controlled depth, multiple puncture apparatus used in the diagnosis of tuberculosis. See *tuberculin test, Sterneedle,* under *tests.*

sternen (ster′nen)   pertaining to the sternum alone.

stern(o)- [L. *sternum,* q.v.]   a combining form denoting relationship to the sternum.

sternoclavicular (ster″no-klah-vik′u-lar)   pertaining to the sternum and clavicle.

sternoclavicularis (ster″no-klah-vik″u-la′ris) [L.]   sternoclavicular.

sternocleidal (ster″no-kli′dal) [*sterno-* + Gr. *kleis* key]   sternoclavicular.

sternocleidomastoid (ster″no-kli″do-mas′toid)   pertaining to the sternum, clavicle, and mastoid process.

sternocostal (ster″no-kos′tal) [*sterno-* + L. *costa* rib]   pertaining to the sternum and ribs.

sternodymia (ster″no-dim′e-ah)   the union of two fetuses by the anterior wall of the chest.

sternodymus (ster-nod′ĭ-mus) [*sterno-* + Gr. *didymos* twin]   a pair of twin fetuses united by the anterior wall of the chest.

sternodynia (ster″no-din′e-ah)   sternalgia.

sternogoniometer (ster″no-go″ne-om′ĕ-ter)   an instrument for measuring the sternal angle.

sternohyoid (ster″no-hi′oid)   pertaining to the sternum and to the hyoid bone.

sternoid (ster′noid)   resembling the sternum.

sternomastoid (ster″no-mas′toid)   pertaining to the sternum and the mastoid process of the temporal bone.

sternopagia (ster″no-pa′je-ah)   sternodymia.

sternopagus (ster-nop′ah-gus) [Gr. *sternon* sternum + *pagos* thing fixed]   sternodymus.

sternopericardial (ster″no-per″ĭ-kar′de-al)   pertaining to the sternum and the pericardium.

sternoscapular (ster″no-skap′u-lar)   pertaining to the sternum and the scapula.

sternoschisis (ster-nos′kĭ-sis) [*sterno-* + Gr. *schisis* cleft]   a developmental anomaly characterized by a fissure of the sternum.

sternothyreoideus (ster″no-thi″re-oi′de-us) [L.]   sternothyroid.

sternothyroid (ster″no-thi′roid)   pertaining to the sternum and to the thyroid cartilage or gland.

sternotomy (ster-not′o-me) [*sterno-* + Gr. *tomē* a cutting]   the operation of cutting through the sternum.

sternotracheal (ster″no-tra′ke-al) [*sterno-* + *trachea*]   pertaining to the sternum and to the trachea.

sternotrypesis (ster″no-tri-pe′sis) [*sterno-* + Gr. *trypēsis* trephination]   surgical perforation of the sternum.

sternovertebral (ster″no-ver′te-bral)   pertaining to the sternum and vertebrae.

sternoxiphopagus (ster″no-zi-fop′ah-gus) [*sterno-* + *xiphoid* process + Gr. *pagus* thing fixed]   a double fetus consisting of two similar components united in the frontal plane, in the region of the sternum and xiphoid process.

sternum (ster′num) [L.; Gr. *sternon*] [NA]   a longitudinal unpaired plate of bone forming the middle of the anterior wall of the thorax, and articulating above with the clavicles and along the sides with the cartilages of the first seven ribs. It consists of three portions, the manubrium, the body, and the xiphoid process.   **cleft s.,** a sternum which is longitudinally fissured.

sternutatio (ster″nu-ta′she-o) [L.]   sternutation.   **s. convulsi′va,** paroxysmal and convulsive sneezing.

sternutation (ster″nu-ta′shun) [L. *sternutatio*]   the act of sneezing; a sneeze.

sternutator (ster″nu-ta″tor)   a gas or other substance that causes sneezing.

sternutatory (ster-nu″tah-tor″e) [L. *sternutatorius*]   1. producing or causing sneezing.   2. an agent that causes sneezing.

sternzellen (stern′tsel-en) [Ger. "star cells"]   Kupffer's cells.

steroid (ste′roid)   a group name for lipids that contain a hydrogenated cyclopentanoperhydrophenanthrene ring system Some of the substances included in this group are progesterone, adrenocortical hormones, the gonadal hormones, cardiac aglycones, bile acids, sterols (such as cholesterol), toad poisons, saponins, and some of the carcinogenic hydrocarbons.   **anabolic s.,** any of a group of synthetic derivatives of testosterone, having pronounced anabolic properties and relatively weak androgenic properties, which are used clinically mainly to promote growth and repair of body tissues in senility, debilitating illness, and convalescence.

steroid 11β-monooxygenase (ster′oid mon″o-ok′sĭ-jĕ-nās) [EC 1.14.15.4]   an enzyme of the oxidoreductase class that catalyzes the reaction steroid + reduced adrenal ferredoxin + O_2 = 11β-hydroxysteroid + oxidized adrenal ferredoxin + H_2O in the synthesis of steroid hormones. Deficient enzyme, an autosomal recessive trait, results in congenital adrenal hyperplasia type IV. Called also *11β-hydroxylase.*

steroid 17α-monooxygenase (ster′oid mon″o-ok′sĭ-jĕ-nās) [EC 1.14.99.9]   an enzyme of the oxidoreductase class that catalyzes the reaction steroid + NAD(P)H + O_2 = 17α-hydroxysteroid + NAD(P)$^+$ + H_2O. The enzyme requires NADH or NADPH and cytochrome *P-450.* The reaction occurs in the synthesis of steroid hormones. Deficient enzyme, an autosomal recessive trait, results in congenital adrenal hyperplasia type V. Called also *17-hydroxylase.*

steroid 21-monooxygenase (ster′oid mon″o-ok′sĭ-jĕ-nas) [EC 1.14.99.10]   an enzyme of the oxidoreductase class that catalyzes the reaction steroid + NAD(P)H + O_2 = 21-hydroxysteroid + NAD$^+$ + H_2O. The system involves a heme-thiolate protein and flavoprotein. It is a part of the steroid hormone synthesis system. Deficiency of the enzyme, an autosomal recessive trait, causes adrenal hyperplasia type III. Called also *21-hydroxylase.*

steroid 5α-reductase (ster′oid re-duk′tās)   5α-reductase.

steroid sulfatase (ster′oid sul′fah-tās)   steryl sulfatase.

steroidogenesis (ste-roi″do-jen′ĕ-sis)   the biosynthesis or production of steroids, as by the adrenal glands.

steroidogenic (ste-roi″do-jen′ik)   producing steroids; giving rise to steroids.

sterol (ste′rol) [Gr. *stereos* solid + *-ol* (L. *oleum* oil)]   steroids with long (8–10 carbons) aliphatic side-chains at position 17 and at least one alcoholic hydroxyl group, usually at position 3. They have lipid-like solubility. Examples are cholesterol and ergosterol.

stertor (ster′tor) [L.]   an act of snoring; stertorous or sonorous breathing.   **hen-cluck s.,** a respiration sound like a hen's cluck in cases of postpharyngeal abscess.

stertorous (ster′to-rus)   characterized by stertor.

steryl sulfatase (ster′il sul′fah-tās) [EC 3.1.6.2]   an enzyme of the hydrolase class that catalyzes the reaction steryl sulfate + H_2O = sterol + sulfate. Deficiency of the enzyme, an x-linked trait, leads to ichthyosis and corneal opacities. Called also *steroid sulfatase.*

stethacoustic (steth″ah-koo′stik)   heard with the stethoscope.

stethalgia (steth-al′je-ah)   pain in the chest or chest wall.

stethemia (steth-e′me-ah) [*steth-* + Gr. *haima* blood + *-ia*]   congestion of the lungs.

stethendoscope (steth-en′do-skōp) [*steth-* + Gr. *endon* within + *skopein* to examine]   a fluoroscope used in examination of the chest.

steth(o)- [Gr. *stēthos* chest]   a combining form denoting relationship to the chest.

stethocyrtograph (steth″o-ser′to-graf)   stethokyrtograph.

stethogoniometer (steth″o-go″ne-om′ĕ-ter) [*stetho-* + Gr. *gōnia* angle + *metron* measure]   an apparatus for measuring the curvature of the chest.

stethograph (steth′o-graf) [stetho- + Gr. graphein to write] an instrument for recording movements of the chest.

stethography (steth-og′rah-fe) 1. use of the stethograph to record movements of the chest. 2. phonocardiography.

stethokyrtograph (steth″o-kir′to-graf) [stetho- + Gr. kyrtos bent + graphein to write] an instrument for recording and measuring the curves of the chest.

stethometer (steth-om′ĕ-ter) [stetho- + Gr. metron measure] an instrument for measuring the circular dimension or expansion of the chest.

Stethomyia (steth″o-mi′yah) a subgenus of anopheline mosquitoes.

stethomyitis (steth″o-mi-i′tis) stethomyositis.

stethomyositis (steth″o-mi″o-si′tis) [stetho + Gr. myos of muscle + -itis] inflammation of the muscles of the chest.

stethoparalysis (steth″o-pah-ral′ĭ-sis) paralysis of the chest muscles.

stethophone (steth′o-fōn) [stetho- + Gr. phōnē voice] 1. an instrument designed to transmit stethoscopic sounds so that many persons can hear them simultaneously. 2. a term proposed as a more accurate name for stethoscope.

stethophonometer (steth″o-fo-nom′ĕ-ter) [stetho- + Gr. phōnē voice + metron measure] an instrument for measuring the intensity of auscultatory sounds.

stethopolyscope (steth″o-pol′ĭ-skōp) [stetho- + Gr. polys many + skopein to examine] a stethoscope for the simultaneous use of several persons.

stethoscope (steth′o-skōp) [stetho- + Gr. skopein to examine] an instrument of various form, size, and material for performing mediate auscultation. By means of this instrument the respiratory, cardiac, pleural, arterial, venous, uterine, fetal, intestinal, and other sounds are conveyed to the ear of the observer. **binaural s.,** one with two adjustable branches, designed for use with both ears. **Cammann's s.,** a binaural stethoscope. **DeLee-Hillis obstetric s.,** a stethoscope worn on the head of the examiner, used for listening to the fetal heart. **differential s.,** one by means of which sounds at two different portions of the body may be compared. **electronic s.,** an electronic amplifier of sounds within the body; selective controls permit tuning for low or high frequency tones. An auxiliary output permits the recording or viewing of audio patterns. **esophageal s.,** one which is positioned within the esophagus to transmit heart and respiratory sounds. **Leff s.,** one for listening to the fetal heart.

stethoscopic (steth″o-skop′ik) pertaining to or performed by means of the stethoscope.

stethoscopy (steth-os′ko-pe) examination by means of the stethoscope.

stethospasm (steth′o-spazm) spasm of the chest muscles.

Stevens-Johnson syndrome (ste′venz-jon′son) [Albert Mason Stevens, 1884–1945, and Frank Chambliss Johnson, 1894–1934, American pediatricians] see under syndrome.

Stewart's purple (stu′artz) [Douglas Hunt Stewart, New York surgeon, 1860–1933] see under purple.

Stewart-Holmes sign (stu′art-hōmz) [Purves Stewart, London physician, 1869–1949; Gordon Holmes, British neurologist] rebound phenomenon.

STH somatotropic (growth) hormone.

sthenia (sthe′ne-ah) [Gr. sthenos + -ia] a condition of strength and activity.

sthenic (sthen′ik) active; strong.

sthen(o)- [Gr. sthenos strength] a combining form denoting relationship to strength.

sthenometer (sthen-om′ĕ-ter) an instrument for measuring the muscular strength of a part.

sthenometry (sthen-om′ĕ-tre) [stheno- + Gr. metron measure] the measurement of bodily strength.

stibamine (stib′ah-min) chemical name: sodium 4-aminobenzenestibonic acid. A brown, amorphous powder, $NH_2C_6H_5SbO(OH)_2$, formerly used in the treatment of leishmaniasis.

stibialism (stib′e-al-izm) [L. stibium antimony] poisoning with antimony.

stibiated (stib′e-āt″ed) containing antimony.

stibiation (stib″e-a′shun) [L. stibium antimony] adminis-

tration of antimonials in large quantities; treatment by bringing the patient under the full influence of antimony.

stibium (stib′e-um) [L.] antimony.

stibocaptate (stib″o-kap′tāt) [BAN] chemical name: 2,2′-(1,2-dicarboxy-1,2-ethanediyl)bis-1,3,2-dithiastibolane-4,5-dicarboxylic acid hexosodium salt. A trivalent antimony compound, $C_{12}H_8Na_6O_{12}S_2Sb$, used as an antischistosomal, administered intramuscularly. Called also antimony dimercaptossiccinate and antimony sodium stibocaptate [INN].

stibogluconate sodium (stib″o-glu′ko-nāt) antimony sodium gluconate.

stibonium (stĭ-bo′ne-um) the radical SbH_4.

stibophen (stib′o-fen) chemical name: bis[4,5-dihydroxy-1,3-benzenedisulfonato(4–)-O⁴,O⁵]antimonato(5–)pentasodium heptahydrate. A trivalent antimony compound, $C_{12}H_4$-$Na_5O_{16}S_4Sb\cdot 7H_2O$, occurring as a white or slightly yellow or pink, crystalline powder; used as an anthelmintic, chiefly in the treatment of schistosomiasis due to Schistosoma mansoni, S. haematobium, and S. japonicum. It is also effective in the treatment of granuloma inguinale, administered intramuscularly and intravenously. Called also neoantimosan.

stichochrome (stik′o-krōm) [Gr. stichos row + chrōma color] any nerve cell having the stainable substance (chromophilic bodies) arranged in more or less regular striae or layers. Cf. arkyochrome, gyrochrome, and perichrome.

Stichotrichina (stik″o-trĭ-ki′nah) [Gr. stichos row + thrix hair] a suborder of mostly free-living ciliate protozoa (order Hypotrichida, subclass Spirotricha) having a generally elongated body with cirri that are often small and inconspicuous, which typically occur in 3 to 12 longitudinal, sometimes spiraled, rows on the ventral surface.

Sticker's disease (stik′erz) [Georg Sticker, German physician, 1860–1960] erythema infectiosum.

Sticta (stik′tah) [Gr. stiktos punctured] a genus of lichens; lungwort.

Stieda's disease, fracture (ste′dahz) [Alfred Stieda, German surgeon, 1869–1945] see Pellegrini's disease, under disease, and see under fracture.

Stieda's process (ste′dahz) [L. Stieda, German anatomist, 1837–1918] processus posterior tali.

Stierlin's symptom (sign) (stēr′linz) [Eduard Stierlin, Munich surgeon, 1878–1919] see under symptom.

stifle (sti′f'l) the part of a horse's limb corresponding to the human knee.

stigma (stig′mah), pl. stigmas or stig′mata [Gr. "mark"] 1. any mental or physical mark or peculiarity which aids in the identification or in the diagnosis of a condition. 2. follicular stigma. 3. purpuric or hemorrhagic lesions of the hands and/or feet, which resemble crucifixion wounds. 4. in botany, the uppermost part of a pistil, which secretes a moist, sticky substance to trap and hold the pollen that reach it. 5. a reddish or brownish red dot or short rod located in the anterior region of chromatophore-bearing protozoa and rarely in colorless forms; its exact nature is unknown. Called also eyespot. **follicular s.,** a spot on the surface of an ovary where the vesicular follicle will rupture and permit passage of the ovum during ovulation. Called also macula folliculi. **Giuffrida-Ruggieri s.,** abnormal shallowness of the glenoid fossa. **malpighian s's,** the points where the smaller veins enter into the larger veins of the spleen.

stigmal (stig′mal) stigmatic.

stigmasterol (stig-mas′tĕ-rol) an unsaturated plant sterol, $C_{29}H_{48}O$, occurring in physostigma, cacao butter, rape oil, soybean oil, and elsewhere. An important starting material for industrial synthesis of steroid hormones.

stigmata (stig′mah-tah) [Gr.] plural of stigma.

Stigmatella (stig″mah-tel′ah) [L., dim. of Gr. stigma mark] a genus of gliding bacteria of the family Cystobacteraceae, order Myxobacterales, found on bark and lichens. The type species is S. auranti′aca.

stigmatic (stig-mat′ik) pertaining to a stigma.

stigmatism (stig′mah-tizm) 1. the condition due to or marked by stigmas. 2. the accurate rendition of points by a lens system.

stigmatometer (stig″mah-tom′ĕ-ter) [Gr. stigma point + -meter] an instrument for testing the refraction of the eye by retinoscopy and for direct ophthalmoscopy.

stijfziekte (stēf-zēk′te) [Dutch] a phosphorus-deficiency disease of the joints of young cattle in South Africa, marked by retardation of growth, skeletal abnormalities, stiffness, and lameness.

stilalgin (stil-al′jin) mephenesin.

Stilbaceae (stil-ba′se-e) a family of imperfect fungi of the order Moniliales, including the genus *Dendrochium*.

stilbazium iodide (stil-baz′ĭ-um) chemical name: 1-ethyl-2,6-bis[2-[4-(1-pyrrolidinyl)phenyl]ethenyl]pyridinium iodide; an anthelmintic, $C_{31}H_{36}IN_3$, reported to be effective against roundworms, threadworms, and whipworms.

stilbene (stil′bēn) toluylene.

stilbestrol (stil-bes′trol) diethylstilbestrol.

stilet (sti-let′) [Fr. *stilette*] stylet.

stilette (sti-let′) [Fr.] stylet.

stili (sti′li) [L.] plural of *stilus*.

Still's disease (stilz) [Sir George Frederick *Still*, English physician, 1868–1941] see under *disease*.

Still-Chauffard syndrome (stil-sho-far′) [Sir G. F. *Still*; Anatole Marie Emile *Chauffard*, French physician, 1855–1932] Chauffard's syndrome.

stillbirth (stil′berth) the delivery of a dead child; see *fetal death*, under *death*.

stillborn (stil′born) born dead.

Stiller's rib (stil′erz) [Berthold *Stiller*, physician in Budapest, 1837–1922] see under *rib*.

stillicidium (stil″ĭ-sid′e-um) [L. *stilla* drop + *cadere* to fall] a dribbling or flowing by drops, as in epiphora. **s. lacrima′rum**, epiphora. **s. na′rium**, coryza. **s. uri′nae**, strangury.

Stilling's canal, column, fibers, fleece, nucleus (stil′ingz) [Benedict *Stilling*, German anatomist 1810–1879] see *canalis hyaloideus* and *columna thoracica* (for column and nucleus), and see under *fiber* and *fleece*.

Stillingia (stil-lin′je-ah) [Benjamin *Stillingfleet*, English botanist, 1702–1771] a genus of euphorbiaceous trees, shrubs, and herbs. The root of *S. sylvat′ica* L., a plant of North America, is sialagogue, diuretic, and laxative.

Stilphostrol (stil-fos′trol) trademark for a preparation of diethylstilbestrol diphosphate.

stilus (sti′lus), pl. *sti′li* [L.] stylus.

stimulant (stim′u-lant) [L. *stimulans*] 1. producing stimulation; especially producing stimulation by causing tension on muscle fiber through the nervous tissue. 2. an agent or remedy that produces stimulation. **cardiac s.**, one which increases the heart's action. **central s.**, a stimulant of the central nervous system. **cerebral s.**, one which exalts the functional activities of the brain. **diffusable s.**, one which acts promptly and strongly, but transiently. **general s.**, one which acts upon the whole body. **genital s.**, an aphrodisiac. **hepatic s.**, one which stimulates the functions of the liver. **intestinal s.**, a cathartic agent. **local s.**, one which affects only, or mainly, that part to which it is applied. **nervous s.**, one which acts mainly upon the nerve centers; a cerebral or a spinal stimulant. **respiratory s.**, one which increases respiratory movements. **spinal s.**, one which acts upon and through the spinal cord. **stomachic s.**, one that promotes the digestion of food in the stomach. **topical s.**, local s. **uterine s.**, an agent which stimulates uterine contraction or menstruation. **vascular s., vasomotor s.**, one which affects the vasomotor centers.

stimulate (stim′u-lāt) to excite to functional activity.

stimulation (stim″u-la′shun) [L. *stimulatio*, from *stimulare* to goad] the act or process of stimulating; the condition of being stimulated. **areal s.**, stimulation of an extended portion of a sense organ. **audio-visual-tactile s.**, the simultaneous rhythmic excitation of the receptors for the senses of hearing, sight, and touch. **nonspecific s.**, stimulation of a sense organ by other than the specific exciting agent. **paradoxical s.**, application of a warm object to one of the cold spots of the body produces a sensation of cold. **paraspecific s.**, nonspecific s. **punctual s.**, excitation of a sense organ by stimulation at a single point.

stimulator (stim″u-la′tor) any agent that excites functional activity. **Bimler s.**, see under *appliance*. **electronic s.**, a device for applying electronic pulses or signals to activate muscles, to identify nerves, to treat muscular disorders, etc. **human thyroid adenylate cyclase**

s's (HTACS), thyroid-stimulating immunoglobulins; see under *immunoglobulin*. **long-acting thyroid s. (LATS)**, the original term applied to the thyroid-stimulating immunoglobulins associated with Graves' disease; the name refers to a mouse bioassay in which LATS thyroid stimulation peaks later than that induced by thyroid stimulating hormone.

stimuli (stim′u-li) plural of *stimulus*.

stimulin (stim′u-lin) a name given by Metchnikoff to an element in the blood serum that stimulates the action of phagocytes.

stimulon (stim′u-lon) a viral antigen postulated to have anti-interferon activity and which therefore promotes the multiplication of other viruses.

stimulus (stim′u-lus), pl. *stim′uli* [L. "goad"] any agent, act, or influence that produces functional or trophic reaction in a receptor or in an irritable tissue. **adequate s.**, a stimulus of the specific form of energy to which the receptor is most sensitive; called also *homologous s.* **aversive s.**, one which, when applied following the occurrence of a response, decreases the strength of that response on later occurrences. **chemical s.**, a chemical substance capable of exciting a response in an organism mediated through specialized nerve endings. **conditioned s.**, a stimulus that acquires the capacity to evoke a particular response by repeated pairing with another stimulus that is naturally capable of eliciting the response. **discriminative s.**, a stimulus associated with reinforcement, which exerts control over a particular form of behavior; the subject discriminates between closely related stimuli and responds positively only in the presence of that stimulus. **electric s.**, a galvanic, induced, or other electric current or shock as applied to a responsive tissue. **eliciting s.**, any stimulus, conditioned or unconditioned, which elicits a response. **heterologous s.**, one which produces an effect or sensation when applied to any part of a nerve tract. **heterotopic s.**, a stimulus to heart contraction arising elsewhere than in the sinoatrial node, the normal pacemaker of the heart. **homologous s.**, adequate s. **liminal s.**, one near the threshold. **mechanical s.**, a stimulant application of mechanical force, as in friction or pinching. **nomotopic s.**, a stimulus to heart contraction arising in the sinoatrial node. **reinforcing s.**, any stimulus that follows a response and that increases the probability of eliciting that response. **subliminal s.**, one well below the threshold. **supraliminal s.**, one well above the threshold. **thermal s.**, application of heat. **threshold s.**, a stimulus that is just strong enough to elicit a response; see also *threshold* (def. 1 and 2). **unconditioned s.**, any stimulus capable of eliciting an unconditioned response.

sting (sting) 1. an injury caused by the venom of a plant or animal (biotoxin) introduced into the individual or with which he has come in contact, together with the mechanical trauma caused by the organ responsible for its introduction. 2. the organ used to inflict such injury. **Irukandji s.**, a clinical syndrome observed in the vicinity of Cairns in Queensland, Australia, attributed to stinging by the carybdeid jellyfish *Carukia barnesi*.

Stintzing's tables (stint′zingz) [Roderich *Stintzing*, Jena internist, 1854–1933] see under *table*.

Stipa viridula (sti′pah vi-rid′u-lah) a grass of the southwestern United States, called *sleepygrass*: poisonous to cattle and horses; said to be a powerful narcotic, diuretic, sudorific, and cardiac poison.

stippling (stip′ling) [Dutch *stippelen* to keep spotting] 1. the appearance of fine light or dark dots, or a spotted appearance. 2. the appearance of the retina as if dotted with light and dark points. 3. see *basophilia*. 4. gingival s. **epiphyseal s.**, the radiographic appearance of punctate opacities in the epiphyses, representing foci of calcification; seen in chrondrodysplasia punctata. **gingival s.**, a condition in which the gingiva presents a minutely lobulated surface, like that of an orange peel, which is a normal adaptive process of the gingiva and its absence or reduction indicates gingival disease. **malarial s.**, the finely granular appearance often seen in stained red blood cells which harbor tertian malarial parasites; the granules are called *Schüffner's dots*. **Maurer's s.**, Maurer's dots. **Schüffner's s.**, malarial s.

stirofos (sti′ro-fos) chemical name: (Z)-2-chloro-1-(2,4,5-trichlorophenyl)ethenyl dimethyl ester phosphoric acid; a veterinary insecticide, $C_{10}H_9Cl_4O_4P$.

stirpicultural (ster″pĭ-kul′tu-ral)   pertaining to stirpiculture.

stirpiculture (ster″pĭ-kul′tūr) [L. *stirps* stock + *culture*] the systematic attempt at improving a stock or race by attention to the laws of breeding.

stirrup (stir′up)   1. a structure or device resembling the stirrup of a saddle, or the portion of an apparatus on which to rest the feet. 2. the stapes. **Finochietto's s.,** an apparatus for exerting skeletal traction in leg fractures, with a U-shaped steel band, passed over the posterior process of the calcaneous and fixed by a cross bar, from which traction is applied.

stitch (stich)   1. to pass lengths of material (thread, catgut, wire, etc.) through tissue by means of a needle, usually to approximate wound edges but also to fix or mobilize an organ or other structure. 2. a single suture. 3. a popular term for a severe pain, generally at the costal margin on one side.

stithe (stīth)   incus.

stizolobin (sti″zo-lo′bin)   the globulin of the Chinese velvet bean.

stochastic (sto-kas′tik) [Gr. *stochastikos* conjecturing]   pertaining to a random process, used particularly to refer to a time series of random variables.

stoechiology (stek″e-ol′o-je)   stoichiology.

Stoerk's blennorrhea (sterks) [Carl *Stoerk*, Austrian laryngologist, 1832–1899]   see under *blennorrhea*.

stoichiology (stoi″ke-ol′o-je) [Gr. *stoicheion* element + *-logy*] the science of elements, especially the physiology of the cellular elements of tissues.

stoichiometry (stoi″ke-om′ĕ-tre) [Gr. *stoicheion* element + *metron* measure]   the study of the numerical relationships of chemical elements and compounds and the mathematical laws of chemical changes; the mathematics of chemistry.

stoke (stōk)   a unit of kinematic viscosity, being that of fluid with a viscosity of 1 poise and a density of 1 gram per cubic centimeter.

Stokes' amputation (operation) [Sir William *Stokes*, Irish surgeon, 1839–1900]   Gritti-Stokes amputation.

Stokes' expectorant, etc. (stōks) [William *Stokes*, Irish physician, 1804–1878]   see under *collar, expectorant, law,* and *syndrome*.

Stokes-Adams disease (syndrome) [William *Stokes*, Irish physician, 1804–1878; Robert *Adams*, Irish physician, 1791–1875]   see *Adams-Stokes disease*, under *disease*.

Stokvis' disease, test (stok′vis) [Barend Joseph E. *Stokvis*, Dutch physician, 1834–1902]   see *enterogenous cyanosis*, under *cyanosis*, and see under *tests*.

Stokvis-Talma syndrome (stok′vis-tal′mah) [B.J.E. *Stokvis*; Sape *Talma*, Dutch physician, 1847–1918]   enterogenous cyanosis.

stoma (sto′mah), pl. *sto′mas* or *sto′mata* [Gr. "mouth"]   1. any minute pore, orifice, or opening on a free surface. 2. the opening established in the abdominal wall by colostomy, ileostomy, etc.; also the opening between two portions of the intestine in an anastomosis.

stomacace (sto-mak′ah-se) [Gr. *stoma* mouth + *kakē* badness]   ulcerative stomatitis.

stomach (stum′ak) [L. *stomachus;* Gr. *stomachos*]   1. the musculomembranous expansion of the alimentary canal between the esophagus and the duodenum. Called also *gaster* [NA] and *ventriculus* [NA alternative]. 2. the midgut of an invertebrate. **aberrant umbilical s.,** an umbilical structure containing gastric mucosa. **bilocular s.,** hourglass s. **cardiac s.,** the portion of the stomach close to the esophagus. **cascade s.,** an atypical form of hourglass stomach, characterized roentgenologically by a drawing up of the posterior wall; an opaque medium first fills the upper sac and then cascades into the lower sac. **cup-and-spill s.,** a roentgenographic finding in which the barium remains for a time in the gastric fundus, before spilling over into the main cavity of the stomach, as a result of pressure by a distended colon. **dumping s.,** a complication that sometimes follows partial gastrectomy and gastroenterostomy, in which food is emptied rapidly from the stomach into the jejunum through the new opening, producing weakness, sweating, palpitation, and varying degrees of syncope. See *dumping syndrome*, under *syndrome*. **hourglass s.,** a stomach

more or less completely and permanently divided into two parts, so that it resembles an hourglass in shape; the deformity is due to scarring which complicates chronic gastric ulcer. **leather bottle s.,** linitis plastica. **miniature s.,** Pavlov's s. **Pavlov's s.,** a portion of the stomach of a dog isolated from communication with the rest of the stomach and opening on to the abdominal wall through a fistula: used in studying gastric secretion. **powdered s.,** the dried and powdered defatted wall of the stomach of the hog, *Sus scrofa*, formerly used in the treatment of anemia. **sclerotic s.,** linitis plastica. **thoracic s.,** a stomach which is situated or drawn up above the level of the diaphragm; i.e., that part of the stomach which has herniated through the diaphragmatic hiatus. **trifid s.,** a stomach with two constrictions, producing three pouches. **upside-down s.,** thoracic s. **waterfall s.,** cascade s. **water-trap s.,** a stomach with an extremely high pylorus, so that it does not readily empty itself.

stomachal (stum′ah-kal)   pertaining to the stomach.

stomachalgia (stum″ah-kal′je-ah)   pain in the stomach.

stomachic (sto-mak′ik) [L. *stomachicus;* Gr. *stomachikos*]   1. pertaining to the stomach. 2. a medicine which promotes the functional activity of the stomach; a stomachic tonic.

stomachodynia (stum″ah-ko-din′e-ah) [*stomach* + Gr. *odynē* pain + *-ia*]   pain in the stomach.

stomadeum (sto″mah-de′um)   stomodeum.

stomal (sto′mal)   pertaining to a stoma or stomata.

stomalgia (sto-mal′je-ah)   stomatalgia.

stomata (sto′mah-tah) [Gr.]   plural of *stoma*.

stomatal (sto′mah-tal)   pertaining to stomata.

stomatalgia (sto″mah-tal′je-ah)   pain in the mouth.

stomatic (sto-mat′ik)   pertaining to the mouth.

stomatitides (sto″mah-tit′ĭ-dēz)   plural of *stomatitis*. A general term applied collectively to inflammatory conditions of the oral mucosa.

stomatitis (sto-mah-ti′tis), pl. *stomatit′ides* [*stomato-* + *-itis*] inflammation of the oral mucosa, due to local or systemic factors, which may involve the buccal and labial mucosa, palate, tongue, floor of the mouth, and the gingivae. **allergic s.,** stomatitis caused by exposure to allergens; stomatitis occurring as a manifestation of an allergic condition. See also *s. venenata*. **angular s.,** perlèche. **aphthobullous s.,** foot-and-mouth disease. **s. aphtho′sa, aphthous s.,** recurrent aphthous s. **s. arsenica′lis** stomatitis due to arsenical poisoning. **bismuth s.,** stomatitis due to bismuth poisoning, consisting of a thin blue-black line in the marginal gingivae (*bismuth line*), pigmentation of the buccal mucosa, sore tongue, metallic taste, and a burning sensation of the mouth. Called also *bismuth gingivitis*. **catarrhal s.,** transitory inflammation of the oral mucosa, sometimes associated with gingivitis, accompanied by erythema, swelling, and occasionally epithelial desquamation; believed to be caused by the oral bacterial flora. **contact s.,** s. venenata. **denture s.,** generalized inflammation of the oral mucosa observed sometimes in patients with new dentures or with old, ill-fitting ones; characterized by redness, swelling, and painfulness of the mucosa coming in contact with the denture. Called also *denture sore mouth*. **epidemic s.,** foot-and-mouth disease. **epizootic s.,** foot-and-mouth disease. **erythematopultaceous s.,** uremic s. **s. exanthemat′ica,** stomatitis secondary to an exanthematous disease. **fusospirochetal s.,** necrotizing ulcerative gingivostomatitis. **gangrenous s.,** noma (def. 1). **gonococcal s.,** gonorrheal s. **gonorrheal s.,** gonorrhea of the oral cavity, usually transmitted by orogenital contact, characterized by a linear or flattened eruption associated with redness, itching, and burning of the mucosa. Called also *gonococcal s.* **herpetic s.,** herpes simplex involving the oral mucosa and lips, characterized by the formation of yellowish vesicles that rupture and produce ragged painful ulcers covered by a gray membrane and surrounded by an erythematous halo. Called also *vesicular s.* **infectious s.,** a general term for a usually mild infection of the oral mucosa, beginning with a circumscribed red, itchy area. **s. intertrop′ica,** stomatitis associated with tropical sprue. **lead s.,** the oral manifestations of lead poisoning, including a bluish line along the free gingival margin, pigmentation of the mucosa in contact with the teeth, metallic taste, excessive salivation, and swelling of the salivary glands. **s.**

medicamento′sa, stomatitis due to an allergic reaction to drugs, ingested, absorbed through the skin or mucosa, or given by hypodermic injection. Principal symptoms include vesicles, erosion, ulcers, erythema, purpura, angioedema, burning, and itching. See also *s. venenata.* **membranous s.,** infection of the oral mucosa, accompanied by the formation of a false membrane. **mercurial s.,** stomatitis due to mercury poisoning; symptoms include necrotic and ulcerative lesions and discoloration similar to lead lines of the gingivae, soreness of gums, strong metallic taste, foul breath, ptyalism, and necrosis of the alveolar process. **mycotic s.,** thrush, def. 1. **s. nicoti′na,** a condition believed to be a variant of oral leukoplakia, observed in smokers, particularly heavy pipe-smokers, and characterized by multiple grayish white nodules or papules with a red spot in the center of each lesion on the palate, representing dilated orifices of accessory palatal salivary glands; thickening, keratinization, and wrinkling of the epithelium with the development of fissures and cracks may occur in later stages. Called also *smokers′ palate* and *smokers′ patches.* **nonspecific s.,** inflammation of the oral mucosa occurring in association with other conditions, such as menstruation, diabetes, or uremia. **recurrent aphthous s.,** a recurrent disease of unknown etiology, characterized by the appearance on the oral mucosa of one or more small round or oval ulcers that are covered by a grayish fibrinous exudate and surrounded by a bright red halo. The lesions usually persist for 7 to 14 days and then heal without scarring. A severe form is known as *periadenitis mucosa necrotica recurrents.* Called also *aphthae, aphthous s.,* and *canker sore.* **s. scarlati′na,** a condition of the oral mucosa seen in scarlatina (scarlet fever), characterized in the early stages by fiery red coloration, congestion, and exudate of the throat, and by strawberry tongue and raspberry tongue in the later stages. **s. scorbu′tica,** stomatitis associated with vitamin C deficiency, characterized by red swollen gums, gingival ulcers and gangrene, periodontal destruction, loose teeth, hemorrhage from the dental pulp, hypoplasia of the dental enamel, arrest of dentin formation, and exaggerated sensitivity of the oral mucosa to irritants. See also *scurvy.* **syphilitic s.,** stomatitis due to systemic syphilis. **tropical s.,** see under *sprue.* **ulcerative s.,** stomatitis characterized by the appearance of shallow ulcers on the cheeks, tongue, and lips. Called also *stomacace* and *stomatocace.* **ulcerative s. of sheep,** contagious ecthyma. **uremic s.,** the oral manifestation of uremia, consisting of azotemic odor of the breath, erythema, exudation, ulcerations, pseudomembrane formation, and burning sensations. Called also *erythematopultaceous s.* **s. venena′ta,** an allergic condition of the oral mucosa resulting from contact with a substance to which the patient is sensitized, including cosmetics, dentifrices, mouthwashes, and dental materials, as well as drugs applied topically; inflammation and edema of the mucosa accompanied by burning and sometimes itching are the principal symptoms. Called also *contact s.* See also *s. medicamentosa.* **vesicular s.,** 1. herpetic s. 2. a vesicular eruption of viral etiology on the oral mucosa, which affects swine, cattle, and horses. In swine, it is accompanied by vesicles on the snout and interdigital spaces, in cattle on the udder and teats, and in horses on the coronary band. It must be distinguished from foot-and-mouth disease. **Vincent's s.,** acute necrotizing ulcerative gingivitis.

stomat(o)- [Gr. *stoma,* gen. *stomatos* mouth] a combining form denoting relationship to the mouth or to the ostium uteri.

stomatocace (sto″mah-tok′ah-se) [*stomato-* + Gr. *kakē* badness] ulcerative stomatitis.

stomatocyte (sto′mah-to-sīt) a form of red blood cell in which a slit or mouthlike area replaces the normal circle of pallor, as seen in a rare form of hemolytic anemia and in liver disease.

stomatocytosis (sto″mah-to-si-to′sis) a rare congenital hemolytic anemia characterized by the presence of stomatocytes in the peripheral blood.

stomatodynia (sto″mah-to-din′e-ah) [*stomato-* + Gr. *odynē* pain + *-ia*] pain in the mouth; sore mouth.

stomatodysodia (sto″mah-to-dis-o′de-ah) [*stomato-* + Gr. *dysōdia* stench] halitosis.

stomatogenesis (sto″mah-to-jen′ĕ-sis) [*stomato-* + Gr. *gennan* to produce] a morphologic process seen in ciliate pro-

tozoa in which all oral structures and associated organelles are formed or existing ones are replaced.

stomatoglossitis (sto″mah-to-glos-si′tis) inflammation involving the oral mucous membranes and the tongue, occurring in nutritional disorders such as pellagra, beriberi, vitamin B complex deficiency, and in infections, etc.

stomatognathic (sto″mah-tog-nath′ik) [*stomato-* + Gr. *gnathos* jaw] denoting the mouth and jaws collectively; see under *system.*

stomatography (sto″mah-tog′rah-fe) [*stomato-* + Gr. *graphein* to write] a description of the mouth.

stomatolalia (sto″mah-to-la′le-ah) speaking through the mouth with the nares closed.

stomatological (sto″mah-to-loj′e-kal) pertaining to stomatology.

stomatologist (sto″mah-tol′o-jist) an expert in stomatology.

stomatology (sto″mah-tol′o-je) [*stomato-* + *-logy*] the branch of medical science concerning the mouth and its diseases, functions, and structure; called also *oralogy. See also dentistry.*

stomatomalacia (sto″mah-to-mah-la′she-ah) [*stomato-* + Gr. *malakia* softness] excessive or abnormal softness of the oral structures.

stomatomenia (sto″mah-to-me′ne-ah) [*stomato-* + Gr. *mēniaia* menses] bleeding from the mucous membrane of the mouth at the time of menstruation.

stomatomy (sto-mat′o-me) [*stoma-* + Gr. *tomē* a cutting] surgical incision of the ostium uteri.

stomatomycosis (sto″mah-to-mi-ko′sis) [*stomato-* + Gr. *mykēs* fungus] any oral disease due to a fungus.

stomatopathy (sto″mah-top′ah-the) [*stomato-* + Gr. *pathos* suffering] any pathological condition of the mouth.

stomatoplastic (sto″mah-to-plas′tik) pertaining to stomatoplasty.

stomatoplasty (sto′mah-to-plas″te) [*stomato-* + Gr. *plassein* to mold] plastic repair of defects of or reconstruction of the mouth.

stomatorrhagia (sto″mah-to-ra′je-ah) [*stomato-* + Gr. *rhēgnynai* to burst forth] hemorrhage from the mouth. **s. gingiva′rum,** hemorrhage from the gingivae.

stomatoschisis (sto″mah-tos′kĭ-sis) [*stomato-* + Gr. *schisis* split] harelip.

stomatoscope (sto-mat′o-skōp) [*stomato-* + Gr. *skopein* to examine] an instrument used in inspecting the mouth.

stomatotomy (sto″mah-tot′o-me) stomatomy.

stomencephalus (sto″men-sef′ah-lus) stomocephalus.

stomion (sto′me-on) [Gr. *stomion,* dim. of *stoma* mouth] a cephalometric landmark, being the midpoint in the oral fissure when the lips are closed.

stom(o)- see *stomat(o)-.*

stomocephalus (sto″mo-sef′ah-lus) [*stomo-* + Gr. *kephalē* head] a fetus with a rudimentary head and jaws, so that the skin hangs in folds about the mouth.

stomodeal (sto″mo-de′al) pertaining to the stomodeum.

stomodeum (sto″mo-de′um) [*stomo-* + Gr. *hodaios* pertaining to a way] an invagination of the ectoderm of the embryo at the point where later the mouth is formed.

stomoschisis (sto-mos′kĭ-sis) [*stomo-* + Gr. *schisis* a splitting] cleft lip.

Stomoxys (sto-mok′sis) a genus of flies of the family Muscidae. **S. bouffar′di,** a species transmitting *Trypanosoma cazalboui,* a parasite of goats in French Guiana. **S. cal′citrans,** the common stable fly; it is annoying to man and beast, and is capable of transmitting anthrax, tetanus, *Trypanosoma evansi,* which causes surra in horses, and infectious anemia of horses. Called also *legsticker.*

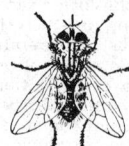

Stomoxys calcitrans.

-stomy (sto′me) [Gr. *stoma* mouth] a word termination denoting the surgical creation of an artificial opening into a hollow organ (colostomy, tracheostomy) or a new opening between two such structures (gastroenterostomy, pyeloureterostomy); also denoting the opening so created.

stone (stōn) 1. a mass of extremely hard and unyielding material, as a gallstone; a calculus. 2. a unit of weight recognized in Great Britain, being the equivalent of 14 pounds (avoirdupois), or about 6.34 kg. (metric). 3. an abrading instrument or tool, such as one used for sharpening instruments. **bladder s.,** vesical calculus. **blue s.,** cupric sulfate. **chalk s.,** articular calculus. **dental s.,** a very strong dental plaster composed chiefly of the α-hemihydrate of gypsum, used for construction of casts of the oral structures. **kidney s.,** renal calculus. **lung s.,** lung calculus. **metabolic s.,** cholesterol calculus. **pulp s.,** denticle, def. 2. **salivary s.,** sialolith. **s.-searcher,** a sound used in searching for calculi in the bladder. **skin s's,** calcareous nodules in the skin. **staghorn s.,** see under *calculus.* **struvite s.,** see under *calculus.* **tear s.,** dacryolith. **vein s.,** phlebolith. **womb s.,** uterine calculus.

Stookey's reflex (stook′ēz) [Byron Polk *Stookey*, New York neurologic surgeon, 1887–1966] see under *reflex.*

stool the fecal discharge from the bowels. **bilious s.,** the yellowish or brownish stools, turning darker on exposure, that are characteristic of bilious diarrhea. **caddy s.,** the stools seen in yellow fever; they look like dark, sandy mud. **fatty s.,** stools containing fat; seen in diseases of the pancreas and in malabsorption syndromes. **lienteric s.,** stool that contains much undigested food. **mucous s.,** stool containing a large amount of mucus; seen in intestinal inflammation or mucous colitis. **pea soup s.,** the characteristic liquid evacuation of typhoid fever. **pipe-stem s.,** stool resembling the shape of a pipe stem, seen in stricture of the lower rectum. **ribbon s.,** a long flattened stool seen in lower rectal stricture. **rice-water s's,** the characteristic and diagnostic watery, light gray to clear evacuations of cholera, containing flecks of mucous material, epithelial cells, and many cholera vibrios. **sago-grain s.,** stools of amebiasis in which the liquid feces contain small flecks of blood-stained mucus. **silver s.,** stools having the color of aluminum or silver paint, due to a mixture of melena and white fatty stools; it occurs in tropical sprue and in children with diarrhea who are given sulfonamides, and is indicative of carcinoma of the ampulla of Vater. **spinach s.,** dark-green stool resembling cooked spinach, resulting from the use of calomel in infants.

stop (stop) 1. to come to a halt. 2. to cease, check, discontinue, or arrest. 3. any device that serves to prevent further progression or advancement. **centric s.,** facies contractus dentis. **occlusal s.,** see under *rest.*

storax (sto′raks) [L. *storax, styrax;* Gr. *styrax*] [USP] a balsam from the trunk of *Liquidambar orientalis* Mill (Levant s.), a tree of western Asia, or of *L. styraciflua* L. (American s.) of North America, occurring as a semiliquid, grayish brown, sticky, opaque mass which deposits on standing a heavy brown layer, or as a semisolid, sometimes solid mass, softened by warming; used as an ingredient of compound benzoin tincture (see under *tincture*). It has been used as an expectorant and topical parasiticide. Called also *styrax.*

storiform (stor′ĭ-form) [L. *storea, storia* a rush mat + *form*] denoting a matted, irregularly whorled pattern, somewhat resembling that of a straw mat; said of the microscopic appearance of fibrous histiocytomas.

storm (storm) an outburst; a temporary and sudden increase in symptoms. **thyroid s., thyrotoxic s.,** see under *crisis.*

Storm van Leeuwen chamber [William *Storm van Leeuwen,* a pharmacist in Leyden, 1882–1933] see under *chamber.*

stoss (stos) [Ger.] see *stosstherapy.*

stosstherapy (stos′ther-ah-pe) [Ger. *stoss* shock, stroke + *therapy*] treatment of a disease by a single massive dose of a therapeutic agent, or by short-term administration of unphysiologically large doses.

Stoxil (stok′sil) trademark for a preparation of idoxuridine.

STP 1. standard temperature and pressure: 0° C and 760 mm Hg. 2. slang term for the hallucinogen 2,5-dimethoxy-4-methamphetamine (DOM).

strabismal (strah-biz′mal) strabismic.

strabismic (strah-biz′mik) pertaining to or of the nature of strabismus.

strabismology (strah″bis-mol′o-je) the study of strabismus.

strabismometer (strah-biz-mom′ĕ-ter) [*strabismus* + *-meter*] an apparatus for measuring strabismus; called also *ophthalmotropometer* and *strabometer.*

strabismometry (strah-biz-mom′ĕ-tree) [*strabismus* + *-metry*] measurement of the amount of strabismus; called also *ophthalmotropometry* and *strabometry.*

strabismus (strah-biz′mus) [Gr. *strabismos* a squinting] deviation of the eye which the patient cannot overcome. The visual axes assume a position relative to each other different from that required by the physiological conditions. The various forms of strabismus are spoken of as tropias, their direction being indicated by the appropriate prefix, as *cyclo*tropia, *eso*tropia, *exo*tropia, *hyper*tropia, and *hypo*tropia. Called also *cast, heterotropia, manifest deviation,* and *squint.* **absolute s.,** that which occurs at all distances of the fixation point; called also *constant s.* **accommodative s.,** that which is due to excessive or deficient accommodative effort. **alternating s., bilateral s., binocular s.,** that which affects each eye alternately. **comitant s., concomitant s.,** that which is due to faulty insertion of the eye muscles, resulting in the same amount of deviation in whatever direction the eyes are looking, because the squinting eye follows the movements of the other eye; called also *muscular s.* and *comitant squint.* **constant s.,** absolute s. **convergent s.,** esotropia. **cyclic s.,** intermittent strabismus that recurs at regular intervals. **s. deor′sum ver′gens,** that in which the visual axis of the squinting eye falls below the fixation point. **divergent s.,** exotropia. **external s.,** exotropia. **incomitant s.,** nonconcomitant s. **intermittent s.,** that which occurs only at intervals. **internal s.,** esotropia. **kinetic s.,** strabismus due to spasm of the muscles controlling ocular movements. **latent s.,** that which occurs only when one eye is occluded. **manifest s.,** strabismus that is evident in binocular vision. **mechanical s.,** that due to pressure or traction on the eye, as by a tumor, producing deflection. **monocular s., monolateral s.,** unilateral s. **muscular s.,** concomitant s. **noncomitant s., nonconcomitant s.,** that in which the amount of deviation of the squinting eye varies according to the direction in which the eyes are turned; called also *incomitant s.* **nonparalytic s.,** concomitant strabismus that is not due to paralysis of the extraocular muscles. **paralytic s.,** that which is due to paralysis of an eye muscle. **s. sur′sum ver′gens,** that in which the visual axis of the squinting eye lies above the fixation point. **unilateral s., uniocular s.,** strabismus affecting only one eye. **vertical s.,** strabismus in which the deviation of the visual axis is in the vertical plane; see *hypertropia* and *hypotropia.*

strabometer (strah-bom′ĕ-ter) strabismometer.

strabometry (strah-bom′ĕ-tre) strabismometry.

strabotome (strab′o-tōm) a knife for performing strabotomy.

strabotomy (strah-bot′o-me) [Gr. *strabos* squinting + *-tomy*] the cutting of the tendon of a muscle of the eye in treatment of strabismus.

strahlen (strah′lin) [Ger. "streaming," "ray"] a large locomotor organelle resembling an axopodium seen in protozoa of the subclass Piroplasmia.

strain (strān) 1. to overexercise; to use to an extreme and harmful degree. 2. to filter or subject to colation. 3. an overstretching or overexertion of some part of the musculature. 4. excessive effort or undue exercise. 5. a group of organisms within a species or variety, characterized by some particular quality, as rough or smooth strains of bacteria. **cell s.,** cells derived from a primary culture or cell line by the selection and cloning of cells having specific properties. **heterologous s.,** a strain of microorganisms different from the strain originally isolated, tested, etc. **high-jumper's s.,** strain of the rotator muscles of the thigh occurring in high jumpers. **homologous s.,** a strain of microorganisms similar to the strain originally isolated, tested, etc. **reference s.,** a strain of bacteria or other microorganisms used as a standard of reference, which appears to meet the criteria of the type strain but is not officially accepted as a neotype. **resistant s.,** a strain of organisms that is resistant to the effects of the agents, such as antibiotics or insecticides, used to control them. **R s.,** the rough strain that results from bacterial dissociation; R colonies have a dull, uneven surface and irregular border, the growth in fluid media tends to flake out, no capsules are seen, and the culture tends to be less virulent. **S s.,** the smooth strain that results from bacterial dissociation. The S colonies have a smooth surface and an unbroken border, growth in fluid media tends to be diffuse, capsules, if present at all, are found in this strain, and the culture tends to be more virulent. **Vi s.,** a strain of bacteria, especially *Salmonella typhi,* that contains the Vi (virulence) antigen of Felix.

strainer (strān′er) an apparatus for straining.

strait (strāt) a narrow passageway. **pelvic s., inferior,** the pelvic outlet. **pelvic s., superior,** the pelvic inlet.

straitjacket (strāt′jak″et) a contrivance for restraining the limbs, especially the arms, of a violently disturbed person; called also *camisole.*

stramonium (strah-mo′ne-um) the dried leaf and flowering or fruiting tops of *Datura stramonium;* used like belladonna and in the treatment of asthma. Called also *thorn apple.*

strand (strand) a thread or fiber. **Billroth's s's,** trabeculae lienis. **lateral enamel s.,** lateral dental lamina.

strangalesthesia (strang″g'l-es-the′ze-ah) [Gr. *strangalizein* to choke + *aisthēsis* perception + *-ia*] zonesthesia.

strangle (strang′g'l) [L. *strangulare*] to choke, or to be choked by compression or other obstruction of the windpipe.

strangles (strang′g'lz) 1. an infectious disease of horses, characterized by a mucopurulent inflammation of the respiratory mucous membrane, with lymph node abscesses, and caused by the *Streptococcus equi.* Called also *colt distemper.* 2. a condition in swine, characterized by infection of the lymph nodes, producing heavily encapsulated abscesses in the region of the pharynx.

strangulated (strang′gu-lāt″ed) [L. *strangulatus*] congested by reason of constriction or hernial stricture, with compromise of the blood supply; see *hernia.*

strangulation (strang″gu-la′shun) [L. *strangulatio*] 1. choking or throttling arrest of respiration, due to occlusion of the air passage. 2. arrest of the circulation in a part, due to compression.

stranguria (strang-gu′re-ah) strangury.

strangury (strang′gu-re) [Gr. *stranx* drop + *ouron* urine] slow and painful discharge of the urine, due to spasm of the urethra and bladder.

strap (strap) 1. a band or strip, as of adhesive tape, used in attaching parts to each other. 2. to bind down tightly. **crib s.,** a strap to be placed around the neck of a horse to prevent cribbing by compressing the windpipe. **Montgomery s's,** straps made of lengths of adhesive tape, used to secure dressings that must be changed frequently. Called also *Montgomery's tapes.*

strapping (strap′ing) the application of strips of adhesive tape, one overlapping the other, to cover and exert pressure upon an extremity or other area of the body; see *accompanying* plate, and see also *bandaging.* **Gibney's s.,** see under *bandage.*

Strasburger's cell plate (strahs-burg′erz) [Eduard Adolf *Strasburger,* German botanist, 1844–1912] midbody.

Strassburg's test (strahs′boorgz) [Gustav Adolf *Strässburg,* German physiologist, born 1848] see under *tests.*

strata (stra′tah) [L.] plural of *stratum.*

stratification (strat″ĭ-fi-ka′shun) [L. *stratum* layer + *facere* to make] disposal in layers.

stratified (strat′ĭ-fīd) disposed in layers.

stratiform (strat′ĭ-form) [L. *stratum* layer + *forma* form] having the form of strata.

stratigram (strat′ĭ-gram) a roentgenogram of a selected layer of the body made by body section roentgenography.

stratigraphy (strah-tig′rah-fe) [L. *stratum* layer + Gr. *graphein* to write] see *body section roentgenography,* under *roentgenography.*

stratum (stra′tum), pl. *stra′ta* [L.] a layer; [NA] a general term for a sheetlike mass of substance of nearly uniform thickness, particularly when the layer is one of several associated layers. **s. adamanti′num,** the enamel of a tooth (enamelum [NA]). **s. al′bum profun′dum cor′poris quadrigem′ini,** a layer of white matter between the corpora quadrigemina and the central gray layer

of the cerebral aqueduct. **s. basa′le,** basal layer: the deepest layer of the endometrium, which contains the blind ends of the uterine glands; the cells of this layer undergo minimal change during the sexual cycle. **s. basa′le epider′midis** [NA], basal layer of epidermis: the deepest stratum of the epidermis, composed of a single layer of deeply basophilic cells. Called also *s. cylindricum epidermidis.* See also *s. germinativum.* **cerebral s. of retina, s. cerebra′le ret′inae** pars nervosa retinae. **s. circula′re gas′tris** [NA], circular layer of muscular tunic of stomach: the layer of circularly coursing fibers in the muscular coat of the stomach; called also *s. circulare ventriculi* [NA alternative]. **s. circula′re membra′nae tym′pani,** circular layer of tympanic membrane: the layer of circularly coursing fibers deep to the mucous layer of the tympanic membrane; it is best developed near the periphery. **s. circula′re tu′nicae muscula′ris co′li** [NA], circular layer of muscular tunic of colon: the inner layer of circularly coursing fibers in the muscular coat of the colon. **s. circula′re tu′nicae muscula′ris intesti′ni ten′uis** [NA], circular layer of muscular tunic of small intestine: the inner layer of circularly coursing fibers in the muscular coat of the small intestine. **s. circula′re tu′nicae muscula′ris rec′ti** [NA], circular layer of muscular tunic of rectum: the inner layer of circularly coursing fibers in the muscular coat of the rectum. **s. circula′re tu′nicae muscula′ris ventric′uli** [NA], circular layer of muscular tunic of stomach: the layer of circularly coursing fibers in the muscular coat of the stomach. **s. circula′re ventric′uli,** NA alternative for *s. circulare gastris.* **stra′ta collic′uli crania′lis,** see *strata grisea et alba colliculi rostralis.* **stra′ta collic′uli rostra′lis,** see *strata grisea et alba colliculi rostralis.* **stra′ta collic′uli superior′is,** see *strata grisea et alba colliculi rostralis.* **s. compac′tum,** compact layer: the layer of the endometrium nearest the surface, which contains the necks of the uterine glands; together with the stratum spongiosum, it forms the *stratum functionale* (q.v.). **connective tissue s. of mesentery,** lamina mesenterii propria. **s. cor′neum epider′midis** [NA], horny layer of epidermis: the outermost layer of the epidermis, consisting of cells that are dead and desquamating. **s. cor′neum un′guis** [NA], horny layer of nail: the outer, compact layer of the nail; called also *nail plate.* **s. cuta′neum membra′nae tym′pani** [NA], cutaneous layer of tympanic membrane: a very thin form of skin that constitutes the lateral layer of the tympanic membrane. **s. cylin′dricum epider′midis,** s. basale epidermidis. **s. ebo′ris,** the dentin of a tooth (dentinum [NA]). **s. exter′num tu′nicae muscula′ris duc′tus deferen′tis,** the outer layer of fibers in the muscular coat of the ductus deferens. **s. exter′num tu′nicae muscula′ris ure′teris,** the outer layer of fibers in the muscular coat of the ureter. **s. exter′num tu′nicae muscula′ris ves′icae urina′riae,** the outer layer of fibers in the muscular coat of the urinary bladder. **s. fibro′sum cap′sulae articula′ris,** NA alternative for *membrana fibrosa capsulae articularis.* **s. fibro′sum vagi′nae ten′dinis** [NA], the fibrous layer of a tendon sheath. **s. functiona′le,** functional layer: the stratum compactum and stratum spongiosum considered together (i.e., all of the endometrium except for the stratum basale), the cells of which are cast off at menstruation and at parturition. It is known as the *decidua* during pregnancy. Called also *pars functionalis.* **s. gangliona′re ner′vi op′tici** ganglionic layer of optic nerve; see under *layer.* **s. gangliona′re ret′inae** ganglionic layer of retina; see under *layer.* **ganglionic s. of optic nerve,** see under *layer.* **ganglionic s. of retina,** see under *layer.* **s. ganglio′sum cerebel′li,** ganglionic layer of cerebellum: the thin middle gray layer of the cortex cerebelli, consisting of a single layer of Purkinje cells; called also *s. Purkinje.* **s. germinativum, s. germinati′vum epider′midis [Malpig′hii],** germinative layer: the stratum basale epidermidis and the stratum spinosum epidermidis considered as a single layer. The term is also sometimes used to designate only the stratum basale epidermidis. Called also *germinative layer of epidermis, malpighian layer or rete, mucous layer,* and *s. Malpighii.* **s. germinati′vum un′guis** [NA], germinative layer of nail: the lower layer of the nail, from which the nail grows; it is continuous with the stratum basale and stratum spinosum of the epidermis. Called also *nail plate.* **s. granulo′sum cerebel′li** [NA], granular layer of cerebellum: the deep layer of the cortex of the cerebellum; it

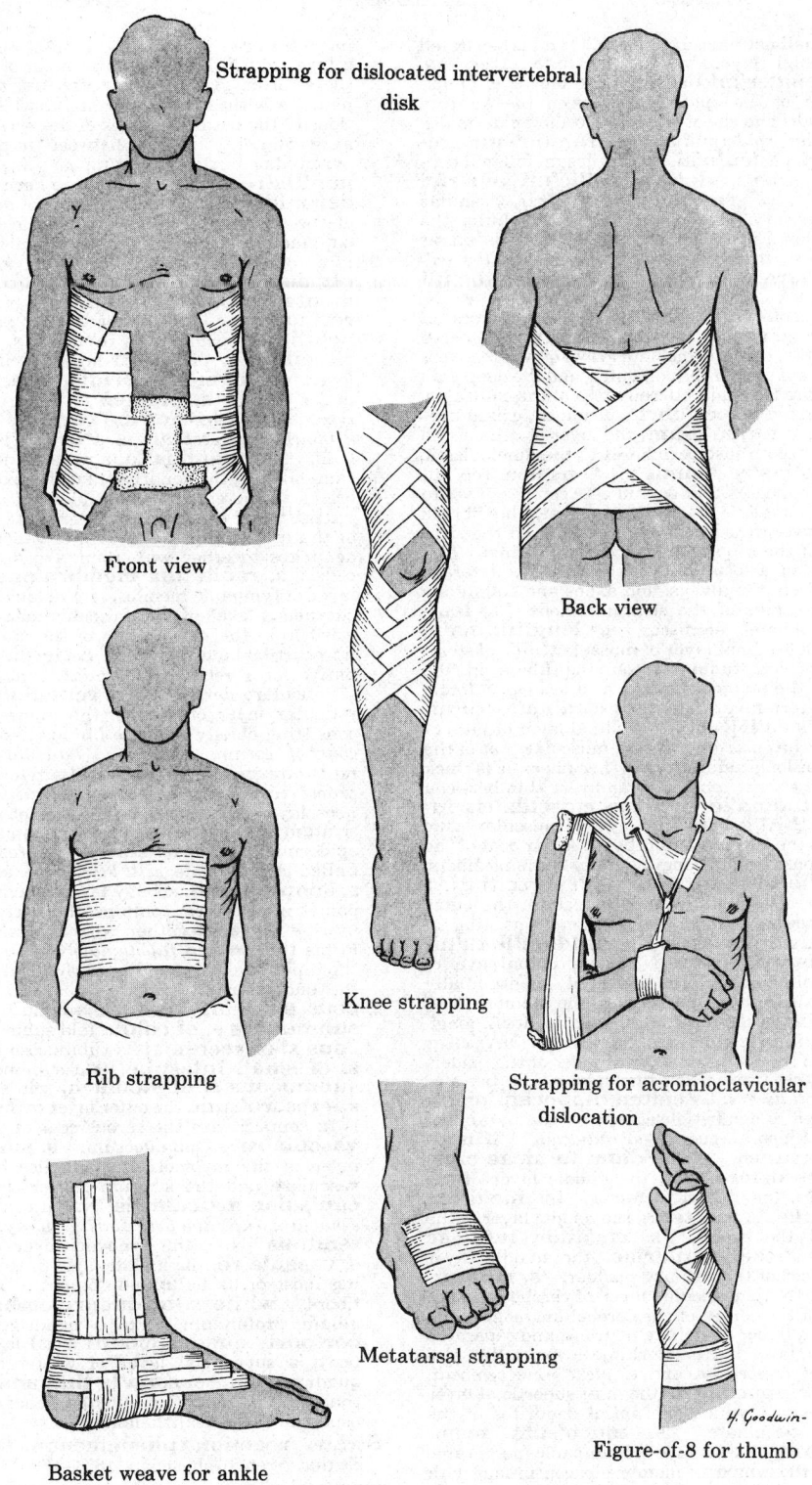

Strapping for dislocated intervertebral disk

Front view

Back view

Rib strapping

Knee strapping

Strapping for acromioclavicular dislocation

Basket weave for ankle

Metatarsal strapping

Figure-of-8 for thumb

H. Goodwin

PLATE 43 — VARIOUS TYPES OF STRAPPING

contains many small neurons (granule cells) and is separated from the molecular layer by the Purkinje layer. **s. granulo′sum epider′midis** [NA], granular layer of epidermis: the layer of the epidermis between the stratum lucidum epidermidis and the stratum spinosum epidermidis. See also *s. corneum epidermidis.* **s. granulo′sum follic′uli ooph′ori vesiculo′si,** s. granulosum folliculi ovarici vesiculosi. **s. granulo′sum follic′uli ova′rici vesiculo′si** [NA], **s. granulo′sum ova′rii,** granular layer of follicle of ovary: the layer of follicle cells lining the theca of a vesicular ovarian follicle. **stra′ta gris′ea et al′ba collic′uli crania′lis,** see *strata (grisea et alba) colliculi rostralis.* **stra′ta (gris′ea et al′ba) collic′uli superio′ris** [NA alternative], (gray and white) layers of rostral colliculus: the four deepest layers of the colliculus, two gray and two white, consisting of nerve cells of various types; the intermediate gray and white layers are the main afferent area of the colliculus, and the deep gray and white layers are the main efferent area of the colliculus. **s. gris′eum centra′le cer′ebri,** substantia grisea centralis cerebri. **s. interme′dium,** the layer of cells of the enamel organ of a tooth just peripheral to the ameloblastic layer. **s. interoliva′re lemnis′ci,** fibers from the nucleus gracilis and cuneatus that ascend between the olives to form the medial lemnisci. **s. lacuno′sum,** the fibrous layer situated between the stratum radiatum and the stratum moleculare of the hippocampus, consisting chiefly of a dense fiber layer in association with Schaffer collaterals, axons ascending from the alveus, and axons and collaterals ascending from neurons of the stratum oriens. **s. lemnis′ci,** s. interolivare lemnisci. **s. longitudina′le gas′tris** [NA], longitudinal layer of muscular tunic of stomach: the layer of longitudinally coursing fibers in the muscular coat of the stomach; called also *s. longitudinale ventriculi* [NA alternative]. **s. longitudina′le tu′nicae muscula′ris co′li** [NA], longitudinal layer of muscular tunic of colon: the outer layer of the muscular coat of the colon, consisting of longitudinally coursing fibers; it is thick in the regions of the three teniae coli and very thin between them. **s. longitudina′le tu′nicae muscula′ris intesti′ni ten′uis** [NA], longitudinal layer of muscular tunic of small intestine: the outer layer of the muscular coat of the small intestine, consisting of longitudinally coursing fibers. **s. longitudina′le tu′nicae muscula′ris rec′ti** [NA], longitudinal layer of muscular tunic of rectum: the outer layer of the muscular coat of the rectum, consisting of longitudinally coursing fibers. **s. longitudina′le tu′nicae muscula′ris ventric′uli** [NA], longitudinal layer of muscular tunic of stomach: the layer of longitudinally coursing fibers in the muscular coat of the stomach. **s. longitudina′le ventric′uli,** NA alternative for *s. longitudinale gastris.* **s. lu′cidum epider′midis** [NA], clear layer of epidermis: the clear translucent layer of the epidermis, just beneath the stratum corneum epidermidis. See also *s. corneum epidermidis.* **s. lu′cidum hippocam′pi,** the cellular (as opposed to dendritic) segment of the pyramidal cell layer of the hippocampus; cf. *s. radiatum.* **s. malpig′hii,** s. germinativum. **s. me′dium tu′nicae muscula′ris duc′tus deferen′tis,** the middle layer of the muscular coat of the ductus deferens. **s. me′dium tu′nicae muscula′ris ure′teris,** the middle layer of the muscular coat of the ureter. **s. me′dium tu′nicae muscula′ris ves′icae urina′riae,** the middle layer of the muscular coat of the urinary bladder. **s. molecula′re cerebel′li** [NA], molecular layer of cerebellum: the superficial layer of the cortex of the cerebellum, containing a relatively small number of stellate neurons, and separated from the granular layer by the Purkinje layer; called also *plexiform layer of cerebellum* and *s. plexiforme cerebelli.* **s. molecula′re hippocam′pi,** the most superficial layer of the hippocampus, in which the apical dendrites of the pyramidal cells terminate. **s. muco′sum membra′nae tym′pani,** mucous layer of tympanic membrane: the inner layer of the tympanic membrane, continuous with the mucosa lining the tympanic cavity. **s. neuroepithelia′le ret′inae** neuroepithelial layer of retina; see under *layer.* **s. neurono′rum pirifor′mium** [NA], the layer of Purkinje neurons situated between the external molecular layer and the internal granular layer of the cerebellar cortex; considered by some to be the deepest layer of the molecular layer. Called also *Purkinje layer* or *Purkinje cell layer.* **s. nuclea′re medul′lae oblonga′tae,** the column of gray substance in the medulla oblongata contain-

ing the nuclei of the lower cranial nerves. **s. op′ticum,** a layer of white fibers in the superior colliculus, just below the stratum griseum. **s. o′riens,** the layer composed of neurons with ascending axons (basket cells), the ramifications of the basal dendrites of the pyramidal cells, and their axon collaterals localized between the alveus and the stratum pyramidale of the hippocampus. **s. papilla′re cor′ii, s. papilla′re cu′tis,** s. papillare dermidis. **s. papilla′re der′midis** [NA], papillary layer of dermis: the outer layer of the dermis, characterized by the presence of ridges or papillae protruding into the epidermis. Called also *papillary layer of corium, s. papillare corii,* and *s. papillare cutis.* **pigmented s. of ciliary body,** see under *layer.* **pigmented s. of iris,** see under *layer.* **pigmented s. of retina,** pars pigmentosa retinae. **s. pigmen′ti bul′bi oc′uli,** pars pigmentosa retinae. **s. pigmen′ti cor′poris cilia′ris,** pigmented layer of ciliary body; see under *layer.* **s. pigmen′ti i′ridis,** pigmented layer of iris; see under *layer.* **s. pigmen′ti ret′inae,** pars pigmentosa retinae. **s. plexifor′me cerebel′li,** NA alternative for *s. moleculare cerebelli.* **s. Purkin′je,** s. gangliosum cerebelli. **s. pyramida′le,** a well-defined double layer of pyramidal cells, the dendrites of which extend from the stratum oriens to the stratum moleculare of the hippocampus. **s. radia′tum,** the superficial part of the pyramidal cell layer of the hippocampus, the bulk of which is formed by apical dendrites together with their axons and a few pyramidal cells. **s. radia′tum membra′nae tym′pani,** radiate layer of tympanic membrane: the layer of fibers beneath the cutaneous layer of the tympanic membrane, radiating outward from the manubrium of the malleus to pass into the fibrocartilaginous ring. **s. reticula′re co′rii,** NA alternative for *s. reticulare dermidis.* **s. reticula′re cu′tis,** s. reticulare dermidis. **s. reticula′re der′midis** [NA], reticular layer of dermis: the inner layer of the dermis, consisting chiefly of dense fibrous tissue. Called also *proper coat of corium* or *dermis, reticular layer of corium, s. reticulare corii* [NA alternative], *s. reticulare cutis,* and *tunica propria corii.* **s. spino′sum epider′midis** [NA], spinous layer of epidermis: the layer of the skin between the stratum granulosum epidermidis and the stratum basale epidermidis characterized by the presence of prickle cells. Called also *prickle cell layer.* See also *s. germinativum.* **s. spongio′sum,** spongy layer: the middle layer of the endometrium, which contains the tortuous portions of the uterine glands; together with the stratum compactum, it forms the *stratum functionale* (q.v.). **s. submuco′sum,** the inner layer of the myometrium, which is in contact with the endometrium; called also *s. subvasculare.* **submucous s. of bladder,** tela submucosa vesicae urinariae. **submucous s. of colon,** tela submucosa coli. **submucous s. of rectum,** tela submucosa recti. **submucous s. of small intestine,** tela submucosa intestini tenuis. **submucous s. of stomach,** tela submucosa ventriculi. **s. subsero′sum,** the outer layer of the myometrium, which is in contact with the serous coat of the uterus. **s. subvascula′re,** s. submucosum. **s. supravascula′re,** the layer of the myometrium that lies between the stratum vasculare and the stratum subserosum. **s. synovia′le cap′sulae articula′ris,** NA alternative for *membrana synovialis capsulae articularis.* **s. synovia′le vagi′nae tendinis** [NA], the synovial layer of a tendon sheath. **s. vascula′re,** the middle layer of the myometrium, forming most of its bulk, and composed of circular and spiral fibers. **white s. of quadrigeminal body, deep,** s. album profundum corporis quadrigemini. **s. zona′le cor′poris quadrigem′ini** zonal layer of quadrigeminal body: a superficial layer of white fibers of the corpora quadrigemina. **s. zona′le thal′ami** [NA], zonal layer of thalamus: a layer of myelinated fibers covering the superior aspect of the dorsal thalamus.

Straus′ reaction (phenomenon, test) (strows) [Isidore *Straus,* French physician, 1854–1896] see under *reaction.*

Strauss′ sign (strows′) [Hermann *Strauss,* physician in Berlin, 1868–1944] see under *sign.*

streak (strēk) a line, stria, striation, or stripe. **angioid s′s,** red to black irregular bands observed in the ocular fundus running outward from the region of the optic disk, which are seen in certain conditions, including pseudoxanthoma elasticum, osteitis deformans, and sickle-cell anemia. The lesions are thought to represent ruptures in Bruch's membrane. **fatty s.,** a small, flat, yellow-gray area, composed mainly of cholesterol, within an artery; possibly an early stage of atherosclerosis. **germinal s.,** primitive s. **Knapp's s's,** lines resembling blood vessels seen occasionally in the retina after hemorrhage. **medullary s.,** the neural groove. **meningeal s.,** tache cérébrale. **primitive s.,** a faint white trace at the caudal end of the embryonic disc, formed by the movement of cells at the beginning of mesoderm formation; it provides the earliest evidence of the embryonic axis.

stream (strēm) a current or flow of water or other fluid. **axial s.,** the core of rapid flow in the center of a channel, as in the lumen of a blood vessel, bordered or surrounded by a zone in which the elements move less rapidly, or are motionless. **blood s.,** see under *B*. **electron s.,** a stream of negatively charged particles (electrons) moving from cathode to anode across a potential difference in a low-pressure gas tube or a vacuum tube. **hair s's,** flumina pilorum.

streblomicrodactyly (streb″lo-mi″kro-dak′tĭ-le) [Gr. *streblos* twisted + *mikros* small + *daktylos* finger] streptomicrodactyly.

stremma (strem′ah) [Gr. "a twist"] a sprain.

strength (strength) the quality or quantity of force, power, concentration, activity, etc. **ionic s.,** a quantity proportional to the amount of electrostatic interaction between ions in solution; equal to $\frac{1}{2} \Sigma_i c_i Z_i^2$, where c_i is the molar concentration of the *i*th species, and Z_i the ionic charge.

strephenopodia (stref″ĕ-no-po′de-ah) [*streph*- + Gr. *en* in + *pous* foot] talipes varus.

strephexopodia (stref″ek-so-po′de-ah) [*streph*- + Gr. *exō* out + *pous* foot] talipes valgus.

streph(o)- [Gr. *strephein* to twist] a combining form meaning twisted.

strephopodia (stref″o-po′de-ah) talipes equinus.

strephosymbolia (stref″o-sim-bo′le-ah) [*strepho*- + Gr. *symbolon* symbol + *-ia*] 1. a disorder of perception in which objects seem reversed, as in a mirror. 2. a reading difficulty inconsistent with a child's general intelligence, beginning with confusion between similar but oppositely oriented letters (b-d, q-p) and a tendency to reverse direction in reading.

strepitus (strep′ĭ-tus) [L.] a noise; a sound heard on auscultation.

strepogenin (strep″o-jen′in) a factor present in casein and certain other proteins which is essential to optimal growth of animals; called also *chick growth factor*.

strepsinema (strep″sĭ-ne′mah) [Gr. *strepsis* a twist + *nēma* thread] the threads of chromatin in the strepsitene stage.

strepsitene (strep′sĭ-tēn) a stage of meiosis, after the diplotene stage, in which the threads become twisted about each other.

streptamine (strep-tam′in) chemical name: 1,3-diamino-2,4,5,6-tetrahydroxycyclohexane. One of the fractions derived from the degradation of streptomycin.

strepticemia (strep″tĭ-se′me-ah) streptococcemia.

streptidine (strep′tĭ-dīn) one of the fractions derived from degradation of streptomycin, the other fraction being streptobiosamine; it is 1,3-diguanido-2,4,5,6-tetrahydroxycyclohexane.

strept(o)- [Gr. *streptos* twisted] a combining form meaning twisted.

streptoangina (strep″to-an′jĭ-nah) a pseudomembranous deposit in the throat due to a streptococcal infection.

streptobacilli (strep″to-bah-sil′i) plural of *streptobacillus*.

Streptobacillus (strep″to-bah-sil′us) [*strepto*- + *bacillus*] a genus of facultatively anaerobic, gram-negative, rod-shaped bacteria of uncertain affiliation, made up of organisms that may be highly pleomorphic, varying from single rods with central swelling to chains or filaments resembling strings of beads. Serum, ascitic fluid, or blood is required for growth. The organisms are found in the throat and nasopharynx of wild and laboratory rats, and they may cause rat-bite fever in humans. The genus contains a single species, *S.* (*Haverhillia*) *moniliformis*. **S. monilifor′mis,** the single species of the genus. Called also *Haverhillia multiformis*.

streptobacillus (strep″to-bah-sil′us) pl. *streptobacil′li*. a bacterium of the genus *Streptobacillus*.

streptobiosamine (strep″to-bi-o′sah-mēn) a disaccharide containing streptose and *N*-methyl-L-glucosamine, a product of the acid hydrolysis of streptomycin in which it is linked glycosidally to streptidine.

streptocerciasis (strep″to-ser-ki′ah-sis) infection with *Mansonella streptocerca*, whose microfilariae produce a pruritic rash resembling that in onchocerciasis; transmitted by midges of the genus *Culicoides*, it occurs in Central Africa.

Streptococcaceae (strep″to-kok-ka′se-e) a family of gram-positive, facultative anaerobic cocci, which are usually nonmotile, and occur in pairs, chains, or tetrads. It includes the genera *Aerococcus*, *Gemella*, *Leuconostoc*, *Pediococcus*, and *Streptococcus*.

streptococcal (strep″to-kok′al) pertaining to or caused by a streptococcus.

streptococcemia (strep″to-kok-se′me-ah) [*streptococcus* + Gr. *haima* blood + *-ia*] the presence of streptococci in the blood; streptococcal infection.

streptococci (strep″to-kok′si) plural of *streptococcus*.

streptococcic (strep″to-kok′sik) streptococcal.

streptococcicide (strep″to-kok′sĭ-sīd) an agent that is destructive to streptococci.

streptococcolysin (strep″to-kok-kol′ĭ-sin) streptolysin.

streptococcosis (strep″to-kou-ko′sis) infection with streptococci.

Streptococcus (strep″to-kok′us) [*strepto*- + Gr. *kokkos* berry] a genus of gram-positive, facultatively anaerobic cocci occurring in pairs or chains, assigned to the family Streptococcaceae. Streptococci are cytochrome-, oxidase-, and catalase-negative organisms that are nonmotile, nonspore forming, and homofermentative. The genus consists of four groups: the *pyogenic* group, the *viridans* group, the *enterococcus* group, and the *lactic* group. The first group includes the β-hemolytic human and animal pathogens, the second includes α-hemolytic, potentially pathogenic organisms occurring as normal flora in the human upper respiratory tract, the third group includes organisms with variable hemolysis that are normal flora of the intestinal tract, and the fourth group includes saprophytic forms associated with the souring of milk. Streptococci are classified according to patterns of hemolysis on blood agar, antigenic composition, and physiologic and biochemical characteristics. See also *hemolytic streptococcus*, under *streptococcus* and *Lancefield classification*, under *classificiation*. **S. acidomi′nimus,** an α-hemolytic species with no group-specific antigen, found in the bovine vagina and in raw milk; it occasionally causes human infection. **S. agalac′tiae,** a β-hemolytic or nonhemolytic species of group B, found in raw milk; it causes mastitis in cattle and is associated with human infection in infants. Called also *S. mastitidis*. **S. anaero′bius,** *Peptostreptococcus anaerobius*. **S. angino′sus,** a species that includes streptococci of both group F and group G. β-Hemolytic strains are found in several human sources and in abscesses. The α-hemolytic and nonhemolytic species (*streptococcus MG*) are associated with primary atypical pneumonia. **S. avi′um,** a species that includes α-hemolytic enterococci of both group D and group Q. It is found primarily in the feces of chickens, and is occasionally associated with human infection. **S. bo′vis,** an α-hemolytic or nonhemolytic species, one of the nonenterococcus group D streptococci. It is found in the bovine alimentary tract and sometimes in human feces; sometimes associated with human endocarditis. **S. cremo′ris,** an α-hemolytic or nonhemolytic species of group N, which is one of the lactic group. It occurs in dairy products; its action on milk results in the production of buttermilk. **S. faecium,** see *S. faecalis*. **S. du′rans,** see *S. faecium*. **S. epidem′icus,** former name for *S. pyogenes*, thought to be disease-specific for epidemic infection of the upper respiratory tract. **S. e′qui,** β-hemolytic streptococci of group C, the specific etiologic agent of strangles in horses; it is nonpathogenic for man. **S. equi′nus,** an α-hemolytic species of the viridans group, which is one of the nonenterococcus group D streptococci. It is found in the alimentary tract of the horse, and is sometimes associated with human infection. **S. equisim′ilis,** a β-hemolytic species of group C, occurring in the upper respiratory tract of humans and animals. It is sometimes associated with erysipelas and puerperal fever. **S. erysipel′atis,** *S. pyogenes*. **S. faeca′lis,** a nonhemolytic species of group D, which is one of the enterococcus group. It is found as a normal inhabitant of the human intestinal tract, and is occasionally associated with urinary tract infections and subacute endocarditis.

Called also *S. liquefaciens.* **S. faeci′um,** α-hemolytic species of group D, which is one of the enterococcus group, found as a normal inhabitant of the human intestinal tract. It may cause urinary tract infections and subacute endocarditis. Called also *S. durans.* **S. foe′tidus,** *Peptostreptococcus anaerobius.* **S. hemolyt′icus,** *S. pyogenes.* **S. lac′ticus, S. lac′tis,** an α-hemolytic or nonhemolytic, nonpathogenic species of group N, which is one of the lactic group. It is found in dairy products and is commonly responsible for the souring of milk. **S. lanceola′tus,** *Peptostreptococcus lanceolatus.* **S. liquefa′ciens,** *S. faecalis.* **S. mastit′idis,** *S. agalactiae.* **S. mi′cros,** *Peptostreptococcus micros.* **S. mi′tis,** an α-hemolytic species of the viridans group, which has no specific group antigen. It is found in the normal human upper respiratory tract and has been associated with subacute bacterial endocarditis. **S. mu′tans,** a group K species of the viridans group with variable hemolysis. It has been implicated in the formation of dental caries. **nonhemolytic s.,** any streptococcus that does not cause a change in the medium when cultured on blood agar. Called also *gamma s.* and *indifferent s.* **S. pneumo′niae,** an α-hemolytic species with no specific group antigen. It is the most common cause of lobar pneumonia; it also causes numerous other serious acute pyogenic disorders, e.g., meningitis, septicemia, empyema, and peritonitis. These lancet-shaped bacteria occur in pairs and are heavily encapsulated in exudates. There are more than 80 serotypes (fewer if some are condensed as subtypes) on the basis of the specificity of the capsular polysaccharides. Called also *Diplococcus pneumoniae* and *pneumococcus.* See also plate accompanying *bacterium* and *pneumococcus polysaccharide,* under *polysaccharide.* **S. pyog′enes,** a species of β-hemolytic, toxigenic pyogenic streptococci of group A, separable into numbered serotypes on the basis of the specificity and combination of the M, R, and T antigens, and causing septic sore throat, scarlet fever, rheumatic fever, puerperal sepsis, acute glomerulonephritis, and other conditions in man. Called also *S. hemolyticus* and *S. scarlatinae.* **S. saliva′rius,** a group k streptococcus with variable hemolysis, making up a part of the normal flora of the upper respiratory tract, and occasionally associated with apical abscesses of the teeth and the subacute form of bacterial endocarditis. **S. san′guis,** an α-hemolytic species of the viridans group, tentatively identified with group H. It is found in humans in dental plaque, in blood, and in subacute bacterial endocarditis. **S. scarlati′nae,** *S. pyogenes.* **S. thermoph′ilus,** an α-hemolytic species of the viridans group, found in milk and milk products. **S. u′beris,** an α-hemolytic or nonhemolytic species with no specific group antigen, found in milk and bovine sources, and occasionally associated with human infections. **S. vir′idans,** a former species name for α-hemolytic streptococci, especially those strains found in human disease; see *hemolytic streptococcus,* under *streptococcus.* **S. zooepidem′icus,** β-hemolytic streptococci of group C, commonly causing pyogenic disease in lower animals and known as "animal pyogenes"; it is rarely found in man.

streptococcus (strep-to-kok′us), pl. *streptococ′ci.* an organism of the genus *Streptococcus.* **alpha s.,** see under *hemolytic s.* **anhemolytic s.,** nonhemolytic s. **Bargen's s.,** (*obs.*) *Streptococcus bovis.* **beta s.,** see under *hemolytic s.* **Fehleisen's s.,** (*obs.*), *Streptococcus pyogenes.* **gamma s.,** nonhemolytic s. **group A, B, C (etc.) streptococci,** a classification of β-hemolytic streptococci based on cell-wall carbohydrate antigens; see *Lancefield classification,* under *classification.* **hemolytic s.,** any streptococcus capable of hemolyzing red blood cells or of producing a zone of hemolysis about the colonies on blood agar. The great majority of streptococci found in pathologic processes belong to this type. The hemolytic streptococci have been classified as the *alpha* (α-hemolytic) or *viridans type,* which produces about the colony on blood agar a zone of greenish discoloration considerably smaller than the clear zone produced by the beta type (see also *viridans s.*); and the *beta* (β-hemolytic) *type,* which produces a clear zone of hemolysis immediately surrounding the colony on blood agar. On immunological grounds, the β-hemolytic streptococci may be divided according to the presence of specific antigenic carbohydrates in the cell wall (C-substance) into Lancefield groups A through T. Those causing human infection are found primarily in groups A through G. See *Lancefield classification,* under *classification.* **indifferent s.,** nonhemolytic s. **s. MG,** any of a strain of biochemically and

antigenically homogeneous, nonhemolytic streptococci of group F agglutinated by the sera of patients with mycoplasmal pneumonia. **viridans s.,** any of a group of α-hemolytic streptococci that have no defined group antigens, found as part of the normal flora of the respiratory tract; streptococci of this group cause dental caries and bacterial endocarditis. See also *hemolytic s.*

streptodornase (strep″to-dor′nās) [*streptococci* + *deoxyribonuclease*] a deoxyribonuclease produced by hemolytic streptococci. **streptokinase-s.,** see under *streptokinase.*

streptoduocin (strep″to-du′o-sin) an antibiotic compound consisting of approximately equal parts of dihydrostreptomycin sulfate and streptomycin sulfate.

streptogenin (strep″to-jen′in) a growth-stimulating factor for certain microorganisms and laboratory animals, found in protein hydrolysates. Since a large number of peptides have streptogenin activity, they may serve simply as an accessible source of amino acids.

streptohemolysin (strep″to-he-mol′ĭ-sin) streptolysin.

streptokinase (strep″to-ki′nās) [*strepto*coccus + *kinase*] a proteolytic enzyme elaborated by hemolytic streptococci, which produces fibrinolysis by activating plasminogen to plasmin; it is used as a thrombolytic agent. See also *kinase,* def. 2. **s.-streptodornase** (SKSD), a mixture of the proteolytic enzymes (streptokinase and streptodornase) produced by hemolytic streptococci; used topically on surface lesions and by instillation in closed body cavities to remove clotted blood or fibrinous or purulent accumulations; also used as a skin test antigen in evaluating generalized cell-mediated immunodeficiency.

streptolysin (strep-tol′ĭ-sin) [*strepto*coccus + *hemolysin*] an exotoxin produced by certain strains of streptococci, particularly those of group A, that lyses red blood cells. **s. O,** an oxygen-labile and antigenic hemolysin produced by most group A streptococci and by some of groups C and G. It is inactive in the oxidized state but is readily activated by treatment with mild reducing agents, such as sulfite. **s. S,** an oxygen-stable and nonantigenic hemolysin and leukocidin produced by many strains of group A streptococci. It is sensitive to treatment with heat or acid, but is not inactivated by oxygen.

streptomicrodactyly (strep″to-mi″kro-dak′tĭ-le) [*strepto* + Gr. *mikros* small + *daktylos* finger] camptodactyly in which the little fingers only are involved.

Streptomyces (strep″to-mi′sēz) [*strepto*- + Gr. *mykēs* fungus] a genus of fungus-like bacteria of the family Streptomycetaceae, order Actinomycetales, consisting of aerobic, nonacid-fast organisms that form a nonfragmented aerial mycelium. The genus is separable into several hundred different species, usually soil forms but occasionally parasitic on plants and animals. Most species produce pigments. More than half of the antibiotics of practical value, including the aminoglycosides, the tetracyclines, and the macrolides, are produced from species of *Streptocmyces.* **S. paraguayen′sis,** a pathogenic species of uncertain status. **S. somalien′sis,** a species commonly found in Africa, North and South America, Israel, and India that is the cause of mycetoma in which the granules in the discharged pus are white to yellow. **S. vina′ceus,** a species that produces vitamin B_{12}. Called also *Actinomyces vinaceus.*

Streptomycetaceae (strep″to-mi″se-ta′se-e) a family of bacteria of the order Actinomycetales. It consists of the genera *Streptomyces, Streptoverticillium, Sporichthya,* and *Microellobosporia.* The only genus containing clinically important species is *Streptomyces.*

streptomycin (strep′to-mi″sin) a bactericidal antibiotic of the aminoglycoside class, which is produced by the soil actinomycete, *Streptomyces griseus,* and is effective against most gram-negative and acid-fast bacteria and some gram-positive forms, but is used chiefly in the treatment of tuberculosis. It causes both inhibition and decreased fidelity in protein synthesis. **s. hydrochloride,** the trihydrochloride salt of streptomycin, $C_{21}H_{39}N_7O_{12}\cdot 3HCl$, having the same actions as the base; it has been used for the same purposes as the sulfate salt. **s. sulfate,** the sesquisulfate salt of streptomycin, $(C_{21}H_{39}N_7O_{12})_2\cdot 3H_2SO_4$, occurring as a white or practically white powder, used primarily as a tuberculostatic, usually concomitantly with another tuberculostatic; it also may be used in certain cases in the treatment of nontuberculous infections due to susceptible organisms, such as plague, tularemia, brucellosis, Klebsiella pneumonia, meningitis, and bacterial endocarditis. It is administered intramuscularly.

streptomycosis (strep″to-mi-ko′sis) infection with bacteria of the genus *Streptomyces*.

streptose (strep′tōs) a pentose found in the streptobiosamine portion of streptomycin.

streptosepticemia (strep″to-sep″tĭ-se′me-ah) septicemia due to a streptococcus.

Streptosporangium (strep″to-spo-ran′je-um) [*strepto-* + Gr. *sporos* seed + *angeion* vessel] a genus of bacteria of the family Actinoplanaceae, order Actinomycetales, made up of mycelium-forming saprophytic microorganisms found in soil and water.

streptothricin (strep″to-thri′sin) an antibiotic substance active against both gram-negative and gram-positive bacteria; it was the first antibiotic isolated, but was found to be too toxic for systemic use.

streptothricosis (strep″to-thri-ko′sis) streptotrichosis.

Streptothrix (strep′to-thriks) [*strepto-* + Gr. *thrix* hair] a genus of sheathed bacteria found in fresh water and activated sludge, made up of gram-negative, thin, rod-shaped cells, occurring in chains enclosed in hyaline sheaths. The type species is *S. hyali′na*. **S. bo′vis,** *Dermatophilus congolensis.* **S. farci′ni,** *Nocardia farcinica.* **S. nocar′dii,** *Nocardia farcinica.*

streptotrichal (strep-tot′rĭ-kal) pertaining to or caused by streptothrix.

streptotrichosis (strep″to-tri-ko′sis) 1. infection with organisms of the former genus *Streptothrix;* see *actinomycosis, nocardiosis* and *streptomycosis.* 2. a former name for dermatophilosis.

Streptoverticillium (strep″to-ver-tĭ-sil′e-um) [*strepto-* + L. *verticillus* whorl] a genus of bacteria of the family Streptomycetaceae, order Actinomycetales, consisting of soil organisms that form an aerial mycelium containing branches in whorls, and bearing chains of spores at the ends of branches. The type species is *S. baldac′cii.*

streptozocin (strep″to-zo′sin) chemical name: 2-deoxy-2-[[(methylnitrosoamino)carbonyl]amino]-D-glucopyranose. An antineoplastic antibiotic, $C_8H_{15}N_3O_7$, derived from *Streptomyces achromogenes* or produced by synthesis; used principally in the treatment of islet-cell tumors of the pancreas and also other endocrine tumors including gastrinomas associated with Zollinger-Ellison syndrome and glucagon-secreting alpha cell of the pancreas; nausea and vomiting and nephrotoxicity are major side effects.

streptozotocin (strep″to-zo-to′sin) streptozocin.

stress (stres) 1. forcibly exerted influence; pressure. In dentistry, the pressure of the upper teeth against the lower in mastication. 2. the sum of the biological reactions to any adverse stimulus, physical, mental, or emotional, internal or external, that tends to disturb the organism's homeostasis; should these compensating reactions be inadequate or inappropriate, they may lead to disorders. The term is also used to refer to the stimuli that elicit the reactions. See also *general adaptation syndrome,* under *syndrome.*

stress-breaker (stres′brāk-er) a device built into a removable partial denture that relieves the abutment teeth from excessive occlusal loads and stresses. Two basic types are recognized: one consisting of a movable joint between the direct retainer and the denture base (*hinge s.*) and the other consisting of a flexible connection between the direct retainer and the denture base or using a movable joint between two major connectors. Called also *stress divider* and *stress equalizer.*

stretcher (strech′er) a litter for carrying the sick or injured.

stria (stri′ah), pl. *stri′ae* [L. "a furrow, groove"] 1. a streak, or line. 2. a narrow bandlike structure; [NA] a general term for such longitudinal collections of nerve fibers in the brain. **acoustic striae,** striae medullares ventriculi quarti. **stri′ae albican′tes,** see *striae atrophicae.* **striae of Amici,** Z band; see under *band.* **stri′ae atro′phicae,** linear, depressed, atrophic, pinkish or purplish, scarlike lesions that later become white (*striae albicantes, lineae albicantes*), occurring on the abdomen, breasts, buttocks, and thighs. They are due to weakening of the elastic tissues, and are associated with pregnancy (*striae gravidarum*), excessive obesity, rapid growth during puberty and adolescence, Cushing's syndrome, or topical or prolonged

treatment with corticosteroids. Called also *striae distensae, lineae atrophicae,* and *linear atrophy.* **auditory striae,** striae medullares ventriculi quarti. **striae of Baillarger,** see *s. laminae granularis interna corticis cerebri* and *s. laminae pyramidalis interna corticis cerebri.* **stri′ae cilia′res,** slight dark ridges running parallel with each other from the teeth of the ora serrata of the retina to the valleys between the ciliary processes. **s. diagona′lis (Broca)** [NA], a band of nerve fibers that forms the caudal zone of the anterior perforated substance where it adjoins the optic tract, which is continuous caudolaterally with the periamygdaloid area and rostromedially passes above the optic chiasm to blend with the paraterminal gyrus; called also *band of Broca, bandaletta diagonalis (Broca), Broca's diagonal band,* and *diagonal band of Broca.* **stri′ae disten′sae,** striae atrophicae. **s. for′nicis** (*obs.*), s. medullaris thalami. **s. of Gennari,** see under *line.* **stri′ae gravida′rum,** see *striae atrophicae.* **habenular s.** (*obs.*), s. medullaris thalami. **s. kaesbekhtere′vi,** Bekhterev's layer. **Knapp's striae,** see under *streak.* **s. lam′inae granula′ris exter′na cor′ticis cer′ebri** [NA], a band of tangentially oriented nerve fibers in the external granular layer of the cerebral cortex. **s. lam′inae granula′ris inter′na cor′ticis cer′ebri** [NA], a band of tangentially oriented white nerve fibers in the internal granular layer of the cerebral cortex. In the region of the calcarine sulcus, this stria is thick and highly visible and here is known as the *line of Gennari* (see also *striate cortex,* under *cortex*). Called also *external* or *outer band, line, stria,* or *stripe of Baillarger.* See also *s. laminae pyramidalis interna corticis cerebri.* **s. lam′inae molecula′ris cor′ticis cer′ebri** [NA], a band of tangentially oriented myelinated nerve fibers in the molecular layer of the cerebral cortex; called also *stria laminae plexiformis corticis cerebri* [NA alternative]. **s. lam′inae plexifor′mis cor′ticis cer′ebri,** NA alternative for *s. laminae molecularis corticis cerebri.* **s. lam′inae pyramida′lis gangliona′ris cor′ticis cer′ebri,** NA alternative for *s. laminae pyramidalis interna corticis cerebri.* **s. lam′inae pyramida′lis inter′na cor′ticis cer′ebri** [NA], a band of tangentially oriented white nerve fibers in the internal pyramidal layer of the cerebral cortex; called also *inner* or *internal band, line, stria,* or *stripe of Baillarger* and *s. laminae pyramidalis ganglionaris corticis cerebri* [NA alternative]. See also *s. laminae granularis interna corticis cerebri.* **s. lancis′ii,** s. longitudinalis medialis corporis callosi. **Langhans' s.,** cytotrophoblast. **Liesgang's striae,** see under *phenomenon.* **longitudinal s. of corpus callosum, lateral,** s. longitudinalis lateralis corporis callosi. **longitudinal s. of corpus callosum, medial,** s. longitudinalis medialis corporis callosi. **s. longitudina′lis latera′lis cor′poris callo′si** [NA], lateral longitudinal stria of corpus callosum: one of two slender bands of myelinated fibers which form longitudinal ridges in the indusium griseum on the superior aspect of each half of the corpus callosum. **s. longitudina′lis media′lis cor′poris callo′si** [NA], medial longitudinal stria of corpus callosum: one of two slender bands of myelinated fibers which form longitudinal ridges in the indusium griseum on the superior aspect of each half of the corpus callosum. **mallear s. of tympanic membrane, s. mallea′ris membra′nae tym′pani** [NA], s. malleola′ris membra′nae tym′pani, a nearly vertical radial band seen on the outer surface of the tympanic membrane; it extends from the umbo upward to the prominentia mallearis and is caused by the manubrium mallei. **stri′ae medulla′res acus′ticae, stri′ae medulla′res fos′sae rhomboi′deae,** striae medullares ventriculi quarti. **s. medulla′ris thal′ami** [NA], medullary stria of thalamus: a fiber bundle that arises from the subcallosal and paraterminal gyri, the preoptic area, and amygdaloid area, and runs backward along the junction of the dorsal and medial surfaces of the thalamus to reach the habenular nucleus. **stri′ae medulla′res ventric′uli quar′ti** [NA], medullary striae of fourth ventricle: bundles of white fibers coursing transversely across the floor of the fourth ventricle; they arise from the arcuate nuclei, pass dorsally close to the midline, and after having reached the fourth ventricle finally enter the inferior cerebellar peduncle. Called also *striae medullares fossae rhomboideae.* **medullary s. of corpus striatum, external,** lamina medullaris corporis striati. **medullary s. of corpus striatum, medial,** lamina medullaris medialis corporis striati. **medullary striae of fourth ventricle, medullary**

striae of rhomboid fossa, striae medullaris ventriculi quarti. **medullary s. of thalamus,** 1. stria medullaris thalami. 2. see *laminae medullares thalami.* **meningitic s.,** tache cérébrale. **Nitabuch's s.,** see under *layer.* **striae olfacto′riae, olfactory striae,** see *intermediate olfactory s.* and *striae olfactoriae medialis et lateralis.* **stri′ae olfacto′riae media′lis et latera′lis** [NA], the radiating fibers of the olfactory tract, which diverge into a lateral and a medial band at the olfactory trigone and border the anterior perforated substance; the bands are covered by the lateral and medial olfactory gyri, respectively. See also *intermediate olfactory s.* **olfactory s., intermediate,** a small band of fibers that pass from the center of the olfactory trigone to penetrate the anterior perforated substance; its presence is variable. See also *striae olfactoriae medialis et lateralis.* **s. pinea′lis** (*obs.*), **s. medullaris thalami. Retzius′ parallel striae,** incremental lines. **Rohr′s s.,** a layer of canalized fibrin in the developing placenta, within the intervillous space at the fetal-maternal junction. **Schreger′s striae,** lines of Schreger. **s. semicircula′ris,** s. terminalis. **s. termina′lis** [NA], a band of fibers along the lateral margin of the ventricular surface of the thalamus, covering the thalamostriate vein and, following the course of the vein, marking the line of separation between the thalamus and the caudate nucleus; it extends from the region of the interventricular foramen to the temporal horn of the lateral ventricle, carrying fibers from the amygdaloid nuclei to the septal, hypothalamic, and thalamic areas. **stri′ae transver′sae cor′poris callo′si,** transverse bands of fibers on the upper surface of the corpus callosum. **s. vascula′ris duc′tus cochlea′ris** [NA], a layer of fibrous vascular tissue covering the outer wall of the cochlear duct, which is thought to secrete the endolymph. **s. ventric′uli ter′tii** (*obs.*), s. medullaris thalami. **Wickham′s striae,** pale grayish dots or lines forming a network on the surface of the papules, characteristic of lichen planus.

striae (stri′e) [L.] plural of *stria.*

striatal (stri-a′tal) pertaining to the corpus striatum.

striate (stri′āt) striated.

striated (stri′āt-ed) [L. *striatus*] striped; marked by striae.

striation (stri-a′shun) 1. the quality of being marked by stripes or striae. 2. a streak or scratch. **tabby cat s., tigroid s.,** a striation or marking on muscle tissue that has undergone marked fatty degeneration; seen especially in degenerated heart muscle.

striatonigral, strionigral (stri″ah-to-ni′gral; stri″o-ni′gral) projecting from the corpus striatum to the substantia nigra.

Striatran (stri′ah-tran) trademark for a preparation of emylcamate.

striatum (stri-a′tum) [L., neuter of *striatus* striped] 1. striped, or grooved. 2. corpus striatum. 3. neostriatum.

stricture (strik′chur) [L. *strictura*] decrease in the caliber of a canal, duct, or other passage, as a result of cicatricial contraction or the deposition of abnormal tissue. **annular s.,** a stricture which encircles the lumen of a tubular structure. **bridle s.,** a fold of membrane stretched across a canal, and partially closing it. **cicatricial s.,** one which follows an operative or traumatic wound, particularly a wound which has been infected. **contractile s.,** one which may be mechanically dilated, but which soon returns to its contracted condition; called also *recurrent s.* **false s., functional s.,** spasmodic s. **Hunner′s s.,** stricture of the ureter due to local inflammation of the wall of the ureter. **impassable s., impermeable s.,** one that does not permit the passage of an instrument. **irritable s.,** one through which the passage or attempted passage of an instrument produces pain. **organic s.,** a stricture due to a structural change in or about a canal. **permanent s.,** one which persists despite treatment. **recurrent s.,** contractile s. **spasmodic s., spastic s.,** one that is due to muscular spasm; called also *false s., functional s.,* and *temporary s.* **temporary s.,** spasmodic s.

stricturization (strik″chur-i-za′shun) the process of decreasing in caliber or of becoming constricted.

stricturotome (strik′chur-o-tōm″) a knife for cutting strictures.

stricturotomy (strik″chur-ot′o-me) incision of a stricture.

strident (stri′dent) stridulous.

stridor (stri′dor) [L.] a harsh, high-pitched respiratory sound such as the inspiratory sound often heard in acute laryngeal obstruction. Cf. *laryngismus stridulus.* **congenital laryngeal s.,** stridor and dyspnea of the newborn due to an indrawing or infolding of a congenitally flabby epiglottis and aryepiglottic folds (laryngomalacia) during inspiration; the condition is usually outgrown in two years. **laryngeal s.,** stridor due to laryngeal obstruction; see also *congenital laryngeal s.* **s. serrat′icus,** a sound like that made by filing a saw, caused by respiration through a tracheostomy tube.

stridulous (strid′u-lus) [L. *stridulus*] attended with stridor; shrill and harsh in sound.

string-halt (string′halt) myoclonus of the hind leg of a horse, causing a gait in which the leg is suddenly raised and then stamped on the ground.

striocellular (stri″o-sel′u-lar) [L. *stria* streak + *cellular*] composed of striated muscle fibers and cells.

striocerebellar (stri″o-ser″e-bel′ar) pertaining to or affecting both the corpus striatum and the cerebellum, as striocerebellar tremor.

striomotor (stri″o-mo′tor) pertaining to or affecting neurons supplying skeletal muscle.

striomuscular (stri″o-mus′ku-lar) pertaining to or composed of striated muscle.

strip (strip) 1. a thin, narrow, comparatively long piece of material. 2. to press the contents from a canal, such as a blood vessel, by running the finger along it. 3. to excise lengths of large veins and competent tributaries by subcutaneous dissection and the use of a stripper. 4. to reduce the mesiodistal width of teeth, usually done to make space to align crowded segments. 5. to remove metal from the inside of a crown electrochemically in order to increase the inside diameter. **abrasive s.,** a linen strip or polymer film having abrasive material, such as silica or garnet, bonded to one side; used for polishing and contouring of the proximal surface of a tooth or denture. Called also *linen s.* **linen s.,** an abrasive strip with a linen backing.

stripe (strīp) a streak or stria. **s′s of Baillarger,** see *stria laminae granularis interna corticis cerebri* and *stria laminae pyramidalis interna corticis cerebri.* **s. of Gennari,** see under *line.* **Hensen′s s.,** a band near the middle of the under surface of the membrana tectoria of the ear. **Mees′ s′s,** diagonal white stripes on the fingernails in arsenic poisoning. **s′s of Retzius,** incremental lines. **Vicq d′Azyr′s s.,** the line of Kaes in the cerebral cortex.

stripper (strip′er) a surgical instrument for excision of veins, consisting of a flexible stainless steel cable with a stripping cup or disk at one end and a guide tip at the other; a rigid type of external stripper is also utilized.

strobila (stro-bi′lah), pl. *strobi′lae* [L.; Gr. *strobilos* anything twisted up] 1. the chain of proglottids constituting the bulk of the body of adult tapeworms; considered by some to include the entire body, including the head, neck, and proglottids. 2. The chain of individuals produced by strobilation, such as the series of buds produced at the oral end of the body of certain jellyfish, which during the process of formation somewhat resemble a pile of plates; each bud is released to form an immature, free-swimming jellyfish.

strobile (stro′bīl) strobila.

strobiloid (stro′bĭ-loid) resembling a row of tapeworm segments.

strobilus (stro-bi′lus) [L.; Gr. *strobilos* anything twisted up] 1. strobila. 2. a cone formed at the tip of a stem by a group of sporophylls.

stroboscope (stro′bo-skōp) [Gr. *strobos* whirl + *skopein* to examine] an instrument by which the successive phases of animal movements may be studied; motion may appear to come to rest.

stroboscopic (stro″bo-skop′ik) pertaining to the stroboscope.

Stroganoff′s (Stroganov′s) treatment (stro-gan′ofs) [Vasilii Vasilovich *Stroganov,* Russian obstetrician, 1857–1938] see under *treatment.*

stroke (strōk) a sudden and severe attack; see *stroke syndrome,* under *syndrome.* **apoplectic s.,** apoplexy (def. 1). **back s.,** 1. the recoil of the ventricles at the time the blood is forced into the aorta. 2. the influence which a peripheral organ of response exerts back upon the nerve center from which the response was generated. **effective s.,** see *cilium* (def. 3). **heat s.,** a condition caused by exposure to excessive heat, natural or artificial, and marked by dry skin, vertigo, headache, thirst, nausea, and muscular cramps; body temperature may be dangerously elevated, contrasting with heat exhaustion in which the body temperature may be subnormal. Called also *heat apoplexy* and *thermoplegia.* Cf. *sunstroke.* **light s.,** a fatal narcosis produced in sensitized mice by exposure to light. **lightning s.,** loss of consciousness and shock with burns, frequently fatal, caused by lightning. **paralytic s.,** a sudden attack of paralysis from injury to the brain or spinal cord. **recovery s.,** see *cilium* (def. 3). **sun s.,** see *sunstroke.*

stroma (stro'mah), pl. *stro'mata* [Gr. *strōma* anything laid out for lying or sitting upon] 1. the supporting tissue or matrix of an organ, as distinguished from its functional element, or parenchyma. 2. the insoluble portion of the erythrocyte remaining after hemolysis, consisting of fragments of the cell membrane. **s. of cornea,** substantia propria corneae. **s. gan'glii** [NA], the endoneurial stroma that permeates the capsule of a neural ganglion and surrounds and supports the neuronal and axonal components of the ganglion. **s. glan'dulae thyreoi'deae, s. glan'dulae thyroi'deae** [NA], stroma of thyroid gland: the tissue that forms the framework of the thyroid gland. **s. i'ridis** [NA], **s. of iris,** the soft mass of connective tissue fibers that make up the major portion of the iris. **s. ova'rii** [NA], **s. of ovary,** the fibrous tissue and smooth muscle composing the framework of the ovary. **Rollet's s.,** that part of a red blood cell which remains after the hemoglobin has been removed. **s. of thyroid gland,** s. glandulae thyroideae. **vitreous s., s. vit'reum** [NA], the framework of firmer material making up the vitreous body of the eye, and enclosing within its meshes the more fluid portion (humor vitreus).

stromal (stro'mal) pertaining to or resembling stroma.

stromatic (stro-mat'ik) stromal.

stromatin (stro'mah-tin) a protein constituent of the stroma of erythrocytes.

stromatogenous (stro″mah-toj'ĕ-nus) [*stroma* + Gr. *gennan* to produce] originating in the stroma or connective tissue of an organ.

stromatolysis (stro″mah-tol'ĭ-sis) [*stroma* + Gr. *lysis* dissolution] destruction of the stroma of a cell, especially that of a red blood cell.

stromatosis (stro″mah-to'sis) adenomyosis in which the invading endometrial substance is stromal and not glandular; stromal adenomyosis.

Stromeyer's cephalhematocele (stro'mi-erz) [Georg Friedrich Ludwig *Stromeyer,* German surgeon, 1804–1876] see under *cephalhematocele.*

stromuhr (strōm'oor) [Ger. "stream clock"] Ludwig's instrument for measuring the velocity of the blood flow (1867).

Strong's bacillus (strongz) [Richard Pearson *Strong,* American physician, 1872–1948] *Shigella flexneri.*

strongyli (stron'jĭ-li) plural of *strongylus.*

strongyliasis (stron″jĭ-li'ah-sis) strongylosis.

strongylid (stron'jĭ-lid) 1. of or pertaining to the superfamily Strongylidae. 2. strongylus.

Strongylidae (stron-jil'ĭ-de) a family of nematodes of the superfamily Strongyloidea, including the genera *Strongylus* and *Oesophagostomum.*

Strongyloidea (stron″jĭ-loi'de-ah) a superfamily of phasmids, including the hookworms and related bursate nematodes. It comprises the families Ancylostomidae, Strongylidae, Trichostrongylidae, Metastrongylidae, and Syngamidae.

Strongyloides (stron″jĭ-loi'dēz) a genus of phasmids belonging to the superfamily Rhabditoidea, widely distributed as intestinal parasites of mammals. In some systems of classification, included in the superfamily Rhabdiasoidea. **S. intestina'lis,** S. stercoralis. **S. papillo'sus,** a species found in cows, pigs, sheep, goats, rabbits, and rats. **S. ranso'mi,** a species found in pigs. **S. rat'ti,** a species found in rats. **S. stercora'lis,** a roundworm occurring widely in tropical and subtropical countries. The female worm and her larvae inhabit the mucosa and submucosa of the small intestine, where they cause diarrhea and ulceration (intestinal strongyloidiasis or Cochin-China diarrhea). The larvae expelled from an infected person with his feces develop

in the soil and penetrate the human skin on contact. They eventually are carried in the bloodstream to the lungs, where they cause hemorrhage (pulmonary strongyloidiasis) when they rupture into the alveoli; from the lungs they reach the intestine via the trachea and esophagus. Massive infections may be seen in patients treated with corticosteroids, immunosuppressive drugs, etc. An endogenous cycle of development may occur, allowing infections to persist for many years. Called also *Anguillula intestinalis, Anguillula stercoralis,* and *Strongyloides intestinalis.*

strongyloidiasis (stron″jĭ-loi-di'ah-sis) infection with *Strongyloides stercoralis* (see under *Strongyloides*).

strongyloidosis (stron″jĭ-loi-do'sis) strongyloidiasis.

strongylosis (stron″jĭ-lo'sis) infection with worms of the genus *Strongylus.*

Strongylus (stron'jĭ-lus) [Gr. *strongylos* round] a genus of parasitic nematode worms of the family Strongylidae. **S. edenta'tus,** a species found in horses. **S. equi'nus,** a worm parasitic in the intestines of horses; called also *palisade worm.* **S. fila'ria,** Dictyocaulus filaria. **S. gibso'ni,** Mecistocirrhus digitatus. **S. gi'gas,** Dioctophyma digitata. **S. longevagina'tus,** Metastrongylus elongatus. **S. micru'rus,** Dictyocaulus viviparus. **S. paradox'us,** Metastrongylus elongatus. **S. rena'lis,** Dioctophyma renale. **S. sub'tilis,** Trichostrongylus colubriformis. **S. vulga'ris,** a species found in horses.

strongylus (stron'jĭ-lus), pl. *stron'gyli.* An individual organism of the genus *Strongylus.*

strontia (stron'she-ah) strontium oxide.

strontium (stron'she-um) [*Strontian* in Scotland] a dark yellowish metal: symbol, Sr; atomic number, 38; atomic weight, 87.62. See also *radiostrontium.* **s. bromide,** a clear, colorless, crystalline substance, $SrBr_2 + 6H_2O$, used like other bromides. **s. hydroxide,** colorless crystals or white powder, $Sr(OH)_2 \cdot 8H_2O$, soluble in 50 parts water and in acids. **s. oxide,** a white, strongly basic substance, SrO, which reacts vigorously with water to give strontium hydroxide; called also *strontia.* **radioactive s.,** radiostrontium. **s. salicylate,** a salt, $(OH \cdot C_6H_4 \cdot CO \cdot O)_2Sr$, in white crystals, soluble in 40 parts of water and freely in alcohol.

strontiuresis (stron″she-u-re'sis) the elimination of strontium from the body by way of the urine.

strontiuretic (stron″she-u-ret'ik) pertaining to, characterized by, or promoting strontiuresis.

strophanthidin (stro-fan'thĭ-din) chemical name: 3β,5,14-trihydroxy-19-oxo-5β-card-20(22)-enolide. An aglycone, $C_{23}H_{32}O_6$, obtained by hydrolysis of glycosides from *Strophanthus kombé* Oliv. (Apocynaceae).

strophanthin (stro-fan'thin) a glycoside or a mixture of steroidal glycosides obtained from *Strophanthus kombé,* occurring as a white or yellowish white powder. It is a cardioactive drug with actions similar to those of ouabain, and is used intravenously when a cardiotonic of rapid onset and short duration is desired. Called also *K-s* or *s.-K.* **G-s., s.-G,** ouabain.

Strophanthus (stro-fan'thus) [Gr. *strophos* a twisted band + *anthos* flower] a genus of apocynaceous shrubs, trees, and woody vines growing especially in tropical Africa, and including several poisonous species. S. gratus (Wall. & Hock.) Baill. yields ouabain; S. hispidus DC. yields pseudostrophanthin; S. kombé Oliv. yields strophanthidin and strophanthin; and S. sarmentosus DC. yields sarmentocymarin, sarmentogenin, and sarmentose.

strophocephalus (strof″o-sef'ah-lus) a fetus exhibiting strophocephaly.

strophocephaly (strof″o-sef'ah-le) [Gr. *strophos* a twisted band + *kephalē* head] a developmental anomaly characterized by distortion of the head and face.

strophosomus (strof″o-so'mus) [Gr. *strophos* a twisted band + *sōma* body] a celosomus, especially in chicks, in which the extremities are reflexed onto the back with the distal ends resting on the head.

strophulus (strof'u-lus) [L.] papular urticaria.

struck (struk) a usually fatal enterotoxemia of young calves, lambs, and piglets, caused by *Clostridium perfringens* type C, occurring chiefly in the winter and spring, apparently throughout the world; it is characterized by hemorrhagic enteritis and peritonitis. It was first reported as a disease of mature sheep in the Romney Marsh district of England. Called also *hemorrhagic enterotoxemia.*

structural (struk′tūr-al)   pertaining to or affecting the structure.

structure (struk′chur) [L. *struere* to build]   the components and their manner of arrangement in constituting a whole. **antigenic s.** (of microorganisms), the mosaic of individual antigens present in cells of a microorganism. **β-s.,** pleated sheet. **covalent s.,** primary s. **denture-supporting s's,** the tissues, either the teeth or residual ridges, or both, which serve as the foundation for removable partial or complete dentures. **fine s.,** ultrastructure. **primary s.,** the amino acid sequence of a polypeptide chain or the base sequence of a nucleic acid strand. Called also *covalent s.* **quaternary s.,** the geometric arrangement of the subunits of a macromolecule. **secondary s.,** aspects of the three-dimensional structure of macromolecules that have a regular geometric pattern, e.g., α-helix or β-sheet regions in proteins, double helix regions in nucleic acids, or the cloverleaf structure of transfer RNAs. **tertiary s.,** the three dimensional structure of a monomeric macromolecule or of a subunit of a multimeric macromolecule.

struma (stroo′mah) [L.]   goiter. **s. aberran′ta,** goiter affecting an accessory thyroid gland. **s. calculo′sa,** a goiter that has undergone calcification. **cast iron s.,** Riedel's s. **s. colloi′des,** colloid goiter. **s. endothora′cica,** intrathoracic goiter. **s. fibro′sa,** fibrous goiter. **s. follicula′ris,** parenchymatous goiter. **s. gelatino′sa,** colloid goiter. **Hashimoto's s.,** see under *disease.* **ligneous s.,** Riedel's s. **s. lipomato′des aberra′ta re′nis,** hypernephroma. **s. lymphat′ica,** status lymphaticus. **s. lymphomato′sa,** Hashimoto's disease. **s. malig′na,** cancer of the thyroid gland. **s. nodo′sa,** adenoma of the thyroid gland. **s. ova′rii,** a rare teratoid tumor of the ovary composed almost entirely of thyroid tissue, with large follicles containing abundant colloid; occasionally there are symptoms of hyperthyroidism. **s. parenchymato′sa,** parenchymatous goiter. **Riedel's s.,** see under *thyroiditis.* **thymus s.,** persistence of the thymus gland beyond the time when it usually atrophies. **s. vasculo′sa,** vascular goiter.

strumectomy (stroo-mek′to-me) [L. *struma* goiter + Gr. *ektomē* excision]   surgical removal of a goiter. **median s.,** surgical removal of the thyroid.

strumitis (stroo-mi′tis)   inflammation of the thyroid gland; thyroiditis.

Strümpell's disease, sign, type (strim′pelz) [Adolf von *Strümpell,* physician in Leipzig, 1853–1925]   see under *disease, sign,* and *type.*

Strümpell-Leichtenstern disease (strim′pel-lik′tenstern) [A. von *Strümpell;* Otto *Leichtenstern,* German physician, 1845–1900]   hemorrhagic encephalitis.

Strümpell-Marie disease (strim′pel-mah-re′) [A. von *Strümpell;* Pierre *Marie,* French physician, 1853–1940]   rheumatoid spondylitis.

Strümpell-Westphal pseudosclerosis (strim′pel-vest′ fawl) [A. von *Strümpell;* Carl Friedrich Otto *Westphal,* German neurologist, 1833–1890]   Wilson's disease.

Strunsky's sign (strun′skēz) [Max *Strunsky,* New York orthopedic surgeon, 1873–1957]   see under *sign.*

Struve's test (stroo′vez) [Heinrich *Struve,* physician in Petrograd]   see under *tests.*

struvite (stroo′vīt)   see under *calculus.*

strychnine (strik′nīn)   an extremely poisonous alkaloid, $C_{21}H_{22}N_2O_2$, obtained chiefly from *Strychnos nux-vomica* and other species of *Strychnos,* which causes excitation of all portions of the central nervous system by blocking postsynaptic inhibition of neural impulses; it has been used as a central nervous system stimulant and was formerly used as a bitter tonic, as a circulatory stimulant, and with cathartic drugs. In veterinary medicine it is occasionally used as a tonic and stimulant. See also *strychninism.* **s. hydrochloride,** a crystalline salt, $C_{21}H_{22}N_2O_2 \cdot HCl + 2H_2O$. **s. nitrate,** a salt, $C_{21}H_{22}N_2O_2 \cdot HNO_3$, occurring as colorless odorless needles or as a white crystalline powder; its medical use is the same as that of strychnine, and its veterinary use is the same as that of strychnine sulfate. **s. phosphate,** a salt, C_{21}- $H_{22}N_2O_2 \cdot H_3PO_4 \cdot 2H_2O$, occurring as colorless or white crystals or as a white powder; its medical use is the same as that of strychnine, and its veterinary use is the same as that of

strychnine sulfate. It was formerly used in compounding iron, quinine, and strychnine phosphates elixir. **s. sulfate,** a salt, $(C_{21}H_{22}N_2O_2)_2 \cdot H_2SO_4 \cdot 5H_2O$, occurring as colorless or white crystals or as a white crystalline powder; used like strychnine. In veterinary medicine it is used in tonics, and in noninflammatory paraplegia, rumen, and intestinal impactions.

strychninism (strik′nin-izm)   a toxic condition due to the misuse of strychnine; chronic strychnine poisoning. Symptoms include increased acuity of hearing, vision, touch, taste, and smell, followed by tonic convulsions and vomiting; in severe cases, it may culminate in respiratory paralysis and death.

strychninization (strik″nin-i-za′shun)   the act of bringing under the influence of strychnine.

strychninomania (strik″nin-o-ma′ne-ah) [*strychnine* + Gr. *mania* madness]   mental aberration due to strychnine poisoning.

strychnism (strik′nizm)   poisoning by strychnine.

strychnize (strik′nīz)   to put under the influence of strychnine.

Strychnos (strik′nos) [Gr. "nightshade"]   a genus of loganiaceous tropical trees. *S. nux-vomica* affords strychnine, curare, brucine, and nux-vomica; *S. ignatii* affords ignatia and brucine.

S.T.S.   serologic test for syphilis, Society of Thoracic Surgeons.

S.T.U.   skin test unit; see under *unit.*

Student's t-test (stoo′dents) [*"Student,"* pseudonym of William Sealy Gossett, British mathematician, 1876–1937]   see *t-test,* under *tests.*

study (stud′e)   a research project. **case-control s.,** retrospective s. **cohort s.,** prospective s. **prospective s.,** an epidemiologic study in which a group of individuals (a cohort), all free of a particular disease and varying in their exposure to a possible risk factor, are followed over a period of time to determine the incidence rates of the disease in the exposed and unexposed groups. Called also *cohort s.* "Prospective" usually implies a cohort selected in the present and followed into the future, but the cohort method can also be applied to existing data such as insurance or medical records: a cohort is identified and classified as to exposure to the risk factor at some date in the past and followed up to the present to determine incidence rates. This is called a historical prospective study, prospective study of past data, or retrospective cohort study. Cf. *retrospective s.* **retrospective s.,** an epidemiologic study in which individuals diagnosed as having a disease (cases) are compared with a group of individuals not having the disease and matched with the cases in respect to certain demographic and other variables (controls) to determine whether the groups differ in their exposure to possible risk factors. As compared to prospective studies, retrospective studies suffer from two drawbacks: only relative risk, not true incidence rates and attributable risk, can be measured, and large biases may be introduced both in the selection of controls and in the recall of past exposure to risk factors. The advantage of the retrospective study is its small scale and its applicability to rare diseases, which would require study of very large cohorts in prospective studies. Cf. *prospective s.*

stump (stump)   the distal end of the limb left after amputation. **conical s.,** a cone-shaped amputation stump produced as a result of undue retraction of the muscles.

stun (stun)   to knock senseless; to render unconscious by a blow or other force; to daze.

stunt (stunt)   to retard the growth of. **bushy s.,** a viral disease of tomatoes marked by stunting and discoloration of the leaves.

stupe (stūp) [L. *stupa* tow]   a cloth, sponge, or the like, for external application, charged with hot water, wrung out nearly dry, and then made irritant or otherwise medicated.

stupefacient (stu″pĕ-fa′shent) [L. *stupefacere* to make senseless]   1. inducing stupor. 2. an agent that induces stupor.

stupefactive (stu″pĕ-fak′tiv)   producing narcosis or stupor.

stupor (stu′por) [L.]   partial or nearly complete unconsciousness, manifested by the subject's responding only to vigorous stimulation. Also, in psychiatry, a disorder marked by reduced responsiveness. **anergic s.,** stupor with immobility. **benign s.,** a condition of stupor sometimes observed in the depressive phase of manic-depressive psychosis. **epileptic s.,** stupor following an epileptic convulsion; called also *postconvulsive s.* **postconvulsive s.,** epileptic s.

stuporous (stu′por-us) affected with or characterized by stupor.

stupp (stup) a poisonous kind of soot which accumulates in the condensers of mercury smelters; it contains metallic mercury in a finely divided condition.

sturdy (stur′de) gid.

Sturge's disease, syndrome (ster′jez) [William Allen *Sturge,* British physician, 1850–1919] Sturge-Weber syndrome.

Sturge-Weber syndrome (sterj-web-er) [W. A. *Sturge;* Frederick Parkes *Weber,* British physician, 1863–1962] see under *syndrome.*

Sturm's conoid, interval (sturmz) [Johann Christoph *Sturm,* German physician, 1635–1703] see under *conoid,* and see *focal interval,* under *interval.*

stuttering (stut′er-ing) a problem of speech behavior involving three definitive factors: (1) speech disfluency, most significantly repetitions of parts of words and whole words, prolongations of sounds, interjections of sounds or words, and unduly prolonged pauses; (2) reactions of the listeners to the speaker's disfluency as evaluated by them as undesirable, abnormal, or unacceptable; and (3) the reactions of the speaker to the listeners' reactions, as well as to his own speech disfluency and to his conception of himself as a stutterer. Stuttering is usually distinguished from *stammering,* which is characterized by blocking or involuntary pauses in speech, sometimes with repetition of sounds. **labiochoreic s.,** labiochorea. **urinary s.,** interruption of the flow during urination.

sty (sti), pl. *sties.* stye.

stycosis (sti-ko′sis) the presence of calcium sulfate in the organs of the body, especially in the lymph nodes.

stye (sti), pl. *styes* [L. *hordeolum*] hordeolum. **meibomian s.,** one involving a meibomian gland, usually draining through the conjunctival surface of the lid. **zeisian s.,** one involving a zeisian gland, occurring on the surface of the skin at the edge of the lid.

style (stīl) stylet.

stylet (sti′let) [L. *stilus;* Gr. *stylos* pillar] 1. a wire run through a catheter or cannula to render it stiff or to remove debris from its lumen. 2. a slender probe.

styliform (sti′lĭ-form) [L. *stilus* stake, pole + *forma* shape] long and pointed; styloid.

styliscus (sti-lis′kus) [L., from Gr. *styliskos* rod] a slender cylindrical tent.

styl(o)- [L. *stilus* a stake, pole] a combining form denoting resemblance to a stake or pole, used especially to denote relationship to the styloid process of the temporal bone.

stylohyal (sti″lo-hi′al) stylohyoid.

stylohyoid (sti″lo-hi′oid) pertaining to the styloid process and to the hyoid bone.

styloid (sti′loid) [Gr. *stylos* pillar + *eidos* form] resembling a pillar; long and pointed; styliform.

styloiditis (sti″loi-di′tis) inflammation of tissues about the styloid process.

stylomandibular (sti″lo-man-dib′u-lar) pertaining to the styloid process and the mandible.

stylomastoid (sti″lo-mas′toid) pertaining to the styloid and mastoid processes.

stylomaxillary (sti″lo-mak′sĭ-ler″e) pertaining to the styloid process and to the maxilla.

stylomyloid (sti″lo-mi′loid) [stylo- + Gr. *mylē* mill + *eidos* form] pertaining to the styloid process and to the region of the lower molar teeth.

stylopodium (sti″lo-po′de-um) see *limb.*

Stylosanthes (sti″lo-san′thēz) [stylo- + Gr. *anthos* flower] a genus of leguminous herbs, chiefly South American. *S. ela′tior,* the pencil-flower of North America, is a uterine sedative.

stylostaphyline (sti″lo-staf′ĭ-lin) pertaining to the styloid process of the temporal bone and the velum palatinum.

stylosteophyte (sti-los′te-o-fīt) a pillar-shaped exostosis.

stylostixis (sti″lo-stik′sis) [stylo- + Gr. *stixis* pricking] acupuncture.

stylus (sti′lus) [L. *stilus*] 1. a stylet. 2. a pencil-shaped medicinal preparation, as a stick of caustic.

stymatosis (sti″mah-to′sis) [Gr. *styma* priapism] priapism with a bloody discharge.

stypage (sti′pij, ste-pahzh′) [Fr.] the application of a stype to produce local anesthesia.

stype (stīp) [Gr. *styppeion* tow] a tampon or pledget.

stypsis (stip′sis) [Gr. *stypsis* contraction] 1. astringency; astringent action. 2. treatment by astringents.

styptic (stip′tik) [Gr. *styptikos*] 1. astringent; arresting hemorrhage by means of an astringent quality. 2. an astringent and hemostatic remedy. **Binelli's s.,** a solution of creosote, formerly used for arresting hemorrhage. **chemical s.,** one which arrests hemorrhage by causing coagulation through chemical action. **mechanical s.,** one which acts by causing coagulation mechanically, as a pledget of cotton. **vascular s.,** one which acts by producing contraction of injured or divided blood vessels of small caliber.

Stypven (stip′ven) trademark for a preparation of Russell's viper venom; used as a hemostatic agent. See also under *tests.*

styramate (stir′ah-māt) chemical name: carbamic acid β-hydroxyphenethyl ester. A crystalline substance, $C_9H_{11}NO_3$, used as a skeletal muscle relaxant.

Styrax (sti′raks) a genus of shrubs and trees of worldwide distribution but growing mainly in Java, Sumatra, and Thailand, various species of which are the source of benzoin (def. 1).

styrax (sti′raks) storax.

styrene (sti′rēn) a fragrant liquid or oil hydrocarbon, vinyl benzene, $C_6H_5CH:CH_2$, from storax; called also *cinnamene, cinnamol,* and *styrol.*

styrol (sti′rol) styrene.

styrolene (sti′ro-lēn) styrene.

styrone (sti′ron) cinnamyl alcohol.

su. abbreviation for L. *su′mat,* let him take.

sub- [L. *sub* under] a prefix meaning under, near, almost, partial, moderately, or subordinate. In chemistry, it denotes a basic compound or a compound containing less of an element or radical than another compound of the same elements.

subabdominal (sub″ab-dom′ĭ-nal) situated below the abdomen.

subabdominoperitoneal (sub″ab-dom″ĭ-no-per″ĭ-to-ne′al) subperitoneal.

subacetabular (sub″as-ĕ-tab′u-lar) situated below the acetabulum.

subacetate (sub-as′ĕ-tāt) any basic acetate.

subacid (sub-as′id) somewhat acid.

subacidity (sub″ah-sid′ĭ-te) deficient acidity.

subacromial (sub″ah-kro′me-al) situated below or beneath the acromion.

subacute (sub″ah-kūt′) somewhat acute; between acute and chronic.

subalimentation (sub″al-ĭ-men-ta′shun) insufficient nourishment.

subanal (sub-a′nal) situated below the anus.

subapical (sub-ap′ĕ-kal) situated below an apex.

subaponeurotic (sub″ap-o-nu-rot′ik) situated beneath an aponeurosis.

subarachnoid (sub″ah-rak′noid) situated or occurring between the arachnoid and the pia mater.

subarcuate (sub-ar′ku-āt) [sub- + L. *arcuatus* arched] somewhat arched or bent.

subareolar (sub″ah-re′o-lar) beneath the areola.

subastragalar (sub″as-trag′ah-lar) situated or occurring under the astragalus (talus).

subastringent (sub″ah-strin′jent) moderately astringent.

subatloidean (sub″at-loi′de-an) situated beneath the atlas.

subatomic (sub″ah-tom′ik) of or pertaining to the constituent parts of an atom as considered under the theory of the nuclear atom; occurring within an atom; smaller than an atom.

subaural (sub-aw′ral) situated beneath the ear.

subaurale (sub″aw-ra′le) an anthropometric landmark, the lowest point on the inferior border of the ear lobule when the subject is looking straight ahead.

subauricular (sub″aw-rik′u-lar) below the pinna (auricle) of the ear.

subaxial (sub-ak′se-al) below an axis.

subaxillary (sub-ak′sĭ-ler″e) below the axilla, or armpit.

subbasal (sub-ba′sal) below a base.

subbrachial (sub-bra′ke-al) relating to the brachium colliculi inferioris.

subbrachycephalic (sub″bra-ke-sĕ-fal′ik) somewhat brachycephalic; having a cephalic index of 78 to 79.

subcalcareous (sub″kal-ka′re-us) slightly calcareous.

subcalcarine (sub-kal′kar-īn) beneath the calcarine fissure.

subcalorism (sub-ka′lor-izm) frigorism.

subcapsular (sub-kap′su-lar) situated below a capsule.

subcapsuloperiosteal (sub-kap″su-lo-per″e-os′te-al) beneath the capsule and the periosteum of a joint.

subcarbonate (sub-kar′bo-nāt) any basic carbonate.

subcartilaginous (sub″kar-tĭ-laj′ĭ-nus) 1. situated beneath a cartilage. 2. partly cartilaginous.

subcentral (sub-sen′tral) located deep to the center.

subception (sub-sep′shun) perception below the level of awareness.

subchloride (sub-klo′rīd) that chloride of any series which contains the smallest proportion of chlorine.

subchondral (sub-kon′dral) beneath a cartilage.

subchordal (sub-kor′dal) situated below the notochord or below the vocal cords.

subchorionic (sub″ko-re-on′ik) situated beneath the chorion.

subchoroidal (sub″ko-roi′dal) beneath the choroid.

subchronic (sub-kron′ik) between chronic and subacute.

subclass (sub′klas) a taxonomic category sometimes established, subordinate to a class and superior to an order.

subclavian (sub-kla′ve-an) situated under the clavicle, as the subclavian artery.

subclavicular (sub″klah-vik′u-lar) situated under the clavicle.

subclinical (sub-klin′ĭ-kal) without clinical manifestations; said of the early stage(s) of an infection or other disease or abnormality before symptoms and signs become apparent or detectable by clinical examination or laboratory tests, or of a very mild form of an infection or other disease or abnormality. See also under *infection*.

subclone (sub′klōn) the progeny of a mutant cell arising in a clone.

subconjunctival (sub″kon-junk-ti′val) situated or occurring beneath the conjunctiva.

subconscious (sub-kon′shus) 1. imperfectly or partially conscious. 2. a term formerly used to include the preconscious and unconscious.

subconsciousness (sub-kon′shus-nes) the state of being partially conscious.

subcoracoid (sub-kor′ah-koid) situated beneath the coracoid process.

subcortex (sub-kor′teks) that part of the brain substance which underlies the cortex.

subcortical (sub-kor′tĭ-kal) situated beneath the cortex.

subcostal (sub-kos′tal) situated beneath a rib.

subcostalis (sub″kos-ta′lis), pl. *subcosta′les* [L.] subcostal.

subcranial (sub-kra′ne-al) beneath the cranium.

subcrepitant (sub-krep′ĭ-tant) pertaining to a rale that is slightly more coarse than a crepitant rale; see under *rale*.

subcrepitation (sub″krep-ĭ-ta′shun) the sound of subcrepitant rales; see under *rale*.

subculture (sub′kul-chur) 1. a culture of bacteria derived from another culture. 2. the act of preparing a fresh culture from an existing one.

subcutaneous (sub″ku-ta′ne-us) beneath the skin.

subcuticular (sub″ku-tik′u-lar) situated beneath the epidermis; subepidermal.

subcutis (sub-ku′tis) [*sub-* + L. *cutis* skin] subcutaneous tissue (tela subcutanea [NA]).

subdelirium (sub″de-lir′e-um) partial or mild delirium.

subdeltoid (sub-del′toid) beneath the deltoid muscle.

subdental (sub-den′tal) [*sub-* + L. *dens* tooth] beneath the teeth.

subdiaphragmatic (sub″di-ah-frag-mat′ik) situated under the diaphragm; subphrenic.

subdorsal (sub-dor′sal) situated below the dorsal region.

subduct (sub-dukt′) [L. *subducere* to lead down] to depress or draw down; see *subduction*.

subduction (sub-duk′shun) infraduction.

subdural (sub-du′ral) situated between the dura mater and the arachnoid.

subendocardial (sub″en-do-kar′de-al) beneath the endocardium.

subendothelial (sub″en-do-the′le-al) situated beneath an endothelium.

subendothelium (sub″en-do-the′le-um) Debove's membrane.

subendymal (sub-en′dĭ-mal) situated beneath the endyma (ependyma).

subependymal (sub″ep-en′dĭ-mal) situated beneath the ependyma.

subependymoma (sub″ep-en″dĭ-mo′mah) an ependymoma in which there is a diffuse proliferation of subependymal fibrillary astrocytes among the ependymal tumor cells.

subepidermal, subepidermic (sub″ep-ĭ-der′mal; sub″-ep-ĭ-der′mik) beneath the epidermis; subcuticular.

subepiglottic (sub″ep-ĭ-glot′ik) below the epiglottis.

subepithelial (sub″ep-ĭ-the′le-al) situated beneath an epithelium.

suberin (soo′ber-in) an insoluble variety of cellulose derived from cork.

suberitin (soo-ber′ĭ-tin) [*Suberites*, a marine sponge (from L. *suber* cork) + chemical suffix -*in*] a toxic substance derived from the marine sponge, *Suberites domunculus*, which, when injected into dogs, produces intestinal hemorrhages and respiratory distress.

suberosis (su″ber-o′sis) [L. *suber* cork + -*osis*] a form of allergic alveolitis due to inhalation of and tissue reaction to moldy cork dust; the offending antigen is from species of *Penicillium*.

subextensibility (sub″eks-ten″sĭ-bil′ĭ-te) decreased extensibility.

subfamily (sub-fam′ĭ-le) a taxonomic category sometimes established, subordinate to a family and superior to a tribe or genus.

subfascial (sub-fash′al) situated beneath a fascia.

subfertile (sub-fer′til) characterized by less than normal fertility.

subfertility (sub″fer-til′ĭ-te) the state of being less than normally fertile; relative sterility.

Sub fin. coct. abbreviation for L. *sub fi′nem coctio′nis*, toward the end of boiling.

subflavous (sub-fla′vus) [*sub-* + L. *flavus* yellow] yellowish.

subfoliar (sub-fo′le-ar) pertaining to a subfolium.

subfolium (sub-fo′le-um) [*sub-* + L. *folium* leaf] any of the elementary divisions of a cerebellar folium.

subgaleal (sub-ga′le-al) situated beneath the galea aponeurotica.

subgallate (sub-gal′āt) a basic gallate.

subgemmal (sub-jem′al) [*sub-* + L. *gemma* bud] situated under a taste bud or other bud.

subgenus (sub-je′nus) a taxonomic category between a genus and a species.

subgerminal (sub-jer′mĭ-nal) below or under the germ.

subgingival (sub-jin′jĭ-val) beneath the gingiva.

subglenoid (sub-gle′noid) situated under the glenoid fossa.

subglossal (sub-glos′al) sublingual.

subglossitis (sub″glos-si′tis) [*sub-* + L. *glossa* tongue + -*itis*] inflammation of the lower surface of the tongue.

subglottic (sub-glot′ik) beneath the glottis.

subgranular (sub-gran′u-lar) somewhat granular.

subgrondation (sub″gron-da′shun) [Fr.] the depression of one fragment of bone beneath another.

subgyrus (sub-ji′rus) any gyrus that is partly concealed or covered by another or by others.

subhepatic (sub″hĕ-pat′ik) situated beneath the liver.

subhumeral (sub-hu′mer-al) below or beneath the humerus.

subhyaloid (sub-hi′ah-loid) situated or occurring beneath the hyaloid membrane.

subhyoid (sub-hi′oid) situated below the hyoid.

subhyoidean (sub″hi-oi′de-an) subhyoid.

subicteric (sub″ik-ter′ik) somewhat jaundiced.

subicular (sŭ-bik′u-lar) of or pertaining to the uncinate gyrus.

subiculum (sŭ-bik′u-lum) [L., from *subicere* to raise, lift] an underlying or supporting structure. **s. cor′nu am-mo′nis, s. hippocam′pi,** gyrus parahippocampalis. **s. promonto′rii ca′vi tym′pani** [NA], **s. of promontory of tympanic cavity,** a ridge of bone bounding the tympanic sinus posteriorly.

subiliac (sub-il′e-ak) below the ilium.

subilium (sub-il′e-um) the lowest portion of the ilium.

subinflammation (sub″in-flah-ma′shun) a slight or mild inflammation.

subinflammatory (sub″in-flam′ah-tor″e) pertaining to or causing only mild inflammation.

subintimal (sub-in′tĭ-mal) beneath the intima (of a vessel).

subintrance (sub-in′trans) recurrence of a paroxysm after a shorter period than usual.

subintrant (sub-in′trant) [L. *subintrans* entering by stealth] 1. beginning before the completion of a previous cycle or paroxysm; anticipating. 2. characterized by recurrence at lessening intervals.

subinvolution (sub″in-vo-lu′shun) incomplete involution; failure of a part to return to its normal size and condition after enlargement due to functional activity, as subinvolution of the uterus after delivery of a baby. **chronic s. of uterus,** a diffuse, symmetrical uterine enlargement commonly associated with painless menorrhagia.

subiodide (sub-i′o-dīd) that iodide of any series which contains the smallest proportion of iodine.

subjacent (sub-ja′sent) [*sub-* + L. *jacere* to lie] lying just beneath or underneath.

subject[1] (sub-jekt′) [L. *subjectare* to throw under] to cause to undergo, or submit to; to render subservient.

subject[2] (sub′jekt) [L. *subjectus* cast under] 1. a person or animal which has been the object of treatment, observation, or experiment. 2. a body for dissection; cadaver.

subjective (sub-jek′tiv) [L. *subjectivus*] pertaining to or perceived only by the affected individual; not perceptible to the senses of another person.

subjectoscope (sub-jek′to-skōp) [*subjective* + *-scope*] an instrument used in the study of subjective visual sensations.

subjee (sub′je) [Hind. *sabzī*, literally, "greenness"] the capsules and larger leaves of *Cannabis indica*.

subjugal (sub-ju′gal) situated below the zygomatic bone.

sublatio (sub-la′she-o) [L.] sublation. **s. re′tinae,** detachment of the retina.

sublation (sub-la′shun) [L. *sublatio*] a lifting up, or elevation.

sublesional (sub-le′zhun-al) performed or occurring beneath a lesion.

sublethal (sub-le′thal) not quite fatal; insufficient to cause death.

sublimate (sub′lĭ-māt) [L. *sublimatum*] 1. a substance obtained or prepared by sublimation. 2. to divert consciously unacceptable instinctual drives into personally and socially acceptable channels through a mechanism operating outside of and beyond conscious awareness. **corrosive s.,** mercury bichloride.

sublimation (sub″lĭ-ma′shun) [L. *sublimatio*] 1. the direct change of state from solid to vapor. 2. an unconscious defense mechanism in which consciously unacceptable instinctual drives are diverted into personally and socially acceptable channels.

Sublimaze (sub′lĭ-māz) trademark for a preparation of fentanyl citrate.

sublime (sub-līm′) [L. *sublimare*] to volatilize a solid body by heat and then to collect it in a purified form as a solid or powder.

subliminal (sub-lim′ĭ-nal) [*sub-* + L. *limen* threshold] below the limen, or threshold, of sensation.

sublimis (sub-li′mis) [L.] superficial.

sublingual (sub-ling′gwal) located beneath the tongue.

sublinguitis (sub″ling-gwi′tis) inflammation of the sublingual gland.

sublobe (sub′lob) a division of a lobe; a lobule.

sublobular (sub-lob′u-lar) situated beneath a lobule.

subluxate (sub-luks′āt) to partially dislocate.

subluxation (sub″luk-sa′shun) [*sub-* + L. *luxatio* dislocation] an incomplete or partial dislocation. **s. of lens,** partial dislocation of lens of the eye. **Volkmann's s.,** a type of tuberculous arthritis marked by flexion contracture of the knee, external rotation of the leg, valgus position of the knee, and bending of the upper third of the tibia.

sublymphemia (sub″lim-fe′me-ah) hypolymphemia.

submammary (sub-mam′ar-e) situated or occurring beneath a mammary gland.

submandibular (sub″man-dib′u-lar) below the mandible.

submarginal (sub-mar′jĭ-nal) situated beneath a margin.

submaxilla (sub″mak-sil′ah) [*sub-* + L. *maxilla* jaw] the mandible.

submaxillaritis (sub-mak″sĭ-ler-i′tis) inflammation of the submaxillary gland.

submaxillary (sub-mak′sĭ-ler″e) situated beneath the maxilla.

submedial, submedian (sub-me′de-al; sub-me′de-an) beneath or near the middle.

submembranous (sub-mem′brah-nus) partly membranous.

submental (sub-men′tal) [*sub-* + L. *mentum* chin] situated below the chin.

submersion (sub-mer′shun) [*sub-* + L. *mergere* to dip] the act of placing or the condition of being under the surface of a liquid.

submetacentric (sub″met-ah-sen′trik) having the centromere more or less equidistant from the center of the chromosome and one end, so that one arm is shorter than the other. Cf. *acrocentric* and *metacentric.*

submicroscopic, submicroscopical (sub-mi″kro-sko-p′ik; sub″mi-kro-skop′ĭ-kal) too small to be visible under the light microscope.

submorphous (sub-mor′fus) neither amorphous nor perfectly crystalline.

submucosa (sub″mu-ko′sah) the layer of areolar tissue situated beneath the mucous membrane; see under *tela* the terms beginning *t. submucosa.*

submucosal (sub″mu-ko′sal) pertaining to the submucosa, or situated beneath the mucous membrane.

submucous (sub-mu′kus) situated or performed beneath the mucous membrane.

subnarcotic (sub″nar-kot′ik) moderately narcotic.

subnasal (sub-na′zal) situated below the nose.

subnasale (sub″na-sa′le) an anthropometric landmark situated at the point at which the nasal septum merges, with the upper lip in the midsagittal plane. Called also *subnasion.*

subnasion (sub-na′ze-on) subnasale.

subnatant (sub-na′tant) 1. situated below or at the bottom of something. 2. the liquid phase situated below a solid phase; it arises when a solid has a lower density than the liquid with which it is in contact.

subneural (sub-nu′ral) situated beneath a nerve, as a subneural apparatus.

subnitrate (sub-ni′trāt) a basic nitrate.

subnormal (sub-nor′mal) below or less than normal; characterized by qualities, such as intelligence, lower than the level usually observed.

subnormality (sub″nor-mal′ĭ-te) the state of being subnormal. **mental s.,** see under *retardation.*

subnotochordal (sub″no-to-kor′dal) situated beneath the notochord.

subnucleus (sub-nu′kle-us) a partial or secondary nucleus into which a large nerve nucleus may be split up.

subnutrition (sub″nu-trish′un) defective nutrition.

suboccipital (sub″ok-sip′ĭ-tal) situated below the occiput.

suborbital (sub-or′bĭ-tal) situated beneath the orbit.

suborder (sub-or′der) a taxonomic category sometimes established, subordinate to an order and superior to a family.

suboxide (sub-ok′sīd) that oxide in any series which contains the smallest proportion of oxygen.

subpapillary (sub-pap′ĭ-lar-e) underlying the stratum papillare of the skin, as the subpapillary layer.

subpapular (sub-pap′u-lar) indistinctly papular.

subparalytic (sub″par-ah-lit′ik) partially paralytic.

subparietal (sub″pah-ri′ĕ-tal) situated below a parietal bone, lobe, etc.

subpatellar (sub″pah-tel′ar) situated below the patella.

subpectoral (sub-pek′tor-al) situated beneath or below the pectoral region or muscles.

subpelviperitoneal (sub-pel″ve-per″ĭ-to-ne′al) situated beneath the pelvic peritoneum.

subpericardial (sub″per-ĭ-kar′de-al) beneath the pericardium.

subperiosteal (sub″per-e-os′te-al) situated beneath the periosteum.

subperiosteocapsular (sub″per-e-os″te-o-kap′su-lar) subcapsuloperiosteal.

subperitoneal (sub″per-ĭ-to-ne′al) situated beneath or deep to the peritoneum, as a subperitoneal abscess.

subperitoneoabdominal (sub″per-ĭ-to-ne″o-ab-dom′ĭ-nal) subperitoneal.

subperitoneopelvic (sub″per-ĭ-to-ne″o-pel′vik) occurring beneath the peritoneum of the pelvis.

subpharyngeal (sub″fah-rin′je-al) situated below the pharynx.

subphrenic (sub-fren′ik) situated under the diaphragm; subdiaphragmatic.

subphyla (sub-fi′lah) plural of *subphylum.*

subphylum (sub-fi′lum) pl. *subphy′la.* A taxonomic category sometimes established, subordinate to a phylum and superior to a class.

subpial (sub-pi′al) situated beneath the pia mater.

subplacenta (sub″plah-sen′tah) the decidua basalis.

subpleural (sub-ploor′al) situated beneath the pleura.

subpreputial (sub″pre-pu′shal) situated beneath the prepuce.

subpubic (sub-pu′bik) situated or performed below the pubic arch.

subpulmonary (sub-pul′mo-ner″e) situated or occurring below the lung, between the lung and the diaphragm.

subpulpal (sub-pul′pal) below the dental pulp.

subpyramidal (sub″pi-ram′ĭ-dal) below a pyramid, as the subpyramidal fossa.

subrectal (sub-rek′tal) below the rectum.

subretinal (sub-ret′ĭ-nal) below the retina.

subscaphocephaly (sub″skaf-o-sef′ah-le) the condition of being moderately scaphocephalic.

subscapular (sub-skap′u-lar) situated below or under the scapula.

subscleral (sub-skle′ral) located or occurring beneath the sclera.

subsclerotic (sub-skle′rot-ik) 1. subscleral. 2. partly sclerosed.

subscription (sub-skrip′shun) that part of a prescription which gives the directions for compounding the ingredients; see *prescription.*

subserosa (sub″sĕ-ro′sah) a layer of tissue situated beneath a serous membrane.

subserous (sub-se′rus) situated beneath a serous membrane.

subsibilant (sub-sib′ĭ-lant) having a muffled, whistling sound.

subsonic (sub-son′ik) infrasonic.

subspecialty (sub-spesh′al-te) a branch of medicine sub-ordinate to a specialty, as gastroenterology is a subspecialty of internal medicine.

subspecies (sub′spe-sēz) a taxonomic category subordinate to a species, whose members differ morphologically from other members of the species but remain capable of interbreeding with them; a variety or race.

subspinale (sub″spi-na′le) the deepest midline point on the maxilla on the concavity between the anterior nasal spine and the prosthion. Called also *point A.*

subspinous (sub-spi′nus) situated below a spinous process.

subsplenial (sub-sple′ne-al) beneath the splenium of the corpus callosum.

substage (sub′stāj) that part of the microscope which is situated beneath the stage.

substance (sub′stans) [L. *substantia*] the material constituting an organ or body; called also *substantia* [NA]. **accessory food s.,** vitamin. **ad s.,** a name given to the substance which effects transmission of a nerve impulse across a synapse. **adamantine s. of tooth,** enamel (enamelum [NA]). **α-s., alpha s.,** reticular s. **antidiuretic s.,** see under *hormone.* **arborescent white s. of cerebellum,** arbor vitae cerebelli. **autacoid s.,** autacoid. **β-s., beta s.,** see *Heinz-Ehrlich bodies.* **black s.,** substantia nigra. **blood group s's,** the antigenic substances responsible for blood group specificities. Those of the ABO and Lewis blood groups are well characterized. They are formed by sequential addition of monosaccharide moieties to any of several different types of precursor substance; addition of one moiety produces the Lewis substance, addition of a second produces the H substance, and addition of a third produces either the A or the B substance. The secreted blood group substances (in individuals having the secretor phenotype) are glycoproteins; the cellular blood group substances (red cell antigens) are glycosphingolipids; the oligosaccharide chains determining blood group specificity are the same in both. **blood grouping specific s's** [USP], a sterile, isotonic solution of the polysaccharide-containing complexes that are capable of reducing the titer of the anti-A and the anti-B isoagglutinins of group O blood. Specific substance A is usually isolated from hog gastric mucin, and specific substance B usually from the glandular portion of horse gastric mucosa. **cement s., cementing s.,** material which serves to hold together the different components of a tissue, as the intercellular substance in endothelium or the interprismatic substance in tooth enamel. **chromidial s.,** granular endoplasmic reticulum. **chromophil s.,** Nissl bodies. **colloid s.,** a jelly-like material formed in colloid degeneration. **compact s. of bones,** substantia compacta ossium. **contact s.,** catalyst. **controlled s.,** any of the drugs regulated under the Controlled Substances Act (see under C). **cortical s. of bone,** substantia corticalis ossium. **cortical s. of kidney,** cortex renis. **cortical s. of lens,** cortex lentis. **cortical s. of lymph nodes,** cortex nodi lymphatici. **cortical s. of suprarenal gland,** the adrenal cortex (cortex glandulae suprarenalis [NA]). **depressor s.,** a substance that tends to decrease activity or blood pressure. **exophthalmos-producing s.,** a substance isolated from crude anterior pituitary extracts which produces exophthalmos in experimental animals; formerly thought to play a part in the ophthalmopathy of Graves' disease. **external s. of suprarenal gland,** cortex glandulae suprarenalis. **gelatinous s., central,** substantia gelatinosa centralis. **gelatinous s. of spinal cord,** substantia gelatinosa. **glandular s. of prostate,** substantia glandularis prostatae. **gray s.,** substantia grisea. **gray s. of cerebrum, central,** substantia grisea centrale cerebri. **gray s. of spinal cord,** substantia grisea medullae spinalis. **ground s.,** the amorphous gel-like material in which connective tissue cells and fibers are embedded. **H s.,** 1. the precursor of the A and B blood group antigens. Normal type O individuals lack enzymes to convert H substance to A or B substances. Rare individuals having the "Bombay phenotype" lack the ability to make H substance and thus are phenotypically type O whether or not they possess A or B genes. 2. (obs.) Lewis's name for the histaminelike substance that is released by minor skin injury and causes the wheal and flare reaction. Called also *released s.* **I s.,** an inhibitory substance which appears in the synapses of the vertebrate central nervous system, which seems generally to act as a hypopolarizer of the postsynaptic junction. **inter-**

fibrillar s. of Flemming, interfilar s., hyaloplasm, def. 1. **intermediate gray s. of spinal cord, central,** substantia intermedia centralis medullae spinalis. **intermediate gray s. of spinal cord, lateral,** substantia intermedia lateralis medullae spinalis. **intermediate s. of suprarenal gland, internal s. of suprarenal gland,** medulla glandulae suprarenalis. **interprismatic s.,** a cementing substance occupying the space between the round or polygonal enamel prisms; it is softer and more plastic than the enamel prism itself. **interspongioplastic s.,** hyaloplasm, def. 1. **interstitial s.,** ground s. **intertubular s. of tooth, ivory s. of tooth,** dentin (dentinum [NA]). **s. of lens,** substantia lentis. **medullary s.,** 1. the white matter of the central nervous system, consisting of axons and their myelin sheaths. 2. the soft, marrow-like substance of the interior of an organ; see under *medulla*. **medullary s. of bone,** medulla ossium. **medullary s. of bone, red,** medulla ossium rubra. **medullary s. of bone, yellow,** medulla ossium flava. **medullary s. of kidney,** medulla renis. **medullary s. of suprarenal gland,** medulla glandulae suprarenalis. **metachromatic s.,** fine particles seen in erythrocytes, especially after supravital staining. **molecular s.,** neuropil. **müllerian inhibiting s.,** a glycoprotein produced by the Sertoli cells of the fetal testis that acts ipsilaterally in the male to suppress the müllerian ducts, consequently preventing development of the uterus and uterine tubes, thus influencing control of the formation of the male phenotype. **muscular s. of prostate,** substantia muscularis prostatae. **neurosecretory s.,** neurosecretion, def. 2. **s. of Nissl,** see *Nissl bodies*. **no-threshold s's,** those substances in the blood which are excreted into the urine in proportion to their absolute amount in the blood. Cf. *threshold s's.* **onychogenic s.,** the nail-forming substance which occurs in parallel fibrils in the nail matrix. **organ-forming s's,** specialized materials that become segregated in definite blastomeres, thus bringing about a mosaic type of development. **s. P,** a peptide composed of 11 amino acids, present in nerve cells scattered throughout the body and in special endocrine cells in the gut; it increases the contractions of gastrointestinal smooth muscle and causes vasodilatation, it is one of the most potent vasoactive substances known, and it seems to be a sensory neurotransmitter mediating pain, touch, and temperature. **P.-P. s., pellagra-preventing s.,** a dietary substance which will prevent or abolish pellagra. **perforated s., anterior,** substantia perforata rostralis. **perforated s., interpeduncular, perforated s., posterior,** substantia perforata interpeduncularis. **perforated s., rostral,** substantia perforata rostralis. **periventricular gray s.,** diffuse collections of small cells immediately surrounding the ependymal lining of the third ventricle of the brain, around the cerebral aqueduct, and in the floor of the fourth ventricle. **prelipid s.,** degenerated nerve tissue which has not yet been converted into fat. **pressor s.,** any substance that tends to increase blood pressure. **proper s. of cornea,** substantia propria corneae. **proper s. of sclera,** substantia propria sclerae. **proper s. of tooth,** dentin (dentinum [NA]). **receptive s.,** a hypothetical substance supposed to exist in muscle tissue, especially near the motor end-plates of the nerves, and to conduct excitation. **red s. of spleen,** pulpa splenica. **Reichert's s.,** the posterior portion of the anterior perforated substance. **Reichstein's s. Fa,** cortisone. **Reichstein's s. M,** hydrocortisone, or cortisol. **released s.,** H s., def. 2. **reticular s.,** the netlike mass of threads seen in erythrocytes after vital staining; called also *alpha s.* and *filar mass.* **reticular s. of medulla oblongata,** formatio reticularis medullae oblongatae. **reticular s., white, of Arnold,** formatio reticularis pontis. **Rolando's gelatinous s.,** substantia gelatinosa. **Rollett's secondary s.,** the transparent material lying in narrow zones on each side of Krause's membranes. **sarcous s.,** the substance composing the sarcous element of muscle. **second visceral s.,** substantia visceralis secundaria. **slow-reacting s., of anaphylaxis,** a substance released in the anaphylactic reaction that induces slow, prolonged contraction of certain smooth muscles. It is composed of a mixture of leukotrienes C_4, D_4, and E_4. **Soemmering's gray s.** (*obs.*), substantia nigra. **specific soluble s. (SSS)** the polysaccharide capsular material of pneumococci (*Streptococcus pneumoniae*), which exhibits type-specific antigenic differences. **spongy s. of bone,** substantia spongiosa ossium.

threshold s's, those substances in the blood, such as glucose, which are excreted into the urine only when their concentration in plasma exceeds a certain value. **thromboplastic s.,** a general term for any material with procoagulant activity. **tigroid s.,** see *Nissl bodies.* **trabecular s. of bone,** substantia spongiosa ossium. **transmitter s.,** neurotransmitter. **white s.,** substantia alba. **white s. of Schwann,** myelin, def. 1. **white s. of spinal cord,** substantia alba medullae spinalis. **zymoplastic s.,** thromboplastic s.

substantia (sub-stan'she-ah), pl. *substan'tiae* [L.] material of which a tissue, organ, or body is composed; used as a general term in nomenclature. Called also *substance.* **s. adamanti'na den'tis,** dental enamel. **s. al'ba** [NA], white substance: the white nervous tissue, constituting the conducting portion of the brain and spinal cord, and composed mostly of myelinated nerve fibers in three funiculi—dorsal, ventral, and lateral. **s. al'ba medul'lae spina'lis** [NA], the white substance of the spinal cord, consisting of long myelinated nerve fibers arranged in parallel longitudinal bundles. **s. cine'rea,** s. grisea. **s. compac'ta os'sium** [NA], compact substance of bone: bone substance which is dense and hard; called also *compact bone.* **s. cortica'lis cerebel'li,** cortex cerebelli. **s. cortica'lis cer'ebri,** old term for cortex cerebri. **s. cortica'lis glan'dulae suprarena'lis,** the adrenal cortex (cortex glandulae suprarenalis [NA]). **s. cortica'lis len'tis,** cortex lentis. **s. cortica'lis lymphoglan'dulae,** cortex nodi lymphatici. **s. cortica'lis os'sium** [NA], cortical substance of bone: the substance comprising the hard outer layer of a bone. **s. cortica'lis re'nis,** cortex renis. **s. ebur'nea den'tis,** dentin (dentinum [NA]). **s. ferrugin'ea,** locus ceruleus. **s. gelatino'sa centra'lis** [NA], central gelatinous substance: the zone of gelatinous-appearing substance consisting chiefly of neuroglia but also containing a few nerve fibers and cells, that encircles the central canal of the spinal cord and is surrounded by the central intermediate gray substance. **s. gelatino'sa** [NA], **s. gelatino'sa (Rolan'di),** gelatinous substance of spinal cord: the gelatinous-appearing cap that forms the dorsal part of the dorsal column of the spinal cord, consisting chiefly of Golgi type II neurons and some layer nerve cells. **s. glandula'ris pro'statae** [NA], glandular substance of prostate: tissue composed of branched tubuloalveolar glands, outgrowths of the tunica mucosa of the urethra, which terminate in excretory ducts opening into the male urethra; it is enclosed in muscular substance and permeated by muscular strands. Called also *corpus glandulare prostatae.* **s. gris'ea** [NA], gray substance: the gray nervous tissue composed of nerve cell bodies, unmyelinated nerve fibers, and supportive tissue. See also *Rexed's laminae,* under *lamina.* **s. gris'ea centra'lis cer'ebri** [NA], central gray substance of cerebrum: the gray substance in the brain surrounding the cerebral aqueduct; called also *stratum griseum centrale cerebri.* **s. gris'ea interme'dia centra'lis medul'lae spina'lis,** s. intermedia centralis medullae spinalis. **s. gris'ea interme'dia latera'lis medul'lae spina'lis,** s. intermedia lateralis medullae spinalis. **s. gris'ea medul'lae spina'lis** [NA], gray substance of the spinal cord: it contains fewer myelinated fibers but more nerve cell bodies, unmyelinated nerve fibers, and blood vessels than the white substance. **s. hyali'na,** the more fluid interstitial part of the protoplasm of a cell. Cf. *s. opaca.* **s. innomina'ta,** nerve tissue immediately caudad to the anterior perforated substance, and ventral to the globus pallidus and ansa lenticularis. Also known as the *s. innominata of Reichert* or *of Reil.* **s. innomina'ta of Reichert, s. innomina'ta of Reil,** s. innominata. **s. interme'dia centra'lis medul'lae spina'lis** [NA], central intermediate substance of spinal cord: the transverse band of gray substance surrounding the central canal of the spinal cord external to the central gelatinous substance which connects the right and left masses of gray substance; called also *central intermediate gray substance of spinal cord, gray commissure,* and *s. grisea intermedia centralis medullae spinalis.* **s. interme'dia latera'lis medul'lae spina'lis** [NA], lateral intermediate substance of spinal cord: the gray substance of the spinal cord that intervenes between the central intermediate substance, the lateral column, and the ventral and dorsal columns; called also *lateral intermediate gray substance of spinal cord* and *s. grisea intermedia lateralis medullae spinalis.* **s. intertubula'ris den'tis,** dentin (dentinum [NA]). **s. len'tis** [NA], the fibrous material making up the bulk of the lens of the eye. **s. medulla′ris glan′dulae suprarena′lis,** medulla glandulae suprarenalis. **s. medulla′ris lymphoglan′dulae,** medulla nodi lymphatici. **s. medulla′ris re′nis,** medulla renis. **s. metachromaticogranula′ris,** see *Heinz-Ehrlich bodies.* **s. muscula′ris pro′statae** [NA], muscular substance of prostate: the muscular stroma of the prostate, which is intimately blended with the fibrous capsule and permeates the glandular substance; called also *musculus prostaticus.* **s. ni′gra** [NA], black substance: the layer of gray substance that separates the dorsal parts of the cerebral peduncles (tegmentum mesencephali) from the ventral parts; it consists of a dorsal compact part with many pigmented cells (*pars compacta*) and a ventral reticular part whose cells contain little pigment (*pars reticularis*). Called also *body of Vicq d'Azyr* and *locus niger.* **s. opa′ca,** the reticulum of the protoplasm of a cell. Cf. *s. hyalina.* **s. perfora′ta ante′rior,** NA alternative for *s. perforata rostralis.* **s. perfora′ta interpeduncula′ris,** interpeduncular perforated substance: the floor of the interpeduncular fossa, between the cerebral peduncles, which is pierced by central branches of the posterior cerebral artery; called also *posterior perforated substance* and *s. perforata posterior* [NA alternative]. **s. perfora′ta poste′rior,** NA alternative for *s. perforata interpeduncularis.* **s. perfora′ta rostra′lis** [NA], rostral perforated substance: an area on the base of the brain, rostral to each optic tract, containing numerous perforations through which small branches of the anterior and middle cerebral arteries are transmitted to deeper structures; called also *anterior perforated substance, olfactory area,* and *s. perforata anterior* [NA alternative]. **s. pro′pria cor′neae** [NA], proper substance of cornea: the fibrous, tough, and transparent main part of the cornea, between the anterior and the posterior limiting lamina; called also *stroma of cornea.* **s. pro′pria scle′rae** [NA], proper substance of sclera: the chief part of the sclera, lying between the lamina fusca and the episcleral lamina, composed of dense bands of fibrous tissue, mostly parallel with the surface, and crossing each other in all directions. It is structurally continuous with the substantia propria corneae. **s. reticula′ris al′ba of Arnold,** formatio reticularis pontis. **s. reticula′ris medul′lae oblonga′tae,** NA alternative for *formatio reticularis medullae oblongatae.* **s. reticulofilamento′sa,** reticular substance. **s. Rolan′di,** *s. gelatinosa.* **s. spongio′sa os′sium** [NA], spongy substance of bone: bone substance made up of thin intersecting lamellae, usually found internal to compact bone; called also *cancellated bone, spongy bone, trabecular substance, s. trabecularis ossium* [NA alternative]. **s. trabecula′ris os′sium,** NA alternative for *s. spongiosa ossium.* **s. viscera′lis secunda′ria** [NA], second visceral substance: the gray substance lying ventral to the central intermediate substance.

substantiae (sub-stan′she-e) plural of *substantia.*

substernal (sub-ster′nal) situated beneath the sternum.

substernomastoid (sub″ster-no-mas′toid) beneath the sternomastoid muscle.

substituent (sub-stich′u-ent) 1. a substitute; especially an atom, radical, or group substituted for another in a compound. 2. of or pertaining to such an atom, radical, or group.

substitute (sub′stĭ-tūt) a material which may be used in place of another. **blood s., plasma s.,** a fluid which may be used instead of whole blood or plasma for replacement of circulating fluid in the body.

substitution (sub″stĭ-tu′shun) [L. *substitutio,* from *sub* under + *statuere* to place] 1. the act of putting one thing in the place of another, especially the chemical replacement of one element or radical by some other. 2. a defense mechanism, operating unconsciously, in which an unattainable or unacceptable goal, emotion, or object is replaced by one that is attainable or acceptable. **creeping s. of bone,** the formation of new bone on the surfaces of necrotic trabeculae by osteoblasts, occurring after the revascularization of an area that has been disrupted by fracture, as at the head of the femur after fracture of the neck has disrupted the blood supply to the head of the bone.

substitutive (sub′stĭ-tu″tive) effecting a change or substitution.

substrate (sub′strāt) [L. *sub* under + *stratum* layer] a substance upon which an enzyme acts.

substratum (sub-stra′tum) [L.] 1. a substrate. 2. a lower layer or stratum.

substructure (sub′struk-chur) 1. a structure that provides a foundation for another structure. 2. a basic underlying or supporting part of an organ or structure. Called also *infrastructure.* 3. implant s. **implant s.,** a metal framework implanted beneath the mucoperiosteum, in contact with bone, that retains, supports, and stabilizes the superstructural part of an implant denture. Called also *implant framework* and *implant infrastructure.*

subsulcus (sub-sul′kus) a sulcus concealed by another.

subsulfate (sub-sul′fāt) a basic sulfate.

subsultus (sub-sul′tus) [L. *subsilire* to spring up] a spasmodic movement. **s. ten′dinum,** a twisting movement of the muscles and tendons such as is observed in a typhoid state.

subsylvian (sub-sil′ve-an) situated deep in the lateral sulcus (fissure of Sylvius).

subtalar (sub-ta′lar) [*sub-* + L. *talus* ankle] beneath the talus, as the subtalar joint.

subtarsal (sub-tar′sal) situated below the tarsus.

subtelocentric (sub-tel″o-sen′trik) having the centromere almost, but not quite, at the telocentric position.

subtemporal (sub-tem′por-al) beneath the temple or any temporal structure or part; see also under *decompression.*

subtenial (sub-te′ne-al) situated beneath a tenia.

subtentorial (sub-ten′to-re-al) situated beneath the tentorium of the cerebellum.

subterminal (sub-ter′mĭ-nal) situated near an end or extremity.

subtetanic (sub″te-tan′ik) mildly tetanic.

subthalamic (sub″thah-lam′ik) situated below the thalamus; pertaining to the subthalamus.

subthalamus (sub-thal′ah-mus) thalamus ventralis.

subtile (sut′′l) [L. *subtilis*] keen and acute.

subtilin (sub′til-in) an antibiotic substance isolated from strains of the soil bacteria *Bacillus subtilis,* which is chiefly effective against gram-positive bacteria and certain acid-fast bacilli.

subtilisin (sub-til′ĭ-sin) a proteolytic enzyme isolated from strains of the soil bacteria *Bacillus subtilis,* which catalyzes the hydrolysis of certain peptide bonds; analysis has shown it to be composed of 274 amino acid residues.

subtle (sut′′l) [L. *subtilis*] 1. very fine. 2. subtile.

subtrapezial (sub″trah-pe′ze-al) situated beneath the trapezius muscle.

subtribe (sub′trīb) a taxonomic category sometimes established, subordinate to a tribe and superior to a genus.

subtrochanteric (sub″tro-kan-ter′ik) situated below a trochanter.

subtrochlear (sub-trok′le-ar) situated beneath the trochlea.

subtuberal (sub-tu′ber-al) situated under a tuber.

subtympanic (sub″tim-pan′ik) 1. below the tympanum. 2. having a somewhat tympanic quality.

subumbilical (sub″um-bil′e-kal) situated beneath the umbilicus.

subungual (sub-ung′gwal) [*sub-* + L. *unguis* nail] situated beneath a nail; hyponychial.

suburethral (sub″u-re′thral) situated or occurring beneath the urethra.

subvaginal (sub-vaj′ĭ-nal) situated under a sheath, or below the vagina.

subvertebral (sub-ver′te-bral) situated on the ventral side of the vertebral column.

subvitrinal (sub-vit′rĭ-nal) situated beneath the vitreous.

subvolution (sub″vo-lu′shun) [*sub-* + L. *volvere* to turn] the operation of reversing a flap; especially the operation of dissecting and turning up a pterygium, so that the outer or cutaneous surface comes in contact with the raw surface of the dissection. It is done to prevent readhesion.

subwaking (sub-wāk′ing) intermediate between waking and sleeping.

subzonal (sub-zo′nal) situated beneath a zone, as below the zona pellucida.

subzygomatic (sub″zi-go-mat′ik) situated below the zygoma.

succagogue (suk′ah-gog) [L. *succus* juice + Gr. *agōgos* leading] 1. inducing glandular secretion. 2. an agent that stimulates glandular secretion.

succedaneous (suk″sĕ-da′ne-us) ensuing; in place of; of the nature of a succedaneum.

succedaneum (suk″sĕ-da′ne-um) [L. *succedaneus* taking another's place] a medicine or material that may be substituted for another of like properties.

succenturiate (suk″sen-tu′re-āt) [L. *succenturiare* to substitute] accessory; serving as a substitute.

succinate (suk′si-nāt) any salt, ester, or anionic form of succinic acid.

succinate-CoA ligase (GDP-forming) (suk′si-nāt li′gās) [EC 6.2.1.4] an enzyme of the ligase class that catalyzes the reaction GDP + succinyl-CoA + orthophosphate = GTP + succinate + CoA. The reversible reaction is part of the citric (tricarboxylic) acid cycle. Called also *succinyl-CoA synthetase*.

succinate dehydrogenase (suk′si nāt de-hi′dro-jĕ-nās) [EC 1.3.99.1] an enzyme of the oxidoreductase class that catalyzes the reaction succinate + ubiquinone = fumarate + ubiquinol. It occurs in mitochondria as a membrane-bound flavoprotein and is part of the citric (tricarboxylic) acid cycle. The electron transfer involves an associated iron-sulfide protein.

succinic acid (suk-sin′ik) 1, 4-butanedioic acid, an intermediate in the tricarboxylic acid cycle (q.v.).

Succinimonas (suk″si-ni-mo′nas) [L. *acidum succinicum* succinic acid + Gr. *monas* unit, from *monos* single] a genus of gram-negative, anaerobic bacteria of the family Bacteroidaceae, made up of motile, short, straight rods with rounded ends that produce large amounts of succinic acid, found in the rumen contents of cattle. The genus contains a single species, S. *amylolytica*.

Succinivibrio (suk″si-ni-vib′re-o) [L. *acidum succinicum* succinic acid + *vibrio*] a genus of gram-negative, anaerobic bacteria of the family Bacteroidaceae, made up of motile curved rods with pointed ends, found in the rumen contents of cattle and sheep. The genus contains a single species, S. *dextrinosol′vens*.

succinoresinol (suk″si-no-rez′i-nol) a resinol from amber, $C_{12}H_{20}O$.

succinous (suk′si-nus) pertaining to amber.

succinyl (suk′si-nil) an acyl radical of succinic acid.

succinylcholine chloride (suk″si-nil-ko′lēn) [USP] chemical name: 2,2′-[(1,4-dioxo-1,4-butanediyl)bis(oxy)]bis-[N,N,N-trimethylethanaminium]dichloride. A neuromuscular blocking agent, $C_{21}H_{22}H_2O_2$, occurring as a white, crystalline powder, which produces skeletal muscle relaxation by blocking transmission at the myoneural junction; used for its muscle relaxant action during shock therapy and such procedures as endotracheal intubation and endoscopy, and as an adjunct to surgical anesthesia, administered intravenously and intramuscularly.

succinyl-CoA (suk′si-nil) a high-energy intermediate formed in the tricarboxylic acid (Krebs) cycle by the oxidation of α-ketoglutaric acid; it then undergoes deacylation to form succinic acid, a step which also involves formation of guanosine triphosphate.

succinyl-CoA synthetase (suk′si-nil sin′thĕ-tās) succinate-CoA ligase (GDP-forming).

succinylcoenzyme A (suk″si-nil-ko′en-zīm) the succinate monothioester of coenzyme A, an intermediate in the tricarboxylic acid cycle.

succinylsulfathiazole (suk″si-nil-sul″fah-thi′ah-zōl) chemical name: 4-oxo-4-[[4-[(2-thiazolylamino) sulfonyl]phenyl]amino]butanoic acid. A sulfonamide, $C_{13}H_{13}N_3O_5S_2$·· H_2O, occurring as a white or yellowish, crystalline powder; used as an antibacterial in patients undergoing gastrointestinal surgery and in the treatment of gastrointestinal infections due to susceptible organisms, administered orally.

succorrhea (suk″o-re′ah) [L. *succus* juice + Gr. *rhoia* flow] an excessive flow of a juice or secretion, as in ptyalism.

succus (suk′us) pl. *suc′ci* [L.] any fluid derived from living tissue; used in anatomical nomenclature as a general term for a bodily secretion or a fluid derived from body tissue; called also *juice*. **s. cera′si,** cherry juice. **s. enter′icus,** intestinal juice: the liquid secreted by the glands in the wall of the small intestine. **s. gas′tricus,** gastric juice: the liquid secretion of the glands of the stomach. **s. pancreat′icus,** pancreatic juice: the liquid secretion of the pancreas, which is discharged into the duodenum. **s. prostat′icus,** the secretion of the prostate gland, which contributes to formation of the semen. **s. ru′bi idae′i,** raspberry juice.

succussion (sŭ-kush′un) [L. *succussio* a shaking from beneath, earthquake] a procedure in which the body is shaken, a splashing sound being indicative of the presence of fluid and air in a body cavity. **hippocratic s.,** succussion to elicit a splashing sound in the chest, usually pathognomonic of pneumohydrothorax.

sucholoalbumin (su″ko-lo-al-bu′min) [L. *sus* pig + Gr. *cholē* bile + *albumin*] a poisonous protein characteristic of hog cholera, and obtained from cultures of the bacillus; it is injected for the purpose of giving immunity to the disease.

suckle (suk′l) to derive or to provide nourishment by feeding at the breast.

Sucostrin (su-kos′trin) trademark for a preparation of succinylcholine.

Sucquet-Hoyer anastomosis (canal) (su-ka′oy-ār) [J. P. *Sucquet;* French anatomist, 1840–1870; Henryk *Hoyer,* Polish anatomist, 1864–1947] segmentum arteriale anastomosias arteriovenae glomeriformis.

sucralfate (soo-kral′făt) chemical name: β-D-fructofuranosylglucopyranoside octakis (hydrogen sulfate) aluminum complex; a gastrointestinal antiulcerative, $C_{12}H_mAl_{16}$-O_nS_8.

sucrase (soo′krās) [EC 3.2.1.48] an enzyme of the hydrolase class that catalyzes the hydrolysis of sucrose and maltose by an α-D-glucosidase type reaction. The enzyme occurs as a complex with α-dextrinase in the intestinal mucosa. Called *sucrose α-glucosidase* in formal EC nomenclature.

sucrate (su′krāt) a compound of a substance with sucrose.

sucre (su′k′r) [Fr.] sugar. **s. actuelle′,** actual sugar. **s. virtuelle′,** virtual sugar.

sucroclastic (su″kro-klas′tik) [Fr. *sucre* sugar + Gr. *klastos* broken] splitting of sugar.

sucrose (su′krōs) [L. *sucrosum*] a disaccharide, $C_{12}H_{22}O_{11}$, obtained from sugar cane, sugar beet, or other sources, crystallizing in prisms, soluble in water, and turning the plane of polarization to the right. By boiling with acids and by the action of certain enzymes it is hydrolyzed and converted into dextrose and fructose. The official preparation conforms to NF specifications. It is extensively used as a food and as a sweetening agent, and is much employed in pharmacy, forming the basis of many pharmaceutical preparations. **s. octaacetate** [NF], a white, almost odorless, hygroscopic powder, having an intensely bitter taste; used as an alcohol denaturant.

sucrose α-D-glucohydrolase (su′krōs gloo″ko-hi′dro-lās) sucrase.

sucrose α-D-glucosidase (soo′krōs gloo-ko′si-dās, gloo′-ko-si-dās) sucrase.

sucrosemia (su″kro-se′me-ah) [*sucrose* + Gr. *haima* blood + *-ia*] the presence of sucrose in the blood.

sucrosuria (su″kro-su′re-ah) [*sucrose* + Gr. *ouron* urine + *-ia*] the presence of sucrose in the urine.

suction (suk′shun) [L. *sugere* to suck] aspiration of gas or fluid by mechanical means. **post-tussive s.,** a sucking sound heard over a lung cavity just after a cough. **Wangensteen s.,** see under *tube*.

Suctoria (suk-to′re-ah) [L. *sugere* to suck] a subclass of protozoa (class Kinetofragminophorea, phylum Ciliophora), characterized by the presence of cilia only during the free-swimming larval stage, the adults bearing suctorial tentacles with haptocysts at the tips used to capture prey. Most suctorians are free-living, unattached or attached to the substrate by a noncontractile stalk, being widespread on marine and freshwater organisms; some are endocommensal in various hosts, including ciliates and vertebrates. It comprises one order: Suctorida.

suctorial (suk-to′re-al) fitted for performing suction.

suctorian (suk-to′re-an) 1. any protozoan of the subclass Suctoria. 2. of or pertaining to the subclass Suctoria.

Suctorida (suk-tor′i-dah) an order of ciliate protozoa (subclass Suctoria, phylum Ciliophora) having characters of the subclass. It comprises three suborders: Exogenina, Endogenina, and Evaginogenina.

sucuuba (soo″koo-oo′bah) the *Plumeria phagedenica*, a medicinal plant of South America.

Sudafed (soo′dah-fed) trademark for preparations of pseudoephedrine hydrochloride.

sudamen (su-da′men), pl. *sudam′ina* [L., from *sudare* to sweat] a whitish vesicle caused by the retention of sweat in the sudorific ducts or the layers of the epidermis. In the plural (*sudamina*), an eruption of such vesicles, known as *miliaria crystallina*.

sudamina (su-dam′ĭ-nah) [L.] plural of *sudamen*.

sudaminal (su-dam′ĭ-nal) pertaining to or resembling sudamina.

Sudan (su-dan′) a group of azo compounds used as stains for fats. **S. G,** S. III. **S. I,** $C_6H_5 \cdot N:N \cdot C_{10}H_6 \cdot OH$. **S. II,** $(CH_3)_2C_6H_3 \cdot N:N \cdot C_{10}H_6 \cdot OH$. **S. III,** chemical name: 1-(*p*-phenylazophenylazo)-2-naphthol. A red fat-soluble azo dye, $C_6H_5 \cdot N \cdot N \cdot C_6H_4 \cdot N:N \cdot C_{10}H_6 \cdot OH$, an important stain for the demonstration of neutral fats. **S. IV,** scarlet red. **S. yellow G,** a brown powder, $C_{12}H_{10}N_2O_2$, used as a stain for fats.

sudanophil (su-dan′o-fil) an element that stains readily with Sudan.

sudanophilia (su-dan″o-fil′e-ah) [*sudan* + Gr. *philein* to love] affinity for Sudan stain.

sudanophilic (su-dan″o-fil′ik) staining readily with Sudan.

sudanophilous (su″dan-of′ĭ-lus) sudanophilic.

sudarium (su-da′re-um) [L.] a sweat bath.

sudarshan shurna (soo-dar′shan shoor′nah) a Hindu febrifuge containing fifty drugs.

sudation (su-da′shun) [L. *sudatio*] the excretion of sweat.

sudatoria (su″dah-to′re-ah) [L.] plural of *sudatorium*.

Sudeck's atrophy (disease), point (soo′deks) [Paul Hermann Martin *Sudeck*, Hamburg surgeon, 1866–1938] see *post-traumatic osteoporosis*, under *osteoporosis*, and see under *point*.

Sudeck-Leriche syndrome (soo′dek-lĕ-rēsh′) [P. H. M. *Sudeck*; René *Leriche*, French surgeon, 1879–1955] see under *syndrome*.

sudogram (su′do-gram) [L. *sudor* sweat + Gr. *gramma* a writing] a graphic representation of the areas of the body on which sweating is present.

sudomotor (su″do-mo′tor) [L. *sudor* sweat + *motor* move] stimulating the sweat glands.

sudor (su′dor) [L.] (*obs.*) sweat, or perspiration. **s. san-guin′eus,** hematidrosis.

sudoresis (su″do-re′sis) diaphoresis.

sudoriferous (su″do-rif′er-us) [L. *sudor* sweat + *ferre* to bear] 1. conveying sweat. 2. sudoriparous.

sudorific (su″do-rif′ik) [L. *sudorificus*] 1. promoting the flow of sweat; diaphoretic. 2. an agent that causes sweating.

sudoriparous (su″do-rip′ah-rus) [L. *sudor* sweat + *parere* to produce] secreting or producing sweat.

sudoxicam (soo-dok′sĭ-kam) chemical name: 4-hydroxy-2-methyl-*N*-2-thiazolyl-1,2-benzothiazine-3-carboxamide; and anti-inflammatory, $C_{13}H_{11}N_3O_4S_2$.

SUDS sudden unexplained death syndrome; see under *syndrome*.

suet (su′et) [L. *sevum*] the fat from the abdominal cavity of a ruminant animal, especially the sheep or ox; used in the preparation of cerates and ointments and as an emollient. The preparation employed in pharmacy is the internal fat of the abdomen of the sheep. **benzoinated s.,** prepared suet 1000, benzoin 30. **prepared s.,** the internal fat of the abdomen of the sheep purified by melting and straining.

sufentanil (su-fen′tah-nil) chemical name: *N*-[4-(methoxy-methyl)-1-[2-(2-thienyl)ethyl]-4-piperidinyl]-*N*-phenylpropanamide; an analgesic, $C_{22}H_{30}N_2O_2S$.

suffocant (suf′o-kant) an agent that causes suffocation.

suffocation (suf″o-ka′shun) [L. *suffocatio*] asphyxiation; the stoppage of respiration, or the asphyxia that results from it.

suffraginis (suf-fraj′ĭ-nis) [L.] the large pastern bone or first phalanx of the horse.

suffusion (sŭ-fu′zhun) [L. *suffusio*] 1. the process of over-spreading, or diffusion. 2. the condition of being moistened or of being permeated through, as by blood.

sugar (shoog′ar) [L. *saccharum*; Gr. *sakcharon*] a sweet carbohydrate of various kinds, and of both animal and vegetable origin. It is an aldehyde or ketone derivative of polyhydric alcohols. The two principal groups of sugars are the disaccharides, having the formula $C_{12}H_{22}O_{11}$, and the monosaccharides, $C_6H_{12}O_6$; all are white, crystallizable solids, soluble in water and dilute alcohol. The disaccharides are sucrose or saccharose (*beet s., cane s., maple s., palm s., malt s.* (maltose), *milk s.* (lactose), and others. The monosaccharides include ordinary dextrose (δ-glucose) (*diabetic s., grape s., liver s., potato s., starch s.*), fructose (*fruit s.*), and inositol (*heart s., muscle s.*). Besides these, a very considerable number of artificial and other sugars are known to chemistry. **actual s.,** (sucre actuelle of Lépine), the free glucose in the blood. **anhydrous s.,** anhydrosugar. **barley s.,** a clear hard form of sugar formed by heating ordinary granulated sugar (sucrose) to 160° F. **beechwood s.,** xylose. **beet s.,** sucrose derived from the root of the beet. **blood s.,** glucose, the form in which carbohydrate is carried in the blood, usually in a concentration of 70–100 mg. per 100 ml. **brain s.,** cerebrose. **burnt s.,** caramel. **cane s.,** sucrose obtained from sugar cane. **collagen s.,** aminoacetic acid. **compressible s.** [NF], a preparation which contains 95–98 per cent sucrose and which may contain starch, dextrin, and invert sugar; used as a sweetening agent and tablet excipient in pharmaceutical preparations. **confectioner's s.** [NF], sucrose ground together with corn starch to a fine powder, containing 95–97 per cent sucrose; used as a sweetening agent and tablet excipient in pharmaceutical preparations. **diabetic s.,** the dextrose found in the urine in diabetes mellitus. **fruit s.,** fructose. **gelatin s.,** aminoacetic acid. **grape s.,** dextrose. **heart s.,** inositol. **invert s.,** the mixture of dextrose and fructose obtained by hydrolysing sucrose; used in solution as a parenteral nutrient. Called also *invertose*. **larch s.,** melezitose. **s. of lead,** lead acetate. **Leo's s.,** laiose. **liver s.,** dextrose from the liver. **malt s.,** maltose. **maple s.,** sucrose from maple sap. **milk s.,** lactose. **muscle s.,** inositol. **oil s.,** eleosaccharum. **palm s.,** sucrose from palm sap. **potato s.,** dextrose from potatoes. **reducing s.,** a sugar which will reduce an alkaline copper tartrate solution. **simple s.,** a monosaccharide. **starch s.,** dextrin. **sulfur s.,** thioglucose. **threshold s.,** the lower limit of hyperglycemia at which dextrose appears in the urine. **virtual s.** (sucre virtuelle of Lépine), sugar in the blood in a colloidal state. **wood s.,** xylose.

sugarin (shoog′ar-in) chemical name: methylbenzoylsulfimide. A crystalline substance said to be 500 times as sweet as sugar.

suggestibility (sug-jes″tĭ-bil′ĭ-te) a condition of enhanced susceptibility to suggestion.

suggestible (sug-jes′tĭ-b'l) highly susceptible to suggestion.

suggestion (sug-jes′chun) [L. *suggestio*] 1. the impartation of an idea to a subject from without. 2. an idea introduced from without. **hypnotic s.,** a suggestion imparted to a person in the hypnotic state, by which he is induced to alter perceptions or memory or to perform actions. **posthypnotic s.,** implantation in the mind of a subject during hypnosis of a suggestion to be acted upon after recovery from the hypnotic state.

suggillation (sug″jĭ-la′shun) [L. *suggillatio*] 1. a bruise or ecchymosis. 2. a mark of postmortem lividity.

suicide (soo′ĭ-sīd) [L. *sui* of himself + *caedere* to kill] the taking of one's own life. **psychic s.,** the termination of one's own life without employment of physical agents.

suint (swint) a fat-like substance derivable from sheep's wool, from which anhydrous lanolin is prepared. Called also *suint de laine*.

suipestifer (soo′ĭ-pes′tĭ-fer) a group of salmonellae (*S. choleraesuis* var. *kuzendorf*, *S. choleraesuis* var. *typhisuis*, *S. enteritidis* serotype *hirschfeldii*) causing paratyphoid gastroenteritis in humans and swine.

suit (sūt) an outer garment covering the entire body. **antiblackout s., anti-G s.,** G suit. **antishock s.,** pneumatic antishock garment. **G s.,** a garment worn by pilots, designed to increase their ability to withstand ill effects of the acceleratory forces experienced in certain aerial maneuvers.

Sulamyd (sul'am-id)   trademark for a preparation of sulfacetamide.

sulazepam (sul-ah'zĕ-pam)   chemical name: 7-chloro-1,3-dihydro-1-methyl-5-phenyl-2*H*-1,4-benzodiazepine-2-thione; a minor tranquilizer, $C_{16}H_{13}ClN_2S$.

sulbenox (sul-ben'oks)   chemical name: (4,5,6,7-tetrahydro-7-oxobenzo[*b*]thien-4-yl)urea; a veterinary growth stimulant, $C_9H_{10}N_2O_2S$.

sulcate (sul'kāt) [L. *sulcatus*]   furrowed or marked with sulci.

sulcation (sul-ka'shun)   the formation of sulci; the state of being marked by sulci.

sulci (sul'si) [L.]   plural of *sulcus*.

sulciform (sul'sĭ-form)   formed like a groove.

sulconazole nitrate (sul-kon'ah-zōl)   chemical name: (+)-1-[2-[[(4-chlorophenyl)methyl]thio]-2-(2,4-dichlorophenyl)ethyl]-1*H*-imidazole mononitrate; an antifungal, $C_{18}H_{15}-CL_3N_2S \cdot HNO_3$.

sulculi (sul'ku-li)   plural of *sulculus*.

sulculus (sul'ku-lus), pl. *sul'culi* [L.]   a small or minute sulcus.

sulcus (sul'kus), pl. *sul'ci* [L.]   1. a groove, trench, or furrow; [NA] a general term for such a depression, especially one of those on the surface of the brain, separating the gyri. Cf. *fissure*. 2. a linear depression or valley in the occlusal surface of a tooth, the sloping sides of which meet at an angle. **alveolabial s.,** the furrow between the dental arch and the lips. **alveolingual s.,** the depression between the dental arch and the tongue. **s. ampulla'ris** [NA], **ampullary s.,** a transverse groove on the membranous ampulla of each semicircular duct, for the ampullary branch of the pars vestibularis nervi octavi. **angular s.,** incisura angularis gastris. **anterolateral s. of medulla oblongata,** s. ventrolateralis medullae oblongatae. **anterolateral s. of spinal cord,** s. ventrolateralis medullae spinalis. **s. anterolatera'lis medul'lae oblonga'tae,** NA alternative for *s. ventrolateralis medullae oblongatae*. **s. anterolatera'lis medul'lae spina'lis,** NA alternative for *s. ventrolateralis medullae spinalis*. **s. anthel'icis transver'sus** [NA], transverse sulcus of anthelix: the depression on the medial surface of the pinna corresponding to the lower crus of the anthelix. **aortic s., s. aor'ticus,** a longitudinal groove on the median surface of the left lung corresponding to the thoracic aorta. **s. arte'riae occipita'lis** [NA], sulcus of occipital artery: the groove just medial to the mastoid notch on the temporal bone, lodging the occipital artery. **s. arte'riae subcla'viae** [NA], sulcus of subclavian artery: a transverse groove on the cranial surface of the first rib, just posterior to the anterior scalene tubercle; it lodges the subclavian artery; called also *s. subclavius*. **s. arte'riae tempora'lis me'diae** [NA], sulcus of middle temporal artery: a nearly vertical groove running just superior to the external acoustic meatus on the external surface of the squamous part of the temporal bone; it lodges the middle temporal artery. **s. arte'riae vertebra'lis atlan'tis** [NA], sulcus of vertebral artery of atlas: the groove on the cranial surface of the posterior arch of the atlas; it lodges the vertebral artery and the first spinal nerve. **sul'ci arterio'si** [NA], grooves on the internal surfaces of the cranial bones for the meningeal arteries; called also *arterial grooves* or *sulci* and *sulci arteriales* [NA alternative]. **sul'ci arteria'les,** NA alternative for *sulci arteriosi*. **atrioventricular s.,** s. coronarius cordis. **s. of auditory tube,** s. tubae auditivae. **s. of auricle, posterior, s. auric'ulae poste'rior** [NA], the slight depression on the pinna that separates the anthelix from the antitragus. **s. of auricular branch of vagus nerve,** s. canaliculi mastoidei. **basilar s. of occipital bone,** s. sinus petrosi inferioris ossis occipitalis. **basilar s. of pons, s. basila'ris pon'tis** [NA], the anteromedian groove in the pons, lodging the basilar artery. **bicipital s., lateral,** s. bicipitalis lateralis. **bicipital s., medial,** s. bicipitalis medialis. **bicipital s., radial,** s. bicipitalis lateralis. **bicipital s., ulnar,** s. bicipitalis medialis. **s. bicipita'lis latera'lis** [NA], lateral bicipital sulcus: a longitudinal groove on the lateral side of the arm which marks the limit between the lateral border of the biceps muscle and the brachialis; called also *lateral* or *radial bicipital groove*,

radial bicipital s., and *s. bicipitalis radialis* [NA alternative]. **s. bicipita'lis media'lis** [NA], medial bicipital sulcus: a longitudinal groove on the medial side of the arm which marks the limit between the medial border of the biceps muscle and the brachialis; called also *medial* or *ulnar bicipital groove, s. bicipitalis ulnaris* [NA alternative], and *ulnar bicipital s.* **s. bicipita'lis radia'lis,** NA alternative for *s. bicipitalis lateralis.* **s. bicipita'lis ulna'ris,** NA alternative for *s. bicipitalis medialis.* **bulbopontine s., s. bulboponti'nus** [NA], a transverse groove in front and on each side of the pons that demarcates it from the medulla oblongata, which is occupied by the abducent, facial, and vestibulocochlear nerves. **calcaneal s., s. calca'nei** [NA], a rough, deep groove on the upper surface of the calcaneus, between the medial and the posterior articular surfaces and giving attachment to the interosseous talocalcaneal ligament. **calcarine s., s. calcari'nus** [NA], a sulcus on the medial surface of the occipital lobe, separating the cuneus from the lingual gyrus; called also *fissura calcarina.* **callosal s.,** s. corporis callosi. **callosomarginal s.,** s. cinguli. **s. callo'sus,** s. corporis callosi. **s. canalic'uli mastoi'dei,** a small groove in the petrous portion of the temporal bone leading to the mastoid canaliculus. **s. cana'lis innomina'tus,** s. nervi petrosi minoris. **s. carot'icus os'sis sphenoida'lis** [NA], **carotid s.,** the groove on the side of the body of the sphenoid bone that lodges the internal carotid artery and the cavernous sinus. **carpal s., s. car'pi** [NA], a broad deep groove on the volar surface of the carpal bones, which transmits the flexor tendons and the median nerve into the palm of the hand. **central s. of cerebrum,** s. centralis cerebri. **s. centra'lis cer'ebri** [NA], central sulcus of cerebrum: a relatively deep, nearly vertical sulcus on the cerebral hemisphere, which separates the frontal from the parietal lobe. **s. centra'lis in'sulae** [NA], a deep, oblique furrow which divides the insula into a larger anterior and a smaller posterior part. **cerebral s., lateral,** s. lateralis cerebri. **sul'ci cer'ebri** [NA], sulci of cerebrum, the furrows between the gyri of the cerebrum. **chiasmatic s., s. chias'matis,** s. prechiasmaticus. **s. cin'guli** [NA], **s. of cingulum,** a long, irregularly shaped sulcus on the medial surface of a hemisphere, which separates the cingulate gyrus below from the medial frontal gyrus and the paracentral lobule above. It may be divided into frontal and marginal portions. Called also *cingulate s.* and *s. cingulatus* [NA alternative]. **s. cingula'tus,** NA alternative for *s. cinguli.* **circular s. of insula, s. circula'ris in'sulae** [NA], a fissure that almost surrounds the insula (lobus insularis [NA]) and separates it from the opercula. **collateral s., s. collatera'lis** [NA], a longitudinal sulcus on the inferior surface of the cerebral hemisphere between the fusiform gyrus and the parahippocampal gyrus; called also *fissura collateralis.* **s. col'li mandib'ulae,** the shallow groove between the ridge of the mandibular neck and the line of attachment of the sphenomandibular ligament. **s. corona'rius cor'dis** [NA], **coronary s. of heart,** a groove on the external surface of the heart, separating the atria from the ventricles; portions of it are occupied by the major arteries and veins of the heart; called also *atrioventricular groove.* **s. cor'poris callo'si** [NA], **s. of corpus callosum,** a sulcus encircling the convex aspect of the corpus callosum at the bottom of the longitudinal cerebral fissure. **s. cos'tae** [NA], **costal s.,** a sulcus that follows the inferior and internal surface of a rib anteriorly from the tubercle, gradually becoming less distinct; it lodges the intercostal vessels and nerves. **costal s., inferior,** s. costae. **s. cru'ris hel'icis** [NA], **s. of crus of helix,** a transverse sulcus on the medial surface of the pinna, corresponding to the crus helicis on the lateral surface. **cuboid, s.,** s. tendinum musculorum peroneorum calcanei. **sul'ci cu'tis** [NA], sulci of skin: the fine depressions on the surface of the skin between the dermal ridges. Called also *skin furrows.* **dorsolateral s. of medulla oblongata,** s. dorsolateralis medullae oblongatae. **dorsolateral s. of spinal cord,** s. dorsolateralis medullae spinalis. **s. dorsolatera'lis medul'lae oblonga'tae** [NA], dorsolateral sulcus of medulla oblongata: an upward extension of the dorsolateral sulcus of the spinal cord; it gives attachment to the fibers of the glossopharyngeal, vagus, and accessory nerves. Called also *posterolateral s.* (or *groove*) *of medulla oblongata, posterior lateral s. of medulla oblongata, s. posterolateralis medullae oblongatae* [NA alternative], and *s. lateralis posterior medullae oblongatae.* **s.**

dorsolatera'lis medul'lae spina'lis [NA], dorsolateral sulcus of spinal cord: a longitudinal sulcus on the dorsolateral surface of the spinal cord; it gives entrance to the dorsal nerve roots and separates the lateral and dorsal funiculi. Called also *posterolateral s.* (or *groove*) *of spinal cord, posterior lateral s. of spinal cord, s. posterolateralis medullae spinalis* [NA alternative], and *s. lateralis posterior medullae spinalis*. **ethmoidal s. of Gegenbaur,** foramen ethmoidale anterius. **ethmoidal s. of nasal bone, s. ethmoida'lis os'sis nasa'lis** [NA], a groove that extends the entire length of the posteromedial surface of the nasal bone and lodges the external nasal branch of the anterior ethmoid nerve. **s. of eustachian tube,** s. tubae auditivae. **frontal s.,** 1. see *s. frontalis inferior* and *s. frontalis superior.* 2. sulcus sinus sagittalis superioris ossis frontalis. **frontal s., inferior,** s. frontalis inferior. **frontal s., superior,** s. frontalis superior. **s. fronta'lis infe'rior** [NA], inferior frontal sulcus: a short longitudinal sulcus that separates the inferior and middle frontal gyri. **s. fronta'lis supe'rior** [NA], superior frontal sulcus: a longitudinal sulcus that separates the middle and superior frontal gyri. **gingival s., s. gingiva'lis** [NA], a shallow V-shaped space around the tooth, bounded by the tooth surface on one side and the epithelium lining the free margin of the gingiva on the other; considered by some authorities to be the same as the gingival crevice and by others to be two separate and distinct entities. **gluteal s., s. glutea'lis** [NA], a curved transverse groove or fold on the back of the upper thigh, separating the upper part of the thigh from the nates; called also *gluteal fold* or *furrow.* **greater palatine s. of maxilla,** s. palatinus major maxillae. **greater palatine s. of palatine bone,** s. palatinus major ossis palatini. **s. of greater petrosal nerve,** s. nervi petrosi majoris. **sulcus of habenula, s. habenu'lae** [NA], **habenular s.,** a groove separating the trigonum habenulae from the upper surface of the thalamus; called also *s. habenularis* [NA alternative]. **s. habenula'ris,** NA alternative for *s. habenulae.* **s. ham'uli pterygoi'dei** [NA], sulcus of pterygoid hamulus: a smooth groove on the lateral surface of the medial pterygoid plate of the sphenoid bone, in the angle at the base of the pterygoid hamulus; it lodges the tendon of the tensor veli palatini muscle. **Harrison's s.,** see under *groove.* **s. hippocam'pi** [NA], the sulcus that extends from the splenium of the corpus callosum almost to the tip of the temporal lobe, and forms the medial boundary of the parahippocampal gyrus; called also *fissura hippocampi* or *hippocampal fissure* and *hippocampal s.* or *s. hippocampalis* [NA alternative]. **s. hippocampa'lis,** NA alternative for *s. hippocampi.* **s. horizonta'lis cerebel'li,** fissura horizontalis cerebelli. **hypothalamic s., s. hypothalam'icus** [NA], **s. hypothalam'icus** [Monro'i], a shallow curved sulcus on the wall of the third ventricle, extending from the interventricular foramen to the cerebral aqueduct. **s. of inferior petrosal sinus of occipital bone,** s. sinus petrosi inferioris ossis occipitalis. **s. of inferior petrosal sinus of temporal bone,** s. sinus petrosi inferioris ossis temporalis. **infraorbital s. of maxilla, s. infraorbita'lis maxil'lae** [NA], a groove in the orbital surface of the maxilla, commencing near the middle of the posterior edge of the surface and running anteriorly for a short distance to become continuous with the infraorbital canal. **infrapalpebral s., s. infrapalpebra'lis** [NA], the furrow below the lower eyelid. **s. of innominate canal,** s. nervi petrosi minoris. **interarticular s. of calcaneus,** s. calcanei. **interarticular s. of talus,** s. tali. **intermediate s. of spinal cord, dorsal,** s. intermedius dorsalis medullae spinalis. **intermediate s. of spinal cord, posterior,** s. intermedius dorsalis medullae spinalis. **s. interme'dius dorsa'lis medul'lae spina'lis** [NA], dorsal intermediate sulcus of spinal cord: a longitudinal sulcus in the cervical and upper thoracic parts of the spinal cord between the fasciculus gracilis and the fasciculus cuneatus. Called also *posterior intermediate* or *posterointermediate s. of spinal cord* and *s. intermedius posterior medullae spinalis* [NA alternative]. **s. interme'dius gastri'cus,** a slight groove in the stomach about 2.5 cm. from the duodenopyloric junction. **s. interme'dius poste'rior medul'lae spina'lis,** NA alternative for *s. intermedius dorsalis medullae spinalis.* **interparietal s., s. interparieta'lis,** s. intraparietalis. **intertubercular s. of humerus, s. intertubercula'ris hu'meri** [NA], a longitudinal groove on the anterior surface of the humerus, lying between the tubercula above

and between the cristae tuberculi farther down, and lodging the tendon of the long head of the biceps muscle. **interventricular s., anterior,** s. interventricularis anterior. **interventricular s., inferior,** s. interventricularis posterior. **interventricular s., posterior,** s. interventricularis posterior. **interventricular s. of heart,** see *s. interventricularis anterior* and *s. interventricularis posterior.* **s. interventricula'ris ante'rior** [NA], anterior interventricular sulcus: a groove on the sternocostal surface of the heart marking the position of the interventricular septum and the line of separation between the ventricles; called also *anterior interventricular groove* and *anterior longitudinal s. of heart.* **s. interventricula'ris cor'dis,** see *s. interventricularis anterior* and *s. interventricularis posterior.* **s. interventricula'ris infe'rior,** s. interventricularis posterior. **s. interventricula'ris poste'rior** [NA], posterior interventricular sulcus: a groove on the diaphragmatic surface of the heart marking the position of the interventricular septum and the line of separation between the ventricles; called also *inferior interventricular groove* or *s., posterior interventricular groove,* and *posterior longitudinal s. of heart.* **intraparietal s., s. intraparieta'lis** [NA], an irregular sulcus on the convex surface of the parietal lobe of the cerebrum and between the inferior and superior parietal lobuli; called also *s. interparietalis* and *Pansch's fissure.* **Jacobson's s.,** 1. sulcus promontorii cavi tympani. 2. sulcus tympanicus ossis temporalis. **labiodental s.,** the arched groove in the embryo which separates off the anterior part of the mandibular process, thus helping to form the lower lip. **lacrimal s. of lacrimal bone,** s. lacrimalis ossis lacrimalis. **lacrimal s. of maxilla,** s. lacrimalis maxillae. **s. lacrima'lis maxil'lae** [NA], lacrimal sulcus of maxilla: a groove directed inferiorly and somewhat posteriorly on the nasal surface of the body of the maxilla, just anterior to the large opening into the maxillary sinus; it is converted into the nasolacrimal canal by the lacrimal bone and inferior nasal concha. **s. lacrima'lis os'sis lacrima'lis** [NA], lacrimal sulcus of lacrimal bone: a deep vertical groove on the anterior part of the lateral surface of the lacrimal bone, which with the maxilla forms the fossa for the lacrimal sac. **lateral s. for lateral sinus of occipital bone,** s. sinus transversi. **lateral s. for lateral sinus of parietal bone,** s. sinus sigmoidei ossis parietalis. **lateral s. of medulla oblongata, anterior,** s. ventrolateralis medullae oblongatae. **lateral s. of medulla oblongata, posterior,** s. dorsolateralis medullae oblongatae. **lateral s. for sigmoidal part of lateral sinus,** s. sinus sigmoidei ossis temporalis. **lateral s. of spinal cord, anterior,** s. ventrolateralis medullae spinalis. **lateral s. of spinal cord, posterior,** s. dorsolateralis medullae spinalis. **s. latera'lis ante'rior medul'lae oblonga'tae,** s. ventrolateralis medullae oblongatae. **s. latera'lis ante'rior medul'lae spina'lis,** s. ventrolateralis medullae spinalis. **s. latera'lis cer'ebri** [NA], lateral cerebral sulcus: a deep cleft beginning at the anterior perforated substance, extending laterally between the temporal and frontal lobes, and turning posteriorly between the temporal and parietal lobes. It divides into posterior, ascending, and anterior branches. Called also *fissure* or *fossa of Sylvius* and *sylvian fissure* or *fossa.* **s. latera'lis mesenceph'ali,** a longitudinal groove on the side of the mesencephalon, separating the crus cerebri from the tegmentum. **s. latera'lis pedun'culi cer'ebri,** s. lateralis mesencephali. **s. latera'lis poste'rior medul'lae oblonga'tae,** s. dorsolateralis medullae oblongatae. **s. latera'lis poste'rior medul'lae spina'lis,** s. dorsolateralis medullae spinalis. **s. of lesser petrosal nerve,** s. nervi petrosi minoris. **s. lim'itans** [NA], a groove midway on the inner surface of each lateral wall of the neural tube, which separates it into a dorsal, alar plate and a ventral, basal plate; called also *s. limitans ventriculorum cerebri.* **s. lim'itans fos'sae rhomboi'deae** [NA], a longitudinal groove on the lateral side of the medial eminence, extending the entire length of the floor of the fourth ventricle. **s. lim'itans in'sulae,** s. circularis insulae. **s. lim'itans ventriculo'rum cer'ebri,** s. limitans. **longitudinal s. of heart,** see *s. interventricularis anterior* and *s. interventricularis posterior.* **lunate s., s. luna'tus** [NA], a small semilunar furrow sometimes seen on the lateral surface of the occipital lobe of the cerebrum; this sulcus is conspicuous in the brain of certain apes and was called by Reidinger *Affenspalte* [Ger. "ape fissure"]. **mallear s. of tem-

poral bone, a groove that runs obliquely downward and forward across the inner aspect of the anterior tympanic ring, which lodges the anterior process of the malleus, chorda tympani, and anterior tympanic artery at birth. Called also *malleolar s. of temporal bone.* **malleolar s. of fibula, s. malleola′ris fib′ulae** [NA], a groove on the posterior surface of the lateral malleolus of the fibula, which lodges the tendons of the peroneal muscles. **malleolar s., of temporal bone,** mallear s. of temporal bone. **malleolar s. of tibia, s. malleola′ris tib′iae** [NA], a short longitudinal groove on the posterior surface of the medial malleolus of the tibia, which lodges the tendons of the posterior tibial muscle and the long flexor muscle of the toes. **mandibular s.,** s. colli mandibulae. **s. of mastoid canaliculus,** s. canaliculi mastoidei. **s. ma′tricis un′guis** [NA], **s. of matrix of nail,** the cutaneous fold in which the proximal part of the nail is embedded. **medial s. of crus cerebri, s. media′lis cru′ris cer′ebri,** s. oculomotorius. **median s. of fourth ventricle,** s. medianus ventriculi quarti. **median s. of medulla oblongata, dorsal,** s. medianus dorsalis medullae oblongatae. **median s. of medulla oblongata, posterior,** s. medianus dorsalis medullae oblongatae. **median s. of spinal cord, dorsal,** s. medianus dorsalis medullae spinalis. **median s. of spinal cord, posterior,** s. medianus dorsalis medullae spinalis. **median s. of tongue, s. media′nus lin′guae** [NA], a shallow groove on the dorsal surface of the tongue in the midline. **s. media′nus dorsa′lis medul′lae oblonga′tae** [NA], dorsal median sulcus of medulla oblongata: a narrow groove present only in the closed part of the medulla oblongata, which is the continuation of the dorsal median sulcus of the spinal cord; it separates the two fasciculi gracili. Called also *dorsal (or posterior) median fissure of medulla oblongata, fissura mediana posterior medullae oblongatae, posterior median s. of medulla oblongata,* and *s. medianus posterior medullae oblongatae* [NA alternative]. **s. media′nus dorsa′lis medul′lae spina′lis** [NA], dorsal median sulcus of spinal cord: a shallow vertical groove on the dorsal surface of the spinal cord in the median place, from which extends the dorsal median septum; it separates the two dorsal funiculi. Called also *dorsal fissure of spinal cord, posterior s. (or fissure) of spinal cord,* and *s. medianus posterior medullae spinalis* [NA alternative]. **s. media′nus poste′rior medul′lae oblonga′tae,** NA alternative for *s. medianus dorsalis medullae oblongatae.* **s. media′nus poste′rior medul′lae spina′lis,** NA alternative for *s. medianus dorsalis medullae spinalis.* **s. media′nus ventric′uli quar′ti** [NA], median sulcus of fourth ventricle: a median groove in the floor of the fourth ventricle. **meningeal sulci,** sulci arteriosi. **mentolabial s., s. mentola′lis** [NA], the depression between the lower lip and the chin. Called also *mentolabial furrow.* **s. mesenceph′ali media′lis,** s. medialis cruris cerebri. **s. of middle temporal artery,** s. arteriae temporalis mediae. **s. of Monro,** s. hypothalamicus. **muscular s. of tympanic cavity,** semicanalis musculi tensoris tympani. **s. mus′culi flexo′ris hal′lucis lon′gi calca′nei,** s. tendinis musculi flexoris hallucis longi calcanei. **s. mus′culi flexo′ris hal′lucis lon′gi ta′li,** s. tendinis musculi flexoris hallucis longi tali. **s. mus′culi perone′i calca′nei,** s. tendinum musculorum peroneorum calcanei. **s. mus′culi perone′i os′sis cuboi′dei,** s. tendinis musculi peronei longi. **s. mus′culi subcla′vii** [NA], sulcus for subclavian muscle: a groove on the inferior surface of the clavicle into which the subclavian muscle is inserted by muscle fibers; called also *subclavian groove.* **mylohyoid s. of mandible, s. mylohyoi′deus mandib′ulae** [NA], a groove on the medial surface of the ramus of the mandible, passing downward and forward from the foramen mandibulae and lodging the mylohyoid artery and nerve. **nasal s., posterior,** meatus nasopharyngeus. **s. of nasal process of maxilla,** s. lacrimalis maxillae. **nasolabial s., s. nasolabia′lis** [NA], the depression between the nose and the upper lip. **s. ner′vi oculomoto′rii,** s. oculomotorius. **s. ner′vi petro′si majo′ris** [NA], sulcus of greater petrosal nerve: a small groove in the floor of the middle cranial fossa, running anteromedially from the hiatus of the facial canal to the foramen lacerum, and lodging the greater petrosal nerve; called also *s. nervi petrosi superficialis majoris.* **s. ner′vi petro′si mino′ris** [NA], sulcus of lesser petrosal nerve: a small groove in the floor of the middle cranial fossa, running

anteromedially just lateral to the sulcus of the greater petrosal nerve, and lodging the lesser petrosal nerve. Called also *s. nervi petrosi superficialis minoris.* **s. ner′vi petro′si superficia′lis majo′ris,** s. nervi petrosi majoris. **s. ner′vi petro′si superficia′lis mino′ris,** s. nervi petrosi minoris. **s. ner′vi radia′lis** [NA], sulcus of radial nerve: a broad oblique groove on the posterior surface of the humerus for the radial nerve and the deep brachial artery; called also *radial groove spiral s.,* and *s. spiralis.* **s. ner′vi spina′lis** [NA], sulcus of spinal nerve: the groove on the upper surface of each transverse process of a cervical vertebra, extending from the foramen transversarium lateralward and separating the anterior and posterior tubercles. It lodges the ventral branch of a cervical nerve. **s. ner′vi ulna′ris** [NA], sulcus of ulnar nerve: a shallow vertical groove on the posterior surface of the medial epicondyle of the humerus for the ulnar nerve; called also *groove of ulnar nerve* or *ulnar groove.* **nymphocaruncular s., nymphohymeneal s.,** a groove between either labium minus and the carunculae hymenales. **obturator s. of pubis, s. obturato′rius os′sis pu′bis** [NA], a groove that obliquely crosses the inferior surface of the superior ramus of the pubis, giving passage to the obturator vessels and nerve. **occipital sulci, lateral,** sulci occipitales laterales. **occipital sulci, superior,** sulci occipitales superiores. **occipital s., transverse,** s. occipitalis transversus. **s. of occipital artery,** s. arteriae occipitalis. **s. occipita′lis ante′rior,** anterior occipital sulcus: a variable, vertically disposed furrow on the convex surface of the cerebrum, which by some is taken as the line of division between the parietal and the occipital lobes. **sul′ci occipita′les latera′les,** lateral occipital sulci: horizontal furrows that divide the lateral occipital gyri into upper and lower portions. **sul′ci occipita′les superio′res,** superior occipital sulci: irregular sulci associated with the superior occipital gyri. **s. occipita′lis transver′sus** [NA], transverse occipital sulcus: a vertical sulcus back of the gyrus angularis, which may help to form the anterior boundary of the occipital lobe or may lie within it. **s. occip′itis,** s. sinus sagittalis superioris ossis occipitalis. **occipitotemporal s., s. occipitotempora′lis** [NA], a longitudinal sulcus on the inferior surface of the temporal lobe that separates the inferior temporal gyrus from the lateral occipitotemporal gyrus; called also *s. temporalis inferior.* **s. oculomoto′rius** [NA], a longitudinal groove on the medial surface of the ventral part of the cerebral peduncle that lodges the oculomotor nerve; called also *medial s. of crus cerebri, s. medialis cruris cerebri,* and *s. nervi oculomotorii.* **s. olfacto′rius lo′bi fronta′lis** [NA], olfactory sulcus of frontal lobe: a straight parasagittal sulcus on the inferior surface of the frontal lobe, lodging the olfactory bulb and tract, and separating the gyrus rectus from the gyri orbitales. **s. olfacto′rius na′si** [NA], olfactory sulcus of nose: a shallow sulcus on the wall of the nasal cavity, passing upward from the level of the anterior end of the middle concha just above the agger nasi to the lamina cribrosa. **olfactory s. of frontal lobe,** s. olfactorius lobi frontalis. **olfactory s. of nose,** s. olfactorius nasi. **optic s.,** s. prechiasmaticus. **orbital sulci of frontal lobe, sul′ci orbita′les lo′bi fronta′lis** [NA], irregular sulci between the orbital gyri of the frontal lobe. **palatine sulci of maxilla, sul′ci palati′ni maxil′lae** [NA], the laterally placed furrows, between the palatine spines on the inferior surface of the hard palate, that lodge the palatine vessels and nerves. **palatinovaginal s., s. palatinovagina′lis** [NA], the groove on the vaginal process of the pterygoid process of the sphenoid bone that participates in formation of the palatinovaginal canal. **s. palati′nus ma′jor maxil′lae** [NA], greater palatine sulcus of maxilla: the sulcus on the nasal surface of the maxilla which, along with the corresponding one on the perpendicular plate of the palatine bone, forms the canal for the greater palatine nerve. **s. palati′nus ma′jor os′sis palati′ni** [NA], greater palatine sulcus of palatine bone: a vertical groove on the maxillary surface of the perpendicular plate of the palatine bone; it articulates with the maxilla to form the canal for the greater palatine nerve; called also *s. pterygopalatinus ossis palatini.* **paracolic sulci, sul′ci paracol′ici** [NA], small, shallow, and variable peritoneal pockets situated lateral to the descending colon; called also *recessus paracolici.* **paraglenoid sulci of hip bone, sul′ci paraglenoida′les os′sis cox′ae,** slight grooves, anterior and inferior to the auricular surface of the ilium, that serve for attachment of the ventral and interosseous sacroiliac ligaments. **parietooccipital s.,** 1. sulcus parietooccipitalis. 2. sulcus intraparietalis. **s. parietooccipita'lis** [NA], parietooccipital sulcus: a sulcus in the medial surface of each cerebral hemisphere, running upward from the calcarine sulcus and marking the boundary between the cuneus and precuneus, and also between the parietal and occipital lobes. Called also *fissura parietooccipitalis*. **s. parolfacto'rius ante'rior,** a sulcus on the medial surface of the cerebral hemisphere, between the area parolfactoria behind and the inferior frontal gyrus in front. **s. parolfacto'rius poste'rior,** a curved sulcus on the medial surface of the cerebral hemisphere, below the splenium of the corpus callosum and between the gyrus paraterminalis and the area parolfactoria. **petrobasilar s.,** s. sinus petrosi inferioris ossis temporalis. **petrosal s. of occipital bone, inferior,** s. sinus petrosi inferioris ossis occipitalis. **petrosal s. of temporal bone, inferior,** s. sinus petrosi inferioris ossis temporalis. **petrosal s. of temporal bone, posterior,** s. sinus petrosi inferioris ossis temporalis. **petrosal s. of temporal bone, superior,** s. sinus petrosi superioris. **s. petro'sus infe'rior os'sis occipita'lis,** s. sinus petrosi inferioris ossis occipitalis. **s. petro'sus infe'rior os'sis tempora'lis,** s. sinus petrosi inferioris ossis temporalis. **s. petro'sus supe'rior os'sis tempora'lis,** s. sinus petrosi superioris. **polar s.,** any of the small fissures which surround the posterior end of the calcarine sulcus. **pontobulbar s.,** the sulcus that separates the pons from the medulla oblongata. **pontopeduncular s.,** the sulcus that separates the pons from the mesencephalon (as represented by the cerebral peduncles). **postcentral s., s. postcentra'lis** [NA], a sulcus on the superolateral surface of the cerebrum, separating the postcentral gyrus from the remainder of the parietal lobe. **postclival s.,** a fissure of the cerebellum between the declive and the folium vermis. **posterointermediate s. of spinal cord,** s. intermedius dorsalis medullae spinalis. **posterolateral s. of medulla oblongata,** s. dorsolateralis medullae oblongatae. **posterolateral s. of spinal cord,** s. dorsolateralis medullae spinalis. **s. posterolatera'lis medul'lae oblonga'tae,** NA alternative for *s. dorsolateralis medullae oblongatae*. **s. posterolatera'lis medul'lae spina'lis,** NA alternative for *s. dorsolateralis medullae spinalis*. **postnodular s.,** a sulcus on the underside of the cerebellum between the nodule and the uvula. **postpyramidal s.,** a sulcus on the underside of the cerebellum between the pyramid and the tuber vermis. **s. praecentra'lis,** s. precentralis. **precentral s., s. precentra'lis** [NA], a vertical sulcus on the convex surface of a cerebral hemisphere, separating the precentral gyrus from the remainder of the frontal lobe. **prechiasmatic s., s. prechiasmat'icus** [NA], **s. prechias'matis,** a furrow on the superior surface of the sphenoid bone, located just anterior to the tuberculum sellae; it lodges the optic chiasm. Called also *chiasmatic s., s. chiasmatis, optic groove,* and *optic s.* **preclival s.,** a fissure of the cerebellum between the culmen and the declive. **prepyramidal s.,** a sulcus on the inferior surface of the cerebellum between the uvula and the pyramid. **prerolandic s.,** s. precentralis. **s. promonto'rii ca'vi tym'pani** [NA], a groove in the surface of the promontory of the tympanic cavity, lodging the tympanic nerve. **s. of pterygoid hamulus,** s. hamuli pterygoidei. **pterygoid s. of pterygoid process,** s. pterygopalatinus processus pterygoidei. **pterygopalatine s. of palatine bone,** s. palatinus major ossis palatini. **pterygopalatine s. of pterygoid process,** s. pterygopalatinus processus pterygoidei. **s. pterygopalati'nus os'sis palati'ni,** s. palatinus major ossis palatini. **s. pterygopalati'nus proces'sus pterygoi'dei** [NA], pterygopalatine sulcus of pterygoid process: a small groove on the inferior surface of the vaginal process of the medial pterygoid plate of the sphenoid bone, forming part of the wall of the vomerovaginal canal. **s. pulmona'lis thora'cis** [NA], **pulmonary s. of thorax,** a large vertical groove in the posterior part of the chest cavity, one on either side of the bodies of the vertebrae posterior to the level of their ventral surface, lodging the posterior, bulky portion of the lung. **radial s. of humerus, s. of radial nerve,** s. nervi radialis. **Reil's s.,** s. circularis insulae. **retrocentral s.,** s. postcentralis. **rhinal s., s. rhina'lis** [NA], a fissure on the inferior surface of the hemisphere, separating the anterior part of the parahippocampal gyrus from the rest of the temporal lobe. **sagittal s.,** s. sinus sagittalis superioris.

s. scle'rae [NA], **scleral s., sclercorneal s.,** the groove at the junction of the sclera and cornea. **s. of semicanal of humerus,** s. intertubercularis humeri. **s. of semicanal of vidian nerve,** s. nervi petrosi majoris. **semilunar s. of radius,** incisura ulnaris radii. **sigmoid s., s. of sigmoid sinus,** s. sinus sigmoidei. **s. of sigmoid sinus of occipital bone,** s. sinus sigmoidei ossis occipitalis. **s. of sigmoid sinus of parietal bone,** s. sinus sigmoidei ossis parietalis. **s. of sigmoid sinus of temporal bone,** s. sinus sigmoidei ossis temporalis. **s. sigmoi'deus os'sis tempora'lis,** s. sinus sigmoidei ossis temporalis. **s. si'nus petro'si inferio'ris os'sis occipita'lis** [NA], sulcus of inferior petrosal sinus of occipital bone: the groove in the floor of the posterior cranial fossa at the line of junction between the basilar part of the occipital and the petrous portion of the temporal bone; it lodges the inferior petrosal sinus. Called also *s. petrosus inferior ossis occipitalis*. **s. si'nus petro'si inferio'ris os'sis tempora'lis** [NA], sulcus of inferior petrosal sinus of temporal bone: a groove on the posteromedial edge of the internal surface of the petrous portion of the temporal bone, which, with a corresponding groove on the adjacent basilar part of the occipital bone, lodges the inferior petrosal sinus. Called also *s. petrosus inferior ossis temporalis*. **s. si'nus petro'si superio'ris** [NA], sulcus of superior petrosal sinus: a small posterolaterally directed sulcus that runs along the internal surface of the petrous part of the temporal bone on the angle separating the posterior and middle cranial fossae; it lodges the superior petrosal sinus. Called also *s. petrosus superior ossis temporalis*. **s. si'nus sagitta'lis supe'rioris** [NA], sulcus for superior sagittal sinus: a groove on the frontal, parietal, and occipital bones that lodges the superior sagittal sinus; called also *sagittal groove* and *sagittal s.* **s. si'nus sigmoi'dei** [NA], sulcus of sigmoid sinus: an S-shaped sulcus beginning on the internal surface of the posteroinferior edge of the parietal bone and continuous with the lateral end of the sulcus of the transverse sinus; it passes onto the internal surface of the mastoid part of the temporal bone, where it bends inferiorly and medially to continue onto the lateral portion of the occipital bone, ending at the jugular foramen. It lodges the sigmoid sinus. **s. si'nus sigmoi'dei os'sis occipita'lis** [NA], sulcus of sigmoid sinus of occipital bone: the portion of the sulcus of the sigmoid sinus found on the occipital bone. **s. si'nus sigmoi'dei os'sis parieta'lis** [NA], sulcus of sigmoid sinus of parietal bone: a short groove on the internal surface of the posteroinferior angle of the parietal bone, continuous with both the sulcus for the sigmoid sinus on the temporal bone and the sulcus for the transverse sinus on the occipital bone; it lodges the superior part of the sigmoid sinus. Called also *s. transversus ossis parietalis*. **s. si'nus sigmoi'dei os'sis tempora'lis** [NA], sulcus of sigmoid sinus of temporal bone: the portion of the sulcus of the sigmoid sinus found on the temporal bone; called also *s. sigmoideus ossis temporalis*. **s. si'nus transver'si** [NA], sulcus of transverse sinus: a wide groove that passes horizontally, lateralward and forward from the internal occipital protuberance to the parietal bone, where it becomes continuous with the sulcus of the sigmoid sinus; it lodges the transverse sinus. Called also *s. transversus ossis occipitalis*. **sulci of skin,** sulci cutis. **s. of spinal nerve,** s. nervi spinalis. **spiral s.,** 1. see *s. spiralis externus* and *s. spiralis internus.* 2. s. nervi radialis. **spiral s., external,** s. spiralis externus. **spiral s., internal,** s. spiralis internus. **spiral s. of humerus,** s. nervi radialis. **s. spira'lis,** 1. see *s. spiralis externus* and *s. spiralis internus.* 2. s. nervi radialis. **s. spira'lis exter'nus** [NA], external spiral sulcus: a concavity within the cochlear duct immediately above the basilar crest. **s. spira'lis inter'nus** [NA], internal spiral sulcus: the C-shaped concavity within the cochlear duct formed by the limbus laminae spiralis and its tympanic and vestibular labia along the edge of the osseous spiral lamina. **s. subcla'viae,** s. arteriae subclaviae. **subclavian s.,** s. arteriae subclaviae. **subclavian s. of lung,** s. subclavius pulmonis. **s. of subclavian artery,** s. arteriae subclaviae. **s. for subclavian muscle,** s. musculi subclavii. **s. of subclavian vein,** s. venae subclaviae. **s. subcla'vius,** s. arteriae subclaviae. **s. subcla'vius pulmo'nis,** subclavian sulcus of lung: a broad, shallow, transverse groove across the top of the lung, lodging the subclavian artery. **subparietal s., s. subparieta'lis** [NA], a sulcus on the medial surface of a cerebral hemisphere, above the splenium of the corpus callosum, separating the precuneus from the cingulate gyrus. **s. of superior petrosal sinus,** s. sinus petrosi superioris. **supra-acetabular s., s. supra-acetabula′ris** [NA], supra-acetabular groove: a sulcus located posterosuperior to the margin of the acetabulum, which is the site of attachment of the reflexed head of the rectus femoris muscle. **supraorbital s.,** foramen supraorbitalis. **suprasplenial s.,** s. subparietalis. **s. Syl′vii,** fossa lateralis cerebri. **s. ta′li** [NA], **s. of talus,** a transverse groove on the inferior surface of the talus, between the medial and the posterior articular surface, which helps to form the sinus tarsi. **temporal s., inferior, temporal s., middle,** s. temporalis inferior [NA]. **temporal s., superior,** s. temporalis superior. **temporal sulci, transverse,** sulci temporales transversi. **temporal s. of temporal bone,** s. arteriae temporalis mediae. **s. tempora′lis infe′rior,** 1. [NA] inferior temporal sulcus: a longitudinal sulcus on the lateral surface of the temporal lobe, separating the middle and the inferior temporal gyri. Formerly called *s. temporalis medius.* 2. sulcus occipitotemporalis. **s. tempora′lis me′dius,** s. temporalis inferior. **s. tempora′lis supe′rior** [NA], superior temporal sulcus: a longitudinal sulcus on the lateral surface of a cerebral hemisphere, passing downward and forward from the gyrus angularis to the temporal pole and separating the superior and the middle temporal gyri. **sul′ci tempora′les transver′si** [NA], transverse temporal sulci: irregularly vertical sulci in the part of the temporal lobe that lies within the lateral sulcus. **s. ten′dinis mus′culi flexo′ris hal′lucis lon′gi calca′nei** [NA], sulcus of tendon of flexor hallucis longus of calcaneus: a groove on the inferior surface of the sustentaculum tali of the calcaneus, lodging the tendon of the flexoris hallucis longus muscle; called also *s. musculi flexoris hallucis longi calcanei.* **s. ten′dinis mus′culi flexo′ris hal′lucis lon′gi ta′li** [NA], sulcus of tendon of flexor hallucis longus of talus: the sagittal groove on the posterior surface of the body of the talus that transmits the tendon of the flexor hallucis longus muscle; called also *s. musculi flexoris hallucis longi tali.* **s. ten′dinis mus′culi perone′i lon′gi** [NA], sulcus of tendon of peroneus longus muscle: a deep groove on the inferior surface of the cuboid bone, which in certain foot positions lodges the tendon of the peroneus longus muscle; called also *s. musculi peronaei ossis cuboidei.* **s. ten′dinum musculo′rum fibula′rium calca′nei,** NA alternative for *s. tendinum musculorum peroneorum calcanei.* **s. ten′dinum musculo′rum peroneo′rum calca′nei** [NA], sulcus of tendons of peroneus muscles: a slight groove on the inferior part of the lateral surface of the calcaneus, lodging the tendons of the peroneus longus and brevis muscles; called also *s. musculi peronaei calcanei.* **s. of tendon of flexor hallucis longus muscle of calcaneus,** s. tendinis musculi flexoris hallucis longi calcanei. **s. of tendon of flexor hallucis longus muscle of talus,** s. tendinis musculi flexoris hallucis longi tali. **s. of tendons of peroneus muscles,** s. tendinum musculorum peroneorum calcanei. **s. of tendon of peroneus longus muscle,** s. tendinis musculi peronei longi. **terminal s. of right atrium,** s. terminalis atrii dextri. **terminal s. of tongue,** s. terminalis linguae. **s. termina′lis a′trii dex′tri** [NA], terminal sulcus of right atrium: a shallow groove on the external surface of the right atrium of the heart between the superior and inferior venae cavae; it represents the junction of the sinus venosus with the primitive atrium in the embryo, and corresponds to a ridge on the internal surface, the crista terminalis. **s. termina′lis lin′guae** [NA], terminal sulcus of tongue: a more or less distinct groove on the tongue, extending from the foramen cecum forward and lateralward to the margin of the tongue on either side, and dividing the dorsum of the tongue from the root. It is marked by a row of vallate papillae. **s. of tongue,** see *s. medianus linguae* and *s. terminalis linguae.* **transverse s. of anthelix,** s. anthelicis transversus. **transverse s. of heart,** s. coronarius cordis. **transverse s. of occipital bone,** s. sinus transversi. **transverse s. of parietal bone,** s. sinus sigmoidei ossis parietalis. **s. of transverse sinus,** s. sinus transversi. **transverse s. of temporal bone,** s. sinus sigmoidei ossis temporalis. **s. transver′sus os′sis occipita′lis,** s. sinus transversi. **s. transver′sus os′sis parieta′lis,** s. sinus sigmoidei ossis parietalis. **s. tu′bae auditi′vae** [NA], **s. tu′bae audito′riae,** sulcus of auditory tube: a groove on the medial part of the base of the spine of the sphenoid bone; it lodges a portion of the cartilaginous part of

the auditory tube. **Turner's s.,** s. intraparietalis. **tympanic s. of temporal bone, s. tympan′icus os′sis tempora′lis** [NA], a narrow groove in the medial part of the external acoustic meatus of the temporal bone, into which the tympanic membrane fits; it is deficient above. **s. of ulnar nerve,** s. nervi ulnaris. **s. of umbilical vein,** s. venae umbilicalis. **sulci for veins,** sulci venosi. **s. of vena cava, s. ve′nae ca′vae** [NA], a groove on the upper part of the posteroinferior surface of the liver, separating the right lobe from the caudate lobe and lodging the inferior vena cava; called also *fossa venae cavae.* **s. ve′nae subcla′viae** [NA], sulcus of subclavian vein: a transverse groove on the cranial surface of the first rib, just anterior to the anterior scalene tubercle; it lodges the subclavian vein. **s. ve′nae umbilica′lis** [NA], sulcus of umbilical vein: the impression on the visceral surface of the liver in the fetus, which lodges the umbilical vein. **sul′ci veno′si** [NA], **venous sulci,** grooves on the internal surfaces of the cranial bones for the meningeal veins; called also *venous grooves.* **s. ventra′lis medul′lae spina′lis,** fissura mediana ventralis medullae spinalis. **ventrolateral s. of spinal cord,** s. ventrolateralis medullae spinalis. **s. ventrolatera′lis medul′lae oblonga′tae** [NA], ventrolateral sulcus of medulla oblongata: a longitudinal sulcus on the ventral surface of the medulla oblongata, lateral to the pyramid, from which emerge the fibers of the hypoglossal nerve. Called also *anterolateral s.* (or groove) *of medulla oblongata, anterior lateral s. of medulla oblongata, s. anterolateralis medullae oblongatae* [NA alternative], and *s. lateralis anterior medullae oblongatae.* **s. ventrolatera′lis medul′lae spina′lis** [NA], ventrolateral sulcus of spinal cord: the longitudinal groove on the ventrolateral surface of the spinal cord, from which the ventral nerve roots emerge; it separates the ventral and lateral funiculi. Called also *anterolateral s.* (or groove) *of spinal cord, anterior lateral s. of spinal cord, s. anterolateralis medullae spinalis* [NA alternative], and *s. lateralis anterior medullae spinalis.* **vermicular s.,** a fissure between the vermis and the hemisphere of the cerebellum. **s. of vertebral artery of atlas,** s. arteriae vertebralis atlantis. **vertical s.,** s. precentralis. **vomeral s., s. vo′meris** [NA], vomeral groove: the cleft in the inferior half on the anterior border of the vomer that receives the inferior border of the septal cartilage of the nose. **vomerovaginal s., s. vomerovagina′lis** [NA], the groove on the vaginal process of the pterygoid process of the sphenoid bone that helps form the vomerovaginal canal. **Waldeyer's s.,** see *s. spiralis externus* and *s. spiralis internus.* **s. of wrist,** s. carpi.

sulfabenzamide (sul″fah-benz′ah-mīd) chemical name: N-[(4-aminophenyl)sulfonyl]benzamide; an antibacterial, $C_{13}H_{12}N_2O_3S$.

sulfacetamide (sul″fah-set′ah-mīd) chemical name: N-sulfanilylacetamide. A sulfonamide, $C_8H_{10}N_2O_3S$, occurring as a white crystalline powder, which has been used in the treatment of urinary tract infections. **s. sodium** [USP], the sodium salt monohydrate of sulfacetamide, $C_8H_9N_2NaO_3S$; applied topically to the conjunctiva in the treatment of sulfonamide-responsive eye infections.

sulfacid (sulf-as′id) thio acid.

sulfacytine (sul″fah-si′tēn) chemical name: 4-amino-N-(1-ethyl-1-2,-dihydro-2-oxo-4-pyrimidinyl)benzenesulfonamide. A short-acting sulfonamide, $C_{12}H_{14}N_4O_3S$, used orally in the treatment of acute urinary tract infections when due to susceptible strains of *Escherichia coli, Klebsiella-Enterobacter* group, *Staphylococcus aureus, Proteus mirabilis,* and *P. vulgaris.*

sulfadiazine (sul″fah-di′ah-zēn) [USP] chemical name: 4-amino-N-2-pyrimidinylbenzenesulfonamide. A sulfonamide, $C_{10}H_{10}N_4O_2S$, occurring as a white or slightly yellow powder; frequently used in combination with other sulfonamides in the treatment of infections due to susceptible organisms, including meningitis caused by *Haemophilus influenzae,* chancroid, acute urinary tract infections, early manifestations of lymphogranuloma venereum, and falciparum malaria caused by chloroquine-resistant plasmodia. It is administered orally. **s. silver,** the silver derivative of sulfadiazine, $C_{10}H_9AgN_4O_2S$, used as a topical antibacterial to prevent wound sepsis in the treatment of second and third degree burns. **s. sodium** [USP], the monosodium salt of sulfadiazine, $C_{10}H_9N_4NaO_2S$, occurring as a white powder, having the same actions and uses as the base; administered subcutaneously and intravenously.

sulfadimethoxine (sul″fah-di″mĕ-thoks′ēn) chemical name: 4-amino-N-(2,6-dimethoxy-4-pyrimidinyl)benzenesulfonamide. A long-acting sulfonamide, $C_{12}H_{14}N_4O_4S$, occurring as an almost white, crystalline powder; used as an antibacterial in a variety of infections, administered orally.

sulfadimetine (sul″fah-di′mĕ-tēn) sulfisomidine.

sulfadimidine (sul″fah-di′mĭ-dēn) sulfamethazine.

sulfadoxine (sul″ ĕn) chemical name: 4-amino-N-(5,6-dimethoxy-4-pyrimidinyl)benzenesulfonamide. A long-acting sulfonamide, $C_{12}H_{14}N_4O_4S$, which has been used in the treatment of leprosy and falciparum malaria.

sulfaethidole (sul″fah-eth′ĭ-dōl) chemical name: 4-amino-N-(5-ethyl-1,3,4-thiadiazol-2-yl)benzenesulfonamide. A short-acting sulfonamide, $C_{10}H_{12}N_4O_2S_2$, occurring as a white to yellowish white, crystalline powder; used principally as a urinary antiseptic, administered orally.

sulfafurazole (sul″fah-fu′rah-zōl) sulfisoxazole.

sulfaguanidine (sul″fah-gwan′ĭ-dēn) chemical name: 4-amino-N-(aminoiminomethyl)benzenesulfonamide. A sulfonamide, $C_7H_{10}N_4O_2S$, occurring as a white to yellowish white, crystalline powder; used as an antibacterial in the treatment of gastrointestinal infections, especially bacillary dysentery, administered orally.

sulfalene (sul′fah-lēn) chemical name: 4-amino-N-(3-methoxypyrazinyl)-benzenesulfonamide. A long-acting sulfonamide, $C_{11}H_{12}N_4O_3S$, used as an antibacterial, especially in the treatment of urinary tract infections.

sulfamerazine (sul″fah-mer′ah-zēn) [USP] chemical name: 4-amino-N-(4-methyl-2-pyrimidinyl)benzenesulfonamide. A readily absorbed antibacterial substance, $C_{11}H_{12}N_4O_2S$, usually used in combination with other sulfonamides. Called also *sulfamethyldiazine*.

sulfameter (sul′fah-me″ter) chemical name: 4-amino-N-(5-methoxy-2-pyrimidinyl)benzenesulfonamide. A long-acting sulfonamide, $C_{11}H_{12}N_4O_3S$, occurring as a fine, white to yellowish-white, powder; used as an antibacterial, especially in the treatment of acute and chronic urinary tract infections, administered orally.

sulfamethazine (sul″fah-meth′ah-zēn) [USP] chemical name: 4-amino-N-(4,6-dimethyl-2-pyrimidinyl)benzenesulfonamide. A sulfonamide, $C_{12}H_{14}N_4O_2S$, occurring as a white to yellowish white powder; used as an antibacterial in a variety of infections, usually, in the United States, in combination with other sulfonamides. It is administered orally. Called also *sulfadimidine*.

sulfamethizole (sul″fah-meth′ĭ-zōl) [USP] chemical name: N^1-(5-methyl-1,3,4-thiadiazol-2-yl)sulfanilamide. A compound, $C_9H_{10}N_4O_2S_2$, occurring as white crystals or powder, used as an antibacterial agent mainly in the treatment of infections of the urinary tract. Called also *sulfamethylthiadiazole*.

sulfamethoxazole (sul″fah-meth-oks′ah-zōl) [USP] chemical name: 4-amino-N-(5-methyl-3-isoxazolyl)benzenesulfonamide. A sulfonamide, $C_{10}H_{11}N_3O_3S$, occurring as a white to off-white, crystalline powder; used as an antibacterial, especially for the prophylaxis and treatment of acute urinary tract infections and of pyodermata and infections of wounds and soft tissues, administered orally.

sulfamethoxypyridazine (sul″fah-meth-ok′se-pi-rid′ah-zēn) chemical name: 4-amino-N-(6-methoxy-3-pyridazinyl)benzenesulfonamide. A compound, $C_{11}H_{12}N_4O_3S$, used as an antibacterial agent in the treatment of infections of the urinary tract and other infections.

sulfamethyldiazine (sul″fah-meth″il-di′ah-zēn) sulfamerazine.

sulfamethylthiadiazole (sul″fah-meth″il-thi″ah-di′ah-zōl) sulfamethizole.

Sulfamezathine (sul″fah-mez′ah-thēn) trademark for a preparation of sulfamethazine.

sulfamido (sul-fam′ĭ-do) one of a group of compounds containing an aminosulfone group, $SO_2 \cdot NH_2$.

sulfamidochrysoidine (sul-fam″ĭ-do-krĭ-soi′dēn) chemical name: p-[(2,4-diaminophenyl)azo] benzenesulfonamide. A compound, $C_{12}H_{13}N_5O_2S$, the hydrochloride salt of which (*Prontosil*) was the forerunner of the sulfonamide drugs.

sulfamine (sul-fam′in) the univalent radical, —SO_2NH_2.

sulfamonomethoxine (sul″fah-mon″o-mĕ-thoks′ēn) chemical name: 4-amino-N-(6-methoxy-4-pyrimidinyl)benzenesulfonamide; an antibacterial sulfonamide, $C_{11}H_{12}N_4O_3S$.

sulfamoxole (sul″fah-moks′ōl) chemical name: 4-amino-N-(4,5-dimethyl-2-oxazolyl)benzenesulfonamide; an antibacterial sulfonamide, $C_{11}H_{13}N_3O_3S$.

Sulfamylon (sul″fah-mi′lon) trademark for preparations of mafenide.

sulfanilamide (sul″fah-nil′ah-mīd) chemical name: p-aminobenzenesulfonamide. A potent antibacterial compound, $NH_2 \cdot C_6H_4 \cdot SO_2NH_2$, the first of the sulfonamides discovered. Formerly used in the treatment of various infections, it has been replaced by more effective and less toxic derivatives, and by antibiotics.

sulfanilate (sulf-an′ĭ-lāt) a salt of sulfanilic acid.

sulfanilic acid (sul″fah-nil′ik) trivial name for p-aminobenzenesulfonic acid.

sulfanitran (sul″fah-ni′tran) chemical name: N-[4-[[(4-nitrophenyl)amino]sulfonyl]phenyl]acetamide; an antibacterial sulfonamide and coccidiostat for poultry, $C_{14}H_{13}N_3O_5S$.

sulfanuria (sulf″ah-nu′re-ah) anuria resulting from the use of sulfonamide drugs.

sulfapyridine (sul″fah-pir′ĭ-dēn) [USP] chemical name: N^1-2-pyridylsulfanilamide. An antibacterial compound, $C_{11}H_{11}N_3O_2S$, occurring as white or faintly yellowish white granules, crystals, or powder; used as an oral suppressant for dermatitis herpetiformis. It was formerly used in the treatment of pneumonia and streptococcal infections.

sulfaquinoxaline (sul″fah-kwin-ok′sah-lēn) chemical name: 4-amino-N-2-quinoxalinylbenzenesulfonamide. An antibacterial sulfonamide, $C_{14}H_{12}N_4S$, used in the treatment of fowl cholera, fowl typhoid, infectious enteritis of swine, shipping dysentery of lambs, and foot rot of cattle, and as a coccidiostat for poultry and an additive to veterinary foodstuffs.

sulfarsphenamine (sulf″ar-sfen′ah-mēn) chemical name: [1,2-diarsenediylbis[(6-hydroxy-3,1-phenylene) imino]]bismethanesulfonic acid disodium salt; an arsenical, $C_{14}H_{14}As_2N_2Na_2O_8S_2$, formerly used as an antisyphilitic.

sulfasalazine (sul″fah-sal′ah-zēn) [USP] chemical name: 2-hydroxy-5-[[4-[(2-pyridinylamino) sulfonyl] phenyl] azo] benzoic acid. An antibacterial sulfonamide derivative, $C_{18}H_{14}N_4O_5S$, occurring as a bright yellow to brownish yellow powder; used orally in the treatment of mild to moderate ulcerative colitis and as adjunctive therapy in severe ulcerative colitis due to susceptible organisms, administered orally. Called also *salazosulfapyridine* and *salicylazosulfapyridine*.

Sulfasuxidine (sul″fah-suk′sĭ-dēn) trademark for preparations of succinylsulfathiazole.

sulfatase (sul′fah-tās) [EC 3.1.6] sulfuric ester hydrolase; one of a sub-subclass of enzymes of the hydrolase class that catalyzes the hydrolysis of an organic sulfate to an alcohol and inorganic sulfate. **multiple s. deficiency,** a lysosomal storage disease, an autosomal recessive trait, combining the infantile form of metachromatic leukodystrophy and a mucopolysaccharidosis; the affected child learns neither to walk nor to talk and shows ichthyosis, coarse facies, hepatosplenomegaly, spinal deformities, and mucopolysacchariduria. Called also *mucosulfatidosis*.

sulfate (sul′fāt) [L. *sulphas*] any salt of sulfuric acid. **acid s.,** one in which only one half of the hydrogen of the sulfuric acid is replaced; a bisulfate. **basic s.,** one in which the normal sulfate of the base is combined with a hydroxide of the same base; a subsulfate. **chondroitin s.,** see *chondroitin*. **conjugated s's,** aromatic substances, such as phenol, scatoxyl, and indoxyl, which occur in the urine along with mineral sulfates. **cupric s.** [USP], the pentahydrate sulfate salt of copper, $CuSO_4 \cdot 5H_2O$, occurring as deep blue, triclinic crystals or as blue crystalline granules or powder, which is a powerful emetic; used orally as an antidote to phosphorus poisoning. Topical application of a 1 per cent solution is used in the treatment of phosphorus burns of the skin. It is also used as a catalyst with iron in the treatment of iron deficiency anemia. In 1:1,000,000 concentration it is used to prevent growth of algae in ponds, reservoirs, and swimming pools. Called also *blue vetriol*, *copper sulfate*, and *bluestone*. **dermatan s.,** chondroitin sulfate B; see *chondroitin*. **ethereal s's,** conjugated s's. **mineral s's,** sulfates in the urine which are combinations of sulfuric acid with mineral substances such as sodium, potassium, calcium, and magnesium. **neutral s., nor-**

mal s., one in which all the hydrogen of the sulfuric acid is replaced. **preformed s's,** mineral s's.

sulfatemia (sul″fāt-e′me-ah) the presence of sulfates in the blood.

Sulfathalidine (sul″fah-thal′ĭ-dēn) trademark for phthalylsulfathiazole.

sulfathiazole (sul″fah-thi′ah-zōl) chemical name: 4-amino-N-2-thiazoylbenzenesulfonamide. A compound, $C_9H_9N_3O_2S_2$, once widely used as an antibacterial agent but replaced by less toxic sulfonamides and antibiotics. Called also *M & B 760* and *norsulfazole.*

sulfatidase (sul-fah-tĭ′dās) arylsulfatase.

sulfatide (sul′fah-tīd) one of a class of cerebroside sulfuric esters; they are found largely in the medullated nerve fibers, and may accumulate in the white matter of the brain in metachromatic leukodystrophy.

sulfazamet (sul-faz′ah-met) chemical name: 4-amino-N-(3-methyl-1-phenyl-1H-pyrazel-5-yl)benzenesulfonamide; an antibacterial sulfonamide for use in veterinary medicine, $C_{16}H_{16}N_4O_2S$.

sulfhemoglobin (sulf″he-mo-glo′bin) sulfmethemoglobin.

sulfhemoglobinemia (sulf″he-mo-glo″bin-e′me-ah) the presence of sulfmethemoglobin in the blood.

sulfhydrate (sulf-hi′drāt) the HS⁻ anion or a salt containing this ion.

sulfhydryl (sulf-hi′dril) the univalent radical, —SH.

sulfide (sul′fīd) any binary compound of sulfur; a compound of sulfur with another element or radical or base. **mercuric s.,** a brilliant scarlet powder, HgS, formerly used in the treatment of syphilis.

sulfindigotate (sul-fin′dĭ-go-tāt) any salt of sulfindigotic acid.

sulfinic acid (sul-fin′ik) an organic compound containing an —SO₂H group bonded to a carbon atom.

sulfinpyrazone (sul″fin-pi′rah-zōn) [USP] chemical name: 1,2-diphenyl-4-[2-(phenylsulfinyl)ethyl]3,5-pyrazolidinedione. A sulfoxide analogue of phenybutazone, $C_{23}H_{20}N_2O_3S$, used as a uricosuric agent in treatment of gout; administered orally. It also prolongs platelet survival and inhibits platelet adherence to subendothelial cells and prostaglandin synthesis and has been studied as an antithrombotic agent.

sulfinyl (sul′fĭ-nil) the bivalent radical, —SO—.

sulfisomidine (sul-fĭ-som′ĭ-dēn) chemical name: 4-amino-N-(2,6-dimethyl-4-pyrimidinyl)benzenesulfonamide. A structural isomer of sulfamethazine, used as an antibacterial agent in the treatment of systemic and urinary tract infections. Called also *sulfadimetine.*

sulfisoxazole (sul″fĭ-sok′sah-zōl) [USP] chemical name: 4-amino-N-(3,4-dimethyl-5-isoxazolyl)benzenesulfonamide. A short-acting sulfonamide, $C_{11}H_{13}N_3O_3S$, occurring as a white to slightly yellowish, crystalline powder; used as an antibacterial in the treatment of a wide variety of infections, administered orally. Called also *sulfafurazole.* **s. acetyl** [USP], chemical name: N-[(4-aminophenyl)sulfonyl]-N-(3,4-dimethyl-5-isoxazolyl)acetamide. A tasteless derivative of sulfisoxazole, $C_{13}H_{15}N_3O_4S$, having the same actions and uses as the base; usually used in infants and children; administered orally. **s. diolamine** [USP], the diethanolamine salt of sulfisoxazole, $C_{11}H_{13}N_3O_3S \cdot C_4H_{11}NO_2$, having the same actions and uses as the base; administered intramuscularly and intravenously. It is also used in the topical treatment of susceptible eye infections.

sulfite (sul′fīt) [L. *sulfis*] any salt of sulfurous acid.

sulfite oxidase (sul′fīt ok/sĭ-dās) [EC 1.8.3.1] an enzyme of the oxidoreductase class that catalyzes the reaction sulfite + 2 cytochrome c + H₂O = sulfate + 2 reduced cytochrome c. The enzyme is a mitochondrial molybdohemoprotein important in brain function. Congenital deficiency of the enzyme causes severe neurological impairment.

sulfmethemoglobin (sulf″met-he″mo-glo′bin) a greenish substance formed by treating blood with hydrogen sulfide or by the absorption of this gas from the intestinal tract; it is the cause of the greenish color seen in the abdominal walls and along the vessels of cadavers. Called also *sulfhemoglobin.*

sulf(o)- a prefix used in naming chemical compounds, indicating the presence of divalent sulfur or of the group SO₂OH.

sulfoacid (sul″fo-as′id) sulfonic acid.

sulfobromophthalein (sul″fo-bro″mo-thal′e-in) chemical name: 3,3′-(tetrabromophthalidylidene) bis[6-hydroxybenzenesulfonate]. Its disodium salt [USP], a white odorless crystalline powder, $C_{20}H_8Br_4Na_2O_{10}S_2$, is soluble in water and is used as a hepatic function determinant.

sulfoconjugation (sul″fo-kon″ju-ga′shun) the formation of conjugated sulfates.

sulfocyanate (sul″fo-si′ah-nāt) thiocyanate.

sulfocyanic acid (sul″fo-si-an′ic) thiocyanic acid.

sulfogel (sul′fo-jel) a gel in which sulfuric acid is the medium instead of water.

N-sulfoglucosamine sulfohydrolase (sul″fo-gloo-kōs′ah-mēn sul″fo-hi′dro-lās) [EC 3.10.1.1] an enzyme of the hydrolase class that catalyzes the reaction N-sulfo-D-glucosamine + H₂O = D-glucosamine + sulfate. The enzyme may be identical with the heparan N-sulfatase that catalyzes the hydrolysis of glucosamine sulfate units in heparan, the absence of which causes Sanfilippo syndrome, type A.

sulfohydrate (sul″fo-hi′drāt) sulfhydrate.

sulfoiduronate sulfatase (sul″fo-id″u-ron′āt sul′fa-tās) iduronate sulfatase.

sulfolipid (sul″fo-lip′id) a lipid which on hydrolysis yields sulfuric acid.

sulfolithocholylglycine (sul″fo-lith″o-ko″lil-gli′sēn) a bile salt, the sulfate ester at C-3 of lithocholylglycine.

sulfolithocholyltaurine (sul″fo-lith″o-ko″lil-taw′rēn) a bile salt, the sulfate ester at C-3 of lithocholyltaurine.

Sulfolobus (sul″fo-lo′bus) [sulfo- + L. *lobus* lobe] a genus of gram-negative chemolithotrophic bacteria of uncertain affiliation, occurring as spherical cells with lobes, that use elemental sulfur as an energy source and have a temperature optimum at 70 to 75° C. They are considered to be members of the archaeobacteria because they lack peptidoglycan in their cell walls and differ from other bacteria in ribosomal RNA and cell lipid structures. They are found in hot acid soils and water. The type species is *S. acidocalda′rius.*

sulfolysis (sul-fol′ĭ-sis) [sulfo- + Gr. *lysis* dissolution] a double decomposition, similar to hydrolysis, but in which sulfuric acid takes the place of water.

sulfomucin (sul″fo-mu′sin) a glucoprotein found in cartilage, cornea, and gastrointestinal mucosa, which contains sulfuric acid, uronic acid, and chondrosamine or glucosamine.

sulfonamide (sul-fon′ah-mīd) the chemical group SO₂-NH₂. The sulfonamides, or sulfa drugs, are derivatives of sulfanilamide, which competitively inhibit folic acid synthesis in microorganisms, and are bacteriostatic against gram-positive cocci (streptococci and pneumococci), gram-negative cocci (meningococci and gonococci), gram-negative bacilli (*Escherichia coli* and shigellae), and a wide variety of other bacteria. Sulfonamides have been largely supplanted by more effective and less toxic antibiotics.

sulfonamidemia (sul″fon-am″ĭ-de′me-ah) the presence of a sulfonamide compound in the blood.

sulfonamidocholia (sul″fon-am″ĭ-do-ko′le-ah) the presence of a sulfonamide compound in the bile.

sulfonamidotherapy (sul″fon-am″ĭ-do-ther′ah-pe) treatment with sulfonamide compounds.

sulfonamiduria (sul″fon-am″ĭ-du′re-ah) the presence of a sulfonamide compound in the urine.

sulfonate (sul′fo-nāt) a salt, ester, or anion of a sulfonic acid.

sulfone (sul′fōn) 1. the radical SO₂. 2. any compound containing two hydrocarbon radicals attached to the radical SO₂, especially dapsone (4,4′-sulfonylbisbenzenamine) and its derivatives, which are potent antibacterials effective against many gram-positive and gram-negative organisms, and are widely used as leprostatics. **Angeli's s.,** glucosulfone sodium.

sulfonethylmethane (sul″fon-eth″il-meth′ān) chemical name: 2,2-bis(ethylsulfonyl)butane; a hypnotic, $C_8H_{18}O_4S_2$.

sulfonic (sul-fon′ik) indicating chemical compounds containing the monovalent —SO₂OH or —SO₃H radical.

sulfonic acid (sul-fon′ik) an organic compound containing an S—SO₃H group bonded to a carbon atom.

sulfonmethane (sul″fon-meth′ān) chemical name: 2,2-bis(ethylsulfonyl)propane. A white, crystalline compound, $(CH_3)_2C(SO_2C_2H_5)_2$, readily soluble in alcohol and slowly in

100 parts of water. It has moderate hypnotic properties, and was formerly used in insomnia of functional origin.

Sulfonsol (sul-fon′sol) trademark for trisulfapyrimidines oral suspension; see under *suspension.*

sulfonterol hydrochloride (sul-fon′ter-ōl) chemical name: α-[[(1,1-dimethylethyl)amino]methyl]-4-hydroxy-3-[(methylsulfonyl)methyl]benzenemethanol hydrochloride; a bronchodilator, $C_{14}H_{23}NO_4S \cdot HCl$.

sulfonyl (sul′fo-nil) the bivalent radical, —SO_2—.

sulfoprotein (sul″fo-pro′te-in) any of a series of albumins containing loosely combined sulfur.

sulfosalicylic acid (sul″fo-sal″ĭ-sil′ik) 3-carboxy-4-hydroxybenzenesulfonic acid, a protein precipitant used in qualitative tests for protein in urine and cerebrospinal fluid. Called also *salicylsulfonic acid.*

sulfosalt (sul′fo-sawlt) a salt of sulfonic acid.

Sulfose (sul′fōs) trademark for preparations of trisulfapyrimidines.

sulfosol (sul′fo-sol) a sol in which sulfuric acid is the dispersion medium.

sulfotransferase (sul″fo-trans′fer-ās) [EC 2.8.2] a subsubclass of enzymes of the transferase class that transfers a sulfate group.

sulfoxide (sul-fok′sīd) 1. the bivalent radical =SO. 2. any member of a group of compounds intermediate between the sulfides and the sulfones.

sulfoxism (sul-fok′sizm) sulfuric acid poisoning.

sulfoxone sodium (sul-foks′on) [USP] chemical name: [sulfonylbis(1,4-phenyleneimino)]bismethanesulfinic acid disodium salt. An antibacterial derivative of dapsone, $C_{14}H_{14}N_2Na_2O_6S_3$, having actions similar to those of the parent compound, occurring as a white to pale yellow powder; used primarily as a leprostatic in the treatment of lepromatous and tuberculoid leprosy, administered orally.

sulfur (sul′fur), gen. *sul′furis* [L.] a nonmetallic element existing in many allotropic forms; symbol, S; atomic number, 16; atomic weight, 32.064. It occurs in protein, being a constituent of the amino acids cysteine and methionine. Sulfur is a laxative and diaphoretic and is used in diseases of the skin and formerly in the treatment of a wide variety of diseases. **colloidal s.,** sulfur in a state of extremely fine division; milk of sulfur. **s. dioxide** [NF], a colorless, nonflammable gas, SO_2, having a strong, suffocating odor; used as an antioxidant in pharmaceutical preparations. Dry sulfur dioxide is often used to kill fleas, mosquitoes, flies, rats, and other vermin. Called also *sulfurous anhydride.* **flower of s.,** sublimed s. **hepar s.,** sulfurated potash. **s. hydride,** H_2S, a poisonous gas having the smell of rotten eggs. **s. iodide,** a binary compound, S_2I_2, which has been used externally in the treatment of various diseases of the skin, and, internally, in the treatment of human glanders. **lac s.,** precipitated s. **liver of s.,** sulfurated potash. **s. lo′tum,** washed s. **milk of s.,** sulfur in a state of extremely fine division; colloidal sulfur. **s. monochloride,** a lacrimating war gas, S_2Cl_2. **precipitated s.** [USP], a very fine, pale yellow, amorphous or microcrystalline powder, containing not less than 99.5 per cent sulfur, obtained by adding acid to a solution containing a polysulfide and a thiosulfate; used topically as a scabicide, and also used in various dermatologic formulations for its antiparasitic, antifungal, and keratolytic effects. Called also *lac sulfuris* and *milk of sulfur.* **radioactive s.,** radiosulfur. **roll s.,** sulfur melted and cast in the form of rods or cylinders. **sublimed s.** [USP], a fine yellow powder, containing not less than 99.5 per cent sulfur, obtained by subliming elemental sulfur and condensing the vapor. It is used topically as a scabicide and parasiticide. Called also *flores sulfuris* and *flowers of sulfur.* **vegetable s.,** lycopodium. **washed s.,** sublimed sulfur purified by washing with water.

sulfuraria (sul″fu-ra′re-ah) a yellow powder, the sediment from certain springs in Italy, said to contain sulfur, calcium sulfide, strontium sulfate, silica, etc.; used in skin diseases.

sulfurated, sulfureted (sul′fu-rāt″ed; sul′fu-ret″ed) combined or charged with sulfur.

sulfurator (sul′fu-ra″tor) an apparatus for applying fumes of sulfur dioxide, used for disinfecting.

sulfuret (sul′fu-ret) sulfide.

sulfuric acid (sul-fūr′ik) a strong mineral acid, H_2SO_4, that is a strong oxidizing agent and is extremely corrosive to skin and mucous membranes; concentrated sulfuric acid can cause severe skin burns.

sulfurize (sul′fu-rīz) to cause to combine with sulfur.

sulfurous acid (sul-fūr-us) the chemical species H_2SO_3, which is formed in aqueous solutions of sulfur dioxide, SO_2; its salts are sulfites.

sulfurtransferase (sul″fur-trans′fer-ās) [EC 2.8.1] a subsubclass of enzymes of the transferase class that transfers sulfur atoms.

sulfuryl (sul′fu-ril) the radical SO_2.

sulfydryl (sul-fi′dril) sulfhydryl.

sulindac (sul-in′dak) [USP] chemical name: (Z)-5-fluoro-2-methyl-1-[[4-(methylsulfinyl)phenyl]methylene]-1H-indene-3-acetic acid; a nonsteroidal anti-inflammatory, analgesic, and antipyretic, $C_{20}H_{17}FO_3S$, used in the treatment of osteoarthritis, rheumatoid arthritis, ankylosing spondylitis, acute painful shoulder, and acute gouty arthritis.

sulisobenzone (sul″ĭ-so-ben′zōn) chemical name: 5-benzoyl-4-hydroxy-2-methoxybenzenesulfonic acid; an ultraviolet screen, $C_{14}H_{12}O_6S$.

Sulkowitch's test (sul′ko-wich″ez) [Hirsh Wolf *Sulkowitch,* American physician, born 1906] see under *tests.*

Sulla (sul′ah) trademark for a preparation of sulfameter.

sullage (sul′ij) sewage.

Sullivan's test (sul′ĭ-vanz) [Michael Xavier *Sullivan,* American physician, born 1875] see under *tests.*

sulnidazole (sul-nĭd′ah-zōl) chemical name: [2-(2-ethyl-5-nitro-1H-imidazol-1-yl)ethyl]carbamothioic acid O-methyl ester; an antiprotozoal, $C_9H_{14}N_4O_3S$, effective against *Trichomonas.*

suloctidil (sul-ok′tĭ-dil) chemical name: (R*,S*)-4-[(1-methylethyl)thio]-α-[1-(octylamino)ethyl]benzenemethanol; a peripheral vasodilator, $C_{20}H_{35}NOS$.

suloxifen oxalate (sul-ok′sĭ-fen) chemical name: N-[2-(diethylamino)ethyl]-S,S-diphenylsulfoximine ethanedioate (1:1); a bronchodilator, $C_{18}H_{24}N_2OS \cdot C_2H_2O_4$.

sulph- for words beginning thus, see those beginning *sulf-.*

sulpiride (sul′pĭ-rīd) chemical name: N-[(1-ethyl-2-pyrrolidinyl)methyl]-5-sulfamoyl-o-anisamide; an antidepressant, $C_{15}H_{23}N_3O_4S$.

sulprostone (sul-pros′tōn) chemical name: [1R-[1α(Z),-2β(1E,3R*),3α]]-7-[3-hydroxy-2-(3-hydroxy-4-phenoxy-1-butenyl)-5-oxocyclopentyl]-N-(methylsulfonyl)-heptenamide; a prostaglandin, $C_{23}H_{31}NO_7S$.

Sul-Spansion (sul-span′shun) trademark for a preparation of sulfaethidole.

sulthiame (sul-thi′ām) chemical name: 4-(tetrahydro-2H-1,2-thiazin-2-yl)benzenesulfonamide S,S-dioxide. A carbonic anhydrase inhibitor, $C_{10}H_{14}N_2O_4S_2$, used as an anticonvulsant in the treatment of all forms of epilepsy except petit mal.

Sulzberger-Garbe syndrome (sulz-ber′ger gar′be) [Marion Baldur *Sulzberger,* American dermatologist, born 1895; William *Garbe,* Canadian dermatologist, born 1908] exudative discoid and lichenoid dermatitis.

sum. abbreviation for L. *su′mat,* let him take; or *sumen′dum,* to be taken.

sumac (soo′mak) a name of various species of *Rhus,* applied principally to the nonpoisonous species. **poison s., swamp s.,** a species, *R. vernix,* usually found in swamps, which causes an itching rash on contact with the skin.

summation (sum-ma′shun) [L. *summa* total] the accumulative effects of a number of stimuli applied to a muscle, nerve, or reflex arc. **central s.,** the condition in which successive subliminal stimuli accumulate in a reflex center until they finally produce a reflex discharge.

summit (sum′it) [L. *summus,* superlative of *superus*] the highest point. **s. of bladder,** apex vesicae urinariae. **s. of nose,** radix nasi.

Sumner (sum′ner) James Batcheller, 1887–1955; co-winner, with Wendell Meredith Stanley and John Howard Northrop, of the Nobel prize for chemistry in 1946 for isolating and crystallizing an enzyme, urease, and showing it to be a protein.

Sumner's method, reagent (sum′nerz) [James Batcheller *Sumner*] see under *method* and *reagent.*

Sumner's sign (sum′nerz) [F.W. *Sumner,* British surgeon] see under *sign.*

Sumycin (soo-mi′sin) trademark for preparations of tetracycline hydrochloride.

sunburn (sun′bern) injury to the skin, with erythema, tenderness, and sometimes blistering, following excessive exposure to sunlight, and produced by ultraviolet rays, which are not filtered out by clouds or water.

suncillin sodium (sun-sil′in) chemical name: 3,3-dimethyl-7-oxo-6-[2-phenyl-D-2-(sulfoamino)acetamido]-4-thia-1-azabicyclo[3.2.0]heptane-2-carboxylic acid disodium salt; an antibacterial, $C_{16}H_{17}N_3Na_2O_7S_2$.

SunDare (sun′dār) trademark for preparations of cinoxate.

sunstroke (sun′strōk) insolation, or thermic fever; a condition produced by exposure to the sun, and marked by convulsions, coma, and a high temperature of the skin. Cf. *heat exhaustion* and *heat stroke*.

super- [L. *super* above] a prefix meaning above, more than normal, excessive, or next above in rank. Cf. *hyper-*.

superabduction (soo″per-ab-duk′shun) extreme or excessive abduction.

superacid (soo″per-as′id) excessively acid.

superacidity (soo″per-ah-sid′ĭ-te) excessive acidity.

superacromial (soo″per-ah-kro′me-al) supra-acromial.

superactivity (soo″per-ak-tiv′ĭ-te) activity greater than normal; hyperactivity.

superacute (soo″per-ah-kūt′) extremely acute.

superalimentation (soo″per-al″ĭ-men-ta′shun) therapeutic treatment by excessive feeding beyond the requirements of the appetite: employed in wasting diseases; called also *gavage*.

superalkalinity (soo″per-al″kah-lin′ĭ-te) excessive alkalinity.

superaurale (soo″per-aw-ra′le) an anthropometric landmark, the highest point on the superior border of the helix of the ear.

supercarbonate (soo″per-kar′bon-āt) bicarbonate.

supercentral (soo″per-sen′tral) above a center.

supercilia (soo″per-sil′e-ah) [L., pl. of *supercilium*] [NA] the hairs growing on the transverse elevation at the junction of the forehead and the upper lid of either eye; called also *eyebrow*.

superciliary (soo″per-sil′e-a-re) pertaining to the eyebrow.

supercilium (soo″per-sil′e-um), pl. *superci′lia* [L.] [NA] the transverse elevation at the junction of the forehead and the upper eyelid; see *eyebrow* (def. 1), and see also *supercilia*.

superclass (su′per-klas) a taxonomic category sometimes established, subordinate to a phylum and superior to a class.

supercoil (su′per-koil) a shape assumed by chromosomes when they have attained their maximum length during interphase, resembling a "zig-zag" pattern with broad turns.

superdistention (soo″per-dis-ten′shun) excessive distention.

superduct (soo″per-dukt′) [*super-* + L. *ducere* to draw] to carry up or elevate.

superduction (soo″per-duk′shun) supraduction.

superego (soo″per-e′go) [*super-* + *ego*] in psychoanalytic theory, the aspect of the personality acting as a monitor and evaluator of ego functioning, comparing it with ideal standard (see *ego ideal*, under *ideal*) and including psychic functions expressed as social attitudes, self-criticism, and a concept of right and wrong (conscience or morality). Cf. *ego* and *id* (def. 2).

superexcitation (soo″per-ek″si-ta′shun) [*super-* + L. *excitatio* excitement] extreme or excessive excitement.

superextended (soo″per-eks-tend′ed) extended beyond the normal.

superextension (soo″per-eks-ten′shun) excessive extension.

superfamily (soo″per-fam′ĭ-le) a taxonomic category sometimes established, subordinate to an order and superior to a family.

superfecundation (soo″per-fe″kun-da′shun) [*super-* + L. *fecundare* to fertilize] fertilization of two or more ova during the same ovulatory cycle by separate coital acts.

superfetation (soo″per-fe-ta′shun) [*super-* + *fetus*] the fertilization and subsequent development of an ovum when a fetus is already present in the uterus, a result of fertilization of ova during different ovulatory cycles and yielding fetuses of different ages.

superficial (soo″per-fish′al) [L. *superficialis*] pertaining to or situated near the surface.

superficialis (soo″per-fish″e-a′lis) superficial; [NA] a term used to designate a structure situated closer than another to the surface of the body.

superficies (soo″per-fish′e-ēz) [L.] an outer surface.

superflexion (soo″per-flek′shun) extreme or excessive flexion.

superfunction (soo″per-funk′shun) excessive activity of an organ or structure; hyperfunction.

supergenual (soo″per-jen′u-al) above the knee.

superimpregnation (soo″per-im″preg-na′shun) [*super-* + *impregnation*] superfetation.

superinduce (soo″per-in-dūs′) to induce or bring on in addition to some already existing condition.

superinfection (soo″per-in-fek′shun) a new infection complicating the course of antimicrobial therapy of an existing infectious process, and resulting from invasion by bacteria or fungi resistant to the drug(s) in use. It may occur at the site of the original infection or at a remote site.

superinvolution (soo″per-in″vo-lu′shun) prolonged involution of the uterus after delivery, to a size much smaller than the normal, occurring in nursing mothers. Called also *hyperinvolution*.

superior (soo-pe′re-or) [L. "upper"; neut. *superius*] situated above, or directed upward; [NA] a term used in reference to a structure occupying a position nearer the vertex.

superjacent (soo″per-ja′sent) located immediately above; overlying.

superlactation (soo″per-lak-ta′shun) hyperlactation.

superlethal (soo″per-le′thal) more than sufficient to cause death.

supermaxilla (soo″per-mak-sil′ah) the maxilla.

supermedial (soo″per-me′de-al) situated above the middle.

supermotility (soo″per-mo-til′ĭ-te) excessive motility.

supernatant (soo″per-na′tant) [*super-* + L. *natare* to swim] 1. situated above or on top of something. 2. the overlying liquid after precipitation of a solid component of a system.

supernate (soo′per-nāt) supernatant, def. 2.

supernormal (soo″per-nor′mal) more than normal.

supernumerary (soo″per-nu′mer-ar″e) [L. *supernumerarius*] in excess of the regular or normal number.

supernutrition (soo″per-nu-trish′un) excessive nutrition.

superoccipital (soo″per-ok-sip′ĭ-tal) supraoccipital.

superolateral (soo″per-o-lat′er-al) above and at the side.

superovulation (soo″per-ov″u-la′shun) extraordinary acceleration of ovulation.

superoxide (soo″per-ok′sīd) any compound containing the highly reactive superoxide radical, O_2^-, which is produced by reduction of molecular oxygen in many biological oxidations; this highly toxic free radical is continuously removed by the enzyme superoxide dismutase.

superoxide dismutase (soo″per-ok′sīd dis-mu′tas) [EC 1.5.1.1] an enzyme of the oxidoreductase class that catalyzes the reaction O_2^- (superoxide) + O_2^- (superoxide) + 2 H^+ = O_2 + H_2O_2. The enzyme protects cells against dangerous levels of superoxide.

superparasite (soo″per-par′ah-sīt) 1. a parasite involved in superparasitism. 2. hyperparasite.

superparasitism (soo″per-par′ah-si″tizm) 1. infestation with more parasites of one species than the host can support or bring to maturity. 2. hyperparasitic.

superphosphate (soo″per-fos′fāt) any acid phosphate, especially calcium superphosphate (see *calcium phosphate, monobasic*).

super-regeneration (soo″per-re-jen″ĕ-ra′shun) the development of superfluous tissue, organs, or parts as a result of regeneration.

supersalt (soo′per-sawlt) any salt obtained by reaction with an excess of acid; a persalt or acid salt.

supersaturate (soo″per-sat′u-rāt) to add more of an ingredient than can be held in solution permanently.

superscription (soo″per-skrip′shun) [L. *superscriptio*]   the sign ℞ before a prescription; see *prescription*.

supersecretion (soo″per-se-kre′shun)   excessive secretion.

supersedent (soo″per-se′dent)   a remedy which cures or prevents a disease in a part.

supersensitivity (soo″per-sen″sĭ-tiv′ĭ-te)   abnormally increased sensitivity.   **disuse s.,** increased activity of a neural pathway following chronic exposure to an antagonist drug caused by changes in postsynaptic receptors.

supersensitization (soo″per-sen″sĭ-ti-za′shun)   hypersensitization.

supersoft (soo″per-soft′)   extremely soft; applied to roentgen rays of extremely long wavelengths, large absorption coefficients, and low penetrating power.

supersonic (soo″per-son′ik) [*super-* + L. *sonus* sound]   1. having a speed greater than the velocity of sound, that is, faster than approximately one-fifth mile per second (or 720 miles an hour) in air.   2. ultrasonic.

supersonics (soo″per-son′iks)   the general science relating to phenomena associated with speed greater than the velocity of sound (as in case of aircraft and projectiles traveling faster than sound).

supersphenoid (soo″per-sfe′noid)   above the sphenoid bone.

superstructure (soo″per-struk′chur)   1. any structure built on something else.   2. the overlying or visible portion of a structure.   3. implant s.   **implant s.,** a removable denture retained, supported, and stabilized by an abutment post protruding from the substructure of an implanted framework.

supervascularization (soo″per-vas″ku-lar-i-za′shun)   in radiotherapy, the relative increase in vascularity that occurs when tumor cells are destroyed so that the remaining tumor cells are better supplied by the (uninjured) capillary stroma.

supervenosity (soo″per-ve-nos′ĭ-te)   an abnormally diminished level of oxygen in venous blood.

supervention (soo″per-ven′shun)   the development of some condition in addition to an already existing one.

superversion (soo″per-ver′zhun)   sursumversion.

supervisor (soo′per-viz″er)   an individual who oversees the activities of others, such as a nurse who oversees the nursing activities in a specific ward or department of a hospital.

supervitaminosis (soo″per-vi″tah-min-o′sis)   hypervitaminosis.

supervoltage (soo′per-vol″tij)   very high voltage. In x-ray therapy, it is generally considered to be voltage in the range of 500 kilovolts, as contrasted with orthovoltage (140 to 400 kilovolts) and with megavoltage (greater than 1 megavolt).

supinate (soo′pĭ-nāt)   to assume or place in a supine position.

supination (soo″pĭ-na′shun) [L. *supinatio*]   the act of assuming the supine position, or the state of being supine. Applied to the hand, the act of turning the palm forward (anteriorly) or upward, performed by lateral rotation of the forearm. Applied to the foot, it generally implies movements resulting in raising of the medial margin of the foot, hence of the longitudinal arch. Cf. *pronation*.

supine (soo′pīn) [L. *supinus* lying on the back, face upward]   lying with the face upward; see also *supination*.

suppedania (sup″ĕ-da′ne-ah) [L. *sub* under + *pes* foot]   local applications to the soles of the feet.

supplemental (sup″lĕ-men′tal)   serving as a supplement or addition.

support (sup-port′)   1. a device or appliance that helps maintain a part or structure.   2. the foundation upon which a denture rests.

suppository (sup-poz′ĭ-to-re) [L. *suppositorium*]   a medicated mass adapted for introduction into the rectal, vaginal, or urethral orifice of the body; suppository bases are solid at room temperature but melt or dissolve at body temperature. Commonly used bases are cocoa butter, glycerinated gelatin, hydrogenated vegetable oils, polyethylene glycols of various molecular weights, and fatty acid esters of polyethylene glycol.   **glycerin s.** [NF]   a suppository made up of a mixture of glycerin and sodium stearate; used as a rectal evacuant.

suppressant (sŭ-pres′sant)   1. inducing suppression.   2. an agent that stops secretion, excretion, or normal discharge.

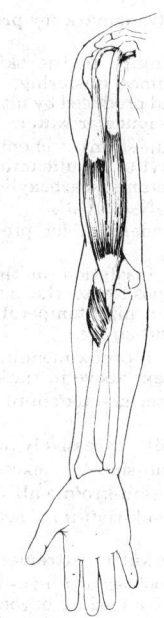

Supinators contracted; forearm, hand supinated.

suppression (sŭ-presh′un) [L. *suppressio*]   the sudden stoppage of a secretion, excretion, or normal discharge.   2. in psychiatry, conscious inhibition of an unacceptable impulse or idea as contrasted with repression, which is unconscious.   3. in genetics, a second mutation occurring at a site different from the first mutation site and able to mask or suppress the phenotypic expression of the first mutation; the organism appears to be reverted but is in fact doubly mutant. Called also *suppressor mutation*. See also *reversion*, def. 2.

suppurant (sup′u-rant) [L. *suppurans*]   1. characterized by suppuration.   2. an agent that causes suppuration.

suppurantia (sup′u-ran′she-ah)   substances that cause suppuration.

suppuration (sup″u-ra′shun) [L. *sub* under + *puris* pus]   the formation of pus; the act of becoming converted into and discharging pus.   **alveodental s.,** periodontitis with the formation of pus.

suppurative (sup′u-ra″tiv)   producing pus, or associated with suppuration.

supra- [L. "above"]   a prefix signifying above or over.

supra-acromial (soo″prah-ah-kro′me-al)   situated above or over the acromion.

supra-anal (soo-prah-a′nal)   situated above the anus.

supra-auricular (soo″prah-aw-rik′u-lar)   situated above the ear.

supra-axillary (soo″prah-ak′sĭ-ler″e)   situated above the axilla.

suprabuccal (soo″prah-buk′al)   above the buccal region.

suprabulge (su′prah-bulj)   the surface or the crown of a tooth sloping toward the occlusal surface from the height of contour or survey line. Cf. *infrabulge*.

suprachoroid (soo″prah-ko′roid)   situated above or upon the choroid.

suprachoroidea (soo″prah-ko-roi′de-ah)   lamina suprachoroidea.

supraciliary (soo″prah-sil′e-er″e)   superciliary.

supraclavicular (soo″prah-klah-vik′u-lar)   situated above the clavicle.

supraclavicularis (soo″prah-klah-vik″u-la′ris) [L.]   supraclavicular.

supraclusion (soo″prah-kloo′zhun)   the condition in which the occluding surface of a tooth extends beyond the normal occlusal plane. Called also *overeruption* and *supraocclusion*.

supracondylar (soo″prah-kon′dǐ-lar) situated above a condyle or condyles.

supracondyloid (soo″prah-kon′dǐ-loid) supracondylar.

supracostal (soo″prah-kos′tal) situated above or upon a rib or ribs.

supracotyloid (soo″prah-kot′ǐ-loid) situated above the acetabulum.

supracranial (soo″prah-kra′ne-al) on the upper surface of the cranium.

supradiaphragmatic (soo″prah-di″ah-frag-mat′ik) situated above the diaphragm.

supraduction (soo″prah-duk′shun) [*supra-* + L. *duction*] 1. the upward rotation of an eye around its horizontal axis. 2. the upward rotation of one eye independent of the other by a basedown prism in testing for vertical divergence. See also *sursumversion*. Called also *superduction, sursumduction, supravergence,* and *sursumvergence.*

supraepicondylar (soo″prah-ep″ǐ-kon′dǐ-lar) situated above an epicondyle.

supraepitrochlear (soo″prah-ep″ǐ-trok′le-ar) situated above the medial epicondyle of the humerus.

supraglenoid (soo″prah-gle′noid) situated above the glenoid cavity.

supraglottic (soo″prah-glot′ik) situated above the glottis.

suprahepatic (soo″prah-he-pat′ik) situated above the liver.

suprahyoid (soo″prah-hi′oid) situated above the hyoid bone.

suprainguinal (soo″prah-in′gwǐ-nal) situated above the groin.

supraintestinal (soo″prah-in-tes′tǐ-nal) situated above the intestine.

supraliminal (soo″prah-lim′ǐ-nal) above the limen of sensation; more than just perceptible.

supralumbar (soo″prah-lum′bar) situated above the loin.

supramalleolar (soo″prah-mah-le′o-lar) situated above a malleolus.

supramammary (soo″prah-mam′ah-re) situated above a mammary gland.

supramandibular (soo″prah-man-dib′u-lar) situated above the mandible.

supramarginal (soo″prah-mar′jǐ-nal) situated above a margin.

supramastoid (soo″prah-mas′toid) situated above the mastoid portion of the temporal bone.

supramaxilla (soo″prah-mak-sil′ah) the maxilla.

supramaxillary (soo″prah-mak′sǐ-ler″e) 1. pertaining to the upper jaw. 2. situated above the maxilla.

supramaximal (soo″prah-mak′sǐ-mal) above the maximum.

suprameatal (soo″prah-me-a′tal) situated above a meatus.

supramental (soo″prah-men′tal) [*supra-* + L. *mentum* chin] situated above the chin.

supramentale (su″prah-men-ta′le) in roentgenographic cephalometry, the most posterior midline point in the concavity between the infradentale and pogonium, determined on the lateral head film.

supranasal (soo″prah-na′zal) above the nose.

supranormal (soo″prah-nor′mal) greater than normal; present or occurring in excess of normal amounts or values.

supranuclear (soo″prah-nu′kle-ar) situated or occurring above or on the cortical side or surface of a nucleus; see also under *paralysis.*

supraoccipital (soo″prah-ok-sip′ǐ-tal) situated above or in the upper portion of the occiput.

supraocclusion (soo″prah-ŏ-kloo′zhun) supraclusion.

supraocular (soo″prah-ok′u-lar) above the eye.

supraoptimal (soo″prah-op′tǐ-mal) greater than optimal.

supraoptimum (soo″prah-op′tǐ-mum) a condition or quantity exceeding the optimum.

supraorbital (soo″prah-or′bǐ-tal) situated above the orbit.

suprapatellar (soo″prah-pah-tel′ar) situated above the patella.

suprapelvic (soo″prah-pel′vik) situated above the pelvis.

suprapharmacologic (soo″prah-fahr″mah-ko-loj′ik) much greater than the usual therapeutic dose or pharmacologic concentration of a drug.

suprapontine (soo″prah-pon′tīn) situated above or in the upper part of the pons.

suprapubic (soo″prah-pu′bik) situated or performed above the pubic arch.

suprarenal (soo″prah-re′nal) [*supra-* + L. *ren* kidney] situated above a kidney; pertaining to the suprarenal (adrenal) gland.

suprarenalectomy (soo″prah-re″nal-ek′to-me) [*suprarenal* + Gr. *ektomē* excision] adrenalectomy; excision of the adrenal gland.

suprarenalism (soo″prah-re′nal-izm) the condition produced by abnormal adrenal activity.

suprarenalopathy (soo″prah-re″nal-op′ah-the) [*suprarenal* + Gr. *pathos* disease] a disorder due to derangement of the adrenal gland.

suprarene (soo″prah-rēn′) [*supra* + L. *ren* kidney] an adrenal gland.

Suprarenin (soo″prah-ren′in) trademark for a preparation of epinephrine.

suprarenogenic (soo″prah-re″no-jen′ik) originating in the adrenal gland; due to abnormal adrenal activity.

suprarenopathy (soo″prah-re-nop′ah-the) suprarenalopathy.

suprarenotropic (soo″prah-re″no-trop′ik) having an influence on the adrenal gland; adrenotropic.

suprascapular (soo″prah-skap′u-lar) situated on the upper part of the scapula.

suprascleral (soo″prah-skle′ral) on the outer surface of the sclera.

suprasellar (soo″prah-sel′ar) above the sella turcica.

supraseptal (soo″prah-sep′tal) situated above a septum.

suprasonics (soo″prah-son′iks) ultrasonics.

supraspinal (soo″prah-spi′nal) situated upon or above a spine.

supraspinous (soo″prah-spi′nus) situated above a spine or a spinous process.

suprastapedial (soo″prah-stah-pe′de-al) situated above the stapes.

suprasternal (soo″prah-ster′nal) situated above the sternum.

suprasterol (soo″prah-ster′ol) an isomer of ergosterol.

suprasylvian (soo″prah-sil′ve-an) situated above the sylvian fissure.

supratemporal (soo″prah-tem′po-ral) situated above the temporal bone, fossa, or region.

supratentorial (soo″prah-ten-to′re-al) above the tentorium of the cerebellum.

suprathoracic (soo″prah-tho-ras′ik) situated above, or cephalad of, the thorax.

supratip (soo″prah-tip″) above the tip of the nose.

supratonsillar (soo″prah-ton′sǐ-lar) situated above a tonsil.

supratrochlear (soo″prah-trok′le-ar) situated above the trochlea.

supratympanic (soo″prah-tim-pan′ik) above the tympanum.

supraumbilical (soo″prah-um-bil′ǐ-kal) situated above the umbilicus.

supravaginal (soo″prah-vaj′ǐ-nal) situated above or outside of a sheath, specifically above the vagina.

supraventricular (soo″prah-ven-trik′u-lar) situated or occurring above the ventricles, especially in an atrium or atrioventricular node.

supravergence (soo″prah-ver′jens) [*supra-* + *vergence*] disjunctive reciprocal movement of the eyes in which one eye rotates upward while the other one remains still; called also *sursumvergence.*

supraversion (su″prah-ver′zhun) [*supra-* + L. *versio* a turning] 1. malocclusion in which a tooth or other maxillary or mandibular structure extends further away from the alveolus than normal, the occluding surfaces of the teeth extending beyond the normal occlusal line. 2. sursumversion.

supravital (soo″prah-vi′tal) denoting a staining method in which the dye is added to a medium of cells already removed from the living organism.

supraxiphoid (soo″prah-zi′foid) above the xiphoid process.

suprofen (soo-pro′fen) chemical name: α-methyl-4-(2-thienylcarbonyl)-benzeneacetic acid; a prostaglandin inhibitor, $C_{14}H_{12}O_3S$, having anti-inflammatory activity.

sura (su′rah) [L.] [NA] the muscular posterior portion of the leg; called also *calf* and *regio suralis* [NA alternative].

Suragina (su-rah-ji′nah) a genus of flies of the family Rhagionidae. *S. longipes* of Mexico is a vicious biter.

sural (su′ral) pertaining to the calf of the leg.

suralimentation (sur″al-ĭ-men-ta′shun) superalimentation.

suramin sodium (soo′rah-min) chemical name: 8,8′-[carbonylbis [imino-3, 1-phenylenecarbonylimino(4-methyl-3,1-phenylene) carbonylimino]] bis - 1, 3, 5- naphthalenesulfonic acid hexasodium salt. An antitrypanosomal and antifilarial agent, $C_{51}H_{34}N_6Na_6O_{23}S_6$, occurring as a white or slightly pink powder; used in the treatment of African trypanosomiasis, especially that due to *Trypanosoma gambiense*, and of onchocerciasis, administered intravenously.

surdimute (sur′dĭ-mūt) [L. *surdus* deaf + *mutus* mute] 1. both deaf and mute. 2. a deaf-mute.

surdimutism (sur″dĭ-mu′tizm) deaf-mutism.

surdimutitas (sur″dĭ-mu′tĭ-tas) [L. *surdus* deaf + *mutus* unable to speak + *-tas* state] deaf-mutism.

surditas (sur′dĭ-tas) [L.] deafness. **s. congen′ita,** congenital deafness.

surdity (sur′dĭ-te) [L. *surditas*] deafness.

surexcitation (sur″ek-si-ta′shun) [L. *super* over + *excitation*] excessive excitation.

Surfacaine (sur′fah-kān) trademark for preparations of cyclomethycaine.

surface (sur′fis) the outer part or an external aspect of an object. For names included in official anatomical nomenclature, see under *facies*. **alveolar s. of maxilla,** arcus alveolaris maxillae. **anterior s.,** that surface which is toward the front of the body (on or nearest the ventral aspect) in man (*facies anterior* [NA]), or toward the head in quadrupeds; in dentistry, the proximal surface of any tooth that is closest to the midline of the dental arch. **anterior s. of manubrium and gladiolus,** planum sternale. **anterior s. of sacral bone,** facies pelvica ossis sacri. **anterior s. of scapula,** facies costalis scapulae. **anterior s. of stomach,** paries anterior ventriculi. **articular s.,** that surface of a bone or cartilage which forms a joint with another (*facies articularis* [NA]). **articular s. of acetabulum,** facies lunata acetabuli. **articular s. of sacral bone, lateral,** facies auricularis ossis sacri. **axial s.,** any surface parallel with an axis; in dentistry, any surface of a tooth which is parallel with its long axis, including the buccal, distal, labial, lingual, and medial surfaces. **basal s.,** that surface of a denture the detail of which is determined by the impression and which rests upon the supporting tissues of the mouth. Called also *foundation s.* and *impression s.* **buccal s.,** the vestibular (or facial) surface of the premolars and molars that faces the cheek; called also *facies buccalis dentis.* Cf. *labial s.* **condyloid s. of tibia,** facies articularis superior tibiae. **contact s.,** see under *area.* **costal s. of scapula,** facies costalis scapulae. **diaphragmatic s.,** the surface of an organ of the thoracic or abdominal cavity that is directed toward the diaphragm (*facies diaphragmatica* [NA]). **distal s.,** that surface of a structure which is farther from a point of reference; in dentistry, the proximal or contact surface of a tooth farthest from the midline of the dental arch (*lateral s.* or *posterior s.*). **dorsal s.,** the aspect of a structure that is toward the back of the body. In man, synonymous with posterior surface (*facies dorsalis, facies posterior* [NA]). **dorsal s. of scapula,** facies posterior scapulae. **extensor s.,** the aspect of a joint of a limb (such as the knee or the elbow) on the side toward which the movement of extension is directed. **facial s.,** facies vestibularis dentus. **flexor s.,** the aspect of a joint of a limb (such as the knee or the elbow) on the side toward which the movement of flexion is directed. **foun-**

dation s., basal s. **impression s.,** basal s. **incisal s.,** the cutting edges of the anterior teeth, the incisors and canines, which come into contact with those of the opposite teeth during the act of protrusive occlusion, in which they assume an edge-to-edge relationship. See also *facies occlusalis dentis.* **inferior s.,** that surface which is lower (directed away from the head, in man) (*facies inferior* [NA]). **infratemporal s. of maxilla,** facies infratemporalis maxillae. **labial s.,** the vestibular or facial surface of the incisors and canines that faces the lips; called also *facies labialis dentis.* Cf. *buccal s.* **lateral s.,** a surface nearer to or directed toward the side of the body (*facies lateralis* [NA]); in dentistry, the proximal surface of an incisor or canine tooth that is farthest from the midline of the dental arch. **left s. of heart,** facies pulmonis cordis. **lingual s.,** facies lingualis dentis. The surface of a tooth (or of a denture) which faces the tongue [NA]. **masticatory s.,** 1. occlusal surface, working. 2. facies occlusalis dentis. **medial s.,** a surface nearer to or directed toward the midline of the body (*facies medialis* [NA]); mesial s. **mesial s.,** in dentistry, the proximal or contact surface of the incisor or canine teeth that is closest to the midline of the dental arch; medial s. **morsal s's,** the occlusal surfaces of the mandibular and maxillary teeth which make contact in centric occlusion. **occlusal s. of teeth,** 1. facies occlusalis dentis. 2. see *incisal s.* and *occlusal s., working.* **occlusal s., working,** the occlusal surfaces of the teeth engaged in the masticatory activities; called also *masticatory s.* and *facies masticatoria dentis.* **oral s.,** facies lingualis dentis. **polished s.,** one that is smoothed to a fine finish; in dentistry, that portion of the surface of a denture that is usually polished, including the palatal surface, and the buccal and lingual surfaces of the teeth. **posterior s.,** that surface which is toward the back of the body (on or nearest the dorsal aspect) in man (*facies posterior, facies dorsalis* [NA]), or toward the tail in quadrupeds; in dentistry, the surface of any tooth that is farthest from the midline of the dental arch. **posterior s. of sacral bone,** facies dorsalis ossis sacri. **posterior s. of scapula,** facies posterior scapulae. **posterior s. of stomach,** paries posterior ventriculi. **proximal s., proximate s.,** 1. any surface nearer to a point of reference. 2. the surface of a tooth facing an adjoining tooth in the same dental arch. The proximal surface facing toward the median line is the *mesial surface;* that facing away from the median line is the *distal surface.* **s. of heart, right,** margo dexter cordis. **sacropelvic s. of the ilium,** facies sacropelvina ossis ilii. **subocclusal s.,** a portion of the surface of a tooth which is directed toward but does not make contact with the occlusal surface of its opposite number in the other jaw. **superior s.,** that surface which is upper or higher (toward the head, in man) (*facies superior* [NA]). **superior articular s. of atlas,** fovea articularis superior atlantis. **tentorial s.,** the portion of the cerebral surface that is in contact with the tentorium cerebelli. **ventral s.,** 1. the anterior surface, in man. 2. that surface which is lower, or on or nearest the abdominal aspect in quadrupeds. **ventral s. of scapula,** facies costalis scapulae. **vestibular s.,** facies vestibularis dentis.

surfactant (sur-fak′tant) a surface-active agent, such as soap or a synthetic detergent. In pulmonary physiology, a mixture of phospholipids (chiefly lecithin and sphingomyelin) secreted by the alveolar type II cells into the alveoli and respiratory air passages, which reduces the surface tension of pulmonary fluids and thus contributes to the elastic properties of pulmonary tissue.

Surfak (sur′fak) trademark for a preparation of docusate calcium.

surgeon (sur′jun) [L. *chirurgio;* Fr. *chirurgien*] 1. a physician who specializes in surgery. 2. the senior medical officer of a military unit. **acting assistant s.,** contract s. **barber s.,** formerly a barber who was authorized to practice minor surgery, including bloodletting. **contract s.,** in the U.S. Army a physician or dentist engaged for temporary service in the medical department; called also *acting assistant surgeon.* **s. general,** 1. the chief of medical services in one of the armed forces. 2. the chief medical officer of the United States Bureau of Public Health, or of a state public health agency. 3. a member of the medical staff of the British Army. **house s.,** a surgeon who is an employee of a hospital and available there when on duty. **post s.,** the surgeon of an established army post.

surgery (sur′jer-e) [L. *chirurgia*, from Gr. *cheir* hand + *ergon* work] 1. that branch of medicine which treats diseases, injuries, and deformities by manual or operative methods. 2. the place in a hospital or doctor's or dentist's office where surgery is performed. 3. in Great Britain, a room or office where a doctor sees and treats patients. 4. the work performed by a surgeon. **abdominal s.,** surgery of the abdominal viscera. **antiseptic s.,** surgery conducted in accordance with antiseptic principles. **aseptic s.,** surgery performed in an environment so free from microorganisms that significant infection or suppuration does not supervene. **aural s.,** the surgical treatment of diseases of the ear. **bench s.,** surgery performed on an organ that has been removed from the body, after which it is reimplanted. **cardiac s.,** surgery of the heart. **cineplastic s.,** creation of a skin-lined tunnel through a muscle adjacent to the stump of an amputated limb, to permit use of the muscle in operating a prosthesis. **clinical s.,** the study of surgical disease by symptomatic analysis, examination, and observation. **conservative s.,** surgery designed to preserve, or to remove with minimal risk, diseased or injured organs, tissues, or extremities. Cf. *radical s.* **cosmetic s.,** that department of plastic surgery which deals with procedures designed to improve the patient's appearance by plastic restoration, correction, removal of blemishes, etc. **dental s.,** oral and maxillofacial surgery. **dentofacial s.,** that branch of the healing arts which deals with the surgical and adjunctive treatment of diseases, injuries, and defects involving the face and structures of the mouth. **general s.,** that which deals with surgical problems of all kinds, rather than those in restricted area, as in a surgical specialty such as neurosurgery. **major s.,** surgery which involves the more important, difficult, and hazardous operations. **minor s.,** surgery restricted to the management of minor problems and injuries. **open heart s.,** surgery that involves incision into one or more chambers of the heart. **operative s.,** the operative or mechanical aspect of surgery; that which deals with manual and manipulative methods or procedures. **oral s.,** oral and maxillofacial s. **oral and maxillofacial s.,** that branch of dental practice that deals with the diagnosis and the surgical and adjunctive treatment of diseases, injuries, and defects of the human mouth and dental structures. Called also *maxillofacial s.* and formerly *dental s.* and *oral s.* **orthopedic s.,** that branch of surgery which deals with the correction of deformities of the musculoskeletal system; orthopedics. **plastic s.,** surgery concerned with the restoration, reconstruction, correction, or improvement in the shape and appearance of body structures that are defective, damaged, or misshapen by injury, disease, or growth and development. **psychiatric s.,** brain surgery performed for treatment of psychiatric disorders. **radical s.,** surgery designed to extirpate all areas of locally extensive disease and adjacent zones of lymphatic drainage; cf. *conservative s.* **reconstructive s.,** plastic s. **sonic s.,** the use of focused ultrasonic waves to produce precisely circumscribed alterations within tissues at predetermined sites. **stereotactic s., stereotaxic s.,** a technique for the production of sharply circumscribed lesions in specific groups of cells in deep-seated brain structures after locating the discrete structure by means of three-dimensional coordinates; the lesions are made by such agents as heat, cold, x-ray or ultrasonic radiation, etc. Called also *stereoencephalotomy.* **structural s.,** surgery devoted to the correction of morphologic abnormalities. **veterinary s.,** the surgery of domestic animals.

surgibone (sur′ji-bōn) bone and cartilage obtained from bovine embryos and young calves, subjected to special processing to reduce antigenicity; it has been used as an internal bone splint in orthopedic and reconstructive surgery, but is used rarely now because of foreign body reaction.

surgical (sur′je-kal) of, pertaining to, or correctable by surgery.

Surgicel (sur′ji-sel) trademark for an absorbable knitted fabric prepared by controlled oxidation of cellulose, used as a hemostatic agent to control intraoperative hemorrhage when other conventional methods are impractical or ineffective.

surinamine (su-rin′ah-min) chemical name: paraoxyphenyl-alphamethylamino-propionic acid. A methyl tyrosine, $OH \cdot C_6H_4 \cdot CH_2 \cdot CH(COOH) \cdot NH \cdot CH_3$, found in many plants.

Surital (sur′i-tal) trademark for preparations of sodium thiamylal.

surma (sur′mah) a lead sulfide (originally antimony sulfide) traditionally applied to the eyelids in India for cosmetic and medical purposes; it can be a source of lead poisoning.

surra (soor′ah) [Indic (Marathi) *sūra* wheezing] any trypanosomiasis of domestic animals, e.g., equines, camels, elephants, pigs, goats, and dogs, cause by *Trypanosoma evansi*, usually transmitted by tabanid flies, and occurring in the Far and Middle East, North Africa, and certain parts of Central and South America; in the latter regions the vampire bat is also a vector, and the disease (known as *murrina* or *derrengadera*) is usually seen in horses. Common symptoms include fever, anemia, edema, progressive emaciation and weakness, and death.

surrogate (sur′o-gāt) [L. *surrogatus* substituted] substitute; one put into the place of another.

sursanure (sur-sān′ūr) an old name for a sore healed outwardly, but not inwardly.

sursumduction (sur″sum-duk′shun) supraduction.

sursumvergence (sur″sum-ver′jens) supravergence.

sursumversion (sur″sum-ver′zhun) [L. *sursum* upward + *version*] binocular conjugate upward rotation of both eyes; called also *supraversion* and *superversion.*

suruçucu (soo″roo-soo′koo) the bushmaster, *Lachesis muta,* a venomous snake of South America.

surveillance (sur-vāl′ans) 1. watching or monitoring. 2. a procedure used instead of quarantine to control the spread of infectious disease, involving close supervision during the incubation period of possible contacts of individuals exposed to an infectious disease. **immune s., immunological s.,** a hypothesized monitoring function by which the immune system protects against cancer; according to the theory, tumor cells constantly arise throughout life by malignant transformation of normal cells but almost all are recognized and destroyed by the immune system, only a few somehow escaping or circumventing immune surveillance to grow and become clinically detectable cancers.

susceptibility (sus-sep″ti-bil′i-te) the state of being readily affected or acted upon; lack of immunity. **differential s.,** nonhomogeneity in response by the various regions of an embryo when subjected to a diffusely applied injurious agent.

susceptible (sus-sep′ti-b'l) 1. capable of impression; readily acted on. 2. not having immunity to an infectious disease and thus at risk of infection.

suscitate (sus′i-tāt) to arouse to greater activity.

suscitation (sus″i-ta′shun) [L. *suscitatio*] an arousal or excitation.

suspenopsia (sus″pen-op′se-ah) [L. *suspensio* wavering + *-opsia*] a condition of frequently occurring momentary suppression of attention in the visual cortex to impulses arising in the central retinal areas.

suspensiometer (sus-pen″se-om′ĕ-ter) nephelometer.

suspension (sus-pen′shun) [L. *suspensio*] 1. a condition of temporary cessation, as of animation, of pain, or of any vital process. 2. a preparation of a finely divided drug intended to be incorporated (suspended) in some suitable liquid vehicle before it is used, or already incorporated in such a vehicle. **alumina and magnesia oral s.** [USP], a mixture of variable amounts of aluminum oxide, in the form of aluminum hydroxide and hydrated aluminum oxide, and magnesium hydroxide, which contains, on a weight/weight basis, the equivalent of 3.6 to 4 per cent aluminum oxide, 1.7 to 2.2 per cent magnesium hydroxide, and 5.3 to 6.2 per cent combined aluminum oxide and magnesium hydroxide; used as an antacid. **ampicillin for oral s.** [USP], a suspension containing 90 to 120 per cent of the labeled amount of ampicillin (anhydrous or as the trihydrate); used as an antibacterial against gram-negative bacteria. **betamethasone sodium phosphate and betamethasone acetate s., sterile** [USP], a sterile preparation of betamethasone sodium phosphate in solution and betamethasone acetate in suspension in water for injection, containing betamethasone sodium phosphate equivalent to 90 to 115 per cent of the labeled amount of betamethasone and 90 to 115 per cent of the labeled amount of betamethasone acetate; used as an anti-inflammatory glucocorticoid for intramuscular, intra-articular, intrasynovial, or intralesional administration. **chloramphenicol palmitate oral s.** [USP], a suspension containing 90 to 120 per cent of the labeled amount of chloramphenicol palmitate; used as an antibacterial and antirickettsial. **chlorothiazide oral s.** [USP], a suspension containing 90–110 per cent of the labeled amount of chlorothiazide; used as a diuretic administered in the treatment of renal, hepatic, and drug-induced edema, edema and toxemia of pregnancy, and fluid retention associated with premenstrual tension. **cholestyramine for oral s.** [USP], a mixture of cholestyramine resin, containing 85–115 per cent of the labeled amount of dried cholestyramine resin; used as an ion-exchange resin for bile salts for the relief of pruritus associated with cholestasis occurring in partial biliary obstruction and as adjunctive therapy to diet in the management of elevated cholesterol due to primary type II hyperlipoproteinemia (patients with pure hypercholesterolemia). **colistin sulfate for oral s.** [USP], a preparation containing colistin sulfate equivalent to 90–120 per cent of the labeled amount of colistin activity; used in the treatment of *Shigella* and intestinal *Pseudomonas* infections, and infant diarrhea due to *Escherichia coli* and susceptible gram-negative organisms. **colloid s.**, a suspension in which the suspended particles are very small. **corticotropin zinc hydroxide s., sterile** [USP], a sterile suspension of corticotropin with prolonged action, adsorbed on zinc hydroxide; administered intramuscularly for diagnostic testing of adrenocortical function and to stimulate adrenal cortex activity. **cortisone acetate s., sterile** [USP], a sterile suspension of cortisone acetate in a suitable aqueous medium, containing 90 to 110 per cent of the labeled amount of total steroids, calculated as cortisone acetate; administered intramuscularly as an anti-inflammatory adrenocortical steroid. **cortisone acetate ophthalmic s.** [USP], a sterile suspension of cortisone acetate in an aqueous medium containing a suitable antimicrobial agent and 90 to 110 per cent of the labeled amount of total steroids, calculated as cortisone acetate; applied topically to the conjunctiva as an anti-inflammatory adrenocortical steroid. **demeclocycline oral s.** [USP], a suspension containing demeclocycline equivalent to not less than 85 per cent of the labeled amount of demeclocycline hydrochloride; used as an antibacterial, administered orally. **desoxycorticosterone pivalate s., sterile** [USP], a sterile suspension containing 90 to 110 per cent of the labeled amount of desoxycorticosterone pivalate in an aqueous medium; used as a mineralocorticoid for replacement therapy in adrenocortical insufficiency in Addison's disease and in the treatment of salt-losing adrenogenital syndrome, administered intramuscularly. **dicloxacillin sodium for oral s.** [USP], a dry mixture containing the equivalent of 90–120 per cent of the labeled amount of dicloxacillin; used as an antibacterial, primarily in the treatment of penicillinase-resistant staphylococci. **diphenylhydantoin oral s.**, phenytoin oral s. **epinephrine oil s., sterile** [USP], a sterile suspension of epinephrine in a suitable vegetable oil, containing, in each milliliter, 1.8 to 2.4 mg. of epinephrine; an adrenergic used as a bronchodilator. **estradiol s., sterile** [USP], a sterile suspension containing 90 to 110 per cent of the labeled amount of estradiol in water for injection; used as an estrogen. **hydrocortisone acetate s., sterile** [USP], a sterile suspension containing 90–100 per cent of total steroids, calculated as hydrocortisone acetate, in a suitable aqueous medium; used in various conditions responsive to the anti-inflammatory action of glucocorticoids, administered by intra-articular injection or soft-tissue infiltration. **hydrocortisone acetate ophthalmic s.** [USP], a sterile suspension of hydrocortisone acetate in an aqueous medium containing a suitable antimicrobial agent and 90 to 110 per cent of the labeled amount of total steroids, calculated as hydrocortisone acetate; used in the treatment of eye infections responsive to the anti-inflammatory actions of glucocorticoids, applied topically to the conjunctiva. **hydrocortisone cypionate oral s.** [NF], a preparation containing hydrocortisone cypionate equivalent to 90–110 per cent of the labeled amount of hydrocortisone; used in the treatment of various conditions responsive to the anti-inflammatory action of glucocorticoids. **hydroxyzine pamoate oral s.** [USP], a suspension containing hydroxyzine pamoate equivalent to 90 to 110 per cent of the labeled amount of hydroxyzine hydrochloride; used as a minor tranquilizer. **ipodate calcium for oral s.** [USP], a dry mixture of calcium ipodate and one or more suitable suspending, dispersing, or flavoring agents; used as a radiopaque medium in cholecystography. **levopropoxyphene napsylate oral s.** [USP], a preparation containing an amount of levopropoxyphene napsylate equivalent to 90–110 per cent of the

labeled amount of levopropoxyphene; used as an antitussive. **magaldrate oral s.** [USP], a suspension containing the equivalent of 2.5 to 3.0 per cent (w/w) of magnesium oxide and the equivalent of 1.5 to 2.0 per cent (w/w) of aluminum oxide; used as an antacid. **magnesia and alumina oral s.** [USP], a mixture containing magnesium hydroxide, and variable amounts of aluminum oxide in the form of aluminum hydroxide and hydrated aluminum oxide; used as an antacid. **medroxyprogesterone acetate s., sterile** [USP], a sterile suspension in a suitable aqueous medium containing 90 to 110 per cent of the labeled amount of medroxyprogesterone acetate; used as a progestin in the treatment of endometriosis, uterine cancer, habitual and threatened abortion, and menstrual disorders, administered intramuscularly. **medrysone ophthalmic s.** [USP], a sterile suspension containing 90–115 per cent of the labeled amount of medrysone in a buffered aqueous medium; used as a topical anti-inflammatory in allergic and inflammatory eye conditions, such as episcleritis, allergic and vernal conjunctivitis, and epinephrine sensitivity. **meprobamate oral s.** [USP], a suspension containing 95 to 110 per cent of the labeled amount of meprobamate; used as a sedative. **methacycline hydrochloride oral s.** [USP], a suspension containing 90 to 125 per cent of the labeled amount of methacycline base and one or more suitable and harmless buffers, dispersants, colorings, flavorings, and preservatives; used as an antibacterial. **methenamine mandelate oral s.** [USP], a suspension of methenamine mandelate in vegetable oil, containing 90 to 110 per cent of the labeled amount of methenamine mandelate; used as a urinary antibacterial. **methylprednisolone acetate s., sterile** [USP], a sterile solution containing 90–110 per cent of the labeled amount of methylprednisolone acetate in a suitable aqueous medium; used as an anti-inflammatory in the treatment of various glucocorticoid-responsive conditions; administered intra-articularly and intramuscularly. **neomycin and polymyxin B sulfates and hydrocortisone otic s.** [USP], a sterile suspension containing not less than 90 and not more than 130 per cent of the labeled amounts of neomycin and of polymyxin B and also containing 10 mg of hydrocortisone per ml. **nitrofurantoin oral s.** [USP], a suspension of nitrofurantoin in a suitable aqueous vehicle, containing, in each 100 ml., 460 to 540 mg. of nitrofurantoin; used as a urinary antibacterial. **novobiocin calcium oral s.**, a suspension of novobiocin calcium in an aqueous vehicle, containing, in each 100 ml., novobiocin calcium equivalent to 2.25–3 gm. of novobiocin (as the free acid), one or more suitable suspending agents, colors, flavors, and preservatives; used as an antibacterial, chiefly in the treatment of infections in children due to staphylococci and other gram-positive organisms resistant to other antibiotics. **oxytetracycline calcium oral s.** [NF], a suspension containing 90–120 per cent of the labeled amount of oxytetracycline calcium in an aqueous vehicle containing one or more suitable suspending agents, flavors, colors, and preservatives; used as an antibacterial in various tetracycline-responsive conditions. **penicillin G benzathine s., sterile** [USP], a sterile suspension of penicillin G benzathine in water for injection with one or more suitable dispersing agents, buffers, and antimicrobial agents; used as an antibacterial in the treatment of infections due to penicillin G–susceptible organisms, administered intramuscularly. **penicillin G procaine s., sterile** [USP], a sterile suspension of procaine penicillin G in water for injection and one or more suitable suspending or dispersing agents and buffers; administered intramuscularly as an antibacterial in the treatment of infections due to penicillin G–susceptible organisms. **penicillin G procaine with aluminum stearate s., sterile** [USP], a sterile suspension of procaine penicillin G in refined peanut oil or sesame oil that has been gelled with 2 per cent of aluminum monostearate; used as an antibacterial in penicillin G–susceptible organisms, administered intramuscularly. **penicillin V benzathine oral s.** [USP], a preparation containing penicillin V benzathine equivalent to not less than 85 per cent of the labeled amount of penicillin V; used as an antibacterial in infections due to penicillin-susceptible organisms. **penicillin V hydrabamine oral s.** [USP], a preparation containing penicillin V hydrabamine equivalent to 90–125 per cent of the labeled amount of penicillin V; used as an antibacterial in the treatment of infections due to penicillin-susceptible organisms. **penicillin V for oral s.** [USP], a dry mixture containing 90–120 per cent of the labeled amount of penicillin units; used as an antibacterial in infections due to penicillin-susceptible organisms. **penicillin V potassium for oral s.** [USP], a dry mixture containing 90–135 per cent of the labeled amount of penicillin V; used as an antibacterial in infections due to penicillin-susceptible organisms. **phensuximide oral s.** [USP], a suspension containing 90–110 per cent of the labeled amount of phensuximide; used as an anticonvulsant, mainly in the treatment of petit mal epilepsy. **phenytoin oral s.** [USP], a suspension containing 90–110 per cent of the labeled amount of phenytoin in a suitable medium; used as an anticonvulsant in the treatment of all forms of epilepsy except petit mal. Called also *diphenylhydantoin oral s.* **prednisolone acetate s., sterile** [USP], a sterile suspension of prednisolone acetate in a suitable aqueous medium, containing 90 to 110 per cent of the labeled amount of prednisolone acetate; used as an anti-inflammatory in the treatment of various glucocorticoid-responsive conditions, administered intra-articularly or intramuscularly. **primidone oral s.** [USP], a suspension of primidone in a suitable aqueous vehicle, containing, in each 100 ml., 4.5–5.5 gm. of primidone; used as an anticonvulsant in controlling grand mal, focal, and psychomotor epileptic seizures. **progesterone s., sterile** [USP], a sterile suspension containing 93 to 107 per cent of the labeled amount of progesterone in water for injection; used as a progestin in the treatment of functional uterine bleeding, menstrual disorders, and threatened abortion, administered intramuscularly. **propoxyphene napsylate oral s.** [USP], a preparation containing 90–110 per cent of the labeled amount of propoxyphene napsylate; used as an analgesic. **propyliodone s., sterile,** a sterile suspension of propyliodone in water for injection, containing 47.5 to 52.5 per cent of propyliodone and a suitable suspending or dispersing agent; used as a radiopaque medium in bronchography, administered intratracheally. **propyliodone oil s., sterile** [USP], a sterile suspension of propyliodone in peanut oil, containing 57 to 63 per cent of propyliodone; used as a radiopaque medium in bronchography, administered intratracheally. **protamine zinc insulin s.** [USP], a sterile suspension of insulin modified by the addition of zinc chloride and protamine, containing 40, 80, or 100 USP insulin units per ml., having a gradual and prolonged action; administered subcutaneously as a hypoglycemic in the treatment of diabetes mellitus. Abbreviated PZI. **pyrantel pamoate oral s.** [USP], a suspension containing 90–110 per cent of the labeled amount of pyrantel in a suitable aqueous vehicle; used as an anthelmintic in the treatment of ascariasis and enterobiasis. **pyrvinium pamoate oral s.** [USP], a suspension containing, in each 100 ml., an amount of pyrvinium pamoate equivalent to 0.90 to 1.10 gm. of pyrvinium; used as an anthelmintic in the treatment of enterobiasis. **salicylamide oral s.,** a suspension containing 93 to 107 per cent of the labeled amount of salicylamide; used as an analgesic. **selenium sulfide detergent s.,** an aqueous, stabilized suspension of selenium sulfide containing a suitable dispersing agent, buffer, and detergent, and containing between 90 and 110 per cent selenium sulfide; used as an antiseborrheic shampoo to control seborrheic dermatitis and dandruff. **simethicone oral s.** [USP], a suspension containing 90–110 per cent of the labeled amount of dimethicone; used as an antiflatulent. **sitosterols s.,** a suspension containing 90 to 110 per cent of the labeled amount of sitosterols; used as an anticholesterolemic. **sulfacetamide, sulfadiazine, and sulfamerazine oral s.,** a suspension containing 90 to 110 per cent of the labeled amounts of sulfacetamide, sulfadiazine, and sulfamerazine; used as an antibacterial. **sulfadimethoxine oral s.** [USP], a suspension containing 93 to 107 per cent of the labeled amount of sulfadimethoxine; used as an antibacterial. **sulfamethizole oral s.** [USP], a buffered aqueous suspension containing 90 to 110 per cent of the labeled amount of sulfamethizole; used as an antibacterial. **sulfamethoxazole oral s.** [USP], a suspension containing 95–100 per cent of the labeled amount of sulfamethoxazole; used as an antibacterial, especially for the prophylaxis and treatment of urinary tract infections and of pyodermata and infections of wounds and soft tissues due to sulfonamide-susceptible organisms. **sulfisoxazole acetyl oral s.** [USP], a suspension containing sulfisoxazole acetyl equivalent to 93 to 107 per cent of the labeled amount of sulfisoxazole; used as an antibacterial in a wide variety of infections due to sulfonamide-susceptible organisms, usually given to infants and children. **testolactone s., sterile** [USP], a suspension containing 90–110 per cent of the labeled amount of testolactone in a suitable aqueous medium; used as an antineoplastic agent for adjunctive therapy in the palliative treatment of advanced or disseminated breast cancer in postmenopausal women; administered orally or by intramuscular injection. **testosterone s., sterile** [USP], a sterile suspension containing 90 to 110 per cent of the labeled amount of testosterone in an aqueous medium; used as an androgen chiefly in the treatment of male hypogonadism, cryptorchidism, and the symptoms of the male climacteric; administered intramuscularly. **tetracycline hydrochloride ophthalmic s.** [USP], a sterile suspension of tetracycline hydrochloride in oil, containing not less than 85 per cent of the labeled amount of tetracycline hydrochloride; used as an antibacterial in the treatment of infections due to susceptible organisms, applied topically to the conjunctiva. **tetracycline oral s.** [USP], tetracycline suspended in one or more suitable suspending and dispersing agents, containing 90 to 120 per cent of the labeled amount of tetracycline hydrochloride; used as an antiamebic, antibacterial, and antirickettsial. **thiabendazole oral s.** [USP], a suspension containing 90 to 110 per cent of the labeled amount of thiabendazole; used as an anthelmintic in the treatment of pinworm, threadworm, whipworm, roundworm, and hookworm infections, and in cutaneous larva migrans. **triamcinolone acetonide s., sterile** [USP], a sterile suspension of triamcinolone acetonide in a suitable aqueous medium, containing 90 to 115 per cent of the labeled amount of triamcinolone acetonide; administered by intra-articular, intrabursal, intradermal, and intramuscular injection in conditions responsive to the anti-inflammatory actions of glucocorticoids. **triamcinolone diacetate s., sterile** [USP], a sterile suspension containing 90–115 per cent of the labeled amount of triamcinolone diacetate in a suitable aqueous medium; administered by intramuscular, intra-articular, and soft tissue injection in conditions responsive to the anti-inflammatory actions of glucocorticoids. **triamcinolone hexacetonide s., sterile** [USP], a sterile suspension of triamcinolone hexacetonide in a suitable aqueous medium, containing 90–115 per cent of the labeled amount of triamcinolone hexacetonide; administered by intra-articular, intralesional, and sublesional injection in conditions responsive to the anti-inflammatory action of glucocorticoids. **trisulfapyrimidines oral s.** [USP], a suspension of sulfadiazine, sulfamerazine, and sulfamethazine, used as an antibacterial in various sulfonamide-responsive infections. **troleandomycin oral s.,** a suspension containing 90 to 120 per cent of the labeled amount of troleandomycin and one or more suitable suspending and dispersing agents, colors, flavors, buffers, and preservatives in an aqueous vehicle; used as an antibacterial, chiefly in the treatment of infections due to staphylococci and other gram-positive bacteria resistant to other systemic antibiotics.

suspensoid (sus-pen′soid) suspension colloid.

suspensorius (sus″pen-so′re-us) [L.] suspensory.

suspensory (sus-pen′so-re) [L. *suspensorius*] 1. serving to hold up a part. 2. a ligament, bone, muscle, sling, or bandage which serves to hold up a part.

Sus-Phrine (sus′frin) trademark for a preparation of epinephrine.

suspirious (sus-pi′re-us) breathing heavily; sighing.

sustentacular (sus′ten-tak′u-lar) [L. *sustentare* to support] pertaining to a sustentaculum; serving to support; see *supporting cells,* under cell, and see under *tissue.*

sustentaculum (sus″ten-tak′u-lum), pl. *sustentac′ula* [L.] a support. **s. lie′nis,** ligamentum phrenicolienale. **s. ta′li** [NA], **s. of talus,** a process of the calcaneus which supports the talus.

susto (soos′to) culture-specific syndrome seen in Latin America consisting of panic reactions due to fear of the evil eye, black magic, and spirit possession.

susurrus (su-sur′us) [L.] murmur.

Sutherland (suth′er-land) Earl Wilbur, Jr. American pharmacologist, 1915–1974; winner of the Nobel prize for medicine or physiology in 1971 for isolation of cyclic AMP in the formation of ATP.

sutika (su′tik-ah) a disease of pregnant women of Bengal, marked by digestive troubles and fever during pregnancy, with progressive pernicious anemia occurring after delivery.

sutilains (soo′tĭ-lāns) [USP] a substance containing proteolytic enzymes derived from *Bacillus subtilis*, occurring as a cream-colored powder; used as a proteolytic agent for débridement of wounds.

Sutton's disease (sut′onz) 1. [Richard Lightburn *Sutton*, American dermatologist, 1878–1952] halo nevus. 2. [R. L. *Sutton*] *periadenitis mucosa necrotica recurrens.* 3. [Richard L. *Sutton*, Jr., American dermatologist, born 1908] granuloma fissuratum.

Sutton's nevus (disease) (sut′onz) [R. L. *Sutton*] halo nevus.

sutura (su-tu′rah), pl. *sutu′rae* [L. "a seam"] [NA] a type of fibrous joint in which the apposed bony surfaces are so closely united by a very thin layer of fibrous connective tissue that no movement can occur; found only in the skull. Called also *suture, sutura vera,* and *true suture.* **s. corona′lis** [NA], coronal suture: the line of junction of the frontal bone with the two parietal bones. **sutu′rae crania′les,** NA alternative for *s. cranii.* **sutu′rae cra′nii** [NA], cranial sutures: the sutures between the various bones of the skull, named generally for the specific components participating in their formation; called also *suturae craniales* [NA alternative]. **s. denta′ta,** s. serrata. **s. ethmoidolacrima′lis** [NA], ethmoidolacrimal suture: the vertical line of junction, on the medial wall of the orbit, between the lacrimal bone and the orbital plate of the ethmoid bone; called also *lacrimoethmoidal suture.* **s. ethmoidomaxilla′ris** [NA], ethmoidomaxillary suture: the line of junction between the orbital lamina of the ethmoid bone and the orbital surface of the maxilla. **s. fronta′lis** [NA], frontal suture: the usually transient line of junction between the right and left halves of the frontal bone. The inferior part often persists in the adult, in which case it is called the *metopic suture (sutura metopica* [NA alternative]). **s. fronto-ethmoida′lis** [NA], frontoethmoidal suture: the line of junction in the anterior cranial fossa between the frontal bone and the cribriform plate of the ethmoid bone. **s. frontolacrima′lis** [NA], frontolacrimal suture: the line of junction between the upper edge of the lacrimal bone and the orbital part of the frontal bone. **s. frontomaxilla′ris** [NA], frontomaxillary suture: the line of junction between the frontal bone and the frontal process of the maxilla. **s. frontonasa′lis** [NA], frontonasal suture: the line of junction between the frontal and the two nasal bones; called also *s. nasofrontalis* or *nasofrontal suture.* **s. frontozygomat′ica** [NA], frontozygomatic suture: the line of junction between the zygomatic bone and the zygomatic process of the frontal bone; called also *s. zygomaticofrontalis,* or *zygomaticofrontal suture.* **s. harmo′nia,** s. plana. **s. incisi′va** [NA], incisive suture: an indistinct suture sometimes seen extending laterally from the incisive fossa to the space between the canine tooth and the lateral incisor, indicating the line of fusion between the premaxilla and the maxilla. **s. infraorbita′lis,** infraorbital suture: a suture sometimes seen extending from the infraorbital foramen to the infraorbital groove. **s. intermaxilla′ris** [NA], intermaxillary suture: the line of junction between the maxillary bones of either side, just below the anterior nasal spine. **s. internasa′lis** [NA], internasal suture: the line of junction between the two nasal bones. **s. lacrimoconcha′lis** [NA], lacrimoconchal suture: the line of junction between the lacrimal bone and the inferior nasal concha. **s. lacrimomaxilla′ris** [NA], lacrimomaxillary suture: a suture on the inner wall of the orbit, between the lacrimal bone and the maxilla. **s. lambdoi′dea** [NA], lambdoid suture: the line of junction between the occipital and parietal bones, shaped like the Greek letter lambda. **s. limbo′sa,** a type of suture in which there is interlocking of the beveled surfaces of the bones. **s. meto′pica** [NA], see *s. frontalis.* **s. nasofronta′lis,** s. frontonasalis. **s. nasomaxilla′ris** [NA], nasomaxillary suture: the line of junction between the lateral edge of the nasal bone and the frontal process of the maxilla. **s. no′tha,** a type of suture formed by apposition of the roughened surfaces of the two participating bones. **s. occipitomastoi′dea** [NA], occipitomastoid suture: an extension of the lambdoid suture between the occipital bone and the posterior edge of the mastoid portion of the temporal bone. **s. palati′na media′na** [NA], median palatine suture: the line of junction between the horizontal part of the palatine bones of either side. **s. palati′na transver′sa** [NA], transverse palatine suture: the line of junction between the palatine processes of the maxillae and the horizontal parts of the palatine bones.

s. palato-ethmoida′lis [NA], palatoethmoidal suture: the line of junction between the orbital process of the palatine bone and the orbital lamina of the ethmoid bone. **s. palatomaxilla′ris** [NA], palatomaxillary suture: the suture in the floor of the orbit, between the orbital processes of the palatine bone and the orbital portion of the maxilla. **s. parietomastoi′dea** [NA], parietomastoid suture: the line of junction between the posterior inferior angle of the parietal bone and the mastoid process of the temporal bone. **s. pla′na** [NA], flat suture: a type of suture in which there is simple apposition of the contiguous surfaces, with no interlocking of the edges of the participating bones. **s. sag′ittalis** [NA], sagittal suture: the line of junction between the two parietal bones. **s. serra′ta** [NA], serrated suture: a type of suture in which the participating bones are united by interlocking processes resembling the teeth of a saw. **s. spheno-ethmoida′lis** [NA], sphenoethmoidal suture: the line of junction between the body of the sphenoid bone and the orbital lamina of the ethmoid bone. **s. sphenofronta′lis** [NA], sphenofrontal suture: a long suture joining the orbital part of the frontal bone to the greater and lesser wings of the sphenoid bone on either side of the skull. **s. sphenomaxilla′ris** [NA], sphenomaxillary suture: a suture occasionally seen between the pterygoid process of the sphenoid bone and the maxilla. **s. sphenoorbi′talis,** spheno-orbital suture: the line or junction between the orbital process of the palatine bone and the body of the sphenoid bone. **s. sphenoparieta′lis** [NA], sphenoparietal suture: the line of junction between the great wing of the sphenoid bone and the parietal bone. **s. sphenosquamo′sa** [NA], sphenosquamous suture: the line of junction between the great wing of the sphenoid bone and the squamous part of the temporal bone. **s. sphenovomeria′na** [NA] sphenovomerine suture: the line of junction between the vaginal processes of the medial pterygoid plates of the sphenoid and the ala of the vomer. **s. sphenozygomat′ica** [NA], sphenozygomatic suture: the line of junction between the great wing of the sphenoid bone and the zygomatic bone. **s. squamo′sa** [NA], squamous suture: a type of suture formed by overlapping of the broad beveled edges of the participating bones. **s. squamo′sa cra′nii** [NA], squamous suture of cranium: the suture between the squamous part of the temporal bone and the parietal bone. **s. squamosomastoi′dea** [NA], squamosomastoid suture: a suture existing early in life between the squamous and mastoid portions of the temporal bone. **s. temporozygomat′ica** [NA], temporozygomatic suture: the line of junction between the zygomatic process of the temporal bone and the temporal process of the zygomatic bone; called also *s. zygomaticotemporalis.* **s. ve′ra,** a true suture, in which no movement of the participating bones can occur. See *sutura.* **s. zygomaticofronta′lis,** s. frontozygomatica. **s. zygomaticomaxilla′ris** [NA], zygomaticomaxillary suture: the line of junction between the zygomatic bone and the zygomatic process of the maxilla. **s. zygomaticotempora′lis,** s. temporozygomatica.

suturae (su-tu′re) plural of *sutura.*

sutural (su′tu-ral) of or pertaining to a suture.

suturation (su″tu-ra′shun) the act or process of suturing.

suture (su′chur) [L. *sutura* a seam] 1. a type of fibrous joint in which the opposed surfaces are closely united, as in the skull; see *sutura.* 2. material used in closing a surgical or traumatic wound with stitches. 3. a stitch or series of stitches made to secure apposition of the edges of a surgical or accidental wound; used also as a verb to indicate the application of such stitches. 4. the act or process of uniting a wound by stitches. **absorbable s.,** a strand of material used for closing wounds which is subsequently either digested by proteolytic enzymes derived from inflammatory cells or hydrolyzed by water. **absorbable surgical s.** [USP], a sterile strand of catgut or synthetic material available in various diameters and tensile strengths and capable of being absorbed by living mammalian tissue. It may be treated to modify its resistance to absorption. It may be impregnated with a suitable antimicrobial agent, and may be colored by an additive approved by the federal Food and Drug Administration. **Albert's s.,** a form of Czerny suture in which the first row of stitches is passed through the entire thickness of the intestine. **Appolito's s.,** Gély's s. **apposition s.,** a superficial suture used for the exact approximation of the cutaneous edges of a wound. **approxima-**

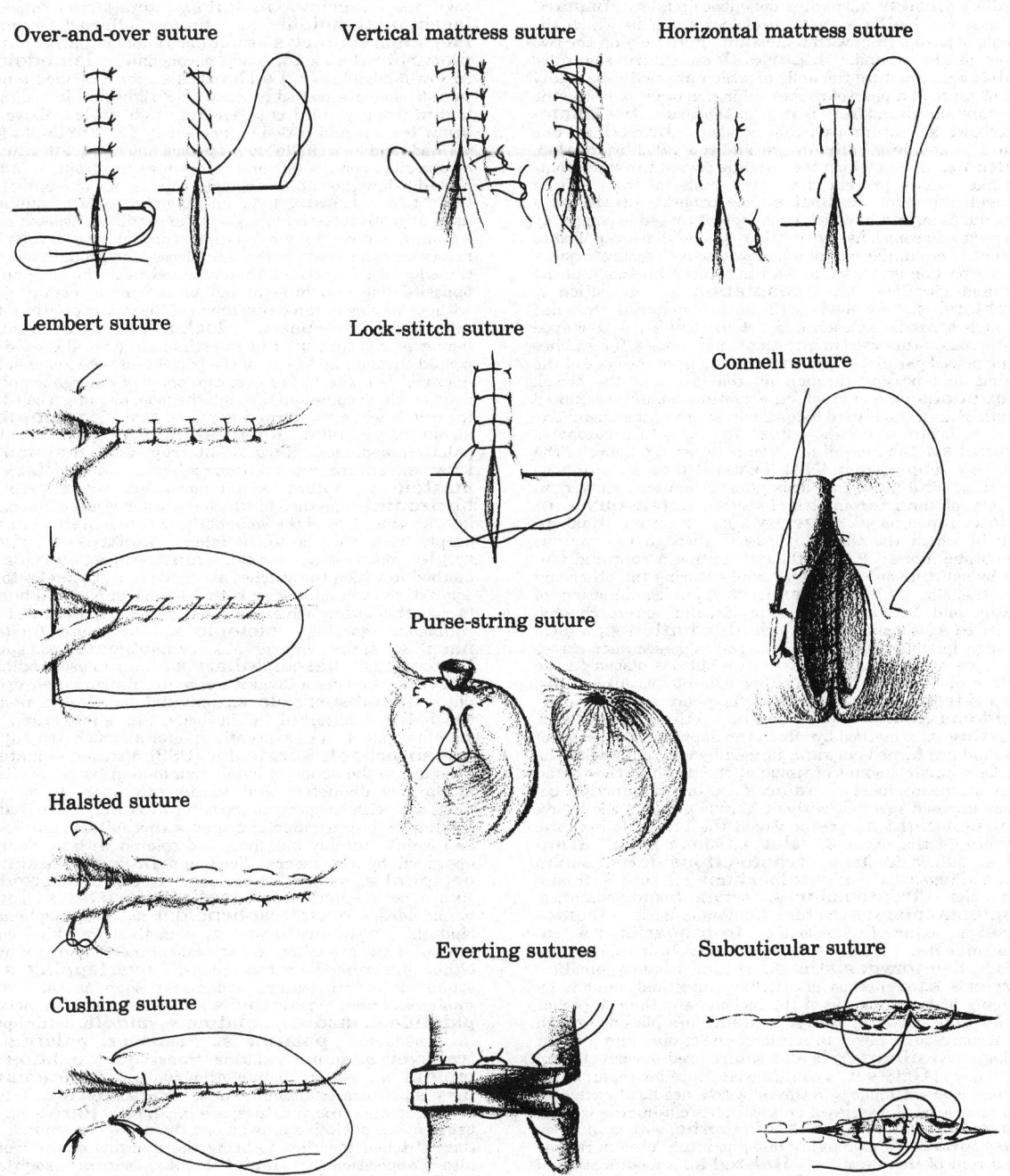

Over-and-over suture

Vertical mattress suture

Horizontal mattress suture

Lembert suture

Lock-stitch suture

Connell suture

Purse-string suture

Halsted suture

Cushing suture

Everting sutures

Subcuticular suture

PLATE 44 — VARIOUS TYPES OF SUTURES AND KNOTS

tion s., a deep suture for securing apposition of the deep tissues of a wound. **arcuate s.,** sutura coronalis. **atraumatic s.,** a suture fused into the end of a small eyeless needle. **basilar s.,** fissura sphenooccipitalis. **bastard s.,** false s. **Bell's s.,** a form of lock-stitch in which the needle is passed from within outward alternately on the two edges of the wound. **biparietal s.,** sutura sagittalis. **bolster s.,** a suture the ends of which are tied over a tiny roll of gauze or a piece of rubber tubing, in order to lessen the pressure on the skin. **bony s.,** sutura. **bregmato-mastoid s.,** sutura parietomastoidea. **buried s.,** one that is placed deep in the tissues and concealed by the skin. **button s.,** one in which the stitch is passed through a button-like disk to prevent the suture material from cutting through the skin. **catgut s.,** see *catgut.* **chain s.,** a continuous suture in which each loop of thread is caught by the next adjacent loop. **circular s.,** one that is applied to the entire circumference of a hollow viscus to secure closure, or to a portion of a visceral wall to achieve inversion of the enclosed circular area. **coaptation s.,** apposition s. **cobblers' s.,** one made with suture material threaded through a needle at each end. **Connell s.,** a U-shaped continuous suture used in intestinal anastomosis, the stitches being placed parallel to and about 4 mm. from the edge of the wound, and passing through all the layers of the bowel. **continuous s.,** one in which a continuous, uninterrupted length of material is used to approximate the cut edges of one or more layers of tissues. **coronal s.,** sutura coronalis. **cranial s's,** the lines of junction between the bones of the skull; see *suturae cranii* [NA]. **Cushing s.,** a continuous inverting suture used for closing the seromuscular layers in surgery of the gastrointestinal tract. **cutaneous s. of palate,** raphe palati. **Czerny's s.,** 1. an intestinal suture in which the thread is passed through the mucous membrane alone. 2. a method of uniting a ruptured tendon by splitting one of the ends and suturing the other end into the slit. **Czerny-Lembert s.,** a combination of Czerny and Lembert sutures in circular enterorrhaphy. **dentate s.,** sutura serrata. **double-button s.,** a form of stitch in which the suture material is passed deep across the edges of the wound, between two buttons placed on the surface of the skin, one on either side of the suture line. **Dupuytren's s.,** a continuous Lembert suture. **ethmoidomaxillary s.,** sutura ethmoidomaxillaris. **everting s.,** a method by which the approximated edges of a wound are turned outward; formed by encircling with the needle a larger amount of tissue at the depth of the wound than at the periphery. **false s.,** a line of junction between apposed surfaces, without fibrous union of the bones. **figure-of-eight s.,** one in which the thread follows the contours of the figure 8. **flat s.,** sutura plana. **frontal s.,** sutura frontalis. **fronto-ethmoidal s.,** sutura fronto-ethmoidalis. **frontolacrimal s.,** sutura fronto-lacrimalis. **frontomalar s.,** sutura frontozygomatica. **frontomaxillary s.,** sutura frontomaxillaris. **fronto-nasal s.,** sutura frontonasalis. **frontoparietal s.,** sutura coronalis. **frontosphenoid s.,** sutura sphenofrontalis. **frontozygomatic s.,** sutura frontozygomatica. **furrier's s.,** a method of stitching intestinal wounds by piercing first one margin of the incision and then the other from within outward; overlying sutures are placed through the seromuscular layers to reinforce the closure and prevent leakage. **Gaillard-Arlt s.,** a suture used in correction of entropion. **Gély's s.,** a continuous suture for repair of intestinal wounds, made by a thread with a needle at each end, and consisting of a series of cross-stitches closing the wound. **glover's s.,** lock-stitch s. **s. of Goethe,** sutura incisiva. **Gussenbauer's s.,** a figure-of-eight suture used in repairing a rent of the intestine. **Halsted s.,** a modification of the Lembert suture, consisting of a stitch parallel to the wound on one side, with the two free ends of the material emerging on the other side, where they are tied. **harelip s.,** a figure-of-eight suture used in the correction of cleft lip. **hemostatic s's,** sutures used to control oozing of blood from raw areas. **incisive s.,** sutura incisiva. **infraorbital s.,** sutura infraorbitalis. **interendognathic s.,** sutura palatina mediana. **intermaxillary s.,** a sutura intermaxillaris. **internasal s.,** sutura internasalis. **interparietal s.,** sutura sagittalis. **interrupted s.,** a noncontinuous suture; one in which each stitch is made with a separate piece of material. **intradermic s.,** a suture applied parallel with the edges of the wound, but within the layers of the skin, usually a continuous stitch. **inverting**

s., a seromuscular stitch used in intestinal anastomosis to appose and invert the serosal surfaces of the two segments, as in the Cushing or Lembert suture. **jugal s.,** sutura sagittalis. **lacrimoconchal s.,** sutura lacrimoconchalis. **lacrimo-ethmoidal s.,** sutura ethmoidolacrimalis. **lacrimomaxillary s.,** sutura lacrimomaxillaris. **lacrimoturbinal s.,** sutura lacrimoconchalis. **lambdoid s.,** sutura lambdoidea. **Le Dentu's s.,** for a divided tendon: two stitches are passed on each side, right and left, and are tied in front; a third is taken from right to left above and below the cut and is tied on one side. **Le Fort's s.,** for a divided tendon: a single loop is passed above the cut, entering at one side, coming out and going in at the front; it is then passed below the cut at each side, coming out in front, and is there tied. **Lembert s.,** an inverting suture commonly used in gastrointestinal surgery: the needle is inserted about 2.5 mm. lateral to the incision, through the serous and muscular tunics but not the submucosa, and brought out near the edge of the incision, then inserted near the edge on the opposite side and brought out at the more distant point, without having entered the lumen of the gut. It may be either interrupted or continuous. **lock-stitch s.,** a continuous hemostatic suture used in intestinal surgery: the needle is passed through all layers of the bowel and the loop of suture material is made to fall over the point of emergence of the needle, which comes up through the loop, forming a self-locking stitch when the strand is pulled taut. **longitudinal s.,** sutura sagittalis. **longitudinal s. of palate,** sutura palatina mediana. **loop s.,** interrupted s. **malomaxillary s.,** sutura zygomaticomaxillaris. **mamillary s., mastoid s.,** sutura occipitomastoidea. **mattress s., horizontal,** a method in which the stitches are made parallel with the edges of the wound, the suture material crossing deeply from one side to the other. **mattress s., right-angle,** mattress s., vertical. **mattress s., vertical,** a method in which the stitches are made at right angles to the edges of the wound, taking both deep and superficial bites of tissue, the latter achieving more exact apposition of the cutaneous margins. **metopic s.,** see *sutura frontalis.* **nasal s.,** sutura internasalis. **nasofrontal s.,** sutura frontonasalis. **nasomaxillary s.,** sutura nasomaxillaris. **nerve s.,** uniting a divided nerve by suturing; neurorrhaphy. **nonabsorbable s.,** material for closing wounds which is not absorbed in the body, e.g., silk, cotton, and stainless steel, or synthetic material such as nylon. **nonabsorbable surgical s.** [USP], a strand of material resistant to the action of living mammalian tissue, available in various diameters and tensile strengths. It may be modified with respect to body or texture, or to reduce capillarity, impregnated or coated with a suitable antimicrobial agent, suitably bleached, and colored with an additive approved by the federal Food and Drug Administration. **occipital s.,** sutura lambdoidea. **occipitomastoid s.,** sutura occipitomastoidea. **occipitoparietal s.,** sutura lambdoidea. **occipitosphenoidal s.,** fissura sphenooccipitalis. **over-and-over s.,** a method in which equal bites of tissue are taken on each side of the wound; it may be either interrupted or continuous. **overlapping s.,** a squamous suture (sutura squamosa), such as the sutura squamosa cranii. **palatine s., anterior,** sutura incisiva. **palatine s., median, palatine s., middle,** sutura palatina mediana. **palatine s., posterior, palatine s., transverse,** sutura palatina transversa. **palato-ethmoidal s.,** sutura palato-ethmoidalis. **palatomaxillary s.,** sutura palatomaxillaris. **Pancoast's s.,** a form of tongue-and-groove suture; see *plastic s.* **Paré's s.,** the use of strips of cloth applied along the edges of a wound, and then stitched together to bring the margins of the wound into apposition. **parietal s.,** sutura sagittalis. **parietomastoid s.,** sutura parietomastoidea. **parietooccipital s.,** sutura lambdoidea. **petrobasilar s., petrosphenobasilar s.,** synchondrosis petrooccipitalis. **petrosphenooccipital s. of Gruber,** fissura petrooccipitalis. **petrosquamous s.,** fissura petrosquamosa. **plastic s.,** a method in which a tongue is cut in one lip of the wound and a groove in the other, the tongue and groove then being stitched together, and the ends of the thread tied over a roll of adhesive plaster. **premaxillary s.,** sutura incisiva. **presection s.,** a stitch or series of stitches placed in the tissues before an incision is made. **primary s.,** prompt surgical closure of a wound. **pursestring s.,** a continuous suture placed around a circular opening that is to be inverted; commonly used for the stump of the appendix or a hernia sac. **quilt s., quilted s.,** a continuous mattress suture. **relaxation s.,** any suture placed to close a wound but so formed that it may be loosened in order to relieve the tension should it become too great. **retention s.,** a reinforcing suture for abdominal wounds, utilizing exceptionally strong material like braided silk or stainless steel, and including a large amount of tissue in each stitch; intended to relieve pressure on the primary suture line and prevent postoperative wound disruption evisceration. **rhabdoid s.,** sutura sagittalis. **sagittal s.,** sutura sagittalis. **scaly s.,** sutura squamosa. **secondary s.,** 1. delayed closure of an operative or accidental wound, usually because of the presence or expectation of infection. 2. resuture of an operative wound following disruption. **seroserous s.,** a suture which apposes two serous surfaces. **serrated s.,** sutura serrata. **shotted s.,** one in which the two ends of the suture wire are passed through a split or perforated lead shot, which is then compressed. **Sims's s.,** a shotted suture. **s's of skull,** suturae cranii. **spheno-ethmoidal s.,** 1. sutura spheno-ethmoidalis. 2. a craniometric landmark, being the most superior point of the sutura sphenoethmoidalis. Called also *point SE.* Abbreviated SE. **sphenofrontal s.,** sutura sphenofrontalis. **sphenomalar s.,** sutura sphenozygomatica. **sphenomaxillary s.,** sutura sphenomaxillaris. **sphenooccipital s.,** fissura sphenooccipitalis. **sphenoorbital s.,** sutura sphenoorbitalis. **sphenoparietal s.,** sutura sphenoparietalis. **sphenopetrosal s.,** synchondrosis petrooccipitalis. **sphenosquamous s., sphenotemporal s.,** sutura sphenosquamosa. **sphenovomerine s.,** sutura sphenovomeriana. **sphenozygomatic s.,** sutura sphenozygomatica. **squamosomastoid s.,** sutura squamosomastoidea. **squamosoparietal s.,** sutura squamosa cranii. **squamososphenoid s.,** sutura sphenosquamosa. **squamous s.,** sutura squamosa. **squamous s. of cranium,** sutura squamosa cranii. **subcuticular s.,** a method of skin closure involving placement of stitches in the subcuticular tissues parallel with the line of the wound; continuous or interrupted sutures may be used. **superficial s.,** one that is placed through the superficial fascia only. **temporal s.,** sutura squamosa cranii. **temporomalar s., temporozygomatic s.,** sutura temporozygomatica. **tongue-and-groove s.,** plastic s. **transverse s. of Krause,** sutura infraorbitalis. **true s.,** sutura vera. **uninterrupted s.,** continuous s. **zygomaticofrontal s.,** sutura frontozygomatica. **zygomaticomaxillary s.,** sutura zygomaticomaxillaris. **zygomaticotemporal s.,** sutura temporozygomatica.

suxamethonium chloride (suk″sah-mě-tho′ne-um) succinylcholine chloride.

Sux-Cert (suks′sert) trademark for preparations of succinylcholine chloride.

suxemerid sulfate (suk-sem′ĕ-rid) chemical name: bis(1,2,2,6,6-pentamethyl-4-piperidyl)succinate sulfate (1:2); an antitussive, $C_{24}H_{44}N_2O_4 \cdot 2H_2SO_4$.

Suzanne's gland (soo-zanz′) [Jean Georges *Suzanne,* French physician, born 1859] see under *gland.*

SV stroke volume; sinus venosus; simian virus.

SV40 simian virus 40; see *vacuolating virus,* under *virus.*

Sv sievert.

s.v. abbreviation for L. *spir′itus vi′ni,* alcoholic spirit.

svedberg (sfed′berg) Svedberg unit.

Svedberg unit, flotation unit (sfed′berg) [Theodor *Svedberg,* Swedish chemist, 1884–1971, inventor of the ultracentrifuge and winner of the Nobel prize for chemistry in 1926 for his work on disperse systems] see under *unit.*

s.v.r. abbreviation for L. *spir′itus vi′ni rectifica′tus,* rectified spirit of wine.

s.v.t. abbreviation for L. *spir′itus vi′ni ten′uis,* proof spirit.

swab (swahb) a wad of cotton or other absorbent material firmly attached to the end of a wire or stick, used for applying medication, removing material, collecting bacteriological material, etc.

swaddler (swahd′ler) a swaddling-suit for infants. **silver s.,** swaddling composed of polyester laminated on the inside surface with a thin layer of aluminum, used to prevent hypothermia in the newborn.

swage (swāj) 1. to shape metal by hammering or by adapting it to a die. 2. to fuse suture material to a needle, espe-

cially an eyeless needle. 3. a tool or form, often one of a pair, for shaping metal by pressure.

swager (swāj′er) a device or apparatus for shaping metal to a desired form by using simultaneous pressures from various angles.

swallowing (swahl′o-ing) the taking in of a substance through the mouth and pharynx, past the cricopharyngeal constriction through the esophagus and into the stomach. The oral phase is a voluntary act, whereas the remainder is a reflex act mediated by an integrating swallowing center in the medulla oblongata.

swarming (sworm′ing) spreading in a swarm; a term applied to bacteria, especially *Proteus* species, which spread over the surface of the colony.

swayback (swa′bak) 1. abnormal downward curvature of the spinal column in the dorsal region in horses. 2. see *lordosis.* 3. enzootic ataxia.

sweat (swet) the perspiration; the liquid secreted by the sweat glands (glandulae sudoriferae), having a salty taste and a pH that varies from 4.5 to 7.5. Sweat produced by the eccrine sweat glands is clear with a faint characteristic odor, and contains water, sodium chloride, and traces of albumin, urea, and other compounds; its composition varies with many factors, e.g., fluid intake, external temperature and humidity, and some hormonal activity. Sweat produced by the larger, deeper, apocrine sweat glands of the axillae contains, in addition, organic material which on bacterial decomposition produces an offensive odor. **bloody s.,** hematidrosis. **blue s.,** chromhidrosis in which the sweat has a blue color; it may occur in copper workers. **fetid s.,** bromhidrosis. **green s.,** a greenish sweating seen among workers in copper. **night s.,** sweating during sleep, a symptom frequently occurring in tuberculosis. **phosphorescent s.,** phosphorescent perspiration, sometimes observed in miliaria and after the eating of phosphorescent fish.

Swediaur's disease (swa″de-aw′erz) [François Xavier *Swediaur,* Austrian physician, 1748–1824] see under *disease.*

sweeny (swe′ne) shoulder slip.

Sweet's syndrome (swētz) [Robert Douglas *Sweet,* English dermatologist, 20th century] acute febrile neutrophilic dermatosis.

swellhead (swel′hed) 1. lechuguilla fever. 2. swelled head.

swelling (swel′ing) 1. a transient abnormal enlargement or increase in volume of a body part or area not caused by proliferation of cells. 2. an eminence, or elevation. **albuminous s.,** cloudy s. **arytenoid s.,** an eminence on each side of the embryonic laryngeal orifice that presages the future larynx. **blennorrhagic s.,** swelling of the knee in gonorrheal synovitis. **Calabar s's,** edematous areas, up to several centimeters in diameter, appearing suddenly on various portions of the body, and lasting only 2 or 3 days; fever, pruritus, and urticaria may occur. It is caused by infection with *Loa loa.* Called also *ambulant edema* and *Calabar edema.* **capsular s.,** the development of a swollen appearance of capsulated pneumococci on exposure to type-specific antibody, due to the binding of antibody with capsular polysaccharide; called also *Neufeld's reaction.* **cloudy s.,** an early stage of toxic degenerative changes, especially in the protein constituents of organs in infectious diseases. The tissues appear swollen, parboiled and opaque but revert to normal when the cause is removed. At the cellular level, it is characterized by slight swelling of the cell and granularity and cloudiness of the cytoplasm. Called also *albuminous degeneration.* **fugitive s.,** an extremely short-lived swelling. **genital s.,** an elevation on each side of the embryonic phallus that becomes either a labial (labia majora) or a scrotal swelling. **glassy s.,** amyloid degeneration. **hunger s.,** edematous swellings in wet beriberi. **Kamerun s's,** Calabar s's. **labial s.,** the primordium of a labium majus. **labioscrotal s.,** genital s. **scrotal s.,** the primordium of one-half of the scrotum. **Soemmerring's crystalline s.,** annular edema of the lower portion of the lens capsule after the removal of a cataractous lens. **tropical s's,** Calabar s's. **tympanic s.,** intumescentia tympanica. **white s.,** former name for the swelling produced by tuberculous arthritis. Called also *tumor albus.*

Swift's disease (swifts) [H. *Swift,* Australian physician] acrodynia.

swinepox (swīn-poks) an acute infectious, eruptive disease of piglets, marked by lesions of the skin of the abdomen, flanks, head, and behind the ears, caused by a poxvirus; it usually runs a mild course but on occasion may be fatal.

switch (swich) 1. a transfer, shift, or change. 2. a device that makes or breaks an electric circuit. **class s.**, the mechanism by which a B cell or plasma cell switches from production of IgM to production of IgG, IgA, or IgE. See *immunoglobulin genes*, under *gene*.

swoon (swoon) syncope.

Swyer-James syndrome (swi′er jāmz) [Paul R. *Swyer*, English physician in Canada, born 1921; G. C. W. *James*, American physician] see under *syndrome*.

sycephalus (si-sef′ah-lus) syncephalus.

sychnuria (sik-nu′re-ah) [Gr. *sychnos* frequent + *ouron* urine + *-ia*] pollakiuria.

sycosiform (si-ko′si-form) resembling sycosis.

sycosis (si-ko′sis) [Gr. *sykōsis*, from *sykon* fig] 1. a disease marked by inflammation of the hair follicles, especially of the beard. 2. a kind of ulcer on the eyelids. **s. bar′bae**, bacterial folliculitis involving the bearded region, usually caused by *Staphylococcus aureus*, in which the primary lesion is a pinhead-sized pustule, pierced by a hair, which may, if neglected, lead to impetiginization and crust formation and become chronic. Called also *barber's itch, folliculitis barbae,* and *s. vulgaris.* See also *pseudofolliculitis.* **lupoid s.**, a chronic, scarring form of deep sycosis vulgaris, characterized by a persistent, slowly enlarging circinate patch with follicular papulopustules in the active, advancing border, and healing with scarring occurring in the central area. **s. nu′chae**, dermatitis papillaris capillitii. **s. tar′si**, blepharitis. **s. vulga′ris**, s. barbae.

Sydenham's chorea, cough (sid′en-hams) [Thomas *Sydenham*, a celebrated English physician, sometimes called the "English Hippocrates," 1624–1689] see under *chorea* and *cough.*

syllabize (sil′ah-bīz) to divide speech sounds into syllables.

syllabus (sil′ah-bus) [L., a collection] an outline of a course of lectures.

syllepsiology (si-lep″se-ol′o-je) [Gr. *syllēpsis* conception + *-logy*] the sum of knowledge regarding conception or pregnancy.

syllepsis (sil-lep′sis) conception, or pregnancy.

sylvan (sil′van) 1. a liquid obtained along with tetrol from distillation of pine wood. 2. sylvatic.

sylvatic (sil-vat′ik) sylvan; pertaining to, located in, or living in the woods. See under *plague.*

Sylvest's disease (sil-vests′) [Ejnar *Sylvest*, Norwegian physician, 1880–1931] epidemic pleurodynia.

sylvian (sil′ve-an) described by or named for Franciscus Sylvius de la Böe, 1614–1672, a Dutch anatomist, as the *sylvian artery* (arteria cerebri media), *fissure* (sulcus lateralis cerebri), *fossa* (fossa lateralis cerebri and sulcus lateralis cerebri), *line, point,* and *vein* (vena cerebri media superficialis); see also *angle of Sylvius* and *valve of Sylvius* (valvula venae cavae inferioris). The name has also been ascribed to Jacobus *Sylvius* (Jacques Dubois), 1478–1555, a French anatomist who was a teacher of Vesalius (*sylvian aqueduct* or *aqueduct of Sylvius* [aqueductus mesencephali]).

symballophone (sim-bal′o-fōn) [Gr. *syn* together + *ballein* to throw + *phōnē* sound] a special type of double stethoscope making possible the comparison of sounds and detection of their direction.

symbiology (sim″bi-ol′o-je) the scientific study of symbiosis and symbiotic organisms.

symbion (sim′bi-on) symbiont.

symbionic (sim-bi-on′ik) pertaining to or characterized by symbiosis.

symbiont (sim′bi-ont, sim′be-ont) [Gr. *syn* together + *bioun* to live] an organism which lives in a state of symbiosis.

symbiosis (sim″bi-o′sis) [Gr. *symbiōsis*] 1. in parasitology, the living together or close association of two dissimilar organisms, each of the organisms being known as a *symbiont.* The association may be beneficial to both (mutualism), beneficial to one without effect on the other (commensalism), beneficial to one and detrimental to the other (parasitism), detrimental to one without effect on the other (amensalism), or detrimental to both (synnecrosis). 2. in psychiatry, a mutually reinforcing relationship between two persons who are dependent on each other; a normal characteristic of the relationship between the mother and infant child. 3. see *symbiotic psychosis,* under *psychosis.* **antagonistic s., antipathetic s.**, an association between two organisms which is to the disadvantage of one of them; parasitism. **conjunctive s.**, association between two different organisms, with bodily union between them. **constructive s.**, an association between two organisms which is of benefit to the physiologic processes of one of them. **disjunctive s.**, symbiosis without actual union of the organisms.

symbiote (sim′bi-ōt) symbiont.

symbiotic (sim″bi-ot′ik) associated in symbiosis; living together.

symblepharon (sim-blef′ah-ron) [Gr. *syn* together + *blepharon* eyelid] an adhesion between the tarsal conjunctiva and the bulbar conjunctiva. **anterior s.**, attachment of the lid to the eyeball by fibrous bands. **posterior s.**, adhesion between the lid and the eyeball extending into the fornix. **total s.**, adhesion of the entire conjunctival surface between the lid and the eyeball.

symblepharopterygium (sim-blef″ah-ro-ter-ij′e-um) a combination of symblepharon and pterygium; a form of symblepharon in which the lid is joined to the eyeball by a cicatricial band resembling a pterygium.

symbol (sim′bul) [Gr. *symbolon,* from *symballein* to interpret] a mark or character representing some quality or relation. In chemistry, a symbol is a letter or combination of letters representing an atom or a group of atoms. In psychiatry, a representation or perception that replaces unconscious mental content. **phallic s.**, in psychoanalysis, any pointed or upright object which may represent the phallus or penis.

symbolia (sim-bo′le-ah) ability to recognize the nature of objects by the sense of touch.

symbolism (sim′bol-izm) 1. an abnormal mental condition in which every occurrence is conceived of as a symbol of the patient's own thoughts. 2. in psychoanalysis, a mechanism of unconscious thinking, usually of a sexual nature, whereby the real meaning becomes transformed so as not to be recognized as sexual by the super-ego.

symbolization (sim″bol-i-za′shun) an unconscious defense mechanism in which one idea or object comes to represent another because of similarity or association between them.

symbrachydactylia (sim-brak″e-dak-til′e-ah) symbrachydactyly.

symbrachydactylism (sim-brak″e-dak′til-izm) symbrachydactyly.

symbrachydactyly (sim-brak″e-dak′ti-le) [Gr. *syn* together + *brachys* short + *daktylos* finger] a condition in which the fingers or toes are short and adherent; webbed fingers or toes.

symclosene (sim′klo-sēn) chemical name: 1,3,5-trichloro-s-triazine-2,4,6($1H,3H,5H$)trione; a topical anti-infective, $C_3Cl_3O_3$.

Syme's amputation (sīmz) [James *Syme*, Scottish surgeon, 1799–1870] see under *amputation.*

symelus (sim′ĕ-lus) symmelus.

Symington's body (si′ming-tonz) [Johnson *Symington*, Scottish anatomist, 1851–1924] the anococcygeal body; see under *body.*

symmelia (sim-me′le-ah) [Gr. *syn* together + *melos* limb + *-ia*] a developmental anomaly characterized by an apparent fusion of the lower limbs. There may be three feet (*tripodial s.*), two feet (*dipodial s.*), one foot (*monopodial s.*), or no feet (*apodial s.*).

symmelus (sim′e-lus) a fetus exhibiting symmelia.

Symmers' disease (sim′merz) [Douglas *Symmers*, American physician, 1879–1952] nodular lymphoma.

Symmetrel (sim′ĕ-trel) trademark for a preparation of amantadine hydrochloride.

symmetrical (sĭ-met′re-kal) [Gr. *symmetrikos*] pertaining to or exhibiting symmetry; in chemistry, denoting compounds which contain atoms or groups at equal intervals in the molecule.

symmetry (sim′ĕ-tre) [Gr. *symmetria; syn* with + *metron* measure] the similar arrangement in form and relationships of parts around a common axis, or on each side of a plane of the body. **bilateral s.**, the configuration of an irregularly shaped body (as the human body or that of higher animals) which can be divided by a longitudinal plane into halves that are mirror images of each other. **inverse s.,** correspondence as between an object and its mirror image, in which one side of one object corresponds with the opposite side of another. **radial s.,** symmetry in which the body parts are arranged regularly around a central axis.

sympathectomize (sim″pah-thek′to-mīz) to subject to sympathectomy.

sympathectomy (sim″pah-thek′to-me) [*sympathetic* + Gr. *ektomē* excision] the transection, resection, or other interruption of some portion of the sympathetic nervous pathways. Operations may be named according to the topographic location of the nerve, ganglion, or plexus operated on, as *cervical, dorsal, lumbar,* or *thoracolumbar s.,* or in reference to the diaphragm, as *subdiaphragmatic, supradiaphragmatic,* or *transdiaphragmatic s.* **chemical s.,** suppression of the activity of the sympathetic nervous system by appropriate drugs.

sympathetectomy (sim″pah-thĕ-tek′to-me) sympathectomy.

sympathetic (sim″pah-thet′ik) [Gr. *sympathētikos*] 1. pertaining to, caused by, or exhibiting sympathy. 2. a sympathetic nerve or the sympathetic nervous system; see under *system.*

sympatheticomimetic (sim″pah-thet″ĭ-ko-mi-met′ik) [*sympathetic* + Gr. *mimētikos* imitative] sympathomimetic.

sympatheticoparalytic (sim″pah-thet″ĭ-ko-par″ah-lit′ik) due to or affected with paralysis of the sympathetic nervous system.

sympatheticotonia (sim″pah-thet″ĭ-ko-to′ne-ah) a condition in which the sympathetic nervous system dominates the general functioning of the body organs, characterized by vascular spasm, heightened blood pressure, dermographic formation of goose flesh, and activity of the ciliospinal reflex.

sympatheticotonic (sim″pah-thet″ĭ-ko-ton′ik) [*sympathetic* + Gr. *tonos* tension] pertaining to or characterized by sympatheticotonia.

sympathetoblast (sim″pah-thet′o-blast) one of the embryonic nerve cells from the sympathetic system which develops into a sympathetic cell.

sympathic (sim-path′ik) sympathetic.

sympathicectomy (sim-path″ĭ-sek′to-me) sympathectomy.

sympathicoblast (sim-path′ĭ-ko-blast″) the primitive pluripotential undifferentiated cell which develops into a sympathetic nerve cell.

sympathicoblastoma (sim-path″ĭ-ko-blas-to′mah) a malignant tumor containing sympathicoblasts; see *neuroblastoma.*

sympathicogonioma (sim-path″ĭ-ko-go″ne-o′mah) sympathicoblastoma.

sympathicolytic (sim-path″ĭ-ko-lit′ik) sympatholytic.

sympathicomimetic (sim-path″ĭ-ko-mi-met′ik) sympathomimetic.

sympathicopathy (sim-path″ĭ-kop′ah-the) any disease due to disorder of the sympathetic nervous system.

sympathicotonia (sim-path″ĭ-ko-to′ne-ah) sympatheticotonia.

sympathicotonic (sim-path″ĭ-ko-ton′ik) sympatheticotonic.

sympathicotripsy (sim-path″ĭ-ko-trip′se) [*sympathetic ganglion* + Gr. *tribein* to crush] the surgical crushing of a nerve, ganglion, or plexus of the sympathetic nervous system.

sympathicotrope (sim-path′ĭ-ko-trōp) sympathicotropic.

sympathicotropic (sim-path″ĭ-ko-trop′ik) [*sympathetic* + Gr. *tropikos* turning] 1. having an affinity for the sympathetic nervous system. 2. an agent that has an affinity for or exerts its principal effect upon the sympathetic nervous system.

sympathicus (sim-path′ĭ-kus) the sympathetic nervous system.

sympathin (sim′pah-thin) a neurohormonal mediator of nerve impulses at sympathetic nerve synapses. The two most important mediators are epinephrine and norepinephrine, the term sympathin being used only when the nature of the mediator is unknown.

sympathism (sim′pah-thizm) susceptibility to hypnotic

influence; suggestibility; the alleged transfer of feelings from one person to another.

sympathist (sim′pah-thist) one susceptible to sympathism.

sympathoadrenal (sim″path-o-ah-dre′nal) 1. pertaining to the sympathetic nervous system and the adrenal medulla. 2. involving the sympathetic nervous system and the adrenal glands, especially increased sympathetic activity that causes increased secretion of epinephrine by the adrenal medulla and of norepinephrine by the postganglionic sympathetic nerve endings.

sympathoblast (sim-path′o-blast) [*sympathetic* + Gr. *blastos* germ] sympathicoblast.

sympathoblastoma (sim″pah-tho-blas-to′mah) sympathicoblastoma.

sympathogone (sim″pah-tho-gōn′) sympathogonium.

sympathogonia (sim″pah-tho-go′ne-ah) [pl., *sympathetic* + Gr. *gonē* seed] undifferentiated embryonic cells which develop into sympathetic cells.

sympathogonioma (sim″pah-tho-go″ne-o′mah) sympathicoblastoma.

sympathogonium (sim″pah-tho-go′ne-um) singular of *sympathogonia.*

sympatholytic (sim″pah-tho-lit′ik) [*sympathetic* + Gr. *lytikos* dissolving] 1. opposing the effects of impulses conveyed by adrenergic postganglionic fibers of the sympathetic nervous system. 2. an agent that opposes the effects of impulses conveyed by adrenergic postganglionic fibers of the sympathetic nervous system; called also *antiadrenergic.*

sympathomimetic (sim″pah-tho-mi-met′ik) [*sympathetic* + Gr. *mimētikos* imitative] 1. mimicking the effects of impulses conveyed by adrenergic postganglionic fibers of the sympathetic nervous system. 2. an agent that produces effects similar to those of impulses conveyed by adrenergic postganglionic fibers of the sympathetic nervous system. Called also *adrenergic.*

sympathy (sim′pah-the) [Gr. *sympatheia*] 1. sharing of a compassion for another person's thoughts, feelings, and experiences; cf. *empathy.* 2. an influence produced in any organ by disease or disorder in another part. 3. a relation which exists between the mind and the body, causing the one to be affected by the other. 4. the influence exerted by one individual upon another, or received by one from another, and the effects thus produced, as seen in hypnotism, in yawning, and in the transfer of hysterical symptoms.

sympectothiene (sim-pek″to-thi′ēn) ergothioneine.

sympectothion (sim-pek″to-thi′on) [Gr. *syn* together + *pexis* fixation + *theion* sulfur] ergothioneine.

sympexion (sim-pek′se-on), pl. *sympex′ia* [Gr. *sympēxis* condensation, coagulation + *on* neuter ending] a concretion.

symphalangia (sim″fah-lan′je-ah) [Gr. *syn* together + *phalanges* + *-ia*] congenital end-to-end fusion of contiguous phalanges of a digit, usually associated with other deformity of the hand or foot.

symphalangism (sim-fal′an-jizm) symphalangia.

symphoricarpus (sim″fōr-ĭ-kar′pus) [Gr. *symphorein* to bear together + *karpos* fruit] a homeopathic preparation of the fruit of *Symphoricarpos racemosus,* or snowberry, a shrub of North America.

Symphoromyia (sim″for-o-mi′yah) a genus of flies (snipe flies) of the family Rhagionidae, some of which are severe biters of man and animals.

Symphyacanthida (sim″fe-ah-kan′thĭ-dah) [Gr. *syn* together + *phyein* to grow + *akantha* thorn, prickle] an order of marine protozoa (class Acantharea, superclass Actinopoda), characterized by the presence of 20 radial spines fused in the cell center or forming there a small sphere by apposition of their basal pyramids, and the capsular membrane situated far outside of the central cell mass.

symphyocephalus (sim″fe-o-sef′ah-lus) [Gr. *syn* together + *phyein* to grow + *kephalē* head] a twin fetus joined at the head.

symphyseal (sim-fiz′e-al) pertaining to a symphysis.

symphyseorrhaphy (sim-fiz″e-or′ah-fe) symphysiorrhaphy.

symphyses (sim′fĭ-sēz) [Gr.] plural of *symphysis.*

symphysial (sim-fiz′e-al) symphyseal.

symphysic (sim-fiz′ik) characterized by abnormal fusion of adjacent parts.

symphysiolysis (sim-fiz″e-ol′ĭ-sis) [*symphysis* + Gr. *lysis* dissolution] separation or slipping of symphyses, especially the symphysis pubis.

symphysiorrhaphy (sim-fiz″e-or′ah-fe) [*symphysis* + Gr. *rhaphē* suture] the suture of a divided symphysis.

symphysiotome (sim-fiz′e-o-tōm) a knife used in performing symphysiotomy.

symphysiotomy (sim-fiz″e-ot′o-me) [*symphysis* + Gr. *tomē* a cutting] the division of the fibrocartilage of the symphysis pubis, in order to facilitate delivery, by increasing the diameter of the pelvis.

symphysis (sim′fĭ-sis), pl. *sym′physes* [Gr. "a growing together, natural junction"] [NA] a type of cartilaginous joint in which the apposed bony surfaces are firmly united by a plate of fibrocartilage; called also *fibrocartilaginous joint*. **intervertebral s., s. intervertebra′lis** [NA], the union between the vertebral bodies, consisting of the anterior and posterior longitudinal ligaments, and the intervertebral disks. **s. mandib′ulae, mandibular s., s. men′ti,** s. mentalis. **manubriosternal s., s. manubriosterna′lis** [NA], the joint uniting the manubrium with the body of the sternum, which begins as a synchondrosis (*synchondrosis manubriosternalis* [NA]) and later becomes a symphysis. **s. menta′lis** [NA], the line of fusion in the median plane of the mandible that marks the union of the two halves of the mandible; called also *s. mandibulae, mandibular s.,* and *s. menti.* **s. os′sium pu′bis, pubic s.,** s. pubica. **s. pu′bica** [NA], **s. pu′bis,** the joint formed by union of the bodies of the pubic bones in the median plane by a thick mass of fibrocartilage; called also *s. ossium pubis* and *pubic s.* **s. sacrococcyg′ea, sacrococcygeal s.,** articulatio sacrococcygea. **sacroiliac s.,** articulatio sacroiliaca.

symphysodactyly (sim″fĭ-so-dak′tĭ-le) [Gr. *symphysis* a growing together + *daktylos* finger] fusion of the fingers or toes.

Symphytum (sim′fĭ-tum) [L.; Gr. *symphyton*] a genus of boraginaceous plants; *S. officinale* L., common comfrey, is the comfrey of Europe and North America; its roots and leaves are demulcent and astringent.

symphytum (sim′fĭ-tum) a demulcent and astringent homeopathic preparation of *Symphytum officinale.*

symplasm (sim′plazm) tissue in which there is no cellular structure.

symplasmatic (sim″plaz-mat′ik) marked by union of protoplasm.

symplast (sim′plast) symplasm.

symplex (sim′pleks) a chemical compound in which a high molecular substance is bound by residual valencies; included are activators, adsorbents, hemoglobin, and toxin-antitoxin.

sympodia (sim-po′de-ah) [Gr. *syn* together + *pous* foot + *-ia*] fusion of the lower extremities. Cf. *sirenomelus* and *sympus.*

symport (sim′port) a mechanism of transporting two compounds simultaneously across a cell membrane in the same direction, one compound being transported down a concentration gradient, the other against a gradient.

symptom (simp′tum) [L. *symptoma*; Gr. *symptōma* anything that has befallen one] any subjective evidence of disease or of a patient's condition, i.e., such evidence as perceived by the patient; a change in a patient's condition indicative of some bodily or mental state. See also *sign.* **abstinence s′s,** withdrawal (def. 2). **accessory s.,** any symptom not pathognomonic. **Anton's s.,** denial of, and usually unawareness of, one's own blindness, with resort to confabulation, as seen in cortical blindness due to bilateral infarction of the occipital lobes; called also *Anton's syndrome.* **assident s.,** accessory s. **Bárány's s.,** 1. in disturbances of equilibrium of the vestibular apparatus, the direction of the fall is influenced by changing the position of the patient's head. 2. see *caloric test,* under *test.* **Baumés's s.,** see under *sign.* **Béhier-Hardy s.,** see under *sign.* **Bekhterev's s.,** paralysis of the facial muscles for automatic movements. **Berger's s.,** see under *sign.* **Bonhoeffer's s.,** loss of normal muscle tonus in chorea. **Brauch-Romberg s.,** see *Romberg's sign,* under *sign.* **Buerger's s.,** in thromboangiitis obliterans, the pain in the affected leg when the patient is lying down is relieved only by lying with the leg hung over the side of the bed. **Burghart's s.,** fine rales over the anterior inferior edge of the

lung; an early sign of pulmonary tuberculosis. **Cardarelli's s.,** see under *sign.* **cardinal s.,** 1. a symptom of greatest significance to the physician, establishing the identity of the illness. 2. [pl.] the symptoms shown in the pulse, temperature, and respiration. **Castellani-Low s.,** a fine tremor of the tongue seen in sleeping sickness. **characteristic s.,** a symptom that is almost universally associated with a particular disease or condition. **Chvostek's s.,** see under *sign.* **Colliver's s.,** a peculiar twitching, tremulous, or convulsive movement of the limbs, face, jaw, and sometimes of the entire body, seen in the preparalytic stage of poliomyelitis. **concomitant s.,** a symptom not essential to a disease, but which may have an accessory value in its diagnosis. **consecutive s.,** a symptom appearing during convalescence from a disease, but having no connection with the disease. **constitutional s.,** a symptom which is indicative of or due to disorder of the whole body. **crossbar s. of Fraenkel,** blocking of the peristaltic wave on the lesser curvature of the stomach at the site of an ulcer, on fluoroscopy of the stomach. **deficiency s.,** a symptom which is due to a deficiency of the secretion of some endocrine gland. **delayed s.,** one which does not appear for some time after the occurrence of the causes which produce it. **direct s.,** one which is directly caused by the disease. **dissociation s.,** anesthesia to pain and to heat and cold without loss of tactile sensibility; seen in syringomyelia. **endothelial s.,** see *Rumpel-Leede phenomenon,* under *phenomenon.* **Epstein's s.,** a symptom seen in nervous infants, consisting of failure of the upper lid to move downward, giving the child a frightened expression. **equivocal s.,** a symptom which may be produced by several different diseases. **esophagosalivary s.,** excessive flow of saliva in patients with cancer of the esophagus. **general s.,** constitutional s. **Goldthwait's s.,** see under *sign.* **Griesinger's s.,** see under *sign.* **guiding s.,** characteristic s. **Haenel s.,** in tabes there is a lack of sensation on pressure over the eyeballs. **halo s.,** the seeing of colored rings around an individual light source; indicative of glaucoma. **Huchard's s.,** see under *sign.* **incarceration s.,** periodically recurring symptoms of displaced kidney, such as nephralgia, gastralgia, and severe collapse; called also *Dietl's crisis.* **indirect s.,** a symptom which points to a condition that may or may not be due to a particular disease or lesion. **induced s.,** one produced intentionally. **Jellinek's s.,** see under *sign.* **Kerandel's s.,** see under *sign.* **Kocher's s.,** see under *sign.* **Kussmaul's s.,** see under *sign* (def. 2). **labyrinthine s′s,** a group of symptoms indicating disease of the internal ear. **Liebreich's s.,** a symptom of red-green color blindness in which light effects appear red and shadows green. **local s.,** one due to local disease or to a particular lesion. **localizing s′s,** symptoms that indicate the location of a lesion. **Magendie's s.,** skew deviation. **Magnan's s.,** a sensation as of a round body beneath the skin, sometimes experienced in chronic cocainism. **neighborhood s.,** a symptom produced in an organ by disease in a neighboring organ, as by pressure of a tumor in one organ on an organ adjacent to it. **nostril s.,** dilatation of the nostrils during expiration and dropping during inspiration. **objective s.,** one that is obvious to the senses of the observer; see *sign.* **Oehler's s.,** coldness and pallor of the feet in intermittent claudication. **passive s.,** static s. **pathognomonic s.,** one that establishes with certainty the diagnosis of the disease. **Pel-Ebstein s.,** see under *fever.* **precursory s., premonitory s.,** signal s. **presenting s.,** the symptom or group of symptoms of which the patient complains the most or from which he seeks relief. **rainbow s.,** halo s. **rational s.,** subjective s. **reflex s.,** a symptom occurring in a part remote from that which is affected by the disease. **Remak's s.,** polyesthesia; also a prolongation of the lapse of time before a painful impression is perceived; both are noted in tabes dorsalis. **Roger's s.,** a temperature below the normal in the third stage of tuberculous meningitis. **Romberg-Howship s.,** see under *sign.* **Séguin's signal s.,** the involuntary contraction of the muscles just before an epileptic attack. **signal s.,** a sensation, aura, or other subjective experience that gives warning of the approach of an epileptic or other seizure. **Sklowsky's s.,** when light pressure with the index finger is made upon the healthy skin near, and then over, a vesicle in varicella, the wall of the vesicle easily collapses and the contents are discharged. **static s.,** a condition indicative of the state of some particular organ independent of the rest of the body; called also *passive s.* **Stellwag's s.,** see under *sign.* **Stierlin's s.,** indurating and ulcerative processes, especially tuberculosis of the cecum and ascending colon, are shown in the roentgen plate by absence of the normal shadow following a contrast meal. **subjective s.,** one that is perceptible to the patient only. **sympathetic s.,** one due to sympathy, as when pain or other disorder affects a part when some other part is the seat of the disease proper. **Tar's s.,** in health the lower borders of the lungs are situated as deeply in the lying down position with moderate exhalation as in the upright position with deep inhalation; in infiltrating process of the lungs this is not the case. **Trendelenburg's s.,** a waddling gait due to paralysis of the gluteal muscles; see also *Trendelenburg's test,* def. 2, under *tests.* **Wartenberg's s.,** 1. itching of the nostrils and tip of the nose indicative of cerebral tumor. 2. flexion of the thumb occurring on flexion of the other fingers against resistance; seen in pyramidal lesions. **Weber's s.,** see under *sign.* **Wernicke's s.,** hemiopic pupillary reaction. **Westphal's s.,** see under *sign.* **withdrawal s's,** withdrawal (def. 2).

symptomatic (simp″to-mat′ik) [Gr. *symptōmatikos*] 1. pertaining to or of the nature of a symptom. 2. indicative (of a particular disease or disorder). 3. exhibiting the symptoms of a particular disease but having a different cause. 4. directed at the allaying of symptoms, as symptomatic treatment.

symptomatology (simp″tom-ah-tol′o-je) 1. that branch of medicine which treats of symptoms; the systematic discussion of symptoms. 2. the combined symptoms of a disease.

symptomatolytic (simp″to-mah-to-lit′ik) [*symptom* + Gr. *lytikos* dissolving] causing the disappearance of symptoms.

symptome (samp-tōm′) [Fr.] symptom. **s's complice′** [Fr. "symptom complex"], a group of symptoms characteristic of a certain condition.

symptomolytic (simp″to-mo-lit′ik) symptomatolytic.

symptosis (simp-to′sis) [Gr. *syn* together + *ptōsis* fall] the gradual wasting of the whole body or of any organ.

sympus (sim′pus) [Gr. *syn* together + *pous* foot] a fetus exhibiting fusion of the lower limbs. Cf. *sirenomelus.* **s. a′pus,** sirenomelus. **s. di′pus,** a form in which both feet are present. **s. mo′nopus,** a form in which one foot is present.

Syms's tractor (simz′ez) [Parker *Syms,* American surgeon, 1860–1933] see under *tractor.*

syn- [Gr. *syn* with, together] a prefix signifying union or association.

synadelphus (sin″ah-del′fus) [*syn-* + Gr. *adelphos* brother] a monster with a single body and eight limbs.

synaetion (sin-e′te-on) [Gr. *synaitios* being a joint cause] the secondary or cooperative cause of a disease.

Synalar (sin′ah-lar) trademark for a preparation of fluocinolone acetonide.

synalbumin (sin″al-bu′min) a postulated competitive inhibitor of insulin, an insulin B chain bound to albumin; of doubtful significance in human diabetes mellitus.

synalgia (sin-al′je-ah) pain experienced in one place as the result of a lesion in another.

synalgic (sin-al′jik) affected with or of the nature of synalgia.

synanche (sin-an′ke) cynanche.

Synangium (sin-an′je-um) in former systems of classification, a genus of bacteria made up of organisms now classified as *Chondromyces.*

synanthrin (sin-an′thrin) inulin.

synanthrose (sin-an′thrōs) levulin.

synaphymenitis (sin-af″ĭ-men-i′tis) conjunctivitis.

synapse (sin′aps) [Gr. *synapsis* a conjunction, connection] the site of functional apposition between neurons, at which an impulse is transmitted from one neuron to another by either electrical (see *ephapse*) or chemical means. In the typical synapse, the impulse is transmitted by a neurotransmitter (e.g., acetylcholine, norepinephrine, etc.) released by the axon terminal of the excited (presynaptic) cell, which diffuses across the synaptic cleft to bind with receptors on the postsynaptic cell membrane, and thereby effects electrical changes in the postsynaptic cell which result in depolarization (excitation) or hyperpolarization (inhibition). Synapses also occur at sites of apposition between nerve endings and

effector organs (e.g., the neuromuscular junction). **axoaxonic s.,** one between the axon of one neuron and the axon of another neuron. **axodendritic s.,** one between the axon of one neuron and dendrites of another. **axodendrosomatic s.,** one between the axon of one neuron and the dendrites and body (soma) of another, as in motoneurons. **axosomatic s.,** one between the axon of one neuron and the body (soma) of another. **dendrodendritic s.,** one from a dendrite of one cell to a dendrite of another. **electrotonic s.,** see *gap junction,* under *junction.* **en passant s.,** synaptic contact characterized by a crossing of cells with similar fiber membranes lying alongside one another, as in coelenterates. **loop s.,** one having a relatively long area of contact of fiber membranes, as in many invertebrates.

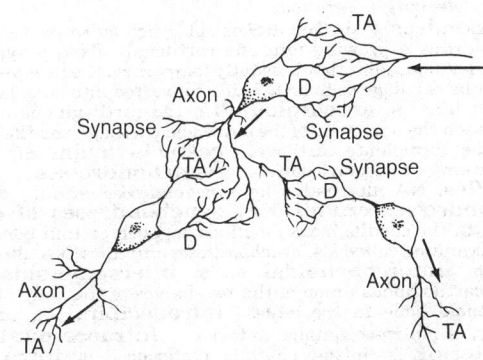

Diagram of three synapses. Nerve impulse is indicated by arrows, showing that the direction of passage is from the terminal arborization (TA) or nerve endings of the axon of one neuron to the dendrites (D) of another neuron.

synapsis (sĭ-nap′sis) [Gr. "conjunction"] the pairing off in point-for-point association of homologous chromosomes from the male and female pronuclei during the early prophase of meiosis.

synaptene (sĭ-nap′tēn) amphitene.

synaptic (sĭ-nap′tik) pertaining to or affecting a synapse; pertaining to synapsis.

synaptology (sin″ap-tol′o-je) that branch of neurology which deals with the synaptic correlations of the nervous system.

synaptosome (sin-ap′to-sōm″) any of the membrane-bound sacs that break away from axon terminals at a synapse after brain tissue has been homogenized in sugar solution; it contains synaptic vessels and mitochondria.

synarthrodia (sin″ar-thro′de-ah) [*syn-* + Gr. *arthrōdia* joint] synarthrosis.

synarthrodial (sin″ar-thro′de-al) pertaining to a synarthrosis.

synarthrophysis (sin″ar-thro-fi′sis) [*syn-* + Gr. *arthron* joint + *physis* growth] any ankylosing process; progressive ankylosis of joints.

synarthroses (sin″ar-thro′sēz) [Gr.] plural of *synarthrosis.*

synarthrosis (sin″ar-thro′sis), pl. *synarthro′ses* [*syn-* + Gr. *arthrōsis* joint] any fibrous joint; see *articulationes fibrosae* [NA], under *articulatio.*

synathresis (sin″ath-re′sis) synathroisis.

synathroisis (sin″ath-roi′sis) [*syn-* + Gr. *athroisis* collection] local hyperemia or congestion.

syncaine (sin-ka′in) procaine hydrochloride.

syncanthus (sin-kan′thus) [*syn-* + Gr. *kanthos* canthus] adhesion of the eyeball to the orbital structures.

syncaryon (sin-kar′e-on) [*syn-* + Gr. *karyon* nucleus] the nucleus formed by fusion of two pronuclei.

syncelom (sin-se′lom) the perivisceral cavities of the body considered as one structure, including the pleural, cardiac, and peritoneal cavities, and tunica vaginalis.

syncephalus (sin-sef′ah-lus) [*syn-* + Gr. *kephalē* head] a double monster with one head, there being a single face with four ears, two on the back of the head.

synchesis (sin′ke-sis) synchysis.

synchilia (sin-ki′le-ah) [*syn-* + Gr. *cheilos* lip + *-ia*] congenital adhesion of the lips.

synchiria (sin-ki′re-ah) [*syn-* + Gr. *cheir* hand + *-ia*] a condition in which the sensation produced by a stimulus applied to one side of the body is referred to both sides.

syncholia (sin-ko′le-ah) [*syn-* + Gr. *cholē* bile + *-ia*] the secretion of substances of exogenous origin in the bile.

synchondrectomy (sin″kon-drek′to-me) [*synchondrosis* + Gr. *ektomē* excision] surgical excision of a synchondrosis, especially of the symphysis of the pubic bone.

synchondroseotomy (sin″kon-dro″se-ot′o-me) [*synchondrosis* + Gr. *tomē* a cutting] an operation for exstrophy of the bladder done by cutting through the sacroiliac ligaments and forcibly drawing together the pelvic bones; called also *Trendelenburg's operation*.

synchondrosis (sin″kon-dro′sis), pl. *synchondro′ses* [Gr. *synchondrōsis* a growing into one cartilage] [NA] a type of cartilaginous joint that is usually temporary, the intervening hyaline cartilage ordinarily being converted into bone before adult life. **s. arycornicula′ta,** the cartilaginous union between the upper end of the arytenoid cartilage and the base of the corniculate cartilage. **costoclavicular s.,** ligamentum costoclaviculare. **synchondro′ses cra-nia′les,** NA alternative for *synchondroses cranii.* **synchondro′ses cra′nii** [NA], **synchondroses of cranium,** the cartilaginous junctions between certain bones of the cranium; called also *synchondroses craniales* [NA alternative]. **intersphenoidal s., s. intersphenoida′lis,** the cartilaginous union of the two halves of the body of the sphenoid bone in the fetus. **intraoccipital s., anterior,** s. intra-occipitalis anterior. **intraoccipital s., posterior,** s. intra-occipitalis posterior. **s. intra-occipita′lis ante′rior** [NA], anterior intraoccipital synchondrosis: the cartilaginous union of the pars basilaris with the partes laterales of the occipital bone in the newborn. **s. intra-occipita′lis poste′rior** [NA], posterior intraoccipital synchondrosis: the cartilaginous union of the squama with the partes laterales of the occipital bone in the newborn. **manubriosternal s., s. manubriosterna′lis** [NA], the joint uniting the manubrium with the body of the sternum, which begins as a synchondrosis and later becomes a symphysis (*symphysis manubriosternalis* [NA]). **petro-occipital s., s. petro-occipita′lis** [NA], the plate of cartilage in the petrooccipital fissure which helps to unite the basilar portion of the occipital bone and the petrous portion of the temporal bone. **pubic s., s. pu′bis,** symphysis pubica. **sacrococcygeal s.,** junctura sacrococcygea. **synchondroses of skull,** synchondroses cranii. **sphenobasilar s.,** s. spheno-occipitalis. **sphenoethmoidal s., s. spheno-ethmoida′lis** [NA], the cartilaginous union between the body of the sphenoid and the labyrinth of the ethmoid bone. **spheno-occipital s.,** 1. s. spheno-occipitalis. 2. in cephalography, the uppermost point of the synchondrosis spheno-occipitalis. Called also *point S₀.* Abbreviated S₀. **s. spheno-occipita′lis** [NA], the cartilaginous union of the anterior end of the basilar portion of the occipital bone with the posterior surface of the body of the sphenoid bone. **s. sphenopetro′sa,** [NA], **sphenopetrosal s.,** the cartilaginous union of the lower border of the great wing of the sphenoid bone with the petrous portion of the temporal bone in the sphenopetrosal fissure. **sternal s., s. sterna′lis** [NA], the cartilaginous union between the manubrium and the body of the sternum.

synchondrotomy (sin″kon-drot′o-me) [*synchondrosis* + Gr. *tomē* a cutting] the division of the symphysis pubis or of any other synchondrosis.

synchorial (sin-ko′re-al) sharing a common placenta; said of multiple fetuses.

synchronia (sin-kro′ne-ah) 1. synchronism. 2. the formation of parts or tissues at the usual time. Cf. *heterochronia* (def. 1).

synchronism (sin′kro-nizm) occurrence at the same time; the quality of being synchronous.

synchronous (sin′kro-nus) [*syn-* + Gr. *chronos* time] occurring at the same time.

synchrotron (sin′kro-tron) a machine for generating high-speed electrons or protons. It combines features of the cyclotron and betatron and will produce 70 million volts.

synchysis (sin′kĭ-sis) [Gr. "a mixing together"] a softening or fluid condition of the vitreous body of the eye; synchysis corporis vitrei. **s. scintil′lans,** cholesterol crystals in the vitreous that develop as a degenerative change following inflammation or other ocular diseases.

syncinesis (sin″si-ne′sis) synkinesis.

synciput (sin′sĭ-put) sinciput.

synclinal (sin-kli′nal) [Gr. *synklinein* to lean together] bent or inclined together.

synclitic (sin-klit′ik) pertaining to or marked by synclitism.

synclitism, syncliticism (sin′klit-izm; sin-klit′ĭ-sizm) [Gr. *synklinein* to lean together] 1. parallelism between the planes of the fetal head and those of the pelvis. 2. normal, synchronous maturation of the nucleus and cytoplasm of blood cells. Cf. *asynclitism.*

synclonus (sin′klo-nus) [*syn-* + Gr. *klonos* turmoil] 1. muscular tremor, or the successive clonic contraction of various muscles together. 2. any disease characterized by muscular tremors. **s. beriber′ica,** muscular tremors associated with beriberi.

syncopal (sin′ko-pal) pertaining to or characterized by syncope.

syncope (sin′ko-pe) [Gr. *synkopē*] a temporary suspension of consciousness due to generalized cerebral ischemia; a faint or swoon. **Adams-Stokes s.,** see under *disease.* **s. angino′sa,** fainting with an episode of coronary insufficiency. **cardiac s.,** sudden loss of consciousness, with momentary or no premonitory symptoms, due to cerebral anemia caused by ventricular asystole, extreme bradycardia, or ventricular fibrillation. **carotid sinus s.,** carotid sinus syndrome. **cough s.,** tussive s. **digital s.,** a sudden temporary loss of strength in the fingers. **laryngeal s.,** tussive s. **micturition s.,** brief loss of consciousness during or immediately after micturition, associated with rising from bed at night to urinate; it may be a form of orthostatic hypotension. **postural s.,** that resulting from orthostatic hypotension. **stretching s.,** syncope associated with stretching the arms upward with the spine extended. **swallow s.,** syncope associated with swallowing, a disorder of atrioventricular conduction mediated by the vagus nerve. **tussive s.,** brief loss of consciousness associated with vigorous and explosive paroxysms of coughing, usually seen in men; called also *cough s., laryngeal s.,* and *laryngeal vertigo.* **vasodepressor s.,** vasovagal attack. **vasovagal s.,** see under *attack.*

syncopic (sin-kop′ik) syncopal.

syncretio (sin-kre′she-o) [L.] a growing together or adhesion, as between inflamed serous surfaces in contact.

Syncurine (sin′ku-rēn) trademark for a preparation of decamethonium bromide.

syncytial (sin-sish′al) of, pertaining to, or producing a syncytium.

syncytiolysin (sin″sit-e-ol′ĭ-sin) a lysin destructive to the syncytium; formed in the blood of an animal into which matter from the placenta of another animal has been injected.

syncytioma (sin-sit″e-o′mah) syncytial endometritis. **s. malig′num,** choriocarcinoma.

syncytiotoxin (sin-sit″e-o-tok′sin) a toxin that has a specific action on the placenta.

syncytiotrophoblast (sin-sit″e-o-trof′o-blast) the outer syncytial layer of the trophoblast; called also *syntrophoblast.*

syncytium (sin-sish′e-um) a multinucleate mass of protoplasm produced by the merging of cells.

syncytoid (sin′sĭ-toid) resembling a syncytium.

syndactylia (sin″dak-til′e-ah) syndactyly.

syndactylism (sin-dak′tĭ-lizm) syndactyly.

syndactylous (sin-dak′tĭ-lus) pertaining to or characterized by syndactyly.

syndactylus (sin-dak′tĭ-lus) an individual exhibiting syndactyly.

syndactyly (sin-dak′tĭ-le) [*syn-* + *daktylos* finger] an autosomal dominant trait, the most common congenital anomaly of the hand or foot, marked by persistence of the webbing between adjacent digits, so they are more or less completely attached. **complete s.,** syndactyly in which the connection extends from the base of the involved digits to the tip.

complicated s., syndactyly in which the bones or nails of the involved digits are fused. **double s.,** syndactyly involving three digits (two webs). **partial s.,** syndactyly in which the connecting web extends only part way up from the base of the involved digits. **simple s.,** syndactyly in which the connecting web consists only of skin. **single s.,** syndactyly involving two digits (a single web). **triple s.,** syndactyly involving four digits (three webs).

syndectomy (sin-dek'to-me) peritectomy.

syndelphus (sin-del'fus) synadelphus.

syndesis (sin'dĕ-sis, sin-de'sis) [syn- + Gr. *desis* binding] 1. arthrodesis. 2. synapsis.

syndesmectomy (sin"des-mek'to-me) [syndesmo- + Gr. *ektomē* excision] excision or resection of a ligament.

syndesmectopia (sin"des-mek-to'pe-ah) [syndesmo- + Gr. *ektopos* out of place + -ia] unusual situation of a ligament.

syndesmitis (sin"des-mi'tis) [syndesmo- + -itis] 1. inflammation of a ligament or ligaments. 2. conjunctivitis. **s. metatar'sea,** inflammation of the metatarsal ligaments occurring during strenuous marches; called also *march tumor.*

syndesm(o)- [Gr. *syndesmos* band or ligament] a combining form denoting relationship to connective tissue, particularly the ligaments.

syndesmochorial (sin"des-mo-ko're-al) a type of placentation, occurring in ruminants, characterized by limited destruction of the endometrial epithelium.

syndesmography (sin"des-mog'rah-fe) [syndesmo- + Gr. *graphein* to write] a description of the ligaments.

syndesmologia (sin"des-mo-lo'je-ah) arthrologia.

syndesmology (sin"des-mol'o-je) [syndesmo- + Gr. *logos* treatise] arthrology.

syndesmoma (sin"des-mo'mah) a connective tissue tumor.

syndesmo-odontoid (sin-des"mo-o-don'toid) the posterior of the two atloaxoid articulations formed between the anterior surface of the transverse ligaments and the back of the odontoid process.

syndesmopexy (sin-des'mo-pek"se) [syndesmo- + Gr. *pēxis* fixation] the operative fixation of a dislocation by reattachment of the ligaments.

syndesmophyte (sin-des'mo-fīt) [syndesmo- + Gr. *phyton* plant] an osseous excrescence, or bony outgrowth, from a ligament.

syndesmoplasty (sin-des'mo-plas"te) [syndesmo- + Gr. *plassein* to form] plastic operation on a ligament.

syndesmorrhaphy (sin"des-mor'ah-fe) [syndesmo- + Gr. *rhaphē* suture] suture or repair of ligaments.

syndesmosis (sin"des-mo'sis) pl. *syndesmo'ses* [Gr. *syndesmos* band] [NA] a type of fibrous joint in which the intervening fibrous connective tissue forms an interosseous membrane or ligament. **radioulnar s., s. radio-ulna'ris** [NA], the fibrous union of the radius and ulna, which consists of the interosseous membrane of the forearm and the oblique cord of the elbow; called also *articulatio radio-ulnaris* [NA alternative] and *radioulnar articulation.* **tibiofibular s., s. tibiofibula'ris** [NA], inferior tibiofibular articulation: a firm fibrous union formed at the distal ends of the tibia and fibula between the fibular notch of the tibia and a roughened triangular surface on the fibula, which frequently contains a synovial prolongation of the cavity of the talocrural articulation. Called also *articulatio tibiofibularis* [NA alternative]. **s. tympanostape'dia** [NA], **tympanostapedial s.,** the connection of the base of the stapes with the secondary membrane in the fenestra vestibuli.

syndesmotomy (sin"des-mot'o-me) [syndesmo- + Gr. *tomē* a cutting] the dissection or cutting of a ligament.

syndrome (sin'drōm) [Gr. *syndromē* concurrence] a set of symptoms which occur together; the sum of signs of any morbid state; a symptom complex. In genetics, a pattern of multiple malformations thought to be pathogenetically related. **Aarskog s., Aarskog-Scott s.,** an X-linked syndrome characterized by ocular hypertelorism, anteverted nostrils, broad upper lip, peculiar scrotal "shawl" above the penis, and small hands. Called also *faciogenital dysplasia* and *faciodigitogenital s.* **Aase s.,** a familial syndrome characterized by mild growth retardation, hypoplastic anemia, variable leukocytopenia, triphalangeal thumbs, narrow

shoulders, and late closure of fontanels, and occasionally by cleft lip, cleft palate, retinopathy, and web neck. A recessive mode of inheritance has been suggested. **Abercrombie's s.,** amyloid degeneration. **abstinence s.,** withdrawal (def. 2). **Achard s.,** arachnodactyly associated with receding mandible and joint laxity limited to the hands and feet. **Achard-Thiers s.,** an association of diabetes, hirsutism, and other masculinizing features in postmenopausal women resulting from overproduction of adrenocortical androgens. **acquired immune deficiency s., acquired immunodeficiency s. (AIDS),** an epidemic, transmissible retroviral disease due to infection with human immunodeficiency virus (HIV), manifested in severe cases as profound depression of cell-mediated immunity, and affecting certain recognized risk groups, including homosexual or bisexual males, intravenous drug abusers, hemophiliacs and other blood transfusion recipients, female sexual contacts of males in at-risk groups, and newborn infants of individuals at risk for AIDS. The criteria established by the Centers for Disease Control for the diagnosis of AIDS (CDC/AIDS) comprise: the presence of reliably diagnosed disease that is at least moderately indicative of an underlying defect in cell-mediated immunity (e.g., Kaposi sarcoma in an individual less than 60 years of age, or Pneumocystis pneumonia or other life-threatening opportunistic infection), occurring in the absence of known causes of underlying immunodeficiency or of any other host defense defects reported to be associated with that disease (e.g., iatrogenic immunosuppression or lymphoreticular malignancies). See also *AIDS-related complex,* under *complex.* **acute brain s., acute organic brain s.,** see *organic brain s.* **acute radiation s.,** a syndrome caused by exposure to a whole-body dose of over 1 gray of ionizing radiation. Symptoms, whose severity and time of onset depend on the size of the dose, include erythema, nausea and vomiting, fatigue, diarrhea, fever, petechiae, bleeding from the mucous membranes, reduction in the number of lymphocytes, granulocytes, and platelets, gastrointestinal hemorrhage, epilation, hypotension, tachycardia, and dehydration; death may occur within hours or weeks of exposure. **Adair-Dighton s.,** van der Hoeve's s. **Adams-Stokes s.,** see under *disease.* **addisonian s.,** the complex of symptoms resulting from adrenal insufficiency; see *Addison's disease,* under *disease.* **Adie's s.,** a syndrome consisting of a pathological pupil reaction (tonic pupil), the most important element of which is a myotonic condition on accommodation; the pupil on the affected side contracts on near vision more slowly than does the pupil on the opposite side, and it also dilates more slowly. The affected pupil does not usually react to direct or indirect light, but it may do so in an abnormal fashion. Certain tendon reflexes are absent or diminished, but there are no motor or sensory disturbances, nor demonstrable changes indicative of disease of the nervous system. Called also *Holmes-Adie s.* **adiposogenital s.,** adiposogenital dystrophy. **adrenogenital s.,** hyperfunction of the adrenal cortex, associated with any of five enzymatic defects, that results in pseudohermaphroditism and virilism in the female, usually evident at birth, and precocious sexual development (epiphyseal syndrome) in the male, usually not appearing until three or four years after birth; the clinical findings are due to deficient production of cortisol and consequent hypersecretion of pituitary ACTH, resulting in excessive production of androgen. Called also *congenital adrenal hyperplasia.* **adult respiratory distress s. (ARDS),** fulminant pulmonary interstitial and alveolar edema, which usually develops a few days after the initiating trauma, thought to result from a massive sympathetic discharge due to brain injury or hypoxia and from increased capillary permeability. Called also *shock lung.* **afferent loop s.,** chronic partial obstruction of the proximal loop of duodenum and jejunum after partial gastrectomy and gastrojejunostomy, resulting in duodenal distention, pain, and nausea following ingestion of food. **aglossia-adactylia s.,** hypoglossia-adactylia s. **Ahumada-del Castillo s.,** a nonpuerperal triad consisting of galactorrhea, amenorrhea, and low gonadotropin secretion. **Aicardi's s.,** a syndrome affecting female infants, characterized by agenesis of the corpus callosum, large discrete areas of chorioretinopathy, spasms and tonic seizures, and mental retardation. **Alajouanine's s.,** symmetric lesions of the sixth and seventh cranial nerves with bilateral facial paralysis and bilateral lateral rectus palsy of the eyeball, associated with bilateral clubfoot. **Albright's s., Albright-McCune-Sternberg s.,** polyostotic fibrous dysplasia, patchy dermal pigmentation, and endocrine dysfunction. Called also *Albright's disease* and *McCune-Albright* s. **Aldrich's s.,** Wiskott-Aldrich s. **Alezzandrini's s.,** unilateral tapetoretinal degeneration followed by facial vitiligo and poliosis on the same side, sometimes associated with deafness. **"Alice in Wonderland" s.,** a delusional state manifested by depersonalization, disturbance of body image, alteration in the sense of the passage of time, and other delusions or illusions. It may be associated with schizophrenia, epilepsy, migraine, diseases of the parietal lobe, hypnogogic states, or the use of hallucinogenic drugs. **Allemann's s.,** the association of double kidney and clubbed fingers, sometimes associated with facial asymmetry and degeneration of various motor nerves. **Alport's s.,** a hereditary disorder characterized by progressive sensorineural hearing loss, progressive pyelonephritis or glomerulonephritis, and, occasionally, ocular defects. It is transmitted as an autosomal dominant trait. **Alström s.,** an autosomal recessive syndrome of retinitis pigmentosa with nystagmus and early loss of central vision, deafness, obesity, and diabetes mellitus. **amnesic s.,** amnestic s. **amnestic s.** [DSM III-R], an organic mental disorder characterized by impairment of memory, both anterograde and retrograde amnesia, occurring in a normal state of consciousness; i.e., the syndrome does not include the memory impairment seen in dementia or delirium. Disorientation, confabulation, and a lack of insight into the memory deficit are often present but are not invariable features. The most common cause is thiamine deficiency associated with chronic alcohol abuse (alcohol amnestic disorder, Wernicke-Korsakoff syndrome), but the syndrome may result from any pathological process causing bilateral damage to certain structures in the medial temporal lobe and diencephalon (e.g., the hippocampal formations, mamillary bodies, and dorsal medial nuclei of the thalamus). Causes include head trauma, brain tumors, infarction, cerebral hypoxia, carbon monoxide poisoning, and herpes simplex encephalitis. Called also *amnesic s., amnestic-confabulatory s., dysmnesic s.,* and *Korsakoff's s.* **amnestic-confabulatory s.,** amnestic s. **amniotic infection s. of Blane,** a syndrome in which fetal sepsis follows swallowing and at times aspiration of contaminated amniotic fluid. **amyostatic s.,** Wilson's disease. **Andersen's s.,** bronchiectasis, cystic fibrosis of the pancreas, and vitamin A deficiency. **Angelucci s.,** excitable temperament, palpitation, and vasomotor disturbance in patients with vernal conjunctivitis. **anorexia-cachexia s.,** a systemic response to cancer occurring as a result of a poorly understood relationship between anorexia and cachexia, manifested by malnutrition, weight loss, muscular weakness, acidosis, and toxemia. The basis of the anorexia may be a multifactorial severe metabolic disturbance that contributes to the development of cachectic wasting, which in turn reinforces the anorexia by the release from the tumor of an anorexigenic humoral product that stimulates the satiety center in the hypothalamus, producing appetite loss. **anterior abdominal wall s.,** continuous pain in the anterior abdominal wall, affecting either the left or right lower quadrant or the superior margins of the upper quadrant area; etiology unknown. **anterior chamber cleavage s.,** a term for several types of mesenchymal dysgenesis affecting neural crest derivatives in the iris, trabeculum, and cornea. In ascending severity these disorders are: *posterior embryotoxon, Axenfeld's anomaly, Axenfeld's syndrome, Rieger's anomaly,* and *Rieger's syndrome.* **anterior cord s.,** localized injury to the anterior portion of the spinal cord, characterized by complete paralysis and hypalgesia and hypesthesia to the level of the lesion, but with relative preservation of posterior column sensations of touch, position, and vibration. **anterior cornual s.,** muscular atrophy due to lesions of the anterior horns of the spinal cord. **anterior tibial compartment s.,** rapid swelling, increased tension, pain, and ischemic necrosis of the muscles of the anterior tibial compartment of the leg; the skin becomes glossy, erythematous, and edematous as the necrosis occurs. The cause is unknown, but usually there is a history of excessive exertion. **anticholinergic s.,** the central and peripheral effects produced by overdosage or abnormal reaction to clinical dosage of anticholinergic drugs, e.g., atropine, phenothiazines, antihistamines, and tricyclic antidepressants; signs and symptoms include anxiety, delirium, disorientation, hallucinations, seizures, tachycardia, hyperpyrexia, mydriasis, vasodilation, gastric and urinary retention, and decreased salivary, sweat, bronchial, and nasopha-

ryngeal secretions. **Anton's s.,** see under *symptom.* **anxiety s.,** the physical symptoms accompanying anxiety, such as palpitation of the heart, rapid and shallow respiration, sweating, pallor, and a feeling of panic. **aortic arch s.,** any of a group of disorders leading to occlusion of the arteries arising from the aortic arch; such occlusion may be caused by atherosclerosis, arterial embolism, syphilitic or tuberculous arteritis, etc. See also *pulseless disease,* under *disease.* **Apert s.,** acrocephalosyndactyly. **Apert's s.,** acrocephalosyndactyly. **argentaffinoma s.,** carcinoid s. **Arnold's nerve reflex cough s.,** a reflex cough due to irritation of the area supplied by Arnold's nerve (the auricular branch of the vagus nerve); this area is the posterior and inferior portion of the external auditory canal and the posterior half of the tympanic membrane. **Arnold-Chiari s.,** see under *deformity.* **Ascher s.,** blepharochalasis occurring with goiter (adenoma of the thyroid) and redundancy of the mucous membrane and submucous tissue of the upper lip. **Asherman's s.,** persistent amenorrhea and secondary sterility due to intrauterine adhesions and synechiae, usually occurring as a result of uterine curettage. **Asherson's s.,** a syndrome of dysphagia due to neuromuscular incoordination and achalasia of the cricopharyngeal sphincter with failure of relaxation of the cricopharyngeal muscle during the third stage of swallowing. It causes diversion of liquids into the air passages, precipitating paroxysms of coughing. Called also *cricopharyngeal achalasia s.* **asplenia s.,** Ivemark's s. **ataxia-telangiectasia s.,** see under *ataxia.* **auriculotemporal s.,** the appearance of a red area and of sweating on the cheek in connection with eating; seen in lesions of the parotid gland and due to some involvement of the auriculotemporal nerve. **autoerythrocyte sensitization s.,** painful bruising s. **autoimmune polyendocrine-candidiasis s.,** polyendocrine autoimmune disease, type I. **Avellis' s.,** ipsilateral paralysis of vocal cord and soft palate, loss of pain and temperature sensibility in contralateral leg, trunk, arm, and neck, and in the skin over the scalp; called also *ambiguospinothalamic paralysis.* **Axenfeld's s.,** Axenfeld's anomaly with glaucoma and with defective development of the corneoscleral trabecular meshwork and other angle structures. See also *anterior chamber cleavage s.* **Ayerza's s.,** pulmonary hypertension with dilatation of the pulmonary arteries, related to disease of the lungs; formerly attributed to syphilis. **Baastrup's s.,** kissing spine. **Babinski's s.,** the association of cardiac and arterial disorders with chronic syphilitic meningitis, tabes dorsalis, paralytic dementia, and other late syphilitic manifestations. **Babinski-Fröhlich s.,** adiposogenital dystrophy. **s. of Babinski-Nageotte,** a syndrome due to multiple lesions affecting the pyramid and sensory tracts, the cerebellar peduncle, and the reticular formation, and marked by contralateral hemiplegia and hemianesthesia (usually only of the pain and temperature senses), ipsilateral hemiasynergia, hemiataxia, and Horner's syndrome. **Babinski-Vaquez s.,** Babinski's s. **BADS s.,** a syndrome whose acronym stands for *b*lack locks, oculocutaneous *a*lbinism, and *d*eafness of the *s*ensorineural type; see *oculocutaneous albinism.* **Bäfverstedt's s.,** lymphocytoma cutis. **Balint's s.,** cortical paralysis of visual fixation, optic ataxia, and disturbance of visual attention, with preservation of spontaneous and reflex eye movements. The parieto-occipital lesions are bilateral. **Baller-Gerold s.,** an autosomal recessive syndrome characterized by craniosynostosis and radial aplasia. Called also *craniosynostosis–radial aplasia s.* **Bannwarth's s.,** the European term for the meningopolyneuritis that may occur in Lyme disease. **Banti's s.,** congestive splenomegaly. **Bardet-Biedl s.,** an autosomal recessive disorder characterized by mental retardation, pigmentary retinopathy, obesity, polydactyly, and hypogonadism; cf. *Lawrence-Moon s.* and *Biemond's s., II.* **Barlow s.,** mitral valve prolapse s. **Barraquer-Simons' s.,** partial lipodystrophy. **Barré-Guillain s.,** acute febrile polyneuritis. **Barrett's s.,** peptic ulcer of the lower esophagus, often with stricture, due to the presence of columnar-lined epithelium, which may contain functional mucous cells, parietal cells, or chief cells, in the esophagus instead of normal squamous cell epithelium. Called also *Barrett's esophagus.* **Bart's s.,** a form of epidermolysis bullosa dystrophica inherited as an autosomal dominant trait, characterized by congenital localized absence of the skin with blister formation as a result of mechanical trauma and nail dystrophy. **Bartter's s.,** hypertrophy and hyperplasia of the juxtaglomerular cells, producing hypokalemic alkalosis and hyperaldosteronism, characterized by absence of hypertension in the presence of markedly increased plasma renin concentrations, and by insensitivity to the pressor effects of angiotensin. It usually affects children, is perhaps hereditary, and may be associated with other anomalies, such as mental retardation and short stature. Called also *juxtaglomerular cell hyperplasia.* **basal cell nevus s.,** an autosomal dominant syndrome characterized by the development in early life of numerous basal cell carcinomas, occurring in association with abnormalities of the skin (especially an unusual erythematous pitting edema of the hands and feet), bone, nervous system, eyes, and reproductive tract. Called also *Gorlin's s., Gorlin-Goltz s., nevoid basal cell carcinoma s.,* and *nevoid basali oma s.* **Bassen-Kornzweig s.,** abetalipoproteinemia; see *familial lipoprotein deficiency.* **battered-child s.,** unexplained or inappropriately explained physical trauma and other manifestations of severe, repeated physical abuse of children, usually by a parent. **Bazex's s.,** eczematous and psoriasiform lesions on the ears, nose, cheeks, hands, feet, and knees in patients with carcinomas of the upper respiratory and digestive tracts. Called also *paraneoplastic acrokeratosis.* **Beals' s.,** see *congenital contractural arachnodactyly,* under *arachnodactyly.* **Bearn-Kunkel s., Bearn-Kunkel-Slater s.,** lupoid hepatitis. **Beau's s.,** asystole. **Beckwith's s.,** a hereditary disorder marked by extreme cytomegaly of the fetal adrenal cortex, omphalocele, macroglossia, hyperplasia of the kidney and pancreas, Leydig-cell hyperplasia, and postnatal gigantism. **Beckwith-Wiedemann s.,** a congenital autosomal dominant syndrome with variable expressivity characterized by exomphalos, macroglossia, and gigantism, often associated with visceromegaly, adrenocortical cytomegaly, and dysplasia of the renal medulla. Called also *EMG s.* and *exomphalos-macroglossia-gigantism s.* **Behçet's s.,** a chronic inflammatory disorder involving the small blood vessels, which is of unknown etiology, and is characterized by recurrent aphthous ulceration of the oral and pharyngeal mucous membranes and the genitalia, skin lesions, severe uveitis, retinal vasculitis, and optic atrophy. It frequently also involves the joints, gastrointestinal system, and central nervous system. Called also *Behçet's disease.* **s. of Benedikt,** a syndrome consisting of ipsilateral oculomotor paralysis, contralateral hyperkinesia, contralateral tremor and paresis of the arm and leg, and ipsilateral ataxia; caused by lesions that damage the third nerve and involve the nucleus ruber and corticospinal tract. **Bernard's s., Bernard-Horner s.,** Horner's s. **Bernard-Sergent s.,** diarrhea, vomiting, and collapse characteristic of Addison's disease. **Bernard-Soulier s. (BSS),** see under *disease.* **Bernhardt-Roth s.,** meralgia paraesthetica. **Bernheim's s.,** right heart failure with absence of dyspnea or pulmonary congestion, in the presence of gross left ventricular hypertrophy, sometimes attributed to impairment of right ventricular capacity and filling. **Bertolotti's s.,** sacralization of the fifth lumbar vertebra together with sciatica and scoliosis. **Bianchi's s.,** a sensory aphasic syndrome with apraxia and alexia, seen in lesions of the left parietal lobe. **Biemond s., II,** an autosomal recessive disorder characterized by iris coloboma, obesity, mental retardation, hypogonadism, and postaxial polydactyly; cf. *Bardet-Biedl s.* and *Laurence-Moon s.* **Björnstad's s.,** an autosomal recessive disorder characterized by congenital sensorineural deafness and pili torti. **Blatin's s.,** hydatid thrill. **blind loop s.,** a syndrome resulting from alterations in the anatomy of the small intestine, as by strictures or after surgery, in which a loop is disconnected from the main stream or when intestinal contents may gain access to it but not readily egress from it; it is associated with bacterial overgrowth, particularly anaerobic organisms, with resultant malabsorption of vitamin B_{12}, steatorrhea, and anemia. **Bloch-Sulzberger s.,** incontinentia pigmenti. **Bloom s.,** an autosomal recessive syndrome developing during infancy, consisting of erythema and telangiectasia in a butterfly distribution on the face, photosensitivity, and dwarfism of prenatal onset. Abnormalities in chromosome structure (sister chromatid exchange, q.v.) and in immunoglobulins are present, and there is a high incidence of malignancy, especially leukemia. About one-half of the patients are of Jewish ancestry. **blue diaper s.,** a defect of tryptophan absorption in which, because of intestinal bacterial action on the tryptophan, the urine contains abnormal indoles, giving it a blue color. It is similar to Hartnup's disease. **Blum's s.,** hypochloremic azotemia.

body of Luys s., hemiballismus. **Boerhaave's s.,** spontaneous rupture of the esophagus. **Bonnier's s.,** a series of symptoms due to lesion of Deiters' nucleus or of the vestibular tracts related thereto; it consists of vertigo, pallor, and various aural and ocular disturbances. **Böök's s.,** PHC s. **Börjeson's s., Börjeson-Forssman-Lehmann s.,** an X-linked syndrome characterized by severe mental retardation, epilepsy, hypogonadism, hypometabolism, marked obesity, swelling of the subcutaneous tissues of the face, and large ears. **Bouillaud's s.,** the coincidence of pericarditis and endocarditis in acute articular rheumatism. **Bouveret's s.,** paroxysmal tachycardia. **brachial s.,** a morbid condition resulting from compression or irritation of nerves of the brachial plexus. **Brachmann-de Lange s.,** de Lange's s. **bradycardia-tachycardia s.,** episodic or repetitive tachycardia of short duration followed by transient or protracted heart standstill, sometimes accentuated by quinidine. **Brennemann's s.,** mesenteric and retroperitoneal lymphadenitis as a sequel of throat infections. **Briquet's s.,** hysteria (q.v.), especially that characterized by multiple symptoms, many visits to physicians, and often much unnecessary medical treatment; now called *somatization disorder.* **Brissaud-Marie s.,** hysterical glossolabial hemispasm. **Brissaud-Sicard s.,** spasmodic hemiplegia caused by lesions of the pons. **Bristowe's s.,** a series of ingravescent symptoms characteristic of tumor of the corpus callosum: (1) gradual onset of hemiplegia; (2) association of hemiplegia on one side, vague hemiplegic symptoms on the other; (3) stupor and drowsiness, difficulty of swallowing, and speechlessness; (4) absence of direct implication of the cranial nerves; (5) death from coma. **brittle bone s.,** osteogenesis imperfecta. **brittle cornea s.,** an X-linked, recessively inherited syndrome, characterized by brittle cornea, blue sclerae, and red hair. **Brock s.,** middle lobe s. **Brown's vertical retraction s.,** adhesion of the muscles of the eye in the fetus. **Brown-Séquard s.,** a syndrome due to damage of one half of the spinal cord, resulting in ipsilateral paralysis and loss of discriminatory and joint sensation, and contralateral loss of pain and temperature sensation. Called also *Brown-Séquard's disease, paralysis,* or *sign.* **Bruns' s.,** intermittent headache, vertigo, vomiting, and visual disturbances on sudden movement of the head, characteristic of cysticercus infection of the fourth ventricle, lesion of the fourth ventricle, or tumors of the midline of the cerebellum and third or lateral ventricles; called also *Bruns' sign.* **Brunsting's s.,** a recurrent eruptive syndrome usually affecting middle-aged men, in which grouped, vesicular lesions occur about the head and neck, and result in scarring. **Brushfield-Wyatt s.,** a congenital syndrome consisting of extensive unilateral nevus flammeus, hemianopia affecting the right or left halves of the visual fields of both eyes, contralateral hemiplegia, cerebral angioma, and mental retardation; it is probably related to the Sturge-Weber syndrome. **Buckley's s.,** hyperimmunoglobulinemia E s. **Budd-Chiari s.,** symptomatic obstruction or occlusion of the hepatic veins, causing hepatomegaly, abdominal pain and tenderness, intractable ascites, mild jaundice, and, eventually, portal hypertension and liver failure; the obstruction is caused by thrombi or fibrous obliteration of the veins and has been associated with coagulation disorders, myeloproliferative disorders, invasion of hepatic veins by hepatic, renal, or adrenal carcinoma, and with abdominal trauma. Onset may be acute with death occurring within days in cases of complete occlusion; more often there is a chronic course with survival for months or years. Called also *Budd-Chiari disease, Chiari's disease* or *syndrome,* and *endophlebitis hepatica obliterans.* Cf. *veno-occlusive disease of liver.* **bulbar s.,** Dejerine's syndrome, def. 2. **Bürger-Grütz s.,** familial hyperlipoproteinemia, type I. **Burnett's s.,** milk-alkali s. **burning feet s.,** Gopalan's s. **Buschke-Ollendorff s.,** dermatofibrosis lenticularis disseminata. **Bywaters' s.,** crush s. **Caffey's s., Caffey-Silverman s.,** infantile cortical hyperostosis. **callosal s.,** an association of symptoms thought to result from a lesion of the corpus callosum. **camptomelic s.,** osteochondrodysplasia associated with flat facies, bowed tibiae with skin dimpling, hypoplastic scapulae, and short vertebrae. **Canada-Cronkhite s.,** Cronkhite-Canada s. **Capgras' s.,** the delusion that other persons in the patient's environment are not their real selves but doubles. **Caplan's s.,** pneumoconiosis associated with rheumatoid arthritis. Radiographically, multiple spherical nodular lesions with clearly demarcated borders are found throughout both lungs. Called also *rheumatoid pneumoconiosis*. **capsular thrombosis s.,** hemiplegia due to thrombosis of a blood vessel supplying the internal capsule. **capsulothalamic s.,** hemiplegia, hemianopia, and perverted pain perception due to lesions of the thalamus and internal capsule. **carcinoid s.,** a symptom complex associated with carcinoid tumors (argentaffinoma) and characterized by attacks of severe cyanotic flushing of the skin lasting from minutes to days and by diarrheal watery stools, bronchoconstrictive attacks, sudden drops in blood pressure, edema, and ascites. Symptoms are caused by secretion by the tumor of serotonin, prostaglandins, and other biologically active substances. Called also *argentaffinoma s.* **cardiofacial s.,** a syndrome of congenital heart disease associated with unilateral partial lower facial paresis, the latter being transient or persistent. **carotid sinus s.,** syncope sometimes associated with convulsive seizures due to overactivity of the carotid sinus reflex when pressure is applied to one or both carotid sinuses. **carpal tunnel s.,** a complex of symptoms resulting from compression of the median nerve in the carpal tunnel, with pain and burning or tingling paresthesias in the fingers and hand, sometimes extending to the elbow. **Carpenter's s.,** acrocephalopolysyndactyly, type II. **cat's cry s.,** cri du chat s. **cat-eye s., cat's eye s.,** an association of coloboma of the iris and anal atresia; there may also be many other anomalies, including preauricular skin tags or fistulas, hypertelorism, congenital heart disease, skeletal abnormalities, and renal malformations. It is associated with partial trisomy 22, i.e., the presence of an additional, deleted chromosome 22. **cauda equina s.,** dull aching pain of the perineum, bladder, and sacrum, generally radiating in a sciatic fashion, with associated paresthesias and areflexic paralysis, due to compression of the spinal nerve roots. **caudal dysplasia s., caudal regression s.,** failure of formation of part or all of the coccygeal, sacral, and occasionally lumbar vertebral units and the corresponding segments of the caudal spinal cord, with resulting neurogenic dysfunction of bowel and bladder; called also *sacral agenesis*. **cavernous sinus s.,** edema of the conjunctiva, proptosis, edema of upper lid and root of the nose, together with paralysis of the third, fourth, and sixth nerves, due to thrombosis of the cavernous sinus. **celiac s.,** see under *disease*. **central cord s.,** injury to the central portion of the cervical spinal cord resulting in disproportionately more weakness or paralysis in the upper extremities than in the lower; pathological change is caused by hemorrhage or edema. **centroposterior s.,** syringomyelic dissociation of sensibility and vasomotor disorders, due to lesions of the centroposterior portion of the gray matter of the spinal cord. **cerebellar s.,** hereditary cerebellar ataxia. **cerebrocardiac s.,** Krishaber's disease. **cerebrohepatorenal s.,** an autosomal recessive disorder characterized by craniofacial abnormalities, hypotonia, hepatomegaly, polycystic kidneys, jaundice, and death in early infancy, and associated with absence of peroxisomes in the liver and kidneys; called also *Zellweger s.* **cervical s.,** a condition caused by irritation or compression of the cervical nerve roots, marked by pain in the neck radiating into the shoulder, arm, or forearm, depending on which nerve root is affected. **cervical rib s., cervicobrachial s.,** scalenus s. **Cestan's s., s. of Cestan-Chenais,** an association of contralateral hemiplegia, contralateral hemianesthesia, ipsilateral lateropulsion and hemiasynergia, Horner's syndrome, and ipsilateral laryngoplegia, due to scattered lesions of the pyramid, sensory tract, inferior cerebellar peduncle, nucleus ambiguus, and oculopupillary center. **Cestan-Raymond s.,** Raymond-Cestan s. **chancriform s.,** primary extrapulmonary coccidioidomycosis. **Charcot's s.,** 1. amyotrophic lateral sclerosis. 2. intermittent claudication. 3. intermittent hepatic fever, due to cholangitis. **Charcot-Weiss-Baker s.,** carotid sinus s. **Charlin's s.,** pain, iritis, neuritis, rhinorrhea, and tenderness along the nose in eye disturbance of nasal origin. **Chauffard's s., Chauffard-Still s.,** polyarthritis with fever and enlargement of the spleen and lymph nodes in persons infected with nonhuman tuberculosis. **Chédiak-Higashi s.,** a lethal autosomal recessive syndrome associated with oculocutaneous albinism, massive leukocyte inclusions (giant lysosomes), histiocytic infiltration of multiple body organs, development of pancytopenia, hepatosplenomegaly, recurrent or persistent bacterial infections, and a possible predisposition to development of malignant lymphoma. Called also *Beguez*

César disease and *Chédiak-Higashi anomaly*. **Chiari's s.,** Budd-Chiari s. **Chiari-Arnold s.,** Arnold-Chiari deformity. **Chiari-Frommel s.,** galactorrhea-amenorrhea syndrome occurring after pregnancy; called also *Frommel-Chiari s.*, *Chiari-Frommel disease*, and *Frommel's disease*. **chiasma s., chiasmatic s.,** a syndrome indicative of lesion affecting the optic chiasma: impairment of vision, limitations of the field of vision, central scotoma, headache, vertigo, and syncope. **Chilaiditi s.,** 1. interposition of the colon between the liver and diaphragm. Usually the condition is asymptomatic in adults, but symptoms are evident in children and include vomiting, abdominal pain, anorexia, constipation, aerophagia. Signs include abdominal distention and absence of liver dullness. 2. hepatoptosis (def. 2). **Chinese restaurant s. (CRS),** a transient syndrome associated with arterial dilatation, due to ingestion of monosodium glutamate, which is used liberally in seasoning Chinese food; it is characterized by throbbing of the head, lightheadedness, tightness of the jaw, neck, and shoulders, and backache. **Chotzen's s.,** an autosomal dominant disorder characterized by acrocephalosyndactyly in which the syndactyly is mild and by hypertelorism, ptosis, and sometimes mental retardation. Called also *acrocephalosyndactyly type III* and *Saethre-Chotzen s.* **Christian's s.,** Hand-Schüller-Christian disease. **Christ-Siemens-Touraine s.,** anhidrotic ectodermal dysplasia. **chronic brain s., chronic organic brain s.,** see *organic brain s.* **Churg-Strauss s.,** allergic granulomatosis angiitis. **Citelli's s.,** mental backwardness, loss of power of concentration, drowsiness or insomnia; seen in persons with adenoids or sinus infection. **Clarke-Hadefield s.,** congenital pancreatic disease with infantilism; with enlarged liver, bulky fatty stools, and extensive atrophy of pancreas in undersized and underweight child. **Claude's s.,** paralysis of the third (oculomotor) nerve on one side and asynergia on the other side, together with dysarthria; called also *inferior s. of red nucleus* and *rubrospinal cerebellar peduncle s.* **Claude Bernard–Horner s.,** Horner's s. **click s.,** a left ventricular abnormality marked by apical midsystolic click and late murmur, with inversion of T waves. **closed head s.,** the complex of symptoms characteristic of cerebral injury without cranial penetration. **Clough and Richter's s.,** anemia in which the red corpuscles exhibit a severe degree of autoagglutination. **Clouston's s.,** hidrotic ectodermal dysplasia. **Cockayne's s.,** a hereditary syndrome transmitted as an autosomal recessive trait, consisting of dwarfism with retinal atrophy and deafness, associated with progeria, prognathism, mental retardation, and photosensitivity. **Cogan's s.,** nonsyphilitic keratitis with vestibuloauditory symptoms. **cold agglutinin s.,** the presence of circulating antibodies, usually IgM, that can agglutinate red cells and do so most efficiently at temperatures below 37 °C. The cold agglutinins are directed against three types of polysaccharide red cell antigens. "I antigens," expressed primarily on adult red cells, "i antigens," expressed primarily on cells of fetuses and infants, and "Pr antigens," which, unlike I and i antigens, are protease sensitive. The primary clinical manifestations are intravascular hemolysis in exposed extremities and mild hemolytic anemia due to complement fixation, both occurring only upon exposure to cold. There are two major types: chronic cold agglutinin disease of the elderly, a condition with gradual onset and chronic course, and postinfectious cold agglutinin syndrome, usually following *Mycoplasma pneumoniae* infection or infectious mononucleosis and lasting a few months. The syndrome can also develop secondary to malignancy. **Collet's s., Collet-Sicard s.,** glossolaryngoscapulopharyngeal hemiplegia due to complete lesion of the ninth, tenth, eleventh and twelfth cranial nerves. **combined immunodeficiency s.,** see immunodeficiency. **compartmental s.,** a condition in which increased tissue pressure in a confined anatomical space causes decreased blood flow leading to ischemia and dysfunction of contained myoneural elements, marked by pain, muscle weakness, sensory loss, and palpable tenseness in the involved compartment. Ischemia can lead to necrosis resulting in permanent impairment of function. **compression s.,** shock with hematuria and oliguria following long continued pressure on a limb, as in bombed buildings. **concussion s.,** encephalopathy due to trauma; see *postconcussional s.* **congenital rubella s.,** transplacental infection of the fetus with rubella usually in the first trimester of pregnancy, as a consequence of maternal infection (which may or may not be clinically apparent), resulting in various developmental abnormalities in the newborn infant. They include cardiac and ocular lesions, deafness, microcephaly, mental retardation, and generalized growth retardation, which may be associated with acute self-limited conditions such as thrombocytopenic purpura anemia, hepatitis, encephalitis, and radiolucencies of long bones. Infected infants may shed virus to all contacts for extended periods of time. Called also *rubella s.* **Conn's s.,** primary aldosteronism. **Conradi's s.,** chondrodysplasia punctata. **Conradi-Hünermann s.,** an autosomal dominant form of chondrodysplasia punctata, characterized by asymmetric shortening of the extremities and scoliosis; intelligence and life expectancy are normal. The syndrome is also associated with maternal use of warfarin sodium during pregnancy. **contiguous gene s.,** any syndrome known to be caused by the involvement of contiguous genes on a chromosome, e.g., aniridia-Wilms tumor association, which may also have genitourinary tract abnormalities, gonadoblastoma, and mental retardation. **Cornelia de Lange's s.,** de Lange's s. **s. of corpus striatum,** Vogt's s. **Costen's s.,** temporomandibular dysfunction s. **costoclavicular s.,** pain or other difficulties in the arm and/or hand, apparently due to pressure, stretching, or friction on the nerves or vessels at the cervicobrachial outlet. **Cotard's s.,** paranoia with delusions of negation, a suicidal tendency, and sensory disturbances. **Courvoisier-Terrier s.,** dilatation of the gallbladder, retention jaundice, and discoloration of the feces, indicating obstruction due to a tumor of the ampulla of Vater. **couvade s.,** the occurrence in the mate of a pregnant woman of symptoms that are related to pregnancy, such as nausea, vomiting, and abdominal pain. **Cowden's s.,** see under *disease.* **craniosynostosis–radial aplasia s.,** Baller-Gerold s. **CREST s.,** a form of systemic scleroderma usually less severe than other forms, consisting of calcinosis cutis, Raynaud's phenomenon, esophageal dysfunction, sclerodactyly, and telangiectasia. That in which esophageal dysfunction is not prominent is known as *CRST s.* **Creutzfeldt-Jakob s.,** see under *disease.* **cricopharyngeal achalasia s.,** Asherson's s. **cri du chat s.,** a hereditary congenital syndrome characterized by hypertelorism, microcephaly, severe mental deficiency, and a plaintive catlike cry, due to deletion of the short arm of chromosome 5. Called also *cat's cry s.* **Crigler-Najjar s.,** an autosomal recessive form of nonhemolytic jaundice due to the absence of the hepatic enzyme glucuronosyltransferase. It is characterized by the presence in the blood of excessive amounts of unconjugated bilirubin and by kernicterus and severe disorders of the central nervous system. Called also *congenital hyperbilirubinemia* and *congenital nonhemolytic jaundice.* **s. of crocodile tears,** spontaneous lacrimation occurring parallel with the normal salivation of eating. It follows facial paralysis and seems to be due to straying of the regenerating nerve fibers, some of those destined for the salivary glands going to the lacrimal glands. **Cronkhite-Canada s.,** allergic granulomatosis angiitis. Called also *Canada-Cronkhite s.* **Cross s., Cross-McKusick-Breen s.,** an autosomal recessive syndrome marked by oculocutaneous albinism, microphthalmus, small opaque corneas, oligophrenia with spasticity, high-arched palate, gingival hypertrophy, and scoliosis. Called also *oculocerebral-hypopigmentation s.* **CRST s.,** see *CREST s.* **crush s.,** the edema, oliguria, and other symptoms of renal failure which follow the crushing of a part, especially a large muscle mass; see *lower nephron nephrosis,* under *nephrosis.* **Cruveilhier-Baumgarten s.,** cirrhosis of the liver with portal hypertension, associated with congenital patency of the umbilical or paraumbilical veins. It is characterized by hematemesis, ascites, splenomegaly, hypersplenism, esophageal varices, caput medusae, large tortuous veins in the abdominal wall, and a venous hum, often accompanied by a thrill, usually heard over the region of the xiphoid process. Called also *Cruveilhier-Baumgarten cirrhosis.* **cryptophthalmos s.,** an autosomal recessive abnormality, characterized by absence of the palpebral apertures, disorganization of one or both ocular globes, malformed ears, cleft palate, laryngeal stenosis, syndactyly, meningoencephalocele, imperforate anus, cardiac defects, and maldeveloped kidneys. **cubital tunnel s.,** a complex of symptoms resulting from injury or compression of the ulnar nerve at the elbow, with pain and numbness along the ulnar aspect of the hand and forearm, and weakness of the hand. **culture-specific s.,** a form of disturbed behavior highly specific to certain

cultural systems and that does not conform to Western nosologic entities; examples are amok, koro, piblokto, and windigo. **Curtius' s.,** hypertrophy of one side of the entire body or a portion of one side of the body, as of the face; called also *hemihypertrophy.* **Cushing's s.,** 1. a condition, more commonly seen in females, due to hyperadrenocorticism resulting from neoplasms of the adrenal cortex or the anterior lobe of the pituitary, or to prolonged excessive intake of glucocorticoids for therapeutic purposes (*Cushing's s. medicamentosus* or *iatrogenic Cushing's s.*). The symptoms and signs may include rapidly developing adiposity of the face, neck, and trunk, kyphosis caused by osteoporosis of the spine, hypertension, diabetes mellitus, amenorrhea, hypertrichosis (in females), impotence (in males), dusky complexion with purple markings (striae), polycythemia, pain in the abdomen and back, and muscular wasting and weakness. When secondary to excessive pituitary secretion of adrenocorticotropin, it is known as Cushing's disease. Called also *Cushing's basophilism,* and *pituitary basophilism.* 2. in tumors of the cerebellopontine angle and acoustic tumors: subjective noises, impairment of hearing, ipsilateral cerebellar ataxia, and eventually ipsilateral impairment of the sixth and seventh nerve function together with elevated intracranial pressure. **Cushing's s. medicamentosus,** see *Cushing's s.,* def. 1. **Cyriax's s.,** a syndrome due to slipped rib cartilages pressing on the nerves at the interchondral joint, resulting in pain in the region of the cartilage, radiation of pain to the shoulder and arm, or pain similar to that of angina pectoris. **DaCosta's s.,** neurocirculatory asthenia. **Danbolt-Closs s.,** acrodermatitis enteropathica. **Dandy-Walker s.,** congenital hydrocephalus due to obstruction of the foramina of Magendie and Luschka; called also *Dandy-Walker deformity.* **Danlos' s.,** Ehlers-Danlos s. **Debré-Sémélaigne s.,** autosomal recessive athyrotic cretinism associated with myotonia and muscular pseudohypertrophy. Called also *Kocher-Debré-Sémélaigne s.* **defibrination s.,** diffuse intravascular coagulation. **Degos' s.,** malignant atrophic papulosis. **Dejerine's s.,** 1. a syndrome in cortical sensory disturbances characterized by impairment of sensory discrimination (astereognosis), judgment of intensity and recognition of differences. 2. of bulbar lesions, those in the upper part of the bulb produce paralysis of the twelfth nerve of the side of the lesion and hemiplegia on the opposite side; lesions in the lower part of the bulb cause paralysis of the larynx and soft palate. 3. symptoms of radiculitis; namely, distribution of the pain, motor and sensory defects in the region of the radicular or segmental disturbance of the nerve roots rather than along the course of the peripheral nerve. 4. a syndrome resembling tabes dorsalis, with deep sensibility depressed but tactile sense normal. It is due to lesion of the long root fibers of the posterior column. **Dejerine-Klumpke s.,** Klumpke's paralysis. **s. of Dejerine-Roussy,** thalamic s. **Dejerine-Sottas s.,** progressive hypertrophic interstitial neuropathy. **de Lange's s.,** a congenital syndrome in which severe mental retardation is associated with many abnormalities, including short stature (Amsterdam dwarf), brachycephaly, low-set ears, webbed neck, carp mouth, depressed bridge of the nose with the end tilted up and forward-directed nostrils, bushy eyebrows meeting at the midline, unruly coarse hair growing low on the forehead and neck, and flat spadelike hands with short tapering fingers. Called also *Brachmann-de Lange s., Cornelia de Lange's s.,* and *typus degenerativus amstelodamensis.* **del Castillo's s.,** galactorrhea-amenorrhea syndrome not associated with pregnancy. **dengue shock s.,** see *hemorrhagic dengue,* under *dengue.* **Dennie-Marfan s.,** spastic paralysis and mental retardation in association with congenital syphilis. **depersonalization s.,** see under *disorder.* **depressive s.,** see *major depressive episode,* under *episode.* **De Sanctis-Cacchione s.,** a hereditary syndrome, transmitted as an autosomal recessive trait, consisting of xeroderma pigmentosum associated with mental retardation, retarded growth, gonadal hypoplasia, and sometimes with neurologic complications and photosensitivity; called also *xerodermic idiocy.* **de Toni-Fanconi s.,** see *Fanconi's s.,* def. 2. **Diamond-Blackfan s.,** congenital hypoplastic anemia. **diencephalic s.,** failure to thrive, emaciation, and sometimes nevus unius lateris. **DiGeorge s.,** a congenital disorder in which defective development of the third and fourth pharyngeal pouches results in hypoplasia or aplasia of the thymus and parathyroid glands, often associated with congenital heart defects, anomalies of the great vessels, esophageal atresia, and abnormalities of facial structures. Depending on the degree of parathyroid and thymic hypoplasia, there is hypocalcemic tetany or seizures due to lack of parathyroid hormone and deficiency of cell-mediated immunity resulting in increased susceptibility to low-grade and opportunistic pathogens, e.g., fungi, viruses, and *Pneumocystis carinii.* Called also *thymic aplasia* or *hypoplasia* and *pharyngeal pouch syndrome.* **Dighton-Adair s.,** van der Hoeve's s. **Di Guglielmo s.,** erythroleukemia. **Donohue's s.,** leprechaunism. **Down s.,** a chromosome disorder characterized by a small, anteroposteriorly flattened skull, short, flat-bridge nose, epicanthal fold, short phalanges, widened spaces between the first and second digits of hands and feet, and moderate to severe mental retardation, with Alzheimer's disease developing in the fourth or fifth decade. The chromosomal aberration is trisomy of chromosome 21 associated with late maternal age. Called also *trisomy 21* and *nondisjunction;* formerly called *mongolism.* **Dresbach's s.,** elliptocytosis. **Dressler's s.,** postmyocardial infarction s. **Duane's s.,** a hereditary congenital syndrome in which the affected eye shows limitation or absence of abduction, restriction of adduction, retraction of the globe on adduction, narrowing of the palpebral fissure on adduction and widening on abduction, and deficient convergence. It is transmitted as an autosomal dominant trait. Called also *retraction s.* and *Stilling-Turk-Duane s.* **Dubin-Johnson s.,** a familial chronic form of nonhemolytic jaundice thought to be due to a defect in the excretion of conjugated bilirubin and certain other organic anions (e.g., sulfobromophthalein) by the liver. It is characterized by the presence of a brown, coarsely granular pigment in the hepatic cells, which is pathognomonic of the condition. **Dubin-Sprinz s.,** Dubin-Johnson s. **Dubreuil-Chambardel s.,** dental caries of the incisors, in most instances only the upper ones, usually appearing during adolescence; within a few years the teeth are irreparably damaged. Some authorities do not consider this syndrome a legitimate entity. **Duchenne's s.,** the collective signs of bulbar paralysis. **Duchenne-Erb s.,** see under *paralysis.* **dumping s.,** a complex reaction thought to be secondary to excessively rapid emptying of the gastric contents into the jejunum, manifested by nausea, weakness, sweating, palpitation, varying degrees of syncope, often a sensation of warmth, and sometimes diarrhea, occurring after ingestion of food by patients who have had partial gastrectomy and gastrojejunostomy. Called also *jejunal s.* and *postgastrectomy s.* **Duncan's s.,** X-linked lymphoproliferative s. **Duplay's s.,** (obs.), subacromial or subdeltoid bursitis; see *calcific tendinitis,* under *tendinitis.* **Dupré's s.,** meningism, def. 1. **Dyke-Davidoff s.,** a syndrome possibly due to injury to or severe disease affecting one side of the brain during the neonatal period, characterized by mental retardation, asymmetry of the face, and varying degrees of hemiplegia, neurological impairment, and atrophy of the side of the body contralateral to the lesion. **dysmnesic s.,** amnestic s. **dysplasia oculodentodigitalis s.,** oculodentodigital dysplasia. **dysplastic nevus s.,** the occurrence of dysplastic nevi in persons with or at risk for familial or nonfamilial malignant melanoma. **Eaton-Lambert s.,** a myasthenia-like syndrome in which the weakness usually affects the limbs, and ocular and bulbar muscles are spared; there is reduced muscle action potential on stimulation of its nerve but with repetitive stimulation it becomes augmented. It is often associated with oat-cell carcinoma of the lung. Called also *myasthenic s.* **ectopic ACTH s.,** a condition in which tumors arising from nonendocrine tissue produce ACTH. Depending on its duration, the syndrome may be subtle, resemble true Cushing's disease, but hypokalemic alkalosis and weakness are often the dominant manifestations. **ectopic-hypercalcemia s.,** hypercalcemia resulting from ectopic production by a pancreatic islet-cell or other (lung, kidney) tumor of a polypeptide with activity like that of parathyroid hormone. **ectrodactyly-ectodermal dysplasia-clefting s.,** EEC s. **Edwards' s.,** trisomy 18 s. **EEC s.,** a congenital syndrome inherited as an autosomal dominant trait involving both ectodermal and mesodermal tissues, which consists of ectodermal dysplasia associated with hypopigmentation of the skin and hair, scanty hair and eyebrows, absence of lashes, nail dystrophy, hypo- and microdontia, ectrodactyly, and cleft lip and palate. Called also *ectrodactyly-ectodermal dysplasia-clefting s.* **effort s.,** neurocirculatory asthenia. **egg-white s.,** biotin deficiency; see *biotin.* **Ehlers-Danlos s.,** a group of

inherited disorders of the connective tissue, occurring in many types based on clinical, genetic, and biochemical evidence, varying in severity from mild to lethal, and transmitted genetically as autosomal recessive, autosomal dominant, or X-linked recessive traits. The major manifestations include hyperextensible skin and joints, easy bruisability, friability of tissues with bleeding and poor wound healing, calcified subcutaneous spheroids and pseudotumors, and cardiovascular, gastrointestinal, orthopedic, and ocular defects. Called also *cutis elastica* or *hyperelastica, Danlos s., Danlos* or *Ehlers-Danlos disease,* and *elastic* or *India rubber skin.* **Eisenmenger's s.,** ventricular septal defect with pulmonary hypertension and cyanosis due to right-to-left (reversed) shunt of blood. Sometimes defined as pulmonary hypertension (pulmonary vascular disease) and cyanosis with the shunt being at the atrial, ventricular, or great vessel area. **Ekbom s.,** restless legs s. **elfin facies s.,** Williams s. **Ellis-van Creveld s.,** chondroectodermal dysplasia. **embryonic testicular regression s.,** vanishing testes s. **EMG s.,** (acronym for exomphalos-macroglossia-gigantism) Beckwith-Wiedemann s. **empty-sella s.,** a syndrome diagnosed radiologically in which the diaphragma sellae is vestigial, the sella turcica forms an extension of the subarachnoid space and is filled with cerebrospinal fluid, and the pituitary fossa appears to be empty, although the pituitary gland is present in a flattened form. Pituitary hormone secretion may be normal, deficient, or excessive. **encephalotrigeminal vascular s.,** the combination of multiple angiomas of the brain and vascular nevi in the trigeminal region. **epiphyseal s.,** precocious development of external genitalia and sexual function, precocious abnormal growth of long bones, appearance of signs of internal hydrocephalus, in the absence of all other motor and sensory symptoms indicating a lesion of the pineal body. Called also *Pellizzi's s., pineal s.,* and *macrogenitosomia precox.* **Epstein's s.,** nephrotic s. **Erb's s.,** the totality of signs of myasthenia gravis. **erythrocyte autosensitization s.,** painful bruising s. **euthyroid sick s.,** the simulation of hypothyroidism as assessed by thyroid-function tests in a euthyroid patient suffering from systemic illness. **Evans's s.,** acquired hemolytic anemia and thrombocytopenia. **exomphalos-macroglossia-gigantism s.,** Beckwith-Wiedemann s. **extrapyramidal s.,** any of a group of clinical disorders characterized by abnormal involuntary movements, including parkinsonism, athetosis, and chorea. **Faber's s.,** hypochromic anemia. **faciodigitogenital s.,** Aarskog-Scott s. **Fallot's s.,** tetralogy of Fallot. **Fanconi's s.,** 1. a rare recessive disorder, with a poor prognosis, characterized by pancytopenia, hypoplasia of the bone marrow, and patchy brown discoloration of the skin due to the deposition of melanin, and associated with multiple congenital anomalies of the musculoskeletal and genitourinary systems. Called also *Fanconi's pancytopenia, pancytopenia-dysmelia s., congenital hypoplastic anemia, constitutional infantile panmyelopathy, Fanconi's anemia,* and *congenital pancytopenia.* 2. a general term for a group of diseases marked by dysfunction of the proximal renal tubules, with generalized hyperaminoaciduria, renal glycosuria, hyperphosphaturia, and bicarbonate and water loss; the most common cause is cystinosis (q.v.), but it is also associated with other genetic diseases and occurs in idiopathic and acquired forms. When unassociated with cystinosis, the disorder is also called *de Toni-Fanconi syndrome.* **Farber s., Farber-Uzman s.,** Farber disease. **Favre-Racouchot s.,** nodular elastoidosis of Favre-Racouchot. **Felty's s.,** a combination of chronic (rheumatoid) arthritis, splenomegaly, leukopenia, pigmented spots on the skin of the lower extremities, and other inconsistent evidence of hypersplenism, namely, anemia and thrombocytopenia. **feminizing testes s.,** testicular feminization s. **fertile eunuch s.,** a syndrome of eunuchoidism, with variable secondary sexual development, associated with normal spermatogenesis, normal levels of follicle-stimulating hormone, and variably low levels of luteinizing hormone. **fetal alcohol s.,** a syndrome of altered prenatal growth and morphogenesis occurring in infants born of women who were chronically alcoholic during pregnancy; it includes maxillary hypoplasia, prominence of the forehead and mandible, short palpebral fissures, microphthalmia, epicanthal folds, severe growth retardation, mental retardation, and microcephaly. **fetal face s.,** Robinow's s. **fetal hydantoin s.,** a symptom complex characterized by poor growth and development with craniofacial and skeletal abnormalities, produced by prenatal exposure to hydantoin analogues, including phenytoin. **Fèvre-Languepin s.,** popliteal webbing associated with cleft lip and palate, fistula of the lower lip, syndactyly, onychodysplasia, and pes equinovarus. Called also *popliteal pterygium s.* **Fiessinger-Leroy-Reiter s.,** Reiter's syndrome. **first arch s.,** malformations including macrostomia, hemignathia, and deformities of the external ear, resulting from an inhibitory process occurring toward the seventh week of embryonic life and affecting the facial bones derived from the first branchial arch. **Fitz-Hugh–Curtis s.,** perihepatitis occurring as a complication of gonorrhea in women, marked by fever, upper quadrant pain, tenderness and spasm of the abdominal wall, and occasionally by friction rub over the liver. **floppy infant s.,** a congenital myopathy of infants, characterized clinically by hypotonia and muscle weakness. The pathologic changes in skeletal muscle include numerous eosinophilic intranuclear crystals, characteristic crystal morphology, myofibrillar fragmentation, sarcoplasmic crystals, and expansion of the Z bands. **floppy valve s.,** mitral valve prolapse s. **focal dermal hypoplasia s.,** a hereditary congenital syndrome of extensive ectodermal and mesodermal dysplasia, chiefly of skin and bones, with linear or serpiginous patches (especially on the buttocks and thighs), telangiectases, pigmentation, and orificial papillomas, often with syndactyly, oligodactyly, or adactyly. An X-linked dominant trait, lethal in the male, is believed responsible. Called also *Goltz's s.* and *Goltz-Gorlin s.* **Forbes-Albright s.,** galactorrhea-amenorrhea syndrome not associated with pregnancy; usually a pituitary tumor is present. **Forsius-Eriksson s.,** an X-linked ocular albinism differing from the Nettleship type in that the males show hypoplastic foveas, axial myopia, and protanomaly and the females show slightly defective color discrimination and latent nystagmus, but no mosaic pigment pattern in the fundus. Called also *ocular albinism, OA2, Forsius-Eriksson type ocular albinism,* and *Åland eye disease.* **Foster Kennedy s.,** Kennedy's s. **four-day s.,** respiratory distress syndrome of newborn; so called because the infant usually recovers or dies within four days. **Foville's s.,** a syndrome similar to the Millard-Gubler syndrome (q.v.), except that, in addition to paralysis of the outward movement of the eye, there is paralysis of conjugate movement. **fragile X s.,** an X-linked syndrome associated with fragile site on the long arm of the X chromosome at q27–28, associated with mental retardation, enlarged testes, high forehead, big jaw, and long ears in most males and mild mental retardation in many heterozygous females. In some families, unaffected transmitting males have occurred. **Franceschetti s.,** mandibulofacial dysostosis. **Franceschetti-Jadassohn s.,** an autosomal dominant disorder characterized by the presence of slate-gray to brown reticular pigmentation beginning after infancy without preceding inflammatory changes, and associated with palmoplantar hyperkeratosis, vasomotor changes with hypohidrosis, and yellowing of the dental enamel. Called also *chromatophore, nevus of Naegeli, Naegeli syndrome,* and *Naegeli's incontentia pigmenti.* Cf. *incontentia pigmenti.* **François' s.,** oculomandibulofacial s. **Freeman-Sheldon s.,** craniocarpotarsal dystrophy. **Frey's s.,** auriculotemporal s. **Friderichsen-Waterhouse s.,** Waterhouse-Friderichsen s. **Friedmann's vasomotor s.,** a train or cycle of symptoms due to a progressive subacute encephalitis of traumatic origin, including a sense of fullness in the head, headache, vertigo, irritability, insomnia, easy fatigability, and defect of memory. **Fröhlich's s.,** adiposogenital dystrophy. **Froin's s.,** a condition of the lumbar spinal fluid consisting of a transparent clear yellow color (xanthochromia), with the finding of large amounts of protein, rapid coagulation, and the absence of an increased number of cells. It is seen in certain organic nervous diseases in which the lumbar fluid is cut off from communication with the fluid in the ventricles. Called also *loculation s.* **Frommel-Chiari s.,** Chiari-Frommel s. **Fuchs' s.,** unilateral heterochromia, fine keratic precipitates, and secondary cataract. **functional prepubertal castrate s.,** vanishing testes s. **G s.,** hypertelorism-hypospadias s. **Gailliard's s.,** dextrocardia from retraction of lungs and pleura to the right. **Gaisböck's s.,** stress polycythemia. **galactorrhea-amenorrhea s.,** amenorrhea and galactorrhea associated with increased levels of prolactin usually produced by a pituitary adenoma. **Ganser s.,** the giving of approximate answers to questions, commonly associated with amnesia,

disorientation, perceptual disturbances, fugue, and conversion symptoms. **Gardner's s.,** familial polyposis of the large bowel (with malignant potential), supernumerary teeth, fibrous dysplasia of the skull, osteomas, fibromas, and epithelial cysts. **Gardner-Diamond s.,** painful bruising s. **Gasser's s.,** hemolytic-uremic s. **gay bowel s.,** an assortment of sexually transmitted bowel and rectal diseases affecting homosexual males, caused by a wide variety of infectious agents. **Gee-Herter-Heubner s.,** the infantile form of nontropical sprue. **Gélineau's s.,** narcolepsy. **gender dysphoria s.,** a group of psychological problems associated with discrepancy between the physical sex assignment and the psychological gender identity. **general adaptation s.,** the total of all nonspecific systemic reactions of the body to long-continued exposure to systemic stress. **Gerhardt's s.,** bilateral abductor paralysis of the vocal cords causing inspiratory dyspnea. **Gerlier's s.,** Gerlier's disease. **Gerstmann's s.,** a combination of finger agnosia, right-left disorientation, agraphia, acalculia, and often constructional apraxia, due to a lesion in the angular gyrus of the dominant hemisphere. **Gianotti-Crosti s.,** a generally benign and self-limited disease of young children representing a primary natural infection with hepatitis B virus, characterized by the appearance of crops of monomorphous, usually nonpruritic, dusky or coppery red, flat-topped, firm papules forming a symmetrical eruption on the face, buttocks, and limbs, including the palms and soles, and associated with malaise, low-grade fever, and few other constitutional symptoms. Called also *acrodermatitis papulosa infantum, infantile papular acrodermatitis,* and *papular acrodermatitis of childhood.* **giant platelet s.,** Bernard-Soulier disease. **Gilbert s.,** an inborn error of bilirubin metabolism, probably autosomal dominant, a benign elevation of unconjugated bilirubin with no liver damage or hematologic abnormalities. Called also *constitutional hepatic dysfunction, familial cholemia, hyperbilirubinemia I, constitutional hyperbilirubinemia, familial nonhemolytic jaundice,* and *Gilbert cholemia* or *disease.* **Gilles de la Tourette's s.,** a syndrome of facial and vocal tics with onset in childhood, progressing to generalized jerking movements in any part of the body, with echolalia and coprolalia; once thought to have an unfavorable prognosis but recently shown to be responsive to treatment with butyrophenones. **glioma-polyposis s.,** Turcot s. **glucagonoma s.,** a glucagon-secreting tumor of the alpha cells of the pancreas (glucagonoma) occurring in association with increased serum levels of glucagon, mild diabetes mellitus, weight loss, anemia, glossitis, stomatitis, angular cheilitis, blepharitis, and necrolytic migrating erythema (q.v.). **Goldenhar's s.,** oculoauriculovertebral dysplasia. **Goltz s.,** focal dermal hypoplasia. **Good's s.,** immunodeficiency with thymoma. **Goodman s.,** acrocephalopolysyndactyly, type IV. **Goodpasture's s.,** glomerulonephritis associated with pulmonary hemorrhage and circulating antibodies against basement membrane antigens, a condition occurring most frequently in young men and usually having a course of rapidly progressing renal failure with hemoptysis, pulmonary infiltrates, and dyspnea. Cf. *anti–glomerular basement membrane antibody disease,* under *disease.* **Gopalan's s.,** a symptom complex resulting from malnutrition, with signs suggestive of riboflavin deficiency, a burning sensation in the extremities, a feeling of "pins and needles" in the distal parts, and hyperhidrosis. **Gorlin's s.,** 1. basal cell nevus s. 2. Gorlin-Chaudhry-Moss s. **Gorlin-Goltz s.,** basal cell nevus s. **Gougerot-Carteaud s.,** confluent and reticulated papillomatosis. **Gougerot-Nulock-Houwer s.,** Sjögren's s. **Gowers' s.,** vasovagal attack. **Gradenigo's s.,** palsy of the sixth nerve and unilateral headache in suppurative disease of the middle ear, caused by involvement of the abducens and trigeminal nerves by direct spread of the infection. **Graham Little s.,** a syndrome characterized by the presence of cicatricial patches of alopecia of the scalp with prominent follicular plugging and follicular keratoses involving the trunk and extremities, sometimes associated with noncicatricial alopecia of the axillae, pubes, trunk, and extremities. **gray s.,** a potentially fatal condition seen in neonates, particularly premature infants, due to a reaction to chloramphenicol, characterized by an ashen gray cyanosis, listlessness, weakness, and hypotension. **gray spinal s.,** muscular atrophy, syringomyelic disturbances of sensation, and vasomotor troubles, due to lesions of the gray matter of the spinal cord. **Greig's s.,** ocular hypertelorism. **Gris-**

celli s., an albinoidism of autosomal recessive inheritance, marked by hypomelanosis, frequent pyogenic infection, hepatosplenomegaly, neutro- and thrombopenia, and possible immunodeficiency. Called also *hypopigmentation-immunodeficiency disease.* **Grönblad-Strandberg s.,** angioid streaks in the retina together with pseudoxanthoma elasticum of the skin. **Gruber's s.,** Meckel's s. **Guillain-Barré s.,** acute febrile polyneuritis. **Gunn's s.,** unilateral ptosis of the eyelid, with the association of movements of the affected upper eyelid with those of the jaw; called also *jaw-winking s.* **gustatory sweating s.,** auriculotemporal s. **Hadefield-Clarke s.,** Clarke-Hadefield s. **Hakim's s.,** normal-pressure hydrocephalus. **Hallermann-Streiff s., Hallermann-Streiff-François s.,** oculomandibulofacial s. **Hallervorden-Spatz s.,** a hereditary disorder characterized by marked reduction in the number of the myelin sheaths of the globus pallidus and substantia nigra, with accumulations of iron pigment, progressive rigidity beginning in the legs, choreoathetoid movements, dysarthria, and progressive mental deterioration. Transmitted as an autosomal recessive trait, it usually begins in the first or second decade, with death usually occurring before the thirtieth year. Called also *Hallervorden-Spatz disease, status dysmyelinatus,* and *status dysmyelinisatus.* **Hamman's s.,** pneumomediastinum. **Hamman-Rich s.,** see *idiopathic pulmonary fibrosis,* under *fibrosis.* **hand-foot-and-mouth s.,** see under *disease.* **hand-foot-uterus s.,** a congenital syndrome consisting of small feet with unusually short great toes, abnormal thumbs, and, in females, duplication of the genital tract. **Hand-Schüller-Christian s.,** the triad of exopthalmos, diabetes insipidus, and bone destruction, sometimes found in Langerhans cell granulomatosis. **hand-shoulder s.,** reflex sympathetic dystrophy of the upper extremity; see under *dystrophy.* **Hanhart's s.,** a congenital syndrome characterized chiefly by severe micrognathia, high nose root, small eyelid fissures, low-set ears, and variable absence of digits or limbs, usually below the elbow or knee. **Hanot's s.,** 1. primary biliary cirrhosis. 2. secondary biliary cirrhosis. **Hanot-Chauffard s.,** hypertrophic cirrhosis with pigmentation and diabetes mellitus. **Harada's s.,** bilateral diffuse exudative choroiditis and retinal detachment occurring in association with headache, vomiting, an increase of lymphocytes in the cerebrospinal fluid, and temporary or permanent deafness; alopecia, vitiligo, and poliosis may be transient features. Called also *Harada's disease.* Cf. *Vogt-Kayanagi s.* **Hare's s.,** Pancoast's s., def. 1. **Harris' s.,** hyperinsulinism due to organic endogenous factors, such as insulinoma, manifested by hypoglycemia, weakness, perspiration, jitteriness, tachycardia, mental confusion, and disturbances of vision. **Hartnup s.,** see under *disease.* **Hayem-Widal s.,** hemolytic anemia. **heart-hand s.,** Holt-Oram s. **Heerfordt's s.,** an occasional manifestation of sarcoidosis consisting of enlargement of the parotid and lacrimal glands, anterior uveitis, Bell's palsy, and fever. Called also *Heerfordt's disease* and *uveoparotid fever.* **Heidenhain's s.,** a rapidly progressive degenerative disease manifested by cortical blindness, presenile dementia, dysarthria, ataxia, athetoid movements, and generalized rigidity. **hemangioma-thrombocytopenia s.,** Kasabach-Merritt s. **hemohistioblastic s.,** reticuloendotheliosis. **hemolytic-uremic s.,** a rare syndrome of unknown etiology occurring mainly in children under 4 years of age, characterized by renal failure, microangiopathic hemolytic anemia, and severe thrombocytopenia and purpura. **hemopleuropneumonic s.,** dyspnea, hemoptysis, tachycardia, and fever, with dullness at the base of the chest and tubular respiration over the middle zone of the chest; indicative of pneumonia and hydrothorax in puncture wounds of the chest. **Hench-Rosenberg s.,** palindromic rheumatism. **Henoch-Schönlein s.,** Schönlein-Henoch purpura. **hepatorenal s.,** functional renal failure, oliguria, and low urinary sodium concentration, without pathological renal changes, associated with cirrhosis and ascites or with obstructive jaundice. **hereditary benign intraepithelial dyskeratosis s.,** a syndrome characterized by plaques of the bulbar conjunctiva and by oral mucosal thickenings clinically similar to white-folded hypertrophy (white sponge nevus of Cannon); it is inherited as an autosomal dominant trait with a high degree of penetrance. **Hermansky-Pudlak s.,** an autosomal recessive form of tyrosinase-positive oculocutaneous albinism (ty-pos OCA) with a hemorrhagic diathesis secondary to a

platelet defect, and accumulation of a ceroid-like substance in the reticuloendothelial system, oral mucosa, and urine. **Hines-Bannick s.,** intermittent attacks of low temperature and disabling sweating. **Hoffmann-Werdnig s.,** Werdnig-Hoffmann paralysis. **holiday heart s.,** paroxysms of arrhythmias, most commonly atrial fibrillation, in alcoholic patients without overt cardiomyopathy after a weekend bout of alcoholic consumption, especially during the year-end holiday season. **Holmes-Adie s.,** Adie's s. **Holt-Oram s.,** autosomal heart disease of varying severity, usually an atrial or ventricular septal defect, associated with skeletal malformation (hypoplastic thumb and short forearm). Called also *heart-hand s.* **Homén's s.,** a genetically determined disease of the nervous system with prominent abnormalities in the lenticular nucleus, marked by vertigo, ataxia, dysarthria, gradually increasing dementia, with rigidity of the body, especially the legs. **Horner's s., Horner-Bernard s.,** sinking in of the eyeball, ptosis of the upper eyelid, slight elevation of the lower lid, constriction of the pupil, narrowing of the palpebral fissure, anhidrosis and flushing of the affected side of the face; caused by paralysis of the cervical sympathetic nerves. Called also *Bernard's s., Bernard-Horner s.,* and *Horner's ptosis.* **Horton's s.,** 1. migrainous neuralgia. 2. temporal arteritis. **Howel-Evans' s.,** diffuse palmoplantar keratoderma occurring between the ages of 5 and 15 and associated with the development of esophageal cancer later in life. **Hunt's s.,** Ramsay Hunt s. **Hunter's s., Hunter-Hurler s.,** a mucopolysaccharidosis caused by deficient iduronate sulfatase, characterized biochemically by excretion of dermatan sulfate and heparan sulfate in the urine, and differing clinically from the Hurler syndrome by (1) X-linked inheritance; (2) slower progression, lesser severity, and longer survival (thus resembling the Hurler-Scheie syndrome); and (3) absence of corneal clouding. Two clinical forms exist: *mucopolysaccharidosis II-XR, severe* or *MPS IIA* has Hurler-Scheie–like symptoms with death before 15, usually from heart disease; *mucopolysaccharidosis II-XR, mild* or *MPS IIB* has onset in first decade, dwarfism, dysostosis multiplex, joint stiffness, visceromegaly, cardiac disease, nerve entrapment, and normal or nearly normal intelligence and life span. **Hurler s.,** the prototype of the mucopolysaccharidoses and the gravest of the three allelic disorders of mucopolysaccharidosis I, specifically marked by corneal clouding and death by 10 years old. Onset is after the first year with progressive physical and mental deterioration. Further symptoms include gargoyle-like facies with hypertelorism, depressed nasal bridge, large tongue, and widely spaced teeth; dwarfism; severe somatic and skeletal changes, including short neck and trunk, scaphocephaly, and kyphosis with gibbus; short broad hands with short fingers; progressive opacities of the cornea; deafness; cardiovascular defects; hepatosplenomegaly; and joint contractures. Death is usually caused by respiratory infection and heart failure. Called also α-L-iduronidase deficiency, Hurler type, and *mucopolysaccharidosis IH.* **Hurler-Scheie s.,** one of the three allelic disorders of mucopolysaccharidosis I, with clinical features intermediate between the Hurler and the Scheie syndromes, specifically characterized by receding chin (micrognathism). Symptoms include mental retardation, dwarfism, dysostosis multiplex, corneal clouding, deafness, hernia, stiff joints (claw hand), and valvular heart disease. Patients survive till their late teens or twenties. Called also *mucopolysaccharidosis I H/S, Hurler-Scheie compound, α-L-iduronidase deficiency, Hurler-Scheie type.* **Hutchinson's s.,** see under *triad.* **Hutchinson-Gilford s.,** progeria. **Hutchison s.,** see under *type.* **hyaline membrane s.,** see *respiratory distress s. of newborn.* **17-hydroxylase deficiency s.,** congenital adrenal hyperplasia resulting from a deficiency of the enzyme 17-α-hydroxylase, leading to a deficiency of estrogen and androgen and consequent sexual infantilism; the compensatory increase in secretion of deoxycorticosterone and corticosterone results in hypokalemic alkalosis and hypertension. **hyperabduction s.,** thoracic outlet syndrome due to compression of the brachial plexus trunk roots and axillary vessels by the pectoralis minor muscle and the coracoid process when the arms are stretched above the head, as during sleep. **hyperactive child s.,** attention-deficit hyperactivity disorder. **hypercalcemia s.,** milk-alkali s. **hypereosinophilic s.,** a massive increase in the number of eosinophils in the blood, mimicking leukemia, and characterized by eosinophilic infiltration of the heart, brain, liver, and lungs and by a progressively fatal course. **hyperimmuno-globulinemia E s.,** a primary immunodeficiency disorder characterized by recurrent staphylococcal abscesses of skin, lungs, joints, and other sites, pruritic dermatitis, very high serum IgE levels, normal levels of IgG, IgA, and IgM, blood and sputum eosinophilia, low anamnestic antibody responses to booster immunization, and poor antibody and cell-mediated responses to neoantigens. Called also *Buckley's s.* **hyperkinetic s.,** attention-deficit hyperactivity disorder. **hyperkinetic heart s.,** increased cardiac output of unknown cause associated with slightly elevated systolic and pulse pressures, normal mean arterial pressure, and low systemic vascular resistance. **hyperlucent lung s.,** a syndrome simulating localized emphysema, but due to congenital absence or hypoplasia of pulmonary arteries; there may be lobar or segmental agenesis, and accessory lungs, lobes, or segments are not unusual. **hypersomnia-bulimia s.,** Kleine-Levin s. **hypertelorism-hypospadias s.,** a congenital condition consisting of hypertelorism associated with hypospadias and a neuromuscular abnormality of the esophagus and swallowing mechanism. Called also *G s.* **hyperventilation s.,** a complex of symptoms that accompany hypocapnia caused by hyperventilation, including palpitations, a feeling of shortness of breath or air hunger, lightheadedness or giddiness, profuse perspiration, and tingling sensations in the fingertips, face, or toes; prolonged overbreathing may result in vasomotor collapse and loss of consciousness. Hyperventilation unrecognized by the patient is a common cause of the subjective somatic symptoms associated with chronic anxiety or panic attacks. **hyperviscosity s.,** any syndrome associated with increased viscosity of the blood. In the *syndrome of serum hyperviscosity,* there is spontaneous bleeding and neurologic and ocular disorders. The *syndrome of polycythemic hyperviscosity,* in which increased viscosity is due to large numbers of red cells, is marked by retarded blood flow, organ congestion, reduced capillary perfusion, and increased cardiac effort. *Syndromes of sclerocythemic hyperviscosity* comprise those in which the deformability of erythrocytes is impaired, as in sickle cell anemia. **hypoglossia-hypodactyly s.,** partial to complete absence of the tongue associated with partial to complete absence of the digits or limbs affecting one or more limbs; it occurs sporadically. Called also *aglossia-adactylia s.* **hypoplastic left-heart s.,** a congenital malformation consisting of hypoplasia or atresia of the left ventricle and of the aorta or mitral valve or both, and characterized by respiratory distress and extreme cyanosis, with cardiac failure and death in early infancy. **idiopathic postprandial s.,** the repeated occurrence of the clinical manifestations of hypoglycemia after meals; a controversial disease entity. **Imerslund s., Imerslund-Graesbeck s.,** familial megaloblastic anemia. **immotile-cilia s.,** a hereditary syndrome of delayed or absent mucociliary clearance from airways and lack of motion of sperm; Kartagener's syndrome is one variety. **immunodeficiency s.,** see under *disease.* **s. of inappropriate antidiuretic hormone (SIADH),** persistent hyponatremia, an inappropriately elevated urine osmolality, and no discernible stimulus for ADH release; it may occur with neoplasms (especially oat cell carcinoma of the lung or pancreatic carcinoma, with ectopic production of ADH by the tumor), pulmonary disorders, and central nervous system diseases, including head trauma. **inferior s. of red nucleus,** Claude's s. **inhibitory s.,** the manifestations produced by a somatostatinoma, including diabetes mellitus, cholecystolithiasis, steatorrhea, indigestion, hypochlorhydria, and occasionally anemia. **inspissated bile s.,** biliary obstruction caused by plugging of the outflow tract. **intrauterine parabiotic s.,** placental transfusion s. **irritable bowel s., irritable colon s.,** a chronic noninflammatory disease characterized by abdominal pain, altered bowel habits consisting of diarrhea or constipation or both, and no detectable pathologic change; a variant form is characterized by painless diarrhea. It is a common disorder with a psychophysiologic basis. Called also *spastic* or *irritable colon.* **Ivemark's s.,** congenital splenic agenesis, cardiac defects, and partial situs inversus viscerum; called also *asplenia s.* and *Polhemus-Schafer- Ivemark s.* **Jaccoud's s.,** chronic arthritis occurring after rheumatic fever, usually after repeated attacks, and characterized by fibrous changes in the joint capsules and tendons, leading to deformities that may resemble rheumatoid arthritis (especially ulnar deviation of fingers); the joints may be painful and rheumatic nodules are

often present. **Jackson's s.,** paralysis of the tenth, eleventh, and twelfth cranial nerves, with paralysis of the soft palate, larynx, and one half of the tongue, associated with paralysis of the sternomastoid and trapezius muscles. **Jadassohn-Lewandowsky s.,** pachyonychia congenita. **Jaffe-Lichtenstein s.,** fibrous dysplasia. **Jahnke's s.,** a variant of the Sturge-Weber syndrome in which glaucoma is absent. **jaw-winking s.,** Gunn's s. **jejunal s.,** dumping syndrome. **Jervell and Lange-Nielsen s.,** a syndrome characterized by attacks of syncope and by sudden death in patients with congenital deafness and electrocardiographic anomalies, especially a prolonged Q-T interval. **Jeune's s.,** asphyxiating thoracic dystrophy. **Job s.,** an autosomal recessive disorder of neutrophils, characterized by the presence of abnormal or absent chemotactic responses, which leads to repeated development of cold staphylococcal abscesses and eczema, and by hyperimmunoglobulinemia E. It is usually associated with red hair and fair skin. Most cases reported have been in girls. **jugular foramen s.,** Vernet's s. **Kallmann's s.,** hypogonadotropic eunuchoidism. **Kanner's s.,** autistic disorder. **Karroo s.,** a condition observed in youth among Afrikaners in the Karroo region, consisting of high fever, alimentary tract disturbance, and tenderness in the lymph glands of the neck. **Kartagener's s.,** a hereditary disorder involving a combination of dextrocardia (situs inversus), bronchiectasis, and sinusitis, transmitted as an autosomal recessive trait. **Kasabach-Merritt s.,** a syndrome usually occurring in the first few months of life in which severe thrombocytopenia and other evidence of intravascular coagulation occur in infants with rapidly expanding hemangiomas of the trunk, extremities, and abdominal viscera, and may be associated with bleeding and anemia. Bleeding is thought to be due to trapping and destruction of platelets within the tumor and depletion of circulating clotting factors. Called also *hemangioma-thrombocytopenia s.* **Kast's s.,** Maffucci's s. **Kawasaki s.,** mucocutaneous lymph node s. **Kearns-Sayre s.,** progressive ophthalmoplegia, pigmentary degeneration of the retina, myopathy, ataxia, and cardiac conduction defect; inherited as an autosomal dominant trait, with onset before age 15. **Kennedy's s.,** retrobulbar optic neuritis, central scotoma, optic atrophy on the side of the lesion and papilledema on the opposite side, occurring in tumors of the frontal lobe of the brain which press downward. **Kiloh-Nevin s.,** ocular myopathy in patients with ptosis and progressive external ophthalmoplegia. **Kimmelstiel-Wilson s.,** intercapillary glomerulosclerosis. **kinky-hair s.,** Menkes' s. **Kinsbourne s.,** myoclonic encephalopathy of childhood; see under *encephalopathy.* **kleeblattschädel (cloverleaf skull) s.,** a congenital disorder, characterized by synostosis of multiple or all cranial sutures, hydrocephalus, and in some cases facial dysostosis and long bone anomalies. **Klein-Waardenburg s.,** Waardenburg s., def. 2. **Kleine-Levin s.,** episodic periods of excessive sleep and overeating lasting for several weeks, usually in adolescent boys. **Klinefelter's s.,** a condition characterized by small testes with hyalinization of the seminiferous tubules, variable degrees of masculinization, azoospermia and infertility, and increased urinary excretion of gonadotropin; patients tend to be tall, with long legs, and about half have gynecomastia. It is associated typically with an XXY chromosome complement, although variants include XXYY, XXXY, XXXXY, and several mosaic patterns (XY/XXY, XXY, XXXY, etc.). **Klippel-Feil s.,** a condition characterized by shortness of the neck resulting from reduction in the number of cervical vertebrae or the fusion of multiple hemivertebrae into one osseous mass; the hairline is low and motion of the neck is limited. **Klippel-Trenaunay s., Klippel-Trenaunay-Weber s.,** a rare condition usually affecting one extremity, characterized by hypertrophy of the bone and related soft tissues, large cutaneous hemangiomas, persistent nevus flammeus (see *port-wine stain,* under *stain*), and skin varices. **Klumpke-Dejerine s.,** Klumpke's paralysis. **Klüver-Bucy s.,** bizarre behavior disturbances following bilateral temporal lobectomy which destroys important limbic structures; it is characterized by a tendency to examine objects orally, depression of drive and emotional reactions, hypermetamorphosis, and lack of sexual inhibitions. **Kocher-Debré-Sémélaigne s.,** Debré-Sémélaigne s. **Koerber-Salus-Elschnig s.,** sylvian s. **König's s.,** constipation alternating with diarrhea and attended with abdominal pain, meteorism, and gurgling sounds in the right iliac fossa. **Korsakoff's s.,** a syndrome of anterograde and retrograde amnesia with confabulation associated with alcoholic or nonalcoholic polyneuritis described as "cerebropathia psychica toxemica" by Korsakoff; currently used synonymously with "amnestic syndrome" or, more narrowly, to refer to the amnestic component of the Wernicke-Korsakoff syndrome, i.e., an amnestic syndrome resulting from thiamine deficiency. Called also *Korsakoff's psychosis.* See also *amnestic s.* and *Wernicke-Korsakoff s.* **Kostmann's s.,** infantile genetic agranulocytosis. **Krause's s.,** a retinal and cerebral dysplasia found in premature infants several months after birth, characterized by malformations of the choroid, retina, and optic nerve, and possible blindness, cataract, coloboma, glaucoma, and microphthalmos. Cerebral symptoms include aplasia, hyperplasia, and hypertrophy of the brain, hydrocephaly, microcephaly, and mental retardation. Called also *encephalo-ophthalmic dysplasia.* **Kunkel's s.,** lupoid hepatitis. **Ladd's s.,** congenital obstruction of the duodenum due to peritoneal bands resulting from a malrotated cecum. **Lambert-Eaton s.,** Eaton-Lambert s. **Landry's s.,** acute febrile polyneuritis. **Larsen's s.,** cleft palate, flattened facies, multiple congenital dislocations, and foot deformities. **Laubry-Soulle s.,** abnormal localized collections of gas in the colon (splenic flexure) and stomach following acute myocardial infarction. **Launois' s.,** gigantism due to excessive pituitary secretion, occurring before puberty and before the epiphyses close; it is most often caused by eosinophilic cell hyperplasia or an eosinophilic adenoma, but sometimes results from a chromophobe adenoma. Called also *hyperpituitary* or *pituitary gigantism.* **Laurence-Moon s.,** an autosomal recessive disorder characterized by mental retardation, pigmentary retinopathy, hypogonadism, and spastic paraplegia; cf. *Bardet-Biedl s.* and *Biemond s., II.* **Läwen-Roth s.,** dwarfism with stippled epiphyses and thyroid deficiency; congenital hypothyroidism or cretinism. **Lawford's s.,** a variant of the Sturge-Weber syndrome in which there is glaucoma but without an increase in the size of the eye. **Lawrence-Seip s.,** total lipodystrophy. **lazy leukocyte s.,** a syndrome occurring in children, marked by recurrent low-grade infections, associated with a defect in neutrophil chemotaxis and deficient random mobility of neutrophils. **Legg-Calvé-Perthes s.,** osteochondrosis of the capitular epiphysis. **Leigh s.,** subacute necrotizing encephalomyelopathy. **Lennox s.,** a childhood epileptic encephalopathy characterized electroencephalographically by diffuse slow spike waves. **Lenz's s.,** a hereditary syndrome, transmitted as an X-linked trait, consisting of microphthalmia or anophthalmos, unilateral or bilateral, and digital anomalies; narrow shoulders, double thumbs, and other skeletal abnormalities; dental, urogenital, and cardiovascular defects may also occur. **leopard s.,** a hereditary syndrome transmitted as an autosomal dominant trait, consisting of multiple lentigines, asymptomatic cardiac defects, and typical coarse facies; it may also be associated with pulmonary stenosis, sensorineural deafness, skeletal changes, ocular hypertelorism, and abnormalities of the genitalia. Called also *multiple lentigines s.* **Leredde's s.,** severe dyspnea on exertion dating from early life, combined with advanced emphysema, recurrent attacks of acute febrile bronchitis; it is a remote sequel of syphilis, usually congenital. **Leriche's s.,** a syndrome caused by obstruction of the terminal aorta, usually occurring in males and characterized by fatigue in the hips, thighs, or calves on exercising, absence of pulsation in the femoral arteries, and impotence, and often pallor and coldness of the lower extremities. **Lermoyez's s.,** tinnitus and hearing loss preceding an attack of vertigo and then subsiding after the vertigo has become established. **Lesch-Nyhan s.,** a rare X-linked disorder of purine metabolism due to deficient hypoxanthine-guanine phosphoribosyltransferase, characterized by physical and mental retardation, compulsive self-mutilation of the fingers and lips by biting, choreoathetosis, spastic cerebral palsy, impaired renal function; and by excessive purine synthesis and consequent hyperuricemia and uricaciduria. Called also *hypoxanthine-guanine phosphoribosyltransferase (HGPRT, HPRT) deficiency.* **levator s.,** episodic pain and a sensation of fullness and pressure in the rectum and sacrococcygeal area; attributed to spasm of the levator ani muscle. **Lévy-Roussy s.,** Roussy-Lévy s. **Leyden-Moebius s.,** limb-girdle muscular dystrophy; see under *dystrophy.* **Lhermitte and McAlpine s.,** combined pyramidal and extrapyramidal system disease.

Libman-Sacks s., atypical verrucous endocarditis. **Lichtheim's s.,** subacute combined degeneration of the spinal cord; see under *degeneration.* **Lightwood's s.,** renal tubular acidosis. **Lignac's s., Lignac-Fanconi s.,** cystinosis. **liver-kidney s.,** hepatorenal s. **Lobstein's s.,** see *osteogenesis imperfecta.* **"locked-in" s.,** a condition of complete paralysis, except for some form of voluntary eye movement, due to bilateral lesions of motor pathways of the lower cranial nerves and limbs. **loculation s.,** Froin's s. **Löffler's s.,** a condition characterized by transient infiltrations of the lungs, accompanied by cough, fever, dyspnea, and eosinophilia. **Looser-Milkman s.,** Milkman s. **Louis-Bar s.,** ataxia-telangiectasia. **Lowe s.,Lowe-Terrey-MacLachlan s.,**oculocerebrorenal s. **lower radicular s.,** Klumpke's paralysis. **Lown-Ganong-Levine s.,** an electrocardiographic abnormality characterized by a short P-R interval with a normal QRS complex, accompanied by atrial tachycardia. **Lucey-Driscoll s.,** a syndrome of retention jaundice due to defective bilirubin conjugation, occurring in infants; apparently the result of an unidentified factor, presumably a steroid in maternal blood, transmitted to the infant. **lupus-like s.,** see *systemic lupus erythematosus,* under *lupus.* **Lutembacher's s.,** atrial septal defect associated with mitral stenosis. Called also *Lutembacher's disease* or *complex.* **Lyell's s.,** toxic epidermal necrolysis. **lymphadenopathy s.,** a condition occurring in a large number of male homosexuals, characterized by the presence of unexplained lymphadenopathy for 3 or more months involving extrainguinal sites, which on biopsy reveal nonspecific lymphoid hyperplasia; considered by some authorities to be a prodrome of acquired immune deficiency syndrome. See also *AIDS-related complex,* under *complex.* **lymphoproliferative s.,** see *lymphoproliferative.* **lymphoreticular s's** see *lymphoreticular.* **McArdle s.,** glycogen storage disease (type V). **McCune-Albright s.,** Albright's s. **Mackenzie's s.,** associated paralysis of the tongue, soft palate, and vocal cord on the same side. **Macleod's s.,** Swyer-James s. **Maffucci's s.,** enchondromatosis associated with multiple cutaneous or visceral hemangiomas. Called also *Kast's s.* **malabsorption s.,** a group of disorders in which there is subnormal absorption of dietary constituents, and thus excessive loss of nonabsorbed substances in the stool; the malabsorption may be due to an intraluminal (digestive) defect (e.g., pancreatic insufficiency), a mucosal abnormality (celiac disease or disaccharidase deficiency), or a lymphatic obstruction (intestinal lymphangiectasia). Unless there is a specific enzyme or transport defect, steatorrhea is usually present. Deficiency syndromes may result from excessive loss of vitamins, electrolytes, iron, calcium, etc. **malarial hyperreactive spleen s.,** tropical splenomegaly s. **Malin's s.,** anemia in which the red cells are ingested by the leukocytes; called also *autoerythrophagocytosis.* **Mallory-Weiss s.,** hematemesis or melena that follows typically upon many hours or days of severe vomiting and retching, traceable to one or several slitlike lacerations of the gastric mucosa, longitudinally placed at or slightly below the esophagogastric junction. **manic s.,** see *manic episode,* under *episode.* **Marchesani's s.,** Weill-Marchesani s. **Marchiafava-Bignami s.,** see under *disease.* **Marchiafava-Micheli s.,** paroxysmal nocturnal hemoglobinuria; see under *hemoglobinuria.* **Marcus Gunn's s.,** Gunn's s. **Marfan s.,** a congenital disorder of connective tissue characterized by abnormal length of the extremities, especially of fingers and toes, subluxation of the lens, cardiovascular abnormalities (commonly dilatation of the ascending aorta), and other deformities. It is an autosomal dominant with variable degree of expression. **Marie s.,** hypertrophic pulmonary osteoarthropathy. **Marie-Bamberger s.,** hypertrophic pulmonary osteoarthropathy. **Marie-Robinson s.,** melancholia, insomnia, and impotence in a form of levulosuria. **Marinesco-Sjögren's s.,** a hereditary syndrome transmitted as an autosomal recessive trait, consisting of cerebellar ataxia, mental and somatic growth retardation, congenital cataracts, inability to chew, thin brittle fingernails, and sparse, incompletely keratinized hair. **Maroteaux-Lamy s.,** a mucopolysaccharidosis caused by deficient N-acetylgalactosamine-4-sulfatase (arylsulfatase B), and characterized biochemically by the predominance of dermatan sulfate in the urine and the presence of coarse metachromatic granules in the leukocytes, and clinically by Hurler-like signs with normal intelligence. There are three clinical forms: the severe or classic form shows Hurler-like symptoms; the intermediate form has the same phenotype as mucolipidosis III (pseudo-Hurler polydystrophy); the mild form is difficult to distinguish from the Scheie syndrome. Called also *mucopolysaccharidosis VI*, N-*acetylgalactosamine-4-sulfatase* and *arylsulfatase B* (ARSB) *deficiency*. **Martorell's s.,** pulseless disease. **mastocytosis s.,** an episodic syndrome occurring in certain patients with systemic mastocytosis, usually those with skin lesions, bone lesions, and hepatosplenomegaly, presumably associated with histamine release from degranulation of mast cells, and characterized mainly by intense pruritus, flushing, headache, tachycardia, hypotension, and syncope. **maternal deprivation s.,** growth failure, autistic behavior, and retarded mental development resulting from loss or absence of the mother or lack of proper mothering. **Mauriac s.,** dwarfism, hepatomegaly, obesity, and retarded sexual maturation, in association with diabetes mellitus. **Mayer-Rokitansky-Küster-Hauser s.,** lack of müllerian development, congenital absence of the vagina and a rudimentary uterus (typically bicornuate remnants), with normal uterine tubes, ovaries, and secondary female sex characteristics and normal growth. Called also *Rokitansky-Küster-Hauser s.* **Meckel's s., Meckel-Gruber s.,** a hereditary syndrome, transmitted as an autosomal recessive trait, most frequently characterized by sloping forehead, posterior meningoencephalocele, polydactyly, and polycystic kidneys, with death occurring in the perinatal period. Called also *Gruber's s.* and *dysencephalia splanchnocystica*. **meconium plug s.,** a syndrome of intestinal obstruction caused by unusually thick or hard meconium in which neither enzymatic nor ganglion cell deficiency can be demonstrated. **megacystis-megaureter s.,** chronic ureteral dilatation (megaureter) associated with hypotonia and dilatation of the bladder (megacystis) and gaping of ureteral orifices, permitting vesicoureteral reflux of urine, and resulting in chronic pyelonephritis. **Meigs' s.,** ascites and hydrothorax associated with ovarian fibroma or other pelvic tumor. **Melkersson's s., Melkersson-Rosenthal s.,** a hereditary syndrome transmitted as an autosomal dominant trait, most often beginning in childhood or adolescence, and characterized chiefly by chronic noninflammatory facial swelling (usually confined to the lips), recurrent peripheral facial palsy, and sometimes fissured tongue. Associated ophthalmic symptoms may include lagophthalmos, burning sensation of the eyes, blepharochalasis, swelling of the eyelids, corneal opacities, retrobulbar neuritis, and bilateral recurrent exophthalmos. **Mendelson's s.,** pulmonary acid aspiration syndrome. **Mengert's shock s.,** a condition resembling shock that sometimes occurs when pregnant women in the late antepartum period lie in the supine position; it is due to the pressure of the uterus on the vena cava. **Meniere's s.,** see under *disease*. **Menkes' s.,** a hereditary abnormality in copper absorption marked by severe cerebral degeneration and arterial changes resulting in death in infancy and by sparse, brittle scalp hair with a twisted appearance microscopically. It is transmitted as an X-linked recessive trait. Called also *Menkes' disease* and *kinky*- or *steely-hair s.* **metameric s.,** segmentary s. **methionine malabsorption s.,** an autosomal recessive disorder of methionine absorption in which the urine has a characteristic odor resembling that of the interior of an oasthouse, due to alpha-hydroxybutyric acid formed by bacterial action on the unabsorbed methionine; it is characterized by white hair, mental retardation, convulsions, and attacks of hyperpnea. Called also *oasthouse urine disease* and *Smith-Strang disease*. **Meyer-Schwickerath and Weyers s.,** oculodentodigital dysplasia. **middle lobe s.,** atelectasis of the right middle pulmonary lobe, with chronic pneumonitis; called also *Brock's s.* **Mikulicz's s.,** a chronic bilateral hypertrophy of the lacrimal, parotid, and salivary glands, associated with decreased or absent lacrimation and xerostomia, and often accompanied by chronic lymphocytic infiltration. It may be associated with other diseases, such as Sjögren's syndrome, sarcoidosis, lupus erythematosus, leukemia, lymphoma, and tuberculosis. See also under *disease*. **milk-alkali s.,** a syndrome characterized by hypercalcemia without hypercalciuria or hypophosphatemia, with only mild alkalosis, normal serum phosphatase, severe renal insufficiency with hyperazotemia, and calcinosis, attributed to ingestion of milk and absorbable alkali for long periods of time; called also *Burnett's s.* and *hypercalcemia s.* **Milkman's s.,** a generalized bone disease marked by multiple transparent stripes of

absorption in the long and flat bones; called also *Looser-Milkman s.* **Millard-Gubler s.,** crossed paralysis, affecting the limbs on one side of the body and the face on the opposite side, together with paralysis of outward movement of the eye; it is due to infarction of the pons, involving the sixth and seventh cranial nerves and the fibers of the corticospinal tract. Called also *Millard-Gubler paralysis*. Cf. *Foville's s.* **Minkowski-Chauffard s.,** hereditary spherocytosis. **Minot-von Willebrand s.,** von Willebrand's disease. **mitral valve prolapse s.,** prolapse of the mitral valve, often with regurgitation, associated with myxomatous proliferation of the leaflets of the mitral valve, a common, usually benign, often asymptomatic condition characterized by mid-systolic clicks and late systolic murmurs on auscultation. Palpitations and chest discomfort may occur, and in some cases progressive mitral regurgitation necessitates valve replacement. Called also *Barlow s.* and *floppy valve s.* **Möbius' s.,** agenesis or aplasia of the motor nuclei of the cranial nerves characterized by congenital bilateral facial palsy in various combinations, with unilateral or bilateral paralysis of the abductors of the eye, sometimes associated with involvement of the cranial nerves, particularly the oculomotor, trigeminal, and hypoglossal, and anomalies of the extremities. Called also *akinesia algera, congenital facial diplegia, nuclear agenesis* or *aplasia, congenital abducens-facial paralysis*, and *congenital oculofacial paralysis*. **Mohr s.,** an autosomal recessive disorder characterized by brachydactyly, clinodactyly, polydactyly, syndactyly, and bilateral hallucal polysyndactyly; by cranial, facial, lingual, palatal, and mandibular anomalies; and by episodic neuromuscular disturbances. Called also *oral-facial-digital* (OFD) *s., type II, orodigitofacial dysostosis, orofaciodigital* (OFD) *s., type II*. See also *oral-facial-digital s., type I*. **Monakow's s.,** hemiplegia on the side opposite the lesion in occlusion of the anterior choroidal artery, sometimes with hemianesthesia and hemianopia. **Moore's s.,** abdominal epilepsy. **Morel's s.,** hyperostosis frontalis interna. **Morgagni's s.,** hyperostosis frontalis interna. **Morgagni-Adams-Stokes s.,** Adams-Stokes disease. **Morgagni-Stewart-Morel s.,** hyperostosis frontalis interna. **morning glory s.,** a coloboma in which there is a funnel-shaped optic nerve head with a dot of whitish, fluffy material in the center, an elevated ring of pigment around the disk, and vessels radiating from the ring like spokes. Vision is severely affected. **Morquio s.,** two biochemically distinct, but clinically nearly indistinguishable, forms of mucopolysaccharidosis characterized by excretion of keratan sulfate in the urine. Clinical features, affecting primarily the skeletal and secondarily the nervous system, include genu valgum, pectus carinatum, progressive platyspondyly, short neck and trunk, normal but broad-mouthed facies with spacing between the teeth, progressive deafness, and very mild corneal clouding. Intelligence is normal. The two enzymatic types are: *type A*, the severe form, caused by N-acetylgalactosamine-6-sulfate deficiency (patients do not survive their thirties); and *type B*, caused by β-galactosidase deficiency (patients may live into their sixties). Called also *mucopolysaccharidosis IV* and *keratansulfaturia*. **Morquio-Ullrich s.,** Morquio's s. **Morton's s.,** a congenital insufficiency of the first metatarsal segment of the foot, characterized by metatarsalgia due to shortening or relaxation of the part. **Morvan's s.,** 1. syringomyelia. 2. manifestation of syringomyelia marked by thickening of the subcutaneous tissues of the hands, which become edematous, soft, swollen, cyanotic, and cold (*main succulente,* or *Marinesco's succulent hand*) associated with analgesic ulceration of the tips of the fingers and paresthesia and atrophy of the hands and forearms. Called also *analgesic panaris* and *Morvan's disease*. **Mosse's s.,** polycythemia vera with cirrhosis of the liver. **Moynahan s.,** 1. multiple symmetric lentigines, congenital mitral valve stenosis, dwarfism, genital hypoplasia, and mental retardation. Called also *progressive cardiomyopathic lentiginosis*. 2. a familial congenital syndrome consisting of delayed hair growth on the scalp, epilepsy, mental retardation, and unusual electroencephalogram. **Muckle-Wells s.,** an autosomal dominant syndrome characterized by amyloidosis involving the kidneys and causing nephritis, recurrent urticaria, deafness, and pain in the extremities. **mucocutaneous lymph node s. (MLNS),** a syndrome of unknown etiology affecting most commonly infants and young children, and marked by fever, conjunctival injection, reddening of the lips and oral cavity, ulcerative gingivitis, enlarged cervical lymph nodes, and maculoerythematous skin eruption that becomes confluent and bright red in a glove-and-sock distribution, the skin becoming indurated and edematous and desquamating from the fingers and toes. It has been observed in Japan since 1967, but has recently been reported in the U.S. with some frequency. Called also *Kawasaki disease.* **mucosal neuroma s.,** multiple endocrine neoplasia, Type III. **multiple glandular deficiency s.,** primary failure of any combination of endocrine glands, including adrenals, thyroid, gonads, parathyroids, and endocrine pancreas, often accompanied by nonendocrine autoimmune abnormalities. **multiple hamartoma s.,** Cowden's disease. **multiple lentigines s.,** leopard s. **Munchausen s.,** a condition characterized by habitual presentation for hospital treatment of an apparent acute illness, the patient giving a plausible and dramatic history, all of which is false; called *chronic factitious disorder with physical symptoms* in DSM III. **Murchison-Sanderson s.,** Hodgkin's disease. **myasthenia gravis s.,** Erb's s. **myasthenic s.,** Eaton-Lambert s. **myelofibrosis-osteosclerosis s.,** a form of myeloproliferative disease characterized by fibrosis of the bone marrow, splenomegaly, extramedullary hematopoiesis, and leukoerythroblastosis. **myeloproliferatives,** see *myeloproliferative.* **Naegeli s.,** Franceschetti-Jadassohn s. **Naffziger's s.,** scalenus s. **nail-patella s.,** onycho-osteodysplasia. **Nelson's s.,** the development of an ACTH-producing pituitary tumor after bilateral adrenalectomy in Cushing's syndrome; it is characterized by aggressive growth of the tumor and hyperpigmentation of the skin. **neostriatal s.,** Hunt's striatal s., def. 2. **nephrotic s.,** a condition characterized by massive edema, heavy proteinuria, hypoalbuminemia, and peculiar susceptibility to intercurrent infections; called also *Epstein's s.* **Netherton's s.,** a congenital syndrome consisting of lamellar ichthyosis or ichthyosis linearis circumflexa, hair shaft defects, atopic diathesis, and sometimes mental retardation and aminoaciduria. It is believed to be autosomal recessive. **neurocutaneous s.,** phakomatosis. **neuroleptic malignant s.,** a rare, sometimes fatal reaction to neuroleptic drugs, characterized by hyperthermia, rigidity, and coma. **nevoid basal cell carcinoma s., nevoid basalioma s.,** basal cell nevus s. **Nezelof s.,** a heterogeneous group of immunodeficiency disorders characterized by profoundly deficient cellular immunity and varying degrees of humoral immunodeficiency. Immunoglobulin levels may be normal or increased, but antibody response to immunization may be absent. Patients are highly susceptible to life-threatening infections with low-grade or opportunistic pathogens, such as *Candida albicans, Pneumocystis carinii,* and cytomegalovirus. Both autosomal recessive and X-linked inheritance have been described. Called also *cellular immunodeficiency with immunoglobulins.* **nitritoid s.,** nitritoid crisis. **Noack's s.,** acrocephalopolysyndactyly (type I). **Nonne's s.,** hereditary cerebellar ataxia. **Nonne-Milroy-Meige s.,** Milroy's disease. **nonsense s.,** Ganser s. **Noonan's s.,** webbed neck, ptosis, hypogonadism, congenital heart disease, and short stature, that is, the phenotype of Turner's syndrome without gonadal dysgenesis; formerly called male Turner's syndrome until the female counterpart was identified. Called also *Ullrich-Turner s.* **Nothnagel's s.,** unilateral oculomotor paralysis combined with cerebellar ataxia, in lesions of the cerebral peduncles. **OAV s.,** oculoauriculovertebral dysplasia. **oculocerebral-hypopigmentation s.,** Cross s. **oculocerebrorenal s.,** an X-linked disorder characterized by vitamin D–refractory rickets, hydrophthalmia, congenital glaucoma and cataracts, mental retardation, and tubule reabsorption dysfunction as evidenced by hypophosphatemia, acidosis, and aminoaciduria. Called also *Lowe disease* and *Lowe-Terrey-Maclachlan s.* **oculodento-osseous s.,** oculodentodigital dysplasia. **oculomandibulofacial s.,** a syndrome principally characterized by dyscephaly (usually brachycephaly), parrot nose, mandibular hypoplasia, proportionate nanism, hypotrichosis, bilateral congenital cataracts, and microphthalmia; called also *Hallermann-Streiff s., Hallermann-Streiff-François s., François' s.,* and *mandibulo-oculofacial dyscephaly.* **OFD s.,** oral-facial-digital s. **Ogilvie's s.,** a condition simulating colonic obstruction, with persistent contraction of intestinal musculature, but without evidence of organic disease of the colon, occurring as a result of a defect in the sympathetic nerve supply. Called also *false colonic obstruction.* **Oldfield's s.,** familial polyposis of the colon associated with extensive sebaceous cysts.

OMM s., ophthalmomandibulomelic dysplasia; see under *dysplasia.* **Oppenheim's s.,** see under *disease.* **oral-facial-digital (OFD) s., type I,** a male-lethal X-linked dominant disorder characterized by camptodactyly, polydactyly, and syndactyly; by cranial, facial, lingual, and dental anomalies; and by mental retardation, familial trembling, alopecia, and seborrhea of the face and milia. Called also *orodigitofacial dysostosis, orofaciodigital s., type I.* See also *Mohr s.* **oral-facial-digital (OFD) s., type II,** Mohr s. **oral-facial-digital (OFD) s., type III,** an autosomal recessive disorder characterized by postaxial hexadactyly of the hands and feet, by ocular, lingual, and dental anomalies, and by profound mental retardation. Called also *orodigitofacial dysostosis, orofaciodigital s., type III.* **organic anxiety s.** [DSM III-R], an organic mental syndrome characterized by prominent, recurrent panic attacks or generalized anxiety caused by a specific organic factor and not associated with delirium. Causes include such endocrine disorders as hyperthyroidism, hypothyroidism, pheochromocytoma, fasting hypoglycemia, and hypercortisolism or the use of psychoactive substances. **organic brain s.,** see *organic mental s.* **organic delusional s.** [DSM III-R], an organic brain syndrome characterized by the presence of delusions caused by a specific organic factor and not associated with delirium. Causes include substances such as amphetamines, cannabis, and hallucinogens and other organic diseases such as temporal lobe epilepsy, head trauma or cerebral lesions, and Huntington's chorea. The substance-induced syndromes are named as "disorders," e.g., "cannabis delusional disorder." **organic mental s.** [DSM III-R], a constellation of psychological or behavioral signs and symptoms associated with one or more specific organic etiologic factors. DSM III-R includes six specific organic brain syndromes, *delirium and dementia; amnestic syndrome or organic hallucinosis; organic delusional syndrome, organic mood syndrome,* and *organic anxiety syndrome; organic personality syndrome; intoxication and withdrawal;* and a residual category, *organic mental syndrome not otherwise specified.* When the etiologic factor is a psychoactive substance, the name of the substance is given, the word "organic" is dropped, and "syndrome" is changed to "disorder," e.g., "alcohol amnestic disorder" or "cannabis delusional disorder." Previous nomenclature classified all organic brain syndromes as "psychotic" or "nonpsychotic" and as "acute" (reversible) or "chronic" (irreversible), the latter pair of terms being used with meanings not in accord with general medical usage. **organic mood s.** [DSM III-R], an organic brain syndrome characterized by the presence of manic or depressive mood disturbance caused by a specific organic factor and not associated with delirium. Common causes are drugs and other psychoactive substances, notably reserpine, methyldopa, and certain hallucinogens; endocrine disorders, notably Cushing's syndrome, Addison's disease, hypothyroidism, and hyperparathyroidism; and viral infections. The substance-induced syndromes are named as "disorders," e.g., hallucinogen mood disorder. **organic personality s.** [DSM III-R] an organic brain syndrome characterized by a marked change in behavior or personality, e.g., emotional lability, marked apathy, impaired impulse control, or paranoid ideation, caused by a specific organic factor and not associated with delirium or dementia. The most common causes are space-occupying lesions of the brain, head trauma, and cerebrovascular disease. **orofaciodigital (OFD) s., type I,** oral-facial-digital s., type I. **orofaciodigital s., type II,** Mohr s. **Ostrum-Furst s.,** congenital synostosis of the neck, platybasia, and Sprengel's deformity. **outlet s.,** brachial s. **ovarian-remnant s.,** pelvic pain, sometimes cyclic, typically occurring several weeks or months after oophorectomy, usually associated with a pelvic mass, most frequently a corpus-luteum cyst, which sometimes leads to unilateral ureteral obstruction. It is due to survival of an ovarian fragment after the operation. **ovarian vein s.,** obstruction of the ureter due to compression by an enlarged or varicose ovarian vein; typically the vein becomes enlarged during pregnancy, the symptoms being those of obstruction or infection of the upper urinary tract. The right side is usually affected. **pain dysfunction s.,** temporomandibular joint s. **painful arc s.,** shoulder pain occurring at a particular portion of the arc described when the arm is abducted from the side to the fully raised position, as in inflammation of the tendons of the supraspinatus muscle. **painful bruising s.,** a purpuric reaction almost always seen in young to middle-aged women in which spontaneous, chronic recurring painful ecchymoses, single or multiple, occur on the body without antecedent trauma or after insufficient trauma, and may be precipitated by emotional stress. Based on studies that show that certain patients exhibit autoerythrocyte sensitization in which intradermal injection of their own erythrocytes produces a painful ecchymosis, the etiology of the condition has been ascribed by some to an autosensitivity to a component of the erythrocyte membrane; others consider it to be of psychosomatic or factitious origin. Called also *autoerythrocyte sensitization s.*, *erythrocyte autosensitization s.*, and *Gardner-Diamond s.* Cf. *psychogenic purpura.* **palcostriatal s.**, juvenile paralysis agitans (of Hunt). **pallidal s.**, juvenile paralysis agitans (of Hunt). **pallidomesencephalic s.**, a syndrome made up of rigidity, poverty of movement, and bradykinesia, amounting to a parkinsonian state. **Pancoast's s.**, 1. roentgenographic shadow at apex of lung, neuritic pain in the arm, atrophy of the muscles of the arm and hand, and Horner's syndrome, observed in tumor near the apex of the lung and due to involvement of the brachial plexus. 2. osteolysis in the posterior part of one or more ribs and sometimes also involving the corresponding vertebra. **pancreaticohepatic s.**, extensive destruction of pancreatic tissue and fatty metamorphosis of the liver. **pancytopenia-dysmelia s.**, Fanconi's s., def. 1. **Papillon-Lefèvre s.**, an autosomal recessive disorder occurring between the first and fifth years of life, characterized by psoriasiform palmoplantar keratoderma, which may also involve the elbows, knees, tibias, external malleoli, and other areas; ectopic calcifications of the skull; and periodontitis and premature shedding of both the deciduous and permanent teeth. **paraneoplastic s.**, a symptom-complex arising in a cancer-bearing patient that cannot be explained by local or distant spread of the tumor. **paratrigeminal s.**, paroxysmal neuralgic pain in the face associated with sympathetic palsy (Horner's syndrome). **Parinaud's s.**, paralysis of conjugate upward movement of the eyes without paralysis of convergence, associated with lesions of the midbrain, such as a tumor of the pineal gland. **Parinaud's oculoglandular s.**, a general term applied to conjunctivitis, most often unilateral, usually of the follicular type, followed by tenderness and enlargement of the preauricular lymph nodes; it is often caused by infection with a leptothrix, or may be associated with other infections, such as cat-scratch fever, lymphogranuloma venereum, and tularemia. **parkinsonian s.**, a form of parkinsonism due to idiopathic degeneration of the corpus striatum or substantia nigra, frequently occurring as a sequel of lethargic encephalitis, although cerebral arteriosclerosis, toxins, neurosyphilis, and trauma have also been implicated. It is characterized by muscular rigidity, immobile facies (Parkinson's facies), slow involuntary tremor (present at rest but tending to disappear during sleep and on volitional movement), abolition of associated automatic movements, festinating gait, stooped posture, and salivation. Called also *postencephalitic parkinsonism.* See also *paralysis agitans.* **Parry-Romberg s.**, facial hemiatrophy. **Patau's s.**, trisomy 13 s. **Paterson's s.**, **Paterson-Brown-Kelly s.**, **Paterson-Kelly s.**, Plummer-Vinson s. **Pellegrini-Stieda s.**, calcification of the medial collateral ligament of the knee. **Pellizzi's s.**, epiphyseal s. **Pendred's s.**, a hereditary syndrome of congenital bilateral nerve deafness associated with development of goiter without hypothyroidism in middle childhood; the main biochemical feature is a partial defect in thyroxine biosynthesis. **pericolic-membrane s.**, symptoms resembling those of chronic appendicitis due to the pressure of pericolic membranes. **persistent müllerian duct s.**, the persistence, in otherwise normal males, of müllerian structures as well as male genital ducts, with undescended testes and bilateral uterine tubes, a uterus, and an upper vagina. There may be unilateral cryptorchidism with contralateral inguinal hernia containing a testis, uterus, and uterine tube (*hernia uteri inguinale*). The disorder is heritable; fertility has been described. **pertussis s.**, 1. pertussis-like s. 2. pertussis. **pertussis-like s.**, a syndrome clinically indistinguishable from pertussis but in which there is no evidence of infection with *Bordetella pertussis* or *B. parapertussis*, although evidence of other infectious agents, such as adenoviruses types 1, 2, 3, 5, and 6, can be demonstrated. Called also *pertussis s.* Cf. *parapertussis.* **Peutz s.**, hereditary intestinal polyposis. **Peutz-Jeghers s.**, a hereditary syndrome characterized by gastrointestinal polyposis (usually hamartomas of the small bowel)

associated with excessive melanin pigmentation of the skin and mucous membranes; gastrointestinal bleeding and intussusception are common complications. It is transmitted as an autosomal dominant trait. **Pfeiffer's s.**, an autosomal dominant disorder characterized by acroecephalosyndactyly associated with broad short thumbs and big toes. Called also *acrocephalosyndactyly type V.* **pharyngeal pouch s.**, DiGeorge syndrome. **PHC s.**, an autosomal dominant syndrome consisting of premolar aplasia, hyperhidrosis, and premature canities. Called also *Böök s.* **Picchini's s.**, inflammation of the three serous membranes connected with the diaphragm, sometimes involving the meninges, synovial sheaths, and tunica vaginalis of the testicle; caused by a trypanosome. **Pick's s.**, 1. Pick's disease (def. 2). 2. (*obs.*) palpitation of the heart: a feeling of oppression on the chest, dyspnea, cyanosis, and dropsical phenomena; seen in certain heart diseases. **pickwickian s.**, the complex of obesity, somnolence, hypoventilation, and erythrocytosis. **Pierre Robin s.**, an autosomal recessive disorder characterized by brachygnathia and cleft palate, often associated with glossoptosis, backward and upward displacement of the larynx, and angulation of the manubrium sterni; cleft palate makes sucking and swallowing difficult, permitting easy access of fluids into the larynx. It may appear in several syndromes or as an isolated hypoplasia. Called also *Robin's s.* and *Robin's anomalad.* **pineal s.**, epiphyseal s. **placental dysfunction s.**, malnutrition and hypoxia of the fetus due to degenerative changes in the placenta; in the full-blown condition the nails, skin, and vernix are stained a bright yellow and the umbilical cord a yellow-green. Called also *yellow vernix s.* **placental transfusion s.**, the birth of one anemic and one plethoric twin due to the forcing of blood of one fetal twin into the circulation of the other via interconnections between their blood vessels; called also *intrauterine parabiotic s.* **Plummer-Vinson s.**, a syndrome usually occurring in middle-aged women with hypochromic anemia, chiefly characterized by cracks or fissures at the corners of the mouth, painful tongue with atrophy of the filiform and later the fungiform papillae, and dysphagia due to esophageal stenosis or webs. Called also *Paterson's s.*, *Paterson-Brown Kelly s.*, *Paterson-Kelly s.*, *sideropenic dysphagia*, and *Vinson's s.* **Poland's s.**, unilateral absence of the sternocostal head of the pectoralis major muscle and ipsilateral syndactyly; called also *Poland's anomaly.* **Polhemus-Schafer-Ivemark s.**, Ivemark's s. **polycystic ovary s.**, Stein-Leventhal s. **pontine s.**, Raymond-Cestan s. **popliteal pterygium s.**, 1. popliteal web s. 2. Fèvre-Languepin s. **popliteal web s.**, a congenital syndrome consisting chiefly of popliteal webs, cleft palate, lower lip pits, and dysplasia of the toenails; a wide variety of other abnormalities may be associated. Called also *popliteal pterygium s.* **postcardiotomy psychosis s.**, anxiety, confusion, and perceptual disturbances occurring 2 to 5 days after an operation using cardiopulmonary bypass. **postcholecystectomy s.**, the persistence or recurrence of abdominal pain or jaundice following cholecystectomy; it may be due to an incorrect preoperative diagnosis, a retained stone in the common bile duct, or to other physical or psychic abnormalities which are not apparent. **postcommissurotomy s.**, postpericardiotomy s. **postconcussional s.**, amnesia, headache, dizziness, tinnitus, irritability, fatigability, sweating, palpitations of the heart, insomnia, and difficulty in concentrating, occurring after concussion of the brain. **posterior cord s.**, sensory and ataxic phenomena derived from a lesion of the posterior columns of the spinal cord, as in locomotor ataxia. **posterolateral s.**, an ataxic and spasmodic condition due to lesions of the posterolateral elements of the spinal cord. **postgastrectomy s.**, dumping s. **postirradiation s.**, a symptom complex caused by massive irradiation, with hemorrhage, anemia, and malnutrition. **post–lumbar puncture s.**, headache in the erect posture, sometimes with nuchal pain, nausea, vomiting, diaphoresis, and malaise, all relieved by recumbency, occurring several hours after lumbar puncture and lasting a few days; it is due to lowering of intracranial pressure by leakage of cerebrospinal fluid through the needle tract. **postmaturity s.**, placental dysfunction syndrome occurring in postmature fetuses. **postmyocardial infarction s.**, pericarditis with fever, leukocytosis, pleurisy, and pneumonia occurring after myocardial infarction; called also *Dressler's s.* **postperfusion s.**, cytomegalovirus mononucleosis occurring about 3 to 6 weeks after extracorporeal circulation or multiple blood transfusions in open heart or other surgical procedures. Called also *post-transfusion s.* and *post-transfusion mononucleosis.* **postpericardiotomy s.,** delayed pericardial or pleural reaction following opening of the pericardium, characterized by fever, chest pain, and signs of pleural and/or pericardial inflammation. **postphlebitic s.,** the various complications associated with deep vein thrombosis which are caused by greatly increased pressure in the deep and communicating veins, resulting in chronic venous insufficiency, and principally characterized by persistent edema, pain, purpura and increased cutaneous pigmentation, eczematoid dermatitis, pruritus, ulceration, and indurated cellulitis. Called also *post-thrombotic s.* **post-thrombotic s.,** postphlebitic s. **post-transfusion s.,** postperfusion s. **post-traumatic brain s.,** a general term denoting all the symptoms occurring after a head injury; see *concussion of the brain, contusion of the brain,* and *postconcussional s.* **Potter's s.,** a rare condition combining a characteristic facial appearance with renal agenesis or hypoplasia and other defects. The face is flattened and features may include widely spaced eyes, epicanthal folds, a crease below the lower lids, large, low-set, floppy ears, micrognathia, and skin crease on the lower chin; skeletal abnormalities, such as clubbed feet and contracted joints, are frequent. Infants die shortly after birth. **Prader-Willi s.,** a congenital disorder characterized by rounded face, almond-shaped eyes, strabismus, low forehead, hypogonadism, hypotonia, insatiable appetite, and mental retardation. **preexcitation s.,** Wolff-Parkinson-White s. **premenstrual s.,** a syndrome of unknown cause sometimes marked by bloating, edema, emotional lability, headache, changes in appetite or cravings for selected foods, breast swelling and tenderness, constipation, and decreased ability to concentrate; called also *premenstrual tension.* **premotor s.,** the association of spastic hemiplegia with increased reflexes, disturbances of skilled movements, forced grasping and transient vasomotor disturbance; occurring in lesions of the premotor cortex. **Profichet's s.,** a gradual growth of calcareous nodules in the subcutaneous tissues (skin stones) especially about the larger joints, with a tendency to ulceration or cicatrization and attended by atrophic and nervous symptoms. **prune-belly s.,** a syndrome in which the lower part of the rectus abdominis muscle and the lower and medial parts of the oblique muscles are absent, the bladder and ureters are usually greatly dilated, the kidneys are small and dysplastic, with hydronephrosis, and the testes are undescended. The abdomen is protruding and thin-walled, with wrinkled skin, giving the syndrome its name. **pseudoclaudication s.,** a condition in which symptoms similar to those of intermittent claudication result from compression of the cauda equina owing to hypertrophic ridging or a herniated lumbar disk. **pulmonary acid aspiration s.,** the disorder produced, as a complication of anesthesia, by inhalation of gastric content with a pH of less than 2.5, including bronchoconstriction and destruction of tracheal mucosa, progressing to a syndrome resembling acute respiratory distress syndrome. Called also *Mendelson's s.* **pulmonary dysmaturity s.,** Wilson-Mikity s. **Putnam-Dana s.,** subacute combined degeneration of spinal cord (see under *degeneration*). **QT s.,** a combination of prolonged QT interval and torsades de pointes; it may be congenital or acquired, the latter usually the result of drug administration. **radicular s.,** a syndrome due to lesion of the roots of the spinal nerves, consisting of restricted mobility of the spine and root pain. **Ramsay Hunt s.,** 1. herpes zoster involving the facial and auditory nerves associated with ipsilateral facial paralysis, usually transitory, and herpetic vesicles of the external ear or tympanic membrane, which also may or may not be associated with tinnitus, vertigo, and hearing disorders. Called also *geniculate neuralgia, herpes zoster auricularis* or *oticus,* and *Hunt's disease* or *neuralgia.* 2. juvenile paralysis agitans (of Hunt). 3. dyssynergia cerebellaris progressiva. **Raymond-Cestan s.,** a syndrome due to obstruction of twigs of the basilar artery causing lesions of the pontine region; it is characterized by quadriplegia, anesthesia, and nystagmus. **Refsum's s.,** see under *disease.* **Reichmann's s.,** gastrosuccorrhea. **Reifenstein's s.,** a syndrome of male hypergonadotropic hypogonadism, due to an inherited defect of androgen receptors and consequent insensitivity to testosterone, with hypospadias, gynecomastia, primary hypogonadism, and postpubertal testicular atrophy and azoospermia. **Reiter's s.,** a triad of symptoms of unknown etiology comprising urethritis, conjunctivitis, and arthritis (the dominant feature), appearing concomitantly or sequentially associated with mucocutaneous manifestations of keratoderma blennorrhagicum, circinate balanitis, and stomatitis, chiefly affecting young men, and usually running a self-limited but relapsing course. Most affected patients have increased levels of the histocompatibility antigen HLA-B27. It possibly represents an abnormal immune response to certain infections, perhaps related to hereditary susceptibility. Epidemiologic studies reveal that there are venereal, or postvenereal, and dysenteric, or postdysenteric forms. The former occurs mainly in the United States and Great Britain, possibly related to infection with *Chlamydia* or *Ureaplasma urealyticum;* and the latter in Asia, continental Europe, and North Africa, possibly related to *Shigella, Salmonella, Yersinia,* or *Campylobacter fetus* infection. Called also *Fiessinger-Leroy-Reiter s.* and *Reiter's disease.* **Rendu-Osler-Weber s.,** hereditary hemorrhagic telangiectasia. **respiratory distress s. of newborn,** a condition of the newborn marked by dyspnea with cyanosis, heralded by such prodromal signs as dilatation of the alae nasi, expiratory grunt, and retraction of the suprasternal notch or costal margins, most frequently occurring in premature infants, children of diabetic mothers, and infants delivered by cesarean section, and sometimes with no apparent predisposing cause. The syndrome includes two patterns: (*a*) *hyaline membrane disease* or *syndrome,* in which affected infants frequently die of respiratory distress in the first few days of life and at autopsy have eosinophilic hyaline material lining the alveoli, alveolar ducts, and bronchioles, and (*b*) *idiopathic respiratory distress of newborn* in which the affected infants may live, but in those that die, only resorption atelectasis is seen and there is no formation of a hyaline membrane. Called also *congenital alveolar dysplasia* and *congenital aspiration pneumonia.* **restless legs s.,** unpleasant deep discomfort inside the calves when sitting or lying down, especially just before sleep, producing an irresistible urge to move the legs. **retraction s.,** Duane's s. **s. of retroparotid space,** Villaret's s. **Rett s.,** a progressive disorder affecting the gray matter of the brain, occurring exclusively in females and present from birth; it is characterized by autistic behavior, ataxia, dementia, seizures, and loss of purposeful use of the hands, with cerebral atrophy, mild hyperammonemia, and decreased levels of biogenic amines. Called also *cerebroatrophic hyperammonemia.* **Reye's s.,** a rare, acute, and sometimes fatal disease of childhood, most often occurring as a sequel of varicella or a viral upper respiratory infection. It is marked by recurrent vomiting and elevated serum transaminase levels, with distinctive changes in the liver and other viscera; an encephalopathic phase with acute brain swelling, disturbances of consciousness, and seizures may follow. **Rh-null s.,** chronic hemolytic anemia affecting individuals who lack all Rh factors (Rh_{null}); it is marked by spherocytosis, stomatocytosis, and increased osmotic fragility. **Richards-Rundle s.,** a congenital syndrome consisting of ketoaciduria, mental retardation, underdevelopment of secondary sex characteristics, deafness, ataxia, and peripheral muscular wasting which progresses during childhood but eventually becomes static. **Richter's s.,** chronic lymphocytic leukemia with diffuse histiocytic lymphoma. **Rieger's s.,** Rieger's anomaly appearing with hypodontia, anal stenosis, hypertelorism, mental deficiency, and agenesis of the facial bones. See also *anterior chamber cleavage syndrome,* under *syndrome.* **Riley-Day s.,** dysautonomia. **Riley-Smith s.,** macrocephaly without hydrocephalus, multiple hemangiomas, and pseudopapilledema; presumed to be transmitted as an autosomal dominant trait. **Robert's s.,** a hereditary syndrome, transmitted as an autosomal recessive trait, consisting of imperfect development of the long bones of the limbs associated with cleft palate and lip and other anomalies. **Robin s.,** Pierre Robin s. **Robinow's s.,** dwarfism associated with increased interorbital distance, malaligned teeth, bulging forehead, depressed nasal bridge, and short limbs. Called also *Robinow's dwarfism* and *fetal face s.* **Roger's s.,** a continuous excessive secretion of saliva as the result of cancer in the esophagus, or other esophageal irritation. **Rokitansky-Küster-Hauser s.,** Mayer-Rokitansky-Küster-Hauser s. **rolandic vein s.,** hemiplegia resulting from interference with the cerebral venous circulation. **Romano-Ward s.,** prolonged Q-t interval and syncope, sometimes with ventricular fibrillation and sudden death; inherited as an autosomal dominant trait. **Rosenbach's s.,** paroxysmal tachycardia with gastric and respiratory complications. **Rosenthal s.,** a hereditary hemorrhagic diathesis clinically similar to hemophilia but due to deficiency of coagulation Factor XI. **Rosenthal-Kloepfer s.,** corneal leukomata, acromegaloid appearance, and cutis verticis gyrata. **Rosewater's s.,** a mild form of familial primary hypogonadism in the male of unknown pathogenesis, marked only by sterility and gynecomastia. **Rot's s., Rot-Bernhardt s.,** meralgia paresthetica. **Roth's s., Roth-Bernhardt s.,** meralgia paresthetica. **Rothmann-Makai s.,** idiopathic circumscribed panniculitis with fat cell necrosis, lipophagic granuloma, and cyst formation; it usually subsides spontaneously. **Rothmund-Thomson s.,** an autosomal recessive syndrome occurring principally in females, characterized by the presence of reticulated, atrophic, hyperpigmented, telangiectatic cutaneous plaques, often accompanied by juvenile cataracts, saddle nose, congenital bone defects, disturbances in the growth of hair, nails, and teeth, and hypogonadism. Called also *poikiloderma congenitale.* Cf. *Thomson disease.* **Rotor's s.,** chronic familial nonhemolytic jaundice differing from Dubin-Johnson syndrome in the lack of liver pigmentation. **Roussy-Dejerine s.,** thalamic s. **Roussy-Lévy s.,** a slowly progressive hereditary disorder, transmitted as an autosomal dominant trait, in which sensory ataxia is associated with areflexia, atrophy of the muscles of the distal extremities, especially the peroneal muscles, static tremor of the hands, pes cavus or clawfoot, and sometimes kyphoscoliosis. Called also *hereditary areflexic dystasia, Roussy-Lévy disease,* and *Roussy-Lévy hereditary areflexic dystasia.* **Rovsing s.,** horseshoe kidney with nausea, abdominal discomfort, and pain on hyperextension. **rubella s.,** congenital rubella s. **Rubinstein's s., Rubinstein-Taybi s.,** a congenital condition characterized by mental and motor retardation, broad thumbs and great toes, short stature, characteristic facies, including high-arched palate and straight or beaked nose, various eye abnormalities, pulmonary stenosis, keloid formation in surgical scars, large foramen magnum, and abnormalities of the vertebra and sternum. **rubrospinal cerebellar peduncle s.,** Claude's s. **Rud's s.,** congenital syndrome consisting of ichthyosis simplex, mental deficiency, epilepsy, and infantilism. **rudimentary testis s.,** vanishing testis s. **runting s.,** graft-vs.-host reaction characterized by diarrhea, dermatitis, hepatosplenomegaly, hemolytic anemia, and pancytopenia. **Russell's s.,** Silver's s. **Rust's s.,** stiff neck, stiff carriage of the head, with the necessity of grasping the head with both hands in lying down or rising up from a horizontal posture, occurring in tuberculosis, cancer, fracture of the spine, rheumatic or arthritic processes, or syphilitic periostitis. **Sabin-Feldman s.,** chorioretinitis and cerebral calcifications, similar to the manifestations of toxoplasmosis, but having all tests for toxoplasmosis negative. **Saethre-Chotzen s.,** Chotzen's s. **Sakati-Nyhan s.,** acrocephalopolysyndactyly, type III. **salt-depletion s.,** salt-losing s. **salt-losing s.,** vomiting, dehydration, hypotension, and sudden death due to very large sodium losses from the body. It may be seen in abnormal losses of sodium into the urine (as in congenital adrenal hyperplasia, adrenocortical insufficiency, or one of the forms of salt-losing nephritis) or in large extrarenal sodium losses, usually from the gastrointestinal tract. Called also *salt-depletion crisis, salt-depletion syndrome, salt-losing crisis,* and *salt-losing defect.* **Sanfilippo's s.,** four heterogeneous, biochemically distinct, but clinically indistinguishable, forms of mucopolysaccharidosis characterized biochemically by excretion of heparan sulfate in the urine and clinically by severe, rapid mental deterioration and relatively mild somatic symptoms. Onset is from 2 to 6 years of age; the head is large, height normal; Hurler-like features (dysostosis multiplex, hepatomegaly) are mild; hirsutism is generalized; death usually occurs before 20 years of age. The four enzymatic types are: type *A,* the severest, due to defective heparan *N*-sulfatase; type *B,* due to defective *N*-acetyl-α-D-glucosaminidase; type *C* due to defective acetyl CoA:α-glucosaminide-*N*-acetyltransferase; and type *D,* due to defective *N*-acetyl-α-D-glucosaminide-β-sulfatase. Called also *mucopolysaccharidosis III.* **scalded skin s., non-staphylococcal,** toxic epidermal necrolysis. **scalded skin s., staphylococcal,** an infectious disease of infants and young children and rarely of older children and adults occurring following infection with certain strains of *Staphylococcus aureus* (phage group II), which elaborate exfoliatin (q.v.), an epidermolytic, erythrogen endotoxin that causes a

clinical spectrum ranging from a localized bullous eruption to widespread development of easily ruptured fine vesicles and bullae resulting in exfoliation of large sheets of skin, leaving raw, denuded areas that make the skin surface look scalded. Called also *dermatitis exfoliativa neonatorum* and *Ritter's disease.* Cf. *toxic epidermic necrolysis.* **scalenus s., scalenus anticus s.,** pain over the shoulder, often extending down the arm (cervicobrachial s.) or radiating up the back of the neck due to compression of the nerves and vessels between a cervical rib and the scalenus anticus muscle; called also *Naffziger's s.* and *cervical rib s.* **scapulocostal s.,** pain in the superior or posterior aspect of the shoulder girdle, radiating to contiguous regions, as a result of long-standing alteration of the relationship of the scapula and the posterior thoracic wall. **Schafer's s.,** pachyonychia congenita associated with retardation of physical and mental development. **Schanz's s.,** a series of symptoms indicating spinal weakness, consisting of a sense of fatigue, pain on pressure over the spinous processes, pain on lying prone, and indications of spinal curvature. **Schaumann's s.,** sarcoidosis. **Scheie's s.,** a relatively mild allelic variant of the Hurler syndrome and the mildest of the three allelic disorders of mucopolysaccharidosis I, characterized by corneal clouding, claw hand, involvement of the aortic valve, somewhat coarse facies with a broad mouth, genu valgum, and pes cavus. Stature, intelligence, and life span are normal. Called also *α-L-iduronidase deficiency, Scheie type,* and *mucopolysaccharidosis IS;* formerly called *mucopolysaccharidosis V.* **Schirmer's s.,** a variant of the Sturge-Weber syndrome in which glaucoma occurs early in the course of the disease. **Schmidt's s.,** 1. [A. Schmidt] paralysis on one side, affecting the vocal cord, the velum palati, the trapezius muscle, and the sternocleidomastoid muscle, due to a lesion of the nucleus ambiguus and nucleus accessorius. 2. [M. B. Schmidt] hypofunction of more than one endocrine gland, including the thyroid, adrenals, gonads, parathyroids, and endocrine pancreas, in any combination, along with nonendocrine abnormalities of presumed autoimmune origin, such as vitiligo, alopecia, and pernicious anemia; it occurs primarily in adult females. Originally, primary failure of the adrenals and thyroid only. Called also *polyendocrine autoimmune disease,* type II. **Schönlein-Henoch s.,** see under *purpura.* **Schüller's s., Schüller-Christian s.,** Hand-Schüller-Christian disease. **Schultz s.,** agranulocytosis. **scimitar s.,** complete or partial venous drainage of the right lung into the inferior vena cava, usually with hypoplasia of the right lung; the name is derived from the convex shadow of the anomalous vein to the right of the lower border of the heart in the chest roentgenogram. **s. of sea-blue histiocyte,** a rare disorder characterized by the presence of a morphologically distinct, sea-blue, granulated histiocyte and by splenomegaly. Clinically, the disorder may range from a relatively benign course with mild purpura secondary to thrombocytopenia, to progressive hepatic cirrhosis, hepatic failure, and death. **Seabright bantam s.,** pseudohypoparathyroidism. **Seckel's s.,** see *bird-headed dwarf,* under *dwarf.* **segmentary s.,** a syndrome produced by a lesion of the gray matter of the spinal cord, and marked by weakness and wasting in the affected segment; called also *metameric s.* **Selye s.,** general adaptation s. **Senear-Usher s.,** pemphigus erythematosus. **s. of sensory dissociation with brachial amyotrophy,** see *syringomyelia.* **Sertoli-cell-only s.,** congenital absence of the germinal epithelium of the testes, the seminiferous tubules containing only Sertoli cells, characterized by testes which are slightly smaller than normal, azoospermia, and elevated titers of follicle-stimulating hormone and sometimes of luteinizing hormone. **serum sickness-like s.,** see *serum sickness,* under *sickness.* **Sézary s.,** a form of cutaneous T-cell lymphoma manifested by generalized exfoliative erythroderma, intense pruritus, peripheral lymphadenopathy, and abnormal hyperchromatic mononuclear cells in the skin, lymph nodes, and peripheral blood (*Sézary cells*). Called also *Sézary erythroderma.* **Sheehan's s.,** postpartum pituitary necrosis. **short-bowel s., short-gut s.,** any of the malabsorption conditions resulting from massive resection of the small bowel, the degree and kind of malabsorption depending on the site and extent of the resection; it is characterized by diarrhea, steatorrhea, and malnutrition. **shoulder-hand s.,** a clinical disorder of the upper extremity, characterized by pain and stiffness in the shoulder, with puffy swelling and pain in the ipsilateral hand, sometimes occurring after myocardial infarction but also produced by other known or unknown causes. **Shwachman s., Shwachman-Diamond s.,** primary pancreatic insufficiency and bone marrow failure, characterized by normal sweat chloride values, pancreatic insufficiency, and neutropenia; it may be associated with dwarfism and metaphyseal dysostosis of the hips. **Shy-Drager s.,** a progressive disorder of unknown cause that results in severe disability or death, beginning with symptoms of autonomic insufficiency including impotence (in males), constipation, urinary urgency or retention, anhidrosis, and the hallmark of the disorder, orthostatic hypotension, followed by signs of generalized neurologic dysfunction, such as parkinsonian-like disturbances, cerebellar incoordination, muscle wasting and fasciculations, and coarse tremors of the legs. **Sicard's s.,** Collet's s. **sicca s.,** keratoconjunctivitis and xerostomia without connective tissue disease; cf. *Sjögren's s.* **sick sinus s.,** a complex cardiac arrhythmia manifested as severe sinus bradycardia alone, sinus bradycardia alternating with tachycardia, or sinus bradycardia with atrioventricular block. **Silver's s.,** a congenital syndrome consisting of low birth weight despite normal duration of gestation, short stature, lateral asymmetry, slight to moderate increase in excretion of gonadotropins, which may be associated with incurved fifth fingers, café-au-lait spots, syndactyly, triangular-shaped face, turned down corners of the mouth, and precocious puberty. Cf. *Russell's s.* **Silverskiöld's s.,** a form of eccentro-osteochondrodysplasia in which the skeletal changes are chiefly in the extremities and which is inherited as a dominant character. **Silvestrini-Corda s.,** eunuchoid body type, absence of body hair, deficient libido, atrophy of the testes, sterility, and gynecomastia: a syndrome indicative of abnormally high estrogenic activity, due to failure of the liver to inactivate the circulating estrogens. **Simmonds' s.,** see *panhypopituitarism.* **Sipple's s.,** multiple endocrine neoplasia, type IIA. **Sjögren's s.,** a symptom complex of unknown etiology, usually occurring in middle-aged or older women, marked by the triad of keratoconjunctivitis sicca with or without lacrimal gland-enlargement, xerostomia with or without salivary gland-enlargement, and the presence of a connective tissue disease, usually rheumatoid arthritis but sometimes systemic lupus erythematosus, scleroderma, or polymyositis. An abnormal immune response has been implicated. See also *sicca s.* Called also *Sjögren's disease.* **Sjögren-Larsson s.,** congenital oligophrenia, ichthyosis, and spastic pyramidal symptoms. **sleep apnea s.,** episodes of cessation of breathing occurring at the transition from NREM to REM sleep, with repeated wakening and excessive daytime sleepiness; it occurs most frequently in middle-aged obese males and is thought to have several causes, one being collapse or obstruction of the airway with the inhibition of muscle tone that characterizes REM sleep. **SLE-like s.,** see *systemic lupus erythematosus,* under *lupus.* **Sluder's s.,** see under *neuralgia.* **Sly s.,** a mucopolysaccharidosis caused by deficient β-glucuronidase and characterized biochemically by excretion of dermatan sulfate and heparan sulfate in the urine and by granular inclusions in granulocytes. Onset is between 1 and 2 years with mild to moderate Hurler-like features including dysostosis multiplex, pectus carinatum, visceromegaly, cardiac murmurs, short stature, and moderate mental retardation. Milder forms exist. Called also *mucopolysaccharidosis VII, β-glucuronidase (GUSB) deficiency.* **Smith-Lemli-Opitz s.,** a hereditary syndrome, transmitted as an autosomal recessive trait, characterized by multiple congenital anomalies, including microcephaly, mental retardation, hypotonia, incomplete development of male genitalia, short nose with anteverted nostrils, syndactyly of second and third toes, etc. **social breakdown s.,** symptoms of a mental patient that are due to the effects of long-term institutionalization, rather than the primary illness; they include excessive passivity, assumption of the chronic sick role, and atrophy of work and social skills. **Sohval-Soffer s.,** a congenital syndrome consisting of male hypogonadism associated with multiple skeletal abnormalities of the cervical spine and ribs and mental retardation. **somnolence s.,** a transient condition of drowsiness, lethargy, anorexia, and irritability with electroencephalographic changes, occurring in children after irradiation of the head in acute leukemia or non-Hodgkin's lymphoma. **Sorsby's s.,** a congenital condition consisting of bilateral macular coloboma associated with apical dystrophy of the hands and feet, usually brachydactyly confined to the distal two phalanges. **Sotos' s., Sotos' s.**

of cerebral gigantism, cerebral gigantism. **space adaptation s.,** a form of motion sickness occurring in a weightless environment during space flight, with nausea, vomiting, anorexia, headache, malaise, drowsiness, and lethargy. It is probably caused by conflicting signals concerning motion from the otolith (whose proper function depends on the presence of gravity) and the visual system (which affects the autonomic nervous system). Called also *space sickness.* **Spens's s.,** Adams-Stokes disease. **spherophakia-brachymorphia s.,** Weill-Marchesani s. **splenic flexure s.,** discomfort in the left upper abdominal quadrant, which may give rise to pain in the precordium and left shoulder and arm, simulating angina. **split-brain s.,** an association of symptoms produced by disruption of or interference with the connection between the hemispheres of the brain. **Sprinz-Dubin s., Sprinz-Nelson s.,** Dubin-Johnson s. **Spurway s.,** osteogenesis imperfecta associated with blue sclerae. **Steele-Richardson-Olszewski s.,** a progressive neurological disorder, having onset during the sixth decade, characterized by supranuclear ophthalmoplegia, especially paralysis of the downward gaze, pseudobulbar palsy, dysarthria, dystonic rigidity of the neck and trunk, and dementia. **steely-hair s.,** Menkes' s. **Stein-Leventhal s.,** a clinical symptom complex characterized by oligomenorrhea or amenorrhea, anovulation (hence infertility), and hirsutism, and regularly associated with bilateral polycystic ovaries; excretion of follicle-stimulating hormone and 17-ketosteroids is essentially normal. Called also *polycystic ovary disease* or *syndrome.* **Steinbrocker's s.,** shoulder-hand s. **Steiner's s.,** Curtius' s. **Stevens-Johnson s.,** a sometimes fatal form of erythema multiforme presenting with a flulike prodrome, and characterized by systemic as well as more severe mucocutaneous lesions. The oronasal and anogenital mucous membranes may become involved with a characteristic gray or white pseudomembrane; hemorrhagic crusts often occur on the lips; ocular lesions vary from injected conjunctivitis, iritis, uveitis, corneal vesicles, erosions, and perforation, which may result in corneal opacities and blindness; and pulmonary, gastrointestinal, cardiac, and renal involvement occur. Called also *ectodermosis erosiva pluriorificialis, erythema multiforme exudativum, erythema multiforme major,* and *Johnson-Stevens disease.* **Stewart-Morel s.,** hyperostosis frontalis interna. **Stewart-Treves s.,** lymphangiosarcoma which occurs as a late complication of severe lymphedema of the arm following excision of lymph nodes, usually associated with radical mastectomy. **"stiff heart" s.,** any cardiac disease characterized by restrictive hemodynamics; it may result from any pathologic process that renders the myocardial fibers abnormally rigid or that externally applies a constricting pressure and as a consequence impedes flow of blood into the ventricular cavities. **stiff-man s.,** a condition of unknown etiology characterized by progressive fluctuating rigidity of axial and limb muscles in the absence of signs of cerebral and spinal cord disease but with continuous electromyographic activity. **Still-Chauffard s.,** Chauffard's s. **Stilling s., Stilling-Turk-Duane s.,** Duane s. **Stokes's s., Stokes-Adams s.,** Adams-Stokes disease. **Stokvis-Talma s.,** enterogenous cyanosis. **straight back s.,** a skeletal deformity characterized by loss of the anterior concavity of the vertebral column in the upper thoracic region, with consequent reduction in the anteroposterior diameter of the thorax and compression of the heart between the dorsal spine and the sternum. **stroke s.,** a condition with sudden onset caused by acute vascular lesions of the brain, such as hemorrhage, embolism, thrombosis, or rupturing aneurysm, which may be marked by hemiplegia or hemiparesis, vertigo, numbness, aphasia, and dysarthria; it is often followed by permanent neurologic damage. Called also *cerebrovascular accident* and *stroke.* **Sturge's s., Sturge-Kalischer-Weber s.,** Sturge-Weber s. **Sturge-Weber s.,** a congenital syndrome of unknown etiology consisting of a port-wine stain type of nevus flammeus distributed over the trigeminal nerve accompanied by a similiar vascular disorder of the underlying meninges and cerebral cortex; it usually occurs unilaterally. Called also *encephalofacial* or *encephalotrigeminal angiomatosis, Sturge's* or *Sturge-Kalischer-Weber s.,* and *Sturge's* or *Weber's disease.* **subclavian steal s.,** cerebral or brain stem ischemia resulting from diversion of blood flow from the basilar artery to the subclavian artery, in the presence of occlusive disease of the proximal portion of the subclavian artery. **sudden infant death s.,** the sudden and unexpected death of an apparently healthy infant, typically occurring between the ages of three weeks and five months, and not explained by careful postmortem studies; called also *crib* or *cot death.* Abbreviated SIDS. **sudden unexplained death s.,** death for which no underlying cause can be found of a person 2 years old or older of Southeast Asian origin; abbreviated SUDS. **Sudeck-Leriche s.,** posttraumatic osteoporosis associated with vasospasm. **Sulzberger-Garbe s.,** exudative discoid and lichenoid dermatitis. **superior mesenteric artery s.,** compression of the third, or transverse, portion of the duodenum against the aorta by the superior mesenteric artery, resulting in complete or partial obstruction that may be chronic, intermittent, or acute; symptoms range from mild to severe, including nausea and vomiting, pain, and extreme distention of the stomach and duodenum. **superior orbital fissure s.,** deep orbital and unilateral frontal headache with progressive sixth, third, and fourth cranial nerve palsies, occurring as a rare complication of sphenoid sinusitis and caused by extension of the infection to the structures of the superior orbital fissure. **superior sulcus tumor s.,** Pancoast's s., def. 1. **superior vena cava s.,** suffusion and brawny edema of the face, neck, or upper arms due to increased venous pressure incident to compression of the superior vena cava, most commonly caused by primary bronchial tumors or metastatic mediastinal lymph nodes in lung cancer. **supraspinatus s.,** tenderness over the supraspinatus tendon, a painful arc on movement of the arm, and a reversal of scapulohumeral rhythm. **sweat retention s.,** 1. a dermatologic condition due to occlusion of sweat ducts, which may result in symptoms ranging from pruritus, scratch dermatitis, and miliaria to very persistent inflammatory changes depending upon the extent of the blockage, environmental temperature, and duration of sweating stimulus. 2. tropical anhidrotic asthenia. **Sweet's s.,** acute febrile neutrophilic dermatosis. **Swyer-James s.,** acquired unilateral hyperlucent lung, with severe airway obstruction during expiration, oligemia, and a small hilum; called also *Macleod s.* **sylvian s., sylvian aqueduct s.,** impairment of vertical gaze, retraction nystagmus, convergence nystagmus, convergence spasms, and poor or absent reaction of the pupils (which are usually of normal size) to light or near vision. It is caused by a neoplasm, inflammation, or vascular lesion adjacent to the periductal gray matter of the aqueduct of Sylvius. Called also *Koerber-Salus-Elschnig s.* and *nystagmus refractorius.* **syringomelic s.,** see *syringomelia.* **Takayasu's s.,** pulseless disease. **Tapia's s.,** unilateral paralysis of the tongue and larynx, the velum palati being unaffected. **tarsal tunnel s.,** a complex of symptoms resulting from compression of the posterior tibial nerve or of the plantar nerves in the tarsal tunnel, with pain, numbness, and tingling paresthesia of the sole of the foot. **Taussig-Bing s.,** a rare congenital malformation of the heart characterized by transposition of the great vessels and a ventricular septal defect straddled by a large pulmonary artery; hemodynamically it is characterized by pulmonary hypertension, pulmonary plethora, cyanosis, and greater O_2 saturation of blood in the pulmonary artery than in the aorta. **tegmental s.,** hemiplegia, alternating with disordered eye movements, indicative of lesions of the tegmentum. **temporomandibular dysfunction s., temporomandibular joint s.,** a symptom complex described as consisting of partial deafness, stuffy sensation in the ear; tinnitus, clicking and snapping in the temporomandibular joint, dizziness, headache, and burning pain in the ear, throat, tongue, and nose. Numerous causes have been proposed, such as mandibular overclosure, lesions of the temporomandibular joint, and stress, but some researchers feel that the anatomical and physiological evidence to justify this syndrome is lacking. Called also *Costen's s.* and *myofascial pain dysfunction.* **Terry's s.,** retrolental fibroplasia. **Terson's s.,** hemorrhage into the vitreous. **testicular feminization s.,** an extreme form of male pseudohermaphroditism, with female external development, including secondary sex characteristics, but with presence of testes and absence of uterus and tubes; it is due to end-organ resistance to the action of 5α-testosterone. **tethered cord s.,** an abnormally low conus medullaris tethered by one or more forms of intradural abnormality such as a short, thickened filum terminale, fibrous bands or adhesions, or an intradural lipoma. **thalamic s.,** a combination of the following symptoms: (1) superficial persistent hemianesthesia; (2) mild hemiplegia; (3) mild hemiataxia and more or less complete astereognosis; (4) severe and persistent pains in the hemiplegic side; (5) choreoathetoid movements in the members of the paralyzed side. Called also *Dejerine-Roussy s.* and *thalamic hyperesthetic anesthesia.* **Thibierge-Weissenbach s.,** calcinosis. **Thiele s.,** tenderness and pain in the region of the lower portion of the sacrum and coccyx, or in contiguous soft tissues and muscles. **Thiemann's s.,** see under *disease.* **thoracic outlet s.,** compression of the brachial plexus nerve trunks, characterized by pain in arms, paresthesia of fingers, vasomotor symptoms (pallor, acrocyanosis, secondary Raynaud's phenomenon, etc.), and weakness and wasting of the small muscles of the hand; it may be caused by drooping shoulder girdle, a cervical rib or fibrous band, an abnormal first rib, continual hyperabduction of the arm (see *hyperabduction s.*), or (rarely) compression of the edge of the scalenus anterior muscle. **Thorn's s.,** see *salt-losing s.* **thrombocytopenia–absent radius (TAR) s.,** an autosomal recessive syndrome consisting of thrombocytopenia associated with absence or hypoplasia of the radius and sometimes congenital heart disease and renal anomalies. **thromboembolic s.,** the association between the formation of thrombi in the deep veins of the leg and pulmonary embolism. **Tietze's s.,** 1. [Alexander *Tietze*] idiopathic painful nonsuppurative swellings of one or more costal cartilages, especially of the second rib; the anterior chest pain may mimic that of coronary artery disease. Called also *costal chondritis* and *Tietze's disease.* 2. albinism, except for normal eye pigment, deaf-mutism, and hypoplasia of the eyebrows. **tired housewife s.,** a form of mild hypothyroidism manifested in symptoms such as mild lassitude, fatigue, slight anemia, constipation, apathy, slight cold intolerance, menstrual irregularities, inability to conceive, dry skin, some loss of hair, and slight to moderate weight gain. **Tolosa-Hunt s.,** unilateral ophthalmoplegia associated with pain behind the orbit and in the area supplied by the first division of the trigeminal nerve; it is thought to be due to nonspecific inflammation and granulation tissue in the superior orbital fissure or cavernous sinus. **Tommaselli's s.,** see under *disease.* **Torres's s.,** multiple carcinomas, primarily of the gastrointestinal tract, in association with a large number of sebaceous gland neoplasms. **Touraine-Solente-Golé s.,** pachydermoperiostosis. **toxic fat s.,** a condition occurring in 3- to 10-week old chickens that have been fed fat-supplemented diets, marked by edema of the pericardium and abdomen, waddling gait, and sudden death; called also *water belly.* **toxic shock s.,** a severe illness characterized by high fever of sudden onset, vomiting, diarrhea, and myalgia, followed by hypotension and, in severe cases, shock; a sunburn-like rash with peeling of the skin, especially of the palms and soles, occurs during the acute phase. The syndrome affects almost exclusively menstruating women using tampons, although a few women who do not use tampons and a few males have been affected. It is thought to be caused by infection with *Staphylococcus aureus.* **transfusion s.,** placental transfusion s. **translocation Down s.,** Down syndrome in which the excess chromosomal material (the long arm of chromosome 21) is translocated to another acrocentric chromosome (in standard trisomy 21 there is an additional chromosome 21). A carrier of the translocation chromosome has 45 chromosomes including the translocation chromosome and may be at increased risk of having a child with Down syndrome. **Treacher Collins s., Treacher Collins-Franceschetti s.,** mandibulofacial dysostosis. **trichorhinophalangeal s.,** an autosomal recessive syndrome consisting of sparse, slowly growing hair, pear-shaped nose with high philtrum, and brachyphalangia with deformity of the fingers and wedge-shaped epiphyses. **triparanol s.,** alopecia, poliosis, ichthyosis, irreversible cataracts, and impotence, due to the use of triparanol, a drug formerly used to depress the synthesis of cholesterol. **trisomy C s.,** trisomy 8 s. **trisomy D s.,** trisomy 13 s. **trisomy E s.,** trisomy 18 s. **trisomy 8 s.,** a syndrome associated with an extra chromosome 8, usually mosaic (trisomy 8/normal), characterized by mild to severe mental retardation, prominent forehead, deep-set eyes, thick lips, prominent ears, and camptodactyly. **trisomy 13 s.,** a chromosome aberration in which an extra chromosome 13 causes central nervous system defects and mental retardation, together with cleft palate and lip, polydactyly, dermal pattern anomalies, and abnormalities of the heart, viscera, and genitalia. Called also *Patau s.* **trisomy 18 s.,** a condition characterized by mental retardation, scaphocephaly or other skull abnormality, micrognathia, blepharoptosis, low-set ears, corneal opacities, deafness, webbed neck, short digits, ventricular septal defects, Meckel's diverticulum, and other deformities. It is due to the presence of an extra chromosome 18. Called also *Edwards' s.* and *trisomy E s.* **trisomy 21 s.,** Down's s. **trisomy 22 s.,** a syndrome due to an extra chromosome 22, characterized typically by mental and growth retardation, microcephaly, low-set or malformed ears, micrognathia, long philtrum, preauricular skin tag or sinus, and congenital heart disease. In males, there is small penis and/or undescended testes. **Troisier's s.,** bronzed cachexia occurring in the diabetes associated with hemochromatosis. **tropical splenomegaly s.,** a condition seen in endemic malarious areas that is said to be due to an aberrant immunological response to malaria, characterized by massive splenomegaly, hepatomegaly, anemia with increased reticulocyte count, and lymphocytic infiltration of the hepatic sinusoids. Patients often have elevated malaria antibody titers and serum IgM levels. Malaria prophylaxis usually causes the condition to improve. Called also *malarial hyperreactive spleen s.* See also *visceral leishmaniasis,* under *leishmaniasis.* **Trousseau's s.,** spontaneous venous thrombosis of upper and lower extremities occurring in association with visceral carcinoma. **tumor lysis s.,** severe hyperphosphatemia, hyperkalemia, hyperuricemia, and hypocalcemia occurring after effective induction chemotherapy of rapidly growing malignant neoplasms, thought to be due to release of intracellular products after cell lysis. **Turcot s.,** familial polyposis of the colon associated with malignant tumors (gliomas) of the central nervous system. **Turner's s.,** a disorder of gonadal differentiation, marked by short stature, undifferentiated (streak) gonads, and variable abnormalities that may include webbing of the neck, low posterior hair line, increased carrying angle of the elbow, cubitus valgus, and cardiac defects; it is typically associated with absence of the second sex chromosome (XO, or 45, X), although structural abnormality of one X chromosome or mosaicism (e.g., XX/XX or X/XXX) may also be responsible. The phenotype is female; patients are usually sterile. Called also *gonadal dysgenesis.* **Turner's s., male,** Noonan's s. **Ullrich-Feichtiger s.,** a condition of micrognathia, hexadactyly, and genital abnormalities, with depressed nose, small eyes, hypertelorism, and protuberant ears, along with other defects. **Ullrich-Turner s.,** Noonan's s. **unilateral nevoid telangiectasia s.,** generalized essential telangiectasia representing a latent vascular nevus that becomes manifest under the possible influence of estrogens (pregnancy, menarche) or increased venous pressure (liver disease). Called also *unilateral nevoid telangiectasia.* **Unna-Thost s.,** diffuse palmoplantar keratoderma. **Unverricht's s.,** myoclonus epilepsy. **urethral s.,** suprapubic aching and cramping, urinary frequency, and such bladder complaints as dysuria, urinary tenesmus, and low back pain, without evidence of urinary infection. **vagoaccessory s.,** Schmidt's s. **van Buchem's s.,** hyperostosis corticalis generalisata. **van der Hoeve's s.,** a hereditary syndrome consisting of blue scleras, osteogenesis imperfecta, and otosclerotic deafness, usually transmitted as an autosomal dominant trait. Called also *Adair-Dighton s.* and *Dighton-Adair s.* See *osteogenesis imperfecta.* **Van der Woude's s.,** a hereditary syndrome, transmitted as an autosomal dominant trait, consisting of cleft lip and/or cleft palate occurring in association with cysts of the lower lip. **vanishing testes s.,** a disorder characterized by the absence of gonadal tissue, a small penis, and no adolescent virilization; the testes are thought to have been present in the embryo but to have "vanished" before completion of male sexual differentiation. The chromosome pattern is XY (male). **vascular s.,** any syndrome due to occlusion or stenosis of vessels supplying the nervous system. **Verner-Morrison s.,** a rare syndrome of profuse watery diarrhea, hypokalemia, and achlorhydria, usually due to a beta cell neoplasm of pancreatic islets and associated with excess levels of vasoactive intestinal polypeptide; called also *pancreatic cholera* and *WDHA syndrome.* **Vernet's s.,** paralysis of the ninth, tenth, and eleventh cranial nerves due to a lesion in the region of the jugular foramen, and marked by paralysis of the superior constriction of the pharynx and difficulty in swallowing solids; paralysis of the soft palate and fauces with anesthesia of these parts and of the pharynx, and loss of taste in the posterior third of the tongue; paralysis of the vocal cords and anesthesia of the larynx; paralysis of the sternocleidomastoid and trapezius muscles. Called also *jugular foramen s.* **Vil-**

laret's s., unilateral paralysis of the ninth, tenth, eleventh, and twelfth cranial nerves and sometimes the seventh, due to a lesion in the retroparotid space, and characterized by paralysis of the superior constriction of the pharynx and difficulty in swallowing solids; paralysis of soft palate and fauces with anesthesia of these parts and of the pharynx; loss of taste in the posterior third of the tongue; paralysis of the vocal cords and anesthesia of the larynx; paralysis of the sternocleidomastoid and trapezius; and paralysis of the cervical sympathetic nerves (*Horner's syndrome*). Called also *s. of retroparotid space.* **Vinson's s.,** Plummer-Vinson s. **Vogt's s.,** a syndrome frequently associated with birth trauma, characterized by bilateral athetosis, walking difficulties, spasmodic outbursts of laughing or crying, speech disorders, excessive myelination of the nerve fibers of the corpus striatum, giving it a marbled appearance (*status marmoratus*), and sometimes mental deficiency. Called also *Vogt's disease* and *s. of corpus striatum.* **Vogt-Koyanagi s.,** uveomeningitis characterized by exudative iridocyclitis and choroiditis associated with patchy depigmentation of the skin and hair; the lashes and eyebrows also become whitened, and there may also be retinal detachment and associated deafness and tinnitus. Cf. *Harada s.* **Vohwinkel's s.,** keratoma hereditarium mutilans. **Volkmann's s.,** post-traumatic muscular hypertonia and degenerative neuritis; Volkmann's contracture. **Waardenburg's s.,** 1. an autosomal dominant disorder characterized by wide bridge of the nose due to lateral displacement of the inner canthi and puncta, pigmentary disturbances, including white forelock, heterochromia iridis, white eyelashes, leukoderma, and sometimes cochlear deafness. 2. an autosomal dominant disorder characterized by acrocephaly, orbital and facial deformities, and brachydactyly with mild soft tissue syndactyly; cleft palate, hydrophthalmos, cardiac malformation, and contractures of the elbows and knees may also be present. Called also *acrocephalosyndactyly type IV* and *Klein-Waardenburg s.* **Wallenberg's s.,** a syndrome due to occlusion of the posterior inferior cerebellar artery, marked by ipsilateral loss of temperature and pain sensations of the face and contralateral loss of these sensations of the extremities and trunk, ipsilateral ataxia, dysphagia, dysarthria, and nystagmus. **Ward-Romano s.,** Romano-Ward s. **Waterhouse-Friderichsen s.,** the malignant or fulminating form of epidemic cerebrospinal meningitis, marked by sudden onset and short course, fever, coma, and collapse, cyanosis, petechial hemorrhages of the skin and mucous membranes, and bilateral adrenal hemorrhage. **WDHA s.** [*watery diarrhea, hypokalemia, achlorhydria*], Verner-Morrison s. **s. of Weber,** paralysis of the oculomotor nerve on the same side as the lesion, producing ptosis, strabismus, and loss of light reflex and of accommodation; also spastic hemiplegia on the side opposite the lesion with increased reflexes and loss of superficial reflexes. Called also *alternating oculomotor hemiplegia* and *Weber's paralysis.* **Weber-Christian s.,** relapsing febrile nodular nonsuppurative panniculitis. **Weber-Cockayne s.,** localized epidermolysis bullosa simplex. **Weber-Dubler s.,** s. of Weber. **Wegener's s.,** see under *granulomatosis.* **Weil's s.,** a severe form of leptospirosis (q.v.) characterized by jaundice usually accompanied by azotemia, hemorrhages, anemia, disturbances of consciousness, and continued fever. It is usually due to *Leptospira interrogans* serogroup *icterohaemorrhagiae* but may be caused by other serogroups such as *bataviae.* The disease has been known by various eponymous and clinically descriptive names, including *Fiedler's, Lancereaux-Mathieu-Weil, Landouzy's,* and *Weil's disease; infectious, infective, leptospiral,* and *spirochetal jaundice;* and *leptospirosis icterohaemorrhagica.* **Weill-Marchesani s.,** a congenital disorder of connective tissue transmitted as an autosomal dominant or recessive trait, characterized by brachycephaly, brachydactyly, short stature with a broad chest and heavy musculature, reduced joint mobility, spherophakia, ectopia lentis, myopia, and glaucoma; called also *dystrophia mesodermalis congenita hyperplastica, Marchesani's s.,* and *spherophakia-brachymorphia s.* **Weingarten's s.,** tropical eosinophilia. **Wermer's s.,** multiple endocrine neoplasia, type I. **Werner s.,** premature aging in the adult, transmitted as an autosomal recessive trait, and characterized principally by scleroderma-like skin changes, involving especially the extremities, cataracts, subcutaneous calcification, muscular atrophy, a tendency to diabetes mellitus, aged appearance of the face, canities and baldness, and a high incidence of neoplasm. **Wernicke's** s., see under *encephalopathy*. **Wernicke-Korsakoff s.,** the neuropsychiatric disorder caused by thiamine deficiency, most commonly due to chronic alcohol abuse and associated with other nutritional polyneuropathies. Wernicke's encephalopathy (confusion, ataxia of gait, nystagmus, and ophthalmoplegia) occurs as an acute attack and is reversible, except for some residual ataxia or nystagmus, by administration of thiamine; Korsakoff's syndrome (severe anterograde and retrograde amnesia) may occur in conjunction with Wernicke's encephalopathy or may become apparent later; only about 20 per cent of patients recover completely from the amnesia. See also *Korsakoff's s.* and *Wernicke's encephalopathy*, under *encephalopathy*. **Woyors' oligodactyly s.,** a congenital syndrome consisting of deficiency of the ulna and ulnar rays, antecubital pterygia, reduced sternal segments, malformations of the kidney and spleen, and cleft lip and palate. **whiplash shake s.,** a constellation of injuries to the brain and eye that may occur when a child less than 3 years old, usually less than 1 year old, is shaken vigorously while being held by the trunk or limbs with the head unsupported. This causes stretching and tearing of the cerebral vessels and brain substance, commonly leading to subdural hematomas and retinal hemorrhages, and sometimes associated with cerebral contusion. It may result in paralysis, blindness and other visual disturbances, convulsions, and death. **whistling face s., whistling face–windmill vane hand s.,** craniocarpotarsal dystrophy. **Widal s.,** icteroanemia. **Willebrand's s.,** von Willebrand's disease. **Williams s.,** supravalvular aortic stenosis, mental retardation, elfin facies, and transient hypercalcemia in infancy. Called also *elfin facies s.* **Williams-Campbell s.,** congenital bronchomalacia due to absence of annular cartilage distal to the first division of the peripheral bronchi; it is marked by bronchiectasis. **Wilson's s.,** see under *disease*. **Wilson-Mikity s.,** a rare form of pulmonary insufficiency in low-birth-weight infants, marked by hyperpnea and cyanosis of insidious onset during the first month of life and often resulting in death. Radiographically, there are multiple cystlike foci of hyperaeration throughout the lung with coarse thickening of the interstitial supporting structures. The disorder has been attributed to disparity of maturation of parenchymal elements, especially of alveoli proliferation, and hence has been called *pulmonary dysmaturity*. **Winter's s.,** a congenital syndrome consisting of renal hypoplasia or aplasia, anomalies of the internal genitalia, especially vaginal atresia, and anomaly of the ossicles of the middle ear. **Wiskott-Aldrich s.,** an X-linked immunodeficiency syndrome characterized by eczema, thrombocytopenia, and recurrent pyogenic infection. There is an inability to produce antibodies to polysaccharide antigens and increased susceptibility to infection with encapsulated bacteria (*Hemophilus influenzae*, meningococcus, pneumococcus). Typically IgM is low and IgA and IgE are elevated; cutaneous anergy is common. There is also a high incidence of lymphoreticular malignant disease. Called also *Aldrich syndrome* and *immunodeficiency with thrombocytopenia and eczema*. **withdrawal s.,** withdrawal (def. 2.) **Wolf-Hirschhorn s.,** a syndrome associated with partial deletion of the short arm of chromosome 4, characterized by microcephaly, ocular hypertelorism, epicanthus, cleft palate, micrognathia, low-set ears simplified in form, cryptorchidism, and hypospadias. **Wolff-Parkinson-White s.,** the association of paroxysmal tachycardia (or atrial fibrillation) and preexcitation, in which the electrocardiogram displays a short P-R interval and a wide QRS complex which characteristically shows an early QRS vector (delta wave); called also *anomalous atrioventricular excitation*. **Wolfram s.,** a hereditary association of diabetes mellitus, diabetes insipidus, optic atrophy, and neural deafness. **Woringer-Kolopp s.,** pagetoid reticulosis. **Wright's s.,** 1. (Irving S. Wright) a neurovascular syndrome caused by hyperabduction of the arm. Such hyperabduction may cause occlusion of the subclavian artery, leading to gangrene, or may produce sensory symptoms due to stretching of the brachial plexus. 2. a condition marked by multifocal areas of osteitis fibrosa, patchy cutaneous pigmentation, and precocious puberty. **X-linked lymphoproliferative s.,** an immunodeficiency disorder characterized by defective cellular or humoral immune response to Epstein-Barr virus (EBV). Fulminant infectious mononucleosis, fatal B cell malignancies, or hypogammaglobulinemia may follow EBV infection. Called also *X-linked lymphoproliferative disease* and *Duncan's disease* or *syndrome*. **XXY s.,**

Klinefelter's s. **yellow nail s.,** a syndrome associated with lymphedema, especially of the legs, consisting of a yellowish to greenish discoloration of the nails, which may be smooth, thickened, excessively curved on the long axis, and slow growing, and may become loose and be shed. **yellow vernix s.,** placental dysfunction s. **Young's s.,** obstructive azoospermia and chronic sinopulmonary infections. **Zellweger s.,** cerebrohepatorenal s. **Zieve s.,** hypercholesterolemia, hepatosplenomegaly, fatty infiltration of the liver, hemolytic anemia, and hypertriglyceridemia following the ingestion of large amounts of ethanol. **Zinsser-Cole-Engman s.,** dyskeratosis congenita. **Zollinger-Ellison s.,** a triad comprising (1) intractable, sometimes fulminating, and in many ways atypical peptic ulcers; (2) extreme gastric hyperacidity; and (3) gastrin-secreting, non-beta islet cell tumors of the pancreas, which may be single or multiple, small or large, benign or malignant. The gastrinoma sometimes occurs in sites (e.g., the duodenum) other than the pancreas. See also *multiple endocrine neoplasia*.

syndromic (sin-drom′ik)   occurring as a syndrome.

syndromology (sin″drom-ol′o-je)   the field concerned with the taxonomy, etiology, and patterns of congenital malformations.

Syndrox (sin′droks)   trademark for preparations of methamphetamine hydrochloride.

synechia (sĭ-nek′e-ah), pl. *synech′iae* [Gr. *synecheia* continuity]   adhesion of parts, especially adhesion of the iris to the cornea or to the lens. **annular s.,** adhesion of the whole rim of the iris to the lens. **anterior s.,** adhesion of the base of the iris to the cornea, producing occlusion of the chamber angle; it may be caused by glaucoma, cataract, intraocular tumors, or after perforation resulting from keratitis, iridocylitis, trauma, or surgery. **circular s.,** annular s. **s. pericar′dii,** concretio cordis. **posterior s.,** adhesion of the iris to the capsule of the lens or to the surface of the vitreous body, producing an irregularly shaped pupil. **total anterior s.,** adhesion of the entire surface of the iris to the cornea. **total posterior s.,** adhesion of the entire surface of the iris to the lens. **s. vul′ vae,** fused vulva: a congenital condition in which the labia minora are sealed in the midline, with only a small opening below the clitoris through which urination and menstruation may occur.

synechiae (sĭ-nek′e-e)   plural of *synechia*.

synechotome (sin-ek′o-tōm)   a cutting instrument for use in synechotomy.

synechotomy (sin″ĕ-kot′o-me) [*synechia* + *-tomy*]   the operation of cutting a synechia.

synechtenterotomy (sin″ek-ten″ter-ot′o-me) [Gr. *synechēs* joined together + *enteron* bowel + *tomē* a cutting]   division of an intestinal adhesion.

synecology (sin″ĕ-kol′o-je)   the study of the environment of organisms in the mass, as distinguished from *autoecology*.

Synemol (sin′ĕ-mol)   trademark for a preparation of fluocinolone acetonide.

synencephalocele (sin″en-sef′ah-lo-sēl″) [*syn-* + Gr. *enkephalos* brain + *kēlē* tumor]   encephalocele with adhesions to the adjoining parts.

synencephalus (sin″en-sef′ah-lus)   a monster exhibiting synencephaly.

synencephaly (sin″en-sef′ah-le) [*syn-* + Gr. *enkephalos* brain]   a developmental anomaly in which there are two bodies and one head.

syneresis (sĭ-ner′ĕ-sis) [Gr. *synairesis* a taking or drawing together]   a drawing together of the particles of the dispersed phase of a gel, with separation of some of the disperse medium and shrinkage of the gel, such as occurs in the clotting of blood.

synergenesis (sin″er-jen′ĕ-sis)   the doctrine that every cell transmits its protoplasm to every generation of cells derived from it.

synergetic (sin″er-jet′ik)   working together; said of muscles which cooperate in performing an action.

synergia (sin-er′je-ah)   synergy.

synergic (sin-er′jik)   acting together or in harmony.

synergism (sin′er-jizm)   the joint action of agents so that their combined effect is greater than the algebraic sum of their individual effects.

synergist (sin′er-jist)   1. a medicine that aids or cooperates with another; an adjuvant.   2. an organ that acts in concert with another.

synergistic (sin″er-jis′tik)   acting together; enhancing the effect of another force or agent.

synergy (sin′er-je) [L. *synergia;* Gr. *syn* together + *ergon* work]   correlated action or cooperation on the part of two or more structures or drugs. In neurology, the faculty by which movements are properly grouped for the performance of acts requiring special adjustments.

synesthesia (sin″es-the′ze-ah) [*syn-* + Gr. *aisthēsis* perception + *-ia*]   a secondary sensation accompanying an actual perception; the experiencing of a sensation in one place, due to stimulation applied to another place; also the condition in which a stimulus of one sense is perceived as sensation of a different sense, as when a sound produces a sensation of color. **s. al′gica,** a painful synesthesia.

synesthesialgia (sin″es-the′ze-al′je-ah)   a condition in which a stimulus produces pain on the affected side but no sensation or even a pleasant one on the normal side of the body.

synezesis (sin′e-ze′sis)   synizesis.

Syngamidae (sin-gam′ĭ-de)   a family of nematodes of the superfamily Strongyloidea, which includes the genera *Syngamus* and *Stephanurus.*

syngamous (sin′gah-mus) [*syn-* + Gr. *gamos* marriage]   1. pertaining to or characterized by syngamy.   2. having the sex of the individual determined at the time when the ovum is fertilized.

Syngamus (sin′gah-mus)   a genus of nematode worms of the family Syngamidae that are parasitic in fowl and other birds.   **S. tra′chea,** the gapeworm, a species of worms which are parasitic in chickens, pheasants, turkeys, and various wild birds, inhabiting the trachea and interfering with respiration when present in large numbers; it is the etiologic agent of gapes.

syngamy (sing′gah-me) [*syn-* + Gr. *gamos* marriage]   1. sexual reproduction.   2. the union of two gametes in fertilization to form a zygote.

syngeneic (sin″jĕ-ne′ik)   in transplantation biology, denoting individuals or tissues that have identical genotypes, i.e., identical twins or animals of the same inbred strain, or their tissues. Called also *isogeneic.*

syngenesioplastic (sin″jĕ-ne″ze-o-plas′tik) [*syn-* + Gr. *genesis* origin + *plassein* to form]   denoting transplantation of tissue from one individual to a related individual of the same species, as from a mother to her child, or from a brother to a sister.

syngenesiotransplantation (sin″jĕ-ne″ze-o-trans″planta′shun)   syngenesioplastic transplantation.

syngenesis (sin-jen′ĕ-sis)   1. the origin of an individual from a germ cell derived from both parents and not from either one alone, as occurs in mammals.   2. the state of having descended from a common ancestor.

syngnathia (sin-na′the-ah) [*syn-* + *gnath-* + *-ia*]   a congenital condition characterized by the presence of fibrous bands extending from the maxilla to the mandible.

syngonic (sin-gon′ik) [*syn-* + Gr. *gonē* seed]   having the sex of the individual determined at the time when the ovum is fertilized.

syngraft (sin′graft)   a graft between genetically identical individuals. Typically, syngrafts are grafts between identical twins, between animals of a single highly inbred strain, or between F₁ hybrids produced by crossing inbred strains. Called also *isogeneic graft* and *isograft.*

Synhymeniida (sin″hi-mĕ-ne′ĭ-dah) [*syn-* + Gr. *hymēn* membrane]   an order of free-living, often cylindrical ciliate protozoa (superorder Nassulidea, subclass Hypostomatia) characterized by the presence of a synhymenium, bipolar kineties, and complete somatic ciliation.

synhymenium (sin″hi-men′e-um)   a structure formed by fusion of parts of the hypostomial frange; characteristic of ciliate protozoa of the order Synhymenida.

synizesis (sin″ĭ-ze′sis) [Gr. *synizēsis*]   1. occlusion.   2. a stage in mitosis in which the nuclear chromatin is massed. **s. pupil′lae,** occlusion of the pupil.

synkainogenesis (sin″ki-no-jen′ĕ-sis) [*syn-* + Gr. *kainos* new + *genesis* production]   the process of developing a new formation simultaneously with another formation.

synkaryon (sin-kar′e-on) [*syn-* + Gr. *karyon* nucleus]   the nucleus produced by the fusion of two pronuclei in karyogamy; the fertilization nucleus.

Synkayvite (sin′ka-vīt)   trademark for preparations of menadiol sodium diphosphate.

synkinesia (sin″ki-ne′ze-ah)   synkinesis.

synkinesis (sin″ki-ne′sis) [*syn-* + Gr. *kinēsis* movement]   an associated movement; an unintentional movement accompanying a volitional movement.   **imitative s.,** an involuntary movement on the healthy side accompanying an attempt at movement on the paralyzed side.   **mouth-and-hand s.,** see *Saunders' sign,* under *sign.*   **spasmodic s.,** a movement on the paralyzed side attending a voluntary movement on the healthy side.

synkinetic (sin″ki-net′ik)   pertaining to or of the nature of synkinesis.

synnecrosis (sin″nĕ-kro′sis) [*syn-* + Gr. *nekrōsis* a state of death]   a relationship between populations (or individuals) resulting in mutual depression or death.

synneurosis (sin″nu-ro′sis) [Gr. *synneurosis* union by sinews]   syndesmosis.

synocha (sin′o-kah) [L.; Gr. *synochos* jointed together]   a continued fever.

synochal (sin′o-kal)   of or pertaining to synocha.

synochus (sin′o-kus)   synocha.

synonychia (sin″o-nik′e-ah) [*syn-* + Gr. *onyx* nail + *-ia*]   fusion of the nails of two or more digits in complicated syndactyly.

synophridia (sin″of-rid′e-ah)   synophrys.

synophrys (sin-of′ris) [Gr. "with meeting eyebrows"]   the condition in which the eyebrows grow together.

synophthalmia (sin″of-thal′me-ah) [*syn-* + Gr. *ophthalmos* eye + *-ia*]   the usual form of cyclopia, in which the two eyes are more or less completely fused into one.

synophthalmus (sin″of-thal′mus)   cyclops.

Synophylate (sin″o-fi′lāt)   trademark for preparations of theophylline sodium glycinate.

synoptophore (sin-op′to-fōr) [*syn-* + *opto-* + Gr. *phora* movement, range]   an instrument for diagnosing strabismus and for treating it by orthoptic methods.

synorchidism (sin-or′kĭ-dizm)   synorchism.

synorchism (sin′or-kizm) [*syn-* + Gr. *orchis* testicle]   fusion of the two testes into one mass, which may be located in the scrotum or in the abdomen.

synoscheos (sin-os′ke-os) [*syn-* + Gr. *oscheon* scrotum]   adhesion between the penis and scrotum.

synosteology (sin″os-te-ol′o-je) [*syn-* + Gr. *osteon* bone + *-logy*]   the sum of knowledge regarding the joints and articulations.

synosteosis (sin″os-te-o′sis)   synostosis.

synosteotic (sin″os-te-ot′ik)   pertaining to or marked by synosteosis.

synosteotomy (sin″os-te-ot′o-me) [*syn-* + Gr. *osteon* bone + *tomē* a cutting]   the dissection of the joints.

synostosis (sin″os-to′sis), pl. *synosto′ses* [*syn-* + Gr. *osteon* bone]   1. [NA] a union between adjacent bones or parts of a single bone formed by osseous material, such as ossified connecting cartilage or fibrous tissue.   2. the osseous union of bones that are normally distinct.   **radioulnar s.,** bony fusion of the proximal ends of the radius and ulna.   **sagittal s.,** scaphocephaly.   **tarsal s.,** fusion of various tarsal bones.   **tribasilar s.,** fusion in infancy of the three bones at the base of the skull, producing mental retardation.

synostotic (sin″os-tot′ik)   synosteotic.

synotia (si-no′she-ah) [*syn-* + Gr. *ous* ear]   a developmental anomaly characterized by persistence of the ears in their horizontal position beneath the mandible.

synotus (si-no′tus) [*syn-* + Gr. *ous* ear]   fetus exhibiting synotia.

synovectomy (sin″o-vek′to-me) [*synovia* + Gr. *ektomē* excision]   excision of a synovial membrane, as of that lining the capsule of the knee joint, performed in treatment of rheumatoid arthritis of the knee, or of the synovial sheath of a tendon.   **radioisotope s.,** synoviorthesis.

synovia (sĭ-no′ve-ah) [L.; Gr. *syn* with + *ōon* egg] [NA]   a transparent alkaline viscid fluid, resembling the white of an egg, secreted by the synovial membrane, and contained in joint cavities, bursae, and tendon sheaths; called also *synovial fluid.*

synovial (sĭ-no′ve-al) [L. *synovialis*] of, pertaining to, or secreting synovia.

synovialis (sĭ-no″ve-a′lis) [L.] synovial.

synovialoma (sĭ-no″ve-ah-lo′mah) synovioma.

synovianalysis (sĭ-no″ve-ah-nal′ĭ-sis) the laboratory examination of joint fluid (synovia).

synovin (sin′o-vin) the mucin found in synovia.

synovi(o)- [L. *synovia*, q.v.] a combining form denoting relationship to the synovia, or to the synovium.

synovioblast (sĭ-no′ve-o-blast) a fibroblast of synovial membrane.

synoviocyte (sĭ-no′ve-o-sīt) a cell of the synovial membrane.

synovioma (sĭ-no″ve-o′mah) a tumor of synovial membrane origin. **benign s.,** giant cell tumor of tendon sheath. **malignant s.,** synoviosarcoma.

synoviorthese (sĭ-no″ve-or-thez) [Fr.] synoviorthesis.

synoviorthesis (sĭ-no″ve-or-the′sis) [*synovi-* + Gr. *orthos* straight] irradiation of the synovium by intra-articular injection of radiocolloids to destroy inflamed synovial tissue.

synoviosarcoma (sĭ-no″ve-o-sar-ko′mah) a malignant neoplasm arising in the synovial membrane of the joints and also in synovial cells of tendons and bursae; called also *malignant synovioma* and *synovial sarcoma.*

synoviparous (sin″o-vip′ah-rus) [*synovia* + L. *parere* to produce] producing synovia.

synovitis (sin″o-vi′tis) inflammation of a synovial membrane. It is usually painful, particularly on motion, and is characterized by a fluctuating swelling due to effusion within a synovial sac. Synovitis is qualified as *fibrinous, gonorrheal, hyperplastic, lipomatous, metritic, puerperal, rheumatic, scarlatinal, syphilitic, tuberculous, urethral,* etc. **bursal s.,** bursitis. **dendritic s.,** that in which villous growths are developed within the synovial sac. **dry s.,** synovitis with but little effusion. **fungous s.,** arthritis fungosa. **localized nodular s.,** lesions of the tendon sheaths that give histological evidence of evolution from a number of smaller nodules, or from villous structures. **pigmented villonodular s.,** synovial proliferation forming brown nodular masses, probably caused by hemangiomas of synovial membrane that become traumatized, resulting in synovial hyperplasia and inflammation; it is characterized by episodic monoarticular pain and swelling, with joint locking and hemorrhagic effusions. **purulent s.,** that in which there is an effusion of pus in a synovial sac. **serous s.,** synovitis with copious nonpurulent effusion. **s. sic′ca,** dry s. **simple s.,** that in which the effusion is clear or but slightly turbid. **tendinous s.,** inflammation of a tendon sheath. **vaginal s.,** tendinous s. **vibration s.,** synovitis produced by the passage of a missile through the tissues near a joint, but without actually wounding the joint. **villonodular s.,** proliferation of synovial tissue, especially of the knee joint, composed of synovial villi and fibrous nodules infiltrated by giant cells and by macrophages containing lipids and hemosiderin.

synovium (sĭ-no′ve-um) a synovial membrane.

synphalangism (sin-fal′an-jizm) symphalangia.

synpneumonic (sin″nu-mon′ik) occurring in association with pneumonia.

synreflexia (sin″re-flek′se-ah) the association existing between various reflexes.

syntactic (sin-tak′tik) pertaining to or affecting syntax, or the proper arrangement of words in speech.

syntaxis (sin-tak′sis) [Gr. "a putting together in order"] articulation.

syntectic (sin-tek′tik) pertaining to or characterized by syntexis.

syntenic (sin-ten′ik) pertaining or relating to synteny.

syntenosis (sin″tĕ-no′sis) [*syn-* + Gr. *tenōn* tendon] a hinge joint surrounded by tendons.

synteny (sin′tĕ-ne) [*syn-* + Gr. *tainia* ribbon] the presence together on the same chromosome of two or more gene loci whether or not in such proximity that they may be subject to linkage (q.v., def. 2).

synteresis (sin″ter-e′sis) [*syn-* + Gr. *tērein* to watch over] preventive treatment; prophylaxis.

synteretic (sin″ter-et′ik) prophylactic.

syntexis (sin-tek′sis) [Gr. *syntēxis* colliquation] wasting or emaciation.

synthase (sin-thās) [EC 4] lyase; a trivial name for enzymes of the lyase class that catalyze the joining together of two molecules in a reaction not involving cleavage of a pyrophosphate bond.

synthermal (sin-ther′mal) [*syn-* + Gr. *thermē* heat] having the same temperature.

synthescope (sin′thĕ-skōp) [Gr. *synthesis* placing together + *skopein* to examine] an instrument for observing the visible effect of placing two liquids in contact.

synthesis (sin′thĕ-sis) [Gr. "a putting together, composition"] 1. the artificial building up of a chemical compound, by the union of its elements or from other suitable starting materials. 2. in psychiatry, the integration of the various elements of the personality; the opposite of analysis. **s. of continuity,** union of the edges of a wound or the ends of a fractured bone. **inducible enzyme s.,** increased formation of an enzyme within a cell in the presence of a metabolite, often its substrate or a precursor of the substrate. The process occurs in procaryotes by operon control of gene transcription (phenotypic adaptation). Called also *enzymatic adaptation.* **morphologic s.,** histogenesis.

synthesize (sin″thĕ-sīz′) to produce by means of synthesis.

synthetase (sin″thĕ-tās) [EC 6] ligase; a trivial name for enzymes of the ligase class that catalyze the joining together of two molecules with concomitant hydrolysis of a pyrophosphate bond in ATP or a similar triphosphate.

synthetic (sin-thet′ik) [L. *syntheticus;* Gr. *synthetikos*] 1. pertaining to, of the nature of, or participating in synthesis. 2. produced by synthesis; artificial.

synthorax (sin-tho′raks) thoracopagus.

Synthroid (sin′throid) trademark for a preparation of levothyroxine sodium.

Syntocinon (sin-to′sĭ-non) trademark for a solution of synthetic oxytocin.

syntonin (sin′to-nin) an acid metaprotein which precipitates from a gastric digestion mixture at or near the neutral point.

syntopie, syntopy (sin′to-pe) [*syn-* + Gr. *topos* place] the position of an organ in relation to neighboring organs.

syntripsis (sin-trip′sis) [*syn-* + Gr. *tribein* to rub] the comminution or crushing of a bone; comminuted fracture.

Syntropan (sin′tro-pan) trademark for a preparation of amprotropine phosphate.

syntrophism (sin′trŏf-izm) [*syn-* + Gr. *trophē* nourishment] crossfeeding; the stimulation of growth of a cell or organ by a factor released by another cell or organ; especially, growth stimulation of a bacterium resulting from admixture with or nearness of another strain or species, e.g., the growth of *Haemophilus influenzae* as satellite colonies of *Staphylococcus.*

syntrophoblast (sin-trof′o-blast) syncytiotrophoblast.

syntropic (sin-trop′ik) [*syn-* + Gr. *trepein* to turn] 1. turning or pointing in the same direction, as the ribs or the vertebral spines. 2. denoting the correlation of several factors, as the relation of one disease to the development or incidence of another disease.

syntropy (sin′tro-pe) [*syn-* + Gr. *tropos* a turning] the state of being syntropic.

synulosis (sin″u-lo′sis) [Gr. *synoulōsis*] complete cicatrization.

synulotic (sin″u-lot′ik) [Gr. *synoulōtikos*] 1. promoting cicatrization. 2. an agent that promotes cicatrization.

Synura (sin-u′rah) [*syn-* + G. *oura* tail] a genus of freeswimming, colonial, plantlike biflagellate freshwater protozoa (order Chrysomonadida, class Phytomastigophorea), which may impart an unpleasant taste to drinking water.

synxenic (sin-zen′ik) [*syn-* + Gr. *xenos* a guest-friend, stranger] associated with a known number of microbic species; applied to laboratory animals whose microfauna and microflora are known (gnotobiotes).

Syphacia (si-fa′se-ah) a nematode parasite found in the intestines of rodents. **S. obvela′ta,** a common cecal parasite of laboratory rats that has been reported occasionally in infants.

syphilid (sif′ĭ-lid) a general term for the skin lesions of secondary syphilis, appearing (usually between six weeks and two years after infection) in a series of crops lasting a few days to a few years, and becoming progressively more severe and conspicuous, more persistent, and less widely generalized, in successive outbreaks. The serologic test for syphilis (STS) is invariably positive. Mucous membrane lesions in this stage are typically teeming with *Treponema pallidum* and are clinically the most contagious lesions of the disease. Syphilids are variously qualified by their shape (annular s.), site (plantar s.), and so on.

syphilide (sif′ĭ-līd), pl. syphil′ides [Fr.]   syphilid.

syphilis (sif′ĭ-lis) [*Syphilus*, the name of a shepherd infected with the disease in the poem of Fracastorius (1530), in which the term first appears. Derived perhaps from Gr. *syn* together + *philein* to love, or from Gr. *siphlos* crippled, maimed]   a subacute to chronic infectious disease caused by the spirochete *Treponema pallidum*, which is usually transmitted by sexual contact, both homosexual and heterosexual, or acquired in utero but can be contracted by direct contact with infected tissues and blood or contaminated fomites. Basically, untreated syphilis progresses through three clinical stages: primary, secondary, and tertiary, with a latent period intervening between the first two and the last. The time of duration of each stage varies. In the first stage (*primary s.*), a painless primary lesion appears at the site of inoculation (see *chancre*, def. 1) and is associated with regional adenopathy (*bubo*). The second stage (*secondary s.*) is characterized chiefly by the presence of widespread mucocutaneous lesions (see *syphilid*) and generalized regional lymphadenopathy. A period of latency follows (*latent s.*), which may last for many years, and in which the only evidence of infection is a reactive serologic test for syphilis. This period is divided into *early latent* and *late latent syphilis*. In the early latent form, which comprises the 2 years from the time of infection, relapse of secondary lesions may occur. The late latent form is usually infectious only in the pregnant woman, who may infect the fetus. The last stage (*tertiary*, or *late, s.*) may develop soon after the lesions of secondary syphilis resolve or many years later, and is marked by destructive lesions involving many organs and tissues. This stage occurs in three principal forms: cardiovascular and late benign syphilis and meningovascular or parenchymatous neurosyphilis. Formerly called *lues* and *pox*. See also *general paresis*, under *paresis*, and *tabes dorsalis*. Cf. *endemic s.* **cardiovascular s.**, a form of tertiary syphilis in which aortic insufficiency and aortic aneurysm, usually of the ascending aorta, occur as a result of obliterative endarteritis of the vasa vasorum, causing damage to the intima and media of the great vessels, and may result in congestive heart failure. **cerebrospinal s.**, Erb's spastic paraplegia. **congenital s.**, syphilis acquired in utero, and manifested variously by any of several characteristic malformations of the teeth or bones known as stigmata and by active mucocutaneous syphilis at the time of birth or shortly afterward, ocular changes, such as interstitial keratitis, or neurologic changes, such as deafness. **early s.**, the stage comprising primary, secondary, and early latent syphilis. **early latent s.**, see *syphilis*. **endemic s.**, a chronic, inflammatory, non-sexually transmitted treponemal infection caused by an organism indistinguishable morphologically from *Treponema pallidum*, *T. pertenue*, and *T. caroteum*, mainly affecting children in arid, dry regions, especially of the Middle East, North Africa, and Eastern Mediterranean, and characterized by early mucous patches of the secondary type localized to the oral and faucial mucosa, followed by the appearance of moist papules in the axilla and skin folds, a latent period, and late complications, including osseous and cutaneous gummata. Called also *bejel* and *nonvenereal s.* **equine s.**, dourine. **gummatous s.**, late benign s. **horse s.**, dourine. **late s.**, see *syphilis*. **late benign s.**, a form of tertiary syphilis that responds very rapidly to treatment and is therefore relatively benign, in which the typical lesion is the gumma (q.v.). Called also *gumma* and *gummatous s.* **late latent s.**, see *syphilis*. **latent s.**, see *syphilis*. **meningovascular s.**, see under *neurosyphilis*. **nonvenereal s.**, endemic s. **parenchymatous s.**, see under *neurosyphilis*. **primary s.**, see *syphilis*. **rabbit s.**, a naturally occurring disease in rabbits caused by *Treponema cuniculi*. **secondary s.**, see *syphilis*. **tertiary s.**, see *syphilis*.

syphilitic (sif′ĭ-lit′ik) [L. *syphiliticus*]   affected with, caused by, or pertaining to syphilis.

syphiloma (sif′ĭ-lo′mah)   gumma.

syphilomania (sif″ĭ-lo-ma′ne-ah) [*syphilis* + Gr. *mania* madness]   syphilophobia.

syphilophobia (sif″ĭ-lo-fo′be-ah) [*syphilis* + Gr. *phobein* to be affrighted by]   1. irrational fear of syphilis.   2. the delusion of being infected with syphilis.

syphilous (sif′ĭ-lus)   syphilitic.

Syr.   abbreviation for L. *syrupus*, syrup.

syrigmophonia (sir″ig-mo-fo′ne-ah) [Gr. *syrigmos* a shrill piping sound + *phōnē* voice + *-ia*]   a high, whistling sound of the voice.

syrigmus (sĭ-rig′mus) [Gr. *syrigmos* a shrill piping sound]   a ringing in the ears.

syringe (sĭ-rinj′, sir′inj) [L. *syrinxe*; Gr. *syrinx*]   an instrument for injecting liquids into or withdrawing them from any vessel or cavity.   **air s.**, a small fine-nozzled syringe connected by a hose to the compressed air tank in the dental unit; used to direct a current of air into a tooth cavity during excavation, to remove the small chips detached from the teeth, or to dry the cavity. Called also *chip s.*   **Anel's s.**, a delicate syringe for the treatment of the lacrimal passages.   **chip s.**, air s.   **dental s.**, a small syringe into which is fitted a hermetically sealed cartridge which contains an anesthetic solution; used for intraoral injection anesthesia.   **fountain s.**, an apparatus which injects a liquid by the action of gravity.   **hypodermic s.**, a syringe, usually of small caliber, by means of which drugs in solution or other liquids are injected through a hollow needle of small bore into the subcutaneous tissues.   **Luer's s., Luer-Lok s.**, a glass syringe for intravenous and hypodermic use, with a metallic tip and locking device to hold the needle firmly in place.   **probe s.**, a syringe whose point may be used also as a probe; used mostly in treating the lacrimal passages.   **water s.**, a syringe that is part of the dental unit, designed to permit controlled spraying of water in a desired area.

syringectomy (sir″in-jek′to-me) [*syringo-* + Gr. *ektomē* excision]   excision of the walls of a fistula.

syringin (sĭ-rin′jin)   chemical name: 4-(3-hydroxypropenyl)-2,6-dimethoxyphenyl D-glucoside. A white, crystalline glycoside, $C_{17}H_{24}O_9$, soluble in hot water and in hot alcohol, from the bark of lilac, *Syringa vulgaris*; formerly used as an antiperiodic. Called also *ligustrin* and *lilacin*.

syringitis (sir″in-ji′tis)   inflammation of the auditory tube.

syring(o)- [Gr. *syrinx* pipe, tube, fistula]   a combining form denoting relationship to a tube or a fistula.

syringoadenoma (sĭ-ring″go-ad″ĕ-no′mah)   syringocystadenoma.

syringobulbia (sĭ-ring″go-bul′be-ah) [*syringo-* + Gr. *bolbos* bulb + *-ia*]   syringomyelia in which the cavity extends to involve the medulla oblongata. Cf *hydromyelia*.

syringocarcinoma (sĭ-ring″go-kar″sĭ-no′mah)   carcinoma of a sweat gland.

syringocele (sĭ-ring′go-sēl)   a cavity-containing herniation of the spinal cord through the bony defect in spina bifida.

syringocoele (sĭ-ring′go-sēl) [*syringo-* + Gr. *koilia* hollow]   the central canal of the spinal cord (canalis centralis medullae spinalis [NA]).

syringocystadenoma (sĭ-ring″go-sis″tad-ĕ-no′mah) [*syringo-* + *cystadenoma*]   adenoma of the sweat glands; a skin disease marked by an eruption of small, hard papules; called also *hidradenoma* and *adenoma hidradenoides*.   **s. papillif′erum**, hamartoma of an apocrine sweat gland, the lesion being a circumscribed, firm, rose-red papule usually on the shoulder, axilla, genitals, inguinal region, or scalp.

syringocystoma (sĭ-ring″go-sis-to′mah) [*syringo-* + Gr. *kystis* cyst + *-oma*]   a cystic tumor of the sweat glands.

syringoencephalia (sĭ-ring″go-en″sĕ-fa′le-ah) [*syringo-* + Gr. *enkephalos* brain + *-ia*]   the formation of abnormal cavities in the brain substance.

syringoencephalomyelia (sĭ-ring″go-en-sef″ah-lo-mi-e′le-ah) [*syringo-* + Gr. *enkephalos* brain + *myelos* marrow + *-ia*]   the existence of cavities in the substance of the brain and spinal cord.

syringoid (sĭ-ring′goid) [L. *syringoides*, from Gr. *syrinx* pipe + *eidos* form]   resembling a pipe or tube; fistulous.

syringoma (sir″ing-go′mah)   adenoma of the sweat glands.

syringomeningocele (sĭ-ring″go-mĕ-nin′go-sēl) [*syringo-* + Gr. *mēninx* membrane + *kēlē* tumor]   a meningocele resembling a syringomyelocele.

syringomyelia (sǐ-ring″go-mi-e′le-ah) [*syringo-* + *myel-* + *-ia*] a slowly progressive syndrome in which cavitation occurs in the central segments of the spinal cord, generally involving the cervical region, but the lesions may extend up into the medulla oblongata (*syringobulbia*) or down into the thoracic region; it may be of developmental origin, arise secondary to tumor, trauma, infarction, or hemorrhage, or be without known cause. It results in neurological deficits that generally consist of segmental muscular weakness and atrophy accompanied by a dissociated sensory loss (loss of pain and temperature sensation, with preservation of the sense of touch), and thoracic scoliosis is often present. Sometimes, the use of the term *syringomyelia* is restricted to the condition, with the terms *segmental sensory dissociation with brachial muscular atrophy*, and *syndrome of sensory dissociation with brachial amyotrophy* being used to denote a similar clinical condition that may be associated with other pathological lesions or states. Called also *Morvan's disease* or *syndrome* and *myelosyringosis*. See also *Morvan's syndrome* (def. 2), under *syndrome*. Cf. hydromyelia. **traumatic s.,** Kienböck's disease, def. 2.

syringomyelitis (sǐ-ring″go-mi″ě-li′tis) inflammation of the spinal cord, with the formation of cavities in its substance.

syringomyelocele (sǐ-ring″go-mi′ě-lo-sēl″) [*syringo-* + Gr. *myelos* marrow + *kēlē* tumor] hernial protrusion of the spinal cord through the bony defect in spina bifida, the mass containing a cavity connected with the central canal of the spinal cord.

syringomyelus (sǐ-ring″go-mi′ě-lus) dilatation of the central canal of the spinal cord, the gray matter being converted into connective tissue.

syringopontia (sǐ-ring″go-pon′she-ah) a condition in which cavities exist in the pons.

Syringospora (si″ring-gos′po-rah) former name of a genus of fungi now called *Candida*.

syringotome (sǐ-ring′go-tōm) a knife for cutting a fistula.

syringotomy (sir″in-got′o-me) [*syringo-* + Gr. *tomē* a cutting] incision of a fistula, particularly an anal fistula.

syrinx (sir′inks) [Gr. "a pipe"] 1. a tube or pipe; also a fistula. 2. the lower or posterior part of the trachea of birds in which vocal sounds are produced.

syrosingopine (si″ro-sing′go-pīn) chemical name: methyl carbethoxysyringoyl reserpate. A crystalline substance, $C_{35}H_{42}N_2O_{11}$, used as an antihypertensive agent.

Syrphidae (sir′phǐ-de) a family of flies, the hover flies, of the order Diptera, including the genera *Eristalis* and *Helophilus*.

syrup (sir′up) [L. *syrupus*; Arabic *sharāb*] a concentrated solution of a sugar, such as sucrose, in water or other aqueous liquid, sometimes with some medicinal substance added. The official preparation [NF] is a solution of sucrose in purified water, and is used as a flavored vehicle in pharmaceutical preparations. **acacia s.** [NF], a preparation of powdered acacia, sodium benzoate, vanilla tincture, sucrose, and water, used as a vehicle for drugs. **amantadine hydrochloride s.** [USP], a preparation containing 95 to 105 per cent of the labeled amount of amantadine hydrochloride; used as an antiviral agent for the prophylaxis of Asian (A_2) influenza. **aminocaproic acid s.** [USP], a preparation containing, in 5 ml., 1.25 gm. of aminocaproic acid; used as a hemostatic. **bromides s.,** a preparation containing potassium, sodium, ammonium, calcium, and lithium bromides, formerly used as a central nervous system depressant. **cacao s.,** cocoa s. **cherry s.,** a mixture of cherry juice, sucrose, alcohol, and purified water, used as a flavored vehicle for drugs. **chloral hydrate s.** [USP], a syrup containing 95 to 110 per cent chloral hydrate; used as a hypnotic and sedative. **chlorpheniramine maleate s.,** [USP], a preparation containing 36–44 mg. of chlorpheniramine maleate in each 100 ml., in a hydroalcoholic vehicle; used as an antihistaminic. Formerly called *chlorpheniramine maleate elixir*. **chlorpromazine hydrochloride s.** [USP], a liquid preparation containing between 190 and 210 mg. of chlorpromazine hydrochloride per 100 ml.; used as an antiemetic and tranquilizer. **citric acid s.,** a preparation of lemon tincture, hydrous citric acid, and purified water, in syrup, used as a flavored vehicle for drugs. **cocoa s.** [NF], a preparation of cocoa, sucrose, liquid glucose, glycerin, sodium chloride, vanillin, sodium benzoate, and purified water; used as a flavored vehicle for drugs. Called also *cacao s.* **cypro-**

heptadine hydrochloride s. [USP], a preparation containing 90 to 110 per cent of the labeled amount of cyproheptadine hydrochloride; used as an antihistaminic for relief of symptoms associated with allergy and as an antipruritic for relief of itching associated with skin disorders. **demethylchlortetracycline s.,** demeclocycline oral suspension. **dexchlorpheniramine maleate s.** [USP], a preparation containing 90 to 110 per cent of the labeled amount of dexchlorpheniramine maleate; used as an antihistaminic. **dextromethorphan hydrobromide s.** [USP], a preparation containing 95–105 per cent of the labeled amount of dextromethorphan hydrobromide; used as an antitussive. **dicyclomine hydrochloride s.** [USP], a preparation containing 95 to 105 per cent of the labeled amount of dicyclomine hydrochloride; used as an antispasmodic in functional gastrointestinal disorders. **dihydrocodeinone bitartrate s.,** hydrocodone bitartrate s. **dimenhydrinate s.** [USP], a liquid preparation of dimenhydrinate, containing between 295 and 330 mg. of dimenhydrinate in each 100 ml.; used as an antiemetic. **dimethindene maleate s.,** a preparation containing 95 to 105 per cent of the labeled amount of dimethindene maleate; used as an antihistaminic. **dioctyl sodium sulfosuccinate s.,** docusate sodium s. **docusate sodium s.** [USP], a preparation containing 95 to 105 per cent of the labeled amount of dioctyl sodium sulfosuccinate; used as a fecal matter softener. Called also *dioctyl sodium sulfosuccinate s.* **doxylamine succinate s.** [USP], a preparation containing 90–110 per cent of the labeled amount of doxylamine succinate; used as an antihistaminic. **ephedrine sulfate s.** [USP], a preparation containing 360–440 mg. of ephedrine sulfate in each 100 ml.; used as a bronchodilator. **eriodictyon s., aromatic** [NF], a solution of eriodictyon fluidextract, potassium hydroxide solution, compound cardamom tincture, sassafras oil, lemon oil, clove oil, alcohol, sucrose, and magnesium carbonate, in purified water; used as a vehicle for drugs. **ferrous iodide s.,** a solution of iron, iodine, hypophosphorous acid, and sucrose, in purified water, used as a hematinic. **ferrous sulfate s.** [USP], a mixture of ferrous sulfate, hydrous citric acid, peppermint spirit, sucrose, and purified water, each 100 ml. of which contains 3.75–4.25 gm. of ferrous sulfate; used as an iron supplement. **glyceryl guaiacolate s.,** guaifenesin s. **glycyrrhiza s.,** a mixture of glycyrrhiza fluidextract, fennel and anise oil, and syrup, used as a flavored vehicle in compounding prescriptions. **guaifenesin s.** [USP], a preparation containing 95–105 per cent of the labeled amount of guaifenesin; used as an expectorant. Called also *glyceryl guaiacolate s.* **hydriodic acid s.,** a solution of diluted hydriodic acid and dextrose in purified water, each 100 ml. of which contains 1.3–1.5 gm. of HI; used as an expectorant. **hydrocodone bitartrate s.,** a preparation of hydrocodon bitartrate and cherry syrup in purified water, containing 90 to 110 per cent of hydrocodone bitartrate; used as an antitussive. **hydroxyzine hydrochloride s.** [USP], a preparation containing 90 to 110 per cent of the labeled amount of hydroxyzine hydrochloride; used as a tranquilizer and antihistamine. **ipecac s.** [USP], a mixture of ipecac fluidextract, glycerin, and syrup, used as an emetic. **isoniazid s.** [USP], a preparation, each 100 ml. of which contains 0.93 to 1.10 gm. of isoniazid; used as a tuberculostatic. **licorice s.,** glycyrrhiza s. **medicated s.,** one to which a medicinal substance has been added. **meperidine hydrochloride s.** [NF], a preparation containing 95 to 105 per cent of the labeled amount of meperidine hydrochloride; used as a narcotic analgesic. **methapyrilene fumarate s.** [USP], a preparation containing 90–110 per cent of the labeled amount of methapyrilene fumarate; used as an antihistaminic in the treatment of allergic manifestations, nausea and vomiting of pregnancy, and insomnia. **methdilazine hydrochloride s.** [USP], a preparation containing 93 to 107 per cent of the labeled amount of methdilazine hydrochloride; used as an antipruritic in the treatment of various dermatoses. **minocycline hydrochloride s.,** see under *suspension*. **orange s.** [NF], a preparation of sweet orange peel tincture, citric acid, talc, and sucrose, in purified water, used as a flavored vehicle for drugs. **phenindamine tartrate s.,** a syrup containing between 190 and 220 mg. of phenindamine tartrate in each 100 ml.; used as an antihistaminic. **piperazine citrate s.** [USP], a syrup containing 10–12 gm. of anhydrous piperazine citrate in each 100 ml.; used as an anthelmintic in the treatment of intestinal pinworm and roundworm infections. **prochlorperazine edisylate s.,** [USP], a syrup containing in each 100 ml. an amount of prochlorperazine edisylate equivalent to 95 to 105 mg. of prochlorperazine; used as an antiemetic and tranquilizer. **promazine hydrochloride s.** [USP], a preparation containing 95 to 110 per cent of the labeled amount of promazine hydrochloride; used mainly as an antipsychotic agent. **promethazine hydrochloride s.** [USP], a syrup containing 112–138 mg. of promethazine hydrochloride in each 100 ml.; used for its antihistaminic effect to provide sedation, to potentiate the action of central depressants, and to manage nausea and vomiting. **pseudoephedrine hydrochloride s.** [USP], a preparation containing 90 to 110 per cent of the labeled amount of $C_{10}H_{15}NO \cdot HCl$; used as a nasal decongestant and bronchodilator. **pyridostigmine bromide s.** [USP], a preparation, each 100 ml. of which contains 1.08 to 1.32 gm. of pyridostigmine bromide; used as an anticholinergic in the treatment of myasthenia gravis. **raspberry s.,** a syrup consisting of raspberry juice, sucrose, and alcohol, in purified water, used as a flavored vehicle for drugs. **sarsaparilla s., compound,** a solution of sarsaparilla and glycyrrhiza fluidextracts, sassafras and anise oils, methyl salicylate, alcohol, and syrup; used as a vehicle for drugs. **senna s.** [USP], a solution of senna fluidextract, coriander oil, sucrose, and purified water, used as a cathartic. **simple s.,** one compounded from purified water and sucrose. **s. of tolu,** tolu balsam s. **tolu balsam s.** [NF], a mixture of tolu balsam tincture, magnesium carbonate, sucrose, and purified water, used as a flavored vehicle for drugs. **triamcinolone diacetate s.** [USP], a preparation containing 90 to 110 per cent of the labeled amount of triamcinolone diacetate; used as an anti-inflammatory glucocorticoid. **trifluoperazine hydrochloride s.** [USP], a preparation containing trifluoperazine hydrochloride equivalent to 93–107 per cent of the labeled amount of trifluoperazine; used as an antipsychotic agent. **trimeprazine tartrate s.** [NF], a preparation containing trimeprazine tartrate equivalent to 90 to 110 per cent of the labeled amount of trimeprazine; used as an antipruritic. **triprolidine hydrochloride s.** [USP], a preparation containing 90–110 per cent of the labeled amount of triprolidine hydrochloride; used as an antihistaminic in the treatment of various allergic conditions and their manifestations. **white pine s., compound,** a solution containing coarsely powdered white pine, wild cherry, aralia, poplar bud, sanguinaria, and sassafras, combined with amaranth solution, chloroform, sucrose, glycerin, alcohol, and water; used as an antitussive and as a vehicle for other drugs. **white pine s., compound, with codeine,** compound white pine syrup combined with codeine phosphate dissolved in purified water, used as an antitussive. **wild cherry s.,** a mixture of a percolate of wild cherry, glycerin, sucrose, alcohol, and water; used as a flavored vehicle. **Yerba santa s., aromatic,** eriodictyon s., aromatic.

syrupus (sir′up-us) [L.] syrup. **s. auran′tii,** orange syrup. **s. cera′si,** cherry syrup. **s. cor′rigens,** aromatic eriodictyon syrup. **s. pi′ni al′bae compos′itus,** compound white pine syrup. **s. pi′ni al′bae compos′itus cum co′deina,** compound white pine syrup with codeine. **s. ru′bi ida′ei,** raspberry syrup. **s. sarsaparil′lae compos′itus,** compound sarsaparilla syrup.

syssarcosic (sis″sar-ko′sik) syssarcotic.

syssarcosis (sis″sar-ko′sis) [Gr. *syn* together + *sarkōsis* fleshy growth] the union or connection of bones by means of muscle, as the connection between the hyoid bone and the lower jaw, the scapula, and the breast bone.

syssarcotic (sis″sar-kot′ik) pertaining to or of the nature of a syssarcosis.

syssomus (sis-so′mus) [Gr. *syn* with + *sōma* body] a double monster with two heads and with the bodies united.

systaltic (sis-tal′tik) [Gr. *systaltikos* drawing together] alternately contracting and expanding; pulsating.

systatic (sis-tat′ik) affecting several of the sensory faculties at the same time.

system (sis′tem) [Gr. *systēma* a complex or organized whole] 1. a set or series of interconnected or interdependent parts or entities (objects, organs, or organisms) that function together in a common purpose or produce results impossible of achievement by one of them acting or operating alone. 2. a school or method of practice based on a specific set of principles, as the eclectic or galenic school. **absorbent**

s., lymphatic s. **accessory portal s. of Sappey,** small compensatory blood vessels formed around the liver and gallbladder in cases of cirrhosis of the liver. **adipose s.,** the fatty tissue of the body, considered collectively. **alimentary s.,** the organs concerned with the ingestion, digestion, and absorption of food or nutritional elements; see *apparatus digestorius*. **association s.,** the tracts of fibers in the brain by means of which perceptions are associated and thought rendered possible. **autonomic nervous s.,** the portion of the nervous system concerned with regulation of the activity of cardiac muscle, smooth muscle, and glands; usually restricted to the two visceral efferent peripheral components, the pars sympathica systematis nervosi autonomici (thoracolumbar part, or sympathetic nervous system) and the pars parasympathica systemis nervosi autonomici (craniosacral part, or parasympathetic nervous system). Called also *pars autonomica systematis nervosi* [NA], *systema nervosum autonomicum* [NA alternative], *systema nervosum sympatheticum,* and *sympathetic nervous system.* **biological s.,** a system composed of living material; such systems range from a collection of separate molecules to an assemblage of separate organisms. **blood group s.,** see *blood group.* **blood-vascular s.,** the blood vessels of the body. **brain cooling s.,** thermoregulated equipment for sensing and controlling brain temperature in neurophysiological and neuropsychological applications. **buffer s.,** see *buffer.* **bulbospiral s.,** muscle bundles in the heart which arise in and are attached to the conus arteriosus and the root of the aorta. **cardiovascular s.,** the heart and blood vessels, by which blood is pumped and circulated through the body. **case s.,** a method of teaching based on the logical analysis of, and deductions formed from, reported cases of disease. **centimeter-gram-second s.,** see *C.G.S.* **central nervous s. (CNS),** that portion of the nervous system consisting of the brain and spinal cord (pars centralis systematis nervosi [NA] and systema nervosum centrale [NA alternative]). **centrencephalic s.,** the system of neurons located in the central core of the upper brain stem from the thalamus down to the medulla oblongata, and connecting the two hemispheres of the brain. **cerebrospinal s.,** central nervous s. **chemoreceptor s.,** the system of body structures, principally the carotid body, the aortic pulmonary bodies, and the glomus jugulare, that respond to variations in oxygen tension and carbon dioxide tension of the blood and may play a role in the regulation of respiration. **chromaffin s.,** the chromaffin cells of the body, which characteristically stain strongly with chromium salts, considered collectively; they occur along the sympathetic nerves, in the adrenal, carotid, and coccygeal glands, and in various other organs. **circulatory s.,** the channels through which the nutrient fluids of the body circulate; often restricted to the vessels conveying blood. **complement s.,** see *complement.* **conducting s. of heart, conduction s. of heart,** systema conducens cordis. **coordinate s.,** a method by which a point, a line, a plane, or a geometric solid can be located in space by a set of numbers. **dentinal s.,** all the tubules radiating from a single pulp cavity. **dermal s., dermoid s.,** the skin and its appendages, including both the hair and the nails. See *integumentum commune.* **digestive s.,** the organs associated with the ingestion, digestion, and absorption of food; see *apparatus digestorius* [NA]. **dioptric s.,** a system of lenses or of different media for refracting light. **disperse s., dispersion s.,** a colloid solution. **dosimetric s.,** a regular and determinate system of administration of a therapeutic agent. **ecological s.,** see *ecosystem.* **endocrine s.,** the system of glands and other structures that elaborate internal secretions (hormones) which are released directly into the circulatory system and which influence metabolism and other body processes. Organs having endocrine function include the hypothalamus, pituitary, thyroid, parathyroid, and adrenal glands, the gonads, the pancreas, the paraganglia, and perhaps the pineal body. The gut and the lung also secrete substances that have hormonal functions. The thymus is no longer considered to perform an endocrine function. See Plate accompanying *gland.* **endothelial s.,** see *reticuloendothelial s.* **exteroceptive nervous s.,** that portion of the afferent elements of the somatic nervous system which is sensitive to stimuli originating outside the body. **exterofective s.,** a little used term referring to the central nervous system, exclusive of the autonomic portion, as viewed in its function of maintaining homeostasis. Cf. *interofective s.*

THE AUTONOMIC NERVES

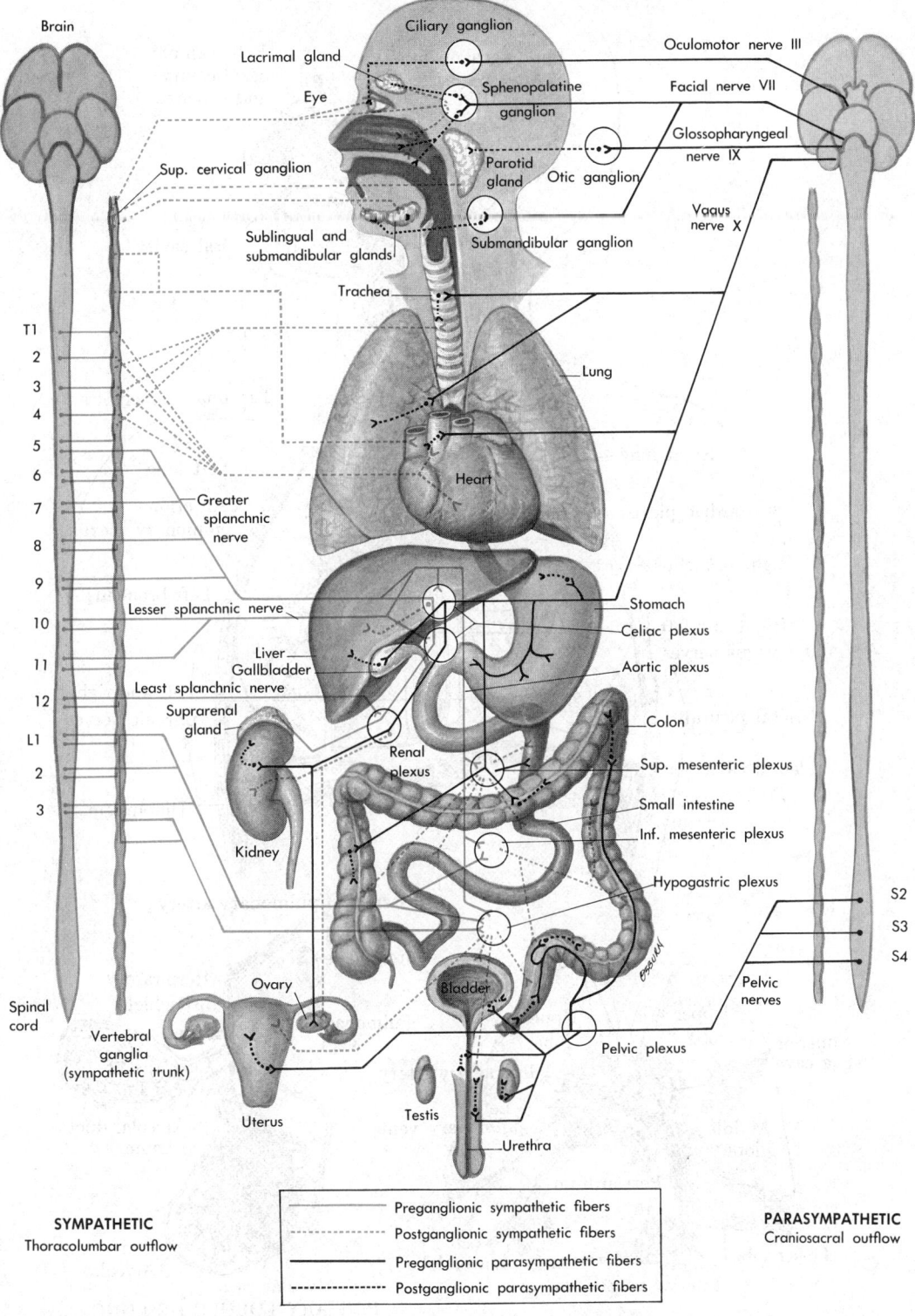

Brain

Ciliary ganglion

Lacrimal gland

Oculomotor nerve III

Eye

Sphenopalatine ganglion

Facial nerve VII

Sup. cervical ganglion

Glossopharyngeal nerve IX

Parotid gland

Otic ganglion

Vagus nerve X

Sublingual and submandibular glands

Submandibular ganglion

Trachea

T1
2
3
4
5
6
7
8
9
10
11
12
L1
2
3

Lung

Heart

Greater splanchnic nerve

Stomach

Celiac plexus

Lesser splanchnic nerve

Aortic plexus

Liver
Gallbladder

Least splanchnic nerve

Colon

Suprarenal gland

Renal plexus

Sup. mesenteric plexus

Small intestine

Inf. mesenteric plexus

Kidney

Hypogastric plexus

S2
S3
S4

Spinal cord

Pelvic nerves

Vertebral ganglia (sympathetic trunk)

Ovary

Bladder

Pelvic plexus

Uterus

Testis

Urethra

SYMPATHETIC
Thoracolumbar outflow

Preganglionic sympathetic fibers
Postganglionic sympathetic fibers
Preganglionic parasympathetic fibers
Postganglionic parasympathetic fibers

PARASYMPATHETIC
Craniosacral outflow

PLATE 45 — AUTONOMIC NERVOUS SYSTEM

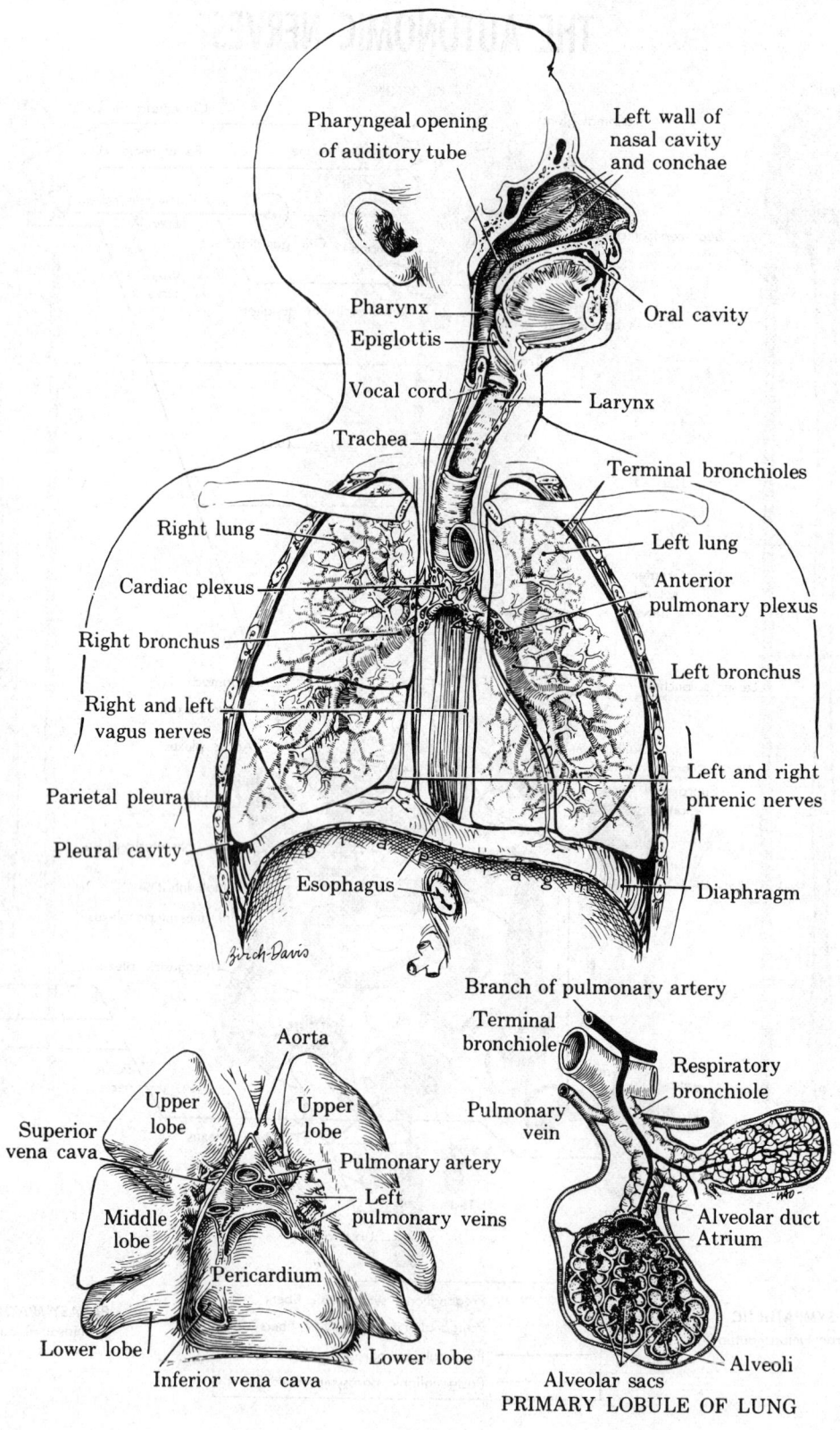

Pharyngeal opening
of auditory tube

Left wall of
nasal cavity
and conchae

Pharynx

Oral cavity

Epiglottis

Vocal cord

Larynx

Trachea

Terminal bronchioles

Right lung

Left lung

Cardiac plexus

Anterior
pulmonary plexus

Right bronchus

Left bronchus

Right and left
vagus nerves

Parietal pleura

Left and right
phrenic nerves

Pleural cavity

Esophagus

Diaphragm

Branch of pulmonary artery

Terminal
bronchiole

Respiratory
bronchiole

Aorta

Upper
lobe

Upper
lobe

Pulmonary
vein

Superior
vena cava

Pulmonary artery

Middle
lobe

Left
pulmonary veins

Alveolar duct
Atrium

Pericardium

Lower lobe

Lower lobe

Alveoli

Inferior vena cava

Alveolar sacs

PRIMARY LOBULE OF LUNG

PLATE 46 — ORGANS OF THE RESPIRATORY SYSTEM

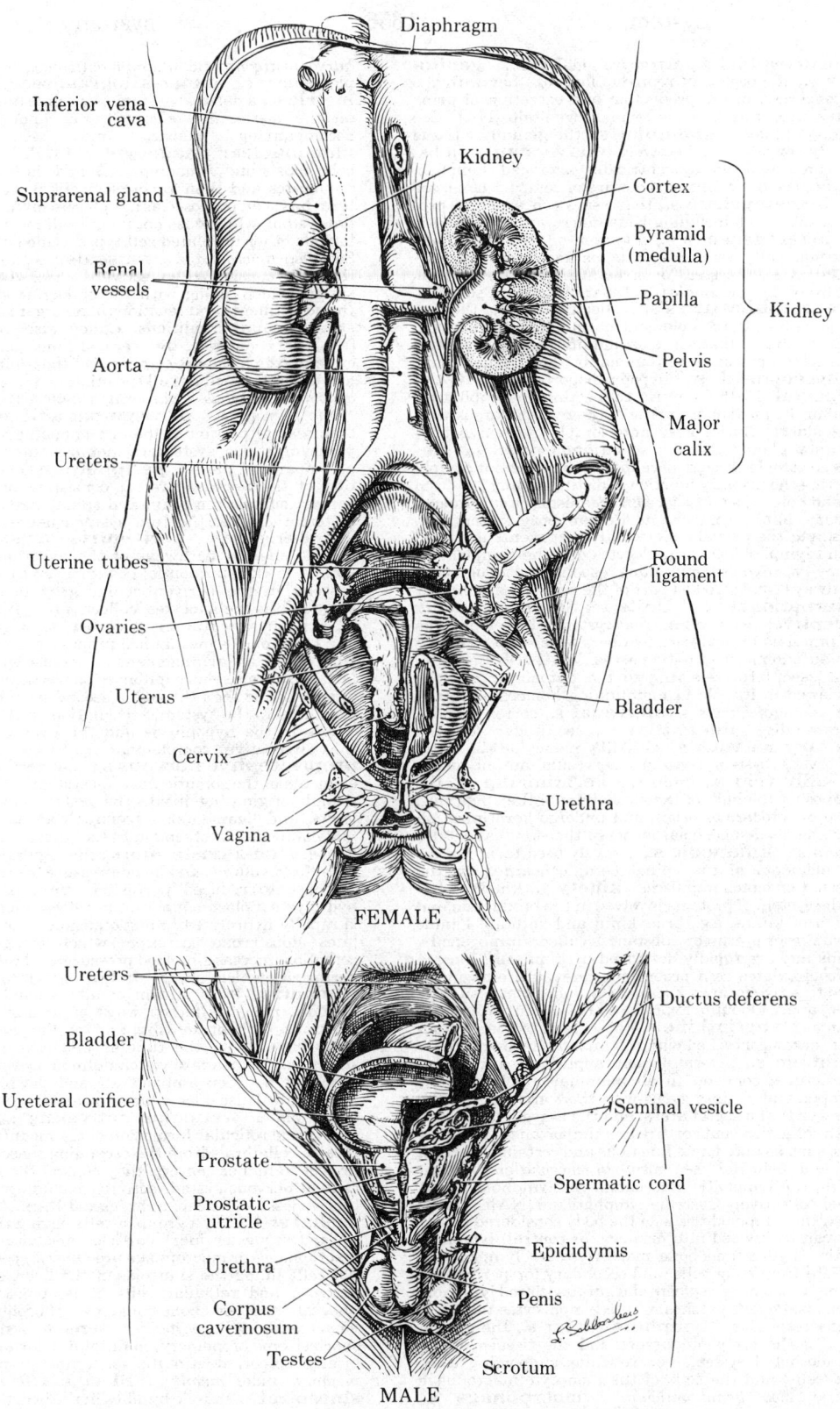

Diaphragm

Inferior vena cava

Suprarenal gland

Renal vessels

Aorta

Ureters

Uterine tubes

Ovaries

Uterus

Cervix

Vagina

Kidney

Cortex

Pyramid (medulla)

Papilla

Pelvis

Major calix

} Kidney

Round ligament

Bladder

Urethra

FEMALE

Ureters

Bladder

Ureteral orifice

Prostate

Prostatic utricle

Urethra

Corpus cavernosum

Testes

Ductus deferens

Seminal vesicle

Spermatic cord

Epididymis

Penis

Scrotum

MALE

PLATE 47 — ORGANS OF THE UROGENITAL SYSTEM

extracorticospinal s., extrapyramidal tract. **genito-urinary s.,** the organs of reproduction, together with the organs concerned in the production and excretion of urine (apparatus urogenitalis or systema urogenitale [NA]). See accompanying plate. **glandular s.,** the glandular tissue of the body considered collectively. **haversian s.,** a haversian canal and its concentrically arranged lamellae, constituting the basic unit of structure of compact bone; see *osteon.* **hematopoietic s.,** the tissues concerned in production of the blood, including bone marrow and lymphatic tissue. **heterogeneous s.,** a system or structure made up of mechanically separable parts, as an emulsion. **homogeneous s.,** a system or structure made up of parts which cannot be mechanically separated, as a solution. **humoral amplification s's,** a collective term for the four enzyme cascades—the complement, coagulation, fibrinolytic, and kinin systems—that serve as amplification and control mechanisms in hemostasis, inflammation, and tissue repair. **hypophyseoportal s.,** hypophysioportal s. **hypophysioportal s.,** the venules connecting the capillaries (gomitoli) in the median eminence of the hypothalamus with the sinusoidal capillaries of the anterior lobe of the hypophysis (pituitary gland). Called also *pituitary portal s.* **immune s.,** a complex system of cellular and molecular components having the primary function of distinguishing self from not self and defense against foreign organisms or substances; the primary cellular components are lymphocytes and macrophages, and the primary molecular components are antibodies and lymphokines; granulocytes and the complement system are also involved in immune responses, although they are not always considered as part of the immune system per se. **International S. of Units,** see *SI unit,* under *unit.* **interoceptive nervous s.,** that system which transmits afferent impulses from viscera by fibers which run centrally either in autonomic or somatic nerves. **interofective s.,** a seldom used term referring to the autonomic nervous system viewed in its role in maintaining homeostasis from within. Cf. *exterofective s.* **interrenal s.,** cortex glandulae suprarenalis. **interstitial s.,** see under *lamella.* **involuntary nervous s.,** Gaskill's name for the autonomic nervous system (systema nervosum autonomicum [NA]). **kallikrein s.,** kinin s. **keratinizing s.,** the cells composing the bulk of the epithelium of the epidermis, which are of ectodermal origin and undergo keratinization and form the dead superficial layers of the skin; called also *malpighian s.* **kinesiodic s.,** a rarely used term for the efferent elements of the spinal cord, concerned in the transmission of motor impulses. **kinety s.,** kinety. **kinin s.,** the system of proteins involved in the production and destruction of kinins, e.g., bradykinin and kallidin. Kinins are cleaved from precursor substances called kininogens by kallikreins and are rapidly destroyed by kininases. Plasma kallikrein circulates as a proenzyme (prekallikrein) and is converted to active form by Factor XIIa, which cleaves HMW kininogen, an α2-globulin, to produce bradykinin. Called also *kallikrein s.* **labyrinthine s.,** those parts of the vestibulocochlear organ concerned with the maintenance of equilibrium. **limbic s.,** a term loosely applied to a group of brain structures common to all mammals (including the hippocampus and dentate gyrus with their archicortex, the cingulate gyrus and septal areas, and the amygdala), associated with olfaction but of greater importance in other activities, such as autonomic functions and certain aspects of emotion and behavior; see also *rhinencephalon.* **lymphatic s.,** the lymphatic vessels and the lymphoid tissue, considered collectively (systema lymphaticum [NA]). **lymphoid s.,** the lymphoid tissue of the body considered collectively; it can be divided into primary (or central) lymphoid tissues, the thymus and bone marrow where lymphocytes differentiate from stem cells, and secondary (or peripheral) tissues, the lymph nodes, spleen, and gut-associated lymphoid tissue (tonsils, Peyer's patches) where lymphocytes take part in immune responses. **lymphoreticular s.,** the system consisting of the lymphoid tissues and the tissues of the reticuloendothelial system, i.e., reticular supporting cells, lymphoid cells, and the cells of the monocyte-macrophage series. See also *lymphoreticular.* **macrophage s.,** mononuclear phagocyte. **malpighian s.,** keratinizing s. **masticatory s.,** see under *apparatus.* **mastigont s.,** an ultrastructural complex characteristic of mastigophorans, comprising all of the organelles associated with the flagella, including basal bodies, axostyle, and Golgi body; it may or may not be associated with a nucleus (see also

karyomastigont and *akaryomastigont*). **melanocyte s.,** pigmentary s. **meter-kilogram-second s.,** see *M.K.S.* **metric s.,** a decimal system of weights and measures based on the meter. See also *SI unit,* under *unit;* see table accompanying *metric,* and see Appendix 1. **mononuclear phagocyte s. (MPS),** the collection of cells consisting of macrophages and their precursors (blood monocytes and their precursor cells in bone marrow). The term has been proposed as a replacement for reticuloendothelial system, which does not include all macrophages and does include other unrelated cell types. Called also *macrophage s.* See also *macrophage.* **muscular s.,** all the muscles of the body considered collectively. **nervous s.,** the organ system which, along with the endocrine system, correlates the adjustments and reactions of an organism to internal and environmental conditions. Called also *systema nervosum* [NA]. It comprises the central and peripheral nervous systems: the former is composed of the brain and spinal cord, and the latter includes all the other neural elements. See also *autonomic nervous s., parasympathetic nervous s.,* and *sympathetic nervous s.* **parasympathetic nervous s.,** the craniosacral portion of the autonomic nervous system (pars parasympathica systematis nervosi autonomici [NA]). See accompanying plate. **peripheral nervous s.,** that portion of the nervous system consisting of the nerves and ganglia outside the brain and spinal cord (pars peripherica systematis nervosi [NA] and systema nervosum periphericum [NA alternative]). **periventricular s.,** collective name for the efferent pathways of the hypothalamus that arise mainly in the supraoptic, posterior, and tuberal nuclei and descend in the periventricular gray matter. **pigmentary s.,** the melanocytes, collectively. **pituitary portal s.,** hypophysioportal s. **plenum s.,** a system of ventilation based on the mechanical propulsion of air into the room. **portal s.,** an arrangement of vessels whereby blood collected from one set of capillaries passes through a large vessel or vessels and then through a second set of capillaries before it returns to the systemic circulation; such an arrangement occurs in the hypophysis and the liver. **properdin s.,** the alternative complement pathway; see *complement.* **proprioceptive nervous s.,** that portion of the afferent elements of the somatic nervous system which is sensitive to stimuli originating inside the body (from muscles, bones, joints, and ligaments). **pyramidal s.,** fasciculus pyramidalis medullae oblongatae; see under *tract.* **renin-angiotension-aldosterone s.,** the regulation of sodium balance, fluid volume, and blood pressure by renal secretions: in response to reduced perfusion, renin is secreted, which hydrolyzes a plasma globulin to release angiotensin I, which is rapidly hydrolyzed to angiotensin II; this in turn stimulates aldosterone secretion, which brings about sodium retention, increase in blood pressure, and restoration of renal perfusion, which shuts off the signal for renin release. **resonating s.,** a system of atoms bonded together that includes many different ways of arranging the external electrons without moving any of the constituent atoms. **respiratory s.,** the tubular and cavernous organs and structures by means of which pulmonary ventilation and gas exchange between ambient air and the blood are brought about; called also *apparatus respiratorius* [NA]. See accompanying plate. **reticular activating s.,** the system of cells of the reticular formation of the medulla oblongata that receive collaterals from the ascending sensory pathways and project to higher centers; they control the overall degree of central nervous system activity, including wakefulness, attentiveness, and sleep; abbreviated RAS. **reticuloendothelial s. (RES),** a group of cells having the ability to take up and sequester inert particles and vital dyes, including macrophages or macrophage precursors, specialized endothelial cells lining the sinusoids of the liver, spleen, and bone marrow, and reticular cells of lymphatic tissue (macrophages) and of bone marrow (fibroblasts). See also *mononuclear phagocyte s.* **sensory storage s.,** the shortest type of memory, maintaining for less than a second briefly perceived stimuli; see *echoic memory* and *iconic memory,* under *memory.* **SI s.,** see *SI unit,* under *unit.* **sinospiral s.,** muscle bundles in the heart which arise from and are inserted into the region of the sinus venosus. **skeletal s.,** systema skeletale. **somatic nervous s.,** the elements of the nervous system concerned with the transmission of impulses to and from the nonvisceral components of the body, such as the skeletal muscles, bones, joints, ligaments, skin, and eye and ear. **stomatognathic s.,** the structures of the mouth and jaws, considered collectively, as they subserve the functions of mastication, deglutition, respiration, and speech. See also *masticatory apparatus,* under *apparatus.* **sympathetic nervous s.,** 1. pars sympathica systematis nervosi autonomici. See Plate showing the autonomic nervous system. 2. autonomic nervous system (pars centralis systematis nervosi [NA]). **T s.,** a system of transverse tubular invaginations (*T,* or *transverse, tubules*) of the sarcolemma, each of which penetrates deep into the muscle fiber. In mammalian skeletal muscle, they are located at the junction of the A band with the I band, and in mammalian cardiac muscle at the level of the Z band; the system plays a role in the excitation and relaxation of muscle and provides an important additional surface for the exchange of metabolites between muscle and the extracellular space. Called also *triad s.* See also *triad of skeletal muscle; terminal cisterns,* under *cistern;* and *T tubule,* under *tubule.* **triad s., T s. urogenital s.,** the organs concerned in the production and excretion of urine, together with the organs of reproduction; see *apparatus urogenitalis* [NA]. See Plate 47. **urinary s., uropoietic s.,** the organs concerned in secretion of urine; see *organa urinaria* [NA]. **vascular s.,** the vessels of the body, especially the blood vessels. **vasomotor s.,** the part of the nervous system that controls the caliber of the blood vessels. **vegetative nervous s.,** an old term for the autonomic nervous system (systema nervosum autonomicum [NA]). **vestibular s.,** labyrinthine s. **visceral nervous s.,** autonomic nervous s. **Waring's s.,** see under *method.*

systema (sis-te′mah) [Gr. *systēma* a complex or organized whole] system: a series of interconnected or interdependent organs which together accomplish a specific function. **s. condu′cens cor′dis** [NA], conducting system of heart: a system of specialized muscle fibers that rapidly transmit cardiac impulses and serve to coordinate contractions, comprising the sinoatrial node, atrioventricular node, atrioventricular bundle and its right and left limbs, and the subendocardial branches (*rami subendocardiales*) of Purkinje fibers. Called also *cardionector.* **s. digesto′rium,** NA alternative for *apparatus digestorius.* **s. lymphat′icum** [NA], lymphatic system: the lymphatic vessels and the lymphoid tissue, considered collectively. **s. nervo′sum** [NA], the nervous system: the chief organ system that correlates the adjustments and reactions of the organism to internal and environmental conditions, composed of the central and the peripheral nervous system; the former comprises the brain and spinal cord, and the latter includes all other neural elements. **s. nervo′sum autonom′icum,** NA alternative for *pars autonomica systematis nervosi:* the portion of the nervous system concerned with regulation of the activity of cardiac muscle, smooth muscle, and glands. See *autonomic nervous system,* under *system,* and see accompanying plate. **s. nervo′sum centra′le,** NA alternative for *pars centralis systematis nervosi:* the central nervous system, i.e., the portion of the nervous system consisting of the brain and spinal cord. **s. nervo′sum peripher′icum,** NA alternative for *pars peripherica systematis nervosi:* the peripheral nervous system, i.e., the portion of the nervous system consisting of the nerves and ganglia outside the brain and spinal cord. **s. nervo′sum sympathet′icum,** 1. sympathetic nervous system (pars sympathica systematis nervosi autonomici [NA]). 2. systema nervosum autonomicum (pars autonomica systematis nervosi [NA]). **s. respirato′rium,** NA alternative for *apparatus respiratorius.* **s. skeleta′le** [NA], skeletal system: the bones (*pars ossea systematis skeletalis*) and cartilages (*pars cartilaginea systematis skeletalis*) of the body. **s. urogenita′le,** NA alternative for *apparatus urogenitalis.* **s. vaso′rum,** the

blood and lymph vessels of the body and all their ramifications, considered collectively.

systematic (sis″te-mat′ik) [Gr. *systēmatikos*] pertaining or according to a system.

systematization (sis-tem″ah-ti-za′shun) arrangement according to a system. In psychiatry, the arrangement of ideas into a logical sequence, or of delusions into a superficially coherent system.

systematized (sis′te-mah-tīzd) made systematic or arranged according to a system.

systematology (sis″tĕ-mah-tol′o-je) [Gr. *systēma* system + *-logy*] the science of classification.

système sécant (sis-tem′ sa-kahn′) [Fr. "cutting system"] one of the suture lines seen in ciliate protozoa where fields of kineties from different body areas converge.

systemic (sis-tem′ik) pertaining to or affecting the body as a whole.

systemoid (sis′tĕ-moid) [Gr. *systēma* system + *eidos* form] 1. resembling a system. 2. denoting tumors made up of various kinds of tissue.

systogene (sis′to-jēn) tyramine.

systole (sis′to-le) [Gr. *systolē* a drawing together, contraction] the contraction, or period of contraction, of the heart, especially that of the ventricles; sometimes divided into components, as pre-ejection and ejection periods, or isovolumic, ejection, and relaxation periods. **aborted s.,** a systole, usually premature, not associated with pulsation of a peripheral artery. **atrial s.,** the contraction of the atria by which blood is propelled from them into the ventricles. **extra s.,** extrasystole. **frustrate s.,** aborted s. **hemic s.** (*obs.*), an independently occurring systole of a ventricle. **ventricular s.,** the contraction of the ventricles of the heart by which the blood is forced into the aorta and the pulmonary trunk.

systolic (sis-tol′ik) pertaining to or produced by the systole; occurring along with the ventricular systole.

systolometer (sis″to-lom′ĕ-ter) [Gr. *systolē* systole + *metron* measure] an instrument for determining the quality of the heart sounds.

systremma (sis-trem′ah) [Gr. "anything twisted up together"] a cramp in the muscles of the calf of the leg.

Sytobex (si′to-beks) trademark for preparations of cyanocobalamin.

syzygial (sĭ-zij′e-al) pertaining to syzygy.

syzygiology (sĭ-zij″e-ol′o-je) [Gr. *syzygia* yoke + *-logy*] the study of the relationship of the whole as contrasted to that of isolated parts and functions.

Syzygium (sĭ-zij′e-um) a genus of tropical myrtaceous trees. S. *jambolanum,* DC., the jambul tree of India, is astringent.

syzygium (sĭ-zij′e-um) syzygy.

syzygy (siz′ĭ-je) [Gr. *syzygia* a union of branches with the trunk] 1. the conjunction and fusion of organs without loss of identity. 2. the temporary association (end-to-end or side-to-side) of gamonts prior to the formation of gametocysts and gametes; applied especially to gregarine protozoa.

Szabo's test (sah′bōz) [Dionys *Szabo,* Budapest physician, 1856–1918] see under *tests.*

Szent-Györgyi (sent′jur-jĭ) Albert. Hungarian-born American physician and biochemist, 1893–1986; winner of the Nobel prize for medicine or physiology in 1937 for his studies in biological combustion and for his discovery of the catalytic properties of ascorbic acid in the adrenal glands.

Szent-Györgyi reaction (sent′jur-jĭ) [Albert *Szent-Györgyi*] see under *reaction.*

T symbol for *tesla, tera-, thymine* or *thymidine* (in nucleic acids), *thoracic vertebrae* (T-1 through T-12), and *intraocular tension*. Normal intraocular tension is indicated by the symbol Tn, while T + 1, T + 2, etc., indicate stages of increased tension, and T − 1, T − 2, etc., indicate stages of decreased tension.

T symbol for *absolute temperature* and *transmittance.*

T$_m$ tubular maximum (of the kidneys); a notation used in reporting kidney function studies, with inferior letters representing the substance used in the test, as T$_{m_{PAH}}$ (tubular maximum for para-aminohippuric acid).

T$\frac{1}{2}$, t$\frac{1}{2}$ half-life.

T$\frac{1}{2}$ symbol for *half-life* or *half-time.*

T$_3$ symbol for *triiodothyronine.*

T$_4$ symbol for *thyroxine.*

t in genetics, symbol for translocation.

t symbol for *time* and *temperature* (measured on a customary scale). See *t-test* under *tests.*

t$\frac{1}{2}$ symbol for *half-life* or *half-time.*

Θ, θ theta, the eighth letter of the Greek alphabet.

τ tau, the nineteenth letter of the Greek alphabet.

T-1824 Evans blue.

2,4,5-T a toxic chlorphenoxy herbicide (2,4,5-trichlorophenoxyacetic acid) that acts as a growth-regulating hormone killing broadleaf plants by overstimulation.

T.A. toxin-antitoxin.

Ta chemical symbol for *tantalum.*

tabacin (tab′ah-sin) a glycoside occurring in tobacco.

tabacism (tab′ah-sizm) tabacosis.

tabacosis (tab″ah-ko′sis) poisoning by tobacco, and chiefly by the inhalation of tobacco dust; also a form of pneumoconiosis attributed to tobacco dust (*t. pulmo′num*).

tabacum (tab′ah-kum) [L., from Amerindian] tobacco.

tabagism (tab′ah-jizm) the condition produced by excessive use of tobacco; nicotinism.

tabanid (tab′ah-nid) any gadfly of the family Tabanidae, of which the genus *Tabanus* is the type. Other genera are *Chrysops, Goniops, Silvius, Chrysozona,* and *Diachlorus.* Many of the species inflict painful bites upon men and animals, and some species are mechanical vectors of diseases.

Tabanus (tah-ba′nus) [L. "gadfly"] a genus of bloodsucking biting flies; the horseflies or gadflies. They transmit trypanosomes and anthrax to various animals. **T. atra′tus,** the common black horsefly of North America. **T. bovi′nus,** the gadfly of cattle in Asia, Africa, and South America. **T. ditaenia′tus, T. fascia′tus, T. gra′tus,** the Seroot

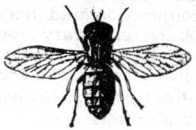

Tabanus bovinus.

flies of the Sudan, which are very troublesome to man and beast.

tabardillo (tab″ar-dēl′yo) [Sp.] murine typhus.

tabatière anatomique (tah-bah″te-ār′ ah-nah-to-mēk′) [Fr. "anatomical snuffbox"] the hollow on the back of the hand and at the base of the thumb, between the tendons of the extensor pollicis longus and extensor pollicis brevis muscles.

tabella (tah-bel′ah), pl. *tabel′lae* [L.] a medicated tablet or troche.

tabernanthine (tab″er-nan′thēn) an alkaloid, C$_{20}$H$_{26}$N$_2$O, isolated from the root of *Tabernanthe iboga* Baill. (Apocynaceae), which has both analgesic and serotonin antagonist properties. It is isomeric with ibogaine.

tabes (ta′bēz) [L. "wasting away, decay, melting"] 1. any wasting of the body; progressive atrophy of the body or a part of it. 2. tabes dorsalis. **diabetic t.,** a peripheral neurop-

athy occurring in diabetic patients with symptoms of tabes dorsalis. **t. dorsa′lis,** parenchymatous neurosyphilis in which there is slowly progressive degeneration of the posterior columns and posterior roots and ganglia of the spinal cord, occurring 15 to 20 years after the initial infection of syphilis, characterized by lancinating lightning pains, urinary incontinence, ataxia, impaired position and vibratory sense, optic atrophy, hypotonia, hyperreflexia, and trophic joint degeneration (Charcot's joints). Called also *Duchenne's disease, locomotor ataxia, posterior* or *posterior spinal sclerosis, tabetic neurosyphilis, tabes,* and *t. spinalis.* **t. ergot′ica,** a condition resembling tabes dorsalis, due to ergotism. **Friedreich's t.,** Friedreich's ataxia. **t. infan′tum,** tabes as seen in infants with congenital syphilis. **t. mesenter′ica, t. mesara′ica,** tuberculosis of the mesenteric glands in children, resulting in digestive derangement and wasting of the body; called also *pedatrophia, pedatrophy,* and *atrophia mesenterica.* **peripheral t.,** pseudotabes. **t. spina′lis,** t. dorsalis.

tabescent (tah-bes′ent) [L. *tabescere* to waste away] wasting away; shriveling.

tabetic (tah-bet′ik) pertaining to or affected with tabes.

tabetiform (tah-bet′ĭ-form) resembling tabes.

tabic (tab′ik) tabetic.

tabid (tab′id) [L. *tabidus* melting, dissolving] tabetic; wasting away.

tabification (tab″ĭ-fi-ka′shun) [L. *tabes* wasting away + *facere* to make] the process of wasting away.

tablature (tab′lah-chūr) the separation of the chief cranial bones into inner and outer tables, which are separated by a diploë.

table (ta′b'l) [L. *tabula*] 1. a flat surface. 2. an arrangement of data in rows and columns. **Aub-Dubois t.,** a table of normal basal metabolic rates for persons of various ages. **cohort life t.,** a table giving the survival data of a cohort of individuals in a clinical study or trial, i.e., the number alive and under observation (not lost to follow-up) at the beginning of each year, the number dying in each year, the conditional probability of survival for each year, and the cumulative probabilities of survival from the beginning of the study to the end of each year. See *survival curve,* under *curve.* **contingency t.,** a table used to display statistical data according to two characteristics, each having a number of mutually inclusive categories; categories of one characteristic are listed in rows and categories of the other characteristic are listed in columns. Statistical analysis (often using chi-squared tests) can be readily applied to the rows and columns of the table. **demographic life t.,** a table giving age-specific mortality rates for each age group in one calendar year, used in the calculation of life expectancy (based on the assumption of unchanging mortality rates). Called also *mortality t.* **Gaffky t.,** see under *scale.* **inner t. of skull,** lamina interna cranii. **inner t. of frontal bone,** facies interna ossis frontalis. **Mendeleev's t.,** periodic t. **mortality t.,** demographic life t. **outer t. of frontal bone,** facies externa ossis frontalis. **outer t. of skull,** lamina externa cranii. **periodic t.,** an ordering of all the known chemical elements in the form of a chart according to the periodic law, in which corresponding elements from the several periods form groups with similar properties; called also *Mendeleev's t.* **Reuss' t's,** see under *chart.* **Stintzing's t's,** tables showing the average value of the normal electric excitability of the muscles and nerves. **vitreous t.,** lamina interna ossium cranii. **water t.,** the upper surface of the impervious strata on which the ground water lies deep to the surface of the earth.

tablespoon (ta′b'l-spoōn) a household unit of capacity, approximately equivalent to 4 fluid drams, or 15 milliliters.

tablet (tab′let) a solid dosage form of varying weight, size, and shape, which may be molded or compressed, and which contains a medicinal substance in pure or diluted form. Cf. *pill.* **buccal t.,** a small, flat, oval tablet to be held between the cheek and gum, permitting direct absorption through the oral mucosa of the medicinal substance contained therein. **dispensing t.,** a compressed or molded tablet containing a large quantity of a drug, used by dispensing pharmacists in compounding prescriptions. **enteric-coated t.,** one coated with material that delays release of the medication until after it leaves the stomach. **hypodermic t.,** one to be dissolved in water, containing a medicinal substance for hypodermic injection. **sublingual t.,** a small, flat, oval tablet to be held beneath the tongue, permitting direct absorption of the medicinal substance contained therein. **t. triturate,** a small, usually cylindrical, molded disk containing a medicinal substance diluted with a mixture of lactose and powdered sucrose, in varying proportions, with a moistening agent.

taboo (tah-boo′) any of the negative traditions and behaviors that are generally regarded as harmful to social welfare. Cf. *mores.*

taboparalysis (ta″bo-pah-ral′ĭ-sis) taboparesis.

taboparesis (ta″bo-pah-re′sis, ta″bo-par′e-sis) dementia paralytica occurring concomitantly with tabes dorsalis.

tabula (tab′u-lah), gen. and pl. *tab′ulae* [L.] table. **t. exter′na os′sis cra′nii,** lamina externa ossium cranii. **t. inter′na os′sis cra′nii, t. vit′rea,** lamina interna ossium cranii.

tabular (tab′u-lar) [L. *tabula* a board or table] resembling or shaped like a table.

tacahout (tak″ah-hoot′) [Arabic] a kind of gall from tamarisk trees; a source of gallic acid.

tacamahac (tak′ah-ma-hak″) a resin or gum derived from various trees, e.g., *Bursera gummifer* L. (Burseraceae) of tropical America; it is medicinally considered to be diaphoretic, diuretic, and purgative.

Tacaryl (tak′ah-ril) trademark for preparations of methdilazine.

TACE (tās) trademark for preparations of chlorotrianisene.

tache (tahsh) [Fr.] a spot or blemish. **t. blanche** (blahnsh) [Fr. "white spot"], a white spot on the liver in certain infectious diseases. **t's bleuâtres** (bluh-ahtr′) [Fr. "bluish spots"], maculae caeruleae. **t. cérébrale** (sa-ra-brahl′) [Fr. "cerebral spot"], a congested streak produced by drawing the nail across the skin: a concomitant of various nervous or cerebral diseases. Called also *t. méningéale.* **t's laiteuses** (la-tēz′) [Fr. "milky spots"], small spots, of a milky appearance in the omentum, made up of lymphoid cells and macrophages and especially prominent in the rabbit. **t. méningéale** (ma-nin-zha-al′) [Fr. "meningeal spot"], t. cérébrale. **t. motrice** (mo-trēs′) [Fr. "motor spot"], a kind of motor nerve ending in which the nerve fibril passes to a muscle cell, where it ends in a slight enlargement. **t. noire** (nwahr) [Fr. "black spot"], an ulcer covered with a black adherent crust, a characteristic local reaction occurring at the presumed site of the infective bite in certain tick-borne rickettsioses, such as scrub typhus or boutonneuse fever. **t. spinale** (spe-nahl′) [Fr. "spinal spot"], a bulla resembling a burn, and due to a spinal cord disease.

tachistoscope (tah-kis′to-skōp) [Gr. *tachistos* swiftest + -*scope*] a device used in physiological psychology to demonstrate iconic memory; it displays images for controlled times, usually less than one-tenth of a second.

tach(o)- [Gr. *tachos* speed] a combining form denoting relationship to speed.

tachogram (tak′o-gram) [*tacho-* + Gr. *gramma* mark] a graphic record of the movement and velocity of the blood current.

tachography (tah-kog′rah-fe) [*tacho-* + Gr. *graphein* to write] the recording of the speed of the blood current.

tachy- [Gr. *tachys* swift] a combining form meaning swift or rapid.

tachyalimentation (tak″e-al″ĭ-men-ta′shun) [*tachy-* + *alimentation*] hypoglycemia occurring postprandially after gastric resection or gastroenterostomy, due to the accelerated passage of glucose into the small intestine, from which it enters the bloodstream at an increased rate, stimulating the production of insulin by the β-cells of the pancreas. It is a manifestation of the dumping syndrome.

tachyarrhythmia (tak″e-ah-rith′me-ah) [*tachy-* + *a* neg. + Gr. *rhythmos* rhythm] tachycardia associated with an irregularity in the normal heart rhythm.

tachyauxesis (tak″e-awk-ze′sis) [*tachy-* + Gr. *auxēsis* growth] heterauxesis in which the part grows more rapidly than the whole.

tachycardia (tak″e-kar′de-ah) [*tachy-* + Gr. *kardia* heart]

excessive rapidity in the action of the heart; the term is usually applied to a heart rate above 100 per minute and may be qualified as atrial, junctional (nodal), or ventricular, and as paroxysmal. **atrial t.,** a rapid cardiac rate, usually between 160 and 190 per minute, originating from an atrial locus. **double t.,** the occurrence of two types of ectopic tachycardia, e.g., nodal and ventricular tachycardia, at the same time. **ectopic t.,** abnormally rapid heart action in response to impulses arising outside the sinoatrial node. **junctional t.,** that arising in response to impulses originating in the atrioventricular junction, i.e., in the atrioventricular node. **nodal t.,** tachycardia in response to impulses originating in or near the atrioventricular node; called also *atrioventricular nodal t.* **orthostatic t.,** disproportionate rapidity of the heart rate on rising from a reclining to a standing position. **paroxysmal t.,** a condition marked by attacks of rapid action of the heart having sudden onset and cessation; called also *Bouveret's disease* or *syndrome.* **reflex t.,** rapid action of the heart initiated through a relatively simple nerve pathway by an event occurring elsewhere in the body. **sinus t.,** simple tachycardia with origin in the sinus node. **t. strumo′sa exophthal′mica,** Graves' disease. **supraventricular t.,** a combination of junctional tachycardia and atrial tachycardia. **ventricular t.,** an abnormally rapid ventricular rhythm with aberrant ventricular excitation (wide QRS complexes), usually in excess of 150 per minute, which is generated within the ventricle and is most commonly associated with atrioventricular dissociation. Minor irregularities of rate may also occur. Evidence implicates a reentrant pathway as the usual cause.

tachycardiac (tak″e-kar′de-ak) 1. pertaining to, characterized by, or causing tachycardia. 2. an agent that acts to accelerate the pulse.

tachycardic (tak″e-kar′dik) tachycardiac.

tachygastria (tak″e-gas′tre-ah) the occurrence of a sequence of electric potentials at abnormally high frequencies in the gastric antrum.

tachygenesis (tak″e-jen′ĕ-sis) [*tachy-* + Gr. *genesis* production] the acceleration and compression of ancestral stages in embryonic development.

tachymeter (tah-kim′ĕ-ter) [*tachy-* + Gr. *metron* measure] any instrument for measuring rapidity of motion of any body.

tachyphagia (tak″e-fa′je-ah) [*tachy-* + Gr. *phagein* to eat + -*ia*] rapid or hasty eating.

tachyphylaxis (tak″e-fi-lak′sis) [*tachy-* + Gr. *phylaxis* protection] 1. rapid immunization against the effect of toxic doses of an extract or serum by previous injection of small doses. 2. rapidly decreasing response to a drug or physiologically active agent after administration of a few doses.

tachypnea (tak″ip-ne′ah) [*tachy-* + Gr. *pnoia* breath] excessive rapidity of respiration; a respiratory neurosis marked by quick, shallow breathing.

tachyrhythmia (tak″e-rith′me-ah) [*tachy-* + Gr. *rhythmos* rhythm + -*ia*] tachycardia, especially when the mechanism is obscure.

tachysterol (tak-is′te-rol) an isomer of ergosterol produced by irradiation.

tachytrophism (tak″e-tro′fizm) [*tachy-* + Gr. *trophē* nutrition] rapid metabolism.

tachyzoite (tak″e-zo′īt) [*tachy-* + Gr. *zōon*] the crescent or oval, quickly multiplying trophozoite of *Toxoplasma gondii,* found in all tissues except non-nucleated erythrocytes during the acute stage of toxoplasmosis. Called also *endozoite.* Cf. *bradyzoite* and *pseudocyst* (def. 2).

taclamine hydrochloride (tah′klah-mēn) chemical name: 2,3,4,4a,8,9,13b,14-octahydro-1*H*-benzo[6,7]cyclohepta[1,2,3-*de*]pyrido[2,1-*a*]isoquinoline; a minor tranquilizer, $C_{21}H_{23}N \cdot HCl$.

tactic (tak′tik) 1. exhibiting tacticity. 2. pertaining to or characterized by taxis.

tacticity (tak-ti′sĭ-te) the condition of having a regular chemical arrangement of the units making up the main chain of a polymer.

tactile (tak′til) [L. *tactilis*] pertaining to the touch.

tactilogical (tak″tĭ-loj′e-kal) pertaining to touch: tactual.

taction (tak′shun) [L. *tactio*] 1. a touch; an act of touching. 2. the sense of touch; perception by the touch.

tactometer (tak-tom′ĕ-ter) [L. *tactus* touch + *metrum* mea-

sure] an instrument for measuring the acuteness of the sense of touch; an esthesiometer.

tactor (tak′tor) a tactile end-organ.

tactual (tak′tu-al) [L. *tactus* touch] pertaining to or accomplished by the touch.

tactus (tak′tus) [L.] touch. **t. erudi′tus** [L. "trained touch"], delicacy of touch acquired by practice. **t. ex′pertus** [L. "experienced touch"], t. eruditus.

TAD a regimen of 6-thioguanine, ara-C (cytarabine), and daunomycin, used in cancer chemotherapy.

Taenia (te′ne-ah) [L. "a flat band," "bandage," "tape"] a genus of large tapeworms of the family Taeniidae. **T. africa′na**, *T. saginata*. **T. antarc′tica**, a species from dogs in Antarctic regions. **T. balan′iceps**, a species from dogs and bobcats in Nevada and New Mexico. **T. brachyso′ma**, a species infesting dogs in Italy. **T. brem′neri**, *T. confusa*. **T. cer′vi**, a species from dogs in Denmark. **T. confu′sa**, a species found in the Mississippi Valley and in East Africa, believed by some to be a variant of *T. saginata*. Called also *T. bremneri*. **T. cras′siceps**, a cestode parasite of foxes in Alaska and Canada, found in rodents as an intermediate host. **T. crassicol′lis**, *T. taeniaeformis*. **T. cucurbiti′na**, *T. saginata*. **T. demararien′sis**, *Raillietina demarariensis*. **T. echinococ′cus**, *Echinococcus granulosus*. **T. ellip′tica**, *Dipylidium caninum*. **T. hydati′gena**, a tapeworm that is parasitic in dogs and wild carnivora; the larval stage (cysticercus) is found in the liver and abdominal cavity of various ruminants and rodents and occasionally in other animals, including man. Called also *T. marginata*. **T. krab′bei**, a cestode parasite found in the bobcat, dog, and wolf in the northern United States, Canada, Alaska, and Iceland. **T. madagascarien′sis**, *Raillietina madagascariensis*. **T. margina′ta**, *T. hydatigena*. **T. mediocanella′ta**, *T. saginata*. **T. na′na**, *Hymenolepis nana*. **T. o′vis**, a species parasitic in dogs; found in the musculature of sheep and goats as intermediate hosts. **T. philippi′na**, *T. saginata*. **T. pisifor′mis**, a tapeworm commonly found in dogs; also parasitic in cats, foxes, wolves, and other animals; the cysticercus (larval stage) is found in the liver and peritoneal cavity of rabbits. **T. sagina′ta**, the commonest of the large tapeworms of man, a species 12 to 25 feet long, found in the adult form in the human intestine. The cysticerci (larval stage) develop in the muscles and other tissues of cattle and other ruminants. Human infection usually results from eating raw or rare beef. Called also *beef* or *unarmed tapeworm* and *T. africana*. **T. so′lium**, the pork tapeworm, a species 3 to 6 feet long found in the adult form in the human intestine; the cysticerci (larval stage) occur most often in the muscle and various tissues of the pig, but are also found in man, monkeys, camels, sheep, and dogs. It gains access to the human intestine through ingestion of inadequately cooked or measly pork (see *cysticercosis*) It is rare in the United States. Called also *armed* or *measly tapeworm*. **T. taeniaefor′mis**, a cestode parasite commonly found in cats, and more rarely in dogs, foxes, and other animals, having rats, mice, and other rodents as intermediate hosts. Called also *T. crassicollis*.

taenia (te′ne-ah), pl. *tae′niae* [L. "a flat band," "bandage," "tape"] 1. [NA] a flat band or strip of soft tissue; called also *tenia* [NA alternative]. 2. an individual organism of the genus *Taenia*; called also *tenia*. **tae′niae acus′ticae**, striae medullares ventriculi quarti. **t. choroi′dea** [NA], the line of attachment of the lateral choroid plexus to the medial wall of the cerebral hemisphere; specifically, the line of attachment of the ependyma of the ventricle to the ependyma of the choroid plexus; called also *t. telae*. **t. cine′rea**, a band of gray substance on the floor of the fourth ventricle outside the striae medullares ventriculi quarti. **tae′niae co′li** [NA], three thickened bands, about ¼ inch wide and one-sixth shorter than the colon, formed by the longitudinal fibers in the muscular tunic of the large intestine, and extending from the root of the vermiform appendix to the rectum, where the fibers spread out and form a continuous layer encircling the tube; they include the *t. libera*, *t. mesocolica*, and *t. omentalis*. Called also *taeniae of Valsalva*. **t. fim′briae**, the line of attachment of the choroid plexus of the lateral ventricle to the fimbria of the hippocampus; see *taenia fornicis* [NA]. **t. for′nicis** [NA], **t. of fornix**, the line of attachment of the choroid plexus of the lateral ventricle to the fornix, including the line of its attachment to the fimbria of the hippocampus (taenia

fimbriae). **t. of fourth ventricle**, t. ventriculi quarti. **t. hippocam′pi**, fimbria hippocampi. **t. li′bera** [NA], the thickened band formed by anterior longitudinal muscle fibers of the large intestine, almost equidistant from the taenia mesocolica and the taenia omentalis. **t. medulla′ris thal′ami op′tici, medullary t. of thalamus**, t. thalami. **t. mesoco′lica** [NA], the thickened band of longitudinal muscle fibers of the large intestine along the site of attachment of the mesocolon. **t. omenta′lis** [NA] the band of longitudinal muscle fibers of the large intestine along the site of attachment of the greater omentum. **t. pon′tis**, a bundle of fibers sometimes found on the cerebral peduncle along the rostral border of the pons, running an isolated course to the cerebellum between the superior and middle cerebellar peduncles. **tae′niae pylo′ri**, ligamenta pylori. **t. semicircula′ris cor′poris stria′ti**, stria terminalis. **t. tec′tae**, stria longitudinalis lateralis corporis callosi. **t. te′lae**, t. choroidea. **t. termina′lis**, 1. t. fimbriae. 2. crista terminalis atrii dextri. **t. thal′ami**, [NA], **t. of thalamus**, the line of attachment of the ependymal cells of the roof of the third ventricle to the dorsal margin of the thalamus; called also *medullary t. of thalamus*, *t. medullaris thalami*, and *t. of third ventricle*. **t. of third ventricle**, t. thalami. **t. tu′bae**, a thickened band of peritoneum along the upper border of the uterine tube. **taeniae of Valsalva**, taeniae coli. **t. ventric′uli quar′ti**, [NA], taeniae of fourth ventricle: the line of attachment of the ependymal cells of the choroid plexus to the ependyma along the edge of the caudal part of the fourth ventricle. **t. ventric′uli ter′tii**, t. thalami.

taenia- [L. *taenia* tape] a combining form denoting relationship to tapeworms or to bands or strips of soft tissue. See also *tenia-*, and words beginning thus.

taeniacide (te′ne-ah-sīd″) [L. *taenia* tapeworm + *caedere* to kill] 1. destructive to tapeworms. 2. an agent that destroys tapeworms.

taeniae (te′ne-e) genitive and plural of *taenia*.

taeniafugal (te″ne-ah-fu′gal) expelling tapeworms.

taeniafuge (te′ne-ah-fūj″) [*taenia* + L. *fugare* to put to flight] an agent that expels tapeworms.

taenial (te′ne-al) 1. of or pertaining to tapeworms of the genus *Taenia*. 2. tenial (def. 1).

Taeniarhynchus (te″ne-ah-ring′kus) a genus name formerly given to beef tapeworms; see *Taenia confusa* and *T. saginata*.

taeniasis (te-ni′ah-sis) infection with any of the tapeworms of the genus *Taenia*.

taeniform (ten′ĭ-form) [*taenia* + L. *forma* shape] resembling the organism *Taenia*, or a tapeworm.

Taeniidae (te-ni′ĭ-de) a family of medium-sized or large tapeworms of the order Cyclophyllidea, subclass Cestoda, which are parasitic in mammals, including man; three medically important genera are *Taenia*, *Multiceps*, and *Echinococcus*.

taeniola (te-ni′o-lah) [L., dim of *taenia*] a slender bandlike structure. **t. cine′rea**, taenia cinerea. **t. cor′poris callo′si of Reil**, lamina rostralis.

Taeniorhynchus (te″ne-o-ring′kus) a genus of mosquitoes now called *Mansonia*.

tag (tag) 1. a small appendage, flap, or polyp. 2. label. **auricular t's**, rudimentary appendages of auricular tissue occurring on the face along the line of union of the first branchial arch. **cutaneous t.**, acrochordon. **radioactive t.**, a radioisotope that has been incorporated within a biological chemical by metabolic or other processes. **skin t.**, acrochordon.

Tagamet (tag′ah-met) trademark for preparations of cimetidine.

tagatose (tag′ah-tōs) a ketohexose, $CH_2OH(CHOH)_3 \cdot CO \cdot CH_2OH$, isomeric with fructose.

tagliacotian rhinoplasty or **operation** (tah″le-ah-ko′she-an) see under *rhinoplasty*.

taiga (tī′ga) [Russian] the northern coniferous forest biome, found primarily in Canada, northern Europe, and Siberia.

tail (tāl) [L. *cauda*; Gr. *oura*] 1. any slender appendage; called also *cauda* [NA]. 2. the appendage that extends from the posterior trunk of animals. **axillary t.**, processus lateralis glandulae mammariae. **t. of caudate nucleus,** cauda nuclei caudati. **t. of epididymis,** cauda epididymidis. **occult t.,** supernumerary segments of the coccyx, present in the buttock. **t. of pancreas,** cauda pancreatis. **polyadenylate (polyA) t.,** a sequence of up to 200 adenylate residues that is added to the 3′ end of many primary mRNA transcripts during post-transcriptional processing in eukaryotes. Its function seems to be protection of the mRNA from enzymatic degradation in the cytosol. **t. of Spence,** the projection of mammary glandular tissue extending into the axillary region, sometimes forming a visible mass which may enlarge premenstrually or during lactation. **t. of spleen,** extremitas anterior lienis. **t. of spermatozoon,** the flagellum of a spermatozoon, which contains the axonema; it presents four regions: the *neck, middle piece, principal piece,* and *end piece.*

tailgut (tāl′gut) a prolongation of the hindgut into the tail of the early embryo.

Taillefer's valve (tah″u-fārs′) [Louis Auguste Horace Sydney Timeléon *Taillefer,* French physician, 1802–1868] see under *valve.*

Taka-diastase (tah′kah di′as-tās) [Jokichi *Takamine,* Japanese chemist in New York, 1854–1922] trademark for an amylolytic enzyme formed by the action of the spores of the fungus *Aspergillus oryzae* on the bran of wheat; used as a digestant.

Takata's reagent (tak-ah′tahz) [Maki *Takata,* Japanese pathologist, born 1892] see under *reagent.*

Tal. abbreviation for L. *tal′is,* such a one.

talalgia (tal-al′je-ah) pain in the heel or ankle.

talampicillin hydrochloride (tal-amp″ĭ-sil′in) chemical name: [2S-[2α,5α,6β(S*)]]-6-[(aminophenylacetyl)-amino]-3,3-dimethyl-7-oxo-4-thia-1-azabicyclo[3.2.0]heptane-2-carboxylic acid 1,3-dihydro-3-oxo-1-isobenzofuranyl ester monohydrochloride. The monohydrochloride salt of the phthalidyl ester of ampicillin, $C_{24}H_{23}N_3O_6S \cdot HCl$, having the actions and uses of ampicillin (q.v.).

talantropia (tal″an-tro′pe-ah) [Gr. *talanton* balance + *tropos* a turning + *-ia*] nystagmus.

talar (ta′lar) of or pertaining to the talus.

Talauma elegans (tal-aw′mah el′e-gans) a plant of Java, valued as a stomachic, antispasmodic, and antihysteric remedy.

talbutal (tal′bu-tal) [USP] chemical name: 5-(1-methylpropyl)-5-(2-propenyl)-2,4-6(1H,3H,5H)-pyrimidinetrione. An intermediate-acting barbiturate, $C_{11}H_{16}N_2O_3$, occurring as a white, crystalline powder; used as a sedative and hypnotic, administered orally.

talc (talk) [USP] a native, hydrous magnesium silicate, sometimes containing a small proportion of aluminum silicate, used as a dusting powder; called also *purified talc.*

talcosis (tal-ko′sis) a morbid condition resulting from the inhalation or implantation in the body of talc. **pulmonary t.,** pneumoconiosis resulting from inhalation of particles of talc.

talcum (tal′kum) [L.] talc.

taleranol (tah-ler′ah-nōl) chemical name: [3S-(3R*,7R*)]-3,4,5,6,7,8,9,10,11,12-decahydro-7,14,16-trihydroxy-3-methyl-1H-2-benzoxacyclotetradecin-1-one; an enzyme that inhibits gonadotropin, $C_{18}H_{26}O_5$.

tali (ta′li) genitive and plural of *talus.*

taliacotian (tal″e-ah-ko′shan) tagliacotian.

taliped (tal′ĭ-ped) 1. clubfooted. 2. a clubfooted person.

talipedic (tal″ĭ-pe′dik) clubfooted.

talipes (tal′ĭ-pēz) [L. "clubfoot"] a congenital deformity of the foot, which is twisted out of shape or position; called also *clubfoot.* See also under *pes.* **t. calcaneoval′gus,** a deformity of the foot in which the heel is turned outward from the midline of the body and the anterior part of the foot is elevated. **t. calcaneova′rus,** a deformity of the foot in which the heel is turned toward the midline of the body and the anterior part is elevated. **t. calca′neus,** a deformity in which the foot is dorsiflexed. **t. cavoval′gus,** a deformity in which the longitudinal arch of the foot is abnormally high, and the heel is turned outward from the midline of the body. **t. ca′vus,** a deformity in which the longitudinal arch of the foot is abnormally high. **t. equinoval′gus,** a deformity of the foot in which the heel is elevated and turned outward from the midline of the body. **t. equinova′rus,** a deformity of the foot in which the heel is turned inward from the midline of the leg and the foot is plantar flexed. This

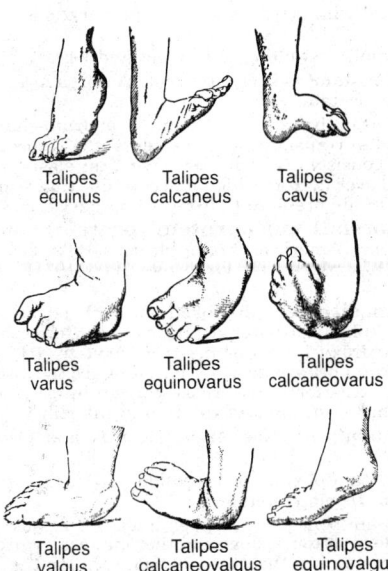

Talipes equinus — Talipes calcaneus — Talipes cavus
Talipes varus — Talipes equinovarus — Talipes calcaneovarus
Talipes valgus — Talipes calcaneovalgus — Talipes equinovalgus

is associated with the raising of the inner border of the foot (supination) and displacement of the anterior part of the foot so that it lies medially to the vertical axis of the leg (adduction). With this type of foot the arch is higher (cavus) and the foot is in equinus (plantar flexion). This is a typical clubfoot. **t. equi′nus,** a deformity in which the foot is plantar flexed, causing the person to walk on the toes without touching the heel. **t. planoval′gus,** a deformity of the foot in which the heel is turned outward from the midline of the leg and the outer border of the anterior part of the foot is higher than the inner border. This results in a lowering of the longitudinal arch. The condition may be congenital and permanent, or it may be spasmodic as a result of reflex spasm of the muscles controlling the foot. **t. val′gus,** a deformity of the foot in which the heel is turned outward from the midline of the leg. **t. va′rus,** a deformity of the foot in which the heel is turned inward from the midline of the leg.

talipomanus (tal″ĭ-pom′ah-nus) [L. *talipes* clubfoot + *manus* hand] a congenital deformity of the hand; see *clubhand.*

tallow (tal′o) suet.

Tallqvist's scale (tahl′kvists) [Theodor Waldemar *Tallqvist,* Finnish physician, 1871–1927] see under *scale.*

Talma's disease, operation (tal′mahz) [Sape *Talma,* physician in Utrecht, 1847–1918] see *myotonia acquisita,* and see under *operation.*

talocalcaneal (ta″lo-kal-ka′ne-al) pertaining to the talus and calcaneus.

talocalcanean (ta″lo-kal-ka′ne-an) talocalcaneal.

talocrural (ta″lo-kroo′ral) [L. *talus* ankle + *crus* leg] pertaining to the talus and the bones of the leg.

talofibular (ta″lo-fib′u-lar) pertaining to the talus and the fibula.

talon (tal′on) [L. "bird's claw"] 1. the claw of a bird of prey or other predatory animal. 2. a talonlike structure or part. **t. noir** (nwahr) [F. "black claw"], black heel.

talonavicular (ta″lo-nah-vik′u-lar) pertaining to the talus and the navicular bone.

talopram hydrochloride (tal′o-pram) chemical name: 1,3-dihydro-N,3,3-trimethyl-1-phenyl-1-isobenzofuran propanamine hydrochloride; a catecholamine potentiator, $C_{20}H_{25}NO \cdot HCl$.

taloscaphoid (ta″lo-skaf′oid) talonavicular.

talose (ta′lōs) an aldehyde hexose, $CH_2OH(CHOH)_4CHO$, an isomer of glucose.

talotibial (ta″lo-tib′e-al) pertaining to the talus and the tibia.

talus (ta′lus), pl. *ta′li* [L. "ankle"] [NA] the highest of the tarsal bones and the one which articulates with the tibia and fibula to form the ankle joint; called also *ankle, ankle bone, astragalus, astragaloid bone,* and *os tarsi tibialis.*

Talwin (tal′win) trademark for preparations of pentazocine.

tama (ta′mah) swelling of the feet and legs.

Tambocor (tam′bo-kor) trademark for a preparation of flecainide acetate.

tambour (tam-boor′) [Fr. "drum"] a drum-shaped appliance used in transmitting movements in a recording instrument. It consists of a cylinder having an elastic membrane stretched over it, from which passes a tube that transmits the changes in air pressure to a recording device.

Tamm-Horsfall mucoprotein (protein) (tam hors′fal) [Igor *Tamm*, American virologist, born 1922; Frank Lappin *Horsfall*, Jr., American virologist, 1906–1971] see under *mucoprotein*.

tamoxifen citrate (tah-moks′ĭ-fen) chemical name: (Z)-2-[4-(1,2-diphenyl-1-butenyl)phenoxy]-N,N-dimethylethanamine 2-hydroxy-1,2,3-propanetricarboxylate (1:1). A nonsteroidal oral antiestrogen, $C_{26}H_{29}NO \cdot C_6H_8O_7$, used in the palliative treatment of breast cancer in postmenopausal women and to stimulate ovulation in infertility.

tampan (tam′pan) see *Argas persicus* and *Ornithodorus moubata*.

tampicin (tam′pĭ-sin) a glycoside, $C_{34}H_{54}O_{14}$, from Tampico jalap, *Ipomoea simulans*.

tampon (tam′pon) [Fr. "stopper, plug"] a pack; a pad or plug made of cotton, sponge, or other material; variously used in surgery to plug the nose, vagina, etc., for the control of hemorrhage or the absorption of secretions.

tamponade (tam″pon-ād′) [Fr. *tamponner* to stop up] surgical use of a tampon; also pathologic compression of a part, as compression of the heart by pericardial fluid (see *cardiac t.*). **balloon t.**, esophagogastric tamponade by means of a device with a triple-lumen tube and two inflatable balloons, the third lumen providing for aspiration of blood clots. **cardiac t.**, acute compression of the heart which is due to effusion of the fluid into the pericardium or to the collection of blood in the pericardium from rupture of the heart or penetrating trauma. **chronic t.**, chronic compression of the heart caused by chronic pericardial effusion and pericardial thickening. **esophagogastric t.**, the exertion of direct pressure against bleeding esophageal varices by insertion of a tube with a sausage-shaped balloon in the esophagus and a globular one in the stomach and inflating the balloons. **heart t.**, cardiac t.

tamponage (tam-po-nahzh′) tamponade.

tamponing (tam′pon-ing) tamponade.

tamponment (tam-pon′ment) the act of plugging with a tampon.

Tamus (ta′mus) [L.] a genus of dioscoreaceous plants. *T. communis* L. is an old-world plant called black bryony, used homeopathically; the root is considered to be rubifacient and diuretic.

tan (tan) 1. to brown or become brown from exposure to sun or to ultraviolet light. 2. the brownish color of the skin acquired by such exposure, resulting from darkening of preformed melanin (Meirowsky phenomenon), accelerated formation of new melanin, and retention of melanin in the epidermis as a result of retardation of keratinization.

tandamine hydrochloride (tan′dah-mēn) chemical name: 9-ethyl-1,3,4,9-tetrahydro-N,N,1-trimethylthiopyrano[3,4-*b*]indole-1-ethanamine monohydrochloride; an antidepressant, $C_{18}H_{26}N_2S \cdot HCl$.

Tandearil (tan-de′ah-ril) trademark for a preparation of oxyphenbutazone.

tangentiality (tan-jen″she-al′ĭ-te) a pattern of speech characterized by oblique, digressive, or irrelevant replies to questions; the responses never approach the point of the questions. It differs from *circumstantiality*, in which the responder eventually reaches the point. The term is roughly synonymous with *loosening of associations*.

tanghin (tan′gēn) the apocynaceous tree, *Cerbera tanghin*, of Madagascar, and its exceedingly poisonous seed; also an extract prepared from it, which is used as an arrow poison.

Tangier disease (tan-jēr′) [*Tangier* Island, in Chesapeake Bay, where the disease was first discovered] see under *disease*.

tangle (tang′g'l) a knot or snarl. **neurofibrillary t's**, intracellular knots or clumps of neurofibrils seen in the cerebral cortex in Alzheimer's disease.

tangoreceptor (tang″go-re-sep′tor) [L. *tangere* to touch + *receptor*] a sense organ that responds only to physical contact, such as touch.

tank (tank) an artificial receptacle for liquids. **activated sludge t.**, a tank for the aerobic digestion of sewage. Screened and sedimented raw sewage, treated with an inoculum of activated sludge (q.v.), flows slowly or intermittently through the tank while being aerated vigorously. The process oxidizes much of the organic material in the sewage, thus reducing the biological oxygen demand. **digestion t.**, a deep septic tank in which sludge is separated and submitted to anaerobic bacterial action to reduce the mass of material and produce a less offensive product. **Dortmund t.**, a deep vertical flow settling tank for removing sludge from sewage. **Emsher t.**, digestion t. **Hubbard t.**, a tank in which a patient may be immersed for the purpose of permitting him to take underwater exercise. **Imhoff t.**, digestion t. **septic t.**, a tank for the receipt of raw sewage, in which putrefaction occurs owing to the presence of anaerobic bacteria, and solid material settles to the bottom. **settling t.**, a basin in which the rate of flow of the sewage is reduced and the sludge allowed to settle out.

tannal (tan′al) aluminum tannate. **insoluble t.**, basic aluminum tannate, a brown-yellow astringent powder, $Al_2(OH)_4(C_{14}H_9O_9)_2 + 10H_2O$.

tannalin (tan′al-in) a formaldehyde solution.

tannase (tan′ās) an esterase found in various tannin-bearing plants and produced in cultures by *Aspergillus niger* and *Penicillium glaucum*, which catalyzes the hydrolysis of various ester linkages in gallic acid compounds.

tannate (tan′āt) [L. *tannas*] any salt of tannic acid; all the tannates are astringent.

tannic acid (tan′ik) [USP] a tannin obtained from nutgalls and used as an astringent for the mucous membranes of the mouth and throat and as suppositories for the treatment of hemorrhoids; it is no longer used to treat burns because of the possibility of severe liver damage. Called also *gallotannic acid*, *tannin*, and, erroneously, *digallic acid*.

tannin (tan′in) tannic acid. **diacetyl t., t. diacetylate**, acetyltannic acid. **pathologic t.**, any tannin derived from galls, or vegetable excrescences due to a local disease of the plant. **physiologic t.**, any tannin normally produced by a healthy plant.

Tanret's reagent, test (reaction) (tahn-rāz′) [Charles *Tanret*, French chemist, 1847–1917] see under *reagent* and *tests*.

tantalum (tan′tah-lum) a rare metallic element: symbol, Ta; atomic number, 73; atomic weight, 180.948. It is a noncorrosive and malleable metal which has been used for plates or disks to replace cranial defects, for wire sutures, and for making prosthetic appliances.

tantrum (tan′trum) a violent display of bad temper.

tanycyte (tan′ĭ-sīt) [Gr. *tanyein* to stretch + *-cyte*] a modified ependymal cell of the median eminence, having a body that lies near the third ventricle and sending out processes that extend to the capillary plexus of the portal circulation. Its function is unknown, but it may transport hormones from the cerebrospinal fluid into the portal circulation or from hypothalamic neurons to the cerebrospinal fluid.

TAO (ta′o) trademark for preparations of troleandomycin.

taon (tah-on′) infantile beriberi occurring in the Philippine Islands.

tap (tap) 1. a quick, light blow. 2. to drain off fluid by paracentesis. **bloody t.**, a lumbar puncture in which the fluid obtained is bloody or pinkish. **front t.**, a tap on the muscles of the front of the leg, producing contraction of the muscles of the calf in spinal irritability. **heel t.**, reflex movement of the toes on tapping the heel, occurring in pyramidal tract damage. **spinal t.**, lumbar puncture.

Tapazole (tap′ah-zol) trademark for a preparation of methimazole.

tape (tāp) a long, narrow strip of fabric or other flexible material. **adhesive t.** [USP], a strip of fabric and/or film evenly coated on one side with a pressure-sensitive, adhesive mixture, the whole having high tensile strength, used for the application of dressings and sometimes to produce immobilization; formerly called *adhesive plaster*. **adhesive t., sterile**, adhesive tape, the adhesive surface of which is covered by strips of a protective material of equal width, and which is sterilized after packaging; formerly called *sterile adhesive plaster*. **Montgomery's t's,** see under *strap*.

tapeinocephalic (tap″ĭ-no-sĕ-fal′ik) characterized by tapeinocephaly.

tapeinocephaly (tap″ĭ-no-sef′ah-le) [Gr. *tapeinos* low-lying + *kephalē* head] a low form of the skull, which is also flattened at front, having a vertical index below 72.

tapetal (tah-pe′tal) pertaining to a tapetum, especially to the tapetum lucidum.

tapetum (tah-pe′tum), pl. *tape′ta* [L.; Gr. *tapētion*, dim. of *tapēs* a carpet, rug] 1. a covering structure, or layer of cells. 2. t. corporis callosi. **t. cellulo′sum,** a type of tapetum lucidum, being the more complex, more cellular type found in all but two species of the order Carnivora and in the seals. **t. choroi′deae,** t. lucidum. **t. cor′poris cal-lo′si** [NA], a stratum of commissural fibers of the corpus callosum on the superolateral aspect of the occipital horn of the lateral ventricle. **t. fibro′sum,** a type of tapetum lucidum, being the simpler, fibrous type found almost exclusively in hoofed animals, in a few fish, and in marsupials, elephants, and whales. **t. lu′cidum,** the iridescent pigment epithelium of the choroid of animals which gives their eyes the property of shining in the dark; called also *t. choroideae*. **t. ni′grum,** stratum pigmenti bulbi oculi. **t. o′culi,** stratum pigmenti retinae. **t. ventric′uli,** fasciculus longitudinalis superior cerebri.

tapeworm (tāp′werm) a parasitic intestinal cestode worm having a flattened, bandlike form. Those infecting man are principally of the genera *Taenia, Diphyllobothrium, Hymenolepis, Echinococcus,* and *Dipylidium*. The eggs of tapeworms are ingested by the intermediate host, whence they make their way into the tissues, where the larval stages are produced (see *plerocercoid; cysticercus;* and *hydatid cyst,* under *cyst*). When the flesh of the intermediate host is eaten, the larvae develop within the alimentary canal of the definitive host into adult tapeworms, which consists of an attachment organ, or scolex, an undifferentiated neck, and a strobila made up of a variable number of separate segments, or proglottids, each of which is hermaphroditic and produces eggs. **African t.,** *Taenia saginata.* **armed t.,** *Taenia solium.* **beef t.,** *Taenia saginata.* **broad t.,** *Diphyllobothrium latum.* **dog t.,** 1. *Echinococcus granulosus.* 2. *Dipylidium caninum.* **double-pored dog t.,** *Dipylidium caninum.* **dwarf t.,** *Hymenolepis nana.* **fish t.,** *Diphyllobothrium latum.* **fringed t.,** *Thysanosoma actinioides.* **heart-headed t.,** *Diphyllobothrium cordatum.* **hydatid t.,** *Echinococcus granulosus.* **Madagascar t.,** *Raillietina madagascariensis.* **Manson's larval t.,** *Diphyllobothrium mansonoides.* **measly t.,** *Taenia solium.* **pork t.,** *Taenia solium.* **rat t.,** *Hymenolepis diminuta.* **Swiss t.,** *Diphyllobothrium latum.* **unarmed t.,** *Taenia saginata.*

taphephobia (taf″ĕ-fo′be-ah) [Gr. *taphos* grave + *phobia*] irrational fear of being buried alive.

Tapia's syndrome (tap′e-ahz) [Antonio Garcia *Tapia*, Spanish otolaryngologist, 1875–1950] see under *syndrome*.

tapinocephalic (tap″ĭ-no-se-fal′ik) tapeinocephalic.

tapinocephaly (tap″ĭ-no-sef′ah-le) tapeinocephaly.

tapioca (tap″e-o′kah) a fecula, or starch, derived from the root of *Jatropha manihot*, or manioc; used as a food.

tapiroid (ta′pĭ-roid) resembling the snout of a tapir.

tapotage (tah-po-tahzh′) coughing and expectoration following percussion in the supraclavicular region: a sign sometimes obtained in pulmonary tuberculosis.

tapotement (tah-pōt-maw′) [Fr.] a tapping or percussing movement in massage; it includes clapping, beating, and punctation.

tar (tahr) a dark-brown or black, viscid liquid, obtained by roasting the wood of various species of pine, or as a by-product of the destructive distillation of bituminous coal. It is a mixture of complex composition, and is the source of a number of substances, such as cresol, creosol, guaiacol, naphthalene, paraffin, phenol, toluene, and xylene. Once used in chronic bronchitis, diarrhea, and diseases of the urinary organs, it now has only limited use in certain skin diseases, notably psoriasis and chronic eczematous disorders. **coal t.** [USP], tar obtained as a by-product of the destructive distillation of bituminous coal, used as a topical antieczematic and antipsoriatic. **gas t.,** a coal tar derived from the coal, rosin, petroleum, and other material used in gas

works. **juniper t.** [USP], the volatile oil obtained from the woody portions of *Juniperus oxycedrus,* L. (Pinaceae), occurring as a thick brown liquid with a bitter taste; used as a pharmaceutic necessity, and for the topical therapy of dermatoses. Called also *cade oil, Haarlem oil, silver balsam,* and *oleum juniperi empyrheumaticum.* **pine t.** [USP], a viscid, blackish brown liquid obtained by destructive distillation of the wood of various pine trees; used as a local antieczematic and rubefacient, applied topically, and has been used as a stimulating expectorant incorporated in syrups.

Tar's symptom (tahrz) [Aloys *Tar*, Budapest physician, born 1886] see under *symptom*.

Taractan (tar-ak′tan) trademark for a preparation of chlorprothixene.

Taraktogenos kurzii King (tar″ak-toj′e-nos kur′ze-e) a tropical tree whose seeds are a source of chaulmoogra oil; called also *Hydnocarpus heterophyllus* Kurz.

tarantula (tah-ran′tu-lah) a venomous spider whose bite causes local inflammation and pain, usually not to a severe extent. **American t.,** a large, dark, ferocious looking spider, *Eurypelma hentzii,* having a poisonous bite. **black t.,** a venomous spider of Panama, *Sericopelma communis.* **European t.,** the true tarantula, the large European wolf spider, *Lycosa tarentula,* the bite of which was believed to cause death.

Taraxacum (tah-rak′sah-kum) [L.] a genus of composite-flowered plants. The dried root of *T. officinale* Weber, the common dandelion or lion's tooth, contains taraxerol, choline, inulin, levulin, and pectin, and is a simple bitter.

tarbadillo (tahr″bah-dēl′yo) [Sp.] tabardillo.

tarbagan (tahr′bah-gan) marmot.

Tardieu's spots, test (tar-dyuz′) [Auguste Ambroise *Tardieu*, French physician, 1818–1879] see under *spot* and *tests*.

tardive (tahr′div) [Fr. "tardy, late"] marked by lateness, late; said of a disease in which the characteristic lesion is late in appearing.

tare (tār) 1. the weight of the vessel in which a substance is weighed. 2. to take the weight of a vessel which is to contain a substance, in order to allow for it when the vessel and the substance are weighed together.

tarentula (tah-ren′tu-lah) tarantula.

target (tahr′get) 1. an object or area toward which something is directed, such as the metal or plate of a roentgen ray tube on which the electrons impinge and from which the roentgen rays are sent out. 2. denoting a cell or organ that is selectively affected by a particular agent, e.g., a hormone or drug.

tarichatoxin (tar″ik-ah-tok′sin) a neurotoxin from the newt (*Taricha*), identical with tetrodotoxin (q.v.).

Tarin, Tarini, Tarinus (tah-rã′, tah-ri′ni, tah-ri′nus), Pierre. A French anatomist and encyclopedist (1700–1761) who wrote a history of anatomy and described many anatomical structures.

tariric acid (tar-ir′ik) 6-octadecynoic acid, a rare fatty acid containing a triple bond found in *Picramnia*, a genus of South American shrubs.

Tarnier's forceps (tar-ne-āz′) [Etienne Stéphene *Tarnier*, French obstetrician, 1828–1897] see under *forceps*.

tarsadenitis (tahr″sad-ĕ-ni′tis) an inflammation of the tarsus of the eyelid and of the meibomian glands.

tarsal (tahr′sal) [L. *tarsalis*] 1. pertaining to the tarsus of an eyelid or to the instep. 2. any of the bones of the tarsus.

tarsalgia (tahr-sal′je-ah) pain in the ankle or foot.

tarsalia (tar-sa′le-ah) the bones of the tarsus.

tarsalis (tahr-sa′lis) [L.] tarsal.

tarsectomy (tahr-sek′to-me) [*tarso-* + Gr. *ektomē* excision] 1. excision of the tarsus, or a part of it. 2. excision of a tarsal cartilage.

tarsectopia (tahr″sek-to′pe-ah) [*tarso-* + Gr. *ektopos* out of place + *-ia*] dislocation of the tarsus.

tarsitis (tahr-si′tis) inflammation of the tarsus, or margin of an eyelid; blepharitis.

tars(o)- [Gr. *tarsos* a broad flat surface] a combining form denoting relationship to the edge of the eyelid, or to the instep of the foot.

tarsocheiloplasty (tahr″so-ki′lo-plas″te) [tarso- + cheilo- + -plasty] a plastic operation upon the edge of the eyelid, as in treatment of trichiasis.

tarsoclasis (tahr-sok′lah-sis) [tarso- + Gr. klasis breaking] the operation of fracturing the tarsus of the foot.

tarsomalacia (tahr″so-mah-la′she-ah) [tarso- + malacia] softening of the tarsus of an eyelid.

tarsomegaly (tahr″so-meg′ah-le) enlargement of the os calcis.

tarsometatarsal (tahr″so-met″ah-tahr′sal) pertaining to the tarsus and the metatarsus.

tarso-orbital (tahr″so-or′bǐ-tal) pertaining to the tarsus of the eyelid and to the orbit.

tarsophalangeal (tahr″so-fah-lan′je-al) pertaining to the tarsus and the phalanges of the toes.

tarsophyma (tahr″so-fi′mah) [tarso- + Gr. phyma growth] any tarsal tumor.

tarsoplasia (tahr″so-pla′ze-ah) tarsoplasty.

tarsoplasty (tahr′so-plas″te) [tarso- + Gr. plassein to form] plastic surgery of the tarsus of an eyelid.

tarsoptosis (tahr″sop-to′sis) [tarso- + Gr. ptōsis falling] falling of the tarsus; flatfoot.

tarsorrhaphy (tahr-sor′ah-fe) [tarso- + -raphy] the operation of suturing together a portion of (partial t.) or the entire (total t.) upper and lower eyelids for the purpose of shortening or closing entirely the palpebral fissure. The terms external t., median t., and internal t. are used to indicate the portion of the lids brought together in partial tarsorrhaphy. Called also blepharorrhaphy.

tarsotarsal (tahr″so-tahr′sal) pertaining to the articulation between the two rows of tarsal bones.

tarsotibial (tahr″so-tib′e-al) pertaining to the tarsus and the tibia.

tarsotomy (tahr-sot′o-me) [tarso- + -tomy] the operation of incising the tarsus, or an eyelid; blepharotomy.

tarsus (tahr′sus) [L.; Gr. tarsos a frame of wickerwork; any broad flat surface] 1. [NA] the region of the articulation between the foot and the leg; see also tarsus osseus. 2. one of the plates of connective tissue forming the framework of an eyelid; see t. inferior palpebrae and t. superior palpebrae. **bony t.,** t. osseus. **t. infe′rior palpe′brae** [NA], the firm framework of connective tissue that gives shape to the inferior eyelid; called also ciliary, palpebral, or tarsal cartilage. **t. os′seus** [NA], the seven bones constituting the articulation between the foot and the leg: the talus, calcaneus, and navicular, in the proximal row; and the cuboid and the lateral, intermediate, and medial cuneiform bones, in the distal row. Called also bony t. **t. supe′rior palpe′brae** [NA], the firm framework of connective tissue that gives shape to the upper eyelid; called also ciliary, palpebral, or tarsal cartilage.

tartar (tahr′tahr) [L. tartarum; Gr. tartaron] 1. the lees, or sediment, of a wine cask; crude potassium bitartrate. 2. dental calculus. **borated t.,** a white powder prepared by evaporating a solution of 2 parts of sodium borate and 5 parts of potassium bitartrate. **cream of t.,** potassium bitartrate. **t. emetic,** antimony potassium tartrate; see under antimony. **vitriolated t.,** potassium tartrate.

tartarated (tahr′tahr-āt″ed) charged with tartaric acid.

tartaric acid (tar-tar′ik) 2,3-dihydroxybutanedioic acid, HOOC-CHOH-CHOH-COOH; its salts (tartrates) are used in food preparation (cream of Tartar) and have been used as cathartics. Tartaric acid has two asymmetric carbon atoms and has three structural isomers: two enantiomers, d- and l-tartaric acid, and one meso compound, meso-tartaric acid, which is a diastereomer of the other two.

tartarized (tahr′tahr-īzd) tartarated.

tartrate (tahr′trāt) [L. tartras] any salt of tartaric acid. **acid t.,** a bitartrate; any salt of tartaric acid in which one atom only of hydrogen is replaced by a base. **normal t.,** one in which two hydrogen atoms are replaced; various tartrates are employed as remedial agents.

tartrated (tahr′trāt-ed) [L. tartratus] containing tartar of tartaric acid.

tartrobismuthate (tahr″tro-biz′mu-thāt) bismuthotartrate.

tastant (tās′tant) any substance, e.g., salt, capable of eliciting gustatory excitation, i.e., stimulating the sense of taste.

taste (tāst) [L. gustus] the peculiar sensation caused by the contact of soluble substances with the tongue; the sense effected by the tongue, the gustatory and other nerves, and the gustation center. Four qualities are distinguished by taste: sweet, sour, salty, and bitter. **color t.,** pseudogeusesthesia. **franklinic t.,** a sour taste produced by stimulating the tongue with static electricity.

taste-blindness (tāst-blīnd′nes) inability to taste certain substances, such as phenylthiocarbamide.

taster (tās′ter) an individual capable of tasting a particular test substance, such as phenylthiocarbamide, used in certain genetic studies.

TAT thematic apperception test.

T.A.T. toxin-antitoxin.

Tatlockia micda′dei (tat-lok′e-ah mik-da′de-i) a waterborne legionellalike organism implicated as an etiologic agent of pneumonia, which is probably transmitted by aersols, direct inoculation into the lung during medical procedures involving the respiratory tract, and aspiration. Called also Pittsburgh pneumonia agent.

tätte melk (tet′ĕ melk) a food article in Sweden, prepared by inoculating milk with leaves of Pinguicula vulgaris, the butterwort, or bog violet.

tattooing (tah-too′ing) the insertion of permanent colors in the skin by introducing them through punctures. **t. of the cornea,** the permanent coloring of the cornea chiefly to conceal leukomatous spots.

Tatum (ta′tum), Edward Lawrie. American biochemist, 1909–1975; co-winner, with George Wells Beadle and Joshua Lederberg, of the Nobel prize for medicine or physiology in 1958 for proving that genes in bread mold transmit hereditary characteristics by controlling particular chemical reactions.

Tatumella (ta″tŭ-mel′ah) [Harvey Tatum, American bacteriologist] a genus of gram-negative, facultatively anaerobic, rod-shaped bacteria of the family Enterobacteriaceae, isolated from human clinical specimens, primarily from the respiratory tract. It is probably an infrequent opportunistic pathogen. The type species is T. pty′seos.

tau (tou, taw) [T, τ] the nineteenth letter of the Greek alphabet.

taurine (taw′rēn taw′rin) a strong organic acid, 2-aminoethanesulfonic acid, $H_2NCH_2CH_2SO_3H$, occurring in bile salts.

taur(o)- [L. taurus bull] a combining form denoting relationship to a bull, or to taurine.

taurochenodeoxycholate (taw″ro-ke″no-de-ok″se-ko′lāt) chenodeoxycholyltaurine.

taurochenodeoxycholic acid (taw″ro-ke″no-de-ok″se-ko′lik) chenodeoxycholyltaurine.

taurocholaneresis (taw″ro-ko″lan-er′ĕ-sis) [taurocholic acid + Gr. hairesis a taking] increase in the output or elimination of taurocholic acid in the bile. Cf. cholaneresis.

taurocholanopoiesis (taw″ro-ko-lan″o-poi-e′sis) synthesis of taurocholic acid by the liver.

taurocholate (taw″ro-ko′lāt) cholyltaurine.

taurocholemia (taw″ro-ko-le′me-ah) the presence of taurocholic acid in the blood.

taurocholic acid (taw″ro-ko′lik) cholytaurine.

taurodontism (taw″ro-don′tizm) [Gr. tauros bull + odont- + -ism] a variation in tooth form characterized by prism-shaped molars with large pulp spaces, resulting from branching of the root only in the middle (mesotaurodontism), or in the apical third or not at all (hypertaurodontism).

Taussig-Bing syndrome (taw′sig-bing) [Helen Brooke Taussig, American pediatrician, 1898–1986; Richard J. Bing, American surgeon, 1909–1986;] see under syndrome.

taut(o)- [Gr. tautos from to auto the same] a combining form meaning the same.

tautomenial (taw″to-me′ne-al) [tauto- + Gr. mēniaia menses] pertaining to the same menstrual period.

tautomer (taw′to-mer) a chemical compound exhibiting, or capable of exhibiting, tautomerism.

tautomeral (taw-tom′er-al) [tauto- + Gr. meros part] pertaining to the same part, especially sending processes to help in the formation of the white matter in the same side of the spinal cord; said of certain neurons and neuroblasts. See tautomeral cells, under cell.

tautomerase (taw-tom′er-ās) [EC 5.3.2] an enzyme of the isomerase class that catalyzes tautomeric reactions.

tautomeric (taw″to-mer′ik) exhibiting, or capable of exhibiting, tautomerism.

tautomerism (taw-tom′er-izm) [*tauto-* + Gr. *meros* part] the relationship that exists between two structural isomers that are in chemical equilibrium and freely change from one form to the other. **enol-keto t.**, tautomerism between two compounds, one an enol and the other a ketone, that equilibrate by transfer of a proton. The keto form usually predominates except where the enol form is stabilized by conjugation with other double bonds. See structural formulas at *enol*. **proton t.**, tautomerism in which an acidic proton is transferred from one position to another in the same molecule, e.g., enol-keto tautomerism. Called also *prototropy*. **ring-chain t.**, tautomerism involving open-chain and ring forms, as occurs with sugars. See *mutarotation*.

Tawara's node (tah-wah′rah) [Sunao *Tawara*, Japanese pathologist, 1873–1952] nodus atrioventricularis.

taxa (tak′sah) plural of *taxon*.

taxine (tak′sēn) an alkaloidal mixture obtainable from the yew, *Taxus baccata* L. (Taxaceae), and responsible for its poisonous properties.

taxis (tak′sis) [Gr. "a drawing up in rank and file"] 1. an orientation movement of a motile organism in response to an external stimulus. Such a response may be either positive (toward) or negative (away from the stimulus). Used also as a word termination, affixed to a stem denoting the nature of the stimulus (e.g., chemotaxis, phototaxis). Cf. *tropism*. 2. exertion of force in the manual replacement of a displaced or injured organ or structure, as in the reduction of a fracture or dislocation, or the replacement of a protruded intestine in hernia.

Taxodium distichum (L.) Rich. (Taxodiaceae) (taks-o′de-um dis′tik-um) the cypress, a timber tree of North America. The resin was formerly used in rheumatism.

taxology (taks-ol′o-je) taxonomy.

taxon (tak′son), pl. *tax′a* [Gr. *taxis* a drawing up in rank and file + *on* neuter ending] a particular group (category) into which related organisms are classified; the main categories are (in ascending order): species, genus, family, order, class, phylum, and kingdom.

taxonomic (tak″so-nom′ik) pertaining to taxonomy.

taxonomist (taks-on′o-mist) a specialist in taxonomy.

taxonomy (tak-son′o-me) [L. *taxinomia*; Gr. *taxis* a drawing up in rank and file + *nomos* law] the orderly classification of organisms into appropriate categories (taxa) on the basis of relationships among them, with the application of suitable and correct names. **numerical t.**, an arithmetic method of classifying larger numbers of bacterial strains on the basis of their overall similarity to one another, according to the number of phenotypic characters they share, each character being given equal weight. Called also *adansonian*, or *numerical, classification*.

Taxopodida (tak″so-po′dĭ-dah) [*taxis* + Gr. *pous* foot] an order of bilaterally symmetrical, small biflagellate, planktonic marine protozoa (class Heliozoa, superclass Actinopoda) having siliceous spines and swimming by the rowing action of axopodia arranged in parallel longitudinal rows.

Tay's choroiditis (disease), sign, spot (tāz) [Warren *Tay*, English physician, 1843–1927] see under *choroiditis*, and see *cherry-red spot*, under *spot*.

Tay-Sachs disease (ta saks′) [Warren *Tay*; Bernard (Barney) *Sachs*, New York neurologist, 1858–1944] see under disease.

Taylor splint (apparatus) (ta′ler) [Charles Fayette *Taylor*, orthopedic surgeon in New York, 1827–1899] see under *splint*.

tazettine (tāz′ĕ-tin) a crystalline alkaloid, $C_{18}H_{21}O_5N$, from the bulbs of daffodils, including *Lycoris radiata* and *Narcissus tazetta*. Called also *sekisanine*.

tazolol hydrochloride (ta′zo-lōl) chemical name: (±)-1-[(1-methylethyl)amino]-3-(2-thiazolyloxy)-2-propanol monohydrochloride. An adrenergic, $C_9H_{16}N_2O_2O_2S \cdot HCl$, having mainly beta$_1$-adrenergic activity; a cardiotonic.

TB see under *tuberculin*.

Tb chemical symbol for *terbium*.

TBG thyroxine-binding globulin.

TBII TSH-binding inhibitory immunoglobulins.

TBP bithionol.

Tc chemical symbol for *technetium*.

TCD$_{50}$ median tissue culture dose; see *TCID$_{50}$*.

TCID$_{50}$ abbreviation for *median tissue culture infective dose:* that quantity of a cytopathogenic agent (virus) that will produce a cytopathic effect in 50 per cent of the cultures inoculated.

TCMI T cell—mediated immunity.

Td tetanus and diphtheria toxoids, adult type.

TD$_{50}$ median toxic dose; a dose that produces a toxic effect in 50 per cent of a population.

TDA TSH-displacing antibody.

TDE a moderately toxic chlorinated hydrocarbon pesticide (tetrachlorodiphenylethane); called also *DDD* (dichlorodiphenyldichlorothane).

t.d.s. abbreviation for L. *ter di′e sumen′dum*, to be taken three times a day.

Te 1. chemical symbol for *tellurium*. 2. tetanus.

TEA tetraethylammonium.

tea (te) [L. *thea*] 1. the dried leaves of *Camellia sinensis* (L.) Kuntze, containing caffeine, theophylline, tannic acid, and a pleasant volatile oil; also a decoction thereof, used as a stimulating beverage and soothing warm drink for various abdominal discomforts. 2. any decoction or infusion. **beef t.**, an infusion of lean beef. **pectoral t.**, an aqueous infusion of expectorant and demulcent herbs and aromatics.

TEAC tetraethylammonium chloride.

Teale's amputation (operation) (tēlz) [Thomas Pridgin *Teale*, Sr., English surgeon, 1801–1868] see under *amputation*.

tear (tār) 1. to pull apart or in pieces by force. 2. to wound or injure, especially by ripping apart or rending; lacerate. 3. laceration. **cemental t., cementum t.,** complete or partial detachment of a fragment of cementum from the root surface of a tooth, especially that occurring in association with occlusal trauma. Called also *cemental* or *cementum fracture*.

tears (tērz) [L. *lacrimae*; Gr. *dakrya*] 1. the watery secretion of the lacrimal glands which serves to moisten the conjunctiva; the secretion is slightly alkaline and saline. 2. small, naturally formed, droplike masses of a gum or resin. **crocodile t.**, lacrimation on chewing and eating; see *syndrome of crocodile tears*.

teart (tert) 1. soil or plants that contain unusual amounts of molybdenum. 2. molybdenosis of farm animals caused by feeding on vegetation grown on soil that contains unusual amounts of molybdenum.

tease (tēz) to pull a tissue apart with needles for microscopical examination.

teaspoon (te′spoon) a household unit of capacity, containing about 5 milliliters.

teat (tēt) the nipple of the mammary gland.

TeBG testosterone-estradiol–binding globulin.

tebutate (teb′u-tāt) USAN contraction for tertiary butyl acetate.

technetium (tek-ne′she-um) a metallic element, atomic number 99, having no stable isotopes or naturally occurring radioactive isotopes; symbol Tc. **t. 99m**, a metastable state of ^{99}Tc having a half-life of 6.03 hours; it decays by isomeric transition emitting gamma rays, primarily 140 keV photons, and is the most commonly used radionuclide in nuclear medicine. **t. Tc 99m aggregated albumin** [USP], a sterile, aqueous suspension of normal human serum that has been denatured to produce aggregates of controlled particle size that are labeled with ^{99m}Tc; used for lung scanning, administered intravenously. Called also *technetated* (^{99m}Tc) *aggregated albumin* (human). **t. Tc 99m etidronate**, a radiopharmaceutical imaging agent used for bone scans; it is a stannous chelate of ^{99m}Tc and etidronate, a diphosphonate compound that localizes in bone tissue and (unlike polyphosphate) is not hydrolyzed by enzymes. **t.-99m pertechnetate**, the ionic form of technetium 99m, Tcat$_4^-$, used in scanning of the brain, thyroid, salivary glands, stomach, heart, and joints and in the preparation of other ^{99m}Tc radiopharmaceuticals.

technic (tek′nik) technique.

technical (tek′nĭ-kal) pertaining to technique.

technician (tek-nish′an) a person trained in and expert in the performance of technical procedures.

technique (tek-nēk′) [Fr.] the method of procedure and the details of any mechanical process or surgical operation. See also under *method, treatment, maneuver, Table of Stains,* etc. **Begg t.,** an orthodontic technique employing a fixed multibanded appliance that incorporates a concept of differential light forces and uses a modified ribbon arch attachment and elastics (Begg appliance). Tipping the crowns of teeth to be moved, rather than moving them laterally, is used in the technique, thereby minimizing the use of orthodontic force. **dilution-filtration t.,** a blood culture technique in which any culture inhibitors present in the blood are diluted out and red blood cells are removed before the sample is filtered and cultured, thereby permitting the identification of organisms in about 24 hours. **Enzyme-Multiplied Immunoassay T.** see *EMIT.* **fluorescent antibody t.,** an immunofluorescence technique in which antigen in tissue sections is located by homologous antibody labeled with fluorochrome (the single-layer technique) or by treating the antigen with unlabeled antibody followed by a second layer of labeled antiglobulin which is reactive with the unlabeled antibody (double-layer technique). Variations include direct, indirect, inhibition, and complement staining techniques. **hanging drop t.,** a method of microscopic examination of organisms suspended in a drop on a special concave microscope slide. **immunoperoxidase t.,** a method of histologic staining in which a peroxidase-labeled antibody that binds to antigen is added to tissue, and the sites of its localization are revealed by addition of a chromogenic substrate system that produces a colored reaction product visible by light microscopy. Cf. *peroxidase-antiperoxidase (PAP) t.* **Jerne plaque t.,** a hemolytic technique for detecting antibody-producing cells: a suspension of presensitized lymphocytes is mixed in an agar gel with erythrocytes; after a period of incubation, complement is added and a clear area of lysis of red cells can be seen around each of the antibody-producing cells. **Kleinschmidt t.,** rupture of the virion by osmotic shock so that viral DNA is exposed. **Kristeller t.,** see under *method.* **Laurell t.,** 1. crossed immunoelectrophoresis (Laurell's first technique). 2. rocket immunoelectrophoresis (Laurell's second technique). **Leboyer t.,** see under *method.* **Mohs′ t.,** a technique of microscopically controlled serial excision of skin cancers in which the tissue to be removed is first fixed in situ with zinc chloride paste (*Mohs′ chemosurgery*), or in which only serial excisions of fresh tissue are used for microscopic analysis (*Mohs′ surgery*). **Oakley-Fulthorpe t.,** double diffusion in one dimension; see under *diffusion.* **Orr t.,** see under *treatment.* **Ouchterlony t.,** double diffusion in two dimensions; see under *diffusion.* **Oudin t.,** a single diffusion (see under *diffusion*) technique in which agar containing antiserum is placed in a test tube and antigen is layered over it; precipitin lines form where the concentrations of each antigen and antibody are equivalent. **peroxidase-antiperoxidase (PAP) t.,** a technique for detecting antigen or antibody in tissue sections. The tissue section is incubated with rabbit antibody specific for the antigen to be detected, followed by an excess of antirabbit IgG. A complex of horseradish peroxidase and rabbit antiperoxidase is added; these are linked to the antigen-bound antibody by the antirabbit IgG. The PAP complexes are then stained by incubation with a chromogenic substrate to produce a colored reaction product. **push-back t.,** a surgical procedure designed to reposition the soft palate posteriorly and reestablish velopharyngeal competence. Called also *push-back procedure.* **Rebuck skin window t.,** a technique used to study the inflammatory process; an area of skin is abraded until capillary bleeding occurs and a coverslip or chamber containing balanced salt solution is applied. This permits direct observation of inflammatory cells migrating into the site; polymorphonuclear leukocytes predominate at about 10 hours; macrophages predominate at about 4 days. **scintillation counting t.,** a method of determining the amount of radioactivity by use of a scintillation crystal and appropriate electronic circuitry. **Seldinger t.,** a technique for percutaneous puncture of arteries or veins, used in angiography and cardiac catheterization. **Southern blot t.,** a technique for transferring DNA fragments separated by agarose gel electrophoresis to a nitrocellulose filter, on which specific DNA fragments can then be detected by their hybridization to radioactive probes. **squash t.,** a method of preparing cells for chromosome study, suspending them in hypotonic solution, then incubating them and exposing them to colchicine for one hour; after fixing and staining, a drop of the stained material is placed on a glass slide and covered with a glass slip, which is then pressed against the slide with one thumb. **time diffusion t.,** a form of spinal anesthesia in which the anesthetic, of low specific gravity, is injected by lumbar puncture, with the patient in the sitting position. The anesthetic is allowed to flow upward for a measured number of seconds and then the patient is placed in the horizontal position. **Trueta t.,** see under *treatment.* **Western blot t.,** a technique for analyzing and identifying protein antigens: the proteins are separated by electrophoresis in polyacrylamide gel, then transferred ("blotted") onto a nitrocellulose membrane or treated paper, where they bind in the same pattern as they formed in the gel. The antigen is overlaid first with antibody, then with anti-immunoglobulin or protein A labeled with a radioisotope, fluorescent dye, or enzyme.

technocausis (tek″no-kaw′sis) [Gr. *technē* art + *kausis* burning] use of the actual cautery.

technologist (tek-nol′o-jist) technician.

technology (tek-nol′o-je) [Gr. *technē* art + *logos* treatise] scientific knowledge; the sum of the study of a technique.

teclozan (tek′lo-zan) chemical name: *N,N′*-[1,4-phenylenebis(methylene)]bis[2,2-dichloro-*N*-(2-ethoxyethyl)acetamide; an antiamebic, $C_{20}H_{28}Cl_4N_2O_4$.

Tectibacter (tek″tĭ-bak′ter) [L. *tectum* covering + -*bacter*] a genus of bacteria of uncertain affiliation that are parasites of paramecia.

tectocephalic (tek″to-sĕ-fal′ik) characterized by tectocephaly.

tectocephaly (tek″to-sef′ah-le) [L. *tectum* roof + Gr. *kephalē* head] scaphocephaly.

tectology (tek-tol′o-je) [Gr. *tektōn* builder + -*logy*] the science which treats of the building up of organisms from structured elements; the doctrine of structure, a division of morphology.

tectorial (tek-to′re-al) [L. *tectum* roof] of the nature of a roof or covering, as the tectorial membrane.

tectorium (tek-to′re-um), pl. *tecto′ria* [L. "roof"] membrana tectoria ductus cochlearis.

tectospinal (tek″to-spi′nal) extending from the tectum mesencephali to the spinal cord; see also under *tract.*

tectum (tek′tum) any rooflike structure. **t. mesenceph′ali** [NA], **t. of mesencephalon,** the roof of the mesencephalon: that part of the tegmentum of the mesencephalon comprising the tectal lamina and the cranial and caudal colliculi.

T.E.D. threshold erythema dose.

teeth (tēth) see *tooth.*

teething (tēth′ing) the entire process which results in the eruption of the teeth.

Teflon (tef′lon) trademark for preparations of polytef (polytetrafluoroethylene). See also *polymer fume fever,* under *fever.*

tegafur (teg′ah-fur) an investigational cancer chemotherapeutic agent, which is 5-fluorouracil (5-FU) attached to a tetrahydrofuran moiety analogous to the ribose and deoxyribose moieties in the active metabolites of 5-FU. It acts like a depot form of 5-FU and potential uses are the same as those of 5-FU.

tegmen (teg′men), pl. *teg′mina* [L. "cover"] any covering, or shelter; used in anatomical nomenclature as a general term to designate a covering structure or roof. **t. an′tri,** t. tympani. **t. cel′lulae,** t. mastoideum. **t. cra′nii,** calvaria. **t. cru′ris,** tegmentum, def. 2. **t. mastoideotympan′icum,** the tegmen mastoideum and tegmen tympani, which together roof over the mastoid cells. **t. mastoid′eum,** the bony roof of the mastoid cells. **t. tym′pani,** 1. [NA] the thin layer of translucent bone, on the petrous part of the temporal bone in the floor of the middle cranial fossa, separating the tympanic antrum from the cranial cavity; called also *roof of tympanum.* 2. paries tegmentalis cavi tympani. **t. ventric′uli quar′ti** [NA], the roof of the fourth ventricle, formed by the superior and inferior medullary vela.

tegmental (teg-men′tal) pertaining to or of the nature of a tegmen or tegmentum.

tegmentum (teg-men′tum), pl. *tegmen′ta* [L.] 1. a covering. 2. t. mesencephali. 3. the dorsal part of each cerebral peduncle; see also *t. mesencephali* and *pedunculus cerebri*. **t. au′ris,** membrana tympani. **hypothalamic t.,** subthalamic t. **t. mesenceph′ali** [NA], **t. of mesencephalon,** the dorsal part of the mesencephalon, formed by continuation of the dorsal parts of the cerebral peduncles across the median plane, and extending on each side from the substantia nigra to the level of the mesencephalic aqueduct. Called also *tegmentum*. **t. of pons,** pars dorsalis pontis. **t. pon′tis,** NA alternative for *pars dorsalis pontis*. **t. rhombenceph′ali,** pars dorsalis pontis. **subthalamic t.,** the portion of the tegmentum of the cerebral peduncle extending beneath the thalamus.

Tegopen (teg′o-pen) trademark for preparations of cloxacillin sodium.

Tegretol (teg′rĕ-tol) trademark for preparations of carbamazepine.

Teichmann's crystals, test (tīk′mahnz) [Ludwig Carl *Teichmann*-Stawiarski, German histologist, 1825–1895] see under *crystal* and *tests*.

teichoic acids (ti-ko′ik as′idz) a diverse group of polymers found in the cell wall and cell membrane of gram-positive bacteria. They have a backbone of sugar alcohol residues linked by phosphodiester bridges. Sugars are attached to the sugar alcohols by glycosidic linkages and may also be a part of the polymer backbone replacing a sugar alcohol. There are two types: glycerol teichoic acids, in which the sugar alcohol is glycerol, and ribitol teichoic acids, in which it is ribitol. The first occurs in both the cell wall and cell membrane, the second only in the cell wall. Several teichoic acids are responsible for antigenic properties of certain bacteria.

teichopsia (ti-kop′se-ah) [Gr. *teichos* wall + *-opsia*] the sensation of a luminous appearance before the eyes, with a zigzag, wall-like outline; called also *fortification spectrum*, *flittering scotoma*, and *scintillating scotoma*.

T-1824 Evans blue.

teinodynia (ti′′no-din′e-ah) tenodynia.

teknocyte (tek′no-sīt) [Gr. *teknon* that which is born + *kytos* cell] a young neutrophil leukocyte.

tektin (tek′tin) any of a group of insoluble structural proteins having elastic properties.

tela (te′lah), pl. *te′lae* [L. "something woven," "web"] any weblike tissue; [NA] a general term for a thin membrane resembling a web. **t. ara′nea,** a spider web. **t. cellulo′sa,** t. conjunctiva. **t. choroi′dea ventric′uli latera′li,** the lateral extension of the tela choroidea ventriculi tertii into the choroid fissure of the lateral ventricle of the brain; from it, vascular folds invaginate the ventricular ependyma to form the choroid plexus of the lateral ventricle. **t. chorioi′dea ventric′uli quar′ti,** t. choroidea ventriculi quarti. **t. chorioi′dea ventric′uli ter′tii,** t. choroidea ventriculi tertii. **t. choroidea of fourth ventricle,** t. choroidea ventriculi quarti. **t. choroidea of third ventricle,** t. choroidea ventriculi tertii. **t. choroi′dea ventric′uli quar′ti** [NA], a double layer or fold of pia mater between the cerebellum and the lower part of the roof of the fourth ventricle; the anterior layer of the fold, together with the ventricular ependyma, contains vascular fringes which comprise the choroid plexus. **t. choroi′dea ventric′uli ter′tii** [NA], a double layer or fold of pia mater which, together with the ventricular ependyma, forms the roof of the third ventricle; from the lower fold two vascular fringes invaginate the roof to form the choroid plexuses. **t. conjuncti′va** [NA], a general term used to designate connective tissue. **t. elas′tica** [NA], a general term used to designate elastic tissue. **t. subcuta′nea** [NA], the layer of loose connective tissue situated directly beneath the skin; called also *hypoderm, hypodermis, subcutaneous fascia,* and *superficial fascia.* **t. submuco′sa** [NA], the layer of loose connective tissue between the lamina muscularis mucosae and the tunica muscularis in most parts of the digestive, respiratory, urinary, and genital tracts. **t. submuco′sa bronchio′rum** [NA], the layer of tissue underlying the tunica mucosa of the bronchi. **t. submuco′sa co′li** [NA], the layer of tissue underlying the tunica mucosa of the colon. **t. submuco′sa esoph′agi,** NA alternative for *t. submucosa oesophagi.* **t. submuco′sa gas′tris** [NA], the tissue underlying the tu-

nica mucosa of the stomach; called also *t. submucosa ventriculi* [NA alternative]. **t. submuco′sa intesti′ni ten′uis** [NA], the submucous layer of the wall of the small intestine. **t. submuco′sa oesoph′agi** [NA], the layer of tissue underlying the tunica mucosa of the esophagus. Written also *t. submucosa esophagi* [NA alternative]. **t. submuco′sa pharyn′gis** [NA], the tissue underlying the tunica mucosa of the pharynx. **t. submuco′sa rec′ti** [NA], the submucous layer of the wall of the rectum. **t. submuco′sa tra′cheae** [NA], the tissue underlying the tunica mucosa of the trachea. **t. submuco′sa tu′bae uteri′nae,** the submucous layer of the wall of the uterus. **t. submuco′sa ventric′uli,** NA alternative for *t. submucosa gastris.* **t. submuco′sa vesi′cae urina′riae** [NA], the submucous layer of the wall of the urinary bladder. **t. subsero′sa** [NA], a layer of loose areolar tissue underlying the tunica serosa of various organs. **t. subsero′sa co′li** [NA], loose areolar tissue underlying the tunica serosa of the colon. **t. subsero′sa gas′tris** [NA], the tissue underlying the tunica serosa of the stomach; called also *t. subserosa ventriculi* [NA alternative]. **t. subsero′sa hep′atis** [NA], loose areolar tissue underlying the tunica serosa of the liver. **t. subsero′sa intesti′ni ten′uis** [NA], the subserous layer of the wall of the small intestine. **t. subsero′sa peritone′i** [NA], a web of loose areolar tissue underlying the tunica serosa of the peritoneum. **t. subsero′sa tu′bae uteri′nae** [NA], the subserous layer of the wall of the uterus; called also *tunica adventitia tubae uterinae.* **t. subsero′sa u′teri** [NA], the areolar tissue underlying the tunica serosa of the uterus. **t. subsero′sa ventric′uli,** NA alternative for *t. subserosa gastris.* **t. subsero′sa vesi′cae bilia′ris** [NA], the tissue underlying the serous coat of the gallbladder; called also *t. subserosa vesicae felleae* [NA alternative]. **t. subsero′sa vesi′cae fel′leae,** NA alternative for *t. subserosa vesicae biliaris.* **t. subsero′sa vesi′cae urina′riae** [NA], the subserous layer of the wall of the urinary bladder.

telae (te′le) [L.] genitive and plural of *tela.*

telalgia (tel-al′je-ah) pain occurring in a part distant from the lesion; referred pain.

telangiectasia (tel-an′′je-ek-ta′ze-ah) [*tele*-(1) + *angi*- + *ectasia*] permanent dilation of preexisting blood vessels (capillaries, arterioles, venules), creating small focal red lesions, usually in the skin or mucous membranes. Called also *telangiectasis.* **generalized essential t.,** that involving the entire body or localized to a large segment of the body; lesions may be discrete or confluent and macular, plaquelike, or retiform. **hereditary hemorrhagic t.,** an autosomal dominant vascular anomaly characterized by the presence of multiple small telangiectases of the skin, mucous membranes, gastrointestinal tract, and other organs, associated with recurrent episodes of bleeding from affected sites and gross or occult melena. Called also *Osler's disease, Osler-Weber-Rendu disease,* and *Rendu-Osler-Weber disease* or *syndrome.* **t. lymphat′ica,** lymphangioma formed by dilatation of the lymph vessels. **t. macula′ris erupti′va per′stans,** a rare form of mastocytosis, usually affecting adults, characterized by the presence of multiple hyperpigmented telangiectatic macules, located primarily on the trunk, but also on the extremities. **spider t.,** vascular spider. **unilateral nevoid t.,** see under *syndrome.*

telangiectasis (tel-an′′je-ek′tah-sis), pl. *telangiec′tases* [*tele*-(1) + *angi*- + *ectasis*] 1. the lesion produced by telangiectasia, which may present as a coarse or fine red line or as a punctum with radiating limbs (spider). 2. telangiectasia. **spider t.,** a focal network of dilated capillaries, radiating from a central arteriole, seen chiefly in pregnancy and in hepatic cirrhosis.

telangiectatic (tel-an′′je-ek-tat′ik) pertaining to or characterized by telangiectasia.

telangiectodes (tel-an′′je-ek-to′dēz) marked by telangiectasia.

telangiitis (tel-an′′je-i′tis) [*tele*-(1) + Gr. *angeion* vessel + *-itis*] inflammation of the capillaries.

telangion (tel-an′je-on) [*tele*-(1) + Gr. *angeion* vessel] a terminal artery.

telangiosis (tel′′an-je-o′sis) [*tele*-(1) + Gr. *angeion* vessel + *-osis*] any disease of the capillary vessels.

telar (te′lar) pertaining to, affecting, or resembling tela.

telarche (te-lar′ke) thelarche.

Teldrin (tel′drin) trademark for a preparation of chlorpheniramine maleate.

tele- 1. [Gr. *telos* end] a combining form denoting relationship to the end. 2. [Gr. *tēle* far off, at a distance] a combining form meaning operating at a distance, or far away.

telebinocular (tel″ĕ-bi-nok′u-lar) a prism-refracting instrument for use in orthoptic training.

telecanthus (tel″e-kan′thus) [*tele*-(1) + L.; Gr. *kanthos* canthus] abnormally increased distance between the medial canthi of the eyelids.

telecardiogram (tel″ĕ-kar′de-o-gram) the tracing obtained by telecardiography.

telecardiography (tel″ĕ-kar″de-og′rah-fe) [*tele*-(2) + Gr. *kardia* heart + *graphein* to write] the recording of an electrocardiogram by transmission of impulses to a site at a distance from the patient.

telecardiophone (tel″ĕ-kar′de-o-fōn″) [*tele*-(2) + Gr. *kardia* heart + *phōnē* voice] an apparatus for rendering heart sounds audible to listeners at a distance from the patient.

teleceptive (tel′ĕ-sep″tiv) pertaining to a teleceptor.

teleceptor (tel′ĕ-sep″tor) [*tele*-(2) + *receptor*] a sensory nerve terminal which is sensitive to stimuli originating at a distance; such nerve endings exist in the eyes, ears, and nose.

telecord (tel′ĕ-kord) an apparatus for attachment to an x-ray machine; by means of it each cardiac phase can be photographed in series.

telecurietherapy (tel″ĕ-ku″re-ther′ah-pe) [*tele*-(2) + *curietherapy*] treatment with a radioactive source, e.g., radium, located at a distance from the body.

teledendrite, teledendron (tel″ĕ-den′drīt′, tel″ĕ-den′dron) telodendron.

telediagnosis (tel″ĕ-di″ag-no′sis) [*tele*-(1) + *diagnosis*] determination of the nature of a disease at a site remote from the patient on the basis of transmitted telemonitoring data or closed-circuit television consultation.

telefluoroscopy (tel″e-floo″or-os′ko-pe) [*tele*-(2) + *fluoroscopy*] television transmission of fluoroscopic images for observation and study at a distant location.

telekinesis (tel″ĕ-ki-ne′sis) [*tele*-(2) + Gr. *kinēsis* movement] the power claimed by certain persons of moving objects without contact with the object moved; also motion produced without contact with a moving body.

telekinetic (tel″ĕ-ki-net′ik) pertaining to telekinesis.

telelectrocardiogram (tel″ĕ-lek″tro-kar′de-o-gram) telecardiogram.

telelectrocardiograph (tel″e-lek″tro-kar′de-o-graf) [*tele*-(2) + *electrocardiograph*] a device for transmission and remote reception of electrocardiographic signals.

telemedicine (tel″e-med′ĭ-sin) [*tele*-(1) + *medicine*] the provision of consultant services by off-site physicians to health care professionals on the scene, as by means of closed-circuit television.

telemetry (tĕ-lem′e-tre) [*tele*-(2) + Gr. *metron* measure] the making of measurements at a distance from the subject, the measurable evidence of the phenomena under investigation being transmitted by radio signals. See *radioelectrocardiography* and *radioencephalography*.

telemnemonike (tel″ĕ-ne-mon′ĭ-ke) [*tele*-(2) + Gr. *mnēmonikos* pertaining to memory] the gaining of consciousness of things in the memory of another person.

telencephal (tel-en′sĕ-fal) telencephalon.

telencephalic (tel″en-sĕ-fal′ik) pertaining to the telencephalon.

telencephalization (tel″en-sef″al-i-za′shun) the transfer to the telencephalon, during the process of evolution, of the direction of the more complex nerve reactions.

telencephalon (tel″en-sef′ah-lon) [*tele*-(1) + Gr. *enkephalos* brain] 1. [NA] the paired cerebral vesicles, which are the anterolateral evaginations of the prosencephalon, together with the median, unpaired portion, the lamina terminalis; from it the cerebral hemispheres are derived. See Plate accompanying *brain*. 2. the anterior of the two vesicles formed by specialization of the prosencephalon in the developing embryo. Called also *endbrain*.

teleneurite (tel″ĕ-nu′rīt) the end expansion of an axon.

teleneuron (tel″ĕ-nu′ron) [*tele*-(1) + Gr. *neuron* nerve] a nerve ending.

teleological (te″le-o-loj′ĭ-kal) 1. pertaining to teleology. 2. serving an ultimate purpose in development.

teleology (tel″e-ol′o-je) [*tele*-(1) + Gr. *logos* treatise] the doctrine of final causes, or of adaptation to a definite purpose.

teleomitosis (tel″e-o-mi-to′sis) [*tele*-(1) + *mitosis*] completed mitosis.

teleonomic (tel″e-o-nom′ik) pertaining to or having evolutionary survival value.

teleonomy (tel″e-on′o-me) [*teleo*- + Gr. *nomos*, law] the doctrine that the existence of a structure or a function in an organism implies that it has had evolutionary survival value.

teleopsia (tel″e-op′se-ah) [*tele*- + *-opsia*] a visual disturbance in which objects appear to be farther away than they actually are.

teleorganic (tel″e-or-gan′ik) necessary to life.

teleoroentgenogram (tel″e-o-rent-gen′o-gram) teleroentgenogram.

teleoroentgenography (tel″e-o-rent″gen-og′rah-fe) teleroentgenography.

teleost (tel′e-ost) a member of the Teleostei, comprising the higher bony fishes.

Telepaque (tel′ĕ-pāk) trademark for a preparation of iopanoic acid.

telepathist (tĕ-lep′ah-thist) a professed mindreader.

telepathize (tĕ-lep′ah-thīz) to affect by sympathetic or other subtle means.

telepathy (tĕ-lep′ah-the) [*tele*-(2) + Gr. *pathos* feeling] extrasensory perception of the mental activity of another person. Cf. *clairvoyance*.

teleradiography (tel″ĕ-ra″de-og′rah-fe) radiography with the radiation source 6 to 7 feet from the subject.

teleradium (tel″ĕ-ra′de-um) [*tele*-(2) + *radium*] a radium source located at a distance from the body.

telergic (tel-er′jik) pertaining to telergy.

telergy (tel′er-je) [*tele*-(2) + Gr. *ergon* work] 1. automatism. 2. a hypothetical action of one brain on another at a distance.

teleroentgenogram (tel″ĕ-rent-gen′o-gram) the picture or film obtained by teleroentgenography.

teleroentgenography (tel″ĕ-rent″gen-og′rah-fe) roentgenography with the x-ray tube 6½ to 7 feet away from the plate in order more nearly to secure parallelism of the rays.

teleroentgentherapy (tel″ĕ-rent″gen-ther′ah-pe) treatment with ionizing radiations from an x-ray source located at a distance from the body.

telesthesia (tel″es-the′ze-ah) [*tele*-(2) + Gr. *aisthēsis* perception + *-ia*] extrasensory perception of objects or conditions.

telesthetoscope (tel″es-thet′o-skōp) [*tele*-(2) + Gr. *aisthēsis* perception + *skopein* to examine] a combination of stethoscope and electrical amplification by which persons at a distance from the patient can hear the heart and lung sounds, as in demonstrating to a class or to a medical audience.

teletactor (tel″ĕ-tak′tor) [*tele*-(2) + L. *tangere* to touch] an instrument for communicating with the deaf by means of touch on a vibrating plate.

teletherapy (tel″ĕ-ther′ah-pe) [*tele*-(2) + Gr. *therapeia* treatment] treatment in which the source of the therapeutic agent, e.g., radiation, is at a distance from the body, as contrasted to contact therapy or brachytherapy.

telethermometer (tel″ĕ-ther-mom′ĕ-ter) an apparatus for determining temperature on which the reading is made at a distance from the object or subject being studied.

telluric (tĕ-lu′rik) 1. pertaining to or originating from the earth. 2. pertaining to the element tellurium.

tellurism (tel′u-rizm) [L. *tellus* earth] the alleged production of disease by emanations from the earth or soil (telluric effluvium, or miasma).

tellurite (tel′u-rīt) any salt of tellurous acid.

tellurium (tĕ-lu′re-um) [L. *tellus* earth] a nonmetallic or metalloid element; symbol, Te; specific gravity, 6.24; atomic weight, 127.60; atomic number, 52.

Tellyesniczky's fluid (mixture) (tel″yets-nits′kēz) [Kálmár *Tellyesniczky*, Budapest anatomist, 1868–1932] see under *fluid*.

tel(o)- [Gr. *telos* end]   a combining form denoting relationship to an end.

telobiosis (tel″o-bi-o′sis) [*telo-* + Gr. *biōsis* way of life]   the end-to-end union of embryos through operative procedures.

telocentric (tel″o-sen′trik)   having the centromere at the extreme end of the replicating chromosome, so that the chromosome consists of only one arm.

telocinesia, telocinesis (tel″o-si-ne′se-ah; tel″o-si-ne′sis)   telophase.

telocoele (tel′o-sēl) [*telo-* + Gr. *koilia* cavity]   the cavity of the telencephalon.

telodendria (tel″o-den′dre-ah)   plural of *telodendrion*.

telodendrion (tel″o-den′dre-on), pl. *teloden′dria*.   Telodendron.

telodendron (tel″o-den′dron) [*telo-* + Gr. *dendron* tree]   one of the many fine twiglike terminal branches of a neuron.

telogen (tel′o-jen)   the quiescent, or resting, phase of the hair cycle, following catagen, the hair having become a club hair and not growing further.

teloglia (tel-og′li-ah)   terminal Schwann cells associated with the motor nerve endings.

telognosis (tel″og-no′sis) [contracted from *telephonic diagnosis*]   diagnosis based on interpretation of roentgenograms transmitted by telephonic or radio communication.

telokinesis (tel″o-ki-ne′sis) [*telo-* + Gr. *kinēsis* motion]   telophase.

telolecithal (tel″o-les′ĭ-thal) [*telo-* + Gr. *lekithos* yolk]   having the yolk concentrated toward one pole which, because of that concentration, is designated the vegetal pole. See under *ovum*. Cf. *eutelolecithal*.

telolemma (tel″o-lem′ah) [*telo-* + Gr. *lemma* rind]   the twofold covering of a motor end-plate, made up of sarcolemma and an extension of Henle's sheath.

telomere (tel′o-mēr) [*telo-* + Gr. *meros* part]   a term applied to each of the extremities of a chromosome, which possess special properties, among them a polarity which prevents their reunion with any fragment after a chromosome has been broken.

telophase (tel′o-fāz) [*telo-* + Gr. *phasis* phase]   the last of the four stages of mitosis and of the two divisions of meiosis; it begins when the chromosomes arrive at the poles of the cell and the division of the cytoplasm starts. In plant cells the new cell wall that separates the daughter cells begins to form during this stage.

telophragma (tel″o-frag′mah) [*telo-* + Gr. *phragmos* a fencing in]   a name given to the Z band; see also *inophragma*.

teloreceptor (te′lo-re-sep″tor)   teleceptor.

telosynapsis (tel″o-sĭ-nap′sis) [*telo-* + Gr. *synapsis* conjunction]   the union of chromosomes end to end during meiosis. Cf. *parasynapsis*.

telotaxis (tel″o-tak′sis)   the tendency of an organism to maintain a constant angle to the source of a stimulus while it moves; observed in the behavior of social insects, such as bees and ants.

telotism (tel′o-tizm)   1. the complete performance of a function. 2. a complete erection of the penis.

telson (tel′son)   an appendage on the terminal segment of some arthropods, especially the stinging organ of a scorpion.

TEM   triethylenemelamine.

Temaril (tem′ah-ril)   trademark for preparations of trimeprazine tartrate.

temazepam (tĕ-maz′ĕ-pam)   chemical name: 7-chloro-1,3-dihydro-3-hydroxy-1-methyl-5-phenyl-2*H*-1,4-benzodiazepin-2-one; a minor tranquilizer, $C_{16}H_{13}ClN_2O_2$.

temefos (tem′ĕ-fos)   chemical name: *O,O′*-(thiodi-4,1-phenylene) *O,O,O′,O′*-trimethyl ester phosphorothioic acid; an organophosphorus insecticide, $C_{16}H_{20}O_6P_2S_3$, used as a veterinary ectoparasiticide.

Temin (te′min)   Howard Martin. American biologist, born 1934; co-winner, with David Baltimore and Renato Dulbecco, of the Nobel prize for medicine and physiology in 1975, for discoveries concerning the interaction between tumor viruses and the genetic material of host cells and the role of reverse transcriptase.

temodex (tem′o-deks)   chemical name: 2-hydroxyethyl ester 3-methyl-2-quinoxalinecarboxylic acid 1,4-dioxide; a veterinary growth stimulant, $C_{12}H_{12}N_2O_5$.

temp. dext.   abbreviation for L. *tem′pori dex′tro*, to the right temple.

temperament (tem′per-ah-ment) [L. *temperamentum* mixture]   an inherent, constitutional predisposition to react to stimuli in a certain way. **atrabilious t.**, melancholic t. **bilious t.**, choleric t. **choleric t.**, that attributed to predominance of yellow bile and characterized by anger and irascibility. **lymphatic t.**, phlegmatic t. **melancholic t.**, that attributed to predominance of black bile and characterized by depression. **phlegmatic t.**, that attributed to predominance of phlegm and characterized by apathy and impassivity. **sanguine t.**, that attributed to predominance of blood and characterized by cheerfulness and optimism.

temperantia (tem″per-an′she-ah)   sedatives.

temperature (tem′per-ah-tūr) [L. *temperatura*]   the degree of sensible heat or cold; the property of a system that determines whether or not the system is in thermal equilibrium with other systems; a measure of the escaping tendency of heat from a system. **absolute t.**, temperature reckoned from absolute zero (−273.15° C. or −459.67° F.), expressed on an absolute scale (Kelvin or Rankine). **body t.**, the temperature of the body: in cold-blooded animals it varies with environmental temperature; in warm-blooded animals it is usually constant within a narrow range. See *normal t.* **body t., basal,** the temperature of the body under conditions of absolute rest. Abbreviated B.B.T. **critical t.**, a temperature below which a gas may be liquefied by increased pressure. **maximum t.**, in bacteriology, the temperature above which growth does not take place. **mean t.**, the average temperature in a locality for a given period of time. **minimum t.**, in bacteriology, temperature below which growth does not take place. **normal t.**, that of the human body in health, about 98.6° F. or 37° C. when measured orally. This is maintained by the thermotaxic nerve mechanism, which maintains a balance between the thermogenetic, or heat-producing, and the thermolytic, or heat-dispelling, processes. **optimum t.**, the temperature promoting the most rapid growth of a given species of microorganism, or the temperature at which a reaction proceeds at maximum velocity. **room t.**, the ordinary temperature of a room, 65°–80° F. **subnormal t.**, temperature below the normal.

template (tem′plat) [Old Fr. *templet* a weaver's bar]   1. a pattern or mold. 2. in genetics, a strand of DNA or RNA (mRNA) that specifies the base sequence of a newly synthesized strand of DNA or RNA, the two strands being complementary. 3. in dentistry, a curved or flat plate used as an aid in setting teeth in a denture. **surgical t.**, a thin transparent resin base shaped to duplicate the form of the impression surface of an immediate denture and used as a guide for surgically shaping the alveolar process and its soft tissue covering to fit an immediate denture.

temple (tem′p'l) [L. *tempula*, dim. of *tempora*, pl. of *tempus*]   the lateral region on either side of the upper part of the head; see *tempora*.

tempolabile (tem″po-la′bīl) [L. *tempus* time + *labilis* unstable]   subject to change with the passage of time.

tempora (tem′po-rah) [L., pl. of *tempus*] [NA]   the temples: the region on either side of the head, above the zygomatic arch.

temporal (tem′po-ral) [L. *temporalis*]   1. pertaining to the lateral region of the head, above the zygomatic arch. 2. pertaining to time; limited as to time; temporary.

temporalis (tem-po-ra′lis) [L.]   pertaining to the lateral region of the head, above the zygomatic arch.

temporoauricular (tem″po-ro-aw-rik′u-lar)   pertaining to the temporal and auricular regions.

temporofacial (tem″po-ro-fa′shal)   pertaining to a temple and the face.

temporofrontal (tem″po-ro-fron′tal)   pertaining to the temporal and frontal bones or regions.

temporohyoid (tem″po-ro-hi′oid)   pertaining to the temporal and hyoid bones.

temporomalar (tem″po-ro-ma′lar)   temporozygomatic.

temporomandibular (tem″po-ro-man-dib′u-lar)   pertaining to the temporal bone and the mandible.

temporomaxillary (tem″po-ro-mak′sĭ-ler″e)   pertaining to the temporal bone, or region, and the maxilla.

temporo-occipital (tem″po-ro-oks-ip′ĭ-tal) pertaining to the temporal and occipital bones or regions.

temporoparietal (tem″po-ro-pah-ri′ĕ-tal) pertaining to the temporal and parietal bones or regions.

temporopontile (tem″po-ro-pon′tĭl) pertaining to or connecting the temporal lobe and the pons.

temporospatial (tem″po-ro-spa′shal) [L. *tempus* time + *spatium* space] pertaining to both time and space.

temporosphenoid (tem″po-ro-sfe′noid) pertaining to the temporal and sphenoid bones.

temporozygomatic (tem″po-ro-zi″go-mat′ik) pertaining to the temporal and zygomatic bones, or to the region of the zygomatic arch.

tempostabile (tem″po-sta′bĭl) [L. *tempus* time + *stabilis* stable] not subject to change with the passage of time.

temp. sinist. abbreviation for L. *tem′pori sinis′tro*, to the left temple.

temuline (tem′u-lēn) an alkaloid contained in seeds of darnel (*Lolium temulentum*) and at one time said to be toxic, though subsequent investigators have said the seeds are not toxic; the question is not yet settled.

tenacious (tĕ-na′shus) [L. *tenax*] holding fast; adhesive.

tenacity (tĕ-nas′ĭ-te) the quality of being tenacious; toughness; the condition of being tough. **cellular t.,** the inherent tendency of all cells to persist in a given form or direction of activity.

tenaculum (tĕ-nak′u-lum) [L.] 1. a hooklike instrument for seizing and holding tissues. 2. any fibrous band for maintaining structures in place. **t. ten′dinum,** retinaculum tendinum.

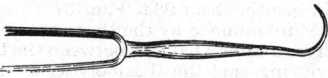

Tenaculum.

tenalgia (te-nal′je-ah) [Gr. *tenōn* tendon + *algos* pain + *-ia*] pain in a tendon.

tenderness (ten′der-nes) abnormal sensitiveness to touch or pressure. **pencil t.,** local tenderness on pressure with the rubber tip of a pencil. **rebound t.,** a sensation of pain felt on the release of pressure.

tendines (ten′dĭ-nēz) plural of *tendo*.

tendinitis (ten″dĭ-ni′tis) inflammation of tendons and of tendon-muscle attachments. **calcific t.,** inflammation and calcification of the subacromial or subdeltoid bursa, resulting in pain, tenderness, and limitation of motion in the shoulder. Called also *calcific bursitis* and *scapulohumeral bursitis*. **t. of horse,** inflammation of the flexor tendons, due to strain of wrenching, and causing great tenderness and lameness. **t. ossif′icans traumat′ica,** a condition in which areas of ossification develop in tendons as a result of trauma. **t. steno′sans, stenosing t.,** stenosing tendovaginitis of the flexor tendons of the finger.

tendinoplasty (ten′dĭ-no-plas″te) [L. *tendo* tendon + Gr. *plassein* to mold] the plastic surgery of the tendons.

tendinosuture (ten″dĭ-no-su′tūr) [L. *tendo* tendon + *sutura* sewing] the suturing of a tendon.

tendinous (ten′dĭ-nus) [L. *tendinosus*] pertaining to, resembling, or of the nature of a tendon.

tendo (ten′do), pl. *ten′dines* [L.] [NA] tendon: a fibrous cord of connective tissue in which the fibers of a muscle end and by which the muscle is attached to a bone or other structure. **t. Achil′lis,** t. calcaneus. **t. calca′neus** [NA], calcaneal tendon: a powerful tendon at the back of the heel which attaches the triceps surae muscle to the tuberosity of the calcaneus; called also *tendo Achillis* or *Achilles tendon*. **t. conjuncti′vus,** NA alternative for *falx inguinalis*. **t. cordifor′mis,** centrum tendineum. **t. cricoesopha′geus** [NA], cricoesophageal tendon: the tendon giving origin to the longitudinal fibers of the esophagus that come from the upper part of the lamina of the cricoid cartilage. **t. infundib′uli** [NA], tendon of infundibulum: a collagenous band connecting the posterior surface of the pulmonary annulus and the muscular infundibulum to the root of the aorta; called also *conus ligament*. **t. oc′uli, t. palpebra′rum,** ligamentum palpebrale mediale.

tendolysis (ten-dol′ĭ-sis) [L. *tendo* tendon + Gr. *lysis* dissolution] tenolysis.

tendomucin (ten″do-mu′sin) a mucin derivable from tendons and closely related to submaxillary mucin.

tendon (ten′dun) [L. *tendo;* Gr. *tenōn*] a fibrous cord by which a muscle is attached; see *tendo*. **Achilles t.,** tendo calcaneus. **calcaneal t.,** tendo calcaneus. **central t. of diaphragm,** centrum tendineum. **central t. of perineum,** centrum tendineum perinei. **common t.,** a tendon that serves more than one muscle. **conjoined t.,** falx inguinalis. **cordiform t. of diaphragm,** centrum tendineum. **coronary t's,** two fibrous rings, one surrounding the cardiac orifice of the aorta and the other the pulmonary trunk orifice; see *annuli fibrosi cordis*. **cricoesophageal t.,** tendo cricoesophageus. **hamstring t.,** see *hamstring*. **t. of Hector, heel t.,** tendo calcaneus. **t. of infundibulum,** tendo infundibuli. **intermediate t. of diaphragm,** centrum tendineum. **membranaceous t.,** aponeurosis. **patellar t., anterior, patellar t., inferior,** ligamentum patellae. **pulled t.,** disruption of the fibers attaching a muscle to its point of origin, occurring as the result of unusual muscular effort. **riders' t.,** injury to the adductor tendons of the thigh incurred in horseback riding. **slipped t.,** perosis. **trefoil t.,** centrum tendineum. **t. of Zinn,** zonula ciliaris.

tendonitis (ten″do-ni′tis) tendinitis.

tendoplasty (ten′do-plas″te) [L. *tendo* tendon + Gr. *plassein* to mold] plastic surgery of the tendons.

tendosynovitis (ten″do-sin″o-vi′tis) tenosynovitis.

tendotome (ten′do-tōm) tenotome.

tendotomy (ten-dot′o-me) tenotomy.

tendovaginal (ten″do-vaj′ĭ-nal) [L. *tendo* tendon + *vagina* sheath] pertaining to a tendon and its sheath.

tendovaginitis (ten″do-vaj″ĭ-ni′tis) 1. inflammation of a tendon and its sheath. 2. tenosynovitis.

tenebrimycin (tĕ-neb″rĭ-mi′sin) tobramycin.

tenectomy (te-nek′to-me) [Gr. *tenōn* tendon + *ektomē* excision] excision of a lesion of a tendon or of a tendon sheath.

tenemycin (ten″ĕ-mi′sin) tobramycin.

Tenericutes (ten″er-ik′u-tēz; te″ner-ĭ-ku′tēz) [L. *tener* soft + *cutis* skin] a division of bacteria of the kingdom Procaryotae made up of organisms that lack a rigid cell wall and do not contain muramic acid. The division, the organisms of which are commonly called the mycoplasmas, includes the class Mollicutes.

tenesmic (te-nez′mik) pertaining to or of the nature of tenesmus.

tenesmus (te-nez′mus) [L.; Gr. *teinesmos*] straining, especially ineffectual and painful straining at stool or in urination. **rectal t.,** painful, long-continued, and ineffective straining at stool. **vesical t.,** that which sometimes accompanies urination.

ten Horn see *Horn*.

tenia (te′ne-ah), pl. *te′niae* [L. *taenia*] 1. NA alternative for *taenia*. 2. taenia (def. 2).

teniacide (te′ne-ah-sīd″) taeniacide.

teniae (te′ne-e) genitive and plural of *tenia*.

teniafugal (ten″e-ah-fu′gal) taeniafugal.

teniafuge (te′ne-ah-fūj″) taeniafuge.

tenial (te′ne-al) 1. pertaining to tenia of anatomical nomenclature. 2. taenial (def. 1).

teniamyotomy (te″ne-ah-mi-ot′o-me) an operation involving a series of transverse incisions of the teniae coli; done in diverticular disease.

teniasis (te-ni′ah-sis) taeniasis.

tenicide (ten′ĭ-sīd) taeniacide.

teniform (ten′ĭ-form) taeniform.

tenifugal (te-nif′u-gal) taeniafugal.

tenifuge (ten′ĭ-fūj) taeniafuge.

tenioid (te′ne-oid) taeniform.

teniola (te-ne′o-lah) [L. *taeniola*] a thin, grayish ridge which separates the striae of the floor of the fourth ventricle from the cochlear part of the acoustic nerve; called also *taeni′ola cine′rea*.

teniotoxin (te″ne-o-tok′sin) a poisonous principle occurring in tapeworms.

teniposide (ten-ĭ-po′sīd) a semisynthetic derivative of podophyllotoxin used as an antineoplastic.

ten(o)-, tenont(o)- [Gr. *tenōn*, gen. *tenontos* tendon, from *teinein* to stretch] combining forms denoting relationship to a tendon.

tenodesis (ten-od′ĕ-sis) [*teno-* + Gr. *desis* a binding together] tendon fixation; suturing of the end of a tendon to a bone.

tenodynia (ten″o-din′e-ah) [*teno-* + Gr. *odynē* pain] pain in a tendon.

tenofibril (ten′o-fi″bril) tonofibril.

tenolysis (ten-ol′ĭ-sis) [*teno-* + Gr. *lysis* dissolution] the operation of freeing a tendon from adhesions; called also *tendolysis*.

tenomyoplasty (ten″o-mi′o-plas″te) [*teno-* + Gr. *mys* muscle + *plassein* to form] a plastic operation involving tendon and muscle.

tenomyotomy (ten″o-mi-ot′o-me) [*teno-* + Gr. *mys* muscle + *tomē* a cutting] excision of a portion of tendon and muscle.

Tenon's capsule (fascia, membrane), space (te′nonz) [Jacques René *Tenon*, French surgeon, 1724–1816] see *vagina bulbi* and *spatium intervaginale*.

tenonectomy (ten″o-nek′to-me) [*teno-* + Gr. *ektomē* excision] excision of a part of a tendon for the purpose of shortening it.

tenonitis (ten″o-ni′tis) 1. tendinitis. 2. inflammation of Tenon's capsule.

tenonometer (ten″o-nom′ĕ-ter) tonometer.

tenonostosis (ten″on-os-to′sis) tenostosis.

tenontagra (ten″on-ta′grah, ten-on′tag-rah) [*tenonto-* + Gr. *agra* seizure] a gouty affection of the tendons.

tenontitis (ten″on-ti′tis) inflammation of a tendon; tendinitis. **t. prolif′era calca′rea,** tendinitis.

tenont(o)- see *ten(o)-*.

tenontodynia (ten″on-to-din′e-ah) [*tenonto-* + Gr. *odynē* pain + *-ia*] pain in the tendons.

tenontography (ten″on-tog′rah-fe) [*tenonto-* + Gr. *graphein* to write] a written description or delineation of the tendons.

tenontolemmitis (ten-on″to-lem-mi′tis) [*tenonto-* + Gr. *lemma* rind + *-itis*] tenosynovitis.

tenontology (ten″on-tol′o-je) the sum of what is known regarding the tendons.

tenontomyoplasty (ten-on″to-mi′o-plas″te) tenomyoplasty.

tenontomyotomy (ten-on″to-mi-ot′o-me) tenomyotomy.

tenontophyma (ten-on″to-fi′mah) [*tenonto-* + Gr. *phyma* growth] a tumorous growth in a tendon.

tenontoplasty (ten-on′to-plas″te) tenoplasty.

tenontothecitis (ten-on″to-the-si′tis) [*tenonto-* + Gr. *thēkē* sheath + *-itis*] inflammation of a tendon sheath.

tenontotomy (ten″on-tot′o-me) tenotomy.

tenophyte (ten′o-fīt) [*teno-* + Gr. *phyton* growth] a growth or concretion in a tendon.

tenoplastic (ten″o-plas′tik) of or relating to tenoplasty.

tenoplasty (ten′o-plas″te) [*teno-* + Gr. *plassein* to shape] plastic surgery of the tendons; operative repair of a defect in a tendon.

tenoreceptor (ten″o-re-sep′tor) [*teno-* + *receptor*] a proprioceptor situated in tendon; such receptors are stimulated by contraction.

Tenormin (ten′or-min) trademark for a preparation of atenolol.

tenorrhaphy (ten-or′ah-fe) [*teno-* + Gr. *rhaphē* suture] the union of a divided tendon by a suture.

tenositis (ten″o-si′tis) tendinitis.

tenostosis (ten″os-to′sis) [*teno-* + Gr. *osteon* bone + *-osis*] ossification of a tendon.

tenosuture (ten″o-su′tūr) [*teno-* + L. *sutura* suture] tenorrhaphy.

tenosynitis (ten″o-si-ni′tis) tendovaginitis.

tenosynovectomy (ten″o-sin″o-vek′to-me) excision or resection of a tendon sheath.

tenosynovitis (ten″o-sin″o-vi′tis) inflammation of a tendon sheath. **t. acu′ta purulen′ta,** tenosynovitis with pus formation. **adhesive t.,** tenosynovitis in which the tendons become bound in an inflammatory mass. **t. crep′itans,** a form accompanied by a crackling sound in the soft tissues on movement. **gonococcic t., gonorrheal t.,** tenosynovitis due to metastatic gonococcal infection. **t. granulo′sa,** tuberculosis of tendon sheaths, which become filled with granulation tissue. **t. hypertroph′ica,** a condition marked by swellings along the tendons and their sheaths. **infectious t.,** a disease of chickens and turkeys caused by a reovirus; the tendons of the legs become infected and inflamed and often rupture; it is primarily egg-transmitted. **nodular t.,** giant cell tumor of tendon sheath; see under *tumor*. **t. sero′sa chron′ica,** tenosynovitis with serous effusion. **t. steno′sans,** a painful condition of the wrist, marked by thickening and narrowing of the tendon sheath of the extensor brevis and abductor longus pollicis (De Quervain). **tuberculous t.,** chronic tuberculous infection of tendon sheaths and bursae. **villonodular t.,** a condition characterized by exaggerated proliferation of synovial membrane cells, producing a solid tumor-like mass, commonly occurring in periarticular soft tissues and less frequently in joints. **villous t.,** chronic infection of tendon sheaths and bursa, with proliferation of villous projections from the surface of the membranes.

tenotome (ten′o-tōm) a cutting instrument used in tenotomy.

tenotomy (ten-ot′o-me) [*teno-* + *-tomy*] the cutting of an extraocular tendon for strabismus. **curb t.,** the operation of cutting an eye muscle in squint and inserting it farther back on the globe of the eye.

tenovaginitis (ten″o-vaj″ĭ-ni′tis) inflammation of a tendon sheath; tenosynovitis.

tense (tens) drawn tight; rigid.

Tensilon (ten′sĭ-lon) trademark for a solution of edrophonium chloride.

tensio-active (ten″se-o-ak′tiv) having an effect on surface tension.

tensiometer (ten″se-om′ĕ-ter) [*tension* + Gr. *metron* measure] an apparatus for measuring the surface tension of liquids.

tension (ten′shun) [L. *tensio*; Gr. *tonos*] 1. the act of stretching. 2. the condition of being stretched or strained; the degree to which anything is stretched or strained. 3. voltage. 4. the partial pressure of a gas in a fluid, e.g., of oxygen in blood. **arterial t.,** blood pressure within an artery; intra-arterial pressure. **electric t.,** electromotive force. **interfacial surface t.,** the tension or resistance to separation possessed by the film of liquid between two well-adapted surfaces, as by the thin film of saliva between the denture base and the tissues. **intraocular t.,** see under *pressure*. **intravenous t.,** venous pressure. **muscular t.,** the condition of moderate contraction produced by stretching a muscle. **oxygen t.,** that concentration of dissolved oxygen at which its partial pressure is in equilibrium with the liquid (solvent). **premenstrual t.,** see under *syndrome*. **surface t.,** the tension or resistance which acts to preserve the integrity of a surface, such as the tension or resistance to rupture possessed by the surface film of a liquid, or the tension or strain upon the surface of a liquid in contact with another substance with which it does not mix. **tissue t.,** a state of equilibrium between tissues and cells which prevents overaction of any part. **wall t.,** the circumferential stretching force in a vessel wall, usually expressed as a function of intraluminal pressure and the radius according to the Laplace equation.

tensometer (tens-om′ĕ-ter) an apparatus by which the tensile strength of materials can be determined.

tensor (ten′sor) [L., "stretcher," "puller"] any muscle that stretches or makes tense.

tent (tent) [L. *tenta*, from *tendere* to stretch] 1. a covering of fabric designed to enclose an open space, especially such an arrangement over a patient's bed for the purpose of administering oxygen or vaporized medication by inhalation. 2. a conical and expansible plug of soft material, as lint, gauze, etc., for dilating an orifice or for keeping a wound open, so as to prevent its healing except at the bottom. **oxygen t.,** a tent erected over a bed into which a constant flow of oxygen can be maintained. **sponge t.,** a slender, cone-shaped piece of compressed sponge used for dilating the ostium uteri. **steam t.,** a tent erected over a bed into which steam is passed; used in certain respiratory conditions.

tentacle (ten′tah-k'l) a slender whiplike appendage in animals that may function in prehension and feeding or as a sense organ.

tentative (ten′tah-tiv) experimental and subject to change.

tenthmeter (tenth-me′ter) one ten-millionth of a meter.

tentoria (ten-to′re-ah) plural of *tentorium*.

tentorial (ten-to′re-al) pertaining to the tentorium of the cerebellum.

tentorium (ten-to′re-um), pl. *tento′ria* [L. "tent"] an anatomical part resembling a tent or a covering. **t. cerebel′li** [NA], **t. of cerebellum,** the process of dura mater that supports the occipital lobes and covers the cerebellum. Its internal border is free and bounds the tentorial notch; its external border is attached to the skull and encloses the transverse sinus behind. **t. of hypophysis,** diaphragma sellae.

tentum (ten′tum) the penis.

Tenuate (ten′u-āt) trademark for preparations of diethylpropion hydrochloride.

tenulin (ten′u-lin) a crystalline principle, $C_{17}H_{22}O_5$, from the bitter weed *Helenium tenuifolium* and other species that is mildly sternutatory and poisonous to fish.

Tepanil (tep′ah-nil) trademark for preparations of diethylpropion hydrochloride.

tephromalacia (tef″ro-mah-la′she-ah) [Gr. *tephros* ash-colored + *malakia* softening] softening of the gray matter of the brain or cord.

tephromyelitis (tef″ro-mi″ĕ-li′tis) [Gr. *tephros* ash-colored + *myelos* marrow + *-itis*] inflammation of the gray substance of the spinal cord.

tephrosis (tef-ro′sis) [Gr. *tephrōsis*] incineration or cremation.

tephrylometer (tef″ril-om′ĕ-ter) [Gr. *tephros* ash-colored + *hylē* matter + *metron* measure] a graduated glass tube for measuring the thickness of the gray matter of the brain.

tepidarium (tep″ĭ-da′re-um) [L., from *tepidus* lukewarm] a warm bath: more correctly, a place for a warm bath.

tepor (te′por) [L. "lukewarmness"] gentle heat.

teprotide (tep′ro-tīd) chemical name: 2-L-tryptophan-3-de-L-leucine-4-de-L-proline-8-L-glutamine-bradykinin potentiator B; a nonapeptide, $C_{53}H_{76}N_{14}O_{12}$, that inhibits the enzyme which converts angiotensin I to the active form (angiotensin II) and thus has antihypertensive properties.

ter- [L. *ter* thrice] a prefix meaning three, three-fold.

tera- [Gr. *teras* monster] a combining form used in naming units of measurement to indicate a quantity one trillion (10^{12}) times the unit specified by the root with which it is combined. Symbol, t.

teras (ter′as), pl. *ter′ata* [L.; Gr.] a monster. **ter′ata anadid′yma,** anadidymus; sometimes applied to a double monster with duplication of the cephalic pole and single toward the podalic pole. **ter′ata kata-anadid′yma,** anakatadidymus. **ter′ata katadid′yma,** katadidymus; sometimes applied to a double monster with duplication of the podalic pole and single toward the cephalic pole.

terata (ter′ah-tah) [Gr.] plural of *teras*.

teratic (ter-at′ik) [Gr. *teratikos*] monstrous; having the characters of a monster.

teratism (ter′ah-tizm) [Gr. *teratisma*] an anomaly of formation or development; the condition of a monster. See under *teras, monster,* and *monstrum,* and names of specific monsters.

terat(o)- [Gr. *teras,* gen. *teratos* monster] a combining form denoting relationship to a monster.

teratoblastoma (ter″ah-to-blas-to′mah) a neoplasm containing embryonic elements and differing from a teratoma in that its tissue does not represent all the germinal layers.

teratocarcinogenesis (ter″ah-to-kar″sĭ-no-jen′ĕ-sis) the production of teratomas.

teratocarcinoma (ter″ah-to-kar″sĭ-no′mah) a malignant neoplasm consisting of elements of teratoma with those of embryonal carcinoma or choriocarcinoma, or both; occurring most often in the testis.

teratogen (ter′ah-to-jen) an agent or factor that causes the production of physical defects in the developing embryo.

teratogenesis (ter″ah-to-jen′ĕ-sis) [*terato-* + Gr. *genesis* production] the production of physical defects in offspring in utero.

teratogenetic (ter″ah-to-jĕ-net′ik) pertaining to teratogenesis.

teratogenic (ter″ah-to-jen′ik) tending to produce anomalies of formation, or teratism.

teratogenous (ter″ah-toj′ĕ-nus) developed from fetal remains.

teratogeny (ter″ah-toj′ĕ-ne) teratogenesis.

teratoid (ter′ah-toid) [*terato-* + Gr. *eidos* form] resembling a monster.

teratologic, teratological (ter″ah-to-loj′ik; ter″ah-to-loj′ĭ-kal) pertaining to teratology.

teratology (ter″ah-tol′o-je) that division of embryology and pathology which deals with abnormal development and congenital malformations.

teratoma (ter″ah-to′mah), pl. *teratomas* or *terato′mata*. A true neoplasm made up of a number of different types of tissue, none of which is native to the area in which it occurs; most often found in the ovary or testis. **benign cystic t., cystic t.,** dermoid cyst, def. 2. **immature t.,** malignant t. **malignant t.,** a solid, malignant ovarian tumor resembling a dermoid cyst but composed of immature embryonal and/or extraembryonal elements derived from all three germ layers. Called also *immature t.* and *solid t.* **mature t.,** dermoid cyst, def. 2. **solid t.,** malignant t.

teratomata (ter″ah-to′mah-tah) plural of *teratoma*.

teratomatous (ter″ah-to′mah-tus) pertaining to or of the nature of teratoma.

teratosis (ter″ah-to′sis) [Gr. *teras* monster + *-osis*] teratism.

teratospermia (ter″ah-to-sper′me-ah) the presence of malformed spermatozoa in the semen.

terbium (ter′be-um) a rare metallic element; symbol, Tb; atomic number, 65; atomic weight, 158.924.

terbutaline sulfate (ter-bu′tah-lēn) [USP] chemical name: 5-[2-[(1,1-dimethylethyl)amino]-1-hydroxyethyl]-1, 3-benzenediol sulfate (2:1) salt. A β-adrenergic receptor agonist, $(C_{12}H_{19}NO_3)_2 \cdot H_2SO_4$, used as a bronchodilator, administered orally, by aerosol inhalation, and subcutaneously.

terchloride (ter-klo′rīd) trichloride.

tere (te′re) rub.

terebene (ter′ĕ-bēn) [L. *terebenum,* from *terebinthus* turpentine] a thin, yellowish, fragrant mixture of terpene hydrocarbons, $C_{10}H_{16}$, obtained from oil of turpentine by the action of sulfuric acid. It is antiseptic and expectorant, and has been used in catarrh, bronchitis, cystitis, fermentative dyspepsia, genitourinary disease, and as an application to gangrenous wounds, etc.

terebenthene (ter″ĕ-ben′thēn) oil of turpentine.

terebinth (ter′ĕ-binth) [L. *terebinthus*] 1. the tree *Pistacia terebinthus,* L. (Anacardiaceae), formerly a source of turpentine. 2. turpentine; it also produces pistacia galls, a source of tannin.

terebinthina (ter″ĕ-bin′thĭ-nah) [L.] turpentine.

terebinthinate (ter″ĕ-bin′thĭ-nāt) resembling or containing turpentine.

terebinthinism (ter″ĕ-bin′thĭ-nizm) poisoning with oil of turpentine; symptoms include hemoglobinemia, pulmonary edema, convulsions, and damage to nervous system and kidneys.

terebrant, terebrating (ter′ĕ-brant; ter′ĕ-brāt″ing) [L. *terebrans* boring] of a boring or piercing quality.

terebration (ter″e-bra′shun) [L. *terebratio*] an act of boring or trephining; also a boring pain.

teres (te′rēz) [L.] long and round, as a muscle.

terfenadine (ter-fen′ah-dēn) chemical name: α-[4-(1,1-dimethylethyl)phenyl]-4-(hydroxydiphenylmethyl)-1-piperidine butanol; an antihistaminic, $C_{32}H_{41}NO_2$.

Terfonyl (ter′fo-nil) trademark for preparations of sulfamethazine, sulfadiazine, and sulfamerazine (trisulfapyrimidines). See *trisulfapyrimidines oral suspension,* under *suspension.*

tergal (ter′gal) [L. *tergum* back] pertaining to the back or the dorsal surface.

ter in die (ter in de′a) [L.] three times a day.

term (term) [L. *terminus,* from Gr. *terma*] 1. a word or combination of words commonly used to designate a specific entity. 2. a limit or boundary. 3. a definite period or specified time of duration, such as the culmination of pregnancy at the end of nine months. **ontogenetic t's,** termini ontogenetici.

terminad (ter'mĭ-nad) [L. *terminus* limit + *ad* to] toward the end or terminus.

terminal (ter'mĭ-nal) [L. *terminalis*] 1. forming or pertaining to an end; placed at the end. 2. a termination, end, or extremity; see *ending.* **C t.,** C-terminal. **N t.,** N-terminal.

terminal addition enzyme DNA nucleotidylexotransferase.

terminal deoxynucleotidyl transferase (de-ok″se-noo″kle-o-ti′dil trans′fer-ās) DNA nucleotidylexotransferase.

terminal deoxyribonucleotidyl transferase (de-ok″se-ri″bo-noo″kle-o-ti′dil trans′fer-ās) DNA nucleotidylexotransferase.

terminatio (ter″mĭ-na′she-o), pl. *terminatio′nes* [L. "a limiting, bounding"] an ending; the site of discontinuation of a structure. **terminatio′nes nervo′rum li′berae** [NA], free nerve endings: those neural receptors having the simplest form, in which the peripheral nerve fiber divides into fine branches that terminate freely in connective tissue or epithelium.

termination (ter″mĭ-na′shun) [L. *terminatio*] a distal end; a cessation.

terminationes (ter″mĭ-na″she-o′nēz) [L.] plural of *terminatio.*

termini (ter'mĭ-ni) [L.] plural of *terminus.*

terminology (ter″mĭ-nol′o-je) [L. *terminus* term + *-logy*] 1. the vocabulary of an art or science. 2. the science which deals with the investigation, arrangement, and construction of terms.

terminus (ter'mĭ-nus), pl. *ter′mini* [L.] an ending. **ter′mini ad extremita′tes spectan′tes,** termini ad membra spectantes. **ter′mini ad mem′bra specta′n′tes,** the NA category embracing terms relating to the upper and lower limbs; called also *termini ad extremitates spectantes.* **ter′mini genera′les,** the NA category embracing general terms (that is, terms not applied exclusively to one specific structure but to all structures belonging to the particular category or to which the term is applicable). **ter′mini ontogenet′ici** [NA], ontogenetic terms: terms relating to development, including those pertaining to the placenta and other fetal membranes or other structures. **ter′mini si′tum et directio′nem par′tium cor′poris indican′tes,** the NA category embracing terms indicating position and direction of parts of the body.

termolecular (ter″mo-lek′u-lar) involving three molecules.

ternary (ter'nah-re) [L. *ternarius*] 1. third in order. 2. made up of three distinct chemical elements.

ternitrate (ter-ni′trāt) a trinitrate.

terodiline hydrochloride (ter″-o-di′lēn) chemical name: *N*-(1,1-dimethylethyl)-α-methyl-γ-phenylbenzepropanamine hydrochloride; a coronary vasodilator, $C_{20}H_{27}N\cdot HCl$, used in the treatment of angina of effort.

teroxide (ter-ok′sīd) [L. *ter* three + *oxide*] trioxide.

terpene (ter'pēn) any hydrocarbon of the formula $C_{10}H_{16}$, derivable chiefly from essential oils, resins, and other vegetable aromatic products. They may be acyclic, bicyclic, or monocyclic, and differ somewhat in physical properties.

terpenism (ter'pen-izm) poisoning with a terpene, resulting in vomiting, convulsions, unconsciousness, pulmonary edema, and tachycardia.

terpin (ter'pin) [L. *terpinum*] a product, $(CH_3)_2C(OH)\cdot C_6H_9\cdot(OH)\cdot CH_3$, obtained by the action of nitric acid on oil of turpentine and alcohol. **t. hydrate** [USP], chemical name: 4-hydroxy-α,α,4-trimethylcyclohexanemethanol

monohydrate. An expectorant, $C_{10}H_{20}O_2\cdot H_2O$, occurring as colorless, lustrous crystals or as a white powder; administered orally.

terpineol (ter-pin′e-ol) chemical name: *p*-menth-1-en-8-ol. An alcohol, $(CH_3)_2\cdot C(OH)\cdot C_6H_8\cdot CH_3$, consisting of a mixture of several isomers occurring in many essential oils; formerly used as an antiseptic, but now used as a perfuming agent.

Terpinol (ter'pĭ-nol) trademark for terpin hydrate.

terra (ter'ah) [L.] earth. **t. al′ba,** white clay, used as an adsorbent. **t. lem′nia,** a yellowish, ferruginous clay. **t. mer′ita,** turmeric. **t. pondero′sa,** barium sulfate, or synthetic baryta. **t. sigilla′ta** [L. "sealed earth" of ancient Lemnos], Armenian bole, sold in masses stamped with a seal. **t. silic′ea purifica′ta,** purified silicious or infusorial earth; silicious earth, boiled, washed, and calcined; it is a fine gray powder and is used in certain pharmaceutical operations.

Terramycin (ter'ah-mi″sin) trademark for preparations of oxytetracycline.

terrein (ter'e-in) a cyclopentane compound, $C_8H_{10}O_2$, formed by the action of *Aspergillus terreus.*

Terridens (ter'rĭ-denz) a genus of nematode worms. **T. diminu′tus,** a parasite frequently present in monkeys and occasionally in man; called also *Triodontophorus diminutus.*

territoriality (ter″ĭ-tor″ĭ-al′ĭ-te) a pattern of behavior in which an individual organism or a group of organisms delineates a territory and vigorously defends it against intrusion by other members of the same or competing species.

terror (ter'er) intense fright. **day t's,** pavor diurnus. **night t's,** pavor nocturnus.

tersulfide (ter-sul′fīd) trisulfide.

tertian (ter'shun) [L. *tertianus*] recurring every third day, counting the day of occurrence as the first day; applied to the type of fever caused by certain forms of malarial parasites. **double t.,** an intermittent fever in which there are two sets of recurrences, each tertian.

tertiary (ter'she-er-e) [L. *tertiarius*] third in order.

tertigravida (ter″she-grav′ĭ-dah) [L. *tertius* third + *gravida* pregnant] a woman pregnant for the third time; also written *gravida III.*

tertipara (ter-ship′ah-rah) [L. *tertius* third + *parere* to bring forth, produce] a woman who has had three pregnancies which resulted in viable offspring; also written *para III* or *III-para.*

tesicam (tes′ĭ-kam) chemical name: *N*-(4-chlorophenyl)-1,2,3,4,-tetrahydro-1,3-dioxo-4-isoquinolinecarboxamide; an anti-inflammatory, $C_{16}H_{11}ClN_2O_3.$

tesimide (tes′ĭ-mīd) chemical name: 5,6,7,8-tetrahydro-4-(phenylmethylene)isoquinolinedione; an anti-inflammatory, $C_{16}H_{15}NO_2.$

tesla (tes′lah) the SI unit of magnetic flux density, calculated as webers per square meter. It replaces the gauss. Abbreviated T.

Teslac (tes′lak) trademark for preparations of testolactone.

teslaization (tes″la-i-za′shun) [named for Nikola *Tesla,* a Serbian inventor in New York, 1856–1943] treatment by Tesla's currents; d'arsonvalism.

Tessalon (tes′sah-lon) trademark for a preparation of benzonatate.

tessellated (tes′el-lāt″ed) [L. *tessellatus; tessella* a square] divided into squares, like a checker board.

test¹ (test) [L. *testum* crucible] 1. an examination or trial. 2. a significant chemical reaction. 3. a reagent. For specific tests, see *Table of Tests.* See also under *method, phenomenon, reaction, reagent, sign,* and *symptom.*

test² (test) [L. *testa* shell] a loose or rigid, secreted or agglutinated, protective shell or shell-like covering or exoskeleton, seen in various invertebrates, including certain protozoa and echinoderms.

A TABLE OF TESTS

(See also under *method, phenomenon, reaction, reagent, sign* and *symptom.*)

abortus Bang ring (ABR) t.: a screening test for brucellosis in cattle; since *Brucella* agglutinins, as well as the organisms, are shed in the milk of infected cattle, a drop of hematoxylin-stained brucellae are mixed in a sample of pooled milk from the herd. After incubation, agglutinated bacteria are adsorbed by the globules of fat that rise to the surface to form a colored ring. Called also *milk-ring t.* and *ring t.*

ABR t., abortus Bang ring t.

acetoacetic acid t., see specific tests, including *Gerhardt's t., Harding and Ruttan's t., Hurtley's t., Lindemann's t.,* and *Nobel's t.* (1). See also *acetoacetic acid, methods for,* under *method.*

acid elution t. (*for fetal hemoglobin*): air-dried blood smears on a glass slide are fixed in 80 per cent methanol and immersed in a buffer at pH 3.3 (citric acid and sodium phosphate); all hemoglobulins are eluted except fetal hemoglobulin, which remains fixed in the red cells and can be detected after staining.

acidified serum t. (*for paroxysmal nocturnal hemoglobinuria*): the patient's washed red cells are incubated at 37° C in acidified normal serum or the patient's acidified serum; after centrifugation the supernatant is examined colorimetrically for hemolysis. In PNH red cells are abnormally susceptible to lysis by complement, which is activated by the alternate pathway in acidified serum, and hemolysis is observed in normal serum and to a lesser degree in the patient's serum. No hemolysis is observed when normal red cells or heat-inactivated serum are used as controls. Called also *Ham's t.*

acid-lability t.: a test to distinguish rhinoviruses from enteroviruses on the basis of their activity at various pH levels, rhinoviruses being inactivated by incubation at pH 3 to 5 for one to three hours.

acoustic reflex t., measurement of the acoustic reflex threshold; used to differentiate between conductive and sensorineural deafness and to diagnose acoustic neuroma.

Addis t.: after the patient is given a dry diet for 24 hours, the specific gravity of the urine is determined; called also *Addis method.*

Adler's t., see *benzidine t.*

Adson's t. (*for thoracic outlet syndrome*): with the patient in a sitting position, his hands resting on thighs, the examiner palpates both radial pulses as the patient rapidly fills his lungs by deep inspiration and, holding his breath, hyperextends his neck and turns his head toward the affected side. If the radial pulse on that side is decidedly or completely obliterated, the result is considered positive. Called also *Adson's maneuver.*

alkali denaturation t.: a moderately sensitive spectrophotometric method for determining the concentration of fetal (F) hemoglobin, which depends on the resistance of the hemoglobin molecule to denaturation of its globin moiety when exposed to alkali.

Allen's t.: 1. (*for glucose in the urine*) add urine to boiling Fehling's solution, and allow it to cool; turbidity will be seen if dextrose is present. (Alfred Henry Allen.) 2. (*for phenol*) to 2 drops of the suspected liquid add 5 drops of hydrochloric acid and 1 of nitric acid. Phenol, if present, will produce a cherry-red color. (Alfred Henry Allen.) 3. (*for strychnine*) extract with ether, concentrate by letting drops fall into a warmed porcelain capsule, cool the residue, and treat with sulfuric acid and manganese dioxide. Strychnine gives a violet color. 4. (*for occlusion of ulnar or radial arteries*) the patient makes a tight fist so as to express the blood from the skin of the palm and fingers; the examiner makes digital compression on either the radial or the ulnar artery. If on opening the hand blood fails to return to the palm and fingers, there is indicated obstruction to the blood flow in the artery that has not been compressed. (Edgar V. Allen.)

Allen-Doisy t. (*for estrogenic substance in laboratory animals*): a positive test is the presence in the vaginal secretion of cornified epithelial cells; a negative test shows only leukocytes in the secretion.

alpha t.: a test of intelligence administered by the U.S. Army in World War I to persons who could read.

alternate binaural loudness balance (ABLB) t., comparison of the intensity levels at which a given pure tone sounds equally loud to the normal ear and the ear with hearing loss; done to determine recruitment with unilateral sensorineural loss.

alternate cover t.: a test for determining the type of tropia and/or phoria done by alternately covering each eye and noting the movement of the uncovered eye.

alternate loudness balance t., a hearing test done with pure tones that compares the loudness perceived in one ear with that perceived in the other, with the frequency kept constant.

Ames t. (*for carcinogenicity*): a mutant strain of *Salmonella typhimurium* that lacks the ability to synthesize histidine is inoculated into a medium deficient in histidine but containing the test compound. If the compound causes DNA damage resulting in mutations, some of the bacteria will regain the ability to synthesize histidine and will proliferate to form colonies. The ability to cause mutations indicates that the substance is carcinogenic.

antiglobulin t. (AGT), a test for the presence of nonagglutinating antibodies against red cells that uses antihuman globulin antibody to agglutinate red cells coated with the nonagglutinating antibody. The *direct antiglobulin test* detects antibodies bound to circulating red cells in vivo. It is used in the evaluation of autoimmune and drug-induced hemolytic anemia and hemolytic disease of the newborn. The *indirect antiglobulin test* detects serum antibodies that bind to red cells in an in vitro incubation step. It is used in typing of erythrocyte antigens and in compatibility testing (cross-match). Called also *Coombs' test.*

antiglobulin consumption t., a test for serum antibodies against cellular antigens. Cells are incubated with the serum sample and then with antiglobulin; any serum antibody that binds to the cells will take up antiglobulin. The amount of antiglobulin consumed is determined by testing the supernatant with antibody-coated red cells; the amount of agglutination is inversely proportional to the antiglobulin consumption.

Apt t. (*for differentiating fetal from adult hemoglobin*): mix the infant's specimen (vomitus or stool) with 5 volumes of water, centrifuge the mixture, and separate the clear pink supernatant. Add 1 ml. 1 per cent sodium hydroxide to 5 ml. of the supernatant. If hemoglobin F is present, the pink color persists for more than 2 minutes (indicating fetal blood). If hemoglobin A is present, it turns from pink to yellow within 2 minutes (indicating swallowed maternal blood).

aptitude t's: tests given to determine aptitude or ability to undertake study or training in a particular field.

Army General Classification t.: an intelligence test whose results are used for placement in the military.

arylsulfatase t. (*for differentiating species of rapid-growing mycobacteria*): a sample from a Tween-albumin broth culture of the suspected organism is incubated with tripotassium phenolphthalein disulfate for three days and then alkalinized. Those species producing arylsulfatase (*Mycobacterium fortuitum* and *M. chelonei*) show a pink to red positive reaction; a colorless reaction is negative.

Aschheim-Zondek t. (*for pregnancy*): the subcutaneous injection of the urine of pregnant women into immature female mice is followed by swelling, congestion, and hemorrhages of the ovaries and premature maturation of the ovarian follicles. Abbreviated AZT and A-Z t.

Aschner's t., Aschner-Danini t., see *Aschner's phenomenon,* under *phenomenon.*

association t.: a test based on associative reaction. It is usually performed by mentioning words to a subject and noting what other words he will give as the ones called up in his mind. The reaction time is also noted.

augmented histamine t. (*of gastric function*): after a 12-hour fast, the residual gastric contents are aspirated. Basal gastric secretion is then collected for 1 hour in divided 15-minute aliquots. Thirty minutes before completion of collection, a suitable dose of antihistamine is given intramuscularly. At conclusion of basal secretion collection, histamine acid phosphate (0.04 mg. per kg. of body weight) is given subcutaneously, and gastric contents collected in 15-minute aliquots for 1 hour. Volume, pH, and titratable acidity are measured for each aliquot. When Histalog (1.7 mg. per kg. of body weight) is used in place of histamine, the antihistamine injection is omitted and 8 (rather than 4) 15-minute aliquots are taken after its injection.

autohemolysis t.: one performed in investigation of certain hemolytic states, particularly the congenital, nonspherocytic hemolytic anemias. Defibrinated blood is incubated at 37° C., under sterile conditions, for 24 and 48 hours, and the amount of spontaneous hemolysis is quantitated.

automated reagin t. (ART), a modification of the rapid plasma reagin (RPR) test for use with automated analyzers used in clinical chemistry.

Ayer's t. (*for spinal block*): with a spinal manometer, the pressure in lumbar puncture and that in a cisterna magna puncture should be identical in the normal subject.

Ayer-Tobey t., see *Tobey-Ayer t.*

Babinski's t., see under *sign.*

Babinski-Weil t.: the patient, with his eyes shut, is made to walk forward and backward ten times in a clear space. A person with labyrinthine disease deviates from the straight path, bends to one side when walking forward and to the other side when walking backward.

bacteriolytic t., see *Pfeiffer's phenomenon,* under *phenomenon.*

Baermann t. *(for extraction of soil nematodes from earth and detecting larvae of Strongyloides stercoralis in feces):* a specimen of soil or feces is suspended over gauze or wire mesh in a water-filled funnel to which a piece of rubber tubing is attached; larval nematodes migrate from the specimen to the water, and collect in the rubber tubing.

Bang t.: milk ring t.

Bárány's t., caloric t.

Bárány's pointing t.: have the patient point at a fixed object alternately with the eyes open and closed; a constant error with the eyes closed indicates a brain lesion.

bar-reading t.: a test for binocular and stereoscopic vision, which consists of holding a ruler midway between the eyes and the printed page. It is also used as an exercise to develop stereoscopic vision; called also *Welland's t.*

Becker's t.: 1. *(for picrotoxin)* Fehling's solution is added and the mixture is warmed; if the alkaloid is present, the solution is reduced. 2. *(for astigmatism)* the patient looks at a test card containing lines radiating in sets of three and points out which seem blurred.

Bekhterev's t.: the patient seated in bed is directed to stretch out both legs; in sciatica he cannot do this, but can stretch out each leg in turn.

Bender Gestalt t., Bender Visual-Motor Gestalt t.: a psychological test used for evaluating perceptual-motor coordination, for assessing personality dynamics, as a test of organic brain impairment, and for measuring neurological maturation. The subject is asked to make free-hand copies of nine simple geometric designs presented separately on cards or sometimes to reproduce the design from memory.

Benedict's t.: 1. *(for dextrose)* 200 gm. of sodium or potassium citrate and 200 gm. crystallized sodium carbonate and 125 gm. of potassium sulfocyanate are dissolved in 800 ml. of boiling water. This is cooled and filtered and 18 gm. copper sulfate dissolved in 100 ml. of water are added and the whole diluted to make 1 liter. To 5 ml. of this reagent, in a test tube, 8 or 10 drops of the solution to be tested are added. Boil for one or two minutes and allow to cool slowly. If dextrose is present the solution will be filled with a precipitate red, yellow, or green in color. 2. *(for urea)* the urea is hydrolyzed to ammonium carbonate by $KHSO_4$ and $ZNSO_4$, made alkaline, and distilled as usual.

bentonite flocculation t., any agglutination test using antigen adsorbed on particles of bentonite; when the antigen is added to serum containing specific antibodies, flocculation occurs.

benzidine t. *(for occult blood in urine or feces)* benzidine, acetic acid, and hydrogen peroxide are added to the specimen; hemoglobin catalyzes the oxidation of benzidine by hydrogen peroxide, giving a blue color. This is the most sensitive screening test for occult blood, but it is seldom used because benzidine is a carcinogen, and its use is restricted.

Bernstein t., esophageal acid infusion test.

beta t.: a test of intelligence administered by the U.S. Army in World War I to persons who could not read or did not speak English.

Bial's t. *(for pentose in urine):* make a reagent consisting of orcinol 1.5 gm., fuming hydrochloric acid 500 gm., and ferric chloride (10 per cent) 20–30 drops. Five ml. of this reagent are boiled in a test tube, and after removal from the flame, several drops of urine are added. A green color appearing at once indicates pentose.

Bielschowsky head-tilting t., tilting the head to the right and the left shoulder with the patient looking at a distance fixation device permits distinction between superior rectus paresis and contralateral superior oblique paresis.

bile solubility t. *(for differentiation of pneumococci from other streptococci):* a sample of a broth culture is incubated at pH 7.4 to 7.6 with sodium deoxycholate. A decrease in turbidity (positive test) indicates lysing of the cells. Pneumococci give a positive result, whereas other viridans streptococci give a negative one.

bilirubin t., see specific tests, including *Fouchet's t., Harrison spot t.,*

binaural distorted speech t's, tests of the capacity of the central nervous system to coordinate two incoming speech patterns, each of which is incomplete.

Binet's t.: a method of testing the mental capacity of children and youth by asking a series of questions adapted to, and

standardized on, the capacity of normal children at various ages. According to the answers given, the mental age of the subject is ascertained.

Binet-Simon t., see *Binet's t.*

Bing t.: a vibrating tuning fork is held to the mastoid process and the auditory meatus is alternately occluded and left open: an increase and decrease in loudness (positive Bing) is perceived by the normal ear and in sensorineural hearing impairment, but in conductive hearing impairment no difference in loudness is perceived (negative Bing).

biuret t.: 1. *(for proteins)* to 2 ml. of unknown solution add 2 ml. of 2 N sodium hydroxide solution and then a few drops of 1 per cent copper sulfate solution. A pinkish-violet color indicates the presence of biuret or of a similar double —CO·NH— grouping. 2. *(for urea)* melt the substance in a dry test tube and gently heat it. Cool, and dissolve in 2 ml. of water. Add 2 ml. of 2 N sodium hydroxide solution, and mix drop by drop with a 1 per cent copper sulfate solution. A pink and finally a bluish color is produced.

Bodal's t.: test of color perception by the use of colored blocks.

bone conduction t.: if a vibrating tuning-fork, when the handle is placed against the skull, is heard more distinctly than when held near the ear, it indicates loss in conduction through the middle ear.

Bozicevich's t.: a serologic test for the detection of trichinosis.

bracelet t.: the production of pain on moderate lateral compression of the lower ends of the radius and ulna; observed in rheumatoid arthritis.

Brenner's t., see under *formula.*

Broadbent's t. *(for cerebral dominance of language function):* different numbers (or words) are presented simultaneously to the two ears; right-handed persons tend to report first the words going into the right ear.

Bromsulphalein t., see *sodium sulfobromophthalein.*

Burchard-Liebermann t., see *Liebermann's t.*

butyric acid t., see *pineapple t.,* and *Noguchi reaction,* under *reaction.*

calcium t., see *Sulkowitch's t.* See also *calcium, methods for,* under *method.*

California mastitis t. (C.M.T.) *(for subclinical mastitis in cows):* equal amounts of milk, bromcresol purple, and an anionic surface-active substance are mixed in four separate cups within a plastic paddle by rapidly rotating the paddle horizontally; a positive reaction is indicated by various degrees of gel formation, according to the degree of abnormality of the milk. Called also *Schalm t.*

Calmette's t. *(obs.),* a tuberculin test in which tuberculin is instilled into the conjunctival sac; a positive response is development of conjunctivitis. Called also *Calmette's ophthalmic reaction* and *Calmette's conjunctival reaction.*

caloric t., irrigation of the normal ear with warm water produces a rotatory nystagmus toward the side of the irrigated ear; irrigation with cold water produces a rotatory nystagmus away from the irrigated side. There is no nystagmus in vestibular disease.

CAMP t. [Christie, *A*tkins, and *M*unch-Petersen, discoverers of the phenomenon] *(for the presumptive identification of Group B beta-hemolytic streptococci):* a culture of streptococcus is streaked on a blood agar plate near a streak of beta-lysin–producing *Staphylococcus aureus.* Group B streptococci produce a substance (CAMP factor) that enlarges the zone of lysis formed by the staphylococcal beta-hemolysin.

Cannabis indica t., see *Gayer t.*

capillary fragility t., capillary resistance t.: apply blood pressure cuff for five minutes tightly enough to obstruct venous return only, or apply a cupping glass, and note the number of petechiae thus produced.

carbohydrate t., see *Moore's t., Schiff's t.* (1).

carbohydrate tolerance t., see *Killian's t.*

carbon monoxide t., see specific tests, including *Dejust's t., Hoppe-Seyler t.* (1), *Katayama's t., Preyer's t., Rubner's t.* (1), *Salkowski's t.* (1), *Wetzel's t., Zaleski's t.*

carotid sinus t. *(for angina pectoris):* on slowing of the heart rate by massage over the right (or left) carotid sinus, the pain of an attack of angina pectoris will lessen or disappear.

Casoni's intradermal t. *(for hydatid disease):* injection into the skin of hydatid fluid followed by the immediate or delayed production of a wheal-and-flare reaction denotes hydatid infection.

catalase t. *(for the production of catalase by bacteria):* a slant culture is treated with hydrogen peroxide. The presence of gas bubbles indicates a positive reaction. Micrococci, staphylococci, most species of *Bacillus*, and anaerobic diphtheroids are catalase-positive; streptococci, pneumococci, and most *Actinomyces* are catalase-negative.

catoptric t.: a test for cataract made by observing the reflections from the cornea and from the surfaces of the crystalline lens.

cephalin-cholesterol flocculation t., a flocculation test formerly used as a test of liver function; a positive result (flocculation when a cephalin-cholesterol emulsion is added to serum) reflects serum protein abnormalities, chiefly, hypergammaglobulinemia or hypoalbuminemia. Called also *Hanger's t.*

chemiluminescence t.: a sensitive test of neutrophil microbicidal function that involves detection of the chemiluminescent energy emitted by unstable and highly reactive oxygen metabolites, e.g., singlet oxygen, produced during the respiratory burst following phagocytosis. It is able to detect heterozygous carriers of chronic granulomatous disease as well as homozygotes and also patients with myeloperoxidase deficiency.

Chick-Martin t.: a test for the efficiency of disinfectants in the presence of organic matter; see under *method*.

Chimani-Moos t.: a test for detecting simulated deafness.

chi-squared (χ^2) **t.:** any statistical hypothesis test that employs the χ^2 distribution (q.v.), especially two tests applied to categorical data: the χ^2-test of goodness of fit, which tests whether an observed frequency distribution fits a specified theoretical model, and the χ^2-test of independence or homogeneity, which tests whether two or more series of frequencies (the rows and columns of a contingency table) are independent. In both cases the test statistic is the sum over all categories of the squared difference between the observed and expected frequencies divided by the expected frequency. The sampling distribution of this χ^2-statistic approaches the χ^2-distribution as the sample size increases.

cholesterol t., see *Liebermann-Burchard t., Obermüller's t., Salkowski's t.* (2), *Schiff's t.* (2), (3), *Schultze's t.* (2), and *Zwenger's t.* (1). See also *cholesterol, methods for,* under *method*.

chromatin t. (*for determination of genetic sex*): examination of somatic cells for presence of the sex chromatin situated at the periphery of the nucleus in normal females but not in normal males; an index of the presence of XX chromosomal constitution.

Chvostek t., see under *sign*.

cis-trans t.: in microbial genetics, a test to determine whether two mutations that have the same phenotypic effect (in a haploid cell or a cell with single phage infection) are located in the same gene (resulting in noncomplementation) or in different genes (resulting in complementation and hence in loss of the mutant defect). The test depends on the independent behavior of two alleles of a gene in a diploid cell or in a cell infected with two phages carrying different alleles.

citrate t. (*for differentiation of organisms of the Enterobacter group of bacteria*): the test organism is grown on a medium containing citrate as its sole carbon source (Simmons citrate agar). The metabolism of citrate (positive reaction) turns the medium from green to blue. The Enterobacteriaceae are mostly positive; *Edwardsiella, Escherichia, Morganella, Shigella,* and *Yersinia* are negative.

Clauberg t.: a formerly used biological assay method for the standardization of corpus luteum preparations or progesterone. Immature rabbits are primed with estrogen and the degree of secretory endometrial development is the end-point.

C.M.T., see *California mastitis t.*

coagulase t.: a test for coagulase activity in which bacteria are added to citrated or oxalated (human or rabbit) blood plasma; in the presence of coagulase, the plasma gels within three hours. Coagulase activity is also demonstrable by mixing bacteria with blood plasma on a slide; if positive, clumping occurs, with fibrin formation.

cocaine t.: after instillation of a cocaine solution in each eye, the pupil of an eye affected by Horner's syndrome remains smaller than that of the normal eye.

coccidioidin t.: an intracutaneous test for coccidioidomycosis; see *coccidioidin*.

Cohn's t.: a test for color perception by the use of variously colored embroidery patterns.

colchicin t., see *Zeisel's t.*

cold pressor t., see *Hines and Brown t.*

collateral circulation t., see specific tests, including *Henle-Coenen t., Korotkoff's t., Pachon's t., tourniquet t.* (2), (3), *Tuffier's t., von Frisch t.*

colloidal gold t., (*for protein—globulin—in the cerebrospinal fluid, and thus for the diagnosis of certain central nervous system disorders, such as neurosyphilis, multiple sclerosis, poliomyelitis, and encephalitis*): progressive dilutions of cerebrospinal fluid are added to ten test tubes containing colloidal gold solution. The extent of precipitation is indicative of various diseases, and the results are interpreted according to the color changes that result. When no color change occurs the reaction is negative, i.e., the deep red colloidal gold color remains unchanged, and is recorded as 0. The appearance of the solution in the tube depends upon the amount of gold precipitated and is scored as 1+ (reddish blue), 2+ (lilac to purple), 3+ (deep blue), 4+ (pale blue), and 5+ (colorless, due to complete precipitation of the gold). Called also *Lange's t.* or *Lange's colloidal gold t.*

color perception t.: see specific tests, including *Bodal's t., Cohn's t., Donders' t., Holmgren's t., Ishihara's t., Jenning's t., lantern t., Mauthner's t., Nagel's t.*

complement fixation t., see under *fixation*.

concentration t. (*for renal function*): the patient is placed under conditions which cause the normal person to elaborate urine containing one or more constituents in high concentration and the results are observed to see whether the patient is able to attain this concentration, as in the *urea concentration t., xylose concentration t.*

conglutinating complement absorption t. (CCAT): a test resembling the complement fixation test (see under *fixation*), using as the indicator of antigen-antibody reaction the disappearance of conglutinin (q.v.) activity.

Congo red t. (*for amyloidosis*): Congo red is injected intravenously; if more than 60 per cent of the dye disappears after one hour, amyloidosis is indicated.

conjunctival t.: the local reaction which occurs when a pollen or an extract of the pollen is instilled into the conjunctival sac of a person sensitive to that pollen.

contact t., see *patch t.*

Coombs' t.: antiglobulin t.

copper t., see *Schönbein's t.* (2).

Corner-Allen t.: a biological method of assay for progesterone or corpus luteum preparations containing it. The rabbits are mated, the ovaries removed eighteen hours later, and the material to be assayed injected. The results are read according to the intensity of the endometrial changes.

cover t., see *alternate cover t.* and *cover-uncover t.*

cover-uncover t.: a test for determining the type of phoria, by covering one eye and noting its movement as it is uncovered.

Crafts' t.: in organic disease of the pyramidal tract, stroking with a blunt point upward over the dorsal surface of the ankle, the leg being extended and the muscles relaxed, produces dorsal extension of the great toe.

Crampton's t.: a test for physical resistance and condition based on the difference between the pulse and blood pressure in the recumbent position and in the standing position. A difference of 75 or more indicates good condition; one of 65 or less shows a poor condition.

creatinine t., see specific tests, including *Jaffé's t.* (1), *Kerner's t., Salkowski's t.* (5), *Thudichum's t., von Maschke's t., Weyl's t.* (1). See also *creatinine, methods for,* under *method*.

cuff t.: a test for angina pectoris by producing ischemia in the left arm for five minutes by raising the pressure in a blood-pressure cuff on the arm to 50 mm. above the usual systolic pressure. This may produce an anginal attack in persons with coronary disease.

Cuignet's t. (*for simulated unilateral blindness*): the bar-reading test used to detect simulated unilateral blindness or malingering.

cysteine t., see specific tests, including *nitroprusside t.* (1), *Sullivan's t.*

cystine t., see *Liebig's t.*

cytosine t., see *Wheeler and Johnson's t.*

dark-adaptation t. (*for vitamin A deficiency*): a test based on the fact that with a deficient intake of vitamin A the ability to see a dimly illuminated object in a dark room is diminished.

darkroom t.: a test to determine the tendency to develop acute angle glaucoma: ocular pressure is measured by the applanation tonometer, the subject is placed in a darkroom for one hour, and applanation tonometry is then repeated.

Davidsohn's t. (*differential test for infectious mononucleosis*): the determination of the agglutination of sheep erythrocytes by the patient's serum after absorption with Forssman antigen (guinea pig kidney or horse kidney) and beef antigen, respectively.

Davidsohn differential absorption t., Paul-Bunnell-Davidsohn t.

Dehio's t.: if bradycardia is relieved by injections of atropine, the condition is caused by increased vagal tone; but if the bradycardia is not relieved, the cause is some affection of the heart muscle.

dehydrocholate t. *(for the speed of blood circulation)*: sodium dehydrocholate solution is injected intravenously; the usual time elapsing until a bitter taste in the mouth occurs is between 10 and 14 seconds.

Denver Developmental Screening t.: a test for identification of infants and preschool children with developmental delay.

deoxyribonuclease (DNase) t. *(for the presence of deoxyribonuclease in bacteria)*: a nutrient agar plate containing deoxyribonucleic acid and toluidine blue is inoculated from a young agar slant; after incubation a red zone around the inoculum indicates the presence of deoxyribonuclease.

deoxyuridine suppression t., a test for folate or cobalamin deficiency, in which lack of 5,10-methylene tetrahydrofolate inhibits incorporation of deoxyuridine into DNA, so that deoxyuridine fails to inhibit incorporation of ^{3}H-thymidine.

dexamethasone suppression t., a test of hypothalamic-pituitary-adrenocortical function; oral administration of dexamethasone causes suppression of adrenal cortisol secretion in normal persons but not in those with Cushing's disease.

dextrose t., see specific tests, including *Allen's t.* (1)., *Benedict's t.*, *Gerrard's t.*, *Hager's t.*, *Haines' t.*, *Heller's t.* (3)., *Horsley's t.*, *hydroxylamine t.*, *Jaffé's t.* (1), *Knapp's t.* (1), *Kowarsky's t.* (1), *Loewe's t.*, *Löwenthal's t.*, *Mathews' t.*, *Maumenét.*, *Molisch's t.* (1), (2), *Moore's t.*, *Mulder's t.* (1), *nitropropiol t.*, *Oliver's t.* (2), *Pavy's t.*, *Pélouse-Moore t.*, *Penzoldt's t.* (2), *Purdy's t.* (1), *Riegler's t.* (3), *Roberts' t.* (2), *Rubner's t.* (2), *saccharimeter t.*, *Sachsse's t.*, *Salkowski's t.* (4), *silver t.*, *Soldaini's t.*, *Tollers' t.* (2), *Trommer's t.*, *von Jaksch's t.* (2), *Wender's t.*, *Worm-Müller t.* See also *glucose (dextrose), methods for*, under *method*.

diabetes t.: see specific tests, including *Bremer's t.*, *Hickey-Hare t.*, *Kowarsky's t.* (2), *Loewi's t.*, *Williamson's blood t.*

diacetyl t. *(for urea)*: the solution to be tested is mixed with concentrated hydrochloric acid and diacetyl monoxime; a yellow color develops on boiling if urea is present.

Dick t. *(for susceptibility to scarlet fever)*: purified erythrogenic toxin from group A streptococci is injected intradermally; appearance within 24 to 48 hours of a small area of reddening of the skin indicates susceptibility of the subject.

differential t. for infectious mononucleosis: a test based on the fact that antisheep agglutinins in infectious mononucleosis are not absorbed by Forssman antigen (whereas as those in serum disease and of normal persons are), but are absorbed by beef cells (whereas those in conditions other than infectious mononucleosis may or may not be).

dilution t. *(for antibiotic sensitivity in bacteria)*: serial dilutions of an antibacterial agent in an agar or broth medium are inoculated with a suspension of a known concentration of a microorganism. Following incubation the lowest concentration at which there is no visible growth is referred to as the minimum inhibitory concentration for the specific antibiotic.

diphtheria t.: see specific tests, including *Schick t.* and *tellurite t.*

disk diffusion t. *(for antibiotic sensitivity in bacteria)*: agar plates are inoculated with a standardized suspension of a microorganism. Antibiotic-containing disks are applied to the agar surface. Following overnight incubation, the diameters of the zones of inhibition or clearing surrounding the disks are measured. Zone diameters are interpreted as sensitive (susceptible), indeterminate (or intermediate), or resistant.

Dolman's t. *(for ocular dominance)*: the patient holds in both hands a card with a hole in it through which to sight at a light.

Donath-Landsteiner t. *(for paroxysmal cold hemoglobinuria)*: a test based on the fact that the blood of patients with this disease contains complement-dependent iso- and autohemolysin which unites with red cells only at low temperatures (2° to 10° C.), hemolysis occurring only after warming to 37° C.

Donders' t.: a color vision test performed by lanterns with sides of colored glass.

double glucagon t. *(for deficiency of amylo-1-6-glucosidase)*: glucagon is administered after a twelve hour fast and again shortly after a meal; if the blood sugar fails to rise after the first administration but has a normal rise after the second, the test is positive.

drinking t. *(for glaucoma)*: one quart of water is ingested as rapidly as possible before breakfast. The intraocular pressure is measured every fifteen minutes. A rise of from 8 to 15 mm. Hg in less than one-half hour indicates glaucoma. Called also *water provocative t.*

Duane's t.: the employment of a candle flame and prisms to measure the degree of ocular heterophoria.

Dugas' t.: a test for the existence of dislocation of the shoulder, made by placing the hand of the affected side on the opposite shoulder and bringing the elbow to the side of the chest. If this cannot be accomplished (Dugas' sign), dislocation of the shoulder exists.

Dukc's t.: a test which measures bleeding time.

dye exclusion t.: the determination of cell viability *in vitro*. Following exposure of a cell preparation to trypan blue or eosin, dead cells take up the dye from the medium whereas living cells remain unstained.

early pregnancy t.: a do-it-yourself immunological test for pregnancy performed in the home as early as nine days after menstruation was expected (missed period). The test materials consist of a mixture of human chorionic gonadotropin (HCG) antiserum and HCG-coated red blood cells in a glass test tube, a vial of water, and a medical dropper. Three drops of urine are placed in the test tube and the vial of water is added. The tube is shaken for 10 seconds and placed in a holder for 2 hours. A brown ring of nonagglutinated red blood cells is positive (indicates pregnancy).

Ehrlich's t.: 1. see *Ehrlich's diazo reaction*, under *reaction*. 2. the benzaldehyde test for urobilinogen.

Ehrmann's t. *(for mydriatic substances)*: the suspected substance is applied to an enucleated frog's eye, dilatation indicating the presence of a mydriatic substance.

Einhorn string t.: a test for determining whether the site of bleeding is in the low esophagus, stomach, or duodenum.

Elek t., see *toxigenicity t.* (*in vitro*).

Elsberg's t.: a method of testing the sense of smell for determining the existence of a brain tumor.

Ely's t.: with the patient prone, if flexion of the leg on the thigh causes the buttocks to arch away from the table and the leg to abduct at the hip joint, there is contracture of the lateral fascia of the thigh.

Erhard's t.: a test for detecting simulated deafness.

Erichsen t., see under *sign*.

erythrocyte protoporphyrin (EP) t., a screening test for lead toxicity, in which erythrocyte protoporphyrin levels are determined by direct fluorometry of whole blood or fluorescence analysis of whole blood extracts; levels are increased in lead poisoning and iron deficiency.

esophageal acid infusion t. *(for diagnosis of gastroesophageal reflux)*: 0.1 N hydrogen chloride infused at a rate of 120 drops per minute produces pain and other symptoms.

euglobulin lysis t.: a test for the presence of plasminogen activator, done by determining the time required to dissolve an incubated clot composed of precipitated plasma euglobulin and exogenous thrombin.

exercise t's, tests for detecting previously undetected coronary artery disease; they are graded tests of coronary fitness in which the subject performs exercise, as by walking a treadmill or pedaling a stationary bicycle, while under continuous electrocardiographic monitoring, usually by means by an oscilloscope, before, during, and after the exercise. Called also *stress t's.* See also *Master 2-step exercise t.*

Fantus t. *(for differentiating between predominant water or salt depletion)*: place 10 drops of urine in a test tube with 1 drop of 20 per cent potassium chromate, then add 2.9 per cent silver nitrate 1 drop at a time, all the while agitating the tube, until there is a sudden color change from yellow to brick red. The number of drops of silver nitrate required to attain this change is the number of grams of chloride per liter in the urine; thus the addition of 4 drops to elicit the end point indicates a urine chloride concentration of 400 mg./100 ml. (4 gm./L.).

Farber's t.: presence of swallowed vernix cells in the meconium of a newborn baby indicates partial intestinal stenosis; their absence indicates intestinal atresia.

Farr t.: a radioimmunoassay for measuring absolute amounts of antibody: antibody is reacted with radiolabelled antigen and precipitated with ammonium sulfate; bound antigen or hapten is precipitated while free antigen remains in solution. This test is based on the capacity of antibody to combine with antigen rather than on such secondary properties as precipitation and therefore measures all immunoglobulin classes and subclasses.

fat t., see specific tests, including *Leffmann-Beam t., Meigs's t., Saathoff's t., Valenta's t.*

FE$_{Na}$ t.: excreted fraction of filtered sodium test, a measure of renal tubular reabsorption of sodium, calculated as follows: $(U/P)Na/(U/P)Cr \times 100$, where U and P represent concentrations of sodium and creatinine in urine and plasma, respectively.

femoral nerve stretch t. *(for lesions of third or fourth lumbar disk)*: passive knee flexion in the prone position causes pain in the back or thighs.

fermentation t. *(for dextrose)*: fill a graduated fermentation tube with the urine or unknown solution, add a small portion of compressed yeast, and incubate for twelve hours; the amount of gas that accumulates in the closed arm indicates the amount of dextrose present.

fern t. *(for estrogen)*: the appearance of a fernlike pattern in dried smears of uterine cervical mucus indicates the presence of estrogen; the level of secretion is determined by the extent of ferning.

ferric chloride t.: 1. *(for thiocyanates in saliva)* add a few drops of dilute ferric chloride to saliva and acidify with hydrochloric acid; red ferric thiocyanate forms, which is decolorized by adding mercury bichloride. 2. *(for salicylic acid)* see *Remont's t.*

finger-to-finger t.: similar to finger-nose test, for testing coordinated movements of the extremities.

finger-nose t. *(for coordinated movements of the extremities)*: with arm extended to one side the patient is asked to slowly try to touch the end of his nose with the point of his index finger.

Fishberg concentration t. *(for renal function)*: the patient is given supper with not more than 200 ml. of fluid and nothing thereafter. Urine voided during the night is discarded. The morning urine is saved, the patient kept in bed, and the urine of one hour later and of two hours later is saved. If the specific gravity of any of these three specimens is less than 1.024 there is impairment of renal function.

Fisher exact t., a statistical hypothesis test of independence of rows and columns in a 2×2 contingency table based on the exact sampling distribution of the observed frequencies.

Fishman-Doubilet t. *(for quick differential diagnosis of acute pancreatitis)*: a minute amount of starch is incubated with serum for 5 minutes. A normal concentration of amylase will leave some of the starch undigested and give a blue color with iodine; a high serum amylase digests all the starch, and the addition of iodine will give only the yellow color of iodine. When the reaction color is yellow, the diagnosis of acute pancreatitis is strongly indicated. Called also *rapid serum amylase t.*

fistula t.: the air in the external auditory canal is compressed or rarefied: if there is erosion of the inner osseous wall of the tympanum exposing the membranous labyrinth, nystagmus will be produced, provided the labyrinth still functions. The site of the fistula is usually in the bony lateral semicircular canal.

Flack t. *(of physical efficiency)*: after a full inspiration the subject blows as long as he can into a mercury manometer with a force of 40 mm. mercury.

flicker t.: see *flicker*.

flocculation t.: 1. any of a variety of nonspecific tests of liver function, now obsolete, in which a precipitating reagent is added to serum, e.g., the cephalin-cholesterol flocculation test or the thymol turbidity test; positive results generally reflect increased gamma and beta globulins and lipoproteins or decreased albumin. 2. any serologic test in which a flocculent agglomerate is formed; usually the term is applied to a variant form of the precipitin reaction, rarely to agglutination reactions.

Fluhmann's t.: a modification of the Allen-Doisy test for estrogenic substance in the body, using mice in which a positive reaction is the mucinification of the vaginal mucosa.

fluorescent treponemal antibody absorption (FTA-ABS) t.: the standard treponemal antigen serologic test for syphilis; patient serum is diluted with an extract of Reiter treponemes to remove nonspecific antibodies, then reacted with the Nichol's strain of *Treponema pallidum* fixed to a glass slide; specific antibodies adhering to the treponemes are demonstrated with fluorescein-labeled antihuman globulin. Positive tests are seen in about 85 per cent of cases of primary syphilis, 100 per cent in secondary syphilis, and 98 per cent in late syphilis.

formaldehyde t., see specific tests, including *Burnam's t., Jorissen's t., Kentmann's t., Leach's t., Lebbin's t., Luebert's t., Schiff's t.* (6).

Foshay's t. *(for tularemia)*: a suspension of *Pasteurella tularensis* is injected into the skin; a positive reaction resembles that in a positive tuberculin test.

Fouchet's t. *(for bilirubin in blood)*: to a sample of the blood serum there is added an equal part of a reagent consisting of 5 gm. trichloracetic acid, 20 ml. water, and 2 ml. ferric chloride; a green color is produced if bilirubin is present.

Fournier t.: the patient is asked to rise on command from a sitting position; he is asked to rise and walk, then stop quickly on command; he is asked to walk and turn around quickly on command. The ataxic gait is thus brought out.

Francis' t.: 1. *(for bile acids in urine)* in a test tube is placed 2 gm. of dextrose in 15 gm. of sulfuric acid and the urine is placed on top of this; a purple color forms if bile acids are present. 2. an intracutaneous test in pneumonia for ascertaining the body response to the infection and whether the specific antibodies are present after treatment with antipneumococcus serum. The homologous pneumococcus polysaccharide is used in the skin test.

Fränkel's t.: examination of the nasal cavity with the patient's head bent down between his knees and rotated so that the side to be examined is turned upward. If pus is seen in the middle meatus, suppuration in some of the anterior accessory sinuses is indicated.

Frei t.: a skin test for lymphogranuloma venereum using material prepared from lymphogranuloma venereum organisms grown in chick embryo yolk sacs; the test is both insensitive and nonspecific and is now rarely used.

Friderichsen's t. *(for vitamin A deficiency)*: determination of the weakest light stimulus which will give rise to an oculomotor reflex. A variation from normal indicates vitamin A deficiency.

Friedman's t., Friedman-Lapham t. *(for pregnancy)*: the injection of the urine of a pregnant woman into female rabbits will cause the formation of corpora lutea and corpora haemorrhagica in the rabbits.

Frohn's t.: the use of the double iodide of bismuth and potassium as a test for alkaloids.

fructose t., see *levulose t.*

FTA-ABS t., fluorescent treponemal antibody absorption t.

fundus reflex t., retinoscopy.

Funkenstein t.: an index of central autonomic reactivity, consisting of observing the response in systolic blood pressure after intramuscular injection of 10 mg. of acetylcholine.

furfurol t. *(for proteins)*: heat the suspected substance with sulfuric acid; if proteins are present, furfurol is formed.

Gaenslen's t., see under *sign*.

Galli Mainini t. *(for pregnancy)*: 10 ml. of urine from the patient is injected into a normal male batrachian (frog or toad); the presence of spermatozoa in a drop of the batrachian's urine indicates the existence of pregnancy.

gastric function t., see specific tests, including *augmented histamine t., chlorophyll t., Rehfuss t., Sahli's t., Sahli's glutoid t., Schwarz's t.* (2).

Gault t. *(for simulated deafness)*: the patient's good ear is closed and a sound is made near the supposed bad ear; a winking motion of the lid on the tested side indicates hearing.

gel diffusion t., see *immunodiffusion*.

Gerhardt's t.: 1. *(for acetone in the urine)* add a solution of ferric chloride and a red color is produced. This test is not reliable (Carl J. Gerhardt). 2. *(for acetoacetic acid in the urine)* filter, in order to remove the phosphates, and add a few drops of a solution of ferric chloride, which produces a deep red color, which disappears when sulfuric acid is added. 3. *(for bile pigments in the urine)* shake urine with an equal measure of chloroform and then add tincture of iodine and potassium hydroxide to the separated chloroform; a yellow or yellowish brown color is produced (Charles Frédéric Gerhardt).

Gerrard's t. *(for dextrose in the urine)*: Fehling's solution is treated with a 5 per cent solution of potassium cyanide until the blue color begins to disappear. The suspected liquid is heated with this mixture, and if there is dextrose present, more or less discoloration takes place.

Gibbon and Landis t. *(for peripheral circulation)*: a pair of extremities (the hands, if the feet are to be tested; the feet, if the hands are to be tested) are immersed in a bath of 43°–45° C. If the temperature in the unimmersed extremities rises, the circulation is normal.

Gies' biuret t. *(for proteins)*: Gies uses the following reagent in making the test: mix 25 ml. of a 3 per cent solution of cupric sulfate and 975 ml. of a 10 per cent solution of potassium hydroxide.

globulin t., see specific tests, including *ammonium sulfate t.* (1), *Gordon's t.*, *Hammarsten's t.* (1), *Kaplan's t.*, *colloidal gold t.*, *Mayerhofer's t.*, *Noguchi's t.* (2), *Nonne-Apelt t.*, *Pándy's t.*, *Pohl's t.*, *Ross-Jones t.*, *Weichbrodt's t.*

glucagon stimulation t. (*for deficiency of growth hormone*): blood samples are taken immediately and at intervals of 1, 2, 2½, and 3 hours after subcutaneous or intramuscular injection of glucagon; radioimmunoassay of the serum is then done by enzyme partition.

glucose t., see *dextrose t.*

glucose tolerance t.: a metabolic test of carbohydrate tolerance; it measures active insulin, a hepatic function based on the power of the normal liver to absorb and store large quantities of glucose, and the effectiveness of intestinal absorption of glucose. Blood sugar should return to normal in two to two and one-half hours after ingesting 100 gm. of glucose into a fasting stomach. See also *Exton and Rose's glucose tolerance t.*

glutoid t., see *Sahli's glutoid t.*

Gluzinski's t.: 1. (*for bile pigments*) boil the solution with solution of formaldehyde until it becomes green; adding a little hydrochloric acid changes the tint to an amethyst violet. 2. (*for differentiation between ulcer and cancer of stomach*) examination of the gastric contents recovered from a fasting patient: (*a*) after a test breakfast consisting of the white of a boiled egg and 200 ml. of water, which is recovered after three quarters of an hour. (*b*) after a test dinner consisting of a beefsteak and 250 ml. of water, which is recovered after three and three-quarters hours. In ulcer, both the breakfast and the dinner give the reaction of free HCl. In beginning cancer, the first meal will give reaction of free HCl, whereas the second meal will show only a slight trace or none at all.

glycerol t., see specific tests, including *hypochlorite-orcinol t.*

glycerophosphate t. (*for renal function*): 500 mg. of sodium glycerophosphate are injected intravenously, and then the free and total phosphorus in the urine collected during the following hour is determined.

glycosylated hemoglobin t.: measurement of the percentage of hemoglobin A molecules that have formed a stable ketoamine linkage between their terminal amino acid position of the β-chains and a glucose group; in normal persons this amounts to about 7 per cent of the total, in diabetics about 14.5 per cent.

glycuronates t., see specific tests, including *Tollens' t.* (4) and *Tollens, Neuberg and Schwket's t.*

glycyltryptophan t. (*for carcinoma of stomach*): filtered gastric contents and glycyltryptophan are placed in a test tube and kept at body temperature for twenty-four hours; if on the addition of a few drops of bromine, a reddish violet color is formed, carcinoma is indicated.

glyoxylic acid t., see *Hopkins-Cole test.*

Gmelin's t. (*for bile pigments*): fuming nitric acid is so added to the suspected urine that it forms a layer under it. Near the junction of the two liquids, rings are formed—a green ring above, and under it a blue, violet-red, and reddish yellow. If the green and violet-red rings are absent, the reaction shows the probable presence of lutein.

gold number t., see *colloidal gold t.*

Goldscheider's t. (*for cutaneous thermal sensibility*) (*obs.*): consists in touching the skin with the slightly pointed end of a metallic cylinder varyingly heated.

gold-sol t., see *colloidal gold t.*

Goodenough draw-a-man t., Goodenough draw-a-person t.: a method of testing the general intelligence of children by asking the subject to draw a picture of a man to the best of his ability.

Goodenough-Harris drawing t.: a revision of the Goodenough draw-a-man test, in which scoring emphasizes the presence or absence of body and clothing detail rather than artistic skill.

Gordon's t. (*for the presence of globulin-albumin in the spinal fluid*): one ml. of spinal fluid is placed in a small test tube and 0.1 ml. of 1 per cent solution of corrosive mercuric chloride in distilled water; the formation of a cloud or precipitate after standing an hour indicates a positive reaction.

Gordon's biological t. (*for Hodgkin's disease*): lymphadenomatous tissue injected intracerebrally into rabbits causes the development of a characteristic lesion in the rabbits' nervous tissues, accompanied by ataxia, spasm, and paralysis.

Göthlin's t.: a test for capillary fragility, done by testing the capillary resistance in the arm.

Graefe's t. (*for heterophoria*): on holding a prism of 10 degrees before one eye, base up or down, two images are formed; one of these images is displaced laterally in heterophoria.

Graham's t.: the intravenous or oral administration of tetraiodophthalein sodium prior to roentgenologic examination of the gallbladder.

Gregerson and Boas' t. (*for blood*): a modification of the benzidine test to make it less sensitive for use in testing feces. Use a 0.5 per cent solution of benzidine instead of a saturated solution and barium peroxide instead of hydrogen peroxide.

Griess t. (*for nitrites in the saliva*): mix it with 5 parts of water; add a few drops of dilute solution of sulfuric acid and a few drops of metadiamidobenzene; this produces a strong yellow color if nitrites are present.

Grigg's t. (*for proteins*): metaphosphoric acid precipitates all proteins except the peptones.

Grocco's t. (*obs.*): in slight cases of purpura and purpura rheumatica, if an elastic ligature is placed around the forearm, punctiform hemorrhages will appear in the bend of the elbow.

Gross' t.: 1. (*for trypsin in feces*) in a mortar, thoroughly rub up a portion of the fecal mass with three times its bulk of 0.1 per cent sodium carbonate solution. Filter. Mix 10 ml. of the filtrate with 100 ml. of a fresh solution consisting of 0.5 gm. Grübler's pure casein, 1 gm. sodium carbonate, and 1000 ml. distilled water. Add a little toluol to prevent bacterial activity and place in an incubator at about 38° C. At intervals remove a few cubic centimeters and test for casein by adding a few drops of acetic acid of about 1 per cent strength. A white cloud appears as long as any casein remains undigested. With the patient on a protein diet, there is normally a sufficient amount of trypsin to digest all the casein in from ten to fifteen hours. Delay or complete failure of digestion shows diminution or absence of trypsin. 2. a color reaction for the diagnosis of carcinoma.

group t.: a test of intelligence or aptitude given to a number of persons at one time.

guaiac t. (*for occult blood*): glacial acetic acid and a solution of gum guaiac are mixed with the specimen; on addition of hydrogen peroxide, the presence of blood is indicated by a blue tint.

guanine t., see *Capranica's t.* (2), (3), and (4).

Gunning's t. (*for acetone in urine*): to a few milliliters of urine or distillate in a test tube, add a few drops of tincture of iodine and of ammonia alternately until a heavy black cloud appears. This cloud will gradually clear up and, if acetone is present, iodoform, usually crystalline, will separate out. The iodoform can be recognized by its odor or by detection of the crystals microscopically. Iodoform crystals are yellowish six-pointed stars or six-sided plates.

Gunning-Lieben t., see *Gunning's t.*

Günzberg's t. (*for hydrochloric acid in the stomach contents*): dissolve 2 gm. of phloroglucin and 1 gm. of vanillin in 30 ml. of alcohol; of this mix 2 drops with 2 drops of filtered gastric juice; heat it slowly in a porcelain cell. Free HCl produces a bright-red color; it is not present if the color is brownish red or brown.

Guthrie t. (*for phenylketonuria*): in the presence of blood containing phenylalanine, β-2-thienylalanine does not inhibit growth of *Bacillus subtilis.*

Gutzeit's t. (*for arsenic*): a paper is moistened with an acidulated silver nitrate solution and exposed to the fumes from the suspected liquid, which is mixed with zinc and dilute sulfuric acid. The formation of a yellow spot on the paper indicates the presence of inorganic arsenic compounds.

Haagensen t.: observation of the contour of the breasts when the patient leans forward as a means of detecting malignant changes in the mammae.

Hager's t., cephalin-cholesterol flocculation t.

Haines' t. (*for dextrose*): copper sulfate, 30 grains; glycerin, ½ fl.oz.; liquor potassae, 5 fl.oz.; water, sufficient to make 6 fl.oz. When boiled and a little urine added, and again boiled, a yellow or reddish yellow precipitate is produced.

Hallion's t., see *Tuffier's t.*

Ham t., acidified serum t.

Hamel's t. (*for slight jaundice*): a little blood is drawn by puncture from the lobe of the ear into a capillary tube and the tube is allowed to stand for a few hours; the serum which collects in the upper part of the tube will be yellow if jaundice is present.

Hamilton's t.: when the shoulder joint is luxated, a rule or straight rod applied to the humerus can be made to touch the outer condyle and the acromion at the same time.

Hammarsten's t.: 1. (*for globulin*) in a neutral solution suspected to contain globulin, dissolve magnesium sulfate to saturation; the globulin will be precipitated and may be filtered out. 2. (*for bile pigment*) to one volume of acid mixture (1 part HNO₃ and 19 parts HCl, each 25 per cent) add four volumes of alcohol, then a few drops of the unknown; a green color indicates biliverdin.

Hammerschlag's t., see under *method.*

Hanger's t. (*for liver cell disease*), see *cephalin-cholesterol flocculation t.*

Hanke and Koessler's t. (*for phenols, hydroxyaromatic acids, and imidazoles*): to 5 ml. of 1.1 per cent sodium carbonate solution add 2 ml. of para-diazobenzene sulfonic acid reagent. Then add 1 ml. of solution to be tested.

hapten inhibition t.: serological characterization of an antigenic determinant by employing known haptens to mask the antigen binding site of antibody specific for it.

Harding and Ruttan's t. (*for acetoacetic acid*): acidify the urine with acetic acid, add 0.5 ml. of N/10 sodium nitroprusside, and then overlay the solution with concentrated aqueous NH₄OH; a violet ring is produced.

Harris and Ray t.: a microtitration for vitamin C in the urine.

Harrison spot t. (*for bilirubin in urine*): add to 10 ml. of urine 5 ml. of a 10 per cent solution of barium chloride, mix, and filter. Spread filter paper on dry filter paper. Add one to two drops of Fouchet's reagent (trichloroacetic acid 25 gm., water 100 ml., and 10 per cent solution of ferric chloride 10 ml.); a positive reaction gives a blue to green color (Godfried).

Hart's t. (*for oxybutyric acid in urine*): remove acetone and diacetic acid by diluting 20 ml. urine with 20 ml. of water, adding a few drops of acetic acid, and boiling down to 10 ml. To this add 10 ml. of water, mix, and divide between two test tubes. To one tube add 1 ml. of hydrogen peroxide, warm gently, and cool. This transforms β-hydroxybutyric acid to acetone. Now apply Lange's test for acetone to each tube. A positive reaction in the tube to which hydrogen peroxide has been added shows the presence of β-oxybutyric acid in the original sample of urine.

hatching t.: a test for the detection of live schistosome eggs in urine or feces, dependent upon the eggs hatching to produce miracidia when placed in water; the miracidia are attracted to light and can readily be identified.

Hay's t. (*for bile salts*): a pinch of sublimated sulfur is dropped in the urine; the sulfur sinks if bile is present, but floats if it is absent.

Heaf t., see *tuberculin t., Sterneedle.*

heel-knee t. (*for coordinated movements of the extremities*): the patient, lying on his back, is asked to touch the knee of one leg with the heel of the other and then to pass the heel slowly down the front of the shin to the ankle.

heel-tap t., see *heel tap,* under *tap.*

Heller's t.: 1. (*for albumin in urine*) stratify cold nitric acid below the urine in a test tube; albumin will form a white coagulum between the urine and the acid. 2. (*for blood in the urine*) add potassium hydroxide solution and heat; the earthy phosphates are precipitated, and if blood is present, they are stained red by hematin. 3. (*for dextrose in urine*) add a solution of potassium hydroxide; sugar will cause a brownish or reddish precipitate.

hemadsorption t.: an *in vitro* test for detecting hemagglutinating viruses based on the adherence of red blood cells to cells of the infected tissue in the presence of hemagglutinin.

hemagglutination inhibition t. (HI, HAI) 1. a highly sensitive procedure for the measurement of soluble antigens in biologic specimens in which the specimen is first incubated with homologous antibody and then incubated with antigen-coated red cells; the amount of hemagglutination reflects the amount of free antibody present after reaction with the specimen and thus varies inversely with the amount of antigen in the specimen. 2. a procedure for the measurement of serum antibodies directed against a hemagglutinating virus; the highest dilution of serum that completely inhibits hemagglutination by a standardized viral preparation is reported as the hemagglutination titer.

hematein t. (*for blood*): to 5 ml. of the unknown add 5 ml. of sodium hydroxide, 2 drops of hematein solution, and 10 drops of hydrogen peroxide. If blood is present the contents will turn rapidly to violet red, then to clear brown, and then to pale yellow. Without blood these changes occur more slowly.

hematin t., see *Schumm's t.* (2).

heme t., see *Schumm's t.* (2).

hemin t. (*for blood*), see *Teichmann's t.*

hemoglobin t., see specific tests, including *alkali denaturation t., Heller's t.* (2), *Katayama's t., Kobert's t., sand t.* See also *hemoglobin, methods for,* under *method.*

hemosiderin t., see specific tests, including *Perl's t.,* and *Rous's t.*

Hench-Aldrich t. (*for the mercury-combining power of saliva*): titrate 5 ml. of saliva with a 5 per cent solution of bichloride of mercury until a drop gives a reddish brown color with a saturated solution of sodium carbonate.

Henle-Coenen t.: the amount of retrograde flow of blood which is obtained from the open end of the distal stump of a divided artery, while the proximal portion is being compressed with a clamp, is a measure (or index) of the adequacy of the collateral circulation.

Hennebert's t., see under *sign.*

Henry's t., Henry's melanoflocculation t. (*for malaria*): an obsolete flocculation test for malaria using melanin from ox eyes as the antigen.

Henshaw t.: a test to aid in the selection of the appropriate homeopathic remedy in a given case of disease. A visible flocculation zone develops in the patient's blood serum when brought into contact with a potentized remedy homeopathically indicated in the case.

hepatic function t., see *liver function t.*

Hering's t.: the subject looks with both eyes through a tube blackened within and having a thread running vertically across the farther end, and a small round body is placed either before or behind the thread—if vision is binocular, the subject is able at once to tell whether the ball is nearer to him than the thread or farther off; but if vision is monocular, he cannot tell whether it is nearer or farther than the thread.

Herter's t.: 1. (*for indole*) to the unknown add 1 drop of a 2 per cent solution of beta-naphtha-quinone-sodium-mono-sulfonate, and then a drop of a 10 per cent solution of potassium hydroxide; a blue or bluish green color indicates indole. 2. (*for skatole*) to the unknown add 1 ml. of an acid solution of para-dimethyl-amino-benzaldehyde and heat to boiling. The purplish blue color is intensified by the addition of hydrochloric acid.

Herzberg's t. (*for free hydrochloric acid in the gastric juice*): moisten a paper with a solution of Congo red and dry it; free HCl colors it blue or bluish black.

Hess capillary t. (*for condition of the capillary walls*), see *tourniquet t.,* def. 1.

heterophile antibody t., see *horse cell t., Paul-Bunnell t.,* and *Paul-Bunnell-Davidsohn t.*

Heynsius' t. (*for albumin*): to a suspected liquid add enough acetic acid to render acidulous, and then boil with a saturated solution of sodium chloride; albumin will form a flocculent precipitate.

Hickey-Hare t. (*for diabetes insipidus*): intravenous infusion of hypertonic saline after establishment of water diuresis induces antidiuresis in normal subjects but not in patients with diabetes insipidus.

Hildebrandt's t. (*for urobilin in urine*): the reagent consists of an unfiltered solution of 10 parts of zinc acetate and 90 parts of absolute alcohol. The reagent is shaken before using, and equal parts of reagent and urine are mixed, the precipitate which forms being filtered off. With increase of urobilin the filtrate shows a distinct green fluorescence, either directly or after the addition of ammonia.

Hindenlang's t. (*for albumin*): to the liquid to be tested add solid metaphosphoric acid; albumin, if present, forms a precipitate.

Hines and Brown t.: cold pressor test; a test which measures the response of the blood pressure to the immersion of one hand in ice water: an excessive increase in pressure (hyperreaction) is said to identify a latent hypertensive state.

Hinton t.: (*obs.*) a nontreponemal antigen serologic test for syphilis.

hippuric acid t., see specific tests, including *Lücke's t., Quick's t.* (1), *Spiro's t.* (2). See also *hippuric acid, methods for,* under *method.*

Histalog t., see *augmented histamine t.*

histamine t.: 1. one ml. of a 0.1 per cent solution of histamine is injected subcutaneously as a stimulant of gastric secretion; see also *augmented histamine t.* 2. (*for lesions of the sympathetic nervous system*) a small area of skin on the wrist, ankle, or knee is cleansed with alcohol, which is allowed to dry. A drop of 1:1000 solution of histamine phosphate is placed on it and introduced into the epidermis by multiple needle punctures in a manner similar to that used for cowpox vaccination. The excess histamine is gently removed. (*a*) A reddish purple spot appears as the result of local capillary dilatation. (*b*) A local wheal succeeds, because of transudation of serum from increased permeability of the capillaries. (*c*) A flare results as the effect of dilatation of the arteries by the reflex of a local axon. The flare being dependent on the integrity of the peripheral nerve, it therefore occurs in hysterical anesthesia and malingering but not in neural lesions. 3. (*for pheochromocytoma*) following rapid intravenous injection of histamine phosphate administered in a standardized dosage of 0.010 to 0.050 mg. of histamine base, normal individuals experience transient headache, flush, and a brief fall in blood pressure, but those with pheochromocytoma, after a fall in blood pressure, experience a marked rise in blood pressure, fear, excitability, etc.

histamine flare t. (*for leprosy and postherpetic neuralgia*): a drop of 1:1000 histamine acid phosphate solution is placed on the skin and a needle puncture is made through it; the test is positive if there is no erythema flare when the puncture is made within the suspected lesion area, or if the flare stops at the border of the lesion when it is made slightly to the outside of it.

histidine loading t. (*for folic acid deficiency*): a loading dose of histidine is given, and the resultant urinary excretion of excess forminiglutamic acid (FIGLU), secondary to decreased amounts of tetrahydrofolic acid, is measured. Called also *FIGLU excretion t.*

Hitzig t. (*for vestibular apparatus*): the positive electrode of a galvanic current is applied just in front of the ear being examined while the negative electrode is held in the patient's hand, the patient standing with feet together and eyes closed. A current of 5 milliamperes causes a leaning toward the positive pole in normal persons.

hock t., spavin t.

Hoffmann's t. (*for tyrosine*): add mercuric nitrate to the suspected liquid and boil it; then add nitric acid with a little nitrous acid. A red color is produced if tyrosine is present, and a red precipitate is seen.

Hofmeister's t.: 1. (*for leucine*) warm the suspected liquid with mercurous nitrate; if leucine is present, metallic mercury is deposited. 2. (*for peptones*) mix phosphotungstic and hydrochloric acids; let the mixture stand twenty-four hours, and filter. With this reagent a solution containing peptones with no albumin will afford a precipitate.

Hogben t., see *Xenopus t.*

Holmgren's t.: the use of skeins of colored worsted as a test of the perception of colors; a skein is given to the subject of the test, and he is asked to match it out of a set of variously colored skeins.

Holten's t.: a creatinine clearance test for renal efficiency.

Hopkins' thiophene t. (*for lactic acid*): add a few drops of stomach contents to 5 ml. of concentrated sulfuric acid containing a little cupric sulfate and heat two minutes. Cool and add a very little thiophene. A cherry-red color indicates lactic acid.

Hopkins-Cole t. (*for protein*): glyoxylic acid is prepared by the action of sodium amalgam on a solution of oxalic acid. A few drops of this solution are added to the protein solution and strong sulfuric acid is poured down the side of the tube. A bluish violet color is produced at the junction of the two fluids due to the presence of tryptophan.

Hoppe-Seyler t.: 1. (*for carbon monoxide in the blood*) add to blood twice its volume of a solution of sodium hydroxide of 1.3 specific gravity: normal blood will form a dingy brown mass with a green shade if spread thin on a white surface; but if carbon monoxide is present, the mass is red, and so is the thin layer. 2. (*for xanthine*) add the substance to be tested to a mixture of chlorinated lime in a porcelain dish; a dark-green ring is formed at first.

hormone t., see specific tests, including *Aschheim Zondek t.* and *Siddall t.*

horse cell t., a modification of the Paul-Bunnell-Davidsohn test (q.v.) for heterophile antibodies associated with infectious mononucleosis that uses horse erythrocytes instead of sheep erythrocytes. No centrifugation step is needed and the whole test is performed in minutes.

Horsley's t. (*for dextrose*): the solution is boiled with potassium hydroxide and potassium chromate; if dextrose is present a green color is produced.

Hotis t. (*for garget or mastitis in cows*): fresh milk containing bromcresol purple is incubated for twenty-four hours; a positive reaction is the formation of yellow flakes on the sides of the test tube.

Howard t. (*for renal function*): both ureters are catheterized and urine collected separately from each kidney; the quantity of urine in each collection and its sodium and creatinine concentrations are then determined. Called also *split-renal function t.*

Howell's t. (*for prothrombin*): a test for the amount of prothrombin in the blood depending on the clotting time of the oxalated plasma treated with calcium chloride and thromboplastin.

Huddleson's t.: an agglutination test for brucellosis in man.

Huhner t.: examination of the secretions aspirated from the vaginal fornix and the endocervical canal after coitus, to determine the number and condition of spermatozoa present and the extent to which they have penetrated the cervical mucus.

Huppert's t. (*for bile pigments*): the suspected solution is treated with lime water or calcium chloride solution and then with a solution of ammonium or sodium carbonate. The precipitate of bile pigments may be removed by shaking with chloroform after washing with water and acidulating with acetic acid. Bilirubin colors the chloroform yellow and the acetic acid solution green.

Huppert-Cole t. (*for bile pigments*): to 50 ml. of the unknown add an excess of baryta water or lime water. To the precipitate add 5 ml. of 95 per cent alcohol, 2 drops of strong sulfuric acid, and 2 drops of a 5 per cent solution of potassium chlorate. Boil, and the supernatant liquid will be emerald or bluish green if bile is present.

Hurtley's t. (*for acetoacetic acid*): to 10 ml. of the unknown add 2 ml. of strong hydrochloric acid and 1 ml. of fresh 1 per cent sodium nitrite solution. Shake and add 15 ml. of concentrated ammonium hydroxide and 5 ml. of 10 per cent ferrous sulfate. A violet or purple color develops slowly if acetoacetic acid is present.

hydrochloric acid t., see specific tests, including *dimethylaminoazobenzene t.*, (1), *Günzburg's t.*, *Herzberg's t.*, *Leo's t.*, *Lütthe's t.*, *Maly's t.* (1), (2), *Mohr's t.*, *Rabuteau's t.* (1), (2), *Riegler's t.* (2), *Scivoletto's t.*, *Szabo's t.*, *Töpfer's t.*, *Uffelmann's t.*, *von Jaksch's t.* (1), (2), *Winckler's t.* (2), *Witz's t.*

hydrogen peroxide t. (*for blood*): a 20 per cent solution of hydrogen peroxide is added to the suspected fluid; if blood is present even in minute proportion, bubbles will rise, forming foam on the surface of the fluid.

hydrostatic t.: floating of the lungs of a dead infant when placed in water indicates that the child was born alive; called also *Raygat's t.*

hydroxyaromatic acid t., see *Hanke and Koessler's t.*

hydroxylamine t. (*for dextrose*), see *Bang's method*, under *method*.

hyperemia t., see *Moschcowitz's t.*

hypochlorite-orcinol t. (*for glycerin*): to 3 ml. of the unknown add 3 drops of N/1 sodium hypochlorite solution and boil one minute to drive off chlorine. Then add an equal volume of strong hydrochloric acid and a little orcinol. Boil, and a violet or greenish blue color indicates glycerine or a sugar, or some substance that can be oxidized to a sugar.

hypothesis t., an abstract procedure for determining whether a set of observations is consistent with a hypothesis under consideration; it is the theoretical basis of most statistical tests. A hypothesis test decides between two hypotheses, one stating that the effect under investigation does not exist (the *null hypothesis, H_0*), and the other that some specified effect does exist (the *alternative hypothesis, H_1*), based on the observed value of a test statistic whose sampling distribution is completely determined by H_0. When the test statistic falls in a set of values known as the critical region, H_0 is rejected. The level of probability of incorrectly rejecting H_0 may be set before the data are collected, usually at 0.05 or 0.01; this is called the *significance level* or α *level*. It is now more common to report the smallest α at which the null hypothesis can be rejected; this is called the *significance probability* or *P value*.

hypoxanthine t., see *Kossel's t.*

Ilimow's t. (*for albumin*): acidulate with acid sodium phosphate, filter, and add a solution of phenol (1:20); a cloudy precipitate indicates albumin.

Ilosvay's t. (*for nitrites*), see under *reagent*.

imidazole t., see *Hanke and Koessler's t.*

immobilizaton t.: detection of antibody based on its ability to inhibit the motility of a bacterial cell or protozoon.

IMViC t. [modified acronym from *i*ndole, *m*ethyl red, *V*oges-Proskauer, *c*itrate] a series of metabolic tests used as standard procedure to differentiate genera of the Enterobacteriaceae. See also the individual tests.

indican t., see specific tests, including *Jaffé's t.* (2), *Jolles' t.* (2), *MacMunn's t., Obermayer's t., Porter's t.* (2), *Wang's t., Weber's t.* (2). See also *indican, methods for,* under *method.*

indigo carmine t. *(for renal permeability)*: a solution of indigo carmine is injected intramuscularly and the time of its appearance in the urine is noted. Normally, it begins to appear in about five minutes. Delay beyond this points to defective renal adequacy.

indigo red t., see *Rosin's t.*

indole t., see specific tests, including *Baeyer's t.* (2), *Herter's t.* (1), *Kondo's t., Legal's t.* (2), *Nencki's t., nitroso-indole-nitrate t., pine wood t., Salkowski's t.* (3). See also *indole, methods for,* under *method.*

indophenol t. *(for the presence of oxidizing enzymes in cells and for detecting the presence of myeloblasts, etc.)*: cover glass films of the cells are fixed in alcohol. Float for ten to twenty minutes, face down, upon a freshly prepared solution of equal parts of 1 per cent aqueous solutions of dimethyl paraphenylenediamine and of alphanaphthol (Nadi's reagent). Rinse and mount in glycerin. The cytoplasm of cells containing oxidase (myeloblasts, myelocytes, polymorphonuclears, and large mononuclears) will be colored blue by indophenol.

inkblot t., see *Rorschach t.*

inoculation t. *(for acute anterior poliomyelitis)*: the cerebrospinal fluid of the suspected patient (i.e., before the appearance of paralytic symptoms) is injected into a monkey. Paralysis will appear in the monkey within seven days if the patient is affected.

inosite t., see specific tests, including *Scherer's t.* (1) and *Seidel's t.*

intelligence t., a set of problems or tasks posed to assess an individual's innate ability to judge, comprehend, and reason.

intracutaneous t.: intradermal t.

intracutaneous tuberculin t., see *Mantoux t.*

intradermal t., a skin test in which the antigen is injected intradermally.

inulin clearance t., see under *inulin.*

iodine t.: 1. *(for starch)* when a compound solution of iodine is added to starch, and especially to an acid or neutral solution of cooked starch paste, a deep-blue color is produced which disappears on heating and reappears on cooling. Erythrodextrin and glycogen give a red color with iodine. 2. see specific tests, including *Lesser's t., Winckler's t.* (3).

iodoform t.: 1. *(for acetone)* see *Gunning's t.* 2. *(for alcohol)* make the unknown alkaline, and add a few drops of iodine solution. Heat gently, and yellow iodoform crystals indicate alcohol or some similar body.

Iowa pressure articulation t.: a test of the ability to produce the consonant sounds in isolated words, particularly the pressure sounds.

irresistible impulse t., see under *impulse.*

irrigation t.: the patient is examined with the bladder full. The anterior urethra is washed out with a warm solution of boric acid (3 per cent), the perineum being compressed to prevent the entrance of the fluid into the posterior urethra. When the washings are perfectly clear, the patient voids his urine and any turbidity must come from the posterior urethra.

Ishihara's t.: a test for color vision made by the use of a series of plates composed of round dots of various sizes and colors.

Ito-Reenstierna t.: *(obs.)* intracutaneous injection of a vaccine of killed *Hemophilus ducreyi* elicits a positive skin reaction in persons who have been infected with chancroid.

Jacoby's t. *(for pepsin)*: the greatest dilution of gastric juice which will clarify an acid solution of ricin in three hours at 38° C. gives the number of peptic units in the juice.

Jacquemin's t. *(for phenol)*: add to the suspected liquid an equal quantity of aniline and some sodium hypochlorite in solution; a blue color is produced.

Jadassohn's t., see *irrigation t.*

Jaffé's t.: 1. *(for creatinine and dextrose)* to the liquid add trinitrophenol and then make alkaline with sodium hydroxide. A red color without heating indicates creatinine; a red color after heating indicates dextrose. 2. *(for indican)* to the suspected liquid are added an equal amount of concentrated hydrochloric acid, 1 ml. of chloroform, and a few drops of a strong solution of chlorinated soda. The chloroform is colored blue if indican is present.

Jaksch's t., see *von Jaksch's t.*

Janet's t. *(for differentiating between functional and organic anesthesia)*: the patient is instructed to say "yes" or "no,"

according as he does or does not feel the examiner's touch. He may say "no" in functional anesthesia, but he will say nothing in cases of organic anesthesia.

Jansen's t. *(for osteoarthritis deformans of the hip)*: the patient is told to cross his legs with a point just above the ankle resting on the opposite knee; this motion is impossible when the disease exists.

Javorski's t., Jaworski's t.: in hourglass stomach a splashing sound will be heard on succussion of the pyloric portion after siphonage.

Jenning's t.: a modification of Holmgren's test for color perception. Small patches of colored worsted are placed so as to be protected from light and dust. The person to be examined indicates his color selection by pricking the record sheet with a pointed pencil.

Jochmann's t., 1. Müller-Jochmann t. 2. antitrypsin t.

Johnson's t. *(for albumin)*: put the urine in a test tube and carefully pour upon it a strong solution of trinitrophenol; a white coagulum of albumin appears at the junction of the liquids, which heating augments.

Jolles' t.: 1. *(for bile pigments in urine)* the urine is shaken with barium chloride solution, chloroform, and a few drops of hydrochloric acid. The precipitate is removed and partially dried. Treatment with 2 drops of strong sulfuric acid will bring out the characteristic colors of the bile pigments. 2. *(for indican)* to the urine add a little alcoholic solution of thymol and fuming hydrochloric acid containing 0.5 per cent of ferric chloride; chloroform shaken with this mixture becomes violet in color.

Jones and Cantarow t., see *urea concentration t.*

Jorissen's t. *(for formaldehyde)*: add 0.5 ml. of a 1 per cent solution of phloroglucinol in 10 per cent sodium hydroxide to 1 ml. of the urine; a bright red color indicates free formaldehyde.

Kantor and Gies' t. *(for proteins)*: test papers, made by dipping them in Gies' reagent (see under *Gies' t.*), drying, and cutting into strips, are used in making biuret test.

Kaplan's t. *(for globulin-albumin in spinal fluid)*: to 0.2 ml. of the fluid in a test tube is added 0.3 ml. of distilled water. This is boiled up twice. Three drops of a 5 per cent solution of butyric acid in physiologic salt solution are added and the mixture carefully underlaid with 0.5 ml. of a saturated aqueous solution of ammonium sulfate. After twenty minutes a definite ring will form at the point of contact if globulin-albumin is present.

Kapsinow's t. *(for bile pigments)*: add Obermayer's reagent to the urine and heat; a green color indicates bile pigments.

Kashiwado's t. *(for pancreatic disease)*: the patient swallows stained nuclei from a calf's thymus mixed with lycopodium grains; these later serve to indicate the portion of the feces which is to be examined.

Kastle's t. *(for raw milk)*: to 5 ml. of the milk add 0.3 ml. of N/10 hydrogen peroxide solution and 1 ml. of a 1 per cent solution of tricresol; raw milk will give a slight yellow color, boiled milk will not.

Kastle-Meyer t., see *phenolphthalein t.*

Katayama's t. *(for carbonyl-hemoglobin)*: to 5 drops of blood add 10 ml. of water, 5 drops of orange-colored ammonium sulfide, and enough acetic acid to make the mixture acid. CO causes a rose-red color; normal blood, a dirty greenish gray.

Kathrein's t., see *Maréchal's t.*

Kato t.: a technique for the quantitative estimation of the worm burden of an individual, based on estimation of a standard 50 mg. sample of fresh feces cleared with glycerine.

Kelling's t.: 1. *(for lactic acid in the stomach)* the stomach contents are diluted with water, and to them are added one or two drops of a 5 per cent watery solution of ferric chloride. A greenish yellow color is formed when lactic acid is present. 2. a test for the presence and location of an esophageal diverticulum by the sound of swallowing. 3. *(for gastric carcinoma)* a test based on the fact that the serum of cancer patients will dissolve the red corpuscles of the hen.

Kentmann's t. *(for formaldehyde)*: dissolve in a test tube 0.1 gm. of morphine in 1 ml. of sulfuric acid; add, without mixing, an equal volume of the liquid to be tested: in a short time the latter will take on a reddish violet color if any formaldehyde is present.

Kerner's t. *(for creatinine)*: acidify the suspected solution and add phosphomolybdic or phosphotungstic acid in solution; if creatinine is present, it will form a crystalline precipitate.

kidney function t., see specific tests, including *amylase t.* (1), *blood-urea clearance t., concentration t., Fishberg concentration t., glycerophosphate t., Holten's t., Howard t., indigo carmine t., inulin clearance t., lactose t.* (1), *Mosenthal's t., Nyiri's t., phenolsulfonphthalein t., phlorhizin t., potassium* iodide t., Pregl's t., radioactive renogram t., radioisotope renal excretion t., Rehberg's t., Simonelli's t., (2), (4), urea concentration t., urine concentration t., xylose absorption or tolerance t.

Killian's t. (*for carbohydrate tolerance*): two hours after a standard breakfast, give the patient 200 ml. of water. One hour later, give 1.75 gm. of dextrose per kilogram of body weight. Determine amount of dextrose in blood specimens taken at hourly intervals and in the twenty-four-hour specimen of urine.

Kinberg's t. (*for liver function*): after a low nitrogen content diet for several days, 50 gm. of gelatin dissolved in hot chocolate is taken fasting; in liver disease there is an increase in the output of amino acids, except in congestion of the liver and catarrhal jaundice.

Kitzmiller t., see *antithrombin t.*

Kjeldahl's t. (*for nitrogen*), see under *method*.

Klein t., see under *reaction*.

Klimow's t. (*for blood in urine*): to a specimen of urine is added an equal quantity of H_2O_2 and a little powdered aloin; formation of a purple color indicates the presence of blood.

Kline t.: (*obs.*) a nontreponemal antigen serologic test for syphilis.

Knapp's t.: 1. (*for sugar in the urine*) ten gm. of mercuric cyanide are dissolved in 100 ml. of a solution of caustic soda and diluted; heated with diabetic urine, metallic mercury is precipitated. 2. (*for organic acids in stomach*) stomach contents are filtered and 1 ml. treated with 5 ml. of ether; the extract is floated on dilute iron solution in test tubes, and the various colored rings formed will indicate the presence of the various acids.

Knott t.: a test for microfilariae or worm larvae in the blood by lysis of the blood in a dilute (2 per cent) formalin solution, centrifugation, and examination of the stained sediment for microfilariae or larvae.

Kober t. (*for estrogens*): when estrogens are treated with a mixture of sulfuric acid and phenolsulfonic acid and then diluted with water, a clear pink color is formed; suitable for qualitative analysis.

Kobert's t. (*for hemoglobin*): the suspected liquid is treated with zinc powder or a solution of zinc sulfate; the resulting precipitate is stained red by alkalis.

Kolmer t.: a modification of the Wassermann test, introduced in 1922, or any of its subsequent improvements; these tests used complement fixation rather than flocculation as the indicator reaction and were once the standard confirmatory tests for syphilis; they are now little used.

Komolgorov-Smirnov t., a statistical test of goodness of fit of a sample to a specified theoretical distribution function, or of whether two samples are drawn from the same population, based on the size of the maximum difference between the cumulative distribution functions of the sample and theoretical distributions, or of the two samples, and using the exact sampling distribution of this difference to determine the significance level.

Kondo's t. (*for indole or skatole*): to 1 ml. of the unknown add 3 drops of solution of formaldehyde and 1 ml. of concentrated sulfuric acid; a violet-red color indicates indole, a yellow or brown color skatole.

Korotkoff's t.: in aneurysm, if the blood pressure in the peripheral circulation remains fairly high while the artery above the aneurysm is compressed, the collateral circulation is good.

Kossel's t. (*for hypoxanthine*): the liquid to be tested is treated with zinc and hydrochloric acid and with sodium hydroxide in excess; if hypoxanthine is present, a ruby-red color is produced.

Kowarsky's t.: 1. (*for dextrose in urine*) in a test tube place 5 drops of pure phenylhydrazine, 10 drops of glacial acetic acid, and 1 ml. of saturated solution of sodium chloride. To the mass which results add 2 or 3 ml. of urine; boil two minutes, and cool. If dextrose is present, crystals of phenylglucosazone will be seen with the microscope. 2. (*blood test for diabetes*) test of the patient's blood based on the reduction of a copper solution by the sugar in the blood to cuprous oxide, and the dissolving of the latter in an acid solution of ferrous sulphate, which causes the separation of an equal amount of ferrous oxide, which is measured by titration with potassium permanganate.

Krokiewicz's t. (*for bile pigment in urine*): 1 ml. of a 1 per cent solution of sodium nitrate and 1 ml. of a 1 per cent solution of sulfanilic acid are mixed and added drop by drop to 0.5 ml. of urine. The amount added must not exceed 10 drops. The mixture becomes bright red, changing to amethyst on the addition of 1 or 2 drops of concentrated hydrochloric acid and a large amount of water.

Kuhlmann's t.: a modification of Binet's test for use in infants.

Külz's t. (*for β-hydroxybutyric acid*): 1. the fermented urine is evaporated to a syrupy consistence, strong sulfuric acid in equal volume is added, and the mixture is distilled. If hydroxybutyric acid is present, α-crotonic acid will be formed, which will crystallize. 2. if, after fermentation, the urine shows dextrorotatory properties, β-hydroxybutyric acid is present.

Kurzrok-Miller t.: an in vitro test of compatibility of cervical mucus and spermatozoa, involving observation, under the microscope, of the behavior of sperm placed beside a sample of mucus taken from the cervical canal at the time of ovulation.

Kveim t. (*for sarcoidosis*): a skin test using antigen from human sarcoid tissue injected intradermally; any palpable nodule developing at the inoculation site within 6 weeks is biopsied, and histopathologic evidence of epithelioid cell granulomas constitutes a positive reaction. The test is positive in about 60 to 80 per cent of patients.

Laborde's t. (*for death*), see *Cloquet's needle sign*, under *sign*.

lactic acid t., see specific tests, including *Hopkins' thiophene t., MacLean t., Uffelmann's t.* See also *lactic acid, methods for*, under *method*.

lactose t.: 1. (*for renal function*) twenty gm. of lactose dissolved in 20 ml. of distilled water are injected under aseptic precautions into a vein at the bend of the elbow. The urine is collected hourly and tested (Nylander's test) until the sugar reaction ceases to be positive. If lactose secretion continues for more than five hours, renal disease is indicated. 2. see specific tests, including *Mathews' t., Moore's t., Rubner's t.* (2).

Ladendorff's t. (*for blood*): treat the suspected liquid with tincture of guaiacum, and afterward with eucalyptus oil; the upper stratum of the mixture is turned violet and the lower blue if blood is present.

Lancefield precipitation t.: a ring precipitation test used to classify and identify streptococci. Group specific antibody reacts *in vitro* with group specific polysaccharide to produce a ring of precipitation where the two reagents react at the interface.

Lang's t. (*for taurine*): the solution to be tested is boiled with freshly prepared mercuric oxide; taurine will cause a white precipitate to appear.

Lange's t., 1. see *colloidal gold t.* 2. (*for acetone in urine*) 15 ml. of urine are mixed with 0.5 to 1 ml. of acetic acid, and a few drops of a freshly prepared concentrated solution of sodium nitroprusside added. The mixture is overlaid with ammonia. At the point of junction a characteristic violet ring is formed.

lantern t.: a test for color blindness made with a set of specially devised lanterns.

latex agglutination t., latex fixation t.: a type of agglutination test using latex particles as passive carriers of adsorbed antigens. The particles agglutinate following the addition of specific antibody. This test has been used extensively for the detection of rheumatoid factor and for the detection of urine human chorionic gonadotropin (hCG) in pregnancy testing.

Leach's t. (*for formaldehyde*): to 10 ml. of milk add 10 ml. of concentrated hydrochloric acid containing 0.02 per cent of ferric chloride. Heat, and if formaldehyde is present a violet color will be produced.

Lebbin's t. (*for formaldehyde in milk*): a small amount of milk is boiled with a mixture of 0.05 gm. of resorcinol and the same quantity of a 5 per cent solution of sodium hydroxide. Change from a yellow to a red color indicates the presence of formaldehyde.

Lechini's t. (*for blood in urine*): ten ml. of urine are treated with 1 drop of acetic acid and 3 ml. of chloroform; with blood the chloroform layer becomes red.

Lee's t. (*for rennin*): add 5 drops of gastric juice to 5 ml. of milk; coagulation should take place in twenty minutes in the incubator.

Legal's t.: 1. (*for acetone*) render the urine acid with HCl and distill it. Solution of sodium hydroxide and sodium nitroprusside added to the distillate produce a ruby-red tint, which acetic acid changes to purple. Creatinine will also produce a red color, but this color disappears when acetic acid is put in. 2. (*for indole*) to the unknown add a few drops of sodium nitroprusside; make alkaline with potassium hydroxide. The violet color changes to blue on the addition of acetic acid.

leishmanin t., intradermal injection of leishmanin (leishmania promastigote antigens); a positive reaction consists of a palpable nodule developing in 48 to 72 hours and indicates delayed hypersensitivity, but not necessarily immunity, to leishmania organisms. The test is not species-specific. It becomes positive early in the course of cutaneous or mucocutaneous leishmaniasis, particularly the New World forms, except in diffuse cutaneous leishmaniasis; it becomes positive only after recovery from visceral leishmaniasis. Called also *Montenegro t.*

Le Nobel's t., see *Nobel's t.*

lentochol t., see *Sachs-Georgi t.*

Leo's t. (*for free hydrochloric acid*): calcium carbonate is added to the solution, which is neutralized if the acidity is due to free acid, but not if due to acid salts.

lepromin t.: intradermal injection of lepromin (a suspension of heat-killed *Mycobacterium leprae*); a positive reaction consists of a tuberculin-type reaction at 48 to 72 hours (*Fernandez reaction*) or a nodular, occasionally ulcerated, lesion at 3 to 4 weeks (*Mitsuda reaction*). The test is not diagnostic; a large fraction of the normal population exhibits lepromin reactivity owing to sensitivity to cross-reacting antigens. In individuals known to have leprosy, lepromin reactivity is indicative of tuberculoid leprosy or borderline leprosy near the tuberculoid end of the spectrum, whereas lepromin anergy is indicative of lepromatous or near-lepromatous disease.

Lesser's t.: any iodine-containing secretion turns yellow when treated with calomel.

leucine t., see specific tests, including *Hofmeister's t.* (1), *Scherer's t.* (2).

Levinson t. (*for tuberculous meningitis and other intracranial conditions*): one ml. of spinal fluid is placed in each of the two test tubes 8 mm. in diameter. To one is added 1 ml. of a 1 per cent solution of mercuric chloride and, to the other, 1 ml. of a 3 per cent solution of sulfosalicylic acid. The tubes are well shaken, stoppered, and allowed to stand at room temperature for forty-eight hours. At the end of twenty-four and forty-eight hours the column of precipitate in each tube is measured in millimeters. When the height of the precipitate in the first test tube is seen to be twice that of the precipitate in the second tube, the result of the test is positive.

levulose t., see *Borchardt's t., methylphenylhydrazine t., Rubner's t.* (2), *Selivanoff's t.*

levulose tolerance t.: a test of hepatic function based on the power of the liver to absorb and store large quantities of levulose.

Lewis and Pickering t.: the employment of a rapid rise of temperature to produce vasodilatation in the part to be tested for the state of the peripheral circulation.

Lichtheim t.: if a patient is able to indicate the number of syllables in a word which he cannot utter, it indicates that the cortex is less involved than the association fibers.

Lieben's t. (*for acetone in urine*): acidulate and distill it, and treat with ammonia and tincture of iodine; if acetone is present, a yellow precipitate of iodoform is produced.

Lieben-Ralfe t. (*for acetone*): boil 1.3 gm. of potassium iodide in 3.75 ml. of solution of potassium hydroxide; float the urine on the surface of the reagent in a test tube: a precipitate of phosphate is formed at the upper surface of the reagent, which, if acetone is present, will be rendered yellow by iodoform.

Liebermann's t. (*for proteins*): a precipitate is made from the urine with alcohol; wash this with ether and heat with strong hydrochloric acid: this produces a fine violet-blue color if proteins are present.

Liebermann-Burchard t. (*for cholesterol*): dissolve the suspected substance in chloroform, add acetic anhydride, and treat with strong sulfuric acid; if cholesterol is present, a violet color is produced, which soon changes to green.

Liebig's t. (*for cystine*): boil the suspected substance with a sodium hydroxide solution and a little lead sulfide; if cystine is present, the lead sulfide will form a black precipitate.

Ligat's t. (*for cutaneous hyperesthesia in abdominal disease*): the skin is pinched between the thumb and forefinger and lifted up from the parts below.

limulus t.: an extract of blood cells from the horseshoe crab (*Limulus polyphemus*) is exposed to a blood sample from a patient; if gram-negative endotoxin is present in the sample, it will produce gelation of the extract of blood cells.

Lindemann's t. (*for acetoacetic acid in urine*): to about 10 ml. of urine add 5 drops of 30 per cent acetic acid, 5 drops Lugol's solution, and 2 or 3 ml. chloroform, and shake. The chloroform does not change color if diacetic acid is present, but becomes reddish violet in its absence. Uric acid also decolorizes iodine, and if much is present double the amount of Lugol's solution should be used.

Lindner's t., see under *sign.*

lipase t.: 1. (*for liver function*) a test based on the fact that lipase is present in the blood plasma of normal persons in a constant amount. Liver injury will cause a rise in the lipase of the blood plasma as measured by the power of the blood to split ethyl butyrate. 2. see specific tests, including *copper soap t., litmus milk t.*

Lipps' t., see *sand t.*

litmus milk t. (*for pancreatic lipase*): add pancreatic lipase to litmus milk, incubate, and note change of color; pancreatic lipase is indicated by a pink coloration.

liver function t., see specific tests, including *Kinberg's t., levulose tolerance t., lipase t., Macdonald's t., nitrogen partition t., phenoltetrachlorophthalein t., Quick's t.* (1), *rose bengal t., Rosenthal's t.* (2), *santonin t., Zappacosta's t.*

Loewe's t. (*for dextrose in urine*): treat the urine with a solution of sodium carbonate containing bismuth subnitrate and glycerine; sugar gives a dark precipitate.

Loewi's t.: three drops of epinephrine chloride solution 1:1000 are instilled into the conjunctival sac, followed in five minutes by 3 more drops. This produces dilatation of the pupil in pancreatic insufficiency, diabetes, and hyperthyroidism.

Lombard's t.: a test for simulated deafness using a noise apparatus.

Löwenthal's t. (*for dextrose not in urine*): boil the suspected substance with a solution of ferric chloride, tartaric acid, and sodium carbonate; if dextrose is present, the liquid becomes dark, and iron oxide is freely precipitated.

Lücke's t. (*for hippuric acid*): add boiling hot nitric acid, evaporate, and heat the dry residue; a strong odor of nitrobenzene proves the presence of hippuric acid.

Luebert's t. (*for formaldehyde in milk*): five gm. of coarsely powdered potassium sulfate are placed in a 100 ml. flask; 5 ml. of suspected milk are put over it by a pipet, and 10 ml. of sulfuric acid (specific gravity, 1.84) are run down the side of the flask. If formaldehyde is present, a violet coloration soon occurs; if none is present, the fluid becomes brown or black.

lupus band t.: an immunofluoresence test to determine the presence and extent of immunoglobulin and complement deposits at the dermal-epidermal junction of skin specimens from patients with systemic lupus erythematosus.

Lüttke's t. (*for free hydrochloric acid in gastric juice*): a quantitative determination in succession of the total chlorides, the chlorine in the fixed chlorides, and then the combined and free HCl.

Lyle and Curtman's t. (*for blood*): boil the stool with acetic acid, extract it with ether, and to the ethereal extract add a little guaiaconic acid in 95 per cent alcohol; a decided green, light-blue, or purple color indicates the presence of blood.

lymphocyte proliferation t., a functional test of the ability of lymphocytes to respond to mitogens, specific antigens, or allogenic cells. Lymphocytes are cultured both with and without the stimulant for several days and then are cultured for several hours with ^{3}H-labeled thymidine. The ratio of the thymidine uptake in the stimulated and control cultures is reported as the "stimulation index" (SI) or "stimulation ratio" (SR). The test with allogenic cells, called a mixed lymphocyte culture (MLC), is commonly performed for transplantation tissue typing; all three types of stimulants are used in investigation of immunodeficiency. Commonly used mitogens are phytohemagglutinin (PHA), concanavalin A (ConA), and pokeweed mitogen (PWM); commonly used antigens are PPD (tuberculin), *Candida* antigen, and streptokinase-streptodornase. Called also *blastogenesis assay* and *lymphocyte proliferation assay.*

Lyon's t., Meltzer-Lyon t.

Macdonald's t. (*for liver function*): inject 2 mg. per kilogram of sodium sulfobromophthalein (Bromsulphalein) and take blood specimens every five minutes for thirty minutes after the injection.

Machado t., Machado-Guerreiro t. (*for Chagas' disease*): a complement-fixation test, using as antigen an extract of the spleen of puppies severely infected with *Trypanosoma cruzi.*

Maclagan's t., see *thymol turbidity t.*

MacLean t. (*for lactic acid in gastric juice*): to 5 ml. of gastric juice add 5 drops of the following reagent: ferric chloride, 5 gm.; concentrated hydrochloric acid, 1.5 ml.; saturated solution of mercury bichloride, 100 ml. Lactic acid is indicated by a yellow coloration.

MacLean-de Wesselow t., see *urea concentration t.*

MacMunn's t. (*for indican*): boil the urine in an equal quantity of hydrochloric acid and a little nitric acid; cool, and shake with chloroform, which becomes violet, and shows one absorption band due to indigo blue and one due to indigo red.

McMurray's t. (*for torn meniscus*): as the patient lies supine with knee fully flexed, the examiner rotates the patient's foot fully outward and the knee is slowly extended; a painful "click" indicates a tear of the medial meniscus of the knee joint. If the click occurs when the foot is rotated inward, the tear is in the lateral meniscus.

MacWilliams' t. (*for albumin*): take 20 ml. of urine and add 2 drops of a saturated solution of salicylsulfonic acid: if albumin is present, a cloudiness or precipitate will be seen; if albumoses or peptones are present, this precipitate will disappear on boiling, but appear again on cooling.

magnesionitric t. (*for albumin in urine*): mix 1 part of nitric acid and 1 part magnesium sulfate; turbidity indicates the presence of albumin.

Magpie's t. (*for salts of mercury*): stannous chloride is added to the suspected solution; a white and gray precipitate is formed, consisting of metallic mercury and mild mercurous chloride.

male frog t., male toad t. (*for pregnancy*): urine or serum of a woman suspected of being pregnant is injected into the dorsal lymph sac of two male frogs (*Rana pipiens*) or male toads (*Bufo marinus*). The presence of spermatozoa in the cloacal fluid of both animals is positive; in one animal, inconclusive; in neither animal, negative.

Malerba's t. (*for acetone*): add a solution of dimethyl-para-phenylenediamine; a fine red or reddish color is seen.

mallein t., see *mallein*.

Malot's t.: a test for the quantitative determination of phosphoric acid in urine by the reaction with cochineal and a uranium salt.

maltose t., see *Rubner's t.* (2).

Maly's t.: 1. (*for free hydrochloric acid in the gastric juice*) a solution of methylene blue is added; the free acid will turn it from a violet to a green or blue tint. 2. (*for free hydrochloric acid in stomach contents*) filter into a glass dish and stain blue with ultramarine; place a piece of lead paper over it and cover; warm the mixture. The free acid will turn the blue to brown and darken the lead paper.

Mann-Whitney t., Mann-Whitney-Wilcoxon t., rank sum t.

Mantoux t.: intracutaneous tuberculin test; the now standard type of tuberculin test in which tuberculin is administered intradermally using a needle and syringe.

Maréchal's t. (*for bile pigments in urine*): drop tincture of iodine carefully into the tube; when the drops touch the urine, a green color is seen.

Maréchal-Rosin t., see *Maréchal's t.*

Marlow's t. (*for heterophoria*): one eye is occluded by a bandage for some time; after the bandage is removed, measurements for heterophoria are made.

Marquardt's t. (*for fusel oil*): add a few drops of dilute potassium permanganate until the light pink color persists. Cork for twenty-four hours. Add more permanganate if necessary to keep the pink color. Note the sickening odor of valeric acid.

Marquis' t. (*for morphine*): evaporate the unknown to dryness on a white porcelain plate and touch with a mixture of 3 ml. of concentrated sulfuric acid and 2 drops of formalin. A purple-red color changing to violet and then to blue indicates morphine.

Marshall's t. (*for urea*): treat the specimen with urease and titrate the ammonia so formed; see under *method*.

Maschke's t., see *von Maschke's t.*

Masset's t. (*for bile pigments in urine*): add 2 or 3 drops of sulfuric acid and a crystal of potassium nitrite; a grass-green color shows the presence of bile pigments.

Master "2-step" exercise t. (*for coronary insufficiency*): an electrocardiographic test, the tracings being recorded while the subject repeatedly ascends and descends two steps, each 9 inches high, immediately after cessation of the climbs, and then 2 and 6 minutes later. The amount of work (number of trips) is standardized for age, weight, and sex.

Matas' t., see *tourniquet t.,* def. 2.

match t.: a screening test of expiration in which a match is held 3 inches from the subject's wide open mouth and several attempts are made to blow it out. Failure after six attempts indicates a maximal breathing capacity below 40 liters per minute and a maximal midexpiratory flow rate below 0.6 liter per second.

Mathews' t. (*for lactose and dextrose*): if both dextrose and lactose are suspected, make a total quantitative test by Benedict's method. Add yeast to the urine and ferment out the dextrose, then make a second quantitative determination. The second determination is or may be lactose; confirm with the osazone test. The difference between the two determinations is dextrose.

Maumené t. (*for dextrose*): heat the urine with a little stannous chloride; if sugar is present, a dark-brown precipitate will be formed.

Mauthner's t.: a method of testing color blindness by the use of small bottles filled with different pigments, some with one only and some with two, the latter containing either pseudoisochromatic or isochromatic solutions.

Mayer's t. (*for alkaloids*): mercuric chloride, $13\frac{1}{2}$ gm., and potassium iodide, 50 gm., are dissolved in 1000 ml. of water: this is used as a test for alkaloid, with which it gives a white precipitate.

Mayerhofer's t.: the reduction of a decinormal solution of potassium permanganate solution by 1 ml. of spinal fluid in an acid medium as an index of the amount of protein substance present in the fluid; used as an indication of the existence of tuberculous meningitis.

Méhu's t. (*for albumin in urine*): add a little nitric acid, and mix with 10 volumes of a solution of 2 parts of alcohol, 1 part of phenol, and 1 part of acetic acid; shake it and a white precipitate appears. This test is said not to be entirely trustworthy.

Meigs's t. (*for fat in milk*): to 10 ml. of milk in a special apparatus add 20 ml. of water, 20 ml. of ethyl ether, and shake. Then add 20 ml. of 95 per cent alcohol. Remove the ethereal layer, evaporate, and weigh.

Meinicke t.: (*obs.*) any of several nontreponemal antigen serologic tests for syphilis.

melanin t., see specific tests, including *Thormählen's t., von Jaksch's t.* (3), *Zeller's t.* (1).

Mendel's t., see *Mantoux t.*

Mendelsohn's t.: a test for efficiency of the heart muscle based on the rapidity of the recovery of the pulse from its acceleration produced by exertion.

meningitis t.: see specific tests, including *Levinson's t., Mayerhofer's t., Takata-Ara t., tryptophan t.* (2).

mercury t., see specific tests, including *Magpie's t., Reinsch's t.* (2), *Vogel and Lee's t.*

Mester's t. (*for rheumatic disease*): blood is withdrawn from the middle finger of the right hand of a fasting patient before and again thirty and sixty minutes after administration of two or three intracutaneous injections of 0.2 ml. each of a sterile 0.1 per cent aqueous solution of salicylic acid, and the number of leukocytes is determined after each withdrawal. The injections are made at the flexor aspect of the right forearm at a distance of about 5 cm. from each other. They are followed by severe pain and burning sensation of short duration and by the formation, at the points of the injections, of wheals which disappear in a few hours. Positive results are shown by transient leukopenia within the first thirty minutes after administration of the injections.

methylphenylhydrazine t. (*for levulose*): add 4 gm. of methylphenylhydrazine to 10 ml. of unknown (containing about 2 gm. of levulose) and enough alcohol to clarify the solution; add 4 ml. of 50 per cent acetic acid and heat from five to ten minutes. Reddish yellow needles of methylphenyl-levulosazone indicate levulose.

methyl red t. (*for differentiation of Enterobacteriaceae*): the organism is inoculated into a buffered glucose-peptone broth containing methyl red. In a positive reaction, the medium remains red after incubation owing to acid metabolic products. Most Enterobacteriaceae are positive; the Klebsielleae are negative and Erwinieae are variable.

Mett's t. (*for estimating pepsin*): tubes (Mett's tubes) of coagulated albumin are introduced into the unknown and into a standard pepsin HCl mixture and the amount of digestion occurring in a given time is noted.

Michailow's t. (*for proteins*): add ferrous sulfate to the solution, underlay it with strong sulfuric acid and a drop or so of nitric acid; a brown ring and red coloration indicate the presence of proteins.

microprecipitation t.: a precipitation test in which a minute quantity of the serum is employed.

MIF t., migration inhibitory factor t.

migration inhibitory factor (MIF) t., an *in vitro* test for the production of MIF by lymphocytes in response to specific antigens; used for evaluation of cell-mediated immunity. MIF production is absent in certain immunodeficiency disorders, e.g., DiGeorge syndrome, Wiskott-Aldrich syndrome, Hodgkin's disease.

milk t., see specific tests, including *Babcock's t.*, *Bauer's t.* (3), *benzidine peroxidase t.*, *dirt t.*, *Kastle's t.*, *Kober t.* (2), *methylene blue t.* (2), *phosphatase t.* (1), *Storck's t.*, *Wilkinson and Peter's t.*

milk ring t., abortus Bang ring t.

Millard's t. (*for albumin*): make a reagent of 2 parts of liquefied carbolic acid, 6 parts of glacial acetic acid, and 22 parts of a solution of potassium hydroxide; this precipitates albumin.

Miller-Kurzrok t.: a laboratory procedure to test the ability of sperm to penetrate the mucus plug in a woman's cervix.

40 millimeter t. (*for athletic efficiency*): the subject sits with nasal respiration occluded with a clamp, and by expiring through a mouthpiece, sustains a column of mercury at the height of 40 mm. as long as he can. The pulse rate is taken meanwhile, every five seconds. In a satisfactory test the pulse rate is unaltered for a minute or more.

Millon's t. (*for proteins and nitrogenous compounds*): a solution is made of 10 gm. of mercury and 20 gm. of nitric acid; this is diluted with an equal volume of water and decanted after standing twenty-four hours. This reagent gives a red color with proteins and other substances, such as tyrosine, phenol, and thymol, which contain the hydroxyphenyl group.

Mills's t. (*for tennis elbow*): with the wrist and fingers fully flexed and the forearm pronated, complete extension of the elbow is painful.

miostagmin t., see under *reaction*.

mirror t.: a mirror is held horizontally above the larynx and the patient instructed to cough. The mirror is thus sprayed with bronchial secretion. Small flecks of secretion on the mirror indicate the nature of the expectoration.

Mitscherlich's t. (*for phosphorus in the stomach*): the contents of the stomach are made acid and distilled in the dark. The condenser will contain a luminous ring. Small amounts of alcohol, ether, or turpentine will prevent the reaction.

Mitsuda t., lepromin t.

Mittelmeyer's t.: the patient is directed to take marching steps on one spot without progressing: in vestibular disorder he will turn to the side ipsilateral to vestibular loss, or contralateral to vestibular excitation.

mixed lymphocyte culture t., see under *culture*, and see *lymphocyte proliferation t.*

Moerner-Sjöqvist t., Sjöqvist method.

Mohr's t. (*for hydrochloric acid in the stomach contents*): dilute to a light-yellow color a solution of iron acetate, free from alkaline acetates; add a few drops of a solution of potassium thiocyanate, and then the filtered contents of the stomach: if they contain the acid, a red coloring ensues, which is destroyed by sodium acetate.

Molisch's t.: 1. (*for dextrose in urine*) add 2 ml. of urine, 2 drops of a 15 per cent solution of thymol, and an equal volume of strong sulfuric acid; a deep-red color results. 2. (*for dextrose in urine*) to 1 ml. of urine add 2 or 3 drops of a 5 per cent solution of alphanaphthol in alcohol, then add 2 ml. of strong sulfuric acid; a deep-violet color is produced, and a violet precipitate follows if water is added. 3. (*for proteins*) the substance is treated with a 15 per cent alcoholic solution of alphanaphthol and then with concentrated sulfuric acid; a violet color is formed if proteins are present.

Moloney t. (*for delayed sensitivity to diphtheria toxoid*): 0.1 ml. of 1:10 dilution of fluid toxoid is injected intradermally on the flexor surface of the forearm; the appearance in 12 to 24 hours of an area of redness with induration of more than 12 mm. in diameter is a positive reaction. Called also *Moloney reaction*.

monaural loudness balance (MLB) t., a test to determine recruitment in bilateral sensorineural hearing loss; the loudness sensation at impaired frequencies is compared with that at normal frequencies.

Montenegro t.: leishmanin t.

Montigne's t.: heat an alcoholic solution of a sterol with silicotungstic acid; a red-brown color appears.

Moore's t. (*for dextrose or any carbohydrate*): boil the suspected solution with sodium or potassium hydroxide; if dextrose or lactose is present, a yellow or brown color is produced.

Morelli's t. (*to differentiate between an exudate and a transudate*): add a few drops of the suspected fluid to a saturated solution of mercuric chloride in a test tube; a flaky precipitate indicates a transudate, a clot indicates an exudate.

Moretti's t. (*for typhoid fever*): 25 ml. of urine are saturated with 20 gm. of crystallized ammonium sulfate. After a quarter of an hour the urine is filtered and diluted to about one third. To 10 ml. of the filtrate one fifth of its volume of a 10 per cent solution of sodium hydroxide is added, and then a drop of 5 per

cent tincture of iodine. The solution is shaken, and if the reaction is positive a persistent golden-yellow color is produced.

Moritz t., see *Rivalta's reaction*, under *reaction*.

Mörner's t.: 1. (*for tyrosine*) to a small quantity of the crystals in a test tube add a few milliliters of Mörner's reagent (solution of formaldehyde, 1 ml.; distilled water, 45 ml.; concentrated sulfuric acid, 55 ml.). Heat gently to the boiling point. A green color shows the presence of tyrosine. 2. see *nitroprusside t.* (1).

Moro t.: an obsolete tuberculin test in which tuberculin was applied to the skin in a lanolin-based ointment.

morphine t., see specific tests, including *Denigès' t.* (3), *Marquis' t.*, *Oliver's t.* (3), *Weppen's t.*

Morton's t.: in metatarsalgia, transverse pressure across the heads of the metatarsals causes a sharp pain, especially between the second and third metatarsals.

Moschcowitz t.: a test for arteriosclerosis made by rendering the lower limb bloodless by means of an Esmarch bandage. This is removed after five minutes have elapsed, when, in a normal limb, the color will return in a few seconds, but in one affected by arteriosclerosis the return of color takes place much more slowly. Called also *hyperemia t.*

Mosenthal's t. (*for kidney function*): with the patient on a prescribed general diet, take samples of urine in two-hour periods during the day and once at night. Examine them for volume, specific gravity, total nitrogen, and chlorides, and compare with normal.

Moynihan's t. (*for hourglass stomach*): the two parts of a Seidlitz powder are given separately; in hourglass stomach two separated protrusions on the abdominal wall can be observed.

Mulder's t.: 1. (*for dextrose*) alkalinize the solution with sodium carbonate; on adding a solution of indigo-carmine and heating, the mixture is decolorized, but becomes blue again when shaken with air. 2. (*for proteins*) treat the suspected substance with nitric acid: proteins are turned yellow by it; alkalinize the substance and it becomes an orange yellow, due to the presence of the phenyl group. Called also *xanthroproteic reaction*.

multiple-puncture t.: an intracutaneous test in which the material used (e.g., tuberculin) is introduced into the skin by pressure of several needles or pointed tines or prongs. See also *tine t.* and *tuberculin t., Sterneedle*.

mumps skin t. (*for immunity to mumps*): an unreliable and little used test consisting of intradermal injection of killed mumps virus, a positive response being development of a tuberculin-type delayed hypersensitivity reaction.

murexide t., see *Weidel's t.* (1).

Murphy's t.: the patient sits with his arms folded in front of him; the examiner's thumb is placed under the twelfth rib and short jabbing movements are made. Thus deep-seated tenderness and muscular rigidity are determined. Called also *Murphy's kidney punch*.

mycobiologic t.: mycologic test.

mycologic t. (*for sugar in urine*): to the specimen of urine an equal quantity of 1 per cent peptone solution is added; this mixture is sown with some species of *Candida*. If sugar is present, gas is developed. Called also *mycobiologic t.*

Myers and Fine t. (*for amylolytic activity*): add decreasing amounts of stomach contents to constant amounts of starch solution and note by means of iodine the amount required to completely hydrolyze the starch.

Mylius' t. (*for bile acids*): to each milliliter of the solution of bile acids add 1 ml. of strong sulfuric acid and 1 drop of furfurol solution; if bile acids are present, a red color is produced, which turns to a bluish violet in the course of a day or so.

Naffziger's t. (*for nerve root compression*): increase or aggravation of pain or sensory disturbance over the distribution of the involved nerve root upon manual compression of the jugular veins bilaterally confirms the presence of an extruded intervertebral disk or other mass.

Nagel's t.: a test for color vision in which one half of the field of an anomaloscope is illuminated with standard yellow and the other half is matched to the yellow by the subject who mixes red and green.

Nagler's t., see under *reaction*.

Nakayama's t. (*for bile pigments*): add 5 ml. of acid urine to the same amount of 10 per cent barium chloride solution and centrifugalize. To the precipitate is added 2 ml. of a reagent consisting of 99 parts of 95 per cent alcohol, 1 part of fuming hydrochloric acid to a liter of which 4 gm. of ferric chloride has been added. The fluid is boiled; a green color is obtained, which, on the addition of yellow nitric acid, becomes violet or red.

NBT t., nitroblue tetrazolium t.

Nencki's t. *(for indole)*: treat the suspected material with nitric acid and a little nitrous acid; a red color follows, and in concentrated solution a red precipitate may appear.

Nessler's t. *(for free ammonia)*, see under *reagent*.

Neubauer and Fischer's t.: the glycyltryptophan test.

Neufeld's t., see under *reaction*.

Neukomm's t. *(for bile acids)*: a drop of the suspected substance is placed on a small white porcelain cover with a drop of dilute cane sugar solution and one of dilute sulfuric acid. The mixture is carefully evaporated over a flame, a violet stain being left if bile acids are present.

neutralization t.: a test for the power of an antiserum or other substance to antagonize the pathogenic properties of a microorganism, toxin, virus, bacteriophage, or toxic substance.

niacin t. *(for Mycobacterium tuberculosis)*: in a chemical hood, add 0.1 ml. of heavy growth from a 10-day-old culture of organisms in Dubos' liquid Tween-albumin medium to 3 ml. of the same medium in a screw-cap tube. Add 1 ml. of 4 per cent aniline in 95 per cent ethanol and 1 ml. of 10 per cent aqueous cyanogen bromide. A distinct yellow color indicates the presence of niacin, a characteristic of human strains of *M. tuberculosis*; bovine strains are doubtful or negative; other strains are negative. Alternatively, add to the culture being tested, 0.5 to 0.1 ml. sterile saline or water, place the tube so that the fluid layers over the colonies, and allow to stand 15 minutes. Remove 0.5 ml. of the aqueous extract to a test tube. Add equal quantities of 4 per cent aniline in 95 per cent ethanol and 10 per cent aqueous cyanogen bromide. If niacin is present, a yellow color will appear.

Nickerson-Kveim t., see *Kveim t.*

Ninhydrin t., see *triketohydrindene hydrate t.*

Nippe's t. *(for blood)*: a modified form of Teichmann's test.

nitrate reduction t. 1. *(for the reduction of nitrate to nitrite by a bacterial culture)* the organism is cultured in a broth containing nitrate. The medium is tested for nitrite by mixing with solutions containing sulfanilic acid and alpha-naphthylamine in 5N acetic acid; a red color indicates the presence of nitrite. The test is useful in identifying doubtful strains of Enterobacteriaceae, mycobacteria, and certain aerobic bacteria. 2. see *Ilosvary's reagent* under *reagent*.

nitric acid t. 1. *(for albumin)* see *Heller's t.* (1). 2. see specific tests, including *Weyl's t.* (2).

nitric acid-magnesium sulfate t. *(for albumin)*, see *Roberts' t.* (1).

nitrites t. *(in saliva)*: to the saliva add 1 or 2 drops of H_2SO_4, a few drops of KI solution, and some starch paste; a blue color indicates nitrites. See also *Griess t., Ilosvay's t., Schaffer's t.*

nitroblue tetrazolium (NBT) t.: a test of neutrophil microbicidal function; neutrophils are incubated with latex particles and NBT. Normally phagocytosis of the particles is accompanied by reduction of NBT to a blue formazan pigment; absence of NBT reduction indicates a defect in some of the metabolic pathways involved in intracellular microbial killing, as seen in chronic granulomatous disease.

nitrogenous compounds t., see *Millon's t.*

nitrogen partition t.: a test of hepatic function based on alterations in the distribution of nitrogen in the various nitrogenous bodies of the blood and urine.

nitropropiol t. *(for sugar in urine)*: the urine is mixed with an alkali and heated with orthonitrophenylpropiolic acid; the indigo blue to green (blue and yellow) color reaction will be seen.

nitroprusside t.: 1. *(for cysteine)* if a protein containing cysteine is dissolved in water and 2 to 4 drops of a 4 or 5 per cent solution of sodium nitroprusside and then a few drops of ammonia are added, a deep purple-red color appears; called also *Mörner's t.* 2. *(for acetone)* see *Legal's t.* (1). 3. *(for indole)* see *Legal's t.* (2). 4. *(for creatinine)* see *Weyl's t.* (1).

nitroso-indole-nitrate t. *(for indole and skatole)*: acidify the unknown with nitric acid and add a few drops of potassium nitrite; a red color or a red precipitate indicates indole, a white turbidity indicates skatole.

nitrous acid t., see *Bertoni-Raymondi t.*

Nobel's t.: 1. *(for aceto-acetic acid and acetone)* stratify ammonium hydroxide on urine acidified with acetic acid and to which a little sodium nitroprusside has been added; a violet ring at the junction indicates acetoacetic acid or acetone. 2. *(for bile pigments)* add zinc chloride and a little of the tincture of iodine; a dichroic coloration follows.

Noguchi's t. *(for globulin)* to 0.5 ml. of Noguchi's reagent add 0.1 ml. of spinal fluid; boil and add 0.1 ml. of N/1 sodium hydroxide. A flocculent precipitate indicates globulin.

Nonne's t., see *Ross-Jones t.*

Nonne-Apelt t., see under *reaction*.

nucleoalbumin t., see *Ott's t.*

Nyiri's t.: a concentration test for kidney function by the use of thiosulfate.

nystagmus t., see *Bárány's symptom*, under *symptom*.

Oakley-Fulthorpe t.: see under *technique*.

Ober's t.: the patient lies on the side opposite that to be tested, with the underneath hip and knee flexed; with the upper knee flexed to a right angle, the upper hip is flexed to 90 degrees, fully abducted, brought into full hyperextension, and allowed to adduct; the angle that the thigh makes above the horizontal is the degree of abduction contracture.

Obermayer's t. *(for indican in urine)*: precipitate the urine with a 1:5 lead acetate solution with care, lest an excess of the reagent be taken; filter and agitate the filtrate with an equal amount of fuming hydrochloric acid containing a little of the solution of ferric chloride; to this add chloroform, which is turned blue by indigo.

Obermüller's t. *(for cholesterin)*: put the substance to be tested in a test tube and melt it with a drop or two of propionic anhydride over a small flame; on cooling, the mass becomes successively blue, green, orange, carmine, and copper colored.

obturator t., see *Cope's t.*

occult blood t., see tests listed under *blood t.*

Oliver's t.: 1. *(for albumin)* underlay the urine with a 1:4 solution of sodium tungstate and a 10:6 solution of citric acid; a white coagulum at the junction of the two layers shows the presence of albumin. 2. *(for sugar)* boil the suspected liquid with indigo carmine; sugar will change the blue to a red or yellow. 3. *(for morphine)* if, to a solution of morphine, a few milliliters of hydrogen peroxide is added and the mixture is stirred with a piece of copper wire, the solution takes on a deep port wine color, with the evolution of gas. 4. *(for bile acids)* to 5 ml. of the unknown add 2 to 3 drops of acetic acid and filter; an equal volume of 1 per cent solution of peptone will produce a precipitate insoluble in excess of acetic acid if bile acids are present.

one-stage prothrombin time t., see *Quick's t.* (2).

one-tailed t., a hypothesis test (q.v.) in which the critical region is one tail of the distribution of the test statistic and the null hypothesis is tested against a *one-sided alternative* that includes deviations from the null hypothesis only in one direction, deviations in the other direction being of no consequence.

ONPG t. *(for β-D-galactosidase in bacteria)*: the organism is grown in a buffered peptone medium containing D-nitrophenyl-β-D-galactopyranoside (ONPG): production of β-galactosidase is indicated by the appearance of a yellow color. Used to differentiate *Salmonella* (positive) from *Arizona* (negative), and *Neisseria lactamicus* (positive) from *N. meningitidis* (negative).

orcinol t. *(for pentose in urine)*, see *Bial's t.*

organic acid t., see *Knapp's t.* (2).

orientation t.: see if patient can give correctly the time of day, the day of the week, month, and year, and the place.

orthotoluidine t. *(for blood)*, see *Ruttan and Hardisty's t.*

osazone t. *(for sugars)*, see *Kowarsky's t.* (1) and *von Jaksch's t.* (2).

Osgood-Haskins t. *(for albumin)*: to 5 ml. of urine add 1 ml. of 50 per cent acetic acid; a precipitate at room temperature indicates bile salts, urates, or resin acids. Add 3 ml. of a saturated solution of sodium chloride; a precipitate suggests Bence Jones protein or globulin. The Bence Jones protein will redissolve on heating.

Osterberg's t. *(for beta-oxybutyric acid)*: to 800 mg. of ammonium sulfate add 0.15 ml. of concentrated ammonium hydroxide solution, 2 drops of a 5 per cent solution of nitroprusside, and 1 ml. of the urine. Dilute to 50 ml. and compare with a standard.

Ott's t. *(for nucleoalbumin in urine)*: to the urine is added an equal volume of saturated solution of sodium chloride, and Almén's reagent (dissolve 5 gm. of tannic acid in 240 ml. of 50 per cent alcohol and add 10 ml. of 25 per cent acetic acid); a precipitate forms when nucleoalbumin is present.

Ouchterlony t.: double diffusion in two dimensions; see under *diffusion*.

Oudin t.: see under *technique*.

ovarian hyperemia t. *(for pregnancy)*: the intraperitoneal injection of urine or blood serum of pregnant women into immature female mice produces a reddened appearance of the ovaries.

oxyphenylsulfonic acid t. *(for albumin in urine)*: dissolve in 20 parts of water 3 parts of oxyphenylsulfonic acid and

1 part of salicylsulfonic acid; add to 1 ml. of urine a drop of the reagent: if albumin is present, a clear white precipitate appears.

Pachon's t.: measuring of the blood pressure for the purpose of determining the state of the collateral circulation in aneurysm.

Paget's t.: a solid tumor is most hard in its center, whereas a cyst is least hard in its center.

palmin t., palmitin t. (*for pancreatic efficiency*): after a test meal containing palmitin, the contents of the stomach are examined for the presence of fatty acids. They will be found in cases in which the pancreas is normal, for the presence of fat in the stomach causes the pylorus to open and admit the pancreatic juice, which splits palmitin into fatty acids.

pancreatic function t., see specific tests, including *Kashiwado's t., litmus milk t., Loewe's t., palmin t., Sahli-Nencki t., secretin t.*

Pándy's t.: a test for globulin in the cerebrospinal fluid. Mix 80 to 100 ml. pure phenol with distilled water, shake, and place in incubator several hours. After several days at room temperature pour off the top watery part, which serves as the reagent. With a Pasteur pipet a drop (0.01 ml.) of the fluid to be tested is deposited on the bottom of a watch crystal filled with the reagent. If no cloudy precipitate forms within five seconds the reaction is negative.

Pap t., Papanicolaou t.: an exfoliative cytological staining procedure for the detection and diagnosis of various conditions, particularly malignant and premalignant conditions of the female genital tract (cancer of the vagina, cervix, and endometrium), in which cells which have been desquamated from the genital epithelium are obtained by smears, fixed and stained, and examined under the microscope for evidence of pathologic changes. Cytologic findings have commonly been expressed in terms of histologic lesions classified as Class I to Class V, but preferably each examination should have an individual histological description. The test is also used in evaluating endocrine function, and in the diagnosis of malignancies of other organs, as of the respiratory tract and lungs, gastrointestinal tract, urinary tract, and breast. See also *Table of Stains.*

paracasein t., see *Leiner's t.*

Parnum's t. (*for albumin*): filter the urine, add one-sixth volume of a saturated solution of magnesium or sodium sulfate, acidulate with acetic acid, and boil; if albumin is present, a white precipitate is formed.

partial thromboplastin time t.: a one-stage clotting test used clinically to detect deficiencies of the components of the intrinsic thromboplastin system; in reality prolonged clotting time may reflect deficiency or absence of coagulation factors I, II, V, and VIII through XII, separately or in combination.

passive cutaneous anaphylaxis t., see *passive cutaneous anaphylaxis.*

passive protection t.: a test in which antiserum is tested for protective antibody by parenteral inoculation of groups of animals with graded doses in constant volume.

passive transfer t., see *Prausnitz-Küstner reaction,* under *reaction.*

patch t's: skin tests, used primarily in the diagnosis of allergies, in which small pieces of gauze or filter paper impregnated with suspected allergens are applied to the skin for a short time period; swelling or redness constitutes a positive reaction.

Patrick's t.: with the patient supine, the thigh and knee are flexed and the external malleolus is placed over the patella of the opposite leg; the knee is depressed, and if pain is produced thereby arthritis of the hip is indicated. Patrick calls this test *fabere sign,* from the initial letters of movements that are necessary to elicit it, namely, flexion, abduction, external rotation, extension.

Patterson's t.: a chemical spot test for the diagnosis of uremia. A drop of Ehrlich's reagent is applied to a drop of blood placed on a white filter paper; if there is greatly increased blood urea, the spot on the filter paper turns a greenish color.

Paul-Bunnell t.: (*for serum heterophile antibodies associated with infectious mononucleosis*): determination of the highest dilution of the patient's serum capable of agglutinating sheep red blood cells.

Paul-Bunnell-Davidsohn t., a modification of the Paul-Bunnell test that differentiates among three types of heterophile sheep erythrocyte agglutinins: those associated with infectious mononucleosis, those associated with serum sickness, and natural antibodies against Forssman antigen. The patient's serum is absorbed with guinea pig kidney cells or with beef erythrocytes and centrifuged. Unabsorbed serum has a high heterophile antibody titer in infectious mononucleosis and serum sickness; a low titer is seen in normal individuals. Absorption with guinea pig kidney removes Forssman antibody and serum sickness heterophile antibody. Absorption with beef erythrocytes removes heterophile antibody associated with infectious mononucleosis or serum sickness. Called also *Davidsohn differential absorption t.*

Pavy's t. (*for dextrose in urine*): prepare a reagent by mixing 120 ml. of Fehling's solution with 200 ml. of ammonia (specific gravity 0.88), 400 ml. of a solution of sodium hydroxide (specific gravity 1.14), and 1000 ml. of water; boil the suspected liquid with this solution: if dextrose is present, the reagent is decolorized.

PCA t., see *passive cutaneous anaphylaxis.*

Pélouse-Moore t. (*for sugar in urine*): boil the urine with a solution of potassa, cool, and add 1 drop of concentrated sulfuric acid; the odor of burnt sugar will be given off.

Penzoldt's t.: 1. (*for acetone*) to the suspected liquid add a warm saturated solution of orthonitrobenzaldehyde, and render it alkaline with sodium hydroxide: if acetone is present, the mixture becomes yellow and then green; thereafter a precipitate forms which, on shaking with chloroform, gives a blue color. 2. (*for dextrose in urine*) add sodium hydroxide solution and a slightly alkaline solution of sodium diazobenzosulfonate; shake the mixture until it foams: a red or yellow-red color is produced, the foam also being red.

Penzoldt-Fischer t. (*for phenol*): alkalinize strongly the substance to be tested and dissolve in a solution of diazobenzolsulfonic acid; phenol, if present, produces a deep-red color.

peppermint t. (*for pulmonary perforation*): the pneumothorax cavity is filled with the vapor of essence of peppermint; if there is a pulmonary perforation the patient will recognize the characteristic smell.

pepsin t., see specific tests, including *Jacoby's t.* and *Mett's t.*

peptide t., see *triketohydrindene hydrate t.*

peptone t., see specific tests, including *Hofmeister's t.* (2), *Ralfe's t.* (2), *Randolph's t., triketohydrindene hydrate t.*

perchloride t.: a port-wine colored reaction obtained by treating the urine of hyperemetic pregnant women with solution of ferric chloride; the intensity of the reaction indicates the gravity of the case.

performance t.: an intelligence test in which the subject is required to carry out certain actions rather than to answer questions.

Peria's t. (*for tyrosine*), see *Piria's t.*

Perls' t.: a test for hemosiderin made by treating the substance with hydrochloric acid and potassium ferrocyanide; the Prussian blue reaction is produced if hemosiderin is present.

permanganate t., see *Weiss' t.*

peroxidase t., see *Arakawa's reagent,* under *reagent,* and *Goodpasture's stain,* under *stain.*

Perthes' t. (*for collateral circulation in varicose veins*), see *tourniquet t.,* def. 3.

Petri's t. (*for proteins*): add diazobenzolsulfonic acid and sodium hydroxide; an orange or brownish color is formed, and on shaking a red froth is produced.

Pettenkofer's t. (*for bile acids in urine*): drop a solution of the suspected material into a mixture of sugar and sulfuric acid; a purplish crimson color is produced. This test is also given by aminomyelin, cephalin, lecithin, and myelin.

Petzetaki's t. (*for typhoid fever*): 15 ml. of urine are placed in a test tube and to this is added a little 5 per cent alcoholic solution of iodine; if the upper part of the urine takes on a golden-yellow color, the test is positive.

phenacetin t. (*in urine*): to the urine add a little concentrated hydrochloric acid, a little 1 per cent solution of sodium nitrate, and a little alkaline alphanaphthol solution; make alkaline and a red color indicates phenacetin.

phenol t., see specific tests, including *Allen's t. Hanke and Koessler's t., Jacquemin's t., Penzoldt-Fischer t., Plugge's t.* See also *phenol, methods for,* under *method.*

phenolphthalein t.: 1. (*for blood*) boil a thin fecal suspension, cool, and add it to half as much reagent (made by dissolving 1 to 2 gm. of phenolphthalein and 25 gm. of potassium hydroxide in water.) Add 10 gm. of metallic zinc and heat until decolorized. A pink color indicates the presence of blood. 2. (*in urine*) make the urine alkaline; a red color indicates phenolphthalein.

phenolsulfonphthalein t. (*for kidney function*): inject 1 ml. of 0.6 per cent solution of the monosodium salt of phenolsulfonphthalein intravenously or intramuscularly and collect the urine at hourly intervals. Make specimens alkaline with sodium hydroxide and match color in colorimeter with standard solution. Usually 60 to 75 per cent of the dye is excreted in two hours; 40 per cent or less indicates impaired function.

phenoltetrachlorophthalein t. (*for liver function*): phenoltetrachlorophthalein is injected intravenously, and normally it appears in the feces, being excreted by the liver with the bile, and giving a bright color to the feces. A decrease in the normal excretion of this substance points to liver injury.

phenylhydrazine t., see specific tests, including *Kowarsky's t.* (1) and *von Jaksch's t.* (2).

phlorhizin t., phlorizin t. (*for renal insufficiency*): the bladder is emptied and a hypodermic injection given of a mixture of 5 to 10 gm. each of sodium carbonate and phlorhizin. Sugar will appear in the urine within half an hour if the kidney is healthy. If only a small quantity of sugar appears, there is probably renal insufficiency; if none at all, then serious kidney disease probably exists.

phosphoric acid t., see specific tests, including *Malot's t.* and *Mitscherlich's t.*

phthalein t., see *phenolsulfonphthalein t.*

picrotoxin t., see *Becker's t.* (1).

Pincus t.: typical colors are produced on heating 17-ketosteroids with concentrated antimony trichloride in glacial acetic acid.

pineapple t. (*for butyric acid in stomach*): a few drops of sulfuric acid and alcohol are added to a dried ethereal extract of the gastric juice; if butyric acid is present, an odor of pineapple will be given off, caused by the formation of ethylbutyrate.

pine wood t. (*for indole*): a pine splinter moistened with concentrated hydrochloric acid is turned cherry red by a solution of indole.

Piotrowski's t., see *biuret t.* (1).

Piria's t. (*for tyrosine*): moisten the suspected material with strong sulfuric acid and warm it; then dilute and warm it again; neutralize it with barium carbonate, filter, and add ferric chloride in dilute solution: if tyrosine is present, a violet color is seen, which is destroyed by an excess of ferric chloride.

Pirquet t.: (*obs.*) a tuberculin test in which the tuberculin is applied by scarification.

P-K t., see under *reaction.*

plantar ischemia t.: a test for circulatory disturbances in the legs and feet, in which the plantar surface of the patient's foot is checked for blanching after he extends and flexes his inclined leg.

Plesch's t. (*for persistent ductus arteriosus*): determination of the amount of oxygen and of carbonic acid in the blood.

Plugge's t. (*for phenol*): a dilute solution containing phenol becomes red on mixture with a mercuric nitrate solution containing a trace of nitrous acid; mercury is also precipitated and the odor of salicylol is given off.

pneumatic t., Hennebert's sign.

Pohl's t. (*for globulins*): these substances are precipitated from solution by ammonium sulfate.

pointing t., see *Bárány's pointing t.*

Politzer's t. (*for deafness in one ear*): when a tuning-fork is placed in front of the nares, it is heard only by an unaffected ear during deglutition.

Pollacci's t. (*for albumin in urine*): dissolve in 100 ml. of water 1 gm. of tartaric acid, 5 gm. of mercuric chloride, and 10 gm. of sodium chloride, and add 5 ml. of solution of formaldehyde; this solution added to urine will cause coagulation of albumin in a white zone.

Porges-Meier t.: a nontreponemal antigen serologic test for syphilis.

porphobilinogen t., see *Watson-Schwartz t.*

Porter's t.: 1. (*for excess of uric acid*) the upper portion of the urine is boiled in a test tube and a few drops of 4 per cent acetic acid added; in a few hours crystals of uric acid will form just below the surface. 2. (*for indican*) 10 ml. of urine is shaken with an equal amount of hydrochloric acid and 5 drops of a 0.5 per cent solution of potassium permanganate; add 5 ml. of chloroform and shake. A purple color with a deposit of blue matter indicates indican.

Porteus maze t.: a performance test in which the subject is required to trace with a pencil through printed mazes of increasing difficulty.

Posner's t.: 1. (*for the source of albumin in urine*) a twenty-four-hour sample of urine is preserved with solution of formaldehyde, shaken, and the leukocytes counted in the blood-counting chamber—100,000 leukocytes per 2 ml. of urine indicate 0.1 per cent of albumin. In this case the albumin is probably due solely to the pus. If albumin is present in greater proportion than this, it is probably due to Bright's disease. 2. (*for proteins*) Posner makes a ring biuret test by mixing the potassium hydroxide solution and the unknown and then stratifying very dilute copper sulfate solution on top of the mixture.

potassium iodide t. (*for renal function*): the patient receives 0.5 gm. of potassium iodide in solution by mouth, and the urine is tested every two hours for iodine; if iodine secretion is prolonged beyond sixty hours, excretion through the renal tubules is indicated.

Prausnitz-Küstner (P-K) t., see under *reaction.*

precipitin t.: any serologic test based on a precipitin reaction (q.v.).

Pregl's t. (*for kidney function*): determine the specific gravity of the urine obtained by catheterization of the ureters. Using Haeser's coefficient, estimate the amount of solid substances excreted, and compare it with the weight of ash. The diseased kidney may excrete the same volume of water, but less solid material. A predominance of mineral substances (ash) over the organic also speaks for a lower function of the kidney.

pregnancy t., see specific tests, including *antitrypsin t., Aschheim-Zondek t., bitterling t., bromine t.* (3), *Brown's t.* (1), *early pregnancy t., Friedman's t., Galli Mainini t., male frog or male toad t., ovarian hyperemia t., pregnanediol t., Prostigmin t., Venning Browne t., Visscher-Bowman t., Xenopus t.*

Preyer's t.: a spectroscopic test for carbon monoxide in the blood.

Proetz t. (*for acuity of sense of smell*): use of a series of substances each in 10 different concentrations in a liter of petroleum of specific gravity 0.880, to determine the least concentration at which the substance can be recognized; termed *olfactory coefficient* or *minimal identifiable odor.*

projective t.: any of various tests in which an individual interprets ambiguous stimulus situations, e.g., a series of inkblots (Rorschach t.), according to his own unconscious dispositions, thus yielding information about his personality structure and its underlying dynamics.

protection t.: serum neutralization t.

protein t., see specific tests, including *biuret t.* (1), *colloidal gold t., Gies' biuret t., Grigg's t., Hopkins-Cole t., Kantor and Gies' t., Liebermann's t., Michailow's t., Millon's t., Molisch's t.* (3), *Mulder's t.* (2), *Petri's t., Posner's t.* (2), *Reichl's t., Schulte's t., Schultze's t.* (3), *Sicard-Cantelouble t., sulfur t., triketohydrindene hydrate t., von Aldor's t.*

proteose t.: proteose does not coagulate on boiling, but gives a ring test with trichloracetic acid. See also *von Aldor's t.*

prothrombin t.: a test for prothrombin based on clotting time; see under *time,* and see *Quick's t.* (2).

prothrombin consumption t.: a test used, for the most part, to measure the formation of intrinsic thromboplastin by determining the residual serum prothrombin after blood coagulation is complete. Because the test is made on whole blood, it also measures, indirectly, the thromboplastic function of platelets.

prothrombin-proconvertin t.: a test used in the control of coumarin-type anticoagulants similar to the Quick method, except that it employs a saline extract of brain as a thromboplastin and requires the presence of excess blood coagulation factor V, usually derived from deprothrombinized ox plasma.

psychological t., any test to measure one's development, achievement, personality, intelligence, thought processes, etc.

psychomotor t., a test that assesses the subject's ability to perceive instructions and perform motor responses, often including measurement of the speed of the reaction.

pulp t.: a diagnostic test to determine tooth pulp vitality or abnormality, usually by means of electric pulp testers or by application of a hot or cold stimulus.

Purdy's t. (*for albumin*): fill a test tube two thirds full of the clear urine, add one sixth of its volume of a saturated solution of sodium chloride and 5 to 10 drops of 50 per cent acetic acid. Gently heat the upper part of the tube and look for a cloud.

purine bodies t., see *purine bodies, methods for,* under *method.*

pus t., see *Vitali's t.* (6).

Pyramidon t. (*for occult blood in urine*): to the urine add tincture of iodine; a yellow ring indicates Pyramidon.

quadriceps t. (*for hyperthyroidism*): the patient sits well forward on the edge of a straight chair and holds the leg out at right angles to the body. Normal persons can hold this position for at least a minute; those with hyperthyroidism can maintain it for only a few seconds.

Queckenstedt's t., see under *sign*.

quellung t., see *Neufeld's reaction*, under *reaction*.

Quick's t.: 1. (*for liver function*) a test based on excretion of hippuric acid following the administration of sodium benzoate. 2. (*one-stage prothrombin time*) by adding an extrinsic thromboplastin such as dried rabbit brain and calcium to oxalated blood the integrity of the prothrombin complex, composed of factors II, V, VII, X, may be defined; used widely to control administration of coumarin-type anticoagulants.

Quick tourniquet t., see *tourniquet t.* (1).

Quinlan's t. (*for bile*): a 3-mm. layer of the suspected liquid is examined by the spectroscope; if bile is present, some of the violet color of the spectrum will be absorbed.

Raabe's t. (*for albumin*): filter the urine into a test tube and drop a crystal of trichloracetic acid into it; albumin will form a white ring about the crystal; uric acid may form a similar ring, but it is not so well defined.

Rabuteau's t.: 1. (*for hydrochloric acid in urine*) add a little indigosulfonic acid to color the urine, and sulfurous acid to decompose what hydrochloric acid may be present; the urine will be decolorized. 2. (*for hydrochloric acid in stomach contents*) one gm. of potassium iodate and 0.5 gm. of potassium iodide are added to 50 ml. of starch mucilage; filtered stomach liquids are added to it; free hydrochloric acid will render the mixture blue.

radioactive renogram t.: an intravenous injection of radioisotopic material is given and its uptake and excretion is monitored by an external scintillation counter over the kidneys.

radioallergosorbent t. (RAST): a test used to measure specific IgE antibodies in serum. Allergen extract is coupled to a solid matrix (paper, cellulose particles); this immunosorbent is reacted with serum and washed and then reacted with radiolabeled anti–human IgE antibody and washed. Uptake of the labeled antibody is proportional to the level of specific serum IgE antibodies to the allergen. RAST is used as an alternative to skin tests to determine sensitivity to suspected allergens.

radioimmunosorbent t. (RIST): a highly sensitive radioimmunoassay for measuring the total IgE antibody concentration in serum; the serum sample is reacted with dilutions of radiolabeled IgE and anti–human IgE antibody coupled to an insoluble support. The amount of labeled IgE bound to the immunosorbent varies inversely with the amount of (unlabeled) IgE present in the sample.

radioisotope renal excretion t. (*for study of renal function*): radioisotopic material diluted with saline is rapidly injected into a well-hydrated patient; urine collected by an indwelling urethral catheter or a ureteral catheter previously inserted into the kidney is collected at known intervals and the radioactivity of each specimen is determined and recorded.

Ralfe's t.: 1. (*for acetone in urine*) boil 4 ml. of solution of potassium hydroxide with 1.5 gm. of potassium iodide; overlay it with 4 ml. of urine; a yellow ring with specks of iodoform appears at the plane of contact. 2. (*for peptones in urine*) put 4 ml. of Fehling's solution in a test tube and overlay it with urine; a rose-colored ring shows the presence of peptones.

Ramon flocculation t.: to a series of tubes containing a constant amount of toxin, e.g., diphtheria toxin, antitoxin is added in increasing amounts; when a zone of flocculation appears, the tube showing it contains a completely neutralized mixture of toxin and antitoxin. The first tube in which flocculation occurs is taken as the end-point.

Randolph's t. (*for peptones in urine*): add 2 drops of a saturated solution of potassium iodide and 3 drops of Millon's reagent to 5 ml. of cold and slightly acid urine; a yellow precipitate shows the presence of peptones.

rank sum t., a nonparametric statistical test of the null hypothesis that two samples are drawn from the same population versus the alternative hypothesis that the two samples are drawn from two populations having probability distributions of the same shape but different locations, based on the value of the rank sum statistic calculated as the sum of the ranks of one sample when the observations in both samples are jointly ranked in ascending order. Called also *Mann-Whitney t.,* *Mann-Whitney-Wilcoxon t., Wilcoxon's t.,* and *Wilcoxon's rank sum t.*

Rantzman's t.: a modification of Lange's test for acetone in which ammonium nitrate is used as a preservative.

rapid plasma reagin (RPR) t's: a group of flocculation tests for syphilis using unheated serum and a modified VDRL antigen containing choline chloride and charcoal particles enabling macroscopic identification of the flocculation; widely used for screening.

rapid serum amylase t., Fishman-Doubilet t.

Raygat's t., see *hydrostatic t.*

Rebuck t., Rebuck skin window technique.

red t., see *phenolsulfonphthalein t.*

red-glass t., a test for ocular deviation using a red glass over the right eye while the patient looks at a light; the position at which the patient sees the red image reveals the affected muscle.

Rees' t. (*for albumin*): small amounts of albumin are precipitated from solution by tannic acid in alcoholic solution.

Rehberg's t.: a test of kidney function based on the excretion of creatinine administered 2 gm. in 500 ml. of water.

Rehfuss' t. (*of gastric secretion*): by means of a specially devised tube (*Rehfuss tube*) inserted into the stomach immediately after an Ewald test meal, a specimen of the contents is drawn off at fifteen-minute intervals until the close of digestion. Each specimen is examined and the results are plotted in a graphic curve, the abscissa of which is the number of minutes at which the gastric contents were removed, and the ordinate the number of milliliters of decinormal sodium hydroxide solution necessary to titrate the free acidity and the total acidity of the gastric contents.

Reichl's t. (*for proteins*): add 2 or 3 drops of an alcoholic solution of benzaldehyde and a quantity of sulfuric acid previously diluted to twice its volume with water; then add a few drops of ferric sulfate solution. The mixture will sooner or later take on a deep-blue color if proteins are present.

Reinsch's t. (*for heavy metals, including arsenic, mercury, bismuth, antimony, and large amounts of selenium, tellurium, and sulfide*): insert a strip of clean copper into the suspected acidified liquid or finely ground tissue, and boil; if one or more heavy metals are present, a coating will form on the copper strip.

Remont's t. (*for salicylic acid*): make the milk acid with sulfuric acid, extract the salicylic acid with ether, and identify it by the purple or violet color produced on the addition of ferric chloride.

renal function t., see *kidney function t.*

rennin t., see individual tests, including *Lee's t.* and *Riegel's t.*

resorcinol-hydrochloric acid t. (*for levulose*), see *Selivanoff's t.*

Reuss' t. (*for atropine*): the substance examined is treated with sulfuric acid and oxidizing agents; if atropine is present, an odor of roses and orange-flowers is given off.

Reynold's t. (*for acetone*): to the liquid to be examined add freshly prepared mercuric oxide, shake and filter, and overlay the filtrate with ammonium sulfide; the liquid turns black if acetone is present.

rheumatoid arthritis t., see specific tests, including *bentonite t., bracelet t., latex agglutination t., sheep cell agglutination t.*

rhubarb t. (*in urine*): make the urine alkaline; a red color indicates rhubarb.

Rideal-Walker t., a test for the bactericidal activity of a disinfectant as compared with that of phenol; see under *method.*

Rieckenberg's t., see under *phenomenon.*

Riegel's t. (*for rennin*): to 10 ml. of milk add 5 ml. of neutral gastric juice and incubate for fifteen minutes; coagulation will occur if rennin is present.

Riegler's t.: 1. (*for albumin*) 10 gm. of betanaphtholsulfonic acid is dissolved in 200 ml. of distilled water and filtered; 5 ml. of urine is treated with 20 to 30 drops of solution. Turbidity shows the presence of albumin. 2. (*for hydrochloric acid in the gastric juice*) Congo red is changed to blue if hydrochloric acid is present. 3. (*for dextrose*) place in a test tube 0.1 gm. of phenyl-hydrazine-hydrochloride, 0.25 gm. of sodium acetate, and 20 drops of the urine. Heat to boiling. Add 10 ml. of a 3 per cent solution of potassium hydroxide and gently shake the tube. A red color indicates sugar.

ring t.: 1. (*for antibiotic activity*) the solution is placed in a ring resting on the surface of seeded agar and the size of the surrounding clear area of inhibition indicates the activity. 2. (*for protein*) see *Heller's t.* (1), *Posner's t.* (2), *Roberts' t.* (1).

Rinne t.: a hearing test made, with the opposite ear masked, with tuning forks of 256, 512, and 1024 Hz; by alternately placing the stem of the vibrating fork on the mastoid process of the temporal bone of the patient and holding it ½ inch from the external auditory meatus until it is no longer heard at one of these positions. When air conduction is greater than bone conduction, it indicates normal hearing or sensorineural hearing loss. When bone conduction is greater than air conduction, it indicates conductive hearing loss.

Rivalta's t., see under *reaction*.

Roberts' t.: 1. (*for albumin*) underlay the urine with a mixture containing 5 parts of saturated solution of magnesium sulfate and 1 part of nitric acid; a white ring or layer forms at the plane of junction. 2. (*for dextrose*) determine the specific gravity of the urine at a certain temperature; add a little tartaric acid and some yeast; after twenty-four hours filter and again find the specific gravity. Each degree of density lost represents a grain of dextrose in a fluidounce of the urine.

Robinson-Kepler t. (*for adrenocortical insufficiency*): a test based on the fact that patients with adrenocortical insufficiency are unable to excrete a large water load at a normal rate, as opposed to normal subjects who will, for example, excrete 50 per cent of 1500 ml. of ingested water within four hours.

Robinson-Kepler-Power water t. (*for sprue*): a test based upon the fact that in sprue there is increased nocturnal elimination of urine, perhaps due to decreased absorption of water.

Romberg t. (*for differentiating between peripheral and cerebellar ataxia*): an increase in clumsiness in all movements and in the width and uncertainty of the gait when the patient's eyes are closed indicates peripheral ataxia; no change indicates the cerebellar type.

Ronchese t. (*for quantitative determination of ammonia in urine*): one based on the action of solution of formaldehyde on the ammonia salts. A 10 per cent solution of sodium carbonate is added, a drop at a time, to the urine until the reaction becomes neutral. The solution of formaldehyde (40 per cent) is neutralized with a one-fourth normal soda solution against phenolphthalein until a slight pink tint develops. Then 25 ml. of the neutral urine and 10 ml. of the neutral solution of formaldehyde are mixed and titrated against decinormal sodium carbonate solution until a deep pink develops. The calculation is simple: 1 ml. of the decinormal sodium carbonate solution for 100 ml. of urine corresponds to 0.017 gm. ammonia in 1000 ml. of urine.

Rorschach t.: a projective test in which the subject is asked to relate his associations to a series of inkblot designs.

Rose's t. (*for blood*): the scrapings from a blood stain are boiled in dilute caustic potash; when examined the liquid will show a greenish color in a thin layer and a red color in a thicker layer.

rose bengal t. (*for liver function*): rose bengal (1 per cent in sodium chloride solution) is injected into the blood stream. Normally it disappears from the blood rapidly; delay in the normal disappearance time points to diminished activity of the liver.

Rose-Waaler t.: an agglutination test for rheumatoid factor (RF) using tanned sheep red blood cells (SRBC) coated with subagglutinating amounts of rabbit anti-SRBC IgG antibody. These cells agglutinate when exposed to RF (anti-IgG autoantibodies) owing to cross-reaction between human and rabbit IgG.

Rosenbach-Gmelin t. (*for bile pigment*): filter the urine through a very small filter, and put a drop of nitric acid with a trace of nitrous acid on the inside of the filter; a pale-yellow spot will appear, surrounded with yellowish red, violet, blue, and green rings.

Rosenheim-Drummond t. (*for vitamin A*): dissolve 1 or 2 drops of cod liver oil in about 5 ml. of an anhydrous fat solvent. Add 1 drop of concentrated sulfuric acid. A temporary deep-violet color indicates vitamin A.

Rosenthal's t.: 1. (*for blood in urine*) add potassium hydroxide solution to the urine, remove the precipitate and dry it; place a small amount on a slide with a crystal of sodium chloride; apply a coverglass and cause a few drops of glacial acetic acid to flow under it; warm the plate. When it is cool hemin crystals will appear if blood is present. 2. (*for liver function*) a modification of the phenoltetrachlorophthalein test based on the amount of the dye which remains in the blood at definite periods after injection of 5 mg. per kilogram of body weight. The normal liver will remove most of the dye from the blood in fifteen minutes and all of it within an hour.

Rosin's t. (*for indigo red*): render the suspected liquid alkaline with sodium carbonate and extract with ether; this is colored red.

Ross-Jones t. (*for excess of globulin in cerebrospinal fluid*): 1 ml. of cerebrospinal fluid is floated over 2 ml. of concentrated ammonium sulfate solution; excess of globulin produces a fine white ring at the line of junction.

Rothera's t. (*for acetone*): to 5 ml. of urine add a little solid ammonium sulfate and add 2 to 3 drops of a fresh 5 per cent solution of sodium nitroprusside and 1 to 2 ml. of ammonium hydroxide; a purple color forms if acetone is present.

Rotter's t. (*for ascorbic acid in the body*): cutaneous injection of 2,6-dichlorphenolindophenol produces colorization of the tissues; decolorization occurring in ten minutes indicates adequate ascorbic acid.

Rous t. (*for hemosiderin*): centrifuge the urine; to the sediment add 5 ml. of a 2 per cent solution of potassium ferrocyanide and 5 ml. of a 1 per cent solution of hydrochloric acid. Hemosiderin granules stain blue.

Roussin's t.: microscopic examination of suspected blood stains.

Rowntree and Geraghty's t., see *phenolsulfonphthalein t.*

RPR t., rapid plasma reagin t.

Rubin's t.: 1. a test for patency of the uterine tubes made by transuterine insufflation with carbon dioxide. If the tubes are patent the gas enters the peritoneal cavity and may be demonstrated by the fluoroscope or roentgenogram. This subphrenic pneumoperitoneum causes pain in one or both shoulders of the patient. If the manometer registers not over 100 mm. Hg the tubes are patent; if between 120 and 130, there may be stenosis or stricture, but not complete occlusion; if it rises to 200, the tubes are completely occluded. 2. a test to detect avian leukosis viruses in egg-culture vaccines; if the viruses are present, they induce a cellular resistance to Rous viruses subsequently inoculated (resistance-inducing factor).

Rubner's t.: 1. (*for carbon monoxide in blood*) shake the blood with 4 or 5 volumes of lead acetate in solution: if the blood contains CO, it will retain its bright color; if not, it becomes a chocolate brown. 2. (*for lactose, dextrose, maltose, and levulose in urine*) add lead acetate to the urine, boil, and then add an excess of ammonium hydroxide: lactose gives a brick-red color, dextrose a coffee-brown color, maltose a light-yellow color, and levulose no color at all.

Ruhemann's t. (*for uric acid in urine*), see under *method*.

ruler t., see *Hamilton's test*.

Rumpel-Leede t., see under *phenomenon*.

Russo's t., see under *reaction*.

Ruttan and Hardisty's t. (*for blood*): blood in the presence of a 4 per cent glacial acetic acid solution of orthotoluidine and hydrogen peroxide gives a bluish color.

Saathoff's t. (*for fat in stools*): rub up the feces with sudan and warm; fat droplets stain yellow to red.

Sabin-Feldman dye t.: a serologic test for the diagnosis of toxoplasmosis, based on the failure of living toxoplasmas, in the presence of specific antibody and accessory factor, to take up methylene blue dye.

saccharimeter t.: dextrose in solution rotates the plane of polarized light to the right, while levulose turns it to the left.

Sachs-Georgi t.: (*obs.*) a nontreponemal antigen serologic test for syphilis.

Sachsse's t. (*for sugar in the urine*): a solution of 18 gm. of red mercuric iodide, 25 gm. of potassium iodide, 80 gm. of potassium hydroxide, in water enough to make a liter; sugar, if present, causes a black precipitate.

Sahli's t. (*for motive and digestive power of stomach*): the patient is fed a soup made of definite amounts of water, flour, butter, and salt, and in an hour the stomach contents are removed. The amount of fat present shows how much of the meal has been digested, and the acidity indicates how much the stomach has secreted.

Sahli's desmoid t., see *desmoid reaction*, under *reaction*.

Sahli's glutoid t. (*for digestive function*): a glutoid capsule containing 0.15 gm. of iodoform is taken with an Ewald breakfast. The capsule is not digested by the stomach fluid, but is readily digested by pancreatic juice. Appearance of iodine in the saliva and urine within four to six hours indicates normal gastric motility, normal intestinal digestion, and normal absorption. Glutoid capsules are prepared by soaking gelatin capsules in solution of formaldehyde.

Sahli-Nencki t. (*for lipolytic activity of the pancreas*): phenyl salicylate (salol) is administered: it is excreted as salicylic acid when pancreatic activity is normal.

Sakaguchi t. (*for arginine*): a reddish or wine color is produced in the presence of arginine when a tissue section is treated with an alkaline mixture of α-naphthol and sodium hypochlorite.

salicylic acid t., see specific tests, including *Remont's t., Siebold and Bradbury's t.*

Salkowski's t.: 1. (*for CO in the blood*) add to the blood 20 volumes of water and sodium hydroxide in solution (specific gravity, 1.34). If CO is present, it becomes cloudy and then red; flakes of red afterward float on the surface. 2. (*for cholesterol*) dissolve in chloroform and add an equal volume of strong sulfuric acid: if cholesterol is present, the solution becomes bluish red, and slowly changes to a violet red, the sulfuric acid becomes red, with a green fluorescence. 3. (*for indole*) to the solution to be tested add a little nitric acid, and drop in slowly a solution of potassium nitrite (2 per cent): a red color shows that indole is present, and a red precipitate is afterward formed. 4. (*for dextrose*) a modified form of Trommer's test. 5. (*for creatinine*) to the yellow solution obtained in Weyl's test add an excess of acetic acid and heat; a green color results, which turns to blue.

Salkowski-Ludwig t. (*for uric acid*): a solution of silver ammonionitrate and ammonium and magnesium chlorides precipitates uric acid.

Salkowski and Schipper's t. (*for bile pigments*): to 10 ml. of the unknown add 5 drops of a 20 per cent solution of sodium carbonate and 10 drops of a 20 per cent solution of calcium chloride. To the precipitate add 3 ml. of alcohol containing 5 per cent of strong hydrochloric acid and a few drops of sodium nitrite. Heat. A green color indicates bile pigments.

salol t., see *Sahli-Nencki t.*

Salomon's t.: test the stomach washing by means of Esbach's reagent, after twenty-four hours without protein food; the presence of albumin indicates ulcerative cancer.

sand t. (*for bile and hemoglobin in urine*): a layer of white sand is spread on a plate and on this is poured some of the urine; if the urine contains pigments, a spot is left on the sand, which is brown with hemoglobin and greenish with bile pigment. Called also *Lipps' t.*

Sandrock t. (*for thrombosis*): vigorous friction is applied to the part; the degree of hyperemia which follows is an indication of the condition of the circulation.

Sanford's t.: prepare a series of dilutions of salt from 0.28 to 0.5 per cent; add 1 drop of blood to each dilution, mix, allow to settle, and note the tubes which show hemolysis.

santonin t.: 1. (*for the antitoxic efficiency of the liver*) the patient is given 0.02 gm. of santonin on a fasting stomach; the urine is examined hourly for oxysantonin by treating it with a dilute sodium hydroxide solution which will produce a red color with oxysantonin. 2. see *Daclin t.*

Saundby's t. (*for blood in feces*): to a small quantity of feces in a test tube 10 drops of a saturated benzidine solution is added; to this is added 30 drops of hydrogen peroxide solution. A dark blue color will develop if blood is present.

scarification t., a skin test in which the antigen is introduced by scarification, e.g., the Pirquet test.

Schaffer's t. (*for nitrites in urine*): decolorize 4 ml. of urine with animal charcoal and add to it 4 ml. of 10 per cent acetic acid and 3 drops of 5 per cent solution of potassium ferrocyanide; an intense yellow color indicates nitrites.

Schalfijew's t. (*for blood*): treat defibrinated blood with excess of glacial acetic acid, heat to 80° C., cool, and examine for hemin crystals.

Schalm t., see *California mastitis t.*

Scherer's t.: 1. (*for inosite*) evaporate on platinum foil with nitric acid, add ammonia water and a single drop of calcium chloride in solution, and reevaporate to dryness; a rose-red coloration indicates the presence of inosite. 2. (*for pure leucine*) a small portion of leucine with a few drops of nitric acid are evaporated on platinum foil. The transparent residue turns a brownish color on the addition of a sodium hydroxide solution. When the mixture is concentrated an oil-like drop is obtained. 3. (*for tyrosine*) treat with nitric acid and dry with care on platinum foil; the formation of nitrotyrosine nitrate renders it yellow, and sodium hydroxide solution changes the color to reddish yellow.

Schick t.: intradermal injection of a quantity of diphtheria toxin equal to one-fiftieth of the guinea pig minimal lethal dose in one arm (the test site) and of an equal quantity of heat-inactivated diphtheria toxin in the other arm (the control site). A positive reaction, which consists of an area of redness that appears in 24 to 36 hours at the test site only and persists for 4 to 5 days, leaving an area of brownish pigmentation, indicates a lack of immunity to diphtheria. A pseudoreaction, which consists of an area of redness appearing at both sites and usually disappearing in 48 hours without residual pigmentation, or a negative reaction indicates immunity.

Schiff's t.: 1. (*for carbohydrates in urine*) warm and add sulfuric acid; expose to the fumes of the urine a paper dipped in a mixture of equal volumes of xylidine and glacial acetic acid with alcohol and then dried: the paper becomes red if carbohydrates are present. 2. (*for cholesterol*) add a reagent composed of 2 parts of sulfuric acid with 1 part of a dilute solution

of ferric chloride; evaporate to dryness and a violet color is produced. 3. (*for cholesterol*) evaporate with nitric acid and add ammonia water; a red color not changed by alkalis is produced. 4. (*for allantoin and urea*) add a solution of furfurol in hydrochloric acid; a yellow color appears, turning to purple and then to a brownish black. 5. (*for uric acid*) treat silver nitrate paper with an alkaline solution of the suspected substance; a brown stain shows the presence of uric acid. 6. (*for formaldehyde in milk*) the solution consists of an aqueous solution of magenta, 40 ml.; distilled water, 250 ml.; aqueous solution of sodium bisulfite, 10 ml.; and pure concentrated sulfuric acid, 10 ml., which is allowed to stand until it is colorless; 2 ml. of this solution is added to a test tube two thirds full of milk. If formaldehyde is present, a pink or lilac color will appear in from thirty to sixty seconds.

Schiller's t. (*for cancer of cervix*): a test for early squamous cell cancer by treating the tissue with a solution of 1 gm. of pure iodine and 2 gm. of potassium iodide in 300 ml. of water: if the cervix is healthy, the surface turns brown; if there is cancer, the treated area turns white or yellow, because cancer cells do not contain glycogen and therefore do not stain with iodine.

Schilling t. (*for gastrointestinal absorption of vitamin B_{12}*): a measured amount of radioactive vitamin B_{12} is given orally, followed by a parenteral flushing dose of the nonradioactive vitamin, and the percentage of radioactivity is determined in the urine excreted over a 24-hour period.

Schirmer's t. (*for keratoconjunctivitis sicca*): a test of tear production in which a piece of filter paper is inserted over the conjunctival sac of the lower lid, with the end of the paper hanging down on the outside. The range of normal wetting, determined by measuring the area of moisture on the projecting paper, depends on age and sex.

Schlesinger's t. (*for urobilin*): to about 5 ml. of the urine in a test tube, add a few drops of Lugol's solution to transform the chromogen into the pigment. Now add 4 or 5 ml. of a saturated solution of zinc chloride in absolute alcohol and filter. A greenish fluorescence, best seen when the tube is viewed against a black background and the light is concentrated upon it with a lens, shows the presence of urobilin. Bile pigment, if present, should be removed by adding about one fifth volume of 10 per cent calcium chloride solution and filtering.

Schlichter t., serum bactericidal activity t.

Schönbein's t.: 1. (*for blood*) blue coloration obtained by adding solution of hydrogen peroxide to tincture of guaiac mixed with suspected blood. 2. (*for copper*) a solution containing a copper salt becomes blue if potassium cyanide and tincture of guaiac are added.

Schopfer's t.: minute amounts of vitamin B in the blood catalyze the mold *Phycomyces blaksleeanus.*

Schroeder's t. (*for urea*): add a crystal of the substance to a solution of bromine in chloroform; the urea will decompose and gas will be formed.

Schulte's t. (*for proteins*): remove all coagulable protein, precipitate with six volumes of absolute alcohol, dissolve the precipitate in water, and apply the biuret test.

Schultz-Charlton t., see under *reaction.*

Schultze's t.: 1. (*for cellulose*) iodine is dissolved to saturation in a zinc chloride solution (specific gravity, 1.8), and 6 parts of potassium iodide are added: this reagent colors cellulose blue. 2. (*for cholesterol*) evaporate with nitric acid, using a porcelain dish and water bath; if cholesterol is present, a yellow deposit is formed, which changes to yellowish red when ammonia is added. 3. (*for proteins*) to a suspected solution add a very little of a dilute solution of cane sugar and concentrated sulfuric acid; keep it at 60° C., and a bluish red coloration is produced.

Schultze's indophenol oxydase t., see *indophenol t.*

Schumm's t.: 1. see *benzidine t.* 2. (*for heme in plasma*) a given volume of plasma is covered with a layer of ether; one-tenth the volume of concentrated ammonium sulfide (analar) is then run in with a pipette and subsequently mixed by shaking. A positive reaction is indicated by the appearance of a hemochromogen with a sharply defined α band at 558 mμ in a depth up to 4 cm. of plasma.

Schwabach t.: a hearing test made, with the opposite ear masked, with tuning forks of 256, 512, 1024, and 2048 Hz, alternately placing the stem of the vibrating fork on the mastoid process of the temporal bone of the patient and that of the examiner (whose hearing should be normal) until it is no longer heard by one of them. The result is expressed as "Schwabach prolonged" if heard longer by the patient (indicative of conductive hearing impairment), as "Schwabach shortened or diminished" if heard longer by the examiner (indicative of sensorineural hearing impairment), and as "Schwabach normal" if heard for the same time by both.

Scivoletto's t. (*for hydrochloric acid in urine*): dip filter paper in starch paste and dry; sprinkle it with urine and dry; hang it in a flask containing strontium acetate in solution: a blue color indicates the presence of the acid.

scleroscope t.: a test to determine the hardness of materials by dropping a steel ball of standard weight from a specific height onto the material being tested and measuring the height of rebound. See also *hardness number*, under *number*.

scratch t., a skin test in which the antigen is applied on a superficial scratch.

screen t.: 1. alternate cover t. 2. cover-uncover t.

screening t., any test used to eliminate those who are definitely not affected by the disease in question, the remainder (those with positive reactions) being subjected to more refined diagnostic tests.

secretin t.: a test for pancreatic function done by examining the pancreatic secretion produced by the intravenous injection of secretin.

Seidel's t. (*for inosite*): evaporate in a platinum crucible with nitric acid, and treat with ammonia and strontium acetate in solution; inosite, if present, causes a green coloration and a violet precipitate.

Seidlitz powder t. (*for diaphragmatic hernia*): the stomach is distended by the administration of a Seidlitz powder, which will enable roentgen visualization of a herniated stomach loop.

Selivanoff's t., Seliwanow's t. (*for fructose in urine*): to the urine is added an equal volume of hydrochloric acid containing resorcinol in the following proportion: 5 mg. resorcinol, 5 ml. water, and 5 ml. 25 per cent concentrated hydrochloric acid. Formation of a burgundy-red color after boiling for 10 seconds indicates fructose.

semen t., see specific tests, including *Barberio's t., Florence t., Huhner t., serum t.*

senna t. (*in urine*): make the urine alkaline; a red color indicates senna.

Sereny t. (*to determine invasiveness of bacteria*): the organism is inoculated into the eye of a guinea pig; invasiveness is determined by the organism's ability to produce conjunctivitis. The test is used particularly for determining the invasiveness of strains of *Escherichia coli* and *Listeria monocytogenes*.

serologic t.: any laboratory test involving serologic reactions (precipitin reaction, agglutination, complement fixation, etc.), especially any such test measuring serum antibody titer.

serologic t. for syphilis (STS): any test for serum antibodies indicative of *Treponema pallidum* infection. There are two types: *Nontreponemal antigen tests* detect antibodies to substance (reagin) derived from host tissues, now known to consist of the phospholipids cardiolipin and lecithin; they originated with the Wassermann test and are now represented by the VDRL and RPR (rapid plasma reagin) tests. *Treponemal antigen tests* detect specific antitreponemal antibodies; they originated with the TPI (*T. pallidum* immobilization) test and are represented by the FTA-ABS (fluorescent treponemal antibody absorption) test, the MHA-TP (microhemagglutination assay—*T. pallidum*), and assays using ELISA (enzyme-linked immunosorbent assay) methods. The term "serologic tests for syphilis" is occasionally used with reference only to nontreponemal antigen tests.

serum bactericidal activity t., determination, by serial dilution, of the titer of serum that will, in combination with the antibiotic in serum, kill 99.9 per cent of the starting inoculum mixed with the serum sample; used to monitor antibiotic therapy in endocarditis, osteomyelitis, and other serious bacterial infections.

serum neutralization t.: a test of the antimicrobial activity of a serum done by inoculating a mixture of the serum and the virus or other microorganism being tested into a susceptible animal; called also *protection t.*

shadow t.: retinoscopy.

Shear's t. (*for vitamin D*): to the oil add an equal volume of acid aniline (1 part concentrated HCl and 15 parts aniline). Mix and boil. A green color changing to red indicates vitamin D.

sheep cell agglutination t. (SCAT), any agglutination test using sheep red blood cells, e.g., the Rose-Waaler test.

short increment sensitivity index (SISI) t., see under *index.*

Sia t. (*for macroglobulinemia*): a simple screening test performed by adding a drop of serum to 10 to 100 ml. of cold distilled water; a positive reaction is indicated by the formation of a heaving cloud of precipitate at the bottom of the container.

It is not diagnostic, because it may be positive in other conditions, as in rheumatoid arthritis.

Sicard-Cantelouble t.: place 4 ml. of spinal fluid in a specially graduated tube, add 12 drops of a 33 per cent trichloracetic acid, mix, and read the amount of protein precipitated after twenty-four hours' sedimentation.

sickling t.: a method to demonstrate hemoglobin S and the sickling phenomenon in erythrocytes, particularly in the heterozygous state, performed by reducing the environmental oxygen to which the red cells are exposed. This may be done by simply sealing a drop of blood under a coverslip or, to hasten the morphologic change, by adding 2 per cent sodium metabisulfite or sodium dithionite to the preparation.

Siebold and Bradbury's t. (*for salicylic acid in urine*): alkalinize with potassium carbonate, add a solution of lead nitrate in excess, filter, and add a dilute solution of ferric chloride; a violet color will be produced.

sign t., a nonparametric statistical test of the null hypothesis that a sample is drawn from a population with median 0 based on the number of observations having positive signs (which under the null hypothesis has a binomial distribution with p = 0.5).

signed rank t., a nonparametric statistical test of the null hypothesis that a sample is drawn from a population with median 0 (or that the median difference between matched pairs in two populations is 0) versus the alternative hypothesis that the median is nonzero based on the signed rank statistic calculated as the sum of the ranks of the positive sample observations (or positive differences between matched pairs) when all of the observations (differences) are arranged in order by absolute value. Called also *Wilcoxon's signed rank t.*

silver t. (*for dextrose in the urine*): boil the urine with silver nitrate solution and an excess of ammonia; metallic silver will be deposited. Tartaric acid and aldehyde also produce this reaction.

Simonelli's t. (*for renal inadequacy*): iodine is administered and the urine and saliva tested for iodine; if iodine does not appear in the urine at the same time as in the saliva, the kidneys are diseased.

Sims' t.: a postcoital test for the ability of the spermatozoa to penetrate the cervical mucus.

skatole t., see specific tests, including *Herter's t.* (2), *Kondo's t., nitroso-indole-nitrate t.*

skin t., any test in which an antigen is applied to the skin in order to observe the response of the patient, described according to method of application as patch tests, scratch tests, and intradermal tests. Skin tests are used to determine immunity to infectious diseases (e.g., tuberculin test), to identify allergens producing allergic reactions, and to assess ability to mount a cellular immune response (using a battery of antigens that give positive tests in most normal individuals).

skin window t., Rebuck skin window technique.

smear t., see *Papanicolaou's stain*, under *Table of Stains.*

Smith's t. (*for bile pigments*): overlay the suspected liquid with tincture of iodine diluted 1:10; a green ring or plane appears at the junction of the two liquids in the tube.

Snellen's t.: 1. (*for pretended blindness in one eye*) the patient is requested to look at alternate red and green letters; the admittedly sound eye is covered with a red glass and if the green letters are read, evidence of fraud is present. 2. determination of visual acuity by means of Snellen test types.

Snider match t. (*a screening test for pulmonary ventilation*): an ordinary book match which is burned nearly half way is held 6 inches from the mouth of the patient, who attempts to extinguish it by exhaling, after taking as deep a breath as possible, and without bringing the lips together.

sniff t.: when a patient sniffs, the paralyzed half of the diaphragm is seen to rise and the intact half to descend, as observed by fluoroscopy.

Soldaini's t. (*for glucose in the urine*): dissolve 15 gm. of copper carbonate and 416 gm. of potassium bicarbonate in 1400 ml. of water for a reagent; 2 parts of urine are boiled with 1 part of the reagent. A yellow precipitate of cupric oxide shows the presence of dextrose.

Solera's t. (*for thiocyanates*): saturate filter paper with 0.5 per cent starch paste containing 1 per cent of iodic acid; dry and preserve as test paper. A piece of this paper moistened with saliva will turn blue if thiocyanate is present.

solubility t. see *bile solubility t.*

Sonnenschein's t. (*for strychnine*): the suspected substance is dissolved in a drop of sulfuric acid, some cerosoceric oxide is added, and stirred with a glass rod; a deep-blue color is formed, changing to violet, and finally to cherry red in the presence of strychnine.

soy bean t., see *urease t.*

spavin t.: a test for spavin in horses made by holding up the limb with the hock bent sharply; the horse is then started suddenly, and in cases of spavin the first steps are very lame. Called also *hock t.*

specific gravity t., see specific tests, including *Fishberg concentration t., urine concentration t., Volhard's t.* (2). See also *specific gravity, methods for,* under *method.*

sphenopalatine t.: the sphenopalatine ganglion is anesthetized with Novocain in order to determine whether the efferent current which is motivating a symptom is routed through either sphenopalatine ganglion, and if so, whether the left one or the right one.

Spiegler's t. (*for albumin*): acidulate with acetic acid and filter; prepare a reagent with 8 gm. of mercuric chloride, 10 gm. of sodium chloride, and 4 gm. of tartaric acid in 200 ml. of water and 20 ml. of glycerin; overlay the reagent with the filtrate. If albumin is present, a white ring appears at the junction of the liquids.

Spiro's t.: 1. a test for the determination of ammonia and urea, embracing a combination of Folin's method for urea and the Sjöqvist method for urea. 2. (*for hippuric acid*) warm the unknown with acetic anhydride, anhydrous sodium acetate, and benzaldehyde. Cool, and crystals of phenylaminocinnamic acid–lactimide form.

split-renal function t., see *Howard t.*

sponge t.: a test performed by passing a hot sponge up and down the spine; if any lesion of the spine is present, pain is felt as the sponge passes over its locality.

Stanford-Binet t.: a modification of Binet's test, translated, adapted, and standardized on children in the United States.

starch t., see *iodine t.* (1).

station t.: a test for disturbances of coordination, made by placing the patient in an erect posture, with the heels and toes of the two feet together; if the swaying of the body is beyond normal, coordination may be defective.

Staub-Traugott t., see under *effect.*

steapsin t., see *ethyl butyrate t.*

Stein's t.: inability to stand on one foot with the eyes shut; seen in disease of the labyrinth.

Steinle-Kahlenberg t.: heat a chloroform solution of a sterol with antimony pentachloride; the purple color changes to cobalt blue in the light.

Stenger t.: a test for detecting simulated unilateral hearing loss: a signal is presented at an intensity less than the admitted threshold to the affected ear and a less intense signal of the same frequency is presented simultaneously to the unaffected ear. If the subject is feigning a loss of hearing, the subject will not be able to detect the signal in the unaffected ear.

Stock t. (*for acetone in urine*): the distillate of the urine is used; 50 to 100 ml. of urine is made acid by the addition of either acetic, hydrochloric, or sulfuric acid. The first 10 ml. of distillate will contain all the possible acetone. About 1 inch of the distillate is placed in a test tube; a drop or two of a 10 per cent solution of hydroxylamine hydrochloride is added, and sufficient sodium hydroxide or carbonate solution to render the solution alkaline to liberate hydroxylamine; the mixture is shaken and a couple of drops of pyridine is added and the mixture shaken again; then 1 inch of ether is added and the mixture shaken. Bromine water is then added drop by drop, with mixing, until the ether layer becomes yellow; then a few drops of strong hydrogen peroxide is added; if acetone is present the ether will turn a distinctive green blue.

Stokvis' t. (*for bile pigment*): with 25 ml. of urine mix 8 ml. of a 1:5 zinc acetate solution; wash the precipitate in water on a filter, and dissolve in ammonia water. Filter again, and in a short time the filtrate shows a bluish green tint.

Stoll t.: a technique for the quantitative estimation of the worm burden of an individual based on collection of a 24-hour stool specimen and counting the number of ova present in an aliquot.

Storck's t. (*for human milk*): catalase present in human milk will decompose hydrogen dioxide.

Strange's t., see *Henderson's t.*

Strassburg's t. (*for bile acids in albumin-free urine*): add cane sugar to the urine; dip filter paper into it and dry; a drop of sulfuric acid on the paper will cause a red or violet spot if bile acids are present.

Straus's biological t. (*for glanders*), see *Straus' reaction*, under *reaction.*

stress t's, exercise t's.

Struve's t. (*for blood in the urine*): alkalinize the urine and add tannic and acetic acids until the reaction becomes acid and a dark precipitate is formed. When this is dried, crystals of hemin may be obtained from it by adding ammonium chloride and glacial acetic acid.

strychnine t., see specific tests, including *Allen's t.* (3), *Brieger's t.* (2), *Sonnenschein's t., Wenzell's t.*

Student's *t*-t., see *t-t.*

Stypven time t.: a test similar to the Quick one-stage prothrombin time test, but performed with Russell's viper venom (Stypven) as the thromboplastic agent; useful in defining deficiencies of blood coagulation Factor X.

sucrose lysis t. (*for paroxysmal nocturnal hemoglobinuria*): the patient's whole blood is mixed with isotonic sucrose solution, which promotes binding of complement to red cells, incubated, and examined for hemolysis; greater than 10 per cent hemolysis is indicative of PNH.

sugar t., see tests listed under *dextrose t., levulose t.,* and *maltose t.*

sulfur t. (*for protein*): the suspected liquid is heated with an excess of sodium hydroxide and a small quantity of acetate of lead; if proteins are present, a black precipitate of lead sulfide is formed.

Sulkowitch's t. (*for calcium in urine*): the precipitation of calcium in urine as an oxalate with use of a reagent consisting of 2.5 gm. of oxalic acid, 2.5 gm. of ammonium oxalate, and 5 ml. of glacial acetic acid dissolved in 150 ml. of distilled water.

Sullivan's t. (*for cysteine*): to 1 or 2 ml. of the unknown solution add 1 to 2 drops of a 0.5 per cent solution of 1,2-naphthoquinone-4-sodium sulfonate and then 5 ml. of a 20 per cent sodium thiosulfate made up in 0.25 normal sodium hydroxide. A brilliant red color indicates a free SH group, cysteine rather than cystine.

susceptibility t. (*for testing the susceptibility of pathogenic bacteria to antibiotics*): see *dilution t.* and *disk diffusion t.*

syphilis t., see *serologic t. for syphilis.*

Szabo's t. (*for HCl in the stomach contents*): add to the suspected liquid a reagent containing equal parts of a 0.5 per cent solution of sodioferric tartrate and ammonium thiocyanate; if HCl is present, the reagent is changed from a pale yellow to a brownish red.

t-t., a statistical hypothesis test based on the *t*-distribution (q.v.) used to test for a difference between the means of two groups. Called also *Student's t-t.*

tannic acid t. (*for nucleoalbumin*), see *Ott's t.*

Tanret's t. (*for albumin*): Tanret's reagent gives a white precipitate with albumin. See under *reagent.*

Tardieu's t. (*for infanticide*): presence of air bubbles in gastric mucosa after establishment of fetal respiration.

taurine t., see *Lang's t.*

Taylor's t.: a modification of Schönbein's test for blood, the blue precipitate forming a deep sapphire blue solution when taken up by alcohol or ether.

Teichmann's t. (*for blood*): the suspected liquid is put under a coverglass with a crystal of sodium chloride and a little glacial acetic acid; heat carefully without boiling and then cool. If blood is present, rhombic crystals of hemin will appear.

Tensilon t. (*for myasthenia gravis*): after administration of Tensilon (edrophonium chloride), the patient's eye signs (ptosis and extraocular muscle abnormalities) markedly decrease.

Terman t.: the Stanford modification of the Binet test.

thalleioquin t. (*for quinine*): a neutralized solution of the suspected liquid is treated with chlorine, or bromine water, and then with an excess of ammonia; a green substance, thalleioquin, will be formed.

thematic apperception t. (TAT): a projective test in which the subject tells a story based on each of a series of standard ambiguous pictures, so that his responses reflect a projection of some aspect of his personality and current psychological preoccupations and conflicts.

thermoagglutination t.: a test to detect antigenic variants, in which slightly rough strains may be detected by their agglutination upon boiling saline for two hours.

thiamine t., see *thiochrome t.*

thiochrome t. (*for thiamine*): oxidize the thiamine to thiochrome and then recognize the latter by its blue-violet fluorescence in ultraviolet radiation.

thiocyanate t., see *ferric chloride t.* (1), *Solera's t.*

Thomas t.: with the patient supine, when one leg is flexed so that the knee touches the chest and the lumbar spine is flattened, the angle taken by the other hip is the degree of flexion deformity.

Thompson's t. (*for gonorrhea*), see *two-glass t.*

Thormählen's t. (*for melanin in urine*): treat urine with a solution of sodium nitroprusside, potassium hydroxide, and acetic acid; if melanin is present, a deep-blue color will form.

three-glass t.: on arising in the morning the patient urinates successively into three glass receptacles labeled I, II, and III. In acute anterior urethritis the urine in I will be turbid from pus, while II and III will be clear; but in posterior urethritis the urine in all three glasses will be turbid. Blood in I only comes from the anterior urethra, but if it comes from the posterior urethra all three will contain blood. Shreds in glass III point to chronic prostatitis.

thromboplastin generation t.: a sensitive test for delineation of defects in formation of intrinsic thromboplastin (prothrombinase, intrinsic prothrombin-converting principle) and hence deficiencies of the factors involved. Patient plasma, serum, calcium chloride, and autologous platelets or platelet lipid substitute are incubated concurrently, and, at appropriate intervals, the clotting times of normal citrated plasma substrate, to which aliquots of the incubation mixture are added in sequential fashion, are determined.

Thudichum's t. (*for creatinine*): add to the suspected substance a dilute solution of ferric chloride; a dark-red color indicates the presence of creatinine.

thumb-nail t. (*for fractured patella*): the examiner's thumbnail is passed over the subcutaneous surface of the patella; a fracture will be felt as a sharp crevice.

thymol turbidity t.: a flocculation test formerly used as a test of liver function; a positive result (formation of a precipitate when a supersaturated thymol solution is added to serum) reflects serum protein abnormalities, chiefly elevated levels of gamma or beta globulins.

thyroid function t.: see specific tests, including *acetonitrile t., Kottmann's t., Loewi's t., quadriceps t.* See also *thyroid function reaction*, under *reaction*, and *thyroid activity, method for*, under *method*.

thyroid suppression t. (*for hyperthyroidism*): after administration of liothyronine for several days, radioactive iodine uptake is decreased in normal persons but not in those with hyperthyroidism.

Tidy's t. (*for albumin in urine*): 1. add equal volumes of phenol and glacial acetic acids; albumin will form a white precipitate. 2. add 15 drops of alcohol and 15 drops of phenol; albumin will form a white precipitate.

tine t., tine tuberculin t. (Rosenthal): four tines or prongs 2 mm. long, attached to a plastic handle and coated with dip-dried Old tuberculin (O.T.) are pressed into the skin of the volar surface of the forearm, where they deposit a dose of the tuberculin in the outer layer. The skin is checked 48 to 72 hours later for the presence of palpable induration; if the induration around one or more of the puncture wounds is 2 mm. or more in diameter, the test is considered positive.

Tizzoni's t. (*for iron in tissues*): treat a section of tissue with a 2 per cent solution of potassium ferrocyanide, and then with a 0.5 per cent solution of HCl; the tissue will be stained a blue color if iron is present.

TNT t., see *Webster's t.*

toad t., 1. see *male frog* or *male toad t.* 2. see *Xenopus t.*

Tobey-Ayer t. (*in the diagnosis of lateral sinus thrombosis*): after spinal puncture a manometer is attached to the puncture needle: compression on both jugular veins causes the fluid to rise in the manometer; pressure on one jugular vein alone, causes a rise in spinal fluid pressure if the lateral sinus is normal but little or no rise if there is thrombosis of the sinus on the same side as compression of the vein. The significance of the test is greater on the right side than on the left.

tolerance t.: 1. an exercise test to determine the efficiency of the circulation. 2. a test to determine the body's ability to metabolize a substance or to endure administration of a drug.

Tollens, Neuberg, and Schwket's t. (*for glycuronic acid*): extract the glycuronic acid from acidified urine with ether, add water, evaporate the ether, and make orcinol test.

tone decay t., an audiometer test in which the patient is asked to raise his hand as long as he hears a continuous tone at his threshold level and to lower it when it becomes inaudible; whenever he lowers it before 60 seconds, the intensity is raised by 5 decibels and the amount of tone decay from the initial threshold level in decibels is determined.

tongue t., see under *phenomenon.*

Töpfer's t's: quantitative tests for hydrochloric acid in gastric contents. 1. (*for total acidity*) 1 per cent solution of phenolphthalein is used as the indicator. 2. (*for free HCl*) 0.5 per

cent alcoholic solution of *p*-dimethylaminoazobenzene is used as the indicator. 3. (*for combined HCl*) 1 per cent aqueous solution of sodium alizarin sulfonate is used as the indicator.

Torquay's t. (*for bile*): a small amount of the suspected liquid is added to a test tube containing an aqueous solution of methyl violet, 1:2000. Bile will change the blue color to red.

tourniquet t.: 1. (*for capillary fragility*) after application of pressure midway between diastolic and systolic for 5 minutes by a manometer cuff, the petechiae are counted in a previously marked area, 2.5 cm. in diameter, on the inner aspect of the forearm, about 4 cm. below the crease of the elbow. A number between 10 and 20 is marginal, above 20, abnormal. Called also *Hess capillary t.* 2. (*for collateral circulation*) after hyperemia of the limb has been artificially produced by application of the tourniquet, the tourniquet is removed and the extent of collateral circulation is determined by compressing the main artery. Called also *Matas' t.* 3. (*for collateral circulation in patients with varicose veins*) a bandage is applied to the upper part of the leg below the knee and the patient walks around with it on; varicose veins of the leg will become evacuated from continuous compression if there is sufficient collateral circulation in the deep veins. Called also *Perthes' t.*

toxigenicity t. (*in vitro*) (*for detection of toxigenic strains of* Corynebacterium diphtheriae): a primary culture is streaked onto a plate of tellurite agar containing a strip of filter paper perfused with diphtheria antitoxin. The exotoxin produced by the bacteria forms a band of precipitation with antitoxin diffusing from the filter paper. Called also *Elek t.*

TPI t., *Treponema pallidum* immobilization t.

trapeze t.: when the patient hangs from a trapeze, a spinal deformity will disappear if the deformity is postural but will remain if it is structural.

Trendelenburg's t.: 1. raise the leg above the level of the heart until the veins are empty, then lower it quickly. If the veins become distended at once, varicosity and incompetence of the valves are indicated. 2. the patient, standing erect, stripped, with back to the examiner, is told to lift one leg and then the other: when weight is supported by the affected limb, the pelvis on the sound side falls instead of rising; seen in disturbances of the gluteus medius mechanism, as in deformity of the femoral neck, dislocated hip joint, and weakness or paralysis of the gluteus medius muscle.

Treponema pallidum complement fixation t's: nontreponemal antigen serologic tests for syphilis using complement fixation rather than flocculation as the indicator reaction. Once widely used to confirm positive results of flocculation procedures, they have now been replaced by treponemal antigen tests.

Treponema pallidum immobilization (TPI) t.: the first treponemal antigen serologic test for syphilis, introduced in 1949, now little used; live *T. pallidum* is mixed with patient serum and complement and examined microscopically to determine the proportion of treponemes that are immobilized by specific antibodies in the serum.

Tretop's t.: to fresh urine in a test tube a few drops of 40 per cent formalin are added; albumin in the urine is coagulated.

Triboulet's t. (*for tuberculous ulceration of the intestines*): a lump of feces as large as a walnut is dissolved in 20 ml. of distilled water and filtered; 3 ml. of the filtrate is diluted with 12 ml. of distilled water; 20 minims of Triboulet's reagent (sublimate 3.5, acetic acid 1, distilled water 100) are added. As a control the same solution is prepared without Triboulet's reagent. The test tubes containing the two solutions are well shaken, and are compared after five and twenty-four hours. A positive reaction is indicated by a cloudy gray or brown deposit.

trichophytin t. (*for trichophyton infection*): when filtrates of the fungus are injected into persons who have been infected with the disease, a reaction is produced somewhat resembling the tuberculin reaction.

tricresol peroxidase t. (*for raw milk*), see *Kastle's t.*

triketohydrindene hydrate t.: to 25 ml. of water add 10 mg. of aminoacetic acid. To 1 ml. of this solution add a solution of 50 mg. of sodium acid in 2 ml. of water, then add 0.2 ml. of a solution of 5 mg. of triketohydrindene hydrate (Ninhydrin) in 1 ml. of water. Add the suspected matter and boil for 1–2 minutes. A violet color indicates a free carboxyl and alpha-amino group in proteins, peptones, peptides, or amino acids.

Trommer's t. (*for dextrose in the urine*): to 2 parts of urine add 1 part of potassium or sodium hydroxide, then add a very dilute solution of copper sulfate drop by drop, and boil the whole. Sugar, if present, causes precipitation of an orange-red deposit.

Trousseau's t. (*for bile in urine*): tincture of iodine diluted with 10 parts of alcohol is added to urine in a test tube; a green ring is formed where the liquids touch if bilirubin is present.

Tsuchiya's t. (*for albumin*): a modified test in which Tsuchiya's reagent is used instead of Esbach's reagent.

tuberculin t.: any of a large number of skin tests for tuberculosis using a variety of different types of tuberculin and methods of application. The most reliable procedure, now standard, is intradermal injection (the Mantoux test) of PPD (purified protein derivative); a positive result consists of a palpable and visible area of erythema and induration greater than 10 mm in diameter developing around the site of injection 48 to 72 hours after the injection. Intermediate strength tuberculin (5 TU) is generally used to test adults; a positive result is virtually diagnostic of a previous or current infection with *Mycobacterium tuberculosis*. Persons with a negative test are retested with second strength tuberculin (250 TU); in this test a positive reaction is frequently due to atypical mycobacteria infection and is thus nonspecific; a negative result indicates either absence of tuberculosis or the presence of cutaneous anergy due to overwhelming tuberculosis infection or to an associated immunosuppressive illness, e.g., Hodgkin's disease or sarcoidosis.

tuberculin t., Sterneedle: the needle points of the Sterneedle are dipped into 1 to 2 drops of tuberculin P.P.D. and then placed on the forearm, where the six needle points are caused to penetrate the skin (by means of a spring device in the handle), through the P.P.D. solution, to a depth of 1 mm., thus depositing tuberculin in the outer layer of the skin. Palpable, coalescing induration (edema) extending more than 5 mm. around the puncture wounds in three to seven days indicates a positive reaction. In England, it is known as the *Heaf test.*

tuberculosis t., see specific tests, including *Craig's t., Mantoux t., mirror t., niacin t.* (1), (2), *Römer's t., tine t., Triboulet's t., tuberculin t., tuberculin t., Sterneedle, urorosein t., Vollmer's t.* See also *tuberculosis reaction,* under *reaction.*

Tuffier's t.: in aneurysm, when the main artery and vein of a limb are compressed, swelling of the veins of the hand or foot will occur only if the collateral circulation is free.

two-glass t. (*for urethritis*): the patient collects his urine on rising, the first part in one glass and the second part in a separate glass. If he has anterior urethritis the first portion will be turbid and the second portion clear; if he has both anterior and posterior urethritis both portions will be turbid.

two-stage prothrombin t.: a method of quantitating prothrombin after tissue thromboplastin and excess Factor V have converted it to thrombin, by determining the clotting time of a standard fibrinogen solution to which the previously generated thrombin has been added.

two-tailed t., a hypothesis test (q.v.) in which the critical region comprises both tails of the distribution of the test statistic and the null hypothesis is tested against a two-sided alternative that includes deviation from the null hypothesis in both directions.

typhoid fever t., see specific tests, including *Ehrlich's t.* (1), *miostagmin t., Moretti's t., Petzetaki's t., urorosein t.* See also *typhoid fever reaction,* under *reaction.*

tyrosine t., see specific tests, including *Hoffmann's t., Mörner's t.* (1), *Piria's t., Scherer's t.* (3), *Udránszky's t.* (2), *Wurster's t.* (2).

Tyson's t. (*for bile acids in urine*): 180 to 240 ml. of urine are evaporated to dryness on the water bath. The residue is extracted with absolute alcohol, and to the extract 12 to 14 volumes of ether are added. The bile acids are precipitated, then are filtered off, dissolved in water, and the aqueous solution decolorized with animal charcoal.

Tzanck t.: examination of tissue from the floor of a lesion, in vesicular or bullous diseases, to discover the type of cell present as a means of diagnosing the disease. Multinucleated giant cells are pathognomonic of varicella, herpes simplex, herpes zoster, or pemphigus.

Udránszky's t.: 1. (*for bile acids*) take 1 ml. of a solution of the suspected substance, add a drop of 0.1 per cent solution of furfurol in water, underlay with strong sulfuric acid, and cool; if bile is present, a bluish-red color is formed. 2. (*for tyrosine*) take 1 ml. of the suspected substance in solution, add a drop of 0.5 per cent aqueous solution of furfurol, and underlay with 1 ml. of concentrated sulfuric acid; a pink color shows the presence of tyrosine.

Uffelmann's t. (*for hydrochloric acid and lactic acid in the gastric contents*): to a quantity of material taken from the stomach add a few drops of a reagent containing 3 drops of a solution of ferric chloride, 3 drops of a concentrated solution of phenol, and 20 ml. of water; hydrochloric acid, if present, decolorizes this solution, while lactic acid turns it yellow.

Ulrich's t. (*for albumin*): the reagent consists of saturated solution of common salt, 98 ml.; glacial acetic acid, 2 ml. It must be perfectly clear. Boil a few milliliters of this fluid in a test tube, and immediately overlay with the urine. Albumin and globulin give a white ring at the zone of contact.

Ultzmann's t. (*for bile pigments*): to 10 ml. of the urine to be tested add 3 or 4 ml. of a 1:3 solution of potassium hydroxide, and an excess of HCl; bile pigments will cause an emerald-green coloration.

Umber's t. (*for scarlet fever*): to a small quantity of urine add 2 drops of a solution made with 30 ml. concentrated hydrochloric acid, 2 gm. of paradimethylaminobenzaldehyde and 70 ml. of water; a red reaction indicates scarlet fever.

unheated serum reagin (USR) t.: a modification of the VDRL test using unheated serum, used primarily for screening.

uracil t., see *Wheeler and Johnson's t.*

urea t., see specific tests, including *Benedict's t.* (2), *biuret t.* (2), *diacetyl t., Marshall's t., Schiff's t.* (4), *Schroeder's t., Spiro's t.* (1), *urease t., Van Slyke t.* (2). See also *urea, methods for,* under *method.*

urea clearance t., see *blood-urea clearance t.*

urea concentration t. (*for renal efficiency*): a test based on the fact that urea is absorbed rapidly from the stomach into the blood, and is excreted unaltered by the kidneys: 15 gm. of urea is given with 100 ml. of fluid, and the urine which is collected at the end of two hours is tested for urea concentration. Called also *MacLean-de Wesselow t.* and *Jones and Cantarow t.*

urease t., 1. a test for urea based on the conversion of urea into ammonium carbonate by the urease of soybean; see *Marshall's method* and *urease, methods for,* under *method.* 2. (*for the production of urease by bacteria*) a peptone agar medium containing urea concentrate and phenol red is prepared in slants. After inoculation of the surface and incubation, urease-positive cultures produce an alkaline reaction (red color) in the medium. *Proteus* cultures show an early urease-positive reaction; other genera may have a delayed response.

Urecholine supersensitivity t. (*for neurogenic bladder*): administer 2.5 mg. of Urecholine (bethanechol) subcutaneously; the bladder is neurogenic if it exhibits a rise in intravesical pressure more than 15 cm. greater than that of a control.

uric acid t., see specific tests, including *Porter's t.* (1), *Salkowski-Ludwig t., Schiff's t.* (5), *von Jaksch's t.* (4), *Weidel's t.* (1). See also *uric acid, methods for,* under *method.*

urine concentration t.: under a controlled diet the specific gravity of the urine should reach 1.18 or more at certain times.

urobilin t., see specific tests, including *Hildebrandt's t., Schlesinger's t.* See also *urobilinogen, methods for,* under *method.*

urochromogen t., see *Weiss' t.*

urorosein t., urorrhodin t.: add to the urine half as much concentrated hydrochloric acid and a few drops of a 1 per cent solution of potassium nitrate; a red color indicates urorosein (urorrhodin); seen in typhoid fever, nephritis, pulmonary tuberculosis, and other diseases.

USR t., unheated serum reagin t.

Valenta's t. (*for foreign fats in butter*): the butter is heated with an equal amount of glacial acetic acid and then cooled. If opacity begins to show at 96° F., there is adulteration; if opacity is not observed until about 62° F., the butter is pure.

Valsalva's t. (*for pneumothorax*): after a deep inspiration, the mouth and nose are held tightly closed, and a strong attempt at expiration is made.

van den Bergh t.: a test for bilirubin in which diazotized serum or plasma is compared with a standard solution of diazotized bilirubin.

van den Velden's t., see *Maly's t.*

Van Slyke t.: 1. (*for amino-nitrogen*) nitrous acid acting on amino-nitrogen sets free nitrogen gas, which is collected and its volume determined. 2. (*for urea*) treat the sample with urease, pass the ammonia so formed into fiftieth normal acid, and titrate the excess of acid.

Van Slyke and Cullen's t., see under *method.*

Vaughan and Novy's t. (*for tyrotoxicon*): adding 2 or 3 drops each of sulfuric and carbolic acids and a few drops of an aqueous solution of the suspected substance to tyrotoxicon gives a yellow or orange-red color.

VDRL [Venereal Disease Research Laboratory] **t.:** the standard nontreponemal antigen serologic test for syphilis, a slide flocculation test using heat-inactivated serum and VDRL antigen, a standardized mixture of cardiolipin, lecithin, and cholesterol. Positive tests are seen in about 70 per cent of cases in primary syphilis, 100 per cent in secondary syphilis, and 70 per cent in tertiary syphilis. There is a 20 to 40 per cent false positive rate; see *biologic false-positive* under *false-positive.*

ventilation t.: measurement of the quantity of air expired by a person during a period of exercise.

Visscher-Bowman t. (*for pregnancy*): a chemical test for pregnancy, depending on the presence of anterior pituitary hormones in the urine.

Vitali's t.: 1. (*for alkaloids*) evaporate with fuming nitric acid and add a drop of potassium hydroxide; color reactions will occur. For atropine the color is violet, turning to red. 2. (*for alkaloids*) add sulfuric acid, potassium chlorate, and an alkaline sulfide; various color reactions will follow. 3. (*for bile pigments*) add a few drops of potassium nitrate in solution and dilute sulfuric acid. The color reactions are green, followed by blue or red and yellow. 4. (*for bile pigments*) add quinine bisulfate in solution and follow with ammonia water, sulfuric acid, a crystal of sugar, and alcohol; a violet color results. 5. (*for thymol*) distill, and pass the vapor through a mixture of chloroform and potassium hydroxide solution; a red color results. 6. (*for pus in the urine*) the urine is acidified with acetic acid and filtered. On the filter paper thus obtained a small quantity of guaiacum is dropped. The paper will turn a dark blue if pus is present.

vitamin t., see specific tests, including *Carr-Price t., Fearon's t., Gothlin's t., Harris and Ray t., Jendrasic's t., Rosenheim-Drummond t., Rotter's t., Schopfer's t., Shear's t., thiochrome t.*

Voelcker and Joseph's t., see *indigo carmine t.*

Vogel and Lee's t. (*for mercury*): add 3 per cent of hydrochloric acid and concentrate the urine to one fifth its original volume. Add a piece of clean copper wire. A silvery film indicates mercury. To confirm, place the wire in a tube with a plug of gold foil and distill the mercury over onto the gold. Sublime a crystal of iodine onto the mercury and form the red iodide of mercury.

Voges-Proskauer t. (*for differentiation of Enterobacteriaceae*): a test for the production of acetylmethylcarbinol from glucose in bacterial cultures. An appropriate culture is treated with a solution of potassium hydroxide and creatine. Development of a red color indicates a positive reaction. *Enterobacter, Klebsiella,* and *Serratia* are V-P positive; *Erwinia, Pectobacterium,* and *Yersinia* are variable; *Escherichia* and other genera of Enterobacteriaceae are V-P negative.

Vollmer t.: (*obs.*) a tuberculin patch test.

von Aldor's t. (*for proteoses*): precipitate the urine with phosphotungstic acid, wash the precipitate with alcohol, bring into solution with potassium hydroxide, and apply the biuret test.

von Jaksch's t.: 1. (*for free HCl in gastric juice*) a test paper prepared with benzopurpurine B takes on a fine violet color if HCl is present. If present in considerable amount, it becomes dark blue. 2. (*for dextrose in urine*) add to the urine a mixture of 3 parts of sodium acetate and 2 parts of phenylhydrazine hydrochloride, warm it, and put the test tube in hot water for half an hour. On cooling, yellow needles of phenylglucosazone are seen as a precipitate. 3. (*for melanin*) add to the suspected liquid a few drops of a solution of ferric chloride. If melanin is present, a gray appearance is produced. After precipitation add more ferric chloride, and the precipitate will be redissolved. 4. (*for uric acid*) heat the powder slowly on a glass dish with a few drops of bromine water or chlorine water; the substance becomes red. After cooling, add ammonia, and it becomes purplish red.

von Maschke's t. (*for creatinine*): to the suspected solution add a few drops of Fehling's solution, after mixing with a cold solution of sodium carbonate; an amorphous, flocculent precipitate proves the presence of creatinine.

von Pirquet t., Pirquet t.

von Recklinghausen's t. (*of heart function*): a test based on the proposition that the product of the frequency of the pulse and the amplitude of the blood pressure is equal to the amount of blood expelled by the heart in a second, divided by the distensibility of the circulatory system.

von Zeynek and Mencki's t. (*for blood*): precipitate the urine with acetone, extract the precipitate with acidified acetone, and examine the colored extract under the microscope for small hemin crystals.

Waaler-Rose t., Rose-Waaler t.

Wada t. (*for cerebral dominance of language function*): amobarbital is injected into an internal carotid artery to produce transient hemiparesis of the contralateral limbs. Injection into the artery of the hemisphere dominant for language produces a transient aphasia, into that of the nondominant hemisphere does not interfere with language function.

Wagner's t. (*for occult blood*), see *benzidine t.*

Walter's bromide t.: a test based on the fact that in normal persons the ratio of the amount of bromide in the blood and cerebrospinal fluid is constant; in persons with mental disorder the ratio may vary.

Wang's t. (*quantitative test for indican*): the indican is converted into indigosulfuric acid and titrated by means of a potassium permanganate solution.

Warren's t., see *Trommer's t.*

Wassermann t., the original (1906) nontreponemal antigen serologic test for syphilis.

water-gurgle t. (*for stricture of the esophagus*): the swallowing of water causes a peculiar gurgle heard on auscultation.

water provocative t.: drinking t.

Watson-Schwartz t.: a simple qualitative procedure, depending upon the chloroform- and butanol-insolubility of porphobilinogen aldehyde, for differentiating porphobilinogen from urobilinogen and other Ehrlich reactors; it is of value in the diagnosis of acute porphyria.

Weber's t.: 1. (*for differentiating between hearing impairment of conductive or sensorineural origin*) the stem of a vibrating tuning fork is placed on the vertex or midline of the forehead; if the sound is heard best in the affected ear, the impairment is probably of the conductive type; if heard best in the normal ear, the impairment is probably of the sensorineural type. (Friedrich Eugen Weber.) 2. (*for indican*) boil 30 ml. of suspected urine with an equal volume of hydrochloric acid containing a little nitric acid; cool it, and shake with ether; if indican is present, the ether will become red or violet and the froth will be blue. (Ernest Heinrich Weber.) 3. (*for blood*) mix the sample with 30 per cent acetic acid and extract with ether; to the ethereal extract add an alcoholic solution of guaiac and hydrogen peroxide. A blue color indicates blood. (Ernest Heinrich Weber.)

Webster's t. (*for TNT in urine*): the urine is extracted with ether, then acidified with a mineral acid, and again extracted with ether. In the latter extract the presence of the azoxy-compound formed from TNT is shown by the development of a violet tint on the addition of alcoholic potash.

Weichbrodt's t. (*for globulin*): to 0.7 ml. of spinal fluid add 0.3 ml. of a 1 per cent solution of mercuric bichloride; a cloudiness or opalescence indicates globulin.

Weidel's t.: 1. (*for uric acid*) the substance tested is treated with nitric acid, evaporated, and moistened with ammonia water; if uric acid is present, murexide will be formed, and a purple color is produced. Called also *murexide t.* 2. (*for xanthine*) warm with freshly prepared chlorine water containing a trace of nitric acid until gas ceases to be produced; contact with gaseous ammonia develops a pink or purple color. 3. (*for xanthine bodies*) dissolve in warm chlorine water, evaporate, and treat with ammonia water; a pink or purple color will form, changing to violet on the addition of sodium or potassium hydroxide solution.

Weil-Felix t. (*for diagnosis of typhus and certain other rickettsial diseases*): the blood serum of a patient with suspected rickettsial disease is tested against certain strains of *Proteus vulgaris* (OX-2, OX-19, OX-K). The agglutination reactions, based on antigens common to both organisms, determine the presence and type of rickettsial infection.

Weiss permanganate t., see *Weiss' t.*

Weiss' t. (*for urochromogen*): to 2 ml. of the urine add 4 ml. of distilled water and 3 drops of a 1:1000 solution of potassium permanganate; a canary yellow color indicates urochromogen.

Welland's t.: bar-reading t.

Wender's t. (*for dextrose*): make a reagent by dissolving 1 part of methylene blue in 300 parts of distilled water; alkalinize this with potassium hydroxide and heat with a suspected solution; dextrose, if present, will decolorize it.

Wenzell's t. (*for strychnine*): treat the suspected material with a solution of 1 part of potassium permanganate in 2000 parts of sulfuric acid; strychnine, even in very small proportion, will cause color reactions.

Weppen's t. (*for morphine*): treat with sugar, bromine, and sulfuric acid; a red color shows the presence of morphine.

Wernicke's t., see *hemiopic pupillary reaction*, under *reaction.*

Wetzel's t. *(for carbon monoxide in blood)*: to the blood to be examined add 4 volumes of water and treat with 3 volumes of a 1 per cent tannin solution. If CO is present, the blood becomes carmine red; normal blood slowly assumes a grayish hue.

Weyl's t.: 1. *(for creatinine)* to the suspected solution add a little of a dilute solution of sodium nitroprusside, and then carefully put in a few drops of a weak solution of sodium hydroxide; a ruby-red color results, changing to blue on warming with acetic acid. 2. *(for nitric acid in the urine)* distill 200 ml. of urine with 0.2 part of sulfuric or hydrochloric acid, receiving the distillate in a potassium hydroxide solution. If metaphenyl-diamine is added, a yellow color will form; if there is added pyrogallic acid in aqueous solution with a little sulfuric acid, the color will be brown; but sulfanilic acid in solution, followed in ten minutes by naphthylamine hydrochlorate, produces a red tint.

Wheeler and Johnson's t. *(for uracil and cytosine)*: to the unknown solution add bromine water until the color is permanent, but avoid excess. Then add an excess of barium hydroxide. A purple color indicates one of these substances.

Whipple's t., see *lipase t.* (1), *phenoltetrachlorophthalein t.*

Whiteside t.: a test for the detection of subclinical mastitis in cows as indicated by an excessively high leukocyte count of the milk. Mix 2 ml. of a normal solution of sodium hydroxide with 10 ml. of milk; the development of a viscous mass is positive. A modified version consists in mixing 1 drop of milk with 5 drops of normal sodium hydroxide solution on a glass plate, and stirring for about 20 seconds with a glass rod. No changes in consistency—negative; threads, clumps, or flakes of coagulated material—positive; the development of a viscous mass with separation of a clear whey— strongly positive.

Widal's t., Widal's serum t. *(for typhoid fever)*: a test for the presence of agglutinins to O and H antigens of *Salmonella typhi* and *Salmonella paratyphi* in the serum of patients with suspected Salmonella infection.

Wideroe's t.: a test for the character of puncture fluids. A few drops of Millon's reagent is placed in a water glass, and 1 drop of the fluid to be tested is placed on the surface. A film of coagulated protein at once forms. If this film is coherent and can be lifted readily, the exudate is tuberculous; if less readily, it is inflammatory; if it breaks up so that it cannot be lifted at all, it is a transudate.

Widmark's t.: a blood test for the diagnosis of alcoholic intoxication.

Wijs' t.: an iodine number test which employs Wijs iodine solution; see *iodine number,* under *number.*

Wilbrand's prism t.: a small circle of white paper is placed upon a black surface, and the patient is seated before it with one eye bandaged. He is directed to look at the spot, and a strong prism is placed before the eye in such a way that the image of the spot is thrown upon the blind half of the retina. It is noticed if the eye at once moves to find the object again, and whether the movement is reversed when the prism is withdrawn. The presence of this reaction places the lesion in the cerebrum; the absence of the reaction locates it in the tract.

Wilcoxon's rank sum t., rank sum t.

Wilcoxon's signed rank t., signed rank t.

Wilkinson and Peter's t. *(for raw milk)*: benzidine and hydrogen peroxide give a blue color in raw milk, but not in heated milk.

Williamson's blood t.: in a narrow test tube 4 ml. of water and 2 ml. of blood are placed; to this are added 1 ml. of methylene blue (1:6000) and 4 ml. of solution of potassium hydroxide. The tube is placed in a pot of boiling water. If the blood is from a diabetic patient, the blue soon disappears, but not otherwise.

Winckler t.: 1. *(for alkaloids)* a solution of mercuric chloride with an excess of potassium iodide is added; alkaloids will cause a white precipitate. 2. *(for free HCl in the gastric juice)* filter the juice into a porcelain cell with a few drops of the 5 per cent alcoholic solution of alphanaphthol containing 1 per cent or less of dextrose. Heat carefully, and a bluish-violet zone will appear, which rapidly grows darker. 3. *(for iodine)* sodium nitrate is mixed with a starch paste; iodine gives a blue color with it.

Winslow's t.: test for respiration in doubtful death by observing a vessel of water placed at the bottom of the chest.

Wishart t. *(for acetonemia)*: a few drops of plasma are placed in a small test tube. Enough dry powdered ammonium sulfate is added to supersaturate, so that at the end of the test there will still be some of the solid sulfate in the bottom of the tube. A couple of drops of a fresh solution of sodium nitroprus-

side are next added and shaken, and finally 1 or 2 drops of ordinary ammonia water. On shaking, a purple color develops, a little more slowly than in the case of urine. The intensity of the color indicates the degree of acetonemia.

Witz's t. *(for hydrochloric acid in the gastric juice)*: a 1:48 aqueous solution of methyl violet causes a violet color, changing to blue and then green.

Woldman's t.: a test for gastrointestinal lesion based on the principle that free phenolphthalein may pass through a lesion in the gastrointestinal mucosa and appear in the urine.

Wolff-Junghans t. *(for gastric cancer)*: quantitative estimation of the soluble albumin in the gastric extracts after giving a test meal; marked increase of dissolved albumin indicating malignant disease.

Woodbury's t. *(for alcohol in the urine)*: to 2 ml. of urine 1 ml. of sulfuric acid is added, and a crystal of potassium dichromate; a green color will soon form.

Worm-Müller t. *(for dextrose in the urine)*: a test made by boiling in a test tube 0.33 ml. of a 2.5 per cent solution of copper sulfate and 2.5 ml. of a solution of potassium hydroxide. Boil each and mix, and a yellowish or red precipitate will be formed.

Wormley's t. *(for alkaloids)*: 1. made by treating with an alcoholic solution of picric acid; a yellow precipitate will be formed. 2. made by treating with a solution of 1 part of iodine and 2 parts of potassium iodide in 60 parts of water; a colored precipitate will be formed.

worsted t., see *Holmgren's t.*

Wurster's t.: 1. *(for hydrogen peroxide)* test paper is saturated with the solution of tetramethylparaphenylenediamine; hydrogen peroxide turns it to a blue-violet color. 2. *(for tyrosine)* the suspected material is dissolved in boiling water and a little quinone; a ruby-red color will form, changing slowly to brown.

X² t., chi-square t.

xanthine t., see specific tests, including *Hoppe-Seyler t.* (2), *Weidel's t.* (2), (3).

xanthoproteic t., see *Mulder's t.* (2).

Xenopus t. *(for pregnancy)*: a female African toad (*Xenopus laevis*) is injected with 2 ml. of urine, or 1 ml. of an extract, into the dorsal lymph sac; a deposit of 5–6 or more eggs within four to twelve hours indicates pregnancy.

xylidine t., see *Schiff's t.* (1).

D-xylose absorption t., D-xylose tolerance t. *(for differential diagnosis in malabsorption syndromes)*: after the oral administration of 25 gm. (sometimes 5 gm. is used) of D-xylose dissolved in 250 ml. of water, followed immediately by an additional 250 ml. of water, to a fasting adult, the amount excreted in the urine during a five-hour period is determined. Since poor renal function may also result in low xylose absorption, blood levels are also determined at two hours. Normally, more than 4.0 gm. of xylose should be excreted over the five-hour period; less than this amount suggests intestinal malabsorption. Blood values are normally more than 25 mg. xylose per 100 ml. of blood.

Young's t. *(for cataract)*: on a disk with a varied number of pinholes in different portions, the patient's ability to recognize the number of holes is a test of the integrity of macular function.

Zaleski's t. *(for carbon monoxide in blood)*: to 2 ml. of blood add an equal volume of water and 3 drops of a one-third saturated solution of copper sulfate: if carbon monoxide is present, a brick-red deposit is thrown down; otherwise the precipitate is greenish brown.

Zappacosta's t. *(for liver function)*: glycocyamine is injected intravenously; if in one quarter of an hour after the injection the substance is still present in the blood, liver function is impaired.

Zeisel's t. *(for colchicine)*: dissolve in hydrochloric acid, boil with ferric chloride, and shake with chloroform; a brown or dark-red layer will form at the bottom.

zinc fluorescence t. *(for urobilin)*, see *Schlesinger's t.*

Zondek-Aschheim t., see *Aschheim-Zondek t.*

Zouchlos' t. *(for albumin in the urine)*: 1. precipitate the urine with a mixture of 1 part of acetic acid and 6 parts of a 10 per cent solution of mercuric chloride. 2. prepare a reagent with 100 parts of a 10 per cent solution of potassium thiocyanate and 20 parts of acetic acid; drop it slowly into the urine until the albumin appears as a white cloudiness. 3. add equal parts of succinic acid and potassium thiocyanate; albumin, if present, will be precipitated.

Zsigmondy's gold number t., see *colloidal gold t.*

Zwenger's t.: 1. (*for cholesterol*) a crystal of cholesterol with 5 parts of sulfuric acid and 1 part water gives a red ring changing to violet. 2. see *Liebermann's t.*

---

testa (tes′tah) [L. "shell"] test².

Testacea (tes-ta′she-ah) [L. *testa* shell] Arcellinida.

Testacealobosia (tes″tah-se″ah-lo-bo′se-ah) [Gr. *testa* shell + L. *lobus* lobe] a subclass of ameboid protozoa (class Lobosea, superclass Rhizopoda), characterized by a body enclosed in a test, tectum, or other complex membrane external to the plasma membrane and glycocalyx. It includes two orders: Arcellinida and Trichosida.

testacean (tes-ta′she-an) 1. any protozoan of the subclass Testacealobosia. 2. pertaining to protozoa of the subclass Testacealobosia.

testaceous (tes-ta′she-us) [L. *testa* shell] of the nature of shell; having a shell.

Testacida (tes-tas′ĭ-dah) [Gr. *testa* shell] Arcellinida.

testalgia (tes-tal′je-ah) [*testis* + *-algia*] pain in the testicle.

Tes-Tape (tes′tāp) trademark for a test strip impregnated with glucose oxidase, peroxidase, and orthotolidine; used for determining the approximate concentration of glucose in urine.

testate (tes′tāt) having a test or covered by a test or similar structure; said of ameboid protozoa of the subclass Testacealobosia.

test card (test kard) a card printed with various letters or symbols, used in testing vision. **stigmometric t. c.,** a card with dots and squares arranged in groups, for testing vision (Fridenberg).

testectomy (tes-tek′to-me) [*testis* + Gr. *ektomē* excision] orchiectomy.

testes (tes′tēz) [L.] plural of *testis.*

testicle (tes′tĭ-k'l) [L. *testiculus*] the testis.

testicond (tes′tĭ-kond) [*testis* + L. *condere* to hide] having the testes retained within the abdominal cavity, as occurs normally in many mammals, such as the elephant and armadillo.

testicular (tes-tik′u-lar) pertaining to a testis.

testiculi (tes-tĭ′cu-li) [L.] genitive and plural of *testiculus.*

testiculoma (tes-tik″u-lo′mah) a testicular tumor. **t. ova′rii,** arrhenoblastoma.

testiculus (tes-tik′u-lus), gen. and pl. *testi′culi* [L., dim. of *testis*] testis.

testis (tes′tis), pl. *tes′tes* [L.] [NA] the male gonad; either of the paired egg-shaped glands normally situated in the scrotum; each testis is surrounded by an outer mesothelial layer (tunica vaginalis) and an inner white capsule (tunica albuginea), and is composed of compartments (lobuli testis) which contain the seminiferous tubules, wherein the spermatozoa are produced. Specialized interstitial cells (Leydig cells) secrete testosterone. Called also *orchis* [NA alternative] and *testicle*. **Cooper's irritable t.,** a testis affected with neuralgia. **ectopic t.,** a testis which has become lodged in some abnormal location. **inverted t.,** a testis whose position in the scrotum is reversed, the epididymis being attached to the anterior instead of the posterior surface. **t. mulie′bris,** an ovary. **obstructed t.,** a testis whose descent has been prevented by a fascial sheet at the entrance to the scrotum. **pulpy t.,** a testis affected with medullary sarcoma. **t. re′dux,** a testis which tends to be drawn to the upper part of the scrotum. **retained t.,** undescended t., see *cryptorchidism.* **undescended t.,** a testis which has failed to descend into the scrotum, but remains in the inguinal canal, and the condition so produced; called also *cryptorchism* or *cryptorchidism.*

testitis (tes-ti′tis) orchitis.

test letter (test let′er) see *test type.*

test meal (test mēl) a meal containing material given for the specific purpose for aiding diagnostic examination of the stomach, as by roentgenoscopy or by chemical analysis later of the stomach contents. See also *meal.* **Boyden t. m.,** a motor meal for testing the evacuation of the gallbladder, containing three or four egg yolks combined with milk and seasoned with sugar, port wine, etc. **motor t. m.,** a meal or drink containing a radiopaque substance, permitting roentgenoscopic observation of its progress through the stomach, pylorus, and other portions of the gastrointestinal tract.

testoid (tes′toid) an older term applied to testicular hormones and other natural or synthetic androgens.

testolactone (tes-to-lak′tōn) [USP] chemical name: D-homo-17α-oxaandrosta-1,4-diene-3,17-dione. An antineoplastic agent, $C_{19}H_{24}O_3$, occurring as a white to off-white, crystalline powder, which may be prepared from testosterone or progesterone. It is used as adjunctive therapy in the palliative treatment of advanced or disseminated breast cancer in postmenopausal women; administered orally or by intramuscular injection.

testopathy (tes-top′ah-the) [*testes* + Gr. *pathos* disease] any disease of the testes.

testosterone (tes-tos′tĕ-rōn) chemical name: 17β-hydroxy-androst-4-en-3-one. 1. the principal and most potent androgenic hormone, $C_{19}H_{28}O_2$, produced by the interstitial (Leydig) cells of the testes in response to stimulation by the luteinizing hormone of the anterior pituitary gland; it is thought to be responsible for regulation of gonadotropic secretion, spermatogenesis, and wolffian duct differentiation (formation of the epididymis, vas deferens, and seminal vesicle). It is also responsible for other male characteristics after its conversion to dihydrotestosterone (q.v.) by 5α-reductase in peripheral tissue. In addition, testosterone possesses protein anabolic properties, manifested by retention of nitrogen, calcium, phosphorus, and potassium, and is important in maintaining muscle mass and bone tissue in the adult male. It is also converted by aromatization to estradiol in peripheral tissue. See also *anabolic steroid,* under *steroid.* 2. [USP] the same principle prepared synthetically from cholesterol or isolated from bull testes, occurring as white or slightly creamy white crystals or crystalline powder; used in the form of various esters in treating male hypogonadism, cryptorchidism, and the symptoms of the male climacteric, and may be used for its anabolic properties; administered by subcutaneous implantation or intramuscular injection or buccally. **t. cyclopentylpropionate,** t. cypionate. **t. cypionate** [USP], an ester of testosterone, $C_{27}H_{40}O_3$, occurring as a white or creamy white, crystalline powder, having the same actions as the free alcohol but a prolonged duration of effect; used chiefly in the treatment of male hypogonadism, frigidity, and inoperable female breast cancer, to suppress lactation, and as an anabolic agent, administered by intramuscular injection. Called also *t. cyclopentylpropionate.* **t. enanthate** [USP], an ester of testosterone, $C_{26}H_{40}O_3$, occurring as a white or creamy white, crystalline powder, having the same actions as the free alcohol but a prolonged duration of effect; used chiefly in the treatment of male hypogonadism, oligospermia, and the symptoms of male climacteric, administered by intramuscular injection. Called also *t. heptanoate.* **ethinyl t.,** ethisterone. **t. heptanoate,** t. enanthate. **t. ketolaurate,** an ester of testosterone, having the same actions as the other esters. **methyl t.,** see *methyltestosterone.* **t. phenylacetate,** an ester of testosterone, $C_{28}H_{38}O_3$, occurring as a white to almost white, crystalline powder, having the same actions as the free alcohol but a prolonged duration of effect; administered by subcutaneous and intramuscular injection. **t. propionate,** an ester of testosterone, $C_{22}H_{32}O_3$, occurring as white or creamy white crystals or crystalline powder, having the same actions as the free alcohol but with a relatively short duration of effect; used chiefly in the treatment of male hypogonadism, symptoms of male climacteric, postpubertal cryptorchidism, and inoperable female breast cancer, and to prevent postpartum breast engorgement; administered buccally or intramuscularly.

Testryl (tes′tril) trademark for a suspension of pure crystalline testosterone.

test type (test tīp) printed letters of varying size, used in the testing of visual acuity; see also under *chart.* **Jaeger's t. t.,** ordinary printer's type of seven different sizes imprinted on a card; used in testing near vision. **Snellen's t. t.,** block letters used in testing visual acuity, so designed that the whole letter subtends, at the appropriate distance, a visual angle usually of 5 minutes, and each component part subtends an angle of 1 minute. See also *Snellen's chart.*

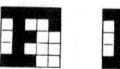

Two of Snellen's test types.

tetanic (tĕ-tan′ik) [Gr. *tetanikos*] 1. pertaining to or of the nature of tetanus. 2. producing tetanus.

tetaniform (tĕ-tan′ĭ-form) [*tetanus* + L. *forma* shape] like or resembling tetanus or tetany; tetanoid.

tetanigenous (tet″ah-nij′ĕ-nus) [*tetanus* + Gr. *gennan* to produce] producing tetanus or tetanic spasms.

tetanization (tet″ah-ni-za′shun) the act of tetanizing a muscle.

tetanize (tet′ah-nīz) to stimulate a muscle at progressively higher frequencies until successive contractions fuse and cannot be distinguished from one another; see *tetanus,* def. 2.

tetanocannabin (tet″ah-no-kan′ah-bin) a poisonous principle sometimes found in hemp; it resembles strychnine in its action.

tetanode (tet′ah-nōd″) the unexcited stage occurring between the tetanic contractions in tetanus.

tetanoid (tet′ah-noid) [*tetanus* + Gr. *eidos* form] like or resembling tetanus or tetany; tetaniform.

tetanolysin (tet″ah-nol′ĭ-sin) [*tetanus* + *lysin*] the hemolytic exotoxin produced by *Clostridium tetani,* the etiologic agent of tetanus; it may or may not contribute to the pathogenicity of the organism. Cf. *tetanospasmin.*

tetanometer (tet″ah-nom′ĕ-ter) [*tetanus* + Gr. *metron* measure] an apparatus for measurement and analysis of tetanus.

tetanospasmin (tet″ah-no-spaz′min) [*tetanus* + L. *spasmus* spasm + *-in* chemical suffix] the neurotoxic component of the exotoxin (tetanus toxin) produced by *Clostridium tetani,* a highly potent protein that binds to gangliosides and blocks the synaptic terminals of the central nervous system, causing the typical muscle spasms of tetanus. It is one of the most powerful poisons known. See also *tetanolysin.*

tetanus (tet′ah-nus) [Gr. *tetanos,* from *teinein* to stretch] 1. an acute, often fatal infectious disease caused by the anaerobic, spore-forming bacillus *Clostridium tetani;* the agent most often enters the body through contaminated puncture wounds (e.g., those caused by metal nails, wood splinters, or insect bites), although other portals of entry include burns, surgical wounds, cutaneous ulcers, injection sites of drug abusers, the umbilical stump of neonates (*t. neonatorum*), and the postpartum uterus. The clinical manifestations of tetanus are due to tetanospasmin, which is a potent neurotoxin elaborated by the germinating spores of *C. tetani. Generalized tetanus* is characterized by tetanic muscular contractions and hyperreflexia, resulting in trismus (lockjaw), glottal spasm, generalized muscle spasm, opisthotonus, respiratory spasm, seizures, and paralysis. *Localized tetanus* may be mild, with localized muscular twitching and spasm of muscle groups near the site of injury, or it may progress to the generalized form. 2. physiological tetanus; a state of sustained muscular contraction without periods of relaxation caused by repetitive stimulation of the motor nerve trunk at frequencies so high that individual muscle twitches are fused and cannot be distinguished from one another; called also *tonic spasm* and *tetany.* **cephalic t.,** a rare disease developing after injuries to the scalp, face, or neck, associated with palsies of cranial nerves 3, 4, 6, 7, 9, 10, and 12, and invariably associated with some degree of trismus. **cephalic t., cerebral t.,** a rare form of infectious tetanus with an extremely poor prognosis that may occur after an injury to the head or face or in association with otitis media in which *Clostridium tetani* is a constituent of the flora of the middle ear; it is characterized by isolated or combined dysfunction of the cranial nerves, especially the seventh cranial, and may remain localized or progress to generalized tetanus. Called also *cephalotetanus.* **cryptogenic t.,** tetanus which occurs without any wound or other ascertainable cause. **neonatal t., t. neonato′rum,** a severe form of infectious tetanus occurring during the first few days of life caused by such factors as unhygienic practice in dressing the umbilical

stump or in circumcising male infants and the lack of maternal immunization. **physiological t.,** tetanus, def. 2.

tetany (tet′ah-ne) 1. hyperexcitability of nerves and muscles due to decrease in concentration of extracellular ionized calcium, which may be associated with such conditions as parathyroid hypofunction, vitamin D deficiency, and alkalosis or result from ingestion of alkaline salts; it is characterized by carpopedal spasm, muscular twitching and cramps, laryngospasm with inspiratory stridor, hyperreflexia, and choreiform movements. 2. tetanus, def. 2. **duration t.,** a continuous tetanic contraction in response to a very strong continuous current; it occurs especially in degenerated muscles; abbreviated Dt. **gastric t.,** a severe form due to disease of the stomach, attended by difficult respiration and painful tonic spasms of the extremities. **grass t.,** an often fatal condition that may be produced in "fresh" cows that are turned out into lush pastures; it is apparently due to a deficiency of magnesium in the diet. **hyperventilation t.,** tetany produced by forced inspiration and expiration continued for a considerable time. **lactation t.,** grass tetany. **latent t.,** tetany elicited by the application of electrical and mechanical stimulation. **neonatal t., t. of newborn,** hypocalcemic tetany occurring in the first few days of life, often marked by irritability, muscular twitchings, jitteriness, tremors, and convulsions, and less frequently by laryngospasm and carpopedal spasm. **parathyroid t., parathyroprival t.,** tetany due to removal of the parathyroids. **transit t., transport t.,** a condition usually affecting well-fed cows and ewes in advanced pregnancy and in lactating mares that have been shipped long distances, which may result in paralysis, unconsciousness, and death unless treatment is begun early in the course of the disease. The etiology is unknown, but may be due to acute hypocalcium associated with improper care and feeding. Called also *railroad disease* or *sickness.*

tetartanope (tet-ar′tah-nōp) a person with tetartanopia.

tetartanopia (tet″ar-tah-no′pe-ah) [Gr. *tetartos* fourth + *an* neg. + *-opia*] 1. quadrantanopia. 2. a rare dichromasy of doubtful existence characterized by retention of the sensory mechanism for two hues only (red and green), and lacking that for blue and yellow, which are replaced in the spectrum by an achromatic (gray) band.

tetartanopic (tet″ar-tah-nop′ik) pertaining to or characterized by tetartanopia.

tetartanopsia (tet″ar-tah-nop′se-ah) tetartanopia.

tetiothalein sodium (te″she-o-thal′e-in so′de-um) iodophthalein sodium.

tetmil (tet′mil) ten millimeters taken as a unit of measurement.

tetra- [Gr. *tetra-* a combining form meaning four] a combining form meaning *four.*

tetrabasic (tet″rah-ba′sik) [*tetra-* + Gr. *basis* base] containing four atoms of replaceable hydrogen.

tetrablastic (tet″rah-blas′tik) having four germ layers.

tetraboric acid (tet″rah-bor′ik) pyroboric acid.

tetrabrachius (tet″rah-bra′ke-us) [*tetra-* + Gr. *brachiōn* arm] a double monster having four arms.

tetrabromofluorescein (tet″rah-bro″mo-floo″o-res′e-in) eosin.

tetrabromophenolphthalein (tet″rah-bro″mo-fe″nol-thal′e-in) an indicator, $C_6H_4 \cdot CO \cdot O \cdot C(C_6H_2Br_2OH)_2$, which is colorless with acids and violet with alkalis.

tetrabromophthalein sodium (tet″rah-bro″mo-thal′e-in so′de-um) the sodium salt of tetrabromophenolphthalein, $NaOOC \cdot C_6H_4 \cdot C:C_6H_2Br_2O \cdot C_6H_2Br_2ONa$, used for roentgenological examination of the gallbladder, in which organ it appears after intravenous injection.

tetracaine (tet′rah-kān) [USP] chemical name: 4-(butylamino)benzoic acid 2-(dimethylamino)ethyl ester. A local anesthetic, $C_{15}H_{24}N_2O_2$, occurring as a white or light yellow, waxy solid; applied topically to the eyeball and conjunctiva. **t. hydrochloride** [USP], a fine, white, crystalline powder, applied topically to the conjunctiva and eyeball, to the mucous membranes of the nose, throat, and respiratory tract, and to the skin to produce surface anesthesia and also used parenterally for conduction and infiltration anesthesia. Called also *amethocaine hydrochloride.*

tetracetate (tet-ras′ĕ-tāt) [*tetra-* + *acetate*] a compound of a base with four acetic acid molecules.

tetrachirus (tet″rah-ki′rus) [*tetra-* + Gr. *cheir* hand] a fetus having four hands.

tetrachlorethane (tet″rah-klōr-eth′ān) acetylene tetrachloride, $CHCl_2 \cdot CHCl_2$, formed by the action of chlorine on acetylene; it is anthelmintic, and is used as a solvent and in dry cleaning. Called also *cellon*.

tetrachloride (tet″rah-klo′rīd) a compound of a radical with four atoms of chlorine.

tetrachlormethane (tet″rah-klōr-meth′ān) carbon tetrachloride, CCl_4.

tetrachloroethylene (tet″rah-klor″o-eth′ĭ-lēn) a moderately toxic chlorinated hydrocarbon, $CCl_2{=}CCl_2$, used as a dry-cleaning solvent and for other industrial uses; called also *perchloroethylene*. Tetrachloroethylene [USP] has been used for treatment of hookworm and is used for treatment of fasciolopsiasis.

tetrachlorphenoxide (tet″rah-klōr′fen-ok′sīd) a fungicide used for the preservation of lumber: it may cause a dermatitis in workmen.

tetrachromic (tet″rah-kro′mik) [*tetra-* + Gr. *chrōma* color] 1. pertaining to or exhibiting four colors. 2. able to distinguish only four of the seven colors of the spectrum according to the Eldridge-Green classification of color blindness.

tetracid (tet′ras-id) capable of replacing four atoms of hydrogen in an acid, or having four atoms of hydrogen replaceable by acid radicals.

tetracosanoic acid (tet′rah-ko″sah-no′ik) lignoceric acid.

tetracrotic (tet″rah-krot′ik) [*tetra-* + Gr. *krotos* beat] showing four elevations in the sphygmographic tracing of the pulse.

tetracycline (tet″rah-si′klēn) 1. any of a group of biosynthetic antibiotics isolated from certain species of *Streptomyces* or produced semisynthetically by catalytic hydrogenation of chlortetracycline or oxytetracycline. The tetracyclines, e.g., chlortetracycline (the first of the group to be discovered), oxytetracycline, tetracycline (see def. 2), demeclocycline, rolitetracycline, methacycline, doxycycline, and minocycline, are effective against a wide variety of organisms, including gram-positive and gram-negative bacteria, rickettsias, mycoplasmas, chlamydias, and certain viruses, protozoa, and actinomycetes. 2 [USP] chemical name: [4S-(4α,4aα,5aα,6β,12aα)]-4-(dimethylamino)-1,4,4a,5,5a,6,11,12a-octahydro-3,-6,10,12,12a-pentahydroxy-6-methyl-1,11-dioxa-2-naphthacenecarboxamide. A semisynthetic antibiotic, $C_{22}H_{24}N_2O_8$, occurring as a yellow, crystalline powder having the same wide spectrum of antimicrobial activity as the other tetracyclines (see def. 1), used as an antibacterial, antiamebic, and antirickettsial, administered orally. **t. hydrochloride** [USP], the monohydrochloride salt of tetracycline, $C_{22}H_{24}N_2O_8 \cdot HCl$, occurring as a yellow crystalline powder, having the same actions and uses as the base; administered orally, intramuscularly, or intravenously, or applied topically to the conjunctiva or eyelid. **t. phosphate complex** [NF], a phosphate complex salt of tetracycline, prepared by the addition of a solution of sodium metaphosphate to a solution of tetracycline or tetracycline hydrochloride; used as an antibacterial, administered orally, intramuscularly, or intravenously.

Tetracyn (tet′rah-sin) trademark for preparations of tetracycline.

tetrad (tet′rad) [Gr. *tetra-* four] a group of four similar or related entities, as (1) any element or radical having a valence, or combining power, of four; (2) a group of four chromosomal elements formed in the pachytene state of the first meiotic prophase; (3) a square of cells produced by the division into two planes of certain cocci (*Sarcina*). **Fallot's t.,** tetralogy of Fallot.

tetradactylous (tet″rah-dak′tĭ-lus) pertaining to or characterized by tetradactyly.

tetradactyly (tet″rah-dak′tĭ-le) [*tetra-* + Gr. *daktylos* finger] the condition of having four digits on the hand or foot.

tetraene (tet′rah-ēn) a chemical compound in which there are four conjugated double bonds.

tetraerythrin (tet″rah-er′ĭ-thrin) crustaceorubin.

tetraethylammonium (tet″rah-eth″il-ah-mo′ne-um) the radical $(C_2H_5)_4N$; the bromide and chloride salts are short acting quaternary ammonium ganglion-blocking agents that have been used in the treatment of acute hypertension, peripheral vascular diseases, and other disorders of the peripheral circulation. They are now seldom employed, having been replaced by more effective drugs. Abbreviated TEA.

tetraethylthiuram disulfide (tet″rah-eth″il-thi′u-ram″) disulfiram.

tetrafilcon A (tet″rah-fil′kon) a hydrophilic contact lens material.

tetragonum (tet″rah-go′num) [L.; Gr. *tetragōnon*] a square or quadrant; a quadrangular area or space. **t. lumba′le,** the quadrangular space bounded by the four lumbar muscles—by the serratus posterior inferior above, the internal oblique below, the erector spinae internally, and the external oblique externally.

tetragonus (tet″rah-go′nus) the platysma.

tetrahydric (tet″rah-hi′drik) containing four atoms of replaceable hydrogen: said of an acid or alcohol.

tetrahydrocannabinol (tet″rah-hi″dro-kah-nab′ĭ-nol) the active principle of cannabis, $C_{21}H_{30}O_2$, occurring in two isomeric forms: Δ^1-3,4-*trans* and Δ^6-3,4-*trans* tetrahydrocannabinol, both considered psychomimetically active. Abbreviated THC.

tetrahydrofolate (tet″rah-hi″dro-fo′lāt) an ester or dissociated form of tetrahydrofolic acid.

tetrahydrofolate dehydrogenase (tĕ″trah-hi″dro-fo′lāt de-hi′dro-jĕ-nās) dihydrofolate reductase.

tetrahydrofolic acid (tet″rah-hi″dro-fol′ik) the reduced form of folic acid that is a coenzyme in one-carbon transfer reactions.

tetrahydropalmatine (tet″rah-hi″dro-pal′mah-tin) a crystalline, berberine type alkaloid, $C_{21}H_{25}NO_4$, from the roots of *Corydalis tuberosa* DC. (Fumariaceae).

tetrahydropteroylglutamate methyltransferase (tĕ″trah-hi″dro-ter″o-il-gloo′tah-māt meth″il-trans′fer-ās) 5-methyltetrahydrofolate-homocysteine methyltransferase.

tetrahydrozoline hydrochloride (tet″rah-hi-dro′zo-lēn) [USP] chemical name: 4,5-dihydro-2-(1,2,3,4-tetrahydro-1-naphthalenyl)-1H-imidazole monohydrochloride. An adrenergic, $C_{13}H_{16}N_2 \cdot HCl$, occurring as a white solid; applied topically to the nasal mucosa and to the conjunctiva to produce vasoconstriction.

Tetrahymena (tet″rah-hi′mĕ-nah) [*tetra-* Gr. *hymēn* membrane] a genus of ciliate protozoa (suborder Tetrahymenina, order Hymenostomatida) used extensively in physiologic and genetic studies; they have been shown to be capable of parasitic existence when experimentally injected into various hosts. *T limacis* and *T. pyriformis* are representative species.

Tetrahymenina (tet″trah-hi′mĕ-ni′nah) a suborder of ciliate protozoa (order Hymenostomatida, subclass Hymenostomatia), characterized by the presence of uniform ciliation, three oral membranelles on the left and an undulating or paroral membrane on the right, and mucocysts. Most are free-living in fresh water, but a few species are symbiotic, mainly in invertebrates. *Tetrahymena* is a representative genus.

tetraiodophenolphthalein (tet″rah-i″o-do-fe″nol-thal′e-in) chemical name: 3′,3″,5′,5″-tetraiodophenolphthalein. A dye, $C_8H_4 \cdot CO \cdot O \cdot C(C_6H_2I_2OH)_2$, which after intravenous injection is excreted in the bile in sufficient amount to make possible roentgenography of the gallbladder; it was once used in treating typhoid fever carriers.

tetraiodophthalein sodium (tet″rah-i″o-do-thal′e-in) iodophthalein sodium.

tetraiodothyronine (tet″rah-i″o-do-thi′ro-nēn) thyroxine; so called because it is formed by the conjugation of two molecules of diiodotyrosine.

tetralogy (tĕ-tral′o-je) a combination of four elements or factors, such as four concurrent symptoms or defects. **t. of Eisenmenger,** Eisenmenger's complex. **t. of Fallot,** a combination of congenital cardiac defects consisting of pulmonary stenosis, interventricular septal defect, dextroposition of the aorta so that it overrides the interventricular septum and receives venous as well as arterial blood, and right ventricular hypertrophy. See illustration.

tetramastigote (tet″rah-mas′tĭ-gōt) [*tetra-* + Gr. *mastix* lash] 1. having four flagella. 2. an organism having four flagella.

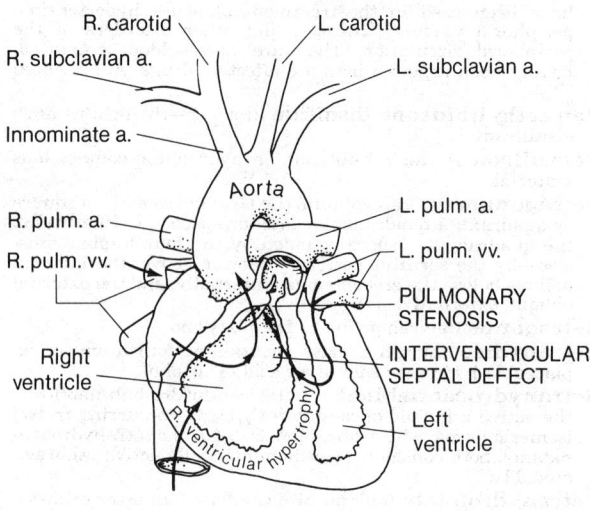

Tetralogy of Fallot.

Labels on figure: R. carotid, L. carotid, R. subclavian a., L. subclavian a., Innominate a., Aorta, R. pulm. a., L. pulm. a., R. pulm. vv., L. pulm. vv., PULMONARY STENOSIS, Right ventricle, INTERVENTRICULAR SEPTAL DEFECT, R. ventricular hypertrophy, Left ventricle

tetramazia (tet″rah-ma′ze-ah) [*tetra-* + Gr. *mazos* breast + *-ia*] the condition of having four mammary glands.

Tetrameres (tĕ-tram′er-ēz) a genus of nematode worms parasitic in the alimentary tract of chickens and other fowl. **T. america′na,** a parasite of the proventriculus of chickens and other birds.

tetrameric (tet″rah-mer′ik) having four parts.

tetramethyl (tet″rah-meth′il) a chemical compound each molecule of which contains four methyl groups.

tetramethylammonium hydroxide (tet″rah-meth″il-ah-mo′ne-um hi-drok′sīd) a toxic fraction, $N(CH_3)_4OH$, isolated from the sea anemone, *Actinia equina*, and from the salivary glands of whelks.

tetramethylenediamine (tet″rah-meth″il-ēn-di′am-in) putrescine.

tetramethylputrescine (tet″rah-meth″il-pu-tres′in) an extremely poisonous crystalline base, $N(CH_3)_2(CH_2)_4N(CH_3)_2$, derivable from putrescine; it produces symptoms like those of muscarine poisoning.

tetramine (tet′rah-mēn) tetramethylammonium hydroxide.

tetramisole hydrochloride (tĕ-tram′ĭ-sōl) chemical name: (±)-2,3,5,6-tetrahydro-6-phenylimidazo[2,1-*b*]-thiazol monohydrochloride; an anthelmintic, $C_{11}H_{12}N_2S \cdot HCl$, effective against roundworms, hookworms, and strongyloids.

Tetramitus mesnili (tĕ-tram′ĭ-tus mes-ni′le) *Chilomastix mesnili.*

tetranitrol (tet″rah-ni′trol) erythrityl tetranitrate.

tetranophthalmos (tet″ran-of-thal′mos) [*tetra-* + Gr. *ophthalmos* eye] a monster having four eyes.

tetranopsia (tet″ran-op′se-ah) quadrantanopia.

tetranucleotide (tet″rah-nu′kle-o-tīd) former name for nucleic acid, which was thought by Levene to be a polymer of four mononucleotides.

Tetranychus (tet-ran′ĭ-kus) [*tetra-* + Gr. *onyx* nail] a genus of mites. **T. autumna′lis,** *Trombicula autumnalis.* **T. molestis′simus,** an acarid attacking man and causing severe itching. **T. tela′rius,** the spider mite, which sometimes infests man.

Tetraodontoidea (tet-ra″o-don-toi′de-ah) a suborder of bony tropical marine fish, including puffers and sunfish; see also *tetrodotoxin* and *tetrodotoxism.*

tetraodontoxin (tet-ra″o-don-tok′sin) [*Tetraodon*, from Gr. *tetra* four + *odous* tooth, a puffer fish + *toxikon* poison] tetrodotoxin.

tetraodontoxism (tet-ra″o-don-tok′sizm) tetrodotoxism.

tetraotus (tet″rah-o′tus) [Gr. *tetraōtos* four-eared] a mon-

ster with two nearly separate heads, two faces, four eyes, and four ears.

tetraparesis (tet″rah-par′e-sis) muscular weakness affecting all four extremities.

tetrapeptide (tet″rah-pep′tid) a peptide which on hydrolysis yields four amino acids.

Tetraphyllidea (tet″rah-fil-lid′e-ah) an order of moderate-sized cestodes possessing four leaf-, trumpet-, or earlike sucking outgrowths on the scolex; the adults are intestinal parasites of elasmobranch fishes.

tetraplegia (tet″rah-ple′je-ah) [*tetra-* + Gr. *plēgē* stroke + *-ia*] paralysis of all four extremities; quadriplegia.

tetraploid (tet″rah-ploid) 1. pertaining to or characterized by tetraploidy. 2. an individual or cell having four sets of chromosomes.

tetraploidy (tet′rah-ploi″de) the state of having four sets of chromosomes (4n).

tetrapodisis (tet″rah-po-di′sis) locomotion on four feet; quadruped locomotion, as in young children.

tetrapus (tet′rah-pus) [*tetra-* + Gr. *pous* foot] a human fetus having four feet.

tetrasaccharide (tet″rah-sak′ah-rid) a carbohydrate composed of four monosaccharide groups, $C_{24}H_{42}O_{21}$.

tetrascelus (tet-ras′e-lus) [*tetra-* + Gr. *skelos* leg] a human fetus having four legs.

tetrasomic (tet″rah-so′mik) pertaining to or characterized by tetrasomy.

tetrasomy (tet″rah-so″me) [*tetra-* + Gr. *sōma* body] the presence of two additional chromosomes of one type in an otherwise diploid cell (2n + 2).

tetraspore (tet′rah-spōr) 1. a haploid asexual spore in the red algae, which is meiotically produced, usually in groups of four, from the carpospore. 2. in fungi, one of the spores of a four-spored basidium.

tetraster (tet-ras′ter) [*tetra-* + Gr. *astēr* star] a figure in abnormal mitosis characterized by four centrosomal centers or asters.

tetrastichiasis (tet″rah-stĭ-ki′ah-sis) [*tetra-* + Gr. *stichos* row + *-iasis*] an extremely rare condition in which there are four rows of eyelashes.

tetratomic (tet″rah-tom′ik) 1. consisting of four atoms. 2. having four replaceable atoms.

Tetratrichomonas buccalis (tet″rah-trik-om′o-nas buk-ka′lis) *Trichomonas tenax.*

tetravalent (tet-rav′ah-lent) having a valence of four.

tetrodonic acid (tĕ″tro-don′ik) a poisonous acid from various fishes of the genus *Tetraodon.*

tetrodotoxin (tet″ro-do-tok′sin) a pure, crystalline, highly lethal neurotoxic substance, $C_{11}H_{17}N_3O_3$, present in numerous species of puffer fish of the suborder Tetraodontoidea and in newts of the genus *Taricha* (in which it is called tarichatoxin). Ingestion results, within minutes, in malaise, dizziness, and tingling about the mouth, which may be followed by ataxia, convulsions, respiratory paralysis, and death.

tetrodotoxism (tet″ro-do-tok′sizm) [*Tetraodon*, from Gr. *tetra* four + *odous* tooth, a puffer fish + *toxikon* poison] the most severe form of ichthyosarcotoxism, produced by ingestion of puffer fish which contain tetrodotoxin (q.v.).

tetronal (tet′ro-nal) diethylsulfondiethylmethane, $(C_2H_5)_2 \cdot C \cdot (SO_2C_2H_5)_2$, occurring in the form of colorless scales; it is a hypnotic.

tetronerythrin (tet″ron-er′ĭ-thrin) a pigment from certain birds' feathers, mullets, and many invertebrates, e.g., lobsters.

tetrophthalmos (tet″rof-thal′mos) [*tetra-* + Gr. *ophthalmos* eye] a double-faced monster with two ears and four eyes.

tetrose (tet′rōs) a monosaccharide containing four carbon atoms in a molecule.

tetrotus (tet-ro′tus) tetraotus.

tetroxide (tĕ-trok′sīd) a compound of an element or a radical with four oxygen atoms, as osmium tetroxide.

tetrydamine (tet-tri′dah-mēn) chemical name: 4,5,6,7-tetrahydro-2-methyl-3-(methylamino)-2*H*-indazole; an analgesic and anti-inflammatory, $C_9H_{15}N_3$.

tetryl (tet′ril) an organic explosive and expellant, tetra-nitro-methyl-aniline, $(NO_2)_3C_6H_2N(NO)_2CH_3$, which may cause an industrial dermatitis.

tetter (tet′er) 1. a once popular name for various eczematous skin diseases. 2. a skin disease of animals communicable to man, and characterized by intense itching. **milky t.,** crusta lactea.

tetterwort (tet′ter-wort) *Sanguinaria canadensis* L. (Papaveraceae).

teucrin (tu′krin) a crystalline glycoside, $C_{21}H_{24}O_{11}$, from *Teucrium fruticans* L. (Labiatae).

Teucrium (tu′kre-um) [Gr. *teukrion* an herb of the germander kind] a genus of labiate plants called germander; generally used for their aromatic qualities.

teutlose (tūt′lōs) [Gr. *teutlon* beet] a kind of sugar found in beet root.

tewfikose (tu′fĭ-kōs) a sugar occurring in the milk of the Egyptian buffalo, *Bos bubalus.*

texis (tek′sis) [L., from Gr. *tiktein* to bear] child-bearing.

textiform (teks′tĭ-form) [L. *textum* any material put together + *forma* form] formed like a tissue, network, or web.

textoblastic (teks″to-blas′tik) [L. *textum* any material put together + Gr. *blastos* germ] forming adult tissue; regenerative: said of cells.

textometer (teks″to-me′ter) [L. *textum* any material put together + Gr. *mētēr* mother] protoplasm regarded as the mother of tissues.

Textulariina (teks″tu-lah-ri′ĭ-nah) a suborder of protozoa (order Foraminiferida, class Granuloreticulosea) having an agglutinated test containing foreign matter held together by various cements. Fossil and recent species are known.

textural (teks′tu-ral) pertaining to the texture, or constitution, of the tissues.

texture (teks′tūr) [L. *textura*] the structure or organization of a tissue or organ.

textus (teks′tus), gen. and pl. *tex′tus* [L., from *texere* to weave] a tissue.

TF transfer factor.

T-group training group; see *sensitivity group,* under *group.*

6-TG 6-thioguanine.

TGT thromboplastin generation test.

Th chemical symbol for *thorium.*

thalamectomy (thal″ah-mek′to-me) [*thalamus* + Gr. *tomē* a cutting] thalamotomy.

thalamencephalic (thal″ah-men″sĕ-fal′ik) pertaining to the thalamencephalon.

thalamencephalon (thal″ah-men-sef′ah-lon) [NA] the part of the diencephalon that comprises the thalamus, metathalamus, and epithalamus.

thalami (thal′ah-mi) [L.] genitive and plural of *thalamus.*

thalamic (thah-lam′ik) pertaining to the thalamus.

thalamocoele (thal′ah-mo-sēl″) [Gr. *thalamos* inner chamber + *koilia* hollow] the third ventricle of the brain (ventriculus tertius cerebri [NA]).

thalamocortical (thal″ah-mo-kor′tĭ-kal) pertaining to the thalamus and cerebral cortex.

thalamolenticular (thal″ah-mo-len-tik′u-lar) pertaining to the thalamus and the lenticular nucleus.

thalamomamillary (thal″ah-mo-mam′ĭ-ler″e) pertaining to the thalamus and mamillary bodies.

thalamotegmental (thal″ah-mo-teg-men′tal) pertaining to the thalamus and tegmentum.

thalamotomy (thal″ah-mot′o-me) [*thalamus* + Gr. *tomē* a cutting] a stereotaxic surgical technique for the discrete destruction of specific groups of cells within the thalamus, as for the relief of pain or for relief of tremor and rigidity in Parkinson's disease. **anterior t.,** production of lesions in the anterior nucleus of the thalamus. **dorsomedial t.,** production of lesions in the dorsomedial nucleus of the thalamus.

thalamus (thal′ah-mus), pl. *thal′ami* [L.; Gr. *thalamos* inner chamber] [NA] either of two large, ovoid masses, consisting chiefly of gray substance, situated one on each side of and forming part of the lateral wall of the third ventricle. It is divided into two major parts: dorsal and ventral, each of which contains many nuclei. When the term *thalamus* is used without a modifying term, it usually designates the *thalamus dorsalis.* **dorsal t., t. dorsa′lis** [NA], the region of the

dorsal part of the diencephalon forming most of each lateral wall of the third ventricle, composed chiefly of gray substance and associated laminae of white substance. It is divided into anterior, medial, and lateral parts, each part containing groups of nuclei that function as relay centers for sensory impulses and cerebellar and basal ganglia projections to the cerebral cortex. The main groups of thalamic nuclei are the reticular, anterior, median, medial, medullary, intralaminar, ventrolateral, and posterior nuclei. See also *thalamus.* **optic t.,** corpus geniculatum laterale. **t. ventra′lis** [NA], the region of the ventral part of the diencephalon interposed between the dorsal thalamus, hypothalamus, and tegmentum of the mesencephalon, which contains the nuclei of the lateral and medial geniculate bodies, subthalamic and reticular nuclei, zona incerta, and nuclei of areae H (Forel's fields); called also *subthalamus.*

thalassanemia (thah-las″sah-ne′me-ah) thalassemia.

thalassemia (thal″ah-se′me-ah) [Gr. *thalassa* sea (because it was observed originally in persons of Mediterranean stock) + *haima* blood + *-ia*] a heterogeneous group of hereditary hemolytic anemias which have in common a decreased rate of synthesis of one or more hemoglobin polypeptide chains and are classified according to the chain involved (α, β, δ); the two major categories are α- and β-thalassemia. It is manifested in homozygotes by profound anemia or death in utero, and in heterozygotes by relatively mild red cell anomalies. α-**t.,** that caused by decreased rate of synthesis of the alpha chains of hemoglobin. The *homozygous* form is incompatible with life, the stillborn infant displaying severe hydrops fetalis. The *heterozygous* form may be asymptomatic or marked by mild anemia. β-**t.,** that caused by diminished synthesis of beta chains of hemoglobin. The *homozygous* form (Cooley's anemia; Mediterranean anemia; erythroblastic anemia of childhood; thalassemia major), in which hemoglobin A is completely absent and which appears in the newborn period, is a severe form marked by a hemolytic, hypochromic microcytic anemia, pronounced hepatosplenomegaly, skeletal deformation, mongoloid facies, and cardiac enlargement. The *heterozygous* form (thalassemia minor), in which hemoglobin A synthesis usually is retarded, is asymptomatic, but there is sometimes moderate anemia and splenomegaly. δ-**t.,** that involving suppression of the delta chains of hemoglobin, but having no clinical significance. δ β-**t.,** a form of heterozygous thalassemia in which synthesis of both delta and beta chains of hemoglobin is decreased; clinically it resembles β-thalassemia. **hemoglobin C-t.,** see under *disease.* **hemoglobin E-t.,** see under *disease.* **hemoglobin S-t.,** sickle cell–thalassemia disease. **t. interme′dia,** that which clinically appears to be intermediate between homozygous and heterozygous β-thalassemia. **t. major,** see β-t. **t. minor,** see β-t. **sickle cell-t.,** see under *disease.*

thalassin (thah-las′sin) a toxic substance derived from tentacles of the sea anemone, *Anemonia sulcata,* which, when injected into dogs, produces allergic symptoms.

thalassoposia (thah-las″so-po′ze-ah) [Gr. *thalassa* sea + *posis* drinking + *-ia*] the ingestion of sea water.

thalassotherapy (thah-las″so-ther′ah-pe) [Gr. *thalassa* sea + *therapeia* treatment] the treatment of disease by sea bathing, sea voyages, and sea air.

thalgrain (thal′grān) grain mixed with thallium sulfate; used as a poison for rodents.

thalidomide (thah-lid′o-mīd) chemical name: 2-(2,6-dioxo-3-piperidenyl)-1*H*-isoindole-1,3(2*H*)-dione. A sedative and hypnotic, $C_{13}H_{10}O_4$, commonly used in Europe in the late 1950's and early 1960's. Its use was discontinued because it was discovered to cause serious congenital anomalies in the fetus, notably amelia and phocomelia, when taken by a woman during early pregnancy. Thalidomide has been shown to be very effective in relieving severe pain associated with acute lepra reactions; it should not be used when pregnancy is possible.

thalleioquin (thal-i′o-kwin) a greenish, resinous substance, produced in a test for quinine; see under *tests.*

thallitoxicosis (thal″ĭ-tok″sĭ-ko′sis) poisoning by thallium or thallium-containing substances.

thallium (thal′e-um) [Gr. *thallos* green shoot] a heavy, soft, bluish white metal; symbol, Tl; atomic number, 81; atomic weight, 204.37; specific gravity, 11.85; its salts are active poisons. **t.-201,** a radioactive isotope of thallium having a half-life of 73.5 hours; used as a diagnostic aid in the form of thallous chloride (q.v.).

thall(o)- [Gr. *thallos* green shoot] a combining form denoting a relationship to a branch or shoot, or to thallium.

Thallobacteria (thal″o-bak-te′re-ah) [*thallo-* + *bacteria*] a class of bacteria of the Firmicutes, kingdom Procaryotae, made up of gram-positive organisms that show a branching habit. It comprises the actinomycetes and related organisms.

Thallophyta (tha-lof′ĭ-tah) [*thallo-* + Gr. *phyton* plant] in former classifications, a taxonomic division of the plant kingdom comprising the fungi and algae, i.e., organisms possessing a thallus, and sometimes including bacteria and slime molds.

thallophyte (thal′o-fīt) [*thallo-* + Gr. *phyton* plant] an individual of the Thallophyta.

thallospore (thal′o-spōr) [*thallo-* + *spore*] a thallus modified to serve as an organ of reproduction.

thallotoxicosis (thal″o-tok″sĭ-ko′sis) thallitoxicosis.

thallous chloride Tl 201 (thal′us) the form in which thallium-201 in solution is injected intravenously as a diagnostic aid in scintillation scanning in myocardial disease. Called also *thallium chloride* (*201TlCl*).

thallus (thal′us) 1. a simple plant body not differentiated into root, stem, and leaf, which is characteristic of mycelial fungi and some algae. 2. the actively growing vegetative organism as distinguished from reproductive or resting portions, as in fungi.

thalposis (thal-po′sis) [Gr. *thalpos* warmth] warmth sense; the sense which perceives warmth.

thalpotic (thal-pot′ik) pertaining to thalposis.

THAM tromethamine.

Thamnidium (tham-nid′e-um) [Gr. *thamnos* bush] a genus of molds of the family Mucoraceae, order Mucorales, which resembles *Mucor* and which is often found growing on meat in cold storage. It can grow at 28° F. and forms a profuse hairy growth. The species most frequently found are *T. elegans* and *T. chaetocladioides.*

thamuria (tham-u′re-ah) [Gr. *thamys* often + *ouron* urine + *-ia*] frequency of urination.

thanat(o)- [Gr. *thanatos* death] a combining form denoting death.

thanatobiologic (than″ah-to-bi″o-loj′ik) [*thanato-* + Gr. *bios* life + *-logy*] pertaining to death and life.

thanatognomonic (than″ah-to-no-mon′ik) [*thanato-* + Gr. *gnōmonikos* decisive] indicating the approach of death.

thanatoid (than′ah-toid) [*thanato-* + Gr. *eidos* form] resembling death.

thanatology (than″ah-tol′o-je) the medicolegal study of death and conditions affecting dead bodies.

thanatometer (than″ah-tom′ĕ-ter) [*thanato-* + Gr. *metron* measure] a thermometer used to prove the occurrence of death by registering the reduction of the bodily temperature.

thanatophidia (than″ah-to-fid′e-ah) [*thanato-* + Gr. *ophis* snake] the venomous snakes collectively; toxicophidia.

thanatophidial (than″ah-to-fid′e-al) pertaining to venomous snakes.

thanatophobia (than″ah-to-fo′be-ah) [*thanato-* + *phobia*] irrational fear of death.

thanatophoric (than″ah-to-fōr′ik) [*thanato-* + Gr. *pherein* to bear] deadly; lethal.

thanatopsia, thanatopsy (than″ah-top′se-ah; than′-ah-top″se) [*thanato-* + Gr. *opsis* view] necropsy.

thanatosis (than″ah-to′sis) gangrene or necrosis.

Thane's method (thānz) [Sir George Dancer *Thane*, British anatomist, 1850–1930] see under *method.*

Thapsia (thap′se-ah) [L.; Gr. *thapsia*; named from the isle of *Thapsus*] a genus of umbelliferous plants. *T. garganica* L. (Umbelliferae), of Northern Africa, affords an irritant resin somewhat used in plasters; the plant is locally employed as a polychrest remedy.

thaumatropy (thaw-mat′ro-pe) [Gr. *thauma* wonder + *tropos* a turning] the transformation of an organ or structure into another organ or structure.

thaumaturgic (thaw″mah-ter′jik) [Gr. *thauma* wonder + *ergon* work] working wonders; magical; miraculous.

Thaysen's disease (thi′senz) [Thornwald Einar Hess *Thaysen*, Copenhagen physician, 1883–1936] nontropical sprue.

THC tetrahydrocannabinol.

thea (the′ah) [L.] tea.

theaism (the′ah-izm) a morbid condition resulting from ingestion of excessive quantities of tea.

thebaic (the-ba′ik) [L. *Thebaicus* Theban, named for Thebes, where opium was once prepared] pertaining to or derived from opium.

thebaine (the-ba′in) a crystalline, poisonous, and anodyne alkaloid from opium, $C_{19}H_{21}NO_3$, having properties similar to those of strychnine; called also *dimethyl morphine.*

thebesian (the-be′ze-an) named for or described by Adam Christian *Thebesius*, German physician, 1686–1732, as *thebesian foramen* (foramina venarum minimarum cordis), *thebesian valve* (valvula sinus coronarii), and *thebesian veins* (venae cordis minimae).

theca (the′kah), pl. *the′cae* [L.; Gr. *thēkē*] an enclosing case or sheath, as of an ovarian follicle or tendon. **t. cor′dis,** pericardium. **t. exter′na,** tunica externa thecae folliculi. **t. of follicle,** t. folliculi. **t. of follicle of von Baer,** tunica externa thecae folliculi. **t. follic′uli** [NA], an envelope of condensed connective tissue surrounding a vesicular ovarian follicle, comprising an internal vascular layer and an external fibrous layer. **t. inter′na,** tunica interna thecae folliculi. **t. medulla′re spina′lis,** dura mater of the spinal cord. **t. vertebra′lis,** dura mater of the spinal cord.

thecae (the′se) [L.] genitive and plural of *theca.*

thecal (the′kal) pertaining to a theca.

Thecina (thĕ-si′nah) [L., from Gr. *thēkē* a sheath] a suborder of ameboid protozoa (order Amoebida, subclass Gymnamoebia), characterized by a body that is flattened and often oblong, ovate, or flabellate with a pellicle-like layer that may be distinctly wrinkled.

thecitis (the-si′tis) inflammation of the sheath of a tendon; tenosynovitis.

thecodont (the′ko-dont) [Gr. *thēkē* sheath + *odous* tooth] having the teeth inserted in sockets or alveoli.

thecoma (the-ko′mah) a theca cell tumor.

thecomatosis (the″ko-mah-to′sis) diffuse hyperplasia of the ovarian stroma.

thecostegnosis (the″ko-steg-no′sis) [Gr. *thēkē* sheath + *stegnōsis* narrowing] contraction of a tendon sheath.

Theden's bandage (ta′denz) [Johann Christian Anton *Theden*, German surgeon, 1714–1797] see under *bandage.*

Theelin (the′lin) trademark for preparations of estrone.

Theile's canal, glands (ti′lez) [Friedrich Wilhelm *Theile*, German anatomist, 1801–1879] see under *canal* and *gland.*

Theiler (ti′ler) Max. South African-born American physician and microbiologist, 1899–1972; winner of the Nobel prize for medicine or physiology in 1951 for developing a vaccine for yellow fever.

Theiler's disease, virus [Max *Theiler*] see under *disease* and *virus.*

Theileria (thi-le′re-ah) [Sir Arnold *Theiler*, Swiss microbiologist, 1867–1936] a genus of minute tickborne protozoa (order Piroplasmida, subclass Piroplasmia) parasitic in the erythrocytes, lymphocytes, and endothelial cells of mammals. Certain species cause economically important diseases in cattle, sheep, and goats. See *theileriasis.* **T. annula′ta,** a species causing tropical theileriasis in cattle, transmitted by ticks of the genus *Hyalomma.* Called also *T. dispar.* **T. dis′par,** *T. annulata.* **T. hir′ci,** a species found in North Africa, the southern USSR, eastern Europe, India, and Asia Minor, causing a highly fatal disease in adult sheep and goats; the vector is unknown. **T. lawren′cei,** the etiologic agent of corridor disease in African cattle, which is antigenically related to and may be a variant of *T. parva.* **T. mu′tans,** a species parasitic in African cattle and African and Indian water buffaloes, which is usually nonpathogenic or only mildly so but has been known to cause a severe form of theileriasis known as Tzaneen disease. **T. o′vis,** a species parasitic in sheep and goats in Africa, Europe, the USSR, India, Sri Lanka, and western Asia, which is nonpathogenic or may cause a mild disease manifested by fever, lymphadenopathy at site of the tick bite, and slight anemia. **T. par′va,** the etiologic agent of East Coast fever, a highly fatal disease of African cattle, transmitted by ticks of the genera *Physicephalus* and *Hyalomma.*

theileriasis (thi″lĕ-ri′ah-sis) a group of diseases due to protozoa of the genus *Theileria*, which results in an acute or chronic febrile infection. Called also *theileriosis*. **bovine t.,** 1. East Coast fever. 2. any of various febrile diseases of cattle caused by species of *Theileria*. **tropical t.,** an infection in cattle similar to but milder than East Coast fever, caused by *Theileria annulata*, transmitted by *Hyalomma* spp., and occurring in North Africa, Mediterranean coastal regions, Asia, India, the Middle East, and the southern USSR. Called also *Mediterranean Coast fever*, and *tropical piroplasmosis*.

theileriosis (thi-lēr″ĭ-o′sis) theileriasis.

theine (the′in) the alkaloid of tea, isomeric with caffeine.

theinism (the′in-izm) theaism.

thelalgia (the-lal′je-ah) [*thel-* + *-algia*] pain in the nipple.

thelarche (the-lar′ke) [*thel-* + Gr. *archē* beginning] the beginning of development of the breasts at puberty.

Thelazia (the-la′ze-ah) a genus of nematode worms of the superfamily Spiruroidea, which are allied to Filaria. Several species (*T. callipaeda, T. californiensis*) are parasitic in the eyes of animals.

thelaziasis (the″la-zi′ah-sis) infection of the eye with *Thelazia*.

thele-, thel(o)- [Gr. *thēlē* nipple] a combining form denoting a relationship to the nipple or to a nipple-like structure.

theleplasty (the′le-plas″te) [*thele-* + *-plasty*] a plastic operation upon the nipple.

thelerethism (thel-er′ĕ-thizm) [*thēlē-* + *erethisma* a stirring up] erection or protrusion of the nipple.

theliolymphocyte (the″le-o-lim′fo-sīt) intraepithelial lymphocyte; a small lymphocyte found within the epithelium, especially intestinal epithelium.

thelitis (the-li′tis) [*thel-* + *-itis*] inflammation of a nipple; mamillitis.

thelium (the′le-um), pl. *the′lia* [L.] 1. a papilla. 2. a nipple.

thel(o)- see *thele-*.

Thelohania (the″lo-ha′ne-ah) a genus of protozoa (suborder Pansporoblastina, order Microsporida) parasitic in the larvae of certain culicine and anopheline mosquitoes and crane flies and in the brains of rodents.

thelorrhagia (the″lo-ra′je-ah) [*thelo-* + *-rrhagia*] hemorrhage from the nipple.

thelothism, thelotism (the′lo-thizm; the′lo-tizm) thelerethism.

thelyblast (thel′e-blast) [Gr. *thēlys* female + *blastos* germ] the female pronucleus.

thelyblastic (thel″e-blas′tik) pertaining to or of the nature of a thelyblast (female pronucleus).

thelygenic (the″le-jen′ik) [Gr. *thēlys* female + *gennan* to produce] producing only female offspring.

thelykinin (the″le-ki′nin) an obsolete term for estrone.

thelytocia (thel″e-to′she-ah) [Gr. *thēlys* female + *tokos* birth] normal parthenogenesis producing females only.

thelytocous (the-lit′o-kus) pertaining to or characterized by thelytocia.

thelytoky (the-lit′o-ke) thelytocia.

Themison (them′ĭ-son) **of Laodicea** (1st century B.C.) a Greek physician who founded the Methodist school of medicine.

thenad (the′nad) toward the thenar eminence or toward the palm.

thenal (the′nal) pertaining to the palm or thenar.

thenar (the′nar) [Gr.] 1. [NA] the mound on the palm at the base of the thumb; called also *eminentia thenaris* [NA alternative] and *thenar eminence*. 2. pertaining to the palm.

thenium closylate (then′ĭ-um klo′sĭ-lāt) chemical name: N,N-dimethyl-N-(2-phenoxyethyl)-2-thiophenemethanaminium salt with 4-chlorobenzenesulfonic acid (1:1); a veterinary anthelmintic, $C_{21}H_{24}ClNO_4S_2$.

thenyldiamine hydrochloride (then″il-di′ah-mēn) chemical name: N,N-dimethyl-N′-2-pyridinyl-N′-(3-thienylmethyl)-1,2-ethanediamine hydrochloride. An antihistamine, $C_{14}H_{19}N_3S \cdot HCl$, used for preoperative sedation, to control postoperative nausea, and to potentiate the action of analgesics.

Thenylene (then′ĭ-lēn) trademark for a preparation of methapyrilene.

thenylpyramine (then″il-pir′ah-mēn) methapyrilene.

Theobaldia (the″o-bal′de-ah) [Frederic Vincent *Theobald*, British zoologist, 1868–1930] *Culiseta*.

Theobroma (the″o-bro′mah) [Gr. *theos* god + *brōma* food] a genus of sterculiaceous plants; the cacao. The seeds of *T. cacao* L. (called theobroma and cacao) contain the alkaloid theobromine, and are used in the preparation of cacao and chocolate.

theobromine (the″o-bro′min) chemical name: 3,7-dihydro-3,7-dimethyl-1H-purine-2,6-dione. A white crystalline alkaloid, $C_7H_8N_4O_2$, prepared from the dried ripe seed of *Theobroma cacao*, or made synthetically from xanthine. It has physiologic properties similar to those of caffeine, and is used as a diuretic and smooth muscle relaxant and as a myocardial stimulant and vasodilator. Derivatives such as t. calcium salicylate, t. sodium acetate, t. sodium salicylate, t. sodium formate, and t. salicylate are available for use.

Theoglycinate (the″o-gli′sĭ-nāt) trademark for a preparation of theophylline sodium glycinate.

theolin (the′o-lin) a colorless, volatile liquid hydrocarbon, heptane, C_7H_{16}, obtainable from petroleum, etc.; it resembles benzine and has similar uses.

theophylline (the-of′ĭ-lin) [USP] chemical name: 3,7-dihydro-1,3-dimethyl-1H-purine-2,6-dione. A xanthine derivative, $C_7H_8N_4 \cdot H_2O$, found in tea leaves and prepared synthetically; it is a smooth muscle relaxant, used chiefly as a diuretic; administered orally. **t. aminoisobutanol,** ambuphylline. **t. cholinate,** oxtriphylline. **t. ethanolamine,** t. olamine. **t. ethylenediamine,** aminophylline. **t. monoethanolamine,** t. olamine. **t. olamine** [USP], a compound containing theophylline (about 75 per cent) and monoethanolamine; used chiefly for its smooth muscle relaxant activity in the treatment of acute bronchial asthma and bronchospasm associated with chronic bronchitis and emphysema, administered rectally. Called also *t. ethanolamine* and *t. monoethanolamine*. **t. sodium acetate,** a hydrated mixture containing theophylline sodium and sodium acetate in approximately equimolecular proportions, and yielding 55 to 65 per cent of anhydrous theophylline; used as a smooth muscle relaxant and also as a diuretic. **t. sodium glycinate** [USP], an equilibrium mixture containing theophylline sodium and aminoacetic acid in approximately equal proportions, and yielding 49 to 52 per cent theophylline; used chiefly as a smooth muscle relaxant for the symptomatic treatment of bronchial asthma, administered orally.

Theorell (the″o-rel′), Axel Hugo Teodor. Swedish biochemist, born 1903; winner of the Nobel prize in medicine or physiology for 1955, for his discoveries concerning the nature and mode of action of oxidation enzymes.

theorem (the′o-rem) [Gr. *theorēma* a principle arrived at by speculation] a proposition capable of demonstration. **Bayes' t.,** a theorem used to interconvert conditional probabilities:

$$P(B|A) = \frac{P(A|B)\,P(B)}{P(A|B)\,P(B) + P(A \text{ not } B)P(\text{not } B)}$$

where $P(A)$ and $P(B)$ are the probabilities of two events, A and B and $P(A|B)$ and $P(B|A)$ are the conditional probabilities of A given B and of B given A. For example, if A denotes a positive laboratory test result and B denotes the actual presence of disease in a tested patient, then $P(A|B)$ is the "diagnostic sensitivity" of the test (true positive rate) and $P(B)$ is the prevalence of the disease ($P(A)$ is the frequency of positive test results). $P(B|A)$ is the "predictive value of a positive test," the probability that a patient testing positive will actually have the disease. **central limit t.,** if random samples of size n are taken from a population having a normally distributed variable with mean μ and standard deviation σ, the distribution of the sample means is normal, with mean μ and standard deviation $\sigma/\sqrt{n}$; if the variable in the population is not normally distributed, the sampling distribution of means approximates the normal distribution and the approximation gets better as the sample size increases. **Gibbs's t.,** substances which lower the surface tension of the pure dispersion medium tend to collect on its surface.

theory (the′o-re) [Gr. *theōria* speculation as opposed to practice] 1. the doctrine or the principles underlying an art as distinguished from the practice of that particular art. 2. a formulated hypothesis, or, loosely speaking, any hypothesis or opinion not based upon actual knowledge. **aging t. of atherosclerosis,** a theory that atherosclerosis is an inevitable consequence of aging and therefore an irreversible process. **Altmann's t.,** a theory that protoplasm is made up of granular particles (bioblasts) grouped in masses and enclosed in indifferent matter. **apposition t.,** the theory that tissues grow by the deposit of cells from without. **Arrhenius' t.,** the theory of electrolytic dissociation, proposed in 1887, which explained the properties of electrolytes based on the presence of free ions in solution and also defined acids and bases as compounds that dissociate to release hydrogen and hydroxide ions, respectively, in solution. **atomic t.,** the theory that the molecules of a substance are made up of one or more atoms, each representing a definite amount of the element, which amount does not vary in the molecule, whatever combinations the molecule may enter. **avalanche t.,** the theory that nervous influence increases in force as it descends along an efferent nerve. **Bolk's retardation t.,** the theory that man, in his development, is at a stage which, in the higher primates, is still a fetal stage. **Bowman's t.** (*of urinary secretion*), the theory that water and inorganic salts are secreted by the glomeruli, whereas the urea and related bodies are secreted by the epithelial cells in the convoluted tubes. Cf. *Ludwig's t.* **Buergi's t.,** two different substances causing identical therapeutic manifestations when combined are increased in their effects if they possess identical pharmacologic points of attack. **cell t.,** the doctrine that all living matter is composed of cells and that cell activity is the essential process of life. **cell-chain t.,** the theory that the nerve fiber consists of a chain of special cells which have only secondarily been brought into relation with the central cell. **cellular immunity t.,** Metchnikoff's cellular immunity. **clonal deletion t.,** a theory of immunologic tolerance to self antigens according to which "forbidden clones" of immunocytes, those reactive with self antigens, are eliminated on contact with antigen during fetal life. The terms "clonal abortion," "clonal anergy," "clonal silencing," and "clonal purging" have also been used for this phenomenon. See also *clonal selection t.* **clonal-selection t.,** a modification of the natural selection theory (q.v.): there are in each adult several million clones of antibody-producing cells, each programmed to make antibody of a single specificity and bearing cell-surface receptors capable of reacting with specific antigens; exposure to antigen induces cells of antigen-reactive clones to proliferate and differentiate to produce large quantities of specific antibody. This theory has been found to be essentially correct. See *clonal deletion t.* and *recombinational germline t.* **closed circulation t.,** one of the theories explaining how the blood in the spleen gets from the arteries to the venous sinuses; it holds that the capillaries empty directly into the venous sinuses. Cf. *open circulation t.* and *closed-open circulation t.* Called also *fast circulation t.* **closed-open circulation t.,** the theory that both an open and a closed circulation are present in the spleen; e.g., a closed circulation in a contracted spleen may become an open circulation when the organ is distended. Cf. *closed circulation t.* and *open circulation t.* **Cohnheim's t.,** 1. the theory, proposed in 1873, that inflammation results from the local action of a noxious agent, which allows blood cells to enter tissues. 2. the theory that tumors develop from embryonic rests which do not participate in the formation of normal surrounding tissue. **contractile ring t.,** a theory advanced to explain the formation of a furrow in a dividing cell. According to this theory, the gelated ring in the cortex of the dividing cell contracts (cortical gel contraction) like the nonmotile portion of an amoeba, and, therefore, decreases the surface area. Actually, however, before division the surface increases by about 26 per cent. **convergence-projection t.,** a theory advanced as an explanation for reference of pain, according to which some visceral afferent nerve fibers converge with cutaneous pain afferents to end upon the same neuron at some point in the sensory pathway. **core conductor t.,** a theory regarding the development of electrotonic potentials and their associated currents along nerve fibers, according to which the nerve fibers are considered to be core conductors, i.e., cylinders of conducting fluid material with a sheath of high electrical resistance, surrounded by a layer of conducting medium. **darwinian t.,** see *darwinism.* **Dieulafoy's**

t., the theory that appendicitis is always due to the appendix becoming a closed cavity. **dimer t.,** the theory that the tooth organ of primates is composed of two halves, each of which is a representative of an independent tooth in the lower orders of animals. **dualistic t.,** the theory that the blood cells arise from two distinct types of primitive cells, the myeloblasts and lymphoblasts. Cf. *monophyletic t.*, *polyphyletic t.*, and *trialistic t.* **ectopic focus t.,** a theory advanced by Rothberger, which states that atrial fibrillation arises as a result of rapid discharges from an ectopic focus. **Ehrlich's biochemical t.,** the theory that specific chemical affinity exists between the substance of specific living cells and specific chemical substances. **Ehrlich's side-chain t.,** the first (1896) comprehensive theory of antibody production, which proposed that antibody-producing cells have surface molecules (side chains) that can bind to antigens and that binding to a specific side chain causes the cell to produce more of the same side chain and to release these side chains into the serum as antibodies. Two of Ehrlich's postulates, that antibodies are identical to the antigen receptors and that antigen binding triggers the synthesis of antibody with the same specificity as the receptor, are now known to be essentially correct. Cf. *clonal-selection t.* **electron t.,** all bodies are complex structures composed of small particles called atoms together with still smaller particles called electrons. **emergency t.,** Cannon's theory that the adrenal medulla is stimulated to secrete by activity on the part of the sympathetic nervous system in conditions of emotional excitement, pain, etc.; or, in other words, to meet bodily emergencies. **emigration t.,** Cohnheim's t., def. 1. **encrustation t.,** a theory advanced by Rokitansky, which states that fibrinous material derived from the blood is deposited on the inner surface of the intima of vessels and that fatty metamorphosis occurs secondarily in this deposit. **equilibrium t.,** a theory that the number of breeding species in a biome is a result of the rate of immigration of new species and the rate of extinction. **expanding surface t.,** a theory of cell division which postulates that a nuclear substance is liberated, probably from chromosomes, which causes expansion of the cellular membrane at the poles; as the polar areas expand, the equator contracts, leading to division. **fast circulation t.,** closed circulation t. **frequency t.,** a theory which postulates that the pattern of excitation of auditory nerve fibers is more important in perception of pitch than is the excitation of any of the fibers in any particular area of the cochlear basilar membrane. Cf. *place t.* **Frerichs' t.,** the theory that uremia is really a poisoning by ammonium carbonate formed by the action on urea of an enzyme contained in the blood. **gate t., gate-control t.,** neural impulses generated by noxious painful stimuli and transmitted to the spinal cord by small-diameter C-fibers and A-delta fibers are blocked at their synapses in the dorsal horn by the simultaneous stimulation of large-diameter myelinated A-fibers, thus inhibiting pain by preventing pain impulses from reaching higher levels of the central nervous system. Called also *gate hypothesis.* **germ t.,** the doctrine that infectious diseases are of microbic origin. **germ layer t.,** the teaching that the embryo develops three primary germ layers, each of which gives rise to definite organ derivatives. **gestalt t.,** see *gestaltism.* **Golgi's t.,** the theory that the neurons communicate by the axons of Golgi's cells and the collaterals of the axons of Deiters' cells. **Goltz's t.,** the theory that the function of the semicircular canals is to transmit sensations of position, and thus materially aid in the sense of equilibrium. **Helmholtz t.,** a theory of sound perception: each basilar fiber responds sympathetically to a definite tone and stimulates the hair cells of Corti's organ, which rest upon the fiber. The nerve impulse from this stimulation of the hair cells is carried to the brain. **Hering's t.,** the doctrine that color sensation depends on decomposition and restitution of the visual substance: disassimilation producing red, yellow, and white, and restitution producing blue, green, and black. Called also *opponent colors t.* **hit t.,** target t. **humoral t.,** see *humoralism.* **incasement t.,** the formerly advocated theory that all animals and plants develop from preexisting germs, and that they encase the germs of all future generations, one within another. **information t.,** a system for analyzing, chiefly by statistical methods, the characteristics of communicated messages and the systems that encode, transmit, distort, receive, and decode them. **instructive t.,** template t. **ionic t.,** a theory that, on going into solution, the molecules of an electrolyte either completely or partially break up or dissociate into two or more portions, these portions being positively and negatively charged electrically, the positively charged portions being different chemically from those negatively charged. When an electric current is passed through the solution of an electrolyte the positively charged portions are attracted by the negative pole or electrode, and move toward it; the negatively charged portions are attracted by and migrate toward the positive electrode. From this property of moving toward one of the electrodes, these charged molecular fractions of electrolytes are called ions, from the Greek verb meaning "to move." **Kern plasma relation t.,** the theory that for each cell there exists a definite size relation of nuclear mass to cell mass. **Ladd-Franklin t.,** a theory of the evolution of color vision: first, light stimulates a substance in the visual cells, producing a sensation of white light; next, molecular changes from the first reaction produce two reactive products, one for each end of the spectrum, for blue and yellow; finally, the reactive product from the yellow becomes two products for red and green. Dichromasies and anomalous trichromasies are considered to be incomplete recapitulations of the evolutionary development. **Lamarck's t.,** the theory that acquired characteristics may be transmitted. **Liebig's t.,** the hydrocarbons which oxidize easily are the foods which produce animal heat. **local circuit t.,** in neurophysiology, the theory that current flows from the unstimulated, positively charged areas of the cell membrane of a neuron to the stimulated, depolarized or negative portion, and that as each new area becomes depolarized or negative, it in turn acts as the sink toward which the current flows from the adjacent area, which results in progressive depolarization, or reversal charge, along the neuron from the point of stimulation; the source of the current is the flow of Na^+ into the cell. **Ludwig's t.** (*of urinary secretion*), the theory that urine is formed by the simple process of filtration in the glomeruli and that reabsorption occurs in the urinary tubules by the process of diffusion. Cf. *Bowman's t.* **membrane ionic t.,** the theory that the resting potential difference between the inside and outside of the cell is related to (1) the thin, electrically insulating membrane between the cytoplasm and the interstitial conducting medium, which is poorly and variably permeable to diverse ions; (2) the presence of a metabolic cellular pump that promotes the efflux of sodium ions from the cell interior to the outside against its electrochemical gradient and, coupled with this, the influx of potassium ions into the cell against its ionic concentration gradient. **mendelian t.,** see *Mendel's law,* under *law.* **metabolic t. of atherosclerosis,** a theory that atherosclerosis is caused by a disturbance in lipid metabolism, specifically cholesterol metabolism. **Metchnikoff's (Mechnikov's) cellular immunity t.,** the theory, proposed in the 1880s, that phagocytosis by macrophages and polymorphonuclear leukocytes is the main mechanism of host defense against bacterial infection and that inflammation is the result of the enzymatic digestion process occurring with phagocytosis. **migration t.** (*obs.*), the theory that sympathetic ophthalmia is produced by migration of the pathogenic agent through the lymph channels of the optic nerve. **Monakow's t.,** the theory of diaschisis; see *diaschisis.* **monophyletic t.,** the theory that all forms of blood cells, both red and white, have their origin in one and the same form of primordial blood cell (hemocytoblast), the several types of cells arising by a process of differentiation. Called also *unitarian t.* Cf. *dualistic t., polyphyletic t.,* and *trialistic t.* **myogenic t.,** the theory that the muscle fibers of the heart possess in themselves the power of originating and maintaining the contraction of the heart. **natural selection t.,** the first selective theory of antibody formation, according to which about a million different antibody molecules are constantly being produced at low levels; when an antibody combines with a complementary antigen the complex is taken up by antibody-producing cells and the antibody is replicated. This theory explained many features of the immune response but incorrectly located immunologic memory in serum rather than cells. See *clonal selection t.* **neuron t.** (Waldeyer, 1801), the obsolete theory that the nervous system consists of innumerable neurons in contiguity, but not in continuity. See *neuron.* **open circulation t.,** one of the theories explaining how the blood in the spleen gets from the arteries to the venous sinuses; it holds that the capillaries open directly into the pulp reticulum, and that the blood gradually filters back into the venous sinuses.

Called also *slow circulation t.* Cf. *closed circulation t.* and *closed-open circulation t.* **open-closed circulation t.,** see *closed-open circulation t.* **opponent colors t.,** Hering's t. **overproduction t.,** see *Weigert's law,* under *law.* **paralytic t.,** the doctrine that hyperemia is the most essential fact of inflammation, and is caused by paralysis of the vasomotor nerves. **Pasteur's t.,** the theory that the immunity secured by an attack of a disease is caused by the exhaustion of material needed for the growth of the organism of the disease; called also *t. of exhaustion of the medium.* **phlogiston t.,** see *phlogiston.* **pithecoid t.,** the theory that man is descended from apelike ancestors. **place t.,** a theory of pitch perception which postulates that excitation of specific areas of the basilar membrane of the cochlea determine the pitch that is perceived. Cf. *frequency t.* **Planck's t.,** quantum t. **polarization-membrane t.,** the theory that living, resting cells are surrounded by a semipermeable membrane lined by a series of electrical doublets, or dipoles, with negative charges on the inner and positive charges on the outer surface. When the membrane is electrically intact, its entire surface is surrounded by doublets, and is said to be polarized. **polyphyletic t.,** the theory that the various corpuscles and cells of the blood have their origin from two or more distinct varieties of primordial (mother) cells. Cf. *dualistic t., monophyletic t.,* and *trialistic t.* **P. O. U. t.,** Ishihara's theory of the placenta-ovary-uterus production of internal secretion. **preformation t.,** the outmoded theory that the individuals of successive generations are contained, completely formed, within the reproductive cell of one of the parents. **quantum t.,** the theory that the radiation and absorption of energy take place in definite quantities called quanta (E) which vary in size and are defined by the equation $E = h\nu$, in which h is Planck's constant and ν is the frequency of the radiation. **recapitulation t.,** ontogeny recapitulates phylogeny; that is, an organism in the course of its development goes through the same successive stages as did the species in developing from the lower to the higher forms of animal life. Called also *biogenetic law* and *Haeckel's law.* **recombinational germline t.,** a theory of the origin of antibody diversity, according to which the DNA coding for a single immunoglobulin chain is assembled by a somatic recombinational event from two genes, one a unique constant region gene and the other one of several million variable region genes. The first theory to propose that two genes might code for a single polypeptide chain, it is now known to be essentially correct, although more than two types of genes are actually involved. Called also *Dreyer and Bennett hypothesis.* **t. of reentry,** the theory that the sinus impulse preceding the premature beat activates the heart, but the activation wave is delayed in an area of diminished irritability; see *reentry.* **resonance t.,** 1. Helmholtz theory. 2. the theory of specificity which assumes that the surface forces of reacting substances must harmonize. **Ribbert's t.,** a tumor is formed from the development of cell rests owing to reduced tension in the surrounding tissues. **Schiefferdecker's symbiosis t.,** the theory that among the tissues of the body there is a sort of symbiosis, so that the products of metabolism in one tissue serve as a stimulus to the activities of other tissues. **Schön's t.,** the theory (of ocular accommodation) that the ciliary muscle exerts on the lens the same effect as is produced on a rubber ball held in both hands and compressed by the fingers. **side-chain t.,** Ehrlich's side-chain t. **single hit t.,** the theory that hemolysis results from a single complement-induced lesion of the erythrocyte surface, rather than that lesions at several sites are necessary. **sliding filament t.,** 1. a theory which postulates that the thin and thick filaments of a myofibril slide past each other, while maintaining their length, during muscle contraction. 2. a theory that postulates that contraction of cilia involves a sliding of filaments (microtubules) in a manner comparable to the sliding filament mechanism for the contraction of muscle (see def. 1). **slow circulation t.,** open circulation t. **spindle elongation t.,** the theory which suggests that the spindle and asters have a decisive role in cell division. The theory is based on the observation that the elongation of the cell at anaphase is accompanied by a shrinkage at the equator. The centers are believed to be pushed apart by the spindle tubules, since the spindles and asters appear to be rigid structures. **Spitzer's t.,** the formation of the septa in the heart are teleologically conditioned, phylogenetically brought about, and mechanically achieved by the appearance and development of the lungs through phylogeny. **target t.,** the theory advanced to explain some biological effects of radiation on the basis of ionization occurring in a very small sensitive region within the cell, which postulates that one or more ionizing events, or "hits," within the sensitive volume are necessary to bring about the biological end-effect; called also *hit t.* **template t.,** a theory of the mechanism of antibody specificity, current during the 1930s and 40s, which proposed that the shape of an antibody molecule is determined as it is synthesized by being molded on an antigen molecule. The antigen thus "instructs" a cell to make specific antibody. Called also *instructive t.* **thermostat t.,** a theory which suggests that the feeding and satiety centers of the brain, like the thermoregulatory centers, are sensitive to body temperature; a decrease in body temperature activates the feeding center and depresses the satiety center, whereas increased temperature acts on the centers in the opposite way. **Traube's resonance t.,** resonance t., def. 2. **trialistic t.,** the theory that the blood cells arise from three distinct types of primitive cells, the myeloblasts, lymphoblasts, and monocytes. Cf. *dualistic t., monophyletic t.,* and *polyphyletic t.* **undulatory t.,** wave t. **unitarian t.,** monophyletic t. **unitary t.,** the theory that disease is single in its nature and is not made up of separate and distinct morbid entities. **wave t.,** the theory that light, heat, and electricity are transmitted through space in the form of waves. **Weismann's t.,** see *weismannism.* **Woods-Fildes t.,** the theory that the antibacterial activity of at least some chemotherapeutic drugs (especially the sulfonamides) is a consequence of a competitive inhibition of essential metabolic reactions of the microorganism. **Young-Helmholtz t.,** the doctrine that color vision depends on three sets of retinal fibers, corresponding to the colors red, green, and violet. **Zuntz's t.,** a theory of muscle contraction.

theotherapy (the"o-ther'ah-pe) [Gr. *theos* god + *therapy*] the treatment of disease by prayer and religious exercises.

Thephorin (thef'o-rin) trademark for preparations of phenindamine tartrate.

theque (těk) [Fr. a "box or small chest"] a round or oval collection, or nest, of melanin-containing nevus cells occurring at the dermoepidermal junction of the skin or in the dermis proper.

therapeusis (ther"ah-pu'sis) therapeutics.

therapeutic (ther"ah-pu'tik) [Gr. *therapeutikos* inclined to serve] 1. pertaining to therapeutics, or to the art of healing. 2. curative.

therapeutics (ther"ah-pu'tiks) 1. the science and art of healing. 2. a scientific account of the treatment of disease.

therapeutist (ther"ah-pu'tist) therapist.

Theraphosidae (ther"ah-fo'sĭ-de) a family of very large hairy spiders (suborder Orthognatha) found in temperate and tropical areas. *Sericopelma communis* is the only species whose venom has a harmful effect on man, but some are capable of inflicting painful bites. The members of this family are sometimes improperly called tarantulas.

therapia (ther"ah-pi'ah) [L., from Gr.] therapy. **t. sterili'sans mag'na,** Ehrlich's procedure of treatment by the use of some chemical agent which will destroy the parasites in the body of a patient without being seriously toxic for the patient.

therapist (ther'ah-pist) [Gr. *therapeutēs* one who attends to the sick] a person skilled in the treatment of disease; often combined with a term indicating the specific type of disorder treated (as *speech therapist*) or a particular type of treatment rendered (as *physical therapist*). **physical t.,** a person skilled in the techniques of physical therapy and qualified to administer treatments prescribed by a physician and under his supervision; called also *physiotherapist.* **speech t.,** a person specially trained and qualified to assist patients in overcoming speech and language disorders.

therapy (ther'ah-pe) [Gr. *therapeia* service done to the sick] the treatment of disease; therapeutics. See also under *treatment.* **anticoagulant t.,** the use of drugs to render the blood sufficiently incoagulable to discourage thrombosis. **autoserum t.,** treatment of disease by the injection of the patient's own blood serum. **aversion t.,** therapy directed at associating an undesirable behavior pattern with unpleasant stimulation or at making the unpleasant stimulation a consequence of the undesirable behavior. **beam t.,** 1. treatment by exposure to light from one of the colors of the spectrum. 2. treatment by radiation emitted from a source

located at a distance from the body. **behavior t.,** a therapeutic approach in which the focus is on the patient's observable behavior, rather than on conflicts and unconscious processes presumed to underlie his maladaptive behavior. This is accomplished through systematic manipulation of the environmental and behavioral variables related to the specific behavior to be modified; operant conditioning, systematic desensitization, token economy, aversive control, flooding, and implosion are examples of techniques that may be used in behavior therapy. Called also *behavior modification* and *conditioning therapy.* **biological t.,** treatment of disease by the injection of the substances which produce a biological reaction in the organism. The term includes the use of sera, antitoxins, vaccines, and nonspecific proteins. **buffer t.,** intravenous injection of buffer substances, such as sodium bicarbonate, with the object of lowering the hydrogen ion concentration. **carbon dioxide t.,** a form of (rarely used) shock therapy employed for the treatment of withdrawn psychotic patients, in which unconsciousness is induced by the administration of carbon dioxide gas by inhalation. **Chaoul t.,** short source-to-tissue distance, low-voltage roentgen therapy; see also under *tube.* **collapse t.,** treatment of pulmonary tuberculosis by operative collapse of the diseased lung. **conditioning t.,** behavior t. **convulsive t.,** treatment of mental disorders, primarily depression, by induction of convulsions. The type now almost universally used is electroconvulsive therapy (ECT), in which the convulsions are induced by electic current. In the original convulsive therapy the convulsions were induced pharmacologically, at first by pentylenetetrazol (Metrazol) and later by flurothyl (Indoklon). Formerly called *shock t.* **corrective t.,** the planning and administration of progressive physical exercise and activities most effective in improving or maintaining general physical and emotional health, through individual or group participation. **Curie t.,** treatment with a radioactive source, e.g., radium. **deep roentgen-ray t.,** treatment by x-radiations generated by at least 150 kilovolts and capable of penetrating significantly below the skin level. **deleading t.,** the use of chelating agents in the mobilization and excretion from the body of heavy metals, such as lead, radium, etc. **diathermic t.,** treatment by thermopenetration; see *diathermy.* **duplex t.,** treatment by diathermic and galvanic currents in combination, both currents being passed through the body at the same time by way of the same two electrodes. **electric convulsive t. (ECT), electric shock t. (EST),** electroconvulsive t. **electroconvulsive t. (ECT),** a treatment for mental disorders, primarily depression, in which convulsions and loss of consciousness are induced by application of low-voltage alternating current to the brain via scalp electrodes for a fraction of a second; a muscle relaxant, generally succinylcholine, is used to prevent injury during the seizure. The coma lasts about 5 minutes and is followed by an acute confusional state lasting about an hour; some memory impairment may be present for several weeks after treatment. ECT produces a therapeutic response in a majority of cases of major depression; it has also been used in schizophrenia, primarily in treatment of acute schizophrenic episodes. **electroshock t. (EST),** electroconvulsive t. **emanation t.,** treatment by ionizing radiations emitted by a radioactive source. **family t.,** group therapy of the members of a family, with exploration of family relationships and processes as potential causes of mental disorder in one or more members of the family. **fever t.,** treatment of disease by induction of high body temperature, accomplished by physical means or by injection of fever-producing vaccines. **Fliess t.,** see under *treatment.* **grid t.,** therapeutic application of ionizing radiations through a metal grid having a pattern of small, evenly spaced perforations. **group t.,** psychotherapy carried out with a group of patients or the relatives of patients or both, which includes utilization of interactions of members of the group to effect changes in maladaptive behavior of the individual members, under the guidance of a single therapist. Called also *group psychotherapy.* **heterovaccine t.,** bacterial vaccine therapy by the use of some infectious agent other than the specific one causing the disease. **high-voltage roentgen t.,** treatment by deeply penetrating x-rays generated by voltages of over 300 kilovolts. **humidification t.,** the use of air supersaturated with moisture in congestive conditions of the upper and lower respiratory tract. **hunger t.,** limotherapy. **immunization t.,** treatment with antiserum and with actively antigenic substances, e.g., vaccines. **immu-**

nosuppressive t., treatment with agents, such as x-rays, corticosteroids, and cytotoxic chemicals, which suppress the immune response to antigen(s); it is used in various conditions, including autoimmune disease, allergy, multiple myeloma, chronic nephritis, and in organ transplantation. **Indoklon convulsive t.,** see *convulsive t.* **inhalation t.,** treatment aimed at restoring toward normal any pathophysiologic alterations of gas exchange in the cardiopulmonary system, as by the use of respirators, aerosol-producing devices, and the therapeutic use of oxygen, helium-oxygen, and carbon dioxide mixtures. **insulin coma t. (ICT), insulin shock t. (IST),** a treatment, now obsolete, used in acute or early schizophrenia; sufficient insulin is administered to place the patient in a deep hypoglycemic coma; the coma is reversed by administration of glucose; generally a course of 20 to 60 treatments is given. **intraosseous t.,** the infusion of blood or other solutions into the circulation by injection through the bone marrow. **intravenous t.,** the introduction of therapeutic liquid agents directly into the venous circulation. **irritation t.,** stimulation t. **light t.,** the therapeutic application of radiation in the visible spectrum. **liquid air t.,** see *refrigeration.* **metatrophic t.,** administration of a diet that acts as an adjunct to the drug taken. **Metrazol shock t.,** see *convulsive t.* **milieu t.,** treatment, usually in a psychiatric hospital, that emphasizes the provision of an environment and activities appropriate to the patient's emotional and interpersonal needs. **Morita t.,** a school of psychotherapy originating in Japan, based on the essential elements of conduct in Zen Buddhism. It emphasizes the combating of egocentricity and the correction of alienation from nature. **myofunctional t.,** training of the orofacial musculature, including modification of habits, in edentulous conditions, malocclusion, or temporomandibular joint disorders. **narcosis t.,** treatment of certain intense anxiety reactions, exhaustion, and severe agitation by inducing prolonged sleep (18 to 20 hours a day for about two weeks) with drugs, usually barbiturates; called also *sleep t.* **nonspecific t.,** treatment of infections by the injection of nonspecific substances, such as proteins, proteoses, bacterial vaccines, etc., which produce a general and nonspecific effect on cellular activity. **occupational t.,** the therapeutic use of self-care, work, and play activities to increase function, enhance development, and prevent disability; it may include modification of tasks or the environment to enable the patient to achieve maximum independence and to enhance the quality of the patient's life. **opsonic t.,** nonspecific therapy with bacterial vaccines to increase the opsonic index of the blood; called also *vaccine t.* **orthomolecular t.,** treatment of disease, especially psychiatric disorders, based on the theory that restoration of optimal concentrations of substances normally present in the body will effect a cure. **oxygen t.,** treatment by means of oxygen inhalation. **paraspecific t.,** nonspecific t. **pharmacological convulsive t.,** see *convulsive t.* **photodynamic t.,** intravenous administration of hematoporphyrin derivative, which concentrates selectively in metabolically active tumor tissue, followed by exposure of the tumor tissue to red laser light of a specific wavelength, to bring about production of cytotoxic free radicals that selectively destroy hematoporphyrin-containing tissue. Called also *photoradiation.* **physical t.,** 1. treatment by physical means. 2. the health profession concerned with the promotion of health, with the prevention of physical disability, with the evaluation and rehabilitation of patients disabled by pain, disease, or injury, and with treatment using physical therapeutic measures as opposed to medical, surgical, or radiologic measures. **play t.,** a method of psychotherapy used in treating emotional disorders in children, in which play is used to a considerable extent as a substitute for verbal communication between the patient and therapist. **primal t.,** psychotherapy in which the patient is encouraged to relive his early traumatic experiences. **protective t.,** sparing t. **protein t., protein-shock t.,** injection of foreign proteins by the parenteral route in inflammatory and venereal disease; nonspecific therapy. **pulp canal t.,** root canal t. **radium t.,** the treatment of disease by means of radium. **radium beam t.,** see *beam t.,* def. 2. **reflex t.,** treatment by producing a reflex action called also *reflexotherapy.* **replacement t.,** treatment to replace deficient formation or loss of body products by administration of the natural body products or synthetic substitutes. **root canal t.,** that aspect of endodontics dealing with the treatment of diseases of the dental pulp, consisting of partial

(pulpotomy) or complete (pulpectomy) extirpation of the diseased pulp, cleaning and sterilization of the empty canal, enlarging and shaping the canal to receive sealing material, and obturation of the canal with a nonirritating hermetic sealing agent. Called also *pulp canal t.* **rotation t.,** in radiotherapy, circular movement of the patient or of the radiation source and beam around a fixed anatomical axis during a treatment exposure; it may entail complete, partial, or skip-field exposure. **serum t.,** see *serotherapy.* **shock t.,** an obsolete term for psychiatric treatments involving induced convulsions or loss of consciousness, i.e., electroconvulsive therapy, pharmacological convulsive therapies, and insulin coma therapy. **short wave t.,** short wave diathermy. **sleep t.,** narcosis t. **solar t.,** heliotherapy. **sparing t.,** treatment directed to the protecting and sparing of an organ by allowing it to rest as much as possible. Called also *protective t.* **specific t.,** treatment by a remedy which acts directly against the cause of the disease, as of malaria by quinine. **speech t.,** the use of special techniques for correction of speech and language disorders. **stimulation t.,** treatment by the parenteral injection of certain substances with the result that the nervous vascular systems of the body function more vigorously and the metabolism is increased: called also *irritation t.* **subcoma insulin t.,** administration of insulin to produce mild hypoglycemia, sedation, and weight gain, formerly used to treat neurotic disorders and schizophrenia. **substitution t.,** the administration of a hormone to compensate for deficiency of that gland. **substitutive t.,** see *substitutive medication,* under *medication.* **suggestion t.,** the treatment of disease by hypnotic suggestion. **vaccine t.,** active immunization against a disease by the injection of the infectious agents of the disease or their products directly into a patient. **zomo t.,** treatment by the administration of meat juice. **zone t.,** treatment of disorder by mechanical stimulation of a body area located in the same longitudinal zone as the disorder; called also *Fitz Gerald method* or *treatment.*

Theria (the′rĭ-ah) [Gr. *thērion* beast, animal] in some systems of classification, a subclass of the Mammalia, including the infraclasses Eutheria and Metatheria, the members of which are viviparous.

theriac (ther′e-ak) theriaca.

theriaca (the-ri′ah-kah) [Gr. *thēriaka* antidotes to the poison of wild animals, from *thērion* wild animal] a mixture regarded as effective against bites by poisonous animals; it contained at one time 60 to 70 substances which were pulverized and made into an electuary with honey.

theriatrics (the″re-at′riks) [Gr. *thērion* beast + *iatrikē* surgery, medicine] veterinary medicine.

Theridiidae (ther″ĭ-di′ĭ-de) a family of small, dark, comb-footed spiders (suborder Labidognatha), including the genus *Latrodectus,* whose venomous bite sometimes causes death in human beings.

theriogenologic (the″re-o″jen-o-loj′ik) pertaining or relating to theriogenology.

theriogenological (the″re-o-jen″o-loj′ĭ-kal) pertaining or relating to theriogenology; of or affecting the reproductive processes of animals.

theriogenologist (the″reo″jen-ol′o-jist) one who specializes in theriogenology.

theriogenology (the″re-o″jen-ol′o-je) [Gr. *thērion* beast + *gennan* to produce + *-logy*] that branch of veterinary medicine which deals with reproduction, including the physiology and pathology of male and female reproductive systems and the clinical practice of veterinary obstetrics, gynecology, and semenology.

theriotherapy (the″re-o-ther′ah-pe) [Gr. *thērion* beast + *therapeia* treatment] treatment of the diseases of lower animals.

therm (therm) [Gr. *thermē* heat] a unit of heat. The word has been used as equivalent to (*a*) large calorie; (*b*) small calorie; (*c*) 1000 large calories; (*d*) 100,000 British thermal units.

thermacogenesis (ther″mah-ko-jen′ĕ-sis) [Gr. *thermē* heat + *genesis* production] the action of a drug in elevating the body temperature.

thermae (ther′me) [L., pl.; Gr. *thermē* heat] 1. warm springs or warm baths. 2. establishments for the therapeutic use of warm medicinal springs.

thermaerotherapy (therm-a″er-o-ther′ah-pe) [*therm-* + Gr. *aēr* air + *therapeia* treatment] treatment by the application of hot air.

thermal (ther′mal) pertaining to or characterized by heat.

thermalgesia (ther″mal-je′ze-ah) [*therm-* + Gr. *algēsis* sense of pain + *-ia*] a condition in which the application of heat produces pain.

thermalgia (ther-mal′je-ah) [*therm-* + Gr. *algos* pain + *-ia*] a condition marked by sensations of intense burning pain; causalgia.

thermanalgesia (therm″an-al-je′se-ah) absence of pain on application of heat.

thermanesthesia (therm″an-es-the′ze-ah) [*therm-* + *an-* neg. + Gr. *aisthēsis* perception + *-ia*] inability to recognize sensations of heat and cold; absence of the heat sense.

thermatology (ther″mah-tol′o-je) the scientific study of heat as a therapeutic agent.

thermelometer (ther″mel-om′ĕ-ter) an electric thermometer.

thermesthesia (therm″es-the′ze-ah) [*therm-* + Gr. *aisthēsis* perception + *-ia*] ability to recognize heat and cold; the temperature sense.

thermesthesiometer (therm″es-the″ze-om′ĕ-ter) [*thermesthesia* + *metron* measure] an instrument for measuring sensibility to heat.

thermhyperesthesia (therm″hi-per-es-the′ze-ah) excessive sensitiveness to high temperatures.

thermhypesthesia (therm″hi-pes-the′ze-ah) [*therm-* + Gr. *hypo* under + *aisthēsis* perception + *-ia*] decrease in the normal sensitiveness to heat.

thermic (ther′mik) of or pertaining to heat.

thermion (ther′me-on) a particle containing an electric charge emitted by an incandescent substance; such as the electrons emitted from the cathode in a Coolidge tube.

thermionics (ther″me-on′iks) the science of the phenomena exhibited by thermions.

thermistor (ther-mis′tor) a thermometer whose impedance varies with the ambient temperature and so is able to measure extremely small changes in temperature.

therm(o)- [Gr. *thermē* heat] a combining form denoting relationship to heat.

Thermoactinomyces (ther″mo-ak″tĭ-no-mi′sēz) [*thermo-* + Gr. *aktis, aktinos* a ray + *mykēs* fungus] a genus of bacteria of the family Micromonosporaceae, order Actinomycetales, consisting of thermophilic (45° to 60° C) organisms having single spores on the aerial and substrate mycelia. They occur as soil and water saprophytes. **T. vulga′ris,** a species isolated from soils, manure, and hay; one of the causative organisms of farmer's lung.

thermoaesthesia (ther″mo-es-the′ze-ah) thermesthesia.

thermoalgesia (ther″mo-al-je′ze-ah) thermalgesia.

thermoanalgesia (ther″mo-an″al-je′ze-ah) thermanalgesia.

thermoanesthesia (ther″mo-an″es-the′ze-ah) thermanesthesia.

thermocauterectomy (ther″mo-kaw″ter-ek′to-me) [*thermocautery* + Gr. *ektomē* exision] excision of an organ by thermocautery.

thermocautery (ther″mo-kaw′ter-e) cauterization by means of a hot wire or point.

thermochemistry (ther″mo-kem′is-tre) the aspect of physical chemistry dealing with heat changes that accompany chemical reactions.

thermochroic (ther″mo-kro′ik) [*thermo-* + Gr. *chroa* color] reflecting some of the heat rays and absorbing or transmitting others.

thermochroism, thermochrosis (ther-mok′ro-izm; ther″mo-kro′sis) the state or condition of being thermochroic.

thermocoagulation (ther″mo-ko-ag″u-la′shun) coagulation of tissue by the action of high-frequency currents; used in removal of growths and also used to produce stereotactic lesions in the brain.

thermocouple (ther′mo-kup″l) a pair of dissimilar electrical conductors (such as platinum and platinum-rhodium, or copper and constantan), so joined that an electromotive force is developed by the thermoelectric effects when the junctions are at different temperatures; used for measuring temperature differences.

thermocurrent (ther″mo-kur′ent) a thermoelectric current.

thermodiffusion (ther″mo-dĭ-fu′zhun) diffusion under the influence of a temperature gradient.

thermodilution (ther″mo-di-lu′shun) a method of measuring ventricular blood volume and cardiac output in which a cold or cool indicator, such as a saline solution or distilled water, is injected and sampled by a thermistor.

thermoduric (ther″mo-du′rik) [*thermo-* + L. *durus* enduring] capable of withstanding high temperature.

thermodynamics (ther″mo-di-nam′iks) [*thermo-* + Gr. *dynamis* power] the branch of science which deals with heat, energy, and the interconversion of these, and with related problems. See also under *law*. **equilibrium t.,** that dealing with the application of the laws of thermodynamics to systems in equilibrium states, or undergoing transformations between two equilibrium states. **laws of t.,** see under *law*. **nonequilibrium t.,** that dealing with steady states and irreversible processes.

thermoelectric (ther″mo-e-lek′trik) pertaining to electricity generated by heat.

thermoelectricity (ther″mo-e″lek-tris′ĭ-te) electricity generated by heat.

thermoesthesia (ther″mo-es-the′ze-ah) thermesthesia.

thermoesthesiometer (ther″mo-es-the″ze-om′ĕ-ter) thermesthesiometer.

thermoexcitory (ther″mo-ek-si′tor-e) exciting or stimulating the production of heat in the body.

thermogenesis (ther″mo-jen′ĕ-sis) [*thermo-* + Gr. *genesis* production] the production of heat, especially within the animal body.

thermogenetic (ther″mo-jĕ-net′ik) pertaining to the production of heat.

thermogenic (ther″mo-jen′ik) producing heat.

thermogenics (ther″mo-jen′iks) the science relating to heat production.

thermogenous (ther-moj′ĕ-nus) caused by elevation of temperature, or by heat.

thermogram (ther′mo-gram) 1. a graphic record of variations in temperature (heat). 2. the visual record obtained by thermography.

thermograph (ther′mo-graf) 1. an instrument for recording variations in temperature (heat). 2. a thermogram (def. 2). 3. the apparatus or device employed in thermography. **continuous scan t.,** a thermograph that presents a continuous scan image of the thermal pattern (thermogram) of a patient or object on cathode ray tube.

thermographic (ther″mo-graf′ik) pertaining to a thermogram or to thermography.

thermography (ther-mog′rah-fe) [*thermo-* + Gr. *graphein* to write] a technique wherein an infrared camera is used to photographically portray the surface temperatures of the body, based on the self-emanating infrared radiation; sometimes employed as a means of diagnosing underlying pathologic processes, such as breast tumors.

thermogravimeter (ther″mo-grah-vim′ĕ-ter) an analytical instrument for measuring change in mass of a substance at changing temperature.

thermohyperalgesia (ther″mo-hi″per-al-je′ze-ah) a condition in which the application of moderate heat causes extreme pain.

thermohyperesthesia (ther″mo-hi″per-es-the′ze-ah) extreme sensitiveness to high temperatures.

thermohypesthesia (ther″mo-hi″pes-the′ze-ah) a state of diminished sensitiveness to high temperatures.

thermohypoesthesia (ther″mo-hi″po-es-the′ze-ah) thermohypesthesia.

thermoinactivation (ther″mo-in-ak″tĭ-va′shun) destruction of the power to act by exposure to heat.

thermoinhibitory (ther″mo-in-hib′ĭ-tor″e) inhibiting or retarding the production of bodily heat.

thermointegrator (ther″mo-in″te-gra′tor) an apparatus for recording environmental warmth.

thermolabile (ther″mo-la′bil) easily altered or decomposed by heat; called also *heat labile*.

thermolamp (ther'mo-lamp) [thermo- + Gr. lampē torch] a lamp for heating.

thermology (ther-mol'o-je) [thermo- + -logy] the science of heat.

thermoluminescence (ther"mo-lu-mĭ-nes'ens) the production of light by a substance when its temperature is increased.

thermolysis (ther-mol'ĭ-sis) [thermo- + Gr. lysis dissolution] 1. chemical dissociation by means of heat. 2. the dissipation of bodily heat by means of radiation, evaporation, etc.

thermolytic (ther"mo-lit'ik) [thermo- + Gr. lytikos dissolving] pertaining to, characterized by, or promoting thermolysis.

thermomassage (ther"mo-mah-sahzh') massage with heat.

thermomastography (ther"mo-mas-tog'rah-fe) the use of thermography in the diagnosis of lesions of the breast.

thermometer (ther-mom'ĕ-ter) [thermo- + Gr. metron measure] an instrument for determining temperatures. In principle, it makes use of some substance with a physical property that varies in magnitude with temperature, to determine a value of temperature on some defined scale. See also under *scale*. **air t.,** one in which the expansible material is air. **alcohol t.,** a liquid-in-glass thermometer in which alcohol is the liquid used. **axilla t.,** a surface thermometer to be used in the axilla. **Beckmann t.,** a thermometer with a large bulb and fine bore stem for measurement of small differences in temperature. **bimetal t.,** one made of two metals of dissimilar temperature coefficients of expansion so bonded together that a change in temperature causes it to curl. **Celsius t.,** a thermometer employing the Celsius scale (q.v.). **centigrade t.,** one employing the Celsius scale (q.v.), that is, having the interval between the two established reference points divided into 100 units. **clinical t.,** one for use in determining temperature of the human body. **depth t.,** a thermometer whose sensitive element may be introduced into the tissues, for registering the actual temperature of a tissue. **differential t.,** one for measuring small differences in temperature. **Fahrenheit t.,** a thermometer employing the Fahrenheit scale (q.v.). **fever t.,** clinical t. **gas t.,** one in which the expansible material is a gas, such as air, carbon dioxide, helium, neon, nitrogen, or oxygen. **half-minute t.,** a clinical thermometer with a short time lag. **kata t.,** see *katathermometer*. **Kelvin t.,** a thermometer employing the Kelvin scale (q.v.). **liquid-in-glass t.,** the common type of thermometer, containing a liquid which expands with increase in temperature; most of the liquid is in a bulb, but its free surface is in a capillary tube graduated to indicate the degree of temperature causing expansion to each particular point. **maximum t.,** one which registers the highest temperature to which it has been exposed. **mercurial t.,** a liquid-in-glass thermometer in which mercury is the liquid used. **metallic t.,** one in which some solid metal is used as the expansible element. **metastatic t.,** one which indicates minute changes of temperature. **minimum t.,** one which registers the lowest temperature to which it has been exposed. **oral t.,** a clinical thermometer which is placed under the tongue, to record the temperature in the mouth; characteristically the bulb containing the mercury is elongated. **Rankine t.,** a thermometer employing the Rankine scale (q.v.). **Réaumur t.,** a thermometer employing the Réaumur scale (q.v.). **recording t.,** a temperature-sensitive instrument by which the temperature to which it has been exposed is continuously recorded on a specially designed chart. **rectal t.,** a clinical thermometer which is inserted in the rectum, for determining body temperature; characteristically the bulb containing the mercury is pear shaped. **resistance t.,** a thermometer which uses the electric resistance of metals for determining temperature; it consists of a resistance bulb of platinum or other metal wire, and uses a Wheatstone bridge. **self-registering t.,** recording t. **surface t.,** a clinical thermometer for determining the temperature on the surface of the body. **thermocouple t.,** a combination of a thermocouple with some device for measuring its electromotive force, such as a potentiometer; in use the thermocouple's reference junction is kept at a reference temperature (such as the ice point) and its measuring junction at the temperature being measured.

thermometric (ther"mo-met'rik) pertaining to a thermometer or to the measurement of degrees of temperature.

thermometry (ther-mom'ĕ-tre) the measurement of temperatures.

Thermomicrobium (ther"mo-mi-kro'be-um) [thermo- + micro- + bios] a genus of gram-negative, aerobic, rod-shaped bacteria of uncertain affiliation, made up of nonmotile cells with an optimal growth temperature of 70° to 75° C, occurring in hot springs. The type species is *T. ro'seum*.

Thermomonospora (ther"mo-mo-nos'pōr-ah) [thermo- + Gr. monas unit, from monos single + spora seed] a genus of bacteria of the family Micromonosporaceae, order Actinomycetales, consisting of thermophilic organisms found in soil, hay, and manure, that form single spores on an aerial mycelium. The type species is *T. curva'ta*.

thermoneurosis (ther"mo-nu-ro'sis) pyrexia of vasomotor origin.

thermonuclear (ther"mo-nu'kle-or) of, pertaining to, or derived from nuclear reactions (e.g., the fusion of hydrogen nuclei) in which the energy required for the reaction is in the form of extraordinarily high temperatures.

thermopalpation (ther"mo-pal-pa'shun) palpation for the purpose of determining differences of temperature at different portions of the body.

thermopenetration (ther"mo-pen"ĕ-tra'shun) application of currents of low tension and high amperage, which produce warmth in the deeper parts of the body; medical diathermy.

thermophile (ther'mo-fīl) 1. an organism that grows best at elevated temperatures. 2. a bacterium with an optimal growth temperature of 50° to 70° C.

thermophilic (ther"mo-fil'ik) [thermo- + Gr. philein to love] growing best at or having a fondness for high temperatures. Cf. *mesophilic* and *psychrophilic*.

thermophore (ther'mo-fōr) [thermo- + Gr. pherein to bear] 1. a device or apparatus for retaining heat. 2. an instrument for estimating heat sensibility.

thermopile (ther'mo-pīl) [thermo + L. pila pillar, pile] a number of thermocouples in series; used to increase the sensitivity for a temperature-measuring device, or for the direct conversion of heat into electric energy.

thermoplacentography (ther"mo-plas"en-tog'rah-fe) the use of thermography for determining the site of placental attachment.

Thermoplasma (ther"mo-plaz'mah) [thermo- + plasma] a genus of bacteria of the order Mycoplasmatales. The organisms are saprophytes found in burning coal refuse and in acid hot springs. They differ in many important respects from other members of the order, and are generally considered to be one of the archaeobacteria.

thermoplastic (ther"mo-plas'tik) softening under heat and capable of being molded into shape with pressure, then hardening on cooling without undergoing chemical change.

thermoplegia (ther"mo-ple'je-ah) [thermo- + Gr. plēgē stroke + -ia] heat stroke or sunstroke (thermic fever).

thermopolypnea (ther"mo-pol"ip-ne'ah) [thermo- + Gr. polys many + pnoia breath] a quickening of the respiration due to great heat or high temperature.

thermopolypneic (ther"mo-pol"ip-ne'ik) pertaining to or characterized by the thermopolypnea.

thermoprecipitation (ther"mo-pre-sip"ĭ-ta'shun) precipitation by heat.

thermoradiotherapy (ther"mo-ra"de-o-ther'ah-pe) application of ionizing radiation to an anatomical site whose tissue-temperature has been elevated by artificial means on the theory of increasing its radiosensitivity.

thermoreceptor (ther"mo-re-sep'tor) a nerve ending that is sensitive to stimulation by heat.

thermoregulation (ther"mo-reg'u-la'shun) heat regulation.

thermoregulator (ther"mo-reg'u-la"tor) 1. controlling or regulating heat. 2. thermostat.

thermoresistance (ther"mo-re-zis'tans) the quality of being little affected by heat.

thermoresistant (ther"mo-re-zis'tant) not greatly affected by heat.

thermoscope (ther'mo-skōp) [thermo- + Gr. skopein to examine] a differential thermometer.

thermostabile (ther″mo-sta′bil) unaffected by heat; able to withstand the effects of heat without undergoing change; in immunology, the term usually refers to substances that are not inactivated by heating to 56°C for 30 minutes, which inactivates complement. Called also *heat stable.*

thermostability (ther″mo-stah-bil′ĭ-te) the quality of withstanding the effects of heat without undergoing change.

thermostasis (ther″mo-sta′sis) [*thermo-* + Gr. *stasis* a placing, setting] the maintenance of body temperature in warm-blooded animals.

thermostat (ther′mo-stat) [*thermo-* + Gr. *histanai* to halt] a device interposed in a heating system by which the temperature can be automatically maintained between certain levels. **hypothalamic t.,** the mechanism for control of body temperature, which involves two thermoregulatory centers of the hypothalamus: the preoptic area of the anterior hypothalamus, which senses core temperature and compares it to the set-point, and an area in the posterior hypothalamus that integrates signals from the preoptic area and from cold and warmth receptors in the skin and controls mechanisms of heat dissipation (skin vasodilation, sweating) and production and conservation (skin vasoconstriction, release of epinephrine and thyroid hormones, sympathetic stimulation).

thermosteresis (ther″mo-stĕ-re′sis) [*thermo-* + Gr. *sterēsis* deprivation] the deprivation of heat.

thermostromuhr (ther″mo-strŏm′oor) an instrument for measuring the amount of blood flowing in a blood vessel.

thermosystaltic (ther″mo-sis-tal′tik) [*thermo-* + Gr. *systellein* to contract] contracting under the influence or stimulus of heat; pertaining to thermosystaltism.

thermosystaltism (ther″mo-sis′tal-tizm) [*thermo-* + Gr. *systellein* to contract] muscular contraction in response to temperature changes.

thermotactic (ther″mo-tak′tik) pertaining to thermotaxis.

thermotaxic (ther″mo-tak′sik) thermotactic.

thermotaxis (ther″mo-tak′sis) [*thermo-* + Gr. *taxis* arrangement] 1. the normal adjustment of the bodily temperature. 2. taxis in response to an increase in temperature.

thermotherapy (ther″mo-ther′ah-pe) [*thermo-* + Gr. *therapeia* treatment] treatment of disease by the application of heat.

thermotics (ther-mot′iks) the science of heat.

thermotolerant (ther″mo-tol′er-ant) enduring heat; said of bacteria whose activity is not checked by high temperature.

thermotonometer (ther″mo-to-nom′ĕ-ter) [*thermo-* + Gr. *tonos* tension + *metron* measure] an instrument for measuring the amount of muscular contraction caused by heat.

thermotropic (ther″mo-tro′pik) pertaining to or exhibiting thermotropism; called also *caloritropic.*

thermotropism (ther-mot′ro-pizm) [*thermo-* + Gr. *tropē* turn] tropism of an organism in response to an increase in temperature.

Thermus (ther′mus) [Gr. "hot"] a genus of gram-negative, aerobic, rod-shaped and filamentous bacteria of uncertain affiliation, made up of nonmotile cells producing yellow to bright orange pigments, with a temperature optimum of 70° to 72° C. They are found in hot springs and waters, and thermally polluted rivers. The type species is *T. aqua′ticus.*

theroid (the′roid) [Gr. *thēriōdēs* beast-like] resembling an animal of a lower order.

theromorph (the′ro-morf) [Gr. *thēr* wild beast + *morphē* form] a morphologic part of an organism or individual with supernumerary, teratic, or absent parts, giving it a resemblance to a lower animal.

theromorphism (the″ro-mor′fizm) the abnormal resemblance of some part of the organism to the normal structure of the corresponding part of an animal of lower type.

Theromyzon (ther-o′mĭ-zon) a genus of leeches of the family Gnathobdellidae.

theront (the′ront) [Gr. *thēr* wild beast + *on, ontos* being] the free-swimming stage or form in the life cycle of certain ciliate protozoa that arises from a tomite and searches ("hunts") for a new host or food source necessary for the development into the trophont.

thesaurismosis (the-saw″riz-mo′sis) [Gr. *thēsauros* treasure] an obsolete term for storage disease (q.v.). **amyloid t.,** amyloidosis. **calcium t.,** calcinosis. **cholesterol t.,** Hand-Schüller-Christian disease. **lipoid t.,** lipoidosis. **urate t.,** gout. **water t.,** edema.

thesaurosis (the″saw-ro′sis) an obsolete term for storage disease (q.v.).

Thessalus (thes′ah-lus) **of Cos** (4th century B.C.) a Greek physician; the son of Hippocrates, whose teachings he followed.

Thessalus (thes′ah-lus) **of Tralles** (1st century A.D.) a Greek physician of the Methodist school and a pupil of Themison.

theta (tha′tah) [Θ, θ] the eighth letter of the Greek alphabet.

Θ the Greek capital letter theta.

θ theta, the eighth letter of the Greek alphabet.

thiabendazole (thi″ah-ben′dah-zōl) [USP] chemical name: 2-(4-thiazolyl)-1*H*-benzimidazole. a broad-spectrum anthelmintic, $C_{10}H_7N_3S$, with vermicidal activity against roundworm, pinworm, threadworm, whipworm, and hookworm; used in the treatment of enterobiasis, strongyloidiasis, ascariasis, uncinariasis, trichuriasus, and creeping larva migrans; it is most commonly used for *Strongyloides stercoralis* and *Trichostrongylus* spp. infections.

thiacetazone (thi-ah-set′ah-zōn) chemical name: *N*-[4-[[(aminothioxomethyl)hydrazono]methylene]phenyl]acetamide; an antibacterial, $C_{10}H_{12}N_3OS$, with tuberculostatic and antileprotic properties. Called also *amithiozone.*

thiadiazide, thiadiazine (thi″ah-di′ah-zīd; thi″ah-di′ah-zēn) thiazide.

thiamazole (thi-am′ah-zōl) methimazole.

thiamin (thi′ah-min) thiamine.

thiaminase (thi-am′ĭ-nās) [EC 3.5.99.2] 1. an enzyme of the hydrolase class that catalyzes the reaction thiamine + H_2O = 2-methyl-4-amino-5- hydroxymethyl-pyrimidine + 4-methyl-5-(2-hydroxyethyl)-thiazole, present in intestinal microorganisms. Called also *thiaminase II.* 2. thiamin pyridinylase.

thiamine (thi′ah-min) 3-[(4-amino-2-methyl-5-pyrimidinyl)methyl]-5-(2-hydroxyethy)-4-methylthiazolium. A water-soluble component of the B complex of vitamins, first isolated in 1926; present in beans, green vegetables, sweet corn, egg yolk, liver, corn meal, and brown rice, and found in blood plasma and cerebrospinal fluid in the free state. Its active form is thiamine pyrophosphate (q.v.). Deficiency of this vitamin results in beriberi. Called also *vitamin B₁* and also written *thiamin.* See also *phosphorylated t.* **t. hydrochloride** [USP], the monohydrochloride salt of thiamine, $C_{12}H_{17}ClN_4OS·HCl$, occurring as white crystals or crystalline powder; administered orally and intramuscularly for the prophylaxis and treatment of thiamine deficiency states. **t. mononitrate** [USP], the mononitrate salt of thiamine, $C_{12}H_{17}N_5O_4S$, occurring as white crystals or crystalline powder; used in the preparation of various multivitamin dosage forms. **phosphorylated t., t. pyrophosphate,** the active form of thiamine, which serves as a coenzyme in reactions involving oxidative decarboxylation of certain important intermediates in carbohydrate metabolism. Called also *cocarboxylase.*

thiamin pyridinylase (thi′ah-min pir-ĭ-dīn′il-ās) [EC 2.5.1.2] an enzyme catalyzing the reaction thiamine + acceptor = 2-methyl-4-amino-5-(methylene-acceptor)-pyrimidine + 4-methyl-5-(2-hydroxyethyl)thiazole. The enzyme occurs in the gastrointestinal tract of many fresh water animals and was responsible for thiamine deficiency in captive foxes and minks fed fish. Also called *thiaminase I.*

thiamphenicol (thi-am-fen′ĭ-kōl) chemical name: [*R*-(*R**, *R**)]-2,2-dichloro-*N*-[2-hydroxy-1-(hydroxymethyl)-2-[4-(methylsulfonyl)phenyl]ethyl]acetamide. A broad-spectrum antibacterial, $C_{12}H_{15}Cl_2NO_5S$, effective against a wide range of gram-positive and gram-negative organisms.

thiamylal sodium (thi-am′ĭ-lal) chemical name: dihydro-5-(1-methylbutyl)-5-(2-propenyl)-2-thioxo-4,6-(1*H*,5*H*)-pyrimidinedione monosodium salt. A very short-acting barbiturate, $C_{12}H_{17}N_2NaO_2S$. A preparation suitable for injection [NF] is administered intravenously to produce general anesthesia of brief duration, for induction of anesthesia, to supplement other anesthetics, or to induce hypnosis.

Thiara (thi-ah′rah) a genus of widely distributed, freshwater snails (family Meloniidae), species of which, such as *T.*

granifera and *T. tuberculata*, act as the main snail hosts of various trematode parasites, including *Paragonimus, Metagonimus,* and *Haplorchis.*

thiasine (thi′ah-sin) ergothioneine.

thiazide (thi′ah-zīd) any of a group of benzothiadiazenesulfonamide derivatives, typified by chlorothiazide, that act as diuretics by inhibiting the reabsorption of sodium in the proximal renal tubule and stimulating chloride excretion, with resultant increase in excretion of water. They also increase the excretion of potassium, which can cause hypokalemia requiring potassium supplementation, and some increase in bicarbonate excretion. Thiazides are used for the treatment of edema due to congestive heart failure or chronic hepatic or renal disease and, alone or in combination with other drugs, in the treatment of hypertension. Called also *benzothiadiazide, benzothiadiazine, thiadiazide,* and *thiadiazine.*

-thiazide a suffix indicating a thiazide diuretic.

thiazole (thi′ah-zōl) the chemical ring:

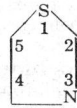

Thiele's syndrome (thēlz) [George Henry *Thiele*, American proctologist, born 1896] see under *syndrome.*

thiemia (thi-e′me-ah) [Gr. *theion* sulfur + *haima* blood + *-ia*] an excess of sulfur in the blood.

Thiersch's graft operation (tērsh′ez) [Karl *Thiersch*, German surgeon, 1822–1895] see *Ollier-Thiersch graft,* under *graft,* and see under *operation.*

thiethylperazine (thi-eth″il-per′ah-zēn) chemical name: 2-(ethylthio)-10-[3-(4-methyl-1-piperazinyl)propyl]phenothiazine. A phenothiazine derivative, $C_{22}H_{29}N_3S_2$. **t. malate** [USP], a slightly yellow, voluminous powder, having the same actions and uses as the maleate salt; administered by intramuscular injection. **t. maleate** [USP], the maleate salt of thiethylperazine, $C_{22}H_{29}N_3S_2 \cdot 2C_4H_4O_4$, occurring as a white to faintly yellow, crystalline powder; used as an antiemetic. It is useful in reducing nausea and vomiting associated with the use of general anesthesia and that following the use of radiation and mustard therapy and is possibly effective in the treatment of vertigo; administered orally or rectally.

thigh (thi) the portion of the lower extremity situated between the hip above and the knee below; called also *femur.* **cricket t.,** rupture of some of the fibers of the rectus femoris, which may occur in playing cricket or football; sometimes the tendon of the quadriceps or that of the patella is also ruptured. **drivers' t.,** sciatic neuralgia caused by pressure from the use of the accelerator in driving an automobile. **Heilbronner's t.,** broadening and flattening of the thigh; seen in cases of organic paralysis when the patient lies on his back on a hard mattress; it does not appear in hysterical paralysis.

thigmesthesia (thig″mes-the′ze-ah) [Gr. *thigma* touch + *aisthēsis* perception + *-ia*] tactile sensibility.

thigm(o)- [Gr. *thigma* touch] a combining form denoting relationship to touch or physical contact.

thigmotactic (thig″mo-tak′tik) pertaining to, characterized by, or causing thigmotaxis.

thigmotaxis (thig″mo-tak′sis) [thigmo- + taxis] taxis of an organism in response to the stimulus of contact or touch; called also *stereotaxis.*

Thigmotrichina (thig″mo-tri-ki′nah) [thigmo- + Gr. *thrix* hair] a suborder of usually heavily ciliated and laterally compressed, parasitic protozoa (order Scuticociliatida, subclass Hymenostomatia), characterized by the presence of a prominent thigmotactic region, typically located anteriorly, and a cytosome often at or near the posterior end; a prominent sucker at the anterior end occurs in some species, and the posterior segment of the paroral membrane may be indistinct.

thigmotropic (thig″mo-trop′ik) pertaining to or exhibiting thigmotropism; responding to the stimulus of contact or touch; called also *stereotropic.*

thigmotropism (thig-mot′ro-pizm) [thigmo- + tropism] tropism of an organism elicited by touch or direct contact with a solid or rigid surface; called also *stereotropism.*

thihexinol methylbromide (thi-hek′sĭ-nōl) chemical name: α-[4-(diethylamino)cyclohexyl]-α-2-thienyl-2-thiophene methanol methyl bromide. An anticholinergic, $C_{18}H_{26}BrNOS_2$, claimed to inhibit intestinal hypermotility.

thimble (thim′b'l) coping.

thimerosal (thi-mer′o-sal) [USP] chemical name: ethyl(2-mercaptobenzoato-S)mercury sodium salt. An organomercurial antiseptic, $C_9H_9HgNaO_2S$, occurring as a light cream-colored, crystalline powder, which is actively antifungal and bacteriostatic for many nonsporulating bacteria; used as a topical anti-infective and as a preservative in pharmaceutical preparations. Called also *thiomersalate.*

thimethaphan camphorsulfonate (thi-meth′ah-fan) trimethaphan camsylate.

thinking (thingk′ing) ideational mental activity (in contrast to emotional activity); the flow of ideas, symbols, and associations that brings forth concepts and reasons. **autistic t.,** autism (def. 1). **dereistic t.,** dereism.

thi(o)- [Gr. *theion* sulfur] a prefix denoting the presence of sulfur. In systematic chemical nomenclature, it indicates the replacement of oxygen by sulfur as in thiophosphoric acid (H_3PSO_3) or ethanethio (CH_3CH_2SH).

thio-acid (thi′′o-as′id) an organic compound produced by replacement of one of the oxygens of the carboxyl group by divalent sulfur.

thioalbumose (thi′′o-al′bu-mōs) an albumose that has a large sulfur content.

thioalcohol (thi′′o-al′ko-hol) mercaptan.

thioarsenite (thi′′o-ar′se-nīt) any compound of sulfur and arsenic of the type K_3AsS_3.

Thiobacillus (thi′′o-bah-sil′us) [thio- + L. *bacillus* little rod] a genus of gram-negative chemolithotrophic bacteria of uncertain affiliation, occurring as small, rod-shaped cells that oxidize sulfur compounds. The organisms are found in soil and waters near sulfur deposits. The type species is *T. thio′parus.*

Thiobacteriaceae (thi′′o-bak-te′′re-a′se-e) in former systems of classification, a family of gram-negative chemolithotrophic bacteria that oxidize sulfur compounds. It included the genera *Thiobacillus, Thiobacterium, Thiospira,* and *Thiovulum.*

Thiobacterium (thi′′o-bak-te′re-um) [thio- + Gr. *baktērion* little rod] a genus of gram-negative chemolithotrophic bacteria of uncertain affiliation, occurring as rod-shaped cells that oxidize sulfur compounds and deposit free sulfur droplets inside the cells. They are found in sulfurous brackish and marine waters. The type species is *T. bovis′ta.*

thiobarbital (thi′′o-bar′bĭ-tal) chemical name: 5,5-diethyl-2-thio-barbituric acid. A salt of thiobarbituric acid, $C_8H_{12}N_2O_2S$, used as a thyroid depressant.

thiobarbiturate (thi′′o-bar-bit′u-rāt) a salt or derivative of thiobarbituric acid.

thiobarbituric acid (thi′′o-bahr′′bĭ-tu′rik) a condensation of malonic acid and thiourea, $C_6H_4N_2O_2S$, differing from barbituric acid only by the presence of a sulfur atom instead of an oxygen atom at the number 2 carbon; it is the parent compound of a class of drugs, thiobarbiturates. Thiobarbiturates and barbiturates are analogous in their effects.

Thiocapsa (thi′′o-kap′sah) [thio- + L. *capsa* box] a genus of aquatic phototrophic bacteria of the family Chromatiaceae, order Rhodospirillales, consisting of spherical nonmotile cells that do not contain gas vacuoles. The organisms fix carbon dioxide in the presence of hydrogen sulfide. Cell suspensions are orange-brown to pink and purple. The type species is *T. roseopersici′na.*

thiocarbamide (thi′′o-kar′bah-mīd) thiourea.

thiochrome (thi′′o-krōm) the fluorescent yellow coloring matter of yeast, $C_{12}H_{14}ON_4S$, resulting from the oxidation of thiamine.

thioctic acid (thi-ok′tic) lipoic acid.

thiocyanate (thi′′o-si′ah-nāt) 1. the $S=C=N^-$ anion or a salt containing this ion. Thiocyanate is produced in the metabolism of cysteine and detoxification of cyanide and is excreted in the urine. 2. an ester $R—S=C=N$, of thiocyanic acid.

thiocyanic acid (thi″o-si-an′ik) the molecular species H—S=C=N; aqueous solutions are an equilibrium mixture of thiocyanic and isothiocyanic acid and are very strong acids. Called also *sulfocyanic acid.*

thiocyanide (thi″o-si′ah-nīd) thiocyanate (1).

Thiocystis (thi″o-sis′tis) [*thio-* + Gr. *kystis* sac, bladder] a genus of aquatic, phototrophic bacteria of the family Chromatiaceae, order Rhodospirillales, consisting of spherical motile cells that do not contain gas vacuoles. The organisms fix carbon dioxide in the presence of hydrogen sulfide. Cell suspensions are brown to purple. The type species is *T. viola′cea.* Called also *Thiothece.*

Thiodendron (thi″o-den′dron) [*thio-* + Gr. *dendron* tree] a genus of appendaged bacteria found in water and mud, made up of vibrio-shaped cells that produce thin stalks at one or both ends and require hydrogen sulfide for growth. The type species is *T. la′tens.*

Thioderma (thi″o-der′mah) [*thio-* + Gr. *derma* skin] a name formerly given a genus of sulfur bacteria.

Thiodictyon (thi″o-dik′te-on) [*thio-* + Gr. *diktyon* net] a genus of aquatic phototrophic bacteria of the family Chromatiaceae, order Rhodospirillales, consisting of rod-shaped nonmotile cells that contain gas vacuoles and fix carbon dioxide in the presence of hydrogen sulfide. Cell suspensions are purple to violet. The type species is *T. e′legans.*

thiodiphenylamine (thi″o-di-fen″il-am′in) phenothiazine.

thiodotherapy (thi″o-do-ther′ah-pe) [*thio-* + *iodine* + *therapy*] combined sulfur and iodine therapy.

thioether (thi″o-e′ther) a sulfur ether; an ether in which sulfur replaces oxygen.

thioethylamine (thi″o-eth″il-am′in) an amine, SH(CH₂)₂-NH₂, formed from cysteine by the loss of CO₂.

thioflavine (thi″o-fla′vin) [*thio-* + *flavine*] a yellow dye, methyl dehydrothio-*p*-toluidine sulfonate.

thiogenic (thi″o-jen′ik) [*thio-* + Gr. *gennan* to produce] able to convert hydrogen sulfide into higher sulfur compounds.

thioglucose (thi″o-glu′kōs) a synthetic glucose that contains a sulfhydryl group which replaces the oxygen in the aldehyde group.

thioguanine (thi″o-gwah′nēn) [USP] chemical name: 2-amino-1,7-dihydro-6*H*-purine-6-thione. An antineoplastic derived from mercaptopurine, C₅H₅N₅S·xH₂O, occurring as a pale yellow, crystalline powder; used in the treatment of acute leukemia, administered orally.

thiokinase (thi″o-ki′nās) [EC 6.2.1] any enzyme of the ligase class that catalyzes the joining of an acid and a thiol (—SH) group coupled with the cleavage of a pyrophosphate bond in ATP or a similar triphosphate, such as enzymes synthesizing acyl-CoA derivatives.

thiol (thi′ol) 1. sulfhydryl. 2. any organic compound containing the —SH group; the analogue of an alcohol, which contains the —OH group.

thiolase (thi′o-lās) an enzyme that cleaves a carbon-carbon bond of a thiol compound to form a thiolester. See *acetyl-CoA acetyltransferase, acetyl-CoA acyltransferase.*

thiolhistidine (thi″ol-his′tĭ-din) the sulfur derivative of histidine occurring in the betaine form as ergothioneine.

thiomersalate (thi″o-mer′sah-lāt) thimerosal.

thioneine (thi″o-ne′in) [Gr. *theion* sulfur + *neos* new] ergothioneine.

thionic (thi-on′ik) 1. pertaining to sulfur. 2. see under *acid.*

thionin (thi′o-nin) a dark-green powder, NH₂·C₆H₃(NS)··C₆H₃·NH₂, giving a purple color in solution, and used as a metachromatic stain in microscopy. Called also *Lauth's violet.*

thionyl (thi′o-nil) the radical SO.

thiopanic acid (thi″o-pan′ik) pantoyltaurine.

thiopectic (thi″o-pek′tik) fixing sulfur.

Thiopedia (thi″o-pe′de-ah) [*thio-* + Gr. *pedion* a plain] a genus of aquatic phototrophic bacteria of the family Chromatiaceae, order Rhodospirillales, consisting of spherical to ovoid nonmotile cells that contain gas vacuoles and fix carbon dioxide in the presence of hydrogen sulfide. All suspensions are pink to purple. The type species is *T. ro′sea.*

thiopental sodium (thi″o-pen′tal) [USP] chemical name: 5-ethyldihydro-5-(1-methylbutyl)-2-thioxo-4,6(1*H*,5*H*)pyrimidinedione monosodium salt. An ultra–short-acting barbiturate, C₁₁H₁₇N₂NaO₂S, occurring as a white to off-white, crystalline powder, or yellowish, hygroscopic powder; administered intravenously to produce general anesthesia of brief duration, for induction of anesthesia prior to administration of other anesthetics, to supplement regional anesthesia, as an anticonvulsive, and for narcoanalysis and narcosynthesis in psychiatric disorders.

thiopentone (thi″o-pen′tōn) thiopental.

thiopexic (thi″o-pek′sik) thiopectic.

thiopexy (thi″o-pek′se) [*thio-* + Gr. *pēxis* fixation] the fixation of sulfur.

Thioploca (thi″o-plo′kah) [*thio-* + Gr. *plokē* anything twisted] a genus of gliding bacteria of the family Beggiatoaceae, order Cytophagales, found in mud, made up of numerous flexible segments in braided filaments, generally with sulfur inclusions. The type species is *T. schmid′lei.*

Thiopolycoccus (thi″o-pol″e-kok′us) [*thio-* + Gr. *polys* many + *kokkos* berry] a genus of sulfur bacteria of uncertain affiliation, probably belonging to the genus *Thiocapsa* or *Thiocystis.*

thiopropazate hydrochloride (thi″o-pro′pah-zāt) chemical name: 4-[3-(2-chlorophenothiazine-10-yl)propyl]-1-piperazineethanol acetate dihydrochloride. A phenothiazine tranquilizer, C₂₃H₂₈ClN₃O₂·2HCl, occurring as a white, crystalline powder; used in the treatment of psychoses and to suppress involuntary muscular activity in Huntington's chorea, administered orally.

Thiorhodaceae (thi″o-ro-da′se-e) Chromatiaceae.

thioridazine hydrochloride (thi″o-rid′ah-zēn) [USP] chemical name: 10-[2-(1-methyl-2-piperidyl)ethyl]-2-(methylthio)phenothiazine monohydrochloride. A tranquilizer, with sedative and behavioral effects, C₂₁H₂₆N₂S₂·HCl, occurring as a white to slightly yellow, granular powder; administered orally.

Thiosarcina (thi″o-sar-si′nah) [*thio-* + L. *sarcina* package, bundle] a genus of aquatic phototrophic bacteria of the family Chromatiaceae, order Rhodospirillales, consisting of spherical to ovoid motile cells that do not contain gas vacuoles. The organisms fix carbon dioxide in the presence of hydrogen sulfide. Cell suspensions are purple to red. The type species is *T. ro′sea.*

thiosinamine (thi″o-sin′ah-min) a bitter, crystalline substance, (NH₂)CS·NHCH₂CH:CH₂, from oil of mustard and ammonia; it has been used to promote absorption of fibrous tissue. Called also *allyl thiocarbamide, allyl sulfocarbamide,* and *allyl thiourea.*

Thiospira (thi″o-spi′rah) [*thio-* + Gr. *speira* coil] a genus of gram-negative chemolithotrophic bacteria of uncertain affiliation, occurring as colorless, spiral-shaped cells that oxidize sulfur compounds and contain sulfur globules. They are found in sulfurous marine and brackish waters. The type species is *T. winograd′sky.*

Thiospirillopsis (thi″o-spi″ril-lop′sis) a genus of sulfur bacteria of uncertain status.

Thiospirillum (thi″o-spi-ril′lum) [thio- + L. *spirillum* dim. of *spira* coil] a genus of aquatic phototrophic bacteria of the family Chromatiaceae, order Rhodospirillales, consisting of spiral motile cells that do not contain gas vacuoles. The organisms fix carbon dioxide in the presence of hydrogen sulfide. Cell suspensions are brown to purple. The type species is *T. sangui′neum.*

thiosulfate (thi″o-sul′fāt) the SSO₃²⁻ anion or a salt containing this ion. Thiosulfate is produced in the metabolism of cysteine and excreted in the urine. It has also been used as a tracer for measuring extracellular fluid volume and is a commonly used reducing agent in laboratory chemistry and photography. Called also *hyposulfite.* See also *sodium thiosulfate.*

Thiosulfil (thi″o-sul′fil) trademark for preparations of sulfamethizole.

thiosulfuric acid (thi″o-sul-fūr′ik) the molecular species H₂S₂O₃.

thiotepa (thi″o-tep′ah) [USP] chemical name: 1,1′,1″-phosphinothioylidynetris-azeridine. A cytotoxic alkylating agent of the ethylenimine group, used as an antineoplastic; now largely supplanted by cyclophosphamide and other nitrogen mustards; it is still used by intracavitary administration for malignant pleural or pericardial effusions. Called also *triethylenethiophosphoramide* (TEPA).

Thiothece (thi″o-the′se) *Thiocystis.*

thiothixene (thi″o-thiks′ēn) [USP] chemical name: (Z)-N, N-dimethyl-9-[3-(4-methyl-1-piperazinyl) propylidene]-9H-thioxanthene-2-sulfonamide. An antipsychotic, $C_{23}H_{29}N_3O_2$-S_2, occurring as white to tan crystals; administered orally. **t. hydrochloride** [USP], the dihydrate dihydrochloride salt of thiothixene, $C_{23}H_{29}N_3O_2S_2 \cdot 2HCl \cdot 2H_2O$, occurring as a white, or nearly white, crystalline powder, having the same uses as the base; administered orally and intramuscularly.

Thiothrix (thi′o-thriks) [*thio-* + Gr. *thrix* hair] a genus of gliding bacteria of the family Leucotrichaceae, order Cytophagales, found attached to solid substrates in water, made up of short, colorless cells growing in long filaments, containing sulfur granules. The type species is *T. ni′vea.*

thiouracil (thi″o-u′rah-sil) chemical name: 2-mercapto-4-hydroxypyrimidine. A thiourea derivative, $C_4H_4N_2OS$, which affects adversely the synthesis of the thyroid hormones. It has been used as an antithyroid agent in hyperthyroidism, and in angina pectoris and congestive heart failure.

thiourea (thi″o-u′re-ah) urea in which the oxygen is replaced by sulfur, H_2HCSNH_2; it inhibits the function of the thyroid gland, and was formerly used as an antithyroid agent. Called also *thiocarbamide.*

Thiovulum (thi-o′vu-lum) [*thio-* + L. *ovum* egg] a genus of gram-negative chemolithotrophic bacteria of uncertain affiliation, occurring as round to ovoid cells that oxidize sulfur compounds and deposit sulfur inclusions inside the cell. They are found in fresh and marine waters at the interface of sulfur- and oxygen-bearing layers. The type species is *T. ma′jus.*

thioxanthene (thi″o-zan′thēn) any of a class of structurally related antipsychotic agents that includes thiothixene and chlorprothixene.

thiozine (thi′o-zin) ergothioneine.

thiphenamil hydrochloride (thi-fen′ah-mil) chemical name: α-phenylbenzene ethanethioic acid S-[2-(diethylamino)ethyl]ester hydrochloride. An anticholinergic, $C_{20}H_{26}$-ClNOS, having potent antispasmodic and smooth muscle relaxant properties; used to relieve pain and discomfort due to smooth muscle spasm associated with gastrointestinal disorders, administered orally.

thiram (thi′ram) chemical name: tetramethylthioperoxydicarbonic diamide; a topical antifungal, $C_6H_{12}N_2S_4$.

thirst (therst) [L. *sitis*, Gr. *dipsa*] a sensation, often referred to the mouth and throat, associated with a craving for drink; ordinarily interpreted as a desire for water. **insensible t.**, subliminal t. **real t.**, true t. **subliminal t.**, a sensation of need for water which is insufficient to prompt the ingestion of water but is at times sufficient to maintain drinking once it is initiated. **true t.**, thirst which is associated with a bodily need for water and is satisfied by the ingestion of water. **twilight t.**, subliminal t.

Thiry's fistula (thi′rēz) [Ludwig *Thiry*, Austrian physiologist, 1817–1897] see under *fistula.*

thixolabile (thik″so-la′bil) easily affected by shaking or stirring.

thixotropic (thik″so-trop′ik) pertaining to or characterized by thixotropy.

thixotropism (thik-sot′ro-pizm) thixotropy.

thixotropy (thik-sot′ro-pe) [Gr. *thixis* a touch + *tropos* a turning] the property, exhibited by certain gels, of becoming fluid when shaken or stirred, and then becoming semisolid again.

thlipsencephalus (thlip″sen-sef′ah-lus) [Gr. *thlipsis* pressure + *enkephalos* brain] a monster with a deficient skull, or with the upper part of the skull lacking.

Thoma's ampulla, fluid (to′mahz) [Richard *Thoma*, German histologist, 1847–1923] see under *ampulla* and *fluid.*

Thoma-Zeiss counting chamber (cell) (to′mah-zīs) [Richard *Thoma;* Carl *Zeiss*, German optician, 1816–1888] see under *chamber.*

Thomas' splint, test (tom′as) [Hugh Owen *Thomas*, orthopedic surgeon in Liverpool, 1834–1891] see under *splint* and *test.*

Thompson's test (tom′sonz) [Sir Henry *Thompson*, English surgeon, 1820–1904] two-glass test.

Thomsen's disease (tom′senz) [Asmus Julius Thomas *Thomsen*, Danish physician, 1815–1896] myotonia congenita.

Thomson's disease (tom′sons) [Mathew Sidney *Thomson*, English dermatologist, 1894–1969] see under *disease.*

Thomson scattering (tom′son) [Sir Joseph John *Thomson*, English physicist, 1856–1940] see under *scattering.*

Thomson's sign (tom′sunz) [Frederick Holland *Thomson*, British physician, 1867–1938] Pastia's lines.

thonzonium bromide (thon-zo′ni-um) chemical name: N-[2-[[(4-methoxyphenyl) methyl]-2-pyrimidinylamino] ethyl]-N, N-dimethyl-1-hexadecanaminium bromide; a cationic detergent, $C_{32}H_{55}BrN_4O.$

thonzylamine hydrochloride (thon-zil′ah-mĕn) chemical name: N-[(4-methoxyphenyl)methyl]-N′,N′-dimethyl-N-2-pyrimidinyl-1,2-ethanediamine monohydrochloride; an antihistaminic, $C_{16}H_{22}N_4O \cdot HCl.$

thoracal (tho′rah-kal) thoracic.

thoracalgia (tho″rah-kal′je-ah) pain in the chest wall.

thoracectomy (tho″rah-sek′to-me) [*thoraco-* + Gr. *ektomē* excision] thoracotomy with resection of a portion of a rib.

thoracentesis (tho″rah-sen-te′sis) [*thoraco-* + Gr. *kentēsis* puncture] surgical puncture of the chest wall into the parietal cavity for aspiration of fluids; called also *pleurocentesis* and *thoracocentesis.*

thoracic (tho-ras′ik) [L. *thoracicus;* Gr. *thōrakikos*] pertaining to or affecting the chest.

thoracicoabdominal (tho-ras″ĭ-ko-ab-dom′ĭ-nal) pertaining to the thorax and abdomen.

thoracicohumeral (tho-ras″ĭ-ko-hu′mer-al) pertaining to the thorax and the humerus.

thoracispinal (tho-ras″ĭ-spi′nal) pertaining to the thoracic portion of the spinal column.

thorac(o)- [Gr. *thōrax*, gen. *thōrakos* chest] a combining form denoting relationship to the chest.

thoracoabdominal (tho″rah-ko-ab-dom′ĭ-nal) pertaining to the thorax and the abdomen.

thoracoacromial (tho″rah-ko-ah-kro′me-al) pertaining to the chest and acromion.

thoracoceloschisis (tho″rah-ko-se-los′kĭ-sis) [*thoraco-* + Gr. *koilia* belly + *schisis* fissure] congenital fissure of the thorax and abdomen.

thoracocentesis (tho″rah-ko-sen-te′sis) thoracentesis.

thoracocyllosis (tho″rah-ko-si-lo′sis) [*thoraco-* + Gr. *kyllōsis* crippling] deformity of the chest.

thoracocyrtosis (tho″rah-ko-sir-to′sis) [*thoraco-* + Gr. *kyrtōsis* a being humpbacked] abnormal curvature of the thorax, or unusual prominence of the chest.

thoracodelphus (tho″rah-ko-del′fus) [*thoraco-* + Gr. *adelphos* brother] a double monster with one head, two arms, and four legs, the bodies being joined above the navel.

thoracodidymus (tho″rah-ko-did′ĭ-mus) [*thoraco-* + Gr. *didymos* twin] conjoined twins united at the thorax.

thoracodynia (tho″rah-ko-din′e-ah) [*thoraco-* + Gr. *odynē* pain] pain in the chest.

thoracogastrodidymus (tho″rah-ko-gas″tro-did′ĭ-mus) [*thoraco-* + Gr. *gastēr* belly + *didymos* twin] conjoined twins united at the belly and chest.

thoracogastroschisis (tho″rah-ko-gas-tros′kĭ-sis) [*thoraco-* + Gr. *gastēr* belly + *schisis* fissure] fissure of the thorax and abdomen.

thoracograph (tho-rak′o-graf) [*thoraco-* + Gr. *graphein* to write] thoracopneumograph.

thoracolaparotomy (tho″rah-ko-lap″ah-rot′o-me) [*thoraco-* + Gr. *lapara* loin + *tomē* a cutting] incision through both the thorax and abdomen to gain access to the subphrenic space and adjoining regions.

thoracolumbar (tho″rah-ko-lum′bar) pertaining to the thoracic and lumbar parts of the spine.

thoracolysis (tho″rah-kol′ĭ-sis) [*thoraco-* + Gr. *lysis* dissolution] the freeing of adhesions of the chest wall.

thoracomelus (tho″rah-kom′e-lus) [*thoraco-* + Gr. *melos* limb] a monster with a supernumerary arm or leg attached to the thorax.

thoracometer (tho″rah-kom′ĕ-ter) [*thoraco-* + Gr. *metron* measure] stethometer.

thoracometry (tho″rah-kom′ĕ-tre) measurement of the thorax.

thoracomyodynia (tho″rah-ko-mi″o-din′e-ah) [*thoraco-* + Gr. *mys* muscle + *odynē* pain] pain in the muscles of the chest.

thoracopagus (tho″rah-kop′ah-gus) [*thoraco-* + Gr. *pagos* thing fixed] a double monster consisting of two nearly complete individuals joined in or near the sternal region, so the two components are face to face. **t. epigas′tricus,** an asymmetrical double monster in which the parasitic component is attached to the epigastric region of the autosite. **t. parasit′icus,** an asymmetrical double monster in which the parasitic component is attached to the thorax of the autosite.

thoracoparacephalus (tho″rah-ko-par″ah-sef′ah-lus) [*thoraco-* + Gr. *para* beside + *kephalē* head] asymmetrical conjoined twins, a parasite with rudimentary head being attached to the thorax of the autosite.

thoracopathy (tho″rah-kop′ah-the) [*thoraco-* + Gr. *pathos* disease] any disorder of the thorax or of the thoracic organs.

thoracoplasty (tho″rah-ko-plas′te) [*thoraco-* + Gr. *plassein* to mold] surgical removal of ribs, allowing the chest wall to move inward and collapse a diseased lung. **costoversion t.,** removal of several ribs and their replacement "inside out," occasionally with one rib placed vertically as a strut, providing a concave bony framework, to prevent paradoxical movement during the healing of the chest wall with the lung in the collapsed position.

thoracopneumograph (tho″rah-ko-nu″mo-graf) [*thoraco-* + Gr. *pneuma* breath + *graphein* to write] an instrument for recording the respiratory movements of the chest.

thoracoschisis (tho″rah-kos′kĭ-sis) [*thoraco-* + Gr. *schisis* fissure] congenital fissure of the chest, which may result in herniation of lung tissue.

thoracoscope (tho-ra′ko-skōp) an endoscope for examining the pleural cavity; it is inserted into the cavity through a skin incision into an intercostal space.

thoracoscopy (tho″rah-kos′ko-pe) [*thoraco-* + Gr. *skopein* to examine] the diagnostic examination of the chest, specifically the direct examination of the pleural cavity by means of the endoscope; pleural endoscopy.

thoracostenosis (tho″rah-ko-stĕ-no′sis) [*thoraco-* + Gr. *stenōsis* contraction] abnormal contraction of the chest wall.

thoracostomy (tho″rah-kos′to-me) [*thoraco-* + Gr. *stomoun* to provide with an opening, or mouth] surgical creation of an opening in the wall of the chest for the purpose of drainage; also, the opening so created. **tube t.,** thoracostomy with insertion of a chest tube for drainage of air or fluid from the pleural space.

thoracotomy (tho″rah-kot′o-me) [*thoraco-* + Gr. *tomē* a cutting] surgical incision of the wall of the chest.

thoradelphus (tho″rah-del′fus) thoracodelphus.

thorax (tho′raks), pl. *tho′races* [Gr. *thōrax*] [NA] the part of the body between the neck and the respiratory diaphragm, encased by the ribs; the chest. **amazon t.,** a chest with only one mammary gland, or breast. **t. asthen′icus,** t. paralyticus. **barrel-shaped t.,** a malformed chest which is rounded like a barrel; seen in advanced pulmonary emphysema. **cholesterol t.,** accumulation in the pleural cavities of fluid with a high cholesterol content. **t. paralyt′icus,** the long flat thorax of patients with constitutional visceroptosis. **Peyrot's t.,** a chest that is obliquely oval; seen in large pleural effusions. **pyriform t.,** a pear-shaped thorax, large above, small below.

Thorazine (thor′ah-zēn) trademark for preparations of chlorpromazine hydrochloride.

Thorel's bundle (to′relz) [Christen *Thorel*, German physician, 1880–1935] see under *bundle*.

thoriagram (tho′re-ah-gram) [*thorium* + Gr. *gramma* mark] a photograph made with thorium.

thorium (tho′re-um) [*Thor*, a Norse deity] a rare, heavy gray metal, atomic number, 90; atomic weight, 232.038; symbol, Th. It is a radioactive metal with a half-life on the order of 10¹⁰ years, and the parent element of a radioactive disintegration series. Because of its radiopacity, various compounds of thorium have been used to facilitate visualization in roentgenography. **t. D,** the last element of the dis-

integration series derived from thorium, a stable isotope of lead with an atomic weight of 208. **t. dioxide,** ThO₂, used in roentgenography of the alimentary tract. **radioactive t.,** radiothorium. **sodium t. tartrate,** used in roentgenography, especially of the gastrointestinal tract. **t. X,** a radioactive element produced by disintegration of thorium, and an isotope of radium with a half-life of about 3⅔ days; formerly used in treatment of superficial skin conditions, but replaced now by soft x-rays and grenz rays.

Thormählen's test (tor′ma-lenz) [Johann *Thormählen*, German physician] see under *tests*.

Thornton's sign (thorn′tonz) [Knowsley *Thornton*, British physician, 1845–1904] see under *sign*.

Thornwaldt see *Tornwaldt*.

thoron (tho′ron) thorium emanation.

thoroughpin (thur′o-pin) a distention of the synovial sheath of the flexor perforans tendon of the horse at the hock joint; also a similar distention on the carpal joint of the foreleg.

thought broadcasting (thawt brawd′kas-ting) the feeling that one's thoughts are being broadcast to the environment.

thought insertion (thawt in-ser′shun) the delusion that thoughts that are not one's own are being inserted into one's mind.

thought withdrawal (thawt with-draw′al) the delusion that someone or something is removing thoughts from one's mind.

thozalinone (tho-zal′ĭ-nōn) chemical name: 2-(dimethylamino)-5-phenyl-2-oxazolin-4-one; an antidepressant, $C_{11}H_{12}N_2O_2$.

Thr threonine.

thread (thred) a long slender structure, such as a continuous filament of some substance used as suture material. **t's of Golgi-Rezzonico,** threads of nerve tissue in the incisure of Lanterman surrounding the axon spiral arrangement. **Simonart's t.,** a band formed by the stretching of adhesions between the amnion and fetus when the amniotic cavity is distended with its proper fluid.

threadworm (thred′wurm) any long slender nematode, especially *Enterobius vermicularis*.

thremmatology (threm″ah-tol′o-je) [Gr. *thremma* nursling + *logos* treatise] the science of the laws of heredity and variation.

threonine (thre′o-nin) alpha-amino-beta-hydroxy butyric acid, $CH_3 \cdot CH(OH) \cdot CH(NH_2) \cdot COOH$; a natural amino acid essential for optimal growth in infants and for nitrogen equilibrium in adults.

threonyl (thre′o-nil) the acyl radical of threonine.

threose (thre′ōs) a sugar, $C_4H_8O_4$, isomeric with erythrose.

threpsis (threp′sis) [Gr.] nutrition.

threpsology (threp-sol′o-je) [Gr. *threpsis* nutrition + *-logy*] the sum of what is known concerning nutrition; the science of nutrition.

threptic (threp′tik) pertaining to nutrition; pertaining to the nurturing of offspring by the parents, especially in certain insect species.

threshold (thresh′old) 1. that value at which a stimulus just produces a sensation, is just appreciable, or comes just within the limits of perception; see also *absolute t.* and *difference t.* 2. a hypothetical barrier that stimuli must pass to enter the mind. 3. that degree of concentration of a substance in the blood plasma above which the substance is excreted by the kidneys and below which it is not excreted; such a substance is called a *threshold substance.* 4. limen. **absolute t.,** the lowest possible limit of stimulation that is capable of producing sensation; called also *stimulus t.* **achromatic t.,** the least intensity of the spectrum that produces a sensation of color; reduction of intensity below this point produces a sensation of brightness only, without any color distinction. **auditory t.,** the *mini′mum au-dib′ile,* or slightest perceptible sound. **t. of consciousness,** the *mini′mum sensib′ile,* or lowest limit of sensibility; the point of consciousness at which a stimulus is barely perceived. **convulsant t.,** the minimum amount of electric current or drug required to produce a convulsion in convulsive therapy. **differential t.,** the lowest limit of discriminative sensibility; the ratio which the difference of two stimuli must bear to half their sum in order that their difference may be just perceptible. **displacement t.,** the threshold of perception of a break in the continuity of a contour or of a border; called also *Vernier acuity.* **double point t.,** the smallest distance apart at which two stimuli of touch are felt as distinct. **erythema t.,** the size of the radiation dose that is required to cause erythema of the skin. **flicker fusion t.,** the frequency at which a flickering light just appears to be continuous; see *flicker.* **galvanic t.,** rheobase. **neuron t.,** that degree of stimulation of a neuron which just suffices to call forth a fruitful excitation (sensation, movement, or the like) in a neuron. **t. of nose,** limen nasi. **relational t.,** the ratio which two stimuli must have to each other in order that the difference between them may be just perceptible. **renal t.,** that concentration of a substance in plasma at which it begins to be excreted in the urine. **renal t. for glucose,** the point of sugar (glucose) concentration in the blood (180 mg. per ml. in the normal) at which the kidney will excrete sugar (glucosuria); called also *leak point.* **resolution t.,** t. of consciousness. **sensitivity t., stimulus t.,** absolute t. **swallowing t.,** the minimal stimulation necessary to elicit the reflex action that leads to swallowing. **t. of visual sensation,** the least possible amount of stimulus that gives rise to the sensation of sight.

thrill (thril) a sensation of vibration felt by the examiner on palpation of the body, as over an incompetent heart valve. **aneurysmal t.,** the vibratory sensation felt on the palpation of an aneurysm. **aortic t.,** a thrill perceptible over the aortic orifice in disease of its valves. **diastolic t.,** the vibratory sensation felt over the precordium in advanced aortic insufficiency. **fat t.,** a peculiar thrill sometimes felt in abdominal examinations due to excessive fatness of the parietes. **hydatid t.,** a tremulous impulse sometimes felt on palpation of the body surface over a hydatid cyst; called also *hydatid fremitus.* **presystolic t.,** a thrill felt just before the systole by the hand placed over the apex of the heart. **purring t.,** a thrill of a quality suggesting the purring of a cat. **systolic t.,** a thrill felt on systole over the precordium, as in aortic stenosis, pulmonary stenosis, and ventricular septal defect.

thrix (thriks) [Gr.] hair; used as a word termination denoting a resemblance or a relationship to hair.

throat (thrōt) 1. the pharynx. 2. the fauces. 3. the anterior part of the neck. **sore t.,** see *sore throat,* under S.

throb (throb) a pulsating movement or sensation.

throbbing (throb'ing) beating; attended with a rhythmic beating sensation.

Throckmorton's reflex [Thomas Bentley *Throckmorton,* American neurologist, 1885–1961] see under *reflex.*

throe (thro) a severe pain or paroxysm.

thrombapheresis (throm″bah-fĕ-re′-sis) thrombocytapheresis.

thrombase (throm′bās) thrombin.

thrombasthenia (throm″bas-the′ne-ah) [*thrombocyte* + Gr. *astheneia* weakness] a platelet abnormality characterized by defective clot retraction, abnormal glass adhesion, impaired aggregation to ADP, collagen, and thrombin, and prolonged bleeding time; it is manifested clinically as Glanzmann's disease, with epistaxis, inappropriate bruising, and excessive bleeding, as during surgery. **Glanzmann's t.,** see *thrombasthenia.*

thrombectomy (throm-bek′to-me) [Gr. *thrombos* clot + *ektomē* excision] excision of a thrombus from a blood vessel.

thrombembolia (throm″bem-bo′le-ah) thromboembolism.

thrombi (throm′bi) plural of *thrombus.*

thrombin (throm′bin) 1. the enzyme derived from prothrombin which converts fibrinogen to fibrin; called also *fibrinoginase* and *thrombase.* 2. [USP] a pharmaceutical preparation (*topical t.*), a sterile protein substance prepared from prothrombin of bovine origin through interaction with added thromboplastin in the presence of calcium is used therapeutically as a local hemostatic.

thrombinogen (throm-bin′o-jen) prothrombin.

thromb(o)- [Gr. *thrombos* clot] a combining form denoting relationship to a clot, or thrombus.

thromboagglutinin (throm″bo-ah-gloo′tĭ-nin) platelet agglutinin.

thromboangiitis (throm″bo-an″je-i′tis) [*thrombo-* + Gr. *angeion* vessel + *-itis*] inflammation of a blood vessel with

thrombosis. **t. oblit′erans,** an inflammatory and obliterative disease of the blood vessels of the extremities, primarily the lower extremities, occurring chiefly in young men and leading to ischemia of the tissues and gangrene; called also *Buerger's disease.*

thromboarteritis (throm″bo-ar″ter-i′tis) thrombosis occurring in association with inflammation of an artery. **t. purulen′ta,** purulent softening of an arterial thrombosis, with infiltration of the artery walls.

thromboasthenia (throm″bo-as-the′ne-ah) thrombasthenia.

thromboclasis (throm-bok′lah-sis) [*thrombo-* + Gr. *klasis* a breaking] thrombolysis.

thromboclastic (throm″bo-klas′tik) thrombolytic.

thrombocyst (throm′bo-sist) [*thrombo-* + Gr. *kystis* cyst] the chronic sac which may form around a thrombus in a hematoma.

thrombocystis (throm″bo-sis′tis) thrombocyst.

thrombocytapheresis (throm″bo-sīt″ah-fĕ-re′sis) [*thrombocyte* + Gr. *aphairesis* removal] the selective separation and removal of thrombocytes (platelets) from withdrawn blood, the remainder of the blood then being retransfused into the donor. Called also *plateletpheresis* and *thrombapheresis.*

thrombocyte (throm′bo-sīt) [*thrombo-* + Gr. *kytos* hollow vessel] a blood platelet.

thrombocythemia (throm″bo-sĭ-the′me-ah) [*thrombocyte* + Gr. *haima* blood + *-ia*] a fixed increase in the number of circulating blood platelets; called also *piastrinemia.* **essential t.,** hemorrhagic t. **hemorrhagic t.,** a clinical syndrome characterized by repeated spontaneous hemorrhages, either external or into the tissues, and a remarkable increase in the number of circulating platelets; regarded as one of the myeloproliferative syndromes. Called also *essential, idiopathic,* or *primary thrombocythemia,* and *megakaryocytic leukemia.* **idiopathic t., primary t.,** hemorrhagic t.

thrombocytic (throm″bo-sit′ik) 1. pertaining to, characterized by, or of the nature of a blood platelet (thrombocyte). 2. pertaining to the thrombocytic series.

thrombocytin (throm″bo-si′tin) serotonin.

thrombocytocrit (throm″bo-si′to-krit) [*thrombocyte* + Gr. *krinein* to separate] the volume of packed blood platelets in a given quantity of blood; the instrument used to measure the platelet volume.

thrombocytolysis (throm″bo-si-tol′ĭ-sis) destruction of blood platelets (thrombocytes).

thrombocytopathia (throm″bo-si″to-path′ĕ-ah) a heterogeneous hemorrhagic disorder characterized by platelets with defective clot-promoting (platelet factor 3) activity.

thrombocytopathic (throm″bo-si″to-path′ik) pertaining to or characterized by thrombocytopathy.

thrombocytopathy (throm″bo-si-top′ah-the) a general term applied to a qualitative disorder of the blood platelets, due mainly to deficiency of platelet factor 3 (PF-3). **constitutional t.,** Glanzmann's thrombasthenia.

thrombocytopenia (throm″bo-si″to-pe′ne-ah) [*thrombocyte* + Gr. *penia* poverty] decrease in the number of blood platelets. **essential t.,** idiopathic thrombocytopenic purpura. **immune t.,** that associated with the presence of anti-platelet antibodies (IgG). **malignant t.,** an old term for aleukia hemorrhagica.

thrombocytopoiesis (throm″bo-si″to-poi-e′sis) [*thrombocyte* + Gr. *poiēsis* a making, creation] the production of blood platelets.

thrombocytopoietic (throm″bo-si″to-poi-et′ik) concerned in the formation of blood platelets.

thrombocytosis (throm″bo-si-to′sis) increased numbers of platelets in the peripheral blood.

thromboelastogram (throm″bo-e-las′to-gram) the graphic record of the values determined by thromboelastography.

thromboelastograph (throm″bo-e-las′to-graf) an apparatus used in study of the rigidity of blood or plasma during coagulation.

thromboelastography (throm″bo-e″las-tog′rah-fe) determination of the rigidity of the blood or plasma during coagulation, by use of the thromboelastograph.

thromboembolia (throm″bo-em-bo′le-ah) thromboembolism.

thromboembolism (throm″bo-em′bo-lizm) obstruction of a blood vessel with thrombotic material carried by the blood stream from the site of origin to plug another vessel.

thromboendarterectomy (throm″bo-end″ar-ter-ek′to-me) [*thrombo-* + Gr. *endon* within + *artēria* artery + *ektomē* excision] removal of thrombus and atherosclerotic inner lining from an obstructed artery.

thromboendarteritis (throm″bo-end-ar″ter-i′tis) inflammation of the innermost coat of an artery, with thrombus formation.

thromboendocarditis (throm″bo-en″do-kar-di′tis) 1. formation of a thrombus on a heart valve which has previously been eroded. 2. an infectious disease of rabbits.

thrombogenesis (throm″bo-jen′ĕ-sis) the formation of blood clots.

thrombogenic (throm″bo-jen′ik) [*thrombo-* + Gr. *gennan* to produce] producing a clot, curd, or coagulum.

thromboid (throm′boid) [Gr. *thromboeidēs*] resembling a thrombus.

thrombokinase (throm″bo-kin′ās) activated Factor X; see *coagulation factors,* under *factor.*

thrombokinesis (throm″bo-ki-ne′sis) [*thrombo-* + Gr. *kinēsis* motion] the formation of a blood clot; clotting of blood.

thrombokinetics (throm″bo-ki-net′iks) the dynamics of blood coagulation.

thrombolymphangitis (throm″bo-lim″fan-ji′tis) inflammation of a lymph vessel due to a thrombus.

Thrombolysin (throm-bol′ĭ-sin) trademark for a preparation of fibrinolysin.

thrombolysis (throm-bol′ĭ-sis) [*thrombo-* + Gr. *lysis* dissolution] the phenomenon by which preformed thrombi are lysed by a complex series of events, the most important of which involves the local action of plasmin confined within the substance of the thrombus.

thrombolytic (throm″bo-lit′ik) 1. dissolving or splitting up a thrombus. 2. a thrombolytic agent.

thrombon (throm′bon) [*thrombo-* + Gr. *on* neuter ending] the element of the blood consisting of the platelets and their precursors; it is the counterpart of erythron and leukon.

thrombopathia (throm″bo-path′e-ah) a blood coagulation disorder due to failure of the platelets to release ADP in response to aggregating agents (collagen, epinephrine, thrombin).

thrombopathy (throm-bop′ah-the) see *thrombopathia.*

thrombopenia (throm″bo-pe′ne-ah) thrombocytopenia. **essential t.,** idiopathic thrombocytopenic purpura.

thrombopeny (throm′bo-pe″ne) thrombocytopenia.

thrombophilia (throm″bo-fil′e-ah) [*thrombo-* + Gr. *philein* to love] a tendency to the occurrence of thrombosis.

thrombophlebitis (throm″bo-fle-bi′tis) [*thrombo-* + Gr. *phleps* vein + *-itis*] inflammation of a vein associated with thrombus formation. Cf. *phlebothrombosis.* **iliofemoral t., postpartum,** thrombophlebitis of the iliofemoral vein following childbirth; called also *phlegmasia alba dolens puerperarum.* **t. mi′grans,** a recurring phlebitis usually affecting segments of superficial peripheral veins, and sometimes involving major and visceral veins; it may occur in multiple sites simultaneously or at intervals. **t. purulen′ta,** thrombophlebitis with purulent softening of the thrombus, and infiltration of the wall of the vessel.

thromboplastic (throm″bo-plas′tik) [*thrombo-* + Gr. *plassein* to form] causing or accelerating clot formation in the blood.

thromboplastid (throm″bo-plas′tid) a blood platelet.

thromboplastin (throm″bo-plas′tin) a substance having procoagulant properties or activity. **extrinsic t.,** the prothrombin activator formed as the result of interaction of coagulation Factors III, VII, and X which, with Factor IV, aids in the formation of thrombin: called *extrinsic* because not all of the components required for its production (e.g., Factor III, or tissue thromboplastin) are derived from intravascular sources. **intrinsic t.,** the prothrombin activator formed as the result of interaction of coagulation Factors V, VIII, IX, X, XI, and XII and platelet factor 3 (PF-3) which, with Factor IV, aids in the conversion of prothrombin to thrombin: called *intrinsic* because the components required for its production

are derived from intravascular sources. **tissue t.,** Factor III; see *coagulation factors,* under *factor.* So called because it is released by or derived from extravascular tissues.

thromboplastinogen (throm″bo-plas-tin′o-jen) former term for Factor VIII; see *coagulation factors,* under *factor.*

thrombopoiesis (throm″bo-poi-e′sis) 1. thrombogenesis. 2. thrombocytopoiesis.

thrombopoietic (throm″bo-poi-et′ik) pertaining to or characterized by thrombopoiesis.

thrombopoietin (throm″bo-poi-e′tin) a hypothetical substance(s) believed to serve as the humoral regulator of the production of blood platelets.

thrombosed (throm′bōsd) affected with thrombosis.

thrombosinusitis (throm″bo-si″nu-si′tis) thrombosis of a sinus of the dura mater.

thrombosis (throm-bo′sis) [Gr. *thrombōsis*] the formation, development, or presence of a thrombus. **agonal t.,** clotting of blood in the heart and great vessels before death (Ribbert, 1916). **atrophic t.,** marasmic t. **cardiac t.,** thrombosis in the heart. **cavernous sinus t.,** thrombosis affecting the cavernous sinus. **cerebral t.,** thrombosis of a cerebral vessel, which may result in cerebral infarction. **coronary t.,** development of an obstructive thrombus in a coronary artery, often causing sudden death or a myocardial infarction. **creeping t.,** thrombosis gradually involving one portion of a vein after another. **dilatation t.,** thrombosis due to the slowing of circulation on account of dilatation of a vein. **infective t.,** that which is associated with a bacterial infection. **marantic t., marasmic t.,** thrombosis, chiefly of the longitudinal sinus, occurring in the wasting diseases of infancy and of old age; called also *atrophic t.* **mesenteric t.,** formation of a clot in an artery or arteriole of the mesentery. **placental t.,** 1. a normal formation of thrombi in the placenta. 2. an abnormal extension of the placental thrombus formation to the veins of the uterus. **plate t., platelet t.,** an aggregation of blood platelets forming the nidus of a thrombus; see also *white thrombus,* under *thrombus.* **propagating t.,** progressive clot formation on an occlusive thrombus, producing an elongated mass sometimes extending into other blood vessels. **puerperal t.,** coagulation of blood in the veins (thrombophlebitis) occurring after childbirth. **Ribbert's t.,** agonal t. **sinus t.,** thrombosis of a venous sinus. **traumatic t.,** thrombosis following injury to a part. **venous t.,** the presence of a thrombus in a vein; phlebothrombosis.

thrombostasis (throm-bos′tah-sis) stasis of blood in a part, attended with the formation of a thrombus.

thrombosthenin (throm″bo-sthe′nin) [*thrombo-* + Gr. *sthenos* strength + *-in* chemical suffix] a contractile protein of platelets, active in clot retraction.

thrombotest (throm′bo-test) a test similar to the one-stage prothrombin test except that it is supposedly sensitive to depression of blood coagulation Factor IX and hence has an advantage over the one-stage test in controlling anticoagulant therapy; such superiority, however, has not been demonstrated.

thrombotic (throm-bot′ik) pertaining to or affected with thrombosis.

thrombotonin (throm″bo-to′nin) serotonin.

thromboxane (throm-boks′ān) [*thrombocyte* + *oxane* ring] either of two compounds, thromboxane A_2 (TXA₂) or thromboxane B_2 (TXB₂); TXA₂ is an extremely potent inducer of platelet aggregation and platelet release reactions and is also a vasoconstrictor; it is thus a physiologic antagonist of prostacyclin. It is synthesized by platelets and is very unstable, undergoing nonenzymatic hydrolysis to TXB₂, which is inactive, with a half-life of 30 seconds.

thrombus (throm′bus), pl. *throm′bi* [Gr. *thrombos* clot] an aggregation of blood factors, primarily platelets and fibrin with entrapment of cellular elements, frequently causing vascular obstruction at the point of its formation. Some authorities thus differentiate thrombus formation from simple coagulation or clot formation. Cf. *embolism.* **agonal t., agony t.,** a clot formed in the heart during the process of dying. **annular t.,** one which has an opening through its center, while the circumference is attached to the wall of the vessel. **antemortem t.,** a thrombus or a clot formed in the heart or in a large vessel before death. **ball t.,** a roughly spherical, organized thrombus which may obstruct an orifice (usually the mitral valve) intermittently like a ball valve. **bile t.,** a plug in one of the intrahepatic bile ducts, causing cholestasis. **blood plate t., blood platelet t.,** one formed by an abnormal accumulation of blood platelets. **calcified t.,** a phlebolith. **coral t.,** a red clot formed by coagulated fibrin enclosing red corpuscles. **currant jelly t.,** a soft, reddish, jelly-like clot. **fibrin t.,** a thrombus composed mainly of fibrin, and attached to the walls of a blood vessel. **hyaline t.,** a thrombus composed of erythrocytes which have lost their hemoglobin, forming a colorless translucent mass. **infective t.,** a thrombus associated with an infective agent. **laminated t.,** a thrombus whose substance is disposed in layers, suggesting different periods of formation. **lateral t.,** a clot attached to the side of a vessel, incompletely obstructing the blood current. **marantic t., marasmic t.,** a form associated with severe wasting diseases, often a terminal event; see also under *thrombosis.* **milk t.,** an accumulation of curdled milk in a lactiferous duct. **mixed t.,** laminated t. **mural t.,** a thrombus attached to the wall of the heart, the endocardium in the area being diseased. **obstructive t.,** one which plugs the lumen of the vessel at its site. **occluding t., occlusive t.,** one that occupies the entire lumen of a vessel and obstructs blood flow. **organized t.,** one which has been invaded by fibroblasts and thereby changed to loose fibrous tissue with varying degrees of vascularity. **pale t.,** a dull-white thrombus. **parasitic t.,** an accumulation of the pigmented bodies of free malarial parasites and their spores in the capillaries of the brain, and causing a condition known as *cerebral malaria.* **parietal t.,** one attached to the wall of a vessel. **phagocytic t.,** an accumulation of melaniferous leukocytes in the capillaries of the brain. **pigmentary t.,** an accumulation of free pigment in the capillaries of the brain. **plate t., platelet t.,** one formed by an abnormal accumulation of blood platelets. Called also *blood plate t.* or *blood platelet t.* **postmortem t.,** a thrombus or clot of blood formed in the heart or in a large vessel after death. **primary t.,** one which remains at the place of its origin. **propagated t.,** one which has grown beyond its original limits. **red t.,** a thrombus of a dark-red color formed by the coagulation of blood. **stratified t.,** one made up of layers of different colors. **traumatic t.,** one which results from an injury. **white t.,** 1. one which contains few or no red cells. 2. one composed chiefly of leukocytes. 3. one composed chiefly of platelets and fibrin, usually seen in arterial thrombosis.

thrush (thrush) 1. candidiasis of the oral mucosa, most frequently involving the buccal mucosa and tongue, but the palate, gingivae, and floor of the mouth may also be affected. It is characterized by the development of creamy, white, slightly elevated plaques made up of soft, creamy or crumbly material resembling milk curds, which may be stripped off from the surface of the tissue, leaving a raw bleeding surface. Thrush usually affects sick, weak infants and elderly individuals in poor health. Called also *mycotic stomatitis.* 2. a disease of the horse's foot characterized by a fetid discharge.

thrust (thrust) a sudden forceful movement forward. **paraspinal t.,** the same as spinal thrust, except that the therapist's hands are placed on either side of the spinous processes, the fingers pointing toward the head. **spinal t.,** with the patient in the prone position on the examining table, the physician stands on the patient's right, facing him, places his right palm over the patient's lumbosacral joint perpendicular to the spinal axis, and using the left hand as reinforcement makes a series of short rapid thrusts downward and toward the head, progressing along each interspace to the midthoracic spine; done for relief of lumbosacral strain. **tongue t.,** the infantile pattern of the suckle-swallow in which the tongue is placed between the incisor teeth or alveolar ridges during the initial stages of deglutition, resulting sometimes in anterior open bite, deformation of the jaws, and abnormal function.

thrypsis (thrip′sis) [Gr. "a breaking in small pieces"] a comminuted fracture.

Thudichum's test (too′de-koomz) [John Lewis William *Thudichum,* London physician of German birth, 1829–1901] see under *tests.*

Thuja (thu′jah) [L.; Gr. *thyia*] a genus of coniferous trees, also called *arbor vitae;* secretions of the leafy twigs of *T. occidentalis* are poisonous to man on ingestion.

thuja (thu′jah) fresh tops of *Thuja occidentalis,* white cedar: diuretic, antipyretic, sudorific, and emmenagogue.

thujone (thu′jōn) an aromatic terpene ketone present in many essential oils. It is $CH_3 \cdot C_6H_6O \cdot CH(CH_3)_2$.

thulium (thu′le-um) [*Thule,* ancient name of Shetland] a very rare metallic element; symbol, Tm; atomic number, 69; atomic weight, 168.934.

thumb (thum) [L. *pollex, pollux*] the first digit of the hand, being the most preaxial of the five fingers, having only two phalanges, and being apposable to the four other fingers of the hand. Called also *pollex* [NA]. **bifid t.,** a deformed thumb in which the distal phalanx is divided or bifurcated. **tennis t.,** tendinitis with calcification in the flexor pollicis longus, resulting from repeated friction experienced in playing tennis.

thumbprinting (thum′print-ing) a roentgenographic sign appearing as smooth indentations on the barium-filled colon, as though made by depression with the thumb; seen in various disorders of the colon, especially ischemic colitis.

thumps (thumps) 1. a disease of swine caused by *Ascaris* larvae in the lungs. 2. a kind of singultus, or hiccup, of horses, due to spasm of the diaphragm.

thylakoid (thi′lah-koid) [Gr. *thylakon* a small sac, a seed pouch + *eidos* form] any of the membranous sacs which are the widened portions of lamellae of chloroplasts and which are arranged in stacks to form grana; thylakoids contain the photosynthetic pigments of chloroplasts and the enzymes that catalyze light-dependent reactions.

thyme (tīm) [L. *thymus;* Gr. *thymos*] a plant of the genus *Thymus.* The *Thymus vulgaris* L. (Labiatae), or garden thyme, contains a volatile oil, which is aromatic and carminative. It also contains *thymol, thymene,* and *cumene.* **creeping t., wild t.,** *Thymus serpyllum,* which contains a volatile oil similar to that of *Thymus vulgaris* L.

thymectomize (thi-mek′to-mīz) to remove the thymus gland.

thymectomy (thi-mek′to-me) [Gr. *thymos* thymus + *ektomē* excision] surgical removal of the thymus gland.

thymelcosis (thi″mel-ko′sis) [Gr. *thymos* thymus + *helkōsis* ulceration] ulceration of the thymus.

thymene (thi′mēn) a clear, oily hydrocarbon, $C_{10}H_{16}$, from the oil of thyme.

-thymia [Gr. *thymos* mind + *-ia*] a word termination denoting a condition of mind.

thymian (thim′e-an, tim′e-an) [Ger.] thyme.

thymic (thi′mik) [L. *thymicus*] 1. pertaining to the thymus. 2. contained in or derived from thyme.

thymicolymphatic (thi″mĭ-ko-lim-fat′ik) pertaining to the thymus and the lymphatic glands.

thymidine (thi′mĭ-dēn) a nucleoside, thymine β-D-ribofuranoside; symbol T. The term is commonly used as a synonym for deoxythymidine (dT), for it was thought that thymidine ribosides do not exist, which would make the prefix deoxy- unnecessary. However, it is now known that thymine, produced by post-transcriptional methylation of uracil, occurs as a rare base in rRNAs and tRNAs; therefore the term should be restricted to ribonucleosides.

thymidylate (thi″mĭ-dil′āt) a dissociated form of thymidylic acid.

thymidylate synthase (thi′mĭ-dĭ′lāt sin′thās) [EC 2.1.1.45] an enzyme of the transferase class that catalyzes the reaction 5,10-methylenetetrahydrofolate + dUMP = dihydrofolate + dTMP in the synthesis of thymidine triphosphate. Improperly called thymidylate synthetase in older literature.

thymidylic acid (thi″mĭ-dil′ik) thymidine monophosphate.

thymidylyl (thi″mĭ-dil′il) the radical formed by removal of OH from the phosphate group of thymidine monophosphate.

thymin (thi′min) thymopoietin.

thymine (thi′min) a pyrimidine base, 5-methyl uracil, $C_5H_6N_2O$, found in deoxyribonucleic acid.

thyminic acid (thi-min′ik) an acid formed by the splitting up of deoxyribonucleic acid.

thymion (thim′e-on) [Gr.] a cutaneous wart.

thymiosis (thim″e-o′sis) yaws.

thymitis (thi-mi′tis) inflammation of the thymus.

thym(o)- 1. [Gr. *thymos* thymus] a combining form denoting relationship to the thymus gland. 2. [Gr. *thymos* mind, spirit.] a combining form denoting relationship to the soul or emotions.

thymocyte (thi'mo-sīt) [thymo-(1) + -cyte] a lymphocyte found in the thymus; about 10 per cent are mature T cells, and the rest are immature precursors in various stages of maturation. See table accompanying *T lymphocyte*, under *lymphocyte*.

thymoform (thi'mo-form) a yellowish, antiseptic powder, thymoloform, CH$_2$[C$_6$H$_3$(CH)$_3$(C$_3$H$_7$)O]$_2$, prepared from formaldehyde and thymol.

thymohydroquinone (thi''mo-hi''dro-kwin-ōn') chemical name: 2,5-dihydroxy-p-cymene. A compound, CH$_3$·C$_6$H$_2$-(OH)$_2$CH(CH$_3$)$_2$, occurring in the urine after the administration of thymol, and also found in various essential oils.

thymokesis (thi''mo-ke'sis) enlargement of the remnant of the thymus that is found in the adult.

thymokinetic (thi''mo-ki-net'ik) tending to stimulate the thymus.

thymol (thi'mol) [NF] chemical name: 5-methyl-2-(1-methylethyl)phenol. A phenol, C$_{10}$H$_{14}$O, occurring as colorless, often large, crystals, or white, crystalline powder, obtained from thyme oil or other volatile oils; used as a stabilizer in pharmaceutical preparations. It has been used for its antiseptic, antibacterial, and antifungal actions, and was formerly used as a vermifuge. **t. iodide,** a mixture of iodine derivatives of thymol, principally dithymol diiodide, (C$_6$H$_2$·CH$_3$·C$_3$H$_7$·OI)$_2$, occurring as a reddish brown or reddish yellow bulky powder, formerly used as an antifungal and antibacterial agent. **t. phthalein,** see *thymolphthalein*.

thymoleptic (thi''mo-lep'tik) [thymo-(2) + Gr. *lēpsis* a taking hold] any drug that favorably modifies mood in serious affective disorders such as depression or mania; the main categories of thymoleptics include the tricyclic antidepressants, monoamine oxidase inhibitors and lithium compounds. Also called antidepressants.

thymolize (thi'mo-līz) to treat with thymol.

thymolphthalein (thi''mol-thal'e-in) an indicator, C$_6$H$_4$·-CO·O·C(C$_6$H$_2$·CH$_3$·C$_3$H$_7$·OH)$_2$, with a pH range of 9.3 to 10.5, being colorless at 9.3 and blue at 10.5.

thymolysis (thi-mol'ĭ-sis) [thymo-(1) + Gr. *lysis* dissolution] involution or dissolution of the thymus.

thymolytic (thi''mo-lit'ik) pertaining to, characterized by, or promoting thymolysis.

thymoma (thi-mo'mah) [thymo-(1) + -oma] a tumor derived from the epithelial or lymphoid elements of the thymus.

thymometastasis (thi''mo-mĕ-tas'tah-sis) a metastasis from the thymus.

thymonucleic acid, thymus nucleic acid (thi''mo-noo-kle'ik, thi'mus noo-kle'ik) deoxyribonucleic acid.

thymopathic (thi''mo-path'ik) pertaining to, characterized by, or causing thymopathy.

thymopathy (thi-mop'ah-the) any disease of the thymus.

thymopentin (thi''mo-pen'tin) a pentapeptide immunostimulant, corresponding to amino acids 32–36 of thymopoietin; it is effective against certain primary immunodeficiencies, such as DiGeorge syndrome and primary T cell defects.

thymopoietin (thi''mo-poi'ĕ-tin) a 5500-dalton polypeptide hormone secreted by thymic epithelial cells that induces differentiation of precursor lymphocytes into thymocytes. Formerly called *thymin*.

thymoprivic (thi''mo-priv'ik) thymoprivous.

thymoprivous (thi-mop'rĭ-vus) [thymo-(1) + L. *privus* without] pertaining to or caused by removal or atrophy of the thymus.

thymosin (thi'mo-sin) a thymic humoral factor separable into several fractions, the most active being thymosin α_1, a 3100-dalton polypeptide; it is secreted by thymic epithelial cells and restores T cell function in thymectomized animals.

thymotoxic (thi''mo-tok'sik) toxic for thymus tissue.

thymotoxin (thi''mo-tok'sin) an element that exerts a deleterious effect on the thymus.

thymotrophic (thi''mo-trōf'ik) having an influence on the thymus.

Thymus (thi'mus) a genus of herbs (family Labiatae) native to south central Europe and grown extensively in other countries. See *thyme*.

thymus (thi'mus) [L., from Gr. *thymos*] [NA] a bilaterally symmetric lymphoid organ consisting of two pyramidal lobes situated in the anterior superior mediastinum. It develops as an outgrowth of the epithelium of the third branchial pouch, which is invaded by lymphoid stem cells that migrate via the blood from the yolk sac and later from the bone marrow. Each lobe is surrounded by a fibrous capsule from which septa penetrate to divide the parenchyma into lobules; each lobule consists of an outer zone, the cortex, relatively rich in lymphocytes (thymocytes), and an inner zone, the medulla, relatively rich in epithelial cells. The thymus is the site of production of T lymphocytes. Precursor cells migrate into the outer cortex, where they actively proliferate. As they mature and acquire T cell surface markers they move through the inner cortex, where approximately 90 per cent die (possibly as part of the acquisition of self-tolerance). The remainder move on to the medulla, become mature T cells, and enter the circulation. T cell maturation is regulated by hormones, including thymopoietin and thymosin, produced by thymic epithelial cells. Congenital athymia or neonatal thymectomy results in complete lack of functional T cells. The thymus reaches its maximal development at about puberty and then undergoes a gradual process of involution (replacement of parenchyma by fat and fibrous tissue), resulting in a slow decline of immune function throughout adulthood. **accessory t.,** a separated portion of the thymus gland which may be found occasionally. **persistent t., t. persis'-tens hyperplas'tica,** a thymus which persists into adult life, sometimes even becoming hypertrophied.

thymus-dependent (thi''mus-de-pen'dent) pertaining to T lymphocytes (see under *lymphocyte*). See also under *area*.

thymusectomy (thi''mus-ek'to-me) [thymus + Gr. *ektomē* excision] excision of the thymus.

thymus-independent (thi'mus-in-de-pen'dent) pertaining to B lymphocytes (see under *lymphocyte*). See also under *area*.

thynnin (thin'in) a protamine from the sperm of the tunny fish, *Thunnus thynnus*.

Thyrar (thi'rar) trademark for a preparation of thyroid (def. 3).

thyratron (thi'rah-tron) a form of discharge tube containing mercury vapor and a multiplicity of electrodes, used as an electric valve to rectify alternating current.

thyre(o)- for other words beginning thus, see also those beginning *thyr(o)-*.

thyr(o)- a combining form denoting relationship to the thyroid gland.

thyroactive (thi''ro-ak'tiv) 1. having a metabolic effect similar to thyroid hormone. 2. stimulating activity of the thyroid gland.

thyroadenitis (thi''ro-ad''ĕ-ni'tis) [thyro- + Gr. *adēn* gland + -*itis*] inflammation of the thyroid gland.

thyroaplasia (thi''ro-ah-pla'ze-ah) [thyro- + *a* neg. + Gr. *plasis* molding + -*ia*] defective development of the thyroid gland with deficient activity of its secretion.

thyroarytenoid (thi''ro-ar''ĭ-te'noid) pertaining to the thyroid and arytenoid cartilages.

thyrocalcitonin (thi''ro-kal''sĭ-to'nin) calcitonin.

thyrocardiac (thi''ro-kar'de-ak) pertaining to actions of the thyroid hormones on the heart.

thyrocele (thi'ro-sēl) [thyro- + Gr. *kēlē* tumor] a tumor of the thyroid gland; goiter.

thyrochondrotomy (thi''ro-kon-drot'o-me) [thyro- + Gr. *chondros* cartilage + *tomē* a cutting] surgical incision of the thyroid cartilage.

thyrocolloid (thi''ro-kol'oid) the colloid matter of the thyroid gland.

thyrocricotomy (thi''ro-kri-kot'o-me) incision of the cricothyroid membrane.

thyroepiglottic (thi''ro-ep''ĭ-glot'ik) pertaining to the thyroid and to the epiglottis.

thyrofissure (thi''ro-fish'ur) the operation of making an opening through the thyroid cartilage for the purpose of gaining access to the interior of the larynx.

thyrogenic (thi''ro-jen'ik) thyrogenous.

thyrogenous (thi-roj'ĕ-nus) [thyro- + Gr. *gennan* to produce] originating in the thyroid gland.

thyroglobulin (thi-ro-glob'u-lin) 1. an iodine-containing glycoprotein of high molecular weight occurring in the colloid of the follicles of the thyroid gland; the iodinated tyrosine moieties of thyroglobulin form the active hormones thyroxine and triiodothyronine, which are released into the blood on proteolysis of thyroglobulin. 2. [USP] a substance obtained by fractionation of thyroid glands from the hog, *Sus scrofa* var. *domesticus*, containing not less than 0.7 per cent of total iodine, occurring as a cream to tan-colored, free-flowing powder; formerly administered orally as a thyroid supplement in the treatment of hypothyroidism.

thyroglossal (thi″ro-glos′al)   pertaining to the thyroid gland and the tongue.

thyrohyal (thi″ro-hi′al)   1. pertaining to the thyroid cartilage and the hyoid bone. 2. cornu majus ossis hyoidei.

thyrohyoid (thi″ro-hi′oid)   pertaining to the thyroid gland or cartilage and the hyoid bone.

thyroid (thi′roid) [Gr. *thyreoeidēs; thyreos* shield + *eidos* form]   1. resembling a shield; scutiform. 2. the thyroid gland (glandula thyroidea [NA]); see under *gland*. 3. [USP] the cleaned, dried, and powdered thyroid gland previously deprived of connective tissue and fat, obtained from domesticated animals that are used for food by man, containing 0.17–0.23 per cent of iodine in thyroid combination, occurring as a yellowish to buff-colored amorphous powder; formerly used as a source of thyroid hormones in the treatment of hypothyroidism. **aberrant t.,** a mass of thyroid tissue situated in an abnormal location. **accessory t.,** an exclave or detached portion of thyroid tissue. **ectopic t.,** aberrant t. **intrathoracic t.,** a mass of thyroid tissue that is located within the thoracic cavity. **lingual t.,** thyroid tissue located at the base of the tongue, between the foramen cecum and the hyoid bone. It may project into the pharynx from the dorsum of the tongue, or be entirely within the tongue or located just beneath it; it may also be accessory to a normally located thyroid gland, or be the only thyroid tissue present. **retrosternal t., substernal t.,** a mass of thyroid tissue situated in the thorax behind the sternum.

thyroidea (thi-roi′de-ah)   the thyroid gland. **t. accesso′ria, t. i′ma,** accessory thyroid.

thyroidectomize (thi″roi-dek′to-mīz)   to remove the thyroid gland surgically.

thyroidectomy (thi″roi-dek′to-me) [*thyroid* + Gr. *ektomē* excision]   surgical removal of the thyroid gland. **medical t.,** diminution of thyroid function by the use of drugs.

thyroiditis (thi″roi-di′tis)   inflammation of the thyroid gland. **acute t.,** painful inflammation of the thyroid gland caused by staphylococcic, streptococcic, or other infection, with suppuration and abscess formation, and progressing to the subacute stage. **autoimmune t.,** thyroiditis produced by autoimmune processes, i.e., Hashimoto's thyroiditis and several experimental animal models. **chronic t., chronic fibrous t.,** Riedel's t. **chronic lymphadenoid t., chronic lymphocytic t.,** Hashimoto's disease. **de Quervain's t.,** subacute granulomatous t. **giant cell t., giant follicular t.,** subacute granulomatous t. **granulomatous t.,** subacute granulomatous t. **Hashimoto's t.,** see under *disease*. **invasive t., ligneous t.,** Riedel's t. **lymphocytic t., lymphoid t.,** Hashimoto's disease. **pseudotuberculous t.,** subacute granulomatous t. **Riedel's t.,** a rare, chronic proliferating, fibrosing, inflammatory process of unknown etiology involving usually one but sometimes both lobes of the thyroid gland, as well as the trachea and other structures adjacent to the gland; called also *Riedel's disease, Riedel's struma,* and invasive, iron-hand, and *ligneous thyroiditis.* **subacute granulomatous t.,** a condition characterized by fever and painful enlargement of the thyroid gland, often following a viral infection, especially of the respiratory tract, with granulomas in the gland consisting of masses of colloid surrounded by giant cells and mononuclear cells, and a moderate amount of fibrosis. **subacute lymphocytic t.,** painless, self-limited hyperthyroidism without the nonthyroidal features of Graves' disease; there is lymphocytic infiltration of the thyroid gland. **woody t.,** Riedel's t.

thyroidization (thi″roid-i-za′shun)   1. treatment with a preparation of the thyroid. 2. in histopathology, the thyroid-like appearance of a tissue.

thyroidotherapy (thi″roid-o-ther′ah-pe)   thyrotherapy.

thyroidotomy (thi″roi-dot′o-me) [*thyroid* + Gr. *tomē* a cutting]   thyrotomy.

thyroidotoxin (thi″roid-o-tok′sin)   a toxin specific for thyroid tissue.

thyroid peroxidase (thi′roid per-ok′sĭ-dās)   iodide peroxidase.

thyrointoxication (thi″ro-in-tok″sĭ-ka′shun)   thyrotoxicosis.

Thyrolar (thi′ro-lar)   trademark for a preparation of liotrix.

thyrolytic (thi″ro-lit′ik) [*thyroid* + Gr. *lysis* dissolution]   destructive to thyroid tissue.

thyromegaly (thi″ro-meg′ah-le) [*thyro-* + Gr. *megaleia* bigness]   enlargement of the thyroid gland; goiter.

thyromimetic (thi″ro-mi-met′ik)   producing effects similar to those of thyroid hormones or the thyroid gland.

thyronucleoalbumin (thi″ro-nu″kle-o-al-bu′min)   a nucleoalbumin present in the thyroid gland.

thyro-oxyindole (thi″ro-ok″se-in′dol)   thyroxine.

thyroparathyroidectomy (thi″ro-par″ah-thi″roi-dek′to-me) [*thyroid* + *parathyroid* + Gr. *ektomē* excision]   excision of the thyroid and parathyroids.

thyroparathyroprivic (thi″ro-par″ah-thi″ro-priv′ik)   lacking thyroid and parathyroid glands or secretions.

thyropathy (thi-rop′ah-the) [*thyroid* + Gr. *pathos* disease]   any disease of the thyroid.

thyroprival (thi″ro-pri′val) [*thyroid* + L. *privus* without]   pertaining to, characterized by, or resulting from deprivation or loss of thyroid function.

thyroprivia (thi″ro-priv′e-ah) [*thyroid* + L. *privus* without]   hypothyroidism: the condition resulting from lack of thyroid hormone, as a consequence of removal of the thyroid gland or suppression of its functions.

thyroprivic, thyroprivous (thi″ro-priv′ik; thi-rop′rĭ-vus)   thyroprival.

thyroptosis (thi″rop-to′sis) [*thyroid* + Gr. *ptōsis* fall]   downward displacement of the thyroid gland into the thorax.

thyrotherapy (thi″ro-ther′ah-pe)   treatment of disease by preparations of the thyroid glands of domestic animals used for food by man.

thyrotome (thi′ro-tōm)   an instrument for cutting the thyroid cartilage.

thyrotomy (thi-rot′o-me) [*thyroid* + Gr. *tomē* a cutting]   1. the surgical division of the thyroid cartilage. 2. the operation of cutting the thyroid gland. 3. biopsy of the thyroid gland.

thyrotoxemia (thi″ro-tok-se′me-ah)   thyrotoxicosis.

thyrotoxic (thi″ro-tok′sik)   1. marked by the effects of presentation to the tissues of excessive quantities of the thyroid hormones. 2. describing a patient suffering from thyrotoxicosis.

thyrotoxicosis (thi″ro-tok″sĭ-ko′sis)   the condition resulting from presentation to the tissues of excessive quantities of the thyroid hormones, whether the excess results from overproduction by the thyroid gland (as in Graves' disease), originates outside the thyroid, or is due to loss of storage function and leakage from the gland. **t. facti′tia,** a factitious disorder resulting from self-administration of thyroid hormone.

thyrotoxin (thi″ro-tok′sin)   a toxic substance produced in the thyroid.

thyrotrope (thi′ro-trōp)   thyrotroph.

thyrotroph (thi′ro-trōf)   any of the basophils (beta cells) of the adenohypophysis that secrete thyrotropin; called also *beta basophil.*

thyrotrophic (thi″ro-trōf′ik)   thyrotropic.

thyrotrophin (thi″ro-trōf′in)   thyrotropin.

thyrotropic (thi″ro-trop′ik)   having an influence on the thyroid gland.

thyrotropin (thi-rot′ro-pin)   a glycoprotein hormone (28,000 daltons) of the anterior pituitary that has affinity for and specifically promotes the growth of, sustains, and stimulates the hormonal secretion of the thyroid gland.

thyroxin (thi-rok′sin)   thyroxine.

thyroxine (thi-rok′sin)   a crystalline iodine-containing hormone, L-3,5,3′,5′-tetraiodothyronine, considered the major hormone elaborated by the thyroid, formed from thyroglobulin and transported mainly in the blood serum thyroxine-binding globulin. Its chief function is to increase the rate of cell metabolism. Thyroxine is deiodinated in peripheral tissues (liver, kidney, and heart) to form triiodothyronine, presumably the active "tissue" form of thyroid hormone, which is much more biologically active. Originally isolated by Kendall from the thyroid gland and later prepared synthetically, it is used in the treatment of hypothyroidism. Symbol T_4. **levo t.,** see *levothyroxine*, under L.

thyroxinic (thi″rok-sin′ik) pertaining to thyroxine.

thyrsus (thir′sus) [Gr. *thyrsos* Bacchic wand] the penis.

Thysanosoma (this″ah-no-so′mah) a genus of the family Anoplocephalidae. **T. actinioi′des,** the fringed tapeworm, found in the bile ducts and small intestine of sheep, cattle, antelope, and deer, in western and southwestern United States and in Africa.

Thytropar (thi′tro-par) trademark for a preparation of thyrotropin.

Ti chemical symbol for *titanium*.

TIA transient ischemic attack.

tiamenidine hydrochloride (ti″ah-men′ĭ-dēn) chemical name: *N*-(2-chloro-4-methyl-3-thienyl)-4,5-dihydro-1*H*-imidazol-2-amine monohydrochloride; an antihypertensive, $C_8H_{10}ClN_3S \cdot HCl$.

tiazuril (ti-az′ur-il) chemical name: 2-[4-[(4-chlorophenyl)-thio]-3,5-dimethylphenyl]-1,2,4-triazine-3,5(2*H*,4*H*)-dione; a coccidiostat for poultry, $C_{17}H_{14}ClN_3O_2S$.

tibia (tib′e-ah) [L. "a pipe, flute"] [NA] the shin bone: the inner and larger bone of the leg below the knee; it articulates with the femur and head of the fibula above and with the talus below. See plate accompanying *skeleton*. **saber t., saber-shaped t.,** a tibia curved outward as a result of gummatous periostitis. **t. val′ga,** a bowing of the leg in which the angulation is away from the midline of the body. **t. va′ra,** medial angulation of the tibia in the metaphyseal region, due to a growth disturbance of the medial aspect of the proximal tibial epiphysis; there is an infantile and an adolescent type. Called also *Blount's disease* and *osteochondrosis deformans tibiae.*

tibiad (tib′e-ad) toward the tibial aspect.

tibial (tib′e-al) [L. *tibialis*] pertaining to the tibia.

tibiale (tib″e-a′le) a bone on the tibial side of the tarsus of the embryo, partly represented in the adult by the astragalus. **t. exter′num, t. posti′cum,** a sesamoid bone found in the tendon of the tibialis posterior muscle.

tibialgia (tib″e-al′je-ah) painful shin, with lymphocytosis and eosinophilia (von Schrötter, 1916).

tibialis (tib″e-a′lis) tibial; [NA] a term designating relationship to the tibia.

tibien (tib′e-en) pertaining to the tibia alone or in itself.

tibiocalcanean (tib″e-o-kal-ka′ne-an) pertaining to the tibia and the calcaneus.

tibiofemoral (tib″e-o-fem′or-al) pertaining to the tibia and the femur.

tibiofibular (tib″e-o-fib′u-lar) pertaining to the tibia and the fibula.

tibionavicular (tib″e-o-nah-vik′u-lar) pertaining to the tibia and the navicular bone.

tibioperoneal (tib″e-o-per″o-ne′al) tibiofibular.

tibioscaphoid (tib″e-o-skaf′oid) tibionavicular.

tibiotarsal (tib″e-o-tar′sal) pertaining to the tibia and the tarsus.

tibolone (tĭ′bo-lōn) chemical name: 17-hydroxy-7α-methyl-19-nor-17α-pregn-5(10)-en-20-yn-3-one; an anabolic steroid, $C_{21}H_{28}O_2$.

tibric acid (ti′brik) an antihyperlipidemic with the same uses as chlofibrate.

tic (tik) [Fr.] an involuntary, compulsive, repetitive, stereotyped movement, resembling a purposeful movement because it is coordinated and involves muscles in their normal synergistic relationships; tics usually involve the face and shoulders. **bowing t.,** nodding spasm. **convulsive t.,** spasm of those parts of the face supplied by the seventh nerve. **degenerative t.,** tic occurring in connection with degeneration of the central nervous system. **t. de pensée** (de pah-sa′), the habit of involuntarily expressing any thought that happens to come to mind. **diaphragmatic t.,** spasmodic twitching movements of the diaphragm; called also *respiratory t.* **t. douloureux** (doo-loo-roo′), trigeminal neuralgia. **facial t.,** spasm of the facial muscles. **ges-**

ticulatory t., that marked by spasmodic movements resembling the gestures of an orator or an actor. **t. de Guinon,** Gilles de la Tourette syndrome. **laryngeal t.,** that marked by a noisy expulsion of air through the glottis. **local t.,** a tic affecting only a limited locality, as the eye. **mimic t.,** facial tic. **motor t.,** a tic which is marked only by the spasmodic movement without mental disturbance; it includes facial spasm, rotatory spasm, blepharospasm, and diaphragmatic, laryngeal, and other varieties of tic. **t. nondouloureux,** myoclonus. **progressive choreic t.,** a chronic disease beginning in early life, marked by spasms which at first affect the neck muscles, but, as the disease advances, spread to the rest of the body. The disease ends fatally. **respiratory t.,** diaphragmatic t. **rotatory t.,** rotatory spasm. **saltatory t.,** saltatory spasm. **t. de sommeil,** an involuntary movement of the head during sleep. **spasmodic t.,** a condition marked by spasmodic movements of groups of muscles occurring at irregular intervals.

Ticar (ti′kar) trademark for a preparation of ticarcillin disodium.

ticarbodine (ti-kar′bo-dēn) chemical name: 2,6-dimethyl-*N*-[3-(trifluoromethyl)phenyl]-1-piperidinecarbothioamide; an anthelmintic, $C_{15}H_{19}F_3N_2S$.

ticarcillin (ti″kar-sil′in) chemical name: 6-[(carboxy-3-thienylacetyl)amino]-3,3-dimethyl-7-oxo-4-thia-1-azabicyclo-[3.2.0]-heptane-2-carboxylic acid. A semisynthetic penicillin bactericidal effective against both gram-negative and gram-positive organisms. **t. cresyl sodium,** a salt of ticarcillin, $C_{22}H_{21}N_2NaO_6S_2$. **t. disodium, t. sodium,** the disodium salt of ticarcillin, $C_{15}H_{14}N_2Na_2O_6S_2$, used primarily in the treatment of severe systemic infections and septicemia and infections of the genitourinary and respiratory tracts and of the soft tissues due to susceptible strains of *Pseudomonas aeruginosa, Proteus* species, and *Escherichia coli;* administered intramuscularly and intravenously. Sterile ticarcillin disodium conforms to USP specifications for antibiotics.

tick (tik) a blood-sucking acarid parasite of the suborder Ixodides, superfamily Ixodoidea. The ticks are larger than their relatives, the mites. There are two families: the Argasidae, or soft ticks, and the Ixodidae, or hard ticks. The former includes the genera *Antricola, Argas, Otobius,* and *Ornithodoros;* the latter the genera *Amblyomma, Anocenter, Aponomma, Boophilus, Dermacentor, Haemaphysalis, Hyalomma, Ixodes, Margaropus, Rhipicephalus,* and *Rhipicentor.* **adobe t.,** *Argas persicus.* **American dog t.,** *Dermacentor variabilis.* **bandicoot t.,** *Haemaphysalis humerosa.* **beady-legged winter horse t.,** *Margaropus winthemi.* **black pitted t.,** *Rhipicephalus simus.* **bont t.,** *Amblyomma hebraeum.* **British dog t.,** *Ixodes canisuga.* **brown dog t.,** *Rhipicephalus sanguineus.* **castor bean t.,** *Ixodes ricinus.* **cattle t.,** *Boophilus annulatus.* **dog t.,** 1. *Haemaphysalis leachi.* 2. *Dermacentor variabilis.* 3. *Rhipicephalus sanguineus.* **ear t.,** *Otobius megnini.* **Gulf Coast t.,** *Amblyomma maculatum.* **hard t., hard-bodied t.,** an individual of the family Ixodidae. **Kenya t.,** *Rhipicephalus appendiculatus.* **Lone Star t.,** *Amblyomma americanum.* **miana t.,** *Argas persicus.* **Pacific coast dog t.,** *Dermacentor occidentalis.* **pajaroello t.,** *Ornithodoros coriaceus.* **pigeon t.,** *Argas reflexus.* **rabbit t.,** *Haemaphysalis leporus-palustris.* **Rocky Mountain wood t.,** *Dermacentor andersoni.* **russet t.,** *Ixodes pilosus.* **scrub t.,** *Ixodes holocyclus.* **seed t.,** the young six-legged larva of a tick: after moulting it emerges as an eight-legged nymph. **sheep t.,** *Melophagus ovinus.* **soft t., soft-bodied t.,** an individual of the family Argasidae. **spinous ear t.,** *Otobius megnini.* **taiga t.,** *Ixodes persulcatus.* **tampan t.,** 1. *Ornithodoros moubata.* 2. *Argas persicus.* **winter t.,** *Dermacentor albipictus.* **wood t.,** *Dermacentor andersoni.*

tickling (tik′ling) light stimulation of a surface, and its reflex effect, such as involuntary laughter, etc.

ticlatone (tik′lah-tōn) chemical name: 6-chloro-1,2-benzisothiazolin-3(2*H*)-one; an antibacterial and antifungal, C_7H_4ClNOS.

ticlopidine hydrochloride (ti-klo′pĭ-dēn) chemical name: 5-[(2-chlorophenyl)methyl]-4,5,6,7-tetrahydrothieno-[3,2-c]pyridine hydrochloride; a platelet inhibitor, $C_{14}H_{14}ClNS \cdot HCl$.

ticpolonga (tik″po-long′ah) an extremely venomous ser-

pent of Ceylon and India, *Vipera russelli;* called also *Russell's viper* and *cobra-monil.*

ticrynafen (ti-krin′ah-fen)   a uricosuric diuretic; withdrawn because of hepatotoxic effects.

tictology (tik-tol′o-je) [Gr. *tiktein* to give birth + *logos* treatise]   obstetrics.

t.i.d.   abbreviation for L. *ter in di′e,* three times a day.

tide (tīd)   a physiological variation or increase of a certain constituent in body fluids.   **acid t.,** temporary increase in the acidity of the urine which sometimes follows fasting. **alkaline t.,** temporary increase in the alkalinity of the urine during gastric digestion.   **fat t.,** the increase of fat in the lymph and blood following a meal.

Tidy's test (ti′dēz) [Charles Meymott *Tidy,* English physician, 1843–1892]   see under *tests.*

Tiedemann's nerve (te′dĕ-manz) [Friedrich *Tiedemann,* German physician, 1781–1861]   see under *nerve.*

tienilic acid (ti″en-il′ik)   ticrynafen.

Tietze's syndrome (disease) (tēt′sez) [Alexander *Tietze,* Breslau surgeon, 1864–1927]   see under *syndrome.*

Tigan (ti′gan)   trademark for preparations of trimethobenzamide hydrochloride.

tigestol (ti-jes′tōl)   chemical name: 19-nor-17α-pregn-5(10)-en-20-yn-17-ol; a progestin, $C_{20}H_{28}O$.

tiglic acid (tig′lik)   an unsaturated fatty acid, *trans*-2-methyl-2-butenoic acid, occurring in triglycerides in croton oil.

tiglium (tig′le-um), gen. *tig′lii* [L.]   the croton oil plant, *Croton tiglium* L. (Euphorbiaceae).

tigogenin (tig-oj′ĕ-nin)   a complex aglycone, $C_{27}H_{44}O_3$, from tigonin.

tigonin (tig′o-nin)   a saponin, $C_{56}H_{92}O_{27}$, from *Digitalis purpurea* L. and *D. lanata* Ehrh. (Schrophulariaceae). On hydrolysis, it yields tigogenin, glucose, galactose, and rhamnose.

tigroid (ti′groid) [Gr. *tigroeidēs* tiger-spotted]   marked like a tiger; a term applied to Nissl bodies or masses of deeply staining substance in the protoplasm of neurons.

tigrolysis (ti-grol′ĭ-sis)   chromatolysis, def. 2.

tikitiki (te″ke-te′ke)   the Japanese name for rice polishings; see *polishing,* def. 2.

tiletamine hydrochloride (ti-let′ah-mēn)   chemical name: 2-(ethylamino)-2-(2-thienyl)cyclohexanone hydrochloride; an anesthetic and anticonvulsant, $C_{12}H_{17}NOS \cdot HCl$.

tilidine hydrochloride (til′ĭ-dēn)   chemical name: (*trans*)-(±)-2-(dimethylamino)-1-phenyl-3-cyclohexene-1-carboxylic acid ethyl ester hydrochloride; a narcotic analgesic, $C_{17}H_{23}NO_2 \cdot HCl$.

Tillaux's disease (te-yōz′) [Paul Jules *Tillaux,* French physician, 1834–1904]   see under *disease.*

Tilletia (til-le′she-ah)   a genus of basidiomycetous fungi of the order Ustilaginales, family Tilletiaceae, causing smut on cereals. *T. caries* causes stinking smut of wheat.

Tilletiaceae (til-le″she-a′se-e)   a family of basidiomycetous fungi of the subclass Heterobasidiomycetidae, order Ustilaginales, including the genera *Tilletia* and *Urocystis.*

tilmus (til′mus) [Gr. *tilmos* a plucking]   carphology.

tilorone (til′or-ōn)   a low-molecular-weight aromatic amine that stimulates the production of interferon in serum.   **t. hydrochloride,** chemical name: 2,7-bis[2-(diethylamino)ethoxy]-9*H*-fluoren-9-one dihydrochloride; an antiviral agent, $C_{25}H_{34}N_2O_3 \cdot 2HCl$.

tiltometer (til-tom′ĕ-ter)   an instrument for measuring the degree of tilting of the operating table in spinal anesthesia and other procedures.

timbre (tim′ber, tam′br) [Fr.]   a musical quality in a tone or sound.   **t. métallique,** a high-pitched tympanic second sound heard in dilatation of the aorta. When heard in persons under fifty-five years of age it has been considered suggestive of syphilitic aortitis. Called also *Potain's sign* and *bruit de tabourka.*

time (tim) [Gr. *chronos;* L. *tempus*]   a measure of duration.   **apex t.,** the interval at which the apex of the summated twitches of a muscle succeeds the second stimulus applied to the same muscle.   **bleeding t.,** the period of duration of bleeding that follows controlled, standardized puncture of the earlobe (Duke method) or forearm (Ivy method); a relatively

inconsistent measure of capillary and platelet function. **bleeding t., secondary,** the time required for the arrest of bleeding when the crust is removed from a traumatized area 24 hours after the original injury; this is generally prolonged in patients with Factor VIII deficiency (hemophilia) and with related hemophilioid states.   **chromoscopy t.,** the time elapsing between the intramuscular injection of a dye and its appearance in the gastric secretion. **circulation t.,** the time required for blood to flow between two designated points, as arm-to-tongue time.   **clot retraction t.,** the time required for 50 per cent of a blood clot (coagulum) to retract from the wall of the vessel containing it; a semiquantitative measure of this phenomenon is available.   **clotting t.,** coagulation t.   **coagulation t.,** the time required for blood to clot in a glass tube.   **decimal reduction t.,** the time of heat sterilization required for a 10-fold reduction of viable microorganisms. Called also *D value.*   **dextrinizing t.,** the time required for saliva to convert starch into sugar.   **doubling t.,** generation t., def. 3.   **generation t.,** 1. the period of time between the receipt of an infection by a host and the maximal infectivity of that host.   2. the time elapsing from one generation to the next.   3. the time required for all components of a cell culture to multiply by two. Called also *doubling t.*   **inertia t.,** the time required to overcome the inertia of a muscle after the reception of a stimulus from a nerve.   **prothrombin t.,** the time required for clot formation after thromboplastin (brain extract) and calcium have been added to blood plasma.   **reaction t.,** the time elapsing between the application of a stimulus and the resulting reaction. **recalcification t.,** the interval required for clot formation when calcium ion is replaced in anticoagulated platelet-rich plasma; an insensitive measure of hemostasis.   **sedimentation t.,** see *erythrocyte sedimentation rate,* under *rate.* **thermal death t.,** the time required at a given temperature to destroy a population of microorganisms with heat.

timer (tīm′er)   a clock mechanism which may be set to automatically signal the expiration of a given interval of time or to activate or cut off certain other apparatus at the desired time.

timolol maleate (ti′mo-lōl)   chemical name: (S)-1-[(1,1-dimethylethyl)amino]-3-[[4-(4-morpholinyl)-1,2,5-thiadiazol-3-yl]oxy]-2-propanol(Z)-2-butanedioate (1:1) (salt).   A beta-adrenergic blocking agent, $C_{13}H_{24}N_4O_3S \cdot C_4H_4O_4$, with antihypertensive and antiarrhythmic properties; it is used topically to lower intraocular pressure in glaucoma, by decreasing the formation of aqueous humor.

tin (tin) [L. *stannum*]   a white, metallic element, atomic number, 50; atomic weight, 118.69; valence 2 or 4; symbol, Sn. Some of its salts are reagents, others are stains, while some of its compounds, particularly the oxide, have been tried in medicine. Its organic compounds exhibit moderate but variable toxicity.   **t. chloride,** a compound, $SnCl_2 + 2H_2O$, or stannous chloride; used as a test reagent.   **t. oxide,** stannic oxide.

Tinactin (tin-ak′tin)   trademark for preparations of tolnaftate.

Tinbergen (tin′berg-en)   Nikolaas. Dutch-born British zoologist, born 1907; co-winner, with Karl von Frisch and Konrad Lorenz, of the Nobel prize for medicine or physiology in 1973, for his work on animal behavior.

tinct.   abbreviation for *tincture,* or *tinctura.*

tinctable (tink′tah-b'l)   stainable or tingible.

tinction (tink′shun) [L. *tingere* to dye]   1. the act of staining.   2. the addition of coloring or flavoring agents to a prescription.

tinctorial (tink-to′re-al)   pertaining to dyeing or staining.

tinctura (tink-tu′rah), gen. and pl. *tinctu′rae* [L.]   tincture.

tincturation (tink″tu-ra′shun)   the preparation of a tincture; the treatment of a drug with a menstruum, such as alcohol or ether, for the purpose of preparing a tincture.

tincture (tink′tūr) [L. *tingere* to wet, to moisten]   an alcoholic or hydroalcoholic solution prepared from animal or vegetable drugs or from chemical substances.   **arnica t.,** a preparation of powdered arnica in equal parts of alcohol and water, formerly used as a local irritant.   **belladonna t.** [USP], an alcoholic preparation of belladonna leaf, containing, in each 100 ml., 27–33 mg. of the alkaloids of belladonna leaf; used as an anticholinergic for the same purposes as atropine and hyoscyamine.   **benzethonium chloride**

t. [USP], a preparation containing 97–103 per cent of benzethonium chloride, calculated on a dried basis; used as a topical anti-infective. **benzoin t., compound** [USP], a preparation of benzoin, aloe, storax, and tolu balsam in alcohol, used as a topical protectant. Called also *friar's balsam*. **camphorated opium t.**, former name for paregoric. **capsicum t.**, a preparation of powdered capsicum in equal parts of alcohol and water; used as an irritant and carminative. **cardamom t., compound**, a preparation of powdered cardamom seed, cinnamon, caraway, and cochineal in glycerin and diluted alcohol; used as a flavoring agent. **digitalis t.**, finely powdered digitalis in a menstruum of alcohol and water, used as a cardiotonic. **ferric chloride t.**, a hydroalcoholic solution of ferric chloride, formerly used as a hematinic in the treatment of iron-deficiency anemias; it has also been used as a topical astringent and styptic. **ferric citrochloride t.**, a hydroalcoholic solution of ferric chloride and sodium citrate, used as a hematinic. **gentian t., compound**, a preparation of powdered gentian, bitter orange peel, and cardamom seed in a menstruum of glycerin, alcohol, and water; formerly used as a bitter. **green soap t.** [USP], a preparation of green soap, lavender oil, and alcohol used as a skin detergent; called also *medicinal soft soap liniment* and *linimentum saponis mollis*. **hyoscyamus t.**, a preparation of powdered hyoscyamus in alcohol and water; formerly used as an anticholinergic for the same purposes as atropine. **iodine t.** [USP], a preparation of iodine and sodium iodide in diluted alcohol, each 100 ml. of which contains 1.8–2.2 gm. of iodine and 2.1–2.6 gm. of sodium iodide; used as an anti-infective on the skin. **iodine t., strong**, an alcoholic solution of iodine and potassium iodide, each 100 ml. of which contains 6.8–7.5 gm. of iodine and 4.7–5.5 gm. of potassium iodide; used as an irritant, antibacterial, and antifungal agent. **lemon t.** [USP], **lemon peel t.**, a preparation of lemon peel in alcohol used as a flavoring agent. **myrrh t.**, a preparation of powdered myrrh in alcohol used as a protective. **nitromersol t.** [USP], a preparation of nitromersol, sodium hydroxide, and acetone, in alcohol and purified water; used as a local anti-infective, applied topically. **nux vomica t.**, a preparation of powdered nux vomica in equal parts of alcohol, hydrochloric acid, and water; used as a bitter. **opium t.** [USP], a preparation, obtained by percolation of granulated opium and concentration of the product, each 100 ml. of which yields 0.95–1.05 gm. of anhydrous morphine; used as an antiperistaltic. Called also *deodorized opium t.* **opium t., camphorated**, paregoric. **opium t., deodorized**, opium t. **rhubarb t., aromatic**, a preparation of powdered rhubarb, cinnamon, clove, and myristica in glycerin, alcohol, and water; used as a cathartic. **stramonium t.**, a hydroalcoholic solution of powdered stramonium formerly used as a parasympatholytic. **sweet orange peel t.** [USP], a preparation produced by the maceration in alcohol of the outer rind of the nonartificially colored fresh ripe fruit of *Citrus sinensis;* used as a flavoring agent. **thimerosal t.** [USP], a preparation of thimerosal, alcohol, acetone, ethylenediamine solution, and monoethanolamine in water; used as a local anti-infective, applied topically to the skin. **tolu balsam t.** [NF], a preparation of tolu balsam in alcohol; used as a flavor and as ingredient of *tolu balsam syrup*. **vanilla t.** [NF], a preparation of vanilla and sucrose in equal parts of diluted alcohol and water; used as a flavor and as an ingredient of *acacia syrup*.

Tindal (tin′dal) trademark for a preparation of acetophenazine maleate.

tinea (tin′e-ah) [L. "grub," "moth larva," "worm"] a term used to describe various dermatophytoses, the specific type usually being designated by a modifying term depending on characteristic appearance of the lesions, etiologic agent, or site. Popularly called *ringworm*. **t. amianta′cea, asbestos-like t.**, a nonfungal condition of the scalp, characterized by a dense concentration on its surface of silvery-white or gray scales which extend up on the hair shafts to form an asbestos-like encasement. Called also *pityriasis amiantacea*. **t. axilla′ris**, trichomycosis axillaris. **t. bar′bae**, tinea involving the bearded area of the face and neck, occurring in three types: in the *inflammatory type*, usually caused by *Trichophyton mentagrophytes* and *T. verrucosum*, the typical lesions are kerion-like swellings and nodular swellings and may produce marked crusting; in the *ringworm type*, the annular lesions resemble those of ring-

worm of nonhairy skin; and in the *sycosiform type* (*t. sycosis*); caused usually by *Trichophyton violaceum* and less often by *T. rubrum*, the lesions are follicular pustules, each containing a hair that may break off and leave a stub or become epilated. Called also *barber's itch* and *ringworm of the beard*. **t. cap′itis**, ringworm of the scalp, caused by species of *Microsporum* and *Trichophyton*, which may occasionally also involve the eyebrows and eyelashes, sometimes occurring in epidemics. Depending upon the etiologic agent, it may vary from a benign scaly noninflammatory subclinical infection to an inflammatory disease marked by scaly, erythematous papular eruptions with loose and broken off hairs causing areas of alopecia that may become severely inflamed with the formation of deep, ulcerative kerions that often result in keloid formation, scarring, and permanent alopecia. Called also *t. tonsurans*. See also *black-dot ringworm* and *gray-patch ringworm*, under *ringworm*. **t. cilio′rum**, fungal infection of the scalp, involving the eyelashes. **t. circina′ta**, t. corporis. **t. corpo′ris**, tinea involving the glabrous skin (excluding infection of the bearded area, scalp, groin, hands, and feet), most commonly caused by *Microsporum canis*, *Trichophyton rubrum*, or *T. mentagrophytes*, although any dermatophyte can be the etiologic agent. It is typically characterized by the presence of one or more well-demarcated erythematous, scaly macules with slighted raised borders and central healing, producing annular outlines. Various other types of lesions may also occur, including those that are vesicular, eczematous, psoriasiform, verrucous, plaquelike, or deep. Called also *ringworm of the body*, *t. circinata*, and *glabrose*. **t. cru′ris**, acute or chronic tinea, generally seen in males, involving the groin, perineum, and perineal regions and sometimes spreading to contiguous areas, which most often accompanies tinea pedis, so that the etiologic agent is usually the same for both infections. It is characterized by severely pruritic, sharply demarcated lesions with a raised erythematous margin and thin, dry scaling. Called also *eczema marginatum*, *jock itch*, and *ringworm of the groin*. **t. facia′le, t. fa′ciei**, tinea of the face (other than on the bearded area) in which the lesion(s) presents as a red slightly scaling patch with an indistinct border instead of as the typical lesion with a ringworm configuration. Called also *ringworm of the face*. **t. favo′sa**, favus. **t. gal′li**, favus of fowl. **t. glabro′sa**, t. corporis. **t. imbrica′ta**, a chronic tropical type of tinea due to *Trichophyton concentricum*, geographically restricted to certain regions of the Pacific islands of Oceania, Southeast Asia, and Central and South America, being seen almost exclusively in Indonesians and Polynesians and their descendents, and characterized by confluent polycyclic concentric rings of papulosquamous patches of scales distributed over and frequently covering large areas of the body. Called also *tokelau* and known also by various local names. **t. ma′nus, t. ma′nuum**, tinea involving the interdigital spaces and palmar surfaces of hands almost always accompanying tinea pedis, so that the etiologic agent is usually the same for both infections. The most common manifestation is hyperkeratosis of the palms and fingers, usually unilaterally, but it may also present as crescentic exfoliation of the skin, vesicular, circumscribed patches, discrete, red papulofollicular patches, and red scaly sheets on the dorsum. Called also *ringworm of the hand*. **t. ni′gra**, a minor fungal infection, caused by *Cladosporium mansoni* or *C. wernecki*, producing strikingly dark lesions with the appearance of stains of spattered silver nitrate on the skin of the hands or, rarely, on other areas. **t. nodo′sa**, piedra. **t. pe′dis**, tinea involving the feet, particularly the interdigital spaces and soles, most often caused by *Trichophyton rubrum*, *T. mentagrophytes*, or *Epidermophyton floccosum*, and characterized by intensely pruritic lesions varying from mild, chronic, and scaling to acute exfoliative, pustular, and bullous. Called also *athlete's foot* and *ringworm of the feet*. See also *t. cruris* and *t. manus*. **t. profun′da**, trichophytic granuloma. **t. syco′sis**, the sycosiform type of tinea barbae. **t. tar′si**, blepharitis ulcerosa. **t. tonsu′rans**, t. capitis. **t. un′guium**, tinea involving the nails in which the invasion is restricted to white patches or pits on the nail surface or the lateral or distal edges of the nail are first involved, followed by establishment of the infection beneath the nail plate. Called also *dermatophytic onychomycosis*, *onychomycosis*, and *ringworm of the nail*. **t. versic′olor**, a common chronic, noninflammatory and usually symptomless disorder, characterized only by occurrence of multiple macular patches, of all sizes and shapes, varying from whitish in pigmented skin to fawn-colored or brown in pale skin; seen most frequently in hot, humid tropical regions, and caused by *Pityrosporon orbiculare.* Called also *pityriasis versicolor.*

Tinel's sign (tin-elz') [Jules *Tinel,* French neurologist, 1879–1952] see under *sign.*

tinfoil (tin'foil) tin foil.

tingibility (tin″jĭ-bil'ĭ-te) the quality of being tingible.

tingible (tin'jĭ-b'l) [L. *tingere* to stain] susceptible of being tinged or stained.

tingling (ting'gling) a pricklike thrill, caused by cold or by striking a nerve, or as a result of various diseases of the central or peripheral nervous system. **distal t. on percussion,** see *Tinel's sign,* under *sign.*

tinidazole (ti-nid'ah-zōl) chemical name: 1-[2-(ethylsulfonyl)ethyl]-2-methyl-5-nitroimidazole; an antiprotozoal, $C_8H_{13}N_3O_4S$, effective against *Trichomonas vaginalis, Entamoeba histolytica,* and *Giardia intestinalis.*

tinkle (ting'k'l) an auscultatory sound like the ringing of a small bell, sometimes heard over large pulmonary cavities and in pneumothorax. **metallic t.,** a ringing sound, as of a metallic object, sometimes heard in connection with other respiratory sounds.

tinnitus (tĭ-ni'tus) [L. "a ringing"] a noise in the ears, as ringing, buzzing, roaring, clicking, etc. Such sounds may at times be heard by others than the patient. **t. aurium,** a subjective sensation of noises in the ears. **clicking t.,** a clicking sound occurring in the ear in chronic catarrhal otitis media; it may be heard by others than the patient. **Leudet's t.,** a crackling sound in the ear, audible also to an observer, produced by involuntary contraction of an internal muscle, coinciding with a tic of some of the fibers of the mandibular division of the trigeminal (fifth cranial) nerve. **nervous t.,** that which arises from some disturbance of the otic nerve or its central connection. **nonvibratory t.,** tinnitus produced by biochemical changes occurring in the nerve mechanism of hearing. **objective t.,** abnormal or pathological sounds originating within the body of the patient, in the region of the ear, which are audible to others than the patient. **vibratory t.,** tinnitus resulting from transmission to the cochlea of vibrations originating in adjacent tissues of the body.

Tinospora (tin-os'po-rah) a genus of menispermaceous vines; the stalk and root of *T. cordifolia* Miers. are used in snakebite, indigestion, ulcers, and fevers.

tint B a color shown by the pastille in an x-ray–measuring instrument that denotes the amount of radiation which will cause depilation.

Tintinnina (tin″tĭ-ni'nah) [L. *tintinnabulum* bell] a suborder of ciliate, mainly pelagic, loricate protozoa (order Oligotrichida, subclass Spirotrichida), characterized by the presence of an adoral zone of membranelles dominating the ciliature, always forming a closed ring; reduced somatic ciliature; and a highly contractile, cylindrical or cone-shaped body.

tintometer (tin-tom'ĕ-ter) [*tint* + Gr. *metron* measure] an instrument used in determining the relative proportion of coloring matter in a liquid.

tintometric (tin″to-met'rik) pertaining to tintometry.

tintometry (tin-tom'ĕ-tre) the use of the tintometer.

tiodonium chloride (ti″o-do'ne-um) chemical name: (4-chlorophenyl)-2-thienyliodonium chloride; an antibacterial, $C_{10}H_7Cl_2IS$.

tioperidone hydrochloride (ti″o-per'ĭ-dōn) chemical name: 3-[4-[4-[2-(propylthio)phenyl]-1-piperazinyl]butyl]-2,4(1H,3H)-quinazolinedione monohydrochloride; a tranquilizer, $C_{25}H_{32}N_4O_2S \cdot HCl$.

tiopinac (ti-o'pĭ-nak) chemical name: 6,11-dihydro-11-oxodibenzo[b,e]thiepin-3-acetic acid; an anti-inflammatory, analgesic, and antipyretic, $C_{16}H_{12}O_3S$.

tioxidazole (ti″ok-si'dah-zōl) chemical name: (6-propoxy-2-benzothiazolyl)carbamic acid methyl ester; an anthelmintic, $C_{12}H_{14}N_2O_3S$.

tip (tip) a pointed extremity of a body part; called also *apex.* **t. of nose,** apex nasi. **t. of sacral bone,** apex ossis sacri. **t. of tongue,** apex linguae. **Woolner's t.,** tuberculum auriculae.

tipping (tip'ing) 1. a tooth movement in which its vertical position is altered, either occurring spontaneously or as a

result of orthodontic therapy. See also *uprighting.* 2. cusp restoration.

tiprenolol hydrochloride (ti-pren'o-lōl) chemical name: 1-[(1-methylethyl)amino]-3-[2-(methylthio)phenoxy]-2-propanol hydrochloride; an antiadrenergic (β-receptor), $C_{13}H_{21}NO_2S \cdot HCl$.

tiqueur (te-ker') [Fr.] a person subject to a tic.

tiquinamide hydrochloride (ti-kwin'ah-mīd) chemical name: 5,6,7,8-tetrahydro-3-methyl-8-quinoline carbothioamide monohydrochloride; a gastric anticholinergic, $C_{11}H_{14}N_2S \cdot HCl$.

tirebal (tēr-bahl') [Fr.] (*obs.*) an instrument resembling a corkscrew, for extracting bullets.

tirefond (tēr-fo') [Fr.] (*obs.*) an instrument like a corkscrew, for raising depressed portions of a bone.

tires (tīrz) trembles.

tiring (tīr'ing) the operation of passing a wire around a fractured patella, like a tire around a wheel; cerclage.

Tiselius apparatus (te-sa'le-us) [Arne Wilhelm Kaurin *Tiselius,* biochemist in Uppsala, Sweden, 1902–1971, winner of the Nobel prize for chemistry in 1948] see under *apparatus.*

tissue (tish'u) [Fr. *tissu*] an aggregation of similarly specialized cells united in the performance of a particular function. **accidental t.,** a tissue growing in or upon a part to which it is foreign; it is either analogous or heterologous. **adenoid t.,** lymphoid t. **adipose t.,** fatty tissue; connective tissue made up of fat cells in a meshwork of areolar tissue. **adipose t., brown,** a thermogenic type of adipose tissue containing a dark pigment, and arising during embryonic life in certain specific areas in many mammals, including man; it is prominent in the newborn of all species in which it occurs and remains a distinct and conspicuous tissue in the adults of certain species, especially those that hibernate. Called also *brown fat.* Cf. *white adipose t.* **adipose t., white, adipose t., yellow,** the adipose tissue comprising the bulk of the body fat. Cf. *brown adipose t.* **adrenogenic t.,** the inner zone of the cortex of an adrenal gland which begins to involute shortly after birth, usually referred to as the fetal cortex. **analogous t.,** an accidental tissue similar to one found normally in other parts of the body. **areolar t.,** connective tissue made up largely of interlacing fibers. **areolar connective t.,** see *connective t.* **basement t.,** the substance of a basement membrane. **bony t.,** bone, whether normal or of a soft tissue, which has become ossified. **brown fat t.,** fatty tissue in various regions of the body of some mammals which contains a dark pigment. Called also *moruloid* or *mulberry fat.* The masses have been called interscapular gland, hibernating gland, and Bonnot's gland. **bursa-equivalent t., bursal equivalent t.,** a hypothesized lymphoid tissue in nonavian vertebrates equivalent to the bursa of Fabricius in birds: the site of B lymphocyte maturation. It now appears that B cell maturation occurs primarily in the bone marrow. **cancellous t.,** the loose spongy tissue of the interior and articular ends of bone. **cartilaginous t.,** the substance of the cartilages. **cavernous t.,** erectile t. **cellular t.,** loose connective tissue with large interspaces. **chondroid t.,** an embryonic form of cartilage composed of vesicular cells provided with elastic capsules and having collagenous fibers in its interstitial substance. **chordal t.,** the tissue of the notochord. **chromaffin t.,** a tissue composed largely of chromaffin cells, well supplied with nerves and vessels; it occurs in the adrenal medulla and also forms the paraganglia of the body. **cicatricial t.,** the dense fibrous tissue forming a scar or cicatrix and derived directly from granulation tissue; called also *scar t.* **compact t.,** the hard external portion of a bone. **connective t.,** the tissue which binds together and is the support of the various structures of the body. It is made up of fibroblasts, fibroglia, collagen fibrils, and elastic fibrils. It is derived from the mesoderm and in a broad sense includes the collagenous, elastic, mucous, reticular, osseous, and cartilaginous tissue. Some also include the blood in this group of tissues. Cf. *fibroblast.* Connective tissue is classified according to concentration of fibers as loose (areolar) and dense, the latter having more abundant fibers than the former. **cribriform t.,** areolar t. **dartoid t.,** that which resembles the dartos in structure. **elastic t., elastic t., yellow,** connective tissue made up of yellow, elastic fibers, frequently massed into sheets. **endothelial t.,** endothelium. **episcleral t.,**

the loose connective tissue over the sclera, between it and the conjunctiva. **epithelial t.,** epithelium. **epivaginal connective t.,** connective tissue surrounding the sheath of the optic nerve. **erectile t.,** tissue containing large venous spaces with which arteries communicate directly, as in the penis and clitoris. Another type formed of dilated venules occurs in the nasal mucosa. The smooth muscle of the nipples constitutes another erectile organ. **extracellular t.,** the total of tissues and body fluids outside the cells, including the plasma volume and all plasma components, the extracellular fluid volume and its components, plus the intercellular and extracellular tissue solids, most notably the collagen, cartilage, bone, elastin, and other connective tissues of the body framework and viscera. **extraperitoneal t.,** fascia extraperitonealis. **fatty t.,** adipose t. **fibrohyaline t.,** chondroid t. **fibrous t.,** the ordinary connective tissue of the body, made up largely of yellow or white fibers. **fibrous t., white,** that which is composed almost wholly of collagenous fibers. **Gamgee t.,** a surgical dressing consisting of a thick layer of absorbent cotton between two layers of absorbent gauze. **gelatiginous t.,** that which yields gelatin on boiling with water. **gelatinous t.,** mucous tissue. **glandular t.,** an aggregation of epithelial cells that elaborate secretions. **granulation t.,** the newly formed vascular tissue normally produced in the healing of wounds of soft tissue and ultimately forming the cicatrix; it consists of small, translucent, red, nodular masses or granulations that have a velvety appearance. **gut-associated lymphoid t. (GALT),** lymphoid tissue associated with the gut, including the tonsils, Peyer's patches, lamina propria of the gastrointestinal tract, and appendix. **hematopoietic t.,** tissue that takes part in the production of the formed elements of the blood. **heterologous t.,** tissue unlike any other that is normal to the organism. **heterotopic t.,** choristoma. **homologous t.,** tissue identical with another tissue in structural type. **hylic t.,** Adami's term for embryonic tissues constituting the body of an organ, in contrast to lining (lepidic) tissue; see also *hylic.* **hyperplastic t.,** 1. tissue affected by hyperplasia. 2. in dentistry, an overgrowth of tissue about the maxilla or mandible that is excessively movable, or more readily displaced than is normal. **indifferent t.,** undifferentiated embryonic tissue. **interrenal t.,** the tissue composing the adrenal cortex. **interstitial t.,** the connective tissue between the cellular elements of a body; the stroma. **junctional t.,** the bridge between the atrium and ventricle of the heart formed by the atrioventricular node and the atrioventricular bundle. **Kuhnt's intermediary t.,** glial tissue surrounding the optic nerve and separating it from the retina. **lardaceous t.,** tissue charged with lardacein as a result of a degenerative process. **lepidic t.,** the lining membrane tissue of the embryo. Cf. *hylic t.* **loose connective t.,** see *connective t.* **lymphadenoid t.,** tissue resembling that of the lymph nodes, found in the spleen, bone marrow, tonsils, and other organs. **lymphatic t.,** lymphoid t. **lymphoid t.,** a lattice work of reticular tissue the interspaces of which contain lymphocytes; lymphoid tissue may be diffuse, or densely aggregated as in lymph nodules and nodes. See also *lymphoid system,* under *system.* **mesenchymal t.,** embryonic connective tissue composed of stellate cells and a ground substance of coagulable fluid; the mesenchyma. **metanephrogenic t.,** the more caudal nephrogenic tissue that gives rise to the nephrons of the permanent kidney. **mucous t.,** a jelly-like connective tissue, such as occurs in the umbilical cord. **muscular t.,** the substance of a muscle. **myeloid t.,** medulla ossis rubra. **nephrogenic t.,** tissue of the nephrotomes which furnishes the material out of which the three kidney types arise. **nerve t., nervous t.,** the substance of which the nerves and nerve centers are composed. **nodal t.,** tissue made up of nerve and muscle fibers, such as that composing the sinoatrial node of the heart. **osseous t.,** the specialized tissue forming the bones. **osteogenic t.,** that part of the periosteum adjacent to bone and concerned in the formation of osseous tissue; any tissue capable of generating bone. **osteoid t.,** uncalcified bone tissue. **parenchymatous t.,** parenchyma. **primitive pulp t.,** hylic t. **reticular t., reticulated t.,** connective tissue consisting of reticular cells and fibers. **rubber t.,** rubber in sheets for use in surgery. **scar t.,** cicatricial t. **sclerous t's,** the cartilaginous, fibrous, and osseous tissues. **shock t.,** that tissue in the animal body which bears the brunt of the antigen-antibody reaction in anaphylaxis. **skeletal t.,** the bony, ligamentous, fibrous,

and cartilaginous tissue forming the skeleton and its attachments. **splenic t.,** red pulp. **subcutaneous t.,** the layer of loose connective tissue situated directly beneath the skin; called also *tela subcutanea* [NA]. **subcutaneous fatty t.,** panniculus adiposus. **sustentacular t.,** a non-nervous structure of the retina composed of the müllerian fibers of that organ. **symplastic t.,** symplasm. **target t.,** 1. tissue, either *in vivo* or *in vitro*, against which humoral or cell-mediated immunity is directed. 2. the tissue that responds specifically to a given hormone. **tuberculosis granulation t.,** the tissue that forms the characteristic tubercle in pulmonary productive tuberculosis, composed of epithelioid cells in concentric masses, lymphocytes, and often Langhans giant cells. **vesicular supporting t.,** chondroid t.

tissular (tish′u-lar) pertaining to organic tissue.

titanium (ti ta′ne-um) [L., from Gk. *titan* a child of Uranus and Gala] a ᵔark-gray, metallic element of widespread distribution but occurring ᵢₙ small amounts; atomic number, 22; atomic weight, 47.90; symbol, Ti; specific gravity, 4.5; used for fixation of fractures. **t. dioxide** [USP], a white powder, TiO_2, used as a topical protectant against sunburn; it is also used in other protectant preparations and in dusting powders, and as a pigment in the manufacture of artificial teeth.

titer (ti′ter) [Fr. *titre* standard] the quantity of a substance required to produce a reaction with a given volume of another substance, or the amount of one substance required to correspond with a given amount of another substance. **agglutination t.,** the highest dilution of a serum which causes clumping of microorganisms or other particulate antigens. **whole complement t.,** see CH_{50} *assay*, under *assay.*

titillation (tit″ĭ-la′shun) [L. *titillatio*] the act or sensation of tickling.

titrant (ti′trant) the solution of known strength that is added in titration.

titrate (ti′trāt) to determine by titration.

titration (ti-tra′shun) [Fr. *titre* standard] determination of a given component in solution by addition of a liquid reagent of known strength until a given endpoint (e.g., change in color) is reached. **colorimetric t.,** a method of determining hydrogen ion concentration by adding an indicator to the unknown and then comparing the color with a set of tubes containing this same indicator in solutions of known hydrogen ion concentration. **complexometric t.,** titration of a substance (e.g., the calcium in clear serum) with a complexing agent (e.g., EDTA); the end point of the titration is generally observed as a change in color of the solution. **coulometric t.,** titration by determining the amount of electricity required to electrochemically generate a titrant which reacts with the substance in question. If the current is kept constant, as for chloride determination using the Cotlove titrator, the amount of electricity (coulombs) used is proportional to the elapsed time. **Dean and Webb t.,** a test for measuring antibody in which varying dilutions of antigen are mixed with a constant quantity of antiserum; antibody activity is determined by the dilution in which flocculation occurs most rapidly, i.e., the end point. In this dilution, antigen and antibody are together at a ratio of optimal proportions. **formol t.,** see *Sörensen's method,* under *method.* **potentiometric t.,** a method of determining hydrogen ion concentration by placing a hydrogen electrode in unknown solution and measuring the potential developed as compared with some standard electrode by means of a potentiometer.

titre (ti′ter) [Fr.] titer.

titrimetric (tit″rĭ-met′rik) pertaining to analysis by titration.

titrimetry (ti-trim′ĕ-tre) [*titration* + Gr. *metron* measure] analysis by titration.

titubant (tit′u-bant) a person who staggers.

titubation (tit″u-ba′shun) [L. *titubatio*] the act of staggering or reeling; a staggering or stumbling gait with shaking of the trunk and head, commonly seen in cerebellar disease. **lingual t.,** stuttering or stammering.

Tityus serrulatus (tit′e-us ser″u-la′tus) a scorpion of Brazil which inflicts a severe, sometimes fatal, sting.

tixanox (tiks′ah-noks) chemical name: 7-(methylsulfinyl)-

9-oxo-9H-xanthene-2-carboxylic acid; an antiallergic, C_{15}-$H_{10}O_5S$.

Tizzoni's test (tid-zo′nēz) [Guido *Tizzoni*, Italian physician, 1853–1932] see under *tests*.

tjettek (tyet′ek) a deadly poison prepared by the Javanese from the root of *Strychnos tieute*.

TKD tokodynamometer.

TKG tokodynagraph.

Tl chemical symbol for *thallium*.

TLC total lung capacity.

Tm chemical symbol for *thulium*.

TMV tobacco mosaic virus.

TNF tumor necrosis factor.

TNM see under *staging*.

TNT trinitrotoluene.

TO abbreviation for *tinctura opii*, tincture of opium.

toadskin (tōd′skin) follicular hyperkeratosis.

toadstool (tōd′stul) a popular name for a poisonous mushroom.

tobacco (to-bak′o) [L. *tabacum*] the dried and prepared leaves of *Nicotiana tabacum* L. (Solanaceae), a solanaceous plant. Tobacco contains various alkaloids, the principal one being *nicotine*, and unites the qualities of a sedative narcotic with those of an emetic and diuretic. It is also a heart depressant and antispasmodic. **mountain t.,** arnica. **poison t.,** hyoscyamus.

tobaccoism (to-bak′o-izm) a morbid condition due to excessive use of tobacco; nicotinism.

Tobey-Ayer test (to′be a′er) [George Loring *Tobey*, Jr., Boston otolaryngologist, 1881–1947; James Bourne *Ayer*, Boston neurologist, born 1882] see under *tests*.

tobramycin (to″brah-mi′sin) [USP] chemical name: *O*-3-amino-3-deoxy-α-D-glucopyranosyl-(1→6)-*O*-[2,2-diamino-2,3,6-trideoxy-α-D-*ribo*-hexopyranosyl-(1→4)]-2-deoxy-D-streptamine. A purified fraction of an aminoglycoside antibiotic complex (see *nebramycin*) produced by *Streptomyces tenebrarius*, $C_{18}H_{37}N_5O_9$, bactericidal against many gram-negative and some gram-positive organisms. Administered intravenously or intramuscularly, as the sulfate salt, in the treatment of septicemia and neonatal sepsis, and in central nervous system, lower respiratory, gastrointestinal, skin, bone, and soft-tissue infections due to susceptible strains of *Pseudomonas aeruginosa*, *Escherichia coli*, indole-negative and indole-positive *Proteus, Providencia, Klebsiella-Enterobacter-Serratia* group, *Citrobacter*, and staphylococci, including coagulase-positive and coagulase-negative *S. aureus*. Called also *tenebrimycin* and *tenemycin*.

tocainide (to-ka′nīd) chemical name: 2-amino-*N*-(2,6-dimethylphenyl)propanamide; a cardiac depressant (antiarrhythmic), $C_{11}H_{16}N_2O$.

tocamphyl (to-kam′fil) chemical name: 1,2,2-trimethyl-1,3-cyclopentanedicarboxylic acid 1-[1-(4-methylphenyl)-ethyl] ester compound with 2,2′-iminobis[ethanol](1:1); a cholerectic obtained from tumeric, $C_{19}H_{26}O_4 \cdot C_4H_{11}NO_2$.

Toclase (to′klās) trademark for preparations of carbetapentane citrate.

toc(o)- [Gr. *tokos* childbirth] a combining form denoting relationship to childbirth, or labor; see also words beginning *tok(o)-*.

tocodynagraph (to″ko-di′nah-graf) tokodynagraph.

tocodynamometer (to″ko-di″nah-mom′ĕ-ter) tokodynamometer.

tocograph (tok′o-graf) a recording tokodynamometer.

tocography (to-kog′rah-fe) [*toco-* + Gr. *graphein* to write] the graphic recording of uterine contractions.

tocokinin (tok″o-kin′in) [*toco-* + Gr. *kinein* to move] an extract from yeast and certain vegetables which has the properties of an estral hormone.

tocology (to-kol′o-je) obstetrics.

tocolysis (to-kol′ĭ-sis) [*toco-* + *lysis*] inhibition of uterine contractions in premature labor.

tocometer (to-kom′ĕ-ter) [*toco-* + Gr. *metron* measure] tokodynamometer.

tocopherol (to-kof′er-ol) [*toco-* + Gr. *pherein* to carry] an alcohol which has the properties of vitamin E; isolated from the oil of the germ of wheat kernel, or produced synthetically. **α-t., alpha-t.,** vitamin E.

tocophobia (to″ko-fo′be-ah) [*toco-* + Gr. *phobein* to be affrighted by] abnormal dread of childbirth.

tocus (to′kus) [L.; Gr. *tokos*] labor; childbirth.

Todd bodies (tod) [John Launcelot *Todd*, Canadian physician, 1876–1949] see under *body*.

Todd's cirrhosis, paralysis (palsy), process (todz) [Robert Bentley *Todd*, English physician, 1809–1860] see under *paralysis*, see *primary biliary cirrhosis*, under *cirrhosis*, and see *fibrae intercrurales*.

Toddalia (to-dal′e-ah) a genus of rutaceous shrubs. The root of *T. aculeata* Pers., of the East Indies, is an aromatic stomachic. The bark is used in India as a source of yellow dye. The rootbark is considered to be antimalarial, and possesses antiperiodic and antipyretic properties.

toddy (tod′e) [Hind. *tāre, tādi*] 1. the fermented sap of various palm trees. 2. a drink prepared from gin or whisky, sugar, and water.

toe (to) any of the five digits of the foot. See also *ossa digitorum pedis*, under os[3]. **curly t's,** a condition affecting chicks, in which the toes curl underneath the feet, due to a deficiency of riboflavin. **great t.,** the first digit of the foot; called also *hallux* [NA]. **hammer t.,** a condition in which the proximal phalanx of a toe—most often that of the second toe—is extended and the second and distal phalanges are flexed, causing a clawlike appearance. **little t.,** the fifth digit of the foot; called also *digitus minimum pedis*. **mallet t.,** flexion contracture of the distal interphalangeal joint of any of the lesser toes. **Morton's t.,** a form of metatarsalgia due to compression of a branch of the plantar nerve by the metatarsal heads; chronic compression may lead to formation of a neuroma. Called also *Morton's disease, foot,* or *neuralgia*. **pigeon t.,** a permanent toeing-in position of the feet. **seedy t.,** a disease of horses' feet marked by a fungous growth of a horny, honeycombed texture between the coffin bone and the wall of the hoof. **tennis t.,** painful great toe associated with subungual hematoma, which, in the absence of treatment, may lead to subungual abscess; it usually develops after a vigorous tennis game, especially when tennis shoes with protective tips are worn. **webbed t's,** toes abnormally joined by strands of tissue at their base.

toenail (to′nāl) the nail on any of the digits of the foot. See *unguis* [NA]. **ingrowing t.,** ingrown nail. **ingrown t.,** aberrant growth of a toenail, with one (usually the outer) margin or, less often, both lateral margins growing deeply into the nail groove and surrounding tissues.

Toepfer (tep′fer) see *Töpfer*.

tofenacin hydrochloride (to-fen′ah-sin) chemical name: *N*-methyl-2-[(2-methylphenyl)phenylmethoxy]ethanamine hydrochloride; an anticholinergic, $C_{17}H_{21}NO \cdot HCl$, with antidepressant properties.

Tofranil (to-fra′nil) trademark for preparations of imipramine hydrochloride.

tofu (to′foo) a Japanese food preparation from the soy bean, in white tablets.

tofukasu (to-foo-kah′soo) a Japanese food prepared from soy beans.

togavirus (to″gah-vi′rus) a subgroup of arboviruses, including mosquito-borne and tickborne viruses that cause hemorrhagic fever; they are RNA viruses with envelopes (or "togas").

toilet (toi′let) cleansing, as of an accidental wound and the surrounding skin, or of an obstetrical patient after childbirth.

Toison's solution (fluid) (twah-zawz′) [J. *Toison*, French histologist, 1858–1900] see under *solution*.

tokelau (to-ke-lah′oo) [*Tokelau*, a South Pacific atoll] tinea imbricata.

tok(o)- [Gr. *tokos* childbirth] for words beginning thus, see also those beginning *toc(o)-*.

tokodynagraph (to″ko-di′nah-graf) [Gr. *tokos* childbirth + *graphein* to write] the record obtained with a tokodynamometer. Abbreviated TKG.

tokodynamometer (to″ko-di″nah-mom′ĕ-ter) [Gr. *tokos* childbirth + *dynamis* power + *metron* measure] an instrument for measuring the expulsive force of the uterine contractions in labor. Abbreviated TKD.

tolamolol (to-lah′mo-lōl) chemical name: 4-[2-[[2-hydroxy-3-(2-methylphenoxy)propyl] amino] ethoxy] benzamide. A beta-adrenergic blocking agent, $C_{19}H_{24}N_2O_4$, which has been used as a coronary vasodilator in the treatment of angina of effort and as a cardiac depressant in the treatment of arrhythmias.

tolazamide (tol-az′ah-mīd) [USP] chemical name: *N*-[[(hexahydro-1*H*-azepin-1-yl) amino] carbonyl]-4-methylbenzene sulfonamide An orally effective hypoglycemic sulfonylurea, $C_{14}H_{21}N_3O_3S$, occurring as a white to off-white, crystalline powder; used in the treatment of diabetes mellitus.

tolazoline hydrochloride (tol-az′o-lēn) [USP] chemical name: 4,5-dihydro-2-(phenylmethyl)-1*H*-imidazole monohydrochloride. An adrenergic blocking agent and peripheral vasodilator, $C_{10}H_{12}N_2 \cdot HCl$, occurring as a white to off-white, crystalline powder; used in the treatment of peripheral vascular disorders due to vasospasm, administered orally.

tolbutamide (tol-bu′tah-mīd) [USP] chemical name: *N*-[(butylamino)carbonyl]-4-methylbenzenesulfonamide. An orally effective hypoglycemic sulfonylurea, $C_{12}H_{18}N_2O_3S$, occurring as a white, or practically white, crystalline powder; used in the treatment of diabetes mellitus. **t. sodium** [USP], the monosodium salt of tolbutamide, $C_{12}H_{17}N_2NaO_3S$, occurring as a white to off-white, crystalline powder, having the same actions as the base; used as a diagnostic test for diabetes mellitus, administered intravenously.

tolciclate (tōl-si′klāt) chemical name: *O*-1,2,3,4-tetrahydro-1,4-methanonaphthalen-6-yl)ester methyl(3-methylphenyl)carbamothioic acid; a topical antifungal, $C_{20}H_{21}NOS$.

Tolectin (tol′ek-tin) trademark for a preparation of tolmetin sodium.

tolerance (tol′er-ans) [L. *tolerantia*] 1. the ability to endure unusually large doses of a drug or toxin. 2. acquired drug tolerance; a decreasing response to repeated constant doses of a drug or the need for increasing doses to maintain a constant response. 3. immunologic tolerance. **acquired t.,** the increasing resistance to the usual effects of a drug due to continued use. **adoptive t.,** immunological tolerance induced by the passive transfer to an irradiated recipient animal of lymphoid cells from a donor rendered tolerant to an antigen. **alkali t.,** ability of the body to endure the administration of alkalis, measured by the amount of alkali that must be given to cause an alkaline urine; this forms a rough measure of the degree of acidosis. **crossed t.,** the lessened susceptibility which persons who have acquired a tolerance for one drug or poison may thereafter exhibit toward another drug. **drug t.,** progressive diminution of susceptibility to the effects of a drug, resulting from its continued administration. **glucose t.,** ability of the body to properly metabolize an administered glucose load. **high-dose t., high-zone t.,** see *immunologic t.* **immunologic t.,** an immunologic response consisting of the development of specific nonreactivity of the lymphoid tissues to a given antigen that in other circumstances can induce cell-mediated or humoral immunity; it results from previous contact with the antigen and has no effect on the response to non–cross-reacting antigens. Tolerance is readily induced by administrator of antigen to immunologically immature animals (fetuses, neonates). In adults tolerance may be induced by repeated administration of very large doses of antigen (*high-dose* or *high-zone t.*), or of small doses that are below the threshold required for stimulation of an immune response (*low-dose* or *low-zone t.*). Tolerance is most readily induced by soluble antigens administered intravenously; immunosuppression also facilitates the induction of tolerance. **impaired glucose t. (IGT),** a term denoting values of fasting blood glucose or results of an oral glucose tolerance test that are abnormal but not high enough to be diagnostic of diabetes mellitus. Formerly called *chemical, latent, preclinical,* or *subclinical diabetes.* **low-dose t., low-zone t.,** see *immunologic t.* **self t.,** immunologic unresponsiveness to autoantigens (self antigens), acquired during fetal life by a process of "self recognition." Theories of tolerance induction include deletion of antigen-responsive clones of B cells, antigen-induced inactivation of B or T cells, and induction of antigen-specific T suppressor cells. **split t.,** 1. following induction of immunologic tolerance to allogeneic cells, tolerance to an antigen or group of antigens on the cell surface occurs, while there is an immune response to other antigens on the cell surface. 2. immunologic tolerance that affects either the humoral immune system or the cell-mediated immune system, but not both simultaneously. Called also *immunodeviation.*

tolerant (tol′er-ant) able to endure, without effect, the action of any particular drug or other agent; exhibiting tolerance.

toleration (tol″er-a′shun) tolerance.

tolerogen (tol′er-o-jen) an antigen used to introduce tolerance, particularly a form of an antigen (usually a soluble form) that induces tolerance, as distinguished from an immunogen, another form (usually an insoluble form) that induces immunity.

tolerogenesis (tol″er-o-jen′ĕ-sis) induction of immunologic tolerance.

tolerogenic (tol″er-o-jen′ik) capable of inducing immunologic tolerance.

tolindate (to-lin′dāt) chemical name: *O*-2,3-dihydro-1*H*-inden-5-yl) ester carbamothioic acid; an antifungal, $C_{18}H_{19}$-NOS.

Tolinase (tōl′in-ās) trademark for a preparation of tolazamide.

toliodium chloride (to-li′o-de-um) chemical name: bis(4-methylphenyl)iodonium chloride; a veterinary food additive, $C_{14}H_{14}ClI$.

Tollens' test (tol′enz) [Bernhard Christian Gottfried *Tollens,* German chemist, 1841–1918] see under *tests.*

tolmetin sodium (tol′met-in) [USP] chemical name: 1-methyl-5-(4-methylbenzoyl)-1*H*-pyrrole-2-acetic acid. An anti-inflammatory, analgesic, and antipyretic, $C_{15}H_{14}NNaO_3 \cdot 2H_2O$, used in the treatment of osteoarthritis and rheumatoid arthritis, administered orally.

tolnaftate (tol-naf′tāt) [USP] chemical name: *O*-2-naphthalenyl ester carbamothioic acid. A synthetic antifungal, $C_{19}H_{17}NOS$, occurring as a white to creamy white, fine powder; used topically in the treatment of various forms of tinea of the skin.

tolonium chloride (to-lo′ne-um) chemical name: 3-amino-7-(dimethylamino)-2-methylphenothiazin-5-ium chloride. An antiheparin compound, $C_{15}H_{16}ClN_3S$, which has been used in the treatment of idiopathic functional uterine bleeding and menorrhagia, topically to detect and delineate oral and cervical neoplasia, and intravenously to stain the parathyroid glands. Called also *toluidine blue O.*

Tolserol (tol′ser-ol) trademark for preparations of mephenesin.

toluene (tol′u-ēn) the hydrocarbon methylbenzene, C_6H_5-CH_3; a colorless liquid obtainable from tolu and other resins and from coal tar. It is an organic solvent used in rubber and plastic cements, paint removers, etc. Poisoning may result from ingesting the solvent or inhaling its concentrated vapors. Called also *toluol* and *methyl benzene.*

toluidine (tol-u′ĭ-din) a compound, 2-amino-toluene, CH_3-$C_6H_4 \cdot NH_2$, made by reducing nitrotoluene. It is homologous with aniline. **t. blue O,** tolonium chloride.

toluol (tol′u-ol) toluene.

tolusafranine (tol″u-saf′rah-nin) a dibenzoparadiazine dye, $NH_2(CH_3) \cdot C_6H_3 \cdot N_2 \cdot (C_6H_5)Cl \cdot C_6H_3(CH_3) \cdot NH_2$, the chief constituent of safranin.

toluyl (tol′u-il) the univalent acid radical, $CH_3 \cdot C_6H_4$.

toluylene (tol-u′ĭ-lēn) the hydrocarbon, diphenyl ethylene, $C_6H_5 \cdot CH:CH \cdot C_6H_5$; called also *stilbene.*

tolyl (tol′il) the univalent radical, $CH_3 \cdot C_6H_4$, isomeric with benzyl. **t. hydroxide,** cresol.

tomatin (to-ma′tin) an antibiotic substance with antifungal properties, isolated from tomato plants affected with wilt.

-tome [Gr. *tomē* a cutting] a word termination signifying (*a*) an instrument for cutting or (*b*) a segment.

tomentum (to-men′tum) a little used term for a network of minute blood vessels of the pia mater and the cortex cerebri; called also *t. cerebri.*

Tomes' fiber, fibril, layer, process (tōmz) [Sir John *Tomes,* English anatomist and dentist, 1815–1895] see *process of odontoblast* (for *fiber, fibril,* and *process*), and see *granular layer of Tomes,* under *layer.*

Tomes' process (tōmz) [Charles Sissmore *Tomes,* English anatomist and dentist, 1846–1928] see under *process* (def. 1).

tomite (to′mīt) [*tom-* + Gr. *mitos* thread] the free-swimming nonfeeding stage or form in the life cycle of certain ciliate protozoa, produced by a tomont and, depending on the species, developing into a phoront, theront, or trophont.

Tommaselli's disease (syndrome) (tom″ah-sel′ēz) [Salvatore *Tommaselli*, Italian physician, 1834–1906] see under *disease*.

tom(o)- [Gr. *tomē* a cutting] a combining form denoting relationship to a cutting, or to a designated layer, as might be achieved by cutting or slicing.

tomogram (to′mo-gram) a roentgenogram of a selected layer of the body made by tomography.

tomograph (to′mo-graf) an apparatus for moving an x-ray source in one direction as the film is moved in the opposite direction, thus showing in detail a predetermined plane of tissue while blurring or eliminating detail in other planes.

tomography (to-mog′rah-fe) [*tomo-* + Gr. *graphein* to write] the recording of internal body images at a predetermined plane by means of the tomograph; called also *body section roentgenography*. **computed t.,** computerized axial t. **computerized axial t. (CAT),** that in which the emergent x-ray beam is measured by a scintillation counter; the electronic impulses are recorded on a magnetic disk and then are processed by a mini-computer for reconstruction display of the body in cross-section on a cathode ray tube. Called also *computed t.* and *CAT scan.* **hypocycloidal t.,** tomography in which the path of the x-ray source is a hypocycloid, i.e., the path traced by a point on one circle rolling along inside the circumferance of another circle. **positron emission t. (PET),** that accomplished by detection of gamma rays emitted from tissues after administration of a natural biochemical substance (e.g., glucose, fatty acids) into which positron-emitting isotopes have been incorporated. The paths of the gamma rays, which result from collisions of positrons and electrons, are interpreted by a computer, and the resultant tomogram represents local concentrations of the isotope-containing substance. **ultrasonic t.,** the ultrasonographic visualization of a cross-section of a predetermined plane of the body by linear scanning with an ultrasonic probe across the desired site and displaying on a B-scan.

tomont (to′mont) [*tom-* + Gr. *ontos* beings] the nonfeeding, dividing stage or form in the life cycle of certain protozoa that typically encysts and produces tomites by fission.

-tomy [Gr. *tomē* a cutting] a word termination signifying the operation of cutting, or incision.

tonaphasia (ton″ah-fa′ze-ah) inability to recall a familiar tune; musical aphasia.

tone (tōn) [Gr. *tonos;* L. *tonus*] 1. the normal degree of vigor and tension; in muscle, the resistance to passive elongation or stretch; tonus. 2. a particular quality of sound or of voice. 3. to make permanent, or to change, the color of silver stain by chemical treatment, usually with a heavy metal. **feeling t.,** the condition or state of mind and feeling which accompanies every thought or act. **heart t's,** the sounds heard in the auscultation of the heart. **jecoral t.,** the sound produced by percussion over the liver. **plastic t.,** the posture-maintaining mechanism of muscle by virtue of which a limb passively placed in any position tends to maintain that position. **Traube's double t.,** a double heart sound heard in aortic regurgitation. **Williams' tracheal t.,** see under *sign*, def. 1.

tonga (tong′gah) a native name for yaws in New Caledonia and the Loyalty Islands.

tongs (tongs) an instrument for grasping and holding, consisting of two arms joined by a hinge or pivot. **skull t.,** tongs used to exert traction on the skull, as in surgery for fractures of cervical vertebrae; many forms are available, including Crutchfield t., Gardner-Wells t., Barton t., and Vinke t.

tongue (tung) [L. *lingua,* Gr. *glōssa*] 1. the movable, muscular organ on the floor of the mouth, subserving the special sense of taste and aiding in mastication, deglutition, and the articulation of sound. Called also *lingua* [NA]. 2. any structure or part having a shape similar to that of the oral organ of the same name. Called also *lingula* [NA]. **adherent t.,** ankyloglossia. **amyloid t.,** enlargement of the tongue due to amyloidosis. **antibiotic t.,** glossitis caused by sensitivity to an antibiotic. **baked t.,** the dry, brown tongue of typhoid fever. **bald t.,** Moeller's glossitis. **beefy t.,** erythematous and/or atrophic glossitis, characterized by red, irregular ulcerations on the dorsal surface of the tongue. **bifid t.,** a tongue that is divided in its anterior part by a longitudinal fissure; called also *cleft t.* **black t., black hairy t.,** hairy tongue (q.v.) in which the hypertrophied filiform papillae are brown or black. Called

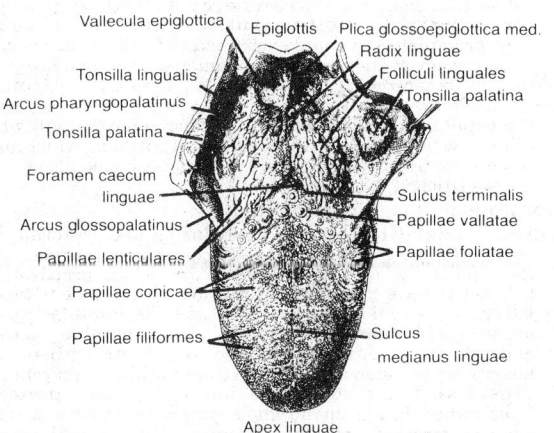

The tongue, showing principal structures.

also *anthracosis linguae, glossophytia, keratomycosis linguae, lingua nigra, lingua villosa nigra, melanoglossia, melanotrichia linguae,* and *nigrities linguae.* **blue t.,** a disease of sheep and cattle in South Africa, caused by a virus, and characterized by hyperemia, erosions, and edema of the lips, tongue, and oral mucosa. **burning t.,** glossopyrosis. **cardinal t.,** a tongue whose surface is denuded of epithelium, giving it a bright red appearance. **cerebriform t.,** fissured t. **choreic t.,** abrupt, snakelike protrusion and withdrawal of the tongue occurring in chorea. **cleft t.,** bifid t. **coated t.,** a tongue covered with a whitish or yellowish layer consisting of desquamated epithelium, debris, bacteria, fungi, or other material, which is readily removed by scraping. **cobble-stone t.,** a condition marked by interstitial glossitis with hypertrophy of the papillae and a verrucous white coating on the tongue, such as seen in riboflavin deficiency. **crocodile t.,** fissured t. **dotted t.,** stippled t. **double t.,** bifid t. **earthy t.,** a tongue that is coated with a deposit of rough, calcareous matter. **encrusted t.,** a heavily coated tongue. **fern leaf t.,** a tongue with a central furrow having lateral branches. **filmy t.,** one marked with symmetrical whitish patches. **fissured t.,** a sometimes familial condition characterized by the presence on the dorsal surface of the tongue of numerous furrows, which may radiate outwardly from the median raphe. Called also *cerebriform t., crocodile t., furrowed t., grooved t., plicated t., scrotal t., sulcated t., wrinkled t.,* and *lingua plicata.* **flat t.,** a condition in which the borders of the tongue cannot be rolled; it is due to paralysis of the transverse lingual muscles occurring as a result of congenital syphilis. **furred t.,** a tongue with papillae so changed as to give the mucous membrane the appearance of whitish fur. **furrowed t.,** fissured t. **geographic t.,** benign migratory glossitis. **grooved t.,** fissured t. **hairy t.,** a benign condition of the tongue characterized by hypertrophy of the filiform papillae that gives the dorsum of the tongue a furry appearance. The color of the elongated papillae varies from yellowish white to brown or black (*black t.* or *black hairy t.*), depending upon staining by substances such as tobacco, foods, or drugs. Called also *glossotrichia* and *trichoglossia.* **lobulated t.,** a congenital condition marked by a secondary lobe arising from the surface of the tongue. **magenta t.,** the magenta-colored tongue seen in cases of riboflavin deficiency. **mappy t.,** benign migratory glossitis. **parrot t.,** the dry, horny tongue of low fever, which cannot be protruded. **plicated t.,** fissured t. **raspberry t.,** the beefy red tongue with a glistening smooth surface and prominent filiform papillae seen after desquamation of the white coating on the tongue characteristic of the early stage of scarlet fever; called also *red strawberry t.* Cf. *white strawberry t.* **Sandwith's bald t.,** an extremely clean tongue sometimes seen in the late stages of pellagra. **scrotal t.,** fissured t. **smokers' t.,** oral leukoplakia of the tongue. **t. of sphenoid bone,** lingula sphenoidalis. **split t.,** bifid t. **stippled t.,** a tongue on which each papilla is covered with a separate white patch of epithelium;

Labels on figure: Vallecula epiglottica; Epiglottis; Plica glossoepiglottica med.; Tonsilla lingualis; Radix linguae; Folliculi linguales; Arcus pharyngopalatinus; Tonsilla palatina; Tonsilla palatina; Foramen caecum linguae; Arcus glossopalatinus; Sulcus terminalis; Papillae vallatae; Papillae lenticulares; Papillae foliatae; Papillae conicae; Papillae filiformes; Sulcus medianus linguae; Apex linguae called also *dotted t.* **strawberry t., red,** raspberry t. **strawberry t., white,** white, the white-coated tongue with prominent red papillae characteristic of the early stage of scarlet fever; the coating desquamates, leaving a beefy red tongue (*raspberry t.*). **sulcated t.,** fissured t. **timber t.,** wooden t. **white t.,** a condition in which all or part of the papillae and epithelium of the tongue have a dull white color. **wooden t.,** actinobacillosis of cattle in which hard tumor-like nodules form inside the tongue; called also *timber t.* **wrinkled t.,** fissured t.

tongue-tie (tung′ti) ankyloglossia.

tonic (ton′ik) [Gr. *tonikos*] 1. producing and restoring the normal tone. 2. characterized by continuous tension. 3. a term formerly used for a class of medicinal preparations believed to have the power of restoring normal tone to tissue. **bitter t.,** a tonic of bitter taste, used for stimulating the appetite and improving digestion, such as quinine, quassia, and gentian. **cardiac t.,** one which strengthens the heart's action, such as digitalis, strophanthin, or strychnine. **digestive t.,** an intestinal or stomachic tonic. **general t.,** one which braces up the whole system; cold baths, electricity, and exercise are general tonics. **intestinal t.,** one that improves the tone of the intestinal tract. **stomachic t.,** one which aids the functions of the stomach; here are classed the alcoholic stimulants, vegetable bitters, hydrochloric and nitrohydrochloric acids. **vascular t.,** one which increases the tone of the blood vessels; among them are belladonna, digitalis, ergot, and strychnine.

tonicity (to-nis′ĭ-te) the state of tissue tone or tension; in body fluid physiology, the effective osmotic pressure equivalent.

tonicize (ton′ĭ-sīz) 1. to improve the tone of a part. 2. to induce tonic contraction of a muscle.

tonicoclonic (ton″ĭ-ko-klon′ik) tonoclonic.

tonka bean (tong′kah bēn) the seed of *Dipteryx odorata* Willd. (Leguminosae), a North America tree; it affords coumarin, and has been used as a flavoring agent and to disguise odors in pharmaceutical and tobacco.

ton(o)- [Gr. *tonos* tension] a combining form denoting relationship to tone or tension.

tonoclonic (ton″o-klon′ik) both tonic and clonic; said of a spasm consisting of a convulsive twitching of the muscles.

tonofibril (ton′o-fi″bril) a bundle of fine filaments (tonofilaments) in certain cells, especially epithelial cells, the individual strands of which transverse the cytoplasm in all directions and extend into the cell processes to converge and insert on the desmosomes; they are thought to have a supportive or cytoskeletal function and, in keratinizing epithelia, to be the principal precursor of keratin.

tonofilament (ton″o-fil′ah-ment) any of the fine filaments of a tonofibril.

tonogram (to′no-gram) the record produced by tonography.

tonograph (to′no-graf) [tono- + -*graph*] a recording tonometer.

tonography (to-nog′rah-fe) [tono- + -*graphy*] the recording of changes in intraocular pressure produced by the constant application of a known weight on the globe of the eye, reflecting the facility of outflow of the aqueous humor from the anterior chamber. **carotid compression t.,** a test for occlusion of the carotid artery by measuring ocular pressure and pulse before, during, and after the proximal portion of the carotid artery is compressed by the fingers.

tonometer (to-nom′ĕ-ter) [tono- + -*metry*] an instrument for measuring tension or pressure; usually used specifically in reference to an instrument by which intraocular pressure is measured; called also *ophthalmotonometer.* **air-puff t.,** an instrument for measuring intraocular pressure; it does not touch the eye, but rather senses deflections of the cornea in reaction to a puff of pressurized air. **applanation t.,** an instrument that measures intraocular pressure by determination of the force necessary to flatten a corneal surface of constant size. **electronic t.,** one having an electronic readout. **Gärtner's t.,** an instrument for measuring blood pressure by means of a compressing ring applied to the finger. **Goldmann's applanation t.,** an instrument for measuring intraocular pressure which eliminates the effects of scleral resistance. **impression t., indentation t.,** an instrument that measures direct pressure on the eyeball, such as the Schiøtz, McLean, or MacKay-Marg

electronic tonometer. **MacKay-Marg electronic t.,** an electronic applanation tonometer equipped with a flat plunger which measures intraocular pressure by direct application to the cornea. **McLean t.,** impression t. **Musken's t.,** an instrument for measuring the tonicity of the Achilles tendon. **Recklinghausen's t.,** an instrument for observing oscillatory blood pressure. **Schiøtz' t.,** an instrument that registers intraocular pressure by direct application to the cornea, the reading on the scale being translated into millimeters of mercury by means of a conversion table.

tonometry (to-nom′ĕ-tre) [tono- + -*metry*] 1. the measurement of tension or pressure. 2. ophthalmotonometry. **digital t.,** estimation of the degree of intraocular pressure by pressure exerted on the eyeball by the finger of the examiner.

tonophant (ton′o-fant) [tono- + Gr. *phainein* to show] (*obs.*) an instrument for rendering acoustic vibrations visible.

tonoplast (ton′o-plast) [tono- + Gr. *plassein* to form] a small intracellular body which forms powerful osmotic substances within itself and thus swells up to form a small vacuole (De Vries, 1885). The term is now applied to the limiting membrane of an intracellular vacuole, the vacuole membrane.

tonoscope (ton′o-skop) [tono- + Gr. *skopein* to examine] (*obs.*) 1. an apparatus for rendering sound visible by registering the vibrations on a screen. 2. a device for examining the head or brain by means of sound. 3. tonometer.

tonotopic (ton″o-top′ik) having a spatial arrangement such that certain tone frequencies are transmitted along a particular portion of the structure, as in the cochlear nuclei.

tonotopicity (ton″o-top-is′ĭ-te) the property of being tonotopic.

tonsil (ton′sil) a small rounded mass of tissue, especially of lymphoid tissue. The term is often used without qualification to designate the palatine tonsil. Called also *tonsilla.* **adenoid t.,** tonsilla pharyngealis. **buried t.,** submerged t. **t. of cerebellum,** tonsilla cerebelli. **eustachian t.,** see *noduli lymphatici tubarii tubae auditivae.* **faucial t.,** see *palatine t.* **Gerlach's t.,** see *noduli lymphatici tubarii tubae auditivae.* **intestinal t.,** see *folliculi lymphatici aggregati.* **lingual t.,** tonsilla lingualis. **Luschka's t.,** tonsilla pharyngea. **palatine t.,** either of two small, almond-shaped masses located between the palatoglossal and palatopharyngeal arches, one or either side of the oropharynx, composed mainly of lymphoid tissue, covered with mucous membrane, and containing various crypts and many lymph follicles; believed to act as sources for supply to the mouth and pharynx of phagocytes which destroy bacteria entering the mouth. Called also *tonsilla palatina* [NA]. **pharyngeal t.,** tonsilla pharyngealis. **submerged t.,** a palatine tonsil that is shrunken and atrophied and is partly or entirely hidden by the palatoglossal arch. **third t.,** tonsilla pharyngealis. **t. of torus tubarius,** tonsilla tubaria. **tubal t's,** noduli lymphatici tubarii tubae auditivae.

tonsilla (ton-sil′ah), pl. *tonsil′lae* [L.] tonsil: [NA] a general term for a small rounded mass of tissue, especially of lymphoid tissue. **t. adenoi′dea,** NA alternative for *t. pharyngealis.* **t. cerebel′li** [NA], **t. of cerebellum,** a rounded mass forming part of the candal lobe of the hemisphere of the cerebellum continuous with the uvula of the vermis; called also *amygdala of cerebellum.* **t. intestina′lis,** see *folliculi lymphatici aggregati.* **t. lingua′lis** [NA], lingual tonsil: an aggregation of lymph follicles on the floor of the oropharyngeal passageway, at the root of the tongue. **t. palati′na** [NA], a small, almond-shaped mass between the palatoglossal and palatopharyngeal arches on either side; see *palatine tonsil.* **t. pharyngea′lis pharyngea′lis** [NA], pharyngeal tonsil: the diffuse lymphoid tissue and follicles in the roof and posterior wall of the nasopharynx; called also *adenoid tonsil* and *t. adenoidea* [NA alternative]. See also *adenoid* (def. 2). **t. tuba′ria** [NA], lymphoid tissue associated with the opening of the auditory tube; called also *tonsil of torus tubarius.*

tonsillar (ton′sĭ-lar) [L. *tonsillaris*] of or pertaining to a tonsil; amygdaline.

tonsillectome (ton″sĭ-lek′tōm) an instrument for performing tonsillectomy.

tonsillectomy (ton″sĭ-lek′to-me) [L. *tonsilla* tonsil + Gr. *ektomē* excision] surgical removal of a tonsil or tonsils.

tonsillith (ton′sĭ-lith) tonsillolith.

tonsillitic (ton″sĭ-lit′ik) pertaining to or affected with tonsillitis.

tonsillitis (ton″sĭ-li′tis) [L. *tonsilla* tonsil + *-itis*] inflammation of the tonsils, especially the palatine tonsils. **caseous t.,** lacunar t. **catarrhal t., acute,** a form associated with acute catarrhal pharyngitis, in which the tonsils are red and swollen; called also *erythematous t.* **catarrhal t., chronic,** a form attended by permanent hypertrophy, and usually requiring tonsillectomy. **diphtherial t.,** diphtheria (q.v.) involving the tonsil(s). **erythematous t.,** catarrhal t., acute. **follicular t.,** that which especially affects the crypts (once referred to as follicles). **herpetic t.,** a local manifestation of herpes on the tonsil. **lacunar t.,** tonsillitis in which the crypts of the tonsils are filled with plugs of caseous matter; called also *caseous t.* **t. len′ta,** chronic inflammation of the tonsils producing a prolonged chronic sepsis. **lingual t.,** inflammation of a lymphoid mass at the base of the tongue. **mycotic t.,** a form due to fungi. **parenchymatous t., acute,** inflammation of the whole substance of the tonsil. **preglottic t.,** inflammation of the lingual tonsil. **pustular t.,** that which is characterized by the formation of pustules. **streptococcal t.,** see *septic sore throat,* under *sore throat.* **superficial t.,** inflammation of the mucous membrane over a tonsil. **suppurative t.,** parenchymatous t., acute. **Vincent's t.,** acute necrotizing gingivitis involving only the tonsils.

tonsill(o)- [L. *tonsilla,* q.v.] a combining form denoting relationship to a tonsil or to the tonsils.

tonsilloadenoidectomy (ton″sil-o-ad″ĕ-noi-dek′to-me) excision of palatine tonsils and adenoids.

tonsillohemisporosis (ton″sĭ-lo-hem″ĭ-spo-ro′sis) infection of the tonsil with *Hemispora.*

tonsillolith (ton-sil′o-lith) [tonsil + Gr. *lithos* stone] a concretion or calculus in a tonsil.

tonsillomoniliasis (ton-sil″o-mo″nĭ-li′ah-sis) infection of the tonsil with *Monilia* (*Candida*).

tonsillomycosis (ton-sil″o-mi-ko′sis) any mycotic infection of the tonsils.

tonsillo-oidiosis (ton-sil″o-o-id″e-o′sis) infection of the tonsil with *Oidium* (*Candida*).

tonsillopathy (ton″sĭ-lop′ah-the) [tonsil + Gr. *pathos* disease] any disease of the tonsil.

tonsillotome (ton-sil′o-tōm) a knife used in tonsillectomy or tonsillotomy.

tonsillotomy (ton″sĭ-lot′o-me) [L. *tonsilla* tonsil + Gr. *tomē* a cutting] incision of a tonsil; the surgical removal of a part of a tonsil.

tonsillotyphoid (ton″sĭ-lo-ti′foid) pharyngotyphoid.

tonsolith (ton′so-lith) tonsillolith.

tonus (to′nus) [L.; Gr. *tonos*] the slight, continuous contraction of muscle, which in skeletal muscles aids in the maintenance of posture and in the return of blood to the heart. See *tone.* **acerebral t.,** tonic contraction of muscles after removal of the cerebrum. **chemical t.,** the state of slight but continuous chemical activity in muscles when at rest. **myogenic t.,** tonic contraction of muscle dependent upon some property of the muscle itself or of its intrinsic nerve cells. **neurogenic t.,** tonic contraction of muscle due to stimulation received through the nervous system.

tooth (tōōth), pl. **teeth** [L. *dens;* Gr. *odous*] any of the hard calcified structures set in the alveolar processes of the mandible and maxilla for mastication of food, or a similar structure. In humans, there are two sets of teeth (*dentes* [NA]), *deciduous* and *permanent.* Each tooth consists of three parts—the *crown,* the portion exposed above the gingival line, having a central cavity which contains the dental pulp; the *neck,* the constricted region between the crown and the root; and the *root,* the portion embedded within the alveolus and attached to the periodontal membrane. The solid part includes *dentin,* forming most of the tooth and resembling true bone; *enamel,* a very hard inorganic substance, covering the crown; and *cementum,* covering the root. The soft tissue, the *dental pulp,* is composed of richly vascularized and innervated connective tissue. See also *dentition.* **abutment t.,** one selected to support a bridge on the basis of the total surface area of a healthy attachment apparatus. See also *abutment,* def. 2. **accessional teeth,** the permanent molars, so called because they do not supplant any deciduous predecessors in the dental arch. Cf. *succedaneous teeth.* **anatomic teeth,** 1. artificial teeth that duplicate the anatomic forms of natural teeth. 2. teeth that have prominent pointed or rounded cusps on the masticating surfaces and are designed to occlude with the teeth of the opposing denture or natural dentition. **ankylosed t.,** submerged t. **anterior teeth,** teeth in the anterior portion of each dental arch; the four incisors (two central and two lateral incisors) and the two canines in either jaw. Called also *labial teeth* and *morsal teeth.* **artificial t.,** one fabricated for use as a substitute for a natural tooth in a prosthesis, usually made of porcelain or resin. See also *denture.* **auditory teeth of Huschke,** dentes acustici. **t. of axis,** dens axis. **baby teeth,** deciduous teeth. **bicuspid teeth,** premolar teeth (dentes premolares [NA]). **buccal teeth,** posterior teeth. **canine teeth,** the four teeth, one on either side in each jaw, immediately lateral to the lateral, or second, incisors; they have a long conical crown

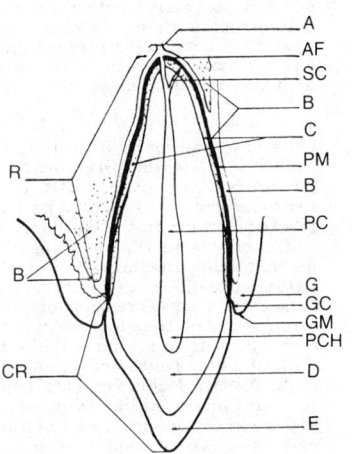

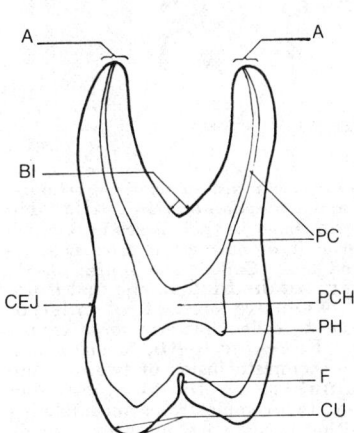

Schematic cross section of an anterior and a posterior tooth in the maxilla. *Left,* Anterior tooth: *A,* apex; *AF,* apical foramen; *SC,* supplementary canal; *C,* cementum; *PM,* periodontal membrane; *B,* bone; *PC,* pulp canal; *G,* gingiva; *GC,* gingival sulcus; *GM,* gingival margin; *PCH,* pulp chamber; *D,* dentin; *E,* enamel; *CR,* crown; *R,* root. *Right,* Posterior tooth: *A,* apices; *PC,* pulp canal; *PCH,* pulp chamber; *PH,* pulp horn; *F,* fissure; *CU,* cusp; *CEJ,* cemento-enamel junction; *BI,* bifurcation of roots.

and the longest, most powerful root of all the teeth. Called also *dentes canini* [NA]. **cheek teeth,** posterior teeth. **conical t.,** peg t. **connate t.,** geminate t. **corner t.,** the third incisor on either side of each jaw in the horse. **cross-bite teeth,** artificial posterior teeth designed to permit positioning of the modified buccal cusps of the upper teeth in the fossae of the lower teeth. **cross-pin teeth,** artificial teeth in which the pins are inserted horizontally. **cuspid teeth,** canine teeth (dentes canini [NA]). **cuspless t.,** any tooth deprived of a cusp; particularly an artificial tooth designed without cuspal prominences on the occlusal surface. **deciduous teeth,** the 20 teeth of the first dentition, which are shed and replaced by the permanent teeth. They begin to calcify at about the fourth month of fetal life, and near the end of the sixth month they all have begun to develop. The first incisors appear at about the age of 6 1/2 months; they are followed by the second incisors 1/2 month later; and, within 1 1/2 months, by the maxillary incisors. The deciduous molars begin eruption at 1 year, and the deciduous canines approximately 4 months later. All the deciduous teeth are expected to erupt by the time the child is 2 1/2 years of age. The deciduous dentition formula (one side) is as follows:

$$I\frac{2}{2} \; C\frac{1}{1} \; M\frac{2}{2} = 10$$

where I = *incisor;* C = *canine;* M = *molar.* Called also *baby,*

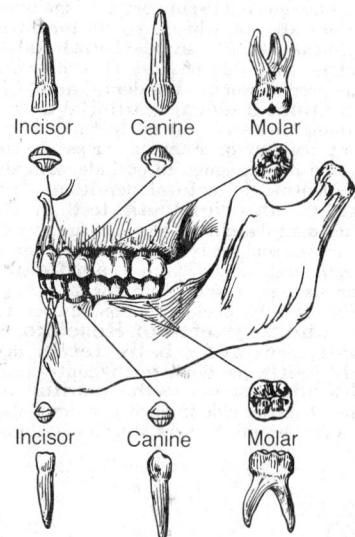

Incisor   Canine   Molar

Incisor   Canine   Molar

Typical deciduous teeth.

milk, primary, or *temporary teeth; deciduous, first, primary,* or *temporary dentition;* and *dentes decidui* [NA]. **diatoric teeth,** artificial teeth with holes in their bases into which the denture base material flows and, when processed, attaches the teeth to the base. Called also *pinless teeth.* **drifting t.,** wandering t. **embedded t.,** one that is unerupted because of lack of eruptive force. **t. of epistropheus,** dens axis. **eye t.,** colloquial term for a canine tooth of the upper jaw. **Fournier teeth,** Moon's teeth. **fused teeth,** partial or complete fusion of two or more individual teeth. **geminate t.,** a tooth with a single root and root canal, but with two completely or incompletely separated crowns, resulting from invagination of a single tooth germ, causing incomplete formation of two teeth. Called also *connate t.* **Goslee t.,** an interchangeable artificial tooth attached to a metal base. **hag teeth,** upper medial incisors that are widely separated. **hair teeth,** dentes acustici. **Horner's teeth,** incisor teeth that are horizontally grooved owing to a deficiency of enamel. **Hutchinson's teeth,** a tooth abnormality seen in congenital syphilis, in which the permanent incisors have a screwdriver-like shape, sometimes associated with notching of the

incisal edges or depressions in the labial surfaces above the cutting edge. Called also *Hutchinson's incisors* and *screwdriver teeth.* **impacted t.,** one prevented from erupting by a physical barrier. See also *unerupted t.* **incisor teeth,** the four front teeth, two on each side of the midline in each jaw; the cutting teeth, each with one long root. Called also *dentes incisivi* [NA]. See *incisor.* **labial teeth,** anterior teeth. **lion's t.** [Fr. *dent-de-lion* dandelion], *Taraxacum officinale* Weber. (Compositae). **malacotic teeth,** teeth that are soft in structure and are abnormally susceptible to caries. **malposed t.,** a tooth out of its normal position. **mandibular teeth,** the teeth of the mandible, or lower jaw. **maxillary teeth,** the teeth of the maxilla, or upper jaw. **metal insert t.,** an artificial tooth, usually of acrylic resin, containing an inserted ribbon of metal or a cutting blade in the occlusal surface, with one edge exposed; sometimes used in removable dentures. **milk t.,** 1. predeciduous t. 2. neonatal t. 3. deciduous t. **molar teeth** [L. *molaris* pertaining to grinding], the most posterior teeth on either side in each jaw, totaling 8 in the deciduous dentition (2 on each side, upper and lower), and usually 12 in the permanent dentition (3 on each side, upper and lower). They are the grinding teeth, having large crowns with broad chewing surfaces. The upper molars characteristically have 4 major cusps and three roots. The lower first molars characteristically have 5 cusps, and the remaining lower molars 4 cusps. Normally all lower molars have two roots. The third molars ("wisdom teeth") are often malformed, but when developed normally their crown and root form corresponds in general with neighboring molars in the same jaw. Called also *dentes molares* [NA]. **Moon's teeth,** small, domed first molars observed in patients with congenital syphilis. **morsal teeth** [L. *morsus* a seizing], anterior teeth. **mottled teeth,** see under *enamel.* **mulberry t.,** mulberry molar. **natal t.,** predeciduous t. **neonatal t.,** one that erupts within the first month of life. Called also *milk t.* **nonanatomic teeth,** a term applied to artificial teeth the occlusal surfaces of which are especially designed on the basis of engineering concepts, without regard to the features of natural teeth. **peg t., peg-shaped t.,** one having a conical form, whose sides converge or taper together incisally, instead of being parallel or diverging mesially and distally; a condition frequently observed in the maxillary lateral incisor. Called also *conical t.* **permanent teeth,** the 32 teeth of the second dentition, which begin to appear in humans at about 6 years of age. The first molars appear first, followed by the mandibular central and lateral incisors, maxillary central incisors, maxillary lateral incisors, mandibular canines, first premolars, second premolars, maxillary canines, second molars, and third molars. They take their position posterior to the deciduous teeth and erupt in succession, whenever the jaws grow sufficiently to accommodate them. Exfoliation of the deciduous teeth is brought about by resorption of their roots, and the succedaneous permanent teeth take their place. The permanent dentition formula (one side) is as follows:

$$I\frac{2}{2} \; C\frac{1}{1} \; P\frac{2}{2} \; M\frac{3}{3} = 16$$

where I = *incisor;* C = *canine;* P = *premolar;* M = *molar.* Called also *dentes permanentes* [NA], and *permanent* or *secondary dentition.* **pink t. of Mummery,** internal tooth resorption (def. 1). **pinless teeth,** diatoric teeth. **posterior teeth,** the teeth on either side in each jaw, distal to the canine teeth, including the premolar (bicuspid) and molar teeth; called also *buccal* or *cheek teeth.* **predeciduous t.,** teeth present at birth, which may be normal in all respects or may represent hornified epithelial rootless structures, found on the gingivae over the crest of the ridge before eruption of the deciduous teeth. Called also *dentia praecox, milk* or *natal teeth,* and *predeciduous dentition.* **premature teeth,** deciduous teeth that erupt prior to the end of the third month of life, or permanent teeth that erupt prior to the end of the fourth year of life. Called also *dentia praecox* and *precocious* or *premature dentition.* See also *predeciduous teeth.* **premolar teeth,** the eight permanent teeth, two on either side in each jaw, between the canine teeth and the molars; the upper premolars have two cusps (bicuspid), but the lower have from one to three. They are succedaneous to the deciduous molar teeth. Called also *dentes premolares* [NA], *bicuspids,* and *bicuspid teeth.* In zoology, those teeth which succeed the deciduous molars regardless of the number to be succeeded. **primary teeth,** deciduous teeth. **pulpless t.,** a tooth from which the pulp has been extir-

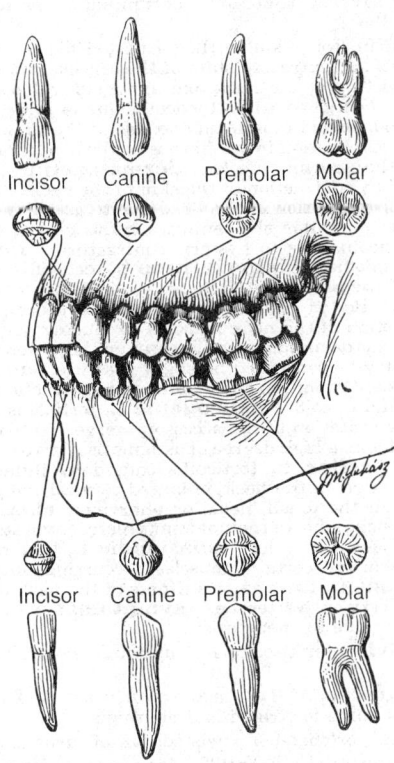

Incisor   Canine   Premolar   Molar

Incisor   Canine   Premolar   Molar

Typical permanent teeth.

pated. **rake teeth,** teeth that are widely separated. **rootless teeth,** dentin dysplasia. **sclerotic teeth,** teeth that are hard in structure and resistant to caries. **screwdriver teeth,** Hutchinson's teeth. **shell t.,** a condition characterized by dysplasia of the dentin, associated with essentially normal enamel, thus resulting in an extremely large pulp chamber and root canal that give the affected tooth the appearance of a shell. **snaggle t.,** a tooth out of proper line with the others. **stomach t.,** a canine tooth of the lower jaw, or mandible. **straight-pin teeth,** artificial teeth in which the pins are inserted vertically. **submerged t.,** a deciduous tooth, usually a second mandibular molar, that has undergone resorption and has become ankylosed to the bone, thus preventing its exfoliation and subsequent replacement by a permanent tooth; it appears to be submerged below the level of occlusion in relation to the adjacent permanent teeth. Called also *ankylosed t.* **succedaneous teeth, successional teeth,** the permanent teeth that have deciduous predecessors in the dental arch. Cf. *accessional teeth.* **superior teeth,** the teeth of the upper jaw, or maxilla. **supernumerary teeth, supplemental teeth,** natural teeth in excess of the number normally present in the jaw. **temporary teeth,** deciduous teeth (dentes decidui [NA]). **tube teeth,** artificial teeth having a vertical, cylindrical aperture from the center of the base up into the body of the tooth, into which a pin may be placed or cast for attachment of the tooth to the denture base. **Turner's t.,** enamel hypoplasia of a single tooth, most commonly one of the permanent maxillary incisors or a maxillary or mandibular premolar, resulting from local infection or trauma. Called also *Turner's hypoplasia.* **unerupted t.,** one that failed to erupt; the presence of multiple unerupted permanent teeth is sometimes referred to as *pseudoanodontia.* See also *embedded t.* and *impacted t.* **vital teeth,** teeth to which the nerve and vascular supply is intact. **wandering t.,** a tooth that drifts from its normal position in the dental arch. Called also *drifting t.* **wisdom t.,** the third molar tooth,

the tooth most distal to the medial line on either side in each jaw, so called because it is the last of the permanent dentition to erupt, usually at the age of 17 to 21 years. Called also *dens serotinus* [NA]. **wolf t.,** a vestigial first premolar tooth sometimes present in the jaw of a horse. **zero degree teeth,** artificial teeth which have no cusp angles in relation to the horizontal on their occlusal surfaces.

toothache (tooth′āk) pain in a tooth. Called also *dentagra, dentalgia,* and *odontalgia.*

Tooth's atrophy, disease, type (tooths) [Howard Henry *Tooth,* English physician, 1856–1925] progressive neuropathic (peroneal) muscular atrophy.

tooth-borne (tōōth′born) supported entirely by the teeth; said of a prosthesis or part of a prosthesis entirely supported by the abutment teeth.

topagnosia (top″ag-no′ze-ah) 1. loss of touch localization. 2. loss of ability to recognize familiar surroundings.

topagnosis (top″ag-no′sis) [Gr. *topos* place + *a* neg. + *gnōsis* recognition] loss of touch localization.

topalgia (to-pal′je-ah) [*top-* + *alg-* + *-ia*] pain fixed in one spot, a common feature of pain without organic basis, as seen in conversion disorder.

topectomy (to-pek′to-me) [*topo-* + Gr. *ektomē* excision] ablation of a small and specific area of the frontal cortex in the treatment of mental illness.

topesthesia (top″es-the′ze-ah) [Gr. *topos* place + *aisthēsis* perception + *-ia*] the power of localizing a tactile sensation.

Töpfer's test (tep′ferz) [Alfred Edouard *Töpfer,* German physician, born 1858] see under *tests.*

tophaceous (to-fa′shus) [L. *tophaceus: tophus* porous stone] hard or gritty; of the nature of or characterized by tophi.

tophi (to′fi) [L.] plural of *tophus.*

topholipoma (tof″o-li-po′mah) a lipoma containing tophi.

tophus (to′fus), pl. *to′phi* [L. "porous stone"] a chalky deposit of sodium urate occurring in gout; tophi form most often around joints in cartilage, bone, bursae, and subcutaneous tissue and in the external ear, producing a chronic, foreign-body inflammatory response. **auricular t.,** a tophus on the ear. **dental t.,** dental calculus. **t. syphilit′icus,** a syphilitic node.

topical (top′e-kal) [Gr. *topikos*] pertaining to a particular surface area, as a topical anti-infective applied to a certain area of the skin and affecting only the area to which it is applied.

Topicort (top′ĭ-kort) trademark for a preparation of desoximetasone.

Topicycline (top″ĭ-si′klēn) trademark for a topical preparation of tetracycline hydrochloride; used in treatment of acne.

Topinard's angle, line (top″e-närz′) [Paul *Topinard,* French physician and anthropologist, 1830–1911] see *ophryospinal angle,* under *angle,* and see under *line.*

top(o)- [Gr. *topos* place] a combining form meaning place.

topoalgia (top″o-al′je-ah) topalgia.

topoanesthesia (top″o-an″es-the′ze-ah) loss of power to localize a tactile sensation.

topochemistry (top″o-kem′is-tre) the chemical composition at specific sites of a structure, as at the surface membrane of a cell.

topodysesthesia (top″o-dis″es-the′ze-ah) localized dysesthesia.

topognosis (top″og-no′sis) [*topo-* + Gr. *gnōsis* recognition] topesthesia.

topographic (top″o-graf′ik) describing or pertaining to special regions.

topographical (top″o-graf′ĭ-kal) pertaining to topography.

topography (to-pog′rah-fe) [*topo-* + Gr. *graphein* to write] the description of an anatomical region or of a special part.

topology (to-pol′o-je) [*topo-* + *-logy*] the relation between the presenting part of the fetus and the birth canal.

toponarcosis (top″o-nar-ko′sis) [*topo-* + Gr. *narkōsis* benumbing] localized anesthesia.

toponym (top′o-nim) the name of a region as distinguished from an organ.

toponymy (to-pon'ĭ-me) [*topo-* + Gr. *onoma* name] terminology pertaining to the regions of the body.

topoparesthesia (top″o-par″es-the′ze-ah) localized paresthesia.

topothermesthesiometer (top″o-therm″es-the-ze-om′ĕ-ter) [*topo-* + Gr. *thermē* heat + *aisthēsis* perception + *metron* measure] an apparatus for measuring the local temperature sense.

Topsyn (top′sin) trademark for a preparation of fluocinonide.

topterone (top′tĕ-rōn) chemical name: 17β-hydroxy-17-propylandrost-4-en-one; an antiestrogen, $C_{22}H_{34}O_2$.

TOPV poliovirus vaccine live oral trivalent.

torcular (tor′ku-lar) [L. "wine-press"] a hollow, or expanded area. **t. Heroph′ili,** confluens sinuum.

Torecan (tor′ĕ-kān) trademark for preparations of thiethylperazine.

Torek operation (to′rek) [Franz J. A. *Torek*, New York surgeon (born in Breslau), 1861–1938] see under *operation*.

tori (to′ri) [L.] plural of *torus*.

toric (to′rik) pertaining to or resembling a torus.

Torkildsen's operation (tor′kild-senz) [Arne *Torkildsen*, Norwegian neurosurgeon, born 1899] see under *operation*.

tormina (tor′mĭ-nah) [L.] colic, def. 2.

torminal (tor′mĭ-nal) pertaining to or characterized by griping pain, or colic.

Tornwaldt's (Thornwaldt's) bursa, bursitis (disease) (torn′vahlts) [Gustav Ludwig *Tornwaldt*, 1843–1910] see *bursa pharyngea*, and see under *bursitis*.

torose, torous (to′rōs; to′rus) [L. *torosus* muscular, brawny] bulging or knobby.

torpent (tor′pent) [L. *torpere* to be sluggish] 1. inactive; in abeyance. 2. an agent that reduces irritation.

torpid (tor′pid) [L. *torpidus* numb, sluggish] not acting with normal vigor and facility.

torpidity (tor-pid′ĭ-te) sluggishness; inactivity, slowness.

torpor (tor′por) [L.] lack of response to normal or ordinary stimuli. **t. re′tinae,** a condition in which the retina is excited to action only by stimuli of considerable luminous power.

torque (tork) [L. *torquēre* to twist] 1. a rotatory force causing a part of a structure to twist about an axis. 2. the rotation of a tooth on its long axis, especially moving the root apex in a buccal or lingual direction through the application of force produced by torsion within the arch wire. See also *torsion*.

torquing (tork′ing) the twisting of a tooth into position, as in the correction of malposition.

torr (tor) [after Evangelista *Torr*icelli, Italian mathematician and physicist, 1608–1647] a unit of pressure equal to exactly $\frac{1}{760}$ atmosphere, equal to one millimeter of mercury (mm Hg) to within one part in 7 million.

torrefaction (tor″ĕ-fak′shun) [L. *torrefactio*] the act of roasting or parching.

torrefy (tor′e-fi) [L. *torrefacere*] to parch, roast, or dry by the aid of heat.

torricellian (to″re-chel′e-an) named for Evangelista *Torri*-*celli*, Italian mathematician, 1608–1647; see under *vacuum*.

torsades de pointes (tōr-sahd′ dĕ pwahnt) [Fr. "fringe of pointed tips"] an atypical rapid ventricular tachycardia with periodic waxing and waning of amplitude of the QRS complexes on the electrocardiogram; it may be self-limited or may progress to ventricular fibrillation.

torsion (tor′shun) [L. *torsio*, from *torquēre* to twist] 1. the act or process of twisting; turning or rotating about an axis. 2. a type of mechanical stress, whereby the external forces (load) twist an object about its axis. See also *torque*. 3. in ophthalmology, any rotation of the vertical corneal meridans. **negative t.,** rotation in a counterclockwise direction. **positive t.,** rotation in a clockwise direction.

torsionometer (tor″shun-om′ĕ-ter) [*torsion* + Gr. *metron* measure] an apparatus for estimating the degree of rotation of the spinal column.

torsive (tor′siv) twisted.

torsiversion (tor″sĭ-ver′zhun) [L. *torquere* to twist + *vertere* to turn] the turning or rotation of a tooth on its long axis.

torso (tor′so) the trunk without the head or extremities.

torticollar (tor″tĭ-kol′ar) pertaining to or affected with torticollis.

torticollis (tor″tĭ-kol′is) [L. *tortus* twisted + *collum* neck] wryneck; a contracted state of the cervical muscles, producing twisting of the neck and an unnatural position of the head. **congenital t.,** torticollis due to injury to the sternocleidomastoid muscle on one side at the time of birth and its transformation into a fibrous cord which cannot lengthen with the growing neck. **dermatogenic t.,** torticollis caused by contraction of the skin of the neck. **fixed t.,** an unnatural position of the head due to actual and persistent organic muscular shortening. **hysteric t., hysterical t.,** torticollis due to hysteric contracture. **intermittent t.,** spasmodic t. **labyrinthine t.,** torticollis due to irritation of the semicircular canals on one side. **mental t.,** a form of tic, or habit spasm, in which there is spasmodic contraction of the neck muscles, producing deviation of the head. This deviation usually ceases on the patient lying down, or it may be controlled by slight pressure. **myogenic t.,** a transient condition due to muscular contraction in rheumatism, and to cold. **neurogenic t.,** torticollis due to pressure or irritation of the accessory nerve. **ocular t.,** torticollis due to a high degree of astigmatism or to ocular muscle palsy. **reflex t.,** torticollis caused by inflammation or suppuration in the neck, enlarged cervical lymph nodes, or tumor in the tonsil, neck, or pharynx. **rheumatoid t.,** that which is due to rheumatism, chiefly of the sternomastoid and adjacent muscles. **spasmodic t.,** that which is due to spasm of certain muscles, occurring intermittently. **spurious t.,** twisting or stiffness of the neck due to caries of the cervical vertebrae. **symptomatic t.,** stiffness of the neck due to rheumatism.

tortipelvis (tor″tĭ-pel′vis) dystonia musculorum deformans.

tortua (tor′tu-ah) [L.] agony; torture. **t. fa′cies,** Avicenna's name for trigeminal neuralgia.

tortuous (tor′choo-us) twisted; full of turns and twists.

Torula (tor′u-lah) [L. "roll"] former name for *Cryptococcus*. **T. capsula′tus, T. histolyt′ica,** *Cryptococcus neoformans*.

toruli (tor′u-li) [L.] plural of *torulus*.

torulin (tor′u-lin) thiamine.

toruloma (tor-u-lo′mah) a tumor or nodule which is one of the lesions of cryptococcosis (torulosis).

Torulopsis (tor″u-lop′sis) a genus of imperfect fungi of the family Cryptococcaceae, order Moniliales, which are morphologically similar to *Cryptococcus* but do not have a capsule, and are normal inhabitants of the respiratory and gastrointestinal tracts and urogenital region. **T. glabra′ta,** an opportunistic organism, an etiologic agent of torulopsosis and other infections, such as meningitis, pneumonia, cystitis, and fungemia; it is part of the normal flora of the mouth, gut, and urinary tract. **T. histolyt′ica,** *Cryptococcus neoformans*. **T. pintolope′sii,** a species similar to *T. glabrata*, found in the mouse alimentary tract.

torulopsosis (tor″u-lop′so-sis) an infection of the tissues resembling histoplasmosis, caused by *Torulopsis glabrata*.

torulosis (tor″u-lo′sis) cryptococcosis.

torulus (tor′u-lus), pl. *tor′uli* [L., dim. of *torus*] a small elevation; a papilla. **tor′uli tac′tiles** [NA], the small elevations on the skin of the palm and the sole, richly supplied with sensory nerve endings; called also *tactile elevations*.

torus (to′rus), pl. *to′ri* [L. "a round swelling," "protuberance"] 1. a bulging projection, a swelling; [NA] a general term for such a protuberance. 2. the doughnut-shaped geometric figure produced by rotating a circle about an axis that lies in the same plane as the circle but does not cut the circle. **t. fronta′lis,** a protuberance in the middle line of the root of the nose, on the external surface of the skull. **t. levato′rius** [NA], the mucosal fold covering the levator veli palatini muscle in the lateral wall of the nasal part of the pharynx. **t. mandib′ulae** [NA], a prominence sometimes seen on the lingual aspect of the mandible at the base of its alveolar part, adjacent to the postcanine teeth. **t. occipita′lis,** a rounded edge occasionally seen on the occipital bone in the region of the superior nuchal line. **t. palati′nus** [NA], a bony protuberance sometimes found on the hard palate at the junction of the intermaxillary and transverse palatine sutures. **t. tuba′rius** [NA], the projecting posterior lip of the pharyngeal opening of the auditory tube. **t. ureter′icus,** interureteric ridge (plica interureterica [NA]).

tosifen (to′sĭ-fen) chemical name: (S)-4-methyl-N-[[(1-methyl -2- phenylethyl)amino]carbonyl]benzenesulfonamide; an antianginal, $C_{17}H_{20}N_2O_3S$.

tosylate (to′sĭ-lāt) USAN contraction for p-toluenesulfonate.

Totacillin (to″tah-sil′in) trademark for preparations of ampicillin.

Toti's operation (to′tēz) [Addeo *Toti,* Italian ophthalmologist, born 1861] dacryocystorhinostomy.

totipotency (to″te-po′ten-se) [L. *totus* all + *potentia* power] the ability of a part to develop in any manner, or of a cell to develop into any type of cell.

totipotent (to-tip′o-tent) totipotential.

totipotential (to″te-po-ten′shal) [L. *totus* all + *potentia* power] characterized by ability to develop in any direction; said of cells which can give rise to cells of all orders, i.e., to the complete individual. Cf. *unipotential.*

totipotentiality (to″tĭ-po-ten″she-al′ĭ-te) the ability to differentiate along any line or into any type of cell.

touch (tuch) [L. *tactus*] 1. the sense by which contact with objects gives evidence as to certain of their qualities. 2. palpation or exploration with the finger. **abdominal t.,** digital palpation of the abdomen. **double t.,** digital examination of the rectum and vagina at the same time. **rectal t.,** exploration of the rectum with the finger. **royal t.,** the touching or tapping of a person with scrofula; once practiced by the kings of England and France as a supposedly curative measure; called also *adenochirapsology.* **vaginal t.,** digital exploration of the vagina. **vesical t.,** digital examination of the bladder.

Touraine-Solente-Golé syndrome (too-ren′ so-lahnt′ go-la′) [Albert *Touraine,* French dermatologist, 1883–1961; G. *Solente* French (?) physician; L. *Golé,* French physician] pachydermoperiostosis.

Tourette's syndrome (disease) (too-retz′) see *Gilles de la Tourette* (for biographical note) and see *Gilles de la Tourette syndrome,* under *syndrome.*

tournesol (tur′nĕ-sol) litmus.

tourniquet (toor′nĭ-ket) [Fr.] an instrument for the compression of a blood vessel by application around an extremity to control the circulation and prevent the flow of blood to or from the distal area. Tourniquets are of various kinds, named chiefly for their inventors. **automatic rotating t.,** a system consisting of a motor, air compressor, and four blood pressure cuffs for application to the extremities; the cuffs are inflated and deflated in series and in sequence for treatment of acute pulmonary edema. **Esmarch's t.,** a tourniquet consisting of a piece of strong, flat rubber bandage, which, after the blood has been forced from the limb by gravity or compression, is wound about the proximal part of the limb to arrest the circulation. **garrote t.,** Spanish windlass. **pneumatic t.,** a narrow rubber bag to be wound around a limb, pressure being applied by pumping air into the inflatable cuff. **scalp t.,** a tourniquet placed around the scalp with enough pressure to occlude the superficial blood vessels and thereby to lessen the risk of drug-induced alopecia. **Spanish t., torcular t.,** Spanish windlass.

tousey (tow′ze) [Sinclair *Tousey,* New York radiologist, 1864–1937] a unit of roentgen-ray power; being the radiance which will produce on a photographic film an effect equal to that produced by a one-candlepower incandescent electric light.

Touton giant cell (toot′on) [Karl *Touton,* German dermatologist, 1858–1934] see under *cell.*

Townsend ionization (town′zend) [John *Townsend,* Irish physicist, 1868–1957] see *avalanche ionization,* under *ionization.*

toxalbumin (tok″sal-bu′min) (*obs.*) any poisonous albumin, including those found in plant juices (abrin, ricin, phallin), serpent venoms, etc. See *toxin.*

toxanemia (tok″sah-ne′me-ah) anemia due to a poison.

toxaphene (toks′ah-fēn) a chlorinated hydrocarbon, $C_{10}H_{10}Cl_8$, used as an agricultural insecticide.

Toxascaris (tok-sas′kah-ris) a genus of parasitic nematodes of the superfamily Ascaridoidea. **T. leoni′na,** a species found commonly in lions, tigers, and other large

Felidae; found also in dogs and cats, but usually only in older animals. Its larvae differ from those of *Toxocara canis* and *Toxocara cati* by not passing through the lungs of the infected animal.

toxemia (tok-se′me-ah) [*toxin* + Gr. *haima* blood + *-ia*] 1. the condition resulting from the spread of bacterial products (toxins) by the bloodstream. 2. a condition resulting from metabolic disturbances, e.g., toxemia of pregnancy. **alimentary t.,** toxemia due to absorption from the alimentary canal of chemical poisons generated therein; a form of autointoxication. **eclamptic t., eclamptogenic t.,** t. of pregnancy. **hydatid t.,** toxemia with urticaria caused by hydatid fluid which has escaped into the peritoneal cavity. **preeclamptic t.,** see *preeclampsia.* **t. of pregnancy,** a group of pathologic conditions, essentially metabolic disturbances, occurring in pregnant women, and manifested by preeclampsia and fully developed eclampsia. **pregnancy t. in ewes,** an acute disorder leading to impaired nervous function, coma, and death, occurring during the last few weeks of pregnancy in ewes that are typically carrying twins, triplets, or a particularly large single lamb; the principal predisposing cause is undernutrition association with stress. Called also *pregnancy disease, twin-lamb disease,* and *lambing paralysis.*

toxemic (toks-e′mik) pertaining to or caused by toxemia.

toxenzyme (toks-en′zīm) any poisonous enzyme.

toxi- see *toxi(o)-.*

toxic (tok′sik) pertaining to, due to, or of the nature of a poison or toxin; manifesting the symptoms of severe infection.

toxicant (toks′ĭ-kant) [L. *toxicans* poisoning] 1. poisonous. 2. a poisonous agent.

toxication (tok″sĭ-ka′shun) poisoning.

toxicemia (toks″ĭ-se′me-ah) toxemia.

toxicide (tok′sĭ-sīd) [*toxin* + L. *caedere* to kill] a drug capable of overcoming toxic agents.

toxicity (tok-sis′ĭ-te) the quality of being poisonous, especially the degree of virulence of a toxic microbe or of a poison. **O₂ t., oxygen t.,** serious, sometimes irreversible, damage to the pulmonary capillary endothelium associated with breathing high partial pressures of oxygen for prolonged periods. Called also O_2 or *oxygen poisoning.*

toxic(o)- [Gr. *toxikon (pharmakon)* arrow (poison), from *toxon* bow] a combining form meaning poisonous or denoting relationship to poison.

toxicodendrol (tok″sĭ-ko-den′drol) a poisonous, nonvolatile oil found in certain plants of the genus *Rhus (Toxicodendron).*

Toxicodendron (tok″sĭ-ko-den′dron) [*toxico-* + Gr. *dendron* tree] *Rhus.*

toxicogenic (tok″sĭ-ko-jen′ik) [*toxico-* + Gr. *gennan* to produce] producing or elaborating toxins.

toxicohemia (tok″sĭ-ko-he′me-ah) toxemia.

toxicoid (tok′sĭ-koid) [*toxico-* + Gr. *eidos* form] resembling a poison.

toxicologic (tok″sĭ-ko-loj′ik) pertaining to toxicology.

toxicologist (tok″sĭ-kol′o-jist) an individual who specializes in toxicology.

toxicology (tok″sĭ-kol′o-je) the sum of what is known regarding poisons; the scientific study of poisons, their actions, their detection, and the treatment of the conditions produced by them.

toxicopathic (tok″sĭ-ko-path′ik) pertaining to toxicopathy.

toxicopathy (tok″sĭ-kop′ah-the) [*toxico-* + Gr. *pathos* disease] any disease induced by a poison.

toxicopectic (tok″sĭ-ko-pek′tik) pertaining to, characterized by, or promoting toxicopexis.

toxicopexic (tok″sĭ-ko-pek′sik) toxicopectic.

toxicopexis (tok″sĭ-ko-pek′sis) [*toxico-* + Gr. *pēxis* fixation] the fixing or neutralizing of a poison in the body.

toxicopexy (tok″sĭ-ko-pek″se) toxicopexis.

toxicophidia (tok″sĭ-ko-fid′e-ah) [*toxico-* + Gr. *ophis* snake] thanatophidia.

toxicophobia (tok″sĭ-ko-fo′be-ah) [*toxico-* + *phobia*] irrational fear of being poisoned.

toxicosis (tok″sĭ-ko′sis) [Gr. *toxikon* poison + *-osis*] any disease condition due to poisoning. **endogenic t.,** autointoxication. **exogenic t.,** poisoning by the ingestion of toxic material, as in the food. See *food poisoning,* under *poisoning.* **gestational t.,** gestosis. **hemorrhagic capillary t.,** Frank's name for a hemorrhagic condition attributed to capillary weakening from some toxic action; see *Henoch's purpura,* under *purpura.* **proteinogenous t.,** an acute and fatal intoxication which appears in white mice which are fed an exclusive diet of various proteins. **retention t.,** that which is due to the nonexcretion of noxious waste products.

toxicyst (tok′sĭ-sist) [*toxi-* + *cyst*] one of the numerous toxic subpellicular organelles occurring as slender extrusible tubular structures located apically in certain ciliate protozoa, especially certain of the Kinetofragminophorea, with which the organism penetrates the body of and cytolyzes its prey. Cf. *trichocyst.*

toxiferous (tok-sif′er-us) [*toxin* + L. *ferre* to bear] conveying or producing a poison.

toxigenic (tok″sĭ-jen′ik) toxicogenic.

toxigenicity (tok″sĭ-jĕ-nis′ĭ-te) the disease-producing virulence of a parasite which acts by virtue of a soluble toxin.

toxignomic (toks″ig-nom′ik) [*toxin* + Gr. *gnōmē* a means of knowing] characteristic of the toxic action of a poison.

toxin (tok′sin) [Gr. *toxikon* arrow poison, from Gr. *toxikos* of or for a bow] a poison; frequently used to refer specifically to a protein produced by some higher plants, certain animals, and pathogenic bacteria, which is highly toxic for other living organisms. Such substances are differentiated from the simple chemical poisons and the vegetable alkaloids by their high molecular weight and antigenicity. **amanita t.,** a toxin from *Amanita phalloides.* **animal t.,** one produced by an animal; a zootoxin. **anthrax t.,** an exotoxin produced by most strains of *Bacillus anthracis* that is immunogenic, produces edema, and is lethal for mice. It consists of three heat-labile, antigenically distinct components: edema factor (EF, factor I), protective antigen (PA, factor II), and lethal factor (LF, factor III). **bacterial t's,** toxic substances produced by bacteria, including exotoxins, endotoxins, enterotoxins, neurotoxins, and toxic enzymes. **botulinus t.,** an exotoxin produced by germinating spores and growing cells of *Clostridium botulinum.* The toxin binds to presynaptic terminals of the central nervous system and blocks the release of acetylcholine, leading to paralysis. There are seven immunologically distinct types (A–G). Type A is one of the most powerful poisons known. **cholera t.,** an exotoxin produced by *Vibrio cholerae;* a protein enterotoxin that binds to the membrane of enteric cells and stimulates the adenylcyclase system, causing the hypersecretion of chloride and bicarbonate ions, resulting in increased fluid secretion and the severe diarrhea of cholera. **clostridial t.,** one elaborated by species of *Clostridium,* including those causing botulism (*botulinus t.*), gas gangrene (*gas gangrene t.*), and tetanus (*tetanus t.*). In addition, *C. difficile* produces an exotoxin causing severe intestinal necrosis. *C. perfringens* produces a number of exotoxins causing gas gangrene, intestinal necrosis, and hemolysis, some with cardiotoxic, deoxyribonuclease, and hyaluronidase activity, and an enterotoxin causing acute food poisoning. **Dick t.,** streptococcal erythrogenic toxin; used in the Dick test. **diphtheria t.,** a protein exotoxin produced by virulent (lysogenic) strains of *Corynebacterium diphtheriae* that is primarily responsible for the pathogenesis of diphtheritic infection. It is an enzyme that inhibits protein synthesis by inactivating a factor (EF-2) required for the transfer of polypeptidyl-tRNA from acceptor to donor sites on ribosomes. **diphtheria t., diagnostic,** diphtheria t. for Schick test. **diphtheria t., inactivated diagnostic,** Schick test control. **diptheria t. for Schick test** [USP], a standardized preparation of diphtheria toxin used in the Schick test (q.v.). Formerly called *diagnostic diphtheria toxin.* **dysentery t.,** an exotoxin produced by various species of *Shigella.* That formed by *Shigella dysenteriae* serotype 1 (Shiga toxin) is a soluble protein with hemorrhagic and paralytic properties. It is a highly potent neurotoxin. **erythrogenic t.,** an exotoxin produced by many, but not all, strains of *Streptococcus pyogenes,* which produces an erythematous reaction on intradermal inoculation in man and to a lesser extent in the rabbit, and is responsible for the scarlatiniform rash of scarlet fever. **extracellular t.,** a toxin excreted by a bacterial cell; an exotoxin. **fatigue t.,** a toxin formed in the body as a result of muscular effort; a kenotoxin. **fugu**

t., tetrodotoxin. **fusarial t.,** any mycotoxin produced by molds of the genus *Fusarium.* **gas gangrene t.,** an exotoxin produced by *Clostridium perfringens* and associated with gas gangrene. At least 10 types have been identified. The α toxin is a lethal, necrotizing lecithinase (phospholipase-C) that splits lecithin in cell membranes, is hemolytic, and causes capillary damage. *Clostridium novyi* and *C. septicum* produce similar toxins causing gas gangrene. **intracellular t.,** a toxin developed and retained within the bacterial cell; an endotoxin. **plague t.,** a necrotizing exotoxin produced by *Yersinia pestis;* its significance in the pathology of plague is unclear. **plant t.,** one produced by a plant; a phytotoxin. **pseudomonal t.,** an exotoxin produced by *Pseudomonas aeruginosa.* It is a protein, lethal for mice and rats and toxic for fibroblast cultures, which inhibits protein synthesis by inactivating elongation factor EF₂. **Shiga t.,** the exotoxin formed by *Shigella dysenteriae* type 1. **soluble t.,** exotoxin. **staphylococcal t.,** a mixture of exotoxins produced by *Staphylococcus aureus.* There are four chemically and serologically distinct hemolysins (α, β, γ, and δ) having also dermonecrotic activity (α-hemolysin), sphingomyelinase activity (β-hemolysin), necrotizing activity (γ-hemolysin), and leukocidin activity (δ-hemolysin). Other toxins produced are leukocidal and exfoliative (causing scalded skin syndrome). Strains of *Staphylococcus aureus* also produce five serologically distinct enterotoxins: types A and D are major factors in staphylococcal food poisoning. **streptococcal t.,** a mixture of exotoxins formed by *Streptococcus pyogenes,* including two distinct hemolysins (*streptolysin O* and *streptolysin S*), an erythrogenic toxin (causing scarlet fever rash), and a DPNase that is cardiotoxic. **tetanus t.,** the potent exotoxin produced by *Clostridium tetani,* consisting of two components, one a neurotoxin (*tetanospasmin*) and the other a hemolysin (*tetanolysin*). **whooping cough t.,** a dermonecrotic exotoxin produced by *Bordetella pertussis* that appears to be associated with the pathogenicity of the organism in whooping cough.

toxin-antitoxin (tok″sin-an′tĭ-tok″sin) a nearly neutral mixture of diphtheria toxin with its antitoxin; formerly used for immunization against diphtheria.

toxinemia (tok″sĭ-ne′me-ah) [*toxin* + Gr. *haima* blood + *-ia*] poisoning of the blood.

toxinology (tok″sin-ol′o-je) the science dealing with the toxins produced by certain higher plants and animals and by pathogenic bacteria.

toxinosis (tok″sĭ-no′sis) any disease condition due to the presence of a toxin.

toxipathy (tok-sip′ah-the) toxicosis.

toxiphobia (tok″sĭ-fo′be-ah) toxicophobia.

toxiresin (tok″sĭ-rez′in) a poisonous resinous substance obtainable from digitoxin.

toxisterol (tok-sis′ter-ol) [*toxin* + *sterol*] a poisonous isomer of ergosterol, produced by ultraviolet radiation of the latter.

toxitabellae (tok″sĭ-tah-bel′e) poison tablets.

tox(o)- a combining form denoting relationship to a toxin, or poison.

Toxocara (tok″so-ka′rah) a genus of nematode worms of the superfamily Ascaridoidea. **T. ca′nis,** a nematode worm parasitic in the intestine of dogs; migrating larvae may cause lesions of the lung, liver, kidney, brain, and eye. In human infections, the larvae do not complete their cycle but cause visceral larva migrans (see under *larva*). **T. ca′ti,** a species closely related to *T. canis* but commonly found in cats; it has also been reported from man, both as an accidental intestinal parasite and as causing visceral larva migrans (see under *larva*). Called also *T. mystax.* **T. mys′tax,** *T. cati.*

toxocaral (tok″so-kār′al) pertaining to or caused by *Toxocara.*

toxocariasis (tok″so-kār-i′ah-sis) infection by roundworms of the genus *Toxocara.* **human t.,** infection with the cat or dog ascarid *Toxocara cati* or *T. canis;* visceral larva migrans (see under *larva*).

toxogen (tok′so-jen) something that produces a poison.

toxoglobulin (tok″so-glob′u-lin) a poisonous globulin.

toxoid (tok′soid) [*toxo-* + Gr. *eidos* form] a modified or inactivated bacterial exotoxin that has lost toxicity but retains the properties of combining with, or stimulating the formation of, antitoxin. **Clostridium perfringens t.,** see under *bacterin-toxoid*. **diphtheria t.,** the formaldehyde-inactivated toxin of *Corynebacterium diphtheriae*, used for immunization against diphtheria; both fluid and adsorbed (on alum, aluminum phosphate, or aluminum hydroxide) forms are available. It is generally used in mixtures with tetanus toxoid and pertussis vaccine (DTP) or with tetanus toxoid alone (DT for pediatric use and Td, which contains 5- to 10-fold less diphtheria toxoid, for other use). DTP (adsorbed) is recommended for routine immunization of all children under 6 years of age, except when pertussis vaccine is contraindicated, in which case DT (adsorbed) is used. Td (adsorbed) is used for all others. Official names [USP] are *diphtheria toxoid, diphtheria toxoid adsorbed, diphtheria and tetanus toxoids* (DT), *diphtheria and tetanus toxoids adsorbed, diphtheria and tetanus toxoids and pertussis vaccine* (DTP), *diphtheria and tetanus toxoids and pertussis vaccine adsorbed,* and *tetanus and diphtheria toxoids adsorbed for adult use* (Td). **tetanus t.,** the formaldehyde-inactivated toxins of *Clostridium tetani*, used for immunization against tetanus; both fluid and adsorbed (on alum, aluminum hydroxide, or aluminum phosphate) forms are available. It is used in mixtures with diphtheria toxoid and pertussis vaccine (DTP, DT, and Td; see under *diphtheria t.*) or by itself (T). DTP (adsorbed) and DT (adsorbed) are used for routine immunization of children under 6 years of age. Td (adsorbed) and T (adsorbed) are used for all others. Official names [USP] are *tetanus toxoid* (T), *tetanus toxoid adsorbed, tetanus and diphtheria toxoids adsorbed for adult use* (Td), *diphtheria and tetanus toxoids* (DT), *diphtheria and tetanus toxoids adsorbed, diphtheria and tetanus toxoids and pertussis vaccine* (DTP) *and diphtheria and tetanus toxoids and pertussis vaccine adsorbed.*

toxoid-antitoxoid (tok″soid-an′tĭ-tok″soid)   a toxoid mixed with an equivalent amount of antitoxic serum, the precipitate being suspended in saline.

toxolecithid (tok″so-les′ĭ-thid)   toxolecithin.

toxolecithin (tok″so-les′ĭ-thin)   a lecithin compounded with a toxin, as cobra venom.

toxoneme (tok′so-nēm)   rhoptry.

toxonosis (tok″so-no′sis)   toxicosis.

toxopexic (tok″so-peks′ik) [*toxo-* + Gr. *pēxis* fixation]   toxicopectic.

toxophil (tok′so-fil) [*toxo-* + Gr. *philein* to love]   having an affinity for toxins.

toxophilic (tok″so-fil′ik) [*toxo-* + Gr. *philein* to love]   easily susceptible to a poison; having an affinity for toxins (like certain haptophore groups).

toxophilous (toks-of′ĭ-lus)   toxophilic.

toxophore (tok′so-fōr) [*toxin* + Gr. *phoros* bearing]   the group of atoms in the molecule of a toxin that is responsible for the toxic effect.

toxophorous (tok-sof′o-rus)   pertaining to the toxophore group of a toxin molecule.

Toxoplasma (toks″o-plaz′mah) [*toxo-* + *plasma*]   a genus of coccidian protozoa (suborder Eimeriina, order Eucoccidiida) comprising intracellular parasites of many organs and tissues of birds and mammals, including humans. See *toxoplasmosis*. The only known complete hosts are cats and other Felidae, in which both asexual and sexual developmental cycles occur in the intestinal epithelium, culminating in the passage of oocysts in the feces. The intestinal stages do not occur in other hosts. **T. cunic′uli,** *T. gondii.* **T. gon′dii,** an obligate intracellar species found in a wide range of hosts, including humans and other mammals and birds. The sexual cycle of the organism takes place in the intestinal epithelium of the cat, which is the definitive host. It exists in three forms: tachyzoite, tissue cysts (pseudocysts), and oocysts. Infection (see *toxoplasmosis*) occurs chiefly by ingestion of oocytes shed in cat feces or by ingestion of cysts in raw or uncooked meat.

toxoplasmin (tok″so-plaz′min)   a preparation of *Toxoplasma* antigens formerly used in a skin test for toxoplasmosis.

toxoplasmosis (tok″so-plaz-mo′sis) [*toxo-* + *plasma* + *-osis*]   an acute or chronic, widespread disease of animals and humans caused by the obligate intracellular protozoon *Toxoplasma gondii*, transmitted by oocysts containing the pathogen in the feces of cats (the definitive host), usually by contaminated soil, direct exposure to infected feces, tissue cysts in infected meat, or tachyzoites (proliferating forms) in blood. Most human infections are asymptomatic, but when symptoms occur they may range from a mild, self-limited disease clinically resembling mononucleosis to a fulminating, disseminated disease that may cause extensive damage to the brain, eyes, skeletal and cardiac muscles, liver, and lungs. Severe manifestations are seen principally in immunocompromised patients and when the fetus is infected transplacentally as a result of maternal infection. Chorioretinitis (retinochoroiditis) may be associated with all forms, but it is usually a late sequel of congenital toxoplasmosis. **ocular t.,** toxoplasmic chorioretinitis.

toxoprotein (tok″so-pro′te-in)   a toxic protein or a mixture of a toxin and a protein.

Toxothrix (tok′so-thriks) [Gr. *toxon* a bow + *thrix* hair]   a genus of gliding bacteria of uncertain affiliation, made up of colorless, cylindrical cells forming a filament that is often U-shaped. The cells deposit oxidized iron and are found in cold waters containing ferrous iron. The type species is *T. tricho′genes.*

toxuria (toks-u′re-ah)   uremia.

Toynbee's corpuscles, experiment, law, ligament, otoscope (toin′bēz) [Joseph *Toynbee*, English otologist, 1815–1866]   see under *experiment, law,* and *otoscope,* see *corneal corpuscles,* under *corpuscle,* and see *musculus tensor tympani.*

TPHA   *Treponema pallidum* hemagglutination assay.

TPN   1. total parenteral nutrition; see *parenteral hyperalimentation,* under *hyperalimentation.*   2. triphosphopyridine nucleotide; the former name for *nicotinamide-adenine dinucleotide phosphate.*

TPNH   reduced triphosphopyridine nucleotide, the former name for the reduced form of nicotinamide-adenine dinucleotide phosphate.

trabecula (trah-bek′u-lah), pl. *trabec′ulae* [L., dim. of *trabs*]   a little beam; [NA] a general term for a supporting or anchoring strand of connective tissue, as such a strand extending from a capsule into the substance of the enclosed organ.   **arachnoid trabeculae,** delicate fibrous threads connecting the inner surface of the arachnoid to the pia mater.   **trabeculae of bone,** anastomosing bony spicules in cancellous bone which form a meshwork of intercommunicating spaces that are filled with bone marrow.   **trabec′ulae car′neae cor′dis** [NA], muscular ridges covering a great part of the interior of the walls of the ventricles of the heart; they may stand out in relief only, or be attached as bundles at both ends and free in the middle.   **trabec′ulae cor′dis,** trabeculae carneae cordis.   **trabeculae of corpora cavernosa of penis, trabec′ulae cor′porum cavernoso′rum pe′nis** [NA], numerous bands and cords of fibromuscular tissue traversing the interior of the corpora cavernosa of the penis, attached to the tunica albuginea and to the septum and creating the cavernous spaces that become filled with blood during erection.   **trabeculae of corpus spongiosum of penis, trabec′ulae cor′poris spongio′si pe′nis** [NA], numerous bands and cords of fibromuscular tissue traversing the interior of the corpus spongiosum of the penis, creating the cavernous spaces that give the structure its spongy character.   **trabec′ulae cra′nii,** a pair of longitudinal cranial bars of cartilage in the embryo, bounding the pituitary space that becomes the sella turcica.   **fleshy trabeculae of heart,** trabeculae carneae cordis.   **trabec′ulae lie′nis,** NA alternative for trabeculae splenicae.   **Rathke's trabeculae,** trabeculae cranii.   **septomarginal t., t. septomargina′lis** [NA], a bundle of muscle at the apical end of the right ventricle of the heart, connecting the base of the anterior papillary muscle to the interventricular septum; it usually contains a branch of the atrioventricular bundle.   **trabeculae of spleen, trabec′ulae sple′nicae** [NA], fibrous bands that pass into the spleen from the tunica fibrosa and form the supporting framework of the organ; called also *trabeculae lienis* [NA alternative].

trabeculae (trah-bek′u-le) [L.]   plural of *trabecula.*

trabecular (trah-bek′u-lar)   pertaining to a trabecula.

trabecularism (trah-bek′u-lar-izm)   the condition of having a trabecular structure.

trabeculate (trah-bek′u-lāt) [L. *trabecula* a small beam or bar]   marked with transverse or radiating bars or trabeculae.

trabeculation (trah-bek″u-la′shun)   the formation of trabeculae in a part.

trabeculoplasty (trah-bek′u-lo-plas″te)   plastic surgery of a trabecula.   **laser t.,** an operation for open-angle glaucoma, in which surface burns are placed in the trabecular meshwork of the eye to lower intraocular pressure.

trabes (tra-bez) [L.]   plural of *trabs.*

trabs (trabs), pl. *tra′bes* [L. "a beam"]   a supporting or anchoring strand or structure.   **tra′bes car′neae,** trabeculae carneae cordis.

tracer (trās′er)   1. a dissecting instrument for isolating vessels and nerves.   2. a mechanical device by which the outline of an object or the direction and extent of movement of a part may be graphically recorded; see also *tracing.*   3. a means or agent by which certain substances or structures can be identified or followed, as a radioactive tracer.   **arrow-point t.,** needle-point t.   **needle-point t.,** a mechanical device used in recording jaw movements, in which the tracing is made on a horizontal plate by a weighted or a spring-loaded needle attached to the jaw. Called also *arrow-point t.* and *stylus t.* See also under *tracing.*   **radioactive t.,** a radioactive isotope replacing a stable chemical element in a compound introduced into the body, permitting study of the metabolism, distribution, and passage through the body of the labeled compound by means of a radiation detector.   **stylus t.,** needle-point t.

trachea (tra′ke-ah), pl. *tra′cheae* [L.; Gr. *tracheia artēria*] [NA]   1. the cartilaginous and membranous tube descending from the larynx and branching into the right and left main bronchi. It is kept patent by a series of about twenty transverse horseshoe-shaped cartilages. 2. one of a system of minute tubes ramifying throughout the body of a terrestrial arthropod and delivering air to the tissues; called also *tracheal tubule.* See also *tracheole.*   **scabbard t.,** a trachea which is flattened by approximation of its lateral walls.

tracheae (tra′ke-e) [L.]   plural of *trachea.*

tracheaectasy (tra″ke-ah-ek′tah-se)   dilatation of the trachea.

tracheal (tra′ke-al) [L. *trachealis*]   pertaining to the trachea.

trachealgia (tra″ke-al′je-ah) [*trachea* + Gr. *algos* pain + *-ia*]   pain in the trachea.

tracheid (tra′ke-id) [Gr. *tracheia* rough, rugged]   any of the elongate, tapering conducting and supportive cells of the xylem of plant tissue, having thick, pitted walls without true perforations.

tracheitis (tra″ke-i′tis)   inflammation of the trachea.

trachelagra (tra″ke-lag′rah, tra-kel′ah-grah) [Gr. *trachēlos* neck + *agra* seizure]   gout in the neck.

trachelectomy (tra″ke-lek′to-me) [Gr. *trachēlos* neck + *ektomē* excision]   cervicectomy.

trachelematoma (tra″ke-lem″ah-to′mah)   a hematoma situated in the sternocleidomastoid muscle.

trachelism, trachelismus (tra′kĕ-lizm; tra″kĕ-liz′mus) [Gr. *trachēlismos*]   spasm of the neck muscles; spasmodic retraction of the head in epilepsy.

trachelitis (tra″kĕ-li′tis)   cervicitis.

trachel(o)- [Gr. *trachēlos* neck]   a combining form denoting relationship to the neck or to a necklike structure.

trachelocele (trak′ĕ-lo-sēl)   tracheocele.

trachelocyllosis (tra″kĕ-lo-si-lo′sis) [*trachelo-* + Gr. *kyllōsis* crooking]   torticollis.

trachelocyrtosis (tra″kĕ-lo-sir-to′sis) [*trachelo-* + Gr. *kyrtos* curved + *-osis*]   trachelokyphosis.

trachelocystitis (tra″kĕ-lo-sis-ti′tis) [*trachelo-* + Gr. *kystis* bladder + *-itis*]   inflammation of the neck of the bladder.

trachelodynia (tra″kĕ-lo-din′e-ah) [*trachelo-* + Gr. *odynē* pain + *-ia*]   pain in the neck.

trachelokyphosis (tra″kĕ-lo-ki-fo′sis) [*trachelo-* + *kyphosis*]   abnormal curvature of the cervical portion of the spine.

trachelologist (tra″ke-lol′o-jist)   one skilled in trachelology.

trachelology (tra″kĕ-lol′o-je) [*trachelo-* + *-logy*]   the study of the neck and its diseases and injuries.

trachelomyitis (tra″kĕ-lo-mi-i′tis) [*trachelo-* + Gr. *mys* muscle + *-itis*]   inflammation of the muscles of the neck.

trachelopexy (tra′kĕ-lo-pek″se) [*trachelo-* + Gr. *pēxis* fixation]   surgical fixation of the neck of the uterus to some other part.

tracheloplasty (tra′kĕ-lo-plas″te) [*trachelo-* + Gr. *plassein* to mold]   plastic repair of the cervix uteri.

trachelorrhaphy (tra″kĕ-lor′ah-fe) [*trachelo-* + Gr. *rhaphē* suture]   suture of the lacerated cervix uteri.

tracheloschisis (tra″kĕ-los′kĭ-sis) [*trachelo-* + Gr. *schisis* fissure]   congenital fissure of the neck.

trachelosyringorrhaphy (tra″kĕ-lo-sir″ing-gor′ah-fe) [*trachelo-* + Gr. *syrinx* pipe + *rhaphē* suture]   trachelorrhaphy for fistula of the vagina.

trachelotomy (tra″kĕ-lot′o-me) [*trachelo-* + Gr. *tomē* a cutting]   incision of the cervix uteri.

trache(o)-   a combining form denoting relationship to the trachea.

tracheoaerocele (tra″ke-o-a′er-o-sēl) [*tracheo-* + Gr. *aēr* air + *kēlē* hernia]   a tracheal hernia containing air.

tracheobronchial (tra″ke-o-brong′ke-al)   pertaining to the trachea and bronchi.

tracheobronchitis (tra″ke-o-brong-ki′tis)   inflammation of the trachea and bronchi.

tracheobronchomegaly (tra″ke-o-brong″ko-meg′ah-le)   a rare and probably congenital condition characterized by great enlargement of the lumen of the trachea and the larger bronchi.

tracheobronchoscopy (tra″ke-o-brong-kos′ko-pe)   inspection of the interior of the trachea and bronchi.

tracheocele (tra′ke-o-sēl″) [*tracheo-* + Gr. *kēlē* hernia]   hernial protrusion of the tracheal mucous membrane.

tracheoesophageal (tra″ke-o-e-sof′ah-je-al)   pertaining to or communicating with both the trachea and esophagus.

tracheofistulization (tra″ke-o-fis″tu-li-za′shun)   an operation to create a permanent opening in the trachea communicating with the cervical skin.

tracheogenic (tra″ke-o-jen′ik)   originating in the trachea.

tracheolaryngeal (tra″ke-o-lah-rin′je-al)   pertaining to the trachea and larynx.

tracheole (tra′ke-ōl)   one of the minute, fluid-filled tubules in which the tracheae of a terrestrial arthropod terminate, which contain air cells and permeate all the body tissues.

tracheomalacia (tra″ke-o-mah-la′she-ah)   softening of the tracheal cartilages.

tracheopathia (tra″ke-o-path′e-ah) [*tracheo-* + Gr. *pathos* disease]   disease of the trachea.   **t. osteoplas′tica,** a condition marked by the formation of a bony and cartilaginous deposit in the tracheal mucosa.

tracheopathy (tra″ke-op′ah-the)   tracheopathia.

tracheopharyngeal (tra″ke-o-fah-rin′je-al)   pertaining to the trachea and pharynx.

Tracheophilus cymbius (tra″ke-of′ĭ-lus sim′be-us)   a trematode parasitic in the trachea of ducks in Europe and Asia.

tracheophonesis (tra″ke-o-fo-ne′sis) [*tracheo-* + Gr. *phōnēsis* sounding]   auscultation of the heart at the sternal notch.

tracheophony (tra″ke-of′o-ne) [*tracheo-* + Gr. *phōnē* voice]   a sound heard in auscultation over the trachea.

tracheophyte (tra′ke-o-fīt″) [*tracheo-* + Gr. *phyton* plant]   a vascular plant containing both phloem and xylem.

tracheoplasty (tra′ke-o-plas″te) [*tracheo-* + Gr. *plassein* to mold]   plastic repair of the trachea.

tracheopyosis (tra″ke-o-pi-o′sis) [*tracheo-* + Gr. *pyon* pus]   purulent tracheitis.

tracheorrhagia (tra″ke-o-ra′je-ah) [*tracheo-* + Gr. *rhēgnynai* to burst forth]   hemorrhage from the trachea.

tracheorrhaphy (tra″ke-or′ah-fe) [*tracheo-* + Gr. *rhaphē* suture]   repair of an incised or wounded trachea.

tracheoschisis (tra″ke-os′kĭ-sis) [*tracheo-* + Gr. *schisis* fissure]   fissure of the trachea.

tracheoscopic (tra″ke-o-skop′ik)   pertaining to or of the character of tracheoscopy.

tracheoscopy (tra″ke-os′ko-pe) [*tracheo-* + Gr. *skopein* to examine]   the inspection of the interior of the trachea.

tracheostenosis (tra″ke-o-stĕ-no′sis) [*tracheo-* + Gr. *stenōsis* narrowing]   contraction or narrowing of the trachea.

tracheostoma (tra″ke-os′to-mah) [*tracheo-* + Gr. *stoma* mouth] an opening into the trachea through the neck.

tracheostomize (tra″ke-os′to-mīz) to perform tracheostomy upon.

tracheostomy (tra″ke-os′to-me) [*tracheo-* + Gr. *stomoun* to furnish with an opening or mouth] the surgical creation of an opening into the trachea through the neck, with the tracheal mucosa being brought into continuity with the skin; also, the opening so created. The term is also used to refer to creation of an opening in the anterior trachea for insertion of a tube to relieve upper airway obstruction and to facilitate ventilation.

tracheotome (tra′ke-o-tōm) an instrument for use in incising the trachea.

tracheotomize (tra′ke-ot′o-mīz) to perform tracheotomy upon.

tracheotomy (tra″ke-ot′o-me) [*tracheo-* + Gr. *tomē* a cutting] incision of the trachea. **inferior t.,** incision of the trachea through the neck, below the isthmus of the thyroid. **superior t.,** incision of the trachea through the neck, above the isthmus of the thyroid.

trachitis (trah-ki′tis) tracheitis.

trachoma (trah-ko′mah), pl. *trachomata* [Gr. *trachōma* roughness] a chronic infectious disease of the conjunctiva and cornea, producing photophobia, pain, and lacrimation, caused by an organism once thought to be a virus but now classified as a strain of the bacteria *Chlamydia trachomatis.* Clinically, it can be divided into four stages (MacCallan): (1) mild infection marked by tiny follicles on the eyelid conjunctiva and subepithelial infiltration; (2) enlargement of the follicles and inflammatory changes forming hard red papillae, usually with vascular invasion of the cornea marking the onset of pannus; (3) severe scarring and contraction resulting in symblepharon, entropion, trichiasis, and corneal scarring which may result in blindness; (4) complete arrest with permanent scarring, entropion, and symblepharon. Called also *Arlt's t., Egyptian, granular,* or *trachomatous conjunctivitis, Egyptian* or *granular ophthalmia,* and *granular lids.* **Arlt's t.,** trachoma. **Türck's t.,** chronic catarrhal laryngitis. **t. of vocal bands,** development of nodular swellings on the vocal cords.

trachomata (trah-ko′mah-tah) [Gr.] plural of *trachoma.*

trachomatous (trah-ko′mah-tus) pertaining to, affected with, or of the nature of trachoma.

Trachybdella bistriata (tra″ke-del′ah bis″tre-ah′tah) a leech found in Brazil which attacks man and other animals.

trachychromatic (tra″ke-kro-mat′ik) [Gr. *trachys* rough + *chrōma* color] strongly or deeply staining.

trachyphonia (tra″ke-fo′ne-ah) [Gr. *trachys* rough + *phōnē* voice + *-ia*] roughness of the voice; hoarseness.

tracing (trās′ing) 1. the act or process of drawing by following lines visible through a transparent paper, or producing an exact graphic replica by mechanical means. 2. a replica so produced. 3. a record of movements of the mandible produced by a tracer; the shape of the tracing depends on the relative location of the marking point and the tracing plate, and the apex of a properly made tracing is considered to indicate the most retruded unstrained position of the mandible in relation to the maxilla (centric jaw relation). 4. cephalometric t. **arrow-point t.,** needle-point t. **cephalometric t.,** a line drawing of structural outlines of craniofacial landmarks and facial bones made directly from a cephalometric roentgenogram. **extraoral t.,** a tracing of mandibular movements made outside the oral cavity. **Gothic arch t.,** needle-point t. **intraoral t.,** a tracing of condylar direction made within the oral cavity. **needle-point t.,** a tracing of the movements of the mandible, resembling an arrowhead or a Gothic arch, made by means of a device attached to the opposing arches, the exact shape depending on the location of the marking point relative to the tracing table; the apex of the tracing is considered as an indication of the centric relation. Called also *arrow point t., Gothic arch t.,* and *stylus t.* See also under *tracer.* **stylus t.,** needle-point t.

track (trak) the path along which something moves, or the mark left by its movement. **fog t.,** the visible trail or track left when an electron or other particle passes through a supersaturated Wilson chamber. It consists of droplets of condensed moisture which can be photographed. **ionization t.,** see under *path.*

tract (trakt) [L. *tractus*] a region, principally one of some length; specifically a collection or bundle of nerve fibers having the same origin, function, and termination (tractus [NA]), or a number of organs, arranged in series, subserving a common function. **alimentary t.,** digestive t. **ascending t.,** any bundle of nerve fibers that conveys impulses toward the brain. **Bekhterev's t.,** tractus tegmentalis centralis. **biliary t.,** the organs, ducts, etc., which participate in the secretion, storage, and delivery of bile into the duodenum. **Bruce's t., t of Bruce and Muir,** fasciculus septomarginalis. **bulbar t.,** any of the bundles of nerve fibers of the medulla oblongata. **bulboreticulospinal t.,** tractus bulboreticulospinalis. **Burdach's t.,** fasciculus cuneatus medullae spinalis. **central t. of auditory nerve,** fibers that pass from the cochlear nuclei to the superior olive, to the lateral lemniscus on the same and the opposite side and then up through the brachium of the inferior colliculus into the medial geniculate body and from there to the cortex of the transverse temporal gyri. **central t. of cranial nerves,** fibers from several cranial nerves which pass upward to the thalamus closely associated with the medial lemniscus. **central t. of thymus,** tractus centralis thymi. **central t. of trigeminal nerve,** a more or less distinct bundle of fibers from the trigeminal nerve which passes upward to the thalamus on the dorsal side of the medial lemniscus. **cerebellorubral t.,** tractus cerebellorubralis. **cerebellorubrospinal t.,** fibers passing from one dentate nucleus of the cerebellum to the contralateral red nucleus, and thence to the spinal cord. **cerebellospinal t.,** uncinate fasciculus of the cerebellum, from the fastigial nucleus to the cervical cord. **cerebellotegmental t's of bulb,** fastigiobulbar t's. **cerebellothalamic t.,** tractus dentatothalamicus. **comma t. of Schultze,** fasciculus interfascicularis. **conariohypophyseal t.,** a portion of the cavity of the embryonic brain connecting the pineal body and the pituitary gland. **cornucommissural t.,** fibers in the anterior part of the posterior column of the spinal cord, extending through the sacral and lumbar regions. **corticobulbar t.,** tractus corticonuclearis. **corticocerebellar t's,** corticopontile t's. **corticohypothalamic t.,** tractus corticohypothalamicus. **corticonuclear t.,** tractus corticonuclearis. **corticopontine t.,** see *fibrae corticopontinae.* **corticorubral t.,** fibers passing from the cerebral cortex to the red nucleus. **corticospinal t., anterior,** tractus corticospinalis ventralis. **corticospinal t., crossed,** tractus corticospinalis lateralis. **corticospinal t., direct,** tractus corticospinalis ventralis. **corticospinal t., lateral,** tractus corticospinalis lateralis. **corticospinal t. of medulla oblongata,** fasciculus pyramidalis [NA]; see *pyramidal t.* **corticospinal t's of spinal cord,** see *tractus corticospinalis lateralis* and *tractus corticospinalis ventralis.* **corticospinal t., ventral,** tractus corticospinalis ventralis. **Deiters' t.,** tractus vestibulospinalis. **dentatothalamic t.,** tractus dentatothalamicus. **descending t.,** any bundle of nerve fibers that conveys impulses from the brain toward the periphery. **digestive t.,** the part of the digestive apparatus formed by the esophagus, stomach, small and large intestines; called also *alimentary canal, alimentary t., canalis alimentarius, digestive canal, digestive tube,* and *tubus digestorius.* **dorsolateral t.,** tractus dorsolateralis. **extracorticospinal t.,** extrapyramidal t. **extrapyramidal t.,** extrapyramidal system. **fastigiobulbar t's,** bundles of efferent fibers running from the nucleus fastigii to the medulla oblongata. **fiber t's of spinal cord,** distinct bundles in the white substance of the spinal cord, made up of fibers which have the same origin, termination, and function. **Flechsig's t.,** tractus spinocerebellaris posterior. **flow t. of the heart,** see *flow track,* under *F.* **foraminous spiral t.,** tractus spiralis foraminosus. **gastrointestinal t.,** the stomach and intestines in continuity. **geniculocalcarine t.,** radiatio optica. **genitourinary t.,** apparatus urogenitalis. **Goll's t.,** fasciculus gracilis medullae spinalis. **Gowers' t.,** tractus spinocerebellaris ventralis. **habenulointerpeduncular t., habenulopeduncular t.,** tractus habenulo-interpeduncularis. **Helweg's t.,** tractus olivospinalis. **hypothalamicohypophysial t.,** tractus hypothalamicohypophysialis. **iliopubic t.,** tractus iliopubicus. **iliotibial t.,** tractus iliotibialis. **intermediolateral t.,** columna lateralis medullae spinalis. **internuncial t.,** a fiber tract connecting two nuclei or centers. **intersegmental t's of spinal cord,** fasciculi proprii medullae spinalis.

intersegmental t's of spinal cord, anterior, fasciculi proprii ventrales medullae spinalis. **intersegmental t's of spinal cord, dorsal,** fasciculi proprii dorsales medullae spinalis. **intersegmental t's of spinal cord, lateral,** fasciculi proprii laterales medullae spinalis. **intersegmental t's of spinal cord, posterior,** fasciculi proprii dorsales medullae spinalis. **intersegmental t's of spinal cord, ventral,** fasciculi proprii ventrales medullae spinalis. **intestinal t.,** the small and large intestines in continuity. **Lissauer's t.,** tractus dorsolateralis. **Löwenthal's t.,** tractus tectospinalis. **Maissiat's t.,** tractus iliotibialis. **mamillopeduncular t.,** a fiber tract from the mamillary body to nuclei in the interpeduncular fossa. **mamillotegmental t.,** fasciculus mamillotegmentalis. **mamillothalamic t.,** fasciculus mamillothalamicus. **Marchi's t.,** tractus tectospinalis. **marginal t., crossed,** tractus dorsolateralis. **mesencephalic t. of trigeminal nerve,** tractus mesencephalicus nervi trigemini. **Meynert's t.,** tractus habenulo-interpeduncularis. **Monakow's t.,** tractus rubrospinalis. **motor t.,** any bundle of nerve fibers conveying motor impulses from the central nervous system to a muscle. **occipitopontine t.,** see *fibrae corticopontine.* **olfactory t.,** tractus olfactorius. **olivocerebellar t.,** tractus olivocerebellaris. **olivocochlear t.,** tractus olivocochlearis. **olivospinal t.,** tractus olivospinalis. **optic t.,** tractus opticus. **parietopontine t.,** see *fibrae parietotemporopontinae.* **peduncular t., transverse,** a small band of fibers which passes from the brachium of the inferior colliculus to the sulcus medialis cruris cerebri. **t. of Philippe-Gombault,** Gombault-Philippe triangle. **pontoreticulospinal t.,** tractus pontoreticulospinalis. **pyramidal t., pyramidal t. of medulla oblongata,** a term applied to two groups of fibers (corticonuclear and corticospinal) arising chiefly in the sensorimotor regions of the cerebral cortex and descending in the internal capsule, cerebral peduncle, and pons to the medulla oblongata, the corticonuclear fibers synapsing with motor nuclei throughout the brain stem. Most of the corticospinal fibers cross in the decussation of the pyramids and descend in the spinal cord as the lateral corticospinal tract; most of the uncrossed fibers form the ventral corticospinal tract; both end by synapsing with internuncial and motor neurons. The pyramidal tract is a phylogenetically new tract, most prominent in man, which provides for direct cortical control and initiation of skilled movements, especially those related to speech and involving the hand and fingers. Called also *corticospinal tract of medulla oblongata, fasciculus pyramidalis medullae oblongatae* [NA], *pyramidal fasciculus of medulla oblongata, pyramidal system,* and *tractus pyramidalis.* **pyramidal t., anterior,** tractus corticospinalis ventralis. **pyramidal t., crossed,** tractus corticospinalis lateralis. **pyramidal t., direct,** tractus corticospinalis ventralis. **pyramidal t., lateral,** tractus corticospinalis lateralis. **pyramidal t's of spinal cord,** see *tractus corticospinalis lateralis* and *tractus corticospinalis ventralis.* **respiratory t.,** apparatus respiratorius. **reticulospinal t., reticulospinal t., anterior, reticulospinal t., ventral,** tractus reticulospinalis. **rubroreticular t.,** fibers from the red nucleus to the reticular formation of the pons and medulla oblongata. **rubrospinal t.,** tractus rubrospinalis. **Schultze's t., semilunar t.,** fasciculus interfascicularis. **sensory t.,** any bundle of nerve fibers conveying sensory impulses from a peripheral receptor to the central nervous system. **septomarginal t.,** fasciculus septomarginalis. **solitary t. of medulla oblongata,** tractus solitarius medullae oblongatae. **spinal t. of trigeminal nerve,** tractus spinalis nervi trigemini. **spinocerebellar t., anterior,** tractus spinocerebellaris ventralis. **spinocerebellar t., direct, spinocerebellar t., dorsal, spinocerebellar t., posterior,** tractus spinocerebellaris posterior. **spinocerebellar t., ventral,** tractus spinocerebellaris ventralis. **spinocervicothalamic t.,** a tract ascending uncrossed in the dorsal part of the lateral funiculus to the lateral cervical nucleus, which relays to the thalamus by way of the opposite medial lemniscus. **spino-olivary t.,** tractus spino-olivarius. **spinoreticular t.,** tractus spinoreticularis. **spinotectal t.,** tractus spinotectalis. **spinothalamic t., anterior,** tractus spinothalamicus ventralis. **spinothalamic t., lateral,** tractus spinothalamicus lateralis. **spinothalamic t., ventral,** tractus spinothalamicus ventralis. **spiral t., foraminous,** tractus spiralis foramino-

sus. **Spitzka's t., Spitzka-Lissauer t.,** tractus dorsolateralis. **strionigral t.,** a bundle of fibers from the corpus striatum to the substantia nigra. **sulcomarginal t.,** fasciculus sulcomarginalis. **supraopticohypophysial t.,** tractus supraopticohypophysialis. **tectobulbar t.,** tractus tectobulbaris. **tectocerebellar t.,** a bundle of fibers from the tectum of the mesencephalon to the cerebellum. **tectospinal t.,** tractus tectospinalis. **tegmental t.,** a tract of fibers in the tegmentum, back of the nucleus posterior corporis trapezoidei, believed to connect the latter with the midbrain. **tegmental t., central,** tractus tegmentalis centralis. **tegmentospinal t.,** tractus reticulospinalis. **temporopontine t.,** see *fibrae parietotemporopontinae.* **thalamo-occipital t.,** radiatio optica. **thalamo-olivary t.,** a bundle of fibers descending from the thalamus to the olivary nucleus. **triangular t.,** tractus olivospinalis. **triangular t. of Philippe-Gombault,** Gombault-Philippe triangle. **trigeminothalamic t.,** lemniscus trigeminalis. **tuberohypophysial t., tuberoinfundibular t.,** the nerve fibers that arise in the cells of the infundibular nucleus and related nuclei of the intermediate hypothalamic region, which is believed to provide a neurosecretory pathway associated with the neurocontrol of secretory activity by the anterior lobe of the pituitary gland. **urinary t.,** the organs and ducts which participate in the secretion and elimination of the urine. **uveal t.,** the vascular tunic of the eye, comprising the choroid, ciliary body, and iris; called also *tunica vasculosa bulbi* [NA]. **vestibulocerebellar t.,** fibers of the pars vestibularis nervi octavi passing to the cortex of the cerebellum. **vestibulospinal t.,** tractus vestibulospinalis. **t. of Vicq d'Azyr,** fasciculus mamillothalamicus.

tractate (trak′tāt) to attract or to tend to come together.

tractellum (trak-tel′um), pl. *tractel′la* [L.] an anterior locomotive flagellum.

traction (trak′shun) [L. *tractio*] the act of drawing or exerting a pulling force, as along the long axis of a structure. **axis t.,** traction along an axis, as of the pelvis in obstetrics. **Bryant's t.,** overhead vertical traction for fracture of the femoral shaft. **elastic t.,** traction by an elastic force or by means of an elastic appliance. **external t.,** traction applied by means of a fixed anchorage (as by a headgear) outside the oral cavity; used principally in the management of midfacial fractures. **halo-pelvic t.,** traction applied to the spine by means of two metal hoops, one (the halo) applied to the skull and the other to the pelvis, connected by four extension rods which can be lengthened by turn screws. **intermaxillary t.,** maxillomandibular t. **internal t.,** traction applied by using one of the cranial bones above the point of fracture for anchorage; used in the management of facial fractures. **maxillomandibular t.,** traction applied by means of elastic or wire ligatures and interdental wiring and/or splints; called also *intermaxillary t.* **Russell t.,** traction incorporating a sling beneath the knee that is connected to an overhead pulley. **skeletal t.,** traction applied directly upon the long bones by means of pins, Kirschner's wire, etc. **skin t.,** traction on a body part maintained by an apparatus affixed by dressings to the body surface. **tongue t.,** 1. a remedial procedure which has been used as a cardiac stimulant. 2. the pulling forward of the tongue to improve the airway.

tractor (trak′tor) [L. "drawer"] an instrument for applying traction. **prostatic t.,** a straight instrument with blades operated by a knob that draws the prostate into view in perineal prostatectomy. **Syms' t.,** a tube with an inflatable rubber bag at the end; used to bring down a prostate into the perineal incision. **urethral t.,** a curved instrument with blades operated by a knob that is inserted through the urethra into the bladder in perineal prostatectomy.

tractotomy (trak-tot′o-me) the operation of severing or incising a nerve tract. **mesencephalic t.,** surgical division of nerve tracts in the mesencephalon.

tractus (trak′tus), pl. *tractus* [L. "a track," "trail"] a tract: a region, principally one of some length; [NA] a general term, especially for a collection or bundle of nerve fibers having the same origin and termination, and serving the same function. See also *fasciculus.* **t. bulboreticulospina′lis** [NA], bulboreticulospinal tract: a group of reticulospinal nerve fibers in the lateral funiculus of the spinal cord, the axons of which are derived from nerve cells of the medulla oblongata. **t. centra′lis thy′mi,** central tract of thymus: the medullary core of the thymus; an irregular fibrous bundle carrying the blood vessels and giving attachment to the lobules of the gland. **t. cerebellorubra′lis** [NA], cerebellorubral tract: fibers arising chiefly in the dentate nucleus of the cerebellum and projecting to the opposite red nucleus via the superior cerebellar peduncle; impulses are then relayed to the reticular formation and spinal cord. **t. cerebello-thalam′icus,** t. dentatothalamicus. **t. corticohypo-thalam′icus** [NA], corticohypothalamic tract: a diffuse collection of fibers that arise from various parts of the frontal lobe and are distributed directly to the hypothalamus. **t. corticonuclea′ris** [NA], corticonuclear tract: the nerve fiber tract formed by fibers (corticonuclear fibers) of the pyramidal tract (q.v.) that arise in the cerebral cortex, descend in the internal capsule, and synapse in the various motor nuclei of the mesencephalon, pons, and medulla oblongata. Called also *corticobulbar tract.* **t. cor-ticopon′tinus,** see *fibrae corticopontinae.* **t. cortico-spina′lis ante′rior,** NA alternative for *t. corticospinalis ventralis.* **t. corticospina′lis latera′lis** [NA], lateral corticospinal tract: a group of nerve fibers in the lateral funiculus of the spinal cord, originating in the cerebral cortex; called also *crossed corticospinal* or *pyramidal tract, lateral pyramidal tract,* and *t. pyramidalis lateralis.* See also *pyramidal tract,* under *tract.* **t. corticospina′lis ven-tra′lis** [NA], ventral corticospinal tract: a group of nerve fibers in the ventral funiculus of the spinal cord, originating in the cerebral cortex; called also *anterior* or *direct corticospinal* or *pyramidal tract, t. corticospinalis anterior* [NA alternative] and *t. pyramidalis anterior.* See also *pyramidal tract,* under *tract.* **t. dentatothalam′icus** [NA], dentato-thalamic tract: fibers arising chiefly in the dentate nucleus of the cerebellum and projecting to the ventral lateral nucleus of the opposite thalamus via the cranial cerebellar peduncle; impulses are then relayed to the frontal lobe. Called also *cerebellothalamic tract* and *t. cerebellothalamicus.* **t. dor-solatera′lis** [NA], dorsolateral tract: a group of nerve fibers in the lateral funiculus of the spinal cord dorsal to the dorsal column, composed in part of primary pain and temperature fibers which enter the spinal cord, travel the distance of a few segments in the dorsolateral tract, and then synapse in the dorsal column. Called also *dorsolateral fasciculus* and *Lissauer's marginal zone.* **t. frontoponti′nus** [NA], fronto-pontine tract: the nerve fiber tract formed by fibers (fronto-pontine fibers) in the frontal lobe of the cerebral hemisphere and traverse the internal capsule and end in the pontine nuclei. **t. habenulo-interpeduncula′ris** [NA], habenulointerpeduncular tract: a bundle of nerve fibers arising in the habenular nuclei and extending rostroven-trally to the interpeduncular nucleus to relay fibers to the reticular formation of the mesencephalon; called also *fasciculus retroflexus, habenulopeduncular tract,* and *Meynert's bundle, fasciculus,* or *tract.* **t. hypothalamohypo-physia′lis** [NA], hypothalamicohypophysial tract: the nerve fibers that make up the efferent pathways of the hypothalamus, which arise in the hypothalamic nuclei and end at various levels in the median eminence, infundibulum, and posterior lobe of the pituitary gland. It contains sets of fibers; see *t. paraventriculohypophysialis, t. supraopticohypo-physialis.* See also *tuberohypophysial tract.* **t. ili-opu′bicus,** iliopubic tract: a thickened band of tissue that strengthens the lower part of the deep inguinal ring and forms the base of the internal spermatic fascia. **t. ili-otibia′lis** [NA], **t. iliotibia′lis [Maissia′ti],** iliotibial tract: a thickened longitudinal band of fascia lata extending from the tensor muscle downward along the lateral side of the thigh to the lateral condyle of the tibia. **t. mesenceph-al′icus ner′vi trigem′ini** [NA], mesencephalic tract of trigeminal nerve: sensory fibers of the entering trigeminal nerve that continue rostrally along the medial aspect of the superior cerebellar peduncle, their cell bodies being located in the nucleus of the mesencephalic tract, which accompanies it. Called also *radix descendens* [*mesencephalica*] *nervi trigem-ini.* **t. occipitopon′tinus,** see *fibrae corticopontinae.* **t. olfacto′rius** [NA], olfactory tract: a narrow triangular band in the olfactory sulcus of the frontal lobe, which arises from the olfactory bulb and extends posteriorly, to end by dividing into medial and lateral olfactory striae, the latter ending in the primary olfactory cortex. **t. olivocerebel-la′ris** [NA], olivocerebellar tract: a fiber tract that arises from the olive, crosses to the opposite side to pierce the other olive, and enters the cerebellum through its inferior pedun-cle. **t. olivocochlea′ris** [NA], olivocochlear tract: fibers derived from the nucleus of the superior olive that terminate

in relation to the hair cells in the spiral organ of the cochlea; called also *olivocochlear fasciculus.* **t. olivospina′lis** [NA], olivospinal tract: a group of nerve fibers in the lateral funiculus, seen as a triangular area in transverse section of the spinal cord, descending from the olivary nucleus to the upper cervical segments; called also *Helweg's t.* or *bundle* and *triangular t.* **t. op′ticus** [NA], optic tract: the tract aris-ing from the optic chiasma, proceeding backward, around the cerebral peduncle, and dividing into a lateral and a medial root; the roots end in the cranial colliculus and lateral geniculate body, respectively. **t. paraventriculohypo-physia′lis** [NA], paraventriculohypophyseal tract: the fi-bers of the hypothalamicohypophysial tract that arise in the paraventricular nucleus of the hypothalamus, some of which end in the infundibulum and others reach the posterior lobe of the pituitary gland, where their neurosecretory material is stored as oxytocin before being released into the systemic circulation. See also *t. supraopticohypophysialis.* **t. parietopon′tinus,** see *fibrae parietotemporopontinae.* **t. pontoreticulospina′lis** [NA], pontoreticulospinal tract: a group of reticulospinal nerve fibers in the lateral funiculus of the spinal cord, arising in the pontobulbar region. **t. pyramida′lis,** fasciculus pyramidalis medul-lae oblongatae; see *pyramidal tract,* under tract. **t. pyramida′lis ante′rior,** t. corticospinalis ventralis. **t. pyramida′lis latera′lis,** t. corticospinalis lateralis. **t. reticulospina′lis** [NA], **t. reticulospina′lis an-te′rior, t. reticulospina′lis ventra′lis,** reticulospinal tract: a group of fibers arising mostly from the reticular formation of the pons and medulla oblongata; chiefly homo-lateral, the fibers descend in the ventral and lateral funiculi to most levels of the spinal cord; called also *anterior* or *ventral reticulospinal tract.* **t. rubrospina′lis** [NA], rubrospinal tract: a group of nerve fibers in the lateral funiculus of the spinal cord, arising in the large cells of the red nucleus of the mesencephalon. **t. solita′rius medul′lae oblon-ga′tae** [NA], solitary tract of medulla oblongata: a descend-ing tract in the medulla oblongata, ventrolateral to the caudal part of the fourth ventricle, near the dorsal nucleus of the vagus and glossopharyngeal nerves, and comprising primary visceral afferent fibers from the facial, glossophar-yngeal, and vagus nerves. **t. spina′lis ner′vi trigem′ini** [NA], spinal tract of trigeminal nerve: a de-scending tract of the trigeminal nerve that extends from the level of entrance of the sensory root of the trigeminal nerves into the pons to the upper cervical segments of the spinal cord. Lying lateral to the nucleus of the spinal tract of the trigeminal nerve, in which its fibers synapse, this tract carries mainly pain and temperature impulses from the face. **t. spinocerebella′ris ante′rior,** NA alternative for *t. spinocerebellaris ventralis.* **t. spinocerebella′ris dor-sa′lis** [NA], dorsal spinocerebellar tract: a group of nerve fibers in the lateral funiculus of the spinal cord; arising chiefly from the columna thoracica and activated by skin, muscle, tendon, and joint endings, they ascend to the cerebellum by way of the dorsal part of the lateral funiculus and then the inferior cerebellar peduncle. Called also *direct* or *posterior spinocerebellar tract* and *t. spinocerebellaris posterior* [NA alternative]. **t. spinocerebella′ris pos-te′rior,** NA alternative for *t. spinocerebellaris dorsalis.* **t. spinocerebella′ris ventra′lis** [NA], ventral spinocer-ebellar tract: a group of nerve fibers in the lateral funiculus of the spinal cord; arising mostly in the opposite gray matter, and activated by skin, muscle, tendon, and joint endings, they ascend to the cerebellum by way of the anterior part of the lateral funiculus and then the superior cerebellar peduncle. Called also *anterior spinocerebellar t., Gowers' column, fasci-culus,* or *tract,* and *t. spinocerebellaris anterior* [NA alterna-tive]. **t. spino-oliva′ris** [NA], spino-olivary tract: an as-cending tract of nerve fibers in the lateral funiculus of the spinal cord, arising from the dorsal gray columns of the spinal cord and running to the olivary nucleus. **t. spinoreticula′ris** [NA], spinoreticular tract: an ascending tract of nerve fibers in the lateral funiculus of the spinal cord, passing to the reticular formation of the brain stem. **t. spinotecta′lis** [NA], spinotectal tract: a group of nerve fibers in the lateral funiculus of the spinal cord, mostly crossed from their origin, which ascend to the superior and inferior colliculi and carry somatic sensory impulses. **t. spinothalam′icus ante′rior,** NA alternative for *t. spino-thalamicus ventralis.* **t. spinothalam′icus latera′lis** [NA], lateral spinothalamic tract: a group of nerve fibers in the lateral funiculus of the spinal cord, which arise in the opposite gray matter; carrying impulses activated by pain and temperature, they ascend to the thalamus, running with the lateral lemniscus in the brain stem. **t. spinothalam'icus ventra'lis** [NA], ventral spinothalamic tract: a group of nerve fibers in the ventral funiculus of the spinal cord, continuous with the lateral spinothalamic tract, which arise in the contralateral gray substance carrying impulses activated by light touch, they ascend to the thalamus, joining the medial lemniscus in the brain stem. Called also *anterior spinothalamic tract* and *t. spinothalamicus anterior* [NA alternative]. **t. spira'lis foramino'sus** [NA], foraminous spiral tract: a spiral area on the fundus of the internal acoustic meatus, below the crista transversa and in front of the area vestibularis inferior; it corresponds to the base of the cochlea and is perforated with numerous holes for the passage of branches of the vestibulocochlear nerve. **t. subarcua'tus,** an area of small cell structure under the arch of the superior semicircular canal. **t. supraopticohypophysia'lis** [NA], supraopticohypophysial tract: the fibers of the hypothalamicohypophysial tract that arise in the supraoptic nucleus of the thalamus, some of which descend to end in the infundibulum and others of which reach the posterior lobe of the pituitary gland, where their neurosecretory material is stored as antidiuretic hormone before being released into the systemic circulation. The term has also been used to denote all of the fibers of the hypothalamicohypophysial tract that enter the infundibulum without regard to their point of termination and also to denote the fibers of the hypothalamicohypophysial tract that arise in both the supraoptic nucleus and the paraventricular nucleus (see *t. paraventriculohypophysialis*). **t. tectobulba'ris,** tectobulbar tract: fibers arising mostly in the cranial colliculus; they descend to the lower border of the pons and end in the nuclei of the brain stem and in the reticular formation. **t. tectospina'lis** [NA], tectospinal tract: a group of nerve fibers, chiefly crossed, which arise mostly in the cranial colliculus and descend to the cervical cord, where they lie in the ventral funiculus. **t. tegmenta'lis centra'lis** [NA], central tegmental tract: a composite nerve tract arising from the midbrain tegmentum, periaqueductal gray matter, and red nucleus; it descends in the tegmentum and reticular formation to end in the inferior olivary complex. The tract includes an ascending component from the reticular formation. Called also *Bekhterev's tract.* **t. temporopon'tinus** see *fibrae parietotemporopontinae.* **t. triangula'ris,** olivospinal tract. **t. trigeminothalam'icus,** NA alternative for *lemniscus trigeminalis.* **t. vestibulospina'lis** [NA], vestibulospinal tract: nerve fibers arising from the lateral vestibular nucleus which descend uncrossed, chiefly in the ventral part of the lateral funiculus, throughout most levels of the spinal cord; some fibers to the caudal spinal segments lie in the ventral funiculus. More than one such tract is considered to exist in some species, including humans.

tragacanth (trag'ah-kanth) [NF]　the dried gummy exudation from *Astragalus gummifer* or other species of *Astragalus;* used as a suspending agent for drugs. Called also *gum tragacanth.*

tragal (tra'gal)　pertaining to the tragus.

tragi (tra'ji) [L., pl. of *tragus*] [NA]　hair growing on the pinna of the external ear, especially on the cartilaginous projection anterior to the external opening (tragus).

Tragia (tra'je-ah)　a genus of poisonous euphorbiaceous plants; several species (*T. urens,* etc.) are weeds of the southern United States.

tragion (traj'e-on)　a cephalometric landmark located at the superior margin of the tragus of the ear.

tragomaschalia (trag"o-mas-kal'e-ah) [Gr. *tragos* goat + *maschalē* the armpit]　bromidrosis.

tragophonia (trag"o-fo'ne-ah)　egophony.

tragophony (trah-gof'o-ne) [Gr. *tragos* goat + *phōne* voice]　egophony.

tragopodia (trag"o-po'de-ah) [Gr. *tragos* goat + *pous* foot]　genu valgum.

tragus (tra'gus), pl. *tra'gi* [L.; Gr. *tragos* goat] [NA]　the cartilaginous projection anterior to the external opening of the ear; see also *tragi.*

trainable (tra'nah-b'l)　capable of being trained; used to describe persons with moderate mental retardation (IQ 35 to 50) who are unlikely to progress beyond the second grade level in academic skills but can profit from vocational training and can take care of themselves under supervision. Cf. *educable.*

training (trān'ing)　a system of instruction or teaching; preparation by instruction and practice. **assertiveness t.,** a form of behavior therapy in which individuals are taught appropriate interpersonal responses, involving expression of their feelings, both negative and positive. Called also *expressive t.* **expressive t.,** assertiveness t.

trait (trāt)　1. any genetically determined characteristic. 2. commonly used in medicine to designate the condition prevailing in the heterozygous state of a recessive disorder, as in sickle cell anemia. 3. a distinctive behavior pattern. **sickle cell t.,** the condition, usually asymptomatic, caused by heterozygosity for hemoglobin S.

trajector (trah-jek'tor)　an instrument for locating a bullet in a wound.

Tral (tral)　trademark for preparations of hexocyclium methylsulfate.

Trallianus, Alexander　see *Alexander of Tralles.*

tralonide (tra'lo-nīd)　chemical name: 9,11β-dichloro-6α,21-difluoro-16α,17-[(1-methylethylidene)bis(oxy)]pregna-1,4-diene-3,20-dione; a glucocorticoid, $C_{24}H_{28}Cl_2F_2O_4$.

tramadol hydrochloride (trah'mah-dōl)　chemical name: *trans*-(±)-2-[(dimethylamino)-methyl]-1-(3-methoxyphenyl)cyclohexanol hydrochloride; an analgesic, $C_{16}H_{25}$-$NO_2 \cdot HCl$.

tramazoline hydrochloride (trah-maz'o-lēn)　chemical name: 4,5-dihydro-*N*-(5,6,7,8-tetrahydro-1-naphthalenyl)-1*H*-imidazol-2-amine monohydrochloride; an adrenergic, $C_{13}H_{17}N_3 \cdot HCl$, with nasal decongestant properties.

tramitis (tram-i'tis) [L. *trama* woof + *-itis*]　a condition of the pulmonary tissue in early tuberculosis seen in the roentgenogram as pleural adhesions, deviated mediastinum, sclerosed bands, calcified nodes, and areas of increased density.

trance (trans)　a state of altered consciousness characterized by heightened focal awareness and reduced peripheral awareness; a sleeplike state of reduced consciousness and activity. **hypnotic t.,** the state induced by hypnosis.

Trancopal (tran'ko-pal)　trademark for a preparation of chlormezanone.

Trandate (tran'dāt)　trademark for a preparation of labetalol hydrochloride.

tranexamic acid (tran-ek-sam'ik)　an antifibrinolytic that acts by competitively inhibiting plasminogen; it is used as a hemostatic in the treatment of severe hemorrhage associated with excessive fibrinolysis.

tranquilizer (tran"kwĭ-līz'er) [L. *tranquillus* quiet, calm + *-ize* verb ending meaning to make + *-er* agent]　a drug with a calming, soothing effect. **major t.,** antipsychotic agent; see *antipsychotic.* **minor t.,** antianxiety agent; see *antianxiety.*

trans (tranz) [L., through]　in organic chemistry, having certain atoms or radicals on opposite sides; in genetics, having one of the two mutant genes of a pseudoallele on each homologous chromosome.

trans- [L. *trans* through]　1. a prefix meaning through, across, or beyond.　2. in organic chemistry, denoting the presence of certain atoms or radicals on opposite sides of the molecule.　3. in genetics, having one of the two mutant genes at each of two loci on each homologous chromosome. Cf. *cis-.*

transabdominal (trans"ab-dom'ĭ-nal)　through the abdominal wall.

transacetylase (trans-as'ě-til-ās, trans-ah-set'il-ās)　acyltransferase.

transacetylation (trans-as"ě-til-a'shun)　a chemical reaction involving the transfer of the acetyl group CH_3—C—. It

$$\overset{\|}{O}$$

occurs in many metabolic reactions.

transacylase (trans-ās'ĭ-lās)　an enzyme that catalyzes transacylation.

transacylation (trans-as"ĭ-la'shun)　a chemical reaction involving the transfer of the acyl radical between acetic and higher carboxylic acids.

transaldolase (trans-al'do-lās) [EC 2.2.1.2]　an enzyme of the transferase class that catalyzes the reaction sedoheptulose 7-phosphate + D-glyceraldehyde 3-phosphate = D-erythrose 4-phosphate + D-fructose 6-phosphate in the pentose-phosphate pathway.

transaminase (trans-am′ĭ-nās) aminotransferase.

transamination (trans″am-i-na′shun) the reversible transfer of an amino group from an amino acid to what was originally an α-keto acid, forming a new keto acid and a new amino acid, without the appearance of ammonia in the free state.

transanimation (trans-an″ĭ-ma′shun) [*trans-* + L. *anima* breath] resuscitation by mouth-to-mouth breathing; see *mouth-to-mouth method of artificial respiration,* under *respiration.*

transaortic (trans″a-or′tik) performed through the aorta; used especially in reference to surgical procedures on the aortic valve, performed through an incision in the wall of the aorta.

transatrial (trans-a′tre-al) performed through the atrium; used especially in reference to surgical procedures on a cardiac valve, performed through an incision in the wall of the atrium.

transaudient (trans-aw′de-ent) permitting passage of the mechanical vibrations perceived as sound.

transaxial (trans-ak′se-al) directed at right angles to the long axis of the body or a part.

transbasal (trans-ba′sal) through the base, as a surgical approach through the base of the skull.

transcalent (trans-ka′lent) [*trans-* + L. *calere* to be hot] permitting the passage of radiant heat.

transcalvarial (trans″kal-vār′e-al) through or across the calvaria.

transcarbamoylase (trans-kar″bah-mo″′l-ās) carbamoyltransferase.

transcarboxylase (trans″kar-bok′sĭ-lās) carboxyltransferase.

transcatheter (trans-kath′ĕ-ter) performed through the lumen of a catheter.

transcervical (trans-ser′vĭ-kal) performed through the cervical opening of the uterus.

transclomiphene (trans-clo′mĭ-fēn) zuclomiphene.

transcobalamin (trans″ko-bal′ah-min) either of two plasma proteins, transcobalamin I (mol. wt., 121,000) and transcobalamin II (mol. wt. 35,000), that bind and transport cobalamins (vitamin B₁₂). B₁₂ appears to enter cells by receptor-mediated endocytosis bound to transcobalamin II. Deficiency of transcobalamin II results in failure of immunoglobulin production, megaloblastic anemia, granulocytopenia, thrombocytopenia, and intestinal villous atrophy: correctable by vitamin B₁₂ therapy.

transcondyloid (trans-kon′dĭ-loid) through the condyles.

transcortical (trans-kor′tĭ-kal) connecting two different parts of the cerebral cortex; also, dependent on disease of the tracts connecting different parts of the cerebral cortex.

transcortin (trans-kor′tin) an α-globulin that specifically and avidly binds and transports in plasma the unconjugated and presumably biologically active cortisol making up less than 5 per cent of the circulating steroid; called also *corticosteroid-binding globulin* and *cortisol-binding globulin* (CBG).

transcricothyroid (trans-kri″ko-thi′roid) through or across the cricothyroid membrane.

transcript (trans′kript) a strand of nucleic acid that has been synthesized using another nucleic acid strand as a template. **primary t.,** the first RNA transcript of a gene, containing introns as well as exons.

transcriptase (trans-krip′tās) DNA-directed RNA polymerase. **reverse t.,** RNA-directed DNA polymerase.

transcription (trans-krip′shun) [L. *transcriptio* transfer, copy] the process by which a single-stranded RNA with a base sequence complementary to one strand of a double-stranded DNA is synthesized. The enzymes involved are called DNA-dependent RNA polymerases (see under *polymerase*).

transcutaneous (trans″ku-ta′ne-us) transdermal.

transdermal (trans-der′mal) entering through the dermis, or skin, as in administration of a drug applied to the skin in ointment or patch form.

transducer (trans-du′ser) a device that translates one form of energy to another, e.g., the pressure, temperature, or pulse to an electrical signal. **neuroendocrine t.,** a neuron having the properties of both nerve and gland, such as a neurohypophysial neuron, that on stimulation secretes a hormone, thereby translating neural information into endocrine information, with consequent inhibition or stimulation of hormonal secretion.

transduction (trans-duk′shun) [L. *transducere* to lead across] a method of genetic recombination in bacteria, in which DNA from a lysed bacterium is transferred to another bacterium by bacteriophage, thereby changing the genetic constitution of the second organism.

transdural (trans-du′ral) through or across the dura mater.

transection (tran-sek′shun) [*trans-* + L. *sectio* a cut] a section made across a long axis; a cross section; division by cutting transversely.

transepidermal (trans″ep-ĭ-der′mal) occurring through or across the epidermis.

transfaunation (trans″faw-na′shun) the transfer of animal parasites from one host organism to another.

transfection (trans-fek′shun) the artificial infection of animal or bacterial cells by uptake of nucleic acid isolated from virus or bacteriophage, resulting in the production of mature virus or phage particles.

transfectoma (tranz″fek-to′mah) lymphoid cells transfected with immunoglobulin genes; they are capable of producing antibody molecules separate from the specificity encoded by their own genes.

transfer (trans′fer) [*trans-* + L. *ferre* to carry] the conveyance of something from one place to another. **linear energy t.,** see *LET.* **passive t.,** the conferring of immunity to a nonimmune host by injection of antibody or lymphocytes from an immune or sensitized donor. **tendon t.,** surgical relocation of the insertion of a tendon of a normal muscle to a different site to take over the function of a muscle inactivated by trauma or disease.

transferase (trans′fer-ās) [EC 2] a class of enzymes that transfer a chemical group from one compound (the donor) to another compound (the acceptor).

transference (trans-fer′ens) 1. the passage or conveyance of a symptom or disorder from one part of the body to another. 2. in psychotherapy, the unconscious tendency to assign to others in one's present environment feelings and attitudes associated with significant persons in one's early life, especially the patient's transfer to the therapist of feelings and attitudes associated with a parent. The feelings may be affectionate (*positive t.*) or hostile (*negative t.*). **counter t.,** see *countertransference.*

transferrin (trans-fer′rin) [*trans-* + L. *ferrum* iron + *-in* chemical suffix] serum β-globulin that binds and transports iron. Several types (e.g., C, B, D, and many others) have been distinguished on the basis of electrophoretic mobility and related as the products of corresponding dominant somatic genes, Tf^C, Tf^B, and Tf^D. Called also *siderophilin.*

transfix (trans′fiks) [*trans-* + L. *figere* to fix] to pierce through and through.

transfixion (trans-fik′shun) a cutting through from within outward, as in amputation.

transformation (trans″for-ma′shun) [*trans-* + L. *formatio* formation] change of form or structure; conversion from one form to another. In oncology, the change that a normal cell undergoes as it becomes malignant. In eukaryotes, the conversion of normal cells to malignant cells in cell culture. **asbestos t.,** the deposition of extraneous fibers in hyaline cartilage, which gives it a silky, glossy appearance. **bacterial t.,** the exchange of genetic material between strains of bacteria by the transfer of a fragment of naked DNA from a donor cell to a recipient cell, followed by recombination in the recipient chromosome. **lymphocyte t.,** the morphologic changes accompanying lymphocyte activation, in which small, resting lymphocytes are transformed into large, active lymphocytes (lymphoblasts).

transfructosylase (trans-frook″to-sil′ās) fructosyltransferase.

transfusion (trans-fu′zhun) [L. *transfusio*] the introduction of whole blood or blood component directly into the blood stream. Cf. *infusion.* **autologous t.,** autotransfusion. **direct t.,** immediate t. **exchange t.,** repetitive withdrawal of small amounts of blood and replacement with donor blood, until a large proportion of the blood volume has been exchanged; used in newborn infants with erythroblastosis and in patients with severe uremia. **exsanguination t.,** exchange t. **fetomaternal t.,** transplacental passage of fetal blood into the circulation of the maternal organism. **immediate t.,** the transfer of blood from one person to another without use of an intermediate container or anticoagulant. **indirect t.,** transfer of blood from a donor to a flask or other container, and then to the recipient. **intraperitoneal t.,** infusion of blood into the peritoneal cavity; see *intrauterine t.* **intrauterine t.,** transfusion of Rh-negative blood into the peritoneal cavity of an unborn infant in the treatment of erythroblastosis fetalis *in utero.* **mediate t.,** indirect t. **placental t.,** return to the newborn, after birth, and through the umbilical vessels, of some of the blood contained in the fetal placenta. **replacement t., substitution t.,** exchange t.

transglucosylase (trans″gloo-ko-sil′ās) glucosyltransferase.

transglutaminase (tranz″gloo-tam′in-ās) protein-glutamine γ-glutamyltransferase.

transglycosidation (trans-gli″ko-si-da′shun) the formation of complex sugars by the transfer of monosaccharide units once glycosidic linkages are formed.

transglycosylase (trans″gli-ko′sil-ās) glycosyltransferase.

transhiatal (trans″hi-a′tal) across or through a hiatus.

transiliac (trans-il′e-ak) across or between the two ilia.

transilient (tran-sil′e-ent) [*trans-* + L. *salire* to leap] leaping or passing across.

transillumination (trans″ĭ-lu″mĭ-na′shun) the passage of light through body tissues for the purpose of examination, the object or part under examination being interposed between the observer and the light source; diaphanoscopy.

transinsular (trans-in′su-lar) across the insula; crossing the insula.

transischiac (trans-is′ke-ak) between the two ischia.

transisthmian (trans-is′me-an) across an isthmus, especially the isthmus of the gyrus fornicatus.

transistor (trans-is′tor) a small wafer of semiconducting material having three electrodes, called the emitter, base, and collector, which perform functions similar to those of the cathode, grid, and plate of a vacuum tube.

transition (tran-zish′un) [L. *transitio* crossing over] in molecular genetics, a point mutation in which a purine base replaces a purine base or a pyrimidine base replaces a pyrimidine base. Cf. *transversion.*

transketolase (trans-ke′to-lās) [EC 2.2.1.1] an enzyme of the transferase class that catalyzes the reaction sedoheptulose 7-phosphate + D-glyceraldehyde 3-phosphate = D-ribose 5-phosphate + D-xylulose 5-phosphate in the pentose phosphate pathway.

translateral (trans-lat′er-al) from side to side; in roentgenography, referring to the view obtained with the patient supine and the radiation directed horizontally.

translation (trans-la′shun) [L. *translatio* transfer] in genetics, the process by which polypeptide chains are synthesized, the amino acid sequence being completely determined by the sequence of bases in a messenger RNA (mRNA), which in turn is determined by the sequence of bases in the DNA of the gene from which it was transcribed.

translocation (trans″lo-ka′shun) [*trans-* + L. *locus* place] a structural chromosome aberration in which one segment of a chromosome is transferred to a nonhomologous chromosome, the result of breakage of both chromosomes with repair in abnormal arrangement. Called also *interchange.* Abbreviated t. See also *chromosome aberration,* under *aberration,* and see *insertion,* def. 2. **balanced t.,** reciprocal translocation which results in no more or no less than the normal diploid or haploid genetic material. The phenotype is normal, but there will be partial aneuploidy in a percentage of the gametes, with a risk of unbalanced offspring. **reciprocal t.,** the complete exchange of fragments between two broken nonhomologous chromosomes, one part of one uniting with part of the other, with no fragments left over. Abbreviated *rcp.* **robertsonian t.,** translocation involving two of the acrocentric chromosomes (13, 14, 15, 21, and 22), which fuse at the centromere region and lose their heterochromatic short arms. A carrier of a balanced Robertsonian translocation involving chromosome 14 and 21 has a virtually complete chromosomal complement but only 45 chromosomes

(including the translocation chromosome), is phenotypically normal, but risks producing offspring with trisomy 21 (translation Down syndrome).

translucent (trans-lu′sent) [*trans-* + L. *lucens* shining] transmitting light, but diffusing it so that objects beyond are not clearly distinguished.

transmethylase (trans-meth′ĭ-lās) methyltransferase.

transmethylation (trans″meth-ĭ-la′shun) the transfer of a methyl group (CH_3—) from the molecules of one compound to those of another.

transmigration (trans″mi-gra′shun) [*trans-* + L. *migratio* migration] 1. a wandering, especially a change of place from one side of the body to the other. 2. diapedesis. **external t.,** the passage of an ovum from one ovary to the uterine tube of the other side without going through its own oviduct. **internal t.,** the passage of an ovum from one oviduct to the other by way of the uterus.

transmissible (trans-mis′ĭ-b'l) capable of being transmitted from one individual or one species to another.

transmission (trans-mish′un) [*trans-* + L. *missio* a sending] 1. a passage or transfer, as of a disease from one individual to another, or of neural impulses from one neuron to another. 2. the communication of inheritable qualities from parent to offspring. **duplex t.,** the transmission of neural impulses in two directions along a nerve. **ephaptic t.,** the conduction of a nerve impulse across an ephapse, as opposed to synaptic transmission. **horizontal t.,** the spread of an infectious agent from one individual to another, usually through contact with excreta, e.g., sputum, etc., containing the agent; cf. *vertical t.* **neurochemical t.,** transmission of an impulse across a synaptic junction through the medium of a chemical substance (neurotransmitter). Called also *neurohumoral t.* **neurohumoral t.,** neurochemical t. **neuromuscular t.,** the chemically mediated transmission of an action potential from nerve to muscle across the myoneural junction. **synaptic t.,** the communication of a neural impulse from one neuron to another neuron, a muscle fiber, or a gland across a synapse. **vertical t.,** transmission from one generation to another. The term is restricted by some to genetic transmission and extended by others to include also transmission of infection from one generation to the next, as by milk or through the placenta. Cf. *horizontal h.*

transmittance (trans-mit′ans) 1. in analytical chemistry, the ratio I/I_0 of the light intensity transmitted by the solution under analysis (I) to that transmitted by the pure solvent or other reference solution (I_0). 2. in physics, the ratio (I/I_0) of the radiant energy transmitted by an object divided by the incident radiant energy. Symbol T.

transmitter (trans-mit′er) something that transmits; see also *substance;* see also *neurotransmitter.*

transmural (trans-mu′ral) [*trans-* + L. *muralis,* from *murus* wall] through the wall of an organ; extending through or affecting the entire thickness of the wall of an organ or cavity.

transmutation (trans″mu-ta′shun) 1. evolutionary change of one species into another. 2. the change of one chemical element into another; nucleonics, the changing of an atomic nucleus to one of a different atomic number by nuclear bombardment, causing rearrangement of the protons and neutrons.

transocular (trans-ok′u-lar) across the eye.

transonance (tran′so-nans) [*trans-* + L. *sonans* sounding] transmission of a sound originating in one organ through the substance of another organ.

transovarial (trans″o-va′re-al) through the ovary; referring to transmission of pathogens from the maternal organism, by invasion of the ovary and infection of eggs, to individuals of the next generation, as may occur in infections of arthropods, especially mites and ticks.

transovarian (trans″o-va′re-an) transovarial.

transpalatal (trans-pal′ah-tal) performed through the roof of the mouth, or palate.

transparent (trans-par′ent) [*trans-* + L. *parere* to appear] permitting the passage of rays of light, so that objects may be seen through the substance.

transparietal (trans″pah-ri′ĕ-tal) [*trans-* + L. *paries* wall] through or across a wall, as through the intact body wall.

transperitoneal (trans″per-ĭ-to-ne′al) through or across the peritoneum.

transphosphorylase (trans″fos-for′ĭ-lās) see *phospho-transferase, phosphorylase.*

transphosphorylation (trans-fos″for-ĭ-la′shun) the exchange of phosphate groups between organic phosphates, without their going through the stage of inorganic phosphate.

transpiration (tran″spĭ-ra′shun) [*trans-* + L. *spiratio* exhalation] the discharge of air, sweat, or vapor through the skin; insensible perspiration. **pulmonary t.,** the exhalation of water vapor from the blood circulating through the lungs.

transplacental (trans″plah-sen′tal) through the placenta.

transplant 1. (trans-plant′) to transfer tissue from one part to another. 2. (trans′plant) an organ or tissue taken from the body for grafting into another area of the same body or into another individual. **Gallie t.,** strips of fascia lata employed as sutures in the repair of hernias.

transplantar (trans-plan′tar) [*trans-* + L. *planta* sole] across the sole.

transplantation (trans″plan-ta′shun) [*trans-* + L. *plantare* to plant] the grafting of tissues taken from the patient's own body or from another. See also entries under *graft.* **allogeneic t.,** transplantation of tissue between genetically dissimilar animals of the same species. **heterotopic t.,** transplantation of tissue typical of one area to a different recipient site. **homotopic t.,** orthotopic t. **orthotopic t.,** transplantation of tissue from a donor into its normal anatomical position in the recipient. **syngeneic t.,** transplantation of tissues between animals in the same pure line, e.g., within an inbred strain. **syngenesioplastic t.,** transplantation of tissue from one individual to a related individual of the same species, as from a mother to her child, or from a brother to a sister. **tendon t.,** 1. surgical replacement of a damaged segment of tendon by a free tendon graft. 2. tendon transfer. **tooth t.,** the insertion into a prepared dental alveolus of an autogenous or homologous tooth; it may be a developing tooth germ from the same mouth, a homologous transplant, or a tooth with or without vital pulp, or one having had endodontic treatment, transplanted from one site to another in the same individual or from one individual to another.

transpleural (trans-ploor′al) through the pleura; by way of the pleural sac.

transport (trans′port) [L. *transportare* to carry across] the movement of materials in biological systems, particularly into and out of cells and across epithelial layers. **active t.,** the movement of materials across cell membranes and epithelial layers resulting directly from the expenditure of metabolic energy. **bulk t.,** the uptake by or extrusion from a cell of fluid and of particles too large to cross the cell membrane by diffusion or active transport, accomplished by invagination and vacuole formation (uptake) or by evagination (extrusion); it includes endocytosis, phagocytosis, pinocytosis, and exocytosis.

transposition (trans″po-zish′un) [*trans-* + L. *positio* placement] 1. displacement of a viscus to the opposite side. 2. the operation of carrying a tissue flap from one situation to another without severing its connection entirely until it is united at its new location. 3. the exchange of position of two atoms within a molecule. **corrected t. of great vessels,** a developmental cardiac anomaly characterized by transposition of the great vessels with inversion of the ventricles and atrioventricular valves; termed "corrected" because the inverted ventricles compensate for the transposition, producing a mirror-image blood flow in the heart. Called also *mixed levocardia.* **t. of great vessels,** a congenital cardiovascular malformation in which the aorta arises entirely from the right ventricle and the pulmonary artery from the left ventricle, so that the venous return from the peripheral circulation is recirculated by the right ventricle via the aorta to the systemic circulation without being oxygenated in the lungs. Life then depends on a crossflow of blood between blood in the right heart and that in the left heart, as through a ventricular septal defect or a patent duct arteriosus. Cyanosis is the chief symptom. **partial t. of great vessels,** Taussig-Bing syndrome.

transposon (tranz-po′zon) a discrete DNA sequence that transposes blocks of genetic material back and forth within a bacterial cell from the chromosome to plasmids or bacteriophage particles, by which the material may be transferred to another cell. Transposons frequently carry genes for resistance to antibiotics.

transpubic (trans-pu′bik) performed through the pubic bone after removal of a segment of the bone.

transsacral (trans-sa′kral) through or across the sacrum.

transsection (trans-sek′shun) transection.

transsegmental (trans″seg-men′tal) extending across a segment.

transseptal (trans-sep′tal) through or across a septum.

transsexual (trans-seks′u-al) 1. a person affected by transsexualism. 2. a person whose external anatomy has been changed to that of the opposite sex.

transsexualism (trans-seks′u-ah-lizm) a disturbance of gender identity in which the affected person has overwhelming desire to change anatomic sex stemming from the fixed conviction that he or she is a member of the opposite sex; such persons often seek hormonal and surgical treatment to bring their anatomy into conformity with their belief. Cf. *transvestism.*

transsphenoidal (trans″sfe-noi′dal) performed through the sphenoid bone.

transsternal (trans-ster′nal) through the sternum.

transsuccinylase (trans-suk-sĭ′nĭ-lās) dihydrolipoamide succinyltransferase.

transtemporal (trans-tem′por-al) crossing the temporal lobe.

transthalamic (trans″thah-lam′ik) crossing the thalamus.

transthermia (trans-ther′me-ah) [*trans-* + Gr. *therme* heat] thermopenetration.

transthoracic (trans″tho-ras′ik) performed through the wall of the thorax, or through the thoracic cavity.

transtracheal (trans-tra′ke-al) performed by passage through the wall of the trachea.

transtympanic (trans″tim-pan′ik) across the tympanic membrane or the cavity of the middle ear.

transudate (trans′u-dāt) [*trans-* + L. *sudare* to sweat] a fluid substance which has passed through a membrane or been extruded from a tissue, sometimes as a result of inflammation. A transudate, in contrast to an exudate, is characterized by high fluidity and a low content of protein, cells, or of solid materials derived from cells.

transudation (trans″u-da′shun) 1. the passage of serum or other body fluid through a membrane or tissue surface, which may or may not be the result of inflammation. 2. transudate.

transuranium (trans″u-ra′ne-um) beyond uranium; see *transuranic elements,* under *element.*

transureteroureterostomy (trans″u-re″ter-o-u-re″ter-os′to-me) anastomosis of the proximal portion of one ureter to the ureter of the opposite side.

transurethral (trans″u-re′thral) performed through the urethra.

transvaginal (trans-vaj′ĭ-nal) performed through the vagina.

transvaterian (trans″vah-te′re-an) through the papilla of Vater.

transvector (trans-vek′tor) an organism that conveys or transmits a poison which is not generated in its own body but is obtained from another source, such as the mussel, *Mytilus,* which serves as a transvector of paralytic shellfish poison derived from the dinoflagellate *Gonyaulax.*

transventricular (trans″ven-trik′u-lar) performed through the ventricle.

transversalis (trans″ver-sa′lis) [*trans-* + L. *vertere, versum* to turn] transverse; [NA] a term designating a structure situated at a right angle to the long axis of the body or of an organ.

transverse (trans-vers′) [L. *transversus*] placed crosswise; situated at right angles to the long axis of a part.

transversectomy (trans″ver-sek′to-me) [*transverse* + Gr. *ektome* excision] surgical removal of the transverse process of a vertebra.

transversion (trans-ver′zhun) [L. *transvertere* to turn away] 1. displacement of a tooth from its proper numerical position in the jaw. 2. in molecular genetics, a point mutation in which a purine base replaces a pyrimidine base or vice versa. Cf. *transition.*

transversocostal (trans-ver″so-kos′tal) costotransverse.

transversotomy (trans″ver-sot′o-me) [*transverse* + Gr. *tomē* a cutting] the operation of cutting the transverse process of a vertebra.

transversourethralis (trans-ver″so-u″re-thra′lis) the transverse fibers of the sphincter urethrae muscle.

transversus (trans-ver′sus) transverse; [NA] a general term designating a position at right angles to a long axis.

transvesical (trans-ves′ĭ-kal) through the bladder.

transvestism (trans-ves′tizm) [*trans-* + L. *vestitus* clothed] cross-dressing; the practice of wearing articles of clothing of the opposite sex. Called *transvestic fetishism* in DSM III-R.

transvestite (trans-ves′tīt) an individual exhibiting transvestism.

transvestitism (trans-ves′tĭ-tizm) transvestism.

Trantas' dots (tran′tas) [Alexios *Trantas*, Greek ophthalmologist, born 1867] see under *dot*.

Tranxene (tran′zēn) trademark for a preparation of clorazepate dipotassium.

tranylcypromine sulfate (tran″il-si′pro-mēn) [USP] chemical name: (+)-*trans*-2-phenylcyclopropylamine sulfate. A monoamine oxidase inhibitor, $(C_9H_{11}N)_2 \cdot H_2SO_4$, occurring as a white crystalline powder; used as an antidepressant, administered orally.

trapezial (trah-pe′ze-al) pertaining to a trapezium.

trapeziform (trah-pez′ĭ-form) trapezoid.

trapeziometacarpal (trah-pe″ze-o-met″ah-kar′pal) pertaining to or connecting the trapezium and the metacarpus.

trapezium (trah-pe′ze-um) [L.; Gr. *trapezion*] an irregular four-sided figure; see *os trapezium*.

trapezoid (trap′e-zoid) [L. *trapezoides*; Gr. *trapezoeidēs* table shaped] 1. having the shape of a four-sided plane, with two sides parallel and two diverging. 2. the os trapezoideum.

Trapp's formula (coefficient) (traps) [Julius *Trapp*, Russian pharmacist, 1814–1908] see under *formula*.

Trasentine (tras′en-tin) trademark for preparations of adiphenine hydrochloride.

Trasylol (tras′ĭ-lol) trademark for a preparation of aprotinin.

Traube's curves, etc. (trow′bez) [Ludwig *Traube*, German physician, 1818–1876] see under *curve, dyspnea, heart, membrane,* and *space,* and see *gallop rhythm,* under *rhythm*.

Traube-Hering curves, waves (trow′be-her′ing) [Ludwig *Traube*; Ewald *Hering,* physiologist in Leipzig, 1834–1918] see Traube's *curve,* under *curve,* and see under *wave*.

trauma (traw′mah), pl. *traumas* or *trau′mata* [L.; Gr.] a wound or injury, whether physical or psychic. **birth t.,** an injury to the infant received in or due to the process of being born. In some psychiatric theories, the psychic shock produced in an infant by the experience of being born. **occlusal t.,** injury to any part of the masticatory system as a result of occlusal dysfunction. See also *traumatic occlusion,* under *occlusion.* **potential t.,** in dentistry, an alteration in tissue that may occur at any time as a result of an existing dental disharmony. **psychic t.,** an emotional shock that produces an emotional or mental disorder.

traumasthenia (traw″mas-the′ne-ah) [*trauma* + *a* neg. + Gr. *sthenos* strength + *-ia*] traumatic neurasthenia.

traumata (traw′mah-tah) [Gr.] plural of *trauma*.

traumatherapy (traw″mah-ther′ah-pe) [*trauma* + Gr. *therapeia* treatment] treatment of wounds and injuries.

traumatic (traw-mat′ik) [Gr. *traumatikos*] pertaining to, occurring as the result of, or causing trauma.

traumatic acid (traw-mat′ik) *trans*-2-dodecenoic acid, a plant wound hormone that stimulates the production of wound periderm.

traumatin (traw′mah-tin) a substance which stimulates the growth of plant tissues; it may be identical with wound hormone.

traumatism (traw′mah-tizm) [Gr. *traumatismos*] 1. the physical or psychic state resulting from an injury or wound. 2. a wound.

traumat(o)- [Gr. *trauma,* gen. *traumatos* wound] a combining form denoting relationship to trauma, or to a wound or injury.

traumatogenic (traw″mah-to-jen′ik) [*traumato-* + Gr. *gen-*

nan to produce] 1. caused by or due to a wound or wounds. 2. capable of causing trauma.

traumatologist (traw″mah-tol′o-jist) a surgeon experienced in treating accidental injuries.

traumatology (traw″mah-tol′o-je) [*traumato-* + *-logy*] the branch of surgery which deals with wounds and disability from injuries.

traumatopathy (traw″mah-top′ah-the) [*traumato-* + Gr. *pathos* disease] any pathological condition due to wound or injury.

traumatophilia (traw″mah-to-fil′e-ah) [*traumato-* + *-philia*] a condition in which a person finds unconscious gratification in being injured or undergoing surgical operations.

traumatopnea (traw″mah-top-ne′ah) [*traumato-* + Gr. *pnoia* breath] a condition of partial asphyxia with collapse caused by traumatic opening of the pleural space (open pneumothorax).

traumatosis (traw″mah-to′sis) traumatism.

traumatotherapy (traw″mah-to-ther′ah-pe) traumatherapy.

traumatropism (traw-mat′ro-pizm) [*trauma* + Gr. *tropos* a turning] the growth or movement of organisms in relation to injury.

travail (trav′āl) childbirth; see *labor*.

Travasol (trav′ah-sol) trademark for a crystalline amino acid solution for intravenous administration, containing a mixture of essential and nonessential amino acids but no peptides.

tray (tra) a flat-surfaced utensil for the conveyance of various objects or material. **acrylic resin t.,** an impression tray made of acrylic resin. **impression t.,** a horseshoe-shaped receptacle made of metal or other suitable material used to carry the impression material to the mouth, to confine the material in apposition to the surfaces to be recorded, and to control the impression material while it sets to form the impression.

trazodone hydrochloride (tra′zo-dōn) chemical name: 2-[3-[4-(3-chlorophenyl)-1-piperazinyl] propyl]-1,2,4-triazolo-[4,3-*a*]pyridin-3-(2*H*)-one monohydrochloride; an antidepressant, tranquilizer, and hypotensive, $C_{19}H_{22}ClN_5O \cdot HCl$.

TRBF total renal blood flow; see under *flow*.

treacle (tre′k′l) [Gr. *thēriaka*] a syrupy substance or mixture; molasses.

tread (tred) injury of the coronet of a horse's hoof, due to striking with the shoe of the opposite side.

treatment (trēt′ment) the management and care of a patient for the purpose of combating disease or disorder. See also under *maneuver, method, technique, tests,* and *therapy*. **active t.,** that which is directed immediately to the cure of a disease or injury. **Albertini's t.,** complete rest and abstinence from food in aneurysm of the aorta. **Allen's t.,** treatment by certain days of fasting, followed by a restricted diet and attended by a careful determination of the quantity of food which the patient can consume without producing glycosuria and glycemia. Called also *starvation t.* **Balfour's t.,** treatment of aneurysm by potassium iodide. **Beard's t.,** treatment of cancer by trypsin. **Bell t.,** treatment of cancer by injections of a preparation of colloidal lead. **Bergonié's t.,** the application of general faradization for the reduction of corpulence. **Bird's t.,** treatment of decubitus ulcer by mild galvanic currents. **Bouchardat's t.,** treatment of diabetes by use of a diet that excludes substances rich in carbohydrates. **Brehmer's t.,** treatment of pulmonary tuberculosis by the use of dietetic and physical measures. **Brown-Séquard t.,** organotherapy. **carbon dioxide t.,** see under *therapy.* **Carrel's t., Carrel-Dakin t.,** treatment of wounds, based on thorough exposure of the wound, removal of all foreign material and devitalized tissue, meticulous cleansing, and repeated irrigation with a dilute sodium hypochlorite solution. The adjacent skin is protected with petrolatum gauze. **causal t.,** treatment that is directed against the cause of a disease. **choline t.,** treatment of cancer by the intravenous injection of borate of choline in connection with the use of radioactive substances. **Coffey-Humber t.,** treatment of cancer by injection of an extract of adrenal cortex of sheep. **conservative t.,** treatment designed to avoid radical medical therapeutic measures or operative procedures; often reserved for elderly or debilitated patients. **curative t.,** active treatment designed to cure an existing disease, as opposed to *palliative t.* **Dancel's t.,** treatment of obesity by a diet containing as little water as possible. **Debove's t.,** treatment of tuberculosis by a special form of forced feeding. **dietetic t.,** treatment of disease by regulation of the diet. **drug t.,** treatment with drugs, as distinguished from treatment with physical means, such as diet, exercise, electricity, etc. **Ehrlich-Hata t.,** see *arsphenamine.* **electroconvulsive t., electroshock t.,** see under *therapy.* **empiric t.,** treatment by means which experience has proved to be beneficial. **eventration t.,** application of ionizing irradiation to internal anatomical tissues through an open laparotomy wound. **expectant t.,** treatment designed only to relieve untoward symptoms, leaving the cure mainly to nature. **fever t.,** pyretotherapy. **Fichera's t.,** treatment of cancer by hypodermic injection of autolyzed human fetal tissue. **Fitz Gerald t.,** zone therapy. **Fliess' t.,** anesthetization of the nasal conchae for the relief of pain in dysmenorrhea and in nervous stomach pains. **foam t.,** treatment with the foam produced by blowing a current of air through water containing saponin solution. **Fränkel's t.,** the use of strophanthin in cardiac failure. **Frenkel's t.,** see under *movement.* **Girard's t.,** treatment of seasickness by hypodermic or oral administration of atropine sulfate and strychnine sulfate. **Goeckerman t.,** treatment of psoriasis by applying ointments of tar followed by irradiation with ultraviolet light. **Guinard's t.,** application of calcium carbide to ulcerating tumors. **Hartel's t.,** alcoholic injection for trigeminal neuralgia in which the needle is passed through the mouth into the region of the foramen ovale of the sphenoid bone. **high-frequency t.,** diathermy. **hygienic t.,** that directed to the restoration or maintenance of hygienic conditions. **insulin coma t., insulin shock t.,** see under *therapy.* **Jacquet's biokinetic t.,** active gymnastics of the hand and fingers. **Jarotzky's (Jarotsky's) t.,** treatment of gastric ulcer by a diet of whites of eggs, fresh butter with bread, and milk or noodles. **Kenny t.,** a treatment formerly used for poliomyelitis consisting of wrapping of the back and limbs in hot cloths, followed, after pain has subsided, by passive exercise and instruction of the patient in exercise of the muscles. **Killgren t.,** a system of medical gymnastics combined with passive exercise, friction, and vibrations, and laying special emphasis on the mechanical treatment of the nerves. **Kittel's t.,** massage and manipulation for the dispersion of the uratic deposits in gouty joints. **Klapp's creeping t.,** treatment of scoliosis by having the patient creep about on the floor, with exaggerated movements of the spine. **Koga t.,** treatment of thromboangiitis obliterans by diluting the blood by hypodermoclysis with normal salt solution. **Korányi's t.,** former method of treating leukemia by the use of benzol (benzene). **La Porte t.,** treatment of chronic osteomyelitis by application over the infected areas of aluminum potassium nitrate in an oatmeal poultice. **Larat's t.,** treatment of diphtheritic paralysis of the palate by faradism. **Lerich's t.** (*of strains*), infiltration of the periarticular tissues with a 0.5–2 per cent solution of procaine. **light t.,** phototherapy. **McPheeters' t.,** treatment of varicose ulcer by bandaging a rubber sponge over the ulcerated area and directing the patient to walk as much as possible; called *venous heart treatment.* **Matas' t.,** treatment of neuralgia by the injection of alcohol under the nerve ganglions at the base of the skull. **medicinal t.,** that in which the treatment is mainly accomplished by the use of remedies. **Minot-Murphy t.,** the treatment of pernicious anemia by the addition to the diet of raw liver or liver extract. **Mitchell t.,** see *Weir Mitchell t.* **Nauheim t.,** Schott's t. **Neuendorf t.,** treatment of rheumatoid arthritis by the mud baths of Neuendorf, Germany. **Noorden t.,** oatmeal t. **Nordach t.,** treatment of pulmonary tuberculosis by fresh air, rest, and an abundance of nourishing food. **oatmeal t.,** treatment of diabetes by restricting the protein of the diet and limiting the carbohydrates to oatmeal. **Ochsner t.,** treatment of appendicitis by securing peristaltic rest so that peritoneal adhesions may form; this is achieved by abstention from food by mouth, gastric suction, and an inlying rectal tube to facilitate the escape of gas. **Oertel's t.,** treatment of heart disease, circulatory diseases, obesity, etc., by regulation of diet, diminution of fluid elements in the food, mountain climbing and other systematic exercises, and by massage and Swedish movements. **Orr t.,** treatment of compound fractures and osteomyelitis by débridement of the wound, alignment of fracture, drainage with petrolatum gauze, and immobilization of limb in a plaster cast which is left on until the wound discharge has softened the plaster. **palliative t.,** treatment which is designed to relieve pain and distress, but which does not attempt a cure. **Paul's t.,** the therapeutic use of lymph for cutaneous therapy of chronic rheumatism. **Petrén's t.,** see under *diet.* **Playfair's t.,** treatment by rest and feeding. **Potter t.,** treatment of intestinal fistulas by administration of tenth normal solution of hydrochloric acid to neutralize the alkalinity of the pancreatic juice, thus preventing tryptic activity. **preventive t., prophylactic t.,** that in which the aim is to prevent the occurrence of the disease; prophylaxis. **rational t.,** treatment based upon a knowledge of disease and the action of the remedies employed. **Retan's t.,** treatment of intussusception by distending the colon with a barium mixture, followed by manipulations. **Rollier t.,** treatment of surgical tuberculosis by systematic exposure of the part to the rays of the sun. **salicyl t.,** treatment of rheumatism with salicylic acid or its derivatives. **sand t.,** treatment with sand baths. **Schlösser's t.,** treatment of trigeminal neuralgia by injections of alcohol into the foramen from which the nerve emerges. **Schott's t.,** treatment of heart disease by use of warm saline baths of Nauheim and systematically conducted exercise. **Schroth's t.** (*obs.*), treatment of obesity by the exclusion of water in any form as far as possible. **sewage t.,** the processing of sewage to remove or so alter some of its constituents as to render it less offensive or dangerous and more fit to discharge into a public water course. **shock t.,** see under *therapy.* **Sippy t.,** a regimen of treatment of peptic ulcer based on neutralization of hydrochloric acid by frequent feedings and the use of alkalies in carefully regulated but adequate quantities. See under *diet.* **slush t.,** the treatment of acne by the application of a mixture of carbon dioxide snow, acetone, and sulfur. **solar t.,** heliotherapy. **specific t.,** treatment that is particularly adapted to the special disease being treated. **starvation t.,** Allen t. **Stoker's t.,** treatment in bronchiectasis by continuous inhalation of oxygen. **subcoma insulin t.,** see under *therapy.* **supporting t.,** that which is mainly directed to sustaining the strength of the patient. **surgical t.,** that in which surgical methods are those chiefly employed. **symptomatic t.,** expectant t. **Tallerman t.,** the localized application of superheated dry air in rheumatism, gout, sprains, neuritis, eczema, etc. See also under *apparatus.* **teleradium t.,** treatment by a radium source located at a distance from the body. **terrain t.,** treatment of weak heart, neurasthenia, corpulence, etc., by regular exercise, mountain climbing, regulation of diet, etc. **thymus t.,** treatment of progressive muscular atrophy by extracts from the thymus gland. **tonic t.,** 1. treatment with tonics. 2. treatment of syphilis with small doses of mercury continued for a long period. **Trueta t.,** immediate treatment of fractures as follows: (1) adopt surgical treatment as soon as possible; (2) thoroughly wash wound and entire limb with water, soap, and a nail brush, shave hair, paint surrounding skin with weak alcoholic solution of iodine, avoiding the wound; (3) débride wound; (4) open neighboring cellular spaces and remove hematomas; (5) remove completely denuded or displaced bone fragments and all foreign matter; (6) reduce fracture; (7) dress wound with sterile gauze and immobilize with plaster, including two adjacent joints if possible; (8) give injection of tetanus antitoxin. **Tuffnell's t.,** treatment of aneurysm by absolute rest and starvation diet. **underwater t.,** treatment of poliomyelitis patients by permitting active movements in the water of a bath or pool. **venous heart t.,** McPheeters' t. **Wagner-Jauregg t.,** treatment of dementia paralytica by infection of the patient with malaria. **Weir Mitchell t.,** a formerly used method of treating neurasthenia, hysteria, etc., by absolute rest in bed, frequent and abundant feeding, and the systematic use of massage and electricity; called also *rest cure.* **Yeo's t.,** treatment of obesity by giving large amounts of hot drinks and withholding carbohydrates.

trebenzomine hydochloride (trĕ-ben′zo-mēn) chemical name: (*cis* or *trans*)-(+)-3,4-dihydro-*N,N*, 2- trimethyl- 2*H*-1-benzopyran -3- amine hydrochloride; an antidepressant, $C_{12}H_{17}NO \cdot HCl$.

tree (tre) 1. a perennial of the plant kingdom characterized by having a main stem or trunk and numerous branches. 2. an anatomical structure with branches resembling a tree.

bronchial t., arbor bronchialis. **tracheobronchial t.,** the trachea, bronchi, and their branching structures.

trehala (tre-ha′lah) a mannitol-like substance deposited by an insect (*Larinus maculatus*) upon an Asiatic plant of the genus *Echinops*.

trehalose (tre-ha′lōs) a disaccharide, $C_{12}H_{22}O_{11}$, from the cocoons of certain beetles (*Trehala manna*) and yeast; it is not digestible, but yields glucose when hydrolyzed with acids.

Treitz's arch, fossa, hernia, muscle (ligament) (trīts) [Wenzel *Treitz*, Austrian physician, 1819–1872] see under *arch* and *hernia*, see *musculus suspensorius duodeni*, and see *recessus duodenalis superior*.

treloxinate (trĕ-loks′ĭ-nāt) chemical name: 2,10-dichloromethyl ester 12*H*-dibenzo[*d,g*] [1,3]dioxocin-6-carboxylic acid; an anticholesteremic, $C_{16}H_{12}Cl_2O_4$.

Trematoda (trem″ah-to′dah) [Gr. *trēmatōdēs* pierced] a class of the Platyhelminthes which includes the flukes. The trematodes or flukes are parasitic in man and animals, infection generally resulting from the ingestion of uncooked or insufficiently cooked fish, crustaceans, and vegetation. All flukes require a mollusk as their first intermediate host, in which a complex developmental cycle takes place. The larval stage, which escapes from the mollusk, may then enter a second intermediate host (fish, crustacean, or another mollusk), encyst on vegetation, or penetrate directly into the skin of the definitive host. The important trematodes of man belong to the genera (1) BLOOD: *Schistosoma.* (2) INTESTINE: *Echinostoma, Fasciolopsis, Gastrodiscoides, Heterophyes, Metagonimus.* (3) LIVER: *Clonorchis, Fasciola, Dicrocoelium, Opisthorchis.* (4) LUNG: *Paragonimus.*

trematode (trem′ah-tōd) any parasitic animal organism belonging to the class Trematoda.

trematodiasis (trem″ah-to-di′ah-sis) infection with trematodes.

trembles (trem′b'lz) poisoning in cattle and sheep that feed on the white snakeroot (*Eupatorium rugosum*) and the rayless goldenrod (*Haplopappus heterophyllus*), in which the animal has muscular tremors and becomes weak and may suddenly stumble and fall. Persons made ill by milk, milk products, or flesh from an animal so affected are said to have milk sickness (q.v.), which may be fatal.

tremelloid, tremellose (trem′ĕ-loid; trem′ĕ-lōs) like jelly.

tremetol (trem′ĕ-tol) chemical name: 2-isopropenyl-2,3-dihydro-5-acetylbenzofuran. A toxin, $C_{13}H_{14}O_2$, in the white snakeroot, *Eupatorium rugosum* (*E. urticaefolium*, and the rayless goldenrod, *Haplopappus heterophyllus*, which causes trembles in cattle and sheep and milk sickness in man. Called also *tremetone*.

tremetone (trem′ĕ-tōn) tremetol.

Tremin (trem′in) trademark for a preparation of trihexyphenidyl hydrochloride.

tremogram (tre′mo-gram) [*tremor* + Gr. *gramma* mark] the tracing or record made by a tremograph; a graphic tracing of a tremor. See *ataxiameter*.

tremograph (tre′mo-graf) [*tremor* + Gr. *graphein* to write] an instrument for recording tremors.

tremolabile (tre″mo-la′bil) [*tremor* + L. *labilis* unstable] susceptible to shaking; easily inactivated by shaking; said of a ferment.

tremor (trem′or, tre′mor) [L., from *tremere* to shake] an involuntary trembling or quivering. **action t.,** rhythmic, oscillatory, involuntary movements of the outstretched upper limb, as when writing or lifting a cup; it may also affect the voice and other parts. **arsenic t.,** a tremor resulting from arsenic poisoning. **coarse t.,** a tremor in which the vibrations are slow. **continuous t.,** a persistent tremor resembling that of paralysis agitans. **t. cor′dis,** palpitation of the heart. **darkness t.,** involuntary movements of the eyes, resembling nystagmus, which occur in young animals kept in the dark. **epidemic t.,** avian encephalomyelitis. **epileptoid t.,** intermitting clonic spasm with tremor. **essential t.,** a familial tremor with onset at varying ages, usually at about 50 years of age, beginning with a fine rapid tremor (as distinct from that of parkinsonism) of the hands, followed by tremor of the arms, tongue, heads, legs, and trunk; it is aggravated by emotional factors, is accentuated by volitional movement, and is temporarily improved by alcohol. Called also *familial t., heredofamilial t.,* and *hereditary essential t.* **familial t.,** essential t. **fib-**

rillary t., a fine rhythmical trembling due to alternate contraction of the different fibrils of a muscle; fibrillation. **fine t.,** a tremor in which the vibrations are rapid. **flapping t.,** asterixis. **forced t.,** a movement persisting after voluntary motion, due to intermittent stimulation of the nerve centers. **hereditary essential t.,** essential t. **heredofamilial t.,** essential t. **Hunt's t.,** the tremor attending every voluntary movement which is characteristic of cerebellar lesions. **intention t.,** a tremor which arises or which is intensified when a voluntary, coordinated movement is attempted. **intermittent t.,** tremor seen in hemiplegia or when attempts at voluntary movement are made. **kinetic t.,** a tremor occurring in a limb during active movement. **t. lin′guae,** trembling of the tongue, as seen in alcoholism, typhoid fever, and paretic dementia. **t. mercuria′lis,** tremor due to mercurial poisoning. **metallic t.,** a tremor seen in various metallic poisonings. **motofacient t.,** a tremor in muscles which participate in an action. **t. opiophago′rum,** the tremor of opium users. **passive t.,** a tremor occurring only when the patient is at rest. **persistent t.,** a tremor occurring whether the patient is at rest or in motion. **t. potato′rum** ["trembling of drinkers"], delirium tremens. **purring t.,** a thrill, like the purring of a cat, felt by the hand placed over the heart. **rest t.,** tremor occurring in a relaxed and supported limb, as in parkinsonism. **senile t.,** a tremor resulting from the infirmities of age. **static t.,** a tremor occurring on effort to hold one of the limbs in a definite position. **striocerebellar t.,** a combined form of tremor with both striatal and cerebellar components, usually due to diffuse degeneration of the central nervous system. **t. ten′dinum** ["trembling of the tendons"], subsultus tendinum. **toxic t.,** a tremor seen in states of chronic poisoning. **trombone t. of tongue,** Magnan's movement. **volitional t.,** a trembling of the entire body during voluntary effort; seen in multiple sclerosis.

tremorgram (trem′or-gram) tremogram.

tremulor (trem′u-lor) a machine for the administration of vibratory treatment.

tremulous (trem′u-lus) [L. *tremulus*] shaking, trembling, or quivering.

trend (trend) inclination in a particular direction or course.

Trendelenburg operation, etc. (tren-del′en-berg) [Friedrich *Trendelenburg*, surgeon in Leipzig, 1844–1924] see under *operation, position, symptom,* and *tests.*

trendscriber (trend′skrīb-er) the apparatus used in trendscription.

trendscription (trend′skrip″shun) a programmed method of continuous electrocardiographic monitoring, wherein the tracing is condensed on a rotating drum recorder and the program permits selective sampling of rhythm data.

trepan (trĕ-pan′) [Gr. *trypanon* auger] 1. an obsolete form of the trephine, resembling a carpenter's bit and brace. 2. to trephine.

trepanation (trep″ah-na′shun) [L. *trepanatio*] an operation with the trepan; trephination.

trepanner (tre-pan′er) one who performs a trepanation; trephiner.

trephination (tref″ĭ-na′shun) the operation of trephining. **corneoscleral t.,** Elliot's operation. **dental t.,** surgical creation of a fistula by puncturing the soft tissue and cortical bone overlying the root apex to provide drainage. Called also *apicostomy.*

trephine (trĕ-fīn′, trĕ-fēn′) [L. *trephina*] 1. a saw for removing a circular disk of bone, chiefly from the skull. 2. an instrument for removing a circular area of cornea, as in corneal transplant operations. 3. to operate upon with the trephine.

trephinement (tre-fīn′ment) the act or process of trephining.

trephiner (tre-fīn′er) one who performs the operation of trephining.

trephocyte (tref′o-sīt) [Gr. *trephein* to feed + *kytos* cell] a cell that furnishes nutrition to other cells, as a Sertoli cell.

trepidant (trep′ĭ-dant) [L. *trepidans* trembling] characterized by tremor.

trepidatio (trep″ĭ-da′she-o) [L.] trepidation. **t. cor′dis,** palpitation of the heart.

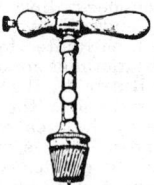

Trephine.

trepidation (trep″ĭ-da′shun) [L. *trepidatio*] 1. a trembling or oscillatory movement. 2. nervous anxiety and fear.

trepo- [Gr. *trepein* to turn] a combining form denoting a relationship to a turning movement.

Trepomonas (trep″o-mo′nas) [*trepo-* + Gr. *monas* unit, from *monos* single] a genus of flagellate protozoa (suborder Diplomonadina, order Diplomonadida) free-living in fresh water, coprophilic, or parasitic in amphibians, fish, and turtles, and characterized by the presence of one long and three short flagella on each side of the body.

Treponema (trep″o-ne′mah) [*trepo-* + Gr. *nēma* thread] a genus of bacteria of the family Spirochaetaceae, order Spirochaetales, consisting of gram-negative, microaerophilic, spiral microorganisms that exhibit motility with a flexing, bending, snapping motion and divide by transverse fission. The outer surfaces have polar flagella (axial filaments) that wind around the organism. They are found in the oral, intestinal, and genital mucosa. Pathogenic species, causing syphilis, yaws, and pinta, have not been cultured in vitro. **T. bucca′le,** a species of uncertain status isolated from the human oral cavity. Called also *Borrelia buccalis*. **T. calligy′rum,** *T. refringens*. **T. cara′teum,** the causative agent of pinta (carate). Called also *T. herrejoni*. **T. cunic′uli,** *T. paraluiscuniculi*. **T. denti′cola,** a nonpathogenic species found in the oral cavity of humans and chimpanzees, usually in calculus occurring at the gingival margin. **T. genita′lis,** *T. refringens*. **T. herrejo′ni,** *T. carateum*. **T. hyodysente′riae,** a species causing diarrheal disease in swine. **T. macroden′tium,** a nonpathogenic species found in the gingival crevices of humans. **T. microden′tium,** *T. denticola*. **T. muco′sum,** a species of uncertain status found in the oral cavity of a human with periodontitis. **T. pal′lidum,** the causative agent of venereal, nonvenereal, and cogenital syphilis in humans. **T. pal′lidum** subsp. **perten′ue,** the causative agent of yaws in humans. **T. paraluiscuni′culi,** a species causing syphilis in guinea pigs and rabbits; not pathogenic for humans. Called also *T. cuniculi*. **T. perten′ue,** *T. pallidum* subsp. *pertenue*. **T. phagede′nis,** a nonpathogenic species found in the genital regions of humans and chimpanzees. Called also *T. reiteri*. **T. refrin′gens,** a nonpathogenic species that is part of the normal flora of male and female genitalia. Called also *T. calligyrum* and *T. genitalis*. **T. reite′ri,** *T. phagedenis*. **T. vincen′tii,** a species isolated from the human oral cavity, especially in acute necrotizing gingivitis in association with *Fusobacterium nucleatum*. Called also *Borrelia vincentii* and *spirillum of Vincent*.

treponema (trep″o-ne′mah) an organism of the genus *Treponema*.

treponemal (trep″o-ne′mal) of, pertaining to, or caused by treponemas.

Treponemataceae (trep″o-ne″mah-ta′se-e) in former systems of classification, a family of spirochetes, including the genera *Borrelia*, *Leptospira*, and *Treponema*, which are now classified in the family Spirochaetaceae.

treponematosis (trep″o-ne-mah-to′sis) an infection with treponema.

treponeme (trep′o-nēm) an organism of the genus *Treponema*.

treponemiasis (trep″o-ne-mi′ah-sis) infection with treponema; syphilis.

treponemicidal (trep″o-ne″mĭ-si′dal) destructive to organisms of the genus *Treponema*.

trepopnea (tre″pop-ne′ah) [Gr. *trepein* to turn + *pnoia* breath] a condition in which breathing is most comfortable with the patient turned in a definite recumbent position.

treppe (trep′ĕ) [Ger. "staircase"] the phenomenon of grad-

ual increase in the extent of muscular contraction following rapidly repeated stimulation (H. P. Bowditch, 1871). Also called *staircase phenomenon*.

Tresilian's sign (tre-sil′e-anz) [Frederick James *Tresilian*, English physician, 1862–1926] see under *sign*.

tresis (tre′sis) [Gr. *trēsis*] perforation.

Trest (trest) trademark for a preparation of methixene hydrochloride.

trestolone acetate (tres′to-lōn) chemical name: 17β-hydroxy-7α-methylestr-4-en-3-one acetate; an antineoplastic and androgenic steroid, $C_{21}H_{30}O_3$.

tretinoin (tret″ĭ-noin) [USP] all-*trans*-retinoic acid, $C_{20}H_{28}O_2$, used topically for treatment of cases of acne vulgaris in which comedones, pustules, and papules predominate; it prevents comedone formation and suppresses keratin synthesis; common adverse effects are erythema and desquamation. Called also *retinoic acid* and *vitamin A acid*.

Treves fold (trēvs) [Sir Frederick *Treves*, English surgeon, 1853–1923] see *plica ileocecalis*.

TRF thyrotropin releasing factor; see under *hormone*.

TRH thyrotropin releasing hormone.

tri- [Gr. *treis*; L. *tres* three] a prefix meaning *three* or *thrice*.

triacetate (tri-as′ĕ-tāt) an acetate which contains three molecules of the acetic acid radical.

triacetin (tri-as′ĕ-tin) [USP] chemical name: 1,2,3-propanetriol. An antifungal agent, $C_9H_4O_6$, occurring as a colorless or pale straw-colored liquid; used topically in the treatment of superficial fungal infections of the skin. Called also *glyceryl triacetate*.

triacetyloleandomycin (tri-as″ĕ-til-o″le-an″do-mi′sin) troleandomycin.

triacid (tri-as′id) a base capable of neutralizing three equivalents of monobasic acid.

Triactinomyxon (tri″ak-tĭ″no-mik′son) [*tri-* + *actino-* + Gr. *myxa* mucus] a genus of parasitic protozoa (order Actinomyxida, subclass Actinomyxia) found in oligochetes.

triacylglycerol (tri-as″il-glis′er-ol) a term proposed to replace triglyceride.

triacylglycerol lipase (tri-ā″sil-glis′er-ol li′pās) [EC 3.1.1.3] an enzyme of the hydrolase class that catalyzes the reaction triacylglycerol + H_2O = diacyl glycerol + a fatty acid anion. It is produced by glands on the tongue and by the pancreas and initiates the digestion of dietary fats. Called also *lipase*.

triad (tri′ad) [L. *trias*; Gr. *trias* group of three] 1. any trivalent element. 2. a group of three entities or objects, as an association of three symptoms. **acute compression t.,** Beck's t. **adrenomedullary t.,** the symptoms produced by activation of the adrenal medulla: tachycardia, vasoconstriction, and sweating. **Andersen's t.,** see under *syndrome*. **Beck's t.,** three symptoms characteristic of cardiac compression: (1) a high venous pressure, (2) a low arterial pressure, and (3) a small quiet heart. **Bezold's t.,** prolonged bone conduction and lessened perception of low tones, indicating otosclerosis. **Charcot's t.,** 1. nystagmus, intention tremor, and staccato speech, often seen in multiple sclerosis. 2. the symptom complex of biliary colic, jaundice, and fever and chills characteristic of intermittent cholangitis. **Dieulafoy's t.,** hypersensitiveness of the skin, reflex muscular contraction, and tenderness at McBurney's point in appendicitis. **Grancher's t.,** lessened vesicular quality of breathing, skodaic resonance, and increased vocal fremitus; seen in early pulmonary tuberculosis. **hepatic t's,** the grouping of the tributaries of the hepatic artery, vein, and bile duct at the angles of the lobules of the liver. **Hutchinson's t.,** diffuse interstitial keratitis, labyrinthine disease, and Hutchinson teeth, seen in inherited syphilis. **Kartagener's t.,** see under *syndrome*. **t. of Luciani,** asthenia, atonia, and astasia, the three major symptoms of cerebellar disease. **Osler's t.,** telangiectasis, capillary fragility, and hereditary hemorrhagic diathesis. **portal t's,** hepatic t's. **t. of retinal cone,** the tip of two horizontal cell dendrites and one midget cell dendrite, enclosed in a synaptic invagination of a retinal cone pedicle. **Saint's t.,** hiatus hernia, colonic diverticula, and cholelithiasis, occurring concomitantly. **t. of Schultz,** jaundice, gangrenous stomatitis, and leukopenia. **t. of skeletal muscle,** a pair of terminal cisterns in close apposition to the T tubule, running transversely across a myofibril of skeletal muscle; in mammalian muscle there are two triads to each sarcomere, situated at the A band–I band junction. See also *T system*, under *system* and *T tubule*, under *tubule*. **Whipple's t.,** the essential clinical features of insulin-producing tumors: (1) spontaneous hypoglycemia (blood sugar levels below 50 mg. per 100 ml.), (2) accompanied by central nervous or vasomotor system symptoms, and (3) relief of symptoms by the oral or intravenous administration of glucose.

triaditis (tri″ad-i′tis) inflammation of three elements taken as a unit. **portal t.,** inflammation of the connective tissue around the hepatic artery, portal vein, and bile duct of the portal tract.

triafungin (tri″ah-fun′jin) chemical name: 3-(phenylmethyl)pyrido[3,4-*e*]-1,2,4-triazine; an antifungal, $C_{13}H_{10}N_4$.

triage (tre-ahzh′) [Fr. "sorting"] the sorting out and classification of casualties of war or other disaster, to determine priority of need and proper place of treatment.

trial (tri′al, tril) a test or experiment. **Bernoulli t's,** in statistics, a series of independent trials, each having only two mutually exclusive outcomes, commonly called "success" and "failure," in which the probability of success remains the same throughout the trials. Cf. *Bernoulli distribution*, under *distribution*. **clinical t.,** an experiment performed on human beings in order to evaluate the comparative efficacy of two or more therapies. The *randomized controlled trial*, which uses an appropriate control group (placebo or sham treatment or the standard well-established therapy) for comparison with the experimental therapy and random allocation of patients to the experimental and control groups, is generally considered to yield the strongest scientific evidence of any well-designed trial. Another element of well-designed trials is blinding or masking; when possible, the knowledge as to whether a patient is in the experimental or control group is hidden from the patient (a *single blind trial*), both the patient and the therapists (a *double blind trial*), or the patient, therapists, and treatment evaluators (a *triple blind trial*). **crossover t.,** a clinical trial in which each patient is exposed first to one treatment and then to the other, but in random order.

trialism (tri′al-izm) trialistic theory; see under *theory*.

triallylamine (tri″al-il-am′in) a volatile, oily, liquid amine, $(CH_2:CH \cdot CH_2)_3N$.

triamcinolone (tri″am-sin′o-lōn) [USP] chemical name: 9-fluoro-11β,16α,17, 21-tetrahydroxypregna-1,4-diene-3,20-dione. A potent synthetic glucocorticoid, $C_{21}H_{27}FO_6$, occurring as a white or almost white, crystalline powder, having practically no mineralocorticoid activity; used in the treatment of various conditions responsive to the anti-inflammatory action of glucocorticoids, administered orally. **t. acetonide** [USP], the acetonide ester of triamcinolone, $C_{24}H_{31}FO_6$, occurring as a white to cream-colored, crystalline powder; applied topically to the skin and oral mucosa or administered by intra-articular, intrabursal, intramuscular, and intradermal injection. **t. acetonide sodium phosphate,** the 21-disodium phosphate salt of triamcinolone acetonide, $C_{24}H_{30}FNa_2O_9P$, having anti-inflammatory actions similar to those of the base. **t. diacetate** [USP], the diacetate ester of triamcinolone, $C_{25}H_{31}FO_8$, occurring as a fine, white to off-white, crystalline powder; administered orally and by intramuscular, intra-articular, and soft tissue injection. **t. hexacetonide** [USP], the hexacetonide ester of triamcinolone, $C_{30}H_{41}FO_7$, occurring as a white to cream-colored powder; it is administered by intra-articular or by intralesional or sublesional injection for treatment of arthritis or of inflammatory skin lesions, respectively.

triamine (tri-am′in) a compound containing three amino (—NH_2) groups.

triamterene (tri-am′ter-ēn) [USP] chemical name: 6-phenyl-2,4,7-pteridinetriamine. A potassium-sparing diuretic, $C_{12}H_{11}N_7$, used to treat edema and, usually in combination with hydrochlorothiazide, to treat hypertension.

triamylose (tri-am′ĭ-lōs) a polymerized anhydride of glucose, $(C_6H_{10}O_5)_3$, isolable from the amylopectin of starch.

triangle (tri′ang-g′l) [L. *triangulum; tres* three + *angulus* angle] a three-cornered area, figure, or object; see also *trigone* and *trigonum*. **Alsberg's t.,** an equilateral triangle with its apex upward, formed by a line passing through the long axis of the femur, a second line passing through the long axis of the neck of the femur, and a third line on a plane passing through the base of the head of the femur. The angle at the apex is known as *Alsberg's angle*, or *angle of elevation*. **Assézat's t.,** facial t. **auditory t.,** area vestibularis.

auricular t., one bounded by lines drawn from the tip of the auricle and the two ends of its base of insertion. **t. of auscultation,** the area limited by the lower edge of the trapezius muscle, the latissimus dorsi, and the medial margin of the scapula. **axillary t.,** the triangular area formed by the inner aspect of the arm, the axilla, and the pectoral region. **Béclard's t.,** the area lying between the posterior edge of the hyoglossal muscle, the posterior belly of the digastric muscle, and the greater cornu of the hyoid bone. **Bolton t.,** the triangle formed by drawing a line from the nasion to the sella turcica to the Bolton point. **Bonwill t.,** one formed by a line connecting the centers of the mandibular condyles and lines connecting either center with the mesial contact area of the mandibular medial incisors, each side being approximately 4 inches long. **brachial t.,** axillary t. **Burger's scalene t.,** a triangle providing a reference frame to represent the quantitative relationships between the electromotive forces of the heart and the extremity leads of the electrocardiograph. As compared to Einthoven's triangle, the lines representing leads I and II are considerably shortened. **Calot's t.,** the triangle formed by the cystic artery superiorly, the cystic duct inferiorly, and the hepatic duct medially; called also *cystohepatic t.* **cardiohepatic t.,** the triangular region in the fifth intercostal space of the right side, separating the heart from the upper edge of the liver. **carotid t.,** trigonum caroticum. **carotid t., inferior,** trigonum musculare. **carotid t., superior,** trigonum caroticum. **cephalic t.,** one on the anteroposterior plane of the skull, between the lines from the occiput to the forehead and to the chin, and a third line extending from the chin to the forehead. **cervical t.,** trigonum cervicale. **clavipectoral t.,** trigonum clavepectorale. **Codman's t.,** a triangular area visible roentgenographically where the periosteum, elevated by a bone tumor, rejoins the cortex of normal bone. **color t.,** a plane figure with red, green, and blue located at the three apices, and gray at the center, with lines drawn from side to side, as a guide to the color mixing equation needed to produce any intermediate hue. **crural t.,** the triangular area formed by the inner aspect of the thigh and the lower abdominal, inguinal, and genital regions. **cystohepatic t.,** Calot's t. **digastric t.,** trigonum submandibulare. **Dunham's t's,** see under *fan*. **Einthoven's t.,** an equilateral triangle used as a mathematical model of the standard electrocardiographic limb leads, in which the instantaneous heart vector in the frontal plane may be projected on the sides of the triangle thereby demonstrating that the algebraic sum of the potential differences as recorded in electrocardiographic leads I and III will equal that potential difference recorded in lead II. See *Einthoven's formula*, under *formula*. **t. of elbow,** a triangular area on the front of the elbow, having the brachioradialis muscle on the lateral side and the pronator teres on the medial side, the base being toward the humerus. **extravesical t.,** Pawlik's t. **facial t.,** a triangular area whose points are the basion, the alveolar point, and the nasion; called also *Assézat's t.* **Farabeuf's t.,** one on the upper part of the neck, its sides being formed by the internal jugular vein and the facial vein, and its base by the hypoglossal nerve. **femoral t.,** trigonum femorale. **fetal t.,** a triangular space made by the side of the fetal trunk, the thigh above, and the arm below. **frontal t.,** one bounded by the maximum frontal diameter and lines from either end of this diameter to the glabella. **Garland's t.,** a triangular area of relative resonance in the lower back, close to the spine on the diseased side; seen in pleurisy with effusion. **Gerhardt's t.,** a triangular area of dullness to percussion above the third left rib, an inconstant sign in patent ductus arteriosus. **Gombault-Philippe t.,** a triangular field formed in the conus medullaris by the fibers of the septomarginal tract. **Grocco's t.,** see *Grocco's sign* (def. 1), under *sign*. **Grynfeltt's t., t. of Grynfeltt and Lesgaft,** Lesgaft's space. **Henke's t.,** a triangular area between the descending portion of the inguinal fold, the lateral portion of the inguinal fold, and the lateral border of the rectus muscle. **Hesselbach's t.,** trigonum inguinale. **hypoglossohyoid t.,** the triangular space in the subhyoid region, bounded above by the hypoglossal nerve, in front by the posterior border of the mylohyoid muscle, and behind and below by the tendon of the digastric muscle. Called also *Pinaud's t.* and *Pirogoff's t.* **iliofemoral t.,** a triangular area bounded by Nélaton's line, a line through the superior iliac spine, and one extending from this spine to the great trochanter. **infra-**

clavicular t., fossa infraclavicularis. **inguinal t.,** 1. trigonum inguinale. 2. trigonum femorale. **Jackson's safety t.,** a triangular space bounded above by the lower end of the thyroid cartilage, its apex in the suprasternal notch, and its sides the inner edges of the sternocleidomastoid muscle; so called because it marks the limits of the area through which the trachea may safely be incised in tracheostomy. **Kanavel's t.,** a triangular area in the middle of the palm beneath which lies the common tendon sheath of the digital flexor tendons. **Korányi-Grocco t.,** see *Grocco's sign* (def. 1), under *sign*. **Labbé's t.,** one included between a horizontal line along the lower border of the cartilage of the ninth rib, the line of the false ribs, and the line of the liver, being the area where the stomach lies in contact with the anterior abdominal wall. **Langenbeck's t.,** one having its apex at the anterior superior spine of the ilium, its base along the anatomical neck of the femur, and its external side by the external face of the great trochanter. **Lesgaft's t.,** see under *space*. **Lesser's t.,** one bounded by the hypoglossal nerve above and the two bellies of the digastricus muscle on the other two sides. **Lieutaud's t.,** trigonum vesicae. **Livingston's t.,** a triangular area bounded by lines from the umbilicus to the crest of the ilium, from the latter to the right pubic spine, and from there to the umbilicus, marking an area which is hypersensitive to palpation in appendicitis. **lumbocostoabdominal t.,** a space between the obliquus externus abdominis muscle, the serratus posterior inferior, the erector spinae, and the obliquus internus abdominis. **lymphoid t.,** see *Waldeyer's tonsillar ring*, under *ring*. **Macewen's t.,** mastoid fossa of temporal bone. **Malgaigne's t.,** superior carotid t. **mesenteric t.,** a triangular space between the two layers of the mesentery as they diverge to enclose the intestine. **Minor's t.,** an angular defect posterior to the anus, produced by attachment of the superficial portion of the external sphincter to the coccyx. **Mohrenheim's t.,** fossa infraclavicularis. **muscular t.,** trigonum musculare. **t's of neck,** see *trigonum cervicale*. **occipital t.,** the area bounded by the sternocleidomastoid muscle anteriorly, the trapezius muscle posteriorly, and the omohyoid muscle inferiorly. **occipital t., inferior,** a triangular area having a line between the two mastoid processes as its base and the inion as its apex. **omotracheal t.,** trigonum musculare. **palatal t.,** one limited by the greatest transverse diameter of the palate and lines from either end of this diameter to the alveolar point. **paravertebral t.,** see *Grocco's sign* (def. 1), under *sign*. **Pawlik's t.,** one within the vagina corresponding exactly with the trigonum vesicae, and bounded laterally by Pawlik's folds. **Petit's t.,** trigonum lumbare. **Pinaud's t. Pirogoff's t.,** hypoglossohyoid t. **popliteal t. of femur,** facies poplitea femoris. **pubourethral t.,** one in the perineum bounded externally by the ischiocavernosus muscle, internally by the bulbocavernosus, and posteriorly by the transversus perinei superficialis. **Rauchfuss' t.,** see *Grocco's sign* (def. 1), under *sign*. **Reil's t.,** trigonum lemnisci. **retromandibular t.,** retromolar t. **retromolar t.,** a triangular shallow fossa on the mandible posterior to the third molar. **sacral t.,** a shallow triangular depression overlying the sacrum. **t. of safety,** the fifth or sixth left intercostal space, considered a safe site for pericardial aspiration. **Scarpa's t.,** trigonum femorale. **sternocostal t.,** trigonum sternocostale. **subclavian t.,** trigonum omoclaviculare. **subinguinal t.,** 1. hiatus saphenus. 2. trigonum femorale. **submandibular t., submaxillary t.,** trigonum submandibulare. **submental t.,** trigonum submentale. **suboccipital t.,** a triangular area lying between the rectus capitis posterior major and the obliquus capitis superior and obliquus capitis inferior muscles. **suprameatal t.,** mastoid fossa of temporal bone. **surgical t.,** any triangular area or region in which certain nerves, vessels, or organs are located; established for reference in surgical operations. **Trautmann's t.,** a space with its anterior angle at the prominence containing the labyrinth, bounded posteriorly by the transverse sinus and superiorly by the inferior temporal line. When the bone is removed, the superior petrosal sinus will be encountered at the superior posterior angle of this triangle. **Tweed t.,** a triangle defined by facial and dental landmarks on a lateral cephalometric film, using the Frankfort horizontal plane as a base. **umbilicomammillary t.,** one having its base formed by the line joining the nipples and its apex at the umbilicus. **urogenital t.,** diaphragma urogenitale.

vaginal t., Pawlik's t. **vesical t.,** trigonum vesicae. **von Weber's t.,** one on the sole of the foot formed by lines connecting the head of the first metatarsal, the head of the fifth metatarsal, and the center of the undersurface of the heel. **Ward's t.,** the space formed by the angle of the trabeculae in the neck of the femur; a vulnerable point for fracture. **Wernicke's t.,** the area within the posterior limb on the internal capsule in which the optic radiation, having just left the lateral geniculate body, comes into close proximity to the auditory and somesthetic radiations.

triangular (tri-ang′gu-lar) [L. *triangularis*] having three angles or corners.

triangularis (tri-ang″gu-la′ris) [L.] triangular.

triantebrachia (tri″an-te-bra′ke-ah) [*tri-* + *antebrachium* + *-ia*] a developmental anomaly characterized by tripling of the forearm.

Triatoma (tri-at′o-mah) a genus of bugs of the family Reduviidae, called the cone-nosed bugs, important in medicine as vectors of *Trypanosoma cruzi*, the etiologic agent of Chagas' disease. **T. megis′ta,** former name for *Panstrongylus megistus*. **T. sanguisu′ga,** the blood-sucking cone-nose or Mexican bedbug of the southern United States. Its bite is painful and causes irritation, swelling, and nausea. Other species which are vectors of *Trypanosoma cruzi* are: *T. dimidia′ta*, of Central America; *T. genicula′ta* (*Panstrongylus geniculatus*), which inhabits the burrows of the armadillo; *T. gerstaeck′eri* of Texas; *T. infes′tans* (*Panstrongylus infes′tans*), the unchuca or great black bug of the Argentine and Paraguay; *T. mexica′na*, found in Mexico; *T. nigrova′rius*, widely distributed in South America; *T. protrac′ta*, of the southern United States; *T. recur′va* and *T. rubi′da* of Arizona; *T. (Entriatoma) sor′dida* of São Paulo; and *T. vit′ticeps*, of Rio de Janeiro.

triatomic (tri″ah-tom′ik) made up of three atoms.

triazene (tri′ah-zēn) 1. the chemical species HN=N—NH₂. 2. a group of cytotoxic alkylating agents containing this moiety, typified by dacarbazine.

triazolam (tri-a′zo-lam) chemical name: 8-chloro-6-(2-chlorophenyl)-1-methyl-4*H*-[1,2,4]triazolo[4,3-*a*] [1,4]benzodiazepine; a tranquilizer, $C_{17}H_{12}Cl_2N_4$.

tribadism (trib′ah-dizm) [Gr. *tribein* to rub] 1. lesbianism in which heterosexual intercourse is simulated; sometimes used to refer to the use of an artificial penis. 2. mutual friction of the genitals between women.

tribasic (tri-ba′sik) [*tri-* + L. *basis* base] having three replaceable hydrogen atoms.

tribe (trīb) a taxonomic category subordinate to a family (or subfamily) and superior to a genus (or subtribe).

tribenoside (tri-ben′o-sīd) chemical name: ethyl-3,5,6-tri-*O*-benzyl-D-glucofuranoside; a sclerosing agent, $C_{29}H_{34}O_6$, which has been used in inflammatory and varicose disorders of the veins.

Tribolium (tri-bo′le-um) a genus of small beetles that live in and are very destructive to flour and other cereal products. The two most common species, *T. confu′sum* and *T. casta′neum*, are reddish brown in color and 3.5 mm. in length.

tribology (tri-bol′o-je) [Gr. *tribē* a rubbing + *-logy*] the study of the lubrication, friction, and wear of the joints.

triboluminescence (tri″bo-lu″mi-nes′ens) [Gr. *tribein* to rub + *luminescence*] luminescence produced by mechanical energy, as by the grinding, rubbing, or breaking of certain crystals.

tribrachia (tri-bra′ke-ah) [*tri-* + Gr. *brachion* arm + *-ia*] a developmental anomaly characterized by tripling of an arm.

tribrachius (tri-bra′ke-us) 1. a monster exhibiting tribrachia. 2. a monster consisting of conjoined twins having only three arms.

tribromaloin (tri″brōm-al′o-in) a yellow, crystalline compound, $C_{17}H_{15}Br_3O_7$, or bromine and barbaloin.

tribromethanol (tri″brōm-eth′ah-nol) tribromoethanol.

tribromide (tri-bro′mīd) a bromine compound containing three atoms of bromine to one of the base.

tribromoethanol (tri-bro′mo-eth′ah-nol) chemical name: tribromoethyl alcohol. An anesthetic, $C_2H_3Br_3O$, occurring as a white, crystalline powder; administered by inhalation. Called also *ethobrom*. See also *solution*.

tribromsalan (tri-brom′sah-lan) chemical name: 3,5-dibromo-*N*-(4-bromophenyl)-2-hydroxybenzamide. A disinfectant with antibacterial and antifungal activities, $C_{13}H_8Br_3NO_2$, used mainly in medicated soaps.

tribulosis (trib″u-lo′sis) poisoning in sheep in South Africa, caused by wilted plants of the species *Tribulus terrestris*.

Triburon (trib′u-ron) trademark for preparations of triclobisonium chloride.

tributyrin (tri-bu′tir-in) a colorless fat, $C_3H_5(OCOCH_2CH_2CH_3)_3$, found in cows' milk.

tributyrinase (tri″bu-tir′ĭ-nās) triacylglycerol lipase.

TRIC (trik) acronym for *tr*achoma *i*nclusion *c*onjunctivitis (group of organisms); see *Chlamydia*.

tricalcic (tri-kal′sik) containing three atoms of calcium.

tricellular (tri-sel′u-lar) three celled.

tricephalus (tri-sef′ah-lus) [*tri-* + Gr. *kephalē* head] a monster having three heads.

triceps (tri′seps) [L., from *tri-* + *caput* head] having three heads, as a triceps muscle. **t. su′rae,** see *Table of Musculi.*

triceptor (tri-sep′tor) an intermediary having three combining groups.

tricheiria (tri-ki′re-ah) [*tri-* + Gr. *cheir* hand + *-ia*] a developmental anomaly characterized by tripling of a hand.

trichesthesia (trik″es-the′ze-ah) trichoesthesia.

trichiasis (trĭ-ki′ah-sis) [Gr.] 1. a condition of ingrowing hairs about an orifice, or of ingrowing eyelashes. 2. the appearance of hairlike filaments in the urine.

Trichiida (trĭ-ki′ĭ-dah) [Gr. *thrix* hair] an order of ameboid protozoa (subclass Myxogastria, class Eumycetozoa), the organisms of which have a spore mass that is usually light colored and a true capitillium composed of a system of uniform threads with spiral or annular thickenings.

trichilemmoma (trik″ĭ-lem-o′mah) a benign neoplasm of the lower outer root sheath of the hair.

Trichina (trĭ-ki′nah) *Trichinella.*

trichina (trĭ-ki′nah), pl. *trichi′nae.* an individual organism of the genus *Trichinella.*

trichinae (trĭ-ki′ne) plural of *trichina.*

Trichinella (trik″ĭ-nel′ah) [Gr. *trichinos* of hair] a genus of nematode parasites of the superfamily Trichuroidea. **T. spira′lis,** the etiologic agent of trichinosis, one of the smallest of the parasitic nematodes, being only about 1.5 mm. in length. It is found coiled in a cyst in the muscles of the bear, rat, pig, and man. When infected meat is eaten without proper cooking the cyst dissolves, the parasite matures, deposits its larvae in the deep mucosa, whence they enter the lymphatics, are carried to all parts of the body, and again encyst. An extract of *Trichinella* larvae is used in an intradermal skin test for trichinosis. Called also *pork worm.*

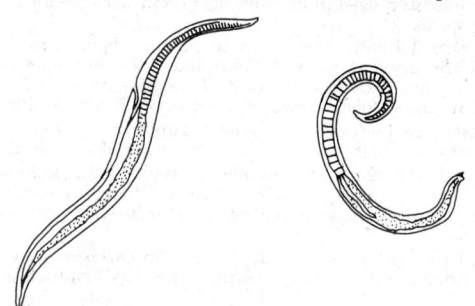

Trichinella spiralis, female (*left*) and male (*right*).

trichinelliasis (trik″ĭ-nel-li′ah-sis) trichinosis.

trichinellosis (trik″ĭ-nel-lo′sis) trichinosis.

trichiniasis (trik″ĭ-ni′ah-sis) trichinosis.

trichiniferous (trik″ĭ-nif′er-us) [*trichina* + L. *ferre* to bear] containing trichinae.

trichinization (trik″ĭ-ni-za′shun) infection with *Trichinella spiralis;* trichinosis.

trichinosis (trik″ĭ-no′sis) a disease due to infection with trichinae. It is produced by eating undercooked meat containing *Trichinella spiralis.* It is attended in the early stages by diarrhea, nausea, colic, and fever, and later by stiffness, pain,

swelling of the muscles, fever, eosinophilia, circumorbital edema, splinter hemorrhages, sweating, and insomnia.

trichinous (trik′ĭ-nus) affected with or containing trichinae.

trichion (trik′e-on), pl. *trich′ia* [Gr.] an anthropometric landmark, the point at which the midsagittal plane of the head intersects the hairline.

trichite (tri′kīt) [Gr. *thrix* hair] 1. one of the radially arranged needle-shaped crystals composing a starch grain. 2. trichocyst. 3. nematodesma. 4. a hollow, rodlike, subpellicular component of the skeleton of oligotrich ciliates.

trichlorfon (tri-klor′fon) a highly toxic organophosphorous insecticide, used also as an antischistosomal agent (see *metrifonate*).

trichloride (tri-klo′rīd) any combination of three atoms of chlorine with one of another element.

trichlormethiazide (tri-klor″mĕ-thi′ah-zīd) [USP] chemical name: 6-chloro-3-(dichloromethyl)-3,4-dihydro-2*H*-1,2,4-benzothiadiazine-7-sulfonamide 1,1-dioxide. A thiazide diuretic, $C_8H_8Cl_3N_3O_4S_2$, used to treat hypertension and edema.

trichloroacetaldehyde (tri-klo″ro-as″et-al′de-hīd) chloral.

trichloroacetic acid (tri-klor″o-ah-se′tik) [USP] a strong acid used as a protein precipitant in clinical chemistry and also as a caustic for removing warts.

trichloroethylene (tri″klo-ro-eth′ĭ-lēn) chemical name: trichloroethene; a clear, colorless liquid, $CHCl=CCl_2$, widely used as an industrial solvent; formerly used as an inhalation anesthetic.

trichloromethylchloroformate (tri-klo″ro-meth″il-klo″-ro-for′māt) a chlorine-containing gas which is irritating to lung tissue.

trichloromonofluoromethane (tri-klo″ro-mon″o-floor-o-meth′ān) [NF] chemical name: trichlorofluoromethane. A clear, colorless gas having a faint, ethereal odor, CCl_3F, used as an aerosol propellant.

trichlorophenol (tri″klor-o-fe′nol) a disinfectant and external antiseptic.

2,4,5-trichlorophenoxyacetic acid (tri-klor″o-fen-ok″se-ah-se′tik) 2,4,5-T.

trichlorotrivinylarsine (tri-klo″ro-tri-vi″nil-ar′sin) a sternutatory war gas $(CHCl:CH)_3As$.

trichlorphon (tri-klŏr′fon) metrifonate.

trich(o)- [Gr. *thrix*, gen. *trichos*, hair] a prefix denoting relationship to hair.

trichoaesthesia (trik″o-es-the′ze-ah) trichoesthesia.

trichoanesthesia (trik″o-an″es-the′ze-ah) loss of hair sensibility.

trichobacteria (trik″o-bak-te′re-ah) [*tricho-* + Gr. *baktērion* rod] 1. a group of bacteria including those forms which possess flagella. 2. the filamentous or threadlike bacteria.

trichobasalioma hyalinicum (trik″o-ba-sal″e-o′mah hi″ah-lĭ′nĭ-kum) cylindroma, def. 2.

trichobezoar (trik″o-be′zōr) [*tricho-* + *bezoar*] a hairball; a concretion within the stomach or intestines formed of hairs.

Trichobilharzia (trik″o-bil-har′ze-ah) a genus of flukes. **T. ocella′ta,** a blood fluke parasitic in European ducks.

trichocardia (trik″o-kar′de-ah) [*tricho-* + Gr. *kardia* heart] cor villosum, or hairy heart.

trichocephaliasis (trik″o-sef″ah-li′ah-sis) trichuriasis.

trichocephalosis (trik″o-sef″ah-lo′sis) trichuriasis.

Trichocephalus (trik″o-sef′ah-lus) [*tricho-* + Gr. *kephalē* head] former name for a genus of nematodes now called *Trichuris.*

trichoclasia (trik″o-kla′se-ah) trichorrhexis nodosa.

trichoclasis (trik-ok′lah-sis) [*tricho-* + Gr. *klasis* fracture] trichorrhexis nodosa.

trichocyst (trik′o-sist) [*tricho-* + Gr. *kystis* bladder] one of the extrusible and explosive, nontoxic, spindle-shaped subpellicular organelles occurring in many protozoa, which can discharge long, striated, fibrous shafts. Its true function is unknown, but it may serve to anchor the organism during feeding, serve an offensive or defensive function, or serve in prey capture. Called also *trichite.*

Trichodectes (trik″o-dek′tēz) [*tricho-* + Gr. *dēktēs* biter] a genus of parasitic insects of the order Mallophaga, the biting lice. **T. can′is,** a biting louse that parasitizes dogs and is an intermediate host of *Dipylidium caninum.* **T. cli′max,** *Damalinia caprae.* **T. e′qui,** *Damalinia equi.* **T. herm′si,** *Damalinia hermsi.* **T. la′tus,** the dog louse, found on dogs, especially puppies. **T. pilo′sus,** *Damalinia pilosus.* **T. retu′sis,** a biting louse that infests ranch-raised mink. **T. sphaeroceph′alus,** the red-headed sheep louse, found in the wool of sheep in Europe and America.

Trichoderma (trik-o-der′mah) [*tricho* + *derma* skin] a genus of soil fungi (family Moniliaceae, order Moniliales), some species of which cause alimentary toxic aleukia.

trichoepithelioma (trik″o-ep″ĭ-the-le-o′mah) a benign skin tumor whose cell growth starts in the follicles of the lanugo; it may occur as a dominantly inherited condition characterized by multiple tumors (sometimes called *trichoepithelioma papillosum multiplex*) or as a solitary lesion. **t. papillo′sum mul′tiplex,** hereditary multiple trichoepithelioma; see *trichoepithelioma.* Called also *acanthoma adenoides cysticum, Brooke's disease* or *tumor,* and *epithelioma adenoides cysticum.*

trichoesthesia (trik″o-es-the′ze-ah) [*tricho-* + Gr. *aisthēsis* perception + *-ia*] the sense by which one perceives when one of the hairs of the skin has been touched; hair sensibility.

trichoesthesiometer (trik″o-es-the″ze-om′ĕ-ter) [*tricho-* + Gr. *aisthēsis* perception + *metron* measure] an electric apparatus for measuring the hair sensibility, or the sensitiveness of the scalp by means of the hairs.

trichoglossia (trik″o-glos′e-ah) [*tricho-* + *gloss-* + *-ia*] hairy tongue.

trichographism (tri-kog′rah-fizm) pilomotor reflex.

trichohyalin (trik″o-hi′ah-lin) [*tricho-* + *hyalin*] a keratohyaline-like substance occurring in granules in the cytoplasm of the cells of Huxley's layer of a hair follicle.

trichoid (trik′oid) [*tricho-* + Gr. *eidos* form] like or resembling a hair, or the hair.

tricholeukocyte (trik″o-lu′ko-sīt) hairy cell.

tricholith (trik′o-lith) [*tricho-* + Gr. *lithos* stone] a hairy concretion.

trichologia (trik″o-lo′je-ah) [*tricho-* + Gr. *legein* to pick out + *-ia*] trichotillomania.

trichology (tri-kol′o-je) the study of hair, or the sum of what is known about the hair.

trichoma (tri-ko′mah) entropion.

trichomania (trik″o-ma′ne-ah) trichotillomania.

trichomatous (trĭ-kom′ah-tus) affected with, of the nature of, or pertaining to trichoma (entropion).

trichome (tri′kōm) [Gr. *trichōma* a growth of hair, hair generally] 1. a filamentous or hairlike structure. 2. a colony of filamentous blue-green algae in which the member cells grow end-to-end to form a chain-like structure.

trichomegaly (trik″o-meg′ah-le) [*tricho-* + Gr. *megalē* large] a congenital syndrome consisting of excessive growth of the eyelashes and brow hair associated with dwarfism, mental retardation, and pigmentary degeneration of the retina.

trichomonacidal (trik″o-mo′nah-si′dal) destructive to trichomonads.

trichomonacide (trik″o-mo′nah-sīd) an agent destructive to trichomonads.

trichomonad (trik″o-mo′nad, trik″o-mon′ad) [*tricho-* + Gr. *monas* unit, from *monas* single] any protozoan of the order Trichomonadida.

Trichomonadida (trik″o-mo-nad′ĭ-dah) an order of chiefly parasitic protozoa (superorder Parabasalidea, class Zoomastigophora), typically characterized by the presence of karyomastigonts with four to six flagella, one of which is recurrent or free or has a proximal segment or the entire length adherent to the body surface; an undulating membrane (if present) associated with adherent segments of recurrent flagellum; and a pelta and noncontractile axostyle in each mastigont. Representative genera include *Dientamoeba, Histomonas, Monocercomonas,* and *Trichomonas.*

trichomonal (trik″o-mo′nal, trik″o-mon′al) pertaining to or caused by trichomonads.

Trichomonas (trik″o-mo′nas, trik″o-mon′as, trĭ-kom′o-nas) [*tricho-* + Gr. *monas* unit, from *monas* single] a genus of parasitic flagellated protozoa (superorder Parabasalidea, class Zoomastigophorea) found in the intestinal and genito-urinary tracts of various invertebrates and vertebrates, including humans, and characterized by the presence of three to five anterior flagella (in some systems of classification, the former has been assigned to a separate genus, *Tritrichomonas,* and the latter to *Pentatrichomonas*) and a pelta, axostyle, and undulating membrane. **T. bucca′lis,** *T. tenax.* **T. foe′tus,** a species with three anterior flagella found in the genital tract of cattle, in which it causes a contagious venereal disease transmitted from bulls to cows by coitus or by artificial insemination, and characterized by early abortion, pyometra, and sterility. **T. gal′linae,** a species with four anterior flagella found in the upper digestive tract and associated structures and in other organs, especially the liver, of domestic pigeons and various other birds, in which it causes a form of avian trichomoniasis. Infection varies from mild to a rapidly fatal disease manifested by caseous accumulations and necrosis in involved tissues and severe weight loss. **T. gallina′rum,** a species with four anterior flagella found in the lower digestive tract of chickens, turkeys, and other domestic birds in which it causes sometimes a fatal form of avian trichomoniasis. Infection is manifested by lesions of the cecum and liver, diarrhea, and loss of appetite and weight. **T. hom′inis,** a species with five flagella that is one of the most common enteric flagellates seen in humans, in whom it may be present in large numbers but is generally considered to be nonpathogenic. Called also *T. intestinalis.* **T. te′nax,** a commensal species with four anterior flagella found in the mouth of primates, including humans, where it is most often seen in the tartar around teeth, cavities of carious teeth, pockets associated with periodontal disease, and tonsillar crypts. Called also *T. buccalis.* **T. vagina′lis,** a species with four flagella found in the vagina and male genital tract, usually transmitted by coitus. Vaginal trichomoniasis may be asymptomatic or it may be manifested by severe vaginitis associated with discharge, burning, pruritus, and chafing; infection in the male may produce urethritis, enlargement of the prostate, and epididymitis.

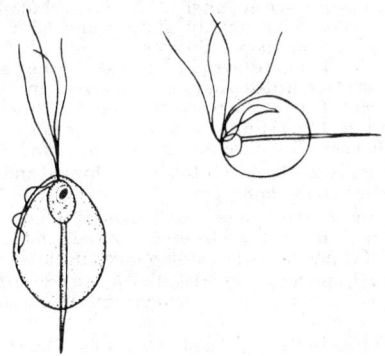

Trichomonas vaginalis.

trichomoniasis (trik″o-mo-ni′ah-sis) infection with *Trichomonas.* **avian t.,** trichomoniasis in birds and poultry, especially pigeons, caused by *Trichomonas gallinae* or *T. gallinarum.* **bovine t.,** venereal trichomoniasis in cattle caused by *Trichomonas foetus.* **t. vagina′lis,** human trichomoniasis caused by *Trichomonas vaginalis.*

Trichomycetes (trik″o-mi-se′tēs) [*tricho-* + Gr. *mykēs* fungus] a group of organisms with a simple or branched thallus attached by a basal cell to the digestive tract or external cuticle of living arthropods. In some classifications, they are included in the Phycomycetes, and are also called *Microsiphonales.*

trichomycosis (trik″o-mi-ko′sis) [*tricho-* + Gr. *mykēs* fungus] any disease of the hair due to infection by a fungus. **t. axilla′ris,** a superficial infection of the axillary or pubic hair in which yellow, black, or red nodular concretions form around the hair shaft; it is caused by *Corynebacterium tenuis,* a nocardia-like microorganism of uncertain affiliation that was formerly thought to be a fungus.

trichon (trik′on) an autolyzed preparation of the fungi of the genus *Trichophyton.*

trichonodosis (trik″o-no-do′sis) a rare condition characterized by apparent or actual knotting of the hair, thought to be the result of inability of new hairs to grow freely from their follicles, because of toughness of the surrounding tissues.

Trichonympha (trik″o-nim′fah) [tricho- + nymph] a genus of multiflagellated, cellulose-digesting, parasitic protozoa (suborder Trichonymphina, order Hypermastigida) found in the gut of termites and woodroaches, and characterized by the presence of flagella arranged in longitudinal rows on the anterior end of the body. Species parasitic in woodroaches reproduce asexually when the host molts.

Trichonymphina (trik″o-nim′fah) a suborder of multiflagellated, cellulose-digesting, parasitic protozoa (order Hypermastigida, class Zoomastigophorea) found in the gut of termites and woodroaches, and characteristically having a bell shape with flagella covering only the anterior (narrow) end of the body. Certain species reproduce sexually when the host insect molts. Representative genera include *Barbulanympha, Spirotrichonympha,* and *Trichonympha.*

trichopathic (trik″o-path′ik) pertaining to disease of the hair.

trichopathy (trĭ-kop′ah-the) [tricho- + Gr. *pathos* disease] disease of the hair.

trichophagia (trik″o-fa′je-ah) [tricho- + Gr. *phagein* to eat] the practice or habit of eating hair.

trichophagy (trĭ-kof′ah-je) trichophagia.

trichophytic (trik″o-fit′ik) pertaining to trichophytosis.

trichophytid (trĭ-kof′ĭ-tid) [*Trichophyton* + *-id*] a dermatophytid associated with trichophytosis; applied especially to allergic manifestations of any ringworm infection.

trichophytin (trĭ-kof′ĭ-tin) the soluble broth culture products of various species of *Trichophyton;* used in the trichophytin test.

trichophytobezoar (trik″o-fi′to-be′zōr) [tricho- + Gr. *phyton* plant + *bezoar*] a bezoar composed of animal hair and vegetable fibers.

Trichophyton (tri-kof′ĭ-ton) [tricho- + Gr. *phyton* plant] a genus of imperfect fungi of the order Moniliales, family Moniliaceae, consisting of flat, branched filaments and various types of spores. Species of *Trichophyton* attack the skin, nails, and hair (dermatophytes). As the perfect (sexual) stages are identified they are classified in the genus *Arthroderma.* The common species include *T. mentagrophy′tes, T. ru′brum, T. ton′surans, T. schoenlei′nii, T. concen′tricum, T. ferrugin′eum, T. viola′ceum, T. galli′nae,* and *T. sim′ii.*

trichophytosis (trik″o-fi-to′sis) a fungal infection caused by species of *Trichophyton.*

Trichoptera (tri-kop′ter-ah) [tricho- + Gr. *pteron* wing] an order of flies, the caddis flies. The hair and scales from the wings may produce allergic symptoms in susceptible persons.

trichoptilosis (trik″o-tĭ-lo′sis) [tricho- + Gr. *ptilon* feather + *-osis*] the condition in which the hairs are split and feather-like.

trichorrhexis (trik″o-rek′sis) [tricho- + Gr. *rhēxis* fracture] a condition in which the hairs break. **t. nodo′sa,** a condition characterized by what appear to be white nodes on the hairs but are actually sites where the cortex of the shaft has fractured and split into strands, weakening the hairs so they break at these nodes. Called also *bamboo hair, clastothrix, trichoclasia,* and *trichoclasis.*

trichoschisis (trik-os′kĭ-sis) [tricho- + Gr. *schisis* fissure] splitting of the hairs.

trichoscopy (trĭ-kos′ko-pe) [tricho- + Gr. *skopein* to examine] examination of the hair.

Trichosida (trĭ-ko′sĭ-dah) [Gr. *thrix, trichos* hair] an order of ameboid protozoa (subclass Testacealobosia, class Lobosia), characterized by the presence of a test composed of a fibrous sheath with calcareous spicules and multiple apertures through which short, conical pseudopodia protrude.

trichosiderin (trik″o-sid′er-in) [tricho- + Gr. *sidēros* iron] an iron-containing brown pigment found in normal human red hair.

trichosis (tri-ko′sis) [Gr. *trichōsis*] any disease or abnormal growth of the hair. **t. carun′culae,** abnormal development of the hair on the lacrimal caruncle.

Trichosoma (trik″o-so′mah) [tricho- + Gr. *sōma* body] *Capillaria.* **T. contor′tum,** *Capillaria contorta.*

Trichosomoides (trik″o-so-moi′dēz) a genus of nematode

parasites. **T. crassicau′da,** a nematode parasite of rats; the male is much smaller than the female, and is parasitic in the rat vagina or uterus.

Trichosporon (tri-kos′po-ron) [tricho- + Gr. *sporos* seed] a genus of imperfect fungi of the family Cryptococcaceae, order Moniliales, which are normal flora of the respiratory and digestive tract of man and animals, and may infect the hair. **T. beigel′ii,** *T. cutaneum.* **T. cuta′neum,** the etiologic agent of white piedra. It is a normal inhabitant of the skin and the respiratory and intestinal tracts, and rarely an opportunistic agent in debilitated patients, causing a fatal systemic infection. Called also *T. biegelii* and *T. giganteum.* **T. gigan′teum,** *T. cutaneum.* **T. pedrosia′num,** *Fonsecaea pedrosoi.*

trichosporosis (trik″o-spo-ro′sis) infection with fungi of the genus *Trichosporon;* see *white piedra, piedra.*

Trichosporum (tri-kos′po-rum) *Trichosporon.*

trichostasis spinulosa (trĭ-kos′tah-sis spin″u-lo′sa) [tricho- + Gr. *stasis* a standing + L. *spinulosus* thorny] a condition in which the hair follicles contain a dark, horny, comedo-like keratin plug, which contains a bundle of villus hair.

Trichostomatida (trik″o-sto-mat′ĭ-dah) [tricho- + Gr. *stoma* mouth] an order of ciliate protozoa (subclass Vestibuliferia, class Kenetofragminophorea), many of which are endocommensals in vertebrates; most have uniform somatic ciliature, sometimes asymmetrical, and no buccal ciliature in the oral region is present. It comprises two suborders: Trichostomatina and Blepharocorythina.

Trichostomatina (trik″o-sto″mah-ti′nah) a suborder of ciliate protozoa (order Trichostomatida, subclass Vestibuliferia) in which the somatic ciliature is not reduced. *Balantidium* and *Isotricha* are representative genera.

trichostrongyliasis (trik″o-stron′jĭ-li′ah-sis) infection by nematodes of the genus *Trichostrongylus,* whose eggs are often mistaken for those of the hookworm. It is usually asymptomatic, but diarrhea may occur.

Trichostrongylidae (trik″o-stron-jil′ĭ-de) a family of nematodes of the superfamily Strongyloidea, including the genera *Trichostrongylus, Haemonchus, Nippostrongylus,* and *Nematodirus.*

trichostrongylosis (trik″o-stron″jĭ-lo′sis) infestation with *Trichostrongylus.*

Trichostrongylus (trik″o-stron′jĭ-lus) a genus of nematode worms (family Trichostrongylidae), comprising some of the species formerly included in the genus *Strongylus.* Adult worms are small and embed their heads in the mucosa of the small intestine; their eggs are often mistaken for those of the hookworm. Infection is usually asymptomatic. **T. caprico′la,** a species commonly found in ruminants. **T. colubriform′is,** a species frequently present in sheep and goats and occasionally in man; called also *Strongylus subtilis* and *T. instabilis.* **T. insta′bilis,** *T. colubriformis.* **T. orienta′lis,** a species found in man in Asia. **T. probolu′rus,** a species found in sheep, mountain goats, dromedaries, gazelles, and occasionally man in Europe, Africa, and North America. **T. vitri′nus,** a species found in sheep, goats, dromedaries, and occasionally in man.

Trichothecium (trik″o-the′se-um) [tricho- + Gr. *thēkē* case] a genus of imperfect fungi of the order Moniliales, family Moniliaceae. **T. ro′seum,** a species causing pinkrot of apples, lumber, etc., and very rarely recovered from otitis externa and mycotic keratitis.

trichotillomania (trik″o-til″o-ma′ne-ah) [tricho- + Gr. *tillein* to pull + *mania* madness] compulsive pulling out of one's hair.

trichotomous (tri-kot′o-mus) [Gr. *tricha* three-fold + *tomē* a cutting] divided into three parts.

trichotoxin (tri″ko-tok′sin) an antibody that has a toxic action on epithelial cells.

trichroic (tri-kro′ik) pertaining to or characterized by trichroism.

trichroism (tri′kro-izm) [tri- + Gr. *chroa* color] the exhibition of three different colors in three different aspects.

trichromasy (tri-kro′mah-se) [tri- + Gr. *chrōma* color] 1. ability to distinguish the three primary colors, red, yellow, and blue, and mixtures thereof. 2. normal color vision; 91.2 per cent of white males and 99.6 per cent of white females have normal color vision. **anomalous t.,** defective color vision in which the patient has all three cone pigments, one of which is deficient or anomalous, but not absent. There are three types of anomalous trichromasy—protanomaly, deuteranomaly, and tritanomaly, and they may be: (1) *acquired*, resulting from a retinal, cerebral, systemic, or toxic disorder; or (2) *congenital* and inherited as an X-linked recessive trait. Called also *anomalous trichromatism*.

trichromat (tri′kro-mat)   a person with trichromasy.

trichromatic (tri″kro-mat′ik)   trichromic.

trichromatism (tri-kro′mah-tizm)   trichroism. **anomalous t.,** anomalous trichromasy.

trichromatopsia (tri″kro-mah-top′se-ah)   trichromasy.

trichromic (tri-kro′mik) [*tri-* + Gr. *chrōma* color]   1. pertaining to or exhibiting three colors.   2. able to distinguish the three primary colors (red, blue, green); having normal color vision.

trichterbrust (trich′ter-broost) [Ger.]   funnel chest.

trichuriasis (trik″u-ri′ah-sis)   the state of being infected with nematodes of the genus *Trichuris*.

Trichuris (trik-u′ris) [*tricho-* + Gr. *oura* a tail]   a genus of intestinal nematode parasites of the superfamily Trichuroidea.   **T. trichiu′ra,** the species that principally infects man. It is about 2 inches in length, the front portion of its body, the esophageal zone, being hairlike in slimness. It inhabits the large intestine, and may cause diarrhea, vomiting, and rectal prolapse in children heavily infected, although it usually produces no symptoms. Also known as *whipworm*.

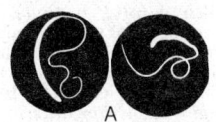 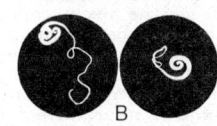

Trichuris trichiura: A, females; *B,* males. The posterior portion of the male is usually coiled as shown in *B.*

Trichuroidea (trik″u-roi′de-ah)   a superfamily of aphasmid nematodes including the genera *Capillaria, Trichinella,* and *Trichuris*.

tricipital (tri-sip′ĭ-tal) [L. *tricipitis*]   1. pertaining to the triceps muscle.   2. having three heads.

triclobisonium chloride (tri″klo-bĭ-so′ne-um)   chemical name: N,N,N′,N′-trimethyl-N,N′-bis[1-methyl-3-(2,2,6-trimethylcyclohexyl)propyl]-1,6-hexanediaminium dichloride. A quaternary ammonium compound, $C_{36}H_{74}Cl_2N_2$, occurring as a white, crystalline powder; used as a local anti-infective, primarily in the treatment of vulvitis, vaginitis, and other gynecological conditions due to *Trichomonas vaginalis, Candida albicans,* and *Haemophilus vaginalis* or to staphylococci and streptococci, administered intravaginally.

triclocarban (tri″klo-kar′ban)   chemical name: N-(4-chlorophenyl)-N′-(3,4-dichlorophenyl)urea. A disinfectant, $C_{13}H_9$-Cl_3N_2O, effective against gram-positive bacteria and to a lesser extent against gram-negative bacteria and against fungi; used in the preparation of soaps and other cleansing products and dermatological compositions to control skin infections.

triclofenol piperazine (tri-klo′fen-ōl)   chemical name: 2,4,5-trichlorophenol compound with piperazine (2:1); an anthelmintic, $C_4H_{10}N_2 \cdot 2C_6H_3Cl_3O$, effective against roundworms and hookworms.

triclofos sodium (tri′klo-fōs)   chemical name: 2,2,2-trichloroethanol dihydrogen phosphate monosodium salt; an oral hypnotic and sedative, $C_2H_3Cl_3NaO_4P$, used especially to induce sleep in the treatment of insomnia. It may also be used as premedication for sleep induction in electroencephalography.

triclonide (tri-klo′nīd)   chemical name: 9,11β,21-trichloro -6α- fluoro- 16α,17- [(1- methylethylidene) bis(oxy)] pregna-1,4-diene-3,20-dione; an anti-inflammatory, $C_{24}H_{28}$-Cl_3FO_4.

Triclos (tri′klōs)   trademark for a preparation of triclofos sodium.

triclosan (tri-klo′san)   chemical name: 5-chloro-2-(2,4-dichlorophenoxy)phenol. An antibacterial, $C_{12}H_7Cl_3O_2$, effective against gram-positive and most gram-negative organ-isms and exhibiting slight activity against yeasts and fungi; used as a detergent in surgical scrubs, soaps, and deodorants.

Tricofuron (tri″ko-fu′ron)   trademark for preparations of furazolidone.

Tricoloid (tri′ko-loid)   trademark for a preparation of tricyclamol chloride.

tricorn (tri′korn) [*tri-* + L. *cornu* horn]   a lateral ventricle of the brain.

tricornute (tri-kor′nūt) [*tri-* + L. *cornutus* horned]   having three horns, cornua, or processes.

tricresol (tri-kre′sol)   cresol.

tricrotic (tri-krot′ik) [Gr. *trikrotos* rowed with a triple stroke; triple beating]   pertaining to or characterized by tricrotism.

tricrotism (tri′kro-tizm)   the quality of having three sphygmographic waves or elevations to one beat of the pulse.

tricuspid (tri-kus′pid) [L. *tricuspis*]   1. having three points or cusps.   2. pertaining to the tricuspid valves of the heart.

tricyclamol chloride (tri-si′klah-mol)   chemical name: 1-(3-cyclohexyl-3-hydroxy-3-phenylpropyl)-1-methyl pyrrolidinium chloride. A quaternary ammonium anticholinergic derived from procyclidine, $C_{20}H_{32}ClNO$, which inhibits gastrointestinal hypermotility and reduces secretion of gastric juices; it has been used in the treatment of peptic ulcer and as a gastrointestinal antispasmodic.

tricyclic (tri-sik′lik)   containing three fused rings or closed chains in the molecular structure; see also under *antidepressant*.

Trid.   abbreviation for L. *trid′uum,* three days.

tridactylism (tri-dak′tĭ-lizm) [*tri-* + Gr. *daktylos* finger]   the condition of having only three digits on one hand or foot.

tridactylous (tri-dak′tĭ-lus)   pertaining to or characterized by tridactylism.

trident, tridentate (tri′dent; tri-den′tāt)   three pronged.

tridermic (tri-der′mik) [*tri-* + Gr. *derma* skin]   derived from the ectoderm, endoderm, and mesoderm.

tridermogenesis (tri″der-mo-jen′ĕ-sis) [*tri-* + Gr. *derma* skin + *genesis* production]   the formation of the three germ layers and, by extension, the stage in embryonic development during which it occurs.

tridermoma (tri″der-mo′mah) [*tri-* + Gr. *derma* skin + *-oma*]   a teratoma containing representatives of all three germ layers.

Tridesilon (tri-des′ĭ-lon)   trademark for preparations of desonide.

tridihexethyl chloride (tri″di-heks-eth′il) [USP]   chemical name: γ-cyclohexyl-N,N,N-triethyl-γ-hydroxybenzenepropanaminium. A quaternary ammonium anticholinergic, $C_{21}H_{36}ClNO$, occurring as a white, crystalline powder, which inhibits gastrointestinal hypermotility and spasms and reduces secretion of gastric juices; used as adjunctive therapy in the treatment of peptic ulcer and in the irritable bowel syndrome, administered orally and parenterally.

Tridione (tri-di′ōn)   trademark for preparations of trimethadione.

tridymite (trid′ĭ-mīt)   a rare crystalline form of silica, SiO_2, obtainable from quartz by heating.

triencephalus (tri″en-sef′ah-lus) [*tri-* + Gr. *enkephalos* brain]   a monster having no organs of sight, hearing, or smell.

-triene (tri′ēn)   a chemical suffix indicating the presence of three double bonds.

triester (tri′es-ter)   a compound containing three ester groups.

triethanolamine (tri″eth-ah-nōl′ah-mēn)   1. an alkanolamine produced by ammonolysis of ethylene oxide.   2. trolamine.

triethylamine (tri″eth-il-am′in)   a somewhat poisonous, oily liquid ptomaine, $N(C_2H_5)_3$, with an ammoniacal smell, derived from decaying fish.

triethylenemelamine (tri-eth″ĭ-lēn-mel′ah-mēn)   TEM; a cytotoxic alkylating agent of the ethylenimine group, no longer commercially available.

triethylenethiophosphoramide (tri-eth″ĭ-lēn-thi″o-fos-fōr′ah-mīd)   thiotepa.

trifacial (tri-fa′shal) [L. *trifacialis*]   designating the fifth cranial nerve (nervus trigeminus [NA]).

trifid (tri'fid) [L. *trifidus*, from *tres* three + *findere* to split] split into three parts.

triflocin (tri-flo'sin) chemical name: 4-[[3-(trifluoromethyl)phenyl]amino]-3-pyridinecarboxylic acid; a diuretic, $C_{13}H_9F_3N_2O$.

triflumidate (tri-floo'mĭ-dāt) chemical name: 3-(benzoylphenyl)[(trifluoromethyl)sulfonyl]carbamic acid ethyl ester; an anti-inflammatory, $C_{17}H_{14}F_3NO_5S$.

trifluoperazine hydrochloride (tri″floo-o-păr'ah-zēn) [USP] chemical name: 10-[3-(4-methyl-1-piperazinyl)propyl]-2-(trifluoromethyl)-10*H*-phenothiazine dihydrochloride. An antipsychotic agent, $C_{21}H_{24}F_3N_3S \cdot 2HCl$, occurring as a white to pale yellow, crystalline powder; administered orally and intramuscularly.

trifluperidol (tri-flu-per'ĭ-dol) chemical name: 4'-fluoro-4-[4-hydroxy-4-(α,α,α-trifluoro-*m*-tolyl)piperidino]butyrophenone; a tranquilizer, $C_{22}H_{23}F_4NO_2$, which has been used in the treatment of mania and schizophrenia.

triflupromazine (tri″floo-pro'mah-zēn) [USP] chemical name: *N,N*-dimethyl-2-(trifluoromethyl)-10*H*-phenothiazine-10-propanamine. An antipsycotic agent, $C_{18}H_{19}F_3N_2S \cdot HCl$, occurring as a viscous, light amber-colored, oily liquid, which crystalizes on long standing to large irregular crystals; administered orally. **t. hydrochloride** [USP], the monohydrochloride salt of triflupromazine, $C_{18}H_{19}F_3N_2S \cdot HCl$, occurring as a white to pale tan, crystalline powder; administered orally and intramuscularly.

trifluridine (tri-floor'ĭ-den) chemical name: α,α,α-trifluorothymidine; an antiviral for use in ophthalmology, $C_{10}H_{11}F_3N_2O_5$.

trifluromethylthiazide (tri-floor″o-meth″il-thi'ah-zīd) flumethiazide.

trifoliosis (tri″fo-le-o'sis) a disease of horses marked by irritation of the skin and of the mucous membrane of the mouth and by general disturbance; attributed to the eating of hybrid clover.

trifurcation (tri″fur-ka'shun) [*tri-* + L. *furca* fork] division into three branches.

trigastric (tri-gas'trik) [*tri-* + Gr. *gastēr* belly] having three bellies; said of a muscle.

trigeminal (tri-jem'ĭ-nal) [*tri-* + L. *geminus* twin] 1. triple. 2. pertaining to the fifth cranial nerve (nervus trigeminus [NA]).

trigeminus (tri-jem'ĭ-nus) [L.] triple; see *nervus trigeminus*.

trigeminy (tri-jem'ĭ-ne) the condition of occurring in threes, especially the occurrence of three pulse beats in rapid succession; see *trigeminal pulse*, under *pulse*.

triglyceride (tri-glis'er-īd) a compound consisting of three molecules of fatty acid esterified to glycerol; it is a neutral fat synthesized from carbohydrates for storage in animal adipose cells. On enzymatic hydrolysis, it releases free fatty acids in the blood.

trigocephalus (tri″go-sef'ah-lus) trigonocephalus.

trigona (tri-go'nah) [L.] plural of *trigonum*.

trigonal (tri'go-nal) triangular; pertaining to a trigone.

trigone (tri'gōn) 1. a triangular area (trigonum [NA]); see also *triangle*. 2. the first three cusps of an upper molar tooth; see *hypocone*, *paracone*, and *protocone*. **t. of bladder**, trigonum vesicae. **carotid t.**, trigonum caroticum. **cerebral t.**, fornix cerebri. **clavipectoral t.**, trigonum clavipectorale. **collateral t., of lateral ventricle**, trigonum collaterale ventriculi lateralis. **collateral t. of fourth ventricle**, trigonum nervi vagi. **femoral t.**, trigonum femorale. **fibrous t. of heart, left**, trigonum fibrosum sinistrum cordis. **fibrous t., of heart, right**, trigonum fibrosum dextrum cordis. **t. of habenula, habenular t.**, trigonum habenulae. **Henke's t.**, Henke's triangle. **hypoglossal t., t. of hypoglossal nerve**, trigonum nervi hypoglossi. **iliopectineal t.**, fossa iliopectinea. **inguinal t.**, trigonum inguinale. **interpeduncular t.**, fossa interpeduncularis. **lumbar t.**, trigonum lumbare. **muscular t.**, trigonum musculare. **olfactory t.**, trigonum olfactorium. **omoclavicular t.**, trigonum omoclaviculare. **Pawlik's t.**, Pawlik's triangle. **pontocerebellar t.**, trigonum pontocerebellare. **t. of Reil**, trigonum lemnisci. **submandibular t.**, trigonum submandibulare. **submental t.**, trigonum submentale. **urogenital t.**, diaphragma urogenitale. **vagal t., t. of**

vagus nerve, trigonum nervi vagi. **vesical t.,** trigonum vesicae.

trigonectomy (tri″gōn-ek'to-me) [trigone + Gr. *ektomē* excision] excision of the base of the bladder (trigonum vesicae).

trigonelline (trig″o-nel'in) an alkaloid, $C_7H_7NO_2$, found in fenugreek, cannabis, strophanthus, and various other plants, in sea urchins and jellyfish, and also in the urine after administration of nicotinic acid. It is a betaine of methyl nicotinic acid.

trigonid (tri-gon'id) the first three cusps of a lower molar tooth. See *hypoconid*, *paraconid*, and *protoconid*.

trigonitis (trig″o-ni'tis) [trigone + *-itis*] inflammation or localized hyperemia of the trigone of the bladder.

trigonocephalia (trig″o-no-sĕ-fa'le-ah) trigonocephaly.

trigonocephalic (trig″o-no-sĕ-fal'ik) pertaining to or characterized by trigonocephaly.

trigonocephalus (trig″o-no-sef'ah-lus) an individual exhibiting trigonocephaly.

trigonocephaly (tri-go″no-sef'ah-le) [Gr. *trigonos* triangular + *kephalē* head] a deformity of the head characterized by sharp angulation ventrad of the squamous portion of the frontal bones at the site of the suture between them.

trigonum (tri-go'num), pl. *trigo'na* [L.; Gr. *trigōnon* triangle] a three-cornered area; [NA] a general term for a triangular area. Called also *triangle* and *trigone*. **t. acus'tici**, area vestibularis. **t. carot'icum** [NA], carotid trigone: the triangular region bounded by the posterior belly of the digastric muscle, the sternocleidomastoid muscle, and the anterior midline of the neck; called also *carotid triangle, fossa carotica*, and *superior triangle*. **t. cerebra'le**, fornix cerebri. **t. cervica'le**, cervical triangle: any of the triangles of the neck; see *t. caroticum, t. musculare, t. omoclaviculare, t submandibulare*, and *t. submentale*. **t. cervica'le ante'rius**, NA alternative for *regio cervicalis anterior*. **t. cervica'le poste'rius**, NA alternative for *regio cervicalis lateralis*. **t. clavipectora'le** [NA], clavipectoral trigone: the triangular region separating the upper border of the pectoralis minor muscle from the clavicle, which contains the clavipectoral fascia; called also *clavipectoral triangle*. **t. collatera'le ventric'uli latera'le** [NA], collateral trigone of lateral ventricle; the triangular area in the floor of the lateral ventricle between the diverging temporal and occipital horns. **t. collatera'le ventric'uli quar'ti**, nervi vagi. **t. col'li latera'le**, regio cervicalis lateralis. **t. coracoacromia'le**, a triangle bounded by the coracoid process, the apex of the acromion, and the concave border of the clavicle. **t. deltoideopectora'le**, fossa infraclavicularis. **t. femora'le** [NA], femoral trigone: a triangular area bounded superiorly by the inguinal ligament, laterally by the sartorius muscle, and medially by the adductor longus muscle; called also *Scarpa's triangle*. **t. fibro'sum dex'trum cor'dis** [NA], right fibrous trigone of heart: a thickened, irregularly triangular portion of the fibrous skeleton of the base of the heart, located between the right and left atrioventricular fibrous rings, posterior to the aortic orifice. Called also *central fibrous body of heart*. **t. fibro'sum sinis'trum cor'dis** [NA], left fibrous trigone of heart: a thickened and irregularly triangular portion of the fibrous skeleton of the base of the heart, located between the left atrioventricular fibrous ring and the left posterior margin of the aortic fibrous ring. **t. haben'ulae** [NA], trigone of habenula: the small, depressed triangular area on the dorsomedial aspect of the posterior part of the thalamus which contains the habenular nuclei and marks the habenular commissure. Called also *habenular trigone* and *t. habenularis*. **t. habenula'ris**, NA alternative for *t. habenulae*. **t. hypoglossa'le**, NA alternative for *t. nervi hypoglossi*. **t. inguina'le** [NA], inguinal trigone: the area on the inferoanterior abdominal wall bounded by the rectus abdominis muscle, the inguinal ligament, and the inferior epigastric vessels: the site in which a direct inguinal hernia begins. **t. interpeduncula're**, fossa interpeduncularis. **t. lemnis'ci**, [NA], a small, more or less distinct triangular area on the side of the isthmus just lateral to the caudal colliculus, bounded below by the cranial cerebellar peduncle, dorsomedially by the brachium of the caudal colliculus, and ventrolaterally by the lateral sulcus of the mesencephalon. **t. lumba're** [NA], **t. lumba're** [Peti'ti], lumbar trigone: a small triangular interval between the inferolateral margin of the latissimus dorsi muscle and the external oblique muscle of the abdomen, just above the ilium; called also *Petit's triangle.* **t. lumbocosta′le,** a triangular opening of variable size between the lateral lumbocostal arch and the pars costalis diaphragmatis. **t. muscula′re** [NA], muscular trigone: the part of the trigonum caroticum medial to the omohyoid muscle; called also *t. omotracheale* [NA alternative], *inferior carotid triangle, muscular triangle,* and *omotracheal triangle.* **t. ner′vi hypoglos′si** [NA], trigone of hypoglossal nerve: the tapering lower end of the medial eminence of the rhomboid fossa just superficial to the position of the hypoglossal nucleus. Called also *hypoglossal trigone* and *t. hypoglossale* [NA alternative]. **t. ner′vi va′gi** [NA], trigone of vagus nerve: an area in the floor of the fourth ventricle immediately lateral to the trigonum nervi hypoglossi; beneath it lies the dorsal nucleus of the vagus nerve. Called also *ala cinerea, t. vagale* [NA alternative], and *vagal trigone.* **t. olfacto′rium** [NA], olfactory trigone: the area of the anterior perforated substance between the diverging lateral and medial olfactory striae, and bounded posteriorly by the diagonal band. **t. omoclavicula′re** [NA], omoclavicular trigone: a deep region of the neck, corresponding to the fossa supraclavicularis major on the surface, in which the brachial plexus may be palpated, and by downward pressure the subclavian artery can be compressed against the first rib; called also *subclavian triangle.* **t. omotrachea′le,** NA alternative for *t. musculare.* **t. pontocerebella′re** [NA], pontocerebellar trigone: the angular depression between the inferior border of the pons, the interior cerebellar peduncle, and the flocculus of the cerebellum. **t. sternocosta′le,** sternocostal triangle: a triangular opening between the pars costalis and the pars sternalis diaphragmatis; beyond this point the internal thoracic vessels become the superior epigastric vessels. Called also *Larrey's cleft.* **t. submandibula′re** [NA], submandibular trigone: the triangular region of the neck bounded by the mandible, the stylohyoid muscle and posterior belly of the digastric muscle, and the anterior belly of the digastric muscle; called also *regio submaxilaris.* **t. submenta′le** [NA], submental trigone: a triangle bounded on either side by the anterior belly of the digastric muscle and below by the hyoid bone; called also *submental triangle.* **t. urogenita′le,** diaphragma urogenitale. **t. vaga′le,** NA alternative for *t. nervi vagi.* **t. va′gi,** t. nervi vagi. **t. ventric′uli latera′lis,** t. collaterale. **t. vesi′cae** [NA], **t. vesi′cae** [Lieutau′di], trigone of bladder: a smooth triangular portion of the mucous membrane at the base of the bladder; it is bounded behind by the interureteric fold and ends in front in the uvula of the bladder.

trihexosylceramide galactosylhydrolase (tri-hek″so-sil-ser′ah-mīd gah-lak′to-sil-hi′dro-lās) ceramide trihexosidase.

trihexyphenidyl hydrochloride (tri-hek″se-fen′ĭ-dil) [USP] chemical name: α-cyclohexyl-α-phenyl-1-piperidinepropanol hydrochloride. An anticholinergic, $C_{20}H_{31}NO \cdot HCl$, occurring as a white or slightly off-white crystalline powder, having atropine-like actions; used as an oral antiparkinsonian agent.

trihybrid (tri-hi′brid) [tri- + *hybrid*] a hybrid offspring of parents differing in three mendelian characters.

trihydrate (tri-hi′drāt) trihydroxide; a compound containing three hydroxyl groups.

trihydric (tri-hi′drik) containing three hydrogen atoms that are replaceable by bases.

trihydrol (tri-hi′drol) the associated water or ice molecule, $(H_2O)_3$.

trihydroxide (tri″hi-drok′sīd) trihydrate.

trihydroxyestrin (tri″hi-drok″se-es′trin) estriol.

tri-iniodymus (tri″in-e-od′ĭ-mus) [tri- + Gr. *inion* nape of the neck + *didymos* twin] a monster with a single body and three heads united posteriorly.

triiodide (tri-i′o-dīd) a compound containing three atoms of iodine to one of another element.

triiodoethionic acid (tri-i″o-do-eth″e-on′ik) iophenoxic acid.

triiodomethane (tri-i″o-do-meth′ān) iodoform.

triiodothyronine (tri″i-o″do-thi′ro-nēn) L-3,5,3′-triiodothyronine, one of the thyroid hormones: an organic iodine-containing compound liberated from thyroglobulin by hydrolysis, and thought to be formed by the conjugation of

one molecule each of monoiodotyrosine and diiodotyrosine, and by the partial deiodination of thyroxine intrathyroidally and in the periphery. It has several times the biological activity of thyroxine and is thought by some to be the "tissue-active" form of thyroid hormone. Symbol T_3. **reverse t. (rT$_3$),** L-3,3′,5′-triiodothyronine, a thyroid principle detectable in human serum, having weak hormonal activity; mainly derived from peripheral diodination of thyroxine (q.v.), it is secreted in minute quantities by the thyroid. Serum values are elevated in thyrotoxicosis and low in myxedema.

triketohydrindene hydrate (tri-ke″to-hi-drin′dēn) chemical name: 1,2,3-indantrione monohydrate. A compound, $C_9H_4O_3 \cdot H_2O$, occurring as white to brownish white crystals or crystalline powder, used as a reagent. See under *tests.*

triketopurine (tri″ke-to-pu′rin) uric acid.

trilabe (tri′lāb) [tri- + Gr. *labē* a handle] a three-pronged instrument for taking calculi from the bladder.

Trilafon (tri′lah-fon) trademark for preparations of perphenazine.

trilaminar (tri-lam′ĭ-nar) consisting of three layers.

trilateral (tri-lat′er-al) [tri- + L. *latus* side] having or pertaining to three sides.

trilaurin (tri-law′rin) a crystalline glyceride, $C_3H_5(OC_{12}H_{23}O)_3$, forming the principal constituent of coconut oil, and found in bayberry oil and palm nut oil.

Trilene (tri′lēn) trademark for a preparation of trichloroethylene.

trilinolein (tri″lin-o′le-in) a glyceride, $C_3H_5(OC_{18}H_{32}O)_3$, found in linseed oil, hempseed oil, sunflower oil, etc.

Trilisate (tril′ĭ-sāt) trademark for choline magnesium trisalicylate.

trilliin (tril′e-in) a concentration prepared from *Trillium erectum* L. (Liliaceae), a North American plant.

Trillium (tril′e-um) a genus of liliaceous plants. **T. erec′tum** L., wake-robin; the rhizome contains trilliin.

trilobate (tri-lo′bāt) [tri- + L. *lobus* lobe] having three lobes.

trilobed (tri′lōbd) trilobate.

trilocular (tri-lok′u-lar) [tri- + L. *loculus* cell] having three compartments or cells.

trilogy (tril′o-je) a combination of three elements, such as three concurrent defects or symptoms. **t. of Fallot,** a term sometimes applied to the combination of pulmonic stenosis, atrial septal defect, and right ventricular hypertrophy.

trilostane (tri′lo-stān) chemical name: 4α,5-epoxy-17β-hydroxy-3-oxo-5α-androstane-2α-carbonitrile; an adrenocortical suppressant, $C_{20}H_{27}NO_3$.

trimastigote (tri-mas′tĭ-gōt) 1. having three flagella. 2. a cell having three flagella.

trimazosin hydrochloride (tri-ma′zo-sin) chemical name: 4-(4-amino-6,7,8-trimethoxy-2-quinazolinyl)-1-piperazine carboxylic acid 2-hydroxy-2-methylpropyl ester monohydrochloride monohydrate; an antihypertensive, $C_{20}H_{29}N_5O_6 \cdot HCl \cdot H_2O$.

trimedoxime (tri″mĕ-dok′sēm) a cholinesterase reactivator used for treatment of organophosphate poisoning. Available as *trimedoxime bromide.*

trimenon (tri-me′non) [tri- + Gr. *mēn* month + *on* neuter ending] trimester.

trimensual (tri-men′su-al) occurring every three months.

trimeprazine tartrate (tri-mep′rah-zēn) [USP] chemical name: *N,N,β*-trimethyl-10*H*-phenothiazine-10-propanamine [R-(R*,R*)]-2,3-dihydroxybutanedioate (2:1). A phenothiazine derivative, $(C_{18}H_{22}N_2S)_2 \cdot C_4H_6O_6$, occurring as a white to off-white, crystalline powder, having mild central nervous system depressant, moderate antiemetic and anticonvulsant properties, and powerful antihistaminic actions; used as an antipruritic, administered orally.

trimer (tri′mer) 1. a compound formed by combination of three identical simpler molecules. 2. a capsomere having three structural units.

trimercuric (tri″mer-ku′rik) containing three atoms of bivalent mercury.

Trimeresurus (trim″ĕ-rē-su′rus) a genus of venomous pit vipers of East and Southeast Asia, which are usually green and possess a prehensile tail. *T. flavorvi′ridis* is the habu.

trimeric (tri′mer-ik)   exhibiting the characteristics of a trimer.

trimester (tri-mes′ter)   a period of three months.

trimethadione (tri″meth-ah-di′ōn) [USP]   chemical name: 3,5,5-trimethyl-2,4-oxazolidinedione. An anticonvulsant with analgesic properties, $C_6H_9NO_3$, occurring as white, crystalline granules; used for the control of petit mal seizures, administered orally. In veterinary medicine, used as an anticonvulsant-analgesic for cats. Called also troxidone.

trimethaphan camsylate (tri-meth′ah-fan) [USP]   chemical name: decahydro-2-oxo-1,3-bis(phenylmethyl)-thieno[1′,2′:1,2]thieno[3,4]imidazol-5-ium salt with (±)-7-7-dimethyl-2-oxobicyclo[2.2.1]heptane-1-methanesulfonic acid (1:1). A short-acting ganglionic blocking agent with direct vasodilator action, $C_{32}H_{40}N_2O_5S_2$, occurring as white crystals or white, crystalline powder; used as an antihypertensive to produce controlled hypotension during surgery and for the emergency treatment of hypertensive crises and pulmonary edema due to hypertension, administered by intravenous infusion. Called also t. camphorsulfonate.

trimethidinium methosulfate (tri-meth″i-din′e-um)   chemical name: 1,3,8,8-tetramethyl-3-[3-(trimethylammonio) propyl]-3-azoniabicyclo[3.2.1]octane bis(methyl sulfate). A quaternary ammonium ganglion blocking agent, $C_{19}H_{46}N_2$-O_8S_2, occurring as a white, hygroscopic powder, used as an oral antihypertensive in the treatment of moderate to severe hypertension in certain patients.

trimethobenzamide hydrochloride (tri-meth″o-ben′-zah-mīd) [USP]   chemical name: N-[[4-[2-(dimethylamino)-oxy]phenyl]methyl]-3,4,5-trimethoxybenzamide monohydrochloride. An antiemetic, $C_{21}H_{28}N_2O_5 \cdot HCl$, occurring as a white, crystalline powder; administered orally, intramuscularly, or rectally.

trimethoprim (tri-meth′o-prim) [USP]   chemical name: 5-[3,4,5-trimethoxyphenyl)methyl]-2,4-pyrimidinediamine. An antibacterial, $C_{14}H_{18}N_4O_3$, closely related to the antimalarial pyrimethamine; administered orally, in combination with a sulfonamide because the two drugs markedly potentiate each other, in the treatment of urinary tract infections due to Escherichia coli, Klebsiella-Enterobacter group, Proteus vulgaris, P. mirabilis, and P. morganii, and in Pneumocystis carinii pneumonitis in children with reduced host defenses. In certain countries, it is used alone as an antimalarial.

trimethylamine (tri″meth-il-am′in)   a colorless gaseous (boiling point 3.2°–3.8° C.) tertiary amine, $(CH_3)_3N$, with an ammoniacal, fishy odor, from beet sugar residue and herring brine. In the body it probably results from the decomposition of choline; it has been reported in menstrual blood.

trimethylene (tri-meth′ĭ-lēn)   cyclopropane.

trimethylxanthine (tri-meth″il-zan′thin)   caffeine.

trimetozine (tri-met′o-zēn)   chemical name: 4-(3,4,5-trimethoxybenzoyl)morpholine; a sedative, $C_{14}H_{19}NO_5$.

trimipramine (tri-mip′rah-mēn)   chemical name: 10,11-dihydro-N,N,β-trimethyl-5H-dibenz[b,f]azepine-5-propanamine; a tricyclic antidepressant, $C_{20}H_{26}N_2$. **t. maleate,** the maleate salt of trimipramine, $C_{20}H_{26}N_2 \cdot C_4H_4O_4$, having the same actions as the base.

trimorphous (tri-mor′fus) [tri- + Gr. morphē form]   existing in three different forms.

trimopam maleate (tri′mo-pam)   chemical name: (+)-2,3,4,5-tetrahydro-7,8-dimethoxy-3-methyl-1-phenyl-1H-3-benzazepine (Z)-2-butenedioate (1:1); a tranquilizer, $C_{19}H_{23}$-$NO_2 \cdot C_4H_4O_4$.

trinegative (tri-neg′ah-tiv)   having three negative valences or charges.

trineural (tri-nu′ral)   pertaining to three nerves.

trineuric (tri-nu′rik)   pertaining to or having three neurons.

trinitrate (tri-ni′trāt)   a nitrate which contains three radicals of nitric acid, as glycerol trinitrate.

trinitrin (tri-ni′trin)   nitroglycerin.

trinitrocellulose (tri″ni-tro-sel′u-lōs)   pyroxylin.

trinitrocresol (tri″ni-tro-kre′sol)   an antiseptic and highly explosive compound, $(NO_2)_3C_6H(CH_3)OH$, formed by the action of concentrated nitric acid on coal tar cresol.

trinitroglycerin (tri-ni″tro-glis′er-in)   nitroglycerin.

trinitroglycerol (tri-ni′tro-glis′er-ol)   nitroglycerin.

trinitrophenol (tri″ni-tro-fe′nol)   a yellow, crystalline, bitter-tasting substance, $C_6H_2(NO_2)_3OH$, sparingly soluble in water; it is used as a dye and a tissue fixative and as an antiseptic, astringent, and stimulant of epithelialization. It can be detonated by percussion or heating above 300° C. Called also carbazotic, nitroxanthic, picric, and picronitric acid.

trinitrotoluene (tri″ni-tro-tol′u-ēn)   a high explosive, C_6-$H_2(NO_2)_3CH_3$, obtained by nitrating toluene; called also TNT.

trinomial (tri-no′me-al) [tri- + L. nomen name]   composed of three names or terms.

trinucleate (tri-nu′kle-āt)   having three nuclei.

trinucleotide (tri-nu′kle-o-tīd)   a polymer made up of three mononucleotides.

triocephalus (tri″o-sef′ah-lus) [tri- + Gr. kephalē head]   a monster in which the structures of the mouth, nose, and eyes are wanting, the head being nearly a shapeless mass.

Triodontophorus diminutus (tri″o-don-tof′o-rus dim-ĭ-nu′tus)   Territans diminutus.

triolein (tri-o′le-in)   olein.

triolism (tri′o-lizm)   sexual interests or practices involving three persons, two of one sex and one of the opposite sex.

triophthalmos (tri″of-thal′mos) [tri- + Gr. ophthalmos eye]   a double-faced monster with three eyes.

triopodymus (tri″o-pod′ĭ-mus) [tri- + Gr. ops face + didymos twin]   a monster having a fused head with three faces.

triorchid (tri-or′kid) [tri- + Gr. orchis testis]   an individual with three testes.

triorchidism (tri-or′kĭ-dizm)   the condition of having three testes.

triorchis (tri-or′kis)   triorchid.

triorchism (tri-or′kizm)   triorchidism.

triose (tri′ōs)   a monosaccharide containing three carbon atoms in a molecule.

triosephosphate dehydrogenase (tri′ōs fos′fāt de-hi′-dro-jen-ās)   glyceraldehyde-3-phosphate dehydrogenase.

triosephosphate isomerase (trī″ōs-fos′fāt i-som′er-ās) [EC 5.3.1.1]   an enzyme of the isomerase class that catalyzes the reaction D-glyceraldehyde 3-phosphate = dihydroxyacetone phosphate in the Embden-Meyerhof pathway. Deficiency of the enzyme, an autosomal recessive trait, causes hemolytic anemia, neuromuscular dysfunction, and susceptibility to infection.

triotus (tri-o′tus) [tri- + Gr. ous ear]   an individual with a supernumerary ear.

trioxide (tri-ok′sīd)   a compound containing three atoms of oxygen to one of another element.

trioxsalen (tri-ok′sah-len) [USP]   chemical name: 2,5,9-trimethyl-7H-furo[3.2-g][1]benzopyran-7-one. A synthetic psoralen, $C_{14}H_{12}O_3$, used orally in conjunction with exposure to ultraviolet light to facilitate repigmentation in vitiligo, and also as a suntan accelerator and sun protectant.

trioxypurine (tri″ok-se-pu′rin)   uric acid.

tripalmitin (tri-pal′mĭ-tin)   palmitin.

tripara (trip′ah-rah) [tri- + L. parere to bring forth, produce]   a woman who has had three pregnancies which resulted in viable offspring; also written para III.

triparanol (tri-par′ah-nol)   chemical name: 1-[p-(2-diethylaminoethoxy)phenyl]-1-(p-tolyl)-2-(p-chlorophenyl)ethanol. A crystalline substance, $C_{27}H_{32}ClNO_2$, formerly used as a cholesterol biosynthesis inhibitor but withdrawn from the market because of association with irreversible cataracts, baldness, and impotence.

tripartite (tri-par′tīt)   having three parts.

tripelennamine (tri″pĕ-len′ah-min)   chemical name: N,N-dimethyl-N′-(phenylmethyl)-N′-2-pyridinyl-1,2-ethanediamine. A histamine antagonist, $C_{16}H_{21}N_3$. **t. citrate** [USP], the citrate salt of tripelennamine, $C_{16}H_{21}N_3 \cdot C_6H_8O_7$, occurring as a white, crystalline powder; used as antihistaminic in the symptomatic treatment of allergic disorders, administered orally. **t. hydrochloride** [USP], the monohydrochloride salt of tripelennamine, $C_{16}H_{21}N_3 \cdot HCl$, have the same appearance, actions, and uses as the citrate salt; administered orally, parenterally, and topically.

tripeptide (tri-pep′tid)   a peptide which on hydrolysis yields three amino acids.

Triperidol (tri-per′ĭ-dol) trademark for a preparation of trifluperidol.

triphalangeal (tri″fah-lan′je-al) pertaining to or characterized by triphalangia.

triphalangia (tri″fah-lan′je-ah) triphalangism.

triphalangism (tri-fal′an-jizm) the presence of three phalanges in the longitudinal axis of a digit normally composed of only two.

triphasic (tri-fa′zik) [tri- + Gr. phasis phase] triply varied or triply phasic; used in describing the electromotive actions of muscles. Cf. diphasic and monophasic.

triphenylethylene (tri-fen″il-eth′i-len) a synthetic estrogen, $C_{20}H_{16}$ (alpha-phenyl-stilbene), not related to naturally occurring estrogens with the phenanthrene nucleus.

triphenylmethane (tri-fen″il-meth′ān) a substance from coal tar, $(C_6H_5)_3CH$, the basis of various dyes and stains, including aurin, rosaniline, basic fuchsin, and gentian violet.

triphosphate (tri-fos′fāt) a salt containing three phosphate radicals.

triphosphopyridine nucleotide (tri-fos″fo-pir′ĭ-dēn) TPN; former name for nicotinamide-adenine dinucleotide phosphate (NADP).

triphthemia (trif-the′me-ah) [Gr. tribein to wear out + haima blood + -ia] the retention of waste products in the blood.

Tripier's amputation (trip″e-āz) [Léon Tripier, French surgeon, 1842–1891] see under amputation.

triple-angle (trip′l ang′g′l) having three angles; a dental instrument having three angulations in the shank connecting the handle, or shaft, with the working portion of the instrument, known as the blade, or nib. Cf. binangle, monangle, and quadrangle (def. 2).

triple blind (trip′l blind) pertaining to a clinical trial or other experiment in which neither the subject nor the person administering treatment nor the person evaluating the response to treatment knows which treatment any particular subject is receiving.

triplegia (tri-ple′je-ah) [tri- + Gr. plēgē stroke] paralysis of three of the extremities.

triplet (trip′let) 1. one of three individuals having coextensive gestation periods and produced at the same birth. 2. a combination of three objects or entities occurring or acting together, as three lenses constituting a microscope eyepiece or objective. 3. codon.

triplex (tri′pleks) [Gr. triploos triple] triple or three-fold.

triploblastic (trip″lo-blas′tik) [Gr. triploos triple + blastos germ] having three germ layers or blastodermic membranes; said of an embryo.

triploid (trip′loid) 1. pertaining to or characterized by triploidy. 2. an individual or cell having three sets of chromosomes.

triploidy (trip′loi-de) the presence in humans of 69 chromosomes, or three full sets, a frequent finding in abortuses.

triplokoria (trip″lo-ko′re-ah) [Gr. triploos triple + korē pupil + -ia] the presence of three pupils in one eye.

triplopia (trip-lo′pe-ah) [Gr. triploos triple + -opia] the perception of three images of a single object; triple vision.

tripod (tri′pod) [Gr. treis three + pous foot] anything having three feet or supports. **Haller's t.,** truncus celiacus. **t. of life, vital t.,** the brain, heart, and lungs regarded as the triple support of life.

tripodia (tri-po′de-ah) [Gr. treis three + pous foot] a type of symmelia characterized by the presence of three feet.

tripoding (tri′pod-ing) the use of three points of support, as adopted by paralyzed patients when changing from a sitting or standing position. See also tripod position, under position.

tripoli (trip′o-le) [Tripoli, Libya] a granulated porous siliceous rock originally mined in North Africa and presently produced from silica; used as a dental polishing agent.

tripositive (tri-pos′ĭ-tiv) having three positive valences or charges.

triprolidine hydrochloride (tri-pro′lĭ-dēn) [USP] chemical name: (E)-2-[1-(4-methylphenyl)-3-(1-pyrrolidinyl)-1-propenyl]pyridine monohydrochloride monohydrate. An antihistaminic, $C_{19}H_{22}N_2 \cdot HCl \cdot H_2O$, occurring as a white, crystalline powder; used in the treatment of various

allergic conditions and their manifestations, administered orally.

triprosopus (tri″pro-so′pus) [Gr. treis three + prosōpon face] a monster having a triple face.

tripsis (trip′sis) [Gr. tripsis rubbing] 1. a trituration; the process of trituration. 2. the act of shampooing or of massage.

-tripsy [Gr. tripsis a rubbing, friction] a word termination designating a surgical procedure in which a structure is intentionally crushed.

triptokoria (trip″to-ko′re-ah) triplokoria.

tripus (tri′pus) [Gr. treis three + pous foot] 1. a tripod. 2. a conjoined twin monster having three feet. **t. hal′leri,** truncus celiacus.

triquetrous (tri-kwe′trus) [L. triquetrus] triangular; three cornered.

triquetrum (tri-kwe′trum) [L.] three cornered; see os triquetrum.

triradial, triradiate (tri-ra′de-al; tri-ra′de-āt) [tri- + L. radiatus rayed] having three rays; radiating in three directions.

triradiation (tri″ra-de-a′shun) radiation in three directions.

TRIS tris(hydroxymethyl)aminomethane; see tromethamine.

trisaccharide (tri-sak′ah-rid) a carbohydrate, $C_{18}H_{32}O_{16}$, composed of three saccharide groups.

tris(hydroxymethyl)-aminomethane (tris″hi-drok″se-meth″il-am″ĭ-no-meth′ān) tromethamine.

trismic (triz′mik) of the nature of or pertaining to trismus.

trismus (triz′mus) [Gr. trismos grating, grinding] motor disturbance of the trigeminal nerve, especially spasm of the masticatory muscles, with difficulty in opening the mouth; a characteristic early symptom of tetanus. Called also lockjaw.

trisnitrate (tris-ni′trāt) trinitrate.

trisomia (tri-so′me-ah) trisomy.

trisomic (tri-so′mik) pertaining to or characterized by trisomy.

trisomy (tri′so-me) [tri + Gr. sōma body] the presence of an extra chromosome of one type in an otherwise diploid cell (2n +1): trisomy 13 results in trisomy 13 syndrome; trisomy 18 results in trisomy 18 syndrome; trisomy 21 results in Down syndrome. See these anomalies under syndrome.

Trisoralen (tri-sor′ah-len) trademark for a preparation of trioxsalen.

trisplanchnic (tri-splangk′nik) [Gr. treis three + splanchna viscera] pertaining to or supplying the three great body cavities and their viscera.

tristearin (tri-ste′ah-rin) a white, crystalline fat, glyceryl tristearate, $C_3H_5(C_{18}H_{35}O_2)_3$, found in the harder fats, such as tallow; called also stearin.

tristichia (tri-stik′e-ah) [Gr. treis three + stichos row] the existence of three rows of eyelashes.

trisubstituted (tri-sub′stĭ-tūt″ed) having three molecules or atoms replaced by three other molecules or atoms.

trisulcate (tri-sul′kāt) having three furrows.

trisulfapyrimidines (tri-sul″fah-pi-rim″ĭ-dēnz) preparations containing a mixture of the sulfonamides sulfadiazine, sulfamerazine, and sulfamethazine.

trisulfate (tri-sul′fāt) a binary compound containing three sulfate (SO_4) groups in the molecule.

trisulfide (tri-sul′fīd) a sulfur compound containing three atoms of sulfur to one of the base.

Trit. abbreviation for L. tri′tura, triturate.

tritan (tri′tan) 1. pertaining to tritanomaly or tritanopia. 2. a person with tritanomaly or tritanopia.

tritanomal (tri″tah-nom′al) a person with tritanomaly.

tritanomalous (tri″tah-nom′ah-lus) pertaining to or characterized by tritanomaly.

tritanomaly (tri″tah-nom′ahle) [Gr. tritos third + anomaly] a very rare anomalous trichromasy in which the third, blue-sensitive, cones have decreased sensitivity; therefore a greater than normal proportion of blue light to green light is required to match a blue-green stimulus. Tritanomaly is an X-linked trait and occurs in about 0.0001 per cent of white males; it is therefore of little clinical importance.

tritanope (tri′tah-nōp″)   an individual exhibiting tritanopia.

tritanopia (tri″tah-no′pe-ah) [Gr. *tritos* third + *an-* neg. + *-opia*] a rare dichromasy characterized by retention of the sensory mechanism for two hues only (red and green) of the normal 4-primary quota, and lacking blue and yellow, with loss of luminance and shift of brightness and hue curves toward the long-wave end of the spectrum. Often associated with drug administration, retinal detachment, or diseases of the nervous system.

tritanopic (tri″tah-nop′ik)   pertaining to or characterized by tritanopia.

tritanopsia (tri″tah-nop′se-ah)   tritanopia.

tritiate (trit′e-āt)   to treat with tritium.

triticeous (tri-tish′us) [L. *triticeus*] resembling a grain of wheat.

triticeum (tri-tis′e-um) [L.] cartilago triticea.

triticin (trit′ĭ-sin) a fructose polysaccharide, $(C_6H_{10}O_5)_n$, which occurs in the rhizome of couch grass, *Agropyron repens* (L.) Beauv. (Gramineae).

Triticum (trit′ĭ-kum) [L.] a genus of grasses, including wheat. *T. (Agropyron) repens* (L.) Beauv., or couch grass, is diuretic; formerly used in the treatment of cystitis and as a nutritive agent in the form of a decoction.

triticum (trit′ĭ-kum) the dried rhizome and roots of couch grass, *Agropyron (Triticum) repens* (L.) Beauv. (Gramineae), which has diuretic properties, and was formerly used in the treatment of cystitis; it was also used as a nutritive agent in the form of a decoction. Called also *agropyrum*.

tritium (trit′e-um, trish′e-um) [Gr. *tritos* third] the mass three isotope of hydrogen, ³H, a radioactive gas obtained by bombardment of beryllium in the cyclotron with deuterium ions. It has a half-life of about 31 years and is used as an indicator or tracer in metabolic studies. Cf. *deuterium* and *protium*.

tritol (tri′tol) any emulsion of the extract of filix mas with the diastasic extract of malt.

triton (tri′ton) trinitrotoluene.

tritotoxin (tri″to-tok′sin) *(obs.)* a toxin which unites less easily with the antitoxin than the prototoxin and deuterotoxin. See *deuterotoxin, hemotoxin, heterotoxin, prototoxin*.

Tritrichomonas (tri″trik-o-mo′nas, tri″trik-o-mon′as) [*tri-* + *tricho-* + Gr. *monas* unit, from *monos* single] in some systems of classification, a genus established to include the species of *Trichomonas* having three anterior flagella, i.e., *T. foetus*.

triturable (trich′er-ah-bel) susceptible of being triturated.

triturate (trich′ĕ-rāt) 1. to rub to a powder. 2. a triturated substance.

trituration (trich″ĕ-ra′shun) [L. *tritura* the treading out of corn] 1. the reduction of solid bodies to a powder by continuous rubbing. 2. a triturated drug, especially one rubbed up with milk sugar. 3. the creation of a homogeneous whole by mixing, as the combining of particles of an alloy with mercury to form dental amalgam; called also *amalgamation*.

triturator (trit′u-ra′tor) an apparatus in which substances can be continuously rubbed, as in the process of amalgamating an alloy with mercury.

trivalence (triv′ah-lens) the condition or quality of being trivalent.

trivalent (triv′ah-lent) [*tri-* + L. *valens* powerful] having a valence of three.

trivalve (tri′valv) having three valves or three blades, as a speculum.

trizonal (tri-zo′nal) arranged in three zones.

tRNA transfer-RNA; see *ribonucleic acid*, under *acid*.

Trobicin (tro-bi′sin) trademark for a preparation of spectinomycin hydrochloride.

trocar (tro′kar) [Fr. *trois quarts* three quarters] a sharp-pointed instrument equipped with a cannula, used to puncture the wall of a body cavity and withdraw fluid.

troch. trochiscus.

trochanter (tro-kan′ter) [L.; Gr. *trochantēr*] either of the two processes below the neck of the femur. **greater t.,** t. major. **lesser t.,** t. minor. **t. ma′jor** [NA], greater trochanter: a broad, flat process at the upper end of the lateral

surface of the femur, to which several muscles are attached. **t. mi′nor** [NA], lesser trochanter: a short conical process projecting medially from the lower part of the posterior border of the base of the neck of the femur. **rudimentary t.,** t. tertius. **small t.,** t. minor. **t. ter′tius** [NA], **third t.,** a term applied to the gluteal tuberosity of the femur when it is unusually prominent.

trochanterian (tro″kan-ter′e-an) trochanteric.

trochanteric (tro″kan-ter′ik) pertaining to a trochanter.

trochanterplasty (tro-kan′ter-plas″te) surgical excision of a ridge of bone to form a new femoral neck.

trochantin (tro-kan′tin) trochanter minor.

trochantinian (tro″kan-tin′e-an) pertaining to the lesser trochanter.

troche (tro′ke) [Gr. *trochos* a round cake] a small circular or oblong tablet usually for solution in the mouth, especially for medication of the throat, consisting of an active ingredient incorporated in a mass made up of sugar and mucilage or fruit base, and air dried. Called also *lozenge, morsulus, rotula,* and *trochiscus*.

trochin (tro′kin) [L. *trochinus*] tuberculum minus humeri.

trochiscus (tro-kis′kus) pl. *trochis′chi* [L.; Gr. *trochiskos*, dim. of *trochos*, a small wheel or disk] a medicated tablet; a troche.

trochiter (trok′ĭ-ter) 1. trochanter major. 2. tuberculum majus humeri.

trochiterian (trok″ĭ-te′re-an) pertaining to the trochiter.

trochlea (trok′le-ah), pl. *troch′leae* [L.; Gr. *trochilia* pulley] a pulley-shaped part or structure; [NA] a general term for such a structure. **t. fibula′ris calca′nei,** NA alternative for *t. peronealis calcanei*. **t. hu′meri** [NA], **t. of humerus,** the pulley-like medial portion of the distal end of the humerus for articulation with the semilunar notch of the ulna; called also *trochlear eminence*. **t. labyrin′thi,** cochlea, def. 2. **muscular t., t. muscula′ris** [NA], an anatomical part that serves to change the direction of pull of a tendon; it may be fibrous or bony. **t. mus′culi obli′qui superio′ris bul′bi** [NA], **t. mus′culi obli′qui superio′ris o′culi,** the fibrocartilaginous pulley near the internal angular process of the frontal bone, through which the tendon of the superior oblique muscle of the eyeball passes; called also *t. of superior oblique muscle*. **peroneal t. of calcaneus, t. peronea′lis calca′nei** [NA], a small eminence on the lateral surface of the calcaneus, separating the tendons of the peroneus brevis and longus muscles; called also *processus trochlearis calcanei* and *t. fibularis calcanei* [NA alternative]. **t. phalan′gis digito′rum ma′nus,** NA alternative for *caput phalangis digitorum manus*. **t. phalan′gis digito′rum pe′dis,** caput phalangis digitorum pedis. **t. of superior oblique muscle,** t. musculi obliqui superioris bulbi. **t. ta′li** [NA], **t. of talus,** the surface of the talus for articulation with the tibia and fibula.

trochlear (trok′le-ar) [L. *trochlearis*] 1. of the nature of or resembling a pulley. 2. pertaining to a trochlea.

trochleariform (trok″le-ar′ĭ-form) pulley-shaped.

trochlearis (trok″le-a′ris) [L.] trochlear.

trochocephalia (tro″ko-sĕ-fa′le-ah) trochocephaly.

trochocephaly (tro″ko-sef′ah-le) [Gr. *trochos* wheel + *kephalē* head] a rounded appearance of the head caused by synostosis of the frontal and parietal bones.

trochoid (tro′koid) [Gr. *trochos* wheel + *eidos* form] resembling a pivot or a pulley.

trochoides (tro-koi′dēz) [Gr. *trochoeidēs*, from *trochos* wheel + *eidos* form] articulatio trochoidea.

trochophore (tro′ko-fōr) [Gr. *trochos* wheel + *phoros* bearing] the pear- or top-shaped larva of certain mollusks and annelids that bears a girdle of cilia (prototroch).

Trocinate (tro′sĭ-nāt) trademark for a preparation of thiphenamil hydrochloride.

Troglotrema (trog″lo-tre′mah) a genus of flukes. **T. salmin′cola,** a parasite found in the kidney and under the skin of various fish, especially salmon and trout, and which serves as a vector of *Neorickettsia helminthoeca*, the etiologic agent of salmon poisoning (q.v.). It is transmitted to man, dogs, cats, foxes, bears, mink, hogs, and other animals by the ingestion of raw, infected fish. Called also *Nanophyetus salmincola*.

troilism (troi′lizm) [Fr. *trois* three] triolism.

Troisier's ganglion, node, sign, syndrome (trwah-ze-āz′) [Charles Emile *Troisier*, French physician, 1844–1919] see under *ganglion*, *sign*, and *syndrome*, and see *sentinel node*, under *node*.

trolamine (tro′lah-mēn) 1. [NF] chemical name: 2,2′,2″-nitrilotrisethanal. A mixture of alkanolamines, $C_6H_{15}NO_3$, consisting largely of triethanolamine and containing some di- and monoethanolamine; used as an alkalizing agent in pharmaceutical preparations. Called also *triethanolamine*. 2. USAN contraction for triethanolamine.

troland (tro′land) [for Leonard Thompson *Troland*, American psychologist and physicist, 1889–1932] the retinal illuminance produced by the image of an object the luminance of which is 1 lumen per square meter for an area of the entrance pupil of 1 square millimeter.

Trolard's plexus (net), vein (tro-lardz′) [Paulin *Trolard*, French anatomist, 1842–1910] see *plexus venosus canalis* and *vena anastomotica inferior*.

troleandomycin (tro″le-an-do-mi′sin) the triacetyl ester of oleandomycin, $C_{41}H_{67}NO_{14}$, occurring as a white, odorless powder; used as an antibacterial, chiefly in the treatment of infections due to staphylococci and other gram-positive bacteria resistant to other systemic antibiotics, administered orally. Called also *triacetyloleandomycin*.

trolnitrate phosphate (trol-ni′trāt) chemical name: 2,2′2″-nitrilotrisethanol trinitrate (ester) phosphate (1:2) (salt). An organic nitrate, $C_6H_{12}N_4O_9$, occurring as a white, crystalline powder, having vasodilating actions; used to reduce the frequency and severity of anginal attacks, administered orally.

Tröltsch's corpuscles, recesses (spaces) (trel′ches) [Anton Friedrich von *Tröltsch*, German otologist, 1829–1890] see under *corpuscle*, and see *recessus membranae tympani anterior* and *recessus membranae tympani posterior*.

Trombicula (trom-bik′u-lah) a genus of acarine mites of the family Trombiculidae. **T. akamu′shi,** the kedani mite, whose larvae (chiggers) transmit *Rickettsia tsutsuga-*

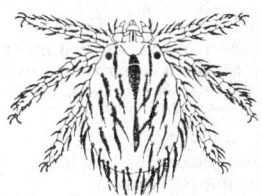

Trombicula akamushi.

mushi, the etiologic agent of scrub typhus; it is the chief vector in Japan. Called also *Microtrombidium akamushi*. **T. alfreddugè′si,** *Eutrombicula alfreddugèsi*; see also under *chigger*. **T. autumna′lis,** the autumnal chigger of Europe whose larvae cause lesions of the skin in man and animals; formerly called *Leptus autumnalis*. **T. delien′-sis,** a species whose larvae transmit *Rickettsia tsutsugamushi,* the etiologic agent of scrub typhus; it is believed to be the chief vector outside of Japan. **T. fletch′eri,** a carrier of *Rickettsia tsutsugamushi,* the causative agent of scrub typhus. **T. holoseri′ceum,** *T. autumnalis*. **T. interme′dia,** a carrier of *Rickettsia tsutsugamushi,* the causative agent of scrub typhus. **T. ir′ritans,** *Eutrombicula alfreddugèsi*. **T. mus′cae domes′ticae,** a red acarid parasite on the housefly. **T. musca′rum,** *T. muscae domesticae*. **T. pal′lida,** a carrier of *Rickettsia tsutsugamushi,* the causative agent of scrub typhus. **T. scutella′ris,** a carrier of *Rickettsia tsutsugamushi,* the causative agent of scrub typhus. **T. tsalsahua′tl,** *Eutrombicula alfreddugèsi*.

trombiculiasis (trom-bik″u-li′ah-sis) infestation with *Trombicula*.

Trombiculidae (trom-bik′u-li″de) a family of mites which is cosmopolitan in distribution, ranging from Alaska and Labrador to New Zealand, and from sea level to an altitude of more than 16,000 feet in the Andes. The parasitic larvae of the mites infest vertebrates. The single genus of medical significance is *Trombicula*, with subgenera *Eutrombicula* and *Leptotrombidium*.

trombidiiasis (trom-bid″e-i′ah-sis) trombiculiasis.

trombidiosis (trom-bid″e-o′sis) trombiculiasis.

Trombidium (trom-bid′e-um) a name formerly given a genus of mites, now included in the genus *Trombicula*.

tromethamine (tro-meth′ah-mēn) [USP] chemical name: 2-amino-2-(hydromethyl)-1,3-propanediol. An amine base, $C_4H_{11}NO_3$, occurring as a white crystalline powder; used intravenously as an alkalizer for the correction of metabolic acidosis. Called also *THAM, TRIS* and *tris(hydroxymethyl)-aminomethane*.

Trommer's test (trom′erz) [Karl August *Trommer*, German chemist, 1806–1879] see under *tests*.

Trömner's sign (Ernest L. O. *Trömner*, German neurologist, 1868–1949] Hoffmann's sign, def. 2.

tromomania (trom″o-ma′ne-ah) [Gr. *tromos* trembling + Gr. *mania* madness] delirium tremens.

tromophonia (trom″o-fo′ne-ah) a form of dysphonia characterized by a tremulous voice.

trona (tro′nah) [possible anagram of *natron*] a crude sodium salt.

tronchado (tron-kah′do) a name in Central America and Mexico for a fatal paralytic disease in cattle.

Tronothane (tron′o-thān) trademark for preparations of pramoxine.

tropate (tro′pāt) a salt of tropic acid.

tropesis (tro-pe′sis) [Gr. *tropos* a turning] Haekel's term for the tendency to action shown by every substance.

trophectoderm (trof-ek′to-derm) [*tropho-* + *ectoderm*] the outer layer of cells of the early blastodermic vesicle; the earliest trophoblast.

trophedema (trof″ĕ-de′mah) [*tropho-* + *edema*] a disease marked by permanent edema of the feet or legs. **congenital t., hereditary t.,** Milroy's disease.

trophesial, trophesic (tro-fe′ze-al; tro-fe′sik) pertaining to or characterized by trophesy.

trophesy (trof′ĕ-se) defective nutrition due to disorder of the trophic nerves.

trophic (trof′ik) [Gr. *trophikos*] of or pertaining to nutrition.

-trophic, -trophin [Gr. *trophikos* nourishing] word terminations denoting relationship to nutrition.

trophicity (tro-fis′ĭ-te) a trophic function or relation.

-trophin see *-tropin*.

trophism (trof′izm) direct trophic influence.

troph(o)- [Gr. *trophē* nutrition] a combining form denoting relationship to food or nourishment.

trophoblast (trof′o-blast) [*tropho-* + Gr. *blastos* germ] a layer of extraembryonic ectodermal tissue on the outside of the blastocyst. It attaches the ovum to the uterine wall and supplies nutrition to the embryo. From it are derived the chorion and amnion. The inner cellular layer of the trophoblast covering a chorionic villus is called *cytotrophoblast* and its outer syncytial layer *syncytiotrophoblast*. The mesoblast, once thought to be trophoblastic, is now traced, in primates, to the caudal end of the primitive streak.

trophoblastic (trof″o-blas′tik) pertaining to the trophoblast.

trophoblastoma (trof″o-blas-to′mah) choriocarcinoma.

trophochromatin (trof″o-kro′mah-tin) trophochromidia.

trophochromidia (trof″o-kro-mid′e-ah) chromatin concerned with the nutrition of the cell rather than with reproduction. Cf. *idiochromidia*.

trophocyte (trof′o-sīt) a lower type of cell which furnishes nourishment to a higher type of cell of a tissue. Cf. *trophospongium* (def. 1).

trophoderm (trof′o-derm) [*tropho-* + Gr. *derma* skin] trophoblast.

trophodermatoneurosis (trof″o-der″mah-to-nu-ro′sis) acrodynia.

trophodynamics (trof″o-di-nam′iks) the study of the forces engaged in nutrition.

trophoedema (trof″o-ĕ-de′mah) trophedema.

tropholecithal (trof″o-les′ĭ-thal) pertaining to the tropholecithus.

tropholecithus (trof″o-les′ĭ-thus) [*tropho-* + Gr. *lekithos* yolk] the food yolk of a meroblastic egg.

trophology (tro-fol′o-je)   the science of nutrition of the body.

trophon (trof′on)   the nutritive non-neural element of the neuron.

trophoneurosis (trof″o-nu-ro′sis)   any functional nervous disease due to the failure of nutrition from defective nerve influence. **facial t.,** facial hemiatrophy. **lingual t.,** progressive hemiatrophy of the tongue. **muscular t.,** trophic alteration of muscular tissue, dependent on nervous derangement. **t. of Romberg,** facial hemiatrophy.

trophoneurotic (trof″o-nu-rot′ik)   pertaining to or of the nature of a trophoneurosis.

trophonosis (trof″o-no′sis) [*tropho-* + Gr. *nosos* disease] any disease or disorder due to nutritional causes.

trophont (tro′font) [*troph-* + Gr. *on, ontos* being]   the active, motile, feeding stage or form in the life cycle of certain ciliate protozoa, especially that produced by a tomite and developing into a theront. Cf. *trophozoite.*

trophonucleus (trof″o-nu′kle-us)   macronucleus.

trophopathia (trof″o-path′e-ah)   trophopathy.

trophopathy (tro-fop′ah-the) [*tropho-* + Gr. *pathos* disease] any derangement of nutrition.

trophoplast (trof′o-plast) [*tropho-* + Gr. *plastos* formed]   a granular protoplasmic body; a plastid.

trophospongia (trof″o-spon′je-ah)   plural of *trophospongium.*

trophospongium (trof″o-spon′je-um), pl. *trophospon′gia* [*tropho-* + Gr. *spongion* sponge] 1. a canalicular network in the cytoplasm of certain cells which was once believed to be instrumental in the circulation of nutritive material. 2. (pl.) the vascular endometrium between the myometrium and the trophoblast.

trophotaxis (tro″fo-tak′sis) [*tropho-* + *taxis*]   chemotaxis of an organism in response to nutritive material.

trophotherapy (trof″o-ther′ah-pe)   treatment of disease by dietetic measures.

trophotropism (tro″fo-tro′pizm) [*tropho-* + *tropism*]   chemotropism of an organism in response to nutritive material.

trophozoite (trof″o-zo′īt) [*tropho-* + Gr. *zōon* animal]   the active, motile, feeding stage of a protozoan organism, as contrasted with the nonmotile encysted stage. In the malarial parasite, it is the stage between the merozoite and the mature schizont. Trophozoites of *Toxoplasma gondii* (tachyzoites) are found in the tissues during the acute stage of toxoplasmosis. Cf. *trophont.*

-trophy [Gr. *trophē* nutrition]   a word termination denoting food or nutrition.

tropia (tro′pe-ah) [Gr. *tropē* a turning]   a manifest deviation of an eye from the normal position when both eyes are open and uncovered; strabismus, or squint. See *cyclotropia, esotropia, exotropia, hypertropia,* and *hypotropia.*

-tropic [Gr. *tropikos* turning]   a word termination denoting turning toward, changing, or tending to turn or change; see *tropism.*

tropic acid (tro′pik)   2-phenyl-3-hydroxypropanoic acid, a constituent of atropine and scopolamine.

tropical (trop′e-kal) [Gr. *tropikos* turning]   pertaining to the regions of the earth bounded by the parallels of latitude 23° 27′ north and south of the equator.

tropicamide (tro-pik′ah-mīd) [USP]   chemical name: *N*-ethyl-α-(hydroxymethyl)-*N*-(4-pyridenylmethyl)benzene acetamide. An anticholinergic, $C_{17}H_{20}N_2O_2$, occurring as a white to practically white, crystalline powder, applied topically to the conjunctiva to produce mydriasis and cycloplegia.

tropidine (trop′ĭ-din)   an oily, liquid base, $CH_3 \cdot N:C_6H_9:CH$, with an odor like that of coniine, formed by the dehydration of tropine.

tropin (tro′pin)   opsonin.

-tropin [Gr. *tropos* a turning]   a word termination denoting an affinity for the structure or thing indicated by the stem to which it is affixed, as gonadotropin.

tropine (tro′pin)   a crystalline alkaloid, $C_8H_{15}NO$, with a smell like tobacco, derivable from atropine and from various plants.

tropism (tro′pizm) [Gr. *tropē* a turn, turning]   the turning, bending, movement, or growth of an organism or part of an organism in response to an external stimulus. Such response may be either positive (toward) or negative (away from the stimulus). By extension, used as a word termination affixed to a stem denoting the nature of the stimulus (phototropism) or the material or entity for which an organism or substance shows a special affinity (neurotropism), usually applied to nonmotile organisms. Cf. *taxis,* def. 1.

tropochrome (tro′po-krōm″) [*tropo-* + Gr. *chrōma* color] refusing to stain with mucin stains after formol-bichromate fixation, as applied to certain serous cells of the salivary nonmotile organisms. Cf. *taxis,* def. 1.

tropocollagen (tro″po-kol′ah-jen) [Gr. *tropē* a turning + *collagen*]   the molecular unit of collagen fibrils, about 1.4 nm. wide and 280 nm. long. It is a helical structure consisting of three polypeptide chains, each chain composed of about a thousand amino acids coiled around each other to form a spiral; tropocollagen is rich in glycine, proline, and hydroxyproline and hydroxylysine, all types of collagen being formed by interaction of these units.

tropoelastin (tro″po-e-las′tin)   the precursor of elastin.

tropometer (tro-pom′ě-ter) [Gr. *tropē* a turning + *-meter*]   an instrument for measuring the twist or torsion of a long bone.

tropomyosin (tro″po-mi′o-sin)   muscle protein of the I band that inhibits contraction unless its position is modified by troponin so that the myosin molecules can make contact with the actin molecules. **t. A,** paramyosin.

tropon (trop′on)   a brownish powder prepared from vegetable and animal albumins; nutrient.

troponin (tro′po-nin)   a complex of globular muscle proteins of the I band that inhibits contraction by blocking the interaction of actin and myosin; when combined with Ca^{++}, it so modifies the position of the tropomyosin molecules that interaction takes place.

trotyl (tro′til)   trinitrotoluene.

trough (trof)   a shallow longitudinal depression or channel. **synaptic t's,** primary synaptic clefts.

Trousseau's phenomenon, sign, spot, twitching (troo-sōz′) [Armand *Trousseau,* French physician, 1801–1867] see under *phenomenon, sign,* and *twitching,* and see *tache cérébrale.*

troxidone (trok′sĭ-dōn)   trimethadione.

troy (troi)   a system of weights commonly used in England and the United States for expressing quantities of gold and silver; for equivalents see *tables of weights and measures.*

Trp   tryptophan.

TRU   see under *unit.*

true (troo)   actually existing; not false; real; meeting all the criteria establishing its identity.

Trueta treatment (method, technique) (troo-a′tah) [José *Trueta,* Spanish surgeon in England, born 1897]   see under *treatment.*

truncal (trun′kal)   pertaining to the trunk.

truncate (trun′kāt) [L. *truncare, truncatus*]   having the end cut squarely off.

trunci (trun′si) [L.]   plural of *truncus.*

truncus (trun′kus), pl. *trun′ci* [L. "trunk"]   the main part, a stem; [NA] a general term for the main part of the body, to which the head and limbs are attached, or a major, undivided, and usually short portion of a nerve or of a blood or lymphatic vessel or other duct. **t. arterio′sus,** an arterial trunk, especially the artery connected with the fetal heart, which gives off the aortic arches and develops into the aortic and pulmonary arteries. **t. arterio′sus, persistent,** a congenital anomaly, characterized by a single arterial trunk arising from the heart, receiving blood from both ventricles and supplying blood to the coronary, pulmonary, and systemic circulations; sometimes classified according to the arrangement of the arteries supplying the lungs. **t. brachiocephal′icus** [NA], brachiocephalic trunk: the first branch of the arch of the aorta, which behind the right sternoclavicular joint divides into the right common carotid and right subclavian arteries, with distribution to the right side of the head and neck and to the right arm; the lowest thyroid artery may arise from this trunk. Called also *arteria anonyma* or *innominate artery.* **t. bronchomediastina′lis dex′ter/sinis′ter** [NA], right and left bronchomediastinal trunk: either of the two lymphatic vessels, right and left, draining the pulmonary, bronchopulmonary, tracheobronchial, tracheal, and parasternal lymph nodes: that on the right side into the right lymphatic duct or subclavian vein, and that on the left into the thoracic duct or the subclavian vein. **t. coeli′acus** [NA], celiac trunk: the arterial trunk that arises from the abdominal aorta, gives off the left gastric, common hepatic, and splenic arteries, and supplies the esophagus, stomach, duodenum, spleen, pancreas, liver, and gallbladder. **t. cor′poris callo′si** [NA], trunk of corpus callosum: the main central portion of the corpus callosum as distinguished from the rostrum and the splenium. **t. costocervica′lis** [NA], costocervical trunk: an artery that arises from the back of the subclavian artery, arches backward, and at the neck of the first rib divides into the deep cervical and highest intercostal arteries, thus supplying blood to the structures of the first two intercostal spaces, the vertebral column, the muscles of the back, and the deep neck muscles. **t. encephal′icus** [NA], encephalic trunk: the stemlike portion of the brain connecting the cerebral hemispheres with the spinal cord and comprising the pons, medulla oblongata, and mesencephalon; the diencephalon is considered part of the truncus encephalicus by some. Called also *brain stem.* **t. fascic′uli atrioventricula′ris** [NA], the undivided portion of the atrioventricular bundle, from its origin at the atrioventricular node to the point of division into right and left branches at the superior end of the muscular part of the interventricular septum. **t. infe′rior plex′us brachia′lis** [NA], inferior trunk of brachial plexus: the trunk of the brachial plexus that is formed by the ventral branches of the eighth cervical and first thoracic nerves; medial pectoral nerves may arise from it. Its anterior division becomes the medial cord of the plexus, and its posterior division helps form the posterior cord; *modality,* general sensory and motor. **trun′ci intestina′les** [NA], intestinal trunks: short lymphatic vessels which leave the gastrointestinal tract and participate in formation of the thoracic duct. **t. jugula′ris dex′ter/sinis′ter** [NA], right and left jugular trunk: either of the two vessels, right and left, draining the deep cervical lymph nodes: on the right side, into the right lymphatic duct or subclavian vein, and on the left side, into the thoracic duct or subclavian vein. **t. linguofacia′lis** [NA], linguofacial trunk: the common trunk by which the facial and lingual arteries often arise from the external carotid artery. **trun′ci lumba′les**, see *t. lumbaris dexter/sinister.* **t. lumba′ris dex′ter/sinis′ter** [NA], right and left lumbar trunk: either of the two lymphatic vessels, right and left, draining lymph upward from the lumbar lymph nodes and helping form the thoracic duct. **t. lumbosacra′lis** [NA], lumbosacral trunk: a trunk formed by union of the lower division of the ventral branch of the fourth lumbar nerve with the ventral branch of the fifth lumbar nerve. **trun′ci lymphat′ici** [NA], lymphatic trunks: the lymphatic vessels (right or left lumbar, intestinal, right or left bronchomediastinal, right or left subclavian, and right or left jugular trunks) that drain lymph from various regions of the body into the right lymphatic or thoracic duct. **t. me′dius plex′us brachia′lis** [NA], middle trunk of brachial plexus: the trunk of the brachial plexus that is formed by the ventral branch of the seventh cervical nerve. Its anterior division, from which lateral pectoral nerves may arise, helps form the lateral cord of the plexus, and its posterior division helps form the posterior cord; *modality,* general sensory and motor. **t. ner′vi accesso′rii** [NA], trunk of accessory nerve: the nerve trunk formed by the cranial and spinal roots of the accessory nerve, which separates into an internal and external terminal branch. See also *nervus accessorius.* **t. ner′vi spina′lis** [NA], trunk of spinal nerve: the usually very short nerve trunk formed by the ventral and dorsal roots of a spinal nerve. **trun′ci plex′us brachia′lis** [NA], trunks of brachial plexus: the three trunks (superior, medial, and inferior) of the brachial plexus, arising from the ventral branches of the lower four cervical nerves and the first thoracic nerve near the lateral border of the scalenus anterior muscle; they continue laterally and downward, above and behind the subclavian artery, and near the clavicle each splits into a ventral and a dorsal division. The ventral divisions of the superior and medial trunks unite to form the lateral fasciculus and that of the inferior trunk forms the medial fasiciculus of the plexus; and the dorsal divisions of the three trunks form the posterior fasciculus of the plexus. **t. pulmona′lis** [NA], pulmonary trunk: the vessel arising from the conus arteriosus of the right ventricle, extending upward obliquely to divide into the right and left pulmonary arteries beneath the arch of the aorta, and conveying unaerated blood toward the lungs.

Called also *arteria pulmonalis* or *pulmonary artery.* **t. subcla′vius dex′ter/sinis′ter** [NA], right and left subclavian trunk: either of two lymphatic vessels, right and left, draining the axillary lymph nodes; that on the right into the right lymphatic duct or subclavian vein, that on the left into the thoracic duct or the subclavian vein. **t. supe′rior plex′us brachia′lis** [NA], superior trunk of brachial plexus: the trunk of the brachial plexus that is formed by the ventral branches of the fifth and sixth cervical nerves. Its anterior division helps form the lateral cord of the plexus, its posterior division helps form the posterior cord, and it gives rise directly to the suprascapular and subclavian nerves; *modality,* general sensory and motor. **t. sympathet′icus**, NA alternative for *t. sympathicus.* **t. sympath′icus** [NA], sympathetic trunk: two long nerve strands, one on each side of the vertebral column, extending from the base of the skull to the coccyx. Interconnected by nerve strands, each has cervical, thoracic, lumbar, and sacral sympathetic ganglia. These receive preganglionic fibers from thoracic and upper lumbar ventral roots by way of rami communicantes, send postganglionic fibers to ventral roots by rami communicantes, and give branches to prevertebral plexuses and adjacent viscera and blood vessels. Called also *t. sympatheticus* [NA alternative]. **t. thyreocervica′lis, t. thyrocervica′lis** [NA], thyrocervical trunk: a short artery that arises from the convex side of the subclavian artery just medial to the anterior scalene muscle and at once divides into the inferior thyroid, transverse cervical, and suprascapular arteries, supplying thyroid, neck, and scapular regions. **t. vaga′lis ante′rior** [NA], anterior vagal trunk: a nerve trunk (or trunks) formed by fibers from both left and right vagus nerves, collected from the anterior part of the esophageal plexus; it descends through the esophageal opening of the diaphragm to supply branches to the anterior surface of the stomach. **t. vaga′lis poste′rior** [NA], posterior vagal trunk: a nerve trunk or trunks formed by fibers from both left and right vagus nerves, collected from the posterior part of the esophageal plexus; it descends through the esophageal opening of the diaphragm to supply branches to the posterior surface of the stomach.

trunk (trunk) [L. *truncus* the stem or trunk of a tree] 1. the main part of the body, to which head and limbs are attached. 2. a major, undivided and usually short, portion of a nerve or of a blood or lymphatic vessel, or other duct. See also *truncus.* **t. of accessory n.,** truncus nervi accessorii. **t. of atrioventricular bundle,** truncus fasciculi atrioventricularis. **basilar t.,** arteria basilaris. **t′s of brachial plexus,** trunci plexus brachialis. **brachiocephalic t.,** truncus brachiocephalicus. **bronchomediastinal t.,** see *truncus bronchomediastinalis.* **celiac t.,** truncus coeliacus. **t. of corpus callosum,** truncus corporis callosi. **costocervical t.,** truncus costocervicalis. **encephalic t.,** truncus encephalicus. **inferior t. of brachial plexus,** truncus inferior plexus brachialis. **intestinal t′s,** trunci intestinales. **jugular t.,** see *truncus jugularis.* **linguofacial t.,** truncus linguofacialis. **lumbar t.,** see *truncus lumbaris.* **lumbosacral t.,** truncus lumbosacralis. **lymphatic t′s,** trunci lymphatici. **middle t. of brachial plexus,** truncus medius plexus brachialis. **pulmonary t.,** truncus pulmonalis. **t. of spinal nerve,** truncus nervi spinalis. **subclavian t.,** see *truncus subclavius.* **superior t. of brachial plexus,** truncus superior plexus brachialis. **sympathetic t.,** truncus sympathicus. **thyrocervical t.,** truncus thyrocervicalis. **vagal t., anterior,** truncus vagalis anterior. **vagal t., posterior,** truncus vagalis posterior.

truss (trus) an elastic, canvas, or metallic device for retaining a hernia reduced within the abdominal cavity. **nasal t.,** a trusslike support for fractured nasal bones.

truxilline (truks′ĭ-lin) an amorphous alkaloid prepared from coca leaves or made synthetically.

try-in (tri′in) a preliminary insertion of a dental prosthesis or orthodontic appliance to determine its fit and suitability.

trypaflavine (trip″ah-fla′vin) acriflavine hydrochloride.

trypanblau (tri′pan-blaw″) [Ger.] trypan blue; see under *blue.*

trypanid (tri′pan-id) trypanosomid.

trypanocidal (tri-pan″o-si′dal) trypanosomicidal.

trypanocide (tri-pan′o-sīd) trypanosomicide.

trypanolysis (tri″pan-ol′ĭ-sis) the destruction of trypanosomes.

trypanolytic (tri″pan-o-lit′ik) destructive to trypanosomes.

Trypanoplasma (tri″pan-o-plaz′mah) [Gr. *trypanon* borer + *plasma* anything formed or molded] *Cryptobia.*

Trypanosoma (tri″pan-o-so′mah) [Gr. *trypanon* borer + *sōma* body] a genus of protozoa (suborder Trypanosomatina, order Kinetoplastida) comprising hemoflagellates parasitic in invertebrates and vertebrates, including humans, some of which are pathogenic. The life cycle of trypanosomes involves amastigote, promastigote, epimastigote, and trypomastigote stages; the first three stages are found in the vector (usually a bloodsucking invertebrate) and the last in the vertebrate (definitive) host. In some systems of classification, trypanosomes are categorized in two groups or sections according to the localization of their development in the digestive system of the vector: *salivaria,* including the subgenera *Duttonella, Nannomonas,* and *Trypanozoon;* and *stercoraria,* including the subgenera *Megatrypanum, Herpetosoma,* and *Schizotrypanum.* Another system of classifying trypanosomes is one in which the organisms are placed in one of four groups based on biological similarities: (1) *lewisi* group, including *T. lewisi, T. duttoni, T. theileri, T. cruzi, T. nabiasi, T. melophagium,* and *T. rangeli;* (2) *vivax* group, including *T. vivax* and *T. uniforme;* (3) *congolense* group, including *T. congolense, T. dimorphon,* and *T. simiae;* and (4) *brucei* group, including *T. brucei, T. gambiense, T. rhodesiense, T. evansi, T. equinum,* and *T. epiperdum.* **T. bru′cei,** a salivarian species widely distributed in Africa where it is transmitted by the bites of tsetse flies (*Glossina* spp.) from a reservoir in wild animals, in which it causes a relatively mild infection, to various domestic animals, especially cattle, in which it causes a severe, often fatal disease (see *nagana*). Some systems of classification consider *T. brucei* to consist of three morphologically indistinguishable subspecies or varieties: *T. brucei brucei,* which causes trypanosomiasis in animals; *T. brucei gambiense,* the etiologic agent of Gambian trypanosomiasis; and *T. brucei rhodesiense,* the cause of Rhodesian trypanosomiasis. Other authorities prefer to grant specific status to *T. gambiense* and *T. rhodesiense* because of their biologic and epidemiologic differences. **T. congolen′se,** a tsetse fly–transmitted salivarian species found in Central Africa that is a cause of nagana in domestic animals, which is especially severe in cattle. Called also *T nanum.* **T. cru′zi,** a stercorarian species commonly infecting many wild and domestic animals throughout North, Central, and South America, with armadillos, cats, dogs, bats, rodents, and other mammals serving as reservoir hosts, and usually transmitted by reduviid bugs of the genera *Panstrongylus, Triatoma,* and *Rhodnius.* It is the etiologic agent of Chagas' disease in humans. Called also *T. triatomae* and *Schizotympanum cruzi.* **T. dimor′phon,** a tsetse fly–transmitted salivarian species widely distributed in Central Africa, which was formerly thought to be identical with *T. congolense* but has been shown to be a distinct species. It is found in horses, pigs, goats, sheep, cattle, and dogs, in the latter three of which it has been shown to be more pathogenic than *T. congolense.* **T. equi′num,** a salivarian species transmitted mechanically primarily by tabanid flies and causing mal de caderas in horses in Central and South America. Except for the absence of a kinetoplast it is identical with *T. evansi.* **T. equiper′dum,** a salivarian species structurally indistinguishable from *T. evansi* that causes the venereal disease dourine in horses in Africa, Asia, and certain regions of Europe and North and South America. Called also *T. rougeti.* **T. evan′si,** a salivarian species transmitted mechanically usually by tabanid flies in the Far and Middle East, in North Africa outside of tsetse fly–inhabiting areas, and in certain parts of Central and South America where the vampire bat is also a vector. *T. evansi* causes surra, which is an economically important disease in domestic animals such as camels, equines, cattle, elephants, and dogs. Called also *T. hippicum.* **T. gambien′se,** a polymorphic salivarian species causing the chronic or Gambian form of trypanosomiasis in West and Central Africa, transmitted by the bites of infected tsetse flies, chiefly *Glossina palpalis, G. tachinoides,* and *G. fucipes,* with humans being the only important natural reservoir. Called also *T. hominis* and *T. ugandense.* See also *T. brucei.* **T. hip′picum,** *T. evansi.* **T. hom′inis,** *T. gambiense.* **T. lew′isi,** a stercorarian species commonly found in the blood of rats worldwide, usually nonpathogenic in adults but causing lethal infection in sucklings, and transmitted by the rat flea, *Nosophyllus fasciatus.* The species is much used in laboratory research. **T. melopha′gium,** a nonpathogenic stercorarian species commonly found in sheep worldwide and transmitted by the sheep ked, *Melophagus ovinus.* **T. na′num,** *T. congolense.* **T. neoto′mae,** a species found in woodrats in California, possibly identical with *T. cruzi.* **T. rangel′i,** a nonpathogenic, stercorarian species infecting humans and various animals, especially cats and dogs, primarily in Venezuela, Brazil, Colombia, Costa Rica, El Salvador, Guatemala, and Panama, and usually transmitted by reduviid flies of the genus *Rhodnius.* **T. rhodesien′se,** a salivarian species causing acute or Rhodesian trypanosomiasis throughout East Africa, transmitted by the bites of infected tsetse flies, chiefly *Glossina pallidipes, G. morsitans,* and *G. swynnertoni.* Although many animals can become infected, the only important wild animal reservoirs are antelopes (particularly the bushbuck and hartebeast), with cattle being the only proven domestic animal reservoir. Humans are only incidentally infected. See also *T. brucei.* **T. rotato′rium,** the type species of the genus, and found in the blood of several species of frogs. **T. rouge′ti,** *T. equiperdum.* **T. sim′iae,** a salivarian species found especially in East Africa and the eastern Congo, first reported from the monkey although its natural reservoir is the warthog, and usually transmitted by tsetse flies (*Glossina* spp.) but sometimes also by bloodsucking flies. It is highly pathogenic for camels and sheep, in which it causes death in several days; mildly pathogenic for sheep and goats; and apparently nonpathogenic for cattle, horses, and dogs. **T. thei′leri,** a large stercorarian species found in the blood of cattle worldwide, transmitted by tabanid flies, and usually nonpathogenic although under stressful conditions it may be associated with illness and perhaps death. **T. theodo′ri,** a nonpathogenic, stercorarian species similar to (and perhaps the same as) *T. melophagium* that is found in goats and has the hippoboscid *Lipoptena caprina* as an intermediate host. **T. tria′tomae,** *T. cruzi.* **T. uganden′se,** *T. gambiense.* **T. unifor′me,** a tsetse fly-transmitted salivarian species similar to but smaller than *T. vivax* that is a cause of nagana in cattle, goats, sheep, and antelopes in Zaire. **T. vi′vax,** a tsetse fly–transmitted salivarian species found in many animals, including cattle, sheep, goats, camels, horses, antelopes, and giraffes in Africa, Central and South America, the West Indies, and Mauritius. It is a cause of nagana, the severity of which depends on the species affected, being fatal in certain types of cattle in certain areas.

trypanosomal (tri-pan″o-so′mal) 1. pertaining to or caused by trypanosomes. 2. see *trypomastigote.*

trypanosomatid (tri″pan-o-so′mah-tid) 1. any protozoan of the suborder Trypanosomatina. 2. pertaining to or caused by a protozoan of the suborder Trypanosomatina.

Trypanosomatina (tri″pan-o-so″mah-ti′nah) a suborder of parasitic protozoa (order Kinetoplastida, class Zoomastigophorea) comprising the hemoflagellates, which are found in the hosts' blood, lymph, and tissues, and are characterized by a leaflike or rounded body with one nucleus, one flagellum that is free or attached to the body by an undulating membrane, and a relatively small compact kinetoplast. All trypanosomatids have morphologically distinct stages in their life cycles during which the organisms of one genus may pass through forms characteristic of other genera of the suborder. These forms include: amastigote, choanomastigote, epimastigote, opithomastigote, promastigote, and trypomastigote. Not all species pass through all of the stages, but all have at least two such forms during their development. Representative genera include *Blastocrithidia, Crithidia, Leishmania, Leptomonas,* and *Trypanosoma.*

trypanosomatotropic (tri-pan″o-so″mah-to-trop′ik) having a selective affinity for trypanosomes.

trypanosome (tri-pan′o-sōm) 1. any protozoan of the genus *Trypanosoma* or of the suborder Trypanosomatina. 2. denoting a morphologic stage in the development of certain trypanosomatid protozoa; see *trypomastigote.*

trypanosomiasis (tri-pan″o-so-mi′ah-sis) the state of being infected with protozoa of the genus *Trypanosoma.* Trypanosomal infections of man include the Gambian and Rhodesian forms of African trypanosomiasis, and Chagas' disease. **African t.,** human trypanosomiasis endemic in tsetse fly–infested areas of tropical Africa. The early stage is manifested by hemolymphatic involvement with intermittent fever, anemia, rash, and transitory, localized edema. Later, invasion of the central nervous system occurs, with resultant meningoencephalitis, leading to extreme mental and physical lethargy, tremors, convulsions, and eventually coma and death. The disease occurs in two forms: *Gambian* (chronic) and *Rhodesian* (acute). Called also *African sleeping sickness.* **American t.,** Chagas' disease. **Cruz t.,** Chagas' disease. **East African t.,** Rhodesian t. **Gambian t.,** the usually chronic and less severe form of African trypanosomiasis, occurring in Central and West Africa, caused by *Trypanosoma gambiense,* and transmitted by the bites of infected tsetse flies, chiefly *Glossina palpalis, G. tachinoides,* and *G. fucipes.* This form differs from Rhodesian trypanosomiasis in that the duration of the chronic disease is several months to years and central nervous system involvement usually occurs later in its course. Called also *Gambian sleeping sickness* and *West African t.* **Rhodesian t.,** the usually acute, more severe, and fatal form of African trypanosomiasis, occurring in East Africa, caused by *Trypanosoma rhodesiense,* transmitted by the bites of infected tsetse flies, chiefly *Glossina pallidipes, G. morsitans,* and *G. swynnertoni.* This form differs from Gambian trypanosomiasis in that the acute form has a duration of 3 to 9 months and central nervous system involvement occurs earlier in its course. Called also *East African t.* and *Rhodesian sleeping sickness.* **South American t.,** Chagas' disease. **West African t.,** Gambian t.

trypanosomicidal (tri-pan″o-so″mĭ-si′dal) destructive to trypanosomes.

trypanosomicide (tri-pan″o-so′mĭ-sīd) [*trypanosome* + L. *caedere* to kill] 1. destructive to trypanosomes. 2. a substance which destroys trypanosomes.

trypanosomid (tri-pan′o-so-mid) a skin eruption occurring in trypanosomiasis; called also *trypanid.*

Trypanozoon (tri-pan″o-zo′on) [Gr. *trypanon* borer + *zoon* animal] in some systems of classification, a subgenus of salivarian trypanosomes, including *Trypanosoma brucei, T. rhodesiense, T. gambiense, T. evansi, T. equinum,* and *T. equiperdum.*

trypanroth (tri′pan-roth) [Ger.] trypan red.

tryparosan (tri-par′o-san) a preparation formed by introducing a halogen radical (e.g., chlorine) into the parafuchsin molecule; used by injection in trypanosomiasis.

tryparsamide (trip-ar′sah-mīd) chemical name: monosodium *N*-(carbamoylmethyl) arsanilate. An antitrypanosomal agent, $C_8H_{10}AsN_2NaO_4 \cdot \frac{1}{2}H_2O$, occurring as a white crystalline powder, used in the treatment of African trypanosomiasis. Called also *tryponarsyl* and *trypotan.*

trypasafrol (tri′pah-saf′rol) one of the safranine group of aniline dyes; believed to be useful in trypanosomiasis.

trypesis (tri-pe′sis) [Gr. *trypēsis*] trephination.

trypomastigote (tri″po-mas′tĭ-gōt) [Gr. *trypanon* borer + *mastix* whip] any of the bodies representing the morphologic (trypanosomal) stage in the life cycle of certain trypanosomatid protozoa, resembling the typical adult form of members of the genus *Trypanosome,* in which the slender elongate cell has a kinetoplast and basal body located at the posterior end and a flagellum running anteriorly along an undulating membrane to become a free-flowing structure. Cf. *amastigote, choanomastigote, epimastigote, opisthomastigote,* and *promastigote.*

tryponarsyl (tri″po-nar′sil) tryparsamide.

trypotan (tri′po-tan) tryparsamide.

trypsin (trip′sin) [EC 3.4.21.4] an enzyme of the hydrolase class that catalyzes the cleavage of peptide linkages involving the carboxyl group of either arginine or lysine. It is secreted by the pancreas as trypsinogen and converted to the active form in the small intestine. **crystallized t.** [USP], a purified, crystallized preparation from an extract of the pancreas of the ox, *Bos taurus,* occurring as a white to yellowish white, crystalline or amorphous powder; used topically for its proteolytic effect in the debridement of necrotic wounds and ulcers, abscesses, fistulas, and sinuses, and in the treatment of empyema.

trypsinogen (trip-sin′o-jen) the crystallizable pre-enzyme occurring in the pancreas, from which trypsin is formed when it comes into contact with enterokinase.

Tryptar (trip′tar) trademark for a preparation of crystallized trypsin.

tryptic (trip″tik) relating to or produced as a result of digestion by trypsin.

tryptone (trip′tōn) a peptone produced by proteolytic digestion with trypsin.

tryptophan (trip′to-făn) an amino acid, $C_8H_6N \cdot CH_2 \cdot CH \cdot NH_2COOH$, or α-amino-β-3-indole propionic acid, existing in proteins, from which it is set free by tryptic digestion; essential for optimal growth in infants and for nitrogen equilibrium in human adults. It is a precursor of serotonin. Adequate levels of tryptophan in the diet may compensate deficiencies of niacin and thus mitigate pellagra. Before the name tryptophan was accepted, *proteinochromagen* was also suggested, both names being derived from the color produced in tests.

tryptophanase (trip′to-făn-ās) tryptophan 2,3-dioxygenase.

tryptophan 2,3-dioxygenase (trip′to-făn di-ok′sĭ-jen-ās) [EC 1.13.11.11] an enzyme of the oxidoreductase class that catalyzes the reaction L-tryptophan + O_2 = L-formylkynurenine, the first step in tryptophan catabolism. The enzyme is a heme protein.

tryptophane (trip′to-făn) an earlier spelling of tryptophan.

tryptophanuria (trip″to-făn-u′re-ah) the presence of excessive amounts of tryptophan in the urine; the symptoms resemble those of pellagra.

tryptophyl (trip′to-fil) the acyl radical of tryptophan.

T.S. test solution.

TSA tumor-specific antigen.

Tsa (sah) denoting a virus mutant that can effect abortive malignant transformation of a cell but not stable transformation.

tsalsahuatl (tsal″sa-whaht′′l) *Eutrombicula alfreddugèsi.*

tsetse (tset′se) an African fly of the genus *Glossina.*

TSH thyroid-stimulating hormone; see *thyrotropin.*

TSH-RF thyroid-stimulating hormone releasing factor; see *thyrotropin releasing hormone,* under *hormone.*

TSTA tumor-specific transplantation antigen.

Tsuga (tsoo′gah) a genus of coniferous trees. **T. canden′sis** (L.) Carr. (Pinaceae), the eastern hemlock tree, affords Canada pitch, oil of spruce, and an astringent extract.

TU tuberculin unit.

Tuamine (too′ah-min) trademark for preparations of tuaminoheptane.

tuaminoheptane (too-am″ĭ-no-hep′tān) [USP] chemical name: 2-heptanamine. An adrenergic, $C_7H_{17}N$, occurring as a volatile, colorless to pale yellow liquid; administered by inhalation to produce vasoconstriction of the nasal mucosa for relief of congestion. **t. sulfate** [USP], the sulfate of tuaminoheptane, $(C_7H_{17}N)_2 \cdot H_2SO_4$, occurring as a white, odorless powder, having the same actions and uses as the base; applied topically to the nasal mucosa.

tuba (too′bah), pl. *tu′bae* [L. "trumpet"] a tube: an elongated hollow cylindrical organ; [NA] a general term for such a structure. **t. acus′tica,** t. auditiva. **t. auditi′va** [NA], auditory tube: a channel, about 36 mm. long, lined with mucous membrane, that establishes communication between the tympanic cavity and the nasopharynx and serves to adjust the pressure of air in the cavity to the external pressure. It comprises a pars ossea, located in the temporal bone, and a pars cartilaginea, ending in the nasopharynx. Called also *eustachian tube* and *t. auditoria* [NA alternative]. **t. audito′ria,** NA alternative for *t. auditiva.* **t. uteri′na** [NA], **t. uteri′na** [Fallop′pii], uterine tube: a long slender tube that extends from the upper lateral cornu of the uterus to the region of the ovary of the same side; it is attached to the broad ligament by the mesosalpinx, and consists of an ampulla, an infundibulum, an isthmus, two ostia, and a pars uterina. Called also *fallopian tube* and *salpinx* [NA alternative].

Tubadil (too′bah-dil) trademark for a preparation of tubocurarine chloride.

tubae (too′be) plural of *tuba.*

tubal (too′bal) pertaining to or occurring in a tube, as a tubal pregnancy.

Tubarine (too′bah-rin) trademark for a preparation of tubocurarine chloride.

tubatorsion (tu″bah-tor′shun) torsion or twisting of the uterine tube.

tube (tūb) [L. *tubus*] an elongated hollow cylindrical organ or instrument. **Abbott-Miller t.,** Miller-Abbott t. **Abbott-Rawson t.,** a double barrelled tube through which fluid may be both injected and aspirated; it may be used for lavage or decompression of the stomach. **air t.,** any tubular passage of the respiratory apparatus. **auditory t.,** the channel that establishes communication between the tympanic cavity and the nasopharynx; see *tuba auditiva* [NA]. **Bouchut's t's,** a set of tubes for use in the intubation of the larynx. **Bowman's t's,** tubes formed artificially between the lamellae of the cornea in the process of injection; called also *corneal t's.* **buccal t.,** see *end t.* **Cantor t.,** a mercury-weighted tube for intestinal intubation. **cathode-ray t.,** a vacuum tube in which the cathode rays are accelerated as a beam to form luminous spots on a fluorescent screen. **Celestin's t.,** a plastic tube used to keep the esophagus open in inoperable esophageal carcinoma. **cerebromedullary t.,** neural t. **Chaoul t.,** a low voltage x-ray tube so designed as to permit the anode to be located at 2 cm. from the body, thus permitting intense but very superficial tissue penetration of the ionizing radiation beam. **collecting t's,** tubuli renales recti. **Coolidge t.,** a vacuum tube for the generation of roentgen rays in which the cathode consists of a spiral filament of incandescent tungsten and the anode (the target) of massive tungsten. **corneal t.,** Bowman's t. **corneal t's,** Bowman's t's. **Craigies t.** (*for separating motile from nonmotile bacteria*): a length of glass tubing with slanted bottom is inserted into a tube of semisolid culture medium so that the top protrudes above the medium. The medium is inoculated by stab inside the glass tube. Organisms isolated from the medium outside the tubing are motile; nonmotile types remain inside. **Crookes' t.,** an early form of vacuum tube by the use of which the roentgen rays were discovered. **digestive t.,** see under *tract.* **discharge t.,** a vessel of insulating material (usually glass) provided with metal electrodes which is exhausted to a low gas pressure and permits the passage of electricity through the residual gas when a moderately high voltage is applied to the electrodes. **drainage t.,** a tube used in surgery to facilitate the escape of fluids. **Durham's t.,** 1. [Arthur Edward *Durham*] a jointed tracheostomy tube. 2. [Herbert Edward *Durham*] a small inverted test tube used in determining bacterial gas production. **empyema t.,** a tube for draining purulent fluid from thoracic cavity. **end t.,** an orthodontic attachment on the buccal surface of a terminal banded molar; often referred to as *buccal tube* when using an edgewise arch mechanism. **endobronchial t.,** a double-lumen tube inserted into the bronchus of one lung and permitting the complete deflation of the other lung; used in anesthesia and thoracic surgery. **endotracheal t.,** an airway catheter inserted in the trachea in endotracheal intubation. **esophageal t.,** a soft, flexible tube for lavage of the stomach and artificial forced feeding. **eustachian t.,** tuba auditiva. **Ewald t.,** a tube of large bore used to evacuate the stomach. **fallopian t.,** tuba uterina. **feeding t.,** a tube for introducing fluids of high caloric value into the stomach. **fermentation t.,** a U-shaped tube with one arm closed for determining gas production by bacteria. **Ferrein's t's,** the convoluted uriniferous tubules. **fusion t's,** heteroscope. **gas t.,** a roentgen-ray tube which depends for its action on the presence of residual gas; the cathode is not heated and the target is usually connected electrically to the anode. **Geissler's t., Geissler-Pluecker t.,** a discharge tube for showing the luminous effects of discharges through rarefied gases. **Harris t.,** a single-lumen tube with a mercury weight, used as a diagnostic aid in the study of the small intestine; similar to the Miller-Abbott tube. **Hittorf t.,** Crookes' t. **horizontal t.,** a metal tube attachment placed in a horizontal position on the buccal surface of each anchor molar. **hot-cathode t.,** a vacuum tube in which the cathode is electrically heated to incandescence and in which the stream of electrons depends on the temperature of the cathode. **Kobelt's t's,** the remains of the tubules of the mesonephros in the paroophoron. **Kuhn's t.,** a flexible tube of metal for use in intratracheal anesthesia. **Leonard t.,** cathode-ray t. **Levin t.,** a gastric catheter that is passed through the nose. **medullary t.,** neural t. **Mett's t's,** small glass tubes filled with coagulated egg white for testing peptic activity; see under *tests.* **Miescher's t.,** sarcocyst. **Miller-Abbott t.,** a double-channel intestinal tube with an inflatable balloon at its distal end, for use in the treatment of obstruction of the small intestine; occasionally useful also as a diagnostic aid. **nasogastric t.,** a tube of soft rubber or plastic inserted through a nostril and into the stomach, for instilling liquid foods or other substances, or for withdrawing gastric contents. **nephrostomy t.,** a tube inserted through the abdominal wall into the pelvis of the kidney, for direct drainage of the urine. **neural t.,** the epithelial tube developed from the neural plate and forming the central nervous system of the embryo; called also *medullary t.* and *cerebromedullary t.* **Olshevsky t.,** a roentgen-ray tube constructed to use only the stronger rays which pass through the target and armoring the rest of the tube. **otopharyngeal t.,** tuba auditiva. **ovarian t's,** groups of cells which grow down and are cut off from the much thickened surface layer of the ovary; they differentiate into primary oocytes, each with a follicular layer. Called also *Pflüger's t's.* **Paul-Mixter t.,** a large-calibered, flanged drainage tube of glass used for temporary intestinal decompression. **Pflüger's t's,** the ovarian tubes. **pharyngotympanic t.,** tuba auditiva. **photomultiplier t.,** a vacuum tube that converts electromagnetic radiation signals into electrical pulses, consisting of a light-sensitive surface that emits electrons when light is incident on it, the electrons then passing through successive stages with electron multiplication at each stage. **polar t.,** a hollow, extensible, filamentous tubular organelle found coiled in the spore of microsporidan protozoa, through which the sacroplasm is injected into the host's tissues. Called also *polar filament.* 2. polar filament, def. 1. **pus t.,** pyosalpinx. **Rainey's t.,** sarcocyst. **Rehfuss' t.,** a specially designed stomach tube used in making the Rehfuss test. **Roida's t.,** a tube designed for the separation of motile from nonmotile bacteria; the motile organisms make their way through sand, glass-wool, and other obstructions. **roll t.,** see *roll tube culture,* under *culture.* **Ruysch's t.,** a very small tubular opening on the nasal septum, just anterior and inferior to the nasopalatine foramen: it is a relic of the fetal Jacobson's organ. **Ryle's t.,** a thin rubber tube with an olive-shaped end used in giving a test meal. **Schachowa's spiral t's,** tubuli renales. **Sengstaken-Blakemore t.,** a multilumen tube used for the tamponade of bleeding esophageal varices: one lumen leads to a balloon which is inflated in the stomach, to retain the instrument in place, and to compress the vessels around the cardia; another leads to a long narrow balloon by which pressure is exerted against the varices in the wall of the esophagus; and a third provides for aspirating contents of the stomach. **Shiner's t.,** a flexible plastic radiopaque tube for obtaining biopsy material from the jejunum under fluoroscopic control; the jejunal mucosa is drawn by suction into a small aperture in the knife cylinder head at the end of the tube, and a portion is excised. **sieve t.,** the conductive element of phloem. **Souttar's t.,** a flexible metal tube used to keep the esophagus open in inoperable esophageal carcinoma. **sputum t.,** a graduated capillary tube for containing sputum to be rotated in the centrifuge. **stomach t.,** a tube for feeding or for irrigation of the stomach. **T t.,** a self-retaining drainage tube in the shape of a T. **tampon t.,** a piece of stout rubber tubing wound with iodoform gauze, used in plugging the rectum to control oozing and at the same time to allow the escape of gas. **test t.,** a tube of thin glass closed at one end, used for various procedures in chemistry and for observing the growth of bacterial cultures. **thoracostomy t.,** a tube inserted through an opening in the chest wall, for application of suction to the pleural cavity; used to reexpand the lung in pneumothorax or to drain fluid or blood. **tracheostomy t.,** a curved tube to be inserted into the trachea through the opening made in tracheostomy. **uterine t.,** tuba uterina. **vacuum t.,** a glass tube from which the air has been exhausted to a high degree of vacuum; see *Crookes's t.* and *Geissler's t.* **valve t.,** a vacuum tube used to rectify an alternating current. **Veillon t.,** a piece of glass tubing with a rubber cork at one end and a plug of cotton at the other, used in bacterial culture work. **vertical t.,** an orthodontic attachment usually placed on the lingual surface of the anchor band to allow for the insertion of the lingual arch wire. **Wangensteen t.,** a small tube passed through the nose into the stomach and connected with a special suction apparatus to maintain gastric and duodenal decompression; called also *Wangensteen's apparatus.* **x-ray t.,** a glass vacuum bulb containing two electrodes. Electrons are obtained either from gas in the tube or from a heated cathode. When suitable potential is applied, electrons travel at high velocity from cathode to anode, where they are suddenly arrested, giving rise to x-rays.

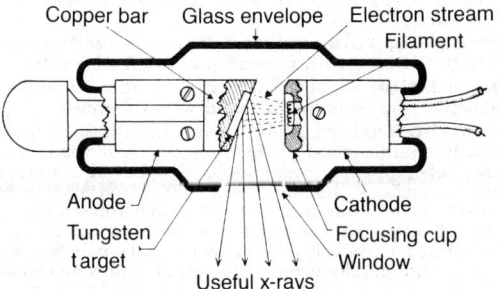

Standard stationary anode x-ray tube; diagram in longitudinal section.

tubectomy (too-bek'to-me) excision of a portion of the uterine tube.

tuber (too'ber), pl. *tubers* or *tu'bera* [L.] 1. a swelling or protuberance; [NA] the general term for such a structure. 2. the essential lesion of tuberous sclerosis, presenting as a pale, firm, nodular phakomalike glial hamartomatous brain lesion that sometimes becomes calcified, which develops predominantly in the cerebral hemispheres, cerebellum, medulla, and spinal cord. **t. ante'rius hypothal'ami,** t. cinereum. **t. calca'nei** [NA], the posteroinferior projection of the calcaneus that forms the heel; called also *tuberosity of calcaneus.* **t. cine'reum,** 1. [NA] a layer of gray matter which is part of the hypothalamus; forming a part of the floor of the third ventricle, it lies in front of and between the corpora mamillaria and merges anteriorly into the infundibulum; called also *gray tubercle* and *tuberculum cinereum.* 2. tuberculum trigeminale. **t. coch'leae,** promontorium tympani. **eustachian t.,** an eminence on the medial wall of the tympanum, below the vestibular window. **external t. of Henle,** tuberculum mentale mandibulae. **frontal t., t. fronta'le** [NA], one of the slight rounded prominences on the frontal bone on either side above the eyes, forming the most prominent portions of the forehead; called also *eminentia frontale* [NA alternative] and *frontal eminence.* **iliopubic t.,** eminentia iliopubica. **t. ischia'dicum** [NA], tuberosity of ischium: a large elongated mass on the inferior part of the posterior margin of the body of the ischium, to which several muscles are attached. Called also *ischial tuberosity* and *t. ischiale* [NA alternative]. **t. ischia'le,** NA alternative for *t. ischiadicum.* **t. maxil'lae** [NA], **t. maxilla're, maxillary t.,** a rounded eminence at the posteroinferior angle of the infratemporal surface of the maxilla; called also *eminence of maxilla, eminentia maxillae,* and *tuberosity of maxilla.* **mental t.,** tuberculum mentale mandibulae. **omental t. of liver,** t. omentale hepatis. **omental t. of pancreas,** t. omentale pancreatis. **t. omenta'le hep'atis** [NA], omental tuber of liver: the rounded prominence on the posteroinferior surface of the left lobe of the liver, just cranial to the lesser curvature of the stomach. **t. omenta'le pancrea'tis** [NA], omental tuber of pancreas: a rounded prominence chiefly on the anterior surface of the neck of the pancreas. **papillary t. of liver,** processus papillaris hepatis. **parietal t., t. parieta'le** [NA], the somewhat laterally bulging prominence just superior to the superior temporal line on the external surface of the parietal bone. **t. ra'dii, t. of radius,** tuberositas radii. **sciatic t.,** t. ischiadicum. **t. val'vulae cerebel'li,** t. vermis. **t. ver'mis** [NA], the part of the vermis of the cerebellum between the folium vermis and the pyramids. **t. zygomat'icum,** tuberculum articulare ossis temporalis.

tubera (too'ber-ah) [L.] plural of *tuber.*

tubercle (too'ber-k'l) 1. any of the small, rounded, granulomatous lesions produced by infection with *Mycobacterium tuberculosis;* it is the characteristic lesion of tuberculosis, and consists of a translucent mass, gray in color, made up of a collection of modified macrophages resembling epithelial cells (*epithelioid cells*), surrounded by a rim of mononuclear cells, principally lymphocytes, and sometimes a center of

giant multinucleate cells (*Langhans' giant cells*). Called also *gray t.* 2. a nodule, or small eminence, such as a rough, rounded eminence on a bone; called also *tuberculum* [NA]. 3. dental t. See also *tuber, tuberositas,* and *tuberosity.* **acoustic t.,** auditory t. **adductor t. of femur,** tuberculum adductorium femoris. **amygdaloid t. of Schwalbe,** area vestibularis. **anatomical t.,** tuberculosis verrucosa cutis. **t. of anterior scalene muscle,** tuberculum musculi scaleni anterioris. **articular t. of temporal bone,** tuberculum articulare ossis temporalis. **t. of atlas, anterior,** tuberculum anterius atlantis. **t. of atlas, posterior,** tuberculum posterius atlantis. **auditory t.,** an eminence in the lateral recess of the fourth ventricle, formed by an extension of the vestibular area and the underlying dorsal nucleus and the cochlear part of the vestibulocochlear nerve; called also *acoustic t.* **auricular t.,** tuberculum auriculae. **Babès' t's,** cellular aggregations around degenerated neurons in the medulla oblongata and the spinal ganglia in cases of rabies and other types of encephalitis. **brachial t. of humerus,** processus supracondylaris humeri. **calcaneal t.,** tuberculum calcanei. **Carabelli t.,** see under *cusp.* **caseous t.,** a yellowish mass of cheesy material, thought to represent a typical lesion of tuberculosis that has undergone degeneration. **caudal t. of liver,** processus caudatus hepatis. **cervical t's,** two small eminences on the femur, a *superior* on the upper and anterior part of the neck at its junction with the greater trochanter, and an *inferior* at the junction with the lesser trochanter. **t. of cervical vertebrae, anterior,** tuberculum anterius vertebrarum cervicalium. **t. of cervical vertebrae, posterior,** tuberculum posterius vertebrarum cervicalium. **Chassaignac's t.,** tuberculum caroticum vertebrae cervicalis VI. **condyloid t.,** an eminence on the condylar process of the mandible for attachment of the lateral ligament of the temporomandibular articulation. **conglomerate t.,** a mass made up of an aggregation of many smaller nodules. **conoid t.,** tuberculum conoideum. **corniculate t.,** tuberculum corniculatum. **crude t.,** caseous t. **t. of cuneate nucleus,** tuberculum cuneatum. **cuneiform t.,** tuberculum cuneiforme. **darwinian t.,** tuberculum auriculae. **deltoid t.,** 1. a prominence on the clavicle for attachment of the deltoid muscle. 2. tuberositas deltoidea humeri. **dental t.,** 1. tuberculum dentale. 2. cuspis dentalis. **dorsal t. of radius,** an easily palpable prominence on the distal, dorsal aspect of the radius, which is grooved by the tendon of the extensor pollicis longus muscle; called also *Lister's t.* **epiglottic t.,** tuberculum epiglotticum. **Farre's t's,** masses beneath the capsule of the liver, felt on palpation in certain cases of hepatic cancer. **fibrous t.,** a tubercle of bacillary origin which contains connective tissue elements. **t. of fibula, posterior,** apex capitis fibulae. **genial t.,** tuberculum mentale mandibulae. **genital t.,** an eminence in front of the cloaca in the early embryo, which becomes the penis or the clitoris. **Ghon t.,** see under *focus.* **gracile t.,** tuberculum nuclei gracilis. **gray t.,** 1. the typical lesion of tuberculosis; see *tubercle* (def. 2). 2. tuberculum trigeminale. 3. tuber cinereum. **greater t. of calcaneus,** processus medialis tuberis calcanei. **t. of greater multangular bone,** tuberculum ossis trapezii. **hard t.,** naked t. **hippocampal t.,** an expansion of the hippocampus at its lower end, separating the fimbria from the gyrus dentatus. **His' t.,** a small prominence on the posteroinferior part of the pinna. **t. of humerus,** capitulum humeri. **t. of humerus, anterior, of Meckel,** tuberculum majus humeri. **t. of humerus, anterior, of Weber,** tuberculum minus humeri. **t. of humerus, external,** tuberculum majus humeri. **t. of humerus, greater,** tuberculum majus humeri. **t. of humerus, internal,** tuberculum minus humeri. **t. of humerus, lesser,** tuberculum minus humeri. **t. of humerus, posterior,** tuberculum majus humeri. **iliac t.,** tuberculum iliacum. **iliopectineal t., iliopubic t.,** eminentia iliopubica. **inferior t. of Humphrey,** processus accessorius vertebrarum lumbalium. **infraglenoid t.,** tuberculum infraglenoidale. **intercolumnar t.,** organum subfornicale. **intercondylar t.,** eminentia intercondylaris. **intercondylar t., lateral,** tuberculum intercondylare laterale. **intercondylar t., medial,** tuberculum intercondylare mediale. **intervenous t.,** tuberculum intervenosum. **intravascular t.,** a tubercle in the intima of a blood vessel. **jugular t. of occipital bone,** tuberculum jugulare ossis occipitalis. **labial t.,** tuberculum labii superioris. **lacrimal t.,** papilla lacrimalis. **lateral orbital t.,** Whitnall's t. **lateral palpebral t.,** Whitnall's t. **lesser t. of calcaneus,** processus lateralis tuberis calcanei. **Lisfranc's t.,** tuberculum musculi scaleni anterioris. **Lister's t.,** dorsal t. of radius. **Lower's t.,** tuberculum intervenosum. **Luschka's t.,** carina urethralis vaginae. **lymphoid t.,** a lesion of tuberculosis consisting of lymphoid cells. **mamillary t.,** processus mamillaris. **mamillary t. of hypothalamus,** corpus mamillare. **marginal t. of zygomatic bone,** tuberculum marginale ossis zygomatici. **mental t.,** tuberculum mentale mandibulae. **mental t., external,** protuberantia mentalis. **mental t. of mandible,** tuberculum mentale mandibulae. **miliary t.,** one of the many minute tubercles formed in many organs in acute miliary tuberculosis. **Montgomery's t's,** greatly enlarged sebaceous glands (Morgagni's tubercles) observed on the surface of the areola of the mammary gland during pregnancy. **Morgagni's t.,** 1. bulbus olfactorius. 2. one of the small nodules on the surface of the areola of the mammary gland produced by the superficially situated large sebaceous glands. **Müller's t.,** a protrusion into the urogenital sinus caused by the downward-growing mesonephric and paramesonephric ducts. **muscular t. of atlas,** tuberculum anterius atlantis. **naked t.,** the characteristic lesion of sarcoidosis, composed of discrete aggregations of large, pale-staining, noncaseating epithelioid cells intermingled with histiocytes, lymphocytes, and Langhans giant cells, sometimes surrounded by a narrow band of lymphocytes; when necrosis is present, it is minimal. Similar lesions may be seen in association with foreign bodies in the tissues and in such conditions as tuberculoid leprosy, cutaneous leishmaniasis, and deep fungal infections. Called also *hard t.* **t. of navicular bone,** tuberculum ossis scaphoidei. **nuchal t.,** the prominence formed by the spinous process of the seventh cervical vertebra. **t. of nucleus cuneatus,** tuberculum nuclei cuneati. **t. of nucleus gracilis,** tuberculum nuclei gracilis. **obturator t., anterior,** tuberculum obturatorium anterius. **obturator t., posterior,** tuberculum obturatorium posterius. **olfactory t.,** bulbus olfactorius. **papillary t.,** processus papillaris hepatis. **pharyngeal t.,** tuberculum pharyngeum. **plantar t.,** tuberositas ossis metatarsalis I. **t. of posterior process of talus, lateral,** tuberculum laterale processus posterioris tali. **t. of posterior process of talus, medial,** tuberculum mediale processus posterioris tali. **pterygoid t.,** tuberositas pterygoidea mandibulae. **pubic t. of pubic bone,** tuberculum pubicum ossis pubis. **rabic t's,** Babès' t's. **t. of rib,** tuberculum costae. **t. of Rolando,** tuberculum trigeminale. **t. of root of zygoma,** tuberculum articulare ossis temporalis. **t. of Santorini,** tuberculum corniculatum. **scalene t.,** tuberculum musculi scaleni anterioris. **t. of scaphoid bone,** tuberculum ossis scaphoidei. **t. of sella turcica,** tuberculum sellae turcicae. **t. of sixth cervical vertebra, anterior,** or **t. of sixth cervical vertebra, carotid,** tuberculum anterius vertebrae cervicalis sextae. **t. of sixth cervical vertebra, posterior,** tuberculum posterius vertebrae cervicalis sextae. **superior t. of Henle,** tuberculum obturatorium posterius. **superior t. of Humphrey,** processus mamillaris vertebrarum. **supraglenoid t.,** tuberculum supraglenoidalis. **supratragic t.,** tuberculum supratragicum. **t. of thalamus, anterior,** tuberculum anterius thalami. **t. of thalamus, posterior,** pulvinar. **thyroid t., inferior,** tuberculum thyroideum inferius. **thyroid t., superior,** tuberculum thyroideum superius. **t. of tibia,** eminentia intercondylaris. **transverse t. of fourth tarsal bone,** tuberositas ossis cuboidei. **t. of trapezium,** tuberculum ossis trapezii. **trochlear t.,** spina trochlearis. **t. of ulna,** tuberositas ulnae. **t. of upper lip,** tuberculum labii superioris. **t's of vertebra,** three elevations (*superior, inferior,* and *external*) upon the transverse process of the last thoracic vertebra, and represented on the lumbar vertebrae by more or less rudimentary structures. **Whitnall's t.,** a small eminence on the internal aspect of the middle of the orbital surface of the zygomatic bone; called also *lateral orbital* or *palpebral t.* **Wrisberg's t.,** tuberculum cuneiforme. **yellow t.,** caseous t. **t. of zygoma, zygomatic t.,** tuberculum articulare ossis temporalis.

tubercula (too-ber′ku-lah) [L.] plural of *tuberculum.*

tubercular (too-ber′ku-lar) of, pertaining to, or resembling tubercles or nodules. Cf. *tuberculous.*

Tuberculariaceae (too-ber″ku-lar″ĭ-a′se-e) a family of Fungi Imperfecti of the order Moniliales, including the genus *Fusarium.*

tuberculate, tuberculated (too-ber′ku-lāt″; too-ber′ku-lāt″ed) covered with tubercles; affected with tubercle.

tuberculation (too-ber″ku-la′shun) the development of tubercles; the becoming affected with tubercles.

tuberculid (too-ber′ku-lid) recurrent eruptions of the skin usually characterized by spontaneous involution. Some believe tuberculids to occur as local hyperergic reactions to mycobacteria or their antigens that are spread hematogenously to the skin from foci of active tuberculosis, while others believe that the lesions are unrelated to tuberculosis. Considered to comprise erythema induratum, lichen scrofulosorum, and papulonecrotic tuberculid, and sometimes lupus miliaris disseminatus faciei. **micronodular t.,** granulomatous rosacea. **papulonecrotic t.,** a grouped symmetric eruption of symptom-less papules appearing in successive crops and healing spontaneously with superficially depressed scars, which occur chiefly on the extensor surface of the extremities in infants, children, and young adults. Called also *acne scrofulosorum* and *papulonecrotic tuberculosis.* **rosacea-like t.,** granulomatous rosacea.

tuberculin (too-ber′ku-lin) [USP] a sterile solution containing growth products of the tubercle bacillus (*Mycobacterium tuberculosis* or *M. bovis*) used in skin tests for tuberculosis (see *tuberculin test,* under *tests*); also commonly used antigen in laboratory immunology. Tuberculin was introduced in 1890 by Koch as a cure for tuberculosis, but proved to be an ineffective and dangerous treatment. Although many different tuberculin preparations have been devised, all are now obsolete except old tuberculin (OT) and purified protein derivative (PPD). Dosages are expressed in tuberculin units (TU), which measure biologic activity as compared with a standard tuberculin preparation. Three dosages are used: first strength tuberculin (1 TU), used for young children or persons in whom extreme hypersensitivity is expected, intermediate strength tuberculin (5 TU), the standard test dose, and second strength tuberculin (250 TU), used for retests. **albumose-free (A.F.) t.,** tuberculin free from albumose, used for the subcutaneous tuberculin test. Called also *Tuberculin Albumose Frei (T.A.F.).* **T. Albumose Frei (T.A.F.),** albumose-free t. **alkaline t.,** a preparation obtained from tubercle bacilli by extracting with $\frac{1}{10}$ normal soda solution; much the same as the original tuberculin. **autogenous t.,** autotuberculin. **bacillary emulsion (B.E.) t. (T.B.E.),** tubercle cultures are dried, ground, and suspended (1 gm.) in equal parts of water and glycerol (200 ml.). It differs from New tuberculin in that the tubercle bacilli are not washed nor is the supernatant fluid from the first centrifugalization discarded. **Behring's t.,** 1. tuberculase. 2. tulase. **Béraneck's t.,** cultures of tubercle bacilli grown on a nonpeptonized, 5 per cent glycerin bouillon are filtered and the microorganisms are extracted in 1 per cent orthophosphoric acid by long-continued shaking. This extract (basiotoxin) is mixed with an equal volume of the filtrate (acidotoxin) for use. **t. bouillon filtrate (B.F.),** the clear glycerin bouillon in which tubercle cultures have been grown and from which they have been filtered out. It is not heated or concentrated. Called also *Denys' tuberculin.* **Calmette's t.,** purified tuberculin, prepared by precipitating Old tuberculin with alcohol, washing, dissolving in water, and filtering. When instilled in the conjunctiva of persons affected with tuberculosis or typhoid fever it produces a severe local reaction. Called also *tuberculin precipitation (T.P.).* See also *ophthalmic reaction,* under *reaction.* **t. contagious (T.C.),** von Behring's name for tuberculin which is said to be taken up by the cells of the body and there transformed into an integral part of those cells; in this form it is called *TX.* **Denys' t.,** t. bouillon filtrate. **Dixon's t.,** a tuberculin prepared by treating living tubercle cultures with ether and extracting in salt solution. **t. filtrate (T.F.),** a tuberculin preparation made by precipitating and filtering the dissolved precipitate separately. **Hirschfelder's t.,** oxytuberculin. **Klebs' t.,** tuberculocidin. **Klemperer's t.,** a tuberculin prepared from cultures of bovine tuberculosis. **Koch's t.,** old t. **Maragliano's t.,** a tuberculin containing all the extracts of the tubercle bacillus that are soluble in water. **Maréchal's t.,** a mixture of Old tuberculin and guaiacol. **Moro's t.,** diagnostic t. **New t.,** a suspension of the fragments of tubercle bacilli, freed from all soluble materials and with glycerin added: tubercle bacilli are triturated to a fine consistency and suspended in distilled water or physiological salt solution. Centrifugation results in separation into a translucent supernatant (TO, *tuberculin ober*) and a muddy sediment (TR, *tuberculin rest*). This sediment is dried, again triturated, and suspended and centrifuged. The process is repeated until only an opalescent fluid is obtained. The addition of a sufficient quantity of glycerin to make a 20 per cent solution renders the preparation ready for use. Called also *Koch's t.*, *original t.* (T.O.), *residue t.*, and *t. residue* (T.R.). **Old t. (O.T.),** a heat-concentrated filtrate of tubercle bacillus culture grown on a special medium, used for tuberculin tests. Called also *Koch's t.* **perlsucht t., Perlsucht T. Original (P.T.O.),** Spengler's t. **purified t.,** Calmette's t. **purified protein derivative (PPD) t.,** a soluble purified protein fraction precipitated by trichloracetic acid from filtrate of tubercle bacillus culture grown on a special medium, used for tuberculin tests. **residual t., t. residue (T.R.),** New t. **Rosenbach's t.,** tuberculin prepared from cultures which have been infected with *Trichophyton holosericum-album*, which reduces the toxicity of the tubercle bacilli. **Ruck's watery extract t.,** tubercle cultures are concentrated in vacuo at 55° C. to one tenth volume and filtered. The filtrate is precipitated with an acid solution of sodium bismuth iodide. Filter, neutralize the filtrate, and filter again. Precipitate the filtrate with enough absolute alcohol to make 90 per cent alcohol, filter, and make a 1 per cent aqueous solution of the dry precipitate. **Seibert's t.,** 1. purified protein derivative of t. 2. a purified tuberculin used intradermally as a test for tuberculosis. **Selter's t.,** vital t. **Spengler's t.,** a preparation from the bacilli of bovine tuberculosis; called also *perlsucht t.* and *Perlsucht Tuberculin Original (P.T.O.).* **Thamm's t.,** tuberculoalbumin. **vacuum t. (V.T.),** Old tuberculin reduced in a vacuum to much less than its original volume. **Vaudremer's t.,** tuberculin prepared by macerating it in the ground up mycelia of *Aspergillus fumigatus*, which renders the tuberculin nearly free from toxicity. **vital t.,** a tuberculin prepared by triturating moist attenuated human tubercle bacilli; the preparation contains a few living tubercle bacilli of very slight virulence. **t. pristi′num,** Old tuberculin.

tuberculitis (too″ber-ku-li′tis) [*tubercle* + *-itis*] inflammation of or near a tubercle.

tuberculization (too-ber″ku-li-za′shun) 1. treatment with tuberculin or its modifications. 2. the formation of or conversion into tubercles.

tuberculocele (too-ber′ku-lo-sēl″) [*tubercle* + Gr. *kēlē* tumor] tuberculous disease of the testis.

tuberculocidal (too-ber″ku-lo-si′dal) lethal to *Mycobacterium tuberculosis.*

tuberculocidin (too-ber″ku-lo-si′din) an albumose derived from tuberculin by treating it with platinum chloride. It is used like tuberculin, but is said to be free from the objectionable characters of the latter.

tuberculoderma (too-ber″ku-lo-der′mah) [*tuberculo-* + Gr. *derma* skin] 1. any tuberculous condition or disease of the skin. 2. a tuberculous lesion of the skin.

tuberculofibroid (too-ber″ku-lo-fi′broid) characterized by a tubercle that has undergone a fibroid degeneration.

tuberculoid (too-ber′ku-loid) resembling a tubercle or tuberculosis.

tuberculoidin (too-ber″ku-loi′din) a form of modified tuberculin cleared of its bacilli by treatment with alcohol.

tuberculoma (too-ber″ku-lo′mah) a tumor-like mass resulting from enlargement of a caseous tubercle. **t. en plaque,** a flat plaque on the surface of the frontoparietal cortex in tuberculous meningoencephalitis, producing the symptoms of brain tumor.

tuberculoprotein (too-ber″ku-lo-pro′te-in) protein derived from the bodies of tubercle bacilli.

tuberculosilicosis (too-ber″ku-lo-sil″ĭ-ko′sis) silicosis complicated by pulmonary tuberculosis.

tuberculosis (too-ber″ku-lo′sis) any of the infectious diseases of man and animals caused by species of *Mycobacterium* and characterized by the formation of tubercles and caseous necrosis in the tissues. The common causative species are *M. tuberculosis* and *M. bovis*, but the disease is also caused by other mycobacteria ("atypical" or anonymous mycobacteria), including *M. avium-intracellulare*, *M. kansasii*, *M. simiae*, and *M. szulgai*. Tuberculosis varies widely in its manifestations and has a tendency to great chronicity. Any organ may be affected, although in man the lung is the major seat of the disease and the usual portal through which the infection reaches other organs. **adult t.,** see *postprimary t.* and *primary t.* **aerogenic t.,** inhalation t. **anthracotic t.,** tuberculosis associated with pneumoconiosis of coal workers. **atypical t.,** mycobacteriosis. **avian t.,** a variety of tuberculosis affecting various birds, including chickens and ducks, caused by *Mycobacterium avium*, and characterized by tubercles consisting principally of epithelioid cells. It may be communicated to other animals and man. **basal t.,** tuberculosis situated in the lower part of the affected lung. **t. of bones and joints,** tuberculosis involving the bones and joints, producing strumous arthritis, or white swelling, and cold abscess. **bovine t.,** an infection of cattle caused by *Mycobacterium bovis*, transmissible to man and other animals. **cerebral t.,** tuberculous meningitis. **cestodic t.,** a disease simulating tuberculosis, but due to excessive infestation with cestode parasites. **chicken t.,** avian tuberculosis occurring in chickens. **childhood t.,** primary t. **t. colliquati′va,** 1. scrofuloderma. 2. tuberculous gumma. **t. colliquati′va cu′tis,** 1. scrofuloderma. 2. tuberculous gumma. **t. cu′tis,** tuberculosis of the skin, occurring as a result of exogenous (e.g., autoinoculation) or endogenous (e.g., by extension of an existing infection) infection or by lymphatic or hematogenous spread of infection, presenting in a large variety of clinical expressions, including lupus vulgaris, tuberculosis verrucosa cutis, scrofuloderma, tuberculous chancre, and papulonecrotic tuberculid. **t. cu′tis indurati′va,** erythema induratum. **t. cu′tis lichenoi′des,** lichen scrofulosorum. **t. cu′tis milia′ris dissemina′ta,** t. miliaris disseminatus. **t. cu′tis orificia′lis,** tuberculous infection of the mucosal orifices and adjacent skin (nose, mouth, especially the tongue, anus, vulva, penis), usually associated with a direct hematogenous or lymphatic extension of infection from an internal organ involvement or inoculation, which is characterized clinically by the presence of a nodule that breaks down to form a painful, shallow oval ulcer with undermined bluish edges. It generally occurs as a manifestation of advanced systemic disease in middle-aged and elderly males. Called also *orificial t.* and *t. ulcerosa.* **disseminated t.,** 1. hematogenous or lymphohematogenous spread of tubercle bacilli from a primary focus of infection. 2. miliary t. **exudative t.,** the simplest form of pulmonary tuberculosis, frequently the earliest reaction to infection, in which the alveolar spaces and the smaller bronchi become filled with a cellular exudate consisting mainly of large mononuclear cells; called also *tuberculous pneumonia.* **fowl t.,** avian tuberculosis occurring in fowl. **genital t.,** tuberculosis of the genital tract, e.g., tuberculous endometritis. **genitourinary t.,** tuberculosis involving the genitourinary tract, often the result of hemic dissemination of pulmonary tuberculosis. **hematogenous t.,** infection with *Mycobacterium tuberculosis* carried through the bloodstream to other organs from the primary site of infection. **hilus t.,** tuberculosis involving the hilus of the lung. **t. indurati′va,** erythema induratum. **inhalation t.,** tuberculosis caused by aspiration of the tubercle bacilli into the lungs. **t. of intestines,** tuberculosis involving the intestines, marked by formation of spreading ulcers, especially of the lymphoid tissue; attended by diarrhea, and sometimes resulting in cicatricial stricture. **t. of kidney,** renal t. **t. of larynx,** tuberculosis involving the larynx, producing ulceration of the vocal cords and elsewhere on the mucosa, and commonly attended by hoarseness, cough, pain on swallowing, and hemoptysis. **t. lichenoi′des,** lichen scrofulosorum. **t. of lungs,** infection of the lungs caused by *Mycobacterium tuberculosis.* Characteristically, the course of the untreated disease is as follows: tuberculous pneumonia, formation of tuberculous granulation tissue, caseous necrosis, calcification, and cavity formation. It may spread to other lung segments via the bronchi, or to other organs via the blood or lymph vessels. Symptoms may include weight loss, lassitude and fatigue, night sweats, and wasting, with purulent sputum, hemoptysis, and chest pain. **t. milia′ris dissemina′ta,** a severe form of acute miliary tuberculosis involving the skin, seen especially in children, occurring as an acute generalized cutaneous eruption consisting of indolent, brownish red, acuminate papules that become necrotic, and may form numerous minute, circular ulcers with a dull red border and a pale granulating base covered by a seropurulent exudate. It may occur in immunosuppressed patients, or following an exanthematous disease or some other type of serious infection. Called also *t. cutis miliaris disseminata.* **miliary t.,** a form of tuberculosis varying from a chronic, slowly progressive debilitating infection to a fulminating acute and overwhelming disease, caused by hematogenous or lymphohematogenous dissemination of infected caseous material into the bloodstream, and resulting in seeding of many organs with numerous millet seed–like tubercles. Called also *disseminated t.* See also *t. miliaris disseminata.* **open t.,** 1. tuberculosis in which there are lesions from which the tubercle bacilli are being discharged out of the body. 2. tuberculosis of the lungs with cavitation. **oral t.,** a rare condition usually occurring as a blood-borne complication of pulmonary tuberculosis, most often involving the gingivae and tongue, and characterized by the presence of small, crateriform, painless ulcers that bleed readily and are surrounded by edema or reddish nodules. See also *tuberculosis gingivitis,* under *gingivitis.* **orificial t.,** t. cutis orificialis. **papulonecrotic t.,** see under *tuberculid.* **postprimary t.,** pulmonary tuberculosis, formerly known as the adult type, that is typical of a fresh infection (a reinfection) of the lungs of a person who has had an earlier and probably subclinical attack of tuberculosis; it is distinguished by caseation and cavitation and by healing that results in fibrosis. Called also *reinfection t.* **primary t.,** tuberculosis of the lungs, formerly known as the childhood type, occurring when the individual is first infected with the disease. In children, it results in tuberculous pneumonia and is characterized by the formation of a primary complex, consisting of a parenchymal pulmonary lesion with a corresponding lymph node focus. In adults, it is more likely to be marked by a small subapical focus. **primary inoculation t.,** the cutaneous reaction at the site of inoculation of tubercle bacilli in individuals with no previous exposure to *Mycobacterium tuberculosis,* associated with prominent involvement of regional lymph nodes, and manifested by a chancriform (tuberculous chancre, the most common manifestation), impetiginous, or ecthymatous lesion. Called also *primary inoculation complex* and *primary tuberculous complex.* **productive t.,** pulmonary tuberculosis in which a new type of tissue—tuberculosis granulation tissue, consisting of epithelioid cells in concentric masses, lymphocytes, and often Langhans giant cells—appears at the site of infection. **pulmonary t.,** t. of lungs. **reinfection t.,** postprimary t. **t. of serous membranes,** tuberculosis involving the pleura, peritoneum, pericardium, and cerebral meninges, producing inflammation of those structures. **t. of skin,** t. cutis. **spinal t., t. of spine,** osteitis or caries of the vertebrae, usually occurring as a complication of tuberculosis of the lungs; it is marked by stiffness of the vertebral column, pain on motion, tenderness on pressure, prominence of certain of the vertebral spines, and occasionally abdominal pain, abscess formation, and paralysis. Called also *David's disease, dorsal phthisis, Pott's disease, spondylitis tuberculosa,* and *tuberculous spondylitis.* **surgical t.,** tuberculosis which is amenable to treatment by surgical means. **tracheobronchial t.,** productive tuberculous involvement of the bronchi, characterized by wheezing, mucosal redness and edema, granulation tissue, and sometimes ulceration and bronchial stricture due to cicatrization. **t. ulcero′sa,** t. cutis orificialis. **t. verruco′sa cu′tis,** a tuberculous warty granulomatous lesion acquired accidentally by inoculation, from an infected source, of an individual having a certain degree of immunity or tuberculin sensitivity owing to previous infection or contact with *Mycobacterium* spp., and occurring often as a result of occupational inoculation (e.g., in pathologists, surgeons, postmortem attendants, or farmers) or as a consequence of autoinoculation or of superinfection from contact with tuberculous sputum. Called also *anatomical tubercle* or *wart, necrogenic, postmortem, prosector's,* or *tuberculous wart, verruca necrogenica,* and *warty tuberculosis.* **warty t.,** t. verrucosa cutis.

tuberculostatic (too-ber″ku-lo-stat′ik) inhibiting the growth of *Mycobacterium tuberculosis.*

tuberculostearic acid (tu-ber″ku-lo-ste′ah-rik as′id) an acid isolated from the acetone-soluble lipid of tubercle bacilli.

tuberculotic (too-ber″ku-lot′ik) pertaining to or affected with tuberculosis.

tuberculous (too-ber′ku-lus) pertaining to or affected

with tuberculosis: tuberculotic; caused by the *Mycobacterium tuberculosis.* Cf. *tubercular.*

tuberculum (too-ber′ku-lum), pl. *tuber′cula* [L., dim. of *tuber*] a tubercle, nodule, or small eminence; [NA] general term for such a structure. See also *tubercle, tuber, tuberositas,* and *tuberosity.* **t. adducto′rium fem′oris** [NA], adductor tubercle of femur: a small projection from the upper part of the medial epicondyle of the femur, to which the tendon of the adductor magnus muscle is attached. **t. ante′rius atlan′tis** [NA], anterior tubercle of atlas: the conical eminence on the front of the anterior arch of the atlas. **t. ante′rius thal′ami** [NA], anterior tubercle of thalamus: a distinct enlargement on the dorsal surface of the most rostral part of the thalamus; it contains the anterior nuclear group. **t. ante′rius ver′tebrae cervica′lis sex′tae** [NA], anterior tubercle of sixth cervical vertebra: the large anterior tubercle of the transverse process of the sixth cervical vertebra, which lies lateral to and at a slightly higher level than the posterior tubercle. Called also *carotid tubercle of sixth cervical vertebra* and *t. caroticum vertebrae cervicalis sextae.* **t. ante′rius vertebra′rum cervica′lium,** anterior tubercle of cervical vertebrae: a tubercle on the anterior part of the extremity of each transverse process, lying lateral to the posterior tubercle and at a slightly higher level in all except the sixth vertebra, to which are attached the scalenus anterior, longus capitis, and longus colli muscles. **t. arthrit′icum,** a gouty concretion in a joint. **t. articula′re os′sis tempora′lis** [NA], articular tubercle of temporal bone: an enlargement of the inferior border of the zygomatic process of the temporal bone, forming the anterior boundary of the mandibular fossa and part of the anterior root of the zygoma; it gives attachment to the lateral ligament of the temporomandibular articulation. Called also *tubercle of root of zygoma.* **t. auric′ulae** [NA], **t. auric′ulae [Darwin′i],** auricular tubercle: a small projection sometimes found on the edge of the helix, and conjectured by some to be a relic of a simioid ancestry. **t. calca′nei** [NA], calcaneal tubercle: the eminence, often double, on the inferior surface of the calcaneus at the anterior extremity of the rough area for the attachment of the long plantar ligament. **t. carot′icum ver′tebrae cervica′lis sextae,** t. anterius vertebrae cervicalis sextae. **t. cine′reum,** 1. t. trigeminale. 2. tuber cinereum. **t. conoi′deum** [NA], conoid tubercle: a prominent elevation on the inferior aspect of the lateral part of the clavicle, to which the conoid part of the coracoclavicular ligament is attached. **t. cornicula′tum** [NA], **t. cornicula′tum [Santorin′i],** corniculate tubercle: a rounded eminence near the posterior end of the aryepiglottic fold, posterior to the cuneiform tubercle, corresponding to the corniculate cartilage. **t. coro′nae,** tubercle of crown of tooth: any of the projections on the crown of a tooth; called also *dental cusp* and *dental tubercle.* **t. cos′tae** [NA], tubercle of rib: a small eminence on the posterior surface of a rib where the neck and body join; it protrudes inferiorly and posteriorly, and bears on its medial part a surface that articulates with the transverse process of the corresponding vertebra. **t. cunea′tum** [NA], an enlargement of the fasciculus cuneatus in the medulla oblongata, just lateral to the tuberculum gracile, produced by the underlying nucleus cuneatus; called also *tubercle of cuneate nucleus* and *t. nuclei cuneati.* **t. cuneifor′me** [NA], **t. cuneifor′me [Wrisber′gi],** cuneiform tubercle: a rounded eminence in the posterior portion of the aryepiglottic fold, anterior to the corniculate tubercle, corresponding to the cuneiform cartilage; called also *Wrisberg's tubercle.* **t. denta′le** [NA], dental tubercle: a small elevation of indiscriminate size on some portion of the crown of a tooth, produced by extra formation of enamel; called also *t. coronae.* See also *cuspis dentalis.* **t. doloro′sum,** a painful nodule or tubercle, such as one situated in the subcutaneous tissue near a joint, produced by enlargement of the end of a sensory nerve. **t. epiglot′ticum** [NA], epiglottic tubercle: a posterior projection on the inferior part of the posterior surface of the epiglottic cartilage. **t. genia′le** t. mentale mandibulae. **t. gra′cile** [NA], an enlargement of the nucleus gracilis in the medulla oblongata, forming the lower lateral border of the posterior part of the fourth ventricle, produced by the underlying nucleus gracilis; called also *tubercle of nucleus gracilis* and *t. nuclei gracilis.* **t. hypoglos′si,** trigonum nervi hypoglossi. **t. ilia′cum** [NA], iliac tubercle: a prominence on the iliac crest about 5 cm behind the anterior superior iliac spine. **t. im′par,** a small tubercle in the midline on the floor of the pharynx of the embryo, between the ends of the mandibular and hyoid arches, which is the primordium of the tongue. **t. infraglenoida′le** [NA], infraglenoid tubercle: a roughened area, just below the glenoid cavity of the scapula, that gives origin to the long head of the triceps muscle; called also *tuberositas infraglenoidalis* or *infraglenoid tuberosity*. **t. intercondyla′re latera′le** [NA], lateral intercondylar tubercle: a lateral spur projecting upward from the intercondylar eminence at the proximal end of the tibia; called also *t. intercondyloideum laterale*. **t. intercondyla′re media′le** [NA], medial intercondylar tubercle: a medial spur projecting upward from the intercondylar eminence at the proximal end of the tibia; called also *t. intercondyloideum mediale*. **t. intercondyloi′deum**, eminentia intercondylaris. **t. intercondyloi′deum latera′le**, t. intercondylare laterale. **t. intercondyloi′deum media′le**, t. intercondylare mediale. **t. interveno′sum** [NA], **t. interveno′sum [Low′eri]**, intervenous tubercle: a more or less distinct ridge across the inner surface of the right atrium between the openings of the venae cavae. **t. jugula′re os′sis occipita′lis** [NA], jugular tubercle of occipital bone: a smooth eminence overlying the hypoglossal canal on the superior surface of the lateral part of the occipital bone. **t. la′bii superio′ris** [NA], the central prominence of the upper border between the skin and the mucous membrane of the upper lip, marking the distal termination of the philtrum. Called also *procheilon, tubercle of upper lip*, and *labial tubercle*. **t. latera′le proces′sus posterio′ris ta′li** [NA], the lateral tubercle or eminence of the posterior process of the talus. **t. Low′eri**, t. intervenosum. **t. ma′jus hu′meri** [NA], greater tubercle of humerus: a large flattened prominence at the upper end of the lateral surface of the humerus, just lateral to the highest part of the anatomical neck, giving attachment to the infraspinatus, the supraspinatus, and the teres minor muscles. **t. margina′le os′sis zygomat′ici** [NA], marginal tubercle of zygomatic bone: a process on the superior part of the temporal border of the zygomatic bone to which a strong slip of the temporal fascia is attached; called also *processus marginalis ossis zygomatici*. **t. media′le proces′sus posterio′ris ta′li** [NA], the medial tubercle or eminence of the posterior process of the talus. **t. menta′le mandib′ulae** [NA], mental tubercle of mandible: a more or less distinct prominence on the inferior border of either side of the mental protuberance of the mandible. **t. mi′nus hu′meri** [NA], lesser tubercle of humerus: a distinct prominence at the proximal end of the anterior surface of the humerus, just lateral to the anatomical neck; it gives insertion to the subscapular muscle. **t. mus′culi scale′ni anterio′ris** [NA], tubercle of anterior scalene muscle: the tubercle on the cranial surface of the first rib for the insertion of the anterior scalene muscle; called also *t. scaleni [Lisfranci]*. **t. nu′clei cunea′ti**, t. cuneatum. **t. nu′clei gra′cilis, t. of nucleus gracilis**, t. gracile. **t. obturato′rium ante′rius** [NA], anterior obturator tubercle: a small spur sometimes present on the margin of the obturator foramen, projecting from the superior ramus of the pubis. **t. obturato′rium poste′rius** [NA], posterior obturator tubercle: a small protuberance often present on the margin of the obturator foramen, projecting from the free edge of the acetabular fossa near the junction of the pubis and ischium. **t. os′sis multan′guli majo′ris**, t. ossis trapezii. **t. os′sis navicula′ris**, t. ossis scaphoidei. **t. os′sis scaphoi′dei** [NA], tubercle of scaphoid bone: a projection on the volar surface of the scaphoid bone of the wrist, giving attachment to the transverse carpal ligament; called also *t. ossis navicularis*. **t. os′sis trape′zii** [NA], tubercle of trapezium: a prominent ridge on the volar surface of the trapezium bone, forming the lateral margin of the groove that transmits the tendon of the flexor carpi radialis muscle; called also *t. ossis multanguli*. **t. pharyn′geum** [NA], pharyngeal tubercle: a midline eminence on the inferior surface of the basilar part of the occipital bone, for attachment of the pharynx (superior constrictor and pharyngeal raphe). **t. poste′rius atlan′tis** [NA], posterior tubercle of atlas: a variable prominence on the posterior surface of the posterior arch of the atlas, which represents a spinous process and gives attachment to the rectus capitis posterior minor muscle. **t. poste′rius thal′ami**, pulvinar. **t. poste′rius ver′tebrae cervica′lis sex′tae** [NA], posterior tubercle of sixth cervical vertebra: the rounded posterior tubercle of the transverse process of the sixth cervical vertebra, which lies lateral to and at a slightly lower level

than the anterior tubercle. **t. poste′rius verte-bra′rum cervica′lium**, posterior tubercle of cervical vertebrae: a tubercle on the posterior part of the extremity of each transverse process of the cervical vertebra, lying lateral to the anterior tubercle and at a slightly lower level in all except the sixth vertebra, to which are attached the splenius, longissimus and iliocostalis cervicis, levator scapulae, and scalenus posterior and medius muscles. **t. pu′bicum os′sis pu′bis** [NA], pubic tubercle of pubic bone: a prominent tubercle situated at the lateral end of the pubic crest and at the medial end of the superior border of the superior ramus of the pubic bone; it is the anterior medial terminal of the obturator crest and of the pecten of the pubic bone. **t. retroloba′re**, His′ tubercle. **t. Santori′ni**, t. corniculatum. **t. scale′ni [Lisfran′ci]**, t. musculi scaleni anterioris. **t. sel′lae os′sis sphenoida′lis**, t. sellae turcicae. **t. sel′lae tur′cicae** [NA], tubercle of sella turcica: a transverse ridge on the upper surface of the body of the sphenoid bone; it is in front of the sella turcica, back of the sulcus chiasmatis, and between the anterior clinoid processes. **t. sep′ti**, a tubercle or prominence on the superior anterior part of the nasal septum. **t. supraglenoida′le** [NA], supraglenoid tubercle: a raised roughened area, just superior to the glenoid cavity of the scapula, that gives attachment to the long head of the biceps muscle of the arm; called also *tuberositas supraglenoidalis scapulae*. **t. supratra′gicum** [NA], supratragic tubercle: a small tubercle sometimes seen on the pinna just superior to the tragus. **t. thyreoi′deum infe′rius**, t. thyroideum inferius. **t. thyreoi′deum supe′rius**, t. thyroideum superius. **t. thyroi′deum infe′rius** [NA], inferior thyroid tubercle: a more or less distinct tubercle at the inferior end of the oblique line of the thyroid cartilage; called also *t. thyreoideum inferius*. **t. thyroi′deum supe′rius** [NA], superior thyroid tubercle: a more or less distinct tubercle at the superior extremity of the oblique line of the thyroid cartilage; called also *t. thyreoideum superius*. **t. trigemina′le** [NA], trigeminal tubercle: an elevation in the caudal part of the posterior surface of the medulla oblongata located between the fasciculus cuneatus and the roots of the accessory nerve, produced by the descending spinal tract of the trigeminal nerve and the caudal (inferior) cerebellar peduncle. Called also *gray tubercle, tubercle of Rolando, tuber cinereum*, and *tuberculum cinereum*.

tuberin (too′ber-in) a simple globulin from potatoes.

tuberosis (too″ber-o′sis) a condition characterized by the development of nodules.

tuberositas (too″bĕ-ros′ĭ-tas), pl. *tuberosita′tes* [L.] tuberosity: an elevation or protuberance; [NA] a general term for such a structure. See also *tuber, tubercle*, and *tuberculum*. **t. coracoi′dea**, see *tuberculum conoideum* and *linea trapezoidea*. **t. cos′tae II**, t. musculi serrati anterioris. **t. costa′lis clavic′ulae**, impressio ligamenti costoclavicularis. **t. deltoi′dea hu′meri** deltoid tuberosity of humerus: a rough, triangular elevation, about the middle of the anterolateral border of the shaft of the humerus, for attachment of the deltoid muscle. **t. fem′oris exter′na**, epicondylus lateralis femoris. **t. fem′oris inter′na**, epicondylus medialis femoris. **t. glu′tea fem′oris** [NA], gluteal tuberosity of femur: an elevation on the upper part of the shaft of the femur for attachment of the gluteus maximus muscle. **t. ili′aca** [NA], iliac tuberosity: a roughened area on the sacropelvic surface of the ilium, between the iliac crest and the auricular surface, for the attachment of muscles and ligaments. **t. infraglenoida′lis**, tuberculum infraglenoidale. **t. masseter′ica** [NA], masseteric tuberosity: an elongated, raised and roughened area on the lateral side of the angle of the mandible, for the insertion of tendinous bundles of the masseter muscles. **t. mus′culi serra′ti anterio′ris** [NA], tuberosity for serratus anterior muscle: a roughened, raised area on the second rib that gives attachment to a slip of the anterior serratus muscle; called also *t. costae II*. **t. os′sis cuboi′dei** [NA], tuberosity of cuboid bone: a transverse ridge on the lower surface of the cuboid bone over which the tendon of the peroneus longus muscle plays. **t. os′sis metatarsa′lis pri′mi** [NA], tuberosity of first metatarsal bone: a blunt process projecting downward and laterally from the lower surface of the base of the first metatarsal bone, to which the tendon of the peroneus longus muscle is attached. **t. os′sis metatarsa′lis quin′ti** [NA], tuberosity of fifth metatarsal bone: a large conical protuberance projecting backward and laterally from the base of the fifth metatarsal bone, to which the tendon of the peroneus brevis muscle is attached. **t. os'sis navicula'ris** [NA], tuberosity of navicular bone: a rough protuberance on the navicular bone of the foot, projecting downward and medially, and giving attachment to the tendon of the posterior tibial muscle. **t. patella'ris,** t. tibiae. **t. phalan'gis dista'lis ma'nus** [NA], distal tuberosity of fingers: a roughened, raised bony mass on the palmar surface of the tip of a distal phalanx of the hand; called also *t. unguicularis manus.* **t. phalan'gis dista'lis pe'dis** [NA], distal tuberosity of toes: a roughened, raised bony mass on the plantar surface of the tip of a distal phalanx of the foot; called also *t. unguicularis pedis.* **t. pterygoi'dea mandib'ulae** [NA], pterygoid tuberosity of mandible: a roughened area on the inner side of the angle of the mandible for the insertion of the internal pterygoid muscle; called also *pterygoid tubercle.* **t. ra'dii** [NA], radial tuberosity: the tuberosity on the anterior inner surface of the neck of the radius, for the insertion of the tendon of the biceps muscle. **t. sacra'lis** [NA], sacral tuberosity: a roughened area on the pars lateralis of the sacrum, on the dorsal surface between the lateral sacral crest and the auricular surface, which gives attachment to the sacroiliac ligaments. **t. supraglenoida'lis scapulae,** tuberculum supraglenoidale. **t. tib'iae** [NA], tuberosity of tibia: a longitudinally elongated, raised and roughened area on the anterior crest of the tibia, located just distal to the intercondylar eminence, and giving attachment to the patellar ligament. **t. tib'iae exter'na,** condylus lateralis tibiae. **t. tib'iae inter'na,** condylus medialis tibiae. **t. ul'nae** [NA], tuberosity of ulna: a large roughened area on the volar surface of the ulna, located just distal to the coronoid process, and giving attachment to the brachialis muscle. **t. unguicula'ris ma'nus,** t. phalangis distalis manus. **t. unguicula'ris pe'dis,** t. phalangis distalis pedis.

tuberositates (too″ber-os″ĭ-tah'tēs) [L.] plural of *tuberositas.*

tuberosity (too″bĕ-ros'ĭ-te) an elevation or protuberance; called also *tuberositas.* **t. for anterior serratus muscle,** tuberositas musculi serrati anterioris. **bicipital t.,** tuberositas radii. **t. of calcaneus,** tuber calcanei. **t. of clavicle,** impressio ligamenti costoclavicularis. **coracoid t.,** see *tuberculum conoideum* and *linea trapezoidea.* **costal t. of clavicle,** impressio ligamenti costoclavicularis. **t. of cuboid bone,** tuberositas ossis cuboidei. **deltoid t. of humerus,** tuberositas deltoidea humeri. **distal t. of fingers,** tuberositas phalangis distalis manus. **distal t. of toes,** tuberositas phalangis distalis pedis. **t. of femur, external,** epicondylus lateralis femoris. **t. of femur, internal,** epicondylus medialis femoris. **t. of femur, lateral,** epicondylus lateralis femoris. **t. of femur, medial,** epicondylus medialis femoris. **t. of fifth metatarsal,** tuberositas metatarsalis quinti. **t. of first carpal bone,** tuberculum ossis scaphoidei. **t. of first metatarsal,** tuberositas metatarsalis primi. **t. of fourth tarsal bone,** tuberositas ossis cuboidei. **gluteal t. of femur,** tuberositas glutea femoris. **greater t. of humerus,** tuberculum majus humeri. **t. of greater multangular bone,** tuberculum ossis trapezii. **t's of humerus,** the three elevations on the humerus; see *tuberculum majus humeri, tuberculum minus humeri,* and *tuberositas deltoidea humeri.* **iliac t.,** tuberositas iliaca. **infraglenoid t.,** tuberculum infraglenoidale. **ischial t., t. of ischium,** tuber ischiadicum. **lesser t. of humerus,** tuberculum minus humeri. **malar t.,** the prominence of the zygomatic bone. **masseteric t.,** tuberositas masseterica. **t. of maxilla,** tuber maxillae. **t. of navicular bone,** tuberositas ossis navicularis. **patellar t.,** tuberositas tibiae. **pterygoid t. of mandible,** tuberositas pterygoidea mandibulae. **t. of pubic bone,** tuberculum pubicum ossis pubis. **pyramidal t. of palatine bone,** processus pyramidalis ossis palatini. **radial t., t of radius,** tuberositas radii. **sacral t.,** tuberositas sacralis. **t. of scaphoid bone,** 1. tuberculum ossis scaphoidei. 2. tuberositas ossis navicularis. **scapular t. of Henle,** processus coracoideus scapulae. **t. of second rib, t. for serratus anterior muscle,** tuberositas musculi serrati anterioris. **supraglenoid t.,** tuberculum supraglenoidale. **t. of tibia,** tuberositas tibiae. **t. of tibia, external,** condylus lateralis tibiae. **t. of tibia, internal,** condylus medialis tibiae. **t. of trapezium,** tuberculum ossis trapezii. **t. of ulna,** tuberositas ulnae. **un**

gual t., unguicular t., see *tuberositas phalangis distalis manus* and *tuberositas phalangis distalis pedis.*

tuberous (too'ber-us) covered with tubers; knobby. See also under *sclerosis.*

tubi (too'bi) [L.] genitive and plural of *tubus.*

Tubifera (too-bif'er-ah) *Eristalis.*

tubiferous (too-bif'er-us) [L. *tuber* + *ferre* to bear] having tubers; tuberous.

tuboabdominal (too″bo-ab-dom'ĭ-nal) pertaining to the oviduct and the abdomen.

tuboadnexopexy (too″bo-ad-nek′so-pek″se) the operation of suturing the uterine adnexa in a fixed position.

tubocurarine (too″bo-ku-rah'rin) an alkaloid isolated from the bark and stems of *Chondodendron tomentosum* R. & P. (Menispermaceae); it is the active principle of curare (q.v.). **t. chloride** [USP], chemical name: 7′,12′-dihydroxy-6,6′-dimethoxy-2,2′,2′-trimethyltubocuraranium chloride hydrochloride pentahydrate. A neuromuscular blocking agent, $C_{37}H_{41}ClN_2O_6 \cdot HCl \cdot 5H_2O$, occurring as a white or yellowish white to grayish white, crystalline powder; administered intravenously to relax skeletal muscles in surgery, tetanus, and shock therapy, and may be used for diagnosis of myasthenia gravis in certain cases. **dimethyl t. iodide,** metocurine iodide.

tuboligamentous (too″bo-lig″ah-men'tus) pertaining to a uterine tube and a broad ligament.

tubo-ovarian (too″bo-o-va're-an) of or pertaining to a uterine tube and ovary.

tubo-ovariotomy (too″bo-o-va″re-ot'o-me) salpingo-oophorectomy.

tubo-ovaritis (too″bo-o″vah-ri'tis) salpingo-oophoritis.

tuboperitoneal (too″bo-per″ĭ-to-ne'al) pertaining to a uterine tube and the peritoneum.

tuboplasty (too′bo-plas″te) plastic repair of a tube, such as the uterine tube or the auditory tube; see also *salpingoplasty.* **eustachian t.,** plastic repair of the eustachian tube.

tuborrhea (too″bo-re'ah) [*tube* + Gr. *rhoia* flow] a condition marked by a discharge from the auditory tube.

tubotorsion (too″bo-tor'shun) a twisting of a tube, especially of the auditory tube.

tubotympanal (too″bo-tim'pah-nal) pertaining to the auditory tube and the tympanic cavity.

tubotympanum (too″bo-tim'pah-num) the auditory tube and tympanic cavity considered together.

tubouterine (too″bo-u'ter-īn) pertaining to a uterine tube and the uterus.

tubovaginal (too″bo-vaj'ĭ-nal) pertaining to a uterine tube and the vagina.

tubular (too'bu-lar) [L. *tubularis*] shaped like a tube; of or pertaining to a tubule.

tubulature (too'bu-lah-tūr) [L. *tuba* tube] the tube of a receiver or retort.

tubule (too'būl) a small tube; called also *tubulus.* **Albarrán's t's,** small branching tubules in the cervical part of the prostate gland. **Bellini's t's,** tubuli renales recti. **biliferous t.,** any small channel conveying bile. **caroticotympanic t's,** canaliculi caroticotympanici. **collecting t's,** channels through which fluids pass from the secreting cells; see *tubuli renales recti.* **connecting t's,** channels connecting other tubules, such as the arching portion of a renal tubule that connects the distal convoluted tubule with the straight tubule. **convoluted t's,** channels which follow a tortuous course; see *tubuli renales contorti* and *tubuli seminiferi contorti.* **convoluted t., distal,** see *tubuli renales contorti.* **convoluted t., proximal,** see *tubuli renales contorti.* **dental t's, dentinal t's,** canaliculi dentales. **discharging t's,** channels by which a fluid is discharged from the substance of the gland or organ in which it is secreted; see *tubuli renales recti.* **Ferrein's t's,** the portions of the renal tubules making up the pars radiata of the lobules of the renal cortex. **galactophorous t's,** ductus lactiferi. **Henle's t's,** the straight ascending and descending portions of a renal tubule forming Henle's loop; called also *straight tubules.* **Kobelt's t's,** 1. the outer series of tubules in the epoöphoron. 2. a similar series of tubules in the paradidymis of the male. **lactiferous t's,** ductus lactiferi. **malpighian t.,** one of the tubular or hairlike excretory organs arising from the midgut-hindgut junction of many arthropods; two to several hundred such tubules may be present. **mesonephric t's,** the tubules comprising the mesonephros, or temporary kidney of amniotes. **metanephric t's,** the tubules comprising the permanent kidney of amniotes. **Miescher's t.,** sarcocyst. **paraurethral t's,** ductus paraurethrales. **pronephric t's,** the tubules comprising the primitive kidney of vertebrates, rudimentary in amniotes. **Rainey's t.,** sarcocyst. **renal t's,** tubuli renales. **renal t's, convoluted,** tubuli renales contorti. **renal t's, straight,** 1. tubuli renales recti. 2. see *Henle's t's.* **segmental t's,** the tubules of the mesonephros. **seminiferous t's,** channels in the testis in which the spermatozoa develop and through which they leave the gland; see *tubuli seminiferi contorti* and *tubuli seminiferi recti.* **seminiferous t's, convoluted,** tubuli seminiferi contorti. **seminiferous t's, straight,** tubuli seminiferi recti. **Skene's t's,** ductus paraurethrales urethrae femininae. **spiral t's,** channels which follow a spiral course; see *tubuli renales contorti.* **straight t's,** channels which follow a comparatively straight course; see *tubuli renales recti* and *tubuli seminiferi recti.* **subtracheal t.,** ductus thyroglossus. **T t's,** the transverse intracellular tubules invaginating from the cell membrane and surrounding the myofibrils of the T system of skeletal and cardiac muscle, serving as a pathway for the spread of electrical excitation within a muscle cell, enabling the nearly simultaneous activation of all myofibrils; in skeletal muscle, a T tubule is the intermediate element of a triad of tubular structures, the other elements being a pair of terminal cisterns. See also *T system,* under *system; terminal cistern,* under *cistern;* and *triad of skeletal muscle.* **tracheal t.,** trachea (def. 2). **transverse t.,** T t. **uriniferous t's, uriniparous t's,** channels for the passage of urine; see *tubuli renales.* **vertical t's,** the inner set of tubules in the epoophoron.

tubuli (too'bu-li) [L.] plural of *tubulus.*

tubulin (too'bu-lin) the constituent protein of microtubules; thought to be involved in phagocyte motility.

Tubulina (too"bu-li'nah) [L. *tubulus,* dim. of *tubus* tube] a suborder of ameboid protozoa (order Amoebida, subclass Gymnamoebia) having a branched or unbranched cylindrical body. Representative genera include *Amoeba* and *Entamoeba.*

tubulization (too"bu-li-za'shun) a method of treating injured nerves by isolating the nerve stump in an absorbable cylinder which serves as a guide for new growth.

tubuloacinar (too"bu-lo-as'ĭ-nar) composed of tubular acini, as a tubuloacinar gland.

tubulocyst (too'bu-lo-sist) any cystic dilatation of a vestigial canal or functionless duct.

tubuloracemose (too"bu-lo-ras'ĕ-mōs) both tubular and racemose.

tubulorrhexis (too"bu-lo-rek'sis) [*tubule* + Gr. *rhēxis* a breaking] disruption of continuity of kidney tubules, the basement membrane being suddenly interrupted, or disintegrated into fibrils.

tubulosaccular (too"bu-lo-sak'u-lar) both tubular and saccular.

tubulous (too'bu-lus) containing tubules.

tubulus (too'bu-lus), pl. *tu'buli* [L., dim. of *tubus*] a tubule or a small tube; [NA] a general term for such a structure. **t. bilif'erus,** a channel for conveying bile; see *ductus cysticus.* **tu'buli contor'ti,** convoluted tubules; see *tubuli renales contorti* and *tubuli seminiferi contorti.* **tu'buli rec'ti,** straight tubules; see *tubuli renales recti* and *tubuli seminiferi recti.* **tu'buli rena'les** [NA], renal tubules: the minute, reabsorptive, secretory, and collecting canals, made up of basement membrane lined with epithelium, that form the substance of the kidneys. See also *nephron.* See plate accompanying *kidney.* **tu'buli rena'les contor'ti** [NA], convoluted renal tubules: the convoluted reabsorptive and secretory portions of the renal tubules, found in the renal cortex. The *proximal convoluted tubule* begins at the renal corpuscle and is continuous with the descending portion of Henle's loop; after passing back near the point of origin of the tubule, the ascending portion of the loop is continuous with the *distal convoluted tubule.* **tu'buli rena'les rec'ti** [NA], straight renal tubules: the excretory or collecting portions of the renal tubules, each of which descends from the distal convoluted tubule through the medulla, joining with

others to form a common duct that opens at the apex of a renal papilla. **tu'buli seminif'eri contor'ti** [NA], convoluted seminiferous tubules: the numerous delicate, contorted canals within each lobule of the testis, from whose epithelial linings the spermatozoa are formed. **tu'buli seminif'eri rec'ti** [NA], straight seminiferous tubules: the straight terminal portions of the seminiferous tubules, which form the rete testis.

tubus (too'bus), gen. and pl. *tu'bi* [L.] tube; used as a general term in anatomical nomenclature. **t. digesto'rius,** digestive tract.

Tuerck see *Türck.*

Tuffier's method, test (te'fe-āz) [Marin Théodore *Tuffier,* surgeon in Paris, 1857–1929] see under *method* and *tests.*

Tuffnell's treatment (tuf'nelz) [Thomas Joliffe *Tuffnell,* English surgeon, 1819–1885] see under *treatment.*

tuft (tuft) a small clump or cluster; a coil. **enamel t's,** bunches of tuftlike structures extending from the dentinoenamel junction through about one third of the thickness of the enamel, representing defects in mineralization; confined to the innermost 20–30 per cent of the enamel. **hair t's,** groups of several hairs from one follicle, consisting of one main hair and some secondary hairs. **malpighian t's, renal t's,** glomeruli renis. **synovial t's,** villi synoviales.

tuftsin (tuft'sin) [*Tufts* University + *-in*] a tetrapeptide (Thr-Lys-Pro-Arg) cleaved from IgG that stimulates phagocytosis by neutrophils. It is produced primarily in the spleen; hereditary tuftsin deficiency and tuftsin deficiency following splenectomy result in increased susceptibility to certain infections.

tugging (tug'ing) a pulling sensation. **tracheal t.,** a pulling sensation in the trachea, due to aneurysm of the arch of the aorta; it is most apparent when the head is extended and a finger is placed on the thyroid cartilage. Called also *Oliver's* or *Porter's sign.*

tularemia (too"lah-re'me-ah) [*Tulare* a county in California, where the disease was first described] an infectious, plaguelike, zoonotic disease found primarily in rodents but also affecting humans and many kinds of wildlife, with rabbits, squirrels, and muskrats being the primary source of infection by the etiologic agent, the bacillus *Francisella tularensis.* It is transmitted by the bites of deer flies, fleas, and ticks, as a result of handling contaminated animals or their products, by inhalation of aerosolized *F. tularensis,* or by ingestion of contaminated food or water. In addition to a marked reaction at the portal of entry of the pathogen, which has led to classification of the various forms of tularemia, most cases are characterized by abrupt onset of fever, chills, weakness, headache, backache, and malaise. Called also *deer fly fever, Francis' disease, Pahvant Valley fever* or *plague, rabbit fever,* and in Japan *Ohara's disease* and *Yatobyo.* **gastrointestinal t.,** a rare form of tularemia due to ingestion of large numbers of *Francisella tularensis,* characterized by cramping abdominal pain, acute watery diarrhea, fever, and, infrequently, superficial ulcerations of the colon resulting in bloody diarrhea or acute hemorrhage with minimal diarrhea. **glandular t.,** tularemia identical to the oculoglandular type except that there is no visible primary lesion. **oculoglandular t.,** a form of tularemia in which the primary site of entry of *Francisella tularensis* is the conjunctival sac, characterized by conjunctivitis, itching, lacrimation, pain, granulomatous corneal lesions that if untreated may result in perforation of the cornea and optic atrophy, and enlargement of preauricular lymph nodes. **oropharyngeal t.,** typhoidal tularemia, usually seen in children, associated with ulcerative pharyngitis with pustular lesions on the tonsils, with or without membrane formation, cervical lymph node involvement resembling the bull neck of diphtheria, and dysphagia. **pulmonary t., pulmonic t.,** tularemia associated with involvement of the lung(s), caused by lymphohematogenous spread of a primary infection or by inhalation of aerosolized *Francisella tularensis,* and characterized by nonproductive cough, headache, fever, malaise, substernal pain, and bloody, mucoid sputum. **typhoidal t.,** the most serious form of tularemia, which may be caused by swallowing an inoculum of the pathogen or by inhaling the organisms while chewing contaminated food, characterized by abdominal pain, high fever, and other symptoms similar to those of typhoid; oropharyngeal involvement and pneumonia and pleural effusion may be associated in many cases.

ulceroglandular t., the most common form of human tularemia, beginning as a painful, swollen, erythematous papule at the point of inoculation with *Francisella tularensis* that becomes pustular and then ruptures to form a shallow ulcer; mild, generalized lymphadenopathy, hepatosplenomegaly, and pneumonia may be associated.

tulase (too′lās) Von Behring's fluid, used by him in the treatment of tuberculosis.

tulle gras (tool-grah′) [Fr. "fatty tulle"] a close-meshed net cut into squares and impregnated with soft paraffin, Peruvian balsam, and vegetable oil; used in treating raw surfaces.

Tulpius' valve (tul′pe-us) [Nikolaas *Tulpius* (Nicolas *Tulp*), Dutch physician, 1593–1674] valva ileocecalis.

tumefacient (too″me-fa′shent) [L. *tumefaciens*] tending to cause or causing a swelling.

tumefaction (too″me-fak′shun) [L. *tumefactio*] a swelling; the state of being swollen, or the act of swelling; puffiness; edema.

tumentia (too-men′she-ah) [L.] swelling. **vasomotor t.,** irregular partial swelling of the lower limbs, and sometimes of the arms, associated with vasomotor changes.

tumescence (too-mes′ens) 1. the condition of being tumid or swollen. 2. a swelling.

tumeur (too-mer′) [Fr.] tumor. **t. perlée** (too-mer′ per-la′) [Fr. "pearly tumor"], cholesteatoma. **t. pileuse** (too-mer′ pe-luz′) [Fr. "hairy tumor"], trichobezoar.

tumid (too′mid) [L. *tumidus*] swollen or edematous.

tumor (too′mor) [L., from *tumere* to swell] 1. swelling, one of the cardinal signs of inflammation; morbid enlargement. 2. a new growth of tissue in which the multiplication of cells is uncontrolled and progressive; called also *neoplasm.* **Abrikosov's (Abrikossoff's) t.,** granular cell t. **acoustic nerve t.,** a tumor growing from the sheath of the acoustic nerve at the cerebellopontine angle. Called also *acoustic neuroma, acoustic neurilemoma, schwannoma,* and *acoustic neurinoma.* **acute splenic t.,** a swelling resulting from acute splenitis. **adenoid t.,** adenoma. **adenomatoid t.,** a small, circumscribed, benign tumor of the genital tract (the epididymis, tunic of testis, uterine corpus, or uterine tube), composed of small glandlike spaces lined by flattened or cuboidal mesothelium-like cells. **adipose t.,** lipoma. **adrenal rest t.,** lipoid cell t. of ovary. **t. al′bus,** "white swelling"; tuberculosis of a bone or joint. **t. al′bus pyo′genes,** a chronic inflammation of gunshot injuries of the bones and joints marked by great swelling of the capsule of the joint and surrounding soft parts, which become converted into a gelatinous, edematous granulation tissue (A. Tietze). **aniline t.,** cancer appearing in workers in the synthetic aniline dye industry. **benign t.,** one that lacks the properties of invasion and metastasis and that is usually surrounded by a fibrous capsule; its cells also show a lesser degree of anaplasia than those of malignant tumors. **blood t.,** 1. hematoma. 2. aneurysm. **Brenner t.,** a tumor of the ovary whose structure consists of groups of epithelial cells lying in a fibrous connecting tissue stroma. When small the tumor may be solid, resembling fibroma; when large it may appear like a cystadenoma with nodular masses of the tumor (Brenner nodules) in the cyst wall. Called by Brenner *oophoroma folliculare.* **Brooke's t.,** trichoepithelioma papillosum multiplex. **brown t.,** a giant-cell granuloma produced in and replacing bone, occurring in osteitis fibrosa cystica and due to hyperparathyroidism. **Brown-Pearce t.,** a transplantable anaplastic carcinoma that forms a soft, friable, necrotic, hemorrhagic lesion at the site of inoculation. **Burkitt's t.,** see under *lymphoma.* **Buschke-Löwenstein t.,** a destructive tumor clinically resembling squamous cell carcinoma but microscopically representing a form of condyloma acuminatum usually occurring on the uncircumcised penis, but also seen elsewhere in the anogenital area such as about the anus and vulva. It presents as a large verrucous to fungating, cauliflower-like mass that erodes the involved skin and progresses to penetrate and destroy the deeper tissues. Called also *giant condyloma acuminatum.* **butyroid t.,** a collection of material in the mammary gland closely resembling butter. **carcinoid t. of bronchus,** a highly vascular tumor of the bronchus similar to carcinoid (argentaffinoma) of the gastrointestinal tract. **carotid body t.,** an invariably benign, encapsulated, firm round mass at the bifurcation of the common carotid artery, with nests of large polyhedral cells in alveolar or organoid arrangement; usually asymptomatic,

but sometimes causing dizziness and nausea or vomiting. It is a form of chemodectoma. **cartilaginous t.,** a chondroma or an enchondroma. **cavernous t.,** angioma cavernosum. **cellular t.,** a tumor made up chiefly of cells in a homogeneous stroma. **chromaffin-cell t.,** pheochromocytoma. **Codman's t.,** chondroblastoma. **t. col′li,** a tumor in the neck. **colloid t.,** myxoma. **connective-tissue t.,** any tumor developed from some structure of the connective tissue, such as a lipoma, fibroma, glioma, chondroma, or sarcoma. **craniopharyngeal duct t.,** craniopharyngioma. **cystic t.,** one not solid, but more or less hollow. **dermoid t.,** a teratoma which contains fatty cutaneous elements, and sometimes hair, nails, etc.; such tumors are usually benign, but solid dermoids are more often malignant than cystic ones (dermoid cysts). Called also *teratoid t.* **desmoid t.,** desmoid. **dumb-bell t.,** hourglass t. **eiloid t.,** a skin tumor having the look of a coil of intestine. **embryonal t.,** embryoma. **embryoplastic t.,** one due to the growth of persistent embryo cells. **encysted t.,** a tumor enclosed in a membranous sac. **epithelial t.,** a tumor containing epithelium; an organized tumor. **erectile t.,** hemangioma cavernosum. **Ewing's t.,** a malignant tumor of the bone which always arises in medullary tissue, occurring more often in cylindrical bones, with pain, fever, and leukocytosis as prominent symptoms; called also *Ewing's sarcoma.* **false t.,** one due to extravasations, exudation, echinococcus, or retained sebaceous matter. **fatty t.,** lipoma. **fecal t.,** stercoroma. **fibrocellular t.,** fibroma. **fibroid t.,** fibroma. **fibroplastic t.,** a fibroma or a fibrosarcoma. **fungating t.,** a tumor with exuberant granulation. **gelatinous t.,** myxoma. **germinal t.,** a tumor of germ cell origin. **giant cell t. of bone,** a bone tumor composed of cellular spindle cell stroma containing scattered multinucleated giant cells resembling osteoclasts; symptoms may include local pain and tenderness, functional disability, and, occasionally, pathologic fractures. The tumors range from benign to frankly malignant lesions. Called also *osteoclastoma.* **giant cell t. of tendon sheath,** a benign tumor-like lesion of tendon sheath origin forming a small, yellow, discrete nodule, most commonly of the wrist and fingers, or ankle and toes; the tissue is laden with lipophages and contains multinucleated giant cells. Called also *benign synovioma* and *nodular tenosynovitis.* **glomus t.,** a blue-red, extremely painful chemodectoma involving a glomeriform arteriovenous anastomosis (glomus body), which may be found anywhere in the skin, most often in the distal portion of the fingers and toes, especially beneath the nail. Such tumors may also occur in the stomach and nasal cavity. Called also *glomangioma.* **glomus jugulare t.,** a chemodectoma involving the tympanic body (glomus jugulare). **granular cell t.,** a relatively common and usually benign neoplasm that is only rarely malignant, although multiple tumors may occur. It can be found anywhere in the body but is most often seen in the oral cavity, especially in the tongue. The tumor cells have a granular appearance by light microscopy. Originally, it was called *granular cell myoblastoma,* but ultrastructural studies have excluded a muscle cell origin. The histiogenesis is uncertain, but Schwann cell derivation is favored. Called also *Abrikosov's t.* and *granular cell schwannoma.* See also *congenital epulis,* under *epulis.* **granulation t.,** a granuloma. **granulosa t., granulosa cell t.,** an ovarian tumor originating in the cells of the primordial membrana granulosa; it may be associated with excessive production of estrin, inducing endometrial hyperplasia with menorrhagia. Called also *folliculoma* and *granulosa cell carcinoma.* **granulosa-theca cell t.,** an ovarian tumor predominantly composed of either granulosa cells (follicular cells) or theca cells, and often associated with excessive production of estrogen, with hyperplasia of the breast and endometrium, and carcinoma of the endometrium. When luteinized, i.e., having cells resembling those of the corpus luteum, it is known as luteoma. **Grawitz's t's,** hypernephroma; the tumors formerly known as adenomas of the kidney, but which Grawitz thought to be an overgrowth of fetal inclusion in the midst of the kidney substance or particles of suprarenal glandular tissue: now considered carcinoma of the renal parenchyma. **Gubler's t.,** a tumor on the back of the wrist, with paralysis of the extensors of the hand, in cases of lead poisoning. **gummy t.,** gumma. **heterologous t.,** one made up of tissue which differs from that in which it grows. **heterotypic t.,** heterologous t. **hilar cell t.,** a rare benign neoplasm of the hilus of the ovary, histologically resembling Leydig cell tumor of the testis; it may cause virilization. **histioid t.,** one which is formed of a single tissue resembling that of the surrounding parts. **homoiotypic t., homologous t.,** a tumor which resembles the surrounding parts in its structure. **Hortega cell t.,** a cellular tumor of the lymphoreticular system arising in the central nervous system. **hourglass t.,** a spinal tumor made up of intradural and extradural masses joined by a narrow pedicle passing through an enlarged intervertebral foramen. **Hürthle cell t.,** a new growth of the thyroid gland composed wholly or predominantly of large cells (Hürthle cells) having abundant granular, eosinophilic cytoplasm. Such tumors are usually benign (Hürthle cell adenoma) but on occasion may be locally invasive or may rarely metastasize (Hürthle cell carcinoma, or malignant Hürthle cell tumor). **infiltrating t.,** a tumor which is not clearly marked off from the surrounding tissue. **innocent t.,** benign t. **islet cell t.,** a tumor of the islets of Langerhans; such tumors may result in hyperinsulinism or in Zollinger-Ellison syndrome. **ivory-like t.,** osteoma durum. **Jensen's t.,** see under *sarcoma*. **Krompecher's t.,** rodent ulcer. **Krukenberg's t.,** a special type of carcinoma of the ovary, usually metastatic from cancer of the gastrointestinal tract, especially of the stomach. It is characterized by areas of mucoid degeneration and the presence of signet-ring–like cells. Called also *carcinoma mucocellulare*. **lacteal t.,** 1. mammary abscess. 2. galactocele. **Leydig cell t.,** the most common nongerminal tumor of the testis, derived from the Leydig cells of the testis; such tumors are rarely malignant. **t. lie′nis,** enlargement of the spleen less in degree than splenomegaly. **lipoid cell t. of ovary,** a rare, usually benign, ovarian tumor composed of eosinophilic cells or cells with lipoid vacuoles, arising from ovarian cells or embryonic rest cells of the adrenals; it causes masculinization. Called also *adrenal rest t.* and *masculinovoblastoma.* **luteinized granulosa-theca cell t.,** luteoma. **malignant t.,** one that has the properties of invasion and metastasis and that shows a greater degree of anaplasia than do benign tumors. **march t.,** syndesmitis metatarsea. **margaroid t.,** a cholesteatoma. **mast cell t.,** mastocytoma. **melanotic neuroectodermal t.,** a benign, rapidly growing, deeply pigmented tumor of the jaw and occasionally of other sites, consisting of an infiltrating mass of cells arranged in an alveolar pattern, and occurring almost exclusively in infants. Its source of origin is in dispute, the various theories giving rise to its several names. Called also *melanoameloblastoma, melanotic ameloblastoma, pigmented ameloblastoma, melanotic progonoma,* and *retinal anlage tumor.* **migrated t., migratory t.,** a tumor arising from a portion of a primary tumor which has become detached from its original location and fixed in some other place or lies free in a cavity. **mixed t.,** a tumor composed of more than one type of neoplastic tissue; especially "a complex embryonal tumor of local origin, which reproduces the normal development of the tissues and organs of the affected part" (Ewing). **mucous t.,** a myxoma. **muscular t.,** a myoma. **Nélaton's t.,** a dermoid tumor of the wall of the abdomen. **neuroepithelial t.,** a highly malignant tumor of peripheral nerves, developed from elements derived from the neural crest and resembling tumors of the central nervous system. **oozing t.,** a rare disease, consisting of a large, flat tumor on one or both labia majora, divided with deep fissures, and discharging a large amount of acrid, offensive fluid. **organoid t.,** a teratoma. **oxyphil cell t.,** Hürthle cell t. **Pancoast's t.,** pulmonary sulcus t. **papillary t.,** a papilloma. **pearl t., pearly t.,** cholesteatoma. **Perlmann's t.,** a benign multiloculated cystic tumor of the kidney, surrounded by a dense fibrous capsule and showing a yellow-blue-gray color on its cut surface. **plasma cell t.,** plasmacytoma. **potato t.,** chemodectoma of the carotid body. **Pott's puffy t.,** a circumscribed area of edema surrounding lesions of osteomyelitis of the skull. **pregnancy t.,** tumorous gingivitis histologically and clinically identical to angiogranuloma or to pyogenic granuloma seen in pregnant women, especially after the third trimester, and occurring as a result of minor trauma or irritation probably intensified by the endocrine alternation during pregnancy. It may or may not regress after delivery. Identical lesions are also seen in men and in nonpregnant women. **premalignant fibroepithelial t.,** premalignant fibroepithelioma. **pseudointraligamentous t.,** a kind of ovarian tumor simulating intraligamentous tumors, but in reality adherent to the posterior surface of the broad ligament. **pulmonary sulcus t.,** one at the apex of the lung, extending outward to destroy the ribs and vertebrae and invading the brachial plexus; called also *Pancoast's t.* **Rathke's t., Rathke's pouch t.,** craniopharyngioma. **Recklinghausen's t.,** adenoleiomyofibroma of the posterior uterine wall or of the wall of an oviduct. **recurring digital fibrous t's of childhood,** infantile digital fibromatosis. **retinal anlage t.,** melanotic neuroectodermal tumor. **sacrococcygeal t.,** a form of spina bifida containing teratomatous tissue. **sand t.,** psammoma. **Schmincke t.,** lymphoepithel*i*oma. **Schwann-cell t.,** a neoplasm of a nerve sheath (Schwann's sheath); schwannoma. **Sertoli cell t.,** androblastoma, def. 1. **Sertoli-Leydig cell t.,** arrhenoblastoma. **sheath t.,** a tumor of the sheaths of the brain or peripheral nerves, including meningioma, acoustic nerve tumor, and schwannoma. **Steiner's t's,** Jeanselme's nodules. **stercoral t.,** stercoroma. **superior sulcus t.,** pulmonary sulcus t. **teratoid t.,** teratoma. **theca cell t.,** a fibroid-like tumor of the ovary containing yellow areas of lipoid material derived from theca cells. It may be associated with excessive production of estrogen and have a tendency to cystic degeneration. The tumor is rarely composed entirely of theca cells; commonly both theca and follicular cells (granulosa cells) are found. Called also *thecoma* and *fibroma thecocellulare xanthomatodes.* See also *granulosa-theca cell t.* **transition t.,** one which recurs after removal and then shows malignant characters. **tridermic t.,** a teratoma. **true t.,** a neoplasm. **turban t.,** a term used to describe the gross appearance of multiple cylindromas of the scalp. See *cylindroma,* def. 1. **varicose t.,** a swelling, composed of dilated veins. **vascular t.,** 1. a tumor of blood vessel elements; an angioma. 2. any tumor with a copious blood supply. **villous t.,** papilloma. **Warthin's t.,** papillary adenocystoma lymphomatosum. **white t.,** chronic tuberculous arthritis. **Wilms' t.,** a rapidly developing malignant mixed tumor of the kidneys, made up of embryonal elements; it usually affects children before the fifth year, but may occur in the fetus and rarely in later life. Called also *embryonal adenomyosarcoma, carcinosarcoma,* or *nephroma,* and *nephroblastoma.* **yolk sac t.,** mesonephroma (type 2).

tumoraffin (too″mor-af′in) [*tumor* + L. *affinis* related] having a special affinity for tumor cells; oncotropic.

tumoricidal (too″mor-ĭ-si′dal)   destructive to cancer cells.

tumorigenesis (too″mor-ĭ-jen′ĕ-sis)   the production of tumors.

tumorigenic (too″mor-ĭ-jen′ik)   giving rise to tumors; said especially of a cell or group of cells capable of producing a tumor. Cf. *oncogenic.*

tumorous (too′mor-us)   of the nature of a tumor.

tumultus (too-mul′tus) [L.]   excessive organic action or motility.

Tunga (tung′gah)   a genus of fleas of the family Hectopsyllidae. **T. pen′etrans,** a species widely distributed in the tropical and subtropical regions of America and Africa; called *Dermatophilus penetrans.* See *chigoe.*

tungiasis (tung-gi′ah-sis)   infestation of the skin with *Tunga penetrans.* Called also *dermatophiliasis.* See *chigoe.*

tungsten (tung′sten) [Swed. "heavy stone"]   the chemical element of atomic number 74, symbol W, and atomic weight 183.85; used in electric light filaments and in steel alloys to secure hardness.

tunic (too′nik)   a covering or coat; see *tunica.* **Bichat's t.,** tunica intima vasorum. **Brücke's t.,** tunica nervea of Brücke. **fibrous t.,** tunica fibrosa. **fibrous t. of eyeball,** tunica fibrosa bulbi. **fibrous t. of liver,** tunica fibrosa hepatis. **mucous t.,** tunica mucosa. **muscular t.,** tunica muscularis. **pharyngeal t., pharyngobasilar t.,** fascia pharyngobasilaris. **proper t.,** tunica propria. **Ruysch's t.,** lamina choriocapillaris. **serous t.,** tunica serosa. **t's of spermatic cord,** tunicae funiculi spermatici.

tunica (too′nĭ-kah), pl. *tu′nicae* [L.]   a covering or coat; [NA] a general term for a membrane or other structure covering or lining a body part or organ. Called also *tunic.* **t. abdomina′lis,** the aponeurosis of the abdominal muscles in certain quadrupeds, as the horse. **t. adna′ta o′culi,** tunica conjunctiva; sometimes applied specifically to the tunica conjunctiva bulbi. **t. adna′ta tes′tis,** lamina parietalis tunicae vaginalis testis. **t. adventi′tia** [NA], the outer coat of various tubular structures, made up of connective tissue and elastic fibers. **t. adventi'tia duc'tus deferen'tis** [NA], the adventitious coat of the ductus deferens. **t. adventi'tia esoph'agi**, NA alternative for *t. adventitia oesophagi*. **t. adventi'tia oesoph'agi** [NA], the adventitious coat of the esophagus. Written also *t. adventitia esophagi* [NA alternative]. **t. adventi'tia tu'bae uteri'nae**, tela subserosa tubae uterinae. **t. adventi'tia ure'teris** [NA], the adventitious coat of the ureter. **t. adventi'tia vaso'rum**, t. externa vasorum. **t. adventi'tia vesic'ulae semina'lis** [NA], the adventitious coat of the seminal vesicle. **t. albugin'ea** [NA], a dense, white, fibrous sheath enclosing a part or organ. **t. albugin'ea cor'poris spongio'si** [NA], the dense, white, fibroelastic sheath that encloses the corpus spongiosum of the penis. **t. albugin'ea corpo'rum caverno'rum** [NA], the dense, white, fibroelastic sheath that encloses the corpora cavernosa penis. Its superficial, longitudinal fibers form a tunic surrounding both corpora, and the deep circularly coursing fibers surround them separately, uniting medially to form the septum of the penis. **t. albugin'ea ova'rii** [NA], the layer of dense connective tissue beneath the germinal epithelium of the ovary. **t. albugin'ea tes'tis** [NA], the dense, white, inelastic tissue immediately covering the testis, beneath the visceral layer of the tunica vaginalis. **t. conjuncti'va** [NA], the thin, transparent mucous membrane lining the eyelids and covering the front surface of the eyeball; called also *conjunctiva*. It comprises the tunica conjunctiva bulbi and the tunica conjunctiva palpebrarum. **t. conjuncti'va bul'bi** [NA], **t. conjuncti'va bul'bi o'culi**, bulbar conjunctiva: the portion of the tunica conjunctiva covering the cornea and front part of the sclera, appearing white because of the sclera behind it. **t. conjuncti'va palpebra'rum** [NA], palpebral conjunctiva: the portion of the tunica conjunctiva lining the eyelids, appearing red because of its great vascularity. **t. dar'tos** 1. [NA] the thin layer of subcutaneous tissue underlying the skin of the scrotum, consisting mainly of nonstriated muscle fibers (*musculus dartos*). Called also *dartos* and *dartos muscle*. 2. musculus dartos. **t. elas'tica inter'na**, t. intima vasorum. **t. ex'terna the'cae follic'uli** [NA], the external, fibrous layer of the theca folliculi. **t. exter'na vaso'rum** [NA], **t. exter'na vaso'rum [adventi'tia]**, the outer, fibroelastic coat of a blood vessel. **t. fibro'sa** [NA], fibrous tunic or coat: an enveloping fibrous membrane. **t. fibro'sa bul'bi** [NA], fibrous tunic of eyeball: the outer of the three tunics of the eye, comprising the cornea and the sclera; called also *t. fibrosa oculi*. **t. fibro'sa hep'atis** [NA], fibrous tunic of liver: the fibroelastic layer that surrounds the liver beneath the peritoneum; it is continuous at the hepatic portal with the perivascular fibrous capsule. **t. fibro'sa lie'nis**, NA alternative for *t. fibrosa splenis*. **t. fibro'sa o'culi**, t. fibrosa bulbi. **t. fibro'sa re'nis**, capsula fibrosa renis. **t. fibro'sa sple'nis** [NA], the fibroelastic coat of the spleen; called also *t. fibrosa lienis* [NA alternative]. **tu'nicae funic'uli spermat'ici** [NA], tunics of spermatic cord: the coverings of the spermatic cord, comprising the external spermatic fascia, the cremasteric muscle and fascia, the internal spermatic fascia, and the tunica vaginalis testis. **t. inter'na bul'bi** [NA], the internal nervous tunic of the eye; called also *t. sensoria bulbi* [NA alternative]. See *retina*. **t. inter'na the'cae follic'uli** [NA], the inner, vascular layer of secretory cells of the theca folliculi; called also *theca interna* and *internal coat of capsule of graafian follicle*. **t. in'tima vaso'rum** [NA], the inner coat of the blood vessels, made up of endothelial cells surrounded by longitudinal elastic fibers and connective tissue. **t. me'dia vaso'rum** [NA], the middle coat of the blood vessels, made up of transverse elastic and muscle fibers. **t. muco'sa** [NA], mucous tunic or coat: the mucous membrane lining of various tubular structures, comprising the epithelium, basement membrane, lamina propria mucosae, and lamina muscularis mucosae. **t. muco'sa bronchio'rum** [NA], the mucous membrane lining the bronchi. **t. muco'sa cavita'tis tympan'icae** [NA], the mucous membrane covering the walls and much of the contents of the tympanic cavity; called also *t. mucosa tympanica* and *mucous coat of tympanic cavity*. **t. muco'sa co'li** [NA], the mucous coat of the colon. **t. muco'sa duc'tus deferen'tis** [NA], the mucous coat of the ductus deferens. **t. muco'sa esoph'agi**, NA alternative for *t. mucosa oesophagi*. **t. muco'sa gas'tris**

[NA], the mucous coat of the stomach; called also *t. mucosa ventriculi* [NA alternative]. **t. muco'sa intesti'ni rec'ti**, t. mucosa recti. **t. muco'sa intesti'ni ten'uis** [NA], the mucous coat of the small intestine. **t. muco'sa laryn'gis** [NA], the mucous coat of the larynx. **t. muco'sa lin'guae** [NA], the mucous membrane covering the tongue. **t. muco'sa na'si** [NA], the mucous membrane lining the nasal cavity; called also *membrana mucosa nasi*. See also *regio olfactoria* and *regio respiratoria*. **t. muco'sa oesophagi** [NA], the mucous coat of the esophagus. Written also *t. mucosa esophagi* [NA alternative]. **t. muco'sa o'ris** [NA], the tunica mucosa of the mouth. **t. muco'sa pharyn'gis** [NA], the mucous coat of the pharynx. **t. muco'sa rec'ti** [NA], the mucous coat of the rectum; called also *t. mucosa intestini recti*. **t. muco'sa tra'cheae** [NA], the mucous coat of the trachea. **t. muco'sa tu'bae auditi'vae** [NA], the mucous membrane lining the auditory tube. **t. muco'sa tu'bae uteri'nae** [NA], the mucous coat of the uterine tube. **t. muco'sa tympan'ica**, t. mucosa cavitatis tympanicae. **t. muco'sa ure'teris** [NA], the mucous coat of the ureter. **t. muco'sa ure'thrae femini'nae** [NA], **t. muco'sa ure'thrae mulie'bris**, the mucous coat of the female urethra. **t. muco'sa u'teri** [NA], the mucous membrane lining the uterus, the thickness and structure of which vary with the phase of the menstrual cycle. See also *endometrium* [NA alternative]. **t. muco'sa vagi'nae** [NA], the mucous coat of the vagina. **t. muco'sa ventric'uli**, NA alternative for *t. mucosa gastris*. **t. muco'sa vesi'cae bilia'ris** [NA], the mucous coat of the gallbladder; called also *t. mucosa vesicae felleae* [NA alternative]. **t. muco'sa vesi'cae fel'leae**, NA alternative for *t. mucosa vesicae biliaris*. **t. muco'sa vesi'cae urina'riae** [NA], the mucous coat of the urinary bladder. **t. muco'sa vesic'ulae semina'lis** [NA], the mucous coat of the seminal vesicle. **t. muscula'ris** [NA], muscular tunic or coat: the muscular coat or layer surrounding the tela submucosa in most portions of the digestive, respiratory, urinary, and genital tracts. **t. muscula'ris bronchio'rum** [NA], the muscular coat of the bronchi. **t. muscula'ris coli** [NA], the muscular coat of the colon, consisting of layers of longitudinally and circularly coursing fibers. **t. muscula'ris duc'tus deferen'tis** [NA], the muscular coat of the ductus deferens. **t. muscula'ris esoph'agi**, t. muscularis oesophagi. **t. muscula'ris gas'tris** [NA], the muscular coat of the stomach, composed of longitudinal, circular, and oblique fibers; called also *t. muscularis ventriculi* [NA alternative]. **t. muscula'ris intesti'ni ten'uis** [NA], the muscular coat of the small intestine, consisting of an inner circular and an outer longitudinal layer. **t. muscula'ris oesoph'agi** [NA], the muscular coat of the esophagus. **t. muscula'ris pharyn'gis** [NA], the muscular coat of the pharynx, consisting primarily of the pharyngeal constrictor muscles. **t. muscula'ris rec'ti** [NA], the muscular coat of the rectum, consisting of an outer longitudinal and an inner circular layer. **t. muscula'ris tra'cheae** [NA], the muscular coat of the trachea. **t. muscula'ris tu'bae uteri'nae** [NA], the muscular coat of the uterine tube. **t. muscula'ris ure'teris** [NA], the muscular coat of the ureter. **t. muscula'ris ure'thrae femini'nae** [NA], **t. muscula'ris ure'thrae mulie'bris**, the muscular coat of the female urethra. **t. muscula'ris u'teri** [NA], the smooth muscle coat of the uterus, which forms the mass of the organ; called also *myometrium* [NA alternative] and *mesometrium*. **t. muscula'ris vagi'nae** [NA], the muscular coat of the vagina. **t. muscula'ris ventric'uli**, NA alternative for *t. muscularis gastris*. **t. muscula'ris vesi'cae bilia'ris** [NA], the muscular coat of the gallbladder; called also *t. muscularis vesicae felleae* [NA alternative]. **t. muscula'ris vesi'cae fel'leae**, NA alternative for *t. muscularis vesicae biliaris*. **t. muscula'ris vesi'cae urina'riae** [NA], the smooth muscle coat of the urinary bladder. **t. muscula'ris vesic'ulae semina'lis** [NA], the muscular coat of the seminal vesicle. **t. ner'vea of Brücke**, the cerebral layer of the retina, exclusive of the rod and cone layer with its fibers and nuclei. **t. pro'pria** [NA], proper tunic: a general term in anatomical nomenclature for the proper coat or layer of a part, as distinguished from an investing membrane. **t. pro'pria co'rii**, stratum reticulare dermidis. **t. pro'pria tu'buli tes'tis**, the proper coat of the seminiferous tubules. **t. ruyschia'na**, lamina choriocapillaris. **t. senso'ria bul'bi**, NA alternative for *t.*

interna bulbi. **t. sero′sa** [NA], the membrane lining the external walls of the body cavities and reflected over the surfaces of protruding organs; it consists of mesothelium lying upon a connective tissue layer, and it secretes a watery exudate; called also *serous coat, membrane,* or *tunic.* **t. sero′sa co′li** [NA], the serous coat of the colon. **t. sero′sa gas′tris** [NA], the serous coat of the stomach; called also *t. serosa ventriculi* [NA alternative]. **t. sero′sa hep′atis** [NA], the serous coat of the liver. **t. sero′sa intesti′ni ten′uis** [NA], the serous coat of the small intestine. **t. sero′sa lie′nis,** NA alternative for *tunica serosa splenis.* **t. sero′sa peritone′i** [NA], the serous coat of the peritoneum. **t. sero′sa sple′nis** [NA], the serous coat of the spleen; called also *t. serosa lienis* [NA alternative]. **t. sero′sa tes′tis,** lamina visceralis tunicae vaginalis testis. **t. sero′sa tu′bae uteri′nae** [NA], the serous coat of the uterine tube. **t. sero′sa u′teri** [NA], the serous coat of the uterus; called also *perimetrium* [NA alternative]. **t. sero′sa ventric′uli,** NA alternative for *t. serosa gastris.* **t. sero′sa vesi′cae bilia′ris** [NA], the serous coat of the gallbladder; called also *t. serosa vesicae felleae* [NA alternative]. **t. sero′sa vesi′cae fel′leae,** NA alternative for *t. serosa vesicae biliaris.* **t. sero′sa vesi′cae urina′riae** [NA], the serous coat of the urinary bladder. **t. spongio′sa ure′thrae femini′nae** [NA], a thin layer of spongiose erectile tissue located just beneath the mucous coat of the female urethra, which contains a plexus of large veins. **t. spongio′sa vagi′nae** [NA], a thin layer of spongiose erectile tissue located between the muscular and mucous coats of the vagina, which contains a large plexus of blood vessels. **t. submuco′sa ure′thrae mulie′bris,** the submucous coat of the female urethra. **tu′nicae tes′tis** [NA], the coverings of the testis; see *tunicae funiculi spermatici.* **t. u′vea,** t. vasculosa bulbi. **t. vagina′lis tes′tis** [NA], the serous membrane covering the front and sides of the testis and epididymis, composed of a visceral and a parietal layer. **t. vasculo′sa,** a vascular coat, or a layer well supplied with blood vessels. **t. vasculo′sa bul′bi** [NA], vascular tunic of the eye: the middle, pigmented, vascular coat of the eyeball, comprising the choroid, the ciliary body, and the iris; called also *uvea* and *uveal tract.* **t. vasculo′sa len′tis,** the vascular envelope which encloses and nourishes the developing lens of the fetus; it consists of the *pupillary membrane* in the region of the pupil, the *capsulopupillary membrane* around the edge of the lens, and the *capsular membrane* at the back of the lens. **t. vasculo′sa oc′uli,** t. vasculosa bulbi.

tunicary (too′nĭ-ker″e) pertaining to or possessing a tunic or enveloping membrane.

Tunicata (too″nĭ-ka′tah) [L. "clothed with a tunic"] Urochordata.

tunicate (too′nĭ-kāt) an animal belonging to the Urochordata (Tunicata), a urochordate.

tunicin (too′nĭ-sin) a substance resembling cellulose occurring in the body covering of some of the lowest vertebrates, such as the tunicates or ascidians; animal cellulose.

tuning fork (toon′ing fork) a two-tined forklike instrument of steel or aluminum, the tines of which when struck give off a musical note.

tunnel (tun′el) a passageway of varying length, through a solid body, completely enclosed except for the open ends, permitting entrance and exit. **aortico-left ventricular t.,** a congenital communication between the ascending aorta just above the coronary arteries, and the left ventricle. **carpal t.,** the osseofibrous passage for the median nerve and the flexor tendons, formed by the flexor retinaculum and the carpal bones. Called also *canalis carpi* [NA]. **cervical t's,** small tubular canals which are extensions of the clefts in the uterine endocervical mucosa. **Corti's t.,** inner t. **cubital t.,** the opening between the two heads of the flexor carpi ulnaris muscle through which the ulnar nerve enters the forearm. **flexor t.,** carpal t. **inner t.,** a canal extending the length of the cochlea, formed by the pillar cells of the organ of Corti; called also *canal of Corti* and *Corti's t.* **outer t.,** Nuel's space. **tarsal t.,** the osseofibrous passage for the posterior tibial vessels, tibial nerve, and flexor tendons, formed by the flexor retinaculum and tarsal bones.

turacin (too′rah-sin) a red or crimson pigment, a copper salt of uroporphyrin.

turacoporphyrin (too″rah-ko-por′fĭ-rin) a derivative from turacin; nearly identical with hematoporphyrin.

turanose (too′rah-nōs) a reducing disaccharide, $C_{12}H_{22}O_{11}$, obtained by partially hydrolyzing melezitose.

Turbatrix (tur-ba′triks) a genus of nematodes. **T. aceti,** a minute nematode found in vinegar, where it helps form "mother of vinegar"; it sometimes occurs in the urine of patients who have used vinegar douches. It may also occur in sour paste and fermenting vegetable substances. Formerly called *Anguillula aceti.*

Turbellaria (tur″be-la′re-ah) a class of platyhelminths, usually found in fresh or salt water, although some are terrestrial.

turbid (tur′bid) [L. *turba* a tumult] cloudy; showing turbidity.

turbidimeter (tur″bĭ-dim′ĕ-ter) an instrument that measures the turbidity of a solution by measuring the loss of intensity of a beam of light in passing through the solution. Cf. *nephelometer.*

turbidimetric (tur″bid-ĭ-met′rik) performed by the turbidimeter.

turbidimetry (tur″bĭ-dim′ĕ-tre) the measurement of the tubidity of a fluid.

turbidity (tur-bid′ĭ-te) cloudiness of a solution caused by the scattering of light by colloidal particles or by suspended precipitate or sediment.

turbinal (tur′bĭ-nal) [L. *turbinalis,* from *turbo* a child's top] 1. shaped like a top; turbinate. 2. a turbinate bone.

turbinate (tur′bĭ-nāt) [L. *turbineus*] 1. shaped like a top. 2. a turbinate bone (concha nasalis). **sphenoid t.,** concha sphenoidalis.

turbinated (tur′bĭ-nāt″ed) shaped like a top.

turbinectomy (tur″bĭ-nek′to-me) [*turbinate* + Gr. *ektomē* excision] the surgical removal of a turbinate bone.

turbinotome (tur-bin′o-tōm) a cutting instrument for use in the removal or cutting of a turbinate bone.

turbinotomy (tur″bĭ-not′o-me) [*turbinate* + Gr. *tomē* a cutting] the surgical cutting of a turbinate bone.

Türck's bundle, cell, column, degeneration, fasciculus (column), trachoma (tĕrks) [Ludwig *Türck,* neurologist and laryngologist in Vienna, 1810–1868] see under the nouns.

Turck's zone (turks) [Fenton Benedict *Turck,* New York physician, 1857–1932] see *zona transformans.*

turgescence (tur-jes′ens) [L. *turgescens* swelling] the distention or swelling of a part.

turgescent (tur-jes′ent) [L. *turgescens*] swelling or beginning to swell.

turgid (tur′jid) [L. *turgidus*] swollen and congested.

turgidization (tur″jid-i-za′shun) the creation of turgor in a tissue by the injection of fluid.

turgometer (tur-gom′ĕ-ter) [L. *turgor* swelling + *metrum* measure] an instrument for measuring the amount of turgescence.

turgor (tur′gor) [L.] the condition of being turgid; normal or other fullness. **t. vita′lis,** the normal consistency of living tissue.

turista (tu-rēs′tah) [Sp.] Mexican name for traveler's diarrhea.

Türk's cell (irradiation leukocyte) (tĕrks) [Wilhelm *Türk,* Austrian physician, 1871–1916] see under *cell.*

turmeric (tur′mer-ik) the rhizome of *Curcuma longa* L. (Zingiberaceae), a plant of India, China, and East Indies. It contains curcumin, an orange-yellow coloring principle, and several aromatic principles that give it a pepper-like and bitter taste; used as a coloring agent, chemical indicator, and condiment (as curry powder).

turmschadel (torm′sha-del) [Ger.] a developmental anomaly in which the skull is high and rounded, due to early synostosis of the three major sutures of the skull.

Turner's sign (tur′nerz) [George Grey *Turner,* English surgeon, 1877–1951] see under *sign.*

Turner's sulcus (tur′nerz) [William Aldren *Turner,* British neurologist, born 1864] sulcus intraparietalis.

Turner's syndrome (tur′nerz) [Henry Hubert *Turner,* American endocrinologist, 1892–1970] see under *syndrome.*

Turner tooth (hypoplasia) (tur′ner) [Joseph George *Turner,* British dentist, died 1955] see under *tooth.*

turnera (tur'ner-ah) damiana.

turnover (turn'o-ver) the movement of something into, through, and out of a place; the rate at which a thing is depleted and replaced. **erythrocyte iron t. (EIT),** the rate at which iron moves from the bone marrow into circulating red cells, calculated as: plasma iron turnover (PIT) × red cell utilization (RCU). Called also *red blood cell iron turnover*. **plasma iron t. (PIT),** the rate at which iron leaves the blood plasma to the bone marrow or other tissues, calculated as: plasma iron concentration × plasma volume × 0.693 ÷ the plasma iron clearance half-time, expressed in mg/day. **red blood cell iron t. (RBC IT),** erythrocyte iron t.

turnsick, turnsickness (turn'sik, turn'sik-nes) gid.

turnsol (turn'sol) litmus.

TURP transurethral prostatic resection.

turpentine (tur'pen-tīn) [L. *terebinthina*] the concrete oleoresin obtained from *Pinus palustris* Mill. (Pinaceae) and other species of *Pinus*. It contains a volatile oil, to which its properties are due, and in which form it is generally used; see under *oil*.

turricephaly (tur''ĭ-sef'ah-le) oxycephaly.

turunda (tu-run'dah) [L.] 1. tent (def. 2). 2. a suppository.

Turyn's sign (too'rinz) [Felix *Turyn*, Warsaw physician, born 1899] see under *sign*.

tus. abbreviation for L. *tus'sis*, a cough.

tussal (tus'al) [L. *tussis* cough] pertaining to a cough.

tussicula (tŭ-sik'u-lah) [L., dim. of *tussis* cough] a slight cough.

tussicular (tŭ-sik'u-lar) [L. *tussicula*] of or relating to a cough.

tussiculation (tŭ-sik''u-la'shun) a short, hacking cough.

tussigenic (tus''ĭ-jen'ik) [L. *tussis* cough + Gr. *gennan* to produce] causing cough.

tussis (tus'is) [L.] cough.

tussive (tus'iv) pertaining to or due to a cough.

tutamen (tu-ta'men), pl. *tuta'mina* [L.] a protective covering or structure. **tuta'mina o'culi** ["defenses of the eye"], the appendages of the eye: the eyelids, lashes, etc. (organa oculi accessoria [NA]).

tutamina (tu-tam'ĭ-nah) [L.] plural of *tutamen*.

Tuttle's proctoscope (tut'l'z) [James Percival *Tuttle*, surgeon in New York, 1857–1912] see under *proctoscope*.

Tween (twēn) trademark for preparations of polysorbates, used with a numerical suffix; e.g., *Tween 80* is a trademark for polysorbate 80.

tween-brain (twēn'brān) diencephalon.

twig in anatomy, a final ramification, as of branches of nerves or blood vessels.

twin (twin) one of two offspring produced in the same pregnancy and developed from one ovum (monozygotic) or from two ova (dizygotic) fertilized at the same time. **acardiac t.,** acardius. **allantoidoangiopagous t's,** twins joined by the vessels of the umbilical cord only; called also *omphaloangiopagous t's*. **binovular t's,** dizygotic t's. **conjoined t's,** monozygotic twins ranging from two well-developed individuals joined by a superficial connection of varying extent, usually in the frontal, transverse, or sagittal body plane (*symmetrical* or *equal conjoined t's*), to those in which only a small part of the body is duplicated or one small and incompletely developed component, the parasite, is attached to a much larger and more fully developed one, the autosite (*asymmetrical* or *unequal t's*). Called also *Siamese t's*. **conjoined t's, asymmetrical,** see *conjoined t's*. **conjoined t's, equal,** see *conjoined t's*. **conjoined t's, symmetrical,** see *conjoined t's*. **conjoined t's, unequal,** see *conjoined t's*. **dichorial t's, dichorionic t's,** dizygotic t's. **dissimilar t's,** dizygotic t's. **dizygotic t's,** two offspring developed from two separate ova fertilized at the same time; they may be of the same or different sex, and they have different genomes. Called also *binovular, dichorial, dichorionic, dissimilar, false, fraternal, heterologous, hetero-ovular, two-egg,* and *unlike t's*. **enzygotic t's,** monozygotic t's. **false t's,** dizygotic t's. **fraternal t's,** dizygotic t's. **heterologous t's,** dizygotic t's. **hetero-ovular t's,** dizygotic t's. **identical t's,** monozygotic t's. **impacted t's,** twins so situated during delivery that the pressure of one against the other prevents simultaneous engagement of both. **monoamniotic t's,** twins developing within a single amniotic cavity; they are always monozygotic. **monochorial t's, monochorionic t's,** monozygotic t's. **mono-ovular t's, monovular t's,** monozygotic t's. **monozygotic t's,** two offspring developed from one zygote or fertilized ovum, and therefore having identical genomes. Called also *enzygotic, identical, monochorial, monochorionic, mono-ovular, similar, true,* and *uniovular t's*. **omphaloangiopagous t's,** allantoidoangiopagous t's. **one-egg t's,** monozygotic t's. **Siamese t's,** conjoined t's. **similar t's,** monozygotic t's. **true t's,** monozygotic t's. **two-egg t's,** dizygotic t's. **uniovular t's,** monozygotic t's. **unlike t's,** dizygotic t's.

twinge (twinj) a short, sharp pain.

twinning (twin'ing) 1. the simultaneous production of two (or more) offspring. 2. the production of symmetrical structures or parts by division. **experimental t.,** embryonic duplication produced by purposeful external intervention. **spontaneous t.,** embryonic duplication without external intervention, as occurs in nature.

twinship (twin'ship) the state of being a twin.

Twiston (twis'ton) trademark for preparations of rotoxamine tartrate.

twitch (twich) 1. a brief contractile response of a skeletal muscle elicited by a single maximal volley of impulses in the motor neurons supplying it. 2. a noose passed through a perforation in a board, used for compressing a part, as the lip of a horse, during slight operations.

twitching (twich'ing) the occurrence of a single contraction or a series of contractions of a muscle; see *twitch*. **fascicular t.,** repetitive brief contraction of large groups of bundles of muscle fibers. **fibrillar t.,** repetitive brief contraction of single bundles of muscle fibers. **Trousseau's t.,** repetitive brief contraction involving muscles of the face.

Twort-d'Herelle phenomenon (twort-dĕ-rel') [Frederick William *Twort*, British bacteriologist, 1877–1950; Felix Hubert d'Herelle of the Pasteur Institute, Paris, 1873–1949] see under *phenomenon*.

TXA₂, TXB₂ thromboxanes A_2 and B_2; see *thromboxane*.

tybamate (ti'bah-māt) chemical name: butylcarbamic acid 2-[[(aminocarbonyl)oxy]methyl]-2-methylpentyl ester. A minor tranquilizer, $C_{13}H_{26}N_2O_4$, occurring as a clear, viscous liquid; administered orally.

tylectomy (ti-lek'to-me) [Gr. *tylos* knot + *ektomē* excision] lumpectomy.

Tylenol (ti'lĕ-nol) trademark for preparations of acetaminophen.

tylion (til'e-on) [Gr. *tyleion* cushion] the point on the anterior edge of the optic groove in the median line.

tyloma (ti-lo'mah) [Gr. *tylōma*] a callus or callosity. Cf. *hyperkeratosis* (def. 1), *keratoderma*, *keratoma* (def. 1), *keratosis*, and *tylosis*.

Tylophora asthmatica Wight et Arn. (ti-lof'o-rah az-mat'ĭ-kah) [Gr. *tylos* knot + *pherein* to bear] an asclepiadaceous plant of South Asia; it is the source of tylophorine.

tylophorine (ti-lof'o-rin) chemical name: 9,11,12,13,-13a, 14-hexahydro-2,3,6,7-tetramethoxydibenzo[*f,h*] pyrrolo-[1,2-*b*]isoquinoline. A crystalline alkaloid, $C_{24}H_{27}O_4N$, from *Tylophora asthmatica* Wight et Arn. (Asclepiadaceae); it is emetic, and is useful in dysentery and asthma.

tylosis (ti-lo'sis) [Gr. *tylōs* a knob or callus] the formation of a callus or callosity. Cf. *hyperkeratosis* (def. 1), *keratoderma*, *keratoma* (def. 1), *keratosis*, and *tyloma*. **t. cilia'ris,** thickening of the eyelids due to long-term ulcerative blepharitis. **t. palma'ris et planta'ris,** keratosis palmaris et plantaris.

tylotic (ti-lot'ik) pertaining to or affected with tylosis.

tyloxapol (ti-loks'ah-pōl) [USP] chemical name: 4-(1,1,3,3-tetramethylbutyl)phenol polymer with formaldehyde and oxirane. A nonionic liquid polymer of the alkyl aryl polyether alcohol type; used as a surfactant to aid liquefaction and removal of mucopurulent bronchopulmonary secretions, administered by inhalation through a nebulizer or with a stream of oxygen.

tympanal (tim'pah-nal) pertaining to the tympanic cavity or to the tympanic membrane.

tympanectomy (tim″pah-nek′to-me) [*tympanum* + Gr. *ektomē* excision] excision of the tympanic membrane.

tympania (tim-pan′e-ah) tympanites.

tympanic (tim-pan′ik) [L. *tympanicus*] 1. of or pertaining to the tympanic cavity or the tympanic membrane. 2. bell-like; resonant.

tympanicity (tim″pah-nis′ĭ-te) a tympanic quality.

tympanion (tim-pan′e-on) [Gr.] a point at either end of the vertical diameter of the annulus tympanicus. **lower t.**, the lowest point on the annulus tympanicus. **upper t.**, the highest point on the annulus tympanicus.

tympanism (tim′pah nizm) [Gr. *tympanon* drum] distention with gas; tympanites.

tympanites (tim″pah-ni′tēz) [Gr. *tympanitēs*, from *tympanon* drum] distention of the abdomen, due to the presence of gas or air in the intestine or in the peritoneal cavity, as in peritonitis and typhoid fever. **false t.**, pseudotympanites. **uterine t.**, physometra.

tympanitic (tim″pah-nit′ik) 1. pertaining to or affected with tympanites. 2. bell-like, or tympanic.

tympanitis (tim″pah-ni′tis) otitis media.

tympan(o)- [Gr. *tympanon* drum] a combining form denoting relationship to the tympanic cavity or to the tympanic membrane.

tympanocentesis (tim″pah-no-sen-te′sis) surgical puncture of the membrana tympani for removal of fluid from the middle ear; called also *myringotomy*.

tympanoeustachian (tim″pah-no-u-sta′ke-an) pertaining to the tympanic cavity and auditory tube.

tympanogenic (tim″pah-no-jen′ik) [*tympanum* + Gr. *gennan* to produce] arising from the tympanic cavity.

tympanogram (tim-pan′o-gram″) [*tympanum* + Gr. *metron* measure] a graphic representation of the relative compliance and impedance of the tympanic membrane and ossicles of the middle ear obtained by tympanometry.

tympanohyal (tim″pah-no-hi′al) 1. pertaining to the tympanic cavity and the hyoid arch. 2. a small bone or cartilage at the base of the styloid process; in early life it becomes a part of the temporal bone.

tympanolabyrinthopexy (tim″pah-no-lab″ĭ-rin′tho-pek″se) Sourdille's operation of uniting a neotympanic system to a labyrinthine fistula for the cure of progressive hearing loss from otosclerosis; of historical interest.

tympanomalleal (tim″pah-no-mal′e-al) pertaining to the tympanic membrane and the malleus.

tympanomastoiditis (tim″pah-no-mas″toi-di′tis) inflammation of the tympanic cavity and the pneumatic cells of the mastoid process.

tympanometric (tim″pan-o-met′rik) pertaining to tympanometry.

tympanometry (tim″pah-nom′ĕ-tre) indirect measurement of the compliance (mobility) and impedance of the tympanic membrane and ossicles of the middle ear; it is done by subjecting the external acoustic meatus to positive, normal, and negative air pressure and monitoring the resultant sound energy flow.

tympanoplastic (tim″pah-no-plas′tik) relating to tympanoplasty.

tympanoplasty (tim″pah-no-plas′te) [*tympanum* + Gr. *plassein* to form] surgical reconstruction of the hearing mechanism of the middle ear, with restoration of the drum membrane to protect the round window from sound pressure, and establishment of ossicular continuity between the tympanic membrane and the oval window. See also *myringoplasty*.

tympanosclerosis (tim″pah-no-sklĕ-ro′sis) a condition characterized by the presence of masses of hard, dense connective tissue around the auditory ossicles in the tympanic cavity.

tympanosquamosal (tim″pah-no-skwah-mo′sal) pertaining to the pars tympanica and pars squamosa of the temporal bone.

tympanostapedial (tim″pah-no-stă-pe′de-al) pertaining to the tympanic cavity and the stapes.

tympanosympathectomy (tim″pah-no-sim″pah-thek′to-me) surgical excision of, or chemical suppression of impulses at, the tympanic plexus for the relief of tinnitus aurium.

tympanotemporal (tim″pah-no-tem′po-ral) pertaining to the tympanic cavity and the region over the temporal bone or region.

tympanotomy (tim″pah-not′o-me) [*tympanum* + Gr. *tomē* a cutting] 1. tympanocentesis. 2. surgical opening of the middle ear.

tympanous (tim′pah-nus) pertaining to or marked by tympanites; distended with gas.

tympanum (tim′pah-num) [L.; Gr. *tympanon* drum] 1. loosely, the tympanic membrane (*membrana tympani* [NA]). 2. the tympanic cavity (*cavitas tympanica* [NA]).

tympany (tim′pah-ne) [Gr. *tympanias*] 1. tympanites. 2. a tympanic, or bell-like, percussion note. **bell t.**, a modified tympanitic note heard on percussion of the chest in some cases of pneumothorax. **Skoda's t., skodaic t.**, skodaic resonance. **t. of the stomach**, a kind of indigestion in cattle and sheep, marked by an abnormal collection of gas in the first stomach; called also *bloat*.

Tyndall light, phenomenon (effect) (tin′dal) [John *Tyndall*, British physicist, 1820–1893] see under *light* and *phenomenon*.

tyndallization (tyn″dal-i-za′shun) [John *Tyndall*] fractional sterilization.

type (tīp) [L. *typus*; Gr. *typos* mark] the general or prevailing character of any particular case of disease, person, substance, etc. Cf. *constitution* and *diathesis*. **amyostatic-kinetic t.**, a type of epidemic encephalitis marked by apathy, rigidity, akinesis, slowing of movement, and sometimes tremor. **asthenic t.**, a constitutional type marked by a slender body, long neck, long, flat chest and abdomen, and poor muscular development. **athletic t.**, a constitutional type marked by broad shoulders, deep chest, flat abdomen, thick neck, and good muscular development. **Aztec t., bird's head t.**, see *microcephalic idiocy*, under *idiocy*. **blood t's**, see *blood group*, under B. **body t.**, constitutional t. **buffalo t.**, obesity confined to the neck, head, and trunk; seen in Cushing's syndrome (def. 1). **Charcot-Marie t., Charcot-Marie-Tooth t.**, see *progressive neuropathic (peroneal) muscular atrophy*, under *atrophy*. **constitutional t.**, a constellation of traits related to body build. **Dejerine t.**, amyotrophic lateral sclerosis. **Dejerine-Landouzy t.**, Landouzy-Dejerine dystrophy. **Duchenne's t.**, pseudohypertrophic muscular dystrophy. **Duchenne-Aran t.**, spinal muscular atrophy. **Duchenne-Landouzy t.**, Landouzy-Dejerine dystrophy. **dysplastic t.**, any constitutional type that differs from the asthenic, the athletic, and the pyknic types. **Eichhorst's t.**, see under *atrophy*. **Erb-Zimmerlin t.**, the juvenile scapular type of primary muscular dystrophy. **Fazio-Londe t.**, the bulbofacial type of familial infantile progressive spinal muscular atrophy. **Hutchison t.**, neuroblastoma with cranial metastases. **Kalmuck t., Kalmuk t.**, Down's syndrome. **Kretschmer t's**, types of physique related to personality or temperamental traits; asthenic, athletic, dysplastic, and pyknic t's. **Landouzy's t., Landouzy-Dejerine t.**, Landouzy-Dejerine dystrophy. **leg t.**, progressive hereditary muscular atrophy. **Leichtenstern's t.**, hemorrhagic encephalitis. **Levi-Lorain t.**, hypophysial infantilism. **Leyden-Möbius t.**, limb-girdle muscular dystrophy. **Lorain t.**, hypophysial infantilism. **mating t.**, in ciliate protozoa, certain bacteria, and certain fungi, the equivalent of a sex; as many as eight sexes are present in some species of protozoa. **Nothnagel's t.**, see under *acroparesthesia*. **Pepper's t.**, see under *syndrome*. **phage t.**, an intraspecies type of bacterium demonstrated by phage typing (see under *typing*); called also *phagotype*. **Putnam's t.**, subacute combined degeneration of spinal cord; see under *degeneration*. **pyknic t.**, a constitutional type marked by a rounded body, large chest, thick shoulders, broad head, and short neck. **Raymond's t. of apoplexy**, see under *apoplexy*. **Remak's t.**, see under *paralysis*. **Runeberg's t.**, see under *anemia*. **scapulohumeral t.**, progressive spinal muscular atrophy beginning in the shoulder. **Schultze's t.**, see under *acroparesthesia*. **Simmerlin t.**, Leyden-Möbius dystrophy. **Strümpell's t.**, see under *disease*, def. 1. **sympatheticotonic t.**, a type of physical constitution characterized by sympathicotonia. **test t.**, see *test type*. **Tooth's t.**, progressive neuropathic (peroneal) muscular atrophy. **Werdnig-Hoffmann t.**, see under *paralysis*. **Wernicke-Mann t.**, see under *hemiplegia*. **wild t.**, in genetics, the standard phenotype for any experimental organism; also a gene that determines a standard phenotypic trait. **Zimmerlin's t.,** see under *atrophy*.

typhlectasis (tif-lek'tah-sis) [Gr. *typhlon* cecum + *ektasis* distention] distention of the cecum.

typhlectomy (tif-lek'to-me) cecectomy.

typhlenteritis (tif‴len-ter-i'tis) [Gr. *typhlon* cecum + Gr. *enteron* intestine] cecitis.

typhlitis (tif-li'tis) [Gr. *typhlon* cecum + -*itis*] inflammation of the cecum; the term was formerly used for the condition now called *appendicitis*.

typhl(o)- 1. [Gr. *typhlon* cecum] a combining form denoting relationship to the cecum. 2. [Gr. *typhlos* blind] a combining form denoting relationship to blindness.

Typhlocoelum (tif‴lo-se'lum) a genus of trematode parasites. **T. cucumeri'num,** a trematode parasitic in the trachea, esophagus, and thoracic cavity of chicks in Brazil and certain ducks and wild aquatic birds in Madagascar.

typhlocolitis (tif‴lo-ko-li'tis) [*typhlo-*(1) + *colitis*] colitis in the region of the cecum.

typhlodicliditis (tif‴lo-dik‴lĭ-di'tis) [*typhlo-*(1) + Gr. *diklis* door + -*itis*] inflammation of the ileocecal valve.

typhloempyema (tif‴lo-em‴pi-e'mah) [*typhlo-*(1) + *empyema*] appendicular abscess.

typhloenteritis (tif‴lo-en‴ter-i'tis) cecitis.

typhlolexia (tif‴lo-lek'se-ah) [*typhlo-*(2) + Gr. *lexis* speech + -*ia*] alexia.

typhlolithiasis (tif‴lo-lĭ-thi'ah-sis) [*typhlo-*(1) + Gr. *lithos* stone + -*ia*] the presence of calculi in the cecum.

typhlology (tif-lol'o-je [*typhlo-*(2) + -*logy*] the sum of what is known in regard to blindness.

typhlomegaly (tif‴lo-meg'ah-le) [*typhlo-*(1) + Gr. *megas* large] abnormal enlargement of the cecum.

typhlon (tif'lon) [Gr.] the cecum.

typhlopexy (tif'lo-pek″se) [*typhlo-*(1) + Gr. *pēxis* fixation] operative suspension and fixation of the cecum.

typhloptosis (tif‴lo-to'sis) [*typhlo-*(1) + Gr. *ptōsis* falling] cecoptosis.

typhlorrhaphy (tif-lor'ah-fe) cecorrhaphy.

typhlosis (tif-lo'sis) [Gr. *typhlōsis* a making blind] blindness.

typhlostenosis (tif‴lo-stĕ-no'sis) [*typhlo-*(1) + Gr. *stenōsis* narrowing] contraction of the cecum.

typhlostomy (tif-los'to-me) [*typhlo-*(1) + Gr. *stomoun* to provide with an opening, or mouth] cecostomy.

typhloteritis (tif‴lo-ter-i'tis) cecitis.

typhlotomy (tif-lot'o-me) [*typhlo-*(1) + Gr. *tomē* a cutting] cecotomy.

typhobacterin (ti″fo-bak'ter-in) typhoid vaccine.

typhoid (ti'foid) [Gr. *typhōdes* like smoke; delirious] 1. typhus-like 2. see under *fever*. 3. typhoidal. **fowl t.,** an acute infectious disease of fowl caused by *Salmonella gallinarum*, marked by drowsiness, anorexia, extreme weakness, and usually diarrhea, finally ending in death in four days to two weeks after onset. Called also *Klein's disease*. **provocation t.,** the systemic reaction to the endotoxin of killed typhoid bacilli in typhoid vaccine.

typhoidal (ti-foid'al) pertaining or relating to or resembling typhoid fever; typhoid. See also *enteric fever*, under *fever*.

Typhonium trilobatum (L.) Schott. (Araceae) (ti-fo'ne-um tri″lo-ba'tum) [L.] an Asiatic plant, highly valued in oriental practice as a polychrest remedy.

typhous (ti'fus) pertaining to or resembling typhus.

typhus (ti'fus) [Gr. *typhos* stupor arising from fever] a group of acute, arthropod-borne infections caused by rickettsiae that are closely related clinically and pathologically but differ in the intensity of certain signs and symptoms, severity, and fatality rate; all are characterized by severe headache, chills, high fever, stupor, and a macular, maculopapular, petechial, or papulovesicular eruption. The three clinical and epidemiologic entities making up the group are *epidemic* (classic or louse-borne) *typhus*, its recrudescent form (Brill-Zinsser disease), and *murine* (endemic or flea-borne) *typhus*. Called also *typhus fever*. In English-speaking countries, often used alone to refer to epidemic typhus, whereas in several European languages it refers to typhoid

fever. **Australian tick t.,** Queensland tick t. **canine t.,** Stuttgart disease. **classic t.,** epidemic t. **endemic t.,** murine t. **epidemic t.,** the classic, louse-borne form of typhus, caused by *Rickettsia prowazekii*, which is transmitted from person to person by the human body louse, *Pediculus humanus corporis*, although the organism can also grow in the head louse, *P. humanus capitis*. It is characterized chiefly by abrupt onset with chills, fever, malaise, headache that progresses in severity, backache, and generalized myalgia; followed by the appearance of an eruption that may be macular, maculopapular, or petechial and spreads from the trunk to cover the entire body except for the face, palms, and soles, and accompanied by central nervous system involvement that progresses from dullness to stupor and sometimes coma and death. Recrudescences occur (see *Brill-Zinsser disease*, under *disease*). Epidemic typhus has been known by various names, including camp, *jail, hospital, prison, ship,* and *war fever, European t., exanthematous t., fleckfieber,* and *t. exanthematique.* **European t.,** epidemic t. **exanthematic t. of São Paulo,** Rocky Mountain spotted fever. **t. exanthematique, exanthematous t.,** epidemic t. **flea-borne t.,** murine t. **Gubler-Robin t.,** the renal form of typhus. **Indian tick t.,** see *boutonneuse fever,* under *fever*. **Kenya tick t.,** see *boutonneuse fever,* under *fever*. **latent t.,** Brill-Zinsser disease. **louse-borne t.,** epidemic t. **Manchurian t.,** murine t. **Mexican t.,** murine t. **mite-borne t.,** scrub t. **Moscow t.,** murine t. **murine t.,** an acute, flea-borne endemic infectious disease clinically similar to epidemic typhus except that it is milder, caused by *Rickettsia typhi* (*mooseri*), which is transmitted from rats to humans chiefly by the rat flea, *Xenopsylla cheopis*, although *R. typhi* (*mooseri*) multiplies in other fleas and in certain lice. Infections identical or nearly identical to murine typhus have been known by various names, including *Congo red fever, Manchurian, Mexican,* or *Moscow t.,* and *tabardillo* or *tarbadillo.* See also *Toulon t.* and *urban t.* **North Asian tick t.,** Siberian tick t. **North Queensland tick t.,** Queensland tick t. **Queensland tick t.,** an acute, febrile, exanthematous disease marked by a primary lesion (tache noire), caused by *Rickettsia australis*, and transmitted by the Australian ticks *Ixodes holocyclus* and *I. tasmani*. Called also *Australian* and *North Queensland tick t.* **recrudescent t.,** Brill-Zinsser disease. **São Paulo t.,** Rocky Mountain spotted fever. **scrub t.,** an acute typhus-like infectious disease caused by *Rickettsia tsutsugamushi*, transmitted by the bite of infected larval trombiculid mites (chiggers), occurring chiefly in Asia and the southern and western Pacific, and characterized chiefly by the formation of a pathognomonic primary cutaneous lesion or eschar at the site of inoculation (tache noire) accompanied by regional lymphadenopathy, fever, and a maculopapular rash. It has many synonyms and local names, including *akamushi, shimamushi, island,* or *tsutsugamushi disease; miteborne* or *tropical t.;* and *tsutsugamushi, Japanese flood* or *river, Kedani, inundation, island,* or *Mossman fever.* **shop t.,** urban t. **Siberian tick t.,** a relatively mild, acutely febrile, spotted fever, characterized by headache, malaise, conjunctival injection, a maculopapular rash, and a primary ulcerative lesion at the site of the tick bite; it occurs in north, central, and east Asia. The causative agent is *Rickettsia siberica*, which is transmitted by ticks of the genera *Dermacentor* and *Haemaphysalis*. Called also *North Asian tick t.* **tick t., tickborne t.,** Rocky Mountain spotted fever; also, any tickborne infectious disease (see *tick fever,* under *fever*). **Toulon t.,** a mild form of murine typhus occurring in the Mediterranean region. **tropical t.,** scrub t. **urban t.,** a mild form of murine typhus, usually observed in indoor workers in Malaya and the Mediterranean regions; called also *shop t.*

typical (tip'ĭ-kal) [Gr. *typikos*] presenting the distinctive features of any type.

typing (tip'ing) determination of the type category to which an individual, object, or other entity belongs; e.g., bacteria, blood cells, cell cultures, or tissues. **t. of blood,** classification of the blood with reference to various erythrocytic membrane antigens. See *blood type*. **HLA t.,** determination of the HLA antigens possessed by an individual. Class I antigens (HLA-A, -B, and -C) are detected by lymphocyte microcytotoxicity assay using standard typing sera. Class II antigens are detected by one-way mixed lymphocyte reactions (MLR) using panels of homozygous typing cells (HTC); they may also be identified by primed lymphocyte typing (PLT). DR Class II antigens are also detected by lymphocyte microtoxicity assay using B-lymphocytes and anti-DR antibody types. HLA typing is used to identify compatible donors and recipients for transplantation or platelet or granulocyte transfusion, to establish associations of HLA antigens with diseases, and in paternity testing. **phage t.,** characterization of bacteria, extending to strain differences, by demonstration of susceptibility to one or more (a spectrum) races of bacteriophage; widely applied to staphylococci, typhoid bacilli, etc., for epidemiological purposes. **primed lymphocyte t. (PLT),** a technique used for typing of Class II HLA antigens: unknown cells are exposed to a panel of lymphocytes primed against specific HLA antigens by prior coculture with stimulator cells that matched the primed cells at all but one HLA locus; when restimulated by the same HLA antigen the primed cells give a secondary proliferative response, which shows that the unknown cells bear the same antigen as the stimulator cells. **tissue t.,** HLA t.

typodont (ti′po-dont) an artificial model that contains artificial teeth or natural teeth that are used for teaching exercises.

typology (ti-pol′o-je) the study of types; the science of classifying, as bacteria according to type.

typoscope (ti′po-skōp) [Gr. *typos* type + *-scope*] an instrument to aid amblyopia and cataract patients in reading.

typus (ti′pus) [L.] type. **t. degenerati′vus amstelodamen′sis,** de Lange's syndrome.

Tyr tyrosine.

tyramine (ti′rah-mēn) a decarboxylation product of tyrosine, which may be converted to cresol and phenol; closely related structurally to epinephrine and norepinephrine, it has a similar but weaker action. It is found in decayed animal tissue, ripe cheese, and ergot.

tyramine oxidase (ti′rah-mēn, tir′ah-mēn ok′sĭ-dās) amine oxidase (flavin-containing).

tyrannism (tir′ah-nizm) [Gr. *tyrrhanos* tyrant] morbid cruelty.

tyrein (ti′re-in) the coagulated casein of milk.

tyresin (ti-re′sin) a principle derivable from the venom of serpents and from the juice of mushrooms; it was thought to be an antidote for snake poisoning.

tyr(o)- [Gr. *tyros* cheese] a combining form denoting relationship to cheese.

tyrocidin (ti″ro-si′din) tyrocidine.

tyrocidine (ti″ro-si′din) a crystalline polypeptide antibiotic substance which is the major component of tyrothricin, the lesser component being gramicidin.

Tyrode's solution (ti′rōdz) [Maurice Vejux *Tyrode,* American pharmacologist, 1878–1930] see under *solution.*

tyrogenous (ti-roj′ĕ-nus) [*tyro-* + Gr. *gennan* to produce] originating in cheese.

Tyroglyphus (ti-rog′lĭ-fus) [*tyro-* + Gr. *glyphein* to carve] *Tyrophagus.* **T. castella′ni,** *Tyrophagus castellani.* **T. fari′nae,** *Tyrophagus farinae.* **T. lon′gior,** *Tyrophagus longior.* **T. si′ro,** *Acarus siro.*

tyroid (ti′roid) [*tyro-* + Gr. *eidos* form] caseous; resembling cheese.

tyroma (ti-ro′mah) a caseous tumor; a new growth or nodule of cheesy material.

tyromatosis (ti″ro-mah-to′sis) a condition characterized by caseous degeneration.

tyropanoate sodium (ti″ro-pah-no′āt) chemical name: α-ethyl-2,4,6-triiodo-3-[(1-oxobutyl)amino]benzene propanoic acid monosodium salt; a diagnostic radiopaque medium for use in cholecystography, $C_{15}H_{17}I_3NNaO_3$.

Tyrophagus (ti-rof′ah-gus) a genus of pale, soft-bodied mites, the meal mites; called also *Tyroglyphus.* **T. castella′ni,** the copra mite, the species that causes copra itch. **T. fari′nae,** the flour mite, found in flour mills and granaries. **T. lon′gior,** the cheese mite, which has been reported from both the urinary and digestive tracts and may be found in the stools. **T. si′ro,** *Acarus siro.*

tyrosamine (ti-ros′ah-mēn) tyramine.

tyrosinase (ti-ro′sin-ās) monophenol monooxygenase.

tyrosine (ti′ro-sēn) a crystallizable amino acid, *p*-hydroxyphenylalanine, $C_9H_{11}O_3N$, found in most proteins and synthesized metabolically from phenylalanine; it is a precursor

of thyroid hormones, catecholamines, and melanin. Sometimes called *oxyphenylaminopropionic acid.*

tyrosine aminotransferase (ti′ro-sēn ah-me″no-trans′-fer-ās) [EC 2.6.1.5] an enzyme of the transferase class that catalyzes the reaction L-tyrosine + 2-ketoglutarate = 4-hydroxyphenylpyruvate + L-glutamate, the first step in the use of tyrosine as a fuel. Deficiency of the enzyme, an autosomal recessive trait, causes tyrosinemia type II.

tyrosine aminotransferase deficiency tyrosinemia, type II.

tyrosinemia (ti″ro-sĭ-ne′me-ah) [*tyrosine* + *-emia*] an aminoacidopathy of tyrosine metabolism occurring in several types: *Type I* shows an excess of tyrosine and an accumulation of succinylacetoacetone and succinylacetone, inhibiting some hepatic enzymes and renal tubular function. It occurs in two forms, acute and chronic: the acute form has onset in the first few weeks or months after birth and is marked by anorexia, vomiting, diarrhea, and a cabbage-like odor; death from liver failure occurs in six to eight months; the chronic form has similar, but milder, features, with possible de Toni-Fanconi syndrome, vitamin D–resistant rickets, and porphyria-like symptoms; death usually occurs in the first decade. Called also *hepatorenal* or *hereditary t., tyrosinosis,* and *hypermethioninemia. Type II* is an oculocutaneous syndrome due to defective hepatic tyrosine aminotransferase (TAT) and clinically marked by the crystallization of the accumulated tyrosine in the epidermis as palmoplantar hyperkeratoses and in the corneas as herpetiform ulcers and by frequent mental retardation; a low-tyrosine, low-phenylalanine diet is curative. Called also *Richner-Hanbart syndrome* and *tyrosine aminotransferase deficiency. Neonatal tyrosinemia* is an asymptomatic condition found in up to 10 per cent of neonates; dietary restriction of protein quickly reduces plasma tyrosine to normal. There are probably no long-term consequences except, possibly, mild mental retardation and impaired psycholinguistic ability. See also *hyperphenylalaninemia.*

tyrosinosis (ti″ro-sĭ-no′sis) 1. a condition characterized by a faulty metabolism of tyrosine in which an intermediate product, parahydroxyphenyl pyruvic acid, appears in the urine and gives it an abnormal reducing power. 2. tyrosinemia, type I.

tyrosinuria (ti″ro-sĭ-nu′re-ah) [*tyrosine* + Gr. *ouron* urine + *-ia*] the presence of tyrosine in urine, as in tyrosinemia.

tyrosis (ti-ro′sis) caseation, def. 2.

tyrosyl (ti′ro-sil) the acyl radical of tyrosine.

tyrosyluria (ti″ro-sil-u′re-ah) the increased urinary excretion of para-hydroxyphenyl compounds derived from tyrosine, as in tyrosinemia.

tyrothricin (ti″ro-thri′sin) an antibiotic substance isolated from the soil bacillus *Bacillus brevis,* occurring as a white, grayish white, or brownish white powder, consisting principally of two polypeptides, the major one being tyrocidine and the other gramicidin. It is effective against many gram-positive bacteria, and is applied topically in pyodermic, ocular, and other localized infections due to susceptible organisms.

tyrotoxicon (ti″ro-tok′sĭ-kon) chemical name: benzenediazonium hydroxide. A poisonous crystalline compound, $C_6H_5N(:N)OH$, sometimes occurring in stale milk, cheese, and ice cream.

tyrotoxicosis (ti″ro-tok″sĭ-ko′sis) a morbid condition resulting from ingestion of tyrotoxicon; marked by vertigo, headache, vomiting, chills, muscular cramps, purging, prostration, and death. Called also *cheese poisoning.*

tyrotoxism (ti″ro-toks′izm) poisoning resulting from ingestion of contaminated cheese; see *tyrotoxicosis.*

Tyrrell's fascia, hook (tir′elz) [Frederick *Tyrrell,* English anatomist, 1793–1843] see *septum rectovesicale,* and see under *hook.*

Tyson's crypts, glands (ti′sunz) [Edward *Tyson,* English physician and anatomist, 1650–1708] glandulae preputiales.

tysonian (ti-so′ne-an) named for Edward *Tyson.*

tysonitis (ti″son-i′tis) inflammation of Tyson's glands.

tyvelose (ti′vel-ōs) an unusual sugar found in the lipopolysaccharides of certain serotypes of *Salmonella.* It is the determinant of somatic (O) antigen factor 9 of group D salmonellae.

Tyzine (ti′zēn) trademark for preparations of tetrahydrozoline hydrochloride.

Tyzzeria (ti-ze′re-ah) a genus of coccidian protozoa (suborder Eimeriina, order Eucoccidiida), characterized by the presence of oocysts containing eight naked sporozoites. It includes *T. perniciosa*, which is highly pathogenic for domestic ducklings, being parasitic in the small intestine, especially in the upper half.

Tzanck cell, test (tsank) [Arnault *Tzanck*, Russian dermatologist in Paris, 1886–1954] see under *cell* and *tests*.

tzetze (set′se) tsetse.

U

U chemical symbol for *uranium;* symbol for *uracil* or *uridine* (in nucleic acids) and for *International Unit* (of enzyme activity).

ubiquinol (u-bik′wĭ-nol) the reduced form of a ubiquinone.

ubiquinol-cytochrome c reductase (u-bik′wĭ-nol si′to-krōm rĕ-duk′tās) [E.C. 1.10.2.2] an enzyme complex of the inner mitochondrial membrane that catalyzes the reaction ubiquinol + 2 ferricytochrome c = ubiquinone + 2 ferrocytochrome. It contains cytochromes 6 and an iron-sulfide protein and is associated with the pumping of protons and resultant phosphorylation of ADP to ATP. The reaction is part of the terminal electron transport scheme by which oxygen is utilized for fuel combustion. Also called *ubiquinol dehydrogenase.*

ubiquinol dehydrogenase (u-bik′wĭ-nol de-hi′dro-jen-ās) ubiquinol-cytochrome c reductase.

ubiquinone (u-bik′wĭ-nōn) a group of quinones with multiprenyl side chains, occurring in the lipid core of inner mitochondrial membranes and functioning in electron transfer reactions coupled to phosphorylation. Formerly called *coenzyme Q.*

udder (ud′er) the mammary organ of cattle and certain other mammals; within the large baglike envelope are two or more glands, each having a teat.

UDP uridine diphosphate.

UDP-*N*-acetylglucosamine-lysosomal-enzyme *N*-acetylglucosaminephosphotransferase (as-ĕ-tēl″gloo-kōs′ah-mēn li″so-so′mal en′zīm as-ĕ-tēl″gloo-kōs′ah-mēn-fos″fo-trans′feras) [EC 2.7.8.17] an enzyme of the transferase class that catalyzes the reaction UDP-*N*-acetyl-D-glucosamine + lysosomal-enzyme-D-mannose = UMP + lysosomal-enzyme N-acetyl-D-glucosaminyl-phospho-D-mannose, required for the synthesis of mannose-6-phosphate lysosomal enzymes. Deficiency of the enzyme, an autosomal recessive trait, causes mucolipidosis types I and II. Called also *N-acetylglucosaminylphosphotransferase.*

UDPbilirubin glucuronosyltransferase (bil″ē-roo′bin gloo″ku-ron″o-sil-trans′fer-ās) glucuronosyltransferase.

UDPgalactose 4-epimerase (gah-lak′tōs ĕ-pim′er-ās) UDP glucose 4-epimerase.

UDPglucose 4-epimerase (gloo′kōs ĕ-pim′er-ās) [EC 5.1.3.2] an enzyme of the isomerase class that catalyzes the reaction UDPglucose = UDPgalactose in circulating red blood cells; it requires NAD as a cofactor. Deficiency of the enzyme, an autosomal recessive trait, causes accumulation of galactose-1-phosphate in red cells. Formerly called *galactowaldenase.*

UDP glucose-hexose-1-phosphate uridylyltransferase (gloo″kos hek″sōs fos″fāt u″rĭ-dil-il-trans′fer-ās) [EC 2.7.7.12] an enzyme of the transferase class that catalyzes the reaction UDP glucose + α-D-galactose 1-phosphate = α-D-glucose 1-phosphate + UDP-galactose, the second step in the utilization of galactose as a fuel. Deficiency of the enzyme, an autosomal recessive trait, causes galactosemia. Called also *galactose-1-phosphate uridyltransferase, hexose-1-phosphate uridylyltransferase.*

UDPglucose pyrophosphorylase (gloo′kōs pi″ro-fos-for′i-lās) UTP glucose-1-phosphate uridylyltransferase.

UDPglucuronate-bilirubin-glucuronosyltransferase (gloo-ku′ro-nāt bil″i-roo′bin gloo″ku-ron″o-sil-trans′fer-ās) glucuronosyltransferase.

UDPglucuronyl transferase (gloo-ku′ron-il trans′fer-ās) glucuronosyltransferase.

Udránszky's test (oo-dran′skēz) [László *Udránszky,* Budapest physiologist, 1862–1914] see under *tests.*

Uffelmann's test (reagent) (oof′el-mahnz) [Jules *Uffelmann,* German physician, 1837–1894] see under *tests.*

Uhthoff's sign (oot′hofs) [Wilhelm *Uhthoff,* ophthalmologist in Breslau, 1853–1927] see under *sign.*

Ulacort (u′lah-kort) trademark for preparations of prednisolone.

ulalgia (u-lal′je-ah) [*ul-* (2) + *algos* pain + *-ia*] gingivalgia.

ulatrophy (u-lat′ro-fe) [*ul-* (2) + *atrophy*] atrophy of the gingiva associated with its recession and exposure of the root portion of the tooth. **afunctional u.,** ulatrophy occurring in congenital malocclusion. **atrophic u.,** ischemic u. **calcic u.,** ulatrophy that is caused by the presence of salivary concretions. **ischemic u.,** ulatrophy due to deficient blood supply. Called also *atrophic u.* **traumatic u.,** ulatrophy due to gingival trauma.

ulcer (ul′ser) [L. *ulcus;* Gr. *helkōsis*] a local defect, or excavation, of the surface of an organ or tissue, which is produced by the sloughing of inflammatory necrotic tissue. **Aden u.,** a local name for *cutaneous leishmaniasis.* **amebic u.,** the ulcerous lesion of amebiasis cutis. **amputating u.,** ulceration which encircles a part and destroys the tissues to the bone. **anastomotic u.,** ulcer at the anastomotic site occurring as a complication after gastroenterostomy performed for duodenal ulcer. **aphthous u.,** the ulcerative lesion of recurrent aphthous stomatitis. **atheromatous u.,** a loss of intima over an atheroma, often giving rise to thrombus formation and/or emboli. **atonic u.,** a chronic ulcer with unhealthy granulations. **Barrett's u.,** chronic peptic ulcer of the esophagus, usually associated with heterotopic gastric mucosa and stricture formation; it is usually a late complication of peptic esophagitis. **burrowing phagedenic u.,** 1. progressive synergistic gangrene. 2. Meleney's u., def. 1. **Buruli u.** [named for the *Buruli* district of Uganda], a cutaneous infection caused by *Mycobacterium ulcerans,* manifested by a small, firm, painless, movable subcutaneous nodule that enlarges and becomes fluctuant and ulcerates, leaving an undermined edge, and occurring principally in Uganda and Zaire but also seen in most countries in Central Africa, in Southeast Asia, in Australia, and sometimes in Central and South America. **catarrhal corneal u.,** an ulcer near the corneal limbus occurring in catarrhal conjunctivitis. **chicle u., chiclero u.,** an endemic, zoonotic forest disease, a form of cutaneous leishmaniasis of the New World, found chiefly in Yucatan, Mexico, Belize, and Guatemala, especially in forest workers in endemic areas. It is caused by *Leishmania mexicana mexicana,* transmitted by *Lutzomyia olmeca,* and characterized by the presence of one or a few lesions that are usually self-limited and heal within 6 months, except when the pinna of the ear is involved, in which case over a period of many years the chronic lesion invades and slowly destroys the cartilage of the ear. **chrome u.,** an ulcer produced by chromium or its salts; seen in tanners and others working in chromium. Called also *tanner's u.* **concealed u.,** destructive inflammation affecting some internal tissue. **Cruveilhier's u.,** simple gastric ulcer. **Curling's u.,** acute ulceration of the stomach or duodenum following a severe burn upon the surface of the body. **Cushing's u.,** a peptic ulcer associated with manifest or occult lesions of the central nervous system. **Cushing-Rokitansky u.,** Rokitansky-Cushing u. **decubital u., decubitus u.,** an ulceration caused by prolonged pressure in a patient allowed to lie too still in bed for a long period of time; called also *decubitus, bed sore,* and *pressure sore.* **dendriform u., dendritic u.,** ulcer of the cornea branching in various directions, usually caused by herpes simplex infection. **dia-**

betic u., an ulcer, usually of the lower extremities, associated with diabetes mellitus. **diphtheritic u.,** one the surface of which is partly or entirely covered by a dirty grayish membrane; it is sometimes, but not always, produced by diphtheria of the skin. **duodenal u.,** a peptic ulcer situated in the duodenum. **elusive u.,** Hunner's u. **Fenwick-Hunner u.,** Hunner's u. **fistulous u.,** the ulcerated superficial end of a fistula. **flask u.,** an ulcer of the intestine in amebic dysentery. **follicular u.,** a small ulcer on the mucous membrane having its origin in a lymph follicle. **gastric u.,** an ulcer of the gastric mucosa. **giant peptic u's,** very large, uncommon, peptic ulcers with characteristic clinical and radiological manifestations. **girdle u.,** a tuberculous ulcer that spreads along the wall of the intestine in an encircling manner. **gouty u.,** a superficial ulcer occurring over a gouty joint. **gummatous u.,** a broken-down superficial gumma. **Hunner's u.,** a lesion occurring in chronic interstitial cystitis, involving all the layers of the bladder wall, and appearing as a small brownish red patch on the mucosa; it tends to heal superficially and is notoriously difficult to detect. **hypertensive ischemic u.,** a manifestation of infarction of the skin due to arteriolar occlusion as part of a long-standing vascular disease, occurring especially in women between the ages of 50 and 70, and presenting as a red painful plaque on the leg or ankle, which breaks down into a superficial ulcer surrounded by a zone of purpuric erythema. **hypopyon u.,** a corneal ulcer accompanied by hypopyon. **Jacob's u.,** rodent ulcer, especially that of an eyelid. **jejunal u.,** an ulcer of the jejunum; such an ulcer developing after gastroenterostomy is called *secondary jejunal u.* **kissing u's,** ulcers on directly opposing surfaces of the stomach, as on opposite sides of the lesser curvature. **Kocher's dilatation u.,** ulceration occurring in a greatly distended intestine or in the course of ileus. **Lipschütz u.,** ulcus vulvae acutum. **lupoid u.,** a skin ulcer that simulates or resembles lupus. **Malabar u.,** tropical phagedenic u. **Mann-Williamson u.,** progressive peptic ulcer produced in experimental animals by the performance of gastric resection or gastroenterostomy. **marginal u.,** a gastric ulcer in the jejunal mucosa near the site of a gastrojejunal anastomosis; called also *stoma u.* **Marjolin's u.,** an ulcer seated upon an old cicatrix; it may degenerate into a squamous cell carcinoma with a propensity for metastasis. **Meleney's u., Meleney's chronic undermining u.,** 1. progressive synergistic gangrene associated with the formation of burrowing cutaneous fissures and sinus tracts that open at distant sites. Called also *burrowing phagedenic u.* and *undermining u.* 2. progressive synergistic gangrene. **Mooren's u.,** chronic serpiginous ulceration, usually bilateral, of the marginal cornea, seen in elderly individuals; it is of unknown etiology. **neurogenic u., neurotrophic u.,** an ulcer resulting from separation of tissue from its nerve supply, as in sensory neuropathy. **penetrating u.,** an ulcerative lesion which involves also the wall or substance of an adjacent organ. **peptic u.,** an ulceration of the mucous membrane of the esophagus, stomach, or duodenum, caused by the action of the acid gastric juice. **perambulating u.,** phagedenic u., def. 1. **perforating u.,** an ulcer which involves the entire thickness of an organ, as the foot, or the wall of the stomach or intestine, creating an opening on both surfaces. **phagedenic u.,** 1. any of a group of conditions due to secondary bacterial invasion of a preexisting cutaneous lesion or the intact skin of a person with impaired resistance as a result of a systemic disease; it is characterized by necrotic ulceration associated with prominent tissue destruction. The group includes desert sore, Meleney's ulcers, and tropical phagedenic ulcer. Called also *perambulatory u.* and *sloughing u.* 2. tropical phagedenic u. **pneumococcus u.,** ulcus serpens corneae. **pudendal u.,** granuloma inguinale. **ring u.,** fusion of foci of ulceration in the cornea to form a peripheral ring of ulceration. **rodent u.,** ulcerating basal cell carcinoma of the skin. **Rokitansky-Cushing u's,** an occasional ulcerative accompaniment of severe lesions of the central nervous system, affecting the lower third of the esophagus, the fundus of the stomach, or the duodenum. **round u.,** a peptic ulcer of the stomach. **Saemisch's u.,** ulcus serpens corneae. **sea anemone u.,** an intestinal ulcer in amebiasis, with a deep crater and partly necrotic undermined edges which are raised above the level of the surrounding mucosa. **secondary jejunal u.,** see *jejunal u.* **serpiginous corneal u.,** ulcus serpens corneae. **simple**

u., a mild form of ulcer which is neither of septic origin nor the expression of a general disease. **sloughing u.,** phagedenic u., def. 1. **soft u.,** chancroid. **stasis u.,** ulceration on the ankle due to venous stasis or insufficiency. **stercoraceous u.,** stercoral u. **stercoral u.,** an ulcer caused by the pressure of impacted feces; also a fistulous ulcer through which fecal matter escapes. **stoma u., stomal u.,** marginal u. **stress u.,** peptic ulcer, usually gastric, resulting from stress; possible predisposing factors include changes in the microcirculation of the gastric mucosa, increased permeability of the gastric mucosa barrier to H^+, and impaired cell proliferation. **sublingual u.,** an ulcer on the frenum of the tongue. **submucous u.,** Hunner's u.; so called because of the tendency of the lesion to heal superficially. **symptomatic u.,** an ulcer that indicates some general disease. **tanner's u.,** chrome u. **trophic u.,** an ulcer due to imperfect nutrition of the part. **trophoneurotic u.,** neurotrophic u. **tropical u.,** 1. a lesion of cutaneous leishmaniasis. 2. tropical phagedenic u. **tropical phagedenic u.,** a chronic, painful phagedenic ulcer usually occurring on the lower extremities of malnourished children in the tropics; the etiology is unknown but spirochetes, fusiform bacilli, and other bacteria are often present in the developing lesion, and protein and vitamin deficiency with lowered resistance to infection may play a role in the etiology. Called also *phagedenic u.* and *tropical u.,* and also known by various native names and by names having only geographical significance, such as *Malabar u.* and *Naga sore.* **undermining burrowing u.,** 1. progressive synergistic gangrene. 2. Meleney's u., def. 1. **varicose u.,** one that is due to varicose veins, as a stasis ulcer. **venereal u.,** a disease marked by the formation of ulcers about the vulvae of women who have not been exposed to venereal disease; the ulcers resemble chancre or chancroid.

ulcera (ul′ser-ah) [L.] plural of *ulcus.*

ulcerate (ul′sĕ-rāt) [L. *ulcerare, ulceratus*] to become affected with ulceration.

ulceration (ul″sĕ-ra′shun) [L. *ulceratio*] 1. the formation or development of an ulcer. 2. an ulcer. **u. of Daguet,** ulceration of the uvula and other parts of the throat, seen in typhoid fever.

ulcerative (ul′ser-a″tiv) pertaining to or characterized by ulceration.

ulcerogangrenous (ul″ser-o-gang′grĕ-nus) characterized by both ulceration and gangrene; pertaining to a gangrenous ulcer.

ulcerogenic (ul″ser-o-jen′ik) causing ulceration; leading to the production of ulcers.

ulcerogranuloma (ul″ser-o-gran″u-lo′mah) a granuloma developing on an ulcer.

ulceromembranous (ul″ser-o-mem″brah-nus) characterized by ulceration and by a membranous exudation.

ulcerous (ul′ser-us) [L. *ulcerosus*] 1. of the nature of an ulcer. 2. affected with ulceration.

ulcus (ul′kus), pl. *ul′cera* [L.] ulcer. **u. am′bulans,** phagedenic ulcer. **u. cancro′sum,** rodent ulcer. **u. ex′edens,** rodent ulcer. **u. interdigita′le,** keratolysis of the horny layer of the skin between the toes, a disease similar to cracked heel. **u. pen′etrans,** one that penetrates not into the peritoneal cavity but into an abutting organ. **u. ro′dens,** rodent ulcer. **u. ser′pens cor′neae,** an ulcer of the cornea; a creeping central suppurative ulcer of the cornea due usually to pneumococcus. Called also *pneumococcus ulcer, Saemisch's ulcer, serpiginous corneal ulcer.* **u. sim′plex vesi′cae,** Hunner's ulcer. **u. ventric′uli,** gastric ulcer. **u. vul′vae acu′tum,** a nonvenereal rapidly growing lesion of the vulva. The etiology is uncertain, but *Bacillus crassus,* a normally nonpathogenic species sometimes found in vaginal cultures, has been implicated. Called also *Lipschütz disease* or *ulcer.*

uldazepam (ul-da′zah-pam) chemical name: 7-chloro-5-(2-chlorophenyl)-N-(2-propenyloxy)-3H-1,4-benzodiazepam-2-amine; a tranquilizer, $C_{18}H_{15}Cl_2N_3O$.

ule- see *ulo-.*

ulectomy (u-lek′to-me) 1. [*ul-*(1) + *ectomy*] excision of scar tissue. 2. [*ul-*(2) + *ectomy*] gingivectomy.

ulegyria (u″le-ji′re-ah) [Gr. *oulē* scar + *gyrus* + *-ia*] a condition in which the cerebral gyri are narrow and distorted by scars, resulting from lesions existing in fetal life or early infancy.

ulemorrhagia (u″lem-o-ra′je-ah) [ul- (2) + rrhagia] gingival hemorrhage.

ulerythema (u″ler-ĭ-the′mah) [Gr. oulē scar + erythēma redness] an erythematous disease of the skin characterized by the formation of cicatrices and by atrophy. **u. ophryo′genes,** keratosis pilaris affecting the follicles of the eyebrow hairs of young men, associated with erythema, and leading to scarring and atrophy; it is transmitted as an autosomal dominant trait.

Ulex europaeus L. (Leguminosae) (u′leks u-ro′pe-us) a leguminous shrub, common gorse or furze, which is a source of cytisine (ulexine).

ulexine (u-leks′ēn) cytisine.

uliginous (u-lij′ĭ-nus) [L. uliginosus moist] muddy or slimy.

ulitis (u-li′tis) [Gr. oulon gum + -itis] inflammation of the gums; gingivitis.

ullem (ul′em) a kind of dyspepsia occurring in Lapland.

Ullmann's line (ul′manz) [Emerich Ullmann, Hungarian surgeon, 1861–1937] see under line.

Ulmus (ul′mus) [L. "elm"] a genus of ulmaceous trees; the elms. **U. ful′va Michx.,** the slippery elm, the inner bark of which is mucilaginous and demulcent.

ulna (ul′nah), pl. ul′nae [L. "the arm"] [NA] the inner and larger bone of the forearm, on the side opposite that of the thumb; it articulates with the humerus and with the head of the radius at its proximal end; with the radius and bones of the carpus at the distal end. See Plate 42.

ulnad (ul′nad) toward the ulna.

ulnar (ul′nar) [L. ulnaris] pertaining to the ulna or to the ulnar (medial) aspect of the arm as compared to the radial (lateral) aspect.

ulnare (ul-na′re) [L.] os triquetrum.

ulnaris (ul-na′ris) ulnar; in official anatomical nomenclature, designating relationship to the ulna.

ulnen (ul′nen) pertaining to the ulna alone.

ulnocarpal (ul″no-kar′pal) pertaining to the ulna and carpus.

ulnoradial (ul″no-ra′de-al) pertaining to the ulna and radius.

ULO trademark for a preparation of chlophedianol hydrochloride.

ul(o)- 1. [Gr. oulē scar] a combining form denoting relationship to a scar, or cicatrix. 2. [Gr. oulon gum] a combining form denoting relationship to the gingivae.

ulocace (u-lok′ah-se) [ulo-(2) + Gr. kakē badness] ulceration of the gingivae.

ulocarcinoma (u″lo-kar″sĭ-no′mah) [ulo-(2) + carcinoma] carcinoma of the gums.

uloglossitis (u″lo-glos-si′tis) [ulo-(2) + Gr. glōssa tongue + -itis] inflammation of the gums and the tongue.

ulorrhagia (u″lo-ra′je-ah) [ulo-(2) + Gr. rhēgnynai to burst forth] a sudden or free discharge of blood from the gingivae.

ulorrhea (u″lo-re′ah) [ulo-(2) + Gr. rhoia flow] an oozing of blood from the gingivae.

ulotomy (u-lot′o-me) 1. [ulo-(1) + -tomy] the cutting or division of scar tissue. 2. [ulo-(2) + -tomy] incision of the gingivae.

ulotripsis (u″lo-trip′sis) [ulo-(2) + Gr. tripsis rubbing] revitalization of the gingivae by massage.

ultimate (ul′tĭ-māt) [L. ultimus last] the last or farthest; final or most remote.

ultimisternal (ul″tĭ-mĭ-ster′nal) pertaining to the xiphoid process.

ultimum moriens (ul′tĭ-mum mo′re-enz) [L. "last to die"] 1. the right atrium; said to be the last part of the body to cease moving in death. 2. the upper part of the trapezius muscle.

ult. praes. abbreviation for L. ul′timum praescriptus, last prescribed.

ultra- [L. "beyond"] a prefix denoting excess, or beyond.

ultrabrachycephalic (ul″trah-brak″e-sĕ-fal′ik) [ultra- + Gr. brachys short + kephalē head] pertaining to or char-

acterized by an extremely broad, short skull, with a cephalic index of more than 90.0.

ultracentrifugation (ul″trah-sen-trif″u-ga′shun) subjection to the action of an ultracentrifuge.

ultracentrifuge (ul″trah-sen′trĭ-fūj) a centrifuge with an exceedingly high rate of rotation which will separate and sediment the molecules of a substance.

ultradian (ul-tra′de-an) [ultra + L. dies day] pertaining to the rhythmic repetition of certain phenomena in living organisms occurring in cycles of greater frequency than circadian, that is, more frequently than once a day. Cf. circadian and infradian.

ultradolicocephalic (ul″trah-dol″ĭ-ko-sĕ-fal′ik) [ultra- + Gr. dolichos long + kephalē head] pertaining to or characterized by an extremely long, narrow head, with a cephalic index of not more than 64.9.

ultrafilter (ul″trah-fil′ter) an apparatus for performing ultrafiltration; a semipermeable membrane.

ultrafiltrate (ul″trah-fil′trāt) the liquid that has passed through an ultrafilter.

ultrafiltration (ul″trah-fil-tra′shun) filtration through filters with minute pores, thus allowing the separation of extremely minute particles. Ultrafiltration occurs naturally, as in the filtration of plasma at the capillary membrane, and it is performed in the laboratory, especially to separate a substance in colloidal solution from its dispersion medium, and usually under pressure in order to accelerate the process.

ultragaseous (ul″trah-gas′e-us) having the properties of gas at one millionth of atmospheric pressure; see radiant matter, under matter.

ultramicrochemistry (ul″trah-mi″kro-kem′is-tre) the chemical study of materials in extremely minute quantities.

ultramicron (ul″trah-mi′kron) an individual element of the dispersed phase of a colloid.

ultramicropipet (ul″trah-mi″kro-pi-pet′) a pipet designed to handle extremely small quantities of liquid (0.002 to 0.005 ml.).

ultramicroscope (ul″trah-mi′kro-skōp) a special darkfield microscope for the examination of particles of colloidal size. See darkfield illumination, under illumination, and darkfield microscope, under microscope.

ultramicroscopic (ul″trah-mi′kro-skop′ik) 1. pertaining to the ultramicroscope. 2. too small to be seen with an ordinary microscope.

ultramicroscopy (ul″trah-mi-kros′ko-pe) the employment of the ultramicroscope.

ultramicrotome (ul″trah-mi′kro-tōm) an instrument for making very thin tissue sections for electron microscopy.

Ultran (ul′tran) trademark for preparations of phenaglycodol.

ultraphagocytosis (ul″trah-fag″o-si-to′sis) ingestion of particles of submicroscopic dimensions.

ultraprophylaxis (ul″trah-pro″fi-lak′sis) prophylaxis directed toward the prevention of diseased or abnormal children by regulation of the marriage of the unfit.

ultraquinine (ul″trah-kwin′in) an alkaloid from cuprea bark.

ultra-red (ul″trah-red′) infrared.

ultrasonic (ul″trah-son′ik) [ultra- + L. sonus sound] pertaining to mechanical radiant energy having a frequency beyond the upper limit of perception by the human ear, that is, beyond about 20,000 Hz (cycles per second); see ultrasonics.

ultrasonics (ul″trah-son′iks) that part of the science of acoustics dealing with the frequency range beyond the upper limit of perception by the human ear (beyond 20 kilocycles per second), but usually restricted to frequencies above 500 kilocycles per second. Ultrasonic radiation is injurious to tissues because of its thermal effects when absorbed by living matter, but in controlled doses it is used therapeutically to selectively break down pathologic tissues, as in treatment of arthritis and lesions of the nervous system, and also as a diagnostic aid by visually displaying echoes received from irradiated tissues, as in echocardiography and echoencephalography.

ultrasonogram (ul″trah-son′o-gram) the record obtained by ultrasonography.

ultrasonographic (ul″trah-son″o-graf′ik) pertaining to or accomplished by ultrasonography; called also sonographic.

ultrasonography (ul″trah-son-og′rah-fe) the visualization of deep structures of the body by recording the reflections of (echoes of) pulses of ultrasonic waves directed into the tissues. Diagnostic ultrasonography, as in echocardiography and echoencephalography, utilizes a frequency range of 1 million to 10 million hertz (cycles per second), or 1 to 10 MHz. Such sound waves are transmissible only in liquids and solids. Called also *echography* and *sonography*. **Doppler u.,** that in which measurement and a visual record are made of the shift in frequency of a continuous ultrasonic wave proportional to the blood-flow velocity in underlying vessels; used in diagnosis of extracranial occlusive vascular disease. It is also used in detection of the fetal heart beat or of the velocity of movement of a structure such as the beating heart. **endoscopic u.,** ultrasonography in which the ultrasound transducer is incorporated into the tip of a fiberoptic endoscope that is inserted into the esophagus, stomach, or duodenum to provide views of the mediastinum or abdominal organs. **gray-scale u.,** a B-scan technique in which a television video-scan converter amplifies and processes echoes according to their strength into a visual display ranging from white for the strongest echoes to varying shades of gray.

ultrasonometry (ul″trah-so-nom′ĕ-tre) the measurement of certain physical properties of biologic fluids by means of ultrasound.

ultrasound (ul′trah-sownd) mechanical radiant energy (see *sound*), with a frequency greater than 20,000 cycles per second; see *ultrasonics*.

ultrastructure (ul′trah-struk″chur) the arrangement of the smallest elements making up a body; the structure beyond the resolution power of the light microscope, i.e., the structure visible only under the ultramicroscope and electron microscope. Called also *fine structure*.

Ultratard (ul′trah-tard) trademark for preparations of extended insulin zinc suspension.

ultraviolet (ul″trah-vi′o-let) beyond the violet end of the spectrum; said of electromagnetic rays or radiation between the violet rays and the roentgen rays, that is, with wavelengths between 4 and 400 nm. These rays have powerful actinic and chemical properties, inducing sunburn and tanning of the skin and producing ergocalciferol (vitamin D_2) by their action on ergosterol in the skin. **far u.,** ultraviolet radiation of shortest wavelength, between 200 and 300 nm. **near u.,** that portion of the ultraviolet near the visible spectrum, that is, with wavelengths between 300 and 400 nm.

ultravirus (ul″trah-vi′rus) (*obs.*) an extremely small pathogenic agent; see *filterable virus*, under *virus*.

ultravisible (ul″trah-viz′ĭ-b'l) ultramicroscopic.

ultromotivity (ul″tro-mo-tiv′ĭ-te) ability to move spontaneously.

Ultzmann's test (ooltz′mahnz) [Robert *Ultzmann*, German urologist, 1842–1889] see under *tests*.

umbauzonen (um″bou-zo′nen) [Ger., "rebuilding zones"] Looser's transformation zones; see under *zone*.

umbelliferone (um″bel-lif′er-ōn) 7-hydroxycoumarin, a substance present in many plants, particularly those of the Umbelliferae family; used to absorb ultraviolet rays in sunscreen creams and lotions.

umber (um′ber) a natural earth containing chiefly manganese, iron oxide, and silica; used as a pigment.

Umber's test (um′berz) [Friedrich *Umber*, German physician, 1871–1946] see under *tests*.

umbilical (um-bil′ĭ-kal) [L. *umbilicalis*] pertaining to the umbilicus.

umbilicate (um-bil′ĭ-kāt) [L. *umbilicatus*] shaped like or resembling the umbilicus.

umbilicated (um-bil′ĭ-kāt″ed) marked by depressed areas resembling the umbilicus.

umbilication (um″bil-ĭ-ka′shun) a pit or depression resembling the umbilicus.

umbilicus (um-bil′ĭ-kus, um″bĭ-li′kus) [L.] [NA] the navel: the cicatrix marking the site of attachment of the umbilical cord in the fetus. **amniotic u.,** the oval aperture formed by converging amnion folds. **decidual u.,** a small cicatricial mark over the human blastocyst shortly after its migration through the uterine epithelium into the stroma, marking the place of the closure of the decidua capsularis. **posterior u.,** pilonidal sinus.

umbo (um′bo), gen. *umbo′nis*, pl. *umbo′nes* [L. "a boss"] a round projection; the projecting center of any rounded surface. **u. membra′nae tym′pani** [NA], **u. of tympanic membrane,** the slight projection at the center of the outer surface of the tympanic membrane, corresponding to the point of attachment of the tip of the manubrium of the malleus.

umbonate (um′bo-nāt) [L. *umbo* a knob] knoblike; button-like; having a button-like, raised center.

umbones (um-bo′nēz) [L.] plural of *umbo*.

umbrascopy (um-bras′ko-pe) retinoscopy.

UMP uridine monophosphate.

unazotized (un a′zo tīzd) containing no nitrogen.

unbalance (un-bal′ans) lack or loss of normal balance.

uncal (ung′kal) of or pertaining to the uncus.

Uncaria (un-ka′re-ah) [L.] a genus of rubiaceous shrubs native to Asia. **U. gam′bier, U. gam′bir** [Hunter] Roxb., Rubiaceae, a species of southeastern Asia, which is the source of gambir and catechin.

uncarthrosis (unk″ar-thro′sis) bone disease involving the uncinate processes of vertebrae.

unci (un′si) [L.] genitive and plural of *uncus*.

uncia (un′se-ah), pl. *un′ciae* [L.] 1. ounce. 2. inch.

unciform (un′sĭ-form) [L. *uncus* hook + *forma* form] shaped like a hook, as the unciform bone.

unciforme (un″sĭ-for′me) [L.] hooked; see *os hamatum*.

uncinal (un′sĭ-nal) uncinate.

Uncinaria (un″sĭ-na′re-ah) [L. *uncus* hook] a genus of nematode worms of the family Ancylostomidae. **U. america′na,** *Necator americanus*. **U. duodena′lis,** *Ancylostoma duodenale*. **U. stenoceph′ala,** a hookworm commonly causing hookworm disease in dogs; also parasitic in foxes, cats, and other carnivores.

uncinariasis (un″sin-ah-ri′ah-sis) the state of being infected with worms of the genus *Uncinaria*. See *hookworm disease*, under *disease*.

uncinariatic (un″sĭ-na″re-at′ik) pertaining to or exhibiting uncinariasis (hookworm disease).

uncinate (un′sĭ-nāt) 1. hooked or barbed, as the uncinate bone. 2. relating to or affecting the uncinate gyrus, as in uncinate epilepsy.

uncinatum (un″sĭ-na′tum) [L.] hooked; see *os hamatum*.

uncipressure (un′sĭ-presh″ur) [L. *uncus* hook + *pressura* pressure] pressure with a hook to control hemorrhage.

uncomplemented (un-kom′ple-ment″ed) not joined with complement, and therefore not active.

unconscious (un-kon′shus) 1. insensible; incapable of responding to sensory stimuli and of having subjective experiences. 2. the part of the mind that is not readily accessible to conscious awareness by ordinary means but whose existence may be manifested in symptom formation, in dreams, or under the influence of drugs; it is one of the systems of Freud's topographic model of the mind. Cf. *conscious* and *preconscious*. **collective u.,** in jungian psychology, the elements of the unconscious that are theoretically common to all mankind.

unco-ossified (un″ko-os′ĭ-fīd) not united into one bone.

uncotomy (ung-kot′o-me) [*uncus* + Gr. *tomē* a cutting] the production of a circumscribed lesion in the uncus in the treatment of psychotic states.

uncovertebral (un″ko-ver′tĕ-bral) pertaining to or affecting the uncinate processes of a vertebra.

unction (ungk′shun) [L. *unctio*] 1. an ointment. 2. the application of an ointment or salve; inunction.

unctuous (ungk′chu-us) greasy or oily; oleaginous.

uncus (ung′kus) [L. "hook"] 1. any hook-shaped structure. 2. [NA] the medially curved anterior end of the parahippocampal gyrus; called also *u. gyri fornicati*. *u. gyri hippocampi*, and *u. gyri parahippocampalis*. **u. cor′poris** [NA], a hooklike projection on each side of the superior surface of the third to seventh cervical vertebral bodies. **u. of hamate bone,** hamulus ossis hamati.

undecane (un′de-kān) a colorless petroleum hydrocarbon, $CH_3(CH_2)_9CH_3$.

undecenoic acid (un-dek″e-no′ik) systematic name for undecylenic acid.

undecylenic acid (un″de-sil-en′ik) [USP] a fungicide (against *Epidermophyton, Trichophyton,* and *Microsporum* spp.) applied topically either alone or with zinc undecylenate.

undercut (un′der-kut) 1. that portion of a tooth which lies between the survey line (height of contour) and the gingivae. 2. the contour of a cross-section of a residual ridge or dental arch which would prevent the insertion of a denture. 3. the contour of flasking stone which interlocks in such a way as to prevent the separation of the parts. 4. a depressed or intaglio irregularity in the wall of a prepared tooth that prevents the ready withdrawl and seating of a wax pattern and the metal alloy casting.

underhorn (un′der-horn) cornu inferius ventriculi lateralis.

undernutrition (un″der-nu-trish′un) improper nutrition due to inadequate food supply or to failure to ingest, assimilate, or utilize any or all of the necessary food elements.

understain (un′der-stān) to stain less deeply than usual.

undertoe (un′der-to) a condition in which the great toe is displaced under the others.

Underwood's disease (un′der-woodz)[Michael *Underwood,* London obstetrician and pediatrician, 1737–1820] sclerema.

undifferentiation (un″dif-er-en″she-a′shun) absence of normal differentiation; anaplasia.

undine (un-dēn′, un′dīn) [L. *unda* wave, water] a small glass flask for irrigating the eye.

undinism (un′din-izm)[*Undine* a water nymph, from L. *unda* wave] the association of sexual ideas with water, including urine and urination.

undulant (un′du-lant) [L. *unda* wave] characterized by wavelike fluctuations; see also under *fever.*

undulate (un′joo-lit) [L. *undulatus,* from *unda* wave] having a wavy, curved border; said of a colony of microorganisms.

undulation (un″du-la′shun) [L. *undulatio*] a wavelike motion in any medium; a vibration. **jugular u.,** venous pulse. **respiratory u.,** the variation of the blood pressure curve due to respiration.

ung. abbreviation for L. *unguen′tum,* ointment.

ungual (ung′gwal) [L. *unguis* nail] pertaining to the nails.

unguent (ung′gwent) [L. *unguentum*] an ointment, salve, or cerate.

unguentum (ung-gwen′tum), gen. *unguen′ti,* pl. *unguen′ta* [L.] ointment. **u. ac′idi bo′rici,** boric acid ointment. **u. ac′idi undecylen′ici compos′itum,** compound undecylenic acid ointment. **u. aeth′ylis aminobenzoa′tis,** benzocaine ointment. **u. al′bum,** white ointment. **u. a′quae ro′sae,** rose water ointment. **u. a′quae ro′sae petrola′tum,** petrolatum rose water ointment. **u. belladon′nae,** belladonna ointment. **u. calami′nae,** calamine ointment. **u. epinephri′nae bitartra′tis ophthal′micum,** epinephrine bitartrate ophthalmic ointment. **u. fla′vum,** yellow ointment. **u. glycol′is polyethyle′ni,** polyethylene glycol ointment. **u. hydrar′gyri biochlo′ridi,** mercury bichloride ointment. **u. hydrar′gyri chlori′di mi′tis,** calomel ointment. **u. hydrar′gyri mi′te,** mild mercurial ointment. **u. hydrar′gyri ox′idi fla′vi,** yellow mercuric oxide ophthalmic ointment. **u. hydrophil′icum,** hydrophilic ointment. **u. ichthammol′lis,** ichthammol ointment. **u. menthol′is compos′itum,** compound menthol ointment. **u. nitrofurazo′ni,** nitrofurazone ointment. **u. pi′cis carbo′nis,** coal tar ointment. **u. pi′cis pi′ni,** pine tar ointment. **u. resorcinol′is compos′itum,** compound resorcinol ointment. **u. sulfacetami′di so′dici,** sodium sulfacetamide ointment. **u. sulfu′ris,** sulfur ointment. **u. zin′ci ox′idi,** zinc oxide ointment.

ungues (ung′gwēz) [L.] plural of *unguis.*

unguiculate (ung-gwik′u-lāt) provided with claws or nails; resembling a claw.

unguiculus (ung-gwik′u-lus) [L., dim. of *unguis*] a small nail or claw.

unguis (ung′gwis), pl. *un′gues* [L.] 1. [NA] the horny cutaneous plate on the dorsal surface of the distal end of the terminal phalanx of a finger or toe, made up of flattened epithelial scales developed from the stratum lucidum of the skin. Called also *nail* (q.v.). 2. a collection of pus in the cornea; an onyx. 3. a nail-like part or structure. **u. incar-**

na′tus, ingrown nail; see under *nail.* **u. ventric′uli latera′lis cer′ebri,** calcar avis.

ungula (ung′gu-lah) [L. "hoof," "claw," "talon"] the hoof of an animal.

ungulate (ung′gu-lāt) [L. *ungula* hoof] a hoofed mammal.

unguligrade (ung′gu-lĭ-grād″) [L. *ungula* hoof + *gradi* to walk] characterized by standing or walking on the tips of the toes (hooves); applied to certain quadrupeds (e.g., horses, cows, pigs) known as *ungulates.* Cf. *digitigrade.*

uni- [L. *unus* one] a prefix meaning one.

uniarticular (u″ne-ar-tik′u-lar) [*uni-* + L. *articulus* joint] pertaining to a single joint.

uniaural (u″ne-aw′ral) monaural.

uniaxial (u″ne-ak′se-al) [*uni-* + L. *axis* axis] 1. having but one axis. 2. developing in an axial direction only, as a uniaxial organism.

unibasal (u″nĭ-ba′sal) [*uni-* + L. *basis* base] having only one base.

unicameral (u″nĭ-kam′er-al) [*uni-* + L. *camera* chamber] having only one cavity or compartment.

unicellular (u″nĭ-sel′u-lar) [*uni-* + L. *cellula* cell] made up of but a single cell, as the bacteria.

unicentral (u″nĭ-sen′tral) [*uni-* + L. *centrum* center] pertaining to or having a single center.

unicentric (u″nĭ-sen′trik) unicentral.

uniceps (u″nĭ-seps) [*uni-* + L. *caput* head] having one head or origin; said of a muscle.

unicornous (u″nĭ-kor′nus) [L. *unicornis*] having only one horn or cornu.

unicuspid (u″nĭ-kus′pid) a tooth with only one cusp.

unicuspidate (u″nĭ-kus′pĭ-dāt) having only one cusp.

unidirectional (u″nĭ-di-rek′shun-al) flowing in only one direction.

uniflagellate (u″nĭ-flaj′ĕ-lāt) having one flagellum.

unifocal (u″nĭ-fo′kal) arising from or pertaining to a single focus.

uniforate (u″nĭ-fo′rāt) [*uni-* + L. *foratus* pierced] having only one opening.

unigeminal (u″nĭ-jem′ĭ-nal) [*uni-* + L. *geminus* twin] pertaining to or affecting one twin of a pair.

unigerminal (u″nĭ-jer′mĭ-nal) 1. pertaining to a single germ or ovum. 2. monozygotic.

uniglandular (u″nĭ-glan′du-lar) pertaining to or affecting only one gland.

unigravida (u″nĭ-grav′ĭ-dah) primigravida.

unilaminar (u″nĭ-lam′ĭ-nar) having only one layer or lamina.

unilateral (u″nĭ-lat′er-al) [*uni-* + L. *latus* side] affecting but one side.

unilobar (u″nĭ-lo′bar) having only one lobe; consisting of a single lobe.

unilocular (u″nĭ-lok′u-lar) [*uni-* + L. *loculus*] having but one loculus or compartment.

unimodal (u″nĭ-mo′dal) having only one mode.

uninuclear (u″nĭ-nu′kle-ar) pertaining to a single nucleus; mononuclear.

uninucleated (u″nĭ-nu′kle-āt″ed) having but one nucleus; mononuclear; mononucleate.

uniocular (u″ne-ok′u-lar) pertaining to or affecting only one eye.

union (ūn′yun) [L. *unio*] the process of healing; the renewal of continuity in a broken bone or between the edges of a wound. See *healing.* **faulty u.,** an ununited fracture. **primary u.,** healing by first intention. **vicious u.,** union of the ends of a fractured bone so as to produce deformity.

uniovular (u″ne-ov′u-lar) [*uni-* + L. *ovum* egg] monozygotic; monovular.

unipara (u-nip′ah-rah) primipara.

uniparental (u″nĭ-pah-ren′tal) pertaining to one of the parents only.

uniparous (u-nip′ah-rus) [*uni-* + L. *parere* to bring forth, produce] 1. producing only one ovum or offspring at one time. 2. primiparous.

Unipen (u′nĭ-pen) trademark for preparations of nafcillin sodium.

unipolar (u″nĭ-po′lar) [*uni-* + L. *polus* pole] 1. having but a single pole or process, as a nerve cell. 2. pertaining to mood disorders in which only depressive episodes occur.

unipotency (u″nĭ-po′ten-se) [L. *unus* one + *potentia* power] the ability of a part to develop in one manner only, or of a cell to develop into only one type of cell.

unipotent (u-nip′o-tent) unipotential.

unipotential (u″nĭ-po-ten′shal) [*uni-* + L. *potens* able] capable in one way only; said of cells which have had their fates determined and can give rise to cells of one order only. Cf. *totipotential*.

unirritable (un-ir′ĭ-tah-b'l) not irritable; not capable of being stimulated.

uniseptate (u″ne-sep′tāt) having only one septum.

unisexual (u″nĭ-seks′u-al) [*uni-* + L. *sexus* sex] of only one sex; having the sexual organs of one sex only.

unit (u′nit) [L. *unus* one] 1. a single thing. 2. a quantity assumed as a standard of measurement. 3. a gene. **Allen-Doisy u.,** see *mouse u.* and *rat u.* **amboceptor u.,** in complement fixation tests, the smallest amount of anti-RBC antibody (amboceptor) that produces complete red cell lysis in the presence of an excess of complement. **American Drug Manufacturers' Association u.,** one tenth of the Steenbock unit. **Angström u.,** the unit of wavelength of electromagnetic and corpuscular radiations, equal to 10^{-7} mm. Called also *angstrom*. Abbreviated A., Å., or A.U. **Ansbacher u.,** a unit of vitamin K dosage. **antigen u.,** in complement fixation tests, the smallest amount of antigen that will fix one unit of complement. **antitoxic u.,** a unit for expressing the strength of an antitoxin. The unit of diphtheria antitoxin is approximately the amount of antitoxin which will preserve the life of a guinea pig weighing 250 gm. for at least four days after it is injected subcutaneously with a mixture of 100 times the minimum lethal dose of diphtheria toxin. Practically, it is the equivalent of a standard unit preserved in Washington. The unit of tetanus antitoxin is approximately ten times the amount of tetanus antitoxin which will preserve the life of a guinea pig weighing 350 gm. for at least ninety-six hours after injection of a mixture with 100 minimum lethal doses of tetanus toxin. The U.S. Public Health Service unit for scarlet fever antitoxin neutralizes 50 skin test doses of scarlet fever toxin. Abbreviated A.E. (Ger. *antitoxineinheit*). **atomic mass u.,** the unit mass equal to $\frac{1}{12}$ the mass of the nuclide of carbon-12, equivalent to 1.657×10^{-24} gm.; abbreviated amu. Called also *atomic weight u.* and *dalton*. **atomic weight u.,** atomic mass u. **Behnken's u.,** a unit of roentgen-ray exposure, being that quantity which, when applied in 1 cc. of air at 18° C. and 760 mm. Hg of pressure, engenders sufficient electric conductivity to equal one electrostatic unit, as measured by the saturation current. **Bethesda u.,** a measure of the level of inhibitor to factor VIII; equal to the amount of inhibitor in patient plasma that will inactivate 50 per cent of Factor VIII in an equal volume normal plasma following a 2-hour incubation period. **Bodansky u.,** the quantity of phosphatase in 100 ml. of serum required to liberate 1 mg. of phosphorus as phosphate ion from sodium β-glycerophosphate in 1 hour at 37° C. and under other standardized conditions. **British thermal u.,** the amount of heat necessary to raise the temperature of 1 pound of water from 39° F. to 40° F., abbreviated B.T.U. **cat u.,** that amount of digitalis calculated per kilogram of weight of a cat which is just sufficient to kill when slowly and continuously injected into the vein (Hatcher). **C. G. S. u.,** any unit in the centimeter-gram-second system. **clinical u.,** a unit of estrogenic activity equal to approximately one sixth of the international unit. **Collip u.,** a unit of dosage of parathyroid extract: it is one one-hundredth of the amount required to increase by 5 mg. the quantity of calcium in 100 ml. of blood at the end of fifteen hours in a dog of 20 kg. weight. **colony-forming u.,** 1. any of several hematopoietic stem cells identified by their ability to give rise to monoclonal colonies in the spleen when transplanted into isogeneic, lethally irradiated mice, including pluripotent myeloid stem cells and the precursors of neutrophils and monocytes, eosinophils, erythrocytes, and megakaryocytes. See also *stem cell* (def. 2), under *cell*. 2. in microbiology, estimation of the number of bacteria or yeasts by counting the colonies on a solid medium, with one bacterium being considered equal to one colony; some colonies develop from two or more organisms attached to or lying close to each other

when inoculated. **complement u.,** in complement fixation tests, the smallest amount of complement or serum that will produce complete hemolysis of sensitized red cells. Called also *hemolytic u.* **Corner-Allen u.,** a unit of progestin dosage. **coronary care u.,** a specially designed and equipped hospital area containing a small number of private rooms, with all facilities necessary for constant observation and possible emergency treatment of patients with severe heart disease. **u. of current,** see *ampere*. **dental u.,** 1. a masticatory unit consisting of a single tooth and its adnexa. 2. a mobile or fixed article of dental equipment, which may be combined with a chair, consisting of items and attachments needed for dental examination and operations, and housing the electrical, mechanical, and plumbing facilities needed to operate the equipment and fixtures of the unit. **digitalis u.,** any of several units once used in bioassay of digitalis preparations and named according to the animal in which it was determined, as cat unit, etc. **electromagnetic u's,** that system of units based on the fundamental definition of a unit magnetic pole as one which will repel an exactly similar pole with a force of one dyne when the poles are 1 cm. apart. **electrostatic u's,** that system of units based on the fundamental definition of a unit charge as one which will repel an equal and like charge with a force of one dyne when the two charges are 1 cm. apart in a vacuum. Abbreviated E.S.E. (Ger., *elektrostatische Einheit*) and *e.s.u.* **enzyme u.,** see *international u. of enzyme activity*, under *unit*. **Felton's u.,** a mouse protective unit of antipneumococcic serum; it is that quantity of antibody capable of protecting a white Swiss mouse against one million fatal doses of a standard pneumococcus culture of the corresponding type. Frequently, it is considered to be the equivalent of the National Institutes of Health control serum (P-11). **Florey u.** (*obs.*), Oxford u. **u. of force,** see *dyne*. **Hampson u.,** a unit of roentgen-ray exposure; it is one quarter of the erythema dose. **u. of heat,** the quantity of heat required to raise the temperature of a kilogram of water 1° C. See *calorie* and *British thermal u.* **hemolytic u.,** complement u. **hemorrhagin u.,** the amount of snake venom necessary to produce hemorrhages in the vascular network of a three-day-old chick embryo. **Hounsfield u.,** a unit of x-ray attenuation used for CT scans, each pixel being assigned a value on a scale on which air is −1000, water is 0, and compact bone is +1000. **intensive care u.,** a hospital unit in which are concentrated special equipment and skilled personnel for the care of seriously ill patients requiring immediate and continuous attention; abbreviated ICU. **International u.,** a unit of biological material, as of enzymes, hormones, vitamins, etc., established by the International Conference for the Unification of Formulas. **international u. of enzyme activity (IU),** that amount of an enzyme that will catalyze the transformation of 1 micromole of substrate per minute under standard conditions of temperature, optimal pH, and optimal substrate concentration. **international u. of estrogenic activity,** the estrus-producing activity represented in 0.1 microgram of the international standard estrone. **international u. of gonadotrophic activity,** the specific gonadotrophic activity of 0.1 mg. of the standard material preserved at and distributed from the National Institute for Medical Research, Hampstead, London. It is derived from pregnancy urine and it is approximately the amount required to produce cornification of the vaginal epithelium of the immature rat. **international insulin u.,** one twenty-second of a milligram of the pure crystalline product now adopted as the standard. **international u. of male hormone,** a previously used standard equal to the androgenic activity represented in 0.1 mg. of crystalline androsterone. **international u. of penicillin,** the specific penicillin activity contained in 0.6 microgram of the international standard sodium salt of II or G penicillin. **international u. of vitamin A,** activity equivalent to 0.6 microgram of pure beta-carotene. **international u. of vitamin D,** the activity of 1 mg. of the international standard solution of irradiated ergosterol (1 mg. in 10 ml. of olive oil). One mg. given daily to rachitic rats for eight consecutive days should produce a wide calcium line. **Kienböck u.,** a unit of roentgen-ray exposure equal to 0.1 erythema dose; symbol X. **King u., King-Armstrong u.,** the amount of phosphatase which, when allowed to act upon an excess of disodium phenylphosphate at a pH of 9 for 30 minutes at 37.5° C., will liberate 1 mg. of phenol. **Lf u.,** that amount of diphtheria toxin or toxoid which gives the most rapid flocculation with one standard unit of diphtheria antitoxin when mixed and incubated *in vitro*. **light u.,** see *footcandle*. **Mache u.,** a German unit for expressing the concentration of radium emanation in solution; it is equivalent to 3.64 eman. Abbreviated M.u. **map u.,** centimorgan. **motor u.,** the unit of motor activity formed by a motor nerve cell and its many innervated muscle fibers. **mouse u.,** the least amount of estrus-producing hormone (estrogen) that causes in a spayed mouse cornification of the vaginal epithelium. Abbreviated m.u. **Noon pollen u.,** the activity present in the saline extract from one millionth of a grain of pollen. **Oxford u.,** that amount of penicillin which, when dissolved in 50 ml. of meat extract broth, just inhibits completely a test strain of *Staphylococcus aureus*. **pepsin u.,** a unit for measuring the proportion of pepsin in the gastric juice. **peripheral resistance u. (PRU),** a conventional unit of vascular resistance equal to the resistance that produces a pressure difference of 1 mm Hg corresponding to a blood flow of 1 ml/sec. **physiologic u.,** see *micelle*. **pilosebaceous u.,** the hair follicle and the associated apocrine gland. **quantum u.,** see *Planck's constant*, under *constant*. **rat u.,** the highest dilution (i.e., least amount) of an estrus-producing hormone (estrogen) that when given to a mature spayed rat in three injections at four-hour intervals during the first day produces cornification and desquamation of the vaginal epithelium. Abbreviated R.U. **u. of resistance,** see *ohm*. **Sherman u.** (*for vitamin A*), see *Sherman-Munsell u. of vitamin A*. **Sherman-Bourquin u. of vitamin B₂,** that amount of riboflavin which fed daily to a standard test rat for eight weeks will give a gain of 3 gm. a week. **Sherman-Munsell u. of vitamin A,** that amount of vitamin A which when fed daily just suffices to support a rate of gain of 3 gm. per week for eight weeks in a standard rat previously depleted of vitamin A. **SI u.,** any of the units of the Système International d'Unités, or International System of Units, adopted in 1960 at the Eleventh General Conference of Weights and Measures. SI units comprise the basic units *meter* (length), *kilogram* (mass), *second* (time), *ampere* (electric current), *kelvin* (temperature [absolute]), *candela* (luminous intensity), and *mole* (amount of substance); supplementary units *radian* (plane angle) and *steradian* (solid angle); and derived units, which are stated in terms of the basic units, *newton* (force), *pascal* (pressure), *joule* (energy), *watt* (power), *volt* (electric potential), *coulomb* (electric charge), *farad* (capacitance), *ohm* (electric resistance), *siemens* (electric conductance), *weber* (magnetic flux), *tesla* (magnetic flux density), *henry* (inductance), *hertz* (frequency), and *degree Celsius* (temperature). For multiples and submultiples of these units formed by the use of prefixes, see Appendices 2 and 3. **Somogyi u.,** that amount of amylase that will liberate reducing equivalents equal to 1 mg of glucose per 30 minutes under defined conditions. **specific smell u.,** the smallest amount in substance in grams per liter which can be detected by smell. **Steenbock u. of vitamin D,** the total amount of vitamin D which will produce a narrow line of calcium deposit in the rachitic metaphyses of the distal ends of the radii and ulnae of standard rachitic rats within ten days. **sudanophobic u.,** the smallest amount of corticotropic hormone which will cause the disappearance of the sudanophobic zone of the adrenal cortex in at least two or three hypophysectomized rats when they are injected morning and evening on eight consecutive days. **Svedberg u.,** a unit equal to 10⁻¹³ second used for expressing sedimentation coefficients (q.v.) of macromolecules. Symbol, S. **Svedberg flotation u.,** a unit equal to 10⁻¹³ second used for expressing negative sedimentation coefficients of macromolecules that float rather than sink in a centrifuge; e.g., lipoproteins. Symbol, Sf. **Thayer-Doisy u.,** a unit of vitamin K activity, being equivalent to the activity of 1 μg. of pure vitamin K₁. **toxic u., toxin u.,** the smallest dose of toxin which will kill a guinea pig weighing about 250 gm. in three to four days. **tuberculin u. (TU),** an arbitrary unit of tuberculin dosage defined by comparison of clinical response with a standard preparation of PPD tuberculin. **turbidity reducing u.,** the amount of hyaluronidase which is just sufficient to reduce the turbidity produced by 0.2 mg. of hyaluronate to that produced by 0.1 mg. after addition of acidified horse serum. **urotoxic u.,** the smallest quantity of urotoxin which will kill an animal weighing 1 gm. **U.S.P. u.,** one used in the United States Pharmacopeia in expressing the potency of antibiotic, pharmacodynamic, and endocrine preparations, as well as most of the sera, toxins, vaccines, and related

products, corresponding to units established internationally, by the Food and Drug Administration, or by the National Institutes of Health. **vitamin A u.,** see *international u. of vitamin A*, and *Sherman-Munsell u. of vitamin A*. **u. of vitamin B₁,** the antineuritic activity of 3 micrograms of the international standard preparation deposited at the National Institute for Medical Research, Hampstead. **vitamin D u.,** see *international u. of vitamin D, Steenbock u. of vitamin D* and *American Drug Manufacturers' Association u. of vitamin D*. **vitamin G u.,** see *Sherman-Bourquin u. of vitamin B₂*. **x-ray u.,** Kienböck u.

unitage (u′nit-ij)   a statement of the unit quantity in any system of measurement.

unitary (u′nĭ-ter″e) [L. *unitas* oneness]   composed of or pertaining to a single unit.

United States Pharmacopeia   see *U.S.P.*

Unitensen (u″nĭ-ten′sen)   trademark for a preparation of cryptenamine acetates or cryptenamine tannates.

uniterminal (u″nĭ-ter′mĭ-nal)   monoterminal.

univalence (u″nĭ-va′lens)   the state or condition of being univalent.

univalent (u″nĭ-va′lent)   monovalent.

univitelline (u″nĭ-vi-tel′in)   pertaining to or derived from a single ovum.

unmedullated (un-med′u-lāt″ed)   not possessing a medulla or myelin sheath; said of a nerve fiber.

unmyelinated (un-mi′ĕ-li-nāt″ed)   not possessing a myelin sheath; said of a nerve fiber.

Unna's boot, etc. (oo′nahz) [Paul Gerson *Unna*, dermatologist in Hamburg, 1850–1929]   see under *boot, cell, dermatosis*, and *Table of Stains*.

Unna-Pappenheim stain (oo′nah-pahp′en-hīm) [Paul Gerson *Unna*; Artur *Pappenheim*, German physician, 1870–1916]   see *Table of Stains*.

Unna-Thost disease, syndrome (oo′nah tost) [Paul Gerson *Unna*; Arthur *Thost*, German physician, born 1854]   diffuse palmoplantar keratoderma.

unorganized (un-or′gan-īzd)   not developed into an organic structure; not having organs.

unorientation (un″o-re-en-tā′shun)   extreme disorder of memory in which the person loses the ideas of place and time; disorientation.

unphysiologic (un″fiz-e-o-loj′ik)   not physiologic in character.

unrest (un-rest′)   a state of uneasiness, or restlessness. **peristaltic u.,** a state of disturbed peristalsis of the stomach or intestine.

unsaturated (un-sat′u-rāt″ed)   not saturated; applied to (1) a chemical compound in which two or more atoms are united by double or triple bonds. These bonds have two or three pairs of shared electrons characterized by pi-electrons (π-electrons) with orbital overlap. Such compounds may still add atoms or groups to the unsaturated bonding atoms up to a limit of bonding power or saturation. Most commonly refers to carbon-carbon bonds, as in unsaturated fatty acids. (2) a solution in which more solute may still be dissolved under stated conditions.

Unschuld's sign (oon′shooldz) [Paul *Unschuld*, German internist, 1835–c. 1905]   see under *sign*.

unsex (un-seks′)   to deprive of the sex glands, or gonads.

unstriated (un-stri′āt-ed)   having no striations or striae; see under *muscle*.

Unverricht's disease (syndrome) (oon′fer-ikts) [Heinrich *Unverricht*, German physician, 1853–1912]   myoclonus epilepsy.

uprighting (up′rīt-ing)   tipping inclined teeth to a more vertical axial inclination. See also *tipping*, def. 1.

upsiloid (up′sĭ-loid) [Gr. υ + *eidos* form]   shaped like the Greek upsilon (υ or Υ); see *hyoid* (def. 1) and *hypsiloid*.

upsilon (up′si-lon) [Υ, υ]   the twentieth letter of the Greek alphabet.

uptake (up′tāk)   absorption and incorporation of a substance by living tissue, as of iodine by the thyroid gland.

urachal (u′rah-kal)   pertaining to the urachus.

urachovesical (u″rah-ko-ves′ĭ-kal)   pertaining to the urachus and the bladder.

urachus (u′rah-kus) [Gr. *ourachos*] [NA]   a canal in the fetus that connects the bladder with the allantois; it persists throughout life as a cord (the median umbilical ligament) into which a patent canal may extend for part of the distance to the umbilicus.

uracil (u′rah-sil) a pyrimidine component, $(C_4H_4O_2N_2)$, found in nucleic acid. **5-methyl u.,** see *thymine*.

uracrasia (u″rah-kra′se-ah) [*ur-* + Gr. *akrasia* bad mixture] a disordered state of the urine.

uracratia (u″rah-kra′she-ah) [*ur-* + Gr. *akrateia* lack of self control] urinary incontinence.

uragogue (u′rah-gog) [*ur-* + Gr. *agōgos* leading] 1. increasing urinary volume flow; diuretic. 2. an agent that increases production of urine.

uramil (u′rah-mil) a white crystalline pyrimidine derivative, $CO(NH \cdot CO)_2CH \cdot NH_2$, dialuramide, or 5-aminobarbituric acid, obtainable from uric acid, alloxantin, and other substances.

uranidin (u-ran′ĭ-din) any one of a group of yellow animal pigments found in sponges, corals, medusae, and worms.

uranin (u′rah-nin) the sodium or potassium salt of fluorescein; see *sodium fluorescein*.

uranisc(o)- [Gr. *ouraniskos*, the roof of the mouth] a combining form denoting relationship to the palate; see also *uran(o)-*.

uraniscochasma (u″rah-nis″ko-kaz′mah) [*uranisco-* + Gr. *chasma* cleft] cleft palate.

uraniscolalia (u″rah-nis″ko-la′le-ah) [*uranisco-* + Gr. *lalia* talking] a speech defect due to cleft palate.

uraniscoplasty (u″rah-nis′ko-plas″te) palatoplasty.

uraniscorrhaphy (u″rah-nis-kor′ah-fe) [*uranisco-* + Gr. *rhaphē* suture] staphylorrhaphy.

uraniscus (u″rah-nis′kus) [Gr. *ouraniskos*, dim. of *ouranos*] the palate.

uranium (u-ra′ne-um) [L. *Uranus* a planet] a hard and heavy radioactive metallic element; symbol, U; atomic number, 92; atomic weight, 238.03; specific gravity, 18.68. Some of its compounds are medicinal. Naturally occurring uranium is composed of three isotopes of mass numbers 234, 235, and 238, respectively. Uranium 235 separated from U 238 undergoes fission with slow neutrons, giving up neutrons which can join the nucleus of U 238 to form neptunium, which in turn decays by beta particle emission to form plutonium. Cf. *neptunium* and *plutonium*.

uran(o)- [Gr. *ouranos* the sky, the vault of heaven or of a ceiling, the roof of the mouth or palate] a combining form denoting relationship to the palate; sometimes used in reference to the sky, or heaven.

uranoplasty (u′rah-no-plas″te) [*urano-* + Gr. *plassein* to mold] palatoplasty.

uranoplegia (u″rah-no-ple′je-ah) [*urano-* + Gr. *plēge* stroke + *-ia*] palatoplegia.

uranorrhaphy (u″rah-nor′ah-fe) [*urano-* + Gr. *rhaphē* suture] staphylorrhaphy.

uranoschisis (u″rah-nos′kĭ-sis) [*urano-* + Gr. *schisis* fissure] cleft palate.

uranoschism (u-ran′o-skizm) [*urano-* + Gr. *schisma* cleft] cleft palate.

uranostaphyloplasty (u″rah-no-staf″ĭ-lo-plas″te) an operation for repairing a defect of both the soft and hard palate. See also *palatoplasty*.

uranostaphylorrhaphy (u″rah-no-staf″ĭ-lor′ah-fe) [*urano-* + Gr. *staphylē* uvula + *rhaphē* suture] suture of both the soft and hard palate. See also *palatorrhaphy*.

uranostaphyloschisis (u″rah-no-staf″ĭ-los′kĭ-sis) cleft palate involving both the soft palate and the hard palate.

Uranotaenia (u″rah-no-te′ne-ah) a genus of culicine mosquitoes. **U. sappari′nus,** a species occurring in the eastern United States.

uranyl (u′rah-nil) the UO_2^{++} ion, as in uranyl sulfate, UO_2SO_4. **u. acetate,** a yellow crystalline compound, $UO_2(C_2H_3O_2)_2 \cdot 2H_2O$, used in coryza.

urapostema (u″rah-pos-te′mah) [*ur-* + Gr. *apostēma* abscess] an abscess which contains urine.

urarthritis (u″rar-thri′tis) gouty arthritis.

urate (ūr′āt) any salt or anion of uric acid (q.v.).

urate oxidase (u′rāt ok′sĭ-dās) [EC 1.7.3.3] an enzyme of the oxidoreductase class that catalyzes the oxidation of uric

acid to allantoin with liberation of CO_2 and H_2O_2. It is a copper enzyme, found in most mammals but not in primates. Called also *uricase*.

uratemia (u″rah-te′me-ah) [*urate* + Gr. *haima* blood + *-ia*] the presence of urates in the blood.

uratic (u-rat′ik) pertaining to urates or to gout.

uratohistechia (u″rah-to-his-tek′e-ah) [*urate* + Gr. *histos* tissue + *echein* to hold] the presence of an excessive amount of urate, urea, or uric acid in a tissue.

uratoma (u″rah-to′mah) a tophus or concretion made up of urates.

uratosis (u″rah-to′sis) the deposition of crystalline urates in the tissues.

uraturia (u″rah-tu′re-ah) [*urate* + Gr. *ouron* urine + *-ia*] the presence of an excess of urates in the urine; lithuria.

urazin, urazine (u′rah-zin) diurea.

urazole (u′rah-zōl) a crystalline compound, 1,2,4-triazolidine-3,5-dione, $(NH \cdot CO)_2NH$, formed by heating urea or biuret with hydrazine sulfate.

Urbach-Wiethe disease (ur′bak vēt′ĕ) [Erich *Urbach*, American dermatologist, 1893–1946; Camillo *Wiethe*, Austrian otologist, 1888–1949] lipoid proteinosis.

urceiform (ur-se′ĭ-form) [L. *urceus* pitcher + *forma* shape] pitcher-shaped.

urceolate (ur-se′o-lāt) urceiform.

urea (u-re′ah) a compound, $CO(NH_2)_2$, that is formed in the liver via the urea cycle from ammonia produced by the deamination of amino acids and is excreted by the kidney; it is the principal end product of protein catabolism and constitutes about one half of the total urinary solids. Elevation of the blood levels of urea and other nitrogenous compounds (azotemia) occurs with decreased glomerular filtration rate due to inadequate renal perfusion, acute or chronic renal disease, or urinary tract obstruction (see *uremia*). *Urea* [USP] administered intravenously is used as an osmotic diuretic to reduce intracranial or intraocular pressure. It is also used in topical preparations to moisten and soften rough dry skin. Called also *carbamide*. **u. nitrogen,** the urea concentration of blood or serum stated in terms of nitrogen content; converted to urea concentration by multiplying by 60/28 or 2.14. The serum or plasma urea nitrogen is traditionally referred to as *blood urea nitrogen* (BUN).

ureagenetic (u-re″ah-jĕ-net′ik) [*urea* + Gr. *gennan* to produce] forming or producing urea.

ureal (u′re-al) pertaining to urea.

ureametry (u″re-am′ĕ-tre) the measurement of the urea present in the urine.

Ureaphil (u-re′ah-fil) trademark for a preparation of urea.

Ureaplasma (u-re′ah-plaz″ma) [*urea* + Gr. *plasma* anything formed or molded] a genus of bacteria of the family Mycoplasmataceae, order Mycoplasmatales, class Mollicutes, made up of pleomorphic, gram-negative organisms that lack a cell wall and that hydrolyze urea. Called also *T-mycoplasma* and *T-strain mycoplasma* (T for *tiny*).

ureapoiesis (u-re″ah-poi-e′sis) [*urea* + Gr. *poiein* to make] the formation of urea.

urease (u′re-ās) [EC 3.5.1.5] an enzyme of the hydrolase class that catalyzes the reaction urea + H_2O = CO_2 + $2 NH_3$, a nickel protein found in microorganisms and the first enzyme prepared in the crystalline state.

urecchysis (u-rek′ĭ-sis) [*uro-* + Gr. *ekchysis* a pouring out] the effusion of urine into the cellular tissue.

Urechites (u-rek′ĭ-tēz) a genus of plants. **U. suberec′ta,** Savannah flower, an apocynaceous plant of tropical America with poisonous and antipyretic leaves.

urechitin (u-rek′ĭ-tin) a poisonous glycoside, $C_{28}H_{42}O_8$ + xH_2O, from *Urechites suberecta*.

urechitoxin (u-rek′ĭ-tok′sin) a poisonous glycoside, $C_{13}H_{20}O_5$, from *Urechites suberecta*.

Urecholine (u″re-ko′lin) trademark for a preparation of bethanechol chloride.

uredema (u″rĕ-de′mah) [*uro-* + Gr. *oidēma* swelling] a puffy condition of the tissues caused by infiltration of extravasated urine.

uredofos (u-re′do-fos) chemical name: [[[2-[[[[(4-methylphenyl)sulfonyl]amino]carbonyl]amino]phenyl]amino]thioxomethyl]phosphoramidic acid diethyl ester; a veterinary anti-helmintic, $C_{19}H_{25}N_4O_6PS_2$.

ureide (u're-id) a compound of urea and an acid or alde-hyde formed by the elimination of water. Those from one molecule of urea, as alloxan, are monoureides; those derived from two, as uric acid, are diureides.

urein (u-re'in) a yellowish, oily substance isolated from the urine, and said to be the principal organic constituent and the true cause of uremia. It has a specific gravity of 1.27, and mixes freely with water and alcohol.

urelcosis (u″rel-ko'sis) [uro- + Gr. *helkōsis* ulceration] 1. ulceration of the urinary passages. 2. an ulcer due to de-rangement of the urinary apparatus.

uremia (u-re'me-ah) [Gr. *ouron* urine + *haima* blood + -ia] 1. an excess in the blood of urea, creatinine, and other nitrogenous end products of protein and amino acid metabo-lism; more correctly referred to as *azotemia*. 2. in current usage the entire constellation of signs and symptoms of chronic renal failure, including nausea, vomiting, anorexia, a metallic taste in the mouth, a uremic odor of the breath, pruritus, uremic frost on the skin, neuromuscular disorders, pain and twitching in the muscles, hypertension, edema, mental confusion, and acid-base and electrolyte inbalances.

uremic (u-re'mik) pertaining to or characterized by ure-mia.

uremigenic (u-re″mĭ-jen'ik) 1. caused by or due to ure-mia. 2. causing uremia.

ure(o)- [*urea*, q.v.] for words beginning thus, see also those beginning *urea-*.

ureolysis (u″re-ol'ĭ-sis) [*urea* + Gr. *lysis* a loosing, setting free] the decomposition of urea to carbon dioxide and am-monia.

ureolytic (u″re-o-lit'ik) pertaining to, characterized by, or promoting ureolysis.

ureometry (u″re-om'ĕ-tre) ureametry.

ureotelic (u″re-o-tel'ik) [*urea* + Gr. *telikos* belonging to the completion, or end] having urea as the chief excretory product of nitrogen metabolism.

uresiesthesis (u-re″se-es-the'sis) [*uresis* + Gr. *aisthēsis* per-ception + -ia] the normal impulse to pass the urine.

uresis (u-re'sis) [Gr. *ourēsis*] the passage of urine; urina-tion. Sometimes used as a word termination denoting excre-tion in the urine of the substance indicated by the stem to which it is affixed, as chloruresis, cupruresis, saluresis.

uret (u'ret) the chemical group CH_2NO.

uretal (u-re'tal) ureteral.

ureter (u-re'ter) [Gr. *ourētēr*] [NA] the fibromuscular tube which conveys the urine from the kidney to the bladder. It begins with the pelvis of the kidney, a funnel-like dilatation, and empties into the base of the bladder, being 16 to 18 inches long. It is divided into a pars abdominalis and a pars pelvina. See Plate accompanying *urogenital system*, under *system*. **circumcaval u.,** postcaval u. **ectopic u.,** a ureter which opens elsewhere than in the bladder wall, usually arising from the upper segment of a double kidney, and, in the female, opening in the vestibule, terminal urethra, vagina, cervix, or uterine cavity; in the male it invariably enters the genital or urinary tract above the level of the external sphincter. **postcaval u.,** a congenital anomaly in which the right ureter passes behind the inferior vena cava and curves round this vessel to regain its anterior position as it descends to the bladder; called also *circumcaval u.* and *retrocaval u.* **retrocaval u.,** postcaval u. **retroiliac u.,** a congenital anomaly in which a ureter passes behind the iliac artery.

ureteral (u-re'ter-al) pertaining to or used upon the ure-ter.

ureteralgia (u″re-ter-al'je-ah) pain in the ureter; neural-gia of the ureter.

ureterectasia (u-re″ter-ek-ta'se-ah) ureterectasis.

ureterectasis (u-re″ter-ek'tah-sis) [*ureter* + Gr. *ektasis* dis-tention] distention of the ureter.

ureterectomy (u″re-ter-ek'to-me) [*ureter* + Gr. *ektomē* exci-sion] the surgical removal of a ureter or of a part of it.

ureteric (u″rĕ-ter'ik) ureteral.

ureteritis (u″re-ter-i'tis) inflammation of a ureter. **u. cys'tica,** ureteritis characterized by the formation of multi-ple submucosal cysts. **u. glandula'ris,** ureteritis char-

acterized by the conversion of transitional mucosal into cylindrical epithelium, with formation of glandular acini.

ureter(o)- [*ureter*, q.v.] a combining form denoting rela-tionship to the ureter.

ureterocele (u-re'ter-o-sēl″) [uretero- + Gr. *kēlē* hernia] sacculation of the terminal portion of the ureter into the bladder, as a result of stenosis of the ureteral meatus. **ectopic u.,** one which is located distal to the trigone of the bladder and which may extend into the urethra.

ureterocelectomy (u-re″ter-o-se-lek'to-me) excision of a ureterocele.

ureterocervical (u-re″ter-o-ser'vĭ-kal) pertaining to a ur-eter and to the cervix uteri.

ureterocolostomy (u-re″ter-o-ko-los'to-me) [uretero- + Gr. *kōlon* colon + *stomoun* to provide with an opening, or mouth] anastomosis of a ureter to the colon.

ureterocutaneostomy (u-re″ter-o-ku-ta″ne-os'to-me) surgical creation of a ureteral opening on the skin, permit-ting drainage of urine directly to the exterior of the body.

ureterocystanastomosis (u-re″ter-o-sis″tah-nas″to-mo'sis) ureteroneocystostomy.

ureterocystoneostomy (u-re″ter-o-sis″to-ne-os'to-me) [uretero- + Gr. *kystis* bladder + *neos* new + *stomoun* to provide with an opening, or mouth] ureteroneocystostomy.

ureterocystoscope (u-re″ter-o-sis'to-skōp) [uretero- + *cysto-scope*] a cystoscope designed for catheterizing the ureters.

ureterocystostomy (u-re″ter-o-sis-tos'to-me) [uretero- + Gr. *kystis* bladder + *stomoun* to provide with an opening, or mouth] ureteroneocystostomy.

ureterodialysis (u-re″ter-o-di-al'ĭ-sis) [uretero- + Gr. *dialy-sis* separation] rupture of a ureter.

ureteroduodenal (u-re″ter-o-du″o-de'nal) pertaining to or communicating with a ureter and the duodenum, as a ureteroduodenal fistula.

ureteroenteric (u-re″ter-o-en-ter'ik) pertaining to or con-necting the ureter and the intestine.

ureteroenteroanastomosis (u-re″ter-o-en″ter-o-ah-nas″to-mo'sis) ureteroenterostomy.

ureteroenterostomy (u-re″ter-o-en″ter-os'to-me) [uretero- + Gr. *enteron* bowel + *stomoun* to provide with an opening, or mouth] surgical creation of an opening between a ure-ter and the intestine.

ureterogram (u-re'ter-o-gram) a radiograph of the ureter.

ureterography (u-re″ter-og'rah-fe) [uretero- + Gr. *graphein* to write] radiography of the ureter after injection of an opaque medium into the ureter.

ureteroileostomy (u-re″ter-o-il″e-os'to-me) anastomosis of the ureters to an isolated loop of the ileum, drained through a stoma on the abdominal wall.

ureterointestinal (u-re″ter-o-in-tes'tĭ-nal) pertaining to or connecting the ureter and intestine.

ureterolith (u-re'ter-o-lith″) [uretero- + Gr. *lithos* stone] a calculus lodged or formed in a ureter.

ureterolithiasis (u-re″ter-o-lĭ-thi'ah-sis) the formation of a calculus in the ureter.

ureterolithotomy (u-re″ter-o-lĭ-thot'o-me) [uretero- + Gr. *lithos* stone + *tomē* a cutting] the removal of a calculus from the ureter by incision.

ureterolysis (u-re″ter-ol'ĭ-sis) [uretero- + Gr. *lysis* dissolu-tion] 1. rupture of the ureter. 2. paralysis of the ureter. 3. the operation of freeing the ureter from adhesions.

ureteromeatotomy (u-re″ter-o-me″ah-tot'o-me) incision of the opening of the ureter in the bladder wall.

ureteroneocystostomy (u-re″ter-o-ne″o-sis-tos'to-me) [uretero- + Gr. *neos* new + *kystis* bladder + *stomoun* to provide with an opening, or mouth] surgical transplanta-tion of the ureter to a different site in the bladder.

ureteroneopyelostomy (u-re″ter-o-ne″o-pi″ĕ-los'to-me) [uretero- + Gr. *neos* new + *pyelos* pelvis + *stomoun* to provide with an opening, or mouth] ureteropyeloneos-tomy.

ureteronephrectomy (u-re″ter-o-nĕ-frek'to-me) [uretero- + Gr. *nephros* kidney + *ektomē* excision] extirpation of a kidney and its ureter.

ureteropathy (u-re″ter-op'ah-the) [uretero- + Gr. *pathos* dis-ease] any disease of the ureter.

ureteropelvic (u-re″ter-o-pel′vik)   pertaining to or affecting the ureter and the renal pelvis.

ureteropelvioneostomy (u-re″ter-o-pel″ve-o-ne-os′to-me)   ureteropyeloneostomy.

ureteropelvioplasty (u-re″ter-o-pel′ve-o-plas″te)   surgical reconstruction of the junction of the ureter and renal pelvis. **Culp-DeWeerd u.,** ureteropelvioplasty in which a spiral pelvic flap is turned down and incorporated into the adjacent ureter. **Foley Y-V u.,** an operation using a pelvic flap for correction of obstructive, congenital high insertion of the ureter into the renal pelvis. **Scardino-Prince u.,** ureteropelvioplasty in which a vertical pelvic flap is turned down and incorporated into the adjacent ureter.

ureterophlegma (u-re″ter-o-fleg′mah) [*uretero-* + Gr. *phlegma* phlegm]   the presence of mucus in the ureter.

ureteroplasty (u-re′ter-o-plas″te) [*uretero-* + Gr. *plassein* to form]   plastic surgery of a ureter.

ureteroproctostomy (u-re″ter-o-prok-tos′to-me) [*uretero-* + Gr. *prōktos* anus + *stomoun* to provide with an opening, or mouth]   surgical creation of an anastomosis between a ureter and the lower rectum.

ureteropyelitis (u-re″ter-o-pi-ĕ-li′tis) [*uretero-* + Gr. *pyelos* pelvis]   inflammation of a ureter and of the pelvis of a kidney.

ureteropyelography (u-re″ter-o-pi-ĕ-log′rah-fe)   roentgenography of the ureter and pelvis of the kidney.

ureteropyeloneostomy (u-re″ter-o-pi″ĕ-lo-ne-os′to-me) [*uretero-* + Gr. *pyelos* pelvis + *neos* new + *stomoun* to provide with an opening, or mouth]   surgical formation of a new passage from the pelvis of a kidney to the ureter.

ureteropyelonephritis (u-re″ter-o-pi″ĕ-lo-nĕ-fri′tis) [*uretero-* + Gr. *pyelos* pelvis + *nephros* kidney + *-itis*]   inflammation of the ureter and the pelvis of the kidney.

ureteropyelonephrostomy (u-re″ter-o-pi″ĕ-lo-nĕ-fros′to-me)   operative anastomosis of the ureter and the pelvis of the kidney.

ureteropyeloplasty (u-re″ter-o-pi′ĕ-lo-plas″te)   any plastic operation on the ureter and renal pelvis.

ureteropyelostomy (u-re″ter-o-pi″ĕ-los′to-me)   ureteropyeloneostomy.

ureteropyosis (u-re″ter-o-pi-o′sis) [*uretero-* + Gr. *pyon* pus + *-osis*]   suppurative inflammation of the ureter.

ureterorectal (u-re″ter-o-rek′tal)   pertaining to or communicating with a ureter and the rectum, as a ureterorectal fistula.

ureterorectoneostomy (u-re″ter-o-rek″to-ne-os′to-me)   ureteroproctostomy.

ureterorectostomy (u-re″ter-o-rek-tos′to-me)   ureteroproctostomy.

ureterorenoscope (u-re″ter-o-re′no-skōp)   a fiberoptic endoscope used in uterorenoscopy.

ureterorenoscopy (u-re″ter-o-re-nos′ko-pe)   visual inspection of the interior of the ureter and kidney by means of a fiberoptic endoscope for such purposes as biopsy, removal or crushing of stones, etc.

ureterorrhagia (u-re″ter-o-ra′je-ah) [*uretero-* + Gr. *rhēgnynai* to burst forth]   a discharge of blood from the ureter.

ureterorrhaphy (u″re-ter-or′ah-fe) [*uretero-* + Gr. *rhaphē* suture]   suture of a ureter.

ureterosigmoidostomy (u-re″ter-o-sig″moi-dos′to-me)   the operation of implanting the ureter into the sigmoid colon.

ureterostegnosis (u-re″ter-o-steg-no′sis) [*uretero-* + Gr. *stegnōsis* contraction]   ureterostenosis.

ureterostenoma (u-re″ter-o-stĕ-no′mah) [*uretero-* + Gr. *stenōma* stricture]   ureterostenosis.

ureterostenosis (u-re″ter-o-stĕ-no′sis) [*uretero-* + Gr. *stenōsis* narrowing]   stricture of the ureter.

ureterostoma (u″re-ter-os′to-mah) [*uretero-* + Gr. *stoma* mouth]   1. the vesical orifice of the ureter (ostium ureteris [NA]). 2. a ureteral fistula.

ureterostomy (u″re-ter-os′to-me) [*uretero-* + Gr. *stomoun* to provide with an opening, or mouth]   surgical formation of a fistula through which a ureter may discharge its contents. **cutaneous u.,** the operation of bringing the ureter to the skin through an incision in the iliac region; ureterocutaneostomy.

ureterotomy (u″re-ter-ot′o-me) [*uretero-* + Gr. *tomē* a cutting]   surgical incision of a ureter.

ureterotrigonoenterostomy (u-re″ter-o-tri-go″no-en″ter-os′to-me)   implantation into the intestine of the ureter with the part of the bladder wall surrounding its termination.

ureterotrigonosigmoidostomy (u-re″ter-o-tri-go″no-sig″moi-dos′to-me)   implantation of the ureter with the part of the bladder wall into the sigmoid colon.

ureteroureteral (u-re″ter-o-u-re′ter-al)   connecting two parts of the ureter.

ureteroureterostomy (u-re″ter-o-u-re″ter-os′to-me)   end-to-end anastomosis of the two portions of a transected ureter; see also *transureteroureterostomy.*

ureterouterine (u-re″ter-o-u′ter-in)   pertaining to or communicating with a ureter and the uterus.

ureterovaginal (u-re″ter-o-vaj′ĭ-nal)   pertaining to or communicating with a ureter and the vagina.

ureterovesical (u-re″ter-o-ves′ĭ-kal)   pertaining to a ureter and the bladder.

ureterovesicoplasty (u-re″ter-o-ves′ĭ-ko-plas′te)   plastic repair of the ureterovesical junction for correction of ureterovesical reflux or obstruction.

ureterovesicostomy (u-re″ter-o-ves″ĭ-kos′to-me)   the operation of reimplanting the ureter at a different site in the bladder wall.

urethan (u′rĕ-than) [NF]   chemical name: carbamic acid ethyl ester. An antineoplastic, $C_3H_7NO_2$, occurring as white crystals or white, granular powder; it has been used in the treatment of myeloid and lymphatic leukemia and plasma cell myeloma, but has been replaced largely by superior drugs.

urethane (u′rĕ-thān)   urethan.

urethra (u-re′thrah) [Gr. *ourēthra*]   the membranous canal conveying urine from the bladder to the exterior of the body. See Plate accompanying *urogenital system,* under *system.* **anterior u.,** the portion of the male urethra extending from the bulb to the meatus on the summit of the glans penis, tunneling the corpus spongiosum; it consists of three parts, the bulbous, the pendulous, and the most distal, glandular part. **double u.,** congenital complete or partial reduplication of the urethra; the urethral openings may be side by side or one above the other. **female u., u. femini′na** [NA], a canal, about 3.7 cm. long, extending from the neck of the bladder, running above the anterior vaginal wall and piercing the urogenital diaphragm, to reach the urinary meatus; called also *u. muliebris.* **male u., u. mas-culi′na** [NA], a canal extending from the neck of the bladder to the urinary meatus, measuring about 20 cm. in length, and presenting a double curve when the penis is flaccid; it is divided into a *pars prostatica, pars membranacea,* and *pars spongiosa.* Called also *u. virilis.* **u. mulie′bris,** u. femin-ina. **posterior u.,** the portion of the male urethra, extending from the bladder to the bulb, and consisting of the membranous and prostatic parts. **u. viri′lis,** u. mascu-lina.

urethral (u-re′thral)   pertaining to the urethra.

urethralgia (u″rĕ-thral′je-ah)   pain in the urethra.

urethrascope (u-re′thrah-skōp)   urethroscope.

urethratresia (u-re″thrah-tre′ze-ah)   imperforation of the urethra.

urethrectomy (u″rĕ-threk′to-me) [*urethra* + Gr. *ektomē* excision]   the surgical removal of the urethra or a part of it.

urethremphraxis (u″rĕ-threm-frak′sis) [*urethra* + Gr. *emphraxis* stoppage]   obstruction of the urethra.

urethreurynter (u-rēth″roo-rin′ter) [*urethra* + Gr. *eurynein* to make wide]   an instrument for dilating the urethra.

urethrism (u′rĕ-thrizm) [L. *urethrismus*]   irritability or chronic spasm of the urethra.

urethritis (u″rĕ-thri′tis)   inflammation of the urethra. **u. cys′tica,** inflammation of the urethra, with the formation of multiple submucosal cysts. **u. glandula′ris,** inflammation of the urethra, with conversion of transitional mucosal lining to cylindrical epithelium, with formation of glandular acini. **gonococcal u., gonorrheal u.,** gonorrhea in the male. **gouty u.,** urethritis due to gout. **u. granulo′sa,** urethritis in which the anterior urethra is filled with granulations. **nongonococcal u., nonspecific u.,** urethritis without evidence of gonococcal infection, as, for example, that caused by *Chlamydia trachomatis;* called also *simple u.* **u. orifi′cii exter′ni,** inflammation and ulceration of the external urethral meatus. **u. petrif′icans,** urethritis with the formation of calcareous matter in the urethral wall. **prophylactic u.,** a mild urethritis that sometimes follows irrigations used to prevent venereal infections. **simple u.,** nongonococcal u. **specific u.,** that due to infection with the gonococcus. **u. vene′rea,** gonorrhea.

urethr(o)- [*urethra,* q.v.] a combining form denoting relationship to the urethra.

urethroblennorrhea (u-re″thro-blen″o-re′ah) a purulent discharge from the urethra.

urethrobulbar (u-re″thro-bul′bar) pertaining to the urethra and the bulbus penis.

urethrocele (u-re′thro-sēl) [*urethro-* + Gr. *kēlē* tumor] 1. prolapse of the female urethra through the meatus urinarius. 2. a diverticulum of the urethral walls encroaching upon the vaginal canal.

urethrocystitis (u-re″thro-sis-ti′tis) inflammation of the urethra and bladder.

urethrocystogram (u-re″thro-sis′to-gram) a roentgenogram of the urethra and bladder.

urethrocystography (u-re″thro-sis-tog′rah-fe) [*urethro-* + Gr. *kystis* bladder + *graphein* to write] roentgenography of the urethra and bladder after the injection of a contrast medium.

urethrocystopexy (u-re″thro-sis′to-pek″se) [*urethro-* + Gr. *kystis* bladder + *pēxis* fixation] surgical fixation of the urethrovesical junction, and the area of the bladder just above it, to the back of the pubic bones, for relief of stress incontinence.

urethrodynia (u-re″thro-din′e-ah) [*urethro-* + Gr. *odynē* pain] pain in the urethra; urethralgia.

urethrograph (u-re′thro-graf) an instrument for recording graphically the caliber of the urethra.

urethrography (u″rě-throg′rah-fe) roentgenography of the urethra after the injection of an opaque medium.

urethrometer (u″rě-throm′ě-ter) [*urethro-* + Gr. *metron* measure] an instrument for measuring the urethra.

urethrometry (u″rě-throm′ě-tre) 1. determination of the resistance of various segments of the urethra to retrograde flow of fluid. 2. measurement of the urethra.

urethropenile (u-re″thro-pe′nīl) pertaining to the urethra and the penis.

urethroperineal (u-re″thro-per″ĭ-ne′al) pertaining to or communicating with the urethra and the perineum.

urethroperineoscrotal (u-re″thro-per-in″e-o-skro′tal) pertaining to the urethra, perineum, and scrotum.

urethropexy (u-re′thro-pek″se) [*urethro-* + Gr. *pēxis* fixation] surgical fixation of the urethra to the overlying symphysis pubis and fascia of the rectus abdominis muscle, in correction of stress incontinence in the female.

urethrophraxis (u-re″thro-frak′sis) [*urethro-* + Gr. *phrassein* to stop up] obstruction of the urethra.

urethrophyma (u-re″thro-fi′mah) [*urethro-* + Gr. *phyma* growth] a tumor or growth in the urethra.

urethroplasty (u-re′thro-plas″te) [*urethro-* + Gr. *plassein* to form] plastic surgery of the urethra.

urethroprostatic (u-re″thro-pros-tat′ik) pertaining to the urethra and the prostate.

urethrorectal (u-re″thro-rek′tal) pertaining to or communicating with the urethra and the rectum.

urethrorrhagia (u-re″thro-ra′je-ah) [*urethro-* + Gr. *rhēgnynai* to burst forth] a flow of blood from the urethra.

urethrorrhaphy (u″rě-thror′ah-fe) [*urethro-* + Gr. *rhaphē* seam] suture of the urethra.

urethrorrhea (u-re″thro-re′ah) [*urethro-* + Gr. *rhoia* flow] an abnormal discharge from the urethra.

urethroscope (u-re′thro-skōp) [*urethro-* + Gr. *skopein* to examine] an instrument for viewing the interior of the urethra.

urethroscopic (u-re″thro-skop′ik) pertaining to the urethroscope or urethroscopy.

urethroscopy (u″rě-thros′ko-pe) [*urethro-* + Gr. *skopein* to examine] visual inspection of the interior of the urethra.

urethroscrotal (u-re″thro-skro′tal) pertaining to or communicating with the urethra and scrotum, as a urethroscrotal fistula.

urethrospasm (u-re′thro-spazm) [*urethro-* + Gr. *spasmos* spasm] spasm of the muscular tissue of the urethra.

urethrostaxis (u-re″thro-stak′sis) [*urethro-* + Gr. *staxis* dropping] oozing of blood from the urethra.

urethrostenosis (u-re″thro-stě-no′sis) [*urethro-* + Gr. *stenōsis* stricture] stricture or stenosis of the urethra.

urethrostomy (u″rě-thros′to-me) [*urethro-* + Gr. *stomoun* to provide with an opening, or mouth] surgical formation of a permanent opening of the urethra at the perineal surface.

urethrotome (u-re′thro-tōm) an instrument for cutting a urethral stricture. **Maisonneuve′s u.,** a urethrotome in which the knife is concealed until it reaches the stricture.

urethrotomy (u″rě-throt′o-me) [*urethro-* + Gr. *tomē* a cutting] incision of the urethra for relief of stricture. **external u.,** incision of the urethra through the perineum. **internal u.,** incision of the urethra from within, either blindly or with an instrument that permits direct visualization.

urethrotrigonitis (u-re″thro-tri″go-ni′tis) inflammation of the urethra and trigone of the bladder.

urethrovaginal (u-re″thro-vaj′ĭ-nal) pertaining to or communicating with the urethra and the vagina.

urethrovesical (u-re″thro-ves′ĭ-kal) pertaining to or communicating with the urethra and the bladder.

uretic (u-ret′ik) [L. *ureticus;* Gr. *ourētikos*] 1. pertaining to the urine. 2. diuretic.

Urex (u′reks) trademark for a preparation of methenamine hippurate.

urgency (ur′jen-se) the sudden compelling urge to urinate.

Urginea (ur-jin′e-ah) [L.] a genus of liliaceous plants. *U. marit′ima* (L.) Baker, the Mediterranean or white variety, and *U. indica* Kunth., the Indian variety, afford squill (q.v.).

urhidrosis (ur″hid-ro′sis) [*ur-* + Gr. *hidrōs* sweat] the presence in the sweat of urinous materials, such as uric acid, urea, etc. Called also *uridrosis.* **u. crystal′lina,** a form in which crystals of uric acid are deposited upon the skin. Called also *urea frost.*

-uria [Gr. *ouron* urine + *-ia* state] a word termination denoting a characteristic or constituent of the urine, indicated by the stem to which it is affixed, as oliguria, proteinuria.

urian (u′re-an) urochrome.

uric (u′rik) [Gr. *ourikos*] of or pertaining to the urine; see also under *acid.*

uric acid (ūr′ik) 2,6,8-trioxopurine, the end-product of purine catabolism in primates. Urate is very insoluble in water and disorders of purine metabolism produce gout, deposition of sodium urate crystals (tophi) in the joints and skin followed by a foreign-body inflammatory response. Called also *lithic acid.*

uricacidemia (u″rik-as″ĭ-de′me-ah) hyperuricemia.

uricaciduria (u″rik-as″ĭ-du′re-ah) hyperuricuria.

uricase (u′rĭ-kās) urate oxidase.

uricemia (u″rĭ-se′me-ah) uricacidemia.

uric(o)- [Gr. *ouron* urine] of or pertaining to the urine or to uric acid.

uricocholia (u″rĭ-ko-ko′le-ah) [*uric* acid + Gr. *cholē* bile] the presence of uric acid in the bile.

uricolysis (u″rĭ-kol′ĭ-sis) [*uric* acid + Gr. *lysis* dissolution] the cleavage of uric acid or of urates.

uricolytic (u″rĭ-ko-lit′ik) pertaining to, characterized by, or promoting uricolysis.

uricometer (u″rĭ-kom′ě-ter) [*uric* acid + Gr. *metron* measure] an instrument for measuring the amount of uric acid in the urine. **Ruhemann′s u.,** one based on the principle that uric acid will absorb iodine.

uricopoiesis (u″rĭ-ko-poi-e′sis) the formation of uric acid.

uricosuria (u″rĭ-ko-su′re-ah) the excretion of uric acid in the urine.

uricosuric (u″rĭ-ko-su′rik) 1. pertaining to, characterized by, or promoting uricosuria. 2. an agent that promotes uricosuria.

uricotelic (u″rĭ-ko-tel′ik) [*uric* acid + Gr. *telikos* belonging to the completion, or end] having uric acid as the chief excretory product of nitrogen metabolism, as in reptiles and birds.

uricotelism (u″rĭ-ko-te′lizm) the excretion of uric acid as the end product of nitrogen metabolism, as in reptiles and birds.

Uricult (u′rĭ-kult) trademark for a bacterial culture device, consisting of a glass slide in a sterile plastic container. On one face of the slide a 13 sq. cm. area is coated with MacConkey's medium, on the other a similar area is coated with nutrient agar. The slide is dipped into freshly voided urine, removed, and replaced in the container, where growth takes place.

uridine (u′rĭ-dēn, u′rĭ-din) a nucleoside (pentoside) from nucleic acid, uracil β-D-ribofuranoside, on hydrolysis it yields uracil and ribose. Symbol U. **u. diphosphate (UDP),** a nucleotide, uridine 5′-pyrophosphate, which serves as a carrier for hexoses, hexosamines, and hexuronic acids in the synthesis of glycogen, glycoproteins, and glycosaminoglycans. UDP-glucose and UDP-N-acetylglucosamine are formed by transfer of a uridylyl (UMP) group from UTP to glucose 1-phosphate or N-acetylglucosamine 1-phosphate. UDP-galactose, UDP-glucuronic acid, UDP-xylose, UDP-iduronic acid, and UDP-N-acetylgalactosamine are then produced by epimerization or oxidation. **u. diphosphoglucuronate,** a nucleotide formed by the oxidation of UDPglucose; it serves in the synthesis of mucopolysaccharides. Abbreviated UDPglucuronate. **u. monophosphate (UMP),** a nucleotide, uridine 5′-phosphate. Called also *uridylic acid.* **u. triphosphate (UTP),** a nucleotide, uridine 5′-triphosphate, required for RNA synthesis and as a source of UDPhexoses involved in glycogen and glycoprotein metabolism.

uridine diphosphogalactose-4-epimerase (u′rĭ-dēn di-fos″fo-gal-ak′tōs ĕ-pim′er-ās) UDPglucose 4-epimerase.

uridrosis (u″rĭ-dro′sis) urhidrosis.

uridylate (ur″ĭ-dil′āt) a dissociated form of uridylic acid.

uridylic acid (ur″ĭ-dil′ik) uridine monophosphate.

uridyl transferase (u′rĭ-dil trans′fer-ās) UDPglucose-hexose-1-phosphate uridylyltransferase.

uridylyl (ur″ĭ-dil′il) the radical formed by removal of OH from the phosphate group of uridine monophosphate.

uriesthesis (u″re-es′the-sis) uresiesthesis.

urina (u-ri′nah) [L.] urine. **u. chy′li, u. ci′bi** ["urine of food"], the urine secreted after a full meal. **u. cruen′ta,** bloody urine; see *hematuria.* **u. galacto′des,** milky urine. **u. jumento′sa,** cloudy urine. **u. po′tus** ["urine of drink"], urine secreted after copious drinking. **u. san′guinis** ["urine of the blood"], urine passed after a night's rest, and so not influenced by food or drink.

urinable (u′rin-ah-b'l) capable of being excreted in the urine.

urinaccelerator (u″rin-ak-sel′er-a″tor) musculus bulbospongiosus.

urinacidometer (u″rin-as″ĭ-dom′ĕ-ter) an instrument for estimating the pH of urine.

urinaemia (u″rĭ-ne′me-ah) uremia.

urinal (u′rĭ-nal) [L. *urinalis* urinary] a vessel or other receptacle for urine.

urinalysis (u″rĭ-nal′ĭ-sis) physical, chemical, or microscopic analysis or examination of urine.

urinary (u′rĭ-ner″e) pertaining to the urine; containing or secreting urine.

urinate (u′rĭ-nāt) to void or discharge urine.

urination (u″rĭ-na′shun) the discharge or passage of urine. **precipitant u.,** a sudden and strong desire to urinate. **stuttering u.,** an intermittent flow of urine, due to vesical spasm.

urinative (u′rĭ-na″tiv) diuretic.

urine (u′rin) [L. *urina;* Gr. *ouron*] the fluid excreted by the kidneys, passed through the ureters, stored in the bladder, and discharged through the urethra. Urine, in health, has an amber color, a slight acid reaction, a peculiar odor, and a bitter, saline taste. The average quantity excreted under ordinary dietary conditions in twenty-four hours is about 1000 to 2000 ml. Specific gravity, about 1.024, varying from 1.005 to 1.030. One thousand parts of healthy urine contain about 960 parts of water and 40 parts of solutes, which consist chiefly of urea, 23 parts; sodium chloride, 11 parts; phosphoric acid, 2.3 parts; sulfuric acid, 1.3 parts; uric acid, 0.5 part; also hippuric acid, leukomaines, urobilin, and certain organic salts. The abnormal matters found in the urine in various conditions include ketone bodies, proteins, proteoses, bile, blood, cystine, glucose, hemoglobin, fat, pus, spermatozoa, epithelial cells, mucous casts, and crystals of sulfanilamide derivatives (crystalluria). **Bence Jones u.,** see *Bence Jones protein,* under *protein.* **black u.,** urine colored black by melanin (melanuria), or by derivatives of homogentisic acid (ochronosis). **chylous u.,** urine of a milky color from the presence of chyle or fat; chyluria. **cloudy u.,** urine having a cloudy appearance, usually due to phosphaturia or uraturia, but may be caused by pyuria; called also *nebulous u.* and *urina jumentosa.* **crude u.,** light-colored, watery urine, which deposits little sediment. **diabetic u.,** that which contains an excess of glucose. **dyspeptic u.,** the urine in dyspepsia, frequently containing calcium oxalate crystals. **febrile u.,** strong, odorous, high-colored, concentrated urine, such as is secreted in fever. **gouty u.,** scanty, high-colored urine containing large quantities of urates. **milky u.,** urine having a milky appearance, which may be due to chyluria or pyuria; called also *urina galactodes.* **nebulous u.,** cloudy u. **residual u.,** the urine that remains in the bladder after urination in disease of the bladder and hypertrophy of the prostate.

urinemia (u″rĭ-ne′me-ah) [urine + Gr. *haima* blood + -ia] uremia.

urine-mucoid (u″rin-mu′koid) a mucinlike substance found in the urine.

urinidrosis (u″rin-ĭ-dro′sis) urhidrosis.

uriniferous (u″rĭ-nif′er-us) [urine + L. *ferre* to bear] transporting or conveying the urine.

urinific (u″rĭ-nif′ik) uriniparous.

uriniparous (u″rĭ-nip′ah-rus) [urine + L. *parere* to produce] producing or elaborating urine.

urin(o)- [L. *urina,* q.v.] a combining form denoting relationship to urine; see also *ur(o)-.*

urinocryoscopy (u-ri″no-kri-os′ko-pe) cryoscopy of the urine.

urinogenital (u″rĭ-no-jen′ĭ-tal) genitourinary; urogenital.

urinogenous (u″rĭ-noj′ĕ-nus) of urinary origin.

urinoglucosometer (u″rĭ-no-gloo″ko-som′ĕ-ter) an instrument for measuring the glucose in the urine.

urinologist (u″rĭ-nol′o-jist) urologist.

urinology (u″rĭ-nol′o-je) urology.

urinoma (u″rĭ-no′mah) a cyst containing urine.

urinometer (u″rĭ-nom′ĕ-ter) [urino- + Gr. *metron* measure] an instrument for determining the specific gravity of the urine.

urinometry (u″rĭ-nom′ĕ-tre) the ascertainment of the specific gravity of the urine.

urinophilous (u″rĭ-nof′ĭ-lus) [urino- + Gr. *philein* to love] having an affinity for urine, as a microorganism that grows best in urine.

urinoscopy (u″rĭ-nos′ko-pe) uroscopy.

urinosexual (u″rĭ-no-seks′u-al) genitourinary; urogenital.

urinous (u′rĭ-nus) pertaining to the urine; containing elements commonly excreted in the urine.

uriposia (u″rĭ-po′ze-ah) [urine + Gr. *posis* drinking + -ia] the drinking of urine.

urishiol (u-rish′e-ol) an extremely allergenically active mixture of catechol derivatives forming the major constituent of the irritant resin of poison ivy and other members of Anacardiaceae.

Urispas (u′rĭ-spaz) trademark for a preparation of flavoxate hydrochloride.

Uritone (u′rĭ-tōn) trademark for preparations of methenamine.

uro-, uron(o)- [Gr. *ouron* urine] combining forms denoting relationship to urine, the urinary tract, or urination.

uroacidimeter (u″ro-as″ĭ-dim′ĕ-ter) an instrument for measuring the acidity of the urine.

uroammoniac (u″ro-ah-mo′ne-ak) containing uric acid and ammonia.

uroanthelone (u″ro-an′thĕ-lōn) urogastrone.

uroazotometer (u″ro-az″o-tom′ĕ-ter) an apparatus for measuring the nitrogenous matter of the urine.

urobenzoic acid (ūr-o-ben-zo′ik) hippuric a.

urobilin (u″ro-bi′lin) [uro- + L. *bilis* bile] an amorphous, brownish pigment, $C_{35}H_{44}O_8N_4$, an oxidized form of urobilinogen, found in the feces and sometimes in urine left standing in the air.

urobilinemia (u″ro-bil″ĭ-ne′me-ah) [*urobilin* + Gr. *haima* blood + *-ia*] the presence of urobilin in the blood.

urobilinogen (u″ro-bi-lin′o-jen) [*urobilin* + Gr. *gennan* to produce] a colorless compound formed in the intestines by the reduction of bilirubin. Some is excreted in the feces, where by oxidation it becomes urobilin; some is reabsorbed, and re-excreted in the bile as bilirubin, or at times in the urine, where it may be later oxidized to urobilin.

urobilinogenemia (u″ro-bi-lin″o-jĕ-ne′me-ah) the presence of urobilinogen in the blood.

urobilinogenuria (u″ro-bi-lin″o-jĕ-nu′re-ah) the presence of urobilinogen in the urine.

urobilinoid (u″ro-bil′ĭ-noid) resembling urobilin.

urobilinoiden (u″ro-bil′ĭ-noi′din) a reduction product of hematin, resembling urobilin, sometimes found in the urine.

urobilinuria (u″ro-bil″ĭ-nu′re-ah) [*urobilin* + Gr. *ouron* urine + *-ia*] the presence of an excess of urobilin in the urine, as in cirrhosis of the liver.

urocanase (u″ro-kan′ās) urocanate hydratase.

urocanate (u″ro-kan′āt) 4-imidazoleacrylic acid, produced by the deamination of histidine.

urocanate hydratase (u′ro-kan′āt hi′drah-tās) [EC 4.2.1.49] an enzyme of the lyase class that catalyzes the reaction urocanate + O_2 = 4-imidazolone-5-propionate in the catabolism of histidine. Called also *urocanase*.

urocanic acid (ūr″o-kan′ik) a product of the direct deamination of histidine, one of the pathways of histidine catabolism.

urocele (u′ro-sēl) [*uro-* + Gr. *kēlē* hernia] distention of the scrotum with extravasated urine.

urocheras (u-rok′er-as) [*uro-* + Gr. *cheras* gravel] uropsammus.

urochezia (u″ro-ke′ze-ah) [*uro-* + Gr. *chezein* to defecate + *-ia*] the discharge of urine in the feces.

Urochordata (u″ro-kor′da-tah) [Gr. *oura* tail + L. *chorda* string] a subphylum of chordates intermediate between the invertebrates and true vertebrates, including the sea squirts and their allies, the members of which have a saclike body and a leathery tunic; the notochord is present only during the larval stage. Called also *Tunicata*.

urochordate (u-ro-kor′dāt) any member of the Urochordata; a tunicate.

urochrome (u′ro-krōm) [*uro-* + Gr. *chrōma* color] a yellow, amorphous pigment of the urine, which gives the urine its yellow color.

urochromogen (u″ro-kro′mo-gen) a low oxidation product found in the urine, which on further oxidation becomes urochrome.

urocinetic (u″ro-si-net′ik) urokinetic.

uroclepsia (u″ro-klep′se-ah) [*uro-* + Gr. *kleptein* to steal] the unconscious escape of urine.

urocoproporphyria (u″ro-kop″ro-por-fir′e-ah) porphyria cutanea tarda symptomatica.

urocrisia (u″ro-kriz′e-ah) [*uro-* + Gr. *krinein* to judge] diagnosis by observing or examining the urine.

urocriterion (u″ro-kri-te′re-on) [*uro-* + Gr. *kritērion* test] an indication of disease observed in examination of the urine.

urocyanin (u-ro-si′ah-nin) [*uro-* + Gr. *kyanos* blue] uroglaucin.

urocyanogen (u″ro-si-an′o-jen) [*uro-* + Gr. *kyanos* blue + *gennan* to produce] a blue pigment of the urine, especially of that of cholera patients.

urocyanosis (u″ro-si″ah-no′sis) [*uro-* + Gr. *kyanos* blue] indicanuria.

urocyst (u′ro-sist) [*uro-* + Gr. *kystis* bladder] the urinary bladder (vesica urinaria [NA]).

urocystic (u″ro-sis′tik) pertaining to the urinary bladder.

Urocystis (u″ro-sis′tis) a genus of basidiomycetous fungi of the order Ustilaginales, family Tilletiaceae. **U. trit′ici,** a fungus which causes flag smut of wheat in Australia, China, and southern Asia.

urocystis (u″ro-sis′tis) [L.] the urinary bladder.

urocystitis (u″ro-sis-ti′tis) inflammation of the urinary bladder.

urodeum (u″ro-de′um) [*uro-* + Gr. *hodaios* on the way] the portion of the cloaca into which the ureters and genital ducts empty.

urodialysis (u″ro-di-al′ĭ-sis) [*uro-* + Gr. *dialysis* cessation] partial or complete suppression of the urine.

urodochium (u″ro-do′ke-um, u″ro-do-ki′um) [*uro-* + Gr. *docheion* holder] a urinal.

urodynamic (u″ro-di-nam′ik) pertaining to the flow and motion of liquids in the urinary tract.

urodynamics (u″ro-di-nam′iks) the dynamics of the propulsion and flow of urine in the urinary tract.

urodynia (u″ro-din′e-ah) [*uro-* + Gr. *odynē* pain + *-ia*] pain accompanying urination.

uroedema (u″ro-ĕ-de′mah″) edema due to infiltration of urine.

uroenterone (u″ro-en′ter-ōn) urogastrone.

uroerythrin (u″ro-er′ĭ-thrin) [*uro-* + Gr. *erythros* red] a dark reddish coloring matter found in the urine; it gives the red color seen in deposits of urates. Called also *purpurin*.

uroflavin (u″ro-fla′vin) a fluorescent compound closely related to riboflavin, excreted in the urine.

uroflometer, uroflowmeter (u″ro-flo′me-ter) a device for the continuous recording of urine flow in milliliters per second, consisting of a cylinder placed on a transducer that weighs the urine entering the cylinder and records it on a time scale.

urofuscin (u″ro-fus′in) [*uro-* + L. *fuscus* tawny] a pigment of the urine which is the precursor of hematoporphyrin.

urofuscohematin (u″ro-fus″ko-hem′ah-tin) a red-brown pigment in the urine in certain diseases.

urogaster (u″ro-gas′ter) [*uro-* + Gr. *gastēr* stomach] the urinary intestine; a part of the allantoic cavity of the embryo.

urogastrone (u″ro-gas′trōn) a polypeptide secreted by the salivary glands and by Brunner's glands, which is a potent inhibitor of gastric acid secretion; it is obtainable from the normal and pregnancy urine of man and other mammals; called also *anthelone U.*

urogenital (u″ro-jen′ĭ-tal) pertaining to the urinary and genital apparatus; genitourinary. See under *system*.

urogenous (u-roj′ĕ-nus) [*uro-* + Gr. *gennan* to produce] producing urine; also produced from or in the urine.

uroglaucin (u″ro-glaw′sin) [*uro-* + Gr. *glaukos* green] indigo blue occurring in the urine; it is due to oxidation of a colorless chromogen in the urine, and is seen in conditions such as scarlet fever.

urogram (u′ro-gram) a roentgenogram of part of the urinary tract.

urography (u-rog′rah-fe) roentgenography of a part of the urinary tract which has been rendered opaque by some opaque medium. **ascending u.,** retrograde u. **cystoscopic u.,** retrograde u. **descending u., excretion u., excretory u., intravenous u.,** roentgen examination of the urinary tract after the intravenous injection of an opaque medium that is rapidly excreted in the urine. **oral u.,** urography in which the opaque medium is given by the mouth. **retrograde u.,** urography in which the contrast medium is injected into the bladder through the urethra.

urogravimeter (u″ro-grah-vim′ĕ-ter) [*uro-* + L. *gravis* heavy + *metrum* measure] urinometer.

urohematin (u″ro-hem′ah-tin) the coloring matter or pigments of the urine; regarded as identical with heme.

urohematonephrosis (u″ro-hem″ah-to-ne-fro′sis) distention of the kidney with urine and blood.

urohematoporphyrin (u″ro-hem″ah-to-por′fĭ-rin) hematoporphyrin derived from the urine.

urohypertensin (u″ro-hi-per-ten′sin) a mixture of bases obtained from the urine which acts as a pressor substance.

urokinase (u″ro-ki′nās) [EC 3.4.21.31] an enzyme of the hydrolase class that catalyzes the conversion of plasminogen to plasmin by preferential cleavage at an arginine-valine bond; it is produced in the kidney and excreted in the urine. Called also *plasminogen activator*.

urokinetic (u″ro-ki-net′ik) [*uro-* + Gr. *kinēsis* movement] caused by a reflex from the urinary organs; said of a form of dyspepsia.

urokymography (u″ro-ki-mog′rah-fe)   kymography applied to study of the urogenital system.

urolagnia (u″ro-lag′ne-ah) [*uro-* + Gr. *lagneia* lust]   a form of paraphilia in which sexual excitement is associated with the sight or thought of urine or urination.

urolith (u′ro-lith) [*uro-* + Gr. *lithos* stone]   a urinary calculus or stone.

urolithiasis (u″ro-lĭ-thi′ah-sis)   1. the formation of urinary calculi. 2. the diseased condition associated with the presence of urinary calculi.

urolithic (u″ro-lith′ik)   pertaining to urinary calculi.

urolithology (u″ro-lĭ-thol′o-je)   the sum of knowledge regarding urinary calculi.

urologic, urological (u″ro-loj′ik; u″ro-loj′ĭ-kal)   pertaining to urology.

urologist (u-rol′o-jist)   a physician who specializes in urology.

urology (u-rol′o-je)   that branch of medicine which concerns itself with the urinary tract in both male and female, and with the genital organs in the male.

urolutein (u″ro-lu′te-in) [*uro-* + L. *luteus* yellow]   a yellow pigment of the urine.

uromancy (u′ro-man″se) [*uro-* + Gr. *manteia* a divination]   prognosis based on examination of urine.

uromantia (u″ro-man′she-ah)   uromancy.

uromelanin (u″ro-mel′ah-nin) [*uro-* + Gr. *melas* black]   a black pigment, $C_{18}H_{43}N_7O_{10}$, sometimes found in urine; it results from the decomposition of urochrome.

uromelus (u-rom′e-lus) [Gr. *oura* tail + *melos* limb]   a monster with fused legs and a single foot.

urometer (u-rom′ě-ter) [*uro-* + Gr. *metron* measure]   urinometer.

urometric (u″ro-met′rik)   pertaining to urometry.

urometry (u-rom′e-tre)   the measurement and recording of pressure changes caused by contraction of the ureter during ureteral peristalsis.

uromucoid (u″ro-mu′koid)   an insoluble mucoprotein found in urine.

uronate (u′ro-nāt)   a sugar in which the terminal alcohol group is oxidized to a carboxylate group.

uroncus (u-rong′kus) [*uro-* + Gr. *onkos* mass]   a swelling containing urine.

uronephrosis (u″ro-ně-fro′sis)   abnormal distention of the pelvis and tubules of the kidney with urine.

uronic acid (ūr-on′ik)   a sugar acid produced by oxidation of the terminal -CH$_2$OH group in a sugar farthest from the carbonyl group to a carboxyl (=COOH) group, e.g., glucuronic acid.

uron(o)-   see *ur(o)-*.

uronology (u″ro-nol′o-je)   urology.

urononcometry (u″ron-on-kom′ě-tre) [*urono-* + Gr. *onkos* mass + *metron* measure]   the measurement of the quantity of urine excreted in twenty-four hours.

uronoscopy (u″ro-nos′ko-pe)   examination of the urine.

uropathogen (u″ro-path′o-jen)   a microorganism which causes diseases of the urinary tract.

uropathy (u-rop′ah-the) [*uro-* + Gr. *pathos* disease]   any pathologic change in the urinary tract. **obstructive u.,** any pathologic change in the urinary tract due to obstruction.

uropenia (u″ro-pe′ne-ah) [*uro-* + Gr. *penia* poverty]   deficiency of urine or urinary secretion.

uropepsinogen (u″ro-pep-sin′o-jen)   pepsinogen occurring in the urine.

urophanic (u″ro-fan′ik) [*uro-* + Gr. *phainein* to show]   appearing in the urine.

urophein (u″ro-fe′in) [*uro-* + Gr. *phaios* gray]   an odoriferous gray pigment of the urine.

urophilia (u″ro-fil′e-ah) [*uro* + *philia*]   a paraphilia involving the use of urine.

urophobia (u″ro-fo′be-ah)   irrational fear of passing urine.

urophosphometer (u″ro-fos-fom′ě-ter)   an instrument for measuring the quantity of phosphorus in the urine.

uropittin (u″ro-pit′in) [*uro-* + Gr. *pitta* pitch]   a resinous product, $C_9H_{10}N_2O_3$, of the decomposition of urochrome.

uroplania (u″ro-pla′ne-ah) [*uro-* + Gr. *planē* wandering + *-ia*]   the presence of urine in, or its discharge from, organs not of the urogenital tract.

uropod (ur′o-pod) [Gr. *oura* tail + *pous* foot]   the cytoplasmic footlike process that trails behind locomoting leukocytes producing a characteristic "hand mirror" shape. The uropod serves as a point of attachment to the substrate and may also be involved in cell-cell interactions.

uropoiesis (u″ro-poi-e′sis) [*uro-* + Gr. *poiein* to make]   the production of the urine.

uropoietic (u″ro-poi-et′ik)   pertaining to or concerned in the production of the urine.

uroporphyria (u″ro-por-fir′e-ah)   porphyria in which there is excessive excretion of uroporphyrin. **erythropoietic u.,** congenital erythropoietic porphyria.

uroporphyrin (u″ro-por′fĭ-rin)   the porphyrin (q.v.) produced by oxidation of the methylene bridges in uroporphyrinogen. Excessive amounts of uroporphyrin I are excreted in congenital erythropoietic porphyria.

uroporphyrinogen (u″ro-por″fĭ-rin′o-jen)   a porphyrinogen (q.v.) in which each pyrrole ring has one acetate side chain and one propionate side chain. The type III isomer, formed by the condensation of four molecules of porphobilinogen, is an intermediate in the biosynthesis of heme.

uroporphyrinogen decarboxylase (u″ro por″fĭ-rin′o-jen, u″ro-por-frin′o-jen de-kar-bok′sĭ-lās) [EC 4.1.1.37]   an enzyme of the lyase class that catalyzes the reaction uroporphyrinogen III = coproporphyrinogen + 4 CO$_2$. Deficiency in the enzyme, an autosomal dominant trait, causes familial porphyria cutanea tarda.

uroporphyrinogen III synthase (u″ro-por″fĭ-rin′o-jen, u″ro-por-frin′o-jen sin′thās) [EC 4.2.1.75]   an enzyme of the lyase class that catalyzes the reaction hydroxymethylbilane = uroporphyrinogen III + H$_2$O. It, together with porphobilinogen deaminase, will convert porphobilinogen to uroporphyrinogen directly. Deficiency of the enzyme, an autosomal recessive trait, causes congenital erythropoietic porphyria.

uropsammus (u″ro-sam′us) [*uro-* + Gr. *psammos* sand]   sediment or gravel in the urine.

uropterin (u-rop′ter-in)   a pigment, identical with xanthopterin, isolated from human urine; see *pterin*.

uropyonephrosis (u″ro-pi″o-ně-fro′sis)   the presence of urine and pus in the pelvis of the kidney.

uropyoureter (u″ro-pi″o-u-re′ter) [*uro-* + Gr. *pyon* pus + *oureter* ureter]   a collection of urine and pus in the ureter.

uroradiology (u″ro-ra″de-ol′o-je)   radiology of the urinary tract.

urorhythmography (u″ro-rith-mog′rah-fe) [*uro-* + Gr. *rhythmos* rhythm + *graphein* to write]   graphic registration of the ejaculation of the urine from the ureteral orifices.

urorosein (u″ro-ro′ze-in)   urorrhodin.

uroroseinogen (u″ro-ro″se-in′o-jen)   urorrhodinogen.

urorrhagia (u″ro-ra′je-ah) [*uro-* + Gr. *rhēgnynai* to burst forth]   an excessive flow of urine; diabetes.

urorrhea (u″ro-re′ah) [*uro-* + Gr. *rhoia* flow]   an involuntary discharge of urine; enuresis.

urorrhodin (u″ro-ro′din) [*uro-* + Gr. *rhodon* rose]   a rose-colored pigment found in the urine in typhoid fever, nephritis, pulmonary tuberculosis, and other diseases. See under *tests*.

urorrhodinogen (u″ro-ro-din′o-jen) [*urorrhodin* + Gr. *gennan* to produce]   a chromogen in the urine which, on decomposition, yields urorrhodin.

urorubin (u″ro-roo′bin) [*uro-* + L. *ruber* red]   a red pigment derivable from the urine by the action of hydrochloric acid.

urorubinogen (u″ro-roo-bin′o-jen)   a chromogen from which urorubin is derived.

urorubrohematin (u″ro-roo″bro-hem′ah-tin) [*uro-* + L. *ruber* red + *hematin*]   a red pigment rarely found in the urine in certain constitutional diseases, as leprosy.

urosaccharometry (u″ro-sak″ah-rom′ě-tre)   the measurement or estimation of sugar in the urine.

urosacin (u-ro′sa-sin)   urorrhodin.

uroscheocele (u-ros′ke-o-sēl″) [*uro-* + Gr. *oscheon* scrotum + *kēlē* tumor]   urocele.

uroschesis (u-ros'kĕ-sis) [*uro-* + Gr. *schesis* holding] retention of the urine.

uroscopic (u"ro-skop'ik) pertaining to uroscopy.

uroscopy (u-ros'ko-pe) [*uro-* + Gr. *skopein* to examine] diagnostic examination of the urine.

urosemiology (u"ro-se"me-ol'o-je) diagnostic study of the urine.

urosepsin (u"ro-sep'sin) a septic poison arising from urine in the tissues.

urosepsis (u"ro-sep'sis) [*uro-* + Gr. *sēpsis* decay] septic poisoning from the absorption and decomposition of urinary substances in the tissues.

uroseptic (u"ro-sep'tik) pertaining to or marked by urosepsis.

urosis (u-ro'sis) any disease of the urinary apparatus.

urospectrin (u"ro-spek'trin) [*uro-* + L. *spectrum* image] one of the pigments of normal urine; a substance obtainable from certain specimens of urine, allied to hematoporphyrin.

Urosporidium (u"ro-spo-rid'e-um) [*uro-* + *spore*] a genus of parasitic protozoa (order Balanosporida, class Stellatosporea) found in the coelom of polychetes.

urostalagmometry (u"ro-stal"ag-mom'ĕ-tre) the use of the stalagmometer in the study of the urine.

urostealith (u"ro-ste'ah-lith) [*uro-* + Gr. *stear* fat + *lithos* stone] a fatty constituent of certain urinary calculi; a urinary calculus having fatty constituents.

urothelial (u"ro-the'le-al) pertaining to the urothelium.

urothelium (u"ro-the'le-um) the epithelium of the urinary bladder.

urotoxia (u"ro-tok'se-ah) [*uro-* + Gr. *toxikon* poison] 1. the toxicity of the urine. 2. the toxic substances of the urine. 3. the unit of the toxicity of the urine or a quantity sufficient to kill 1 kg. of living substance.

urotoxic (u"ro-tok'sik) pertaining to the toxic materials of the urine.

urotoxicity (u"ro-toks-is'ĭ-te) the toxic quality of the urine.

urotoxin (u"ro-tok'sin) the toxic or poisonous constituents of the urine.

urotoxy (u'ro-tok"se) urotoxia.

Urotropin (u-rot'ro-pin) trademark for a preparation of methenamine.

uroureter (u"ro-u-re'ter) distention of the ureter with urine.

uroxanthin (u"ro-zan'thin) [*uro-* + Gr. *xanthos* yellow] a yellow pigment of normal urine convertible into indigo blue.

uroxin (u-rok'sin) alloxantin.

urrhodin (u-ro'din) urorrhodin.

ursodeoxycholate (ur"so-de-ok"se-ko'lāt) the dissociated form of lithocholic acid.

ursodeoxycholic acid (ur"so-de-ok"se-ko'lik) a secondary bile acid, 3α, 7β-dihydroxy-5β-cholanic acid.

ursodeoxycholylglycine (ur"so-de-ok"se-ko"lil-gli'sēn) a bile salt, the glycine conjugate of ursodeoxycholic acid.

ursodeoxycholyltaurine (ur"so-de-ok"se-ko"lil-taw'rēn) a bile salt, the taurine conjugate of ursodeoxycholic acid.

ursone (ur'sōn) ursolic acid; a crystallizable triterpene, $C_{30}H_{48}O_3$, from waxlike coatings of fruits (e.g., apples and pears) and leaves (e.g., rhododendron and uva ursi).

Urtica (ur-ti'kah) [L.] a genus of plants, including the true or typical nettles; plants covered with stinging hairs and secreting a poisonous fluid. **U. dio'ica,** a stinging nettle of temperate regions having stimulant, diuretic, and hemostatic properties.

urtica (ur-ti'kah), pl. *urti'cae* [L., "a stinging nettle"] (*obs.*) a wheal or pomphus.

urticant (ur'tĭ-kant) causing an itching or stinging sensation, or creating a wheal, or both.

urticaria (ur"tĭ-kār'e-ah) [L. *urtica* stinging nettle + *-ia*] a vascular reaction, usually transient, involving the upper dermis, representing localized edema caused by dilatation and increased permeability of the capillaries, and marked by the development of wheals. Many different stimuli are capable of inducing an urticarial reaction, and it may be classified according to precipitating causes as: immune-mediated, complement-mediated (involving either immunologic or nonimmunologic mechanisms), urticariogenic material–induced, physical agent–induced, stress-induced, or idiopathic. The condition may also be designated acute or chronic (depending on duration of an attack); the former evolves over a period of days or several weeks, whereas the latter is continuous or persists episodically for at least 6 weeks, and generally longer. Angioedema (q.v.) is the same physiological response in the deep dermis or subcutaneous or submucosal tissues. Called also *hives*. **acute u.,** see *urticaria*. **aquagenic u.,** contact urticaria that may be due to a combination of water and sweat or sebum, regardless of the temperature, which produces urticariogenic substances, and characterized by the development of small perifollicular wheals with surrounding erythema. **u. bullo'sa, bullous u.,** that in which bullae are superimposed on the characteristic wheals. **cholinergic u.,** that characterized by the presence of distinctive punctate wheals surrounded by areas of erythema, thought to be a nonimmunologic hypersensitivity reaction in which acetylcholine released from parasympathetic or motor nerve terminals induces release of mediators from mast cells, and evoked by conditions of exertion, stress, or increased environmental heat. Cf. *heat u.* **chronic u.,** see *urticaria*. **cold u.,** urticaria precipitated by cold air, water, or objects, occurring in two forms: In the autosomal dominant form, which is associated with fever, arthralgias, and leukocytosis, the lesions present as erythematous, burning papules and macules. The more common acquired form is usually idiopathic and self-limited. **contact u.,** a localized or generalized, transient wheal-and-flare response elicited by exposure to rapidly absorbable urticariogenic agents. **giant u.,** angioedema. **heat u.,** localized or generalized urticaria produced by application of heat to the skin or by exposure to high environmental temperature, sometimes associated with cramps, weakness, flushing, salivation, and collapse, which is probably mediated by acetylcholine. Cf. *cholinergic u.* **light u.,** solar u. **u. medicamento'sa,** a drug eruption manifested by the development of wheals. **u. multifor'mis endem'ica,** harara. **papular u.,** a persistent cutaneous eruption representing a hypersensitivity reaction to insect bites (e.g., mites, fleas, bedbugs, gnats, mosquitoes, animal lice), seen primarily in atopic children, and characterized by crops of small urticarial papules and wheals and transitional forms of these lesions, which may become secondarily infected or lichenified owing to rubbing and excoriation. Called also *lichen urticatus, prurigo chronica multiformis, prurigo simplex,* and *strophulus*. **u. pigmento'sa,** the most common form of mastocytosis, occurring primarily in children, typically characterized by multiple persistent small, reddish brown, hyperpigmented, pruritic macules and papules, located most commonly on the trunk but also seen on the extremities, head, and neck, which tend to urticate upon mild mechanical trauma or chemical irritation (Darier's sign). See also *mastocytoma*. **pressure u.,** urticaria of unknown cause occurring hours after local pressure on the skin, most often seen on the feet after walking and on the buttocks after sitting, and associated with pain. **solar u., u. sola'ris,** rapidly developing urticaria occurring on brief exposure to sunlight. Called also *light u.*

urticarial (ur"tĭ-ka're-al) pertaining to, characterized by, or of the nature of urticaria. Called also *urticarious*.

urticariogenic (ur"tĭ-ka"re-o-jen'ik) causing urticaria.

urticarious (ur"tĭ-ka're-us) urticarial.

urticate (ur'tĭ-kāt) 1. marked by the presence of wheals. 2. to produce urtication.

urtication (ur"tĭ-ka'shun) [L. *urtica* a stinging nettle] 1. the development or formation of urticaria. 2. a burning sensation as of stinging with nettles.

urushiol (u-roo'she-ol) the chief constituent of the irritant oil of *Rhus radicans* L. (*Toxicodendron radicans* L.) (poison ivy), *R. diversiloba* L. (poison oak), *R. vernix* L., and related plants, consisting of a mixture of several oleoresins.

USAN (u'san) acronym for *United States Adopted Names*, a nonproprietary designation for any compound used as a drug, established by negotiation between the manufacturer of the compound and a nomenclature committee known as the USAN Council, which is sponsored jointly by the American Medical Association, the American Pharmaceutical Association, and The United States Pharmacopeial Convention. A liaison representative of the United States Food and Drug Administration sits on the USAN Council. The term is currently limited to names adopted by the Council since June, 1961. These names will appear as the monograph titles in the official compendia, U.S.P. and N.F., when and if the respective drugs are admitted to either compendium.

U.S.D.A. United States Department of Agriculture.

Usnea barbata (us′ne-ah bar-ba′tah) a large lichen growing on forest trees; also its homeopathic preparation. The active ingredients include usnic acid (usnein), $C_{18}H_{16}O_7$, which has antibacterial activity. The crude plant is used as a dressing for wounds.

usnein (us′ne-in) usnic acid.

U.S.P. the United States Pharmacopeia, a legally recognized compendium of standards for drugs, published by The United States Pharmacopeial Convention, Inc., and revised periodically. It includes also assays and tests for the determination of strength, quality, and purity.

U.S.P.H.S. United States Public Health Service.

Ustilaginales (us″tĭ-laj″ĭ-na′lēz) an order of basidiomycetous fungi of the subclass Heterobasidiomycetidae, which includes the family Tilletiaceae.

ustilaginism (us″tĭ-laj′ĭ-nizm) a condition resembling ergotism caused by eating maize containing *Ustilago maydis*.

Ustilago (us″tĭ-la′go) [L.] a genus of basidiomycetous fungi of the order Ustilaginales, family Ustilaginaceae, called smuts, parasitic on plants. **U. may′dis,** a fungus causing corn smut; the ingestion of infected seeds causes ustilaginism, a condition similar to ergotism.

ustion (us′chun) [L. *ustio*] burning with the actual cautery.

ustulation (us″tu-la′shun) [L. *ustulare* to scorch] the drying of a moist drug by heat.

ustus (us′tus) [L.] burnt; calcined.

usustatus (u-su′sta-tus) [L. *usus* use + *status* position] the ordinary erect or standing posture usual to an animal.

uta (oo′tah) a form of cutaneous leishmaniasis of the New World occurring in the Peruvian Andes, caused by *Leishmania peruviana*, which is found only at 900 to 3000 meters, probably transmitted by *Lutzomyia verrucarum* and *Lutzomyia peruensis*, and characterized by the presence of a single or a few ulcer-like, self-limited lesions.

Ut dict. abbreviation for L. *ut dic′tum*, as directed.

Utend. abbreviation for L. *uten′dus*, to be used.

uteralgia (u″ter-al′je-ah) metralgia or metrodynia.

uteri (u′ter-i) [L.] genitive and plural of *uterus*.

uterine (u′ter-ĭn) [L. *uterinus*] of or pertaining to the uterus.

uter(o)- [L. *uterus*] a combining form denoting relationship to the uterus. See also words beginning with *hyster(o)-, metra-,* and *metr(o)-.*

uteroabdominal (u″ter-o-ab-dom′ĭ-nal) pertaining to the uterus and the abdomen.

uterocervical (u″ter-o-ser′vĭ-kal) pertaining to the uterus and the cervix uteri.

uterodynia (u″ter-o-din′e-ah) metralgia or metrodynia.

uterofixation (u″ter-o-fik-sa′shun) hysteropexy.

uterogenic (u″ter-o-jen′ik) formed in the uterus.

uterogestation (u″ter-o-jes-ta′shun) [*uterus* + L. *gestatio* a carrying] 1. uterine pregnancy; any pregnancy which is not extrauterine. 2. the full period of time of normal pregnancy.

uteroglobulin (u″ter-o-glob′u-lin) blastokinin.

uterography (u″ter-og′rah-fe) hysterography.

uterolith (u′ter-o-lith″) [*uterus* + Gr. *lithos* stone] a hysterolith.

uterometer (u″ter-om′ĕ-ter) an instrument for measuring the uterus.

uterometry (u″ter-om′ĕ-tre) measurement of the uterus.

utero-ovarian (u″ter-o-o-va′re-an) pertaining to the uterus and ovary.

uteropexy (u′ter-o-pek″se) hysteropexy.

uteroplacental (u″ter-o-plah-sen′tal) pertaining to the uterus and the placenta.

uteroplasty (u′ter-o-plas″te) any plastic operation on the uterus.

uterorectal (u″ter-o-rek′tal) pertaining to the uterus and rectum, or communicating with the uterine cavity and rectum, as a uterorectal fistula.

uterosacral (u″ter-o-sa′kral) pertaining to the uterus and the sacrum.

uterosalpingography (u″ter-o-sal″ping-gog′rah-fe) hysterosalpingography.

uterosclerosis (u″ter-o-sklĕ-ro′sis) sclerosis of the uterus.

uteroscope (u′ter-o-skōp″) [*uterus* + Gr. *skopein* to examine] hysteroscope.

uterothermometry (u″ter-o-ther-mom′ĕ-tre) the measurement of the temperature in the uterus.

uterotomy (u″ter-ot′o-me) hysterotomy.

uterotonic (u″ter-o-ton′ik) 1. giving muscular tone to the uterus. 2. an agent that increases the tonus of the uterine muscle.

uterotropic (u″ter-o-trop′ik) having a special affinity for or exerting its principal influence upon the uterus.

uterotubal (u″ter-o-tu′bal) pertaining to the uterus and the oviducts.

uterotubography (u″ter-o-tu-bog′rah-fe) hysterosalpingography.

uterovaginal (u″ter-o-vaj′ĭ-nal) pertaining to the uterus and the vagina.

uteroventral (u″ter-o-ven′tral) pertaining to the uterus and the cavity of the abdomen.

uteroverdin (u″ter-o-ver′din) a term once applied to biliverdin when occurring in the placenta or in the eggs of some birds.

uterovesical (u″ter-o-ves′ĭ-kal) pertaining to the uterus and the bladder.

uterus (u′ter-us), pl. *u′teri* [L.; Gr. *hystera*] [NA] the hollow muscular organ in female mammals in which the fertilized ovum normally becomes embedded and in which the developing embryo and fetus is nourished. In the nongravid human, it is a pear-shaped structure, about 3 inches in length, consisting of a body, fundus, isthmus, and cervix. Its cavity opens into the vagina below, and into the uterine tube on either side at the cornu. It is supported by direct attachment to the vagina and by indirect attachment to various other nearby pelvic structures. Called also *metra.* **u. acol′lis,** a uterus in which the vaginal portion is absent. **u. arcua′tus,** a uterus with a depressed fundus. **u. bicamera′tus vetula′rum,** a uterus in which the cervical orifices are closed by adhesions, resulting in distention of the cervix and corpus uteri. **u. bicor′nis,** a uterus which has two horns, or cornua. **u. bicor′nis bicol′lis,** a uterus with two horns and two cervices. **u. bicor′nis unicol′lis,** a uterus with two horns and a single cervix. **u. bif′oris,** a uterus in which the external os is divided by a septum. **u. bilocula′ris,** a uterus the cavity of which is divided into two parts by a partition. **u. biparti′tus,** u. bilocularis. **cochleate u.,** a small adult uterus with a conical cervix and body which is small, globular, and acutely flexed. **u. cordifor′mis,** a heart-shaped uterus. **Couvelaire u.,** see *uteroplacental apoplexy,* under *apoplexy.* **u. didel′phys,** either of two distinct uteri occurring side by side in the same individual. **duplex u., u. du′plex,** a double uterus; normal in marsupial mammals, and rarely seen in the human subject. **fetal u.,** a uterus in which the cervical canal is longer than the cavity of the corpus. **gravid u.,** the pregnant uterus. **u. incudifor′mis,** a uterus bicornis which is broad between the two horns. **infantile u.,** pubescent u. **u. masculi′nus,** utriculus prostaticus. **u. parvicol′lis,** a uterus in which the cervical portion is very small, but the corpus is of normal size. **u. planifor′lis,** u. incudiformis. **pubescent u.,** one which is adult in type but is undeveloped; called also *infantile u.* **ribbon u.,** an aplastic uterus found as a transverse ribbon of fibromuscular tissue between the blind ends of the uterine tubes and the bladder. **u. rudimenta′rius,** a hypoplastic uterus measuring 1 to 3 cm. in length; affected women are amenorrheic and sterile. **saddle-shaped u.,** u. arcuatus. **u. sep′tus,** u. bilocularis. **u. simplex,** one that is single throughout its length, as in the human. **u. subsep′tus,** u. bicornis. **u. triangula′ris,** u. incudiformis. **u. unicor′nis,** one with only one cornu, one lateral half being undeveloped or imperfectly developed.

Utibid (u′tĭ-bid) trademark for a preparation of oxolinic acid.

Uticillin VK (u″tĭ-sil′in) trademark for a preparation of penicillin V potassium.

utilization (u″til-ĭ-za′shun)   the use or employment of something.   **red cell u. (RCU),** the fraction of iron leaving the blood plasma that is incorporated in circulating red cells; iron-59 bound to the patient's own transferrin is administered, and the RCU is calculated as: radioactivity/ml blood 10–14 days later ÷ extrapolated radioactivity/ml blood at time zero × 100 per cent.

UTP   uridine triphosphate.

UTP–glucose-1-phosphate   uridylyltransferase (gloo′kōs fos′fāt u″rĭ-dil-il-trans′fer-ās) [EC 2.7.7.9]   an enzyme of the transferase class that catalyzes the reaction UTP + α-D-glucose 1-phosphate = pyrophosphate + UDP-glucose, a reaction in the glycogen storage mechanism. Called also *UDPglucose pyrophosphorylase.*

utricle (u′tre-k'l) [L. *utriculus*]   1. any small sac.   2. the larger of the two divisions of the membranous labyrinth; see *utriculus,* def. 2.   **prostatic u., urethral u.,** utriculus prostaticus.

utricular (u-trik′u-lar)   1. pertaining to a utricle.   2. resembling a bladder.

utriculi (u-trik′u-li) [L.]   genitive and plural of *utriculus.*

utriculitis (u-trik″u-li′tis)   inflammation of the prostatic utricle or of the utricle of the ear.

utriculosaccular (u-trik″u-lo-sak′u-lar)   pertaining to the utricle and saccule of the labyrinth.

utriculus (u-trik′u-lus), pl. *utric′uli* [L., dim. of *uter*]   1. a small sac.   2. [NA] the larger of the two divisions of the membranous labyrinth, located in the posterosuperior region of the vestibule. It is the major organ of the vestibular system, which gives information about position and movements of the head. Called also *utricle* and *utriculus vestibuli.*   **u. mas-culi′nus,** u. prostaticus.   **u. prostat′icus** [NA], prostatic utricle: the remains of the lower part of the paramesonephric duct in the male; it is a small blind pouch arising in the prostatic substance and opening onto the seminal colliculus.   **u. vestib′uli,** utriculus (def. 2).

utriform (u′trĭ-form)   having the shape of a bottle.

uva (u′vah), pl. *u′vae* [L. "grape"]   the raisin; the dried fruit of *Vitis vinifera* L. (Vitaceae), grape vine.   **u. ur′si** L. (Ericaceae) [L. "bear's grapes"], the leaves of *Arctostaphylos uva-ursi,* or bearberry, a trailing ericaceous shrub; used medicinally as astringent, diuretic tea.

Uval (u′val)   trademark for preparations of sulisobenzone.

uvea (u′ve-ah)   the vascular middle coat of the eye, comprising the iris, ciliary body, and choroid (tunica vasculosa bulbi [NA]).

uveal (u′ve-al)   pertaining to the uvea.

uveitic (u″ve-it′ik)   pertaining to uveitis.

uveitis (u″ve-i′tis) [*uvea* + *-itis*]   an inflammation of part or all of the uvea, the middle (vascular) tunic of the eye, and commonly involving the other tunics (the sclera and cornea, and the retina).   **anterior u.,** uveitis involving the structures of the iris and/or ciliary body, including iritis, cyclitis, and iridocyclitis.   **Förster's u.,** syphilitic involvement of the entire uvea.   **granulomatous u.,** uveitis of any part of the uveal tract but particularly the posterior portion, characterized by nodular collections of epithelioid cells and giant cells surrounded by lymphocytes.   **heterochromic u.,** see under *iridocyclitis.*   **lens-induced u.,** three disorders—phacoantigenic uveitis, phacotoxic uveitis, and phacolytic glaucoma—of greater or lesser severity caused by autoimmune response to lens protein leaking through the capsule. The leakage may be from hypermature cataract, capsular rupture, extracapsular lens extraction, or other trauma.   **nongranulomatous u.,** inflammation of the anterior portion of the uveal tract (iris and ciliary body).   **phacoantigenic u.,** one of the lens-induced uveitides, it is a severe anterior uveitis, similar to sympathetic ophthalmia,

observed weeks or even months after extracapsular lens surgery or other trauma to the capsule. Called also *phacoanaphylactic endophthalmitis.*   **phacotoxic u.,** an extremely rare lens-induced uveitis that is a low-grade reaction to lens protein, and not a separate disease entity.   **posterior u.,** uveitis involving the posterior segment of the eye, including choroiditis and chorioretinitis.   **sympathetic u.,** see under *ophthalmia.*   **toxoplasmic u.,** chorioretinitis as a complication of toxoplasmosis.   **tuberculous u.,** granulomatous uveitis due to infection with the tubercle bacillus, usually a severe caseating granulomatous chorioretinitis.

uveomeningitis (u′ve-o-men″in-ji′tis)   a disorder characterized by lesions of the uvea accompanied by meningeal signs; see *Harada's disease* and *Vogt-Koyanagi syndrome.*

uveoparotid (u″ve-o-pah-rot′id)   affecting the uvea and the parotid gland; see under *fever.*

uveoscleritis (u″ve-o-skle-ri′tis)   scleritis resulting from an extension of the inflammation from the uvea to the sclera.

uviform (u′vĭ-form) [L. *uva* grape + *forma* form]   having the form of a grape.

uviofast (u′ve-o-fast″)   uvioresistant.

uviolize (u′ve-o-līz)   to subject to the action of ultraviolet rays.

uviometer (u″ve-om′ĕ-ter)   an instrument for measuring ultraviolet emanation.

uvioresistant (u″ve-o-re-zis′tant)   resistant to or not affected by ultraviolet rays.

uviosensitive (u″ve-o-sen′sĭ-tiv)   sensitive to ultraviolet rays.

uvula (u′vu-lah), pl. *u′vulae* [L. "little grape"]   a pendent, fleshy mass; used as a general term in anatomical terminology. Usually used alone to designate the *uvula palatina.*   **bifid u.,** bifurcation of the uvula, considered to be an incomplete form of cleft palate. Called also *cleft u., u. fissa, forked u.,* and *split u.*   **u. of bladder,** u. vesicae.   **u. cerebel′li, u. of cerebellum,** u. vermis.   **cleft u.,** bifid u.   **u. fis′sura, forked u.,** bifid u.   **Lieutaud's u.,** u. vesicae.   **u. palati′na** [NA], **palatine u.,** the small, fleshy mass hanging from the soft palate above the root of the tongue, composed of the levator and tensor palati muscles and the muscle of the uvula, connective tissue, and mucous membrane.   **split u.,** bifid u.   **u. ver′mis** [NA], the part of the vermis of the cerebellum between the pyramis and the nodulus; called also *u. of cerebellum.*   **u. vesi′cae** [NA], a rounded elevation at the neck of the bladder, formed by convergence of many fibers of the trigonal muscle as they pass through the encircling musculus sphincter vesicae to terminate in the urethra. Called also *u. of bladder.*

uvular (u′vu-lar)   pertaining to the uvula; staphyline.

uvularis (u″vu-la′ris) [L., from *uvula*]   uvular.

uvulectomy (u″vu-lek′to-me) [*uvula* + Gr. *ektomē* excision]   excision of the uvula; cionectomy.

uvulitis (u″vu-li′tis) [*uvula* + *-itis*]   inflammation of the uvula; staphylitis.

uvuloptosis (u″vu-lop-to′sis) [*uvula* + Gr. *ptōsis* falling]   a relaxed and pendulous condition of the palate; staphyloptosis; cionoptosis.

uvulotome (u′vu-lo-tōm)   an instrument for cutting the uvula; staphylotome.

uvulotomy (u″vu-lot′o-me) [*uvula* + Gr. *tomē* a cutting]   the operation of cutting off the uvula or a part of it; cionotomy; staphylotomy.

uzara (u-zah′rah)   the dried root of a species of *Gomphocarpus* (Asclepiadaceae), an African plant; used by certain natives in diarrhea and dysentery. It is the source of uzarin.

uzarin (u-zar′in)   a constituent of uzara, $C_{35}H_{54}O_{14}$, which has antidiarrheal properties.

V chemical symbol for *vanadium;* symbol for *volt.*

V symbol for *velocity, voltage,* or *volume.*

v. abbreviation for L. *vena* vein.

V$_{max}$ symbol for the maximum velocity of an enzyme-catalyzed reaction; see *Michaelis-Menten equation* under *equation.*

V$_T$ symbol for *tidal volume* (in pulmonary ventilation).

VA visual acuity.

V.A. Veterans Administration.

VAC a regimen of vincristine, dactinomycin, and cyclophosphamide, used in cancer chemotherapy.

vaccenic acid (vak-sen′ik) *cis*-11-octadecenoic acid, an unsaturated fatty acid found in butterfat.

vaccina (vak-si′nah) vaccinia.

vaccinal (vak′sĭ-nal) [L. *vaccinus*] 1. pertaining to vaccinia, to vaccine, or to vaccination. 2. having protective qualities when used by way of inoculation.

vaccinate (vak′sĭ-nāt) to inoculate with vaccine for the purpose of producing immunity.

vaccination (vak″sĭ-na′shun) [L. *vacca* cow] the introduction of vaccine into the body for the purpose of inducing immunity. Coined originally to apply to the injection of smallpox vaccine, the term has come to mean any immunizing procedure in which vaccine is injected.

vaccinator (vak′sĭ-na″tor) 1. one who vaccinates. 2. an instrument for use in vaccination.

vaccine (vak′sēn) [L. *vaccinus*] a suspension of attenuated or killed microorganisms (bacteria, viruses, or rickettsiae), administered for the prevention, amelioration, or treatment of infectious diseases. **anaplasmosis v.,** a killed vaccine consisting of inactivated and lyophilized *Anaplasma marginale* organisms, used for prevention of clinical symptoms of bovine anaplasmosis. **anthrax v.,** a cell-free protein extract of cultures of *Bacillus anthracis,* used for immunization of persons with occupational exposure to anthrax, e.g., workers with imported animal hides or hair. **anthrax spore v.,** a live vaccine consisting of *Bacillus anthracis* spores in saponified diluent, used for vaccination of domestic farm animals against anthrax. **attenuated v.,** a vaccine prepared from live microorganisms or viruses cultured under adverse conditions leading to loss of their virulence but retention of their ability to induce protective immunity. **autogenous v.,** a vaccine prepared from microorganisms which have been freshly isolated from the lesion of the patient who is to be treated with it. **avian encephalomyelitis v.,** a live virus vaccine of chick embryo origin, used for immunization of layer or breeder replacement pullets against avian encephalomyelitis. **bacterial v.,** a preparation of killed or attenuated bacteria used as an active immunizing agent. Called also *bacterin.* **BCG v.** (bacille Calmette-Guérin) [USP], a vaccine made from the Calmette-Guérin strain of *Mycobacterium bovis,* which was made avirulent by culture by Calmette and Guérin for many years on a medium enriched in beef bile; it is administered by intradermal injection or scarification to tuberculin-negative individuals for prevention of tuberculosis. It is used for routine vaccination of children only in regions where there is a high incidence of tuberculosis. In the United States it is recommended only for immunization of high-risk individuals. BCG vaccine is also used in cancer immunotherapy, particularly in malignant melanoma; it is thought to act as a nonspecific stimulator of cell-mediated immunity. **bluetongue v.,** a live virus vaccine of bovine tissue culture origin, used for prevention of bluetongue in sheep. **bovine rhinotracheitis v.,** a modified live virus vaccine of tissue culture origin used for immunization of healthy cattle against infectious bovine rhinotracheitis. **bovine virus diarrhea v.,** a modified live virus vaccine of tissue culture origin, used for immunization of cattle against bovine virus diarrhea. **bronchitis v.,** a live virus vaccine of chick embryo origin prepared from the Massachusetts or Connecticut variant strains of bronchitis virus, used for prevention of infectious bronchitis in chickens and other birds. **Brucella abortus v.,** a live virus vaccine of *B. abortus* strain 19, used for immunization of healthy calves against brucello-sis. **bursal disease v.,** a modified live virus of chick embryo origin, used for immunization of chicks against infectious bursal disease. **Calmette's v.,** BCG v. **canine distemper v.,** a modified live virus vaccine consisting of an attenuated strain of canine distemper virus propagated in tissue culture, used for immunization of dogs against canine distemper. **cholera v.** [USP], a killed bacteria vaccine containing equal portions of the Inaba and Ogawa strains of *Vibrio cholerae,* used for immunization against cholera. It enhances protection in adults for about six months, but does not reduce fecal shedding of bacteria or reduce disease transmission. **coccidiosis v.,** live sporulated oocysts of chicken origin, used to introduce subclinical coccidial infection in chickens in order to establish immunity against clinical infections. **Cox v.,** typhus v. **distemper v.–mink,** a modified live virus vaccine of chick embryo of tissue culture origin, used for prevention of canine distemper in mink. **duck embryo v.,** vaccine prepared from embryonate duck eggs infected with inactivated fixed virus. **duck virus enteritis v.,** a modified live virus vaccine of chick embryo origin, used for prevention of duck virus enteritis. **duck virus hepatitis v.,** a modified live virus vaccine of chick embryo origin, used for prevention of duck virus hepatitis. **encephalomyelitis v.,** a bivalent killed virus vaccine of chicken tissue culture origin, used for immunization of horses against Eastern and Western equine encephalomyelitis. **equine influenza v.,** a bivalent killed virus vaccine of chick embryo origin, used for immunization of horses against equine influenza due to influenza virus A equine strains 1 and 2. **equine rhinopneumonitis v.,** an attenuated live virus vaccine of tissue culture origin or a killed virus vaccine, used for immunization of horses against equine viral rhinopneumonitis due to equine herpesvirus type 1. **Erysipelothrix rhusiopathiae v.,** an avirulent live culture of *E. rhusiopathiae,* used for prevention of erysipelas in swine. **feline panleukopenia v.,** a modified live virus vaccine or killed virus vaccine of tissue culture origin, used for immunization of cats against feline panleukopenia. **feline pneumonitis v.,** a modified live vaccine of chick embryo origin, used for immunization of cats against *Chlamydia psittaci.* **feline rhinotracheitis v.,** a modified live virus vaccine of tissue culture origin, used for immunization of cats against feline rhinotracheitis. **fowl laryngotracheitis v.,** a modified live virus vaccine of chick embryo origin, used for prevention of laryngotracheitis in chickens. **fowl pox v.,** a modified live virus vaccine of chicken embryo or tissue culture origin, used to immunize chickens and turkeys against fowl pox. **hepatitis B v.,** formalin-treated hepatitis B surface antigen isolated from plasma of human carriers of hepatitis B, used for immunization of persons at high risk, e.g., medical and dental personnel, immunocompromised patients and patients requiring hemodialysis or frequent transfusions, residents and staff of closed institutions, contacts of carriers, and male homosexuals. **heterologous v.,** a vaccine that confers protective immunity against a pathogen not present in the vaccine, because it contains microorganisms that possess cross-reacting antigens which they share in common with that pathogen. For example, vaccinia virus protects against smallpox. Called also *heterotypic v.* **heterotypic v.,** heterologous v. **influenza virus v.** [USP], a killed virus vaccine; both whole virion and subvirion vaccines are available. The composition of the vaccine is changed each year in response to antigenic shifts and changes in prevalence of influenza virus strains; the vaccine is usually bivalent or trivalent, containing one or two influenza virus A strains and one influenza virus B strain. Annual immunization before November is recommended for high-risk individuals (persons over 65 years of age and persons with chronic disease). **live v.,** a vaccine prepared from live microorganisms or viruses that have been attenuated but that retain their immunogenic properties. **Marek's disease v.,** a live turkey herpesvirus vaccine of tissue culture origin, used for immunization of 1-day-old chicks against Marek's disease. **measles v.,** a modified live virus vaccine of canine tissue culture origin, used to induce resistance to canine distemper in 3- to 6-week-old puppies in which response to canine distemper vaccine would be neutralized because of interference by maternal antibody. **measles virus v. live,** a live attenuated virus vaccine of chick embryo origin, used for routine immunization of children and for immunization of adolescents and adults who have not had measles or been immunized with live measles vaccine and have no serum antibodies against measles. Children are usually immunized with measles-mumps-rubella (MMR) combination vaccine. Official names [USP] are *measles virus vaccine live, measles, mumps, and rubella virus vaccine live,* and *measles and rubella virus vaccine live.* **meningococcal polysaccharide v.,** a preparation of the capsular polysaccharide antigen of *Neisseria meningitidis,* types A, C, Y, or W-135; monovalent group A or C, bivalent group A and C, and quadrivalent vaccines are available. The vaccine is administered to persons over 2 years of age at risk in event of an epidemic of meningococcal disease caused by these serotypes and routinely only to military recruits. **mink enteritis v.,** a killed virus vaccine of feline tissue culture origin, used for immunization of mink against mink viral enteritis. **mixed v.,** polyvalent v. **mumps virus v. live,** a live attenuated virus vaccine of chick embryo origin, used for routine immunization of children and for immunization of adolescents and adults who have not had mumps or been immunized with live mumps vaccine. Children are usually immunized with measles-mumps-rubella (MMR) combination vaccine. Official names [USP] are *mumps virus vaccine live, measles and mumps virus vaccine live, measles, mumps, and rubella virus vaccine live,* and *rubella and mumps virus vaccine live.* **Newcastle disease v.,** live virus vaccine or chemically inactivated, adsorbed killed virus vaccine, both of chick embryo origin, used for immunization of chickens against Newcastle disease, the live vaccine for mass immunization in drinking water, aerosol spray, or eyedrops, the killed vaccine for immunization by injection. **ovine ecthyma v.,** a live virus vaccine of ovine origin, used for immunization of sheep and goats against contagious ecthyma (orf). **Pasteurella multocida v.,** a live bacterial vaccine, used for prevention of pasteurellosis in turkeys due to *P. multocida,* types 3 and 4. **pertussis v.,** a suspension of killed *Bordetella pertussis* organisms, used for immunization against pertussis (whooping cough); both fluid and adsorbed (on alum, aluminum hydroxide, or aluminum phosphate) forms are available. It is generally used in a mixture with diphtheria and tetanus toxoids (DTP). Routine pertussis immunization is recommended for all children under 6, except when a specific contraindication exists. Official names [USP] are *pertussis vaccine, pertussis vaccine adsorbed, diphtheria and tetanus toxoids and pertussis vaccine* (DTP), and *diphtheria and tetanus toxoids and pertussis vaccine adsorbed.* **pigeon pox v.,** a live virus vaccine of chick embryo origin, used for prevention of fowl pox in chickens and turkeys. **plague v.** [USP], a suspension of killed *Yersinia pestis* bacilli, used for immunization of persons having occupational or avocational exposure to wild rodents in plague enzootic areas. **pneumococcal polysaccharide v.,** a 23-valent vaccine containing capsular polysaccharide of *Streptococcus pneumoniae* types 1–5, 8, 9, 12, 14, 17, 19, 20, 22, 23, 26, 34, 43, 51, 54, 56, 57, 68, and 70, which are responsible for about 90 per cent of pneumococcal disease in the United States; used for immunization of persons over 2 years of age having chronic cardiac, pulmonary, hepatic, or renal disease, diabetes mellitus, sickle cell anemia, or anatomic or functional asplenia, and persons in nursing homes or other institutions where there is high risk of pneumococcal disease. **poliomyelitis v.,** poliovirus vaccine inactivated. **poliovirus v. inactivated (IPV)** [USP], a suspension of formalin-inactivated poliovirus, types I, II, and III, grown in monkey kidney cell tissue culture, used in the United States only for immunization of immunologically deficient patients and for primary immunization of unimmunized adults at risk. Called also *Salk v.* and (formerly) *poliomyelitis v.* **poliovirus v. live oral (OPV)** [USP], **poliovirus v. live oral trivalent (TOPV),** a live vaccine containing attenuated poliovirus, types I, II, and III, grown in monkey kidney cell tissue culture, used for routine immunization of children against polio. OPV induces long-lasting intestinal and humoral immunity; IPV (killed vaccine) induces only humoral immunity. OPV should not be administered to immunocompromised individuals or their household contacts. Called also *Sabin v.* **polyvalent v.,** a vaccine prepared from cultures or antigens of more than one strain or species. **pseudorabies v.,** a modified live virus vaccine of porcine

tissue culture origin, used for immunization of swine against pseudorabies. **rabies v.** [USP], a killed virus vaccine, used for preexposure immunization to persons at high risk of exposure, e.g., veterinarians, and in conjunction with rabies immune globulin, for postexposure prophylaxis. The current *human diploid cell vaccine* (HDC), produced from rabies virus grown in cultures of human diploid embryo lung cells, has a much lower incidence of adverse reactions than the previously used *duck embryo vaccine* (DEV). **reo-corona viral calf diarrhea v.,** a modified live virus vaccine of bovine tissue culture origin, used for immunization of newborn calves against enteric disease caused by reoviruses and coronaviruses. **replicative v.,** any vaccine containing organisms that are able to reproduce, including live and attenuated viruses and bacteria. **Rocky Mountain spotted fever v.** [USP], a killed rickettsia vaccine produced from *Rickettsia rickettsi* grown in yolk sacs of embryonated chicken eggs; it had limited effectiveness and is no longer available. A new chick embryo cell culture vaccine is under investigation. **rubella virus v. live,** a live attenuated virus vaccine of duck embryo or human diploid cell tissue culture origin, used for routine immunization of children and for immunization of nonpregnant adolescent and adult females of childbearing age who are unimmunized and do not have serum antibodies to rubella. Children are usually immunized with measles-mumps-rubella (MMR) combination vaccine. Official names [USP] are *measles and rubella virus live, measles, mumps, and rubella virus vaccine live, rubella virus vaccine live,* and *rubella and mumps virus vaccine live.* **Sabin v.,** poliovirus v. live oral. **Salk v.,** poliovirus v. inactivated. **Semple v.,** a phenol-inactivated rabbit nerve tissue vaccine, formerly used for rabies treatment. **smallpox v.** [USP], a live vaccina virus vaccine of calf lymph or chick embryo origin, used for immunization against smallpox. Now recommended only for laboratory workers exposed to smallpox virus; certain countries continue to vaccinate those in the military forces. Complications that result from smallpox vaccination include vaccinia, secondary bacterial infections, and encephalomyelitis. **split-virus v.,** subunit v. **streptococcus group E v.,** an oral modified live virus vaccine of Lancefield group E streptococcus, used for prevention of streptococcal lymphadenitis (jowl or cervical abscesses) in swine. **subunit v.,** a vaccine produced from specific protein subunits of a virus and thus having less risk of adverse reactions than live or killed whole virus vaccines, e.g., hepatitis B vaccine and some influenza vaccines. Called also *split-virus v.,* and *subvirion v.* **subvirion v.,** subunit v. **tenosynovitis v.,** an oral modified live virus vaccine of chick embryo origin, administered to broiler-breeder replacement chickens for prevention of infectious tenosynovitis. **transmissible gastroenteritis v.,** a modified live virus vaccine of porcine tissue culture origin, used for prevention of transmissible gastroenteritis in swine. **tuberculosis v.,** BCG v. **typhoid v.** [USP], a killed bacteria vaccine, either acetone-dried or phenol-inactivated, used for immunization against typhoid fever. It confers about 70 per cent protection, which can be overcome by a large challenge. Immunization is recommended only for exposure due to travel, epidemic, or household contact with a carrier. A new live oral vaccine consisting of a mutant strain (*Salmonella typhi* Ty 21a) of high antigenicity and limited viability in man is under investigation. **typhoid and paratyphoid v.,** a killed bacteria vaccine containing typhoid bacilli and paratyphoid strains A and B bacilli; no longer used because of lack of effectiveness of the paratyphoid component. **typhus v.** [USP], a formalin-inactivated vaccine of chick embryo origin, used for immunization against epidemic (*Rickettsia prowazeki*) typhus. Efficacy of this vaccine has not been established and it is no longer available in the United States. A live vaccine containing the attenuated Madrid E strain of *R. prowazeki* is protective but can cause mild symptomatic infection; it also is not generally available. **yellow fever v.,** a live attenuated virus vaccine of chick embryo origin, used for prevention of yellow fever; recommended for immunization of persons residing or traveling in endemic areas of Africa and South America.

vaccinia (vak-sin′e-ah) [L., from *vacca* cow] the cutaneous and sometimes systemic reactions associated with vaccination with smallpox vaccine. Cf. *cowpox* and *paravaccinia.* **fetal v.,** vaccinia of the fetus due to bloodborne dissemination of vaccinia virus in the pregnant woman after primary smallpox vaccination; it is frequently lethal to the fetus.

v. gangreno'sa, progressive v. **generalized v.,** a usually self-limited skin eruption resembling smallpox, sometimes occurring after primary smallpox vaccination, caused by transient viremia with localization of the virus in the skin. **progressive v.,** a rare but often fatal complication of smallpox vaccination in those with deficient immune mechanisms or receiving immunosuppressive therapy, characterized by tissue necrosis that spreads from the inoculation site, which may result in metastatic vaccinial lesions in the skin, bones, and viscera. Called also *v. gangrenosa.*

vaccinial (vak-sin'e-al) pertaining to or characteristic of vaccinia.

vacciniform (vak-sin'ĭ-form) resembling vaccinia.

vaccinization (vak"sin-i-za'shun) vaccination persistently repeated until the virus has no perceptible effect.

vaccinogen (vak-sin'o-jen) a source from which vaccine is derived.

vaccinogenous (vak"sĭ-noj'ĕ-nus) producing vaccine.

vaccinostyle (vak-sin'o-stīl) a small lance used in vaccination.

vaccinotherapy (vak"sĭ-no-ther'ah-pe) therapeutic use of vaccines.

VACTERL an acronym for *v*ertebral, *a*nal, *c*ardiac, *t*racheal, *e*sophageal, *r*enal, and *l*imb; used to designate a pattern of congenital anomalies.

vacuolar (vak'u-o"lar) pertaining to a vacuole; characterized by the presence of vacuoles.

vacuolate (vak'u-o-lāt") to form small spaces, or vacuoles.

vacuolated (vak'u-o-lāt"ed) pertaining to or characterized by vacuoles.

vacuolation (vak"u-o-la'shun) the process of forming vacuoles; the condition of being vacuolated.

vacuole (vak'u-ōl) [L. *vacuus* empty + -*ole* diminutive ending] any small space or cavity formed in the protoplasm of a cell. **autophagic v.,** autoplasmosome. **condensing v's,** membrane-bound spherical vacuoles in the Golgi complex of secretory cells, which contain secretory product in varying degrees of condensation and which mature, pass to the cell surface as secretory granules or droplets, and discharge their contents. **contractile v.,** an osmoregulatory organelle of protozoa and sponges that alternately fills with water extracted from the adjacent cytoplasm and then ejects the water to the outside; thus it acts as a pumping mechanism to remove excess water from the cell. Called also *water expulsion vesicle.* **digestive v.,** secondary lysosome. **food v.,** a fluid-containing intracytoplasmic space in which food material is suspended; it occurs in holozoic protozoa. **heterophagic v.,** heterophagosome. **plasmocrine v.,** a small cavity containing crystalloids in a secretory cell. **rhagiocrine v.,** a small cavity containing colloids in a secretory cell. **water v.,** a small drop of water within the protoplasm of a cell.

vacuolization (vak"u-o-li-za'shun) vacuolation.

vacuome (vak'u-ōm) the system of vacuoles in a cell which stain with neutral red.

vacuum (vak'u-um) [L.] a space devoid of air or of other gas; a space from which the air has been exhausted. **high v.,** a vacuum in which the attenuation is extreme. **torricellian v.,** the vacuum in a barometric tube.

vadum (va'dum) [L. "a shallow"] an occasional elevation from the bottom of a cerebral sulcus, rendering the sulcus more or less shallow.

vagal (va'gal) pertaining to the vagus nerve.

vagectomy (va-jek'to-me) surgical excision of a segment of the vagal nerve.

vagi (va'ji) [L.] genitive and plural of *vagus.*

vagina (vah-ji'nah), pl. *vagi'nae* [L.] 1. a sheath, or sheathlike structure; used as a general term in anatomical nomenclature. 2. [NA] the canal in the female, extending from the vulva to the cervix uteri, which receives the penis in copulation. **v. bul'bi** [NA], connective tissue that forms the capsule enclosing the posterior part of the eyeball, extending anteriorly to the conjunctival fornix, and continuous with the muscular fascia of the eye; called also *bulbar fascia, capsula bulbi, fascia bulbi* [Tenoni], *bulbar sheath, sheath of eyeball,* and Bonnet's, *ocular,* or *Tenon's capsule.* **v. carot'ica fas'ciae cervica'lis** [NA], the portion of the cervical fascia that encloses the carotid vessels and vagus

nerve. **v. commu'nis musculo'rum flexo'rum** [NA], the common synovial sheath for the flexor tendons as they pass through osteofibrous canals of the fingers; called also *v. synovialis communis musculorum flexorum.* **v. cor'dis,** pericardium. **v. exter'na ner'vi op'tici** [NA], the thick outer sheath of the optic nerve, continuous with the dura mater and connecting it with the sclera; called also *external* or *fibrous sheath of optic nerve.* **v. fem'o-ris,** fascia lata femoris. **vagi'nae fibro'sae digito'-rum ma'nus** [NA], strong fibrous, semicylindrical sheaths investing the grooved palmar surface of the proximal and middle phalanges of the fingers; called also *ligamenta vaginalia digitorum manus* and *fibrous sheaths of fingers.* **vagi'nae fibro'sae digito'rum pe'dis** [NA], more or less complete fascial sheaths surrounding the phalanges of the toes, for attachment of the tendons and their synovial membranes; called also *ligamenta vaginalia digitorum pedis* and *fibrous sheaths of toes.* **v. fibro'sa ten'dinis** [NA], the fibrous sheath of a tendon, usually confining it to an osseous groove. **v. inter'na ner'vi op'tici** [NA], the inner sheath of the optic nerve, continuous with the pia mater; called also *internal sheath of optic nerve.* **v. mas-culi'na,** utriculus prostaticus. **vagi'nae muco'sae,** vaginae synoviales. **v. muco'sa ten'dinis,** v. synovialis tendinis. **v. mulie'bris,** the organ of copulation in the female; see *vagina,* def. 2. **v. musculo'rum fibula'rium commu'nis,** NA alternative for *v. musculo-rum peroneorum communis.* **v. musculo'rum peroneo'rum commu'nis** [NA], the double tendon sheath for the long and short peroneal muscles; called also *v. musculorum fibularium communis* [NA alternative], *v. syno-vialis musculorum fibularium communis,* and *v. synovialis musculorum peroneorum communis.* **v. mus'culi rec'ti abdo'minis** [NA], a sheath formed by the aponeuroses of other abdominal muscles, within which the rectus abdominis can move. **vagi'nae ner'vi op'tici,** the internal and external meningeal sheaths of the optic nerve within the orbit, continuous with the meninges of the brain. See *v. externa nervi optici* and *v. interna nervi optici.* Called also *sheaths of optic nerve.* **v. o'culi,** v. bulbi. **v. proces'-sus styloi'dei,** a ridge on the lower surface of the temporal bone, partly enclosing the base of the styloid process; called also *sheath of styloid process.* **vagi'nae synovia'les** [NA], double-layered, fluid-filled sheaths such as those that usually surround tendons running in osseofibrous tunnels. **v. synovia'lis commu'nis musculo'rum flexo'rum,** v. communis musculorum flexorum. **vagi'nae syno-via'les digito'rum ma'nus** [NA], the synovial sheaths of the tendons of the fingers. **vagi'nae synovia'les digito'rum pe'dis** [NA], the synovial sheaths of the ten-dons of the toes. **v. synovia'lis intertubercula'ris** [NA], the synovial membrane that surrounds the long head of the biceps brachii muscle as it passes through the intertubercular sulcus; called also *synovial sheath of inter-tubercular groove.* **v. synovia'lis musculo'rum fibula'rium commu'nis,** v. musculorum fibularium communis. **v. synovia'lis mus'culi obli'qui su-perio'ris,** v. tendinis musculi obliqui superioris. **v. synovia'lis musculo'rum peroneo'rum com-mu'nis,** v. musculorum peroneorum communis. **v. synovia'lis ten'dinis** [NA], a double-layered, fibrous sheath usually found surrounding a tendon running in an osteofibrous canal, with synovial fluid present between the layers; called also *v. mucosa tendinis* and *synovial sheath of tendon.* **vagi'nae synovia'les ten'dinum digito'-rum ma'nus,** vaginae tendinum digitorum manus. **vagi'nae synovia'les ten'dinum digito'rum pe'-dis,** vaginae tendinum digitorum pedis. **v. synovia'lis ten'dinis mus'culi flexo'ris car'pi radia'lis,** v. ten-dinis musculi flexoris carpi radialis. **v. synovia'lis ten'dinis mus'culi flexo'ris hal'lucis lon'gi,** v. ten-dinis musculi flexoris hallucis longi. **v. synovia'lis ten'dinis mus'culi tibia'lis posterio'ris,** v. tendinis musculi tibialis posterioris. **v. ten'dinis** [NA] a sheath of a tendon; a fibrous or synovial tendon sheath. **vagi'-nae ten'dinum digita'les ma'nus,** vaginae synoviales tendinum digitorum manus. **vagi'nae ten'dinum digito'rum ma'nus** [NA], the tendon sheaths of the long and short flexors of the fingers; called also *vaginae synoviales tendinum digitorum manus.* **vagi'nae ten'dinum digito'rum pe'dis** [NA], the synovial sheaths of the ten-dons of the toes; called also *vaginae synoviales tendinum digitorum pedis.* **v. ten'dinum musculo'rum ab-**

ducto'ris lon'gi et extenso'ris bre'vis pol'licis [NA], the tendon sheath of the long abductor and short extensor muscles of the thumb. **v. ten'dinum muscu-lo'rum extenso'rum car'pi radia'lium** [NA], the tendon sheath of the short and long extensor carpi radialis muscles. **v. ten'dinis mus'culi extenso'ris car'pi ulna'ris** [NA], the tendon sheath of the extensor carpi ulnaris muscle. **v. ten'dinum musculo'rum extenso'ris digito'rum commu'nis et extenso'ris in'dicis,** v. tendinum musculorum extensoris digitorum et extensoris indicis. **v. ten'dinum musculo'rum extenso'ris digito'rum et extenso'ris in'dicis** [NA], the tendon sheath of the extensor digitorum and extensor indicis muscles. **v. ten'dinis mus'culi extenso'ris dig'iti min'mimi** [NA], the tendon sheath of the extensor digiti minimi muscle. **vagi'nae ten'dinum mus'culi extenso'ris digito'rum pe'dis lon'gi** [NA], the tendon sheaths of the extensor digitorum longus muscle, running from the cruciate ligament to the intermediate cuneiform bone. **v. ten'dinis mus'culi extenso'ris hal'lucis lon'gi** [NA], the tendon sheath of the extensor hallucis longus muscle, extending from the cruciate ligament to the dorsal fascia of the foot. **v. ten'dinis mus'culi extenso'ris pol'licis lon'gi** [NA], the sheath of the extensor pollicis longus tendon. **v. ten'dinis mus'culi fibula'-ris lon'gi planta'ris,** NA alternative for *v. tendinis musculi peronei longi plantaris.* **v. ten'dinis mus'culi flexo'ris car'pi radia'lis** [NA], the tendon sheath of the flexor carpi radialis muscle; called also *v. synovialis musculi flexoris carpi radialis.* **vagi'nae ten'dinum mus'culi flexo'ris digito'rum pe'dis lon'gi** [NA], the tendon sheaths of the flexor digitorum longus muscle, extending from the medial malleolus to below the navicular bone. **v. ten'dinis mus'culi flexo'ris hal'lucis lon'gi** [NA], the tendon sheath of the flexor hallucis longus muscle, extending from the medial malleolus to where it crosses the tendon of the flexor digitorum longus; called also *v. synovialis tendinis musculi flexoris hallucis longi.* **v. ten'dinis mus'culi flexo'ris pol'licis lon'gi** [NA], the tendon sheath for the long flexor muscle of the thumb in the wrist and palm. **v. ten'dinis mus'culi obli'qui superio'ris** [NA], the synovial sheath of the superior oblique muscle, particularly where its tendon passes through the trochlea; called also *synovial bursa of trochlea, trochlear synovial bursa,* and *v. synovialis musculi obliqui superioris.* **v. ten'dinis mus'culi perone'i lon'gi planta'ris** [NA], the tendon sheath of the peroneus longus muscle, beginning in the peroneal groove of the cuboid bone. **v. ten'dinis mus'culi tibia'lis anterio'ris** [NA], the tendon sheath of the tibialis anterior muscle, extending from the transverse crural ligament to the talonavicular joint. **v. ten'dinis mus'culi tibia'lis posterio'ris** [NA], the tendon sheath of the tibialis posterior muscle, beginning at the medial malleolus and extending into the foot; called also *v. synovialis tendinis musculi tibialis posterioris.* **v. vaso'rum** [NA], a fibrous sheath that encloses certain arteries, sometimes along with their veins and nerves.

vaginae (vah-ji'ne) genitive and plural of *vagina.*

vaginal (vaj'ĭ-nal) 1. of the nature of a sheath; ensheathing. 2. pertaining to the vagina. 3. pertaining to the tunica vaginalis testis.

vaginalectomy (vaj''ĭ-nah-lek'to-me) vaginectomy.

vaginalitis (vaj''ĭ-nah-li'tis) inflammation of the tunica vaginalis testis. **plastic v.,** pachyvaginalitis.

vaginapexy (vaj''ĭ-nah-pek'se) vaginofixation.

vaginate (vaj''ĭ-nāt) [L. *vaginatus* sheathed] provided with a sheath.

vaginectomy (vaj''ĭ-nek'to-me) excision of the vagina.

vaginiperineotomy (vaj''ĭ-nĭ-per''ĭ-ne-ot'o-me) paravaginal incision.

vaginismus (vaj''ĭ-niz'mus) [L.] painful spasm of the vagina due to involuntary contraction of the vaginal musculature severe enough to prevent intercourse; the cause may be organic or psychogenic.

vaginitis (vaj''ĭ-ni'tis) 1. inflammation of the vagina; it is marked by pain and by a purulent discharge. Called also *colpitis.* 2. inflammation of a sheath. **v. adhaesi'va, adhesive v.,** see *atrophic v.* **atrophic v.,** vaginitis occurring in postmenopausal women and associated with estrogen deficiency. The common types are: *senile vulvovaginitis,* in which there is intense itching around the vagina,

often with burning, almost complete lack of vaginal secretions, and evidence of tissue atrophy; and *senile vaginitis* or *adhesive vaginitis,* marked by the formation of superficial erosions, which often adhere to opposed surfaces, sometimes causing obliteration of the vaginal canal. **desquamative inflammatory v.,** vaginitis of unknown etiology, resembling atrophic vaginitis clinically and microscopically, but occurring in the absence of estrogen deficiency, and characterized chiefly by recrudescent reddened superficial ulcerations. **diphtheritic v.,** diphtheritic inflammation of the vagina. **v. emphysemato'sa, emphysematous v.,** inflammation of the vagina and adjacent cervix, characterized by numerous, asymptomatic, gas-filled cystlike lesions; the gas filling the lesions has been shown to have a carbon dioxide content. **granular v.,** the most common variety, in which the papillae are enlarged and infiltrated with small cells. **senile v.,** see *atrophic v.* **v. tes'tis,** perididymitis. **trichomonas v.,** vaginitis produced by *Trichomonas.*

vaginoabdominal (vaj''ĭ-no-ab-dom'ĭ-nal) pertaining to the vagina and the abdomen.

vaginocele (vaj''ĭ-no-sēl'') [L. *vagina* sheath + Gr. *kēlē* tumor] 1. hernia into the vagina. 2. polapse or falling of the vagina.

vaginocutaneous (vaj''ĭ-no-ku-ta'ne-us) pertaining to the vagina and skin, or communicating with the vagina and the cutaneous surface of the body, as a vaginocutaneous fistula.

vaginodynia (vaj''ĭ-no-din'e-ah) [L. *vagina* sheath + Gr. *odynē* pain + *-ia*] pain in the vagina; colpodynia.

vaginofixation (vaj''ĭ-no-fiks-a'shun) suture of the vagina to the abdominal wall.

vaginogram (vah-ji'no-gram) a roentgenogram of the vagina.

vaginography (vaj''ĭ-nog'rah-fe) roentgenography of the vagina.

vaginolabial (vaj''ĭ-no-la'be-al) pertaining to the vagina and the labia.

vaginometer (vaj''ĭ-nom'ĕ-ter) [*vagina* + Gr. *metron* measure] an instrument for measuring the length and diameter of the vagina.

vaginomycosis (vaj''ĭ-no-mi-ko'sis) [*vagina* + Gr. *mykēs* fungus] fungal disease of the vagina.

vaginopathy (vaj''ĭ-nop'ah-the) [*vagina* + Gr. *pathos* disease] any disease of the vagina.

vaginoperineal (vaj''ĭ-no-per''ĭ-ne'al) pertaining to the vagina and perineum.

vaginoperineoplasty (vaj''ĭ-no-per''ĭ-ne'o-plas''te) [*vagino-* + *perineoplasty*] plastic surgery of the vagina and perineum.

vaginoperineorrhaphy (vaj''ĭ-no-per''ĭ-ne-or'ah-fe) suture repair of the vagina and perineum.

vaginoperineotomy (vaj''ĭ-no-per''ĭ-ne-ot'o-me) paravaginal incision.

vaginoperitoneal (vaj''ĭ-no-per''ĭ-to-ne'al) pertaining to the vagina and peritoneum.

vaginopexy (vah-ji'no-pek''se) [*vagina* + Gr. *pēxis* fixation] vaginofixation.

vaginoplasty (vah-ji'no-plas''te) [*vagina* + Gr. *plassein* to form] plastic surgery of the vagina; called also *colpoplasty.*

vaginoscope (vaj'ĭ-no-skōp) [*vagina* + Gr. *skopein* to examine] a vaginal speculum; colposcope.

vaginoscopy (vaj''ĭ-nos'ko-pe) [*vagina* + Gr. *skopein* to examine] inspection of the vagina; colposcopy.

vaginosis (vaj''ĭ-no'sis) a disease of the vagina. **bacterial v.,** a nonspecific vaginitis associated with positive cultures for *Gardnerella vaginalis,* characterized by increased malodorous vaginal discharge that cannot be attributed to other cause.

vaginotomy (vaj''ĭ-not'o-me) [*vagina* + Gr. *tomē* a cutting] colpotomy.

vaginovesical (vaj''ĭ-no-ves'ĭ-kal) pertaining to the vagina and bladder.

vaginovulvar (vaj''ĭ-no-vul'var) vulvovaginal.

vagitus (vah-ji'tus) [L.] the cry of an infant. **v. uteri'nus,** the crying of a child in the uterus. **v. vagina'lis,** the crying of a child while its head is still within the vagina.

vagoaccessorius (va″go-ak″ses-so′re-us) [L.] the vagus nerve and the cranial root of the accessory nerves regarded as together forming one nerve.

vagoglossopharyngeal (va″go-glos″o-fah-rin′je-al) pertaining to the vagus and glossopharyngeal nerves.

vagogram (va′go-gram) [*vagus* + Gr. *gramma* mark] a tracing showing the electrical variations of the vagus nerve; called also *electrovagogram*.

vagolysis (va-gol′ĭ-sis) [*vagus* + Gr. *lysis* dissolution] surgical destruction of the vagus nerve.

vagolytic (va″go-lit′ik) having an effect resembling that produced by interruption of impulses transmitted by the vagus nerve; parasympatholytic.

vagomimetic (va″go-mi-met′ik) having an effect which resembles that produced by vagal stimulation.

vagosplanchnic (va″go-splank′nik) vagosympathetic.

vagosympathetic (va″go-sim″pah-thet′ik) pertaining to both the vagus and sympathetic innervation.

vagotomy (va-got′o-me) [*vagus* + Gr. *tomē* a cutting] interruption of the impulses carried by the vagus nerve or nerves. **bilateral v.,** transection of the right and left vagus nerves. **highly selective v.,** division of only those vagal fibers supplying the acid-secreting glands of the stomach, with preservation of those supplying the antrum as well as the hepatic and celiac branches. **medical v.,** interruption of the impulses carried by the vagus nerve by administration of suitable drugs; vagus block. **parietal cell v.,** selective severing of the vagus nerve fibers supplying the proximal two-thirds (parietal area) of the stomach; done for duodenal ulcer. **selective v.,** division of the vagal fibers to the stomach with preservation of the hepatic and celiac branches. **surgical v.,** transection of the vagus nerve by surgical means. **truncal v.,** surgical division of the two main trunks of the abdominal vagus nerve as they emerge through the esophageal hiatus.

vagotonia (va″go-to′ne-ah) [*vagus* + Gr. *tonos* tension + *-ia*] hyperexcitability of the vagus nerve; a condition in which the vagus nerve dominates in the general functioning of the body organs. It is marked by vasomotor instability, constipation, sweating, and involuntary motor spasms with pain.

vagotonic (va″go-ton′ik) pertaining to or characterized by vagotonia.

vagotony (va-got′o-ne) vagotonia.

vagotrope (va′go-trōp) vagotropic.

vagotropic (va″go-trop′ik) having an effect on the vagus nerve.

vagotropism (va-got′ro-pizm) [*vagus* + Gr. *tropos* a turning] affinity of a drug or poison for the vagus nerve.

vagovagal (va″go-va′gal) arising as a result of afferent and efferent impulses which are both mediated through the vagus nerve.

vagrant (va′grant) [L. *vagrans,* from *vagare* to wander] 1. wandering; moving from one place to another. 2. a vagabond.

vagus (va′gus), pl. *va′gi* [L. "wandering"] designating the tenth cranial nerve; see *nervus vagus*.

vagusstoff (va′gus-stof) [*vagus* + Ger. *Stoff* stuff, substance] a substance liberated by the vagus nerve endings that inhibits cardiac activity; it is identical to acetylcholine.

Vahlkampfia (vahl-kamp′fe-ah) a genus of freshwater or parasitic ameboid protozoa (suborder Schizopyrenida, subclass Gymnamoeba), characterized by the presence of one broad pseudopodium.

Val valine.

valamin (val′ah-min) the valerian ester of amylene hydrate, $(CH_3)_2 \cdot C_2H_5 \cdot CO \cdot O \cdot C_5H_9$, formerly used as a hypnotic and sedative.

valence (va′lens) [L. *valēre* to be strong] 1. a positive number that represents the combining power of an element in a chemical compound, i.e., the number of bonds each atom of that element makes with other atoms. In this most general sense "valence" has been superseded by the concept "oxidation number." However, "valence" is still used to indicate (*a*) the number of covalent bonds formed by an atom in a covalent compound or (*b*) the charge on a monoatomic or polyatomic molecule. 2. in immunology, the number of antigen binding sites possessed by an antibody molecule, two per immunoglobulin monomer, or the number of antigenic

determinants possessed by an antigen, usually a large number.

valency (va′len-se) [L. *valentia*] 1. strength; ability. 2. valence.

Valentin's corpuscles, ganglion (pseudoganglion) (val′en-tēnz) [Gabriel Gustav *Valentin,* German physician, 1810–1883] see under *corpuscle,* and see *intumescentia tympanica.*

Valentine's position (val′en-tīnz) [Ferdinand C. *Valentine,* surgeon in New York, 1851–1909] see under *position.*

valerian (va-le′re-an) [L. *valeriana*] any plant of the genus *Valeriana.* The dried roots and rhizome of *V. officinalis* L. (Valerianaceae) of Europe are antispasmodic and nerve stimulant and have been used in nervousness and hysteria. **Greek v.,** the European plant *Polemonium caeruleum* L. (Polemoniaceae), or Jacob's ladder, used as a topical application to ulcers.

valerianic acid (vah-ler-e′-an′ik) valeric acid.

valeric acid (vah-ler′ik) trivial name for pentanoic acid, $CH_3(CH_2)_3COOH$.

valethamate bromide (val-eth′ah-māt) chemical name: *N,N*-diethyl-*N*-methyl-2-[(3-methyl-1-oxo-2-phenylpentyl)-oxy]ethanaminium bromide. A quaternary ammonium anticholinergic, $C_{19}H_{32}BrNO_2$, occurring as a white, crystalline powder; used as an antispasmodic in the treatment of hypermotility and spasm of the gastrointestinal, genitourinary, and biliary tracts, administered orally, intramuscularly, or intravenously.

valetudinarian (val″e-tu″dĭ-na′re-an) [L. *valetudinarius* sickly] an invalid; a feeble person.

valetudinarianism (val″e-tu″dĭ-na′re-an-izm) an infirm or feeble habit of body.

valgus (val′gus) [L.] bent outward, twisted; denoting a deformity in which the angulation of the part is away from the midline of the body, as in *talipes valgus.* The term valgus is an adjective and should be used only in connection with the noun it describes, as talipes valgus, genu valgum, coxa valga. The meanings of *valgus* and *varus* are often reversed, so that genu valgum is knock-knee, not bowleg. Cf. *varus.*

validity (vah-lid′ĭ-te) 1. the extent to which a measurement, test, or study measures what it purports to measure. 2. occasionally, accuracy (q.v.).

valine (val′in) an essential amino acid, alpha-amino-isovaleric acid, $(CH_3)_2 \cdot CH \cdot CH(NH_2) \cdot COOH$, produced by the digestion or hydrolytic decomposition of proteins; it is essential for optimal growth in infants and for nitrogen equilibrium in human adults. Called also *2-aminoisovaleric acid* and *isopropyl-aminoacetic acid.*

valinemia (val″ĭ-ne′me-ah) hypervalinemia.

Valisone (val′ĭ-sōn) trademark for preparations of betamethasone valerate.

Valium (val′e-um) trademark for a preparation of diazepam.

vallate (val′āt) [L. *vallatus* walled] having a wall or rim; cup-shaped.

vallecula (vah-lek′u-lah), pl. *vallec′ulae* [dim. of L. *valles* a hollow] a depression or furrow; used as a general term in anatomical nomenclature. Sometimes used alone to designate the *vallecula epiglottica.* **v. cerebel′li** [NA], the longitudinal hollow on the inferior surface of the cerebellum, between the hemispheres, in which the medulla oblongata rests. **v. epiglot′tica,** a depression between the lateral and median glossoepiglottic folds on each side. **v. ova′ta,** fossa vesicae felleae. **v. for petrosal ganglion,** fossula petrosa. **v. syl′vii,** fossa lateralis cerebri. **v. un′guis,** sulcus matricis unguis.

vallecular (vah-lek′u-lar) pertaining to or affecting a vallecula.

Valleix's points (vahl-lāz′) [François Louis Isidore *Valleix,* French physician, 1807–1855] see under *point.*

Vallestril (val-les′tril) trademark for a preparation of methallenestril.

valley (val′e) a small hollow. **v. of cerebellum,** vallecula cerebelli.

Valli-Ritter law (val″e-rit′er) [Eusebio *Valli,* Italian physiologist, 1755–1816; Johann Wilhelm *Ritter,* German physicist, 1776–1810] see *Ritter-Valli law,* under *law.*

vallicepobufagin (vah-lis″ĕ-po-bu′fah-jin) a cardiac poison, $C_{26}H_{38}O_5$, from the skin glands of the toad, *Bufo valliceps*.

vallis (val′is) [L. "valley"] vallecula cerebelli.

vallum (val′um), gen. *val′li*, pl. *val′la* [L. "rampart"] a mound, or wall. **v. un′guis** [NA], the fold of skin overlapping the sides and the proximal end of a nail; called also *nail wall*.

Valmid (val′mid) trademark for a preparation of ethinamate.

valnoctamide (val-nok′tah-mīd) chemical name: 2-ethyl-3-methylvaleramide; a tranquilizer, $C_8H_{17}NO$.

Valpin (val′pin) trademark for preparations of anisotropine methylbromide.

valproate sodium (val-pro′āt) chemical name: 2-propylpentanoic acid sodium salt. It is the sodium salt, $C_8H_{15}NaO_2$, of valproic acid, a simple eight-carbon branched-chain fatty acid and is used as an antiepileptic especially for control of absence seizures.

Valsalva's ligaments, maneuver (experiment), sinus, zone (val-sal′vahz) [Antonio Maria *Valsalva*, Italian anatomist, 1666–1723] see under *maneuver*, and see *ligamenta auricularia, lamina basilaris ductus cochlearis*, and *sinus aortae*.

value (val′u) a measure of worth or efficiency; a quantitative measurement of the activity, concentration, etc., of specific substances (see *normal v's*). **acetyl v.,** acetyl number. **acid v.,** acid number. **buffer v.,** a numerical expression of the degree of change in pH of a solution in response to the addition of acid or alkali. **cryocrit v.,** the per cent volume of sedimented cryoglobulin after cold centrifugation of serum kept at 4° to 5° C. **D v.,** decimal reduction time. See under *time*. **fuel v.,** the potential heat energy of a food. **Hehner's v.,** the percentage of insoluble (nonvolatile) fatty acids that are yielded by a saponified fat. **liminal v.,** that intensity of a stimulus which produces a just noticeable impression. **mean clinical v.,** see *MCV*. **normal v's,** the range in concentration of specific substances found in normal healthy tissues, secretions, etc. **P v.,** the smallest level at which the sample results are significant. **predictive v.,** the conditional probability that a clinical test result correctly identifies a patient as having or not having a disease, i.e., the predictive value of a positive test is the probability that a person with a positive test is a true positive (i.e., does have the disease) and the predictive value of a negative test is the probability that a person with a negative test does not have the disease. Cf. *sensitivity* and *specificity*. The predictive value of a screening test is determined by the sensitivity and specificity of the test, and by the prevalence of the condition for which the test is used. **reference v's,** a set of values of a quantity measured in the clinical laboratory that characterize a specified population in a defined state of health. The values obtained from a statistical sample are used to establish a *reference interval* that covers 95 percent of the values of the healthy general population or of specific subpopulations differing in age and sex. These concepts were originally and are still widely referred to as "normal values" and the "normal range," but the use of these terms is now discouraged because of their implication that value falling outside of the reference interval are "abnormal" or "unhealthy," which has led to much confusion. It must be remembered that, by definition, 5 per cent of healthy individuals fall outside of the reference interval. **saponification v.,** saponification number. **threshold v.,** liminal v. **valence v.,** the number obtained by multiplying the lowering of the freezing point in degrees by the amount of urine in milliliters.

valva (val′vah), pl. *val′vae* [sing. of L. *valvae* folding doors] [NA] a valve: a membranous fold in a canal or passage, which prevents the reflux of the contents passing through it. **v. aor′tae** [NA], **v. aor′tica,** aortic valve: a valve composed of three semilunar cusps or segments (posterior, right, and left), guarding the aortic orifice in the left ventricle of the heart; it prevents backflow into the left ventricle. Called also *valvulae semilunares aortae* and *semilunar valve*. **v. atrioventricula′ris dex′tra** [NA], right atrioventricular valve: the valve between the right atrium and right ventricle of the heart; it usually has three cusps (anterior, posterior, and septal), but additional small cusps may be present. Called also *valvula tricuspidalis* or *tricuspid valve*. **v. atrioventricula′ris sinis′tra** [NA], left atrioventricular valve: the valve between the left atrium and left ventricle of

the heart; it usually has two cusps (anterior and posterior), but additional small cusps may be present. Called also *valvula bicuspidalis* [*mitralis*] and *bicuspid* or *mitral valve*. **v. ilea′lis,** NA alternative for *v. ileocaecalis*. **v. ileocaeca′lis** [NA], ileocecal valve: a so-called valve formed by the flaps or lips, one above and one below, of the ileocecal opening. In the cadaver the flaps project into the lumen of the large intestine as thickened folds, but in the living individual the ileum forms a conical or papillary projection (papilla ileocaecalis). Called also *ileocolic valve, v. ilealis* or *v. ileocecalis* [NA alternatives], and *valvula ileocolica*. **v. mitra′lis,** NA alternative for *v. atrioventricularis sinistra*. **v. pulmona′ria,** v. trunci pulmonalis. **v. tricuspida′lis,** v. atrioventricularis dextra. **v. trun′ci pulmona′lis** [NA], valve of pulmonary trunk: a valve composed of three semilunar segments (anterior, right, and left), guarding the pulmonary orifice in the right ventricle of the heart; it prevents backflow of blood into the right ventricle. Called also *pulmonary valve, semilunar valve*, and *v. pulmonaria*.

valval, valvar (val′val; val′var) pertaining to a valve.

valvate (val′vāt) pertaining to or having valves.

valve (valv) a membranous fold in a canal or passage, which prevents the reflux of the contents passing through it; see also *valva* and *valvula*. **anal v's,** valvulae anales. **v. of aorta, aortic v.,** valva aortae. **artificial v.,** artificial cardiac v. **atrioventricular v., left,** valva atrioventricularis sinistra. **atrioventricular v., right,** valva atrioventricularis dextra. **auriculoventricular v., left,** valva atrioventricularis sinistra. **auriculoventricular v., right,** valva atrioventricularis dextra. **Ball's v's,** valvulae anales. **Bauer v.,** a piece of unglazed porcelain fused into the wall of a gas tube by means of which air can be admitted as needed. **Bauhin's v.,** valva ileocaecalis. **Béraud's v.,** a fold of mucous membrane sometimes found at the junction of the lacrimal sac and the nasolacrimal duct; called also *Arnold's fold* and *Krause's valve*. **Bianchi's v.,** plica lacrimalis. **bicuspid v.,** valva atrioventricularis sinistra. **Bjork-Shiley v.,** a tilting disk valve containing a disk made of pyrolytic carbon that opens to an angle of 60 degrees. **Bochdalek's v.,** a

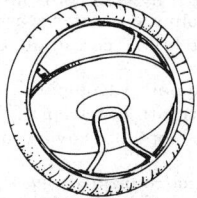

Bjork-Shiley valve.

fold within the lacrimal duct near the punctum lacrimale. **caged-ball v.,** a heart valve prosthesis consisting of a sewing ring attached to a cage composed of struts that contains a ball that floats free to allow passage of blood and occlusion of the orifice to prevent reflux. **cardiac v's,** valves that

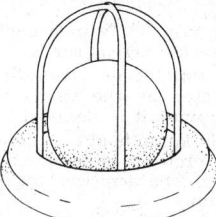

Caged-ball valve.

control the flow of blood through and from the heart; they are the atrioventricular, aortic, and pulmonary trunk valves. **cardiac v., artificial,** a substitute, mechanical or composed of tissue, for a cardiac valve. **Carpentier-Edwards v.,** a porcine valve mounted on a stent made of an alloy of spring steel. **caval v.,** valvula venae cavae inferioris. **coronary v., v. of coronary sinus,** valvula sinus coronarii. **eustachian v.,** valvula venae cavae inferioris. **fallopian v.,** valva ileocaecalis. **flair v.,** a cardiac valve having a cusp that has lost its normal support (as in ruptured chordae tendineae) and flutters in the blood stream. **Foltz's v.,** a fold of membrane at the lacrimal canaliculus. **v. of foramen ovale,** 1. valvula foraminis ovalis. 2. the septum primum of the fetal heart. **Gerlach's v.,** valvula processus vermiformis. **Guérin's v.,** valvula fossae navicularis. **Hancock v.,** a porcine valve mounted on a semiflexible stent made of a stellite ring and flexible struts of polypropylene. **Hasner's v.,** plica lacrimalis. **heart v's,** cardiac v's. **heart v., artificial,** artificial cardiac v. **Heister's v.,** plica spiralis. **Hoboken's v's,** foldlike thickenings of the media of the umbilical arteries which protrude into the lumen of the arteries. **Houston's v's,** plicae transversales recti. **Huschke's v.,** plica lacrimalis. **hymenal v. of male urethra,** valvula fossae navicularis. **ileocecal v., ileocolic v.,** valva ileocaecalis. **v. of inferior vena cava,** valvula venae cavae inferioris. **interauricular v.,** 1. limbus fossae ovalis. 2. valvula foraminis ovalis (def. 1). **Ionescu v.,** a cardiac valve substitute composed of bovine pericardium constructed as a three-cusp valve mounted on a Dacron-covered titanium frame. **Kerckring's v's,** plicae circulares. **Kohlrausch's v's,** plicae transversales recti. **Krause's v.,** Béraud's v. **lymphatic v.,** valvula lymphaticum. **v. of Macalister,** valva ileocaecalis. **Mercier's v.,** interureteric ridge (plica interureterica [NA]). **mitral v.,** valva atrioventricularis sinistra. **Morgagni's v's,** valvulae anales. **v. of navicular fossa,** valvula fossae navicularis. **O'Beirne's v.,** see under *sphincter*. **porcine v.,** a cardiac valve substitute made from a pig aortic valve cured in glutaraldehyde. **pulmonary v., pulmonary trunk v., v. of pulmonary trunk,** valva trunci pulmonalis. **pyloric v.,** valvula pylori. **Rosenmüller's v.,** plica lacrimalis. **semilunar v.,** a valve having semilunar cusps, i.e., the aortic valve and the pulmonary valve. The term is sometimes used to designate the semilunar cusps composing these valves; see entries beginning *valvula semilunaris*. **semilunar v's of colon,** plicae semilunares coli. **semilunar v's of Morgagni,** sinus anales. **sigmoid v's of colon,** plicae semilunares coli. **spiral v. of cystic duct, spiral v. of Heister,** plica spiralis. **Starr-Edwards v.,** a caged-ball heart valve prosthesis consisting of a retaining cage containing a Silastic ball. **v. of Sylvius,** valvula venae cavae inferioris. **Taillefer's v.,** a fold of the mucous membrane of the nasolacrimal duct near the middle of its course. **Tarinus' v.,** velum medullare inferius. **thebesian v.,** valvula sinus coronarii. **tilting-disk v.,** a heart valve prosthesis consisting of a sewing ring and a valve housing containing a suspended disk that swings between closed and open positions. **tricuspid v.,** valva atrioventricularis dextra. **v. of Tulpius,** valva ileocaecalis. **ureteral v.,** a congenital transverse fold across the lumen of the ureter, composed of redundant mucosa prominent by circular muscle fibers; it usually disappears in time but may rarely cause urinary obstruction. Pathological valves or kinks also occur. **v. of Varolius,** valva ileocaecalis. **v. of veins,** valvula venosa. **v. of vermiform appendix,** valvula processus vermiformis. **v. of Vieussens, Willis' v.,** velum medullare superius.

valved (valvd) having valves; opening by valves.

valviform (val′vĭ-form) [L. *valva* valve + *forma* shape] shaped like a valve.

valvotome (val′vo-tōm) a surgical instrument for incising a heart valve.

valvotomy (val-vot′o-me) [L. *valva* valve + Gr. *tomē* a cutting] incision of a valve, such as a valve of the heart. **mitral v.,** dilation of the left atrioventricular (mitral) valve, the commissures being split with or without the aid of a knife or a mechanical dilator. **pulmonary v.,** incision of the pulmonary valve to correct valvular stenosis. **transventricular closed v.,** correction of pulmonary valvular stenosis by passage of a valvulotome through the wall of the right ventricle into the pulmonary artery to open the valve; called also *Brock's operation*.

valvula (val′vu-lah), pl. *val′vulae* [L., dim of *valva*] a small valve; once used in official nomenclature as a general term to designate a valve, such as in the heart, but in NA restricted to designation of a cusp of the aortic valve or of the valve of the pulmonary trunk, or the valves of the anus, foramen ovale, navicular fossa, coronary sinus, inferior vena cava, or of the lymphatic vessels and veins. **val′vulae ana′les** [NA], anal valves: archlike folds of mucous membrane connecting the caudal ends of the anal columns. **v. biscuspida′lis [mitra′lis],** valva atrioventricularis sinistra. **val′vulae conniven′tes** [L. "closing valves"], plicae circu-

lares. v. fora′minis ova′lis, 1. [NA] valve of foramen ovale: in the adult, a crescentic ridge on the left side of the interatrial septum, representing the edge of what was the septum primum before fusion of the septum; called also *falx septi* [NA alternative]. 2. the septum primum of the fetal heart. **v. fos′sae navicula′ris** [NA], valve of navicular fossa: a fold of mucous membrane occasionally occurring in the roof of the fossa navicularis of the urethra. **v. ileocol′ica,** valva ileocaecalis. **v. lymphat′icum** [NA], a lymphatic valve: any of the usually doubled cusps in the collecting lymphatic vessels, serving to ensure flow in only one direction. **v. mitra′lis,** valva atrioventricularis sinistra. **v. proces′sus vermifor′mis,** an inconstant fold of mucous membrane at the opening into the cecum of the canal of the vermiform appendix. **v. pylo′ri,** pyloric valve: a prominent circular fold of mucous membrane at the pyloric orifice of the stomach; called also *Haller's circle*. **v. semiluna′ris,** a semilunar cusp. **v. semiluna′ris ante′rior arte′riae pulmona′lis,** v. semilunaris anterior trunci pulmonalis. **v. semiluna′ris ante′rior trun′ci pulmona′lis** [NA], the anterior cusp of the valve of the pulmonary trunk. **val′vulae semiluna′res aor′tae,** valva aortae. **v. semiluna′ris dex′tra aor′tae** [NA], the right cusp of the aortic valve. **v. semiluna′ris dex′tra arte′riae pulmona′lis,** v. semilunaris dextra trunci pulmonalis. **v. semiluna′ris dex′tra trun′ci pulmona′lis** [NA], the right cusp of the valve of the pulmonary trunk. **v. semiluna′ris poste′rior aor′tae** [NA], the posterior cusp of the aortic valve. **v. semiluna′ris sinis′tra aor′tae** [NA], the left cusp of the aortic valve. **v. semiluna′ris sinis′tra arte′riae pulmona′lis,** v. semilunaris sinistra trunci pulmonalis. **v. semiluna′ris sinis′tra trun′ci pulmona′lis** [NA], the left cusp of the valve of the pulmonary trunk. **v. si′nus corona′rii** [NA], **v. si′nus corona′rii [Thebe′sii],** valve of coronary sinus: a fold of endocardium along the right margin of the opening of the coronary sinus into the right atrium of the heart, which covers the lower part of the sinus. **v. spira′lis [Heis′teri],** plica spiralis. **v. tricuspida′lis,** valva atrioventricularis dextra. **v. ve′nae ca′vae inferio′ris** [NA], **v. ve′nae ca′vae inferio′ris [Eusta′chii],** valve of inferior vena cava: the variably sized crescentic fold of endocardial and subendocardial tissue that is attached to the anterior margin of the opening of the inferior vena cava into the right atrium of the heart. **v. veno′sa** [NA], valve of veins: any of the small cusps or folds of the tunica intima found in many veins, serving to prevent the backflow of blood. **v. vestib′uli,** either of the two thin folds bordering the opening of the sinus reuniens into the right atrium of the embryonic heart; they develop into the valves of the inferior vena cava and coronary sinus.

valvulae (val′vu-le) [L.] genitive and plural of *valvula.*

valvular (val′vu-lar) pertaining to, affecting, or of the nature of a valve.

valvulitis (val″vu-li′tis) inflammation of a valve or valvula, especially a valve of the heart. **rheumatic v.,** involvement of a cardiac valve by the rheumatic process; endocarditis.

valvuloplasty (val′vu-lo-plas″te) plastic repair of a valve.

valvulotome (val′vu-lo-tōm″) an instrument for splitting a stenotic valve.

valvulotomy (val″vu-lot′o-me) valvotomy.

valyl (val′il, va′lil) the acyl radical of valine.

valylene (val′ĭ-lēn) a hydrocarbon, C_5H_6.

VAMP a regimen of vincristine, methotrexate, 6-mercaptopurine, and prednisone, used in cancer chemotherapy.

vampire (vam′pīr) a neotropical bat belonging to the genera *Desmodus, Diaemus,* and *Diphylla.*

Vampirovibrio (vam-pi″ro-vib′re-o) [Fr. *vampire* vampire + *vibrio*] a genus of small, aerobic, motile, vibrioid, gram-negative bacteria that are obligate parasites of *Chlorella* algae, growing on the outside of the host cell. The type species is *V. chlorellavo′rus.*

vanadate (van′ah-dāt) any salt of vanadic acid.

vanadic acid (vah-nad′ik) an inorganic acid produced by dissolving vanadium pentoxide in water; there are various degrees of hydration, HVO_3, H_3VO_4, $H_4V_2O_7$, etc., seen in salts (vanadates).

vanadium (vah-na′de-um) [*Vanadis,* a Norse deity] a rare, gray, metallic element; symbol, V; atomic number, 23; atomic weight, 50.942. Its salts have been used in treating various diseases. See also *vanadiumism*.

vanadiumism (vah-na′de-um-izm″) a chronic intoxication caused by absorption of vanadium compounds, usually via the lungs; symptoms include irritation of the respiratory tract, pneumonitis, conjunctivitis, and anemia.

van Buren's disease (van-bu′renz) [William Holme *van Buren*, American surgeon, 1819–1883] Peyronie's disease.

Vancocin (van′ko-sin) trademark for a preparation of vancomycin hydrochloride.

vancomycin hydrochloride (van′ko-mi″sin) [USP] an antibiotic produced by the soil bacillus *Streptomyces orientalis*, which is highly effective against cocci, especially staphylococci, and other gram-positive bacteria, occurring as a tan to brown, free-flowing powder; used in the treatment of severe staphylococcal infections resistant to other antibiotics, administered intravenously or by intravenous infusion.

van Deen's test (van dēnz) [Izaak Abramson *van Deen*, Dutch physician, 1804–1869] see *Deen's test*, under *tests*.

Van de Graaff machine (van de grahf) [Robert Jemison *Van de Graaff*, American physicist, 1901–1967] see under *machine*.

van den Bergh's disease, test (van den bergz′) [A. A. Hijmans (Hymans) *van den Bergh*, Dutch physician, 1869–1943] see *enterogenous cyanosis*, under *cyanosis*, and see under *tests*.

van der Velden's test (van der vel′denz) [Reinhardt *van der Velden*, German physician, 1851–1903] *Maly's test*.

Vane (vān) John Robert. British pharmacologist, born 1927; co-winner, with Sune Bergström and Bengt Ingemar Samuelsson, of the Nobel prize for medicine or physiology in 1982 for their discovery of prostaglandins and related substances.

van Gehuchten's cells, method (van-ga-hook′tenz) [Arthur *van Gehuchten*, Belgian anatomist, 1861–1914] see *Golgi type II neurons*, under *neuron*, and see under *method*.

Vanghetti's prosthesis (vahn-get′ēz) [Giuliano *Vanghetti*, Italian surgeon, 1861–1940] see under *prosthesis*.

van Gieson's stain (van-ge′sonz) [Ira *van Gieson*, New York neuropathologist, 1865–1913] see *Table of Stains*.

van Helmont's mirror (van hel′monts) [Johannes Baptista *van Helmont*, Belgian physician, 1577–1644] the central tendon of the diaphragm (centrum tendineum [NA]).

van Hook's operation (van hooks′) [Weller *van Hook*, Chicago surgeon, 1862–1933] ureteroureterostomy.

van Hoorne's canal (van hornz) [Jean *van Hoorne*, Dutch anatomist, 1621–1670] the thoracic duct (ductus thoracicus [NA]).

Vanilla (vah-nil′ah) [L.] a genus of climbing orchidaceous plants of hot climates. The fruit of *V. planifolia* Andr. (Orchidaceae) or of *V. tahitensis* Moor. (Orchidaceae), of Mexico, are the vanilla beans, which contain vanilla and are used as a flavor and a mild stimulant; said to be aphrodisiac.

vanilla (vah-nil′ah) [NF] the cured, full-grown, unripe fruit of *Vanilla planifolia* Andr. (Mexican or Bourbon v.) or of *V. tahitensis* Moor. (Tahiti v.), used in medicine as a flavoring agent, usually in the form of a tincture.

vanillal (vah-nil′lal) ethyl vanillin.

vanillic acid (vah-nil′ik) 4-hydroxy-3-methoxybenzoic acid, obtained by oxidation of vanillin. **v. a. diethylamide,** ethamivan.

vanillin (van′ĭ-lin, vah-nil′in) [NF] chemical name: 4-hydroxy-3-methoxybenzaldehyde. A constituent of vanilla and other plants, which also may be prepared synthetically, $C_8H_8O_3$, occurring as fine fluffy white to yellow crystals, usually needle-like; used as a flavor in pharmaceutical preparations. **ethyl v.** [NF], chemical name: 3-ethoxy-4-hydroxybenzaldehyde. Fine white or slightly yellowish crystals, $C_9H_{10}O_3$; used as a flavor in pharmaceutical preparations.

vanillism (vah-nil′izm) symptoms of dermatitis, coryza, and malaise seen in those handling raw vanilla and caused by the mite *Acarus siro*.

vanillylmandelic acid (vah-nil′il-man-del′ik) VMA; 4-hydroxy-3-methoxymandelic acid, the primary end-product of catecholamine metabolism excreted in the urine. Urinary VMA levels are used in screening patients for pheochromocytoma.

Vanogel (van′o-jel) trademark for an aqueous suspension of aluminum hydroxide gel.

Vansil (van′sil) trademark for a preparation of oxamniquine.

Van Slyke's formula, etc. (van-slīks′) [Donald Dexter *Van Slyke*, American biochemist, 1883–1971] see under *formula*, *method*, and *tests*.

Van Slyke-Cullen method (test) (van-slik′-kul′en) [Donald D. *Van Slyke*; Glenn Ernest *Cullen*, American biochemist, 1890–1940] see under *method*.

Van Slyke-Fitz method (van-slik′fitz) [Donald D. *Van Slyke*; Reginald *Fitz*, American physician, 1885–1953] see under *method*.

van't Hoff's law, rule (vant hofs) [Jacobus Hendricus *van't Hoff*, Dutch chemist, 1852–1911; winner of the Nobel prize for chemistry in 1901] see under *law* and *rule*.

Vanzetti's sign (vahn-tset′ēz) [Tito *Vanzetti*, Italian surgeon, 1809–1888] see under *sign*.

vapor (va′por), pl. *vapo′res*, *va′pors* [L.] steam, gas, or exhalation.

vaporarium (va″po-rār′e-um) [L.] an establishment or apparatus for treating certain diseases by the use of vapors.

vaporium (va-po′re-um) [L.] vaporarium.

vaporization (va″por-i-za′shun) 1. the conversion of a solid or liquid into a vapor without chemical change; distillation. 2. treatment by vapors.

vaporize (va′por-īz) to convert into vapor or to be transformed into vapor.

vaporizer (va″por-i′zer) a device for producing an aerosol or mist, as from a solution containing a medication to ease breathing.

vapors (va′porz) an old term for hypochondriasis or hysterical depression.

vapotherapy (va″po-ther′ah-pe) the therapeutic use of vapor, steam, or spray.

Vaquez's disease (vak-āz′) [Louis Henri *Vaquez*, French physician, 1860–1936] polycythemia vera.

var. variety.

variability (var″e-ah-bil′ĭ-te) the state of being variable.

variable (va′re-ah-b′l) [L. *variare* to change] 1. changing from time to time. 2. in mathematics, a symbol that represents an arbitrary number or an arbitrary element of a set. **random v.,** an outcome of a random process that has a numerical value.

variance (vār′e-ans) in statistics, a measure of the variation shown by a set of observations: the average of the squared deviations from the mean; it is the square of the standard deviation (q.v.). Symbol σ^2.

variant (vār′e-ant) 1. something that differs in some characteristic from the class to which it belongs, as a variant of a disease, trait, species, etc. 2. exhibiting such variation. **L-phase v.,** a variant phase of certain bacteria, induced by osmotic shock, temperature shock, or the presence of antibiotics, and consisting of a spherical or ellipsoidal body without a rigid cell wall. The cells are capable of growth and multiplication; they may be stable or may revert to a normal bacterial cell. Called also *L-form*.

variate (va′re-āt) a variable or random variable.

variation (va″re-a′shun) in genetics, deviation in characters in an individual from those typical of the group to which it belongs; also, deviation in characters of the offspring from those of its parents. **allotypic v.,** the antigenic differences that characterize immunoglobulin allotypes. **antigenic v.,** 1. a mechanism whereby parasites, such as trypanosomes, plasmodia, and *Borrelia*, are enabled to escape immune surveillance of a host by modifying or completely altering their surface antigens. 2. a phenomenon occurring in the influenza virus, in which the virus spontaneously exhibits both slow antigenic drift and sharp antigenic changes at intervals. **continuous v.,** phenotypic differences so numerous and minute that the values selected for observation form a continuous spectrum, and no one phenotype or group of phenotypes predominates. **discontinuous v.,** phenotypic differences that are marked, do not grade into one another, and form two or more separate, discontinuous classes. **idiotypic v.,** the antigenic differences that characterize the different amino acid sequences and structures of immunoglobulin variable regions (idiotypes) and corresponding differences in antigen specificity. **impressed v.,** differences among individuals or groups arising from a particular environmental, nongenetic stimulus. **inborn v.,** one which arises from changes in the germ cells and not from the somatic cells. **isotypic v.,** the antigenic differences that characterize the immunoglobulin classes and subclasses (isotypes). **meristic v.,** variation in the number of parts in the offspring. **microbial v.,** the range of characteristics within a species used in identification and differentiation. **phenotypic v.,** the total range of variation, of whatever cause, observed in one character. **quasicontinuous v.,** variation in which the underlying distribution of variability is continuous but a threshold effect makes it appear discontinuous. **saltatory v.,** halmatogenesis. **smooth-rough (S-R) v.,** a genetic mutation or an adaptation seen in bacteria, most often evidenced by a change in the surface of colonies from smooth (S, glossy) to rough (R, dull). The change correlates with pathogenicity, S strains being generally more virulent and R strains less so. The cells in S colonies have polysaccharide capsules and are more antigenically complete; R cells contain little or no capsule. The term may also refer to changes in other cell structures such as flagella and somatic antigens, as well as susceptibility to bacteriophage. Variations are often reversible and tend to result in mixed types on repeated subculture. See also *bacterial dissociation*, under *dissociation*.

varication (var″ĭ-ka′shun) 1. the formation of a varix. 2. a varicose condition; a varicosity.

variceal (var″ĭ-se′al) pertaining to or caused by a varix.

varicella (var″ĭ-sel′ah) [L.] chickenpox. **v. gangreno′sa,** a rare form of chickenpox in which the eruption leads to a gangrenous ulceration, occurring mainly in children with leukemia or other severe underlying disease.

varicelliform (var″ĭ-sel′ĭ-form) resembling chickenpox (varicella); varicelloid.

varicelloid (var″ĭ-sel′oid) [*varicella* + Gr. *eidos* form] varicelliform.

varices (vār′ĭ-sēz) [L.] plural of *varix*.

variciform (var-is′ĭ-form) [*varix* + L. *forma* form] resembling a varix; varicose.

varic(o)- [L. *varix* a varicose vein] a combining form denoting relationship to a varix, or meaning twisted and swollen.

varicoblepharon (var″ĭ-ko-blef′ah-ron) [*varico-* + Gr. *blepharon* eyelid] a varicose swelling of the eyelid.

varicocele (var′ĭ-ko-sēl″) [*varico-* + Gr. *kēlē* tumor] a varicose condition of the veins of the pampiniform plexus, forming a swelling that feels like a "bag of worms," appearing bluish through the skin of the scrotum, and accompanied by a constant pulling, dragging, or dull pain in the scrotum. **ovarian v., pelvic v.,** a varicose condition of the veins of the broad ligament. **utero-ovarian v.,** a varicose condition of the veins of the pampiniform plexus of the female.

varicocelectomy (var″ĭ-ko-sĕ-lek′to-me) [*varicocele* + Gr. *ektomē* excision] ligation and excision of the enlarged veins for varicocele.

varicography (var″ĭ-kog′rah-fe) [*varico-* + Gr. *graphein* to write] roentgenological visualization of varicose veins.

varicoid (var′ĭ-koid) [*varico-* + Gr. *eidos* form] resembling a varix.

varicole (var′ĭ-kōl) varicocele.

varicomphalus (var″ĭ-kom′fah-lus) [*varico-* + Gr. *omphalos* navel] a varicose tumor at the umbilicus.

varicophlebitis (var″ĭ-ko-fle-bi′tis) varicose veins with inflammation.

varicose (var′ĭ-kōs) [L. *varicosus*] of the nature of or pertaining to a varix; unnaturally and permanently distended: said of a vein; variciform.

varicosis (var″ĭ-ko′sis) [L.] a varicose condition of the veins of any part.

varicosity (var″ĭ-kos′ĭ-te) 1. a varicose condition; the quality or fact of being varicose; varication. 2. a varix or varicose vein.

varicotomy (var″ĭ-kot′o-me) [*varico-* + Gr. *tomē* a cutting] incision into a varix or a varicose vein.

varicula (vah-rik′u-lah) [L.] a varix of the conjunctiva.

Varidase (var′ĭ-dās) trademark for preparations of streptokinase-streptodornase.

variety (vah-ri′ĕ-te) in taxonomy, a subcategory of a species.

variola (vah-ri′o-lah) [L.] smallpox. **v. capri′na,** goatpox. **v. haemorha′gica,** hemorrhagic smallpox. **v. ma′jor,** the classic severe form of smallpox, characterized by a very high case fatality rate (about 20 to 50%), cf. *v. minor.* **v. mi′nor,** a mild form of smallpox confined to certain parts of the world such as South America and West Africa, associated with a much lower case fatality (about 1 to 2%) rate than classic smallpox (*v. major*). It has many synonyms and local names, including *alastrim, cottonpox, Cuban itch, milk pox,* and *whitepox.* **v. ovi′na,** sheeppox. **v. si′ne eruptio′ne,** modified smallpox in which no rash is present.

variolar (vah-ri′o-lar) pertaining to smallpox; variolic.

Variolaria amara (va″re-o-la′re-ah ah-ma′rah) a febrifugal and anthelmintic lichen of the Old World, which is a source of litmus.

variolate (va′re-o-lāt) 1. having the nature or appearance of smallpox. 2. to inoculate with smallpox virus.

variolation (va″re-o-la′shun) deliberate inoculation with the virus of unmodified smallpox to produce immunity to the naturally occurring disease. As practiced in the Orient in ancient times, the dried crusts of smallpox lesions were applied to the skin or nasal mucous membranes, or were ingested. The method employed in Europe in the eighteenth century consisted in subcutaneous injection of material from the lesions. Variolation is now used only experimentally in animals. **bovine v.** (*obs.*), inoculation of a calf with smallpox.

variolic (var″e-ol′ik) variolar.

varioliform (va″re-ol′ĭ-form) resembling smallpox.

variolization (va″re-o-li-za′shun) variolation.

varioloid (va′re-o-loid″) 1. modified small pox. 2. resembling smallpox; varioliform.

variolous (vah-ri′o-lus) pertaining to or of the nature of smallpox.

variolovaccine (vah-ri″o-lo-vak′sēn) (*obs.*) a vaccine obtained by vaccinating heifers with smallpox.

variolovaccinia (vah-ri″o-lo-vak-sin′e-ah) cowpox in the heifer caused by inoculation with smallpox.

varistor (va-ris′tor) a voltage-variable resistor; a resistor, usually a semiconductor, designed to change its resistance with the voltage applied across it.

varix (vār′iks), pl. *var′ices* [L.] an enlarged and tortuous vein, artery, or lymphatic vessel. **anastomotic v.,** a varix composed of intercommunicating channels. **aneurysmal v., aneurysmoid v.,** a markedly dilated tortuous vessel; sometimes used to denote a form of arteriovenous aneurysm in which the blood flows directly into a neighboring vein without the intervention of a connecting sac. Called also *Pott's aneurysm.* **arterial v.,** a racemose aneurysm or varicose artery. **cirsoid v.,** racemose aneurysm. **esophageal v.,** varicosities of the branches of the azygos vein which anastomose with tributaries of the portal vein in the lower esophagus, occurring in patients with portal hypertension. **lymph v., v. lymphat′icus,** a soft, lobulated swelling of a lymph node, resulting from obstruction and dilatation of the lymphatic vessels.

varnish (var′nish) 1. a solution of resin or of natural gum, such as copal or rosin, in a suitable solvent, such as acetone, ether, or chloroform, which is capable of hardening into a thin film. 2. cavity v. **cavity v.,** a cavity lining agent consisting of a solution of one or more natural or synthetic resins, gums, and rosin in an organic solvent such as chloroform, ethanol, acetone, or benzene; applied to the floor and walls of the prepared cavity.

varolian (vah-ro′le-an) 1. described by or named for Costanzo *Varolius* (Varoli, Varolio), Italian anatomist and surgeon, 1543–1575. 2. pertaining to the pons.

Varolius' bridge, valve (vah-ro′le-us) [Costanzo *Varolius* (Varoli, Varolio), Italian anatomist, 1543–1575] see *pons* (def. 2) and *valva ileocecalis.*

varus (va′rus) [L. "knock-kneed"] bent inward; denoting a deformity in which the angulation of the part is toward the midline of the body, as talipes varus. The term varus is an adjective and should be used only in connection with the noun it describes, as talipes varus, genu varum, coxa vara. The meanings of *varus* and *valgus* are often reversed, so that genu verum is bowleg, not knock-knee. Cf. *valgus*.

vas (vas), pl. *va′sa* [L.]   a vessel: any canal for carrying a fluid; [NA] a general term for such channels, especially those carrying blood, lymph, or spermatozoa. **v. aber′rans,** 1. a blind tubule sometimes connected with the epididymis; it is a vestigial mesonephric tubule.   2. any anomalous or unusual vessel. **va′sa aberran′tis hep′atis,** numerous vessels found in the inconstant fibrous appendix and in the capsule of the liver. **v. aber′rans of Roth,** see *ductuli aberrantes.* **va′sa afferen′tia,** vessels that convey fluid to a structure or part. **v. af′ferens glomer′uli,** NA alternative *arteriola glomerularis afferens.* **va′sa afferen′-tia lymphoglan′dulae,** vasa afferentia nodi lymphatici. **va′sa afferen′tia no′di lymphat′ici** [NA], afferent vessels of lymph node: lymphatic vessels that carry lymph to a lymph node, entering through the capsule. **v. anas-tomot′icum** [NA], anastomotic vessel: a vessel that serves to interconnect other vessels; such communications are present in the palm of the hand, sole of the foot, base of the brain, and other regions. **va′sa au′ris inter′nae** [NA], vessels of the internal ear. **va′sa bre′via,** arteriae gastricae breves. **v. capilla′re** [NA], a capillary: any of the minute vessels connecting the arterioles and the venules, forming networks found in nearly all parts of the body. Their walls act as semipermeable membranes for the interchange of various substances between the blood and tissue fluid. See also *continuous capillaries* and *fenestrated capillaries,* under *capillary.* **v. collatera′le** [NA], collateral vessel: a vessel that parallels another vessel, nerve, or other structure. **v. def′erens,** ductus deferens. **va′sa efferen′tia,** efferent vessels: vessels that convey fluid away from a structure or part; see *vasa efferentia nodi lymphatici* and *ductuli efferentes testis.* **v. ef′ferens glomer′uli,** NA alternative for *arteriola glomerularis efferens.* **va′sa efferen′tia lymphoglan′dulae,** vasa efferentia nodi lymphatici. **va′sa efferen′tia no′di lymphat′ici** [NA], efferent vessels of lymph node: lymphatic vessels that carry lymph away from a lymph node, emerging at the hilus. **v. epididym′idis,** ductus epididymidis. **va′sa intesti′ni ten′uis,** arteriae intestinales. **v. lymphat′icum** [NA], a vessel that conveys lymph; pl. **va′sa lymphat′ica** [NA], lymphatic vessels: collectively, the lymphocapillary vessels, collecting vessels, and trunks which collect lymph from the tissues and through which the lymph passes to reach the bloodstream. **v. lymphat′icum profun′dum** [NA], deep lymphatic vessel: any lymphatic vessel that drains lymph from deep body structures; deep lymphatic vessels accompany the deeply placed blood vessels. **v. lym-phat′icum superficia′le** [NA], superficial lymphatic vessel: any lymphatic vessel located under the skin and superficial fascia, in the submucous areolar tissue of the digestive, respiratory, and genitourinary tracts, and in the subserous tissue of the walls of the abdomen and thorax. **v. lym-phocapilla′re** [NA] lymphocapillary vessel: one of the minute vessels of the lymphatic system, having a caliber greater than a blood capillary; they form closed networks (sing. *rete lymphocapillare*) by which they communicate freely with one another. **va′sa nervo′rum,** blood vessels supplying the nerves. **va′sa nutri′tia,** see *vasa vasorum.* **va′sa prae′via,** presentation, in front of the fetal head during labor, of the blood vessels of the umbilical cord where they enter the placenta. **v. prom′inens duc′tus cochlea′ris** [NA], a small vessel often seen deep to the spiral prominence in the cochlear duct. **va′sa pro′pria of Jungbluth,** vessels situated beneath the amnion of the early embryo. **va′sa rec′ta** [L. "straight vessels"], NA alternative for *arteriolae rectae renis.* **va′sa sanguin′ea integumen′ti commu′nis,** the blood vessels of the skin, or common integument. **va′sa san-gui′nea re′tinae,** the blood vessels of the retina, including all the arterioles, derived from the central artery of the retina, and the venules, which return blood to the central vein. **v. sinusoi′deum** [NA], sinusoidal vessel: a thin-walled vascular channel of larger caliber and more tortuous than a capillary; it has a lining of reticuloendothelium but little or no adventitia; such vessels are found instead of capillaries in such organs as the liver, spleen, bone marrow, carotid and coccygeal bodies, adenohypophysis, adrenal cortex, and parathyroid glands, and are also found in the heart. Called also *sinusoid* and *sinusoidal capillary.* **v. spira′le** [NA], a prominent vessel in the basilar mem-

brane near the osseous spiral lamina. **va′sa vaso′rum** [NA], the small nutrient arteries and the veins in the walls of the larger blood vessels. **va′sa vortico′sa,** venae vorticosae.

vasa (va′sah) [L.]   plural of *vas.*

Vasal (vas′al)   trademark for a preparation of papaverine hydrochloride.

vasal (va′sal)   pertaining to a vas or to a vessel.

vasalgia (vah-sal′je-ah)   pain in vessels.

vasalium (vah-sa′le-um)   true vascular tissue, such as is found in closed or vascular organs.

Vascoray (vas′ko-ra)   trademark for a preparation of iothalamate meglumine and iothalamate sodium.

vascular (vas′ku-lar)   pertaining to blood vessels or indicative of a copious blood supply.

vascularity (vas″ku-lar′ĭ-te)   the condition of being vascular.

vascularization (vas″ku-lar-ĭ-za′shun)   the process of becoming vascular, or the natural or surgically induced development of vessels in a tissue.

vascularize (vas′ku-lar″īz)   to supply with vessels.

vasculature (vas′ku-lah-tūr)   the vascular system of the body or any part of it.

vasculitic (vas″ku-lit′ik)   pertaining to vasculitis.

vasculitis (vas″ku-li′tis) [L. *vasculum* vessel + *-itis*]   inflammation of a vessel; angiitis. **allergic v.,** hypersensitivity v. **hypersensitivity v.,** a group of systemic necrotizing vasculitides thought to represent hypersensitivity to an antigenic stimulus, such as a drug, infectious agent, or exogenous or endogenous protein; all disorders in this group involve the small vessels. Called also *allergic* or *leukocytoclastic v.* and *leukocytoclastic angiitis.* **leukocytoclastic v.,** hypersensitivity v. **livedo v.,** segmented hyalinizing v. **necrotizing v.,** any of a group of disorders characterized by inflammation and necrosis of blood vessels occurring in a broad spectrum of cutaneous and systemic disorders. Called also *necrotizing angiitis.* **nodular v.,** a chronic vasculitis of unknown etiology found predominantly below the knees, especially on the calves in young and middle-aged women, which is characterized by the presence of painful, reddish blue nodular lesions that may ulcerate, leaving scars, or resorb, leaving atrophic depressions. In the late stages, there is replacement of the subcutaneous fat by fibrosis and atrophy (*wucher atrophy*). See also *erythema induratum.* **segmented hyalinizing v.,** chronic relapsing vasculitis of the lower legs, the lesions being nodular or purpuric, or both, at the onset and later becoming superficially ulcerated, resulting in scars; histologically, endothelial proliferations, hyaline degeneration, and thrombosis are seen in the mid and lower dermis. It usually affects middle-aged persons with circulatory difficulties. Called also *livedo v.*

vasculogenesis (vas″ku-lo-jen′ĕ-sis) [L. *vasculum* vessel + Gr. *genesis* production]   the development of the vascular system.

vasculogenic (vas″ku-lo-jen′ik)   inducing vascularization.

vasculolymphatic (vas″ku-lo-lim-fat′ik)   pertaining to blood or lymph vessels.

vasculomotor (vas″ku-lo-mo′tor)   vasomotor.

vasculopathy (vas″ku-lop′ah-the)   any disorder of blood vessels.

vasculotoxic (vas″ku-lo-tok′sik)   pertaining to or characterized by a deleterious or toxic effect on the vessels of the body.

vasculum (vas′ku-lum), gen. *vas′culi,* [L., dim. of *vas*]   a small vessel. **v. aber′rans,** vas aberrans.

vasectomized (vas-ek′to-mīzd)   having undergone removal of the ductus deferentes (vasa deferentia) by surgical means.

vasectomy (vah-sek′to-me) [*vas* + Gr. *ektomē* excision]   surgical removal of the ductus (vas) deferens, or of a portion of it; done in association with prostatectomy, or to induce infertility. **cross-over v.,** vasectomy in which the right and the left vas deferens are transected, the lower portion of each (the portions still attached to the epididymis) then being tied together. The technique prevents recanalization while allowing surgical reconstruction.

vasifactive (vas″ĭ-fak′tiv) [*vas* + L. *facere* to make]   vasoformative.

vasiform (vas'ĭ-form) [*vas* + L. *forma* form] having the appearance of a vessel.

vasitis (vah-si'tis) inflammation of the ductus (vas) deferens.

vas(o)- [L. *vas* vessel] a combining form denoting relationship to a vessel or to a duct.

vasoactive (vas''o-ak'tiv) exerting an effect upon the caliber of blood vessels.

vasoconstriction (vas''o-kon-strik'shun) the diminution of the caliber of vessels, especially constriction of arterioles leading to decreased blood flow to a part.

vasoconstrictive (vas''o-kon-strik'tiv) pertaining to, characterized by, or producing vasoconstriction.

vasoconstrictor (vas''o-kon-strik'tor) 1. causing constriction of the blood vessels. 2. an agent (motor nerve or chemical compound) that causes constriction of the blood vessels.

vasocorona (vas''o-ko-ro'nah) [*vaso-* + L. *corona* crown] the arterial vessels which pass radially from the spinal cord to its periphery.

vasodentin (vas''o-den'tin) [*vaso-* + L. *dens* tooth] dentin provided with blood vessels, as in the teeth of some fishes.

vasodepression (vas''o-de-presh'un) decrease in vascular resistance with hypotension.

vasodepressor (vas''o-de-pres'sor) 1. having the effect of lowering the blood pressure through reduction in peripheral resistance. 2. an agent that causes vasodepression.

Vasodilan (vas''o-di'lan) trademark for preparations of isoxsuprine hydrochloride.

vasodilatation (vas''o-di-lah-ta'shun) a state of increased caliber of the blood vessels.

vasodilatin (vas''o-di-la'tin) (*obs.*) a substance obtained from tissue extracts, causing vasodilation and stimulating gastric secretion; possibly identical with *histamine*.

vasodilation (vas''o-di-la'shun) dilation of a vessel, especially dilation of arterioles leading to increased blood flow to a part. **reflex v.,** vasodilation occurring as a reflex response to stimuli applied elsewhere, or subsequent to an initial vasoconstrictive response.

vasodilative (vas''o-di'la-tiv) pertaining to, characterized by, or producing vasodilatation.

vasodilator (vas''o-di-lāt'or) 1. causing dilation of the blood vessels. 2. an agent (motor nerve or chemical compound) that causes dilation of the blood vessels.

vasoepididymography (vas''o-ep''ĭ-did''ĭ-mog'rah-fe) radiography of the vas deferens and epididymis after injection of a contrast medium.

vasoepididymostomy (vas''o-ep''ĭ-did-ĭ-mos'to-me) operative formation of a communication between the ductus (vas) deferens and the epididymis.

vasofactive (vas''o-fak'tiv) vasoformative.

vasoformative (vas''o-for'mah-tiv) pertaining to or promoting the formation of blood vessels.

vasoganglion (vas''o-gang'gle-on) any vascular ganglion or rete.

vasography (vah-sog'rah-fe) [*vaso-* + Gr. *graphein* to write] roentgenography of the blood vessels.

vasohypertonic (vas''o-hi''per-ton'ik) vasoconstrictor.

vasohypotonic (vas''o-hi''po-ton'ik) vasodilator.

vasoinert (vas''o-in-ert') exerting no effect on the caliber of blood vessels.

vasoinhibitor (vas''o-in-hib'ĭ-tor) an agent that inhibits the action of the vasomotor nerves.

vasoinhibitory (vas''o-in-hib'ĭ-tor-e) hindering the action of the vasomotor nerves.

vasoligation (vas''o-li-ga'shun) ligation of the ductus (vas) deferens.

vasomotion (vas''o-mo'shun) [*vaso-* + L. *motio* movement] change in the caliber of a vessel, especially of a blood vessel.

vasomotor (vas-o-mo'tor) [*vaso-* + L. *motor* mover] 1. affecting the caliber of a vessel, especially of a blood vessel. 2. any element or agent that affects the caliber of a blood vessel.

vasomotorial (vas''o-mo-to're-al) 1. pertaining to the vasomotorium. 2. pertaining to the change in caliber of a blood vessel.

vasomotoricity (vas''o-mo-tor-is'ĭ-te) the power of producing change in the caliber of blood vessels.

vasomotorium (vas''o-mo-to're-um) the vasomotor system of the body, i.e., the part of the nervous system that controls the caliber of blood vessels.

vasomotory (vas''o-mo'tor-e) affecting the caliber of a vessel, especially a blood vessel.

vasoneuropathy (vas''o-nu-rop'ah-the) a combined vascular and neurologic defect, the lesions being caused by simultaneous action of both the vascular and the nervous systems, or by the interaction of the two systems.

vasoneurosis (vas''o-nu-ro'sis) angioneuropathy.

vaso-orchidostomy (vas''o-or''kid-os'to-me) the operation of suturing tubules of the epididymis to the ductus (vas) deferens.

vasoparesis (vas''o-pah-re'sis) [*vaso-* + Gr. *paresis* relaxation] partial paralysis of vasomotor nerves.

vasopermeability (vas''o-per''me-ah-bil'ĭ-te) the permeability of a blood vessel; the extent to which a blood vessel is permeable.

vasopressin (vas''o-pres'in) 1. one of two octapeptide hormones formed by the neuronal cells of the hypothalamic nuclei and stored in the posterior lobe of the pituitary gland (neurohypophysis), the other being oxytocin. It stimulates the contraction of the muscular tissue of the capillaries and arterioles, raising the blood pressure. It promotes contraction of the intestinal musculature and increases peristalsis, and also exerts some contractile influence on the uterus. It also has a specific effect on the epithelial cells of the distal portion of the uriniferous tubule, augmenting resorption of water independently of solutes, resulting in concentration of urine and dilution of blood serum. Its rate of secretion is regulated chiefly by the osmolarity of the plasma. 2. [USP], a pharmaceutical preparation of the same principle, prepared synthetically or obtained from the posterior pituitary of healthy domestic animals used for food by man; used mainly as an antidiuretic in the treatment of acute or chronic diabetes insipidus, administered intravenously, intramuscularly, or subcutaneously or by nasal inhalation or topical application to the nasal mucosa. It is also administered intramuscularly as a test of hypothalamo-neurohypophysial-renal function in distinguishing central from nephrogenic diabetes insipidus; it may also be used to stimulate smooth muscle tissue, especially to induce vasoconstriction in the presence of hemorrhage. Called also *antidiuretic hormone* (*ADH*) and formerly *beta-hypophamine*.

vasopressor (vas''o-pres'or) 1. stimulating contraction of the muscular tissue of the capillaries and arteries. 2. an agent that stimulates contraction of the muscular tissue of the capillaries and arteries.

vasopuncture (vas''o-punk'tūr) puncture of the ductus (vas) deferens.

vasoreflex (vas''o-re'flex) a reflex of a blood vessel.

vasorelaxation (vas''o-re-lak-sa'shun) decrease of vascular pressure.

vasoresection (vas''o-re-sek'shun) resection of the ductus (vas) deferens.

vasorrhaphy (vas-or'ah-fe) suture of the ductus (vas) deferens.

vasosection (vas''o-sek'shun) [*vaso-* + L. *sectio* a cutting] the severing of a vessel or vessels, especially of the ductus deferentes (vasa deferentia).

vasosensory (vas''o-sen'so-re) supplying sensory filaments to the vessels.

vasospasm (vas'o-spazm) spasm of the blood vessels, resulting in decrease in their caliber.

vasospasmolytic (vas''o-spaz''mo-lit'ik) arresting spasm of the vessels.

vasospastic (vas''o-spas'tik) producing or affected by vagospasm.

vasostimulant (vas''o-stim'u-lant) stimulating or arousing vasomotor action.

vasostomy (vah-sos'to-me) [*vas* deferens + Gr. *stomoun* to provide with an opening, or mouth] the operation of forming an opening into the ductus (vas) deferens.

vasotocin (vas''o-to'sin) a nonapeptide hormone having the properties of both vasopressin and oxytocin, occurring in the supraoptico-neurohypophysical unit of birds, amphibians, and fishes.

vasotomy (vah-sot′o-me) [*vaso-* + Gr. *tomē* a cutting] incision into or cutting of the ductus (vas) deferens.

vasotonia (vas″o-to′ne-ah) [*vaso-* + Gr. *tonos* tone + *-ia*] tone or tension of the vessels; called also *angiotonia*.

vasotonic (vas″o-ton′ic) pertaining to, characterized by, or promoting vasotonia.

vasotribe (vas′o-trīb) angiotribe.

vasotripsy (vas′o-trip″se) angiotripsy.

vasotrophic (vas″o-trof′ik) [*vaso-* + Gr. *trophē* nutrition] affecting nutrition through the alteration of the caliber of the blood vessels.

vasotropic (vas″o-trop′ik) tending to act on blood vessels.

vasovagal (vas″o-va′gal) vascular and vagal; see *vasovagal attack*, under *attack*.

vasovasostomy (vas″o-vah-sos′to-me) anastomosis of the ends of the severed ductus (vas) deferens; done to restore fertility in vasectomized males.

vasovesiculectomy (vas″o-ve-sik″u-lek′to-me) excision of the ductus (vas) deferens and seminal vesicles.

vasovesiculitis (vas″o-ve-sik″u-li′tis) inflammation of the ductus deferentes (vasa deferentia) and seminal vesicles.

Vasoxyl (vas-ok′sil) trademark for preparations of methoxamine hydrochloride.

vastus (vas′tus) [L.] great or vast; description of muscles, as musculus vastus lateralis.

VATER an acronym for *v*ertebral defects, imperforate *a*nus, *t*racheoesophageal fistula, and *r*adial and *r*enal dysplasia, which together form a nonrandom association of congenital defects.

Vater's ampulla, corpuscles, duct, papilla (fah′terz) [Abraham *Vater*, German anatomist, 1684–1751] see *ampulla hepatopancreatica, corpuscula lamellosa, ductus thyroglossalis,* and *papilla duodeni major.*

Vater-Pacini corpuscles (fah′ter-pa-se′ne) [Abraham *Vater*: Filippo *Pacini*, Italian anatomist, 1812–1883] corpuscula lamellosa.

Vateria (vah-te′re-ah) [named for A. *Vater*] a genus of Asian trees of the family Dipterocarpaceae. **V. in′dica** L., an East Indian tree which yields Indian copal, piny varnish, white dammar, or Indian anime; used as a varnish, candle-stuff, and medicine.

Vaughan-Novy's test [Victor Clarence *Vaughan,* American pathologist, 1851–1929; Frederick George *Novy,* American bacteriologist, 1864–1957] see under *tests.*

vault (vawlt) 1. any arched or domelike structure. See also *fornix.* 2. the longest palatal border obtainable through a coronal section of the maxilla. 3. a cavity or a prepared area within a bone for an implant. **v. of pharynx,** fornix pharyngis.

VC vital capacity.

VCG vectorcardiogram.

V-Cillin (ve-sil′in) trademark for preparations of penicillin V.

V.D. venereal disease; see also *sexually transmitted disease,* under *disease.*

VDEL Venereal Disease Experimental Laboratory.

V.D.H. valvular disease of the heart.

VDRL Venereal Disease Research Laboratories; see also under *antigen* and *test.*

vection (vek′shun) [L. *vectio* a carrying] the carrying of disease germs from an infected person to a well person. It is *circumferential, indirect,* or *mediate* when pathogens are carried by an intermediate host; *direct, immediate,* and *radial* when transferred directly from one person to another.

vectis (vek′tis) [L. from *vehere* to carry] a curved lever for making traction upon the fetal head in labor.

vector (vek′tor) [L. "one who carries," from *vehere* to carry] 1. a carrier, especially the animal (usually an arthropod) that transfers an infective agent from one host to another. 2. a plasmid or viral chromosome into whose genome a fragment of foreign DNA is inserted, used to introduce the foreign DNA into a host cell in the cloning of DNA. 3. a quantity possessing magnitude, direction, and sense (positivity or negativity), and commonly represented by a straight line resembling an arrow: the length of the line denotes magnitude, the

arrowhead denotes sense, and the position of the line with respect to an axis of reference denotes direction. **biological v.,** an animal vector in whose body the pathogenic organism develops and multiplies before being transmitted to the next host. **cloning v.,** a plasmid or viral chromosome so constructed that it will accept insertion of a foreign DNA fragment while retaining the ability to replicate. **mechanical v.,** an animal vector not essential to the life cycle of the parasite. **recombinant v.,** a vector into which a foreign DNA fragment has been inserted. **spatial v.,** one representing a three-dimensional force; see *vectorcardiography.*

vector-borne (vek′tor-born″) spread or transmitted from one host to another by a vector, as an infectious disease.

vectorcardiogram (vek″tor-kar′de-o-gram″) the record, usually a photograph, of the loop formed on the oscilloscope in vectorcardiography, the inscribed loop representing the ends of the instantaneous vectors.

vectorcardiograph (vek″tor-kar′de-o-graf) the instrument used in vectorcardiography.

vectorcardiography (vek″tor-kar″de-og′rah-fe) the registration, usually by formation of a loop display on an oscilloscope, of the direction and magnitude (vector) of the moment-to-moment electromotive forces of the heart during one complete cycle, as transmitted by electrocardiographic leads. **spatial v.,** that in which the potential vectors of cardiac excitation are projected upon three mutually perpendicular coordinates, usually designated X, Y, and Z, where X is the transverse (right or left), Y the vertical (up or down), and Z the sagittal (anterior or posterior).

vectorial (vek-to′re-al) pertaining to a vector.

vectorscope (vek′tor-skōp) a device utilized in viewing vectorcardiograms.

Vectrin (vek′trin) trademark for preparations of minocycline hydrochloride.

Vedder's culture medium (agar), sign (ved′erz) [Col. Edward Bright *Vedder,* U.S. Army Surgeon, 1878–1952] see under *culture medium,* and see under *sign.*

VEE Venezuelan equine encephalomyelitis.

Veetids (ve′tidz) trademark for a preparation of penicillin V potassium.

vegan (vej′an, ve′gan) an extreme vegetarian who excludes all animal protein from his diet.

veganism (vej′ah-nizm, ve′gah-nizm) strict limitation to a vegetable diet, with exclusion of all protein of animal origin.

vegetable (vej′e-tah-b′l) [L. *vegetabilis* quickening] 1. pertaining to or derived from plants. 2. any plant or species of plant, especially one cultivated as a source of food.

vegetal (vej′e-tal) 1. pertaining to plants or to a plant. 2. vegetative.

vegetality (vej″e-tal′ĭ-te) the aggregate of phenomena that are common to plants.

vegetarian (vej″e-tār′e-an) one whose food is exclusively of vegetable origin.

vegetarianism (vej″e-tār′e-ah-nizm″) restriction of the diet to food substances of vegetable origin.

vegetation (vej″e-ta′shun) [L. *vegetatio*] any plantlike fungoid neoplasm or growth; a luxuriant fungus-like growth of pathologic tissue. **adenoid v.,** fungus-like growths of lymphoid tissue in the nasopharynx. **bacterial v′s,** irregular excrescences on the cardiac valves or endocardium formed by bacteria. **dendritic v.,** 1. the shaggy appearance of a villous cancer. 2. the arachnoidal tufts and villous neoplasms on the pleura and other serous membranes. **verrucous v′s,** small irregular excrescences on the cardiac valves.

vegetative (vej′e-ta″tiv) 1. concerned with growth and with nutrition. 2. functioning involuntarily or unconsciously, as the vegetative nervous system; see under *system.* 3. resting; denoting the portion of a cell cycle during which the cell is not involved in replication. 4. of, pertaining to, or characteristic of plants. 5. of or pertaining to asexual reproduction, as by budding or fission.

vegetoanimal (vej″e-to-an′ĭ-mal) common to plants and animals.

vehicle (ve′ĭ-k′l) [L. *vehiculum*] 1. an excipient. 2. any medium through which an impulse is propagated.

veil (vāl) 1. a covering structure; see *velum.* 2. a caul or piece of the amniotic sac occasionally covering the face of a newborn child. 3. a slight huskiness in the voice of a singer. **Fick's v.,** see under *phenomenon.* **Hottentot v.,** see under *apron.* **Jackson's v.,** see under *membrane.* **Sattler's v.,** see *Fick's phenomenon.*

Veillon tube (va-yaw′) [Adrien *Veillon*, Paris bacteriologist, 1864–1931] see under *tube.*

Veillonella (va″yon-el′ah) [Adrien *Veillon*] a genus of bacteria of the family Veillonellaceae made up of small, gram-negative, anaerobic cocci occurring in pairs or short chains. They are found as nonpathogenic parasites in the mouth and intestines of humans and animals. The type species is *V. par′vula.*

Veillonellaceae (va″yon-el-a′se-e) a family of gram-negative, anaerobic, coccoid bacteria occurring in pairs and short chains. They are asporogenous nonmotile organisms found in the alimentary tract of humans, ruminants, rodents, and pigs. The family includes the genera *Acidaminococcus, Megasphaera,* and *Veillonella;* only *Veillonella* is of medical importance.

vein (vān) [L. *vena*] a vessel through which blood passes from various organs or parts back to the heart. Called also *vena* [NA]. All veins except the pulmonary veins carry blood low in oxygen. Veins, like arteries, have three coats, an *inner, middle,* and *outer,* but the coats are not so thick, and they collapse when the vessel is cut. Many have *valves* formed of reduplications of their lining membrane, which prevent the backward flow of blood away from the heart. See Plates accompanying the *Table of Venae,* under *vena.* **ac-**

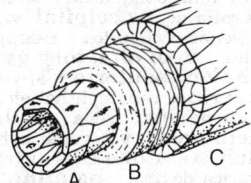

The three coats of a vein: *A,* tunica intima (endothelium); *B,* tunica media; *C,* tunica adventitia.

companying v., vena comitans. **accompanying v. of hypoglossal nerve,** vena comitans nervi hypoglossi. **adrenal v's,** venae suprarenales. **afferent v's,** veins that carry blood to an organ. **allantoic v's,** paired vessels that accompany the allantois, growing out from the primitive hindgut and entering the body stalk of the early embryo; they fuse later into one vessel, the umbilical vein. **anastomotic v., inferior,** vena anastomotica inferior. **anastomotic v., superior,** vena anastomotica superior. **angular v.,** vena angularis. **anonymous v's,** venae brachiocephalicae [dextra et sinistra]. **antebrachial v., median,** vena intermedia antebrachii. **appendicular v.,** vena appendicularis. **v. of aqueduct of cochlea,** vena aqueductus cochleae. **v. of aqueduct of vestibule,** vena aqueductus vestibuli. **aqueous v's,** microscopic, blood vessel–like pathways on the surface of the eye, containing aqueous humor or diluted blood and connecting the sinus venosus sclerae (Schlemm's canal) with conjunctival or subconjunctival veins. **arciform v's, arcuate v's of kidney,** venae arcuatae renis. **arterial v.,** truncus pulmonalis. **arterial v. of Soemmering,** vena portae. **articular v's,** venae articulares. **ascending v's of Rosenthal,** venae cerebri inferiores. **atrial v's of heart,** venae atriales cordis. **atrial v., lateral,** vena lateralis atrii. **atrial v., medial,** vena medialis atrii. **atrioventricular v's of heart,** venae atrioventriculares cordis. **auditory v's, internal,** venae labyrinthi. **auricular v's, anterior,** venae auriculares anteriores. **auricular v., posterior,** vena auricularis posterior. **axillary v.,** vena axillaris. **azygos v.,** vena azygos. **azygos v., left,** vena hemiazygos. **azygos v., lesser superior,** vena hemiazygos accessoria. **basal v.,** vena basilis. **basilic v.,** vena intermedia basilica. **basilic v., median,** vena intermedia basilica. **basivertebral v's,** venae basivertebrales. **brachial v's,** venae brachiales. **brachiocephalic v's,** venae brachiocephalicae [dextra et sinistra]. **Breschet's v's,** venae diploicae. **bronchial v's,** venae bronchiales. **Browning's v.,** the upper portion of the inferior anastomotic vein. **v. of bulb of penis,** vena bulbi penis. **v. of bulb of vestibule,** vena bulbi vestibuli. **Burow's v.,** a vessel formed

by the two inferior epigastric veins and a branch from the bladder; it joins the portal vein. **v. of canaliculus of cochlea,** vena canaliculi cochleae. **cardiac v's,** venae cordis. **cardiac v's, anterior,** venae cardiacae anteriores. **cardiac v., great,** vena cardiaca magna. **cardiac v., middle,** vena cardiaca media. **cardiac v., small,** vena cardiaca parva. **cardiac v's, smallest,** venae cardiacae minimae. **cardinal v's,** embryonic vessels that include the precardinal and postcardinal veins and the ducts of Cuvier (common cardinal veins). **carotid v., external,** vena retromandibularis. **v's of caudate nucleus,** venae nuclei caudati. **cavernous v's of penis,** venae cavernosae penis. **central v.,** a vein that occupies the axis of an organ. **central v's of hepatic lobules, central v's of liver,** venae centrales hepatis. **central v. of retina,** vena centralis retinae. **central v. of suprarenal gland,** vena centralis glandulae suprarenalis. **cephalic v.,** vena cephalica. **cephalic v., accessory,** vena cephalica accessoria. **cephalic v., median,** vena intermedia cephalica. **cerebellar v's,** venae cerebelli. **cerebellar v's, inferior,** see *venae cerebelli.* **cerebellar v's, superior,** see *venae cerebelli.* **v's of cerebellar hemisphere, inferior,** venae inferiores hemispherii cerebelli. **v's of cerebellar hemisphere, superior,** venae superiores hemispherii cerebelli. **cerebral v's,** venae cerebri. **cerebral v's, anterior,** vena anteriores cerebri. **cerebral v's, deep,** venae profundae cerebri. **cerebral v., great,** vena magna cerebri. **cerebral v's, inferior,** venae inferiores cerebri. **cerebral v's, internal,** venae internae cerebri. **cerebral v., middle, deep,** vena media profunda cerebri. **cerebral v., middle, superficial,** vena media superficialis cerebri. **cerebral v's, superficial,** venae superficiales cerebri. **cerebral v's, superior,** venae superiores cerebri. **cervical v., deep,** vena cervicalis profunda. **cervical v's, transverse,** venae transversae cervici. **choroid v., inferior,** vena choroidea inferior. **choroid v., superior,** vena choroidea superior. **ciliary v's,** venae ciliares. **ciliary v's, anterior,** see *venae ciliares.* **ciliary v's, posterior,** 1. see *venae ciliares.* 2. venae vorticosae. **circumflex femoral v's, lateral,** venae circumflexae laterales femoris. **circumflex femoral v's, medial,** venae circumflexae mediales femoris. **circumflex iliac v., deep,** vena circumflexa profunda iliaca. **circumflex iliac v., superficial,** vena circumflexa superficialis ilium. **v. of cochlear canaliculus,** vena aqueductus cochleae. **colic v., left,** vena colica sinistra. **colic v., middle,** vena colica media. **colic v., right,** vena colica dextra. **communicating v's,** perforating v's. **conjunctival v's,** venae conjunctivales. **coronary v., left,** vena cordis magna. **v. of corpus callosum, dorsal,** vena dorsalis corporis callosi. **v. of corpus callosum, posterior,** vena posterior corporis callosi. **costoaxillary v's,** venae costoaxillares. **cubital v., median,** vena intermedia cubiti. **cutaneous v.,** vena cutanea. **cutaneous v., ulnar,** vena basilica. **cystic v.,** vena cystica. **deep v.,** vena profunda. **deep v's of clitoris,** venae profundae clitoridis. **deep v's of penis,** venae profundae penis. **deep v. of thigh,** vena profunda femoris. **deep v. of tongue,** vena profunda linguae. **digital v's, palmar,** venae digitales palmares. **digital v's, plantar,** venae digitales plantares. **digital v's of foot, common,** venae digitales communes pedis. **digital v's of foot, dorsal,** venae digitales dorsales pedis. **diploic v's,** venae diploicae. **diploic v., frontal,** vena diploica frontalis. **diploic v., occipital,** vena diploica occipitalis. **diploic v., temporal, anterior,** vena diploica temporalis anterior. **diploic v., temporal, posterior,** vena diploica temporalis posterior. **dorsal v. of clitoris, deep,** vena dorsalis profunda clitoridis. **dorsal v's of clitoris, superficial,** venae dorsales superficiales clitoridis. **dorsal v. of penis, deep,** vena dorsalis profunda penis. **dorsal v's of penis, superficial,** venae dorsales superficiales penis. **dorsal v's of tongue,** venae dorsales linguae. **dorsispinal v's,** see *plexus venosi vertebrales externi [anterior et posterior].* **duodenal v's,** venae duodenales. **emissary v.,** one passing through a foramen of the skull and draining blood from a cerebral sinus into a vessel outside the skull; called also *vena emissaria* [NA]. **emissary v., condylar,** vena emissaria condylaris. **emissary v., mastoid,** vena emissaria mastoidea. **emissary v., occipital,** vena emissaria occipitalis. **emissary v., parietal,** vena emissaria parietalis.

emulgent v., the portion of the left spermatic vein near its termination in the left renal vein. **v's of encephalic trunk,** venae trunci encephalici. **epigastric v., inferior,** vena epigastrica inferior. **epigastric v., superficial,** vena epigastrica superficialis. **epigastric v's, superior,** venae epigastricae superiores. **epiploic v., left,** vena gastro-omentalis sinistra. **epiploic v., right,** vena gastro-omentalis dextra. **episcleral v's,** venae episclerales. **esophageal v's,** venae oesophageales. **ethmoidal v's,** venae ethmoidales. **facial v.,** vena facialis. **facial v., anterior, facial v., common,** see *vena facialis.* **facial v., deep,** vena profunda faciei. **facial v., posterior,** vena retromandibularis. **facial v., transverse,** vena transversa faciei. **femoral v.,** vena femoralis. **femoral v., deep,** vena profunda femoris. **femoropopliteal v.,** vena femoropoplitea. **fibular v's,** venae fibulares. **frontal v's,** 1. venae frontales. 2. venae supratrochleares. **Galen's v's,** 1. venae cerebri internae. 2. vena cerebri magna. **gastric v., left,** vena gastrica sinistra. **gastric v., right,** vena gastrica dextra. **gastric v's, short,** venae gastricae breves. **gastroepiploic v., left,** vena gastro-omentalis sinistra. **gastroepiploic v., right,** vena gastro-omentalis dextra. **gastro-omental v., left,** vena gastro-omentalis sinistra. **gastro-omental v., right,** vena gastro-omentalis dextra. **genicular v's,** venae geniculares. **gluteal v's, inferior,** venae gluteae inferiores. **gluteal v's, superior,** venae gluteae superiores. **hemiazygos v.,** vena hemiazygos. **hemiazygos v., accessory,** vena hemiazygos accessoria. **hemorrhoidal v's, inferior,** venae rectales inferiores. **hemorrhoidal v's, middle,** venae rectales mediae. **hemorrhoidal v., superior,** vena rectalis superior. **hepatic v's, intermediate,** venae hepaticae intermediae. **hepatic v's, middle,** venae hepaticae intermediae. **hypogastric v.,** vena iliaca interna. **hypophyseoportal v's,** a system of venules connecting capillaries in the hypothalamus with sinusoidal capillaries in the anterior lobe of the hypophysis. **ileal v's,** venae ileales. **ileocolic v.,** vena ileocolica. **iliac v., common,** vena iliaca communis. **iliac v., external,** vena iliaca externa. **iliac v., internal,** vena iliaca interna. **iliolumbar v.,** vena iliolumbalis. **v's of inferior member, deep,** venae profundae membri inferioris. **v's of inferior member, superficial,** venae superficiales membri inferioris. **infralobar v.,** pars infralobaris. **infrasegmental v.,** pars intersegmentalis. **innominate v's,** venae brachiocephalicae [dextra et sinistra]. **insular v's,** venae insulares. **intercapitular v's of foot,** venae intercapitulares pedis. **intercapitular v's of hand,** venae intercapitulares manus. **intercostal v's, anterior,** venae intercostales anteriores. **intercostal v., highest,** vena intercostalis suprema. **intercostal v's, posterior,** venae intercostales posteriores. **intercostal v., superior, left,** vena intercostalis superior sinistra. **intercostal v., superior, right,** vena intercostalis superior dextra. **interlobar v's of kidney,** venae interlobares renis. **interlobular v's of kidney,** venae interlobulares renis. **interlobular v's of liver,** venae interlobulares hepatis. **intermediate v.,** vena colica media. **interosseous v's of foot, dorsal,** venae metatarseae dorsales. **interosseous metacarpal v's, dorsal,** venae metacarpeae dorsales. **intersegmental v.,** 1. pars intersegmentalis. 2. pars intralobaris. **intervertebral v.,** vena intervertebralis. **jejunal v's,** venae jejunales. **jugular v., anterior,** vena jugularis anterior. **jugular v., anterior horizontal,** arcus venosus juguli. **jugular v., external,** vena jugularis externa. **jugular v., internal,** vena jugularis interna. **v's of kidney,** venae renis. **Kohlrausch v's,** superficial veins passing from the under surface of the penis to the dorsal vein. **Krukenberg's v's,** venae centrales hepatis. **Kuhnt's postcentral v.,** a vein branching from the vena centralis retina, extending posteriorly from the center of the optic nerve, and draining into the canalis opticus. **Labbé's v.,** vena anastomotica inferior. **labial v's, anterior,** venae labiales anteriores. **labial v's, inferior,** venae labiales inferiores. **labial v's, posterior,** venae labiales posteriores. **labial v., superior,** vena labialis superior. **v's of labyrinth,** venae labyrinthi. **lacrimal v.,** vena lacrimalis. **laryngeal v., inferior,** vena laryngea inferior. **laryngeal v., superior,** vena laryngea superior. **lateral direct v's,** venae directae laterales. **v. of lateral recess of fourth ventricle,** vena

recessus lateralis ventriculi quarti. **v. of lateral ventricle, lateral,** vena lateralis atrii. **v. of lateral ventricle, medial,** vena medialis atrii. **lingual v.,** vena lingualis. **lingual v., deep,** vena profunda linguae. **lingual v's, dorsal,** venae dorsales linguae. **v's of lower member, deep,** venae profundae membri inferioris. **v's of lower member, superficial,** venae superficiales membri inferioris. **lumbar v's,** venae lumbales. **lumbar v., ascending,** vena lumbalis ascendens. **mammary v's, external,** venae costoaxillares. **mammary v., internal,** see *venae thoracicae internae.* **v. of Marshall, Marshall's oblique v.,** vena obliqua atrii sinistri. **masseteric v's,** venae massetericae. **maxillary v's,** venae maxillares. **median v. of elbow,** vena intermedia cubiti. **median v. of forearm,** vena intermedia antebrachii. **median v. of neck,** vena mediana colli. **mediastinal v's,** venae mediastinales. **v's of medulla oblongata,** venae medullae oblongatae. **meningeal v's,** venae meningeae. **meningeal v's, middle,** venae meningeae mediae. **mesencephalic v's,** venae trunci encephalici. **mesenteric v., inferior,** vena mesenterica inferior. **mesenteric v., superior,** vena mesenterica superior. **metacarpal v's, dorsal,** venae metacarpales dorsales. **metacarpal v's, palmar,** venae metacarpales palmares. **metatarsal v's, dorsal,** venae metatarsales dorsales. **metatarsal v's, plantar,** venae metatarsales plantares. **muscular v's,** venae musculares. **musculophrenic v's,** venae musculophrenicae. **nasal v's, external,** venae nasales externae. **nasofrontal v.,** vena nasofrontalis. **oblique v. of left atrium,** vena obliqua atrii sinistri. **obturator v's,** venae obturatoriae. **occipital v.,** vena occipitalis. **occipital v's,** venae occipitales. **oesophageal v's,** venae oesophageales. **v. of olfactory gyrus,** vena gyri olfactorii. **omphalomesenteric v's,** vitelline v's. **ophthalmic v., inferior,** vena ophthalmica inferior. **ophthalmic v., superior,** vena ophthalmica superior. **ophthalmomeningeal v.,** vena ophthalmomeningea. **ovarian v., left,** vena ovarica sinistra. **ovarian v., right,** vena ovarica dextra. **palatine v., palatine v., external,** vena palatina. **palpebral v's,** venae palpebrales. **palpebral v's, inferior,** venae palpebrales inferiores. **palpebral v's, superior,** venae palpebrales superiores. **pancreatic v's,** venae pancreaticae. **pancreaticoduodenal v's,** venae pancreaticoduodenales. **paraumbilical v's,** venae paraumbilicales. **parietal v's,** venae parietales. **parietal v. of Santorini,** vena emissaria parietalis. **parotid v's,** venae parotideae. **parotid v's, anterior,** rami parotidei venae facialis. **parotid v's, posterior,** venae parotideae. **parumbilical v's,** venae paraumbilicales. **peduncular v's,** venae pedunculares. **perforating v's,** veins that accompany the perforating arteries and connect superficial and deep veins; they are found in the thigh, lower part of the leg, and foot. Called also *communicating v's.* See also *venae perforantes* [NA]. **pericardiac v's,** venae pericardiales. **pericardiacophrenic v's,** venae pericardiacophrenicae. **peroneal v's,** venae fibulares. **petrosal v.,** vena petrosa. **pharyngeal v's,** venae pharyngeales. **phrenic v's, inferior,** venae phrenicae inferiores. **phrenic v's, superior,** venae pericardiacophrenicae. **v's of pons,** venae pontis. **pontomesencephalic v., anterior,** vena pontomesencephalica anterior. **popliteal v.,** vena poplitea. **portal v., portal v. of liver,** vena porta hepatis. **postcardinal v's,** paired vessels in the embryo caudal to the heart. **posterior v. of left ventricle,** vena posterior ventriculi sinistri cordis. **precardinal v's,** paired venous trunks in the embryo cranial to the heart. **precentral v. of cerebellum,** vena precentralis cerebelli. **prefrontal v's,** venae prefrontales. **prepyloric v.,** vena prepylorica. **primary head v's,** vessels alongside the embryonic brain that continue into the precardinal veins. **v. of pterygoid canal,** vena canalis pterygoidei. **pudendal v's, external,** venae pudendae externae. **pudendal v., internal,** vena pudenda interna. **pulmonary v's,** venae pulmonales. **pulmonary v., left inferior,** vena pulmonalis sinistra inferior. **pulmonary v., left superior,** vena pulmonalis sinistra superior. **pulmonary v., right inferior,** vena pulmonalis dextra inferior. **pulmonary v., right superior,** vena pulmonalis dextra superior. **pulp v's,** vessels draining the venous sinuses of the spleen. **pyloric v.,** vena gastrica dextra. **radial v's,** venae radiales. **radial v., exter-**

nal, of Soemmering, vena cephalica accessoria. **ra-nine v.**, vena sublingualis. **rectal v's, inferior,** venae rectales inferiores. **rectal v's, middle,** venae rectales mediae. **rectal v., superior,** vena rectalis superior. **renal v's,** venae renales. **retromandibular v.,** vena retromandibularis. **Retzius's v's,** veins from the walls of the intestine to the branches of the inferior vena cava. **Rosenthal's v.,** vena basalis. **Ruysch's v's,** venae vorticosae. **sacral v's, lateral,** venae sacrales laterales. **sacral v., middle,** vena sacralis mediana. **salvatella v.,** a small vein of the little finger and dorsum of the hand. **saphenous v., accessory,** vena saphena accessoria. **saphenous v., great,** vena saphena magna. **saphenous v., small,** vena saphena parva. **v's of Sappey,** venae paraumbilicales. **scleral v's,** venae sclerae. **scrotal v's, anterior,** venae scrotales anteriores. **scrotal v's, posterior,** venae scrotales posteriores. **v. of septum pellucidum, anterior,** vena anterior septi pellucidi. **v. of septum pellucidum, posterior,** vena posterior septi pellucidi. **sigmoid v's,** venae sigmoideae. **small v. of heart,** vena cordis parva. **spermatic v.,** vena spermatica. **spinal v's, anterior and posterior,** venae spinales anteriores/posteriores. **spiral v. of modiolus,** vena spiralis modioli. **splenic v.,** vena splenica. **stellate v's of kidney,** venulae stellatae renis. **Stensen's v's,** venae vorticosae. **sternocleido-mastoid v.,** vena sternocleidomastoidea. **striate v's,** venae thalamostriatae inferiores. **stylomastoid v.,** vena stylomastoidea. **subcardinal v's,** paired vessels in the embryo, replacing the postcardinal veins and persisting to some degree as definitive vessels. **subclavian v.,** vena subclavia. **subcostal v.,** vena subcostalis. **subcutaneous v's of abdomen,** venae subcutaneae abdominis. **sublingual v.,** vena sublingualis. **sublobular v's,** tributaries of the hepatic veins that receive the central veins of hepatic lobules. **submental v.,** vena submentalis. **superficial v.,** vena superficialis. **v's of superior member, deep,** venae profundae membri superioris. **v's of superior member, superficial,** venae superficiales membri superioris. **supracardinal v's,** paired vessels in the embryo, developing later than the subcardinal veins and persisting chiefly as the lower segment of the inferior vena cava. **supraorbital v.,** vena supraorbitalis. **suprarenal v., left,** vena suprarenalis sinistra. **suprarenal v., right,** vena suprarenalis dextra. **suprascapular v.,** vena suprascapularis. **supratrochlear v's,** venae supratrochleares. **sylvian v., v. of sylvian fossa,** vena cerebri media superficialis. **temporal v's, deep,** venae temporales profundae. **temporal v., middle,** vena temporalis media. **temporal v's, superficial,** venae temporales superficiales. **temporomandibular articular v's,** venae articulares. **terminal v.,** vena thalamostriata superior. **testicular v., left,** vena testicularis sinistra. **testicular v., right,** vena testicularis dextra. **thalamostriate v's, inferior,** venae thalamostriatae inferiores. **thalamostriate v., superior,** vena thalamostriata superior. **thebesian v's, v's of Thebesius,** venae cordis minimae. **thoracic v's, internal,** venae thoracicae internae. **thoracic v., lateral,** vena thoracica lateralis. **thoracoacromial v.,** vena thoracoacromialis. **thoracoepigastric v's,** venae thoracoepigastricae. **thymic v's,** venae thymicae. **thyroid v., inferior,** vena thyroidea inferior. **thyroid v's, middle,** venae thyroideae mediae. **thyroid v., superior,** vena thyroidea superior. **tibial v's, anterior,** venae tibiales anteriores. **tibial v's, posterior,** venae tibiales posteriores. **trabecular v's,** vessels coursing in splenic trabeculae, formed by tributary pulp veins. **tracheal v's,** venae tracheales. **transverse v. of face,** vena transversa faciei. **transverse v's of neck,** venae transversae colli. **Trolard's v.,** vena anastomotica superior. **tympanic v's,** venae tympanicae. **ulnar v's,** venae ulnares. **umbilical v.,** vena umbilicalis. **umbilical v., left,** vena umbilicalis sinistra. **v. of uncus,** vena unci. **v's of upper member, deep,** venae profundae membri superioris. **v's of upper member, superficial,** venae superficiales membri superioris. **uterine v's,** venae uterinae. **varicose v.,** a dilated tortuous vein, usually in the subcutaneous tissues of the leg; incompetency of the venous valves is associated. **ventricular v's of heart,** venae ventriculares cordis. **ventricular v., inferior,** vena ventricularis inferior. **v. of vermis, inferior,** vena inferior vermis. **v. of vermis,**

superior, vena superior vermis. **vertebral v.,** vena vertebralis. **vertebral v., accessory,** vena vertebralis accessoria. **vertebral v., anterior,** vena vertebralis anterior. **vertebral v's, superficial, v's of vertebral column, external,** see *plexus venosi vertebrales externi* [*anterior et posterior*]. **v's of vertebral column,** venae columnae vertebralis. **vesalian v.,** an emissary vein connecting the cavernous sinus with the pterygoid venous plexus, sometimes passing through an opening in the great wing of the sphenoid bone. **vesical v's,** venae vesicales. **vestibular v's,** venae vestibulares. **vidian v's, v's of Vieussens,** venae canalis pterygoidei. **v's of Vieussens,** venae cordis anteriores. **vitelline v's,** veins that return the blood from the yolk sac to the primitive heart of the early embryo. **vorticose v's,** venae vorticosae.

Veinamine (vān′ah-mēn) trademark for a crystalline amino acid solution for intravenous administration, containing a mixture of essential and nonessential amino acids but no peptides.

vela (ve′lah) [L.] plural of *velum*.

Velacycline (vel″ah-si′klēn) trademark for preparations of rolitetracycline.

velamen (ve-la′men), pl. *vela′mina* [L. "a covering"] a membrane, velum, meninx, or tegument. **v. vul′vae,** Hottentot apron.

velamenta (vel″ah-men′tah) [L.] plural of *velamentum*.

velamentous (vel″ah-men′tus) [L. *velamen* veil] membranous and pendent; like a veil.

velamentum (vel″ah-men′tum), pl. *velamen′ta* [L.] any covering, velum, or envelope. **velamen′ta cer′ebri,** the meninges.

velar (ve′lar) pertaining to a velum, especially to the velum palatinum (palatum molle).

Velban (vel′ban) trademark for a preparation of vinblastine sulfate.

veliform (vel′ĭ-form) velamentous.

Vella's fistula (ve′lahz) [Luigi *Vella,* Italian physiologist, 1825–1886] see under *fistula*.

vellosine (vel-lo′sin) a poisonous alkaloid occurring in yellow crystals, $C_{23}H_{28}N_2O_4$, from the bark of *Geissospermum laeve* (*vellosii*).

vellus (vel′us) [L. "fleece"] the fine hair which succeeds the lanugo over most of the body. **v. oli′vae,** a narrow band of tangential fibers surrounding the olive.

velocimetry (ve″lŏ-sim′ĕ-tre) measurement of speed. **laser-Doppler v.,** measurement of the flow of red cells in a microcirculatory bed by means of laser light delivered to and detected from the region of interest by fiberoptic probes.

velonoskiascopy (ve″lo-no-ski-as′ko-pe) belonoskiascopy.

velopharyngeal (vel″o-fah-rin′je-al) pertaining to the soft palate (velum palatinum) and pharynx; see also under *insufficiency* and *portal*.

Velosef (vel′o-sef) trademark for preparations of cephradine.

Velosulin (ve-lo′soo-lin) trademark for preparations of insulin injection (regular insulin).

Velpeau's bandage, deformity, hernia (vel-pōz′) [Alfred Armand Louis Marie *Velpeau,* surgeon in Paris, 1795–1867] see under *bandage* and *hernia,* and see *silver fork fracture,* under *fracture*.

velum (ve′lum), pl. *ve′la* [L.] a covering; [NA] a general term for a veil or veil-like structure. **artificial v.,** a prosthetic appliance used in correction of a cleft of the soft palate. **Baker's v.,** an obturator used in cleft palate. **v. interpos′itum cer′ebri,** tela choroidea ventriculi tertii. **v. medulla′re ante′rius,** NA alternative for *v. medullare rostralis.* **v. medulla′re cauda′le** [NA], caudal medullary velum: either of two thin layers of white substance, located on each side of the nodule of the vermis, the internal surface of which forms the lower wall of the laterodorsal recess of the fourth ventricle; on the sides it is continuous with the pedunculus flocculi and the taenia and ventrally it is fused with the choroid plexus. Called also *inferior* or *posterior medullary v., v. medullare inferius* [NA alternative], and *v. medullare posterius* [NA alternative]. **v. medulla′re infe′rius, v. medulla′re poste′rius,** NA alternatives for *v. medullare caudale.* **v. medulla′re rostra′lis** [NA], rostral medullary velum: a thin layer of white substance forming the roof of the cranial part of the fourth ventricle, and extending from the tectal lamina in front to the fastigium behind, and between the cranial cerebellar penduncles; called also *anterior, cranial,* or *superior medullary v., v. medullare anterius* [NA alternative], *v. medullaris cranialis,* and *v. medullare superius* [NA alternative]. **v. medulla're supe'rius,** NA alternative for *v. medullare rostralis.* **medullary v., anterior,** v. medullare rostralis. **medullary v., cranial,** v. medullare rostralis. **medullary v., inferior, medullary v., posterior,** v. medullare caudale. **medullary v., rostral, medullary v., superior,** v. medullare rostralis. **v.**

pala'ti, palatum molle. **v. palati'num,** NA alternative for *palatum molle.* **v. pen'dulum pala'ti,** palatum palati. **v. of Tarinus,** v. medullare inferius. **v. transver'sum,** a transverse fold of the tela choroidea marking the boundary between the diencephalon and the telencephalon in the embryonic brain.

vena (ve'nah), pl. *ve'nae* [L.] [NA]   vein: a vessel that conveys blood to or toward the heart, or from the heart itself to the right atrium. See *vein.* For names and descriptions of specific veins, see *Table of Venae* and accompanying Plates.

TABLE OF VENAE

Descriptions of veins are given on NA terms, and include anglicized names of specific veins.

ve'nae advehen'tes, channels in the early embryo that convey blood to the sinusoids of the liver and later become the portal vein.

v. anastomot'ica infe'rior [NA], inferior anastomotic vein: a vein that interconnects the superficial middle cerebral vein and the transverse sinus.

v. anastomot'ica supe'rior [NA], superior anastomotic vein: a vein that interconnects the superficial middle cerebral vein and the superior sagittal sinus.

v. angula'ris [NA], angular vein: a short vein between the eye and the root of the nose; it is formed by union of the supratrochlear and supraorbital veins and continues inferiorly as the facial vein.

ve'nae anon'ymae [dex'tra et sinis'tra], venae brachiocephalicae [dextra et sinistra].

ve'nae anterio'res cer'ebri [NA], anterior cerebral veins: veins that accompany the anterior cerebral artery and join the basal vein; called also *venae cerebri anteriores.*

v. ante'rior sep'ti pellu'cidi [NA], anterior vein of septum pellucidum: a vein that drains the anterior septum pellucidum into the superior thalamostriate vein; called also *v. septi pellucidi anterior.*

v. appendicula'ris [NA], appendicular vein: the vena comitans of the appendicular artery; it unites with the anterior and posterior cecal veins to form the ileocolic vein.

v. aqueduc'tus coch'leae [NA], vein of aqueduct of cochlea: a vein along the aqueduct of the cochlea that empties into the superior bulb of the internal jugular vein; called also *vein of cochlear canaliculus* and *v. canaliculi cochleae.*

v. aqueduc'tus vestib'uli [NA], vein of aqueduct of vestibule: a small vein from the internal ear that passes through the aqueduct of the vestibule and empties into the superior petrosal sinus.

ve'nae arcifor'mes re'nis, venae arcuatae renis.

ve'nae arcua'tae re'nis [NA], arcuate veins of kidney: a series of complete arches across the bases of the pyramids of the kidneys; they are formed by union of the interlobular veins and the venulae rectae and drain into the interlobar veins. Called also *venae arciformes renis.*

ve'nae articula'res temporomandib'ulae, venae articulares.

ve'nae articula'res [NA], articular veins: small vessels that drain the plexus around the temporomandibular articulation into the retromandibular vein; called also *temporomandibular articular veins* and *venae articulares temporomandibulae.*

ve'nae atria'les cor'dis [NA], the veins of the atria of the heart.

v. a'trii latera'lis, v. lateralis atrii.

v. a'trii media'lis, v. medialis atrii.

ve'nae atrioventricula'res cor'dis [NA], the veins that supply the atria and ventricles of the heart.

ve'nae auditi'vae inter'nae, venae labyrinthi.

ve'nae auricula'res anterio'res [NA], anterior auricular veins: branches from the anterior part of the pinna that enter the superficial temporal vein.

v. auricula'ris poste'rior   [NA], posterior auricular vein: a vein that begins in a plexus on the side of the head, passes down behind the pinna, and joins with the retromandibular vein to form the external jugular vein.

v. axilla'ris [NA], axillary vein; the venous trunk of the upper member; it begins at the lower border of the teres major muscle by junction of the basilic and brachial veins, and at the lateral border of the first rib is continuous with the subclavian vein.

v. az'ygos [NA], azygos vein: an intercepting trunk for the right intercostal veins as well as a connecting branch between the superior and inferior venae cavae: it arises from the ascending lumbar vein, passes up in the posterior mediastinum to the level of the fourth thoracic vertebra, where it arches over the root of the right lung (*arcus venae azygou*), and empties into the superior vena cava. See also *lobule of azygos vein.*

v. basa'lis [NA], basal vein: a vein that arises at the anterior perforated substance, passes backward and around the cerebral peduncle, and empties into the internal cerebral vein; called also *v. basalis [Rosenthali]*.

v. basa'lis [Rosentha'li], v. basalis.

v. basil'ica [NA], basilic vein: the superficial vein that arises from the ulnar side of the dorsal rete of the hand, passes up the forearm, and joins with the brachial veins to form the axillary vein.

ve'nae basivertebra'les [NA], basivertebral veins: venous sinuses in the cancellous tissue of the bodies of the vertebrae, which communicate with the plexus of veins on the anterior surface of the vertebrae and with the anterior internal vertebral plexus.

ve'nae brachia'les [NA], brachial veins: the venae comitantes of the brachial artery, which join with the basilic vein to form the axillary vein.

ve'nae brachiocephal'icae (dex'tra/sinis'tra) [NA], brachiocephalic veins: the two veins that drain blood from the head, neck, and upper extremities, and unite to form the superior vena cava. Each is formed at the root of the neck by union of the ipsilateral internal jugular and subclavian veins. The right vein (*v. brachiocephalica dextra*) passes almost vertically downward in front of the brachiocephalic artery, and the left vein (*v. brachiocephalica sinistra*) passes from left to right behind the upper part of the sternum. Each vein receives the vertebral, deep cervical, deep thyroid, and internal thoracic veins. The left vein also receives intercostal, thymic, tracheal, esophageal, phrenic, mediastinal, and pericardiac branches, as well as the thoracic duct. The right vein receives the right lymphatic duct. Called also *venae anonymae [dextra et sinistra]*.

ve'nae bronchia'les [NA], bronchial veins: vessels that drain blood from the larger subdivisions of the bronchi into the azygos vein on the left, and into the hemiazygos or the superior intercostal vein on the right.

ve'nae bronchia'les anterio'res, ve'nae bronchia'les posterio'res, see *venae bronchiales.*

v. bul'bi pe'nis [NA], vein of bulb of penis: a vein draining blood from the bulb of the penis into the internal pudendal vein.

v. bul'bi vestib'uli [NA], vein of bulb of vestibule: a vein draining blood from the bulb of the vestibule of the vagina into the internal pudendal vein.

v. canalic'uli coch'leae, v. aqueductus cochleae.

v. cana'lis pterygoi'dei [NA], vein of pterygoid canal: one of the veins that pass through the pterygoid canal and empty into the pterygoid plexus; called also *v. canalis pterygoidei [Vidii]*.

v. cana'lis pterygoi'dei [Vid'ii], v. canalis pterygoidei.

ve'nae cardi'acae anterio'res [NA], anterior cardiac veins: small vessels from the anterior wall of the right ventricle that empty into the right atrium or join the lesser cardiac vein; called also *venae cordis anteriores.*

v. cardi'aca mag'na [NA], great cardiac vein: a vein that collects blood from the anterior surface of the ventricles, follows the anterior longitudinal sulcus, and empties into the coronary sinus; called also *v. cordis magna.*

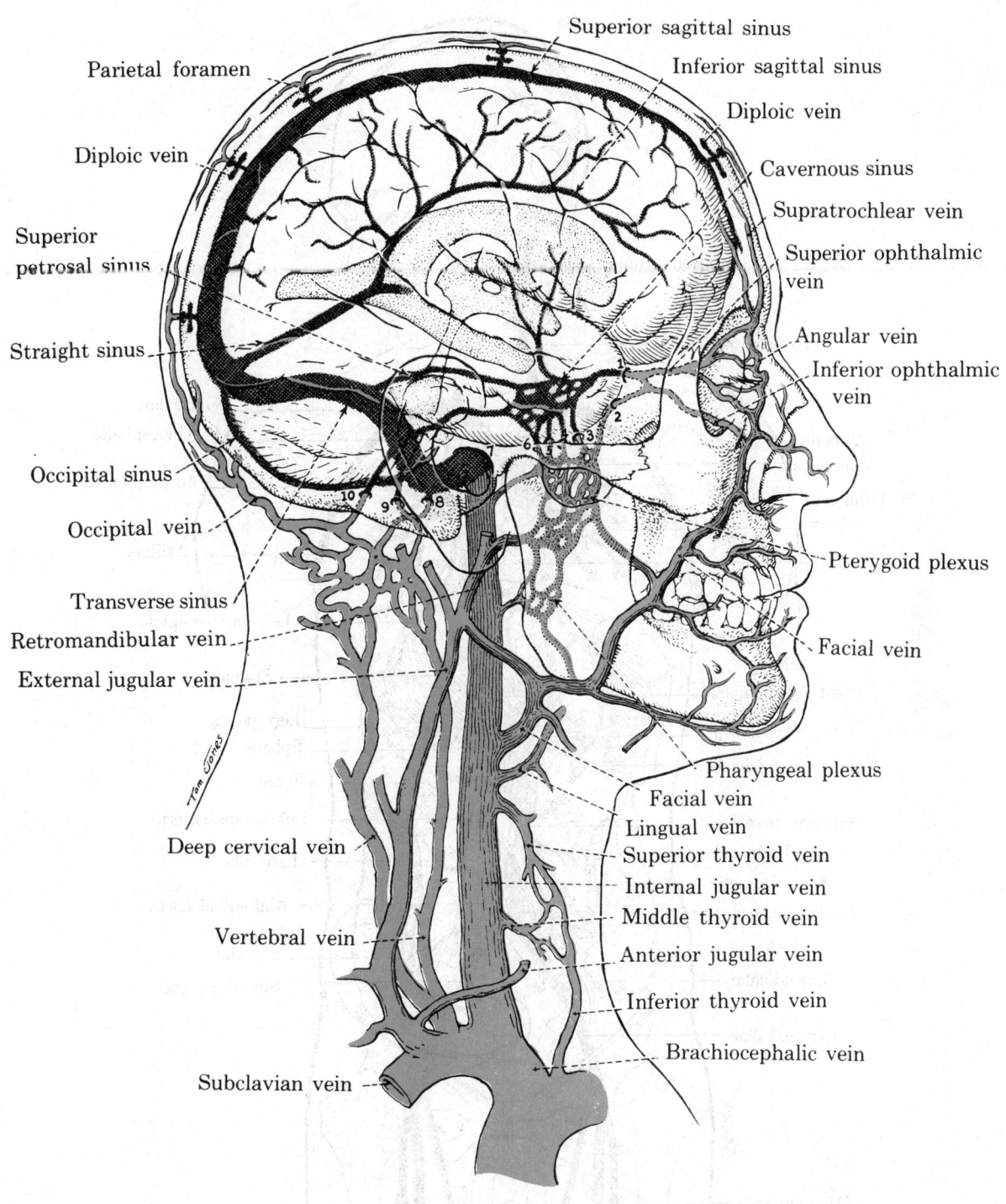

PLATE 48 — VEINS OF THE HEAD AND NECK

1815

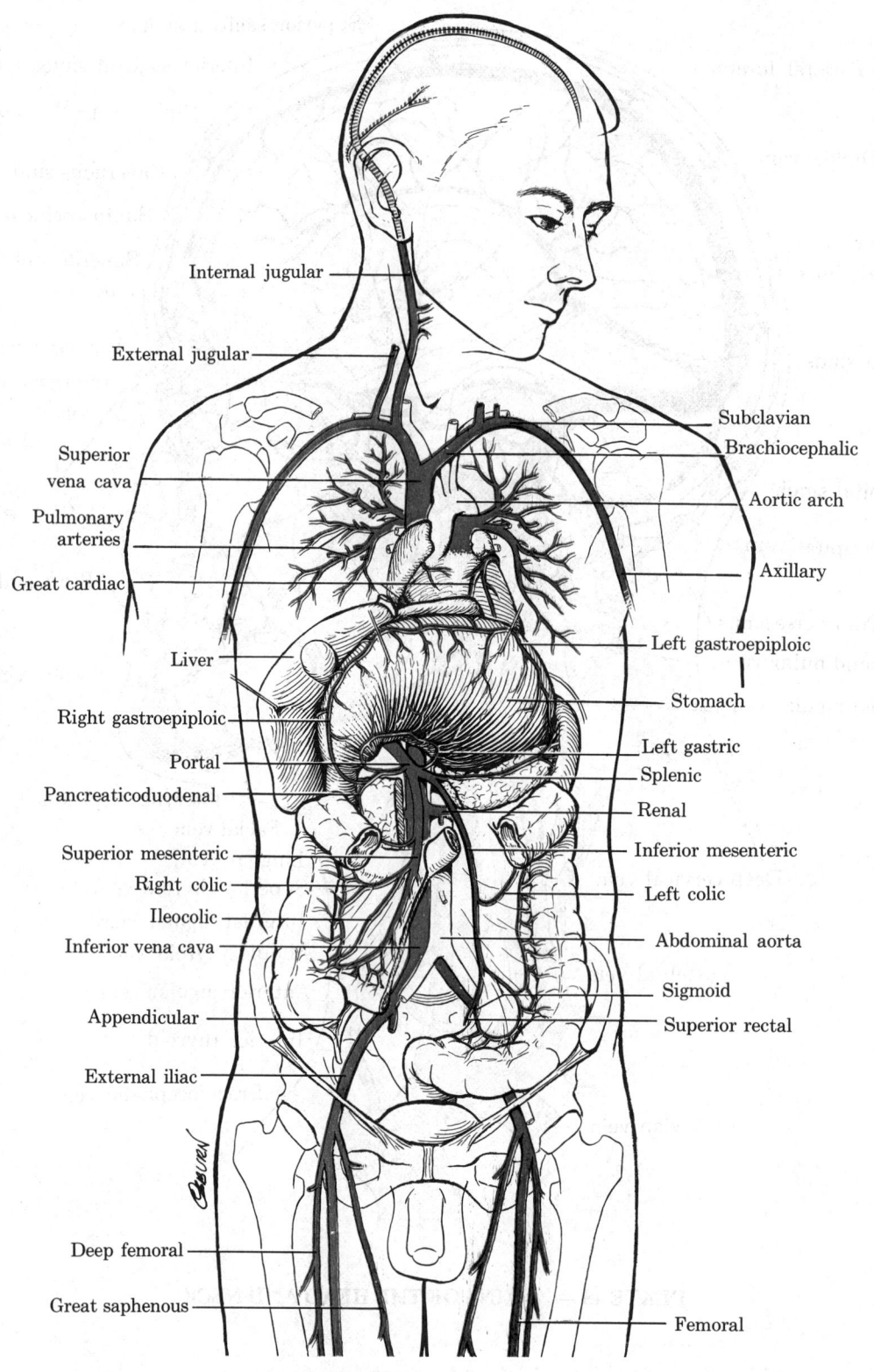

Internal jugular

External jugular

Superior
vena cava

Pulmonary
arteries

Great cardiac

Liver

Right gastroepiploic

Portal

Pancreaticoduodenal

Superior mesenteric

Right colic

Ileocolic

Inferior vena cava

Appendicular

External iliac

Deep femoral

Great saphenous

Subclavian

Brachiocephalic

Aortic arch

Axillary

Left gastroepiploic

Stomach

Left gastric

Splenic

Renal

Inferior mesenteric

Left colic

Abdominal aorta

Sigmoid

Superior rectal

Femoral

PLATE 49 —   PRINCIPAL VEINS OF THE BODY

1816

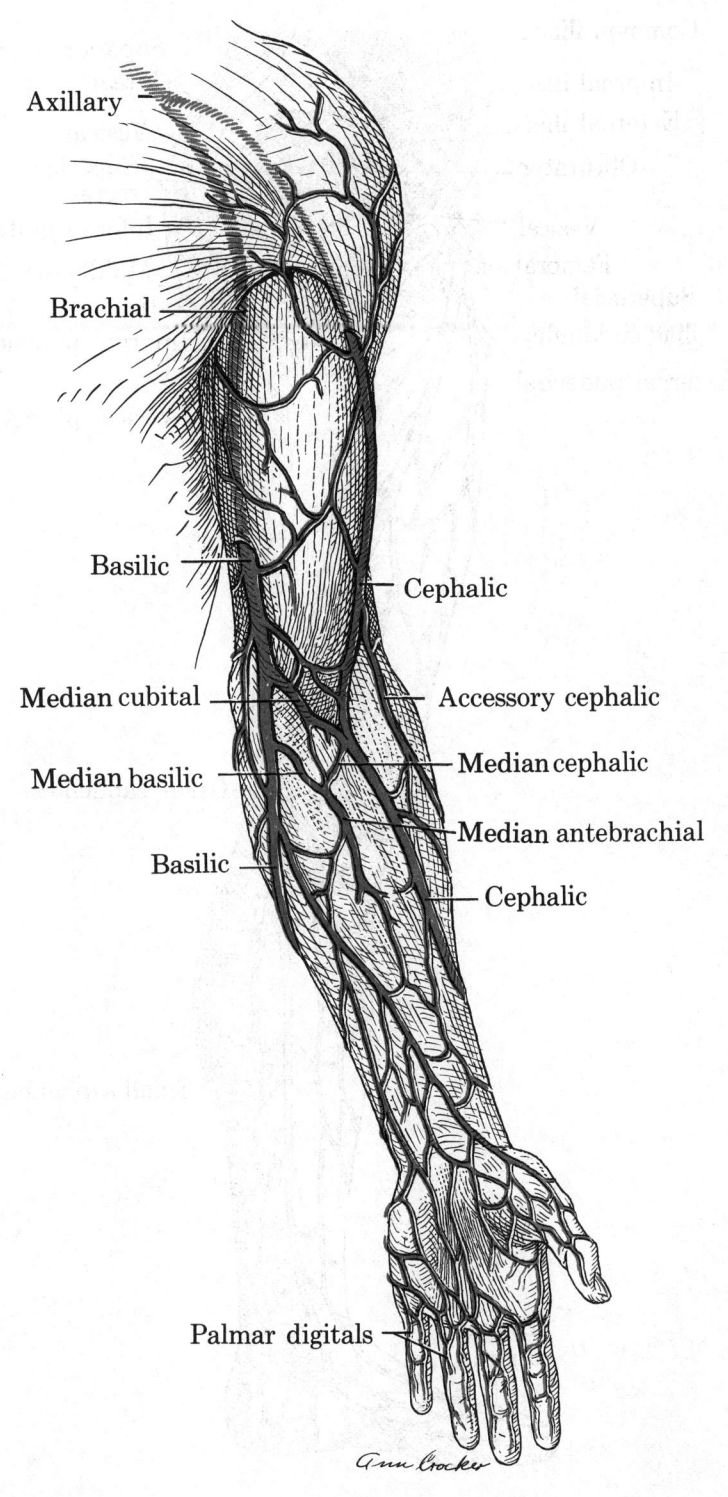

Axillary

Brachial

Basilic

Cephalic

Median cubital

Accessory cephalic

Median basilic

Median cephalic

Median antebrachial

Basilic

Cephalic

Palmar digitals

PLATE 50 — SUPERFICIAL VEINS OF THE UPPER EXTREMITY

1817

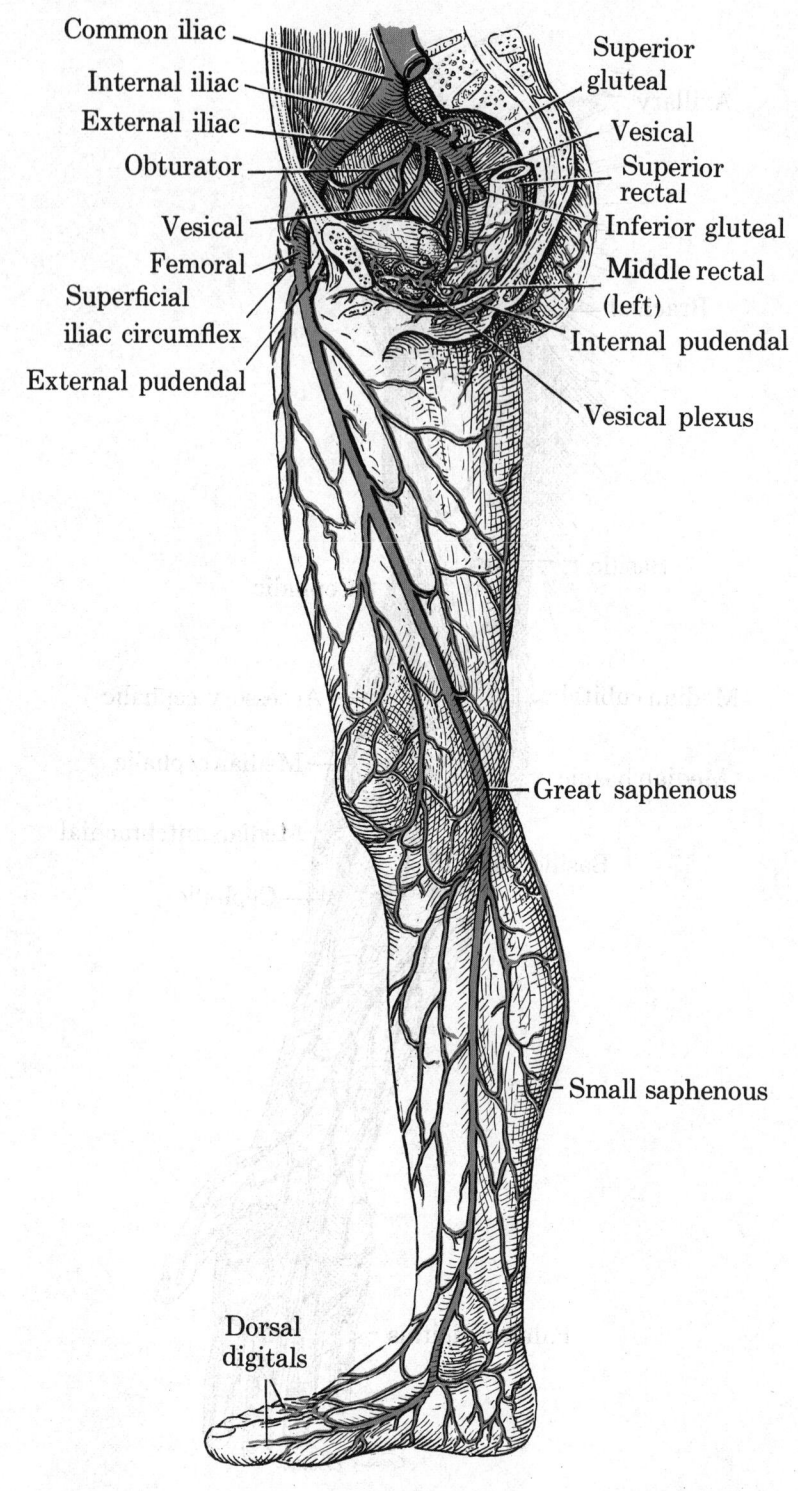

Common iliac

Internal iliac

External iliac

Obturator

Vesical

Femoral

Superficial
iliac circumflex

External pudendal

Superior
gluteal

Vesical

Superior
rectal

Inferior gluteal

Middle rectal
(left)

Internal pudendal

Vesical plexus

Great saphenous

Small saphenous

Dorsal
digitals

PLATE 51 — SUPERFICIAL VEINS OF THE LOWER EXTREMITY

v. cardi′aca me′dia [NA], middle cardiac vein: a vein that collects blood from the diaphragmatic surface of the ventricles, follows the posterior longitudinal sulcus, and empties into the coronary sinus; called also *v. cordis media.*

ve′nae cardi′acae min′imae [NA], smallest cardiac veins: numerous small veins arising in the muscular walls and draining independently into the cavities of the heart, and most readily seen in the atria; called also *venae cordis minimae.*

v. cardi′aca par′va [NA], small cardiac vein: a vein that collects blood from both parts of the right heart, follows the coronary sulcus to the left, and opens into the coronary sinus; called also *v. cordis parva.*

ve′nae ca′vae, the vena cava inferior and superior.

v. ca′va infe′rior [NA], inferior vena cava: the venous trunk for the lower extremities and for the pelvic and abdominal viscera; it begins at the level of the fifth lumbar vertebra by union of the common iliac veins, passes upward on the right of the aorta, and empties into the right atrium of the heart.

v. ca′va supe′rior [NA], superior vena cava: the venous trunk draining blood from the head, neck, upper extremities, and chest; it begins by union of the two brachiocephalic veins, passes directly downward, and empties into the right atrium of the heart.

v. cava superior, persistent left, a developmental anomaly in which the left superior vena cava persists into postnatal life, usually draining into the left atrium; it is due to failure of the upper part of the left anterior cardinal vein to become obliterated. It may be an isolated anomaly or accompany other cardiovascular defects, such as tetralogy of Fallot.

ve′nae caverno′sae pe′nis [NA], cavernous veins of penis: veins that return the blood from the corpora cavernosa to the deep veins and the dorsal vein of the penis.

v. centra′lis glan′dulae suprarena′lis [NA], central vein of suprarenal gland: the large single vein into which the various veins within the substance of the gland empty, and which continues at the hilum as the suprarenal vein.

ve′nae centra′les hep′atis [NA], central veins of liver: veins in the middle of the hepatic lobules, draining into the hepatic vein.

v. centra′lis ret′inae [NA], central vein of retina: the vein that is formed by union of the retinal veins; it passes out of the eyeball in the optic nerve to empty into the superior ophthalmic vein.

v. cephal′ica [NA], cephalic vein: the superficial vein that arises from the radial side of the dorsal rete of the hand, and winds anteriorly to pass along the anterior border of the brachioradialis muscle; above the elbow it ascends along the lateral border of the biceps muscle and the pectoral border of the deltoid muscle, and opens into the axillary vein.

v. cephal′ica accesso′ria [NA], accessory cephalic vein: a vein arising from the dorsal rete of the hand, passing up the forearm to join the cephalic vein just above the elbow.

ve′nae cerebel′li [NA], cerebellar veins: the veins on the surface of the cerebellum; those from the *superior* surface empty into the straight sinus and the great cerebral vein or into the transverse and superior petrosal sinuses; those from the *inferior* surface empty into the transverse, sigmoid, and inferior petrosal sinuses or into the occipital sinus.

ve′nae cer′ebri [NA], cerebral veins: veins that drain the surfaces or inner regions of the cerebral hemispheres; they are divided into superficial and deep groups.

ve′nae cer′ebri ante′riores, venae anteriores cerebri.

ve′nae cer′ebri inferio′res, venae inferiores cerebri.

ve′nae cer′ebri inter′nae, venae internae cerebri.

v. cer′ebri mag′na, v. magna cerebri.

v. cer′ebri me′dia profun′da, v. media profunda cerebri.

ve′nae cer′ebri me′diae superficia′les, venae mediae superficiales cerebri.

ve′nae cer′ebri profun′dae, venae profundae cerebri.

ve′nae cer′ebri superio′res, venae superiores cerebri.

v. cervica′lis profun′da [NA], deep cervical vein: a vein that arises from a plexus in the suboccipital triangle, follows the deep cervical artery down the neck, and empties into the vertebral or the brachiocephalic vein.

v. choroi′dea infe′rior [NA], inferior choroid vein: a vein that drains the inferior choroid plexus into the basal vein.

ve′nae choroi′deae oc′uli, NA alternative for *venae vorticosae.*

v. choroi′dea superior [NA], superior choroid vein: the vein that runs along the whole length of the choroid plexus, draining it and the hippocampus, fornix, and corpus callosum;

it unites with the superior thalamostriate vein to form the internal cerebral vein.

ve′nae cilia′res [NA], ciliary veins: veins that arise inside the eyeball by branches from the ciliary muscle and drain into the superior ophthalmic vein. The *anterior ciliary veins* follow the anterior ciliary arteries, and receive branches from the sinus venosus, sclerae, the episcleral veins, and the tunica conjunctiva bulbi. The *posterior ciliary veins* follow the posterior ciliary arteries and empty also into the inferior ophthalmic vein.

ve′nae circumflex′ae fem′oris latera′les, venae circumflexae laterales femoris.

ve′nae circumflex′ae fem′oris media′les, venae circumflexae mediales femoris.

v. circumflex′a ilia′ca profun′da [NA], deep circumflex iliac vein: a common trunk formed from the venae comitantes of the homonymous artery and emptying into the external iliac vein.

v. circumflex′a il′ium profun′da, v. circumflexa iliaca profunda.

v. circumflex′a il′ium superficia′lis, v. circumflexa superficialis ilium.

ve′nae circumflex′ae latera′les fem′oris [NA], lateral circumflex femoral veins: venae comitantes of the lateral circumflex femoral artery, emptying into the femoral or the deep femoral vein; called also *venae circumflexae femoris laterales.*

ve′nae circumflex′ae media′les fem′oris [NA], medial circumflex femoral veins: venae comitantes of the medial circumflex femoral artery, emptying into the femoral or the deep femoral vein; called also *venae circumflexae femoris mediales.*

v. circumflex′a superficia′lis il′ium [NA], superficial circumflex iliac vein: a vein that follows the homonymous artery and empties into the great saphenous vein; called also *v. circumflexa ilium superficialis.*

v. col′ica dex′tra [NA], right colic vein: a vein that follows the distribution of the right colic artery and empties into the superior mesenteric vein.

v. col′ica interme′dia, NA alternative for *v. colica media.*

v. col′ica me′dia [NA], middle colic vein: a vein that follows the distribution of the middle colic artery and empties into the superior mesenteric vein; called also *intermediate colic vein* and *v. colica intermedia* [NA alternative].

v. col′ica sinis′tra [NA], left colic vein: a vein that follows the left colic artery and opens into the inferior mesenteric vein.

ve′nae colum′nae vertebra′lis [NA], veins of the vertebral column: a plexiform venous network extending the entire length of the vertebral column, outside or inside the vertebral canal; the anterior and posterior external and anterior and posterior internal groups freely anastomose and end in the intervertebral veins. See terms beginning *plexus venosus vertebralis.*

v. com′itans [NA], an accompanying vein: such veins (venae comitantes), usually two in number, closely accompany their homonymous artery and are found especially in the extremities.

ve′nae comitan′tes arte′riae femora′lis, accompanying veins of the femoral artery, which empty into the external iliac vein.

v. com′itans ner′vi hypoglos′si [NA], accompanying vein of hypoglossal nerve: a vessel, formed by union of the vena profunda linguae and the vena sublingualis, that accompanies the hypoglossal nerve; it empties into the facial, lingual, or internal jugular vein.

ve′nae conjunctiva′les [NA], conjunctival veins: small veins that drain blood from the conjunctiva to the superior ophthalmic vein.

ve′nae cor′dis [NA], cardiac veins: the veins of the heart, which drain blood from the various tissues making up the organ.

ve′nae cor′dis anterio′res, venae cardiacae anteriores.

v. cor′dis mag′na, v. cardiaca magna.

v. cor′dis me′dia, v. cardiaca media.

ve′nae cor′dis min′imae, venae cardiacae minimae.

v. cor′dis par′va, v. cardiaca parva.

ve′nae costoaxilla′res, costoaxillary veins: veins that arise from the areolar venous plexus, anastomose with the upper six or seven posterior intercostal veins, and empty into the axillary vein.

1819

v. cuta′nea [NA], cutaneous vein: one of the small veins that begin in the papillae of the skin, form subpapillary plexuses, and open into the subcutaneous veins.

v. cys′tica [NA], cystic vein: a small vein that returns the blood from the gallbladder to the right branch of the portal vein, within the substance of the liver.

ve′nae digita′les commu′nes pe′dis, common digital veins of foot: short veins formed by union of the dorsal digital and the intercapitular veins of the foot.

ve′nae digita′les dorsa′les pe′dis [NA], dorsal digital veins of foot: the veins on the dorsal surfaces of the toes that unite in pairs around each cleft to form the dorsal metatarsal veins; called also *venae digitales pedis dorsales.*

ve′nae digita′les palma′res [NA], palmar digital veins: the venae comitantes of the proper and common palmar digital arteries, which join the superficial palmar venous arch.

ve′nae digita′les pe′dis dorsa′les, venae digitales dorsales pedis.

ve′nae digita′les planta′res [NA], plantar digital veins: veins from the plantar surfaces of the toes which unite at the clefts to form the plantar metatarsal veins of the foot.

ve′nae digita′les vola′res commu′nes, see *venae digitales palmares.*

ve′nae digita′les vola′res pro′priae, see *venae digitales palmares.*

ve′nae diplo′icae [NA], diploic veins: veins of the skull, including the frontal, occipital, anterior temporal, and posterior temporal diploic veins, which form sinuses in the cancellous tissue between the laminae of the cranial bones. They send branches to the external and the internal lamina, the periosteum, and the dura mater, and empty in part inside and in part outside the skull.

v. diplo′ica fronta′lis [NA], frontal diploic vein: a vein that drains the frontal bone, emptying externally into the supraorbital vein or internally into the superior sagittal sinus.

v. diplo′ica occipita′lis [NA], occipital diploic vein: the largest of the diploic veins, which drains blood from the occipital bone and empties into the occipital vein or the transverse sinus.

v. diplo′ica tempora′lis ante′rior [NA], anterior temporal diploic vein: a vein that drains the lateral portion of the frontal and the anterior part of the parietal bone, opening internally into the sphenoparietal sinus and externally into a deep temporal vein.

v. diplo′ica tempora′lis poste′rior [NA], posterior temporal diploic vein: a vein that drains the parietal bone and empties into the transverse sinus.

ve′nae direc′tae latera′les [NA], lateral direct veins: veins of the lateral ventricle, draining into the great cerebral vein.

v. dorsa′lis clitor′idis profun′da, v. dorsalis profunda clitoridis.

ve′nae dorsa′les clitor′idis superficia′les, venae dorsales superficiales clitoridis.

v. dorsa′lis cor′poris callo′si [NA], dorsal vein of corpus callosum: a vein that drains the superior surface of the corpus callosum into the great cerebral vein.

ve′nae dorsa′les lin′guae [NA], dorsal lingual veins: veins that unite with a small vena comitans of the lingual artery and join the main lingual trunk.

v. dorsa′lis pe′nis profun′da, v. dorsalis profunda penis.

ve′nae dorsa′les pe′nis superficia′les, venae dorsales superficiales penis.

v. dorsa′lis profun′da clito′ridis [NA], deep dorsal vein of clitoris: a vein that follows the course of its homonymous artery and opens into the vesical plexus; called also *v. dorsalis clitoridis profunda.*

v. dorsa′lis profun′da pe′nis [NA], deep dorsal vein of penis: a vein lying subfascially in the midline of the penis between the dorsal arteries; it begins in small veins around the corona glandis, is joined by the deep veins of the penis as it passes proximally, and passes between the arcuate pubic and transverse perineal ligaments where it divides into a left and right vein to join the prostatic plexus. Called also *v. dorsalis penis profunda.*

ve′nae dorsa′les superficia′les clito′ridis [NA], superficial dorsal veins of clitoris: veins that collect blood subcutaneously from the clitoris and drain into the external pudendal vein; called also *venae dorsales clitoridis superficiales.*

ve′nae dorsa′les superficia′les pe′nis [NA], superficial dorsal veins of penis: veins that collect blood subcutane-

ously from the penis and drain into the external pudendal vein; called also *venae dorsales penis superficiales.*

v. emissa′ria [NA], emissary vein: one of the small, valveless veins that pass through foramina of the skull, connecting the dural venous sinuses with scalp veins or with deep veins below the base of the skull; called also *emissarium.*

v. emissa′ria condyla′ris [NA], **v. emissa′ria condyloi′dea,** condylar emissary vein: a small vein running through the condylar canal of the skull, connecting the sigmoid sinus with the vertebral or the internal jugular vein; called also *emissarium condyloideum.*

v. emissa′ria mastoi′dea [NA], mastoid emissary vein: a small vein passing through the mastoid foramen of the skull and connecting the sigmoid sinus with the occipital or the posterior auricular vein; called also *emissarium mastoideum.*

v. emissa′ria occipita′lis [NA], occipital emissary vein: an occasional small vein running through a minute foramen in the occipital protuberance of the skull and connecting the confluence of the sinuses with the occipital vein; called also *emissarium occipitale.*

v. emissa′ria parieta′lis [NA], parietal emissary vein: a small vein passing through the parietal foramen of the skull and connecting the superior sagittal sinus with the superficial temporal veins; called also *emissarium parietale.*

v. epigas′trica infe′rior [NA], inferior epigastric vein: a vein that accompanies the inferior epigastric artery and opens into the external iliac vein.

v. epigas′trica superficia′lis [NA], superficial epigastric vein: a vein that follows its homonymous artery and opens into the great saphenous or the femoral vein.

ve′nae epigas′tricae superio′res [NA], superior epigastric veins: the venae comitantes of the superior epigastric artery, which open into the internal thoracic vein.

v. epiplo′ica dex′tra, NA alternative for *v. gastro-omentalis dextra.*

v. epiplo′ica sinis′tra, NA alternative for *v. gastro-omentalis sinistra.*

ve′nae episclera′les [NA], episcleral veins: the veins that ring the cornea and drain into the vorticose and ciliary veins.

ve′nae esopha′geae, venae oesophageales.

ve′nae esophagea′les, NA alternative for *venae oesophageales.*

ve′nae ethmoida′les [NA], ethmoidal veins: veins that follow the anterior and posterior ethmoidal arteries, emerge from the ethmoidal foramina, and empty into the superior ophthalmic vein.

v. ethmoida′lis ante′rior, v. ethmoida′lis poste′rior, see *venae ethmoidales.*

v. facia′lis [NA], facial vein: the vein that begins at the medial angle of the eye as the angular vein, descends behind the facial artery, and usually ends in the internal jugular vein; formerly called the *anterior facial vein* or *vena facialis anterior,* this vessel sometimes joins the retromandibular vein to form a common trunk previously known as the *common facial vein* or *vena facialis communis.*

v. facia′lis ante′rior, v. facia′lis commu′nis, see *v. facialis.*

v. facia′lis poste′rior, v. retromandibularis.

v. facie′i profun′da, profunda faciei.

v. femora′lis [NA], femoral vein: a vein that lies in the proximal two-thirds of the thigh; it is a direct continuation of the popliteal vein, follows the course of the femoral artery, and at the inguinal ligament becomes the external iliac vein. NOTE: Vascular surgeons refer to the portion of the femoral vein proximal to the branching of the deep femoral vein as the *common femoral vein,* and to its continuation distal to the branching as the *superficial femoral vein.*

v. femoroplite′a, femoropopliteal vein: a superficial descending vein draining the lower and back part of the thigh and opening into the small saphenous vein just before it perforates the deep fascia.

ve′nae fibula′res [NA], peroneal veins: the venae comitantes of the peroneal artery, emptying into the posterior tibial vein; called also *venae peroneae* [NA alternative] or *peroneal veins.*

ve′nae fronta′les, 1. frontal veins: superficial superior cerebral veins that drain the frontal cerebral cortex. 2. venae supratrochleares.

ve′nae gas′tricae bre′ves [NA], short gastric veins: small vessels draining the left portion of the greater curvature of the stomach and emptying into the splenic vein.

v. gas′trica dex′tra [NA], right gastric vein: the vena comitans of the right gastric artery, emptying into the portal vein.

v. gas′trica sinis′tra [NA], left gastric vein: the vena comitans of the left gastric artery, emptying into the portal vein.

v. gastroepiplo′ica dex′tra, v. gastro-omentalis dextra.

v. gastroepiplo′ica sinis′tra, v. gastro-omentalis sinistra.

v. gastro-omenta′lis dex′tra [NA], right gastro-omental vein: a vein that follows the distribution of its homonymous artery and empties into the superior mesenteric vein; called also *right epiploic vein, right gastroepiploic vein, v. epiploica dextra* [NA alternative], and *v. gastroepiploica dextra.*

v. gastro-omenta′lis sinis′tra [NA], left gastro-omental vein: a vein that follows the distribution of its homonymous artery and empties into the splenic vein; called also *left epiploic vein, left gastroepiploic vein, v. epiploica sinistra* [NA alternative], and *v. gastroepiploica sinistra.*

ve′nae genicula′res [NA], **ve′nae ge′nus,** genicular veins: veins accompanying the genicular arteries and draining into the popliteal vein.

ve′nae glute′ae inferio′res [NA], inferior gluteal veins: venae comitantes of the inferior gluteal artery; they drain the subcutaneous tissue of the back of the thigh and the muscles of the buttock, unite into a single vein after passing through the greater sciatic foramen, and empty into the internal iliac vein.

ve′nae glute′ae superio′res [NA], superior gluteal veins: venae comitantes of the superior gluteal artery; they drain the muscles of the buttock, pass through the greater sciatic foramen, and empty into the internal iliac vein.

v. gy′ri olfacto′rii [NA], vein of olfactory gyrus: a vein that drains the olfactory gyrus into the basal vein.

ve′nae haemorrhoida′les inferio′res, venae rectales inferiores.

v. haemorrhoida′lis me′dia, see *venae rectales mediae.*

v. haemorrhoida′lis supe′rior, v. rectalis superior.

v. hemiaz′ygos [NA], hemiazygos vein: an intercepting trunk for the lower left posterior intercostal veins; it arises from the ascending lumbar vein, passes up on the left side of the vertebrae to the eighth thoracic vertebra, where it may receive the accessory branch, and crosses over the vertebral column to open into the azygos vein.

v. hemiaz′ygos accesso′ria [NA], accessory hemiazygos vein: the descending intercepting trunk for the upper, often the fourth through the eighth, left posterior intercostal veins. It lies on the left side and at the eighth thoracic vertebra joins the hemiazygos vein or crosses to the right side to join the azygos vein directly; above, it may communicate with the left superior intercostal vein.

ve′nae hemisphe′rii cerebel′li inferio′res, venae inferiores hemispherii cerebelli.

ve′nae hemisphe′rii cerebel′li superio′res, venae superiores hemispherii cerebelli.

ve′nae hepat′icae [NA], hepatic veins: several veins that receive blood from the central veins of the liver; two or three large vessels in an upper group and six to twenty small veins in a lower group form successively larger vessels which ultimately open into the inferior vena cava on the posterior aspect of the liver.

ve′nae hepat′icae dex′trae [NA], the right hepatic veins that drain into the vena cava inferior.

ve′nae hepat′icae interme′diae [NA], the intermediate hepatic veins that drain into the vena cava inferior; called also *middle hepatic veins* and *venae hepaticae mediae.*

ve′nae hepat′icae me′diae, venae hepaticae intermediae.

ve′nae hepat′icae sinis′trae [NA], the left hepatic veins that drain into the vena cava inferior.

v. hypogas′trica, v. iliaca interna.

ve′nae ilea′les [NA], ileal veins: veins draining blood from the ileum into the superior mesenteric vein.

v. ileocol′ica [NA], ileocolic vein: a vein that follows the distribution of its homonymous artery and empties into the vena mesenterica superior.

v. ili′aca commu′nis [NA], common iliac vein: a vein that arises at the sacroiliac articulation by union of the external iliac and the internal iliac veins, and passes upward to the right side of the fifth lumbar vertebra where the two unite to form the inferior vena cava.

v. ili′aca exter′na [NA], external iliac vein: the continuation of the femoral vein from the inguinal ligament to the

sacroiliac articulation, where it joins with the internal iliac vein to form the common iliac vein.

v. ili′aca inter′na [NA], internal iliac vein: a short trunk formed by union of parietal branches; it extends from the greater sciatic notch to the brim of the pelvis, where it joins the external iliac vein to form the common iliac vein; called also *v. hypogastrica.*

v. iliolumba′lis [NA], iliolumbar vein: a vein that follows the distribution of the iliolumbar artery and opens into the internal iliac or the common iliac vein, or it may divide to end in both.

inferior v. cava, v. cava inferior.

ve′nae inferio′res cer′ebri [NA], inferior cerebral veins: rather large superficial cerebral veins that ramify on the base and the inferolateral surface of the brain: those on the inferior surface of the frontal lobe drain into the inferior sagittal sinus and the cavernous sinus; those on the temporal lobe, into the superior petrosal sinus and the transverse sinus; those on the occipital lobe into the straight sinus. Called also *venae cerebri anteriores.*

ve′nae inferio′res hemisphe′rii cerebel′li [NA], inferior veins of cerebellar hemisphere: veins that drain the inferior surface of the cerebellum and empty into the transverse, sigmoid, and inferior petrosal sinuses, or into the occipital sinus; called also *venae hemispherii cerebelli inferiores.*

v. infe′rior ver′mis [NA], inferior vein of vermis: a vein that drains the inferior surface of the cerebellum; it runs backward on the inferior vermis to empty into the straight sinus or one of the sigmoid sinuses; called also *v. vermis inferior.*

ve′nae insula′res [NA], insular veins: veins that drain the insula and join the deep middle cerebral vein.

ve′nae intercapita′les, venae intercapitulares manus.

ve′nae intercapita′les ma′nus, venae intercapitulares manus.

ve′nae intercapitula′res ma′nus [NA], intercapital veins of hand: veins at the clefts of the finger which pass between the heads of the metacarpal bones and establish communication between the dorsal and the palmar venous system of the hand; called also *venae intercapitales manus.*

ve′nae intercapitula′res pe′dis, intercapitular veins of foot: veins at the clefts of the toes which pass between the heads of the metatarsal bones and establish communication between the dorsal and the plantar venous system.

ve′nae intercosta′les, veins that accompany the intercostal arteries; see *venae intercostales anteriores, venae intercostales posteriores, v. intercostalis superior dextra, v. intercostalis superior sinistra,* and *v. intercostalis suprema.*

ve′nae intercosta′les anterio′res [NA], anterior intercostal veins: the twelve paired venae comitantes of the anterior thoracic arteries, which drain into the internal thoracic veins.

ve′nae intercosta′les posterio′res [NA], posterior intercostal veins: the veins that accompany the corresponding intercostal arteries and drain the intercostal spaces posteriorly; the first ends in the brachiocephalic or the vertebral vein, the second and third join the superior intercostal vein, and the fourth to eleventh join the azygos vein on the right and the hemiazygos veins on the left.

v. intercosta′lis supe′rior dex′tra [NA], right superior intercostal vein: a common trunk formed by union of the second, third, and sometimes fourth posterior intercostal veins, which drains into the azygos vein.

v. intercosta′lis supe′rior sinis′tra [NA], left superior intercostal vein: the common trunk formed by union of the second, third, and sometimes fourth posterior intercostal veins, which crosses the arch of the aorta and joins the left brachiocephalic vein.

v. intercosta′lis supre′ma [NA], highest intercostal vein: the first posterior intercostal vein of either side, which passes over the apex of the lung and ends in the brachiocephalic, vertebral, or superior intercostal vein.

ve′nae interloba′res re′nis [NA], interlobar veins of kidney: veins that drain the venous arcades of the kidney, pass down between the pyramids, and unite to form the renal vein.

ve′nae interlobula′res hep′atis [NA], interlobular veins of liver: the veins that arise as tributaries of the portal vein between the hepatic lobules.

ve′nae interlobula′res re′nis [NA], interlobular veins of kidney: veins that collect blood from the capillary network of the cortex and empty into the venous arcades of the kidney.

v. interme′dia antebra′chii [NA], median antebrachial vein: a vein that arises from a palmar venous plexus and passes up the forearm between the cephalic and the basilic veins to the elbow, where it either joins one of these, bifurcates to join both, or joins the median cubital vein; called also *median vein of forearm* and *v. mediana antebrachii*.

v. interme′dia basil′ica [NA], median basilic vein: a vein sometimes present as the medial branch, ending in the basilic vein, of a bifurcation of the median antebrachial vein; called also *v. mediana basilica*.

v. interme′dia cephal′ica [NA], median cephalic vein: a vein sometimes present as the lateral branch, ending in the cephalic vein, formed by bifurcation of the median antebrachial vein; called also *v. mediana cephalica*.

v. interme′dia cu′biti [NA], median cubital vein: the large connecting branch that arises from the cephalic vein below the elbow and passes obliquely upward over the cubital fossa to join the basilic vein; called also *median vein of elbow* and *v. mediana cubiti*.

ve′nae inter′nae cer′ebri [NA], internal cerebral veins: two veins that arise at the interventricular foramen by the union on the thalamostriate and the choroid veins; they pass backward through the tela choroidea, collecting blood from the basal nuclei, and unite at the splenium of the corpus callosum to form the great cerebral vein. Called also *venae cerebri internae*.

ve′na intervertebra′lis [NA], intervertebral vein: any one of the veins that drain the vertebral plexuses, passing out through the intervertebral foramina and emptying into the regional veins: in the neck, into the vertebral; in the thorax, the intercostal; in the abdomen, the lumbar; and in the pelvis, the lateral sacral veins.

ve′nae jejuna′les [NA], jejunal veins: veins draining blood from the jejunum into the superior mesenteric vein.

v. jugula′ris ante′rior [NA], anterior jugular vein: a vein that arises under the chin, passes down the neck, and opens into the external jugular or the subclavian vein or into the jugular venous arch.

v. jugula′ris exter′na [NA], external jugular vein: the vein that begins in the parotid gland behind the angle of the jaw by union of the retromandibular and the posterior auricular vein, passes down the neck, and opens into the subclavian, the internal jugular, or the brachiocephalic vein.

v. jugula′ris inter′na [NA], internal jugular vein: the vein that begins as the superior bulb in the jugular fossa, draining much of the head and neck; it descends with first the internal carotid and then the common carotid artery in the neck, and joins with the subclavian vein to form the brachiocephalic vein.

ve′nae labia′les anterio′res [NA], anterior labial veins: veins that collect blood from the anterior aspect of the labia and drain into the external pudendal vein; they are homologues of the anterior scrotal veins in the male.

ve′nae labia′les inferio′res [NA], inferior labial veins: veins that drain the region of the lower lip into the facial vein.

ve′nae labia′les posterio′res [NA], posterior labial veins: small branches from the labia which open into the vesical venous plexus; they are homologues of the posterior scrotal veins in the male.

v. labia′lis supe′rior [NA], superior labial vein: the vein that drains blood from the region of the upper lip into the facial vein.

ve′nae labyrin′thi [NA], veins of labyrinth: several small veins that pass through the internal acoustic meatus from the cochlea into the inferior petrosal or the transverse sinus; called also *venae auditivae internae*.

v. lacrima′lis [NA], lacrimal vein: the vein that drains blood from the lacrimal gland into the superior ophthalmic vein.

v. laryn′gea infe′rior [NA], inferior laryngeal vein: a vein draining blood from the larynx into the inferior thyroid vein.

v. laryn′gea supe′rior [NA], superior laryngeal vein: a vein that drains blood from the larynx into the superior thyroid vein.

v. latera′lis a′trii [NA], lateral atrial vein: a vein passing through the lateral wall of the lateral ventricle to drain the temporal and parietal lobes into the superior thalamostriate vein; called also *lateral vein of lateral ventricle, v. atrii lateralis,* and *v. ventriculi lateralis lateralis*.

v. liena′lis, v. splenica.

v. lingua′lis [NA], lingual vein: the deep vein that follows the distribution of the lingual artery and empties into the internal jugular vein.

ve′nae lumba′les [NA], lumbar veins: the veins, four or five on each side, that accompany the corresponding lumbar arteries and drain the posterior wall of the abdomen, vertebral

canal, spinal cord, and meninges; the first four usually end in the inferior vena cava, although the first may end in the ascending lumbar vein; the fifth is a tributary of the iliolumbar or of the common iliac vein; and all are generally united by the ascending iliac vein.

v. lumba′lis ascen′dens [NA], ascending lumbar vein: an ascending intercepting vein for the lumbar veins of either side; it begins in the lateral sacral vein and passes up the spine to the first lumbar vertebra, where by union with the subcostal vein it becomes on the right side the azygos vein, and on the left side, the hemiazygos vein.

v. mag′na cer′ebri [NA], great cerebral vein: a short median trunk formed by union of the two internal cerebral veins, which curves around the splenium of the corpus callosum and empties into, or is continued as, the straight sinus; called also *v. cerebri magna*.

v. mamma′ria inter′na, see *venae thoracicae internae*.

ve′nae masseter′icae, masseteric veins: veins from the masseter muscle that empty into the facial vein.

ve′nae maxilla′res [NA], maxillary veins: veins from the pterygoid plexus, usually forming a single short trunk, passing back and uniting with the superficial temporal vein in the parotid gland to form the retromandibular vein.

v. media′lis a′trii [NA], medial atrial vein: a vein passing through the medial wall of the lateral ventricle to drain the parietal and occipital lobes into the internal cerebral or great cerebral vein; called also *medial vein of lateral ventricle, v. atrii medialis,* and *v. ventriculi lateralis medialis*.

v. media′na antebra′chii, v. intermedia antebrachii.

v. media′na basil′ica, v. intermedia basilica.

v. media′na cephal′ica, v. intermedia cephalica.

v. media′na col′li, median vein of neck: a vein formed when the anterior jugular veins unite as they pass down the neck.

v. media′na cu′biti, v. intermedia cubiti.

v. me′dia profun′da cer′ebri [NA], deep middle cerebral vein: the vein that accompanies the middle cerebral artery in the floor of the lateral sulcus, and joins the basal vein; called also *v. cerebri media profunda*.

ve′nae me′diae superficia′les cer′ebri [NA], superficial middle cerebral veins: veins that drain the lateral surface of the cerebrum, follow the lateral cerebral fissure, and empty into the cavernous sinus; called also *venae cerebri mediae superficiales*.

ve′nae mediastina′les [NA], mediastinal veins: numerous small branches that drain blood from the anterior mediastinum into the brachiocephalic vein, azygos vein, or the superior vena cava; called also *venae mediastinales anteriores*.

ve′nae mediastina′les anterio′res, venae mediastinales.

ve′nae medul′lae oblonga′tae [NA] veins of medulla oblongata: the veins that drain the medulla oblongata, which empty into the veins of the spinal cord, the adjacent dural venous sinuses, or along the last four cranial nerves to the inferior petrosal sinus or superior bulb of the jugular vein.

ve′nae menin′geae [NA], meningeal veins: the venae comitantes of the meningeal arteries, which drain the dura mater, communicate with the lateral lacunae, and empty into the regional sinuses and veins.

ve′nae menin′geae me′diae [NA], middle meningeal veins: the venae comitantes of the middle meningeal artery, which end in the pterygoid venous plexus.

ve′nae mesencephal′icae, venae trunci encephalici.

v. mesenter′ica infe′rior [NA], inferior mesenteric vein: a vein that follows the distribution of its homonymous artery and empties into the splenic vein.

v. mesenter′ica supe′rior [NA], superior mesenteric vein: a vein that follows the distribution of its homonymous artery and joins with the splenic vein to form the portal vein.

ve′nae metacarpa′les dorsa′les [NA], dorsal metacarpal veins: veins that arise from the union of dorsal veins of adjacent fingers and pass proximally to join in forming the dorsal venous rete of the hand; called also *venae metacarpeae dorsales*.

ve′nae metacarpa′les palma′res [NA], palmar metacarpal veins: the venae comitantes of the palmar metacarpal arteries, which open into the deep palmar venous arch; called also *venae metacarpeae palmares*.

ve′nae metacar′peae dorsa′les, venae metacarpales dorsales.

ve′nae metacar′peae palma′res, venae metacarpales palmares.

ve′nae metatarsa′les dorsa′les [NA], dorsal metatarsal veins: veins that are formed by the dorsal digital veins of the toes at the clefts of the toes, joining the dorsal venous arch; called also *venae metatarseae dorsales.*

ve′nae metatarsa′les planta′res [NA], plantar metatarsal veins: deep veins of the foot that arise from the plantar digital veins at the clefts of the toes and pass back to open into the plantar venous arch; called also *venae metatarseae plantares.*

ve′nae metatar′seae dorsa′les, venae metatarsales dorsales.

ve′nae metatar′seae planta′res, venae metatarsales plantares.

ve′nae muscula′res, muscular veins: veins that drain blood from the levator palpebrae, superior rectus, superior oblique, and medial rectus muscles into the superior ophthalmic vein.

ve′nae musculophren′icae [NA], musculophrenic veins: the venae comitantes of the musculophrenic artery, draining blood from parts of the diaphragm and from the wall of the thorax and abdomen.

ve′nae nasa′les exter′nae [NA], external nasal veins: small ascending branches from the nose that open into the angular and facial veins.

v. nasofronta′lis [NA], nasofrontal vein: a vein that begins at the supraorbital vein, enters the orbit, and joins the superior ophthalmic vein.

ve′nae nu′clei cauda′ti [NA], the veins of caudate nucleus, which are part of the corpus striatum.

v. obli′qua a′trii sinis′tri [NA], oblique vein of left atrium: a small vein from the left atrium that opens into the coronary sinus; called also *v. obliqua atrii sinistri [Marshalli].*

v. obli′qua a′trii sinis′tri [Marshal′li], v. obliqua atrii sinistri.

ve′nae obturato′riae [NA], obturator veins: veins that drain the hip joint and the regional muscles, enter the pelvis through the obturator canal, and empty into the internal iliac or the inferior epigastric vein, or both.

v. occipita′lis [NA], occipital vein: a vein in the scalp that follows the distribution of the occipital artery and opens under the trapezius muscle into the suboccipital venous plexus; it may continue with the occipital artery and end in the internal jugular vein.

ve′nae occipita′les [NA], occipital veins: superficial superior cerebral veins that drain the occipital cerebral cortex.

ve′nae oesophagea′les [NA], esophageal veins: small veins that drain blood from the esophagus into the hemiazygos and azygos veins, or into the left brachiocephalic vein; called also *venae esophageae* and *venae esophageales* [NA alternative].

v. ophthal′mica infe′rior [NA], inferior ophthalmic vein: a vein formed by confluence of muscular and ciliary branches, and running backward either to join the superior ophthalmic vein or to open directly into the cavernous sinus; it sends a communicating branch through the inferior orbital fissure to join the pterygoid venous plexus.

v. ophthal′mica supe′rior [NA], superior ophthalmic vein: the vein that begins at the medial angle of the eyelid, where it communicates with the frontal, supraorbital, and angular veins; it follows the distribution of the ophthalmic artery, and may be joined by the inferior ophthalmic vein at the superior orbital fissure before opening into the cavernous sinus.

v. ophthalmomenin′gea, ophthalmomeningeal vein: a small inferior meningeal vein that opens usually into the superior ophthalmic vein, or occasionally into the superior petrosal sinus.

v. ova′rica, see *v. ovarica dextra* and *v. ovarica sinistra.*

v. ova′rica dex′tra [NA], right ovarian vein: a vein that drains the pampiniform plexus of the broad ligament on the right into the inferior vena cava.

v. ova′rica sinis′tra [NA], left ovarian vein: a vein that drains the pampiniform plexus of the broad ligament on the left into the left renal vein.

v. palati′na, v. palatina externa.

v. palati′na exter′na [NA], external palatine vein: the vein that drains blood from the tonsils and the soft palate into the facial vein; called also *v. palatina.*

ve′nae palpebra′les [NA], palpebral veins: small branches from the eyelids that open into the superior ophthalmic vein.

ve′nae palpebra′les inferio′res [NA], inferior palpebral veins: branches that drain the blood from the lower eyelid into the facial vein.

ve′nae palpebra′les superio′res [NA], superior palpebral veins: branches that drain the blood from the upper eyelid to the angular vein.

ve′nae pancreat′icae [NA], pancreatic veins: numerous branches from the pancreas which open into the splenic and the superior mesenteric vein.

ve′nae pancreaticoduodena′les [NA], pancreaticoduodenal veins: four veins that drain blood from the pancreas and duodenum, closely following the homonymous arteries. A superior and an inferior vein originate from both an anterior and a posterior venous arcade. The anterior superior vein joins the right gastroepiploic vein; the posterior superior vein joins the portal vein. The anterior and posterior inferior veins join, sometimes as one trunk, the uppermost jejunal vein or the superior mesenteric vein.

ve′nae paraumbilica′les [NA], paraumbilical veins: veins that communicate with the portal vein and anastomose with the superior and inferior epigastric and the superior vesical veins in the region of the umbilicus. They form a part of the collateral circulation of the portal vein in the event of hepatic obstruction. Called also *venae parumbilicales [Sappeyi].*

ve′nae parieta′les [NA], parietal veins: superficial superior cerebral veins that drain the parietal cerebral cortex.

ve′nae paroti′deae [NA], parotid veins: small veins from the parotid gland that open into the superficial temporal vein; called also *venae parotideae posteriores.*

ve′nae paroti′deae anterio′res, rami parotidei venae facialis.

ve′nae paroti′deae posterio′res, venae parotideae.

ve′nae parumbilica′les [Sap′peyi], venae paraumbilicales.

ve′nae pectora′les [NA], collective term for branches of the subclavian vein that drain the pectoral region.

ve′nae peduncula′res [NA], peduncular veins: veins that drain the cerebral peduncle into the basal vein.

ve′nae perforan′tes [NA], perforating veins that empty into the deep femoral vein and by which an anastomosis is established between the deep femoral vein, and the popliteal vein below and the inferior gluteal vein above.

ve′nae pericardi′acae, venae pericardiales.

ve′nae pericardiacophren′icae [NA], pericardiacophrenic veins: small veins that drain blood from the pericardium and diaphragm into the left brachiocephalic vein; called also *venae phrenicae superiores.*

ve′nae pericardia′les [NA], pericardiac veins: numerous small branches that drain blood from the pericardium into the brachiocephalic, inferior thyroid and azygos veins, and the superior vena cava; called also *venae pericardiacae.*

ve′nae perone′ae, NA alternative for *venae fibulares.*

v. petro′sa [NA], petrosal vein: a short trunk arising from the union of four or five cerebellar and pontine veins opposite the middle cerebellar peduncle and terminating in the superior petrosal sinus.

ve′nae pharyn′geae, venae pharyngeales.

ve′nae pharyngea′les [NA], pharyngeal veins: veins that drain the pharyngeal plexus and empty into the internal jugular vein; called also *venae pharyngeae.*

ve′nae phren′icae inferio′res [NA], inferior phrenic veins: veins that follow the homonymous arteries, the one on the right entering the inferior vena cava, and the one on the left entering the left suprarenal or renal vein or the inferior vena cava.

ve′nae phren′icae superio′res, venae pericardiacophrenicae.

ve′nae pon′tis [NA], veins of pons: the veins that drain the pons, which empty into the basal vein, cerebellar veins, petrosal or venous plexus of the foramen ovale.

v. pontomesencephal′ica ante′rior [NA], anterior pontomesencephalic vein: a vein lying on the superior and anterior aspects of the pons in the midline of the interpeduncular fossa, communicating superiorly with the basal vein and inferiorly with the petrosal vein.

v. poplite′a [NA], popliteal vein: a vein following the popliteal artery, and formed by union of the venae comitantes of the anterior and posterior tibial arteries; at the adductor hiatus it becomes continuous with the femoral vein.

v. por′tae hep′atis [NA], **v. porta′lis hep′atis,** portal vein of liver: a short thick trunk formed by union of the superior mesenteric and the splenic vein behind the neck of the pancreas; it passes upward to the right end of the porta hepatis, where it divides into successively smaller branches, following the branches of the hepatic artery, until it forms a capillary-like system of sinusoids that permeates the entire substance of the liver. Called also *portal vein*.

v. poste′rior cor′poris callo′si [NA], posterior vein of corpus callosum: a vein that drains the posterior surface of the corpus callosum into the great cerebral vein.

v. poste′rior sep′ti pellu′cidi [NA], posterior vein of septum pellucidum: a vein that drains the posterior septum pellucidum into the superior thalamostriate vein; called also *v. septi pellucidi posterior*.

v. poste′rior ventric′uli sinis′tri cor′dis [NA], posterior vein of left ventricle: the vein that drains blood from the posterior surface of the left ventricle into the coronary sinus.

v. precentra′lis cerebel′li [NA], precentral vein of cerebellum: a vein arising in the precentral cerebellar fissure and passing anterior and superior to the culmen, terminating in the great cerebral vein.

ve′nae prefronta′les [NA], prefrontal veins: superficial superior cerebral veins that drain the prefrontal cerebral cortex.

v. prepylo′rica [NA], prepyloric vein: a vein that accompanies the prepyloric artery, passing upward over the anterior surface of the junction between the pylorus and the duodenum and emptying into the right gastric vein.

ve′na profun′da [NA], deep vein: any deeply situated vein.

ve′nae profun′dae cer′ebri [NA], deep cerebral veins: the veins that drain the inner regions of the cerebral hemispheres; called also *venae cerebri profundae*.

ve′nae profun′dae clitor′idis [NA], deep veins of clitoris: small veins of the clitoris that drain into the vesical venous plexus.

v. profun′da facia′lis, NA alternative for *v. profunda faciei*.

v. profun′da facie′i [NA], deep facial vein: a vein draining from the pterygoid plexus to the facial vein; called also *v. faciei profunda* and *v. profunda facialis* [NA alternative].

v. profun′da fem′oris [NA], deep femoral vein: a vein that follows the distribution of the deep femoral artery and opens into the femoral vein.

v. profun′da lin′guae [NA], deep lingual vein: a vein that drains blood from the deep aspect of the tongue and joins the sublingual vein to form the vena comitans of the hypoglossal nerve.

ve′nae profun′dae mem′bri inferio′ris [NA], deep veins of inferior, or lower, member: veins that drain the lower limb, found accompanying homonymous arteries, and anastomosing freely with the superficial veins; the principal deep veins are the femoral and popliteal veins.

ve′nae profun′dae mem′bri superio′ris [NA], deep veins of superior, or upper member: veins that drain the upper limb, found accompanying homonymous arteries, and anastomosing freely with the superficial veins; they include the brachial, ulnar, and radial veins, and their tributaries, all of which ultimately drain into the axillary vein.

ve′nae profun′dae pe′nis [NA], deep veins of penis: veins that follow the distribution of the homonymous artery and empty into the dorsal vein of the penis.

ve′nae puden′dae exter′nae [NA], external pudendal veins: veins that follow the distribution of the external pudendal artery and open into the great saphenous vein.

v. puden′da inter′na [NA], internal pudendal vein: a vein that follows the course of the internal pudendal artery, and drains into the internal iliac vein.

ve′nae pulmona′les [NA], pulmonary veins: the four veins, the right and left superior and inferior pulmonary veins, that return aerated blood from the lungs to the left atrium of the heart. See also *segmenta bronchopulmonalis*.

ve′nae pulmona′les dex′trae [NA], see *v. pulmonalis dextra inferior* and *v. pulmonalis dextra superior*.

v. pulmona′lis dex′tra infe′rior [NA], inferior right pulmonary vein: the vein that returns blood from the lower lobe of the right lung (from the superior [apical] branch and from the common, superior, and inferior basal veins) to the left atrium of the heart; called also *v. pulmonalis inferior dextra*.

v. pulmona′lis dex′tra supe′rior [NA], superior right pulmonary vein: the vein that returns blood from the upper and middle lobes of the right lung (from the superior [apical], anterior, and posterior branches and the middle lobar branch) to the left atrium of the heart; called also *v. pulmonalis superior dextra*.

v. pulmona′lis infe′rior dex′tra, v. pulmonalis dextra inferior.

v. pulmona′lis infe′rior sinis′tra, v. pulmonalis sinistra inferior.

ve′nae pulmona′les sinis′trae [NA], see *v. pulmonalis sinistra inferior* and *v. pulmonalis sinistra superior*.

v. pulmona′lis sinis′tra infe′rior [NA], inferior left pulmonary vein: the vein that returns blood from the lower lobe of the left lung (from the superior apical branch and the common basal vein) to the left atrium of the heart; called also *v. pulmonalis inferior sinistra*.

v. pulmona′lis sinis′tra supe′rior [NA], superior left pulmonary vein: the vein that returns blood from the upper lobe of the left lung (from the apicoposterior, anterior, and lingular branches) to the left atrium of the heart; called also *v. pulmonalis superior sinistra*.

v. pulmona′lis supe′rior dex′tra, v. pulmonalis dextra superior.

v. pulmona′lis supe′rior sinis′tra, v. pulmonalis sinistra superior.

ve′nae radia′les [NA], radial veins: the venae comitantes of the radial artery, which open into the brachial veins.

v. reces′sus latera′lis ventric′uli quar′ti [NA] vein of lateral recess of fourth ventricle: a small vein arising in the tonsil of the cerebellum, passing the lateral recess of the fourth ventricle, and terminating in the petrosal vein.

ve′nae recta′les inferio′res [NA], inferior rectal veins: veins that drain the rectal plexus into the internal pudendal vein; called also *venae haemorrhoidales inferiores*.

ve′nae recta′les me′diae [NA], middle rectal veins: veins that drain the rectal plexus and empty into the internal iliac and superior rectal veins.

v. recta′lis supe′rior [NA], superior rectal vein: the vein that drains the upper part of the rectal plexus into the inferior mesenteric vein and thus establishes connection between the portal and the systemic system; called also *v. haemorrhoidalis superior*.

ve′nae rena′les, NA alternative for *venae renis*.

ve′nae re′nis [NA], the veins within the kidney, including the *venae interlobares renis, venae arcuatae renis, venae interlobulares renis, venulae rectae renis,* and *venulae stellatae renis.* Called also *venae renales* [NA alternative].

v. retromandibula′ris [NA], retromandibular vein: the vein that is formed in the upper part of the parotid gland behind the neck of the mandible by union of the maxillary and superficial temporal veins; it passes downward through the gland, communicates with the facial vein, and emerging from the gland joins with the posterior auricular vein to form the external jugular vein. Called also *v. facialis posterior*.

ve′nae revehen′tes, channels in the early embryo that convey blood from the sinusoids of the liver to the sinus venosus and later become the hepatic veins.

ve′nae sacra′les latera′les [NA], lateral sacral veins: veins that follow the homonymous arteries, help to form the lateral sacral plexus, and empty into the internal iliac vein or the superior gluteal veins.

v. sacra′lis me′dia, v. sacralis mediana.

v. sacra′lis media′na [NA], middle sacral vein: a vein that follows the middle sacral artery and opens into the common iliac vein; called also *v. sacralis media*.

v. saphe′na accesso′ria [NA], accessory saphenous vein: a vein that, when present, drains the medial and posterior superficial parts of the thigh and opens into the great saphenous vein.

v. saphe′na mag′na [NA], great saphenous vein: the longest vein in the body, extending from the dorsum of the foot to just below the inguinal ligament, where it opens into the femoral vein.

v. saphe′na par′va [NA], small saphenous vein: the vein that continues the marginal vein from behind the malleolus and passes up the back of the leg to the knee joint, where it opens into the popliteal vein.

v. scapula′ris dorsa′lis [NA], a branch of the subclavian vein.

ve′nae sclera′les [NA], scleral veins: tributaries of the anterior ciliary veins that drain the sclera.

ve′nae scrota′les anterio′res [NA], anterior scrotal veins: veins that collect blood from the anterior aspect of the scrotum and drain into the external pudendal vein.

ve′nae scrota′les posterio′res [NA], posterior scrotal veins: small branches from the scrotum that open into the vesical venous plexus.

v. sep′ti pellu′cidi anterior v. anterior septi pellucidi.

v. sep′ti pellu′cidi posterior, v. posterior septi pellucidi.

ve′nae sigmoi′deae [NA], sigmoid veins: veins from the sigmoid colon that empty into the inferior mesenteric vein.

v. spermat′ica, spermatic vein: the vein that drains blood from the testis and epididymis, forms the pampiniform plexus of the spermatic cord, and accompanies the internal spermatic artery. The vein on the right enters the inferior vena cava; that on the left enters the left renal vein.

ve′nae spina′les anterio′res/posterio′res [NA], anterior and posterior spinal veins: veins that drain the spinal cord into the internal vertebral venous plexuses; they form a tortuous plexus in the pia mater that consists of two median longitudinal veins, one in front of the anterior median fissure and the other behind the posterior median septum of the spinal cord; and two anterolateral veins that run in back of the ventral nerve roots; and two posterolateral veins that run in back of the dorsal nerve roots.

ve′nae spina′les exter′nae anterio′res, small longitudinal veins draining blood from the anterior part of the pia mater of the spinal cord; see *venae spinales.*

ve′nae spina′les exter′nae posterio′res, small longitudinal veins draining blood from the posterior part of the pia mater of the spinal cord; see *venae spinales.*

ve′nae spina′les inter′nae, minute veins draining blood from the substance of the spinal cord; see *venae spinales.*

v. spira′lis modi′oli [NA], spiral vein of modiolus: a small vein in the spiral modiolus, a tributary of the labyrinthine veins.

v. sple′nica [NA], splenic vein: the vein formed by union of several branches at the hilum of the spleen, passing from left to right to the neck of the pancreas, where it joins the superior mesenteric vein to form the portal vein; called also *v. lienalis.*

ve′nae stella′tae re′nis, venulae stellatae renis.

v. sternocleidomastoi′dea [NA], sternocleidomastoid vein: a vein that follows the course of the homonymous artery and opens into the internal jugular vein.

ve′nae stria′tae, venae thalamostriatae inferiores.

v. stylomastoi′dea [NA], stylomastoid vein: a vein following the stylomastoid artery and emptying into the retromandibular vein.

v. subcla′via [NA], subclavian vein: the vein that continues the axillary as the main venous stem of the upper member, follows the subclavian artery, and joins with the internal jugular vein to form the brachiocephalic vein.

v. subcosta′lis [NA], subcostal vein: the vena comitans of the subcostal artery, which joins the ascending lumbar vein to form the azygos or hemiazygos vein, on the right or left side respectively.

ve′nae subcuta′neae abdom′inis [NA], subcutaneous veins of abdomen: the superficial veins of the abdominal wall.

v. sublingua′lis [NA], sublingual vein: a vein that follows the sublingual artery and opens into the lingual vein.

v. submenta′lis [NA], submental vein: a vein that follows the submental artery and opens into the facial vein.

v. superficia′lis [NA], superficial vein: any superficially situated vein.

ve′nae superficia′les cer′ebri [NA], superficial cerebral veins: the veins that drain the surfaces of the cerebral hemispheres, comprising the superior, inferior, and middle superficial cerebral veins and their tributaries; called also *venae cerebri superficiales.*

ve′nae superficia′les mem′bri inferio′ris [NA], superficial veins of inferior, or lower member: veins that drain the lower limb, found immediately beneath the skin, and anastomosing freely with the deep veins; the principal superficial veins are the great and small saphenous veins.

ve′nae superficia′les mem′bri superio′ris [NA], superficial veins of superior, or upper, member: veins that drain the upper limb, found immediately beneath the skin, and anastomosing freely with the deep veins; they include the cephalic, basilic, and median cubital and antebrachial veins, and their tributaries, all of which ultimately drain into the axillary vein.

superior v. cava, v. cava superior.

ve′nae superio′res cer′ebri [NA], superior cerebral veins: the 8 to 12 superficial cerebral veins (prefrontal, frontal, parietal, and occipital) that drain the superior, lateral, and medial surfaces of the cerebrum toward the longitudinal cerebral fissure, where they open into the superior sagittal sinus; called also *venae cerebri superiores.*

ve′nae superio′res hemisphe′rii cerebel′li [NA] superior veins of cerebellar hemisphere: veins that drain the superior surfaces of the cerebellar hemisphere and empty into the transverse or superior petrosal sinuses; called also *venae hemispherii cerebelli superiores.*

v. supe′rior ver′mis [NA], superior vein of vermis: a vein that drains the superior surface of the cerebellum; it runs forward and medially across the superior vermis to empty into the straight sinus or the great cerebral vein; called also *v. vermis superior.*

v. supraorbita′lis [NA], supraorbital vein: the vein that passes down the forehead lateral to the supratrochlear vein, joining it at the root of the nose to form the angular vein.

ve′nae suprarena′les, see *v. suprarenalis dextra* and *v. suprarenalis sinistra.*

v. suprarena′lis dex′tra [NA], right suprarenal vein: a vein that drains the right suprarenal gland into the inferior vena cava.

v. suprarena′lis sinis′tra [NA], left suprarenal vein: the vein that returns blood from the left suprarenal gland to the left renal vein.

v. suprascapula′ris [NA], suprascapular vein: the vein that accompanies the homonymous artery (sometimes as two veins that unite), opening usually into the external jugular, or occasionally into the subclavian vein; called also *v. transversa scapulae.*

ve′nae supratrochlea′res [NA], supratrochlear veins: two veins, each beginning in a venous plexus high up on the forehead and descending to the root of the nose, where it joins with the supraorbital to form the angular vein; called also *venae frontales.*

v. tempora′lis me′dia [NA], middle temporal vein: the vein that arises in the substance of the temporal muscle and passes down under the fascia to the zygoma, where it breaks through to join the superficial temporal vein.

ve′nae tempora′les profun′dae [NA], deep temporal veins: veins that drain the deep portions of the temporal muscle and empty into the pterygoid plexus.

ve′nae tempora′les superficia′les [NA], superficial temporal veins: veins that drain the lateral part of the scalp in the frontal and parietal regions, the tributaries forming a single superficial temporal vein in front of the ear, just above the zygoma. This descending vein receives the middle temporal and transverse facial veins and, entering the parotid gland, unites with the maxillary vein deep to the neck of the mandible to form the retromandibular vein.

v. termina′lis, NA alternative for *v. thalamostriata superior.*

v. testicula′ris, see *v. testicularis dextra* and *v. testicularis sinistra.*

v. testicula′ris dex′tra [NA], right testicular vein: a vein that drains the right pampiniform plexus into the inferior vena cava.

v. testicula′ris sinis′tra [NA], left testicular vein: a vein that drains the left pampiniform plexus into the left renal vein.

ve′nae thalamostria′tae inferio′res [NA], inferior thalamostriate veins: veins that pass through the anterior perforate substance and join the deep middle cerebral and anterior cerebral veins to form the basal vein; called also *striate veins* and *venae striatae.*

v. thalamostria′ta supe′rior [NA], superior thalamostriate vein: a vein that collects blood from the corpus striatum and thalamus, and joins with the choroid vein to form the internal cerebral vein; called also *terminal vein* and *v. terminalis* [NA alternative].

v. thoraca′lis latera′lis, v. thoracica lateralis.

ve′nae thora′cicae inter′nae [NA], internal thoracic veins: two veins formed by junction of the venae comitantes of the internal thoracic artery of either side; each continues along the artery to open into the brachiocephalic vein; called also (sing.) *v. mammaria interna.*

v. thora′cica latera′lis [NA], lateral thoracic vein: a large vein accompanying the lateral thoracic artery and draining into the axillary vein; called also *v. thoracalis lateralis.*

v. thoracoacromia′lis [NA], thoracoacromial vein: the vein that follows the homonymous artery and opens into the subclavian vein.

ve′nae thoracoepigas′tricae [NA], thoracoepigastric veins: long, longitudinal, superficial veins in the anterolateral subcutaneous tissue of the torso, which empty superiorly into the lateral thoracic and inferiorly into the femoral vein.

ve′nae thy′micae [NA], thymic veins: small branches from the thymus gland that open into the left brachiocephalic vein.

v. thyreoi′dea i′ma, an occasional vein formed by high junction of the right and left inferior thyroid veins, and emptying usually into the left brachiocephalic vein.

ve′nae thyreoi′deae inferio′res, see *v. thyroidea inferior.*

ve′nae thyreoi′deae superio′res, 1. see *vena thyroidea superior.* 2. veins draining blood from the upper portion of the thyroid gland into the posterior facial vein.

v. thyroi′dea infe′rior [NA], inferior thyroid vein: either of two veins, left and right, that drain the thyroid plexus into the left and right brachiocephalic veins; occasionally they may unite into a common trunk to empty, usually, into the left brachiocephalic vein.

ve′nae thyroi′deae me′diae [NA], middle thyroid veins: veins that drain blood from the thyroid gland into the internal jugular vein.

v. thyroi′dea supe′rior [NA], superior thyroid vein: a vein arising from the upper part of the thyroid gland on either side, opening into the internal jugular vein, occasionally in common with the facial vein.

ve′nae tibia′les anterio′res [NA], anterior tibial veins: venae comitantes of the anterior tibial artery, which unite with the posterior tibial veins to form the popliteal vein.

ve′nae tibia′les posterio′res [NA], posterior tibial veins: venae comitantes of the posterior tibial artery, which unite with the anterior tibial veins to form the popliteal vein.

ve′nae trachea′les [NA], tracheal veins: small branches that drain blood from the trachea into the brachiocephalic vein.

ve′nae transver′sae cer′vicis [NA], transverse cervical veins: veins that follow the transverse artery of the neck and open into the subclavian vein; called also *venae transversae colli.*

ve′nae transver′sae col′li, venae transversae cervicis.

v. transver′sa facia′lis, NA alternative for *v. transversa faciei.*

v. transver′sa facie′i [NA], transverse facial vein: a vein that passes backward with the transverse facial artery just below the zygomatic arch to join the retromandibular vein; called also *v. transversa facialis* [NA alternative].

v. transver′sa scap′ulae, v. suprascapularis.

ve′nae trun′ci encephal′ici, [NA], veins of encephalic trunk: the veins that drain the brainstem and empty into the basal or great cerebral vein; called also *venae mesencephalicae.* See *venae pontomesencephalicae, venae pontis, venae medullae oblongatae,* and *v. recessus lateralis ventriculi quarti.*

ve′nae tympan′icae [NA], tympanic veins: small veins from the tympanic cavity that pass through the petrotympanic fissure, open into the plexus around the temporomandibular articulation, and finally drain into the retromandibular vein.

ve′nae ulna′res [NA], ulnar veins: the venae comitantes of the ulnar artery, which unite with the radial veins at the elbow to form the brachial veins.

v. umbilica′lis, umbilical vein: former NA term for either of the paired veins that carry blood from the chorion to the sinus venosus and heart in the early embryo; they later fuse and a single vessel persisting in the umbilical cord carries all the blood from the placenta to the ductus venosus of the fetus. See *v. umbilicalis sinistra.*

v. umbilica′lis sinis′tra [NA], left umbilical vein of the fetus, the vein formed by fusion of the atrophied right umbilical vein with the left umbilical vein, which carries all the blood from the placenta to the ductus venosus.

v. un′ci [NA], vein of uncus: a vein that drains the uncus into the ipsilateral inferior cerebral vein.

ve′nae uteri′nae [NA], uterine veins: veins that drain the uterine plexus into the internal iliac veins.

ve′nae vaso′rum, small veins that return blood from the tissues making up the walls of the blood vessels themselves.

ve′nae ventricula′res cor′dis [NA], the veins of the ventricles of the heart.

v. ventricula′ris infe′rior [NA], inferior ventricular vein: a vein that drains the temporal lobe into the basal vein.

v. ventric′uli latera′lis latera′lis, v. lateralis atrii.

v. ventric′uli latera′lis media′lis, v. medialis atrii.

v. ver′mis infe′rior, v. inferior vermis.

v. ver′mis supe′rior, v. superior vermis.

v. vertebra′lis [NA], vertebral vein: a vein that arises from the suboccipital venous plexus, passes with the vertebral artery through the foramina of the transverse processes of the upper six cervical vertebrae, and opens into the brachiocephalic vein.

v. vertebra′lis acceso′ria [NA], accessory vertebral vein: a vein that sometimes arises from a plexus formed around the vertebral artery by the vertebral vein, descends with the vertebral vein, and emerges through the transverse foramen of the seventh cervical vertebra to empty into the brachiocephalic vein.

v. vertebra′lis ante′rior [NA], anterior vertebral vein: a small vein accompanying the ascending cervical artery; it arises in a venous plexus adjacent to the more cranial cervical transverse processes, and descends to end in the vertebral vein.

ve′nae vesica′les [NA], vesical veins: veins passing from the vesical plexus to the internal iliac vein.

ve′nae vestibula′res [NA], vestibular veins: branches draining blood from the vestibule into the labyrinthine veins.

ve′nae vortico′sae [NA], vorticose veins: four veins that pierce the sclera and carry blood from the choroid to the superior ophthalmic vein; called also *posterior ciliary veins* and *venae choroideae oculi* [NA alternative].

---

venacavogram (ve″nah-ka′vo-gram)   the film obtained by venacavography.

venacavography (ve″nah-ka-vog′rah-fe)   radiography of a vena cava, usually of the inferior vena cava.

venae (ve′ne) [L.]   genitive and plural of *vena.*

Vena medinensis (ve′nah med″ĭ-nen′sis)   *Dracunculus medinensis.*

venation (ve-na′shun) [L. *vena* vein]   the manner of distribution of the veins of a part.

venectasia (ve″nek-ta′ze-ah)   phlebectasia; varicosity.

venectomy (ve-nek′to-me)   phlebectomy.

veneer (vĕ-nēr′)   in the construction of crowns or pontics, a layer of tooth-colored material, usually porcelain or acrylic resin, attached to the surface by direct fusion, cementation, or mechanical retention.

venenation (ven″ĕ-na′shun) [L. *venenum* poison]   poisoning; a condition of being poisoned.

veneniferous (ven″ĕ-nif′er-us) [L. *venenum* poison + *ferre* to bear]   carrying poison.

venenific (ven″ĕ-nif′ik) [L. *venenum* poison + *facere* to make]   forming poison.

Venenosa (ven″ĕ-no′sah) [pl., L. *venenosus* poisonous]   a term once used to designate venomous snakes collectively; thanatophidia.

venenosalivary (ven″ĕ-no-sal′ĭ-ver″e)   venomosalivary.

venenosity (ven″ĕ-nos′ĭ-te)   the condition of being venomous.

venenous (ven′ĕ-nus) [L. *venenosus*]   venomous.

venenum (vĕ-ne′num), gen. *vene′ni,* pl. *vene′na* [L.]   a poison.

venepuncture (ven′e-punk″tūr)   venipuncture.

venereal (ve-ne′re-al) [L. *venereus*]   pertaining or related to or transmitted by sexual contact; see *sexually transmitted disease,* under *disease.*

venereologist (ve-ne″re-ol′o-jist)   a specialist in venereology.

venereology (ve-ne″re-ol′o-je)   the branch of medicine that deals with sexually transmitted diseases.

venerupin (ven″er-oo′pin) [*Venerupis* (L. *veneris*) the Venus shell + -*in,* suffix for chemical compounds]   a toxic substance, believed to be an amine, found in certain Japanese pelecypods which were formerly placed in the genus *Venerupis;* this toxin, the exact chemical nature of which is unknown, is entirely distinct from the paralytic shellfish poison found in other bivalves.

venery (ven′er-e) [L. *venereus* pertaining to Venus]   coitus; sexual intercourse.

venesection (ven″ĕ-sek′shun) [L. *vena* vein + *sectio* cutting]   phlebotomy.

venesuture (ven″ĕ-su′tūr)   phleborrhaphy.

veniplex (ven′ĭ-pleks) [L. *vena* vein + *plexus* plexus]   a venous plexus.

venipuncture (ven′ĭ-punk″tūr)   puncture of a vein.

venisection (ven′ĭ-sek′shun)   phlebotomy.

venisuture (ven′ĭ-su′tūr) [L. *vena* vein + *sutura* stitch]   phleborrhaphy.

ven(o)- [L. *vena* vein] a combining form denoting relationship to a vein. See also words beginning *phlebo-*.

venoatrial (ve″no-a′tre-al) pertaining to the vena cava and the right atrium.

venoauricular (ve″no-aw-rik′u-lar) venoatrial.

venoclysis (ve-nok′lĭ-sis) [*vena* + Gr. *klysis* injection] phleboclysis.

venofibrosis (ve″no-fi-bro′sis) a disease of the veins characterized by hyperplasia of the fibrous connective tissue of the median coat of the vein.

venogram (ve′no-gram) 1. phlebogram. 2. a venous-pulse tracing.

venography (ve-nog′rah-fe) phlebography. **intraosseous v.,** roentgenography of the veins after injection of the contrast medium into bone marrow at an appropriate site, such as the iliac crest, ischium, pubic bones, greater trochanter, spinous processes of the vertebrae, or sternum. **portal v.,** portography. **splenic v.,** splenic portography.

venom (ven′um) [L. *venenum* poison] a poison; specifically, a toxic substance normally secreted by a serpent, insect, or other animal. **Russell's viper v.,** the venom of Russell's viper, *Vipera russelli,* which acts *in vitro* as an intrinsic thromboplastin and is useful in defining deficiencies of blood coagulation Factor X. **snake v.,** the poisonous secretion of snakes, containing hemotoxins, hemagglutinins, neurotoxins, leukotoxins, or endotheliotoxins. The venoms of various species have been used as hemostatics. See also *antivenomous serum,* under *serum.* **spider v.,** the venom of a spider such as *Latrodectus, Atrax, Ctenus,* and *Lycosa.*

venomization (ven″um-i-za′shun) treatment of a substance with snake venom.

venomosalivary (ven″o-mo-sal′ĭ-ver″e) secreting a poisonous saliva.

venomotor (ve″no-mo′tor) pertaining to or producing constriction or dilatation of the veins.

venomous (ven′o-mus) secreting venom; poisonous.

veno-occlusive (ve″no-ŏ-kloo′siv) pertaining to or characterized by obstruction of the veins.

venoperitoneostomy (ve″no-per″ĭ-to″ne-os′to-me) [*veno-* + *peritoneum* + Gr. *stomoun* to provide with an opening, mouth] anastomosis of the saphenous vein with the peritoneum for permanent drainage of the peritoneal cavity in ascites.

venopressor (ve-no-pres″or) 1. pertaining to venous blood pressure. 2. an agent that causes venous constriction.

venosclerosis (ve″no-sklĕ-ro′sis) phlebosclerosis.

venose (ve′nōs) provided with veins.

venosinal (ve″no-si′nal) pertaining to the venae cavae and the right atrium of the heart.

venosity (ve-nos′ĭ-te) 1. excess of venous blood in a part. 2. a plentiful supply of blood vessels or of venous blood.

venostasis (ve″no-sta′sis) [*veno-* + Gr. *stasis* stopping] retardation of venous outflow from a part, as from the leg on standing when venous valves are incompetent; see *phlebostasis.*

venotomy (ve-not′o-me) phlebotomy.

venous (ve′nus) [L. *venosus*] of or pertaining to the veins.

venovenostomy (ve″no-ve-nos′to-me) phlebophlebostomy.

vent (vent) [Fr. *fente* slit] 1. any opening or outlet; especially the anus. 2. an opening that discharges pus. 3. cloacal aperture. **pulmonic alveolar v's,** interalveolar pores.

Ventaire (ventār) trademark for a preparation of protokylol hydrochloride.

venter (ven′ter), pl. *ven′tres* [L. "belly"] 1. any belly-shaped part; [NA] a general term for a fleshy contractile part of a muscle. 2. the abdomen or stomach. 3. any hollowed part or cavity. **v. ante′rior mus′culi digas′trici** [NA], anterior belly of digastric muscle: the shorter belly of the digastric muscle, arising from the digastric fossa on the mandible and extending backward to join the posterior belly through an intermediate tendon attached to the hyoid bone. **v. fronta′lis mus′culi occipitofronta′lis** [NA], the frontal belly of the occipitofrontal muscle, originating from the galea aponeurotica and inserting into the skin of the eyebrows and the root of the nose. Called also *musculus frontalis.* **v. il′ii,** the free (pelvic) portion of the sacropel-

vic surface of the ilium. **v. i′mus,** the lowermost of the great body cavities, the abdominal cavity (cavum abdominis). **v. infe′rior mus′culi omohyoi′dei** [NA], the lowermost belly of the omohyoid muscle. **v. me′dius,** the middle of the great body cavities, the thoracic cavity (cavum thoracis). **v. mus′culi** [NA], belly of muscle: the fleshy contractile part of a muscle. **v. occipita′lis mus′culi occipitofronta′lis** [NA], the occipital belly of the occipitofrontal muscle, originating from the highest nuchal line of the occipital bone and inserting into the galea aponeurotica; called also *musculus occipitalis.* **v. poste′rior mus′culi digas′trici** [NA], posterior belly of digastric muscle: the longer belly of the digastric muscle, arising from the mastoid notch of the temporal bone and extending forward to join the anterior belly through an intermediate tendon attached to the hyoid bone. **v. propen′dens,** pendulous abdomen. **v. scap′ulae,** fossa subscapularis. **v. supe′rior mus′culi omohyoi′dei** [NA], the uppermost belly of the omohyoid muscle. **v. supre′mus,** the uppermost of the great body cavities, the cranial cavity.

ventilation (ven″tĭ-la′shun) [L. *ventilatio*] 1. the process or act of supplying a house or room continuously with fresh air. 2. in respiratory physiology, the process of exchange of air between the lungs and the ambient air. *Pulmonary ventilation* (usually measured in liters per minute) refers to the total exchange, whereas *alveolar ventilation* refers to the effective ventilation of the alveoli, in which gas exchange with the blood takes place. 3. in psychiatry, verbalization of one's emotional problems. **alveolar v.,** the amount of gas expelled from the alveoli to the outside of the body per minute. **assist/control mode v.,** mechanical ventilation in which inspiration is assisted; if the spontaneous ventilation rate falls below a preset level, the ventilator enters control-mode ventilation. **control-mode v.,** mechanical ventilation in which the ventilator cycle is not influenced by the patient's efforts at spontaneous ventilation. **downward v.,** that in which the outlets have places lower than those of the inlets. **exhausting v.,** ventilation by means of the exhausting fan or by some other process which withdraws the foul air. **intermittent mandatory v. (IMV),** mechanical ventilation in which the patient breathes spontaneously while the ventilator delivers a positive-pressure breath at preset intervals. **mechanical v.,** ventilation accomplished by extrinsic means, as under positive end-expiratory pressure. **minute v.,** the total amount of gas (in liters) expelled from the lungs per minute. Called also *total ventilation.* **natural v.,** ventilation effected without any special appliance to render it certain. **plenum v.,** the supply of fresh air to a building by fan blowers. **synchronized intermittent mandatory v. (SIMV),** mechanical ventilation in which the patient breathes spontaneously while the ventilator delivers a positive-pressure breath at intervals that are predetermined but synchronized with the patient's breathing. **upward v.,** that which introduces air below the place of its withdrawal. **vacuum v.,** that which is effected by the forced extraction of air.

ventilator (ven″tĭ-la′tor) an apparatus designed to qualify the air that is breathed through it or to assist or control pulmonary ventilation, either intermittently or continuously.

ventouse (vaw-tooz′) [Fr.] a cupping glass.

ventrad (ven′trad) [L. *venter* belly + *ad* to] toward a belly, venter, or ventral aspect.

ventral (ven′tral) [L. *ventralis*] 1. pertaining to the belly or to any venter. 2. denoting a position more toward the belly surface than some other object of reference; same as *anterior* in human anatomy.

ventralis (ven-tra′lis) ventral; [NA] a general term used to designate a position closer to the belly surface. Cf. *anterior.*

ventralward (ven′tral-ward) ventrad.

ventri- see *ventro-.*

ventricle (ven′trĭ-k'l) a small cavity, such as one of the several cavities of the brain, or one of the lower chambers of the heart; called also *ventriculus.* **aortic v. of heart,** ventriculus sinister cordis. **v. of Arantius,** the fossa rhomboidea, especially its lower end; the eponym is also sometimes applied to the cavitas septi pellucidi. **auxiliary v.,** an implanted pumping mechanism designed to assist the left ventricle of the heart in maintaining normal output, rate, and blood pressure; called also *booster heart.*

v's of the brain, the cavities within the brain which are filled with cerebrospinal fluid, including the two lateral, the third, and the fourth ventricles. They are lined by ependyma which, in certain regions, is invaginated by vascular fringes of pia mater to form the choroid plexuses. The cavum septi pellucidi, to which the term ventricle is sometimes applied, is not a true ventricle. **v. of cord,** canalis centralis medullae spinalis. **double-outlet right v.,** incomplete transposition of the great vessels in which both the aorta and the pulmonary artery arise from the right ventricle, associated with a subaortic ventricular septal defect. In type I, the septal defect is posteroinferior to the crista supraventricularis and remote from the pulmonary valve. In type II, it is anterosuperior to the crista and close to the valve. **Duncan's v., fifth v.,** cavitas septi pellucidi. **first v. of cerebrum,** ventriculus lateralis cerebri. **fourth v. of cerebrum,** an irregularly shaped cavity in the rhombencephalon; see *ventriculus quartus cerebri* [NA]. **Galen's v.,** ventriculus laryngis. **v. of heart,** one of a pair of cavities, with thick muscular walls, that make up the bulk of the heart; see *ventriculus dexter cordis* and *ventriculus sinister cordis.* Called also *ventriculus cordis* [NA]. **v. of larynx,** ventriculus laryngis. **lateral v. of cerebrum,** the cavity in each hemisphere, derived (developed) from the cavity of the embryonic neural tube; see *ventriculus lateralis cerebri.* **left v. of heart,** ventriculus sinister cordis. **Morgagni's v.,** ventriculus laryngis. **pineal v.,** recessus pinealis. **right v. of heart,** ventriculus dexter cordis. **second v. of cerebrum,** ventriculus lateralis cerebri. **single v.,** cor triloculare biatriatum. **sixth v.,** Verga's v. **v. of Sylvius,** cavitas septi pellucidi. **terminal v. of spinal cord,** ventriculus terminalis medullae spinalis. **third v. of cerebrum,** ventriculus tertius cerebri. **Verga's v.,** an occasional space between the corpus callosum and the fornix; called also *sixth v.* **Vieussen's v.,** cavitas septi pellucidi.

ventricornu (ven″trĭ-kor′nu) [*ventri-* + L. *cornu* horn] cornu anterius medullae spinalis.

ventricornual (ven″trĭ-kor′nu-al) pertaining to the ventricornu.

ventricose (ven′trĭ-kōs) having an expansion or belly on one side.

ventricular (ven-trik′u-lar) pertaining to a ventricle.

ventriculi (ven-trik′u-li) [L.] genitive and plural of *ventriculus.*

ventriculitis (ven-trik″u-li′tis) inflammation of a ventricle, especially of a ventricle of the brain.

ventricul(o)- [L. *ventriculus,* dim. of *venter* belly] a combining form denoting relationship to a ventricle, of the heart or brain.

ventriculoatriostomy (ven-trik″u-lo-a″tre-os′to-me) ventriculoatrial shunt.

ventriculocisternostomy (ven-trik″u-lo-sis″ter-nos′to-me) surgical establishment of a communication between the third ventricle and the cisterna magna for drainage of cerebrospinal fluid in hydrocephalus; called also *Torkildsen's operation.*

ventriculogram (ven-trik′u-lo-gram) a roentgenogram of the cerebral ventricles or of the ventricles of the heart.

ventriculography (ven-trik″u-log′rah-fe) [*ventriculo-* + Gr. *graphein* to write] 1. roentgenography of the head following removal of cerebrospinal fluid from the cerebral ventricles and its replacement by air or other contrast medium. 2. roentgenography of a ventricle of the heart after injection of a contrast medium.

ventriculometry (ven-trik″u-lom′ĕ-tre) [*ventriculo-* + Gr. *metron* measure] the measurement of the intraventricular (intracranial) pressure.

ventriculomyotomy (ven-trik″u-lo-mi-ot′o-me) incision of the muscular wall of the heart.

ventriculonector (ven-trik″u-lo-nek′ter) [*ventriculo-* + L. *nector* joiner] bundle of His.

ventriculopuncture (ven-trik′u-lo-punk″tūr) puncture of a lateral ventricle of the brain by the insertion of a needle.

ventriculoscope (ven-trik′u-lo-skōp) an endoscope for examining the cerebral ventricles and for cauterizing the choroid plexus.

ventriculoscopy (ven-trik″u-los′ko-pe) [*ventriculo-* + Gr.

skopein to examine] direct examination of the cerebral ventricles by means of an endoscope or cystoscope.

ventriculostium (ven-trik″u-los′tĭ-um) [*ventriculo-* + L. *ostium* mouth] the development of an opening between one of the cerebral ventricles and the external surface of the brain.

ventriculostomy (ven-trik″u-los′to-me) [*ventriculo-* + Gr. *stomoun* to provide with an opening, or mouth] the operation of establishing a free communication between the floor of the third ventricle and the underlying cisterna interpeduncularis; for the treatment of hydrocephalus.

ventriculosubarachnoid (ven-trik″u-lo-sub″ah-rak′-noid) pertaining to the cerebral ventricles and the subarachnoid spaces.

ventriculotomy (ven-trik″u-lot′o-me) [*ventriculo-* + *-tomy*] incision of a ventricle (of the brain or heart).

ventriculovenostomy (ven-trik″u-lo-vĕ-nos′to-me) ventriculovenous shunt.

ventriculus (ven-trik′u-lus), pl. *ventric′uli* [L., dim. of *venter* belly] 1. NA alternative for *gaster* (the stomach). 2. a small, normal cavity in an organ, as in the heart or brain; called also *ventricle.* 3. the midgut of an invertebrate. **v. cor′dis** [NA], ventricle of heart: one of the pair of cavities, with thick muscular walls, that make up the bulk of the heart. See *v. dexter cordis* and *v. sinister cordis.* **v. dex′ter cer′ebri,** the ventriculus lateralis cerebri of the right cerebral hemisphere. **v. dex′ter cor′dis** [NA], right ventricle of heart: the cavity of the heart that propels the blood through the pulmonary trunk and arteries into the lungs. See Plate 19. **v. laryn′gis** [NA], **v. laryn′gis [Morgag′nii]**, ventricle of larynx: a lateral evagination of mucous membrane between the vocal and vestibular folds, reaching nearly to the angle of the thyroid cartilage. **v. latera′lis cer′ebri** [NA], lateral ventricle of cerebrum: the cavity in each cerebral hemisphere, derived (developed) from the cavity of the embryonic neural tube; it consists of a pars centralis and three horns—frontal (anterior), temporal (inferior), and occipital (occipital) in the frontal, temporal, and occipital lobes, respectively. They are separated from each other by the septum pellucidum, and each communicates with the third ventricle by an interventricular foramen through which also the choroid plexuses of the lateral ventricles become continuous with that of the third ventricle. Cerebrospinal fluid formed in the lateral ventricle flows into the third ventricle through the interventricular foramina. **v. quar′tus cer′ebri** [NA], fourth ventricle of cerebrum: an irregularly shaped cavity in the rhombencephalon, between the medulla oblongata, the pons, and the isthmus in front, and the cerebellum behind; it is continuous with the central canal of the cord below and with the cerebral aqueduct above, and through its lateral and median apertures it communicates with the subarachnoid space. **v. sinis′ter cer′ebri,** the ventriculus lateralis cerebri of the left cerebral hemisphere. **v. sinis′ter cor′dis** [NA], left ventricle of heart: the cavity of the heart that propels the blood out through the aorta into the systemic arteries. See Plate 19. **v. termina′lis medul′lae spina′lis** [NA], terminal ventricle of spinal cord: a saclike expansion of the central canal of the spinal cord within the conus medullaris. **v. ter′tius cer′ebri** [NA], third ventricle of cerebrum: a narrow cleft below the corpus callosum, within the diencephalon between the two thalami. Its floor is formed by the hypothalamus, its anterior wall by the lamina terminalis, and its roof by ependyma. It communicates with the lateral ventricles by the interventricular foramina, and with the fourth ventricle by the cerebral aqueduct.

ventricumbent (ven″trĭ-kum′bent) [*ventri-* + L. *cumbere* to lie] lying upon the belly; prone.

ventriduct (ven′trĭ-dukt) [*ventri-* + L. *ducere* to draw] to bring or carry ventrad.

ventriduction (ven″trĭ-duk′shun) the act of drawing a part ventrad.

ventriflexion (ven″trĭ-flek′shun) [*ventri-* + *flexion*] flexion toward the belly or ventral surface.

ventrimesal (ven″trĭ-me′sal) pertaining to the ventrimeson.

ventrimeson (ven-trim′e-son) [*ventri-* + Gr. *meson* middle] the middle line on the ventral surface.

ventr(o)-, ventri- [L. *venter* belly or abdomen] combining forms denoting relationship to the belly, or to the front (anterior) aspect of the body.

ventrocystorrhaphy (ven″tro-sis-tor′ah-fe) the stitching of a cyst, or of the bladder, to the abdominal wall.

ventrodorsad (ven″tro-dor′sad) from the ventral toward the dorsal aspect.

ventrodorsal (ven″tro-dor′sal) pertaining to the ventral and dorsal surfaces.

ventrofixation (ven″tro-fiks-a′shun) [*ventro-* + L. *fixare* to fix] the operation of suspending the retroplaced uterus to the abdominal wall. Cf. *hysteropexy*.

ventrohysteropexy (ven″tro-his′ter-o-pek″se) ventrofixation of the uterus.

ventroinguinal (ven″tro-ing′gwĭ-nal) pertaining to the abdomen and the inguinal region.

ventrolateral (ven″tro-lat′er-al) both ventral and lateral.

ventromedian (ven″tro-me′de-an) both ventral and median.

ventroposterior (ven″tro-pos-te′re-or) both ventral and posterior (caudal).

ventroptosia (ven″trop-to′se-ah) [*ventro-* + Gr. *ptōsis* falling + *-ia*] gastroptosis.

ventroptosis (ven″trop-to′sis) gastroptosis.

ventroscopy (ven-tros′ko-pe) [*ventro-* + Gr. *skopein* to examine] peritoneoscopy.

ventrose (ven′trōs) [L. *ventrosus*] having a belly-like expansion.

ventrosuspension (ven″tro-sus-pen′shun) ventrofixation.

ventrotomy (ven-trot′o-me) [*ventro-* + Gr. *tomē* a cutting] celiotomy.

venturimeter (ven″tu-rim′ĕ-ter) [G. B. *Venturi* (Italian physicist, 1746–1822) + Gr. *metron* measure] an instrument for measuring the flow of liquids, as of the blood in vessels, by relating difference of pressures between a constricted and a nonconstricted portion of a tube through which fluid is flowing.

venula (ven′u-lah), pl. *ven′ulae* [L., dim. of *vena*] [NA] venule: any of the small vessels that collect blood from the capillary plexuses and join to form veins. **v. macula′ris infe′rior** [NA], inferior macular venule: the inferior venule draining blood from the macula retinae. **v. macula′ris supe′rior** [NA], superior macular venule: the superior venule draining blood from the macula retinae. **v. media′lis ret′inae** [NA], medial venule of retina: a small branch draining blood from the central region of the retina to the central retinal vein; called also *v. retinae medialis*. **v. nasa′lis ret′inae infe′rior** [NA], inferior nasal venule of retina: a small vein returning blood from the inferior nasal region of the retina to the central vein. **v. nasa′lis ret′inae supe′rior** [NA], superior nasal venule of retina: a small vein returning blood from the superior nasal region of the retina to the central vein. **ven′ulae rec′tae re′nis** [NA], straight venules of kidney: straight veins from the papillary part of the kidney, emptying into the arcuate veins. **v. ret′inae media′lis**, v. medialis retinae. **ven′ulae stella′tae re′nis** [NA], stellate venules of kidney: veins on the surface of the kidney that collect blood from the superficial parts of the cortex and empty into the interlobular veins; called also *venae stellatae renis*. **v. tempora′lis ret′inae infe′rior** [NA], inferior temporal venule of retina: a small vein returning blood from the inferior temporal region of the retina to the central vein. **v. tempora′lis ret′inae supe′rior** [NA], superior temporal venule of retina: a small vein returning blood from the superior temporal region of the retina to the central vein.

venulae (ven′u-le) [L.] genitive and plural of *venula*.

venular (ven′u-lar) pertaining to, composed of, or affecting venules.

venule (ven′ūl) any of the small vessels that collect blood from the capillary plexuses and join to form veins; called also *venula* [NA]. **high endothelial v's**, postcapillary v's. **macular v., inferior**, venula macularis inferior. **macular v., superior**, venula macularis superior. **medial v. of retina**, venula medialis retinae. **nasal v. of retina, inferior**, venula nasalis retinae inferior. **nasal v. of retina, superior**, venula nasalis retinae superior. **postcapillary v's**, 1. a venous capillary. 2. specialized postcapillary venules with tall cuboidal endothelial cells that are found in lymph nodes and gut-associated lymphoid tissue

and are the sites where lymphocytes recirculate from blood to lymph, binding specifically to the endothelial cells and then passing between them. Called also *high endothelial v's*. **stellate v's of kidney**, venulae stellatae renis. **straight v's of kidney**, venulae rectae renis. **temporal v. of retina, inferior**, venula temporalis retinae inferior. **temporal v. of retina, superior**, venula temporalis retinae superior.

VePesid (ve′pe-sid) trademark for a preparation of etoposide.

Veracillin (ver″ah-sil′in) trademark for a preparation of dicloxacillin sodium.

Veraguth's fold (va′rah-goots) [Otto *Veraguth*, Zurich neurologist, 1870–1940] see under *fold*.

Veralba (ver-al′bah) trademark for a mixture of protoveratrines A and B.

verapamil (ver-ap′ah-mil) chemical name: α-[3-[[2-(3,4-dimethoxyphenyl) ethyl] methylamino] propyl] - 3, 4 - dimethoxy - α - (1-methylethyl)benzeneacetonitrile; a coronary vasodilator, $C_{27}H_{38}N_2O_4$, used in the treatment and prophylaxis of angina of effort.

veratric acid (ve-at′rik) a compound, 3,4-dimethoxybenzoic acid, found in sabadilla seeds.

veratroidine (ver″ah-troi′din) a crystallizable base, $C_{32}H_{53}NO_9$, from the liliacious plants *Veratrum album* L. and *V. viride* Aiton, a powerful nerve stimulant and cardiac inhibitor.

Veratrum (ve-ra′trum) [L.] a genus of poisonous liliaceous plants, including *V. album* L., or European white hellebore, and *V. viride* Aiton, or American or green hellebore, both of which are the source of antihypertensive alkaloids.

verbal (ver′bal) [L. *verbum*] consisting of words; pertaining to words or speech.

verbenol (ver-be′nol) a terpene alcohol, $(CH_3)_2C:C_6H_6-(OH)·CH_3$, from *Boswellia carterii* Birdw. (Burseraceae), a tree of southern Europe, Arabia, and Somali; a source of the biblical frankincense.

verbenone (ver-be′nōn) a terpene ketone, $(CH_3)_2C:C_6H_5O··CH_3$, from *Verbena triphylla*, an American herb.

verbigeration (ver-bij″er-a′shun) [L. *verbigerare* to chatter] stereotyped and meaningless repetition of words and phrases; seen in some cases of schizophrenia. Called also *cataphasia*. Cf. *perseveration*.

verbomania (ver″bo-ma′ne-ah) [L. *verba* word + Gr. *mania* madness] logorrhea.

Vercyte (ver′sīt) trademark for a preparation of pipobroman.

verdigris (ver′dĭ-gris) [Fr., from *vert de Grèce* green of Greece] a blue, hydrated, basic copper acetate, $(CH_3·COO)_2·Cu·Cu·(OH)_2$; astringent.

verdohemin (ver″do-he′min) a compound analogous to hemin, in which one porphyrin ring is open.

verdohemochromogen (ver″do-he″mo-kro′mo-jen) a compound analogous to hemochromogen, in which one porphyrin ring is open.

verdohemoglobin (ver″do-he″mo-glo″bin) a compound analogous to hemoglobin, in which one porphyrin ring is open.

verdoperoxidase (ver″do-per-ok″sĭ-dās) myeloperoxidase.

Verga's lacrimal groove, ventricle (ver′gahz) [Andrea *Verga*, Italian neurologist, 1811–1895] see under *groove* and *ventricle*.

verge (verj) a circumference, or ring. **anal v.**, the external or distal boundary of the anal canal; the line where the walls of the anus come in contact during the normal state of apposition.

vergence (ver′jens) [L. *vergere* to bend] 1. the amount of convergence or divergence of a pencil of rays entering or leaving a lens or mirror, expressed as the reciprocal of the distance from the lens or mirror to the focus of the rays. For rays through a principal focus, the vergence is equal to the focal power of the lens or mirror. See *convergence* (def. 2) and *divergence* (def. 1). 2. a disjunctive reciprocal rotation of both eyes around their horizontal, vertical, or anteroposterior axes such that the axes of fixation are not parallel. The kind of vergence is indicated by a prefix. See *convergence* (def. 3), *divergence* (def. 2), *infravergence*, *supravergence*, *cyclovergence*, and see *duction* and *version* (def. 5).

vergency (ver′jen-se)   vergence.

Verheyen's stars (ver-hi′enz) [Philippe *Verheyen*, Flemish anatomist, 1648–1710]   venulae stellatae renis.

Verhoeff's operation, stain (ver′hefz) [Frederick Herman *Verhoeff*, American ophthalmologist, born 1874]   see under *operation* and *Table of Stains.*

Veriloid (ver′ĭ-loid)   trademark for a preparation of alkavervir.

vermes (ver′mēz) [L.]   plural of *vermis.*

Vermes (ver′mēz)   obsolete term for the group of invertebrates called worms.

vermetoid (ver′mĕ-toid)   wormlike.

vermian (ver′me-an)   pertaining to the vermis of the cerebellum.

Vermicella (ver″mĭ-sel′ah) [L.]   a genus of mildly venomous Australian serpents.

vermicidal (ver″mĭ-si′dal)   destructive to worms.

vermicide (ver″mĭ-sīd) [*vermis* + L. *caedere* to kill]   an anthelmintic drug or medicine destructive to intestinal animal parasites.

vermicular (ver-mik′u-lar) [L. *vermicularis*, from *vermis* worm]   wormlike in shape or appearance.

vermiculation (ver-mik″u-la′shun) [L. *vermiculatio*, from *vermis* worm]   peristaltic or wormlike movements, as of the intestine; peristalsis.

vermicule (ver′mĭ-kūl)   a wormlike structure; see also *ookinete.*

vermiculose (ver-mik′u-lōs)   vermiculous.

vermiculous (ver-mik′u-lus)   1. wormlike.   2. infected with worms.

vermiform (ver′mĭ-form) [L. *vermiformis*, from *vermis* worm + *forma* shape]   shaped like a worm.

vermifugal (ver-mif′u-gal) [*vermis* + L. *fugare* to put to flight]   expelling worms or intestinal animal parasites.

vermifuge (ver′mĭ-fūj)   an agent that expels worms or intestinal animal parasites; an anthelmintic.

vermilion (ver-mil′yun)   cinnabar, or mercuric sulfide, HgS, a red pigment; see also under *border.*

vermilionectomy (ver-mil″yon-ek′to-me)   excision of the vermilion border of the lip, the surgically created defect being resurfaced by advancement of the undermined labial mucosa.

vermin (ver′min) [L. *vermis* worm]   an external animal parasite; animal ectoparasites collectively.

verminal (ver′mĭ-nal)   pertaining to or due to worms; pertaining to or due to vermin.

vermination (ver″mĭ-na′shun) [L. *verminatio*]   infection with worms; infestation with vermin.

verminosis (ver″mĭ-no′sis)   vermination.

verminotic (ver″mĭ-not′ik)   pertaining to or caused by infection with worms; pertaining to or caused by infestation with vermin.

verminous (ver′mĭ-nus) [L. *verminosus*]   pertaining to, due to, or abounding in worms; pertaining to, due to, or abounding in vermin.

vermis (ver′mis) [L.]   a worm or wormlike structure; often used alone to designate the vermis cerebelli.   **v. cerebel′li** [NA], the narrow median part of the cerebellum, between the two lateral hemispheres; the *cranial* or *superior* portion extends from the lingula to the folium vermis, and the *inferior* or *caudal* portion from the tuber vermis to the nodulus. See also *cerebellum.*

vermix (ver′miks)   appendix vermiformis.

vermography (ver-mog′rah-fe)   roentgenography of the vermiform appendix.

Vermox (ver′moks)   trademark for preparations of mebendazole.

vernal (ver′nal) [L. *vernalis* of the spring]   pertaining to or occurring in the spring.

Vernet's syndrome (ver-nāz′) [Maurice *Vernet*, French neurologist, born 1887]   see under *syndrome.*

Verneuil's canals, etc. (ver-na′ez) [Aristide August Stanislaus *Verneuil*, French surgeon, 1823–1895]   see under *canal, disease,* and *neuroma.*

vernier (ver′ne-er) [Pierre *Vernier*, French physicist, 1580–1637]   a finely graduated scale accessory to a more coarsely graduated one for measuring fractions of the divisions of the latter.

vernin (ver′nin)   a pentoside of adenine found in *Vicia* seedlings.

vernix (ver′niks) [L. "sandarac" (resin), from Gr. *Berenikē* (now *Benghazi*) where first made]   varnish.   **v. caseo′sa** ["cheesy varnish"], an unctuous substance composed of sebum and desquamated epithelial cells, which covers the skin of the fetus.

Vernonia anthelmintica Willd. (ver-no′ne-ah an″thel-min′tĭ-kah)   a plant called *somraj* in India; it is anthelmintic. Also used there for skin diseases and leprosy and as an abortifacient.

Verocay bodies (ver′o-ka) [José *Verocay*, Prague pathologist, 1876–1927]   see under *body.*

Veronicella (ve-ron″ĭ-sel′lah)   a genus of slugs.   **V. leydig′i,** an intermediate host of *Angiostrongylus cantonensis* in the Pacific, especially in Tahiti and Hawaii.

verruca (vĕ-roo′kah), gen. and pl. *verru′cae* [L.]   1. a lobulated hyperplastic epidermal lesion with a horny surface caused by a human papillomavirus, transmitted by contact or autoinoculation, and usually occurring on the dorsa of the fingers and hands; called also *common wart, v. vulgaris, verruga,* and *wart.*   2. any of various nonviral, wartlike epidermal proliferations.   **v. acumina′ta,** condyloma acuminatum.   **v. digita′ta,** a wart with finger-like excrescences growing from its surface.   **v. filifor′mis,** a wart with soft, thin, threadlike projections on its surface.   **v. necrogen′ica,** tuberculosis verrucosa cutis.   **v. perua′na, v. peruvia′na,** see *bartonellosis.*   **v. pla′na, v. pla′na juveni′lis,** a small, smooth, usually skin-colored or light brown, slightly raised wart sometimes occurring in great numbers, on the face, neck, back of the hands, wrists, and knees; seen most frequently in children but also in adults. Called also *flat, fugitive, juvenile,* and *plane wart.* See also *epidermodysplasia verruciformis.*   **v. planta′ris,** plantar wart: a viral epidermal tumor on the sole.   **v. seborrhe′ica,** seborrheic keratosis.   **v. vulga′ris,** verruca, def. 1.

verrucae (vĕ-roo′se) [L.]   genitive and plural of *verruca.*

verruciform (vĕ-roo′sĭ-form) [L. *verruca* wart + *forma* form]   resembling or shaped like a verruca, or wart.

verrucose (ver′oo-kōs) [L. *verrucosus*]   verrucous.

verrucosis (ver″oo-ko′sis)   a condition marked by the presence of multiple warts, or verrucae.

verrucous (ver′oo-kus)   rough; warty.

verruga (vĕ-roo′gah) [Sp.]   verruca.   **v. perua′na,** see *bartonellosis.*

Versapen (ver′sah-pen)   trademark for preparations of hetacillin.

versicolor (ver-sik′o-lor) [L. *vertere* to turn + *color* color]   variegated; changing color.

version (ver′zhun) [L. *versio,* turning]   1. the act or process of turning something or of changing direction.   2. the situation of an organ or part in relation to an established normal position.   3. in gynecology, the misalignment or tilting of the uterus; cf. *flexion* (def. 2).   4. in obstetrics, the manual conversion of or changing of the polarity of the fetus with reference to the mother; cf. *presentation.*   5. in ophthalmology, the conjugate rotation of both eyes in the same direction. See *infraversion* and *sursumversion,* and see *duction* and *vergence* (def. 2).   **abdominal v.,** external v.   **bimanual v.,** version done by combined external and internal manipulation, the cervix being open enough to admit the hand; called also *combined v.*   **bipolar v.,** version done by purely external manipulation or by combined internal and external manipulation.   **Braxton Hicks v.,** internal podalic version performed through a partially but not completely dilated cervix; used on a nonviable fetus.   **cephalic v.,** version in which the fetal head is brought down into the maternal pelvis.   **combined v.,** bimanual v.   **Denman's spontaneous v.,** see under *evolution.*   **external v.,** manipulation of the fetal body applied through the abdominal wall of the mother.   **Hicks v.,** Braxton Hicks v.   **internal v.,** turning of the fetus effected by the hand or fingers inserted through the dilated cervix.   **pelvic v.,** version done by manipulating the buttocks of the fetus.   **podalic v.,** version in which one or both legs of the fetus are brought down into the maternal pelvis.   **Potter v.,** podalic version in head presentation when the cervix is fully effaced and dilated. **spontaneous v.,** conversion of an abnormal position of the fetus into a normal or relatively normal one, occurring without the aid of manipulation. **Wigand's v.,** external conversion of a transverse lie into a cephalic presentation, accomplished by pushing the fetal head down with one hand and its buttocks up with the other; called also *Wigand's maneuver.*

vertebra (ver'tĕ-brah), pl. *ver'tebrae* [L.]   any of the thirty-three bones of the spinal column (columna vertebralis), comprising the seven *cervical,* twelve *thoracic,* five *lumbar,* five *sacral,* and four *coccygeal* vertebrae. **abdominal vertebrae,** vertebrae lumbales. **basilar v.,** the lowest or last of the lumbar vertebrae. **caudal vertebrae, caudate vertebrae,** vertebrae coccygeae. **cervical vertebrae, ver'tebrae cervica'les** [NA], the upper seven vertebrae, constituting the skeleton of the neck. **ver'tebrae coccyg'eae** [NA], **coccygeal vertebrae,** the lowest segments of the vertebral column, comprising three to five rudimentary vertebrae which form the coccyx. **ver'tebrae col'li,** vertebrae cervicales. **cranial v.,** the segments of the skull and facial bones, by some regarded as modified vertebrae. **v. denta'ta,** the second cervical vertebra (axis [NA]). **dorsal vertebrae,** vertebrae thoracicae. **false vertebrae,** the vertebrae that become fused, i.e., the sacral and coccygeal vertebrae. **ver'tebrae lumba'les** [NA], **lumbar vertebrae,** the five vertebrae between the thoracic vertebrae and the sacrum. **v. mag'num,** os sacrum. **odontoid v.,** the second cervical vertebra (axis [NA]). **v. pla'na,** a condition of spondylitis in which the body of the vertebra is reduced to a sclerotic disk; often due to eosinophilic granuloma. **v. prom'inens** [NA], **prominent v.,** the seventh cervical vertebra; so called because of the length of its spinous process, although it is only the spine that is prominent. (NOTE: the spinous process of the first thoracic vertebra is often more prominent.) **sacral vertebrae, ver'tebrae sacra'les** [NA], the vertebrae below the lumbar vertebrae (usually five in number), which normally fuse to form the sacrum (os sacrum). **sternal v.,** sternebra. **terminal v., great,** os sacrum. **ver'tebrae thoraca'les, thoracic vertebrae,** vertebrae thoracicae. **ver'tebrae thora'cicae** [NA], thoracic vertebrae: the vertebrae, usually twelve in number, situated between the cervical and the lumbar

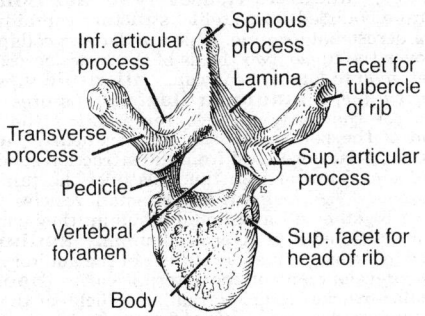

Inf. articular process   Spinous process   Lamina   Facet for tubercle of rib   Transverse process   Sup. articular process   Pedicle   Vertebral foramen   Sup. facet for head of rib   Body

Typical (sixth) thoracic vertebra viewed from above.

vertebrae, giving attachment to the ribs and forming part of the posterior wall of the thorax; called also *vertebrae thoracales.* **tricuspid v.,** the sixth cervical vertebra of quadrupeds. **true vertebrae,** the vertebrae that normally remain unfused throughout life, i.e., the cervical, thoracic, and lumbar vertebrae.

vertebrae, (ver'tĕ-bre) [L.]   genitive and plural of *vertebra.*

vertebral (ver'te-bral) [L. *vertebralis*]   of or pertaining to a vertebra.

vertebrarium (ver"tĕ-bra're-um) [L.]   the vertebral column.

vertebrarterial (ver"tĕ-brar-te're-al)   pertaining to the vertebral artery.

Vertebrata (ver"tĕ-bra'tah)   a subphylum of the Chordata comprising all animals that have a vertebral column, including mammals, birds, reptiles, amphibians, and fishes.

vertebrate (ver'tĕ-brāt) [L. *vertebratus*]   1. having a vertebral column. 2. an animal having a vertebral column; any member of the Vertebrata.

vertebrate collagenase   see *vertebrate* c. under *collagenase.*

vertebrated (ver'tĕ-brāt"ed)   made up of joints resembling the vertebrae.

vertebrectomy (ver"tĕ-brek'to-me) [*vertebro-* + Gr. *ektomē* excision]   excision of a vertebra.

vertebr(o)- [L. *vertebra,* q.v.]   a combining form denoting relationship to a vertebra, or to the vertebral column.

vertebroarterial (ver"tĕ-bro-ar-te're-al)   vertebrarterial.

vertebrobasilar (ver"tĕ-bro-bas'ĭ-lar)   pertaining to or involving the vertebral and basilar arteries.

vertebrochondral (ver"tĕ-bro-kon'dral)   pertaining to a vertebra and a costal cartilage.

vertebrocostal (ver"tĕ-bro-kos'tal) [*vertebro-* + L. *costa* rib]   pertaining to a vertebra and a rib.

vertebrodidymus (ver"tĕ-bro-did'ĭ-mus) [*vertebro-* + Gr. *didymos* twin]   a twin monster united in the region of the spinal column.

vertebrodymus (ver"tĕ-brod'ĭ-mus)   vertebrodidymus.

vertebrofemoral (ver"tĕ-bro-fem'or-al)   relating to the vertebrae and the femur.

vertebrogenic (ver"tĕ-bro-jen'ik)   arising in a vertebra or in the vertebral column.

vertebroiliac (ver"tĕ-bro-il'e-ak)   pertaining to the vertebrae and the ilium.

vertebromammary (ver"tĕ-bro-mam'er-e)   pertaining to or extending between the vertebral column and the pectoral region.

vertebrosacral (ver"tĕ-bro-sa'kral)   pertaining to the vertebrae and the sacrum.

vertebrosternal (ver"tĕ-bro-ster'nal)   pertaining to the vertebrae and the sternum.

vertex (ver'teks), pl. *ver'tices* [L.]   1. a summit or top. 2. [NA] the top or crown of the head; called also *vertex cranii.* **v. of bony cranium,** the highest point of the skull; generally located on the sagittal suture, usually near the midpoint. Called also *v. cranii ossei.* **v. cor'dis,** vortex cordis. **v. of cornea, v. cor'neae** [NA], the central, thinner portion of the cornea. **v. cra'nii** [NA], vertex (def. 2). **v. cra'nii os'sei,** v. of bony cranium. **v. of urinary bladder, v. vesi'cae urina'riae,** apex vesicae urinariae.

vertical (ver-ti-kal)   1. perpendicular to the plane of the horizon. 2. relating to the vertex.

verticalis (ver"tĭ-ka'lis) [L.]   vertical, or perpendicular to the plane of the horizon; [NA] a general term used in reference to structures with the body in the anatomical, that is, upright, position.

verticillate (ver-tis'ĭ-lāt) [L. *vertex* a whorl]   arranged in the form of a whorl.

Verticillium (ver"tĭ-sil'e-um)   a genus of imperfect fungi of the order Moniliales, family Moniliaceae, some species of which cause apple wilt. **V. gra'phii,** a species of uncertain identity, which is considered by some to be a species of *Trichosporon,* sometimes reported in otitis externa and mycotic keratitis.

verticine (ver'tĭ-sin)   a crystalline alkaloid, $C_{27}H_{45}NO_3$, from *Fritillaria verticillata* Willd. (Liliaceae), a bulbous herb.

verticomental (ver"tĭ-ko-men'tal)   pertaining to the vertex and the chin.

vertiginous (ver-tij'ĭ-nus) [L. *vertiginosus*]   pertaining to or affected with vertigo.

vertigo (ver'tĭ-go, ver-ti'go) [L. *vertigo*]   an illusion of movement; a sensation as if the external world were revolving around the patient (*objective vertigo*) or as if he himself were revolving in space (*subjective vertigo*). The term is sometimes erroneously used to mean any form of dizziness. Vertigo may result from diseases of the inner ear or may be due to disturbances of the vestibular centers or pathways in the central nervous system. **v. ab stom'acho lae'so,** stomachal v. **alternobaric v.,** a transient, true, whirling vertigo sometimes affecting those (caisson workers, air crew members, etc.) subjected to large, rapid variations in barometric pressure; called also *pressure v.* **angiopathic v.,** vertigo due to arteriosclerosis of the cerebral vessels. **apoplectic v.,** scotodinia. **arteriosclerotic v.,** angiopathic v. **auditory v., aural v.,** Meniere's disease. **benign paroxysmal positional (or postural) v.,** recurrent vertigo and nystagmus occurring when the head is placed in certain positions, usually not associated with lesions of the central nervous system. **cardiac v.,** vertigo due to some chronic disease of the heart. **cardiovascular v.,** vertigo due to sclerosis of the blood vessels and heart. **central v.,** vertigo due to disease of the central nervous system. **cerebral v.,** that which is due to some brain disease. **disabling positional v.,** constant vertigo or dysequilibrium and nausea in the upright position, without hearing disturbance or loss of vestibular function. **encephalic v.,** a sensation of movement of tissues within the skull, as of the brain turning over and over, or round and round. **endemic paralytic v.,** Gerlier's disease. **epidemic v.,** an epidemic condition characterized chiefly by vertigo but with some nausea and vomiting. See *epidemic nausea,* under *nausea.* Cf. *nausea epidemica.* **epileptic v.,** that which attends or follows an epileptic attack. **essential v.,** a vertigo, often severe, but of no discoverable cause; probably due to some disease or lesion in a brain center. **galvanic v.,** voltanic v. **gastric v.,** a form associated with disease or disorder of the stomach. **height v.,** dizziness (not a true vertigo) felt on looking down from a high location. **horizontal v.,** that which comes on when a person lies down. **hysterical v.,** vertigo associated with hysterical symptoms, often of a bizarre form. **labyrinthine v.,** a form associated with disease of the labyrinth of the ear. See *Meniere's disease,* under *disease.* **laryngeal v.,** tussive syncope. **lateral v.,** that which is caused by rapidly passing a row of similar objects, as a fence or series of pillars. **lithemic v.,** that which is associated with gout and lithemia. **mechanical v.,** vertigo due to long-continued turning or vibration of the body, as in seasickness. **neurasthenic v.,** a subjective form of vertiginous sensation associated with neurasthenia. **nocturnal v.,** a sensation of falling occurring as the subject is going to sleep. **objective v.,** a form in which the objects seen by the patient seem to be moving around him. **ocular v.,** a form due to eye disease, especially to paralysis of or lack of balance in the eye muscles. **organic v.,** vertigo due to vestibular brain disease or to tabes dorsalis. **paralyzing v.,** Gerlier's disease. **peripheral v.,** vestibular v. **pilot's v.,** spatial disorientation. **positional v., postural v.,** vertigo associated with a specific position of the head in space or changes in the position of the head in space; called also *positional v.* **pressure v.,** alternobaric v. **primary v.,** vertigo resulting from a stimulus, e.g., an active disease process, within the vestibular system of the ear, and independent of body movement. **residual v.,** vertigo associated with motion, resulting from hypofunction or absence of vestibular sensory or neural elements; when it occurs only in one plane of movement, it is called *postural v.* **riders' v.,** motion sickness. **rotary v., rotatory v.,** vertigo in which there is a definite feeling of rotation. **sham-movement v.,** vertigo attended by a sensation as if objects were circling around the body. **special sense v.,** aural (Ménière's disease) or ocular v. **stomachal v.,** vertigo associated with a disorder of the digestive system. **subjective v.,** that in which the patient seems to himself to be turning round and round. **systematic v.,** rotary v. **tenebric v.,** scotodinia. **toxemic v., toxic v.,** a form of vertigo which results from poisoning, alcoholism, uremia, or lithemia. **vertical v.,** that which is caused by looking up or down at a distant object. **vestibular v.,** vertigo due to disturbances of the vestibular centers or pathways in the central nervous system; called also *peripheral v.* **villous v.,** that which is caused by a functional derangement of the liver. **voltaic v.,** an inclination of the head toward the shoulder on the side of the positive pole when a galvanic current is applied to the vestibular fibers of the eighth nerve.

vertigraphy (ver-tig′rah-fe) [L. *vertigo* a whirling + Gr. *graphein* to write] see *body section roentgenography,* under *roentgenography.*

verumontanitis (ve″ru-mon″tah-ni′tis) inflammation of the verumontanum (colliculus seminalis).

verumontanum (ve″ru-mon-ta′num) [L. "mountain ridge"] colliculus seminalis.

vesalian (ve-sa′le-an) named in honor of Andreas *Vesalius,* as the vesalian bone (os vesalianum) or vein.

vesalianum (ve-sa″le-a′num) [Andreas *Vesalius*] a name applied to several sesamoid bones: one on the outer border of the foot between the cuboid and fifth metatarsal bone, and one (sometimes more) in the tendon of origin of the gastrocnemius muscle.

Vesalius (ve-sa′le-us), Andreas (1514–1564) a Flemish physician and professor of anatomy of Padua, where in 1543 he produced his *De humani corporis fabrica libri septem* (Seven Books on the Structure of the Human Body) and founded the modern science of anatomy. Following Galen's exhortations to dissect and observe, Vesalius dissected and observed and overthrew Galen's anatomy (which was founded on nonhuman dissection). Vesalius standardized anatomical nomenclature and made important contributions in osteology and myology; in cardiology he rejected Galen's doctrine of the pervious septum. The riot of criticism for the old orthodoxy and against Vesalius drove him from Padua to Spain, where he became physician to Emperor Charles V. See also *foramen venosum,* under *foramen* and under *ligament.*

Vesic. abbreviation for L. *vesic'ula, vesicato'rium,* a blister.

vesica (vĕ-si′kah), pl. *vesi'cae* [L.] a membranous sac or receptacle for a secretion; [NA] a general term for such a structure. Called also *bladder.* **v. bilia'ris,** [NA], the gallbladder: the pear-shaped reservoir for the bile on the posteroinferior surface of the liver between the right and quadrate lobes; called also *cholecyst* and *v. fellea* [NA alternative]. **v. fel'lea,** NA alternative for *v. biliaris.* **v. prostat'ica,** utriculus prostaticus. **v. urina'ria** [NA], urinary bladder: the musculomembranous sac, situated in the anterior part of the pelvic cavity, that serves as a reservoir for urine; it receives the excretory products of the kidneys through the ureters, and expels them through the urethra.

vesicae (ve-si′se) [L.] genitive and plural of *vesica.*

vesical (ves′ĭ-kal) pertaining to the bladder.

vesicant (ves′ĭ-kant) [L. *vesica* blister] 1. causing blisters; blistering. 2. a blistering drug or agent.

vesication (ves″ĭ-ka′shun) 1. the process of blistering. 2. a blistered spot or surface.

vesicatory (ves′ĭ-kah-tor″e) [L. *vesicare* to blister] vesicant.

vesicle (ves′ĭ-k'l) [L. *vesicula,* dim. of *vesica* bladder] 1. a small bladder or sac containing liquid; see also *vesicula.* 2. a small circumscribed epidermal elevation, less than 5 mm. in circumference, usually containing a clear fluid. Cf. *bullae.* 3. the swollen end of a conidiophore from which sterigmata are produced. **acoustic v.,** auditory v. **acrosomal v.,** a membrane-bounded vacuole-like structure containing the enlarging acrosomal granule, which undergoes collapse and spreads over the upper two thirds of the head (acrosome) of a spermatozoon to form a head cap. **allantoic v.,** see under *diverticulum.* **amniocardiac v's,** fissures in the mesoderm of the early embryo representing the paired primordia of the pericardial sac and the heart. **archoplasmic v.,** a sac developed from the attraction sphere of a spermatid and growing into the sheath of the tail of the spermatozoon. **Ascherson's v's,** small vesicles formed by shaking together oil and liquid albumin; they consist of drops of oil enclosed in a layer of albumin. **auditory v.,** a detached ovoid sac formed by closure of the auditory pit, in embryonic development of the internal ear. **Baer's v.,** the vesicular ovarian follicle (graafian follicle) of the ovary with its contained ovum. **blastodermic v.,** the blastocyst. **brain v's,** the five divisions of the closed neural tube in the developing embryo, including, in craniocaudal sequence, the telencephalon, diencephalon, mesencephalon, metencephalon, and myelencephalon. **brain v's, primary,** the three earliest subdivisions of the embryonic neural tube, including the prosencephalon, mesencephalon, and rhombencephalon. **brain v's, secondary,** the four brain vesicles formed by specialization of the prosencephalon (the telencephalon and diencephalon) and of the rhombencephalon (the metencephalon and myelencephalon) in later embryonic development. **cephalic v's, cerebral v's,** brain v's. **cervical v.,** a temporary sac in the cervical region of the embryo formed by the closing off of the cervical sinus. **chorionic v.,** the mammalian chorion. **concentrating v's,** condensing vacuoles. **encephalic v's,** brain v's. **germinal v.,** the fluid-filled nucleus of an oocyte toward the end of prophase of its meiotic division. **graafian v's,** folliculi ovarici vesiculosi. **intermediate v's,** transfer v's. **lens v.,** a vesicle formed from the lens pit of the embryo and developing into the crystalline lens;

called also *lens sac.* **Malpighi's v's,** alveoli pulmonei. **matrix v's,** small membrane-limited structures at sites of calcification of the cartilage matrix. **Naboth's v's,** nabothian follicles. **ocular v.,** vesicula ophthalmica. **olfactory v.,** 1. the vesicle in the embryo which later develops into the olfactory bulb and tract. 2. a bulbous expansion at the distal end of an olfactory cell, from which the olfactory hairs project. **ophthalmic v., optic v.,** vesicula ophthalmica. **otic v.,** auditory v. **phagocytotic v.,** phagosome. **pinocytotic v.,** pinosome. **pituitary v.,** Rathke's pouch. **plasmalemmal v.,** caveola. **prostatic v.,** utriculus prostaticus. **Purkinje's v.,** germinal v. **secretory v's,** condensing vacuoles. **seminal v.,** vesicula seminalis. **sense v.,** the vesicular primordium of a sense organ in the embryo. **spermatic v., false,** utriculus prostaticus. **synaptic v's,** a profusion of small round structures in the end-feet of neurons, believed to contain protein-bound humoral transmitter substance. **transfer v's, transitional v's, transport v's,** small vesicles formed by budding off the granular endoplasmic reticulum, in which secretory material is transferred to the Golgi complex, where it is concentrated in condensing vacuoles (q.v.). Called also *intermediate v's.* **umbilical v.,** the pear-shaped expansion of the yolk sac growing out into the cavity of the chorion at the end of the fourth week of development, and joined to the midgut of the embryo by the yolk stalk. **water expulsion v.,** contractile vacuole.

vesic(o)- [L. *vesica* bladder] a combining form denoting relationship to the bladder, or to a blister.

vesicoabdominal (ves″ĭ-ko-ab-dom′ĭ-nal) pertaining to the urinary bladder and abdomen, or communicating with the bladder and an abdominal viscus, as a vesicoabdominal fistula.

vesicocavernous (ves″ĭ-ko-kav′er-nus) both vesicular and cavernous.

vesicocele (ves′ĭ-ko-sēl″) [*vesico-* + Gr. *kēlē* hernia] hernial protrusion of the bladder.

vesicocervical (ves″ĭ-ko-ser′vĭ-kal) [*vesico-* + L. *cervix* neck] pertaining to the urinary bladder and the cervix uteri, or communicating with the bladder and the cervical canal, as a vesicocervical fistula.

vesicoclysis (ves″ĭ-kok′lĭ-sis) [*vesico-* + Gr. *klysis* washing] the injection of a fluid into the urinary bladder.

vesicocolic (ves″ĭ-ko-kol′ik) vesicocolonic.

vesicocolonic (ves″ĭ-ko-ko-lon′ik) pertaining to or communicating with the urinary bladder and colon, as a vesicocolonic fistula. Called also *vesicocolic.*

vesicoenteric (ves″ĭ-ko-en-ter′ik) vesicointestinal.

vesicofixation (ves″ĭ-ko-fiks-a′shun) the surgical fixation of the urinary bladder; cystopexy.

vesicointestinal (ves″ĭ-ko-in-tes′tĭ-nal) pertaining to or communicating with the urinary bladder and intestine, as a vesicointestinal fistula.

vesicoperineal (ves″ĭ-ko-per″ĭ-ne′al) pertaining to or communicating with the urinary bladder and perineum, as a vesicoperineal fistula.

vesicoprostatic (ves″ĭ-ko-pros-tat′ik) pertaining to the urinary bladder and the prostate.

vesicopubic (ves″ĭ-ko-pu′bik) pertaining to the urinary bladder and the pubes.

vesicopustule (ves″ĭ-ko-pus′tūl) a vesicle which is developing into a pustule by entry of leukocytes into its contents.

vesicorectal (ves″ĭ-ko-rek′tal) pertaining to the urinary bladder and the rectum.

vesicorenal (ves″ĭ-ko-re′nal) pertaining to the urinary bladder and the kidney.

vesicosigmoid (ves″ĭ-ko-sig′moid) pertaining to the urinary bladder and sigmoid flexure.

vesicosigmoidostomy (ves″ĭ-ko-sig″moi-dos′to-me) [L. *vesica* bladder + *sigmoid* + Gr. *stomoun* to provide with an opening or mouth] surgical creation of an opening between the urinary bladder and the sigmoid colon.

vesicospinal (ves″ĭ-ko-spi′nal) pertaining to the urinary bladder and the spine.

vesicostomy (ves″ĭ-kos′to-me) the formation of an opening into the bladder; cystostomy. **cutaneous v.,** surgical anastomosis of the bladder mucosa to an opening in the skin below the umbilicus, creating a stoma for bladder drainage.

vesicotomy (ves″ĭ-kot′o-me) [L. *vesica* bladder + Gr. *tomē* a cutting] incision of the urinary bladder; cystotomy.

vesicoumbilical (ves″ĭ-ko-um-bil′ĭ-kal) pertaining to the umbilicus and the urinary bladder.

vesicourachal (ves″ĭ-ko-u′rah-kal) pertaining to the urinary bladder and the urachus.

vesicoureteral, vesicoureteric (ves″ĭ-ko-u-re′ter-al; ves″ĭ-ko-u″rĕ-ter′ik) pertaining to or communicating with the urinary bladder and the ureter.

vesicourethral (ves″ĭ-ko-u-re′thral) pertaining to or communicating with the urinary bladder and the urethra.

vesicouterine (ves″ĭ-ko-u′ter-īn) pertaining to or communicating with the urinary bladder and the uterus.

vesicouterovaginal (ves″ĭ-ko-u″ter-o-vaj′ĭ-nal) pertaining to or communicating with the urinary bladder, uterus, and vagina.

vesicovaginal (ves″ĭ-ko-vaj′ĭ-nal) pertaining to or communicating with the urinary bladder and vagina.

vesicovaginorectal (ves″ĭ-ko-vaj″ĭ-no-rek′tal) pertaining to or communicating with the urinary bladder, vagina, and rectum.

vesicula (vĕ-sik′u-lah), pl. *vesic′ulae* [L., dim. of *vesica*] a vesicle: a small bladder or sac containing liquid; used as a general term in anatomical nomenclature. **v. bi′lis, v. fel′lea,** vesica biliaris. **v. germinati′va,** germinal vesicle. **vesic′ulae graafia′nae,** folliculi ovarici vesiculosi. **vesic′ulae nabo′thi,** Naboth's follicles. **v. ophthal′mica** [NA], optic vesicle: an evagination developing on either side of the forebrain of the early embryo, from which the percipient parts of the eye are formed. **v. prostat′ica,** utriculus prostaticus. **v. semina′lis** [NA], seminal vesicle: either of the paired, sacculated pouches attached to the posterior part of the urinary bladder; the duct of each joins the ipsilateral ductus deferens to form the ejaculatory duct. Called also *glandula seminalis* [NA alternative] and *seminal gland.* **v. sero′sa,** chorion.

vesiculae (vĕ-sik′u-le) [L.] genitive and plural of *vesicula.*

vesicular (vĕ-sik′u-lar) [L. *vesicula* a little bladder] 1. composed of or relating to small, saclike bodies. 2. pertaining to or made up of vesicles on the skin.

vesiculated (vĕ-sik′u-lāt″ed) marked by the presence of vesicles.

vesiculation (vĕ-sik″u-la′shun) the presence or formation of vesicles.

vesiculectomy (vĕ-sik″u-lek′to-me) [*vesicle* + Gr. *ektomē* excision] excision of a vesicle, especially the seminal vesicle.

vesiculiform (vĕ-sik′u-lĭ-form″) [*vesicle* + L. *forma* form] shaped like a vesicle.

vesiculitis (vĕ-sik″u-li′tis) inflammation of a vesicle, especially of a seminal vesicle.

vesiculobronchial (vĕ-sik″u-lo-brong′ke-al) both vesicular and bronchial; bronchovesicular.

vesiculocavernous (vĕ-sik″u-lo-kav′er-nus) both vesicular and cavernous.

vesiculogram (vĕ-sik′u-lo-gram″) a roentgenogram of the seminal vesicles.

vesiculography (vĕ-sik″u-log′rah-fe) roentgenography of the seminal vesicles.

vesiculopapular (vĕ-sik″u-lo-pap′u-lar) pertaining to or characterized by vesicles and papules.

vesiculopustular (vĕ-sik″u-lo-pus′tu-lar) consisting of or pertaining to vesicles and pustules.

vesiculotomy (vĕ-sik″u-lot′o-me) [*vesicle* + Gr. *tomē* a cutting] incision of a vesicle, especially the seminal vesicle.

vesiculotubular (vĕ-sik″u-lo-tu′bu-lar) having both a vesicular and a tubular quality; said of auscultatory sounds.

vesiculotympanic (vĕ-sik″u-lo-tim-pan′ik) having both a vesicular and tympanic quality; said of percussion sounds.

vesperal (ves′per-al) [L. *vespera* evening] pertaining to or occurring in the evening.

Vesprin (ves′prin) trademark for preparations of triflupromazine.

vessel (ves′el) any channel for carrying a fluid, such as the blood or lymph, see also *vas.* **absorbent v's,** lymphatic vessels. **afferent v. of glomerulus,** arteriola glomerularis afferens. **afferent v's of lymph node,** vasa afferentia nodi lymphatici. **anastomotic v.,** vas anastomoticum. **arterioluminal v's,** small branches of coronary arterioles that lie near the endocardium, and after a short course open directly into the lumen of the heart. **arteriosinusoidal v's,** small branches of coronary arterioles that soon break up into sinusoids that lie between bundles or individual muscle fibers of the heart. **bile v.,** one of the vessels in the liver which conduct bile; called also *ductuli biliferi* [NA]. **blood v.,** any of the vessels conveying the blood, and comprising the arteries, arterioles, capillaries, venules, and veins. **chyliferous v's,** lacteal v's. **collateral v.,** 1. a vessel that parallels another vessel, nerve, or other structure (vas collaterale [NA]). 2. a vessel important in establishing and maintaining a collateral circulation; see under *circulation*. **efferent v. of glomerulus,** anteriola glomerularis efferens. **efferent v's of lymph node,** vasa efferentia nodi lymphatici. **great v's,** the large vessels entering the heart, including the aorta, the pulmonary arteries and veins, and the venae cavae. **hemorrhoidal v's,** veins of the rectum which have become dilated and swollen; see *hemorrhoid*. **Jungbluth's v's,** vasa propria of Jungbluth. **lacteal v's,** any of the intestinal lymphatic vessels that transport chyle (q.v.); so called because during absorption they are white from absorbed fat. Called also *chyliferous v's* and *lacteals*. **lymphatic v.,** vas lymphaticum. **lymphatic v., deep,** vas lymphaticum profundum. **lymphatic v., superficial,** vas lymphaticum superficiale. **lymphocapillary v.,** vas lymphocapillare. **nutrient v's,** vessels that supply nutritive elements to special tissues, such as arteries entering the substance of bone, or supplying walls of the blood vessels themselves. See also *arteria nutricia*. **sinusoidal v.,** vas senusoideum.

vessicnon, vessignon (ves'ik-non, ves″ēn-yaw) [Fr.] windgall.

vestibula (ves-tib'u-lah) [L.] plural of *vestibulum*.

vestibular (ves-tib'u-lar) [L. *vestibularis*] pertaining to or toward a vestibule. In dental anatomy, used to refer to the tooth surface directed toward the vestibule of the mouth; see *facies vestibularis dentis*.

vestibule (ves'tĭ-būl) a space or cavity at the entrance to a canal; called also *vestibulum* [NA]. **v. of aorta,** a space within the left ventricle at the root of the aorta. **buccal v.,** that portion of the vestibule of the mouth which lies between the cheeks and the teeth and gingivae, or the residual alveolar ridges. **v. of ear,** an oval cavity in the middle of the bony larynith; see *vestibulum auris* [NA]. **Gibson's v.,** v. of aorta. **labial v.,** that portion of the vestibule of the mouth which lies between the lips and the teeth and gingivae, or residual alveolar ridges. **v. of larynx,** vestibulum laryngis. **v. of mouth,** vestibulum oris. **v. of nose,** vestibulum nasi. **v. of omental bursa,** vestibulum bursae omentalis. **v. of pharynx,** 1. fauces. 2. oropharynx. **Sibson's v.,** v. of aorta. **v. of vagina, v. of vulva,** vestibulum vaginae.

Vestibuliferia (ves-ti″bu-lĭ-fer′e-ah) [*vestibul-* + Gr. *phŏros* bearing] a subclass of free-living or parasitic (especially in the digestive tract of vertebrates and invertebrates) ciliate protozoa (class Kinetofragminophorea, phylum Ciliophora), characterized by the presence of a cytosome within a groove (vestibulum) bearing distinct ciliature at or near the apical end of the body and a cytopharynx. It comprises three orders: Trichostomatida, Entodiniomorphida, and Colpodida.

vestibulocerebellum (ves-tib″u-lo-ser″ĕ-bel′lum) [*vestibulo-* + *cerebellum*] archeocerebellum.

vestibulogenic (ves-tib″u-lo-jen′ik) arising in a vestibule, as that of the ear.

vestibulo-ocular (ves-tib″u-lo-ok′u-lar) pertaining to the vestibular and oculomotor nerves; or to the maintenance of visual stability during head movements.

vestibuloplasty (ves-tib′u-lo-plas″te) the surgical modification of the gingival–mucous membrane relationships in the vestibule of the mouth, including deepening of the vestibular trough, repositioning of the frenum or muscle attachments, and broadening of the zone of attached gingiva, after periodontal treatment.

vestibulotomy (ves-tib″u-lot′o-me) [*vestibule* + Gr. *tomē* a cutting] surgical opening of the vestibule of the inner ear.

vestibulourethral (ves-tib″u-lo-u-re′thral) pertaining to the vestibulum vaginae and to the urethra.

vestibulum (ves-tib′u-lum), pl. *vestib′ula* [L.] 1. a vesti-

bule: a space or cavity at the entrance to a canal; [NA] a general term for such a structure. 2. a depression, invagination, chamber, or cavity in the body of an organism that gives access to another such space, e.g., as the preoral chamber of certain ciliate protozoa. **v. au′ris** [NA], vestibule of ear: an oval cavity in the middle of the bony labyrinth, communicating anteriorly with the cochlea and posteriorly with the semicircular canals, and containing the sacculus and utriculus. **v. bur′sae omenta′lis** [NA], vestibule of omental bursa: that part of the omental bursa dorsal to the lesser omentum and adjacent to the epiploic foramen. **v. glot′tidis,** v. laryngis. **v. laryn′gis** [NA], vestibule of larynx: the portion of the laryngeal cavity above the vestibular folds. **v. na′si** [NA], vestibule of nose: the anterior part of the nasal cavity situated just inferior to the nares and limited posteriorly by the limen nasi. **v. o′ris** [NA], vestibule of mouth: the portion of the oral cavity bounded on one side by the teeth and gingivae, or the residual alveolar ridges, and on the other side by the lips (*labial vestibule*) and cheeks (*buccal vestibule*); called also *cavitas oris externa, cavum oris externum,* and *external oral cavity*. **v. vagi′nae** [NA], vestibule of vagina: the space between the labia minora into which the urethra and vagina open.

vestige (ves′tij) the remnant of a structure which functioned in a previous stage of species or individual development; called also *vestigium*. **coccygeal v.,** the remnant of the caudal end of the neural tube. **v. of vaginal process,** vestigium processus vaginalis.

vestigia (ves-tij′e-ah) [L.] plural of *vestigium*.

vestigial (ves-tij′e-al) of the nature of a vestige, trace, or relic; rudimentary.

vestigium (ves-tij′e-um), pl. *vestig′ia* [L. "a trace"] a vestige: the remnant of a structure which functioned in a previous stage of species or individual development; used in NA to designate the degenerating remains of any structure which served as a functioning entity in the embryo or fetus. **v. proces′sus vagina′lis** [NA], vestige of vaginal process: a band of connective tissue in the spermatic cord which is that vestige of the processus vaginalis; called also *rudimentum processus vaginalis*.

vesuvin (ve-su′vin) aniline brown.

veta (va′tah) [Sp.] mountain sickness of the Andes; see under *sickness*.

veterinarian (vet″er-ĭ-nār′e-an) a person trained and authorized to practice veterinary medicine and surgery; a doctor of veterinary medicine.

veterinary (vet′er-ĭ-ner″e) [L. *veterinarius*] pertaining to domestic animals and their diseases.

V.F. vocal fremitus.

v.f. field of vision.

via (vi′ah), gen. and pl. *vi′ae* [L.] a way or passage. **vi′ae natura′les,** the natural passages of the body. **pri′mae vi′ae,** canalis alimentarius.

viability (vi″ah-bil′ĭ-te) ability to live after birth.

viable (vi′ah-b'l) capable of living; especially said of a fetus that has reached such a stage of development that it can live outside of the uterus.

Viadril (vi′ah-dril) trademark for a preparation of hydroxydione sodium.

viae (vi′e) [L.] genitive and plural of *via*.

vial (vi′al) [Gr. *phialē*] a small bottle.

vibesate (vi′bĕ-sāt) a modified polyvinyl plastic applied topically as a spray, to form an occlusive dressing for surgical wounds and other surface lesions.

vibex (vi′beks), pl. *vibi′ces* [L. *vibix* mark of a blow] a narrow linear mark or streak; a linear subcutaneous effusion of blood.

vibices (vĭ-bi′sēz) [L.] plural of *vibex*.

Vibramycin (vi-brah-mi′sin) trademark for a preparation of doxycycline.

vibratile (vi′brah-tīl) [L. *vibratilis*] having an oscillatory motion; swaying or moving to and fro.

vibration (vi-bra′shun) [L. *vibratio*, from *vibrare* to shake] 1. a rapid movement to and fro; oscillation. 2. the shaking of the body as a therapeutic measure. 3. a form of massage.

vibrative (vib′rah-tiv) a consonantal sound like that or *r*, produced by so forcing the breath that the margins of a narrow portion of the respiratory canal are made to vibrate, the nasal cavity being shut off.

vibratode (vi′brah-tōd)   the instrument or appliance at the end of a vibratory appliance by which the vibrations are applied to the body.

vibrator (vi′bra-tor)   an instrument for producing vibrations used in the mechanical treatment of disease.

vibratory (vi′brah-tor″e) [L. *vibratorius*]   vibrating or causing vibration.

Vibrio (vib′re-o) [L. *vibrare* to move rapidly, vibrate]   a genus of gram-negative, facultatively anaerobic, straight or curved, rod-shaped bacteria of the family Vibrionaceae. The organisms are actively motile with one or more polar flagella. The species include the cholera vibrios, highly pathogenic for humans; the paracholera or cholera-like marine vibrios, associated with diarrhea; and agents of disease in lower animals. See also *vibrio*.   **V. alginoly′ticus,** a halophilic species found in seawater and seafoods that is sometimes associated with diarrhea, septicemias, and wound infections. **V. anguilla′rum,** the etiologic agent of an epidemic disease of carp and other fish. Called also *V. piscium.*   **V. chol′erae,** the etiologic agent of human Asiatic cholera; some strains produce a milder, cholera-like disease (noncholera vibrios). The organisms are found in the intestinal tract of normal and diseased humans and animals and in water. The species is divided into four biotypes. Six serogroups are based on somatic (O) antigens. Pathogenic, virulent strains produce a potent enterotoxin and agglutinate specific polyvalent 01 antiserum. Serotypes that are not agglutinated by 01 antiserum generally cause a milder diarrheal disease. Called also *V. comma.*   **V. chol′erae** biotype **alben′sis,** a strain that may be luminescent, isolated from fresh water and from human feces and bile specimens, which does not agglutinate 01 serum and is not pathogenic. Called also *V. phosphorescens.*   **V. chol′erae** biotype **chol′erae,** a pathogenic strain producing epidemic and pandemic cholera. It belongs to serogroup 0:1.   **V. chol′erae** biotype **el′tor,** a pathogenic strain first isolated at the El Tor Quarantine Station on the Sinai Peninsula, in 1960–1961, the cause of the present pandemic of cholera. It belongs to serogroup 0:1. Called also *El Tor vibrio* and *V. eltor.*   **V. chol′erae** biotype **pro′teus,** *V. metschnikovii.*   **V. co′li,** *Campylobacter jejuni.*   **V. com′ma,** *V. cholerae.*   **V. dam′sela,** a halophilic species isolated from human clinical specimens. It is oxidase positive and sucrose and lactose negative.   **V. danu′bicus,** see *noncholera vibrios,* under *vibrio.*   **V. el′tor,** *V. cholerae* biotype *eltor.*   **V. fe′tus,** *Campylobacter fetus.*   **V. fluvia′lis,** a halophilic species isolated from human clinical specimens. It is oxidase and sucrose positive and lactose negative.   **V. ghin′da,** see *noncholera vibrios,* under *vibrio.*   **v. group EF-6, v. group F,** a group of vibrios isolated from individuals with diarrheal disease.   **V. har′veyi,** a luminescent species found in sea water and on the surface of dead marine animals. The organisms were formerly classified as a separate genus, *Lucibacterium.*   **V. hol′lisae,** a halophilic species isolated from human clinical specimens. It is oxidase positive and sucrose and lactose negative.   **V. jeju′ni,** *Campylobacter jejuni.*   **V. mas-sau′ah,** see *noncholera vibrios,* under *vibrio.*   **V. metschniko′vii,** a halophilic species found in rivers and sewage and in the intestinal tract or feces of humans and other animals, especially birds. It is pathogenic for humans and guinea pigs, producing gastroenteritis. In fowls it produces an epidemic cholera-like disease. Called also *V. cholerae* biotype *proteus* and *V. proteus.* See also *fowl septicemia,* under *septicemia.*   **V. mim′icus,** a halophilic species isolated from human clinical specimens.   **noncholera v's (NCVs),** microorganisms closely similar to *Vibrio cholerae,* but differing from it immunologically and having variable pathogenic properties. Many such organisms isolated from water and from the feces of persons with mild diarrheal disease have been designated by the name of the place of their discovery, as *V. danu′bicus, V. ghin′da,* and *V. massau′ah.* Called also *paracholera v's.*   **V. parahaemoly′ticus,** a halophilic species that is a major cause of gastroenteritis due to the consumption of raw or improperly cooked fish or seafood, especially in Japan.   **V. phosphores′cens,** *V. cholerae* biotype *albensis.*   **V. pis′cium,** *V. anguillarum.*   **V. pro′teus,** *V. metschnikovii.*   **V. sep′ticus,** *Clostridium septicum.*   **V. succinog′enes,** *Wolinella succinogenes.*   **V. vulnif′icus,** a halophilic species, the strains of which are similar to *V. parahaemolyticus* and *V. alginolyticus*

but differ in that they are able to ferment lactose. Infection causes septicemia and cellulitis in those who have eaten raw seafood, being especially severe and sometimes fatal in persons with preexisting hepatic disease. Wound infection may occur following exposure to sea water or from injury when handling crabs.

vibrio (vib′re-o), pl. *vib′rios* or *vibrio′nes.*   an organism of the genus *Vibrio.*   **Celebes v.,** the pathogenic El Tor biotype of *V. cholerae,* isolated in Celebes (Suluwasi); see *Vibrio cholerae* biotype *eltor.*   **cholera v.,** the etiologic agent of classic (Asiatic) cholera, *Vibrio cholerae.*   **El Tor v.,** see *Vibrio cholerae* biotype *eltor.*   **NAG v's, nonagglutinating v's,** nonpathogenic paracholera vibrios, unrelated to the cholera vibrio O antigenic group.   **paracholera v's,** noncholera v's.

vibriocidal (vib″re-o-si′dal)   destructive to organisms of the genus *Vibrio,* especially *V. cholerae.*

vibrion (ve″bre-on′) [Fr.]   a vibrio, or spiral motile organism.   **v. septique** (ve″bre-on′ sep-tēk′), *Clostridium septicum.*

Vibrionaceae (vib″re-o-na′se-e)   a family of gram-negative, facultatively anaerobic, motile, straight or curved, rod-shaped bacteria. It contains the genera *Aeromonas, Photobacterium, Plesiomonas,* and *Vibrio.*

vibriones (vib″re-o′nēz)   plural of *vibrio.*

vibriosis (vib″re-o′sis)   infection with bacteria of the genus *Vibrio.*   **bovine genital v.,** see under *campylobacteriosis.*   **ovine genital v.,** see under *campylobacteriosis.*

vibrissa (vi-bris′ah), pl. *vibris′sae* [L.]   a long coarse hair, such as those occurring about the nose (muzzle) of an animal, as of the dog or cat. See also *vibrissae.*

vibrissae (vi-bris′e) [L. pl. of *vibrissa*] [NA]   the hairs growing in the vestibular region of the nasal cavity.

vibrocardiogram (vi″bro-kar′de-o-gram″)   the graphic record produced by vibrocardiography.

vibrocardiography (vi″bro-kar″de-og′rah-fe)   the graphic recording of vibrations produced by the heart, usually those in the nonaudible low-frequency range.

vibrolode (vi″bro-lōd)   vibratode.

vibrophonocardiograph (vi″bro-fo″no-kar′de-o-graf″)   an instrument for recording heart vibrations and sounds.

vibrotherapeutics (vi″bro-ther″ah-pu′tiks) [L. *vibrare* to shake + *therapeutics*]   the therapeutic use of vibratory appliances.

Viburnum (vi-bur′num) [L.]   a genus of caprifoliaceous trees and shrubs.   **V. op′ulus,** the high bush or cranberry tree, the dried bark (cramp bark) of which has been used as an antispasmodic, uterine sedative, and antiscorbutic.   **V. prunifo′lium** L., black haw, the dried bark of the root or stem of which has been used as a uterine sedative.

vicarious (vi-kar′e-us) [L. *vicarius*]   acting in the place of another or of something else; occurring at an abnormal site, as vicarious menstruation.

vice (vīs) [L. *vitium*]   1. a blemish, defect, or imperfection.   2. depravity; immorality.

Vicia (vish′e-ah)   a genus of herbs including the vetch and broad bean.   **V. fa′ba** (fa′va), a species whose beans or pollen contain a component that is capable of causing a condition known as *favism* in susceptible individuals; called also *fava, fava bean,* and *broad bean.*

vicianose (vīs′e-ah-nōs)   a disaccharide, $C_{11}H_{20}O_{10}$, which on hydrolysis yields glucose and arabinose; obtained from the seeds of *Vicia angustifolia.*

vicilin (vi′sĭ-lin)   a globulin from lentils and other legumes.

vicine (vi′sin)   a white crystalline glycoside, $C_{10}H_{16}N_4O_8$, found in *Vicia sativa* and other species of vetch; it is a mononucleoside and on hydrolysis yields dextrose.

vicious (vish′us) [L. *vitio′sus*]   1. faulty or defective; malformed.   2. depraved; refractory or unruly.

Vicq d'Azyr's band, etc. (vēk dah-zēr′) [Félix *Vicq d'Azyr,* French anatomist, 1748–1794]   see under *band, body, fasciculus, foramen,* and *stripe.*

Vicryl (vi′kril)   trademark for polyglactin 910.

vidarabine (vi-dār′ah-bēn)   chemical name: 9-β-D-arabinofuranosyl-9H-purin-6-amine monohydrate. A purine analogue that inhibits DNA synthesis, $C_{10}H_{13}N_5O_4H_2O$, used as a topical antiviral agent in the treatment of herpes simplex keratitis and intravenously in the treatment of herpes simplex encephalitis. Sterile vidarabine conforms to USP specifications. Called also *adenine arabinoside* or *ara-A*.

videognosis (vid″e-og-no′sis) [*video-*, from L. *videre* to see + diagnosis] diagnosis based on the interpretation of roentgenograms transmitted by television techniques to a radiologic center.

videomicroscopy (vid″e-o-mi-kros′ko-pe) television microscopy.

vidian artery, canal, nerve (vid′e-an) [Guido Guidi (L. *Vidius*), Italian physician, 1500–1569] see *arteria canalis pterygoidei*, *canalis pterygoideus*, *nervus canalis pterygoidei*, and *nervus petrosus profundus*.

Vieussens' ansa, etc. (ve-uh-sahz′) [Raymond de *Vieussens*, French anatomist, 1641–1715] see under *ansa*, *foramen*, *limbus*, *valve*, *vein*, and *ventricle*.

VIG vaccinia immune globulin.

vigilambulism (vij″il-am′bu-lizm) an ambulatory automatism resembling somnambulism but occurring in the waking state.

vigilance (vij′ĭ-lans) [L. *vigilantia*] wakefulness; watchfulness; arousal.

vigintinormal (vi-jin″tĭ-nor′mal) [L. *viginti* twenty + *norma* rule] having one twentieth the strength of normal, as a solution.

Vignal's cells (vēn-yahlz′) [Guillaume *Vignal*, French physiologist, 1852–1893] see under *cell*.

vignin (vig′nin) a protein from the cow pea.

vigor (vig′or) [L. *vigere* to flourish] a combination of attributes of living organisms which expresses itself in rapid growth, high fertility and fecundity, large size, and long life. **hybrid v.**, heterosis.

Villaret's syndrome (ve-lar-āz′) [Maurice *Villaret*, French neurologist, 1877–1946] see under *syndrome*.

Villarsia nymphaeoides (vil-lar′ze-ah nim″fe-oi′dēz) an old world gentianaceous plant having antiscorbutic properties.

villi (vil′i) [L.] genitive and plural of *villus*.

villiferous (vil-lif′er-us) having or bearing villi.

villikinin (vil″ĭ-ki′nin) [*villi* + Gr. *kinein* to move] a hypothetical hormone said to stimulate villus movement and to be released by action of hydrochloric acid on the mucous membrane of the duodenum.

villitis (vĭ-li′tis) [*villi* + *-itis*] inflammation of the villous tissue of the coronet and of the plantar substance of a horse's foot.

villoma (vĭ-lo′mah) [*villus* + *-oma*] papilloma.

villonodular (vil″o-nod′u-lar) characterized by villous and nodular thickening; said of a proliferative disorder of the synovial tissue.

villose (vil-lōs′) [L. *villosus*] shaggy with soft hairs; covered with villi.

villositis (vil″o-si′tis) a bacterial disease characterized by alterations in the villi of the placenta.

villosity (vĭ-los′ĭ-te) 1. the condition of being covered with villi. 2. a villus.

villous (vil′us) villose.

villus (vil′lus), pl. *vil′li* [L. "tuft of hair"] a small vascular process or protrusion, especially such a protrusion from the free surface of a membrane; [NA] a general term for such a structure. **amniotic v.**, one of the irregular, flat, opaque areas of imperfect skin on the amnion near the distal end of the umbilical cord. **anchoring v.**, a chorionic villus that attaches to the decidua basalis. **arachnoid villi**, 1. granulationes arachnoideales. 2. numerous microscopic projections of the arachnoid into some of the venous sinuses, which are thought by some to enlarge in man with advancing age to become the granulationes arachnoideales (q.v.). **chorionic v.**, one of the threadlike projections growing in tufts on the external surface of the chorion; see *primary*, *secondary*, and *tertiary v.* **free v.**, a chorionic villus that projects into the intervillous space. **intestinal villi, vil′li intestina′les** [NA], the multitudinous threadlike projections that cover the surface of the mucosa of the small intestine and serve as the sites of absorption (by active transport and diffusion) of fluids and nutrients. **lingual villi**, papillae filiformes. **pericardial v.**, one of the threadlike projections on the free surface of the pericardium. **pleural villi, vil′li pleura′les**, the shaggy appendages

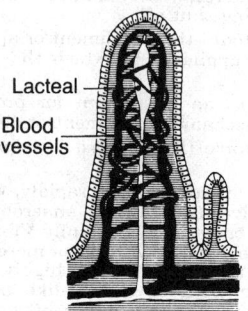

Intestinal villus.

on the surface of the pleura near the costomediastinal sinus. **primary v.**, one of the earliest chorionic villi, composed of trophoblast only. **secondary v.**, an intermediate stage of chorionic villi, having a core of connective tissue (mesoblast) covered with trophoblast. **villi of small intestine**, villi intestinales. **synovial villi, vil′li synovia′les** [NA], slender projections of the synovial membrane from its free inner surface into the joint cavity. **tertiary v.**, one of the definitive type of chorionic villi, having trophoblastic cover, connective tissue (mesoblastic) core, and blood vessels.

villusectomy (vil″us-ek′to-me) synovectomy; excision of a synovial villus.

viloxazine hydrochloride (vĭ-loks′ah-zēn) chemical name: 2-[(2-ethoxyphenyl)methyl]morpholine hydrochloride; an antidepressant, $C_{13}H_{19}NO_3 \cdot HCl$.

Vinactane (vin-ak′tān) trademark for a preparation of viomycin.

vinbarbital (vin-bar′bĭ-tal) chemical name: 5-ethyl-5-(1-methyl-1-butenyl)-2,4,6(1*H*,3*H*,5*H*)-pyrimidinetrione. An intermediate-acting barbiturate, $C_{11}H_{16}N_2O_3$, it has been used as a hypnotic and sedative, administered orally. **sodium v.**, the sodium salt of vinbarbital, $C_{11}H_{15}N_2NaO_3$, having the same actions and uses as the base; administered orally and parenterally.

vinblastine sulfate (vin-blas′tēn) [USP] chemical name: vincaleukoblastine sulfate (1:1) (salt). The sulfate salt of a vinca alkaloid extracted from *Vinca rosea* L. (Apocynaceae), $C_{46}H_{58}N_4O_9 \cdot H_2SO_4$; used as an antineoplastic in the palliative treatment of lymphomas, including generalized Hodgkin's disease, lymphosarcoma, reticulum-cell sarcoma, and advanced mycosis fungoides, and of neuroblastoma, Letterer-Siwe disease, choriocarcinoma resistant to other agents, breast carcinoma resistant to other agents, and embryonal carcinoma of the testis. Administered intravenously. Major side effects are nausea, vomiting, and bone marrow depression.

Vinca (vin′kah) a genus of apocynaceous woody herbs, including the periwinkles. *V. minor* L. is the common, or lesser, periwinkle. *V. rosea* L. (*Catharanthus roseus* G. Don), the Madagascar periwinkle, contains many alkaloids, including vinblastine and vincristine.

vincamine (vin′kah-mēn) a major alkaloid, $C_{21}H_{26}N_2O_3$, obtained from *Vinca minor* L. (Apocynaceae); used to help improve intellectual capacity in patients with cerebrovascular disorders.

Vincent's angina, gingivitis, infection, spirillum, stomatitis, tonsillitis (vin′sents) [Henri *Vincent*, physician in Paris, 1862–1950] see under *angina*, *infection*, *stomatitis*, and *tonsillitis*, and see *acute necrotizing gingivitis*, under *gingivitis*, and *Treponema vincenti*.

vincofos (vin′ko-fos) chemical name: phosphoric acid 2,3-dichloroethenyl methyl octyl ester; an anthelmintic, $C_{11}H_{21}Cl_2O_4P$.

vincristine sulfate (vin-kris′tēn) [USP] chemical name: 22-oxovincaleukoblastine sulfate (1:1) (salt). The sulfate salt of a vinca alkaloid extracted from *Vinca rosea* L. (Apocynaceae), $C_{46}H_{56}N_4O_{10} \cdot H_2SO_4$, used as an antineoplastic agent, primarily as a component of combination chemotherapy regimens for Hodgkin's disease, acute lymphocytic leukemia, and non-Hodgkin's lymphomas, and also in the treatment of Wilm's tumor, neuroblastoma, breast carcinoma, rhabdomyosarcoma and other sarcomas, and certain brain tumors. The major side effect is mixed motor-sensory and autonomic peripheral neuropathy.

vincula (ving′ku-lah) [L.] plural of *vinculum*.

vinculum (ving′ku-lum), pl. *vin′cula* [L.] a band or band-like structure; [NA] a general term for such a structure. **v. bre′ve** [NA], either of two fan-shaped expansions near the ends of the flexor tendons of a finger, one connecting the superficial tendon to the proximal interphalangeal joint and the other connecting the deep tendon to the intermediate interphalangeal joint. **v. lin′guae,** frenulum linguae. **vin′cula lin′gulae cerebel′li,** lateral prolongations of the lingula of the cerebellum. **v. lon′gum** [NA], either of two independent pairs of slender bands in each finger, one connecting the deep flexor tendon to the superficial tendon after the latter becomes subjacent, and the other connecting the superficial tendon to the proximal phalanx. **vin′cula ten′dinum digito′rum ma′nus** [NA], vincula of tendons of fingers: small vascular bands that connect the tendons of the flexor digitorum profundus and flexor digitorum superficialis muscles to the phalanges and interphalangeal articulations of the hand. The tendon blood supply is also carried in them. See *v. breve* and *v. longum*. **vin′cula ten′dinum digito′rum pe′dis** [NA], vincula of tendons of toes: bands connecting the tendons of the flexor digitorum longus and flexor digitorum brevis muscles to the phalanges and interphalangeal articulations of the foot. They are similar to the vincula found in the hand. **vincula of tendons of fingers,** vincula tendinum digitorum manus. **vincula of tendons of toes,** vincula tendinum digitorum pedis.

vindesine (vin′dĕ-sēn) chemical name: 23-amino-O⁴-deacetyl-23-demethoxyvincaleukoblastine; an antineoplastic, $C_{43}H_{55}N_5O_7$.

Vineberg operation (vīn′berg) [Arthur M. *Vineberg*, Canadian surgeon, born 1903] see under *operation*.

vinegar (vin′e-gar) [Fr. *vinaigre* sour wine] 1. a weak and impure dilution of acetic acid; especially a sour liquid consisting chiefly of acetic acid, formed by the fermentation of cider, wine, etc., or by the distillation of wood. 2. a medicinal solution of a drug in dilute acetic acid.

vinegaroon (vin″e-gah-rōon′) the whip-scorpion, *Mastigoproctus giganteus*, so called because it produces an irritating excretion which has an odor resembling that of vinegar.

Vinethene (vin′ĕ-thēn) trademark for vinyl ether; see under *ether*.

vinic (vi′nik) [L. *vinum* wine] pertaining to wine.

vinometer (vi-nom′ĕ-ter) [L. *vinum* wine + L. *metrum* measure] an instrument for estimating the percentage of alcohol in wine.

vinous (vi′nus) [L. *vinosus*, from *vinum* wine] pertaining to or containing wine.

Vinson's syndrome [Porter Paisley *Vinson*, American surgeon, 1890–1959] see *Plummer-Vinson syndrome*, under *syndrome*.

vinum (vi′num), gen. *vi′ni*, pl. *vi′na* [L.] wine.

vinyl (vi′nil) the univalent group CH₂:CH—. **v. acetate,** a vinyl group to which the monovalent radical CH₃COO— is attached, the monomer which polymerizes to polyvinyl acetate. **v. chloride,** a vinyl group to which an atom of chlorine is attached, CH₂·CHCl, the monomer which polymerizes to polyvinyl chloride. **v. ether** [USP], a colorless, volatile, flammable liquid, CH₂=CH—O—CH=CH₂, that is an inhalational anesthetic; now little used because of its flammability.

viocid (vi′o-sid) gentian violet.

Viocin (vi′o-sin) trademark for a preparation of viomycin sulfate.

Vioform (vi′o-form) trademark for preparations of iodochlorhydroxyquin.

Viokase (vi′o-kās) trademark for a preparation of pancreatin.

Viola (vi′o-lah) [L.] a genus of plants (family violaceae), the violets and pansies. **V. odora′ta** L., a sweet-scented violet of Europe and Asia; mainly used in perfumery as a source of oil. **V. tri′color** L., a species with emetic properties; it has been used in skin diseases and as an expectorant in cough preparations.

violacein (vi″o-la′se-in) a violet pigment with antibiotic properties produced by species of *Chromobacter*. It is soluble in ethanol but not in water or chloroform.

Violaquercitrin (vi-o″lah-kwer′sĭ-trin) rutin.

violescent (vi″o-les′ent) somewhat violet in color.

violet (vi′o-let) 1. the hue seen in the most refracted end of the spectrum. 2. a violet-colored dye. **amethyst v.,** a tetraethylphenosafranine used in triple staining, $(C_2H_5)_2N$-$C_6H_3 \cdot N_2Cl(C_6H_5) \cdot C_6H_3 \cdot N(C_2H_5)_2$. Called also *heliotrope B.* and *iris v.* **ammonium oxalate crystal v.,** a type of Gram stain prepared by mixing 2 gm. of crystal violet (90 per cent dye content) and 20 ml. of ethyl alcohol (95 per cent) with 0.8 gm. of ammonium oxalate and 80 ml. of distilled water. **v. 7 B or C,** gentian v.; see under G. **chrome v.,** a tricarboxyl derivative of pararosolic acid, $COONa \cdot C_6H_3(O)C[C_6-H_3(OH)COONa]_2$. **cresyl v., cresylecht v.,** a dye used in pathologic staining. **crystal v.,** gentian v.; see under G. **v. G,** gentian v.; see under G. **gentian v.** see under G. **hexamethyl v.,** gentian v. **Hofmann's v.,** iodine v., dahlia. **iris v.,** amethyst v. **Lauth's v.,** thionine. **methyl v.,** gentian v.; see under G. **methylene v.,** one of the constituents of polychrome methylene blue, $(CH_3)_2N \cdot C_6H_3(SN)CH_3:O$. **neutral v.,** a dye that resembles neutral red, but is more violet in color, $(CH_3)_2N \cdot C_6H_3 \cdot N_2 \cdot C_6H_2 \cdot (NH_2 \cdot HCl) \cdot NH \cdot C_6H_4 \cdot N(CH_3)_2$. **Paris v., pentamethyl v.,** gentian v.; see under G. **visual v.,** iodopsin.

viomycin sulfate (vi′o-mi″sin) the sulfate salt of an antibacterial antibiotic produced by *Streptomyces puniceus, S. floridae,* and *Actinomyces vinaceus,* or by other means, $C_{25}H_{43}N_{13}O_{10} \cdot x H_2SO_4$, occurring as a white to slightly yellow, crystalline powder; used as a tuberculostatic, administered intramuscularly.

viosterol (vi-os′ter-ol) ergocalciferol.

VIP vasoactive intestinal polypeptide.

viper (vi′per) any venomous snake, especially any member of the families Viperidae and Crotalidae. See table accompanying *snake*. **European v.,** a venomous viperine snake, *Vipera berus*, native to Europe, North Africa, and the Near East; it may be red, brown, or gray with dark markings, or black; called also *adder*. **Gaboon v.,** a very deadly, brightly marked, viperine snake, *Bitis gabonica*, of tropical West Africa. **nose-horned v.,** sand v. **palm v.,** any of various small, greenish, arboreal pit vipers of the genera *Bothrops* and *Trimeresurus*, which have prehensile tails that enable them to move from tree to tree. **pit v.,** any of the venomous snakes of the family Crotalidae, having a depression or pit between the nostril and the eye. They include the habu, rattlesnake, copperhead, bushmaster, fer-de-lance, palm viper, and water moccasin. **rhinoceros v.,** a venomous, brightly colored, viperine snake, *Bitis nasicornis*, of tropical Africa, characterized by the presence on the snout of a pair of hornlike growths. **Russell's v.,** the daboia (*Vipera russelli*), an extremely venomous, brightly colored, viperine snake of southeastern Asia, Java, and Sumatra. **sand v.,** a snake, *Vipera ammodytes*, found from southern Europe to Asia Minor, which possesses a hornlike protuberance on the snout for burrowing; called also *nose-horned v.* **true v.,** any one of the snakes of the family Viperidae.

Vipera (vi′per-ah) a genus of venomous snakes of the family Viperidae, including *V. ammodytes,* the sand viper, *V. berus,* the adder or European viper, and *V. russelli,* Russell's viper.

viperid (vi′per-id) viperine.

Viperidae (vi-per′ĭ-de) a family of venomous snakes, the true or Old World vipers, characterized by front, movable, hollow fangs. It includes the European viper, Russell's viper, sand viper, puff adder, Gaboon viper, and rhinoceros viper. Cf. *Crotalidae.*

viperine (vi′per-in, vi′per-īn) 1. any snake of the family Viperidae; a true viper. 2. of or pertaining to the family Viperidae.

vipoma (vĭ-po′mah) [vasoactive *i*ntestinal *p*olypeptide + -*oma*] an endocrine tumor, usually arising in the pancreas, that produces vasoactive intestinal polypeptide, which is the mediator of a syndrome of watery diarrhea, hypokalemia, and hypochlorhydria, leading to renal failure and death.

viraginity (vi″rah-jin′ĭ-te) [L. *virago* a manlike woman] the adoption by a woman of masculine qualities.

viral (vi′ral) pertaining to, caused by, or of the nature of virus.

Virales (vi-ra′lēz) the taxonomic order comprising the viruses; further classification under this taxon has been abandoned. See *virus.*

Virchow (fir′ko), Rudolf Ludwig Karl (1821–1902). German writer and editor, politician and statesman, anthropologist, ethnologist, archaeologist, and pathologist; Virchow's *Cellularpathologie* (1858) finally overthrew humoralism and marked the beginning of modern pathology. Virchow made valuable contributions to anatomy, parasitology, the history of medicine, public health, histology, and morbid anatomy; he regarded the body as a cell-state in which every cell is a citizen, and disease as a civil war brought about by external forces among the cells; he thought all cells arose from other cells (implicitly rejecting spontaneous generation), and that cell theory applied to diseased tissue. Virchow opposed Pasteur's theory of germs, Darwin's of natural selection and evolution, and Semmelweiss's washing of hands to prevent puerperal fever.

Virchow's angle, etc. (fir′kōz) [Rudolf Ludwig Karl *Virchow*, German pathologist, 1821–1902] see under *angle, cell, corpuscle, crystal, degeneration, granulation, line,* and *node,* and see *psammoma.*

Virchow-Robin spaces (fir′ko-ro-ban′) [Rudolf *Virchow*; Charles Philippe *Robin*, French anatomist, 1821–1885] see under *space.*

viremia (vi-re′me-ah) the presence of viruses in the blood, usually characterized by malaise, fever, and aching of the back and extremities.

virgin (vir′jin) [L. *virgo*] a woman or girl who has not had sexual intercourse.

virginal (vir′jĭ-nal) pertaining to a virgin or to virginity.

virginiamycin (ver-jin″yah-mi′sin) an antibiotic produced by *Streptomyces virginiae* or by other means, consisting chiefly of two components, virginiamycin M_1 (factor M_1) and virginiamycin S_1 (factor S); used in animal feedstuffs and feed supplements and in infections due to sensitive organisms, especially gram-positive cocci.

virginity (vir-jin′ĭ-te) [L. *virginitas*] maidenhood; the condition of being a virgin.

virginium (vir-jin′e-um) a former name of the element francium.

viricidal (vir″ĭ-si′dal) virucidal.

viricide (vir′ĭ-sīd) virucide.

viridin (vi-rid′in) 1. an oily principle, $C_{12}H_{19}N$, distilled from bone oil and from coal tar. 2. an antifungal antibiotic, $C_{20}H_{16}O_6$, isolated from *Gliocladium virens.*

viridobufagin (vir″ĭ-do-bu′fah-jin) a cardiac poison, $C_{23}H_{34}O_5$, from the skin glands of the toad, *Bufo viridis.*

virile (vir′il) [L. *virilis*] 1. peculiar to men or the male sex. 2. possessing masculine traits, especially copulative power.

virilescence (vir″ĭ-les′ens) the development of male secondary sex characters in the female; virilization.

virilia (vi-ril′e-ah) [L.] the male genital organs (organa genitalia masculina [NA]).

virilism (vir′ĭ-lizm) [L. *virilis* masculine] masculinity; the development of masculine physical and mental traits in the female (see virilization). **adrenal v.,** virilism due to inappropriate adrenal cortical androgen production; in it the body of a girl, woman, or prepubertal boy changes toward the adult masculine type.

virility (vĭ″-ril′ĭ-te) [L. *virilitas*, from *vir* man] possession of the normal primary sex characters in one of the male sex; maleness.

virilization (vir″ĭ-li-za′shun) the induction or development of male secondary sex characters, especially the induction of such changes in the female, including enlargement of the clitoris, growth of facial and body hair, development of a hairline typical of the male forehead, stimulation of secretion and proliferation of the sebaceous glands (often with acne), and deepening of the voice. Called also *masculinization.*

virion (vi′re-on) the complete viral particle, found extracellularly and capable of surviving in crystalline form and infecting a living cell; it comprises the nucleoid (genetic material) and the capsid. Called also *viral particle.*

viripotent (vi-rip′o-tent) [L. *viripotens; vir* man + *potens* able] sexually mature; said of a male.

virogene (vi′ro-jēn) [*virus* + *gene*] in theoretical genetics, an RNA tumor virus assembled by the normal genetic complement of a cell.

virogenetic (vi″ro-jĕ-net′ik) having a viral origin; caused by a virus.

viroid (vi′roid) any of a class of infectious agents consisting of a small strand of RNA not associated with any protein. The RNA does not code for proteins and is not translated; it is replicated by host cell enzymes. Viroids are known to cause several plant diseases.

virolactia (vi″ro-lak′she-ah) secretion of viruses in the milk.

virologist (vi-rol′o-jist) a microbiologist specializing in virology.

virology (vi-rol′o-je) that branch of microbiology which is concerned with viruses and viral diseases.

viromicrosome (vi″ro-mi′kro-sōm) a name sometimes applied to an incomplete virus particle released by premature disruption of the host cell.

viropexis (vi″ro-pek′sis) [*virus* + Gr. *pēxis* fixation] the fixation of virus to the membrane of an animal cell and its subsequent engulfment by the cell.

viroplasm (vi′ro-plazm) plaques of very fine granular substance that appear in cells before virions are observed and which correspond to the DNA material, as in poxvirus infections.

virose (vi′rōs) [L. *virosus*, from *virus* poison] having poisonous qualities.

virosis (vi-ro′sis), pl. *viro′ses.* a disease caused by a virus.

virostatic (vi″ro-stat′ik) 1. inhibiting the replication of viruses. 2. an agent that inhibits the replication of viruses.

virous (vi′rus) virose.

virtual (vir′tu-al) [L., *virtus* strength] see under *focus.*

virucidal (vi″ru-si′dal) capable of neutralizing or destroying a virus.

virucide (vi′ru-sīd) an agent that neutralizes or destroys a virus.

virulence (vir′u-lens) [L. *virulen′tia*, from *virus* poison] the degree of pathogenicity of a microorganism as indicated by the severity of the disease produced and its ability to invade the tissues of a host. It is measured experimentally by the median lethal dose (LD_{50}) or median infective dose (ID_{50}). By extension, the competence of any infectious agent to produce pathologic effects.

virulent (vir′u-lent) [L. *virulentus*, from *virus* poison] pertaining to or characterized by virulence; exceedingly pathogenic, noxious, or deleterious.

virulicidal (vir″u-lis′ĭ-dal) destructive of virulence; capable of destroying the deleterious potency of a virus or other noxious agent.

viruliferous (vir″u-lif′er-us) [L. *virus* poison + *ferre* to bear] conveying or producing a virus or other noxious agent.

viruria (vīr-u′re-ah) the presence of viruses in the urine.

virus (vi′rus) [L.] one of a group of minute infectious agents, with certain exceptions (e.g., poxviruses) not resolved in the light microscope, and characterized by a lack of independent metabolism and by the ability to replicate only within living host cells. Like living organisms, they are able to reproduce with genetic continuity and the possibility of mutation. They range from 200–300 nm. to 15 nm. in size and are morphologically heterogeneous, occurring as rod-shaped, spherical, or polyhedral, and tadpole-shaped forms; masses of the spherical or polyhedral forms may be made up of orderly arrays, to give a crystalline structure. The individual particle, or virion, consists of nucleic acid (the nucleoid), DNA or RNA (but not both) and a protein shell, or capsid, which contains and protects the nucleic acid and which may be multilayered. Viruses are customarily separated into three subgroups on the basis of host specificity, namely bacterial viruses, animal viruses, and plant viruses. They are also classified as to their origin (e.g., reoviruses), mode of transmission (arboviruses, tickborne viruses), or the manifestations they produce (polioviruses, polyomaviruses, poxviruses). They are sometimes named for the geographical location in which they were first isolated (e.g., coxsackievirus). **acute laryngotracheobronchitis v.,** parainfluenza 2 v.; see *parainfluenza v.* **adeno-associated v.,** a parvovirus that apparently cannot replicate unless associated with an adenovirus. **Amapari v.,** an arenavirus isolated from rodents in Brazil.

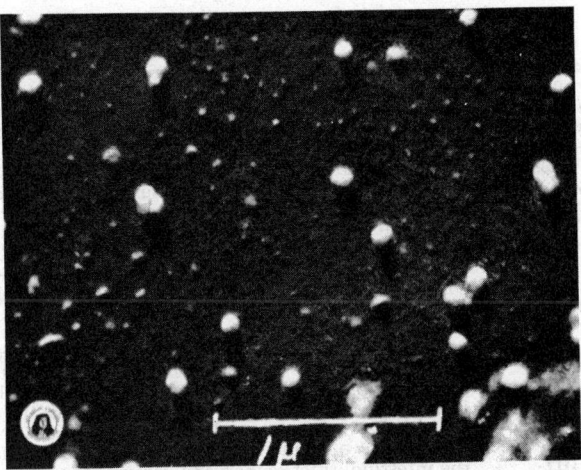

Influenza virus. (Williams and Wyckoff, S.A.B. LS-136.)

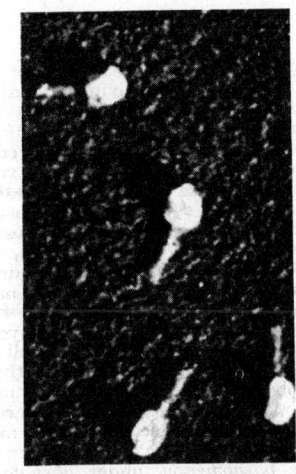

Bacteriophage (T₂) of *Escherichia coli*. (Williams and Frazer, Virology, vol. 2.)

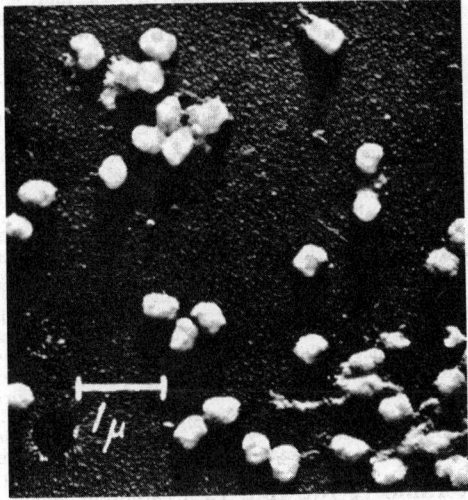

Vaccinia virus. (G. G. Sharp, S.A.B. LS-142.)

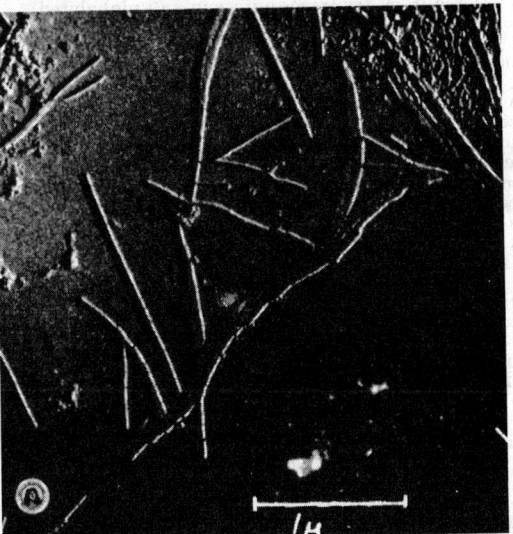

Tobacco mosaic virus. (Williams and Wyckoff, S.A.B. LS-135.)

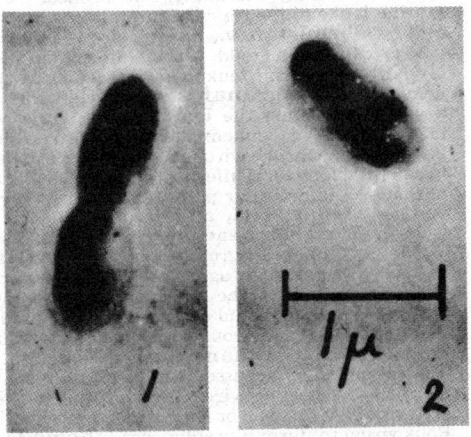

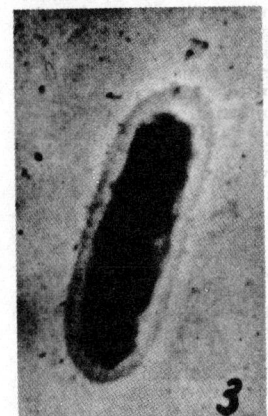

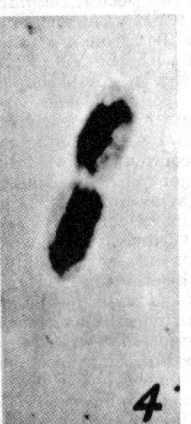

PLATE 52 — ELECTRON MICROGRAPHS OF VIRUSES AND RICKETTSIAE

animal v's, viruses that produce diseases of man and other animals. **v. anima′tum,** a living animal poison. **arbor v's** (*arthropod-borne*), former name for *arbovirus*. **Argentine hemorrhagic fever v.,** Junin v. **attenuated v.,** one whose pathogenicity has been reduced by serial animal passage or by other means. **Australian X disease v.,** see under *disease*. **avian leukosis v.,** any of a complex of leukoviruses causing erythroblastosis, granulomatosis, lymphomatosis, and myelocytomatosis in chickens; see *avian leukosis,* under *leukosis.* **B v.,** a herpesvirus causing a mild disease in monkeys, the natural host, but a severe and usually fatal disease in humans accidentally infected by exposure to infected monkeys. **bacterial v.,** a virus capable of producing transmissible lysis of bacteria; the virus particle attaches to the bacterial cell wall and viral nucleoprotein enters the cell, resulting in the synthesis of virus and its liberation on physical disruption of the cell. Bacterial viruses are usually specific for bacterial species, but they may be strain-specific or may infect more than one species of bacteria. Called also *bacteriophage* or *phage.* See *Twort-d'Herelle phenomenon,* under *phenomenon.* **Bittner v.,** mouse mammary tumor v. **Bolivian hemorrhagic fever v.,** Machupo v. **Brunhilde v.,** the prototype strain of poliovirus type 1. **Bunyamwera v.,** an arbovirus isolated from *Aedes* mosquitoes in an uninhabited part of the Semliki Forest in western Uganda; it causes a mild febrile disease. **bushy stunt v.,** a small spherical plant virus, which causes bushy stunt of tomatoes. **Bwamba fever v.,** an arbovirus, originally isolated from the blood of natives in Bwamba county in Uganda, which causes a mild febrile disease. **C v.,** coxsackievirus. **CA v.** (*croup-associated*), parainfluenza 2 virus. **Cache Valley v.,** an arbovirus, related to the Bunyamwera virus, first isolated from *Culiseta inornata* in the Cache Valley in northern Utah. It has also been found in Brazil, and was isolated from *Aedes scapularis* in Trinidad. **California v.,** a virus isolated in California in 1943 from species of mosquitoes, capable of causing disease in laboratory animals and the probable cause of fatal encephalitis in an infant. **cancer-inducing v.,** a virus that causes uncontrolled proliferation of infected cells, including both RNA and DNA viruses. **Catu v.,** an arbovirus closely related to Guama virus. **CCA v.** (**chimpanzee coryza agent),** respiratory syncytial v. **CELO (chicken-embyro-lethalorphan) v.,** an enteric orphan virus which is lethal for chicken embryos and induces tumors in newborn and weanling hamsters. **Chagres v.,** an arbovirus causing fever associated with malaise, headache, and pains of localized and generalized distribution, in Panama. **Chenuda v.,** an arbovirus closely related to Quaranfil virus. **chikungunya v.,** an alphavirus transmitted chiefly by mosquitoes of the genus *Aedes* that causes chikungunya, a dengue-like disease found principally in Southeast Asia and Africa. **Coe v.,** coxsackievirus type A21. **Colorado tick fever v.,** the etiologic agent of a febrile disease occurring in regions of the Rocky Mountains where the tick vector, *Dermacentor andersoni,* is prevalent. **Columbia SK v.,** an encephalomyocarditis virus originally isolated in 1940 from a monkey which had previously been inoculated with the Yale SK strain of poliovirus. **common cold v's,** a subgroup of rhinoviruses considered to cause the common cold. **Congo-Crimean hemorrhagic fever v.,** an arbovirus transmitted by various species of ticks, by close contact with an infected individual, or by direct contact with viremic domestic animals; it is the etiologic agent of hemorrhagic fever in the Crimea, central Asia, Bulgaria, and West, Central, and East Africa. Called also *Crimean hemorrhagic fever v.* **coryza v.,** rhinovirus. **cowpox v.,** a naturally occurring orthopoxvirus closely related to but antigenically different from the vaccinia virus (q.v.); it is the etiologic agent of cowpox, a vesicular disease on the udders and teats of milk cows that can be transmitted to humans during milking, who in turn can spread the virus among uninfected cows. Cowpox virus is to be distinguished from the *paravaccinia* (pseudocowpox) *virus.* **Coxsackie v.,** coxsackievirus. **Crimean hemorrhagic fever v.,** Congo-Crimean hemorrhagic fever v. **croup-associated v.,** parainfluenza 2 virus. **cytomegalic inclusion disease v.,** see *cytomegalovirus.* **defective v.,** one that cannot be completely replicated or cannot form a protein coat; in some cases replication can proceed if missing gene functions are supplied by other (helper) viruses; see *helper v.* **dengue v.,** a flavivirus existing as four antigenically related but distinct types (designated 1, 2, 3, and 4) that causes

classic dengue and hemorrhagic dengue. **EB v.,** Epstein-Barr v. **Ebola v.,** an unclassified RNA virus, morphologically similar to but antigenically distinct from the Marburg virus, that causes an acute, highly fatal hemorrhagic fever in the Sudan and adjacent areas in northern Zaire; the natural reservoir and mode of transmission of primary infection are unknown, but secondary infection is by direct contact with infected blood and other body secretions and by airborne particles. **ECBO v.,** ecbovirus. **ECDO v.,** ecdovirus. **ECHO v.,** echovirus. **ECHO 28 v.,** echovirus 28. **ECMO v.,** ecmovirus. **ECSO v.,** ecsovirus. **EEE v.,** eastern equine encephalomyelitis v.; see *equine encephalomyelitis v.* **EMC v.,** encephalomyocarditis v. **encephalomyocarditis v.,** an enterovirus found in Africa, South America, and elsewhere, which causes mild aseptic meningitis and encephalomyocarditis; it is represented by four strains which appear to be substantially identical in immunological and other respects. It includes the Columbia SK, Mengo, and MM viruses. **enteric v.,** enterovirus. **enteric orphan v's,** viruses isolated from the intestinal tract of man and various other animals, called orphan viruses because they are often not specifically associated with illness; they include such viruses isolated from cattle (ecboviruses), dogs (ecdoviruses), man (echoviruses), monkeys (ecmoviruses), and swine (ecsoviruses). **epidemic keratoconjunctivitis v.,** adenovirus type 8. **Epstein-Barr v.** (**EB v.; EBV),** a herpes-like virus that causes infectious mononucleosis and is associated with Burkitt's lymphoma and nasopharyngeal carcinoma. **equine encephalomyelitis v.,** a group of arboviruses causing encephalomyelitis in horses, mules, and man, with a reservoir of infection in birds, and transmitted by mosquitoes. The group includes *eastern equine encephalomyelitis virus* (*EEE v.*), the cause of equine encephalomyelitis in a region extending from New Hampshire to Texas, and as far west as Wisconsin in the United States, and also in Canada, the Caribbean, Mexico, and parts of Central and South America; *Venezuelan equine encephalomyelitis virus* (*VEE v.*), the cause of equine encephalomyelitis in Venezuela and other South American countries, and Mexico and Florida; and *western equine encephalomyelitis virus* (*WEE v.*), the cause of equine encephalomyelitis in the United States west of the Mississippi (with evidence suggesting its presence also in the Atlantic and Gulf Coast states), transmitted primarily by *Culex tarsalis.* **exanthematous disease v.,** any of a group of dermotropic viruses, including poxviruses, causing exanthematous disease in man and lower animals. **FA v.,** a strain of virus causing encephalomyelitis of mice. **filterable v., filtrable v.,** a pathogenic agent capable of passing through fine filters of diatomite or unglazed porcelain; ultravirus. **v. fixé, fixed v.,** rabies virus whose virulence and incubation period have been stabilized by serial passage and remain fixed during further transmission; used for inoculating animals from which rabies vaccine is prepared. **fowl plague v.,** a virus causing a disease of fowl in northern Italy, Germany, and France. **Friend v.,** a murine leukemia virus causing malignant reticulopathy in mice. **Germistan v.,** an arbovirus of the Bunyamwera group, causing a mild febrile disease in South Africa. **Graffi v.,** a murine leukemia virus which causes chloroleukemia in mice. **granulosis v.,** baculovirus. **Gross v.,** a virus resembling the Rous sarcoma virus, which causes many kinds of leukemia in newborn mice and rats. **Guama v.,** an arbovirus isolated in the Belem region of Brazil from foresters suffering from hyperthermia, headache, muscular and articular pains, and occasionally nausea and vertigo. **Guaroa v.,** an arbovirus isolated in Colombia from the blood of patients with a febrile disease; a member of the Bunyamwera group of viruses. **Hantaan (Hataan) v.,** the etiologic agent of epidemic hemorrhagic fever, which is believed to be transmitted by contact, direct or indirect, with saliva and excreta of infected rodents such as the field mouse and ground vole; called also *Korean hemorrhagic fever v.* **Hataan v.,** see *Hantaan v.* **helper v.,** a virus (e.g., the Rous-associated virus) that aids the development of a defective virus by supplying or restoring the activity of a viral gene or enabling a defective virus (e.g., the Rous virus) to form a protein coat. **hemadsorption v., type 1 (HA1),** parainfluenza 3 virus. **hemadsorption v., type 2 (HA2),** a parainfluenza 1 virus isolated from children with febrile respiratory disease. **hemagglutinating v. of Japan,** Sendai v. **hepatitis A v. (HAV),** an RNA virus, possibly an enterovirus, having virions 27–29 nm in diameter and a single-stranded genome; the etiologic agent of hepatitis A. **hepatitis B v. (HBV),** an unclassified DNA virus having complex, double-layered virions 42 nm in diameter, a double-stranded genome, and three major.antigens, the hepatitis B core antigen (HBcAg), surface antigen (HBsAg), and e antigen (HBeAg). It is the etiologic agent of hepatitis B. **hepatitis C v.,** an unclassified virus with virions 27 nm in diameter; the etiologic agent of non-A, non-B hepatitis. Called also *non-A, non-B hepatitis v.* **hepatitis delta v.,** a defective RNA viral agent that can replicate only in the presence of hepatitis B virus and is transmitted like it; the etiologic agent of delta hepatitis. Called also *delta agent.* **herpangina v.,** one of the viruses of the coxsackievirus A group, causing a febrile disease, usually of children, characterized by small herpes-like lesions on the soft palate or in the faucial area. **herpes v.,** see *herpesvirus.* **human immunodeficiency v. (HIV),** a human T-cell leukemia/lymphoma virus that is the agent of acquired immune deficiency syndrome. HIV has a selective affinity for helper T-cells; in vitro infection of helper T-cells results in cytopathic effects and cell lysis. Called also *human T-cell leukemia/lymphoma v. Type III, human T-cell lymphotrophic v. Type III* and *lymphadenopathy-associated v.* **human T-cell leukemia/lymphoma v., human T-cell lymphotrophic v., (HTLV),** a family of retroviruses that are lymphocytotrophic with a selective affinity for T lymphocytes of the inducer/helper subset, which have been isolated from unusual and epidemiologically distinct T-cell leukemias and lymphomas; one type, human immunodeficiency virus (HIV), is the agent of acquired immune deficiency syndrome. **Ilheus v.,** an arbovirus first isolated from species of *Aedes* and *Psorophora* in Brazil; and also found in Panama, where birds may be hosts. It is related to St. Louis encephalitis virus, Japanese B encephalitis virus, and West Nile virus. **infectious porcine encephalomyelitis v.,** Teschen v. **infectious wart v.,** a papillomavirus that causes warts in man. **influenza v.,** any of a group of myxoviruses that cause influenza, including at least three serotypes (A, B, and C) and several antigenic variations, classified on the basis of their surface antigens (hemagglutinin and neuraminidase) as H_1N_1, H_2N_2, etc. Serotype A viruses are subject to major antigenic changes (antigenic shifts) as well as minor gradual antigenic changes (antigenic drift) and cause the major pandemics. Serotype B viruses appear to undergo only minor antigenic changes (antigenic drift) and cause more localized epidemics. Serotype C viruses appear to be antigenically stable and cause only sporadic disease. **insect v's,** viruses capable of causing disease in insects. **iridescent v.,** iridovirus. **Japanese B encephalitis v.,** the causative agent of Japanese B encephalitis, closely similar to the various agents causing the different types of equine encephalomyelitis and St. Louis encephalitis, but having a wider range of pathogenicity for experimental animals. **JH v.,** echovirus 28. **Junin v.,** an arenavirus, first isolated in 1958 during an epidemic of hemorrhagic fever in the northwestern area of the province of Buenos Aires, Argentina, that is serologically related to the Machupo virus. It is the etiologic agent of Argentine hemorrhagic fever, transmitted by contact with infected rodents, especially of the genus *Calomys.* Called also *Argentine hemorrhagic fever v.* **K v.,** a nononcogenic polyomavirus that produces fatal pneumonia on inoculation into newborn mice. **Kemerova v.,** an arbovirus (tickborne) responsible for a benign febrile disease in western Siberia. **Korean hemorrhagic fever v.,** Hantaan v. **Kumba v.,** a virus isolated from mosquitoes in the Kumba region of Cameroon; antigenically identical with the Semliki Forest virus. **Kyasanur Forest disease v.,** a flavivirus transmitted by ticks of the genus *Haemophysalis,* especially *H. spingera,* first isolated in an epidemic of hemorrhagic fever among forest workers and monkeys in the Kyasanur Forest in Mysore State, India; it is antigenically related to the Omsk hemorrhagic fever virus. **Langat v.,** a tickborne arbovirus that causes encephalitis in man and in mice. **Lansing v.,** the prototype strain of poliovirus type 2. **Lassa fever v.,** an extremely virulent arenavirus, originally isolated in Lassa, Nigeria, in 1969, which causes an acute, febrile disease with high fatality rate; it morphologically resembles the viruses of lymphocytic choriomeningitis and the Tacaribe-Junin-Machupo group. **latent v.,** masked v. **Latino v.,** an arenavirus isolated from rodents in Bolivia. **LCM v.,** lymphocytic choriomeningitis v. **Leon v.,** the prototype strain of poliovirus

type 3. **louping ill v.,** a virus transmitted by the tick, *Ixodes ricinus;* it causes louping ill of sheep, is transmissible to man, and is closely related to Russian spring-summer encephalitis virus. **Lunyo v.,** a neurotropic variant of Rift Valley fever virus. **lymphadenopathy-associated v. (LAV),** human immunodeficiency virus. **lymphocytic choriomeningitis (LCM) v.,** an arenavirus, the etiologic agent of lymphocytic choriomeningitis that occurs naturally in mice, dogs, and monkeys. **lytic v.,** one that is replicated in the host cell and causes death and lysis of the cell. **M-25 v.,** a virus with the properties of a myxovirus, although antigenically unrelated; isolated from a person with upper respiratory illness. **Machupo v.,** an arenavirus, first isolated during an epidemic of hemorrhagic fever in Bolivia in 1959, that is the etiologic agent of Bolivian hemorrhagic fever, transmitted by contact with virus-infected rodents; indistinguishable from the Junin virus by complement fixation, but distinct by the neutralization test. Called also *Bolivian hemorrhagic fever v.* **Makonde v.,** an arbovirus isolated along with the chikungunya virus in the region of the Makonde plateau in Tanzania. **mammary tumor v.,** mouse mammary tumor v. **Marburg v.,** an unclassified RNA virus that causes Marburg disease, an acute, highly fatal type of hemorrhagic fever, first reported in Marburg and Frankfurt, West Germany, and Belgrade, Yugoslavia, in laboratory workers who handled infected African green monkeys or their organs; secondary infection is acquired by direct physical contact with infected patients. **masked v.,** a virus which ordinarily occurs in a noninfective state and is demonstrable by indirect methods which activate it, as by blind passage in experimental animals. **Mayaro v.,** an arbovirus found in Mayaro county, Trinidad, and in the region of the Guama River in Brazil as an etiologic agent of febrile disease; closely related to and possibly identical with Semliki Forest virus. **measles v.,** a paramyxovirus, the etiologic agent of measles. **Mengo v.,** an encephalomyocarditis virus isolated originally in 1948 from a captive monkey in Uganda and later from mosquitoes and a mongoose of the same area; identified also as the cause of an epizootic disease of swine in Panama. **milker's node v.,** paravaccinia v. **MM v.,** an encephalomyocarditis virus originally isolated in 1943 from the brain of a hamster that was previously inoculated with material from a human case of paralytic disease. **molluscum contagiosum v.,** a poxvirus that causes molluscum contagiosum. **Moloney v.,** a murine leukemia virus which causes lymphoid leukemia in mice. **monkeypox v.,** an orthopoxvirus that produces a mild, epidemic exanthematous disease in monkeys and a smallpox-like disease in humans. **Mossuril v.,** a mosquito-borne arbovirus. **mouse mammary tumor v.,** a virus causing mammary adenocarcinoma in mice of certain genotype and influenced by estrogenic stimulation; it is usually transmitted from the mother to her offspring through the milk. Called also *Bittner agent, Bittner v., mammary tumor agent, milk agent* or *factor.* **mumps v.,** a paramyxovirus that causes mumps and, in some cases, tenderness and swelling of the testes, pancreas, ovaries, or other organs. **murine leukemia v.,** any of a group of leukoviruses causing leukemia and solid tumors in rats, mice, hamsters, and other animals; the group includes the Gross, Rauscher, Friend, Moloney, and Graffi viruses. **Murray Valley encephalitis v.,** a virus closely resembling the Japanese B encephalitis virus; see under *encephalitis.* **Nakiwogo v.,** Semunya v. **neurotropic v.,** one that has a predilection for and causes infection in nervous tissues, e.g., the rabies virus. **newborn pneumonitis v.,** Sendai v. **Newcastle disease v.,** a virus causing disease in chickens and occasionally in man; related to the influenza viruses. Abbreviated NDV. **non-A, non-B hepatitis v.,** hepatitis C virus. **nononcogenic v.,** one that does not cause cancer. **Norwalk v.** [*Norwalk,* Ohio], a common cause of epidemics of acute gastroenteritis, with diarrhea and vomiting lasting 24 to 48 hours. **Ntaya v.,** a virus originally isolated in 1943 from various species of mosquitoes, including *Culex* and *Aedes,* in the Ntaya Swamp in western Uganda; it is fatal to mice infected by intracerebral inoculation. **Omsk hemorrhagic fever v.,** a flavivirus transmitted by ticks of the genus *Dermacentor,* isolated from patients with hemorrhagic fever in a forested region of Siberia; it is antigenically related to the Kyasanur Forest hemorrhagic fever virus. **oncogenic v.,** a cancer-inducing virus. **O'nyong-nyong v.,** an alphavirus that causes a febrile disease that clinically resembles dengue and chikungunya in Uganda, Kenya, Tanzania, Malawi, and Senegal; it is transmitted by anapheline mosquitoes. **Oropouche v.,** an arbovirus isolated from a patient with febrile disease in Trinidad; related to the Simbu virus. **orphan v's,** viruses which when isolated originally in tissue culture showed no specific association with disease, such as the enteric orphan viruses; some have since been found to occur in association with human disease. **papilloma v.,** papillomavirus. **pappataci fever v.,** the etiological agent of phlebotomus (pappataci) fever, transmitted by *Phlebotomus,* and occurring as two serotypes, the Naples and Sicilian types. **parainfluenza v.,** a group of viruses isolated from patients with upper respiratory tract disease of varying severity. Parainfluenza viruses are classified as: *Parainfluenza 1 v.,* comprising two immunologically related but not identical viruses, *Sendai virus* and *hemadsorption type 2 (HA2) virus; Parainfluenza 2 v.,* a virus isolated from patients with acute laryngotracheobronchitis; called also *CA v.* or *croup-associated v.; Parainfluenza 3 v.,* a virus causing bronchitis and pneumonia, especially in children; called also *hemadsorption v., type 1 (HA1 v.); Parainfluenza 4 v.,* a virus associated with respiratory disease in children. **Parana v.,** an arenavirus isolated from rodents in Paraguay. **paravaccinia v.,** a parapoxvirus that produces nodular lesions similar to those of cowpox and orf on the udders and teats of milk cows and the oral mucosa of suckling calves (paravaccinia), which can be transmitted to humans during milking. Called also *milker's node v.* and *pseudocowpox v.* **pharyngoconjunctival fever v.,** adenovirus type 3. **Pichinde v.,** an arenavirus infecting rodents in Colombia, and isolated from human subclinical infections. **Piry v.,** an arbovirus isolated from East African patients with an acute febrile syndrome. **plant v's,** viruses that replicate in and may produce diseases of higher plants. **poliomyelitis v.,** see *poliovirus.* **polyoma v.,** polyomavirus. **Pongola v.,** an arbovirus causing a febrile disease in Africa. **Powassan v.,** a tickborne virus isolated from a fatal case of encephalitis in Ontario, Canada; closely related to Russian spring-summer encephalitis virus. **pox v.,** see *poxvirus.* **pseudocowpox v.,** paravaccinia v. **Quaranfil v.,** an arbovirus found in Egypt, where it was isolated from the blood of children with febrile disease, from the blood of young egrets, and from ticks (*Argas arboreus* and *A. hermanni*). **rabbit fibroma v.,** a poxvirus closely related to the rabbit myxoma virus, which causes rabbit fibroma. **rabbit myxoma v.,** a poxvirus, closely related to the rabbit fibroma virus, which causes infectious myxomatosis in rabbits. **rabbit papilloma v.,** a papillomavirus virus, morphologically the same as the infectious wart virus, which causes rabbit papilloma. **rabies v.,** the etiological agent of rabies, one of the most neurotropic of the viruses; it is a bullet-shaped RNA virus of the rhabdovirus group. **Rauscher leukemia v.,** a murine leukemia virus that causes lymphoid leukemia in mice. **respiratory syncytial v.,** a paramyxovirus resembling the influenza virus; it is the cause of an epidemic acute respiratory disease that is more serious in children, in whom it causes bronchopneumonia and bronchiolitis. In tissue cultures, the virus causes syncytium formation. First isolated from chimpanzees with symptoms of respiratory disease. Called also *chimpanzee coryza agent (CCA),* and *RS v.* **Rift Valley fever v.,** a bunyavirus of the phlebotomus subgroup, which is the etiologic agent of Rift Valley fever in domestic animals and humans, first seen in the Rift Valley of Kenya, but now widespread in southern and eastern Africa to Egypt; transmitted by mosquitoes of the species *Aedes, Culex,* and *Erethmapodites* or by contact with tissues and secretions of infected animals. **Rous-associated v. (RAV),** a helper virus in whose presence a defective Rous sarcoma virus is able to form a protein coat. **Rous sarcoma v.,** a leukovirus producing fibrosarcoma in fowl, especially chickens; some strains have been shown to produce tumors in other animals. See *Rous sarcoma,* under *sarcoma.* **RS v.,** respiratory syncytial v. **Russian spring-summer encephalitis v.,** a tickborne virus which causes spring-summer encephalitis in the Soviet Union and Central Europe. **SA v.,** a virus isolated from the hamster brain following inoculation with a chick embryo allantoic culture of nasal washings from a person with acute upper respiratory infection. **St. Louis encephalitis v.,** the etiologic agent of St. Louis encephalitis, with a distribution similar to that of western equine encephalomyelitis virus, but differing from it immunologically. **salivary gland v.,** cytomegalovirus.

satellite v., a strain of virus unable to replicate except in the presence of helper virus; considered to be deficient in coding for capsid formation. **Schwartz leukemia v.,** a virus that causes lymphoid leukemia in Swiss mice. **Semliki Forest v.,** an arbovirus isolated from mosquitoes of the Semliki Forest of western Uganda; it is pathogenic for laboratory animals and man. **Semunya v.,** an arbovirus isolated from East African patients with an acute febrile syndrome; called also *Nakiwogo v.* **Sendai v.,** a parainfluenza 1 virus, which seems to have been the etiologic agent of a highly fatal epidemic pneumonitis of newborn infants in Japan, and has been found in infants in Germany and the Soviet Union. It is related to the mumps virus. **sigma v.,** a virus that induces carbon dioxide sensitivity in *Drosophila melanogaster* and other fruit flies. **Simbu v.,** a virus isolated from a species of mosquitoes (*Aedes circumluteolis*) in Africa. **simian v's,** viruses that have been recovered from monkeys; they belong to many different groups, including adenoviruses, enteroviruses, herpesviruses, and reoviruses. **simian v. 40 (SV40),** vacuolating v. **Sindbis v.,** an alphavirus transmitted by mosquitoes of the genus *Culex,* which causes Sinbis fever in southern and eastern Africa, Egypt, Israel, India, the Philippines, and eastern Australia. **slow v.,** any virus causing a disease characterized by a very long preclinical course and very gradual progression once the symptoms appear. **Spondweni v.,** an arbovirus originally isolated in 1955 from South African mosquitoes, which may cause a short-term febrile illness in man. **street v.,** rabies virus from a naturally infected animal, as opposed to a laboratory-adapted strain of the virus. **Tacaribe v.,** an arenavirus, isolated from bats in Trinidad, which is immunologically related to the Junin and Machupo viruses. **Tahyna v.,** a virus serologically related to the California virus, isolated in various European countries; it is suspected of causing human and animal disease. **Tamiami v.,** an arenavirus isolated from rodents in Florida. **temperate v.,** see under *bacteriophage.* **Teschen v.,** the etiologic agent of infectious porcine encephalomyelitis (Teschen disease). **Theiler's v.,** the etiologic agent of a spontaneous encephalomyelitis of mice (Theiler's disease); it resembles human polioviruses but is immunologically distinct from them. **tickborne v's,** viruses that are transmitted by ticks. **tobacco mosaic v.,** a plant virus containing RNA which causes mosaic disease of tobacco. **tumor v.,** a cancer-inducing v. **Turlock v.,** a mosquito-borne virus isolated from *Culex tarsalis* in California; it is unrelated to other arthropod-borne viruses and is not known to cause human disease. **2060 v.,** echovirus 28. **U v.,** a virus resembling the parainfluenza 2 virus but of uncertain status, found in children with subglottic laryngitis; called also *Uppsala v.* **Uganda S v.,** an arbovirus first isolated from species of *Aedes* in Bwamba county in Uganda. It causes mild febrile disease in certain areas in Africa, especially in Nigeria. **Uppsala v.,** U v. **Uruma v.,** an arbovirus causing epidemic febrile disease in Colombia. **vaccinia v.,** an orthopoxvirus that does not occur in nature, being only propagated in the laboratory for use as an active vaccine against smallpox. The present virus is derived from the original one used by Jenner, obtained from the lesions of cowpox, but the origin of the original virus remains unclear. Some believe that vaccinia virus is a derivative of the immunologically similar but antigenically different viruses of cowpox and variola (smallpox), while others think that it may be a recombinant of these viruses. **vacuolating v.,** a polyomavirus isolated from *Rhesus* monkey kidney tissue, which produces malignancy in human and newborn hamster kidney cell cultures and tumors on inoculation into newborn hamsters; called also *simian v. 40.* **VEE v.,** Venezuelan equine encephalomyelitis v.; see *equine encephalomyelitis v.* **vesicular stomatitis v.,** a rhabdovirus, the etiologic agent of vesicular stomatitis of swine, cattle, and horses. **wart v.,** see *infectious wart v.* **WEE v.,** western equine encephalomyelitis v.; see *equine encephalomyelitis v.* **Wesselsbron v.,** an arbovirus repeatedly isolated in South Africa from mosquitoes and from sheep and man, in whom it causes a mild febrile disease. **West Nile v.,** an arbovirus related to Japanese encephalitis B virus and St. Louis encephalitis virus, which causes a mild disease in humans; it was first isolated in Uganda, but is widespread in Africa and has been observed in Israel. *Culex uvivittatus* is the most probable vector. **Wyeomyia v.,** a virus of the Bunyamwera group originally isolated in Colombia from the mosquito *Wyeomyia melanocephala* and later from man in Panama; it produces encephalitis in the infant mouse after intracerebral inoculation. **Yaba v.,** a virus that produces superficial benign tumors in the monkey. **Yale SK v.,** a strain of poliovirus. **yellow fever v.,** a mosquito-borne flavivirus that causes yellow fever in Central and South America and Africa. **Zika v.,** an arbovirus originally isolated in 1947 from monkeys in the Zika Forest, Uganda, and later found to infect *Aedes africanus;* human infection also occurs. **Zimmermann v.,** a neurotropic arbovirus of the tickborne encephalitis group.

virusemia (vi″rus-e′me-ah) viremia.

virustatic (vir″u-stat′ik) [*virus* + Gr. *statikos* bringing to a standstill] inhibiting the replication of viruses.

vis (vis), gen. *vi′ris*, pl. *vi′res* [L.] force; energy. **v. a ter′go,** the factor of pressure transmitted through the capillaries to the veins by the blood pumped into the arteries by the heart. **v. conserva′trix,** the natural power of the organism to resist injury and disease. **v. formati′va,** energy manifesting itself in the formation of new tissue to replace that which has been destroyed. **v. in si′tu,** power or force inherent in a particular tissue. **v. medica′trix natu′rae,** the healing power of nature; the natural curative power inherent in the organism. **v. vi′tae, v. vita′lis,** the vital, or life, force.

viscera (vis′er-ah) [L.] plural of *viscus.*

viscerad (vis′er-ad) toward the viscera.

visceral (vis′er-al) [L. *visceralis,* from *viscus* a viscus] pertaining to a viscus.

visceralgia (vis″er-al′je-ah) [L. *viscus* viscus + Gr. *algos* pain + *-ia*] pain in the viscera or in any bodily organ.

visceralism (vis′er-al-izm) the opinion that the viscera are the principal seats of disease.

viscerimotor (vis″er-ĭ-mo′tor) [L. *viscus* viscus + *motor* mover] conveying motor impulses to a viscus.

viscer(o)- [L. *viscus,* gen. *visceris*] a combining form denoting relationship to the organs (viscera) of the body.

viscerocranium (vis″er-o-kra′ne-um) that part of the skull which is derived from the branchial arches.

viscerography (vis″er-og′rah-fe) roentgenography of the viscera.

visceroinhibitory (vis″er-o-in-hib′ĭ-tor″e) inhibiting the essential movements of any viscus or organ.

visceromegaly (vis″er-o-meg′ah-le) [*viscero-* + Gr. *megas* large] enlargement of the viscera; organomegaly.

visceromotor (vis″er-o-mo′tor) concerned in the essential movements of the viscera.

visceroparietal (vis″er-o-pah-ri′ĕ-tal) pertaining to the viscera and the abdominal wall.

visceroperitoneal (vis″er-o-per″ĭ-to-ne′al) pertaining to the viscera and the peritoneum.

visceropleural (vis″er-o-ploor′al) pertaining to both the viscera and the pleura.

visceroptosis (vis″er-op-to′sis) [L. *viscus* viscus + Gr. *ptōsis* fall] splanchnoptosis.

viscerosensory (vis″er-o-sen′so-re) pertaining to sensation in the viscera.

visceroskeletal (vis″er-o-skel′e-tal) pertaining to the visceral skeleton.

viscerosomatic (vis″er-o-so-mat′ik) pertaining to the viscera and body.

viscerotome (vis′er-o-tōm) 1. an instrument designed for obtaining specimens of liver tissue from cadavers by simple puncture. 2. an area on an abdominal viscus which is supplied with afferent nerve fibers by a single posterior root.

viscerotomy (vis″er-ot′o-me) [*viscero-* + Gr. *tomē* a cutting] incision of an organ, especially postmortem excision of a portion of the liver.

viscerotonia (vis″er-o-to′ne-ah) [*viscero-* + *ton-* + *-ia*] a temperament type characterized by love of physical comfort, sociability, tolerance for others, and extroversion; the behavioral counterpart of endomorphy.

viscerotrophic (vis″er-o-trof′ik) trophic and dependent upon the viscera.

viscerotropic (vis″er-o-trop′ik) [*viscero-* + Gr. *tropos* a turning] primarily acting on the viscera; having a predilection for the abdominal or thoracic viscera.

viscid (vis′id) [L. *viscidus*] glutinous or sticky.

viscidity (vĭ-sid′ĭ-te) the quality of being viscid.

viscin (vis′in) [L. *viscum* mistletoe] a glutinous principle obtainable from mistletoe.

viscogel (vis′ko-jel) a gel which on melting gives a sol of high viscosity. Cf. *liquogel.*

viscometer (vis-kom′ĕ-ter) viscosimeter.

viscometry (vis-kom′ĕ-tre) viscosimetry.

viscose (vis′kōs) 1. viscous. 2. a form of cellulose acetate, used in dialysis membranes, etc.

viscosimeter (vis″ko-sim′ĕ-ter) an apparatus used in determination of the viscosity of a substance. **Ostwald v.,** one which measures relative viscosity by comparing the time required for the meniscus of the solution under study to move a fixed distance with the time required for a meniscus of water to move the same distance. **Stormer v.,** an apparatus for determining viscosity by measurement of the time required, under controlled conditions, for a definite number of revolutions of a rotating cylinder immersed in the substance to be tested.

viscosimetry (vis″ko-sim′ĕ-tre) the measurement of the viscosity of a substance.

viscosity (vis-kos′ĭ-te) a physical property of fluids that determines the internal resistance to shear forces. **absolute v.,** the frictional resistance generated in a fluid when two parallel planes are flowing at different velocities, defined as the frictional force per unit area times the separation of the planes divided by the relative velocity of the planes; measured in poises. Called also *dynamic v.* Symbol, η **dynamic v.,** absolute v. **kinematic v.,** absolute viscosity divided by the density of the fluid; measured in stokes. Symbol, ν

viscous (vis′kus) [L. *viscosus*] characterized by a high degree of friction between component molecules as they slide by each other.

viscus (vis′kus), pl. *vis′cera* [L.] any large interior organ in any one of the three great cavities of the body, especially in the abdomen; see accompanying plate.

visibility (viz″ĭ-bil′ĭ-te) [L. *visibilitas*] the quality of being visible.

visible (viz′ĭ-b'l) [L. *visibilis*] capable of being seen; perceptible by the sight.

visile (viz′īl) pertaining to vision; understanding or recalling most readily what has been seen. Cf. *audile.*

Visine (vi′sēn) trademark for a preparation of tetrahydrozoline hydrochloride.

vision (vizh′un) [L. *visio,* from *vidēre* to see] 1. the act or faculty of seeing; sight. 2. an apparition; a subjective sensation of vision not elicited by actual visual stimuli. 3. visual acuity; symbol V. **achromatic v.,** monochromatism. **binocular v.,** the use of both eyes together without diplopia. **central v.,** that which is elicited by stimuli impinging directly on the macula retinae. **chromatic v.,** color v. **color v.,** 1. perception of the different colors making up the spectrum of visible light; it is mediated by the cones of the retina. 2. chromatopsia. **day v.,** visual perception in the daylight, or under conditions of bright illumination; see also *light adaptation.* **dichromatic v.,** dichromacy. **direct v.,** central v. **double v.,** diplopia. **facial v.,** the ability, formerly thought to be possessed by some blind people, to judge distance, direction, etc., of objects in one's environment by sensation felt in the skin of the face. **foveal v.,** central v. **halo v.,** perception of a colored halo about a light source, one of the symptoms of glaucoma, punctate cataract, and sometimes conjunctivitis. **haploscopic v.,** stereoscopic v. **indirect v.,** peripheral v. **low v.,** impairment of vision such that there is significant visual handicap but also significant usable residual vision; such impairment may involve visual acuity, visual fields, or ocular motility. **monocular v.,** vision with one eye. **multiple v.,** polyopia. **night v.,** visual perception in the darkness of night, or under conditions of reduced illumination; see also *dark adaptation.* **v. null,** the existence of scotomas in the field of vision of which the patient is not aware. **v. obscure,** the existence of scotomas in the field of vision of which the patient is aware. **oscillating v.,** oscillopsia. **peripheral v.,** that which is elicited by stimuli falling on areas of the retina distant from the macula. **photopic v.,** day v. **Pick's v.,** a visual condition in which objects lose their normal horizontal-vertical alignment and converge toward or diverge from one another.

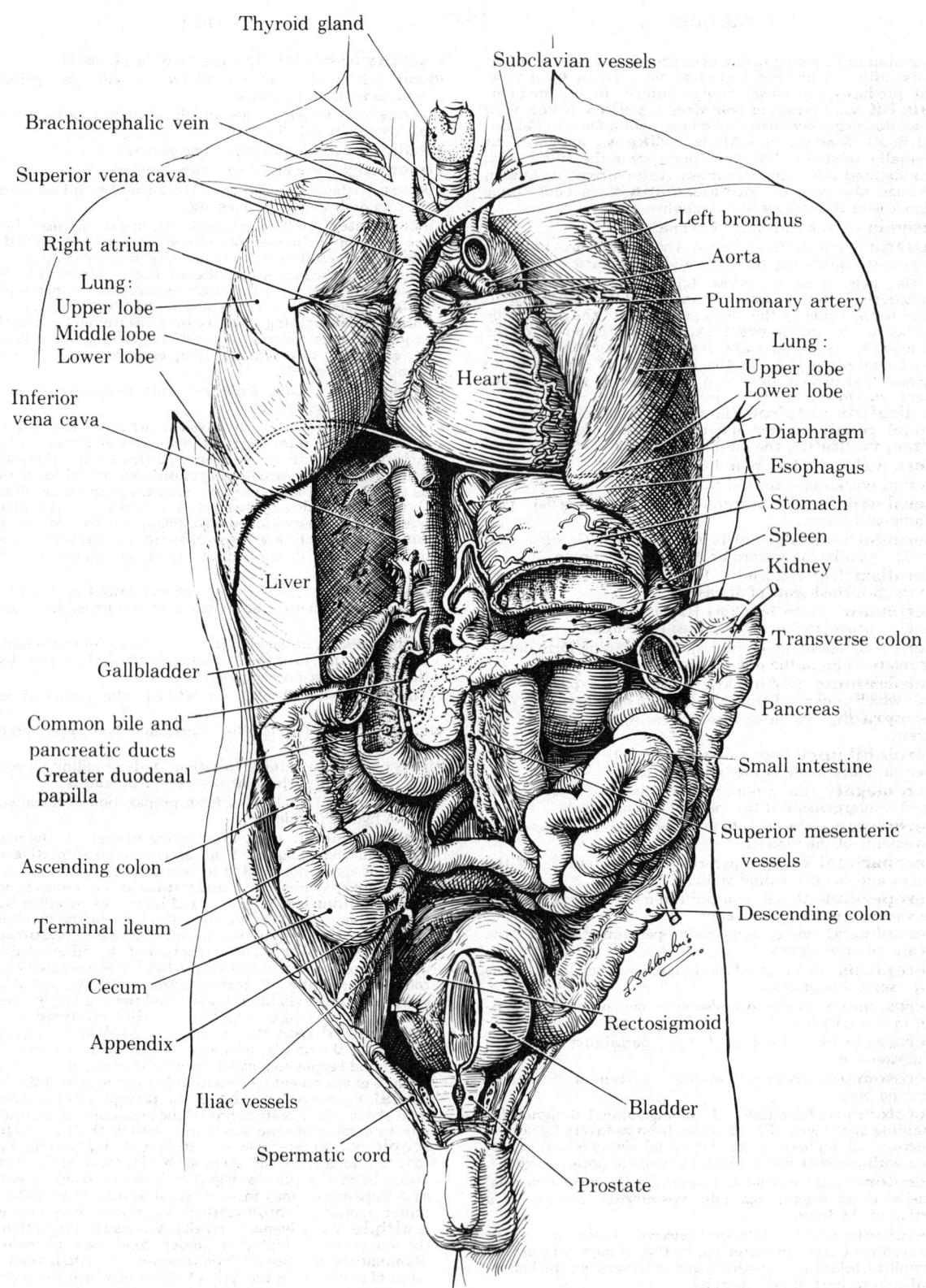

Thyroid gland

Subclavian vessels

Brachiocephalic vein

Superior vena cava

Left bronchus

Right atrium

Aorta

Lung:
Upper lobe
Middle lobe
Lower lobe

Pulmonary artery

Heart

Lung:
Upper lobe
Lower lobe

Inferior
vena cava

Diaphragm

Esophagus

Stomach

Spleen

Kidney

Liver

Transverse colon

Gallbladder

Pancreas

Common bile and
pancreatic ducts

Small intestine

Greater duodenal
papilla

Superior mesenteric
vessels

Ascending colon

Descending colon

Terminal ileum

Cecum

Rectosigmoid

Appendix

Iliac vessels

Bladder

Spermatic cord

Prostate

PLATE 53 — THORACIC AND ABDOMINAL VISCERA

1844

pseudoscopic v., the reverse of stereoscopic vision, an illusion produced by reversing the pictures in a stereoscope, with apparent reversal of concavity and convexity, near and far, etc. **rainbow v.,** halo v. **rod v.,** vision in which the cones of the retina play little or no part, as in night vision. **scotopic v.,** night v. **solid v., stereoscopic v.,** perception of the relief of objects or of their depth; vision in which objects are perceived as having three dimensions, and not merely as two-dimensional pictures. **triple v.,** triplopia. **tubular v.,** 1. a symptom of malingering or conversion hysteria in which the area of the visual field is the same regardless of the testing distance. In normal persons the visual field area is proportional to the square of the testing distance. 2. tunnel vision. **tunnel v.,** 1. that in which the visual fields are severely constricted to about ten degrees from the fixation point; common in retinitis pigmentosa and advanced chronic glaucoma. 2. tubular vision. **twilight v.,** night v. **violet v.,** ianthinopsia. **word v.,** the ability to perceive printed or written words. **yellow v.,** xanthopsia.

visna (vis′nah) a viral disease of sheep affecting primarily the central nervous system, characterized by insidious onset and paresis of the hind limbs which progresses to total paralysis and death.

Vistaril (vis′tah-ril) trademark for preparations of hydroxyzine.

visual (vizh′u-al) [L. *visualis,* from *videre* to see] pertaining to vision or sight.

visualization (vizh″u-al-i-za′shun) the act of viewing, or of achieving a complete visual impression of an object, as by roentgenography. **double contrast v.,** see *mucosal relief roentgenography,* under *roentgenography.*

visualize (vizh′u-al-īz) 1. to achieve a complete view of; to become visible. 2. to picture in the mind.

visuoauditory (vizh″u-o-aw′dĭ-tor″e) audiovisual.

visuognosis (vizh″u-og-no′sis) [L. *visus* sight + Gr. *gnōsis* knowledge] the recognition and interpretation of visual impressions.

visuopsychic (vizh″u-o-si′kik) visual and psychic; a term applied to that area of the cerebral cortex concerned in the judgment of visual sensations.

visuosensory (vizh″u-o-sen′sor-e) pertaining to the perception of stimuli giving rise to visual impressions.

vitagonist (vi-tag′o-nist) a vitamin antagonist; a substance that produces deficiency of a given vitamin.

vital (vi′tal) [L. *vitalis,* from *vita* life] 1. necessary to or pertaining to life. 2. (pl.) the parts and organs necessary to life.

Vitali's test (ve-tal′ēz) [Dioscoride *Vitali,* Italian physician, 1832–1917] see under *tests.*

vitalism (vi′tah-lizm) [L. *vita* life] the theory, opposed to mechanism (def. 3), that biological activities are due to a vital force or principle distinct from physical and chemical forces.

vitalist (vi′tal-ist) a believer in vitalism.

vitalistic (vi″tal-is′tik) pertaining to vitalism.

vitality (vi-tal′ĭ-te) 1. the life principle. 2. the condition of being alive.

vitalize (vi′tal-iz) to give life to.

Vitallium (vi-tal′e-um) trademark for a cobalt-chromium alloy used in dentures and in surgical appliances, prostheses, and instruments.

vitamer (vi′tah-mer) any of a number of compounds that possess a given vitamin activity, i.e., that act to overcome a given vitamin deficiency in one or another organism, plant or animal. Thus, there are biotin vitamers, niacin vitamers, thiamine vitamers, pyridoxin vitamers, A vitamers, D vitamers, K vitamers, etc. (Dean Burk).

vitameter (vi-tam′ĕ-ter) an intrument for assaying vitamins.

vitamin (vi′tah-min) [L. *vita* life + *amine*] a general term for a number of unrelated organic substances that occur in many foods in small amounts and that are necessary in trace amounts for the normal metabolic functioning of the body. They may be water-soluble or fat-soluble. See *Table of Vitamins.* **anticanitic v.,** a substance that counteracts or prevents graying of the hair; see *para-aminobenzoic acid.* **antihemorrhagic v.,** a substance that counteracts a hemorrhagic tendency; see *vitamin K* in *Table of Vitamins.* **anti-infection v.,** one that is useful in preventing infection; see *vitamin A* in *Table of Vitamins.* **antineuritic v.,** thiamine. **antipellagra v.,** niacin. **antiscorbutic v.,** ascorbic acid. **antisterility v.,** a substance that promotes fertility; see *vitamin E* in *Table of Vitamins.* **antixerophthalmic v.,** a substance that counteracts xerophthalmia; see *vitamin A* in *Table of Vitamins.* **fat-soluble v's,** those (vitamins A, D, E, and K) that are soluble in fat solvents and are absorbed along with dietary fats; they are not normally excreted in the urine and tend to be stored in the body in moderate amounts. **permeability v.,** a substance necessary to insure integrity of the capillary walls. **water-soluble v's,** all the vitamins soluble in water (i.e., all but vitamins A, D, E, and K); they are excreted in the urine and are not stored in the body in appreciable quantities.

TABLE OF VITAMINS

Individual vitamins are listed here under their different designations (letters and subscript numbers or letters), with description or cross reference to the name of the specific compound.

v. A, a fat-soluble vitamin occurring in nature in two forms: retinol and dehydroretinol. Deficiency in the diet causes (*a*) inadequate production and regeneration of the visual purple of the retina with resulting night blindness and (*b*) disturbances in epithelial tissue resulting in keratomalacia, xerophthalmia, and lessened resistance to infections through the epithelial surfaces. Vitamin A is present in the liver oils of the cod and other fish, in butter, egg yolk, cheese, and liver as well as in tomatoes and many other vegetable foods in most of which it exists in precursor form as carotene. Vitamin A is toxic when taken in excess; see *hypervitaminosis A.* The term vitamin A is used sometimes to mean retinol alone. See *retinol* and *dehydroretinol.*

v. A₁, retinol.

v. A₂, dehydroretinol.

v. B, a member of the vitamin B complex.

v. B complex, a group of water-soluble substances including thiamine, riboflavin, niacin (nicotinic acid), niacinamide (nicotinamide), the vitamin B₆ group (including pyridoxine, pyridoxal, pyridoxamine), biotin, pantothenic acid, folic acid, possibly para-aminobenzoic acid, inositol, vitamin B₁₂, and possibly choline. Niacin and niancinamide are also known, together, as the pellagra-preventing factor, P.-P. factor, or antipellagra factor.

v. B₁, thiamine.

v. B₂, riboflavin.

v. B₆, water-soluble substances (including pyridoxine, pyridoxal, and pyridoxamine) found in most foods, especially meats, liver, vegetables, whole grain cereals, and egg yolk, and concerned in the metabolism of amino acids, in the degradation of tryptophan, and in the breakdown of glycogen to glucose-1-phosphate.

v. B₁₂, cyanocobalamin.

v. B₁₂ᵦ, hydroxocobalamin.

v. Bᴄ, folic acid.

v. Bᴄ conjugate, polyglutamic acid conjugates of folic acid.

v. C, ascorbic acid.

v. D, any one of several fat-soluble compounds, including cholecalciferol and ergocalciferol, which have antirachitic properties. Known collectively as *calciferol,* they may be produced artificially by the irradiation of ergosterol and a few related sterols. See *ergosterol.* Deficiency of vitamin D tends to cause rickets in children and osteomalacia and osteoporosis in adults. It is present in the liver oils of various fish, in butter and egg yolk, and is produced in the body on exposure to sunlight. Ingestion of excess amounts of vitamin D leads to hypercalcemia, weakness, loss of weight, and other symptoms.

v. D₂, ergocalciferol.

v. D₃, cholecalciferol.

v. E, a fat-soluble vitamin necessary in the diet of many species for normal reproduction, normal development of muscles, normal resistance of erythrocytes to hemolysis, and various other biochemical functions. Chemically it is alpha-tocopherol, one of the three tocopherols (alpha, beta, and gamma) occurring in wheat germ oil, cereals, egg yolk, and beef liver. It is also prepared synthetically. Tocopherols act as antioxidants.

v. G, riboflavin.

v. H, biotin.

v. K, a group of fat-soluble vitamins (see *v. K₁, v. K₂, v. K₃*) which promote clotting of the blood by increasing the synthesis of prothrombin by the liver. They occur naturally in alfalfa, spinach, cabbage, putrefied fish meal, hog-liver fat, egg yolk, and hempseed. Vitamin K and its synthetic analogues have an antihemorrhagic activity with a specific effect on prothrombin deficiency. They are used in obstructive jaundice, in hemor-

rhagic states associated with intestinal diseases and with disease of the liver, in the hypoprothrombinemia of the newborn, administered parenterally to the infant or to the mother during labor.

v. K₁, phytonadione.

v. K₂, menaquinone.

v. K₃, menadione.

v. L, a factor necessary for lactation in rats, L₁ is found in beef-liver extract, L₂ in yeast.

v. M, folic acid.

---

vitamin A acid tretinoin.

vitaminogenic (vi-tam″ĭ-no-jen′ik) caused by or due to a vitamin.

vitaminoid (vi′tah-min-oid) 1. resembling a vitamin. 2. a substance having vitamin-like activity, e.g., a bioflavonoid.

vitaminology (vi″tah-min-ol′o-je) the study of vitamins.

vitaminoscope (vi″tah-min′o-skōp) [*vitamin* + Gr. *skopein* to examine] an instrument for measuring the time required for recovery from glare as an indication of the vitamin A reserve of the body.

vitanition (vi″tan-ish′un) nutritional disorder due to vitamin deficiency.

vitellarium (vit″ĕ-lār′e-um) an accessory genital gland found in flukes and tapeworms which secretes the yolk and shell for the fertilized egg; called also *vitelline gland*.

vitellary (vit′ĕ-lār″e) pertaining to the vitellus, or yolk.

vitellicle (vi-tel′ĭ-k′l) [L. *vitellus* yolk] the yolk sac.

vitellin (vi-tel′in) [L. *vitellus* yolk] a phosphoprotein found in the yolk of eggs.

vitelline (vi-tel′in) [L. *vitellus* yolk] resembling or pertaining to the yolk of an egg or ovum.

vitellogenesis (vi″tel-o-jen′ĕ-sis) production of yolk.

vitellolutein (vi″tel-o-lu′te-in) [L. *vitellus* yolk + *luteus* yellow] a yellow pigment obtainable from lutein.

vitellorubin (vi″tel-o-ru′bin) [L. *vitellus* yolk + *ruber* red] 1. a reddish pigment obtainable from lutein. 2. crustaceorubin.

vitellose (vi-tel′ōs) a form of proteose derived from vitellin.

vitellus (vi-tel′us) [L.] the yolk of an egg, or of an ovum.

vitiatin (vi-ti′ah-tin) a compound sometimes occurring in the urine along with creatine and creatinine; it is a homologue of choline.

vitiation (vish″e-a′shun) [L. *vitiatio*] impairment of efficiency; the perversion of any process so as to render it faulty or ineffective.

vitiligines (vit″ĭ-lij′ĭ-nēz) [pl. of *vitiligo*] depigmented areas of the skin, as those occurring in vitiligo, or the whitened lines of striae atrophicae.

vitiliginous (vit″ĭ-lij′ĭ-nus) relating to or affected with vitiligo.

vitiligo (vit″ĭ-li′go) [L.] a usually progressive, chronic pigmentary anomaly of the skin manifested by depigmented white patches that may be surrounded by a hyperpigmented border; it is associated with a dominantly inherited predisposition, and it has been speculated that autoimmune mechanisms are involved in the etiology. Cf. *leukoderma* and *piebaldism.* **v. i′ridis,** depigmentation of the iris.

Vitis (vi′tis) [L.] a genus of plants of the family Vitaceae, including various species of grape or grape vine. **V. vinif′era,** L., a species affording most of the more valuable varieties of cultivated and wine-producing grapes. Various preparations of the fruit have numerous medicinal uses by the laity.

vitium (vish′e-um), pl. *vi′tia* [L.] fault, defect. **v. conformatio′nis,** a defect in shape; a malformation. **v. cor′dis,** an organic heart defect. **v. pri′mae formatio′nis,** a developmental anomaly.

vitochemical (vi″to-kem′ĭ-kal) organic; pertaining to organic chemistry.

vit. ov. sol. abbreviation for L. *vitel′lo o′vi solu′tus,* dissolved in yolk of egg.

vitrectomy (vĭ-trek′to-me) [*vitreum* + *ectomy*] surgical extraction usually via the pars plana of the contents of the

vitreous chamber of the eye.

vitreocapsulitis (vit″re-o-kap″su-li′tis) [L. *vitreus* glassy + *capsula* capsule + *-itis*] inflammation of the capsule enclosing the vitreous; hyalitis.

vitreoretinal (vit″re-o-ret″ĭ-nal) of or pertaining to the vitreous and retina.

Vitreoscilla (vit″re-os-sil′ah) [L. *vitreus* glassy + *oscillum* swing] a genus of gliding bacteria of the family Beggiatoaceae, order Cytophagales, made up of colorless filaments. The type species is *V. beggiatoi′des*.

Vitreoscillaceae (vit″re-os″sil-la′se-e) in former systems of classification, a family of gliding bacteria, now included in the families Beggiatoaceae and Cytophagaceae.

vitreous (vit′re-us) glasslike or hyaline; often used alone to designate the vitreous body of the eye (corpus vitreum [NA]). **detached v.,** vitreous separated from its attachments, as from the retina. **primary v.,** the earliest vitreous in the embryo, formed from a mass of ectodermal and mesodermal fibrils and vascularized by the proliferating hyaloid system. It ceases to be formed when the hyaline capsule of the lens is formed, and is then enveloped by secondary vitreous. **primary persistent hyperplastic v.,** a congenital anomaly, usually unilateral, due to persistence of embryonic remnants of the fibromuscular tunic of the eye and part of the hyaloid vascular system. Clinically, there is a white pupil, elongated ciliary processes, and often microphthalmia; the lens, although clear initially, may become completely opaque. **secondary v.,** embryonic vitreous composed of densely packed fine fibrils formed around the primary vitreous by the inner layer of the optic cup. **tertiary v.,** embryonic zonular fibers derived from the primary vitreous and the basement membrane of the nonpigmented epithelium of the ciliary body; the fibers eventually attach to the lens capsule, giving rise to the zonule of Zinn.

vitreum (vit′re-um) the vitreous body of the eye (corpus vitreum [NA]).

vitrina (vĭ-tri′nah) [L. *vitrum* glass] a translucent or glassy material. **v. audito′ria, v. au′ris,** endolympha. **v. ocula′ris, v. o′culi,** corpus vitreum.

vitriol (vit′re-ol) [L. *vitriolum*] any crystalline sulfate. **blue v.,** the pentahydrate form of cupric sulfate. **elixir of v.,** aromatic sulfuric acid. **green v.,** ferrous sulfate. **oil of v.,** sulfuric acid. **white v., zinc v.,** zinc sulfate.

vitriolated (vit′re-o-lāt″ed) containing vitriol; containing sulfuric acid.

vitrum (vit′rum) [L.] glass.

Vivactil (vi-vak′til) trademark for a preparation of protriptyline hydrochloride.

vivi- [L. *vivus* alive] a combining form meaning alive or denoting relationship to life.

vividialysis (viv″ĭ-di-al′ĭ-sis) removal by dialysis through a living membrane (the peritoneum). Cf. *peritoneal lavage,* under *lavage*.

vividiffusion (viv″ĭ-dĭ-fu′zhun) removal of diffusible substances from the circulating blood of living subjects by dialysis, performed by the continuous passage of the blood from an artery through a system of tubes made of celloidin immersed in saline solution, and its return to a vein, thus yielding by dialysis certain of its constituents to the fluid surrounding the tubes.

vivification (viv″ĭ-fi-ka′shun) [L. *vivificatio,* from *vivus* living + *facere* to make] the conversion of lifeless into living protein matter in the process of assimilation.

viviparity (viv″ĭ-par′ĭ-te) the quality of being viviparous.

viviparous (vi-vip′ah-rus) [*vivi-* + L. *parere* to bring forth, produce] bearing living young which derive nutrition directly from the maternal organism.

Viviparus (vi-vip′ah-rus) a genus of fresh-water snails. **V. javan′icus,** a second intermediate host of the fluke *Echinostoma ilocanum* in Java.

vivipation (viv″ĭ-pa′shun) the form of reproduction in which the embryo develops within and derives nutrition directly from the maternal organism.

viviperception (viv″ĭ-per-sep′shun) the study of the vital processes of the living organism.

vivisection (viv″ĭ-sek′shun) the performance of surgical procedures upon living animals for purposes of research.

vivisectionist (viv″ĭ-sek′shun-ist) one who practices or defends vivisection.

vivosphere (vi′vo-sfēr) [L. *vivus* alive + *atmosphere*] the region between the atmosphere above and the petrosphere below, in which life is found most abundantly; biosphere.

Vladimiroff-Mikulicz amputation (vlad″ĭ-mēr′of mik′u-lich) [Alexander A. *Vladimiroff;* Johann von *Mikulicz*-Radecki, Polish surgeon, 1850–1905] see under *amputation.*

Vladimiroff's operation (vlad″ĭ-mēr′ofs) [Alexander A. *Vladimiroff,* Russian surgeon, 1837–1903] see *Mikulicz's operation,* def. 3, under *operation.*

VLDL very low-density lipoprotein.

V.M.D. Doctor of Veterinary Medicine [L. *Veterinariae Medicinae Doctor*].

vocal (vo′kal) [L. *vocalis,* from *vox* voice] pertaining to the voice.

Voges-Proskauer test (reaction) [O. *Voges,* German physician; Bernhard *Proskauer,* German hygienist, 1851–1915] see under *tests.*

Vogt's angle (fōgts) [Karl *Vogt,* German naturalist and physiologist, 1817–1895] see under *angle.*

Vogt's point (fōgts) [Paul Frederick Emmanuel *Vogt,* surgeon in Greifswald, 1844–1885] see under *point.*

Vogt's syndrome (disease) (fōgts) [Oskar *Vogt,* German neurologist, 1870–1959] see under *syndrome.*

Vogt-Hueter point (fōgt-he′ter) [P. F. E. *Vogt;* Karl *Hueter,* German surgeon, 1838–1882] see Vogt's *point,* under *point.*

Vohwinkel's syndrome (fo-vink′el) [Karl Hermann *Vohwinkel,* German dermatologist, 20th century] keratoma hereditarium mutilans.

voice (vois) [L. *vox* voice] a sound produced by the larynx and modified by the vocal tract. **amphoric v.,** cavernous v. **cavernous v.,** a hollow sound heard on auscultation when the patient speaks; it indicates a cavity in the lung. **double v.,** diphonia. **eunuchoid v.,** a high falsetto voice in a man, resembling that of a eunuch or a woman. **whispered v.,** the transmission of a whisper to the auscultating ear, heard in pulmonary consolidation.

void (void) to cast out as waste matter.

Voigt's boundary lines (voits) [Christian August *Voigt,* Austrian anatomist, 1809–1890] see under *line.*

Voillemier's point (vwal-me-āz′) [Léon Clémont *Voillemier,* French urologist] see under *point.*

Voit's nucleus (foits) [Carl von *Voit,* physiologist in Munich, 1831–1908] see under *nucleus.*

voix (vwah) [Fr.] voice. **v. de polichinelle** (vwah″dĕ-pol″ish-ĭ-nel′) [Fr. "voice of Punch"], a variety of egophony.

vola (vo′lah), gen. and pl. *vo′lae* [L.] a concave or hollow surface. **v. ma′nus,** the hollow of the hand (palma manus [NA]). **v. pe′dis,** the hollow of the foot (planta pedis [NA]).

volar (vo′lar) pertaining to the palm or sole; plantar; indicating the flexor surface of the forearm, wrist, or hand.

volardorsal (vo″lar-dor′sal) from the volar to the dorsal surface.

volaris (vo-la′ris) palmar; designating relationship to the palm of the hand.

volatile (vol′ah-til) [L. *volatilis,* from *volare* to fly] tending to evaporate rapidly.

volatilization (vol″ah-til-i-za′shun) the conversion into vapor or gas without chemical change.

volatilize (vol′ah-til-īz) to convert into vapor.

volatilizer (vol′ah-til-īz″er) an apparatus for producing volatilization.

Volhard's test (fōl′harts) [Franz *Volhard,* German internist, 1872–1905] see under *tests.*

volition (vo-lish′un) [L. *velle* to will] the act or power of willing.

volitional (vo-lish′un-al) pertaining to the will.

Volkmann's canal, membrane (fōlk′mahnz) [Alfred Wilhelm *Volkmann,* German physiologist, 1800–1877] see under *canal* and *membrane.*

Volkmann's contracture, etc. (fōlk′mahnz) [Richard von *Volkmann,* German surgeon, 1830–1889] see under *contracture, disease, paralysis,* and *spoon.*

volley (vol′e) a rhythmical succession of muscular twitches artificially induced; the aggregate of nerve impulses set up by a single stimulus. **antidromic v.,** the backfire excitation traveling centrad through the anterior root during the reflex arc.

volsella (vol-sel′ah) [L.] vulsella.

volt (vōlt) [Alessandro *Volta,* Italian physiologist and physicist, 1745–1827] the SI unit of electric potential or electromotive force equal to one joule per coulomb or one ampere-ohm. Symbol, V. **electron v., (eV, ev),** the energy acquired by an electron accelerated through a potential difference of one volt, equal to 1.6022×10^{-19} joule. Larger units, used for specifying rest masses and kinetic energies of particles, are obtained by attaching SI prefixes, giving *kilo electron volt* (keV = 10^3 eV), *mega electron volt* (MeV = 10^6 eV), and *giga electron volt* (GeV = 10^9 eV).

voltage (vōl′tij) electromotive force measured in volts.

voltaic (vol-ta′ik) galvanic (def. 2).

voltaism (vol′tah-izm) galvanism.

voltammeter (vōlt-am′me-ter) an instrument for measuring both volts and amperes.

voltampere (vōlt-am′pēr) the product of multiplying a volt by a milliampere.

voltmeter (vōlt′me-ter) an instrument for measuring electromotive force in volts.

Voltolini's disease, tube (vol″to-le′nēz) [Frederic Edward Rudolf *Voltolini,* rhinologist and otologist in Breslau, 1819–1889] see under *disease* and *tube.*

volume (vol′ūm) the measure of the quantity or capacity of a substance. **atomic v.,** the value obtained by dividing the atomic weight of an element by its specific gravity in the solid condition. **blood v.,** the sum of the red cell volume and the plasma volume. **circulation v., v. of circulation,** the amount of blood pumped through the lungs and out to all the organs of the body by the heart, expressed in liters of blood flow per minute. **v. of distribution,** a dilution method for determining the volume of fluids, e.g., plasma, in a body fluid compartment. A solute (e.g., inulin) is injected into the compartment and, after it is equally distributed, a sample is taken. Then the quantity of solute removed (as by metabolism, excretion, etc.) is subtracted from the quantity administered, and the result is divided by the concentration per milliliter in the sample. **end-diastolic v.,** the volume of blood in each ventricle at the end of diastole, usually about 120–130 ml. but sometimes reaching 200–250 ml. in the normal heart. **end-systolic v.,** the volume of blood remaining in each ventricle at the end of systole, usually about 50–60 ml. but sometimes as little as 10–30 ml. in the normal heart. **expiratory reserve v.,** the maximal amount of gas that can be expired from the resting end-expiratory level. Abbreviated ERV. See illustration accompanying *capacity.* **inspiratory reserve v.,** the maximal amount of gas that can be inspired from the end-inspiratory position. Abbreviated IRV. **mean corpuscular v.,** see *MCV.* **minute v.,** the quantity of gas expelled from the lungs per minute. Abbreviated MV. **packed-cell v. (PCV), volume of packed red cells (VPRC),** the venous hematocrit determined by centrifugation; the number of packed red cells in milliliters per 100 ml. of centrifuged blood. Abbreviated PCV. **plasma v.,** the total volume of blood plasma, i.e., the extracellular fluid volume of the vascular space, measured by tracer dilution using ^{125}I- or ^{131}I-labeled albumin or T-1824 Evans blue dye as the tracer. **red cell v.,** the total volume of red cells in the body measured by isotopic dilution methods, usually with ^{51}Cr-labeled autologous red cells. **residual v.,** the amount of gas remaining in the lung at the end of a maximal expiration. Abbreviated RV. See illustration accompanying *capacity.* **stroke v.,** the amount of blood ejected from a ventricle at each beat of the heart.

tidal v., the amount of gas that is inspired and expired (i.e., ventilation) during one respiratory cycle. Abbreviated V$_T$. See illustration accompanying *capacity.*

volumenometer (vol″ūm-nom′ĕ-ter) volumometer.

volumetric (vol″u-met′rik) [*volume + metric*] pertaining to or accomplished by measurement in volumes.

volumette (vol″u-met′) an instrument for delivering repeatedly quantities of fluid in accurate predetermined amounts.

volumometer (vol″u-mom′ĕ-ter) [*volume* + Gr. *metron* measure] an instrument for measuring volume or changes in volume.

voluntary (vol′un-tār″e) [L. *voluntas* will] accomplished in accordance with the will.

voluntomotory (vo″lun-to-mo′tor-e) [L. *voluntas* will + *motor* mover] subject to voluntary motor influence.

volute (vo-lūt′) rolled up.

volutin (vo-lu′tin) a complex molecule containing large amounts of orthophosphate polymers, nucleoprotein, and lipid, occurring as cytoplasmic granular inclusions (granules) in certain bacteria, yeasts, yeastlike fungi, and protozoa, and serving as an intracellular phosphate reserve. Because volutin granules stain red with blue basic dyes they are sometimes called *metachromatic granules.*

Volvocida (vol-vos′ĭ-dah) [L. *volvere* to twist around] an order of plantlike, flagellate, chiefly freshwater protozoa (class Phytomastigophorea, subphylum Mastigophora) having two or four equal apical flagella, a cellulose wall, and pale green chloroplasts. Most members are colonial, forming platelike or spherical aggregations. Representative genera include *Chlamydomonas* and *Volvox.*

Volvox (vol′voks) a genus of plantlike, biflagellate protozoa (order Volvocida, class Phytomastigophorea), the members of which form colonies that are large hollow spheres, each of which moves through the water by rotation.

volvulate (vol′vu-lāt) [L. *volvere* to twist round] to twist or form a knot (volvulus).

volvulosis (vol″vu-lo′sis) onchocerciasis caused by *Onchocerca volvulus* (q.v.).

volvulus (vol′vu-lus) [L. *volvere* to twist round] intestinal obstruction due to a knotting and twisting of the bowel. **v. neonato′rum,** volvulus occurring in the newborn.

vomer (vo′mer) [L. "plowshare"] [NA] the unpaired flat bone that forms the inferior and posterior part of the nasal septum.

vomerine (vo′mer-īn) of or pertaining to the vomer.

vomerobasilar (vo″mer-o-bas′ĭ-lar) pertaining to the vomer and to the basilar portion of the cranium.

vomeronasal (vo″mer-o-na′sal) pertaining to the vomer and the nasal bone.

vomica (vom′ĭ-kah), pl. *vom′icae* [L. "abscess"] 1. the profuse and sudden expectoration of pus and putrescent matter. 2. an abnormal cavity in an organ, especially in the lung, caused by suppuration and the breaking down of tissue.

vomicose (vom′ĭ-kōs) full of ulcers; ulcerous.

vomit (vom′it) [L. *vomitare*] 1. to cast up from the stomach by the mouth. 2. matter cast up from the stomach; vomited matter. 3. an emetic. **Barcoo v.,** vomiting and nausea, with bulimia, occurring in southern Australia. **bilious v.,** vomited matter stained with bile. **black v.,** blackish matter consisting of blood which has been acted upon by the gastric juice, cast up from the stomach in yellow fever and other conditions in which blood collects in the stomach. **coffee-ground v.,** vomit containing dark altered blood mixed with stomach contents; see *black v.*

vomiting (vom′it-ing) the forcible expulsion of the contents of the stomach through the mouth. **cerebral v.,** spontaneous vomiting without nausea, frequently seen in intracranial disease. **cyclic v.,** vomiting recurring at irregular intervals, especially in children; called also *periodic v.* and *recurrent v.* **dry v.,** nausea with attempts at vomiting, but with the ejection of nothing but gas. **fecal v.,** stercoraceous v. **hysterical v.,** vomiting accompanying an attack of hysteria. **nervous v.,** vomiting as a symptom of gastric neurosis. **periodic v.,** cyclic v. **pernicious v.,** vomiting in pregnancy, so severe as to threaten the life of the mother. **v. of pregnancy,** vomiting occurring in pregnancy, especially the early morning vomiting common in that condition. **projectile v.,** vomiting in which the

vomitus is ejected with force. **recurrent v.,** cyclic v. **stercoraceous v.,** the vomiting of fecal matter; it is seen in intestinal obstruction, appendicitis, etc., when bacterial overgrowth in the upper intestine has modified the intestinal contents.

vomitive (vom′ĭ-tiv) emetic.

vomito (vom′ĭ-to) [Sp.] vomit. **v. negro** (vom′ĭ-to na′gro) [Sp.], black vomit.

vomitory (vom′ĭ-tor″e) an emetic.

vomiturition (vom″it-u-rish′un) repeated ineffectual attempts at vomiting.

vomitus (vom′ĭ-tus) [L.] 1. vomiting. 2. matter vomited. **v. cruen′tus,** bloody vomit. **v. matuti′nus,** the morning vomiting of chronic gastric catarrh.

von Behring see *Behring.*

von Bekhterev see *Bekhterev.*

von Bergmann see *Bergmann.*

von Bezold see *Bezold.*

von Ebner see *Ebner.*

von Economo see *Economo.*

von Frisch see *Frisch.*

von Gierke see *Gierke.*

von Graefe see *Graefe.*

von Haller see *Haller.*

von Hippel see *Hippel.*

von Jaksch see *Jaksch.*

von Kossa see *Kossa.*

von Langenbeck see *Langenbeck.*

von Leyden see *Leyden.*

von Mikulicz see *Mikulicz.*

von Monakow see *Monakow.*

von Pirquet see *Pirquet.*

von Recklinghausen see *Recklinghausen.*

von Ruck see *Ruck.*

von Wahl see *Wahl.*

von Willebrand see *Willebrand.*

von Zenker see *Zenker.*

von Zumbusch see *Zumbusch.*

Vontrol (von-trōl′) trademark for preparations of diphenidol.

Voorhees' bag (voor′ēz) [James Ditmars *Voorhees,* obstetrician in New York, 1869–1929] see under *bag.*

Voranil (vor′ah-nil) trademark for a preparation of clortermine hydrochloride.

Voronoff's operation (vo′ro-nofs) [Serge *Voronoff,* Russian physician in Paris, 1866–1951] see under *operation.*

vortex (vor′teks), pl. *vor′tices* [L. "whirl"] a whorled arrangement, design, or pattern, as of muscle fibers, or of the ridges or hairs on the skin; [NA] a general term for a structure having a whorled arrangement, design, or pattern. **coccygeal v., v. coccyg′eus,** a spiral arrangement of hairs over the region of the coccyx. **v. cor′dis** [NA], **v. of heart,** the whorled arrangement of muscle fibers at the apex, in the left ventricle of the heart, through which the more superficial fibers pass to the interior of the left ventricle toward the base. **Fleischer's v.,** a rare congenital opacity characterized by ochre-colored whorls which radiate from the center of the cornea at the level of Bowman's membrane; called also *cornea verticillata.* **v. len′tis,** a spiral figure on the surface of the lens of the eye produced by the concentric arrangement of the fibers composing it; called also *nuclear arc* or *zone.* **vor′tices pilo′rum** [NA], whorled patterns of hair growth on the body, as that on the crown of the head.

vortices (vor′tĭ-sēz) [L.] plural of *vortex.*

v. o. s. abbreviation for L. *vitel′lo o′vi solu′tus,* dissolved in yolk of egg.

Vossius lenticular ring (vos′e-us) [Adolf *Vossius,* German ophthalmologist, 1855–1925] see under *ring.*

vox (voks), gen. *vo′cis,* pl. *vo′ces* [L.] voice. **v. choler′ica,** the faint, sometimes inaudible, high-pitched voice of patients with severe cholera.

voyeur (voi-yer′) a person who practices voyeurism.

voyeurism (voi′yer-izm) [DSM III-R] a paraphilia characterized by recurrent, intense sexual urges or sexually arousing fantasies involving watching unsuspecting people who are naked, disrobing, or engaging in sexual activity.

VPRC volume of packed red cells.

V.R. vocal resonance.

V.S. volumetric solution.

v.s. vibration seconds (the unit of measurement of sound waves.)

vuerometer (vu″er-om′ĕ-ter) [Fr. *vue* sight + *-meter*] an instrument for measuring the interpupillary distance.

vulcanize (vul′kah-nīz) to subject caoutchouc, in the presence of sulfur, to heat and high steam pressure, producing a flexible or hard rubber, as desired.

vulgaris (vul-ga′ris) [L.] ordinary; common. See *acne vulgaris, lupus vulgaris*, etc.

vulnerability (vul″ner-ah-bil′ĭ-te) susceptibility to injury or to contagion.

vulnerant (vul′ner-ant) 1. inflicting injury or causing a wound. 2. an agent that causes injury.

vulnerary (vul′ner-er″e) [L. *vulnerarius*, from *vulnus* wound] 1. pertaining to wounds or the healing of wounds. 2. an agent that promotes the healing of wounds.

vulnerate (vul′ner-āt) [L. *vulnerare*] to wound.

vulnus (vul′nus), pl. *vul′nera* [L.] a wound.

Vulpian's atrophy (vul′pe-anz) [Edme Felix Alfred *Vulpian*, French physician, 1826–1887] see under *atrophy*.

vulsella, vulsellum (vul-sel′ah, vul-sel′um) [L.] a forceps with clawlike hooks at the extremity of each blade.

vulva (vul′vah) [L.] the region of the external genital organs of the female, including the labia majora, labia minora, mons pubis, bulb of the vestibule, vestibule of the vagina, greater and lesser vestibular glands, and vaginal orifice. See *pudendum femininum* [NA]. **fused v.**, synechia vulvae.

vulval, vulvar (vul′val; vul′var) pertaining to the vulva.

vulvectomy (vul-vek′to-me) excision of the vulva.

vulvismus (vul-viz′mus) vaginismus.

vulvitis (vul-vi′tis) [*vulva* + *-itis*] inflammation of the vulva. **diabetic v.**, vulvitis occurring in diabetes. **eczematiform v.**, vulvitis marked by the formation of vesicular pustules. **erosive v.**, a condition due to mixed microbial infection in which gangrenous ulcerations similar to the lesions seen in noma of the oral tissues affect one labium majus and then the other. Called also *noma vulvae* and *phlegmonous v.* **leukoplakic v.**, kraurosis vulvae. **phlegmonous v.**, erosive v. **plasma cell v., v. plasmocellula′ris**, the counterpart of balanitis circumscripta plasmacellularis in women, in which the vulva has a lacquer-like appearance; erosions, punctate hemorrhage, synechiae, and a slate- to ochre-colored pigmentation may supervene. **pseudoleukoplakic v.**, vulvitis in which the mucosa is whitish and opaque, resembling leukoplakia. **ulcerative v.**, a form with ulceration, pain, and lymphangitis.

vulvocrural (vul-vo-kroo′ral) pertaining to the vulva and the thigh.

vulvopathy (vul-vop′ah-the) [*vulva* + Gr. *pathos* disease] any disease of the vulva.

vulvorectal (vul″vo-rek′tal) pertaining to or communicating with the vulva and rectum, as a vulvorectal fistula.

vulvouterine (vul″vo-u′ter-in) pertaining to the vulva and uterus.

vulvovaginal (vul″vo-vaj′ĭ-nal) pertaining to the vulva and vagina.

vulvovaginitis (vul″vo-vaj″ĭ-ni′tis) inflammation of the vulva and vagina, or of the vulvovaginal glands. **infectious pustular v.**, an acute contagious nonvenereal viral disease of cattle characterized by inflammation, necrosis, and pustule formation of varying degree in the vulva and vagina; in the male, similar lesions occur on the skin of the penis. **senile v.**, see *atrophic vaginitis*.

vv. abbreviation for L. *ve′nae* (veins).

v/v volume (of solute) per volume (of solvent).

V.W. vessel wall.

V-Y plasty V-Y procedure.

VZIG varicella-zoster immune globulin.

W

W chemical symbol for *tungsten* [Ger. *Wolfram*]; symbol for *watt*.

Waardenburg's syndrome (var′den-bergz) [Petrus Johannes *Waardenburg*, Dutch ophthalmologist, born 1886] see under *syndrome*.

Wachendorf's membrane (vahk′en-dorfs) [Eberhard Jacob *Wachendorf*, German anatomist, 1702–1758] see under *membrane*.

Wagner's corpuscles, spot (vahg′nerz) [Rudolf *Wagner*, German physiologist, 1805–1864] see *corpuscula tactus*, and see under *spot*.

Wagner's hammer (vahg′nerz) [Johann Philip *Wagner*, German physicist, 1799–1879] Neef's hammer.

Wagner's theory (vahg′nerz) [Moritz *Wagner*, German zoologist, 1813–1887] see *migration theory*, under *theory*.

Wagner-Jauregg treatment (vahg′ner-yow′rek) [Julius *Wagner-Jauregg*] see under *treatment*.

Wagstaffe's fracture (wag′stafs) [William Warwick *Wagstaffe*, English surgeon, 1843–1910] see under *fracture*.

waist (wāst) the portion of the body between the thorax and the hips.

wakamba (wa-kam′bah) an African arrow poison.

wakefulness (wāk′ful-nes) a state marked by indisposition to sleep; sleeplessness; arousal.

Waksman (waks′man), Selman Abraham. Russian-born American microbiologist, 1888–1973; winner of the Nobel prize for medicine or physiology in 1952 for his discovery of streptomycin and its effectiveness against tuberculosis.

Wald (wahld) George. American biologist, born 1906; cowinner, with Ragnar Arthur Granit and Haldan Keffer Hartline, of the Nobel prize for medicine or physiology in 1967 for discoveries regarding the molecular basis of visual excitation.

Waldenburg's apparatus (vahl′den-boorgz) [Louis *Waldenburg*, German physician, 1837–1881] see under *apparatus*.

Waldenström's disease (vahl′den-stremz) [Johan Henning *Waldenström*, orthopedic surgeon in Stockholm, born 1877] see *osteochondrosis*.

Waldenström's macroglobulinemia (vahl′den-stremz) [Jan *Waldenström*, Swedish biochemist, born 1906] see under *macroglobulinemia*.

Waldeyer's fluid, etc. (vahl′di-erz) [Heinrich Wilhelm Gottfried von *Waldeyer*, anatomist in Berlin, 1836–1921] see under *fluid, fossa, gland, layer, ring*, and *sulcus*.

walk (wok) 1. to move on foot. 2. the manner in which one moves on foot; see also *gait* and *walking*.

walking (wok′ing) progressing on foot, or the manner in which one moves on foot. **chromosome w.**, in molecular genetics, the sequential isolation of clones carrying overlapping DNA sequences so that the isolation "walks" along part of a chromosome. **heel w.,** a gait marked by walking on the heels to avoid the pain of pressure upon the hyperalgesic soles of the feet in cases of peripheral neuritis. **sleep w.,** somnambulism.

wall (wawl) the limiting structure of a space, as of the chest, abdomen, or hollow organ, or of a definitive mass of material. For official names of specific walls of various anatomical structures, see under *paries.* **axial w.,** a cavity wall approximating the pulp tissue, parallel with the long axis of the tooth. **cavity w.,** the walls of a prepared cavity, named according to the surface of a tooth toward which they are placed, extracoronal walls being named after surfaces that have been reduced, and intracoronal ones after surfaces from which they derive. **cell w.,** a rigid structure that lies just outside of and is joined to the plasma membrane of plant cells and most prokaryotic cells; it protects the cell and maintains its shape. **germ w.,** a ringlike thickening around the blastoderm of the bird, consisting of the advancing boundary zone at its margin. **gingival w.,** a peripheral cavity wall near the apical end of the crown of the tooth. **nail w.,** vallum unguis. **parietal w.,** somatopleure. **periotic w.,** the wall of the otic vesicle. **pulpal w.,** the cavity wall on the occlusal surface that covers the pulp in a plane at right angles to the long axis of the tooth. **splanchnic w.,** splanchnopleure. **subpulpal w.,** the floor of a prepared cavity formed when the pulp is removed and the cavity is extended to include the pulp chamber.

Wallenberg's syndrome (vahl′en-bergz) [Adolf *Wallenberg,* German physician, 1862–1949] see under *syndrome.*

wallerian degeneration, law (wahl-le′re-an) [Augustus Volney *Waller,* English physician, 1816–1870] see under *degeneration* and *law.*

walleye (wahl′i) 1. leukoma of the cornea. 2. exotropia.

Wallhauser-Whitehead method [A. *Wallhauser;* J. M. *Whitehead,* American physicians] see under *method.*

Walter's bromide test (vahl′terz) [Friedrich Karl *Walter,* Bremen neurologist, 1881–1935] see under *tests.*

Walthard's islets (cell rests, inclusions) [Max *Walthard,* Swiss gynecologist, 1867–1933] see under *islet.*

Walther's ducts, oblique ligament (vahl′terz) [August Friedrich *Walther,* German anatomist, 1688–1746] see *ductus sublinguales minores* and *ligamentum talofibulare posterius.*

wambles (wahm′b'lz) milk sickness.

wandering (wahn′der-ing) moving about freely, as a wandering cell; abnormally movable; too loosely attached. **pathologic tooth w.,** see under *migration.*

Wang's test (wangz) [*Wang* Chung Tik, Chinese physician, 1888–1931] see under *tests.*

Wangensteen drainage, tube (apparatus, suction) (wan′gen-stēn) [Owen Harding *Wangensteen,* American surgeon, born 1898] see under *drainage* and *tube.*

Wanscher's mask (vahn′sherz) [Oscar *Wanscher,* Danish physician, 1846–1906] see under *mask.*

warbles (war′b'lz) see *Hypoderma.* **ox w.,** larvae of flies of the genus *Hypoderma* (*H. bovis* and *H. lineatum*) which infest cattle of the Northern Hemisphere.

Warburg's coenzyme (var′boorks) [Otto Heinrich *Warburg*] see *nicotinamide-adenine dinucleotide phosphate,* under *dinucleotide.*

ward (ward) a large room in a hospital for the accommodation of several patients.

warfarin (war′fah-rin) [named for *Wisconsin Alumni Research Foundation*] chemical name: 4-hydroxy-3-oxo-1-phenylbutyl-2H-1-benzopyran-2-one. One of the synthetic coumarin anticoagulants, $C_{19}H_{16}O_4$. **w. potassium** [USP] the potassium salt of warfarin, $C_{19}H_{15}KO_4$, occurring as a white crystalline powder, having anticoagulant actions and uses similar to those of the sodium salt; administered orally. **sodium w.** [USP] the sodium salt of warfarin, $C_{19}H_{15}NaO_4$, occurring as a white, amorphous or crystalline powder, the anticoagulant action of which is of intermediate duration and cumulative; administered orally, intravenously, or intramuscularly. It is also used as a rodenticide.

Waring's method (system) (wār′ings) [George Edward

Waring, American sanitarian, 1833–1898] see under *method.*

Warren's incision (war′enz) [John Collins *Warren,* Boston surgeon, 1778–1856] see under *incision.*

wart (wort) [L. *verruca*] verruca. **acuminate w.,** condyloma acuminatum. **anatomical w.,** tuberculosis verrucosa cutis. **cattle w.,** a condition of viral origin in cattle, characterized by development of nodular tumors, usually in the skin of the head, neck, and shoulders, and often on the udder. **common w.,** verruca (def. 1). **digitate w.,** verruca digitata. **flat w.,** verruca plana. **filiform w.,** verruca filiformis. **fugitive w.,** verruca plana. **Hassall-Henle w's,** hyaline excrescences in the periphery of Descemet's membrane (lamina limitans posterior corneae) occurring with advancing age. **juvenile w.,** verruca plana. **moist w.,** condyloma latum. **mosaic w.,** an irregularly shaped lesion on the sole of the foot, with a granular surface, formed by an aggregation of contiguous plantar warts. **necrogenic w.,** tuberculosis verrucosa cutis. **peruvian w.,** see bartonellosis. **pitch w's,** precancerous, keratotic, epidermal tumors occurring in individuals who work in gas, tar, pitch, or various oils derived from coal. **plane w.,** verruca plana. **plantar w.,** verruca plantaris. **pointed w.,** condyloma acuminatum. **postmortem w., prosector's w.,** tuberculosis verrucosa cutis. **seborrheic w.,** seborrheic keratosis. **seed w.,** verruca or common wart; so called because of the minute black specks or "seeds" within it, which are actually thrombosed elongated capillary loops extending up into the substance of the wart. **soot w.,** chimney-sweeps' cancer. **telangiectatic w.,** a misnomer for the verrucous papule of angiokeratoma. **tuberculous w.,** tuberculosis verrucosa cutis. **venereal w.,** condyloma acuminatum.

Wartenberg's disease, etc. (wor′ten-bergz) [Robert *Wartenberg,* American neurologist, 1887–1956] see under *disease, sign,* and *symptom.*

wash (wosh) a solution used for cleansing or bathing a part, as an eye or the mouth. **eye w.,** collyrium. **mouth w.,** see mouthwash.

wasp (wosp) [L. *vespa*] any stinging hymenopterous insect of the family Vespidae, of which the genus *Vespa* is the type. Its venom contains histamine, 5-hydroxytryptamine, etc.

wasserhelle (vos′er-hel″lĕ) [Ger. "water-clear"] see water-clear cells, under *cell.*

Wassermann test (reaction) (wos′er-man) [August Paul von *Wassermann,* bacteriologist in Berlin, 1866–1925] see under *test.*

Wassermann-fast (wos′er-man fast″) showing a persistent positive Wassermann reaction despite antisyphilitic treatment.

waste (wāst) 1. gradual loss, decay, or diminution of bulk. 2. useless and effete material, unfit for further use within the organism. 3. to pine away or dwindle. **phonetic w. of the breath,** a too rapid expiratory act, due to paralysis of a lateral cricoarytenoid muscle.

water (wah′ter) 1. a tasteless, odorless, colorless liquid, $(H_2O)_n$, used as the standard of specific gravity and of specific heat. It freezes at 32° F. (0° C.) and boils at 212° F. (100° C.). It is present in all organic tissues and in many other substances, and is the most universal of the solvents. 2. aromatic water. 3. purified water. **ammonia w.,** diluted ammonia solution. **ammonia w., stronger,** strong ammonia solution. **aromatic w.,** a solution, usually saturated, of a volatile oil or other aromatic or volatile substance in purified water, prepared by distillation or solution; called also *aqua aromatica.* **bound w.,** water in the tissues of the body bound to macromolecules or organelles. **capillary w.,** the water contained in the soil above the water table of the ground water. **carbon dioxide-free w.,** purified water which has been boiled vigorously for 5 minutes or more and protected from absorption of carbon dioxide from the atmosphere while it is cooling. **chlorine w.,** a saturated solution of chlorine in water. **cinnamon w.,** a clear, saturated solution of cinnamon oil in purified water, used as a flavored vehicle in pharmaceutical preparations; called also *aqua cinnamomi.* **w. of combustion,** metabolic w. **w. of crystallization,** that which is an ingredient of many salts, forming a structural part of the crystal. **distilled w.,** water which has been purified by distillation; called also *aqua distillata.* **egg w.,** 1. water that has bathed eggs of various invertebrates and acquired one or another substance detectable by a physiological reaction; e.g., oyster egg water may stimulate spawning of male oysters. 2. water containing fertilizin exuded from the ripe eggs of sea urchins and other aquatic animals, by which the spermatozoa are agglutinated.　**free w.,** that portion of the water in body tissues which is not bound by macromolecules or organelles.　**Goulard's w.,** diluted lead subacetate solution.　**ground w.,** the water which lies in the depth of soils, being carried along underground over impervious strata.　**hamamelis w.,** an astringent solution prepared by maceration in water of cut dormant twigs of *Hamamelis virginiana*; called also *aqua hamamelidis* and *witch-hazel water*.　**hard w.,** water that contains salts of calcium or magnesium, which resist the action of soap, so that it does not readily form lather.　**heavy w.,** a compound analogous to water, but containing deuterium, the mass two isotope of hydrogen, the formula being D_2O or ^2H_2O. It differs from ordinary water in having a higher freezing point (3.8° C.) and boiling point (101.4° C.), and in the fact that it is incapable of supporting life. It is the stable isotope used as a moderator in nuclear reactors. Called also *deuterium oxide*.　**w. for injection** [USP], water for parenteral use, prepared by distillation, and meeting certain standards as to sterility and clarity.　**w. for injection, bacteriostatic** [USP], sterile water for injection, containing one or more suitable antimicrobial agents.　**w. for injection, sterile** [USP], water for injection that has been sterilized and suitably packaged.　**lead w.,** diluted lead subacetate solution.　**lime w.,** calcium hydroxide solution.　**metabolic w.,** water in the body derived from metabolism of a food element such as starch, glucose, or fat; called also *w. of combustion*.　**mineral w.,** water containing mineral salts in solution in sufficient quantity to give it special properties and taste.　**orange flower w.** [NF], a saturated solution of the odoriferous principles of the flowers of *Citrus aurantium* Linné, used as a vehicle, flavor, and perfume in pharmaceutical preparations; called also *aqua aurantii florum*.　**peppermint w.** [NF], a clear, saturated solution of peppermint oil in purified water; used as a vehicle in pharmaceutical preparations; called also *aqua menthae piperitae*.　**potable w.,** water that is suitable for drinking purposes.　**purified w.** [USP], water obtained by distillation or de-ionization, used for pharmaceutical or other purposes requiring mineral-free water.　**rose w.,** a solution prepared by diluting stronger rose water with an equal volume of purified water; used as a perfuming agent in pharmaceutical preparations.　**rose w., stronger** [NF], a saturated solution of the odoriferous principles of the flowers of *Rosa centifolia* Linné, used as a perfuming agent in pharmaceutical preparations; called also *aqua rosae fortior*.　**saline w.,** water which contains neutral salts.　**soft w.,** water that contains little or no mineral matter.　**witch-hazel w.,** hamamelis w.

water-borne (wah′ter-born″)　conveyed or spread by water, as an infectious disease; see under *infection*.

water brash (wah′ter brash′)　heartburn with regurgitation of sour fluid or almost tasteless saliva into the mouth.

Waterhouse-Friderichsen syndrome (wah′ter-hous frid″er-ik′sen) [Rupert *Waterhouse*, British physician, 1873–1958; Carl *Friderichsen*, Danish physician, born 1886]　see under *syndrome*.

watermelon (wah″ter-mel′on)　the edible fruit of the plant *Citrullus vulgaris* (Curcurbitaceae), whose seeds are the source of cucurbitol and cucurbocitrin.

waters (wah′terz)　a popular name for the amniotic fluid.

watershed (wah′ter-shed)　a ridge which directs drainage toward either side.　**abdominal w's,** the ridges formed in the supine position by the forward projection of the lumbar vertebrae and the projecting brim of the pelvis, causing free effusions to gravitate into the lumbar fossae and pelvis.

Watkins' operation (wot′kinz) [Thomas James *Watkins*, gynecologist in Chicago, 1863–1925]　see under *operation*.

Watson (wot′son), James Dewey.　American biochemist, born 1928; co-winner, with Maurice Hugh Frederick Wilkins and Francis Harry Compton Crick, of the Nobel prize for medicine or physiology in 1962 for the discovery of the molecular structure of nuclear acids and its significance for information transfer in living material.

Watson-Crick helix (wat′son-krik) [James Dewey *Watson*; Francis Harry Compton *Crick*]　see under *helix*.

Watson-Schwartz test (wot′son-shwarts) [Cecil James

Watson, American physician, born 1901; Samuel *Schwartz*, American physician, born 1916]　see under *tests*.

Watsonius watsoni (wot-so′ne-us wot-so′ni) [Malcolm *Watson*, British physician, 1873–1955]　a pear-shaped amphistome trematode found in the intestines of man and monkeys in Africa; called also *Amphistoma watsoni*.

watt (wot) [after James *Watt*, 1736–1819]　a unit of electric power, being the work done at the rate of 1 joule per second. It is equivalent to a current of 1 ampere under a pressure of 1 volt.

wattage (wot′ij)　the power output or consumption of an electrical device expressed in watts.

watt-hour (wot′our)　a unit of electrical work or energy, equal to the wattage multiplied by the time in hours.

wattmeter (wot′me-ter)　an instrument for measuring electric activity in watts.

wave (wāv)　a uniformly advancing disturbance in which the parts moved undergo a double oscillation; any wavelike pattern.　**a w.,** see *phlebogram*.　**alpha w's,** brain waves in the electroencephalogram which have a frequency of 8 to 13 per second; they are typical of the normal person awake and in a quiet resting state, and occur principally in the occipital region.　**anacrotic w., anadicrotic w.,** see under *pulse*.　**beta w's,** brain waves in the electroencephalogram, which have a frequency of 18 to 30 per second; they are typical during periods of intense activity of the nervous system, and occur principally in the parietal and frontal regions.　**brain w's,** the fluctuations of electrical potential in the brain, as recorded by electroencephalography. See *alpha*, *beta*, *delta*, and *theta w's*. Some observers distinguish three types of waves: (1) *trains*, which correspond to alpha waves; (2) *spindles*, short series with a frequency of 14 per second; and (3) *random w's*, irregular changes of potential with no fixed frequency which appear at the beginning of sleep.　**c w.,** see *phlebogram*.　**catacrotic w., catadicrotic w.,** see under *pulse*.　**contraction w.,** the wave of progression of the contraction in a muscle from the point of stimulation; also the graphic representation of a contracting muscle.　**delta w's,** 1. waves in the electroencephalogram which have a frequency below 3½ per second; they are typical in deep sleep, in infancy, and in serious brain disorders. 2. an early QRS vector in the electrocardiogram characteristic of Wolff-Parkinson-White syndrome.　**dicrotic w.,** 1. the second portion of the arterial pulse or arterial pressure recording after the dicrotic notch and aortic valve closure. 2. recoil wave.　**electroencephalographic w's,** see *brain w's*.　**electromagnetic w's,** the entire series of ethereal waves which are similar in character, and which move with the velocity of light, but which vary enormously in wavelength. The unbroken series is known from the hertzian waves used in radio transmission which may be miles in length (one mile equals 1.6×10^5 cm.) through heat and light, the ultraviolet, roentgen rays, and the gamma rays of radium to the cosmic rays, the wavelength of which may be as short as 0.0004 of an Angström unit (4×10^{-12} cm.).　**Erb's w's,** undulations in a muscle stimulated by a moderately powerful constant current; sometimes seen in myotonia congenita.　**excitation w.,** an electric wave flowing from a muscle just previous to its contraction.　**F w's,** a series of rapid minute waves in the venous pulse in atrial flutter.　**fibrillary w's,** small irregular deflections in the electrocardiogram in atrial fibrillation.　**h w.,** see *phlebogram*.　**hertzian w's,** electromagnetic waves resembling light waves, but having greater wavelength; they are used in wireless telegraphy.　**Liesegang's w's,** see under *phenomenon*.　**light w's,** the electromagnetic waves that produce sensations in the retina; see *light*.　**longitudinal w.,** one in which the oscillatory motion is parallel to the direction of propagation of the wave.　**P w.,** a deflection in the electrocardiogram produced by excitation of the atria; see *electrocardiogram*.　**papillary w., percussion w.,** the chief ascending portion of a sphygmographic tracing.　**phrenic w.,** see *diaphragm phenomenon*, under *phenomenon*.　**pulse w.,** the elevation of the pulse felt by the finger or shown graphically in a recording of pulse or pressure.　**Q w.,** in the QRS complex, the initial downward (negative) deflection, related to the initial phase of depolarization (excitation) of the ventricular myocardium; see *electrocardiogram*.　**R w.,** the initial upward deflection of the QRS complex, following the Q wave in the normal electrocardiogram. See *electrocardiogram*.　**radio w's,** electromagnetic radiation of wavelength between 10^{-1} and 10^6 cm. and frequency of about 10^{11} to 10^4 cps. **random w's,** see *brain w's.* **recoil w.,** the second of the two principal waves of a dicrotic pulse, attributed to the reflected impulse of the closure of the aortic valves. **S w.,** a downward deflection of the QRS complex following the R wave in the normal electrocardiogram. See *electrocardiogram.* **short w.,** a wave having a wavelength of 60 meters or less. **sine w.,** the wave form of an alternating current characterized by a rise from zero to maximum positive potential, descending back through zero to its maximum negative value, and then rising back to zero. **sonic w's,** audible sound waves. **stimulus w.,** the wave which passes along a muscle as a result of a stimulus applied at a certain point. **supersonic w's,** a term applied to waves similar to ordinary sound waves but of frequencies from 200,000 to 1,500,000 cycles per second; they are highly destructive to some organisms and some chemical substances. **T w.,** the second major deflection of the normal electrocardiogram, reflecting the potential variations occurring with repolarization of the ventricles; see *electrocardiogram.* **theta w's,** brain waves in the electroencephalogram which have a frequency of 4 to 7 per second; they occur mainly in children but also in adults during periods of emotional stress. **tidal w.,** the sphygmographic wave next after the percussion wave; the second elevation of the sphygmographic tracing between the percussion wave and the dicrotic elevation. **transverse w.,** one in which the oscillatory motion is perpendicular to the direction of propagation of the wave. **Traube-Hering w's,** rhythmical rises and falls in the arterial pressure, attributed to rhythmical activity of the vasoconstrictor center. **tricrotic w.,** a third wave in the sphygmographic curve in addition to the tidal and dicrotic waves, occurring during systole. **U w.,** see *electrocardiogram.* **ultrashort w.,** an electromagnetic wave of wavelength of less than 10 meters; called also *microwave.* **ultrasonic w's,** waves similar to sound waves but of such high frequency that the human ear does not perceive them as sound; see *ultrasonics.* **v w.,** see *phlebogram.* **ventricular w.,** the part of the tracing of the venous pulse occurring during ventricular systole. **x w.,** see *phlebogram.* **y w.,** see *phlebogram.*

wavelength (wāv'length) the distance between the top of one wave and the identical phase of the succeeding one. **effective w., equivalent w.,** in radiology, the wavelength of monochromatic x-rays which would undergo the same percentage attenuation in a specified absorber as the heterogeneous beam under consideration. **minimum w.,** the shortest wavelength in an x-ray spectrum.

wax (waks) [L. *cera*] a plastic substance deposited by insects or obtained from plants. Waxes are esters of various fatty acids with higher, usually monohydric alcohols. The wax of pharmacy is principally yellow wax (beeswax), the material of which honeycomb is made. It consists chiefly of cerotic acid and myricin and is used in making ointments, cerates, etc. When yellow wax is bleached it becomes white (*white w.*). **baseplate w.,** a dental wax containing about 75% paraffin or ceresin with additions of beeswax and other waxes and resins; used chiefly to establish the initial arch form in making trial plates for the construction of complete dentures. Called also *try-in w.* **blockout w.,** a dental wax used as a blockout (q.v.) material to eliminate undercuts on master casts prior to duplication. **bone w.,** a waxy substance used for packing small bone cavities, as in bones of the skull, and for controlling bleeding from them. **boxing w.,** a dental wax used for boxing (q.v.) impressions in the fabrication of restorations and appliances. **candelilla w.,** a wax obtained from the plant *Euphorbia antisyphilitica* Zucc. (Euphorbiaceae), and used as a substitute for beeswax. **carding w.,** dental wax used as a base for mounting artificial teeth, organized by standard sizes, shades, and so forth. **carnauba w.** [NF], a wax obtained from the leaves of *Copernic'ia cerif'era* Mart., a palm of South America; used as a tablet coating agent. **casting w.,** a mixture of several dental waxes; used for making patterns to determine the shape of the metallic framework and other parts of removable partial dentures. **cetyl esters w.** [NF], a mixture consisting primarily of esters of saturated fatty alcohols and saturated fatty acids; used as a stiffening agent in pharmaceutical preparations. Called also *synthetic spermaceti.* **Chinese w.,** a hard white wax deposited by certain insects on trees, such as the Chinese ash, *Fraxinus chinensis;* also a similar wax from the plant *Ligustrum madra.* **dental**

w., a mixture of two or more natural and synthetic waxes, resins, coloring agents, and other additives; used for pattern making for casting purposes and in the construction of nonmetallic denture bases, for registering jaw relations, and as aids in laboratory work. **dental inlay casting w.,** a wax used to make a pattern for an inlay (wax pattern), usually containing paraffin, carnauba, ceresin, and candelilla waxes, beeswax, and gum dammar; synthetic waxes are sometimes used to replace the carnauba wax. Called also *inlay casting w.* and *inlay pattern w.* **ear w.,** cerumen. **emulsifying w.** [NF], a waxy solid prepared from cetostearyl alcohol, containing a polyoxyethylene derivative of a fatty acid ester of sorbitan; used as an emulsifying and stiffening agent in pharmaceutical preparations. **grave w.,** adipocere. **Horsley's w.,** a bone wax composed of wax, petrolatum, and phenol. **inlay casting w., inlay pattern w.,** dental inlay casting w. **Japan w.,** a fat from the fruit of *Myri'ca cerif'era* L. (Myricaceae) and other species of the same genus. **palm w.,** 1. carnauba wax. 2. a wax from *Ceroxylon andicola,* a South American palm. **set-up w.,** a dental wax used in laboratories to align artificial teeth in dentures. **sticky w.,** adhesive w. **try-in w.,** baseplate w. **tubercle bacillus w.,** a high-molecular-weight phosphatidic glycolipid extracted from the cell walls of *Mycobacterium tuberculosis,* made up of arabinoglycans and mycolic and muramic acids. It is used as an adjuvant to enhance the immunogenicity of tuberculin preparations. Called also *w. D.* **utility w.,** a soft, pliable, adhesive dental wax used for various purposes in the laboratory, such as to give the desired contour to a perforated tray to be used with hydrocolloids. **vegetable w.,** a waxy substance, resembling beeswax, derived from various vegetable sources. **white w.** [NF], the bleached, purified wax from the honeycomb of the bee, *Apis mellifera,* used as an ingredient in several ointments. **yellow w.** [NF], the purified wax from the honeycomb of the bee *Apis mellifera;* used as a stiffening agent in pharmaceutical preparations and as an ingredient of yellow ointment. It was formerly used internally, in the treatment of diarrhea. Called also *beeswax* and *cera flava.*

waxing (wak'sing) the contouring of a wax pattern or the wax base of a trial denture into the desired shape. Called also *waxing up.*

waxing up (wak'sing up) waxing.

Wb weber.

W.B.C. white blood cell; white blood [cell] count (see *blood count,* under *count*).

wean (wēn) to discontinue the breast feeding of an infant, with substitution of other feeding habits.

weanling (wēn'ling) 1. newly changed to nourishment other than breast feeding. 2. an animal newly changed to other forms of nourishment than breast feeding.

web (web) a tissue or membrane. **esophageal w.,** a fibrous, weblike, circumferential fold of the mucous membrane of the esophagus. The term is sometimes used interchangeably with *esophageal ring.* **laryngeal w.,** the most common congenital malformation of the larynx, it may be a thin, translucent diaphragm or thicker and more fibrotic; it is spread between the vocal folds near the anterior commissure and may cause obstruction, hoarseness, aphonia, etc. **subsynaptic w.,** a system of filaments or fine canaliculi which have been observed to penetrate at a varying distance into the postsynaptic cell. **terminal w.,** a feltwork of fine filaments in the cytoplasm immediately beneath the free surface of certain epithelial cells, especially those with a brush border of microvilli, such as the absorptive cells of the intestines and the hair cells of the inner ear; it is thought to have a supportive or cytoskeletal function.

webbed (webd) connected by a membrane.

weber (web'er) a unit of magnetic flux which, linking a circuit of one turn, produces in it an electromotive force of one volt as it is reduced to zero at a uniform rate in one second. In SI, it replaces the maxwell. Abbreviated Wb.

Weber's corpuscle (organ), glands, zone (va'berz) [Moritz Ignatz *Weber,* German anatomist, 1795–1875] see under *gland,* and see *utriculus prostaticus* and *zona orbicularis articulationis coxae.*

Weber's disease (web'erz) [Frederick Parkes *Weber,* British physician, 1863–1962] Sturge-Weber syndrome.

Weber's law, paradox, test (va'berz) [Ernest Heinrich

Weber, German anatomist and physiologist, 1795–1878] see under *law*, *paradox*, and *tests* (def. 2 and 3).

Weber's sign (symptom), syndrome (paralysis) (web′erz) [Sir Hermann David *Weber*, London physician, 1823–1918]   see under *sign* and *syndrome*.

Weber's test (va′berz) [Friedrich Eugen *Weber*, German otologist, 1832–1891]   see under *tests*, def. 1.

Weber-Christian disease, panniculitis, syndrome (web′er-kris′chan) [F. P. *Weber*; Henry Asbury *Christian*, American physician, 1876–1951]   relapsing febrile nodular nonsuppurative panniculitis.

Weber-Cockayne syndrome (web′er kok′ān) [F.P. *Weber*; Edward Alfred *Cockayne*, English physician, 1880–1956] localized epidermolysis bullosa.

Weber-Fechner law (va′ber-fek′ner) [Ernest Heinrich *Weber*; Gustav Theodor *Fechner*, Prussian natural philosopher, 1801– 1887]   see under *law*.

Webster's operation (web′sterz) [John Clarence *Webster*, American gynecologist, 1863–1950]   see under *operation*.

Webster's test (web′sterz) [John *Webster*, London chemist, 1878–1927]   see under *tests*.

wedge (wej) [A.S. *wecg*]   a piece of material thick at one end and tapering to a thin edge at the other end.   **step w.**, penetrometer; a block of an absorber, usually aluminum, machined in steps of increasing thickness, used to measure the penetrability of roentgen rays.

WEE   western equine encephalomyelitis.

Weeks' bacillus (wēks) [John Elmer *Weeks*, New York ophthalmologist, 1853–1949]   *Hemophilus aegyptius*.

weep (wēp)   1. to shed tears. Called also *cry*.   2. to ooze serum.

Wegener's granulomatosis (veg′ĕ-nerz) [F. *Wegener*, German pathologist, 20th century]   see under *granulomatosis*.

Wegner's disease, sign (veg′nerz) [Friedrich Rudolf Georg *Wegner*, German pathologist, 1843–1917]   see under *disease* and *sign*.

wehnelt (va′nelt)   the unit of hardness or penetrating ability of roentgen rays. Abbreviated W.

Weichardt's antikenotoxin (vi′karts) [Wolfgang *Weichardt*, German pathologist, 1875–1945]   see *antikenotoxin*.

Weichbrodt's reaction, test (vīk′brōts) [Raphael *Weichbrodt*, Frankfurt neurologist, born 1886]   see under *reaction* and *tests*.

Weichselbaum's diplococcus (vīk′sel-bawm″) [Anton *Weichselbaum*, Austrian pathologist, 1845–1920]   *Neisseria meningitidis*.

Weidel's test (vi′delz) [Hugo *Weidel*, Austrian chemist, 1849–1899]   see under *tests*.

Weigert's law, stain (method) (vi′gerts) [Karl *Weigert*, German pathologist, 1845–1904]   see under *law*, and *Table of Stains*.

weight (wāt)   heaviness; the degree to which a body is drawn toward the earth by gravity. See tables of weights and measures (Appendix 3).   **apothecaries′ w.**, a system of weights used in compounding prescriptions based on the grain (equivalent 64.8 mg.). Its units are the scruple (20 grains), dram (3 scruples), ounce (8 drams), and pound (12 ounces).   **atomic w.**, the weight of an atom of a substance as compared with the weight of an atom of carbon-12 isotope, which is taken as 12.00000; see also *mass*. Abbreviated At. wt.   **avoirdupois w.**, the system of weight commonly used for ordinary commodities in English-speaking countries; its units are the dram (27.344 grains), ounce (16 drams), and pound (16 ounces).   **combining w.**, the relative weight, compared with that of hydrogen (which is considered as 1), of an element that enters into combination with other elements.   **equivalent w.**, the weight in grams of a substance which is equivalent in a chemical reaction to 1.008 gm. of hydrogen.   **gram molecular w.**, a quantity of a substance which has a weight in grams numerically equivalent to its molecular weight. See *mole*, def. 3.   **molecular w.**, the weight of a molecule of a substance as compared with that of an atom of carbon-12; it is equal to the sum of the atomic weights of its constituent atoms. Abbreviated Mol. wt.   **troy w.**, a system of weights used by jewelers for gold and precious stones.

weights and measures   see *Tables of Weights and Measures*.

Weil's basal layer (zone) (vīlz) [L. A. *Weil*, German dentist, 1849–1895]   see under *layer*.

Weil's stain (wīlz) [Arthur *Weil*, American neuropathologist, born 1887]   see *Table of Stains*.

Weil's syndrome (disease) (vīlz) [Adolf *Weil*, physician in Wiesbaden, 1848–1916]   see under *syndrome*.

Weil-Felix reaction (test) (vīl-fa′liks) [Edmund *Weil*, German physician in Prague, 1880–1922; Arthur *Felix*, Prague bacteriologist, 1887–1956]   see under *reaction*.

Weill's sign (vēlz) [Edmond *Weill*, French pediatrician, 1858–1924]   see under *sign*.

Weinmannia (wīn-man′e-ah)   a genus of saxifragaceous plants with an astringent medicinal bark.

Weir Mitchell treatment (wēr-mich′el)   see *Mitchell*, and under *treatment*.

Weisbach's angle (vīs′bahks) [Albin *Weisbach*, Austrian anthropologist, 1837–1914]   see under *angle*.

Weismann's theory (vīs′manz) [August Friedrich Leopold *Weismann*, German biologist, 1834–1914]   weismannism.

weismannism (wīs′man-izm) [named for August *Weismann*]   the doctrine of the noninheritance of acquired characters.

Weiss′ reflex (vīs′) [Leopold *Weiss*, Austrian oculist, 1848–1901]   see under *reflex*.

Weiss′ sign (vīs′) [Nathan *Weiss*, physician in Vienna, 1851–1883]   Chvostek's sign.

Weiss′ test (vīs′) [Moriz *Weiss*, Vienna physician]   see under *tests*.

Weitbrecht's cord (ligament), foramen (vīt′brekts) [Josias *Weitbrecht*, German anatomist in Petrograd, 1702–1747]   see *chorda obliqua membranae interosseae antebrachii*, and see under *foramen*.

Welch's bacillus (welch′ez) [William Henry *Welch*, pathologist in Baltimore, 1850–1934]   *Clostridium perfringens*.

Welcker's method (vel′kerz) [Hermann *Welcker*, German physician, 1822–1897]   see under *method*.

Weller (wel′er), Thomas Huckle.   American physician and parasitologist, born 1915; co-winner, with John Franklin Enders and Frederick Chapman Robbins, of the Nobel prize for medicine or physiology in 1954 for the discovery that viruses (specifically, poliomyelitis viruses) can be grown in tissue culture and thereby isolated and studied, making possible the production of vaccines.

welt (welt)   wheal.

wen (wen)   1. epidermal cyst.   2. pilar cyst.

Wenckebach's disease, period (ven′kĕ-bahks) [Karel Frederik *Wenckebach*, Dutch internist in Vienna, 1864–1940]   see *cardioptosis*, and see under *period*.

Wender's test (ven′derz) [Neumann *Wender*, Austrian chemist]   see under *tests*.

Wenzell's test (wen′zelz) [William Theodore *Wenzell*, American physician, 1829–1913]   see under *tests*.

Werdnig-Hoffmann paralysis (atrophy, disease, syndrome, type) (verd′nig-hof′man) [Guido *Werdnig*, Austrian neurologist; Johann *Hoffmann*, German neurologist, 1857–1919]   see under *paralysis*.

Werlhof's disease (verl′hofs) [Paul Gottlieb *Werlhof*, German physician, 1699–1767]   idiopathic thrombocytopenic purpura.

Werner's syndrome (ver′nerz) [Otto *Werner*, German physician, born 1879]   see under *syndrome*.

Werner-His disease (ver′ner-his′) [Heinrich *Werner*, German physician, 1874–1946; Wilhelm *His*, Jr., German physician, 1863–1934]   trench fever.

Wernicke's encephalopathy (disease, syndrome), etc. (ver′nĭ-kez) [Karl *Wernicke*, German neurologist, 1848–1905]   see under *aphasia*, *area*, *dementia*, *encephalopathy*, *fissure*, and *triangle* and see *hemiopic pupillary reaction*, under *reaction*.

Wernicke-Korsakoff syndrome (ver′nĭ-kĕ kor-sak′of) [Karl *Wernicke*; Sergei Sergeivich *Korsakoff*, Russian neurologist, 1854–1900]   see under *syndrome*.

Wernicke-Mann hemiplegia (type) (ver′nĭ-kĕ-mahn) [Karl *Wernicke*; Ludwig *Mann*, German neurologist, 1866–1936]   see under *hemiplegia*.

Wertheim's operation (vert′himz) [Ernst *Wertheim*, gynecologist in Vienna, 1864–1920]   see under *operation*.

Westberg's space (vest′bergz) [Friedrich *Westberg*, German physician of the 19th century]   see under *space*.

Westergren method (west′er-gren) [Alf *Westergren*, Swedish physician, born 1891]   see under *method*.

Westermark's sign (ves′ter-mark) [N. *Westermark*, Swedish radiologist]   see under *sign*.

Westphal's nucleus, sign (phenomenon, symptom) (vest′fahls) [Carl Friedrich Otto *Westphal*, German neurologist, 1833–1890]   see under *sign*, and see *nucleus accessorius*.

Westphal's phenomenon, pupillary reflex (vest′fahlz) [Alexander Karl Otto *Westphal*, Austrian neurologist, 1863–1941]   orbicularis pupillary reflex.

Westphal-Piltz phenomenon, reflex (vest′fahl-pilts′) [A. K. O. *Westphal*; Jan *Piltz*, Austrian neurologist, 1871–1930]   orbicularis pupillary reflex.

Westphal-Strümpell disease, pseudosclerosis (vest′-fahl-strim′p'l) [C. F. O. *Westphal*; Ernst Adolf Gustav Gottfried von *Strümpell*, physician in Leipzig, 1853–1925]   Wilson's disease.

wet-nurse (wet′nurs)   a woman who nurses the child of another at her own breast.

wetpox (wet′poks)   a disease resembling fowlpox, with lesions occurring in the mouth and frequently causing death by suffocation.

wet-scald (wet′skahld)   eczema in sheep.

Wetzel's grid (wet′selz) [Norman Carl *Wetzel*, Cleveland pediatrician, born 1897]   see under *grid*.

Wetzel's test (vet′selz) [Georg *Wetzel*, German anatomist, 1871–1951]   see under *tests*.

Weyl's test (vīlz) [Theodor *Weyl*, German chemist 1851–1913]   see under *tests*.

Wharton's duct, jelly (gelatin) (hwar′tunz) [Thomas *Wharton*, English physician and anatomist, 1614–1673]   see *ductus submandibularis*, and see under *jelly*.

wheal (hwēl, wēl)   a smooth, slightly elevated area on the body surface, which is redder or paler than the surrounding skin; it is often attended with severe itching, and is usually evanescent, changing its size or shape, or disappearing, within a few hours. It is the typical lesion of urticaria, the dermal evidence of allergy, and in sensitive persons may be provoked by mechanical irritation of the skin. Called also *hive* and *welt*.

wheat (hwēt)   the plant *Triticum vulgare* and its cereal grain. The grain is a source of energy and of protein which is of lower biological value than animal protein; the bran and germ of the grain contain iron, phosphorus, and vitamins of the B complex, which are lost when wheat is highly milled.

wheel (wēl) [A.S. *hwēol*]   1. a circular frame or disk designed to revolve around a central axis.   2. any of various round, engine-driven cutting or polishing dental instruments that may be of uniform thickness or knife-edge.   **rag w.,** a dental disk made up of several layers of cloth stitched together and wetted down with pumice; used to polish dentures. Called also *cloth disk*.

wheeze (hwēz)   a whistling sound made in breathing.   **asthmatoid w.,** a sound similar to the wheezing heard when the ear is placed close to the mouth of an asthmatic; heard in cases of foreign body in the trachea or bronchus. Called also *Jackson's sign*.

whelp (hwelp)   1. an unweaned puppy.   2. to give birth to; said of the female dog.

whey (hwa)   the thin serum of milk remaining after the curd and cream have been removed.   **alum w.,** a whey prepared by boiling milk with a piece of alum and removing the curd by straining.   **wine w.,** a preparation of milk coagulated with white wine, strained from the curd, and sweetened with sugar.

whiplash (hwip′lash)   a popular term for an acute cervical sprain; acceleration extension injury of the cervical spine.

Whipple (hwip′el)   George Hoyt. American pathologist, 1878–1976; co-winner, with George R. Minot and William P. Murphy, of the Nobel prize for medicine or physiology in 1934 for their research into the therapeutic value of liver in cases of pernicious anemia and in the regeneration of hemoglobin.

Whipple's disease, tests (hwip′elz) [George Hoyt *Whipple*]   see *intestinal lipodystrophy*, under *lipodystrophy*, and see under *tests*.

Whipple's operation, triad (hwip′elz) [Allen O. *Whipple*, American surgeon, 1881–1963]   see under *operation and triad*.

whipworm (hwip′werm)   *Trichuris trichiura*.

whisper (hwis′per)   a soft, low, sibilant breathing sound produced by the unvoiced passage of the breath through the glottis.

White (hwīt), Charles (1728–1813).   English surgeon and obstetrician, whose *Treatise on the Management of Pregnant and Lying-in Women* (1773) antedated the work of Semmelweis in its appeal for surgical cleanliness to combat puerperal fever.

white (hwīt) [A.S. *hwīt*]   reflecting all the rays of the spectrum; the opposite of black.   **Spanish w.,** bismuth subnitrate.   **visual w.,** exhausted or decolorized rhodopsin; called also *leukopsin*.

White's operation (hwīts) [J. William *White*, Philadelphia surgeon, 1850–1916]   see under *operation*.

whitecomb (hwīt′kōm)   favus of fowl.

Whitehead's operation (hwīt′hedz) [Walter *Whitehead*, English surgeon, 1840–1913]   see under *operation*.

whitehead (hwīt′hed)   milium.

Whitehorn's method (hwīt′hornz) [John Clare *Whitehorn*, American biochemist, born 1894]   see under *method*.

whiteleg (hwīt′leg)   phlegmasia alba dolens.

whitepox (hwīt′poks)   variola minor.

Whitfield's ointment (hwit′fēldz) [Arthur *Whitfield*, British dermatologist, 1868–1946]   benzoic and salicylic acid ointment.

whitlow (hwit′lo)   a felon.   **herpetic w.,** a primary herpes simplex infection of the terminal segment of a finger, usually occurring in persons exposed to infected oral or respiratory secretions (such as dentists, physicians, nurses). It begins with intense itching and pain, followed by the formation of deep coalescing vesicles. The process is associated with much tissue destruction and may be accompanied by systemic symptoms. A similar lesion may occur as a result of nail biting during the course of primary herpetic gingivostomatitis. Called also *herpetic paronychia*.   **melanotic w.,** see *acral-lentiginous melanoma*, under *melanoma*.   **thecal w.,** suppurative tenosynovitis of the terminal phalanx of a finger.

Whitman's operation (hwit′mahnz) [Royal *Whitman*, New York orthopedic surgeon, 1857–1946]   see under *operation*.

Whitmore's bacillus, disease (fever) (hwit′mōrz) [Major Alfred *Whitmore*, of the Indian Medical Service]   see *Pseudomonas pseudomallei* and *melioidosis*.

W.H.O.   World Health Organization, an international agency associated with the United Nations and based in Geneva.

whoop (hoōp)   the sonorous and convulsive inspiration of pertussis (whooping cough).

whooping cough (hoōp′ing kawf)   pertussis.

whorl (hwerl)   a spiral turn or twist, such as one of the turns of the cochlea of the ear, the arrangement of muscle fibers in the heart (*vortex*), or a spiral arrangement of the ridges apparent in a finger print.   **bone w.,** an enostosis.

Whytt's disease (hwits) [Robert *Whytt*, Scottish physician, 1714–1766]   see under *disease*.

Wichmann's asthma (vik′mahnz) [Johann Ernst *Wichmann*, German physician, 1740–1802]   laryngismus stridulus.

Wickersheimer's fluid (medium) (vik′er-shi″merz) [J. *Wickersheimer*, anatomist in Berlin, 1832–1896]   see under *fluid*.

Wickham's striae (wik′amz) [Louis-Frédéric *Wickham*, Paris dermatologist, 1861–1913]   see under *stria*.

Widal's syndrome, test (reaction, serum test) (ve-dahz′) [Georges Fernand Isidore *Widal*, French physician, 1862–1929]   see *icteroanemia*, and see under *tests*.

Widal-Abrami disease (ve-dahl′-ah-brahm′e) [G. F. I. *Widal*; Pierre *Abrami*, French physician, 1879–1943]   acquired hemolytic anemia.

Wiesel (ve′z′l)   Tolsten Nils. Swedish physician residing in the United States, born 1924; co-winner, with David Hunter Hubel and Roger Wolcott Sperry, of the Nobel prize for medicine or physiology in 1981 for their research on information processing in the visual system.

Wigand's version (maneuver) (ve′gants) [Justus Heinrich *Wigand*, German gynecologist, 1769–1817]   see under *version*.

Wilbur-Addis test (wil′ber-ad′is) [Ray Lyman *Wilbur*, San Francisco physician, 1875–1949; Thomas *Addis*, San Francisco physician, 1881–1949]   Schneider's test, def. 2.

Wilcoxon's rank sum test, signed rank test (wil-kok′-sonz) [Frank *Wilcoxon*, American chemist and statistician, born 1892]   see *rank sum test* and *signed rank test*, under *tests*.

Wildbolz test (reaction) (vilt′bōlts) [Hans *Wildbolz*, Swiss urologist, 1873–1940]   autourine test.

Wilde's cords (wīldz) [Sir William Robert Wills *Wilde*, Irish surgeon, 1815–1876]   see *striae transversae corporis callosi*.

Wilder's diet (wīl′derz) [Russell Morse *Wilder*, Sr., American physician, 1885–1959]   see under *diet*.

Wilder's law of initial value (wīl′derz) [Joseph *Wilder*, neuropsychiatrist in New York, born 1895]   see under *law*.

Wilder's sign (wīl′derz) [William Hamlin *Wilder*, ophthalmologist in Chicago, 1860–1935]   see under *sign*.

Wildermuth's ear (vil′der-moots) [Hermann A. *Wildermuth*, alienist in Stuttgart, 1852–1907]   see under *ear*.

Wilkins (wil′kinz), Maurice Hugh Frederick.   British biochemist, born 1916; co-winner, with Francis Harry Compton Crick and James Dewey Watson, of the Nobel prize for medicine or physiology in 1962 for the discovery of the molecular structure of nuclear acids and its significance for information transfer in living material.

Willan's lepra (wil′anz) [Robert *Willan*, English physician, 1757–1812]   psoriasis.

Willebrand disease, factor (vil′ĕ-brahnt) [Erik Adolf von *Willebrand*, Finnish physician, 1870–1949]   von Willebrand disease, factor; see under *disease* and *factor*.

Willett forceps (clamp) (wil′et) [J. Abernethy *Willett*, London obstetrician, died 1932]   see under *forceps*.

Willia (wil′e-ah)   former name for *Hansenula*.

Williams' sign (tracheal tone) (wil′yamz) [Charles J. B. *Williams*, English physician, 1805–1889]   see under *sign*, def. 1.

Williams syndrome (wil′yamz) [J.C.P. *Williams*, New Zealand cardiologist, 20th century]   see under *syndrome*.

Williamson's blood test (wil′yam-sunz) [Richard Thomas *Williamson*, English physician, 1862–1937]   see under *tests*.

Williamson's sign (wil′yam-sunz) [Oliver K. *Williamson*, London physician, 1866–1941]   see under *sign*.

Willis' antrum, circle, cords, nerve, paracusis (wil′is) [Thomas *Willis*, English anatomist and physician, 1621–1675]   see *antrum pyloricum*, *circulus arteriosus cerebri*, and *nervus accessorius*, and see under *cord* and *paracusis*.

Wilms' tumor (vilmz) [Max *Wilms*, German surgeon, 1867–1918]   see under *tumor*.

Wilson's muscle (wil′sunz) [James *Wilson*, English surgeon, 1765–1821]   musculus sphincter urethrae.

wilt (wilt)   a disease of plants characterized by plugging of the conducting tissues by a fungus, resulting in wilting; potato wilt is caused by *Fusarium solanae*, banana wilt by *Fusarium oxysporum*, and apple wilt by species of *Verticillium*.

Wimshurst machine (wimz′hurst) [James *Wimshurst*, English engineer, 1832–1903]   see under *machine*.

Winckel's disease (ving′kelz) [Franz Karl Ludwig Wilhelm von *Winckel*, gynecologist in Munich, 1837–1911]   see under *disease*.

windburn (wind′burn)   chapping of the skin caused by excessive exposure to wind.

windchill (wind′chil)   loss of heat from bodies subjected to wind.

windgall (wind′gawl)   a distention of the joint capsule, or of a tendon sheath in the region of the fetlock of a horse.

windigo (wind′dĭ-go) [Ojibwa]   a cannibalistic monster of the mythology of Eskimos and certain American Indians; also, a culture-specific syndrome characterized by delusions of being possessed by the windigo, with fears of becoming cannibalistic, sometimes actual cannibalistic behavior, and agitated depression. Called also *witigo*.

windlass, Spanish (wind′las)   an improvised tourniquet consisting of a handkerchief tied around a part and twisted by a stick passed under it.

window (win′do) [L. *fenestra*]   a circumscribed opening in a plane surface. **aortic w.,** a transparent region below the aortic arch formed by the bifurcation of the trachea, visible in the left anterior oblique roentgenogram of the heart and adjacent vessels. **aorticopulmonary w.,** aortic septal defect. **oval w.,** fenestra vestibuli. **round w.,** fenestra cochleae. **skin w.,** see under *technique*.

windpipe (wind′pīp)   the trachea.

windpuff (wind′puf)   a swelling just below the fetlock joint of a horse, caused by a collection of synovial fluid between the tendons of the leg.

wind-sucking (wind′suk-ing)   cribbing.

wing (wing) [L. *ala*]   1. either of the paired anterior appendages of birds, which are modified for flight.   2. a structure or part resembling the wing of a bird; called also *ala*. **ash-like w.,** trigonum nervi vagi. **great w. of sphenoid bone, greater w. of sphenoid bone,** ala major ossis sphenoidalis. **w. of ilium,** ala ossis ilii. **w's of Ingrassias,** w's of sphenoid bone. **lateral w. of sacrum,** pars lateralis ossis sacri. **lateral w. of sphenoid bone,** ala major ossis sphenoidalis. **lesser w. of sphenoid bone,** ala minor ossis sphenoidalis. **major w. of sphenoid bone,** ala major ossis sphenoidalis. **minor w. of sphenoid bone,** ala minor ossis sphenoidalis. **w. of nose,** ala nasi. **orbital w. of sphenoid bone, small w. of sphenoid bone,** ala minor ossis sphenoidalis. **w's of sphenoid bone,** the laterally projecting processes of the sphenoid bone; see *ala major ossis sphenoidalis* and *ala minor ossis sphenoidalis*. **superior w. of sphenoid bone,** ala minor ossis sphenoidalis. **temporal w. of sphenoid bone,** ala major ossis sphenoidalis. **w. of vomer,** ala vomeris.

WinGel (win′jel)   trademark for a preparation of alumina and magnesia.

winking (wingk′ing) [A.S. *wincian*]   quick closing and opening of the eyelids, particularly of only one eye. **jaw w.,** involuntary closing movements of the eyelid occasionally associated with movements of the jaw; see *Gunn's syndrome*, under *syndrome*.

Winkler's disease (vink′lerz) [Max *Winkler*, Swiss physician, 1875–1952]   chondrodermatitis nodularis chronica helicis.

Winslow's foramen, etc. (winz′lōz) [Jacob Benignus *Winslow*, anatomist in Paris, 1669–1760]   see under *foramen, ligament, pancreas*, and *star*.

Winstrol (win′strol)   trademark for a preparation of stanozolol.

Winterbottom's sign (win′ter-bot″umz) [Thomas Masterman *Winterbottom*, English physician, 1765–1859]   see under *sign*.

wintergreen (win′ter-grēn)   *Gaultheria procumbens*.

Winternitz's sound (vin′ter-nits″ez) [Wilhelm *Winternitz*, physician in Vienna, 1835–1917]   see under *sound*.

Wintrich's sign (vin′triks) [Anton *Wintrich*, German physician, 1812–1882]   see under *sign*.

Wintrobe hematocrit, method (win′trōb) [Maxwell M. *Wintrobe*, American hematologist, born 1901]   see under *hematocrit* and *method*.

wire (wīr)   1. a long, slender, flexible structure of metal, used in surgery and dentistry.   2. to insert wires into a body structure, as into a broken bone to immobilize the fragments, or into an aneurysm to promote the formation of clots. **arch w.,** a wire attached to molar bands or an orthodontic appliance and applied around the dental arch to control and force tooth movement in orthodontic therapy. Called also *orthodontic w.* **arch w., ideal,** the configuration of an arch wire that conforms as closely as possible to the desired ultimate shape of the arch for a particular individual. **Kirschner w.,** a steel wire for skeletal fixation of fractured bones and for obtaining skeletal traction in fractures; it is inserted through the soft tissues and the bone. **ligature w.,** a soft thin wire used to tie an arch wire to band attachments or brackets in an orthodontic appliance. **orthodontic w.,** arch w. **separating w.,** a brass wire threaded between two teeth having tight contact in an effort to wedge them slightly apart before fitting a band in the application of an orthodontic appliance. **twin w.,** see under *appliance*.

wireworm (wīr'werm) *Haemonchus contortus.*

wiring (wīr'ing) the fixing into position by means of wire, as of segments of fractured bone. **circumferential w.,** a technique for fixation of mandibular fractures in which wires are passed around a section of bone with the ends exiting into the oral cavity and then around a fixed intraoral splint. **continuous loop w.,** wiring of the teeth for the reduction and fixation of fractures, by using a single length of wire to form wire loops on both the maxillary and mandibular teeth, over which intermaxillary elastics can be placed; called also *Stout w.* **craniofacial suspension w.,** wiring of noncontiguous areas of bone (piriform aperture, zygomatic arch, zygomatic process of the frontal bone) for the support of fractured jaw segments. **Gilmer w.,** a method of intermaxillary fixation in which single opposing teeth are wired circumferentially and the wires twisted together. **Ivy loop w.,** wiring of adjacent teeth in groups of two to provide an attachment for intermaxillary elastics. **perialveolar w.,** the fixing of a splint to the maxillary arch by passing a wire through the alveolar process from the buccal plate to the palate. **piriform aperture w.,** wiring through the nasal bones at the piriform aperture for the stabilization of fractures of the jaws. **Stout w.,** continuous loop w.

Wirsung's canal, duct (vēr'soongz) [Johann Georg *Wirsung*, German physician, 1600–1643] ductus pancreaticus.

Wishart test (wish'art) [Mary B. *Wishart*] see under *tests.*

Wiskott-Aldrich syndrome (vis'kot al'drich) [Alfred *Wiskott*, German pediatrician, born 1898; Robert Anderson *Aldrich*, American pediatrician, born 1917] see under *syndrome.*

withdrawal (with-draw'al) 1. a pathological retreat from interpersonal contact and social involvement, as may occur in schizophrenia, depression, or schizoid avoidant and schizotypal personality disorders. 2. [DSM III-R] a substance-specific organic brain syndrome that follows the cessation of use or reduction in intake of a psychoactive substance that had been regularly used to induce a state of intoxication. DSM III-R includes specific withdrawal syndromes for alcohol, amphetamines or similarly acting sympathomimetics, cocaine, nicotine, opioids, and sedatives, hypnotics, or anxiolytics. Called also *substance withdrawal, withdrawal symptoms* or *syndrome,* and *abstinence symptoms* or *syndrome.*

withers (with'erz) the top of the shoulders of the horse. **fistulous w.,** a name applied to a condition occurring in horses after a dual infection of the supraspinous bursa by *Brucella* and *Actinomyces,* leading to distention and sometimes to rupture of the bursa, with suppuration.

witigo (wǐ-ti'go) windigo.

witkop (wit'kop) [Afrikaans "whitehead"] the name for favus among black South Africans. Called also *dikwakwadi* and *white head.*

Witzel gastrostomy (operation) (vit'sel) [Friedrich Oskar *Witzel,* German surgeon, 1856–1925] see under *gastrostomy.*

witzelsucht (vit'sel-zōōkt) [Ger.] a mental condition characteristic of frontal lobe lesions and marked by the making of poor jokes and puns and the telling of pointless stories, at which the patient himself is intensely amused.

WMA World Medical Association.

wobble (wob'l) to move unsteadily or unsurely back and forth or from side to side. See under *hypothesis.*

wobbles (wob'b'lz) posterior incoordination in the horse, beginning with a slight swaying action of the hindquarters, or stumbling, with worsening of the condition until the animal cannot trot without rolling from side to side and falling; it is usually associated with spinal cord malacia but the cause is unknown.

Wohlfahrtia (vōl-fahr'te-ah) a genus of flies of the family Sarcophagidae. **W. magnif'ica,** a very common flesh fly of the Old World; its larvae may produce wound myiasis in man and animals. **W. o'paca,** a North American species; its larvae cause cutaneous myiasis in man and animals, especially foxes and mink. **W. vig'il,** a North American species; its larvae may produce cutaneous myiasis in man and animals.

Wolbachia (wol-bak'e-ah) [Simeon Burt *Wolbach,* American physician, 1880–1954] a genus of bacteria of the tribe Wolbachieae, family Rickettsiaceae, order Rickettsiales, made up of rickettsia-like microorganisms associated with

arthropods but not pathogenic for vertebrates. The type species is *W. pipien'tis.*

Wolbachieae (wol''bah-ki'e-e) [S. B. *Wolbach*] a tribe of bacteria of the family Rickettsiaceae, order Rickettsiales, made up of rickettsia-like organisms occurring symbiotically or parasitically within the cells of arthropod hosts. It includes the genera *Rickettsiella* and *Wolbachia.*

Woldman's test (wold'manz) [Edward Elbert *Woldman,* American physician, born 1897] see under *tests.*

Wolfe's graft (woolfs) [John Reissberg *Wolfe,* Scottish ophthalmologist, 1824–1904] Krause-Wolfe graft.

Wolfe-Krause graft (wolfe-krowz) [J. R. *Wolfe;* Fedor *Krause,* German surgeon, 1857–1937] Krause-Wolfe graft.

Wolfenden's position (wol'fen-denz) [Richard Norris *Wolfenden,* British laryngologist, 1854–1925] see under *position.*

Wolff's law (volfs) [Julius *Wolff,* German anatomist, 1836–1902] see under *law.*

Wolff-Eisner reaction (test) (volf īz'ner) [Alfred *Wolff-Eisner,* German serologist, 1877–1948] see *ophthalmic reaction,* under *reaction.*

Wolff-Parkinson-White syndrome [Louis *Wolff,* American cardiologist, born 1898; Sir John *Parkinson,* British physician, born 1885; Paul Dudley *White,* American cardiologist, 1886–1973] see under *syndrome.*

wolffian (woolf'e-an) described by Kaspar Friedrich *Wolff,* German anatomist and embryologist, 1733–1794, as wolffian body (mesonephros), cyst, duct (ductus mesonephricus), and ridge (mesonephric ridge).

Wölfler's operation (vel'flerz) [Anton *Wölfler,* surgeon in Prague, 1850–1917] see under *operation.*

wolfram (wool'fram) tungsten.

wolframium (wolf-ra'me-um) [L. "wolfram"] (obs.) tungsten.

Wolfring's glands (vōlf'ringz) [Emilij Franzevic von *Wolfring,* Polish ophthalmologist, 1832–1906] see under *gland.*

wolfsbane (wolfs'bān) 1. *Arnica.* 2. *Aconitum napellus.*

Wolinella (wo''lǐ-nel'ah) [M.J. *Wolin,* American bacteriologist] a genus of gram-negative, anaerobic, helical, curved or straight, rod-shaped bacteria of the family Bacteroidaceae, motile with a polar flagellum, found in cattle and the human oral cavity. **W. rec'ta,** a species isolated from human gum tissue, from oral pockets in periodontal disease, and from dental root canal infections. **W. succinog'enes,** a species found in the bovine rumen. Called also *Vibrio succinogenes.*

Wollaston's doublet (wool'as-tonz) [William Hyde *Wollaston,* English physician, 1766–1828] see under *doublet.*

womb (wōōm) the uterus.

Wong's method (wongz) [San Yin *Wong,* Chinese biochemist, born 1894] see under *method.*

Wood's light (filter, glass) (woodz) [Robert Williams *Wood,* American physicist, 1868–1953] see under *light.*

wool (wool) [L. *lana*] the hair of sheep and lambs; by extension applied to any material existing as fine threads. **collodion w.,** pyroxylin. **lumpy w.,** dermatophilosis of sheep, characterized by erythematous, exudative, scaling lesions of the skin which develop into pyramidal scabby masses; called also *wool rot.*

Woolner's tip (wool'nerz) [Thomas *Woolner,* English sculptor and poet, 1826–1892] tuberculum auriculae.

word salad (werd sal'ad) a meaningless mixture of words and phrases characteristic of advanced schizophrenia; called also *schizophasia.*

work-up (werk'up) the procedures done to arrive at a diagnosis, including history taking, laboratory tests, x-rays, and so on.

World Health Organization (WHO) an agency of the United Nations, devoted to attainment of the highest level of health by all peoples of the world; the permanent secretariat is located in Geneva, Switzerland.

worm (werm) [L. *vermis*] 1. any of the soft-bodied, naked, elongated invertebrates of the phyla Platyhelminthes, Annelida, Acanthocephala, and Aschelminthes. Formerly classified as Vermes. 2. any anatomical structure resembling a worm; see *vermis.* 3. the spiral tube of a distilling apparatus. **bilharzia w.,** *Schistosoma.* **bladder w.,** a cysticercus; bladder worms exist in various parenchymatous tissues of a host; being then transferred to the stomach of another host, they develop into tapeworms. **case w.,** *Echinococcus.* **cayor w.,** the larva of *Cordylobia anthropophaga.* **w. of cerebellum,** vermis cerebelli. **dragon w.,** *Dracunculus medinensis.* **eel w.,** *Ascaris.* **eye w.,** *Loa loa.* **flat w.,** any member of the Platyhelminthes. **fluke w.,** see *fluke.* **guinea w.,** *Dracunculus medinensis.* **heart w.,** *Dirofilaria immitis.* **horsehair w.,** *Gordius.* **kidney w.,** *Dioctophyma renale.* **lung w.,** see *lungworm.* **maw w.,** *Ascaris.* **meal w.,** *Asopia farinalis, Tenebrio molitor,* and other grain beetles. **Medina w.,** *Dracunculus medinensis.* **palisade w.,** *Strongylus equinus.* **pork w.,** *Trichinella spiralis.* **ribbon w.,** see *Rhynchocoela.* **screw w.,** see *screwworm.* **serpent w.,** *Dracunculus medinensis.* **spinyheaded w.,** Acanthocephala. **stomach w.,** *Haemonchus contortus.* **thorny-headed w.,** Acanthocephala. **tongue w.,** Pentastomida. **trichina w.,** *Trichinella.*

Worm-Müller's test (vorm-mil′erz) [Jacob *Worm-Müller,* Norwegian physician, 1834–1889] see under *tests.*

wormian bones (wer′me-an) [Olaus *Worm,* Danish anatomist, 1588–1654] ossa suturarum.

Wormley's test (worm′lēz) [Theodore George *Wormley,* Philadelphia chemist, 1826–1897] see under *tests.*

wormseed (werm′sēd) 1. santonica. 2. *Chenopodium.*

wormwood (werm′wood) absinthium.

Woulfe's bottle (woolfs) [Peter *Woulfe,* English chemist, 1727–1803] see under *bottle.*

wound (woōnd) [L. *vulnus*] a bodily injury caused by physical means, with disruption of the normal continuity of structures. **aseptic w.,** one which is not infected with pathogens. **blowing w.,** open pneumothorax. **contused w.,** a wound in which the skin is unbroken. **incised w.,** one made by a cutting instrument. **lacerated w.,** laceration. **nonpenetrating w.,** one in which there is no disruption of the skin but there is injury to underlying structures. **open w.,** one that communicates with the atmosphere by direct exposure. **penetrating w.,** one caused by a sharp, usually slender object, such as a nail or ice pick, which passes through the skin into the underlying tissues. **perforating w.,** a penetrating wound which extends into a viscus or bodily cavity. **puncture w.,** one made by a pointed instrument; penetrating wound. **septic w.,** one that is infected with pathogens. **seton w.,** one which enters and exits on the same side of the injured part. **subcutaneous w.,** one which involves only the skin and subcutaneous tissue. **sucking w.,** a penetrating wound of the chest through which air is drawn in and out. **summer w's,** see *esponja, habronemiasis,* and *summer sores,* under *sore.* **tangential w.,** an oblique glancing wound which results in one edge being undercut. **traumatopneic w.,** sucking w.

W-plasty a technique in plastic surgery used mainly in the repair of straight scars that require the redistribution of tension. It consists in excising a series of consecutive small triangular areas of tissue on each side of the wound or scar, and imbricating the resultant triangular flaps.

W.R. Wassermann reaction.

wreath (rēth) an encircling structure, resembling a circlet of flowers or leaves such as may be worn about the head.

daughter w., the amphiaster as viewed from its surface.

Wreden's sign (vra′denz) [Robert Robertovich *Wreden,* otologist in Petrograd, 1837–1893] see under *sign.*

Wright's stain (rīts) [James Homer *Wright,* Boston pathologist, 1871–1928] see under *Table of Stains.*

Wright's syndrome (rīts) [Irving Sherwood *Wright,* New York physician, born 1901] see under *syndrome.*

Wrisberg's cartilage, etc. (ris′bergz) [Heinrich August *Wrisberg,* German anatomist, 1739–1808] see under *cartilage, ganglion, ligament, line, nerve,* and *tubercle.*

wrist (rist) 1. the part of the upper limb between the forearm and hand, in the region of the wrist joint. Called also *carpus* [NA]. The term is also applied to the corresponding part in the thoracic limb of quadrupeds. 2. articulatio radiocarpalis. **tennis w.,** tenovaginitis of the tendons of the wrist in tennis players.

wristdrop (rist′drop) a condition resulting from paralysis of the extensor muscles of the hand and fingers. Called also *carpoptosis* and *drop hand.*

writing (rīt′ing) the inscription of letters or other symbols, and of words, phrases, and sentences, so that they may be perceived by the eyes or, by the blind, through the fingertips. **mirror w.,** writing in which the right and left relationships of letters and words are reversed, as if seen in a mirror.

wryneck (ri′neck) torticollis.

wt. weight.

wucheratrophie (voo″ker-at′ro-fe) [Ger. "proliferation atrophy"] wucher atrophy.

Wuchereria (voo″ker-e′re-ah) [Otto *Wucherer,* German physician in Brazil, 1820–1873] a genus of filarial nematodes (roundworms) indigenous in various countries of warmer regions of the world. **W. bancrof′ti,** a white threadlike worm which causes elephantiasis, lymphangitis, and chyluria by interfering with the lymphatic circulation. The immature forms, or microfilariae (*microfilaria bancrofti*), are found in the circulating blood, especially at night, and are carried by *Culex* and other mosquitoes. In the Pacific form of *W. bancrofti,* sometimes called *W. bancrofti* var. *pacifica,* the microfilariae do not show the nocturnal periodicity seen elsewhere. **W. ma′layi,** *Brugia malayi.*

wuchereriasis (voo-ker″e-ri′ah-sis) infection with worms of the genus *Wuchereria.*

Wunderlich's curve (voon′der-liks) [Carl Reinhold August *Wunderlich,* German physician, 1815–1877] see under *curve.*

Wundt's tetanus (voonts) [Wilhelm *Wundt,* German physiologist, 1832–1920] see under *tetanus.*

Wurster's test (vurs′terz) [Casimir *Wurster,* Dresden physiologist, 1856–1913] see under *tests.*

w./v. weight (of solute) per volume (of solvent).

Wyamine (wi′ah-min) trademark for preparations of mephentermine.

Wycillin (wi-sil′lin) trademark for preparations of penicillin G procaine.

Wydase (wi′dās) trademark for preparations of hyaluronidase for injection.

Wyeomyia (we″o-mi′yah) a genus of culicine mosquitoes.

Wynn method (win) [Sidney Keith *Wynn,* American plastic surgeon, born 1917] see under *method.*

X

X 1. symbol for *Kienbock's unit.* 2. symbol for xanthosine (in nucleotides).

Ξ the Greek capital letter xi.

ξ xi, the fourteenth letter of the Greek alphabet.

Xanax (zan′aks) trademark for a preparation of alprazolam.

xanchromatic (zan″kro-mat′ik) xanthochromic.

xanoxate sodium (zah-noks′āt) chemical name: 7-(1-methylethoxy)-9-oxo-9*H*-xanthene-2-carboxylic acid sodium salt; a bronchodilator, $C_{17}H_{13}NaO_5$.

xanthate (zan′thāt) any salt of xanthic acid.

xanthelasma (zan″thel-az′mah) [*xanth-* + Gr. *elasma* plate] 1. planar xanthoma involving the eyelid(s). Called also *x. palpebrarum* and *xanthoma palpebrarum.* 2. xanthoma.

xanthelasmatosis (zan″thel-az″mah-to′sis) xanthomatosis.

xanthematin (zan-them′ah-tin) an ill-defined yellow substance derivable from hematin, sometimes by the action of nitric acid.

xanthemia (zan-the′me-ah) [*xanth-* + *-emia*] carotenemia.

xanthene (zan′thēn) the compound, $(C_6H_4)_2(O)CH_2$, or dibenzpyran, from which the xanthene dyes and indicators are derived.

xanthic (zan'thik) 1. yellow. 2. pertaining to xanthine.

xanthin (zan'thin) any of the yellow pigments obtained from yellow flowers and other plants, probably consisting of oxygen-containing carotenoids.

xanthine (zan'thēn) [Gr. *xanthos* yellow: named from the yellow color of its nitrate] a white, amorphous base, 2,6-dioxypurine, $C_5H_4N_4O_2$, from most of the body tissues and fluids, urinary calculi, and certain plants. It is formed by the oxidation of hypoxanthine and may be oxidized to uric acid. It is insoluble in cold water, but freely soluble in dilute acid and alkaline solutions. It possesses stimulant properties to muscle tissue, especially that of the heart. The three derivatives of xanthine most used in medicine are caffeine, theobromine, and theophylline and their derivatives.

xanthine oxidase (zan'thēn ok'sĭ-dās) [EC 1.1.3.22] an enzyme of the oxidoreductase class that catalyzes the reaction xanthine + H_2O + O_2 = urate + O_2, the final step in the degradation of purines to urate. It is an iron-molybdenum flavoprotein containing FAD. Deficient enzyme, an autosomal recessive trait, causes xanthinuria.

xanthinin (zan'thĭ-nin) 1. a white, crystalline substance, $C_4H_9N_3O_2$, formed by heating ammonium thionurate. 2. a keto-lactone from leaves of *Xanthium pennsylvanicum*, or cocklebur.

xanthinuria (zan"thin-u're-ah) [*xanthine* + Gr. *ouron* urine] a rare hereditary disorder of purine metabolism due to deficiency of the enzyme xanthine oxidase, which results in excessive urinary secretion of xanthine and hypoxanthine, in place of uric acid, and may lead to the formation of xanthine calculi in the urinary tract.

xanthinuric (zan"thin-u'-rik) pertaining to or resulting from xanthinuria.

xanthism (zan'thizm) rufous albinism; see *oculocutaneous albinism*, under *albinism*.

xanthiuria (zan"the-u're-ah) xanthinuria.

xanth(o)- [Gr. *xanthos* yellow] a combining form meaning yellow.

Xanthobacter (zan"tho-bak'ter) [*xantho-* + Gr. *baktron* a rod] a genus of gram-negative, aerobic, coccoid to rod-shaped bacteria of uncertain affiliation, made up of chemolithotrophic or chemo-organotrophic, nitrogen-fixing organisms occurring in wet soils and water. The type species is *X-autotroph'icus*.

xanthochromatic (zan"tho-kro-mat'ik) xanthochromic.

xanthochromia (zan"tho-kro'me-ah) [*xantho-* + Gr. *chrōma* color + *-ia*] any yellowish discoloration, as of the skin or of the spinal fluid. **x. stria'ta palma'ris,** planar xanthoma involving the volar creases of the palms and finger joints, manifested by yellowish brown discoloration of the creases of the palmar aspect of the hands, which is assumed by some to gradually progress to xanthoma striatum palmare.

xanthochromic (zan"tho-kro'mik) having a yellow color; applied almost exclusively to cerebrospinal fluid.

xanthocyanopsia (zan"tho-si"ah-nop'se-ah) [*xantho-* + Gr. *kyanos* blue + *opsis* vision + *-ia*] ability to discern yellow and blue tints, but not red or green.

xanthocystine (zan"tho-sis'tin) a substance found in tubercles from a dead body.

xanthocyte (zan'tho-sīt) a cell that contains yellow pigment.

xanthoderma (zan"tho-der-mah) [*xantho-* + *derma*] any yellowish discoloration of the skin. For example, see *carotenemia, jaundice*, and *xanthochromia*.

xanthoerythrodermia (zan"tho-ĕ-rith"ro-der'me-ah) a yellowish red coloration of the skin. **x. per'stans,** small plaque parapsoriasis.

xanthofibroma thecocellulare (zan"tho-fi-bro'mah the"ko-sel"u-lah're) dermatofibroma.

xanthogranuloma (zan"tho-gran"u-lo'mah) a tumor having the histologic characteristics of both granuloma and xanthoma. **juvenile x.,** a benign, self-limited disorder of infants and children, usually present at birth, manifested by the development of single or multiple papules or nodules, which may be yellow, pink, orange, or reddish brown in color, found typically on the scalp, face, proximal extremities, or trunk; involvement of mucous membranes, viscera, eye, and

other organs may also occur. Mature lesions are characterized histologically by a dermal infiltrate of lipid-laden histiocytes, admixed inflammatory cells, and Touton giant cells. Most lesions regress spontaneously during the first few years of life. Formerly called *nevoxanthoendothelioma*.

xanthokyanopy (zan"tho-ki-an'o-pe) xanthocyanopsia.

xanthoma (zan-tho'mah) [*xanth-* + *-oma*] a tumor composed of lipid-laden foam cells, which are histiocytes containing cytoplasmic lipid material. See also *xanthomatosis*. Called also *xanthelasma*. **craniohypophyseal x.,** deposits of cholesterol esters in bones around the hypophysis in Hand-Schüller-Christian disease. **diabetic x., x. diabetico'rum,** eruptive x. **disseminated x., x. dissemina'tum,** a rare form of normolipoproteinemic xanthomatosis manifested by the development of reddish yellow to brown papules and nodules that may coalesce to form furrowed plaques, and have a predilection for flexural creases, mucous membranes of the mouth and respiratory tract, cornea, sclera, and central nervous system, including the pituitary gland, the involvement of which often produces diabetes insipidus. Called also *x. multiplex*. **eruptive x., x. erupti'vum,** a form characterized by the sudden onset of crops of small yellowish orange or yellow papules, surrounded by an erythematous halo, occurring principally on the buttocks, posterior thighs, knees, and elbows, which may be intensely pruritic and may ulcerate. It is caused by high concentrations of plasma triglycerides, especially that associated with uncontrolled diabetes mellitus, the correction of which usually results in disappearance of the lesions. Called also *diabetic x.* and *x. diabeticorum*. See also *tuberoeruptive x.* **x. mul'tiplex,** disseminated x. **planar x., plane x., x. pla'num,** a form manifested as soft yellowish, tannish, or dark red flat macules or slightly raised plaques, sometimes having a white central area, which may be localized or generalized, often occurring in association with other types of xanthomas and certain types of hyperlipoproteinemia, and may be associated with lymphoma and multiple myeloma. **x. stria'tum palma're,** planar xanthoma involving the creases of the palms and volar finger joints, manifested by linear, slightly elevated papules in the palmar creases, especially of the fingers; assumed by some authorities to be a gradual transition from xanthochromia striata palmaris. **tendinous x., x tendino'sum,** a form manifested by the presence of freely movable papules or nodules in the tendons, ligaments, fascia, and periosteum, especially on the dorsum of the hands, fingers, elbows, knees, and heels, which occurs in association with certain types of hyperlipoproteinemia, tuberous xanthoma, xanthelasma, and cerebrotendinous xanthomatosis. **tuberoeruptive x.,** a form in which the lesions of eruptive xanthoma develop in association with already existing lesions of the tuberous form and have a tendency to coalesce, and usually occur in combination with hyperlipoproteinemia (type III). **x. tubero'sum, x. tubero'sum mul'tiplex, tuberous x.,** a form manifested by the development of large flat or elevated and rounded, grouped, yellowish or orange indurated nodules on the extensor surfaces and areas subjected to trauma, particularly on the elbows and knees, which show a tendency to coalesce, and seen in association with such conditions as certain types of hyperlipoproteinemias, biliary cirrhosis, and myxedema. See also *tuberoeruptive x.*

xanthomatosis (zan"tho-mah-to'sis) a condition characterized by the presence of xanthomas. Called also *xanthelasmatosis*. See also *xanthoma*. **biliary hypercholesterolemic x.,** widespread xanthomatosis resulting from hypercholesterolemia due to biliary tract obstruction. **x. bul'bi,** fatty degeneration of the cornea. **cerebrotendinous x.,** a lipid storage disease, inherited as an autosomal recessive trait, chacterized by xanthomas of the tendons, the white matter of the brain, and the lungs and by spasticity, ataxia, pyramidal paresis, mental retardation, dementia, early cataracts, and atherosclerosis. It is associated with elevated plasma and tissue levels of cholestanol and defective bile synthesis, with the deposition of cholestanol in the central nervous system and in the myelin of peripheral nerves. The lesions contain cholesterol and dehydrocholesterol. **chronic idiopathic x.,** Hand-Schüller-Christian disease. **x. cor'neae,** dystrophia adiposa corneae. **x. generalisa'ta os'sium,** lipid granulomatosis of the bones. **x. i'ridis,** the formation of yellow patches in the discolored iris of an eye blinded as the result of protracted iritis or glaucoma. **primary familial x.,** Wolman disease. **Wolman x.,** Wolman disease.

xanthomatous (zan-tho'mah-tus) pertaining to or of the nature of xanthoma.

Xanthomonas (zan"tho-mo'nas) [Gr. *xanthos* yellow + Gr. *monas* unit, from *monos* single] a genus of gram-negative, aerobic, rod-shaped bacteria of the family Pseudomonadaceae. The organisms produce a yellow pigment; most species are plant pathogens.

xanthone (zan'thōn) xanthene ketone, CO:(C$_6$H$_4$)$_2$:O, a derivative of xanthine.

xanthophore (zan'tho-fōr) [*xantho-* + Gr. *phoros* bearing] a chromatophore of cold-blooded animals containing granules of yellow-red pigment.

xanthophose (zan'tho-fōz) [*xantho-* + Gr. *phōs* light] any yellow or yellowish phose.

xanthophyll (zan'tho-fil) [*xantho-* + Gr. *phyllon* leaf] a yellow coloring matter of plants, one of a group of oxygenated carotenoids, e.g., 3,3-dihydroxy alpha-carotene, C$_{40}$H$_{56}$O$_2$, occurring along with carotene in green leaves, grass, and other vegetable matter.

xanthopia (zan-tho'pe-ah) xanthopsia.

xanthoproteic (zan"tho-pro-te'ik) pertaining to xanthoprotein.

xanthoproteic acid (zan"tho-pro-te'ik) the product of treating protein with nitric acid.

xanthoprotein (zan"tho-pro'te-in) an orange pigment produced by heating proteins with nitric acid.

xanthopsia (zan-thop'se-ah) [*xantho-* + Gr. *opsis* vision + *-ia*] a form of chromatopia in which objects looked at appear yellow.

xanthopsin (zan-thop'sin) all-*trans* retinal; see *retinal.*

xanthopsis (zan-thop'sis) [*xantho-* + Gr. *opsis* appearance] a yellow pigment or pigmentation in cancers.

xanthopterin (zan-thop'ter-in) [*xantho-* + Gr. *pteron* wing] chemical name: 2-amino-4,6-pteridinediol. A yellow pigment, C$_6$H$_5$N$_5$O$_2$, from the integument of wasps and hornets and from butterfly wings, which has some hematopoietic activity in anemic animals. It is an inhibitor of xanthine oxidase. See *pterin.*

xanthopuccine (zan"tho-puk'sin) [*xantho-* + *puccoon*, Algonquin name for plants used as pigments] an alkaloid from *Hydrastis canadensis* L. (Ranunculaceae), the goldenseal.

xanthorhamnin (zan"tho-ram'nin) chemical name: 3,3', 4',5-tetrahydroxy-7-methoxyflavone-3-rhamninoside. A yellow glycoside, C$_{34}$H$_{42}$O$_{20}$, from the fruit of several species of *Rhamnus.*

xanthosarcoma (zan"tho-sar-ko'mah) giant cell tumor of the tendon sheath; see under *tumor.*

xanthosine (zan'tho-sēn) a nucleoside, xanthine-9-ribofuranoside, C$_{10}$H$_{12}$O$_6$N$_4$, which on hydrolysis yields xanthine and ribose. **x. monophosphate (XMP),** a nucleotide, xanthosine 5'-phosphate, that is an intermediate in the synthesis of guanosine monophosphate (GMP).

xanthosis (zan-tho'sis) a yellowish discoloration; degeneration with yellowish pigmentation. **x. of septum nasi,** yellow pigmentation of the mucous membrane of the nose, due to degeneration of the blood after hemorrhage.

xanthous (zan'thus) yellow or yellowish.

xanthurenic acid (zanth"u-ren'ik) 4,8-dihydroxyquinaldic acid; a minor catabolite of tryptophan present in increased amounts in the urine in vitamin B$_6$ deficiency.

xanthuria (zan-thu're-ah) [*xanthine* + Gr. *ouron* urine + *-ia*] xanthinuria.

xanthyl (zan'thil) the monovalent radical C$_{13}$H$_9$O.

xanthylic (zan-thil'ik) pertaining to xanthine.

xanthylic acid (zan-thil'ik) xanthosine monophosphate.

X-bite crossbite

Xe chemical symbol for *xenon.*

xenembole (zen-em'bo-le) [*xeno-* + Gr. *embolē* insertion] the introduction of foreign substances into the system.

xenenthesis (zen"en-the'sis) [*xeno-* + Gr. *enthesis* putting in] xenembole.

xenia (ze'ne-ah) [Gr. "a friendly relation between two foreigners"] the appearance in the endosperm (seed) resulting from cross-pollination of dominant characters inherited from the male (pollen) plant.

xen(o)- [Gr. *xenos* strange, foreign] a combining form meaning strange, or denoting relationship to foreign material.

xenoantigen (zen"o-an'tĭ-gen) an antigen occurring in organisms of more than one species, e.g., the A and B antigens of the ABO blood group.

xenobiotic (zen"o-bi-ot'ik) a chemical foreign to the biologic system.

xenocytophilic (zen"o-si"to-fil'ik) [*xeno-* + Gr. *kytos* hollow vessel + *philein* to love] having an affinity for cells derived from a different species.

xenodiagnosis (zen"o-di-ag-no'sis) [*xeno-* + *diagnosis*] a method of animal inoculation using laboratory-bred bugs and animals in the diagnosis of certain parasitic infections when it is not possible to demonstrate the infecting organism in blood films. Originally used in the diagnosis of *Trypanosoma cruzi* (Chagas' disease), the method is also used in *Trichinella spiralis* infections. In the original method, bugs are fed or offered the patient's blood through a membrane, and the feces or intestinal contents are examined later for the presence of the organisms. For the diagnosis of trichinosis muscle tissue from patient's is fed to laboratory rats to detect larvae of the parasite.

xenodiagnostic (zen"o-di"ag-nos'tik) pertaining to xenodiagnosis.

xenogeneic (zen"o-jen-a'ik) [*xeno-* + *gennan* to produce] in transplantation biology, denoting individuals or tissues from individuals of different species and hence of disparate cell type; called also *heterologous.* See *allogeneic.*

xenogenesis (zen"o-jen'ĕ-sis) 1. alternation of generation; heterogenesis. 2. the hypothetical production of offspring unlike either parent.

xenogenous (zen-oj'ĕ-nus) [*xeno-* + Gr. *gennan* to produce] caused by a foreign body, or originating outside the organism.

xenograft (zen'o-graft) a graft of tissue transplanted between animals of different species. Called also *heterograft, heterologous graft,* and *heteroplastic graft.* **Hancock porcine x.,** see under *valve.*

xenology (ze-nol'o-je) the science of the relations of parasites to their hosts.

xenomenia (zen"o-me'ne-ah) [*xeno-* + Gr. *mēniaia* menses] vicarious menstruation.

xenon (ze'non) [Gr. *xenos* stranger] a chemically unreactive gaseous element found in the atmosphere; atomic number, 54; atomic weight, 131.30; symbol, Xe.

xenoparasite (zen"o-par'ah-sīt) an organism not usually parasitic on the host, but which becomes so because of a weakened condition of the host.

xenophobia (zen"o-fo'be-ah) [*xeno-* + *phobia*] irrational fear of strangers.

xenophonia (zen"o-fo'ne-ah) [*xeno-* + Gr. *phōnē* voice + *-ia*] alteration of the accent and intonation of a person's speech.

xenophthalmia (zen"of-thal'me-ah) [*xeno-* + Gr. *ophthalmia* ophthalmia] ophthalmia caused by a foreign body in the eye.

Xenophyophorea (ze"no-fi"o-fo're-ah) [*xeno-* + Gr. *phyein* to beget + *phōros* bearing] a class of ameboid marine protozoa (superclass Rhizopoda, subphylum Sarcodina), occurring as multinucleate plasmodia enclosed in a branched tube system composed of a transparent organic substance, and characterized by the presence of numerous barite crystals in the cytoplasm, fecal pellets retained outside of the tube system as conspicuous, dark masses, and a test composed of foreign matter surrounding the tube system and the fecal pellets. It includes two orders: Psamminida and Stannomida.

Xenopsylla (zen"op-sil'ah) [*xeno-* + Gr. *psylla* flea] a genus of fleas, including more than 30 species, many of which transmit disease-producing microorganisms. **X. as'tia,** a rat flea of parts of Ceylon and India that has been implicated in the transmission of plague. **X. brasilien'sis,** a rat flea of Africa, Brazil, and India, a transmitter of plague. **X. che'opis,** a rat flea of worldwide distribution, which transmits plague and murine typhus; called also *Pulex cheopis* and *Asiatic rat flea.* **X. hawaiien'sis,** X. *vexabilis.* **X. vexabil'is,** a species infesting field rats in the Hawaiian islands; called also *X. hawaiiensis.*

Xenopus (zen'o-pus) a genus of amphibians. **X. lae'vis,**

the South African clawed toad; see *Xenopus test*, under *tests*.

xenorexia (zen″o-rek′se-ah) [*xeno-* + *orexis* appetite + *-ia*] perversion of appetite leading to the repeated swallowing of foreign bodies not ordinarily ingested.

Xenorhabdus (ze″no-rab′dus) [*xeno-* + Gr. *rhabdus* rod] a genus of gram-negative, facultatively anaerobic, rod-shaped bacteria of the family Enterobacteriaceae, isolated from nematodes and from the insect larvae they parasitize. The type species is *X. nematoph′ilus*.

xenyl (zen′il) the univalent chemical group, $C_6H_5 \cdot C_6H_4$—.

xerantic (ze-ran′tik) causing dryness; siccative.

xer(o)- [Gr. *xēros* dry] a combining form meaning dry, or denoting relationship to dryness.

xerocollyrium (ze″ro-ko-lir′e-um) [*xero-* + Gr. *kollyrion* collyrium] a dry collyrium; an eye salve.

xeroderma (ze″ro-der′mah) [*xero-* + Gr. *derma* skin] a mild form of ichthyosis, marked by a dry, rough, discolored state of the skin, with the formation of a scaly desquamation. **x. pigmento′sum,** a rare pigmentary and atrophic autosomal recessive disease affecting all races, in which there is extreme cutaneous photosensitivity to ultraviolet light, as a result of a deficient enzyme in the excisional repair of ultraviolet-damaged DNA. It begins in childhood with the early development of senile changes in sun-exposed skin, including excessive freckling, telangiectases, keratoses, papillomas, and malignancies; and of severe ophthalmologic abnormalities, including photophobia, lacrimation, keratitis, opacities, and tumors of the lid and cornea. Mental retardation, areflexia, and other neurological disorders may be associated. Subtypes of the disorder have been identified based on the capacity for excisional DNA repair. See also *pigmented xerodermoid*, under *xerodermoid*.

xerodermatic (ze″ro-der-mat′ik) pertaining to or of the nature of xeroderma.

xerodermia (ze″ro-der′me-ah) xeroderma.

xerodermoid (ze″ro-der′moid) [*xeroderma* + *-oid*] resembling xeroderma. **pigmented x.,** a condition considered to be a variant of xeroderma pigmentosum in which there is no defect in the excisional repair of ultraviolet-damaged DNA; it is characterized by a late onset, associated with prolonged exposure to the sun, with freckling appearing in the second decade and no skin cancers until age 40.

xerogel (ze′ro-jel) a gel containing little liquid. Cf. *lyogel*.

xerography (ze-rog′rah-fe) xeroradiography.

xeroma (ze-ro′mah) an abnormally dry condition of the conjunctiva; xerophthalmia.

xeromammography (ze″ro-mam-mog′rah-fe) xeroradiography of the breast.

xeromenia (ze″ro-me′ne-ah) [*xero-* + Gr. *mēniaia* menses] a condition in which the bodily symptoms of menstruation occur without any bloody flow.

xeromycteria (ze″ro-mik-te′re-ah) [*xero-* + Gr. *myktēr* nose] dryness of the nasal mucous membrane.

xerophthalmia (ze″rof-thal′me-ah) [*xero-* + Gr. *ophthalmos* eye + *-ia*] dryness of the conjunctiva and cornea due to vitamin A deficiency. The condition begins with night blindness and conjunctival xerosis and progresses to corneal xerosis and, in the late stages, to keratomalacia.

xerophthalmus (ze″rof-thal′mus) xerophthalmia.

xeroradiography (ze″ro-ra″de-og′rah-fe) a dry, totally photoelectric process for recording x-ray images, using metal plates coated with a semiconductor, such as selenium.

xerosialography (ze″ro-si″ah-log′rah-fe) sialography in which the images are recorded by xeroradiography.

xerosis (ze-ro′sis) [Gr. *xērosis*] abnormal dryness, as of the eye, skin, or mouth. **x. conjuncti′vae, conjunctival x.,** dryness of the conjunctiva. When associated with Bitot's spots, it is due to vitamin A deficiency and may progress to xerophthalmia and keratomalacia. **x. cor′neae, corneal x.,** dryness of the cornea, giving it a hazy or milky appearance; see *xerophthalmia*. **x. cu′tis,** xerotic eczema. **x. parenchymato′sa,** xerophthalmia due to trachoma. **x. superficia′lis,** xerophthalmia due to abnormal exposure of the eyeball to the air.

xerostomia (ze″ro-sto′me-ah) [*xero-* + Gr. *stoma* mouth + *-ia*] dryness of the mouth from salivary gland dysfunction, as in Sjögren's syndrome.

xerotes (zer′o-tēz) [Gr. *xērotēs*] dryness.

xerotic (ze-rot′ik) characterized by xerosis or dryness.

xerotomography (ze″ro-to-mog′rah-fe) tomography in which the images are recorded by xeroradiography.

xerotripsis (ze″ro-trip′sis) [*xero-* + Gr. *tripsis* friction] dry friction.

xi (zi, kse) [Ξ, ξ] the fourteenth letter of the Greek alphabet.

xilobam (zi′lo-bam) chemical name: N-(2,6-dimethylphenyl)-N′-(1-methyl-2-pyrrolidinylidene)urea; a muscle relaxant, $C_{14}H_{19}N_3O$.

Ximenia (zi-me′ne-ah) a genus of African olacineous trees; the drupes of some species are edible and aromatic.

xipamide (zip′ah-mīd) chemical name: 5-(aminosulfonyl)-4-chloro-N-(2,6-dimethylphenyl)-2-hydroxybenzamide; a diuretic and antihypertensive, $C_{15}H_{15}ClN_2O_4S$.

xiphi- see *xiph(o)-*.

xiphin (zif′in) a protamine from the sperm of the swordfish, *Xiphias gladius*.

xiphisternal (zif″ĭ-ster′nal) pertaining to the xiphisternum.

xiphisternum (zif″ĭ-ster′num) [*xiphi-* + Gr. *sternon* sternum] the xiphoid process (processus xiphoideus [NA]).

xiph(o)-, xiphi- [Gr. *xiphos* sword] combining forms denoting relationship to the xiphoid process.

xiphocostal (zif″o-kos′tal) [*xipho-* + L. *costa* rib] pertaining to the xiphoid process and the ribs.

xiphodidymus (zif″o-did′ĭ-mus) [*xipho-* + Gr. *didymos* twin] xiphopagus.

xiphodymus (zi-fod′ĭ-mus) xiphopagus.

xiphodynia (zif″o-din′e-ah) [*xipho-* + Gr. *odynē* pain + *-ia*] pain in the xiphoid process.

xiphoid (zif′oid) [*xipho-* + Gr. *eidos* form] 1. shaped like a sword. 2. the xiphoid process (processus xiphoideus [NA]).

xiphoiditis (zif″oi-di′tis) inflammation of the xiphoid process.

xiphopagus (zi-fop′ah-gus) [*xipho-* + Gr. *pagos* thing fixed] symmetrical conjoined twins fused in the region of the xiphoid process.

X-linked (eks′linkt) see under *gene*.

XMP xanthosine monophosphate.

XO an unapproved but widely used symbol to indicate the presence of only one sex chromosome, the other X or the Y chromosome being absent.

X-Prep (eks′prep) trademark for a preparation of senna.

x-ray (eks′ra) roentgen ray; see under *ray*. **spark x-r's,** brush discharge.

xylazine hydrochloride (zi′lah-zēn) chemical name: N-(2,6-dimethylphenyl)-5,6-dihydro-4H-1,3-thiazin-2-amine monohydrochloride; an analgesic, sedative, and muscle relaxant, $C_{12}H_{16}N_2S \cdot HCl$, used in veterinary medicine.

xylem (zi′lem) [Gr. *xylon* wood] the tissue in woody plants which conducts water and dissolved salts up from the roots, characterized by the presence of tracheids. In bulk it forms wood. Cf. *phloem*.

xylene (zi′lēn) 1. dimethylbenzene; an antiseptic hydrocarbon from methyl alcohol or coal tar; used in microscopy as a solvent and clarifier. 2. a group of hydrocarbons of the benzene series.

xylenol (zi′lĕ-nol) any of a series of colorless, crystalline substances, $(CH_3)_2C_6H_3OH$, resembling phenol. **x. salicylate,** a white antirheumatic powder, $OH \cdot C_6H_4 \cdot CO \cdot O \cdot C_6H_3(CH_3)_2$.

xylidine (zi′lĭ-din) a compound, dimethylaniline $(CH_3)_2C_6H_3 \cdot NH_2$, used as a dyestuff intermediate and for blending gasoline.

xylitol (zi′lĭ-tol) an alcohol, $CH_2OH(CHOH):CH_2OH$, from xylose.

xylitol dehydrogenase (zi′lĭ-tol de-hi′dro-jĕ-nās) xylulose reductase.

xylitone (zi′lĭ-tōn) an oil, $C_{12}H_{18}O$, formed by treating acetone with hydrochloric acid.

xyl(o)- [Gr. *xylon* wood] a combining form denoting relationship to wood.

Xylocaine (zi′lo-kān) trademark for preparations of lidocaine.

xylogen (zi′lo-jen) lignin.

xyloidin (zi-loid′in) [*xylo-* + Gr. *eidos* form] a white, explosive substance, $C_6H_9(NO_2)O_5$, prepared from starch by the action of nitric acid.

xyloketose (zi″lo-ke′tōs) xylulose.

xyloketosuria (zi″lo-ke″to-su′re-ah) essential pentosuria.

xylol (zi′lol) [Gr. *xylon* wood] xylene.

xyloma (zi-lo′mah) a woody tumor on a tree or plant.

xylometazoline hydrochloride (zi″lo-met″ah-zo′lēn) [USP] chemical name: 2[[4-(1,1-dimethylethyl)-2,6-dimethylphenyl]methyl]-4,5-dihydro-1*H*-imidazole monohydrochloride. An adrenergic, $C_{16}H_{24}N_2 \cdot HCl$, occuring as a white, crystalline powder; used topically as a vasoconstrictor to reduce swelling and congestion of the nasal mucosa.

xylonite (zi′lo-nīt) a substance which resembles celluloid manufactured from pyroxylin.

xylopyranose (zi″lo-pi′rah-nōs) xylose in the cyclic pyranose form.

xylosazone (zi-lo′sa-zōn) the phenyl-osazone of xylose.

xylose (zi′lōs) a pentose, $CH_2OH(CHOH)_3CHO$, in a pyranose form, occurring in mucopolysaccharides of connective tissue and sometimes in the urine (see *xylosuria*); also obtained from vegetable gums, beechwood, and jute. The official preparation is used as a diagnostic aid in determining intestinal function.

xyloside (zi-lo-sīd) a glycoside of xylose.

xylosidoglucose (zi″lo-sid″o-gloo′kōs) primaverose.

xylosuria (zi″lo-su′re-ah) presence of xylose in the urine. A form of alimentary pentosuria reportedly occurring after ingestion of certain fruits, e.g., cherries, plums, and grapes; the identity of the urinary pentose(s) has not been crisply established. It is to be distinguished from essential pentosuria, which results from a genetic defect.

xylotherapy (zi″lo-ther′ah-pe) [*xylo-* + Gr. *therapeia* treatment] medical treatment by the application of certain woods to the body.

xylulose (zi′lu-lōs) a pentose sugar, $CH_2OH(CHOH)_2CO\text{-}CH_2OH$, occurring in two forms: L-xylulose, one of the few L sugars found in nature and sometimes excreted in the urine (see *pentosuria*), and D-xylulose.

xylulose reductase (zi′lu-lōs re-duk′tās) [EC 1.1.1.10] an enzyme of the oxidoreductase class that catalyzes the reaction L-xylulose + NADPH = xylitol + NADP$^+$. Deficiency in the enzyme, an autosomal recessive trait, leads to pentosuria.

L-xylulosuria (zi″lu-lo-su′re-a) a pentosuria.

xylyl (zi′lil) the hydrocarbon radical, $CH_3C_6H_4CH_2$.

xyphoid (zi′foid) xiphoid.

xysma (zis′mah) [Gr. "that which is scraped or shaved off"] a material, like bits of membrane, seen in the stools of diarrhea.

xyster (zis′ter) [Gr. *xystēr* a scraper] a surgeon's file or raspatory.

Y

Y chemical symbol for *yttrium*.

Υ the Greek capital letter upsilon.

υ upsilon, the twentieth letter of the Greek alphabet.

Yalow (yal′o) Rosalyn Sussman. American medical physicist, born 1921; co-winner, with Roger Charles Louis Guillemin and Andrew Victor Schally, of the Nobel prize for medicine or physiology in 1977 for her work in endocrinology and the development of the radioimmunoassay technique.

yard (yard) a unit of linear measure, 3 feet, or 36 inches, being the equivalent of 86.44 cm.

yaw (yaw) a lesion of yaws (q.v.). **guinea corn y.,** a lesion of yaws which resembles a grain of maize. **mother y.,** the initial cutaneous lesion of yaws; called also *frambesioma* and *framboesioma.* **ringworm y.,** a circular or ring-shaped lesion of yaws.

yawning (yawn′ing) a deep, involuntary inspiration with the mouth open, often accompanied by the act of stretching. Cf. *pandiculation.*

yaws (yawz) an endemic, infectious, tropical disease caused by *Treponema pertenue,* usually affecting persons under the age of 15, and spread by direct contact with skin lesions or by contaminated fomites. It is characterized by the appearance at the site of inoculation of the spirochete, which enters the body through abraded or otherwise compromised skin, of a painless papule that grows into a papilloma (mother yaw). This heals, leaving a scar, which is followed by crops of generalized secondary granulomatous papules that may relapse repeatedly. Late manifestations include destructive and deforming lesions of the skin, bones, and joints. Called also *Breda's disease, Charlouis' disease, frambesia, frambesia tropica, framboesia, granuloma tropicum, polypapilloma tropicum,* and *thymiosis.* Also known by numerous local names, e.g., *bouba, parangi, pian,* and *tonga.* **crab y.,** yaws characterized by hyperkeratosis with fissuring and ulceration of the soles of the feet, and less commonly involving the palms of the hands. **forest y.,** pian bois.

Ya Yan Tzu the Chinese species of the simaroubaceous plant of the genus *Brucea,* e.g., *B. antidysenterica* J.F. Mill., the seeds of which are used in treating amebic dysentery.

Yb chemical symbol for *ytterbium.*

yd. yard.

yeast (yēst) a general term including single-celled, usually rounded fungi that produce by budding (blastospore formation). Some yeasts transform to a mycelial (mold) stage under certain environmental conditions, while others always remain single-celled. The perfect yeasts are included in the class Ascomycetes, subclass Hemiascomycetes, order Endomycetales, and the imperfect yeasts in the class Deuteromycetes, order Moniliales, family Cryptococcaceae. A few are pathogenic for man. **bakers' y., brewers' y.,** *Saccharomyces cerevisiae,* used in brewing beer, making alcoholic liquors, and baking bread. **dried y.,** the dry cells of any suitable strain of *Saccharomyces cerevisiae,* usually a by-product of the brewing industry; used as a natural source of protein and B-complex vitamins. **imperfect y.,** one whose perfect (sexual) stage is unknown. **perfect y.,** one whose perfect (sexual) stage is known.

yeast nucleic acid (yēst noo-kle′ik) ribonucleic a.

yellow (yel′o) 1. one of the primary colors of wavelength of 571.5 to 578.5 millimicrons. 2. a dye or stain that produces a yellow color. **acid y.,** fast y. **alizarin y.,** an indicator used in the determination of hydrogen ion concentration with a pH range of 10.1–12.1. **brilliant y.,** an indicator used in determining hydrogen ion concentration, with a pH range of 6–8. **butter y.,** *p*-dimethylaminoazobenzene. **chrome y.,** lead chromate, $PbCrO_4$, used in paints and injection masses. **corallin y.,** yellow corallin. **fast y.,** a yellow, acid azo dye, $(N\cdot C_6H_4\cdot SO_2ONa)_2NH_2$, used in staining bone. **imperial y.,** aurantia. **Manchester y., Martius y.,** a poisonous, yellow, azo dye, $C_6H_5(NO_2)_2OH$, used as a stain and in the preparation of light filters. **metanil y., metaniline y. (extra),** an indicator used in the determination of hydrogen ion concentration, with a pH range of 1.2–2.3. **naphthol y.,** Manchester y. **Philadelphia y.,** phosphine, def. 2. **visual y.,** all-*trans* retinal; see *retinal.*

yellows (yel′ōz) 1. a form of canine leptospirosis resembling leptospiral jaundice in man, caused by *Leptospira interrogans* serogroup *icterohaemorrhagiae.* 2. a disease affecting sheep and cattle in Scotland during June and July; it is marked by photosensitization and jaundice after ingestion of clover or alfalfa followed by exposure to sunlight; called also *headgrit.*

Yeo's treatment (ye′ōz) [Isaac Burney *Yeo,* London physician, 1835–1914] see under *treatment.*

yerba (yer′bah) [Sp.] herb. **y. santa** (yer′bah sahn′tah) [Sp. "sacred herb"], *Eriodictyon.*

yerbine (yer′bin) an alkaloid resembling caffeine, obtained from *Ilex paraguayensis,* a holly tree of Brazil, Argentina, and Paraguay.

Yerkes discrimination box (yer′kēz) [Robert M. *Yerkes,* Boston psychobiologist, 1876–1956] see under *box.*

Yersinia (yer-sin′e-ah) [A.J.E. *Yersin,* Swiss bacteriologist in

Paris, 1863–1943] a genus of gram-negative, facultatively anaerobic, rod-shaped to ovoid bacteria of the family Enterobacteriaceae. It contains the organism responsible for bubonic plague (see *Y. pestis*) and other species that cause gastroenteritis and mesenteric lymphadenitis. Numerous serotypes based on the presence of an O antigen have been described. **Y. enterocolit′ica,** a ubiquitous species isolated from mammals, birds, and frogs, and from material contaminated by feces. The organisms cause acute gastroenteritis and mesenteric lymphadenitis, especially in young children, and arthritis, septicemia, and erythema nodosum in adults. It is transmitted by infected food and water and by person-to-person contact. **Y. frederiksen′ii,** an opportunistic pathogen, a species that resembles *Y. enterocolitica* except that it ferments L-rhamnose. **Y. interme′dia,** an opportunistic pathogen, a species that resembles *Y. enterocolitica* except that it ferments L-rhamnose, raffinose, and melibiose. **Y. kristensen′ii,** an opportunistic pathogen, a species that resembles *Y. enterocolitica* except that it does not ferment sucrose. **Y. pes′tis,** the etiologic agent of bubonic and pneumonic plague in humans and rats, ground squirrels, and other rodents, transmitted from rat to rat and from rat to man by the rat flea, and from man to man by the human body louse; pathogenic for mice, guinea pigs, and rabbits. Formerly called *Bacterium pestis* and *Pasteurella pestis.* **Y. pseudotuberculo′sis,** a species found in the intestinal tract of birds, rodents, and other animals. It is pathogenic, causing mesenteric lymphadenitis in humans and pseudotuberculosis in guinea pigs, white rats, rabbits, and occasionally other animals. Human infection occurs from contact with infected food or animals. Formerly called *Pasteurella pseudotuberculosis.* **Y. ruck′eri,** a species that resembles *Y. enterocolitica* except that it does not ferment cellobiose. It is found in fresh waters, and can cause red mouth disease in fish.

Yersinieae (yer-sin′e-e) in some systems of classification, a tribe of gram-negative, facultatively anaerobic, rod-shaped bacteria of the family Enterobacteriaceae, consisting of the single genus *Yersinia.*

-yl [Gr. *hylē* matter, substance] a chemical suffix signifying a radical, particularly a univalent hydrocarbon radical.

-ylene a suffix used in chemistry to denote a bivalent hydrocarbon radical.

Yodoxin (yo-dok′sin) trademark for preparations of iodoquinol.

yogurt (yo′goort) a form of curdled milk, produced by fermentation with organisms of the genus *Lactobacillus.*

yohimbine (yo-him′bēn) an alkaloid, $C_{21}H_{26}N_2O_3$, from *Corynanthe johimbe* K. Schum. (Rubiaceae) and from *Rauwolfia serpentina* L. Benth. (Apocynaceae). It possesses adrenergic blocking properties and is used in arteriosclerosis and angina pectoris, and formerly as a local anesthetic and mydriatic and for its purported aphrodisiac properties.

yoke (yōk) a connecting structure; a depression or ridge connecting two structures. Called also *jugum.* **aleolar y′s of mandible,** juga alveolaria mandibulae. **alveolar y′s of maxilla,** juga alveolaria maxillae. **cerebral y′s of bone of cranium,** juga cerebralia ossium cranii. **sphenoidal y.,** jugum sphenoidale.

yolk (yōk) [L. *vitellus*] 1. the stored nutrient of the ovum. 2. crude wool fat or suint. **accessory y.,** the part of the yolk that serves for the nutrition of the formative portion. **egg y.,** the yellow portion of the egg of a bird. **formative y.,** that part of the ovum from which the embryo is developed. **nutritive y.,** accessory y.

Yomesan (yo′me-san) trademark for preparations of niclosamide.

Young's operation (yungz) [Hugh Hampton *Young*, Baltimore urologist, 1870–1945] see under *operation.*

Young's rule (yungz) [Thomas *Young,* English physician, physicist, mathematician, and philologist, 1773–1829, the "father of physiologic optics"] see under *rule.*

Young-Helmholtz theory (yung-helm′hōlts) [Thomas *Young;* H. L. F. von *Helmholtz,* German physician, 1821–1894] see under *theory.*

yperite (i′per-īt) dichlorodiethyl sulfide.

ypsiliform (ip-sil′ĭ-form) upsiloid.

ypsiloid (ip′sĭ-loid) upsiloid.

ytterbium (ĭ-ter′be-um) [from *Ytterby,* in Sweden] a very rare metal; symbol, Yb; atomic number, 70; atomic weight, 173.04.

yttrium (ĭ′tre-um) [from *Ytterby,* in Sweden] a very rare metal, allied to cerium; symbol Y; atomic number, 39, atomic weight, 88.905.

Z

Z symbol for *atomic number, impedence, ionic charge number.*

Z- [Ger. *zusammen* together] a stereodescriptor used to specify the absolute configuration of compounds having double bonds. See *E-.*

ζ zeta, the sixth letter of the Greek alphabet.

Zactane (zak′tān) trademark for a preparation of ethoheptazine citrate.

Zahn's lines (ribs) (zahnz) [Friedrich Wilhelm *Zahn,* Swiss pathologist, 1845–1904] see under *line.*

Zander apparatus (zan′der) [Jonas Gustaf Wilhelm *Zander,* Swedish physician, 1835–1917] see under *apparatus.*

Zang's space (zangz) [Christoph Bonifacius *Zang,* German surgeon, 1772–1835] fossa supraclavicularis minor.

Zanosar (zan′o-sar) trademark for preparations of streptozocin.

Zappert's chamber (tsap′ertz) [Julius *Zappert,* physician in Vienna, 1867–1942] see under *chamber.*

Zarontin (zah-ron′tin) trademark for a preparation of ethosuximide.

Zaroxolyn (zah-roks′o-lin) trademark for a preparation of metolazone.

Zaufal's sign (tsow′fahlz) [Emanuel *Zaufal,* Prague rhinologist, 1833–1910] saddle nose.

Zea (ze′ah) 1. maize. 2. corn-silk, the fresh styles and stigmas of the flowers of American corn, *Zea mays* L. (Gramineae). Formerly used in the treatment of cystitis and urethritis.

zeatin (ze′ă-tin) [from *Zea mays,* the generic name for corn] a cytokinin, or growth-stimulating factor of plants, 6-(4-hydroxy-3-methyl-*trans*-2-butenylamino)purine, first isolated from young kernels of sweetcorn but now known to occur in peas and spinach as well.

zeaxanthin (ze″ah-zan′thin) [zea + Gr. *xanthos* yellow] a carotinoid, $C_{40}H_{56}O_2$, from yellow corn, egg yolk, and *Fucus vesiculosus,* a seaweed of the North Atlantic Ocean.

zedoary (zed′o-a″re) [L. *zedoaria*] the rhizome of *Curcuma zedoaria,* a plant of India, which resembles ginger; used medicinally as an aromatic stimulant and carminative.

Zeeman effect (tse′man) [Pieter *Zeeman,* Dutch physicist, 1865–1943] see under *effect.*

zein (ze′in) a yellowish prolamin obtainable from corn; molecular weight is about 40,000. It does not contain tryptophan or lysine.

zeinolysis (ze″in-ol′ĭ-sis) [zein + Gr. *lysis* dissolution] the decomposition or splitting up of zein.

zeinolytic (ze″in-o-lit′ik) pertaining to, characterized by, or promoting zeinolysis.

zeiosis (zi-o′sis) [Gr. *zeiein* to boil, seethe + *-osis*] bubbling or blebbing activity, giving the appearance of boiling in slow motion, observed at the periphery of cells cultured in artificial media.

zeisian gland, stye (zi′se-an) [Edourd *Zeis,* Dresden ophthalmologist, 1807–1868] see *glandulae sebaceae conjunctivales,* and see *external hordeolum,* under *hordeolum.*

zeism (ze′izm) [L. *zea* maize, corn] any condition attributed to excessive use of maize in the diet, principally pellagra.

zeismus (ze-is′mus) zeism.

zeistic (ze-is′tik) pertaining to maize.

Zellweger syndrome (zel'weg-er) [Hans Ulrich *Zellweger*, American pediatrician, born 1909] see *cerebrohepatorenal syndrome*, under *syndrome*.

Zenker's crystals, degeneration (necrosis), diverticulum (zeng'kerz) [Friedrich Albert von *Zenker*, German pathologist, 1825–1898] see *Charcot-Leyden crystals* under *crystal*, and see under *degeneration* and *diverticulum*.

Zenker's fixative (fluid, solution) (zeng'kerz) [Konrad *Zenker*, German histologist, died 1894] see under *fixative*.

zenkerism (zeng'ker-izm) [F. A. *Zenker*] Zenker's degeneration; see under *degeneration*.

zenkerize (zeng'ker-īs) [K. *Zenker*] to treat with Zenker's fixative.

zeolite (ze'o-lit) a hydrated double silicate with ion-exchange properties; probably the active constituent in permutit.

zeoscope (ze'o-skōp) [Gr. *zeein* to boil, seethe + *skopein* to examine] an apparatus for determining the alcoholic strength of a liquid by means of its boiling point.

Zephiran (zef'ĭ-ran) trademark for preparations of benzalkonium.

zeranol (zer'ah-nōl) chemical name: (3S,7X)-3,4,5,6,7,8,9,10, 11,12-decahydro-7,14,16-trihydroxy-3-methyl-1*H*-2-benzoxacyclotetradecin-1-one; anabolic-estrogenic agent, $C_{18}H_{26}O_5$, which has been used for estrogen replacement in human subjects, but is used chiefly in veterinary medicine.

zero (ze'ro) [Ital. "naught"] the point on a thermometer scale at which the graduation begins; the ice point on the Celsius and Réaumur scales and 32° below the ice point on the Fahrenheit. **absolute z.,** the lowest possible temperature, designated as 0 on the Kelvin or Rankine scale; by definition this is equivalent –273.15° C. or –459.67° F. **limes z.,** limes nul dose. **physiologic z.,** the temperature at which a thermal stimulus ceases to cause a sensation.

zerumbet (ze-rum'bet) [East Indian] a spice or drug, the dried rhizome of a species of ginger, *Zingiber zerumbet* (L.) Smith (Zingiberaceae), now little used.

zestocausis (zes"to-kaw'sis) [Gr. *zestos* boiling hot + *kausis* burning] the therapeutic application of a tube containing superheated steam.

zestocautery (zes"to-kaw'ter-e) a tube or appliance used in zestocausis.

zeta (za'tah) [Z, ζ] the sixth letter of the Greek alphabet.

zetacrit (za'tah-krit) see *zeta sedimentation ratio* under *ratio*.

Zetafuge (za'tah-fūj) trademark for a device used in determination of the zeta sedimentation ratio.

zeugopodium (zu"go-po'de-um) zygopodium (see *limb*).

zidometacin (zi"do-met'ah-sin) chemical name: 1-4(4-azidobenzoyl)-5-methoxy-2-methyl-1*H*-indole-3-acetic acid; an anti-inflammatory, $C_{19}H_{16}N_4O_4$.

zidovudine (zi-do'vu-dēn) azidothymidine.

Ziegler's operation (zēg'lerz) [Samuel Louis *Ziegler*, ophthalmologist in Philadelphia, 1861–1926] see under *operation*.

Ziehen's test (ze'henz) [Georg Theodor *Ziehen*, German neurologist, born 1862] see under *tests*.

Ziehen-Oppenheim disease (ze'hen-op'en-hīm) [Georg Theodor *Ziehen*, German neurologist, 1862–1950; Herman *Oppenheim*, German neurologist, 1858–1919] dystonia musculorum deformans.

Ziehl's carbolfuchsin stain, solution (zēlz) [Franz *Ziehl*, German bacteriologist, 1857–1926] carbolfuchsin stain; see *Table of Stains*.

Ziehl-Neelsen carbolfuchsin method, stain (zēl-nēl'senz) [Franz *Ziehl*; German bacteriologist, 1857–1926; Friederich Karl Adolf *Neelsen*, 1854–1894] see *acid-fast stain* and *carbolfuchsin stain* in *Table of Stains*.

Ziemssen's motor points (zēm'senz) [Hugo Wilhelm von *Ziemssen*, physician in Munich, 1829–1902] see under *point*.

zigzagplasty (zig'zag-plas"te) the surgical technique of minimizing the visual impact of a long linear scar by breaking it up into short irregular segments at right or acute angles to each another.

zilantel (zil-an'tel) chemical name: (diethoxyphosphinyl)-carbonimidodithioic acid 1,2-ethanediyl bis(phenylmethyl)ester; an anthelmintic, $C_{26}H_{38}N_2O_6P_2S_4$.

zimelidine hydrochloride (zĭ-mel'ĭ-dēn) chemical name: (Z)-3-(4-bromophenyl)-*N*,*N*-dimethyl-3-(3-pyridinyl-2-propen-1-amine dihydrochloride monohydrate; an antidepressant, $C_{16}H_{17}BrN_2 \cdot 2HCl \cdot H_2O$.

Zimmerlin's atrophy (type) (zim'er-linz) [Franz *Zimmerlin*, Swiss physician, 1858–1932] see under *atrophy*.

Zimmermann's arch, corpuscle (zim'er-mahnz) [Karl Wilhelm *Zimmermann*, German histologist, 1861–1935] see under *arch*, and see *achromocyte*.

Zimmermann's pericyte (zim'er-mahnz) [Karl Wilhelm Bruno *Zimmermann*, Bern anatomist, born 1900] pericyte.

zinc (zingk) [L. *zincum*] a blue-white metal, many of whose salts are used in medicine; symbol, Zn; atomic number, 30; atomic weight, 65.37. Zinc is necessary in trace amounts in the body (and hence in the diet); it forms an essential part of many enzymes (e.g., carbonic anhydrase, important in carbon dioxide metabolism), and plays an important role in protein synthesis and in cell division. Deficiency in zinc is associated with anemia, short stature, hypogonadism, impaired wound healing, and geophagia. Zinc salts are often poisonous when absorbed by the system, producing a chronic poisoning resembling that caused by lead. **z. acetate,** [USP], a salt, $Zn(C_2H_3O_2)_2 \cdot 2H_2O$, produced by the reaction of zinc oxide with acetic acid, used as a pharmaceutic necessity for zinc-eugenol cement and as an astringent, styptic, and formerly as an emetic. **z. carbonate,** a salt, $2Zn-CO_3 \cdot 3Zn(OH)_2$, used as a dusting powder or in the form of a cerate. **z. chloride** [USP], a white, or nearly white, odorless crystalline powder, $ZnCl_2$, used topically as an astringent and desensitizer for dentin. It is also used topically as a caustic antiseptic, and deodorant. **z. hydroxide,** a white powder, $Zn(OH)_2$, an ingredient of medicinal zinc peroxide. **z. iodide,** a white, granular powder, ZnI_2, which has been used as a topical antiseptic and astringent. **z. oxide** [USP], a very fine, odorless, amorphous, white or yellowish white powder, ZnO, used topically as an astringent and protectant in various cutaneous conditions. Called also *white z*. **z. permanganate,** a salt, $Zn(MnO_4)_2 \cdot 6H_2O$, in violet crystals, formerly used in solution as an astringent and antiseptic in the treatment of urethritis. **z. peroxide,** a white to yellowish white odorless powder, ZnO_2, used in pharmaceuticals. **z. peroxide, medicinal,** a mixture of zinc peroxide, zinc carbonate, and zinc hydroxide, used topically in a 40 per cent solution as a local anti-infective and oxidant. It is also used as an astringent and deodorant. **z. phenolsulfonate,** chemical name: *p*-hydroxybenzenesulfonic acid zinc salt. A colorless, crystalline salt, $(HO \cdot C_6H_4 \cdot SO_3)_2Zn \cdot 8H_2O$, formerly used as an antiseptic and astringent, and in the manufacture of insecticides. Called also *z. sulfocarbolate*. **z. pyrithione,** chemical name: bis[1-hydroxy-2(1*H*)-pyridinethionato]zinc. A compound, $C_{10}H_8N_2O_2S_2Zn$, used as an antibacterial, topical antifungal, and antiseborrheic. **z. salicylate,** a salt in colorless crystals, $(C_7H_5O_3)_2Zn \cdot 3H_2O$, which has been used as an antiseptic and astringent. **z. stearate** [USP], a compound of zinc with variable proportions of stearic acid and palmitic acid, containing 12.5 to 14.0 per cent of zinc oxide; used as a dusting powder. **z. sulfanilate,** chemical name: zinc sulfanilate tetrahydrate; an antibacterial, $C_{12}H_{12}N_2O_6S_2Zn \cdot 4H_2O$. **z. sulfate** [USP], the heptahydrate zinc salt of sulfuric acid, $ZnSO_47H_2O$, occurring as colorless, transparent prisms, or small needles; used as an astringent for the mucous membranes, especially for those of the eye, being considered specific for conjunctivitis due to *Haemophilus duplex*. It has also been used in various dermatological preparations, and internally as an antiemetic, especially in the treatment of poisoning. Called also *white vitriol* and *z. vitriol*. **z. sulfocarbolate,** z. phenolsulfonate. **z. undecylenate** [USP], see *undecylenic acid*. **z. vitriol,** z. sulfate. **white z.,** z. oxide.

zincalism (zingk'al-izm) zinc poisoning; symptoms include fever, chills, myalgia, vomiting, headache, and pneumonitis.

zincative (zingk'ah-tiv) electrically negative, i.e., like the zinc in a Daniell cell.

zinciferous (zing-kif'er-us) containing zinc.

zincoid (zing'koid) [L. *zincum* + Gr. *eidos* form] pertaining to or resembling zinc.

zincum (zing'kum), gen. *zin'ci* [L.] zinc.

Zinn's artery, etc. (zinz) [Johann Gottfried *Zinn*, German anatomist, 1727–1759] see *annulus tendineus communis* (for *ligament* and *ring*); *arteria centralis retinae* (for *artery*);

circulus vasculosus nervi optici (for *circle*); *fibrae zonulares* (for *aponeurosis*); and *zonula ciliaris* (for *zone*); and see under *cap.*

Zinsser-Cole-Engman syndrome (zin′ser kōl eng′man) [Ferdinand *Zinsser*, German dermatologist, 1865–1952; Harold Newton *Cole*, American dermatologist, 1884–1966; Martin Feeney *Engman*, American dermatologist, 1869–1953] dyskeratosis congenita.

zinterol hydrochloride (zin′tĕ-rōl) chemical name: *N*-[5-[2-[(1,1,-dimethyl-2-phenylethyl)amino]-1-hydroxyethyl]-2-hydroxyphenyl]methanesulfonamide monohydrochloride; a bronchodilator, $C_{19}H_{26}N_2O_4S \cdot HCl$.

zipp (zip) a paste made by grinding together 1 part of zinc oxide, 2 parts of iodoform, and 2 to 3 parts of liquid paraffin; it is applied to wounds in veterinary surgery.

zirconium (zir-ko′ne-um) a rather rare metallic element; symbol Zr; atomic number, 40; atomic weight, 91.22; chiefly obtained from a mineral called zircon.

zisp (zisp) a modified form of zipp in which zinc peroxide is used in place of zinc oxide.

Zn chemical symbol for zinc.

ZnSO₄ zinc sulfate.

zoacanthosis (zo″ak-an-tho′sis) any dermatitis caused by the retention of animal structures, such as bristles, stings, hairs, etc.

zoanthropic (zo″an-throp′ik) pertaining to or characterized by zoanthropy.

zoanthropy (zo-an′thro-pe) [Gr. *zōon* animal + *anthrōpos* man] the delusion that one has become an animal.

zoescope (zo′ĕ-skōp) [Gr. *zōē* life + *skopein* to examine] stroboscope.

zoetic (zo-et′ik) [Gr. *zōē* life] pertaining to life.

zoetrope (zo′ĕ-trōp) [Gr. *zōē* life + *trepein* to turn] an apparatus which affords pictures of objects apparently moving as in life.

zoic (zo′ik) [Gr. *zōikos* of or proper to animals] pertaining to or characterized by animal life.

zolamine hydrochloride (zo′lah-mēn) chemical name: *N*-[(4-methoxyphenyl)methyl]-*N′*,*N′*-dimethyl-*N*-2-thiazolyl-1,2-ethanediamine monohydrochloride. An antihistaminic with local anesthetic action, $C_{15}H_{21}N_3OS \cdot HCl$, which has been used as a topical anesthetic in the treatment of earache associated with otitis media and in the treatment of hemorrhoids.

Zollinger-Ellison syndrome (zol′lin-jer-el′lǐ-son) [Robert Milton *Zollinger*, American physician, born 1903; Edwin H. *Ellison*, American physician, 1918–1970] see under *syndrome.*

Zöllner's lines (figures) (zel′nerz) [Johann Carl Friedrich *Zöllner*, German physicist, 1834–1882] see under *line.*

Zomax (zo′maks) trademark for preparations of zomepirac sodium.

zomepirac sodium (zo″mĕ-pēr′ak) chemical name: 5-(4-chlorobenzoyl)-1,4-dimethyl-1*H*-pyrrole-2-acetic acid sodium salt dihydrate; an analgesic and anti-inflammatory, $C_{15}H_{13}$-$ClNNaO_3 \cdot 2H_2O$.

zometapine (zo-met′ah-pēn) chemical name: 4-(3-chlorophenyl)-1,6,7,8-tetrahydro-1,3-dimethylpyrazolo[3,4-*e*][1,4]-diazepine; an antidepressant, $C_{14}H_{15}ClN_4$.

zomidin (zo′mǐ-din) [Gr. *zōmos* broth] a constituent of meat extract.

zomotherapy (zo″mo-ther′ah-pe) [Gr. *zōmos* broth + *therapeia* service done to the sick] the treatment of disease by muscle plasma, meat juice, or by meat diet.

zona (zo′nah), pl. *zo′nae* [L. "a girdle"] 1. a zone: an encircling region or area; [NA] a general term for an area with a specific boundary or characteristics. 2. herpes zoster. **z. arcua′ta,** canal of Corti. **z. cartilagin′ea,** limbus laminae spiralis osseae. **z. cilia′ris,** ciliary zone. **z. denticula′ta,** denticulate zone: the inner zone of the lamina basilaris ductus cochlearis with the limbus of the osseous spiral lamina. **z. dermat′ica,** an elevation of thick skin around the protruding mass in spina bifida. **z. epithelioseró′sa,** an area of membranous tissue inside the zona dermatica. **z. fascicula′ta,** fascicular zone: the thick middle layer of the cortex of the suprarenal gland. **z. gangliona′ris,** a mass of ganglion tissue on the pars cochlearis nervi octavi. **z. glomerulo′sa,** glomerular zone:

the thin outer layer of the cortex of the suprarenal gland, which is contiguous with the capsule. **z. granulo′sa,** the peripheral stratified cuboidal epithelium of the ovarian follicle. **z. hemorrhoida′lis,** hemorrhoidal zone: that part of the anal canal extending from the anal valves to the anus and containing the rectal venous plexus; called also *annulus haemorrhoidalis.* **z. incer′ta** [NA], a narrow layer of gray matter extending throughout most of the diencephalon, ventral to and separated from the thalamus by the thalamic fasciculus and laterally continuous with the reticular nucleus of the thalamus. See also *fields of Forel,* under *field.* **z. ophthal′mica,** herpes zoster ophthalmicus. **z. orbicula′ris articulatio′nis cox′ae** [NA], orbicular zone of hip joint: circular fibers of the articular capsule of the hip joint which form a ring around the neck of the femur; they are especially prominent at the inferior and posterior part of the capsule. **z. pectina′ta,** pectinate zone: the outer part of the lamina basilaris ductus cochlearis running from the rods of Corti to the spiral ligament. **z. pellu′cida,** 1. pellucid zone: a thick, transparent, noncellular layer or envelope of uniform thickness surrounding an oocyte; called also *oolemma.* Under the light microscope, it appears as a radially striated layer, which can be seen to be microvillous under the electron microscope, and is therefore called *zona radiata, zona striata,* or *striated membrane.* 2. area pellucida. **z. perfora′ta,** the inner portion of the lamina basilaris ductus cochlearis. **z. radia′ta,** see *Z. pellucida,* def. 1. **z. reticula′ris,** reticular zone: the inner layer of the cortex of the suprarenal gland, consisting of cells arranged as clearly anastomosing cords, and abutting on the medulla. **z. rolan′dica,** the motor area of the cerebral cortex. **z. spongio′sa,** apex cornus posterioris medullae spinalis. **z. stria′ta,** see *z. pellucida,* def. 1. **z. tec′ta,** canal of Corti. **zo′nae tendino′sae cor′dis,** annuli fibrosi cordis. **z. transfor′mans,** transformation zone: the connective tissue layer of the intestinal wall where bacteria penetrating from the intestine are destroyed; called also *Turck's zone.* **z. Valsal′vae,** lamina basilaris ductus cochlearis. **z. vasculo′sa,** vascular zone: a region in the supramastoid fossa containing many foramina for the passage of blood vessels. **z. Web′eri,** z. orbicularis articulationis coxae.

zonae (zo′ne) [L.] genitive and plural of *zona.*

zonal (zo′nal) [L. *zona′lis*] of the nature of a zone.

zonary (zo′ner-e) zonal.

Zondek-Aschheim test (tson′dek-ash′hīm) [Bernhardt *Zondek,* German gynecologist, 1891–1966; Selmar *Aschheim,* German gynecologist, 1878–1965] Aschheim-Zondek test.

zone (zōn) [Gr. *zōnē* a belt, girdle] an encircling region or area; by extension any area with specific characteristics or boundary; called also *zona.* **abdominal z's,** regiones abdominales. Three zones into which the surface of the abdomen is divided by transverse lines. These zones are the *subcostal* or *epigastric*—that above the subcostal line; the *mesogastric*—that between the subcostal and intertubercular lines; and the *hypogastric*—that below the intertubercular line. **androgenic z.,** the provisional cortex of the embryonic suprarenal gland, which is possessed of certain testicular hormonal functions. **anelectrotonic z.,** polar z. **z. of antibody excess,** in a precipitin reaction, the region of relatively high antibody concentration, in which soluble complexes are formed and the reaction is inhibited. Called also *prezone* and *prozone.* **z. of antigen excess,** in a precipitin reaction, the region of relatively high antigen concentration, in which soluble complexes are formed and the reaction is inhibited. Called also *postzone.* **apical z.,** a narrow area along the mucous membrane over the apexes of the roots of the teeth. **arcuate z.,** canal of Corti. **biokinetic z.,** the range of temperatures within which the living cell carries on its life activities, lying approximately between 10° and 45° C. **border z.,** a zone at the boundary of two contiguous structures, as that where the trophoblast and the endometrium meet. **cervical z.,** that third of the coronal zone which is nearest the cervix of the tooth, marked by the cementoenamel junction of crown and root. **ciliary z.,** the outer of the two regions into which the anterior surface of the iris is divided by the angular line. Cf. *pupillary z.* **comfort z.,** an environmental temperature between 13° and 21° C. (55°–70° F.) with a humidity of 30 to 55 per cent. **contact area z.,** the zone which includes the contact area of adjoining teeth; usually it is in the middle third of the coronal zone between the occlusal and the cervical zone. **cornuradicular z.,** the outer part of the fasciculus cuneatus medullae spinalis. **coronal z.,** the entire enamel area of the tooth crown above the cementoenamel junction, the demarcation between crown and root. The coronal zone is subdivided horizontally into three areas; the occlusal zone, the contact area zone, and the cervical zone. These divisions are also spoken of as the occlusal third, the middle third, and the cervical third. **Cozzolino's z.,** fissula ante fenestram. **denticulate z.,** zona denticulata. **dentofacial z.,** the entire lower part of the face; the region of the face overlying the teeth and the alveolar processes of the jaws. **z's of discontinuity,** zones of varying optic density, seen with the slit lamp, in the lens of the eye; these zones are formed at particular periods in the prenatal development of the lens. **dolorogenic z.,** an area stimulation of which produces pain, or excites an attack of neuralgia. **dorsal z. of His,** the smaller upper thickening of the dorsal portion of the embryonic spinal cord projecting into the central canal. **entry z.,** the area of the spinal cord where the dorsal roots enter. **ependymal z.,** see under *layer*. **epigastric z.,** see *abdominal z's*. **epileptogenic z., epileptogenous z.,** an area, stimulation of which may bring on an epileptic attack. **z. of equivalence,** z. of optimal proportions. **erogenous z., erotogenic z.,** a portion of the body, such as the genitals, urethra, lips, anus, and breasts, whose stimulation produces erotic excitation. **z. of exclusion** the area of the cytoplasm devoid of all cytoplasmic components except the Golgi complex. **extravisual z's,** those dioptric surfaces and media outside the visual zone that are practically incapable of accurately focusing light. **fascicular z.,** zona fasciculata. **Flechsig's primordial z's,** the cortex of the ascending frontal gyrus and the ascending parietal gyrus of the brain. **glomerular z.,** zona glomerulosa. **Golgi z.,** the intracellular zone close to the nucleus and containing the Golgi complex; in most secretory cells, it is between the nucleus and the apical surface through which expulsion of the secretion occurs. **Head's z's,** areas of cutaneous sensitiveness associated with diseases of the viscera; called also *z's of hyperalgesia*. **hemorrhoidal z.,** zona hemorrhoidalis. **His's z's,** four thickenings which run the entire length of the embryonic spinal cord. **z's of hyperalgesia,** Head's z's. **hyperesthetic z.,** a region of the body surface marked by abnormal sensibility. **hypogastric z.,** see *abdominal z's*. **hysterogenic z., hysterogenous z.,** a region of the body on which pressure may elicit a hysterical attack. **interpalpebral z.,** the part of the cornea not covered by the eyelids when the eye is open. **keratogenous z.,** the zone immediately above the dome of the dermal papilla, in which the cellular components of a hair follicle undergo keratinization and form the hair shaft. **language z.,** a general term referring to all cortical areas concerned with language mechanisms; usually in the dominant hemisphere. **Lissauer's marginal z.,** tractus dorsolateralis. **Looser's transformation z's,** dark lines seen on roentgenograms of bones, thought to represent pathological healing phases of fatigue fractures occurring in certain bone diseases. **mantle z.,** see under *layer*. **marginal z.,** 1. border zone. 2. see under *layer*. **median root z.,** oval fasciculus. **mesogastric z.,** see *abdominal z's*. **motor z.,** an area of the cortex of the brain which, when electrically stimulated, causes contraction of voluntary muscles. **nephrogenic z.,** the subcapsular layer of the kidney. **neutral z.,** the potential space between the lips and cheeks on one side and the tongue on the other, natural or artificial teeth in this zone being subject to equal and opposite forces from the surrounding musculature. **neutral z. of His,** a thickening of the dorsal portion of the embryonic spinal cord projecting into the central canal. **Nitabuch z.,** see under *layer*. **nuclear z.,** vortex lentis. **Obersteiner-Redlich z.,** see under *area*. **occlusal z.,** that third of the coronal zone of the teeth which is nearest the occlusal plane. **z. of optimal proportions,** in a precipitin reaction, the region of maximal precipitation, the antigen and antibody combining to form a cross-linked lattice. Called also *z. of equivalence*. **orbicular z. of hip joint,** zona orbicularis articulationis coxae. **z. of oval nuclei,** a narrow band of sustentacular cells with oval nuclei in the olfactory mucosa. **pectinate z.,** zona pectinata. **pellucid z.,** zona pellucida. **peripolar z.,** the region surrounding a polar zone. **placental z.,** the area of the uterus to which the placenta is attached. **polar z.,** the region immediately around an electrode applied to the body. **pupillary z.,** the inner of the two regions into which the anterior surface of the iris is divided by the angular line. Cf. *ciliary z.* **reticular z.,** zona reticularis. **Rolando's z.,** the motor area of the cerebral cortex. **root z.,** those parts of the spinal cord to which dorsal and ventral roots are attached. **z. of round nuclei,** a broad band of olfactory cells with round nuclei in the olfactory mucosa. **rugae z.,** see under *area*. **z's of Schreger,** see under *line*. **segmental z.,** a zone of undifferentiated mesoderm between somites already formed and the primitive knot, from which additional somites will be produced. **subcostal z.,** see *abdominal z's*. **sudanophobic z.,** a broad zone of cells which appears in the adrenal cortex of rats following hypophysectomy, and which does not stain with Sudan. **tendinous z's of heart,** annuli fibrosi cordis. **thymus-dependent z.,** see under *area*. **thymus-independent z.,** see under *area*. **transformation z.,** zona transformans. **transition z., transitional z.,** any anatomical region that marks the point at which the constituents of a structure change from one type to another; for example, the circle in the equator of the ocular lens in which epithelial fibers are developed into lens fibers, or the zone (*anocutaneous line*) that marks the junction of stratified squamous epithelium with columnar epithelium. **trigger z.,** dolorogenic z. **Turck's z.,** zona transformans. **umbau z's** [Ger.], Looser's transformation z's. **Valsalva's z.,** lamina basilaris ductus cochlearis. **vascular z.,** zona vasculosa. **visual z.,** those dioptric surfaces and media around an optic axis in which there is practically no aberration of light rays. **Weber's z.,** zona orbicularis articulationis coxae. **Weil's basal z.,** see under *layer*. **Wernicke's z.,** see under *area*. **Westphal's z.,** a zone of the posterior gray column of the spinal cord in the lumbar region; it is said to contain the exodic fibers concerned in the patellar reflex. **X z.,** androgenic z. **z. of Zinn,** zonula ciliaris.

zonesthesia (zo″nes-the′ze-ah) [Gr. *zōnē* girdle + *aisthēsis* perception + *-ia*] a sensation of constriction, as by a girdle.

zonifugal (zo-nif′u-gal) [L. *zona* zone + *fugere* to flee from] passing outward from any area or region.

zoning (zōn′ing) the occurrence of a stronger fixation of complement in a lesser amount of suspected serum.

zonipetal (zo-nip′ĕ-tal) [L. *zona* zone + *petere* to seek] passing from outside into any area or region.

zonoskeleton (zōn″o-skel′ĕ-ton) see *limb*.

zonula (zōn′u-lah), pl. *zon′ulae* [L., dim. of *zona*] a small zone, or zonule. **z. adher′ens,** that portion of the junctional complex of columnar epithelial cells, just deep to the zonula occludens, where the cell membranes diverge to form an intercellular space 150 to 200 Å wide and are supported on their inner aspect by moderately dense filamentous material forming a continuous band parallel to the zonula occludens. **z. cilia′ris** [NA], **z. cilia′ris** [Zin′nii], ciliary zonule: a system of fibers extending between the ciliary body and the equator of the lens, holding the lens in place; called also *Zinn's membrane*, or *tendon* or *zonule of Zinn*. **z. occlu′dens,** that portion of the junctional complex of columnar epithelial cells, just beneath the free surface, where the intercellular space is obliterated; it extends completely around the cell perimeter, above the zonula adherens. Called also *tight junction*.

zonulae (zon′u-le) [L.] genitive and plural of *zonula*.

zonular (zon′u-lar) pertaining to a zonule.

zonule (zōn′ul) a small zone; called also *zonula*. **ciliary z.,** zonula ciliaris. **lens z.,** zonula ciliaris. **z. of Zinn,** zonula ciliaris.

zonulitis (zōn″u-li′tis) inflammation of the ciliary zonule.

zonulolysis (zon″u-lol′i-sis) [*zonule* + *lysis*] dissolution of the zonule of Zinn (zonula ciliaris) in surgery by means of enzymes such as alpha-chymotrypsin.

zonulotomy (zon″u-lot′o-me) [*zonule* + *-tomy*] incision of the ciliary zonule.

zonulysis (zon″u-li′sis) zonulolysis.

zo(o)- [Gr. *zōon* animal] a combining form denoting relationship to an animal.

zoo-agglutinin (zo″o-ah-gloo′tĭ-nin) a substance in animal poisons having the power of agglutinating red blood cells.

zooamylon (zo″o-am′ĭ-lon) [*zoo-* + Gr. *amylon* starch] (*obs.*) glycogen.

zoobiology (zo″o-bi-ol′o-je) [zoo- + Gr. *bios* life + -*logy*] the biology of animals.

zoobiotism (zo″o-bi′o-tizm) biotics.

zooblast (zo′o-blast) [zoo- + Gr. *blastos* germ] an animal cell.

zoochemical (zo″o-kem′ĭ-kal) pertaining to zoochemistry.

zoochemistry (zo″o-kem′is-tre) the study of the chemical reactions occurring in animal tissues.

zoodermic (zo″o-der′mik) [zoo- + Gr. *derma* skin] performed with the skin of an animal; said of skin grafting in which the grafts are from the skin of an animal.

zoodetritus (zo″o-de-tri′tus) biodetritus produced by the disintegration and decomposition of animal organisms. Cf. *phytodetritus.*

zoodynamic (zo″o-di-nam′ik) pertaining to zoodynamics (animal physiology).

zoodynamics (zo″o-di-nam′iks) [zoo- + Gr. *dynamis* power] animal physiology.

zooerastia (zo″o-e-ras′te-ah) [zoo- + Gr. *erastēs* lover] bestiality.

zooflagellate (zo″o-flaj′ĕ-lāt) [zoo- + L. *flagellum* whip] an animal-like flagellate protozoan of the class Zoomastigophorea. Cf. *phytoflagellate.*

zoofulvin (zo″o-ful′vin) a yellow pigment from the feathers of certain birds.

zoogenesis (zo″o-jen′ĕ-sis) zoogeny.

zoogenous (zo-oj′ĕ-nus) 1. acquired from animals. 2. viviparous.

zoogeny (zo-oj′ĕ-ne) [zoo- + Gr. *gennan* to produce] the development and evolution of animals.

zoogeography (zo″o-je-og′rah-fe) the study of the distribution of animal life on the earth.

zooglea (zo″o-gle′ah), pl. *zoogle′ae* [zoo- + Gr. *gloios* gum] 1. any microorganism of the genus *Zoogloea.* 2. (*obs.*) a colony of bacteria embedded in a jelly-like mass. Called also *zoogloea.*

zoogleal (zo″o-gle′al) pertaining to or characterized by the presence of zooglea.

Zoogloea (zo″o-gle′ah) a genus of gram-negative, aerobic, rod-shaped bacteria of the family Pseudomonadaceae, occurring in gelatinous macroscopic flocs, and found in water and sewage.

zoogloea (zo″o-gle′ah) zooglea.

zoogonous (zo-og′o-nus) viviparous.

zoogony (zo-og′o-ne) [zoo- + Gr. *gonē* offspring] the production of living young from within the body.

zoografting (zo′o-graft″ing) the grafting of animal tissue.

zoography (zo-og′rah-fe) [zoo- + Gr. *graphein* to write] a treatise on animals.

zoohormone (zo″o-hor′mōn) an animal hormone.

zooid (zo′oid) [zoo- + Gr. *eidos* form] 1. resembling an animal. 2. an object or form which resembles an animal. 3. one of the individuals in a united colony of animals. See *blastozooid* and *oozooid.*

zoolagnia (zo″o-lag′ne-ah) [zoo- + Gr. *lagneia* lust] sexual attraction toward animals.

zoology (zo-ol′o-je) [zoo- + Gr. *logos* treatise] the biology of animals; the sum of what is known regarding animals. **experimental z.,** the study of animals by means of experiments performed upon them.

zoomania (zo″o-ma′ne-ah) [zoo- + Gr. *mania* madness] an abnormal love of animals.

Zoomastigophora (zo″o-mas″tĭ-gof′o-rah) Zoomastigophorea.

Zoomastigophorea (zo″o-mas″tĭ-gof′o-re′ah) [zoo- + Gr. *mastix* whip + *phōros* bearing] a class comprising all of the animal-like, as opposed to plantlike, protozoa (subphylum Mastigophora, phylum Sarcomastigophora), collectively called zooflagellates. Zoomastigophoreans lack chromatophores and are heterotrophic, and most are either commensal or parasitic. They have one to many flagella and some are capable of ameboid movement with or without flagella. It comprises one superorder, Parabasilidea, and six orders: Choanoflagellida, Kinetoplastida, Proteromonadina, Retortamonadida, Diplomonadida, and Oxymonadida. Cf. *Phytomastigophorea.*

zoomastigophorean (zo″o-mas″tĭ-gof″o-re′an) a protozoan of the class Zoomastigophorea.

Zoon's erythroplasia (zōnz) [Johannes Jacobus *Zoon,* Dutch dermatologist, born 1902] balanitis circumscripta plasmacellularis.

zoonerythrin (zo″on-er′ĭ-thrin) [zoo- + Gr. *erythros* red] crustaceorubin.

zoonite (zo′o-nīt) a cerebrospinal metamere.

zoonomy (zo-on′o-me) [zoo- + Gr. *nomos* law] zoobiology.

zoonoses (zo″o-no′sēz) plural of *zoonosis.*

zoonosis (zo″o-no′sis, zo-on′ĕ-sis), pl. *zoono′ses* [zoo- + Gr. *nosos* disease] a disease of animals that may be transmitted to man under natural conditions (e.g., brucellosis, rabies).

zoonosology (zo″o-no-sol′o-je) [zoo- + Gr. *nosos* disease + *logos* treatise] the classification of diseases of animals.

zoonotic (zo″o-not′ik) transmissible from animals to man under natural conditions; pertaining to or constituting a zoonosis.

zooparasite (zo″o-par′ah-sīt) any parasitic animal organism or species; see *animal parasite,* under *parasite.*

zooparasitic (zo″o-par″ah-sit′ik) pertaining to or produced by zooparasites.

zoopathology (zo″o-pah-thol′o-je) animal pathology; the study of the diseases of animals.

zooperal (zo-op′er-al) pertaining to zoopery.

zoopery (zo-op′er-e) [zoo- + Gr. *peiran* to experiment] the performing of experiments on animals.

zoophagous (zo-of′ah-gus) [zoo- + Gr. *phagein* to eat] subsisting upon animal food.

zoopharmacology (zo″o-fahr″mah-kol′o-je) veterinary pharmacology.

zoopharmacy (zo-o-fahr′mah-se) veterinary pharmacy.

zoophile (zo′o-fīl) [zoo- + Gr. *philein* to love] 1. zoophilic. 2. an antivivisectionist.

zoophilia (zo″o-fil′e-ah) 1. abnormal fondness for animals. 2. [DSM III] a paraphilia in which intercourse or other sexual activity with animals is the preferred method of achieving sexual excitement.

zoophilic (zo″o-fil′ik) preferring animals to man; said of certain mosquitoes. Cf. *anthropophilic* and *anthropozoophilic.*

zoophilism (zo-of′ĭ-lizm) 1. fondness for animals; antivivisection. 2. the state of being zoophilic. **erotic z.,** sexual pleasure experienced in the fondling of animals.

zoophilous (zo-of′ĭ-lus) zoophilic.

zoophobia (zo″o-fo′be-ah) [zoo- + *phobia*] irrational fear of animals.

zoophysiology (zo″o-fiz″e-ol′o-je) animal physiology.

zoophyte (zo′o-fīt) [zoo- + Gr. *phyton* plant] any plantlike animal, such as sponges or hydroids.

zooplankton (zo″o-plank′ton) [zoo- + Gr. *planktos* wandering] the minute animal organisms which, with those of the vegetable kingdom (phytoplankton), make up the plankton of natural waters.

zooplasty (zo′o-plast″te) [zoo- + Gr. *plassein* to form] zoografting.

zooprecipitin (zo″o-pre-sip′ĭ-tin) a precipitin obtained by injections of protein substances of animal origin.

zooprophylaxis (zo″o-pro″fi-lak′sis) 1. prophylaxis applied to animals; veterinary prophylaxis. 2. the prevention or amelioration of disease (e.g., smallpox) in man as a result of previous exposure to heterologous infection of animal origin (e.g., cowpox). 3. protection of man from bites of mosquitoes by providing cattle or other animals for the mosquitoes to feed on.

zoopsia (zo-op′se-ah) [zoo- + Gr. *opsis* vision + -*ia*] a hallucination in which the patient thinks he sees animals.

zoopsychology (zo″o-si-kol′o-je) animal psychology.

zoosadism (zo″o-sa′dizm) sadism directed toward animals.

zoosis (zo-o′sis) [zoo- + -*osis*] any disease due to animal agents.

zoosperm (zo′o-sperm) [zoo- + Gr. *sperma* seed] spermatozoon.

zoospermia (zo″o-sper′me-ah) the presence of live spermatozoa in the ejaculated semen.

zoosporangia (zo″o-spo-ran′je-ah) plural of *zoosporangium.*

zoosporangium (zo″o-spo-ran′je-um), pl. *zoosporan′gia* [*zoo-* + Gr. *angeion* vessel] the structure in which zoospores are developed. See *spore.*

zoospore (zo′o-spōr) [*zoo-* + *spore*] a motile spore, such as an asexual flagellate of certain algae and lower fungi, or a minute sexual or asexual flagellate or ameboid spore produced by certain protozoa.

zoosteroid (zo″o-ste′roid) any steroid of animal origin.

zoosterol (zo″o-ste′rol) any sterol of animal origin.

zootechnics (zo″o-tek′niks) [*zoo-* + Gr. *technē* art] the art of breeding, keeping, and handling animals in domestication or captivity.

zootic (zo-ot′ik) pertaining to the lower animals. Cf. *demic.*

zootomist (zo-ot′o-mist) a comparative anatomist.

zootomy (zo-ot′o-me) [*zoo-* + Gr. *tomē* a cutting] 1. the dissection of animals. 2. the anatomy of animals.

zootoxin (zo″o-tok′sin) [*zoo-* + Gr. *toxikon* poison] a toxic substance of animal origin, such as the venoms of snakes, spiders, and scorpions.

zootrophic (zo″o-trof′ik) [*zoo-* + Gr. *trophē* nutrition] pertaining to the nutrition of animals.

zootrophotoxism (zo″o-trof″o-tok′sizm) [*zoo-* + Gr. *trophē* nutrition + *toxikon* poison] poisoning with animal foods.

zooxanthella (zo″o-zan-thel′ah), pl. *zooxanthel′lae* [*zoo-* + Gr. *xanthos* yellow] minute, photosynthetic, yellow-brown or yellow-green unicellular marine organisms, considered by some to be algae and by others a stage of certain dinoflagellates, living endosymbiotically with certain marine invertebrates, such as corals and certain marine planktonic protozoa.

zooxanthellae (zo″o-zan-thel′e) plural of *zooxanthella.*

Zopfius (zop′fe-us) in former systems of classification, a genus of bacteria made up of organisms now classified as *Kurthia.*

zorbamycin (zor-bah-mi′sin) an antibacterial antibiotic derived from a variant of *Streptomyces bikiniensis.*

zorubicin hydrochloride (zo-ru′bǐ-sin) chemical name: (2S-*cis*)-benzoic acid[1-[4-[(3-amino-2,3,6-trideoxy-α-L-lyxo-hexopyranosyl)oxy]-1,2,3,4,6,11-hexahydro-2,5,12-trihydroxy-7-methoxy-6,11-dioxo-2-naphthacenyl]ethylidene]hydrazide; an antineoplastic, $C_{34}H_{35}N_3O_{10} \cdot HCl$.

zoster (zos′ter) [Gr. *zōstēr* a girdle] herpes zoster. **z. si′ne eruptio′ne, z. si′ne her′pete,** pain typical of herpes zoster in an appropriate sensory area but not followed by the development of characteristic lesions. **ophthalmic z.,** herpes zoster ophthalmicus.

Zostera marina (zos′ter-ah mah-ri′nah) seawrack or eelgrass, a marine plant.

zosteriform (zos-ter′ǐ-form) resembling herpes zoster.

zosteroid (zos′ter-oid) resembling herpes zoster.

Zovirax (zo′vir-aks) trademark for preparations of acyclovir.

zoxazolamine (zok″sah-zol′ah-mēn) chemical name: 2-amino-5-chlorobenzoxazole. A plate-like substance, $C_7H_{15}Cl-N_2O$, occasionally used as a skeletal muscle relaxant and uricosuric agent in gout.

Z-plasty (ze-plas′te) a plastic operation for the relaxation of contractures, in which a Z-shaped incision is made, the middle bar of the Z being over the contracted scar, and the triangular flaps rotated so that their apices cross the line of contracture.

Zr chemical symbol for *zirconium.*

Zsigmondy's gold number method, test (sig-mon′dēz) [Richard Adolf *Zsigmondy*, German chemist, 1865–1929; winner of the Nobel prize in chemistry for 1925, for his work on colloids; inventor of the ultramicroscope in 1903] colloidal gold test.

Zuberella (zu″ber-el′ah) in former systems of classification, a genus of bacteria made up of organisms now classified in the genera *Bacteroides* and *Fusobacterium.*

zuckergussdarm (tsook′er-goos″darm) [Ger. "sugar-icing intestine"] peritonitis chronica fibrosa encapsulans.

zuckergussleber (tsook′er-goos″la-ber) [Ger. "sugar-icing liver"] perihepatitis chronica hyperplastica.

Zuckerkandl's body, convolution, gland, organs

(tsook′er-kan″d'lz) [Emil *Zuckerkandl*, German anatomist, 1849–1910] see under *body, gland,* and *organ,* and see *gyrus paraterminalis.*

zuclomiphene (zoo-klo′mǐ-fēn) chemical name: (Z)-2-[4-(2-chloro-1,2-diphenylethenyl)phenoxy]-N,N-diethylethanamine; the *trans*-isomer of the gonad-stimulating principle clomiphene citrate (q.v.), $C_{26}H_{28}ClNO$. Called also *transclomiphene.* Cf. *enclomiphene.*

Zumbusch's psoriasis (tsoom′bushs) [Leo von *Zumbusch*] generalized pustular psoriasis.

Zuntz's theory (zoont′zes) [Nathan *Zuntz*, Berlin physician, 1847–1920] see under *theory.*

zwieback (tsve′bak) pieces of bread made of rich dough and heated in the oven until they are deep yellow in color.

Zwischenferment (tsvish″en-fer′ment) glucose 6-phosphate dehydrogenase.

zwitterion (tsvit′er-i″on) a dipolar ion, i.e., an ion that has both positive and negative regions of charge; amino acids, for example, occur as zwitterions in neutral solution, and the pH value at which the zwitterion state is at a maximum is the isoelectric point.

zwölffingerdarm (tsvelf-fing′ger-darm) [Ger. *zwölf* twelve + *finger* finger + *darm* bowel] the duodenum.

zygadenine (zi-gad′ě-nin) a crystalline alkaloid, $C_{39}H_{63}-NO_{10}$, from the plant *Zygadenus intermedius.*

zygal (zi′gal) [Gr. *zygon* yoke] shaped like a yoke.

zygapophyseal (zi″gah-po-fiz′e-al) pertaining to an articular process of a vertebra (zygapophysis).

zygapophysis (zi″gah-pof′ǐ-sis), pl. *zygapoph′yses.* An articular process of a vertebra; see *processus articularis inferior vertebrarum* (z. *inferior* [NA alternative]) and *processus articularis superior vertebrarum* (z. *superior* [NA alternative]).

zygia (zij′e-ah) plural of *zygion.*

zygion (zij′e-on), pl. *zyg′ia* [Gr.] a craniometric and cephalometric landmark, being the most laterally situated point on either zygomatic arch.

zyg(o)- [Gr. *zygon* yoke] a combining form meaning yoked or joined, or denoting relationship to a junction.

Zygocotyle lunatum (zi″go-ko′tǐ-le lu-na′tum) a trematode parasitic in the intestine of a variety of hosts, including rats, cattle, and ducks in North America.

zygocyte (zi′go-sīt) see *zygote.*

zygodactyly (zi″go-dak′tǐ-le) [*zygo-* + Gr. *daktylos* finger] a term sometimes used to designate simple syndactyly, as distinguished from syndactyly in which there is bony fusion between the phalanges of the digits involved; usually occurring in the hand between the third and fourth digits, and in the foot between the fourth and fifth.

zygoite (zi′go-īt) an organism formed by zygosis; a zygote.

zygoma (zi-go′mah) [Gr. *zygōma* bolt or bar] 1. processus zygomaticus temporalis. 2. arcus zygomaticus. 3. a term sometimes applied to os zygomaticum.

zygomatic (zi″go-mat′ik) pertaining to the zygoma.

zygomaticofacial (zi″go-mat″ǐ-ko-fa′shal) pertaining to the zygoma and the face.

zygomaticofrontal (zi″go-mat″ǐ-ko-fron′tal) pertaining to the zygoma and the frontal bone.

zygomaticomaxillary (zi″go-mat″ǐ-ko-mak′sǐ-ler″e) pertaining to the zygoma and the maxilla.

zygomatico-orbital (zi″go-mat″ǐ-ko-or′bǐ-tal) pertaining to the zygoma and the orbit.

zygomaticosphenoid (zi″go-mat″ǐ-ko-sfe′noid) pertaining to the zygoma and the sphenoid bone.

zygomaticotemporal (zi″go-mat″ǐ-ko-tem′por-al) pertaining to the zygoma and the temporal bone.

zygomaxillare (zi″go-mak′sǐ-la″re) [L.] a craniometric point at the lower end of the zygomatic suture.

zygomaxillary (zi″go-mak′sǐ-ler″e) pertaining to the zygoma and the maxilla.

Zygomycetes (zi″go-mi-se′tēz) a subclass of phycomycetous fungi, including the orders Mucorales and Entomophthorales.

zygon (zi′gon) [Gr.] the bar or stem connecting the two branches of a zygal fissure.

zygopodium (zi″go-po′de-um) see *limb.*

zygosis (zi-go′sis) [Gr. *zygōsis* a balancing] conjugation; the sexual union of two unicellular organisms.

zygosity (zi-gos′ĭ-te) [Gr. *zygon* yoke + *-ity* state or condition] the condition relating to conjugation, or to the zygote, as (*a*) the state of a cell or individual in regard to the alleles determining a specific character, whether identical (homozygosity) or different (heterozygosity); or (*b*), in the case of twins, whether developing from one zygote (monozygosity) or two (dizygosity). Often used as a word termination affixed to a root descriptive of the condition.

zygosperm (zi′go-sperm) zygospore.

zygosphere (zi′go-sfēr) a gamete arising from a zygophore which unites with another to form a zygospore.

zygospore (zi′go-spōr) a spore formed by the conjugation of two cells (isogametes) which are morphologically identical, or in the Zygomycetes, from the fusion of like gametangia. See *spore*.

zygostyle (zi′go-stīl) the last coccygeal vertebra.

zygote (zi′gōt) [Gr. *zygōtos* yoked together] the cell resulting from union of a male and a female gamete, until it divides; the fertilized ovum. More precisely, the cell after synapsis at the completion of fertilization until first cleavage. Also, used loosely to refer to the fertilized ovum and derivatives for an indefinite period, extending even to birth. Cf. *conceptus*.

zygotene (zi′go-tēn) [Gr. *zygōtos* yoked together] the synaptic stage of the first meiotic prophase in which the two leptotene chromosomes undergo pairing by the formation of synaptonemal complexes to form a bivalent structure. See also *diplotene, leptotene,* and *pachytene.* Called also *amphitene.*

zygotic (zi-got′ik) pertaining to a zygote.

zylonite (zi′lo-nīt) [Gr. *xylon* wood] xylonite.

Zyloprim (zi′lo-prim) trademark for a preparation of allopurinol.

zymase (zi′mās) [Gr. *zymē* leaven + *-ase*] 1. an enzyme. 2. the intracellular enzymes of yeast by which alcoholic fermentation is produced; called also *Buchner's z.*

zymasis (zi′mah-sis) the excretion of the active substance of yeast by hydraulic pressure.

zyme (zīm) [Gr. *zymē* leaven] enzyme.

zymin (zi′min) zyme.

zym(o)- [Gr. *zymē* leaven] a combining form denoting relationship to an enzyme, or to fermentation.

zymochemistry (zi″mo-kem′is-tre) the chemistry of fermentation.

zymogen (zi′mo-jen) proenzyme.

zymogenic (zi″mo-jen′ik) 1. causing a fermentation. 2. pertaining to a fermentation.

zymogenous (zi-moj′ĕ-nus) zymogenic.

zymogic (zi-moj′ik) zymogenic.

zymoid (zi′moid) [*zymo-* + Gr. *eidos* form] 1. resembling an enzyme. 2. any poison derived from a decaying tissue that has lost its power of decomposing the substratum, but not its power of uniting with it.

Zymomonas (zi″mo-mo′nas) [*zyme* + Gr. *monas* unit, from *monos* single] a genus of facultatively anaerobic, gram-negative, rod-shaped bacteria that are motile with polar flagella, occurring as a spoiler in beer and cider, as fermenting agents in plant saps, on bees, and in ripening honey. The type species is *Z. mo′bilis.*

Zymonema (zi″mo-ne′mah) [*zymo-* + Gr. *nēma* thread] a name formerly given a genus of fungi. **Z. al′bicans,** *Candida albicans.* **Z. capsula′tum, Z. dermatit′idis, Z. gilchris′ti,** *Blastomyces dermatitidis.* **Z. farcimino′sum,** *Histoplasma farciminosus.*

zymophosphate (zi″mo-fos′fāt) hexosephosphoric acid occurring in yeast; it may accumulate in large amounts.

zymosan (zi′mo-san) a mixture of polysaccharides, proteins, and ash, of variable concentration, derived from the cell walls, or the entire cell, of yeast, commonly *Saccharomyces cerevisiae.* It is anticomplementary, absorbing the C3 component of complement, and is used in assaying properdin.

zymoscope (zi′mo-skōp) [*zymo-* + Gr. *skopein* to examine] an apparatus for determining the zymotic (fermentative) power of yeast.

zymosterol (zi-mos′ter-ol) mycosterol; a sterol, $C_{27}H_{44}O$, occurring in fungi and molds, which is second to ergosterol in abundance in yeast fat.

Zz. abbreviation for L. *zin′giber,* ginger.

Z.Z.′Z.″ increasing degrees of contraction.

Appendices

1. CELSIUS (CENTIGRADE) AND FAHRENHEIT TEMPERATURE EQUIVALENTS

CELSIUS—FAHRENHEIT

°C	°F	°C	°F	°C	°F
−40	−40.0	9	48.2	58	136.4
−39	−38.2	10	50.0	59	138.2
−38	−36.4	11	51.8	60	140.0
−37	−34.6	12	53.6	61	141.8
−36	−32.8	13	55.4	62	143.6
−35	−31.0	14	57.2	63	145.4
−34	−29.2	15	59.0	64	147.2
−33	−27.4	16	60.8	65	149.0
−32	−25.6	17	62.6	66	150.8
−31	−23.8	18	64.4	67	152.6
−30	−22.0	19	66.2	68	154.4
−29	−20.2	20	68.0	69	156.2
−28	−18.4	21	69.8	70	158.0
−27	−16.6	22	71.6	71	159.8
−26	−14.8	23	73.4	72	161.6
−25	−13.0	24	75.2	73	163.4
−24	−11.2	25	77.0	74	165.2
−23	−9.4	26	78.8	75	167.0
−22	−7.6	27	80.6	76	168.8
−21	−5.8	28	82.4	77	170.6
−20	−4.0	29	84.2	78	172.4
−19	−2.2	30	86.0	79	174.2
−18	−0.4	31	87.8	80	176.0
−17	+1.4	32	89.6	81	177.8
−16	3.2	33	91.4	82	179.6
−15	5.0	34	93.2	83	181.4
−14	6.8	35	95.0	84	183.2
−13	8.6	36	96.8	85	185.0
−12	10.4	37	98.6	86	186.8
−11	12.2	38	100.4	87	188.6
−10	14.0	39	102.2	88	190.4
−9	15.8	40	104.0	89	192.2
−8	17.6	41	105.8	90	194.0
−7	19.4	42	107.6	91	195.8
−6	21.2	43	109.4	92	197.6
−5	23.0	44	111.2	93	199.4
−4	24.8	45	113.0	94	201.2
−3	26.6	46	114.8	95	203.0
−2	28.4	47	116.6	96	204.8
−1	30.2	48	118.4	97	206.6
0	32.0	49	120.2	98	208.4
+1	33.8	50	122.0	99	210.2
2	35.6	51	123.8	100	212.0
3	37.4	52	125.6	101	213.8
4	39.2	53	127.4	102	215.6
5	41.0	54	129.2	103	217.4
6	42.8	55	131.0	104	219.2
7	44.6	56	132.8	105	221.0
8	46.4	57	134.6	106	222.8

FAHRENHEIT—CELSIUS

°F	°C	°F	°C	°F	°C
−40	−40	55	12.7	146	63.3
−39	−39.4	60	15.5	147	63.8
−38	−38.9	65	18.3	148	64.4
−37	−38.3	70	21.1	149	65.0
−36	−37.8	75	23.8	150	65.5
−35	−37.2	80	26.6	151	66.1
−34	−36.7	85	29.4	152	66.6
−33	−36.1	86	30.0	153	67.2
−32	−35.6	87	30.5	154	67.7
−31	−35.0	88	31.0	155	68.3
−30	−34.4	89	31.6	156	68.8
−29	−33.9	90	32.2	157	69.4
−28	−33.3	91	32.7	158	70.0
−27	−32.8	92	33.3	159	70.5
−26	−32.2	93	33.8	160	71.1
−25	−31.7	94	34.4	161	71.6
−24	−31.1	95	35.0	162	72.2
−23	−30.6	96	35.5	163	72.7
−22	−30.0	97	36.1	164	73.3
−21	−29.4	98	36.6	165	73.8
−20	−28.9	98.6	37.0	166	74.4
−19	−28.3	99	37.2	167	75.0
−18	−27.8	100	37.7	168	75.5
−17	−27.2	101	38.3	169	76.1
−16	−26.7	102	38.8	170	76.6
−15	−26.1	103	39.4	171	77.2
−14	−25.6	104	40.0	172	77.7
−13	−25.0	105	40.5	173	78.3
−12	−24.4	106	41.1	174	78.8
−11	−23.9	107	41.6	175	79.4
−10	−23.3	108	42.2	176	80.0
−9	−22.8	109	42.7	177	80.5
−8	−22.2	110	43.3	178	81.1
−7	−21.7	111	43.8	179	81.6
−6	−21.1	112	44.4	180	82.2
−5	−20.6	113	45.0	181	82.7
−4	−20.0	114	45.5	182	83.3
−3	−19.4	115	46.1	183	83.8
−2	−18.9	116	46.6	184	84.4
−1	−18.3	117	47.2	185	85.0
0	−17.8	118	47.7	186	85.5
+1	−17.2	119	48.3	187	86.1
5	−15.0	120	48.8	188	86.6
10	−12.2	121	49.4	189	87.2
15	−9.4	122	50.0	190	87.7
20	−6.6	123	50.5	191	88.3
25	−3.8	124	51.1	192	88.8
30	−1.1	125	51.6	193	89.4
31	−0.5	126	52.2	194	90.0
32	0	127	52.7	195	90.5
33	+0.5	128	53.3	196	91.1
34	1.1	129	53.8	197	91.6
35	1.6	130	54.4	198	92.2
36	2.2	131	55.0	199	92.7
37	2.7	132	55.5	200	93.3
38	3.3	133	56.1	201	93.8
39	3.8	134	56.6	202	94.4
40	4.4	135	57.2	203	95.0
41	5.0	136	57.7	204	95.5
42	5.5	137	58.3	205	96.1
43	6.1	138	58.8	206	96.6
44	6.6	139	59.4	207	97.2
45	7.2	140	60.0	208	97.7
46	7.7	141	60.5	209	98.3
47	8.3	142	61.1	210	98.8
48	8.8	143	61.6	211	99.4
49	9.4	144	62.2	212	100.0
50	10.0	145	62.7	213	100.5

2. MULTIPLES AND SUBMULTIPLES OF THE METRIC SYSTEM

MULTIPLES AND SUBMULTIPLES		PREFIX	SYMBOL
1,000,000,000,000	(10^{12})	tera-	T
1,000,000,000	(10^9)	giga-	G
1,000,000	(10^6)	mega-	M
1,000	(10^3)	kilo-	k
100	(10^2)	hecto-	h
10	(10)	deka-	da
0.1	(10^{-1})	deci-	d
0.01	(10^{-2})	centi-	c
0.001	(10^{-3})	milli-	m
0.000 001	(10^{-6})	micro-	μ
0.000 000 001	(10^{-9})	nano-	n
0.000 000 000 001	(10^{-12})	pico-	p
0.000 000 000 000 001	(10^{-15})	femto-	f
0.000 000 000 000 000 001	(10^{-18})	atto-	a

3. TABLES OF WEIGHTS AND MEASURES

MEASURES OF MASS

AVOIRDUPOIS WEIGHT

GRAINS	DRAMS	OUNCES	POUNDS	METRIC EQUIVALENTS (grams)
1	0.0366	0.0023	0.00014	0.0647989
27.34	1	0.0625	0.0039	1.772
437.5	16	1	0.0625	28.350
7000	256	16	1	453.5924277

APOTHECARIES' WEIGHT

GRAINS	SCRUPLES (℈)	DRAMS (ℨ)	OUNCES (℥)	POUNDS (℔)	METRIC EQUIVALENTS (grams)
1	0.05	0.0167	0.0021	0.00017	0.0647989
20	1	0.333	0.042	0.0035	1.296
60	3	1	0.125	0.0104	3.888
480	24	8	1	0.0833	31.103
5760	288	96	12	1	373.24177

METRIC WEIGHT

MICRO-GRAM	MILLI-GRAM	CENTI-GRAM	DECI-GRAM	GRAM	DECA-GRAM	HECTO-GRAM	KILO-GRAM	METRIC TON	EQUIVALENTS Avoirdupois	Apothecaries'
1	—	—	—	—	—	—	—	—	0.000015 gr	
10^3	1	—	—	—	—	—	—	—	0.015432 gr	
10^4	10	1	—	—	—	—	—	—	0.154323 gr	
10^5	100	10	1	—	—	—	—	—	1.543235 gr	
10^6	1000	100	10	1	—	—	—	—	15.432356 gr	
10^7	10^4	1000	100	10	1	—	—	—	5.6438 dr	7.7162 scr
10^8	10^5	10^4	1000	100	10	1	—	—	3.527 oz	3.215 oz
10^9	10^6	10^5	10^4	1000	100	10	1	—	2.2046 lb	2.6792 lb
10^{12}	10^9	10^8	10^7	10^6	10^5	10^4	1000	1	2204.6223 lb	2679.2285 lb

TROY WEIGHT

GRAINS	PENNYWEIGHTS	OUNCES	POUNDS	METRIC EQUIVALENTS (grams)
1	0.042	0.002	0.00017	0.0647989
24	1	0.05	0.0042	1.555
480	20	1	0.083	31.103
5760	240	12	1	373.24177

MEASURES OF CAPACITY

APOTHECARIES' (WINE) MEASURE

| MINIMS | FLUID DRAMS | FLUID OUNCES | GILLS | PINTS | QUARTS | GALLONS | EQUIVALENTS | | |
							Cubic Inches	Milliliters	Cubic Centimeters
1	0.0166	0.002	0.0005	0.00013	—	—	0.00376	0.06161	0.06161
60	1	0.125	0.0312	0.0078	0.0039	—	0.22558	3.6967	3.6967
480	8	1	0.25	0.0625	0.0312	0.0078	1.80468	29.5737	29.5737
1920	32	4	1	0.25	0.125	0.0312	7.21875	118.2948	118.2948
7680	128	16	4	1	0.5	0.125	28.875	473.179	473.179
15360	256	32	8	2	1	0.25	57.75	946.358	946.358
61440	1024	128	32	8	4	1	231	3785.434	3785.434

METRIC MEASURE

MICRO- LITER	MILLI- LITER	CENTI- LITER	DECI- LITER	LITER	DEKA- LITER	HECTO- LITER	KILO- LITER	MEGA- LITER	EQUIVALENTS (Apothecaries' Fluid)
1	—	—	—	—	—	—	—	—	0.01623108 min
10^3	1	—	—	—	—	—	—	—	16.23 min
10^4	10	1	—	—	—	—	—	—	2.7 fl dr
10^5	100	10	1	—	—	—	—	—	3.38 fl oz
10^6	10^3	100	10	1	—	—	—	—	2.11 pts
10^7	10^4	10^3	100	10	1	—	—	—	2.64 gal
10^8	10^5	10^4	10^3	100	10	1	—	—	26.418 gals
10^9	10^6	10^5	10^4	10^3	100	10	1	—	264.18 gals
10^{12}	10^9	10^8	10^7	10^6	10^5	10^4	10^3	1	26418 gals

1 liter = 2.113363738 pints (Apothecaries')

MEASURES OF LENGTH

METRIC MEASURE

MICRO- METER	MILLI- METER	CENTI- METER	DECI- METER	METER	DEKA- METER	HECTO- METER	KILO- METER	MEGA- METER	EQUIVALENTS
1	0.001	10^{-4}	—	—	—	—	—	—	0.000039 inch
10^3	1	10^{-1}	—	—	—	—	—	—	0.03937 inch
10^4	10	1	—	—	—	—	—	—	0.3937 inch
10^5	100	10	1	—	—	—	—	—	3.937 inches
10^6	1000	100	10	1	—	—	—	—	39.37 inches
10^7	10^4	1000	100	10	1	—	—	—	10.9361 yards
10^8	10^5	10^4	1000	100	10	1	—	—	109.3612 yards
10^9	10^6	10^5	10^4	1000	1000	10	1	—	1093.6121 yards
10^{10}	10^7	10^6	10^5	10^4	1000	100	10	—	6.2137 miles
10^{12}	10^9	10^8	10^7	10^6	10^5	10^4	1000	1	621.370 miles

CONVERSION TABLES

AVOIRDUPOIS—METRIC WEIGHTS

OUNCES	GRAMS	OUNCES	GRAMS	POUNDS	GRAMS	KILOGRAMS
1/16	1.772	7	198.447	1 (16 oz)	453.59	
1/8	3.544	8	226.796	2	907.18	
1/4	7.088	9	255.146	3	1360.78	1.36
1/2	14.175	10	283.495	4	1814.37	1.81
1	28.350	11	311.845	5	2267.96	2.27
2	56.699	12	340.194	6	2721.55	2.72
3	85.049	13	368.544	7	3175.15	3.18
4	113.398	14	396.893	8	3628.74	3.63
5	141.748	15	425.243	9	4082.33	4.08
6	170.097	16 (1 lb)	453.59	10	4535.92	4.54

METRIC—AVOIRDUPOIS WEIGHT

GRAMS	OUNCES	GRAMS	OUNCES	GRAMS	POUNDS
0.001 (1 mg)	0.000035274	1	0.035274	1000 (1 kg)	2.2046

APOTHECARIES'—METRIC WEIGHT

GRAINS	GRAMS	GRAINS	GRAMS	SCRUPLES	GRAMS
1/150	0.0004	2/5	0.03	1	1.296(1.3)
1/120	0.0005	1/2	0.032	2	2.592(2.6)
1/100	0.0006	3/5	0.04	3 (1 ℈)	3.888(3.9)
1/90	0.0007	2/3	0.043	**DRAMS**	**GRAMS**
1/80	0.0008	3/4	0.05	1	3.888
1/64	0.001	7/8	0.057	2	7.776
1/60	0.0011	1	0.065	3	11.664
1/50	0.0013	1 1/2	0.097(0.1)	4	15.552
1/48	0.0014	2	0.12	5	19.440
1/40	0.0016	3	0.20	6	23.328
1/36	0.0018	4	0.24	7	27.216
1/32	0.002	5	0.30	8 (1 ʒ)	31.103
1/30	0.0022	6	0.40	**OUNCES**	**GRAMS**
1/25	0.0026	7	0.45	1	31.103
1/20	0.003	8	0.50	2	62.207
1/16	0.004	9	0.60	3	93.310
1/12	0.005	10	0.65	4	124.414
1/10	0.006	15	1.00	5	155.517
1/9	0.007	20 (1 ℈)	1.30	6	186.621
1/8	0.008	30	2.00	7	217.724
1/7	0.009			8	248.828
1/6	0.01			9	279.931
1/5	0.013			10	311.035
1/4	0.016			11	342.138
1/3	0.02			12 (1 ℔)	373.242

METRIC—APOTHECARIES' WEIGHT

MILLIGRAMS	GRAINS	GRAMS	GRAINS	GRAMS	EQUIVALENTS
1	0.015432	0.1	1.5432	10	2.572 drams
2	0.030864	0.2	3.0864	15	3.858 "
3	0.046296	0.3	4.6296	20	5.144 "
4	0.061728	0.4	6.1728	25	6.430 "
5	0.077160	0.5	7.7160	30	7.716 "
6	0.092592	0.6	9.2592	40	1.286 oz
7	0.108024	0.7	10.8024	45	1.447 "
8	0.123456	0.8	12.3456	50	1.607 "
9	0.138888	0.9	13.8888	100	3.215 "
10	0.154320	1.0	15.4320	200	6.430 "
15	0.231480	1.5	23.1480	300	9.644 "
20	0.308640	2.0	30.8640	400	12.859 "
25	0.385800	2.5	38.5800	500	1.34 lb
30	0.462960	3.0	46.2960	600	1.61 "
35	0.540120	3.5	54.0120	700	1.88 "
40	0.617280	4.0	61.728	800	2.14 "
45	0.694440	4.5	69.444	900	2.41 "
50	0.771600	5.0	77.162	1000	2.68 "
100	1.543240	10.0	154.324		

APOTHECARIES'—METRIC LIQUID MEASURE

MINIMS	MILLILITERS	FLUID DRAMS	MILLILITERS	FLUID OUNCES	MILLILITERS
1	0.06	1	3.70	1	29.57
2	0.12	2	7.39	2	59.15
3	0.19	3	11.09	3	88.72
4	0.25	4	14.79	4	118.29
5	0.31	5	18.48	5	147.87
10	0.62	6	22.18	6	177.44
15	0.92	7	25.88	7	207.01
20	1.23	8 (1 fl oz)	29.57	8	236.58
25	1.54			9	266.16
30	1.85			10	295.73
35	2.16			11	325.30
40	2.46			12	354.88
45	2.77			13	384.45
50	3.08			14	414.02
55	3.39			15	443.59
60 (1 fl dr)	3.70			16 (1 pt)	473.17
				32 (1 qt)	946.33
				128 (1 gal)	3785.32

METRIC—APOTHECARIES' LIQUID MEASURE

MILLILITERS	MINIMS	MILLILITERS	FLUID DRAMS	MILLILITERS	FLUID OUNCES
1	16.231	5	1.35	30	1.01
2	32.5	10	2.71	40	1.35
3	48.7	15	4.06	50	1.69
4	64.9	20	5.4	500	16.91
5	81.1	25	6.76	1000 (1 L)	33.815
		30	7.1		

U.S. AND BRITISH—METRIC LENGTH

INCHES	MILLIMETERS	CENTIMETERS	METERS
1/25	1.00	0.1	0.001
1/8	3.18	0.318	0.00318
1/4	6.35	0.635	0.00635
1/2	12.70	1.27	0.00127
1	25.40	2.54	0.0254
12 (1 foot)	304.80	30.48	0.3048

4. TABLES OF METRIC DOSES WITH APPROXIMATE APOTHECARY EQUIVALENTS

These *approximate* dose equivalents represent the quantities usually prescribed, under identical conditions, by physicians using, respectively, the metric system or the apothecary system of weights and measures. In labeling dosage forms in both the metric and the apothecary systems, if one is the approximate equivalent of the other, the approximate figure shall be enclosed in parentheses.

When prepared dosage forms such as tablets, capsules, pills, etc., are prescribed in the metric system, the pharmacist may dispense the corresponding *approximate* equivalent in the apothecary system, and vice versa, as indicated in the following table.

For the conversion of specific quantities in converting pharmaceutical formulas, equivalents must be used. In the compounding of prescriptions, the exact equivalents, rounded to three significant figures, should be used.

Note—A milliliter (ml) is the *approximate* equivalent of a cubic centimeter (cc).

LIQUID MEASURE

METRIC	APPROXIMATE APOTHECARY EQUIVALENTS	METRIC	APPROXIMATE APOTHECARY EQUIVALENTS
1000 ml	1 quart	3 ml	45 minims
750 ml	1 1/2 pints	2 ml	30 minims
500 ml	1 pint	1 ml	15 minims
250 ml	8 fluid ounces	0.75 ml	12 minims
200 ml	7 fluid ounces	0.6 ml	10 minims
100 ml	3 1/2 fluid ounces	0.5 ml	8 minims
50 ml	1 3/4 fluid ounces	0.3 ml	5 minims
30 ml	1 fluid ounce	0.25 ml	4 minims
15 ml	4 fluid drams	0.2 ml	3 minims
10 ml	2 1/2 fluid drams	0.1 ml	1 1/2 minims
8 ml	2 fluid drams	0.06 ml	1 minims
5 ml	1 1/4 fluid drams	0.05 ml	3/4 minim
4 ml	1 fluid dram	0.03 ml	1/2 minim

WEIGHT

METRIC	APPROXIMATE APOTHECARY EQUIVALENTS	METRIC	APPROXIMATE APOTHECARY EQUIVALENTS
30 g	1 ounce	30 mg	1/2 grain
15 g	4 drams	25 mg	3/8 grain
10 g	2 1/2 drams	20 mg	1/3 grain
7.5 g	2 drams	15 mg	1/4 grain
6 g	90 grains	12 mg	1/5 grain
5 g	75 grains	10 mg	1/6 grain
4 g	60 grains (1 dram)	8 mg	1/8 grain
3 g	45 grains	6 mg	1/10 grain
2 g	30 grains (1/2 dram)	5 mg	1/12 grain
1.5 g	22 grains	4 mg	1/15 grain
1 g	15 grains	3 mg	1/20 grain
750 mg	12 grains	2 mg	1/30 grain
600 mg	10 grains	1.5 mg	1/40 grain
500 mg	7 1/2 grains	1.2 mg	1/50 grain
400 mg	6 grains	1 mg	1/60 grain
300 mg	5 grains	800 µg	1/80 grain
250 mg	4 grains	600 µg	1/100 grain
200 mg	3 grains	500 µg	1/120 grain
150 mg	2 1/2 grains	400 µg	1/150 grain
125 mg	2 grains	300 µg	1/200 grain
100 mg	1 1/2 grains	250 µg	1/250 grain
75 mg	1 1/4 grains	200 µg	1/300 grain
60 mg	1 grain	150 µg	1/400 grain
50 mg	3/4 grain	120 µg	1/500 grain
40 mg	2/3 grain	100 µg	1/600 grain

The above *approximate* dose equivalents have been adopted by the *United States Pharmacopeia* and the *National Formulary*, and these dose equivalents have the approval of the federal Food and Drug Administration

5. LABORATORY VALUES OF CLINICAL IMPORTANCE*

REFERENCE VALUES IN HEMATOLOGY

	CONVENTIONAL UNITS		SI UNITS		NOTES
Acid hemolysis test (Ham)	No hemolysis		No hemolysis		
Alkaline phosphatase, leukocyte	Total score 14–100		Total score 14–100		
Carboxyhemoglobin	Up to 5% of total		0.05 of total		a
Cell counts					
Erythrocytes					
Males	4.6–6.2 million/cu mm		$4.6–6.2 \times 10^{12}$/l		
Females	4.2–5.4 million/cu mm		$4.2–5.4 \times 10^{12}$/l		
Children (varies with age)	4.5–5.1 million/cu mm		$4.5–5.1 \times 10^{12}$/l		
Leukocytes					
Total	4500–11,000/cu mm		$4.5–11.0 \times 10^{9}$/l		
Differential	*Percentage*	*Absolute*			
Myelocytes	0	0/cu mm	0/1		b
Band neutrophils	3–5	150–400/cu mm	$150–400 \times 10^{6}$/l		
Segmented neutrophils	54–62	3000–5800/cu mm	$3000–5800 \times 10^{6}$/l		
Lymphocytes	25–33	1500–3000/cu mm	$1500–3000 \times 10^{6}$/l		
Monocytes	3–7	300–500/cu mm	$300–500 \times 10^{6}$/l		
Eosinophils	1–3	50–250/cu mm	$50–250 \times 10^{6}$/l		
Basophils	0–0.75	15–50/cu mm	$15–50 \times 10^{6}$/l		
Platelets	150,000–350,000/cu mm		$150–350 \times 10^{9}$/l		
Reticulocytes	25,000–75,000/cu mm		$25–75 \times 10^{9}$/l		b
	0.5–1.5% of erythrocytes				

Bone marrow, differential cell count

	Range	Average	Range	Average	
Myeloblasts	0.3–5.0%	2.0%	0.003–0.05	0.02	a
Promyelocytes	1.0–8.0%	5.0%	0.01–0.08	0.05	
Myelocytes: Neutrophilic	5.0–19.0%	12.0%	0.05–0.19	0.12	
Eosinophilic	0.5–3.0%	1.5%	0.005–0.03	0.015	
Basophilic	0.0–0.5%	0.3%	0.00–0.005	0.003	
Metamyelocytes	13.0–32.0%	22.0%	0.13–0.32	0.22	
Polymorphonuclear neutrophils	7.0–30.0%	20.0%	0.07–0.30	0.20	
Polymorphonuclear eosinophils	0.5–4.0%	2.0%	0.005–0.04	0.02	
Polymorphonuclear basophils	0.0–0.7%	0.2%	0.00–0.007	0.002	
Lymphocytes	3.0–17.0%	10.0%	0.03–0.17	0.10	
Plasma cells	0.0–2.0%	0.4%	0.00–0.02	0.004	
Monocytes	0.5–5.0%	2.0%	0.005–0.05	0.02	
Reticulum cells	0.1–2.0%	0.2%	0.001–0.02	0.002	
Megakaryocytes	0.3–3.0%	0.4%	0.003–0.03	0.004	
Pronormoblasts	1.0–8.0%	4.0%	0.01–0.08	0.04	
Normoblasts	7.0–32.0%	18.0%	0.07–0.32	0.18	

Coagulation tests

	CONVENTIONAL UNITS	SI UNITS	NOTES
Antithrombin III (synthetic substrate)	80–120% of normal	0.8–1.2 of normal	
Bleeding time (Duke)	1–5 min	1–5 min	
Bleeding time (Ivy)	Less than 5 min	Less than 5 min	
Bleeding time (template)	2.5–9.5 min	2.5–9.5 min	
Clot retraction, qualitative	Begins in 30–60 min	Begins in 30–60 min	
	Complete in 24 hrs	Complete in 24 h	
Coagulation time (Lee-White)	5–15 min (glass tubes)	5–15 min (glass tubes)	
	19–60 min (siliconized tubes)	19–60 min (siliconized tubes)	
Euglobulin lysis time	2–6 hr at 37°	2–6 h at 37 C	
Factor VIII and other coagulation factors	50–150% of normal	0.50–1.5 of normal	a
Fibrin split products (Thrombo-Wellco test)	Less than 10 mcg/ml	Less than 10 mg/l	

REFERENCE VALUES IN HEMATOLOGY *(Continued)*

	CONVENTIONAL UNITS	SI UNITS	NOTES
Fibrinogen	200–400 mg/dl	5.9–11.7 µmol/l	c
Fibrinolysins	0	0	
Partial thromboplastin time, activated (APTT)	20–35 sec	20–35 sec	
Prothrombin consumption	Over 80% consumed in 1 hr	Over 0.80 consumed in 1 h	a
Prothrombin content	100% (calculated from prothrombin time)	1.0 (calculated from prothrombin time)	a
Prothrombin time (one stage)	12.0–14.0 sec	12.0–14.0 sec	
Tourniquet test	Ten or fewer petechiae in a 2.5 cm circle after 5 min	Ten or fewer petechiae in a 2.5 cm circle after 5 min	
Cold hemolysin test (Donath-Landsteiner)	No hemolysis	No hemolysis	
Coombs' test			
Direct	Negative	Negative	
Indirect	Negative	Negative	
Corpuscular values of erythrocytes (values are for adults; in children, values vary with age)			
MCH (mean corpuscular hemoglobin)	27–31 picogm	0.42–0.48 fmol	d
MCHC (mean corpuscular hemoglobin concentration)	32–36%	0.32–0.36	a
MCV (mean corpuscular volume)	80–96 cu micra	80–96 fl	
Haptoglobin (as hemoglobin binding capacity)	100–200 mg/dl	16–31 µmol/l	d
Hematocrit			
Males	40–54 ml/dl	0.40–0.54	a
Females	37–47 ml/dl	0.37–0.47	
Newborn	49–54 ml/dl	0.49–0.54	
Children (varies with age)	35–49 ml/dl	0.35–0.49	
Hemoglobin			
Males	14.0–18.0 grams/dl	2.17–2.79 mmol/l	d
Females	12.0–16.0 grams/dl	1.86–2.48 mmol/l	
Newborn	16.5–19.5 grams/dl	2.56–3.02 mmol/l	
Children (varies with age)	11.2–16.5 grams/dl	1.74–2.56 mmol/l	
Hemoglobin, fetal	Less than 1% of total	Less than 0.01 of total	a
Hemoglobin A_{1c}	3–5% of total	0.03–0.05 of total	a
Hemoglobin A_2	1.5–3.0% of total	0.015–0.03 of total	a
Hemoglobin, plasma	0–5.0 mg/dl	0–0.8 µmol/l	d
Methemoglobin	0–130 mg/dl	4.7–20 µmol/l	e
Osmotic fragility of erythrocytes	Begins in 0.45–0.39% NaCl	Begins in 77–67 mmol/NaCl	
	Complete in 0.33–0.30% NaCl	Complete in 56–51 mmol/l NaCl	
Sedimentation rate			
Wintrobe: Males	0–5 mm in 1 hr	0–5 mm/h	
Females	0–15 mm in 1 hr	0–15 mm/h	
Westergren: Male	0–15 mm in 1 hr	0–15 mm/h	
Females	0–20 mm in 1 hr	0–20 mm/h	
(May be slightly higher in children and during pregnancy)			

*From Rex B. Conn, Laboratory Values of Clinical Importance. *In* Robert E. Rakel (ed.): Conn's Current Therapy 1988. Philadelphia, W.B. Saunders Company, 1988.

REFERENCE VALUES FOR BLOOD, PLASMA, AND SERUM
(FOR SOME PROCEDURES THE REFERENCE VALUES MAY VARY DEPENDING UPON THE METHOD USED)

	CONVENTIONAL UNITS	SI UNITS	NOTES
Acetoacetate plus acetone, serum			
Qualitative	Negative	Negative	
Quantitative	0.3–2.0 mg/dl	3–20 mg/l	
Adrenocorticotropin (ACTH), plasma			
6 AM	10–80 picogm/ml	10–80 ng/l	
6 PM	Less than 50 picogm/ml	Less than 50 ng/l	
Alanine aminotransferase, *see* Transaminase			
Aldolase, serum	0–11 milliunits/ml (30°)	0–11 units/l (30 C)	f
Aldosterone			
Adult, supine	3–10 nanogm/dl	0.08–0.3 nmol/l	
standing			
male	6–22 nanogm/dl	0.17–0.61 nmol/l	
female	5–30 nanogm/dl	0.14–0.8 nmol/l	
Alpha amino nitrogen, serum	3.0–5.5 mg/dl	2.1–3.9 mmol/l	
Ammonia (nitrogen), plasma	15–49 mcg/dl	11–35 μmol/l	
Amylase, serum	25–125 milliunits/ml	25–125 units/l	
Anion gap	8–16 mEq/liter	8–16 mmol/l	
Ascorbic acid, blood	0.4–1.5 mg/dl	23–85 μmol/l	
Aspartate aminotransferase, *see* Transaminase			
Base excess, blood	0 ± 2 mEq/liter	0 ± 2 mmol/l	
Bicarbonate, serum	23–29 mEq/liter	23–29 mmol/l	
Bile acids, serum	0.3–3.0 mg/dl	3.0–30.0 mg/l	
Bilirubin, serum			
Direct	0.1–0.4 mg/dl	1.7–6.8 μmol/l	
Indirect	0.2–0.7 mg/dl (Total minus direct)	3.4–12 μmol/l (Total minus direct)	
Total	0.3–1.1 mg/dl	5.1–19 μmol/l	a
Calcium, serum	4.5–5.5 mEq/liter	2.25–2.75 mmol/l	
	9.0–11.0 mg/dl		
	(Slightly higher in children)	(Slightly higher in children)	
	(Varies with protein concentration)	(Varies with protein concentration)	
Calcium, ionized, serum	2.1–2.6 mEq/liter	1.05–1.30 mmol/l	
	4.25–5.25 mg/dl		
Carbon dioxide content, serum			
Adults	24–30 mEq/liter	24–30 mmol/l	
Infants	20–28 mEq/liter	20–28 mmol/l	
Carbon dioxide tension (Pco_2), blood	35–45 mm Hg	35–45 mm Hg	g
Carotene, serum	40–200 mcg/dl	0.74–3.72 μmol/l	
Ceruloplasmin, serum	23–44 mg/dl	230–440 mg/l	h
Chloride, serum	96–106 mEq/liter	96–106 mmol/l	
Cholesterol, serum			
Total	150–250 mg/dl	3.9–6.5 mmol/l	
Esters	68–76% of total cholesterol	0.68–0.76 of total cholesterol	a
Cholinesterase			
Serum	0.5–1.3 pH units	0.5–1.3 pH units	f
Erythrocytes	0.5–1.0 pH unit	0.5–1.0 pH unit	f
Copper, serum			
Males	70–140 mcg/dl	11–22 μmol/l	
Females	85–155 mcg/dl	13–24 μmol/l	
Cortisol, plasma			
8 AM	6–23 mcg/dl	170–635 nmol/l	
4 PM	3–15 mcg/dl	82–413 nmol/l	
10 PM	Less than 50% of 8 AM value	Less than 0.5 of 8 AM value	
Creatine, serum	0.2–0.8 mg/dl	15–61 μmol/l	
Creatine kinase, serum (CK, CPK)			
Males	12–80 milliunits/ml (30°)	12–80 units/l (30 C)	f
	55–170 milliunits/ml (37°)	55–170 units/l (37 C)	f
Females	10–55 milliunits/ml (30°)	10–55 units/l (30 C)	f
	30–135 milliunits/ml (37°)	30–135 units/l (37 C)	f
Creatine kinase isoenzymes, serum			
CK-MM	Present	Present	
CK-MB	Absent	Absent	
CK-BB	Absent	Absent	
Creatinine, serum	0.6–1.2 mg/dl	53–106 μmol/l	
Cryoglobulins, serum	0	0	
Fatty acids, total, serum	190–420 mg/dl	7–15 mmol/l	i
nonesterified, serum	8–25 mg/dl	0.30–0.90 mmol/l	

REFERENCE VALUES FOR BLOOD, PLASMA, AND SERUM *(Continued)*
(FOR SOME PROCEDURES THE REFERENCE VALUES MAY VARY DEPENDING UPON THE METHOD USED)

	CONVENTIONAL UNITS	SI UNITS	NOTES
Ferritin, serum	20–200 nanogm/ml	20–200 µg/l	
Fibrinogen, plasma	200–400 mg/100 ml	5.9–11.7 µmol/l	c
Folate, serum	1.8–9.0 nanogm/ml	4.1–20.4 nmol/l	
Erythrocytes	150–450 nanogm/ml	340–1020 nmol/l	
Follicle-stimulating hormone (FSH), plasma			
Males	4–25 milliunits/ml (I.U.)	4–25 IU/l	
Females	4–30 milliunits/ml (I.U.)	4–30 IU/l	
Postmenopausal	40–250 milliunits/ml (I.U.)	40–250 IU/l	
Gamma glutamyltransferase			
Males	6–32 milliunits/ml (30°)	6–32 units/l (30 C)	f
Females	4–18 milliunits/ml (30°)	4–18 units/l (30 C)	f
Gastrin, serum	0–200 picogm/ml	0–200 ng/l	
Glucose (fasting)			
Blood	60–100 ng/dl	3.33–5.55 mmol/l	
Plasma or serum	70–115 mg/dl	3.89–6.38 mmol/l	
Growth hormone, serum	0–10 nanogm/dl	0–10 µg/l	
Haptoglobin, serum	100–200 mg/dl	16–31 µmol/l	d
	(As hemoglobin binding capacity)	(As hemoglobin binding capacity)	
Hydroxybutyric dehydrogenase, serum (HBD)	0–180 milliunits/ml (30°)	0–180 units/l (30 C)	f
17-Hydroxycorticosteroids, plasma	8–18 mcg/dl	0.22–0.50 µmol/l	j
Immunoglobulins, serum			
IgG	550–1900 mg/dl	5.5–19.0 g/l	
IgA	60–333 mg/dl	0.60–3.3 g/l	
IgM	45–145 mg/dl	0.45–1.5 g/l	
IgD	0.5–3.0 mg/dl	5–30 mg/l	
IgE	<500 nanogm/ml	<500 µg/l	
	(Varies with age in children)	(Varies with age in children)	
Insulin, plasma (fasting)	5–25 microunits/ml	36–179 pmol/l	
Iodine, protein bound, serum	3.5–8.0 mcg/dl	0.28–0.63 µmol/l	k
Iron, serum	75–175 mcg/dl	13–31 µmol/l	
Iron binding capacity, serum			
Total	250–410 mcg/dl	45–73 µmol/l	
Saturation	20–55%	0.20–0.55	a
Lactate, blood, venous	4.5–19.8 mg/dl	0.5–2.2 mmol/l	
arterial	4.5–14.4 mg/dl	0.5–1.6 mmol/l	
Lactate dehydrogenase, serum (LD, LDH)	45–90 milliunits/ml (I.U.) (30°)	45–90 units/l (30 C)	f
	100–190 milliunits/ml (37°)	100–190 milliunits/ml (37 C)	
LDH$_1$	22–37% of total	0.22–0.37 of total	
LDH$_2$	30–46% of total	0.30–0.46 of total	a
LDH$_3$	14–29% of total	0.14–0.29 of total	
LDH$_4$	5–11% of total	0.05–0.11 of total	
LDH$_5$	2–11% of total	0.02–0.11 of total	
Leucine aminopeptidase, serum	14–40 milliunits/ml (30°)	14–40 units/l (30 C)	f
Lipase, serum	0–1.5 units (Cherry-Crandall)	0–1.5 units (Cherry-Crandall)	f
Lipids, total, serum	450–850 mg/dl	4.5–8.5 g/l	m
Lipoprotein cholesterol, serum			
LDL cholesterol	60–180 mg/dl	600–1800 mg/l	
HDL cholesterol	30–80 mg/dl	300–800 mg/l	
Luteinizing hormone (LH), serum			
Males	6–18 milliunits/ml (I.U.)	6–18 IU/l	
Females, premenopausal	5–22 milliunits/ml (I.U.)	5–22 IU/l	
midcycle	3 times baseline	3 times baseline	
postmenopausal	Greater than 30 milliunits/ml (I.U.)	Greater than 30 IU/l	
Magnesium, serum	1.5–2.5 mEq/liter	0.75–1.25 mmol/l	
	1.8–3.0 mg/dl		
5′-Nucleotidase, serum	3.5–12.7 milliunits/ml (37°)	3.5–12.5 units/l (37 C)	f
Nitrogen, nonprotein, serum	15–35 mg/dl	10.7–25.0 mmol/l	
Osmolality, serum	285–295 mOsm/kg serum water	285–295 mmol/kg serum water	n
Oxygen, blood			
Capacity	16–24 vol % (varies with hemoglobin)	7.14–10.7 mmol/l (varies with hemoglobin)	o
Content Arterial	15–23 vol %	6.69–10.3 mmol/l	o
Venous	10–16 vol %	4.46–7.14 mmol/l	o
Saturation Arterial	94–100% of capacity	0.94–1.00 of capacity	a
Venous	60–85% of capacity	0.60–0.85 of capacity	a
Tension, PO$_2$ Arterial	75–100 mm Hg	75–100 mg Hg	g

REFERENCE VALUES FOR BLOOD, PLASMA, AND SERUM *(Continued)*
(FOR SOME PROCEDURES THE REFERENCE VALUES MAY VARY DEPENDING UPON THE METHOD USED)

	CONVENTIONAL UNITS	SI UNITS	NOTES
P_{50}, blood	26–27 mm Hg	26–27 mm Hg	g
pH, arterial, blood	7.35–7.45	7.35–7.45	p
Phenylalanine, serum	Less than 3 mg/dl	Less than 0.18 mmol/l	
Phosphatase, acid serum	0.11–0.60 milliunit/ml (37°)	0.11–0.60 units/l	f
	(Roy, Brower, Hayden)		
Phosphatase, alkaline, serum (ALP)	20–90 milliunits/ml (30°)	20–90 units/l (30 C)	f
	(Values are higher in children)	(Values are higher in children)	
Phosphate, inorganic, serum			
Adults	3.0–4.5 mg/dl	1.0–1.5 mmol/l	
Children	4.0–7.0 mg/dl	1.3–2.3 mmol/l	
Phospholipids, serum	6–12 mg/dl	1.9–3.9 mmol/l	
	(As lipid phosphorus)	(As lipid phosphorus)	
Potassium, serum	3.5–5.0 mEq/liter	3.5–5.0 mmol/l	
Prolactin, serum			
Males	1–20 nanogm/ml	1–20 μg/l	
Females	1–25 nanogm/ml	1–25 μg/l	
Protein, serum			
Total	6.0–8.0 grams/dl	60–80 g/l	m
Albumin	3.5–5.5 grams/dl	35–55 g/l	q
	52–68% of total	0.52–0.68 of total	a
Globulin			
Alpha$_1$	0.2–0.4 gram/dl	2–4 g/l	m
	2–5% of total	0.02–0.05% total	a
Alpha$_2$	0.5–0.9 gram/dl	5–9 g/l	m
	7–14% of total	0.07–0.14 of total	a
Beta	0.6–1.1 grams/dl	6–11 g/l	m
	9–15% of total	0.09–0.15 of total	a
Gamma	0.7–1.7 grams/dl	7–17 g/l	m
	11–21% of total	0.11–0.21 of total	a
Protoporphyrin, erythrocyte	27–61 mcg/dl packed RBC	0.48–1.09 μmol/l packed RBC	
Pyruvate, blood	0.3–0.9 mg/dl	0.03–0.10 mmol/l	
Sodium, serum	136–145 mEq/liter	136–145 mmol/l	
Sulfates, inorganic, serum	0.8–1.2 mg/dl	83–125 μmol/l	
Testosterone, plasma			
Males	275–875 nanogm/dl	9.5–30 nmol/l	
Females	23–75 nanogm/dl	0.8–2.6 nmol/l	
Pregnant	38–190 nanogm/dl	1.3–6.6 nmol/l	
Thyroid-stimulating hormone (TSH), serum	0–7 microunits/ml	0–7 milliunits/l	
Thyroxine, free, serum	1.0–2.1 nanogm/dl	13–27 pmol/l	
Thyroxine (T_4), serum	4.4–9.9 mcg/dl	57–128 nmol/l	
Thyroxine binding globulin (TBG), serum (as thyroxine)	10–26 mcg/dl	129–335 nmol/l	
Thyroxine iodine, serum	2.9–6.4 mcg/dl	229–504 nmol/l	k
Triiodothyronine (T_3), serum	150–250 nanogm/dl	2.3–3.9 nmol/l	
Triiodothyronine (T_3) uptake, resin (T_3RU)	25–38% uptake	0.25–0.38 uptake	a
Transaminase, serum			
SGOT (asparate aminotransferase, AST)	8–20 milliunits/ml (30°)	8–20 units/l (30 C)	
	7–40 milliunits/ml (37°)	7–40 units/l (37 C)	
SGPT (alanine aminotransferase, ALT)	8–20 milliunits/ml (30°)	8–20 units/l (30 C)	f
	5–35 milliunits/ml (37°)	5–35 units/l (37 C)	f
Triglycerides, serum	40–150 mg/dl	0.4–1.5 g/l	r
		0.45–1.71 mmol/l	
Urate, serum			
Males	2.5–8.0 mg/dl	0.15–0.48 mmol/l	
Females	1.5–7.0 mg/dl	0.09–0.42 mmol/l	
Urea			
Blood	21–43 mg/dl	3.5–7.3 mmol/l	
Plasma or serum	24–49 mg/dl	4.0–8.3 mmol/l	
Urea nitrogen			
Blood	10–20 mg/dl	7.1–14.3 mmol/l	k
Plasma or serum	11–23 mg/dl	7.9–16.4 mmol/l	
Viscosity, serum	1.4–1.8 times water	1.4–1.8 times water	
Vitamin A, serum	20–80 mcg/dl	0.70–2.8 μmol/l	
Vitamin B$_{12}$, serum	180–900 picogm/ml	133–664 pmol/l	

REFERENCE VALUES FOR URINE
(FOR SOME PROCEDURES THE REFERENCE VALUES MAY VARY DEPENDING UPON THE METHOD USED)

	CONVENTIONAL UNITS	SI UNITS	NOTES
Acetone and acetoacetate, qualitative	Negative	Negative	
Albumin			
Qualitative	Negative	Negative	
Quantitative	10–100 mg/24 hrs	10–100 mg/24 h	q
		0.15–1.5 μmol/24 h	
Aldosterone	3–20 mcg/24 hrs	8.3–55 nmol/24 h	
Alpha amino nitrogen	50–200 mg/24 hrs	3.6–14.3 mmol/24 h	
Ammonia nitrogen	20–70 mEq/24 hrs	20–70 mmol/24 h	
Amylase	1–17 units/hr	1–17 units/h	f
Amylase/creatinine clearance ratio	1–4%	0.01–0.04	
Bilirubin, qualitative	Negative	Negative	
Calcium			
Low Ca diet	Less than 150 mg/24 hrs	Less than 3.8 mmol/24 h	
Usual diet	Less than 250 mg/24 hrs	Less than 6.3 mmol/24 h	
Catecholamines			
Epinephrine	Less than 10 mcg/24 hrs	Less than 55 nmol/24 h	
Norepinephrine	Less than 100 mcg/24 hrs	Less than 590 nmol/24 h	
Total free catecholamines	4–126 mcg/24 hrs	24–745 nmol/24 h	s
Total metanephrines	0.1–1.6 mg/24 hrs	0.5–8.1 μmol/24 h	t
Chloride	110–250 mEq/24 hrs	110–250 mmol/24 h	
	(Varies with intake)	(Varies with intake)	
Chorionic gonadotropin	0	0	
Copper	0–50 mcg/24 hrs	0–0.80 μmol/24 h	
Cortisol, free	10–100 mcg/24 hrs	27.6–276 mmol/24 h	
Creatine			
Males	0–40 mg/24 hrs	0–0.30 mmol/24 h	
Females	0–100 mg/24 hrs	0–0.76 mmol/24 h	
	(Higher in children and during pregnancy)	(Higher in children and during pregnancy)	
Creatinine	15–25 mg/kg body weight/24 hrs	0.13–0.22 mmol·kg⁻¹ body weight/24 h	
Creatinine clearance			
Males	110–150 ml/min	110–150 ml/min	
Females	105–132 ml/min	105–132 ml/min	
	(1.73 sq meter surface area)	(1.73 m² surface area)	
Cystine or cysteine, qualitative	Negative	Negative	
Dehydroepiandrosterone	Less than 15% of total 17-ketosteroids	Less than 0.15 of total 17-ketosteroids	a
Males	0.2–2.0 mg/24 hrs	0.7–6.9 μm/24 h	
Females	0.2–1.8 mg/24 hrs	0.7–6.2 μm/24 h	
Delta aminolevulinic acid	1.3–7.0 mg/24 hrs	10–53 μmol/24 h	
Estrogens			
Males			
Estrone	3–8 μg/24 hrs	11–30 nmol/24 h	
Estradiol	0–6 μg/24 hrs	0–22 nmol/24 h	
Estriol	1–11 μg/24 hrs	3–38 nmol/24 h	
Total	4–25 μg/24 hrs	14–90 nmol/24 h	u
Females			
Estrone	4–31 μg/24 hrs	15–115 nmol/24 h	
Estradiol	0–14 μg/24 hrs	0–51 nmol/24 h	
Estriol	0–72 μg/24 hrs	0–250 nmol/24 h	
Total	5–100 μg/24 hrs	18–360 nmol/24 hr	u
	(Markedly increased during pregnancy)	(Markedly increased during pregnancy)	

REFERENCE VALUES FOR URINE *(Continued)*

(FOR SOME PROCEDURES THE REFERENCE VALUES MAY VARY DEPENDING UPON THE METHOD USED)

	CONVENTIONAL UNITS	SI UNITS	NOTES
Glucose (as reducing substance)	Less than 250 mg/24 hrs	Less than 250 mg/24 h	
Hemoglobin and myoglobin, qualitative	Negative	Negative	
Homogentisic acid, qualitative	Negative	Negative	
17-Hydroxycorticosteroids			
Males	3–9 mg/24 hrs	8.3–25 µmol/24 h	j
Females	2–8 mg/24 hrs	5.5–22 µmol/24 h	
5-Hydroxyindoleacetic acid			
Qualitative	Negative	Negative	
Quantitative	Less than 9 mg/24 hrs	Less than 47 µmol/24 h	
17-Ketosteroids			
Males	6–18 mg/24 hrs	21–62 µmol/24 h	l
Females	4–13 mg/24 hrs	14–45 µmol/24 h	
	(Varies with age)	(Varies with age)	
Magnesium	6.0–8.5 mEq/24 hrs	3.0–4.3 mmol/24 h	
Metanephrines (see Catecholamines)			
Osmolality	38–1400 mOsm/kg water	38–1400 mmol/kg water	n
pH	4.6–8.0, average 6.0	4.6–8.0, average 6.0	p
	(Depends on diet)	(Depends on diet)	
Phenolsulfonphthalein excretion (PSP)	25% or more in 15 min	0.25 or more in 15 min	a
	40% or more in 30 min	0.40 or more in 30 min	
	55% or more in 2 hrs	0.55 or more in 2 h	
	(After injection of 1 ml PSP intravenously)	(After injection of 1 ml PSP intravenously)	
Phenylpyruvic acid, qualitative	Negative	Negative	
Phosphorus	0.9–1.3 gram/24 hrs	29–42 mmol/24 h	
Porphobilinogen			
Qualitative	Negative	Negative	
Quantative	0–0.2 mg/dl	0–0.9 µmol/l	
	Less than 2.0 mg/24 hrs	Less than 9 µmol/24 h	
Porphyrins			
Coproporphyrin	50–250 mcg/24 hrs	77–380 nmol/24 h	
Uroporphyrin	10–30 mcg/24 hrs	12–36 nmol/24 h	
Potassium	25–100 mEq/24 hrs	25–100 mmol/24 h	
	(Varies with intake)	(Varies with intake)	
Pregnanediol			
Males	0.4–1.4 mg/24 hrs	1.2–4.4 µmol/24 h	
Females			
Proliferative phase	0.5–1.5 mg/24 hrs	1.6–4.7 µmol/24 h	
Luteal phase	2.0–7.0 mg/24 hrs	6.2–22 µmol/24 h	
Postmenopausal phase	0.2–1.0 mg/24 hrs	0.6–3.1 µmol/24 h	
Pregnanetriol	Less than 2.5 mg/24 hrs in adults	Less than 7.4 µmol/24 h in adults	
Protein			
Qualitative	Negative	Negative	
Quantitative	10–150 mg/24 hrs	10–150 mg/24 h	m
Sodium	130–260 mEq/24 hrs	130–260 mmol/24 h	
	(Varies with intake)	(Varies with intake)	
Specific gravity	1.003–1.030	1.003–1.030	
Titratable acidity	20–40 mEq/24 hrs	20–40 mmol/24 h	
Urate	200–500 mg/24 hrs	1.2–3.0 mmol/24 h	
	(With normal diet)	(With normal diet)	
Urobilinogen	Up to 1.0 Ehrlich unit/2 hrs	Up to 1.0 Ehrlich unit/2 h	
	(1–3 PM)	(1–3 PM)	
	0–4.0 mg/24 hrs	0–6.8 µmol/24 h	
Vanillylmandelic acid (VMA)	1–8 mg/24 hrs	5–40 µmol/24 h	
(4-hydroxy-3-methoxymandealic acid			

REFERENCE VALUES FOR THERAPEUTIC DRUG MONITORING

DRUG	THERAPEUTIC RANGE	TOXIC LEVELS	PROPRIETARY NAMES
Antibiotics			
Amikacin, serum	15–25 mcg/ml	Peak: >35 mcg/ml	Amikin
		Trough: >5–8 mcg/ml	
Chloramphenicol, serum	10–20 mcg/ml	>25 mcg/ml	Chloromycetin
Gentamicin, serum	5–10 mcg/ml	Peak: >12 mcg/ml	Garamycin
		Trough: >2 mcg/ml	
Tobramycin, serum	5–10 mcg/ml	Peak: >12 mcg/ml	Nebcin
		Trough: >2 mcg/ml	
Anticonvulsants			
Carbamazepine, serum	5–12 mcg/ml	>12 mcg/ml	Tegretol
Ethosuximide, serum	40–100 mcg/ml	>100 mcg/ml	Zarontin
Phenobarbital, serum	10–30 mcg/ml	Vary widely because of developed tolerance	
Phenytoin, serum (diphenyl-hydantoin)	10–20 mcg/ml	>20 mcg/ml	Dilantin
Primidone, serum	5–12 mcg/ml	>15 mcg/ml	Mysoline
Valproic acid, serum	50–100 mcg/ml	>100 mcg/ml	Depakene
Analgesics			
Acetaminophen, serum	10–20 mcg/ml	>250 mcg/ml	Tylenol
			Datril
Salicylate, serum	100–250 mcg/ml	>300 mcg/ml	
Bronchodilator			
Theophylline (aminophylline)	10–20 mcg/ml	>20 mcg/ml	
Cardiovascular drugs			
Digitoxin, serum	15–25 nanogm/ml (Specimen obtained 12–24 hrs after last dose)	>25 nanogm/ml	Crystodigin
Digoxin, serum	0.8–2 nanogm/ml (Specimen obtained 12–24 hrs after last dose)	>2.4 nanogm/ml	Lanoxin
Disopyramide, serum	2–5 mcg/ml	>5 mcg/ml	Norpace
Lidocaine, serum	1.5–5 mcg/ml	>5 nanogm/ml	Anestacon
			Xylocaine
Procainamide, serum	4–10 mcg/ml	>16 mcg/ml	Pronestyl
	*10–30 mcg/ml (*Procainamide + N-Acetyl Procainamide)	*>30 mcg/ml	
Propranolol, serum	50–100 nanogm/ml	Variable	Inderal
Quinidine, serum	2–5 mcg/ml	>10 mcg/ml	Cardioquin
			Quinaglute
			Qunidex
			Quinora
Psychopharmacologic drugs	*120–150 nanogrm/ml	*>500 nanogm/ml	Amitril
Amitriptyline, serum	(*Amitriptyline + Nortriptyline)		Elavil
			Endep
			Etralon
			Limbitrol
			Triavil
Desipramine, serum	*150–300 nanogm/ml (*Desipramine + Imipramine)	*>500 nanogm/ml	Norpramin
			Pertofrane
Imipramine, serum	*150–300 nanogm/ml (*Imipramine + Desipramine)	*>500 nanogm/ml	Antipress
			Imavate
			Janimine
			Presamine
			Tofranil
Lithium, serum	0.8–1.2 mEq/liter (Specimen obtained 12 hrs after last dose)	>2.0 mEq/liter	Lithobid
			Lithotabs
Nortriptyline, serum	50–150 nanogm/ml	>500 nanogm/ml	Aventyl
			Pamelor

REFERENCE VALUES IN TOXICOLOGY

	CONVENTIONAL UNITS	SI UNITS	NOTES
Arsenic, blood	3.5–7.2 mcg/dl	0.47–0.96 μmol/l	
Arsenic, urine	Less than 100 mcg/24 hrs	Less than 1.3 μmol/24 h	
Bromides, serum	0	0	
	Toxic levels: Above 17 mmol/l	Toxic levels: Above 17 mmol/l	
Carbon monoxide, blood	Up to 5% saturation	Up to 0.5 saturation	
	Symptoms occur with 20% saturation	Symptoms occur with 0.20 saturation	a
Ethanol, blood	Less than 0.005%	Less than 1 mmol/l	
Marked intoxication	0.3–0.4%	65–87 mmol/l	
Alcoholic stupor	0.4–0.5% mcg/dl	87–109 mmol/l	
Coma	Above 0.5%	Above 109 mmol/l	
Lead, blood	0–40 mcg/dl	0–2 μmol/l	
Lead, urine	Less than 100 mcg/24 hrs	Less than 0.48 μmol/24 h	
Mercury, urine	Less than 100 mcg/24 hrs	Less than 50 nmol/24 h	

REFERENCE VALUES FOR CEREBROSPINAL FLUID

	CONVENTIONAL UNITS	SI UNITS	NOTES
Cells	Fewer than 5/cu mm; all mononuclear	Fewer than 5/μl; all mononuclear	
Chloride	120–130 mEq/liter	120–130 mmol/l	
	(20 mEq/liter higher than serum)	(20 mmol/l higher than serum)	
Electrophoresis	Predominantly albumin	Predominantly albumin	
Glucose	50–75 mg/dl	2.8–4.2 mmol/l	
	(20 mg/dl less than serum)	(1.1 mmol/less than serum)	
IgG			
Children under 14	Less than 8% of total protein	Less than 0.08 of total protein	a, m
Adults	Less than 14% of total protein	Less than 0.14 of total protein	
Pressure	70–180 mm water	70–180 mm water	g
Protein, total	15–45 mg/dl	0.150–0.450 g/l	m
	(Higher, up to 70 mg/dl, in elderly adults and children)	(Higher, up to 0.70 g/l, in elderly adults and children)	

REFERENCE VALUES FOR GASTRIC ANALYSIS

	CONVENTIONAL UNITS	SI UNITS	NOTES
Basal gastric secretion (1 hour)			
Concentration	(Mean ± 1 S.D.)	(Mean ± 1 S.D.)	
Males	25.8 ± 1.8 mEq/liter	25.8 ± 1.8 mmol/l	
Females	20.3 ± 3.0 mEq/liter	20.3 ± 3.0 mmol/l	
Output	(Mean ± 1 S.D.)	(Mean ± 1 S.D.)	
Males	2.57 ± 0.16 mEq/hr	2.57 ± 0.16 mmol/h	
Females	1.61 ± 0.18 mEq/hr	1.61 ± 0.18 mmol/h	
After histamine stimulation			
Normal	Mean output 11.8 mEq/hr	Mean output 11.8 mmol/h	
Duodenal ulcer	Mean output 15.2 mEq/hr	Mean output 15.2 mmol/h	
After maximal histamine stimulation			
Normal	Mean output 22.6 mEq/hr	Mean output 22.6 mmol/h	
Duodenal ulcer	Mean output 44.6 mEq/hr	Mean output 44.6 mmol/h	
Diagnex blue (Squibb):			
Anacidity	0–0.3 mg in 2 hrs	0–0.03 mg in 2 h	
Doubtful	0.3–0.6 mg in 2 hrs	0.3–0.6 mg in 2 h	
Normal	Greater than 0.6 mg in 2 hrs	Greater than 0.6 mg in 2 h	
Volume, fasting stomach content	50–100 ml	50–100 ml	
Emptying time	3–6 hrs	3–6 h	
Color	Opalescent or colorless	Opalescent or colorless	
Specific gravity	1.006–1.009	1.006–1.009	
pH (adults)	0.9–1.5	0.9–1.5	p

GASTROINTESTINAL ABSORPTION TESTS

	CONVENTIONAL UNITS	SI UNITS
D-Xylose absorption test	After an 8 hour fast, 10 ml/kg body weight of a 0.05 solution of D-xylose is given by mouth. Nothing further by mouth is given until the test has been completed. All urine voided during the following 5 hours is pooled, and blood samples are taken at 0, 60, and 120 minutes. Normally 0.26 (range 0.16–0.33) of ingested xylose is excreted within 5 hours, and the serum xylose reaches a level between 25 and 40 mg/100 dl after 1 hour and is maintained at this level for another 60 minutes.	No change
Vitamin A absorption	A fasting blood specimen is obtained and 200,000 units of vitamin A in oil is given by mouth. Serum vitamin A level should rise to twice fasting level in 3 to 5 hours.	No change

REFERENCE VALUES FOR FECES

	CONVENTIONAL UNITS	SI UNITS	NOTES
Bulk	100–200 grams/24 hrs	100–200 g/24 h	
Dry matter	23–32 grams/24 hrs	23–32 g/24 h	
Fat, total	Less than 6.0 grams/24 hrs	Less than 6.0 g/24 h	
Nitrogen, total	Less than 2.0 grams/24 hrs	Less than 2.0 g/24 hr	
Urobilinogen	40–280 mg/24 hrs	40–280 mg/24 h	
Water	Approximately 65%	Approximately 0.65	a

REFERENCE VALUES FOR IMMUNOLOGIC PROCEDURES

	CONVENTIONAL UNITS
Lymphocyte subsets	
T cells	60–85%
B cells	1–20%
T-helper cells	35–60%
T-suppressor cells	15–30%
T-H/S ratio	1.5–2.5
Complement	
C3	85–175 mg/dl
C4	15–45 mg/dl
CH_{50}	25–55 H_{50} units/ml
Tumor markers	
Carcinoembryonic antigen (CEA)	
(Roche)	Less than 5 nanogm/ml
(Abbott)	Less than 4.1 nanogm/ml
Alpha-fetoprotein (AFP)	Less than 10–30 nanogm/ml (depends on method)

REFERENCE VALUES FOR SEMEN ANALYSIS

	CONVENTIONAL UNITS	SI UNITS	NOTES
Volume	2–5 ml; usually 3–4 ml	2–5 ml; usually 3–4 ml	
Liquefaction	Complete in 15 min	Complete in 15 min	
pH	7.2–8.0; average 7.8	7.2–8.0; average 7.8	p
Leukocytes	Occasional or absent	Occasional or absent	
Count	60–150 million/ml	60–150 million/ml	
	Below 60 million/ml is abnormal	Below 60 million/ml is abnormal	
Motility	80% or more motile	0.80 or more motile	a
Morphology	80–90% normal forms	0.80–0.90 normal forms	a

ORAL GLUCOSE TOLERANCE TEST

The oral glucose tolerance test (OGTT) may be unnecessary if the fasting plasma glucose concentration is elevated (venous plasma ≥140 mg/dl or 7.8 mmol/l) on two occasions. The OGTT should be carried out only on patients who are ambulatory and otherwise healthy and who are known not to be taking agents that elevate the plasma glucose (see reference 10). The test should be conducted in the morning after at least 3 days of unrestricted diet (≥150 grams of carbohydrate) and physical activity. The subject should have fasted for at least 10 hours but no more than 16 hours. Water is permitted during the test period; however, the subject should remain seated and should not smoke throughout the test.

The dose of glucose administered should be 75 grams (1.75 grams per kg of ideal body weight, up to a maximum of 75 grams for children). Commercial preparations containing a suitable carbohydrate load are acceptable. If criteria for gestational diabetes are used, a dose of 100 grams of glucose is required.

A fasting blood sample should be collected, after which the glucose dose is taken within 5 minutes. Blood samples should be collected at 30 minute intervals for 2 hours (for gestational diabetes, fasting 1, 2 and 3 hours). The following diagnostic criteria have been recommended by the National Diabetes Data Group:

Normal OGTT in Nonpregnant Adults	Fasting venous plasma glucose <115 mg/dl (6.4 mmol/l); ½ h, 1 h, and 1½ h OGTT venous plasma glucose <200 mg/dl (11.1 mmol/l); 2 h OGTT venous plasma glucose <140 mg/dl (7.8 mmol/l)
Diabetes Mellitus in Nonpregnant Adults	Both the 2 hour sample *and* some other sample taken between administration of the 75 gram glucose dose and 2 hours later must show a venous plasma glucose ≥200 mg/dl (11.1 mmol/l)
Impaired Glucose Tolerance in Nonpregnant Adults	Three criteria must be met: Fasting venous plasma glucose <140 mg/dl (7.8 mmol/l); ½ h, 1 h, or 1½ h OGTT value ≥200 mg/dl (11.1 mmol/l); 2 h OGTT venous plasma glucose between 140 and 200 mg/dl (7.8 and 11.1 mmol/l)
Gestational Diabetes	Two or more of the following values after a 100 gram oral glucose challenge must be met or exceeded: (values are for venous plasma glucose)

Fasting	105 mg/dl	5.8 mmol/l
1 h	190 mg/dl	10.6 mmol/l
2 h	165 mg/dl	9.2 mmol/l
3 h	145 mg/dl	8.1 mmol/l

NOTES

a. Percentage is expressed as a decimal fraction.

b. Percentage may be expressed as a decimal fraction; however, when the result expressed is itself a variable fraction of another variable, the absolute value is more meaningful. There is no reason, other than custom, for expressing reticulocyte counts and differential leukocyte counts in percentages or decimal fractions rather than in absolute numbers.

c. Molecular weight of fibrinogen equals 341,000.

d. Molecular weight of hemoglobin equals 64,500. Because of disagreement as to whether the monomer or tetramer of hemoglobin should be used in the conversion, it has been recommended that the conventional grams per deciliter be retained. The tetramer is used in the table; values given should be multiplied by 4 to obtain concentration of the monomer.

e. Molecular weight of methemoglobin equals 64,500. See note d above.

f. Enzyme units have not been changed in these tables because the proposed enzyme unit, the katal, has not been universally adopted (1 International Unit equals 16.7 nkat).

g. It has been proposed that pressure be expressed in the pascal (1 mm Hg equals 0.133 kPa); however, this convention has not been universally accepted.

h. Molecular weight of ceruloplasmin equals 151,000.

i. "Fatty acids" includes a mixture of different aliphatic acids of varying molecular weight. A mean molecular weight of 284 has been assumed in calculating the conversion factor.

j. Based upon molecular weight of cortisol 362.47.

k. The practice of expressing concentration of an organic molecule in terms of one of its constituent elements originated when measurements included a heterogeneous class of compounds (nonprotein nitrogenous compounds, iodine-containing compounds bound to serum proteins). It was carried over to expressing measurements of specific substances (urea, thyroxine), but the practice should be discarded. For iodine and nitrogen 1 mole is taken as the monoatomic form, although they occur as diatomic molecules.

l. Based upon molecular weight of dehydroepiandrosterone 288.41.

m. Weight per volume is retained as the unit because of the heterogeneous nature of the material measured.

n. The proposal that osmolality be reported as

freezing point depression using the millikelvin as the unit has not been received with universal enthusiasm. The milliosmole is not an SI unit, and the unit used here is the millimole.

o. Volumes per cent might be converted to a decimal fraction; however, this would not permit direct correlation with hemoglobin content, which is possible when oxygen content and capacity are expressed in molar quantities. One millimole of hemoglobin combines with 4 millimoles of oxygen.

p. Hydrogen ion concentration in SI units would be expressed in nanomoles per liter; however, this change has not received general approval. Conversion can be calculated as antilog ($-$pH).

q. Albumin is expressed in grams per liter to be consistent with units used for other proteins.

Concentration of albumin may be expressed in mmol/l also, an expression that permits assessment of binding capacity of albumin for substances such as bilirubin. Molecular weight of albumin is 65,000.

r. Most techniques for quantitating triglycerides measure the glycerol moiety, and the total mass is calculated using an average molecular weight. The factor given assumes a mean molecular weight of 875 for triglycerides.

s. Calculated as norepinephrine, molecular weight 169.18.

t. Calculated as metanephrine, molecular weight 197.23.

u. Conversion factor calculated from molecular weights of estrone, estradiol, and estriol in proportions of 2:1:2.

Credits

PLATES

Plate 11   Anson, BJ: An Atlas of Human Anatomy. 2nd ed. Philadelphia, WB Saunders Company, 1963.

Plate 12   (*bottom*) King, BG, and Showers, MJ: Human Anatomy and Physiology. 6th ed. Philadelphia, WB Saunders Company, 1969.

Plate 27   Jones, T, and Shepard, WC: Manual of Surgical Anatomy. Philadelphia, WB Saunders Company, 1945.

Plate 28   Jones, T, and Shepard, WC: Manual of Surgical Anatomy. Philadelphia, WB Saunders Company, 1945.

Plate 29   Jones, T, and Shepard, WC: Manual of Surgical Anatomy. Philadelphia, WB Saunders Company, 1945.

Plate 30   Jones, T, and Shepard, WC: Manual of Surgical Anatomy. Philadelphia, WB Saunders Company, 1945.

Plate 31   Jones, T, and Shepard, WC: Manual of Surgical Anatomy. Philadelphia, WB Saunders Company, 1945.

Plate 33   (*top and bottom left*) King, BG, and Showers, MJ: Human Anatomy and Physiology. 6th ed. Philadelphia, WB Saunders Company, 1969. (*bottom right*) Leeson, CR, Leeson, TS, and Paparo, AA: Textbook of Histology. 5th ed. Philadelphia, WB Saunders Company, 1985.

Plate 34   Jones, T, and Shepard, WC: Manual of Surgical Anatomy. Philadelphia, WB Saunders Company, 1945.

Plate 36   Jones, T, and Shepard, WC: Manual of Surgical Anatomy. Philadelphia, WB Saunders Company, 1945.

Plate 38   Jones, T, and Shepard, WC: Manual of Surgical Anatomy. Philadelphia, WB Saunders Company, 1945.

Plate 39   Jones, T, and Shepard, WC: Manual of Surgical Anatomy. Philadelphia, WB Saunders Company, 1945.

Plate 41   Kouwenhofen, WB, Jude, JR, and Knickerbocker, GG: Closed Cardiac Massage. JAMA 173:1064, 1960.

Plate 42   King, BG, and Showers, MJ: Human Anatomy and Physiology. 6th ed. Philadelphia, WB Saunders Company, 1969.

Plate 44   Nealon, TF: Fundamental Skills in Surgery. 3rd ed. Philadelphia, WB Saunders Company, 1979.

ILLUSTRATIONS AND TABLES

Page 21   Dunphy, JE, and Botsford, TW: Physical Examination of the Surgical Patient. 3rd ed. Philadelphia, WB Saunders Company, 1964.

63   Balinsky, BI: An Introduction to Embryology. 5th ed. Philadelphia, Saunders College Publishing, 1981.

332   Courtesy of RG Worton. *In* Thompson, MW: Genetics in Medicine. 4th ed. Philadelphia, WB Saunders Company, 1986.

463   (*left*) Moloy, HC: Clinical and Roentgenologic Evaluation of the Pelvis in Obstetrics. Philadelphia, WB Saunders Company, 1951.

506   Hauser, EDW: Diseases of the Foot. 2nd ed. Philadelphia, WB Saunders Company, 1950.

535   Guyton, AC: Textbook of Medical Physiology. 7th ed. Philadelphia, WB Saunders Company, 1986.

689   Cheng, TC: General Parasitology. New York, Academic Press, 1973.

996   Adapted from Thompson, MW: Genetics in Medicine. 4th ed. Philadelphia, WB Saunders Company, 1986.

1033   Cheng, TC: General Parasitology. New York, Academic Press, 1973.

1043   Villee, C, Walker, WF, and Smith, FE: General Zoology. 2nd ed. Philadelphia, WB Saunders Company, 1963.

1084   Rippon, JW: Medical Mycology. 3rd ed. Philadelphia, WB Saunders Company, 1987.

1350   Greenhill, JP, and Friedman, EA: Biological Principles and Modern Practice of Obstetrics. Philadelphia, WB Saunders Company, 1974.

1364   King, BG, and Showers, MJ: Human Anatomy and Physiology. 6th ed. Philadelphia, WB Saunders Company, 1969.

1409   Gardner, E, Gray, DJ, and O'Rahilly, R: Anatomy: A Regional Study of Human Structure. 4th ed. Philadelphia, WB Saunders Company, 1975.

1433   Redrawn from Terhorst, C, et al, The T-Cell Receptor/T3 Complex. *In* The Year in Immunology, 1985–1986, vol. 3. ed. Cruse, JM, and Lewis, RE, Jr. New York, S Karger, 1986.

1442   Scheie, HG, and Albert, DM, Textbook of Ophthalmology. 9th ed. Philadelphia, WB Saunders Company, 1977.

1535   (*top*) Silvers, DN: *In* Domonkos, AN, Arnold, HR, Jr., and Odom, RB: Andrews' Diseases of the Skin. 7th ed. Philadelphia, WB Saunders Company, 1982.

1538   Hunter, GW, III, Frye, WW, and Swartzwelder, JC: Manual of Tropical Medicine. 3rd ed. Philadelphia, WB Saunders Company, 1960.

1614   King, BG, and Showers, MJ: Human Anatomy and Physiology. 6th ed. Philadelphia, WB Saunders Company, 1969.

1670   Da Costa, JC: Modern Surgery. 9th ed. Philadelphia, WB Saunders Company, 1925.

1732   (*top*) Ash, MM: Wheeler's Dental Anatomy, Physiology, and Occlusion. 6th ed. Philadelphia, WB Saunders Company, 1984.

1753   Markell, EK, Voge, M, and John, DT: Medical Parasitology. 6th ed.–Philadelphia, WB Saunders Company, 1986.

1755   Henry, JB: Todd-Sanford-Davidsohn: Clinical Diagnosis by Laboratory Methods. 17th ed. Philadelphia, WB Saunders Company, 1984.

1767   Meschan, I: Synopsis of Radiologic Anatomy with Computed Tomography. Revised Reprint. Philadelphia, WB Saunders Company, 1980.

1831   King, BG, and Showers, MJ: Human Anatomy and Physiology. 6th ed. Philadelphia, WB Saunders, 1969.